Pcd.

MW00680324

PAK BOOK CORPORATION.
Star Centre, Main Tariq Road,
P.E.C.H.S. Karachi 2513. Ph449129

*Principles and Practice of*
# Pediatrics

*Second Edition*

# *Principles and Practice of*
# Pediatrics

*Editor-in-Chief*

## Frank A. Oski, MD

*Given Professor and Chairman*
*Department of Pediatrics*
*The Johns Hopkins University*
*School of Medicine*
*Director, The Johns Hopkins*
*Children's Center*
*Baltimore, Maryland*

*Editors*

## Catherine D. DeAngelis, MD

*Professor of Pediatrics*
*Senior Associate Dean for Academic Affairs and Faculty*
*The Johns Hopkins University School of Medicine*
*The Johns Hopkins Hospital*
*Baltimore, Maryland*

## Ralph D. Feigin, MD

*J. S. Abercrombie Professor of Pediatrics*
*Chairman, Department of Pediatrics*
*Baylor College of Medicine*
*Physician-in-Chief*
*Texas Children's Hospital*
*Physician-in-Chief, Pediatric Services*
*Ben Taub General Hospital*
*Chief, Pediatric Service*
*The Methodist Hospital*
*Houston, Texas*

## Julia A. McMillan, MD

*Associate Professor of Pediatrics*
*Johns Hopkins University School of Medicine*
*Deputy Director*
*Department of Pediatrics*
*Residency Program Director*
*Johns Hopkins Hospital*
*Baltimore, Maryland*

## Joseph B. Warshaw, MD

*Professor and Chairman*
*Department of Pediatrics*
*Yale University School of Medicine*
*Physician-in-Chief of Pediatrics*
*Children's Hospital at Yale-New Haven*
*New Haven, Connecticut*

*284 Contributors*

**J. B. LIPPINCOTT COMPANY**
Philadelphia

*Acquisitions Editor:* Richard Winters
*Associate Editor:* Kimberley Cox
*Associate Managing Editor:* Elizabeth A. Durand
*Indexer:* Sandra King
*Design Coordinator:* Doug Smock
*Production Manager:* Caren Erlichman
*Production Coordinator:* Kevin P. Johnson
*Compositor:* Tapsco, Inc.
*Printer/Binder:* Courier Book Co./Westford
*Color Insert Printer:* Princeton Polychrome Press

2nd Edition

Copyright © 1994, by J. B. Lippincott Company.
Copyright © 1990 by J. B. Lippincott Company. All rights reserved. No part of this book may
be used or reproduced in any manner whatsoever without written permission except for brief
quotations embodied in critical articles and reviews. Printed in the United States of America.
For information write J. B. Lippincott Company, 227 East Washington Square, Philadelphia,
Pennsylvania 19106.

6   5   4   3   2   1

Library of Congress Cataloging-in-Publication Data

Principles and practice of pediatrics / editor-in-chief, Frank A. Oski;
    editors, Catherine D. DeAngelis . . . [et al.] ; 284 contributors.—
    2nd ed.
        p. cm.
    ISBN 0-397-51221-X
    1. Pediatrics.   I. Oski, Frank A.
    [DNLM:   1. Pediatrics.   WS 100 P9574 1994]
RJ45.P6754   1994
618.92—dc20
DNLM/DLC
for Library of Congress                                             93-31374
                                                                         CIP

The authors and publisher have exerted every effort to ensure that drug selection and dosage
set forth in this text are in accord with current recommendations and practice at the time of
publication. However, in view of ongoing research, changes in government regulations, and
the constant flow of information relating to drug therapy and drug reactions, the reader is
urged to check the package insert for each drug for any change in indications and dosage and
for added warnings and precautions. This is particularly important when the recommended
agent is a new or infrequently employed drug.

We dedicate this book

*To our spouses: Barbara Oski, James Harris, Judith Feigin, Jed Dietz and Cynthia Warshaw;*

*To our children and grandchildren: Jonathan, Jane, Jessica, Sara, and Joshua Oski; Susan, Michael, and Debra Feigin; Edith, Robert, and Elihu Dietz; Debbie Warshaw Gould, Kathy Warshaw Meyer, and Larry Warshaw.*

*To our students and house staff, past and present, who help to generate the excitement and curiosity that make medicine both rewarding and enjoyable; and, To pediatricians everywhere, who work hard each day to make a difference.*

# Preface

The "five books in one" approach to the first edition of *Principles and Practice of Pediatrics* enjoyed success among the readership and we, for the moment, have become hostages to that success. We have changed very little in the organization of the book. In the second edition, we have focused on filling in the omissions from the first edition, which ranged from lead poisoning to roseola infantum, and to bringing all the original material up to date. In the process of bringing you a better, and slightly bigger, textbook, we have also added an additional editor to our masthead, Julia A. McMillan. We hope you find this edition of the book even more helpful and as easy to use as the first edition of *Principles and Practice of Pediatrics*.

*Frank A. Oski*, MD

# Preface
## to the First Edition

*Principles and Practice of Pediatrics* represents a unique departure from current textbooks of pediatrics. Really five books in one, it reflects the way our specialty is learned and practiced today. The book is divided into five parts: "General Pediatrics," "The Fetus and the Newborn," "Ambulatory Pediatrics," "The Sick or Hospitalized Patient," and "The Pediatrician's Companion: Important Things You Forget to Remember."

In Part I, "General Pediatrics," the reader will find the basic topics that are relevant to all aspects of pediatrics, whether the patient is newborn, ambulatory, or acutely ill in the hospital. Examples of these chapters are "The History of Pediatrics," "The Economics of Medicine," "Immunology" "Molecular Genetics," "Ethics," "The Pediatric History and Physical Examination," "The Problem-Oriented Medical Record," "The Diagnostic Process," and even "The Consultation." Such fundamental topics transcend all boundaries and are important to every pediatrics student or practitioner.

Part II, "The Fetus and the Newborn," is a self-contained treatise containing what the physician needs to know once he or she enters a nursery, whether it is a nursery for the normal term infant or a neonatal intensive care unit. The newborn and its problems are discussed from the developmental, physiologic, and pathologic perspectives.

Part III, "Ambulatory Pediatrics," provides the necessary information for the conduct of a comprehensive and satisfying office practice that includes infants and adolescents, the well child, and the child with a chronic illness. Chapters in this part discuss topics such as infant feeding, immunizations, developmental as-

sessment, and psychobehavioral disturbances. Part III includes material on the common acute illnesses and sudden emergencies that confront the pediatrician on a daily basis.

Part IV, "The Sick or Hospitalized Patient," is a detailed presentation of the disturbances that may result in the hospitalization of infants and children. This part is a truly encyclopedic work that has been designed to serve as a core reference for every pediatrician treating a sick or hospitalized patient.

The final part of our book, "The Pediatrician's Companion: Important Things You Forget to Remember," provides you with laboratory values and guidelines on how to interpret them, assistance with the identification of 50 of the more common syndromes, and an illustrated manual of pediatric procedures. Part V concludes with a list of common symptoms and signs and their differential diagnoses. We hope that you will turn to this section frequently and find the answers to your problems.

This book is designed to meet the needs of the student of pediatrics, whether he or she is a medical student, a busy pediatric house officer, or a practitioner of our much-valued discipline. We believe the book is both comprehensive and cohesive. Our goal has been to represent accurately and fully the broad and rich tapestry that is pediatrics today.

My colleagues, Catherine D. DeAngelis, Ralph D. Feigin, and Joseph B. Warshaw, join me in wishing you enjoyment and satisfaction in the use of our book.

*Frank A. Oski, MD*

# Acknowledgments

We wish to acknowledge the help given in the preparation of the second edition of this book and express our gratitude for the able assistance provided by a group of dedicated people. A special thanks to Leslie Burke, Veronica Green, Vanessa Bradley, Carrel Briley, Anita Cecchin and Ann Palmeri. A special acknowledgment also should go to Richard Winters, Kimberley Cox, and Elizabeth Durand of the J. B. Lippincott Company, who helped conceive, promote, edit, and complete this book.

# Contributors

**Pasquale J. Accardo, MD**
Professor of Pediatrics
Saint Louis University School of Medicine
Director, Knights of Columbus
  Developmental Center at Cardinal
  Glennon Children's Hospital
St. Louis, Missouri

**Hoover Adger, Jr., MD**
Associate Professor of Pediatrics
The John Hopkins University School of
  Medicine
Medical Coordinator, Adolescent Program
The Johns Hopkins Hospital
Baltimore, Maryland

**Donald C. Anderson, MD**
Professor, Pediatrics, Microbiology,
  Immunology and Cell Biology
Baylor College of Medicine
Houston, Texas
Executive Director, Discovery Research
Upjohn Laboratories
Kalamazoo, Michigan

**Beth M. Ansel, PhD**
Health Scientist Administrator
Division of Communication Sciences and
  Disorders
National Institute of Deafness and Other
  Communication Disorders
Knoxville, Tennessee

**Billy S. Arant, Jr., MD**
Professor and Chairman
Department of Pediatrics
University of Tennessee College of
  Medicine
Chattanooga Unit
Medical Director
T. C. Thompson Children's Hospital
Chattanooga, Tennessee

**Shai Ashkenazi, MD**
Senior Lecturer
Tel Aviv University Sackler School of
  Medicine
Children's Hospital
Beilinson Medical Center
Petahtikua, Israel

**Carol J. Baker, MD**
Professor of Pediatrics, Microbiology and
  Immunology
Head, Section of Infectious Diseases
Baylor College of Medicine
Attending Physician
Texas Children's Hospital
Houston, Texas

**William F. Balistreri, MD**
Dorothy M.M. Kersten Professor of
  Pediatrics
University of Cincinnati School of
  Medicine
Director, Division of Pediatric
  Gastroenterology and Nutrition
Children's Hospital Medical Center
Cincinnati, Ohio

**Gerald Barber, MD**
Associate Professor of Clinical Pediatrics
New York University Medical Center
New York, New York

**Lewis A. Barness, MD**
Professor of Pediatrics
University of South Florida
College of Medicine
Tampa, Florida
Emeritus Professor
University of Wisconsin
Madison, Wisconsin

**Nancy M. Bauman, MD**
Fellow, Pediatric Otolaryngology
University of Iowa Hospitals and Clinics
Iowa City, Iowa

**William M. Belknap, MD**
Associate Professor of Pediatrics
University of Tennessee College of
  Medicine
Director, Pediatric Gastroenterology and
  Nutrition
T. C. Thompson Children's Hospital
Chattanooga, Tennessee

**Merton Bernfield, MD**
Clement A. Smith Professor of Pediatrics
Professor of Anatomy and Cell Biology
Director, Joint Program in Neonatology
Harvard Medical School
Chief, Division of Newborn Medicine
Children's Hospital
Boston, Massachusetts

**Phillip L. Berry, MD**
Associate Professor of Pediatrics
University of Arkansas for Medical
  Sciences
Director, Pediatric Nephrology
Arkansas Children's Hospital
Little Rock, Arkansas

**Ellen L. Blank, MD**
Assistant Clinical Professor of Pediatrics
Medical College of Wisconsin
Pediatric Gastroenterologist
Children's Hospital of Wisconsin
Milwaukee, Wisconsin

**Marc L. Boom, MD**
Resident in Internal Medicine
Massachusetts General Hospital
Boston, Massachusetts

**Kenneth M. Boyer, MD**
Professor and Associate Chairman
Department of Pediatrics
Rush Medical College
Director, Section of Pediatric Infectious
  Diseases
Rush-Presbyterian-St. Luke's Medical
  Center
Chicago, Illinois

**Ira K. Brandt, MD**
Professor Emeritus of Pediatrics and
  Medical Genetics
Indiana University School of Medicine
Indianapolis, Indiana

**Eileen D. Brewer, MD**
Associate Professor of Pediatrics
Renal Section, Department of Pediatrics
Baylor College of Medicine
Medical Director, Dialysis and Renal
  Transplantation
Texas Children's Hospital
Houston, Texas

**J. Timothy Bricker, MD**
Associate Professor of Pediatrics
Baylor College of Medicine
Chief, Lillie Frank Abercrombie Section of
  Cardiology
Texas Children's Hospital
Houston, Texas

**David A. Bross, MD**
Fellow, Gastroenterology/Nutrition
Combined Program in Pediatric
  Gastroenterology and Nutrition
Children's Hospital
Massachusetts General Hospital
Boston, Massachusetts

**Marilyn R. Brown, MD**
Pediatric Gastroenterologist
Associate Professor of Pediatrics
University of Rochester School of Medicine
Medical Director
Nutrition Support Service
Strong Memorial Hospital
Rochester, New York

**Iley Baker Browning III,** MD
Assistant Professor of Pediatrics
Duke University Medical Center
Training Director, Pediatric Pulmonology
    Fellowship
Director, Pediatric Pulmonary Function
    Laboratory
Co-Director, Duke Cystic Fibrosis Center
Durham, North Carolina

**George R. Buchanan,** MD
Professor of Pediatrics
Director, Division of Pediatric Hematology-
    Oncology
The University of Texas, Southwestern
    Medical Center at Dallas
Children's Medical Center of Dallas
Dallas, Texas

**Rebecca L. Byers,** MD
Assistant Professor of Medicine
University of Wisconsin Medical School
Attending Physician
University of Wisconsin Hospitals
Madison, Wisconsin

**Arnold J. Capute,** MD
Professor of Pediatrics
Division of Child Development
The Johns Hopkins University School of
    Medicine
Director of Training
Kennedy Krieger Institute
Baltimore, Maryland

**Richard O. Carpenter,** MD
Director of Medical Behavioral Unit
Scottish Rite Children's Medical Center
Atlanta, Georgia

**Thomas O. Carpenter,** MD
Associate Professor of Pediatrics
Yale University School of Medicine
Attending Physician
Yale-New Haven Hospital
New Haven, Connecticut

**John L. Carroll,** MD
Assistant Professor of Pediatrics
Pediatric Pulmonary Division
The Johns Hopkins Children's Center
Baltimore, Maryland

**Thomas B. Casale,** MD
Associate Professor and Director
Division of Allergy and Immunology
Department of Internal Medicine
University of Iowa College of Medicine
Iowa City, Iowa

**James F. Casella,** MD
Associate Professor of Pediatrics
The Johns Hopkins University School of
    Medicine
The Johns Hopkins Hospital
Baltimore, Maryland

**William J. Cashore,** MD
Professor of Pediatrics
Brown University School of Medicine
Associate Chief of Pediatrics
Women and Infants Hospital
Providence, Rhode Island

**James T. Cassidy,** MD
Professor of Child Health
Department of Child Health
University of Missouri-Columbia School of
    Medicine
Columbia, Missouri

**Elizabeth A. Catlin,** MD
Assistant Professor of Pediatrics
Harvard Medical School
Chief, Neonatology Unit
Massachusetts General Hospital
Boston, Massachusetts

**Frank Cecchin,** MD
Fellow in Pediatric Cardiology
Baylor College of Medicine
Texas Children's Hospital
Houston, Texas

**Evan Charney,** MD
Professor of Pediatrics
University of Massachusetts Medical
    School
Chairman
Department of Pediatrics
University of Massachusetts Medical
    Center
Worcester, Massachusetts

**John P. Cheatham,** MD
Associate Professor of Pediatrics
D. B. and Paula Varner Professorship in
    Pediatric Cardiology
Section of Pediatric Cardiology
Medical Director
Pediatric Cardiac Catheterization
    Laboratory
Pediatric Non-Invasive Laboratory Heart
    Station
University of Nebraska Medical Center
Medical Director
Cardiac Catheterization Laboratory
Non-Invasive Laboratory
Children's Memorial Hospital
Omaha, Nebraska

**James D. Cherry,** MD
Professor of Pediatrics
Chief, Division of Infectious Diseases
Department of Pediatrics
UCLA Medical Center
UCLA School of Medicine
Los Angeles, California

**Myra L. Chiang,** MD
Assistant Professor of Pediatrics
West Virginia University–Charleston
    Division
Chief, Pediatric Nephrology Section
Charleston Area Medical Center
Charleston, West Virginia

**J. Julian Chisolm, Jr.,** MD
Professor of Pediatrics
Johns Hopkins University School of
    Medicine
Director, Lead Poisoning Prevention
    Program
The Kennedy Krieger Institute
Baltimore, Maryland

**Thomas G. Cleary,** MD
Professor of Pediatrics
Director, Pediatric Infectious Diseases
The University of Texas Medical School at
    Houston
Hermann Hospital
Houston, Texas

**William D. Cochran,** MD
Clinical Associate Professor of Pediatrics
Harvard Medical School
Physician-in-Charge
Newborn Service
Beth Israel Hospital
Boston, Massachusetts

**William J. Cochran,** MD
Clinical Associate Professor
Department of Pediatrics
Jefferson Medical College
Philadelphia, Pennsylvania
Associate in Pediatric Gastroenterology and
    Nutrition
Geisinger Clinic
Danville, Pennsylvania

**Edward V. Colvin,** MD
Assistant Professor of Pediatrics
Director, Pediatric Cardiology
University of Alabama School of Medicine
University of Alabama at Birmingham
University of Alabama Hospital
Birmingham, Alabama

**John D. Crawford,** MD
Professor of Pediatrics, Emeritus
Harvard Medical School
Emeritus Chief, Pediatric Endocrine Unit
Massachusetts General Hospital
Boston, Massachusetts

**Debra A. Cutler,** MD
Private Medical Staff
Texas Children's Hospital
Houston, Texas

**Mary E. D'Alton,** MD
Associate Professor
Chief of Obstetrics and Maternal-Fetal
    Medicine
Tufts University School of Medicine
Chief of Obstetrics and Maternal-Fetal
    Medicine
New England Medical Center
Boston, Massachusetts

**Catherine DeAngelis,** MD
Professor of Pediatrics
Senior Associate Dean for Academic
    Affairs and Faculty
The Johns Hopkins University School of
    Medicine
The Johns Hopkins Hospital
Baltimore, Maryland

**Gail J. Demmler,** MD
Assistant Professor
Departments of Pediatrics, Microbiology,
    Immunology, and Pathology
Baylor College of Medicine
Director, Diagnostic Virology Laboratory
Texas Children's Hospital
Houston, Texas

**Britton M. Devillier,** MD
Post-Doctoral Fellow
Pediatric Emergency Medicine
Baylor College of Medicine
Texas Children's Hospital
Houston, Texas

**Darryl C. DeVivo,** MD
Sidney Carter Professor of Neurology
Professor of Pediatrics
College of Physicians and Surgeons of
    Columbia University
Attending Neurologist and Pediatrician
Presbyterian Hospital
New York, New York

**Michael Dewar,** MD
Assistant Professor of Cardiothoracic
    Surgery
Yale University School of Medicine
New Haven, Connecticut

**Elliot C. Dick, PhD**
Professor of Preventive Medicine
Chief, Respiratory Virus Research
  Laboratory
University of Wisconsin Medical School
Madison, Wisconsin

**Harry C. Dietz, MD**
Assistant Professor of Pediatrics and
  Medicine
The Johns Hopkins University School of
  Medicine
The Johns Hopkins Hospital
Baltimore, Maryland

**Salvatore DiMauro, MD**
Lucy G. Moses Professor of Neurology
Columbia University College of Physicians
  and Surgeons
New York, New York

**Patricia A. Donohoue, MD**
Assistant Professor of Pediatrics
Division of Pediatric Endocrinology
The University of Iowa College of
  Medicine
The University of Iowa Hospitals and
  Clinics
Iowa City, Iowa

**ZoAnn E. Dreyer, MD**
Assistant Professor
Baylor College of Medicine
Attending Physician
Texas Children's Hospital
Houston, Texas

**David J. Driscoll, MD**
Professor of Pediatrics
Mayo Medical School
Head, Section of Pediatric Cardiology
Mayo Foundation
Rochester, Minnesota

**Christopher Duggan, MD**
Fellow
Combined Program in Pediatric
  Gastroenterology and Nutrition
Harvard Medical School
Massachusetts General and Children's
  Hospitals
Boston, Massachusetts

**Lisa M. Dunkle, MD**
Director, Antiviral Clinical Research
Bristol-Myers Squibb Pharmaceutical
  Research Institute
Wallingford, Connecticut

**Morven S. Edwards, MD**
Professor of Pediatrics
Baylor College of Medicine
Active Staff
Texas Children's Hospital
Ben Taub General Hospital
Houston, Texas

**Peyton A. Eggleston, MD**
Professor of Pediatrics
Johns Hopkins University School of
  Medicine
Attending Physician
Johns Hopkins Hospital
Baltimore, Maryland

**Richard A. Ehrenkranz, MD**
Professor of Pediatrics, Obstetrics and
  Gynecology
Yale University School of Medicine
Clinical Director, Newborn Special Care
  Unit
Yale-New Haven Hospital
New Haven, Connecticut

**Galal M. El-Said, MD**
Professor of Cardiology
Cairo University
Kaser El-Aini Hospitals
Cairo, Egypt

**Lamia F. Elerian, MD**
Fellow
Division of Neonatal-Perinatal Medicine
University of Texas Health Science Center
Houston, Texas

**B. Keith English, MD**
Assistant Professor
Department of Pediatrics
University of Tennessee, Memphis
College of Medicine
Member, Division of Infectious Diseases
Department of Pediatrics
Le Bonheur Children's Medical Center
Memphis, Tennessee

**Lawrence K. Epple, Jr., MD**
Instructor in Pediatrics and Family
  Medicine
Thomas Jefferson University Medical
  Center
Philadelphia, Pennsylvania
Instructor and Attending Physician
Underwood Memorial Hospital Family
  Practice
Residency Program
Woodbury, New Jersey

**Jose A. Ettedgui, MD**
Assistant Professor of Pediatrics
University of Pittsburgh
School of Medicine
Children's Hospital of Pittsburgh
Pittsburgh, Pennsylvania

**Ralph D. Feigin, MD**
J. S. Abercrombie Professor of Pediatrics
Chairman, Department of Pediatrics
Baylor College of Medicine
Physician-in-Chief
Texas Children's Hospital
Physician-in-Chief, Pediatric Services
Ben Taub General Hospital
Chief, Pediatric Service
The Methodist Hospital
Houston, Texas

**Donald J. Fernbach, MD**
Professor Emeritus
Baylor College of Medicine
Houston, Texas

**Marvin A. Fishman, MD**
Professor of Pediatrics and Neurology
Director, Section of Child Neurology
Baylor College of Medicine
Chief, Neurology Service
Texas Children's Hospital
Houston, Texas

**David E. Fixler, MD**
Professor of Pediatrics
University of Texas, Southwestern Medical
  Center
Director of Pediatric Cardiology
Children's Medical Center
Dallas, Texas

**Alan R. Fleischman, MD**
Professor of Pediatrics
Professor of Epidemiology and Social
  Medicine
Albert Einstein College of Medicine
Director, Division of Neonatology
Montefiore Medical Center
Bronx, New York

**Samuel Flint, PhD**
Director
Department of Child Health Care Finance
  and Organization
American Academy of Pediatrics
Elk Grove Village, Illinois

**Thomas R. Flynn, DMD**
Clinical Assistant Professor
Department of Oral and Maxillofacial
  Surgery
University of Connecticut
School of Dental Medicine
Farmington, Connecticut
Associate Attending Physician
Section of Oral and Maxillofacial Surgery
Department of Dentistry
Saint Francis Hospital and Medical Center
Hartford, Connecticut

**James D. Fortenberry, MD**
Assistant Professor
Department of Pediatrics
Critical Care Division
Pediatric Intensivist
Henrietta Egleston Children's Hospital
Atlanta, Georgia

**Norman Fost, MD**
Professor and Vice Chairman of Pediatrics
Director, Program in Medical Ethics
University of Wisconsin Medical School
Attending Physician
Department of Pediatrics
University of Wisconsin Hospital
Madison, Wisconsin

**Robert W. Frenck, Jr., MD**
Pediatric Infectious Diseases
Naval Hospital
Oakland, California

**Lisa M. Frenkel, MD**
Assistant Professor of Pediatrics
University of Rochester School of Medicine
  and Dentistry
Attending Physician
Strong Memorial Hospital
Rochester, New York

**Richard A. Friedman, MD**
Assistant Professor of Pediatrics
Baylor College of Medicine
Director of Pacing and Electrophysiology
Texas Children's Hospital
Houston, Texas

**Junichiro Fukushige, MD**
Associate Professor of Pediatrics
Faculty of Medicine
Kyushu University
Chief, Division of Cardiology
Department of Pediatrics
Kyushu University Hospital
Fukuoka, Japan

**Glenn T. Furuta, MD**
Research Fellow
Harvard Medical School
Children's Hospital
Massachusetts General Hospital
Boston, Massachusetts

**Norman F. Gant,** MD
Executive Director
The American Board of Obstetrics and
Gynecology, Inc.
Professor of Obstetrics and Gynecology
The University of Texas Southwestern
Medical School
Parkland Memorial Hospital
Dallas, Texas

**Arthur Garson, Jr.,** MD
Professor of Medicine, Pediatrics and
Public Policy
Associate Vice Chancellor for Health
Affairs
Chief, Pediatric Cardiology
Duke University Medical Center
Durham, North Carolina

**Karen M. Gaudio,** MD
Associate Professor of Pediatrics
Director, Pediatric End-Stage Renal Disease
Program
Yale University School of Medicine
Attending Physician
Yale-New Haven Hospital
New Haven, Connecticut

**Joseph M. Gertner,** MB, MRCP
Professor of Pediatrics
Cornell University Medical College
Program Director, Children's Clinical
Research Center
The New York Hospital-Cornell Medical
Center
New York, New York

**Mark A. Gilger,** MD
Assistant Professor of Pediatrics
Baylor College of Medicine
Director, GI Procedures Suite
Texas Children's Hospital
Houston, Texas

**Daniel G. Glaze,** MD
Associate Professor
Pediatric Neurology
Baylor College of Medicine
Houston, Texas

**W. Paul Glezen,** MD
Professor and Head, Preventive Medicine
Section
Department of Microbiology, Immunology,
and Pediatrics
Baylor College of Medicine
Attending Physician
Harris County Hospital District
Courtesy Staff in Infectious Diseases
Texas Children's Hospital
Houston, Texas

**Julius G. K. Goepp,** MD
Assistant Professor
Pediatrics and International Health
Johns Hopkins University
Assistant Director
Pediatric Emergency Department
Johns Hopkins Hospital
Baltimore, Maryland

**Edmond T. Gonzales, Jr.,** MD
Professor of Urology
Scott Department of Oncology
Baylor College of Medicine
Chief, Urology Service
Head, Department of Surgery
Texas Children's Hospital
Houston, Texas

**Robert J. Gorlin,** DDS
Regents' Professor of Oral Pathology and
Genetics
University of Minnesota School of
Dentistry
Professor of Pathology, Dermatology,
Pediatrics, Obstetrics-Gynecology, and
Otolaryngology
University of Minnesota School of
Medicine
University of Minnesota Hospital and
Clinic
Minneapolis, Minnesota

**Richard J. Grand,** MD
Professor of Pediatrics
Tufts University School of Medicine
Chief, Pediatric Gastroenterology and
Nutrition
New England Medical Center Hospitals
The Boston Floating Hospital for Infants
and Children
Boston, Massachusetts

**Morris Green,** MD
Perry W. Lesh Professor of Pediatrics
Indiana University School of Medicine
Attending Physician
James Whitcomb Riley Hospital for
Children
Indianapolis, Indiana

**John F. Griffith,** MD
Executive Vice President for Health
Sciences
Executive Dean of the School of Medicine
Georgetown University Medical Center
Professor of Pediatrics and Neurology
Georgetown University Hospital
Washington, DC

**Johnny Ray Griggs,** MD
Baylor College of Medicine
Texas Children's Hospital
Houston, Texas

**Charles Grose,** MD
Professor of Pediatrics and Microbiology
University of Iowa College of Medicine
Director, Division of Infectious Diseases
Department of Pediatrics
University of Iowa Hospitals
Iowa City, Iowa

**Ian Gross,** MD
Director of Perinatal Medicine
Professor of Pediatrics
Yale University School of Medicine
Yale-New Haven Hospital
New Haven, Connecticut

**William C. Gruber,** MD
Assistant Professor of Pediatrics
Vanderbilt University School of Medicine
Vanderbilt University Medical Center
Nashville, Tennessee

**Carl H. Gumbiner,** MD
Associate Professor of Pediatrics
Section of Pediatric Cardiology
University of Nebraska Medical Center
Director, Intensive Care
Children's Memorial Hospital
Omaha, Nebraska

**Howard P. Gutgesell,** MD
Professor of Pediatrics
Director, Pediatric Cardiology
University of Virginia Medical Center
Charlottesville, Virginia

**Margaret R. Hammerschlag,** MD
Professor of Pediatrics and Medicine
State University of New York
Health Science Center at Brooklyn
Attending, Pediatric Infectious Diseases
University Hospital of Brooklyn
Active Attending
Kings County Hospital Medical Center
Brooklyn, New York

**Paul E. Hammerschlag,** MD
Associate Clinical Professor
Department of Otolaryngology
New York University School of Medicine
Tisch Hospital
New York University Medical Center
New York, New York

**Brian D. Hanna,** MDCM, PhD
Assistant Professor
Dalhousie Medical School
Attending Cardiologist
I.W.K. Children's Hospital
Halifax, Nova Scotia
Canada

**I. Celine Hanson,** MD
Associate Professor of Pediatrics
Baylor College of Medicine
Texas Children's Hospital
Houston, Texas

**James C. Harris,** MD
Director, Developmental Neuropsychiatry
Associate Professor of Psychiatry,
Pediatrics, and Mental Hygiene
Johns Hopkins University
Director, Developmental Neuropsychiatry
Johns Hopkins Hospital
Baltimore, Maryland

**Brenda S. Harvey,** MD
Assistant Professor of Pediatrics
Section of Neonatology
University of Texas Medical School at
Houston
Houston, Texas

**Edith P. Hawkins,** MD
Professor of Pathology
Associate Professor of Pediatrics
Baylor College of Medicine
Staff Pathologist
Texas Children's Hospital
Houston, Texas

**Hal K. Hawkins,** PhD, MD
Assistant Professor of Pathology and
Pediatrics
Baylor College of Medicine
Pathologist
Texas Children's Hospital
Houston, Texas

**William R. Hayden,** MD
Associate Professor
Department of Pediatrics
Rush Medical College
Director
Rush/Cook County Hospital
Pediatric Critical Care Program
Chicago, Illinois

**Robert A. Herzlinger,** MD
Associate Clinical Professor of Pediatrics
Yale New-Haven Hospital
Director of Neonatology
Bridgeport Hospital
New Haven, Connecticut

Peter W. Hiatt, MD
Assistant Professor of Pediatrics
Department of Pediatrics
Baylor College of Medicine
Houston, Texas

L. Leighton Hill, MD
Professor and Head of Renal Section
Department of Pediatrics
Baylor College of Medicine
Chief, Renal Service
Texas Children's Hospital
Houston, Texas

Lewis B. Holmes, MD
Professor of Pediatrics
Harvard Medical School
Pediatrician and Chief, Embryology/
Teratology Unit
Massachusetts General Hospital
Boston, Massachusetts

Richard Hong, MD
Professor of Pediatrics
University of Vermont Comprehensive
Cancer Center
Attending Physician
Medical Center Hospital of Vermont
Burlington, Vermont

Walter T. Hughes, MD
Chairman, Department of Infectious
Diseases
St. Jude's Children's Research Hospital
Memphis, Tennessee

James C. Huhta, MD
Clinical Professor of Pediatrics, Obstetrics
and Gynecology
University of Pennsylvania School of
Medicine
Chief, Section of Perinatal Cardiology
Pennsylvania Hospital
Philadelphia, Pennsylvania

Richard L. Hurwitz, MD
Assistant Professor
Baylor College of Medicine
Attending Physician
Texas Children's Hospital
Houston, Texas

Nancy Hutton, MD
Assistant Professor of Pediatrics
The Johns Hopkins University School of
Medicine
Director, Pediatric HIV/AIDS Program
Johns Hopkins Children's Center
Baltimore, Maryland

W. Daniel Jackson, MD
Assistant Professor of Pediatrics
University of Utah School of Medicine
Salt Lake City, Utah

Richard F. Jacobs, MD
Horace C. Cabe Professor of Pediatrics
University of Arkansas for Medical
Sciences
Arkansas Children's Hospital
Chief, Pediatric Infectious Diseases
Arkansas Children's Hospital
Little Rock, Arkansas

Joseph Jankovic, MD
Professor of Neurology
Director, Parkinson's Disease Center
Movement Disorder Clinic
Senior Attending
The Methodist Hospital
Houston, Texas

Alain Joffe, MD
Associate Professor of Pediatrics
Director, Adolescent Medicine
Johns Hopkins Medical Institutions
Baltimore, Maryland

Victoria E. Judd, MD
Assistant Clinical Professor of Pediatrics
University of Utah School of Medicine
Primary Children's Medical Center
Director of Electrocardiography
Pediatric Cardiology
Salt Lake City, Utah

Sheldon L. Kaplan, MD
Professor and Vice-Chairman for Clinical
Affairs
Department of Pediatrics
Baylor College of Medicine
Chief, Infectious Disease Service
Texas Children's Hospital
Houston, Texas

Michael Katz, MD
Carpenter Professor Emeritus of Pediatrics
College of Physicians and Surgeons
Columbia University
Vice President for Research and Grants
Administration
Consultant in Pediatrics
Babies Hospital (Presbyterian Hospital)
New York
White Plains, New York

Haig H. Kazazian, Jr., MD
Sutland Professor of Pediatric Genetics
Director, Center for Medical Genetics
Johns Hopkins Hospital
Baltimore, Maryland

James S. Kemp, MD
Assistant Professor
Washington University School of Medicine
Attending Physician
St. Louis Children's Hospital
Medical Director, Respiratory Care
Pulmonary Function Laboratory
St. Louis, Missouri

Kathleen A. Kennedy, MD
Assistant Professor of Pediatrics
University of Texas Southwestern Medical
Center
Medical Director of Nurseries
St. Paul Hospital
Dallas, Texas

Bradley Howard Kessler, MD
Assistant Professor of Pediatrics
Albert Einstein College of Medicine
Attending–Division of Pediatrics GI/
Nutrition
Schemeiden Children's Hospital
Long Island Jewish Medical Center
New Hyde Park, New York

John L. Kirkland, MD
Professor of Pediatrics
Baylor College of Medicine
Chief, Endocrinology and Metabolism
Texas Children's Hospital
Houston, Texas

Rebecca T. Kirkland, MD
Professor of Pediatrics
Chief, Academic Ambulatory Pediatrics
Baylor College of Medicine
Medical Director, Ambulatory Services
Texas Children's Hospital
Houston, Texas

Mark W. Kline, MD
Associate Professor of Pediatrics
Sections of Allergy/Immunology and
Infectious Diseases
Department of Pediatrics
Baylor College of Medicine
Attending Physician
Texas Children's Hospital
Houston, Texas

William J. Klish, MD
Professor of Pediatrics
Baylor College of Medicine
Chief, Nutrition and Gastroenterology
Texas Children's Hospital
Houston, Texas

Edward C. Kohaut, MD
Professor of Pediatrics
Director, Nephrology Division
University of Alabama School of Medicine
Department of Pediatrics
Director, Nephrology Division
The Children's Hospital of Alabama
Birmingham, Alabama

Steve Kohl, MD
Professor of Pediatrics
University of California, San Francisco
Chief of Pediatric Infectious Diseases
Moffitt-Long Hospital
San Francisco General Hospital
San Francisco, California

Gary S. Kopf, MD
Professor of Surgery
Yale University School of Medicine
Director, Pediatric Cardiac Surgery
Yale-New Haven Hospital
New Haven, Connecticut

Andrew J. Kornberg, MB, BS, FRACP
Instructor in Neurology and Pediatrics
Department of Neurology
Washington University School of Medicine
Instructor in Neurology and Pediatrics
St. Louis Children's Hospital
St. Louis, Missouri

Seth Paul Kravitz, MD
Assistant Professor of Pediatrics
Baylor College of Medicine
Renal Attending
Texas Children's Hospital
Houston, Texas

Katherine Kula, DMD
Associate Professor
Departments of Pediatric Dentistry and
Orthodontics
School of Dentistry
University of North Carolina at Chapel
Hill
Chapel Hill, North Carolina

Alan M. Lake, MD
Associate Professor of Pediatrics
Johns Hopkins University School of
Medicine
Attending Gastroenterologist
Johns Hopkins Hospital
Baltimore, Maryland

Rebecca M. Landa, PhD
Assistant Professor of Psychiatry
The Johns Hopkins Hospital
Baltimore, Maryland

Gregory L. Landry, MD
Associate Professor of Pediatrics
University of Wisconsin Medical School
Head, Medical Team Physician
University of Wisconsin-Madison Athletic
Teams
Staff Physician
University of Wisconsin Hospital
Madison, Wisconsin

Claire Langston, MD
Professor of Pathology
Baylor College of Medicine
Director, Anatomic Pathology
Texas Children's Hospital
Houston, Texas

Marc H. Lebel, MD, FRCPC
Assistant Professor of Pediatrics
Department of Pediatrics, Microbiology
and Immunology
University of Montreal
Chief, Section of Infectious Diseases
Hôpital Sainte-Justine
Montreal, Quebec
Canada

Howard M. Lederman, MD, PhD
Associate Professor of Pediatrics
The Johns Hopkins University School of
Medicine
Clinical Director, Immunodeficiency Clinic
The Johns Hopkins Hospital
Baltimore, Maryland

Carlos H. Lifschitz, MD
Associate Professor of Pediatrics
Baylor College of Medicine
Attending Physician, Nutrition and
Gastroenterology
Texas Children's Hospital
Houston, Texas

Sarah S. Long, MD
Professor of Pediatrics
Temple University School of Medicine
Chief, Section of Infectious Diseases
St. Christopher's Hospital for Children
Philadelphia, Pennsylvania

Martin I. Lorin, MD
Professor of Clinical Pediatrics
Baylor College of Medicine
Attending Physician
Ben Taub General Hospital
Texas Children's Hospital
Houston, Texas

Gerald M. Loughlin, MD
Associate Professor of Pediatrics
Johns Hopkins University School of
Medicine
Director
Eudowood Division of Pediatric
Respiratory Sciences
Baltimore, Maryland

Penelope Terhune Louis, MD
Assistant Professor of Pediatrics
Baylor College of Medicine
Critical Care and Emergency Medicine
Services
Texas Children's Hospital
Houston, Texas

Donald H. Mahoney, Jr., MD
Associate Professor of Clinical Pediatrics
Baylor College of Medicine
Houston, Texas

Carole L. Marcus, MBBCh
Assistant Professor of Pediatrics
Division of Pediatric Pulmonology
Johns Hopkins University
Medical Director, Pediatric Sleep
Laboratory
Johns Hopkins Hospital
Baltimore, Maryland

Judith F. Margolin, MD
Postdoctoral Fellow in Pediatric
Hematology and Oncology
University of Pennsylvania School of
Medicine
Children's Hospital of Philadelphia
Philadelphia, Pennsylvania

M. Michele Mariscalco, MD
Assistant Professor of Pediatrics
Baylor College of Medicine
Houston, Texas

Paul L. Martin, MD, PhD
Assistant Professor of Pediatrics
Bowman Gray School of Medicine of Wake
Forest University
Attending Physician
Brenner Children's Hospital
Winston-Salem, North Carolina

Steven R. Martin, MD
Service Division of Pediatric
Gastroenterology and Nutrition
Hôpital Sainte-Justine
University of Montreal
Montreal, Quebec
Canada

Edward O. Mason, Jr., PhD
Professor of Clinical Pediatrics
Assistant Professor of Microbiology and
Immunology
Baylor College of Medicine
Director, Infectious Diseases Laboratory
Texas Children's Hospital
Houston, Texas

John J. Mathewson, PhD
Assistant Professor of Infectious Diseases
University of Texas Medical School and
School of Public Health
Houston, Texas

David O. Matson, MD, PhD
Associate Professor of Pediatrics
Center for Pediatric Research
Eastern Virginia Medical School and
Children's Hospital of the King's
Daughters
Norfolk, Virginia

Irene M. Maumenee, MD
ORT Professor of Ophthalmology
Joint Appointment in Medicine and
Pediatrics
Johns Hopkins Hospital
Baltimore, Maryland

Steven R. Mayfield, MD
Staff Neonatologist
Director, Neonatology Follow-Up Clinic
Boise, Idaho

Edward R. B. McCabe, MD, PhD
Professor and Acting Director
Institute for Molecular Genetics
Professor and Vice Chairman for Research
Department of Pediatrics
Baylor College of Medicine
Houston, Texas

Kenneth L. McClain, MD, PhD
Associate Professor of Pediatrics
Baylor College of Medicine
Hematology/Oncology Section
Texas Children's Hospital
Houston, Texas

Colston F. McEvoy, MD
Instructor
Department of Pediatrics
Yale University School of Medicine
Attending Physician
Yale New-Haven Hospital
New Haven, Connecticut

Julia A. McMillan, MD
Associate Professor of Pediatrics
Johns Hopkins University School of
Medicine
Deputy Director
Department of Pediatrics
Residency Program Director
Johns Hopkins Hospital
Baltimore, Maryland

Dan G. McNamara, MD
Professor of Pediatrics
Baylor College of Medicine
Emeritus Chief of Pediatric Cardiology
Texas Children's Hospital
Houston, Texas

Patricia Mena, MD
Adjunct Instructor of Pediatrics and
Nutrition
Instituto de Nutricion y Tecnologia de los
Alimentos (INTA)
University of Chile
Attending Neonatologist
Hospital Sotero del Rio
Santiago, Chile

Laura R. Ment, MD
Professor, Departments of Pediatrics and
Neurology
Yale University School of Medicine
New Haven, Connecticut

Douglas K. Mitchell, MD
Instructor
Department of Pediatrics
Eastern Virginia Medical School
Children's Hospital of the King's
Daughters
Norfolk, Virginia

John F. Modlin, MD
Professor of Pediatrics and Medicine
Dartmouth Medical School
Attending Physician
Dartmouth-Hitchcock Medical Center
Lebanon, New Hampshire

Mary J. H. Morriss, MD
Associate in Pediatric Cardiology
University of Iowa College of Medicine
Iowa City, Iowa

**W. Robert Morrow,** MD
Associate Professor of Pediatrics
Wayne State University School of Medicine
Director, Cardiac Catheterization
Laboratory
Children's Hospital of Michigan
Detroit, Michigan

**Immanuela R. Moss,** MD, PhD
Professor of Pediatrics
McGill University
Attending Physician
Division of Respiratory Medicine
Montreal Children's Hospital
Montreal, Quebec
Canada

**Kathleen J. Motil,** MD, PhD
Assistant Professor of Medicine
Baylor College of Medicine
Children's Nutrition Research Center
Active Staff
Texas Children's Hospital
Houston, Texas

**Charles E. Mullins,** MD
Professor of Clinical Pediatrics
Baylor College of Medicine
Medical Director, Cardiac Catheterization
Laboratories
Texas Children's Hospital
Houston, Texas

**Prathiba Nanjundiah,** MD
Assistant Professor of Clinical Pediatrics
University of Southern California
Attending Gastroenterologist
Children's Hospital of Los Angeles
Los Angeles, California

**William H. Neches,** MD
Professor of Pediatrics
University of Pittsburgh School of
Medicine
Associate Director, Pediatric Cardiologist
Children's Hospital of Pittsburgh
Pittsburgh, Pennsylvania

**John D. Nelson,** MD
Professor of Pediatrics
University of Texas Southwestern Medical
Center at Dallas
Attending Staff
Parkland Memorial Hospital
Children's Medical Center
Dallas, Texas

**John D. Newman,** PhD
Chief, Section on Developmental
Neuroethology
Laboratory of Comparative Ethology
National Institute of Child Health and
Human Development
National Institutes of Health
Poolesville, Maryland

**Bruce G. Nickerson,** MD
Associate Clinical Professor
Department of Pediatrics
UCLA School of Medicine
Los Angeles, California
Associate Pediatric Pulmonologist
Children's Hospital of Orange County
Orange, California

**Donald A. Novak,** MD
Assistant Professor of Pediatrics
University of Florida
Shands Teaching Hospital
Gainesville, Florida

**Edward J. Novotny, Jr.,** MD
Assistant Professor of Pediatrics and
Neurology
Yale University School of Medicine
Attending Physician in Pediatrics and
Neurology
Yale-New Haven Hospital
New Haven, Connecticut

**Angela A. Ogden,** MD
Assistant Professor of Pediatrics
Baylor College of Medicine
Hematology-Oncology Section
Texas Children's Hospital
Houston, Texas

**Frank A. Oski,** MD
Given Professor of Pediatrics
Department of Pediatrics
Johns Hopkins University School of
Medicine
Pediatrician-in-Chief
Johns Hopkins Children's Center
Baltimore, Maryland

**Frederick B. Palmer,** MD
Associate Professor of Pediatrics
Director, Division of Child Development
The Johns Hopkins University School of
Medicine
Director, Developmental Pediatrics
Kennedy Krieger Institute
Baltimore, Maryland

**Marc Paquet,** MD, FRCPC
Associate Professor
Department of Pediatrics
McGill University
Director, Service of Cardiology
The Montreal Children's Hospital
Montreal, Quebec
Canada

**Stephen M. Paridon,** MD
Assistant Professor of Pediatrics
Wayne State University School of Medicine
Director, Exercise Physiology Laboratory
Children's Hospital of Michigan
Detroit, Michigan

**Sang C. Park,** MD
Professor of Pediatrics
University of Pittsburgh School of
Medicine
Staff Cardiologist
Children's Hospital of Pittsburgh
Pittsburgh, Pennsylvania

**Julie Thorne Parke,** MD
Assistant Professor of Neurology
University of Oklahoma Health Sciences
Center
Pediatric Neurology Service
Children's Hospital of Oklahoma
Oklahoma City, Oklahoma

**Wade P. Parks,** MD, PhD
The Pat and E. John Rosenwald Professor
and Chairman
Department of Pediatrics
New York University School of Medicine
Attending Director of Pediatrics
Bellevue Hospital Center
Tisch Hospital
New York, New York

**Linda D. Parsi**
Baylor College of Medicine
Houston, Texas

**Christian C. Patrick,** MD, PhD
Associate Professor
Department of Pediatrics
University of Tennessee, Memphis College
of Medicine
Associate Member
Department of Infectious Diseases
St. Jude Children's Research Hospital
Memphis, Tennessee

**Lori Ellen Rhodes Patterson,** MD
Director, Pediatric Infectious Disease
East Tennessee Children's Hospital
Knoxville, Tennessee

**Howard A. Pearson,** MD
Professor of Pediatrics
Yale University School of Medicine
Attending
Yale-New Haven Hospital
New Haven, Connecticut

**Alan K. Percy,** MD
Professor and Director
Division of Pediatric Neurology
University of Alabama at Birmingham
The Children's Hospital of Alabama
Birmingham, Alabama

**Larry K. Pickering,** MD
Professor and Vice Chairman for Research
Department of Pediatrics
Eastern Virginia Medical School
Director, Center for Pediatric Research
Eastern Virginia Medical School
Children's Hospital of the King's
Daughters
Norfolk, Virginia

**Joseph F. Piecuch,** DMD, MD
Associate Clinical Professor
University of Connecticut Health Center
Farmington, Connecticut
Senior Attending Surgeon
Hartford Hospital
Hartford, Connecticut

**Leslie P. Plotnick,** MD
Associate Professor of Pediatrics
Johns Hopkins University School of
Medicine
Johns Hopkins Hospital
Baltimore, Maryland

**William J. Pokorny,** MD
Professor of Surgery and Pediatrics
Baylor College of Medicine
Houston, Texas

**David R. Powell,** MD
Associate Professor of Pediatrics
Baylor College of Medicine
Renal Service
Texas Children's Hospital
Houston, Texas

**David Prado,** MD
Associate Professor of Pediatrics
Departamento de Pediatria
Hospital General San Juan de Dios
Guatemala City, Guatemala

**Arthur L. Prensky,** MD
The Allen P. and Josephine B. Green
Professor of Pediatric Neurology
Washington University School of Medicine
Neurologist
St. Louis Children's
Barnes Hospital
St. Louis, Missouri

Guy R. Randolph, MD
Pediatric Resident
Baylor College of Medicine
Texas Children's Hospital
Houston, Texas

Vincent M. Riccardi, MD
Clinical Professor of Pediatrics (Genetics)
University of California, Los Angeles
Los Angeles, California

Donald A. Riopel, MD
Director, Division of Pediatric Cardiology
The Sanger Clinic
Charlotte, North Carolina

John W. Rippon, PhD
Associate Professor Emeritus
Department of Medicine/Dermatology
University of Chicago
Chicago, Illinois

Kenneth B. Roberts, MD
Professor and Vice Chairman of Pediatrics
University of Massachusetts Medical
   School
Director, Inpatient Pediatrics
University of Massachusetts Medical
   Center
Worcester, Massachusetts

Lynne J. Roberts, MD
Associate Professor
Departments of Dermatology and
   Pediatrics
University of Texas Southwestern Medical
   Center
Director of Dermatology
Children's Medical Center at Dallas
Dallas, Texas

Robert J. Roberts, MD, PhD
Professor and Chair
Department of Pediatrics
University of Virginia School of Medicine
Medical Director, Children's Medical
   Center
University of Virginia Hospitals
Charlottesville, Virginia

Carol L. Rosen, MD
Assistant Professor of Pediatrics
Section of Respiratory Medicine
Yale University School of Medicine
Attending Physician-Pediatrics
Yale-New Haven Hospital
New Haven, Connecticut

Leon A. Rosenberg, PhD
Professor of Education with Joint
   Appointment in Pediatrics and
   Psychiatry
The Johns Hopkins University
Affiliate Staff
The Johns Hopkins Hospital
Baltimore, Maryland

Beryl J. Rosenstein, MD
Professor of Pediatrics
Johns Hopkins University School of
   Medicine
Director, Cystic Fibrosis Center
Johns Hopkins Hospital
Baltimore, Maryland

N. Paul Rosman, MD
Professor of Pediatrics and Neurology
Tufts University School of Medicine
Chief, Division of Pediatric Neurology
Floating Hospital for Infants
Director, Center for Children with Special
   Needs
New England Medical Center
Boston, Massachusetts

David R. Roth, MD
Associate Professor of Clinical Urology
Scott Department of Urology
Baylor College of Medicine
Texas Children's Hospital
Houston, Texas

Peter C. Rowe, MD
Associate Professor of Pediatrics
Johns Hopkins University Medical School
Baltimore, Maryland

Guillermo Ruiz-Palacios, MD
Professor and Head
Department of Infectious Diseases
National Institute of Nutrition
Mexico City, Mexico

Hugh A. Sampson, MD
Professor of Pediatrics
Johns Hopkins University School of
   Medicine
Director, Pediatric Clinical Research Center
Johns Hopkins Hospital
Baltimore, Maryland

Pablo J. Sanchez, MD
Assistant Professor
The University of Texas Southwestern
   Medical Center at Dallas
Attending Physician
Parkland Memorial Hospital
Children's Medical Center
Dallas, Texas

Mathuram Santosham, MD
Professor, Department of International
   Health
Director, Center for American Indian and
   Alaskan Native Health
Department of Pediatrics
The Johns Hopkins University School of
   Medicine
Baltimore, Maryland

Herbert Schneiderman, MD
Associate Professor of Pediatrics and
   Rehabilitation Medicine
Medical Director, Spina Bifida Clinic
State University of New York
Health Science Center at Syracuse
Syracuse, New York

Kenneth C. Schuberth, MD
Assistant Professor of Pediatrics
Johns Hopkins University School of
   Medicine
Attending Physician
The Johns Hopkins Hospital
Baltimore, Maryland

Paula J. Schweich, MD
Clinical Associate Professor
University of Washington School of
   Medicine
Emergency Pediatrician
Mary Bridge Children's Hospital
Seattle, Washington

David T. Scott, PhD
Associate Professor of Psychiatry and
   Behavioral Sciences
Child Development and Mental
   Retardation Center
University of Washington School of
   Medicine
University of Washington Medical Center
Seattle, Washington

Gwendolyn B. Scott, MD
Associate Professor of Pediatrics
University of Miami School of Medicine
Attending Physician
Pediatrics and Pediatric Infectious Disease
   Consultant
Children's Hospital Center at Jacksonville
Memorial Hospital
Miami, Florida

Dan K. Seilheimer, MD
Associate Professor of Clinical Pediatrics
Baylor College of Medicine
Chief, Pulmonary Medicine Service
Texas Children's Hospital
Houston, Texas

Bruce K. Shapiro, MD
Associate Professor of Pediatrics
The Johns Hopkins University School of
   Medicine
Director, Center for Learning and Its
   Disorders
Kennedy Krieger Institute
Baltimore, Maryland

Larry J. Shapiro, MD
Professor and Chair
University of California, San Francisco
   School of Medicine
Chief of Pediatric Services
University of California Medical Center
San Francisco, California

Bennett A. Shaywitz, MD
Professor of Pediatrics and Neurology
Yale University School of Medicine
Chief, Pediatric Neurology
Yale-New Haven Hospital
New Haven, Connecticut

William T. Shearer, MD, PhD
Professor of Pediatrics, Microbiology and
   Immunology
Baylor College of Medicine
Chief, Allergy and Immunology Service
Texas Children's Hospital
Houston, Texas

Robert J. Shulman, MD
Associate Professor of Pediatrics
Baylor College of Medicine
Director, Nutritional Support Team
Texas Children's Hospital
Houston, Texas

Jane D. Siegel, MD
Associate Professor of Pediatrics
University of Texas Southwestern Medical
   Center at Dallas
Attending Physician and Infection Control
   Committee Chairman
Children's Medical Center of Dallas
Attending Physician and Medical Director
   of Pediatric Inpatient Services
Parkland Memorial Hospital
Dallas, Texas

Norman J. Siegel, MD
Professor of Pediatrics and Medicine
Director, Section of Pediatric Nephrology
Vice Chairman, Department of Pediatrics
Yale University School of Medicine
Assistant Chief, Pediatrics
Attending Physician
Yale-New Haven Hospital
New Haven, Connecticut

Michael J. Silka, MD
Associate Professor of Pediatrics
Oregon Health Sciences University
Doernbecher Children's Hospital
Portland, Oregon

Richard H. Sills, MD
Associate Professor of Pediatrics
New Jersey Medical School
University of Medicine and Dentistry of
New Jersey
Director, Pediatric Hematology and
Oncology
Children's Hospital of New Jersey
Newark, New Jersey

F. Estelle R. Simons, MD
Professor and Deputy Chairman
Department of Pediatrics and Child Health
Head, Section of Allergy and Clinical
Immunology
The University of Manitoba
Director, Clinical Investigation
Children's Hospital of Winnipeg
Winnipeg, Manitoba
Canada

Frank R. Sinatra, MD
Professor of Pediatrics
University of Southern California School of
Medicine
Head, Division of Pediatric
Gastroenterology and Nutrition
Los Angeles County
University of Southern California Medical
Center
Los Angeles, California

M. Melisse Sloas, MD
Senior Clinical Investigator
Pediatric Branch
National Cancer Institute
National Institutes of Health
Bethesda, Maryland

Richard J. H. Smith, MD
Professor, Pediatric Otolaryngology
Director, Molecular Otolaryngology
Research Laboratory
University of Iowa Hospitals and Clinics
Iowa City, Iowa

C. Wayne Smith, MD
Professor, Department of Pediatrics,
Microbiology, and Immunology
Baylor College of Medicine
Houston, Texas

Marianna M. Sockrider, MD
Associate Professor
Baylor College of Medicine
Pediatric Pulmonologist
Texas Children's Hospital
Houston, Texas

Paul D. Sponseller, MD
Associate Professor, Pediatric Orthopaedics
Johns Hopkins University Medical School
Head, Division of Pediatric Orthopaedics
Johns Hopkins Hospital
Baltimore, Maryland

Barbara H. Starfield, MD
Professor and Head
Division of Health Policy and Joint
Appointment in Pediatrics
The Johns Hopkins University
School of Public Health and Medicine
Medical Staff (Pediatrics)
The Johns Hopkins Hospital
Baltimore, Maryland

Rachel E. Stark-Selz, PhD
Professor, Audiology and Speech Sciences
Purdue University
West Lafayette, Indiana

Jeffrey R. Starke, MD
Assistant Professor of Pediatrics
Baylor College of Medicine
Infection Control Advisor
Texas Children's Hospital
Houston, Texas

Barbara W. Stechenberg, MD
Associate Professor of Pediatrics
Tufts University School of Medicine
Boston, Massachusetts
Director, Pediatric Infectious Diseases
Baystate Medical Center
Springfield, Massachusetts

Fernando Stein, MD
Assistant Professor of Pediatrics
Baylor College of Medicine
Deputy Director, Critical Care Service
Texas Children's Hospital
Houston, Texas

C. Philip Steuber, MD
Professor of Clinical Pediatrics
Baylor College of Medicine
Acting Chief, Hematology/Oncology
Service
Texas Children's Hospital
Houston, Texas

Janette F. Strasburger, MD
Assistant Professor of Pediatrics
Northwestern University
Children's Memorial Hospital
Chicago, Illinois

Frederick J. Suchy, MD
Professor of Pediatrics
Chief, Pediatric Gastroenterology/
Hepatology
Yale Medical School
New Haven, Connecticut

Ciro V. Sumaya, MD
Professor and Associate Medical Dean
University of Texas Health Science Center
at San Antonio
Staff Physician
Bexar County Hospital District
Santa Rosa Children's Hospital
San Antonio, Texas

Larry H. Taber, MD
Professor of Pediatrics
Department of Pediatrics
Baylor College of Medicine
Houston, Texas

Norman S. Talner, MD
Professor of Pediatrics (Pediatric
Cardiology)
Duke University School of Medicine
Attending Pediatric Cardiologist
Duke University Medical Center
Durham, North Carolina

Dan W. Thomas, MD
Associate Professor of Pediatrics
University of Southern California School of
Medicine
Staff Gastroenterology
Children's Hospital of Los Angeles
Los Angeles, California

Jack L. Titus, MD, PhD
Clinical Professor of Pathology
University of Minnesota Medical School
Director, Jesse E. Edwards Registry of
Cardiovascular Disease
United Hospital
St. Paul, Minnesota

Richard G. Topazian, DDS
Professor and Chairman
Department of Oral and Maxillofacial
Surgery
School of Dental Medicine
Professor of Surgery
School of Medicine
University of Connecticut Health Center
Attending Surgeon
John N. Dempsey Hospital
Farmington, Connecticut

Robert James Touloukian, MD
Professor of Surgery and Pediatrics
Chief, Pediatric Surgery
Yale University School of Medicine
Yale-New Haven Hospital
New Haven, Connecticut

Elias I. Traboulsi, MD
Assistant Professor of Ophthalmology and
Pediatrics
The Johns Hopkins School of Medicine
The Johns Hopkins Center for Hereditary
Eye Diseases of the Wilmer Eye Institute
The Johns Hopkins Hospital
Baltimore, Maryland

Theodore F. Tsai, MD
Clinical Microbiology Services
National Institutes of Health
Bethesda, Maryland

Walter W. Tunnessen, Jr., MD
Professor of Pediatrics
University of Pennsylvania School of
Medicine
Associate Chairman for Medical Education
The Children's Hospital of Philadelphia
Philadelphia, Pennsylvania

Jon E. Tyson, MD
Professor of Pediatrics and Obstetrics/
Gynecology
The University of Texas Southwestern
Medical Center at Dallas
Dallas, Texas

**Ricardo Uauy**, MD, PhD
Professor of Pediatrics and Nutrition
Instituto de Nutrician y Tecnologia de los
  Alimentos (INTA)
University of Chile
Attending Neonatologist
Hospital Sotero del Rio
Santiago, Chile

**Jack van Hoff**, MD
Assistant Professor of Pediatrics
Division of Hematology/Oncology
Yale University School of Medicine
Yale-New Haven Hospital
New Haven, Connecticut

**Jon A. Vanderhoof**, MD
Chairman, Department of Pediatrics
Creighton University School of Medicine
Director, Section of Pediatric
  Gastroenterology and Nutrition
Children's University School of Medicine
University of Nebraska Medical Center
Chief of Pediatrics
St. Joseph Hospital
Omaha, Nebraska

**Thomas A. Vargo**, MD
Associate Professor of Pediatrics
Baylor College of Medicine
Associate in Cardiology
Texas Children's Hospital
Houston, Texas

**G. Wesley Vick III**, MD, PhD
Research Assistant Professor
Division of Cardiology
Department of Pediatrics
Baylor College of Medicine
Associate in Pediatric Cardiology
Texas Children's Hospital
Houston, Texas

**Ellen R. Wald**, MD
Professor of Pediatrics
University of Pittsburgh School of
  Medicine
Chief, Pediatric Infectious Diseases
Children's Hospital of Pittsburgh
Pittsburgh, Pennsylvania

**W. Allan Walker**, MD
Professor of Pediatrics
Harvard Medical School
Children's Hospital
Boston, Massachusetts

**David S. Walton**, MD
Associate Clinical Professor in
  Ophthalmology
Harvard Medical School
Surgeon in Ophthalmology
Massachusetts Eye and Ear Infirmary
Boston, Massachusetts

**Rebecca S. Wappner**, MD
Professor of Pediatrics
Indiana University School of Medicine
James Whitcomb Riley Hospital for
  Children
Indianapolis, Indiana

**Kent E. Ward**, MD
Assistant Professor of Pediatrics
University of Oklahoma Health Sciences
  Center
Division of Pediatric Cardiology and
  Critical Care Medicine
Children's Hospital of Oklahoma
Oklahoma City, Oklahoma

**Joseph B. Warshaw**, MD
Professor and Chairman
Department of Pediatrics
Yale University School of Medicine
Physician-in-Chief of Pediatrics
Children's Hospital at Yale-New Haven
New Haven, Connecticut

**David D. Weaver**, MD
Professor
Department of Medical and Molecular
  Genetics
Indiana University School of Medicine
Indianapolis, Indiana

**Steven L. Werlin**, MD
Professor of Pediatrics
Medical College of Wisconsin
Director of Gastroenterology
Children's Hospital of Wisconsin
Milwaukee, Wisconsin

**James A. Wilde**, MD
Fellow
Pediatric Emergency Medicine
Johns Hopkins University School of
  Medicine
Johns Hopkins Children's Center
Baltimore, Maryland

**Robert Lee Williams**, MD
Clinical Instructor in Pediatrics
University of Arizona
St. Joseph's Hospital Children's Health
  Centre
Phoenix, Arizona

**Christopher B. Wilson**, MD
Professor of Pediatrics and Immunology
University of Washington
Head, Division of Immunology and
  Rheumatology
Children's Hospital and Medical Center
Seattle, Washington

**Michele Diane Wilson**, MD
Assistant Professor of Pediatrics
Adolescent Medicine
Director, Teenage Parenting Clinic
The Johns Hopkins University School of
  Medicine
The Johns Hopkins Hospital
Baltimore, Maryland

**Modena Hoover Wilson**, MD
Director, Division of General Pediatrics
Associate Professor of Pediatrics
The Johns Hopkins University School of
  Medicine
Baltimore, Maryland

**Jerry A. Winkelstein**, MD
Professor of Pediatrics
Johns Hopkins University School of
  Medicine
Director, Division of Pediatric Allergy and
  Immunology
Johns Hopkins Hospital
Baltimore, Maryland

**Merrill S. Wise**, MD
Assistant Professor of Pediatrics and
  Neurology
University of Alabama at Birmingham
Children's Hospital of Alabama
Birmingham, Alabama

**Larry S. Wissow**, MD
Associate Professor of Pediatrics
Johns Hopkins University School of
  Medicine
Baltimore, Maryland

**Robert H. Yolken**, MD
Professor of Pediatrics
Johns Hopkins University School of
  Medicine
Director, Division of Pediatric Infectious
  Diseases
Johns Hopkins Hospital
Baltimore, Maryland

**Richard S. K. Young**, MD
Associate Clinical Professor
Pediatrics and Neurology
Yale University School of Medicine
Chairman
Department of Pediatrics
Hospital of Saint Raphael
New Haven, Connecticut

# Contents

## PART IV
## *The Sick or Hospitalized Patient*

Ralph D. Feigin

SECTION I   *Principles of Intensive Care*

SECTION II   *Infectious Diseases*

PART V

*The Pediatrician's Companion:
Important Things You Forget
to Remember*

Frank A. Oski

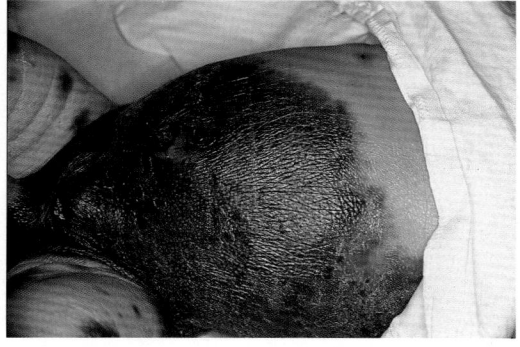

Color Figure 1

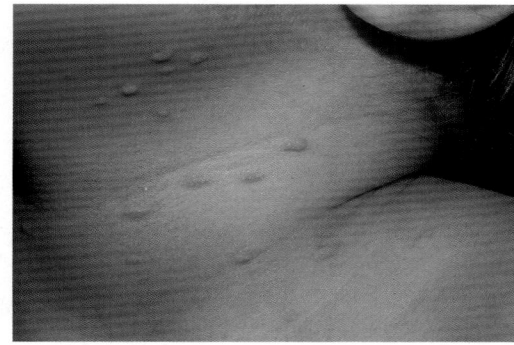

Color Figure 2

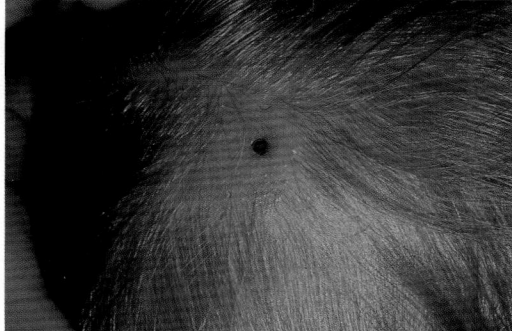

Color Figure 3

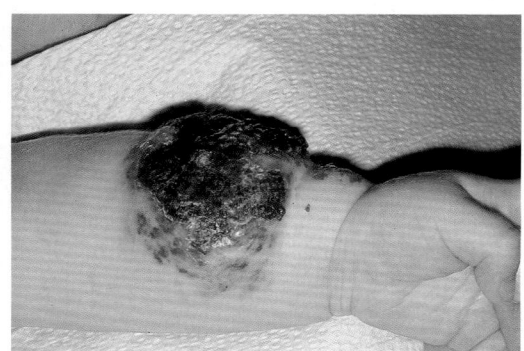

Color Figure 4

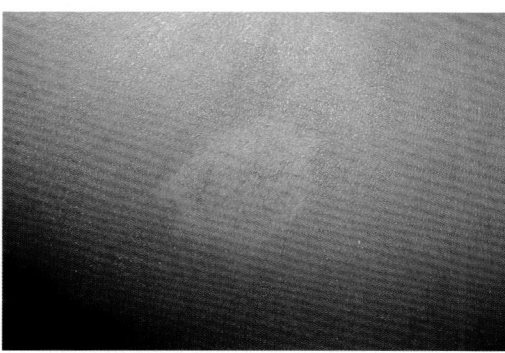

Color Figure 5

**Color Figure 1.** Giant congenital melanocytic nevus with atypical features, including a scalloped border, irregular pigmentation, and variable thickness.

**Color Figure 2.** Multiple pinkish brown papules and nodules of generalized cutaneous mastocytosis.

**Color Figure 3.** Striking yellow-orange, pebbly appearance of a typical nevus sebaceous on the scalp. Note the absence of hair within the lesion. The dark, crusted area is the site of a punch biopsy.

**Color Figure 4.** Large, mixed capillary and cavernous hemangioma on the left forearm with ulceration and crusting. The capillary component is superficial and bright red; the cavernous component is deeper and blue.

**Color Figure 5.** Incipient capillary (strawberry) hemangioma heralded by the central telangiectasia surrounded by an area of pallor.

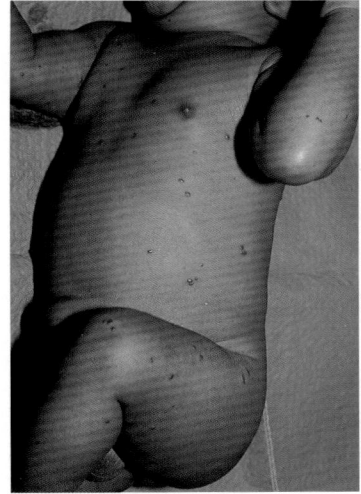

Color Figure 6

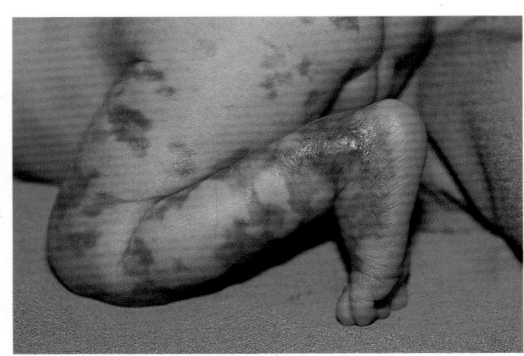

Color Figure 7

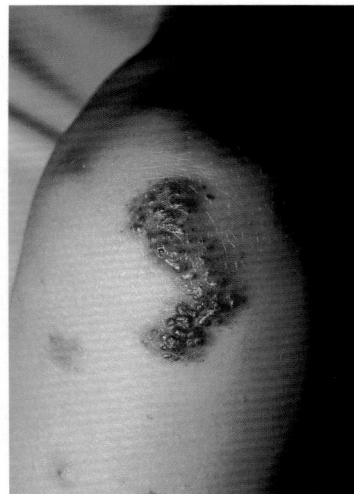

Color Figure 8

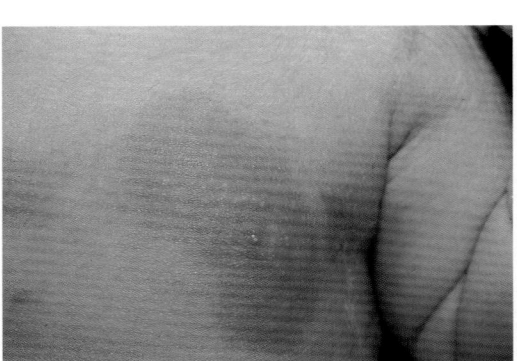

Color Figure 9

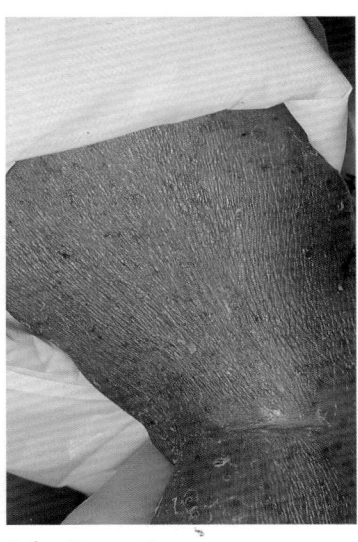

Color Figure 10

**Color Figure 6.**   Newborn with multiple 1- to 4-mm, firm, red, papular capillary hemangiomas of the diffuse neonatal hemangiomatosis syndrome.

**Color Figure 7.**   Reticulated mottling of cutis marmorata telangiectatica congenita with atrophy and telangiectasia of the skin.

**Color Figure 8.**   Lymphangioma circumscriptum with a purple-red hemangiomatous component on the extensor aspect of the elbow.

**Color Figure 9.**   The hallmark splotchy erythema studded with small papules and pustules of erythema toxicum.

**Color Figure 10.**   Hyperpigmented macules of transient neonatal pustular melanosis, many of which are surrounded by a collarette of scale that is the remnant of the roof of the preceding pustule.

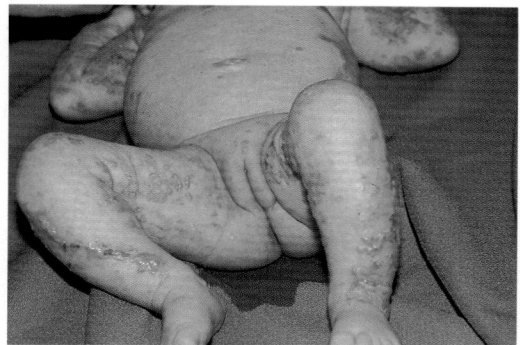

Color Figure 11

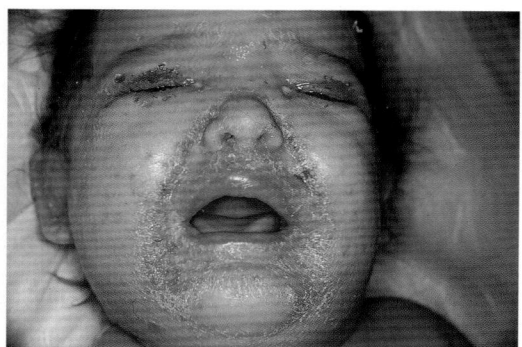

Color Figure 12

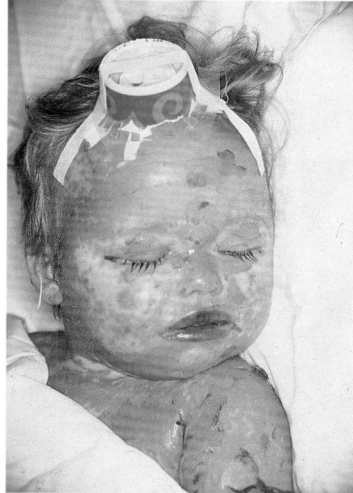

Color Figure 13

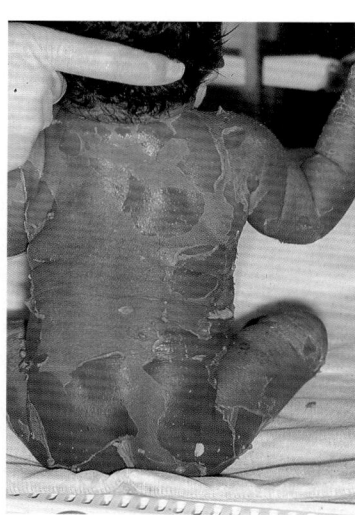

Color Figure 14

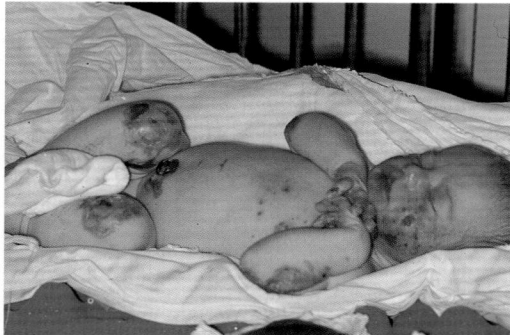

Color Figure 15

**Color Figure 11.** Vesicular stage of incontinentia pigmenti: linear streaks of vesicles on the extremities with less involvement on the trunk.

**Color Figure 12.** Characteristic facial appearance of an infant with staphylococcal scalded skin syndrome with purulent drainage and crusting around the eyes, nose, and mouth.

**Color Figure 13.** Maculopapular erythema, with blister formation on the face and extensive denudation on the arm, in an infant with toxic epidermal necrolysis.

**Color Figure 14.** Newborn with widespread blistering of epidermolytic hyperkeratosis.

**Color Figure 15.** Generalized epidermolysis bullosa simplex with erosions and bullae on the face, elbows, hands, and knees at sites of trauma.

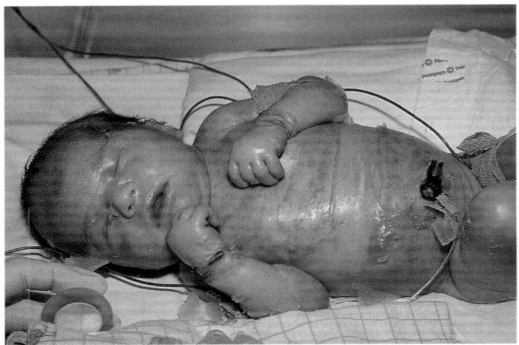

Color Figure 16

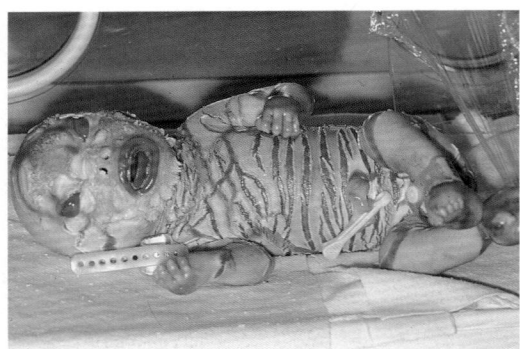

Color Figure 17

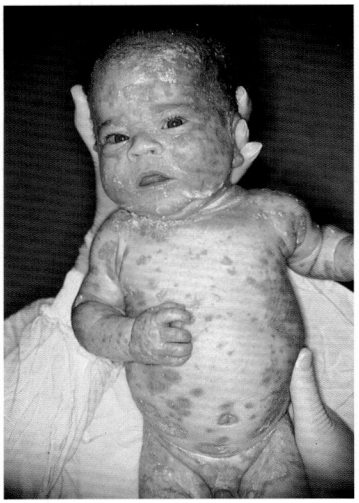

Color Figure 18

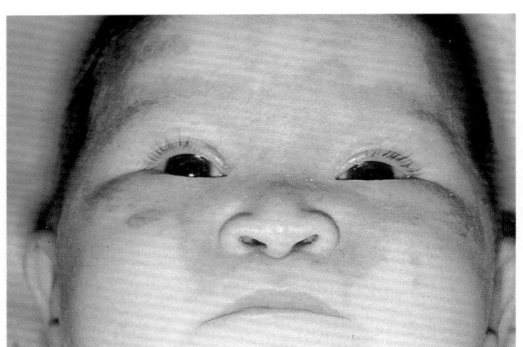

Color Figure 19

**Color Figure 16.**   Collodion baby after partial shedding of the collodion membrane. The hands, arms, legs, and a portion of the abdomen are still encased in a tight, shiny membrane.

**Color Figure 17.**   Harlequin fetus with thick yellow skin traversed by deep fissures, ectropion, eclabium, and mitten deformity of the hands and feet.

**Color Figure 18.**   Beefy red, sharply demarcated, scaling plaques of psoriasis.

**Color Figure 19.**   Characteristic erythematous, scaling plaques over the central face in an infant with neonatal lupus erythematosus.

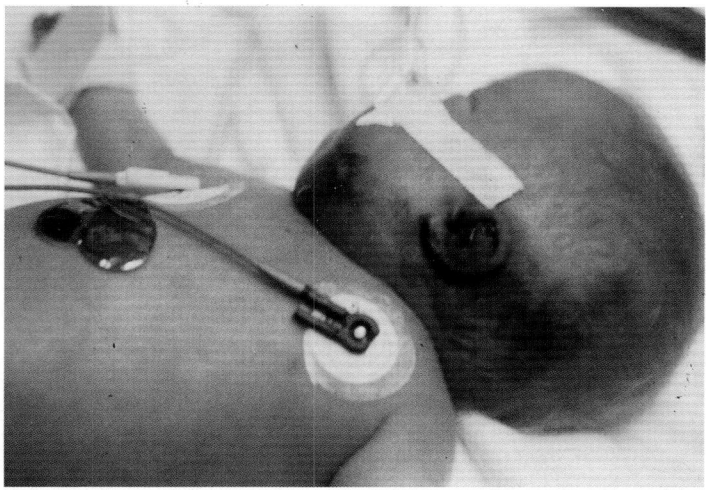

Color Figure 20

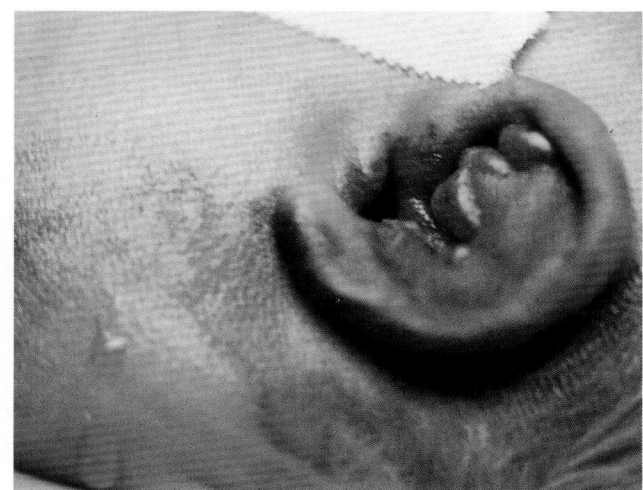

Color Figure 21

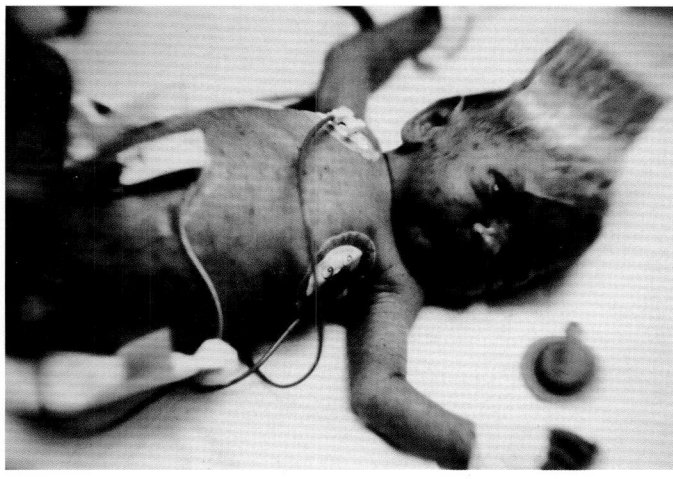

Color Figure 22

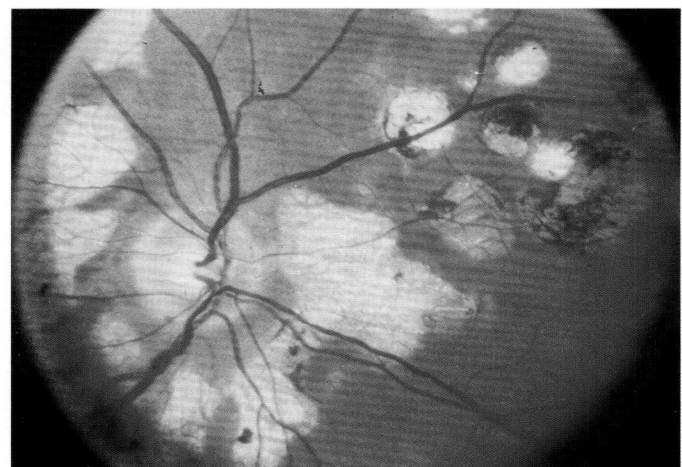

Color Figure 23

**Color Figure 20.**   Necrotizing fasciitis of the submandibular area and pinna in a 3-month-old premature infant with late onset group B streptococcal sepsis.

**Color Figure 21.**   Necrotizing fasciitis of the pinna in a 3-month-old premature infant with late onset group B streptococcal sepsis.

**Color Figure 22.**   "Blueberry muffin spots." Extramedullary dermal erythropoiesis observed in the most severely affected infants with congenital cytomegalovirus infection and congenital rubella.

**Color Figure 23.**   Patchy, yellow-white lesions of chorioretinitis seen with both congenital cytomegalovirus infection and congenital toxoplasmosis. (Courtesy of George H. McCracken, Jr, MD, Dallas, Texas)

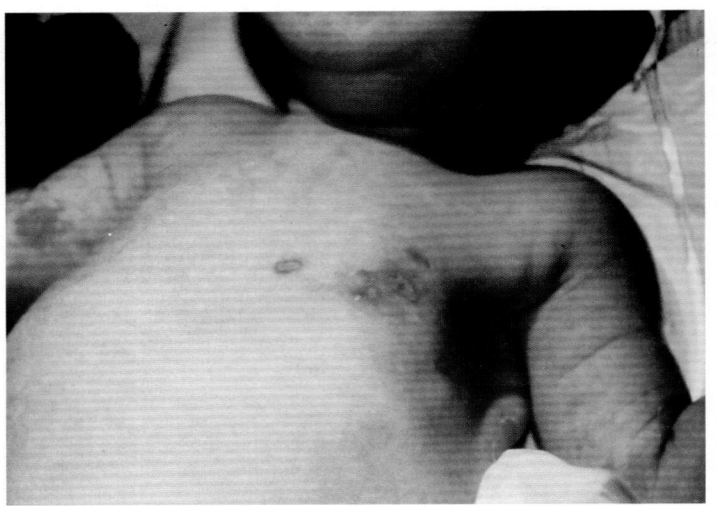

Color Figure 24

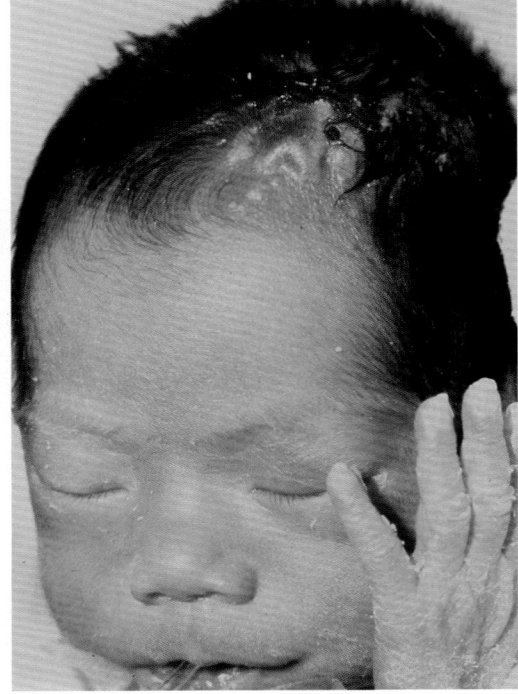

Color Figure 25

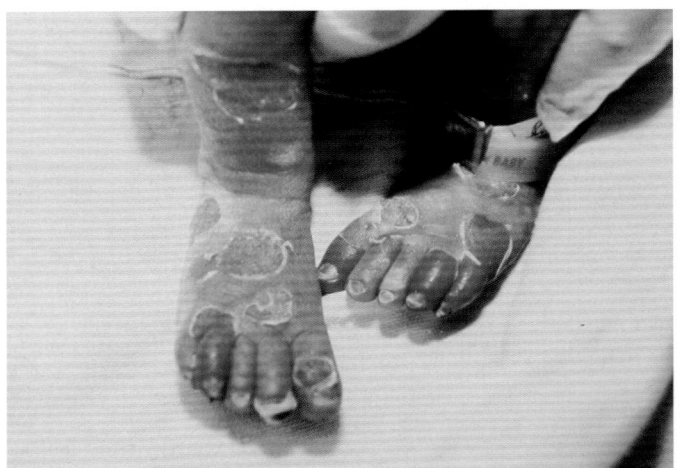

Color Figure 26

**Color Figure 24.** Discrete vesicles on an erythematous base in a neonate with herpes simplex virus infection.

**Color Figure 25.** Vesicular lesion of neonatal herpes simplex virus infection that developed at the site of a scalp electrode placed during labor for monitoring fetal heart rate. (Courtesy of Alec Wittek, MD)

**Color Figure 26.** Pemphigus syphiliticus, a widely disseminated vesiculobullous eruption in an infant with early congenital syphilis. (Courtesy of Charles M. Ginsburg, MD, Dallas, Texas)

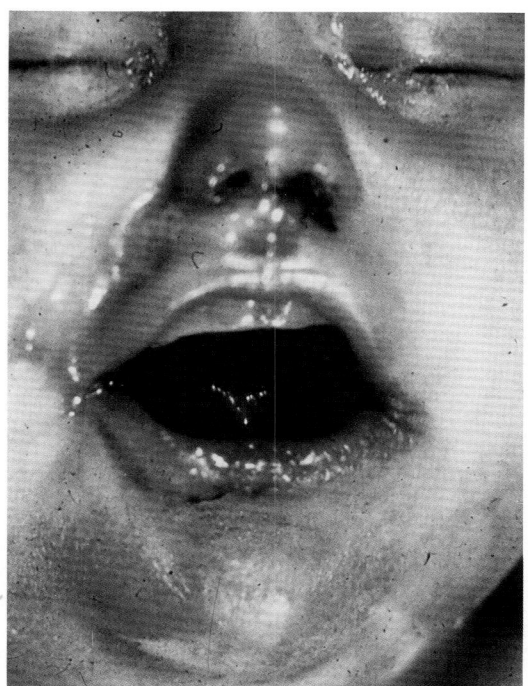

Color Figure 27

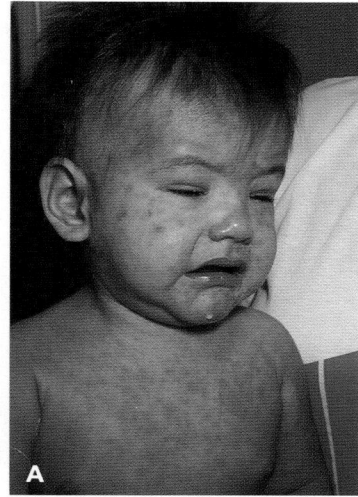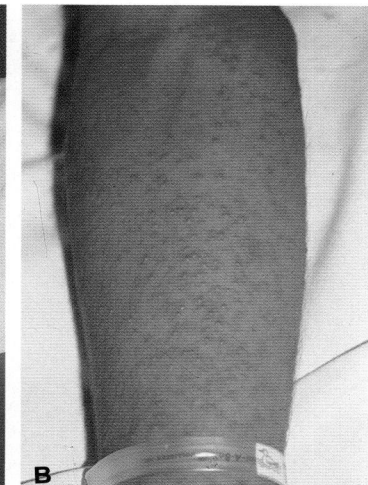

Color Figure 28

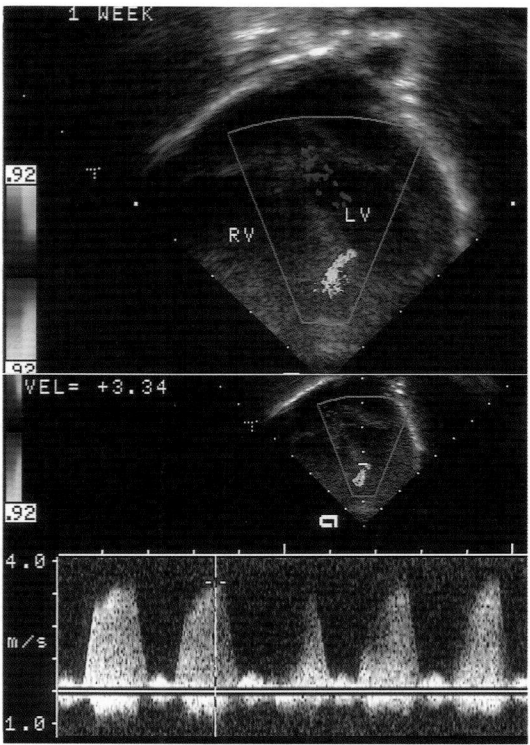

Color Figure 29

**Color Figure 27.** "Sniffles" or rhinitis in an infant with early congenital syphilis. This mucus discharge develops after the first week of life. (Courtesy of George H. McCracken, Jr, MD, Dallas, Texas)

**Color Figure 28.** Maculopapular rash in (*A*) typical measles (courtesy of Gail Demmler, MD) and (*B*) atypical measles.

**Color Figure 29.** Two-dimensional echocardiography and color Doppler show a ventricular septal defect with a right-to-left shunt and a heart murmur in a 1-week-old child. The color jet shows the location and the orientation of the abnormal blood flow (*upper panel*). The peak velocity of the jet was greater than 3.3 meters per second, predicting a gradient from the left to right ventricles of 40 mm Hg (*lower panel*).

# PART

# I

Frank A. Oski, Editor

# *General Pediatrics*

*Principles and Practice of Pediatrics, Second Edition.*
edited by Frank A. Oski et al. J. B. Lippincott Company, Philadelphia © 1994.

# CHAPTER 1
# *The History of Pediatrics in the United States*

## Howard A. Pearson

Pediatrics, or at least the medical care of infants and children, began in America shortly after the founding of the English colonies in the early 17th century. For more than 100 years, medical care of children was handled largely by parents, midwives, and nurses. Folk remedies often were directed by the "doctrine of signatures," based on the ancient belief that the form, shape, and color of plants corresponded to the diseased organs for which they had medicinal value. Hepatica was used for liver diseases and boneset for fractures. Because "like cures like," yellow plants were considered good for jaundice and red ones were good for the blood.

A few colonial "physicians" interested in children's diseases can be identified. Part-time pediatrics was practiced by pastor-physicians exemplified by Thomas Thacher of Boston, who championed smallpox vaccination and who, in 1677, wrote the first medical publication in the English colonies, a broadside on smallpox. Governor-physicians, notably John Winthrop, Jr., of Connecticut, conducted an extensive, if unusual, practice through the colonial mails. The scarcity of physicians and Winthrop's willingness to prescribe free of charge led to his being consulted frequently. Winthrop's medical records, some of which are preserved in Boston's Countway Medical Library, described a wide range of pediatric problems, such as rashes, jaundice, seizures, and diarrhea. There even is a clear description of child abuse. Cotton Mather, the great Massachusetts Puritan preacher, wrote of Winthrop's medical prowess: "Wherever he came the diseased flocked about him as if the healing angel of Bethesda had appeared in the place."

These part-time, nonphysician healers, as well as other colonial physicians who usually were uneducated, poorly trained practitioners, wielded a variety of ineffective remedies and anecdotal treatments against the formidable assaults of disease and death. These were perilous times for children. As Ernest Caulfield, an important American pediatric historian, wrote:

> In addition to diphtheria, dysentery, measles, and scarlet fever, smallpox, influenza and tuberculosis should certainly be included in the list of common diseases of colonial children. A surprisingly large proportion of them had worms. Deaths from falls, burns, and poisonings were frequent. It seems a little surprising that any of them survived.

Although universities and colleges were founded early in the Americas, they emphasized classical and theological curricula. Training in secular subjects such as medicine came much later, with the establishment of colleges of medicine. The first American medical schools were the University of Pennsylvania in Philadelphia (established in 1765), Harvard in Boston (established in 1783), the College of Physicians and Surgeons in New York (established in 1788), and Dartmouth in Hanover, New Hampshire (established in 1798).

Teaching of the diseases of children at most of these early medical schools was done sporadically, if at all, and then under the aegis of physic (medicine) or midwifery (obstetrics). At the University of Pennsylvania, Dr. Benjamin Rush, a preeminent American patriot-physician, a signer of the Declaration of Independence, and a prodigious "bleeder," was a professor of medicine between 1789 and 1813. Rush was the most influential American physician of his day and was designated "the American Sydenham" by European physicians.

Rush's medical lectures included a section on "Diseases peculiar to children." He published articles describing pediatric diseases, including spasmodic asthma, diseases of the mind, and diphtheria. Rush also coined the term *cholera infantum* to describe the lethal summer diarrhea that killed thousands of American children well into the middle of the 20th century.

Dr. William Potts Dewees, also a professor of midwifery at the University of Pennsylvania, in 1825 published a treatise on *The Physical and Medical Treatment of Children*. This text had eight subsequent re-editions and was arguably the first formal American textbook of pediatrics. Dr. John Eberle, Professor of Medicine at Jefferson Medical College, also published a pediatric textbook in 1833.

The first formal medical school course on the diseases of children was given and the first faculty appointment in the diseases of children in the United States was held at Yale University in New Haven, Connecticut by Dr. Eli Ives. For nearly 40 years, between 1813 and 1852, Ives lectured on the diseases of children to an estimated 1500 Yale medical students. Ives' lectures, recorded by hand in student notebooks of the time, are preserved in Yale's Sterling Library archives. They consisted of discourses on subjects ranging from angina to worms. Ives ascribed many medical illnesses to offending substances in the gastrointestinal tract. These had to be removed by inducing vomiting or by purging. Teething either caused or aggravated many diseases during the first 2 years of life and lancing of the gums was considered essential. Ives firmly subscribed to his teacher Benjamin Rush's theory that all diseases were "fevers" brought on by overstimulation of the arteries and, consequently, had to be treated by "depletion" through bloodletting, vomiting, or purging. Although Ives used phlebotomy sparingly, his therapeutic sheet anchors were calomel (mercury) and ipecac, plus a wide variety of herbal remedies. Ives' teachings received little attention outside of Connecticut, and formal instruction in the diseases of children at Yale ceased after his retirement in 1852.

It was nearly 25 years after Ives that American pediatrics began to take on a more defined presence. Children's hospitals were established, the first of these being the New York Nursing and Child Hospital, which opened in 1854; the Children's Hospital of Pennsylvania in Philadelphia, which opened in 1855; and the Boston Children's Hospital, which opened in 1869. Pediatric progress was perhaps most evident in New York City, where Abraham Jacobi and Job Lewis Smith were contemporaries in the latter part of the 19th century.

Jacobi received his medical training at the University of Bonn, Germany. After graduation, he was imprisoned for 2 years as a suspected revolutionary, and then emigrated to New York City in 1853. Although he was a general practitioner, he devoted most of his time to the care of children and their diseases. In 1860, he established a children's clinic at the New York Medical College, where his appointment as Professor of Infantile Pathology and Therapeutics was one of the first academic appointments in pediatrics made in the United States. He later became professor of pediatrics at Columbia's College of Physicians and Surgeons. Among Jacobi's most important contributions were his founding of the Section of Pediatrics of the American Medical Association (AMA) in 1880 and his selection as the first president of the American Pediatric Society (APS) in 1888. He established pediatric services in several New York hospitals and effectively championed causes that promoted the welfare of children. His drive and enthusiasm were instrumental in establishing pediatrics as a separate discipline in the United States.

Job Lewis Smith, who entered practice in Manhattan about the same time as Jacobi, also played a major role in early American pediatrics. Smith worked primarily at the Bellevue Medical School, where he was appointed clinical professor of morbid anatomy in 1861 and clinical professor of diseases of children in 1876. Smith was a prolific writer, publishing papers on infectious disease, rickets, and neonatal tetanus. He was very concerned with the dangers of bottle feeding and vigorously promoted milk sterilization. The appalling consequences of hand (artificial) feeding of foundlings in New York were described poignantly by Smith at the 1889 meeting of the APS: "The steamboat every morning brought foundlings to (Randall's) Island and every afternoon removed an equal number for burial in Potters' Field."

Between 1869 and 1896, Smith also published eight editions of *A Treatise on the Diseases of Infancy and Childhood*. This was an important textbook for medical students and practitioners for 30 years.

One of Smith's signal accomplishments was the organization and founding of the APS. In 1887, following the Pediatric Section of the Ninth International Medical Congress held in Washington, DC, Smith invited a group of physicians whom he knew to be interested in the diseases of children to join him in establishing the APS, an aim that was achieved in the following year. Forty-three American physicians who were interested and involved in pediatrics were elected as the founding members. For fully 50 years, the APS was the premier pediatric organization in the United States. The presentations and discussions that took place at the annual meetings, as noted in the record of society transactions, documented striking progress and advances of the specialty.

The availability of safe, pure milk for infant feeding was an overriding concern in the early days of pediatrics in the United States. Although breast-feeding was advocated strongly, it was recognized that societal pressures and a very high rate of abandonment and orphaning of infants caused artificial feeding to be used widely. In U.S. cities, much of the milk supply was contaminated dangerously and adulterated disgustingly. Between 1870 and 1920, the need for safe milk for infant feeding became a crusade for leaders of American pediatrics, including Jacobi, Smith, Rotch, LaFetra, Schick, Abt, and many others.

Application of the principles of the burgeoning science of bacteriology to infant nutrition in the early 20th century provided a scientific basis for safe infant feeding. That pasteurization of milk could prevent milk-transmitted diseases initially was appreciated about 1895. It was not until 1908, however, that Chicago became the first American city to make the pasteurization of milk mandatory. Soon thereafter, pasteurization became nearly universal, and the lives of many children were saved.

In Boston, pediatrics was taught at Harvard Medical School as early as 1871. In 1893, Thomas Morgan Rotch was appointed a full professor of diseases of children with a chair on the faculty. Rotch is remembered best for his "percentage method" of infant feeding. This system was based upon the concept that cow's milk was relatively indigestible and, therefore, had to be diluted before feeding. Because dilution reduced fat and carbohydrate content, cream and sugar were added to approximate the composition of human milk. However, this surprisingly modern concept became exquisitely convoluted in Rotch's hands. His system mandated complex formulations with varying percentages of protein, fat, and carbohydrates, and changes frequently were made on a day-to-day basis. The system required: "almost the equivalence of an advanced degree in higher mathematics employing algebraic equations to compute the food mixture of a baby."

It has been suggested that Rotch's successes were due more to his insistence on pure milk than to his percentage system. This system was accepted and employed widely by most physicians in the United States during the first decade of the 20th century, but had little acceptance in Europe. Ultimately, the system collapsed under its own complexity. As Oliver Wendell Holmes quipped: "A pair of substantial mammary glands has the advantage over the two hemispheres of the most learned professor's brain in the art of compounding a nutritious fluid for infants."

Jacobi is said to have commented to Rotch at a meeting of the APS, "You can't raise a baby by mathematics." European physicians often have wondered why Americans call a milk mixture for feeding infants a *formula*. This nomenclature derives from the formulas of Dr. Rotch.

By the end of the first decade of the 20th century, physicians in the United States developed and employed much more simplified feeding techniques based on the changing caloric needs of growing infants (calorimetric method) and also on the recognition by Brennemann and Powers that the casein of cow's milk could be made more digestible by simple heating. The increasing availability of evaporated milk and later of commercially prepared infant feeding mixtures reduced the complexities of feeding infants who were not breast-fed. This decreased emphasis on the technicalities of infant feeding resulted in elimination of the term *baby feeders* to describe pediatricians.

The other major concern of pediatricians during this era was infectious diseases. Diphtheria, scarlet fever, measles, whooping cough, and infant diarrhea were epidemic. Diphtheria was particularly lethal because of laryngeal obstruction by the diphtheritic pseudomembrane. Joseph O'Dwyer developed a device for laryngeal intubation—the O'Dwyer tube. Intubation became largely unnecessary, however, when large collaborative studies in 1896 and 1897 conducted by members of the APS demonstrated the effectiveness of diphtheria antitoxin in reducing the mortality of diphtheria, including laryngeal diphtheria. The incidence of diphtheria was reduced greatly by the introduction of the Schick test and active immunization with diphtheria toxoid after 1920.

Infant diarrhea, the "summer complaint" and the *cholera infantum* of Benjamin Rush, was epidemic in the urban areas of the United States well into the 20th century. It had a distressingly high mortality. Therapy, as summarized by Grover Powers, was largely symptomatic: "tea, barley water, protein milk, floating hospitals or country sanatoria." The Boston Floating Hospital had its origin in 1894 when a rented barge was loaded with hundreds of mothers and infants and towed around Boston harbor for a day. It was believed that sick infants would benefit from a day of salt air and cool ocean breezes.

L. Emmett Holt, Sr. of New York can be credited with establishing a scientific basis for pediatrics in the United States. Following his graduation from the College of Physicians and Surgeons in 1878, and a surgical internship, Holt entered private practice in midtown Manhattan. In 1889, he became the medical director of the New York Babies Hospital. This institution was in danger of closing because of financial and staffing problems. Holt threw himself into the task of rebuilding and reshaping the hospital. His efforts culminated in the opening of a new, modern hospital in 1910. In addition to outpatient facilities and 70 inpatient beds, the new Babies Hospital also had a dedicated research laboratory. Holt had no formal biochemical training, but he appointed experienced chemists to his staff. Holt also played a major role in the founding of the Rockefeller Institute. He worked with Rockefeller scientists and published a score of collaborative papers dealing with the chemical analysis of milk and milk proteins, salt and water balance, and absorption of nutrients and electrolytes in diarrheal diseases.

In 1901, Holt succeeded Jacobi as professor of pediatrics at Columbia's School of Physicians and Surgeons. One of his greatest accomplishments was the authorship of the classic pediatric textbook, *The Diseases of Infancy and Childhood*. First published in 1897, it had 11 subsequent editions during Holt's lifetime. It became the standard pediatric textbook and was considered the equal of Osler's *Textbook of Internal Medicine*.

John Howland, one of the greatest figures of pediatrics in the United States, graduated from the Cornell Medical School, studied in Europe, and worked with Holt in New York. He assumed the position of professor and full-time head of the pediatric department at Johns Hopkins in 1912. During the next 14 years, he built and directed the first modern, scientifically based, full-time pediatric department in the United States. The Harriet Lane Home, a freestanding children's hospital, opened in 1912, and Howland ensured that there were well-equipped biochemistry laboratories and a staff of full-time physicians dedicated to the care of infants and children. Howland recognized the importance of biochemical investigations of the diseases of children. He and a group of talented clinician-investigators published a series of classic studies on acidosis, rickets, and tetany. The men Howland trained became leaders in U.S. pediatrics for the next quarter of a century, and included Edwards Park, Kenneth Blackfan, Grover Powers, William McKim Marriott, James Gamble, Alfred Shohl, and Benjamin Kramer.

Edwards A. Park succeeded John Howland as professor of pediatrics at the Johns Hopkins School of Medicine. One of his major achievements was the development of pediatric subspecialty programs. Helen Taussig became one of the first pediatric cardiologists, and Lawson Wilkins became the father of pediatric endocrinology. Johns Hopkins had a profound influence on research, teaching, and patient care in departments of pediatrics throughout the world.

One of Howland's proteges, Kenneth D. Blackfan, became a professor of pediatrics at Harvard and director of the Boston Children's Hospital. Under Blackfan's leadership, James Gamble continued his important research on fluid and electrolyte physiology; Ladd and Gross developed pediatric surgery as a specialty; Louis Diamond established pediatric hematology as a separate discipline; and Sidney Farber, a pediatric pathologist, pioneered chemotherapy for acute lymphatic leukemia and other childhood malignancies.

Humanistic and psychosocial aspects of pediatrics also were recognized and emphasized during the middle of the 20th century. This perhaps was exemplified best by Grover Powers of Yale. Powers was educated and trained at Johns Hopkins School of Medicine under John Howland. In 1921, he accompanied Edwards Park to New Haven, Connecticut, where a new department of pediatrics had been established at Yale. When Park returned to Johns Hopkins in 1926 to become professor and chairman after Howland's death, Powers was appointed chairman of pediatrics at Yale—a position he was to hold for the next 30 years. Among Powers' unique contributions were his clear definition and articulation of the humanistic and social aspects of pediatrics, his initiation of "rooming in" for newborns, and his description of the myriad problems associated with mental retardation. As Powers' colleague at Yale, Daniel Darrow, emphasized, the decreasing mortality and morbidity of infectious diseases made possible by microbiology and by fluid and electrolyte therapy during the 1930s and 1940s resulted in an apparent emergence of the importance of childhood emotional disorders and mental retardation. Powers did much to address these issues.

Concerns over children's health have received national attention intermittently during the 20th century. The first White House Conference on the Care of Dependent Children, convened in 1909 by President Theodore Roosevelt, addressed some of the problems of children. The conference recommended the formation of a federal agency devoted to children. In 1912, President Taft acted on this recommendation, creating the Children's Bureau. The bureau's charge was to:

investigate and report . . . upon all matters pertaining to the welfare of children and child life among all classes of our people and . . . especially [to] investigate the questions of infant mortality, the birth rate, orphanages, juvenile courts, desertion, dangerous occupations, accidents and diseases of children.

Congress appropriated $25,000 for the foundation of the Children's Bureau, but at the same time approved $650,000 for a study of hog cholera! Unfortunately, the bureau was given little administrative or enforcement authority and could do little about high rates of maternal and infant mortality and the unequal access to medical care of poor families. Between 1909 and 1991, nine presidents have convened conferences on children and their health needs. Each conference issued "strong sweeping and perceptive reports which ultimately only gathered dust." The most recent National Commission on Children (1991) has made equally broad recommendations concerning the needs of America's children. Only time will determine whether these pressing needs will be not only acknowledged, but acted upon.

In 1921, Congress enacted the Sheppard-Towner Act authorizing the Children's Bureau to intervene in health problems of infants and children and to provide grants to states for maternal and child health activities. The intent of the act was approved unanimously by the Pediatric Section of the AMA in 1922. On the same day, however, the House of Delegates of the AMA independently passed a resolution condemning the Sheppard-Towner Act as interfering with the private practice of medicine. When news of the Pediatric Section's action was received by the AMA House of Delegates, not only was the Pediatric Section reprimanded, but also a ruling was made that sections could not act independently of AMA policy. The action of the AMA was viewed by many pediatricians as censorship. This became the major impetus for the founding in 1930 of a new pediatric organization independent of the AMA, the American Academy of Pediatrics (AAP). An indication of the growth of pediatrics in the United States can be seen by comparing the 43 pediatricians who were founders of the APS in 1888 with the 304 pediatricians who were charter members of the Academy of Pediatrics in 1930 and the more than 25,000 pediatricians who are members of the AAP in 1993.

Issac Abt of Chicago was the first president of the AAP. In his inaugural address he noted:

It is our desire to build an association so that every qualified pediatrician could seek membership. It will be necessary for the Academy to interest itself in undergraduate and post-graduate instruction and to exert a regulatory influence over hospitals. As an organization it should assist and lead in public health measures in society reform and in hospital and educational administration as they affect the welfare of children.

One of the first actions of the executive committee of the American Academy of Pediatrics was to set in motion an initiative that led to the founding of the American Board of Pediatrics in 1933. Qualifications for board certification included specific training requirements and an examination. Certification by the American Board of Pediatrics, which ensured clinical training and competence, was made a requirement for AAP membership.

As pediatric research increased during the 1920s and 1930s, a need for a research society to complement the APS was perceived. This led to organization of the Eastern Society for Pediatric Research in 1929. Its aim was "to serve the younger members of University groups in Pediatrics." In 1931, it went national, becoming the Society for Pediatric Research (SPR). Requirements for SPR membership were active involvement in pediatric research and age younger than 45 years. The annual scientific meetings of the APS and SPR became the preeminent forums for advances in pediatrics during much of the 20th century. These societies were joined by the Ambulatory Pediatric Society (APA) in 1960 and the Association of Medical School Pediatric Department Chairmen (AMSPDC) in 1967.

The control of many infectious diseases permitted pediatricians increasingly to address other diseases and problems, including genetic, metabolic, mental, and psychiatric diseases. Normal growth and development became well established, permitting comparison with aberrant patterns in disease. Gesell at Yale published important studies describing the normal development of infants and children.

Following a slowdown during World War II, a postwar boom in pediatrics occurred. Full-time departments of pediatrics were established or expanded at most American medical schools. Expansion of pediatric research was fueled largely by federal funds, especially from the National Institutes of Health. The National Institute of Child Health and Human Development (NICHD) was founded in 1960. Under its first director, Robert Aldrich, the NICHD supported investigations of a wide range of child health issues.

The introduction of antibiotics—first penicillin and then a large number of broad-spectrum antibiotics—permitted the successful treatment and prevention of previously lethal infections such as *Haemophilus influenzae* and tuberculous meningitis. More recently, vaccines effective against *H influenzae* are greatly reducing the incidence of bacterial meningitis. The Nobel Prize–winning discovery by John Enders and his colleagues that viruses could be grown successfully in tissue culture resulted in the development of vaccines against poliomyelitis, measles, and rubella that virtually can eliminate these diseases. Unfortunately, many American children still are not immunized. The recurrence of epidemics of measles and pertussis is cause for great pediatric concern.

The use of prophylactic antibiotics for the control of β-hemolytic streptococcal infections was an important factor in the near disappearance of rheumatic fever and carditis in the United States. Pediatric cardiologists, led by Helen Taussig, developed techniques that could differentiate between the various congenital anatomic lesions of the heart during life. This led to the development of procedures to correct many of these disorders surgically. Louis Diamond in Boston continued his lifelong studies of Rh erythroblastosis, which proceeded from clinical and laboratory definition to effective therapy and ultimately to prevention.

Some of the most dramatic developments in pediatrics have been advances in the care of premature infants. Modern incubators, such as the Isolette designed by Chapple in Philadelphia, maintained the premature infant's body temperature and provided oxygenation and isolation from external infections. Because of their efficiency, however, the incubators also often exposed premature infants to high oxygen levels that later were proven to be the cause of retrolental fibroplasia and resultant blindness. Techniques for monitoring oxygen levels sharply reduced the incidence of this iatrogenic disease. Low–birth-weight infants often developed respiratory distress syndrome, also called hyaline membrane disease, because of lung immaturity. Improved procedures for respiratory management, better respirators, and, later, recognition of the role of pulmonary surfactant by Mary Ellen Avery led to the increasing survival of ever smaller premature infants.

However, unforeseen challenges still are being presented to pediatricians. "New" diseases such as Kawasaki disease, Reye's syndrome, and Lyme disease have appeared; fortunately, these conditions have been understood and controlled largely through incisive epidemiologic studies and effective interventions. The last decades of the 20th century have seen the emergence of human immunodeficiency virus infection as the new scourge of children.

As the end of the 20th century nears, a true revolution in bioscience and in pediatrics—the so-called new biology—has occurred. Dazzling new research technologies have made possible the definition of disease at the cellular, subcellular, and molecular levels. Recombinant DNA technology has revolutionized the diagnosis and understanding of many genetic diseases. Techniques such as magnetic resonance imaging and radioimmune assay have enhanced greatly our ability to diagnose many pediatric diseases.

Pediatric subspecialties have multiplied and their special skills have advanced the effective treatment of a wide variety of pediatric disorders. Unfortunately, each specialty has developed its own argot that sometimes makes communication between pediatricians difficult. A plethora of subspecialty societies and subspecialty journals has resulted in the fragmentation of pediatric communication. Even more unfortunate is what appears to be an increasing emphasis on single organ systems or diseases, with resultant neglect of the whole child, the child's community, and the child's family. Perhaps the greatest challenge of U.S. pediatrics today is deciding whether the art, empathy, and concern for the whole child that have characterized this discipline over the last 150 years can be preserved as technologies become ever more complex and the body of scientific knowledge becomes ever larger.

## Selected Readings

Cone TE Jr. History of American pediatrics. Boston: Little Brown, 1979.

Cone TE Jr. History of the care and feeding of the premature infant. Boston: Little Brown, 1985.

Faber K, McIntosh R. History of the American Pediatric Society 1887–1965. New York: McGraw-Hill, 1966.

Pearson HA. Lectures on the diseases of children by Eli Ives, M.D. of Yale and New Haven: America's first academic pediatrician. Pediatrics 1986;77:680.

Pearson HA. The centennial history of the American Pediatric Society. New Haven: American Pediatric Society, 1988.

Veeder S. Pediatric profiles. St Louis: CV Mosby, 1957.

*Principles and Practice of Pediatrics, Second Edition.*
edited by Frank A. Oski et al. J. B. Lippincott Company, Philadelphia © 1994.

## CHAPTER 2
# *The Field of Pediatrics*

Evan Charney

Children are one third of our population and all of our future.*

The field of pediatrics is about children's health or, more precisely, about the threats to their health, both those that become manifest in childhood and those that will impair health in later years. Because habits and practices established in childhood have im-

* Select Panel for the Promotion of Child Health, 1981.

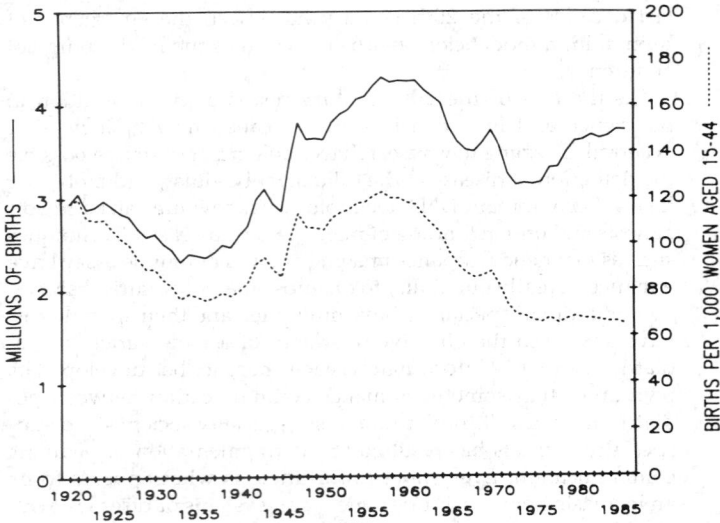

**Figure 2-1.** Live births and fertility rates, United States, 1920 to 1990. (Wegman ME. Annual summary of vital statistics. Pediatrics 1991;88:1081.)

plications for health and illness throughout life, pediatricians have come to adopt a strong preventive orientation.

This chapter describes the childhood population of the United States in terms of both current numbers and future projections. In general, children in this country in the 1990s are healthy, with lower rates of morbidity and mortality than adults and markedly lower rates of ill health than existed in the past. Chronic handicapping conditions are similarly uncommon and are diminishing in frequency.

There are gaps in this rosy picture, however. In 1990, 25% of American children lived in poverty. Children in low-income families have a higher incidence of disease and receive less care than do children in more affluent families. The United States, alone among industrialized countries, still lacks a coordinated system of health services that all people have access to and all can afford. Thirty-seven million Americans have no health insurance, and nearly half of those are children. Preventive services, counseling, and guidance—the cornerstones of pediatrics—are financed less well than are the more procedure-oriented fields of medicine. As one result, immunization rates against common preventable diseases of childhood protect only two thirds of American preschool children and a considerably lower percentage of the poor. In contrast, all Western European countries have markedly higher immunization rates for children (Williams, 1992).

The field of pediatrics also is about pediatricians, and this chapter examines who they are, how they spend their time, and what trends in pediatrics are likely to influence what they will do in the coming years. In the United States today, pediatrics is both a primary care and a subspecialty, consultant discipline. Pediatricians are involved in a wide range of activities, functioning as individual clinicians to children and families, as consultants to health agencies and schools, and as advocates for children at the local, state, and national level.

## THE CHILDHOOD POPULATION OF THE UNITED STATES

In 1990, there were 64 million children under 18 years of age in the United States and 4,179,000 live births. As indicated in Figure 2-1, the birth rate has remained steady over the past decade, at its lowest point in 50 years. The current fertility rate is 70 live births per 1000 women of childbearing age (15 to 44 years). The fact that the total number of births has been increasing since the mid-1970s in the face of this low fertility rate reflects the large

number of women currently in their childbearing years, themselves a product of the "baby boom" of the period from 1945 to 1960.

For the next decade, if the fertility rate is unchanged, we can anticipate a slow decrease in the number of children under 5 years of age as the baby-boom population moves through the childbearing years (Table 2-1). The overall number of individuals less than 24 years of age should remain stable at 90 million to 91 million until the middle of the next century, but with varying proportions of younger and older children and adolescents. However, as Figure 2-1 also documents, predictions about fertility rates and the consequent size of the childhood population are risky; wide swings are the rule. These data have obvious implications for health planning. Because infants and young children require the most frequent care, both for illness and for child health supervision, a small shift in the number of births is reflected promptly in a greater or lesser demand for health care. A variation in the childhood population of 1 million (just 1.1% of 91 million) either up or down translates into the need for 600 more or fewer pediatricians, respectively.

## MORTALITY AND MORBIDITY

Several facts are evident from a review of the causes of childhood mortality in the United States. There are about 30,000 deaths of liveborn infants on the first day of life from immediate perinatal

**TABLE 2-1.  Actual and Projected Population (×10⁶) 0 to 24 Years of Age in the United States**

| Year | 0–4 (%) | 5–13 (%) | 14–17 (%) | 18–24 (%) | Total |
|------|---------|----------|-----------|-----------|-------|
| 1990 | 18.4 | 32.4 | 13.2 | 26.1 | 90.1 |
| 1995 | 17.8 | 33.8 | 14.5 | 24.3 | 90.4 |
| 2000 | 16.9 | 33.5 | 15.3 | 25.2 | 90.9 |
| 2005 | 16.6 | 32.0 | 15.5 | 26.9 | 91.0 |
| 2010 | 16.9 | 31.0 | 14.7 | 27.2 | 89.8 |

*Projections of the population of the United States by age, sex, and race: 1988–2080. Current Population Reports Series p-25, No 1018. U.S. Bureau of the Census, January 1989.*

conditions, congenital anomalies, birth asphyxia, and extreme prematurity. In fact, that number equals the total childhood mortality for the next 15 years of life. Then there is a gradual reduction in mortality to the age of 5 to 15 years, the healthiest decade of life, followed by a steady rise thereafter.

Death from trauma—both unintentional and intentional injury—rapidly assumes first rank between 1 and 4 years of age and is the leading cause of death throughout the remainder of the first 45 years of life (Table 2-2). Indeed, accidental injury accounts for nearly half of all deaths of persons aged 1 to 25 years. Between the ages of 15 and 24 years, the effects of violence on mortality are even more striking. Homicide and suicide rates are about the same, 16.9 and 13.3 per 100,000, respectively, and together equal the mortality for all remaining medical threats to health during adolescence: malignancy, infections, and organ system disease. In 1989, for the first time, human immunodefi-

### TABLE 2-2. Major Causes of Death by Age: United States, 1989

| | Number of Deaths | Rate (Per 100,000) |
|---|---|---|
| **Under 1 Year** | 39,655 | 981 |
| Certain perinatal conditions | 12,572 | 311 |
| Congenital anomalies | 8120 | 201 |
| Sudden infant death syndrome | 5634 | 139 |
| Extreme immaturity | 3931 | 97 |
| Respiratory distress syndrome | 3631 | 90 |
| Anoxia-birth asphyxia | 1158 | 31 |
| Accidents | 996 | 25 |
| **1 to 4 Years** | 7292 | 49.2 |
| Accidents | 2774 | 18.7 |
|    Motor vehicle | 1005 | 6.8 |
|    All others | 1769 | 11.9 |
| Congenital anomalies | 928 | 6.3 |
| Malignant neoplasms | 506 | 3.4 |
| Homicide | 393 | 2.7 |
| Cardiovascular disease | 281 | 1.9 |
| Pneumonia | 228 | 1.5 |
| **5 to 14 Years** | 8914 | 25.4 |
| Accidents | 4090 | 11.6 |
|    Motor vehicle | 2266 | 6.4 |
|    All others | 1824 | 5.2 |
| Malignant neoplasms | 1155 | 3.3 |
| Homicide | 510 | 1.5 |
| Congenital anomalies | 480 | 1.4 |
| Cardiovascular disease | 295 | 0.8 |
| Suicide | 240 | 0.7 |
| **15 to 24 Years** | 36,488 | 99.9 |
| Accidents | 16,738 | 45.8 |
|    Motor vehicle | 12,941 | 35.4 |
|    All others | 3797 | 10.4 |
| Homicide | 6185 | 16.9 |
| Suicide | 4870 | 13.3 |
| Malignant neoplasms | 1851 | 5.1 |
| Cardiovascular disease | 938 | 2.6 |
| Human immunodeficiency virus infection | 613 | 1.7 |

*National Center for Health Statistics. Monthly vital statistics report. 1992;40(Suppl 2).*

### TABLE 2-3. Death Rates by Age, Sex, and Race: United States, 1989

| | Race (Rates Per 100,000) | | |
|---|---|---|---|
| | White | African-American | All |
| **Male** | | | |
| <1 year | 909.4 | 2179 | 1107 |
| 1–4 years | 47.8 | 88.4 | 54.2 |
| 5–9 years | 24.8 | 39.3 | 26.9 |
| 10–14 years | 31.7 | 44.3 | 33.5 |
| 15–19 years | 115.3 | 176.2 | 123.9 |
| 20–24 years | 149.5 | 300.7 | 169.7 |
| **Female** | | | |
| <1 year | 716.0 | 1863.9 | 898.4 |
| 1–4 years | 38.4 | 72.5 | 44.0 |
| 5–9 years | 18.4 | 28.6 | 20.3 |
| 10–14 years | 19.0 | 27.6 | 20.4 |
| 15–19 years | 49.8 | 48.6 | 49.4 |
| 20–24 years | 48.1 | 86.8 | 53.7 |

*National Center for Health Statistics. Monthly vital statistics report. 1992;40(Suppl 2).*

ciency virus infection was listed as the sixth leading cause of death for 15- to 24-year-olds.

Variations in childhood mortality rates by sex and race are listed in Table 2-3. Death rates for boys are about 50% higher than those for girls throughout childhood, with threefold and fourfold higher intentional and unintentional injury rates for boys, respectively, particularly during adolescence. Death rates in African-Americans generally are 1½ to 2 times those for whites under the age of 15 years for most conditions, including all infectious diseases. For homicide, particularly between 15 and 24 years of age, the rate for African-American males is more than five times greater than that for white males (78.2 v 14.4 per 100,000) and has been increasing since 1987. Indeed, homicide is the single greatest cause of death for African-American male adolescents, equalling all other causes combined. In only two major categories do white mortality rates exceed those for African-Americans: accidental injury (largely motor vehicle–related) and suicide, for which the rate in white children is twice that in African-American children. It is noteworthy that racial differences in the rates of malignancy and congenital anomalies are negligible, however, suggesting that social and environmental factors account for the disparity in other areas; unfortunately, racial differences in mortality still largely reflect the disparity in economic status between races in the United States in the 1990s.

## INFANT MORTALITY

The infant mortality rate (defined as deaths in the first year of life per 1000 live births) shows similar race and sex differences. The mortality rate has declined for both races since 1950 (Fig 2-2); however, a significant difference between the races remains. Although the reduction in infant mortality has been remarkable and gratifying, the United States in 1989 still ranked below 20 other countries in this measure. Moreover, the infant mortality rate for whites alone was higher than that in 17 other countries. Our persistently low standing seems paradoxical considering that advances in neonatal intensive care have reduced mortality and morbidity dramatically at each birth weight interval. The salvage rate in the United States at every birth weight interval is among

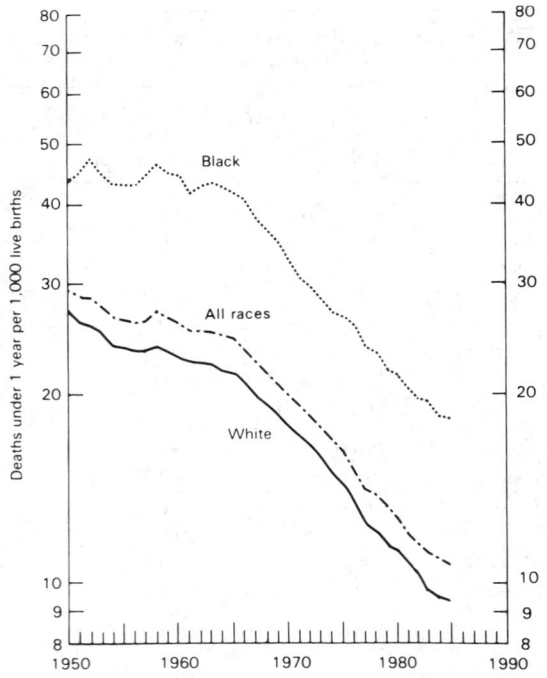

Figure 2-2.  Infant mortality rate by race, United States, 1950 to 1990. (National Center for Health Statistics. Monthly Vital Statistics Report 1992;40(Suppl 2).)

the best in the world, a testimony to the effectiveness of modern neonatal intensive care. What, then, accounts for our relatively low standing? The answer lies in several interrelated issues, including the high incidence of low–birth-weight infants, high rates of teenage pregnancy, and persistent gaps in adequate, comprehensive prenatal care.

The single most powerful correlate of neonatal mortality is birth weight, because most deaths are consequences of extreme immaturity. In 1989, 7% of all newborns weighed less than 2500 g, and a disproportionate number of them were born to teenage mothers who had received inadequate prenatal care. Despite the fact that the teenage pregnancy rate in the United States has declined over the past 15 years (12.8% of all births were to mothers younger than 20 years of age in 1989), it still exceeds that of other industrialized countries: all countries with infant mortality rates below 10 per 1000 births had fewer than 9% of those births to teenage mothers. The third factor, the provision of prenatal care, can be shown to reduce prematurity rates and birth complications. In 1985, however, 5% of pregnant women (10% of African-Americans) received no prenatal care whatsoever. Moreover, 21% of white women and 58% of African-American women lacked prenatal care during the first trimester. In fact, the United States has a higher teenage pregnancy rate, a higher abortion rate, and less adequate prenatal care than do other comparably industrialized countries. Although societal factors have a major influence on these problems, the structure of the health system can be an important ameliorating force. Western European countries with better mortality rates and fewer resources than our own all have well-organized maternity services, which are accessible to pregnant women, with integrated social support programs and no financial barriers to care.

## HEALTH STATUS AND HEALTH NEEDS OF CHILDREN

Despite the health problems that remain, from a historical perspective—looking backward in time—the current statistics are a

triumph. At the beginning of the 20th century, 160 of every 1000 children born did not survive the first year of life, compared to 9 per 1000 at present, a striking reduction in mortality of 94%. The reduction in death rates at other ages has been dramatic also: from 2000 to 50 per 100,000 in 1- to 4-year-olds and from 390 to 20 per 100,000 in 5- to 14-year-olds. Indeed, infant mortality has fallen by 50% since 1970 alone. Death rates in the first 15 years of life have been reduced more dramatically over the past 50 years than have rates at all older ages. However, deaths from injury, childhood malignancy, and congenital anomalies have been reduced only modestly and, therefore, are prime subjects to be addressed in the future.

One of the most comprehensive assessments of the health needs of children is contained in the 1981 report of the Select Panel for the Promotion of Child Health, a study commissioned by Congress. Although based on data now more than a decade old, its insights are pertinent, and its recommendations outline a timely agenda for the 1990s. The Panel outlined three sets of goals:

1. *Ensure access to needed health services for infants, children, adolescents, and pregnant women.* Although the health status of American children has improved dramatically, not all groups have shared equally in the progress. The ability of health care to ameliorate health problems is demonstrable, but because of financial barriers and a lack of coherently organized private and public health services, effective care is not provided universally.
2. *Devise strategies of health promotion that are beyond the reach of personal health services.* To reduce the major causes of childhood (and adult) mortality, strategies aimed at injury control (accident prevention), control of hazards in the physical environment, and promotion of the adoption of healthy living practices require the involvement of the general public, the schools, and the media. Promoting health-relevant behavior is one task of the primary care physician, but school-based and community-based education is essential.
3. *Encourage support of research.* In addition to strong support for fundamental research, the panel urged expanded support for research in epidemiology, prevention, health policy, and environmental risks to health.

As the major threats to child health of the early part of this century have been overcome—principally those related to infectious disease and malnutrition—the conditions that remain are not likely to be solved by medical science alone. As the Select Panel report documents, preventive strategies devised and carried out in collaboration with other groups in society will be more effective than will curative strategies in addressing these problems.

## PEDIATRICIAN DEMOGRAPHICS

The number of pediatricians in the United States has more than doubled between 1970 and 1990, to a total of 40,893 physicians. Table 2-4 lists the number of pediatricians and all physicians in the United States at intervals between 1970 and 1990, identifying the proportion of women in medicine. Women always have been well represented in pediatrics, and their number has continued to increase. In 1991, 58% of the 6731 residents in accredited pediatric training programs were women. It can be anticipated that, by the year 2000, the sexes will be represented equally in pediatrics. There always has been a disproportionately large number of international medical graduates in pediatrics compared to all United States physicians, but this percentage appears to be diminishing. Pediatricians are younger, on average, than are other physicians: in 1990, 29% of pediatricians were less than 35 years of age, compared to 22% of all physicians.

| | All Physicians (%) | | Pediatricians (%) | |
|---|---|---|---|---|
| Year | Total | Women | Total | Women |
| 1970 | 334,028 (100) | 25,507 (7.7) | 18,819 (100) | 3,907 (20.8) |
| 1975 | 393,742 (100) | 35,636 (9.1) | 22,730 (100) | 5,244 (23.1) |
| 1980 | 467,679 (100) | 54,284 (11.6) | 29,462 (100) | 8,314 (28.2) |
| 1985 | 552,716 (100) | 80,725 (14.6) | 35,617 (100) | 12,373 (34.7) |
| 1990 | 615,421 (100) | 104,194 (16.9) | 40,893 (100) | 15,675 (38.3) |

**TABLE 2-4. Number of all US Physicians and Pediatricians**

*Roback F, Randolph L, Seidman B. Physician characteristics and distribution in the U.S. Chicago: American Medical Association, 1992.*

For physicians in office-based practice, there has been a steady, accelerating trend away from solo and into group practice arrangements. In 1991, 30% of pediatricians were in solo practice (a lower proportion than other physicians) and almost half were in groups of four or more physicians. As a harbinger of the future, three fourths of those entering practice since 1980 have joined groups, and the number of physicians in those groups has been increasing as well.

## THE SUPPLY OF PEDIATRICIANS

Between 1970 and 1990, when the number of pediatricians doubled, there was only a 21% increase in the population of children younger than 10 years of age. As a result, the calculated number of children per pediatrician declined from about 3000 in 1970 to 2000 in 1983, and is projected to drop to 1200 by the year 2000. Moreover, in considering staffing needs for children, the role of family practitioners is important: on average, persons under 21 years of age represent one quarter of a typical family practice population. Figure 2-3 depicts these staffing trends between 1970 and 2000.

Data for pediatricians and for the total number of child health providers (pediatricians plus one-quarter the number of family

practitioners) are listed. Current health management organization (HMO) staffing patterns indicate that a pediatrician can provide care to 1500 to 2000 children; by these calculations, there will be an excess of child health providers projected over the next decade. Table 2-5 lists factors that influence future staffing needs, each of which can have an impact on the quantity and quality of health services available to children. However, staffing projections are subject to considerable variation, as discussed below:

- The relatively young average age of pediatricians and the increased number of those completing residency (about double that of 2 decades ago) means that fewer doctors now retire per year than enter practice, which will result in a net gain in physician supply.
- The number of hours worked per week by all physicians, including pediatricians, has been decreasing slowly. In addition, in the past, women physicians have averaged less work time than men, reflecting outside family demands. If those trends continue, the result would be a net reduction in the supply of active pediatricians.
- About one quarter of practicing pediatricians are international medical graduates, a higher proportion than in other primary care disciplines. Because many enter from countries with serious shortages of well-trained physicians, efforts have increased to ensure that they will return to their countries of origin after residency training in the United States. In a climate of potential physician oversupply, those pressures are likely to intensify, which would reduce the number of available physicians.
- Appropriately educated nurse practitioners or child health associates can provide a proportion of pediatric primary care services that are both high-quality and acceptable to families. It was estimated a decade ago that, by 1990, 15% of pediatric primary care would be provided by such allied health personnel. The current figure is under 5%, however, and pediatric nurse practitioner training programs have diminished markedly in recent years. Conversely, the lower costs of such personnel relative to physicians may make their employment economically attractive within managed health care systems.
- The relative roles of pediatricians and family physicians as primary care providers to children also are subject to change. A 1981 study found that each accounted for about 35% of ambulatory visits of persons less than 19 years of age (the remaining 30% were to internists and various surgical

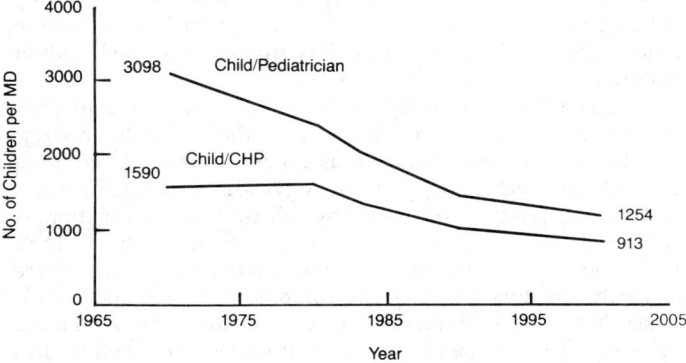

**Figure 2-3.** Actual and projected number of children aged 0 to 19 years per pediatrician or child health physician (*CHP*), 1970 to 2000. (Council on Long Range Planning and Development in cooperation with the American Academy of Pediatrics. The future of pediatrics: Implication of the changing environment of medicine. JAMA 1987;258:240.)

**TABLE 2-5. Supply and Demand Factors That Influence Pediatric Staffing Needs**

| Supply Factors | Demand Factors |
|---|---|
| Number of US medical graduates and proportion entering pediatrics | Size of child population; proportion of care at each age provided by pediatricians |
| Number of foreign medical graduates in pediatrics | Mechanisms and adequacy of payment for health services |
| Number of pediatric residency positions | Health and illness patterns; new diseases |
| Relative proportion of primary care provided by family physicians and pediatricians | Scope of problems seen as appropriate to medical management |
| Relative proportion of pediatricians in primary v subspecialty practice | Site of care: office, hospital, school |
| Role of allied health personnel | Geographic distribution of children |
| Geographic distribution of pediatricians | |

subspecialists). If the increasing proportion of elderly in the American population occupy more of the time of family physicians in the future, they will have less time to devote to children. At present, relative to family practitioners, pediatricians provide a larger proportion of care to infants and young children and considerably less to adolescents. In the decade between 1977 and 1987, pediatricians gradually increased their proportion of the "market" from 38.3% to 49.8% of all visits to children less than 19 years of age. The geographic distributions of family physicians and pediatricians differ as well. Pediatricians are located disproportionately in urban and suburban areas relative to the distribution of children; family practitioners are located more proportionately.

- Hospitalization rates have been reduced, and there may be less demand for acute illness care as children's health continues to improve; new vaccines (eg, against *Haemophilus influenzae B*) should reduce further the risk of serious infection. Conversely, new diseases (eg, the acquired immunodeficiency syndrome) or new disease patterns (eg, bronchopulmonary disease in neonatal intensive care survivors) will increase the demand on ambulatory and hospital services.

In summary, the shortage of physicians in the United States evident in the 1970s has been eliminated, and at least a rough balance in primary care providers for children appears more likely for the future. A number of factors, which are difficult to quantify, will continue to influence this equilibrium. At the present time, serious gaps in health services for children remain. For these to be ameliorated, the organization and financing of services must be changed and an adequate supply of physicians assured.

## THE DUAL IDENTITY OF PEDIATRICS

Pediatrics has a dual identity as both a primary care and a subspecialty discipline, and practitioners divide along those lines. A 1991 American Medical Association survey reported that 87.4% of pediatricians who have completed training and are involved in patient care are office-based primary care providers, and that 10% of these spend a significant part of their time in subspecialty practice. The remaining 12.6% of pediatricians (about 4500) are principally hospital-based subspecialists, with a smaller fraction working in public service positions at the local, state, and national levels. Of those in full-time subspecialty practice, the largest numbers are in neonatology, cardiology, and hematology/oncology, with smaller numbers in allergy, endocrinology, nephrology, gastroenterology, and pulmonology.

It may be helpful to differentiate further the nature of primary and consultant pediatrics. These are clinical disciplines, in the personal rather than the public health sphere. Primary care has several core ingredients. First, it represents the initial contact that the public has with the medical profession. In that regard, it is concerned with defining those aspects of health and illness that are managed appropriately by the family (and child) and the point at which the medical profession's role begins—that is, when and how children become "patients." Second, it implies a longitudinal "contract" with the patient or family to provide care over time, regardless of the presence or absence of disease. Third, it involves a coordinating or integrative role for the physician, who may refer a patient at times for medical or surgical consultation, but who continues to serve as that patient's advocate and interpreter within an increasingly complex and subspecialized health system. The value of this primary care function is recognized for its economic efficiency and patient satisfaction in the rapidly growing health maintenance organization system in the United States.

Secondary and tertiary care can be defined as consultant care provided in either an ambulatory or inpatient setting for problems requiring diagnostic or therapeutic skills or resources not normally available in the primary care setting. This differs from primary care in that the relationship to the patient usually is episodic rather than ongoing, and the conditions treated are less common and more complex.

To summarize the difference in emphasis between primary and consultant care, the primary care physician is identified with a patient and the way in which various factors influence that patient's health over time; the consultant physician is identified with a set of diseases (or technical skills) and the way in which various patients fit into that field of interest over time. For one, the illness is the episode; for the other, the patient is the episode.

## THE PRACTICE OF PEDIATRICS

Most office visits to pediatricians are made by patients previously known to the physician, rather than referred consultations, documenting the primary care nature of pediatric practice. Child health supervision accounts for one third of office visits and closer to one half of the physician's time, because these visits are longer on average than are illness visits. Respiratory tract and ear infections and their complications account for almost one half of all acute illness diagnoses.

However, primary care pediatricians play an important role in the care of children with chronic conditions as well; about 20% of children will have a diagnosed chronic condition over time, including asthma and allergy, vision and hearing impairment, and seizure disorders.

The challenges for primary care pediatrics are to define the boundaries of its responsibilities and to refine the content of its practice. For example, the development of urgent-care facilities, either freestanding or within hospital emergency rooms, appeals to the public demand for easily accessible and immediate medical service, but excludes the longitudinal relationship between patient and doctor, which is an anchor piece of primary care. Another issue to be clarified is the relative role of the generalist and the subspecialist in the care of chronically ill children: how best to combine the skills and knowledge the subspecialist possesses about the disease with the skills and knowledge the generalist possesses about the child and family. Other content areas of particular interest to primary care include child health supervision, particularly selecting screening tests that identify at-risk children at a point when intervention can be effective; providing more refined developmental and behavioral assessment and therapy for common behavioral problems of childhood; and helping children to adopt healthy habits in regard to nutrition and physical activity so as to reduce the cardiovascular hazards of adult life.

Primary care physicians are the only group in society to see children on a regular basis from the time they are born until they enter school at the age of 5 or 6 years. As such, they have a unique opportunity to influence the current and future health of children.

Most pediatric subspecialists have interests similar to their counterparts in internal medicine (eg, cardiology, pulmonology, endocrinology); others function as general consultants within a defined age subgroup (eg, neonatology, adolescent medicine).

Without question, pediatricians will continue to function as subspecialists for the more complex diseases of childhood. They will be located increasingly in regional tertiary hospitals where research and clinical care can be combined. The remarkable advances that have been made in the care of children in such areas as neonatal and pediatric intensive care, prevention and control of infectious disease through vaccines and immunotherapy, and treatment of the organ system diseases of childhood have been of proven value in reducing morbidity and mortality.

In addition to these subspecialty functions, there is a general consultant role for the pediatrician. That role perhaps is most relevant in rural communities and in community hospitals, where major referral centers for children are at a distance or inconvenient. For example, at present, two thirds of the 3.6 million annual hospital admissions of children less than 17 years of age in the United States are made to hospital services without a pediatric house staff or teaching affiliation. The presence of a general consultant pediatrician is of particular value if the child is cared for by a family physician or pediatrician whose experience with hospitalized children may be limited. This "secondary care" pediatrician can oversee inpatient care and identify those children who should be transferred to a regional tertiary care setting where a range of subspecialists is available.

## THE SOCIAL TRANSFORMATION OF MEDICINE

Pediatricians, like all physicians, are involved in what Starr has called the "social transformation of American medicine," the change from a largely entrepreneurial practice by independent physicians to a modern industry. As part of this transformation, the ability of the medical profession to define the nature and terms of practice in largely autonomous fashion almost certainly will be reduced. That degree of autonomy reached its zenith in the United States in the middle years of this century, relative to all other professions and relative to the status of medicine in other countries. The sovereignty the profession has enjoyed in determining how medicine will relate to the public is likely to be curtailed further. For example, decisions regarding the number of individuals allowed to enter the profession, the number and types of specialists and generalists that will be trained, the organization and location of practices, the sites of care used, the extent and nature of technology employed, and the amount of reimbursement allowed for service will be influenced increasingly by public and private agencies and by nonphysician administrators. What still remains to be determined is whether American medicine will be organized and financed principally under private auspices, as are other industries in the United States; under public auspices, as it is in most other industrialized countries; or in some combination unique to our own society.

## THE FUTURE OF PEDIATRICS

The forces that will influence pediatrics and the care of children in the immediate future were summarized in a 1987 joint report by the American Medical Association and the American Academy of Pediatrics. Three factors were identified: demographic trends in the number of children and child care physicians, willingness of third-party payors to reimburse the preventive and counseling services that characterize most of pediatric primary care, and public attitudes toward services for children. Perhaps the pediatrician's most important role will be to help influence those public attitudes. Pediatrics is unique among clinical disciplines in adopting an advocacy role for its patients. Indeed, the stated mission of the American Academy of Pediatrics is a commitment to attaining optimal physical, mental, and social health for all children. Its success in pursuing that goal can be a significant influence on child health in the United States.

## Selected Readings

Better health for our children: A national strategy. Report of the Select Panel for the Promotion of Child Health (4 vols). 1981 DHHS (PHS) Publication No 79–55071.

Charney E. Secondary care: The role of the community hospital in pediatrics. Am J Dis Child 1983;137:902.

Council on Long Range Planning and Development in cooperation with the American Academy of Pediatrics. The future of pediatrics: Implications of the changing environment of medicine. JAMA 1987;258:240.

Martinez G, Ryan A. The pediatric marketplace. Am J Dis Child 1989;143:924.

Miller CA. Maternal health and infant survival. Washington, DC: National Center for Clinical Infant Programs, 1987.

National Center for Health Statistics. Monthly vital statistics report. 1992;40(Suppl 2).

Roback F, Randolph L, Seidman B. Physician characteristics and distribution in the U.S. Chicago: American Medical Association, 1992.

Starfield B. Childhood morbidity: Comparisons, clusters, and trends. Pediatrics 1991;88:519.

Starr P. The social transformation of American medicine. New York: Basic Books, 1982.

Wegman ME. Annual summary of vital statistics. Pediatrics 1991;88:1081.

Williams B, Miller C. Preventive health care for young children. Pediatrics 1992;89(Suppl):5.

*Principles and Practice of Pediatrics, Second Edition.*
edited by Frank A. Oski et al. J. B. Lippincott Company, Philadelphia © 1994.

CHAPTER 3
# The Ethics of Pediatric Medicine

Norman Fost

Every patient presents ethical problems. How much should be disclosed about the side effects of common drugs? How much authority should parents have in determining medical management of their children, for trivial or life-threatening conditions? How much autonomy should be given to adolescents regarding their own health care? How should a pediatrician allocate his or her time, among patients and between practice and personal life?

Many of these problems are generic, in the sense that they arise in any clinical setting. Some are exotic, applying only to small numbers of patients or practitioners. This chapter focuses on problems common in pediatric practice. For discussion of a broader range of ethical problems in health care, the reader is referred to some of the excellent anthologies that are available (Beauchamp and Walters, 1982; Beauchamp and Childress, 1983; Gaylin and Macklin, 1982). There also are excellent readable introductions to ethical theory (Beauchamp and Childress, 1983). A few concepts are so central to pediatric practice that a brief review of them is necessary here.

## AUTONOMY, COMPETENCE, CONSENT, AND PATERNALISM

American health care, and the political and legal milieu in which it exists, is oriented heavily toward autonomy or self-governance. A competent person has an absolute right to decide what shall be done to his or her own body, according to a United States Supreme Court decision made 50 years ago. Any touching done without consent, by a doctor or anyone else, is a battery. Consent can justify touching, but only if it is meaningful consent, requiring at least that it be informed and uncoerced. The legal requirements for informed consent reflect the widely shared moral belief that individuals should be free to make their own decisions, however foolish they may be.

These principles apply to competent patients. The definition and boundaries of competence are controversial, but clearly exclude many, if not most, children. For such individuals, others must be entrusted with authority to make decisions on their behalf. This is called *paternalism*—interfering with someone's liberty on the grounds that it is in his or her interest. To be justified, paternalism requires that the interference be such that the individual is likely to agree with it later on, or plausibly would agree with it if he or she had a moment of lucidity and could see the issue clearly. Given this condition, imposing health care upon people simply on the grounds that it is good for them is not sufficient. If that were the case, consent would be unnecessary.

What are the implications of these principles for pediatrics? For those older adolescents who resemble adults more than they do children (ie, who would meet standard notions of competence), consent is necessary and sufficient for providing health care for the same reasons that apply to other competent patients. For infants and most young children—who would not meet any common notion of competence—proxy consent, motivated by paternalistic impulses, provides a sufficient basis upon which to intervene with standard therapeutic interventions. For children between these extremes, who have an evolving capacity to understand the nature and implications of proposed interventions, there is a growing claim for involvement in the decision-making process.

## SERIOUSLY ILL INFANTS: THE "BABY DOE" PROBLEM

No single ethical issue has so preoccupied American pediatrics in the past decade as the controversy surrounding withholding life-sustaining treatment from handicapped or seriously ill newborns. The practice of allowing such infants to die, or even killing them, is thousands of years old, but it became a national debate in the early 1970s with the public disclosure that routine, standard treatment—such as repair of duodenal atresia—commonly was withheld from infants with birth defects such as Down syndrome. The death of "Baby Doe" in 1982, resulting from untreated esophageal atresia and Down syndrome, triggered a federal statute and regulations requiring that all infants be given medically beneficial treatment, regardless of handicap, unless they are comatose or their death is imminent. Application of these regulations to specific cases, in theory and practice, is controversial.

Whatever the merits or effects of the legal response, the Baby Doe debate appeared to cause a shift in consensus on a fundamental ethical point: that the value to be maximized in considering whether to give or withhold treatment should be the best interest of the infant. This replaced previous notions that parents' wishes should predominate and earlier efforts to rely on distinctions between ordinary and extraordinary means as a basis for making decisions. The "best interest" standard left open questions of how and by whom these interests should be defined and ascertained, but on these matters, too, there has been a growing consensus. In theory and practice, there is increasing agreement that multidisciplinary consultations are more likely to result in ethically sound decisions than is the practice of parents and personal physicians making decisions in private. The growth of hospital ethics committees, also called infant care review committees, has been dramatic, considering that they were not required by federal or state law during their most rapid growth phase. More than 60% of all hospitals that serve children now have such groups. These committees typically do not make decisions, but strive toward

facilitating consensus among providers and parents. One of their most important functions appears to be improving the factual basis for decisions. Good ethics starts with good facts; many of the most controversial Baby Doe decisions were predicated on inadequate information, which could have been corrected if a more deliberate and collaborative process had been employed.

## Case 1

A 700-g newborn has trisomy 13. He has congestive heart failure and chronic renal failure, and is ventilator-dependent with severe bronchopulmonary dysplasia at 5 months of age. His parents ask that the ventilator be discontinued, realizing that he will die.

### Comment

The child is unlikely to leave the nursery. He does not appear to be experiencing any of the pleasures of even neonatal life. His parents' request is consistent with his caretakers' view that continued treatment is likely to bring him prolonged suffering with little prospect of relief until death occurs. If there were disagreement by any of his caretakers or family members, consultation with an ethics committee would be advisable. Otherwise, there seems little reason not to discontinue life support. Withholding and withdrawing life support are morally equivalent, although some believe that withdrawal is preferable because it implies a clinical trial to document better the poor prognosis (President's Commission, 1983).

## Case 2

A newborn with anencephaly is expected to die. The parents ask that he be used as a heart donor.

### Comment

Even more clearly than in Case 1, this child has no discernible interests, either in living or dying. He presumably experiences no pain, so continued intensive care or surgery presents no burdens to him. If he is breathing, he is not brain dead and, therefore, would not be considered legally dead in any state. Brain death is not an essential condition for discontinuation of life support, but it is an essential condition for removal of vital organs. Removal of the heart before documentation of death would be contrary to traditional attitudes and policies of transplantation. It technically would be homicide. Consultation with an ethics committee, the hospital attorney, and, perhaps, a court, should occur before the traditional boundary of using only dead donors is crossed.

## SCREENING

Screening can be defined as the search for occult disease or the potential for disease to develop, in a defined population. The purpose is variably treatment (eg, newborn screening for phenylketonuria [PKU]), counseling (eg, human immunodeficiency virus [HIV] testing in a sexually active adolescent), or research. As with all interventions, benefits should be established and shown to be commensurate with risks before application is made to broad populations. The harms of screening usually are indirect and, therefore, underrecognized. These harms can be organic, such as when a positive test result leads to possibly harmful treatment. This occurred in the early days of widespread PKU testing, when the significance of elevated serum phenylalanine was unknown and the toxicity of a low-phenylalanine diet was not fully understood. Many children were labeled incorrectly as having PKU and were harmed by the diet. Harms more commonly are psychosocial, a result of labeling and stigmatization. This was widespread when mandatory sickle screening laws as a condition of school entry caused parents to believe falsely that their children had a fatal condition or reduced the children's access to life and health insurance. Similar concerns surround HIV testing.

Screening has become such a central part of medical care that it often is not recognized as such, its risks are underestimated, and its benefits are assumed. Such common tests as the Denver Developmental Screening Test or an annual urine culture may result in undesirable and unwanted consequences. The former may cause the child to be labeled, by parents or others, as retarded. The latter may result in a series of costly and possibly toxic studies and therapies of uncertain benefit. When the benefits are clear and the risks trivial, there will be little disagreement. But when the benefits have not been established, or when the risks of stigmatization may be serious, the physician should be cautious about routine screening. At the least, parents or patients should be informed of the likelihood and evidence of claimed benefits, and of the possibility of risks, and they should be given the opportunity to choose. New screening tests should be thought of as experimental until well-designed trials demonstrate their benefits and assess their risks.

## Case 3

A 16-year-old boy is found by his pediatrician to have chlamydia urethritis. The physician suggests "blood tests" to screen for other venereal disease, including an HIV titer, which is reported as Western blot–positive.

### Comment

If HIV infection is discovered, that discovery will have major negative implications for this patient, including the possibility of loss of life insurance or health insurance and exclusion from school, sports, or jobs. His sexual partners may benefit from the information, depending on his willingness to change his behavior or inform his partners. The benefits to him are less clear. Explicit informed consent should be obtained, whether required explicitly by law or not.

## Case 4

The hospital laboratory has a new method for screening newborns for cystic fibrosis, using the same blood taken for PKU screening. The pediatric staff is asked to check and return a form if they want their patients screened.

### Comment

The benefits of presymptomatic detection of cystic fibrosis are unclear. There are costs and organic risks of more frequent treatment and hospitalization for respiratory infections. There may be genetic counseling benefits, depending on the parents' reproductive plans. False-positive test results may have prolonged stigmatizing effects, even when the sweat test is negative. Parents should participate in the decision whether to have their infants screened.

## CONFLICTS OF INTEREST

The pediatrician shares with other physicians the familiar conflicts of interest inherent in charging fees for service, and in balancing patient needs with personal needs and goals. In addition, because children needing health care typically are represented by their parents, the pediatrician often will need to distinguish the parents' needs from those of the children. A mother asking for methods with which to control nocturnal enuresis in a 4-year-old child may be more concerned with her own interests than with her child's. Requests to withhold life-sustaining treatment from a handicapped newborn sometimes are based explicitly on consid-

eration of the welfare of the other family members rather than on the interests of the patient. Contemporary notions of holistic medicine, including advocacy for treating the whole family, compete with traditional ideas of placing the interests of the patient above all others.

The physician who is employed by an institution or by the state has more explicit conflicts. His or her contract implies that his or her primary duty is to the employer.

## Case 5

Dr. Jones is a pediatric sports medicine specialist. He is a paid consultant to the university athletic department, which has asked him to set up a drug-screening program. Athletes with three violations must lose their scholarships and, therefore, for many, their opportunity for an education. Jones does not approve of illegal drug use, but he does not like being a policeman and thinks that his duty to his "patients"—the students—supersedes his duty to the school.

### Comment

Having contracted with the school to test for drugs, Dr. Jones is obliged to fulfill his contract. He could try to change the rule requiring expulsion. He could ask the school to hire an outside consultant to administer the drug program. If these approaches fail, and if Jones does not like the heat, he may have to get out of the kitchen, or at least advise his patients of his conflicting interests so that there is no deception involved.

The state may impose obligations on the pediatrician that compete with his or her duty to serve his or her patients. Requirements for reporting contagious diseases compete with promises of confidentiality and may jeopardize seriously the interests of the patient. This has been most dramatic in cases of HIV infection.

Legal requirements that child abuse be reported may expose children to professionals with other conflicting interests, which may work to the detriment of the child. A physician often feels, sometimes correctly so, that he cannot serve the interests of his or her patients and simultaneously obey the law.

## Case 6

Timmy, 3 years old, is in the emergency room with his third fracture in a year, allegedly caused by falling from a tree. The father is president of Mega, Incorporated. The mother seems distracted, defensive, and not nurturing of her son. Dr. Smith, their private pediatrician, suspects abuse, but believes that it would be best to discuss his concerns in the office when they return for follow-up.

### Comment

Smith's explicit duties are to the child and to the state, not to the parents. He clearly is violating the reporting law and is vulnerable to a charge of breaking another law—negligence. He might claim that the law is a bad one, not deserving of respect, but one of the requirements for justified civil disobedience is openness. As a physician, he has no more claim than any other citizen to decide which laws deserve respect.

## CONFIDENTIALITY

Physicians who work for institutions or under the requirements of state laws may have little choice about disclosing confidential information to authorities, without the consent of the patient or parents. There are many situations, however, in which the decision whether to disclose information is discretionary. The pediatrician who is asked to prescribe contraception or treat venereal disease in a young adolescent clearly is authorized to do so without disclosure to the parents, but still must decide whether he or she can promote the child's interests without including the family. Similarly, the physician who discovers that his or her patient is abusing drugs may feel obliged to inform school or law enforcement officials in order to recruit their assistance in helping the patient. And the physician who discovers HIV infection in a neonate or school-age child may feel obliged to inform foster parents, day-care providers, or school officials because of a concern of contagion. The general rule is that no information obtained in a doctor–patient relationship should be disclosed without the consent of the patient, if he or she is competent, or of his or her guardian, if the patient is not competent. There are two reasons for this ancient rule. First, there is the public health concern that patients will be less likely to seek medical attention if they are not confident that stigmatizing information will be kept confidential. Decreased use of medical resources can impose costs on others, by increasing the spread of contagious diseases, increasing the costs to the community of treating disability, and so on. Second, the presumption that personal information will not be disclosed without consent is so widespread, among professionals as well as the public, as to constitute an implied promise. To break that promise for the benefit of others, without warning the patient beforehand, is to deceive the patient into disclosing information when he or she otherwise would not do so.

As with all principles, there are exceptions. Intervening in suicides and reporting child abuse are the most familiar examples of clinical problems for which nearly everyone supports the disclosure of confidential information. There is a principled basis for such disclosures—when there is a high probability of serious physical harm, a high likelihood of benefit, and no alternatives exist, disclosure may be warranted.

## Case 7

Susan, age 16 years, has gonorrhea. She has been having unprotected intercourse with a 19-year-old man who has used heroin. She refuses HIV testing. Her doctor wants to get her parents involved, but she refuses.

### Comment

Susan came to the doctor under the appropriate assumption that information would not be disclosed to her parents. She is accepting treatment for gonorrhea. She is at risk for HIV infection, but testing has no clear benefit at present. If she were HIV-positive, early treatment might be of help, but it is experimental at present and could not be imposed on her. Her venereal disease will have to be disclosed to the state, as required by law. Disclosure to her parents would not seem to have such a clear benefit as to justify breaking the promise of confidentiality. If the physician's personal sense of morality requires him to disclose the information in spite of Susan's objection, he probably should have forewarned her, although this practice presumably would become known in the community, resulting in a decline in visits for such problems.

## ADOLESCENT SEXUALITY

Competent citizens have a nearly absolute right to decide what shall be done with their own bodies, and age is an imperfect measure of competence. Legal notions of majority, therefore, are only guidelines as to whether an adolescent can consent to any medical care. When a minor is emancipated—living independently of his or her parents—there is a presumption that he or she is competent to consent to medical care. In actual practice, the state is extremely deferential to physician judgment in these

matters; there are virtually no legal risks to treating anyone more than 15 years of age.

When reproductive behavior is involved, the state is even more protective of the adolescent's right to health care, regardless of demonstrated competence. The reason for this is twofold. The first concern is that many patients will not seek medical care if parental consent is required, and will suffer resultant harm. Second, there is broad public concern regarding the epidemic of teenage pregnancy and venereal disease, with its adverse implications for adolescents and their children. Accordingly, such patients are granted broad access to services for birth control, treatment of venereal disease, and abortion. Although everyone favors including parents in such discussions and decisions whenever possible, there will be an irreducible number of patients for whom parental involvement is not possible. It may be the case that treating such patients is not ideal, and possibly not in their interest, but courts consistently have prohibited rules that block access to reproductive services. As stated earlier, the reason may be based more on public health considerations than on the interests of any specific patient. In some sense, this debate centers on an unresolved empiric question; namely, whether access to reproductive services promotes sexual behavior and thereby increases the incidence of adverse consequences of early sexuality.

## TERMINAL CARE

There comes a point at which every person's life no longer is worth living, when the burdens outweigh the benefits. Because medical technology is so successful in prolonging life, it usually becomes necessary to decide whether and when to withhold or withdraw treatment, whether it be resuscitation, ventilation, or more specific therapy. For most patients, these questions arise late in life, and the difficult question of defining the patient's best interest can be answered by each patient in his or her own idiosyncratic way, either at the time decisions must be made, or beforehand through written declarations such as living wills.

Allowing competent patients to participate in such decisions is a recent development in medical practice. Traditionally, physicians treated all patients paternalistically, shielding them from bad news and protecting them from the perceived stress of making hard choices. Similar attitudes persist among some pediatricians, who "protect" parents from active participation in life-or-death decisions and, more commonly, shield children from facts and from discussion of their terminal care. Empirically, there is little support for the notion that patients are well served by this protection. Ethically, such paternalism precludes them from participating in decisions that affect them more than anyone else.

To include parents and patients in such discussions is not to yield all authority to them. Not all decisions are acceptable, and decision making, therefore, must be collaborative, including the physician, the family, and, when appropriate, the pediatric patient. Although controversy abounds over the limits of acceptable decisions, there has been increasing consensus over several issues that once were controversial:

1. *A patient does not have to be brain dead, terminally ill, or comatose to justify discontinuing life support.* There are many children whose interests are not served by prolonged survival. The terminally ill child, by definition, soon will escape the burdens of treatment. It is especially the child who faces a long life of continued suffering, with little prospect for the pleasures that make life worth living, whose interests may not be served by continued existence.

2. *Withholding and withdrawing life support are morally equivalent; indeed, withdrawing may be morally preferable.* If treatment is not serving the interest of the patient, it is irrelevant whether

or not it is contemplated or in progress. Other things being equal, withdrawing treatment has the advantage of a clinical trial, so the judgment that the patient is not thriving is based on some evidence rather than merely on speculation.

3. *Retardation or handicap alone is not a sufficient reason for terminating treatment.* Until recent times, Down syndrome and spina bifida, common malformation syndromes with good prospects for long and happy lives, commonly were considered sufficient reason for allowing a child to die. It is not clear whether the virtual disappearance of such practices is the result of a consensus on ethical issues or a fear of legal repercussions, but the moral issue does not seem to be in dispute.

4. *The child's best interest is the strongest argument for discontinuing treatment, not the family's or the community's interest.* The child's interest is not only a necessary and sufficient reason for discontinuing treatment, it requires such discontinuation. When treatment is not serving the child's interests, it not only is permissible to discontinue treatment, it is obligatory.

5. *When the child is incompetent, the parents generally should make decisions, but when such choices appear not to be in the child's interest, the decisions must be reviewed.* The past decade has seen a rapid trend toward collaborative decision making in such matters, particularly when there is disagreement between the medical staff and the family, or within the family or medical staff. Hospital ethics committees, once rare, now are common and are involved increasingly in consensus development in controversial cases. The ethical basis for such committees is the obligation to ensure that decisions are based on the best available facts, that interests other than the patient's are not playing a dominant role, and that the relevant issues are considered in a dispassionate manner.

## Selected Readings

American Academy of Pediatrics, Infant Bioethics Task Force. Guidelines for infant bioethics committees. Pediatrics 1984;74:306.

Beauchamp TL, Childress JF. Principles of biomedical ethics. New York: Oxford, 1983.

Beauchamp TL, Walters L. Contemporary issues in bioethics, ed 2. Belmont, CA: Wadsworth, 1982.

Christie RJ, Hoffmaster CB. Ethical issues in family medicine. New York: Oxford, 1986.

Fost N. Ethical problems in pediatrics. Curr Probl Pediatr 1976;6:1.

Fost N. Treatment of seriously ill and handicapped newborns. Crit Care Clin 1986;2:149.

Gaylin W, Macklin R. Who speaks for the child. New York: Plenum, 1982.

Holder AR. Legal issues in pediatrics and adolescent medicine, ed 2. New Haven: Yale Press, 1984.

Jonsen AR, Siegler M, Winslade WJ. Clinical ethics, ed 2. New York: Macmillan, 1986.

President's Commission for the Study of Ethical Problems in Medicine and Biomedical Research. Deciding to forego life-sustaining treatment. Washington, DC: US Government Printing Office, 1983.

The rights of children. Harv Ed Rev 1974;44.

Wald M. State intervention on behalf of neglected children. Stanford Law Review 1976;28:623.

*Principles and Practice of Pediatrics, Second Edition.*
edited by Frank A. Oski et al. J. B. Lippincott Company, Philadelphia © 1994.

CHAPTER 4
# *Economics of Medicine*

## Barbara Starfield and Samuel Flint

In the United States, knowledge about the financing and organization of health services requires continual updating. The system of health care is highly volatile and subject to marked change in nature and degree even within short periods of time. The United States is almost unique among industrialized nations in not having a national health system that sets the bounds for the way in which services are paid for and delivered.\* Although a commitment to considering health care a "right" was made almost 3 decades ago through the passage of certain federal legislation, philosophic and ideologic developments since that time have eroded the concept. The lack of commitment to health care as a "right" results in a situation in which a substantial proportion of the population is unable to pay for necessary care, and in which even those who are able to afford services often lack the information and ability to identify the most appropriate care for their needs.

\* This chapter was written before the appointment of President Clinton's Task Force on Health Care Reforms. By 1993 it appears that managed health care may become national policy, but with guarantees for universal coverage by some form of health insurance. The venue for providing that insurance is not yet clear.

Virtually all systems of care in other nations are organized according to the principle of levels of care, in which individuals who need services first seek those services from a generalist physician (a "primary care physician"). That physician either takes care of the problem or, if it is beyond the scope of his or her expertise, refers the patient to a consultant for short-term diagnosis and management ("secondary" care) or for longer-term care (in the case of particularly specialized needs that can be provided only by a "tertiary" care specialist trained for these unusual problems). Thus, in most countries with rational health systems, physicians are trained to be primary physicians, consultants, or specialists. Primary physicians work in local offices or health centers, consultants work in area hospitals or large centers, and specialists work in regional hospitals.

The system of health services in the United States has developed piecemeal, and is largely bipartite, although with considerable overlap of its parts. The system is primarily within the "private" sector, in which physicians generally are self-employed and hospitals may be organized on a profit or nonprofit basis. Some care is provided directly by various levels of government, however; such is the case for members of the military and their dependents, and for certain segments of the population (such as the very poor or Native Americans) who otherwise would face extraordinary barriers to entry into the private system. A substantial amount of care provided in the private sector is paid for by public funds. Until recently, accountability for the expenditure of public funds by the private sector has been relatively loose. Furthermore, there is no clear distinction by level of care; in most places in the country, patients can go directly to specialists without first seeing a primary care physician.

The coalescence of three phenomena is responsible for recent changes in the organization and financing of health care. First, the percentage of the gross national product contributed by health services is far outstripping all other components of national expenditures, and is rising at a rate far higher in this country than elsewhere. Thus, the costs of care are perceived to be on an ever-increasing spiral upward, without any clear bounds. Second, there is increasing evidence of diminishing access to appropriate care, not only for the poor who lack the means to pay for services, but also for the rest of the population, which has increasing difficulty in identifying the most appropriate source of care for problems. Third, there is mounting evidence of wide variation in the use of diagnostic and therapeutic procedures across geographic regions and among hospitals, without any apparent reason for the differences or any evidence of better health resulting from them.

This chapter reviews the existing state of affairs with regard to the organization and financing of health services, and provides a basis for understanding changes that may occur in the near future.

## ORGANIZATION AND FINANCING OF HEALTH SERVICES

Until a few years ago, all but a small proportion (less than 5%) of the civilian population received their medical care from a physician who worked alone or in a small group and charged a fee for each service rendered. Within the decade 1975 to 1985, a plethora of new organizational formats began to assume prominence. The major distinguishing characteristics have to do with the degree to which responsibility for a defined panel of patients is assumed and the method by which services are reimbursed.

### Responsibility for a Defined Panel of Patients

In contrast to the traditional method of delivering services, which involves the provision of care by the physician when patients come to the physician's office, responsibility for care involves a contractual agreement in which both the physician (usually as part of a physician group) and the patient recognize that all care over a defined period of time (usually a year) will be obtained from that physician. Patients generally do not consult specialists without a referral from the primary care physician.

### Method of Reimbursement for Services

In the traditional mode of reimbursement, physicians are paid for seeing the patient and for performing diagnostic and therapeutic procedures. The payment can be made directly by the patient, either immediately or in response to subsequent billing, or it can be reimbursed by insurance companies or other third-party payors (such as state agencies that reimburse for services to certain of their employees or public assistance that is provided for the poor). In most cases, insurance fails to cover a substantial proportion of the costs of care so that patients have additional out-of-pocket expenses.

Over the past 40 years, this traditional method of paying for care has been eroded gradually in favor of prepayment for services. In this form of reimbursement, third-party payors contract with physicians or physician groups, so that these providers of care are at some financial risk. In return for this prepayment, the providers agree to provide a defined package of services according to a contract. In some forms of prepayment, these physicians also are at financial risk of assuming costs of care that results from referrals or hospitalizations, although most arrangements exempt certain "catastrophic" costs over which the physician has no control.

The new organizational arrangements, which often are designated as "managed care" and are assuming increasing importance in the U.S. health care scene, are characterized by various combinations and permutations of organizational format and reimbursement. In the next section, the most important of these forms of care are described briefly.

## Health Maintenance Organizations

The health maintenance organization (HMO) is an organizational format unique to the United States. In 1932, the Commission on the Costs of Medical Care recommended that health care be provided by organized groups of health professionals, preferably in a hospital setting, on a prepayment basis. Although care provided by such organized groups is a feature of many health care systems, it is only in the United States that they are organized within the private sector and reimbursed largely through private insurance mechanisms.

HMOs are distinguished by prepayment for care. The HMO's payment is fixed in advance, depending on the number (and, sometimes, on the type) of patients that are enrolled to receive their care in the HMO, regardless of whether the individual needs care or how much care is needed. The burden is on physicians who work in the HMO to control health care expenditures; if more care is provided than the HMO anticipates, the HMO will run a deficit. On the other hand, if too little care is provided, the HMO could be suspected of not providing necessary care. HMOs are characterized as being one of several types:

1. Staff model: the physicians work directly for the HMO, on salary, but sometimes with a bonus depending on the HMO's earnings.
2. Group model: the HMO contracts with a separate physician group to provide its services. These also are known as prepaid group practices (PPGPs), and physicians may be paid a salary or a "capitation" depending upon how many individuals the physician has on his or her panel of patients. The network model HMO contracts with several independent group practices instead of just one.
3. Individual practice association (IPA): the HMO contracts with individual physicians who are in independent practice, or with a group of physicians, each of whom works independently, usually in solo practice or single specialty groups. A capitation fee is paid to the HMO for each person enrolled. Physicians are reimbursed according to a fixed fee schedule for services rendered; the fees typically are based on a percentage of the physician's usual and customary fee. Usually, a portion of the fee is withheld by the IPA to cover losses at the end of the year. If utilization and costs are in line with expectations, the withheld amount is redistributed to the physicians.

In both the group model and the IPA, the physicians usually are free to see patients outside of the HMO in addition to those patients enrolled in the HMO.

## Managed Indemnity Plans and Preferred Provider Organizations

A managed indemnity plan (MIP) is a conventional (indemnity) insured fee-for-service arrangement in which the use of services and procedures is monitored carefully and there is significant cost-sharing on the part of the patient.

A preferred provider organization (PPO) is an arrangement by which associations of physicians or hospitals contract with employers or insurers to provide services to individuals for a negotiated, generally discounted, fee. In a PPO, patients may use a physician of their choice, regardless of whether the physician participates in the PPO. The patient must pay part of the fee (coinsurance or a deductible) himself or herself, however, when a non-PPO physician is consulted. In an exclusive provider organization (EPO), the use of non-PPO physicians is not covered except in emergency situations. The EPO, therefore, is similar to the IPA, except that the EPO is paid a fee for service by the third-party payor, whereas the IPA is prepaid. In both cases, physicians rendering the services are paid a preset fee for service.

Integral to a PPO is a "managing" organization that provides certain administrative functions that monitor the use of services. These include preadmission certification (wherein patients slated for elective admission to hospitals are reviewed for appropriate admission), second opinions before surgery, certification of treatment plans for certain nonemergency services (such as mental health services), and review of the medical care that is provided.

Table 4-1 summarizes the different ways in which medical services are organized and financed.

## Trends in the Development of New Organizational Formats

Before the late 1920s, most people paid directly for medical care services; those unable to pay either did not receive needed care or relied on charitable organizations and local health department clinics where they existed. Private health insurance became increasingly popular during the late 1920s and 1930s, for those who could afford to purchase it; physicians in the majority of cases, however, were paid a fee for their services. During the 1930s and especially the 1940s, major societal changes made access to medical care a societal priority. During this period, the precursors of PPOs were developed (the first prototype was in 1934) and the forerunners of the IPA were initiated (generally by county medical societies in the form of "foundations" for medical care). Kaiser Industries, faced with the need for medical services to care for the influx of workers in defense industries during World War II, developed the first large-scale PPGP HMO. These alternative delivery systems grew very slowly; in the 1970s, fewer than 5% of the population and physicians were involved in them. Rapidly exploding medical care costs, fueled by a growth in technology in the form of diagnostic and therapeutic tests and procedures, and by a fee-for-service reimbursement system that

simply passed the costs on to patients and their insurers, provided impetus for new thinking about prepayment and cost controls. Federal legislation was passed. The HMO Act of 1973 (implemented in 1976) encouraged the growth of prepaid organizations; in 1982, the Tax Equity and Fiscal Responsibility Act (TEFRA) encouraged the enrollment of the elderly, who had been covered since 1965 for most of their medical services as part of the Social Security Insurance system, in HMOs.

Between 1981 and 1986, the number of HMOs increased 145% (from 243 to 595). HMO enrollment jumped by 130% from 10.3 to 23.7 million people, or about 10% of the population. However, a different pattern emerged during the next 5-year period. Although aggregate enrollment increased by nearly 50% between 1986 and 1991, reaching 35.1 million, the number of operational HMOs decreased to 556.

By the early 1990s, solvency problems receded and enrollment continued to climb. The pattern of strong growth of the IPA type of organization continued into the 1990s. By the middle of 1991, 62% of HMOs were of the IPA type, 12% were of the network type, 8% were of the staff type, and 7% were categorized as being of "mixed" types, which means that they use any combination of the four standard model types (Interstudy 1992).

Before 1983, there were 20 operational PPOs in the United States, whereas by 1986, there were 413 operating in 41 states. From June 1985 to June 1986 alone, the number of PPOs increased by 59%. By the end of 1990, there were 824 PPOs owned by 571 corporate structures. The total number of individuals served by PPOs is unknown, but various estimates have been made. About 38 million employees and about 88 million individuals were eligible to use PPOs by the end of 1990. Thus, by 1991, roughly 50% of the U.S. population had at least some of their health care financed and delivered through an HMO or a PPO, compared to 25% in 1987. Of the 125 million workers eligible for PPOs, about 2.7 million with an additional 3.5 million dependents were associated with EPOs. Almost half of the PPOs (47%) were operated by insurance companies, 16% were independent plans, 9% were physician/hospital joint ventures, and 10% were owned by hospitals or hospital alliances.

**TABLE 4-1. Types of Health Services Organizations, by Method of Payment to Physicians and Source of Payment**

| Source of Payment | Preset Fee | | | | Reimbursed Fee |
| | No Enrollment* | | Enrollment‡ | |
| | Salary | Fee for Service† | | |
|---|---|---|---|---|
| Out-of-pocket | | | Individual contracts for specified types of care (eg, obstetrics, dental) | Traditional ambulatory services, freestanding emergency centers |
| Private insurance | Corporate health centers | PPOs MIPs | HMOs (PPGPs and IPAs) | Most inpatient services, certain ambulatory services |
| Tax revenues | Some governmental health centers, community health centers | PPOs | Prepaid Medicaid programs | Medicaid, CHAMPUS |
| Federal insurance | Veterans Administration facilities | PPOs (through Medicare) | HMOs (special arrangements) | Medicare |

PPO, preferred provider organization; MIP, managed indemnity plan; HMO, health maintenance organization; PPGP, prepaid group practice; IPA, individual practice association; CHAMPUS, Civilian Health and Medical Program of the Uniformed Services.
* For purposes of this table, enrollment means that individual names are provided to physicians, which, in the aggregate, constitute a practice roster.
† Individual physicians paid fee-for-service, although subject to utilization review.
‡ Payments to physician may be made by capitation or salary (as in PPGPs and some IPAs) or by fee for service.
*Starfield B. Primary care: Concept, evaluation, and policy. New York: Oxford University Press, 1992.*

This marked growth in alternative delivery formats has been accompanied by notable shifts in the ownership and management of medical care organizations. Initially, HMOs were established as not-for-profit organizations. The federal Health Maintenance Organization Act of 1973 provided impetus for the development of HMOs by supplying loans; most of the applications were from not-for-profit organizations. Early in the 1980s, the national administration and the TEFRA legislation encouraged a movement toward "marketplace competition"; this resulted in the entry into the health field of entrepreneurs and venture capitalists. The rapid growth of for-profit national health care corporations also spurred the entry into the field of insurance companies, which had to protect their own indemnity plans from the new competition. From 1981 to the end of 1985, the percent of HMOs that were for profit grew from 18% to 51%. Although the majority (54% as of 1986) of PPOs are operated by hospitals and physician groups, it is likely that insurance companies will capture an increasing share of the market so that these organizations, too, will be dominated by a profit motive.

## Financing of Health Services

Insurance coverage for children, who generally are insured as part of family plans, falls far short of covering the costs of medical care, especially when the costs are for outpatient (out-of-hospital) services. At any given time during a year, between 15% and 20% of children in the United States completely lack health insurance. In 1990, nearly 10 million children under 18 years of age (or 15% of the child population) were uninsured. Over a year's time, at least 11% of children lack *any* means of reimbursement for medical care expenses. Furthermore, private insurance fails to cover many important aspects of health care. For children under 18 years of age in general, almost 50% of expenses for health services were paid out-of-pocket in 1987. The proportion of children without insurance and the proportion of expenses covered by insurance have been falling during the most recent decade.

For children in low-income families, the situation is even more acute. Poor children are much more likely to be uninsured for medical care than are other children; those who are most deprived are children in lower-working-class families. In fact, the lower the family income, the higher the percentage of expenses for medical care that have to be paid by the family. Governmental programs (see below) provide a safety net for the poorest children, but one fourth of all poor children (3.4 million) remained uninsured in 1990. The proportion of uninsured children was even greater for children in families with incomes between 100% and 150% of the federally defined poverty level. Nearly 30% (2 million) of these children in low-income families were uninsured in 1990.

Of concern for the future is the fact that the proportion of the child population that is poor is not declining. Slightly more than one in five children in the United States are in families that are poor. The poverty rate for very young children is even higher than that for older children, with about one in four newborns born into poverty in 1990. Poor children are more than three times as likely to be in poor or fair health (more than 6%) than are non-poor children (less than 2%). Despite this fact, they have fewer physician visits: more than 20% made no visits in 1990 compared with 14% for non-poor children. When they do visit a doctor, they are only about half as likely to see a physician in a private office and are twice as likely to be seen in a hospital clinic. They are much less likely to be seen by a pediatrician. The discrepancy in number of visits in a year between poor and non-poor children worsened during the 1980s as compared with the prior decade. One in eight infants in poor families had not visited a physician for routine health care in a year, as compared with 3% for more advantaged infants; in the preschool period, 21%

and 14%, respectively, had not had such a visit, and in the young teenage period (ages 12 to 14 years), 56% and 47%, respectively, had not had such a visit.

The increasing prominence of new organizational formats for providing health services does not bode well for individuals with the greatest health needs. Health care organizations that are competing for enrolled populations at the same time that they are attempting to maximize profits cannot be expected to welcome individuals who are likely to require a relatively large amount of services. Competition encourages nonprofit organizations to take the same stance. HMOs generally adopt techniques to minimize the possibility of adverse risk selection. Such techniques involve excluding certain categories of employment in which risks are relatively high (such as construction firms) and conducting pre-enrollment health screening to detect existing medical conditions. As marginal workers and those working for low wages (and their families) are more likely than others to be excluded for these reasons, low-income children will be at an even greater disadvantage in the future than they have been in the recent past. Chronically ill children, who are poor risks for pre-budgeted health care organizations, also are at a disadvantage. In the past, public agencies have attempted to overcome some of the barriers to care for those in high-risk groups. Whether or not state legislatures will develop new strategies (such as insurance pools supported by a tax on employers) to pay for the care of the uninsured remains to be seen; such options currently are under consideration in several states, and have been adopted in at least 17 states.

The importance of unimpeded access to health services cannot be overemphasized. An extensive review of the evidence regarding the effectiveness of medical care showed how the health of children improved when barriers to access were reduced. Conversely, health status worsens when families are required to pay a coinsurance fee for their medical services. In a large-scale insurance experiment, families were assigned randomly to one of a variety of plans differing in the rate of coinsurance for medical visits; one plan required no fee at all. Both health status and use of services were monitored for several years. As compared with the free plan, children (as well as adults) in the copayment groups were less likely to receive care for conditions for which medical care is effective. The adverse effect of coinsurance was even more striking for poor children than for other children. Poor children whose families were in the coinsurance groups also had poorer health status at the end of the experiment than did poor children in the free-care group.

## TAX-SUPPORTED HEALTH PROGRAMS

Although government always has assumed some responsibility for the medical care of some individuals with no ability to pay for such services, it was the depression of the 1930s that resulted in federal commitment on a large scale. Title V of the Social Security Act of 1935 and various amendments to it provided funds to states to support services for children with certain chronic conditions, maternal and child health clinics, family planning, regionalized prenatal care, and dental care. In 1965, the legislation was amended in a major way. For the first time, federal dollars were appropriated from general tax revenues to pay for care, through the states, to families with dependent children whose incomes were below a certain amount. By 1978, (the latest year for which information is known), public programs contributed 29% of the total expenditures for health care of children under 19 years of age; two thirds of the amount came from the federal government and one third came from states and localities. More than half of these expenditures (55%) were in the form of reimbursement directly to physicians for services rendered; the rest went to federally supported service programs (6%), the Department of Defense (14%), state and local hospitals (2%), and various other programs (3%).

## Medicaid

The Medicaid program was established in 1965 as Title XIX of the Social Security Act. Its intent was to provide medical coverage to welfare recipients who were unable to afford to pay for health care services or to purchase health insurance. Until the late 1980s, children's eligibility for Medicaid was dependent on passing both a categoric test based on factors such as family composition, age, or disability, and an income-based test based on some fraction of the federal poverty standard at a level that is set by the states. Medicaid is financed jointly by state and federal general revenues; therefore, states must determine the scope and design of their programs within broad federal guidelines. (Medicaid's federal share is derived by a formula that is based on state per capita income, with poorer states receiving higher shares.) Medicaid provides generous coverage of mandatory services to its beneficiaries, including inpatient and outpatient hospital care, physician services, laboratory and x-ray services, and nursing home care. States may choose to provide selected optional services, such as coverage for eyeglasses and prescription drugs, and receive matching federal funds. Although the range of covered services is broad, beneficiaries often experience difficulties in accessing the health care system because of factors such as limited physician participation in Medicaid or because the poor often reside in medically underserved communities.

In 1990, Medicaid provided health care coverage for 25 million persons (1 in 10 Americans) and accounted for 11 cents of every health care dollar spent in the United States. In 1991, Medicaid spent $92.1 billion in state and federal funds for the provision of health care services and program administration, an amount that has grown significantly from the $72.5 billion spent in 1990. Two thirds of the Medicaid expenditures pay for institutional care such as inpatient hospital and nursing home services. As a result, although half of Medicaid recipients are children who tend to use less costly ambulatory care, they (individuals under 18 years of age) account for only about 20% percent of Medicaid expenditures.

In the first decade of its existence, the number of Medicaid beneficiaries and expenditures grew at a rapid rate. Beginning in 1976, however, the process was reversed. Despite the economic recessions in the mid-1970s and early 1980s, high levels of unemployment, and increasing poverty, the size of the Medicaid population did not grow substantially, remaining at around 22 million persons.

Legislation in the early 1980s (the Omnibus Reconciliation Act [OBRA] of 1981) reduced federal funding and gave states increased flexibility to reduce eligibility standards; the non-elderly poor experienced the greatest loss of coverage, with the ratio of Medicaid enrollees to the poverty population declining by almost 13%, from 52.1% to 45.5%. Among those families rendered ineligible for Medicaid, about one half were left without any insurance coverage. A national survey of access to medical care showed that use of medical services declined markedly between 1982 and 1985, with poor children, especially those in poor health, suffering the greatest declines. In response to the high rates of infant mortality and the erosion in coverage of children in low-income families, Congress acted to expand coverage of pregnant women and children in the mid and late 1980s, resulting in a rollback of the restrictions imposed by OBRA 1981.

The Deficit Reduction Act of 1984 (DEFRA) and the Consolidated Budget Reconciliation Act of 1985 (COBRA) required all states to provide Medicaid coverage to pregnant women and children to the age of 5 years who reside in families with incomes below the Aid to Families With Dependent Children payment level for a family of comparable size. This expansion of Medicaid eligibility required states to extend benefits to pregnant women and young children ("Ribicoff children") in two-parent families. Before this time, nearly half of the states excluded pregnant women and children, regardless of their income, if two parents were present.

OBRA 1986 gave states the option to cover pregnant women and infants (initially and as they grew to the age of 4 years), and to cover the elderly and disabled with incomes up to 100% of the federal poverty level. In 1988, coverage was made mandatory for all pregnant women and infants up to the federal poverty level. OBRA 1989 raised the eligibility level for all pregnant women and for infants and children up to the age of 6 years to 133% of the poverty level. States also were given the option to cover pregnant women with incomes up to 185% of the poverty level. As of January 1992, 30 states have exceeded the mandated level of 133% and 22 of these states have opted to cover pregnant women and infants up to 185% of the poverty level.

OBRA 1990 expanded coverage to all poor children, but is phasing the coverage in year by year as the originally eligible children become older; all poor children will be covered by the year 2001. In 1990, 60% of poor children and nearly one in five of all American children were covered by Medicaid.

In addition to the expansions in eligibility policy, significant changes have been made in the services and structure of the Medicaid program since its early years. OBRA 1989 required states to cover the treatment of conditions identified through childhood screening via the Early Periodic Screening, Diagnosis and Treatment Program, regardless of whether the services were covered by the state Medicaid plan. As a result, children covered by Medicaid are entitled to have payment made for a broad range of services, although they may not always have them available.

Another important change in Medicaid has been its shift from acting only as a payor of care to becoming a program that also is responsible for the delivery and organization of care. This has come about primarily through the growth of managed care. OBRA 1981 modified existing Medicaid procedures to permit prepayment for care of recipients with a special exemption from the provisions of the original Medicaid legislation that guaranteed freedom of choice of providers. In 1981, only 2% of Medicaid beneficiaries were enrolled in some form of managed care. As of June 1991, more than 10% of Medicaid beneficiaries (close to 2.7 million individuals) were enrolled in 224 managed care programs across the country. It is anticipated that enrollment will increase dramatically in the coming years, particularly for those living in low-income families, as states proceed with the implementation of state-wide mandatory managed care programs.

Most state Medicaid agencies use either one or a combination of three basic models of managed care. The first of these is primary care case management, in which a single provider is assigned to coordinate patient care. In addition to receiving a fee-for-service payment for services rendered, providers often are paid a fee (usually about $3.00/month) to coordinate care. The second model is capitation contracting, in which states contract with an HMO, other providers such as group practices, other preexisting clinics, or community health centers to provide a specific set of services to individuals for an actuarially sound prepayment in lieu of fees for service. This agreement is referred to as a risk contract. Under current Medicaid regulations, payment for the services may not exceed the costs of services under fee-for-service practice. In risk-contracting, the organization accepts the risk that costs may be greater than expected, but it can make a profit if the costs are lower. Capitation may cover either the full range of services or a partial set of services. With full capitation, the bulk of the risk for incurring costs lies with the provider. In partial capitation, the risk is shared with the state. The third model of managed care is health-insuring organizations, in which entities assume the full risk of costs to provide medical care for beneficiaries in exchange for a state-paid premium. Health-insuring organizations do not provide direct services, because they contract with providers. Currently, there are six health-insuring organizations in the United States, and no new ones have been established since 1986 when Congress mandated that they meet HMO standards.

The overarching question regarding managed care is whether it really expands access while controlling costs. States have claimed that managed care systems have stemmed the erosion in provider participation in Medicaid, reduced inappropriate utilization of emergency rooms, and guaranteed access to providers. They also maintain that managed care increases the efficiency of their Medicaid programs by using limited Medicaid dollars more effectively and by permitting them to predict budget needs more accurately through the use of prepaid capitated systems.

Although managed care has found strong support from the states and the federal administration, many advocates have voiced concerns. Of utmost concern is the risk that access to care may be limited because states are attempting to reduce "unnecessary" utilization to a population that has a high need for health care services. Despite these concerns, Congress currently is considering legislation that will eliminate the need for states to obtain waivers to provide managed care and will allow states to make enrollment in managed care mandatory.

Although financing of services for Medicaid-eligible individuals has been expanded greatly, problems of access remain. Because Medicaid is an entitlement program, there is no limit to the amount states and the federal government can pay for services to the low-income, covered population. States have responded to budgetary pressure by limiting income eligibility, reducing coverage of optional groups, and reducing the scope of covered services. In 1992, the average income eligibility standard for a family of three was $5106, or 44% of the federal poverty level, with state-to-state variability ranging from a low of $1786/year, or 15.5% of the federal poverty level, in Alabama to $7956/year, or 69% of the federal poverty level, in California. There also are problems with access to services. Many pediatricians and obstetricians do not agree to see patients covered by Medicaid (Yudkowsky et al, 1990). To ensure that enacted mandatory eligibility expansions were providing the access to care for which they were designed, OBRA 1989 required states to demonstrate annually the availability of private physicians' care for Medicaid beneficiaries. To be in compliance, states must document either that at least half of all pediatric and obstetric providers are full Medicaid participants or that fee-for-service rates for selected commonly used procedures are at least 90% of the average allowance of private insurers, or they must provide other documentation that Medicaid beneficiaries have access to maternal and child health services equal to those available to the general population in all geographic areas.

## Local Health Department Programs

The role of local health departments has waxed and waned. In the early decades of the century, public health efforts to provide both environmental and direct maternal and child health services had a major impact in reducing infant and early childhood mortality. In the 1950s, population migration, particularly from southern rural areas to large municipal areas, found local health departments unprepared; as a result, health statistics such as infant mortality worsened. During the 1960s, the domestic "War on Poverty" rekindled the commitment to the public's health in the form of community health clinics that were supported both by direct federal grants and by state and local dollars. The wave of "privatization" and "marketplace competition" in the early

1980s was accompanied by a declining role for local health departments in the provision of direct health services. Efforts now are concentrated largely on environmental health matters and communicable disease control. Although they often do not provide the services, all states now require children to have basic immunizations as a condition of entry to school and to organized day-care programs. Some also require a physical examination for entry to school and periodically thereafter, and some jurisdictions provide school health services where children otherwise are not able to obtain them.

## Community Health Centers

Initiated in the mid-1960s as an effort to provide comprehensive health services for underserved populations, community health centers have grown into a network of about 800 facilities serving nearly 6 million poor and underserved individuals in 50 states, Puerto Rico, and the District of Columbia. The centers are funded primarily by grants from the federal government through the Program for Community Health Centers, Migrant Health Centers, the National Health Service Corps, the Maternal and Child Health Block grant to states, and the Urban Indian Health Program, although many also try to attract patients with Medicaid or private insurance. However, fewer than one fourth of the country's 25 million medically underserved individuals are reached by existing facilities.

## Maternal and Child Health Services Block Grants

Although maternal and child health services have been provided through federal grants for more than 5 decades, the "New Federalism" policies in the early 1980s resulted in the formation of "block" grants that consolidated funding to the states. The program contains grants for maternal and child health services, Supplemental Security Income for Disabled Children (for children with chronic health problems), lead-based paint poisoning prevention programs, sudden infant death prevention programs, hemophilia treatment centers, and adolescent pregnancy and genetics services grants. In most southern, midwestern, and western states that have large networks of county and local health departments, services often are provided directly through governmental agencies in schools, local health clinics, well child clinics, antenatal clinics, health screening, and immunization services. In other areas, particularly the Northeast, the state maternal and child health agency often contracts with private health centers to provide services.

## Special Education

In 1975, Congress passed the Education for the Handicapped Act (PL 94–142) to provide federal funding for state education departments to assure "free public education" for handicapped children aged 3 to 21 years. More recent legislation (PL 99–457) extended the program to include children from birth to 3 years of age. About 10% of children, including those with deficits such as hearing problems, are served across the country; as yet, however, there is little coordination between educational services and health services for these children.

## Supplemental Program for Women, Infants, and Children

The Supplemental Program for Women, Infants, and Children (WIC) was initiated in 1972 to provide supplemental food and nutrition education to pregnant and postpartum women, nursing mothers, and children from birth to 5 years of age in families whose incomes are below 185% of the federal poverty level. The program is administered by the Department of Agriculture through grants to state health departments.

## Head Start

The Head Start program resulted from legislation passed in the mid-1960s that was designed to improve the developmental level of preschool children in low-income families. It is administered by the Federal Administration for Children, Youth and Families, with support given directly to local Head Start groups.

## Family Planning

Support for family planning comes from a variety of public and private sources, including Planned Parenthood funds, the Maternal and Child Health Block grant, and several other sources deriving from federal legislation. Services are provided through a network of uncoordinated centers located in health clinics, hospitals, and private physicians' offices.

## THE ROLE OF PEDIATRICIANS IN PROVIDING SERVICES TO THE COUNTRY'S CHILDREN

For optimal care, every child should have a physician who serves as the source of primary care, that is, a physician who is contacted first when there is a new problem, is available or arranges for a substitute when he or she is unavailable, provides preventive and illness-related services and refers the child to the hospital or to a specialist when indicated, keeps continuous medical records, and coordinates all the care that the child needs from whatever source it is obtained.

Children who have no regular source of care are less likely to have received all of their required immunizations. Children without a regular source of care are less likely to have had a visit with a physician within a year than are children who do have such a relationship; those with a set place but no specific physician as a regular source of care are less likely to initiate a visit than those who have a relationship with a particular physician.

Having a regular physician provides other benefits as well. It facilitates the follow-up of patients' problems from one visit to the next, reduces the number of visits made overall, increases patients' satisfaction with care, and enhances recognition of patients' psychosocial and behavioral problems. It also reduces the probability that inappropriate procedures will be done.

Although 88% of all children have a regular source of care for when they are sick or need routine health care, poor children are less likely to have such a place and, when they do, the place is more likely to be a hospital clinic or emergency room than a private physician or HMO. For example, between 35% and 40% of poor children in each age group do not have a source of care that is a private physician or HMO; this percentage falls to about 22% among the near-poor, and to about 7% for the non-poor. Although children in central city areas are less likely to have a relationship with a private physician or HMO, there are no consistent differences between rural and other urban children in this regard.

Most medical care for children in nonmetropolitan areas is provided by general/family physicians rather than by pediatricians. In 1981, almost 60% of children in nonmetropolitan areas had a generalist as their regular source of care, whereas only 18% had a pediatrician as this source of care. Moreover, the older children are, the less likely they are to have a pediatrician as their regular source of care. In 1987, 72% of all visits by children under 3 years of age were to pediatricians, as compared with 55% for 3- to 9-year-olds and only 24% for 10- to 19-year-olds.

In contrast to general/family physicians, pediatricians tend to be less accessible to patients because they are more likely to require appointments, and their office locations may be less accessible. They also are less likely to make house calls. The range of the services they offer is somewhat more restricted than that of generalists in that they provide less minor surgery.

Overall, about two thirds of all visits with physicians made by children take place in a physician's office, about one in six occur in a hospital clinic, and another one or two are in some other place (such as another type of clinic). There are marked differences according to family income, however. The greater the family income, the more often visits take place in doctors' offices. In fact, children in families in the lowest income group are twice as likely to be seen in hospital clinics and other clinics as are children in the highest income group.

Where do pediatricians practice? Most of the surveys that periodically request information from physicians do not request information that would reveal the extent to which pediatricians (or other types of physicians) practice within the new types of organizations that were described earlier in this chapter or even in organizations such as community health centers that have been in existence for at least 2 decades. The American Academy of Pediatrics, which includes about 75% of pediatricians in the United States, conducts periodic surveys of its members. Of those respondents who indicate patient care as their primary professional activity, 23% are in solo practice, 33% are in a pediatric group, 10% are in a multi-specialty group, 6% are in an HMO, 12% practice in a university hospital, 8% practice in some other hospital, 4% work in a clinic, and 5% work in some other arrangement (August 1991 *SSP Fellowship Directory* address verification form, 84% response rate).

Do pediatricians spend much time providing care to children in community settings? More than one half of pediatricians (54%) report that they spend some time in community-based activities such as health fairs, child advocacy, or provision of services to indigent children. The amount of time that pediatricians spend in such activities is unknown, because the most recent data on the subject derive from a 1976 survey in which one third of the pediatricians in solo or group practice spent less than 1% of their patient-care time in school or community activities; about one fifth of pediatricians spent 2% to 5% of their time in this way. Less than 10% spent more than 5% of their time in schools and community facilities. (The remainder of the pediatricians did not respond and, presumably, spent no time in these settings.)

Thus, relative to the proportion of child visits in various types of sites, there is underrepresentation of pediatricians in facilities such as community clinics. This "maldistribution" of pediatricians effectively deprives a large proportion of children in lower-income families and children in nonurban areas from receiving their care from pediatricians. As noted above, many features of insurance coverage also reduce the likelihood that poor families will have a physician as their regular source of care.

## HOW ARE PEDIATRICIANS PAID FOR THE CARE THEY PROVIDE?

In 1988, 71% of pediatricians participated in managed care plans of some type. Within that group, 47% had some additional HMO affiliation, with half of those in salaried positions and the other half reimbursed on a fee-for-service basis. Forty-six percent had affiliations with PPOs and 7% had other contract care arrangements, such as MIPs. Only a small percentage of all visits are prepaid, however, even for physicians affiliated with HMOs. For pediatricians with HMO affiliation, 1 in 7 pediatric office visits is prepaid, compared with 1 in 12 office visits for all nonsurgical specialists. For HMO-affiliated pediatricians, 13% (on average) of total income is derived from prepayment, as compared with

10% for all office-based physicians. Therefore, despite the dramatic increase in HMOs and prepayment plans, fee for service continues to be the primary way in which pediatricians and other physicians are paid in the United States.

The American Academy of Pediatrics survey in 1984 provided information on the sources of income for pediatricians primarily in direct patient care. Two thirds of these physicians received their income largely from noncontract fee-for-service practice. Another 10% had their secondary source of income in this category. Eight percent received their primary source of income from contract fee for service, with another 41% having their secondary source in this category. The remainder of their income came from salary (25% as a primary source and 30% as a secondary source) or from some other source (2% and 19%, respectively). More than half (52%) reported that they had more than one type of source of income. The most common combinations of sources were noncontract fee for service and contract fee for service (11% of respondents), and noncontract fee for service and salary (8%). None of the other combinations were reported by more than 4% of the pediatricians.

This general overview indicates the wide variety that exists in types of arrangements for providing care and in sources of payment and coverage for various types of services. This extraordinary organizational and financial disarray of a health services system is virtually unique in the industrialized world. As a result of the disarray, people who need care often lack the information they need to decide where to obtain care and how to pay for it. Moreover, administrative costs of the system are much higher than in more organized systems of care, even those that still are primarily in the private sector (such as Canada). Will more rationality be brought into the system, and will costs be lowered as a result? The answer depends upon whether or not the prevailing emphasis on "marketplace competition" can be tempered by systems more like the national health programs of comparable nations elsewhere in the world.

## QUALITY AND COSTS OF CARE

One of the problems resulting from the great fragmentation of care is difficulty in assigning responsibility for the quality of care while controlling costs. In most other countries, the vast majority of the population has a regular source of care, that is, a particular doctor or place where care is centralized and coordinated. This source of care is known as a "primary care" provider, who usually is a physician. In the United States, family physicians and general practitioners, general internists, and pediatricians also are known as "primary care" physicians, but in contrast to the situation in other countries, the majority of patients do not have to "enroll" on the panel of a physician or physician group, and the majority of physicians do not have a panel of persons for whom they explicitly maintain ongoing responsibility for general care and for referral to specialists when needed.

Since the 1970s and largely as a result of rapidly increasing costs of care, both federal and state governments have initiated a variety of mechanisms to assign responsibility to physicians both for the costs of care and for its quality. In this section, the basis for these efforts and the most important of the mechanisms for controlling costs and quality are reviewed.

### Physician Payment Reform

In the fee-for-service system characteristic of most medical care in the United States, invasive procedures typically are compensated at more than double the rate for interventions such as counseling and advice giving, even when both take the same amount of time. A new compensation system based on the "re-source cost" for medical services (known as RBRVS for resource-based relative value scale) was accepted by Congress in 1989 as the basis for physician payment in the Medicare program, to be phased in starting in 1992. The aim is to encourage the provision of primary care services rather than procedure-intensive specialty services in the country. Some state Medicaid programs also adopted the Medicare RBRVS and private insurers are considering this system for their fee-for-service insurance plans. Given pediatricians' orientation toward provision of these so-called "cognitive" services, adoption of an RBRVS-payment system should increase reimbursement for their services, at least relatively. At the time of its implementation for Medicare, however, the RBRVS system did not include services that were not applicable to the Medicare population, such as newborn care, child health supervision, and obstetric care. Thus, the degree to which this new payment system will improve compensation for pediatric services remains unknown.

## Medical Practice Variations

A series of studies has provided clear evidence that rates of hospitalization and surgery vary widely from one area to another, even within areas as small as counties; similar variability is apparent across larger areas, such as countries. Why should this be the case? In some cases, the differences can be accounted for by variations in population needs. For example, hospitalization rates for children with asthma differ according to the geographic area in which the children live; in poorer areas, where asthma is more severe, hospitalization rates are greater than in non-poor areas. Another possible reason concerns differences in the availability of a mechanism by which to pay for certain services; where a procedure is reimbursed by a third-party payor, it is more likely to be performed. The main reason, however, appears to be physician uncertainty about the effectiveness of diagnostic and therapeutic modalities. Where there is lack of knowledge about effectiveness, or where there is knowledge that is not disseminated widely, certain practice patterns become established in particular geographic areas and are reinforced by common practice within those areas.

Starting in the late 1980s, a national effort to ascertain the relative effectiveness of various methods of clinical management was initiated by the federal government. Known as the Medical Treatment Effectiveness Program, this consists of a program of research to test various modes of management and a concerted effort to develop guidelines for practice based on documented evidence rather than on clinical consensus or common practice. Most major professional organizations, including the American Academy of Pediatrics, are engaging in these efforts to improve the rational basis for and, hence, the quality of, medical care.

## Prospective Payment

One way to reduce the variability in costs of care is to pay for care ahead of time, based upon the projected demand for services, so that the hospital or physician is at risk of financial loss if costs are greater than projected. Many of the following mechanisms to control costs and quality are based upon this principle.

Prospective payment differs from the traditional retrospective reimbursement in establishing a per diem or per-case payment ahead of time based on the diagnosis, instead of after care has been provided. Such an approach has been applied primarily to hospitalizations. The earliest of the approaches to be used on a wide scale were those resulting from state cost review commissions or insurance agencies. In one form of prospective reimbursement, a statewide formula is established to determine the percentage increase in hospital costs from one year to the next. The starting point is the hospital's costs in the previous year; the costs for the current year are those from the previous year, adjusted by the formula for projected increases in labor costs, supplies, technology, and other relatively fixed expenditures. In another type of state rate setting, negotiations are conducted with each hospital individually.

A third form of prospective reimbursement further decouples payment for care from the actual costs incurred. In this form of reimbursement, which began in New Jersey in 1979, hospitals are paid according to their "case-mix," on the assumption that costs should be determined primarily by the problems that are treated. The basis for this approach derives from research on "diagnosis-related groups" (DRGs). In this approach, all diagnoses responsible for hospitalizations were grouped into about 450 categories that are relatively homogeneous with regard to clinical type and length of hospital stay. As costs of care are associated highly with the duration of hospital stays, diagnoses that are similar in their length of stay presumably are similar in their costs of care. In 1983, the amendments to the Social Security Act mandated the use of DRGs as the basis for reimbursement of federally reimbursed care for Medicare. Hospitals are paid according to their case mix, that is, their mix of DRGs. A hospital's compensation is determined by the number of patients in each diagnostic category multiplied by the payment rate for the category summed over all diagnostic categories after adjusting for various other factors such as residency programs and rural/urban locations. Provisions are made for "outliers," that is, patients who have extraordinarily high costs because of unusual circumstances; it is expected that no more than 5% of patients would be outliers. Provisions also are made for increases in costs because of inflation.

Although DRGs initially applied only to patients whose care was reimbursed by Medicare, some private insurers and state Medicaid programs have adopted DRGs or similar systems in an attempt to reduce variability in expenditures across hospitals and overall increases in costs. A separate case-mix classification has been developed for the pediatric age group.

Furthermore, a prospective approach to care provided in ambulatory (outpatient) settings is likely to be adopted in an attempt to control the variability in outpatient physician practices. As noted earlier in this chapter, prospective payment already is a feature of PPGP HMOs. Physicians in the most rapidly growing new forms of organization of services, the IPAs and the PPOs, however, still are paid a fee for service, albeit a negotiated fee. As price competition continues to increase among competing health care financing and delivery systems, the impetus toward greater cost containment will make case-mix–adjusted ambulatory care payments a likely prospect.

When control of the costs of care involves procedures that reduce the use of services, there always is the concern that the reduction will include indicated as well as unnecessary services. As a result of these concerns, there have been periodic attempts to develop procedures to monitor the quality of care. The federal government, which was first to implement cost control on a large scale, also was the first to devise large-scale efforts to deal with the issue of quality of practice.

## Peer Review

In the Social Security Amendments of 1972, Congress established the Professional Standards Review Organizations (PSROs). The legislation mandated that professional organizations assure the quality of care provided in programs that received federal funding. (These included the Medicare program for the elderly, the Medicaid program for the indigent, and the Maternal and Child Health programs.) These organizations were to be nonprofit and composed of physicians. They might be set up on a state level or be local in character; they were funded by grants. The PSRO program was intended to use three mechanisms in pursuit of their mandate.

The first and most well developed was utilization review, wherein admissions to hospitals were reviewed for necessity and where a maximum length of stay was determined. If the admission lasted longer than the set length of stay, the responsible physician had to provide justification. The second function was medical care review, in which the PSROs were required to choose certain diagnoses and review medical records to determine whether the standards of care were met. Re-review after the institution of educational programs to remedy deficits was required. The third function, which never was well developed, was the collection of data to compare care across institutions and develop programs to determine reasons for differences in the "profiles of care" where they were found. Evaluations of the effectiveness of the PSROs generally concluded that the costs of the efforts were about equivalent to the dollars that were saved as a result of them.

Disenchantment with the program and its failure to reduce costs or capture the imagination of the medical profession led to its demise and replacement by the Utilization and Quality Control Peer Review Organizations. This legislation (TEFRA 1982) was prompted by concern that the DRG prospective reimbursement program might compromise the quality of care provided to Medicare recipients, and it mandated that peer review organizations assess the validity of diagnostic information to make sure that the assigned DRG was correct, and that they examine the completeness, accuracy, and quality of care to ensure that underservice was not occurring. The major difference between the PSRO and the peer review programs is the aegis under which they operate. PSROs were nonprofit physician organizations funded by grants; peer review organizations operate on contract (and, hence, under greater surveillance and control) with the federal government, and can be for profit and operated by nonphysician organizations such as fiscal intermediaries and insurers if no satisfactory physician group applies. Little is known of the operations of these agencies or their effectiveness in detecting inadequate patterns of care.

In 1986, Congress passed additional legislation to strengthen peer review by offering immunity from prosecution of peer review groups by physicians whose practices are found deficient. The legislation also mandated the establishment of the National Practitioner Data Bank, which contains information on the names of physicians who have had successful malpractice judgments made against them and descriptions of the acts that led to the claims. The law also mandated the reporting to the data bank of the names of all physicians who have had their licenses revoked or suspended for reasons related to professional incompetence, and the names of physicians who have had their clinical privileges suspended by hospitals, HMOs, or other professional groups. Hospitals must search the database when physicians are considered for medical staff privileges.

Procedures for disclosure to the public of information about practice patterns also has undergone change in the past decade. In creating the peer review organization program, Congress altered the ground rules under which PSROs had been operating, in the direction of increased disclosure. The new regulations, which were published in April of 1986, permit peer review organizations to disclose interpretations and generalizations concerning the quality of care in a particular institution (such as a hospital) as long as no individuals are identifiable. Increasingly, information about differences in practice patterns and about differences in performance as reflected in mortality and morbidity rates are being made available not only to third-party payors, but also to the public. The U.S. Department of Health and Human Services releases about annually a list of the nation's hospitals that have mortality rates that are significantly higher and lower than expected, given the type of the hospital. The department cited the Federal Freedom of Information Act as the justification for releasing the list to the public. Although the rates involve only patients on the Medicare program (those more than 65 years of age), the action sets a precedent for public disclosure of information about the practices of health services facilities in general.

## THE FUTURE OF PEDIATRIC PRACTICE

Pediatric practice, like all physician practices in the United States, may undergo radical change in the near future. Recent directions suggest an increasing "corporatization" of medicine, with the ownership of facilities and control of medical groups being assumed by large for-profit companies that contract with physicians and physician groups to provide care. Concern about expenditures for care are resulting in increasing scrutiny over medical practice and imposition of various types of control over it. Both community-based and hospital-based physicians will be affected; assumption by corporations of ownership of hospitals, including teaching hospitals, occurred at an increasing rate during the early 1980s.

The trend toward "managed care" has several implications for the practice of pediatrics. One advantage of managed plans, for individuals who are enrolled in them, is that they include well child services, immunizations, and other child health supervision services, which are not part of the benefits of most indemnity insurance plans. The proportion of pediatricians, however, and especially of pediatric subspecialists, affiliated with these managed care systems is likely to be considerably less than in the current health system, for various reasons. These systems of care will have an underrepresentation of children at highest risk of illness, and they often substitute nonphysicians for physicians for certain types of services. Moreover, reductions in use will reduce the number of pediatricians that are required. Some estimates indicate that insured children in "managed care" plans require nearly 25% fewer primary care pediatricians than is the case under ordinary circumstances.

Managed care systems provide an opportunity for pediatricians (and for all physicians) to participate in efforts to improve the accuracy and completeness of information systems in practice. Little is known about the extent to which commonly employed procedures actually achieve the purposes for which they are intended. Currently, the imperative of managed care systems is cost control. Clinicians can capitalize on the opportunities in managed care to develop techniques to measure, document, and assess the effectiveness of health services as well as to control their costs.

The number of pediatricians is rising at a significantly faster rate than the growth of the child population. Between 1970 and 1985, the number of pediatricians rose 89%, in contrast to a 21% growth in the number of children. Many analysts have predicted a clear surplus of pediatricians, at least in the early years of the next century. The birth rate has not fallen as far as predicted, however, and actually may be rising, and other medical specialties face similar physician-to-population ratio changes. Pediatricians also may be expanding their role with older children and adolescents, and into different types of care (including the management of developmental and psychosocial problems). Moreover, as this chapter has shown, the revolution in organizational formats for providing care gradually is disenfranchising a growing segment of the population: children of poor and working-class families. Currently, pediatricians provide relatively little care to socioeconomically disadvantaged children and to children in nonurban areas. Responsiveness to community needs always has been a hallmark of pediatric practitioners. As individuals and through their organizations, pediatricians need to find new ways to provide care to those who now lack access to it, to be more available to care for new problems as they arise, to increase the scope of services they provide and to evaluate their effectiveness, and, thus, to work toward reducing barriers to care and improving the health status of all of the country's children.

## Selected Readings

Adams P, Benson V. Current estimates form the National Health Interview Study. National Center for Health Statistics. Vital Health Stat 1991;10(181).
American Academy of Pediatrics. Child health financing report. Elk Grove Village, IL: American Academy of Pediatrics, published periodically.
Employee Benefit Research Institute. Sources of health insurance and characteristics of the uninsured: Analysis of the March 1991 Current Population Survey. Washington, DC: Employee Benefit Research Institute, 1992.
Himmelstein D, Woolhandler S. Cost without benefit: Administrative waste in U.S. health care. N Engl J Med 1986;314:441.
Hsiao W, Braum P, Yntema D, et al. Estimating physicians' work for a resource-based relative value scale. N Engl J Med 1988;319:835.
Levit KR, Lazenby HC, Cowan CA, Letsch SW. National health expenditures, 1990. Health Care Financing Review 1991;13:29.
Lohr KN, Brook RH, Kamberg CJ, Goldberg GA, et al. Use of medical care in the Rand Health Insurance experiment. Diagnosis- and service-specific analyses in a randomized controlled trial. Med Care 1986;24(Suppl 9):S1.
Marion Merrill Dow. Managed care digest, PPO edition. Kansas City MO: Marion Merrill Dow, 1991.
Martinez G, Ryen G. The pediatric marketplace. Am J Dis Child 1989;143:924.
Porter MJ, Ball PA, Kraus N. The InterStudy Competitive Edge, Excelsior, MN: InterStudy, 1992.
Starfield B. Effectiveness of medical care: Validating clinical wisdom. Baltimore: The Johns Hopkins University Press, 1985.
Starfield B. Primary care: Concept, evaluation, and policy. New York: Oxford, 1992.
Steinwachs D, Weiner J, Shapiro S, Batalden P, Coltin K, Wasserman F. A comparison of the requirements for primary care physicians in HMOs with projections made by the GMENAC. N Engl J Med 1986;314:217.
Yudkowsky BK, Cartland JDC, Flint SS. Pediatrician participation in Medicaid: 1978–1989. Pediatrics 1990;85:567.

*Principles and Practice of Pediatrics, Second Edition.*
edited by Frank A. Oski et al. J. B. Lippincott Company, Philadelphia © 1994.

# CHAPTER 5
# *Reading the Medical Literature*

## Kenneth B. Roberts and Lawrence S. Wissow

Although many modes of continuing education are available to the modern practitioner, ranging from seminars to tapes, the most widely relied upon method continues to be reading the medical literature (journals and texts). The printed media provide sources that are convenient, particularly in terms of time, and that permit the reader to proceed at any pace desired. By selecting more than one article or text, a reader can determine what various experts think and whether a consensus exists; with the aid of various computer-assisted searches, such selection can be performed with relative ease and speed. Medical decision making appears to be influenced most strongly by the opinions of experts and by local custom; the medical literature provides a forum through which to link communities, experts, and conventional wisdom.

## USES OF THE MEDICAL LITERATURE

The three main uses of the medical literature for the reader are to answer a particular question, to acquire or maintain knowledge in a specific area, and to acquire or maintain general knowledge.

In order to be answered, a particular question must be stated clearly; the answer to a poorly articulated question is likely to be unsatisfying or misleading. Once the information sought is specified, it must be accessed. This is accomplished most frequently with major general textbooks, such as this one; with specialty texts, such as the American Academy of Pediatrics' "Red Book" (Report of the Committee on Infectious Diseases); or with reference manuals, such as *The Harriet Lane Handbook*.

Practitioners increasingly are using computers to search for journal articles that are relevant to specific clinical issues. A database of journal articles (such as MEDLINE) and the equipment necessary to search for them may be accessed at a library or directly by the physician. Some services provide not only listings of articles, but also abstracts and, in some cases, the article's full text.

In order to conduct a computer search, the clinical question must be translated into the vocabulary of the search software. This usually requires two steps. First, the reader must know what system of key words and logic has been used to index articles in the database. Asking for articles about "newborns" may prove disappointing, for example, if the database knows this population only as "neonates." Most medical indexing systems are based on the *Medical Subject Headings (MeSH) Annotated Alphabetical List*, which is published by the National Library of Medicine and is available in most medical libraries or directly from the United States National Technical Information Service. Second, the reader must know how the search software uses the subject headings to define increasingly narrower areas of interest. Some search programs are mastered more easily than others, but even the most complicated can be mastered with relatively little practice. Texts and training courses on computer searching are widely available.

Conducting computer searches has many advantages over exploring resources that may be at hand or even browsing through a well-stocked library. Computer searches help to sift relevant articles from among thousands of publications spanning many years and several languages. In the end, however, the reader alone must determine which articles appear to be of high quality and which are relevant to the clinical question at hand. Some criteria for judging research articles are listed below.

The medical literature in a specific area of interest is likely to be defined more easily: specialty texts and journals can be identified and accessed, although general interest journals still will need monitoring as well. Review on a regular basis requires discipline, but rewards the reader with a sense of keeping up to date. Delving more deeply into a specific area may involve sources beyond the scope of many medical libraries, such as basic science and social science journals. Networking between libraries or among colleagues eases problems of both identification and availability. Some readers also may wish to set up so-called Selective Dissemination of Information (SDI) plans with a medical library or computer data service. SDIs are individually tailored computer literature searches that can be run on a regular basis (ie, monthly) to retrieve new literature in a predetermined field. Readers with direct access can perform their own SDI by making a regular computer search part of their library reading routine. Publications such as *Current Contents* also allow regular perusal of new titles from selected journals.

Keeping up with medical progress in general and with pediatrics in particular also requires discipline and time committed to the process, plus a few "favorite" sources. In the spring of each year, the *Yearbook of Pediatrics* becomes available, providing abstracts and commentaries on articles published the preceding year. Various newsletters provide such a service on an ongoing basis, usually weekly or biweekly. Journals such as *Pediatrics in Review, Pediatrics, American Journal of Diseases of Children,* and *Contemporary Pediatrics* are geared to readers in general pediatrics. The *New England Journal of Medicine* and *JAMA* are the leading general medical journals in this country.

## READING A JOURNAL ARTICLE

Most frequently, perusal of a journal means scanning of the table of contents and selected abstracts. Before conclusions from particular articles should be permitted to affect decision making, however, a more critical review should be performed. Many readers consider this to be the function of the editor and reviewers in so-called refereed journals, and they presume that publication serves as an endorsement of scientific quality. In relative terms, this undoubtedly is true, as reflected in the low publication rate of studies first presented in abstract form at meetings. The process has limitations, however. Questions of personal relevance and applicability, for example, cannot be answered by the editorial process, nor are the implications of a given study necessarily the same to all readers. The ability to read critically and to analyze a study is a valuable skill; although many physicians are intimidated by the belief that a thorough knowledge of complicated statistics is required, the fact is that the most important analytic tool is, simply, logical reasoning. An organized approach, such as the one presented below, greatly facilitates this process.

After finding an interesting title, some readers make their first test an examination of an article's list of authors, their institutional affiliations, and the study's funding source. Recognizing a name that the reader has seen before on an interesting article may make the present work seem more worthy of being read. In similar fashion, a given institution may be known for the strength of its work (or its access to patients with a particular clinical problem). Funding sources that require competitive application and peer review also may be an indication of a study whose premises and methods have been planned and scrutinized more carefully. The absence of these factors rarely weighs against reading an otherwise interesting paper, but their presence often calls attention to papers the reader otherwise might disregard.

Most readers first turn to a paper's abstract in an attempt to learn what the paper is about. Unfortunately, the abstract is not always clear. Sometimes the problem lies in editorial constraints, usually strict space limitations that make the abstract too brief to be helpful. At times, though, this is the first clue that the authors themselves are not too sure of their paper's take-home message. Most of the time, the abstract only serves to explain the study's general subject matter. One must read further to determine its relevance to one's own interests.

If the general subject matter seems to be of interest, the next step is to define exactly what question the study is designed to address, and whether this is of interest to the reader. The study question should be stated quite explicitly in the paper's introduction section, either as a hypothesis to be tested or as a goal for a descriptive study. Even a review paper should have a clearly stated goal or focus. Again, failure to find such a statement can be an important warning about the value of what is to follow.

The next test of relevance usually requires delving into the "fine print" of an article, that is, the methods section. Of most importance at this stage of reading is whether the study's patient population, clinical tests or procedures, and outcome measures have anything in common with the setting in which the reader works. A paper on screening for anemia, for example, might seem on the surface to be of great interest to the office-based pediatrician, unless it is discovered that the work was carried out on a Caribbean island under technologic constraints that vary greatly from those in the reader's practice.

A final screen for relevance can involve scrutinizing the paper's tables and graphs. These usually summarize major findings in a way that is least influenced by the authors' interpretations. Are the tables understandable? Do they list the variables with which the reader is most concerned? Do they seem to address the same study question that was stated in the introduction?

## READING THE METHODS SECTION

The methods section often can be the most tedious part of the paper to read, but it probably is the most important. The more weight one plans to put on the author's conclusions, the more carefully one must read the methods he or she employed. Various research strategies require attention to particular kinds of problems, but all studies require evaluation of a few key areas:

1. How was the study population assembled?
   Did the authors have an explicit case definition? Did they stick to it and include all qualified patients? Is it a definition that fits with the study's stated goals? Are criteria for exclusion acceptable and reasonable?
   What biases are inherent in the way in which the population was recruited? Is it likely that only more severe cases were included or, conversely, are those studied only those who survived long enough to be enrolled? Have the diagnostic or therapeutic dilemmas been altered by the prior exclusion of patients with similar illnesses, especially those that are common in the reader's practice?
2. If there was a control, normal, or comparison group, how was it assembled? Many of the same problems arise in this process as in the selection of study patients (see below).
3. What was the nature of the test, intervention, or study instrument?
   Was it defined explicitly and applied consistently? Was there any means in the study by which to determine whether the intervention actually was delivered as planned?
   Especially for questionnaires or other kinds of survey instruments and rating scales, is the method one that is accepted in the literature and has been shown to be valid and reliable? If so, were these characteristics ascertained in a population similar to the one in which the instrument now is being used? Has the instrument been modified and, if so, have the authors tested the effect of the modification before performing the study? (Answers to these questions may require further reading. Unfortunately, most methods sections assume that the reader already is an expert in the field.)
4. How were outcome observations made?
   Were there explicitly defined outcome measures and were they as objective as possible?
   Was there sufficient blinding so that those persons assessing outcome were not biased by their beliefs about how the study should turn out?
   What happened to data regarding persons who were lost to follow-up, had incomplete ascertainment of baseline data, or changed classification from study to control group? (Some of this information may be present in the results section.)

## PROBLEM POINTS FOR PARTICULAR TYPES OF STUDIES

It is not always useful to belabor the determination of what particular type of study design is being used, such as case-control, cross-sectional, or clinical trial. Many clinical studies use hybrid designs that cannot be classified easily. Identifying the design, however, even tentatively, may help focus the reader's attention on those pitfalls that are encountered most often.

Individual and series case reports frequently make the earliest observations about a new field, therapy, or illness. Their main importance is to define an issue that requires more extensive and rigorous study. Case reports and case series usually are retrospective (ie, the author realizes that something unusual has happened and looks back at the case, or examines a series of patient charts on which to report). This process has three major pitfalls that must be kept in mind:

1. Was a systematic effort made to find and review all similar cases? Is a consistent case definition being used? If the report describes an unusually good or bad outcome from a common condition, do the patients described fit accepted criteria for the condition being studied? Is it possible that they differed in some way from other patients with similar problems (eg, they had an earlier or later stage of disease or were selected because they lacked certain complicating conditions)?
2. Was all information necessary to the study consistently available, obtained, and recorded from the medical records being reviewed? If information came from other sources (eg, a clinician's recollection), was it confirmed in some way?
3. Are the authors sufficiently careful about the conclusions they have drawn? Most of the time, case studies serve to generate hypotheses for further study rather than reaching any firm conclusions themselves.

Case-control studies are very popular in clinical research because they lend themselves to the examination of relatively rare events and to the use of interview or record review techniques. They are used very often to probe for the etiology of conditions that develop over long periods of time or that ultimately may prove to be multifactorial in nature. To conduct such a study, the researcher assembles a group of cases—individuals with the disease or condition in question—and a group of controls—individuals who are similar to the cases in as many ways as possible with the exception that they do not have the disease. Then, through record review, interviews, or other means, the researcher sees whether there is any difference in exposure or experience in the two groups that may be related to onset of the disease.

Case-control studies risk having all of the common problems discussed above, but two merit particular concern.

1. Selection of control subjects: It often proves difficult to find control subjects who are similar enough to the patients being studied. For example, patients hospitalized for other conditions may come from a different referral population and, thus, have differing socioeconomic status or environmental exposures. Children attending school constitute a special group that is healthier than the group of children who cannot attend school; therefore, they might not be good control subjects for a study of children with chronic illness. Many case-control studies use more than one control group if no single, ideal, group can be found.

   One also must be sure that the control group does not contain individuals who really should be classified as cases. These might be persons who are in the early stages of a condition, or who have a condition that is not diagnosed easily (such as child abuse). The more cases are mixed in with the control subjects, the less likely it is that any differences related to etiology will be found.

2. Bias in obtaining information about past exposures or experience: The term "bias" refers to systematic errors that, if undetected, will alter the apparent results of a study. The greatest risk of bias in case-control studies is that being a case may make one more likely to remember certain past events, or make it more likely that these events have been documented. When reading a paper, it is important to consider ways in which data gathering may have been different in the case and control groups. Did cases get more medical care or have more detailed histories taken on admission to the hospital? Were members of one group interviewed, whereas members of the other only had their records reviewed?

Cohort or prospective studies often are used to determine the prognosis or natural history of a condition. Groups of similar individuals are assembled and followed over time until some specific outcome occurs: relapse, death, cure, and so forth. The outcome of the study usually is some description of the proportion of persons who experience the outcome as a function of time from the study's start.

Again, the general problems discussed earlier apply to accounts of cohort studies. In particular, however, the reader must note the following:

1. The source and homogeneity of the group being observed. Are there differences among members of the group that might relate to their risk of having a particular outcome? Is the group representative of patients whom the reader treats?
2. The definition of "outcome." Is it objective? Is it an outcome that is clinically meaningful to the reader?
3. Analysis of incomplete data. What happens to individuals for whom only incomplete information is available? Are they omitted? Is it likely that those who were lost to follow-up are somehow different from those who remained to be observed?

Clinical trials usually are considered to be the gold standard of medical research, but they are applicable to only a small range of study questions. Clinical trials compare outcomes among two or more groups, one of which is exposed deliberately to a therapy or intervention while the others receive alternative or no interventions. As such, they are used primarily to test the efficacy of new treatments and procedures.

Most clinical trials are randomized and blinded; these techniques add to accuracy, but are not foolproof. Points to watch for in clinical trials include those listed below:

1. *Randomization.* Patients are assigned to treatment or control groups through a mechanism based on chance, such as a random number table, the spinning of a wheel, or throwing dice. The purpose is to eliminate both conscious and unconscious bias in deciding which patients are assigned to which group. Every account of a clinical trial should have a table that shows how well the randomization worked for important factors that can be measured (usually variables such as age, race, and sex). The two groups should be quite similar. If they are not, it could be just by chance, but the data analysis that follows will have to compensate for any noted differences.
2. *Blinding.* Both study subjects and researchers who have a role in carrying out the study protocol or collecting data should be shielded from knowledge of treatment allocations and specific study goals. This also is intended to reduce both conscious and unconscious bias on the part of a study's participants. Blinding is especially important when outcome measures are subjective, or when there are opportunities to change therapy in the course of the study. More elaborate studies include

checks to ensure that blinding is not violated. Some studies use placebos as a means of promoting blinding.

3. *Assessment of unwanted side effects.* Clinical trials are difficult to carry out and usually include the minimum number of patients necessary to prove that a new treatment is effective. This frequently is many fewer patients than would be needed to determine whether the new treatment has any uncommon but dangerous side effects, or side effects that may be delayed beyond the study's period of observation. Thus, clinical trials present only one part of the information needed to decide if a new treatment is worth using.

Studies that examine new diagnostic tests must give clear information about test characteristics such as sensitivity, specificity, and predictive value (see Chap. 164). But even before these are determined, the reader must be assured that the methods used to study the test were sound. Was the test applied properly or in the same way it would be used in everyday practice? What population was used to study the test? Was it representative of patients the reader might encounter? What gold standard was used to measure the new test's performance?

## EVALUATION OF RESULTS

In a well-written paper, the reader should be able to go through the results section and find data addressing each of the study questions posed in the introduction. Ideally, the authors will not just state their findings ("Factor $x$ was associated with disease $y$."), but also will provide the corresponding numeric data. Minimal weight should be placed on findings that the reader cannot trace back to actual study data or methods. Often, this means checking the numbers in a table of results against procedures and numbers given in the methods section. Have all of the eligible patients been included in the analysis?

Results often are couched in statistical terms with which the reader may not be familiar. Statistical techniques have two major uses in data analysis: first, as a way to wrap a large number of observations into a single, summary measure; and second, to help the researcher decide how large a role chance may have played in the results of a study.

In the first case, the simplest summary techniques look at one concept or variable at a time and tell us something about its "central tendency" (average value or overall proportion, for example) and its variation around this central point (standard deviation or confidence limits). More complex techniques such as multiple regression look simultaneously at relationships among many variables. For any of these techniques, the reader's major task is to judge whether the summary provides an adequate picture of the raw data. For single variables, charts or tables can help one decide whether an average is being distorted by a few wildly discrepant values, or whether a proportion is being drawn from observations of only a few patients. With more complex statistical procedures, it may be necessary to consult a statistician to decide if the technique used is selected appropriately and applied properly. A good paper, though, usually will present raw data or some simpler analysis that corroborates at least in part what was obtained using fancier techniques.

In the second case, statistics help estimate the role of chance in the assessment of a single number (such as a mean or a rate) or of the difference between two numbers. For example, statistics may be used to determine how much a given proportion or average might vary, simply by chance, from its observed value. In this case, we usually say that, if we repeated the observation 100 times, 95% of the observations would fall between a set of lower and upper limits, often called confidence limits. Alternatively, statistics may be used to decide how likely two rates are to have differed simply because of chance. If this likelihood is low (usually less than 5%), we are willing to say that the difference has some cause related to the subject under study. Commonly encountered statistical tests of this kind include the chi-squared test (for differences in proportions) and the Student's $t$-test (for differences in averages).

It is important to realize that these measures of statistical significance examine only one attribute of a result's importance. A result may be statistically significant but have little or no clinical significance. As the number of persons enrolled in a study increases, confidence limits narrow and smaller differences will be found to be statistically significant. For example, with very large groups, it might be possible to determine with great confidence that new drug A lowers fever 1 hour sooner than new drug B, but this difference may not be important to our decisions regarding therapy. On the other hand, some very small differences can have great clinical importance, such as a reduction in the time necessary for medical teams to respond to cardiorespiratory arrests.

## TYPE I AND TYPE II ERRORS

Most statistical tests for the difference in two rates or averages are based on what is known as the null hypothesis. One starts with the assumption that there is no difference between the two outcomes, and then seeks to reject this hypothesis by showing that a difference of the size observed is unlikely to have occurred simply by chance. The usual standard for "unlikely" is fewer than 5 chances in 100, or $p < .05$. This leaves up to 5 chances in 100 of rejecting the null hypothesis when, in fact, it should be accepted. In other words, there is a chance as large as 5% that there really is no difference in the two groups. This chance for error is called type I error, and its size is labeled with the Greek letter alpha ($\alpha$).

Many studies forget that, in examining differences, one must consider an alternative hypothesis stating that the observed difference is, in fact, real and not the result of chance. The importance of considering this hypothesis is that testing for a difference of any given magnitude requires a certain minimum number of observations to be made. If this number of observations has been made and no difference is found, then one can have a certain degree of confidence that chance alone was not responsible for the negative results. Researchers usually are more willing to risk rejecting alternative hypotheses—and, thus, committing a so-called type II error—than they are to risk rejecting the null hypothesis. Studies that look at differences usually try to enroll enough research subjects so that there will be no more than 20 chances in 100 that a negative result will occur simply due to chance. The amount of type II error possible in a study often is labeled with the Greek letter beta ($\beta$). Authors sometimes refer to the quantity 1-beta as the power of a study to find a difference of a given size with a given number of patients enrolled. If a study reports negative results or asserts that there is no difference between two groups based on some statistical test (chi-squared or $t$-test, for example), the reader should check the methods section to see if the authors demonstrate sufficient statistical power to find a difference.

## DRAWING CONCLUSIONS

It is rare for a single study to provide such convincing or widely applicable evidence that its results should be used to make major clinical decisions. Even if we are willing to accept a study's methods and analysis, we still have to assess whether its conclusions make sense in light of other available information or in terms of our own clinical experience. Points to consider when weighing a study's conclusions include the following:

1. Does the study show results in the same direction (positive or negative association, helpful or harmful therapy) and of similar magnitude as other studies? Even a result that is not significant statistically may be important if it tends toward the same results as other work. If this study is different, why is it different? Is the intervention really the same? Are the patients very different? Were there simply too few patients studied (a type II error)?
2. Do the study results make both biologic and clinical sense? Are there parallel concepts in other areas of medicine or science that make these new results seem plausible?
3. How extensively have the authors discussed other implications of their findings? If a new therapy is effective, is it any more effective than other therapies that might be less expensive or less risky?

## CHECKING YOUR CONCLUSIONS

Various methods can be used to provide feedback regarding one's assessment or interpretation of a study. In many areas, journal clubs are popular, run either as peer review or with the guidance of a knowledgeable leader. Other strategies include tapes, meetings, local experts, and commentaries in weekly or biweekly newsletters. Letters to the editor often shed valuable additional light on recent studies; this forum is particularly valuable as an opportunity to raise new questions and clarify points of interest. Perhaps the most important ingredient is the experience of disciplined, regular reading of the literature. The cost is commitment of time and attention; the reward is continued growth and stimulation, the ability to find answers to clinical problems, and a feeling of remaining current on medical advances.

## MAINTAINING A PERSONAL FILE OF JOURNAL ARTICLES

Few clinicians leave training without having established often voluminous files of journal articles, course handouts, and other teaching materials. These files quickly become unwieldy and defeat their original purpose: granting rapid access to literature that the reader has selected carefully for both its quality and its relevance. Haynes and coworkers make several suggestions for maintaining usable personal files:

1. Develop a practical and flexible set of subject headings or key words by which to file and cross-reference articles. The table of contents of a favorite text may be adapted, or MeSH headings from the National Library of Medicine could be used. Serious attempts to cross-reference articles probably will require a personal computer if they are not to become too time-consuming, but a set of notes linking related subject headings can work well for a small file.
2. Include only articles that seem to be of high quality or already are known to be "classics." If you do not have time to read the articles before placing them in the file, at least choose those whose methods seem to be most sound. Include review articles only when they are either very recent, have needed citations, or give a particularly clear overview of an area.
3. Periodically clean out the files, throwing out articles that are more than a few years old or that have not proved to be useful. Do not try to duplicate the library's holdings (unless there is none nearby). Keep only those items that will be needed most urgently or most often.

Whatever system is used, it must make sense in terms of the reader's own clinical logic and resource needs. Many clinicians have highly personalized and idiosyncratic ways of classifying articles and maintaining a file. What counts is that an article filed yesterday can be retrieved easily tomorrow.

## Selected Readings

Department of Clinical Epidemiology and Biostatistics, McMaster University Health Sciences Center. How to read clinical journals. Series in Can Med Assoc J.
    I. Why to read them and how to start reading them critically. 1981;124:555.
    II. To learn about a diagnostic test. 1981;124:703.
    III. To learn the clinical course and prognosis of disease. 1981;124:869.
    IV. To determine etiology or causation. 1981;124:985.
    V. To distinguish useful from useless or even harmful therapy. 1981;124:1156.
    VI. To learn about the quality of clinical care. 1984;130:377.
    VII. To understand an economic evaluation (part A). 1984;130:1428.
    VIII. To understand an economic evaluation (part B). 1984;130:1542.
Haynes RB, McKibbon KA, Fitzgerald D, et al. How to keep up with the medical literature. Series in Ann Intern Med.
    I. Why try to keep up and how to get started. 1986;105:149.
    II. Deciding which journals to read regularly. 1986;105:309.
    III. Expanding the number of journals you read regularly. 1986;105:474.
    IV. Using the literature to solve clinical problems. 1986;105:636.
    V. Access by personal computer to the medical literature. 1986;105:810.
    VI. How to store and retrieve articles worth keeping. 1986;105:978.
Menke JA, McClead RE. On-line with Medline: An introduction for the pediatrician. Pediatrics 1987;80:605.
Sackett DL, Haynes RB, Guyatt GH, Tugwell P. Clinical epidemiology: A basic science for clinical medicine, 2nd ed. Boston: Little Brown, 1991.
Wyatt J. Use and sources of medical knowledge. Lancet 1991;338:1368.

*Principles and Practice of Pediatrics, Second Edition.*
edited by Frank A. Oski et al. J. B. Lippincott Company, Philadelphia © 1994.

CHAPTER 6

# The Pediatric History and Physical Examination

Lewis A. Barness

## HISTORY

Obtaining a complete history on a pediatric patient not only is necessary, but also leads to the correct diagnosis in the vast majority of children. The history usually is learned from the parent, the older child, or the caretaker of a sick child. After learning the fundamentals of obtaining and recording historic data, the nuances associated with the giving of information must be interpreted.

For the acutely ill child, a short, rapidly obtained report of the events of the immediate past may suffice temporarily, but as soon as the crisis is controlled, a more complete history is necessary. A convenient method of learning to obtain a meaningful history is to ask systematically and directly all of the questions outlined below. After confidence is gained with experience, questions can be problem-directed and asked in an order designed to elicit more specific information about a suspected disease state or diagnosis. Some psychosocial implications will be obvious. More subtle details often are obtained by asking open-ended questions. Those with organic illness usually have short histories; those with psychosomatic illness have a longer list of symptoms and complaints.

During the interview, it is important to convey to the parent interest in the child as well as the illness. The parent is allowed to talk freely at first and to express concerns in his or her own words. The interviewer should look directly either at the parent or the child intermittently and not only at the writing instruments. A sympathetic listener who addresses the parent and child by name frequently obtains more accurate information than does a harried, distracted interviewer. Careful observation during the interview frequently uncovers stresses and concerns that otherwise are not apparent.

The written record is not only helpful in determining a diagnosis and making decisions, but also is necessary for observing the growth and development of the child. A well-organized record facilitates the retrieval of information and obviates problems if it is required for legal review.

The following guidelines indicate the information needed. If preferred, a number of printed forms are available, which contain similar material, or forms may be modified as long as consistency is maintained.

## General Information

Identifying data include the date, name, age and birth date, sex, race, referral source if pertinent, relationship of the child and informant, and some indication of the mental state or reliability of the informant. It frequently is helpful to include the ethnic or racial background, address, and telephone numbers of the informants.

## Chief Complaint

After the identifying data, the chief complaint should be recorded. Given in the informant's or patient's own words, the chief complaint is a brief statement of the reason why the patient was brought to be seen. It is not unusual that the stated complaint is not the true reason the child was brought for attention. Expanding the question of "Why did you bring him?" to "What concerns you?" allows the informant to focus on the complaint more accurately. Carefully phrased questions can elicit information without prying.

## History of Present Illness

Next, the details of the present illness are recorded in chronologic order. For the sick child, it is helpful to begin: "The child was well until _____ days before this visit." This is followed by a daily documentation of events leading up to the present time, including signs, symptoms, and treatment, if any. Statements should be recorded in number of days before the visit or dates, but not in days of the week, because chronology will be difficult to retrieve even a short time later if days of the week are used. If the child is taking medicine, the amount being taken, the name of the medicine, the frequency of administration, and how well and how long it has been or is being taken are needed.

For the well child, a simple statement such as "No complaints" or "No illness" suffices. A question about school attendance may be pertinent. If the past medical history is significant to the current illness, a brief summary is included. If information is obtained from old records, it should be noted here or may be recorded in the past medical history.

## Past Medical History

Obtaining the past medical history serves not only to provide a record of data that may be significant either now or later to the well-being of the child, but also to provide evidence of children who are at risk for health or psychosocial problems.

### Prenatal History

If a prenatal interview has been held (see below), this information already may be available. Questions to be answered include those regarding the health of the mother during this pregnancy, especially in regard to any infections, other illnesses, vaginal bleeding, toxemia, or care of animals, such as cats, which may induce toxoplasmosis or other animal-borne diseases, all of which can have permanent effects on the embryo and child. The time and type of movements the fetus made in utero should be determined. The number of previous pregnancies and their results, radiographs or medications taken during the pregnancy, results of serology and blood typing of the mother and baby, and results of other tests such as amniocentesis should be recorded. If the mother's weight gain has been excessive or insufficient, this also should be noted.

### Birth History

The duration of pregnancy, the ease or difficulty of labor, and the duration of labor may be important, especially if there is a question of developmental delay. The type of delivery (spontaneous, forceps-assisted, or cesarean section), type of anesthesia or analgesia used during delivery, attendance by other family members at delivery, and presenting part (if known) are recorded. Note this child's birth order (if there have been multiple births) and birth weight.

### Neonatal History

Many informants are aware of Apgar scores at birth and at 5 minutes, any unusual appearance of the child such as cyanosis or respiratory distress, and any resuscitative efforts that took place and their duration. If the mother was delayed in seeing the infant after birth, reasons should be sought. Jaundice, anemia, convulsions, dysmorphic states, and congenital anomalies or infections in the mother or infant are some of the reasons that viewing or handling of the newborn by the mother may be delayed. The time of onset of any of these abnormal states may be significant.

### Feeding History

Note whether the baby was breast- or bottle-fed and how well the baby took the first feeding. Poor sucking at the first feeding may be the result of sleepiness of the baby, but also is a warning sign of neurologic abnormality, which may not become manifest until much later in life. By the second or third feeding, even brain-damaged children usually nurse well.

If the infant has been bottle-fed, inquire about the type of formula used and the amount taken during a 24-hour period. At the same time, ask about the mother's initial reaction to her baby, the nature of bonding and eye-to-eye contact, and the patterns of crying, sleeping, urinating, and defecating. Requirements for supplemental feeding, vomiting, regurgitation, colic, diarrhea, or other gastrointestinal or feeding problems should be noted.

Determine the ages at which solid foods were introduced and supplementation with vitamins or fluoride took place, as well as the age at which weaning occurred and the method used to wean. In addition, note the age at which baby foods, toddlers' foods, and table food were introduced, the response to these, and any evidence of food intolerance or vomiting. If feeding difficulties are present, determine the onset of the problem, methods of feeding, reasons for changes, interval between feedings, amount taken at each feeding, vomiting, crying, and weight changes. With any feeding problem, evaluate the effect on the family by asking, "How did you manage the problem?"

For an older child, ask the informant to supply some breakfast, lunch, and dinner (supper) menus, likes and dislikes, and response of the family to eating problems.

## Developmental History

Estimation of physical growth rate is important. Attempt to ascertain the birth weight and the weights at 6 months, 1 year, 2 years, 5 years, and 10 years. Lengths at similar ages are desirable. These data are plotted on physical growth charts. Any sudden gain or loss in physical growth should be noted particularly, because its onset may correspond to the onset of organic or psychosocial illness. It may be helpful to compare the child's growth with the rate of growth of siblings or parents.

Ages at which major developmental milestones were met aid in indicating deviations from normal. Some such milestones include following a person with the eyes, holding the head erect, smiling responsively, reaching for objects, transferring objects, sitting alone, walking with support and alone, speaking the first words and sentences, and experiencing tooth eruption. Ages of dressing self, tying own shoes, hopping, skipping, and riding a tricycle and bicycle should be noted, as well as grade in school and school performance.

In addition, note should be made of the age at which bowel and bladder control were achieved. If problems exist, the ages at which toilet teaching began also may indicate reasons for problems.

## Behavior History

Amount of sleep and sleep problems, and habits such as pica, smoking, and use of alcohol or drugs should be questioned. The informant should state whether the child is happy or difficult to manage, and should indicate the child's response to new situations, strangers, and school. Temper tantrums, excessive or unprovoked crying, nail biting, and nightmares and night terrors should be recorded. Question the child regarding masturbation, dating, dealing with the opposite sex, and parents' responses to menstruation and sexual development.

## Immunization History

The types of immunizations received, with the number, dates, sites given, and reactions should be recorded as part of the history. In addition, it is helpful to record these immunizations on the front of the chart or in a conveniently obvious place with a lot number for future reference when completing school physical examinations or when determining need for booster immunizations or possible reactions.

## History of Past Illnesses

A general statement should be made about the child's general health before the present encounter, such as weight change, fever, weakness, or mood alterations. Specific inquiry is helpful regarding the results of any screening tests and regarding any history of roseola, rubeola, rubella, pertussis, mumps, varicella, scarlet fever, tuberculosis, anemia, recurrent tonsillitis, otitis media, pneumonia, meningitis, encephalitis or other nervous system disease, gastrointestinal tract disease, or any other illness, as well as specific treatment, results, and residua. The history of each past illness should include dates of onset, course, and termination.

If hospitalization or surgery was necessary, the diagnoses, dates, and name of the hospital should be included. Questions concerning allergies include the occurrence and type of any drug reactions, food allergies, hay fever, and asthma. Accidents, injuries, and poisonings should be noted.

## Review of Systems

The review of systems serves as a checklist for pertinent information that might have been omitted. If information has been obtained previously, simply state, "See history of present illness" or "See history of past illnesses." Questions concerning each system may be introduced with a question such as: "Are there any symptoms related to . . .?"

Head (eg, injuries, headache)

Eyes (eg, visual changes, crossed or tendency to cross, discharge, redness, puffiness, injuries, glasses)

Ears (eg, difficulty with hearing, pain, discharge, ear infections, myringotomy, ventilation tubes)

Nose (eg, discharge, watery or purulent, difficulty in breathing through nose, epistaxis)

Mouth and throat (eg, sore throat or tongue, difficulty in swallowing, dental defects)

Neck (eg, swollen glands, masses, stiffness, symmetry)

Breasts (eg, lumps, pain, symmetry, nipple discharge, embarrassment)

Lungs (eg, shortness of breath, ability to keep up with peers, cough with time of cough and character, hoarseness, wheezing, hemoptysis, pain in chest)

Heart (eg, cyanosis, edema, heart murmurs or "heart trouble," pain over heart)

Gastrointestinal (eg, appetite, nausea, vomiting with relation to feeding, amount, color, blood- or bile-stained, or projectile, bowel movements with number and character, abdominal pain or distention, jaundice)

Genitourinary (eg, dysuria, hematuria, frequency, oliguria, character of urinary stream, enuresis, urethral or vaginal discharge, menstrual history, attitude toward menses and opposite sex, sores, pain, intercourse, venereal disease, abortions, birth control method)

Extremities (eg, weakness, deformities, difficulty in moving extremities or in walking, joint pains and swelling, muscle pains or cramps)

Neurologic (eg, headaches, fainting, dizziness, incoordination, seizures, numbness, tremors)

Skin (eg, rashes, hives, itching, color change, hair and nail growth, color and distribution, easy bruising or bleeding)

Psychiatric (eg, usual mood, nervousness, tension, drug use or abuse)

## Family History

The family history provides evidence for considering familial diseases as well as infections or contagious illnesses.

A genetic type chart is easy to read and very helpful. It should include parents, siblings, and grandparents, with their ages, health, or cause of death. If problems with genetic implications exist, all known relatives should be inquired about. If a genetic type chart is used, pregnancies should be listed in a series and should include the health of the siblings (Fig 6-1).

Family diseases, such as allergy; blood, heart, lung, venereal, or kidney disease; tuberculosis; diabetes; rheumatic fever; convulsions; skin, gastrointestinal, behavioral, or mental disorders; cancer; or other disease the informant mentions should be included. These diseases may have a heritable or contagious effect. Pertinent negatives should be included also.

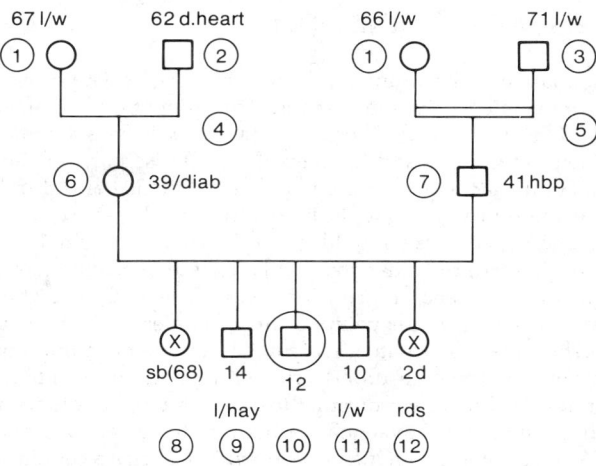

Figure 6-1.   Genetic type chart. (*Circle,* female, *square,* male.) *1,* maternal grandmother, 67 years old, living and well; paternal grandmother, 66, living and well. *2,* Maternal grandfather, died at 62 of heart disease. *3,* Paternal grandfather, 71, living and well. *4, Single horizontal line,* married. *5, Double horizontal line,* consanguineous marriage. *6,* Mother, 39 years old, living, diabetic. *7,* Father, 41 years old, living, hypertensive. *8,* Stillbirth, 1968 (x, died). *9,* Male sibling, 14 years old, living, hay fever. *10,* Patient, 12 years old (note *light circle*). *11,* Brother, 10 years old, living and well. *12,* Female, died at 2 days old of respiratory distress (year can be included).

## Social History

Details of the family unit include the number of people in the habitat and its size, the presence of grandparents, the marital status of the parents, the significant caretaker, the total family income and its source, and whether the mother and father work outside the home. If it is pertinent to the current problems of the child, inquire about the family's attitude toward the child and toward each other, the type of discipline used, and the major disciplinarian. If the problem is psychosocial and only one parent is the informant, it may be necessary to interview the other parent, and to outline a typical day in the life of the child.

## Prenatal History

It is desirable, if feasible, to interview the mother and father before the child is born. Not only can some necessary data be obtained, but also the parents can become acquainted with the doctor who will be seeing them shortly after the arrival of their newborn. The health of the mother, whether she will nurse or bottle-feed the baby and whether the husband supports her choice, the preparation for the baby on arrival home, and whether help will be available can be ascertained. Because the father may feel bypassed by the pregnancy except for the initial event, it is important to direct some questions to him, such as, "Do you want your son circumcised?," and to get the family history of diseases first from him.

## History From the Child

Even young children should be asked about their symptoms and their understanding of their problem. This also provides an opportunity to determine the interaction of the child with the parent. For most adolescents, it is important to take part of the history from the adolescent alone after asking for his or her approval. Regardless of your own opinion, obtain the history objectively without any moral implications, starting with open-ended questions related to the initial complaint and then directing the questions.

## PHYSICAL EXAMINATION

Examination of the infant and young child begins with observing him or her and establishing rapport. The order of the examination should fit the child and the circumstances. It is wise to make no sudden movements and to complete first those parts of the examination that require the child's cooperation. Painful or disagreeable procedures should be deferred to the end of the examination, and these should be explained to the child before proceeding. For the older child and adolescent, examination can begin with the head and conclude with the extremities. The approach is gentle, but expeditious and complete. For the young, apprehensive child, chatter, reassurance, or other communication frequently permits an orderly examination. Some children are best held by the parent during the examination. For others, part of the examination may require restraint by the parent or assistant.

When the complaint includes a report of pain in a certain area, this area should be examined last. If the child has obvious deformities, that area should be examined in a routine fashion without undue emphasis, because extra attention may increase embarrassment or guilt.

Because the entire child is to be examined, at some time all of the clothing must be removed. This does not necessarily mean that it must be removed at the same time. Only the part that is being examined needs to be uncovered and then it can be reclothed. Except during infancy, modesty should be respected and the child should be kept as comfortable as possible.

With practice, the examination of the child can be completed quickly even in most critical emergency states. Only in those with apnea, shock, absence of pulse, or, occasionally, seizures is the complete examination delayed. Although the method of procedure may vary, the record of examination should be in the same format for all children. This provides easy access to needed information later. The description that follows is the usual way of recording the examination and not necessarily its required order. When diseases are given with a sign, these are examples and not a complete differential for that sign. The significance of a previous examination cannot be overstressed. A murmur that was not heard a year ago but now is easily audible has far different significance than does a similar murmur heard many years before.

Completion of the history can be accomplished during the physical examination. Talking to the parent frequently reassures the child. Praising the young child, explaining the parts of the examination to the older child, and reassuring the adolescent of normal findings facilitates the examination. Usually, if the examiner enjoys the spontaneity and responsiveness of children, the examination will be easier and more thorough.

### Measurements (Vital Signs)

Temperature is taken in the axilla or rectum in the young child and by mouth after 5 or 6 years of age, when the child can understand how to hold the thermometer. Electronic thermometer probes inserted as usual or in the ear canal give rapid, accurate determinations. Elevated temperature occurs with infection, excitement, anxiety, exercise, hyperthyroidism, collagen-vascular disease, or tumor. Decreased temperature occurs with chilling, shock, hypothyroidism, or inactivity. Temperature may be decreased after taking certain drugs, with hypocortisolism, or with overwhelming infection.

The pulse rate can be obtained at any peripheral pulse (femoral, radial, or carotid) or by palpation over the heart. The normal rate varies from 70 to 170 beats per minute at birth to 120 to 140 shortly after birth, and ranges from 80 to 140 at 1 to 2 years, from 80 to 120 at 3 years, and from 70 to 115 after 3 years. The sleeping pulse after the age of 2 years normally is about 20 beats per minute less than the awake pulse, but does not decrease with

rheumatic fever or thyrotoxicosis. For each degree of temperature rise, the pulse rate increases about 10 beats per minute. The pulse rate is elevated with excitement, exercise, or hypermetabolic states, and is decreased with hypometabolic states, hypertension, or increased intracranial pressure. Irregularity may be caused by sinus arrhythmia, but can indicate underlying heart disease. Absence of the femoral pulse is a cardinal sign of postductal coarctation of the aorta.

### Respiratory Rate

The respiratory rate should be determined by observing the movement of the chest or abdomen or by auscultating the chest. The normal newborn rate is 30 to 80 breaths per minute; the rate decreases to 20 to 40 in early infancy and childhood and then to 15 to 25 in late childhood and adolescence. Exercise, anxiety, infection, and hypermetabolic states increase the rate; central nervous system lesions, metabolic abnormalities, alkalosis, depressants, and other poisons decrease the rate.

### Blood Pressure

The blood pressure should be measured with a cuff, with the bladder completely encircling the extremity and the width covering one half to two thirds of the length of the upper arm or upper leg. The pressure should be recorded and compared with normal readings (Figs 6-2 through 6-7). High systolic pressure occurs with excitement, anxiety, and hypermetabolic states. High systolic and diastolic pressures occur with renal diseases, pheochromocytoma, adrenal disease, arteritis, or coarctation of the aorta.

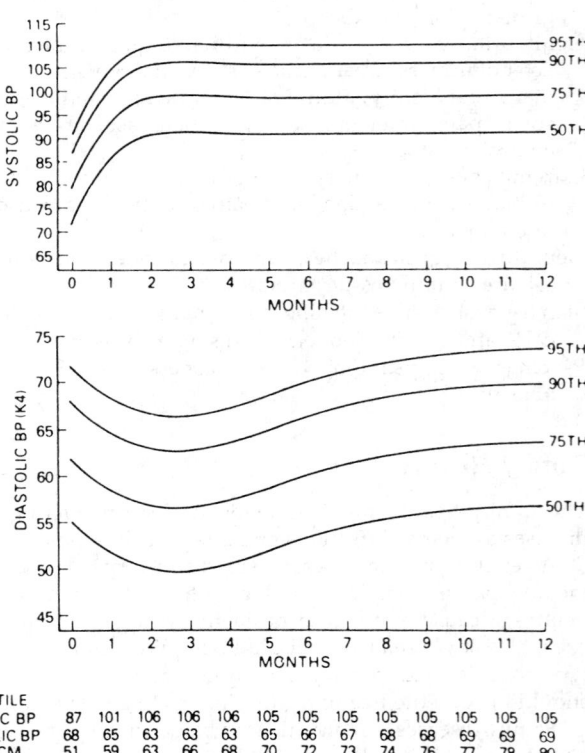

| 90TH PERCENTILE | | | | | | | | | | | | |
|---|---|---|---|---|---|---|---|---|---|---|---|---|
| SYSTOLIC BP | 87 | 101 | 106 | 106 | 106 | 105 | 105 | 105 | 105 | 105 | 105 | 105 | 105 |
| DIASTOLIC BP | 68 | 65 | 63 | 63 | 63 | 65 | 66 | 67 | 68 | 68 | 69 | 69 | 69 |
| HEIGHT CM | 51 | 59 | 63 | 66 | 68 | 70 | 72 | 73 | 74 | 76 | 77 | 78 | 80 |
| WEIGHT KG | 4 | 4 | 5 | 5 | 6 | 7 | 8 | 9 | 9 | 10 | 10 | 11 | 11 |

**Figure 6-2.** Age-specific percentiles of blood pressure (BP) measurements in boys—birth to 12 months of age; Korotkoff phase IV (K4) used for diastolic BP. (American Academy of Pediatrics. Task Force on Blood Pressure. Pediatrics 1987;79:1.)

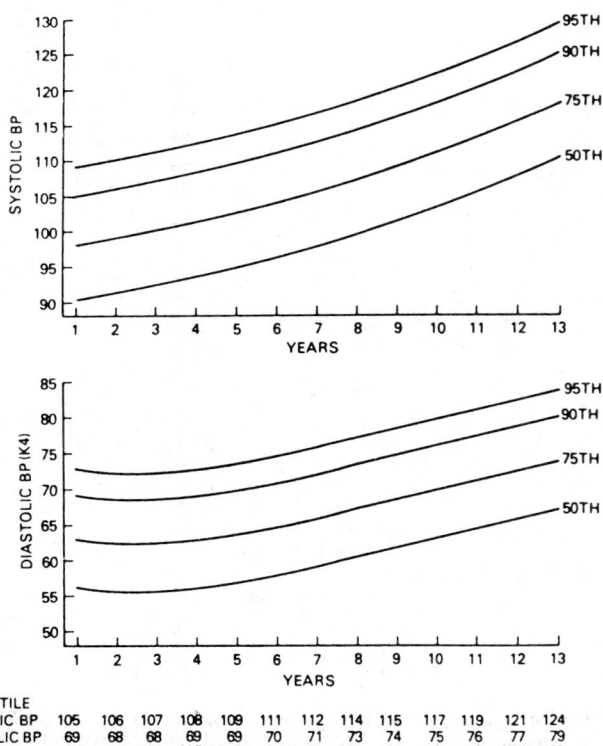

| 90TH PERCENTILE | | | | | | | | | | | | | |
|---|---|---|---|---|---|---|---|---|---|---|---|---|
| SYSTOLIC BP | 105 | 106 | 107 | 108 | 109 | 111 | 112 | 114 | 115 | 117 | 119 | 121 | 124 |
| DIASTOLIC BP | 69 | 68 | 68 | 69 | 69 | 70 | 71 | 73 | 74 | 75 | 76 | 77 | 79 |
| HEIGHT CM | 80 | 91 | 100 | 108 | 115 | 122 | 129 | 135 | 141 | 147 | 153 | 159 | 165 |
| WEIGHT KG | 11 | 14 | 16 | 18 | 22 | 25 | 29 | 34 | 39 | 44 | 50 | 55 | 62 |

**Figure 6-3.** Age-specific percentiles of blood pressure (*BP*) measurements in boys—1 to 13 years of age; Korotkoff phase IV (*K4*) used for diastolic BP. (American Academy of Pediatrics. Task Force on Blood Pressure. Pediatrics 1987;79:1.).

## Height, Weight, Head Circumference

To obtain height and weight recordings, measure the infant supine up to the age of 2 years, and standing thereafter. Measure head circumference in all infants less than 2 years of age and in those with misshapen heads. Record height, weight, and head circumference measurements with percentiles on a chart (Figs 6-8 through 6-15).

Shortness may be caused by malabsorption, chronic illness, psychosocial deprivation, hormonal disorders, familial patterns, or syndromes with dwarfism. Gigantism may be the result of pituitary abnormalities. Compare sitting height and total height in dwarfs to standard measurements to determine the type of syndrome present.

Decreased weight can be caused by conditions similar to those that cause decreased height. In states of malnutrition, weight percentile is less than height percentile; head circumference remains normal unless the condition is severe and persists. Overweight usually is exogenous and associated with increased height until epiphyseal closure. Overweight resulting from endocrine disorders is associated with decreased linear growth.

## Skin Fold Measurements

Skin fold measurements are useful in determining obesity and in identifying and following malnutrition. Skin fold calipers are applied over the mid-triceps.

## General Appearance

A statement should be recorded about the alertness, distress, general development, and nutrition of the child. Mental status,

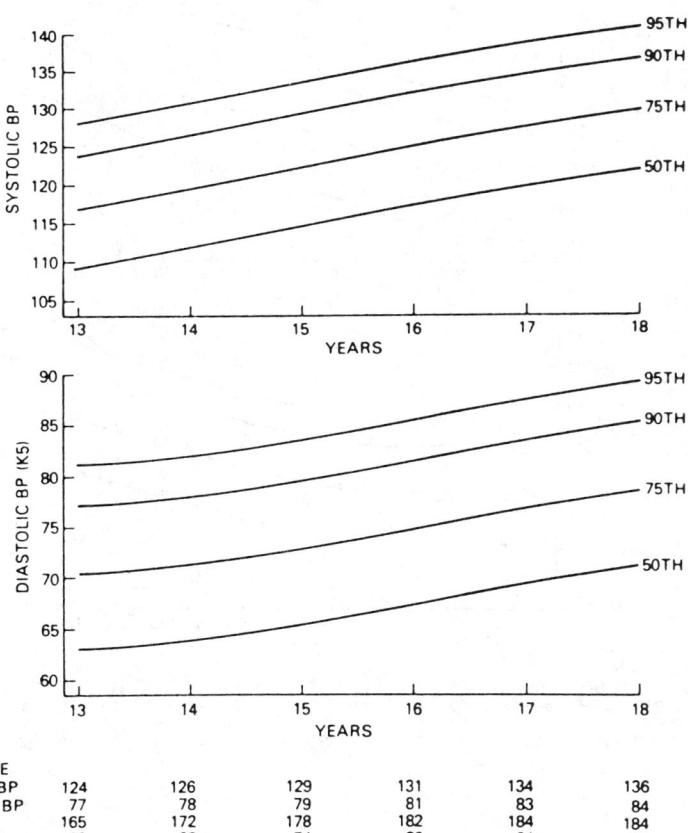

**Figure 6-4.** Age-specific percentiles of blood pressure (*BP*) measurements in boys—13 to 18 years of age; Korotkoff phase V (*K5*) used for diastolic BP. (American Academy of Pediatrics. Task Force on Blood Pressure. Pediatrics 1987;79:1.)

| 90TH PERCENTILE | | | | | | |
|---|---|---|---|---|---|---|
| SYSTOLIC BP | 124 | 126 | 129 | 131 | 134 | 136 |
| DIASTOLIC BP | 77 | 78 | 79 | 81 | 83 | 84 |
| HEIGHT CM | 165 | 172 | 178 | 182 | 184 | 184 |
| WEIGHT KG | 62 | 68 | 74 | 80 | 84 | 86 |

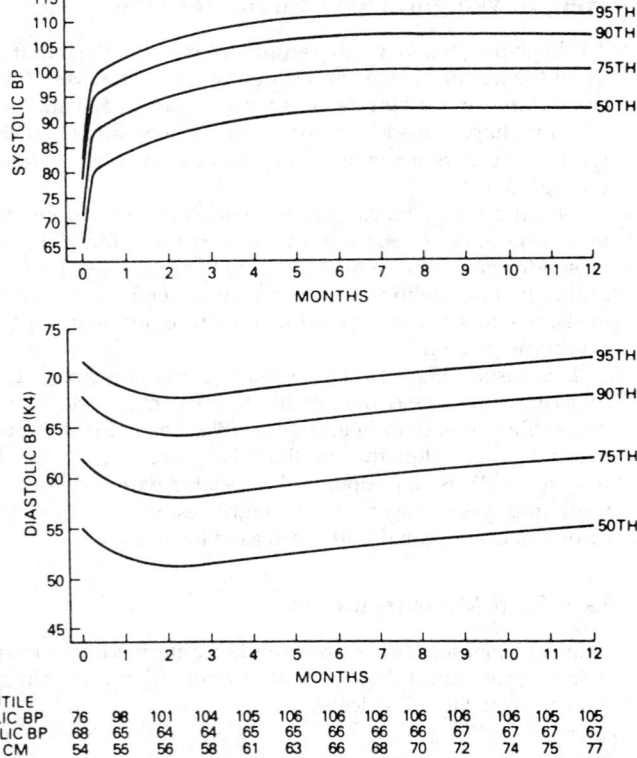

| 90TH PERCENTILE | | | | | | | | | | | | |
|---|---|---|---|---|---|---|---|---|---|---|---|---|
| SYSTOLIC BP | 76 | 98 | 101 | 104 | 105 | 106 | 106 | 106 | 106 | 106 | 106 | 105 | 105 |
| DIASTOLIC BP | 68 | 65 | 64 | 64 | 65 | 65 | 66 | 66 | 66 | 67 | 67 | 67 | 67 |
| HEIGHT CM | 54 | 55 | 56 | 58 | 61 | 63 | 66 | 68 | 70 | 72 | 74 | 75 | 77 |
| WEIGHT KG | 4 | 4 | 4 | 5 | 5 | 6 | 7 | 8 | 9 | 9 | 10 | 10 | 11 |

**Figure 6-5.** Age-specific percentiles of blood pressure (*BP*) measurements in girls—birth to 12 months of age; Korotkoff phase IV (*K4*) used for diastolic BP. (American Academy of Pediatrics. Task Force on Blood Pressure. Pediatrics 1987;79:1.)

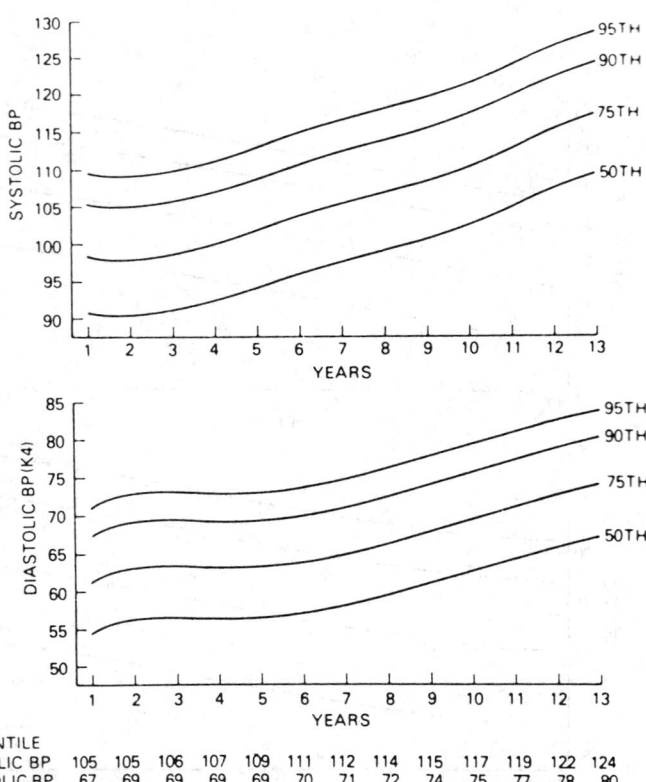

| 90TH PERCENTILE | | | | | | | | | | | | |
|---|---|---|---|---|---|---|---|---|---|---|---|---|
| SYSTOLIC BP | 105 | 105 | 106 | 107 | 109 | 111 | 112 | 114 | 115 | 117 | 119 | 122 | 124 |
| DIASTOLIC BP | 67 | 69 | 69 | 69 | 69 | 70 | 71 | 72 | 74 | 75 | 77 | 78 | 80 |
| HEIGHT CM | 77 | 89 | 98 | 107 | 115 | 122 | 129 | 135 | 142 | 148 | 154 | 160 | 165 |
| WEIGHT KG | 11 | 13 | 15 | 18 | 22 | 25 | 30 | 35 | 40 | 45 | 51 | 58 | 63 |

**Figure 6-6.** Age-specific percentiles of blood pressure (*BP*) measurements in girls—1 to 13 years of age; Korotkoff phase IV (*K4*) used for diastolic BP. (American Academy of Pediatrics. Task Force on Blood Pressure. Pediatrics 1987;79:1.)

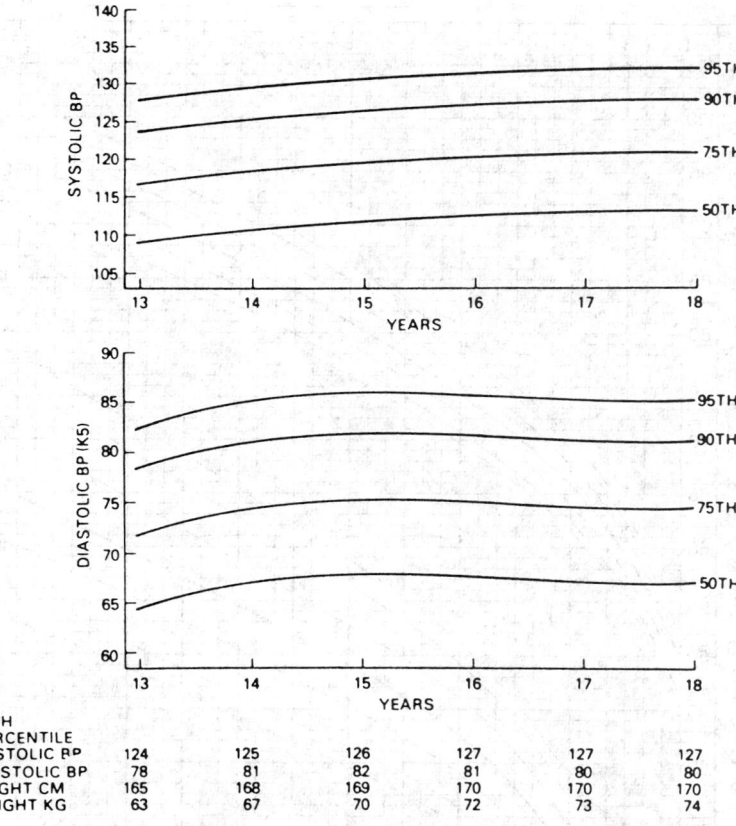

**Figure 6-7.** Age-specific percentiles of blood pressure (*BP*) measurements in girls—13 to 18 years of age; Korotkoff phase V (*K5*) used for diastolic BP. (American Academy of Pediatrics. Task Force on Blood Pressure. Pediatrics 1987;79:1.)

| 90TH PERCENTILE | | | | | | |
|---|---|---|---|---|---|---|
| SYSTOLIC BP | 124 | 125 | 126 | 127 | 127 | 127 |
| DIASTOLIC BP | 78 | 81 | 82 | 81 | 80 | 80 |
| HEIGHT CM | 165 | 168 | 169 | 170 | 170 | 170 |
| WEIGHT KG | 63 | 67 | 70 | 72 | 73 | 74 |

activity, unusual positions, or apprehension or cooperativeness may direct one to consider an acute or chronic illness or no illness at all. The child who lies quietly, staring into space, may be gravely ill. The child who lies quietly but becomes irritable when held by his mother (paradoxic irritability) may have meningitis or pain in motion. Note any unusual odor, which may suggest the presence of a foreign body in one of the orifices or certain metabolic diseases or toxins.

## Skin

In examining the skin, record its color and turgor, the type of any lesions, and the condition of body and scalp hair and nails.

Normal color of the skin is the result of the presence of melanin; depigmented areas are vitiligo; absence of pigment occurs in albinism. Cyanosis is caused by unsaturation of or abnormal forms of hemoglobin; jaundice is caused by excessive bilirubin deposited in the adipose tissue. Note the size and borders of nevi, which usually are darkly pigmented areas, and café au lait spots, which are brownish areas that may signal neurofibromatosis. White spots shaped like a leaf suggest tuberous sclerosis. Ecchymoses or petechiae and scars may indicate abuse.

Swelling may be caused by edema. Lack of turgor occurs with dehydration or recent weight loss. Describe any rashes, many of which are characteristic of viral or bacterial infection.

## Head and Face

Record the shape, symmetry, and any defects of the head; the distribution of hair; and the size and tension of fontanelles. A large head may be an early sign of hydrocephalus or an intracranial mass. A small head may be a result of early closure of sutures or lack of brain development. For any deviation from normal head size, frequent measurements are necessary. The fontanelles normally are flat. The posterior fontanelle closes by 2 months of age, and the anterior fontanelle closes by 12 to 18 months of age. Unusual hair whorls are associated with severe intracranial abnormalities.

The face may appear distinctive for a number of syndromes. For example, unilateral facial paralysis may be associated with congenital heart disease. Coarse facies occur with storage diseases. Epicanthal folds occur in a number of syndromes, including Down and trisomy 21.

## Eyes

Test vision grossly in the young child with brightly colored objects. In the older child, test with Snellen's E chart. Evaluate for strabismus by noting the position of the reflection of light on the cornea from a distant source. Evaluate the range of eye movements and the presence of nystagmus. Both eyelids should open equally. Failure to open is ptosis and may be caused by neurologic or systemic diseases. Upward slanting of the palpebral fissures with covering of the inner canthus (epicanthal folds) is a sign of Down syndrome. The conjunctivae should be pink, but not inflamed; the sclerae should be white. Examine the cornea for haziness (a sign of glaucoma) or opacities. Record the size and shape of the pupils, the color of the iris, and the response of the iris to light and accommodation. In the fundoscopic examination, use a zero lens and note the presence of a red reflex, or hemorrhages or pigmented areas, and the size of the veins compared to the arteries. Any obstruction, such as corneal or lenticular cataract, will obliterate part or all of the red reflex. The disc borders should be sharp. They are blurred with increased intracranial pressure. The macula may not be clear, which is a sign of degenerative diseases. Obtain the corneal reflex by lightly touching the cornea with a piece of cotton. Failure to blink indicates trigeminal or facial nerve injury.

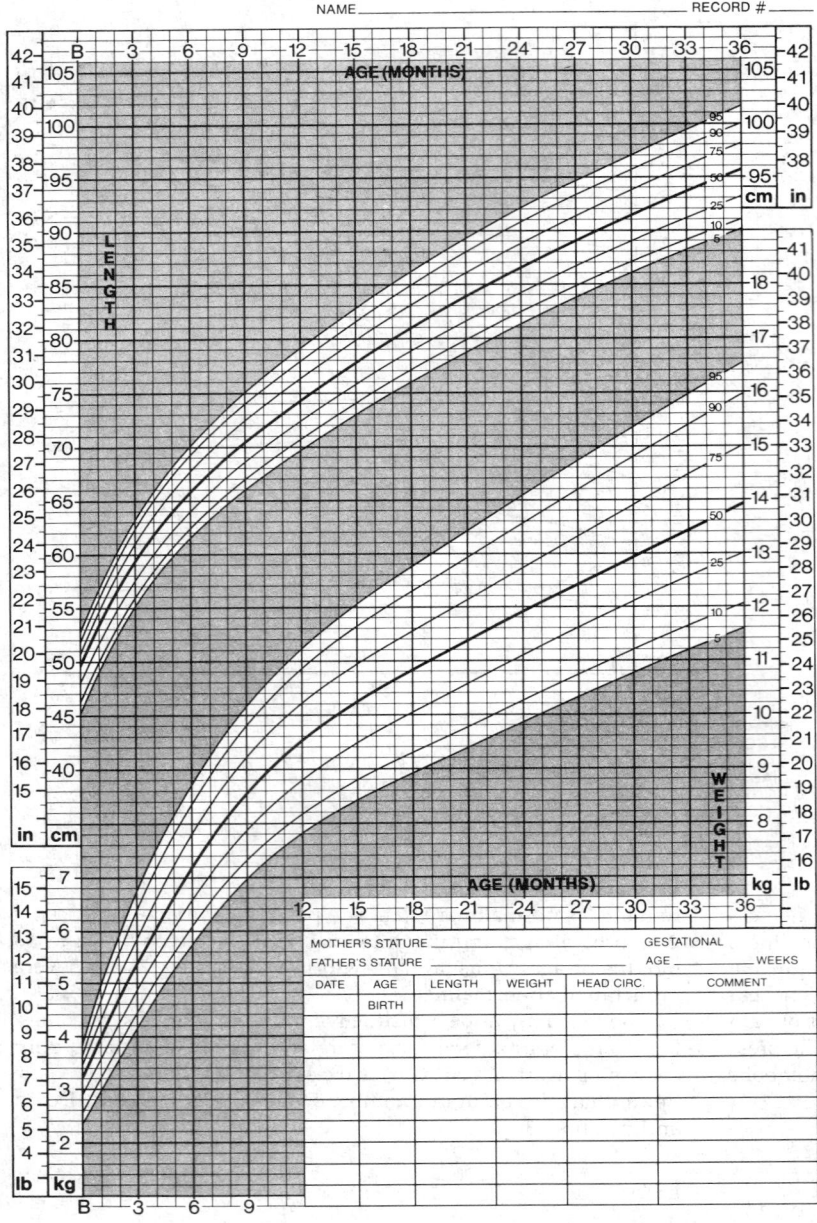

NAME _____ RECORD # _____

**Figure 6-8.** NCHS percentiles of physical growth in girls—birth to 36 months of age. (© 1982 Ross Laboratories, Columbus OH 43216. Adapted from Hamill PVV, Drizd TA, Johnson CL, et al. Physical growth: National Center for Health Statistics percentiles. Am J Clin Nutr 1979;32:607. Data from the Fels Research Institute, Wright State University School of Medicine, Yellow Springs, Ohio.)

## Ears

Note the position of the ears and abnormalities of the external ear, the pinna. Low-set ears may suggest the presence of renal agenesis. Tags and deformities frequently are associated with other minor or major anomalies. Grossly evaluate hearing, then proceed with examination of the inner ear. Pull the earlobe up and anteriorly. Grasp an otoscope equipped with a bright light so that the holding hand rests on the child's head and moves with any movement of the head, and use the largest speculum that will fit into the canal. The canal should be clear, and the drum should be pearly gray in color and concave. A cone of light, the malleus, and sometimes the incus will be identified. If the bones are not visualized, the drum is not gray in color or is infected, or the drum is not concave, fluid may be in the inner ear, which is diagnostic of otitis media.

## Nose

Raise the tip of the nose and look up the nose with a bright light. Deformities of the septum, bleeding, or discharges should be recorded. The normal nasal mucosa is light pink in color. Tap on the maxillary and frontal sinuses for tenderness. Feel for air egress from both nares.

## Mouth and Throat

Examination of the mouth and throat usually is the most resistant part of the examination and should be performed near the end of the examination. The child should be sitting so that the tongue is less likely to obstruct the pharynx. Deformities or infections around the lips are recorded. Count the number and note the condition of the teeth. Similarly, note the condition and color of the tongue, buccal mucosa, palate, tonsils, and posterior pharynx. Normally, these are pink in color. Exudate indicates infection by bacteria, viruses, or fungi, but etiology usually cannot be determined by physical examination alone. Note also the presence of the gag reflex and the voice or cry. If the child seems hoarse, question the parent concerning the normal voice. Laryngitis can lead to airway obstruction. After the age of 2 years, children should not drool. Chronic drooling may suggest mental deficiency,

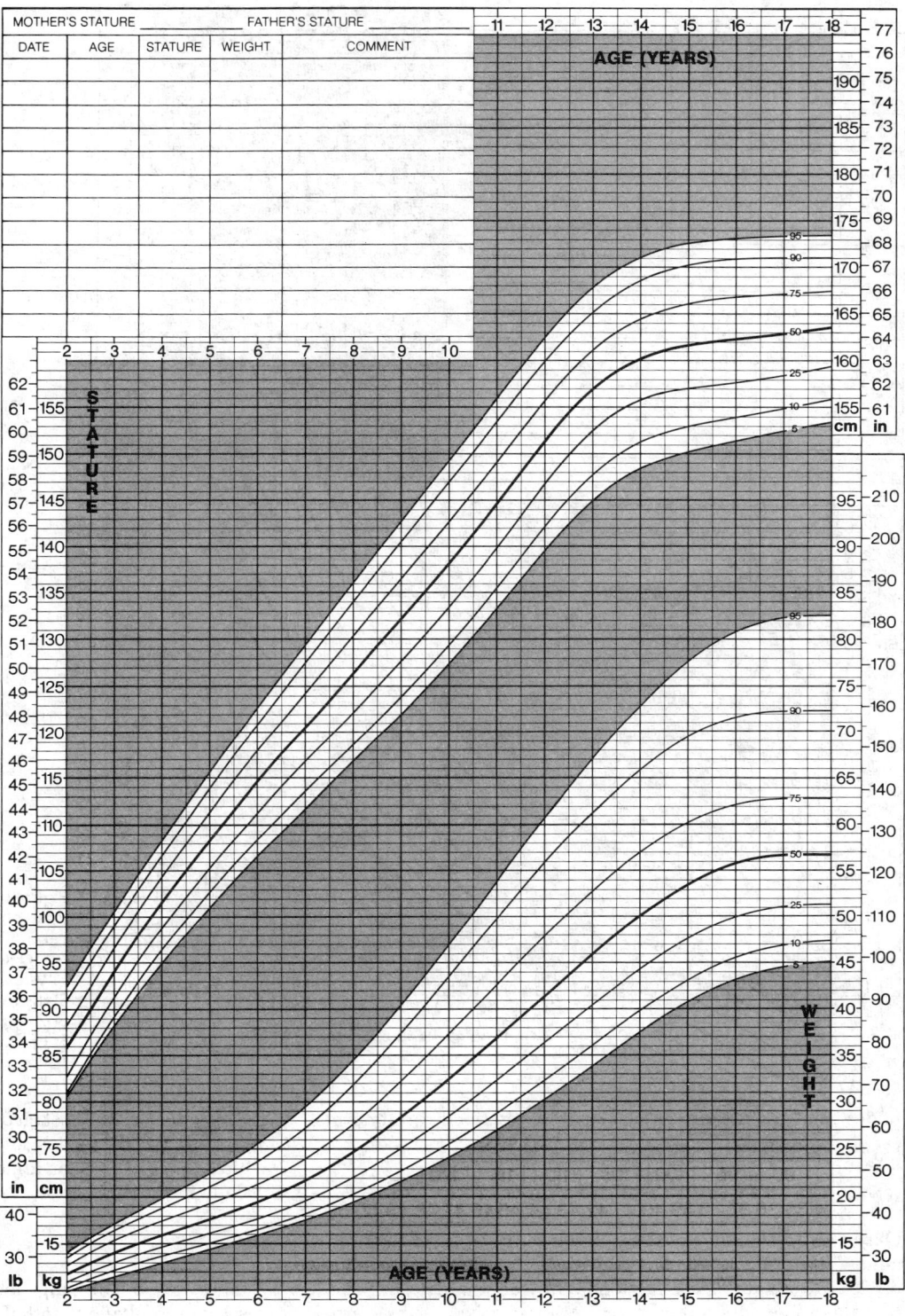

**Figure 6-9.** NCHS percentiles of physical growth in girls—2 to 18 years of age. (© 1982 Ross Laboratories, Columbus OH 43216. Adapted from Hamill PVV, Drizd TA, Johnson CL, et al. Physical growth: National Center for Health Statistics percentiles. Am J Clin Nutr 1979;32:607. Data from the National Center for Health Statistics (NCHS), Hyattsville, Md.)

but acute onset of drooling is a grave sign of epiglottitis or poison ingestion.

## Neck

Feel in the neck for lymph nodes, which normally are nontender and up to 1 cm in diameter in both the anterior and posterior cervical triangles. Larger or tender nodes occur with local or systemic infection or malignancies. Feel the trachea in the midline. The thyroid may not be palpable. Other masses may be present

and are always abnormal. Flex the neck. Resistance to flexion is a cardinal sign of meningitis, but this also occurs with severe infections around the neck or dislocation of the cervical vertebrae.

## Lymph Nodes

In addition to the lymph nodes in the neck, palpate inguinal, epitrochlear, supraclavicular, axillary, and posterior occipital nodes. Normally, inguinal nodes may be up to 1 cm in diameter; the others are nonpalpable or less than 5 mm. Larger or tender

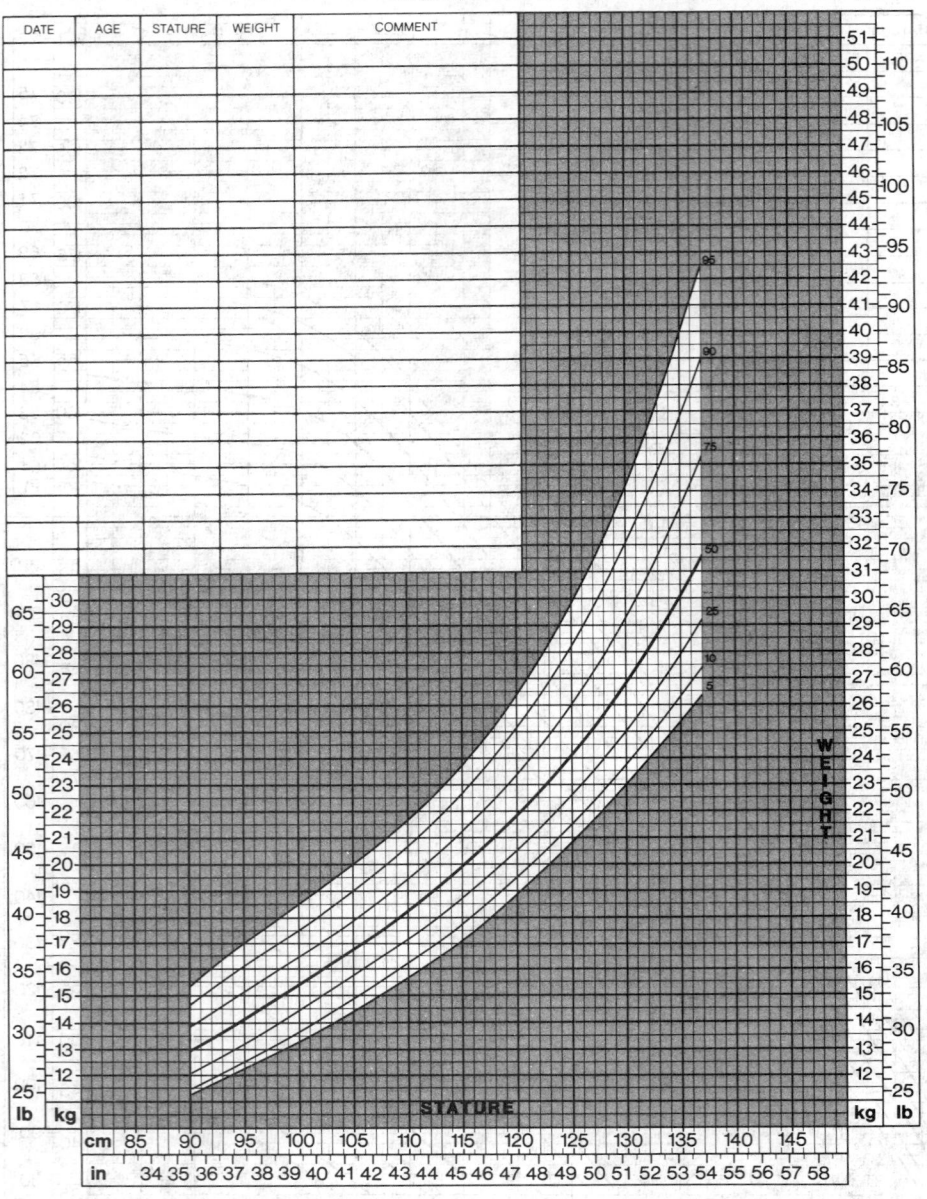

NAME_____   RECORD #_____

**Figure 6-10.**   NCHS percentiles of prepubescent physical growth in girls. (© 1982 Ross Laboratories, Columbus OH 43216. Adapted from Hamill PVV, Drizd TA, Johnson CL, et al. Physical growth: National Center for Health Statistics percentiles. Am J Clin Nutr 1979;32: 607. Data from the National Center for Health Statistics (NCHS), Hyattsville, Md.)

nodes hold significance similar to that described for abnormal cervical glands.

## Chest

Observe the chest for shape and symmetry. The chest wall is almost round in infancy and in children with obstructive lung disease. Respirations are predominantly abdominal until about 6 years of age, when they become thoracic. Note suprasternal, intercostal, and subcostal retractions, which are signs of increased respiratory work. Swelling at the costochondral junctions is an indication of rickets. Edema of the chest wall occurs in children with superior vena cava obstruction. Asymmetry of expansion occurs with diaphragmatic paralysis, pneumothorax, or other intrathoracic abnormalities.

## Breasts

Breasts normally are hypertrophied at birth; they regress within 6 months and develop with the onset of puberty. Development during adolescence is staged. Breast development in both boys and girls usually begins asymmetrically. Palpate for nodules, which may be cysts or tumors. Redness, heat, and tenderness usually indicate infection.

## Lungs

Examination of the lungs includes observation, palpation, percussion, auscultation, and, if indicated, transillumination.

### Observation

Note the type and rate of the child's breathing. The rate of respiration varies, as described previously. Rapid rates, known as tachypnea, are associated with infection, fever, excitement, exercise, heart failure, or intoxicants. Slower rates are characteristic of intracranial lesions, depression caused by sedative drugs, heart block, or alkalosis. Cheyne-Stokes breathing, which is characterized by periods of deep, rapid respirations followed by slow, shallow respirations, is common in premature and newborn infants, and in those with intracranial or metabolic abnormalities.

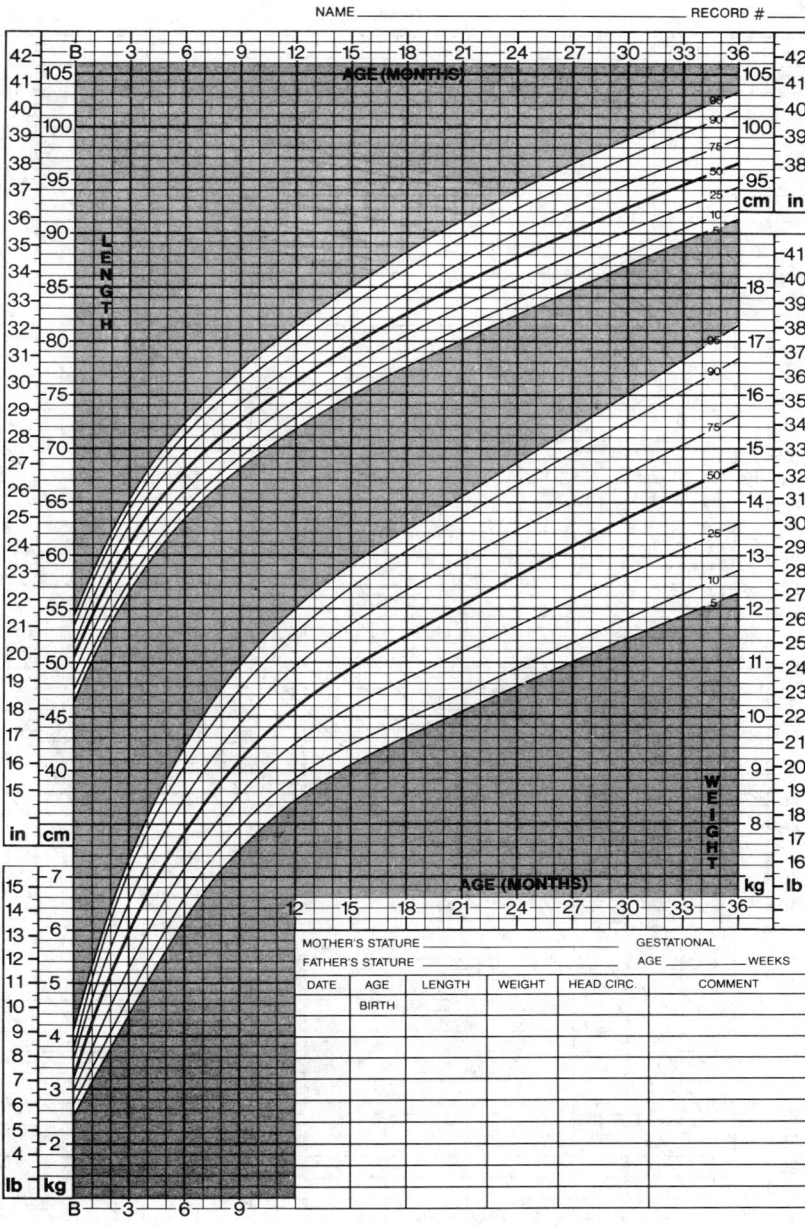

**Figure 6-11.** NCHS percentiles of physical growth in boys—birth to 36 months of age. (© 1982 Ross Laboratories, Columbus OH 43216. Adapted from Hamill PVV, Drizd TA, Johnson CL, et al. Physical growth: National Center for Health Statistics percentiles. Am J Clin Nutr 1979;32:607. Data from the Fels Research Institute, Wright State University School of Medicine, Yellow Springs, Ohio.)

Dyspnea, or distress during breathing, is associated with flaring of the intercostal spaces and nares. Inspiratory dyspnea is more common with obstruction high in the respiratory system and expiratory dyspnea is more common with lower respiratory diseases.

### Palpation

Feel the entire chest with the palms and fingertips. Note masses or areas of tenderness. Tactile fremitus, a vibratory sensation during crying or speaking, normally is felt over the entire chest. Fremitus is absent if the airway is obstructed.

### Percussion

Either direct percussion (tapping the chest wall directly with either the index or middle fingers) or indirect percussion (placing a finger of one hand *firmly* on the chest wall and tapping that finger with the index or middle finger of the opposite hand) may be used in children. The entire chest wall is percussed anteriorly, posteriorly, and along the midaxillary line. A resonant sound will be obtained over most of the chest except over the scapulae, diaphragm, liver, and heart, where dullness is elicited. Dullness detects consolidation in the lungs, as well as the size and position of the liver and heart. Scratch percussion, which involves tapping the chest wall with a finger while listening with a bell stethoscope over the heart and liver, is especially useful in determining heart and liver size. Increased resonance is found with increased trapped air, emphysema, or air in the pleural space (pneumothorax).

### Auscultation

To auscultate the lungs in children, listen with a small bell in small children and with the diaphragm in older children. Normal breath sounds are bronchovesicular and inspiration is twice as long as expiration in young children; breath sounds are vesicular and inspiration is three times as long as expiration in older children. Breath sounds are decreased with consolidation or pleural fluid in the young child and increased with pneumonia in the older child. Fine crackles either in inspiration or expiration (rales) indicate foreign substances, usually fluid, in the alveoli or smaller

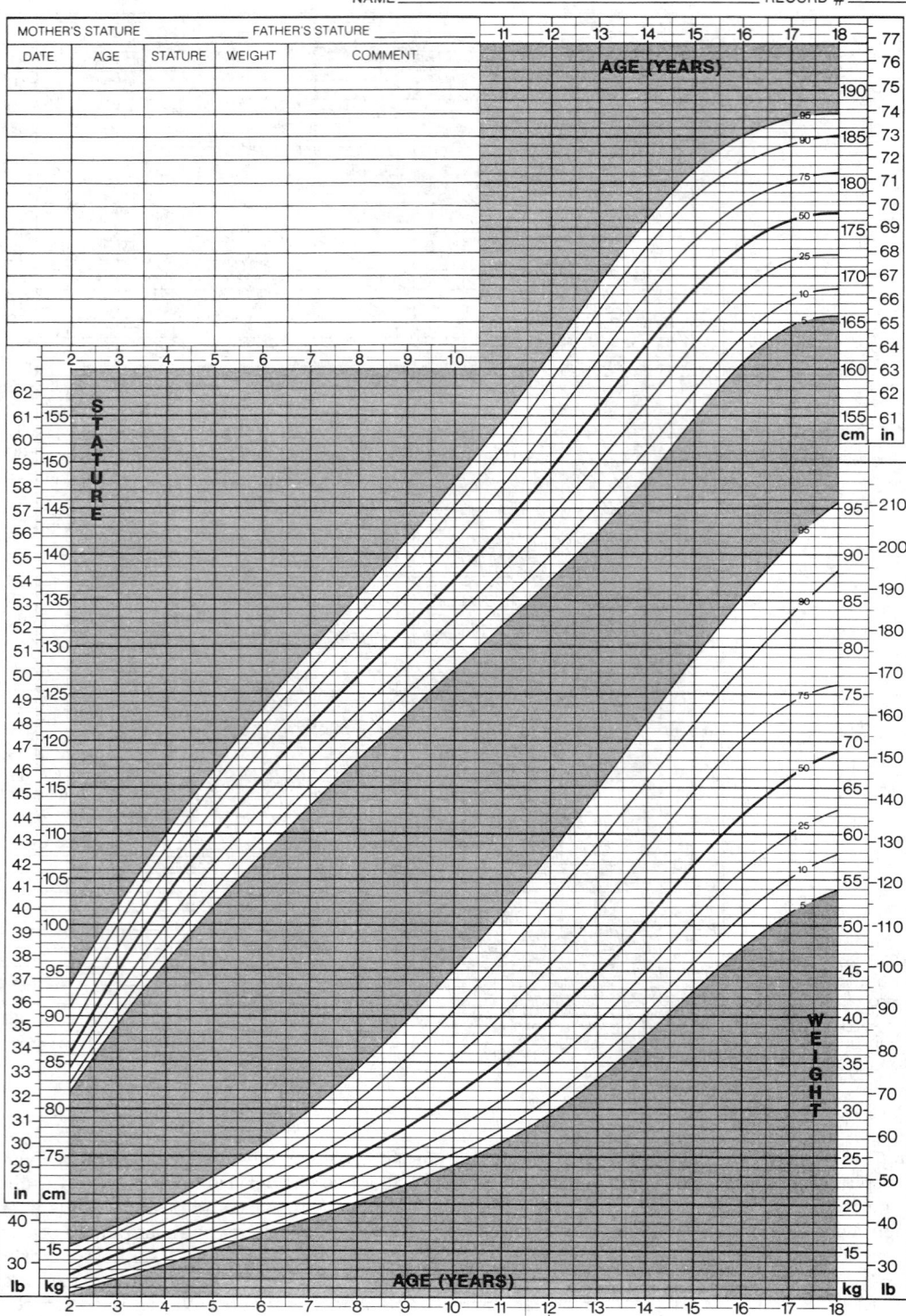

**Figure 6-12.** NCHS percentiles of physical growth in boys—2 to 18 years of age. (© 1982 Ross Laboratories, Columbus OH 43216. Adapted from Hamill PVV, Drizd TA, Johnson CL, et al. Physical growth: National Center for Health Statistics percentiles. Am J Clin Nutr 1979;32: 607. Data from the National Center for Health Statistics (NCHS), Hyattsville, Md.)

bronchi, as occurs in bronchitis, pneumonia, or heart failure. Coarse extraneous sounds (rhonchi) are the result of foreign substances in the larger airways, as in crying or upper respiratory infection. Musical extraneous sounds (wheezes) are caused by airflow through compromised larger airways, as in asthma.

### Transillumination

If pneumothorax is present, the chest will transilluminate. This is especially useful in the newborn.

### Heart

In addition to the heart's rate (pulse) and rhythm, and the blood pressure, note the size, shape, sound quality, and presence of murmurs when examining the heart.

Precordial bulging is a sign of right-sided enlargement. A cardiac impulse may not be noted in a young child, but in a thin, active child, it may suggest the size and position of the heart. An apex beat outside the midclavicular line in the fifth interspace indicates cardiomegaly, which is a significant sign of heart disease

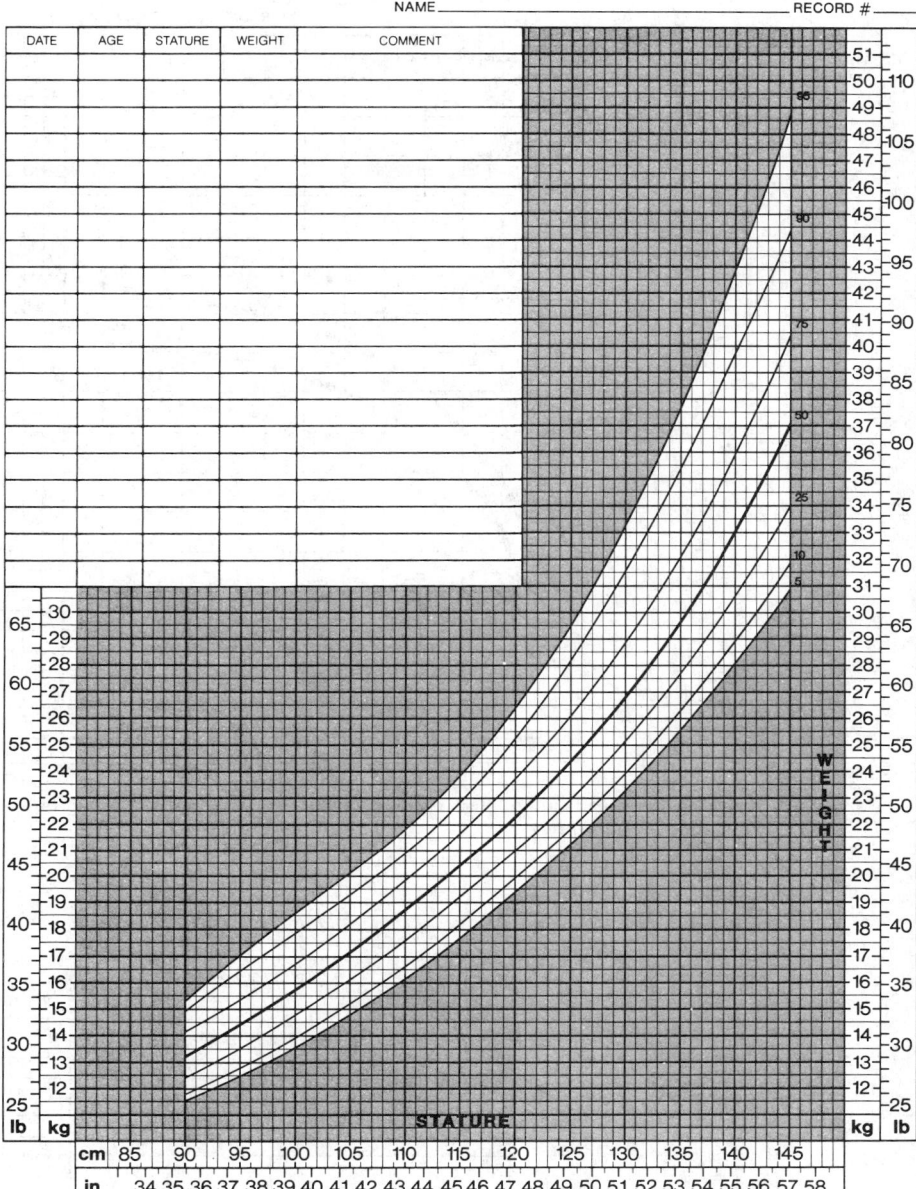

NAME_____ RECORD #_____

**Figure 6-13.** NCHS percentiles of prepubescent physical growth in boys. (© 1982 Ross Laboratories, Columbus OH 43216. Adapted from Hamill PVV, Drizd TA, Johnson CL, et al. Physical growth: National Center for Health Statistics percentiles. Am J Clin Nutr 1979;32: 607. Data from the National Center for Health Statistics (NCHS), Hyattsville, Md.)

or heart failure. Palpation and percussion are described above. Auscultate both in the sitting and the supine position. Determine the heart rate and rhythm if this was not done previously. Auscultate initially over the apex (mitral area), then over the lower right sternal border (tricuspid area), the second left intercostal space at the sternal edge (pulmonary area), and the second right intercostal space at the sternal edge (aortic area). Next, proceed to the remainder of the precordium, the axillae, back, and neck. Note heart sounds and any arrhythmia. A loud first sound at the apex occurs with mitral stenosis, a loud second sound at the pulmonary area occurs with pulmonary hypertension, and a fixed split-second sound in the pulmonary area occurs with an atrial septal defect. Innocent murmurs are systolic, musical, or vibratory and of low intensity, and usually are heard at the second left interspace, just inside the apex, or beneath either clavicle. The latter is a venous hum that may be continuous and that disappears when the patient is supine. Diastolic murmurs are almost always significant. Significant systolic murmurs may be stenotic and are loudest in mid-systole over the aortic or pulmonary areas. Regurgitant murmurs begin immediately after the first sound. Over

the mitral or tricuspid area, they indicate valvular insufficiency. A continuous or uneven systolic murmur along the upper left sternal border indicates patent ductus arteriosus.

## Abdomen

Observe the shape of the abdomen. A flat abdomen may indicate diaphragmatic hernia; a distended abdomen may indicate intestinal obstruction or ascites. Auscultate before percussing or palpating. Normally, peristaltic sounds are heard every 10 to 30 seconds. High-pitched frequent sounds occur with obstruction or peritonitis; absent sounds indicate ileus. Next, palpate gently, beginning in the left lower quadrant and proceeding to the left upper, right upper, right lower, and midline areas. Then palpate more deeply in the same areas and follow with palpation in the same areas with the unused hand, pushing toward the front hand from the child's back. Feel especially for the liver in the right upper quadrant and the spleen in the left upper quadrant, and estimate their size. Any other masses are abnormal. Determine tenderness and attempt to locate the maximum point of any ten-

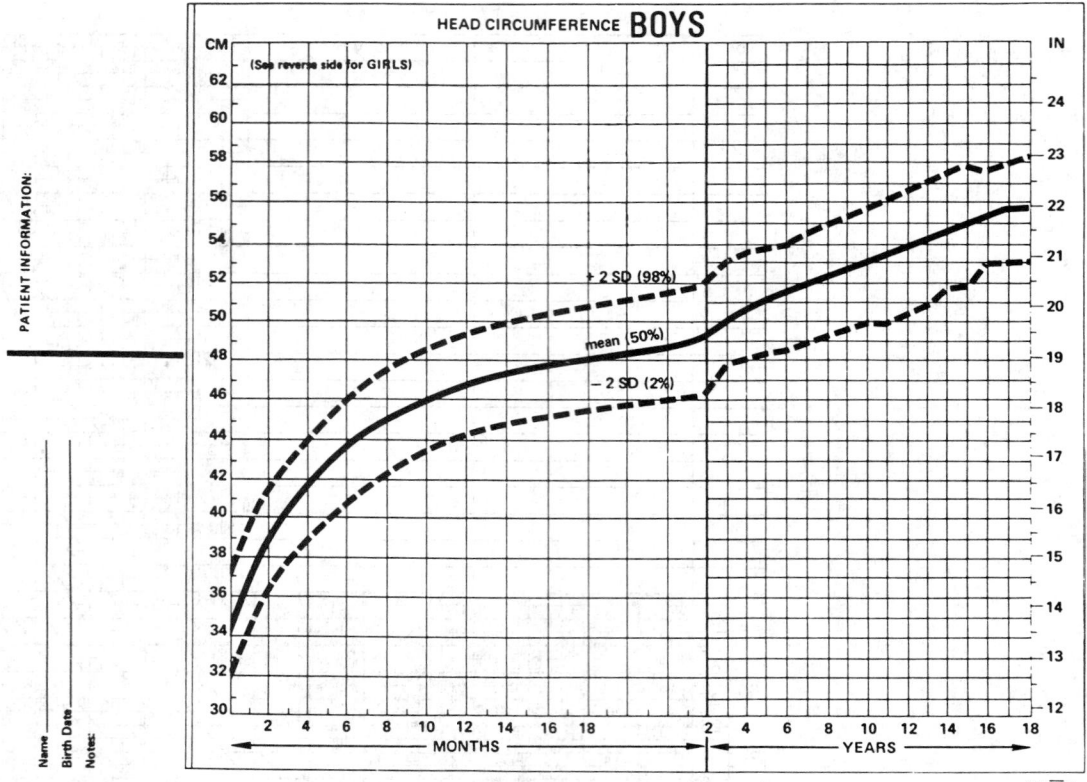

**Figure 6-14.** Head circumference, boys. (Nellhaus G. Composite international and interracial graphs. Pediatrics 1968;41:106.)

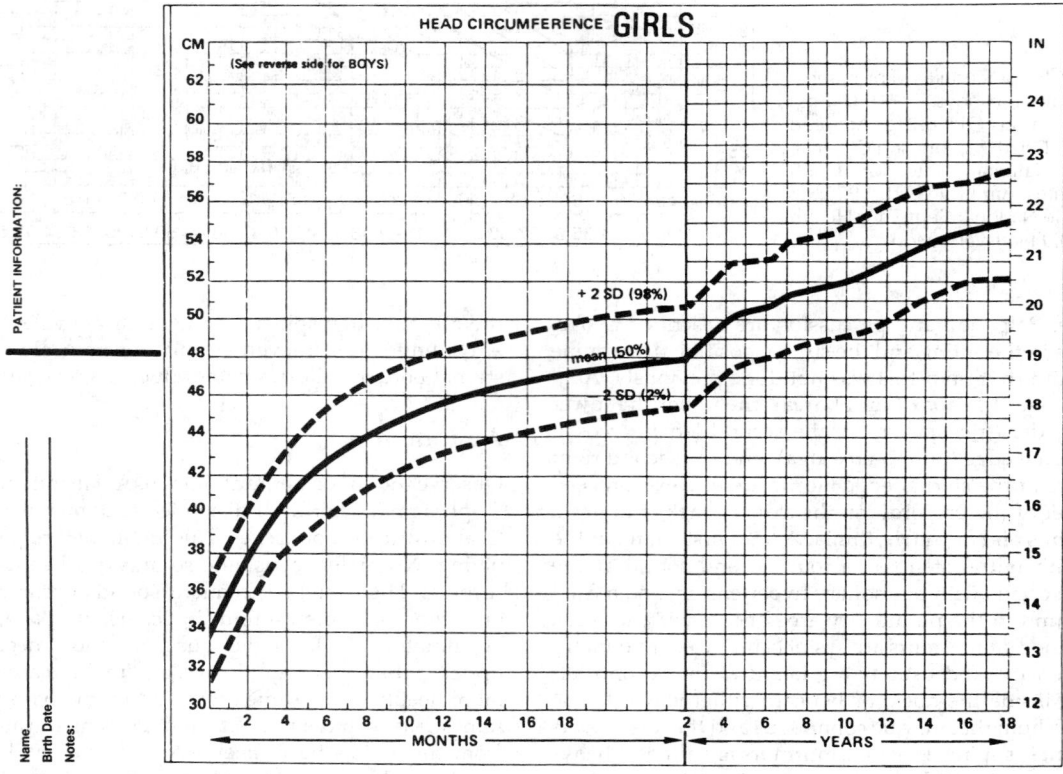

**Figure 6-15.** Head circumference, girls. (Nellhaus G. Composite international and interracial graphs. Pediatrics 1968;41:106.)

derness, which may indicate intra-abdominal infection such as peritonitis, cystitis, or appendicitis, or rapid enlargement of organs, as occurs with enlargement of the liver in heart failure. Percuss to verify findings. Feel in the costovertebral angles to determine kidney size. Tenderness usually indicates pyelonephritis.

## Genitalia

A child's stage of pubertal development is estimated from the presence of pubic hair. Average adolescent development in girls proceeds as follows: breast development after 8 years of age, pubic hair after 12 years of age, increase in height velocity after 12 years of age, and menarche and axillary hair after 13 years of age. Average development in boys proceeds as follows: testicular enlargement at 11.5 years of age, pubic hair at 12.5 years of age, increase in height velocity at 14 years of age, and facial and axillary hair at 14.5 years of age. Variations in order of development suggest hormonal abnormalities. Modesty of the child should be respected during the examination, especially of the genitalia.

Inspect the genitalia for urethral discharges, which are always pathologic and indicate infection anywhere in the genitourinary systems.

In a girl, vaginal bleeding after the newborn period and before puberty may be the result of injury or foreign body. Fused labia minora usually part with hygiene. Imperforate hymen causes hydrocolpos before puberty and hematocolpos after menarche. Vaginal discharge may be the result of injury or foreign body in a young girl, usually is normal at the start of puberty, and suggests infection in an older girl. Adolescents with vaginal discharge, dysuria, lower abdominal pain, irregular bleeding, or sexual activity require a complete vaginal examination. The uterus in a younger child is palpated for size, shape, and tenderness with one hand over the lower abdomen and a finger of the other hand in the rectum. For an older child, the cervix is visualized with a vaginoscope or small speculum, and cultures are obtained.

In boys, testes should be in the scrotum after birth, although active cremasteric reflexes may empty the scrotum temporarily. The meatal opening should be slitlike and the urinary stream should be strong. Hydroceles, which do not reduce and do transilluminate, and hernias, which reduce but do not transilluminate, enlarge the scrotum. Testicular tenderness suggests torsion of the testis or epididymitis.

## Rectal

Inspect the anus for fissures, inflammation, or lack of tone. The latter may indicate child abuse. The rectum is not examined routinely, but is examined in all children with abdominal or gastrointestinal complaints, including diarrhea, constipation, or bleeding from the rectum.

## Extremities and Back

Asymmetry, anomalies, unusual size, pain, tenderness, heat, and swelling deformities of the extremities and back must be distinguished from congenital malformations, osteomyelitis, cellulitis, myositis, or, rarely, rickets and scurvy. Joint heat, tenderness, swelling, effusion, redness, and limitation or pain on motion may indicate arthritis, arthralgia, synovitis or injury, or septic arthritis (which is a medical emergency). Observe as the child walks for the presence of a limp. Clubbing of the fingers is a sign of chronic hypoxemia, as in congenital heart or chronic pulmonary diseases.

The spine should be straight with mild lumbar lordosis. Kyphosis, scoliosis, masses, tenderness, limitation of motion, spina bifida, pilonidal dimples, or cysts may be caused by injury, malformation, infections, or tumors.

Weakness, tenderness, or paresis of the muscles suggests inflammatory muscle disease, congenital or metabolic neuromuscular diseases, or central nervous system abnormalities.

## Neurologic Examination

Mental status and orientation help determine the acuteness of a child's illness, depending on the environmental conditions. Position at rest and abnormal movements such as tremors, twitchings, choreiform movements, and athetosis are characteristic of hyperirritability of the central nervous system. Incoordination of gait usually indicates cerebellar dysfunction. Kernig's sign (inability to extend the leg with the hip flexed) and Brudzinski's sign (flexing the neck with resultant flexion of the hip or knee) are indications of meningeal irritation.

Cranial nerves can be tested. Dysfunction of olfactory nerve I results in anosmia. Nerves II, III, IV, and VI are described briefly under "Eyes" in Chapter 34, and nerve VIII is discussed under "Ears" in Chapters 36.6 and 36.7. Dysfunction of the trigeminal nerve V results in lack of sensation of the face and tongue. With peripheral facial nerve VII paralysis, neither the forehead nor the face moves. With nuclear VII paralysis, the forehead moves. Difficulty in swallowing and loss of pharyngeal reflexes are caused by dysfunction of the glossopharyngeal nerve IX or the vagus nerve X. Patients cannot contract the sternocleidomastoid or trapezius muscles with involvement of the spinal accessory nerve XI. The tongue protrudes to the involved side with hypoglossal nerve XII lesions.

Examination of tendon reflexes (biceps, triceps, patellar, and Achilles) is less important than is observation of general activity. Hyperactive reflexes indicate an upper motor neuron lesion or hypocalcemia. Decreased reflexes are seen in lower motor neuron lesions or the muscular dystrophies.

## NEWBORN EXAMINATION

In the delivery room, a minimal examination is needed. The general appearance is noted and, at 1 and 5 minutes of age, an Apgar score is assigned (Table 6-1). A score of 7 or less indicates that an infant is at risk.

The infant is placed in a warmer. A small catheter is passed through both nares. Secretions are aspirated, and the tube is continued into the stomach and the stomach contents are aspirated. Easy passage of the catheter indicates patency of both nares. Passage into the stomach obviates blind pouch types of tracheoesophageal fistula. The infant may urinate or defecate, indicating patency of these orifices. The mouth is inspected for cleft palate. Gestational age is assessed based on neurodevelopmental signs.

TABLE 6-1.  Apgar Score

| Rating | 0 | 1 | 2 |
|---|---|---|---|
| Appearance | Pale or blue | Body pink, extremities blue | Pink all over |
| Pulse | Absent | 100 | 100 |
| Grimace | None | Weak | Strong |
| Activity (tone) | Limp | Some flexion | Spontaneous movement |
| Respiratory effort | Absent | Hypoventilation, gasping | Coordinated, vigorous cry |

Newborn care then is given and further examination is deferred to the nursery.

Preferably within the first few hours of birth, an admission newborn examination is performed in the presence of the parents. The examiner should develop a routine for the newborn examination so that critical areas are never omitted. In the first few hours of life, the newborn usually is awake, but after 4 hours, he or she may be sleepy. The pressing question to be answered in the first examination is: "Is my child normal?" Although the order of the examination may vary, as with the history, a stereotyped order of recording should be initiated for easy retrieval of information if it is needed later.

## Vital Signs

Vital signs include temperature, heart rate, respiratory rate, blood pressure (using an apparatus for newborns) in an upper and a lower extremity, weight, length, and head, chest, and abdominal circumferences. In addition to recording these, it is essential that they also be plotted on a chart (see Figs 6-8, 6-11).

## General Appearance

Within a few moments, observe the movement of the four extremities, the appearance of the head and neck, body symmetry, and any gross abnormalities.

## Skin

The skin may be covered by a white, greasy, easily removable material called vernix caseosa. Note skin color, consistency, and hydration. Cyanosis, jaundice, eruptions, edema, bruises, petechiae, and pallor are significant abnormalities. Note also hemangiomas and nevi, their size and location. Mongolian (brown) spots over the back are not suggestive of disease, but café au lait spots, if they are numerous, may be a cardinal sign of neurofibromatosis. Papules and pustules must be identified as either normal eruptions or infections.

## Head and Neck

The fontanelle size and head circumference are variable on the first day because of molding. Scalp edema (caput succedaneum) crosses the midline and may be present; this is distinguished from cephalhematoma, which does not cross the midline and is caused by subperiosteal bleeding.

Unusual facies suggests dysmorphic syndromes. Peripheral facial nerve palsies are common. Edema of the eyelids is a result of birth processes or reaction to silver nitrate prophylaxis. Subconjunctival and retinal hemorrhages are found frequently. Red reflex from the fundus, if not visible, indicates some obstruction in the preretinal chambers. Malformation of the pinnae of the ears often is accompanied by severe congenital malformations. If the nose was not found to be patent in the first examination, it should be examined at this time by passing a catheter through both nares. The mouth should be reexamined for cleft palate. The neck should be examined for shortening (as in Klippel-Feil syndrome), redundant skin folds (as in gonadal dysgenesis), vertebral anomalies, cysts, sinuses, and limitation of motion (torticollis).

## Chest

The chest normally is barrel-shaped and smooth at birth, and expands symmetrically with no retractions. Unequal expansion or asymmetry suggests intrathoracic pathology such as cardiac enlargement, pneumothorax, or diaphragmatic hernia. The respiratory rate normally is less than 60 breaths per minute. Occasional irregularities with apnea up to 10 seconds can be normal. Auscultation may reveal adventitious sounds for the first 4 to 6 hours. Percussion is resonant throughout. Maximal cardiac impulse is felt in the fourth interspace close to the sternum. Thrills, if they are present, usually indicate cardiac abnormalities. Murmurs are present in 60% of normal newborns, but the lack of a murmur does not eliminate a diagnosis of congenital heart disease. Brachial and femoral pulses, if they are not of equal intensity, suggest vascular anomalies such as coarctation of the aorta. If chest expansion is unequal, transilluminate the chest. Transillumination occurs with pneumothorax and occasionally with diaphragmatic hernia.

## Abdomen

Distention of the abdomen occurs with sepsis, intestinal or urinary system obstruction, ascites, tumors, or pneumoperitoneum. Scaphoid abdomen suggests a diaphragmatic hernia. Palpate gently. The liver's edge usually is felt 1 to 2 cm below the costal margin and the spleen tip is barely palpable. The bladder, if it is palpable, should be reexamined after voiding. Palpation of the costovertebral angle with ballottement helps to determine the size of the kidneys. The umbilical cord contains two arteries, which are small and thick-walled, and one vein, which is larger and thin-walled. A single umbilical artery is associated with an increased incidence of congenital anomalies. Erythema at the base of the cord suggests omphalitis. Note the patency of the urethral meatus by observing voiding and the patency of the anus either by observing the passage of meconium or by inserting a small rubber catheter.

## Extremities

Asymmetric posturing requires careful palpation of the clavicles, shoulders, and extremities for fractures or brachial plexus injuries. Anomalies of the hands and feet such as webbing, polydactyly, and clubfoot are noted. Abduct both legs to determine any limitation of movement or instability of the hips, which is characteristic of dislocated hips.

## Genitalia

Testes normally are in the scrotum of term infants. Determine the position and size of the urethral meatus. The newborn's penis is greater than 2 cm in length. An enlarged clitoris can be confused with a small penis and requires evaluation for chromosomal sex and other abnormalities of the genitourinary system. The vaginal opening is inspected, and mucosal tags, imperforate hymen, and ambiguous genitalia are sought.

## Neurologic Examination

Assess muscle tone and strength. Extremities normally recoil spontaneously when they are extended from a flexed position and thrash about when they are irritated. Moro's reflex, which is obtained by loud noise or sudden motion, involves abduction of the upper arms and legs, and extension at the elbows and knees, followed by flexion. Absence of this reflex indicates central nervous system depression. Asymmetry suggests extremity fracture or peripheral nerve injury.

## Selected Reading

Barness LA: Manual of Pediatric Physical Diagnosis, 6th ed. St Louis: Mosby-Year Book, 1991.

*Principles and Practice of Pediatrics, Second Edition.*
edited by Frank A. Oski et al. J. B. Lippincott Company, Philadelphia © 1994.

CHAPTER 7

# The Problem-Oriented Medical Record

## Herbert Schneiderman

The problem-oriented medical record (POMR) system was introduced in 1965 by Dr. Lawrence Weed as a means of correcting certain deficiencies in the traditional approach to medical record keeping. Enthusiastically endorsed by many clinicians, it has been used for patient care, student and house officer teaching, and medical audit. In recent years, the POMR system has also been implemented by members of the allied health professions.

## TRADITIONAL APPROACH

Courses in introduction to clinical medicine have employed variants of the traditional scheme shown in Figure 7-1. One takes a history from the patient or a parent and then performs a physical examination. This information provides the basis for producing a differential diagnosis. A differential diagnosis is a mutually exclusive list of diagnoses used to develop a diagnostic plan. The diagnostic plan generates clinical data. Analysis of the data leads to modification of the differential diagnosis, and this process continues until a definitive diagnosis is achieved. At that point, treatment begins.

## DIFFICULTIES WITH THE TRADITIONAL APPROACH

The traditional model is a rough guide to medical decision making that every clinician has learned to modify for practical purposes. As a model, it is heavily oriented toward making a diagnosis. Sometimes, however, a decision must be made in a situation in which the diagnosis is not the primary concern (eg, a routine history of an infant hospitalized with bronchiolitis reveals that he or she has had no immunizations; a child with rheumatoid arthritis is not responding to aspirin therapy). Much of modern inpatient management is directed at patients with complex treatment problems; in the traditional model, these complexities do not receive sufficient recognition or emphasis.

Even when diagnosis is a central concern, the traditional model may present difficulties. It suggests that each patient has a single diagnosis, when, in fact, a child may have concurrent diseases (eg, a child with malabsorption also has pediculosis). Or, while one diagnostic problem is investigated, another is discovered (eg, a child is undergoing evaluation for a pneumonia, and a complete blood count (CBC) reveals a microcytic, hypochromic anemia).

The traditional model is even less helpful when a single disease or diagnosis has multiple components, each of which may present diagnostic problems (eg, a patient with meningomyelocele has hydrocephalus and orthopedic deformities and is not urinating spontaneously).

Because the traditional model emphasizes diagnosis, the phy-

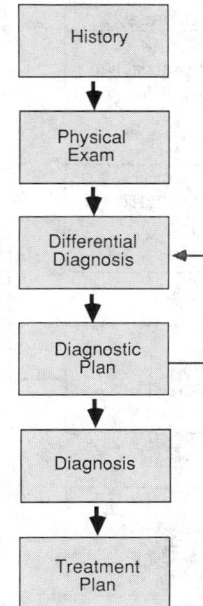

Figure 7-1. The traditional model.

sician may formulate a diagnosis prematurely or ignore abnormal data that do not seem to relate to a current diagnostic formulation. In addition, some conventional diagnostic labels are insufficiently descriptive. The broad term *asthma* is equally likely to refer to the illness of a child who takes medication occasionally for symptoms or to that of another child who has had numerous hospitalizations and requires long-term maintenance on several drugs.

## PROBLEM-ORIENTED MEDICAL RECORD SYSTEM

The problem-oriented medical record (POMR) system, although not perfect, remedies some of the deficiencies of the traditional model. It facilitates identification and tracking of multiple diagnoses, diagnostic investigations, and therapeutic problems.

The POMR system consists of the following components: a database, a problem list, an initial plan, progress notes (which include narrative notes and flow sheets), and discharge notes (Fig 7-2). A database, based partly on a patient's chief complaint, is formulated first. This database leads to the formulation of a complete problem list. Using this list, an initial plan of action is constructed. Progress notes also are structured by the problem list. Information gathered during investigation leads to modification of the problem list, or the patient may develop new problems as a consequence of treatment or the natural course of the disease, and these problems are added to the list. If the patient is hospitalized, the discharge summary also is organized according to the problem list.

### Database

The database includes the history, physical examination, background information, and laboratory data. It is useful to separate data gathering into three groups: inquiry into problem, routine screening, and general background information. Inquiry into problem includes the traditional consideration of the present illness and pertinent parts of the physical examination. Routine screening consists of questions and items of the physical examination regarding problems unsuspected by the patient or parents

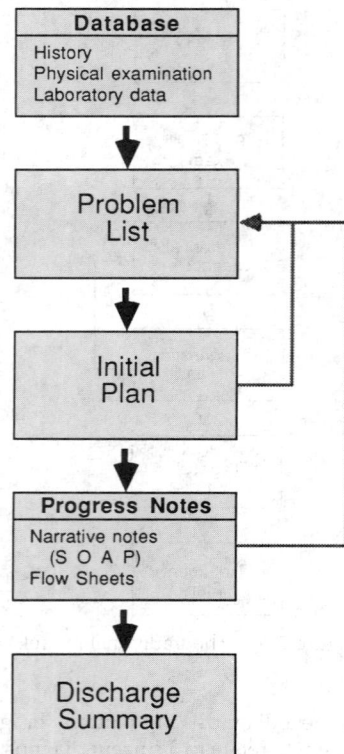

Figure 7-2. The problem-oriented medical record system.

(eg, a child brought in with a running nose is found, after a routine developmental check, to have delayed speech). General background information includes family and social history, hobbies, and so forth.

It is important to distinguish between inquiry and screening. In routine screening, tapping the knees of a healthy 2-year-old child to elicit deep tendon reflexes is of limited use; investigation of gross motor development is much more helpful. Testing for deep tendon reflexes in a comatose 2-year-old, however, is an essential part of an inquiry into the problem.

The content of a structured inquiry into a problem varies with the problem. Similarly, routine screening and background information vary with the age, sex, race, and socioeconomic status and background of the patient. For example, a birth history or information on formula feeding is more useful in evaluating an infant than a husky 14-year-old admitted for a sports injury. Likewise, abduction of the hips with the knees flexed is an important technique used to evaluate infants for hip dysplasia, but it is not particularly helpful in the routine evaluation of a normal 4 year old, for whom gait observation is more useful.

## Problem List

A problem can be medical, psychiatric, psychosocial, or educational. A medical problem can be a diagnosis, a symptom, or a physical or laboratory finding. The problem can be diagnostic or therapeutic. It can be active, inactive, or resolved.

Each of the patient's problems should be numbered and listed in the problem list, as in the following:

1. Pneumonia
2. Hypochromic microcytic anemia
3. Developmental delay by history
4. Behind in immunizations

A problem should be listed in its most definitive form, but it should not be a guess, no matter how inspired, based on incom-

plete data. If the first problem is a suspected meningitis manifesting as a bulging fontanelle, the problem should be listed as "1. Bulging fontanelle." If a lumbar puncture has already been done before the write-up and corroborates your suspicions, the problem should be recorded as "1. Meningitis"; if the culture is positive for *Haemophilus influenzae*, the problem should then be changed to "1. *H influenzae* meningitis," but the number (in this case, 1) should not be changed, for ease in reviewing the chart.

A diagnostic problem may have several manifestations. If the manifestations are minor, they can be listed as part of the same problem. If the manifestations are major and require careful, individual management, they should be treated as separate problems. For example, a single problem could be listed like this:

1. Rheumatic fever with fever, arthritis, and carditis

If the carditis is severe, however, the list would specify two separate problems, as follows:

1. Rheumatic fever with fever and arthritis
2. Carditis secondary to problem 1

The utility of a problem list is apparent when a disease process is complex and several different components each require a decision. The following is an example of a problem list for a patient with meningomyelocele and concomitant illnesses:

1. Meningomyelocele
2. Hydrocephalus secondary to Arnold-Chiari malformation
3. Blocked VP shunt
4. Scoliosis with vertebral and rib abnormalities
5. Restrictive airway disease secondary to 4
6. Feeding difficulty secondary to 5
7. Bilateral equinovarus deformities secondary to 1
8. Neurogenic bladder secondary to 1
9. Family education regarding home care

This breakdown is not the only way to construct this problem list. For example, the Arnold-Chiari malformation could be designated as a separate problem, or problems 2 and 4 could be listed as secondary to 1. Minor variations in constructing a list are unimportant. What *is* important is to have a coherent, complete set of problems that help the clinician think and plan for the patient.

## Initial Plan

In the traditional scheme, a differential diagnosis leads to a diagnostic plan, which results in a diagnosis. Then, a treatment plan is constructed. In real life, diagnostic and treatment decisions are made as soon as initial impressions (including differential diagnosis) are formed, and both types of planning usually continue concurrently. For example, if a lumbar puncture reveals 1000 polymorphonuclear cells, a diagnosis of bacterial meningitis is made. The patient is taken off oral feeding, put on intravenous fluids, confined to bed, and treated with cefotaxime. If *Pneumococcus* grows from blood and spinal fluid when cultures are taken, all antibiotics but penicillin are stopped.

The more complex the case, the more likely it is that the traditional unstructured diagnostic and treatment plans will be incomplete and will omit needed items.

In the POMR system, the problem list serves to organize initial planning efforts, and the plan is numbered to correspond with the problems on the problem list, as shown in this example:

*Problem list*

1. Left lower lobe pneumonia with cough
2. Microcytic, hypochromic anemia
3. Developmental delay revealed by history
4. Behind on immunizations

*Initial plan*

1. Chest radiograph, blood culture, PPD
2. FEP, stool guaiac, detailed nutritional history
3. Do developmental assessment before discharge
4a. Discuss routine health care with parents
4b. Give second DPT and OPV on discharge

Specific plans are of three types: diagnostic, therapeutic, and patient/family education. In this system, "rule-out iron deficiency anemia" is not a diagnosis or a problem, but a plan to establish a diagnosis. The patient/family education component is extremely important and has been insufficiently stressed in medical education. If a problem has several components, it may be useful to categorize planning efforts by type. For example, if the problem is "failure to thrive," the planning efforts for that problem could be listed as follows:

Diagnostic—CBC, BUN, liver function tests, intake and output, nutritional analysis of daily feeding
Therapeutic—regular infant diet
Educational—teach parents parenting and feeding techniques, have social agency follow family

## Progress Notes

Progress notes are of two types, narrative notes and flow sheets.

### Narrative Notes

Narrative notes are organized by the SOAP (*s*ubjective, *o*bjective, *a*ssessment, *p*lan) method. Subjective information, including symptoms, comes from the patient. Objective information, including physical findings and laboratory data, is obtained from and by health professionals. Assessment is the interpretation of subjective and objective data. Plan is the action to be taken, including diagnostic, therapeutic, and educational components, arrangements for services, and other steps.

An example of narrative notes for the problem "1. Sore throat" using the SOAP breakdown follows:

Subjective—patient says throat feels better and she is hungry
Objective—temperature is down to 99°F; throat culture grew β-hemolytic streptococci
Assessment—streptococcal pharyngitis
Plan—continue penicillin for 8 more days

In this case, the problem would now be redefined as "1. Streptococcal pharyngitis."

Entries do not need to be made every day for each SOAP category or each problem, as the following list shows:

1. Left lower lobe pneumonia
    Objective—day 3 on penicillin; patient is coughing less; temperature down to 100°F
4. Behind on immunizations
    Plan—discuss rationale for immunizations with parents; consider ordering a visiting nurse for a home visit after discharge

### Flow Sheets

When variables such as blood urea nitrogen (BUN) or bilirubin are repeated serially, it may be difficult to compare and analyze them from narrative notes, particularly if several types of measurements are being compared.

The flow sheet is an excellent way to record and assess serial observations. (In pediatrics, we have traditionally used variations of flow sheets—head circumference and growth charts—to display and compare data.) This type of record is particularly valuable when several variables, such as laboratory tests, symptoms, and treatment, are monitored simultaneously. Figure 7-3 is an example of a flow sheet for a child with a neurogenic bladder.

## The Discharge Summary

Discharge summaries are potentially excellent self-teaching tools, providing physicians the opportunity to review and analyze a patient's hospitalization, the decisions made, and the outcomes. They are also important sources of information for the community health professionals who will care for the recently hospitalized child.

Unfortunately, discharge summaries are often dictated in a perfunctory manner to meet hospital regulations. Little thought is given to their use, and, consequently, they are too long; contain irrelevant, unstructured, and unassessed material; and lack important information for future health care providers.

The discharge summary should be problem-oriented. This requirement is perhaps less important for a child admitted for a single problem, which was successfully treated and is resolving, than it is for a child with multiple problems, some of which are still active at the time of discharge. All problems, active and inactive, should be listed. It is useful to organize the information related to each problem in the categories of subjective, objective, and therapeutic. Sometimes a problem may be best described by combining elements of the subjective and objective in a concise narrative, as in the following example of a patient with pneumococcal pneumonia:

*The patient was admitted with a 3-day history of coughing and fever. On admission, dullness and rales were apparent posteriorly in the left lower lung field. Other physical findings were normal. The chest film showed LLL pneumonia, and sputum culture grew S. pneumoniae.*

Only those items from the medical history, physical examination, or laboratory data necessary for future analysis or management of the patient should be included. The degree of detail should vary with the types and complications of the problems. An episode of asthma successfully treated with a short course of inhalant bronchodilators and steroids may be described briefly. It is pointless to include a series of all the blood gases taken during the child's hospitalization. These data, useful at the time they are drawn, are of little significance for the future management of the patient. On the other hand, if a child is admitted with a fever of unknown origin and is discharged without a di-

| | January | February | March | April | May |
|---|---|---|---|---|---|
| BUN | 10 | | | 8 | |
| renal scan | | normal | | | |
| VCU | | | normal | | |
| urine culture | E. coli | E.coli | Klebsiella | negative | negative |
| prophylactic antibiotics | | | | trimethoprim/ sulfa | ⟶ |

Figure 7-3.  Sample flow sheet.

agnosis, it is important to list the various x-ray films and laboratory tests that were obtained, even if the results were normal. Here, it is important for a physician to know what studies were done and what they showed at a particular time.

Again, as in the initial plan, a problem-oriented discharge summary makes it easier to record and review complicated management plans. Flow sheets may be useful as part of the discharge summary. Although they cannot be dictated, they can be copied and added to the summary.

## SOME PROBLEMS IN USING THE POMR SYSTEM

Students working with the POMR system occasionally ask about the correct way to chart a situation in which there is interaction between problems, so that treatment for one problem may influence the treatment for or be the same as that for a second problem. There are no hard and fast solutions. One should be clear about what one is planning and not worry excessively about the form. Consider the following example:

*Restrictive airway disease in a small infant may affect the ability to feed. Proper treatment of the airway disease may also alleviate the feeding problem.*

The following are two ways of charting the plan:

4. Restrictive airway disease

5. Feeding difficulty secondary to 4

*Plan*

4. To request ENT consult for tracheotomy and assisted ventilation; this may also alleviate feeding problem
5. See plan for 4

*or*

*Plan*

4 and 5. To request ENT consult for tracheotomy and assisted ventilation; this may also alleviate feeding problem

Another difficulty exists for the isolated user. The POMR system is intended to be used by the entire health team. The intern writes the problem list, and the list is modified by the resident and the attending physician. The resident and attending physician check for completeness and accuracy in formulation of problems, and the intern makes corrections. The same numbering system is used by all the physicians. Consultants, nurses, therapists, and social workers also are expected to stay within the framework for the sake of convenience and coherence.

This scenario may not occur in real life. Some physicians on a ward do not use the system at all; others use their own organization schemes or numbering sequence. It is still worthwhile for the individual student or house officer to use the POMR system to organize his or her thinking and to impose an intelligent order on observations, problems, and plans.

## Selected Readings

Bjorn JC. Problem-oriented pediatric practice. Current problems in pediatrics. Chicago: Year Book Medical Publishers, 1975.
Hurst JW, Walker HK, eds. The problem-oriented system. New York: Medcom Press, 1972.
Walker HK, Hurst JW, Woody MF, eds. Applying the problem-oriented system. New York: Medcom Press, 1973.
Ways PO, Jones JW. Use of the problem-oriented record in pediatrics. Adv Pediatr 1973;20:133.
Weed LL. Medical records that guide and teach. N Engl J Med 1968;278:652.
Weed LL. Medical records, medical education and patient care. The problem-oriented record as a basic tool. Chicago: Year Book Medical Publishers, 1971.

*Principles and Practice of Pediatrics, Second Edition.*
edited by Frank A. Oski et al. J. B. Lippincott Company, Philadelphia © 1994.

# CHAPTER 8
# *The Consultation*

## Alan M. Lake

The concept of medical consultation is traced to roots in Egypt in 2500 BC when self-declared medical specialization was first defined. Over the ages, indications for consultation have been well established (Table 8-1). The first indication is to establish or confirm the diagnosis. The consultant is expected to offer greater experience and wider perspective in the area of concern. Increasingly, the consultant is expected to employ special technology or diagnostic skill. In so doing, this science of consultation threatens to overshadow the former art of consultation.

Foremost in the art of consultation is the consultant's ability to reduce the anxiety of the child, the family, and the referring physician regarding the symptom complex and its significance. The focus on the problem is narrowed, extraneous concerns are discarded, and a plan for evaluation and treatment is devised.

The referring physician often is certain of the diagnosis but wants to share the burden of management and to maximize the sophistication of therapy. With chronic disease concerns, the consultant also provides ready access to the multifaceted team approach of family and patient support systems.

It is crucial for the consultant to provide guidelines as to the future course of a child's problem. Complications of both the disease and its treatment must be anticipated, not merely recognized. To accomplish this, there must be both communication and trust among all four parties—patient, family, primary care provider, and consultant. Without effective communication, this trust will neither develop nor be sustained.

## RESPONSIBILITIES OF THE REFERRING PHYSICIAN

The Committee on Standards of Child Health Care of the American Academy of Pediatrics (1979) has established excellent

**TABLE 8-1.   Indications for Consultation**

Establish or confirm diagnosis.
Reduce patient/family/physician anxiety.
Maximize sophistication of therapy.
Anticipate future course and possible complications.

guidelines for the etiquette and ethics of consultation and referral. The guidelines are summarized in Table 8-2.

The first obligation of the referring physician is knowing when to refer a child for consultation, especially when faced with anxiety in the family. The timing of the consultation is important (Nazarian, 1992). The economic significance of this issue is enhanced by the advent of gatekeeper responsibilities for the primary care provider in health maintenance organizations (HMOs). While trivial referral (the dump or turf) must be discouraged, referral must not be put off until the consultation is seen as an act of despair.

In a 1988 poll conducted by *Contemporary Pediatrics*, the average pediatrician referred between 8 and 10 patients a month to a subspecialist. The rate of referral increases gradually in the first 20 years in practice, then declines slightly. The five most common referrals were for orthopedic surgery, allergy, surgery, neurology, and cardiology. The more complex problems—cancer, cystic fibrosis, hemophilia, and suicide gesture—were nearly always referred to a subspecialist, whereas the more common concerns such as acute otitis, acute urinary tract infection, constipation, or enuresis were rarely referred to subspecialists. The average pediatrician, in turn, is requested to be a consultant for an average of 8 patients a month, usually upon referral from a generalist or obstetrician/gynecologist.

That study, as well as a recent study by Cartland and Yudkowsky (1992), confirms a somewhat lower rate of referral for consultation by physicians in managed care programs. Within an HMO model, the rate of referral is influenced by denial of approval and by pressure to refer within the HMO to subspecialists with training primarily in internal medicine. Within a preferred provider organization (PPO), the reduced rate of referral is influenced by the inconvenience of applying for out-of-plan referral approval. Even within the PPO plan, the subspecialist is, by definition, providing discounted service and hopefully not discounted care.

Providing a choice of consultant is the second obligation of the referring physician. Subspecialists are often intently focused on their areas of expertise, so concerns should be prioritized, especially for the child with obscure multisystem complaints. An orderly progression of referral is vastly superior to a "shotgun" referral process. The primary care provider must remain the ringmaster, discouraging consultants from referring to each other even without gatekeeper restraints. Ideally, the family is offered a choice of competent consultants; in reality, however, the referring physician usually directs the family to one premier authority. Similarly, the primary care provider should steer the family away from a charlatan. A dilemma frequently encountered by the experienced generalist is the need to avoid basing referral on the high likelihood that the consultant will agree with the generalist's advice. For example, most community pediatricians know in advance which orthopedist will cast an infant's turned-in foot and which will preach patience.

The third obligation of the referring physician is to communicate clearly the specific question or concern to be addressed. For inpatients, the consultant's task often is obscured by multiple system failures; for ambulatory patients, communication of necessary information may be obscured because the physician is concentrating on responding to the family's anxiety. Goldbloom (1975) cites how the informality of consultation, so prevalent during residency training, can lead to a depersonalization of referrals and lack of fully informed opinions. To minimize these concerns, the referring physician must provide a concise summary of the thought process applied and evaluations performed.

The fourth obligation of the referring physician is to relate to the consultant how comfortable or experienced the referring physician will be in the ongoing collaborative management of the problem. The referring physician thus avoids the predicament of being asked to perform a task without appropriate preparation. Even in situations as complex as childhood cancer, with its protocol of care, Kisker and associates (1980) demonstrate that 70% of ongoing care could be provided as well by a general pediatrician in communication with the consulting oncologist as by the subspecialists' clinic alone.

Preparing the child and family for the consultation is the final responsibility of the referring physician. In addition to providing the specifics of time, place, and cost, the referring physician should provide the family with some idea of the style of care to expect. Will residents or fellows see the patient first? What materials should be taken with them? Will the consultant discuss the diagnosis and management with them directly or advise only the referring physician?

This concept of extent of transfer of care is critical. There should be direct communication by telephone or letter with the consultant emphasizing extent of concern, degree of urgency, and extent of evaluation performed before referral. With both inpatient and outpatient consultations, the referral should be documented in the medical record.

In the present medico-legal climate, it is also vital to understand the liability issues intrinsic to consultation. These general principles are outlined by Wilde and Pedroni (1991), although differences pertain from state to state.

For the referring physician, there is potential liability in failure to consult if a plaintiff can prove that the sophistication of care required exceeds that of the average pediatrician and that an available specialist promptly called would likely have handled the problem successfully. A second issue for the referring physician is failure to accept a consultant's counsel. While there is often room for reasonable disagreement and the issues should often be resolved by direct communication, the primary care provider is obligated to document in the medical record why a consultant's advice for further testing or specific therapy will not be followed.

Once a physician refers a patient for specialty consultation, he or she is not liable for the negligent acts of that physician. The consultant is an independent contractor and is thus responsible for his or her own negligence. The consultant assumes both the responsibility and liability for a patient's care the moment he or she agrees to do the consultation, even though the patient has not yet been seen.

## RESPONSIBILITIES OF THE CONSULTANT

The obligations of the consultant frequently resemble the Boy Scout creed: ". . . trustworthy, loyal, helpful, friendly. . ." (with increasing significance recently placed on "thrifty"). The consultant should enjoy several luxuries: a known progression of symptoms, a defined set of questions, and a retrospective analysis. There are also burdens, primarily the family's anticipation that the consultant is omnipotent.

The consultant's primary responsibility is to identify the basic issue or appropriate concern (Table 8-3). This requires access to the history, prior evaluation, and reliable physical examination.

| TABLE 8-2. Responsibilities of Referring Physician |
| --- |
| Timing of referral |
| Choice of consultant |
| Identification of specific concerns |
| Indication of level of confidence in management |
| Preparation of patient/family for consultant |

TABLE 8-3. Responsibilities of Consultant

Distinguish appropriate from inappropriate concerns.
Take the time to get complete history and address major concerns.
Avoid the seduction of excessive technology.
Communicate specific assessment and recommendations to referring physician and patient.

Some consultants prefer to start with a clean slate by obtaining their own history and forming their own conclusions before reviewing the results of prior evaluations (Stickler, 1987). This can be done only with excellent histories from patients or families. In most ambulatory circumstances, it helps to have a more structured format to the history, including a series of tasks for the family to complete before their first consultative visit. In addition to bringing x-ray films, record of usual dietary intake, growth data, and records from the referring physician, bringing a symptom diary of at least 1 week's duration helps record objectively the symptoms and their relation to meals or pertinent daily activities.

Ideally, the child is at ease, especially during the history taking. With older children, this is accomplished by taking the time to have a relaxed conversation and to answer honestly their fears of what is to take place. With infants and toddlers, it is best to leave them dressed, sitting on the parent's lap or playing during the history. The consultant must be relaxed and in control no matter how intense the circumstances. Diplomacy and avoidance of self-righteous airs are critical to placing the family and child at ease. Obviously, no single style of interaction is right for everyone.

Most patients and families arrive with predetermined anxieties. These must be acknowledged and addressed, especially in the context of functional concerns. Failure to devote attention to these concerns is a major excuse for "doctor shopping," seeking the consultant "who will listen to us." When Cousins (1985) investigated this concern, he discovered that 85% of patients had either changed physicians or contemplated doing so in the preceding 5 years. There is a built-in seduction here, however, because the consultant may use these anxieties to justify excessive exclusionary procedures. It is very easy to conclude that "I'm the court of last resort, and if I don't do the procedure someone else (less skilled, of course) will do it."

Once the consultant has completed his or her assessment, it must be communicated effectively. By tradition, this is only to the referring physician. Today's educated consumer, however, deserves direct, diplomatic discussion, if only to answer questions required of the consultant (Schwartz, 1984). This must be understood in advance by the referring physician.

The consultant will not always have a specific diagnosis or mandated therapy. In such circumstances, it is critical to be honest and to avoid inconsequential alterations in therapy just to give the impression of change. The consultant must provide a framework of what to do next. The referring physician is left with the choice of options, usually including the option of observation alone.

The report to the referring physician must be written concisely and without ambiguity even when the consultant is perplexed. Three paragraphs suffice: one summarizes the history as of that time, one reports results of procedures and assessment, and one outlines specific recommendations. Follow-up plans must be clearly delineated. The educational responsibility of the consultant also should be addressed by brief comment or reference to enclosed review articles. If dramatic alterations in therapy are indicated, a telephone call is mandated, especially if the assessment or recommendations conflict with those proposed previously by the primary care provider.

The impact of establishing a diagnosis has received little research. In a recent British study of the impact of making the diagnosis of childhood asthma on rates of consultation, Charlton and associates (1991) noted no difference in the overall rates of referral before or after the diagnosis; however, after a diagnosis, a greater proportion of the referrals were generated by the physician than by the family. Whether this truly reduces rates of morbidity for asthma is assumed but unproven.

## RESPONSIBILITIES OF PATIENT AND FAMILY

The patient and family also have responsibilities in this process of consultation (Table 8-4). Most of these have been alluded to in the previous discussion. In preparation for the consultative visit, the family should be responsibly educated consumers. They will encounter no shortage of advice.

It is difficult for parents to be objective about a health concern in their child, but all communication must be as objective as possible. Families must avoid excessive self-analysis and must provide complete background data essential for developing a differential diagnosis.

Specific questions should be prepared by the family in advance. While both parents should be present for the consultation, attending with an array of concerned family members is counterproductive. In a critical situation, the parents may ask (and usually expect) the consultant to speak briefly with immediate relatives. Most communication of this nature, however, is best handled by the attending or primary care physician.

At the end of the consultation, the patient and family should review their understanding of the assessment and recommendations. In most circumstances, the child should be present to avoid the feeling that "something is being kept from me." Often, the child is the key to compliance, that part of the consultation that extends after the visit. The benefits of consultation can be negated by lack of a responsible response to the consultant's recommendations.

## CONCLUDING COMMENTS

A number of factors threaten the system of mutual trust implicit in the process of consultation and will require creative responses in the years ahead.

Berczeller (1991) recently editorialized against the increased use of consultation to create disease-based care by committee as opposed to patient care coordinated by a single physician. He emphasizes that the tradition of personal bedside dialogue with a consultant is neglected and that the inevitable result is an abdication of decision-making responsibility by the primary care provider.

The proliferation of managed health-care systems has several effects. In the gatekeeper system, there is usually a direct financial

TABLE 8-4. Responsibilities of Patient/Family

Be an educated consumer.
Communicate concerns as objectively as possible.
Provide complete background information.
Prepare a list of questions/concerns in advance.
Review recommendations and respond responsibly.

incentive to avoid formal consultation. With preferred provider discounts or capitation systems, the subspecialists have an incentive to provide rapid, discounted service. Consultants are increasingly challenged by the proliferation of telephone consultations, whereby some responsibility, if not liability, is assumed with no immediate likelihood of seeing the patient. Telephone consultations jeopardize long-term relationships with primary care providers.

The greatest influence in pediatrics will come from increased entry of well-trained subspecialists into private, nonacademic practice, potentially in competition with university teaching programs. The ability to incorporate these subspecialists creatively into the teaching programs and continue to attract their hospital admissions to the university will tax the ingenuity of department and division chairpersons. Initially, these subspecialists are expected to compete in urban centers rather than meet rural healthcare needs. Internists with subspecialty training in a competitive market are lowering the age of patients accepted in referral.

The introduction of practice guidelines to formalize review of care and diagnostic undertakings also will affect the process of consultation. Insurers and quality care reviewers will determine the consultant's reimbursement and eligibility for subsequent consultations based on guidelines that may or may not be relevant to the patient's dilemma.

The self-referred patient has long taxed the relationship of consultant and primary care provider. Whereas the Greeks in 400 BC flocked to the temples of Aesculapius, the god of healing, the modern family turns to the Yellow Pages. Whenever possible, the consultant should request that the primary care provider be made aware of the scheduled consultation. The letter of summary and recommendations should be sent to the primary care provider when the family expresses some concern in this regard. When a family has no primary care provider, every effort should be made to locate one to coordinate ongoing care needs.

## Selected Readings

American Academy of Pediatrics. The etiquette and ethics of consultation and referrals standards of child health care, ed 3. Evanston, Ill: American Academy of Pediatrics, 1979:104.

Berczeller P. The malignant consultation syndrome. Hosp Pract 1991 pt:29.

Burnside JW. In: Foreword to Kammerer WS, Gross RJ, eds. Medical consultation. Baltimore: Williams & Wilkins, 1983:3.

Cartland JDC, Yudkowsky BK. Barriers to pediatric referral in managed care systems. Pediatrics 1992;89:183.

Charlton I, Jones K, Bain J. Delay in diagnosis of childhood asthma and its influence on respiratory consultation rates. BMJ 1991;303:633.

Goldbloom RB. The lost art of consultation: a plea for the return of striped trousers. Pediatrics 1975;56:347.

Kisker CT, Strayer F, Wong K. Health outcomes of a community based therapy program for children with cancer: a shared management approach. Pediatrics 1980;66:900.

Nazarian L. On consulting and being consulted. Pediatr Rev 1992;13:124.

Oski FA, ed. The pattern of pediatric referrals. Contemporary Pediatrics 1988;5 (Dec): 20.

Rosenbloom AL. Primary and subspecialty care of diabetes mellitus in children and youth. Pediatr Clin North Am 1984;31:107.

Schwartz RH. Children with chronic asthma: care by the generalist and the specialist. Pediatr Clin North Am 1984;31:87.

Stickler GB. Clinical guidelines for the pediatrician. Pediatrics 1987;80:118.

Wilde JA, Pedrone AT. The do's and don'ts of consultation. Contemporary Pediatrics 1991;7 (May):23.

*Principles and Practice of Pediatrics, Second Edition.*
edited by Frank A. Oski et al. J. B. Lippincott Company, Philadelphia © 1994.

# CHAPTER 9
# *The Diagnostic Process*

Frank A. Oski

Diagnosis is one of the most important tasks of the clinician. Problem solving in medicine has been described, somewhat cynically, as "the process of making adequate decisions with inadequate information."

If the diagnosis is correct and treatment is available, proper care usually follows. If no specific treatment is available, correct diagnosis is still important because it provides a basis for prognosis and advice to patients or parents.

The need for a logical approach to medical diagnosis is vitally important to the economy of the United States, where health costs account for about 10% of the gross national product. Former United States Secretary of Health, Education and Welfare Joseph A. Califano observed that "the physician is the central decision maker for more than 70% of health care services." These decisions include that for hospitalization, duration of hospitalization, medications employed, and diagnostic tests used.

The cognitive processes used in making a diagnosis are not fully understood. Perhaps nowhere else in medicine do the art and the science of medicine blend as imperceptibly as they do in the process of making a diagnosis.

Physicians use four basic approaches to reach a diagnosis: pattern recognition, sampling the universe, clinical algorithms, and hypothesis generation.

*Pattern recognition* is the process by which a diagnosis is made based on physical clues or linkage identification. For example, a diagnosis of Down syndrome can be made by recognizing the physical findings that make up this genetic abnormality. Similarly, the diagnosis of Henoch-Schönlein purpura is immediately apparent if the rash has a characteristic pattern and distribution. Diagnosis by pattern identification requires familiarity with diseases through experience or study. The expression "the more you see, the more you know, and the more you know, the more you see" describes how pattern recognition develops. Linkage identification is a form of pattern recognition. A diagnosis is based on history and physical or laboratory findings. For example, the finding of a micropenis and hypoglycemia in a neonate would result in a prompt diagnosis of congenital hypopituitarism. A history of bloody diarrhea in association with a white blood cell count demonstrating more band forms than mature polymorphonuclear leukocytes would result in an immediate diagnosis of *Shigella* gastroenteritis. Skill in linkage identification, like pattern recognition, is gained by observation and study. The seemingly intuitive diagnosis, often the hallmark of the older physician, is usually a result of linkage identification.

*Sampling the universe* refers to the mindless ordering of laboratory studies in hopes that an abnormality will appear that will result in a diagnosis. This is a diagnostic process to be decried. In the United States, about 27 billion dollars per year are spent on laboratory tests, and another 2 billion dollars per year are spent on chest roentgenograms. An estimated 20% to 60% of these tests are unnecessary. If the estimates are accurate, then 6 to 12 billion dollars per year are spent on procedures that do not aid in the diagnosis or treatment of illness. The amount spent specifically on pediatric patients is unknown.

Laboratory tests should be obtained only to support a hypothesis. If the history and physical diagnosis do not suggest an underlying organic disorder, there is no rationale for ordering a battery of laboratory tests in an attempt to uncover an occult disease. The evaluation of infants and children with failure to thrive is an example of this form of behavior. In a 1978 review of 2607 laboratory studies performed on 185 patients with failure to thrive, Sills found that only 1.4% of the tests were of any positive diagnostic assistance, and all of them were specifically indicated by the history or physical examination.

A *clinical algorithm* is a protocol, presented as a flow chart, that contains branch points that require decisions. The clinical algorithm enables the user to reach a diagnosis. The clinical algorithm is a by-product of computer science and is based on the belief that the medical diagnostic process can be automated. A number of clinical situations have been adapted successfully to algorithms, but the majority have not. An example of a clinical algorithm is depicted in Figure 9-1.

Early algorithms were comprehensive and required many laboratory tests and physical findings. Many of these procedures were found to be unnecessary, and algorithms were simplified. An algorithm is not merely a list of symptoms or diagnostic procedures, but a logical flow chart or decision table that helps clinicians make decisions. They often require a precise yes or no answer; not all clinical questions can be answered so crisply. "Maybe" or any other vague answer blocks the progression in the typical algorithm. Algorithms have not been developed for every clinical situation or patient complaint. Algorithms are not yet a substitute for decision analysis or hypothesis generation in the establishment of a diagnosis.

*Hypothesis generation,* the development of explanations for the patient's problem, is the most common and intellectually satisfying technique for arriving at a diagnosis. The development of hypotheses distinguishes the problem-solving process from mere data collection. The stockpiling of facts, without a hypothesis, has been likened to baseball statisticians with a great number of facts available to them but no way of determining what they really mean.

Hypotheses, or potential diagnoses, are generated early in patient encounters. Studies demonstrate that the competent physician begins to generate hypotheses the moment the chief complaint is heard. The generation of hypotheses continues as the remainder of the history unfolds. These hypotheses guide further inquiry. This immediate hypothesis generation directly contrasts the conventional strategy taught to medical students to defer all hypotheses until history-taking and physical examination are completed.

Many physicians employ a common strategy to analyze presenting complaints. Initially, they interpret complaints anatomically; next, they interpret complaints physiologically; and finally, they interpret major symptoms pathophysiologically.

Fulginiti (1981) lists seven principles used to establish a clinical hypothesis:

1. Common diseases and conditions occur commonly.
2. A single process should be invoked to explain most of the data, if not all of it.
3. Simple problems usually have simple explanations.
4. Hypotheses should derive from the data and not be imposed on them.
5. The hypothesis should be consistent with known pathophysiologic mechanisms.
6. Serious consideration of an individual hypothesis should be based on its probability.
7. Hypotheses may be formulated, accepted, rejected, or modified at any point in the course of problem solving.

As mentioned, research reveals that competent physicians tend to generate hypotheses the moment the chief complaint is heard.

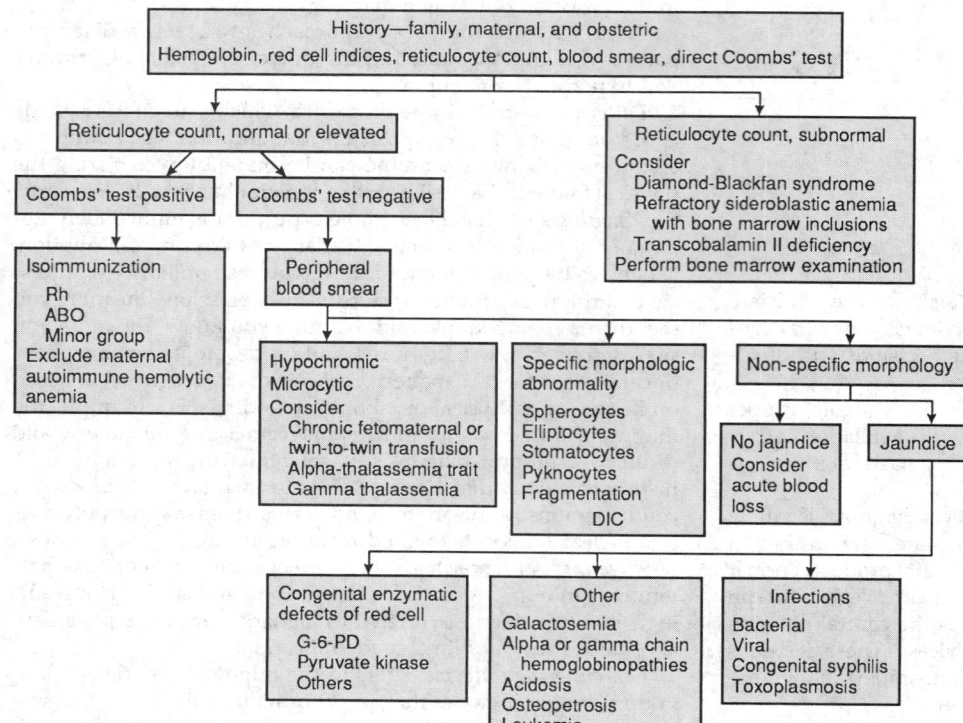

**Figure 9-1.** An approach to the differential diagnosis of anemia in the newborn (Oski FA, Naima JL. Hematologic problems of the newborn. Philadelphia: WB Saunders, 1982:72)

The same research demonstrates that a limited number of hypotheses are entertained simultaneously. It is uncommon for more than five hypotheses to be actively retained, and never are more than seven considered. Investigation often is limited to the hypotheses that survive revisions that occur while the history and physical examination are performed. Several things can go wrong. The physician may retain hypotheses that are too general and often not easily tested. Facts and findings may be ignored because they are inconsistent with a hypothesis. Physicians appear loath to generate new hypotheses after the initial list is formulated, and equally loath to discard an existing one.

The human mind needs to perceive problems as having limited degrees of complexity. We oversimplify by assigning new information to existing hypotheses rather than forming new hypotheses, even when the information does not fit. The labeling of a condition as atypical or as a "form fruste" is an example of the parsimony of the human mind and is responsible for the slow recognition of new diseases.

## SUGGESTED GUIDELINES FOR ESTABLISHING A DIAGNOSIS

1. Always think of a number of diagnostic possibilities that are compatible with the chief complaint or the initial physical findings. Always consider the most common diagnosis first, but always include among your diagnoses those conditions, no matter how rare, for which treatment is available and which, if missed and untreated, would produce irreparable harm or even death to your patient.
2. Form a reasoned plan for testing your hypothesis. Sequence laboratory tests to establish, or rule out, the most common diseases first as well as the diseases requiring urgent treatment.
3. Don't rush to make a diagnosis for which no treatment is available.
4. Never perform a diagnostic procedure that is not related to any of your diagnostic possibilities (eg, a urinalysis in a patient being evaluated for inspiratory stridor).
5. Do not pursue a differential among diagnoses that will not alter your course of action.
6. Always consider the harm that tests might do as well as their costs. Balance the harm and the costs against the information that may be gained.
7. Be constantly aware of the natural tendency to discount, or even disregard, evidence likely to eliminate your favored diagnosis.
8. Never dismiss the possibility that a patient with multiple complaints or problems may have more than one disease. The chances of having two common diseases simultaneously is greater than the chance of having one rare disease.
9. If you cannot rule out the possibility of the presence of a disease that would result in serious harm to the patient if left untreated, then treat the patient as if the disease was present.

Probability and utility should always guide your actions.

## Selected Readings

Cutler P. Problem solving in clinical medicine: from data to diagnosis. Baltimore: Williams & Wilkins, 1979.
Elstein AS, Shulman L, Sprafka SA. Medical problem solving: an analysis of clinical reasoning. Cambridge, Mass: Harvard University Press, 1978.
Fulginiti VA. Pediatric clinical problem solving. Baltimore: Williams & Wilkins, 1981.
Schwartz S, Griffin T. Medical thinking: the psychology of medical judgment and decision making. New York: Springer-Verlag, 1986.
Sills RH. Failure to thrive: the role of clinical and laboratory evaluation. Am J Dis Child 1978;132:967.

*Principles and Practice of Pediatrics, Second Edition.*
edited by Frank A. Oski et al. J. B. Lippincott Company, Philadelphia © 1994.

## CHAPTER 10
# *Pharmacologic Principles of Drug Therapy*

### Robert J. Roberts

An ideal course of drug therapy is to select the appropriate drug of choice, administer at the proper dose and interval, and complete the entire therapy. The essential and critical element of controlled clinical trial for the basis of drug of choice must be satisfied to legitimize related decisions. Physicians should recognize that failure to achieve the anticipated result from drug therapy may be caused by failure to use the drug optimally rather than the drug's failure to work.

Examples of past therapeutic misadventures reinforce the importance of understanding pharmacologic principles in order to optimize therapeutic intervention. When diethylene glycol was used as a vehicle for elixir of sulfonamide in the 1930s, many children died. This tragic situation resulted in the creation of the Food and Drug Administration (FDA) and the requirement for evidence of safety in medication. Children and particularly infants, however, continued to fall victims of drug therapy related toxicity. The gray baby syndrome was the result of inexperience with chloramphenicol dosage in neonates. Chloramphenicol dosages were increased because of apparent clinical deterioration even though drug concentrations in these infants were already inordinately high. Chloramphenicol is largely metabolized before elimination, and infants may metabolize chloramphenicol slowly, resulting in accumulation of toxic concentrations of the drug. This information might have averted the gray syndrome if it had been known. Other adverse effects of drug therapy in neonates might have been prevented if there had been an appreciation of the amounts of "inert ingredients" found in parenteral medications being administered to neonates in NICUs. The "gasping syndrome" believed to be the consequence of benzyl alcohol accumulation is one such example. Benzyl alcohol had been used as a bacteriostatic agent in parenteral drug preparations and was considered safe before it was used in premature neonates. Like chloramphenicol, benzyl alcohol is metabolized and excreted slowly by neonates, resulting in potential accumulation of toxic amounts of the alcohol and its metabolites with repeated administration. The following discussion details important pharmacologic principles that significantly influence the safe and effective uses of therapeutic agents in the management of sick infants.

## SCIENTIFIC BASIS OF PEDIATRIC CLINICAL PHARMACOLOGY

Experience with certain therapies in pediatric patients has resulted in recognition of their potential for producing toxicity. A great deal of therapy has been instituted in the management of pediatric disease without first establishing unequivocally the efficacy of such therapy. The fundamental principle for establishing drug efficacy is based on prospective randomized controlled studies for which there are few examples in pediatric therapeutics. Controlled clinical trials to examine therapeutic efficacy in pediatric patients is complicated and difficult. For example, studies of steroid therapy in chronic lung disease in neonates (bronchopulmonary dysplasia) has been difficult to accomplish because of a range of clinical features within the patient population such as severity of lung disease, other major organ problems, nutritional status, and infectious disease. In addition, striking differences in clinical practice change the baseline for examining the effects and outcomes of variable drug treatment for such patients. Thus, extrapolation from one therapeutic clinical study to another clinical population can be problematic. The ethical issue of experimental studies in pediatrics challenges the pursuit of such knowledge. Consequently, much of the scientific basis for therapy in pediatrics is based on controlled trials in adult populations or clinical experiences in pediatric patients. Although this might be considered acceptable in selected situations, studies in adults of pediatric experiences do not adequately address the fundamental need for a scientific basis for answers to efficacy and toxicity questions in pediatric patients. The power of scientific clinical trials is apparent and cannot be ignored. Ongoing studies of surfactant in management of respiratory distress syndrome (RDS) illustrate the value of examining fundamental questions of efficacy and addressing such issues as definitions of pediatric populations that would benefit most. Attention to such details of therapy through controlled clinical trials will lead to establishing ideal opportunities for effectiveness. Experience teaches us that ineffectiveness of a drug is most notable when toxicity occurs. Such experience is harmful to the professional image and seriously undermines the initiative for therapeutic research. We must maintain a vigilance for requiring the efficacy while seeking evidence for potential toxicity. The following paragraphs deal with important pharmacologic principles, but are based on the premise that issues of efficacy for an individual drug have been determined based on scientific clinical trials.

## PHARMACOLOGIC PRINCIPLES: DOSE, INTERVAL, AND DURATION OF DRUG THERAPY

Examination of the concentration of a drug in relation to pharmacologic response shows how drug dose, interval of administration, and duration of therapy influence the outcome of drug therapy. With rare exception, the concentration of a drug at the site of action relates proportionately to pharmacologic response, either desired (efficacy) or undesired (toxicity) (Fig 10-1).

Each drug and different sites of effect are likely to have a different proportionality between drug concentration and pharmacologic effect. Line A and line B can represent two different drugs or sites of action (see Fig 10-1). Line A reflects greater change in drug response with each change in drug concentration than does line B. If lines A and B are drugs, drug A is more potent than drug B; if lines A and B are sites of drug action, then site A is more responsive than site B.

The physician can manipulate drug concentration at the site of effect. The physician controls variables that affect concentration of drug at the site of effect including dose, interval, and duration of administration. In general, the larger the dose and the more frequent its administration, the greater the drug concentration achieved in the body (Fig 10-2).

Figure 10-2 shows that it is possible to vary drug doses and intervals so equal or very different drug concentrations are achieved at equivalent points of time. This influence by the physician is not always appreciated and can be further complicated by ambiguous drug dosage recommendations such as "100 to 200 mg per day given in divided doses every 6 to 12 hours." In this example, two extremes in dosage can be achieved:

Situation 1 $\frac{100 \text{ mg}}{4 \text{ doses}} = 25$ mg q 6 h

Situation 2 $\frac{200 \text{ mg}}{2 \text{ doses}} = 100$ mg q 12 h

The drug concentration versus time profiles that could result from this example are shown in Figure 10-3. The drug concentration to time relationships are very different in each situation. Therefore, any change in dose or dosing interval that results in a change in the drug concentration versus time profile can potentially alter the efficacy or toxicity of a drug. In situations in which the ability of the drug to clear the body of the neonate

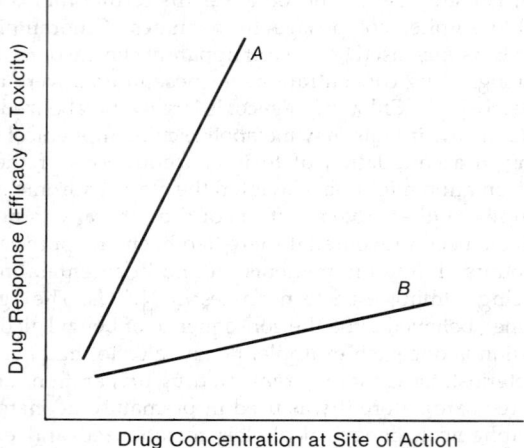

**Figure 10-1.** Relationship between drug concentration and response produced by the drug (efficacy or toxicity), which is proportional to the concentration of drug at the site of action. Each line (A and B) could represent either different drugs or different sites of action.

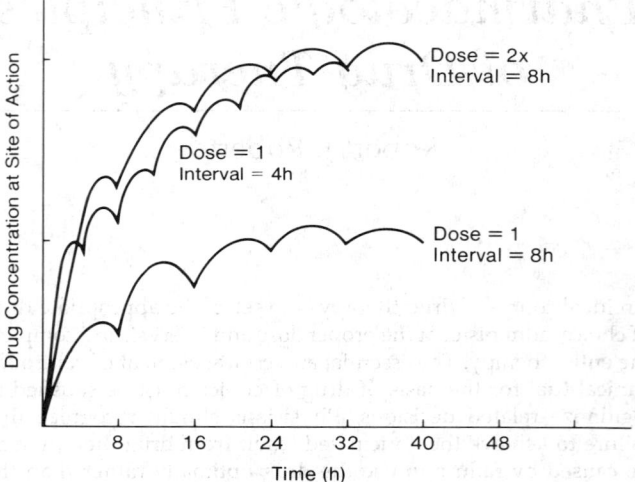

**Figure 10-2.** Influence of drug dose and interval on the concentration of drug at site of action. Doubling the dose or giving the drug twice as often produces the same result in terms of drug concentration.

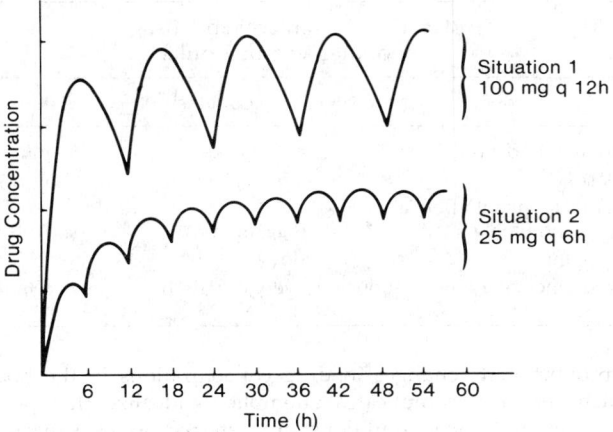

**Figure 10-3.** Example of drug concentration versus time profiles developed from a single dosage recommendation (see text).

reaches a maximum (see section on Biotransformation), the consequences of dosage change (dose or interval) are more complicated and even unpredictable. It is, therefore, critical that physicians employing drug therapy have a working knowledge and understanding of drug disposition and how drug disposition relates to physician-determined variables (dose, interval, and duration of drug therapy).

## PHARMACOLOGIC PRINCIPLES: DRUG DISPOSITION

Ideal drug dosage regimens are accomplished best by understanding the developmental aspects of drug disposition. Drug disposition refers to events associated with drug absorption, distribution, metabolism (biotransformation), and excretion.

### Absorption

The rate and extent of drug absorption depend on elements of pharmaceutics (ie, drug solubility), other physical-chemical features of drug preparation, and physiology. Drug absorption can be fast or slow (Fig 10-4A) and can be complete or incomplete (Fig 10-4B). In Figure 10-4A, although the amounts of drug absorbed are equal, the concentration versus time profiles are very different. The time of peak drug concentration and the drug concentrations achieved at equivalent times differ, which results in differences in the time and quantity of drug effect.

In Figure 10-4B, the differences in completeness of drug absorption are expected to produce the differences illustrated in drug concentrations at respective points in time. The time of peak drug concentration, however, is the same.

Drug failure can result from differences in rate as well as completeness of drug absorption. Different rates of absorption associated with different routes of administration (oral, intramuscular, intravenous, subcutaneous) are well documented. The completeness of drug absorption, particularly as related to developmental concentrations in infants, has been the subject of very few studies. Figure 10-4 shows dramatically different drug concentrations versus time profiles can result from differences in rate and completeness of drug absorption. Disease can also influence both rate and completeness of drug absorption from any site of administration.

Drug concentration versus time profiles differ for the same drug when different routes of administration are used. Different organs, then, are exposed to substantially different concentrations of a drug depending on the route of drug administration. For example, a drug given orally is likely to achieve greater concentrations in the gastrointestinal tissues and the liver before distribution to other tissues. In contrast, intravenous injection of the same drug can result in much higher concentrations of drug throughout the body as a result of bypassing the gastrointestinal tract and hepatic circulation before distribution. Drugs that undergo high first-pass extraction by the liver such as propranolol represent extremes of this principle. High first-pass extraction means the drug is largely removed from the circulation during initial passage through the liver. The dosage differences for propranolol document the significance of this first-pass effect: the oral dose is 0.1 mg/kg versus 0.01 mg/kg if given intravenously.

Narcotic agents are practical examples of the influence that route of administration has on rate and completeness of drug absorption. Subcutaneous or intramuscular administration of morphine is expected to have an onset of action 15 to 20 times slower than a comparable dose given intravenously. An intravenous dose may result in such rapid and high drug concentrations in the central nervous system that respiratory depression results. If circulatory collapse exists, subcutaneous or intramuscular injection of morphine may be useless, a consequence of very slow rate and possibly incomplete absorption of the administered dose into the circulation.

### Distribution

Major controlling factors that influence the distribution of drug to various tissues in the body include the concentration of drug

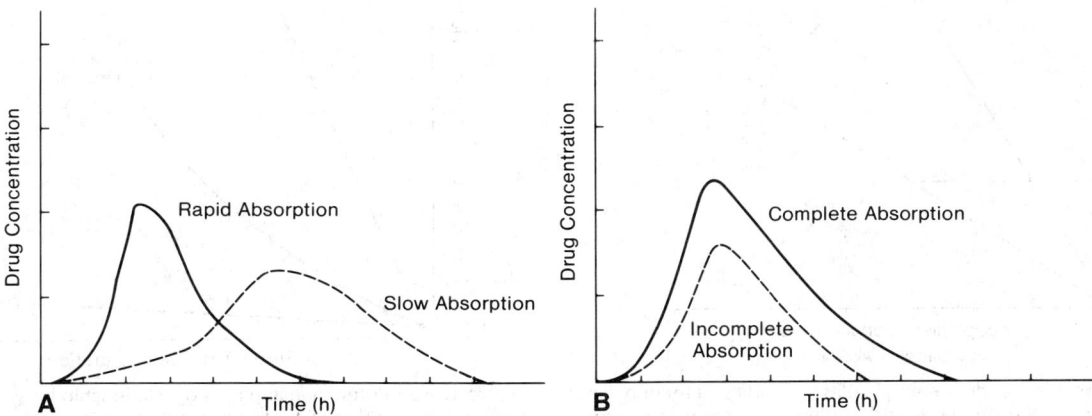

**Figure 10-4.** (**A**) Differences in rate of drug absorption affect both the quantity and time of peak drug concentration. (**B**) Differences in completeness of drug absorption affect only the concentration of drug.

in the blood, the amount of drug bound to serum proteins and to intracellular protein binding sites, blood flow, and the solubility of the drug. Differences in drug protein binding account for major differences in the amount of drug that reaches equilibrium in the blood versus tissues. For example, a drug that is highly bound to serum proteins tends to be trapped in the vascular compartment instead of freely moving into the extravascular compartments. Other drugs are bound more avidly at intracellular sites and are, therefore, highly concentrated outside of the vascular compartment. For example, digoxin can achieve concentrations within the myocardium that are 200 times greater than digoxin concentrations found in the serum.

Theophylline is a good example of a drug with which changes in plasma protein binding influence distribution. Serum concentrations of theophylline reflect tissue concentrations of theophylline. Differences in plasma protein binding of theophylline among patients, however, can render the use of serum drug measurements dangerous. Because of reduced serum protein binding of theophylline in infants, the drug is more likely to escape into extravascular compartments in infants than in adults. Therefore, a serum theophylline concentration of 10 $\mu$g/mL in a neonate is actually associated with a greater tissue concentration of theophylline than an adult with an equal serum theophylline concentration. Thus, a neonate may be expected to achieve a greater drug response than an adult with an equal serum concentration of theophylline (Fig 10-5).

## Biotransformation

Drug metabolism (biotransformation) is a significant factor in influencing drug dosage requirements (dose and interval of administration), as exemplified by the large volume of literature on the topic. Drugs differ remarkably in their ability to be metabolized, including rate and pathway of metabolism. Equally important are the differences between individuals and in rapidly maturing populations, particularly infants, in their abilities to metabolize a given drug. It is, therefore, inappropriate to generalize about drug metabolism, particularly in respect to influence of age. The enzymatic reactions involved in drug metabolism can be limited in regard to the capacity of the process. When a drug dosage exceeds the enzymatic drug-metabolizing capacity, concentrations of drug in the body (eg, serum) based on drug dosage are less predictable. Changes in drug dosage generally result in

| TABLE 10-1.   Gentamicin Dosage in Neonates Versus Adults | | |
|---|---|---|
| | Neonates | Adults |
| Volume of distribution | 400 mL/kg | 350 mL/kg |
| Dose | 2.5 mg/kg | 2.0 mL/kg |
| Plasma concentration achieved (peak) | 6 $\mu$g/mL | 6 $\mu$g/mL |
| Clearance | slow | rapid |
| Frequency of administration | every 8 to 24 h | every 6 h |

disproportionate changes in drug concentrations in the body, which seriously complicates attempts to idealize therapeutic management. Such conditions are referred to as saturation pharmacokinetics.

Infants are regularly characterized as slow metabolizers of drugs, even though some drugs are metabolized more rapidly by infants than adults. Dosage requirements for theophylline, phenobarbital, and phenytoin can be several times greater in infants between 1 and 6 months of age than adults on a per kilogram body weight basis.

## Excretion

Maturation of renal function is associated with a change in the ability to clear drugs from systemic circulation. Drugs that depend heavily on renal elimination require dosage adjustments based on such changes in renal function. Gentamicin is a drug with differing dosage requirements in infants and adults because of differences in disposition (Table 10-1). The greater body distribution (volume of distribution) of gentamicin results in an increased dose requirement in infants to achieve the same serum drug concentration as adults. The rate of elimination of gentamicin by renal mechanisms is slower in infants than in adults, which translates to a longer interval of time between gentamicin dose administration in infants than in adults.

## PHARMACOLOGIC PRINCIPLES: THERAPEUTIC DRUG MONITORING

Therapeutic drug monitoring in pediatric patients is an effective modality for enhancing drug efficacy and minimizing drug tox-

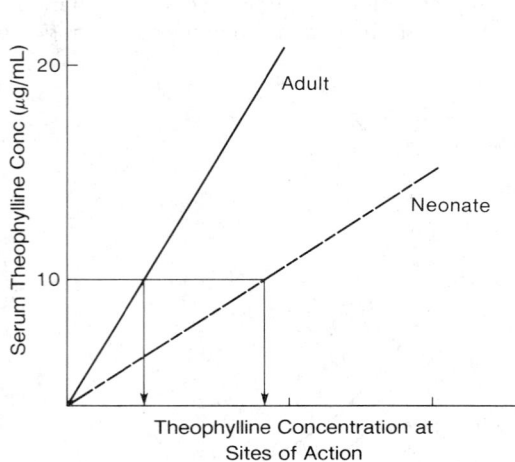

**Figure 10-5.**   The effect of differences in plasma binding of theophylline on drug action between neonates and adults. Because of less serum protein binding of theophylline in neonates, achievement of equal serum theophylline concentrations to those in adults actually delivers more drug to sites of action (*arrows*).

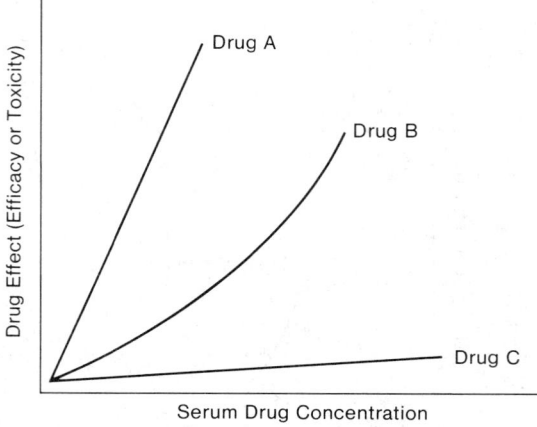

**Figure 10-6.**   Potential usefulness of relationship between serum drug concentration and drug effect. Drug A demonstrates a useful relationship and Drug B a changing, less predictable and useful situation. Drug C illustrates a difficult circumstance where major changes in serum drug concentration reflect very little change in drug effect.

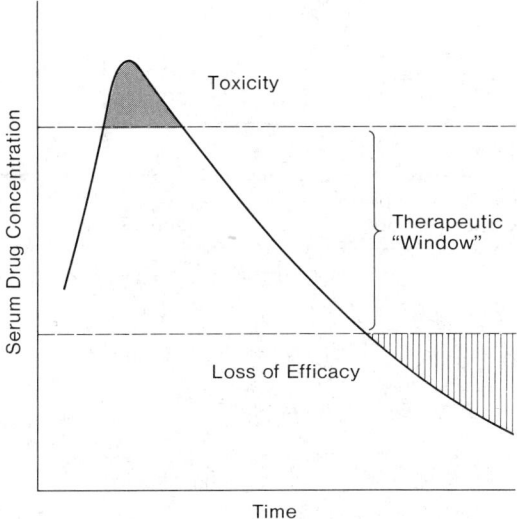

**Figure 10-7.** The concept of therapeutic window, the ideal drug serum concentration above which toxicity is expected and below which efficacy is reduced or lost.

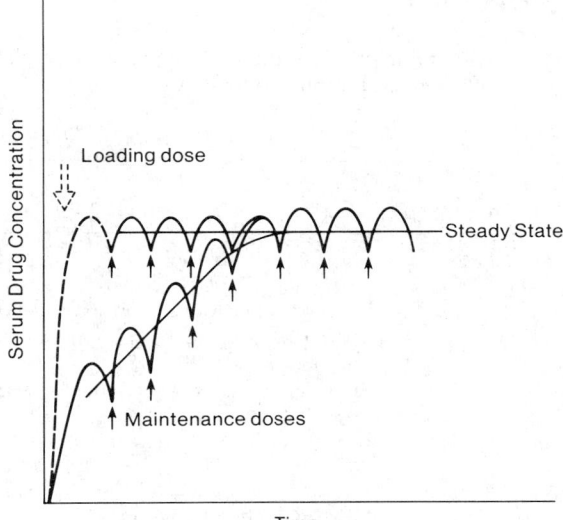

**Figure 10-8.** Steady-state serum concentrations achieved over time with repeated maintenance doses (*solid line*) or more rapidly after a loading dose (*dashed line*).

icity. Differences among individuals in drug disposition and the consequences of dosage changes (dose and frequency) can be determined precisely by monitoring serum drug concentrations. The minimum requirement for use of practical pharmacokinetics, however, is a relationship between drug effect and serum concentration. As illustrated in Figure 10-6, different drugs (A, B, and C) can have different relationships between serum drug concentrations and effect. Drug C represents a difficult working situation because there are proportionately greater changes in drug concentration than in effect compared to drugs A and B. From a predictable relationship between drug concentration and effect, one can identify target concentrations of drug in the serum. Target serum drug concentrations represent an ability to achieve a therapeutic window above which toxicity is expected and below which therapeutic efficacy is compromised (Fig 10-7).

The timing of serum sampling is critical. Peak concentrations of drug in the serum are expected to develop immediately after drug administration and trough concentrations occur just before. It is not always obvious when peak and trough concentrations will be reached. As discussed, rate and completeness of drug absorption are major factors influencing the time and peak of drug concentration. Serious timing problems arise in serum drug sampling, even with intravenous drug administration, because of delays in completion of infusion of the drug into the patient. Less problematic is timing of trough concentrations. Trough serum drug concentrations are invariably present just before administration of the subsequent drug dose.

The concept of steady state (Fig 10-8) with repeated doses of drug is important to appropriate timing of serum sampling in monitoring drug therapy. Blood samples obtained before steady state do not represent or predict drug concentrations at steady state. Dosage adjustments based on such premature data can result in serious dosage errors.

Loading doses of drug may be necessary to achieve adequate therapeutic drug concentrations rapidly, thus reducing the time

required to achieve maximum therapeutic effect. Drugs that use loading dose regimens include digoxin, phenobarbital, theophylline, and chloramphenicol. If saturation pharmacokinetics exist, each dosage change should be about 30% to minimize overcompensation. After a dosage change, steady state should be reestablished before monitoring the effect of the change on serum drug concentration.

## CONCLUSION

The history of drug therapy-related problems should convince physicians that it is important to have a scientific basis (controlled clinical trial) for the expectation of therapeutic efficacy and a working knowledge of the pharmacologic principles outlined here. This knowledge base and an appreciation of drug pharmacology provide the best opportunity to maximize drug efficacy and minimize drug potential for toxicity. Representative examples of dosages specifically for neonates are included in Appendix 10-1.

## Selected Readings

American Academy of Pediatrics Committee on Drugs. Inactive ingredients in pharmaceutical products. Pediatrics 1985;76:635.

Aranda JV, Stern L. Clinical aspects of developmental pharmacology and toxicology. Pharmacol Ther 1983;20:1.

Lang D, Hofstetter R, von Bernuth G. Postmortem tissue and plasma concentrations of digoxin in newborns and infants. Eur J Pediatr 1978;128:151.

Leff RD, Roberts RJ. Practical Aspects of Intravenous Drug Therapy Techniques, ed 2. Bethesda: American Society of Hospital Pharmacists, 1991.

Roberts RJ. Drug therapy in infants: pharmacological principles and clinical experience. Philadelphia: WB Saunders, 1984.

Roberts RJ. Developmental aspects of clinical pharmacology. In: Spector R, ed. The scientific basis of clinical pharmacology: principles and examples. Boston: Little, Brown & Co, 1986:160.

Warner A. Drug use in the neonate: interrelationships of pharmacokinetics, toxicity and biochemical maturity. Clin Chem 1986;32:721.

## APPENDIX 10-1

The following table provides initial dosage recommendations for selected drugs. Dosages for each neonate must be individualized to maximize efficacy and minimize toxicity.

| | Drug Dosages for Neonates | | |
|---|---|---|---|
| Drug | Route; Dose | Therapeutic Serum Concentration | Potential Toxicity |
| Albumin, 5% | IV; 1.0 g/kg slowly | | Hypervolemia, congestive heart failure |
| Ampicillin | Neonates < 7 days IM, IV; 25 mg–50 mg/kg q 12 h; >7 days IM, IV; 25 mg–50 mg/kg q 8 h IM or IV | | |
| Atropine | IV; 0.01 mg/kg, up to maximum total dose of 0.04 mg/kg | | Fever, tachycardia, loss of GI motility |
| Caffeine | PO, IV; Loading dose*: 10 mg/kg; Maintenance dose*: 2.5 mg/kg q 24 h | 5 ng–20 ng/mL | Tachycardia |
| Calcium salts | IV; bolus therapy 1.0 mEq/kg†; continuous infusion | | Bradycardia with rapid infusion, tissue necrosis with infiltration |
| Carbenicillin | Neonates < 7 days, IV; 100 mg/kg initial, then 75 mg/kg q 8 h; >7 days, IV; 100 mg/kg q 6–8 h | | |
| Chloramphenicol | PO, IV; Loading dose: 20 mg/kg; Maintenance dose: PO, IV 2.5 up to 12.5 mg/kg q 6 h | 10 $\mu$g–25 $\mu$g/mL | Blood level monitoring mandatory; hematologic, cardiac toxicity, "gray syndrome" |
| Chlorpromazine | PO, IM, IV; 0.2 mg–0.5 mg/kg q 6 h | | Extrapyramidal symptoms, potentiate sed-hypnotics and narcotics |
| Chlorothiazide | PO; 10 mg–20 mg/kg/q 12 h | | Hypokalemia, hyponatremia |
| Dexamethasone | IM, IV; Loading dose: 0.5–1.0 mg; Maintenance dose: 0.05 mg–0.1 mg/kg/q 6 h | | |
| Diazepam (Valium) | PO; IV; IM<br>Sedative: 0.02 mg–0.3 mg/kg q 6–8 h<br>Seizure: 0.3 mg–1.0 mg/kg slow IV push, use increments of 0.2 mg/kg q 2 min | | Diluted injection may precipitate. IM may result in poor absorption, respiratory depression, hypotension |
| Digoxin | Digitalization dose (TDD): IM or PO‡<br>Prematures < 2.5 kg   Dose 10 $\mu$g–20 $\mu$g/kg<br>Full term to 1 month   40 $\mu$g–60 $\mu$g/kg<br>Maintenance Dose: TDD is given in 3 to 4 divided doses over 24–36 h. ¼ of TDD in 2 divided doses (q 12 h). Usual dose 2.5 $\mu$g–5 $\mu$g/kg q 12 h. (Start maintenance dose 12 h after last digitalization dose.) | 1.5 ng–3.0 ng/mL | Monitoring for cardiotoxicity mandatory. Renal dysfunction requires blood level monitoring. |
| Dopamine | IV 2 $\mu$g–20 $\mu$g/kg/min | | |
| Epinephrine | IV or intratracheal; 1:10,000 (may dilute 1 mL 1:1000 with 9 mL saline) 1 mL–2 mL, repeated as needed. | | Tachycardia |
| Erythromycin (ethylsuccinate) (lactobionate) | PO, IV; 10 mg/kg q h | | IV administration painful |
| Furosemide (Lasix) | PO, IV; 1.0 mg/kg/dose up to 2 mg/kg | | Hypokalemia, hyponatremia, hypochloremia |
| Gentamicin | IV, IM; 2.5 mg/kg q 8–12 | 2 $\mu$g–8 $\mu$g/mL | Blood level monitoring indicated, nephrotoxic, ototoxic |
| Hydrochlorothiazide (Hydrodiuril) | PO; 1 mg–2 mg/kg every 12 h | | |
| Indomethacin (Indocin) | PO, IV; initial dose 0.3 mg/kg then 0.2 mg/kg at 24 h and 48 h as necessary | | Transient renal dysfunction |
| Isoproterenol | IV; 0.05 $\mu$g–0.1 $\mu$g/kg/min, increase to maximum 2 $\mu$g/kg/min | | |
| Meperidine | IV; 0.5 mg/kg/dose q 4 h PRN | | Respiratory depression reversible with naloxone |
| Methicillin (Staphcillin) | Neonate: IV; <7 days, 25 mg/kg q 8–12 h<br>              >7 days, q 6–8 h | | |
| Morphine sulfate | IV; 0.1 mg/kg/dose q 6 h PRN | | Respiratory depression reversible with naloxone |
| Naloxone HCl (Narcan) | IV, IM; 0.1 mg/kg/dose. May repeat as necessary | | |

*(continued)*

## Drug Dosages for Neonates *(Continued)*

| Drug | Route; Dose | Therapeutic Serum Concentration | Potential Toxicity |
|---|---|---|---|
| Nitroprusside (Nipride) | IV; begin 1.0 μg/kg/min, increase as needed to control blood pressure. Should not exceed 2 μg/kg/min | | Profound hypotension possible, requires arterial BP monitoring. Thiocyanate and cyanide toxicity with long-term use |
| Pancuronium | IV; 0.02 mg/kg dose q 1–4 h PRN | | Edema patient requires mechanical ventilation. |
| Paraldehyde | PO, rectal; 0.15 mL/kg. Repeat q 4–6 h | | IM may cause sterile abscess. |
| Phenytoin | Loading dose: IV; 20 mg/kg; Maintenance dose: IV, PO; 4 mg–8 mg/kg q 24 h or up to q 12 or 8 h | 5 μg–15 μg/mL | Therapeutic blood level monitoring indicated, blood dyscrasias, rash, cardiac arrhythmia |
| Penicillin G | IM, IV; aqueous solution 20,000–50,000 units/kg q 8 h<br><br>IM; 20,000 units/kg/divided over 3–15 days (for treatment of congenital syphilis) | | |
| Prostaglandin | IV; 0.05 μg/kg/min initial, may reduce dose to as low as 0.002 μg/kg/min. Do not exceed 0.1 μg/kg/min | | Apnea, seizurelike activity, flushing, hypoglycemia hypotension |
| Phenobarbital | Anticonvulsant: Loading dose: 10 mg–20 mg/kg/ slow IV push. May repeat.<br>Maintenance dose: IV, PO; 2 mg–4 mg/kg q 12 h | 15 μg–40 μg/mL | Therapeutic blood level monitoring indicated, hypersensitivity reactions (rash, blood dyscrasias), CNS depression |
| Priscoline (Tolazoline) | Loading dose: 2 mg/kg IV push<br>Maintenance dose: IV; 2 mg/kg/h | | Hypotension, GI and pulmonary bleeding, renal dysfunction |
| Propranolol (Inderal) | IV; 0.05 mg–0.15 mg/kg infused over 10 min; may be repeated in 10 min, then given every 6 h<br>PO; 0.25 mg/kg q 6–8 h up to maximum daily dose of 4 mg/kg | | Contraindicated in low-output congestive heart failure |
| Sodium bicarbonate | IV; 1 mEq–2 mEq/kg/dose | | Dilute to half strength.<br>Infuse slowly.<br>Monitoring of blood gases is imperative. |
| Spironolactone (Aldactone) | PO; 1 mg–3 mg/kg every 24 h. | | Onset of action is delayed; active metabolite must be formed. |
| THAM (tromethamine) | Total dose (mL) = kg of body weight × base deficit. ¼ dose over 2–5 min; rest according to response. Max. (24 h) 40 mL/kg | | Monitoring of blood gases is imperative. |
| Theophylline | PO, IV; Loading dose: 5 mg/kg<br>Maintenance dose: 1 mg/kg q 8 h to 3.6 mg/kg q 12 h | 4 μg–15 μg/mL | Blood level monitoring is required.<br>Vomiting, tachycardia, seizures |
| Tobramycin | Same as gentamicin | | |
| Vancomycin | IV, PO; 15 mg/kg q 12 h | 25 μg–40 μg/mL | Nephrotoxicity, ototoxicity.<br>Serum-level monitoring is recommended. |

\* Doses are for the free base.
† Use extreme care in calculation of dose volume for various calcium preparations.
‡ IV dose is 75% of IM or PO dose.

*Principles and Practice of Pediatrics, Second Edition.*
edited by Frank A. Oski et al. J. B. Lippincott Company, Philadelphia © 1994.

## CHAPTER 11
# *The Pathophysiology of Body Fluids*

### Norman J. Siegel, Thomas Carpenter, and Karen M. Gaudio

This chapter considers the pathophysiology of body fluids. We will use parenteral fluid therapy as an approach to our understanding of the body's need for fluids and electrolytes. With an understanding of basic physiologic principles that relate to the maintenance of "the sea within us," we will be able to dissect and understand perturbations in fluid volume, electrolyte content, and mineral metabolism. In *From Fish to Philosopher*, Homer Smith put forth the intriguing hypothesis that we have evolved as a higher species and are able to reason and think by virtue of the complexity of our kidney, which allows us to maintain ourselves free from the sea for long periods. As Claude Bernard, the renowned 19th century physiologist noted, we live either in air or in water, the plasma or liquid part of the blood that bathes all our tissues and elements. This chapter is devoted to an understanding, then, of this internal environment from which we achieve a free and independent life, physically and mentally.

## PARENTERAL FLUID THERAPY

Parenteral fluid therapy, the provision of fluids and electrolytes intravenously, long has been the bailiwick of pediatricians. In 1831, O'Shaugnessy conceived the idea that replacing the water and salt lost during cholera might help to decrease the mortality from that disorder. Latta attempted to put O'Shaugnessy's theories into practice and successfully administered fluid and electrolytes to an aging patient in whom all other attempts had failed. It was not until the 20th century, however, that interest in intravenous fluid therapy was revived. By this time, pediatricians had assumed a leading role in advancing our understanding of the pathophysiology of fluids and electrolytes, and had made important observations. Howland and Marriot observed that acidosis occurred as a consequence of dehydration, and Gamble conceived the compartmentalization of body fluids, which still is used as a conceptual framework (Gamble, 1950). During the first half of this century, many pediatricians made additional contributions that have allowed us to become more sophisticated in our use of intravenous fluid and electrolyte therapy.

Partly because of the diffuse interest in this area and partly because no single system can be shown to be markedly superior, a large number of different approaches to parenteral fluid therapy have been advocated. In the final analysis, the majority of these systems are empiric, based on clinical experience, and, in many cases, quite interchangeable. A broad overview provides us with some guiding principles, which actually are common to a variety of different systems for parenteral fluid therapy:

1. Therapy must be individualized for every patient, and a cookbook approach is discouraged.
2. Calculations of the requirements for either fluids or electrolytes always are estimates based largely on empiric observations and cannot be assumed to be definitive.
3. The patient's condition, particularly his or her response to the therapy being administered, is the ultimate determinant of the success of any parenteral fluid therapy program.
4. Simplicity in the design and execution of parenteral fluid therapy is essential for accurate and effective treatment of the patient.

Parenteral fluid therapy is divided into three major components: maintenance therapy designed to maintain a state of hydration until oral feedings or fluids can be reinstituted; deficit therapy designed to replace losses of salt and water that occurred before a physician encountered the patient; and replacement therapy designed to replace ongoing losses after the patient has entered a therapeutic program.

## Maintenance Fluids

We will use maintenance therapy to illustrate the basic principles and as a touchstone for parenteral fluid therapy in infants and children. Conceptually, maintenance therapy is designed to replace the water and electrolytes that are lost under ordinary homeostatic conditions during which the patient is relatively inactive and afebrile. The volume of fluid provided requires minimal renal compensation and assumes that urine will be excreted in an isotonic manner (specific gravity 1.010 or osmolarity 280 to 310 mOsm/L). Fluid requirements for maintenance therapy are related to the metabolic rate and to energy expenditures. Holliday and Segar demonstrated that the rate of caloric expenditure was relatively fixed for infants and children in three weight categories. In children weighing between 1 and 10 kg, the rate was 100 calories/kg; in those weighing between 11 and 20 kg, it was 50 calories/kg; and in those weighing between 21 to 80 kg, it was 20 calories/kg. Many of the initial programs for fluid therapy suggested that water would be expended at a rate of 120 mL/kcal of energy expenditure. These original assumptions did not take into account two endogenous sources of water, however: water of oxidation, which contributes 17 mL/100 kcal; and preformed water, which contributes 3 mL/100 kcal. Thus, as these more complex systems are simplified, it becomes apparent that 100 mL of exogenous water needs to be supplied for every 100 kcal of energy expended. Therefore, a single sliding scale can be used to estimate both a caloric expenditure and total maintenance fluid required (Table 11-1). For example, a child who weighs 13 kg would have an estimated maintenance fluid requirement of 1150 mL/d: 1000 mL would be for the first 10 kg, then 50 mL/kg for the next 3 kg equals 1000 mL plus 150 mL, or a total of 1150 mL/day. Similarly, this same patient would be expected to have a caloric expenditure of about 1,150 kcal/day. In using the sliding scale shown in Table 11-1, it must be recognized that, after 80 kg, the proportion of body weight and water distribution

---

**TABLE 11-1. Estimate of Caloric Expenditure or Volume of Maintenance Fluids\***

| Body Weight (kg) | Caloric Expenditure (kcal/kg/d) Maintenance Fluids (mL/kg/d) |
|---|---|
| 1–10 | 100/kg |
| 11–20 | 1000 + 50/kg more than 10 kg |
| 21–80 | 1500 + 20/kg more than 20 kg |

\* Example: Assume that a child is afebrile and minimally active. A 13-kg child needs 1000 + 50 (13 − 10) = 1150 kcal or mL/d.

diverges significantly, so that calculations extended beyond 80 kg are likely to be a significant overestimate of fluid requirements.

Having made an estimate of the volume of fluid required to maintain a homeostatic condition for the patient, it is important to understand that maintenance fluids will provide for losses from two major sources only: evaporative or insensible losses and urinary losses. Fluids and electrolytes lost from other sources are termed third-space losses.

Fluid lost from the skin and lungs originally was considered insensible because, when attempts were made to account for fluids used in metabolic balance studies, these two sites were not readily apparent. Eventually, it was recognized that water is used for thermal regulation and to humidify inspired air. Evaporative water lost from the skin is not apparent and is lost by the means of convection and conduction to regulate core body temperature. This is not ordinary sweat. Water lost through the lungs is used to humidify the air we breathe so that it is 100% saturated by the time it reaches the bifurcation of the trachea. In the usual environment and under ordinary conditions, insensible or evaporative losses amount to about one third of the calculated maintenance fluids. Clearly, then, ambient temperature and humidity will have a profound effect on the volume of fluid lost. An increase in insensible losses might be anticipated when children are hyperthermic or tachypneic, are placed under a radiant warmer, or otherwise are exposed to a dry or particularly hot environment. For example, a body temperature greater than 38°C will increase insensible fluid losses by 12.5% per degree of fever. In contrast, a significant reduction in evaporative fluid losses might be expected when children are receiving humidified air or when they are hypothermic. The proportion of losses between skin and lungs is about two thirds and one third, respectively. Finally, it is apparent that evaporative fluid losses do not contain solutes and, therefore, the fluid required to replace this volume should be free of electrolytes.

During maintenance fluid therapy, we expect that urinary losses will account for about two thirds of the calculated maintenance requirement and that the patient will be capable of making urine that is isosthenuric. In most clinical situations in which the patient might be expected to make a more dilute urine (diabetes insipidus, prematurity of birth, sickle-cell disease), an appropriate increase in maintenance fluids must be provided. On the other hand, in those clinical situations in which it is not possible to dilute the urine to a specific gravity of 1.010 or an osmolality of 300 mOsm/L (excessive or inappropriate antidiuretic hormone [ADH] release, congestive heart failure), the volume of maintenance fluids must be decreased appropriately.

Early empiric studies determined that about 2 to 3 mEq of sodium and chloride, and 2 to 2.5 mEq of potassium were required for each 100 kcal expended or for each 100 mL of maintenance fluid needed to maintain normal electrolyte homeostasis and allow for growth. The addition of 5 g of dextrose in each 100 mL of fluid would allow for the provision of about 20% of the caloric

need when full maintenance fluid volume could be administered. Therefore, the parenteral fluid solution recommended for maintenance fluid therapy contains 25 to 30 mEq/L of sodium and chloride, 20 mEq/L of potassium, and 50 g/L of dextrose. A number of commercially available solutions meet the requirements for maintenance therapy. Table 11-2 illustrates the composition of various commonly used solutions as they relate to normal saline as a standard. For the purpose of maintenance therapy, a solution of D5 0.2 NS plus 20 mEq/L of potassium would be recommended commonly.

Having made calculations of the volume of fluid to be administered and having chosen an appropriate fluid to meet the objectives of maintenance therapy, it is essential that we return to the bedside and judge the adequacy of these estimates. The major clinical parameters we will use will be a change in body weight, a change in serum sodium concentration, and the overall status of the patient. Because maintenance therapy provides for only 20% of the caloric expenditure, we should anticipate that our patient will lose weight at about 0.5% to 1% per day because of this deficit caloric intake. It must be recognized that, if the volume of fluid being administered is less than full maintenance therapy, the impact on nutrition will be even greater. We also should anticipate that the serum sodium level will remain between 130 and 140 mEq/L if we are providing adequate fluids and electrolytes to meet the ongoing maintenance needs. A gain in weight combined with a fall in serum sodium level or the development of peripheral edema would suggest that our patient is being overhydrated, and we must assess those factors that would reduce either insensible or urinary fluid losses. In contrast, a very rapid loss of weight, a continuing increase in the serum sodium level, or a persistent tachycardia would suggest that we have provided inadequate fluids, and we must assess those factors that would increase fluid losses. Having considered the volume and content of fluid to be given to maintain homeostatic conditions, we now will turn our attention to fluid and electrolyte therapy in disordered states.

## Disorders of Volume Depletion

Small infants and young children are particularly susceptible to volume depletion and concomitant dehydration from common abnormalities such as gastroenteritis, diarrhea, vomiting, and excessive fluid losses. Before the effective development of parenteral fluid therapy, seasonal diarrhea and endemic or epidemic episodes of gastroenteritis were a major cause of significant morbidity and mortality in children. A limited ability of the kidney in the premature infant and young child to concentrate the urine maximally makes these individuals particularly susceptible to dehydration. This limited concentrating ability is the result of intrinsic factors, particularly decreased urea deposition in the medullary portion of the kidney, which limits the concentrating gradient and is a reflection of the normal development of renal function. The lim-

TABLE 11-2.  Electrolyte Composition of Common Parenteral Solutions

| Electrolyte | Normal Saline (NS) | D5 0.5 NS | D5 0.2 NS | Ringer's Lactate | Plasmalyte A |
|---|---|---|---|---|---|
| Na (mEq/L) | 155 | 75 | 35 | 130 | 140 |
| Cl (mEq/L) | 155 | 75 | 35 | 109 | 98 |
| K (mEq/L) | ... | ... | ... | 4 | 5 |
| Glucose (g/L) | ... | 50 | 50 | ... | ... |
| Lactate (mEq/L) | ... | ... | ... | 28 | ... |
| Acetate (mEq/L) | ... | ... | ... | ... | 27 |

ited capacity to conserve water, however, results in a very narrow margin of reserve for these children when they are exposed to fluid losses outside the range of normal expectations.

The expected pathophysiologic response to diminished intravascular volume with concomitant decreases in cardiac output is shown in Figure 11-1. For individuals with an intact cardiovascular system and kidney, a decrease in intravascular volume will result in diminished renal perfusion, stimulation of adrenergic activity, and release of ADH. The intrarenal hemodynamic response to diminished renal plasma flow is to elicit the release of renin and concomitantly to maintain glomerular filtration rate (GFR) by constriction of the efferent arteriole. Because GFR is maintained at relatively normal values while renal plasma flow has diminished (termed an increase in filtration fraction), a greater fraction of the plasma in the glomerular capillary bed has been filtered and the postglomerular capillary will have an increase in protein concentration and a decrease in capillary hydrostatic pressure. This increase in capillary oncotic pressure and decrease in hydrostatic pressure serves to enhance peritubular capillary reabsorption in the proximal tubule. Thus, the quantity of sodium and fluid reabsorbed from the proximal portion of the nephron is enhanced. Salt and water reabsorption in the distal part of the nephron is increased also. Aldosterone secretion by the zona glomerulosa of the adrenal cortex has occurred in response to the circulating angiotensin II, which was produced from the increased renin secretion. Aldosterone stimulates sodium reabsorption in exchange for potassium in the distal tubule and early collecting duct. Finally, the ADH that was released in response to diminished cardiac output will increase the permeability of the collecting duct to water and result in enhanced water reabsorption in this final segment of the nephron. Taken together, each of these factors will maximize the reabsorption of salt and water such that, in a severely dehydrated state, the kidney will excrete less than 0.1% of the filtered sodium and, after maturity, will be able to achieve a urinary osmolarity in excess of 1000 mOsm/L. If the period of excessive volume loss is extensive, these compensatory mechanisms will provide only partial repletion of the intravascular volume and the patient eventually will become dehydrated. When these compensatory mechanisms are limited because of either intrinsic renal disease or immaturity of the kidney, the infant or young child is less able to adapt to states of volume loss and becomes dehydrated more rapidly.

**Deficit Fluid Therapy**

In evaluating a child who is dehydrated, three essential steps must be completed:

1. The degree or severity of the dehydration must be estimated.
2. The type of deficit must be determined.
3. A plan for repair of the deficit must be developed and initiated.

The first step in our assessment requires carefully obtaining the history and performing a clinical evaluation. Unfortunately, no one laboratory finding can determine accurately the severity or degree of dehydration. The only truly objective means of making such a determination is to know precisely the change in body weight that has occurred over a limited period. Therefore, the estimate of the degree of dehydration is made most often on the basis of clinical observation and experience. Table 11-3 lists a number of clinical features that can be used in assessing the degree of dehydration. Similar clinical findings will represent a different degree of dehydration in older children as compared to infants. With mild degrees of volume depletion, the clinical signs are not very remarkable, and one relies largely on a history of excessive fluid losses. When the patient approaches a more moderate state of dehydration, the clinical findings become more apparent and usually are corroborated by the duration of vomiting, diarrhea, or other sources of fluid loss. For patients with severe dehydration, we must consider this a nearly shock-like state, which requires

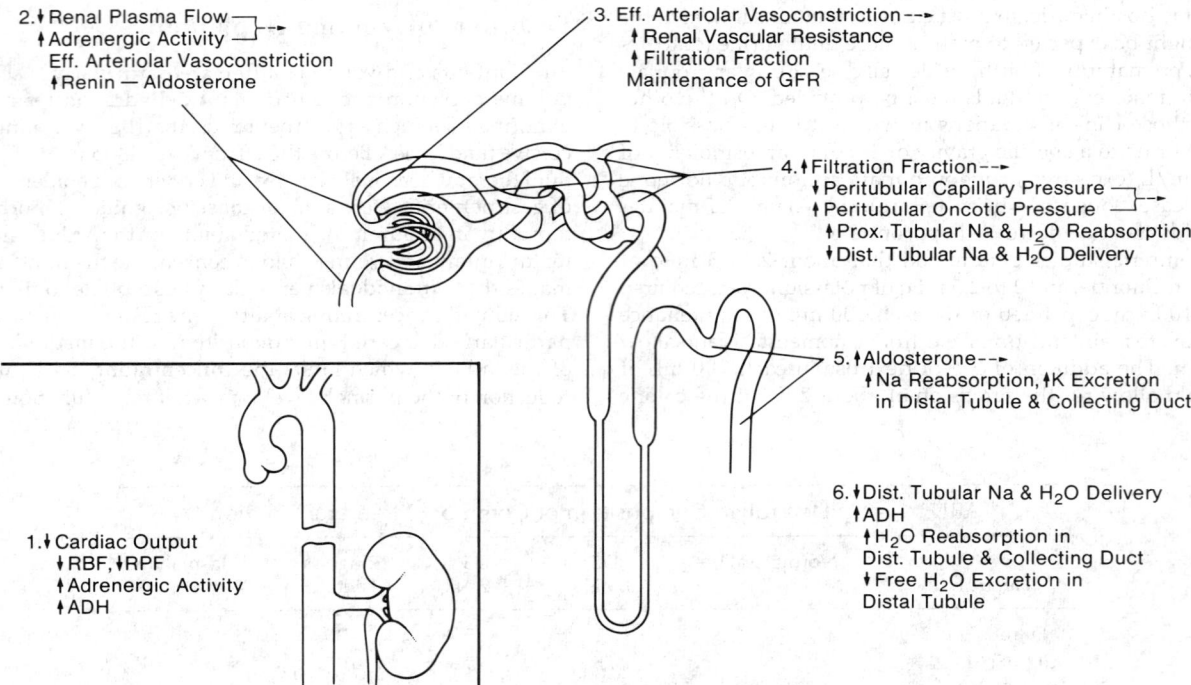

**Figure 11-1.** Pathophysiologic response to decreased cardiac output or diminished renal perfusion. In patients who are volume depleted, this sequence of events will attempt to restore intravascular volume. In patients who are volume overloaded, these responses will result in edema formation. *GFR,* glomerular filtration rate; *Prox,* proximal; *Dist,* distal; *RBF,* renal blood flow; *RPF,* renal plasma flow; *ADH,* antidiuretic hormone; *Eff,* efferent.

TABLE 11-3. Evaluation of Severity of Dehydration

| Examination | Older Child: 3%<br>Infant: 5% | 6%<br>10% | 9%<br>15% |
|---|---|---|---|
| Skin turgor | Normal | Tenting | None |
| Skin—touch | Normal | Dry | Clammy |
| Buccal mucosa/lips | Moist | Dry | Parched/cracked |
| Eyes | Normal | Deep-set | Sunken |
| Crying—tears | Present | Reduced | None |
| Fontanelle | Flat | Soft | Sunken |
| CNS | Consolable | Irritable | Lethargic |
| Pulse | Regular | Slight increased | Tachycardia |
| Urine output | Normal | Decreased | Anuria |

the initiation of resuscitative fluids in an expeditious manner to prevent the development of irreversible metabolic changes. It must be remembered that this initial assessment of the patient, which will provide the basis for developing a plan for rehydration, is almost always subjective, and that the assessment of a given patient by several skilled observers may produce widely varying estimates of the degree of dehydration that is present. Nevertheless, this assessment is essential and, therefore, must be performed and recorded carefully.

Our second objective is to determine the type of dehydration that has occurred. Conventionally, this determination is based on serum electrolyte levels and is defined in three categories: isotonic (serum sodium 130 to 150 mEq/L), hypotonic (serum sodium less than 130 mEq/L), and hypertonic (serum sodium greater than 155 mEq/L). Although these terms are used to define a type of dehydration for the clinical purposes of planning an approach for fluid replacement, the patient's serum electrolyte levels really are a mirror image of the type of losses that have occurred. For example, in a patient who has hypotonic dehydration (ie, a serum sodium level less than 130 mEq/L), it is likely that the losses have consisted of more sodium than water or that their replacement fluid has contained an excess of free water. The pathophysiologic adaptive mechanisms to dehydration (see Fig 11-1) place particular constraints on free water excretion.

Therefore, the patient who is lacking in essential electrolytes and takes in a great deal of fluid will become hypotonic. Similarly, for the patient with hypertonic dehydration (serum sodium greater than 155 mEq/L), it is most likely that the fluid losses have consisted of more water than electrolytes. This is particularly evident in certain types of diarrhea, in which the electrolyte losses may be very low but the water losses quite high, or in situations in which the predominant form of water loss is through an increase in insensible losses because these latter losses are free of electrolytes. For example, the patient who is exposed to a prolonged period of thirsting and fasting essentially has no intake of any type of fluid and will have hypertonic dehydration because of the continued loss of solute-free fluid from the skin and lungs. In large part, patients with isotonic or hypotonic dehydration are treated quite similarly, whereas patients with hypertonic dehydration require special consideration.

The final aspect of deficit fluid therapy is to plan an approach for rehydration (Table 11-4). Just as there are multiple systems for calculating or determining maintenance fluid therapy, there are a number of different approaches to the design of rehydration fluids. In the last analysis, most of these programs are interchangeable; no one approach is superior to any other. With careful attention to the patient and recognition of certain guidelines, effective therapy can be developed in most clinical situations. Our

TABLE 11-4. Programs for Deficit Fluid Therapy

| | Plan I* | Plan II* | Plan III† |
|---|---|---|---|
| **Phase One** | | | |
| Volume | 1%–2% BW/(10–20 mL/kg) | 1%–2% BW/(10–20 mL/kg) | 1%–2% BW/(10–20 mL/kg) |
| Fluid | NS, RL, PLA | NS, RL, PLA | NS, RL, PLA |
| Duration | 1–2 h | 1–2 h | 1–2 h |
| **Phase Two** | | | |
| Volume | Replace entire deficit | ⅓ maintenance + ½ deficit | Maintenance + deficit |
| Fluid | D5 0.5 NS + 20 mEq/L K | D5 0.5 NS + 20 mEq/L K | D5 0.2 NS + 20 mEq/L K |
| Duration | 6 h | 8 h | 24–48 h |
| **Phase Three** | | | |
| Volume | Maintenance + replacement | Maintenance + replacement + residual deficit | Maintenance + replacement |
| Fluid | D5 0.2 NS + 20 mEq/L K | D5 0.2 NS + 20 mEq/L K | D5 0.2 NS + 20 mEq/L K |
| Duration | As required | As required | As required |

BW, body weight; NS, normal saline; RL, Ringer's lactate; PLA, plasmalyte A.
* Plans I and II are used for hypotonic or isotonic dehydration.
† Plan III is used for hypertonic dehydration.

attention should be turned first to the restoration and preservation of cardiovascular function to aid in the perfusion of the brain and kidneys, and to allow the adaptive mechanisms (illustrated in Fig 11-1) to help us in reestablishing intravascular volume. Thus, the first phase of therapy should consist of the rapid infusion of a relatively isotonic fluid. For these purposes, normal saline, Ringer's lactate, or plasmalyte A usually are administered. The rate of infusion is 1% to 2% of body weight (10 to 20 mL/kg) over 1 to 2 hours. This initial rapid infusion of isotonic fluid allows the therapist an opportunity to assess the initial laboratory data and to plan the remainder of rehydration in an orderly manner while preventing the patient from becoming increasingly dehydrated, because it is unlikely that the sources of fluid loss will abate immediately upon initiation of therapy.

The major objective of the second phase of therapy is to replace the deficit of fluids and electrolytes that has occurred. This may be accomplished in several different ways, but certain principles must be observed.

1. Total body repair will require a relatively prolonged period in all types of dehydration.
2. Total body potassium losses cannot be replaced rapidly because potassium is predominantly an intracellular ion. Therefore, potassium should be added to the rehydration solution only after the patient has voided and then in concentrations that generally do not exceed 40 mEq/L or a rate of infusion of 0.5 mEq/kg/h.
3. A solution of half normal saline is used during the period of rehydration because it has been determined empirically that this concentration of sodium is relatively safe for the majority of causes of dehydration in children. This solution provides more sodium than do standard maintenance fluids and more water, proportional to sodium, than is contained in plasma (see Table 11-2). Thus, 0.5 NS serves well to replace the deficits in both salt and water.
4. The patient must be monitored very carefully during the period of rehydration.

Remembering that the initial estimate of the degree of dehydration is based on subjective criteria, we must rely on the patient's clinical response to therapy as an indication of the adequacy of our calculations. After the initiation of deficit therapy, we should note improvement in the patient's general condition over a relatively short period. It is expected that the urine normally will be quite concentrated initially, with specific gravities between 1.020 and 1.030, and that, during the course of rehydration, there will be a progressive decrease in the specific gravity of the urine and a progressive increase in the frequency of urination as intravascular volume is replaced. As illustrated in Table 11-4, there are several different approaches to this second phase of deficit therapy. In small children who are dehydrated mildly to moderately, or for whom intravenous access may be a problem, it is quite feasible to replace the entire deficit in 6 hours (plan I). In some cases, this requires the relatively rapid infusion of large volumes of fluid and, therefore, it generally is not recommended for use in adolescents, patients with diabetic ketoacidosis, or children with more than 10% dehydration. In these circumstances and in older children, it is preferable to embark on a somewhat slower plan for rehydration in which the patient is given one third of the maintenance volume plus one half of the deficit over the first 8 hours of rehydration (plan II). In children who weigh 10 kg or less, the volume of fluid to be administered will be quite similar in both plans I and II. Either of these approaches is quite satisfactory for the rehydration of patients with isotonic or hypotonic dehydration.

Children with hypertonic dehydration represent a very special and complex problem. As illustrated in plan III in Table 11-4, these children must be approached more cautiously and their estimated deficit should be replaced over 24 to 48 hours. These patients require particularly careful reassessment, and the goal should be to lower the serum sodium level by no more than 0.4 to 0.8 mEq/L/h or 10 to 12 mEq/L/d. A more rapid fall in the serum sodium level suggests that the rehydration plan is overzealous and could be associated with the development of significant central nervous system symptoms and seizures. It also must be remembered that hyperglycemia frequently is present in patients with hypertonic dehydration. Therefore, in these patients, the effective serum sodium level is even higher than the measured serum sodium level. Thus, during the first 2 to 3 hours of rehydration, failure of the serum sodium level to correct significantly may represent simply a clearing of the hyperglycemia with a resultant shift of water into cells, rather than underhydration. These children sometimes have hypocalcemia, which will complicate their assessment in terms of neurologic signs and may need specific correction. It also must be recognized that these children have a greater deficit of water than sodium and, therefore, the solution used for rehydration should contain only 30 to 40 mEq/L of sodium as compared to the fluid recommended for children with isotonic or hypotonic dehydration.

In all types of dehydration, this second phase of deficit therapy must be monitored carefully, and its duration will depend on the patient's response to treatment. Although a specific rate of infusion may have been chosen to deliver a specific amount of fluid over a fixed period, this frequently will need to be adjusted according to the patient's clinical response. If the patient has persistent tachycardia and continues to demonstrate the signs of dehydration shown in Table 11-3, it is quite possible that the degree of dehydration was underestimated initially or that the ongoing losses have been substantial enough to prevent adequate rehydration of the patient. In such circumstances, the rate of fluid administration will need to be increased and the appropriateness of the fluids being administered will need to be reevaluated. In situations in which the patient's clinical condition improves rapidly, urine output is brisk, and specific gravity is decreasing progressively, and in which the signs of intravascular volume depletion are diminished, one may choose to switch from phase 2 to phase 3 of deficit therapy earlier than originally estimated.

Phase 3 of deficit therapy essentially is a transition toward maintenance fluid therapy. In addition to the usual maintenance therapy, one must provide for ongoing fluid losses from sources other than evaporative or urinary losses.

### Replacement Therapy

Fluids designed to replenish ongoing losses usually are termed *replacement therapy*. The composition of the electrolytes in various body fluids can vary considerably from patient to patient and may be quite different from the fluids used for either maintenance or deficit therapy. Therefore, in situations in which it is expected that third-space losses will continue for a significant period, it is preferable to measure specifically the electrolyte content of those fluids and then replace them milliequivalent for milliequivalent and milliliter for milliliter. In children receiving parenteral alimentation, there always is a tendency to replace ongoing losses simply by increasing the volume of the intravenous fluid being administered. Such procedures actually may produce paradoxic results and cause significant derangement of serum electrolyte levels. The use of intravenous alimentation solutions to replace ongoing losses may present patients with a renal solute load that will challenge their concentrating capacity and, thereby, obligate sufficient intracellular water to be used for the excretion of excessive solutes. Thus, as the rate of infusion is increased, the patient clinically will appear to become increasingly dehydrated and will be making a large volume of urine, which is concentrated because of the osmolar diuresis induced by the renal solute load.

In some instances, it may be very difficult to judge the magnitude of third-space loss, particularly if patients have an ileus, ascites, burns, or open wounds. In such instances, it may be necessary to monitor central volume to provide a more accurate estimate of these ongoing losses and to allow for a more judicious plan for replacement therapy.

Finally, no discussion of fluid therapy would be complete without a consideration of oral rehydration. The administration of specific fluids and electrolytes by mouth to correct fluid deficits has been of interest for the past 40 years. Traditionally, pediatricians have used a number of commercially available products to provide initial rehydration for children with gastroenteritis. In large measure, these products may have highly variable electrolyte concentrations, but they often have been quite successful, probably because episodes of viral gastroenteritis are of short duration and are self-limited. In the 1940s and 1950s, Darrow and Harrison each formulated specific oral rehydration solutions. Because of untoward side effects of these solutions and others, particularly the development of hypernatremia, there was initial considerable concern about the appropriate sodium concentration for these products. Moreover, the use of ordinary kitchen utensils for the preparation of these solutions frequently led to aberrant electrolyte contents. In the midst of this controversy, Franz and Segar demonstrated that, when the sodium concentration in oral hydration solutions was doubled, there was no difference in the serum sodium level as long as all the children took in an average of 135 mL/kg/d of fluid. This was a particularly important observation, indicating that the volume of fluid being administered probably was more critical than was its specific sodium content. In fact, the World Health Organization has recommended the use of a solution that contains 90 mEq/L of sodium, 20 mEq/L of potassium, and 2 g of glucose per 100 mL of solution. Finberg has raised particular concern about this solution and its administration to young children whose renal function may be immature and whose adaptive mechanisms may not be completely operable. In fact, he has proposed that three different oral hydrating solutions be used during various phases of rehydration. Several workers have defended the solution recommended by the World Health Organization, however, and have pointed out the impracticality of using three different solutions and the potential confusion it presents for parents. Careful scrutiny of the data provided and the types of solutions used previously as well as the current controversies leads to several conclusions:

1. The use of high concentrations of carbohydrate in the past may have resulted in further water losses and prolonged diarrhea because of the rapid transit time, bacterial overgrowth of the small intestine, and disaccharidase deficiencies. Early oral rehydration products contained as much as 8 g of carbohydrate per 100 mL of solution, whereas the most recent recommendation is 2 to 3 g of carbohydrate per 100 mL of solution based on studies that have shown that the maximum absorption of isotonic mixtures of glucose and saline from the gastrointestinal tract occurred when the concentration of glucose was between 56 and 140 mmol/L.
2. It has become apparent that the total amount of fluid ingested is more critical than is the sodium concentration. Because hypotonic fluid usually is lost with diarrhea, and the ongoing body losses of fluids, particularly evaporative losses, also are hypotonic, there is a tendency for the serum sodium level to rise progressively and for the patient to become hypertonic. This can be offset only if the patient takes in an adequate volume of fluid. Consequently, the amount of fluid given is the major determinant of the rise or fall seen in the serum sodium level in patients with diarrhea who are given oral rehydration solutions.
3. Oral rehydration is a particularly personnel-intense program

that requires that the child be given small volumes of fluid at very regular intervals. The cost-benefit ratio of this approach is not likely to prove effective in developed countries. For example, in a study in which oral hydration was given to 100 children in an emergency room, 8 patients required parenteral fluids because of the inability to take oral fluids, 13 returned because of a failure to maintain hydration at home, and the mean emergency room stay for the other patients was 15.5 hours.
4. When oral hydration therapy is feasible, it must be considered as carefully as is parenteral fluid therapy and it requires a prescription as specific and education of parents and care providers as extensive as would be necessary for the initiation of traditional intravenous fluids.

In a randomized, controlled study of 86 infants, 3 to 18 months of age, who were dehydrated mildly to moderately, Pizzaro and associates have shown that oral rehydration solutions containing rice-syrup solids not only promote rehydration and restore fluid volume, but also reduce stool output and volume of diarrhea. These observations suggest that oral hydration therapy may be able to limit the duration of the disease as well as promote the retention of water and electrolytes.

## Disorders of Volume Excess

An excess accumulation of salt and water is termed edema. In states of generalized edema, there is retention of salt and water, and renal regulation of salt and water balance is disturbed. Under usual circumstances, an increase in the intake of sodium would result in the retention of both salt and water, which would increase intravascular volume and, in turn, cause an increase in renal perfusion. Increased intravascular volume leads to a decrease in sodium reabsorption by the kidney and re-regulation of intravascular volume without any net increase in total body salt and water.

Generalized edema usually is a manifestation of either cardiac failure, hepatic cirrhosis, or nephrotic syndrome. Interestingly, in each of these conditions, the pathophysiologic response of the kidney is similar to that which occurs in states of volume depletion. In each of these three clinical disorders, there is either a decrease in cardiac output (congestive heart failure) or a decrease in effective renal perfusion (nephrotic syndrome and hepatic cirrhosis). Once either cardiac output falls or effective renal perfusion is reduced, the sequence of events outlined in Figure 11-1 is set in motion and the kidney responds in a manner designed to increase intravascular volume and to promote increased renal perfusion. Because there are no ongoing excessive losses of salt and water in patients with congestive heart failure, nephrosis, or cirrhosis, this renal response results in a generalized state of salt and water excess, and the eventual development of anasarca.

In patients with congestive heart failure, the decrease in cardiac output is a manifestation of their intrinsic cardiac disease and leads inevitably to a fall in renal plasma flow. If cardiac output is reduced enough, the ability of the efferent arteriole to maintain glomerular filtration will be overridden and a concomitant fall in renal function will occur. A decrease in renal blood flow and the increase in filtration fraction result in maximal stimuli for sodium retention in both the proximal and distal portions of the nephron. Thus, at a time when intravascular volume actually may be expanded, the kidney is responding to further increase salt and water retention and is acting in a manner that is paradoxic to that which would benefit the heart.

In patients with either nephrosis or cirrhosis, there is a decrease in serum albumin because of either a loss of proteins in the urine or diminished protein synthesis by the liver, and, concomitantly, there is a decrease in plasma oncotic pressure. In both conditions, this hypoalbuminemia is associated with decreases in effective renal perfusion and an increase in tubular reabsorption of salt and water. Because of the low plasma oncotic pressure, there is diminished return of interstitial fluid with progressive development of edema, ascites, and, eventually, anasarca. Thus, in a manner analogous to that of congestive heart failure, we find that the kidney is continuing to maximize its reabsorption of salt and water in a physiologic setting in which total body fluid is increased.

The management of edema in each of these disorders is complex and difficult. In patients with congestive heart failure, the most effective form of therapy is to improve their cardiac output, usually with the use of inotropic drugs. In so doing, improved cardiac contractility may result in improved renal perfusion and the sequence of events that leads to salt and water retention effectively can be reversed.

In patients with nephrotic syndrome, the most effective therapy is to reduce their proteinuria, which may be accomplished with corticosteroids in the majority of children with this disorder. If the nephrotic syndrome is persistent, the salt intake must be restricted because the kidney is retaining essentially all the filtered sodium. Remembering that the plasma volume already is reduced slightly in these patients, and that the low plasma oncotic pressure results in a very slow equilibration of fluid from the interstitial to the intravascular space, one must be very cautious with the use of diuretic agents. Overzealous diuresis may diminish plasma volume further and result in significant hypovolemia, decreased GFR, and hypotension. Thus, the primary therapy to limit continued edema formation is restriction of sodium intake.

The management of patients with cirrhosis is equally difficult. Once again, restriction of sodium intake becomes the primary mode of therapy. The use of diuretics may be very complex and result in a stimulation of ammonia production. Because of the diminished plasma oncotic pressure associated with hypoalbuminemia, these patients also are susceptible to severe volume depletion, which can induce the hepatorenal syndrome.

Clearly, in disorders of volume excess, fluid and electrolyte therapy must be undertaken with great caution. Moreover, any therapeutic approach other than allowing patients to regulate their own intake, as long as their thirst mechanism is intact, is likely to result in either fluid or electrolyte abnormalities or a potential worsening of the edema. For these patients, correction of the underlying deficit is the preferred and primary mode of therapy.

## Disorders of Urine Volume

The rate of urine formation is an important index of the clinical stability of children. As demonstrated previously, in euvolemic patients receiving full maintenance therapy, a urine output of 1.5 to 3 mL/kg/h would be expected. Consequently, there is a tendency to assume that changes in urine output must be a direct reflection of renal function. Such assumptions are an oversimplification of complex renal physiology and can be hazardous for patient management. In a mature individual, GFR is about 100 mL/min, which, over a 24-hour period, produces an initial filtrate of 144 L. If each liter contains 145 mEq of sodium, there will be 20,160 mEq (460 g) of sodium entering the proximal tubule each day. The renal tubule and collecting duct reabsorbs 98% to 99% of this filtrate, resulting in a final urine output of about 2 L/d, which contains 4 g of sodium. In most circumstances, the kidney reacts to maintain intravascular volume and plasma tonicity by balancing these processes of filtration, reabsorption, and secretion. The intact kidney, in fact, responds to a variety of stimuli in a reasonably predictable manner, so that an assessment of urinary indices (urinary sodium and urinary osmolarity) can be helpful in evaluating patients with a variety of fluid and electrolyte disorders (Table 11-5). In this context, the urinary sodium concentration will be a good reflection of intravascular volume and renal perfusion. As demonstrated in Figure 11-1, when intravascular volume or renal perfusion is decreased, the sequence of pathophysiologic events results in nearly complete reabsorption of all the filtered sodium. Concomitantly, if renal perfusion is increased or intravascular volume is expanded, there will be a decrease in proximal sodium reabsorption and, consequently, the urinary sodium concentration will be increased. Therefore, a low urinary sodium concentration will occur in those conditions in which renal perfusion is compromised, and an increased urinary sodium concentration will occur either because of expanded intravascular volume or because of a tubular defect in sodium reabsorption. Similarly, the urinary osmolality can be used as an index of the release of ADH, the ability of the collecting duct to respond to this agent, and regulation of serum tonicity.

Because the final urine output is, in fact, the result of the

---

**TABLE 11-5. Clinical Utilization of Urinary Sodium Concentrations and Urine Osmolarity***

| Increased Weight | $U_{Na}$† | $U_{osm}$‡ | Decreased Weight |
|---|---|---|---|
| A. Hypoalbuminemia (nephrosis, cirrhosis, malnutrition)<br>Congestive heart failure<br>Acute glomerulonephritis | <10 | >500 | Dehydration/volume depletion/cystic fibrosis |
| B. Acute volume expansion (water intoxication, excess intravenous fluid) | <10 | <300 | Diabetes insipidus |
| C. Acute renal failure (sepsis, shock, nephrotoxin) | >50 | ≤300 | Adrenal insufficiency; salt-losing nephropathy (interstitial nephritis, cystic disease, or obstructive nephropathy) |
| D. Nonphysiologic ADH secretion | >50 | >500 | Diabetic ketoacidosis; osmotic diuretics |

* Each of the values given represents the most common clinical setting for each condition, and absolute values are applicable to children 1 year of age or older.
† $U_{Na}$ is urinary sodium concentration given in mEq/L.
‡ $U_{osm}$ is urinary osmolarity given in mOsm/L.

processes of filtration, reabsorption, and secretion, it is clear that urine volume alone is not a direct reflection of GFR. For example, if GFR is maintained, the reabsorptive processes are enhanced (as discussed previously in terms of dehydration), there will be an increased volume of tubular fluid reabsorbed, and urine output may be less than expected while glomerular filtration rate actually will be normal. Alternatively, GFR could be reduced severely, but a concomitant reduction in tubular fluid reabsorption would result in a final urine volume that would not be different than expected. For example, if GFR were reduced to 10% of normal values, an initial filtrate of 14.5 L might be expected, and, if tubular reabsorptive mechanisms were reduced similarly, 12.5 L of that filtrate might be reabsorbed, with a final urine output of 2 L. Nonetheless, in this latter circumstance, there would be a normal urine output, but a severely reduced GFR. In essence, then, the only measure of renal function per se is a direct evaluation by determination of either the blood urea nitrogen (BUN) or the serum creatinine value. If more precise estimates are necessary, the clearance of either creatinine or inulin must be relied upon. Moreover, it should be clear that the assessment of altered states of urine output requires evaluation of these processes without making any initial assumptions about the overall status of renal function.

## Assessment of Oliguria

A child or an adolescent who is excreting less than half of the expected urine volume (less than 0.8 mL/kg/h) is considered to have oliguria. Traditionally, this problem has been assessed by determining pre-renal, renal, and post-renal causes. Such a designation, however, although seemingly logical, does not follow physiologic principles and, at times, can be misleading and inaccurate. Therefore, our approach to this problem is to consider first obstruction or occlusion of major anatomic sites: both renal arteries, both renal veins, both ureters, or the bladder outlet. Second, we must evaluate the pathophysiologic causes, which include decreased intravascular volume or impaired renal perfusion, acute renal failure or acute tubular necrosis (ATN), and nonphysiologic or inappropriate ADH secretion (SIADH).

In evaluating the anatomic causes for a reduction in urine output, it is important to remember that oliguria will not occur unless renal artery, renal vein, or ureteral obstruction is bilateral. Therefore, unilateral obstruction at any of these anatomic sites will not produce a perceptible decrease in urine output. The compensatory changes in the contralateral unaffected kidney will compensate physiologically within minutes, and we would not detect unilateral renal artery, renal vein, or ureteral obstruction clinically on the basis of changes in urine volume. On the other hand, bladder outlet obstruction will render the patient significantly oliguric. Therefore, this problem must be evaluated in all children who have a significant decrease in urine volume. Particular attention should be paid to male infants who may have posterior urethral valves. In many instances, the bladder will be palpable, but even if this is not the case, appropriate diagnostic studies, usually a renal ultrasound examination, should be undertaken to rule out the possibility of bladder outlet obstruction. Overall, anatomic causes for decreased urine output will account for only a small proportion of oliguric children.

In evaluating the pathophysiologic causes of oliguria, it should be emphasized that the urinary constituents, especially sodium and osmolality, are characteristic and can be diagnostic when the kidney has not been manipulated pharmacologically with the use of vasodilators or diuretics (see Table 11-5). For example, a decrease in intravascular volume, as discussed previously and outlined in Figure 11-1, has a very predictable renal response. The net result of this pathophysiologic process is to enhance maximally reabsorption of tubular fluid in the proximal and distal segments of the nephron and to release, on a physiologic basis,

ADH. Taken together, these factors act to restore intravascular volume and, therefore, are considered physiologic responses. In these circumstances, the urinary sodium concentration should be quite low, usually less than 10 mEq/L, and the urinary osmolarity should be high, usually greater than 500 mOsm/L. These general guidelines need to be altered when children less than 1 year of age or premature infants are being evaluated. In some situations, the fractional sodium excretion ($FE_{Na}$) provides a more accurate index of renal sodium reabsorption. The $FE_{Na}$ simply is an expression of the amount of sodium excreted in the final urine ($U_{Na} \times$ volume) divided by the amount of sodium filtered (GFR $\times$ plasma sodium). $FE_{Na}$ can be calculated as the urine-to-plasma ratio (U/P) of sodium divided by the U/P of creatinine. This can be determined on a spot urine without the need to collect a timed sample. Similarly, in patients who have significant hypo-osmolarity or hyponatremia, the urine-to-plasma osmolar ratio (U/P Osm) may be a better index of water reabsorption. Generally, a U/P Osm of 1.5 indicates significant water reabsorption. If, for example, a patient had a serum sodium level of 120 mEq/L and a plasma osmolality of 240 mOsm/L, then a urine osmolarity of only 360 mOsm/L would be a significantly concentrated urine, a U/P osmolar ratio of 1.5. In patients with diminished renal perfusion, the term *prerenal azotemia* is encountered frequently, which is used to denote a BUN-to-creatinine ratio greater than 20. If we look at the basic renal physiology, it is apparent that this relationship actually is caused by the pathophysiologic response of the kidney to diminish renal perfusion and is not an artifact of a "pre-renal state." When proximal reabsorption is maximized, there is reabsorption not only of sodium, but of other solutes, including urea. Creatinine is impermeable to the tubule epithelium, however, and is not affected by the forces driving enhanced fluid reabsorption. Therefore, an increased amount of urea is reabsorbed while creatinine remains unchanged and we find that the BUN-to-creatinine ratio rises. Similarly, it is important to remember that, although a low urine sodium level and increased urine osmolarity will be accounted for most often by decreased intravascular volume or renal perfusion from causes such as dehydration or congestive heart failure, similar urinary indices are expected in patients with acute glomerulonephritis. In the latter condition, the inflammatory reaction in the glomerulus provides a high resistance, which diminishes renal perfusion, and the postglomerular capillary bed sees the same hemodynamic factors as are encountered in a patient with volume depletion. Consequently, the tubule response is such that the reabsorption of sodium and water is maximized. Thus, the term *pre-renal* to describe the pathophysiologic response to decreased intravascular volume or diminished renal perfusion is inaccurate and misleading.

The renal response to a fixed or established insult that produces ATN is easily predictable when the kidney has not been exposed to pharmacologic manipulation. The development of ATN is an extremely complex, variable, and dynamic state. From a clinical perspective, however, this condition is characterized by an acute loss of glomerular filtration and essentially a paralysis of tubule function. The abrupt loss of glomerular filtration is accounted for by severe renal vasoconstriction, a back-leak of fluid from the tubular lumen to the capillaries, and intratubular obstruction from sloughed injured epithelial cells. Clinically, this is reflected by a rise in both the BUN and the serum creatinine concentrations. Although GFR falls to negligible values very quickly, the serum creatinine level will rise only 0.5 to 1.5 mg/dL/d. Eventually, the serum creatinine concentration will level off to a value consistent with the degree of residual GFR. It may take several days for this to be accomplished, however, and, in the meantime, the rate of change in the serum creatinine level rather than the actual value itself is the true index of GFR. Because the BUN can be affected by a number of factors, such as catabolic rate, protein load, and medications, the serum creatinine level actually is a better index of GFR in this clinical setting. Although it has been argued that the term *acute tubular necrosis* may be inappropriate from an anatomic perspective, it actually is a very good reflection of tubular function in patients with an acute established renal insult. In this condition, the tubule is not able to continue to carry out its primary functions of sodium and water reabsorption and, therefore, the urinary indices are characterized by a high sodium concentration (usually greater than 50 mEq/L) and an elevated $FE_{Na}$ (usually greater than 2%). Moreover, these patients may excrete small volumes of urine that exhibit isosthenuria, with an osmolarity between 280 and 300 mOsm/L and a U/P Osm of 0.8 to 1.0. Because a great deal of tubule work is consumed in either diluting or concentrating tubule fluid, a dilute urine would be as unexpected as a concentrated urine in patients with acute renal failure. In some circumstances, particularly after the administration of contrast media, acute renal failure can occur in the setting of a low urinary sodium concentration. These circumstances are the exception rather than the rule, however, and probably are a reflection of the specific nephron segment injured.

Finally, it must be remembered that ADH has a powerful effect on water reabsorption from the collecting duct. Secretion of this hormone from the posterior pituitary is regulated closely under homeostatic conditions by osmolar and volume receptors. A 2% increase in plasma osmolarity will result in the release of enough ADH to produce antidiuresis, whereas a 1.2% decrease in plasma osmolarity will suppress ADH secretion. Baroreceptors modulate the release of ADH in response to changes in intravascular volume. A marked increase in water reabsorption from the collecting duct under the influence of this hormone can result in the development of oliguria, particularly in a patient with a low renal solute load. In a clinical setting in which we do not have evidence of stimulation of either osmolar or volume receptors, secretion of this hormone is termed inappropriate or nonphysiologic (SIADH). In patients with SIADH, we find a persistently concentrated urine, even though plasma osmolarity is decreased and intravascular volume is expanded. The water reabsorbed from the collecting duct under the influence of ADH is transmitted to the plasma and results in a dilution of the usual electrolytes. Therefore, evidence for ADH release can be obtained clinically by noting that the urinary osmolarity is greater than 500 mOsm/L and that the U/P Osm is greater than 1.5. Moreover, if the syndrome is regulated nonphysiologically, this would be likely to occur in the face of diluted plasma, with a plasma osmolarity of less than 280 mOsm/L and a serum sodium level less than 135 mEq/L. Additional evidence for intravascular dilution can be obtained by the finding of a low BUN level (usually less than 15 mg/dL) and a low uric acid level (usually less than 2 mg/dL). Continued infusion of the intravascular space with water reabsorbed from the collecting duct results in intravascular volume expansion. The renal response to increased renal blood flow and vascular expansion is to depress proximal tubule sodium reabsorption and to promote a natriuresis. Therefore, in patients with SIADH, we expect to find an elevated urinary sodium level (usually greater than 50 mEq/L) and an increased fractional sodium excretion (usually greater than 2%). Once again, the urinary indices can be of considerable help in establishing this diagnosis (see Table 11–5). When a patient has a persistently concentrated urine despite a fall in the serum sodium level associated with an elevated urinary sodium concentration, the diagnosis of SIADH must be entertained. The condition is considered nonphysiologic because the hypo-osmolarity of the plasma indicates that the osmolar receptors have not been stimulated and the increased urine sodium implies a replete intravascular space; therefore, the baroreceptors should not have been stimulated. In this circumstance, a persistently concentrated urine cannot be accounted for by the known physiologic regulators of ADH release. Clearly,

this syndrome presents not only as a decrease in urine output, but also as hyponatremia.

In many patients, it will not be possible initially to make a specific diagnosis and determine an etiology for declining urine output. After obtaining appropriate laboratory studies from both blood and urine, two approaches can be taken. First, assuming that, on clinical examination, the patient does not have overt evidence of fluid overload, a volume challenge of isotonic fluid can be given (20 mL/kg/h). Because the fluid administered will be isotonic, the potential hyponatremia associated with ATN or SIADH should not be exacerbated and the patient with oliguria secondary to volume depletion should have an increase in urine output. Second, a potent loop-acting diuretic such as furosemide could be given (4 mg/kg intravenously). This would be expected to produce a diuresis in patients with volume depletion, but also might exacerbate the degree of intravascular volume depletion if the urine formed is not replaced adequately. Such treatment would be unlikely to produce a diuresis in patients with established acute renal failure, however. It must be remembered that both of these manipulations will invalidate the use of urinary sodium and osmolarity as an index for the diagnosis of a cause of oliguria (see Table 11-5).

**Assessment of Polyuria**

Although it seems less ominous, the excretion of more than 4 mL/kg/h of urine needs to be evaluated carefully. In general, polyuria may arise from two pathophysiologic sources: in response to the excretion of a volume load, or a tubular defect in salt or water reabsorption. Urinary indices may be quite helpful in evaluating these conditions (see Table 11-5). Generally, patients who are in the midst of excreting a volume load will appear well hydrated clinically and will have either a stable or a slightly increased body weight. The urinary constituents associated with this diuresis will be dependent, to a large extent, on the type of fluid load given. Because of the concomitant intravascular volume expansion, the urinary sodium concentration should be elevated early in a volume diuresis, irrespective of the tonicity of fluid given. If hypertonic solutions are given, then plasma osmolarity should rise and ADH secretion should be stimulated. In this situation, the patient is excreting a large volume of a concentrated urine containing a high solute load. With a large solute diuresis, urinary osmolarity may not be maximum, but still is greater than plasma osmolarity. If the fluid given is isotonic to plasma, the resulting diuresis also will be isotonic. No significant changes in plasma electrolytes should occur, and the urinary constituents generally reveal an iso-osmolar urine with a high sodium concentration. If hypotonic solutions are given, there should be a progressive fall in the serum sodium level concomitant with an increase in intravascular volume. The combination of these factors should result in diminished ADH secretion and, therefore, a large urine volume that is hypotonic to plasma and has a low sodium concentration. Most often, volume overload occurs secondary to overzealous parenteral fluid therapy or attempts to promote good urine output to protect the kidney from potential insults from chemotherapeutic agents or nephrotoxic antibiotics. Moreover, in evaluating patients with volume overload, fluids given enterally must be accounted for and any fluid given intraoperatively must be scrutinized carefully. In these conditions, the simplest therapy is to restrict additional fluid intake until such time as the urine output returns to expected rates.

Polyuria also may arise when the level of GFR exceeds the tubular reabsorptive capacity, and a state of glomerulotubular imbalance occurs. In contrast to patients excreting a volume load, patients in whom there is a tubular defect in sodium or water reabsorption generally will appear dehydrated or will manifest a decrease in body weight. It is important to remember that the tubule is presented each day with 144 L of fluid based on a GFR of 100 mL/min. Therefore, even a small decrease in tubular reabsorptive capacity will result in a marked increase in urine volume. In patients with tubular defects, which may include interstitial nephritis, cystic disease of the kidney, or obstructive nephropathy, there is clinical evidence of intravascular volume depletion, but in the context of a high urinary sodium concentration and a urine that is not concentrated maximally. This represents aberrant tubular responses to volume depletion and results from damage to the tubular epithelium, which occurs in each of these disease states. Usually, the cause will be apparent from associated clinical findings, but some patients will have ATN without oliguria and will have these symptoms, and polyuria is characteristic of the early phase of several different types of nephrotoxicity.

Finally, diabetes insipidus, in which there is either a lack of ADH secretion by the posterior pituitary or a failure of the collecting duct to respond to this hormone, invariably presents with a marked increase in urine output. Because tubular reabsorptive capacity for sodium is intact in these individuals, the marked diuresis they experience is almost purely a water diuresis. Consequently, the urinary sodium concentration usually is low because these patients have some degree of intravascular volume depletion and the urinary osmolarity often is less than that of plasma. In fact, this condition is the mirror image of the SIADH syndrome. These patients have a decrease in intravascular volume with a progressive increase in plasma tonicity, but a persistently dilute urine with a low sodium concentration.

## ELECTROLYTE DISORDERS

### Sodium Disorders

#### Sodium Homeostasis

The total body sodium content is regulated closely by two physiologic processes. The sodium concentration in extracellular fluid is controlled and adjusted largely through the regulation and excretion of water. Because sodium is a major contributor to extracellular osmolarity, the concentration of this ion is affected by osmoregulatory processes, including thirst and secretion of ADH. In counterbalance, total body fluids and volume are regulated closely by the renal handling of sodium, as discussed previously in consideration of disorders of intravascular volume (see Fig 11-1). The kidney responds to subtle changes in intravascular volume by altering the quantity of glomerular filtrate reabsorbed in both the proximal and the distal portions of the nephron. Thus, the serum sodium concentration determined in the laboratory not only is a reflection of total body sodium balance, but actually is an index of the regulation of total body water in the majority of clinical situations. Consequently, determination of the urinary sodium concentration and the urine osmolarity (see Table 11-5) can be of considerable help in assessing patients who have abnormal serum sodium concentrations.

#### Hyponatremia

Hyponatremia, defined as a serum sodium concentration less than 130 mEq/L, is a common electrolyte abnormality. The first step in evaluating children with this disorder is to determine whether the low serum sodium level is an artifact. A low serum sodium level can be found if the blood sample has been drawn through an indwelling catheter that has not been cleared adequately or if the sample is obtained upstream from a rapidly infusing intravenous fluid that is hypotonic. Hyperlipidemia causes an increase in serum solids and, concomitantly, a falsely low serum sodium value will be reported unless the laboratory is aware of the lipid abnormality. Also, hyperglycemia results in fluid shifts into the intravascular space. Consequently, the serum sodium value may not reflect the effective sodium concentration under these conditions. The true serum sodium level in patients with hyperglycemia can be estimated by adding 1.6 mEq/L to the measured serum sodium value for each 100 mg/dL that the serum glucose is above normal values (usually assumed to be 100 mg/dL). For example, if a patient were to have a serum sodium level of 130 mEq/L with a serum glucose level of 600 mg/dL, then the effective serum sodium level would be 138 mEq/L (ie, $1.6 \times 5$ added to the serum sodium of 130 mEq/L). Once it is certain that the serum sodium value obtained is not an artifact, careful systematic evaluation of the patient usually will lead to a specific diagnosis. This evaluation should include an estimation of the patient's state of hydration combined with an assessment of urinary indices (see Table 11-5).

In patients whose weight has decreased, a primary source of salt loss should be searched for. In this clinical setting, sodium could have been lost from urine, sweat, tears, or the gastrointestinal tract. If the salt loss is the result of any condition other than one affecting the kidney, the urinary sodium concentration should be reduced (usually less than 20 mEq/L). In patients with gastrointestinal losses of sodium, the causes frequently are obvious (ie, vomiting or diarrhea). In young children with cystic fibrosis, however, the loss of sodium in sweat can be substantial, and this site of sodium loss may not be evident until the diagnosis is established.

When patients have clinical evidence of volume depletion, but an elevated urinary sodium concentration, either an intrinsic or an extrinsic renal defect should be suspected. Patients with autosomal dominant cystic disease of the kidney or acute interstitial nephritis are not able to conserve sodium appropriately in the setting of volume depletion. Similarly, patients with adrenal insufficiency or those receiving chronic diuretic therapy are susceptible to the development of hyponatremia because of renal sodium losses. Clearly, the combination of hyponatremia, hyperkalemia, and volume depletion always should indicate a diagnosis of adrenal insufficiency. Interestingly, newborn infants with urinary tract obstruction frequently also have these same electrolyte abnormalities.

In patients who have stable weight or manifestations of volume excess such as edema, attention should be turned to searching for a primary defect in water excretion. Five steps are essential for the excretion of free water, and defects in each of these steps can be associated with specific clinical conditions in which hyponatremia is a common finding. For the plasma to be cleared of excess water, glomerular filtration must be maintained so that hypotonic fluid can be presented to the renal tubules. A diminished or limited GFR will impede the rate at which free water excretion occurs and can contribute to the development of hyponatremia. Except in premature and very young infants, it is unusual for a defect in GFR to be responsible for hyponatremia unless GFR is reduced severely. Maximal free water excretion occurs at about 10 mL for every 100 mL of GFR; in the normal adult with a GFR of 100 mL/min, free water can be cleared at a rate of 600 mL/h. Therefore, it is particularly difficult to account for hyponatremia simply by the intake of free water, such as psychogenic water drinking, in older children and adults. In premature and young infants, an intrinsically low GFR contributes substantially to their propensity toward the development of hyponatremia. For example, in a neonate, an uncorrected GFR of 10 mL/min would be within the normally expected values. Concomitantly, free water excretion would be maximal at 1 mL/min or 60 mL/h. Clearly, it is not difficult to conceive of situations in which a small infant may take in more than 2 ounces of hypotonic fluid per hour.

The second major component of free water excretion is the delivery of fluid to the diluting segment of the nephron, the ascending limb of the loop of Henle. This requires that fluid exit the proximal tubule and be available for the processes of urinary dilution in the ascending limb. Therefore, clinical situations in which proximal reabsorption is enhanced can be expected to be associated with diminished free water excretion. As discussed previously (see Fig 11-1), augmented proximal reabsorption is to be expected in clinical situations in which intravascular volume is depleted, such as dehydration, or in which effective renal blood flow is decreased, such as congestive heart failure, cirrhosis, or nephrosis. In each of these disorders, a propensity toward the development of hyponatremia occurs for the following reasons:

Fluid reabsorption in the proximal tubule is isotonic and, there- fore, the hypotonic glomerular filtrate is reabsorbed without a change in osmolarity.

The rate of free water production is diminished because the rate of delivery of tubule fluid to the diluting segment is decreased as a result of the enhanced proximal reabsorption.

The time required to excrete a volume load is increased, making these patients particularly vulnerable to continued intake of hypotonic fluid.

Once fluid has reached the diluting segment of the nephron, electrolytes must be reabsorbed and water left behind in the tu- bule lumen. Therefore, those processes that diminish electrolyte reabsorption in the ascending limb of the loop of Henle will con- tribute to the development of hyponatremia. Such factors may include loop-acting diuretics and intrinsic renal diseases.

Corticosteroids and thyroxine are fundamental for maximal free water excretion. The specific mechanism by which these two hormones participate in the excretion of free water is not com- pletely known.

Finally, once dilute fluid has reached the collecting duct, it is important that the tubule fluid pass into the final urine without the reabsorption of water. ADH increases the permeability of the collecting duct to water; therefore, any condition that causes se- cretion of this hormone will diminish free water excretion and lead to the development of hyponatremia. In states of hypona- tremia, ADH secretion should be reduced because of hypo- osmolar extracellular fluid. If extracellular hypotonicity is com- bined with volume depletion, however, ADH may be released in response to volume receptors. In patients whose weight has not decreased, this response could not be invoked and release of ADH might be occurring in a nonphysiologic or inappropriate manner. It should be noted that patients with the SIADH syn- drome do not manifest edema, although their total body weight may have increased. This appears to be related to the fact that the SIADH syndrome is associated with overhydration of both the extracellular and the intracellular space, along with a shift of sodium ion distribution.

Determining the specific cause for hyponatremia is essential for designing effective therapy. For those patients who are intra- vascularly volume depleted and hyponatremic, the primary ther- apy should be to replace salt and water losses by the adminis- tration of parenteral or enteral fluids, as discussed previously. In patients who have a primary defect in free water excretion, the major aspect of therapy is to restrict fluid intake in order to provide an adequate amount of time for free water to be excreted. Thus, in one group of patients, therapy will concern the provision of additional salt and water, and in the other group, it will concern restriction of fluids. Some patients, albeit a minority, will have central nervous system signs such as a clouded sensorium or seizures because of severe hyponatremia (serum sodium level < 120 mEq/L). In this situation, it may be important to raise the serum sodium level to at least 125 mEq/L by the infusion of hypertonic sodium chloride. The infusion of about 12 mL/kg of a 3% saline solution can be estimated to raise the serum sodium

level about 10 mEq/L. For those patients with severe hypoal- buminemia and markedly enhanced proximal tubule reabsorp- tion, effective therapy may require the infusion of intravenous albumin in order to increase effective renal perfusion and diminish proximal reabsorption. It must be realized, however, that, in pa- tients with nephrosis or cirrhosis, infusion of intravenous albumin is largely a temporizing procedure that may help in correcting electrolyte abnormalities, but that the exogenously administered albumin will be dissipated quickly into either the ascites or the urine.

## Hypernatremia

Hypernatremia, generally defined as a serum sodium level greater than 160 mEq/L, is an important and potentially serious problem that requires careful evaluation. Although the kidney generally will function to maintain both intravascular volume and tonicity, excessive water losses or the intake of salt can result in hyper- natremia. As described previously for patients with hyponatremia, it is helpful to assess the potential causes for hypernatremia rel- ative to the patient's state of hydration. In a patient whose body weight is unchanged or increased slightly, it could be assumed that the hypernatremia is the result of a net increase in total body sodium that has not been accompanied by an appropriate amount of water. Normally, an increase in sodium intake would result in hypertonicity of plasma and stimulation of our thirst mecha- nism and ADH release. Concomitantly, these two factors would act to restore the plasma sodium to relatively normal values. Therefore, in the face of a normally functioning posterior pituitary and hypothalamus, it is unusual for sodium intake to be the pri- mary cause of hypernatremia. In patients who receive large vol- umes of hypertonic sodium-containing solutions such as sodium bicarbonate (which contains 1 mEq/mL) or small children in whom the formula has been compounded inadvertently with sodium chloride rather than sugar, a state of euvolemic hyper- natremia could be encountered. Such a condition would be maintained only to the extent that the offending agent was not recognized or that the patient was unable to respond and request additional free water. Unless the period of salt poisoning has been extensive, appropriate therapy for these patients involves eliminating the sodium intake and providing adequate free water to restore plasma tonicity. In a few patients, hypernatremia will be termed *essential* or will be related to central hypodipsia because of resetting of the osmolar receptors. These are unusual and rare patients who may have extreme hypernatremia without signifi- cant clinical signs. Most often, this is seen in children who have had significant central nervous system insults.

Hypernatremia usually is encountered in the setting of hy- povolemia, and this can occur from the loss of either hypotonic fluid or water alone. Hypotonic fluid losses occur in patients with severe gastroenteritis or excessive sweating, or after the admin- istration of diuretic agents. In each of these clinical settings, hy- pernatremia occurs only when inadequate free water has been provided. For example, in patients placed on diuretic agents, urine usually is excreted in a hypotonic fashion with a sodium con- centration of 75 to 100 mEq/L. Therefore, if a patient receives no fluid intake, the net effect of the diuretic agent should be the development of hypernatremia with concomitant hypovolemia. Similarly, as we have pointed out previously, failure to provide infants with adequate fluid intake, particularly in the course of oral rehydration, will increase markedly their risk of hypernatremia.

Excessive free water losses can occur either because of an enhancement of insensible fluid losses or because of the inability of the kidney to retain water. In patients with high fevers or those in a particularly dry environment, the magnitude of free water lost from the skin and lungs as evaporative and insensible water will be increased significantly. This free water will be removed initially from the extracellular fluid and will result in the development of hypernatremia. Premature infants placed under a radiant warmer are particularly susceptible to the development of hypernatremia. Also, free water can be lost from the kidney either because of a lack of ADH secretion by the posterior pituitary (central diabetes insipidus) or because of the resistance of the collecting duct to respond to ADH (nephrogenic diabetes insipidus). As described above, patients with diabetes insipidus frequently will have polyuria despite significant dehydration (see Assessment of Polyuria, in this chapter). About half of all patients with central diabetes insipidus will not have a definable cause, and the remainder will have this problem because of a suprasellar mass, postinfection encephalopathy, trauma with subsequent anoxic encephalopathy, cerebral edema, or, rarely, either vascular malformations or histiocytosis X. Nephrogenic diabetes insipidus may be either congenital, with onset in infancy manifested by episodes of fever, vomiting, and dehydration combined with a persistently hypotonic urine, or it may be acquired in association with pathologic or pharmacologic insults. The most common reason for children to have nephrogenic diabetes insipidus is intrinsic renal disease. For example, it can be expected that, once GFR is below 40% of normal values, children will not be able to concentrate their urine maximally. In addition, several drugs are known to inhibit the effect of ADH on the collecting duct, including lithium, methoxyflurane, and demeclocycline.

The appropriate treatment for hypernatremia in association with volume depletion has been a matter of concern and controversy. The greatest risk factor for these patients has been the development of cerebral edema as the serum sodium decreases toward normal values. As the extracellular sodium level falls, there is a tendency for water to move into brain cells and cause intracellular overhydration. This paradoxic rebound effect has been attributed to "idiogenic osmoles." Recent studies using nuclear magnetic resonance spectroscopy of the brain have shown that specific osmolytes (trimethylamines, betaine, and phosphoglycerocholine) are produced in response to chronic volume depletion. Consequently, it is possible that the accumulation of these intracellular osmolytes, which are related to sorbitol and aldose reductase metabolism, may be responsible for the paradoxic cerebral edema that is associated with rapid correction of hypernatremia. In this respect, however, it is important to point out that these intracellular osmolytes neither are generated nor are dissipated rapidly. Therefore, it is likely that a patient would have to sustain a prolonged period of hypernatremia, probably greater than 24 hours, in order for these products to be produced; likewise, a slow, cautious rehydration program extended over several days would allow for a progressive decrease in these compounds as extracellular tonicity is returned to normal. Specific protocols for the rehydration of patients with hypertonic dehydration have been discussed previously and are given in Table 11-4.

For patients with central diabetes insipidus, treatment with ADH or the synthetic analogue 1-deamino, 8D-arginine vasopressin can result in effective water reabsorption. Generally, it is advisable to attempt to rehydrate these patients with standard parenteral fluids before the administration of these hormones to avoid rapid volume shifts and the potential development of hyponatremia. Therapy for patients with nephrogenic diabetes insipidus is more complex and may require the use of chronic thiazide diuretics, a low-salt diet, and other attempts to manipulate the renal concentrating mechanisms. For children with congenital or inherited nephrogenic diabetes insipidus, early recognition of this condition and prevention of repeated episodes of hypertonic dehydration may be of crucial importance in preventing developmental delays and learning disabilities.

## Potassium Disorders

### Potassium Homeostasis

Potassium is the most abundant intracellular cation and it plays a fundamental role in cellular homeostasis. A large variety of regulatory mechanisms combine to maintain total body potassium at about 50 mEq/kg of body weight. Ninety-eight percent of total body potassium is intracellular, and this site provides a large sink to accommodate wide fluctuations in potassium intake and excretion. In large part, adaptive mechanisms for the conservation or excretion of potassium take many hours to days because of the need to affect essential transport processes such as sodium potassium, adenosine triphosphatase, and the production of hormones such as aldosterone. Although the kidney is a primary organ with regard to maintaining potassium balance, it is important to recognize that extrarenal adaptive mechanisms contribute significantly to acute loads of potassium. For example, only half of an acute potassium load will appear in the urine within 6 hours after administration. Accordingly, if extrarenal mechanisms were not effective, significant hyperkalemia would ensue. These nonrenal factors include insulin secretion, catecholamines, mineralocorticoids, and acid–base balance.

Potassium handling by the kidney is complex and influenced by a number of both intrinsic and extrinsic factors. About 80% of filtered potassium is reabsorbed in the proximal tubule by both active and passive mechanisms. This proximal reabsorption may be affected by concomitant fluid reabsorption and will be altered markedly by osmotic diuretics, such as mannitol, which inhibit both salt and water movement in the proximal tubule. Potassium appears to be secreted in the descending limb of Henle, but then net reabsorption occurs in the thick ascending limb. Transport of potassium in this area also results in a trapping of potassium in the medulla secondary to the countercurrent mechanism, which, in turn, may facilitate recycling of potassium in this deeper medullary region. The major potassium-secreting segments are the late distal tubule and the collecting duct. A variety of factors will affect the net movement of potassium in this region, including urinary flow rate, plasma potassium concentration, luminal potassium concentration, delivery of sodium, delivery of chloride, availability of non-reabsorbable anions such as sulfate or phosphate, and, finally, diuretic agents.

In evaluating patients with disorders of potassium, it must be remembered that the serum potassium concentration represents an extremely small portion of total body potassium, and that alterations in the serum potassium level may not be a reflection of overall total body potassium balance. Consequently, it is important to look for those factors that can result in a change in serum potassium without having any effect on total body potassium.

### Hypokalemia

Hypokalemia, generally defined as a serum potassium level less than 3.5 mEq/L, requires a systematic approach, which includes the following:

1. An assessment of acid–base status and the possibility that hypokalemia simply is secondary to shifts of potassium from the extracellular to the intracellular space.
2. An evaluation of potential lack of potassium intake, although this would have to be prolonged and fairly severe to produce total body potassium deficiency.
3. An assessment of potential sources of potassium loss through either the gastrointestinal tract or sweating, in which case, the urinary potassium level should be quite low.
4. Excessive losses of potassium through the kidney, in which

case, the urinary potassium concentration should be elevated and other metabolic abnormalities may be present.

Unfortunately, we do not have a practical and effective method for determining total body potassium status. The appearance of U waves on the electrocardiogram is a relatively crude and late-developing index of potassium balance.

Conditions in which hypokalemia will occur without total body potassium loss, but by the movement of potassium from extracellular to intracellular fluid, must be assessed carefully. In patients with alkalosis, hypokalemia occurs because of movement of potassium into cells as hydrogen ions move out of cells in order to buffer the extracellular alkalinity. It has been estimated that the plasma potassium level will drop between 0.2 and 0.4 mEq/L for each 0.1-unit increase in plasma pH. Although this represents a relatively mild change, it should be noted that hypokalemic alkalosis in children usually is associated with vomiting, and the concomitant volume depletion and stimulation of aldosterone secretion will affect potassium loss further. Similarly, insulin will drive potassium into cells from the extracellular fluid and result in an apparent hypokalemia. This is most notable in patients with diabetes mellitus who, during the course of rehydration after an episode of ketoacidosis, are noted to become severely hypokalemic. The hypokalemia in these patients is due in part to the loss of potassium during the period of osmotic diuresis from their hyperglycemia and in part to the effect of insulin and concomitant correction of metabolic acidosis. Catecholamines, which play an important role in the non-renal adaptive mechanisms, also may be stimulated by stress. The release of catecholamines will result in increased potassium removal into skeletal muscle, producing a state of hypokalemia. Similarly, hypokalemia has been associated with hypothermia, barium ingestion, and periodic paralysis.

Hypokalemia in the face of total body potassium depletion will occur because of either inadequate potassium intake or excessive potassium losses. If potassium intake is inadequate, the kidney can reduce potassium excretion to less than 20 mEq/L within 7 days and to less than 10 mEq/L in 10 days. Therefore, patients either must reduce their intake of potassium drastically or they must be kept on potassium-free parenteral fluids for a prolonged period to induce total body potassium deficiency.

Excessive loss of potassium through the gastrointestinal tract, sweat, or the kidney can result in significant hypokalemia. The intestines preferentially secrete potassium bicarbonate into the lumen and reabsorb sodium chloride. Moreover, several liters of fluid enter the gastrointestinal tract daily. Therefore, in the setting of chronic or long-term diarrhea, potassium depletion can become a significant problem. Although hypokalemia frequently is associated with persistent or pernicious vomiting, this is not caused by an excessive loss of potassium in gastric fluid. The alkalosis and volume depletion associated with persistent vomiting both contribute to continued potassium losses.

Although sweat contains only about 10 mEq/L of potassium, losses through this route can be substantial when they are associated with heavy exercise. It is likely, however, that the profound hypokalemia associated with heavy exercise and profuse sweating is contributed to by volume depletion and activation of aldosterone secretion as well as by release of catecholamines.

Potassium losses in the kidney will increase when the peritubular potassium concentration increases or when the luminal potassium concentration decreases. In most clinical situations, it can be anticipated that the major defect in potassium homeostasis will occur in the distal nephron because this is the final regulatory site for potassium homeostasis. For example, an increase in flow through the distal nephron, which can be associated with volume expansion, will increase potassium secretion. Potassium secretion in this segment also is sensitive to sodium and chloride content.

If the luminal chloride concentration is decreased or the luminal sodium concentration is increased, potassium entry into the tubular fluid will be enhanced. Diuretic agents, which increase the flow in the distal nephron, will stimulate potassium secretion by several mechanisms, including increased distal flow rate, increased luminal sodium and chloride concentration, and stimulation of aldosterone secretion. Similarly, corticosteroids, which produce a significant mineralocorticoid effect, can be expected to result in hypokalemia through the stimulation of potassium secretion. Any of the multiple causes of polyuria discussed previously can be associated with hypokalemia (see Polyuria, in this chapter). It should be noted that the concentration of potassium in the urine may be very low in polyuric conditions, but the high flow rate will result in significant potassium losses. Finally, either primary or secondary hypermineralocorticoidism will stimulate sodium reabsorption in exchange for potassium and hydrogen. Primary hyperaldosteronism is relatively rare in children, as is Cushing's syndrome. Aldosterone secretion associated with hyperreninemia, secondary to renal artery stenosis, will result in hypokalemia and hypertension. Congenital adrenal hyperplasia has been associated with hypokalemia, although it is associated more commonly with hyperkalemia. Finally, the rare disorder of Bartter's syndrome, which is characterized by growth failure, muscle weakness, poor feeding, vomiting, polyuria, constipation, and normal blood pressure, must be considered in patients who have severe and continuing hypokalemic metabolic alkalosis. The syndrome is characterized by the combination of persistent potassium wasting, hyperaldosteronism, and hyperreninemia. Despite the hyperreninemia, these patients are relatively resistant to angiotensin II and do not have hypertension. It is important to remember that clinical features of this syndrome can be mimicked easily by surreptitious vomiting, or abuse of laxatives or diuretics.

### Hyperkalemia

Hyperkalemia, generally defined as a serum potassium concentration greater than 6.5 mEq/L, is a potentially life-threatening abnormality. Consequently, humans have evolved complex mechanisms for the deposition of potassium loads. Although the kidney remains the primary site for potassium disposal, non-renal adaptive mechanisms, which include insulin secretion and catecholamines, are important for minimizing elevation of the serum potassium level in response to acute ingestions. In addition, chronic ingestion of a diet high in potassium induces additional adaptive factors, including an increase in sodium potassium adenosine triphosphatase activity, which allows for an even greater tolerance for potassium loads. Thus, the development of hyperkalemia signals a breakdown in both acute and long-term adaptive mechanisms and requires very careful evaluation (Table 11-6).

Because potassium is the dominant intracellular cation, various causes for hyperkalemia involve situations in which potassium is released from the intracellular site to the extracellular fluid. The release of potassium from red cells that are injured during venipuncture can increase the serum potassium concentration significantly. Although one would expect that hemoglobin would be released from the damaged cells, the serum is not always reported as being pink because the concentration of hemoglobin released may be quite small. Because the extracellular potassium level usually is determined based on a serum sample obtained after the blood has clotted, lysis or breakdown of cells during the clotting process also will increase the serum potassium concentration. In patients with marked leukocytosis or very high platelet counts, this can provide a significant contribution to the level of serum potassium reported by the laboratory. Finally, as discussed with respect to hypokalemia, cellular shifts of hydrogen and potassium ions in response to acid–base balance can be sig-

### TABLE 11-6.  Assessment of Hyperkalemia

Spurious
   Mechanical trauma to RBC during venipuncture
   Marked leukocytosis (WBC > $10^5$/mm³)
   Thrombocytosis (platelets > 500,000/mm³)
   Acidosis
Increased intake or tissue breakdown
   Oral or parenteral fluid intake
   Tissue catabolism
   Succinylcholine
Diminished excretion/deposition
   Renal insufficiency/diminished distal nephron function
   Decreased aldosterone effect
   Volume depletion
   Drugs

nificant. It has been estimated that, for every 0.1-unit reduction in the arterial pH, there is an approximate 0.2- to 0.4-mEq/L increase in the plasma potassium concentration. Thus, patients who are significantly acidotic also may appear to have hyperkalemia, even when their total body potassium is normal or depleted. This is particularly important in patients with diabetic ketoacidosis who initially may have markedly elevated serum potassium levels, but whose total body potassium will have been depleted secondary to the osmotic diuresis induced by the hyperglycemia. A spurious cause for hyperkalemia should be suspected when a significantly elevated serum potassium level appears to be unassociated with any change in the patient's clinical condition and there are no notable changes on the electrocardiogram. Significant hyperkalemia can be expected to be associated with a decrease in muscle strength and the development of peaked T waves on the electrocardiogram.

On rare occasions, hyperkalemia can be attributed to an increase in potassium intake or endogenous potassium from tissue catabolism. If renal function and the other adaptive mechanisms related to potassium excretion are intact, it generally is difficult to explain hyperkalemia on the basis of an acute potassium load. For example, mild hyperkalemia is a potent stimulus for aldosterone secretion and results in increased urinary flow rate. Thus, with an intact kidney, an acute potassium load from either oral or parenteral fluids can be excreted relatively efficiently and should not induce severe hyperkalemia. When the rate of tissue breakdown is extremely rapid or is combined with a mild degree of renal dysfunction, hyperkalemia may occur. Examples of this include the rapid hemolysis of red blood cells that is associated with autoimmune hemolytic anemia or an incompatible blood transfusion, the administration of cytotoxic agents to patients with malignant lymphomas, severe tissue damage from trauma or rhabdomyolysis, or the inadvertent administration of potassium-containing antibiotics to small children. In this context, it should be remembered that patients with extensive trauma, neuromuscular disease, or burns may be particularly sensitive to the depolarizing effects of the muscle relaxant succinylcholine.

In large part, the development of significant hyperkalemia should suggest a primary defect in potassium excretion. Patients with renal insufficiency are particularly susceptible to hyperkalemia. Interestingly, potassium balance is maintained relatively well until significant oliguria develops. Therefore, patients with nonoliguric renal failure will tolerate potassium intake considerably better than will those with limited urine output. The plasma level of serum potassium in patients with renal failure also is related to the degree of metabolic acidosis, which is a common feature of chronic renal failure. Children with damage predominantly to the distal part of the nephron, as occurs in cystic dys-

plastic kidneys, reflux nephropathy, and sickle-cell disease, appear to be particularly susceptible to the development of hyperkalemia. This may be because, in these clinical situations, the nephron site, which has a dominant role in potassium disposal, has been primarily affected by the disease process. Moreover, although patients with chronic renal insufficiency are able to achieve potassium balance, their adaptive reserve in response to acute potassium loading is reduced significantly.

As discussed previously, aldosterone plays an important role in maintaining a normal serum potassium level. Consequently, a reduction in aldosterone production or end-organ unresponsiveness to aldosterone will lead to the development of hyperkalemia. The hyperkalemia that is associated with adrenal insufficiency or congenital adrenal hyperplasia is an example of decreased mineralocorticoid availability. In addition, pseudohypoaldosteronism has been described in infants who have been characterized as having sodium wasting, hyperkalemia, and markedly elevated levels of renin and aldosterone. Similarly, the administration of competitive inhibitors of aldosterone such as spironolactone in an attempt to spare potassium losses in association with diuretic administration may make patients more susceptible to hyperkalemia, particularly if they encounter an acute potassium load.

Severe volume depletion also may be associated with the development of hyperkalemia. In situations in which renal perfusion has been diminished markedly, such as severe diarrhea or intractable congestive heart failure, delivery of sodium to the distal site will be decreased significantly. Because potassium excretion into the urine is dependent, to some extent, on exchange for sodium in the tubular lumen in the distal nephron, the diminished delivery of sodium to this nephron site, in turn, will decrease the rate of potassium secretion and make the patient susceptible to hyperkalemia. In these situations, the degree of volume depletion and renal perfusion must be diminished profoundly; consequently, this clinical setting usually is associated with severe metabolic acidosis.

Last, drugs known to cause an impairment in the renin–aldosterone axis have been associated with the development of hyperkalemia. Most notably, the beta-blocking agents that inhibit plasma renin activity and the production of angiotensin II have been associated with this effect. The hyperkalemia associated with these agents generally has been quite mild, however, and of minimal clinical significance. Angiotensin converting enzyme inhibitors have been shown to cause hyperkalemia. Again, this effect probably occurs because of the diminished production of angiotensin II and the lack of stimulation of aldosterone secretion. Finally, the prostaglandin inhibitors also have been associated with diminished aldosterone synthesis and the induction of hyperkalemia. In the majority of these situations, the hyperkalemia is transient and will dissipate once the offending drug has been withdrawn.

## Chloride Disorders

### Chloride Homeostasis

Traditionally, the chloride ion has been assigned a relatively passive role. Because the reabsorption of tubular fluid must be isoelectric (ie, for each positively charged ion, a negatively charged ion also must be reabsorbed to maintain electric neutrality across the tubular epithelium), it has been assumed that chloride and bicarbonate, the major reabsorbable anions, will move passively in response to the active transport of sodium and potassium. Although this concept remains generally applicable to the reabsorption of solute and electrolytes from the proximal tubule, it now is clear that chloride is the dominant and actively transported species in the ascending limb of the loop of Henle. Moreover, the obligatory relationship between chloride and bicarbonate reabsorption inevitably results in acid–base disorders as a consequence of or concomitant with disordered chloride metabolism. When chloride is available in excess in extracellular fluid, there is a decrease in bicarbonate reabsorption and a resultant hyperchloremic metabolic acidosis. Similarly, when there is a deficiency of chloride in body fluids, there is a compensatory increase in bicarbonate reabsorption, particularly in the setting of volume depletion and the development of a hypochloremic metabolic alkalosis.

## Hypochloremia

Hypochloremia, generally defined as serum chloride level less than 95 mEq/L, may develop in a variety of clinical situations either from the loss of chloride or from the inadequate intake of this anion. Interestingly, in both situations, the pathophysiologic response is quite similar. Children with pyloric stenosis represent the prototype of this disorder. Persistent vomiting, the hallmark of pyloric stenosis, results in the loss of fluid and hydrochloric acid from the stomach. It must be remembered that the hydrogen ion that is present in gastric secretions is produced by the action of carbonic anhydrase in the gastric mucosa and results in the production of a bicarbonate ion, which enters the blood. This bicarbonate ion subsequently is unbuffered by its hydrogen equivalent, which is lost in the vomitus. Therefore, a metabolic alkalosis is initiated and is characterized by a rise in the serum bicarbonate level and an increase in the serum pH level. If the process were to stop at this point, the hyperbicarbonatemia would be corrected rapidly because the kidney would maintain a normal bicarbonate threshold and the excess bicarbonate would be excreted in the urine. This normal regulatory process is disrupted, however, because of the decrease in intravascular volume that results from the loss of fluid, which is a concomitant part of this process. The kidney's physiologic response to volume depletion (see Fig 11-1) includes an increase in proximal tubule reabsorption and stimulation of the renin–aldosterone system. Enhanced proximal tubule reabsorption results in increased bicarbonate reabsorption because of the deficiency of chloride in the tubular filtrate and the ability of the proximal tubule to compensate for the lack of this anion by producing bicarbonate from the action of carbonic anhydrase. Because this nephron segment is under a maximal stimulus for reabsorption and the tubular fluid in this segment must be reabsorbed in an isotonic and electrically neutral fashion, the excess bicarbonate that is present in the tubular filtrate is reabsorbed, maintaining the metabolic alkalosis. The rise in the serum bicarbonate level cannot offset the fall in the serum chloride level completely, however, and, therefore, a small excess of sodium remains at the end of the proximal tubule and is displaced into the distal nephron. Concomitantly, the distal tubule is working under the influence of a high level of aldosterone, which will promote the excretion of potassium and hydrogen ions in exchange for sodium. This further exacerbates the metabolic alkalosis by producing hypokalemia and increasing distal bicarbonate reabsorption associated with hydrogen ion secretion. Thus, the metabolic alkalosis associated with hypochloremia is generated by the unopposed entry of bicarbonate into the plasma concomitant with the loss of chloride ions. The alkalosis is maintained and hypokalemia develops because of the kidneys' physiologic response to volume depletion in the setting of a diminished chloride level in extracellular fluid.

This sequence of pathophysiologic events easily can explain the development of metabolic alkalosis and hypokalemia in the setting of chloride depletion. Clinically, this would be seen in patients with persistent vomiting or nasogastric drainage, in whom the chloride and fluid would be lost from gastric secretion; in patients being treated with loop-acting diuretics, which have as their principal mechanism the inhibition of active chloride transport in the ascending limb; in patients with cystic fibrosis, in whom increased chloride losses in sweat can be of significance; and in patients with a rare form of congenital diarrhea in which chloride is lost in the stool, chloridorrhea. In each of these conditions, the deficiency in chloride ion is coupled with a source for continuing fluid loss and the development of volume depletion.

Alternatively, in patients who have hypochloremia without evidence of volume depletion, the proposed pathophysiologic sequence of events is less satisfying. Patients who have received adequate volumes of parenteral fluids deficient in chloride or infants who were fed a chloride-deficient formula have been reported to have a significant hypochloremic, hypokalemic metabolic alkalosis. A better potential understanding of this situation is provided from some recent studies, which have suggested that chloride may have a more active role in the development of metabolic alkalosis. Diminished chloride delivery to the thick ascending limb of the loop of Henle and the macula densa has been demonstrated to stimulate renin release directly. This stimulation may occur in the presence of a normal or expanded intravascular volume; thus, it is proposed that chloride depletion, per se, can result in an increase in the secretion of aldosterone. In addition, it has been suggested that hydrogen secretion in the medullary collecting duct may be stimulated in the absence of luminal chloride. Therefore, the reduced distal delivery of chloride would be expected to promote directly increased bicarbonate reabsorption in the distal segments of the nephron.

Lastly, Bartter's syndrome is characterized by a significant and severe metabolic alkalosis associated with hypokalemia and hypochloremia. Although the specific mechanism responsible for this rare and unusual syndrome is not understood completely, one of the more appealing hypotheses is that diminished chloride reabsorption in the ascending limb plays a dominant role. This certainly is compatible with the observation that, in the face of severe chloride depletion, patients with Bartter's syndrome cannot conserve sodium maximally and characteristically have elevated urinary chloride concentrations. This important point can be used to differentiate patients with Bartter's syndrome from those with surreptitious vomiting or diuretic abuse who can have similar acid–base and electrolyte abnormalities.

For those patients who have hypochloremia associated with a metabolic alkalosis and volume depletion, special consideration must be given to the fluids that are used in deficit therapy. In these circumstances, infusion of fluids that contain acetate or lactate would be inappropriate as part of the initial fluids used for volume expansion. In patients with an intact liver, acetate and lactate are converted to bicarbonate equivalents and would serve to enhance the metabolic alkalosis. Also, in evaluating and treating these patients, it must be recognized that replacement of the chloride ion with concomitant correction of intravascular volume will have a major effect on diminishing the pathophysiologic response that is perpetuating the electrolyte and acid–base abnormalities. Although these patients also will require potassium as a part of their rehydration fluid regimen, only rarely will the infusion of weak acids be needed to correct the metabolic alkalosis. With restoration of the chloride deficit and repletion of intravascular volume, the forces working to maintain the increased bicarbonate reabsorption will be diminished and the metabolic alkalosis will be corrected. Finally, it must be recognized that, in some patients in whom the period of volume depletion has been excessive, the exchangeable pool of intracellular potassium eventually will be depleted and, under the influence of aldosterone, the distal tubule will exchange hydrogen ion for sodium and the patient may have a paradoxic aciduria (ie, an acid urine in the face of an alkaline plasma). This should be recognized as a metabolic emergency because it indicates that total body potassium stores have been depleted to a critical level.

## Hyperchloremia

From a clinical perspective, hyperchloremia, generally defined as a serum chloride level greater than 109 mEq/L, is seen almost inevitably in combination with metabolic acidosis. Excessive chloride ions in extracellular fluid suppress bicarbonate reabsorption and lead to the development of metabolic acidosis. This sequence of events can be complicated further if chloride is ingested in association with sodium or other compounds that increase serum osmolality. In these situations, the thirst mechanism would be enhanced and the concomitant intake of fluid would result in intravascular volume expansion and a further decrease in bicarbonate reabsorption because of decreased proximal reabsorption.

Hyperchloremic metabolic acidosis generally is seen in three clinical settings: increased chloride intake, enhanced chloride reabsorption from the gastrointestinal tract, and renal tubular acidosis. Excessive chloride administration (eg, if a child were to receive normal saline as a sole hydrating solution) inevitably will result in the development of hyperchloremic metabolic acidosis. In these disorders, identification of the offending substance or reduction of the chloride content of parenteral fluid will serve to correct this abnormality.

The epithelial cells of the gastrointestinal tract function, to a certain extent, as inverted renal tubular epithelial cells. Consequently, fluid and electrolyte transport in this organ result in the reabsorption of sodium chloride and the excretion of potassium bicarbonate. Diarrhea is the most common cause of hyperchloremic acidosis. In addition, however, similar electrolyte abnormalities have been reported in patients with small-bowel, biliary, and pancreatic drainage or fistulas. In addition, those patients in whom the urine has been diverted into bowel, either as a ureterosigmoidostomy or as an ileal loop, also may have hyperchloremic metabolic acidosis. In this circumstance, urine is retained in the colon or the ileum. Water and chloride are reabsorbed by the bowel mucosa, with secretion of bicarbonate and potassium resulting in the development of metabolic acidosis with hyperchloremia. If the contact time between the bowel mucosa and the urine is limited, an electrolyte abnormality will not occur. Therefore, the development of hyperchloremia in a patient with an ileal loop suggests the presence of obstruction or a delay in emptying rather than the ileum simply serving as a conduit for the removal of urine.

Finally, hyperchloremic metabolic acidosis without an anion gap that is persistent always must evoke the possibility of renal tubular acidosis. This problem may be caused by a variety of primary or systemic disorders that interfere with the ability of renal tubules to secrete hydrogen ions, to reabsorb bicarbonate ions, or to excrete ammonia maximally. It must be remembered that renal tubular acidosis is a reasonably rare condition and, in the majority of children who have hyperchloremia, the most likely diagnosis will be persistent diarrhea.

# DISORDERS OF MINERAL METABOLISM

## Calcium Disorders

### Calcium Homeostasis

In extracellular fluid, calcium exists in three forms: ionized or free, protein-bound, and complexed to bicarbonate, phosphate, and citrate. Most often, the serum calcium level is measured routinely as the total of each of these components. It is possible using ion-specific electrodes to measure the ionized calcium concentration directly. The total serum concentration will be affected by the plasma level of proteins, particularly albumin, whereas the ionized calcium concentration may be altered by changes in the extracellular pH level. Under stable conditions, serum calcium, particularly the ionized portion, is regulated carefully by the complex interaction of parathyroid hormone (PTH), vitamin D, and bone metabolism. It must be remembered that the mineralized skeleton represents an enormous reserve for the uptake or elaboration of calcium. Therefore, in evaluating the pathophysiologic causes for alterations in serum calcium, we must take into account factors that will affect the measurement itself as well as the evaluation of calciotropic hormones and indices of bone metabolism (Table 11-7).

### Hypocalcemia

Hypocalcemia, generally defined as a serum calcium level less than 9 mg/dL, can be either transient or sustained. Our first

**TABLE 11-7.  Laboratory Assessment of Disorders of Serum Calcium**

| | Serum PO$_4$ | Parathyroid Hormone Level | Serum Alkaline Phosphatase | Serum 1,25(OH)$_2$ D$_3$ |
|---|---|---|---|---|
| **Hypocalcemia** | | | | |
| Hypoparathyroidism | I | D | N | D |
| Pseudohypoparathyroidism | I | I | N or D | D |
| Vitamin D deficiency | N or D | I | I | N, D, or I |
| Dietary calcium deficiency | N or I | N or I | N or I | N or I |
| **Hypercalcemia** | | | | |
| Hyperparathyroidism | D | I | N or I | N, D, or I |
| Familial hypocalciuric hypercalcemia | N | N or I | N | D or N |
| Idiopathic infantile hypercalcemia | N or I | D | N | N or I |
| Vitamin D excess | N, I, or D | D | N or I | N, D, or I |
| Sarcoid | N or I | D | N or I | I |
| Hypophosphatasia | N | D | D | |
| Hypophosphatemic rickets | D | N or I | I | N or D |

N, normal range; I, increased; D, decreased.

approach to this problem is to assess whether the decrease in the serum calcium level is related simply to a decrease in the serum albumin level or an increase in the serum phosphate concentration. The bound portion of serum calcium is related largely to serum albumin. A simple bedside correction can be made by increasing the measured serum calcium value by 1 mg/dL for each gram per deciliter that the serum albumin level is less than normal values (usually considered to be 3.5 g/dL). If hypoproteinemia is the cause for the hypocalcemia, signs and symptoms largely attributable to decreases in ionized calcium, such as the development of tetany or an abnormal QT interval on the electrocardiogram, would not be expected. Also, it must be remembered that there is a tendency to maintain a serum calcium–phosphate product of about 60. Therefore, conditions in which serum phosphate levels are elevated may be associated with decreases in serum calcium levels.

Transient decreases in the serum calcium concentration are seen primarily in the newborn period, but also have been reported under the following circumstances:

In older children who receive large concentrations of citrate, usually from citrated blood products
During the early treatment of rickets, when there is a sudden movement of circulating calcium into bone because of the marked depletion of this mineral
In conditions of severe rhabdomyolysis or acute pancreatitis, in which calcium is deposited in the severely injured tissues.

Finally, hypomagnesemia also may be associated with a transient, and infrequently persistent, fall in the serum calcium level. This occurs because of the complex interrelationship between magnesium, and PTH secretion and activity.

Because the calcified skeleton offers an enormous reserve for calcium, sustained hypocalcemia requires careful assessment of PTH and vitamin D metabolism. Hypoparathyroidism is characterized by a decrease in the serum calcium concentration, an increase in the serum phosphate concentration, and an inappropriately low level of circulating PTH with a normal alkaline phosphatase concentration and diminished urinary phosphorus excretion. In the newborn period, this condition represents congenital hypoplasia of the parathyroid glands, which may occur with dysembryogenesis of the brachial cleft. Classically, these infants have associated cardiac anomalies and impaired cell-mediated immunity. This condition has been termed *DiGeorge syndrome*. In older children, hypoparathyroidism may occur because of removal of the parathyroid glands during thyroid surgery or in association with the syndrome of multiple endocrine deficiencies, which results from an autoimmune destruction of endocrine tissue, frequently associated with moniliasis. Sustained hypocalcemia from hypoparathyroidism also has been reported in patients with thalassemia because of iron overload associated with multiple transfusions, and in children with Wilson's disease. The condition of patients who have decreased serum calcium levels with increased serum phosphorus levels, but increased circulating levels of parathyroidism has been termed *pseudohypoparathyroidism*. These individuals are thought to have impaired end-organ responsiveness to PTH, which results in increased tubule reabsorption of phosphate, a relative hyperphosphatemia, and concomitant hypocalcemia. Persistence of the hypocalcemia in this syndrome has been explained by a defect in bone response to PTH or decreased levels of 1,25(OH)$_2$D. Certain forms of pseudohypoparathyroidism manifest Albright's hereditary osteodystrophy, a phenotype that includes short stature, obesity, round facies, mental retardation, and shortening of the metacarpals. A deficiency of vitamin D, because of either nutritional deprivation or decreased production of one of its active metabolites, will result in sustained hypocalcemia. Intestinal calcium absorption, bone responsiveness to PTH, and normal turnover

of bone all are related to vitamin D. Therefore, a sustained deficiency in this vitamin will result not only in hypocalcemia, but also in altered growth and development of bone characterized by undermineralization of the bone matrix. In the growing child, this manifests as the classic appearance of rickets. Although the fortification of a number of food products with vitamin D largely has eliminated this disorder, rickets still occurs in children whose diets are low in calcium or phosphorus and vitamin D, and in breast-fed infants who do not receive supplemental vitamin D or good exposure to sunlight. Finally, sustained hypocalcemia can be a reflection of inadequate calcium intake. Once again, hypocalcemia would not be expected to occur unless the intake of calcium had been low for a long period, because the stimulation of PTH activity ordinarily would result in the resorption of calcium from bone and the maintenance of a normal serum calcium level, despite a lack of adequate calcium intake. In patients with malabsorptive disorders, however, particularly if there is concomitant malabsorption of vitamin D and calcium, hypocalcemia and the development of nutritional rickets may result from sustained deficiencies of calcium intake.

## Hypercalcemia

Hypercalcemia, generally defined as a serum calcium level greater than 11 mg/dL, can arise from or in association with a number of disorders. These diseases may be characterized as related to abnormalities in PTH or vitamin D metabolism, skeletal disorders in which calcium is mobilized from bone, and miscellaneous disorders in which the specific mechanism is not understood completely (Table 11-8). Hyperparathyroidism can be an inherited condition, in which case it appears in the neonatal period. The dominantly inherited forms occur in various age groups, whereas the recessively inherited form occurs more often in neonates. Hyperplasia of the chief cells of the parathyroid gland results in a sustained hypercalcemia associated with hypercalciuria and hyperphosphaturia, which leads to the complications of renal stone disease and nephrocalcinosis. The serum phosphate level usually is decreased because of the phosphaturic effect of PTH. The presenting signs and symptoms in these children can be very vague and sometimes include anorexia, failure to thrive, and various nonspecific complaints. When serum calcium levels are elevated markedly, decreases in central nervous system function such as stupor and coma can be associated as well. Interestingly, a number of these patients will complain of polyuria because of the effect of hypercalcemia in reducing the responsiveness of

| TABLE 11-8.   Causes of Hypercalcemia |
| --- |
| Related to parathyroid hormone/vitamin D |
|   Hyperparathyroidism |
|   Familial hypocalciuric hypercalcemia |
|   Idiopathic infantile hypercalcemia (Williams syndrome) |
|   Hypervitaminosis D |
|   Sarcoid/granulomatous diseases |
| Skeletal disorders |
|   Hypophosphatasia |
|   Skeletal dysplasia |
|   Immobilization |
|   Malignancy |
| Miscellaneous |
|   Blue diaper syndrome |
|   Hyperthyroidism/hypothyroidism |
|   Thiazide diuretics |
|   Glycogen storage disease |
|   Milk-alkali syndrome |
|   Rhabdomyolysis |
|   Low phosphate intake |
|   Hypervitaminosis A |

collecting ducts to ADH. Hyperparathyroidism also can be a component of the multiple endocrine neoplasia syndrome, which includes an association with pituitary or pancreatic neoplasia, pheochromocytoma, and medullary carcinoma of the thyroid.

The autosomal dominant condition familial hypocalciuric hypercalcemia results in sustained hypercalcemia with minimal clinical symptoms such as polyuria and arthralgias. Although the parathyroid glands frequently show evidence of mild hyperplasia, no improvement has been demonstrated in the hypercalcemia of these patients after subtotal parathyroidectomy. It has been speculated that there is a decreased sensitivity of parathyroid cells to ambient calcium concentrations in this disorder.

Patients with idiopathic infantile hypercalcemia may have elevated serum calcium levels that persist until 3 to 4 years of age. The severe form of infantile hypercalcemia is associated with Williams syndrome, which is characterized by phenotypic features including short stature, elfin facies, cardiac defects (particularly supravalvular aortic stenosis), and, in some cases, mental retardation. These patients frequently are asymptomatic with regard to their hypercalcemia. The specific etiology for this syndrome has not been determined. Experimental data suggest that the syndrome may be related to high doses of vitamin D prenatally, or to abnormal conversion of vitamin D into its metabolically active products.

Hypervitaminosis D can result in the development of severe hypercalcemia. Hyperabsorption of calcium from the gastrointestinal tract under the influence of vitamin D is thought to be the major mechanism responsible for the elevated serum calcium levels in this condition. Native vitamin D is converted readily in the liver to 25-OHD. The final conversion by $1\alpha$-hydroxylation in the kidney is not influenced substantially, however; therefore, the $1,25(OH)_2D$ levels are not elevated. In patients with sarcoidosis or granulomatous diseases, the metabolically active macrophages may convert 25-OHD to $1,25(OH)_2D$, resulting in abnormal elevations of the active metabolite in plasma. Therefore, hypercalcemia occurs in these syndromes as a result of the metabolic activity of the abnormal cells associated with these disorders.

Several disorders are associated with impaired net balance of calcium and bone, which may be related to alterations in bone turnover rather than to the specific activities of vitamin D or PTH. These disorders include infantile hypophosphatasia. This is a rare syndrome in which hypercalcemia occurs in children with hypertonia, failure to thrive, fractures, and craniotabes. There is a rachitic-like deformity of long bones, which can be characteristic. Classically, the alkaline phosphatase level is depressed in these patients and there is thought to be a primary defect in the initiation of the mineralization of bone. Similarly, hypercalcemia has been associated with other rare types of skeletal dysplasia. In this context, however, it is important to remember that prolonged immobilization is associated with the development of hypercalcemia, often associated with osteoporosis. These patients usually will be minimally symptomatic, although polyuria or the development of renal stones as a result of the high urinary calcium excretion may be of concern. It has been proposed that increased bone resorption or decreased accretion of minerals is related to the development of hypercalcemia. Electric forces generated by the tension and compression of bone during exercise or weight bearing may stimulate osteoblast activity. Removal of these forces during immobilization results in a net loss of bone mineral. Interestingly, similar findings with respect to bone mineral metabolism have been observed after prolonged periods of weightlessness in space.

Finally, hypercalcemia may occur as a result of calcium mobilization from bone in patients with malignancies. Although this is considerably more common in adults than in children, this condition may occur because of systemic or local factors that stimulate bone reabsorption. The elaboration of humoral factors by the tumor that have PTH-like activity or the complex interactions of prostaglandins, growth factors, and other products of tumor metabolism are thought to be responsible for these effects.

There are a large number of additional miscellaneous causes associated with hypercalcemia in children (see Table 11-8). It is important to remember that thiazide diuretics will stimulate calcium reabsorption in the ascending limb of the loop of Henle and may contribute to the development of hypercalcemia. The use of these diuretic agents to avoid hypercalciuria associated with furosemide in the newborn infant with chronic pulmonary insufficiency simply may exchange one disorder, nephrocalcinosis and stone formation, for another, hypercalcemia. Hypercalcemia can result from severe phosphate depletion.

## Phosphorus Disorders

### Phosphorus Homeostasis

It must be realized that phosphate, like potassium, is largely an intracellular ion. Therefore, changes in serum phosphate concentration may be a relatively poor reflection of the total body stores. This is particularly relevant because alterations in the serum phosphate level (ie, hyperphosphatemia or hypophosphatemia) usually are associated with mild symptomatology such as muscle weakness. Phosphate depletion, however, indicating a reduction in the total body phosphate stores, may be associated with a number of metabolic derangements. Phosphate is a fundamental component of the mineralization of growth cartilage and nonmineralized bone. It also plays an important role in oxygen–hemoglobin binding through the glycolytic intermediate 2,3-diphosphoglycerate and in maintaining high-energy phosphate compounds. The adenine nucleotides (adenosine triphosphate, adenosine diphosphate, and adenosine monophosphate) are of crucial and central importance to the maintenance of cell function and membrane integrity. Metabolic balance for this mineral is affected by intestinal absorption, bone mineralization, and renal excretion. The normal serum values for phosphate are quite different in young children and adults. This may be because of differences in the maturation of the renal system and the rate of bone growth and turnover. In young infants and children, serum phosphate concentrations between 4 and 7 mg/dL are considered normal, whereas in mature individuals, concentrations between 2.5 and 4.5 mg/dL are normal.

### Hypophosphatemia

In evaluating patients whose serum phosphate level is less than the lower limit of normal for their age, we must consider three possibilities: movement of serum phosphate into intracellular stores or the skeleton, conditions in which excessive renal loss of phosphate is a dominant factor, and conditions in which the absorption of phosphate from the intestinal tract is abnormal. The movement of phosphate from plasma to intracellular sites most likely results in an acute and relatively transient decrease in the serum phosphate concentration. These conditions rarely are associated with alterations in total body phosphate and usually are the result of factors that represent physiologic interactions under homeostatic conditions. For example, a striking decrease in the plasma phosphate level can be seen in patients with chronic malnutrition once parenteral feeding has been initiated. It appears that insulin is an important factor in initiating this decrease in plasma phosphate in malnourished patients, just as it is in the hypophosphatemia that is seen after correction of diabetic acidosis. Acute respiratory alkalosis will stimulate the intracellular uptake of phosphate caused by increased intracellular diffusivity of $CO_2$ and increased use of phosphate for metabolic purposes.

A decrease in phosphate absorption from the intestinal tract also will lead to hypophosphatemia and, eventually, to phosphate depletion. This condition may occur in a number of different clinical settings. Low–birth-weight infants fed predominantly human milk may be deprived substantially of phosphate during the period of early rapid growth, and this can result in the development of nutritional rickets on the basis of phosphate depletion. In these small infants, radiographic evidence of osteomalacia will be seen in the clinical context of a normal or slightly elevated serum calcium level, with markedly reduced serum phosphate and elevated alkaline phosphatase levels. In other situations, dietary deficiency of phosphates is relatively rare because of the prevalence of this divalent ion in most foods. However, the use of antacids that contain aluminum hydroxide can lead to the binding of phosphate in foods and to diminished absorption of this divalent ion.

The renal response to phosphate depletion is to diminish phosphate excretion concomitant with an increase in calcium excretion associated with increased intestinal absorption of calcium, decreased ammonia excretion, and increased production of $1,25(OH)_2D$. Therefore, excessive phosphate excretion, which may occur when these adaptive mechanisms are not intact, will lead to hypophosphatemia. Familial hypophosphatemic rickets, which is the result of a basic defect in the renal tubular reabsorption of phosphate, is a classic example of such a disorder.

As discussed previously, patients with primary hyperparathyroidism would be expected to be hypophosphatemic because of the phosphaturic action of PTH on the proximal tubule. Consequently, any stimulation of PTH secretion from a secondary source, such as vitamin D deficiency or renal transplantation, may be expected to result in an increase in urinary phosphate losses. Finally, syndromes associated with an endogenous renal defect in phosphate reabsorption, such as renal tubular acidosis, potassium deficiency, or Fanconi's syndrome, also can produce significant hypophosphatemia.

## Hyperphosphatemia

Under homeostatic conditions, increased intake of phosphate should lead to a decrease in the serum calcium concentration and an elevation in PTH activity. In turn, PTH should increase urinary phosphate excretion and restore calcium phosphate balance through the multiplicity of interactions between PTH, vitamin D, and bone. Therefore, the causes of hyperphosphatemia must be considered in three categories: decreased renal function, increased phosphate load, and diminished renal tubular phosphate excretion. Because an important component of phosphate excretion is its filtration into tubular fluid, a decrease in GFR can be expected to be associated with an increase in the serum phosphate concentration. This is apparent with both acute and chronic decreases in GFR. The anion gap associated with volume depletion is accounted for in part by the accumulation of phosphate secondary to diminished cardiac output and renal perfusion. In patients with chronic renal insufficiency, GFR usually is reduced to less than 20% of normal values before evidence of phosphate retention is present. Thus, in patients with an elevated serum phosphate level, it is important to determine renal function by measuring BUN and serum creatinine levels.

An increased load of phosphate can occur from either exogenous or endogenous sources. The ingestion of cow's milk, which has a high phosphate content, has been associated with the development of significant hypocalcemia and tetany in young infants. Similarly, phosphate-containing enemas and intravenous phosphate solutions are not recommended for use in children. Because phosphate is an important intracellular ion, cell lysis connected with the destruction of normal cells in association with rhabdomyolysis, infection, hyperthermia, or the cytotoxic treatment of neoplastic disorders can result in significant hyperphosphatemia.

Finally, diminished phosphaturia occurs in association with hypoparathyroidism, pseudohypoparathyroidism, magnesium deficiency, and an uncommon familial syndrome, hyperphosphatemic tumoral calcinosis. Hypogonadism, increased growth hormone or thyroid hormone, and familial intermittent hyperphosphatemia also have been reported as causes for hyperphosphatemia.

## Magnesium Disorders

### Magnesium Homeostasis

Like calcium, magnesium is present in an ionic, protein-bound, and complexed form in plasma. The usual measurement of the serum magnesium level is a determination of the total magnesium. Measurement of the ionized magnesium concentration is not readily available. Alterations in the serum magnesium level frequently are manifest by a concomitant effect on the serum calcium concentration. The normal levels for serum magnesium range between 1.6 and 2.3 mg/dL and are maintained fairly constant.

### Hypomagnesemia

Severe hypomagnesemia is associated almost invariably with hypocalcemia. This phenomenon occurs because magnesium has a complex interaction with PTH. The secretion of PTH is impaired in magnesium deficiency, and end-organ activity of PTH also may be defective in this condition. In large part, when patients have the symptoms of hypocalcemia, particularly tetany, and measurements of the serum calcium level are not excessively low or the patients do not respond to treatment for the hypocalcemia, concomitant hypomagnesemia should be suspected. Depletions in the serum magnesium concentration have been related to diminished intestinal absorption, particularly in patients with chronic diarrhea or malnutrition, but also in those with chronic alcoholism. Moreover, a renal tubular defect for magnesium reabsorption has been described in patients with Bartter's syndrome, the polyuric recovery phase of acute renal failure, and postobstructive diuresis. Magnesium wasting by the kidney is a prominent feature of the chemotherapeutic agent, cisplatin, and the immunosuppressant, cyclosporin A, and of aminoglycoside antibiotics. Hypomagnesemia should be suspected and prevented in patients receiving these drugs. In the majority of situations, assessment of gastrointestinal integrity and the intactness of renal tubular magnesium reabsorption will lead to a diagnosis in patients with hypomagnesemia.

### Hypermagnesemia

Hypermagnesemia is uncommon and usually is iatrogenic. In patients with renal failure, the continued ingestion of compounds or medications high in magnesium, such as antacids, will result in the accumulation of the divalent ion because of diminished renal excretion. Similarly, children born to mothers receiving large amounts of magnesium as therapy for preeclampsia may present with hypotonia, bradycardia, and hypotension.

### *Acknowledgments*

*We would like to dedicate this chapter to Dr. William Lattanzi, who has fostered our interest in parenteral fluid therapy and has been fundamental in our development and teaching of a simplified approach to this complex subject. Also, we are grateful for the excellent secretarial and administrative assistance of Marie Campbell.*

## Selected Readings

Arieff AI, DeFronzo RA, eds. Fluid electrolyte and acid-base disorders, vol I. New York: Churchill Livingstone, 1985.

Chan JCM, Gill JR, eds. Kidney electrolyte disorders. New York: Churchill Livingstone, 1990.

Finberg L, Kravath RE, Fleshman AR. Water and electrolytes in pediatrics, appendix II. Philadelphia: WB Saunders, 1982:241.

Gamble JL. Chemical anatomy, physiology and pathology of extracellular fluid. Cambridge, Mass: Harvard University Press, 1950.

Holliday MA, Segar WE. Maintenance need for water in parenteral fluid therapy. Pediatrics 1957;19:823.

Lattanzi WE, Siegel NJ. A practical guide to fluid and electrolyte therapy. In: Lockhart JD, ed. Current problems in pediatrics. St Louis, Mosby-Year Book, 1986.

Pizzaro D, Posada G, Sandi L, Moran RJ. Rice-based oral electrolyte solutions for the management of infantile diarrhea. N Engl J Med 1991;324:517.

Rose BD, ed. Clinical physiology of acid-base and electrolyte disorders. New York: McGraw-Hill, 1977.

Schrier RW, ed. Renal and electrolyte disorders, ed 2. Boston: Little, Brown & Co, 1980.

Smith HW. From fish to philosopher. Boston: Little, Brown & Co, 1953.

*Principles and Practice of Pediatrics, Second Edition.*
edited by Frank A. Oski et al. J. B. Lippincott Company, Philadelphia © 1994.

# CHAPTER 12
# *Inborn Errors of Metabolism*

## Rebecca S. Wappner and Ira K. Brandt

# *12.1 Introduction to Inborn Errors of Metabolism*

## DEFINITION AND HISTORY

Inborn errors of metabolism are genetically determined abnormalities in the biochemistry of the body whereby a single defect results in the blockage of a metabolic pathway at a specific step. This results in excessive accumulation of immediate or precursor substrates and deficiency of immediate and subsequent products of the reaction normally occurring at that step. Individual disorders are caused by defects in the genome involving point mutations, deletions, and other alterations of the DNA and may involve any of the chromosomes, including the 25th, the mitochondrial chromosome. Although almost always, a single enzyme activity is affected, rarely, a multifunctional enzyme protein or even several enzymes may be involved, and a composite clinical picture incorporating features of several enzyme deficiencies may result. Such is the case in methylmalonic aciduria/homocystinuria, because the enzyme deficiency involves an initial, common step in the conversion of cobalamin to its two cofactor forms. Conversely, identical clinical pictures may result from mutational effects in different proteins. An example of the latter is Sanfilippo syndrome, which may be caused by a deficiency of any one of four different enzymes.

It is of interest that the term *inborn errors of metabolism* first was used by Garrod in the early years of this century. Mendel's law of heredity recently had been rediscovered, and Garrod synthesized this knowledge into a concept that explained the cause of the four disorders he described in 1908 in his landmark published lecture entitled "Inborn Errors of Metabolism." Experience in the years since then has confirmed his concept amply. Although one of the disorders, cystinuria, does not result from the blockage of a metabolic pathway, the defect is a specific genetic one involving a transport system and fits well within the current, expanded concept of the group of disorders. Indeed, it is fair to say that all enzymes, transport systems, and structural proteins are subject to mutation-induced alterations, and the fact that abnormalities for all of them have not been described may be explained either by the lethality of the abnormalities in embryonic or fetal life or by our lack of the technology to enable us to perceive more than the several hundred currently recognized disorders.

## CLINICAL PRESENTATION

Some of these disorders are of no clinical significance. Iminoglycinuria, for example, never has been associated with any abnormalities in the affected homozygotes. These conditions occasionally are confusing diagnostically, however, so mention must be made of them.

Many of the disorders, although they may show no manifestations in a particular individual, may be preclinical in that the individual will become symptomatic later on. A worst-case scenario is a healthy infant with a negative family history who, at 36 hours of age, will go rapidly into coma with severe acidosis because of propionic acidemia with secondary hyperammonemia, and either will succumb or else will survive with heroic treatment only for severe psychomotor retardation to develop. A less dramatic but still devastating scenario is the phenylketonuric child who is considered to be normal until his slowness in development eventually discloses what has become an irreversible, significant, yet preventable psychomotor disability. Such is the argument for newborn screening programs discussed elsewhere. Certainly, a family history of a particular disorder is indication enough for appropriate diagnostic studies, including prenatal diagnosis if available and desired.

Mental and motor retardation, neurologic abnormalities, and other developmental disabilities should alert one to the possibility of an inborn error of metabolism. A minimal diagnostic biochemical screening panel is given in Table 12-1.

Some affected persons will have their disease diagnosed easily on the basis of their clinical picture. The odor of maple syrup in the urine of a newborn who is lethargic, acidotic, and having seizures points toward a diagnosis of branched-chain ketoaci-

| TABLE 12-1.   Screening for Inborn Errors of Metabolism: Urinary Studies |
| --- |
| Odor |
| Ketones (dipstick) |
| Glucose (dipstick) |
| Reducing substances (Clinitest) |
| pH (dipstick) |
| Sulfhydryl groups (cyanide-nitroprusside) |
| Oxo acids ($FeCl_3$, dinitrophenylhydrazine) |
| Glycosaminoglycans (toluidine blue, acid albumin) |
| Auto-oxidation (overnight in open container) |
| Amino acids, qualitative (electrophoresis) |
| Organic acids (gas chromatography, mass spectrometry) |
| Oligosaccharides (thin-layer chromatography) |

TABLE 12-2.   Physical Findings Suggesting an Inborn Error of Metabolism

The following general signs and symptoms are common to many of the inborn errors of metabolism: failure to thrive, lethargy, coma, seizures, cyclic vomiting and dehydration, hypoglycemia, ataxia, hypotonia, hypertonia, spasticity, psychomotor retardation, psychomotor regression, and central nervous system degeneration. The findings listed below are more specific signs and symptoms and their related disorders.

| Finding | Related Disorder(s) |
| --- | --- |
| **Cutaneous** | |
| Absent or reduced pigment | PKU, albinism, sialidoses, Menkes disease |
| Alopecia | Hereditary generalized resistance to 1,25-dihydroxyvitamin D, acrodermatitis enteropathica |
| Angiokeratoma | Fabry disease, fucosidosis, sialidosis, galactosialidosis, mannosidoses |
| Dermatitis | PKU, Hartnup disease, acrodermatitis enteropathica, biotinidase deficiency, prolidase deficiency |
| Edema | $GM_1$ gangliosidosis, prolidase deficiency |
| Hair, light | PKU, homocystinuria, cystinosis |
| Hair, sparse | Biotinidase deficiency, Menkes disease |
| Hair, straightened | MPS, ML, GP |
| Hair, woolly (kinky) | Menkes disease, argininosuccinic aciduria |
| Hirsutism | MPS, ML, GP |
| Hyperpigmentation | Familial hemochromatosis |
| Ichthyosis | Steroid sulfatase deficiency, multiple sulfatase deficiency |
| Jaundice | Galactosemia, hereditary fructose intolerance, tyrosinemia, hemochromatosis |
| Keratosis palmoplantaris | Tyrosine aminotransferase deficiency |
| Masses | Farber disease |
| Photosensitization | Porphyrias |
| Scarring and deformities | Porphyrias |
| Ulceration | Prolidase deficiency |
| Xanthomas | Hyperlipoproteinemias |
| **Head** | |
| Facies, coarse | MPS, ML, GP |
| Macrocephaly | MPS, ML, GP, glutaric acidemia I, Canavan's disease |
| Microcephaly | PKU, fetal PKU, tyrosine aminotransferase deficiency, leukodystrophies |
| **Eyes** | |
| Arcus juvenilis | Hyperlipoproteinemias |
| Cataracts | Fabry, Farber, and Niemann-Pick diseases, $\alpha$-mannosidase deficiency, sialidosis, aspartylglucosaminuria, steroid sulfatase deficiency, lysinuric protein intolerance, Zellweger syndrome and peroxisomal disorders, mitochondrial disorders |
| Cherry-red macular spots | $GM_1$ and $GM_2$ gangliosidosis, Niemann-Pick disease, Farber disease, sialidoses, galactosialidosis, Krabbe disease |
| Corneal clouding | MPS, ML, GP, sialidoses, Tangier disease |
| Corneal opacities | Tangier disease, mitochondrial disorders |
| Ectopia lentis | Homocystinuria, sulfite oxidase deficiency |
| Glaucoma | Zellweger syndrome, homocystinuria |
| Gyrate atrophy of retina | Ornithine aminotransferase deficiency |
| Kayser-Fleischer rings | Wilson disease |
| Keratitis | Tyrosine aminotransferase deficiency |
| Retinitis pigmentosa | Adult Refsum disease, other peroxisomal disorders, abetalipoproteinemia |
| **Ears** | |
| Deafness | Hunter syndrome, SL, PPRP-S overactivity, biotinidase deficiency |
| **Mouth** | |
| Gingival hyperplasia | MPS, ML, GP |
| **Cardiac** | |
| Cardiomyopathy | Pompe disease, fatty acid oxidation defects, 3-methylglutaconic acidemia, tyrosinemia, myoadenylate deaminase deficiency, hemochromatosis, MPS, Fabry disease |
| **Abdomen** | |
| Acute visceral attacks | Hepatic porphyrias, Fabry disease |
| Hepatic dysfunction | Galactosemia, hereditary fructose intolerance, tyrosinemia glycogenoses, Wilson disease, porphyrias, hemochromatosis, cholesteryl ester storage disease, Zellweger syndrome and other peroxisomal disorders, argininosuccinic aciduria, mitochondrial disorders, fatty acid oxidation defects, familial hemochromatosis |
| Hepatosplenomegaly | MPS, ML, Tangier disease, GP, some SL, sialidoses, lipoprotein lipase deficiency |

TABLE 12-2.    *(Continued)*

| Finding | Related Disorder(s) |
| --- | --- |
| Hernias | MPS, ML, homocystinuria |
| Splenomegaly | Gaucher and Tangier diseases |
| **Musculoskeletal** | |
| Arthritis | Gout and other purine disorders, Farber disease |
| Dorsal kyphosis (gibbus) | MPS, ML, $GM_1$ gangliosidosis, multiple sulfatase deficiency |
| Joint motility decrease | MPS, ML, homocystinuria |
| Marfanoid appearance | Homocystinuria |
| Rickets | Familial hypophosphatemia, disorders of vitamin D metabolism, hypophosphatasia, disorders associated with renal tubular dysfunction |
| **Neurologic** | |
| Chaplinesque gait | Homocystinuria |
| Dystonia | Wilson disease, glutaric acidemia I |
| Muscle cramping after exercise | Muscle glycogenoses, myoadenylate deaminase deficiency, fatty acid oxidation defects |
| Myopathy | Pompe disease, muscle glycogenoses, mitochondrial disorders, fatty acid oxidation defects, glycerol kinase deficiency |
| Paresthesia | Fabry disease, sialidosis |
| Peripheral neuropathy | Metachromatic leukodystrophy, peroxisomal disorders, Tangier disease |
| Psychoses | Adult Tay-Sachs disease, porphyrias, purine disorders, homocystinuria |
| Self-mutilation | Lesch-Nyhan, adenylosuccinase deficiency, tyrosine aminotransferase deficiency |
| **Renal** | |
| Renal failure | Fabry disease, disorders associated with stones |
| Renal tubular dysfunction | Galactosemia, hereditary fructose intolerance, tyrosinemia, cystinosis, glycogenosis I |
| Stones | Cystinuria, hyperoxaluria, gout and other purine disorders, orotic aciduria |
| Renal cysts | Glutaric acidemia II, severe CPT II deficiency, Zellweger syndrome |
| **Other** | |
| Adrenal insufficiency | Adrenoleukodystrophy, adrenomyeloneuropathy, glycerol kinase deficiency |
| Immunodeficiency | Adenosine deaminase deficiency, purine nucleoside phosphorylase deficiency |
| Nonspherocytic hemolytic anemia | Adenylate kinase deficiency, pyrimidine-5'-nucleotidase deficiency |
| **Urine and Diaper Coloration** | |
| Black | Homogentisic aciduria |
| Blue | Tryptophan malabsorption |
| Pink | Disorders with hematuria, stone formation |
| Port wine | Porphyrias |
| Yellow-orange | Disorders with increased uric acid |
| **Urine Odor** | |
| Acrid | Glutaric acidemia II |
| Cabbage | Tyrosinemia |
| Cat urine | 3-Methylcrotonyl-CoA carboxylase deficiency |
| Fishy | Trimethylaminuria |
| Maple syrup | Maple syrup urine disease |
| Mouse-like | PKU |
| Sweaty feet | Isovaleric acidemia |
| Sweet | 3-Oxothiolase deficiency |
| Swimming pool | Hawkinsinuria |

*CPT,* carnitine palmityl transferase; *GP,* glycoproteinoses; *MPS,* mucopolysaccharidoses; *ML,* mucolipidoses; *PPRP-S,* phosphoribosylpyrophosphate synthetase; *SL,* sphingolipidoses; *PKU,* phenylketonuria.

demia just as strongly as steamy corneas, coarse features, and hepatosplenomegaly in an 8-month-old child point toward a diagnosis of Hurler syndrome. A number of physical findings suggest inborn errors of metabolism (Table 12-2).

The patient may have acute metabolic disease. In the young infant, this poses two challenges to the physician: ascertainment and timely management. The clinical picture usually is indistinguishable from that of infections, injuries, gut obstructions, and other disorders. Moreover, signs such as anorexia, vomiting, lethargy, drowsiness, hypotonia, spasticity, tachypnea, hyperpnea, dehydration, odd odor, posturing, seizures, stupor, and coma should alert one to the possibility, as should a family history of prior unexplained infant deaths. Without immediate treatment, permanent damage will occur and will result in death or, if the infant survives, in psychomotor retardation and other developmental disabilities.

*Principles and Practice of Pediatrics, Second Edition.*
edited by Frank A. Oski et al. J. B. Lippincott Company, Philadelphia © 1994.

**TABLE 12-3. Acute Metabolic Disease: Initial Procedures**

1. Discontinue feeding of milk and all other foods, particularly those that contain protein, and begin intravenous (or oral, if possible) administration of a balanced electrolyte/glucose solution, maintaining the glucose concentration at a high-normal level.
2. Collect urine. Immediately spot-test for odor, reducing substances (if positive, test for glucose), ketones, specific gravity, pH, and FeCl$_3$, and send remainder to laboratory to be processed for studies of amino acids and organic acids. If all of these cannot be done immediately, the specimen should be fresh-frozen.
3. Blood should be obtained for determination of electrolyte (anion gap), glucose, ammonia, quantitative amino acid, organic and short-chain fatty acid, and lactate levels.

Upon the suspicion of a metabolic disorder, potentially noxious foodstuffs should be interdicted while appropriate specimens are obtained (Table 12-3). It is important to obtain these when the patient is at his worst. The first urine the patient voids is the one most likely to be informative. As the patient comes under metabolic control, the biochemical abnormalities tend to become corrected, particularly because immediate management provides an abundant energy supply (glucose) and the withholding of protein. Both of these are excellent initial therapeutic measures for the vast majority of these disorders. The laboratory results will direct one to the appropriate disorder or group of disorders that should be considered.

It is important to mention that older infants and children may have had previous episodes of vomiting, lethargy, or other symptoms, which resolved spontaneously or with treatment, as outlined previously. *Cyclic vomiting* is an appropriate descriptive term. In this situation, a child with a relatively mild disorder of ammonia or organic acid metabolism may have vomiting and other symptoms when his metabolic requirements (eg, with a fever) exceed his limited metabolic ability. Because routine therapy for vomiting includes discontinuing feedings and administering water, glucose, and electrolytes in corrective and maintenance amounts, the patient may become asymptomatic. He may be discharged from the doctor's supervision while only partially restored to a normal food intake, so that, when he is restored completely to a noxious level of intake at home, the symptoms will recur. This cycle may be repeated, each one potentially additively damaging to the child, even to the point of fatality. The metabolic basis must be determined so that future occurrences may be prevented and appropriate genetic counseling given.

## Selected Readings

Burton BK. Inborn errors of metabolism: The clinical diagnosis in early infancy. Pediatrics 1987;79:359.
Scriver CR, Beaudet AL, Sly WS, Valle D, eds. The metabolic basis of inherited disease, ed 6. New York: McGraw-Hill, 1989.
Waber L. Inborn errors of metabolism. Pediatr Ann 1990;19:105.
Ward JC. Inborn errors of metabolism of acute onset in infancy. Pediatr Rev 1990;11:205.

# 12.2 Disorders of Transport

Although disorders of transport do not fit the definition of "inborn errors of metabolism" originally given by Garrod, their inclusion now is considered entirely appropriate. Transport of a substance across a membrane into the compartment in which it undergoes its metabolic activities obviously is a necessary step in its overall metabolic scheme and, in many instances, the substance can cross the membrane only with the aid of some sort of mechanism that involves a specific polypeptide carrier subject to the same mutational events as is any other class of polypeptides. It is of interest that cystinuria, one of the four disorders described by Garrod as evidence of his concept, is a transport defect rather than a defect in effecting a change in molecular structure.

## CYSTINURIA

Cystinuria is named after the characteristically high cystine concentration found in the urine of affected persons. The very low solubility of the substance encourages its precipitation in the genitourinary tract, resulting in stone formation, which, depending on the site, can produce a variety of symptoms. In those with acute onset, which is more likely to occur in adults but does occur in children, urethral stones will cause very severe, cramp-like pain in the lumbar region extending inferiorly and around to the lower abdomen. Urethral stones may produce severe urgency, frequency, and pain. The stones can pass spontaneously, but they may require urologic intervention. Other findings include hematuria, hydronephrosis, and urinary tract infection. The combination of the mechanical injury and the infection results in permanent structural damage, which, as attacks recur, increases to the extent of bringing about significant reduction in renal function, which can be quite severe.

Patients may be detected who have a milder clinical presentation. Routine urinalysis may reveal cystine crystals in a specimen from a healthy child or from one who has experienced urinary tract infection without having formed a stone large enough to cause colic.

The mechanism of the disorder appears to be a selective deficiency in the low-specificity, high-capacity renal tubular reabsorption transport system for dibasic amino acids, but cystine-creatinine clearance ratios of less than 1 suggest a more complex situation. Figure 12-1 shows that cystine, even though it is a disulfide formed by two molecules of cysteine, resembles the dibasic amino acids lysine, arginine, and ornithine in that the amino groups are about the same distance apart. It is ironic that in this disorder lysine is excreted in much larger amounts than is cystine, but because it is relatively quite soluble and, thus, does not form stones to call attention to its presence, the much less abundant but much less soluble cystine becomes the hallmark of the disorder.

Diagnosis is confirmed most dramatically by analysis of the

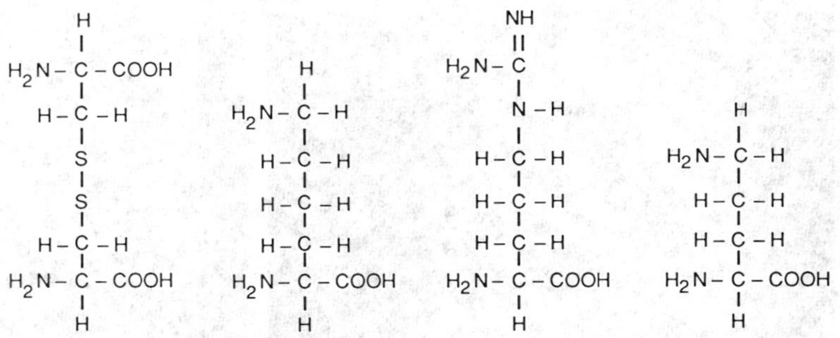

H
|
H₂N – C – COOH
|
H – C – H
|
S
|
S
|
H – C – H
|
H₂N – C – COOH
|
H

**CYSTINE**

H
|
H₂N – C – H
|
H – C – H
|
H – C – H
|
H₂N – C – COOH
|
H

**LYSINE**

NH
‖
H₂N – C
|
N – H
|
H – C – H
|
H – C – H
|
H₂N – C – COOH
|
H

**ARGININE**

H
|
H₂N – C – H
|
H – C – H
|
H – C – H
|
H₂N – C – COOH
|
H

**ORNITHINE**

Figure 12-1. The four amino acids excreted in excess in cystinuria.

excreted stones. There is a caveat, however, in that 10% of all stones (including the first) produced by cystinuric persons are made of calcium oxalate, presumably formed around the nidus of a cystine crystal or a tissue fragment resulting from local injury or infection. The diagnosis may be made with confidence after a patient reaches 6 months of age on the basis of quantitative analysis of the urine, preferably a 24-hour sample, indicating characteristically increased concentrations of the four amino acids. In a patient less than 6 months of age, immaturity of renal tubular transport results in inability to distinguish homozygotes from heterozygotes for other than the type I disorder (see below).

Management involves keeping the urine dilute by encouraging enough intake of liquids to keep the cystine concentration below 300 mg/L, or even lower if the person is a known stone-former. This should be done prophylactically in all patients. Alkalinization of the urine to a pH above 7.5 will increase the solubility of cystine, but this is difficult to achieve. If stones form, the use of D-penicillamine or one of its less toxic homologues, N-acetyl penicillamine and 2-mercaptopropionyl glycine, is indicated. These form a mixed disulfide with cysteinyl residues of cystine; the disulfides are soluble and excreted readily. If repeated insults to the kidney have resulted in severe renal failure, renal transplant may be undertaken with the assurance that the dibasic amino acid transport system in the donor kidney will remain intact if the kidney remains functional.

The disorder is not rare (1:2000 to 1:20,000 in various studies) and is inherited as an autosomal recessive trait. Intestinal transport of dibasic amino acids is affected also, albeit to a clinically insignificant extent. Genetic heterogeneity is revealed by urinary studies of carriers, who, in families designated as having the type I disorder, have normal excretion. Carriers in families with the type II and III disorders have moderately increased renal cystine losses, even to the extent that they occasionally will form stones. Prenatal diagnosis is not available.

## IMINOGLYCINURIA

Iminoglycinuria is a disorder of another one of the low-specificity, high-capacity transport systems of the renal tubule. The system is shared by the two imino acids, proline and hydroxyproline, and glycine. Because there are no clinical manifestations, the disorder is merely a medical curiosity. Diagnosis should be confirmed by the finding of normal or low concentrations of all three acids in the plasma. Disorders resulting in increased plasma proline or hydroxyproline concentrations may cause iminoglycinuria because the specific imino acid will so load the renal tubular reabsorption system as to interfere with reabsorption of the other one and that of glycine.

The disorder is an autosomal recessive one and is manifested in some carriers by selectively increased glycine excretion. Occasionally, normal newborn infants will manifest transient iminoglycinuria.

## HARTNUP DISEASE

Hartnup disease involves the third low-specificity, high-capacity transport system of the renal tubule as well as the gut. The so-called neutral amino acid system transports all of the amino acids except those transported by the dibasic and iminoglycine systems previously discussed and the dicarboxylic amino acids, which have yet another system of their own. Individuals with this disorder have a clinical picture related to the intestinal malabsorption of tryptophan, which results in reduced synthesis of one of its products, nicotinic acid. Because the human body relies on this process for about half of its requirement for nicotinic acid (the other half comes directly from the diet), affected persons will have a syndrome resembling that of pellagra, with dermatitis in exposed areas, neuropsychiatric problems such as cerebellar ataxia and emotional upsets, and diarrhea. The urinary amino acid pattern is diagnostic: excretion of all of the "neutral" amino acids (except proline, hydroxyproline, and glycine) is increased. Management is simple and effective: administration of at least twice the recommended daily allowance of nicotinic acid (as the amide to avoid vascular symptoms). Neurologic complications may not be reversible, however.

This autosomal recessive disorder is not rare, with an incidence of about 1:20,000 in newborn screening programs. It is rare to see patients with clinical manifestations, however, presumably because the relatively high nicotinic acid intake in developed countries is enough to meet the increased requirements of affected persons. Carriers cannot be identified.

## HYPOPHOSPHATEMIC RICKETS

Hypophosphatemic rickets is a disorder of both the proximal renal tubular reabsorption of phosphate and the metabolism of vitamin D. It has a spectrum of clinical manifestations. Extensive surveys of families in which the X-linked dominant disorder is present have demonstrated that as many as 30% of affected individuals, particularly females, may have no manifestation other than a low serum phosphorus concentration and, perhaps, some limb shortness. Others, particularly males, will present with rickets, in some cases quite severe, which does not respond to the usual dose of vitamin D given for nutritional rickets (Fig 12-2). Abnormalities of tooth structure may bring about early and extensive caries. Manifestations of the disorder may appear in early infancy, with slow growth and radiologic evidence of rickets. Later on, weight bearing will result in bowing or other deformities of the lower extremities, which frequently will be of a nature severe enough to require osteotomies. The serum calcium level in an untreated patient is normal, and the phosphorus level is below normal for the patient's age. Active rickets is reflected in the increased activity of alkaline phosphatase in the plasma. Serum calcifediol (25-hydroxyvitamin D) concentration is usually

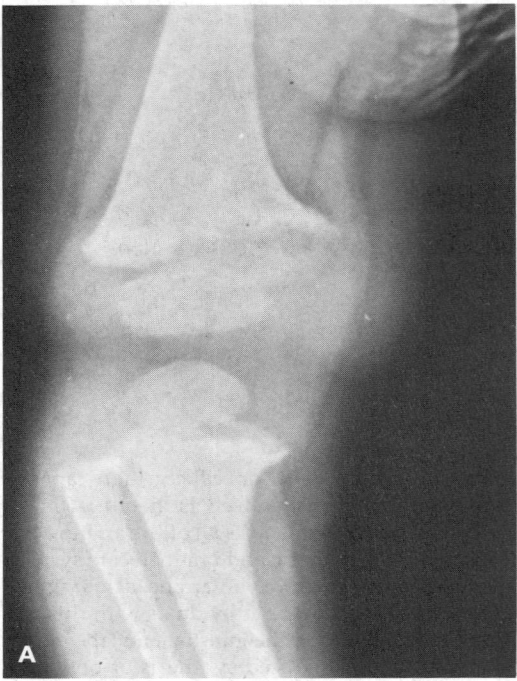
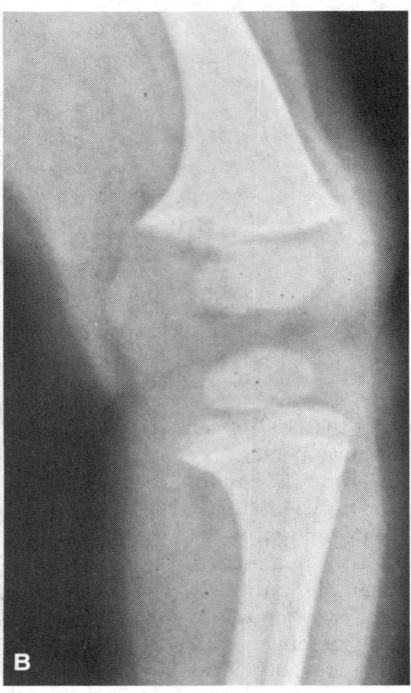

Figure 12-2. Familial hypophosphatemic rickets. (**A**) Right knee radiogram; (**B**) left knee radiogram. Note the moth-eaten appearance of the epiphyses, particularly medially, and the varus deformities of the diaphyses of the tibias and femurs.

normal, although the calcitriol (1,25-dihydroxyvitamin D) may be low-normal or even low. Indeed, studies indicate an inappropriate lack of increased calcitriol synthesis in response to parathormone and to phosphate depletion, and a hyperactive calcitriol catabolism. In contrast to nutritional rickets, in which the serum calcium usually is low, there is no secondary hyperparathyroidism. Parathormone levels commonly are normal, and there is no aminoaciduria. These patients not only have significantly reduced tubular reabsorption of phosphorus in their renal tubules, but there also is evidence that the intestinal absorption of phosphorus is reduced. Management of the disorder consists of increasing the phosphorus intake by the administration of up to 2.0 g of

elemental phosphorus daily divided into five doses given every 4 hours. A sixth dose, which ordinarily would be given in the middle of the night, is omitted to allow the patient to sleep, but it must be recalled that the 8-hour period will allow the phosphorus to become reduced to its pretreatment level. Evaluation for adequacy of treatment must take into consideration the relatively poor absorption of phosphorus from the intestine as well as its abnormally increased renal clearance. Thus, the phosphorus concentration should be measured 4 hours after the previous dose of phosphate was given. Also, because food itself will result in a transient reduction of the serum phosphorus level, it is customary to obtain the monitoring blood specimens 4 hours after

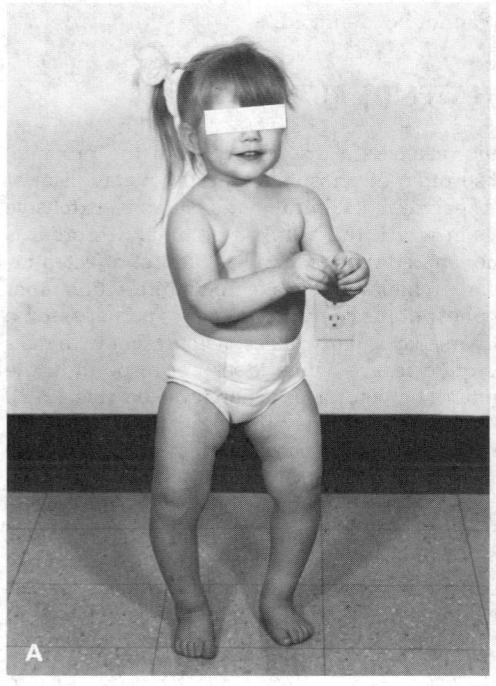
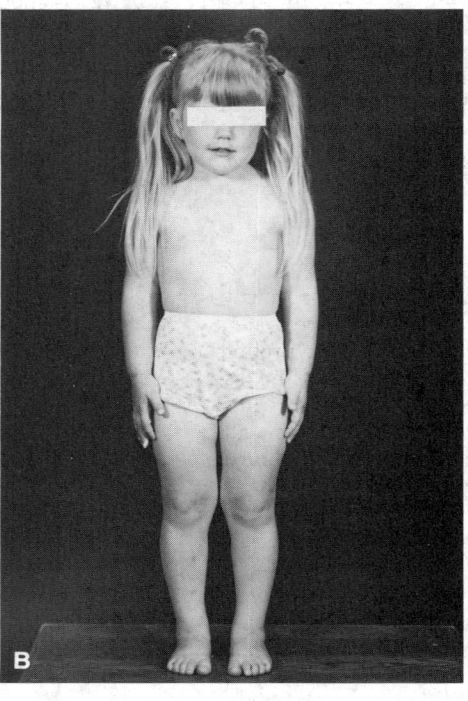

Figure 12-3. Familial hypophosphatemic rickets. (**A**) Before therapy; (**B**) after therapy.

both the previous dose of phosphorus was given and a meal was eaten. Because, even in normal individuals, phosphate is absorbed poorly and, indeed, is used as a cathartic, oral phosphate dosages should be started low and advanced slowly. Patients usually will have diarrhea during the first 2 or 3 weeks of administration; thereafter, the diarrhea will be less prominent, although it is unusual for the stools to return to normal consistency. In addition to phosphorus, one also must supply calcitriol. Calcitriol is required to promote bone mineralization, to promote the intestinal absorption of calcium (incompletely absorbed phosphorus in the gut will trap an appreciable proportion of the dietary calcium), and to inhibit any increase in parathormone production (secondary to a decrease in calcium concentration that might result from trapping by phosphorus in the gut). The initial dose is 0.25 µg/d; this is adjusted upward as indicated. Patients are monitored to make certain that the calcium and parathormone concentrations remain normal, and that the alkaline phosphatase level returns to and stays within normal limits. The increased intake of phosphorus and its trapping effect on the calcium may lead to hypocalcemia, which is corrected rapidly by the parathyroid glands, resulting in a secondary hyperparathyroidism. This must be anticipated, because, if it is allowed to continue, the patient may have a tertiary hyperparathyroidism requiring surgical management. Although there is no question that this management program has been successful (Fig 12-3), it does not appear to be completely so, because many well-managed patients will not reach their full height as predicted by family measurements and may have some deformity of the extremities. Periodic dental examinations should begin in very early childhood. Orthopedic surgeons should be consulted if any bone deformities occur.

Most of the cases appear to be determined genetically on an X-linked dominant basis, although a number appear to be on a sporadic basis or, rarely, inherited by other types of mendelian pattern. Because children of affected individuals run a risk of inheriting the disorder, they should be evaluated in early infancy to determine whether they have the disorder so that treatment may be instituted and shortness and deformities may be minimized, if not prevented completely. Prenatal diagnosis is not available.

## Selected Readings

Pollitt RJ. Amino acid disorders. In: Holton JB, ed. The inherited metabolic diseases. New York: Churchill Livingstone, 1987:96.
Scriver CR, Beaudet AL, Sly WS, Valle D, eds. The metabolic basis of inherited disease, ed 6. New York: McGraw-Hill, 1989.

*Principles and Practice of Pediatrics, Second Edition.*
edited by Frank A. Oski et al. J. B. Lippincott Company, Philadelphia © 1994.

# 12.3 *Disorders of Amino Acid Metabolism*

## DISORDERS OF PHENYLALANINE METABOLISM

Phenylketonuria, the most important paradigm of the inborn errors of metabolism, was discovered in the early 1930s by Folling, who was asked by the parents of two severely retarded children if anything could be done about their musty, mousey, pungent odor, which induced asthma in their father. Folling's finding that a bluish olive color was produced in the patients' urine by the addition of ferric chloride, and his laboratory studies indicating that the color reaction was a result of a high phenylpyruvic acid concentration, led him to believe that a disorder of phenylalanine metabolism was responsible for their clinical picture. He demonstrated on the patients, himself, and others that an oral phenylalanine load resulted in increased phenylpyruvic acid excretion. Later on and in other laboratories, it was learned that the odor was caused by a phenylpyruvic acid oxidation product, phenylacetic acid, and that the metabolic block was in the conversion of phenylalanine to tyrosine (Fig 12-4).

Patients with disorders of phenylalanine metabolism usually appear to be normal at birth. Some of them may have vomiting episodes, occasionally to the point of having a diagnosis and surgical correction of pyloric stenosis. Psychomotor development will be impaired such that, despite normal performance at birth, at the age of 1 year, the intelligence quotient will be about 50 and, at the age of 3 years, it will average about 20. Beginning at several months of age, the patient may manifest the mousey, pungent odor responsible for the disorder first being elucidated. Although the infant's pigmentation at the time of birth will be normal for infants in the family, melanization will not progress as would be expected ("dilute" pigmentation). The majority of affected persons will show poor head growth, and abnormal electroencephalograms and seizures are common. An indolent, eczema-like rash may develop, particularly in the perineal region. Until newborn screening programs were developed, the diagnosis usually was made during the workup of a mentally retarded young child. Dilute pigmentation, rash, and seizures in addition to the retardation helped to indicate phenylketonuria. The urinary findings of increased phenylpyruvic acid and other metabolites of phenylalanine, coupled with a significant increase in the plasma phenylalanine concentration but a low or, at most, normal tyrosine concentration, are diagnostic. Unfortunately, enzyme studies have not been carried out very frequently because the activity is present only in the liver and intestinal tract. The few studies that have been done have shown essentially no enzyme activity in the fully developed classic cases with relatively high phenylalanine concentrations.

Treatment consists of administering a diet that is selectively low in its phenylalanine content. Because phenylalanine is an essential amino acid, controlling the dietary intake will permit the patient to have only that amount of phenylalanine that is necessary for normal protein synthesis. This is achieved by giving one of several commercial formulas that are phenylalanine-poor or phenylalanine-free and supplementing it with a standard formula and low-protein foods. It is imperative that the phenylalanine concentration be monitored at appropriate intervals so that it is maintained within the limits of 2 and 8 mg/dL for optimum results. Although dietary control will not result in the restoration of damaged neurologic function, it will prevent further neurologic deterioration and correct the dilute pigmentation, odor, and skin

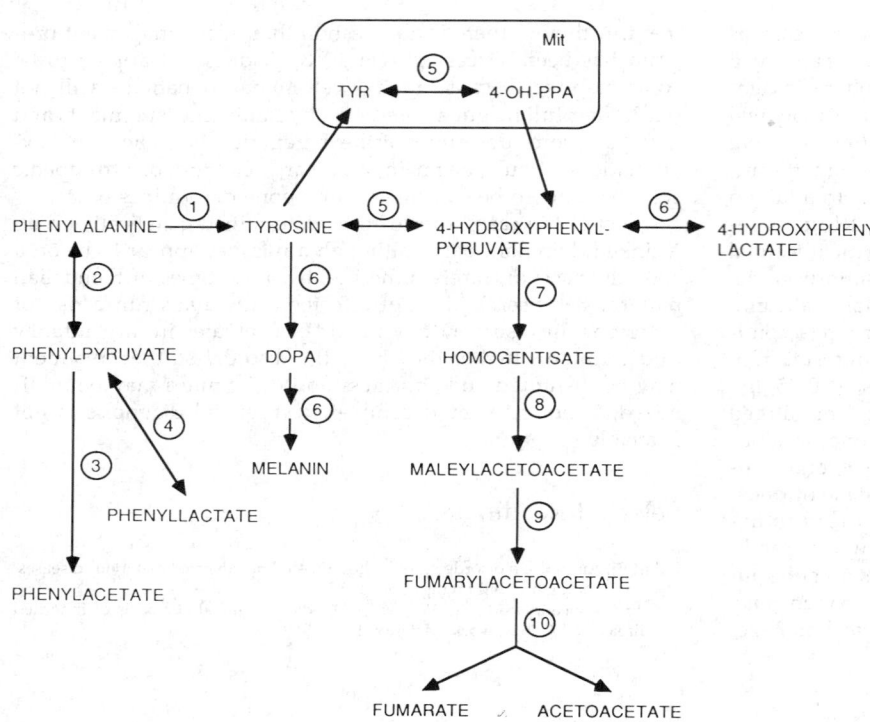

Figure 12-4. The metabolic pathway of phenylalanine and tyrosine. *Mit*, mitochondrion; *1*, phenylalanine hydroxylase; *2*, phenylalanine aminotransferase; *3*, uncertain, *4*, phenyllactate dehydrogenase; *5*, tyrosine aminotransferase; *6*, tyrosinase; *7*, 4-hydroxyphenylpyruvate oxidase; *8*, homogentisic acid oxidase; *9*, maleylacetoacetate isomerase, *10*, fumarylacetoacetate hydrolase.

eruption. The patient should be maintained on the diet for his or her lifetime. This frequently is difficult to achieve, however, after late childhood or adolescence. It is particularly important for females to remain on dietary control.

Fetal hyperphenylalaninemia syndrome caused by maternal phenylketonuria uniformly results from the pregnancy of an untreated phenylketonuric woman. Even though the vast majority of the children of phenylketonuric women do not have phenylketonuria (although all of them are at least carriers), the presence of an abnormally elevated phenylalanine concentration in the mother and the fact that there is a fetal–maternal concentration ratio of about 1.5 almost always results in a fetal phenylalanine concentration that is greater than 15 mg/dL, which is considered toxic to the developing nervous system. Thus, the infants will be born with moderately severe mental retardation, which will not progress after birth because they are able to regulate their own phenylalanine concentrations at a normal level. The teratogenic effect of the hyperphenylalaninemia during embryonic and fetal life will result in a 25% incidence of significant malformations, mostly ventricular septal defects, and a dysmorphology resembling that of the fetal alcohol syndrome. There is some evidence that this may be prevented completely if the mother is on a well-established dietary program such that her phenylalanine concentration does not extend beyond the limits of 2 and 6 mg/dL throughout the entire pregnancy. This is rather difficult to achieve, however, particularly because many of the women seek medical care only after they have become pregnant, and because a significant number of them are unable to conform to the very rigorous dietary control.

Newborn screening programs have been quite successful. After demonstration that the phenylalanine concentration even in phenylketonuric infants is essentially normal at birth, it was hypothesized that, if cases were detected and appropriate treatment instituted in the first days of life, mental retardation and other manifestations would be prevented. This was demonstrated first on siblings of known cases. Further extension of this hypothesis was enabled by the development by Guthrie of an inexpensive test that could be applied to all newborns. At preferably 3 to 5 days of age, the age at which the initial data were obtained, a

few drops of blood are allowed to flow onto a special filter paper. When the blood is dry, the paper can be transported to a laboratory and its phenylalanine concentration determined. When the phenylalanine concentration is above a specified level (in most laboratories, 4 mg/dL), further studies are done and, if the diagnosis is made, a low-phenylalanine diet is instituted immediately, ideally before 2 weeks of age.

Hyperphenylalaninemia is the term used to describe the disorder of individuals whose phenylalanine concentrations, although increased, are not high enough to warrant dietary control. Presumably, the abnormality in the phenylalanine hydroxylase gene has occurred in a region coding for an amino acid that is less critical for enzyme activity. They should be followed, however, to make certain that the levels do not increase at periods when the protein intake is increased and, if the individuals are females, to make certain that their level does not exceed 6 mg/dL during pregnancy.

Phenylketonuria variants make up about 1% or 2% of all patients with high phenylalanine concentrations. These are disorders not of the phenylalanine hydroxylase enzyme per se, but rather in the metabolism of the very important cofactor involved, tetrahydrobiopterin (Fig 12-5). Indeed, the presence of a high phenylalanine concentration is an indication for urinary biopterin studies. These individuals either will not be able to synthesize the tetrahydrobiopterin because of defects in one of the stages of the synthetic pathway (tetrahydrobiopterin synthetase deficiency) or they may not be able to regenerate tetrahydrobiopterin after it has been oxidized to dihydrobiopterin in the course of the phenylalanine hydroxylase reaction (dihydropteridine reductase deficiency). What makes the disorder much more severe than classic phenylketonuria is the fact that tetrahydrobiopterin also is needed for hydroxylation of tryptophan and tyrosine in the brain, and these pathways are equally impaired. This results in decreased production of the corresponding neurotransmitters, serotonin and catecholamines. Thus, the infant, despite good dietary control maintaining the phenylalanine concentration at therapeutic levels, will experience progressive neurologic deterioration resembling Parkinson disease and frequently will die before 1 year of age. Those infants with a tetrahydrobiopterin

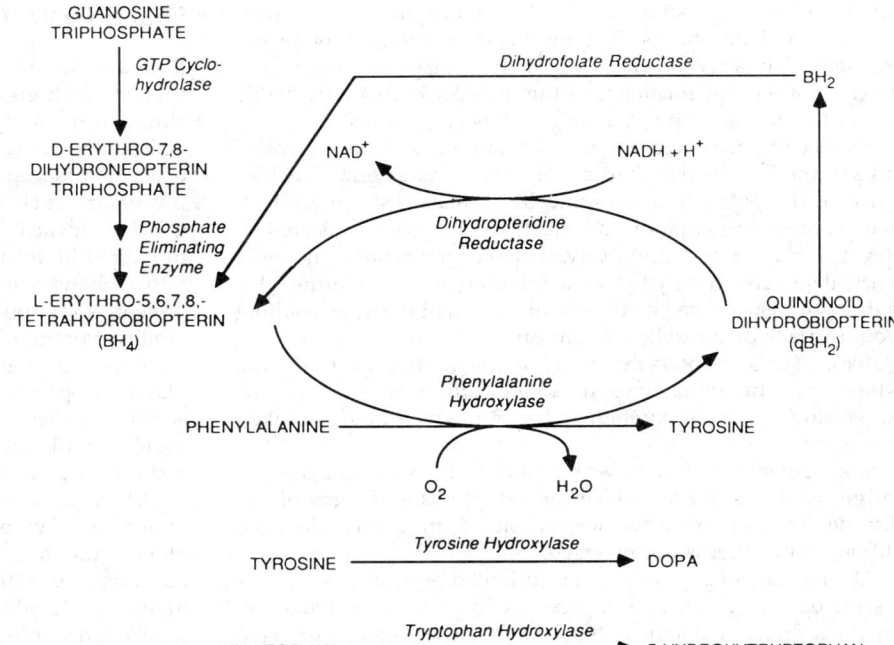

**Figure 12-5.** Hydroxylase reactions and tetra-hydrobiopterin synthesis. *GTP,* guanosine triphosphate; *NAD+,* the oxidized form of nicotinamide-adenine dinucleotide; *NADH,* the reduced form of nicotinamide-adenine dinucleotide.

synthesis defect may respond to very large doses of tetrahydrobiopterin, but because it does not cross the blood–brain barrier readily, dihydroxyphenylalanine (levodopa) and 5-hydroxytryptophan have to be administered (along with carbidopa, to minimize the decarboxylation of the other two substances in the gut and blood). Indeed, it appears that, in most patients, administration of the two neurotransmitter precursors, in carefully controlled quantities to minimize neurologic symptoms, along with a small dose of tetrahydrobiopterin that is enough to provide the liver with adequate cofactor, will result in optimum management of the patient without the need for a low-phenylalanine diet. Supplying adequate quantities of tetrahydrobiopterin to patients who have the dihydropteridine reductase deficiency is more difficult, even for just the phenylalanine hydroxylase, however, because all the administered tetrahydrobiopterin can go through only one cycle of enzyme activity. These patients must be managed with both the neurotransmitter precursors and a low-phenylalanine diet.

All these forms of phenylketonuria are inherited on an autosomal recessive basis. Classic phenylketonuria has its highest incidence of 1:4500 in Celtic peoples, an incidence of about 1:12,000 in mixed populations such as that of the United States, and low to virtually no incidence in Asians, Finns, black Africans, and Ashkenazi Jews. Hyperphenylalaninemia and biopterin disorders are distributed more evenly.

Diagnosis of the carrier state may be achieved by the administration of deuterium-labeled phenylalanine and subsequent measurement of labeled tyrosine in the blood. It is an expensive procedure, however, because of the requirement for a deuterated reagent and the high-resolution mass spectrometry necessary to assay the specimens. More recently, recombinant DNA techniques in informative families have been used for carrier detection and prenatal diagnosis.

## DISORDERS OF TYROSINE METABOLISM

Transient tyrosinemia of the newborn usually is asymptomatic, although some infants may be lethargic and have some feeding problems. Both the serum tyrosine and phenylalanine levels are increased, and cases usually are ascertained on follow-up of a positive newborn screening for phenylketonuria. There has been some association with a high-protein diet; reducing protein intake to that of breast milk or, in some cases, administration of supplements of ascorbic acid (presumably to maximize p-hydroxyphenylpyruvate oxidase activity, see Fig 12-4) are curative. There probably are no long-term residual effects.

Hepatorenal tyrosinemia has been designated type I tyrosinemia and may begin with an acute severe picture in the neonatal period, characterized by vomiting, diarrhea, the odor of rotten cabbage, jaundice, and hepatomegaly, progressing to death. In addition to the usual laboratory findings associated with liver disorders, one finds an increase in the plasma methionine and tyrosine concentrations. The urinary organic acid pattern shows a prominence of 4-hydroxyphenyllactate, and special studies reveal the accumulation of small but abnormal amounts of succinylacetone and succinylacetoacetate (see Fig 12–4). The increase in succinylacetone is considered to be responsible for at least a major share of the toxic effect on the liver, the other enzyme systems, and the renal tubule. Porphyrin metabolism is inhibited at the 5-aminolevulinic acid dehydratase level, so that 5-aminolevulinic acid is increased in the urine. Patients who have the severe neonatal form usually do not survive the neonatal period. The majority of patients, however, first exhibit symptoms later in infancy with failure to thrive associated with cirrhosis, cardiomyopathy, renal tubular dysfunction, and rickets. The diagnosis is made by assay of fumaroylacetoacetate hydrolase (fumarylacetoacetase), the site of the metabolic block, in filter paper blood dots, lymphocytes, and fibroblasts.

Management involves the administration of a diet low in phenylalanine and tyrosine. Although some improvement is recorded, most patients have severe progressive cirrhosis and usually die in the first decade of life. Liver transplantation has been accomplished and, although successful in reversing the manifestations, does not do away with the increase in succinylacetone. The latter presumably is synthesized in other tissues and may have long-term negative effects.

Prenatal diagnosis has been accomplished both by estimation of succinylacetone in the amniotic fluid and by assay of fumarylacetoacetase in cultured amniotic fluid cells and chorionic villi samples. Carrier detection is available by enzyme assay in lymphocytes and fibroblasts. Enzyme heterogeneity, although not frequent, may affect the accuracy of fetal diagnosis and carrier determination. The incidence of the disorder is about 1:100,000 live births, but in French Canadians, it is about 1:700.

Oculocutaneous tyrosinemia, also known as type II tyrosinemia or the Richner-Hanhart syndrome, is characterized by keratosis of the palms and soles and by corneal dystrophy. There may be mental retardation as well. The diagnosis is indicated by elevated plasma and urinary tyrosine concentrations and by a marked increase in 4-hydroxyphenylacetic acid in the urine. This is thought to be caused by the accumulation of tyrosine resulting from the lack of cytosolic tyrosine aminotransferase (see Fig 12-4). Excess tyrosine enters the mitochondria in extrahepatic tissues, where mitochondrial tyrosine aminotransferase catalyzes its conversion to 4-hydroxyphenylpyruvate, which then is broken down further.

Management is by diet, with reduced phenylalanine and tyrosine, which is felt to relieve the symptoms and signs of the disorder and to prevent further neurologic and corneal damage, although the latter is not reversed.

Oculocutaneous tyrosinemia is inherited on an autosomal recessive basis and is found particularly in persons of Italian extraction. Prenatal diagnosis has not been reported, nor have studies for carrier testing.

The progressive darkening of urine as it remains exposed to air characterizes alkaptonuria. This may start in early infancy or be postponed to the third decade of life. Aesthetics aside, there are no problems until middle age, when it is noted that dark brown pigment has accumulated in the sclerae, ears, nose, cheeks, and cartilage. This ochronosis is the result of nonenzymatic polymerization of homogentisate in cartilage and fibrous tissue, and it is secondary to the considerable accumulation of the substance caused by the lack of homogentisic acid oxidase (see Fig 12-4). The accumulated pigment is associated with significant arthritis and other connective tissue problems, partly because of secondary inhibition of lysyl hydroxylase, an important enzyme in collagen synthesis. Homogentisic acid may be identified by organic acid studies of the urine. There is no treatment. This autosomal recessive disorder is relatively rare.

Hawkinsinuria may be asymptomatic or it may be detected as a severe metabolic ketoacidosis in young infants. It is diagnosed by finding increased deaminated tyrosine metabolites, including hawkinsin (a by-product of the incomplete conversion of 4-hydroxyphenylpyruvate to homogentisate caused by a dysfunctional enzyme) in the urine. Patients may have a chlorine-like, swimming pool odor. Treatment is a low-phenylalanine, low-tyrosine diet until the disorder resolves spontaneously, usually at about 1 year of age. It is an autosomal dominant condition.

## DISORDERS OF AMMONIA METABOLISM

Excess dietary or waste nitrogen, remaining after that needed for protein synthesis and tissue maintenance is used, normally is not stored in the body, but is converted into urea by a series of reactions known as the urea cycle (Fig 12-6). Disorders of the urea cycle are associated with the accumulation of ammonia and its precursors, such as glutamine, glutamic acid, aspartic acid, and glycine. Elevated plasma ammonia levels that exceed three times the upper limits of normal are toxic and are associated with cytotoxic changes in the brain and liver. With rising ammonia levels, patients show poor feeding, anorexia, behavioral changes, irritability, vomiting, lethargy, ataxia, and seizures. As the hyperammonemia progresses, the child becomes comatose and ventilatory support may be needed. Circulatory collapse and cerebral edema may occur. The classic cases are neonates who have been asymptomatic for 24 to 48 hours and then have a rapidly progressing course with neurologic deterioration. Milder forms of the disorders may be detected later in the neonatal period, produce intermittent symptoms over a period of years, or be detected in older children or adults as a result of neurologic problems or psychomotor retardation. As a group, they are estimated to occur in about 1:30,000 live births. All the disorders of ammonia metabolism are inherited as autosomal recessive traits, except for ornithine-transcarbamylase (OTC) deficiency, which is associated with an X-linked pattern of inheritance, and transient hyperammonemia of the newborn, which is not genetic in nature.

Diagnosis of a specific urea cycle disorder usually can be made on the basis of the pattern of plasma and urine amino acid abnormalities and the presence or absence of orotic aciduria. Confirmation of specific enzymatic deficiencies requires only erythrocytes or cultured skin fibroblasts for some of the disorders, but necessitates liver biopsy for others. Secondary hyperammonemia, caused by organic acidurias, usually can be excluded by the absence of acidosis, but urinary organic acid determination is suggested to rule out the rare case that might be detected initially with only hyperammonemia.

Treatment of acute hyperammonemia, either as the initial presenting episode or as a subsequent intercurrent episode, is a medical emergency. With the initial episode, blood and urine samples should be collected for diagnostic testing, but treatment should be started immediately, before a specific diagnosis is established. Therapy should include the removal of all exogenous protein sources and the administration of intravenous glucose to prevent protein catabolism. Reduction of markedly elevated plasma ammonia and ammonia precursors is carried out most effectively by hemodialysis. Alternatively, peritoneal dialysis may be employed. If there is a temporary delay in dialysis, exchange transfusion, which is the least effective, may be done. In that the

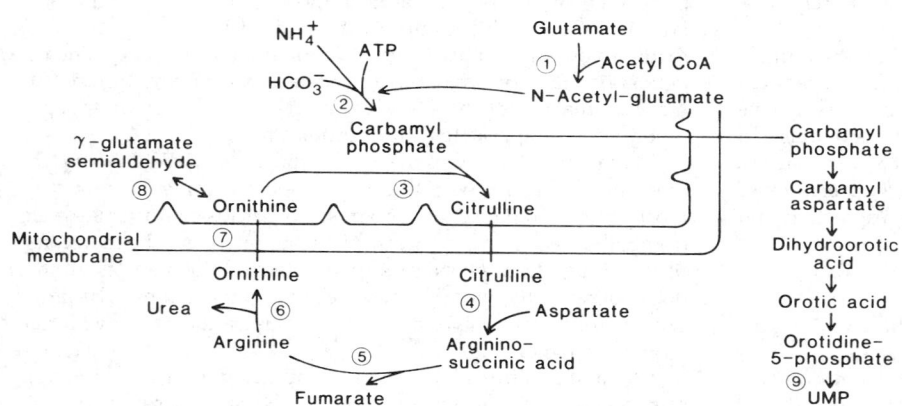

Figure 12-6.  Urea cycle. *1*, N-acetyl-glutamate synthetase (NAGS); *2*, carbamyl phosphate synthetase I (CPS I); *3*, ornithine transcarbamylase (OTC); *4*, argininosuccinate synthetase (AS); *5*, argininosuccinate lyase (AL); *6*, arginase; *7*, mitochondrial ornithine transport defect (HHH); *8*, ornithine aminotransferase; *9*, decarboxylase, site of allopurinol block in pyrimidine pathway. *ATP*, adenosine triphosphate; *CoA*, coenzyme A; *UMP*, uridine monophosphate.

duration of time in coma is related inversely to outcome, prompt referral to a tertiary medical center is indicated if dialysis is not readily available.

Drugs that employ alternate pathways for waste nitrogen excretion, such as sodium benzoate and sodium phenylacetate, may be used intravenously to control acute mild to moderate hyperammonemia (less than 350 $\mu$M). One must be prepared to start dialysis immediately if there is no significant improvement in ammonia levels within a short period after this therapy is instituted, however. These drugs also are used enterally to maintain plasma ammonia levels within the normal range between intercurrent episodes in patients with the more severe forms of the disorders. Sodium benzoate combines with glycine to form hippurate. Sodium phenylacetate combines with glutamine to form phenylacetylglutamine. Sodium phenylbutyrate, which is converted into sodium phenylacetate, also may be used. Both hippurate and phenylacetylglutamine are excreted rapidly by the kidneys and remove a significant amount of nitrogen, the ammonia precursor. Before these drugs were available, many patients with the severe forms of ammonia disorders did not survive past 1 year of age.

Once plasma ammonia levels fall to below 100 $\mu$M, the patient may be started on enteral therapy. Nutritional supplements such as Protein-Free Diet Powder (Mead-Johnson, product #80056) or UCD (Milupa) may be necessary to meet basic caloric and other nutrient needs. Depending on the type of disorder and its severity, a fairly limited protein intake, with or without essential amino acid supplementation, will be needed. Specific amino acid supplementation with L-citrulline or L-arginine also is needed for relative insufficiencies of these amino acids and to "prime" the urea cycle. Intravenous L-arginine hydrochloride is used for the same purpose during hyperammonemic episodes.

Even with prompt and aggressive medical therapy, only 30% to 50% of neonates who have hyperammonemic coma survive the neonatal period. Most of those who do survive have significant neurologic deficits and psychomotor retardation. Seizure disorders, cortical atrophy, and spastic quadriparesis are common. Later acute episodes, usually precipitated by intercurrent infections or excessive protein intake, also may lead to further neurologic sequelae or death.

## CARBAMYL PHOSPHATE SYNTHETASE I DEFICIENCY

Carbamyl phosphate synthetase I (CPS I) is a mitochondrial enzyme that catalyzes the formation of carbamoyl phosphate from ammonia, adenosine triphosphate, and bicarbonate in the presence of N-acetylglutamate. N-acetylglutamate is a critical cofactor for this reaction and is formed from acetyl coenzyme A and glutamate in the presence of N-acetylglutamate synthetase. Inhibition of N-acetylglutamate synthetase by organic acids, such as propionic acid, is thought to be the reason for the secondary hyperammonemia seen with organic acidurias.

Most cases of CPS I deficiency begin with neonatal hyperammonemic coma. Near-zero levels of citrulline and lowered arginine, as well as elevated levels of glutamine, alanine, and glycine, are noted on plasma amino acid determinations. There is no elevation of urinary orotic acid. Less than 10% of normal CPS I activity is noted on liver, rectal, or duodenal biopsy. Partial deficiencies with 10% to 25% of normal enzyme activity have been reported with later onset of symptoms. Treatment includes a fairly restrictive dietary protein intake (0.5 to 0.7 g/kg/d), supplemental essential amino acids and L-citrulline, and either combined sodium benzoate and sodium phenylacetate or high-dose phenylbutyrate. The disorder is inherited as an autosomal reces-

sive trait. Prenatal diagnosis is possible using fetal liver biopsy for enzymatic analysis or DNA probes for restriction fragment length polymorphisms.

N-acetylglutamate synthetase deficiency is a very rare disorder with neonatal presentation. Plasma citrulline and arginine levels and urinary orotic acid levels are normal. Therapy is similar to that of CPS I deficiency, except that arginine, an activator of N-acetylglutamate synthetase, and N-carbamylglutamate, a congener of N-acetylglutamate, are given.

## ORNITHINE-TRANSCARBAMYLASE DEFICIENCY

OTC deficiency probably is the most common of the urea cycle disorders and is inherited as an X-linked trait. Affected males usually have massive hyperammonemia in the neonatal period. Plasma citrulline levels are reduced markedly; plasma glutamine, glycine, and alanine levels are elevated, along with other nonspecific elevations associated with massive hyperammonemia, such as lysine and proline levels. Urinary orotic acid is elevated markedly. Plasma ammonia levels often exceed 1,000 $\mu$M. Even with aggressive management, many patients do not survive the neonatal period. The enzymatic deficiency may be confirmed with liver biopsy. Males with 10% to 25% of normal enzymatic activity and a milder clinical course have been reported. Therapy for those males who survive the neonatal period is similar to that for CPS I deficiency and includes a restricted dietary protein intake (0.4 to 0.7 g/kg/d), supplemental essential amino acids and L-citrulline, use of non-protein caloric and other nutrient supplements, and either combined sodium benzoate and sodium phenylacetate or high-dose phenylbutyrate.

Females who are heterozygous for OTC deficiency have a wide clinical spectrum, ranging from being affected as severely as are hemizygous affected males to being asymptomatic. The degree of relative lyonization (random X chromosome inactivation) in hepatocytes of normal and abnormal OTC genes in the individual female determines the clinical severity of her disease. At least three severely affected females have not survived the neonatal period. More often, affected females have 10% to 20% of normal OTC activity and have the disorder diagnosed initially during childhood with symptoms of intermittent hyperammonemia, such as cyclic vomiting, lethargy, and coma, or with protein intolerance or avoidance. Neurologic problems such as strokes, cerebral atrophy, dementia, or other encephalopathic processes may be seen. Therapy for heterozygous females depends on the degree of severity of their disease.

It is important that female relatives of affected patients be evaluated to determine if they are carriers for OTC deficiency. Approximately two thirds of mothers of affected males will be carriers for the disorder. Carrier detection may allow early identification of females at risk for hyperammonemic episodes and also may be helpful in reproductive planning. Measurement of urinary orotic acid or orotidine while taking allopurinol, which inhibits the pyrimidine pathway beyond orotic acid, will detect most OTC carriers. Urinary orotic acid measurement during protein loading should be avoided in that it is less accurate and carries a risk of producing symptomatic hyperammonemia in partially affected females. DNA probes have been established and are available for both carrier detection and prenatal diagnosis. Using this technique, a few predicted affected males have been treated from birth with varying outcomes. Even with aggressive therapy, some have died with hyperammonemia in the neonatal period. At least four male patients, three of whom were treated from birth, and one severely affected female patient have undergone successful liver transplantation resulting in correction of their urea cycle disorder.

## CITRULLINEMIA

Citrullinemia is associated with deficient activity of argininosuccinate synthetase. Most patients are seen initially in the neonatal period with massive hyperammonemia. Plasma citrulline (greater than 1000 $\mu$M) and urinary citrulline levels are elevated markedly. Plasma argininosuccinic acid is absent; plasma glutamine and alanine are elevated. Urinary orotic acid may be increased, but to a lesser degree than with OTC deficiency. Milder forms with partial argininosuccinate synthetase deficiency have been reported with presentation in early childhood. An adult form has been reported in Japan.

In that citrulline is excreted fairly rapidly in the urine, which is a means for waste nitrogen excretion, this disorder usually is managed more easily than is OTC or CPS I deficiency after the neonatal period. Patients still require a protein-restricted diet (0.8 to 1.5 g/kg/d), supplemental non-protein nutrients, and sodium benzoate and sodium phenylacetate. L-arginine supplementation is employed. The disorder is inherited as an autosomal recessive trait. The diagnosis may be confirmed by measurement of argininosuccinate synthetase in cultured skin fibroblasts or liver. Carrier detection, prenatal diagnosis, and DNA probes are available.

## ARGININOSUCCINIC ACIDURIA

Argininosuccinic aciduria is associated with argininosuccinase (argininosuccinate lyase) deficiency. Plasma and urine argininosuccinic acid levels are elevated markedly. Plasma arginine is reduced markedly; plasma glutamine and alanine are elevated. There is no marked increase in urinary orotic acid.

The disorder presents in the neonatal period, but as late as 1 to 2 weeks of age. Milder cases have presented in childhood or been detected by urinary newborn screening. Many patients have chronic hepatomegaly with fatty infiltration and fibrosis on biopsy. Arginine deficiency may lead to trichorrhexis nodosa with friable hair and erythematous maculopapular rashes, which respond to arginine therapy. In that argininosuccinic acid is excreted rapidly in the urine, this serves as a means for waste nitrogen excretion, as in citrullinemia. Patients also respond well to intravenous and oral L-arginine therapy. Protein restriction may be needed. Intercurrent episodes may require the use of sodium benzoate and sodium phenylacetate, but they usually are not required otherwise. The disorder is inherited as an autosomal recessive trait and may be confirmed by demonstrating deficient activity of argininosuccinate lyase in erythrocytes, cultured skin fibroblasts, or liver. Carrier detection and prenatal diagnosis are available.

## ARGININEMIA

Argininemia is a rare disorder associated with deficient activity of arginase and only modest hyperammonemia (100 to 300 $\mu$M). Patients usually do not have neonatal hyperammonemia. More often, there is a history of episodic vomiting, headache, irritability, seizures, cerebral atrophy, psychomotor retardation, and progressive spastic quadriparesis. Hepatomegaly may be present, with abnormal liver function tests and multifocal hydropic changes notable on biopsy. Plasma and urinary arginine levels are elevated, the former to a concentration greater than 500 $\mu$M. Urinary lysine, cystine, and ornithine may be increased as a result of competition with the large amounts of arginine for renal tubular reabsorption. Urinary orotic acid is increased because of arginine stimulation of N-acetylglutamate synthetase; the amount of carbamoyl phosphate produced is greater than the urea cycle can use, and the excess is channeled into pyrimidine pathways. Therapy includes protein restriction, dietary supplements for other non-protein nutrients, sodium benzoate or sodium phenylacetate, and supplementation of lysine and ornithine. Deficient activity of arginase may be demonstrated in erythrocytes, leukocytes, or the liver. The disorder is inherited as an autosomal recessive trait. Carrier detection is available. Prenatal diagnosis would require fetal liver biopsy or fetal blood sampling because the enzyme is not expressed in cultured fibroblasts.

## LYSINURIC PROTEIN INTOLERANCE

Two disorders associated with the transport of dibasic amino acids, lysinuric protein intolerance and the hyperammonemia-hyperornithinemia-homocitrullinuria syndrome, are associated with hyperammonemia and faulty urea synthesis.

Lysinuric protein intolerance is associated with faulty renal tubular, intestinal, and hepatic transport of dibasic amino acids. Urinary levels of lysine, arginine, and ornithine are elevated. Urinary levels of cystine, another dibasic amino acid, are not elevated, which distinguishes the urinary findings from those noted in cystinuria. Plasma levels of lysine, arginine, and ornithine are low. Plasma citrulline may be elevated. As a result of the low levels of ornithine, urea synthesis is impaired. Modest hyperammonemia (100 to 300 $\mu$M) and orotic aciduria occur. Patients may have signs of intermittent or acute hyperammonemia. They also are noted to have short stature, osteoporosis, hypotonia, lens opacities, hyperelastic skin, hyperextendable joints, friable hair, psychomotor retardation, and hepatosplenomegaly. Pancytopenia may be present. Treatment includes dietary protein restriction and L-citrulline supplementation. The disorder is inherited as an autosomal recessive trait and is most common in persons of Finnish background.

## HYPERAMMONEMIA-HYPERORNITHINEMIA-HOMOCITRULLINURIA SYNDROME

Hyperammonemia-hyperornithinemia-homocitrullinuria syndrome is a rare, autosomal recessive disorder thought to be caused by defective ornithine transport into the mitochondria, which leads to decreased urea synthesis. The plasma ornithine level is elevated moderately (350 to 555 $\mu$M) and the lysine level may be decreased. Urinary orotic acid is increased in one half of the patients. Intermittent increases in levels of urinary cystine, ornithine, arginine, and lysine may occur with episodes of hyperammonemia. There also is increased urinary excretion of homocitrulline, a metabolite of lysine. Plasma ammonia levels usually are elevated only mildly except with intercurrent episodes. Most patients have the syndrome diagnosed initially during the first year of life as a result of symptoms of intermittent hyperammonemia. Therapy includes protein restriction and supplemental ornithine administration.

## ORNITHINE-AMINOTRANSFERASE DEFICIENCY (GYRATE ATROPHY OF THE RETINA)

Ornithine aminotransferase is a mitochondrial, pyridoxal, phosphate-dependent enzyme involved in ornithine synthesis and degradation. Deficient activity of this enzyme is associated with hyperornithinemia without hyperammonemia. Patients may have a dibasic aminoaciduria. There is no increased urinary homocitrulline as is seen with hyperammonemia-hyperornithinemia-homocitrullinuria. The major clinical feature of the disorder is a characteristic gyrate atrophy of the choroid and retina with progressive loss of vision. The onset usually is in childhood, with myopia and decreased peripheral and night vision. Complete loss of vision commonly occurs between 20 and 50 years of age. Therapy includes supplementation with lysine or $\alpha$-aminoisobutyric acid in an attempt to increase renal excretion of ornithine, administration of pyridoxine (to which some patients are responsive), and dietary protein restriction, especially of arginine. The disorder is inherited as an autosomal recessive trait. About one half of all reported cases have occurred in Finnish individuals.

## TRANSIENT HYPERAMMONEMIA OF THE NEWBORN

In contrast to primary disorders of the urea cycle, in which there often is a 1- to 2-day period or longer before the onset of symptoms, patients with transient hyperammonemia of the newborn are seen with symptomatic hyperammonemia during the first 2 days of life. They often are premature infants in whom respiratory distress, lethargy, and coma develop rapidly. Plasma ammonia levels frequently are elevated massively in the range of 2000 to 4000 $\mu$M. Plasma citrulline levels may be normal or elevated mildly. Urinary orotic acid levels usually are normal, but may be elevated mildly for a brief period. The hyperammonemia should be treated promptly and vigorously because the associated mortality and morbidity rates are similar to those for primary urea cycle defects that are seen with neonatal hyperammonemic coma. For individuals who survive, recurrent hyperammonemia is rare, even with a normal protein intake. The etiology for the disorder is unknown, but it may be related to a transient immaturity of the urea cycle. In infants who weigh less than 2500 g at birth, about half may be noted to have plasma ammonia levels that are about twice as high as normal for the first 6 to 8 weeks of life. This usually asymptomatic mild hyperammonemia also is thought to be the result of a transient immaturity of the urea cycle.

## OTHER DISORDERS OF DIBASIC AMINO ACIDS

In glutaric acidemia type I, glutaric acid, a derivative of lysine and tryptophan, accumulates in tissues, cerebrospinal fluid, plasma, and urine. Most patients have a progressive macrocephaly from birth and then, before 2 years of age, have the sudden onset of hypotonia and dystonia after an intercurrent illness. Acute episodes of ketoacidosis with hypoglycemia, hyperammonemia, hepatomegaly, coma, and seizures may occur. Computed tomography and magnetic resonance imaging scans will show neuronal degeneration of the caudate and putamen. Urine organic acids will show elevated glutaric and 3-hydroxyglutaric acids. Deficient activity of glutaryl coenzyme A dehydrogenase may be shown in leukocytes or fibroblasts. Treatment includes pharmacologic doses of riboflavin, which forms the flavin adenine dinucleotide cofactor for glutaryl coenzyme A dehydrogenase. L-carnitine, which serves as a "trap" for the glutaric acid, and a low-protein or low-lysine and low-tryptophan diet. Baclofen or valproic acid may be helpful in controlling the movement disorder. The best outcomes occur in patients who are started on therapy before they develop acute episodes or neurologic involvement. The disorder is inherited on an autosomal recessive basis; carrier detection and prenatal diagnosis are available.

Hyperlysinemia associated with a defect in the bifunctional enzyme lysine-2-oxoglutarate reductase/saccharopine dehydrogenase, saccharopinuria caused by deficient activity of saccharopine dehydrogenase, 2-aminoadipic aciduria resulting from deficient 2-aminoadipate aminotransferase, and 2-oxoadipic aciduria caused by defective 2-oxoadipate dehydrogenase activity are of uncertain clinical significance in that the biochemical abnormalities have been noted in otherwise normal individuals as well as in patients who are being evaluated for biochemical genetic disorders.

## DISORDERS OF HISTIDINE METABOLISM

Histidinemia generally is considered not to be associated with any disabilities, although it is possible that the disorder may potentiate damage as a result of unrelated acute metabolic disturbances. Affected individuals have been ascertained by means of newborn screening programs that measure blood histidine concentrations and by ferric chloride testing of urine. The ferric ion complexes with imidazolepyruvic acid, which accumulates as a result of the transamination of increased quantities of histidine. The disorder is caused by a deficiency of histidase, which catalyzes the first step in the major metabolic pathway of histidine. Diagnosis may be confirmed by finding large amounts of histidine in the blood and urine, increased excretion of imidazolepyruvic acid in the urine, and reduced histidase activity in the liver or in cornified epithelium. A histidine-poor diet will correct the metabolic abnormalities, but rarely is indicated. Histidinemia is inherited on an autosomal recessive basis. In some families, carrier detection may be accomplished by skin histidase assay.

Formiminoglutamic aciduria involves an intermediate in histidine catabolism, formiminoglutamate, which accumulates because of a deficiency of glutamate formiminotransferase activity. Patients may have mild psychomotor retardation and hypotonia, although some from Japan have been reported to have severe neurologic deterioration with cortical atrophy.

## DISORDERS OF SULFUR-CONTAINING AMINO ACIDS

Disorders of sulfur-containing amino acids involve the transsulfuration pathway in which methionine is converted to cysteine in multi-stage forward reactions and the methionine concentration is regulated by a separate return pathway (Fig 12-7).

Homocystinuria is the prototype; the accumulation of homocystine results in a variety of acute and long-term symptoms and signs. The classic patient will be marfanoid in appearance, with dolichostenomelia, subluxated lenses, connective tissue weaknesses producing hernias and scoliosis, and cardiac complications (Fig 12-8). Patients with homocystinuria differ from those with Marfan syndrome, however, in that their joints are enlarged and stiffer than normal rather than hyperextendable. Also, their lenses tend to subluxate downward and inward as opposed to upward and outward as in Marfan syndrome, and patients with homocystinuria have no clinical manifestations of their disorder at birth. Cardiac findings may be similar in that the mitral and aortic valves may be incompetent, but there usually is no aortic dilatation as is seen in Marfan syndrome. Patients with homocystinuria frequently have osteoporosis, especially of the spine. Additional features of the disorder appear to be caused by the secondary effect of the defective collagen in bringing about vascular accidents. Mental retardation, strokes, and heart attacks are thought to be caused by a propensity to vascular thromboses, which may occur at any time of life, even earliest infancy. The pathogenesis is thought to be the result of the increase in homocystine in the body fluids. Homocystine is a disulfide that, in its monosulfide form, homocysteine, will bond covalently and permanently to the allysyl residues of nascent collagen molecules, thus preventing these residues from forming covalent bonds with similar residues on other collagen molecules. Accordingly, the collagen structure is weakened, and this weakening of the con-

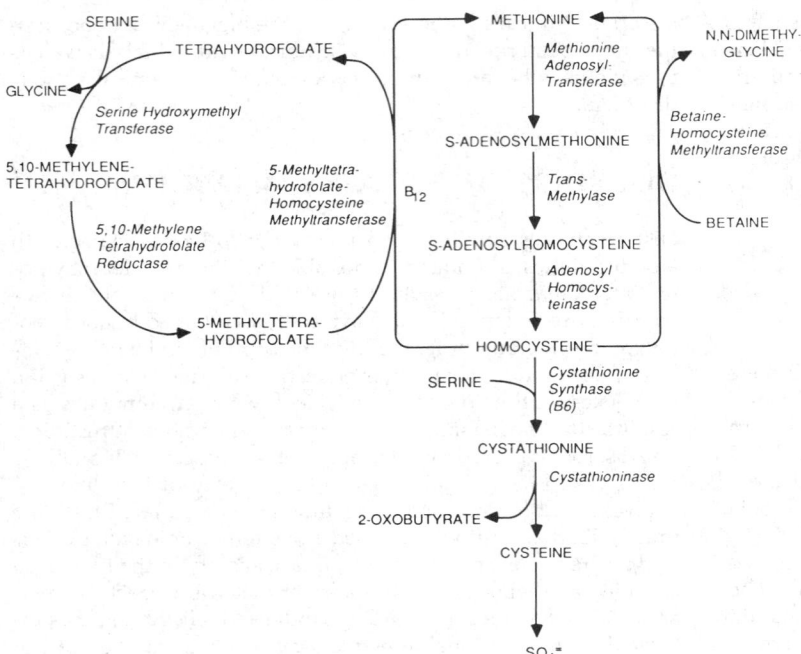

Figure 12-7.   The transsulfuration pathway.

nective tissue results in the structural manifestations of the disorder. Also, because of the poor quality of the connective tissue in the blood vessels, there is relatively poor binding of the endothelial cells to their substrate. The cells detach, exposing the substrate to platelets, which bind to it and form platelet thrombi, resulting in vascular accidents. The mental retardation associated with the disorder is thought to result from these vascular thrombi.

Management is directed toward reducing the homocystine concentration. About half the patients have some residual activity of cystathionine synthase. Administration of pharmacologic doses of pyridoxine, the cofactor of the enzyme, will result in enough of an increase in residual enzyme activity to cause the homocystine concentration to fall to low or undetectable levels. In responsive patients, treatment with a low-protein diet and pyridoxine, along with folic acid (which may become depleted), will be enough to prevent both the progression of the disorder and the vascular accidents. Otherwise, attempts are made to reduce the dietary protein intake or to reduce methionine intake selectively, employing special formulas. Supplementation with cystine is necessary. These attempts rarely, if ever, are completely suc-

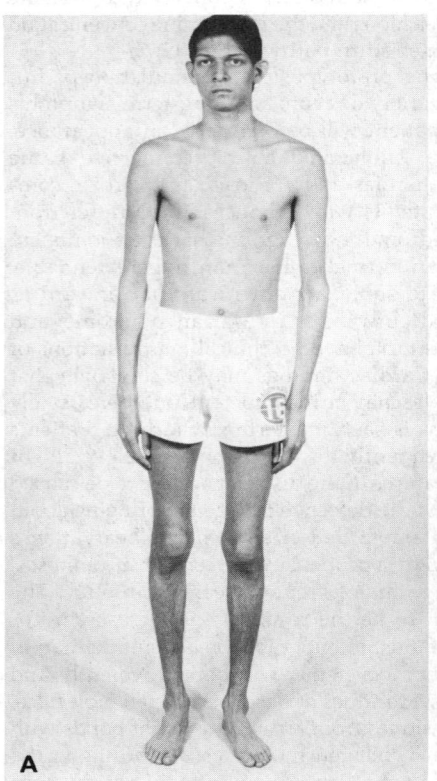

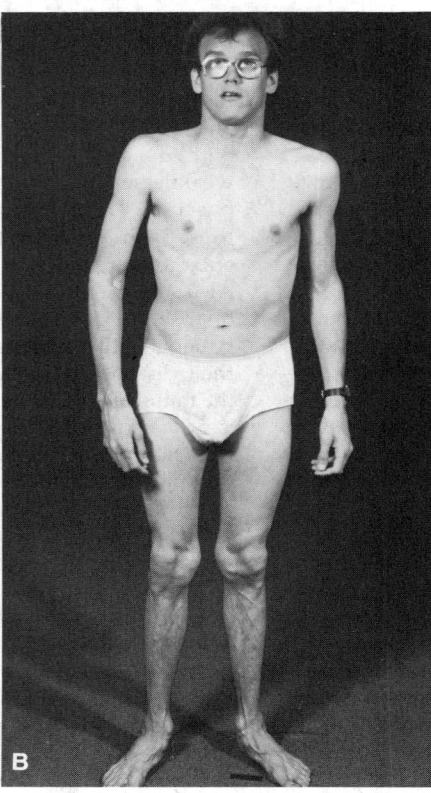

Figure 12-8.   Homocystinuria. (**A**) Teenage boy who presented with a pulmonary embolus; (**B**) young adult.

cessful, however, so aspirin is given to diminish the ability of the platelets to form thrombi, and betaine may be used to promote the remethylation of homocystine to methionine. Precautions are taken to avoid situations such as dehydration or invasive radiographic studies such as cardiac catheterization, which may result in fatal thromboses.

The diagnosis is made by finding increased methionine and homocystine levels and decreased cystine levels in the plasma and urine. Fibroblasts may be used to document reduced activity of cystathionine synthase. Lymphocytes normally do not have cystathionine synthase activity, but, when grown with mitogenic agents, will develop this activity over a period of days and may be used diagnostically.

The disorder has an incidence of 1:335,000 as determined by newborn screening using filter paper blood specimens to measure methionine concentration. The sensitivity is not 100%, however, because some patients do not have increased methionine levels until 1 month of age, so the true incidence is thought to be higher. It is inherited on an autosomal recessive basis; carriers may be defined by enzyme studies, as indicated previously. Prenatal diagnosis is accomplished by assay of cystathionine synthase in cultured amniotic fluid cells.

Hypermethioninemia is a rare disorder in which the first enzyme in the transsulfuration pathway, methionine adenosyl transferase, is defective, resulting in the accumulation of methionine. Affected persons do not appear to have any untoward effects from this disorder, so it remains a curiosity rather than a disease.

Cystathioninuria occurs when there is a deficiency of cystathionase. This is another disorder in which there are no ascertainable ill effects. Presumably, the elevated cystathionine level is not toxic and, even though the metabolic block makes cysteine an essential amino acid (normally, it is synthesized from methionine via the transsulfuration pathway), the latter is obtainable from the diet in adequate quantities.

Homocystinuria variants caused by defects in the remethylation of homocystine will result in the accumulation of homocystine and will give a clinical picture similar to that of the prototype disorder. 5,10-Methylenetetrahydrofolate reductase deficiency, if marked, will produce a severe clinical picture, including symptoms brought about not only by the homocystine accumulation, but also by the trapping of folic acid and methyl groups, which produces central nervous system manifestations. These patients frequently die in early infancy. Those with more enzyme activity will have less severe central nervous system manifestations, but still will be subject to the complications of the homocystine accumulation. Management is difficult, complex, and not entirely successful. 5-Methyltetrahydrofolate-homocysteine methyltransferase deficiency also will result in homocystinuria, but with milder symptoms. A severe disorder may result in individuals with defects in vitamin $B_{12}$ metabolism. Homocystine will accumulate and, if the defect in $B_{12}$ metabolism occurs in the initial processing of the cofactor, there will be not only a deficiency of methylated cobalamin, the cofactor for the 5-methyltetrahydrofolate-homocysteine methyltransferase, but also a deficiency of the 5'-deoxyadenosylated form, the cofactor for the enzyme methylmalonyl-CoA mutase. Thus, the patient will have not only homocystinuria, but also methylmalonic aciduria. Treatment consists of diet modification and the administration of pharmacologic amounts of the cofactors involved, but it frequently is unsuccessful. All these disorders are inherited on an autosomal recessive basis. The enzymes may be assayed in cultured skin fibroblasts and cultured amniotic fluid cells; prenatal diagnosis is available.

Sulfite oxidase deficiency is a very rare disorder associated with severe, progressive, ultimately fatal neurologic problems and subluxation of the lenses. It usually is a result of absence of the molybdenum cofactor. The accumulated sulfite combines with cysteine to give S-sulfocysteine, which is detectable in the urine of patients along with sulfite. The sulfite may be detected by a spot test. No successful therapy is available. It is inherited on an autosomal recessive basis and prenatal diagnosis is possible.

## DISORDERS OF GLYCINE METABOLISM

Nonketotic hyperglycinemia is a devastating disorder manifested in the early neonatal period by progressive lethargy, obtundation, feeding difficulties, and rapid progression to respiratory failure and death. If these infants are maintained on life-support systems and are fed by nasogastric tube, they will recover, over a period of weeks to months, respiratory functions and feeding abilities, in that order. They progress little beyond that, however, and become severely retarded with seizures and spastic tetraplegia. The disorder results from absence of the glycine cleavage enzyme. This enzyme usually is deficient in both the brain and liver of patients, but there have been normal results on assay of liver enzymes in some patients. Its pathogenesis is thought to be the result of the increased concentration of glycine, which leads to complete occupancy of glycine receptors in the neuroinhibitory pathways in the sections of the central nervous system in which glycine functions as a neurotransmitter. Attempts at reducing the glycine concentration have not met with clinical success. Valine has a toxic effect, even to the extent of coma, so a low-protein diet is suggested. The disorder is inherited on an autosomal recessive basis; prenatal diagnosis is available, but difficult. The diagnosis is made by finding markedly increased glycine levels in the plasma and urine. The glycine concentrations may vary, and it has been found that the cerebrospinal fluid-to-plasma glycine concentration ratio gives a more reliable interpretation because this always is elevated.

Sarcosine (N-methylglycine) normally is not demonstrable in the blood. It is an intermediate in the progressive demethylation of betaine. Its accumulation in sarcosinemia does not appear to be responsible for any abnormality in affected homozygotes and is the result of deficient activity of sarcosine dehydrogenase or one of its cofactors.

## DISORDERS OF BRANCHED-CHAIN AMINO ACID METABOLISM

Maple syrup urine disease varies greatly in its degree of severity, which is inversely proportional to the residual activity of the enzyme involved (Fig 12-9). In the severest cases, patients will have acute metabolic disease in the early neonatal period, will progress to seizures, and, if untreated, will die within a matter of days to weeks. Severe acidosis, hypoglycemia, and hyperammonemia occur, and these infants may require dialysis. The characteristic odor of maple syrup, although not present uniformly, has led to the diagnosis in a number of these infants. Milder cases may not be detected until later in infancy or even in childhood when there is an intercurrent illness or some other source of metabolic stress that results in decompensation and the findings of dullness, lethargy, and acidosis of varying degrees. Plasma and urine studies will show an increase in both the branched-chain amino acids leucine, isoleucine, and valine, and their corresponding oxo acids (keto acids). The disorder is caused by reduced activity of branched-chain oxo acid dehydrogenase, which may be demonstrated in cultured skin fibroblasts. Management in patients with milder forms of the disease who have appreciable residual enzyme activity may be accomplished with the administration of thiamine in pharmacologic doses and prescription of a low-protein diet. Severely affected patients will

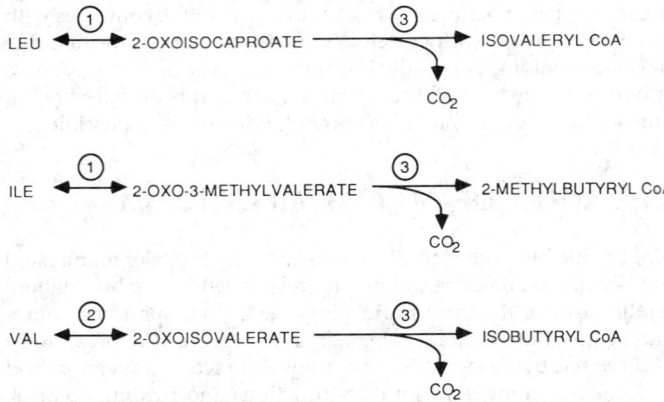

**Figure 12-9.** Maple syrup urine disease. The amino acids accumulate as well as the oxo acids because of the ready reversibility of the transaminases. Note that here are two transaminases; very rare disorders have been associated with each. *1*, leucine-isoleucine transaminase; *2*, valine transaminase; *3*, branched-chain oxo acid dehydrogenase complex, the enzyme deficient in this disorder.)

require a milk substitute that is free of the branched-chain amino acids, with supplementation of small but appropriate amounts of the individual branched-chain amino acids to achieve a normal or near-normal concentration of all amino acids. At initial diagnosis and in times of catabolism, they may require dialysis or special hyperalimentation mixtures to achieve control of their disorder. The isoleucine concentration is the first to change when its intake is varied, but it is felt that the leucine concentration is related most to symptomatology. If all three of the "noxious" amino acids as well as all the other amino acids are not monitored, there tends to be an amino acid imbalance, which may result in severe nutritional difficulties, which of themselves may be a severe and potentially fatal problem.

Prenatal diagnosis has been accomplished using cultured amniotic fluid cells, but carrier detection is not reliable. The disorder has an incidence of about 1:200,000 and is inherited on an autosomal recessive basis. It is felt that the various degrees of severity in different families are caused by different alleles at the same locus. Newborn screening may be carried out using filter paper specimens to measure the blood leucine concentration.

Isovaleric aciduria results from a defect in the catabolic pathway of leucine and may produce a severe acute metabolic disorder in the first days of life. Vomiting, acidosis, and lethargy, progressing to coma and death characterize the severe form of the disorder. In milder forms, the symptoms will be delayed for weeks or even to toddlerhood. Mental retardation to some extent is present in most patients. The odor of isovaleric acid is quite offensive and is described as being similar to that of "sweaty feet." In some patients, the degree of its unpleasant pervasiveness is inversely proportional to the degree of control of the disorder. Finding large amounts of isovalerylglycine in the urine and reduced activity of isovaleryl-CoA dehydrogenase in lymphocytes or cultured skin fibroblasts completes the diagnosis. Management includes prescription of a low-leucine diet, administration of glycine to facilitate conversion of isovaleric acid to isovalerylglycine (a nontoxic, odorless, readily excreted substance), and the administration of carnitine, which has the same mode of action as glycine and is needed to replace excessive isovalerylcarnitine losses. This autosomal recessive disorder has an incidence of less than 1:200,000. Prenatal diagnosis is possible.

3-Methylcrotonylglycinuria is a very rare disorder of leucine catabolism, which may begin with symptoms of acute metabolic disease, acidosis, hypoglycemia, and an odor of tomcat's urine. The disorder is controlled readily with a low-protein diet. Finding

3-methylcrotonylglycine and 3-hydroxisovalerate in the urine is characteristic of this autosomal recessive disorder. 3-Methyl-crotonyl CoA carboxylase deficiency may be demonstrated in lymphocytes and cultured skin fibroblasts. In contrast to multiple carboxylase deficiency, which is discussed below, this disorder is not responsive to biotin therapy.

3-Methylglutaconic aciduria is another rare disorder of leucine catabolism. Its severe form is characterized by the onset in infancy of a slowly progressive encephalopathy with hypotonia, spastic paraparesis, and optic atrophy. A mild form has been reported to be associated with language delay, and a third form beginning with dilated cardiomyopathy and neutropenia has been reported recently. Acute acidotic episodes may occur with intercurrent illnesses in all forms of this disorder. Cultured skin fibroblasts reveal deficient 3-methylglutaconyl-CoA hydratase activity in the mild form; the urine shows 3-methylglutaconate, 3-methylglutarate, and 3-hydroxisovalerate. The defects in the severe and cardiac-neutropenia forms are unknown; the urine reveals 3-methylglu-taconate and 3-methylglutarate, but no 3-hydroxisovalerate. 2-Ethylhydracrylic acid also may be found in the urine with the cardiac-neutropenia form. Treatment with a low-protein or low-leucine diet and L-carnitine may be of benefit.

3-Hydroxy-3-methylglutaric aciduria is a rare disorder of leucine catabolism with a presentation similar to that of Reye's syndrome in neonates or young infants. Nonketotic hypoglycemia and acidosis may lead to coma and death. A few patients have been diagnosed on study for milder symptoms such as hypotonia, but even these eventually to have severe attacks. Hypoglycemia is severe, and the blood ammonia concentration may rise to toxic levels. Although 3-hydroxy-3-methylglutarate is prominent in the urine, a variety of other organic acids are excreted, including 3-methylcrotonylglycine, 3-methylglutaconate, 3-methylglutarate, 3-hydroxisovalerate, and, occasionally, lactate and glutarate. Ketone bodies are characteristically absent. Leukocytes and cultured skin fibroblasts demonstrate reduced 3-hydroxy-3-methylglutaryl-CoA lyase. The enzyme catalyzes the key reaction in the conversion of fat as well as leucine and other ketogenic amino acids to ketones. In that ketones provide an appreciable source of energy for body metabolism, the reduction in ketone formation results in increased use of glucose as an energy source and hypoglycemia with fasting. Management of the acute episodes is as for any acute metabolic disorder, with special efforts directed at the acidosis, hypoglycemia, and hyperammonemia. The hyperammonemia may require dialysis, whereas correction of the accumulation of organic acids may be helped by carnitine administration. Prevention of recurrences involves a leucine- and fat-poor diet, with carbohydrate supplements given to minimize catabolism. Prenatal diagnosis is available both by analysis of amniotic fluid for metabolites and by enzyme assay of chorionic villi or cultured amniocytes. As expected for an autosomal recessive disorder, heterozygotes have intermediate enzyme activity.

Mevalonic aciduria is a very rare disorder in which there is a deficiency of mevalonate kinase, the second step in cholesterol biosynthesis. There is a marked accumulation of urinary mevalonic acid, which is converted to mevalonolactone during routine analytic procedures involving acidic extraction. The clinical picture is characterized by variable degrees of visceromegaly, anemia, thrombocytopenia, hypotonia, and central nervous system involvement. The serum cholesterol concentration is normal or low. There is no effective treatment. Affected individuals and carriers for this autosomal recessive disorder may be ascertained by enzyme assay of fibroblasts or lymphocytes. Prenatal diagnosis may be accomplished by enzyme assay of cultured amniocytes or by measuring the mevalonate concentration in aminotic fluid.

In mitochondrial 2-methylacetoacetyl-CoA thiolase deficiency, also previously called 3-oxothiolase ($\beta$-ketothiolase) deficiency, a block in the isoleucine degradative pathway results in the urinary accumulation of 2-methyl-3-hydroxybutyrate and 2-methylcrotonylglycine (tiglylglycine) as well as the CoA-free immediate substrate 2-methylacetoacetate. Affected infants frequently have episodic vomiting, acidosis, ketosis, a sweet odor, and hyperammonemia. Older children have less dramatic symptoms. Enzyme assay employing cultured skin fibroblasts is diagnostic. Management involves a low-protein diet to minimize isoleucine intake and usually is effective. The disorder is inherited on an autosomal recessive basis. Prenatal diagnosis should be possible employing amniotic fluid cell cultures.

Mitochondrial acetoacetyl-CoA thiolase deficiency, cytosolic acetoacetyl-CoA thiolase deficiency, and succinyl-CoA: 3-oxo acid-CoA transferase deficiency are very rare disorders associated with chronic ketosis, faulty utilization of acetoacetate, and severe neurologic dysfunction. Persistent elevation of $\beta$-hydroxybutyrate and acetoacetate occurs even with normal blood glucose in the non-fasted state. Reduced enzymatic activity may be shown in cultured skin fibroblasts or liver. A high-carbohydrate, low-fat diet may stabilize some patients.

Propionic acidemia is a rare disorder that classically begins with a severe acidosis and hyperammonemia at 2 days of age. There is a rapid increase in the severity of symptoms, starting with a simple anorexia, which progresses to lethargy, obtundation, hyperventilation, seizures, coma, and death if it is not treated. Blood studies reveal neutropenia, increased anion gap, low pH, hyperammonemia, hyperglycinemia, and greatly increased propionic acid concentration. Methylcitrate, 3-hydroxypropionate, propionylglycine, and 3-hydroxyvaleric acid are present in the urine, along with increased quantities of glycine. The disorder is caused by a deficiency in propionyl-CoA carboxylase and results in the accumulation of propionyl-CoA, an intermediate in the distal, common pathway of metabolism of isoleucine, valine, methionine, threonine, and the side chain of cholesterol and other three-carbon fatty acids (Fig 12-10). Propionyl-CoA is an intense inhibitor of the synthesis of N-acetylglutamate, a required cofactor for the initial enzyme in the conversion of ammonia to urea, carbamyl phosphate synthetase; this results in reduced urea synthesis and marked hyperammonemia. Indeed, some of the highest

ammonia concentrations ever recorded have been in patients with this disorder. The accumulated propionyl-CoA is split into coenzyme A and propionic acid; the propionic acid is responsible for the very severe acidosis that may occur. Milder cases may be seen in patients with acidotic episodes in infancy or early childhood. Definitive diagnosis requires enzyme assay using leukocytes or fibroblasts. The initial treatment involves discontinuation of protein intake and administration of glucose, bicarbonate, L-carnitine, and biotin, the cofactor of the enzyme. Dialysis may be required. Biotin never has been truly effective in reversing the disorder, however, so it is necessary to place the infant on a low-protein diet and, in severe cases, to use artificial formulas devoid of the four "noxious" amino acids. It is necessary to monitor carefully the concentrations of those noxious amino acids because they all are "essential" for life. Exacerbations are not uncommon, however, because illness and other stresses will cause increased protein catabolism, thus releasing a greater load of the four noxious amino acids than the patients can handle. The disorder is inherited on an autosomal recessive basis, and prenatal diagnosis may be accomplished by assay of cultured amniotic fluid cells for the enzyme activity and by measurement of methylcitrate levels in amniotic fluid.

Methylmalonic acidemia is another disorder in which the classic case becomes apparent at about 2 days of age, with much the same symptomatology and laboratory findings as are seen in propionicacidemia. This includes an increase in propionic acid in the plasma, as well as hyperammonemia. The distinguishing feature is that large quantities of methylmalonic acid are found in the urine (see Fig 12-10). Treatment is essentially the same as with propionicacidemia, except that the cofactor involved in this disorder is vitamin $B_{12}$, more specifically the 5'-deoxyadenosylated form, and there have been some patients who have been responsive to pharmacologic doses of hydroxyvitamin $B_{12}$ (hydroxocobalamin). Although some cases are associated with a deficiency in methylmalonyl-CoA mutase, others are associated with defects in vitamin $B_{12}$ metabolism.

The incidence is at least 1:50,000. Prenatal diagnosis is available employing enzyme assay on cultured amniotic fluid cells or assaying the amniotic fluid or the mother's urine for methylmalonic acid. Fetuses with the vitamin $B_{12}$–responsive disorder may be treated in utero; administration of vitamin $B_{12}$ in pharmacologic doses to the pregnant woman results in disappearance of methylmalonic acid from her urine. Accurate carrier detection is not available.

S-(2-carboxypropyl) cysteinuria is an extremely rare disorder of valine catabolism in which the deficiency of 3-hydroxyisobutyryl-CoA deacylase results in the accumulation of its penultimate precursor, methylacryly-CoA. The latter not only reacts with cysteine to produce the substance giving a name to the disorder, but also is thought to be teratogenic, in that the patient described died, having manifested multiple malformations and failure to thrive.

## MULTIPLE CARBOXYLASE DEFICIENCY

Multiple carboxylase deficiency involves pyruvate, propionyl-CoA, 3-methylcrotonyl-CoA, and acetyl-CoA carboxylases, all of which require a covalently linked cofactor, biotin, to function.

Holocarboxylase synthase deficiency prevents the covalent linkage of biotin to a lysyl residue of the apoenzyme and, thus, causes severe metabolic disease in earliest infancy with myoclonic seizures, hypotonia, acidosis, vomiting, failure to thrive, alopecia, and an erythematous desquamative rash. The plasma and urinary organic acid pattern reveals ketoacidosis and lactic acidosis. Urinary lactate, 3-hydroxyisovalerate, methylcitrate, 3-methycrotonylglycine, 3-hydroxypropionate, and tiglylglycine are elevated.

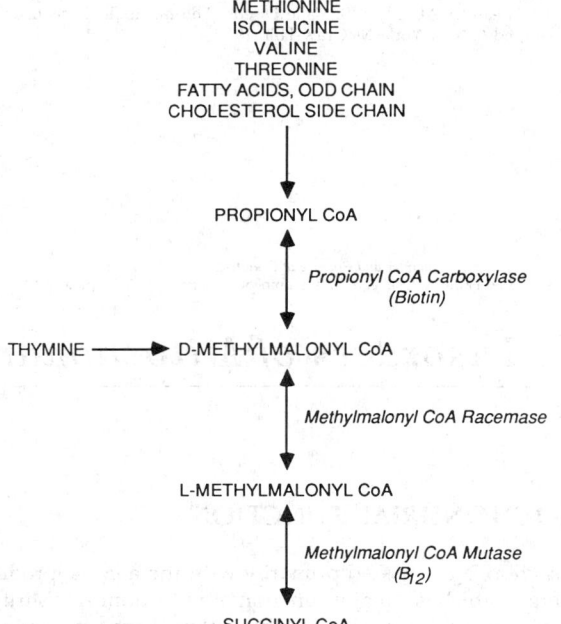

**Figure 12-10.** The metabolism of propionic and methylmalonic acids. *CoA*, coenzyme A.

Mild to moderate hyperammonemia occurs. The diagnosis is confirmed by assay of the synthetase or the carboxylases in leukocytes or fibroblasts. Administration of biotin in large doses usually ameliorates the condition, although some patients may be only partially responsive. Heterozygotes cannot be detected reliably. Prenatal diagnosis may be accomplished by measurement of amniotic fluid metabolite levels or amniotic cell culture enzyme activity. Prenatal therapy by administering biotin to the pregnant woman may be effective.

Biotinidase deficiency results in the same clinical picture as does holocarboxylase synthase deficiency, but is later in onset. Patients also may have optic atrophy, deafness, and immuno-regulatory dysfunction. The enzyme enables salvage of biotin as the holoenzyme is broken down in the course of the normal dynamic equilibrium. Biotinidase splits biotin from its covalent bond with a lysyl residue. In biotinidase deficiency, the biotin-lysine dipeptide (biocytin) is excreted, and the biotin is lost at a greater rate than its normal dietary intake. Administration of biotin in pharmacologic dosage appears to restore most patients completely except for permanent neurologic damage that already has occurred. In some patients, continued nerve degeneration has been noted, however, which may be caused by decreased pyruvate carboxylase activity and lactate accumulation in the brain. Many states have incorporated a test for blood biotinidase activity into their newborn screening programs. Heterozygosity may be determined reliably.

## DISORDERS OF IMINO ACID AND GLUTAMATE METABOLISM

The two types of prolinemia are considered to be innocuous because affected individuals, ascertained for reasons other than having a clinical problem themselves, have been asymptomatic. Both proline oxidase deficiency (type I) and $\Delta$1-pyrroline-5-carboxylate dehydrogenase deficiency (type II) are characterized by increased plasma and urinary proline concentrations. The urine also may contain increased quantities of glycine and hydroxyproline because the excessive proline excretion exceeds the tubular reabsorption capacity of the iminoglycine transport system.

Patients with iminopeptiduria have multiple problems with skin disorders, ulceration and dermatitis being most common, and some have bony deformities and mental retardation. Dipeptides containing proline or hydroxyproline are present in urine and are detected on routine chromatographic studies as well as by determination of bound imino acids. The enzyme involved, proline dipeptidase (prolidase), is demonstrated to be deficient using red blood cells, leukocytes, and cultured skin fibroblasts. The disorder is inherited as an autosomal recessive trait.

In the 5-oxoprolinurias, 5-oxo-L-proline (pyroglutamate) accumulates in persons with glutathione synthetase deficiency or with 5-oxoprolinase deficiency. Glutathione synthetase deficiency is an autosomal recessive disorder that results in glutathione deficiency with associated reduced ability to detoxify oxidants, hemolytic anemia, and chronic metabolic acidosis as a consequence of very high concentrations of 5-oxoproline in the plasma. Psychomotor retardation, cerebellar and cerebral damage become apparent, and some patients succumb in the first year of life. Management is effective in controlling the disorder at least partially and consists of combating acidosis with bicarbonate and avoiding environmental oxidants and drugs such as acetaminophen that require glutathione for detoxification. 5-Oxoprolinase deficiency is associated with lower levels of 5-oxoproline and is of uncertain clinical significance.

4-Hydroxybutyric aciduria may occur in patients with mental retardation, hypotonia, and ataxia, and is caused by succinic semialdehyde dehydrogenase deficiency. No treatment is available. It is inherited as an autosomal recessive disorder; prenatal diagnosis is possible.

## DISORDERS OF β-AMINO ACIDS

Hyper-β-alaninemia is a rare disorder characterized by coma, seizures, and early death. There is no treatment. The disorder is thought to be caused by a deficiency of β-alanyl:2-oxoglutarate aminotransferase. β-Alanine is an inhibitory neurotransmitter; it is presumed that its accumulation interferes with neurologic functions.

Carnosinemia has not been associated consistently with any specific clinical abnormalities and probably is an innocuous metabolic curiosity.

## DISORDERS OF AMINE METABOLISM

Persons with trimethylaminuria have a body odor of rotten fish after ingesting foods containing trimethylamine oxide or choline. Intestinal bacteria convert those substances to trimethyamine (TMA), which is absorbed into the circulation. A lack of hepatic TMA oxidase prevents conversion of TMA to trimethylamine oxide, a nonodorous compound. Treatment consists of dietary avoidance of fish (trimethylamine oxide), or of eggs and liver (choline).

## Selected Readings

Batshaw ML. Hyperammonemia. Curr Probl Pediatr 1984;14:1.

Batshaw ML, Monahan PS. Treatment of urea cycle disorders. Enzyme 1987;38: 242.

Berry GT, Heidenreich R, Kaplan P, et al. Branched chain amino acid-free parenteral nutrition in the treatment of acute metabolic decompensation in patients with maple syrup urine disease. N Engl J Med 1992;324:175.

Chalmers RA. Disorders of organic acid metabolism. In: Holton JB, ed. The inherited metabolic diseases. New York: Churchill Livingstone, 1987:141.

Desnick RJ. Treatment of genetic diseases. Part I. Metabolic therapy. New York: Churchill Livingstone, 1991:1.

Kelly RI, Cheatham JP, Clark BJ, Nigro MA, et al. X-linked cardiomyopathy with neutropenia, growth retardation and 3-meglutaconic aciduria. J Pediatr 1991;119: 738.

Maestri NE, Hauser ER, Bartholomew D, Brusilow SW. Prospective treatment of urea cycle disorders. J Pediatr 1991;119:923.

Nyhan WL, Sakati NA. Diagnostic recognition of genetic disease. Philadelphia: Lea & Febiger, 1987.

Scriver CR, Beaudet AL, Sly WS, Valle D, eds. The metabolic basis of inherited disease, ed 6. New York: McGraw-Hill, 1989.

*Principles and Practice of Pediatrics, Second Edition.*
edited by Frank A. Oski et al. J. B. Lippincott Company, Philadelphia © 1994.

# 12.4 *Disorders of Mitochondria*

## MITOCHONDRIAL FUNCTION

This section is concerned primarily with the aerobic production of energy, which is a major function of mitochondria (Mit); other biochemical reactions taking place within these cytoplasmic organelles are discussed elsewhere. Although Mit have varying sizes and shapes, depending on the specific tissue in which they are located and its particular physiologic state, the prototype is 1 to 2 μm long and roughly cylindric, with rounded ends. The outer surface is bounded by the outer membrane, which is permeable to virtually all compounds of low molecular weight. The inner membrane is much more restrictive, however, and most substances cannot enter or leave the matrix contained within the inner membrane unless a specific transport system is available. Furthermore, the inner membrane is folded narrowly at somewhat regular intervals into cristae, which project more or less deeply into the matrix. The narrow space between the outer and inner membranes is continuous with the narrow space between the two layers of each crista. In general, the areas where the inner membrane is contiguous with the outer membrane primarily have transport functions, whereas those areas of the inner membrane that form the cristae primarily have electron transport/oxidative phosphorylation (OP) functions. The matrix has its own complement of enzymes serving various functions.

It generally is accepted that Mit are the evolutionary descendants of primitive prokaryotic protists, which exist within eukaryotic cells in a symbiotic relationship, donating the apparatus for OP while taking advantage of those of the host cells' functions that they cannot perform themselves. In support of this is the fact that, within each mitochondrion, there are about five copies of the 25th type of human chromosome, also known as the mitochondrial chromosome. The mitochondrial chromosome is a double-stranded, 1-mm (when unfolded) loop that codes for two ribosomal RNAs (more like those of bacteria than those coded for by nuclear DNA), 22 transfer RNAs (unique in structure to the Mit), and 13 messenger RNAs. The messenger RNAs code for 7, 1, 3, and 2 polypeptide subunits of complexes I, III, IV, and V, respectively, of the mitochondrial OP system. There are no introns. It is pertinent that these mitochondrial chromosomes replicate and that their replication is associated with the binary fission process whereby Mit multiply as cell growth and division takes place. Furthermore, because, in human reproduction, any Mit that may be in the sperm do not enter the egg during fertil-

ization, the Mit in the zygote and in the individual who grows from that zygote are derived strictly maternally. This has been borne out by growing evidence that many families with a disorder of OP have a phenotypic heterogeneity thought to be accounted for by mutational events in chromosome 25, which may affect a varying percentage of the typically several hundred Mit per cell. The ultimate phenotype depends on the relative quantity of the different alleles present.

## LACTIC ACIDOSIS

Lactic acid is a relatively strong acid (pKa 3.79 versus 6.11 for carbonic acid) that does not participate directly in any metabolic pathway, but is important because it is interconvertible with pyruvic acid. Pyruvic acid is an intermediary in energy metabolism, but it is not mentioned nearly as frequently as is lactate because its concentration is 15 times lower than that of lactic acid under ordinary circumstances and is even less in anoxic states and other situations of reduced electron transport. The metabolic pathway of anaerobic metabolism goes through pyruvate to lactate, which accumulates. The lactate then will be oxidized back to pyruvate for more efficient utilization when aerobiosis is restored. With respect to inborn errors of metabolism, lactic acidosis may result either if a metabolic pathway distal to pyruvic acid is blocked or if there is an excess accumulation of protons/electrons because of an electron transport block.

Pyruvate dehydrogenase complex deficiency may produce a severe lactic acidosis. This complex catalyzes the conversion of pyruvate to acetyl-CoA and involves three enzymes, pyruvate dehydrogenase (E1), dihydrolipoyltransacetylase (E2), and dihydrolipoyl dehydrogenase (E3), and two cofactors, thiamine pyrophosphate and lipoate (Fig 12-11). The system is complicated further by its control system: stimulation of pyruvate dehydrogenase by a specific phosphatase and inhibition by a specific kinase.

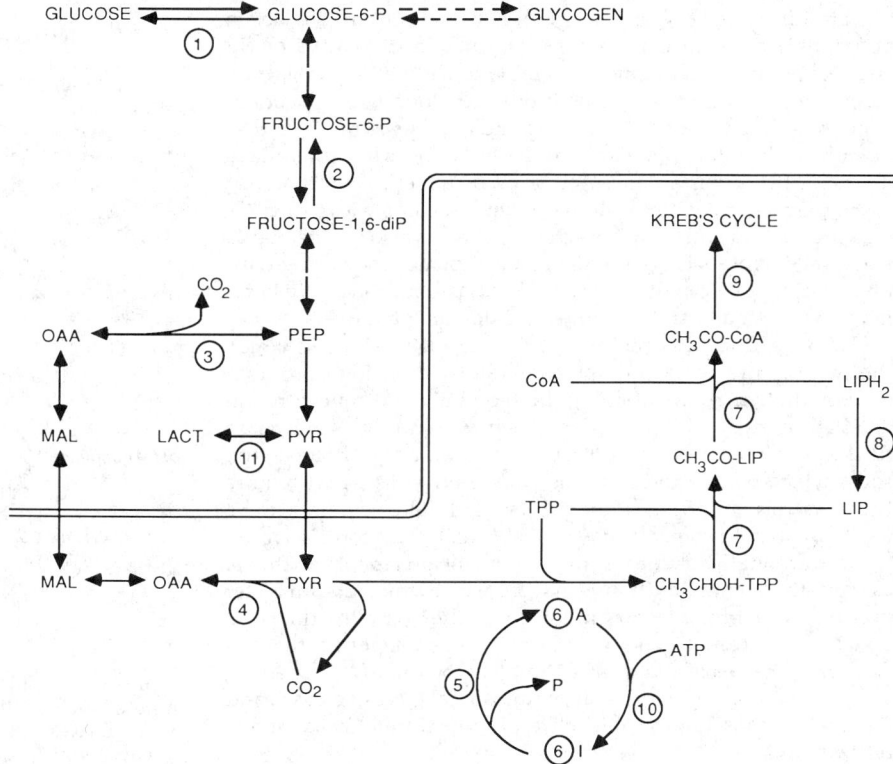

**Figure 12-11.** Pyruvic acid metabolism. *PEP,* phosphoenolpyruvate; *PYR,* pyruvate; *LACT,* lactate; *OAA,* oxaloacetate; *MAL,* malate; *A,* active; *I,* inactive; *Pi,* inorganic phosphate; *TPP,* thiamine pyrophosphate; *LIP,* lipoate; *ATP,* adenosine triphosphate; *CoA,* coenzyme A; *1,* glucose-6-phosphatase; *2,* fructose-1,6-diphosphatase; *3,* phosphoenolpyruvate carboxykinase; *4,* pyruvate carboxylase; *5,* pyruvate dehydrogenase phosphatase; *6,* pyruvate dehydrogenase (E1); *7,* dihydrolipoyltransacetylase (E2); *8,* dihydrolipoyldehydrogenase (E3); *9,* citrate synthase; *10,* pyruvate dehydrogenase kinase; *11,* lactate dehydrogenase.

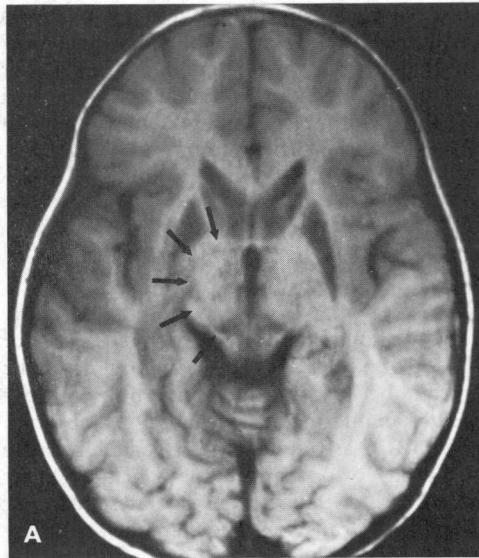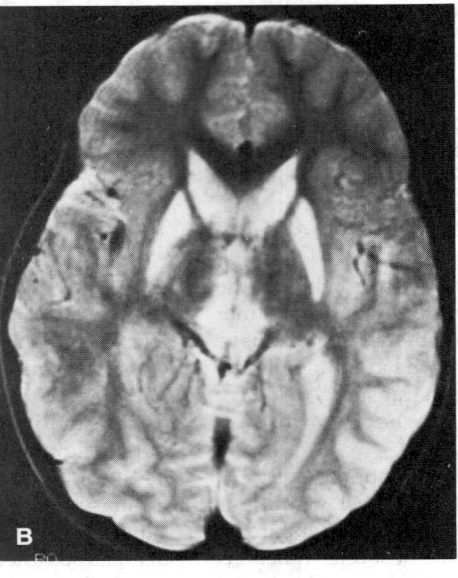

Figure 12-12.   Leigh syndrome. (**A**) MRI, T1-weighted image; (**B**) MRI, T2-weighted image, demonstrating necrotic areas in the basal ganglia.

The disorder may become clinically apparent in the first few days of life and can be extremely severe and even unresponsive to treatment. Alternatively, it may not be manifested for months or even years until it is precipitated by infection, prolonged fasting, or some other stimulus for gluconeogenesis. The patient will manifest the effects of lactate accumulation, acidosis with its attendant hyperpnea, and inadequate energy production, such as hypotonia, ataxia, confusion, lethargy, or coma. Survivors of the initial episode will have evidence of central nervous system damage, which worsens with each recurrence. Some patients will have the Leigh syndrome, with degeneration of basal nuclei (Fig 12-12).

A high anion gap produced by an increase in lactate concentration to more than 4 mmol/L and a normal glucose concentration in a child with a normal tissue oxygen tension should suggest this disorder. Hyperalaninemia essentially will confirm the lactate accumulation because the excess production of pyruvate will channel to some extent into transamination as well as into lactate formation. Ketogenesis may be promoted along with gluconeogenesis as a joint response to fasting and hypoglycemia. No other organic acids will be increased in the blood or urine when E1 is deficient. If there is a deficiency of E2 or E3, enzymes that also form part of two other dehydrogenase complexes, then 2-oxoglutaric acid and branched-chain oxo acids also will be noted. Ultimate diagnosis is accomplished by enzyme assay using lymphocytes, tissues, or cultured skin fibroblasts, although the latter may give normal results in otherwise documented cases.

Therapy involves minimizing gluconeogenesis (for which the major pathway is through pyruvate) with a high-fat, low-carbohydrate diet, maintaining the blood glucose concentration at a high-normal level (excessively high concentrations will cause further channeling of glucose into lactate), and administering sodium bicarbonate and carnitine. More severe cases may require hemodialysis or peritoneal dialysis; special fluids will have to be made up because commercially available dialysates contain lactate as a bicarbonate substitute (the latter will precipitate with the calcium these contain). It also may be worthwhile to administer precursors of the cofactors involved in the complex, thiamine and lipoate. Recent experimental work has suggested that dichloroacetate, a stimulator of E1, may be of value.

The disorder is inherited on an autosomal recessive basis, and prenatal diagnosis is available. Heterozygotes cannot be identified reliably.

Krebs' tricarboxylic acid cycle defects have been described (Fig 12-13). As cited previously, patients with reduced dihydrolipoyltransacetylase (E2) or dihydrolipoyl dehydrogenase (E3) will manifest not only the findings of pyruvate dehydrogenase complex deficiency, but also those of branched-chain oxo acid dehydrogenase and 2-oxoglutarate dehydrogenase deficiencies. Fumarase deficiency has been described.

OP deficiency may result in a broad spectrum of clinical manifestations, befitting the broad spectrum of specific defects reported. Lactic acidosis may be absent to severe, depending on the degree of impairment of the specific OP component relative to the actual energy requirement of the moment. Muscle weakness and other symptoms may be equally varied and may be organ

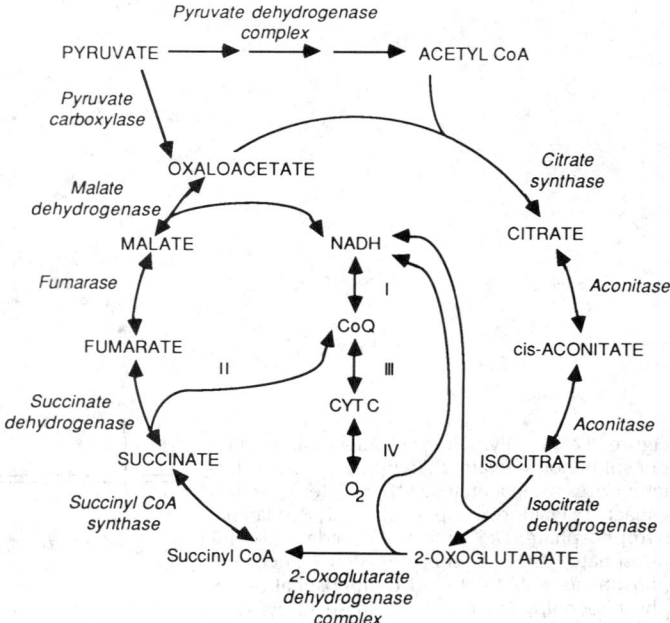

Figure 12-13.   Krebs' cycle. Note that the three dehydrogenases contribute NADH to the electron transport system, whereas succinate dehydrogenase is a part of the pathway and contributes an electron directly to coenzyme Q (*CoQ*). *CoA*, coenzyme A; *CYT C*, cytochrome C.

specific (ie, a documentable enzyme defect limited to striated muscle).

The OP system is composed of five complexes (Fig 12-14), all of which are located in the mitochondrial cristae (see above). These complexes, I, II, III, IV, and V, have the reduced form of nicotinamide-adenine dinucleotide-ubiquinone reductase, succinate-ubiquinone reductase, ubiquinone-cytochrome C reductase, cytochrome oxidase, and F0–F1 adenosine triphosphate synthetase activities, respectively, and are composed of 26, 5, 10, 8, and 11 or 12 polypeptide subunits, of which 7, 0, 1, 3, and 2 are coded for by Mit DNA. Deficiencies of the system's many components, each of which may be affected by many mutations, each one specific for a different site within the polypeptide molecule as well as for tissue-specific penetrance and expression, result in the broad range of symptoms and signs cited previously.

A number of names have been used to designate this group of disorders and some of the symptom complexes it includes. *Mitochondrial cytopathy* has been proposed for an overall designation; it emphasizes the fact that most patients have an increase in Mit, which aggregate in irregular clumps within cells, mainly type I (aerobic) muscle fibers, producing a "ragged-red" appearance in routinely stained light-microscope sections. Another general term is *mitochondrial encephalomyopathy*, which is more clinically descriptive. Two acronyms have been used to describe syndromes associated with OP defects: MERRF (*myoclonic epilepsy with ragged-red fibers*) and MELAS (*mitochondrial myopathy, encephalopathy, lactic acidosis, and stroke-like episodes*). Other syndromes have been described: Kearns-Sayre syndrome (ophthalmoplegia plus), Leigh syndrome (subacute necrotizing encephalomyelopathy), Alpers syndrome (progressive infantile poliodystrophy), Leber's optic atrophy, chronic progressive external ophthalmoplegia, oculo-cranio-somatic neuromuscular disorder, and infantile striatal necrosis.

Findings in various patients have involved a number of organ systems. Eye findings have included ophthalmoplegia, ptosis, corneal opacities, cataracts, glaucoma, and changes in retinal pigment. Neurologic findings have involved facial weakness, moderate mental retardation, dementia, speech disorders, sensory neuropathy, ataxia, pyramidal signs, epilepsy, and deafness. Heart conduction defects, cardiomyopathy, glomerulosclerosis, or Fanconi's syndrome may occur. Endocrine problems noted have been shortness of stature with or without growth hormone deficiency, diabetes mellitus, adrenocorticotropic hormone deficiency, hypogonadism, hypoparathyroidism, hyperthyroidism (Luft syndrome), and hyperaldosteronism. Anemia and hepatopathies also have been noted.

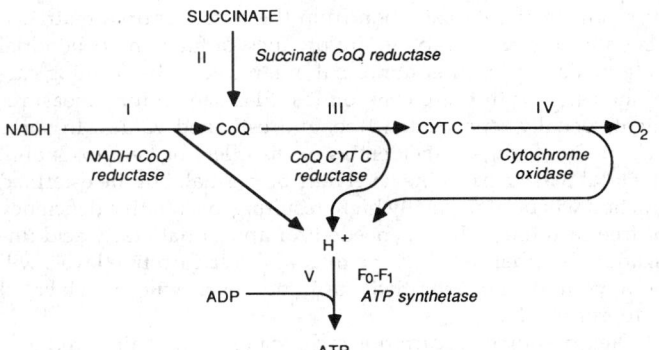

**Figure 12-14.** Electron transport pathway. As an electron passes through complexes I, III, and IV, a proton is discharged from each complex to provide the energy for adenosine triphosphate (*ATP*) synthesis. *ADP*, adenosine diphosphate; *CoQ*, coenzyme Q; *NADH*, the reduced form of nicotinamide-adenine dinucleotide; *CYT C*, cytochrome C.

Laboratory findings have included lactic acidosis with an increased lactate/pyruvate ratio and anion gap, and high creatine kinase, and cerebrospinal fluid protein and lactate levels. Finding abnormal Mit in increased number in muscle biopsy studies is quite suggestive, but assay of the OP system is the definitive procedure. The generation of adenosine triphosphate using succinate and pyruvate as substrates provides evidence of intact complexes II through V and of pyruvate dehydrogenase/Krebs' cycle/complexes I, III, IV, and V, respectively. Failure of succinate to generate adenosine triphosphate with normal results for pyruvate pinpoints the defect to complex II, failure of pyruvate with success of succinate indicates a defect in complex I or one of the antecedent reactions, and failure of both substrates denotes a defect in complex III, IV, or V. Further studies involving immunochemistry and DNA analyses may reveal the actual subunit that is deficient.

Treatment involves keeping the blood glucose concentration at a high-normal, but not elevated, level to minimize gluconeogenesis, administering bicarbonate to minimize acidosis (even between episodes), bypassing a defective complex with an artificial electron transport system, and administering cofactor precursors of the OP enzyme system. Some improvement in the OP system has been noted after giving riboflavin in pharmacologic doses to individuals with complex II or III deficiencies. Ascorbate or ubiquinone may result in some improvement in patients with complex IV deficiency. In the severest (particularly neonatal) cases, even dialysis may be required, though it frequently is to no avail.

Family studies are important in understanding the particular disorders involved. Evidence of maternal inheritance (all siblings and the maternal half-siblings of the index case are affected to some degree) indicates deficiency of a polypeptide subunit normally coded for by the mitochondrial chromosome. A more uniform clinical picture in affected siblings, with the latter constituting 25% of the sibship, indicates autosomal recessive inheritance and, thus, coding by a nuclear chromosome. Heterozygosity cannot be determined reliably. Prenatal diagnosis is possible only if a tissue known to demonstrate the defect in the index case is used and the pattern of inheritance is understood clearly .

Disorders of gluconeogenesis by the reverse Embden-Meyerhof pathway may produce severe lactic acidosis compounded by hypoglycemia. The efficiency of the forward pathway in anaerobic glycolysis as well as the fact that all of the intermediates between glucose and pyruvate are phosphorylated and, thus, cannot leave the cell, means that a block at any step will result in pyruvate (and, thus, lactate) accumulation as long as there is any stimulus to gluconeogenesis. Because glucose concentration is low and is not restored, further stimulation of gluconeogenesis goes on until the vicious cycle is stopped by providing exogenous glucose. Indeed, a clinical picture of cyclic vomiting may characterize these disorders, as discussed in the section on acute metabolic disease.

Pyruvate carboxylase deficiency may be a severe, episodic disorder, as indicated previously. Except for prominent hypoglycemia, these patients' problems are similar to those of patients with pyruvate dehydrogenase deficiency and are managed much the same, particularly because the diagnosis may not be clearcut. Because biotin is the cofactor involved in this enzyme, there may be some advantage to administering it in a dosage of 10 mg daily, although it is unusual to see a significant response. Some patients with Leigh syndrome have been found to have a deficiency of this enzyme.

Definitive diagnosis is based on enzyme studies of liver, leukocytes, or cultured skin fibroblasts. Heterozygosity for this autosomal recessive disorder is not defined reliably, but prenatal diagnosis is available.

Phosphoenolpyruvate carboxykinase deficiency is extremely rare, but manifests as do the others in this group. It is mentioned here because some of the patients have a deficiency of the mitochondrial enzyme, whereas others have a deficiency of the cytosolic enzyme.

Other enzymes further on in the gluconeogenic (reverse Embden-Meyerhof) pathway may be deficient. These are described in the section on carbohydrates.

## DISORDERS OF FATTY ACID OXIDATION

During fasting, mitochondrial beta-oxidation of fatty acids is an important source of energy production. After fatty acids are mobilized from adipose tissue, they are transported bound to albumin to the liver and other tissues, where they are taken across the plasma membrane by fatty acid binding proteins. The fatty acids then are "activated" to their coenzyme A (CoA) esters by cytosolic acyl-CoA synthase, transported across the mitochondrial membrane by a carnitine-mediated system, and oxidized to ketone bodies in the mitochondrial matrix. Thus, the disorders involving mitochondrial beta-oxidation of fatty acids are characterized by faulty formation of ketone bodies, impaired energy production, and the accumulation of partially oxidized fatty acid metabolites during periods of stress and fasting. The disorders have widely varying clinical manifestations. All are thought to be inherited as autosomal recessive traits.

Long-chain (C10 to C18) fatty acids are activated by cytosolic acyl-CoA synthase at the outer aspect of the mitochondrial membrane to form long-chain acyl-CoA esters, which then are trans-esterified with carnitine by carnitine palmityl transferase (CPT) I to form long-chain acyl-carnitine esters at the inner aspect of the outer mitochondrial membrane. The long-chain acyl-carnitines then cross the inner mitochondrial membrane by a process that is mediated by carnitine translocase. At the matrix side of the inner mitochondrial membrane, the long-chain acyl-carnitines are re-esterified to long-chain acyl-CoA esters by CPT II. Medium-chain (C6 to C12) and short-chain (C4 and C6) fatty acids do not appear to need carnitine-mediated transport to enter the mitochondrial matrix, where they are activated to form their acyl-CoA esters. The acyl-CoA esters then enter into the beta-oxidation pathway, as shown in Figure 12-15. With each cycle through the pathway, the fatty acid-CoA ester is reduced in length by two carbons, and an acetyl-CoA group is generated that can be metabolized further to ketone bodies in the liver and kidneys or can enter the tricarboxylic acid cycle. The beta-oxidation pathway includes a series of chain length–specific acyl-CoA dehydrogenases, enoyl-CoA hydratase, 3-hydroxyacyl-CoA dehydrogenase, and 3-ketoacyl-CoA thiolase. The acyl-CoA dehydrogenases are flavoproteins that transfer the electrons that are generated to electron transfer flavoprotein and subsequently to the mitochondrial respiratory chain. Long-chain acyl-CoA dehydrogenase (LCAD) catalyzes the reaction for fatty acid chain lengths of 12 to 18 carbons, medium-chain acyl-CoA dehydrogenase (MCAD) catalyzes the reaction for fatty acid chain lengths of 4 to 14 carbons, and short-chain acyl-CoA dehydrogenase (SCAD) catalyzes the reaction for fatty acid chain lengths of 4 or 6 carbons. Fatty acid acyl-CoA esters with odd chain lengths are oxidized similarly until the three-carbon propionyl-CoA is formed. Unsaturated fatty acids require two additional enzymes, 3-cis, 2-trans-enoyl-CoA isomerase and 2,4-dienoyl-CoA reductase, for complete beta-oxidation of these compounds.

The acetyl-CoA and acyl-CoA esters formed as a result of beta-oxidation exit the mitochondrial matrix by carnitine-mediated transport similar to that for the entrance of long-chain acyl-CoA esters. Acetylcarnitine is formed by carnitine acetyl-

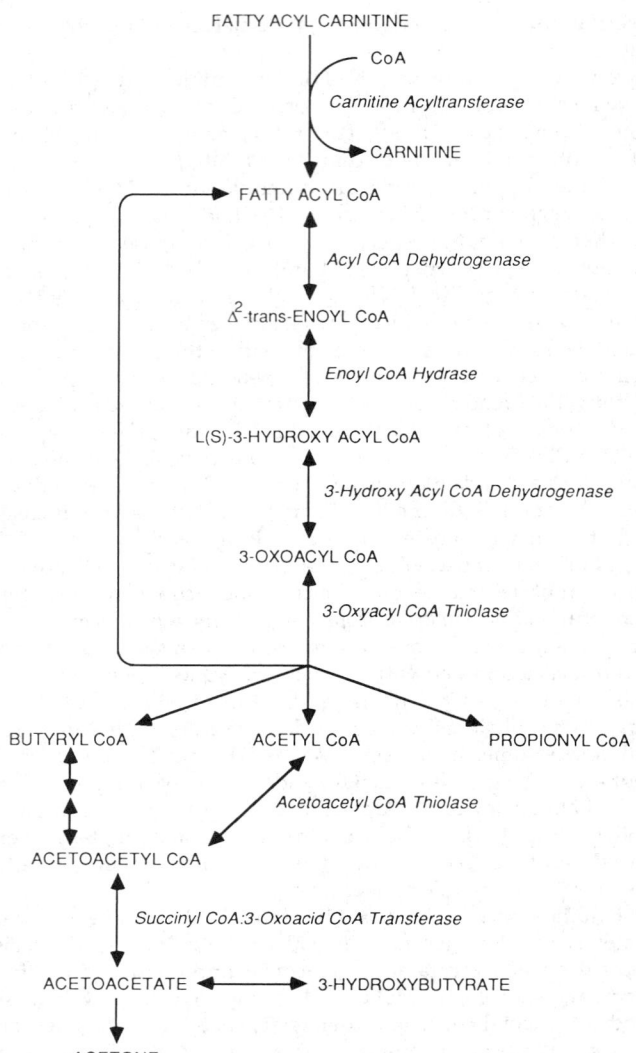

**Figure 12-15.** Hepatic mitochondrial metabolism of fatty acids. *CPT II*, carnitine palmitoyl transferase II; *ETF*, electron transport flavoprotein; *HMG*, 3-hydroxymethylglutaryl; *CoA*, coenzyme A; *FAD*, flavin adenine dinucleotide, *FADH$_2$*, reduced form of FAD.

transferase and is transported by a translocase from the mitochondrial matrix to the cytosol.

Carnitine (L-*carnitine*) is involved in the transport of long-chain fatty acid acyl-CoA esters into the Mit and the transport of products of beta-oxidation from the mitochondrial matrix. It also functions as a "trap" for by-products of faulty mitochondrial beta-oxidation or other abnormal organic acids by forming carnitine esters with these compounds. Plasma carnitine measurements usually report total, free, and esterified values. In some patients with organic acidemias or disorders of beta-oxidation, the total plasma carnitine level may be normal, but the esterified fraction will be abnormally high, resulting in a relative deficiency of free carnitine, which is needed for appropriate fatty acid utilization. In other patients, the total and free carnitine levels will be low and the esterified carnitine level will be elevated inappropriately.

Dietary sources of carnitine include meats and dairy products. Endogenous carnitine can be synthesized from lysine. Deficiency states usually are associated with organic acidemias or faulty beta-oxidation. Secondary deficiencies also may be seen with renal tubular disorders, vitamin C and pyridoxine deficiencies, strict vegetarian diets, total parenteral nutrition, hemodialysis, and valproate anticonvulsant therapy.

Systemic carnitine deficiency, regardless of the etiology, results in faulty fatty acid oxidation and has been associated with inability to tolerate fasting, hypoketotic hypoglycemia, liver dysfunction, hypotonia, myopathies, and cardiomyopathies. In that our knowledge of carnitine deficiency preceded our understanding of fatty acid oxidation, many of the patients reported to have systemic carnitine deficiency in the past subsequently have been found to have defects in fatty acid oxidation.

MCAD deficiency is the most common of the disorders and is estimated to occur in 1:10,000 births. Most patients are seen between 5 and 24 months of age with repeated episodes of vomiting, lethargy, and hypotonia after a decreased carbohydrate intake associated with an intercurrent illness or fasting. Mild hepatomegaly and seizures may occur. Hypoglycemia and mildly elevated ammonia and liver enzyme levels usually are noted. A mild metabolic acidosis may be present. Urine ketones may be absent or present in trace amounts, which has led to the term *hypoketotic hypoglycemia* for this group of disorders. However, some patients are able to make ketone bodies with stress. The amount of ketones produced, though, as determined by plasma $\beta$-hydroxybutyrate levels, is inappropriately low for the degree of hypoglycemia and the marked elevation of plasma free fatty acids mobilized in response to fasting. The pathophysiologic reason for the hypoglycemia is not understood completely, but is thought to result from failure of the normal gluconeogenic response to fasting, which normally occurs as a response to increased acetyl-CoA and ketone body production.

There is wide variability in clinical presentation. Some patients have had the disorder diagnosed in the newborn period, whereas others are asymptomatic and are detected only by family screening. Some patients have a rapidly deteriorating course with an episode that progresses to coma and death from cardiorespiratory collapse or cerebral edema. The accumulation of acyl-CoA compounds, especially those with chain lengths of three carbons or more, is associated with encephalopathies and may result in cerebral edema. The mortality rate is highest between 15 and 26 months of age, when it is reported to be 59%. About 25% of patients die with their first episode, which frequently is unrecognized as being caused by a disorder of fatty acid oxidation until the disorder is diagnosed in a second child in the family. Many of the deaths have been thought to be the result of Reye's syndrome or sudden infant death syndrome. Autopsy findings include fatty infiltration of the liver, which may be macrovesicular or microvesicular in pattern. Mitochondrial changes in the liver on electron microscopy differ from those seen in Reye's syndrome and may show a condensed appearance of the Mit with increased matrix density and intracristal widening, or enlarged and abnormally shaped Mit with an increase in the number of cristae and crystalloids in the matrix.

With episodes, affected individuals accumulate metabolites of medium chain length (C6 to C12), especially octanoic acid and 4-decenoic acid. With the accumulation of fatty acyl-CoA intermediates of medium chain length with the Mit, alternative pathways of microsomal (omega and omega-1) oxidation and peroxisomal beta-oxidation become involved and lead to excessive production of (omega-1)-hydroxy acids and medium-chain dicarboxylic acids such as adipic, suberic, and sebacic acids. These metabolites may be detected in the blood or urine of patients during episodes by organic acid analysis employing gas chromatography-mass spectrometry. Acyl-CoA compounds may be conjugated with glycine as well as carnitine. Abnormal metabolite patterns may be detected by either urinary acyl-glycine profiles (stable isotope dilution gas chromatography-mass spectrometry) or plasma or urine acyl-carnitine profiles (fast atom

bombardment with tandem mass spectrometry). These latter two tests are more sophisticated and sensitive than are routine organic acid measurements, and are available in only a limited number of laboratories. They are indicated in the evaluation of all patients suspected of having a defect in fatty acid oxidation, however, because asymptomatic patients may have normal routine organic acid analysis (gas chromatography-mass spectroscopy) between episodes, but frequently will have abnormal profiles by acyl-glycine or acyl-carnitine techniques. Patients usually have abnormal plasma and urinary carnitine levels, with lowered total and elevated esterified fractions. An oral carnitine load, followed by measurement of urinary acyl-carnitines, may assist in the diagnosis of patients who are carnitine depleted. Patients should not be subjected to a provocative fast because of the possibility of inducing a fatal acute episode. The recent availability of acyl-carnitine profiles from blood filter paper dots will allow retrospective diagnosis in children who have died and will make newborn screening for this group of disorders feasible in the future. Deficient activity of MCAD may be shown in cultured skin fibroblasts or leukocytes. The complementary DNA has been cloned, and DNA diagnosis may be done using blood filter paper dots in most patients. Prenatal diagnosis and carrier detection are available.

The basis for treatment is the avoidance of fasting and lipolysis. Frequent meals or feedings, with a high carbohydrate and relatively lowered fat intake is recommended. MCT (medium-chain triglyceride) oil in any form should be avoided. Treatment should be started as soon as the diagnosis is considered, even if test results are not available yet. L-carnitine supplementation is indicated in symptomatic patients. Only the prescription form of L-carnitine should be used and not the D,L form that is available in health food stores. Episodes should be treated promptly with intravenous glucose and hydration, to which most patients respond. Once the disorder is recognized and treated, many patients do well. However, residual neurologic dysfunction from severe episodes will persist.

LCAD deficiency is a rare disorder. In most cases, the clinical features are similar to those of MCAD deficiency, but the onset is earlier, usually before 6 months of age; the episodes are more severe, with a high mortality rate; and a hypertrophic cardiomyopathy is present. Some patients also have hypotonia and developmental delay. Milder variants have been reported to cause initial symptoms similar to those of MCAD deficiency. Others have begun later in life with recurrent episodes of stress-related myalgias and rhabdomyolysis. Liver biopsies in the severe type may reveal portal fibrosis in addition to steatosis. During episodes, urinary organic acid (gas chromatography-mass spectroscopy) profiles may show elevated long-chain (C12 and C14) as well as medium-chain dicarboxylic acids. Because long-chain acyl-carnitines are not excreted readily in the urine, urinary acyl-carnitine profiles frequently are normal. Urinary acyl-glycine profiles and plasma or blood filter paper dot acyl-carnitine profiles may be abnormal, however. Lowered total and elevated esterified plasma carnitine levels are noted. The disorder is confirmed by demonstrating reduced activity of LCAD in leukocytes or cultured skin fibroblasts. Therapy includes avoidance of fasting and prompt treatment of episodes as for MCAD deficiency. For the infantile-onset types, a high-carbohydrate diet with fat intake restricted to medium-chain triglycerides and essential fatty acids is recommended. For those with rhabdomyolysis, carbohydrate loading is recommended before exercise. Carnitine supplementation may be of benefit to patients with all types of the disorder.

SCAD deficiency is a very rare disorder. In contrast to medium- and LCAD deficiencies, patients with SCAD deficiency are able to tolerate fasting and are capable of ketone body production in that their metabolic block allows the beta-oxidation of medium-

and long-chain fatty acids to proceed. Two patients with an infantile form of the disorder were seen in the neonatal period for poor feeding and metabolic acidosis. One child died at 6 days of age with cerebral edema. Another patient was seen for poor feeding, failure to thrive, microcephaly, developmental delay, hepatomegaly, and progressive hypotonia at 1 year of age. Lipid deposition was noted in the liver of the child that died and on muscle biopsy in the older child with hypotonia. All three patients had abnormal organic acid levels, with elevations in butyric and ethylmalonic acids, among others. SCAD deficiency was documented in cultured skin fibroblasts in these patients. Two adults have been reported to have SCAD deficiency presumably limited to skeletal muscle. Both had episodic weakness; this led to muscle biopsy, which demonstrated lipid deposits in type I fibers. Mitochondria were noted to have osmiophilic inclusions in one patient and were normal in the other. One patient responded to oral riboflavin therapy.

Long-chain 3-hydroxyacyl-CoA dehydrogenase deficiency has been reported in young infants before 9 months of age with clinical features similar to those seen with LCAD deficiency. Patients excrete 3-hydroxydicarboxylic acids and 3-hydroxy-monocarboxylic acids with episodes. Plasma or blood filter paper dot acyl-carnitine profiles are abnormal. Plasma carnitine levels reveal elevated esterified fractions. The defect may be demonstrated in cultured skin fibroblasts. Treatment is similar to that for LCAD deficiency. Other patients with similar clinical symptoms along with chronic progressive liver dysfunction, pigmentary retinopathy, and peripheral neuropathy have been noted to have 3-hydroxydicarboxylic aciduria; the biochemical basis for this disorder is unclear. A "trifunctional enzyme" deficiency also has been noted that involves mitochondrial long-chain 3-hydroxyacyl-CoA dehydrogenase, 2-enoyl-CoA hydratase, and 3-ketoacyl-CoA thiolase deficiencies. Patients have the onset in childhood of clinical features similar to those of LCAD deficiency with a progressive hypotonia and fatty infiltration of the liver. Accumulation of 3-hydroxyacyl-CoA, 2-enoyl-CoA, and 3-ketoacyl-CoA intermediates has been noted in muscle and fibroblast mitochondrial fractions.

Short-chain 3-hydroxyacyl-CoA dehydrogenase deficiency has been reported recently in a 16-year-old girl with recurrent myoglobinuria, hypoketotic hypoglycemic encephalopathy, and hypertrophic cardiomyopathy. The enzymatic defect was noted in muscle, but not in cultured skin fibroblasts.

2,4-Dienoyl-CoA reductase deficiency is unique in that it is the first enzymatic defect to be reported to involve only unsaturated fatty acid oxidation. The only reported case to date was seen in the neonatal period with hypotonia, hyperlysinemia, and lowered total and free carnitine levels. Failure to thrive, microcephaly, and shortened trunk, arms, and fingers also were noted; the patient died at 4 months of age with respiratory acidosis. An unusual acyl-carnitine, 2-*trans*,4-*cis*-decadienoylcarnitine, was noted in the plasma and urine. The reductase was reduced to levels only 40% of those of control subjects in the liver and 17% of those of control subjects in muscle.

Carnitine plasma membrane transporter deficiency is caused by a defect in the carrier protein responsible for sodium-dependent transport of carnitine across plasma membranes. The defect is present in cultured skin fibroblasts, cardiac and skeletal muscle, and kidneys, but not in liver. Plasma and tissue total carnitine levels are markedly low. The majority of patients are seen between 2 and 7 years of age with a progressive cardiomyopathy and skeletal muscle weakness. Other patients may have symptoms similar to those of MCAD deficiency, including hypoglycemia, hyperammonemia, hepatomegaly and liver dysfunction, and decreased ketone body production, between 3 months and 2 years of age, before the development of symptomatic cardiac involvement. Urine organic acid levels are normal. Most patients respond well to carnitine supplementation.

Carnitine translocase deficiency has been reported to be associated with fasting hypoketotic hypoglycemia, coma, chronic hyperammonemia, hypotonia, and cardiomyopathy in early infancy. The plasma carnitine level is low, with an increased esterified fraction. Plasma acyl-carnitine profiles will be abnormal and will reveal both medium- and long-chain dicarboxylic acids.

CPT deficiency appears in three clinical forms. The "hepatic form" is rare and usually is associated with CPT I deficiency in young infants with clinical symptoms similar to those of MCAD deficiency. There usually is no muscle involvement. The "muscular form" is more common and is associated with CPT II deficiency in young adults with recurrent attacks of rhabdomyolysis that are precipitated by fasting, exercise, cold, or infection. There is a higher incidence of anesthetic-related malignant hyperthermia among these patients. A severe lethal neonatal muscular form of CPT II deficiency has been described in one patient with essentially no enzymatic activity compared to the adult form, which usually has 20% to 25% residual activity. An infantile "hepato-cardio-muscle form" with 10% residual activity of CPT II and onset before 6 months of age has been described, with hypoketotic hypoglycemia, metabolic acidosis, hyperammonemia, hypotonia, cardiomyopathy, and, occasionally, cardiac arrhythmias, renal cortical cysts, and brain malformations.

Multiple acyl-CoA dehydrogenase deficiency, or glutaric acidemia type II, is associated with electron transfer flavoprotein or electron transfer flavoprotein-ubiquinone oxidoreductase deficiency. Electron transfer flavoprotein and electron transfer flavoprotein-ubiquinone oxidoreductase are proteins that mediate the transfer of electrons from flavin-containing acyl-CoA dehydrogenases involved in the mitochondrial oxidation of fatty acids and several amino acids to the main respiratory chain. The disorder has three forms. Two are severe and are seen in the neonatal period in patients with or without congenital anomalies. Neonatal patients often are premature infants who, by 2 days of age, are noted to have hypotonia, hepatomegaly, hypoglycemia, metabolic acidosis, hyperammonemia, and an acrid odor (similar to that of sweaty feet) from isovaleric acid. In the patients with anomalies, the dysmorphology is similar to that noted with Zellweger syndrome, with a high forehead, hypoplastic mid-face, hypertelorism, and low-set ears. Rocker-bottom feet, muscular defects of the abdominal wall, anomalies of the external genitalia, enlarged cystic kidneys, and brain malformations have been seen. Most patients with the severe forms die by 1 week of age. A few who have lived longer have had cardiomyopathies. Some patients without anomalies have had only hypoglycemia during the neonatal period and later have had symptoms similar to those of Reye's syndrome. Serum and urine organic acid levels have marked elevations of metabolites of varying chain length, including glutaric, ethylmalonic, 3-hydroxyisovaleric, 2-hydroxyglutaric, 5-hydroxyhexanoic, adipic, suberic, and dodecanedioic acids. Short-chain volatile acids such as isovaleric, isobutyric, and 2-methylbutyric have been noted, as well as isovaleryl-, isobutyryl-, and 2-methylbutyryl-glycine conjugates. A generalized aminoaciduria with elevations of proline and hydroxyproline is common. Ketonuria usually is not present. There is no successful therapy.

The mild form of the disorder, also known as ethylmalonic-adipic aciduria, varies in onset from infancy to adulthood. There is episodic vomiting, hypoglycemia, and acidosis. Some patients have hepatomegaly and myopathy. With episodes, urinary organic acid profiles will show a pattern similar to that of the severe form, although less elevated. Elevated blood and urine sarcosine levels may be noted. Plasma carnitine will have an elevated esterified fraction. Treatment with riboflavin, carnitine, and a diet low in protein and fat is indicated. Episodes should be treated vigorously with intravenous glucose and hydration.

Both electron transfer flavoprotein and electron transfer flavoprotein-ubiquinone oxidoreductase deficiencies have been reported with all types of the disorders. The severe neonatal form with congenital anomalies is more likely to be associated with electron transfer flavoprotein-ubiquinone oxidoreductase deficiency. Some of the patients have not had electron transfer flavoprotein or electron transfer flavoprotein-ubiquinone oxidoreductase deficiency and, although the basis for their disorder is unknown, it is postulated that they may have defects in flavin adenine dinucleotide biosynthesis or transport. Prenatal diagnosis is available for the severe forms.

## Selected Readings

DiMauro S, Bonilla E, Zeviani M, et al. Mitochondrial myopathies. Ann Neurol 1985;17:521.

DiMauro S, Bonilla E, Zeviana M, et al. Mitochondrial myopathies. J Inherited Metab Dis 1987;10(Suppl 1):113.

Egger J, Lake BD, Wilson J. Mitochondrial cytopathy. A multisystem disorder with ragged-red fibers on muscle biopsy. Arch Dis Child 1981;56:741.

Freeman FE, Goodman SI. Glutaric acidemia type II and defects of the mitochondrial respiratory chain. Chapter 34. In: Scriver CR, Beaudet AL, Sly WS, Valle D, eds. The metabolic basis of inherited disease, ed 6. New York: McGraw-Hill, 1989:915.

Robinson B. Lactic acidemia. Chapter 32. In: Scriver CR, Beaudet AL, Sly WS, Valle D, eds. The metabolic basis of inherited disease, ed 6. New York: McGraw-Hill, 1989:869.

Roe CR, Coates PM. Acyl-CoA dehydrogenase deficiencies. Chapter 33. In: Scriver CR, Beaudet AL, Sly WS, Valle D, eds. The metabolic basis of inherited disease, ed 6. New York: McGraw-Hill, 1989:889.

Roe CR, Millington DS, Maltby DA, et al. Recognition of medium-chain acyl-CoA dehydrogenase deficiency in asymptomatic siblings of children dying of sudden infant death or Reye-like syndromes. J Pediatr 1986;108:13.

Schulz H. Oxidation of fatty acids. In: Vance DE, Vance J, eds. Biochemistry of lipids, lipoproteins and membranes. Amsterdam: Elsevier, 1991:87.

Scriver CR, Beaudet AL, Sly WS, Valle D, eds. The metabolic basis of inherited disease, ed 6. New York: McGraw-Hill, 1989.

Tanaka K, Coates PM. Fatty acid oxidation; clinical, biochemical, and molecular aspects. New York: Alan R Liss, 1990.

Tulinius MH, Holme E, Kristiansson B, et al. Mitochondrial encephalomyopathies in childhood. I. Biochemical and morphologic investigations. J Pediatr 1991;119:242.

Tulinius MH, Holme E, Kristiansson B, et al. Mitochondrial encephalomyopathies in childhood. II. Clinical manifestations and syndrome. J Pediatr 1991;119:251.

*Principles and Practice of Pediatrics, Second Edition.*
edited by Frank A. Oski et al. J. B. Lippincott Company, Philadelphia © 1994.

# 12.5 *Defects in Carbohydrate Metabolism*

Dietary carbohydrates include polymeric starch from plant sources, glycogen from animal sources, disaccharides in the form of lactose from milk sources and sucrose from fruit and vegetable sources, and, to a lesser extent, monosaccharides such as glucose, galactose, and fructose. The polymers and disaccharides are hydrolyzed to monosaccharides by enzymes that are present in the brush border of intestinal villi. The free monosaccharides, glucose, galactose, and fructose, are absorbed and transported to the liver,

where they are used rapidly. Carbohydrate metabolism in the liver is concerned primarily with maintenance of the blood-glucose concentration. Glucose may be formed by the metabolism of dietary carbohydrates, galactose, and fructose, from degradation of glycogen, or by gluconeogenesis from amino acids, glycerol, and lactate. Glucose-6-phosphate occupies a central position in the pathways in that all sources for free glucose first must be converted to glucose-6-phosphate except for that resulting from the action of debrancher enzyme on glycogen. In addition to being used for free glucose, glucose-6-phosphate also may be used for glycogen synthesis, for glycolysis and the production of lactate and $CO_2$ by the Embden-Meyerhof pathway, for the production of the reduced form of nicotinamide-adenine dinucleotide and $CO_2$ by entering the pentose cycle, and for glucuronate formation.

The major disorders of carbohydrate metabolism involve the intermediary metabolism of glycogen, galactose, and fructose.

## DISORDERS OF GLYCOGEN SYNTHESIS AND DEGRADATION

### Glycogen Metabolism

Glycogen, the principal storage form of carbohydrate in humans, is found primarily in liver and muscle. It is a high–molecular-weight, highly branched, spherical structure composed of glucosyl residues in $\alpha$-1,4-linkage in the form of linear chains with branch points where the glucosyl residues are in $\alpha$-1,6-linkage. Ten percent of the glucosyl residues are at the non-reducing end of the molecules; 60% of these are on outer branches, making them readily accessible for glycogenolysis. The usual concentration of glycogen in liver is less than 5 g/100 g wet weight.

Glycogen is synthesized from glucose-1-phosphate by the actions of three enzymes (Fig 12-16). Uridine diphosphate (UDP)-glucose pyrophosphorylase converts glucose-1-phosphate to UDP-glucose. Glycogen synthetase catalyzes the transfer of glucosyl residues from the UDP-glucose to glycogen primer in $\alpha$-1,4-linkage, thus lengthening the chains. Finally, the brancher enzyme, amylo-1,4–1,6-transglucosylase, creates the branch points by transferring groups of glucosyl residues in $\alpha$-1,4-linkage from outer chains and attaching them in $\alpha$-1,6-linkage along the linear chains.

Glycogen degradation involves sequential removal of non-reducing terminal glucosyl residues by a phosphorylase system and the debrancher enzyme. Phosphorylase exists in both inactive (b) and active (a) forms. Conversion of the phosphorylase to the active form requires the presence of adenosine triphosphate (ATP) and active phosphorylase kinase. Phosphorylase kinase also exists in inactive (b) and active (a) forms and is activated in the presence of ATP by a protein kinase that is generated in response to increased cyclic adenosine monophosphate (AMP) formation from hormonal and chemical influences on the hepatic parenchymal cell plasma membrane. The activated phosphorylase a cleaves the $\alpha$-1,4-linkages of the outer chains to within four glucosyl residues of the branch points and liberates glucose-1-phosphate. Debrancher enzyme then is needed for further degradation to proceed. Debrancher functions both as a transferase, which moves three glucosyl residues to another linear chain, and as an amylo-1,6-glucosidase, which removes the glucosyl residues in branched $\alpha$-1,6-linkage with liberation of free glucose. In this manner, about 10% free glucose and 90% glucose-1-phosphate is released. The glucose-1-phosphate is converted to glucose-6-phosphate by phosphoglucomutase. Then, glucose-6-phosphate is converted to free glucose by glucose-6-phosphatase.

The synthesis and degradation of hepatic glycogen is regulated

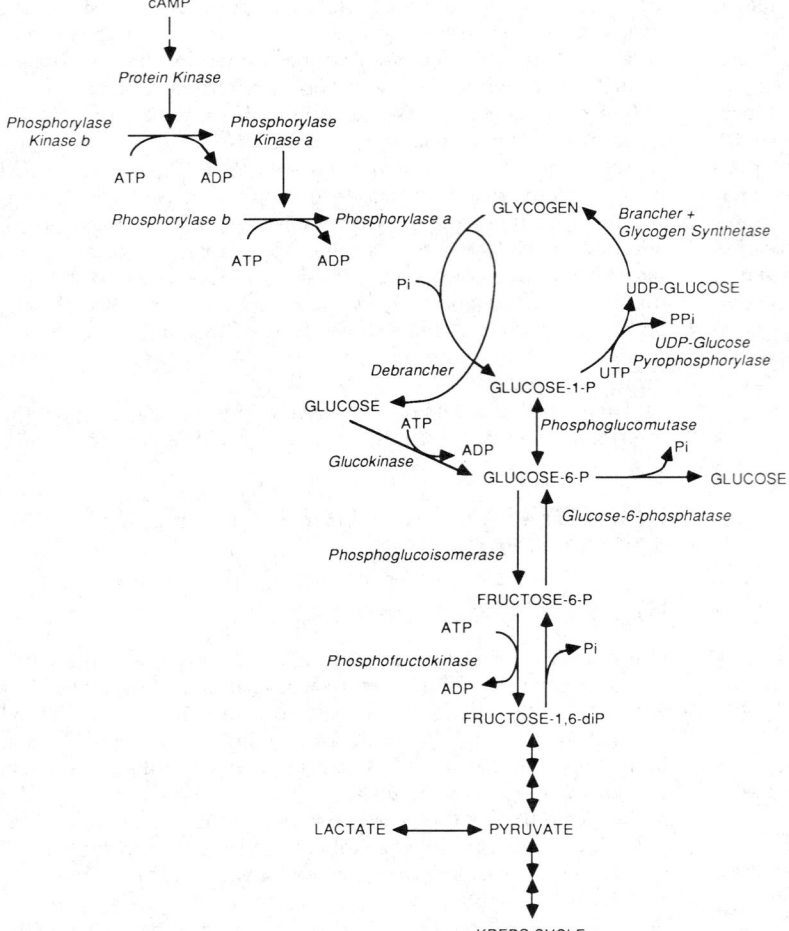

**Figure 12-16.** Glycogen synthesis and degradation. *cAMP,* cyclic adenosine monophosphate; *ATP,* adenosine triphosphate; *ADP,* adenosine diphosphate; *UDP,* uridine diphosphate; *UTP,* uridine triphosphate; *Pi,* inorganic phosphate; *PPi,* pyrophosphate.

primarily by cyclic AMP, glucose, and glycogen. An increased demand for blood glucose results in increased activation of phosphorylase and suppression of glycogen synthetase activity. Hepatic glycogen functions as a reserve for blood glucose. In contrast, muscle glycogen functions mainly as a fuel reserve for ATP generation, which is needed during exercise and usually does not contribute to blood glucose levels. Under anaerobic conditions, muscle glycogen also can be degraded to lactate by glycolysis.

## Classification of Glycogen Storage Disorders

The disorders associated with abnormal synthesis and degradation of glycogen vary widely in their clinical spectrum. Table 12-4 lists the disorders according to their currently accepted type and specific enzymatic defect. The disorders may have primarily hepatic or muscle involvement.

### Hepatic Glycogen Storage Disorders

The frequency of hepatic glycogen storage disorders is estimated to be 1:60,000 births. The pathogenesis of the various disorders often may by predicted by the site of their associated enzymatic defects. All cause some degree of hepatomegaly and usually hypoglycemia. Functional testing may help to distinguish between the disorders. The presence of fasting hypoglycemia, the response to glucagon in the fasting and fed state, the response of blood glucose to the administration of other carbohydrates such as galactose, and the type of glucose response noted with a glucose tolerance test may be used to help differentiate between the disorders. All fasting and tolerance testing should be done with

caution and close observation of the patient. For the severe disorders, the presence of lactic acidosis and hypoglycemia may be considered a relative contraindication to proceeding with fasting, glucagon stimulation, and other tests in the classic fashion. Liver and muscle biopsies may be done to assess the total content of glycogen and the type of glycogen structure present, and to document deficient activity of specific enzymes. Open liver biopsies and muscle biopsies, rather than punch biopsies, are preferred because of the sample size needed for these analyses. Muscle biopsy should be done at the same time as open liver biopsy, regardless of the suspected clinical type of glycogen storage. It is most important that an experienced laboratory be contacted before obtaining the samples to ensure appropriate handling. Because many of the disorders may be documented in leukocytes, erythrocytes, or cultured skin fibroblasts, these less invasive procedures should be done first, if possible.

All the disorders are inherited as autosomal recessive traits except for type IXb, which is inherited as an X-linked trait. Carrier detection and prenatal diagnosis varies depending on the tissue distribution of the enzyme involved in the specific disorder.

*Type Ia Glycogen Storage Disease (von Gierke's Disease).* Type Ia glycogen storage disease (GSD), also known as hepatorenal GSD, is associated with deficient activity of glucose-6-phosphatase in liver, kidney, and intestine. Patients have marked hepatomegaly, lactic acidosis, and hypoglycemia, and the disorder often is diagnosed in the neonatal period. Milder forms may be discovered later with hepatomegaly and short stature. Other clinical features include a doll-like appearance, decreased motor

TABLE 12-4.  Classification of Glycogen Storage Disorders

| Type | Enzyme Affected | Major Tissue Involved | Clinical Features |
|---|---|---|---|
| 0 | Glycogen synthetase | Liver | Hypoglycemia, ketosis, no hepatomegaly |
| Ia | Glucose-6-phosphatase | Liver, kidney, intestine | Hypoglycemia, lacticacidosis, hepatomegaly |
| Ib | Transport defect of glucose-6-phosphate | As in Ia, plus neutrophils | As in Ia, plus Crohn's disease |
| Ic | Transport defect of inorganic phosphate | As in Ia | As in Ia, juvenile diabetes |
| II | Lysosomal α-glucosidase | Muscle, generalized | Lysosomal storage disease |
| III | Debrancher | Liver, muscle | Milder Ia, cirrhosis, ketosis, ± muscle |
| IV | Brancher | Liver, muscle | Hepatomegaly, cirrhosis, ± muscle |
| V | Muscle phosphorylase | Muscle | Weakness, cramps, myoglobinuria |
| VI | Hepatic phoshorylase | Liver | Hepatomegaly |
| VII | Muscle phosphofructokinase | Muscle | Weakness, cramps, myoglobinuria |
| VIII | Loss of activation of phosphorylase | Liver, brain | Hepatomegaly, progressive CNS dysfunction |
| IX | Phosphorylase kinase | Liver, ± muscle | Hepatomegaly, ketosis |
| X | cAMP-dependent kinase | Liver, muscle | Hepatomegaly, ± mild muscle |
| XI | Unknown | Liver, kidney | Hepatomegaly, renal tubular dysfunction |

mass, renal enlargement, failure of maturation in puberty, vomiting, and diarrhea. Many infants are obese as a result of demanding frequent feedings, including nocturnal feedings beyond the time this behavior usually disappears (Fig 12-17).

Fasting hypoglycemia may be profound and often is without clinical symptoms in the untreated patient. This tolerance of hypoglycemia is thought to be the result of the ability of these patients to use alternative substrates for glucose in the brain. Glucose-6-phosphatase is essential for the normal release of hepatic free-glucose, whether it is the product of glycogenolysis or gluconeogenesis. Dietary carbohydrates other than glucose also cannot be converted to glucose because the conversion involves glucose-6-phosphatase as the final step. The fasting hypoglycemia results in activation of phosphorylase and hepatic glycogenolysis, which leads to the formation of glucose-6-phosphate. The glucose-6-phosphate then is metabolized to lactate by glycolysis. Gluconeogenesis also is stimulated, and there occurs a recycling between lactate and glycogen, which results in a net increase in lactate. Stimulation of the glycolytic and gluconeogenic pathways also results in elevated triglyceride, cholesterol, very–low-density lipoprotein, free fatty acid, and uric acid levels. Xanthomas, lipemia retinalis, gout, and uric acid nephropathy may occur. Within the liver parenchyma, adenomatous nodules may appear, which can develop into hepatic carcinoma. Abnormal bleeding tendencies occur; these are thought to be caused by decreased platelet adhesiveness from the hypoglycemia.

In that patients with GSD I frequently become hypoglycemic after 2 to 3 hours of fasting, any tolerance or stimulation test should be done cautiously and with intravenous glucose at hand. Glucose tolerance testing gives a diabetic-type early response. Insulin levels are low. There is no glycemic response to galactose (1 to 2 g/kg of 20% solution, orally or intravenously). Glucagon stimulation (20 to 30 μg/kg intramuscularly or intravenously, maximum dose 1 mg) occasionally will produce a response, which

is defined as a rise in blood glucose of 50% more than baseline. Lactic acid levels will rise with fasting and with glucagon or galactose administration. Glycogen content is elevated in liver, kidney, and intestine. Glycogen structure is normal. On liver biopsy, the hepatocytes are noted to have glycogen in the nuclei and lipid droplets of varying size in the cytoplasm. There are no signs of cirrhosis. The diagnosis may be confirmed by measurement of glucose-6-phosphatase in liver or intestinal biopsy samples. Prenatal diagnosis and carrier detection are not readily available.

Treatment is directed at supplying continuous exogenous glucose. Infants are given a formula with glucose or glucose polymers as the only carbohydrate source. Older children are given similar enteral supplements and are restricted in their intake of natural sources of galactose and fructose. Frequent daily feedings, every 2 to 3 hours, are supplemented with nocturnal nasogastric or gastrostomy drip feeding. Uncooked cornstarch slurries may be used with older children. There is remarkable clinical and laboratory improvement with dietary therapy. Tolerance of hypoglycemia may be present no longer, however, and clinical symptoms of hypoglycemia may occur. The patients continue to be at risk for significant acidosis and hypoglycemia with intercurrent illnesses or if enteral feedings are interrupted.

*Type Ib Glycogen Storage Disease.*    Type Ib GSD is similar in clinical and laboratory findings to type Ia GSD. Patients also have been noted to have abnormalities of neutrophil mobility and neutropenia, Fanconi-type renal dysfunction, and Crohn's disease. The disorder is caused by defective transport of glucose-6-phosphate across the microsomal membrane of hepatocytes and leukocytes. Measurement of glucose-6-phosphatase in frozen liver biopsy samples usually is normal because of disruption of the membrane with freezing. Measurement of specific activity of glucose-6-phosphatase in fresh tissue will demonstrate the defect. Treatment is similar to that for type Ia GSD. In addition,

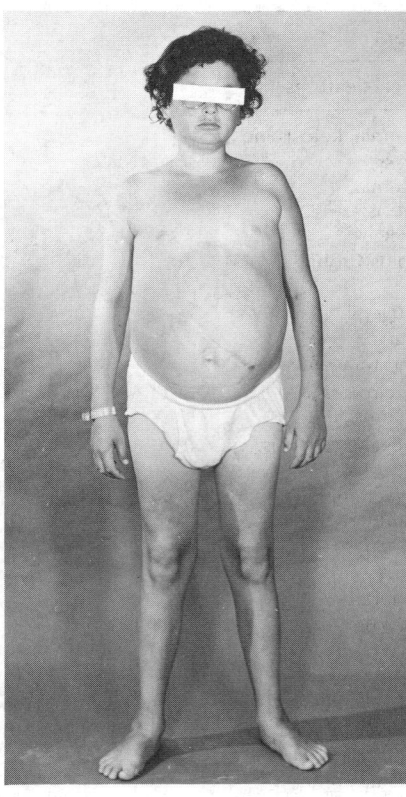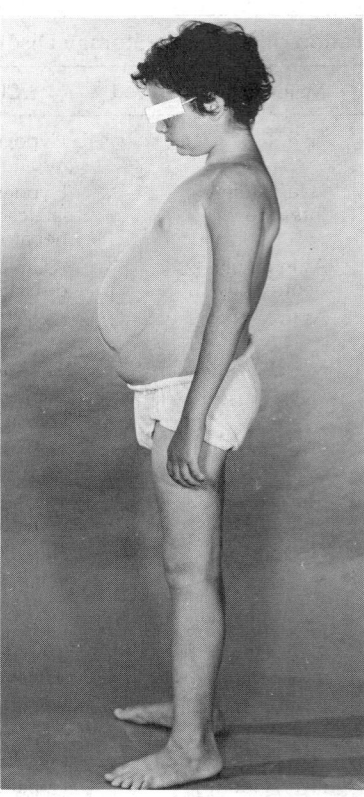

**Figure 12-17.** Glycogen storage disease IA, age 13 years.

the neutropenia usually is responsive to granulocyte colony-stimulating factor. Patients also will need the care of a pediatric hematologist and gastroenterologist.

*Type Ic Glycogen Storage Disease.* One patient with insulin-dependent diabetes and elevated liver glycogen content has been reported to have deficient transport of inorganic phosphate across the microsomal membrane of hepatocytes. The clinical picture is similar to that for type Ia GSD.

*Type II Glycogen Storage Disease (Pompe's Disease).* Pompe's disease is associated with deficient activity of lysosomal $\alpha$-glucosidase (acid maltase) and generalized storage of glycogen. The disorder is discussed with the lysosomal storage disorders.

*Type III Glycogen Storage Disease (Cori's Disease).* Type III GSD is associated with deficient activity of the debrancher enzyme, amylo-1,6-glucosidase. The disorder also is known as limit dextrinosis because glycogen of abnormal structure, similar to limit dextrin with short outer chains, is stored in liver and muscle. Most patients are seen in the first year of life with fasting hypoglycemia, hepatomegaly, and growth retardation. There is no renal enlargement, but renal tubular dysfunction is present occasionally. Mild inflammatory disease of the liver and cirrhosis may occur. Milder cases and cases with hypotonia, muscle wasting, or cardiac involvement are known. The clinical course and laboratory findings are similar to, but milder than, those seen in type Ia GSD. Glucose tolerance testing will reveal a diabetic-type early response. Galactose can be converted readily to glucose. The response to glucagon is variable, but usually is normal in the fed state; no response is seen in the fasted state. Fasting lactate levels commonly are normal, but become elevated after a glucose load. Fasting ketonuria is common. Blood levels of cholesterol and uric acid may be elevated. There is elevation of glycogen content in liver and erythrocytes. The glycogen structure is abnormal. Liver biopsy samples have more nuclear glycogen and

less lipid droplets than are seen with type Ia GSD. Fibrous septa often are present. Deficiency of the debrancher enzyme may be shown in leukocytes and liver. Treatment includes frequent feedings that are high in protein. There is no carbohydrate restriction because gluconeogenesis is intact. Nocturnal drip feedings may be required for hypoglycemia. Many patients improve with age and have a normal adult life.

*Type IV Glycogen Storage Disease (Andersen's Disease).* Type IV GSD is associated with deficiency of the brancher enzyme, amylo-1,4–1,6-transglucosylase. The disorder also is known as amylopectinosis because the glycogen stored has fewer than the normal number of branch points and long outer chains similar to amylopectin. The decreased branching makes the glycogen less soluble. It is thought that the cirrhosis seen in this disease is the result of a foreign-body reaction to the abnormal glycogen. Infants usually are normal at birth, but exhibit hepatomegaly and failure to thrive within a few months. Progressive fibrosis of the liver often leads to cirrhosis, splenomegaly, and liver failure. Some patients also have been seen with poor motor development, hypotonia, muscle atrophy, and absent reflexes as major clinical manifestations. Cardiac involvement occurs occasionally and may be severe. Many of the severely affected patients die by 4 years of age. Patients with milder cases have a longer lifespan, and the condition even improves with age in some. Fasting hypoglycemia may occur and can be treated with frequent feeding. Liver, muscle, and erythrocyte glycogen concentrations usually are normal, but there is the presence of glycogen with an abnormal structure. The enzymatic defect may be demonstrated in leukocytes, cultured skin fibroblasts, and liver. Prenatal diagnosis is available.

*Type VI Glycogen Storage Disease (Hers' Disease).* Type VI GSD is associated with deficient activity of hepatic phosphorylase and hepatomegaly. Hypoglycemia is rare. The hepatomegaly may recede with age. Occasionally, patients have hepatic fibrosis. There may be elevation of serum lipids and transaminases. There usually is no glycemic response to glucagon. There is elevation of liver glycogen content of normal structure. Deficient activity of phosphorylase may be demonstrated in liver. The disorder may be indistinguishable clinically from types IX and X GSD.

*Type VIII Glycogen Storage Disease.* Type VIII GSD is characterized by the onset of hepatomegaly and progressive central nervous system degeneration shortly after birth. There are no clinical problems with glucose homeostasis. Glycogen concentration is increased in the liver and on cerebral biopsy. The particulate matter in brain appears larger than usual on electron microscopy. Liver phosphorylase activity is low and is thought to result from impaired control of phosphorylase activation. The exact biochemical defect is not known.

*Type IX Glycogen Storage Disease.* Type IX GSD is associated with deficient activity of hepatic phosphorylase kinase and is indistinguishable clinically from types VI and X GSD. It exists in three forms. Type IXa GSD, an autosomal recessive trait, and type IXb GSD, an X-linked trait, affect only hepatic phosphorylase kinase. Type IXc GSD, an autosomal recessive trait, involves both hepatic and muscle phosphorylase kinase. All types are associated with massive hepatomegaly, which recedes with age. Fasting hypoglycemia is rare. Fasting lactate levels may be normal or slightly elevated. Fasting ketonuria is common. There is a normal response to glucagon. Most patients do well, but two have been reported to have nodular cirrhosis with portal hypertension in late childhood. There is elevated glycogen of normal structure. Deficient activity of phosphorylase kinase may be demonstrated in liver, leukocytes, and erythrocytes.

*Type X Glycogen Storage Disease.* Type X GSD is associated with failure of activation of hepatic and muscle phosphorylase caused by deficiency of a cyclic AMP–dependent protein kinase needed for activation of phosphorylase kinase. On biopsy, phosphorylase is found only in the b or inactive form. The disorder is similar to types VI and IX GSD. The one reported patient also had minimal muscle symptoms.

*Type XI Glycogen Storage Disease.* Type XI GSD is characterized by marked hepatomegaly, growth retardation, and proximal renal tubular dysfunction of the Fanconi type during childhood. Clinical manifestations improve after puberty. Glycogen content is elevated in liver and kidney, but is normal in muscle. There usually is no response in the blood glucose level to glucagon, although there is increased urinary excretion of cyclic AMP. The blood glucose level increases appropriately after fructose administration, but decreases after galactose administration. A functional deficiency of hepatic phosphoglucomutase has been proposed.

*Type O Glycogen Storage Disease.* Type O GSD is associated with deficient activity of hepatic glycogen synthetase. Patients are seen during the first year of life with fasting hypoglycemia and ketosis. There is no hepatomegaly. The disorder often is difficult to distinguish clinically from ketotic hypoglycemia. Lactate may increase after a glucose load or 12 hours of fasting. The glucose tolerance test is diabetic-type. Hypoglycemia is not responsive to glucagon. The diagnosis is made by confirmation of the enzymatic defect on liver biopsy. The hepatic glycogen concentration is reduced markedly, but is not absent.

### Muscle Glycogen Storage Disorders

Two disorders of glycogen metabolism, types V and VII GSD, affect only muscle. They have a similar clinical presentation and often can be distinguished only by demonstration of the specific enzymatic defect on muscle biopsy. Resting muscle derives its energy from the oxidation of glucose and fatty acids. With exercise, the requirement for ATP may increase several hundredfold, and the demand for substrates for aerobic metabolism may exceed that supplied from the blood. The additional ATP required must come from glycogenolysis. In both disorders, the enzymatic defects occur in the glycolytic pathway, and there is no increase in muscle or blood lactate with exercise. During childhood and adolescence, the patients are noted to have increased fatigability. Between 20 and 40 years of age, severe muscle cramps, myoglobinuria, and elevated blood levels of lactate dehydrogenase, aldolase, and creatine kinase are noted with exercise. After 40 years of age, the cramps and myoglobinuria are less evident, but muscle wasting and weakness appear with increasing severity. Reduced exercise tolerance may be demonstrated by having the patient perform an ischemic exercise test. With a blood pressure cuff on the arm inflated to more than systolic pressure, repeated pressure on a rubber ball by the hand usually will produce severe muscle cramping. Measurement of venous lactate levels in the same arm before and after exercise will fail to show the normal rise. Skeletal muscle biopsy reveals increased glycogen deposits in the cytoplasm beneath the sarcolemma. Treatment involves avoidance of strenuous exercise, which may create myoglobinuria and acute renal failure.

*Type V Glycogen Storage Disease (McArdle Disease).* Type V GSD is associated with deficient activity of muscle phosphorylase. Elevated muscle glycogen content and the enzymatic defect may be demonstrated on muscle biopsy.

*Type VII Glycogen Storage Disease (Tarui Disease).* Type VII GSD is associated with deficient activity of muscle phosphofructokinase, which catalyzes the conversion of fructose-6-phosphate to fructose-1,6-diphosphate. Phosphofructokinase is important in the regulation of glycolysis in muscle and affects the use of both glycogen and glucose in muscle. There is increased glycogen content of muscles secondary to increased stimulation of glycogen synthetase and UDP-glucose pyrophosphorylase. The disorder usually is more severe than is type V GSD. Erythrocyte phosphofructokinase activity also is decreased to about 50% of normal, and patients may have a mild hemolytic anemia. A severe variant of the disorder has been described in a child who died at 6 months of age with respiratory failure. The enzymatic defect may be demonstrated on muscle biopsy.

## DISORDERS OF GALACTOSE METABOLISM

### Galactose Metabolism

Galactose, the major dietary carbohydrate in infants, must be converted to glucose to be used as an energy source. This occurs primarily in hepatocytes by the Leloir pathway (Fig 12-18). Galactose first is phosphorylated to galactose-1-phosphate by a specific galactokinase. The galactose-1-phosphate then reacts with UDP-glucose to form UDP-galactose and glucose-1-phosphate in the presence of galactose-1-phosphate uridyl transferase. UDP-galactose is converted to UDP-glucose by UDP-galactose-4-epimerase. The UDP-glucose formed may reenter the Leloir pathway at the transferase step, react with pyrophosphate to form glucose-1-phosphate, or be used to form glycogen in the presence of glycogen synthetase.

Galactose also may be reduced by a nonspecific aldose reductase in the presence of the reduced form of nicotinamide-adenine dinucleotide to form galactitol. In patients with kinase and transferase deficiencies, elevated galactitol levels lead to osmotic swelling and disruption of lenticular fibers, resulting in

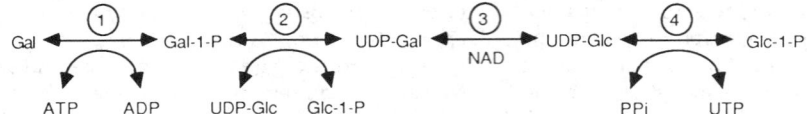

**Figure 12-18.** Disorders of galactose metabolism. *Gal*, galactose; *Glc*, glucose; *ATP*, adenosine triphosphate; *ADP*, adenosine diphosphate; *UDP*, uridine diphosphate; *UTP*, uridine triphosphate; *NAD*, nicotinamide-adenine dinucleotide; *PPi*, pyrophosphate; *1*, galactokinase; *2*, galactose-1-phosphate uridyltransferase; *3*, UDP-galactose-4-epimerase; *4*, UDP-glucose phosphorylase.

cataract formation. Galactose also may be oxidized to galactonic acid, which does not appear to be related to clinical problems, but may be demonstrated in the urine of patients.

UPD-galactose also may be synthesized in the body from glucose-1-phosphate by reversing the pathway described previously. In this manner, UDP-galactosyl residues needed for biosynthesis of macromolecules such as gangliosides may be generated even in the absence of dietary galactose. The UDP-galactose also may be converted to galactose-1-phosphate by pyrophosphorylase, which is thought to be the source of the galactose-1-phosphate that is seen in patients in whom the transferase deficiency is well controlled.

## Galactokinase Deficiency

Galactokinase deficiency is an autosomal recessive trait that occurs in about 1:150,000 births. It is associated with increased galactose in body fluids. The major clinical manifestation is nuclear cataracts, which begin to form after birth and usually are apparent clinically by early infancy if a lactose-containing diet is taken. The cataracts often are not completely reversible and often require surgery. There is no natural aversion to milk or milk products, nor is there the generalized multi-system involvement seen in the other types of galactose metabolic defects.

Urinary galactose and galactonic acid levels are elevated. Urinary galactose may be detected by spot testing for non-glucose reducing sugars. Tests for reducing sugars (ie, Clinitest, Galactostix) will be positive, whereas simultaneous testing specific for glucose (ie, with Combistix, Glucostix) will be negative or only slightly positive. False negatives may occur in patients on galactose-restricted diets and in those with poor intake. False positives may occur in neonates (especially those that are premature), in patients with intestinal lactase deficiency, and in those with severe liver dysfunction. Galactokinase deficiency may be detected with newborn screening programs that detect blood galactose elevation, but not in those programs that detect only galactose-1-phosphate elevation or screen only for the transferase deficiency. The disorder may be confirmed by demonstrating deficient activity of galactokinase in erythrocytes or cultured skin fibroblasts. Treatment consists of strict dietary elimination of all lactose and galactose sources. Milk and milk products must be avoided strictly, as well as other sources of lactose such as medications (vehicles) and prepared foods. Infants should be given a lactose-free formula. Older children may be given lactose-free calcium supplements. Therapy will arrest further cataract formation, but, even with improvement, some visual impairment may remain. Carrier detection is available.

## Galactose-1-Phosphate Uridyl Transferase Deficiency (Classic Galactosemia)

Galactose-1-phosphate uridyl transferase deficiency is the most common group of the disorders of galactose metabolism and is inherited as an autosomal recessive trait. In its classic form, it occurs in about 1:62,000 births. Affected infants appear normal at birth. Shortly after the ingestion of dietary galactose, symptoms appear, which usually are evident by 1 week of age. Failure to thrive, vomiting, diarrhea, and lethargy are noted. There may be prolonged physiologic jaundice or the appearance of hepatotoxic jaundice after 1 week of age with increased direct bilirubin. Exchange transfusion and phototherapy may be indicated. Hepatomegaly and abnormal liver function tests are common. Extrahepatic biliary atresia may have been considered. Nuclear cataracts appear within days or weeks and may become irreversible. Often, the cataracts are evident only on slit-lamp examination. Renal tubular dysfunction with generalized aminoaciduria, proteinuria, and galactosuria develops. Marasmus and increasing central nervous system involvement develop. The symptoms are rapidly progressive, and most untreated infants do not survive past 6 weeks of age. Deaths are due most commonly to liver failure and septicemia, especially with *Escherichia coli*. The cataracts are thought to be the result of lenticular accumulation of galactitol, as with the kinase deficiency. Galactose-1-phosphate levels are elevated markedly in the tissues and are thought to be responsible for the hepatic, renal, and central nervous system manifestations of the disorder.

The presence of non-glucose reducing substances in the urine may be demonstrated, as in galactokinase deficiency. Care should be taken because false-negative results may be obtained in those infants with poor intake, vomiting, or marasmus, or in those receiving a galactose-free diet. Galactose tolerance testing is dangerous and should be avoided. The disorder may be confirmed by demonstrating deficient activity of galactose-1-phosphate uridyl transferase in erythrocytes. If the child has received a transfusion or an exchange transfusion, a falsely elevated level of erythrocyte enzymatic activity may be obtained. The disorder also may be detected by newborn screening programs that test for elevated blood galactose (Paigen test) or galactose-1-phosphate (Paigen test) or screen for the transferase by spot enzyme assay (Beutler test). All screening tests should be confirmed with quantitative enzymatic testing and electrophoresis, which can be done with erythrocytes or cultured skin fibroblasts. Because of the seriousness of the disorder, however, it is recommended that patients who are presumed to be affected based on newborn screening or on clinical grounds be changed promptly to a galactose-free diet while awaiting the results of confirmatory testing. Carrier testing and prenatal diagnosis are available.

Treatment includes strict dietary restriction of all galactose and lactose sources, as for galactokinase deficiency. There is gradual and dramatic improvement when the child is placed on the diet. Markedly elevated galactose-1-phosphate intracellular levels decrease slowly, but may remain elevated for 10 to 15 days. Some persistent mild elevation of erythrocyte galactose-1-phosphate may be seen in well-controlled patients, which is thought to occur as a result of in vivo formation from UDP-galactose. The hepatic and renal manifestations improve slowly and may be reversed entirely. There is significant improvement in the cataracts, but residua may remain, which usually do not interfere with vision. About 50% of patients who are treated early may have later psychomotor difficulties and specific learning disabilities, especially in expressive language, mathematics, and spatial relationships. Behavioral problems with attention deficits and other psychologic problems may occur. Females may have hypergonadotropic hypogonadism with ovarian atrophy, which can occur prenatally or at any later time. Males have normal gonadal function. Because there is no improvement in galactose tolerance with age, the dietary restriction must continue indefinitely. Intermittent erythrocyte galactose-1-phosphate determinations may help to guide clinical management. Failure to comply with dietary restriction also will lead to poor physical growth.

Milder forms of classic galactosemia may present with a less severe clinical picture without failure to thrive and may not be detected until the patient is more than 4 months of age. Some children may present even later in childhood with a history of intermittent milk aversion or partial treatment. The findings of cataracts, hepatic involvement, and psychomotor difficulties should raise the possibility of this diagnosis.

## Variants of Transferase Deficiency

A number of other mutant alleles at the transferase locus are known to be associated with varying enzyme activity (0% to 140%) and starch-gel electrophoretic patterns. Some are associated with clinical manifestations when present in the homozygous state, and others are symptomatic only when present in compound heterozygosity with the classic galactosemia (G) gene. The Duarte (D) variant is the most common one, and it is estimated that 8% to 13% of the population are carriers for the Duarte allele. The Duarte allele produces 50% of normal transferase activity. The compound heterozygote (D/G) for Duarte and classic galactosemia is the most frequent form of transferase abnormality and usually will be detected by newborn screening programs. D/G galactosemia is estimated to occur in about 1:4,000 births. Affected infants have about 25% transferase activity, and most patients have elevated erythrocyte galactose-1-phosphate levels in infancy. Some have clinical signs of galactose toxicity. Dietary galactose restriction is recommended for the first 6 months of life, at which time a controlled oral galactose tolerance test with measurement of plasma and erythrocyte galactose and galactose-1-phosphate levels may be done. About 90% of patients will have normal galactose tolerance by this age. The remainder usually have normal galactose tolerance by 1 year of age. The disorder may be confirmed by quantitative determination of enzymatic activity and a distinctive banding pattern with starch-gel electrophoresis of erythrocyte hydrolysates.

## Uridine Diphosphate Galactose-4-Epimerase Deficiency

Two forms of the autosomal recessive disorder uridine diphosphate galactose-4-epimerase deficiency have been documented. The more common form occurs in about 1:46,000 births. Deficient enzymatic activity occurs only in leukocytes, lymphocytes, and erythrocytes. The overall ability to metabolize galactose is normal, and there are no significant clinical abnormalities. There usually is no galactosemia or galactosuria. There is elevation of erythrocyte galactose-1-phosphate such that the disorder may be detected in newborn screening programs that use this method.

The other form is characterized by a generalized deficiency of epimerase activity in all tissues. The clinical manifestations are similar to those seen with classic galactosemia. There is elevation of blood galactose and erythrocyte galactose-1-phosphate. The disorder should be considered in neonates who have features of classic galactosemia, with positive newborn screening for galactose or galactose-1-phosphate, but who have normal transferase activity levels. Therapy is similar to that for classic galactosemia except that some dietary galactose must be given to supply the UDP-galactose needed for gangliosides during growth. Careful monitoring of erythrocyte galactose-1-phosphate and UDP-galactose levels is indicated. Deficient activity of epimerase may be seen in erythrocytes, cultured skin fibroblasts, and liver.

## DISORDERS OF FRUCTOSE METABOLISM

### Fructose Metabolism

Sucrose, as well as small amounts of fructose and sorbitol, are distributed widely in fruits, vegetables, and other natural and sweetened foods, and comprise a major portion of the daily dietary carbohydrate consumption in Western societies. After hydrolysis of sucrose, a large portion of the ingested fructose is absorbed unchanged in the small intestine and is transported to the liver, the main site of fructose metabolism. Some of the fructose is converted to glucose in the small intestine, and some is metabolized in muscle, adipose tissue, and the kidneys. Ingested sorbitol is converted to fructose by sorbitol dehydrogenase.

Fructose is converted to intermediates of the gluconeogenic and glycolytic pathways, and is metabolized primarily to glucose and lactate (Fig 12-19). Fructokinase catalyzes the phosphorylation of fructose to fructose-1-phosphate. In normal individuals, this is associated with a decrease in intracellular Pi and ATP concentration, and secondary transient mild hyperuricemia, hypermagnesemia, hyperkalemia, hypophosphatemia, and hypoglycemia. It is an exaggeration of this response that is thought to be the basis for the clinical symptoms seen in hereditary fructose intolerance. Fructose-1-phosphate is cleaved to D-glyceraldehyde and dihydroxyacetone phosphate in the presence of aldolase. Aldolase also catalyzes the cleaving of fructose-1,6-diphosphate to D-glyceraldehyde-3-phosphate and dihydroxyacetone phosphate. There are three forms of aldolase with different tissue distributions. Aldolase B is the major form in liver, aldolase A is the major form in muscle, and aldolase C is the major form in brain. Triokinase catalyzes the phosphorylation of D-glyceraldehyde to D-glyceraldehyde-3-phosphate. Other pathways exist for the conversion of D-glyceraldehyde to triose-phosphate intermediates such as D-glyceraldehyde-3-phosphate and phosphoglycerate. Glyceraldehyde-3-phosphate then may be metabolized to pyruvate or it may be condensed with dihydroxyacetone phosphate to form fructose-1,6-diphosphate, which ultimately is converted to glucose and glycogen. Fructose-1,6-diphosphatase, which irreversibly catalyzes the formation of fructose-6-phosphate from fructose-1,6-diphosphate, plays a key role in gluconeogenesis. In glycolysis, phosphofructokinase irreversibly catalyzes this step in reverse order. The products of fructose metabolism may be diverted to gluconeogenesis and glycogen synthesis or into glycolysis and the Krebs' cycle, depending on the metabolic need at the time.

### Hepatic Fructokinase Deficiency (Essential Fructosuria)

The autosomal recessive disorder hepatic fructokinase deficiency occurs in about 1:130,000 individuals. It is benign and is associated with fructosuria detected on routine urinalysis if the procedure includes testing for reducing substances. Fructose probably is metabolized to fructose-6-phosphate in adipose tissue and skeletal muscle.

### Fructose-1-Phosphate Aldolase B Deficiency (Hereditary Fructose Intolerance)

The autosomal recessive disorder fructose-1-phosphate aldolase B deficiency is associated with reduced activity of aldolase B in the liver, renal cortex, and small intestine. There is considerable heterogeneity in residual activity among affected patients, who usually have less than 15% of normal hepatic aldolase B activity. The true incidence of the disorder is unknown; it is estimated to occur in 1:20,000 individuals in Switzerland and also is seen in North America and Europe.

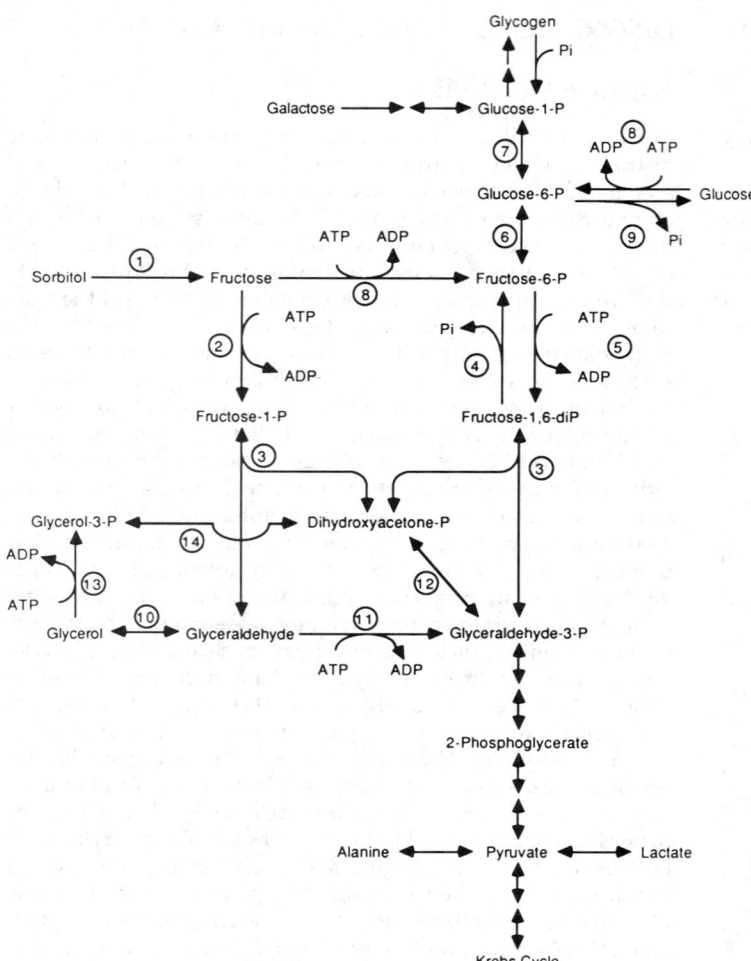

**Figure 12-19.** Pathways of fructose metabolism. *1,* sorbitol dehydrogenase; *2,* fructokinase; *3,* fructoaldolase; *4,* fructose-1,6-diphosphatase; *5,* phosphofructokinase; *6,* phosphohexose isomerase; *7,* phosphoglucomutase; *8,* hexokinase; *9,* glucose-6-phosphatase; *10,* alcohol dehydrogenase; *11,* triokinase; *12,* triose phosphate isomerase; *13,* glycerol kinase; *14,* glycerophosphate dehydrogenase.

The symptoms of this disorder, which occur only after the ingestion of dietary fructose, are related to acute hypoglycemia and chronic hepatic and renal dysfunction. In young infants, the symptoms usually do not start until weaning or the introduction of fruits, vegetables, and juices. Symptoms may occur before this time if the infant is taking a formula with fructose or sucrose as the carbohydrate source. The symptoms of an acute ingestion, which are more severe in young infants than in older children and adults, are associated with hypoglycemia and include sweating, trembling, emesis, lethargy, coma, seizures, and even shock and death. With acute fructose ingestion, there is depletion of intracellular Pi and ATP, and secondary inhibition of gluconeogenesis and glycolysis. More chronic symptoms include poor feeding, failure to thrive, vomiting, diarrhea, irritability, tremors, hepatomegaly, hepatic dysfunction leading to cirrhosis and hepatic failure, and proximal renal tubular dysfunction of the Fanconi type. The accumulation of fructose-1-phosphate in the liver, kidney, and small intestine is thought to be responsible for these manifestations. The pattern of these chronic symptoms with intermittent acute episodes, associated with the ingestion of fructose-containing foods, point to the disorder clinically. Older children and adults will have a nutritional history of avoidance of fructose and may be referred for bizarre eating patterns.

Laboratory findings associated with acute episodes will include hypoglycemia, hypophosphatemia, hypermagnesemia, hyperuricemia, hyperkalemia, lactic acidosis, and fructosemia and fructosuria. The presence of a non-glucose reducing substance in the urine should be confirmed as fructose by sugar chromatography. Fructosuria will not be present in those patients with intake of foods or fluids with other carbohydrate sources and may not be seen in patients with poor intake or those without recent exposure to fructose. Laboratory findings from chronic exposure are those associated with hepatic dysfunction and proximal renal tubular dysfunction. Liver biopsy samples reveal diffuse steatosis, scattered hepatic necrosis, periportal and intralobular fibrosis, and cirrhosis in later stages. Renal biopsy reveals granulation and vacuolization of epithelial cells with dilated proximal tubules. Small-intestinal biopsy samples may exhibit submucosal or serosal hemorrhages.

Treatment with avoidance of all dietary sources of fructose, including foods and medications, should be instituted once the disorder is suspected. There is prompt cessation of symptoms with intravenous glucose in acute episodes. Once a fructose-restricted diet is started, clinical improvement usually is evident within days. Small children may have persistent hepatomegaly, and some in the later stages of liver failure may go on to die. After several weeks of treatment, an intravenous fructose tolerance test with a maximum dose of 200 mg/kg may be done with caution. An oral fructose tolerance test may lead to a severe acute episode and should be avoided. The disorder also can be documented by enzymatic assay of aldolase B in biopsy samples from the liver or small intestine. Because aldolase B is not expressed in cultured skin fibroblasts or amniocytes, carrier and prenatal testing are not available.

## Fructose-1,6-Diphosphatase Deficiency

Fructose-1,6-diphosphatase deficiency is a rare, autosomal recessive disorder associated with deficient activity of fructose-1,6-diphosphatase in the liver, jejunum, and kidney. It is a severe disorder of gluconeogenesis associated with life-threatening episodes of hypoglycemia, lactic acidosis, and ketosis, which are triggered by fasting. About half of the patients are seen in the first 4 days of life with symptoms of hypoglycemia and acidosis. Moderate hepatomegaly and hypotonia may be present. Apnea and cardiac arrest may occur. The episodes usually respond to intravenous glucose and bicarbonate. Later episodes may be triggered by intercurrent infections and other states that increase the metabolic need for glucose, or when the patients are fasted or have repeated vomiting. Laboratory testing at the time of an episode will reveal hypoglycemia, elevated blood and urine lactate levels, pyruvate, alanine, and uric acid. Fructosuria usually is not present.

Treatment includes strict dietary restriction of fructose and the avoidance of fasting. Most patients respond well with regression of hepatomegaly. An intravenous (never oral) fructose tolerance test with a maximum dosage of 200 mg/kg may be done cautiously, but the results will not be as striking as those seen with hereditary fructose intolerance. A cautious fasting test may reveal an increase in lactic acid and ketosis as blood glucose decreases. There usually is a glycemic response to glucagon in the fasting state. There is a glycemic response to glucose or galactose, but not to fructose, glycerol, alanine, or dihydroxyacetone. Deficient activity of fructose-1,6-diphosphatase may be demonstrated in liver and jejunal biopsy samples. There is no carrier testing or prenatal diagnosis available because the enzyme normally is not expressed in cultured skin fibroblasts or amniocytes.

## OTHER DISORDERS OF CARBOHYDRATE METABOLISM

### Pentosuria

Essential pentosuria is a benign, autosomal recessive disorder associated with excessive urinary excretion of 1 to 4 g of L-xylulose daily. It is most common in persons of Jewish heritage and is noted frequently by the finding of a non-glucose reducing substance on urinalysis. It is associated with deficient activity of L-xylulose reductase, which catalyzes the conversion of L-xylulose to xylitol in the glucuronic acid pathway. The L-xylulose may be demonstrated by sugar chromatography.

### Glycerol Kinase Deficiency

Glycerol kinase deficiency is inherited as an X-linked trait and is associated with elevated serum and urine glycerol levels. It may be suspected in individuals found to have a very high triglyceride blood concentration when the laboratory methodology employed involves the measurement of glycerol released with the hydrolysis of triglyceride (pseudo-hypertriglyceridemia). There are three clinical forms of the disorder. Isolated glycerol kinase deficiency, or the juvenile form, is associated with episodic vomiting, lethargy that may progress to coma, and often significant metabolic acidosis that requires intravenous hydration and bicarbonate. Markedly elevated glycerol levels are noted on urinary organic acid testing by gas chromatography-mass spectroscopy and marked pseudo-hypertriglyceridemia is present. Treatment includes a low-glycerol (low-fat) diet and prompt treatment of episodes, which may occur with intercurrent illnesses or times of fasting.

The benign, or adult form, of isolated glycerol kinase deficiency usually is asymptomatic, does not require dietary therapy, and is recognized most often by finding pseudo-hypertriglyceridemia as part of an evaluation for hyperlipidemia.

The microdeletion, or infantile or complex, form of glycerol kinase deficiency is characterized by deletions in the p21 region of the X chromosome, which involve the glycerol kinase gene locus and one or more of the closely linked Xp21 loci for congenital adrenal hypoplasia, Duchenne muscular dystrophy, and ornithine-transcarbamylase deficiency. Boys with one of these disorders should be evaluated for the others. Treatment includes glycerol dietary restriction in addition to any therapy that is indicated for the associated disorder or disorders.

The deficiency of glycerol kinase may be noted in leukocytes, fibroblasts, or transformed lymphoblast cell lines. Molecular genetic studies also should be done to rule out the microdeletion forms.

### Ketotic Hypoglycemia

With fasting, blood glucose levels are maintained initially by breakdown of hepatic glycogen. Adults are able to continue glycogenolysis for as long as 6 to 12 hours, whereas children, who have relatively fewer glycogen stores and a proportionately greater demand for glucose for the central nervous system, may be able to sustain glycogenolysis for only 4 to 6 hours. Glycogenolysis is stimulated by epinephrine and glucagon, which activate the hepatic phosphorylase system. Once hepatic glycogen stores are depleted, gluconeogenesis ensues and is stimulated by growth hormone and adrenocorticotropic hormone–induced cortisol. In adults, about 50% of glucose is derived from amino acid precursors (especially alanine) through breakdown of skeletal muscle, 30% is derived from lactate, and 10% is formed from glycerol from adipose tissue stores. Gluconeogenesis occurs mainly in the liver, but also may occur in the kidney with prolonged fasting. Also, with prolonged fasting, adipose tissue is metabolized to release free fatty acids and glycerol from triglyceride stores. Free fatty acids may be used directly or oxidized in the liver for energy with the resultant formation of the ketone bodies, acetoacetate and 3-hydroxybutyrate. Abnormalities in any of the pathways involved, in the hormonal influences, or in availability of substrates for gluconeogenesis may result in fasting hypoglycemia.

Ketotic hypoglycemia is a common disorder that presents with fasting hypoglycemia and ketosis in patients between 1 and 5 years of age. Most patients are seen between 18 and 24 months of age. It also has been termed *accelerated starvation, idiopathic hypoglycemia,* or *substrate-limited hypoglycemia.* Many patients are not able to fast longer than 8 to 16 hours before symptoms develop. There often is a history of transient hypoglycemia and being small for gestational age in the neonatal period. As young infants, these patients feed frequently; as toddlers, they usually are observed to want to eat immediately on arising or after fasting for what commonly would be considered a short time for their age. They often are thin, not obese, and have relatively smaller muscle mass than would be expected for their age. Episodic hypoglycemia occurs with situations that lead to caloric deprivation, such as intercurrent illnesses with associated decreased intake, missing meals, or sleeping longer than usual. Acute hypoglycemia is associated with the usual signs of lethargy, coma, and seizures. Although the exact biochemical basis for the disorder is unknown, it is felt to be the result of decreased availability or impaired mobilization of muscle amino acids for gluconeogenesis. Plasma alanine levels usually are lowered in fasting states in these patients. Excretion of epinephrine is blunted in response to hypoglycemia induced by insulin or a ketogenic diet. There may be a delay in maturation of adrenal response to hypoglycemia. Because of accelerated starvation, free fatty acid oxidation leads to the markedly elevated levels of plasma and urine ketone bodies, for which the disorder is named. The ability to fast improves with age, and most children "outgrow" their disorder by puberty. This disorder is not inherited and affects males more commonly than females. There has been a gradual decrease in the number of patients with this disorder, which is thought to be a result of the recognition of newer inborn errors of metabolism that have similar clinical findings and improved diagnostic techniques for the organic acidurias.

Treatment during acute episodes requires prompt normalization of blood glucose levels, usually with intravenous glucose administration. Clinical symptoms subside rapidly. Between episodes, a high-protein, high-carbohydrate, frequent feeding diet is given. The parents should be instructed in the measurement of urinary ketones and should be directed to increase glucose sources at those times when ketones are detected or glucose intake decreases. Situations such as surgery or persistent vomiting with intercurrent illness, which require fasting, often will necessitate the use of intravenous glucose administration to maintain normal glucose levels.

The disorder is established by exclusion because many disorders involving hormone deficiencies and defects in metabolic pathways also may present with fasting hypoglycemia with ketosis. Diagnostic testing may be done during an acute episode before glucose therapy or with a carefully monitored provocative fast. Because normal children may become ketotic and hypoglycemic after 24 to 36 hours of fasting, it is important that these children be monitored carefully and that the fast not extend beyond 16 to 24 hours. An intravenous line without glucose, but with electrolytes should be placed in children who have a history of significant hypoglycemia occurring frequently or after only a short period of fasting. Blood glucose levels should be monitored at least every 4 hours for the first 8 hours of fasting, then every 2 hours for the remainder of the test, unless the glucose level is dropping or symptoms occur, in which case, it should be monitored more frequently. Glucose oxidase test strips may be used, but all low values should be confirmed with immediate laboratory blood glucose measurements. It is helpful to monitor urine ketones during the fast because they usually will become positive before hypoglycemia develops. When the glucose drops to 40 mg/dL or below, or at 16 to 24 hours of fasting with urine that is positive for ketones, or at 24 hours, blood and urine sampling should be done. Blood testing (with expected results) should include measurements of glucose (at or less than 40 mg/dL), insulin (low or less than 0.25 to 0.5 of glucose level), growth hormone (elevated), cortisol (elevated), thyroxine (normal), free fatty acids (elevated), $\beta$-hydroxybutyrate (elevated), ketones (elevated), quantitative amino acids (decreased alanine), and carnitine (normal total, esterified fraction less than 40% of total). Liver function testing, electrolytes, pH, and lactate and pyruvate levels also should be obtained if there is concern that a glycogenosis may be present or if hypoglycemia occurs before 8 hours of fasting. Urine should be tested for reducing substances (negative), ketones (markedly positive), and organic acids (elevated ketones only). Additional samples of frozen heparinized plasma (1 mL) and urine (20 mL) should be held in case further studies are needed. Some patients with fatty acid oxidation defects may be able to generate ketone bodies and their symptoms may be similar to those associated with idiopathic ketotic hypoglycemia. The children should be fed or given intravenous glucose after samples are obtained at the termination of the provocative testing, especially if they are symptomatic. In patients with ketotic hypoglycemia, there is no response to glucagon in the fasted state, but a response is present in the fed state. Glucagon stimulation testing is not absolutely necessary unless a glycogenosis is suspected, and should not be done in these patients if symptomatic hypoglycemia has occurred. If the studies are obtained during an acute episode, before treatment, by an astute physician, then provocative fasting may not be necessary. Abnormalities noted that are different from those listed above (ie, failure to note elevated cortisol levels) should be followed up appropriately with further diagnostic testing.

## Selected Readings

Bickel H, Guthrie R, Hammersen G, eds. Neonatal screening for inborn errors of metabolism. New York: Springer-Verlag, 1980.

Burman D, Holton JB, Pennock CA, eds. Inherited disorders of carbohydrate metabolism. Lancaster, England: MTP Press, Ltd, 1980.

Cornblath M, Schwartz R, eds. Disorders of carbohydrate metabolism in infancy, ed 2. Philadelphia: WB Saunders, 1976.

Hsia DJ. Galactosemia. Springfield, Ill: Charles C Thomas, 1969.

La Franchi S. Hypoglycemia of infancy and childhood. Pediatr Clin North Am 1987;34:959.

Scriver CR, Beaudet AL, Sly WS, Valle D, eds. The metabolic basis of inherited disease, ed 6. Chapters 11–14 and 36. New York: McGraw-Hill, 1989:399.

*Principles and Practice of Pediatrics, Second Edition.*
edited by Frank A. Oski et al. J. B. Lippincott Company, Philadelphia © 1994.

# 12.6 Disorders of Lipoproteins

The plasma lipoproteins are particles containing components as shown in Tables 12-5 and 12-6. They are classified according to both density and relative position in an electrophoretic field. Their function in lipid metabolism and relationship to disease states are complex and being elucidated still; an abbreviated outline follows.

Dietary long-chain triglycerides (TGs) and cholesteryl esters are hydrolyzed in the gut and absorbed into the intestinal cells, where the TGs are re-formed and, together with cholesterol and apolipoproteins A and B-48, are packaged into chylomicrons, which are secreted into the circulation via lymph channels. After acquiring apolipoproteins C-II and E from high-density lipoprotein (HDL), local endothelial lipoprotein lipase hydrolyzes many of the TGs out of the chylomicrons; the fatty acids are taken up by the tissues. Next, the chylomicron remnants are taken up, via the receptors on their surface, by liver cells, where the remaining TGs and cholesteryl esters are hydrolyzed; the resulting increase in intracellular cholesterol concentration serves to inhibit the initial step in cholesterol synthesis, catalyzed by 3-hydroxy-3-methylglutaryl (HMG)-CoA reductase. The liver synthesizes TGs, which, along with apolipoprotein B-100, apolipoprotein E, and some other lipid, are packaged into very–low-density lipoprotein (VLDL). In turn, the VLDL acquires apolipoprotein C-II from HDL and their TGs subsequently are hydrolyzed by lipoprotein lipase. The resulting VLDL remnants either are taken up by the liver or are broken down into intermediate-density lipoprotein (IDL) and then LDL. The latter then are taken up by the liver and other tissues via their LDL receptors and are broken down; again, the resulting increase in cholesterol inhibits its own further synthesis. HDL is synthesized in the liver and intestine, and acts in the circulation to esterify cholesterol from peripheral cells, and to take up the esters and transfer them to IDL, which then can be taken up by the liver. Thus, HDL is the agent for "reverse cholesterol transport," which explains its beneficial effect in the prevention of atheromatosis.

Analphalipoproteinemia (also called Tangier disease or apolipoprotein A-I deficiency) may be suspected in a person with large, orange tonsils who may have corneal clouding, hepato-

**TABLE 12-5. Plasma Lipoproteins**

| Class | | Lipids (%) | | | | Apolipoproteins | |
|---|---|---|---|---|---|---|---|
| Dens | Elec | TC | TG | PL | TL | Percent | Types |
| Chyl | Orig | 3 | 90 | 6 | 99 | 1 | A, B-48, C, E |
| VLDL | Pre-β | 22 | 55 | 15 | 92 | 8 | B-100, C, E |
| IDL | Slow Pre-β | 38 | 23 | 19 | 80 | 19 | E, C, B-100 |
| LDL | β | 50 | 5 | 25 | 80 | 20 | B-100 |
| HDL | α | 20 | 5 | 25 | 50 | 50 | A, C, E |

*Chyl*, chylomicrons; *VLDL*, very–low-density lipoproteins; *IDL*, intermediate–density lipoproteins; *LDL*, low-density lipoproteins; *HDL*, high-density lipoproteins; *dens*, density; *elec*, electrophoretic position; *TC*, total cholesterol; *TG*, triglycerides; *PL*, phospholipids; *TL*, total lipids.

megaly or splenomegaly, and neuropathy. The almost complete lack of HDL and cholesteryl esters in the plasma is reflected in the very low plasma total cholesterol level and in the increased storage of cholesteryl esters in tissues. No specific treatment is available for this rare autosomal recessive disorder, which has its highest incidence in a population semi-isolated on the island for which it is named.

Abetalipoproteinemia (Bassen-Kornzweig disease) is characterized by fat malabsorption from birth. Intestinal biopsy demonstrates normal-appearing villi, thus ruling out celiac disease. The plasma has a lack of apolipoprotein B, and of chylomicrons, VLDL, and LDL, all of which require apolipoprotein B as a constituent. Cholesterol and TG levels are very low, and the abnormal lipid status affects the membranes of erythrocytes, causing spiny projections (acanthocytes) to develop on them. Retinitis pigmentosa and cerebellar ataxia complete the clinical picture. Complete absence of apolipoprotein B confirms the diagnosis. Management involves a low-fat diet and supplemental fat-soluble vitamins, particularly vitamin E, the lack of which appears to be related to the neurologic and ophthalmologic problems associated with abetalipoproteinemia. This rare disorder is inherited as an autosomal recessive trait.

Familial hypercholesterolemia may manifest itself during early adult life by the appearance of xanthomas in the skin (Fig 12-20) and tendons and of arcus in the corneas, and by the occurrence of myocardial infarctions. The disorder is one of regulation of

LDL metabolism. Normally, LDL goes through the circulation and is taken up by the liver in a process involving binding to LDL receptors in the cell membranes. These receptors, along with receptors for other ligands, move across the cell membrane until they are retained in a coated pit. Coated pits form continually, invaginate, and then form vesicles, which enter the cytoplasm, carrying with them the receptors, with or without ligands. The receptors release their ligands and in turn are released to return to the membrane; the vesicles containing the ligands then merge with lysosomes. Within the lysosomes, acid hydrolases reduce ligand macromolecules to small–molecular-weight components, which then leave the lysosome. Thus, the LDL proteins are hydrolyzed to amino acids and the cholesteryl esters are hydrolyzed to cholesterol and fatty acids. The freed cholesterol will tend to slow the rate of cholesterol synthesis by inhibiting the key enzyme HMG-CoA reductase, and will tend to stimulate the activity of lecithin-cholesterol acyltransferase and, thus, the esterification of cholesterol. Patients with this disorder have a reduced number of functioning receptors resulting in less intracellular cholesterol and, therefore, less negative feedback, with the result that cholesterol synthesis is accelerated.

The disorder may be suspected in any child with a parent or grandparent who, at or before 55 years of age, has a cholesterol level of 240 mg/dL or greater, coronary atheromatosis, persistent angina, peripheral vascular disease, heart attack, or stroke. Regardless of the family history, measurement of the serum cholesterol is indicated in any child with xanthomas or arcus who is more than 2 years of age. This age is selected because it is the youngest age at which there is general agreement that treatment may be started. Universal screening of persons under 20 years of age was not recommended by the Lauer panel (see Suggested Readings) because of problems with sensitivity and selectivity, and because the universal adoption of modern nutritional guidelines would be the equivalent of the Step-One Diet employed in therapy. Newborn screening may be carried out; the greatest accuracy is obtained by measuring apolipoprotein B.

The diagnosis is made by obtaining a blood specimen after a 12-hour fast and measuring the total cholesterol, HDL-cholesterol, and TG concentrations. The LDL-cholesterol concentration may be determined by subtracting the HDL-cholesterol and one fifth of the TGs (if their concentration is less than 400) from the total. It generally is agreed that diet therapy is indicated for individuals whose total cholesterol concentration is greater than the 95th percentile, which is about 200 mg/dL for all pediatric age groups other than newborns. The threshold for treatment may be higher if the concentration of HDL-cholesterol is high because this fraction is associated with a protective effect. On the other hand, the threshold may be lowered if the LDL-cholesterol is above its 95th

**TABLE 12-6. Apolipoproteins***

| Apo Group | Lipoprotein (in order of prevalence) | Function |
|---|---|---|
| A-I | Chyl, HDL | LCAT cofactor |
| B-48 | Chyl | Secretion of TG from intestine |
| B-100 | LDL, IDL, VLDL | Secretion of TG from liver; binds LDL to receptor |
| C-II | HDL, VLDL, IDL, LDL | LPL cofactor |
| D | HDL | Reverse cholesterol transport |
| E | Chyl, HDL, IDL, VLDL, LDL | Binds LDL to receptor |

* See Table 12-5; *LCAT*, lecithin-cholesterol acyltransferase; *LPL*, lipoprotein lipase; *TG*, triglycerides.

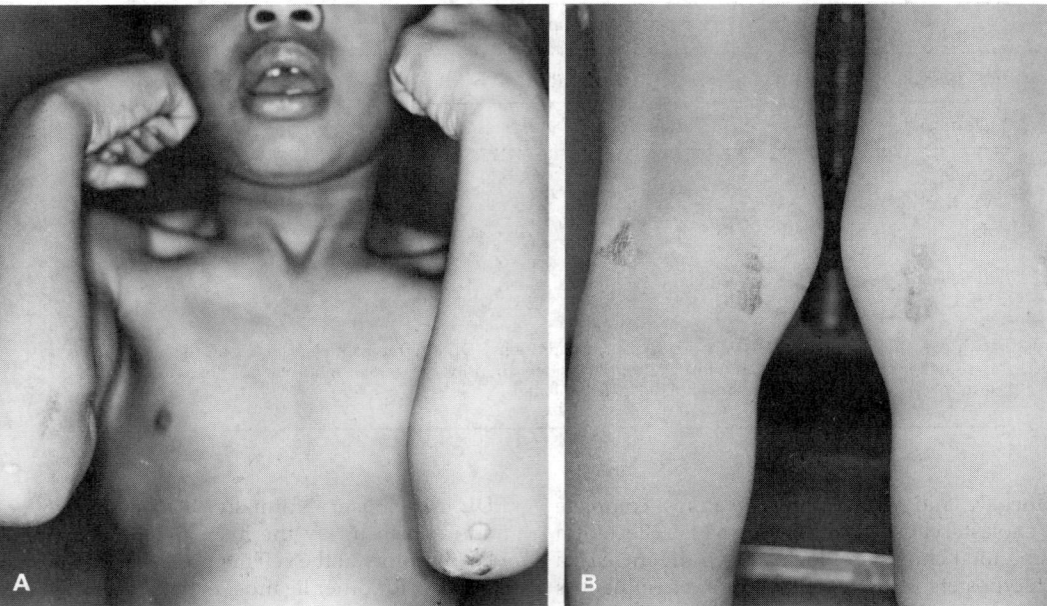

**Figure 12-20.** Homozygous hypercholesterolemia in a 7-year-old boy. Cutaneous xanthomas had been present since the age of 4 years. (**A**) Elbows; (**B**) popliteal fossa.

percentile value of 130 because LDL-cholesterol is considered to be the fraction that induces atheromatosis. Indeed, the diet is considered to be a healthy one for all persons. It involves restriction of cholesterol intake to less than 300 mg/d and limitation of fat intake to less than 30% of the total calories consumed. Additionally, saturated fatty acids and polyunsaturated fatty acids each should comprise less than 10% of the total calories consumed. A wide variety of foods should be included, and the caloric intake should be adequate for growth. Diet should be maintained on a lifetime basis, and its effectiveness should be evaluated by repeated blood studies every month until the levels stabilize. If, after 3 months, the LDL-cholesterol level remains above 130 mg/dL, the Step-Two Diet (maximal daily cholesterol intake less than 200 mg and saturated fatty acid consumption less than 7% of total calories consumed) should be instituted. If the goal of normal or near-normal cholesterol levels is not achieved, additional measures may be indicated. Continued significant elevation of the plasma total cholesterol level is an indication for the addition (not the substitution) of an ion-exchange resin, either cholestyramine or colestipol, to the management program. It usually is given twice daily in gradually increasing dosage with full precautions with respect to technique of administration so as to avoid interference with absorption of vitamins and medications. Several months of monitoring the lipid levels until they are stabilized should be followed by reevaluation to determine whether additional measures should be considered. Nicotinic acid or lovastatin, an inhibitor of HMG-CoA reductase, may be administered. The latter has proven to be effective in adults; it is not approved for use in children, however. The disorder is an autosomal dominant one with a prevalence of 1:500.

Homozygous hypercholesterolemia is a much rarer (1: 1,000,000) and more severe disorder in which the complete absence of LDL receptors results in even greater accumulation of cholesterol, with concentrations in the range of 700 to 1000 mg/ dL or even higher. Untreated, these patients manifest xanthomas and arcus in early childhood, occasionally even prenatally, and will have myocardial infarctions during their teenage years. Management as for the heterozygous condition has helped, but plasmapheresis may be required as well.

Familial combined hyperlipidemia is more common than is hypercholesterolemia. It is characterized by increased plasma cholesterol or TG levels, or both, and is inherited on an autosomal dominant basis. The lipoprotein pattern may vary among affected members of the same family. Affected persons may not have elevation of blood lipids until late adolescence or adulthood. The greatly increased risk of early myocardial infarction is reduced by treatment of the hypercholesterolemia.

Hypercholesterolemia may exist without a single gene pattern. These patients should be treated empirically because the increased risk of myocardial infarction appears to result from the pathophysiologic effects of the blood lipid abnormality per se.

Hypertriglyceridemia occurs frequently as a phenomenon secondary to another disorder. Among the causes are obesity, hypothyroidism, diabetes mellitus, renal disease, alcohol ingestion, and use of oral contraceptives and other medications. The most significant and dramatic inborn errors causing hypertriglyceridemia result from reduced or absent lipoprotein lipase. The latter normally is present in vascular endothelium and, when its cofactor apolipoprotein C-II is present, it degrades chylomicrons. Lipoprotein lipase deficiency and apolipoprotein C-II deficiency occur in the absence of the enzyme or its cofactor, respectively. There is massive accumulation of chylomicrons and their constituents such that the plasma TG concentration will be in the thousands of milligrams per deciliter. An affected child may have abdominal pain, eruptive xanthomas, hepatosplenomegaly, and pancreatitis. A presumptive diagnosis is made by demonstrating very high TG concentrations with normal cholesterol levels and the continued presence of chylomicrons in the plasma in a fasting state. Lipoprotein electrophoresis will show a type I pattern with a dense band at the origin. Definitive diagnosis of lipoprotein lipase deficiency depends on the absence of lipoprotein lipase in the plasma after the administration of heparin, assuming the presence of apolipoprotein C-II. A very–low-fat diet will be of benefit; medium-chain triglycerides may be given because these are absorbed without forming chylomicrons. These autosomal recessive disorders do not increase significantly the risk of atheromatosis.

Type V hyperlipoproteinemia presents the same clinical picture as that of lipoprotein lipase deficiency, with the exceptions that the onset is late in childhood and there is an increased risk of atherosclerosis. There is a marked increase in both chylomicrons and VLDL. The disorder is named after its type of lipoprotein electrophoretic pattern. Weight reduction (if the patient is obese) and reduced carbohydrate intake will be of help. Although an autosomal dominant pattern has been found in some families, it is not present consistently in others; it is expected that this will be clarified when the pathophysiology becomes understood more clearly.

Dysbetalipoproteinemia gives a type III or broad-beta lipoelectrophoretic pattern. The VLDL appears to be electrophoretically abnormal because its apolipoprotein E is a relatively rare allele (ApoE-2) with an amino acid substitution that alters its electrophoretic motility. Both cholesterol and TGs are increased, and affected individuals have premature atherosclerosis as well as the various types of xanthomas, including a specific type, xanthoma striatum palmare (yellow lipid deposits in the palmar creases), but usually not until adult life. Weight control and a diet low in carbohydrates and cholesterol and relatively high in polyunsaturated fat should be of great help. Although the clinical manifestations of the disorder are confined to persons homozygous for the ApoE-2 abnormality, the majority of these homozygotes do not have abnormal plasma lipid levels, indicating that other factors are responsible for bringing about disease.

## Selected Readings

Blades BL, Dudman NPB, Wilken DEL. Screening for familial hypercholesterolemia in 5000 neonates: A recall study. Pediatr Res 1988;23:500.
Bolton CH. Lipid disorders. In: Holton JB, ed. The inherited metabolic diseases. New York: Churchill Livingstone, 1987:358.
Kwiterovich PO Jr. Diagnosis and management of familial dyslipoproteinemia in children and adolescents. Pediatr Clin North Am 1990;37:1489.
Lauer RM, Chairman. Report of the expert panel on blood cholesterol levels in children and adolescents (NIH Publication No 91–2732). Washington, DC: National Institutes of Health, 1991.
Lauer RM, Chairman. Report of the expert panel on blood cholesterol levels in children and adolescents. Pediatrics 1992;89:525.
Marinetti GV. Disorders of lipid metabolism. New York: Plenum Press, 1990.
Scriver CR, Beaudet AL, Sly WS, Valle D, eds. The metabolic basis of inherited disease, ed 6. New York: McGraw-Hill, 1989.
Strong JP. Coronary atherosclerosis in soldiers. A clue to the natural history of atherosclerosis in the young. JAMA 1986;256:2863.
Williams CL, Wynder EL, eds. Hyperlipidemia in childhood and the development of atherosclerosis. Ann N Y Acad Sci 1991;623:1.

*Principles and Practice of Pediatrics, Second Edition.*
edited by Frank A. Oski et al. J. B. Lippincott Company, Philadelphia © 1994.

# 12.7 *Lysosomal Storage Disorders*

Lysosomes are cytoplasmic, single membrane–bound organelles that contain hydrolytic enzymes responsible for the degradation of a variety of compounds, including mucopolysaccharides (MPSs), sphingolipids, and glycoproteins. The substances to be degraded are either exogenous materials, which have been taken into the cell by endocytosis, or endogenous materials contained in cytoplasm, which has been segregated into autophagosomes. Deficient activity of lysosomal acid hydrolases leads to progressive lysosomal enlargement as a result of the accumulation of partially degraded material, which distends the cells and disrupts cellular

function. Deficient activity of a specific acid hydrolase may be the result of genetic mutations at the enzyme locus, which result in lowered specific activity or reduced stability of the enzyme; failure of formation of a protective protein or activator for the enzyme; or failure of formation of a recognition marker on the enzyme, which targets it for lysosomal location. A relatively new class of lysosomal storage disorders exists in which lysosomal storage of material also may be caused by failure of active transport of small molecules from the lysosome.

The pattern of clinical findings seen with the various disorders is related to the type of compound stored and its natural distribution in the body. The disorders usually are classified according to the type of compound stored. All the disorders are inherited as either autosomal recessive or X-linked traits. Carrier testing and prenatal diagnosis are available for most of the disorders, but only in a limited number of experienced laboratories. Exact enzymatic diagnosis is essential for accurate carrier and prenatal studies.

Current therapy consists of symptomatic and supportive therapy for the patient and family. Enzyme replacement therapy is available only for type I Gaucher's disease, but it may be available for other lysosomal storage disorders in the future. Bone marrow transplantation with tissue-typed identical siblings may be considered, especially for those disorders that do not have central nervous system involvement and for the mucopolysaccharidoses. Animal models are available that can be used for the investigation of new therapies. For many of the disorders, the associated genes have been mapped and cloned. Heterogeneity has been noted in the molecular basis for many of the disorders and, at times, has been correlated with varying clinical presentations.

## MUCOPOLYSACCHARIDOSES

The mucopolysaccharidoses are associated with lysosomal accumulation of partially degraded acid MPSs. MPSs, also termed *glycosaminoglycans*, are large molecules composed of repeating sulfated hexuronate or hexosamine disaccharide units attached to a protein core. MPSs normally are degraded by a series of acid hydrolases, which remove the sulfate and carbohydrate residues in a stepwise manner. Deficiency of a specific hydrolase results in partial degradation of the molecules and lysosomal storage of the residual fragments.

The degradation of heparan sulfate, dermatan sulfate, keratan sulfate, or chondroitin sulfate, alone or in combination, may be involved, depending upon the specific hydrolase affected. Disorders associated with heparan sulfate storage usually have central nervous system involvement and progressive mental retardation, those with dermatan sulfate storage usually are associated with visceral and bone involvement, and those with keratan sulfate storage have bone involvement as their major clinical feature.

Radiographs may show a distinct pattern that is termed *dysostosis multiplex*. The skull is enlarged and elongated (dolichocephaly), and the calvarium is thickened. The sella may be J-, wooden-shoe-, or boot-shaped (Fig 12-21). The vertebral bodies in the lower thoracic and upper lumbar areas have a "beaking" of the anterior inferior surface caused by hypoplasia of their anterosuperior areas (Fig 12-22). A dorsal kyphosis, or gibbus deformity, develops. The ribs are thickened, except where they join the spine, and they have an oar-shaped appearance (Fig 12-23). The metacarpals have a proximal narrowing with distal widening, giving them a "baby-bottle" appearance. The distal humerus and ulna may show an abnormal angulation called a *Madelung's deformity* (Fig 12-24). The pelvis may have flaring of the iliac bones, shallow acetabular areas, and progressive coxa valga. The long bones become shortened, thickened, and may have signs of expansion of the medullary cavity. Hypoplasia of the odontoid

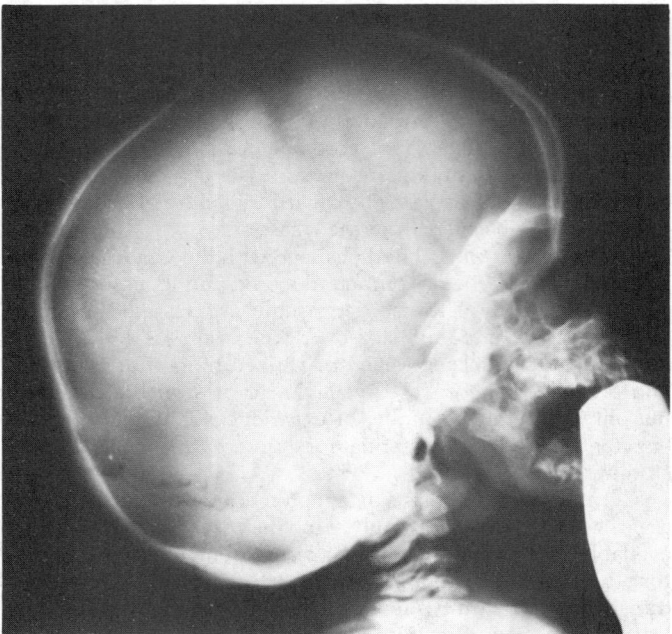

Figure 12-21. Lateral skull radiogram in Hurler syndrome.

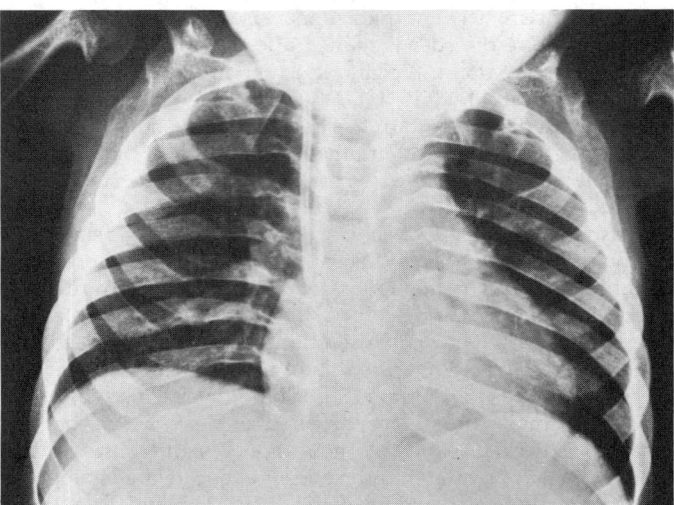

Figure 12-23. AP chest radiogram in Hurler syndrome.

process may occur. Radiographs in Morquio syndrome, which is associated with keratan sulfate and chondroitin-6-sulfate storage, show a different pattern, with platyspondyly, which resembles the spondyloepiphyseal dysplasias (Fig 12-25).

The age of onset, severity, and pattern of clinical and radiographic findings help to distinguish between the various types of mucopolysaccharidoses. Although urinary MPS testing may be helpful in some cases, the diagnosis is made on the basis of enzymatic testing. Demonstration of deficient activity of a specific lysosomal hydrolase may be done with serum or leukocytes for most of the disorders. Cultured skin fibroblasts may be required for others.

## Hurler Syndrome (MPS I-H)

Hurler syndrome is associated with deficient activity of $\alpha$-L-iduronidase and excessive storage of heparan and dermatan sulfates. It is inherited as an autosomal recessive trait and occurs in about 1:100,000 births. Hurler syndrome is considered to be the most severe of the mucopolysaccharidoses and is the prototype for the group.

Children with this disorder appear normal at birth. Between 6 and 12 months of age, they have the onset of gradual coarsening

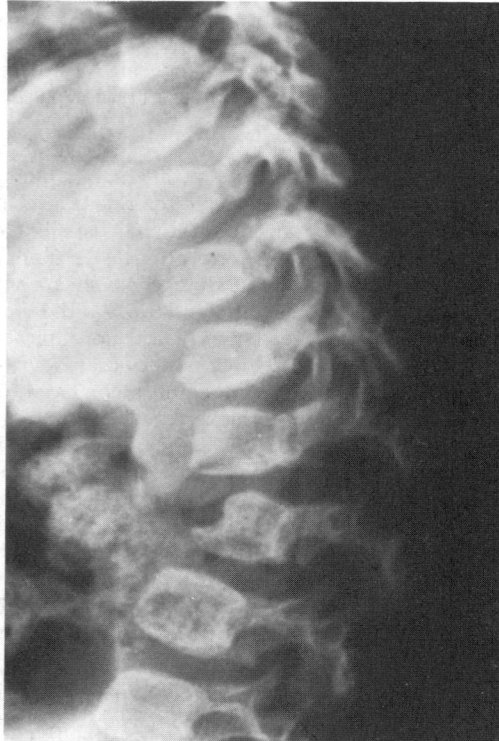

Figure 12-22. Lateral spine radiogram in Hurler syndrome.

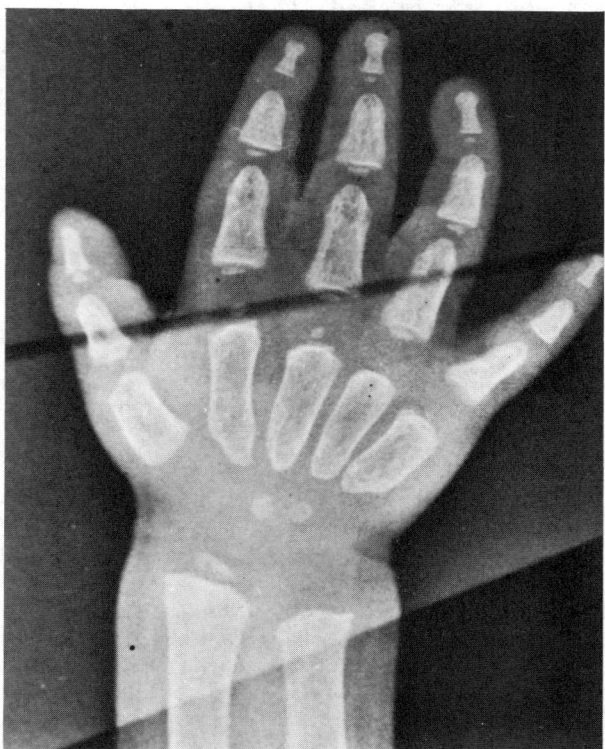

Figure 12-24. AP hand and wrist radiogram in Hurler syndrome.

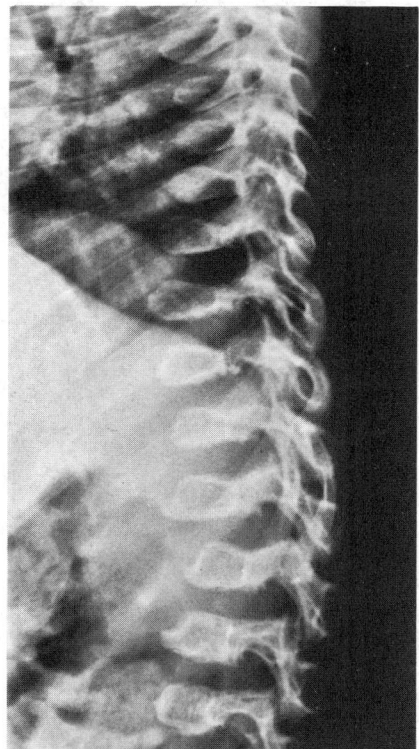

**Figure 12-25.** Lateral spine radiogram in Morquio syndrome.

involvement results from thickening of the soft tissues in the nasal and pharyngeal areas. Initially, the child may have persistent rhinorrhea or noisy breathing. Gradual upper airway obstruction may result in sleep apnea and cor pulmonale. Cardiac involvement usually develops between 2 and 5 years of age, and may result in thickened valve leaflets, pseudo-atheromatosis of the coronary arteries, cardiomyopathy, and congestive heart failure. Hepatosplenomegaly develops during the first year. There usually are no associated physiologic problems except for occasional hypersplenism with thrombocytopenia or pancytopenia. Umbilical and inguinal hernias often require surgical correction (Figs 12-26, 12-27).

Bone growth is delayed and there usually is minimal linear growth after 2 to 3 years of age. The gibbus deformity, a dorsolumbar kyphosis, develops during the first year and may progress. The head becomes enlarged and dolichocephalic, with prominence of the frontal areas and suture lines. Radiographs show a progression of the dysostosis multiplex as described previously.

Overproduction of collagen and elastin may accompany the MPS storage and result in joint stiffness, carpal tunnel syndrome, thickening of the meninges with hydrocephalus, and decreased compliance of the thoracic cage.

Psychomotor development appears normal for the first year, remains on a plateau for 1 to 2 years, then regresses gradually. Physical limitations are noted as a result of the joint stiffness and bone involvement. Contractures in the lower extremities lead to a "jockey stance," and the hands become stiff and claw-like in appearance with limited manual dexterity. Physical therapy may be prescribed, with the restriction that flexion and extension of the neck should not be done because of possible hypoplasia of the odontoid process. Adaptive equipment may be of benefit. Most children eventually become wheelchair-bound and do not live past their early teenage years. Death may occur earlier from cardiopulmonary involvement.

Hurler syndrome may be confirmed by demonstrating deficient

and prominence of the facial features, with flattening of the midfacial areas and widening of the nasal bridge. Clouding of the corneas is present. Gingival hyperplasia and thickening of the alveolar ridge develop. Dental eruption is delayed. Deafness may occur and often is helped transiently by amplification. Respiratory

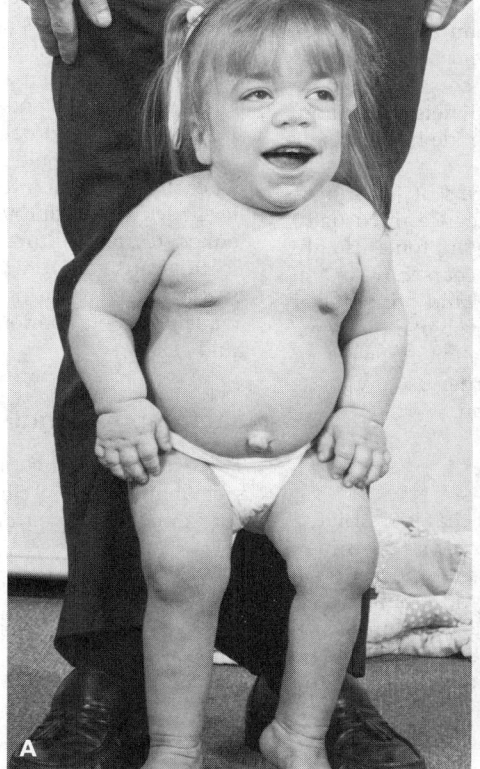
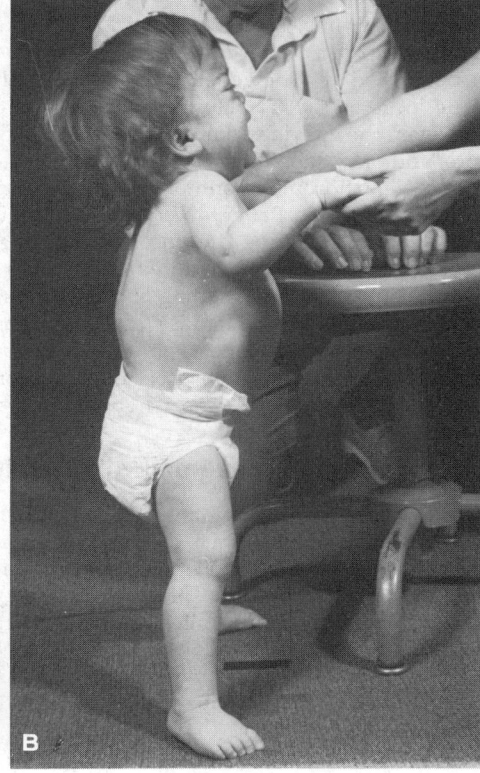

**Figure 12-26.** Children with Hurler syndrome. (**A**) Age 37 months; (**B**) age 27 months. Note the dolichomacrocephaly and dorsal kyphosis.

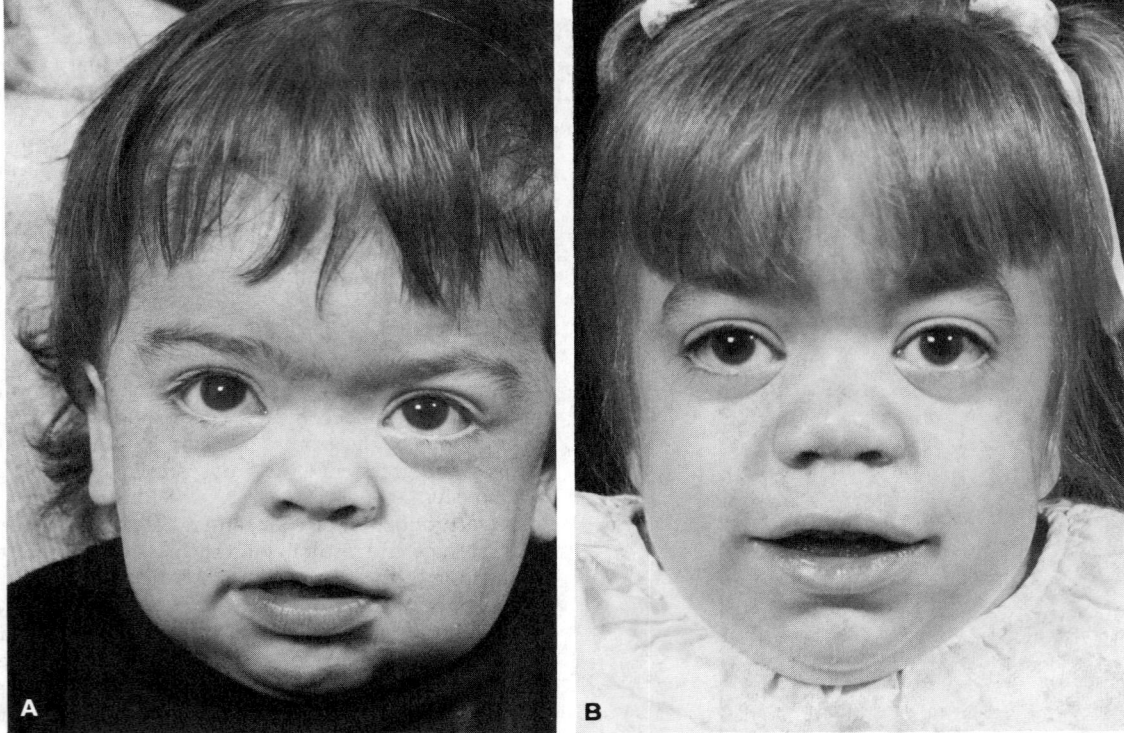

Figure 12-27. Face in Hurler syndrome. (**A**) Age 27 months; (**B**) age 37 months.

activity of α-L-iduronidase in leukocytes or cultured skin fibroblasts. Carrier detection is available, but there is considerable overlap between carriers and noncarriers. Prenatal diagnosis is available with both chorionic villi sampling and cultured amniotic fluid cells.

## Scheie Syndrome (MPS I-S)

Scheie syndrome, formerly called MPS V, is an autosomal recessive disorder that also is associated with deficient activity of α-L-iduronidase. The genetic mutation is allelic, or at the same gene locus as that for Hurler syndrome. In Scheie syndrome, however, the enzyme retains the ability to degrade heparan sulfate, and only dermatan sulfate is stored.

Scheie syndrome is one of the mildest forms of the mucopolysaccharidoses. Patients have normal intelligence and usually are of normal stature. The onset of clinical symptoms usually occurs after 5 years of age and includes mild coarsening of the facial features, severe clouding of the corneas, and pronounced joint involvement in the hands and feet. Aortic valvular problems are common. Carpal tunnel syndrome, degeneration of the retina, glaucoma, and deafness may occur. The disorder usually is associated with a normal or near-normal life span.

## Hurler-Scheie Syndrome (MPS I-H/I-S)

Hurler-Scheie syndrome is a very rare disorder that is associated with deficient activity of α-L-iduronidase. Affected patients may be compound heterozygotes (ie, they may have one gene for Hurler syndrome and the other for Scheie syndrome) or they may represent yet another allelic mutation at the α-L-iduronidase locus. The clinical features are intermediate between those of Hurler and Scheie syndromes. The onset usually is during the first 2 years of life; survival has been reported into the third decade of life.

## Hunter's Syndrome (MPS II)

Hunter's syndrome is associated with deficient activity of iduronosulfate sulfatase and storage of heparan and dermatan sulfate. It is inherited as an X-linked trait. There are both severe (type A) and mild (type B) forms. The clinical features of the severe form are very similar to those of Hurler syndrome except that the onset is between 1 and 2 years of age, the course of the disease is somewhat slower, and there is no corneal clouding (Fig 12-28). Deafness is common. Skin lesions, consisting of ivory raised papules, often are noted on the upper back and on the lateral upper arms and thighs. Patients commonly survive until the second or third decades. The milder type of this disorder is comparable to Scheie's syndrome, with usually normal intelligence and survival into the sixth or seventh decade of life. Deficient activity of iduronosulfate sulfatase may be noted in serum, leukocytes, and cultured skin fibroblasts. Carrier detection is difficult because of lyonization in the female; there is considerable overlap between carriers and noncarriers. Prenatal diagnosis is available using chorionic villi sampling and cultured amniotic fluid cells.

## Sanfilippo's Syndrome (MPS III)

There are four forms of Sanfilippo's syndrome, all of which are indistinguishable in clinical manifestations. All are inherited as autosomal recessive traits and are associated with storage of heparan sulfate. Type A (MPS IIIA) is associated with deficient activity of heparan N-sulfatase (sulfamidase), type B (MPS IIIB) with α-N-acetylglucosaminidase, type C (MPS IIIC) with acetyl-CoA:α-glucosaminide N-acetyltransferase, and type D (MPS IIID) with deficient activity of N-acetylglucosamine-6-sulfatase.

The major clinical finding is that of mental retardation with progressive central nervous system involvement. The onset is between 2 and 4 years of age with developmental delay and

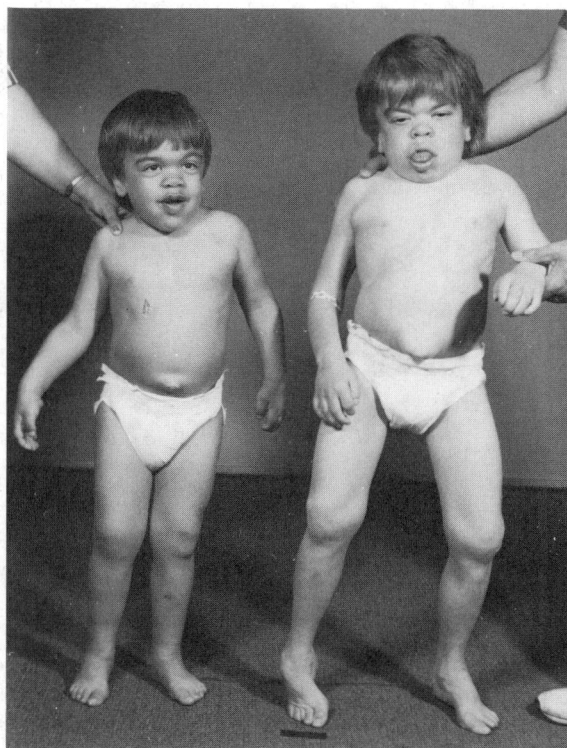

Figure 12-28. Brothers, ages 5 and 15 years, with Hunter's syndrome.

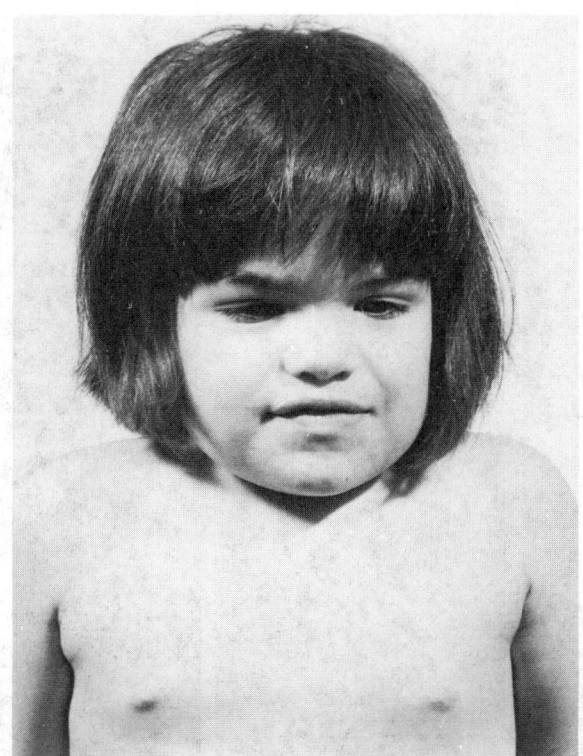

Figure 12-29. Sanfilippo's syndrome, age 6 years.

behavior problems. Patients have hyperactivity that usually is not responsive to therapy. Mild coarsening of the facial features may be noted early in their disease (Fig 12-29). Later, they have joint stiffness, hepatosplenomegaly, hernias, and radiographic findings similar to, but milder than, those seen with Hurler syndrome. They usually do not have corneal clouding, short stature, or cardiac involvement. Most survive into their teenage years.

The specific enzyme deficiencies may be demonstrated in leukocytes and cultured skin fibroblasts for all types. Type B also may be demonstrated in serum. Prenatal diagnosis is available for all types.

## Morquio Syndrome (MPS IV)

Morquio syndrome is associated with keratan sulfate and chondroitin-6-sulfate storage. There are two forms of this disorder. Type A is associated with deficient activity of N-acetylgalactosamine-6-sulfate sulfatase (galactose-6-sulfatase) and type B with β-galactosidase, specific for keratan sulfate. The two forms are very similar in clinical findings and are inherited as autosomal recessive traits.

The major clinical feature is skeletal involvement. Mental retardation usually is not present. The onset of short stature and joint laxity occurs at about 1 year of age. Shortening of the trunk and neck, flaring of the ribs, prominence of the sternum (pectus carinatum), genu valgum, and enlargement and instability of the joints may be noted. Mild corneal clouding and hepatosplenomegaly may be present. Enamel hypoplasia usually is noted in type A Morquio syndrome, but not in type B. Progressive hearing loss, either mixed or sensorineural, occurs and may require hearing aids. Cardiorespiratory problems usually are secondary to the skeletal involvement; valvular heart disease also may be present. Acute or chronic cervical myelopathy is associated with the severe hypoplasia of the odontoid process and with atlantoaxial subluxation. Posterior spinal fusion of the upper cervical spine usually

is required. There are both mild and severe forms of both types. More severely affected patients have minimal linear growth after 6 to 7 years of age and die of cardiorespiratory compromise in their third or fourth decade; patients with mild cases have survived into their seventh decade.

Radiographic findings commonly are evident by 2 years of age and include flattening of the vertebral bodies (platyspondyly), hypoplasia of the odontoid process, irregular metaphyses, shortening of the long bones, and findings similar to those of Hurler syndrome in the wrists and metacarpals. Keratansulfaturia is most marked early in the disease. The two types of this disorder may be confirmed by demonstration of the enzyme deficiencies in cultured skin fibroblasts.

## Maroteaux-Lamy Syndrome (MPS VI)

Maroteaux-Lamy syndrome is associated with dermatan sulfate storage and deficient activity of arylsulfatase B (N-acetylgalactosamine-4-sulfatase). It is inherited as an autosomal recessive trait. There are three forms of this disease: mild, intermediate, and severe. Clinical features of the severe form are very similar to those of Hurler syndrome except that mental retardation usually is not present. Survival is possible into the third decade of life. Hydrocephalus and increased intracranial pressure may occur. Mitral and aortic insufficiency may be present. The milder form resembles Scheie's syndrome except that patients are short in stature. An intermediate type also has been reported (Figs 12-30, 12-31). Deficient activity of arylsulfatase B may be seen in leukocytes or cultured skin fibroblasts. Carrier detection and prenatal diagnosis are available.

## β-Glucuronidase Deficiency (MPS VII)

β-Glucuronidase deficiency, also known as Sly syndrome, is associated with the storage of heparan sulfate, keratan sulfate,

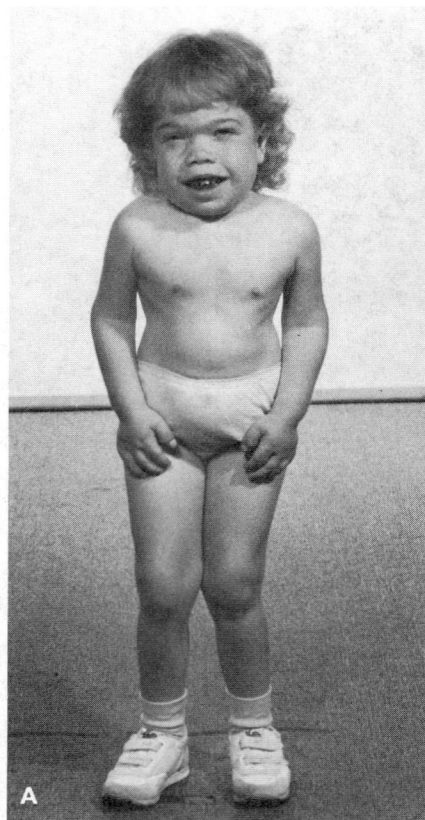
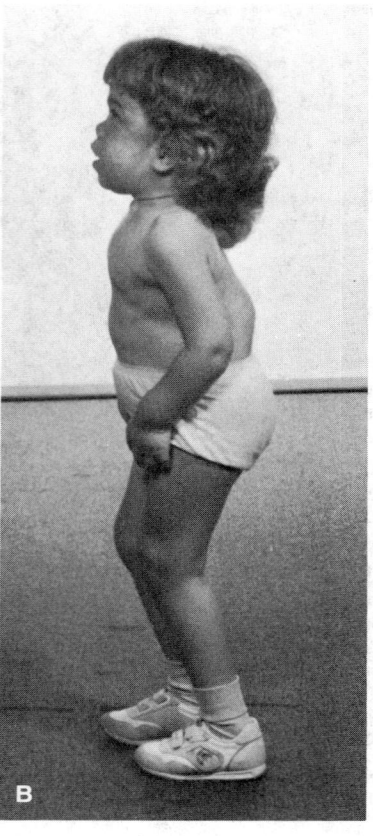

Figure 12-30. Maroteaux-Lamy syndrome, severe form, age 10 years.

chrondroitin-4-sulfate, and chondroitin-6-sulfate. It is inherited as an autosomal recessive trait and is associated with deficient activity of β-glucuronidase. Varying clinical findings have been reported. This disorder may be similar clinically to Hurler syndrome in some patients and milder, without mental retardation, in others, or it might become manifest in the neonatal period with hydrops fetalis along with features of a storage disorder. The enzyme deficiency may be demonstrated in leukocytes and cultured skin fibroblasts.

## THE SPHINGOLIPIDOSES

The sphingolipidoses are associated with lysosomal accumulation of glycosphingolipids, gangliosides, and sphingomyelin. Faulty degradation of the molecules results from deficient activity of lysosomal acid hydrolases as a result of gene mutations at the enzyme loci or a missing sphingolipid activator protein needed for enzyme–lipid stabilization and interaction.

Ceramide, also known as N-acylsphingosine, which is the basic structure for these molecules, is composed of sphingosine to which a long-chain fatty acid, usually C16, has been attached at the

amino group (Fig 12-32). Attachment of neutral carbohydrate groups, in an oligosaccharide chain, occurs at the hydroxyl group of the sphingosine. The attachment of a glucosyl residue, in beta linkage, as the first neutral sugar, leads to a glucosylceramide (glucocerebroside) series of glycosphingolipids. Attachment of a galactosyl residue leads to a galactosylceramide (galactocerebroside) series. The neutral sugars of the oligosaccharide side chain may be in alpha or beta linkage and are derived from glucose, galactose, N-acetyl-galactosamine, or N-acetyl-glucosamine. If the first neutral sugar is a sulfated galactosyl, the compound is called a *sulfatide*. If sialic acid, or N-acetyl-neuraminic acid, is attached to the neutral sugars, the structure is termed a *ganglioside*.

Current nomenclature of the gangliosides, according to the Svennerholm classification, is determined by the number of sialic acid residues that are attached to the oligosaccharide chain (M = mono, D = di, T = tri) and by the number (5 minus $n$) of neutral sugars in the chain. For example, $GM_1$ ganglioside would have one (M = mono) sialic acid residue and four (5 minus 1) neutral sugars in the oligosaccharide chain attached to the ceramide. Degradation of glycosphingolipids involves stepwise removal of the neutral sugars, sulfate, and sialic acid by a series of lysosomal hydrolases (Fig 12-33).

## $GM_1$ Gangliosidoses

$GM_1$ gangliosidoses are inherited as autosomal recessive traits and are associated with acid β-galactosidase deficiency. There are numerous subtypes, which vary widely in clinical spectra and are thought to be the result of different structural mutations at this gene locus. Some of the mutations allow for the retention of compound-specific enzyme activity for the multiple sources that contain β-galactoside residues, such as $GM_1$ ganglioside glycoproteins, oligosaccharides, and keratan sulfate–like MPSs.

Type I (generalized gangliosidosis) (Fig. 12-34) is associated

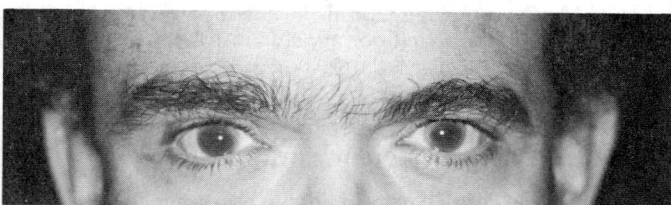

Figure 12-31. Eyes in adult-onset Maroteaux-Lamy syndrome. Note the corneal clouding.

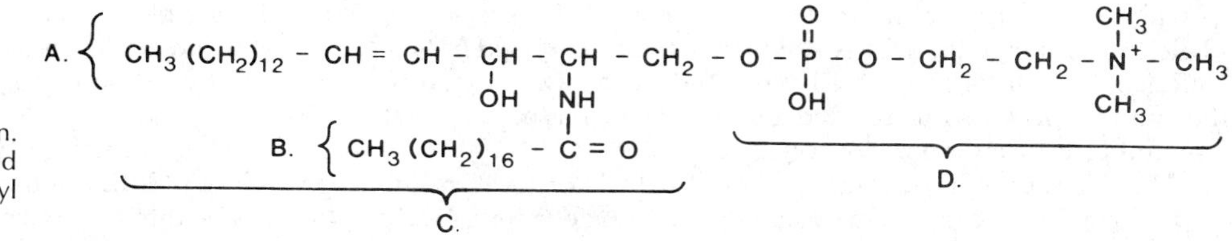

Figure 12-32. Structure of sphingomyelin. *A*, sphingoid (sphingosine); *B*, fatty acid (stearoyl); *C*, ceramide; *D*, phosphoryl choline.

with a complete lack of acid $\beta$-galactosidase activity. Symptoms begin at or shortly after birth and include severe progressive central nervous system degeneration, coarse facial features, macroglossia, gingival hyperplasia, hepatosplenomegaly, hernias, joint stiffness, dorsal kyphosis, and edema of the extremities. Corneal clouding usually is not present. Cherry-red macular spots may be seen in half of the patients. Radiographs show dysostosis multiplex. Foamy histiocytes may be noted in bone marrow and visceral organs. Death usually occurs by 2 years of age.

Type 2 (juvenile GM$_1$ gangliosidosis) is a milder disorder with less severe symptoms of MPS storage. The onset of ataxia between 1 and 2 years of age is followed by progressive mental and motor deterioration, spasticity, seizures, and blindness. Death occurs between 3 and 10 years of age. There usually is no coarsening of the facial features, hepatosplenomegaly, corneal clouding, or macular changes. Radiographs may show mild changes of dysostosis multiplex.

Type 3 (adult GM$_1$ gangliosidosis) is the mildest type of the disorder and manifests with dysarthria, gait disturbance, and a slowly progressive dystonia as early as 4 years of age, but more often in the teenage years. If they are present, intellectual involvement and bone changes are mild. Survival into early adulthood is possible.

## GM$_2$ Gangliosidoses

GM$_2$ gangliosidoses are a group of disorders, inherited as autosomal recessive traits, that are associated with cerebral degeneration secondary to lysosomal storage of GM$_2$ ganglioside and related glycosphingolipids, caused by deficient activity of specific $\beta$-hexosaminidases or a sphingolipid activator protein.

$\beta$-Hexosaminidase has two subunits, $\alpha$ and $\beta$, which are the products of two separate genes on chromosomes 15 and 5, respectively. The isoenzymes of $\beta$-hexosaminidase are comprised of different combinations of these subunits. Hexosaminidase A is composed of one $\alpha$ subunit and two $\beta$ subunits; hexosaminidase B has four $\beta$ subunits. Hexosaminidase A usually comprises 55% to 70% of the total hexosaminidase specific activity, and hexo-

saminidase B comprises 30% to 45%. Genetic mutation at the $\alpha$ subunit gene locus leads to hexosaminidase A deficiency and Tay-Sachs disease. Mutation at the $\beta$ subunit gene locus leads to both hexosaminidase A and hexosaminidase B deficiency, and to Sandhoff disease. There also is a GM$_2$ activator protein, which is needed for stabilization of the substrate–enzyme complex. Other mutations at all these gene sites are responsible for the varying clinical and enzymatic findings in this group of disorders.

### Tay-Sachs Disease, GM$_2$ Gangliosidosis, Type I

Tay-Sachs disease is associated with the storage of GM$_2$ ganglioside in the nervous system. Affected children usually are normal at birth. Between 6 and 12 months of age, hypotonia and psychomotor retardation are noted. Children may display an exaggerated startle response to stimuli that is termed *hyperacusis*. After 1 year of age, there is a steady progression of central nervous system degeneration with spasticity and blindness. Seizures and macrocephaly occur. Cherry-red spots in the macular area may be seen as early as 3 months of age and represent a normal red macular area surrounded by a white area of storage. Later in the disorder, the spots appear darker, with brown coloration, as macular degeneration advances. Most children require nasogastric or gastrostomy feedings and have problems with oral secretions after 18 to 24 months of age. Intercurrent respiratory problems are frequent. Most die between 3 and 4 years of age. The diagnosis can be confirmed by measurement of hexosaminidase A in serum,

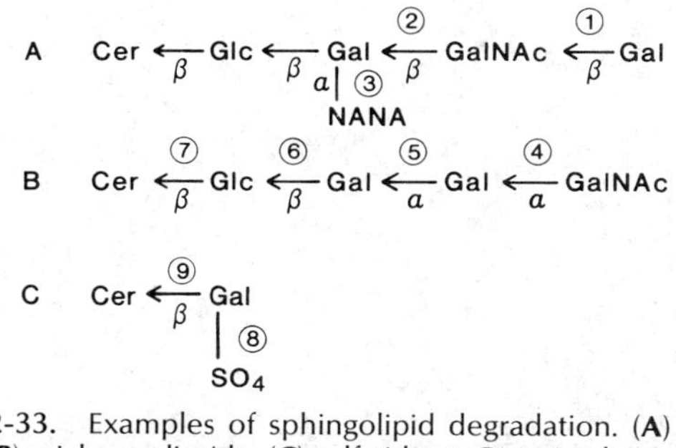

Figure 12-33. Examples of sphingolipid degradation. (**A**) GM1 ganglioside; (**B**) asialoganglioside; (**C**) sulfatide; *1,* GM$_1$-$\beta$-galactosidase (GM$_1$ gangliosidosis); *2,* $\beta$-N-acetylgalactosaminidase, $\beta$-hexosaminidase A and B (GM$_2$ gangliosidoses); *3,* GM$_3$-$\alpha$-neuraminidase; *4,* $\alpha$-N-acetylgalactosaminidase, $\alpha$-galactosidase B; *5,* $\alpha$-galactosidase A (Fabry's disease); *6,* ceramide-lactoside $\beta$-galactosidase (lactosylceramidosis); *7,* $\beta$-glucosidase (Gaucher's disease); *8,* arylsulfatase A (metachromatic leukodystrophy); *9,* $\beta$-galactosidase (Krabbe's leukodystrophy).

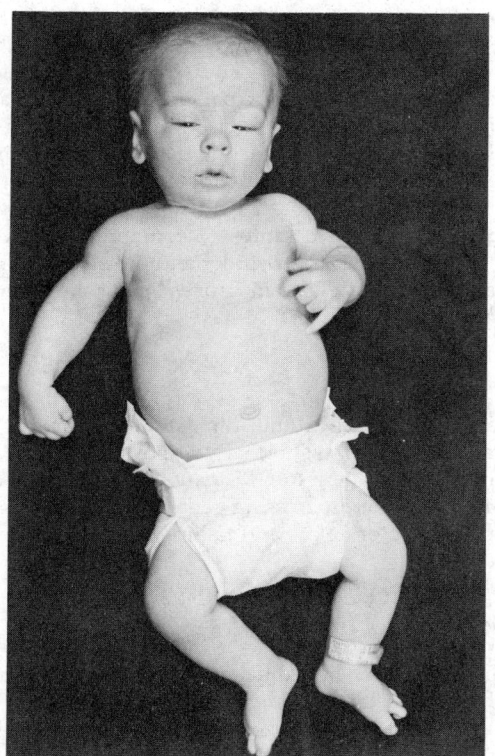

Figure 12-34. Patient with GM$_1$ gangliosidosis.

plasma, leukocytes, or cultured skin fibroblasts. There is severe deficiency of hexosaminidase A, which may be expressed in specific activity units or as a percentage of the total enzyme. Because hexosaminidase B is not affected and may be increased, the total amount of $\beta$-hexosaminidase is normal.

The disorder is most common in individuals of Eastern European Jewish ancestry, among whom the carrier rate is 1:27. Since the 1970s, community education and carrier testing have allowed more than one half million individuals to be tested. At-risk couples, in which both individuals are carriers for Tay-Sachs disease, have been identified before the birth of an affected child. It currently is recommended that all couples of Eastern European Jewish ancestry have carrier testing performed before conception. Because the carrier rate among individuals of other backgrounds is about 1:200, the possibility of Tay-Sachs disease cannot be excluded in non-Jewish families. Prenatal diagnosis is available using chorionic villi sampling or amniocentesis.

### Sandhoff Disease, GM$_2$ Gangliosidosis, Type 2

Sandhoff disease is associated with total deficiency of $\beta$-hexosaminidase and storage in the brain and viscera of GM$_2$ ganglioside, as well as other glycolipids, glycoproteins, and oligosaccharides that contain $\beta$-hexosaminide residues. The clinical features are very similar to those of Tay-Sachs disease. Hepatosplenomegaly and renal storage may be noted. This disorder occurs in children of all backgrounds. Carrier detection and prenatal diagnosis are available.

There are juvenile forms of both Tay-Sachs disease and Sandhoff disease, with the onset between 2 and 6 years of age of ataxia or developmental regression, followed by loss of speech, spasticity, athetosis, and minor motor seizures. Macular changes may not be present, but optic atrophy and retinitis pigmentosa may occur. Death usually occurs between 5 and 15 years of age.

An adult form of Tay-Sachs disease has been reported, which has an atypical spinocerebellar degeneration. Some patients have had psychoses. The onset has varied widely from between 2 and 4 years of age to as late as 16 years of age.

There are affected patients, of all types, who have been reported to have normal enzyme activity when they were tested using the standard methods, which employ artificial substrates. Deficient activity may be demonstrated if they are tested with natural substrates. Some of these patients also have an activator protein deficiency. Rarely, otherwise normal adults have been noted to have absent total hexosaminidase or hexosaminidase A when measured with artificial substrates, but only partially reduced activity when measured with natural substrates. These individuals are thought to represent compound heterozygotes with one gene for the classic disorder and the other for a mutant allele, which does not allow measurement of enzyme activity with artificial substrates.

### GM$_3$ Gangliosidosis

One case of decreased uridine diphosphate-N-acetylgalactosaminyl transferase activity, normally responsible for the conversion of GM$_3$ ganglioside into GM$_2$ ganglioside, was reported in a child with a rapidly progressing generalized hyporeflexia, hypotonia, psychomotor delay, and failure to thrive.

### Fabry's Disease ($\alpha$-Galactosyl-Lactosyl Ceramidosis)

Fabry's disease is an X-linked disorder associated with deficient activity of $\alpha$-galactosidase (formerly referred to as $\alpha$-galactosidase A). Storage of glycosphingolipids with terminal galactosyl residues in $\alpha$ linkage, such as globotriaosylceramide, galabiosylcer-

amide, and blood group B substances, occurs in the eyes, kidneys, skeletal and cardiac muscle, central and autonomic nervous system, and vascular endothelium and smooth muscle throughout the body.

Clinical symptoms usually are evident by 10 years of age and include an almost constant discomfort in the hands and feet, with paresthesia or burning pain (acroparesthesia). Intermittent painful crises, lasting minutes to days, may involve the extremities or the abdomen. Because episodes often are accompanied by a low-grade fever and an elevated erythrocyte sedimentation rate, they may be mistaken for other causes of acute abdominal crises. Low-dose diphenylhydantoin or carbamazepine may improve the acroparesthesia and painful crises.

A characteristic whorl-like corneal dystrophy with spoke-like or propeller-like cataracts may be seen. Angiokeratoma corporis diffusum are punctate, flat to slightly raised, dark red to blue-black, characteristic skin lesions, which usually appear in clusters in areas between the umbilicus and knees (bathing suit area) (Fig 12-35). They also may be seen on the conjunctiva or mucosal surfaces. Hypohidrosis is common.

With advancing age, patients may complain of fatigue, weakness, and poor vision, and they may be hypertensive. Cardiac involvement may lead to myocardial infarction, cardiomyopathies, or conduction defects. Vascular involvement of the central nervous system may lead to aneurysms, vascular occlusion, or hemorrhage. Renal dysfunction, initially evident as proteinuria, progresses to renal failure by 30 to 40 years of age. Renal dialysis or transplantation may be indicated.

Foamy macrophages may be present in bone marrow. Using polarized light, characteristic birefringent crystals with a Maltese cross configuration may be seen in cells of urine sediment. The diagnosis is established by the demonstration of deficient activity of $\alpha$-galactosidase in leukocytes or cultured skin fibroblasts. Carrier detection and prenatal diagnosis are available.

Female carriers for Fabry's disease often have milder, but similar, clinical findings. The most frequent of these is corneal dystrophy. With advancing age, many become symptomatic, and deaths may occur from vascular, renal, or cardiac involvement, as in males.

### Schindler Disease

Schindler disease is an autosomal recessive disorder that is associated with $\alpha$-N-acetylgalactosaminidase deficiency. Patients

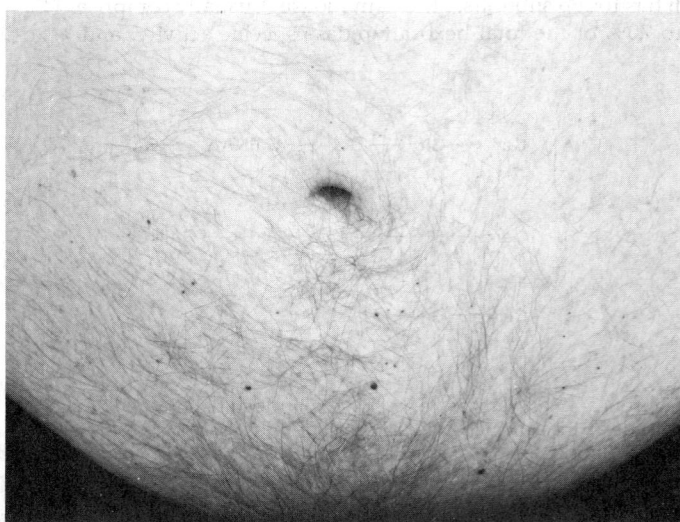

Figure 12-35.   Angiokeratomas in a patient with Fabry's disease.

have severe psychomotor retardation, myoclonic seizures, optic atrophy, and progressive neurologic deterioration in childhood. $\alpha$-N-acetylgalactosaminidase (formerly called $\alpha$-galactosidase, B isoenzyme) cleaves terminal $\alpha$-galactosyl and $\alpha$-N-acetylgalactosaminyl residues in sphingolipids and glycoproteins. Deficient activity may be demonstrated in plasma, leukocytes, and cultured skin fibroblasts.

## Lactosylceramidosis (Ceramide Lactoside Lipidosis)

Lactosylceramidosis is a rare disorder that is associated with deficient activity of neutral $\beta$-galactosidase, which cleaves the terminal $\beta$-galactosyl residues from lactosylceramide. Storage of lactosylceramide occurs in the viscera, brain, connective tissue, and reticuloendothelial system. In one reported patient, delayed development and hypotonia were noted at 30 months of age, after which, psychomotor regression, cerebellar ataxia, optic atrophy, generalized lymphadenopathy, and hepatosplenomegaly developed. The bone marrow contained foamy-looking monocytes. Death occurred at 50 months of age.

## Gaucher's Disease (Glucocerebrosidosis)

Gaucher's disease is an autosomal recessive disorder that is associated with deficient activity of $\beta$-glucocerebrosidase ($\beta$-glucosidase) and storage of sphingolipid with terminal glucosyl residues in $\beta$ linkage, glucocerebroside (glucosylceramide), in the reticuloendothelial system.

Type 1, the adult, chronic, non-neuronopathic form, may have the onset of symptoms at any age. This is the most common of the sphingolipid storage disorders and is found most often among individuals of Eastern European Jewish ancestry. The initial symptoms usually are splenomegaly with pancytopenia from hypersplenism. Hepatomegaly is common, with mildly elevated liver function test results, but usually no significant dysfunction. Infiltration of the bone marrow also interferes with bone growth and mineralization, and may lead to a leukoerythroblastic anemia. Radiographs show an expanded cortex of the distal femur termed an *Erlenmeyer-flask deformity*; bone erosion with cyst-like changes of varying sizes may occur. Patients also may have avascular crises, pseudo-osteomyelitis, and avascular necrosis of the femoral heads. Pulmonary storage may lead to abnormal pulmonary function test results and cor pulmonale. Older patients may have a yellow or brown discoloration of the exposed skin or pingueculae on the conjunctiva. Although central nervous system disease is not common, oculomotor apraxia may occur. The disorder is very slowly progressive, and many patients who are seen initially in childhood live well into adult life.

Bone marrow and other tissues from the reticuloendothelial system have large, lipid-laden, fusiform histiocytes with dense eccentric nuclei and are said to resemble "wrinkled tissue paper" or "crumpled silk" (Gaucher's cells). Serum acid phosphatase levels may be elevated.

Enzyme replacement therapy with intravenous infusions of macrophage-targeted modified glucocerebrosidase (Ceredase) has been commercially available since early 1991 for type I Gaucher's disease. Significant clinical improvement has been noted in the more than 100 patients treated to date, who have experienced no major side effects. Responses in hematologic status and reduction in size of the liver and spleen were noted to occur more rapidly than were skeletal changes. Although it is extremely expensive, enzyme replacement therapy should be considered for any symptomatic patient with type 1 disease. Bone marrow transplantation also has resulted in clinical improvement, but it

is associated with considerable risks when compared to enzyme replacement therapy.

Before enzyme replacement therapy was available, many patients required splenectomy for persistent thrombocytopenia and bleeding diatheses. Post-splenectomy management should include prophylactic antibiotics and immunization, as for other asplenic individuals. Orthopedic problems often difficult are to treat and should be referred to specialists who are experienced with these patients.

Type 2, the acute neuronopathic or infantile form of Gaucher's disease, has its onset between birth and 18 months of age. Hepatosplenomegaly is accompanied by a rapidly progressing central nervous system deterioration. Trismus, strabismus, and retroflexion of the head are pathognomonic. Spasticity, hyperreflexia, and seizures occur. Feeding and respiratory problems are common. Death usually occurs by 2 years of age. Treatment is symptomatic and supportive.

Type 3, the subacute neuronopathic or juvenile form of Gaucher's disease, has features of both types 1 and 2. Most cases are seen in individuals with ancestry from northern Sweden (Norrbottnian type Gaucher's disease). The onset of hepatosplenomegaly in childhood usually precedes the progressive neurologic symptoms. Behavioral changes, oculomotor apraxia, extrapyramidal and cerebellar signs, seizures, and developmental regression are common. Many patients live into early adulthood.

The diagnosis of all three types of Gaucher's disease is established by the demonstration of deficient activity of $\beta$-glucosidase in leukocytes or cultured skin fibroblasts in experienced laboratories. Atypical cases may be associated with a deficient sphingolipid activator protein for $\beta$-glucosidase. Carrier detection and prenatal diagnosis are available. Molecular genetic studies may help to differentiate between type 1 and type 3 disease in young patients.

## Farber Disease (Ceramidosis, Lipogranulomatosis)

Farber disease is inherited as an autosomal recessive trait and is associated with deficient activity of ceramidase (acylsphingosine deacylase). There is storage of ceramide and other gangliosides in the skin, lymph nodes, viscera, and brain, with connective tissue granuloma formation in response to the storage. Type 1, the "classic" and most common form of the disorder, is seen between 2 weeks and 4 months of age. A hoarse cry; swollen, painful joints; periarticular nodules; and pulmonary infiltration are noted. Older patients have more widely distributed skin nodules over pressure points and in the periorbital and perioral regions. There are granulomatous lesions of the conjunctiva. Occasionally, macular changes and corneal or lens opacities are noted. Swallowing and respiration are hindered by granulomas in the pharynx and upper respiratory tract. Valvular cardiac lesions, hepatosplenomegaly, and a generalized lymphadenopathy may occur. Psychomotor development slows; seizures, hypotonia, hyporeflexia, and failure to thrive are noted. Death usually occurs within a few years of onset, but some patients have survived to the late teenage years. Other forms of this rare disorder differ in the age of onset, clinical severity, and degree of visceral involvement. They are termed the type 2 or intermediate form, the type 3 or mild form, the type 4 or neonatal-visceral form, the type 5 or progressive neurologic form, and the type 6 form, which is type 1 combined with Sandhoff disease. Current therapy mainly is supportive.

Tissues in patients with Farber disease show granulomas and lipid-laden macrophages. The diagnosis is established by demonstrating deficient activity of ceramidase in leukocytes or cultured skin fibroblasts. Carrier detection and prenatal diagnosis are available.

# Niemann-Pick Disease (Sphingomyelin-Cholesterol Lipidosis)

Niemann-Pick disease is a group of disorders that are associated with hepatosplenomegaly and the storage of sphingomyelin, $GM_2$ and $GM_3$ gangliosides, cholesterol, bis(monoacylglyceryl)phosphate, and other glycosphingolipids in the reticuloendothelial system, viscera, and brain. All are inherited as autosomal recessive traits. The disorders recently have been reclassified and divided into two groups, types I and II, on the basis of etiology. The types are subdivided further according to the age of onset and the severity into acute (A), subacute (S), and chronic (C) forms. Type I is associated with deficient activity of sphingomyelinase, and with sphingomyelin and cholesterol storage. Type II varies in the material stored, which may include sphingomyelin, cholesterol, glycolipid, or bis(monoacylglyceryl)phosphate. The exact biochemical basis is unknown for many of the type II disorders. Defects in cholesterol esterification have been shown in the forms of type IIS that previously were designated as types C and D. However, tissue-specific sphingomyelinase deficiency, sphingomyelinase isoenzyme deficiencies, or a sphingomyelinase activator protein deficiency also may be involved. Lipid-filled "foam cells" may be noted in the bone marrow, liver, spleen, adrenals, brain, lymph nodes, and lungs. "Sea-blue histiocytes" may be demonstrated with Romanovsky's staining. Deficient activity of sphingomyelinase may be demonstrated in leukocytes or cultured skin fibroblasts for type I Niemann-Pick disease. Defects in cholesterol esterification may be shown in fibroblasts for type IIS. Reliable carrier detection and prenatal diagnosis currently are available only for types IA and IS.

Type IA Niemann-Pick disease, formerly designated as type A, the acute neuronopathic form, is the most common, and many patients are of Eastern European Jewish ancestry. The onset of hepatosplenomegaly between birth and 12 months of age is followed by a rapidly progressing central nervous system deterioration. Lymphadenopathy, pulmonary infiltration, corneal opacifications with brownish discoloration of the anterior lens capsule, a yellow-brown discoloration of the skin, and seizures may be noted. One half of patients have cherry-red spots in the macular areas. Failure to thrive and respiratory problems are common. Most die by 2 to 5 years of age. Patients with type IIA disease clinically resemble those with type IA disease, but their disorder progresses more slowly. They also may have a neonatal hepatitis-like syndrome.

Type IS Niemann-Pick disease, formerly called type B, the chronic non-neuronopathic form, is characterized by the onset of splenomegaly during infancy or childhood. Hepatomegaly, pulmonary infiltration, and lymphadenopathy are noted. Abnormalities may be noted in the macular areas of the fundi, nerve conduction velocities may be prolonged, and varying degrees of central nervous system involvement may be present. Many patients survive into adulthood. Type IS is thought to be a milder allelic variant of type IA.

Type IIS Niemann-Pick disease encompasses patients previously classified as having types C and D disease, as well as those with vertical supranuclear ophthalmoplegia and DAF (down gaze, ataxia, athetosis, foam cell) syndrome. The disease variant formerly called type C, the chronic, neuronopathic, juvenile form, is associated with the onset of behavioral changes, psychomotor delay and regression, myoclonus, incoordination, ataxia, hyperreflexia, hypertonia, seizures, variable hepatosplenomegaly with cholestasis, and lymphadenopathy between 2 and 7 years of age. Many affected individuals die in late childhood or adolescence. The disorder previously referred to as type D clinically resembles type C, but is seen in patients of western Nova Scotian ancestry. A lowered cholesterol intake may be beneficial for patients with type IIS Niemann-Pick disease who have defects in cholesterol esterification.

Type IC Niemann-Pick disease, formerly known as type E, or the adult, non-neuronopathic form, is associated with hepatosplenomegaly and variable neurologic involvement. Type IIC disease is associated with adult onset of dementia, extrapyramidal signs, and variable organomegaly.

# Krabbe's Disease (Globoid Cell Leukodystrophy, Galactosylceramidosis)

Krabbe's disease is associated with deficient activity of the $\beta$-galactosidase specific for removing the terminal $\beta$-galactosyl residue from galactosylceramide (galactosylceramidase). Storage of galactosylceramide (galactocerebroside) occurs in the white matter of the central nervous system and in the peripheral nervous system. "Globoid cells" (globoid bodies) are large, distended, multinucleated, modified macrophages, with a cytoplasm that is positive with periodic acid-Schiff stain and a lacy pink cytoplasm with hematoxylin-eosin stain, which may be found in clusters in the perivascular areas of the white matter.

The infantile type of Krabbe's disease usually manifests before 6 months of age with increased motor tone, irritability, hypersensitivity to external stimuli, episodic hypothermia, optic atrophy, and developmental regression. Thereafter follows a rapidly progressing degeneration of the central and peripheral nervous systems, with hypotonia and loss of vision and hearing. Cherry-red spots may be seen. Seizures and peripheral neuropathy are common. The cerebrospinal fluid protein concentration may be elevated markedly (100 to 500 mg/dL), and there is decreased nerve conduction velocity. There is severe brain atrophy with demyelination and gliosis. Most patients die by 2 years of age.

The late-onset variants of Krabbe's disease (late infantile, juvenile, and adult forms) cause clinical symptoms between 6 months and 35 years of age. Decreased vision with optic atrophy, spastic quadriparesis with pyramidal signs, acute polyneuropathy, ataxia, spinocerebellar degeneration, and psychomotor regression may be seen. Elevated cerebrospinal fluid protein concentrations and decreased nerve conduction velocities are variable.

The disorder is inherited as an autosomal recessive trait and is more common in persons of Scandinavian ancestry. Deficient activity of galactosylceramidase (galactocerebroside $\beta$-galactosidase) may be demonstrated in leukocytes and cultured skin fibroblasts. Carrier detection and prenatal diagnosis are available.

# Metachromatic Leukodystrophy (Sulfatide Lipidosis)

Metachromatic leukodystrophy is associated with the accumulation of galactosyl sulfatide (cerebroside sulfatide) in the white matter of the central nervous system and in the peripheral nervous system. In addition, galactosyl sulfatide and sulfated galactoglyceroolipids accumulate in the kidney, gallbladder, and other visceral organs. Along with the storage of sulfatides, there is demyelination, gliosis, spongy degeneration, and atrophy of the brain. The storage of the acidic sulfatides gives rise to the metachromatic staining noted with acetic acid-cresyl violet stain for which the disorder is named.

Three are three clinical types of metachromatic leukodystrophy classified according to age of onset, although the disorder may manifest at any age. All are inherited as autosomal recessive traits.

The late-infantile type of metachromatic leukodystrophy has its onset between 1 and 2 years of age. Delayed development, ataxia, gait disturbances, weakness, or peripheral neuropathy may be presenting signs. These are followed by a progressive psychomotor regression, and by central and peripheral nervous system deterioration. Weakness, hypotonia, and hyporeflexia progress to dysarthria and loss of speech, optic atrophy and blindness, nystagmus, loss of truncal and limb control, and spasticity. Respiratory and feeding problems are common as a result of bulbar and pseudobulbar palsies. Seizures may occur. A gray discoloration of the macular areas may be present. The cerebrospinal fluid protein concentration is elevated. Nerve conduction velocities are slowed. Computed tomographic scanning of the head may reveal atrophy of the white matter with enlargement of the ventricles and widening of the sulci. Metachromatic granules may be demonstrated in urine sediment. There usually are no specific findings on bone marrow examination. Most children die between 2 and 4 years after the onset of their disease.

The juvenile type of metachromatic leukodystrophy usually becomes apparent between 5 and 7 years of age, but may have its onset as late as 16 to 20 years of age. Changes in personality or school performance, gait disturbances, ataxia, speech problems, or incontinence often are presenting symptoms. The disorder progresses in a manner similar to, but slower than, the late-infantile type. Seizures are more common. Most affected individuals do not live past their teenage years or for more than 4 to 6 years after the onset of the disease.

The adult type of metachromatic leukodystrophy has its onset after puberty. Initial symptoms may be emotional lability, apathy, personality change, weakness, incontinence, dementia, or psychosis. Thereafter follows progressive dementia, ataxia, dystonia, optic atrophy, and spasticity. Most patients live 5 to 10 years after the onset of the disease, but some have had a slower course, with survival for several decades.

Deficient activity of galactosyl-3-sulfate-ceramide sulfatase (cerebroside sulfatase), also termed arylsulfatase A, has been associated with all three types of clinical presentation. The variation is thought to be the result of different allelic mutations, with preservation of some residual activity in the milder forms, which can be demonstrated by radiolabeled sulfatide accumulation in cell culture. Normal activity of arylsulfatase A, but deficiency of a cerebroside sulfatase activator protein (sphingolipid activator protein 1) has been associated with the juvenile and adult clinical types.

Carrier detection and prenatal diagnosis are available, but may require radiolabeled sulfatide accumulation studies. Healthy adults have been reported who have absent or reduced arylsulfatase A activity when tested using artificial substrates, but who do not have abnormal radiolabeled sulfatide accumulation. This pseudo-deficiency is not rare and can be problematic if parents of affected children are not tested before prenatal diagnosis.

## Multiple Sulfatase Deficiency (Mucosulfatidosis, Austin Disease)

Multiple sulfatase deficiency is a rare disorder that is thought to result from impaired production or activation, or from increased degradation of multiple lysosomal and non-lysosomal sulfatases. The enzymes known to be involved and the disorders associated with single deficiency of each include arylsulfatase A (metachromatic leukodystrophy), arylsulfatase B (Maroteaux-Lamy syndrome), arylsulfatase C (steroid sulfatase deficiency), iduronosulfate sulfatase (Hunter's syndrome), heparan sulfamidase (Sanfilippo's syndrome A), N-acetylglucosamine-6-sulfate sulfatase (Sanfilippo's syndrome D), and N-acetylgalactosamine-6-sulfate sulfatase (Morquio syndrome A). All but one of the individual disorders associated with deficient activity of the single enzymes are discussed elsewhere in this chapter. The other, a deficiency of the cytosolic enzyme steroid sulfatase (arylsulfatase C), is associated with X-linked ichthyosis, corneal opacities, and

elevated blood cholesterol sulfate levels in affected males. Carrier females who are carrying an affected male fetus may have low urinary and serum estriol levels and elevated urine and amniotic fluid dehydroepiandrosterone sulfate levels. They may have difficulties with parturition, with delayed onset of labor and relative refractoriness of cervical dilatation and effacement.

Multiple sulfatase deficiency, an autosomal recessive disorder, is associated with clinical manifestations that are a combination of those features seen with late-infantile metachromatic leukodystrophy, the mucopolysaccharidoses, and steroid sulfatase deficiency. Patients usually are seen by 2 years of age with coarsening of the facial features, dysostosis multiplex, hepatosplenomegaly, weakness, deafness, ichthyosis, and psychomotor delay. An early onset, more severe form of the disorder has been noted at birth. There is elevated urinary excretion of dermatan and heparan sulfates, slowed nerve conduction velocities, and increased cerebrospinal fluid protein concentrations. The progression of this disorder is similar to that of late-infantile metachromatic leukodystrophy. Most children do not live past 10 years of age (Fig 12-36).

## DISORDERS OF LYSOSOMAL ENZYME TRANSPORT (MUCOLIPIDOSES)

Before we reached our current biochemical understanding of this group of disorders, it was recognized that affected patients had features of both the mucopolysaccharidoses and the sphingolipidoses; hence, the disorders were called *mucolipidoses*. Of the four previously classified subgroups of mucolipidoses, types I and IV now are known to be associated with α-neuraminidase deficiency and are described with the glycoproteinoses. Types II and III still retain the name *mucolipidosis* and are associated with faulty synthesis of the recognition marker needed for transport of the acid hydrolases into lysosomes. Deficient activity of multiple acid hydrolases occurs.

Lysosomal acid hydrolases are glycoproteins that require posttranslational processing. After leaving the membrane-bound polysomes, they enter the endoplasmic reticulum, where man-

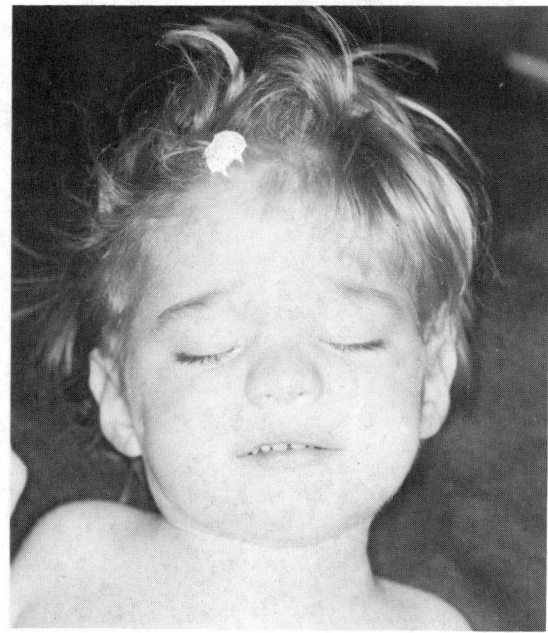

Figure 12-36.    Patient with multiple sulfatase deficiency.

nose-rich oligosaccharide side chains are attached. The enzymes then enter the Golgi apparatus, where the mannose groups are phosphorylated by a series of steps in which N-acetylglucosamine-1-phosphate is attached to the 6-hydroxyl groups of terminal mannose residues by N-acetylglucosamine-1-phosphotransferase. The N-acetylglucosamine then is removed by a phosphodiesterase to expose the mannosyl-6-phosphate. This mannosyl-6-phosphate is the signal for receptor sites in the Golgi cisternae, which transport the enzymes into the lysosomes. Without the mannosyl-6-phosphate signal, the enzymes do not become localized in the lysosomes and are excreted from cells. The enzymes also do not undergo the usual final processing in the lysosome to mature enzymes and have additional sialic residues attached, which alters their biochemical properties.

The defect in most patients with mucolipidoses II and III is failure to phosphorylate the terminal mannose residues because of deficient activity of N-acetylglucosamine-1-phosphotransferase. Patients with mucolipidosis III have some residual activity and, thus, milder disease than do those with mucolipidosis II. In addition, some patients with mucolipidosis III have been found to have normal levels of the phosphotransferase, but defective recognition function. Other patients with mucolipidoses II and III have reduced activity of phosphodiesterase.

In both mucolipidosis II and mucolipidosis III, the specific activity of many lysosomal hydrolases is increased markedly (10 to 20 times normal) in plasma and serum, and is lowered or absent in cultured skin fibroblasts. Leukocytes have normal or decreased activity. Arylsulfatase A, β-galactosidase, β-hexosaminidase, and α-L-iduronidase may be measured to show this effect. Acid phosphatase and β-glucosidase are not affected. Deficient activity of the phosphotransferase may be demonstrated in cultured skin fibroblasts. Both disorders are inherited as autosomal recessive traits. Prenatal diagnosis is available, but carrier detection is not.

## Mucolipidosis II, I-Cell Disease

Most patients with mucolipidosis II are seen shortly after birth with features similar to those associated with Hurler syndrome and GM$_1$ gangliosidosis. There is prominent gingival hypertrophy. Severe dysostosis is present from birth. Most patients do not live past 5 years of age. The disorder is named after the numerous dense inclusions that are seen with phase-contrast microscopy in cultured skin fibroblasts from these patients. Urinary MPS excretion is normal, but sialo-oligosaccharide concentrations may be increased (Figs 12-37 and 12-38).

## Mucolipidosis III, Pseudo-Hurler Polydystrophy

Patients with mucolipidosis III have a milder clinical course than do those with mucolipidosis II, with the onset of stiffness of the large and small joints occurring between 4 and 5 years of age. The disorder is similar to the intermediate form of Maroteaux-Lamy syndrome (MPS VI). They may be mildly mentally handicapped. Cardiac valvular lesions are common. Carpal tunnel syndrome and atlantoaxial subluxation may occur. Many patients have lived to be young adults.

## GLYCOPROTEINOSES

Glycoproteins are characterized by the presence of oligosaccharide chains attached to a peptide core. There are two major classes of glycoproteins that differ in structure because of variations in synthetic pathways. The protein portions of glycoproteins are synthesized on membrane-bound polysomes and then pass to the smooth endoplasmic reticulum and Golgi apparatus, where the carbohydrate side chains are added. In one major class, the glycoprotein oligosaccharide side chains are synthesized by a sugar-

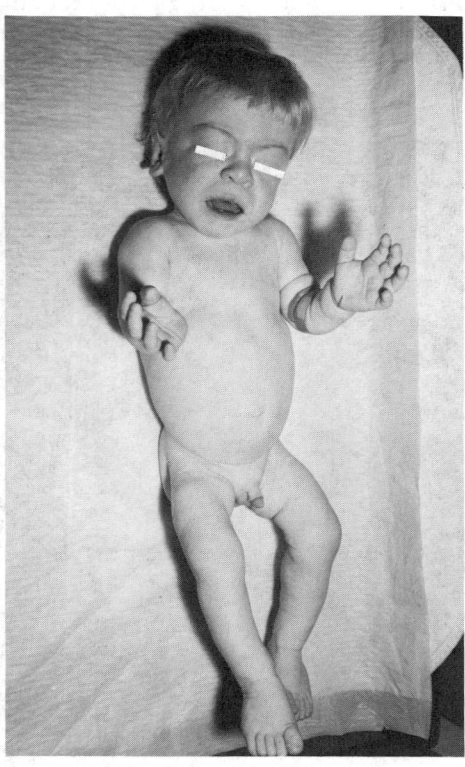

**Figure 12-37.**   Patient with I-cell disease.

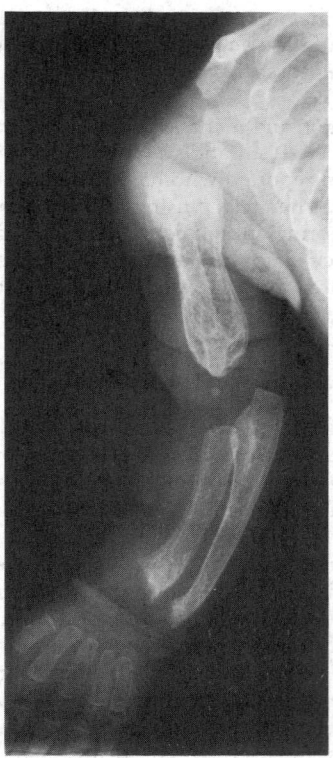

**Figure 12-38.**   Radiogram in a patient with I-cell disease. Note the severe dysostosis multiplex and the "bone within bone" appearance.

nucleotide pathway, which involves the stepwise addition of single sugars from sugar-nucleotides catalyzed by a series of specific glycosyltransferases. The oligosaccharide chains are attached to the protein core by N-acetylgalactosaminyl residues, which bind with the hydroxyl groups of serine or threonine. Examples of this group include blood group substances, IgA, and submaxillary mucins.

Alternatively, the glycoproteins may be synthesized by a dolichol pathway that uses phosphorylated sugar-dolichol intermediates in addition to the sugar-nucleotides. In this synthetic pathway, the oligosaccharide chains are attached to the protein core by N-acetylglucosaminyl residues, which bind with the amino group of asparagine. In addition, as the oligosaccharide chains are formed, they receive a large number of mannosyl residues, which subsequently are "trimmed," and then glucosyl, glucosaminyl, galactosyl, fucosyl, and sialic acid (N-acetyl neuraminic acid) residues are added to form the final complex branched structure (Fig 12-39). Examples of glycoproteins formed by the dolichol pathway include ovalbumin, thyroglobulin, and IgM.

The enzymatic defects in the glycoproteinoses involve failure of sequential removal of specific carbohydrate residues from the oligosaccharide chains as a result of deficient activity of specific lysosomal acid hydrolases. Because oligosaccharide linkages also appear in sphingolipids and MPSs, more than one type of partially degraded material may be stored in the individual disorders. Many of the clinical features of these disorders resemble those described for the mucopolysaccharidoses, mucolipidoses, and sphingolipidoses. There usually is vacuolization of peripheral lymphocytes and increased urinary excretion of oligosaccharides, which contain the specific sugar involved in patients with these disorders.

## FUCOSIDOSIS

Fucosidosis is an autosomal recessive disorder that is associated with α-fucosidase deficiency and the storage of fucose-containing sphingolipids, glycoproteins, and oligosaccharides. Many affected individuals are of Italian and Spanish-American origin. Type I fucosidosis has its onset between 3 and 18 months of age and is characterized by short stature, coarse facial features, macroglossia, hepatosplenomegaly, cardiac involvement, dysostosis multiplex, seizures, and psychomotor retardation. Many patients have elevated sweat chloride levels. Most die in childhood before 10 years of age. Type II fucosidosis is a milder disorder with onset

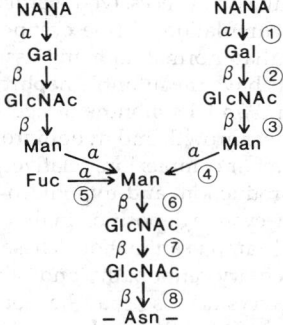

**Figure 12-39.** Degradation of glycoproteins. *NANA*, N-acetylneuraminic acid, sialic acid; *Gal*, galactose; *GlcNAc*, N-acetylglucosamine; *Man*, mannose; *Fuc*, fucose; *Asn*, asparagine; *1*, α-neuraminidase; *2*, β-galactosidase; *3*, β-N-acetylglucosaminidase, β-hexosaminidase A and B; *4*, α-mannosidase; *5*, α-fucosidase; *6*, β-mannosidase; *7*, endo-β-N-acetylglucosaminidase or β-hexosaminidase A and B; *8*, β-aspartylglucosaminidase.

between 1 and 2 years of age and survival to young adulthood. Patients with this variant usually do not have hepatosplenomegaly or elevated sweat chloride levels, but they may have angiokeratomas. Deficient activity of α-fucosidase may be demonstrated in leukocytes or cultured skin fibroblasts. Carrier detection and prenatal diagnosis are available.

## MANNOSIDOSIS (α-MANNOSIDASE DEFICIENCY)

Mannosidosis is an autosomal recessive disease that is associated with deficiency activity of α-mannosidase and storage of mannose-containing glycoproteins. Type I mannosidosis has its onset between 3 and 12 months of age. Clinical findings include coarse facial features, hepatosplenomegaly, psychomotor retardation, mild dysostosis multiplex, posterior spoke-like cataracts, corneal opacities, frequent infections, hearing loss, and hypotonia. Most patients die in childhood between 3 and 10 years of age. Type II mannosidosis is a milder disorder with onset between 1 and 4 years of age and survival to young adult life. Deficient activity of α-mannosidase may be shown in leukocytes and cultured skin fibroblasts. Carrier detection and prenatal diagnosis are available.

## β-MANNOSIDASE DEFICIENCY

Deficient activity of β-mannosidase has been reported both with and without heparan sulfamidase deficiency. Both disorders are thought to be inherited as autosomal recessive traits.

Deficient activity of β-mannosidase was noted in two adult siblings with psychomotor retardation dating from childhood. Angiokeratomas also were present. The facies were normal and there was no visceromegaly. The urine contained mannosyl-β-N-acetylglucosamine. Deficient activity of β-mannosidase was noted in leukocytes, cultured skin fibroblasts, and urine.

One patient also has been reported with deficient activity of both β-mannosidase and heparan sulfaminidase (Sanfilippo syndrome A). Clinical features of this patient resembled those seen with Sanfilippo syndrome. The urine contained mannosyl-β-N-acetylglucosamine and heparan sulfate.

## SIALIDOSES

The sialidoses are autosomal recessive disorders that are associated with deficient activity of the α-neuraminidase, which cleaves the terminal α-N-acetyl-neuraminic acid, or sialic acid, residues from glycoproteins and oligosaccharides. The disorders previously were classified as type I mucolipidoses.

Type I sialidosis, or the normosomatic type, also has been called the "cherry-red-spot-myoclonus syndrome." The onset is between 8 and 25 years of age. There is progressive visual impairment, along with cherry-red macular spots and, occasionally, punctate lenticular opacities. The myoclonus is generalized and debilitating, and it may be difficult to control with medication. A painful neuropathy (as in Fabry's disease), delayed nerve conduction velocities, hyperreflexia, ataxia, nystagmus, and major motor seizures may occur. Most patients die as young adults. The disorder is seen most often in patients of Italian background.

Type II sialidosis, the dysmorphic form, has three subgroups, which vary in age of onset and clinical severity. In addition to the features of type I sialidosis, they also are associated with coarse facial features and dysostosis multiplex. The juvenile form has its onset between 2 and 20 years of age. There usually is no hepatosplenomegaly or renal involvement. Angiokeratomas may be present. Many patients have survived to the fourth or fifth decade of life. This form is most common in Japan. The infantile form has its onset between birth and 12 months of age. Hepatosplenomegaly and renal involvement occur. Most patients die by 10 to 20 years of age. The congenital form may result in stillbirth of an infant with an appearance similar to that of hydrops fetalis. Other infants survive for a few months. Facial edema, ascites, hepatosplenomegaly, inguinal hernias, renal involvement, stippling of the epiphyses, and corneal clouding may be seen.

Deficient activity of $\alpha$-neuraminidase may be noted in cultured skin fibroblasts. Carrier detection and prenatal diagnosis are available.

## OTHER DISORDERS OF $\alpha$-NEURAMINIDASE DEFICIENCY

### Sialolipidosis

Deficient activity of an $\alpha$-neuraminidase specific for ganglioside substrates ($GM_3$ and $GD_2$) has been proposed as the basis for this disorder, but it may not be the primary enzymatic deficiency. Sialolipidosis is associated with the onset of hypotonia and progressive neurologic dysfunction within the first 2 months of life. Corneal clouding is prominent, but hepatosplenomegaly and dysostosis multiplex do not occur. Most patients die in childhood, but some may survive into the third decade of life. This autosomal recessive disease previously was classified as mucolipidosis IV. Lysosomal inclusions may be noted in almost every organ or tissue in the body. Abnormal ganglioside content may be shown in cultured skin fibroblasts. Prenatal diagnosis has been reported.

### Galactosialidosis

Galactosialidosis is an autosomal recessive disorder that is associated with deficiency of both $\alpha$-neuraminidase and $\beta$-galactosidase, as a result of deficiency of a protective protein that complexes with both enzymes. The clinical findings and subtypes are similar to those of sialidosis type II.

### Aspartylglucosaminuria

Aspartylglucosaminuria is an autosomal recessive disorder that is most common in Finland and is associated with deficient activity of aspartylglucosaminidase. Onset occurs between 1 and 5 years of age. Gradual coarsening of the facial features, sagging skin, and psychomotor deterioration are noted. Mild dysostosis multiplex, lenticular opacities, acne, and photosensitivity usually are seen. Some patients also have been noted to have joint laxity, macroglossia, short stature, hypotonia, and spasticity. Many live into the fourth decade of life. Deficient activity of aspartylglucosaminidase may be shown in leukocytes and cultured skin fibroblasts.

### Canavan Disease

Spongy degeneration of the brain, or Canavan disease, is an autosomal recessive disorder most common in individuals of Eastern European Jewish ancestry. A leukodystrophy with optic atrophy, macrocephaly, hyperreflexia, rigidity, and neurologic deterioration starts in early infancy and results in death by 5 years of age. Brain biopsy samples reveal spongy degeneration of myelin. There are excessive amounts of N-acetylaspartic acid in the blood and urine of patients. Deficient activity of aspartoacylase may be demonstrated in cultured skin fibroblasts.

## LYSOSOMAL MEMBRANE TRANSPORT DEFECTS

It recently has been shown that carrier-mediated transport systems are needed for small molecules to pass from the lysosomal space into the cytosol. Systems have been described for monosaccharides and amino acids. Defective transport has been associated with lysosomal storage of free sialic acid and cystine. One patient also has been reported in whom cytosolic vitamin $B_{12}$ deficiency was thought to result from faulty transport of lysosomal cobalamin. Many similar disorders may be recognized in the future.

### Free Sialic Acid Storage Disease

There are two major forms of free sialic acid storage disease—Salla disease, and the more severe infantile free sialic acid storage disease. Both are inherited as autosomal recessive traits. Patients with intermediate forms have been described, as well as patients with a mild clinical presentation but markedly increased urinary excretion of sialic acid comparable to that seen in the severe forms.

Salla disease is most common in the Salla region of Finland. Patients are seen with hypotonia, ataxia, psychomotor retardation, and coarse facies between 3 and 12 months of age. Progressive central nervous system involvement leads to impaired coordination, dysarthrias, dyspraxias, dystonias, seizures, muscle rigidity, and dementia. Affected individuals may live to be adults.

Infantile free sialic acid storage disease, the more generalized sialic acid storage disease, manifests within the first 2 months of life with coarse facies, hepatosplenomegaly, psychomotor retardation, hypopigmentation, anemia, and diarrhea. Ascites may be present in this and the other forms of the disease. Dysostosis multiplex may be noted on radiographs. The disorder is rapidly progressive, and most patients do not live past the first few years of life.

Lysosomal levels of free sialic acid, or N-acetylneuraminic acid, are 10 to 30 times higher than normal in patients with Salla disease and up to 200 times higher than normal in those with the infantile form of the disorder. Urinary excretion of free sialic acid is increased with both disorders, more so in the more severe forms. Activity of neuraminidase is normal. The disorders may be documented by elevated levels of free sialic acid in cultured skin fibroblasts and leukocytes. Prenatal diagnosis is possible. Carrier detection is not.

### Cystinosis

Cystinosis is an autosomal recessive disorder that is associated with lysosomal accumulation of free cystine, with levels 10 to 1000 times higher than normal, in many tissues throughout the body. Most patients have the infantile nephropathic type, which manifests between 3 and 18 months of age with renal Fanconi syndrome. Poor linear growth and hypothyroidism are common. The patients have a fair complexion, relatively light hair because of poor melanin production, and hypohidrosis. Extreme photophobia is caused by cystine deposition in the corneas, which may be evident with slit-lamp examination. These patients may have a peripheral pigmentary retinopathy and other ophthalmologic problems. Cystine crystals also may be noted by electron microscopy in renal interstitial tissues, bone marrow, lymph nodes, and conjunctivae. Before therapy with cysteamine was available, most patients developed renal failure by 10 years of age. There also is an intermediate, adolescent type of cystinosis, with onset between 10 and 20 years of age and slower progression of the disease, and an adult type without significant renal involvement.

The disorder may be documented by showing elevated levels

of free cystine in leukocytes or cultured skin fibroblasts. Carrier detection and prenatal diagnosis are available.

Treatment includes the use of the free thiol cysteamine ($\beta$-mercaptoethylamine) in enteral and eye drop forms; this depletes intracellular cystine by forming a mixed disulfide with the cysteinyl residues of cystine. The disulfide is transported across the lysosomal membrane by a different, unaffected carrier system. Symptomatic therapy for the renal tubular dysfunction is similar to that for primary Fanconi's syndrome. Renal dialysis and transplantation are indicated for those patients in whom renal failure develops. Although cystine storage does not occur in the donor kidney, extrarenal progressive storage of cystine may lead to loss of vision, corneal erosions, diabetes mellitus, and neurologic involvement in transplanted patients as teenagers or adults.

## OTHER DISORDERS OF LYSOSOMES

### Lysosomal $\alpha$-Glucosidase Deficiency

Glycogenosis (glycogen storage disease) type II is associated with deficient activity of lysosomal acid $\alpha$-1,4-glucosidase (acid maltase), which catalyzes the hydrolysis of glucose residues from lysosomal glycogen. The disorder may occur at any age. Three groups have been identified based on clinical severity and age of onset of symptoms.

The classic infantile form of the disorder, also called Pompe's disease or generalized glycogenosis, is seen shortly after birth with a rapidly progressive generalized myopathy and hypertrophic cardiomyopathy. The appearance of a prominent tongue may be the result of macroglossia or the fact that the mouth is held open because of the hypotonia. Hepatomegaly may be present and often is associated with cardiac failure. There usually is no intellectual impairment. Death occurs by 1 year of age from cardiac or respiratory failure. The electrocardiogram shows gigantic QRS complexes in all leads and a shortened PR interval. Echocardiography reveals biventricular hypertrophy with left outflow tract obstruction. Electromyography shows pseudomyotonic discharges, high-frequency discharges, and fibrillations. Hypoglycemia and other biochemical abnormalities noted with defects in cytosolic glycogen metabolism do not occur. Lysosomal accumulation of glycogen occurs in the muscle, heart, liver, and most other tissues of the body.

Less severe forms occur at later ages with muscle wasting and weakness, and little or no cardiac involvement. The juvenile form has its onset in early childhood; most patients die of respiratory failure by 20 years of age. The adult form is characterized by a chronic myopathy with onset between the second and fourth decades of life. Electromyopathic findings in the milder forms are similar to those in the infantile form.

Increased lysosomal glycogen content may be seen in muscle biopsy samples. Deficient activity of $\alpha$-1,4-glucosidase may be noted in muscle or cultured skin fibroblasts. Care should be taken if the enzyme is measured in leukocytes because of the presence of an unaffected renal isoenzyme. The disorder is inherited as an autosomal recessive trait. Carrier testing and prenatal diagnosis are available.

### Lysosomal Acid Lipase Deficiency

Lysosomal acid lipase is needed for hydrolysis of cholesteryl esters and triglycerides. Two allelic autosomal recessive disorders are associated with deficient activity of lysosomal acid lipase, Wolman disease and cholesteryl ester storage disease. These disorders may be confirmed by demonstrating deficient activity of acid lipase in leukocytes or cultured skin fibroblasts. Carrier detection and prenatal diagnosis are available.

Wolman disease is characterized by the onset in the first few weeks of life of vomiting, diarrhea, steatorrhea, abdominal distention, hepatosplenomegaly, and calcification of the adrenal glands. Liver function test results are abnormal. Total plasma cholesterol and triglyceride levels usually are normal; elevated very–low-density lipoprotein levels have been noted in a few cases. Severe failure to thrive usually leads to death by 6 months of age. There is storage of cholesteryl esters and triglycerides in the liver, spleen, adrenals, intestines, lymph nodes, bone marrow, and interstitial tissues throughout the body. Lymphocytes may be vacuolated. Foam cells and "sea-blue histiocytes" may be noted in bone marrow. The liver also may show portal fibrosis.

Cholesteryl ester storage disease is a milder disorder that is associated with hepatomegaly and may not be present until adult life. Splenomegaly, hepatic fibrosis or micronodular cirrhosis, esophageal varices, and intestinal involvement occur in some patients. Hypercholesterolemia with variable hypertriglyceridemia usually is present and atherosclerosis may develop. Adrenal calcification does not occur, and foam cells are not prominent. Treatment with lovastatin may improve the abnormal plasma lipoprotein level.

### Glutamyl Ribose-5-Phosphate Storage Disease

Glutamyl ribose-5-phosphate was purified from the brain and kidney of an 8-year-old boy who died of renal failure and progressive neurologic deterioration. The onset of speech and language delay at 2 years of age was followed by hyporeflexia, hypotonia, mild coarse facies, optic atrophy with granular retinopathy, seizures, microcephaly, cortical atrophy, and failure to thrive. Glomerulosclerosis, occasional foamy glomerular epithelial cells, and lysosomal accumulation of floccular granular material were noted on renal biopsy samples. Glutamyl ribose-5-phosphate is one of the linkage groups connecting poly(ADP-ribose) to histones and proteins, a posttranslational modification of proteins that is important in gene expression and DNA repair. It has been proposed that the disorder is caused by deficient activity of an adenosine diphosphate-ribose protein hydrolase. Because a maternal uncle died at 7 years of age with similar clinical findings, an X-linked pattern of inheritance is suggested.

## Selected Readings

Barton NW, Brady RO, Dambrosia JM, et al. Replacement therapy for inherited enzyme deficiency–macrophage-targeted glucocerebrosidase for Gaucher's disease. N Engl J Med 1991;324:1464.

Gahl WA, Renlund M, Thoene JG. Lysosomal transport disorders: Cystinosis and sialic acid storage disorders. In: Scriver CR, Beaudet AL, Sly WS, Valle D, eds. The metabolic basis of inherited disease, ed 6. Chapter 107. New York: McGraw-Hill, 1989:2619.

Leroy JG. The oligosaccharidoses. In: Emery AEH, Rimoin DL, eds. Principles and practice of medical genetics, vol 2. New York: Churchill Livingstone, 1983.

Pennock CA. Lysosomal storage disorders. In: Holton JB, ed. The inherited metabolic diseases. New York: Churchill Livingstone, 1987:69.

Percy AK. The gangliosidoses and related lipid storage diseases. In: Emery AEH, Rimoin DL, eds. Principles and practice of medical genetics, vol 2. New York: Churchill Livingstone, 1983.

Scriver CR, Beaudet AL, Sly WS, Valle D, eds. The metabolic basis of inherited disease, ed 6. Part 11, Lysosomal enzymes. New York: McGraw-Hill, 1989:1565.

Spranger J. The mucopolysaccharidoses. In: Emery AEH, Rimoin DL, eds. Principles and practice of medical genetics, vol 2. New York: Churchill Livingstone, 1983:1339.

Watts RWE, Gibbs DA, eds. Lysosomal storage diseases: Biochemical and clinical aspects. Philadelphia: Taylor and Francis, 1986.

*Principles and Practice of Pediatrics, Second Edition.*
edited by Frank A. Oski et al. J. B. Lippincott Company, Philadelphia © 1994.

# 12.8 *Peroxisomal Disorders*

## PEROXISOMAL FUNCTION

Peroxisomes are small, single-membrane–bound, electron-dense, subcellular organelles associated with a growing number of recognized biochemical functions and related disorders. Initially termed "microbodies," the name later was changed to peroxisomes when catalase, which reduces hydrogen peroxide to water, and a series of oxidases were found to be localized to this organelle. There are at least 40 enzymatic reactions known to occur in peroxisomes. Abnormalities noted in patients with peroxisomal disorders have included catalase deficiency, reduced beta-oxidation of very–long-chain fatty acids (carbon chain length greater than 22; VLCFAs), reduced biosynthesis of plasmalogens and bile salts, reduced oxidation of phytanic acid and pipecolic acid, and abnormalities in glyoxylate metabolism.

Peroxisomal beta-oxidation of fatty acids differs from that in mitochondria in that the process is not linked to oxidative phosphorylation. Also, the energy produced is not conserved, but is dissipated as heat (Fig 12-40). The peroxisome appears to be the exclusive site for the beta-oxidation of unsaturated VLCFAs and plays a major role in the beta-oxidation of monounsaturated long-chain fatty acids (C22:1). Faulty beta-oxidation of VLCFAs leads to elevated plasma levels and tissue storage of VLCFAs, especially tetracosanoic acid (lignoceric acid; C24:0) and hexacosanoic acid (cerotic acid; C26:0).

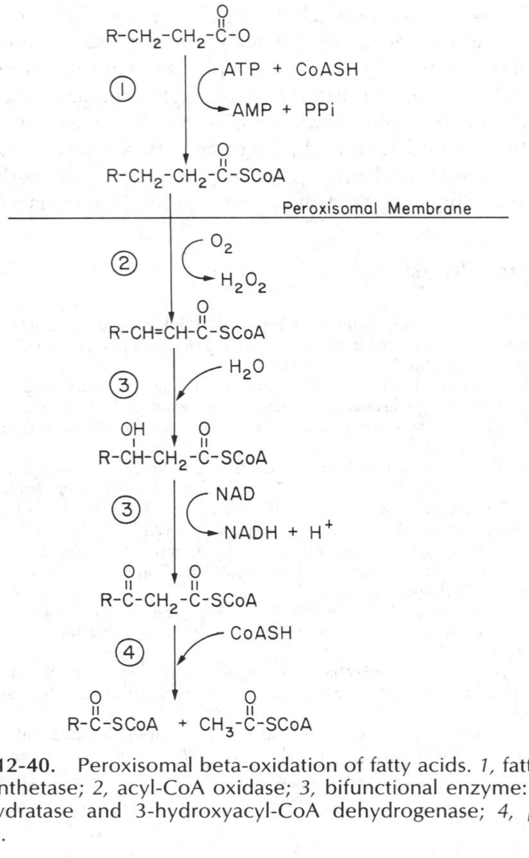

**Figure 12-40.** Peroxisomal beta-oxidation of fatty acids. *1,* fatty acyl-CoA synthetase; *2,* acyl-CoA oxidase; *3,* bifunctional enzyme: enoyl-CoA hydratase and 3-hydroxyacyl-CoA dehydrogenase; *4,* β-keto-thiolase.

Plasmalogens are ether-phospholipids, which are major constituents of cell membranes, myelin, and platelet activating factor. Dihydroxyacetone phosphate acyltransferase and alkyl dihydroxyacetone phosphate synthetase are peroxisomal enzymes involved in plasmalogen synthesis, which have been shown to be deficient in patients with certain peroxisomal disorders.

Biosynthesis of bile acids, chenodeoxycholic and cholic acids, from cholesterol involves a series of peroxisomal reactions similar to those for beta-oxidation of VLCFAs. Faulty biosynthesis leads to the accumulation of bile acid precursors such as dihydroxycholestanoic and trihydroxycholestanoic acids in the serum, urine, and bile.

Phytanic acid, an unusual 20-carbon branched-chain fatty acid mainly of dietary origin, has been noted to be elevated in certain of the peroxisomal disorders as a result of deficient phytanic acid oxidation caused by deficient activity of phytanic acid α-hydroxylase. Pipecolic acid, an intermediary in the degradation of lysine, also has been noted to be elevated in certain disorders as a result of deficient activity of pipecolic acid oxidase.

Alanine:glyoxylate aminotransferase, which is deficient in hyperoxaluria type 1, is peroxisomal in location.

The peroxisomal disorders are classified into three groups according to the presence or absence of intact peroxisomes and whether one or more than one peroxisomal enzyme or function is affected. Group I includes disorders with generalized peroxisomal dysfunction. The number of peroxisomes is reduced markedly or absent, and there is deficient activity of multiple peroxisomal enzymes. The fundamental defect is thought to be failure to form or maintain the peroxisome membrane. The peroxisomal enzymes appear to be transcribed, but probably are degraded or fail to mature without intraperoxisomal localization. This group includes classic and mild Zellweger syndrome, classic and severe neonatal adrenoleukodystrophy (ALD), infantile Refsum disease, and hyperpipecolic acidemia.

Group 2 includes disorders with intact peroxisomes but reduced activity of more than one peroxisomal enzyme or function. The exact pathophysiology of this group still is uncertain. Pseudo-Zellweger syndrome and the rhizomelic form of chondrodysplasia punctata are included.

Group 3 includes disorders with intact peroxisomes with deficient activity of a single peroxisomal enzyme or function. The disorders are thought to result from single gene mutations and include X-linked ALD and adrenomyeloneuropathy (AMN), pseudo-neonatal ALD, adult Refsum disease, hyperoxaluria type I, and acatalasemia.

Table 12-7 summarizes the biochemical findings in the major disorders known to involve peroxisomal function. It is anticipated that other disorders will be added and the classification will be changed as our knowledge expands.

## DISORDERS ASSOCIATED WITH GENERALIZED PEROXISOMAL DYSFUNCTION

Zellweger syndrome (cerebrohepatorenal syndrome) previously was classified as a dysmorphic syndrome affecting almost every organ system. Major dysmorphic features include a flat midfacial area with shallow orbital ridges and epicanthal folding, large fontanelle, flat occiput, high prominent forehead, dolichocephaly, Brushfield's spots, mild micrognathia, external ear anomalies, and transverse palmar creases. Retinitis pigmentosa with impaired vision, hearing problems, hepatomegaly with impaired function and cirrhosis, albuminuria, renal cortical cysts and impaired cortisol response to adrenocorticotropic hormone, or adrenal atrophy usually are noted. Marked generalized hypotonia, present from birth, often is associated with feeding and respiratory problems. Some patients also have had congenital cataracts, glaucoma,

TABLE 12-7.  Biochemical Abnormalities in Peroxisomal Disorders

| | Elevated VLCFAs | Faulty Plasmalogen Synthesis | Faulty Bile Acid Synthesis | Elevated Phytanic Acid | Elevated Pipecolic Acid | Other, not Lipid |
|---|---|---|---|---|---|---|
| **Group 1.  Generalized Peroxisomal Dysfunction** | | | | | | |
| Zellweger syndrome | + | + | + | ± | + | − |
| Neonatal ALD | + | + | + | ± | + | − |
| Infantile Refsum disease | + | + | + | + | + | − |
| Hyperpipecolic acidemia | + | + | + | ± | + | − |
| **Group 2.  Impairment of More Than One Peroxisomal Function** | | | | | | |
| Pseudo-Zellweger syndrome | + | − | + | − | − | − |
| Rhizomelic chondrodysplasia punctata | − | + | − | + | − | − |
| **Group 3.  Impairment of a Single Peroxisomal Function** | | | | | | |
| X-linked ALD/AMN | + | − | − | − | − | − |
| Pseudo-neonatal ALD | + | − | − | − | − | − |
| Adult Refsum disease | − | − | − | + | − | − |
| Hyperoxaluria type I | − | − | − | − | − | + |
| Acatalasemia | − | − | − | − | − | + |

*VLCFAs,* very–long-chain fatty acids; *ALD,* adrenoleukodystrophy; *AMN,* adrenomyeloneuropathy; +, abnormal; −, normal.

punctate mineralization of joints, cardiac defects, and elevated serum iron levels. Abnormal fetal brain development with macrogyria and polymicrogyria, and failure of myelination and white-matter development lead to severe progressive psychomotor retardation and seizures. Most children have marked failure to thrive and do not live past 6 months of age (Fig 12-41).

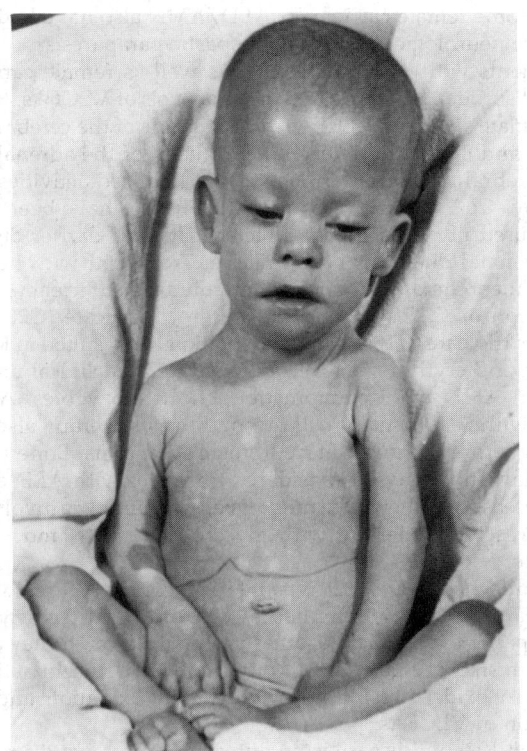

**Figure 12-41.**   Child with Zellweger syndrome at age 8½ months. (The spots are from film processing and are not due to hypopigmentation.)

This disorder is associated with an absence of peroxisomes and generalized peroxisomal dysfunction. Elevated plasma and tissue levels of VLCFAs, phytanic acid, pipecolic acid, and bile salt precursors as well as decreased plasmalogen synthesis are noted. Deficient enzyme activities associated with these findings have been noted. Attempts at induction of peroxisomal formation with clofibrate have not been successful. Glycerolether lipid dietary supplementation has resulted in improved erythrocyte plasmalogen levels in two patients; no improvement in the neurologic findings were noted, however. Current therapy is symptomatic and supportive. The disorder is inherited as an autosomal recessive trait. Prenatal diagnosis is available, but carrier detection is not.

Neonatal ALD, infantile Refsum disease, hyperpipecolic acidemia, and "mild" Zellweger syndrome are very similar in clinical and biochemical features. It has been proposed that they be termed *peroxisomal polydystrophy syndromes.* All are associated with generalized peroxisomal dysfunction, but the defects may be less severe than those seen in classic Zellweger syndrome. Likewise, the clinical features may be milder and later in onset, the dysmorphic features may be variable, and there usually are no renal cysts or chondrodysplasia punctata. Further biochemical and tissue cell line complementation studies will help to clarify this group of similar disorders (Fig 12-42).

## DISORDERS ASSOCIATED WITH INTACT PEROXISOMES AND ABNORMALITIES IN MORE THAN ONE PEROXISOMAL FUNCTION

Pseudo-Zellweger syndrome has been reported in a patient with many of the clinical features of classic Zellweger syndrome, but who had an abundance of hepatic peroxisomes. Abnormalities were noted in two peroxisomal functions, beta-oxidation of VLCFAs and biosynthesis of bile salts. Deficient activity of β-ketothiolase was demonstrated. Some classifications include this

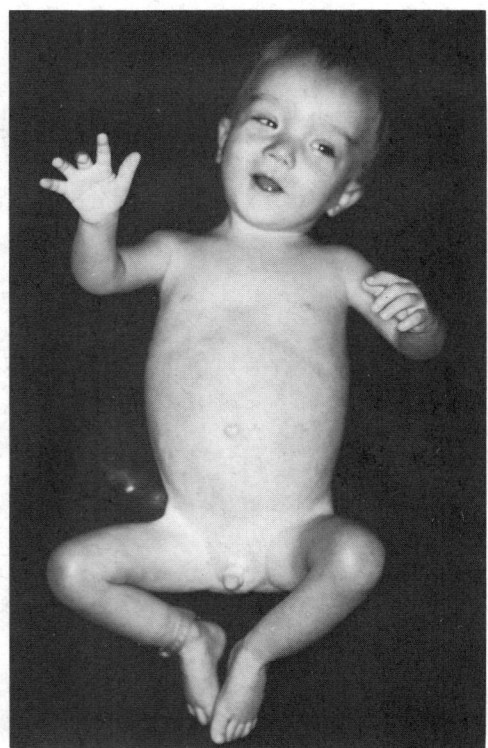

**Figure 12-42.** Child with mild Zellweger syndrome at age 15 months.

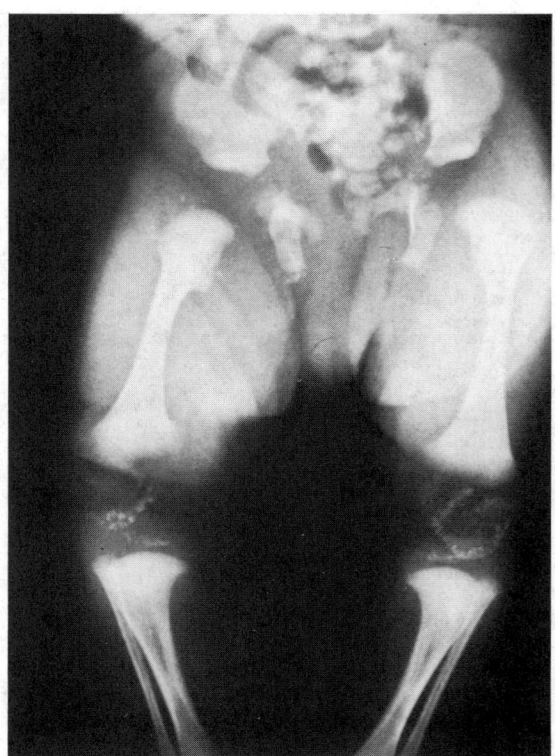

**Figure 12-43.** Radiograph of a patient with the rhizomelic form of chondrodysplasia punctata. Note the extraepiphyseal calcifications.

disorder in group 3 because only one enzyme deficiency has been demonstrated to date.

The rhizomelic form of chondrodysplasia punctata is an autosomal recessive disorder associated with elevated plasma phytanic acid levels and faulty plasmalogen biosynthesis. Clinical features, present from birth, include disproportionate short stature affecting the proximal part of the extremities, abnormal facies with frontal bossing and flat nasal bridge, congenital cataracts, joint contractures, microcephaly, mental retardation, failure to thrive, and death in infancy. Radiographic findings include severe, symmetric epiphyseal and extraepiphyseal calcifications, which spare the vertebral column. There is splaying and metaphyseal cupping as well as shortening of the humeri or femora (Fig 12-43).

## DISORDERS ASSOCIATED WITH INTACT PEROXISOMES AND ABNORMALITIES IN ONLY ONE PEROXISOMAL FUNCTION

X-linked or childhood ALD is characterized by the onset, between 4 and 8 years of age, of changes in behavior; disturbances in vision, hearing, or school performance; abnormalities of gait or coordination; dysarthrias; and dysphagias. Thereafter follows a progressive central and peripheral nervous system demyelination with gradual loss of hearing, vision, and motor and mental abilities, and the development of seizures. Most boys die within 3 to 5 years after the onset of symptoms. Adrenocortical atrophy or insufficiency and a suppressed response to adrenocorticotropic hormone may be noted. Occasionally, a patient will exhibit Addison's disease before the neurologic symptoms are notable.

AMN is an adult variant of ALD that usually occurs in males who are in their twenties and is characterized by progressive spastic paraparesis, sensory deficits, and polyneuropathy. Often,

there is a history of adrenal insufficiency. Primary hypogonadism with low testosterone and elevated follicle-stimulating hormone levels usually occurs. In that both ALD and AMN are inherited as X-linked traits and because both have occurred in the same sibship, AMN is considered to be a milder phenotypic variant of ALD. Some female carriers for ALD/AMN also have had a progressive neurologic disorder with spastic paraparesis.

Patients with ALD and AMN, as well as female carriers of these disorders, have elevated plasma levels of VLCFAs. Patients accumulate saturated VLCFAs in ganglioside of the cerebral white matter and in the cholesteryl ester fraction of the adrenal cortex and cerebral white matter (Fig 12-44). Reduced activities of lignoceroyl-CoA and hexacosanoyl-CoA ligases have been shown in cultured fibroblasts from affected patients. Carrier detection and prenatal diagnosis are available. Treatment with hormone replacement therapy is indicated for adrenal insufficiency. Dietary restriction of C26:0 along with glycerol trierucate (C22:1) and glycerol trioleate (C18:1) supplementation has resulted in lowered plasma and erythrocyte levels of VLCFAs and clinical improvement in AMN and symptomatic ALD heterozygotes. Affected males with ALD usually will respond to this therapy also if it is started before the onset of neurologic symptoms. Bone marrow transplantation may be considered for males with ALD early in their disease or if they have progression of neurologic involvement while receiving therapy with glycerol trierucate and glycerol trioleate.

Pseudo-neonatal ALD is similar in clinical presentation to neonatal ALD and is inherited as an autosomal recessive trait. These patients have peroxisomes present, although they are enlarged in size, and have been found to have deficient activity of acyl-CoA oxidase resulting in faulty beta-oxidation and accumulation of VLCFAs.

Adult Refsum disease is an autosomal recessive disorder associated with deficient activity of phytanic acid $\alpha$-hydroxylase

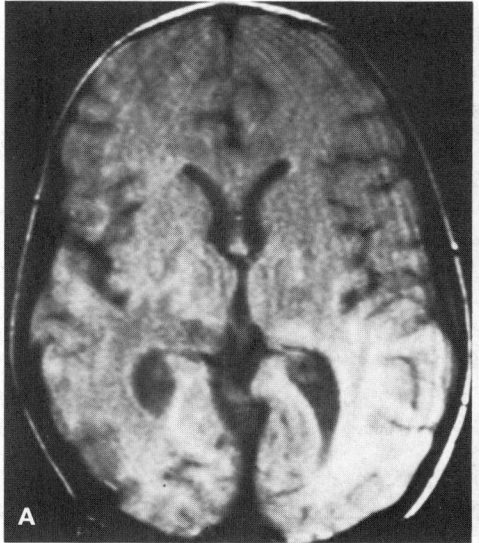 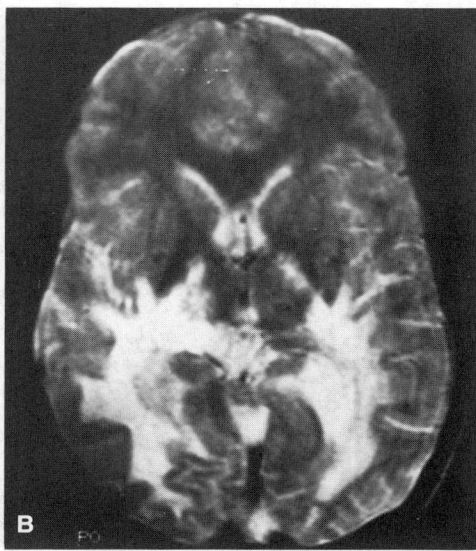

**Figure 12-44.** Adrenoleukodystrophy. (**A**) MRI, T1-weighted image; (**B**) MRI, T2-weighted image. Note the increased periventricular signal in the posterior areas.

and elevated plasma, serum, and tissue levels of phytanic acid. The age of onset is variable, but cerebellar ataxia, peripheral polyneuropathy, retinitis pigmentosa, and elevated spinal fluid protein concentrations are detectable in most patients before 20 years of age. They also may have ichthyosis, anosmia, skeletal abnormalities, sensorineural hearing loss, and cardiac conduction defects. Treatment with strict reduction of dietary phytanic acid sources may result in clinical improvement. Occasionally, plasmapheresis combined with dietary therapy may be needed to reduce phytanic acid stores during initial therapy.

Primary hyperoxaluria type I is characterized by excessive urinary excretion of oxalic, glyoxylic, and glycolic acids, recurrent calcium oxalate nephrolithiasis, nephrocalcinosis, and chronic renal failure. The age of onset and clinical severity are variable, but most patients are symptomatic by the age of 5 years. Initial symptoms may be related to uremia and chronic renal failure. Oxalosis, extrarenal calcium oxalate deposition, usually involves the bones, myocardium, and testes, but may be widespread with advanced disease. Crystals may be seen in the proximal convoluted tubules on renal biopsy. This disorder is inherited as an autosomal recessive trait and is associated with deficient activity of peroxisomal alanine:glyoxylate aminotransferase. Glyoxylate is the immediate precursor of oxalate. Treatment includes the use of pyridoxine in an attempt to reduce oxalate synthesis by stimulating an alternate pathway, the avoidance of dietary sources high in oxalate and ascorbic acid (an oxalate precursor), and the administration of magnesium or phosphate to increase urinary oxalate solubility. Renal transplantation is successful only temporarily in that it does not correct the basic disorder. Combined liver and kidney transplants have been successful, however. Hyperoxaluria type II, which is not classified as a peroxisomal disorder, has a milder clinical presentation, without renal insufficiency, and is associated with excessive urinary excretion of oxalate and L-glyceric acid, and deficient activity of D-glyceric dehydrogenase. Secondary hyperoxaluria also may result from pyridoxine deficiency, ascorbic acid ingestion, ethylene glycol poisoning, increased intake of oxalate or oxalate precursors, and increased absorption with small-bowel disorders and steatorrhea.

Acatalasemia (catalase deficiency), inherited as an autosomal recessive trait, may be associated with varying degrees of ulcerating gangrenous lesions of the oral cavity during childhood, which require medical and dental therapy. Most homozygous persons are asymptomatic, however.

## Selected Readings

Moser HW. New approaches in peroxisomal disorders. Dev Neurosci 1987;9:1.

Moser HW, Auborg P, Cornblath D, Boree J, et al. Therapy for X-linked adrenoleukodystrophy. In: Desnick RJ, ed. Treatment of genetic diseases. New York: Churchill Livingstone, 1991:111.

Naidu S, Moser AE, Moser HW. Phenotypic and genotypic variability of generalized peroxisomal disorders. Pediatr Neurol 1988;4:5.

Schutgens RHB, Wanders RJA, Nijenhuis A, et al. Genetic diseases caused by peroxisomal dysfunction: New findings in clinical and biochemical studies. Enzyme 1987;38:161.

Scriver CR, Beaudet AL, Sly WS, Valle D, eds. The metabolic basis of inherited disease, ed 6. Part 10, Peroxisomes. New York: McGraw-Hill, 1989:1479.

Talwar D, Swaiman KF. Peroxisomal disorders. Clin Pediatr (Phila) 1987;26:497.

*Principles and Practice of Pediatrics, Second Edition.*
edited by Frank A. Oski et al. J. B. Lippincott Company, Philadelphia © 1994.

# 12.9 *Disorders of Purine and Pyrimidine Metabolism*

Purine and pyrimidine nucleotides are important constituents of RNA, DNA, nucleotide sugars, and other high-energy compounds, and of cofactors such as adenosine triphosphate and nicotinamide-adenine dinucleotide. Both purines and pyrimidines may be synthesized de novo from ribose-5-phosphate and carbamyl phosphate, respectively, as shown in Figures 12-45 and 12-46. The nucleosides guanosine, adenosine, cytidine, uridine, and thymidine are formed by the addition of ribose-1-phosphate to their respective purine bases, guanine and adenine, and pyrimidine bases, cytosine, uracil, and thymine. Phosphorylation of the nucleosides results in monophosphate, diphosphate, and triphosphate nucleotides. There is recycling and interconversion of the compounds (salvage pathways), which conserve the nucleotides and nucleosides and exert a negative feedback on de novo synthesis.

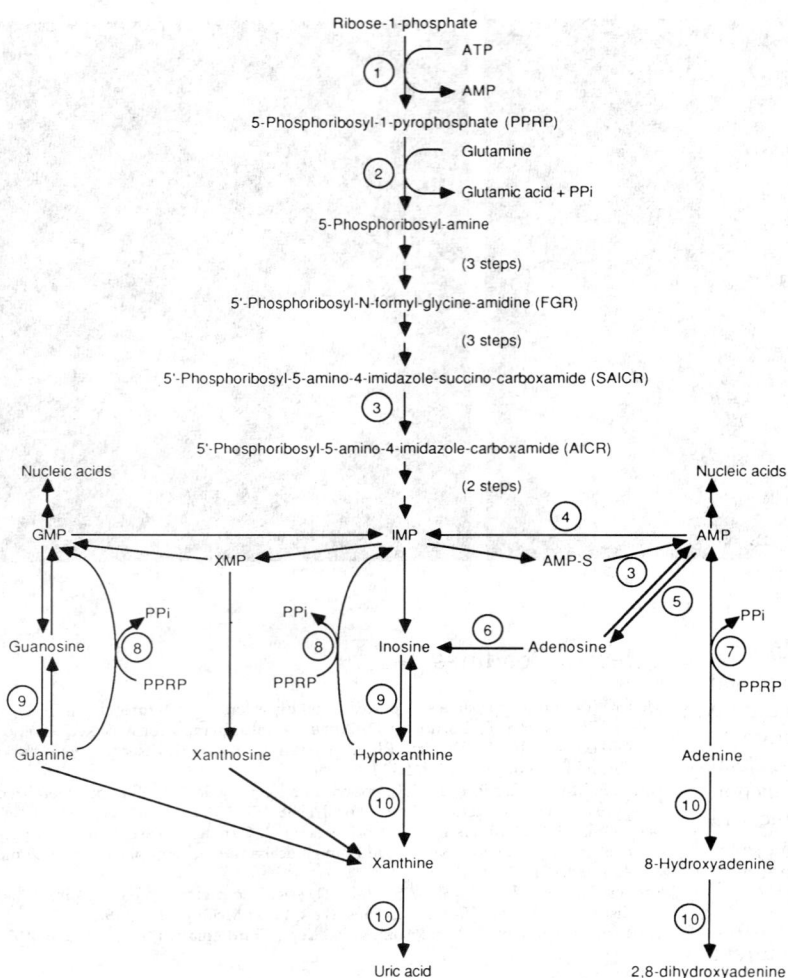

**Figure 12-45.** Purine metabolism. *1,* phosphoribosylpyrophosphate synthetase; *2,* amido-phosphoribosyltransferase; *3,* adenylosuccinate lyase; *4,* adenylate deaminase; *5,* purine-5'-nucleotidase; *6,* adenosine deaminase; *7,* adenine phosphoribosyltransferase (APRT); *8,* hypoxanthine guanine phosphoribosyltransferase (HGPRT); *9,* purine-nucleoside phosphorylase; *10,* xanthine oxidase. Only the ribose forms of the nucleosides and nucleotides are illustrated. The deoxyribose forms follow similar pathways.

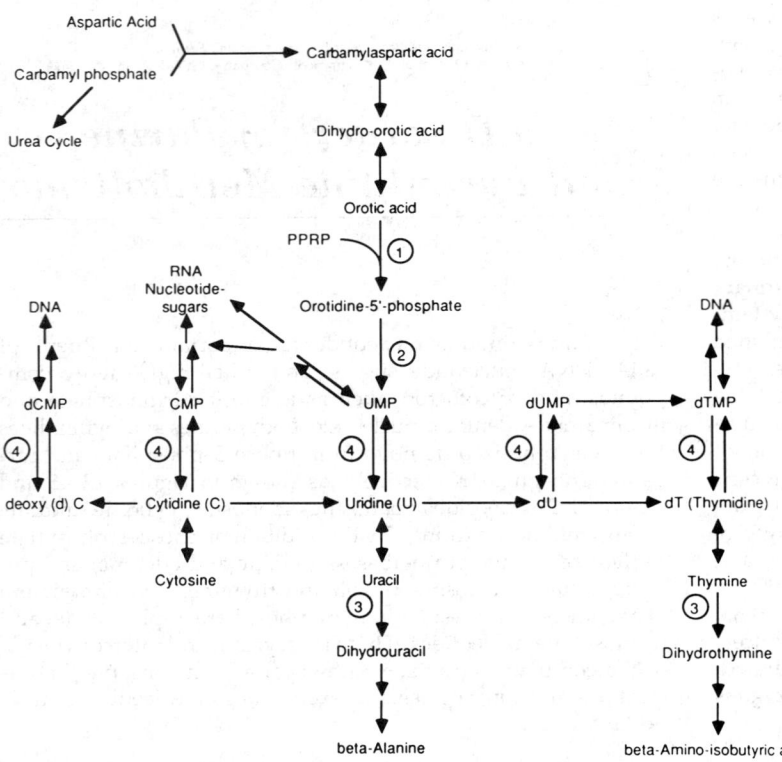

**Figure 12-46.** Pyrimidine metabolism. *1,* orotic acid phosphoribosyltransferase (OPRT); *2,* orotidine phosphate decarboxylase (OPD); *3,* dihydropyrimidine dehydrogenase; *4,* pyrimidine-5'-nucleotidase; *PPRP,* phosphoribosylpyrophosphate.

The disorders of purine and pyrimidine metabolism exhibit a wide array of clinical symptoms, which include renal calculi, neurologic problems, delayed physical and mental development, self-mutilation, hemolytic anemias, and immunodeficiencies.

# DISORDERS OF PURINE METABOLISM

## Gout

Gout is manifested by hyperuricemia, uric acid nephrolithiasis, and arthritis. Primary gout is associated with the overproduction or decreased renal excretion of uric acid. The biochemical basis for the disorders is unknown in most patients, and the disorder is considered to be a polygenic trait. Primary gout also can be seen with the overproduction of uric acid associated with increased activity of phosphoribosylpyrophosphate synthetase (PPRP-S) and deficiency of hypoxanthine guanine phosphoribosyltransferase (HGPRT), inherited disorders that are discussed below. In addition, familial juvenile gout appears to include a group of rare, inherited disorders that occur at younger ages than does primary polygenic gout. Secondary gout may be seen with other disorders in which there is increased production or decreased excretion of uric acid, such as states of starvation, dehydration, lactic acidosis, ketoacidosis, diuretic therapy, renal dysfunction, and those associated with rapid tissue breakdown and accelerated cell turnover, and during treatment of malignancies. Environmental factors may play a role in the pathogenesis of gout in that excessive purine, ethanol, or carbohydrate ingestion appears to be related to increased production of uric acid.

Gouty arthritis results from monosodium urate crystal deposition in joints and surrounding tissues. The presentation usually is monoarticular and peripheral, and the most commonly affected site is the metatarsophalangeal joint of the great toe. Untreated, an acute arthritic attack will resolve spontaneously within a few days to a few weeks. During acute attacks, colchicine, steroids, and nonsteroidal anti-inflammatory agents may be used. Chronic arthritis may lead to joint damage and deformity. The monosodium urate crystals may be noted in joint fluid. Tophi, which are monosodium urate crystal deposits, may occur over the helix of the ears and over points of insertion of tendons at the elbows, knees, and feet. Urolithiasis may occur before or after the onset of the arthritis. Calcium oxalate as well as urate stones may be seen. Uric acid stones are yellow-orange, smooth, hard, and radiolucent, and they crush with difficulty. Renal dysfunction is thought to be caused by underlying hypertension and renal vascular disease, rather than to the hyperuricuria. Treatment consists of the following: allopurinol, which inhibits xanthine oxidase activity and results in reduced purine biosynthesis and reduced excretion of uric acid; probenecid, which increases uric acid clearance and may be used with patients with normal renal function; alkalinization of the urine, which increases uric acid solubility; and increased fluid intake, which decreases the concentration of urinary uric acid. Dietary reduction of purine-containing foods, correction of obesity, and cessation of ethanol ingestion will help to lessen environmentally related causes of hyperuricemia.

## Phosphoribosylpyrophosphate Synthetase (PPRP-S) Overactivity

PPRP-S catalyzes the transfer of the pyrophosphate group of adenosine triphosphate to ribose-5'-phosphate to form pyrophosphate-ribosyl-phosphate (PPRP). PPRP-S is induced by lowered purine nucleotide levels under normal circumstances. The resulting PPRP acts as an inducer of amidophosphoribosyl transferase, the next step in the purine biosynthetic pathway. The increased levels of purine nucleotides that result then act by means of negative feedback to inhibit purine biosynthesis. This X-linked recessive disorder is associated with reduced sensitivity of PPRP-S to nucleotide inhibition and increased specific activity of PPRP-S in vitro. The result is a continuous overproduction of purines by de novo biosynthesis. Patients have hyperuricemia and hyperuricuria, and the disease manifests itself during the teenage or young adult years with severe gout or renal calculi. There is a more severe form of the disorder in which severe psychomotor retardation, autistic features, hypotonia, and nerve deafness occur. Female carriers for the severe form may have deafness.

Elevated PPRP-S levels may be detected in erythrocytes, lymphocytes, and cultured skin fibroblasts. Treatment includes allopurinol, high fluid intake, and alkalinization of the urine.

## Adenylosuccinase Deficiency

Adenylosuccinase is associated with two steps in purine metabolism. In the de novo synthetic pathway, it catalyzes the conversion of succinyl aminoimidazole carboxamide ribotide to aminoimidazole carboxamide ribotide with release of fumarate. In the second reaction, adenylosuccinic acid is converted to adenosine monophosphate, also with release of fumarate. Deficient activity of adenylosuccinase is associated with the accumulation of both substrates for the enzyme in their nucleoside-derivative forms, succinyl aminoimidazole carboxamide riboside and succinyl adenosine. Adenylosuccinase deficiency is a rare disorder with an autosomal recessive pattern of inheritance. Affected children have psychomotor retardation by 2 years of age. Autistic features, hypotonia, self-mutilation, and cerebellar hypoplasia on computed tomographic scanning have been noted. The diagnosis may be established by the finding of elevated levels of succinyl aminoimidazole carboxamide riboside and succinyl adenosine in the plasma, urine, and cerebrospinal fluid. Elevated levels of aspartic acid and glycine also may be noted after acid hydrolysis of body fluids. No therapy is available.

## Myoadenylate Deaminase Deficiency

Adenylate deaminase catalyzes the deamination of adenosine monophosphate to inosine monophosphate and is comprised of multiple isoenzymes that are tissue specific. Deficient activity of muscle adenylate deaminase (myoadenylate deaminase) is associated with muscle cramping and myalgia after exercise. Exercise does not lead to ammonia production, which normally would stimulate glycolysis. Muscle adenosine triphosphate and total purine content fall to a greater extent than normally occurs with exercise. The exact metabolic abnormalities in muscle energy metabolism are not known fully. Increased creatine kinase has been noted in 60% of patients. Some patients also have hypotonia, and a few have been reported to have hyperuricemia and gout. The majority of cases are inherited as an autosomal recessive disorder. A rare, severe, autosomal dominant form has been reported to be associated with progressive skeletal and cardiac myopathies.

Other patients have been reported to have what is thought to be a secondary muscle adenylate deaminase deficiency in association with other neuromuscular disorders such as hypokalemic paralysis, muscular dystrophy, motor neuron disorders, polymyositis, and other collagen vascular diseases. There also appears to be a higher risk for malignant hyperthermia with muscle adenylate deaminase deficiency. In general, there is no specific therapy. Ribose administration has resulted in varying responses.

## Adenosine Deaminase Deficiency

Adenosine deaminase (ADA) catalyzes the deamination of deoxyadenosine to deoxyinosine and, to a lesser extent, the deamination of adenosine to inosine. Under normal circumstances, adenosine usually is converted to adenosine monophosphate by adenylate kinase. Deficiency of ADA is associated with elevated levels of deoxyadenosine and deoxyadenosine nucleotides, especially deoxyadenosine triphosphate. These elevations lead to activation of adenosine monophosphate deaminase and cytoplasmic 5'-nucleotidase, which results in depletion of adenosine triphosphate and other adenosine nucleotides. Elevated levels of deoxyadenosine nucleotides and decreased levels of adenosine nucleotides are noted in plasma, erythrocytes, and platelets of patients. Plasma and urine levels of deoxyadenosine are elevated markedly. The elevated levels of deoxyadenosine also bind with S-adenosyl-homocysteine hydrolase and decrease its specific activity, which results in reduced methylation reactions. Elevated levels of deoxyadenosine, which inhibit ribonucleoside diphosphate reductase and DNA synthesis in T cell and B cell precursors, are thought to be responsible for the severe combined immunodeficiency that is associated with ADA deficiency.

Most patients are seen with symptoms of repeated infections and failure to thrive by 2 years of age. T cell function usually is impaired completely, and B cell function is variable. Mild forms have been reported. This autosomal recessive disorder may be confirmed by the finding of deficient activity of ADA in erythrocytes, plasma, lymphocytes, and cultured skin fibroblasts. Most obligate carriers have about one half normal erythrocyte ADA activity, but there is overlap with normal individuals. Prenatal diagnosis is available.

General treatment is similar to that for other forms of severe combined immunodeficiency. Bone marrow transplantation is the treatment of choice and is indicated if there is an appropriate donor. Treatment with injections of polyethylene glycol–modified bovine ADA has resulted in clinical improvement in all patients treated to date. It is recommended that all patients with severe combined immunodeficiency be tested for ADA deficiency because this disorder may account for 20% to 25% of all cases of severe combined immunodeficiency.

## Purine-Nucleoside Phosphorylase Deficiency

Purine-nucleoside phosphorylase catalyzes the conversion of inosine, deoxyinosine, guanosine, and deoxyguanosine to their corresponding bases. The enzyme has a wide tissue distribution and plays a major role in purine salvage. Deficiency of purine-nucleoside phosphorylase results in elevated levels of the nucleosides, and deoxynucleosides in body fluids and lead to markedly elevated levels of deoxyguanosine triphosphate.

This disorder is associated with defective T cell–mediated immunity. Most patients are seen with failure to thrive and repeated infections during infancy. B cell function usually is normal; serum immunoglobulin levels are normal or elevated. The elevated deoxyguanosine triphosphate levels are thought to lead to inhibition of ribonucleoside diphosphate reductase, which results in decreased synthesis of deoxyribonucleotides and DNA in T cell precursors. Some patients also have been noted to have psychomotor retardation, hypotonia, spastic quadriparesis, and other neurologic symptoms. Others have had a milder disease with familial autoimmune hemolytic anemia.

Patients have elevated plasma and urinary levels of inosine, deoxyinosine, guanosine, and deoxyguanosine. Hypoxanthine and guanine, which have been produced by gut bacterial action, may be found in the urine of severely affected individuals. There is reduced plasma and urine uric acid. Deficiency of purine-nucleoside phosphorylase may be noted in lysed erythrocytes.

The disorder is inherited as an autosomal recessive trait. Carrier detection and prenatal diagnosis are available. Intermittent transfusions of irradiated normal erythrocytes will supply the patient with exogenous enzyme and may result in clinical improvement. Bone marrow transplantation may be considered if there is a suitable donor.

## Adenylate Kinase Deficiency

Deficiency of adenylate kinase is a rare, autosomal recessive disorder, associated with severe, nonspherocytic hemolytic anemia. In that adenylate kinase catalyzes the synthesis of adenosine diphosphate from adenosine monophosphate, interference in the production of adenosine triphosphate may be involved in the pathogenesis of the disorder.

## Adenine Phosphoribosyl Transferase Deficiency

Adenine phosphoribosyl transferase catalyzes the conversion of adenine to adenine monophosphate. With adenine phosphoribosyl deficiency, adenine is not salvaged and is converted to 8-hydroxyadenine and the extremely insoluble 2,8-dihydroxyadenine by xanthine oxidase. This disorder is inherited as an autosomal recessive trait in which there is great clinical heterogeneity among patients. About 15% do not have symptoms. The disorder may appear as early as 2 years of age and as late as the fourth decade. The major clinical findings are related to urinary stone formation, with urinary tract infections, hematuria, crystalluria, renal colic, and renal failure. The renal calculi are soft, creamy gray, and radiolucent, and they crush with ease. Urinary levels of adenine, 8-hydroxyadenine, and 2,8-dihydroxyadenine are elevated. The plasma uric acid level is normal. The enzymatic defect may be noted in erythrocytes, lymphocytes, and cultured skin fibroblasts. A symptomatic variant with partial adenine phosphoribosyl transferase deficiency has been reported in Japan. Treatment includes a high fluid intake, dietary purine restriction, and allopurinol, which will inhibit the conversion of adenine to its metabolites.

## Hypoxanthine Guanine Phosphoribosyl Transferase (HGPRT) Deficiency

HGPRT catalyzes the conversion and salvage of the purine bases guanine and hypoxanthine to their corresponding nucleotides guanosine monophosphate and inosine monophosphate. Under normal circumstances, the nucleotides formed exert a strong negative feedback inhibition on de novo purine biosynthesis. In addition, the salvage of these purines restricts the renal loss of purines in the form of uric acid. Deficiency of HGPRT is associated with loss of inhibition of purine biosynthesis and subsequent overproduction and overexcretion of purines in the form of uric acid.

In complete HGPRT deficiency (Lesch-Nyhan syndrome), the disease manifests itself as early as the first week of life with yellow-orange crystalluria. Renal failure and gout may develop. Hyperuricemia may not be present in young children, but usually is present after puberty. Hyperuricuria occurs at all ages. Patients also have elevated plasma and urinary hypoxanthine levels. Neurologic manifestations usually begin between 6 and 8 months of age and are noted first as athetosis and loss of motor abilities. A movement disorder with choreoathetosis and dystonia develops. Spasticity may be severe and often leads to dislocated hips. Deep tendon reflexes are brisk, and Babinski's signs often are present. The patients usually are not ambulatory. Although mental retardation is prominent and most patients have an estimated intelligence quotient of less than 50, their motor handicaps may limit their performance during testing and innate intelligence actually may be higher. Patients have a compulsive aggressive behavior disorder, which includes self-mutilation. Most commonly, they bite their lips and fingers, experiencing the pain while doing so, and tooth extraction and physical restraints may be required. They also may be aggressive toward caretakers. With age, they become verbally abusive and aggressive. There may be recurrent emesis and failure to thrive.

The disorder is inherited as an X-linked recessive trait. HGPRT deficiency may be noted in erythrocytes or cultured skin fibroblasts. Carrier detection and prenatal diagnosis are available. Treatment consists of careful administration of allopurinol because these patients are very sensitive to this drug. Careful monitoring of urinary xanthine and oxipurinol levels must be done to prevent urolithiasis from these purines. There is no successful treatment for the neurologic manifestations.

Partial deficiency of HGPRT manifests as hyperuricemia, gout, renal dysfunction, and urolithiasis in the teenage years or early adulthood. The severe neurologic manifestations of Lesch-Nyhan syndrome usually are not present. The disorder is inherited as an X-linked recessive disorder, and carrier females occasionally have clinical manifestations. Partial deficiency of HGPRT may be noted in lysed erythrocytes and cultured skin fibroblasts. Treatment is similar to that for primary gout.

An intermediate form of HGPRT deficiency has been reported with manifestations of hyperuricemia and gout similar to those of partial HGPRT deficiency. In addition, the patients are noted to have choreoathetosis and spasticity, but not abnormal behavior or mental retardation.

## Xanthine Oxidase Deficiency

Xanthine oxidase (xanthine dehydrogenase) catalyzes the degradation of hypoxanthine and xanthine to uric acid. This autosomal recessive disorder, known as hereditary xanthinuria, is associated with increased excretion of xanthine and, to a lesser extent, hypoxanthine, and with lowered serum and urine levels of uric acid. About 50% of patients are asymptomatic and usually are detected by routine screening panels on which the lowered level of serum uric acid is noted. Others have symptoms related to the elevated levels of the relatively insoluble xanthine in the urine. Renal colic and calculi, repeated urinary tract infections, hydronephrosis, and renal failure may occur. Xanthine stones are brownish orange, smooth, oval, and radiolucent. There is no specific therapy other than high fluid intake and treatment of the calculi and infections. The enzymatic deficiency may be noted in liver and intestinal mucosal biopsies.

Combined xanthine oxidase and sulfite oxidase deficiencies caused by deficiency of a molybdenum cofactor essential to both enzymes have been reported.

## DISORDERS OF PYRIMIDINE METABOLISM

The biosynthesis and degradation of pyrimidines are illustrated in Figure 12-46.

## Hereditary Orotic aciduria

Hereditary orotic aciduria is associated with deficient activity of both orotate phosphoribosyltransferase and orotidine 5'-monophosphate decarboxylase. The enzymes are thought to exist as a complex, are associated with a multifunctional protein carrier, and catalyze the conversion of orotic acid to uridine monophosphate. The bifunctional enzyme complex is termed uridine monophosphate synthetase. Deficient activity of the enzyme

complex results in interruption of the biosynthesis of pyrimidines and markedly elevated urinary excretion of orotic acid. The disorder becomes apparent during the first year of life with a severe hypochromic anemia with megaloblastic changes in the marrow. Psychomotor retardation, failure to thrive, and cellular immunodeficiency are common. Birth defects and cardiac malformations also have been reported. Crystalluria and, occasionally, urinary tract obstruction may occur with the massive orotic aciduria. Uric acid clearance also is elevated and probably is the result of a uricosuric effect of orotic acid. Many patients die during childhood. The enzymatic defect may be seen in liver, cultured skin fibroblasts, lymphoblasts, erythrocytes, and leukocytes. The administration of uridine results in clinical improvement and reduction in orotic acid excretion. Heterozygotes may have a mild orotic aciduria. Prenatal diagnosis is possible.

Orotic aciduria also can result from defects in the urea cycle and is discussed elsewhere. Orotic aciduria may be seen in association with essential amino acid deficiency, Reye's syndrome, and parenteral nutrition.

## Hereditary Thymine-Uraciluria and Uraciluria

Hereditary thymine-uraciluria and uraciluria are associated with deficient activity of dihydropyrimidine dehydrogenase, which catalyzes the degradation of the pyrimidine bases, uracil and thymine, to $\beta$- alanine and $\beta$-amino isobutyric acid, respectively. Elevated urinary thymine and uracil levels have been noted in most patients. One patient was reported to have elevation of the uracil level alone. Varying clinical manifestations have been reported, including cyanosis and respiratory distress occurring shortly after birth, psychomotor retardation, delayed speech, behavioral problems, sparse fine hair, hypotonia, and microcephaly. The enzymatic defect may be seen in leukocytes or cultured skin fibroblasts. Elevated urine thymine and uracil levels also have been noted with medulloblastoma, neuroblastoma, and adverse reactions to 5-fluorouracil.

## Pyrimidine-5'-Nucleotidase Deficiency

Pyrimidine-5'-nucleotidase is a major enzyme in the pyrimidine salvage pathway that catalyzes the conversion of monophosphated nucleotides to their respective nucleosides. Deficiency of erythrocyte pyrimidine-5'-nucleotidase is inherited as an autosomal recessive trait and is associated with elevated levels of erythrocyte pyrimidine nucleotides uridine triphosphate and cytidine triphosphate. The patients are seen either in childhood or as adults with a nonspherocytic hemolytic anemia. The disorder usually is relatively benign, and transfusions and splenectomy seldom are required.

## Selected Readings

Hershfield MS, Chaffee S. PEG-enzyme replacement therapy for adenosine deaminase deficiency. In: Desnick RJ, ed. Treatment of genetic disease. New York: Churchill Livingstone, 1991:169.

Nyhan W, Sakati N, eds. Diagnostic recognition of genetic disease. Inborn errors of purine metabolism. Philadelphia: Lea & Febiger, 1987:1.

Perignon JL, Durandy A, Peter MO, et al. Early prenatal diagnosis of inherited severe immunodeficiencies linked to enzyme deficiencies. J Pediatr 1987;111: 595.

Scriver CR, Beaudet AL, Sly WS, Valle D, eds. The metabolic basis of inherited disease, ed 6. Part 5, Purines and pyrimidines. New York: McGraw-Hill, 1989: 965.

Seegmiller JE. Disorders of purine and pyrimidine metabolism. In: Emery AEH, Rimoin DL, eds. Principles and practice of medical genetics. New York: Churchill Livingstone, 1983:1286.

Simmonds HA. Purine and pyrimidine disorders. In: Holton JB, ed. The inherited metabolic diseases. New York: Churchill Livingstone, 1987:215.

*Principles and Practice of Pediatrics, Second Edition.*
edited by Frank A. Oski et al. J. B. Lippincott Company, Philadelphia © 1994.

# 12.10 *The Porphyrias*

## HEME BIOSYNTHESIS AND REGULATION

The porphyrias are associated with defects in the biosynthesis of heme and the overproduction of heme precursors (Fig 12-47). Glycine and succinyl-CoA combine to form δ-aminolevulinic acid (ALA) in the presence of mitochondrial ALA synthetase. The ALA then passes to the cytosol, where two molecules combine to form the monopyrrole porphobilinogen (PBG). This reaction is catalyzed by ALA dehydratase (PBG synthetase). Four PBG molecules then combine to form the straight-chain tetrapyrrole hydroxymethylbilane in the presence of PBG deaminase (previously termed uroporphyrinogen I synthetase). The hydroxymethylbilane either can cyclize spontaneously to form uroporphyrinogen I or, in the presence of uroporphyrinogen III cosynthetase, can cyclize to a different isomer uroporphyrinogen III. Of the four possible isomers, only types I and III are seen in humans. Modification of the acetic acid side chains of the cyclic tetrapyrroles by cytosolic uroporphyrinogen decarboxylase and mitochondrial coproporphyrinogen oxidase results in a divinyl tetrapyrrole, protoporphyrinogen IX, which then is oxidized further to protoporphyrin IX. The final step in heme synthesis is catalyzed by ferrochelatase and involves the insertion of iron into the molecule.

Certain physical properties of the porphyrins are important to clinical symptomatology and diagnostic testing. The porphyrinogen precursors described in the biosynthetic pathways are colorless, relatively unstable compounds that may auto-oxidize

to porphyrins within tissues. Thus, with the metabolic blocks, the porphyrin form rather than the porphyrinogen precursor form of specific types of porphyrins may be noted in affected individuals. The water solubility of porphyrins decreases as they proceed down the biosynthetic pathway. ALA and PBG are excreted mainly in urine, the porphyrins and porphyrinogens are excreted in urine and bile, and protoporphyrin usually is excreted only in bile. Metal-free porphyrins and porphyrin chelates with diamagnetic metals (Mg, Zn, Sn) fluoresce, whereas porphyrin chelates with paramagnetic metals (Fe) do not. This fluorescence is related to their function as photodynamic sensitizers when they are present in elevated amounts in patients' skin. The skin porphyrins are deposited from elevated plasma levels and may be of either erythroid or hepatic origin. Upon exposure to ultraviolet light, photodynamic cellular injury occurs, which results in intense itching, erythema, edema, pigmentation, ulceration, and scarring of the skin. With severe photosensitization, hypotension and circulatory collapse may occur.

About 15% of heme is synthesized in the liver, and the remainder is synthesized in the bone marrow. Heme is the prosthetic group for a number of important hemoproteins, such as hemoglobin, myoglobin, the mitochondrial and microsomal cytochromes, and peroxisomal catalase and peroxidase. The biosynthesis of heme in the liver is controlled by the rate of production of mitochondrial ALA synthetase, which is feedback regulated by the intracellular concentration of heme. ALA synthetase activity also can be induced by exogenous drugs and chemicals, and by endogenous natural steroids, which may be related to acute exacerbation of disease in affected patients. Compounds that induce microsomal cytochrome P-450 formation, promote heme catabolism, or inhibit heme synthesis also may induce ALA synthetase activity. Listings of drugs and compounds known to cause this effect are available for patients and physicians. The most commonly offending drugs are barbiturates, other anticonvulsants, sulfonamides, griseofulvin, and synthetic

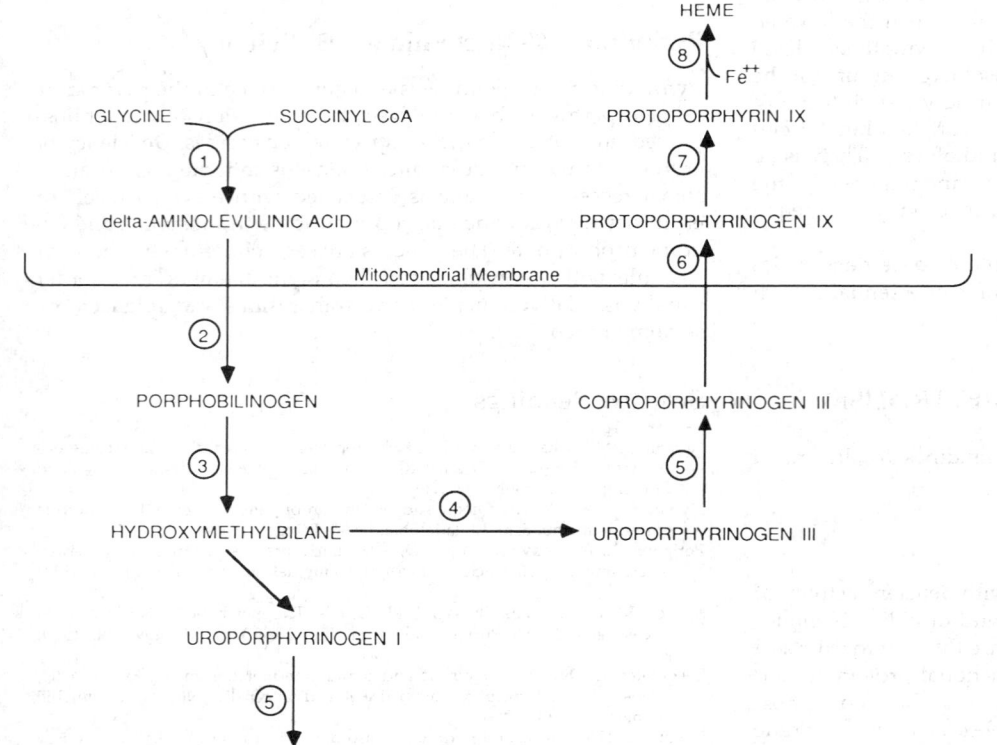

Figure 12-47. Heme biosynthesis. *CoA,* coenzyme A; *1,* delta-aminolevulinic acid (ALA) synthetase; *2,* ALA dehydratase (PBG synthetase); *3,* porphobilinogen (PBG) deaminase; *4,* uroporphyrinogen III cosynthetase; *5,* uroporphyrinogen decarboxylase; *6,* coproporphyrinogen oxidase; *7,* protoporphyrinogen oxidase; *8,* ferrochelatase.

estrogens and progestins. ALA synthetase induction can be blocked by hematin and heme arginate, which may be used in the treatment of patients during acute neurovisceral attacks. Hepatic heme oxygenase, which promotes the degradation of free heme by the production of bilirubin, also is related to the regulation of heme production. Because starvation increases heme oxygenase activity and causes a compensatory increase in ALA synthetase activity, patients with hepatic porphyrias are advised to avoid situations of decreased nutrient intake and to ingest a high-carbohydrate diet.

The disorders of heme biosynthesis are classified as either erythropoietic or hepatic in reference to the major site of overproduction of heme precursors. In all forms, environmental factors, such as exposure to sunlight or chemicals that induce ALA synthetase, play a significant role in the clinical expression of the disorders. The major clinical features are of two types: those associated with cutaneous photosensitivity and those associated with acute attacks involving neurologic and visceral symptoms and elevated urine porphyrin precursors. There are eight recognized disorders. Although most are inherited, except for sporadic and environmentally related cases of porphyria cutanea tarda (PCT), there is great clinical heterogeneity and penetrance of gene expression in persons who have inherited the gene in the autosomal dominant forms. Many such persons have no clinical symptoms and have been termed "latent" cases.

## THE ERYTHROPOIETIC PORPHYRIAS

### Congenital Erythropoietic Porphyria

Congenital erythropoietic porphyria (CEP) is a rare, autosomal recessive disorder associated with reduced activity of uroporphyrinogen III cosynthetase. There is a marked increase of porphyrins in the bone marrow, erythrocytes, spleen, urine, and feces, especially of the type I isomers. There is no increase in ALA or PBG excretion.

The major clinical manifestation is severe cutaneous photosensitivity, which usually is present by 5 years of age. There is blistering and bulla formation in the epidermis. The fluid in the bullous vesicles may fluoresce. Friable skin and hypertrichosis are present. Secondary skin infections are common and may lead to cutaneous scarring and deformities of the eyelids, nose, ears, digits, and corneas. The teeth have a reddish brown erythrodontia. The first clinical manifestation may be reddish brown (burgundy red) urine or diapers in the neonatal period. Some patients have a hemolytic anemia with hypersplenism, which may require splenectomy. Increased hepatic porphyrin concentration and cirrhosis have been reported. Bone marrow examination reveals erythroid hyperplasia, and porphyrin fluorescence may be noted in late normoblasts and early reticulocytes. Reduced levels of uroporphyrinogen III cosynthetase to about 15% of normal may be noted in cultured skin fibroblasts and erythrocytes. Prenatal diagnosis is available.

Therapy includes avoidance of sunlight and the use of sunscreens and oral β-carotene, which may improve light tolerance. Skin infections should be treated aggressively to prevent scarring. Oral activated charcoal or cholestyramine may be used to bind and retard the absorption of endogenous enteral porphyrins from the gut. Repeated transfusions to induce polycythemia and to suppress porphyrin production may be considered.

A mild, adult-onset type of CEP, which is indistinguishable clinically from PCT, has been reported. These patients also have about 15% of normal activity of uroporphyrinogen III cosynthetase.

### Erythropoietic Protoporphyria

Erythropoietic protoporphyria (EPP) is inherited as an autosomal dominant trait and is associated with reduced activity of ferrochelatase. There is overproduction of porphyrins in the bone marrow. Elevated free protoporphyrin IX is noted in liver, erythrocytes, plasma, bile, and stool. Urinary porphyrin levels usually are within normal limits. The clinical manifestations are similar to those seen in CEP, except that the skin findings usually are milder. There is an increased risk for the formation of protoporphyrin-containing gallstones, cirrhosis, and hepatic failure. Reduced activity of ferrochelatase, to 10% to 25% of normal, may be seen in cultured skin fibroblasts and erythrocytes. Treatment is similar to that for CEP. Cholestyramine also may be used to interrupt the enterohepatic circulation of protoporphyrin and to reduce the levels of hepatic protoporphyrin accumulation in those patients with hepatic disease.

Erythrocyte protoporphyrin levels also may be increased in lead poisoning and iron-deficiency anemia; in these conditions, the protoporphyrin IX is present as a zinc chelate. The routine free erythrocyte protoporphyrin test available in most laboratories will detect both the free and the zinc chelate protoporphyrins.

### Erythropoietic Coproporphyria

Erythropoietic coproporphyria has been reported in two patients with clinical features similar to EPP, but with elevated coproporphyrin levels in erythrocytes.

### Hepatoerythropoietic Porphyria

Hepatoerythropoietic porphyria is an autosomal recessive disorder that is associated with marked reduction of uroporphyrinogen decarboxylase activity. Increased porphyrin production occurs in the bone marrow and in the liver. Although there is clinical heterogeneity in expression of the disorder, related to the amount of residual enzyme, most patients have findings similar to those of CEP. There are elevated levels of zinc protoporphyrin in erythrocytes and increased excretion of uroporphyrins, coproporphyrins, carboxyporphyrins, and isocoproporphyrins, as is seen in PCT, the autosomal dominant form of this enzymatic defect. Reduced activity of uroporphyrinogen decarboxylase to 2% to 11% of normal may be noted in erythrocytes. Treatment is similar to that for CEP and EPP.

## THE HEPATIC PORPHYRIAS

### Acute Intermittent Porphyria

Acute intermittent porphyria (AIP) is an autosomal dominant disorder that is associated with reduced activity of PBG deaminase (uroporphyrinogen I synthase) to about 50% of normal. It is one of the most common of the porphyrias. Only about 10% of those individuals who inherited the gene have clinical symptoms, and there are highly variable clinical manifestations, determined in part by environmental influences such as exposure to hormones and drugs, ethanol ingestion, or weight-reducing diets, all of which are known to induce ALA synthetase activity. Symptoms usually begin after puberty, are more common in women than in men, and frequently are associated with an environmental precipitating factor. The acute intermittent attacks develop rapidly and then resolve over a period of days to weeks. These are characterized by the onset of acute, severe abdominal pain, followed by vomiting; pain or discomfort in the chest, back, or extremities; muscle weakness; urinary dysfunction; mental disturbances such as anxiety, depression, or disorientation; seizures; and, occasionally, bulbar and respiratory paralysis, which may result in death. Vomiting or inappropriate secretion of antidiuretic hormone may lead to hyponatremia. In addition, signs of sympathetic overload such as tachycardia and hypertension may occur. The clinical manifestations are caused by a neuropathy, which involves anterior horn cells, dorsal root ganglions, splanchnic motor cells, cranial nerve nuclei, and the hypothalamus. There is neuronal damage and axonal degeneration followed by demyelinization. After a severe attack, there may be residual weakness, and complete or partial improvement may take months to appreciate. Most patients are asymptomatic between attacks, although some have continuing complaints. During attacks, there is a marked increase in urinary excretion of ALA and PBG. PBG excretion usually is greater than is ALA excretion. The urine may turn a brown or reddish color on standing as a result of the polymerization of PBG or other porphyrins and porphobilin. Stool porphyrin levels usually are normal, which helps to differentiate AIP from the other forms of porphyria that manifest with acute attacks. Once the disorder has become clinically symptomatic, patients usually continue to excrete elevated ALA and PBG between acute attacks. The disorder may be confirmed by finding lowered activity of PBG deaminase in erythrocytes. There is some overlap between the normal and affected ranges of erythrocyte enzyme specific activity, however, and this should be accompanied by enzyme measurement in mitogen-stimulated lymphocytes or cultured skin fibroblasts, urinary quantitative porphyrin studies, and pedigree analysis for better ascertainment of asymptomatic gene carriers. Treatment includes avoidance of hormones, drugs, alcohol consumption, starvation, and other factors known to be associated with acute attacks. During acute attacks, oral carbohydrate loading and intravenous glucose may be helpful. β-Adrenergic blockers may be needed for control of tachycardia or hypertension. Medication may be needed for relief of pain and for the emotional manifestations, including anxiety. Folic acid, a cofactor for PBG deaminase, may be given. Intravenous hematin has been shown to result in faster resolution of neurologic symptoms and may be used for acute attacks that are accompanied by severe or progressive neurologic symptoms. Heme arginate, also given by intravenous infusion, has been shown to reduce porphyrin precursor overproduction and the duration of acute attacks. Hemoperfusion for removal of porphyrin precursors also may be considered. Some women who have acute attacks associated with the menstrual cycle may respond to luteinizing hormone–releasing hormone inhibitors or to prophylactic hematin administration.

## Porphyria Cutanea Tarda

PCT is a relatively common form of porphyria associated with reduced activity of uroporphyrinogen decarboxylase. The disorder may be inherited as an autosomal dominant trait, it may occur sporadically, or it may be caused by environmental toxins. The autosomal dominant form is associated with decreased activity, to 40% to 65% of normal, of the decarboxylase in both erythrocytes and liver, whereas the sporadic, and presumably toxic, form is associated with reduced activity only in the liver. Known associated environmental toxins include halogenated hydrocarbons, ethanol, estrogen, and iron. The familial, autosomal dominant form usually manifests before the age of 20 years. There is incomplete penetrance, and not all carriers of the gene become clinically symptomatic. The sporadic or toxic forms often do not become manifest until 40 to 60 years of age. The most common clinical symptoms are related to cutaneous photosensitivity, which

occurs immediately after sunlight exposure. Small white plaques (milia) are followed by vesicles and bullae. There is increased friability of the skin. Occasionally, scarring, hypopigmentation, lichenification, and hypertrichosis occur, but not as frequently as with CEP. Most adults have some form of hepatic disease. Cirrhosis, focal hepatocellular necrosis, and hepatoma may be seen. The prognosis is related to the severity of the associated hepatic disease. The acute attacks seen with AIP do not occur. Treatment includes avoidance of sunlight and the use of sunscreens. Cholestyramine and activated charcoal may be used, as with CEP. Because the majority of patients have some evidence of iron overload, treatment includes repeated phlebotomy to reduce total body iron stores. Low-dose chloroquine also may be considered, especially for those patients who do not respond to phlebotomy. Precipitating environmental factors should be avoided in all forms. The diagnosis is established by the finding of elevated urinary uroporphyrin levels, 5-, 6-, and 7-carboxyporphyrins, and, to a lesser degree, coproporphyrins. The stool has increased levels of isocoproporphyrins and coproporphyrins. Between attacks, urinary and stool porphyrin levels may be normal. Excretion of ALA and PBG, and erythrocyte porphyrin levels are normal. The reduced uroporphyrinogen decarboxylase activity may be demonstrated in erythrocytes for the familial hereditary form and in liver for the sporadic and toxin-related forms.

## Hereditary Coproporphyria

Hereditary coproporphyria (HC) is an autosomal dominant disorder associated with reduced activity of coproporphyrinogen oxidase activity to 48% to 53% of normal. There is variable expression of the disorder, which is similar to, but milder than, AIP. The acute neurovisceral attacks usually have their onset during childhood and often are triggered by the same precipitating factors and drugs as is AIP. About 30% of patients also have cutaneous photosensitivity similar to that seen with PCT. During attacks, urinary ALA and PBG levels are elevated. Urine and stool coproporphyrin III levels are elevated markedly with attacks. Between attacks, stool coproporphyrin III levels may remain elevated and provide a means by which to screen for clinically asymptomatic patients more than 10 years of age. Erythrocyte porphyrin levels are normal. The reduced enzymatic activity may be demonstrated in cultured skin fibroblasts and lymphocytes. Treatment is similar to that for AIP. Cholestyramine or activated charcoal, sunscreens, and avoidance of sunlight also may be helpful for the photosensitivity.

A few cases of homozygous affected patients with 2% of normal coproporphyrinogen oxidase activity and more severe clinical manifestations, including short stature, have been described.

Harderoporphyria, associated with 10% of normal coproporphyrinogen oxidase activity, is caused by a mutation that alters the kinetics of the enzyme so that a tricarboxylic porphyrinogen intermediate, harderoporphyrin, accumulates in addition to the usual pattern seen with HC.

## Variegate Porphyria

Variegate porphyria (VP) is an autosomal dominant disorder associated with reduced activity of protoporphyrinogen oxidase to 43% to 55% of normal. The disorder is most common in South African whites, in whom the incidence is estimated to be 3:1,000. The clinical manifestations include acute neurovisceral attacks, as are seen in AIP. At least 30% of patients have cutaneous photosensitivity similar to that seen with PCT, which may occur both with and without acute neurovisceral attacks. There is little or minimal hepatic dysfunction, which differentiates the disorder from AIP and HC. The same environmental factors may trigger attacks as with AIP and HC. There are increased ALA, PBG, and coproporphyrin III levels in the urine with clinical attacks. Between attacks, ALA and PBG levels may be normal or increased slightly. There is a marked increase in stool protoporphyrin, coproporphyrin III, and X-porphyrin levels, which are porphyrin–peptide conjugates. Erythrocyte porphyrin levels are normal. The reduced enzymatic activity may be seen in cultured skin fibroblasts or lymphocytes. Stool porphyrin levels also may be used to screen asymptomatic relatives of patients after puberty. Treatment is similar to that for AIP. Avoidance of sunlight, use of sunscreens, and therapy with oral $\beta$-carotene and cholestyramine or activated charcoal may be helpful for the photosensitivity.

A homozygous form of this disorder, associated with 14% of normal protoporphyrinogen oxidase activity, has been reported with more severe clinical manifestations, including mental retardation and ocular nystagmus.

## δ-Aminolevulinic Acid Dehydratase Deficiency

δ-Aminolevulinic acid dehydratase deficiency (PBG synthase deficiency) is an autosomal recessive disorder that is associated with marked reduction to 1% to 2% of normal ALA dehydratase activity in erythrocytes. The onset is in the teenage years with acute clinical attacks similar to those associated with AIP. During attacks, elevated urinary ALA and coproporphyrin III levels, but usually not PBG levels, are noted. There are elevated erythrocyte zinc protoporphyrin levels. Stool porphyrin levels are normal. Treatment is similar to that for AIP.

## Selected Readings

Elder GH. The porphyrias. In: Holton JB, ed. The inherited metabolic diseases. New York: Churchill Livingstone, 1987:257.

Herrick A, McColl KEL, McLellan A, et al. Effect of haem arginate therapy on porphyrin metabolism and mixed function oxygenase activity in acute hepatic porphyria. Lancet 1987;2:1178.

Kappas A, Sassa S, Galbraith RA, Nordmann Y. The porphyrias. In: Scriver CR, Beaudet AL, Sly WS, Valle D, eds. The metabolic basis of inherited disease, ed. 6. New York: McGraw-Hill, 1989:1305.

Pimstone NR, Gandhi SN, Mukerji SK. Therapeutic efficacy of oral charcoal in congenital erythropoietic porphyria. N Engl J Med 1987;316:390.

Toback AC, Sassa S, Poh-Fitzpatrick MB, et al. Hepatoerythropoietic porphyria: Clinical, biochemical and enzymatic studies in a three-generation family lineage. N Engl J Med 1987;316:645.

*Principles and Practice of Pediatrics, Second Edition.*
edited by Frank A. Oski et al. J. B. Lippincott Company, Philadelphia © 1994.

# 12.11 *Disorders of Metal Metabolism*

Inorganic metallic cations require carrier-mediated transport mechanisms to cross cell membranes during intestinal absorption and for uptake into tissues. They also require transport proteins to carry them to their sites of tissue utilization or storage. The metals have associated intracellular ligands, such as metallothioneins, that function as a means for storage of the metals, prevent the tissue injury that may result from toxicity of the ions in the free state, and appear to be involved with regulation of the intracellular metabolism of the metals. Inherited defects may occur in any of these mechanisms associated with the absorption, transport, cellular uptake, storage, function, and excretion of cationic metals.

## DISORDERS OF IRON METABOLISM

The body of the normal, healthy adult contains 3 to 5 g of iron. About two thirds of this is found in hemoglobin and myoglobin, and 25% to 30% is stored as ferritin and hemosiderin. The remainder exists in transferrin, heme, and flavin enzymes, and in other iron-containing compounds. Dietary iron is absorbed in the duodenum and upper jejunum. A transferrin-like protein facilitates the carrier-mediated transport through mucosal cells. Plasma iron is bound to transferrin, a transport glycoprotein, in which 30% to 40% of the iron-binding sites usually are saturated. The transferrin apoprotein is synthesized in the liver; the concentration increases with iron deficiency and decreases in states of iron overload. The level also may be elevated with pregnancy and oral contraceptive use, and decreased with malnutrition, nephrosis, protein-losing enteropathies, and hemolysis. The apotransferrin binds with iron in the ferric state. During uptake of the transferrin in erythrocyte precursors, the iron-apotransferrin complex is absorbed to erythrocyte membrane receptors. The transferrin-receptor complex then undergoes endocytosis before the iron is released by an energy-dependent process. Apotransferrin then is released to the plasma for reutilization in the transport of absorbed dietary iron or storage iron that is entering the plasma for redistribution.

Iron is stored in the body in the liver, spleen, skeletal muscle, and bone marrow in the form of ferritin and hemosiderin. Apoferritin is a glycoprotein of large molecular weight that complexes with ferrous ions. The ions are oxidized to the ferric state as they are complexed and exist as ferric oxyhydroxide, which is readily accessible for tissue utilization. Apoferritin is synthesized in response to the presence of tissue iron and is increased in states of iron overload. Thus, plasma ferritin levels reflect the state of body iron storage. Other conditions in which there are increased plasma ferritin levels, unassociated with iron overload, include hepatic damage, inflammatory reactions, and neoplasias. The high ferritin levels seen with hepatic damage are thought to result from the release of stored ferritin, which occurs with tissue necrosis. Hemosiderin is an insoluble storage form of iron that is formed upon partial digestion of ferritin in autophagosomes. Usually, most of the storage iron exists as ferritin, but with increasing iron storage, some of the ferritin is transformed into hemosiderin.

## Familial (Idiopathic) Hemochromatosis

Familial (idiopathic) hemochromatosis is a fairly common disorder that is associated with excessive intestinal uptake and transfer of iron, and progressive storage of hemosiderin in parenchymal cells throughout the body. The exact biochemical defect and pathogenesis are unknown. The intestinal absorption and transfer of iron across the intestinal mucosal cells is disproportionately high for the degree of iron storage in the body. There is a low iron concentration in the intestinal mucosal cells and reticuloendothelial cells, suggesting that a defect in the regulation of iron uptake and transfer may be involved. Because the gene for hemochromatosis is located on chromosome 6 near the human leukocyte antigen region, and because the genes for transferrin and ferritin are located on other chromosomes, it is unlikely that genetic mutations at the transferrin or ferritin locus are directly responsible for this disorder. The major site of hemosiderin deposition is in the parenchymal cells of the liver, pancreas, heart, gonads, skin, and joints. There is minimal storage in the reticuloendothelial system, which is the major site for hemosiderin deposition in other nongenetic forms of hemosiderosis. The mechanism by which tissue damage occurs is unknown, but may be related to increased lysosomal fragility or free radical production in response to elevated levels of hemosiderin.

The disorder is inherited as an autosomal recessive trait and has an incidence of about 1:250 persons. There is great variability in clinical manifestations among affected individuals. Most often, the patient is a male more than 40 years of age. Because of the slow progression of iron storage, the disorder usually is not seen in childhood and is infrequent in women before menopause as a result of the protective effect of body iron loss through menses and with pregnancy.

The clinical manifestations are related to the slowly progressive storage of hemosiderin in parenchymal cells. The classic triad of hepatic cirrhosis, bronze hyperpigmentation of the skin, and diabetes mellitus is characteristic for the later stages of the disorder. In addition, patients may have abdominal pain, hypogonadism, other endocrine abnormalities, myocardial disease, osteoporosis, and arthropathies. Untreated, the majority die within 10 years of their diagnosis from hepatoma, other malignancies, or hepatic or cardiac failure. The reason for the increased risk of malignancies, especially hepatoma and cholangioma, is unknown.

Treatment by repeated phlebotomy is effective in reducing iron stores. It is done weekly initially, for up to 2 years, and must be continued throughout life at periodic intervals. Phlebotomy is more effective than chelators in removing parenchymal hemosiderin storage. With treatment, there is improvement in all clinical signs except advanced cirrhosis with portal hypertension, hypogonadism, arthropathy, and diabetes. The cardiomyopathy usually regresses, and hyperpigmentation disappears.

The diagnosis is established by finding elevated serum iron concentrations, an elevated percentage saturation of transferrin (more than 62%), and elevated serum ferritin levels. Urinary excretion of iron after deferoxamine will be elevated. Liver biopsy samples will reveal hemosiderin deposition and an elevated iron concentration. Heterozygotes may have abnormal serum and urine testing and elevated liver iron stores, but usually not to the extent seen in affected homozygotes. The majority of heterozygotes are unaffected clinically; long-term studies are being conducted to determine if they should take any special precautions with dietary sources of iron, however.

Because relatives, especially siblings, of affected individuals also may be affected, but preclinical in manifestation, it is important to screen them so that treatment may be started before the development of the irreversible features of the disorder. Human leukocyte antigen typing may be helpful, in addition to the usual blood and urine testing described previously.

Secondary hemosiderosis may result from other causes of cirrhosis, increased dietary iron intake, hemolytic anemias, multiple transfusions, and porphyria cutanea tarda. In these forms, the hemosiderin storage usually is in the reticuloendothelial system and less is seen in the parenchymal cells.

## Congenital Atransferrinemia

Congenital atransferrinemia is a rare, autosomal recessive disorder that is associated with a hypochromic, microcytic, iron-resistant anemia. Iron absorption and turnover are elevated. Serum transferrin levels are low or absent and serum iron concentrations are low. Poor growth, infections, and symptoms similar to those of familial hemochromatosis are noted in early childhood. Treatment includes intravenous infusions of transferrin-rich plasma fractions. Reduced transferrin levels also may be noted with protein malnutrition, nephrotic syndrome, protein-losing enteropathies, infection, malignancy, and hepatic disease.

## Idiopathic Neonatal Iron Storage Disease

Idiopathic neonatal iron storage disease is a rare condition that is associated with increased lysosomal storage of iron and clinical findings similar to those of familial hemochromatosis. Affected children usually die by 4 months of age.

## Impaired Uptake of Iron by Reticuloendothelial Cells

Impaired uptake of iron by reticuloendothelial cells has been reported as a rare, autosomal recessive disorder that appears in childhood with microcytic anemia, high serum iron levels, and elevated transferrin saturations. There is essentially no uptake of iron in the reticuloendothelial cells, and there is increased storage of iron in hepatocytes. The defect is presumed to be either in the cell membrane receptors for transferrin or in post-receptor iron transport.

# DISORDERS OF COPPER METABOLISM

Copper is an essential trace mineral that is a component of many biologically important enzymes, such as cytochrome oxidase, superoxide dismutase, tyrosinase, dopamine hydroxylase, lysyl oxidase, and ceruloplasmin. Nutritional copper deficiency is associated with clinical features related to decreased function of the referenced enzymes. Dietary copper is absorbed in the small intestine, and is transported to the liver bound to albumin and, to a lesser extent, to free amino acids. There are at least three hepatic pools of copper. One copper pool, bound to a high–molecular-weight ceruloplasmin-like protein, is destined for homeostatic excretion in bile. A second copper pool exists as the ferroxidase ceruloplasmin. About 90% to 95% of serum copper also is in the form of ceruloplasmin. In the third hepatic pool, copper appears to be stored in association with metallothionein, a low–molecular-weight protein that is involved principally with zinc metabolism and is important in binding excess metal ions in cells throughout the body. This store of copper is bound to heavy lysosomes. Free copper ions are very reactive and toxic, and there probably exist yet-undescribed transport molecules that deliver copper to tissues where it is needed for incorporation into the copper enzymes.

## Wilson's Disease

Wilson's disease (hepatolenticular degeneration) is an autosomal recessive disorder that is associated with progressive intracellular accumulation of copper in the liver and subsequently throughout the body. The basic defect is yet to be characterized, but it appears to occur in the liver and is associated with defective incorporation of copper into apoceruloplasmin and with defective biliary secretion of copper. Similarity of the hepatic copper deposition to that seen in normal neonates has suggested that the defect may be caused by an altered controller gene, which fails to switch the metabolism of copper from that of the fetus to that of the postnatal period. Indeed, recent studies in patients with Wilson's disease have shown a reduction in transcription of the ceruloplasmin gene and also deficiency of a high–molecular-weight ceruloplasmin-like protein, which is responsible for the biliary excretion and decreased intestinal reabsorption of copper in normal individuals.

The major clinical manifestations of Wilson's disease involve the liver and central nervous system. Hepatic dysfunction may occur at any age, but often is the presenting manifestation in children. The onset may occur as early as 4 years of age, but usually is between 8 and 16 years of age. A slow hepatic accumulation of copper begins at birth. Symptoms often are insidious, but they also may occur as acute hepatic and renal failure with hemolysis caused by toxicity from acute hepatic free copper release. These episodes often are difficult to treat, even with plasmapheresis and peritoneal dialysis, and many patients have frank hepatic failure and die. The disorder may be indistinguishable clinically from chronic active hepatitis. Wilson's disease should be considered in any patient who has recurrent episodes of jaundice and hemolysis, and in any child who has cirrhosis after 8 years of age.

Copper storage also is prominent in the brain and results in the gradual onset of dysarthria, dystonia, choreoathetosis, tremors, ataxia, peripheral neuropathy, and seizures. Late in the disorder, intellectual deterioration develops, and pseudobulbar palsies may lead to death. Patients also may have behavioral and psychiatric problems. The neurologic manifestations of Wilson's disease are rare before 14 years of age and are seen most frequently between 20 and 40 years of age. Patients may have degeneration of basal ganglia, cortical atrophy, and ventricular dilatation on computed tomographic scanning. All patients, regardless of whether they experience neurologic symptoms, have elevated hepatic copper stores. The hepatic copper may result in storage in other tissues throughout the body, and anemia, neutropenia, thrombocytopenia, osteoarthropathy, renal calculi, renal tubular acidosis, pancreatic disease, cardiomyopathy, and hypoparathyroidism may develop. Storage of copper in the cornea may result in the pathognomonic Kayser-Fleischer rings, which are brownish green granular copper deposits in Descemet's membrane extending a few millimeters centrally from the corneal limbus. Many may be seen directly, but others require slit-lamp examination. "Sunflower" cataracts also may develop. Patients with neurologic involvement often have Kayser-Fleischer rings; patients with hepatic involvement frequently do not.

The disorder usually is associated with reduced total serum copper levels, reduced ceruloplasmin concentrations, elevated nonceruloplasmin copper levels, and elevated urinary copper excretion, which may be augmented by the administration of D-penicillamine. Ninety-five percent of adult patients and 80% to 85% of affected children may be detected by these tests. Elevation of liver copper levels may be detected with liver biopsy and may be needed to establish the diagnosis. Care should be taken in handling samples because copper contamination may occur if proper containers and technique are not used. Elevated liver copper levels also may occur with other disorders that are associated with hepatic dysfunction and decreased biliary function. Reduced in vitro incorporation of radiolabeled copper into ceruloplasmin is perhaps the most sensitive and accurate testing method available. Partial reduction of incorporation of radiolabeled copper may be noted in heterozygotes and in patients with other liver disorders. About 10% to 20% of heterozygotes will have lowered ceruloplasmin levels; a few also will have reduced total serum copper concentrations and elevated copper excretion with D-penicillamine, electroencephalographic abnormalities, and neurologic manifestations. All siblings of patients should be evaluated thoroughly because they may be affected, but asymptomatic.

Treatment includes the use of D-penicillamine to promote urinary copper excretion and decreased body copper stores. Dosages are determined by monitoring 24-hour urinary copper excretion levels. Pyridoxine supplementation should be given with D-penicillamine due to the known interference with pyridoxal phosphate-dependent enzymes during chelation therapy. Zinc deficiency may result and zinc also should be given to induce the formation of metallothionein, a metal-binding protein, which may help sequester copper in the gut and prevent copper reabsorption. Trientine hydrochloride also may be used for chelation

if significant side effects or toxicity from D-penicillamine occur. Clinical improvement in the neurologic symptoms may be seen in several weeks, but they may take up to 2 years to resolve completely. Hepatic dysfunction also may improve, but more slowly, and cirrhosis and portal hypertension persist. Even with aggressive management, late-stage hepatic dysfunction may continue to progress, and liver transplantation should be considered. Prenatal diagnosis is not possible.

## Menkes' Disease

Menkes' disease is an X-linked recessive disorder with an incidence of about 1:100,000. Although the basic genetic defect is not known, there appears to be faulty transport and cellular accumulation of copper, which results in copper being unavailable to the sites of copper enzyme synthesis. There is decreased intestinal absorption of copper. Serum levels of copper and ceruloplasmin are low. The copper content of brain and liver also are reduced. The copper content of other tissues, however, such as kidney, spleen, pancreas, intestinal mucosa, lung, skeletal muscle, and placenta, is elevated. The copper that accumulates is bound to metallothionein, which also has a high concentration in the tissues. When affected individuals are given parenteral copper, the hepatic formation of ceruloplasmin appears to be normal. Abnormal intracellular accumulation and reduced excretion of copper may be demonstrated with radiolabeled copper studies in cultured skin fibroblasts and amniocytes from affected patients. Such testing may be used for the identification of female heterozygotes and for prenatal diagnosis by experienced laboratories.

Most affected children appear normal at birth, but they may have a history of prematurity, transient hyperbilirubinemia, and hypothermia. They appear normal for the first 2 to 3 months of life and then have failure to thrive, feeding problems, developmental delay and regression, hypotonia, and generalized seizures. Thereafter follows progressive cerebral degeneration, with loss of awareness of environment, loss of vision and hearing, and the development of spasticity. The most characteristic feature of the disorder is the presence of "kinky hair," which is brittle, depigmented, dull, short, and brush-like. The individual hair shafts are twisted on the long axis (pili torti) and have irregular caliber (monilethrix) and node-like fracture points (trichorrhexis nodosa). The children have a characteristic facies, with pudgy cheeks, cupid-bow lips, micrognathia, inexpressive look, and abnormal eyebrows. They also are noted to have pale, lax skin, dolichomicrocephaly, frontal and occipital prominence, high arched palate, and gingival hyperplasia. Bladder diverticula and trabeculation, hydronephrosis and hydroureter, hernias, and undescended testes are common. The arteries are noted to be elongated and tortuous, and to have localized areas of dilatation and narrowing in the brain. Arterial rupture and thrombosis, and subdural hematomas are common. Radiograms of the bones reveal osteoporosis, changes in the long bones similar to those seen with scurvy, and wormian bones in the skull. Electroencephalography will be abnormal, with a multifocal spike pattern and, occasionally, hypsarrhythmia. Computed tomographic scanning will reveal diffuse cerebral and cerebellar atrophy or multiple areas of focal infarctions. Most children have recurrent, often overwhelming, infections and usually die by 3 years of age.

Milder clinical variants of Menkes' disease have been reported. In addition, patients with the occipital horn syndrome have many of the same clinical and biochemical features as do those with mild Menkes' disease. They also have low levels of lysyl oxidase in addition to abnormal radiolabeled copper study results, however, and connective tissue clinical features are more predominant. Radiogram changes are diagnostic and include an ossified occipital horn for which the disorder is named.

The clinical manifestations of Menkes' disease may be related in part to deficiencies of the copper enzymes. Cytochrome oxidase is needed for electron chain transport, superoxidase dismutase for free radical detoxification, tyrosinase for melanin production, dopamine $\beta$-hydroxylase for catecholamine production, and lysyl oxidase for cross-linkage of collagen and elastin. For unknown reasons, patients with Menkes' disease do not have anemia and neutropenia, which is seen in nutritional copper deficiency.

Therapy includes management of seizures and other supportive treatment. The administration of parenteral copper histidinate has provided patients with some improvement in their general condition and has prolonged their lives, but usually has not made appreciable changes in the degeneration of the central nervous system unless it is started early in life.

## Familial Hypoceruloplasminemia

Familial hypoceruloplasminemia is a rare disorder that has not been shown to have associated clinical disease.

# DISORDERS OF ZINC METABOLISM

## Acrodermatitis Enteropathica

Acrodermatitis enteropathica is a rare, autosomal recessive disorder that is associated with severe systemic zinc deficiency caused by impaired intestinal absorption. The basic metabolic defect is unknown, but it may be related to a zinc binding factor or ligand such as metallothionein, which facilitates zinc uptake or transport in intestinal mucosa. There are numerous zinc-dependent enzymes that function in many important biologic pathways, including those involved with nucleic acid and protein synthesis, regulation of cell division, antioxidant activity, stabilization of macromolecules and polymers, and association of hormones with receptors on cell surfaces or in the nuclei. Zinc also appears to be necessary for wound healing and intact chemotaxis in response to infections.

Most affected infants have acrodermatitis, failure to thrive, irritability, anorexia, and diarrhea before 1 year of age. Because breast milk has more bioavailable zinc than do infant formulas, children who are breast-fed are detected later than are those who are fed formula. The clinical manifestations in breast-fed infants often appear after weaning. The earliest sign usually is maceration and fissures at the angles of the mouth. This is associated with a vesicobullous and eczematoid dermatitis, which extends from the mouth to symmetric, well-demarcated lesions on the face and behind the ears. The rash also appears on the distal extremities, which has given the disorder its name. The diaper area, areas subject to irritation, knees, elbows, and trunk may be affected. Initially, the dermatitis is intensely erythematous and erosive, but later it becomes dry, hyperkeratotic, and psoriasis-like in appearance. The hair is sparse, fine, and brittle, and it often has a reddish color. Alopecia is seen frequently. Ocular manifestations include photophobia, conjunctivitis, blepharitis, and a corneal dystrophy, which may be seen with slit-lamp examination. Other features include paronychia, nail dystrophy, person-

ality changes, superficial and systemic moniliasis, repeated bacterial infections, tremor, ataxia, and reversible cerebral atrophy. The failure to thrive is progressive and may lead to marasmus and death if it is not treated. Milder cases with later onset have been reported. Depression, apathy, and paranoia may be seen in older children and adults. Untreated adult females may have a history of miscarriages and children born with anencephaly and congenital skeletal dysplasias.

The diagnosis is established by finding low serum zinc levels. Occasionally, normal zinc levels are noted in clinically affected infants; with therapy, there is improvement in growth, which increases the requirement for zinc and may cause the serum zinc level to decrease, confirming the diagnosis. Alkaline phosphatase, a zinc-requiring enzyme, usually is present in low levels. Plasma ammonia concentrations may be elevated, and a hypobetalipoproteinemia with an altered lipid profile will be noted.

Treatment with oral zinc preparations (sulfate, acetate, or gluconate) in divided doses to total 35 to 150 mg of elemental zinc daily will result in clinical improvement in a matter of days. The dosage must be individualized in accordance with the patient's clinical response and blood levels. Treatment is needed for life. Increased requirements occur at times of increased growth, such as puberty, and with infections. Pregnancies in treated women have resulted in normal infants. There are no means for carrier detection or prenatal diagnosis.

Zinc deficiency also may be seen with malnutrition, synthetic diets, chronic hyperalimentation without zinc supplementation, chronic enteritis, cirrhosis, extensive burns, and chelation therapy for other metals.

## Familial Hyperzincemia

Familial hyperzincemia has been reported in a family with an autosomal dominant pattern of inheritance. Plasma zinc concentrations were elevated up to five times normal. Because the zinc was complexed with albumin, no clinical symptoms were noted.

## Selected Readings

Aggett PJ. Metal disorders. In: Holton JB, ed. The inherited metabolic diseases. New York: Churchill Livingstone, 1987:384.

Baerlocher DE, Steinman B, Rao VH, et al. Menkes' disease: Clinical, therapeutic and biochemical studies. J Inherited Metab Dis 1983;6(Suppl 2):87.

Davison PJ, Stalenhoef AFH, Humphries SE. Molecular studies of ceruloplasmin deficiency in Wilson's disease. J Clin Invest 1987;80:1200.

Dunn A, Blalock TL, Cousins RJ. Minireview. Metallothionein. Proc Soc Exp Biol Med 1987;185:107.

Edwards CQ, Griffen LM, Goldgar D, et al. Prevalence of hemochromatosis among 11,065 presumably healthy blood donors. N Engl J Med 1988;318:1355.

Emery AEH, Rimoin DL, eds. Principles and practice of medical genetics. Chapters 92 and 93. New York: Churchill Livingstone, 1983:1319.

McClain CJ, Shedlofsky SI. Copper toxicity in Wilson's disease; an absorbing problem. J Lab Clin Med 1988;11:261.

Nyhan WL, Sakati NA. Diagnostic recognition of genetic disease, section 5. Philadelphia: Lea & Febiger, 1987:291.

Scriver CR, Beaudet AL, Sly WS, Valle D, eds. The metabolic basis of inherited disease, ed 6. Part 9, Metals. New York: McGraw-Hill, 1989:1411.

Ygengar V, Brewer GI, Dick RD, et al. Studies of cholecystokenin-stimulated biliary secretions reveal a high molecular weight copper-binding substance in normal subjects that is absent in patients with Wilson's disease. J Lab Clin Med 1988;11:267.

*Principles and Practice of Pediatrics, Second Edition.*
edited by Frank A. Oski et al. J. B. Lippincott Company, Philadelphia © 1994.

# 12.12 *Inborn Errors Associated With Faulty Bone Mineralization**

## DISORDERS OF ALKALINE PHOSPHATASE

### Hypophosphatasia

Alkaline phosphatase is contained in membrane-enclosed vesicles located at the sites of mineral deposition in bone matrix and cartilage. The alkaline phosphatase appears to act as a pyrophosphatase, which releases phosphate ions needed for calcification. Deficiency of alkaline phosphatase is associated with a group of disorders characterized by faulty bone mineralization. The types of the disorders vary in age of onset and overlap in clinical severity. All are associated with reduced serum levels of alkaline phosphatase and elevated levels of plasma and urinary pyridoxal-5-phosphate, inorganic pyrophosphate, and phosphoethanolamine, natural substrates for the enzyme. Prenatal diagnosis is available for the severe forms.

The perinatal or lethal form of hypophosphatasia is the most severe and is expressed in utero. There is almost complete lack of skeletal mineralization in most cases. Many affected individuals are stillborn, whereas others live a few days, then succumb in the immediate neonatal period of respiratory insufficiency. This form of the disorder is inherited as an autosomal recessive trait.

The infantile form of hypophosphatasia is a severe, autosomal recessive disorder that presents within the first year of life with generalized skeletal demineralization. Shortened extremities, fractures, failure to thrive, hypercalcemia, hypercalciuria, nephrocalcinosis, premature synostosis of the skull, and respiratory infections are common. Dietary reduction in vitamin D and calcium may be needed to control the hypercalcemia. Reduced exposure to sunlight and use of sunscreens also are required.

The childhood form of hypophosphatasia is characterized by premature loss of deciduous teeth and short stature. There is an increased incidence of scoliosis and fractures. Radiograms show demineralization and rachitic changes. There is a tendency toward hypercalcemia, and treatment is similar to that for the infantile form of the disorder. This form may be inherited as an autosomal dominant or autosomal recessive trait.

Patients with the relatively mild adult form of hypophosphatasia may have a history of repeated fractures or "rickets" in infancy. Some patients are detected on screening blood panels. This form of the disorder may be inherited as an autosomal dominant or autosomal recessive trait. Hypercalcemia usually is not present, and no specific therapy is required.

### Pseudo-Hypophosphatasia

Pseudo-hypophosphatasia has clinical and radiographic findings similar to those of hypophosphatasia, including elevated urinary phosphoethanolamine levels, but serum alkaline phosphatase levels are normal.

* See also the sections on transport disorders and skeletal dysplasias (Chapters 12.2 and 12.13).

## The Hyperphosphatasemias

Serum levels of alkaline phosphatase in children usually are three times those in adults because of an increase in the bone fraction that is associated with active bone growth. Elevations of alkaline phosphatase levels may be seen with fractures, liver dysfunction, growth spurts, and inherited genetic disorders.

Transient hyperphosphatasemia of infancy usually has its onset between 2 months and 3 years of age, although some report occurrences as late as 6 years. Patients are detected most often when screening panels are carried out for some illness, usually an acute infection. Alkaline phosphatase fractionation studies indicate that both bone and liver isoenzymes are elevated. There has been no evidence of bone or liver pathology documented, however, and the alkaline phosphatase activity usually normalizes within 4 months. Occasionally, resolution may take as long as 18 months or more. Nonspecific effects of infection or medication have been cited as possible causes. It is a sporadic, benign condition that requires no therapy.

Familial hyperphosphatasemia also is a benign condition that may be differentiated from transient hyperphosphatasemia of infancy by the fact that it will not resolve. Because it is inherited as an autosomal dominant trait, one of the parents usually also will have hyperphosphatasemia.

Hyperphosphatasemia with osteoectasia is a rare disorder, inherited as an autosomal recessive trait, that is associated with elevated bone alkaline phosphatase levels, severe osteoporosis, and bone fragility leading to progressive skeletal deformities. There are characteristic radiographic findings, with the long bones having a cylindric appearance, pseudocysts, irregular trabeculation, and dilated shafts of bones (osteoectasia). The onset usually occurs between 1 and 3 years of age. Calcitonin therapy may be considered.

## DISORDERS OF VITAMIN D METABOLISM

Vitamin D exists as ergocalciferol (vitamin $D_2$) and cholecalciferol (vitamin $D_3$). In humans, exposure to ultraviolet light results in the photoconversion of 7-dehydrocholesterol to vitamin $D_3$ in the skin and usually is sufficient to supply the daily recommended need. Ergocalciferol is added routinely to commercial milk and infant formulas to prevent dietary vitamin D deficiency as a result of inadequate exposure to sunlight. Both vitamin $D_2$ and vitamin $D_3$ are stored in plasma, muscle, and adipose tissue, and are converted to their active metabolites by hydroxylation. Vitamin D ($D_2$ or $D_3$) is converted to 25-hydroxycalciferol (calcidiol, calcifediol; 25-OH-D) in the liver by microsomal 25-cholecalciferol hydroxylase. The 25-OH-D then is transported to the kidney, where it undergoes a second hydroxylation step by mitochondrial 1-$\alpha$-hydroxylase to form 1,25-dihydroxycholecalciferol (calcitriol; 1,25-diOH-D). 1,25-diOH-D then binds to receptor sites in target organs. The activated vitamin D—receptor complex that is formed is transported to the nucleus of the cell, where it induces translation, which results in the production of specific proteins (eg, calcium-binding protein) that are related to the physiologic actions of activated vitamin D. Defects in hydroxylation, receptor binding, nuclear uptake, and post-receptor processing have been demonstrated in patients and have been associated with autosomal recessive patterns of inheritance.

Clinical manifestations are similar to those seen with dietary vitamin D deficiency. The patients appear well at birth, but rickets develops during the first year of life. Many have hypocalcemic seizures (tetany) by 4 months of age. Hypotonia, repeated respiratory infections, failure to thrive, and delayed motor milestones are common. Radiograms show classic florid rickets with decreased mineralization, fraying and cupping of epiphyseal areas, and fractures and pseudofractures. Widening of the wrists and knees, enlargement of costochondral junctions (rachitic rosary), craniotabes of the skull, frontal bossing, and bowing of long bones may be seen. Occasionally, pseudotumor cerebri develops. The serum calcium concentration is low, the phosphorus concentration may be low, and alkaline phosphatase and parathyroid hormone levels are elevated.

Hereditary deficiency of 1,25-diOH-D is associated with deficient activity of renal 1-$\alpha$-hydroxylase and reduced serum levels of 1,25-diOH-D. Serum 25-OH-D levels are normal or elevated. Treatment is the administration of physiologic quantities of 1,25-diOH-D (calcitriol).

Hereditary generalized resistance of 1,25-diOH-D results from abnormalities in the 1,25-diOH-D-receptor sites in cell membranes in most of the patients. Other, very rare, forms have been associated with defects in post-receptor processing. Serum 25-OH-D levels are normal, and 1,25-diOH-D levels usually are elevated. These patients are affected more severely than are those with 1-$\alpha$-hydroxylase deficiency. Many are seen at birth, and 50% have alopecia totalis. Pharmacologic doses of 1,25-diOH-D are necessary to produce and sustain remission. Some patients have been relatively unresponsive to this therapy, however.

## Selected Readings

Emery AEH, Rimoin DL, eds. Principles and practice of medical genetics. Chapter 25. New York: Churchill Livingstone, 1983:746.

Fomon SJ, ed. Infant nutrition, ed 2. Philadelphia: WB Saunders, 1974.

Nyhan WL, Sakati NA. Diagnostic recognition of genetic disease. Chapters 41, 75, 76. Philadelphia: Lea & Febiger, 1987:253.

Scriver CR, Beaudet AL, Sly WS, Valle D, eds. The metabolic basis of inherited disease, ed 6. Chapters 80, 116. New York: McGraw-Hill, 1989.

*Principles and Practice of Pediatrics, Second Edition.*
edited by Frank A. Oski et al. J. B. Lippincott Company, Philadelphia © 1994.

# 12.13 *Skeletal Dysplasias*

### David D. Weaver

Skeletal dysplasias are a heterogenous group of disorders with a wide variety of clinical and radiographic manifestations. Much of their variation comes from the different combinations of involved bones and the ways in which these bones are affected (eg, differences in their shape, length, and density). Most skeletal dysplasias are inherited and cause disproportionately short stature; as a result, the term *dwarfism* frequently is applied to this category of diseases. Other names include chondrodysplasias, chondrosteodysplasias, osteochondrodysplasias, and bone dysplasias.

## STATEMENT OF RELEVANCE

There are more than 200 recognized types of skeletal dysplasias. Similar to most inborn errors of metabolism, the incidence of any single dysplasia is low. Collectively, however, they are relatively frequent. It is essential, therefore, to recognize these conditions in a fetus or child so that the diagnosis can be established, the prognosis determined, a treatment plan developed, and genetic counseling provided for the parents and family.

The aim of this section is to provide the primary care physician with a basic understanding of skeletal dysplasias and to present the major clinical and radiographic features of the more commonly encountered disorders, as well as the complications that may occur in association with them. The responsibilities of the primary care physician when he or she encounters one of these disorders are to treat any immediate medical problems, become familiar with the particular skeletal dysplasia under consideration, and obtain appropriate and timely consultation. In all cases in which the patient survives the neonatal period, a long-term treatment program should be established.

## FREQUENCY OF SKELETAL DYSPLASIAS

Most skeletal dysplasias appear to be extremely uncommon, although the exact incidence of any one disorder usually is not known. Osteitis deformans, or Paget disease, is estimated to occur in as many as 1:1,500 individuals more than 45 years of age, and in as many as 1:20 individuals more than 75 years of age. Osteogenesis imperfecta type I, which is one of the milder forms of the disorder, has an estimated frequency of 1:20,000, whereas osteogenesis imperfecta type II, the more severe form, affects about 1:50,000. Thanatophoric dysplasia, the most frequently encountered lethal skeletal dysplasia, is seen in about 1:30,000 births. Classic or heterozygous achondroplasia, the most widely known skeletal dysplasia, occurs with a frequency of 2:100,000 or 3:100,000.

The incidence of some skeletal dysplasias may be substantially higher in certain ethnic groups. For instance, the McKusick type of metaphyseal chondrodysplasia, or cartilage hair hypoplasia, is rare in the general population, but is found in 1:1000 or 2:1000 live births among the Amish communities of North America. The higher incidence of certain bone dysplasias in ethnic groups usually is the result of inbreeding.

## DEVELOPMENT AND ANATOMY OF BONE

Bone is formed from either mesodermal or neural crest cells. These cells form mesenchyma, which in turn, forms embryonic connective tissue. For cartilaginous bone, cartilage is formed within the embryonic connective tissue, which then changes to bone. For membranous bone, the bone is formed directly within the connective tissue. The cartilage in cartilaginous bone is formed by chondroblasts, whereas the mineral portion of the bone is derived from osteoblasts in both bone types. The skull (except for its base), the maxilla, mandible, squama portion of the temporalis, nasal bone, and clavicles are membranous bone; all the rest of the skeleton is cartilaginous bone.

The anatomy of long bones is depicted in Figure 12-48. When long bones are growing, the growing end is known as the epiphysis (Fig 12-49A). Below the epiphyseal center is the metaphysis. Longitudinal growth actually occurs at the junction between the epiphysis and the metaphysis, an area called the physis or growth plate. During puberty, the growth plate is obliterated, the epiphysis and metaphysis fuse, and lengthening of the bone ceases.

The shaft of the bone is the diaphysis. Molding of the diaphysis takes place as the bone becomes longer. The diaphysis also thickens with age and in response to stress placed on the bone.

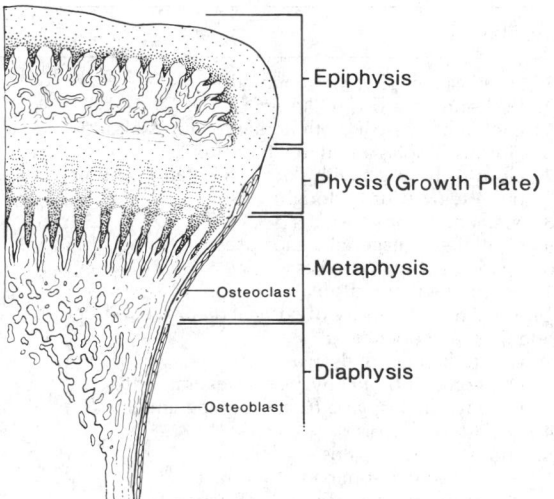

**Figure 12-48.** Anatomy of normal prepubertal tubular bone. Note that the bone is divided into four segments, each of which may be involved in skeletal dysplasias either separately or in combination.

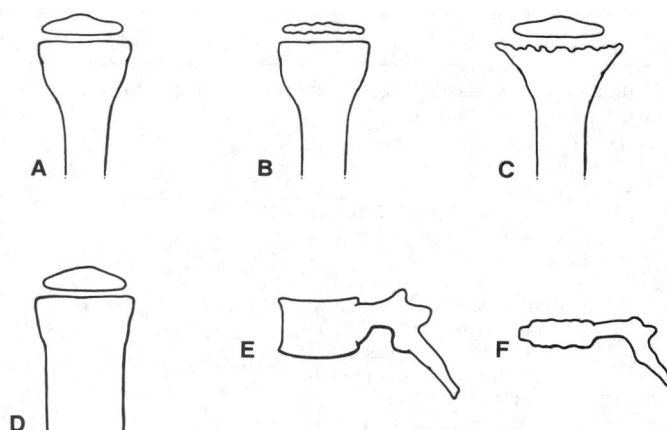

**Figure 12-49.** Diagrammatic representation of various types of bone dysplasias. (**A**) Normal shape of growing long bones. (**B**) Epiphyseal involvement such as in multiple epiphyseal dysplasia; note flattened and irregular epiphysis. (**C**) Metaphyseal involvement that might be seen in achondroplasia; note widening and irregular surface of metaphysis. (**D**) Diaphyseal involvement as seen in craniodiaphyseal dysplasia. (**E**) Normal lateral view of vertebra. (**F**) Vertebral involvement that can be found in spondyloepiphyseal dysplasia congenita; note vertebral body flattening and surface irregularities. (Modified from Rimoin DL, Lachman RS. The chondrodysplasias. In: Emery AEH, Rimoin DL, eds. Principles and practice of medical genetics. New York: Churchill Livingstone, 1990: 895.)

## NOMENCLATURE AND CLASSIFICATION OF SKELETAL DYSPLASIAS

Skeletal dysplasias in general are named after the anatomic parts of the bones that are affected, after the appearance of the bone, or after the individual(s) who described the condition. In some cases, a combination of these methods is used.

An example of the anatomic naming of bone dysplasias is multiple epiphyseal dysplasia (Fig 12-50). In this condition, numerous epiphyses (see Fig 12-49B) are involved, but the spine is affected only minimally. As a result of the involvement of multiple epiphyses, the individual usually is shorter than average and may have arthritis in the affected joints as an adult. Another example of anatomic nomenclature is spondyloepiphyseal dysplasia congenita. Similar to multiple epiphyseal dysplasia, most epiphyses in this disorder are involved, including those of the spine. The clinical picture is one of small, irregular epiphyses,

flattened vertebral bodies (platyspondyly; see Fig 12-49F), and, in some cases, kyphoscoliosis.

Other bone dysplasias are named after the appearance of the bone. Campomelic dysplasia is one example of this nomenclature. In this disorder, there is characteristic bowing of the long bones of the lower extremities. The term *campomelic* is coined from the Greek word meaning *bent limb*. In osteogenesis imperfecta, another skeletal dysplasia, the term *imperfecta* refers to poor mineralization of the bones. In a newly described disorder, schneckenbecken dysplasia, the pelvis is shaped like a snail shell; *schneckenbecken* is German for *snail-shaped*.

The third mechanism for naming bone dysplasias involves

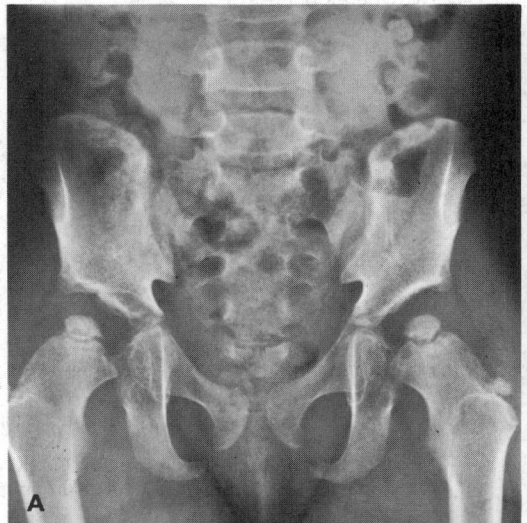
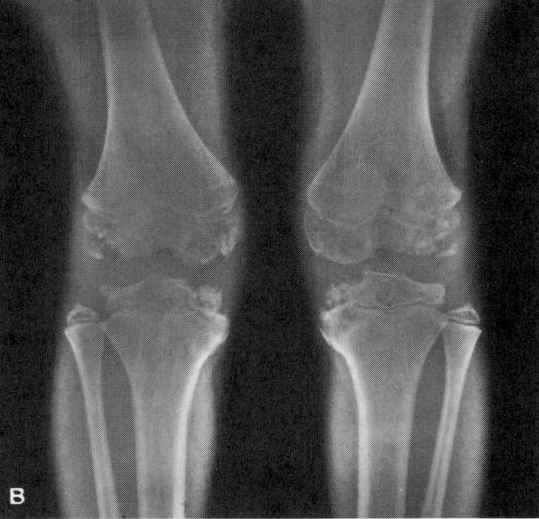

**Figure 12-50.** Radiographs of a patient with multiple epiphyseal dysplasia. (**A**) Pelvis and hips at age 8 years; note small irregular proximal femoral epiphyses and poorly developed acetabular roof. (**B**) Knees of patient at age 10 years; note irregular and mottled epiphyses of the long bones.

## TABLE 12-8. Skeletal Dysplasias

Osteochondrodysplasias (abnormalities of cartilage or bone growth and development)

I. Defects of growth of tubular bones or spine
  A. Identifiable at birth
    1. Achondrogenesis
      a. Type I (Parenti-Fraccaro)
      b. Type II (Langer-Saldino)
    2. Achondroplasia
    3. Acromesomelic dysplasia
    4. Asphyxiating thoracic dysplasia (Jeune)
    5. Atelosteogenesis
    6. Campomelic dysplasia
    7. Chondrodysplasia punctata
      a. Rhizomelic form
      b. Autosomal dominant form
      c. X-linked dominant form
    8. Chondroectodermal dysplasia (Ellis-van Creveld)
    9. Cleidocranial dysplasia
    10. Diastrophic dysplasia
    11. Dyssegmental dysplasia
    12. Fibrochondrogenesis
    13. Hypochondrogenesis
    14. Kniest dysplasia
    15. Kyphomelic dysplasia
    16. Larsen syndrome
    17. Mesomelic dysplasia
      a. Nievergelt type
      b. Langer type (probable homozygous dyschondrosteosis)
      c. Robinow type
      d. Rheinardt type
    18. Metatropic dysplasia (several forms)
    19. Otopalatodigital syndrome
    20. Schneckenbecken dysplasia
    21. Short rib-polydactyly syndrome
      a. Type I (Saldino-Noonan)
      b. Type II (Majewski)
      c. Type III (lethal thoracic dysplasia)
    22. Spondyloepiphyseal dysplasia congenita, Spranger-Wiedemann type
    23. Thanatophoric dysplasia
    24. Thanatophoric dysplasia with cloverleaf skull
  B. Identifiable in later life
    1. Acrodysplasia with retinitis pigmentosa and nephropathy (Saldino-Mainzer)
    2. Arthro-ophthalmopathy (Stickler)
    3. Dyggve-Melchior-Clausen dysplasia
    4. Dyschondrosteosis
    5. Hypochondroplasia
    6. Metaphyseal chondrodysplasia
      a. Jansen type
      b. McKusick type
      c. Schmid type
    7. Metaphyseal chondrodysplasia with exocrine pancreatic insufficiency and cyclic neutropenia
    8. Multiple epiphyseal dysplasia
      a. Fairbanks type
      b. Ribbing type
    9. Myotonic chondrodysplasia (Catel-Schwartz-Jampel)
    10. Parastremmatic dysplasia
    11. Progressive pseudorheumatoid chondrodysplasia
    12. Pseudoachondroplasia
      a. Dominant
      b. Recessive
    13. Spondyloepimetaphyseal dysplasia (several forms)
    14. Spondyloepiphyseal dysplasia, other forms (also see I.A.22)
    15. Spondyloepiphyseal dysplasia tarda
    16. Spondylometaphyseal dysplasia, Kozlowski type
    17. Trichlorhinophalangeal dysplasia
II. Disorganized development of cartilage and fibrous components of skeleton
    1. Acrodysplasia with exostoses (Giedion-Langer)
    2. Cherubism (familial fibrous dysplasia of the jaws)
    3. Dysplasia epiphyseal hemimelia
    4. Enchondromatosis (Ollier)
    5. Enchondromatosis with hemangioma (Maffucci)
    6. Fibrous dysplasia (Jaffe-Lichtenstein)
    7. Fibrous dysplasia with skin pigmentation and precocious puberty (McCune-Albright)
    8. Metachondromatosis
    9. Multiple cartilagenous exostoses
    10. Osteoglophonic dysplasia
    11. Spondyloenchondroplasia
III. Abnormalities of density of cortical diaphyseal structure or metaphyseal modeling
    1. Craniodiaphyseal dysplasia
    2. Craniometaphyseal dysplasia (several forms)
    3. Diaphyseal dysplasia (Camurati-Engelmann)
    4. Dysosteosclerosis
    5. Endosteal hyperostosis
      a. Autosomal dominant (Worth)
      b. Autosomal recessive (van Buchem)
      c. Autosomal recessive (sclerosteosis)
    6. Frontometaphyseal dysplasia
    7. Infantile cortical hyperostosis (Caffey disease, familial type)
    8. Juvenile idiopathic osteoporosis
    9. Melorheostosis
    10. Metaphyseal dysplasia (Pyle)
    11. Oculodentoosseous dysplasia
      a. Mild type
      b. Severe type
    12. Osteodysplasty (Melnick-Needles)
    13. Osteoectasia with hyperphosphatasia
    14. Osteogenesis imperfecta
      a. Type I
      b. Type II
      c. Type III
      d. Type IV
    15. Osteomesopycnosis
    16. Osteopathia striata
    17. Osteopathia striata with cranial stenosis
    18. Osteopetrosis with delayed manifestations (several forms)
    19. Osteopetrosis with precocious manifestations
      a. Autosomal recessive, lethal form
      b. Intermediate recessive form
      c. Autosomal dominant form
      d. Recessive with renal tubular acidosis
    20. Osteopoikilosis
    21. Osteoporosis with pseudoglioma
    22. Osteosclerosis, dominant type (Stanescu)
    23. Pachydermoperiostosis
    24. Pycnodysostosis
    25. Sclerosteosis
    26. Tubular stenosis (Kenny-Caffey)

Dysostoses (Malformation of Individual Bones, Singly or in Combination)

I. Dysostoses with cranial and facial involvement
    1. Acrocephalopolysyndactyly (Carpenter) and others
    2. Acrocephalosyndactyly
      a. Apert type
      b. Chotzen type
      c. Pfeiffer type
    3. Cephalopolysyndactyly (Greig)
    4. Craniofacial dysostosis (Crouzon)
    5. Craniosynostosis (several forms)
    6. First and second branchial arch syndromes
      a. Acrofacial dysostosis (Nager)
      b. Mandibulofacial dysostosis (Treacher Collins, Franceschetti)
      c. Oculoauriculovertebral dysostosis (Goldenhar)
    7. Oculomandibulofacial syndrome (Hallermann-Streiff-Francois)
II. Dysostoses with predominant axial involvement
    1. Cerebrocostomandibular syndrome
    2. Cervicooculoacoustic syndrome (Wildervanck)
    3. Oculovertebral syndrome (Weyers)

## TABLE 12-8.  (Continued)

4. Osteo-onychodysostosis
5. Spondylocostal dysostosis
   a. Dominant form
   b. Recessive forms
6. Sprengel's deformity
7. Vertebral segmentation defects (including Klippel-Feil)
III. Dysostoses with predominant involvement of extremities
1. Acheiria
2. Aglossia-adactyly syndrome (Hanhart)
3. Apodia
4. Blackfan-Diamond anemia with thumb anomalies (Aase)
5. Brachydactyly (several forms)
6. Camptodactyly
7. Cardiomelic syndrome (Holt-Oram and others)
8. Congenital bowing of long bones (see also osteochondrodysplasias)
9. Ectrodactyly syndrome
   a. Ectrodactyly-ectodermal dysplasia cleft palate syndrome (EEC syndrome)
   b. Ectrodactyly with scalp defects
   c. Isolated, autosomal dominant type
10. Familial radioulnar synostosis
11. Femoral focal deficiency (with or without facial anomalies)
12. Focal dermal hypoplasia (Goltz)
13. Hand-foot-genital syndrome
14. Manzke syndrome
15. Multiple synostoses (includes some forms of symphalangism)
16. Orodigitofacial syndrome
    a. Papillon-Leage type
    b. Mohr type
17. Pancytopenia-dysmelia syndrome (Fanconi)
18. Poland syndrome
19. Polydactyly (several forms)
20. Polysyndactyly (several forms)
21. Rubinstein-Taybi syndrome
22. Scapuloiliac dysostosis (Kosenow-Sinios)
23. Symphalangism
24. Syndactyly (several forms)
25. Tetraphocomelia syndrome (pseudothalidomide syndrome, Robert, SC)
26. Thrombocytopenia-radial-aplasia syndrome

### Idiopathic Osteolyses

1. Multicentric
   a. Hajdu-Cheney form
   b. Torg form
   c. Winchester form

2. Phalangeal (several forms)
3. Tarsocarpal
   a. Including Francois form and others
   b. With nephropathy

### Miscellaneous Disorders With Osseous Involvement

1. Cerebrohepatorenal syndrome (Zellweger)
2. Cockayne syndrome
3. Coffin-Lowry syndrome
4. Congenital contractural arachnodactyly (Beals)
5. Early acceleration of skeletal maturation
   a. Marshall-Smith syndrome
   b. Weaver syndrome
6. Epidermal nevus syndrome (Solomon)
7. Fibrodysplasia ossificans congenita
8. Marfan syndrome
9. Multiple congenital fibromatosis
10. Nevoid basal cell carcinoma syndrome
11. Neurofibromatosis

### Chromosomal Aberrations

Individual disorders not listed

### Primary Metabolic Abnormalities

I. Disorders associated with faulty bone mineralization
1. Hypophosphatasia (several forms)
2. Hypophosphatemic rickets
3. Idiopathic hypercalciuria
4. Late rickets (McCance)
5. Pseudohypoparathyroidism (normocalcemic and hypocalcemic forms, include acrodysostosis)
6. Vitamin D dependency or pseudo-deficiency rickets
II. Lysosomal storage disorders
1. Mucopolysaccharidoses
2. Mucolipidoses
3. Glycoproteinoses
4. Sialic acid transport disorders
5. Certain sphingolipidoses
III. Nucleic acids
1. Adenosine-deaminase deficiency and others
IV. Amino acids
1. Homocystinuria and others
V. Metals
1. Menkes kinky hair syndrome and others
2. Occipital horn syndrome (Ehlers-Danlos type IX)

Modified from Maroteaux P, Beighton P, Poznanski AK, et al. International nomenclature of constitutional diseases of bone, with bibliography. Birth Defects 1986;22:1.

the use of eponyms. For example, Kniest dysplasia is a rare, autosomal dominant disorder characterized by short stature and dumbbell-shaped femurs with extremely broad and shortened femoral necks. The condition first was reported by Kniest in 1952.

More frequently, eponyms are used in combination with one of the first two methods of naming skeletal dysplasias, most often to delineate the subtype of dysplasia. For instance, there are two types of achondrogenesis, one known as Parenti-Fraccaro (type I) and the other as Langer-Saldino (type II; Fig 12-51). These two subtypes are not based on differences in the clinical appearance of the affected children, but on radiographic variations. Type I has been subdivided further into type IA, which has rib fractures and spike-shaped femurs, and type IB, which lacks the rib fractures, but has a pelvis that appears to be turned upside down. Type IA also has been denoted as the Houston-Harris type and type IB as the Fraccaro type.

Various systems for classification of the skeletal dysplasias have been devised. One of the earliest of these was based on the relative shortening of the limb or of the spine; for example, was the short stature of the child caused by primary shortening of the extremities with relatively normal length of the spine, or was the spine relatively short compared to the length of the arms and legs? Achondroplasia is one example of a short-limbed skeletal dysplasia. In this condition, the sitting height (ie, the apparent height of an individual when he or she is sitting in a chair) is nearly normal, but the standing height is far less than normal. This reflects the very short legs that are present in achondroplasia. On the other hand, patients with Morquio syndrome (mucopolysaccharidosis type IV) have the opposite characteristics. An individual with this condition has a short trunk and, in relationship to the spinal length, long extremities. The shortening of the spine is a result of platyspondyly.

Another classification system is based on the age at which the first manifestation of the skeletal dysplasia appears. Some disorders can be detected prenatally or at birth (congenita), whereas some do not manifest the changes that allow diagnosis until

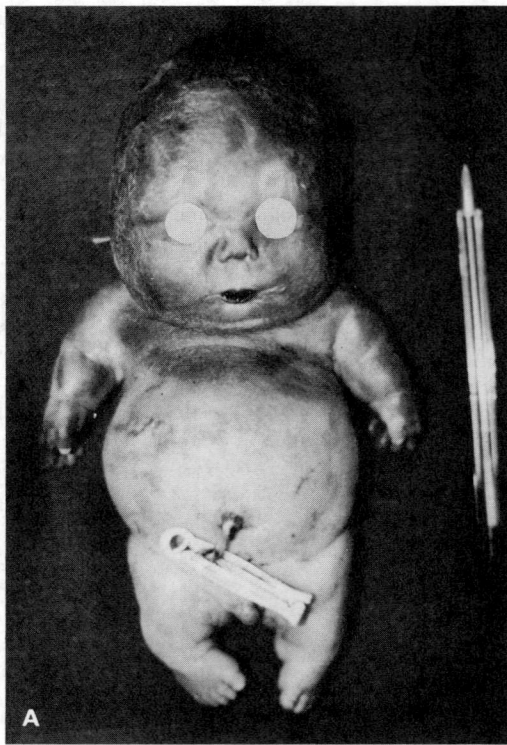
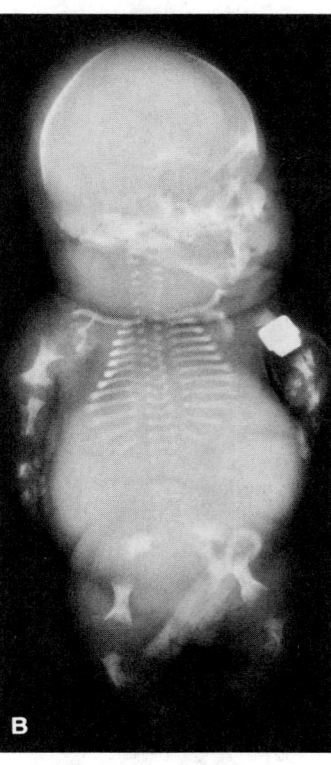

**Figure 12-51.** Achondrogenesis type II in a term newborn. (**A**) Note severe growth deficiency (standard ballpoint pen alongside for comparison), small chest and extremities, and protruding abdomen. This was a postmortem picture. (**B**) Radiograph of the same patient; note the very short, irregularly shaped bones of the extremities, short and horizontal ribs, and poorly calcified vertebral bodies.

months or years after birth (*tarda*). Yet another system is based on the pattern of bone involvement and the type of changes seen in the bones with each skeletal disorder. The International Nomenclature of Constitutional Diseases of Bone (Maroteaux et al., 1986; Table 12-8) uses this approach. In this section, we shall distinguish between lethal and nonlethal dysplasias for reasons that will be presented later.

## DELINEATION OF SKELETAL DYSPLASIAS

The discovery of new skeletal dysplasias has been an ongoing process for the past 50 years. A bewildering number of different disorders are recognized, making diagnosis problematic for the average clinician. Recognition of a specific disorder is made more difficult by the similar appearances of many of these conditions. Furthermore, there may be a spectrum of severity within a single entity, or two conditions may have overlapping features, making arrival at a correct diagnosis exasperating for most physicians and even for experts. In addition, recognition of the particular type of bone dysplasia is complicated further by the fact that these conditions usually become more severe with time. If the condition manifests itself prenatally, it probably will be severe at birth, and even may be fatal. If the disorder is mild or not expressed at birth, it invariably will worsen as the child ages. If the child is seen early in the course of the condition, when the features are not expressed fully, it may be difficult or impossible to make the diagnosis.

An illustration of the identification of new skeletal dysplasia syndromes is depicted in Figure 12-52. In the 1940s, most individuals with disproportionately short statures were classified as having achondroplasia, if the extremities were relatively short, or as having Morquio disease, if the trunk was shortened disproportionately. Since then, a number of skeletal dysplasias have been delineated from each of these disorders. This demarcation has been accomplished by the careful study of clinical, radiographic, and pathologic features, as well as of the inheritance patterns associated with the various skeletal dysplasias.

Another level of delineation of bone dysplasias is by biochemical definition of these disorders. As certain of the biochemical abnormalities for some skeletal dysplasias have been discovered, it has become clear that many previously described single conditions in actuality are composed of many different mutations within the gene that codes for the condition. Thus, individuals with the same apparent clinical condition may have biochemically distinct and, thus, different disorders. This chemical heterogeneity in part accounts for the difference in severity of the "same" clinical condition. Furthermore, because the same mutated gene usually is passed within a family, affected individuals in that family will have the same biochemical defect and, often, similar clinical courses.

## BIOCHEMISTRY OF SKELETAL DYSPLASIAS

For most skeletal dysplasias, the biochemical lesions producing the disorders still are unknown. If biochemical errors are to be found, one would expect to find them in the bone matrix, particularly in its connective tissue component; in the osteoid, the mineral portion of the bone; or in the cartilage. In addition, problems may be found in the function of the osteoblasts, those cells that form bone, or the osteoclasts, those cells that degrade and reshape bone.

The notable exception to the dearth of biochemical understanding, however, is osteogenesis imperfecta type II. This disorder, which invariably leads to the death of the affected child, is produced by a defect in either the procollagen $\alpha$-1 or the procollagen pro-$\alpha$-2 gene. These genes normally produce the polypeptides pro-$\alpha$-1 and pro-$\alpha$-2, respectively. Under normal circumstances, two pro-$\alpha$-1 chains combine with one pro-$\alpha$-2 procollagen in a helical structure to form type I procollagen (Fig 12–53). Portions of type I procollagen molecules then are cleaved to form collagen molecules that are incorporated into the definitive type I collagen fibril. Deletions of one or more amino acids, or the substitutions of amino acids in the pro-$\alpha$-1 or pro-$\alpha$-2 chains

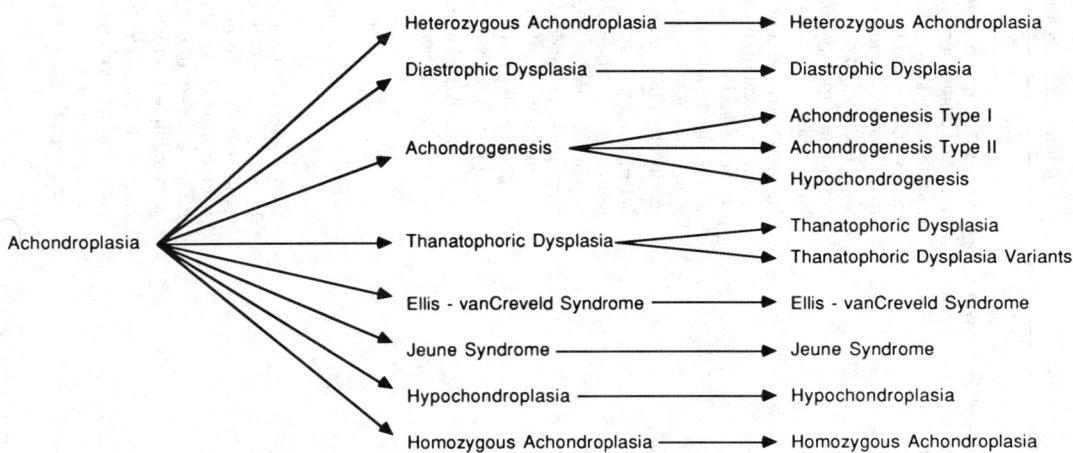

Figure 12-52. Delineation of various skeletal dysplasias from achondroplasia during the past 40 years.

have been found in most patients with osteogenesis imperfecta type II.

When the above defects occur in the pro-$\alpha$-1 or pro-$\alpha$-2 chains, formation of the normal helical structure of the type I procollagen molecule is disrupted (see Fig 12-53). The disruption may lead

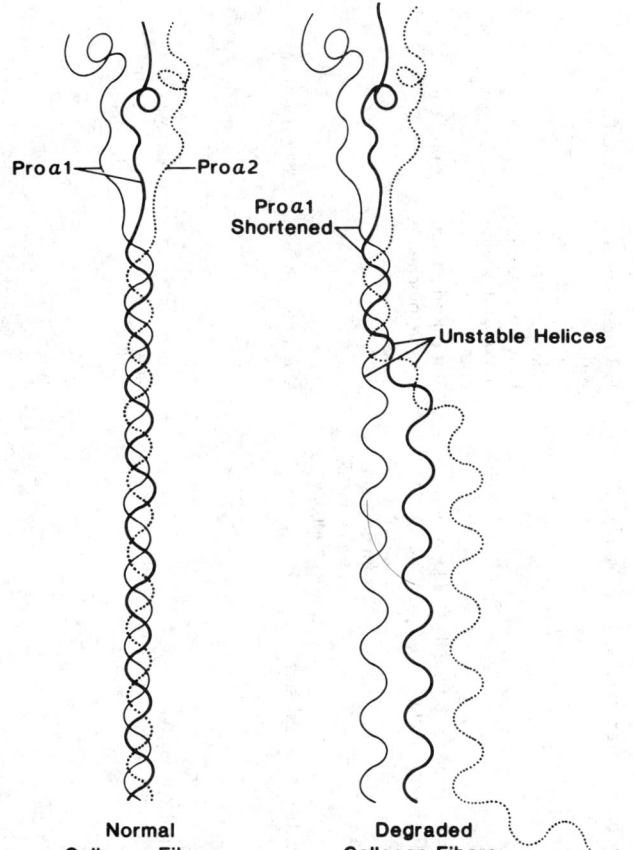

Figure 12-53. Normal type I procollagen molecule on the left showing normal helical formation. The figure on the right depicts the lack of coiling of the polypeptides when there is deletion of one or more amino acids in both pro-$\alpha$-1 chains. One pro-$\alpha$-1 chain in each figure has been thickened for clarity.

to intracellular destruction of the procollagen molecule within the cell, a process called protein suicide, which results in a deficiency of type I collagen and inadequate collagen fibril formation. The lack of collagen in turn leads to the condition. Furthermore, the degree of severity of the osteogenesis imperfecta type II is correlated with the location of the defect within the pro-$\alpha$-1 or pro-$\alpha$-2 chains. In general, when the defect is near the point where coiling of the chains begins, there is little coiling, greater chain degradation, little type I collagen production, and more severe clinical problems. On the other hand, if the defect is located near the end of the chain, little effect on coiling occurs, fewer chains are lost, and the clinical effect is milder.

More than 70 mutations have been identified in the procollagen $\alpha$-1 or $\alpha$-2 genes that result not only in osteogenesis imperfecta type II, but in the other forms of this condition. In some of the variant forms, there may be abnormal types of procollagen produced and secreted by the cell. Because of the ability to detect these abnormal types of procollagen or a deficiency in the production of procollagen, analysis of the procollagen in patients with suspected osteogenesis imperfecta may assist in the diagnosis of this condition.

A few other biochemical defects also are known in other skeletal dysplasias. For instance, there is a deficiency of the pro-$\alpha$-1 messenger RNA in some patients with osteogenesis imperfecta type I. This deficiency leads to a deficiency in the production of type I procollagen and, ultimately, in type I collagen. In some forms of hypophosphatasia, there may be complete or partial deficiency of bone alkaline phosphatase that leads to undermineralized osteoid. Also known is the biochemical defect for most of the storage diseases (see other sections of this text for specific details). Vitamin-, mineral-, and hormone-deficient states also can produce skeletal dysplasias. Probably the most severe bone dysplasia encountered is produced by the total absence of thyroxine. This dysplasia occurs because thyroxine probably is the most important hormone involved in normal bone growth; its deficiency produces a severe delay in osseous maturation.

With the advent and application of the new DNA technologies, identification of the defective genes that result in bone dysplasias will be possible. Such identification will lead to the elucidation of the various biochemical defects in these conditions, reliable and specific methods of diagnosing these disorders prenatally and postnatally, and, ultimately, methods of treating or preventing them.

(Text continues on p. 155.)

TABLE 12-9. Inheritance and Features of Selected Lethal Skeletal Dysplasias

| Name of Condition | Mode of Inheritance | Clinical Features | | | | Radiographic Features |
|---|---|---|---|---|---|---|
| | | Head and Neck | Trunk | Limbs | Other | |
| **Conditions That Usually Are Lethal in the Neonatal Period** | | | | | | |
| Achondrogenesis type I (Parenti-Fraccaro type; subtypes: Houston-Harris, type IA; Fraccaro, type IB) | AR | Round or oval face, membranous skull, short neck | Short, rounded, protruding abdomen | Very short | Hydrops fetalis, growth failure, congenital heart defects | Poor ossification of cranium, vertebral bodies, pelvis, and sacrum; very short tubular bones; platyspondyly; short, thin, beaded, fractured ribs; short ilia, no pubic ossification; multiple spurs of long bones |
| Achondrogenesis type II (Langer-Saldino type)* | AR | Same as above | Same as above | Same as above | Same as above | Same as above except almost absent ossification of vertebrae and sacrum, less severe shortening of tubular bones, and well-developed calcification of cranium |
| Fibrochondrogenesis | AR | Flat face, prominent eyes, cleft palate | Narrow chest | Short, enlarged joints | | Short, dumbbell-shaped tubular bones, short ribs with cupping at anterior ends, platyspondyly, marked coronal cleft of vertebrae, small ilia with narrow sacrosciatic notches |
| Kniest dysplasia (severe neonatal form) | Possibly AR | Flat face, prominent wide-set eyes, broad mouth, cleft palate, frontal flattening, maxillary hypoplasia, shallow orbits | Short | Short limbs, prominent knees, joint contractures | | Dumbbell-shaped long bones, coronal clefts of vertebrae |
| Osteogenesis imperfecta type II (osteogenesis imperfecta congenita) | AD, new mutation, 5%–7% recurrence risk from germline mosaicism; AR occasionally | Soft calvaria, blue sclerae, pinched nose | Small chest | Short, bent limbs; fractures | CNS hemorrhage | Generalized deficiency of bone, wormian bones of the skull, thin ribs with multiple fractures (beading) broad ribbon-shaped tubular bones with multiple fractures |
| Schneckenbecken dysplasia† | AR | Macrocephaly | Narrow thorax | Short limbs | | Dumbbell-shaped long bones, platyspondyly with wide vertebral bodies, characteristic snail-shaped pelvis |
| Short rib-polydactyly type 1 (Saldino-Noonan type) | AR | Round, flattened face | Narrow chest, protuberant abdomen | Markedly short limbs, postaxial polydactyly | Hydrops fetalis; imperforate anus; defects of heart, lungs, kidneys, and GI tract | Very short long bones, metaphyseal spurs, polydactyly; very short horizontal ribs, platyspondyly, wide intervertebral spaces; small ilia, flat acetabulum |

| Condition | Inheritance | Facial/Head | Thorax/Trunk | Limbs | Associated Findings | Radiographic Findings |
|---|---|---|---|---|---|---|
| Short rib–polydactyly type 2 (Majewski type) | AR | Short, flat nose; low-set ears; cleft lip or palate | Same as above | Moderately short limbs, preaxial or postaxial polydactyly | ±PDA, dysplastic kidneys, respiratory tract anomalies, ambiguous genitalia | Stippled epiphyses; short, horizontal ribs; polydactyly; wide coronal clefts of vertebrae; trapezoid ilia; hypoplastic, oval-shaped tibias |
| Spondyloepiphyseal dysplasia congenita (severe lethal forms) | Mostly AD new mutations, some possibly AR | Flat face, cleft palate, short neck | Short trunk, barrel-shaped chest | Short limbs | Respiratory distress | Delayed osseous maturation, platyspondyly, coronal cleft of the vertebrae |
| Spondylohumerofemoral dysplasia (atelosteogenesis) | Unknown, sporadic in all cases | Depressed nasal bridge, cleft palate | | Proximal limb shortening, bowed limbs, dislocated elbows and knees, talipes | | Hypoplastic thoracic vertebral bodies and ribs, delayed ossification of some metacarpals and phalanges, short humeri and femurs with hypoplastic distal segment |
| Thanatophoric dysplasia | Unknown, usually sporadic | Large head with or without cloverleaf configuration of skull, depressed nasal bridge, prominent eyes, large fontanelles, small foramen magnum | Narrow thorax, relatively long trunk, congenital heart defects | Short extremities, extra creases around arms and legs, short fingers with prominent finger creases | | Flat vertebrae that are U-shaped in the thoracic region and inverted U-shaped in the lumbar region; short, bowed long bones; metaphyseal flaring; short ribs; hypoplastic pelvis with narrow sacrosciatic notch |

### Conditions That May Be Lethal in the Neonatal Period

| Condition | Inheritance | Facial/Head | Thorax/Trunk | Limbs | Associated Findings | Radiographic Findings |
|---|---|---|---|---|---|---|
| Achondroplasia, homozygous form | Homozygous dominant, both parents usually have achondroplasia heterozygous type | Large head with frontal bossing, depressed nasal bridge, large anterior fontanelle open sagittal suture | Small thorax, protuberant abdomen | Disproportionately short limbs, extra skin folds, trident hand | | Large calvaria; short narrow base of skull; small foramen magnum, calvarial thickening; short mandibular rami; short ribs with wide, cupped ends; narrow, flat vertebral bodies; unusually wide intervertebral distances; decrease in the lumbar area; short, almost square-shaped ilia; short, bowed long bones with more proximal shortening |
| Asphyxiating thoracic dysplasia (Jeune syndrome) | AR | | Long narrow thorax, respiratory insufficiency, renal disease as adults | Shortening variable, short hands and feet, ±postaxial polydactyly | | Short horizontal ribs; squared, short ilia; flat acetabulum with spur projecting from end; short middle and distal phalanges with markedly cone-shaped epiphyses |
| Campomelic dysplasia | AR? | Large skull; small, flat face; shallow orbits; micrognathia; short palpebral fissures | Small, narrow chest | Short and bowed femurs and tibias, dimples at point of maximum curvature, talipes equinovarus | Sex reversal in some males | Narrow, wavy ribs; hypoplastic cervical vertebral bodies; long, slender, bowed femurs and tibias; short clavicles; hypoplastic scapulas |
| Chondrodysplasia punctata, rhizomelic form | AR | Flat face, depressed nasal bridge and tip of nose, cataract | | Rhizomelic shortening, joint contractures | Ichthyosiform erythroderma | Stippled calcification in multiple epiphyses, wide clefts of vertebral bodies, trapezoid ilia, stippling of ischiopubis, calcification of larynx and trachea |

(continued)

TABLE 12-9. *(Continued)*

| Name of Condition | Mode of Inheritance | Clinical Features — Head and Neck | Trunk | Limbs | Other | Radiographic Features |
|---|---|---|---|---|---|---|
| Chondroectodermal dysplasia (Ellis-van Creveld) | AR | Notching or tenting of the upper lip, natal teeth, teeth abnormalities | Long, narrow chest and abdomen | Postaxial polydactyly of the hand and sometimes feet, shortening of arms and hands, hypoplastic nails | Congenital heart defects (>50%) | Short ribs and narrow chest, squared ilia with hook-like spurs from the acetabulum, acromesomelic shortening, cone-shaped epiphyses, fused hamate and capitate bones |
| Dyssegmental dysplasia | AR | | | Short, bowed limbs | | Coronal vertebral clefts, marked variation in the size of the vertebral bodies, bowed long bones, advanced carpal maturation |
| Hypochondrogenesis | AR | Midfacial hypoplasia with depressed nasal bridge | Ribs not fractured, abdomen prominent | Very short extremities | Respiratory distress | Short, relatively well-proportioned long bones and vertebrae; small but well-sculptured ilia; partial ossification of ischia; femoral shaft straight with flat metaphyseal ends |
| Hypophosphatasia, congenital lethal form | AR | Soft calvaria, globular-shaped head | Respiratory distress | Short, bowed, flaccid extremities | Low levels of serum alkaline phosphatase and raised levels of phosphoethanolamine, death hours or days after birth | Poor mineralization of the calvaria; short, thin ribs and tubular bones; irregular ossification of metaphyses; poor mineralization of other bones |

* Recent evidence indicates that achondrogenesis type II, hypochondrogenesis, spondyloepiphyseal dysplasia congenita, spondyloepimetaphyseal dysplasia, Kniest dysplasia, and arthro-ophthalmopathy (Stickler syndrome) constitute a spectrum of diseases produced by lesions at various locations in the procollagen molecules that produce type II collagen. In achondrogenesis type II, there may be little type I collagen; in the less severe forms (ie, hypochondrogenesis and spondyloepiphyseal dysplasia congenita), there appears to be over-modulated type II collagen.

† Schneckenbecken is German for snail-shaped.

Abbreviations: AR, autosomal recessive; AD, autosomal dominant; CNS, central nervous system; GI, gastrointestinal tract; PDA, patent ductus arteriosus.

Data modified from Rimoin and Lachman, 1983; Scott, 1988; Spranger et al, 1974; and Winter et al, 1988. A more complete history of the lethal skeletal dysplasias can be found in the article by Spranger and Maroteaux, 1990.

## EVALUATION OF PATIENTS WITH SUSPECTED SKELETAL DYSPLASIAS

The diagnosis of a skeletal dysplasia should be considered in any patient who has disproportionately short stature or abnormal development of one or more bones. When such an individual is encountered, he or she should be evaluated fully to determine whether a skeletal dysplasia is present and, if so, which disorder it is. The history should include the pregnancy history with particular reference to any fetal evaluation; birth length, weight, and head circumference; postnatal growth and development; and medical problems. With regard to the family history, one should inquire about short stature and orthopedic problems in other family members, and determine if there is consanguinity between the parents. While performing the physical examination, one should take care to search for nonosseous abnormalities such as cataracts, cleft palate, and congenital heart disease that would be useful in establishing the diagnosis and helpful in formulating a treatment plan. Basic measurements should be obtained, including height, weight, head circumference, arm span, and upper segment-to-lower segment ratio. The latter ratio is determined by measuring the distance from the anterior-superior edge of the pubic symphysis to the floor or the bottom of the feet in infants (lower segment) and subtracting this value from the length or height (upper segment). The upper segment-to-lower segment ratio in normal children varies from 1.6 at birth to 0.93 in older teenagers and adults (McKusick, 1972). Many children with bone dysplasias will have ratios that are greater than normal for their age and are likely to have short lower extremities, whereas children with values less than normal for their age usually will have short trunks.

In addition to the above evaluation, a complete skeletal radiographic series also is essential, because the diagnosis of most skeletal dysplasias can be made only on the basis of the radiographic findings. A complete survey is crucial because an inadequate study may not allow for the diagnosis to be established. Films that should be obtained include anteroposterior and lateral views of the skull and the entire spine; anteroposterior views of the chest, hands, and pelvis; and views of all the long bones, including the elbows, knees, and ankles. In most patients at risk for atlantoaxial instability, extension and flexion views of the cervical vertebrae need to be obtained. If present, atlantoaxial instability may lead to spinal cord compression and loss of nerve function in some individuals. Osseous maturation should be determined from radiographs of the hand or the left hemiskeleton. Finally, other radiographs need to be taken as indicated by the history and findings of the patient.

Laboratory testing is important as an aid in the diagnosis of some skeletal dysplasias and in determining the health status of affected patients. Serum calcium, phosphorus, protein, and alkaline phosphatase levels should be obtained to rule out hypophosphatasia, vitamin D–resistant rickets, vitamin D–dependent rickets, and other disorders. Urine screening for storage and other metabolic diseases also should be completed. A serum thyroxine level needs to be determined on any youngster with short stature, large fontanelles, and retarded bone age to diagnose unrecognized hypothyroidism. Other laboratory testing also should be obtained as dictated by the clinical situation.

## CLASSIFICATION OF SKELETAL DYSPLASIAS

An extensive list of skeletal dysplasias is presented in Table 12-8. The classification system used in this table has been discussed above.

From the management standpoint, however, skeletal dysplasias can be divided conveniently into lethal and nonlethal types.

A lethal bone dysplasia means that most affected infants die of the condition shortly after birth or during the first year or two of life. A nonlethal skeletal dysplasia implies that the dysplasia normally does not lead to the death of the children. The major significance of distinguishing between lethal and nonlethal skeletal dysplasias lies in the fact that the lethal dysplasias frequently require that a decision be made whether to support the affected infants immediately after birth. If the decision is made to support a newborn with a normally lethal skeletal dysplasia, extensive and long-term ventilator care may be required. For instance, it is not uncommon for patients with less severe ''lethal'' skeletal dysplasias to be placed on assisted ventilation after birth and for them to become ventilator-dependent, requiring support for months or years, and then to die. Thus, it also is essential for physicians to recognize when newborns have lethal skeletal dysplasias and when they probably will not survive despite extensive treatment efforts. In these situations, proper evaluation to establish the diagnosis and subsequent appropriate genetic counseling of the parents are essential. On the other hand, physicians also need to be aware that some patients with normally lethal skeletal dysplasias (eg, asphyxiating thoracic dysplasia) may have mild presentations of the condition and will survive with appropriate respiratory and other medical support.

## Lethal Skeletal Dysplasias

Listed in Table 12-9 are the more common lethal skeletal dysplasias. Usually, these conditions are lethal because the infant possesses a small thoracic cage as a direct result of having short ribs. The small chest cage then leads to respiratory insufficiency and death in most cases. The chest circumference-to-abdominal circumference ratio in most of these infants usually is less than 0.85 and reflects the reduction of the chest size. The exact chest size that is associated with the death of the child has not been established, however.

Clinically, lethal bone dysplasias are encountered in three time frames. The first is in the prenatal period, when fetuses are detected with short limbs and small chest circumferences. When the condition is detected in the second trimester, the pregnancy often is terminated. The second situation is when the child is stillborn or is liveborn but dies within minutes or hours after birth regardless of the efforts put forth to support the infant. The last situation is the one that generally causes the greatest distress for everyone involved and entails a child who is born with a skeletal dysplasia and survives when placed on ventilator care. Some of these patients eventually can be weaned from the ventilator, but most cannot. Those children who are weaned successfully tend to survival long-term without much respiratory difficulty. For example, no children with asphyxiating thoracic dysplasia (Fig 12-54) who have managed to live beyond the age of 2 years have been reported to die of respiratory failure. The reason for their survival appears to be the growth of the thoracic cage with age and adequate respiratory function. On the other hand, no children with thanatophoric dysplasia (Fig 12-55) are known to have lived beyond 14 months, even with full respiratory support. Thus, it is critical when dealing with a newborn with a bone dysplasia to establish the diagnosis quickly and then to decide if a child should receive ventilator care. If the decision is made to support the child, the parents need to be made aware of the prolonged nature of the therapy, what it may involve, and the possibility that the child may not survive even though he or she receives full respiratory support.

## Nonlethal Skeletal Dysplasias

In contrast to lethal bone dysplasias, the nonlethal dysplasias (Table 12-10) usually do not require intensive neonatal respiratory

(Text continues on p. 161.)

TABLE 12-10. Inheritance and Features of Selected Nonlethal Skeletal Dysplasias

| Name of Condition | Mode of Inheritance | Clinical Features | | | | Complications | Radiographic Features |
|---|---|---|---|---|---|---|---|
| | | Head and Neck | Trunk | Limbs | Other | | |
| **Conditions Identifiable at Birth** | | | | | | | |
| Achondroplasia, heterozygous type (classic form) | AD, 80% represent new mutations | Large head, depressed nasal bridge, bulging forehead, prominent mandible, small foramen magnum | Stocky, prominent buttocks and abdomen | Short extremities with major shortening proximally, trident hands | Spinal stenosis | Sudden infant death, hydrocephalus, bowed legs, kyphosis, otitis media, nerve root compression | Short vertebral pedicles, decreasing lumbosacral distance between pedicles, square-shaped pelvis, ice cream–shaped proximal femur and humerus in infancy, relative overgrowth of fibula |
| Cleidocranial dysplasia | AD, wide variation in expression of disorder | Large head with large fontanelles and open sutures, delayed closure of fontanelles, persistence of deciduous teeth | Droopy shoulders and narrow chest, occasionally scoliosis | Hyperextensible joints; short, squared fingers | Adult height normal or slightly reduced | Scoliosis; respiratory distress; dislocations of shoulders, head of radius, and hips | Absent or hypoplasia of clavicles, decreased ossification of skull, multiple wormian bones, delayed ossification of many bones |
| Chondrodysplasia punctata, dominant type (Conradi-Hunermann disease) | AD | Flat face, depressed nasal bridge and tip of the nose, cataracts (20%) | ±Scoliosis | Asymmetrical shortening of limbs, joint contractures | | Ichthyosiform erythroderma, alopecia, death in severe cases | Flat facial bones, cleft of vertebral bodies, multiple but variable stippling of epiphyses, vertebrae, and ischiopubis; asymmetry of long bones |
| Diastrophic dysplasia* | AR | Acute swelling of the pinnae leading to a cauliflower-like ear, cleft palate (50%) | Scoliosis, respiratory distress, congenital heart defects, kyphosis | Short limbs with club feet, progressive joint contractures, hitchhiker thumbs, symphalangism | | Severe limitation of joint movement making feeding and walking difficult | Calcium deposit in ears, precocious ossification of rib cartilages, scoliosis, kyphosis, lumbar interpedicular narrowing, shortened long bones, broad metaphyses, delayed epiphyseal ossification |
| Kniest kysplasia | AD | Flat face, widely spaced and prominent eyes, depressed nasal bridge, hearing loss, cleft palate (50%), occasionally myopia and retinal detachment | Short trunk; kyphosis; scoliosis; accentuated lordosis; short broad thorax with sternal prominence | Short stature and extremities, prominent joints, joint contractures | | Chronic otitis media, hearing loss, blindness | Frontal flattening hypoplasia of maxilla, platyspondyly, small ilia, club-like metaphyses |

| | | | | | | | |
|---|---|---|---|---|---|---|---|
| Larsen's syndrome (multiple congenital dislocations) | AD and AR | Prominent forehead with flat face, ocular hypertelorism; ±cleft palate or bifid uvula | Laxity of chest wall during early infancy | Multiple dislocated joints, especially the elbows, hips, and knees; abnormal hands, pes equinovarus | Kyphosis, hypermobility of small vertebra joints | Cord compression, producing apnea and death | Multiple joint dislocations, abnormal curvature of the spine, supernumerary carpal bones |
| Mesomelic dysplasia, Langer type | AR probably homozygous dominant form of dyschondrosteosis | Micrognathia | | Severe mesomelic (forearm and lower leg) shortening | | None | Mandibular hypoplasia; shortening of long bones; more severe shortening of radius, ulna, and tibia; severe hypoplasia of fibula |
| Mesomelic dysplasia, Nievergelt type | AD | | | Severe mesomelic shortening of legs and sometimes arms, clubfoot deformities, limited extension of elbows | | Walking delayed | Short, triangular and rhomboid-shaped tibia; sometimes shortened fibula and ulna; radioulnar and tarsal synostosis |
| Metatropic dysplasia | AD, AR | | Relatively long trunk with narrow chest, frequently tail-like appendage over sacrum, progressive kyphoscoliosis | Prominent joints with restricted range of motion, hyperextensibility of finger joints | | | Marked platyspondyly; kyphoscoliosis; hypoplastic, crescent-shaped ilia; short, broad, club-shaped long bones; marked metaphyseal flaring of long bones; epiphyseal dysplasia |
| Spondyloepiphyseal congenita (Spranger-Wiedemann type) | AD with most cases representing new mutations | Flat face, occasionally ocular hypertelorism, myopia, short neck, ±cleft palate | Short, barrel-shaped chest, pectus carinatum | Short limbs, neck, and spine; genu valgum; clubfeet; normal-sized hands | | Subluxation of C1–C2 and cord compression, detached retina, hearing loss | Pear-shaped vertebrae, ±odontoid hypoplasia, retarded osseous maturation, shortened long bones, moderate kyphoscoliosis with lumbar lordosis |
| **Conditions Identifiable Later in Life** | | | | | | | |
| Arthro-ophthalmopathy (Stickler syndrome) | AD with variable expression and incomplete penetration | Flat facies with ocular hypertelorism, epicanthal folds, and micrognathia; myopia with retinal detachment during the first 2 decades of life; cleft of the hard or soft palate, or both; bifid uvula; conductive hearing loss | | Hypotonia; hyperextensible knees; prominent joints; later in life, joint pain and morning stiffness | | Respiratory distress from glossoptosis, blindness, cataracts, glaucoma, uveitis, normal height | Wedging of thoracic vertebrae; mild epiphyseal dysplasia; degenerative arthropathy, especially of weight-bearing joints |

(continued)

TABLE 12-10. (Continued)

| Name of Condition | Mode of Inheritance | Head and Neck | Trunk | Limbs | Other | Complications | Radiographic Features |
|---|---|---|---|---|---|---|---|
| | | | Clinical Features | | | | |
| Dyggve-Melchior-Clausen dysplasia | AR | Short neck | Short trunk, prominent sternum, excessive lumbar lordosis, scoliosis | Small hands and feet, claw-like hands, waddling gait, enlarged joints | Retardation in most patients | | Platyspondyly; pear-shaped vertebrae; C1–C2 subluxation; short broad ilia; late ossification of femoral epiphyses; shortening of the tubular bones, with irregular epiphyseal and metaphyseal ossification |
| Dyschondrosteosis | AD with more severe expression | | | Mild forearm shortening, subluxation of distal end of ulna (Madelung's deformity) | Mild short stature in some individuals | Occasional pain in wrist | Radius short in relation to ulna, dorsal subluxation of ulna, short tibia |
| Hypochondroplasia | AD | Macrocephaly with frontal prominence (56%) | Normal, with mild lumbar lordosis | Rhizomelic shortening of extremities, limited elbow extension, broad hands, bowed legs that usually do not require treatment | Mild short stature, muscular appearance | | Lumbosacral interpedicular distant narrowing; short pedicles of vertebrae; short, wide long bones; elongated fibula; short, broad femoral neck |
| Metaphyseal chondrodysplasia, Jansen type | AD | Enlarged, broad head with prominent forehead | | Short limbs, enlarged joints, clubfeet, osseous restriction of mobility, ligamentous hyperlaxity | Hypercalcemia | | Generalized demineralization; widened, splayed, frayed metaphyses; severe shortening and abnormal curvature of tubular bones; hyperostosis of skull; sclerosis of the base of the skull |
| Metaphyseal chondrodysplasia, McKusick type (cartilage hair hypoplasia) | AR, with considerable variation in expression | Fine, spare hair, eyebrows, and lashes; hair usually is lightly pigmented | | Short limbs; short, pudgy hands and feet; laxity of ligaments | Hirschsprung's disease | Malabsorption, immune deficiency, sometimes lethal reactions to varicella infection, increased risk of skin cancer | Metaphyseal flaring and irregularities, shortened long bones, disproportionately long fibula, moderate flattening of vertebral bodies during childhood |
| Metaphyseal chondrodysplasia, Schmid type | | | | Short stature with short extremities, waddling gait, and bowed legs | | | Metaphyseal splaying with cupping of all long bones, shortening of long bones, short femoral necks, coxa vara, genu varum |

| Disorder | Inheritance | | | | | |
|---|---|---|---|---|---|---|
| Multiple epiphyseal dysplasia, Fairbanks type | AD | | Kyphoscoliosis, back pain in later life | Pain or arthritis of hips, knees, and ankles; waddling gait | Mild short stature in some | | Small irregularly ossified epiphyses of all joints, end plates of vertebrae irregular |
| Multiple epiphyseal dysplasia, Ribbing type | AD | | | Pain and progressive osteoarthropathy of hips, ±short hands | Mild short stature in some adults | Total hip replacement | Irregular and delayed ossification of epiphyses with more severe involvement in the hips |
| Pseudoachondroplastic dysplasia (pseudoachondroplasia) | AD and AR | Normal skull and face | Disproportionately long trunk; accentuated lumbar lordosis, mild scoliosis | Shortening of limbs similar to that seen in achondroplasia, hypermobile joints except for elbows; genu valgum or varum; small broad hands; waddling gait | Onset 2 years or later | Osteoarthroses especially of hips and knees | Epiphyseal and metaphyseal dysplasia with striking involvement of the hands and feet, shortened long bones, platyspondyly, tongue-like projection from vertebrae anteriorly, hypoplastic ischium and pubis, irregular acetabulum |
| Spondyloepiphyseal dysplasia tarda | XLR | | Short trunk, prominent sternum, broad thorax, small hips | Osteoarthropathy of hips and knees | Short stature | Pain in back, hips, and knees | Hypoplasia or larger epiphyses, premature osteoarthrosis of hips, platyspondyly with hump-shaped central portion of body, hypoplastic iliac wings |
| Spondylometaphyseal dysplasia tarda | AD | Occasional hyperopia | Short trunk, pectus carinatum, kyphoscoliosis | Limitation of movement of larger joints, knee and hip pain, waddling gait | Short stature | Cesarean section for affected female because of narrow pelvis | Platyspondyly, kyphosis, scoliosis, narrow sacrosciatic notches, metaphyseal irregularities, delayed carpal ossification, short tubular bones |
| Spondyloepimetaphyseal dysplasia, Strudwick type | AR | Occasional cleft palate | Pectus carinatum, scoliosis | Short long bones, genu valgum | Short stature | | Short tubular bones; small epiphyses of proximal femur, humerus, and radius; enlarged epiphyses of knees, mild metaphyseal irregularities; excessive down-slanting of ribs; platyspondyly; narrow ilia, hypoplastic acetabulum |

* Diastrophic dysplasia is thought to be a disease of the cartilage in which inflammation occurs with minimal trauma. The inflammation leads to joint fixation and the ear changes seen in this condition.

Abbreviations: AD, autosomal dominant inheritance; AR, autosomal recessive inheritance; XLR, X-linked recessive inheritance; ±, feature may not be present.

Data modified from Rimoin and Lachman, 1983; Scott, 1988; and Spranger et al, 1974.

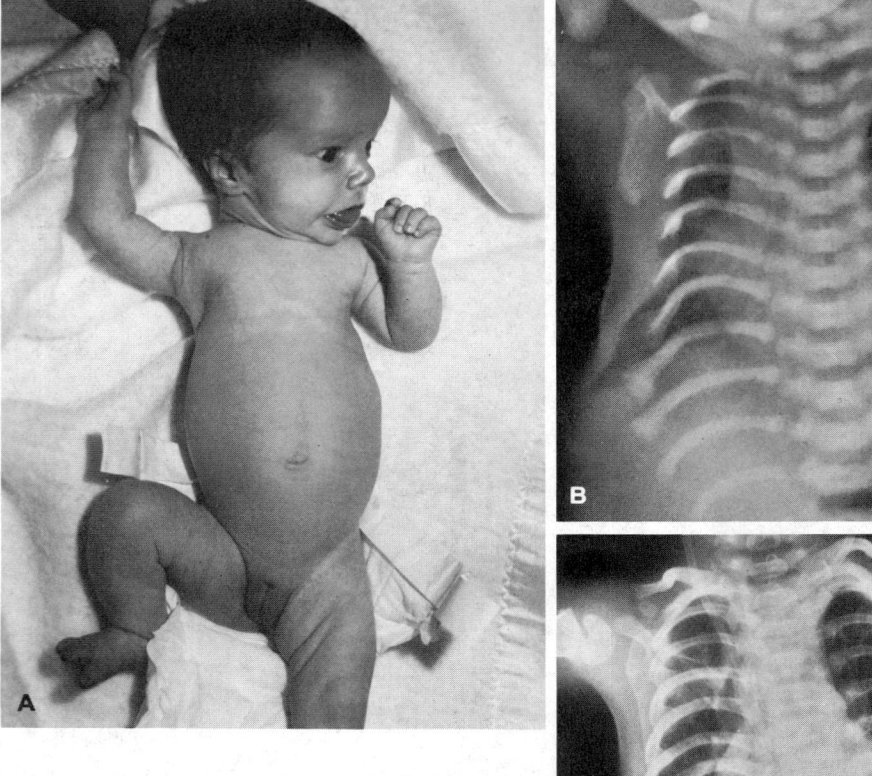

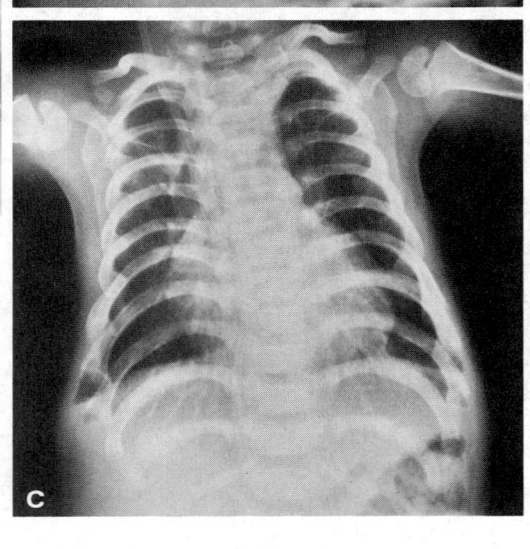

Figure 12-54. Asphyxiating thoracic dysplasia (Jeune syndrome). (A) Six-month-old female infant who had mild respiratory distress, a small rib cage, and relatively normal length of the extremities. (B) Chest radiograph of patient in the newborn period; note the short ribs and small thorax. This child required ventilator support for a few weeks and then nasal oxygen for the rest of the first year. (C) Chest radiograph at about 1 year of age; note enlargement of chest size. Tubes in the picture are nasal oxygen tubes, (Courtesy of Harvey Bender, M.D., University of Notre Dame, South Bend, IN)

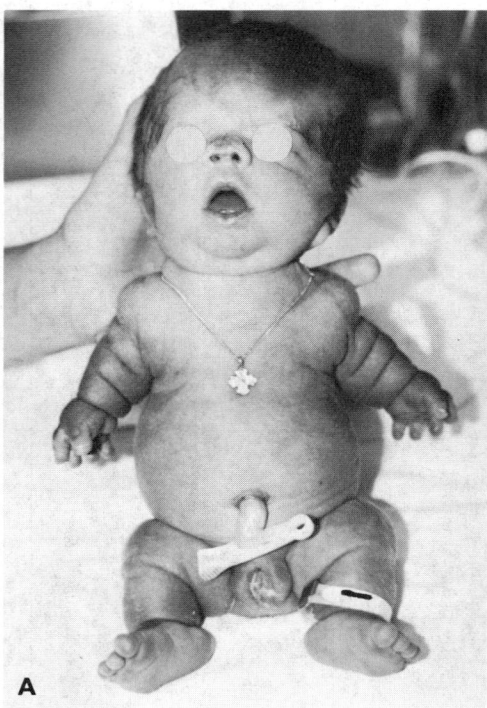

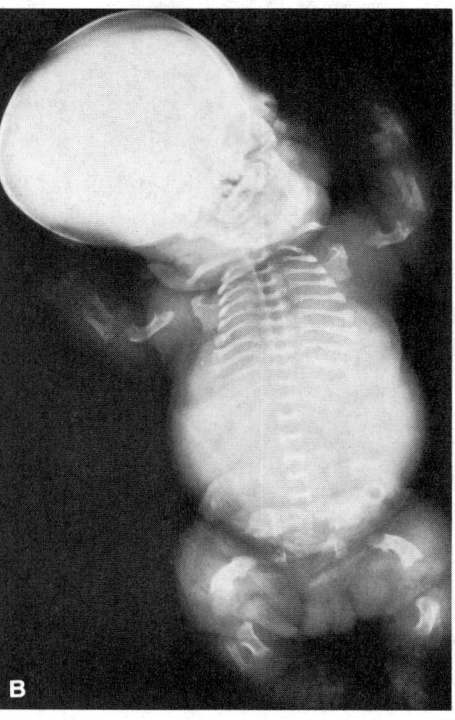

Figure 12-55. Thanatophoric dysplasia. (A) Newborn born at 32 weeks' gestation. Note depressed nasal bridge, short extremities with extra skin fold creases, small chest, and prominent abdomen. The patient died a few hours after the picture was taken. (B) Radiograph of another newborn with thanatophoric dysplasia; note the shortened bowed long bones, the short horizontal ribs, the U-shaped vertebral bodies, and the tiny pelvis.

care, although there may be other problems in the infant such as cleft palate, congenital heart defects, or fractures that will require medical intervention. Instead, these individuals are more likely to require medical, orthopedic, and neurosurgical care as infants, children, and adults. Thus, the spectrum of problems found in the nonlethal skeletal dysplasias usually is quite different from that in the lethal disorders.

Many of the problems encountered in the nonlethal bone dysplasias are chronic and require extensive therapy. Often, they are difficult to treat or resistant to treatment. For example, individuals with achondroplasia typically have small foramina magna that may cause spinal cord compression. If it is severe enough, this problem may result in sudden infant death from apnea during infancy or hydrocephalus at any age. In addition, many individuals with nonlethal skeletal dysplasias may have orthopedic problems, either in the form of malalignment of the legs or back, or in the form of arthritis that requires total joint replacement in some cases.

When providing care for a patient with a nonlethal skeletal dysplasia, the primary care physician needs to become familiar not only with the features of the condition, but also with the associated complications. It is imperative that the physician advise the parents to watch for these complications. Furthermore, the primary care physician should check for the development of these complications on a regular basis. A qualified pediatrician or clinical geneticist and an orthopedic surgeon who is knowledgeable about and experienced in the evaluation and management of these disorders and their complications also should see these children on a regular basis. It should be recognized that, when their disease is managed properly, most individuals with nonlethal bone dysplasias can live relatively normal and productive lives.

## CLINICAL FEATURES OF SKELETAL DYSPLASIAS

Tables 12-9 and 12-10 list the relevant features of the common lethal and nonlethal skeletal dysplasias, respectively. Please refer to the selected readings list at the end of this section for additional information about these disorders.

## PRENATAL DIAGNOSIS OF SKELETAL DYSPLASIAS

Prenatal diagnosis of bone dysplasias can be accomplished for many of the disorders by the use of high-resolution ultrasound. Measurements of long bones and other parts of the fetus may be obtained by the 16th week of gestation. It is possible, therefore, to detect significant shortening of the extremities, a small chest circumference, and, in some cases, the presence of a skeletal dysplasia. If there is no family history of a bone dysplasia, however, there often is no way to diagnose in utero the specific dysplasia that is present.

In the future, prenatal diagnosis of these conditions probably will be made in large part by DNA techniques and will be less equivocal than with current methods. For more specific infor-

**TABLE 12-11. Medical Complications of Both Lethal and Nonlethal Skeletal Dysplasias**

| | |
|---|---|
| Intrauterine | Hydramnios, edema, fractures, hydrocephalus, fetal demise |
| Respiratory | Respiratory distress secondary to small chest and hypoplastic lungs, asphyxiating thoracic dysplasia, small or collapsing trachea, narrowed upper airway and obstruction, snoring, hypoxic episodes |
| Central nervous system | Hydrocephalus, spinal cord compression, nerve damage secondary to instability of cervical vertebrae and stenotic vertebral foramina |
| Skeletal | Kyphosis, scoliosis, excessive lordosis, instability of vertebrae C1 and C2, various vertebral abnormalities, hip dysplasia and dislocated hips, tight and loose joints, joint contracture, osteoarthritis, bowed legs, fractures |
| Muscular | Truncal hypotonia, muscle disease, contractures of the muscles |
| Otolaryngologic | Frequent otitis media, hearing loss (conductive and neurosensory) |
| Dental | Malocclusions, dental crowding, structural abnormalities of teeth |
| Ophthalmologic | Cataracts, severe myopia, retinal detachment, blindness |
| Nutritional | Obesity |
| Obstetric | Constricted birth canal, cephalopelvic disproportions, caesarean required for delivery |

*Modified from Hall JG, Rimoin DL. Medical complications of dwarfing syndromes. Growth Genetics and Hormones 1988;4(2):6.*

**TABLE 12-12. Respiratory Complications That May Be Encountered in Skeletal Dysplasias**

| Pathology | Conditions |
|---|---|
| Small, mechanically abnormal chest | Asphyxiating thoracic dystrophy |
| | Thanatophoric dysplasia |
| | Achondrogenesis types I and II |
| | Hypochondrogenesis |
| | Spondyloepiphyseal dysplasia congenita |
| | Achondroplasia |
| | Achondroplasia, homozygous form |
| | Short rib-polydactyly syndromes |
| | Campomelic dysplasia |
| Upper airway obstruction secondary to retrognathia (Robin sequence) | Arthro-ophthalmopathy |
| | Campomelic dysplasia |
| | Diastrophic dysplasia |
| Upper airway obstruction secondary to basicranial malformations and pharyngeal obstruction | Achondroplasia |
| Laryngeal stenosis | Atelosteogenesis |
| Laryngomalacia | Campomelic dysplasia |
| | Diastrophic dysplasia |
| | Larsen syndrome |
| Tracheobronchomalacia | Campomelic dysplasia |
| | Larsen syndrome |
| | Spondyloepiphyseal dysplasia congenita |
| Central apnea due to medullary compression caused by foramen magnum stenosis | Achondroplasia |
| | Achondroplasia, homozygous form |
| Central apnea due to cervical or medullary compression caused by cervical spine instability | Larsen syndrome |
| | Spondyloepiphyseal dysplasia congenita |

*Modified from Harding CO, Green CG, Perloff WH, Pauli RM. Respiratory complications in children with spondyloepiphyseal dysplasia congenita. Pediatr Pulmonol 1990;9:49.*

mation on current techniques used for the prenatal diagnosis of these disorders, including ultrasound techniques, one should consult the reference by Weaver (1992), a clinical geneticist, or an obstetrician.

## MANAGEMENT OF SKELETAL DYSPLASIAS

Because of the many complications that can arise with the various types of skeletal dysplasias, a number of different specialists should be available for consultation. Those that should be accessible are a pediatrician, a clinical geneticist, and an orthopedic surgeon, as mentioned previously, as well as an ophthalmologist, an otolaryngologist, a psychologist, a neurologist, a neurosurgeon, a dentist, an orthodontist, a dietitian, and physical and occupational therapists. The primary pediatrician or family practitioner caring for the child should coordinate the management and treatment of the child in most cases.

### Complications

Each of the bone dysplasias has a set of recognized complications. The same complications, however, may be encountered in a number of different disorders. Table 12-11 lists many of the recurring medical complications seen in bone dysplasias, and Table 12-12 delineates further the respiratory problems that may be encountered in these disorders.

### Genetic Counseling

Parents of children and adults with skeletal dysplasias need to be informed of the mode of inheritance of their particular disorder and of the degree of risk they face that any further children they may have will be affected. Depending on the inheritance pattern of the condition and whether one or both of the parents is affected, the risk will vary from the general background risk (ie, usually less than 1% to as high as 75%). Parents of a child with an autosomal dominant bone dysplasia who are normal them-

selves most likely do not have an increased risk of having another child with the disorder because their affected child probably is the result of a new mutation. New evidence suggests, however, that in some of these families, one parent may have a germline mosaicism. Germline mosaicism occurs when a clone of germ cells contains a new mutation and, even though the somatic cells of the parent do not carry the mutation, that parent is at increased risk for having another child with the same genetic condition. For example, osteogenesis imperfecta type II (Fig 12-56) previously was thought to be a typical autosomal recessive disorder. Recent evidence, however, indicates that the affected offspring in most families with this disease represents a new autosomal dominant mutation in the heterozygous state. The recurrence risk for parents who previously have had a child with osteogenesis imperfecta type II has been observed to be 5% to 7%, instead of 25%, which is the risk for an autosomal recessive trait, or much less than 1%, which is the risk for a new autosomal dominant mutation. The recurrence of children affected with this condition now is thought to be produced by germline mosaicism for an autosomal dominant trait rather than associated with an autosomal recessive pattern of inheritance. Biochemical evidence supports this contention.

If the skeletal dysplasia in a particular family is X-linked recessive and the mother is a carrier, the recurrence risk in subsequent children of the parents is 25%. If the child's condition is inherited in an autosomal recessive manner, the parents' risk of having future children with the disorder also is 25%. In the latter case, the affected child's risk of having an affected offspring is less than 1%, assuming that his or her mate is not a relative. On the other hand, if one parent has an autosomal dominant skeletal dysplasia, the couple will have a 50% risk of having an affected offspring.

### Psychosocial Counseling

Parents who have given birth to a child with a lethal bone dysplasia need a great deal of emotional support. After the birth of

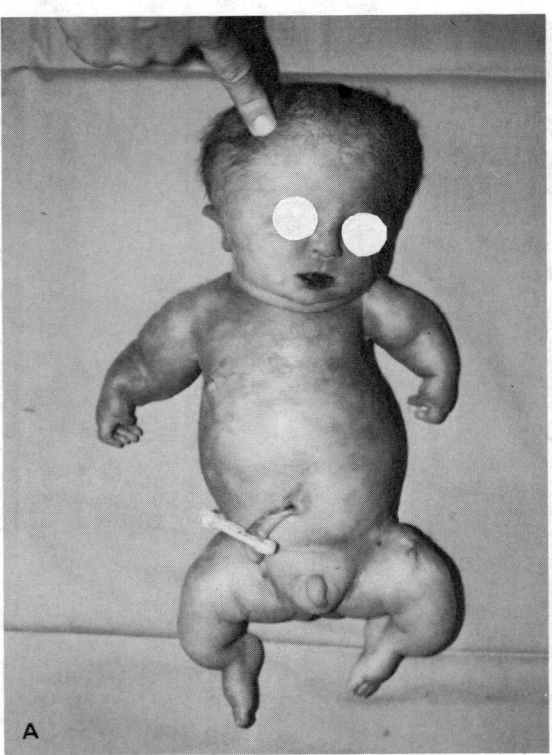
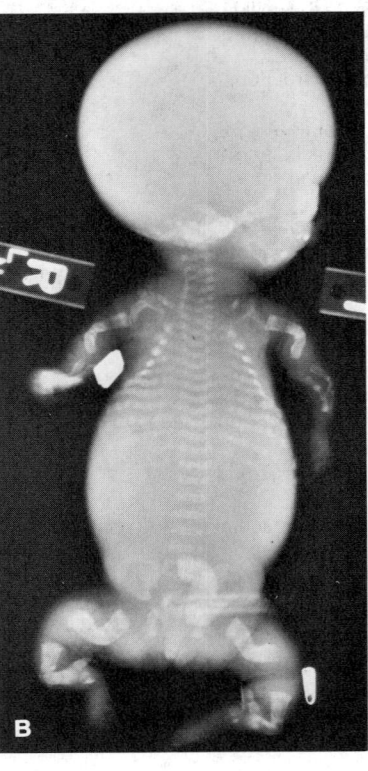

**Figure 12-56.** Osteogenesis imperfecta, type II. (**A**) Newborn who died immediately after birth from respiratory insufficiency; note lack of calcified calvaria (finger easily indenting skull), and bowed arms and legs. (**B**) Radiograph of another patient with this condition; note the demineralization of all bones (particularly the skull), the ribbon shape of the long bones, and the multiple fractures (particularly those of the ribs).

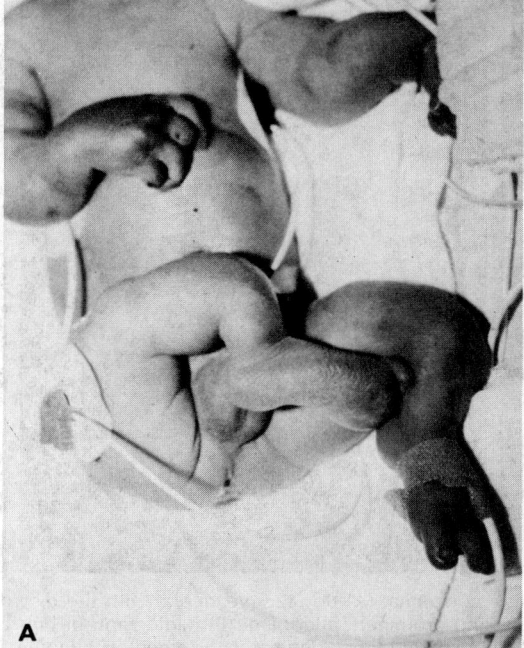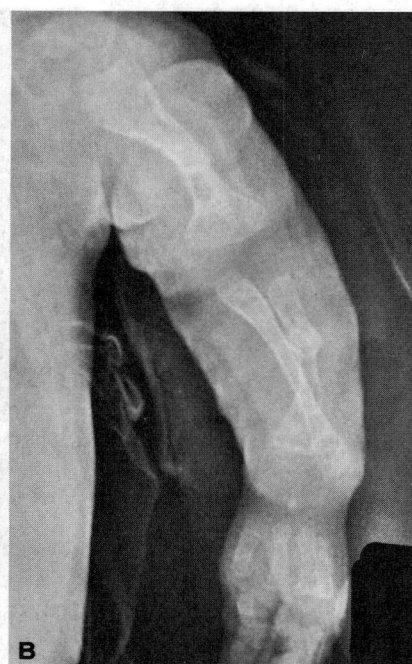

Figure 12-57. Osteogenesis imperfecta type III. (**A**) Extremities and trunk of a newborn who survived; note marked bowing of the extremities. (**B**) Radiograph of another patient (age 1 month) with this condition; note marked osteoporosis, relative thinness, and fractures of the bones.

their affected child, they will go through the various stages of grief that are seen with the birth of any defective child. All caregivers need to be concerned, sympathetic, and available to spend time with the parents discussing their child's condition and their feelings.

Parents who deliver a child with a nonlethal dysplasia also will have similar emotional reactions. In addition, they may be filled with numerous questions, such as how tall their child will be as an adult, what problems the child will have, and whether he or she will be normal intellectually. If the answers are known, they should be provided. Furthermore, at some time, the parents may wish to become involved in a support group such as a local chapter of the Little People of America (LPA National, c/o Jean Elmendorf, PO Box 9897, Washington, DC 20016). Because this organization is composed of parents of children with bone dysplasias, their affected children, and adults with these disorders, these individuals can provide answers, support, and fellowship for these parents and their affected youngsters. From the physician's standpoint, the goals of counseling parents are to have them make the best possible adjustment to their child's condition and to encourage them to foster age-related, not size-related, behavior, social interaction, and independence in their child.

## Medical Management

Appropriate respiratory support, if it is needed, should be undertaken if the decision is made to support a neonate with a skeletal dysplasia. Respiratory therapy may be managed better with a tracheostomy. If the child is weaned from the ventilator and survives, he or she probably will require long-term respiratory management, even if it is only in the form of supplemental nasal oxygen. During infancy, children with skeletal dysplasias, particularly those with achondroplasia, should be evaluated for the development of hydrocephalus. This evaluation should be done by periodic measurement of the head circumference (see Horton et al., 1978 for head circumference graphs of achondroplasia) and, if there is excessive head growth, by ultrasound, computerized axial tomographic, or magnetic resonance imaging assess-

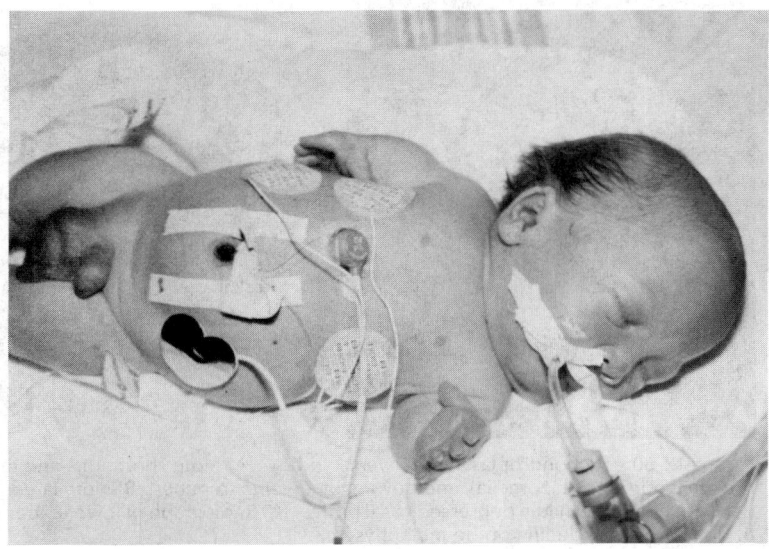

Figure 12-58. Diastrophic dysplasia in a term newborn. Note the short extremities, relatively normal chest size, and normal ears. The ears became inflamed at about 2 weeks of age and developed the typical cauliflower appearance seen in this disorder. The patient had tracheomalacia and respiratory distress during infancy, but now has no significant respiratory problems.

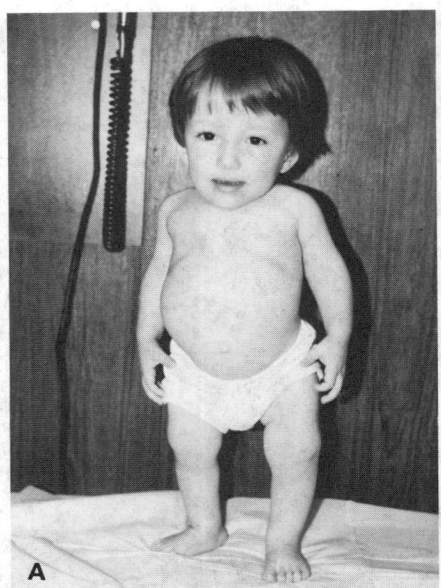
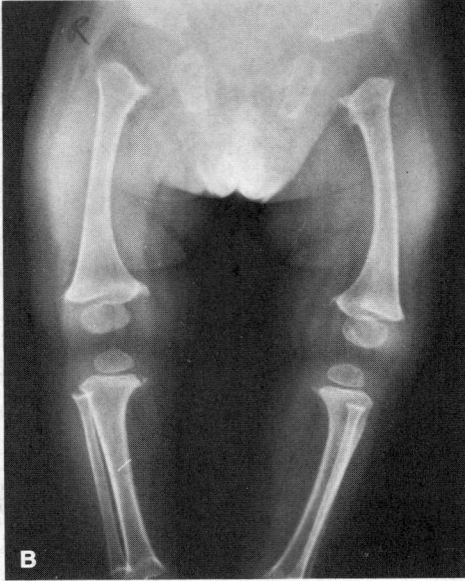
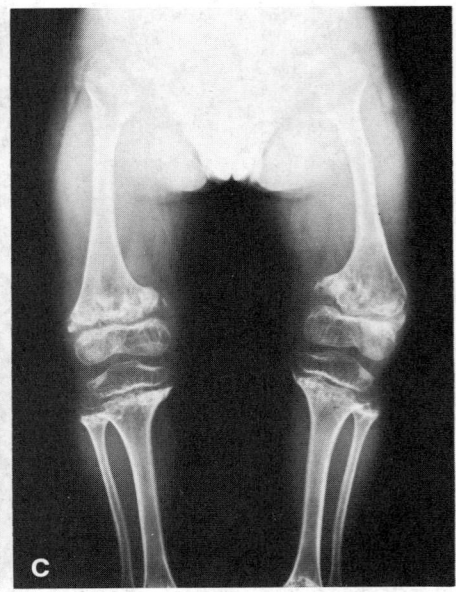

**Figure 12-59.** Spondyloepiphyseal dysplasia congenita. (**A**) Boy (2.5 years old) with the disorder; note short stature, chest deformity, lordosis, and prominent abdomen. (**B**) Radiograph of hips and lower extremities of patient at 9 months of age; note mild metaphyseal involvement. (**C**) Radiograph of patient's hips and legs at 9.5 years of age; note the marked involvement of the metaphyses at this age.

ment of the brain. If there is apnea or other unexplained neurologic problems in any child with a bone dysplasia, the size of the foramen magnum should be assessed, because it may be abnormally small and may be the source of the problems. If this problem is found, decompression by enlarging the foramen should be considered. The size of the foramen magnum probably should be assessed in all newborns or infants who have achondroplasia because as many as 11% have been found to have significant compression of the cord by the foramen. These infants then are in need of prophylactic decompression (Dr. Richard Pauli, personal communications, 1992).

In infancy and childhood, recurrent upper airway infections

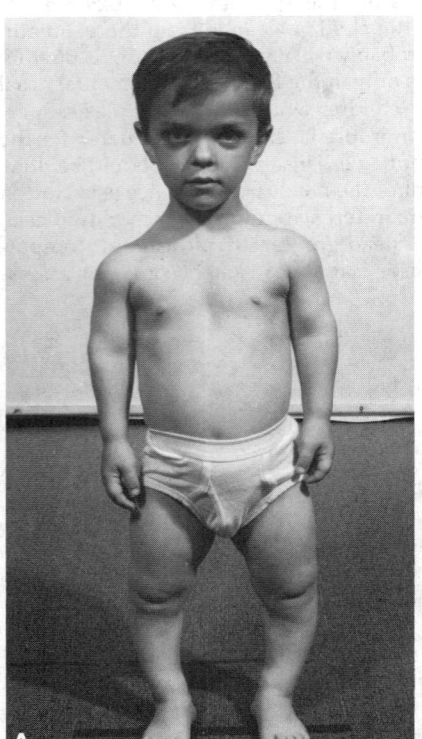
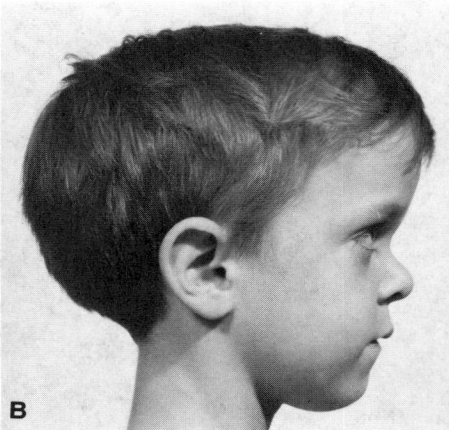
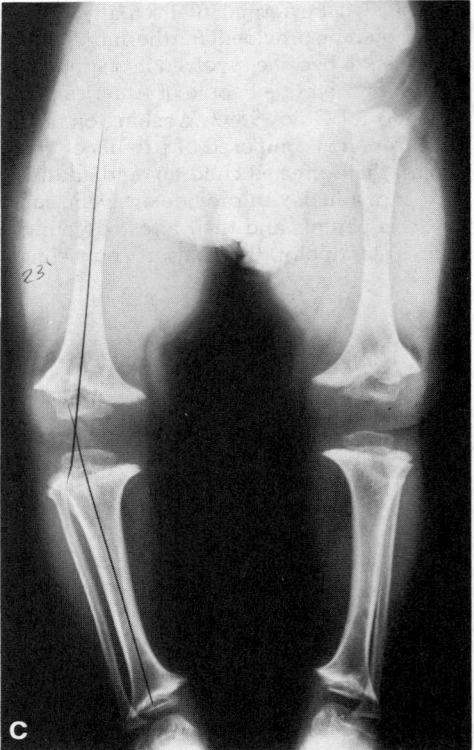

**Figure 12-60.** Achondroplasia in a 7-year-old boy. (**A**) Note short arms and legs, particularly in the proximal portions (rhizomelia), and bowing of lower extremities. (**B**) Note larger than normal dolichocephalic head and mildly depressed nasal bridge. (**C**) Radiograph of lower extremities; note angulation of right leg and widening of the metaphyses.

and otitis media are common. These infections should be treated appropriately and the child's hearing should be checked periodically. Skeletal deformities and malalignment problems also are frequent during childhood and, although they may be amenable to bracing, these problems often require surgical correction. Obesity is common among children and adults with skeletal dysplasias. Good dietary and nutritional habits should be encouraged starting in early childhood.

Exercise should be promoted in children with bone dysplasias to assist in weight control and to develop strength and good tone. These children, however, should avoid strenuous physical activities and contact sports, opting instead for activities such as swimming and bicycling, in which there is less trauma to the joints. Arthritis and neurologic problems are encountered commonly in teenagers and adults with bone dysplasias. Frequently, these problems are more severe in overweight individuals or in those who have been unusually active.

Because medical problems are relatively common and often are serious in individuals with bone dysplasias, both during childhood and later in life, complaints by these people should be taken seriously by medical personnel and investigated thoroughly. When problems are detected, appropriate management must be undertaken to prevent lifelong disabilities and death.

## Surgical Management

Many nonosseous birth defects such as cleft lip and congenital heart disease may be found in infants with skeletal dysplasias, and these problems in themselves may require treatment in infancy or early childhood. As stated previously, skeletal problems frequently develop with age and should be treated at appropriate times and by appropriate means. For instance, bowing of the legs in children with achondroplasia is common and results from the fact that the fibulas grow more rapidly than do the tibias. If one or both of the fibular epiphyses are removed surgically at a judicious time, the child will finish growing with straight legs.

Other skeletal problems commonly found in individuals with skeletal dysplasias that may require surgical intervention include

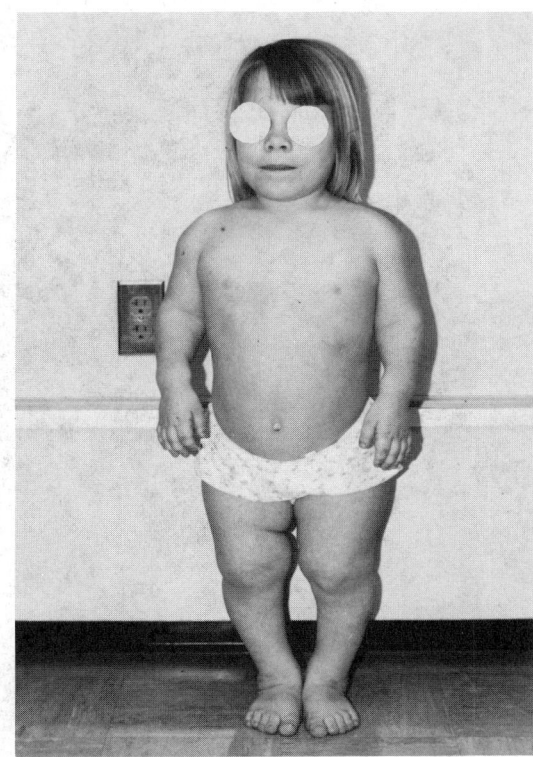

Figure 12-62.  Pseudoachondroplasia in an 11-year-old child; note short stature, short extremities, and normal face. Children and adults with this condition have more osteoarthroses than do individuals with achondroplasia.

scoliosis, kyphosis, hip dysplasia, coxa vara, coxa valga, genu valgum, atlantoaxial instability, arthritis, and spinal or nerve root compression. If arthritis is present and is severe enough to cause either significant pain or immobility, the person may benefit from joint replacement. Many neurologic problems that are encountered in skeletal dysplasias result from abnormal size or shape of the vertebrae or small vertebral foramina. Surgical invention may be functional or lifesaving in these situations.

The surgeon who treats children with bone dysplasias should be experienced in the treatment of these problems. Often, the surgical management of these problems differs from the management of similar orthopedic problems in other patient populations. For example, in diastrophic dysplasia, the cartilage becomes inflamed with minimal trauma, leading to marked joint stiffness and joint fusion. Clubfoot is a common result. Treatment of the foot is not directed at making the foot mobile, but rather at keeping the foot in a functional position, allowing the person to bear weight and ambulate.

## LIVING WITH SKELETAL DYSPLASIAS

The individual with a skeletal dysplasia frequently must cope with medical problems that are associated with his or her disorder. Because of these problems, the affected child or adult may have medical expenses that are higher than usual, may need to see physicians more frequently, and may be more likely to be hospitalized than is the average individual. Furthermore, older children and adults with bone dysplasias often have more aches, pains, and discomfort than do individuals without these conditions.

Being short because of a bone dysplasia poses many other disadvantages to the individual. The living spaces for many so-

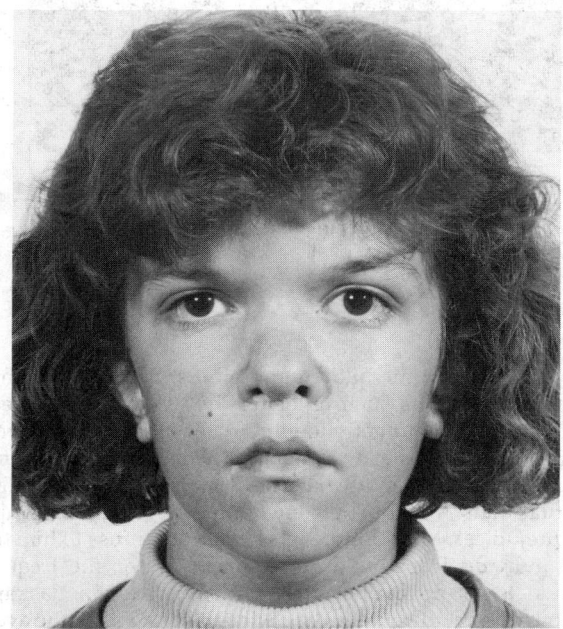

Figure 12-61.  Facial view of a 13-year-old child with achondroplasia; note mild depression of the nose, shortening of the nose, and mild malar hypoplasia.

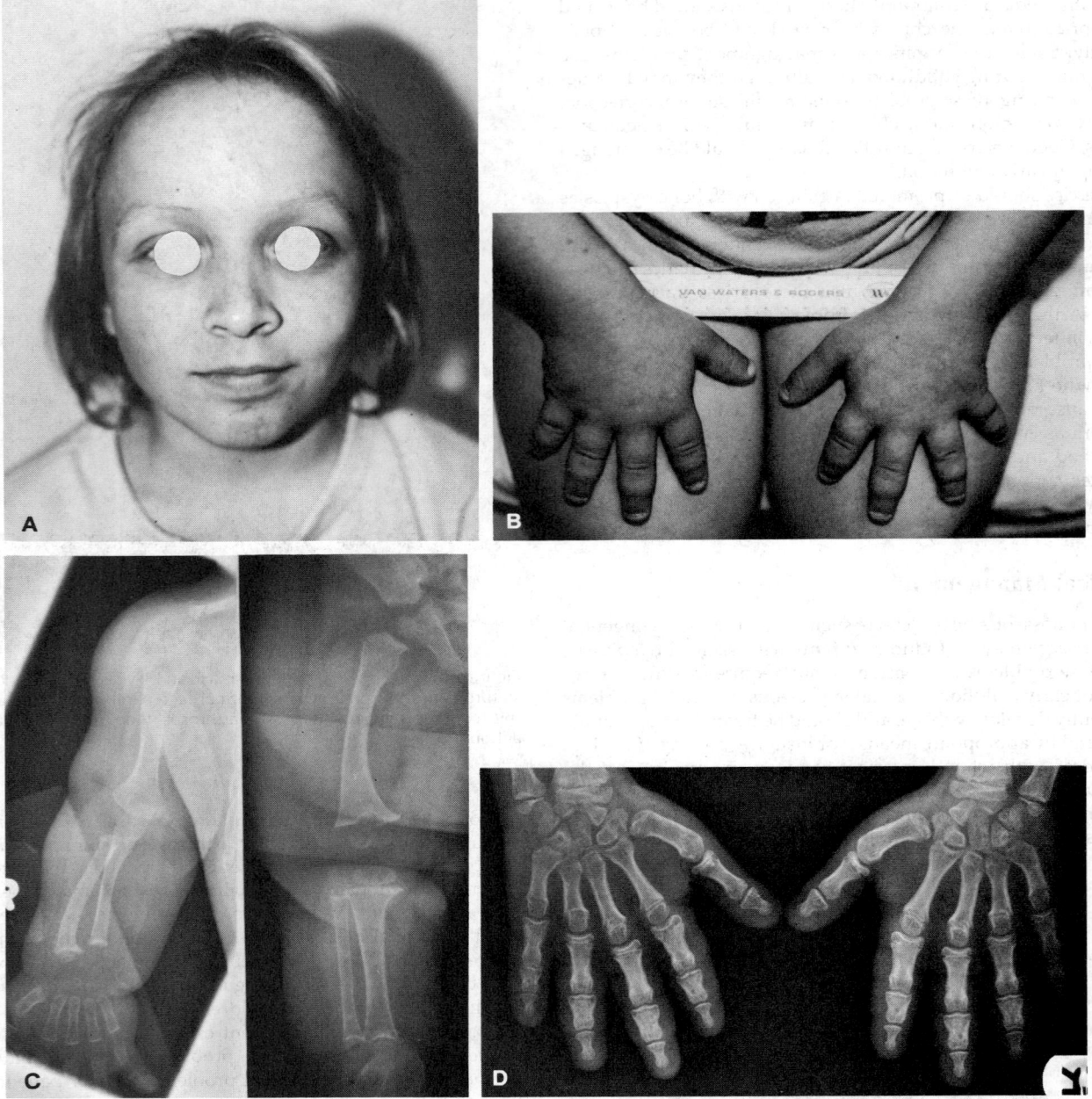

**Figure 12-63.** Metaphyseal dysplasia, McKusick type (cartilage hair hypoplasia). (**A**) 13-year-old girl with the disorder; note thinning of hair and normal facial appearance. (**B**) Hands of the same patient; note short fingers. (**C**) Radiographs of the patient at age 9 months; note bowing of femur and widening of the metaphyses. (**D**) Radiographs of the hands of the patient at age 13 years; note shortening of all tubular bones.

cieties are designed for persons who are at least 154 cm (5 ft) tall. As a result, short individuals find it more difficult to live in a world designed for taller people. Many short people experience prejudice that affects their self-image directly or indirectly, affects their earning power, and affects their acceptance in society. Difficulties encountered by little people include being unable to reach the steering wheel or pedals of an automobile without pillows or pedal extenders, being unable to touch the floor with their legs when sitting in a chair, having to hem or alter most clothing, having people bump into them in public places because they do not see them, and being unable to reach light switches, window latches, or curtain pulls. Emotional situations that little people experience include being teased about their height, being stared

at frequently by both children and adults, being placed in embarrassing situations such as being the "class dwarf," feeling smothered (unable to get enough air) when they are in crowds where everyone is taller, and being leaned upon or patted on top of the head as an animal would be. The most devastating problems that many small people encounter, however, are employment prejudices. Many employers hesitate or refuse to hire them. If the individual does find employment, he or she frequently receives a lower-paying position and does not advance as rapidly as do other, similarly qualified individuals. As a result, the average little person earns less and has a lower standard of living than does the average normal-sized individual in the society.

Physicians and other medical personnel who care for children

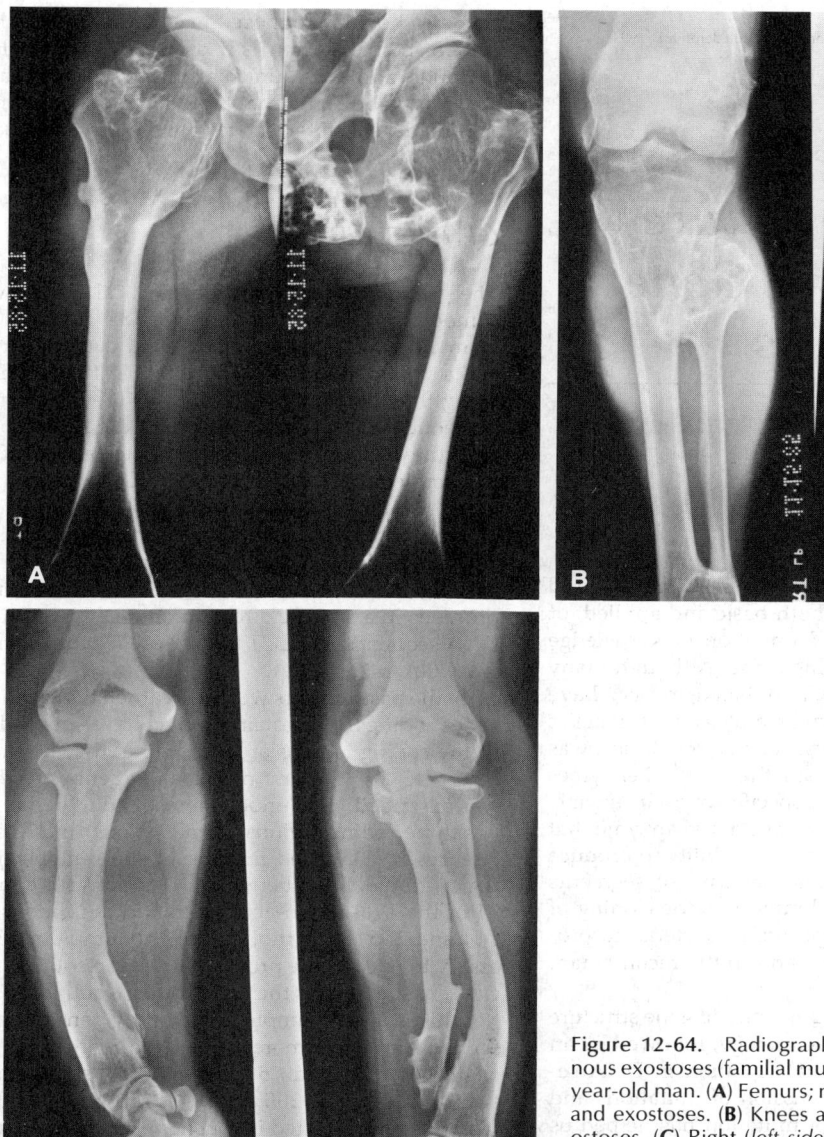

**Figure 12-64.** Radiographs of multiple cartilaginous exostoses (familial multiple exostoses) in a 30-year-old man. (**A**) Femurs; note broadening of neck and exostoses. (**B**) Knees and lower legs; note exostoses. (**C**) Right (*left side*) and left (*right side*) elbows and forearms; note hypoplasia of the ulnae and bowing of the radii.

and adults with skeletal dysplasias need to be sensitive to the physical, social, and emotional problems faced by these individuals. All possible efforts should be made to meet the needs of short people and to make them feel as comfortable as possible in the medical environment where they receive medical care, be it the physician's office, the outpatient clinic at a medical center, or the hospital. Despite all the difficulty that most little people encounter, they learn to accept being short, adjust their living style to compensate for their shortness, and even have a sense of humor about their size. Most are well-adjusted individuals who get along just fine. In addition to providing a good quality of health care, the pediatrician also can help these individuals by being supportive and by attempting to break down the medical, physical, and psychologic barriers that they face.

## PHOTOGRAPHIC ALBUM

Figures 12–57 through 12–64 provide examples of other bone dysplasias.

## Selected Readings

Hall JG, Rimoin DL. Medical complications of dwarfing syndromes. Growth Genetics and Hormones 1988;4(2):6.

Harding CO, Green CG, Perloff WH, Pauli RM. Respiratory complications in children with spondyloepiphyseal dysplasia congenita. Pediatr Pulmonol 1990;9:49.

Horton WA, Rotter JI, Rimoin DL, Scott CI, Hall JG. Standard growth curves for achondroplasia. J Pediatr 1978;93:435.

Maroteaux P, Beighton P, Poznanski AK, et al. International nomenclature of constitutional diseases of bone, with bibliography. Birth Defects 1986;22:1.

McKusick VA. Heritable disorders of connective tissue. Saint Louis: CV Mosby, 1972:72.

Rimoin DL, Lachman RS. The chondrodysplasias. In: Emery AEH, Rimoin DL, eds. Principles and practice of medical genetics. New York: Churchill Livingstone, 1983:703.

Scott CI Jr. Dwarfism. Clin Symp 1988;40:2.

Spranger JW, Langer LO Jr, Wiedemann HR. Bone dysplasia: An atlas of constitutional disorders of skeletal development. Philadelphia: WB Saunders, 1974.

Spranger J, Marateaux P. The lethal osteochondrodysplasias. Adv Hum Genet 1990;19:1.

Weaver DD. Catalog of prenatally diagnosed disorders, 2nd ed. Baltimore: Johns Hopkins University Press, 1992.

Winter RM, Knowles SAS, Bieber FR, Baraitser M. The malformed fetus and stillborn: A diagnostic approach. Chapter 21. New York: John Wiley and Sons, 1988: 183.

*Principles and Practice of Pediatrics, Second Edition.*
edited by Frank A. Oski et al. J. B. Lippincott Company, Philadelphia © 1994.

## CHAPTER 13
# Molecular Genetics: Gene Structure, the Nature of Mutation, and Gene Diagnosis

### Haig H. Kazazian, Jr.

The "golden age" of biology and medical science began around 1945 and can be traced to the work, both basic and applied, of many investigators; they forged the foundation of knowledge now rapidly revolutionizing modern medicine. Although many disciplines, particularly immunology and biochemistry, have participated in this revolution, molecular biology and genetics have played a special role. The catalyst for this revolution was the discovery of restriction endonucleases, the bacterial enzymes that cut DNA at precise recognition sites specific for each enzyme. This discovery, along with that of another bacterial enzyme that ligates two pieces of DNA together, led to the ability to produce recombinant DNA (ie, DNA fragments made up of segments from different species). This ability led rapidly to the cloning of human DNA in vectors known to replicate in bacteria, to production of libraries of DNA fragments, and to the recombinant DNA era.

In this chapter we discuss the basic principles of gene structure and the basics of recombinant DNA technology, followed by an outline of what we know about normal variation in DNA sequences. The chapter ends with a discussion of mutations and how our knowledge of specific sites of mutation has helped us learn which nucleotide sequences are important in gene expres-

sion and how to diagnose the genetic diseases they produce. Included in this section is a discussion of nonclassical forms of mutation and some unusual modes of inheritance. Because of space limitations the chapter touches on only the highlights, and the reader is referred to specialized textbooks for further information.

## GENE STRUCTURE

The genetic material is double-helical DNA, with each strand composed of the deoxyribonucleotides A, G, T, C (adenylic acid, guanylic acid, thymidylic acid, and cytidylic acid, respectively) and a sugar-phosphate backbone (Fig 13-1). This backbone runs along the outside of the helix, and the base components of the nucleotides face into the interior of the helix. In that central portion, the critical hydrogen bonds between A of one strand and its complement T of the other, or G of one strand and C of the other, are formed. The human genome contains about $3 \times 10^9$ of these base pairs. The base-pairing rules (A with T and G with C) are critical in information transfer both during DNA replication and transcription of the DNA code into RNA. Transcription also proceeds in a specific direction on a DNA strand; for example, a DNA sequence 3'-TGCTT-5' is decoded during transcription into 5'-ACGAA-3' in RNA.

In the past 15 years we have learned that nearly all mammalian genes coding for a protein product have split coding regions; that is, the coding regions are discontinuous. The example shown in Figure 13-2 is the first mammalian gene for which this feature was described, the β-globin gene of adult hemoglobin. This gene has three coding regions, termed exons, and two intervening sequences (IVS), called introns. In the β-globin gene the coding regions are divided between the codons for amino acids 30 and 31 of the 146-amino-acid chain and the codons for amino acids 104 and 105. Even though only about 450 nucleotides are necessary to encode the protein (three nucleotides/amino acid), because of the introns the gene contains roughly 1500 nucleotides. Yet this is a very simple gene. Many genes have now been described with ten or more introns (the gene for the pro-α 1 collagen chain has more than 50 introns), and some genes have a total size of more than 200 kilobases (kb) or 200,000 base pairs. In fact, the gene affected in Duchenne muscular dystrophy has between 2.0 and 2.5 million base pairs. On the other hand, certain genes, such as those encoding histones and interferons, are small and do not contain introns. These genes are unexplained exceptions to the split gene rule.

How protein-coding genes are expressed is exemplified by the globins (Fig 13-3). The entire gene, including the two introns, is transcribed into a precursor RNA. This RNA is immediately modified at both its ends (called 5' and 3' ends). The modification at the 5' end is an addition of a methylated G in an unusual triphosphate linkage. This modification, which is specific for messenger RNA, is called 5' capping. The modification at the 3' end is the addition of about 150 A residues (the poly A tail). The 5' cap is thought to be important in translating the RNA into protein, while the 3' poly A tail may have a role in RNA stability. Next, the introns are precisely spliced out of the RNA, thereby approximating the coding region sequences. The precise mechanism and the enzymes involved in RNA splicing are becoming

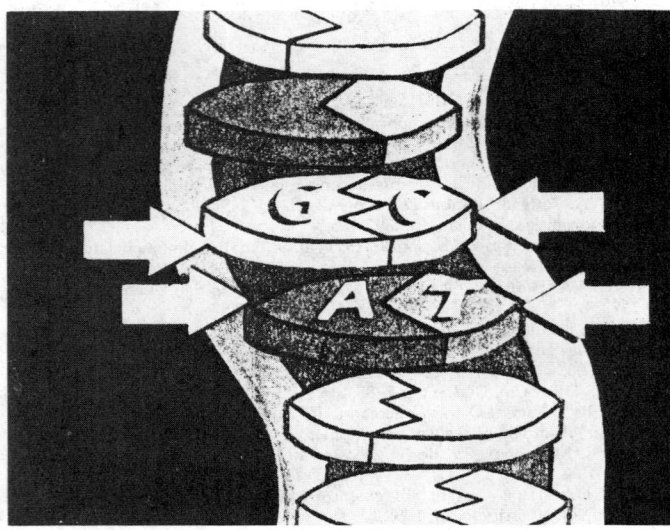

**Figure 13-1.** Base pairing in DNA. As shown, G of one strand pairs by hydrogen bonding with C of the other strand. Likewise, A pairs with T.

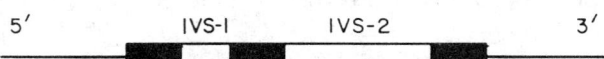

**Figure 13-2.** β-globin gene: a typical split gene coding for a protein. Black areas denote exons or regions encoded into protein; open areas denote introns. This gene is quite simple, with two introns and three exons. *IVS-1,* intron-1; *IVS-2,* intron-2.

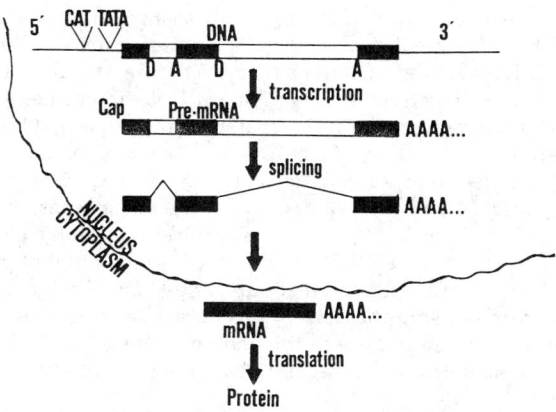

**Figure 13-3.** Gene expression. Steps include (1) transcription of precursor RNA, (2) cap and poly A addition to the ends of the RNA, (3) splicing out of intron sequences, and (4) translation of the mature messenger RNA into protein. CAT and TATA in front of the gene refer to sequences important in transcription, while D and A refer to donor and acceptor splice junctions important in RNA splicing.

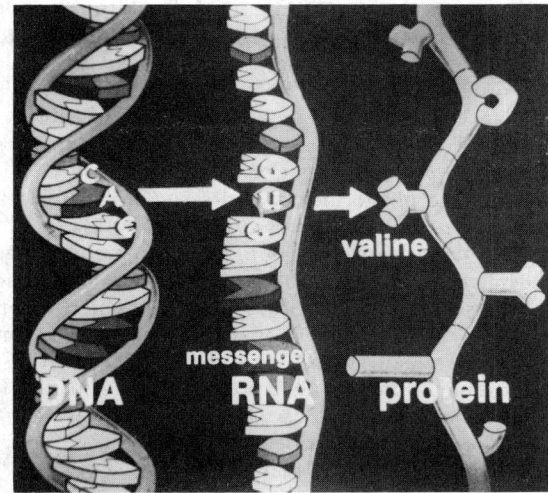

**Figure 13-4.** Relationship between the triplet code in the strand of DNA that is transcribed, the codon in messenger RNA, and the specific amino acid inserted in the polypeptide chain. For instance, CAC in the DNA is transcribed into GUG in RNA and the amino acid inserted is valine. Shown here is the mutant sequence in the β-globin gene for the β^s or sickle hemoglobin chain. The sequence of normal β^A-globin DNA for the strand shown is CTC.

understood. We know that splicing is important in transporting the RNA from the nucleus to the cytoplasm, where it will be translated into protein. We also know that nucleotide sequences near the exon-intron junctions are important in normal splicing. Translation then occurs on the fully processed messenger RNA in the cytoplasm.

The genetic code as found in the messenger RNA is critical to translation. There are 64 possible combinations of a code composed of three nucleotides. One combination, AUG (note that U is substituted for T in RNA) is the initiation codon and always places methionine as the initial amino acid in a protein. Methionine is usually not the first amino acid in the finished protein because it is often removed while the nascent protein is in the early stages of production. The code also contains three terminator codons, UAG, UAA, and UGA. These codons cannot be decoded into an amino acid and, therefore, protein synthesis terminates whenever one of these triplets is present in the reading frame. A mutation in the coding region of a gene that produces a terminator codon is called a nonsense mutation. The remaining 60 codons can be decoded so that an amino acid is inserted into the growing or nascent polypeptide chain. The degeneracy of the genetic code allows for six different codons for leucine and serine, and four codons for many other of the total of 20 amino acids. This degeneracy permits some variation in the coding DNA sequence without necessarily producing a change in the amino acid encoded.

The relationship between the nucleotide triplet in DNA, its complement in messenger RNA, and the amino acid designated by that triplet is demonstrated for the sixth codon of the β-globin chain in Figure 13-4. CTC in DNA is decoded GAG in messenger RNA and glutamate in the protein. A single nucleotide substitution in the codon (T to A) leads to sickle-cell anemia, as discussed later.

## GENOME ORGANIZATION

The reader must understand the environment within the genome in which a gene is located, and this involves the topic of gene families. Again, the example chosen from many known gene families is the β-globin gene cluster. In this family of related genes there are five functional genes, one embryonic (ε), two fetal (Gγ and Aγ), a minor adult (δ), and a major adult (β) (Fig 13-5). These genes account for only about 7500 nucleotides, or 15% of

the roughly 50,000 nucleotides in this cluster. The functional genes are arranged in order of their expression in development (ie, embryonic, fetal, and adult). A single pseudogene sequence, Ψβ1, is also found in this cluster. This pseudogene sequence is very similar to the β-gene sequence, but it contains mutations that prevent gene expression. Pseudogenes may be evolutionary vestiges much like the anatomical appendix.

The function of the roughly 40 kilobases (kb) of flanking sequences in this cluster is unknown, but repeated sequences are interspersed between the functional globin genes. Some of these sequences (designated in Fig 13-5 by an A) are repeated over 500,000 times in the genome. These sequences are called Alu sequences because many of them contain an Alu I restriction endonuclease site (see below). They are about 300 nucleotides long, and when compared to one another are roughly 95% homologous. Another often repeated sequence (a LINE, or long interspersed element) is found in two places in the β-globin gene cluster, 3' to the β-gene and between the δ and Gγ gene. This sequence or an incomplete form of it occurs about 100,000 times in the genome. Some copies of this repeat sequence are transposable elements; they can be transcribed into RNA, reverse-transcribed into DNA, and some of the DNA copies can be reinserted back into the genome in a new location (see below). The occurrence of repeated sequences located in the flanking DNA between functional gene sequences is a general characteristic of the human genome.

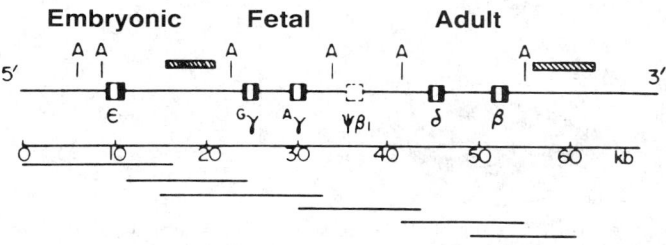

**Figure 13-5.** β-globin gene cluster with repeated sequences designated by A and shaded rectangles. Functional gene sequences are designated ε, Gγ, Aγ, δ, and β. The Ψβ1 sequence is a pseudogene that is similar to a β-globin gene but has mutations that prevent its function.

The lines at the bottom of Figure 13–5 indicate the cloned DNA fragments from this region that have been aligned to determine the organization of the β-gene cluster. These cloned fragments were isolated from a library containing essentially the entire human genome in 15- to 20-kb pieces. This library was developed by Tom Maniatis and his coworkers, who took the bacteriophage λ, which grows in *E coli*, and removed a 17-kb DNA piece of the phage that does not contain sequences important for phage replication and growth by cutting it out with a restriction endonuclease (Fig 13-6). They then partially digested about 200 micrograms of total human genomic DNA (this amount of DNA represents that found in the leukocytes of 2 to 4 mL of whole blood) with a restriction enzyme to generate fragments with an average size of 15 kb. The human fragments were then ligated to the important sequences of the phage to regenerate recombinant phage of about 50 kb (15 kb of which were human in origin). The recombinant phage were then grown in *E coli*, initially in broth and then on agar plates.

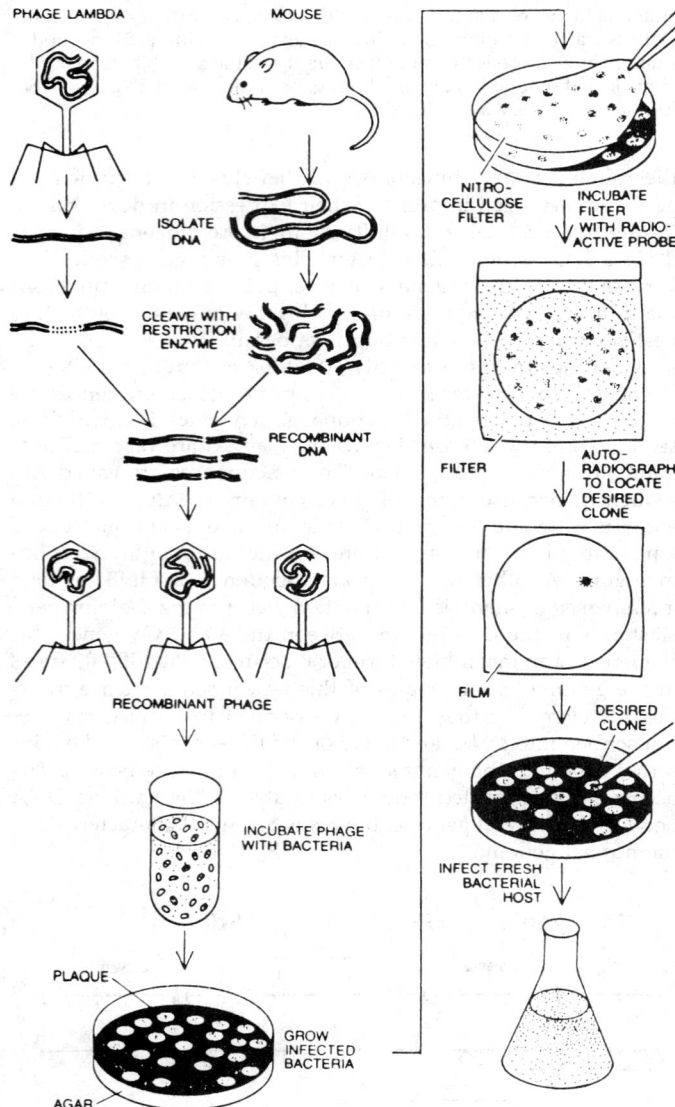

**Figure 13-6.**   Cloning of DNA fragments in bacteriophage λ. The process of cloning DNA fragments from human leukocytes is identical to that shown here in the mouse. Each plaque at the bottom left is derived from a single bacterium containing a single λ phage. The desired clone is isolated as demonstrated on the right half of the figure, and it can be obtained in large amounts.

Each *E coli* bacterium can accept only a single phage molecule; this is the key ingredient to molecular cloning. Thus, each colony of *E coli* has its origin from a single bacterium and contains no more than a single type of recombinant DNA molecule. Not all *E coli* contain phage, and those that do can be detected because they are lysed by phage, forming a clear area or plaque. Since the human genome contains roughly $3 \times 10^9$ base pairs or $3 \times 10^6$ kb of DNA and the average size of the recombinant human fragments is about 15 kb, theoretically the entire human genome could be contained in $3 \times 10^6/15$ or $2 \times 10^5$ recombinant phage. Thus, it is necessary to screen about 200,000 *E coli* colonies containing recombinant phage from this library in order to isolate a sequence found only once in the genome. This is precisely how the sequences from the β-gene cluster represented in Figure 13-5 were isolated.

This library of human DNA fragments was screened for the β-globin gene by using radioactive copies of the β-globin messenger RNA. It was easy to isolate β-globin messenger RNA from human reticulocytes (it makes up about 45% of the messenger RNA in these specialized cells). The β-messenger RNA was then used to make a complementary DNA (cDNA), which is an exact complementary copy of the RNA in which each U is substituted by a T. This copy was made by the enzyme reverse transcriptase of avian myeloblastosis virus in the presence of radioactive deoxynucleoside triphosphates. After the colonies containing recombinant phage were lightly transferred to a filter paper in such a way that any colony containing a recombinant phage of interest could be reisolated from the agar, the filter paper was mixed with the radioactive cDNA under conditions favoring hybridization of complementary DNA sequences. In other words, the β-complementary DNA was used to locate sequences that are homologous to it and stick to them by base pairing. Such hybridizing colonies are then radioactive and can be detected by autoradiography after nonspecific unhybridized radioactivity is washed away. The recombinant phage of positive colonies were then grown in *E coli* and the human DNA fragments were isolated and mapped with restriction enzymes. Many were subjected to nucleotide sequencing. In this way, the human β-globin gene cluster and many other regions of the human genome have been characterized.

Over 2000 human genes have been cloned from various types of gene libraries. New techniques have made it possible to clone all types of genes, even those that are transcribed into a small number of messenger RNA molecules per cell.

Each gene cluster is unique in its organization. For example, the α-globin cluster found on the short arm of chromosome 16 contains two pseudogenes, no fetal genes, one embryonic gene, and two α-genes and spans only about 25 kb of DNA. In addition, the two introns in the α-genes are each only about 150 bp long.

## DNA REARRANGEMENT

The switching in gene expression from embryonic to fetal to adult hemoglobin genes is not a consequence of DNA rearrangement during development. The DNA in both the β- and α-gene clusters appears to be static, and the mechanism of hemoglobin switching remains unknown, although regulatory proteins, generally various transcription factors needed for gene expression, are encoded by genes elsewhere in the genome and have been implicated. In contrast, DNA rearrangement in the immunoglobulin gene clusters plays a critical role in the expression of these important genes.

Immunoglobulin light chains are composed of variable regions (V), short junction regions (J), and constant regions (C) (Fig 13-7). Heavy chains contain a D region between the V and J regions. The DNA sequences coding for the V region of a chain are at some unknown distance from those sequences coding for the D

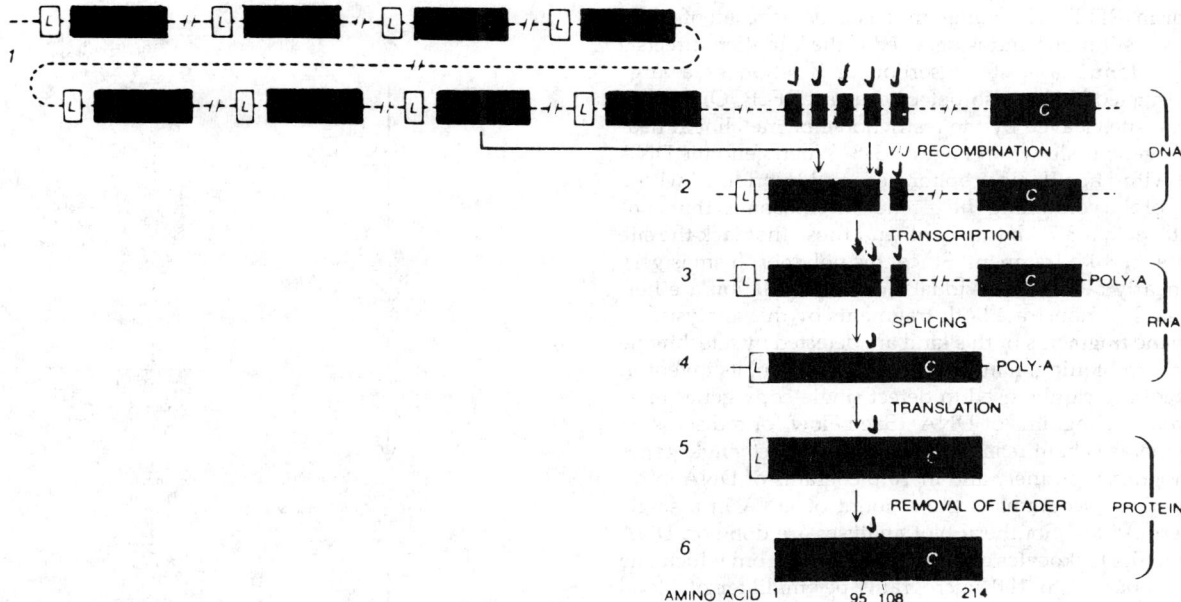

**Figure 13-7.** Immunoglobin light chain production. In 1, many V-region genes preceded by L or leader sequences are at some distance from five J-region genes in undifferentiated cells. In 2, a rearrangement at the DNA level takes place in B-lymphocytes that brings one V-region gene into contiguity with a J-region gene. The gene is then transcribed into RNA and splicing of RNA occurs before the light chain messenger RNA is translated into immunoglobin.

and J regions. During differentiation of B lymphocytes, a DNA rearrangement occurs to make one of many light chain V-region genes contiguous with one of several light chain J-region genes. Transcription produces an RNA that contains a large intron between J and C sequences, which is removed to produce a mature messenger RNA for an entire V-J-C-containing immunoglobulin light chain. In heavy chain synthesis, DNA sequences for V, D, and J regions must be brought into contiguity, and the intron between V and C regions must be removed.

The picture is even more complicated because antibody diversity can be extended through the class switch of heavy chains from $\mu$ to $\gamma$ to $\alpha$ to $\delta$. The class switch occurs through unequal crossing over at the DNA level to place a new C sequence into the position originally occupied by the C$\mu$ gene. Antibody diversity is further achieved through different RNA processing alternatives and additional DNA rearrangements.

Even though our cells are diploid and have two of every au-

tosomal gene, only one particular light chain or heavy chain gene seems to function in any particular B lymphocyte. This is probably because the error rate in DNA rearrangement is so great that only rarely does a functional rearrangement occur on both chromosomal homologues. Thus, the genome, at least as represented by immunoglobulin genes, appears to be in a fluid state.

## NORMAL VARIATION IN DNA

Discussion of mutations and their consequences requires a brief introduction to normal variation. Much has been learned about normal variation at the protein or enzyme level. Now scientists are learning that variation in the DNA is even more extensive than we imagined from protein data. Several types of variation have been found. Originally, common normal variation in DNA was termed DNA polymorphism or restriction fragment length

HINC II POLYMORPHISM

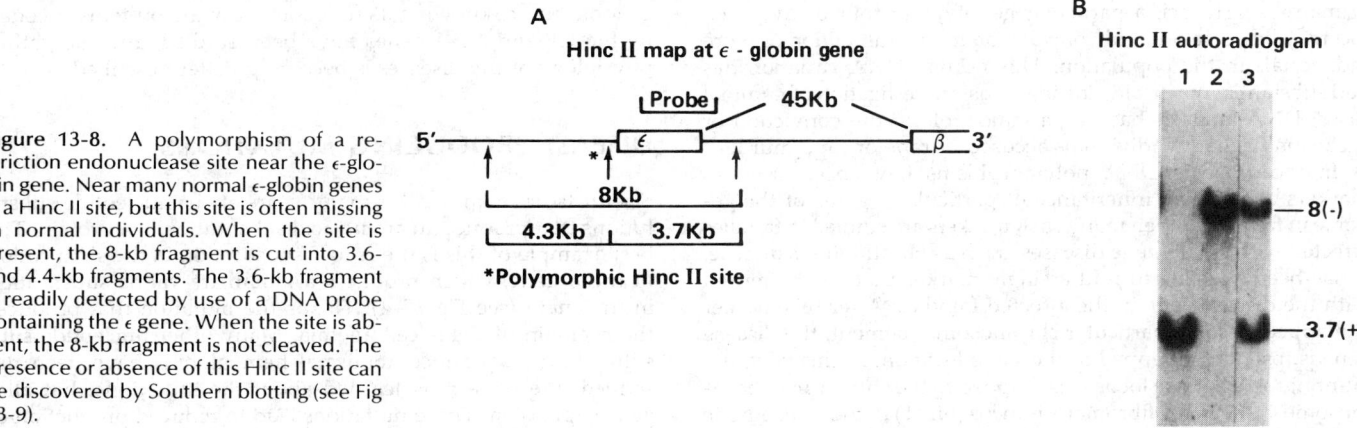

**Figure 13-8.** A polymorphism of a restriction endonuclease site near the ε-globin gene. Near many normal ε-globin genes is a Hinc II site, but this site is often missing in normal individuals. When the site is present, the 8-kb fragment is cut into 3.6- and 4.4-kb fragments. The 3.6-kb fragment is readily detected by use of a DNA probe containing the ε gene. When the site is absent, the 8-kb fragment is not cleaved. The presence or absence of this Hinc II site can be discovered by Southern blotting (see Fig 13-9).

polymorphism (RFLP). This variation is usually the result of single nucleotide substitutions and is detected if the variation affects a restriction endonuclease site. Insertion or deletion of a large number of nucleotides is also detected as an RFLP. One RFLP that affects a site cleaved by the restriction enzyme Hinc II near the $\epsilon$-globin gene is shown in Figure 13-8. When genomic DNA is digested with Hinc II, electrophoresed, and hybridized with a radioactive probe containing the $\epsilon$-gene, chromosomes that contain this site yield a 3.7-kb fragment, and those that lack the site demonstrate an 8-kb fragment. Since this polymorphism is very common, nearly 50% of individuals in the population are heterozygous and demonstrate both fragments by this analysis.

Single-gene fragments of this kind are detected by a technique called Southern blotting, named for E.M. Southern, its inventor. Southern blotting can be used to detect single-copy genes in as little as 3 to 5 micrograms of DNA. (See below for a discussion of the polymerase chain reaction, which can detect single genes in 100 nanograms routinely and in 10 picograms of DNA in research labs. Ten picograms is the amount of DNA in a single human sperm.) Most Southern blot analyses are done on DNA isolated from the leukocytes of peripheral blood, from which one can isolate about 50 to 100 micrograms per milliliter of blood (Fig 13-9). Usually 5 micrograms of genomic DNA of an individual is digested with a specific restriction enzyme, the digested DNA is subjected to electrophoresis in an agarose gel that separates DNA on the basis of size, the DNA is transferred to a nitrocellulose paper, and it is hybridized to a radioactive cloned DNA fragment of interest (the probe). After hybridization with the probe, the filter is washed to remove nonspecific radioactivity, and the washed filter is placed in contact with an x-ray film. After a day or two the film is removed and developed to demonstrate the bands of interest. The procedure is both simple and elegant.

Using this procedure one can find several DNA polymorphisms in the $\beta$-gene cluster and in and around many other genes. Thus, normal variation in DNA is extensive. The reader should realize that the 50,000 nucleotides of the $\beta$-gene cluster derived from his or her father contain 100 or more nucleotide differences from the 50,000 nucleotides of this cluster derived from his or her mother. In total, the haploid DNA derived from one parent contains 3 to 10 million differences (single nucleotide substitutions) from the genetic material derived from one's other parent.

Even more important forms of DNA polymorphisms are variable number of tandem repeats (VNTRs) and simple sequence repeats (SSRs). VNTRs are repeats of 15 to 50 nucleotides; the repeat number at a locus may vary widely (Fig 13-10). SSRs are variations in the number of repeats of very short sequences, usually two to four nucleotides. Often a VNTR locus may contain many possible alleles, perhaps 100 or more, if a population group is studied. SSR loci may contain five to ten alleles. The variation in VNTRs and SSRs contrasts with that of most common RFLPs, which are dimorphisms. Because of the large number of alleles at many VNTR loci, a particular genotype at four or five such loci may be present in only one person in several million or more individuals in the population. This normal DNA variation has had substantial practical value in forensic investigation of criminal cases. DNA analysis has had a major role in the conviction or exclusion of many individuals accused of rape or rape-murder.

In recent years DNA polymorphisms have been used as markers to trace the inheritance of particular regions of the genome in families. When many such markers are studied in families affected with single-gene diseases, such as Huntington's disease, it has been possible to find a single marker that is coinherited with the disease gene in the affected families. After this marker is mapped to some particular chromosome segment, the disease gene is ipso facto mapped to the same location. In this way, the Huntington's disease locus was mapped to the short arm of chromosome 4, the neurofibromatosis locus (NF-1) to the centromeric

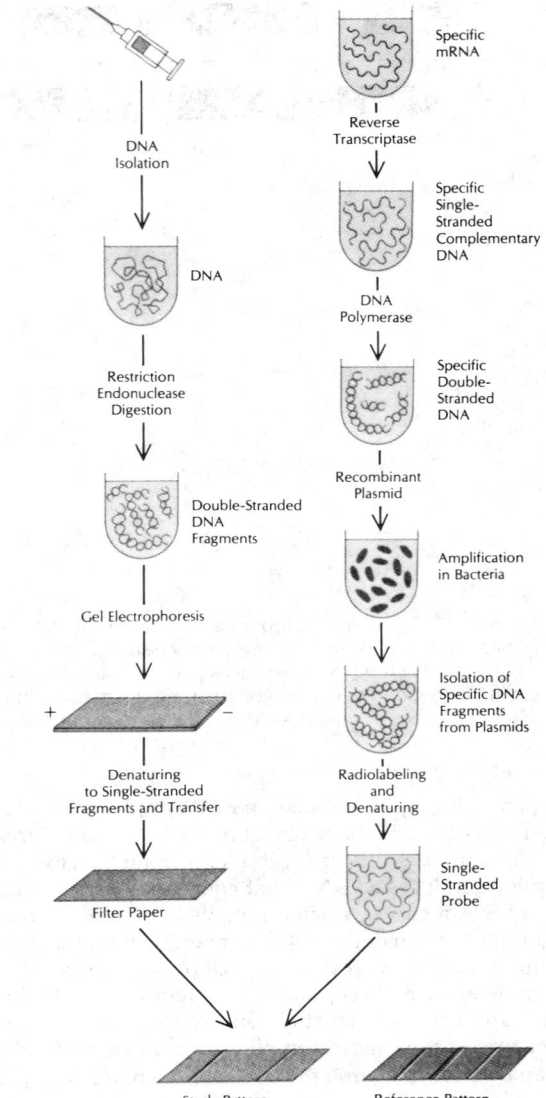

**Figure 13-9.** Southern blotting, or restriction endonuclease analysis. The steps in this procedure are shown beginning with isolation of DNA from leukocytes to discovery of hybridizing fragments (bands) in that DNA with a specific radioactive probe.

region of chromosome 17, and the cystic fibrosis (CF) locus to the long arm of chromosome 7, to name a few successful examples. The genes responsible for these three diseases have now been isolated by this method of finding the gene's location in the genome before knowing its function. Now the proteins encoded by the CF and NF-1 genes have been studied, and the pathophysiology of the diseases is becoming better described.

## DISEASE-PRODUCING MUTATIONS

Scientists have known for many years about nucleotide substitutions that produce an amino acid substitution in a protein. The best example of this is the A to T substitution in the sixth codon of the $\beta$-gene, which produces a glutamate-valine substitution in the chain (see Fig 13-4). This is the mutation that produces the $\beta$-globin of sickle-cell anemia. Many other nucleotide substitutions that produce abnormal hemoglobins have been described. We have now learned about the mutations that alter gene expression. These mutations lead to reduced production of

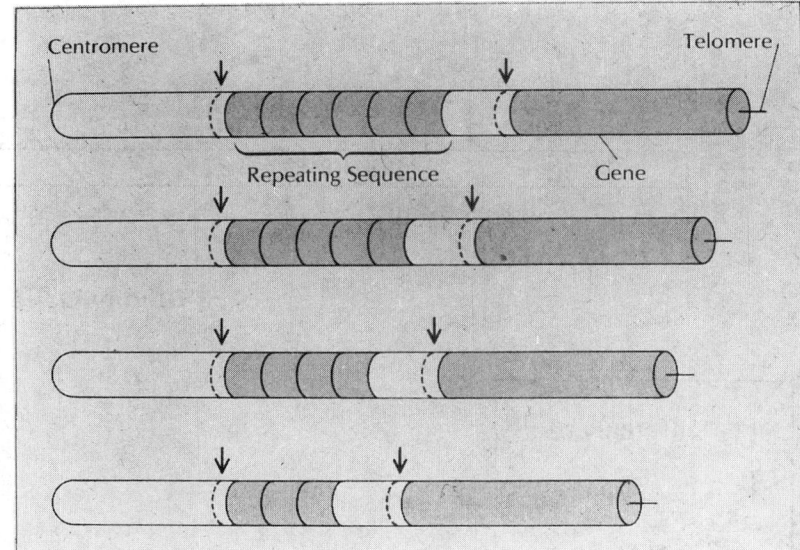

**Figure 13-10.**  A VNTR (variable number of tandem repeats) polymorphism adjacent to a gene. A 30-nucleotide sequence has three repeats, four repeats, five repeats, or six repeats in tandem in different chromosomal homologues. The length variation in this region of the genome can be easily detected by Southern blot analysis or the polymerase chain reaction. In an SSR (simple sequence repeat) polymorphism, the polymorphic repeat sequence would contain two to four nucleotides (eg, the dinucleotide CA).

the encoded protein, and they tell us what sequences within and adjacent to the gene are important in expression. The best examples of such mutations are still the point mutations that produce the $\beta$-thalassemias, inherited disorders of $\beta$-globin gene expression.

## Molecular Defects in $\beta$-Thalassemia

The genetic defects in $\beta$-thalassemia are best reviewed in the context of the normal sequence of events in gene expression (see Fig 13-3). To review, in erythroid cells the $\beta$-globin gene is transcribed by RNA polymerase into a globin RNA precursor that contains two intron sequences. Within the nucleus these introns are excised during RNA processing and the coding blocks (or exons) are ligated together precisely to form the processed mRNA that is transported to the cytoplasm and translated into $\beta$-globin. Genetic lesions that interrupt the normal sequence of events lead to the decreased $\beta$-globin production that defines $\beta$-thalassemia. When no $\beta$-globin protein is synthesized from an affected gene, a $\beta^0$-thalassemia defect is present. When some $\beta$-globin is made, the defect is of the $\beta^+$-variety.

We can consider the defined mutations by the phase of the gene expression pathway that is affected. Nearly all $\beta$-thalassemia defects known to date involve DNA sequences of the $\beta$-globin gene rather than distant nucleotides in the genome. We can consider five classes: sizable deletion of the $\beta$-globin gene, transcription mutations (in flanking regions 5' to the gene), RNA processing mutations (cap site, RNA cleavage, RNA splicing), translation mutations (frameshift and nonsense codons), and posttranslation mutations (producing highly unstable globins). Mutations in all of these classes have been found in $\beta$-thalassemia patients.

The known molecular defects in $\beta$-thalassemia are shown in Figure 13-11. At present, about 100 point mutations and several deletions have been found in various affected ethnic groups. The point mutations are almost all single nucleotide substitutions, about half of which affect RNA processing. Each affected ethnic group, whether Mediterranean, Asian Indian, Chinese, or black, has its own battery of $\beta$-thalassemia alleles, usually four to six common ones and a handful of rare ones.

## Examples of Mutations in Other Single-Gene Disorders

The $\beta$-globin model for types of mutations has been validated by observing the same type of mutation in other single-gene

disorders. The following are some characterized mutations in other inborn errors of metabolism. A common mutation in the phenylalanine hydroxylase gene producing phenylketonuria prevents normal RNA splicing at one exon-intron boundary. The mutation in the low-density-lipoprotein receptor gene producing a common form of familial hypercholesterolemia in Lebanon is a nonsense mutation that blocks translation. One mutation producing Tay-Sachs disease in Ashkenazi Jews prevents normal RNA splicing of the hexosaminidase A precursor RNA. These are a few of the many examples, perhaps thousands, of characterized point mutations in genes producing single-gene disorders.

As mutant genes producing inborn errors of metabolism were characterized, many examples of the types of alleles observed in the $\beta$-thalassemias and hemoglobinopathies were found, but a few surprise defects were also uncovered, as discussed below.

## NONCLASSICAL MUTATIONS PRODUCING GENETIC DISEASE

In recent years nonclassical types of mutation have been described, some of which lead to unusual non-Mendelian inheritance. These mutations are unstable repeat sequences and insertion of transposable elements into new genomic sites. Classical types of mutation have also been associated with unusual inheritance patterns. Two examples of this phenomenon are uniparental disomy (inheritance of two chromosomal homologues from one parent and none from the other) and imprinting as an explanation for one genotype producing two different phenotypes, depending on which parent provides a defective chromosome.

### Unstable Repeat Sequences

Expansion of nucleotide repeat sequences is responsible for the fragile X syndrome, myotonic dystrophy, Huntington's disease, and spinal and bulbar muscular atrophy. Our information on the unstable nature of these sequences is most complete for the fragile X syndrome. This syndrome is one of the most common causes of mental retardation in males (about 1 in 1500 males is affected). When lymphocytes of affected males are grown in folate-deficient medium and their chromosomes are examined, a substantial fraction of X chromosomes contain a break at Xq27 near the

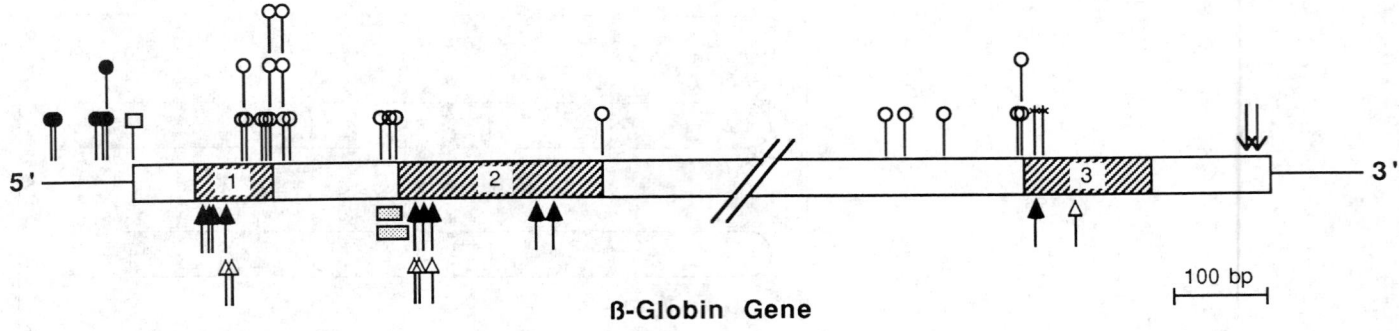

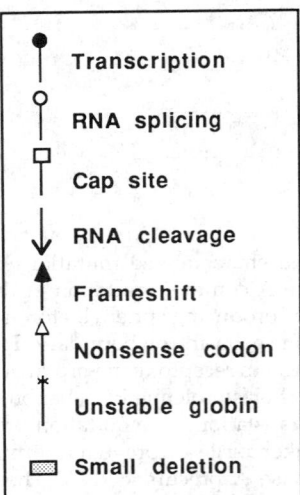

Transcription

○ RNA splicing

□ Cap site

↓ RNA cleavage

▲ Frameshift

△ Nonsense codon

✳ Unstable globin

▦ Small deletion

**β-Globin Gene**

**Figure 13-11.** Point mutations producing β-thalassemia. The β-globin gene is shown with numbered hatched areas representing the coding regions of exons. Boxed open areas between the exons are introns and boxed open areas at the 5' and 3' ends of the gene are untranslated regions that appear in the messenger RNA. The various types of mutations are denoted by different symbols.

distal end of the long arm. This phenotype is associated with lack of expression of a gene (familial mental retardation-1 or FMR-1) and inappropriate methylation of DNA near the 5' end of the gene. In turn, the inappropriate methylation is a secondary effect of a marked expansion of a trinucleotide repeat (CGG) in the 5' coding region of the FMR-1 gene (Fig 13-12).

In normal X chromosomes the repeat number of this trinucleotide is polymorphic, centering around 29 with a normal range of six to 45. In some X chromosomes, the repeat number increases to 52 to 200. These chromosomes carry what is termed a premutation for the fragile X phenotype. This premutation is associated with normal intelligence, normal methylation of nearby sites, and normal expression of the FMR-1 gene. When a male passes the premutation to a female offspring it remains essentially unchanged. However, when a female carrier of a premutation passes this X chromosome to her offspring, there is a significant risk for both sons and daughters that the trinucleotide repeat will expand greatly to 200 to 600 copies. This large number of repeats

**FRAGILE X: Amplification of (CGG)$_n$ in Exon 1 of the FMR-1 Gene**

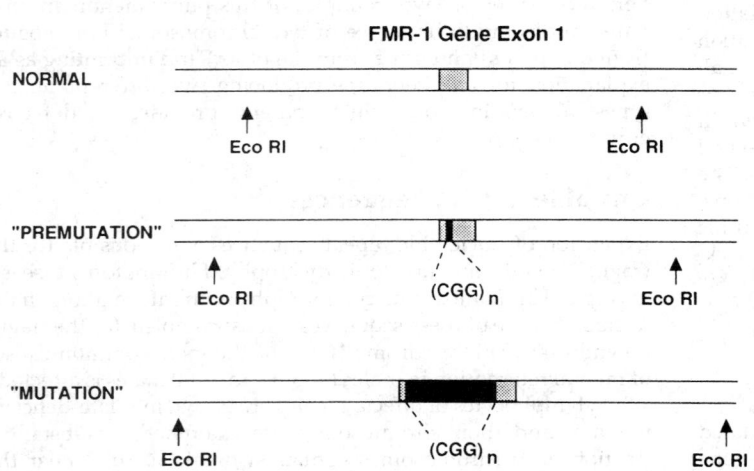

**Figure 13-12.** Expansion of a trinucleotide repeat in the fragile X syndrome. In the normal FMR-1 gene on the long arm of the X chromosome there is a CGG repeat sequence. When this repeat expands in meiosis from the normal six to 45 repeats to 52 to 200 repeats, the premutation is produced. Offspring of females with the premutation are at high risk of further expansion of the repeat in meiosis or early mitotic development. Massive expansion to 200 to 600 copies of the repeat is the full mutation and leads to inactivation of the FMR-1 gene and the fragile X syndrome.

is the full mutation and is associated with inappropriate methylation of nearby DNA and inactivation of the FMR-1 gene. The probability that a premutation will become a full mutation is a function of the size of the repeat in the premutation, being very low if the premutation contains under 60 repeats and approaching 100% if it contains 100 or more repeats. Repeat expansion can occur either in female meiosis or in early mitotic development. In the latter instance, lymphocyte DNA contains the premutation repeat along with full mutation repeats of various sizes.

Myotonic dystrophy, spinal and bulbar muscular atrophy, and Huntington's disease are also caused by expansion of a trinucleotide repeat that inactivates a gene. We expect that other disorders will show this same unusual inheritance pattern, perhaps even some now thought to be multifactorial in nature. For example, some forms of schizophrenia or bipolar affective disorder may be due to the meiotic and mitotic expansion of a trinucleotide repeat that alters the expression of a nearby gene.

## Insertion of Transposable Elements

A second nonclassical type of mutation is insertion of a transposable element, either a LINE or an Alu element. Descriptions of these larger repeated sequences were discussed above. LINE insertions have been observed in the Factor VIII gene producing hemophilia A, in a tumor suppressor gene, APC, in a colon cancer, and in the dystrophia gene, causing muscular dystrophy. Disease-producing Alu I insertions have been found in the neurofibromatosis type 1 gene, the cholinesterase gene, and the Factor IX gene. These insertions are rare causes of de novo mutation. In the case of LINE insertions, these are presumably derived from a small number of active transposable elements that move through an RNA intermediate using a reverse transcriptase encoded by the element (Fig 13-13). Alu elements are transcribed, but require a reverse transcriptase encoded elsewhere, perhaps from an active LINE element, to transpose.

Although these types of mutations probably have only a small impact in producing disease, they have had a major impact throughout evolution in modifying our genome.

## Uniparental Disomy

Uniparental disomy is an unusual inheritance of two chromosomal homologues from one parent and none from the other.

Rarely, both of the chromosomes of a pair are the identical chromosome inherited from one parent. This is called uniparental isodisomy, and it provides a mechanism to explain the rare occurrence of an autosomal recessive disease where only one parent is a carrier. In two cases of cystic fibrosis, the affected child received two copies of the same chromosome 7 containing a cystic fibrosis mutation from one parent and no chromosome 7 from the other parent. These children showed other effects of homozygosity for an entire chromosome, such as short stature and developmental delay. Many mechanisms for the phenomenon are possible, but perhaps the most likely is that the fertilized egg was trisomic for chromosome 7 (two copies from parent 1 and one copy from parent 2) but early in embryonic development the copy of chromosome 7 from parent 2 was lost. Cells containing two copies of chromosome 7 (disomic) were then selected over cells containing three copies (trisomic).

Another example of uniparental disomy is the inheritance in an XY male of both an X chromosome and a Y chromosome from the father and no sex chromosome from the mother. This has been seen in a case of male-to-male transmission of hemophilia A in which the affected son received a mutant X chromosome (along with a Y chromosome) from his affected father.

## Imprinting

Imprinting refers to the situation in which different phenotypes result from the same genotype, depending on whether a mutation-marked chromosome is derived from the mother or the father. An example of the phenomenon already mentioned is seen in inheritance of the fragile X syndrome, in which the expansion from premutation to full mutation can occur only in transmission from a female parent. A more telling example is found in the inheritance of the Prader-Willi and Angelman syndromes, two syndromes in which the affected children have very different dysmorphic features. In Prader-Willi syndrome there is paternal deficiency of chromosome 15q11–q13, while in Angelman syndrome there is maternal deficiency of the same chromosomal region. Of Prader-Willi cases, 70% have a deletion of the paternal chromosome 15q11–q13 and a normal maternal chromosome 15, while 30% have maternal disomy for chromosome 15 and no paternal chromosome 15 (Fig 13-14). Of Angelman syndrome children, 60% have a maternal chromosome 15 with the q11–q13 deletion, a small percentage have paternal disomy for chromosome 15, and the rest have unknown mutations presumably

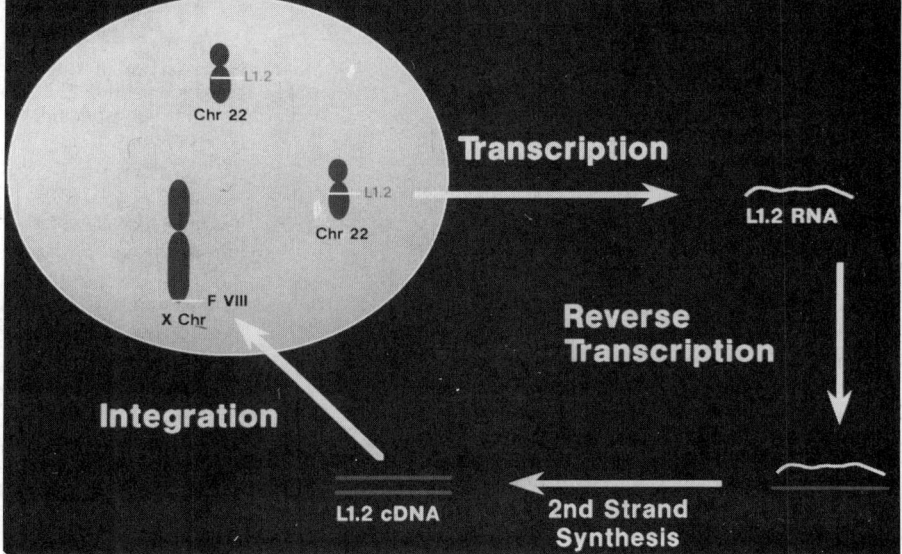

**Figure 13-13.** Transposition of a LINE element (L1.2) from chromosome 22 in the Factor VIII gene on the X chromosome causing de novo hemophilia A. A 6-kb LINE element (L1.2) is present as a gene on chromosome 22. In one parent's germ cell this gene was transcribed into RNA, then reverse transcribed into cDNA, and the double-stranded cDNA was reintegrated back into the genome at the tip of the X chromosome. Note that the L1.2 genes have not themselves moved, but that a new copy of the gene has been placed at a distant location in the patient's genome.

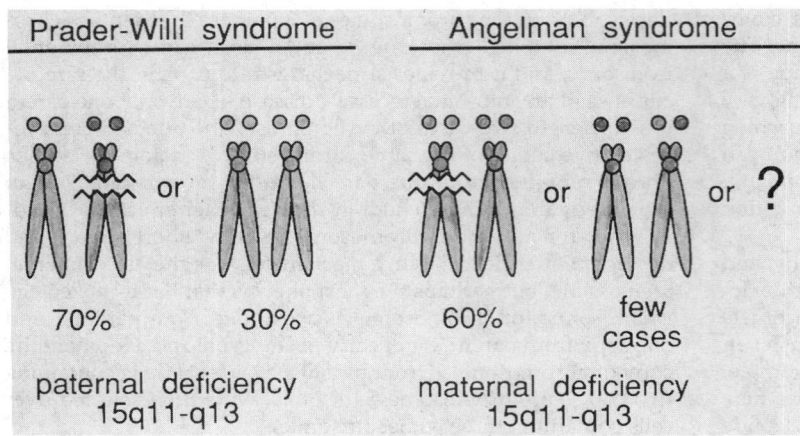

**Figure 13-14.** Imprinting in the Prader-Willi and Angelman syndromes. Deficiency of chromosome 15q11-q13 leads to two different syndromes depending on the parental origin of the deficiency. *Left,* paternal deficiency of 15q11-q13, either through interstitial deletion or maternal disomy (no chromosome 15 donated by the father), produces the Prader-Willi syndrome. *Right,* maternal deficiency of 15q11-13 through interstitial deletion, paternal disomy, or other unknown mechanisms produces the Angelman syndrome. Filled chromosomes are paternally derived; open chromosomes are maternal in origin.

affecting one or more genes in the q11–q13 region of the mother's chromosome 15. The role of methylation in this process is thought to be critical, but the mysterious process of imprinting needs further explanation.

## PRENATAL DIAGNOSIS OF SINGLE-GENE DISORDERS BY DNA ANALYSIS

DNA techniques were first applied to prenatal diagnosis of certain single-gene disorders in 1976. DNA-based tests were first applied on a practical basis to prenatal diagnosis of α-thalassemia in 1978, sickle-cell anemia in 1978, β-thalassemia in 1980, hemophilia A in 1985, hemophilia B in 1984, phenylketonuria in 1985, Duchenne and Becker muscular dystrophy in 1985, cystic fibrosis in 1986, Huntington's disease in 1986, neurofibromatosis in 1989, and fragile X in 1991. This list should give an indication of the recent explosion of knowledge and new diagnostic possibilities. The list of disorders that can be diagnosed by such techniques for couples known to be at risk continues to grow and now includes many of the more common inherited disorders (Table 13-1).

**TABLE 13-1.** Single-gene Disorders Diagnosable by DNA Analysis for Couples Identified as Being at Risk

| Disorder | Direct Detection | RFLP Analysis | % of Pregnancies Diagnosable | Accuracy of Diagnosis |
|---|---|---|---|---|
| $\alpha_1$-antitrypsin deficiency | Yes; oligonucleotide analysis used | Usually not necessary | 99% | 99%–100% |
| Carbamyl phosphate synthetase deficiency | | In most cases | 75% | |
| Cystic fibrosis | Yes, in nearly all cases | Rarely | 99% | 99% |
| Duchenne muscular dystrophy | In about 70%–80% of cases | In many cases | 90% | 94%–99% depending on RFLPs used |
| Fragile X | Yes, in all cases | Not necessary | 100% | 99%–100% |
| Hemophilia A | Rarely used | In most cases | 99% | 95%–99% depending on RFLPs used |
| Hemophilia B | Yes, in nearly all cases | | 99% | 99% |
| Huntington's disease | | Necessary in all cases; currently only used for very specific type of family pedigree | 85% | 98% |
| Myotonic dystrophy | Yes, in nearly all cases | | 100% | 99%–100% |
| Neurofibromatosis | | Necessary in all cases | >80% | >96% |
| Ornithine trans-carbamylase deficiency | | In most cases | 85%–90% | 99% |
| Phenylketonuria (PKU) | | In most cases | 80% | 99% |
| Retinoblastoma | Yes, in many instances | In most cases | >80% | 98%–100% |
| Sickle-cell anemia | Yes, in all cases by Cvn I (or Mst II or Sau I) endonuclease | Not necessary | 100% | 99%–100% |
| α-thalassemia | Yes, in perhaps all cases due to α-globin gene deletion | Not necessary | 100% | 99%–100% |
| β-thalassemia | Yes, in nearly all of cases | Rarely | 99% | 99% |

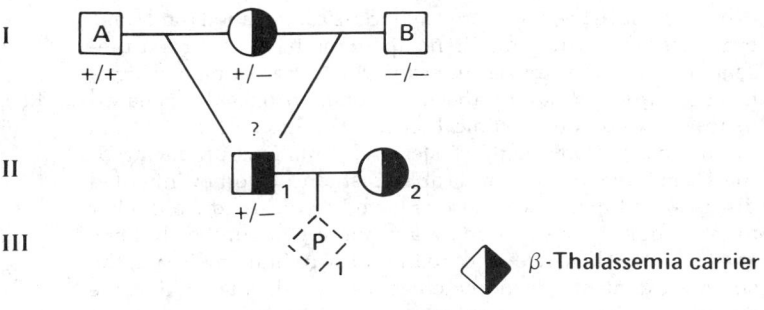

**Figure 13-15.** The problem of misstated paternity in prenatal diagnosis by linkage analysis. In the example shown, a mutant β-globin gene is being tracked using a DNA polymorphism in the β-globin gene cluster. If the paternity is as shown on the left, the β-thalassemia gene in the father (II-1) is marked by the + form of the polymorphism. However, if paternity is as shown on the right, the β-thalassemia gene in the father (II-1) is marked by the − form of the polymorphism. It is clear that an error in paternity can lead to an error in the prenatal diagnosis of β-thalassemia in the case shown.

## DNA Analysis: Current Uses and Limitations

DNA analysis has been well received for several reasons. First, the fetal samples necessary for diagnosis can be obtained by mid-trimester amniocentesis or first-trimester chorion villus sampling. These techniques represent vast improvements over mid-trimester fetoscopy, which, before DNA testing, had been the sole method for diagnosis of the hemoglobinopathies, coagulation disorders, and $\alpha_1$-antitrypsin deficiency. Second, because gene expression is not required for DNA diagnosis, any nucleated cell type in any stage of differentiation is suitable for analysis. Third, DNA analysis permits diagnosis of some disorders for which the primary causative defect is not yet known.

The main limiting factor in the generalized application of prenatal testing for the population at large, whether by DNA techniques or more conventional analyses, is that for many disorders carrier testing is unavailable. Hemophilia A and B and Duchenne muscular dystrophy in the absence of a positive family history are examples of genetic disorders for which generalized screening for detection of carriers does not exist. Pilot programs to test the psychological effect of population screening of cystic fibrosis are underway, and general population screening for cystic fibrosis may occur within 5 years. On the other hand, effective, inexpensive methods for detecting carriers of globin variants, particularly sickle-cell anemia, α-thalassemia, and β-thalassemia, are available through hemoglobin electrophoresis and determination of mean corpuscular volume.

## General Methods of DNA Analysis

At present, several methods are used for diagnosis by DNA analysis, including direct detection of the genetic defect and indirect detection by using polymorphic sites closely linked to the disease-producing mutation. Direct detection can be achieved in three situations: the mutation alters an endonuclease restriction site, as it does in all cases of sickle-cell anemia; the mutation is the result of a gene deletion, as in virtually all cases of hydrops fetalis associated with α-thalassemia and over 50% of cases of Duchenne muscular dystrophy; or the mutation is known, and oligonucleotide probes specific for the mutation can be synthesized (β-thalassemia, $\alpha_1$-antitrypsin deficiency, and cystic fibrosis are often diagnosed by the use of such probes). Many genetic disorders (eg, β-thalassemia) are caused by different mutations, called alleles, at a single locus (β-globin in the case cited). Allele-specific oligonucleotide probes are made to order in the laboratory. Their very short length—about 20 nucleotides—prevents them from hybridizing, under stringent conditions, with any sequence that varies by even as little as a single nucleotide. Thus, an oligonucleotide probe can theoretically be made for any mutation in which the exact nucleotide change is known as well as the DNA sequence of the 19 nucleotides surrounding the mutation.

Direct detection schemes have been greatly aided by the recent development of the polymerase chain reaction (PCR). This simple technique allows one in a few hours to amplify by up to 10

million-fold any particular region of the DNA that has been cloned previously or about which at least some sequence is known. For example, one can take a sample of genomic DNA containing two copies of the β-globin gene per cell (one on each chromosome 11) and within a few hours, after PCR amplification, obtain the equivalent of one to 10 million copies of the β-globin gene per cell in a test tube. This has led to rapid assays for three kinds of mutations: those that alter restriction endonuclease sites, those detected by oligonucleotide hybridization, and those that can be identified by direct nucleotide sequencing of the amplified gene. The PCR technique has also had many applications in research beyond those of gene diagnosis, and indeed has revolutionized work in molecular genetics since its introduction in 1985.

The accuracy of a diagnosis achieved by a direct detection technique theoretically should be close to 100%. However, in diagnoses achieved by an indirect detection technique using DNA polymorphisms physically close to the gene of interest, false assumptions about paternity may allow a misinterpretation of the inheritance patterns between the RFLP and the disease gene (Fig 13-15). A mistake in diagnosis can also occur if the association between the RFLP and the defective gene breaks down as a result of interchromosomal DNA exchange at meiosis (meiotic recombination) (Fig 13-16). The chance of recombination per meiosis is a function of the degree of linkage between the RFLP and the disease gene. This means that the closer the RFLP is to the disease gene and the mutation causing the disease, the smaller the chance of a recombination event producing an error in diagnosis. This biological error rate is determined empirically. RFLPs within the disease gene are in general more tightly linked to the mutation than extragenic RFLPs and thus are more accurate predictors of inheritance of the disease.

## CONCLUSION

In this chapter the salient features of gene structure, genomic organization, normal variation, and mutations affecting gene

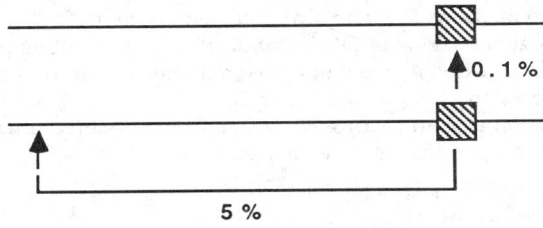

**Figure 13-16.** The problem of meiotic recombination in prenatal diagnosis by linkage analysis. If the polymorphic marker used to track a mutation in the gene shown on the right is within the gene (the arrow in the top drawing), the error rate due of meiotic recombination between the polymorphism (*arrow*) and the mutation within the gene is very low (0.1%). However, when one uses a polymorphic marker at a 5% meiotic recombination distance from the gene of interest (the arrow in the bottom drawing), the error rate for diagnosis due to recombination is 5% for each generation.

expression have been discussed. Nonclassical mutations and some examples of unusual inheritance patterns have also been presented. Prenatal diagnosis and carrier detection of many single-gene disorders, including the most common ones, by gene diagnosis have become a clinical reality. The lessons learned from the normal $\beta$-globin gene cluster and mutations producing $\beta$-thalassemia have been applicable to studies of other inherited diseases, and many new lessons have been learned from other more complex genes. As more and more gene probes become available that have relevance to the study of human disease, the striking extent of genetic heterogeneity producing single-gene disorders in humans is being illuminated. In turn, as we learn more about the molecular basis of many of these disorders, the potential for gene therapy grows.

Progress in human molecular genetics has been phenomenal; indeed, this area currently may be the most productive in all of medical science. On the other hand, our knowledge about how gene expression is regulated in different tissues and at different stages of development is still primitive, but growing rapidly. Gene therapy will be greatly enhanced by further detailed knowledge of how genes are regulated.

## Glossary

**Allele.** An alternative form of a gene; for instance, the $\beta^s$-gene is an allele of the $\beta$-gene.

**Codon.** A group of three nucleotides coding for an amino acid.

**Complementary DNA.** A single-stranded DNA copy of a messenger RNA made with the use of the viral enzyme reverse transcriptase; cDNA contains only the coding sequences of a gene.

**Exon.** DNA sequences that are transcribed into messenger RNA; most exon sequences are also translated into protein.

**5' and 3' ends of DNA fragments.** By convention, the 5' end refers to the left end of a DNA fragment and the 3' end refers to the right end. Biochemically, 5' and 3' refer to the points of attachment of phosphate to ribose on the two ends of the coding strand.

**Genomic DNA.** DNA contained in chromosomes in the nucleus of a cell. Mitochondrial, chloroplast, or synthetic DNA are not genomic DNA.

**Hybridization.** The re-annealing of single-stranded nucleic acid molecules. The formation of double-stranded regions indicates complementary sequences.

**Intervening sequences or intron.** DNA sequences that interrupt coding sequences of a gene.

**Kilobase.** One thousand base (nucleotide) pairs of DNA.

**Linkage.** The close physical association of the specific site in the genome with another on a particular chromosome.

**Plasmid.** A small circular piece of DNA in a bacterium that replicates independently of the bacterial genome.

**Probe.** Radioactive single-stranded nucleic acid used to locate genomic DNA sequences complementary to it.

**Pseudogene.** Region of DNA that displays significant homology to a functional gene but has mutations that prevent its expression.

**Restriction endonucleases.** Bacterial enzymes that recognize and cleave a specific DNA sequence.

## Selected Readings

Caskey CT, Pizzuti A, Fu Y-H, et al. Triple repeat mutations in human disease. Science 1992;256:784.

DiLella AG, Marvit J, Lidsky AS, et al. Tight linkage between a splicing mutation and a specific DNA haplotype in phenylketonuria. Nature 1986;322:799.

Fritsch EF, Lawn RM, Maniatis T. Molecular cloning and characterization of the human $\beta$-like globin gene cluster. Cell 1980;19:959.

Gusella J, Wexler NS, Conneally PM, et al. A polymorphic DNA marker genetically linked to Huntington's disease. Nature 1983;306:234.

Kan YW, Dozy AM. Polymorphism of DNA sequence adjacent to the human $\beta$-globin structural gene: relation to sickle mutation. Proc Natl Acad Sci USA 1978;75:5631.

Kazazian HH Jr. Gene probes: application to prenatal and postnatal diagnosis of genetic disease. Clin Chem 1985;31:1509.

Kerem B-S, Rommens JM, Buchanan JA, et al. Identification of the cystic fibrosis gene: Genetic analysis. Science 1989;245:1073

Leder P. The genetics of antibody diversity. Sci Am 1982;246:102.

Maniatis T, Fritsch ER, Lauer J, Lawn RM. The molecular genetics of human hemoglobin. Ann Rev Genet 1980;14:145.

Orkin SH, Kazazian HH Jr. The mutation and polymorphism of the human $\beta$-globin gene and its surrounding DNA. Ann Rev Genet 1984;18:131.

Southern EM. Detection of specific sequences among DNA fragments separated by gel electrophoresis. J Mol Biol 1975;98:503.

Saiki RK, Gelfand DH, Stoffel S, et al. Primer-directed enzymatic amplification of DNA with a thermostable DNA polymerase. Science 1988;239:487.

Tilghman SM, Tiemeier DC, Seidman JG, et al. Intervening sequences of DNA identified in the structural portion of a mouse $\beta$-globin gene. Proc Natl Acad Sci USA 1978;75:725.

*Principles and Practice of Pediatrics, Second Edition.*
edited by Frank A. Oski et al. J. B. Lippincott Company, Philadelphia © 1994.

# CHAPTER 14
# *Immunology and Allergy*

# *14.1 Immunology*

## *14.1.1 The Primary Immunodeficiency Diseases*

Howard M. Lederman and Jerry A. Winkelstein

The immune system is composed of a variety of cells (B lymphocytes, T lymphocytes, monocytes, and neutrophils) and their secretory products (antibodies, complement, and cytokines), which all recognize foreign antigens and react to them. The first primary immunodeficiency disease, X-linked agammaglobulinemia, was recognized in 1952 by Ogden C. Bruton. Since then, disorders involving nearly all components of the immune system have been identified. This chapter reviews the normal physiology of the immune system, discusses the clinical presentation of immunodeficient patients, and outlines the laboratory tests that are most useful in their diagnosis.

## THE NORMAL IMMUNE SYSTEM

Components of the immune system are found in all parts of the body, but are concentrated in the thymus, bone marrow, lymph nodes, spleen, liver, and blood (Fig 14-1). Successfully integrated and functioning together, B lymphocytes, T lymphocytes,

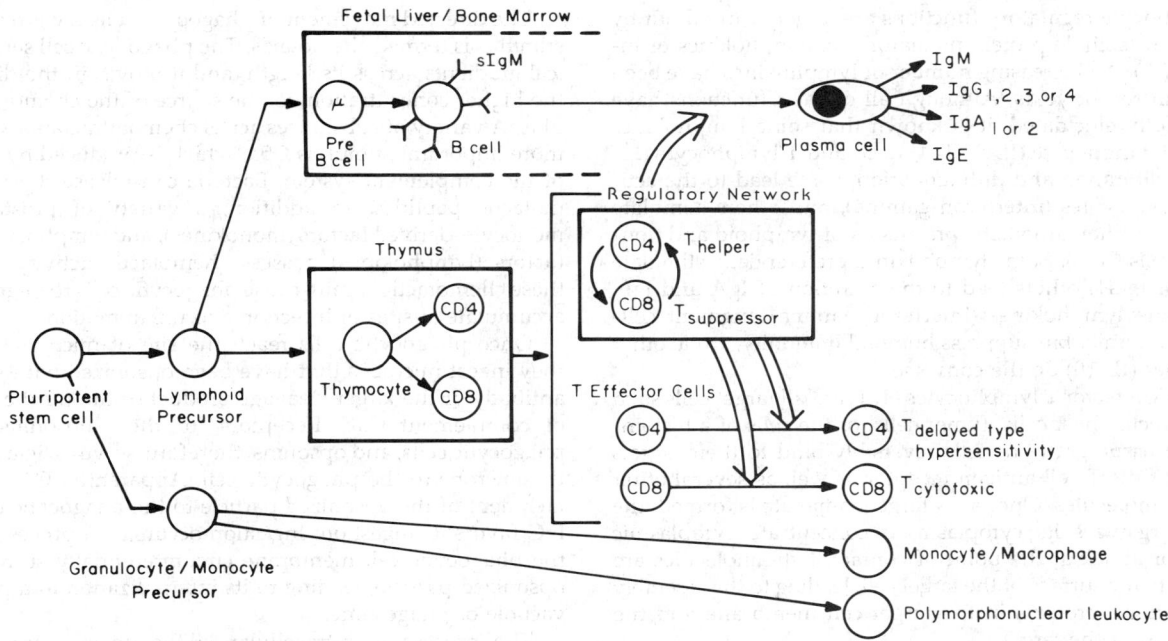

**Figure 14-1.** The cells of the immune system.

phagocytes, and the complement system form an important homeostatic mechanism necessary for the host's defense against infection and the generation of a normal inflammatory response.

## The Lymphoid System

Lymphoid stem cells arise in the fetal yolk sac, then migrate to the bone marrow, liver, and spleen. Their progeny of immature lymphoid precursors differentiate along one of two mutually exclusive pathways to become B or T lymphocytes.

B lymphocytes are the effector cells of antibody-mediated or humoral immunity. Differentiation of B lymphocytes, which largely takes place in the bone marrow and liver, is a two-stage process. In the first stage, an enormous number of B lymphocyte clones are generated by a series of immunoglobulin gene rearrangements that occur irrespective of antigenic stimulation. Once the immunoglobulin heavy chain genes rearrange, cytoplasmic immunoglobulin is expressed and the cells reach the pre-B cell stage. Further differentiation, including the rearrangement of immunoglobulin light chain genes, is associated with expression of surface membrane IgM and IgD. Each such B cell has a unique antigenic specificity, marked by the immunoglobulin receptor on its cell membrane. The second stage of B cell differentiation occurs under the influence of antigen. When antigen binds to the immunoglobulin (antibody) expressed on the surface of one of the B lymphocytes, that cell proliferates to form a clone of progeny cells with identical antibody specificity. These cells then differentiate into plasma cells that secrete IgM, IgG, IgA, or IgE. Most antigens are T-dependent; that is, optimal B cell differentiation into plasma cells requires the presence of T lymphocyte helper cells. There are a few antigens, however, including such clinically important ones as bacterial capsular polysaccharides, that are T-independent and are thus able to trigger terminal B cell differentiation even in the absence of T lymphocytes. In all cases, T helper ($T_H$) and T suppressor ($T_S$) lymphocytes are important modulators of B cell function, influencing the degree, the duration, and the quality (affinity and class distribution) of the antibody response.

There are five major classes of immunoglobulins: IgG, IgM, IgA, IgE, and IgD. Each class has unique structural and functional characteristics. Depending on the class, immunoglobulins function in host defense by opsonization of foreign microorganisms, activation of serum complement, neutralization of toxins and viruses, and inhibition of microbial attachment to mucosal surfaces. IgM is the first immunoglobulin produced in an immune response and is the most efficient activator of complement. IgG is the predominant serum immunoglobulin, is actively transported across the placenta, possesses opsonic activity, and activates complement. IgA, which is the major immunoglobulin secreted onto mucosal surfaces, is largely silent as an inflammatory mediator, but does prevent microbial adherence and penetration across the mucosa, and clears and disposes of antigens. IgE is a mediator of allergic disease; its protective functions, if any, have not been identified.

T lymphocytes are the effectors for cell-mediated immunity. They also serve as important regulators of both the humoral and cell-mediated immune systems, and modulate the activities of nonlymphoid cells such as monocytes. Differentiation of T lymphocytes occurs within the microenvironment of the thymus. Like the B lymphocyte lineage, T lymphocyte clones with a variety of antigenic specificities are generated in the absence of antigen by rearrangements of T cell antigen receptor genes. After these gene rearrangements occur, the T cell antigen receptor is expressed on the surface of the T lymphocyte.

The diverse effector and regulatory functions of T lymphocytes are carried out by distinct lymphocyte subpopulations. A differentiation process, operating in addition to the process that generates antigenic specificity, causes individual T lymphocytes to mature along functionally distinct pathways. These T lymphocyte subpopulations have characteristic patterns of cell surface membrane protein expression that are related to their functional activities. For example, the subset of T lymphocytes that are able to positively modulate immune responses (helper T lymphocytes, $T_H$) bear the cell surface protein CD4. A related but distinct CD4-bearing T lymphocyte subpopulation is responsible for delayed-type hypersensitivity responses ($T_{DTH}$). A subset of T lymphocytes bearing the cell surface protein CD8 can negatively modulate immune responses (suppressor T lymphocytes, $T_S$). Another subset, also bearing CD8, can function as cytotoxic effectors in cell-mediated immunity (cytotoxic T lymphocytes, $T_C$).

T lymphocyte regulatory functions are largely carried out by the release of soluble protein mediators, ie, lymphokines or interleukins (IL). An increasing number of lymphokines have been identified in recent years. Although all of their functions have not been fully elucidated, it is known that some lymphokines stimulate B lymphocyte (IL-2, IL-4, IL-5) and T lymphocyte (IL-2, IL-4) proliferation and differentiation, some lead to the activation of monocytes (interferon gamma), and others stimulate proliferation of hematopoietic precursors of lymphoid and non-lymphoid cells (IL-3). Some lymphokines preferentially stimulate secretion of IgG1; others lead to the secretion of IgA and IgE. Finally, some lymphokines (interferon gamma) augment cell-mediated immunity but suppress humoral immunity, while other lymphokines (IL-10) do the converse.

Cytotoxic effector T lymphocytes ($T_C$) can kill target cells such as virus-infected host cells, tumor cells, or the cells of a histoincompatible tissue graft. $T_C$ cells reversibly bind to their targets by means of the T cell antigen receptor as well as several other cell surface molecules. Once a $T_C$-target conjugate is formed, the $T_C$ cell reorganizes its cytoplasm to concentrate cytoplasmic granules for attack at the point of contact. Lytic molecules are released onto the surface of the target cell, leading to the assembly of pore-forming proteins in the target cell membrane and the eventual lysis of the target.

## Phagocytic Cells

Phagocytic cells ingest foreign antigens and microorganisms. Although many phagocytic cells are mobile and can move from the blood stream through tissues to the site of microbial invasion or inflammation, other phagocytic cells are fixed in the sinusoids of the bloodstream and the lymphatic system where they clear microorganisms and other particulate matter from circulation. A variety of cells possess phagocytic activity, but neutrophils and cells of the monocyte/macrophage system are the most critical to the functions of the immune system.

Neutrophils are large polymorphonuclear leukocytes that arise in the bone marrow, circulate in the bloodstream, and migrate into tissues where they are the first line of defense against local infections and the principal phagocytic cells of the acute inflammatory response. Monocytes also arise from stem cells in the bone marrow, circulate in the bloodstream, and migrate to the tissues where they undergo morphologic and functional maturation to become macrophages. Monocytes/macrophages cannot only participate as effector cells in host defense and inflammation, but present antigen to lymphoid cells and secrete a variety of pro-inflammatory substances (including cytokines and complement components among many others). Monocytes/macrophages thus play an important role in the generation of normal immune responses.

In order to function properly, phagocytic cells must attach to a substrate (adherence), move through tissues toward the site of microbial invasion (chemotaxis), attach to opsonized microbes and ingest them (phagocytosis), and finally kill the microbes (intracellular killing).

Adherence to a substrate is a prerequisite for phagocytic cells to move. For example, phagocytes circulating in the bloodstream must adhere to vascular endothelium before they egress from the bloodstream. Similarly, once in the tissues, phagocytic cells adhere to connective tissue substrate as they crawl toward the site of microbial invasion or inflammation. The adherence of phagocytic cells is mediated by a family of cell surface glycoproteins including CR3 (the receptor for the opsonic fragment of the third component of complement, iC3b), LFA-1, and p150,95. This adherence is enhanced by a number of soluble mediators including C5a, thromboxane $A_2$, leukotrienes, and platelet-activating factor.

The directed movement of phagocytic cells toward a chemical stimulus is termed chemotaxis. The phagocytic cell senses chemical gradients across its length, and it moves in the direction of the higher concentration, ie, the source of the chemotactic stimulus. A variety of substances act as chemoattractants. One of the more important stimuli is C5a, which is produced by activation of the complement system. Bacteria can release their own chemotactic peptides. In addition, a variety of prostaglandins, monocyte-derived factors (monokines), and lymphocyte-derived factors (lymphokines) possess chemotactic activity. Together, these chemotactic stimuli cause phagocytic cells to migrate to and accumulate at sites of infection and inflammation.

Once phagocytic cells reach the site of microbial invasion, they ingest microbes that have been opsonized with either IgG antibody or the larger cleavage product of the third component of complement C3b. Receptors for these opsonins exist on phagocytic cells, and opsonins, therefore, serve as ligands to bind the microbe to the phagocytic cell. Apparently, C3b favors attachment of the opsonized particle to the phagocytic cell, while IgG favors its ingestion. Ingestion occurs by a process in which the phagocytic cell membrane circumferentially surrounds the opsonized particle, leading to its internalization in a phagocytic vacuole or phagosome.

The process of intracellular killing begins soon after the phagosome is internalized. Both primary (azurophilic) and secondary (specific) granules can fuse with the phagosome, and a number of antimicrobial substances are thereby introduced into the phagosome. These substances include lysozyme, lactoferrin, acid hydrolases, and cationic proteins. Perhaps the most important, however, is the myeloperoxidase-$H_2O_2$-halide system. Upon ingestion of microorganisms, molecular oxygen is reduced to superoxide by a series of reactions involving NADPH oxidase. The superoxide, in turn, undergoes further reactions, leading to the generation of reduced oxygen derivatives such as hydrogen peroxide and hydroxyl radicals. Myeloperoxidase catalyzes the reaction of hydrogen peroxide with chloride to create hypochlorite ions. The net effect of these toxic derivatives of reduced molecular oxygen is to kill microorganisms within the phagocytic vacuole.

## The Complement System

The complement system is composed of a number of serum proteins that, when functioning in an ordered and integrated fashion, mediate a variety of defensive and inflammatory reactions. The majority of the biologically significant effects of the complement system are mediated by the third component (C3) and the terminal components (C5–C9). In order to subserve their biologic functions, however, C3 and C5–C9 must first be activated via either the classical or alternative pathway.

In the classical pathway, antigen-antibody complexes composed of either IgG or IgM activate the first component of complement (C1). C1 is a trimolecular complex composed of C1q, C1r, and C1s. The C1q binds to the Fc portion of the immunoglobulin molecule and consequently activates C1r, which activates the C1s. Activated C1s then cleaves C4 and C2, and the larger cleavage products of each combine to form the classical pathway C3-cleaving enzyme, C4b,2a. In contrast to the classical pathway, activation of the alternative pathway can occur in the absence of specific antibody. Fluid phase C3 binds factor B allowing its cleavage by factor D. The larger cleavage product, Bb, then can be associated with C3 to form a low-grade, C3-cleaving enzyme C3,Bb, which is responsible for the continuous generation of small amounts of nascent C3b. Nascent C3b possesses a reactive thiolester that allows it to covalently bind to molecules on the surface of cells. Bound C3b then forms a complex with native factor B, which is cleaved by factor D to create a new and highly

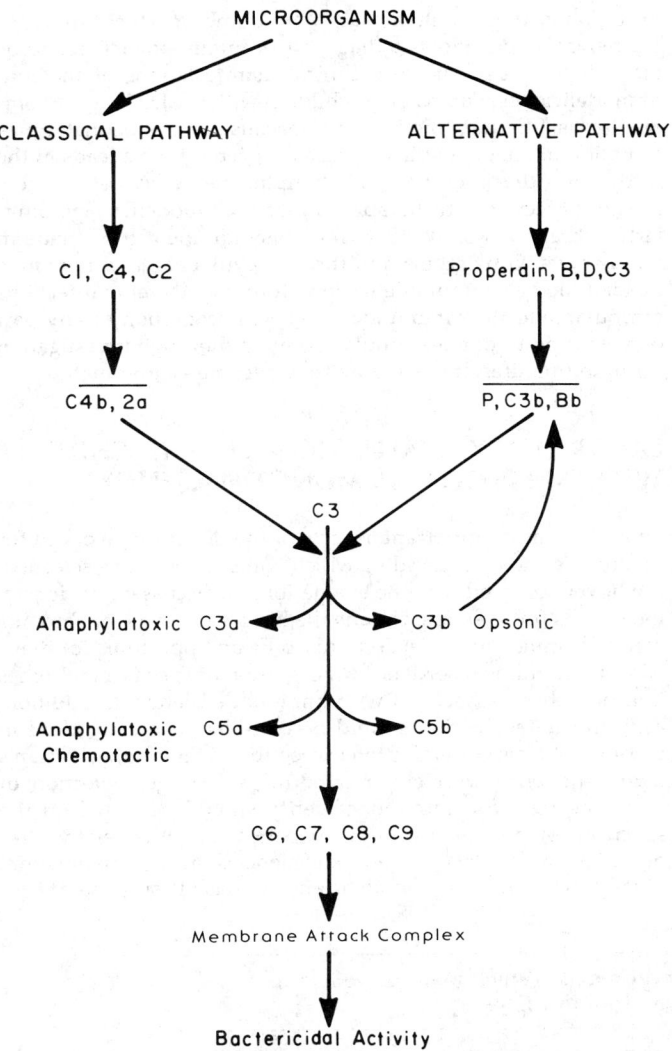

MICROORGANISM

CLASSICAL PATHWAY     ALTERNATIVE PATHWAY

C1, C4, C2     Properdin, B, D, C3

C4b, 2a     P, C3b, Bb

C3

Anaphylatoxic C3a    C3b Opsonic

Anaphylatoxic C5a    C5b
Chemotactic

C6, C7, C8, C9

Membrane Attack Complex

Bactericidal Activity

Figure 14-2. The complement pathway.

efficient particle-bound C3-cleaving enzyme, C3b,Bb. Properdin stabilizes this C3b,Bb complex.

Whether C3 is activated via the classical or alternative pathway, two fragments of unequal size are produced, C3a and C3b. In either case, the activation of C3 represents an amplification step because hundreds of C3 molecules can be cleaved by a single C3-convertase. C3a is released into the fluid phase where it can act as an anaphylatoxin. Most of the C3b is also released into the fluid phase where it is rapidly inactivated by hydrolysis. Some C3b, however, binds covalently to the surface of the activating cells or to the immunoglobulins of the activating immune complex, thereby acting as opsonins or combining with either of the C3-convertases to create C5-convertases. The classical pathway C5-convertase is C4b,2a,3b, while the alternative pathway C5-convertase is $(C3b)_2,Bb$.

Activation of C5 creates a small cleavage product, C5a, and a large cleavage product, C5b. C5a is released into the fluid phase where, like C3a, it can act as an anaphylatoxin. In addition, C5a possesses potent chemotactic activity. C5b can combine with native C6. If it does so while still attached to the C5-convertase, it initiates the formation of a membrane attack complex, a multimolecular assembly of C5b, C6, C7, C8, and C9. This complex inserts into cell membranes and is responsible for the cytolytic and bacteriolytic/bactericidal actions of complement.

Uncontrolled activation of C3 and C5–C9 could result in the

generation of excessive amounts of the phlogistic fragments of complement and immunopathologic damage to the host. A number of mechanisms, however, control the assembly and expression of the C3 and C5 convertases. With respect to the classical pathway, the enzymatic actions of C1r and C1s are inhibited by a control protein, C1 esterase inhibitor. A second inhibitor, C4 binding protein, inhibits the C4b,2a enzyme by limiting the uptake of C2 by C4b, by accelerating the dissociation/decay of the C2a, and by enhancing the ability of yet another regulatory protein, factor I (C3b/C4b inactivator), to cleave and inactivate C4b. With respect to the alternative pathway, two control proteins, factor H and factor I, inhibit the generation and/or expression of the C3 and C5 convertases. Factor H competes with B for binding to C3b and can displace Bb from the $(C3b)_2,Bb$ complex. Factor I inhibits the alternative pathway C3 convertase by inactivating cell-bound C3b through proteolytic cleavage; its rate of inactivation of C3b is accelerated by factor H. Thus, the assembly and expression of the C3 cleaving enzymes usually proceed in a controlled fashion and are limited to the immediate vicinity of the initiating substance.

## THE CLINICAL PRESENTATION OF PRIMARY IMMUNODEFICIENCY DISEASES

The primary immunodeficiency diseases were originally viewed as rare disorders, presenting early in life with severe clinical symptoms. It has become increasingly clear, however, that these diseases are not as uncommon as originally suspected, that their clinical expression can sometimes be mild, and that they may present at any age. Furthermore, although the initial description of patients with primary immunodeficiency diseases focused on their increased susceptibility to infection, these patients may present with a variety of other clinical manifestations. These include autoimmune or chronic inflammatory disorders and syndrome complexes in which immunodeficiency may occur but is often not the presenting feature.

### Increased Susceptibility to Infection

Children with primary immunodeficiency diseases most commonly present with an increased susceptibility to infection. Respiratory tract infections and diarrhea are characteristic, but sepsis, meningitis, and osteomyelitis can occur as well. Individual infections may not be more severe than in a normal host, but the striking clinical feature of immunodeficiency is the chronic or recurring nature of infections. However, not all patients with immunodeficiency are diagnosed after a long series of recurrent infections. In some instances, the initial infection is so severe (eg, pneumonia with empyema) or is caused by such an unusual organism (eg, *Pneumocystis carinii*) that the diagnosis of immunodeficiency is made.

Because each functional compartment of the immune system plays a specialized role in host defense, infections with certain microorganisms are characteristically found in specific immunodeficiency diseases. For example, patients with abnormalities of cell-mediated immunity characteristically develop *P carinii* pneumonia, disseminated fungal infections, mucocutaneous candidiasis, overwhelming viral infections, and severe mycobacterial disease. Conversely, patients with defects of antibody or complement more often have infections with pyogenic encapsulated bacteria. Patients with phagocytic defects develop bacterial and fungal infections of the skin and reticulo-endothelial system. These distinctions may be blurred, however, since the host's defense against any given microorganism depends on the successful integration of all components of the immune system. Thus, a rare patient with an antibody deficiency will develop pneumocystis pneumonia or chronic enteroviral meningitis, while patients with deficiencies of cell-mediated immunity can develop pyogenic bacterial infections. Recurrent infections at a single anatomic site should always prompt consideration of other predisposing conditions such as ciliary dyskinesia, cystic fibrosis, or bronchial obstruction.

## Autoimmune and Inflammatory Disorders

Children with primary immunodeficiency diseases sometimes present with clinical manifestations that do not appear to relate directly to their increased susceptibility to infection. Just as immunodeficiency can lead to defects in the protective functions of the immune system and an increased susceptibility to infection, immunodeficiency can also lead to abnormal immunoregulatory mechanisms with the result being autoimmune or chronic inflammatory diseases. Thus, patients with primary immunodeficiency diseases sometimes present with autoimmune hemolytic anemia or immune thrombocytopenia, autoimmune endocrinopathy, juvenile rheumatoid arthritis, a lupus-like illness, or inflammatory bowel disease. This type of presentation is most often seen in patients with common variable immunodeficiency, selective IgA deficiency, chronic mucocutaneous candidiasis, and deficiencies of the classical complement pathway. Occasionally, a disorder that appears to be autoimmune may be caused by an infectious agent. For example, the dermatomyositis syndrome that is sometimes seen in patients with X-linked agammaglobulinemia is really a manifestation of a chronic enteroviral infection and is not an autoimmune disease.

## Immunodeficiency Syndromes

Immunodeficiency can also be seen as one part of a constellation of signs and symptoms in a syndrome complex (Table 14-1).

Recognition that a patient has a syndrome in which immunodeficiency occurs allows a diagnosis of immunodeficiency to be made before there are any clinical manifestations of that immunodeficiency. For instance, children with the DiGeorge anomaly are usually identified initially because of the neonatal presentation of congenital heart disease or tetany. This leads to the recognition that they have a T lymphocyte defect before there are any infections attributable to that immunodeficiency. Similarly, a diagnosis of Wiskott-Aldrich syndrome can be made in young boys with eczema and thrombocytopenia, and they may be identified as immunodeficient before they develop infections attributable to their immunodeficiency. Recognition of any part of a syndrome complex should prompt a thorough investigation for other manifestations before they become symptomatic.

## LABORATORY EVALUATION OF THE CHILD WITH SUSPECTED IMMUNODEFICIENCY

One of the most important aspects of the diagnostic workup for immunodeficiency is deciding which patients should be screened, not how to proceed with the evaluation. As discussed previously, indications for screening include the history of severe or chronic/recurrent infections, infection caused by an opportunistic organism, autoimmune disorders, or recognition of specific syndromes that have been associated with immunodeficiency. In addition, a diagnostic evaluation should be considered for any child in whom problems with infection exceed the norm for the clinician's own experience with children of the same age. Selection of screening tests for immunodeficiency should be based on the spectrum of problems in a given patient and the relative frequencies of primary immunodeficiencies in the population. Finally, whenever immunodeficiency disease is suspected, con-

| TABLE 14-1. Examples of Congenital Syndromes in Which Immunodeficiency Occurs as Part of a Symptom Complex | | |
|---|---|---|
| Syndrome | Clinical Presentation | Immunologic Abnormality |
| Acrodermatitis enteropathica | Dermatitis<br>Alopecia<br>Diarrhea | Variable B- and T-lymphocyte deficiency |
| Ataxia-telangiectasia | Ataxia<br>Telangiectasia | Variable B- and T-lymphocyte deficiency |
| Autoimmune polyglandular syndrome | Hypofunction of 1 or more endocrine organs | Variable B- and T-lymphocyte deficiency |
| Cartilage hair hypoplasia | Short-limbed dwarfism<br>Sparse hair | Neutropenia<br>T-lymphocyte deficiency |
| Centromeric instability syndrome | Dysmorphic facies<br>Ataxia<br>Developmental delay | Variable B- and T-lymphocyte deficiency |
| Chédiak-Higashi syndrome | Oculocutaneous albinism | Abnormal neutrophil function |
| DiGeorge anomaly | Hypoparathyroidism<br>Congenital heart disease<br>Elfin facies | T-lymphocytic deficiency |
| Hyperimmunoglobulin E syndrome | Coarse facies<br>Eczematoid rashe<br>Elevated IgE | Neutrophil chemotactic defect |
| Ivemark syndrome | Bilateral right-sidedness<br>Bilateral 3-lobed lungs<br>Bilateral morphologic right atria | Congenital asplenia |
| Wiskott-Aldrich syndrome | Thrombocytopenia<br>Eczema | Variable B- and T-lymphocyte deficiency |

sideration must also be given to secondary causes for immuno-deficiency, eg, human immunodeficiency virus (HIV) infection or complications of drug therapy (corticosteroids, trimethoprim/sulfamethoxazole, phenytoin).

## Examination of the Peripheral Blood Smear

The complete blood count with examination of the blood smear is an inexpensive, readily available test that provides important diagnostic information relating to a number of immunodeficiency diseases.

Neutropenia may occur secondary to immunosuppressive drugs, infection, malnutrition, autoimmunity, or as a primary problem (congenital or cyclic neutropenia). A persistent neutro-philia with a predominance of immature forms is characteristic of leukocyte adhesion molecule deficiency, and abnormal cyto-plasmic granules may be seen in the peripheral blood smear of patients with Chédiak-Higashi syndrome.

The blood is predominantly a "T cell organ", ie, the majority (50% to 70%) of peripheral blood lymphocytes are T cells whereas only 5% to 15% are B cells. Therefore, lymphopenia sometimes may be a presenting feature of T cell or combined immunode-ficiency disorders such as severe combined immunodeficiency disease or DiGeorge syndrome.

Thrombocytopenia may occur as a secondary manifestation of immunodeficiency, but is often a presenting manifestation of the Wiskott-Aldrich syndrome. A unique finding in the latter group of patients is an abnormally small platelet volume, a mea-surement that is made easily by automated blood counters.

Examination of red blood cell morphology yields important clues about splenic function. Howell-Jolly bodies may be visible in peripheral blood in cases of splenic dysfunction or asplenia. The converse is not always true, and absence of Howell-Jolly bodies does not guarantee that splenic function is normal.

## Evaluation of Humoral Immunity

Measurement of serum immunoglobulin levels is an important screening test to detect immunodeficiency for three reasons:

1. More than 80% of patients with primary disorders of immunity will have abnormalities of serum immunoglobulins.
2. These measurements yield indirect information about several disparate aspects of the immune system because immuno-globulin synthesis requires the coordinated function of B lym-phocytes, T lymphocytes, and macrophages.
3. The measurement of serum immunoglobulin levels is readily available, highly reliable, and relatively inexpensive.

The initial screening test for humoral immune function is the quantitative measurement of serum immunoglobulins. Neither serum protein electrophoresis nor immunoelectrophoresis is suf-ficiently sensitive or quantitative to be useful for this purpose. Quantitative measurements of serum IgG, IgA, and IgM identify patients with panhypogammaglobulinemia as well as those with deficiencies of an individual class of immunoglobulins, such as selective IgA deficiency. Interpretation of results must be made in view of the marked variations in normal immunoglobulin levels with age. Therefore, age-related normal values must always be used for comparison.

There are four subclasses of IgG, and selective deficiencies of these have been described. $IgG_1$ and $IgG_3$ are the principal sub-classes used for responses to protein antigens; $IgG_2$ is the principal subclass used for responses to polysaccharide antigens. In some instances, the total serum IgG may be normal or near normal, but the patient may still have an IgG subclass deficiency. Thus, in a child whom there is a strong suspicion of humoral immu-

nodeficiency but total serum IgG is normal, quantitative mea-surements of individual IgG subclasses should be performed.

In addition to measurement of immunoglobulin levels, as-sessment of antibody function should always be included as part of the evaluation of humoral immunity. Antibody titers generated in response to childhood immunization with diphtheria and tet-anus toxoids are usually the most convenient to measure. In chil-dren older than ages 18 to 24 months, it is also important to assess the antibody response to polysaccharide antigens, because these responses may be deficient in some patients who can re-spond normally to protein antigens (eg, Wiskott-Aldrich syn-drome or $IgG_2$ subclass deficiency). Antibody can be measured in response to immunization with pneumococcal (Pneumovax) or meningococcal capsular polysaccharide vaccines. Alternatively, because the ABO blood group antigens are polysaccharides, an-tipolysaccharide antibody can be assessed by quantitating isoag-glutinin titers. Their value in the young child is limited, however, because even normal children of this age may not have significant isoagglutinins.

If immunoglobulin levels and antibody titers are decreased, the evaluation should proceed with enumeration of B lympho-cytes in the peripheral blood. Further specialized tests may be necessary to specifically delineate the functional B cell defect. These may include in vitro studies of mitogen or antigen-driven B cell proliferation and immunoglobulin secretion.

## Evaluation of Cell-Mediated Immunity

Testing for defects of cell-mediated immunity is difficult because of the lack of good screening tests. Since T lymphocytes make up 50% to 80% of peripheral blood mononuclear cells, lympho-penia is suggestive of T lymphocyte deficiency. However, lym-phopenia is not always present in patients with T lymphocyte functional defects. Similarly, the lack of a thymus silhouette on chest x-ray is a helpful sign in some T lymphocyte disorders, but the thymus of normal children may involute after stress and may give the appearance of thymic hypoplasia.

Delayed type hypersensitivity skin testing with a panel of an-tigens is an excellent screening method for older children. A standardized panel of antigens prepared for delayed-type hy-persensitivity testing should be used. The presence of one or more positive delayed-type skin tests is generally indicative of intact cell-mediated immunity. There are significant limitations to this testing:

Prior exposure to antigen is a prerequisite.

A positive skin test to some antigens does not ensure that the patient has normal cell-mediated immunity to all antigens (eg, patients with chronic mucocutaneous candidiasis have a la-cunar defect in which cell-mediated immunity is generally intact except for their response to Candida).

Normal patients may have transient depression of delayed-type hypersensitivity with acute viral infections.

Normal children younger than age 12 months frequently are un-responsive to all of the antigens in the panel.

The test is, therefore, least helpful when it is most needed, namely in young infants in whom a congenital abnormality of T lym-phocytes (eg, severe combined immunodeficiency) is suspected. In conclusion, delayed-type hypersensitivity testing has poor positive or negative predictive value when applied to children for evaluation of immunodeficiency.

Indirect information about T cell function may be obtained by enumerating peripheral blood T lymphocytes, using fluores-cein-conjugated monoclonal antibodies to cell surface determi-nants. Total T ($CD2^+$ or $CD3^+$), T helper ($CD4^+$) and T killer/suppressor ($CD8^+$) cells can be quantitated with the appropriate monoclonal antibodies. Patients with severe combined immunodeficiency and DiGeorge anomaly generally have decreased numbers of both CD4[+] and CD8[+] T lymphocytes. Patients infected with the human immunodeficiency virus have decreased T lymphocytes because there are decreased numbers of CD4[+] lymphocytes, whereas patients infected with the Epstein-Barr virus characteristically have elevated numbers of CD8[+] cells.

Other specialized tests of cell-mediated immunity include the measurement of lymphocyte proliferate in vitro after stimulation with mitogens, antigens, or allogeneic cells. Production of lymphokines and cytotoxic effector function can be measured as well.

## Evaluation of Phagocytic Cells

Evaluation of phagocytic cells usually entails assessment of both their number and their function. Disorders that are characterized by a deficiency in phagocytic cell number, such as congenital agranulocytosis or cyclic neutropenia, usually can be detected by using a white blood cell count and differential.

Assessment of phagocytic cell function depends on a variety of assays. In vitro measurement of directed cell motility (chemotaxis), ingestion (phagocytosis), and intracellular killing (bactericidal activity) can be performed. In addition, there are assays that indirectly assess bactericidal activity by measuring the metabolic changes in the cell that accompany or are responsible for intracellular killing. The most readily available tests assess the oxidative metabolic responses of phagocytes by measuring the reduction of nitroblue tetrazolium to formazan (NBT test), the production of reduced forms of molecular oxygen (peroxide, superoxide, hydroxyl radicals), and chemiluminescence. Each of these functions is reduced markedly in disorders of intracellular killing such as chronic granulomatous disease.

## Evaluation of the Complement System

Most of the genetically determined deficiencies of the classical activating pathway of C3 (C1, C4, and C2), of C3 itself, and of the terminal components (C5, C6, C7, C8, and C9) can be detected using antibody sensitized sheep erythrocytes in a total serum hemolytic complement ($CH_{50}$) assay. Since this assay depends on the functional integrity of C1 through C9, a severe deficiency of any of these components leads to a marked reduction or absence of total hemolytic complement activity. Deficiencies of factor H, factor I, and properdin of the alternative pathway can be detected by a hemolytic assay that assesses lysis of rabbit erythrocytes. The serum of patients with deficiencies of C3 or C5–9 is abnormal when tested in the rabbit erythrocyte assay (as well as in the $CH_{50}$ assay), because the lysis of rabbit erythrocytes depends on these components as well as components of the alternative activating pathway.

The identification of the specific component that is deficient usually rests on both functional and immunochemical tests, and highly specific assays have been developed for each of the individual components. In most cases, both functional and immunochemical assessment of the specific component will demonstrate the deficiency. There are some exceptions. For example, one form of C1 inhibitor deficiency and one form of C1q deficiency are characterized by dysfunctional proteins that can be detected by using immunochemical assays but are markedly reduced in functional activity.

## Selected Readings

Cooper MD. B lymphocytes: normal development and function. N Engl J Med 1987;317:1452.

Denny T, Yogev R, Gelman R, et al. Lymphocyte subsets in healthy children during the first 5 years of life. JAMA 1992;267:1484.

Frank MM. The complement system in host defense and inflammation. Review of Infectious Diseases 1979;1:483.

Frank MM. Detection of complement in relation to disease. J Allergy Clin Immunol 1992;89:641.

Hitzig WH. Protean appearances of immunodeficiencies: syndromes and inborn errors involving other systems which express associated primary immunodeficiency. Birth Defects: Original Article Series 1983;19:307.

Huston DP, Kavanaugh AF, Rohane PW, Huston MM. Immunoglobulin deficiency syndromes and therapy. J Allergy Clin Immunol 1991;87:1.

Johnston RB Jr. Recurrent bacterial infections in children. N Engl J Med 1984;310:1237.

Kniker WT, Lesourd BM, McBryde JL, Corriel RN. Cell-mediated immunity assessed by multitest CMI skin testing in infants and preschool children. AJDC 1985;139:840.

Lockey RF, Bukantz SC, eds. Primer on allergic and immunologic diseases, ed 2. JAMA 1987;258:2829.

Malech HL, Gallin JI. Neutrophils in human diseases. N Engl J Med 1987;317:687.

Nossal GJV. The basic components of the immune system. N Engl J Med 1987;316:1320.

Rosen FS, Cooper MD, Wedgwood RJP. The primary immunodeficiencies. N Engl J Med 1984;235:300.

Royer HD, Reinherz EL. T lymphocytes: ontogeny, function and relevance to clinical disorders. N Engl J Med 1987;317:1136.

Shyur S-D, Hill HR. Immunodeficiency in the 1990s. Pediatr Infect Dis J 1991;10:595.

Stiehm ER. Clinical and laboratory evaluation of the child with suspected immunodeficiency. Pediatr Rev 1985;7:53.

Stiehm ER, Fulginiti VA, eds. Immunologic Disorders in Infants and Children, ed 3. Philadelphia: WB Saunders, 1989.

Wheeler JG, Steiner D. Evaluation of humoral responsiveness in children. Pediatr Infect Dis J 1992;11:304.

WHO Scientific Group in Immunodeficiency. Primary immunodeficiency diseases. Immunodefic Rev 1989;1:173.

Winkelstein JA, Colten HR. Genetically determined disorders of complement. In: Scriver CR, Beaudet AL, Sly WS, Valle D, eds. The Metabolic Basis of Inherited Disease, ed 6. New York: McGraw-Hill, 1988.

Wood RA, Sampson HA. The child with frequent infections. Curr Probl Pediatr 1989;19:235.

*Principles and Practice of Pediatrics, Second Edition.*
edited by Frank A. Oski et al. J. B. Lippincott Company, Philadelphia © 1994.

## 14.1.2 *Disorders of Humoral Immunity*

Howard M. Lederman

Antibodies play a critical role in the host's defense against infection. Many of the protective functions of antibody, such as neutralization of viruses and toxins and inhibition of microbial adherence, can be performed without the participation of other components of the immune system. In addition, there are antibody-mediated functions such as the activation of complement and the ability to opsonize foreign particles for phagocytosis that depend on the recruitment of nonspecific host defense mechanisms. Together these effector mechanisms form a defense network that is particularly effective against a variety of extracellular pathogens. Most notably, these include encapsulated bacteria such as *Haemophilus influenzae* and *Streptococcus pneumoniae*. Antibody also participates in host defense against many viruses. Humoral immunity generally is not as important in the host's defense against intracellular bacteria (eg, mycobacteria), fungi, or protozoa. The biologic significance of antibody in host defense against microorganisms is largely defined by recognition of the specific infections that occur in patients with inborn errors of humoral immunity.

## X-Linked Agammaglobulinemia

X-linked agammaglobulinemia (X-LA) is the prototypic disorder of humoral immunity. Males with this disease have severe panhypogammaglobulinemia with little or no humoral immune function, but intact cell-mediated immunity. These patients have B lymphocyte precursors (pre-B cells), but do not have mature B lymphocytes or plasma cells. T lymphocytes and all other components of the immune system are normal.

It appears that X-LA results from a developmental arrest of B lymphocyte maturation, although the precise pathophysiologic basis of this disorder is unknown. The defective gene has been mapped to the X-chromosome, and X-LA, therefore, is not the result of abnormal structural genes on the somatic chromosomes that encode the immunoglobulins. The X-chromosome effect on B lymphocyte differentiation is observed in the female carriers of X-LA, all of whom are immunologically normal. Generally, inactivation of one X-chromosome occurs at random in female cells. However, among carriers for X-LA, all mature B lymphocytes have inactivated the abnormal X-chromosome. Evidently, lack of expression of the normal gene (or possibly expression of the X-LA gene) blocks B-cell differentiation. Analysis of X-chromosome activation patterns of peripheral blood can be used to determine carrier status.

The differential diagnosis of panhypogammaglobulinemia in infancy includes transient hypogammaglobulinemia of infancy, immunoglobulin deficiency with increased IgM, combined immunodeficiency disorders and rare cases of human immunodeficiency virus (HIV) infection. Quantitation of B and T lymphocytes in peripheral blood helps distinguish among these possibilities. Boys with X-LA have normal numbers of T lymphocytes but have no detectable B lymphocytes. In contrast, infants with transient hypogammaglobulinemia or common variable immunodeficiency generally have normal numbers of B and T lymphocytes; children with severe combined immunodeficiency have decreased numbers of T lymphocytes with normal, decreased, or increased numbers of B cells; and children with HIV infection have decreased numbers of CD4$^+$ T lymphocytes.

Boys with X-LA are usually protected by transplacentally acquired maternal IgG for the first 3 to 4 months of life. Thereafter, chronic and recurrent infections are the predominant clinical manifestation of X-LA. Otitis media, pneumonia, diarrhea, and sinusitis occur most often, usually in combination with each other. Clues to the diagnosis of immunodeficiency include the chronic or recurrent nature of infections, and the occurrence of those infections at more than one anatomic site. *S pneumoniae, H influenzae,* and *Staphylococcus aureus* are the most frequently identified bacterial pathogens, but non-typeable *H influenzae, Salmonellae, Pseudomonas,* and mycoplasma infections occur with increased frequency, as do viral infections. Infections are not limited to mucosal surfaces. Bacterial meningitis, sepsis, and osteomyelitis occur in as many as 10% to 15% of untreated patients. Other sentinel symptoms that should prompt consideration of X-LA include the presentation of oligoarticular arthritis or dermatomyositis in a young male.

Patients with X-LA have an increased susceptibility to infections throughout life. Gamma globulin replacement therapy is highly effective in reducing the incidence of systemic bacterial infections such as meningitis and sepsis. It is sometimes less effective in preventing infections along mucosal surfaces. Chronic infections develop in a large proportion of X-LA patients, particularly those who had severe recurrent or chronic infections before the recognition of immune deficiency and initiation of gamma globulin prophylaxis. The respiratory tract and contiguous mucosal surfaces including the paranasal sinuses are the most common sites of chronic disease. Gamma globulin therapy should allow normal or near-normal growth velocity. Persistently impaired linear growth should prompt evaluation of growth hormone levels because X-LA has occurred in association with growth hormone deficiency in a few kindreds.

Enterovirus infections are a particularly difficult problem in X-LA patients. This group of viruses (Coxsackie, ECHO, and polio viruses) tend to cause chronic diarrhea, hepatitis, pneumonitis, and meningoencephalitis in patients with X-LA. In some instances, the infection takes the form of a dermatomyositis-like syndrome consisting of rash, edema of subcutaneous tissue, and muscle weakness. Enterovirus infections often are fatal in X-LA patients, although therapy with huge doses of gamma globulin containing virus-specific antibodies has been helpful.

Therapeutic management of patients with X-LA includes the use of gamma globulin prophylaxis and an aggressive approach to the diagnosis and therapy of febrile or inflammatory illnesses. Early recognition of the disease and adequate gamma globulin replacement leads to a good prognosis in most patients. Although there are no controlled studies, gamma globulin prophylaxis appears to be most effective in patients who have not yet incurred structural damage to target organs of the respiratory or gastrointestinal tract. Most reported deaths of X-LA patients are attributed to recurrent lower respiratory tract infections with resulting chronic pulmonary disease or to chronic enterovirus infections. Early diagnosis is critical to initiate gamma globulin therapy before the onset of any of these problems and to provide families with appropriate genetic counseling.

## Common Variable Immunodeficiency

The phrase common variable immunodeficiency (CVID) describes a heterogeneous group of disorders characterized by hypogammaglobulinemia. In distinction from X-LA, B lymphocytes frequently are found in the peripheral blood of CVID patients, and the hypogammaglobulinemia may be less profound. Additional immunologic abnormalities such as T cell dysfunction and autoimmune diseases are expressed variably. Many patients with CVID appear to have defects intrinsic to the B lymphocyte, but other patients have excessive T lymphocyte suppressor function, inadequate T lymphocyte helper function, or anti-B lymphocyte antibodies. Most patients do not manifest symptoms until after the first decade of life, but some patients present in early childhood or infancy. It has long been assumed that CVID patients have acquired hypogammaglobulinemia, although there are only a few reports in which the acquisition is documented. There is no recognizable pattern of inheritance in most patients, but other disorders of humoral immunity (eg, IgA deficiency and transient hypogammaglobulinemia of infancy) occur at higher frequency among family members of CVID patients than among the general population.

As in X-LA, the most frequent manifestations of CVID are chronic or recurrent infections of the upper and lower respiratory tracts. Recurrent pneumonia, chronic bronchitis, and sinusitis occur in the majority of patients and some eventually develop chronic pulmonary dysfunction. Most of the identified respiratory tract pathogens are encapsulated bacteria. There is an almost equal incidence of obstructive and restrictive lung disease. Somewhat in contrast to patients with X-LA, disease of the gastrointestinal tract occurs with almost equal frequency as disease of the respiratory tract in patients with CVID. As many as 30% to 60% of patients with CVID have chronic diarrhea. An infectious agent is identified in only about half of the patients; many of the others have idiopathic inflammatory bowel diseases. The most frequently documented gastrointestinal pathogen is *Giardia lamblia.* Bacterial overgrowth of the small bowel is another recognized cause of chronic diarrhea in patients with CVID; enteroviruses are less of a problem.

Patients with CVID have a variety of associated disorders for which no infectious etiology has been established. These disorders may be the result of infections caused by unidentified pathogens, but many are believed to be autoimmune in origin, perhaps the result of the same disordered immunoregulation that is presumed to be responsible for the hypogammaglobulinemia in some CVID patients. Gastrointestinal and hematologic disorders predominate. Chronic idiopathic diarrhea is the single biggest problem. Intestinal biopsy samples typically demonstrate nodular lymphoid hyperplasia as well as villous blunting and epithelial atrophy in the small bowel. Inflammatory bowel diseases, achlorhydria, and pernicious anemia occur with significant frequency. Hematologic abnormalities include the development of persistent splenomegaly, immune thrombocytopenia, leukopenia, and autoimmune hemolytic anemia. Curiously, a few patients have developed a clinical picture typical of sarcoidosis with granulomatous lesions and elevated angiotensin converting enzyme levels, although without hypergammaglobulinemia. There appears to be an increased susceptibility to malignancy (particularly thymoma and lymphoma) in adults with CVID, but the risk in children is not known.

Treatment of these patients is the same as for those with X-LA: replacement with gamma globulin and aggressive management of infections.

## Selective IgA Deficiency

The diagnosis of selective IgA deficiency is established when a patient has a serum IgA level less than 5 mg/dL with normal levels of other immunoglobulin classes, normal serum antibody responses, and normal cell mediated immunity. Selective IgA deficiency is the most prevalent primary immunodeficiency disease, occurring in approximately 1 of 600 individuals in the population. Usually, there is no recognized pattern of inheritance, although the incidence of selective IgA deficiency is higher in families with other lymphocyte disorders.

IgA has several unique biological features. Although IgA makes up only 15% of serum immunoglobulins, it is the predominant immunoglobulin class on the mucosal surfaces of the gastrointestinal and respiratory tracts. IgA is secreted onto mucosal surfaces as a macromolecular complex consisting of two IgA molecules joined to a J chain and a secretory component. The majority of patients with IgA deficiency lack both serum and secretory IgA, but there are rare cases in which there is a deficiency of secretory but not serum IgA. Unlike the other major serum immunoglobulin classes IgG and IgM, IgA is largely silent as a mediator of inflammatory responses. IgA is an antimicrobial defense that inhibits microbial adherence and neutralizes virus. It also has an important role in antigen clearance, thus excluding soluble antigens from penetrating the mucosa and entering the systemic circulation. The unique biologic features of IgA may help to explain the clinical associations of IgA deficiency with infection, atopic disease, and rheumatic disorders.

Some patients with selective IgA deficiency are more susceptible to infection, although there is disagreement about the relative risk of infection that IgA deficiency imposes on the host. Among patients referred to tertiary care centers for evaluation of recurrent sinopulmonary infections, the incidence of IgA deficiency is significantly higher compared to that of the general population. Apparently, asymptomatic individuals have been identified as IgA deficient by population-based screening. As might be expected by its role as the predominant secretory immunoglobulin, the most common infections in IgA deficient patients occur on mucosal surfaces. Otitis media, sinusitis, bronchitis, pneumonia, and diarrhea are common; meningitis and bacterial sepsis are rare. In some series, as many as 50% of patients with selective IgA deficiency have chronic respiratory tract infections. A subgroup of IgA deficient patients have additional deficiencies of the IgG subclasses IgG2 and IgG4. Studies suggest that these are the IgA deficient patients who tend to experience the most severe and chronic sinopulmonary infections. Since IgG subclass deficiencies are treatable (see section below), IgG subclass determinations should be included in the workup of all IgA deficient patients. The second major target for infections in IgA deficient patients is the gastrointestinal tract. Chronic diarrhea is often idiopathic. *Giardia* is the most frequently identified pathogen. Gluten sensitive enteropathy, ulcerative colitis, and Crohn's disease have each been associated with selective IgA deficiency.

Atopic diseases such as allergic rhinitis, asthma, urticaria, eczema, and food allergy have been reported to occur in as many as 50% of patients with selective IgA deficiency. It has been postulated that lack of secretory IgA allows inhaled and ingested antigens to penetrate the mucosal epithelium and to elicit antibody responses in the bronchial and gastrointestinal lymphoid tissues. A particularly hazardous allergic reaction in IgA deficient patients is the development of anaphylactic reactions after the infusion of plasma or gamma globulin.

A variety of autoimmune and rheumatic diseases have been associated with selective IgA deficiency. These include juvenile rheumatoid arthritis, systemic lupus erythematosus, thyroiditis, and pernicious anemia. A unifying etiology to explain the association of these disorders with selective IgA deficiency has not been established. It has been hypothesized that penetration of environmental antigens may lead to production of antibodies with specificity for self, or that disordered immunoregulation underlies both IgA deficiency and autoimmune disease.

Children with low but not absent IgA (5 to 10 mg/dL) share many of the same disease manifestations, but they tend to be less severely affected. Furthermore, in longitudinal studies, it has been observed that serum IgA levels increase to within the normal range in more than half of these less severe cases, and concomitantly symptoms cease.

Immunoglobulin therapy is generally contraindicated in selective IgA deficiency. Commercial gamma globulin preparations contain trace amounts of IgA, which are insufficient to provide replacement therapy but are sufficient to sensitize the patient to IgA, thereby inducing an IgG or IgE anti-IgA antibody response. This is a relative and not an absolute contraindication to gamma globulin therapy. Patients with IgA deficiency and associated IgG subclass deficiencies who suffer from recurrent infections may benefit from immunoglobulin prophylaxis. In such cases, an intravenous gamma globulin preparation that contains less than .01 g/L of IgA can be used, but with caution.

## IgG Subclass Deficiencies

There are four subclasses of IgG that differ somewhat in their biologic activities. IgG1, IgG2, and IgG3 fix complement, bind to Fc receptors on monocytes, and participate in antibody-dependent cellular cytotoxicity; IgG4 does not. The IgG response to protein antigens occurs predominantly within the IgG1 and IgG3 subclasses, whereas the IgG response to polysaccharide antigens generally is restricted to the IgG2 and IgG4 subclasses. Because antibodies to the polysaccharide capsules of bacteria such as *S pneumoniae* and *H influenzae* are important for host defense, deficiencies of IgG2 and IgG4 may predispose the host to infections caused by these and other encapsulated bacteria.

Deficiencies of IgG subclasses have been described in association with other primary immunodeficiency diseases such as selective IgA deficiency, ataxia-telangiectasia, and Wiskott-Aldrich syndrome. Isolated IgG subclass deficiencies have been only recently identified. The clue to the diagnosis is often the presence of borderline or low normal total serum IgG levels in a patient with recurrent sinopulmonary infections. In such individuals, further tests should include quantitation of IgG subclasses and measurement of antibody responses to protein (eg, diphtheria and tetanus toxoids) and polysaccharide (eg, pneumococcal) vaccines. Some patients with selective deficiency of IgG2 or deficiencies of IgG3 and IgG4 suffer from recurrent pyogenic infections of the respiratory tract. They may benefit from antibiotic prophylaxis or therapy with gamma globulin, but formal studies documenting efficacy are lacking. Only a small number of patients have been identified with isolated deficiencies of IgG3 or IgG4, and the biologic significance of these deficiencies is uncertain. Isolated IgG1 deficiency has not been reported.

## Immunoglobulin Deficiency With Increased IgM

Patients with this disorder have normal or elevated serum IgM and IgD but are deficient in all other immunoglobulin classes. Early in life, it may be difficult to distinguish this disease from X-linked agammaglobulinemia because IgM is not consistently elevated in the first few months of life. Later, the marked elevation in IgM may mask the IgG deficiency if total gamma globulin is measured only by serum protein electrophoresis.

Immunoglobulin deficiency with increased IgM is thought to be caused by an inability of B cells to switch their immunoglobulin secretion from IgM to IgG or IgA. Patients with this disorder have peripheral blood B cells bearing immunoglobulin on their surface, and plasma cells are present in bone marrow and lymphoid tissues. However, most such cells express surface IgM; IgG and IgA bearing B lymphocytes are decreased. Antibody responses to immunization may be present, but are predominantly or exclusively IgM antibodies. Cell-mediated immunity is intact. Most patients with this disorder demonstrate X-linked inheritance, but autosomal recessive and autosomal dominant inheritance have been described.

The clinical course of the disease is marked by recurrent pyogenic infections. Hematologic disorders, presumed to be autoimmune in origin, are often associated and include neutropenia, hemolytic anemia, thrombocytopenia, and pancytopenia. In some cases malignant lymphoproliferative disorders, particularly of IgM-bearing cells, develop.

## Transient Hypogammaglobulinemia of Infancy

Transient hypogammaglobulinemia is an ill-defined disorder of infants in whom there is delayed acquisition of normal serum immunoglobulins. It is a diagnosis that can be established only in retrospect, after immunoglobulin levels become normal. Some patients who initially appear to have transient hypogammaglobulinemia in infancy continue to have persistent abnormalities of humoral immunity and eventually are classified as having CVID, immunodeficiency with increased IgM, or selective IgA deficiency.

There are two broad groups of infants who have been identified with transient hypogammaglobulinemia. The first includes children who have had serum immunoglobulins measured because they have recurrent infections, chronic diarrhea, or other symptoms attributable to immunodeficiency. The second group are infants who may have had no symptoms attributable to hypogammaglobulinemia, but were evaluated prospectively because they had first degree relatives with immunodeficiency. In addition, there is likely to be a number of unrecognized babies who are clinically healthy but have somewhat delayed acquisition of serum immunoglobulin levels. There is a controversy as to whether transient hypogammaglobulinemia of infancy should be considered an immunodeficiency disease or a developmental variant.

Most symptomatic patients with transient hypogammaglobulinemia have chronic or recurrent infections of the respiratory and gastrointestinal tracts. Bacterial sepsis, meningitis, and other systemic infections are rare. Atopic diseases, including eczema and asthma, have also been reported in some but not all series.

Immunologic evaluation of infants with transient hypogammaglobulinemia discloses a variable degree of panhypogammaglobulinemia and reduced antibody responses, but normal numbers of peripheral blood B lymphocytes. For a period of months or as long as several years, immunoglobulin levels remain low, then eventually rise to within the normal range. Antibody titers to previously administered vaccines (eg, diphtheria and tetanus toxoids) often become detectable and indicate resolution of the transient defect before serum immunoglobulin levels increase.

Almost all children with transient hypogammaglobulinemia of infancy can be managed symptomatically without the need for gamma globulin. Prophylactic antibiotics are sometimes useful for managing recurrent sinopulmonary infections. Chronic diarrhea is often caused by malabsorption, presumed to be the result of a previous acute infection, and is treated most quickly with dietary management. In the rare patient in whom symptoms do not respond to conservative measures, gamma globulin therapy may be considered. More importantly, in that patient the diagnosis should be reconsidered.

## General Principles of Gamma Globulin Therapy

As a general rule, the mainstay of therapy for disorders of humoral immunity is replacement of the missing antibody by gamma globulin. There are several limitations, however, on the extent to which pooled exogenous gamma globulin can replace antibody actively produced by the host. First, the antibodies provided are related to the previous antigenic exposure of the donor pool and do not necessarily reflect the exposure of a particular patient to a particular microorganism. For common organisms such as H influenzae, this may have little therapeutic importance, but for organisms encountered infrequently in the general community, it may represent a major deficiency. The second limitation is inherent in the purification process used to prepare gamma globulin, which results in preparations containing virtually IgG only. These preparations contain insufficient amounts of IgA or IgM to provide replacement, and they contain no secretory IgA. Although there is insufficient IgA to provide replacement, there is enough IgA to serve as an antigen in IgA deficient patients, thus making repeated gamma globulin infusions difficult or dangerous for patients with selective IgA deficiency.

Different gamma globulin preparations are available for intramuscular and for intravenous use. Neither form is inherently more effective than the other; efficacy appears to be a function of serum level attained, regardless of the route or preparation used. Most patients, however, are managed with intravenous preparations because this route allows for higher serum levels and less patient discomfort. There is no widely accepted standard dose. Minimum dosage is 300 to 400 mg/kg/month, but in many patients a larger, more frequent dosage is necessary to provide adequate therapy. Both the dose and dosing interval should be adjusted for each patient to provide adequate prophylaxis of symptoms. For some patients, maintaining a trough serum IgG concentration of 400 mg/dL may be sufficient to control symptoms, but others may require substantially higher levels. In this regard, control of symptoms should be defined in the pediatric population as prophylaxis against infections and maintenance of normal growth velocity. Gamma globulin may additionally be used in the management of antibody-mediated autoimmune diseases, such as immune thrombocytopenia, but substantially higher doses may be necessary.

There are several advantages of intravenous gamma globulin preparations over intramuscular preparations. It is easier to infuse sufficient gamma globulin intravenously to maintain desired serum IgG levels. Intravenous infusion allows rapid attainment of serum levels, prevents local proteolysis, and allows infusion into patients with bleeding disorders. Intravenous infusions are generally preferred by the patients who complain of less discomfort than with intramuscular injections. The disadvantages of the intravenous forms of gamma globulin are the cost (intravenous drug plus infusion may cost more than 10 times as much as the intramuscular preparation) and the time required for infusion.

Regarding safety, gamma globulin has an enviable record. There are no reports of disease transmission from commercially prepared lots in the United States, although there have been rare reports of non-A, non-B hepatitis apparently transmitted by several noncommercial lots of gamma globulin. The plasma fractionation process used to prepare gamma globulin has been tested and approved with regard to its ability to inactivate HIV at concentrations far exceeding those that have been found in any patient's serum.

## Selected Readings

### X-Linked Agammaglobulinemia

Fearon ER, Winkelstein JA, Civin CI, et al. Carrier detection in X-linked agammaglobulinemia by analysis of X-chromosome inactivation. N Engl J Med 1987;316:427.
Lederman HM, Winkelstein JA. X-linked agammaglobulinemia: an analysis of 96 patients. Medicine 1985;64:145.
McKinney RE Jr, Katz SL, Wilfert CM. Chronic enteroviral meningoencephalitis in agammaglobulinemic patients. Review of Infectious Diseases 1987;9:334.

### Common Variable Immunodeficiency

Cunningham-Rundles C. Clinical and immunologic analyses of 103 patients with common variable immunodeficiency. J Clin Immunol 1989;9:22.

Hausser C, Virelizier J-L, Buriot D, Griscelli C. Common variable hypogammaglobulinemia in children: clinical and immunologic observations in 30 patients. Am J Dis Child 1983;137:833.

### Selective IgA Deficiency

Oxelius V-A, Laurell A-B, Lindquist B, et al. IgG subclasses in selective IgA deficiency: importance of IgG2-IgA deficiency. N Engl J Med 1981;304:1476.
Strober W, Sneller MC. IgA deficiency. Ann Allergy 1991;66:363.

### IgG Subclass Deficiency

Schur PH. IgG subclasses—a review. Ann Allergy 1987;58:89.

### Immunodeficiency With Increased IgM

Meyer L, Kwan SP, Thompson C, Ko HS, Chiorazzi N, Waldmann T, Rosen F. Evidence for a defect in "Switch" T cells in patients with immunodeficiency and hyperimmunoglobulinemia M. N Engl J Med 1986;314:409.

### Transient Hypogammaglobulinemia of Infancy

Tiller TL, Buckley RH. Transient hypogammaglobulinemia of infants: review of the literature, clinical and immunologic features of 11 new cases, and long-term follow-up. J Pediatr 1978;92:347.

### General Principles of Gamma Globulin Therapy

Dwyer JM. Manipulating the immune system with immune globulin. N Engl J Med 1992;326:107.
Stiehm ER. Intravenous immunoglobulins as therapeutic agents. Ann Intern Med 1987;107:367.

*Principles and Practice of Pediatrics, Second Edition.*
edited by Frank A. Oski et al. J. B. Lippincott Company, Philadelphia © 1994.

## 14.1.3 Complement Deficiencies

Jerry A. Winkelstein

The complement system is composed of a series of plasma proteins and cellular receptors which, when functioning in an ordered and integrated fashion, serve as important mediators of host defense and inflammation. Although the complement system was first described at the turn of the century, it was not until 1960 that the first patient with a genetically determined complement deficiency was identified. Since then, deficiencies have been described for nearly all components of the complement system (Table 14-2).

## CLINICAL PRESENTATION

Individuals with genetically determined complement deficiencies have a variety of clinical presentations. Most patients present with an increased susceptibility to infection, a variety of rheumatic diseases, or angioedema.

### Increased Susceptibility to Infection

An increased susceptibility to infection is a prominent clinical finding in patients with complement deficiencies. The kinds of infections relate to the biologic functions of those components that are missing. The third component of complement (C3) is an important opsonic ligand. Therefore, patients with a deficiency of C3 or of a component in either of the two pathways that activate C3 are more susceptible to infections caused by encapsulated bacteria for which opsonization is the primary host defense (eg, *Streptococcus pneumoniae*, *Streptococcus pyogenes*, and *Haemophilus influenzae*). Similarly, C5–C9 form the membrane attack complex and are responsible for the bactericidal functions of complement. Patients with deficiencies of C5, C6, C7, C8, or C9 opsonize bacteria normally and are not unduly susceptible to gram-positive bacteria. They are, however, susceptible to gram-negative bacteria, notably *Neisseria* species, because serum bactericidal activity is an important host defense against these organisms.

A number of studies have examined groups of patients with specific infectious diseases to determine the frequency of complement deficiencies and to evaluate the utility of screening for complement deficiencies. Between 5% and 15% of patients with systemic meningococcal infections have a genetically determined complement deficiency. The differing estimates may reflect differences in populations examined. In general, the prevalence is higher if the patient has had recurrent meningococcal disease, if the patient has a positive family history for meningococcal disease, or if the patient is infected with an uncommon meningococcal serotype. Therefore, it seems reasonable to screen children with systemic meningococcal infections for the presence of a complement deficiency. In contrast, many patients with complement deficiencies present with systemic pneumococcal or *H influenzae* infections, but the prevalence of complement deficiencies in patients with these specific infections appears low. Recommending screening for complement deficiencies in patients with bacteremia or meningitis caused by pneumococcus or *H influenzae* is more difficult to justify.

### Rheumatic Diseases

Patients with complement deficiencies also have a variety of clinical conditions that best can be described as rheumatic diseases.

TABLE 14-2.   Genetically Determined
Complement Deficiencies

| Deficiency | Inheritance | Major Clinical Manifestation |
|---|---|---|
| C1q | Autosomal recessive | Rheumatic disorders and pyogenic infections |
| C1r/s | Autosomal recessive | Rheumatic disorders |
| C4 | Autosomal recessive | Rheumatic disorders and pyogenic infections |
| C2 | Autosomal recessive | Rheumatic disorders and pyogenic infections |
| C3 | Autosomal recessive | Pyogenic infections |
| C5 | Autosomal recessive | Meningococcal sepsis and meningitis |
| C6 | Autosomal recessive | Meningococcal sepsis and meningitis |
| C7 | Autosomal recessive | Meningococcal sepsis and meningitis |
| C8 | Autosomal recessive | Meningococcal sepsis and meningitis |
| C9 | Autosomal recessive | Meningococcal sepsis and meningitis |
| Factor I | Autosomal recessive | Pyogenic infections |
| Factor H | Autosomal recessive | Hemolytic uremic syndrome |
| Properdin | X-linked recessive | Meningococcal sepsis and meningitis |
| C1 Inhibitor | Autosomal dominant | Angioedema |

These include a disorder that resembles systemic lupus erythematosus (SLE) as well as glomerulonephritis, dermatomyositis, anaphylactoid purpura, and vasculitis. The prevalence of these inflammatory disorders is highest in those patients with deficiencies of the classical activating pathway (C1, C4, and C2) and of C3. The pathophysiologic basis for the occurrence of these diseases in complement deficient patients is unclear, but may relate in part to the physiologic role of the complement system in processing immune complexes or its role in the induction of a normal humoral immune response.

There are some important differences between the rheumatic diseases seen in complement-deficient patients and their counterparts in "normal" noncomplement-deficient individuals. For example, the SLE-like illness seen in complement-deficient individuals is often characterized by onset in childhood, skin lesions resembling discoid lupus, and relatively limited renal and pleuropericardial involvement. In addition, complement-deficient individuals with the lupus-like syndrome usually have absent or low titers of antinuclear antibodies and negative lupus preparations. In contrast, their incidence of anti-Ro antibodies is significantly higher than in noncomplement-deficient patients with lupus. Thus, clinical manifestations of and serologic findings for complement-deficient patients with the lupus-like syndrome resemble a subgroup of lupus patients who are "ANA-negative" or have subacute, cutaneous lupus.

## SPECIFIC DISORDERS

### C1q Deficiency

There appear to be two distinct forms of C1q deficiency. In one form, C1q cannot be detected by either functional or immunochemical analysis. In the other form, immunochemical C1q is present, but it lacks functional activity; ie, it is dysfunctional. The dysfunctional C1q is antigenically deficient, and it does not interact with either IgG or C1r and C1s. The most common clinical presentation of either form of C1q deficiency has been a lupus-like syndrome. Some patients also have had an increased susceptibility to infection manifested by bacterial sepsis or meningitis.

### C1r/C1s Deficiency

Genetically determined deficiency of C1r is characterized by a marked reduction of C1r (less than 1% of normal) and a moderate reduction of C1s (20% to 50% of normal). The basis for the association of the moderately reduced levels of C1s with the absence of C1r in these patients is unknown. (C1r and C1s are structurally and functionally similar and have close genetic linkage.) The clinical presentation of C1r/C1s deficiency has included both a lupus-like illness and glomerulonephritis.

### C4 Deficiency

There are two loci (C4A and C4B) within the major histocompatibility complex that encode for C4. Although the products of the two loci share some functional, structural, and antigenic characteristics that identify them as C4, other characteristics differ slightly. Patients with total C4 deficiency are homozygous for a double null C4 haplotype and have severely depressed serum levels of both antigenic and functional C4 (less than 1%). Those serum activities that depend on C3 and C5–C9 and can be mediated via activation of the alternative pathway, such as opsonic, chemotactic, and bactericidal activities, are present but reduced because of a lack of an intact classical pathway. The predominant clinical manifestation of complete C4 deficiency has been an SLE-like illness, characterized by photosensitive skin rashes, renal disease, and occasionally arthritis. Although some patients are more susceptible to infection, these are patients in whom the SLE-like illness is also present.

Although complete C4 deficiency is rare, individuals who are homozygous deficient for either C4A or C4B are relatively common. Approximately 1% of the population is deficient in C4A and 3% of the population is deficient in C4B. As mentioned, C4A and C4B differ somewhat in their function; C4A interacts more efficiently with proteins and C4B interacts more efficiently with carbohydrates. Because of these functional differences, it has been suggested that individuals who are deficient in one isotype might be predisposed to certain illnesses. For example, individuals who lack C4A are missing the isotype that interacts most efficiently with proteins. They might not be able to clear protein-containing immune complexes normally and be more susceptible to immune complex diseases such as SLE. The prevalence of C4A deficiency in SLE is between 10% and 15%, a prevalence at least 10 times higher than that in the general population. Individuals who are deficient in C4B lack the isotype that is most efficient in interacting with polysaccharides. They might not be able to assemble the classical pathway C3-cleaving enzyme on bacterial polysaccharide capsules and be more susceptible to blood-borne bacterial infections. In fact, the prevalence of C4B deficiency is increased in children with bacteremia and meningitis.

### C2 Deficiency

A deficiency of C2 is the most common of the inherited complement deficiencies. The frequency of the gene for C2 deficiency is estimated at 1 in 100 with homozygous deficient individuals occurring as frequently as 1 in 10,000. Complement-mediated serum activities such as opsonization and chemotaxis are present in patients with C2 deficiency, presumably because their alternative pathway is intact, although they are not generated as quickly nor to the same degree as in individuals with an intact classical pathway. The clinical manifestations of C2 deficiency vary from individuals who are asymptomatic to individuals who are clinically affected with either an increased susceptibility to infection or rheumatic diseases or both. The infections are mostly blood-borne and systemic (eg, sepsis, meningitis, arthritis, and osteomyelitis), and caused by encapsulated bacteria. A variety of rheumatic diseases are associated with C2 deficiency. The most common are disorders that resemble systemic lupus erythematosus and discoid lupus. Glomerulonephritis, dermatomyositis, anaphylactoid purpura, and vasculitis have also been seen.

## C3 Deficiency

Patients with C3 deficiency generally have less than 1% of the normal amount of C3 in their serum. Those serum activities either directly dependent on C3 (opsonization) or indirectly dependent on C3 because of its role in the activation of C5–C9 (chemotaxis and bactericidal activity) are also markedly reduced. The clinical manifestations of C3 deficiency in man include increased susceptibility to infection and rheumatic disorders. Patients with C3 deficiency have a variety of infections, including pneumonia, bacteremia, meningitis, and osteomyelitis, caused by encapsulated pyogenic bacteria. A number of patients have presented with arthralgias and vasculitic skin rashes and a clinical picture consistent with systemic lupus erythematosus. Renal disease has also been seen in C3 deficient patients. Histologically, the lesions most closely resemble membranoproliferative glomerulonephritis.

## C5 Deficiency

Genetically determined C5 deficiency has been identified in a number of different families. The sera of patients with C5 deficiency have markedly reduced levels of C5 and are unable, therefore, to generate normal amounts of chemotactic or bactericidal activity. Serum opsonic activity is intact because activation of C3 can proceed without participation of C5. Although the initial patient identified as C5 deficient had SLE and membranoproliferative glomerulonephritis, subsequent patients have had either meningococcal meningitis or disseminated gonococcal infections.

## C6 Deficiency

The only abnormality relating to the complement system in C6 deficient patients is a marked deficiency of serum bactericidal activity. The major clinical manifestation of C6 deficiency has been systemic Neisserial infections. While most patients have had meningococcal sepsis and meningitis, a few have had disseminated gonococcal infections.

## C7 Deficiency

Only a few patients with C7 deficiency have been identified. Serum bactericidal activity has been markedly reduced in those patients in whom it has been tested. As with other deficiencies of terminal components, systemic meningococcal infections or disseminated gonococcal infections are predominant.

## C8 Deficiency

Native C8 is composed of three chains (alpha, beta, and gamma). The alpha and gamma chains are covalently joined to form one subunit (C8 alpha-gamma), which is joined to the other subunit composed of the beta chain (C8 beta) by noncovalent bonds. In one form of C8 deficiency, patients lack the C8 alpha-gamma subunit, while in the other form, the C8 beta subunit is deficient.

In either case, C8 functional activity is markedly reduced (less than 1% of normal). The only functional defect in C8 deficient sera is a marked reduction in bactericidal activity. The clinical presentation of C8 deficiency consists of meningococcemia, meningococcal meningitis, and disseminated gonococcal infections. SLE has also rarely been seen.

## C9 Deficiency

Only a few patients with C9 deficiency have been identified. Serum hemolytic activity can be generated by a membrane attack complex composed only of C5b-8, albeit more slowly and to a lesser degree than the C5b-9 complex. Thus, patients with C9 deficiency possess some serum hemolytic and bactericidal activity. Patients with C9 deficiency have an increased susceptibility to systemic meningococcal infections, although probably not to the same degree as patients with deficiencies of the other terminal components.

## Factor I Deficiency

Factor I controls the assembly and expression of the alternative pathway C3-cleaving enzyme. Factor I deficiency is characterized by uncontrolled activation of C3 via the alternative pathway because, in the absence of factor I, there is no control imposed on the formation and expression of the alternative pathway C3 convertase. Patients with factor I deficiency, therefore, have a secondary consumption of C3 resulting in markedly reduced levels of native C3 in their serum. Most of the C3 is not native C3 but rather the cleavage product, C3b. Those serum activities that directly or indirectly depend on C3 (opsonic activity, chemotactic activity, and bactericidal activity) are reduced in patients with factor I deficiency. The most common clinical expression of factor I deficiency is an increased susceptibility to infection. Organisms most commonly responsible for these infections are encapsulated, pyogenic bacteria, organisms for which C3 is an important opsonic ligand.

## Factor H Deficiency

Factor H deficiency has been described in a few families only. Factor H levels in the serum generally are reduced to less than 10% of normal. Both rheumatic disorders and an increased susceptibility to infection have been described in factor H deficiency.

## Properdin Deficiency

Properdin is a control protein that stabilizes the alternative pathway enzymes that activate C3 and C5. Properdin deficiency is inherited as an X-linked recessive disorder. There are at least two forms of properdin deficiency. In one form, patients lack both antigenic and functional properdin in their serum; in the second form, antigenic properdin is present but has no functional activity. The only reported clinical manifestation of properdin deficiency is a marked increased susceptibility to systemic meningococcal infections.

## C1 Inhibitor Deficiency

A genetically determined deficiency of C1 inhibitor (C1-INH) is responsible for the clinical disorder Hereditary Angioedema (HAE). C1 inhibitor deficiency is inherited in an autosomal dominant fashion. There are at least two forms of C1-INH deficiency. In the most common form (Type I), which accounts for about 85% of patients, the serum of affected individuals is deficient in both C1-INH protein (5% to 30% of normal) and C1-INH activity. In the less common form (Type II), a dysfunctional protein is present in normal or elevated concentrations, but its functional activity is markedly reduced. In either case, the level of C4 in serum is commonly reduced both during and between attacks, making it a useful diagnostic clue.

The pathophysiologic mechanisms by which the absence of C1-INH activity leads to the angioedema characteristic of the disorder are still incompletely understood. Neither the mediators responsible for producing the edema nor the mechanisms initiating their production have been clearly identified, although evidence implicates both the complement system and the kinin system in the pathogenesis of the edema.

The clinical symptoms of HAE are the result of submucosal or subcutaneous edema. The lesions are characterized by non-inflammatory edema associated with capillary and venule dilation. The three most prominent areas of involvement are the skin, respiratory tract, and gastrointestinal tract.

Attacks involving the skin may involve an extremity, the face, or genitalia. The edema may vary in size from a few centimeters to involvement of a whole extremity. The lesions are pale rather than red, are usually not warm, and are characteristically non-pruritic. There may be a feeling of tightness in the skin caused by accumulation of subcutaneous fluid. Attacks usually progress for 1 to 2 days and resolve over an additional 2 to 3 days.

Attacks involving the upper respiratory tract represent a serious threat to the patient with HAE. Pharyngeal edema occurs at least once in nearly two thirds of the patients. The patients may initially experience a "tightness" in the throat and swelling of the tongue, buccal mucosa and oropharynx follow. In some instances, laryngeal edema, accompanied by hoarseness and stridor, progresses to respiratory obstruction and represents a life-threatening emergency.

The gastrointestinal tract can be affected by HAE. Symptoms are secondary to edema of the bowel wall and may include anorexia, dull aching of the abdomen, vomiting, and crampy abdominal pain. Abdominal symptoms can occur in the absence of concurrent cutaneous or pharyngeal involvement.

The onset of symptoms referable to HAE occurs in more than half the patients before adolescence, but in some patients, symptoms do not occur until adulthood. Even though trauma, anxiety, and stress are frequently cited as events that initiate attacks, more than half of patients can not clearly identify an event that initiated an attack. Dental extractions and tonsillectomy can initiate edema of the upper airway, and cutaneous edema may follow trauma to an extremity.

Therapy of HAE is divided into two categories: prophylaxis of attacks and treatment of attacks. Long-term prevention of attacks may be indicated in those patients who have had laryngeal obstruction or have suffered frequent and debilitating attacks. Antifibrinolytic agents such as epsilon aminocaproic acid (EACA) or its cyclic analog, tranexamic acid, have been used with some success in the long-term prevention of attacks. More recently, "impeded" androgens such as danazol and stanozolol, which have attenuated androgenic potential, have been found to be useful in long-term prophylaxis of HAE. These agents have not been used extensively in children, however, because of their androgenic effects. Apparently, they act by stimulating the synthesis of functionally intact C1-INH by the normal gene. In some instances, patients may need short-term prophylactic therapy (eg, before oral surgery). In these circumstances, danazol therapy may be initiated 1 week before surgery or EACA the day before surgery.

A number of drugs have been used in an attempt to interrupt an attack of HAE once it has begun. Epinephrine, antihistamines, and corticosteroids are of no proven benefit. Recent trials with partially purified C1-INH are encouraging. Infusion of C1-INH has been accompanied by resolution of edema and symptoms within a few hours.

## Selected Readings

Figueroa JE, Densen P. Infectious diseases associated with complement deficiencies. Clin Microbiol Rev 1991;4:359.

Frank MM. The complement system in host defense and inflammation. Review of Infectious Diseases 1979;1:483.

Frank MM, Gelfand JA, Atkinson JP. Hereditary angioedema: the clinical syndrome and its management. Ann Intern Med 1976;84:580.

Ross SC, Densen P. Complement deficiency states and infections: epidemiology, pathogenesis, and consequences of neisserial and other infections in an immune deficiency. Medicine 1984;63:243.

Rother K, Rother V. Hereditary and acquired complement deficiencies in animals and man. Progress in Allergy 1986; vol. 39.

Schur PH. Inherited complement component abnormalities. Annu Rev Med 1986;37:333.

Winkelstein JA. Complement and natural immunity. Clinics in Allergy and Immunology 1983;3:421.

Winkelstein JA, Colten H. Genetically determined disorders of the complement system. IN: Schriver CR, Beaudet AL, Sly WS, Valle D. The metabolic basis for inherited disease. New York: McGraw-Hill, 1989.

*Principles and Practice of Pediatrics, Second Edition.*
edited by Frank A. Oski et al. J. B. Lippincott Company, Philadelphia © 1994.

## 14.1.4 *Functional Disorders of Granulocytes*

Donald C. Anderson and C. Wayne Smith

Mobile blood granulocytes and monocytes and fixed phagocytic cells of reticuloendothelial tissues function as a first line defense against invasion by bacterial or fungal microorganisms. Impaired granulocyte production as well as functional abnormalities of granulocytes or other professional phagocytes may significantly compromise host defense, thus increasing susceptibility to infection. Early animal studies demonstrated a critical 2- to 4-hour period after cutaneous invasion by pathogenic bacteria during which phagocytes must localize at a site of invasion in order to prevent or suppress an infections process. Recurrent bacterial or fungal infections of the skin or mucous membranes are prominent in patients with quantitative deficiencies of blood granulocytes and in patients with functional deficits of granulocytic cells.

Two broad categories of functional disorders are those typified by impaired motility, recruitment, or localization of granulocytes at or to sites of infection; and those resulting from defective ingestion or intracellular killing of microorganisms by granulocytes and other phagocytic cells. In this latter group of patients, granulocytes accumulate normally in inflamed tissues but are unable to eradicate invading microorganisms. Laboratory studies of representative patients of both categories can be used to define abnormalities of one or more cellular functions (eg, directed migration or chemotaxis, adhesion, ingestion, degranulation, and oxidative intracellular killing) in vitro. In selected disorders, molecular deficits have been defined, which allows important new approaches to the diagnosis or clinical management of disease.

## DISORDERS OF ADHERENCE AND MOTILITY

Several lines of evidence emphasize the critical role of immunospecific adhesion molecules in guiding granulocytes and other leukocytes to sites of inflammation in infected tissues. Early intravital studies showed that granulocytes preferentially adhere to vascular endothelium adjacent to a site of inflammation before migration into surrounding tissues. More recent studies characterize at least three gene families of adhesion molecules expressed on leukocytes and endothelial or other mesenchymal cells that participate in the process of blood leukocyte emigration. These include members of the integrin, immunoglobulin, and selectin gene families, each of which is dynamically regulated by inflammatory mediators and contributes to granulocyte adherence functions. Several clinical entities typified by diminished or enhanced cellular adherence properties have been identified. In selected cases, a molecular pathogenesis of disease has been described.

## Leukocyte Adhesion Deficiency

Leukocyte adhesion deficiency (LAD) is a recently recognized autosomal-recessive trait characterized by recurrent bacterial infections, impaired pus formation and wound healing, and a spectrum of functional abnormalities in granulocytes, monocytes, and lymphoid cells. The molecular basis of LAD has been found to involve a family of structurally and functionally related glycoproteins on the surface of myeloid cells. These glycoproteins occur as noncovalently associated $\alpha$ and $\beta$ subunits with $\alpha_1\beta_1$ stoichiometry. They share an identical $\beta$ subunit ($M_r$ = 95,000) and are distinguished immunologically by distinct $\alpha$ subunits designated Mac-1$\alpha$($\alpha$M) ($M_r$ = 165,000), LFA-1$\alpha$($\alpha$L) ($M_r$ = 177,000), and p150,95$\alpha$($\alpha$X) ($M_r$ = 150,000). The World Health Organization designation for these glycoproteins is CD18 for the beta subunit, CD11a for the $\alpha$L subunits, CD11b for the $\alpha$M subunits, and CD11c for the $\alpha$X subunits. The entire complex is designated CD11/CD18. Biosynthetic studies show that these patients possess heterogeneous abnormalities of the $\beta$(CD18) but not $\alpha$ subunits of the CD11/CD18 glycoproteins. These findings suggested distinct mutations in the CD18 gene, which has been mapped to chromosome 21. Such mutations have been defined in several patients and include point mutations, deletions, or insertions as identified by nucleotide sequence analysis of patient or heterozygote CD18 cDNA or genomic DNA. Although most LAD phenotypes are not defined at the nucleotide level, it is probable that all include mutations of the CD18 gene and that CD18 mutants vary in their ability to complex with the different $\alpha$ subunits, thus determining the relative deficiency of $\alpha\beta$ protein complexes expressed on cell surfaces.

The clinical hallmarks of this disease are recurrent, necrotic, and indolent infections of soft tissues, primarily involving skin, mucous membranes, and intestinal tract. Superficial infections of body surfaces may invade locally or systemically. Typical small, erythematous, nonpustular skin lesions often progress to large, well-demarcated, ulcerative craters (or pyoderma gangrenosa), which heal slowly or with dysplastic eschars. Staphylococcal or gram-negative enteric bacterial organisms may be cultured from such lesions for several weeks despite antimicrobial therapy. Septicemia progressing from omphalitis associated with delayed umbilical cord severance has been observed in several families. Perirectal abscess or cellulitis leading to peritonitis or septicemia has been reported in multiple patients, and facial or deep neck cellulitis has been observed to progress from ulcerative mucous membrane lesions of the oral cavity. Recurrent invasive candidal esophagitis, erosive gastritis, acute appendicitis, and necrotizing enterocolitis have been reported in multiple patients. Recurrent otitis media occurs commonly, and progression to mastoiditis and facial nerve paralysis has been reported. Other common respiratory infections include severe bacterial (pseudomonal) laryngotracheitis, recurrent pneumonitis, and sinusitis. Severe gingivitis or periodontitis is a major feature among all patients who survive

infancy. Acute gingivitis has appeared in all cases with eruption of the primary dentition. Subsequently, these patients develop characteristic features of progressive generalized prepubescent periodontitis, including gingival proliferation, defective recession, mobility, pathologic migration, and advanced alveolar bone loss associated with periodontal pocket formation and partial or total loss of both the deciduous and permanent dentitions.

The recurrent infections observed in affected patients appear to reflect a profound impairment of leukocyte mobilization into extravascular inflammatory sites. "Skin windows" and biopsy samples of infected tissues demonstrate inflammatory infiltrates totally devoid of neutrophils. This histopathologic feature is particularly striking because marked peripheral blood leukocytosis (5 to 20 times normal values) is a constant feature of this disorder. Transfusions of leukocytes result in the appearance of donor neutrophils and monocytes in "skin windows" and in skin chambers. Impaired healing of traumatic or surgical wounds observed in several patients represents a clinical feature not generally observed in patients with neutropenia or dysfunctional neutrophils. Unusual paper-thin or dysplastic cutaneous scars have been found in some patients.

The severity of infectious complications among LAD patients appears to be related directly to the degree of glycoprotein deficiency. Two phenotypes, designated severe and moderate deficiency, have been identified. Severely affected patients have essentially undetectable expression of all three $\alpha\beta$ complexes in their neutrophils. Moderately deficient patients express 2.5% to 6% of all three $\alpha\beta$ complexes. Patients with severe deficiency have either died in infancy or have demonstrated a susceptibility to severe, life-threatening systemic infections (peritonitis, septicemia, pneumonitis, aseptic meningitis). In contrast, among the patients with moderate deficiency, life-threatening infections have been observed infrequently despite a relatively prolonged survival (up to 45 years). In some moderately affected patients, skin lesions may disappear after the first few years of life, recurring only with occasional infections. Severe gingivitis is always observed in these patients and may be the presenting symptom. Delayed umbilical cord separation occurs more frequently in patients with the severe phenotype, but it is not universally found.

Suggested therapeutic guidelines for LAD are based on limited clinical experience. While infectious complications generally are observed on body surfaces, life-threatening systemic infections may occur at any time, especially in individuals with severe disease. Superficial inflammatory lesions must be managed aggressively with local care and antibiotic therapy. This is of special importance because inflammatory signs may be minimal before the development of septicemic episodes. Moreover, impaired healing of superficial wounds appears to allow indolent colonization and subsequent reinfection. The early use of empiric combination therapy with a staphylocidal agent and an aminoglycoside is justified in acutely ill or febrile patients in the absence of localizing findings. The use of prophylactic antibiotics may be advised. Limited clinical experience suggests that the number of systemic infections of LAD patients is considerably diminished by prophylactic regimens. Because of the high incidence of staphylococcal and gram-negative enteric infections, trimethoprim-sulfamethoxazole is a useful agent based on its spectrum of antimicrobial activity. Leukocyte transfusions have been successfully employed in several LAD patients; enhancement of inflammatory functions and clinical resolution of even life-threatening infections have been achieved in a clinical setting where systemic antibiotic or surgical interventions were ineffective.

Bone marrow transplantation with successful engraftment and apparent clinical recovery from disease has been achieved in several patients. Because of inherent risks and expense, this approach should be considered only for patients with the severe phenotype of disease. Among patients undergoing transplantation, recipients of HLA-identical as well as HLA-mismatched (eg, haplotype match) bone marrow have shown successful engraftment. In some cases, mixed but stable chimerism between donor and recipient cells is apparent 3 to 5 years after transplantation. In these cases, normal or slightly diminished blood granulocyte function is observed in vitro, and the patients demonstrate no clinical complications.

The identification in LAD patients of CD18 mutations raises the possibility that the introduction of a normal CD18 gene into hematopoietic cells could cure this disease, especially in light of the encouraging results of bone marrow transplantation. Recent reports document the successful transfection or retroviral-mediated infection of LAD cells or cell lines with a normal CD18 cDNA resulting in normal CD18 protein expression and normal cell adherence properties. Thus, the stage is set for future attempts at somatic cell gene therapy in LAD.

## Specific Granule Deficiency

Neutrophilic granulocytes contain multiple subpopulations of granules. Azurophilic or primary granules appear early in neutrophil development and contain lysosomal enzymes, including lysozyme and myeloperoxidase. Specific or secondary granules develop later. Though they lack myeloperoxidase and other hydrolases, specific granules are capable of the extracellular release of a number of substances that may regulate inflammation. Recent evidence indicates secretory determinants of granulocyte adherence and migratory functions. For example, specific granules represent a major intracellular pool for chemotactic factor receptors and the CD11b/CD18 adherence protein which are transported to the cell surface after chemotactic activation.

The first example of a primary deficiency of neutrophil-specific granules was recognized in 1972. Other cases have been subsequently reported by several laboratories. One patient appears to have had an acquired deficiency (associated with a myeloproliferative syndrome), while all others appear to have genetically determined disease. Each demonstrated susceptibility to recurrent and severe infections of the skin, mucous membranes, and lung, most commonly due to *Staphylococcus aureus, Pseudomonas aeruginosa*, other enteric pathogens, and *Candida albicans*. Infections may progress from superficial sites; otitis media with associated mastoiditis was reported in one patient, and lung abscess formation due to *S aureus* followed the onset of pneumonia in another individual. The occurrence of necrotic oral lesions due to invasion by *Escherichia coli* and species of *Pseudomonas* and *Klebsiella* were reported in another individual, but severe neutropenia recognized in that patient may have accounted for the development of these mucous membrane lesions. Another patient with severe scalp infections due to *Proteus mirabilis* and *S aureus* required prolonged intravenous antibiotic therapy in addition to surgical debridement. Detailed descriptions of the histopathology of infected tissues in all patients are not reported, but "skin window" studies have demonstrated diminished pus formation in tissues of some individuals who were not neutropenic.

Neutrophils from each patient studied have demonstrated morphologic abnormalities, including a severe or total deficiency of specific granules and a variety of nuclear abnormalities including bi-lobed or multi-lobed nuclei or nuclear blebs, clefts, or pockets. Diminished or absent neutrophil lactoferrin content has been confirmed in only three cases, and the membrane marker alkaline phosphatase has been shown to be diminished or absent in neutrophils of all but one reported case. Total cellular content and release of the secondary granule markers (lactoferrin, B$_{12}$ transport protein, cytochrome b, and lysozyme) have been shown to be diminished when assessed in selected patients, although levels of primary granule constituents (myeloperoxidase, β-gluc-

uronidase) are generally normal. Among recognized cases, somewhat heterogeneous abnormalities in cellular functions have been observed. Chemotaxis and intracellular microbicidal activity represent the most consistently reported functional deficits.

Deficiency of specific granules is suggested by a history of recurrent cutaneous, subcutaneous, mucous membrane, or pulmonary infections due to *S aureus*, virulent gram-negative enteric bacteria, or species of *Candida*. Findings of abnormal morphology and abnormally weak cytochemical reactions for alkaline phosphatase are highly suggestive of this disorder. Cytochemical and ultrastructural studies to confirm diminished numbers or abnormal morphology of specific granules and their specific constituents will establish a diagnosis. While most examples of primary specific granule deficiency recognized to date are probably genetic in origin, the mode of transmission of this disorder is uncertain. A prognosis is not well defined, but most individuals have survived the pediatric age group with antimicrobial and supportive therapy.

## Functional Abnormalities in Neonatal Neutrophils

Because specific immunity is limited severely in the immediate postpartum period, the inflammatory functions of phagocytic cells are especially important for host defense against microbial invasion. Both quantitative and qualitative abnormalities of phagocytic cells contribute to the enhanced infectious susceptibility of neonates. Neutropenia is commonly observed in systemically infected neonates, and studies in neonatal animals indicate that exhaustion of a limited reserve pool of bone marrow granulocytes contributes to a depletion of circulating or marginating pools when tissue demand is increased. Among the most consistently observed functional abnormalities thought to contribute to impaired inflammation in neonates are those related to the motility of leukocytes. As shown with "skin windows," inflammatory responses in newborns differ from those in older children and adults in two respects: the shift from the early granulocyte predominance to a predominance of mononuclear cells is slower and less pronounced, and a marked eosinophilia is observed in some infants aged 2 to 21 days. Strikingly diminished leukocyte mobilization in neonatal rats inoculated intraperitoneally with bacteria or chemotactic agents has been demonstrated.

Neonatal neutrophils exhibit impaired chemotactic responses to numerous chemotactic factors including those released by growing *S aureus* and *E coli* and those generated in plasma by antigen-antibody complexes (eg, C5a). Visual assays demonstrate that neonatal cells not only have depressed migration but also are impaired significantly in their ability to orient toward a gradient of chemotactic factors. Depressed chemotaxis has been found in healthy neonates aged 1 to 5 days. In addition, there is diminished generation of chemotactic activity (chemotaxigenesis) by virulent Type III Group B Streptococci in neonatal sera, an abnormality directly related to diminished levels of both type-specific anticapsular antibody and serum complement activity. Thus, impaired generation of chemotactic stimuli as well as abnormal cellular responses appear to account for diminished inflammatory responses observed in even healthy term neonates.

The basis for abnormal migratory functions of neonatal granulocytes is not fully defined but appears to involve defects of stimulated cell adhesion. Induction of surface expression of CD11b/CD18 (MAC-1) by chemotactic agonists is diminished, and basal levels of the L-selectin adherence protein are markedly diminished on cord blood or neonatal granulocytes. The importance of these observations is suggested by findings of diminished transendothelial migration by neonatal neutrophils in vitro. This defect reflects impaired Mac-1-adhesive interactions with the endothelial ligand ICAM-1 and deficits of L-selectin interactions with another endothelial adherence molecule, ELAM-1. Studies in neonatal animal models of inflammation support a role for both neutrophil adhesion determinants in diminished inflammatory exudation.

Because multiple host defense mechanisms are defective or developmentally delayed in human neonates, no precise cause and effect relationship between impaired cellular migration and the occurrence of infectious complications is established. However, neonates are particularly susceptible to the development of cutaneous inflammatory lesions or abscesses at sites of local trauma (for example, circumcision wounds, umbilicus, intertriginous areas, or sites of electrode-monitoring devices). Microorganisms such as *S aureus*, gram negative-enteric organisms, and species of *Candida* represent the most common agents infecting cutaneous or mucous membrane lesions in human neonates. The propensity for systemic invasion and the development of neonatal septicemia by endogenous respiratory or gastrointestinal flora may be related to insufficient infiltration of granulocytes or monocytes into submucosal tissues.

## Chédiak-Higashi Syndrome

The Chédiak-Higashi syndrome is an autosomal recessive disorder of mink, cattle, beige mice, and humans. This condition is characterized clinically by partial oculocutaneous albinism, the presence of giant lysosomal granules in all granular cell types, susceptibility to bacterial infection, variable occurrence of neutropenia and thrombocytopenia, and an accelerated lymphoma-like proliferative phase generally occurring in the first decade of life. Infectious complications are attributable to both neutropenia and functional deficits of neutrophils, monocytes, and natural killer (NK) cells. A comprehensive review in 1972 documented the significance of infectious morbidity and mortality in this syndrome. Among 56 cases reviewed, 33 individuals died before age 10 years; among 27 cases for which a cause of death was determined, infections was the sole cause in 17 and a contributing factor in 9 more cases. Pulmonary, cutaneous, subcutaneous, and upper respiratory infections were observed most. *S aureus* accounted for about 70% of all infections for which an etiologic agent was determined; group A Streptococcus, gram-negative enteric organisms (*Klebsiella, Pseudomonas, Proteus, Shigella* sp), *Aspergillus*, and species of *Candida* represented occasional etiologic agents.

Neutrophils, monocytes, and lymphocytes from these patients demonstrate large intracellular inclusions or granules, which represent the pathologic hallmark of the disease. Although they are most easily demonstrated in leukocytes, they also are present in renal tubular epithelium, gastric mucosa, pancreas, thyroid, neural tissue, and melanocytes. In neutrophils, inclusions contain azurophilic granule markers (myeloperoxidase and acid phosphatase) and are assumed to represent abnormal azurophilic granules. These abnormal granules, however, contain both azurophilic and specific granule markers. Normal-appearing specific granules are present, but normal azurophilic granules have not been seen. Analysis of bone marrow samples from patients with Chédiak-Higashi syndrome suggest that abnormal granules are formed during granulocyte maturation by the progressive aggregation and fusion of azurophilic and specific granules. Such findings are consistent with a proposed membrane abnormality.

Several functional abnormalities of neutrophils, monocytes, and natural killer cells of these patients have been identified. Defective neutrophil and monocyte chemotaxis has been consistently reported, but the molecular determinants of these abnormalities are undefined. Neutrophils demonstrate delayed and diminished intracellular killing of both gram-positive and gram-negative bacterial organisms, despite a normal capacity to ingest these organisms and a normal or elevated oxidative burst. Microbicidal abnormalities are attributed to impaired post-phagocytic phagolysosomal fusion. A selective impairment of the func-

tions of natural killer cells (as opposed to other lymphocyte functions) has been reported. Dysfunction of the natural killer cell system may account for the ultimate development of an aggressive lymphoproliferative syndrome in most patients.

A diagnosis of Chédiak-Higashi syndrome is made by identifying characteristic clinical features of the disorder in addition to characteristic large cytoplasmic inclusions in all granular cells, including peripheral blood granulocytes. Giant melanosomes can be demonstrated from hair of patients. Neutropenia and thrombocytopenia are most characteristic during the accelerated phase of disease. When bone marrow aspirates are examined, common abnormalities include hypercellularity with extensive vacuolization and inclusions in myeloid precursors. Elevated serum lysozyme levels probably reflect intramedullary granulocyte destruction. The accelerated phase of Chédiak-Higashi syndrome is characterized by widespread tissue infiltrates of lymphoid and histiocytic cells, usually without malignant histologic characteristics. Splenomegaly and associated hypersplenism contribute to anemia and thrombocytopenia and may also contribute to neutropenia. Although viral agents and immunologic mechanisms may contribute to the pathogenesis of the accelerated phase, the precise mechanisms are undefined.

Most patients with Chédiak-Higashi syndrome succumb to infectious or infiltrative complications within the first decade of life. Successful bone marrow transplantation with reversal of the defect in natural killer activity has been reported in one case. Definitive preventive or therapeutic strategies await definition of the disease's molecular pathogenesis.

## Type 1b Glycogen Storage Disease

The association of neutropenia, impaired neutrophil migration, and recurrent infection in type 1b glycogen storage disease was first reported in 1980. Most clinical features of type 1b glycogen storage disease are similar to those of type 1a glycogen storage disease, including hepatomegaly, fasting hypoglycemia, lactic acidosis, short stature, hyperlipidemia, and the occurrence of hepatomas with potential for malignant degeneration. Patients with type 1a glycogen storage disease demonstrate a deficiency of glucose-6-phosphatase activity in liver, kidney, and intestine. In contrast, type 1b glycogen storage disease patients demonstrate normal glucose-6-phosphatase activity.

A review of the clinical and laboratory features of 21 patients with type 1b glycogen storage disease indicated that most suffered from a variety of moderate to severe bacterial infections including pneumonitis, recurrent otitis media, subcutaneous abscesses, generalized pyoderma, cellulitis, wound infections, and osteomyelitis, most commonly secondary to *S aureus*. Most patients exhibited chronic neutropenia, which, in some patients, was associated with demonstrable serum inhibitors of myeloid stem cell proliferation, abnormalities of myeloid maturation, and decreased peripheral marginating pools. Functional abnormalities including diminished random or directed migration of neutrophils in vitro were documented in 8 of 11 patients tested, and deficient chemotactic modulation of adherence by chemotactic factors was observed in 2 patients. In contrast, microbicidal activity of neutrophils and phagocytosis-associated oxidative metabolic activity are normal in most patients with type 1b glycogen storage disease.

The biochemical basis for quantitative or qualitative abnormalities of neutrophils or mononuclear leukocytes is uncertain. Studies in one patient identified a defect of glucose-6-phosphatase translocase, one of three integral membrane components of the hepatic microsomal glucose-6-phosphatase system. A physiologic role of glucose-6-phosphate transport in neutrophils is not defined, so a causal relationship between aberrant glucose-6-phosphate transport and impaired neutrophil migration cannot be established yet.

## Mannosidosis

Mannosidosis is a lysosomal storage disease characterized clinically by psychomotor retardation, facial dysmorphology similar to that of Hurler's syndrome, dysostosis multiplex, hepatosplenomegaly, hearing loss, and recurrent soft tissue infections. This autosomal recessive disease is due to a deficiency of acidic $\alpha$-mannosidase A and B activity resulting in mannose-rich oligosaccharide accumulation in lysosomes of circulating leukocytes and in neural and visceral tissues. A defect of neutrophil chemotaxis and phagocytosis in neutrophils and a diminished lymphocyte transformation were described in one child with systemic mannosidosis. It is suggested that these functional defects result from abnormal mannose catabolism, and that partially degraded oligosaccharides, glycopeptides, glycoproteins, and terminal $\alpha$D-mannose residues may bind to leukocyte plasma membranes as well as accumulate in lysosomal granules. In a review of 17 cases, 13 experienced significant or recurrent infections, including chronic otitis media, upper respiratory infections, severe or progressive pneumonia, and cutaneous inflammatory lesions. While the majority of documented infections were bacterial in origin, individuals also were susceptible to viral infections, which partly reflects impairment of cell-mediated immunity in this disease. One patient died of overwhelming adenoviral pneumonia. A diagnosis of mannosidosis as suggested by typical clinical features can be confirmed by the demonstration of deficient acidic $\alpha$-mannosidase activity in plasma, peripheral blood leukocytes, or cultured skin fibroblasts.

## Periodontitis Syndromes

Experimental and clinical evidence documents the important protective role of phagocytic cells and, in particular, neutrophils in oral cavity tissues. The infiltration of neutrophils into gingival tissues early in the development of gingivitis is thought to provide a first-line defense against invasion by pathogenic oral microflora. Individuals with developmental, genetic, or acquired disorders are characterized by quantitative deficiencies of peripheral blood phagocytes or functional abnormalities of neutrophils commonly present with oral complications. Primary or secondary agranulocytosis and cyclic neutropenia syndromes are typified by severe ulceration, necrosis, or chronic inflammation of gingival or periodontal tissues. Patients with severe leukocytopathies such as chronic granulomatous disease, Chédiak-Higashi syndrome, and leukocyte adhesion deficiency present with systemic as well as oral infections while those demonstrating less profound functional deficits such as in localized juvenile periodontitis, post-localized juvenile periodontitis, or generalized juvenile periodontitis present exclusively with periodontal manifestations.

Defective chemotactic responsiveness of neutrophils is thought to represent a major pathogenic mechanism in individuals with periodontitis syndromes. Of 183 patients with localized juvenile periodontitis studied by multiple investigators, 71% are reported to exhibit defective chemotaxis. Most patients exhibit intrinsic cellular defects, but cell-directed serum inhibitors, chemotactic factor inactivators, or abnormalities of chemotaxigenesis are reported in a small proportion of patients tested. The pathogenic mechanisms accounting for impaired chemotaxis have not been defined. The epidemiologic or clinical associations of certain periodontopathic bacterial organisms with some periodontitis syndromes suggest the possibility that cellular constituents or extracellular factors elaborated by these microorganisms may secondarily alter functions of leukocytes. The pathogenic roles of gram-negative oral bacteria including *Actinobacillus actinomycetemcomitans*, species of Bacteroides, and species of Capnocytophaga have been increasingly appreciated. Among the potentially pathogenic products of *A actinomycetemcomitans*, a leukocytotoxin has been identified in vitro which may contribute to diminished chemotactic function. Sera from patients contain IgG antibodies that neutralize leukotoxic activity of *A actinomycetemcomitans*, and serum and gingival crevicular fluids from such patients contain high titers of antibodies to *A actinomycetemcomitans* antigens. Other poorly defined inhibitors of chemotaxis are found in culture filtrates or sonicates of *Bacteroides gingivalis*, *Fusobacterium nucleatum*, and species of Capnocytophaga.

Despite intensive study, the prevalence, natural history, and etiology of juvenile periodontitis remain undefined. The familial aggregation in juvenile periodontitis has prompted a number of researchers to propose a possible genetic basis for this disease. It has not been determined if the familial occurrence of juvenile periodontitis results from a Mendelian inheritance, multifactorial inheritance, or environmental effects. The mode of genetic transmission of specific periodontitis syndromes awaits the identification of molecular markers for disease.

## Schwachman-Diamond Syndrome

Clinical features of a syndrome first described by Schwachman and Diamond include exocrine pancreatic insufficiency, bone marrow hypoplasia with associated neutropenia, metaphyseal chondrodysplasia, growth retardation, and recurrent soft tissue infections. In a series of 21 patients, otitis media, bronchial pneumonia, osteomyelitis, dermatitis, and septicemia occurred in 17 (81%), from which 3 (14% of total series) died. Neutropenia was intermittent in most patients in this and other series. Bone marrow aspirations from patients with this disorder have demonstrated absent myeloid precursors or maturation arrest with variable degrees of hypoplasia. Normal bone marrow aspirates in neutropenic patients have also been described, suggesting that marrow hypoplasia is patchy in distribution. Diminished chemotaxis of neutrophils without other functional abnormalities was found in 12 of 14 patients with this syndrome. Nine of these patients were neutropenic, and 4 demonstrated low levels of serum IgA or IgM without other immunologic abnormalities. Intermediate abnormalities of neutrophil chemotaxis were recognized in parents of some of these individuals, suggesting that the individuals were heterozygous for the abnormality and that the abnormality is inherited as an autosomal recessive trait. A pathogenic basis for hematologic and other features of this multisystem disease is not determined, and the relative contributions of impaired cellular motility as opposed to neutropenia to infectious susceptibility in affected patients is uncertain.

## DISORDERS OF INTRACELLULAR MICROBIAL KILLING

Opsonophagocytosis mediated by specific membrane receptors initiates a sequence of metabolic, biophysical, and cytoskeletal events that promote rapid, efficient killing of intracellular microorganisms by phagocytes. Phagocytosis is associated with a burst of oxidative metabolic activity including the consumption of molecular oxygen and the evolution of superoxide, hydrogen peroxide, or other oxygen radicals. This respiratory burst requires a series of electron transfers using nicotinamide-adenine dinucleotide phosphate (NADPH) as the electron donor. It involves a flavin-adenine dinucleotide-containing flavoprotein and a unique cytochrome b. This oxidase system is associated with the plasma membrane of granulocytes or mononuclear phagocytes. Thus, lethal oxygen radicals are concentrated together with ingested microbes in phagosomes or the extracellular environment of neutrophils. Neutrophil myeloperoxidase (MPO) in the presence of $H_2O_2$ and halide further catalyzes the formation of additional oxidants such as hypochlorous acid and free chlorine in pha-golysosomes. Constituents of both primary and secondary ly-sosomal granules including defensins, elastase, cathepsin G, lac-toferrin, and other proteins significantly contribute to non-oxidative microbicidal activity within phagosomes. Increased understanding of the molecular biology of phagocytes allows the delineation of several clinical disorders of intracellular microbi-cidal functions that are characterized by enhanced susceptibility to recurrent bacterial or fungal infections.

## Chronic Granulomatosis Disease

The chronic granulomatous diseases (CGD) are a genetically het-erogeneous group of disorders of the oxidative metabolism of phagocytes. CGD results in impairment of intracellular killing of catalase-positive bacteria, fungi, or other microbes. CGD occurs at a frequency of 1 in 1 million and is identified most often in males. Most patients with CGD develop recurrent soft tissue in-fections during the first year of life; a high proportion of these become clinically ill before age 3 months. Rarely, individuals may be clinically well until early adolescence or adulthood, pos-sibly reflecting less deleterious genetic phenotypes. Disease-free intervals may increase in some patients with increasing age, but older individuals are still at high risk for life-threatening infec-tions. Improved prophylactic or therapeutic regimens may di-minish mortality rates in CGD. Among 168 cases reviewed by Johnston in 1977, 59 deaths were reported, 45 before the age of 7 years and 50 before the age of 12 years. In some cases, however, considerable longevity has been documented; for example, four brothers with CGD were reported to range in age from 28 to 40 years. The routine use of prophylactic antibiotics and the more recent introduction of interferon gamma in clinical management of CGD is likely to affect significantly the severity of this disease.

The basis for abnormal oxygen-dependent microbicidal activity in CGD cells is related directly to impaired generation of super-oxide anion, $H_2O_2$, and other oxygen intermediates. This abnor-mality is expressed in a number of cell types including neutrophils, macrophages, eosinophils, and lymphocytes. Abnormal NADPH oxidase activity caused by one of several molecular defects rec-ognized among CGD patients represents the fundamental basis for diminished microbicidal function.

Distinct forms of CGD are defined to involve deficits of each of the components NADPH oxidase complex, including the unique membrane associated cytochrome b and soluble cytosolic factors. Such definition is possible because of the availability of cDNAs or monoclonal antibodies reactive with patient mRNA or protein components. Historically, three genetic forms of CGD were described based on inheritance patterns and spectropho-tometric detection of the cytochrome b in phagocytes of affected patients; X-chromosome linked (about 70%), autosomal recessive (about 30%), and autosomal dominant (rare cases).

Current evidence suggests the following types of molecular defects in X-linked patients: subtle mutations in the 91kd cyto-chrome b gene, regulatory defects in mRNA transcription of cy-tochrome b components, structural mutations altering the stability of mRNA for these components, and abnormal assembly of the 91kd cytochrome protein with other components of NADPH oxidase.

The most common form of autosomal disease is a recessive trait in which cytochrome b levels are normal, implying defects of other components of the membrane oxidase complex. A recent study of 25 autosomal recessive CGD patients shows that 22 lacked a 47kd cytosolic protein and 3 lacked a 67kd cytosolic factor. Rare cases of autosomally transmitted CGD demonstrate deficient expression of cytochrome b, which appears to reflect mutations of the gene that encodes the 22kd subunit of this membrane protein. Genotypic heterogeneity appears to account

for the considerable range of clinical severity among CGD kindreds. Precise definition of the molecular lesions in individual patients may even allow prognostic information or unique insights concerning novel therapeutic approaches (eg, somatic cell gene therapy).

Patients with CGD demonstrate a specific predilection for in-fection due to catalase-positive microorganisms that generally do not elaborate $H_2O_2$. S aureus represents the most common in-fecting agent, accounting for 30% to 56% of clinical isolates in reported series of patients. Catalase-positive, gram-negative bac-teria including E coli, Klebsiella, and Enterobacter species, Serratia marcescens, Salmonellae, and Pseudomonas species account for ap-proximately 30% of infections overall. In specific geographic lo-cations, Chromobacterium violacium infections have been recog-nized in several CGD patients. Fungal pathogens also represent frequent and important etiologic agents. Fungal infections oc-curred in 20% of 245 cases reviewed in one report. Aspergillus species accounted for 78% of these; Candida albicans and species of Torulopsis accounted for most of the remaining isolates. Other reports document the pathogenic importance of obligate intra-cellular pathogens such as Pneumocystis carinii and Mycobacterium species. Thus, patients with CGD are susceptible to infection by a variety of endogenous flora as well as ubiquitous organisms.

Clinical infections in CGD largely reflect an inability of cir-culating phagocytes to kill invading bacteria or fungi at sites of heavy colonization on or beneath skin or mucous membranes. Predictable clinical features in CGD are infections on body sur-faces including inflammatory lesions of skin or subcutaneous tis-sues, ulcerative stomatitis, pneumonitis, perianal abscesses, and conjunctivitis. More widespread and deep-seated infections in CGD further reflect the persistence of invading organisms within circulating phagocytes, which allows localized or generalized seeding of tissue macrophages throughout the reticuloendothelial system. As a result, typical granulomas, which constitute the his-topathologic hallmark of this disorder, commonly develop in lymph nodes, lungs, liver, spleen, gastrointestinal tract, bone, and other tissues. Once established, these infections generally remain localized but may overwhelm the reticuloendothelial bar-riers leading to the development of septicemia or meningitis. Prolonged intracellular microbial residence in tissue abscesses or granulomas accounts for the indolent nature of observed clinical infections, considerable difficulties encountered in identifying specific infecting agents, and a delayed or refractory response to antimicrobial, surgical, or other therapeutic regimens in patients with CGD.

A diagnosis of CGD should be considered when a history of recurrent systemic infections or other clinical features beginning in infancy is elicited. Patients with CGD often are referred to tertiary care centers with histories of recurrent or chronic illness or inflammatory disease for which no etiology has been deter-mined despite extensive diagnostic evaluations. They frequently present with fever of unknown origin or carry a presumptive diagnosis of rheumatoid disease, and they may be misdiagnosed as examples of other granulomatous inflammatory disorders such as Crohn's disease or tuberculosis. Particularly typical is a history of sterile tissue aspirates of superficial or deep-seated abscesses. The identification of unusual etiologic agents such as Serratia marcescens or Pseudomonas maltophilia, the occurrence of infec-tions in unusual locations such as osteomyelitic involvement of small bones of hands or feet, and the occurrence of characteristic types of infections such as liver or other deep-seated abscesses should alert the clinician to the possibility of CGD.

Laboratory findings suggestive of CGD include leukocytosis, elevation of erythrocyte sedimentation rate, abnormal chest ra-diographs, and hypergammaglobulinemia. Serum levels of im-munoglobulin G, A, and M generally are elevated, while IgE levels are variably increased or normal. Specific antibody synthesis and delayed hypersensitivity skin test responses generally are normal. Microscopic evaluations of postmortem or biopsy tissues almost uniformly reveal granulomas at sites of infection. Commonly, histiocytes contain pigmented (yellow or tan) lipid material that may result from persistent residence of microorganisms within macrophages.

A definitive diagnostic test for CGD is the demonstration of impaired intracellular bactericidal activity by neutrophils, eosinophils, or mononuclear phagocytes. Because bactericidal assays require special laboratory facilities and experience, other screening tests including the nitroblue tetrazolium (NBT) dye test are applicable for use in the general diagnostic laboratory. Oxidized NBT is colorless. When reduced by superoxide, it precipitates in the cytosol as blue formazan, which can be identified histochemically. Absence of superoxide evolution by CGD neutrophils or monocytes precludes their reduction of formazan in response to soluble oxidative stimulants or during phagocytosis. A modified qualitative NBT slide test employing the stimulant phorbol myristate acetate was originally developed by Newberger to allow a prenatal diagnosis of CGD using fetal blood. This rapid, inexpensive, and highly accurate assay is useful for both the identification of patients and family studies. Employing this technique, essentially no CGD leukocytes demonstrate a normal reduction of NBT, whereas essentially all of those of normal individuals are NBT positive. Heterozygous carriers of X-linked recessive CGD have nearly equal proportions of NBT positive and NBT negative cells.

Other laboratory techniques can be used to demonstrate impairment of the respiratory burst and thereby confirm a diagnosis of CGD. During phagocytosis, normal neutrophils or monocytes produce highly energized and unstable oxygen radicals, which return to more stable intermediates by emission of light energy or chemiluminescence. Chemiluminescence associated with phagocytosis or after stimulation by soluble stimulants can be conveniently measured in a scintillation counter. Leukocytes from patients with CGD generate no or markedly diminished chemiluminescence under most experimental conditions. The chemiluminescence assay may allow recognition of heterozygous CGD carriers in family studies, and it may be used to detect other heritable disorders of leukocyte oxidative metabolism including myeloperoxidase deficiency, G6PD deficiency, and abnormalities of glutathione metabolism, each of which can be confirmed by more specific biochemical assays. Because molecular heterogeneity has been increasingly recognized among identified patients with CGD and their kindreds, more detailed investigations to delineate a precise molecular lesion in selected cases should be performed in specialized laboratories.

The major clinical objectives in the management of CGD include prevention of infection, early identification of infection, and antimicrobial or surgical treatment. Superficial lesions such as furuncles, paronychia, and areas of cellulitis warrant concern, even with no fever or other systemic symptoms. Vigorous efforts should be made to isolate etiologic agents from involved tissues and to promptly initiate antimicrobial therapy. For recognized acute infections, appropriate antibiotics (based on susceptibility studies) should be administered for at least 10 to 14 days, even if the clinical response is prompt and favorable. Longer intervals of administration may be required when delayed defervescence is observed or when leukocytosis, an elevated sedimentation rate, or local inflammatory signs persist. Fever without an obvious site of infection is common. Noninvasive diagnostic procedures such as ultrasonography or radionucleotide scans should be considered early in the management of febrile episodes. The early administration of parenteral antibiotics is justified in febrile patients without localizing findings.

When possible, aggressive and early surgical intervention including incision and drainage of abscesses should be considered.

Antibiotic administration should be continued for about 1 to 2 weeks after complete wound healing, even if a specific and highly sensitive etiologic agent is recovered. Administration of oral antibiotics may be justified for several weeks to several months longer even in the complete absence of clinical signs or laboratory abnormalities. The general rationale for this prolonged therapeutic interval is based on the knowledge that microorganisms are sequestered and not killed within phagocytes defective in microbicidal mechanisms and on the high incidence of relapsing infections in these patients.

The ubiquity of agents infecting patients with CGD precludes measures to diminish or eliminate exposure to most potential pathogens. One preventive measure, however, is for the patient to not smoke marijuana, which may be contaminated heavily with *Aspergillus* or *Salmonella* organisms. Although prolonged prophylactic antibiotic administration is recommended by many centers caring for individuals with CGD, the overall benefit of this approach is unproven. In a review of patients followed at the University of Minnesota Medical Center, disease-free periods were longer in patients administered prophylactic antibiotic therapy compared to those not receiving antibiotics. Forty percent of patients on prophylaxis had disease-free intervals of greater than 12 months, compared to 6.5% of patients who did not receive prophylactic antibiotics. In most cases, dicoxacillin or oxacillin, or less commonly, trimethoprim-sulfamethoxazole (TMP/SMZ) were used. Another retrospective study at the National Institutes of Health documented that disease-free intervals were significantly longer among patients administered prophylactic doses of TMP/SMZ (80 mg/400 mg) or combinations of TMP/SMZ and dicloxacillin. An average interval of 40.4 months between major infections was noted in patients who were on prophylactic agents, compared to 12.0 months in those not receiving prophylactic drugs. During that study, no infections due to organisms resistant to the prophylactic agent were recognized. Some investigators, however, emphasize that prophylactic regimens potentially lead to an increased incidence of *Aspergillus* infections. Prophylactic parenteral antibiotics generally are recommended for patients with CGD before elective surgical or dental procedures. A combination of an antistaphylococcal drug [eg, nafcillin, 2 g (adult) or 200 mg/kg (child) intravenously] in addition to an aminoglycoside [eg, gentamicin, 1.5 mg/kg intramuscularly (adult) or intravenously (child)] provided 30 to 60 minutes before and 8 to 16 hours after the procedure has been suggested. Vancomycin [0.5 g to 1 g (adults) or 20 mg/kg (child) intravenously for 1 hour] can be administered to individuals who are hypersensitive to penicillin.

The use of leukocyte transfusions in selected clinical settings should be considered. Even though several investigators have reported beneficial effects in managing infectious complications, comparative evaluations of the efficacy or possible complications associated with leukocyte transfusions in these patients are lacking. Possible benefits of transfused leukocytes must be weighed against possible complications associated with their use. Foremost is the possibility of sensitization to granulocyte or monocyte antigens in patients who have the McLeod phenotype. Three clinical indications for leukocyte transfusions in CGD include failure of conventional medical and surgical therapy to control infection or inflammation, rapidly progressive or life-threatening infection, and failure to appropriately localize an infectious process or focus, thereby obviating the possibility of conventional medical or surgical approaches.

In addition to the therapeutic and supportive measures described above, the recent availability of recombinant interferon-gamma (INF-$\gamma$) provides a potentially important advantage in the clinical management of CGD. In vitro studies show that INF-$\gamma$ enhances expression of cytochrome b 91kd mRNA and superoxide production in phagocytic cells from normal and some X-linked CGD patients. Administration of subcutaneous INF-γ resulted in enhanced superoxide production and staphylococcal killing (to near normal levels) in association with increased cytochrome b levels when studied in one series of CGD patients. In another report, the enhancement of the 47 kd cytosolic factor and its mRNA as well as increased production of superoxide and mRNA for the 91 kd cytochrome b subunit were evident in INF-γ treated normal macrophages. These findings suggest possible clinical applications of INF-γ in autosomal as well as X-linked phenotypes of CGD.

These in vitro and in vivo findings prompted the recent International CGD Cooperative Study of INF-γ prophylaxis in all forms of CGD. This study comprehensively evaluated the efficacy of subcutaneous INF-γ in decreasing the severity or frequency of serious infections in 128 patients, 67 of whom had X-linked CGD. Although no improvement in neutrophil staphylococcal killing or superoxide production by patient neutrophils was shown, there was a significant clinical benefit noted in the treatment group. In subjects younger than 10 years of age, there was as much as a four-fold increase in the risk for significant infection in the placebo-treated controls when compared with the INF-γ treated subjects. It seems likely that the ameliorative effects of INF-γ in CGD involves immunologic mechanisms unrelated to (or in addition to) the NADPH oxidase complex.

In addition to the management of infections, patients with CGD must be evaluated carefully with respect to their erythrocyte phenotype. Some individuals with CGD lack known antigens from the Kell series, a phenotype termed $K_o$, while others have the McLeod phenotype, characterized by erythrocytes that react weakly with antibodies defining some Kell antigens. Because both phenotypes are rare, these patients are at risk of forming antibodies to antigens on erythrocytes of most blood donors. Thus, transfusion should be avoided in patients who have these rare Kell-associated phenotypes, or their erythrocytes should be stored for possible future use. Additional management involves the identification of a carrier state among family members and the provision of appropriate genetic counseling.

## Glucose-6-Phosphate Dehydrogenase (G6PD) Deficiency

Most variants of heritable G6PD deficiency are characterized clinically by chronic nonspherocytic hemolytic anemia with no features related to leukocyte dysfunction. Rare examples of severe or total deficiency of both erythrocyte and leukocyte G6PD activity associated with impaired leukocyte function and susceptibility to severe and life-threatening infectious complications have been described. Leukocytes of individuals severely deficient (1% to 5% of normal) in G6PD share many characteristics of CGD. Cells of both groups demonstrate diminished intracellular killing of catalase-positive organisms and fail to reduce NBT or generate chemiluminescence, superoxide anion, or $H_2O_2$, and both demonstrate impaired activation of the hexose monophosphate shunt (HMPS) during phagocytosis. Methylene blue does not normalize HMPS shunt activation by G6PD deficient leukocytes as it does with CGD cells. This occurs because G6PD deficient leukocytes contain limited pools of reduced pyridine nucleotides (NADPH), which serve as substrates for methylene blue, even though they do contain normal NADPH oxidase activity.

Patients with severe variants of G6PD deficiency are susceptible to a variety of infectious agents and complications similar to that observed in individuals with CGD. A fatal episode of septicemia due to E coli and Klebsiella pneumonia was reported in a 52-year-old white female with total G6PD deficiency. In another report, granulocytes of three G6PD deficient male siblings of a single kindred demonstrated moderately diminished NBT reduction, HMPS activity, and microbicidal activity for S aureus.

One sibling experienced recurrent granulomatous lymphadenitis due to S aureus and required multiple drainage procedures and prolonged antibiotic therapy. A second sibling experienced a single episode of cervical lymphadenitis, and a third reportedly had no history of infections. A recent report described a Texas child with total G6PD deficiency who died of an overwhelming septicemia-shock syndrome secondary to Chromobacterium violacium. Granulocytes of an identical twin demonstrated severely impaired NBT reduction, HMPS activation, superoxide generation, and impaired microbicidal activity for S aureus and C violacium. This unique infectious complication probably reflected both host defense deficits in this child as well as the selective endemic occurrence of C. violacium in the southeastern United States. Individuals with mild-moderate G6PD deficiency (20% to 50% of normal G6PD) do not demonstrate susceptibility to infections.

## Selected Readings

Anderson DC, Rothlein R, Marlin SD, Krater SS, Smith CW. Impaired transendothelial mMigration by neonatal neutrophils: abnormalities of Mac-1 (CD11b/CD18)-dependent adherence reactions. Blood 1990;78:2613.

Anderson DC, Schmalstieg FC, Goldman AS, et al. The severe and moderate phenotypes of heritable Mac-1, LFA-1, p150,95 deficiency: their quantitative definition and relation to leukocyte dysfunction and clinical features. J Infect Dis 1985;152:688.

Anderson DC, Springer TA. 1987. Leukocyte adhesion deficiency: an inherited defect in the Mac-1, LFA-1 and p150,95 glycoproteins. Annu Rev Med 1987;38:175.

Clark RA. The human neutrophil respiratory burst oxidase. J Infect Dis 1990;161:1140.

Ezekowitz RAB, Izu AE, Kramer SM, Jaffe HS, Gallin JI, Malech HL, et al. A controlled trial of interferon gamma to prevent infection in chronic granulomatous disease. N Engl J Med 1991;324:509.

Johnston RB. Management of patients with chronic granulomatous disease. In Gallin JI, eds. Advances in host defense mechanisms. New York: Raven Press, 1983:77.

Lehrer RI, Ganz T, Selsted ME, Babior BM, Curnutte JT. Neutrophils and host defense. Ann Intern Med 1988;109:127.

Malech HL, Gallin JI. Current concepts: immunology, neutrophils in human diseases. N Engl J Med 1987;317(11):687.

Orkin SH. Molecular genetics of chronic granulomatous disease. Annu Rev Immunol 1989;7:277.

Todd RF III, Freyer DR. The CD11/CD18 leukocyte glycoprotein deficiency. Hematology/Oncology Clinics of North America 1988;2:13.

Wilson JM, Ping AJ, Krauss JC, et al. Correction of CD18-deficient lymphocytes by retrovirus-mediated gene transfer. Science 1990;248:1413.

*Principles and Practice of Pediatrics, Second Edition.*
edited by Frank A. Oski et al. J. B. Lippincott Company, Philadelphia © 1994.

## 14.1.5 Combined Immunodeficiency Diseases

### Richard Hong

The first report of an immunodeficiency disease appeared in 1952 with the description of agammaglobulinemia. During the next dozen years, many other immunodeficiency disorders characterized by recurrent infections were reported. Confusion ensued because the types of infection that dominated the clinical picture in one group of patients appeared to cause few or no problems for patients with a different syndrome. In the 1960s, the immune system was shown to consist of two components with distinct but complementary roles in defense against infectious agents.

Studies in rabbits, mice, and chickens established the presence of these two systems: the T cell, or cellular immune system, and the B cell, or humoral immune system.

Patients with defects in their B-cell system usually experience infections with high-grade encapsulated microorganisms such as *Haemophilus influenzae* and *Streptococcus pneumoniae*. These organisms cause infections ranging in severity from otitis media and pneumonia to septicemia and meningitis. In contrast, patients with abnormal T cell function more frequently experience infections with opportunistic pathogens, resulting in infections such as disseminated fungal infections, *Pneumocystis carinii* pneumonia, mucocutaneous candidiasis, and overwhelming viral infections such as fatal chicken pox or cytomegalovirus infection.

Several of the unique genetic immune deficiency disorders appeared to involve both groups of infectious agents, and patients with these disorders were shown to have defects in both the T cell and the B cell immune systems. These combined or dual system immune deficiency disorders are the focus of this chapter.

## SEVERE COMBINED IMMUNODEFICIENCY (SCID)

Severe combined immunodeficiency is the most extreme form of the inherited or primary immunodeficiency diseases. It is characterized by profound functional defects in both the humoral and the cell-mediated immune systems. A family history of similarly affected relatives occurs in about half the cases. Within the general classification of SCID are several distinct disorders with different modes of inheritance and different patterns of cellular deficiency. Both autosomal-recessive and X-linked inherited forms have been described in SCID. One type is associated with agranulocytosis as well as dual-system immune deficiency. Other forms of SCID are characterized by an absence of all lymphocytes or by an absence of T cells but not B cells. Originally, SCID was seen only in infants because the immune deficit was so severe that patients usually died of infection within the first weeks or months of life. With earlier diagnosis and improved medical care, longevity is no longer so limited, and curative therapy for all patients is now available.

### Clinical Features

Infants with SCID often present with infections within the first months of life. Recurrent pneumonia, failure to thrive, chronic diarrhea, and persistent candidiasis of the mouth, esophagus, and skin of the face and diaper area are common. These infants may have infections with all types of microorganisms, but opportunistic pathogens tend to dominate the clinical picture. Death has occurred from generalized chicken pox, measles with Hecht's (giant cell) pneumonia, disseminated mycobacterial infection, and cytomegalovirus and adenovirus infections. When smallpox vaccination was used routinely, SCID infants regularly developed fatal generalized vaccinia infections. Live attenuated polio vaccine may cause paralytic poliomyelitis in infants with SCID, although it is often tolerated without symptoms in these patients. In addition to infections, many infants with SCID have developed graft-versus-host disease (GVHD) after transfusions of whole blood containing immunocompetent donor T lymphocytes. Maternal lymphocytes entering fetal circulation during labor and delivery or during gestation also have caused GVHD in infants with SCID.

### Immunologic Findings

SCID is classified as a profound dual-system immunodeficiency, meaning that SCID patients essentially have no normal function in either their T- or B-cell systems. Careful laboratory evaluation, however, reveals great heterogeneity within this general diagnostic group with certain cellular components of the immune system preserved in some patients. Serum immunoglobulins vary from panhypogammaglobulinemia to variable partial immunoglobulin deficiency involving only one or two of the major isotypes. Antibody responses, however, almost always are profoundly impaired. B lymphocytes are absent in some SCID patients, whereas other patients have normal or even elevated B-cell numbers. Particularly in the X-linked variety, B cells may account for all of the circulating lymphocytes. Most tests of T-cell function are abnormal. The children are anergic to cutaneous delayed-hypersensitivity skin testing. Usually, the number of T cells in the blood is depressed to less than 10% of normal in more than 80% of SCID patients. In vitro tests show T-cell function is markedly impaired with defective proliferative, cytotoxic, and immunoregulatory activity. Patients occasionally retain some proliferative capacity to respond to allogeneic cells (lymphocytes from a nonidentical twin) or to one or more mitogens. In these patients, however, antigen proliferation is always nil.

### Pathogenesis

SCID is a disease category that includes a heterogeneous group of disorders; no single pathogenic mechanism is common to all patients. Defects that lead to immunodeficiency include failure of differentiation into mature T or B cells, failure to transduce the antigen signal, poor cytokine secretion, and failure to recognize antigen. SCID is inherited as either an autosomal or X-linked recessive disease.

### SCID With Generalized Hematopoietic Hypoplasia (Reticular Dysgenesis)

Reticular dysgenesis is the most severe of the disorders of host defense because it is characterized by agammaglobulinemia, alymphocytosis, and agranulocytosis. Patients die of overwhelming infection within hours or days of birth unless treated as newborns by bone marrow transplantation. It has been suggested that the primitive hematopoietic stem cell precursor of all leukocytes is defective in this condition, so both myeloid and lymphoid lineages fail to develop.

### SCID With Failure of Lymphoid Stem-Cell Development (Swiss Type)

Swiss-type agammaglobulinemia is a type of SCID characterized by the absence of both T and B lymphocytes. It is inherited as an autosomal-recessive disorder and is rare. The receptors for antigen on T cells and B cells are generated by complex events that bring together discontinuous segments of DNA through a process of DNA rearrangement to form a complete functional gene. Both T cells and B cells use the same enzyme for this process of DNA recombination. A defect in this recombinase enzyme could cause this type of SCID because such a defect would prevent the formation of the unique receptors that characterize all immunocompetent lymphocytes. This is the defect of SCID mice, a laboratory analog of the human disease.

### SCID With Normal B Cells

Some patients with SCID have normal or even increased numbers of B lymphocytes despite their profound T-cell deficiency. These patients may produce small amounts of IgM, but are unable to produce specific antibody after antigenic challenge. In tissue culture, the B cells from some of these patients produce immunoglobulin if mixed with T cells from a normal individual. In these patients, the clinical B-cell defect is secondary to a primary abnormality in the development of helper T lymphocytes. Defects at the level of the prethymic T-cell precursor, the intrathymic T cell, and the post-thymic T cell have all been demonstrated. Most of the X-linked SCID patients are of this phenotype.

## SCID With MHC Class-I or MHC Class-II Deficiency (Bare Lymphocyte Syndrome)

A unique type of autosomal-recessive SCID has been found in which the patient's lymphocytes do not express major histocompatibility complex (MHC) antigens on surface membranes. The HLA antigens are coded for by genes located on chromosome 6, but inheritance of this disease is not linked to this chromosome. The defect involves a transacting regulatory gene that is essential for the expression of MHC antigens on the cell surface. Lack of MHC antigens on the lymphocyte membranes can cause immunodeficiency by several mechanisms. B cells recognize antigens directly, whereas T cells "see" antigens after they are processed and then presented in a digested form in association with class-II MHC antigens on the surface of an antigen-presenting cell. The lack of MHC antigens on the cell surface cripples the initial T-cell antigen recognition process. In addition to this initial recognition phase, T cells also interact with MHC antigens during both cytotoxic and immunoregulatory activities. The CD8[+] cells interact with class-I MHC molecules, and CD4[+] cells interact with cells bearing class-II molecules.

## SCID With Adenosine Deaminase Deficiency (ADA[-] SCID)

ADA(-) SCID was the first of the immunodeficiency diseases in which the enzyme defect causing the disease was identified. ADA catalyzes the conversion of adenosine to inosine and deoxyadenosine to deoxyinosine in the normal pathway of purine metabolism and salvage (Fig 14-3). Deoxyadenosine accumulates in high concentrations in the serum and tissues of these patients because ADA is the principal catabolic enzyme for this compound. Although all cells of the body lack the enzyme, lymphocytes are especially susceptible to damage from ADA deficiency, apparently because lymphocytes are the most efficient cells at phosphorylating deoxyadenosine to deoxyATP. DeoxyATP is toxic to cells, interfering with cellular metabolism in several ways. Thus, the lymphocytes in this disorder essentially poison themselves, leading to a dual-system immunodeficiency.

ADA(-) SCID presents with agammaglobulinemia and severe lymphopenia in some patients and with less severe defects in others. In some patients, the immune deficiency worsens with increasing age.

## Other Forms of SCID

SCID has been described in association with a number of other disorders. It has been reported in children with an unusual form of dysostosis resulting in short-limbed dwarfism. It has also been seen in cartilage-hair hypoplasia, a distinctive form of a genetically determined dwarfism (Fig 14-4). A form of SCID may also be observed in infants with acrodermatitis enteropathica; the immune deficiency in these patients may respond dramatically to zinc replacement therapy.

## Treatment of SCID

Development of effective treatment for these desperately ill children is a major challenge to clinical immunology. In 1968, bone marrow transplantation was introduced to clinical medicine when an infant with SCID was given a bone marrow transplant from a histocompatible sibling donor. The transplanted marrow completely reconstituted both the T- and the B-cell immune systems in this infant, and this reconstitution has persisted now for more than 20 years. Although the bone marrow is generally considered to provide a source of stem cells, at least some of the restoration is due to post-thymic T cells and mature B cells that apparently are long-lived and replicating. Overall, 50% to 60% of SCID patients treated by bone marrow transplantation are cured. The percentage would be higher if patients were all in good general health at the time of transplantation.

In many forms of combined immunodeficiency, conditioning of the patient with myeloablative or immunosuppressive drugs or x-ray is not necessary. Occasionally sufficient immunity to reject a marrow is present even in those children with profound deficiencies, and pretransplant conditioning is required. Laboratory tests to identify this variant of combined immunodeficiency precisely are not available yet.

Bone marrow transplantation may cause fatal GVHD because of the disparity of histocompatibility antigens. The donor and recipient must be matched appropriately to minimize this com-

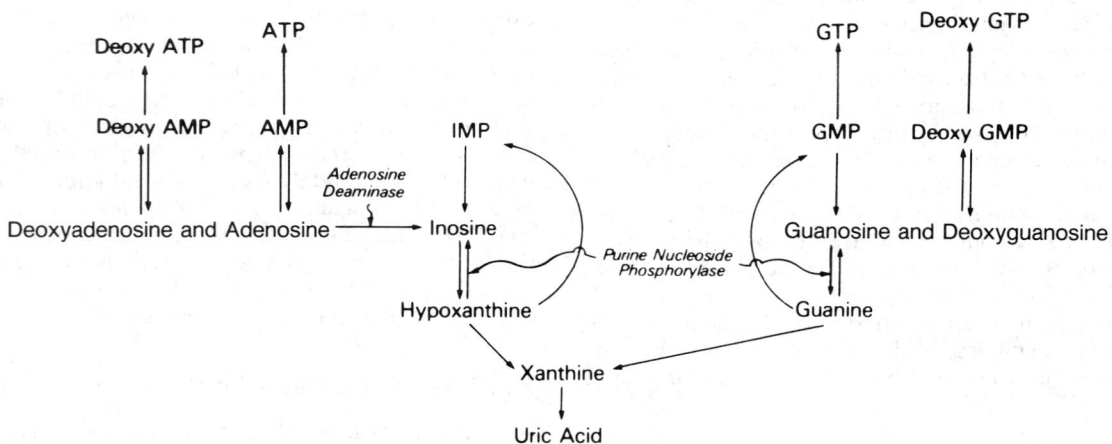

**Figure 14-3.** Purine catabolic pathway showing the positions at which the enzymes adenosine deaminase (ADA) and purine nucleoside phosphorylase (PNP) catalyze their respective reactions. The accumulation of the toxic triphosphates of deoxyadenosine and deoxyguanosine leads to the immunodeficiency in these disorders.

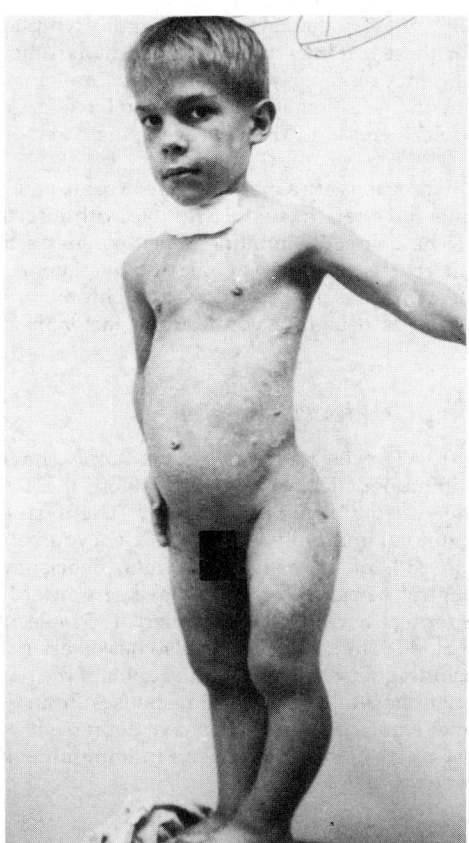

**Figure 14-4.** An 8-year-old boy with cartilage-hair hypoplasia. Disproportionate shortening of extremities is seen, and the hair is fine. Scars from a recent life-threatening episode of varicella are apparent on the trunk, and the bandage covers a tracheostomy required for the treatment of varicella pneumonia. Immune deficiency was unsuspected before the varicella infection.

plication. When donors are matched, prophylaxis for GVHD is unnecessary, and only occasionally is GVHD severe enough to require therapy. The inheritance of the transplantation antigens is such that, except in rare circumstances, only siblings are a match. This event occurs about 25% of the time. With today's small families and the frequency with which first children are affected, the actual number of matched donors available for bone marrow transplantation is slightly less than 25%. Because GVHD primarily is caused by mature T cells, if they are eliminated, bone marrow can be transplanted even from a mismatched donor without fatal GVHD. This strategy enlarges the donor pool. In practice, a parent is used as the donor, because at least 50% of the antigens (haploidentical) including minor antigens that are not assessed by tissue-typing techniques, will match. A haploidentical sibling also is a suitable donor if age and size are not precluding factors.

More than 300 transplantations for SCID using haploidentical bone marrow donors have been performed. The long-term survival rate appears to be equal to that achieved with matched donors. Bone marrow transplantation using haploidentical partners, however, is significantly more complicated. Conditioning is more often necessary, implying that the mature T cells of the nondepleted marrows are actively involved in the engraftment process. Second and third transplants are necessary more often. The B-cell engraftment may be less complete, and the incidence of post-transplant B-cell lymphomas is higher. Nevertheless, haploidentical bone marrow transplantation is the preferred method of treatment if no fully matched sibling or close relative

is available. Strides are being made in understanding and overcoming the problems of haploidentical bone marrow transplantation. Recently, matched unrelated donors (MUD) have been used with success. In this strategy, a national or worldwide search for an individual with closely matched histocompatibility antigens is conducted. A major problem with unrelated transplants is the difficulty in finding donors for minority groups that are underrepresented in the available donor pools.

Alternative forms of treatment have included thymus transplantation, combined thymus and fetal liver transplantation, and intrauterine transplantation. Overall, the results of these transplantations are inferior to those of bone marrow transplantation. A few long-term survivors, however, have impressive degrees of reconstitution.

Bone marrow transplantation has been successful in both ADA(+) and ADA(-) SCID patients. As an alternative to transplantation, enzyme replacement has also been tried in ADA(-) SCID. Initially, exchange transfusions with irradiated whole blood were used because erythrocytes are a rich source of ADA. RBC transfusions have not proven to be effective treatment, although they have resulted in some improvement in lymphocyte function in vitro and in correction of the levels of deoxyadenosine in the blood and deoxyATP in the lymphocytes. Recently, bovine ADA has been conjugated with polyethylene glycol (PEG-ADA) and given as weekly intramuscular injections to ADA(-) SCID patients. The PEG conjugation renders the bovine enzyme less immunogenic and extends the serum half-life of the ADA from minutes to several hours. In the few patients treated with this material, there is a striking increase in lymphocyte numbers in the blood, an improvement in in vitro lymphocyte function tests, and some indication of clinical benefit. Antigen-specific immune responses, however, have not been consistent in treated patients, so PEG-ADA treatment may not result in sustained clinical correction.

ADA deficiency is the first immunodeficiency disease to be treated by gene therapy. Already, T-cell lines established from ADA(-) SCID patients have been "cured" in vitro after successful transfer of the human ADA gene into these cells using a recombinant retrovirus vector gene transfer system. A limited number of children have received monthly infusions of 1 billion transfected cells. After several months of treatment, one child's immunity improved enough to stop infusions; the length of persistent benefit is being assessed. This patient now attends a regular school. Successful transfection of stem cells is the next step.

## PURINE NUCLEOSIDE PHOSPHORYLASE DEFICIENCY (PNP DEFICIENCY)

Deficiency in the enzyme purine nucleoside phosphorylase (PNP) is associated with an immunodeficiency state consisting of severely defective T-cell function. PNP is a trimer of 29,000 dalton subunits encoded by a gene on chromosome 14, and its deficiency is inherited as an autosomal-recessive trait. The enzyme catalyzes the conversion of inosine to hypoxanthine and guanosine to guanine in the pathway of purine catabolism. This is the step in purine degradation immediately after the step catalyzed by adenosine deaminase.

In contrast to ADA deficiency, which is associated with SCID, PNP deficiency usually is associated with a defect in T-cell immunity with preservation of B cell function and immunoglobulin production. These patients have profound T-lymphopenia, skin-test anergy, and defective in vitro lymphocyte function tests. Thymic morphology is intact, as is the ability of the patients to produce isohemagglutinins and antibodies. The serum concentrations of IgM, IgG, and IgA may be normal. Some patients have received live-virus vaccines and multiple blood transfusions without complication. Other patients, however, have developed generalized vaccinia after vaccination and GVHD after blood transfusion. Similar to ADA deficiency, the immune deficiency in PNP deficiency may be progressive with infants being relatively free of infection, then having infectious episodes that increase in severity and frequency. Because PNP catalyzes the degradation of inosine and guanosine, the principal substrates for uric acid production, PNP deficiency usually results in low levels of uric acid in the blood and urine. This provides a simple, convenient screening test for this disorder.

As in ADA deficiency, it is the accumulation of substrates of PNP that seems to cause the problem, rather than a deficiency in a product of PNP enzyme action. In PNP deficiency, it is the accumulation of deoxyGTP as the toxic compound that interferes with T lymphocyte development and function.

Bone marrow transplantation has successfully treated these patients. Repeated red blood cell transfusions that replace enzymes have provided limited benefit in some patients with PNP deficiency.

## ATAXIA-TELANGIECTASIA

Ataxia-telangiectasia (AT) is an autosomal-recessive multisystem disorder characterized by severe cerebellar ataxia, oculocutaneous telangiectasia, variable immunodeficiency, and high incidence of malignancy. The neurologic symptoms usually dominate the clinical picture with onset at about the time the child is learning to walk. The disorder frequently results in profound disability, and the patient becomes almost totally dependent on others for care and feeding.

### Clinical Features

The cerebellar dysfunction is manifested early as ataxia and is followed by choreoathetosis, severe involuntary myoclonic jerking movements, and oculomotor abnormalities. The telangiectasia usually appear first on the bulbar conjunctiva at between 2 and 5 years of age (Fig 14-5). They then begin to appear on the skin of exposed areas and on areas of trauma such as the nasal bridge, ears, and flexor folds on the neck and extremities. Other features involving the skin include cafe-au-lait spots, vitiligo, and prematurely gray hair. Multiple endocrine abnormalities are common, and half of patients have abnormal glucose tolerance tests. Hypoplasia or agenesis of the ovaries is common in females, but hypogonadism is less common in males. Cancer develops in as

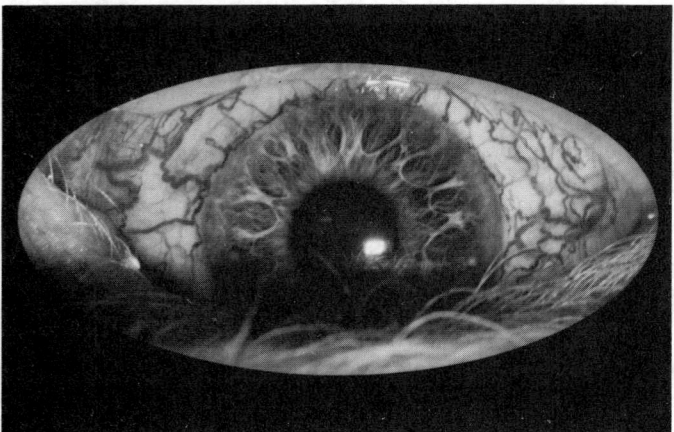

**Figure 14-5.** Striking telangiectasia on the bulbar conjunctiva of a 22-year-old patient with ataxia-telangiectasia. These dilated vessels typically appear between ages 2 and 5 years, first in the eye and later on cutaneous areas of chronic exposure or trauma.

many as 15% of AT patients. Non-Hodgkin's lymphomas predominate in these patients as they do in many other primary immunodeficiency diseases, while carcinomas are more common in older patients. Adult males with AT who have IgA deficiency have a 70-fold increase in risk of developing carcinoma of the stomach.

Recurrent infections are a major feature in some patients, while other patients have relatively little trouble with infections until late in life. The degree of immune deficit correlates to the frequency of infectious episodes experienced by patients. Sinopulmonary infections are most common, and chronic bronchopulmonary disease is usually a contributing factor in a patient's demise.

### Immunologic Defects

Patients with AT, even within the same family, have varying degrees of immunodeficiency. Defects in both the T and the B cell immune systems have been reported. The most consistent defects in humoral immunity are IgA deficiency in 75% and IgE deficiency in 85% of cases. $IgG_2$ and $IgG_4$ deficiency are also common. Eighty percent of patients have serum IgM in a monomeric 7S form rather than the pentameric 19S molecule usually seen in the blood. The T-cell system also has a variety of abnormalities, including skin-test anergy in about half the patients and depressed lymphocyte proliferative responses in an equal proportion. An even higher percentage have depressed cytotoxic T-cell responses, and many have defects in immunoregulatory T-cell function as well.

### Pathogenesis

The fundamental defect underlying the immune system and neurologic dysfunction in AT is unknown. One hypothesis arises from observations that patients are sensitive to ionizing radiation and radiomimetic drugs. Further, cultured fibroblasts from AT patients have a markedly reduced ability to form colonies and grow in vitro after being exposed to x-irradiation. There is presumed to be a major defect in one or more of the repair mechanisms for DNA in these patients, but the precise nature of the defect has not been elucidated. In more than half the cases, the sites of chromosomal breakage involve chromosomes 7 and 14 at the sites of the T-cell receptor genes and the immunoglobulin heavy-chain genes. These are chromosomal regions that regularly undergo DNA rearrangements, deletions, and repair during the course of the generation of the cellular antigen receptors and during heavy-chain class switch.

It has been suggested that normal levels of IgA and IgE and normal numbers of mature T cells with alpha/beta T-cell receptors require an immune system that differentiates efficiently and successfully over a protracted period of time, because more gene rearrangement events are required for their development. With the DNA repair defect in AT patients, the generation of these more "downstream" immune products is less efficient. Thus, the immune deficit is characterized by a lack of IgA, IgE, and alpha/beta T cells. The translocations also are associated with the high tendency for leukemia found in AT patients.

### Treatment

There is no specific useful therapy that corrects both the neurologic and the immunologic defects in this disease. Immunoglobulin replacement therapy and blood transfusions have been associated in some instances with fatal episodes of anaphylaxis in AT patients. These episodes occur because IgA-deficient AT patients may make IgG antibodies to IgA, which then react with IgA in the transfusion and cause a serious anaphylactic reaction.

Administration of any blood product to an AT patient should be done with caution, and treatment for shock should be instituted as soon as any signs of a reaction appear.

## WISKOTT-ALDRICH SYNDROME

Wiskott-Aldrich syndrome (WAS) is an X-linked disorder showing the triad of recurrent infection with all classes of microorganisms, hemorrhage secondary to thrombocytopenia, and eczema of the skin. Bleeding episodes or symptoms due to infection typically begin during the first 6 months of life.

### Clinical Features

WAS is characterized by recurrent infections and a variety of significant clinical abnormalities, which frequently overshadow the infections as management problems. Both high-grade and opportunistic pathogens cause infections. Patients frequently come to medical attention initially with otitis media or pneumonia caused by *S pneumoniae* or *H influenzae*. They also are prone to septicemia or meningitis with these organisms. *Candida albicans*, cytomegalovirus, and *P carinii* are also causes of significant infectious episodes in these children. WAS patients have died of generalized vaccinia after smallpox vaccination, and disseminated herpes simplex has also been reported. Chicken pox has also been lethal to WAS patients, particularly to those treated with corticosteroids (Fig 14-6).

The thrombocytopenia in WAS is unique because the platelets are very small in size and depressed in number, often in the 15,000 to 30,000 range. Small or microthrombocytes are not found regularly in any other thrombocytopenic disease, and their presence is perhaps the best single test to confirm the diagnosis of WAS. Bleeding accounts for about 30% of the mortality in WAS with intracranial hemorrhage being the greatest threat.

The third component of the clinical triad defining WAS is

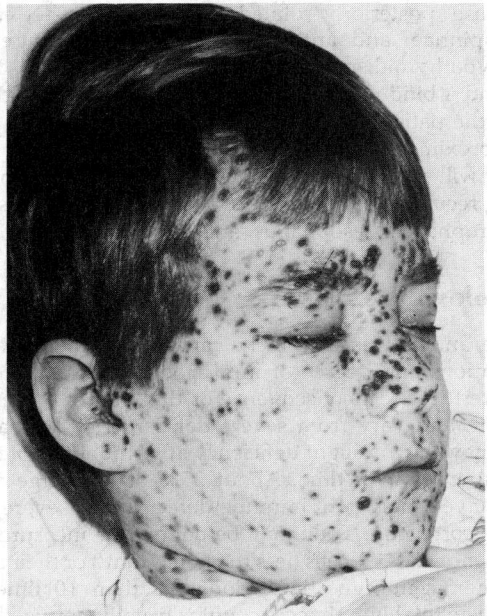

**Figure 14-6.** A Wiskott-Aldrich syndrome (WAS) patient with severe chickenpox covering every square inch of his skin. Patients with combined immunodeficiency are at particular risk for overwhelming varicella infection. This is especially true for WAS patients who are receiving corticosteroid treatment for the autoimmune disease that occasionally complicates management of their WAS disorder.

eczema of the skin. In addition, patients experience a high incidence of severe autoimmune disease. This autoaggressive disorder may take on many forms, including severe Coombs positive or negative hemolytic anemia, a JRA-like disorder with fevers and joint involvement, leukocytoclastic vasculitis usually involving the lower legs, and larger-vessel vasculitis affecting the coronary or cerebral arteries. In addition to their intrinsic thrombocytopenia, patients also develop an ITP-like thrombocytopenia, which is usually only appreciated after their original thrombocytopenia is corrected by splenectomy. This is often seen in association with high levels of circulating immune complexes and may be an ominous sign of clinical deterioration.

Another striking feature of WAS is a high incidence of malignancy. Patients with many of the primary immunodeficiency diseases show an increased frequency of cancer, and WAS patients have been estimated to have a cancer frequency 128 times that in the normal population. Most cancers are non-Hodgkin's lymphomas with the brain involved in more than half of cases. Despite this high incidence of lymphoma, the peripheral lymph nodes almost never contain cancer, although they often becoming markedly enlarged. Since the introduction of routine antibiotic prophylaxis and splenectomy, the incidence of cancer with this disease may be falling.

### Immunologic Defects

Wiskott-Aldrich syndrome is unique among the immunodeficiency diseases because it has selective defects involving each component of the host defense system, rather than having the more global defects seen in diseases like SCID. The patients have variable patterns of immunoglobulins in their serum, with the most typical profile consisting of normal levels of IgG, IgA elevated to about twice normal levels, and IgM at about half the normal level. Antibody responses to many antigens, such as tetanus, are normal, while responses to others are absent. WAS is the only disease that fails to produce antibodies to an entire class of antigens, the polysaccharides. Because of this unique defect, these patients have low or absent isohemagglutinins and do not produce antibody to the capsular polysaccharides of *H. influenzae* or the pneumococci. This immune defect explains patients' susceptibility to infection with encapsulated organisms despite normal or elevated immunoglobulin levels, and their ability to make antibody to protein antigens like tetanus toxoid.

Another abnormality unique to WAS patients is that they hypercatabolize their serum immunoglobulins and albumin at a very rapid rate. The serum half-life of IgM, IgG, IgA, and albumin in WAS patients is only one third to one half of normal rates, so to keep serum levels normal, these proteins are synthesized at far greater than normal rates.

The cellular immune system also has selective defects in many functions. WAS patients are anergic and even have impaired rejection of skin allografts. They do have normal or near normal numbers of T lymphocytes in their blood and a normal ratio of CD4$^+$ to CD8$^+$ T cells. The T cells can proliferate normally to mitogens such as PHA and can produce IL-1, IL-2, gamma interferon, and other cytokines when stimulated appropriately. Nevertheless, cells usually respond poorly to antigens like tetanus and to allogeneic cells in mixed lymphocyte culture (MLC), and they do not develop self-restricted antigen-specific cytotoxic T cells, even to antigens to which they make antibodies, such as influenza.

The monocytes from WAS patients have defects in chemotaxis and cytotoxic function mediated by antibodies (ADCC) and by the endogenous mannosyl-fucosyl membrane receptor. Even the granulocytes from these patients are involved with defective chemotactic responsiveness, a common finding although their bactericidal capacity seems to be normal.

## Pathogenesis

The fundamental defect in WAS that leads to all the diverse manifestations is not known. The selective defects in the function of T cells, B cells, platelets, granulocytes, and monocytes demonstrate that this disorder can not be the result of a defect in the differentiation of a single cellular lineage such as is seen in X-linked agammaglobulinemia. Rather, some more general cellular defect must be present. A cell-membrane glycoprotein, sialophorin, has been shown to be defective on the lymphocytes of WAS patients, as well as on those from other immunodeficient subjects. A different glycoprotein is also abnormal on the platelets from WAS patients. A defect in an X-linked transacting factor involved in cell membrane structure or stability might be the site of the primary defect in this disease. There are at least seven distinct immunodeficiency diseases that are inherited as X-linked traits, and each of those studied has mapped to a different region of the X chromosome. The WAS maps to the short arm of X near the centromere.

As with most X-linked diseases, the female carriers of this genetic defect are immunologically and hematologically normal, displaying none of the abnormalities found in the affected males. Because females are mosaic for genes encoded on their X chromosomes (random X-inactivation–Lyonization–occurs in the embryo), it is expected that some defect in immune or platelet function would be found in the carriers. This would be true unless those precursors whose X-chromosomes bore the defective WAS gene were at a selective disadvantage and not differentiating or developing. Normally, all cell lineages in a female have the same ratio of cells in which each of the parental X chromosomes is active. On the average, half of a female's cells use the paternally derived X chromosome and the other half use the maternally derived X. Skin biopsy samples from WAS carriers show this expected pattern of X inactivation, with roughly half the cells using either the maternally or the paternally derived X chromosome. All T cells, B cells, and granulocytes from these carriers, however, use only one of the two possible X chromosomes, the chromosome carrying the normal WAS gene. This striking unbalanced pattern of X-chromosome inactivation is not seen in normal females, and therefore its presence provides a convenient test to detect carriers of this X-linked disease.

## Treatment

There are several approaches to the treatment of WAS. HLA-matched bone marrow transplantation is the treatment of choice if a matched sibling donor is available. Following transplantation, all of the manifestations of this disease, including the eczema and autoimmune problems, are corrected.

Treatment for patients lacking an HLA-identical sibling donor presents a more difficult decision. T-cell-depleted, haploidentical bone marrow transplantation has been successful depending on the treatment center. There is a high incidence of failure of engraftment, GVHD, and B-cell proliferative disease complicating this form of treatment. There are increasing numbers of success with matched unrelated donors.

Splenectomy cures the thrombocytopenia in more than 90% of patients, has a major impact on the quality of life, and simplifies medical management. It is essential that prophylactic antibiotics or intravenous gamma globulin be used regularly, because these patients are more susceptible to overwhelming sepsis after removal of the spleen. The platelet size also becomes normal after splenectomy.

The autoaggressive syndrome recently recognized as a common complication of this disease may be very difficult to treat. The leukocytoclastic vasculitis usually responds to nonsteroidal anti-inflammatory drugs, but may require systemic corticosteroids. The thrombocytopenia that sometimes occurs after splenectomy usually resolves without specific treatment, although some patients require aggressive treatment with intravenous gamma globulin, steroids, and even vincristine therapy to control this complication. As with all patients with severe T-cell immunodeficiency, all transfusions containing blood cells should be irradiated to prevent the development of GVHD.

Although these patients experience many different and sometimes serious medical problems, the overall prognosis is improving. Several patients treated by splenectomy have reached adulthood, married, and had children; patients treated successfully by bone marrow transplantation should have a nearly normal life expectancy.

## DIGEORGE ANOMALY (THYMIC HYPOPLASIA, THIRD AND FOURTH PHARYNGEAL POUCH SYNDROME)

DiGeorge anomaly (formerly DiGeorge syndrome) is a congenital immunodeficiency disease caused by the maldevelopment of structures derived from the first through sixth branchial pouches during embryonic development. Structures derived from the branchial pouches include portions of the ear and certain facial features, portions of the aortic arch and heart, the parathyroids and thyroid, and the thymus.

### Clinical Features

Patients with DiGeorge anomaly usually present in early infancy with symptoms unrelated to immunodeficiency. Congenital heart lesions, particularly conotruncal defects such as truncus arteriosus and interrupted aortic arch type B, are common presenting problems during the first 2 weeks of life. Abnormal calcium homeostasis because of hypoparathyroidism is seen in nearly all patients, and hypocalcemic tetany is the most common initial problem. Facial abnormalities include microstomia, hypertelorism, upturned nose, posteriorly rotated and small, low-set ears with notched pinnae, and anti-Mongoloid slant of the eyes (Fig 14-7). Hypothyroidism, esophageal atresia, tracheoesophageal fistula, and a bifid uvula also have been described in these patients. If the patients survive the newborn period and they fall in the approximately 25% who have a significant immune deficit, then they will experience an increased susceptibility to infections, including recurrent pneumonia, diarrhea, and candidiasis of the mouth, oropharynx, esophagus, and skin of the diaper area.

### Immunologic Defects

DiGeorge anomaly is extremely variable in extent of clinical manifestations and degree of immunodeficiency. Immunologic defects are the direct consequence of the failure of thymus development, and vary from severe deficiency to normal. Some patients may show a slight deficiency at birth, but improved immune responses with time. About 25% of DiGeorge anomaly patients have a persistent immune defect that is severe enough to require correction. They may be defined by measurement of the number of CD4$^+$ T cells (less than 400/mm$^3$) or their response to phytohemagglutinin stimulation (less than 10 times background). The total lymphocyte count is usually normal, but consists mostly of B cells and non-T cells. The morphology of the spleen and lymph nodes reflects the T-lymphopenia with depletion seen in the usual "thymic-dependent areas." Immunoglobulin production is variable.

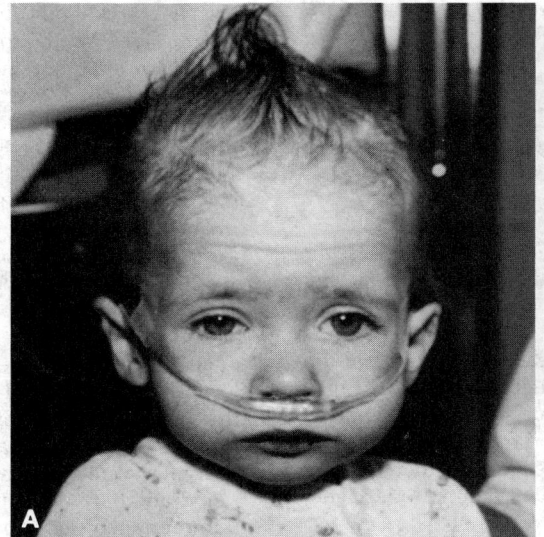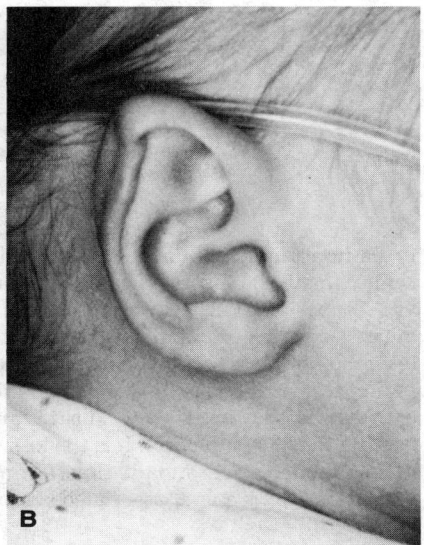

**Figure 14-7.** DiGeorge anomaly is a congenital disorder involving maldevelopment of the structures derived from the first through the sixth pharyngeal pouches during embryonic life. As a consequence, these children often have facial abnormalities, as illustrated in this child by hypertelorism, defective low-set ears, hypoplastic mandible, and upward bowing of the upper lip (**A**). Closeup of the ear shows notched pinna and deficient helix formation (**B**).

## Pathogenesis

The structures affected in the DiGeorge anomaly derive from the pharyngeal pouches. The third pouch gives rise to the parathyroids, the third and fourth produce the thymus, the first and second contribute to the lip and ear, and the sixth produces the pulmonary artery and the ultimobranchial body. These pouch derivatives all depend on a major contribution from the cephalic neural crest. If neural crest development is inhibited, multiple pouches are deprived. Multiple insults can affect the neural crest; in this way, the association of DiGeorge anomaly with many apparently unrelated intrauterine insults is explained. These causes range from teratogen exposure (retinoids, alcohol) to chromosomal abnormalities (monosomy 22) to midline developmental defects such as arrhinencephaly.

## Treatment

The nonimmunologic features of DiGeorge anomaly are often more life-threatening to newborns than is the immunodeficiency. Initial treatment should be directed at controlling the congenital heart disease and the metabolic abnormalities of these infants. Hypoparathyroidism and associated hypocalcemia are treated with vitamin D and calcium, and may require long-term replacement. The congenital heart disease frequently is severe and often requires immediate surgical intervention. Treatment of the heart lesion should not be deferred until after correction of the immune defect. Despite the immune system compromise, patients tolerate the surgical procedures very well. All blood products must be irradiated, however.

When a deficiency state is confirmed, immunologic reconstitution can be accomplished. Thymus transplantation using cultured glands obtained from small children has been successful. Bone marrow transplantation using a matched sibling has been successful.

## Selected Readings

Ammann AJ, Hong R. Disorders of the T-cell system. In: Stiehm ER, ed. Immunological diseases in infants and children, ed 3. Philadelphia: WB Saunders, 1989:257.

Anderson WF. Prospects for human gene therapy. Science 1984;226:401.

Blaese RM, Strober W, Waldmann TA. Immunodeficiency in the Wiskott-Aldrich syndrome. In: Bergsma D, Good RA, Finstad J, Paul NW, eds. Immunodeficiency in man and animals: birth defects. Sunderland, Mass: Sinauer Associates, 1975.

Cooper MD, Peterson RDA, South MA, Good RA. The functions of the thymus system and the bursa system in chickens. J Exp Med 1966;123:75.

Gatti RA, Swift M, eds. Ataxia-telangiectasia: genetics, neuropathology, and immunology of a degenerative disease of childhood. KROC Foundation Series, Vol. 19, 1985.

Higgins EA, Simininovitch KA, Zhuang D, Brockhausen I, Dennis JW. Aberrant O-linked oligosaccharide biosynthesis in lymphocytes and platelets from patients with the Wiskott-Aldrich syndrome. J Biol Chem 1991;266:6280.

Hitzig WG. Protean appearances of immunodeficiencies: syndromes and inborn errors involving other systems which express associated primary immunodeficiency. In: Wedgwood R, Rosen FS, Paul NQW, eds. Primary immunodeficiency diseases. New York: Alan R. Liss, 1983:307.

Hong R. Update on immunodeficiency. Am J Dis Child 1990;144:983.

Hong R. The DiGeorge anomaly. Immunol Rev 1991;3:1.

Moen RC, Horowitz SD, Sondel PM, et al. Immunologic reconstitution after haploidentical bone-marrow transplantation for immune deficiency disorders: treatment of bone-marrow cells with monoclonal antibody CT-2 and complement. Blood 1987;70:664.

Reisner Y, Kapoor N, Kirkpatrick D, et al. Transplantation for severe combined immunodeficiency with HLA-A, B, D, DR-incompatible parental marrow cells fractionated by soybean agglutinin and sheep red cells. Blood 1983;61:341.

Rosen FS, Cooper MD, Wedgwood RJ. The primary immunodeficiencies (1). N Engl J Med 1984;311:235.

Rosen FS, Cooper MD, Wedgwood RJ. The primary immunodeficiencies (2). N Engl J Med 1984;311:311.

Waldmann TA. The arrangement of immunoglobulin and T-cell-receptor genes in human lymphoproliferative disorders. Adv Immunol 1987;40:247.

*Principles and Practice of Pediatrics, Second Edition.*
edited by Frank A. Oski et al. J. B. Lippincott Company, Philadelphia © 1994.

## 14.1.6 *Pediatric AIDS*

Gwendolyn B. Scott and Wade P. Parks

Pediatric acquired immunodeficiency syndrome (AIDS) is a severe clinical manifestation of infection with human immunodeficiency virus, type 1 (HIV-1). Most pediatric HIV-1 infections are transmitted perinatally from infected mothers; as such, pediatric AIDS resembles other sexually transmitted diseases with perinatal consequences, such as syphilis and hepatitis B. The etiologic agent of AIDS, HIV-1, infects and kills thymus-derived lymphocytes bearing the CD4 molecule. It is the loss of these cells that results in immunodeficiency and the clinical consequences thereof. Thus, pediatric AIDS is a viral-associated secondary immunodeficiency.

## ETIOLOGIC AGENT AND PATHOGENESIS

The virus etiologically associated with AIDS is a human retrovirus belonging to the subfamily Lentivirinae. Visna, a neurotropic "slow" virus of sheep, is the prototype of this viral subfamily. A closely related sheep virus, Maedi, is also known as progressive pneumonia virus (PPV); it produces a lymphocytic interstitial pneumonitis (LIP) in sheep. Histologically, the pulmonary lesions caused by PPV are similar to those noted in HIV-1 infected pediatric patients.

HIV-1 infects CD4-bearing lymphocytes via high-affinity binding of the viral envelope to the CD4 receptor molecule. Because the affinity of viral binding to the CD4 receptor is higher than for most HIV-1 neutralizing antibodies, HIV-1 infection is favored over neutralization. A second characteristic of HIV-1 is its ability to replicate in T lymphocytes. Retroviral replication depends on cellular DNA synthesis and cell division. Because lymphocytes generally undergo cell division in response to specific antigenic stimuli or differentiation signals, the virus has a number of accessory genes that regulate viral replication. Genetically, HIV-1 is one of the most complicated retroviruses. This complexity is associated with the unique life cycle of the virus—a combination of tropism for highly differentiated cells such as lymphocytes and the ability of the virus to be transmitted horizontally from person to person. As the virus replicates in the lymphocyte, the CD4$^+$ cells are killed and immunologic dysfunction ensues. Exposure to any body fluid with HIV-1 infected lymphocytes carries a potential for transmission; however, blood has the highest titers. The immune system may control the infection within a host but can not eliminate HIV-1 infected T lymphocytes from the body. The immunologic dysfunction associated with lymphocyte killing eventuates in dysgammaglobulinemia. This is manifest as hypergammaglobulinemia in most cases with about 10% of children having a panhypogammaglobulinemia. Also associated with significant dysfunction is the inability of the host to mount a normal primary immune response to new antigens. This, in turn, is associated with an increased susceptibility to pathogenic bacteria and fungi. Similarly, the virally mediated destruction of CD4$^+$ lymphocytes results in lower numbers of absolute CD4$^+$ lymphocytes, a relatively specific sign of immune dysfunction. The progressive loss of CD4$^+$ lymphocytes is associated with the loss of the ability of the HIV-1 infected host to respond rapidly to primary infections or to regulate latent infections such as herpes viruses.

The host immune response to HIV-1 can be measured by both antigen-binding (serologic) and functional (neutralization of viral infectivity) antibody tests. Antibody responses in children are quantitatively similar to those in adults. In infants, however, particularly in the first 6 months of life, antibody levels may be low and is confounded by the presence of maternal antibody. As in adults, there is evidence that the host immune response partially inhibits replication of HIV-1. In certain clinical disease patterns such as lymphocytic interstitial pneumonitis (LIP), there is a marked lymphocytic inflammatory component. In contrast to the process for most viral infections, the host's immune response does not eliminate virus-infected cells. Virus can usually be recovered from the blood of all infected children. Thus, HIV-1 infection is a chronic, persistent infection directed principally at CD4$^+$ lymphocytes.

HIV-1 evades immune elimination by several mechanisms. Several potentially relevant characteristics of the persistence phenomenon include direct infection and elimination of subsets of T lymphocytes that are important in immune regulation. The external envelope glycoprotein coat of HIV-1 contains more carbohydrate than most human viruses; this may block recognition of immunogenic epitopes of the virus. Also, there is a high error rate of reverse transcription of the viral genome that results in enormous heterogeneity of the protein sequence of the HIV-1 envelope. This causes the immune response to be continually redirected as new B- and T-cell epitopes are generated, particularly in the external glycoprotein gp120. Finally, HIV-1 can infect macrophages. Since macrophages generally divide slowly and present antigen to lymphocytes, HIV-1 infection of macrophages offers an opportunity for the virus to remain latent and to be able to infect CD4$^+$ lymphocytes without having to pass outside the cell and thereby risk destruction by the immune system.

## EPIDEMIOLOGY

Pediatric AIDS and HIV-1 infections generally occur in three settings. First and most common, infection is transmitted perinatally from an infected mother. This may occur in utero, during delivery by exposure to the mother's infected blood, or postpartum, by ingestion of breast milk. There is no evidence of casual transmission of HIV-1 in households, daycare settings, or schools. The perinatally infected child usually exhibits signs of HIV-1 infection in the first 2 years of life, but may asymptomatically harbor virus for years before developing clinical manifestations. Perinatal transmission accounts for more than 80% of pediatric AIDS cases in the United States and all new cases worldwide, nearly all cases occur by the perinatal. The second setting involves blood or blood-product recipients. Pediatric patients who received blood products before March 1985, the time when HIV-1 donor screening began, have a higher risk of HIV-1 infection than do more recent recipients; however, the number of units received is an important variable. Finally, adolescents constitute the third setting in which HIV-1 infection is acquired. At least three factors contribute to adolescent risk. First, adolescent risk behavior in general is high, and exposure to drugs and higher risk sexual behavior is increased. Second, sexually active adolescent women have a 1000-fold higher risk of acquiring any sexually transmitted disease, including HIV-1. Third, male homosexual behavior often begins in the adolescent period, and the opportunity for HIV-1 infection is particularly high in receptive anal intercourse. The incidence of AIDS in adolescents remains relatively low because of the latent period of disease, but the HIV-1 infection rate is likely to be increasing.

The Centers for Disease Control (CDC) pediatric case definition for AIDS forms the basis for the pediatric AIDS surveillance system. This system includes pediatric patients younger than age 13 years and depends on local and state reporting. Approximately

1.7% of overall AIDS incidence in the United States is due to pediatric cases. This proportion is higher in parts of the world where heterosexual transmission of HIV-1 is more common. Pediatric AIDS incidence in the United States parallels the incidence of AIDS in women. The actual number of children with HIV infection in the United States is not known, but it is estimated that 6000 at-risk infants born to mothers with HIV-1 infection were born in the United States in 1990. In addition, more cases are being identified in rural areas. Cases of AIDS in women and children continue to increase, while the incidence in other populations has stabilized.

Clinically asymptomatic women are the major source of perinatal HIV-1 infection. Immunologically, HIV-1 infected women have elevated IgG and lowered absolute levels of CD4$^+$ lymphocytes. Generally, it is only through serologic screening for HIV-1 that women at risk of infecting newborn infants can be identified, because clinically they are often asymptomatic. The major risk factors for mothers appear to be either intravenous drug abuse or heterosexual contact with an HIV-1 infected male. A number of independent studies in different populations indicate that the risk that an infected mother will transmit HIV-1 and infect her infant is 13% to 39%.

The geographical distribution of HIV-1 infected women and children mirrors other aspects of the AIDS epidemic. In general, perinatal pediatric AIDS in the United States has been noted predominantly in east coast urban areas and Puerto Rico. Worldwide, the urban pattern predominates, and areas with an increased incidence of sexually transmitted diseases and intravenous drug abuse (IVDA) are expected to be sources of pediatric AIDS cases. A more specific characteristic of perinatal AIDS in the United States is the preponderance of cases in lower socioeconomic classes and in racial and ethnic minorities. Seventy percent of perinatal AIDS cases are associated with IVDA. The CDC reports a doubling of pediatric AIDS incidence approximately every 16 months.

## CLINICAL MANIFESTATIONS

HIV-1 infection is a chronic, multisystem infection. Thus, the presentation of clinical disease is varied. The CDC has devised a pediatric classification system that outlines the spectrum of clinical disease. A number of nonspecific findings may herald the onset of clinical disease. These include failure to thrive, generalized lymphadenopathy, hepatosplenomegaly, persistent oral candidiasis, recurrent or chronic diarrhea, and rarely, parotitis. Similar findings occur in other congenital infections, primary immunodeficiencies, and other secondary immunodeficiencies, including malnutrition and cancer. Initially, the differential diagnosis is extensive. To shorten the time to diagnosis, consideration should be given to the epidemiologic setting in which such nonspecific findings exist. If the prevalence of HIV-1 infection is high, then appropriate testing should be done early, when clinical signs manifest. Testing should be done with parental consent, counseling, and confidentiality.

*Pneumocystis carinii* pneumonia (PCP) is the most common and serious opportunistic infection in children with AIDS. As a consequence of HIV-1 infection acquired perinatally, PCP usually occurs in the first year of life and is associated with high morbidity and mortality. Onset of the disease may be acute or subacute, with fever and tachypnea as a common presenting sign. Bilateral interstitial perihilar infiltrates develop as the disease progresses. Diagnosis is made by demonstration of the organism in endotracheal aspirates, bronchial washings, or lung tissue. Since other pneumonias can present with a similar picture in immunocompromised hosts, aggressive diagnosis and treatment are necessary. Candida esophagitis is another common opportunistic infection.

Children with poor oral intake, dysphagia, vomiting, and fever associated with oral candidiasis are candidates for diagnostic studies. A barium swallow suggests the diagnosis which can be confirmed by endoscopy with biopsy and appropriate culture. Other opportunistic infections include disseminated cytomegalovirus infection, *Mycobacterium avium* intracellulare complex infection, cryptosporidiosis, recurrent herpes simplex infection, and less commonly cryptococcosis and toxoplasmosis.

LIP occurs in about 30% of HIV-1 infected children and is an AIDS-defining diagnosis. LIP is characterized by the presence of bilateral reticulonodular infiltrates with or without hilar lymphadenopathy. Diagnosis in confirmed by lung biopsy, although in most instances the diagnosis is made presumptively, based on the persistence of typical radiographic findings and a failure to demonstrate infectious agents. The onset of LIP is usually insidious; histologically, the lesions are characterized by the presence of lymphocytes, plasmacytes, and mononuclear cells in the interstitial and peribronchiolar areas. The disease may be static or progressive, resulting in chronic lung disease with the development of hypoxemia and pulmonary hypertension. The pathophysiology of LIP remains unclear although regional immunity of bronchial associated lymphoid tissue is involved.

Recurrent bacterial infections in HIV-1 infected children have been seen with increasing frequency and include infections with *Streptococcus pneumoniae*, *Haemophilus influenzae* type b, *Salmonellae* species, and *Staphylococcus aureus*. The spectrum of infections reported is broad, and includes bacteremia, meningitis, septic arthritis, osteomyelitis, pneumonia, urinary tract infections, otitis media, and deep and superficial abscesses. Gram-negative enteric infections occur, particularly in the chronically ill host. The paradoxically high levels of immunoglobulin G, likely secondary to T-cell dysfunction, mask an associated inability to produce specific antibody to protein and polysaccharide antigens.

Central nervous system (CNS) abnormalities have been described in as many as 50% to 90% of HIV-infected children. Neurodevelopmental abnormalities range from mild developmental delay to progressive encephalopathy. The encephalopathy may be static or progressive, and is characterized by loss of developmental milestones, weakness usually beginning in the lower extremities with extension to the trunk and upper extremities, and secondary microcephaly. Seizures, ataxia, pseudobulbar palsy, myoclonus, and extrapyramidal rigidity are associated findings. The cerebrospinal fluid frequently is normal, but mild pleocytosis or elevated protein may be present. Computed tomography of the brain may show cortical atrophy or calcifications in the basal ganglia. There is increasing evidence that HIV-1 encephalopathy results from direct invasion of HIV-1 into the brain. HIV-1 nucleotide sequences have been demonstrated in the brains of both adults and children at autopsy. HIV-1 also has been cultured from spinal fluid, and intrathecal production of specific antibody has been demonstrated. The mechanism of CNS damage, however, is not clear because the virus does not directly infect neurons. Evidence suggests that some of these effects can be mediated by cytokines.

Nephropathy in children with HIV-1 infection is an important complication. Proteinuria is an early finding and nephrotic syndrome with renal failure has been described. Pathologic lesions in the kidney include glomerulitis with focal segmental sclerosis or mesangial hyperplasia. Cardiomyopathy may occur as an acute or a subacute process. The clinical picture is similar to that in other cardiomyopathies, presenting with signs of heart failure along with cardiac enlargement and evidence of left ventricular hypertrophy with ST-T wave changes. It is not known if this is a direct effect of HIV-1, is secondary to another virus, or is an immune response to HIV-1.

Other associated clinical manifestations include anemia, leukopenia, and thrombocytopenia. Craniofacial dysmorphia has been described in HIV-infected children, but there is controversy whether this is related to HIV-1 or represents the influence of secondary factors such as maternal alcohol or drug abuse during pregnancy, the consequences of immunodeficiency, or other intercurrent processes. A number of cutaneous viral infections such as *Herpes simplex* stomatitis, Herpes zoster, molluscum contagiosum, and condylomata may be presenting, persistent, or recurrent problems. Cutaneous Kaposi's sarcoma (KS) in children has been reported rarely; the limited number of KS cases in infants has been a diffuse lymphadenopathic form of the disease. Malignancies, most commonly B-cell lymphomas, have been reported in about 2% of children with AIDS.

What factors influence clinical expression of disease in children is not understood. In children reported with AIDS, the mortality ranges from 58% to 61%. Of those diagnosed before 1 year of age, there is a 50% mortality rate within 6 months after diagnosis. Survival varies, depending on clinical presentation. Progressive encephalopathy and PCP tend to be associated with a worse outcome than that for children with LIP. Thus, both age at onset of disease and type of clinical disease appear to influence prognosis. In addition, the effect of newer modalities of therapy such as antiretroviral drugs and PCP prophylaxis on survival has not yet been fully assessed. This illness, however, is among the 10 leading causes of death in children of all ages in the United States and has had a significant effect on infant and child mortality. In major urban areas, eg, New York City, AIDS is the leading cause of death in children 2 to 5 years of age.

## DIAGNOSIS

The diagnosis of pediatric HIV infection remains a complicated algorithm. The primary and most successful diagnostic procedure objectively documents infection with HIV-1 by direct virus isolation. Recent studies indicate that virus isolation and polymerase chain reaction (PCR) detection of viral DNA in patient lymphocytes are of comparable sensitivity. Both are positive usually by 2 to 3 months of age if the infant is infected. Serologic tests that measure antibody to HIV-1 reliably indicate either exposure or infection. In the first year of life, serologic tests for HIV-1 remain positive because of the persistence of passively transferred maternal IgG; maternal antibody may persist through age 18 months in some cases. Diagnosis in this age group is most difficult and often rests on viral culture or a combination of clinical findings, documented exposure, or abnormal immunologic findings such as elevated IgG or lowered absolute numbers of CD4$^+$ lymphocytes. HIV-1 core p24 antigen is noted in the serum of symptomatic patients in approximately 25% of cases and is a specific indicator of HIV-1 infection. Recently, more sensitive tests for detection of p24 antigen that dissociate antigen and antibody complexes may increase the usefulness of p24 antigen tests for primary diagnosis. A number of new laboratory tests developed for early diagnosis of HIV infection include polymerase chain reaction, detection of IgA antibody to HIV, use of an immune complex dissociation assay for p24, and in vitro methods detecting antibody production against HIV from lymphocytes isolated from the infant. None of these tests are licensed for use in neonatal diagnosis of HIV. In the research setting, a combination of the tests provides a diagnosis by age 3 to 6 months in most children. Infants born to HIV-1 infected mothers and who show no evidence of infection should be closely followed until at least age 18 months. Precision of detecting HIV-1 infection early continues to improve as new techniques become generally available. When perinatal exposure is suspected, the mother should be studied for evidence of infection. Identification of a maternal-child infection indicates the father and other siblings may be infected and necessitates family counseling.

## TREATMENT

Treatment strategies for HIV-1 infected children have changed dramatically and continue to evolve. Available therapies include antiretroviral drugs and PCP prophylaxis. Selected patients receive intravenous gamma globulin. Supportive treatment and frequent medical monitoring is important. Source of fever and cause of infection should be diagnosed and treated promptly, just as for any severely immunocompromised patient. The immunization schedule for HIV-1 infected or exposed infants includes diphtheria-tetanus-pertussis (DPT), inactivated polio (IPV), measles, mumps, and rubella (MMR), *H influenzae* type b (HIB), and hepatitis B vaccines. Influenza vaccine and pneumococcal polyvalent vaccines are also recommended. Live attenuated oral poliovirus vaccine (OPV) and BCG are not recommended, although the former has been inadvertently administered to hundreds of HIV-1 infected infants without evidence of problems.

Children with HIV-1 infection may have significant B-cell defects, with a resultant inability to form specific antibody. Such children may benefit from intravenous gamma globulin (IVIG) therapy monthly. A recent double-blind placebo controlled study showed that intravenous gamma globulin administered monthly delayed development of serious bacterial infections in children with CD4$^+$ lymphocyte counts more than 200/mm$^3$ but did not affect survival. Thus, children with recurrent serious bacterial infection, recurrent pneumonia, hypogammaglobulinemia, or poor antibody formation are candidates for IVIG therapy.

In 1991, a panel of experts convened to determine guidelines for beginning PCP prophylaxis in infants younger than 15 months at risk for HIV as well as for all children with known HIV infection. The basis for these recommendations included the age distribution of PCP among children, CD4$^+$ lymphocyte counts in children with PCP, the high mortality and normative data on CD4$^+$ lymphocyte counts in healthy children at various ages. The following age-adjusted CD4$^+$ lymphocyte counts are recommended thresholds for beginning PCP prophylaxis: 1 month to 11 months, less than 1500 cells/mm$^3$; 12 months to 23 months, 750 cells/mm$^3$; 24 months through 5 years, less than 500 cells/mm$^3$; 6 years and older, less than 200 cells/mm$^3$. In addition, any infected child with a CD4$^+$ lymphocyte percentage of 20% or less or with a prior episode of PCP should receive prophylaxis. Because of its proven efficacy in prevention of PCP in children with cancer and adults with AIDS, trimethoprim-sulfamethoxazole given three times weekly is the drug of choice for prophylaxis.

Two antiviral agents, zidovudine (ZDV) and dideoxyinosine (DDI), are licensed for use in children. Both are potent inhibitors of HIV-1 replication. ZDV is indicated for children with symptomatic disease at a dose of 180mg/M$^2$/dose given every 6 hours. Anemia and neutropenia are the most common adverse effects. Didanosine (ddI) is licensed for use in children with advanced HIV disease who are intolerant to ZDV or who demonstrate significant immunologic or clinical deterioration while on ZDV. Adverse effects reported with ddI therapy include pancreatitis and neutropenia. The drugs are well tolerated in infants and children, and beneficial effects include weight gain, increased energy, an increase in CD4$^+$ lymphocyte count and a decrease in p24 antigen levels. The effect of combination therapy (ZDV plus ddI) and other antiviral agents, dideoxycytosine (ddc) and nevirapine, and immunomodulators such as alpha interferon are being systematically studied in children.

## PREVENTION

Vaccination appears distant. Although as an adjunct to immune serum globulin and chemotherapy in newborns, vaccines may have a future role, at present the most concrete means of preventing pediatric AIDS is to further reduce the risk of blood or blood-product transfusion by improved testing for HIV-1 in blood donors and voluntary donor deferral. To alter the incidence of perinatal pediatric AIDS, it is first necessary to identify HIV-1 infected women. Second, it is essential to counsel known HIV-1 positive women regarding the risk of perinatal transmission of HIV-1 and offer information regarding contraception and family planning. Breast-feeding by HIV-1 positive women is not recommended. These procedures may be only partially successful, but are integral to any HIV-1 control program.

One important goal is the prevention of perinatal transmission. The timing and mechanism of perinatal transmission is not well understood. Infection of aborted fetal tissue with HIV has been reported as early as 12 weeks of gestation. Studies of twins born to HIV seropositive mothers indicate a higher incidence of infection in twin "A," suggesting perinatal exposure to infected secretions during the birth process. A more recent study found that infection in the infant occurred with a subset of the maternal HIV-1 strain, suggesting that immune factors may be important. Other studies of maternal risk factors for perinatal transmission suggest that maternal stage of disease, maternal immune status, and lack of certain antibodies to specific viral epitopes might promote transmission.

Several approaches to the prevention of perinatal AIDS are being considered. A current study uses chemotherapy with ZDV in second and third trimester pregnant women with CD4+ lymphocyte counts more than 200 and randomizes them to treatment with ZDV or placebo. Their newborns will receive 6 weeks of therapy with the same drug the mother received. The purpose of this approach is to decrease the likelihood of HIV-1 transmission to the fetus. Other drugs, such as hyperimmune globulin to HIV (HIVIG) and soluble CD4 linked to IgG are also candidates for drug trials in this population of HIV-1 infected women. To prevent pediatric AIDS, it is apparent that a combination of approaches by teams of health care workers throughout the world is necessary, and the focus must be the HIV-1 infected or at-risk woman.

*Principles and Practice of Pediatrics, Second Edition.*
edited by Frank A. Oski et al. J. B. Lippincott Company, Philadelphia © 1994.

## 14.2 *Allergy*

### 14.2.1 *General Considerations*

Hugh A. Sampson and Peyton A. Eggleston

In the past 15 years, there has been a virtual explosion in our knowledge of the immunologic and biochemical mechanisms responsible for allergic disorders. Data support the pathogenic role of allergy in many cases of asthma, allergic rhinitis, atopic dermatitis, urticaria/angioedema, adverse food reactions, drug and biologic agent reactions, and stinging insect hypersensitivity. Information is available to approach the diagnosis and treatment of these disorders in a rational medical fashion. Much remains to be learned about allergic disorders, but allergy is now firmly planted on a scientific base.

Allergy may be defined as any untoward physiologic event caused by an immunologically mediated response. This definition has several components that restrict its scope. First, there must be a demonstrable event or disease, which must be both symptomatic and pathologic. This disease must be related to an antigen or environmental factor that could be airborne pollen, ingested foods, industrial chemicals, or a parenterally administered drug. Finally, the disease must have a demonstrable immunologic mechanism and must occur as a result of this immune mechanism.

Atopy, on the other hand, is a constellation of chronic diseases based on an IgE-mediated mechanism and that have a strong genetic predisposition. Coca and Cooke initially coined the term *atopy* in 1923 and later suggested that atopy was made up of asthma, allergic rhinitis, and atopic eczema (or atopic dermatitis). Not all asthma, rhinitis, or eczema is IgE-mediated, which results in considerable semantic confusion.

## CLASSIFICATION OF ALLERGIC DISEASES

Allergic diseases were classified into four types by Gell and Coombs in 1963. The classification is simple and presumes that only one mechanism participates in the pathophysiology of immunologically mediated disease, when diseases usually are associated with diverse immunological responses. Nevertheless, the classification is helpful and is still used. Although there are four types of allergic reactions, this chapter deals primarily with type I reactions.

### Type I (Anaphylactic Reactions)

Type I reactions begin with a response to an antigen that includes IgE antibodies. This class of antibody can bind to the surface of mast cells or circulating basophilic granulocytes. Exposure of these IgE-coated cells to antigen results in cell activation and release of a variety of pharmacologically potent mediators. The interaction of these mediators with blood vessels, bronchi, or mucus-secreting glands causes disease. Examples of this type of allergy include anaphylactic reactions to insect stings, food-induced urticaria, or allergic rhinitis.

### Type II (Cytotoxic Reactions)

In type II reactions, antibodies of the IgG or IgM class are formed by the patient to an environmental antigen or self-antigen (as in autoimmune disease). Upon subsequent exposure, the antigen may adsorb to the surface of a cell (because of certain chemical properties) and result in binding of antibody to the adsorbed antigen. Complement activation may ensue, whereupon the cell is damaged or destroyed by the membrane attack complex. Common clinical examples of this allergic reaction include drug-induced leukopenia, hemolytic anemia, and thrombocytopenia.

### Type III (Arthus or Immune Complex Reactions)

In type III reactions, as in type II responses, IgG and IgM antibodies to an environmental antigen are produced. In this type of reaction, however, the antigen does not bind to cells but circulates in soluble form. The antigen-antibody complexes that are formed may be small, intermediate, or large. Small complexes may remain harmlessly in the circulation, while large complexes are rapidly cleared by the reticuloendothelial system. Intermediate size complexes, however, may become deposited in vessel walls and tissues. Vascular damage is then initiated by activation of complement, granulocytes, platelets, and probably basophils. The most common example of this reaction is classical serum sickness.

## Type IV (Cell-Mediated Reactions)

Type IV reactions do not involve antibody but rather involve T-lymphocytes with specific receptors for an antigen. After primary exposure, these cells respond to subsequent exposure by proliferation, differentiation into cells capable of causing cytolysis (natural killer cells), or by recruiting other cytolytic cells (macrophages). Classic examples of these reactions are contact dermatitis from poison ivy or other chemicals, graft-versus-host reactions, and tuberculin skin tests.

## PATHOGENESIS OF IGE-MEDIATED DISORDERS

By definition, atopic disease is caused by type I, IgE-mediated reactions, although more recent evidence suggests that the classical mast cell-bound IgE-allergen reaction is not the only means by which mast cells and basophils participate in inflammation. IgE is produced primarily by plasma cells in lymphoid tissue lining the respiratory and gastrointestinal tracts and constitutes 0.001% of circulating immunoglobulins in normal individuals. This immunoglobulin class does not activate complement, nor does it cross the placenta. It has the unique property of binding to high-affinity receptors on the surface of mast cells and basophilic granulocytes, and to low-affinity receptors on lymphocytes, monocytes/macrophages, eosinophils, and platelets. The IgE molecule is bound by the Fc terminal end, so the antigen-specific N-terminal end (Fab$_2$) is exposed and confers antigen specificity to the mast cell or basophil (sensitizes). Forty thousand to 90,000 IgE molecules may bind to the plasma cell membrane of a mast cell or basophil.

All mammalian species make IgE antibody, and much of the information regarding its production and regulation is derived from work with rodent models. IgE-producing plasma cells are found in all lymphoid organs, but they are in highest concentration in the lymphoid tissue of the respiratory tract (tonsils and adenoids) and gut (Peyer's patches and lamina propria). IgE-bearing B cells are present in the human fetus by the 11th week of gestation, but IgE production in utero is negligible.

As with other immunoglobulin classes, surface IgM-bearing, virgin B cells differentiate into surface IgE-bearing memory B cells influenced by regulatory CD4$^+$ T helper cells (TH). Recent studies have shown presence of two types of CD4$^+$ cells based on the profile of cytokines they generate: TH$_1$ cells that promote cell-mediated reactions by secreting interleukin-2 (IL-2), interferon gamma, and GM-CSF; and TH$_2$ cells that promote immunoglobulin synthesis, especially IgE synthesis, by secreting IL-4, IL-5, IL-6, IL-10, and GM-CSF. B cells differentiate and mature into IgE-secreting plasma cells in the presence of allergen, antigen-presenting cells (eg, macrophages, dendritic cells, Langerhans cells), and the appropriate T cell-derived cytokines. The nature of the antigen is an important component of IgE antibody response. Certain antigens such as penicillin, ovalbumin, ragweed antigen E, and parasitic proteins stimulate the production of more IgE than IgG antibodies. In general, these proteins are glycoproteins in the 20,000 to 40,000 dalton molecular weight range. Immunization with low doses of these antigens favors IgE production. Exposure to any antigen initiates IgE production in most individuals, but the response normally is "turned off" rapidly by specific suppressor T-lymphocytes. Procedures that eliminate T suppressor cells, such as irradiation or cyclophosphamide, pro-

mote the indefinite production of high-titer IgE antibodies in animal models.

Modulation of IgE antibody is genetically controlled, although development of an IgE immune response occurs only after appropriate environmental exposure. Certain inbred strains of mice preferentially produce IgE antibodies when immunized, while others produce IgG. It appears that control resides primarily with a T helper lymphocyte population that is regulated by IgE-enhancing or IgE-inhibitory factors (cytokines) produced by other T helper or T suppressor lymphocytes, respectively.

The small amount of data available concerning human IgE regulation is compatible with information derived from rodent models. Data from family and twin studies suggest that elevated serum IgE concentrations (more than 100 IU/mL) are inherited as a simple recessive trait. In addition, specific IgE antibody responses more frequently are associated with specific human leukocyte antigen (HLA) specificities. For example, the development of IgE antibody to the Ra5 antigen of ragweed frequently is associated with HLA-DW2, whereas individuals with a response to rye grass pollen have a frequency of HLA-B8 three times higher than expected.

Elevated serum IgE concentrations are not restricted to allergic disorders. Many disease states are associated with elevated levels of IgE (Table 14-3). With atopic disease, the IgE concentration generally is elevated in only 60% to 70% of patients and correlates roughly with disease severity. Individuals with no detectable serum or cell-bound IgE are apparently healthy, which suggests that IgE is not essential in maintaining good health.

Serum containing IgE antibody can transfer sensitivity, but not particular atopic disorders, to normal individuals. The first human example of this was reported in 1919 when a patient with pernicious anemia was transfused with blood from a donor who was allergic to horses. The patient subsequently developed wheezing for the first time while driving behind horses. Before the advent of radioimmunoassays, circulating IgE antibody was detected by its ability to sensitize normal skin (Prausnitz-Kustner reaction); the technique is still useful in animal experiments (passive cutaneous anaphylaxis). Passive sensitization occurs when

**TABLE 14-3.   Pharmacologically Active Mediators From Mast Cells and Basophils**

**Preformed**
Histamine
Eosinophil chemotactic factor of anaphylaxis (ECF-A)
Neutrophil chemotactic factor (NCF)
Kallikrein
Prekallikrein activator
Hageman factor cleaver
Heparin
Tryptase

**Newly Formed**
Leukotriene B$_4$/C$_4$/D$_4$/E$_4$
Prostaglandin D$_2$
Thromboxane B$_2$
HETE
Platelet activating factor

**Secondary**
Bradykinin (serum)
Serotonin (platelets)
Major basic protein (MBP), eosinophils

IgE molecules bind with high avidity to specific receptors found on tissue mast cells and blood basophils. In allergic individuals, a similar process occurs when mast cells and basophils are sensitized by IgE molecules produced by plasma cells and released into the circulation.

Sensitization confers on the mast cell or basophil the ability to respond to an allergen. Once sensitization occurs, allergen exposure causes rapid (in seconds) changes in mast cell phospholipid and calcium metabolism, which results in an energy-dependent secretion of numerous pharmacologically active chemicals (the mediators listed in Table 14-3). Release of these mediators results in an immediate response (within 15 to 30 minutes), which may include vasodilation, increased vascular permeability, and smooth muscle constriction and mucus secretion in the respiratory and gastrointestinal tracts. In addition, thromboxanes and at least two proteins with chemotactic activity (eosinophilic chemotactic factor of anaphylaxis and neutrophil chemotactic factor) are secreted during the immediate phase, which may contribute to the infiltration of inflammatory cells.

In addition to the immediate response, mast cell activation may result in what is termed a late phase reaction (LPR). As shown in Figure 14-8, injection of an allergen causes an immediate wheal-and-flare reaction within 10 to 20 minutes. During the next 2 to 4 hours, the site may remain somewhat erythematous and edematous, but generally is not symptomatic. After 6 to 8 hours, the test site becomes pruritic (sometimes tender), warm, and more edematous and erythematous. This LPR may last 12 to 48 hours, although discoloration caused by extravasation of erythrocytes in severe reactions may persist for days. Histologically, lesions of LPRs show edema and perivascular infiltration of eosinophils and neutrophils. After 48 hours, mononuclear cells predominate in the cellular infiltrate, and the histology is indistinguishable from the classic type IV, cell-mediated response.

Recent studies demonstrate that infiltrating lymphocytes are allergen-specific $CD4^+$ $TH_2$ cells, which would promote further IgE synthesis, upregulation of low-affinity IgE receptors on many cell types, and attract inflammatory cells. In addition to cytokines secreted by lymphocytes, it has been shown that tissue macrophages, mast cells, and eosinophils secrete a variety of cytokines (interleukins) that promote the IgE-allergen-driven inflammatory response.

In the nose, the LPR causes persistent nasal obstruction and hypersecretion. In the lung, it is associated with a persistent airflow obstruction that only responds partially to bronchodilator therapy. Airway hyperirritability (propensity of the airways to obstruct secondary to nonimmunologic stimuli) may persist for weeks after the LPR. Airway hyperirritability can be assessed by measuring pulmonary functions before and after bronchoprovocation with methacholine or histamine (Fig 14-9). In animal models, biopsies of the lung demonstrate an infiltrate similar to that seen in human skin. Although the exact mechanism of the LPR is unknown, it is clearly important to the pathophysiology in chronic allergic disease.

## CLINICAL PRESENTATION OF THE ATOPIC SYNDROME

Atopy is a syndrome of various chronic disorders of the skin and respiratory tree associated with type I mechanisms. These disorders include atopic dermatitis, allergic rhinitis, and asthma. They constitute a syndrome because each has an identifiable IgE-dependent mechanism, and therefore each is frequently associated with one or more of the other disorders. For instance, asthma occurs in 20% to 50% of children with atopic dermatitis, and 80% to 90% of children with asthma have concomitant allergic rhinitis.

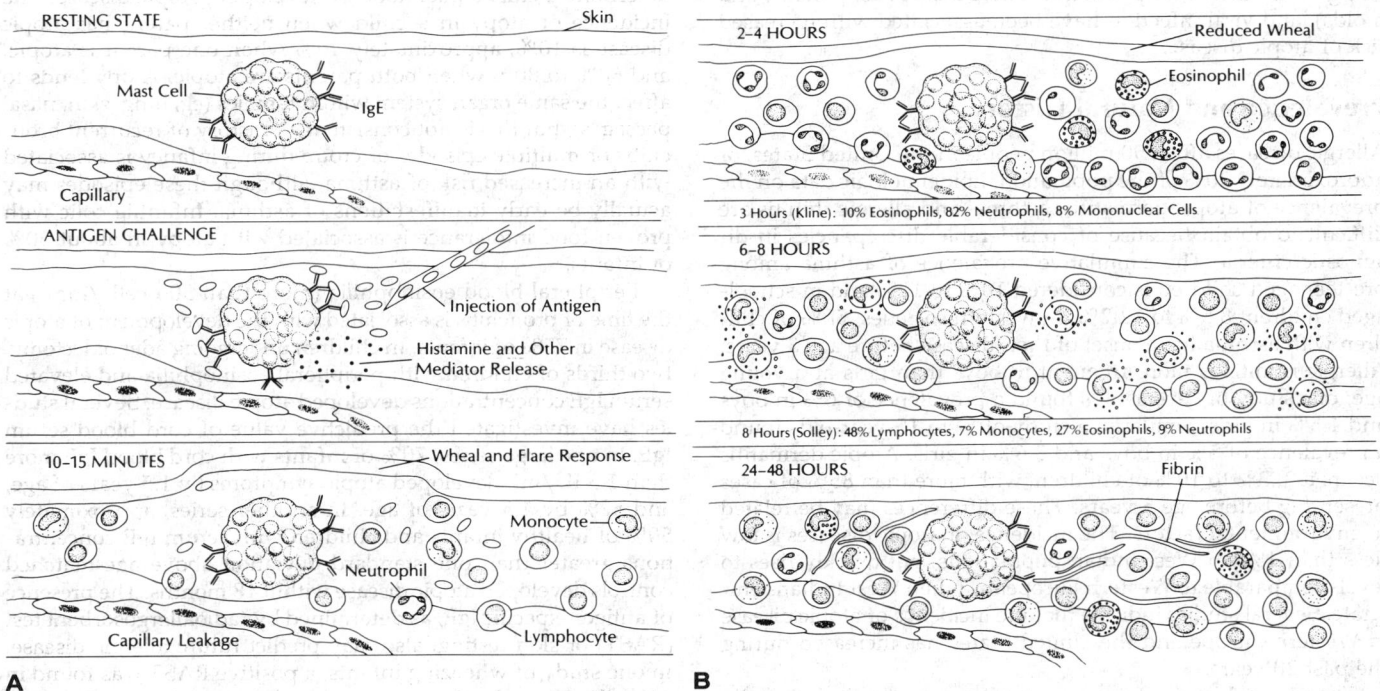

**Figure 14-8.** Biphasic cutaneous response. (**A**) Injected antigen activates mast cells by binding surface-bound IgE. Degranulation with release of histamine and activation of arachidonic acid metabolism with generation of inflammatory mediators occur in the immediate phase. (**B**) In the late phase, neutrophils and eosinophils initially, and then lymphocytes and monocytes, infiltrate the area. (Reproduced with permission. Sampson HA. Late-phase response to food in atopic dermatitis. Hosp Prac 1987;22(12): 112. Illustration by I. Arbel.)

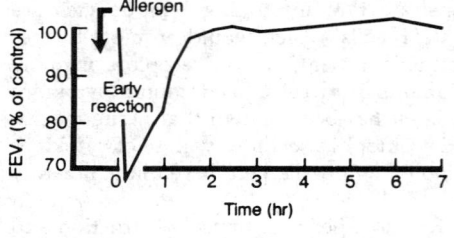
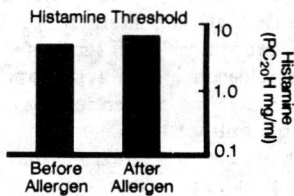
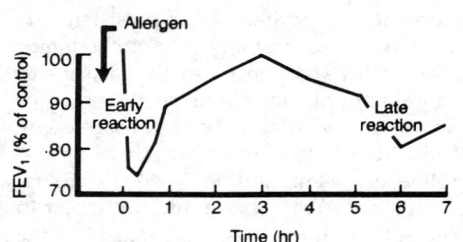
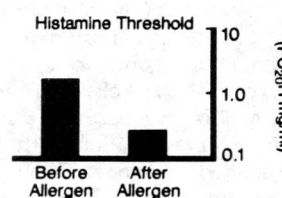

Figure 14-9.  Effect of early and late reactions on bronchial hyperreactivity. Increased bronchial hyperreactivity associated with decrease in $PC_{20}$ and late-phase reaction. (Cockroft DW, Ruffin RE, Dolovich J, et al. Allergen-induced increase in nonallergic bronchial reactivity. Clin Allergy 1977;7:503.)

A number of allergic signs and symptoms are not included in the atopic syndrome, although some occur frequently in atopic individuals. These include food allergy, drug allergy, insect hypersensitivity, urticaria, angioedema, and contact dermatitis. Epidemiologic studies have not confirmed the suggestion that drug allergy, especially allergy to penicillin, occurs more frequently in atopic individuals. Similarly, anaphylactic allergy to stinging insects is not more common in atopic individuals.

Atopic disease has a strong familial tendency. In a study of college-aged persons, the incidence of atopic disease was 15% when no first-degree relative had one of the diseases, 33% when one other relative was atopic, and 68% when two or more relatives were atopic. There is no clear pattern of inheritance, and it is felt to be polygenic. Exposure to several environmental factors such as cigarette smoke, air pollutants, allergens (foods, pollens, and molds), and viral infection have been associated with increased risk of atopic disease.

## Prevalence and Natural History

Allergic diseases affect 50 million people in the United States, or approximately 20% of the population. Epidemiologic data on the prevalence of atopic dermatitis, asthma, and allergic rhinitis are difficult to obtain because of considerable discrepancies in diagnostic criteria. The cumulative prevalence of asthma among pre-teenaged children is considered 10% to 12% and in school-aged children, 8.5% to 12.2%. In western societies, 50% of children with asthma have onset of their disease before age 3 years. Allergic rhinitis is more frequent in boys than girls at a young age; one study of 7-year-olds found a prevalence of 6% in boys and 1.5% in girls. Similarly, a study of 5- to 15-year-olds found a prevalence of 5% in boys and 3.6% in girls. Atopic dermatitis occurs in 8.3% to 10% of children, with more than 85% of cases presenting before age 5 years. These differences may be related to environmental factors. The incidence of atopic diseases is low (less than 1%) in West Indian populations, but quickly rises to levels comparable to Western Europeans when West Indians emigrate. Several studies indicate that the incidence of atopic disease in Western Europe and the United States has increased during the past 20 years.

The natural history of atopic diseases is complex. Each disorder generally appears for the first time at a characteristic age, frequently becomes more severe over a period of months to years, then undergoes a period of prolonged remission. For example, asthma begins by age 4 years in the majority of children and may be "outgrown" by late adolescence, while allergic rhinitis more commonly appears in late adolescence and remits less frequently. Eczema and food allergy appear in the first few months of life and may resolve during the first several years of life.

## Prediction and Prevention

The development of atopic disease depends on sufficient contact between a genetically predisposed host and an allergen. Sensitization may take weeks or years and depends on host genetic factors, allergen dose and time of exposure, and adjuvant factors such as infection. Since external factors are important in the sensitization of a predisposed individual, appropriate identification of subjects at risk and modification of their environment may prevent atopic disease.

Several historical and laboratory parameters may be used to determine a child's likelihood of developing atopic disease. The incidence of atopy in a child when neither parent has atopic disease is 10%, approximately 40% when one parent is atopic, and 60% to 80% when both parents are atopic. Atopy tends to affect the same organ system within families (eg, lung, skin, nasal passages), but this is not consistent. A history of recurrent bronchitis or multiple episodes of croup during infancy is associated with an increased risk of asthma, although these episodes may actually be early manifestations of asthma. Infantile colic with proven food intolerance is associated with atopy in about 50% of infants.

Peripheral blood eosinophilia (more than 500 cells/mm³) at the time of bronchitis is associated with the development of atopic disease in 75% of infants. In children undergoing adenoidectomy, two thirds of children with peripheral eosinophilia and elevated serum IgE concentrations developed atopic disease. Several studies have investigated the predictive value of cord blood serum IgE. In one large series, 70% of infants with cord blood IgE more than 1.3 IU/mL developed atopic symptoms by 1.5 years of age, and 82% by 4.5 years of age. In another series, approximately 50% of healthy infants and children with serum IgE concentrations greater than one standard deviation above age-matched controls developed atopic disease within 18 months. The presence of antigen-specific IgE, as determined by radioallergosorbent test (RAST) or skin testing, also may predict future allergic disease. In one study of wheezing infants, a positive RAST was found in 44% of infants who developed asthma or other allergic symptoms, and in only 3% who remained healthy on follow-up.

Although genetic constitution appears to be of primary importance in developing atopic disease, several environmental factors are major contributors. Because allergen exposure induces specific IgE, avoidance of allergen exposure early in life may reduce the incidence of atopic disease. In general, well-controlled prospective studies demonstrate that breast-feeding exclusively in the first year of life can affect the natural history of atopic disease. Allergic symptoms can be postponed until after the first or second year of life with exclusive breast-feeding for the first 6 months of life. More recent studies suggest that placing a lactating mother of a high-risk infant on a diet free of major allergens (egg, milk, peanut) may be even more protective, because food allergens are transmitted in maternal breast milk. The addition of solid foods to an infant's diet in the first 4 months of life has been directly correlated with increased risk of developing food allergy and atopic disease.

Exposure to inhalant allergens such as animal dander (especially cat dander), molds, and pollens in the first 6 months of life is associated with increased risk for developing atopic disorders. Consequently, measures to diminish exposure to animal products, dust mites, and molds seem justified in high-risk infants. Exposure to irritants or infection also may increase the risk of atopy. Several studies show that infants exposed to tobacco smoke develop higher serum IgE levels, have skin tests more positive to pollens, and develop respiratory disease at an earlier age than do infants in a nonsmoking environment. Furthermore, maternal smoking during pregnancy is associated with a two-fold increased risk of atopy in offspring. A few studies suggest that certain viral infections (eg, RSV, parainfluenza) may act as adjuvants for increased IgE responses to environmental allergens. Further study is needed before strong recommendations can be made about avoiding likely settings of infectious exposures.

Multiple atopic disorders (asthma, allergic rhinitis, atopic dermatitis), one of which being severe, and markedly elevated serum IgE levels (more than 600 IU/mL) are bad prognostic indicators. If patients remove themselves from pertinent allergens by controlling their environment or moving to an area of country free of offending pollen or allergens, they often experience remission. Many will develop sensitivities to new local allergens, so moving is not frequently recommended.

## DIAGNOSTIC EVALUATION

No single historical, physical, or laboratory finding is diagnostic of atopic disease. In fact, practically every symptom or sign of atopic disease can be seen in nonatopic disorders. Although clinical history provides the majority of information, a firm diagnosis must be based on accumulation of historical, physical, and laboratory data.

It is important to develop a clear understanding of the age of onset and progress of symptoms in terms of increasing or decreasing severity. A patient with relatively severe disease that is worsening warrants a more aggressive diagnostic approach than does someone with mild or remitting disease. Symptoms sometimes are related to allergen exposure, but more frequently overt symptoms do not follow contact with an isolated allergen. Recent studies suggest that immediate symptoms experienced by an allergic subject may go unrecognized, as distinct from the chronic disease state. Instead, a late-phase response, which is largely unresponsive to theophylline and beta-agonists, sets up a state of hyperirritability that causes the child to respond to a variety of nonspecific and often minor stimuli. For example, a pollen-sensitive asthmatic may respond to a histamine bronchoprovocation challenge for up to 4 weeks after a single allergen exposure.

A variety of allergens may affect the atopic patient. Pollen-sensitive subjects generally experience seasonal difficulty, so knowledge of local flora helps in making the appropriate diagnosis. In general, most tree pollens are released during early spring (February to March), and in most parts of the country, grass pollens are released from late spring to midsummer. In the eastern and midwestern United States, ragweed is a major source of pollen in late summer and early fall. While pollens are wind-borne during dry weather and are cleared from the air during rainy periods, mold spores are found in high counts in clouds and mist. High humidity provides favorable conditions for mold growth. House dust (composed of dust mites, animal danders, molds, pollens) is nonseasonal and may be increased to high concentrations when cleaning or when a child plays in a closet or under a bed. Domestic animals are common sources of potent allergens, but families often deny that their pet causes symptoms, suggesting that the problem is just pets in the neighborhood. Molds, especially in high concentrations frequently found in basements or around vegetation (hay, cut grass, barns, forests), can be a major source of difficulty. Foods, especially cow's milk, eggs, and peanuts, are frequent causes of allergic symptoms. A complete accounting of a patient's environment (indoors and outdoors), daily activities, and eating habits is necessary to assess potential allergen exposure.

Several features in the physical examination will suggest atopy. Characteristic features of specific atopic disorders is covered more thoroughly in the following chapters. Atopic children without overt atopic dermatitis may have dry skin with follicular prominence, mild scaling, and white dermographism. Children with nasal symptoms frequently have characteristic "allergic facies", with allergic shiners and Dennie-Morgan folds below the eyes due to venous congestion, a transverse crease across the bridge of the nose secondary to the "allergic salute," and persistent mouth breathing with "adenoid facies" characterized by deepened nasolabial folds, high arched palate, and some degree of malocclusion and overbite. Tonsils and adenoids frequently are enlarged in children with atopic disease, presumably in response to allergy and more frequent infection. Serous otitis media also is a common finding in atopic children. Chest deformities are uncommon except in severe, long standing asthma.

Laboratory tests help substantiate clinical impressions formed from a careful history. Peripheral blood eosinophilia (more than 500 cells/mm$^3$) often occurs in atopic patients with asthma and atopic dermatitis, but is seen less commonly in patients with allergic rhinitis. Eosinophilia in respiratory or gastrointestinal secretions highly suggests allergic disease. Secretions may be collected, dried on a microscope slide, and stained with Hansel stain, which stains eosinophils in a few minutes. Both circulating and secretory eosinophils are related directly to the severity of disease, and may be absent when the disease is asymptomatic. A peripheral blood eosinophil count may be elevated with other illnesses such as malignancy, collagen vascular disease, and parasites, but secretory eosinophilia is seen in few other conditions.

Total serum IgE concentration is somewhat useful as a screening test for allergic disease, but levels may be elevated with so many other illnesses that they are even less specific than an eosinophil count. Normal values are age-dependent, with highest levels normally found in late adolescence. Quantitation of IgE usually is performed by radioimmunoassay; values range from 0 to 100 IU/mL in childhood. An IgE concentration of greater than 100 IU/mL in the first year of life is correlated highly to future development of atopic disease.

Specific sensitivity may be confirmed with immediate wheal-and-flare skin tests. These are performed using various epicutaneous methods: prick, puncture, or scratch techniques. The skin is lightly abraded by "catching" the skin with the tip of a needle, pressing a needle onto the skin, or scratching the skin through a drop of allergen solution. An intracutaneous (intradermal) technique is a solution injected into the skin. The size of the resulting wheal using either method is determined at about 15 minutes and is compared to sizes of a positive and a negative control. The magnitude of the wheal and flare response correlates roughly with the severity of symptoms produced by natural exposure to the same allergens, although a positive skin test does not always reflect current clinical sensitivity. The intradermal test is more sensitive but less specific than the epicutaneous methods. Skin tests provide a rapid response and are relatively inexpensive. Disadvantages include moderate patient discomfort, minor risk of anaphylaxis, and suppression by antihistamines (for up to 1 week in some patients taking hydroxyzine).

As an alternative to the skin test, several serologic assays used to measure allergen-specific IgE are available. The RAST was developed first and is used most widely. Other methods are variations of the RAST: enzyme allergosorbent test (EAST), fluorescent allergosorbent test (FAST), multiple-thread allergosorbent test (MAST), and ventrex allergosorbent test (VAST). Although these assays measure circulating allergen-specific IgE antibodies that did not fix to mast cells, blood levels correlate with skin tests quite well. The tests are performed by incubating sera with solid materials to which allergen is chemically coupled. Nonspecific antibody is washed away, and adherent antibody is detected by incubation with a radiolabeled (enzyme-linked or fluorescein-linked) anti-human IgE antibody. The amount of radioactivity (enzyme activity or fluorescence) bound to the solid material directly correlates to the quantity of allergen-specific IgE. Serum can be drawn anywhere and sent to a competent technical facility, there is no risk of anaphylaxis, and patient medications do not interfere with the test. However, the tests are more expensive than skin tests and are somewhat less sensitive, and results are not available immediately.

## TREATMENT

Treatment of allergic diseases falls into three categories: allergen avoidance, drug intervention, and allergen immunotherapy. Allergen avoidance is the treatment of choice and is the most effective. It is often impossible, however, to implement this mode of therapy effectively. Use of drug intervention and allergen immunotherapy depends on the disease state. Effective drug therapy usually is available and practical, but treatment merely provides symptomatic relief. Immunotherapy is time-consuming, expensive, and has risk, but it may abrogate specific hypersensitivities. In some allergic disorders, eg, life-threatening stinging insect allergy, immunotherapy is the preferred treatment.

Allergen avoidance not only reduces symptoms, but sometimes reverses allergic disease activity. Specific IgE antibody production frequently diminishes over time without continued allergen exposure (stimulation). When total avoidance is possible for long periods of time (penicillin allergy, food allergy), re-exposure frequently is possible without risking recurrence of symptoms. For example, in a large series of patients with atopic dermatitis and food hypersensitivity, about one third of food allergies were "lost" after 1 to 2 years on a food allergen elimination diet.

Animal dander from household pets, such as cats and dogs, are potent allergens that frequently lead to allergic symptoms. Removal of the pet from the household is the most effective form of therapy, although it may take months for the allergen content to drop to insignificant levels. Dust mites, the major allergen in house dust, also are a major cause of allergic symptoms. To date, there are no measures known to eradicate dust mites completely, but exposure can be reduced. "Dust-proof" covers can be put on pillows and mattresses, throw rugs and nonwashable bedding can be removed, nonwashable stuffed animals and dolls ("mite farms") can be removed, and electrostatic filters can be used. Because mites thrive in humid environments, room humidifiers may aggravate the problem. These practices should be directed primarily at the child's bedroom, because children spend so much time there. When household molds are a problem, they are best dealt with by installing a dehumidifier, because most available fungicides are only partially effective. Exposure to outdoor allergens is difficult to avoid. Using air conditioning instead of leaving windows open during pollen season decreases exposure significantly.

Drug intervention is the second arm of allergy therapy. Certain drugs prevent IgE-mediated activation of mast cells and basophils. Corticosteroids inhibit mast cell activation and interleukin production and also interfere with the late-phase reaction through direct effects on granulocyte chemotaxis. These drugs are especially important in treating chronic atopic diseases because topically active agents with minimal toxicity are available for use in the airway. Cromolyn interferes with allergen-induced immediate and late-phase reactions through mechanisms that are still poorly defined after 20 years of clinical use. Antihistamines are competitive antagonists that interfere with immediate reaction by blocking the effects of histamine released by mast cells and basophils. Theophylline, beta-adrenergic drugs, atropinic drugs, and decongestants largely attempt to reverse effects of mast cell and basophil mediators. These are discussed in more detail in sections on specific allergic disorders.

Immunotherapy is an attempt to modify immune mechanisms involved in allergic disease. Immunotherapy, or allergy-injection therapy, consists of repeated injections of allergenic material to increase the patient's tolerance of those allergens. Immunotherapy is indicated only for stinging insect hypersensitivity and for allergic rhinitis and asthma (where allergen-related symptoms are implicated by history and laboratory testing). Immunotherapy is begun with subcutaneous injections of very small doses of allergens. The treatment solutions may contain various extracts of windborne pollens, mold spores, or dust mites. There is no evidence to substantiate the effectiveness of use of food or bacterial proteins for immunotherapy. Although immunotherapy with animal dander extracts is effective, it is not generally recommended because removal of the pet from the household is the preferred treatment. Immunotherapy with any allergen extract begins with subcutaneous injection of very dilute solutions. The concentration is gradually increased at weekly intervals until doses approximately 10,000 times higher are tolerated. At these levels, the therapy is extremely effective for allergy to venom of stinging insects and has been shown to be efficacious in treating seasonal allergic rhinitis (hay fever), perennial allergic rhinitis, and extrinsic asthma. The mechanism of this beneficial effect is uncertain, but may relate to the IgG-"blocking" antibodies produced, specific suppressor cell activation, and subsequent decreased IgE production or decreased releasability by mast cells and basophils. Immunotherapy carries a small (1% to 5%) risk of systemic anaphylaxis. Its effectiveness should be analyzed critically, because some individuals do not respond; ineffective treatment should be discontinued within 2 to 3 years.

## UNPROVEN DISEASES AND THERAPY

A variety of disorders affecting every system of the body are attributed to allergy, although most allergists doubt their association. Examples include learning disorders, behavioral problems (especially hyperactivity), depression, schizophrenia, fatigue, insomnia, myalgia, inability to concentrate or think clearly, arthralgia and arthritis, assorted gastrointestinal complaints including obesity, pounding heart, and enuresis. A new subspecialty—Clinical Ecology—has emerged, proponents of which believe that the above symptoms are caused by an accumulation of low-dose exposures to chemicals in the environment and in our food supply. An evaluation includes a variety of unproven tests (eg, sublingual or subcutaneous provocation, leukocyte cytotoxic tests, tests for IgG antibodies or antigen-antibody complexes, and trace metal hair analysis). Although the concept that environmental exposure causing human disease is similar to the concept of allergy, there is no scientific basis for clinical ecology and the methods have never been validated by objective clinical trials.

The tension-fatigue syndrome has received considerable attention in pediatric literature. Proponents consider a large number of emotional symptoms (anxiety, inattention, fatigue, headaches, hyperactivity) are caused by exposure to food or food additives. Many children with severe atopic disorders become irritable, moody, fatigued, secondary to the physical discomfort or sleep deprivation caused by their disease. The concept of tension-fatigue, however, is that symptoms are a direct consequence of allergy. Attempts to validate this syndrome in controlled, blinded clinical trials have failed.

Several therapeutic methods are practiced under the guise of allergy therapy with either no adequate experimental support or clear experimental evidence that the method is not effective. These include administration of low doses of inhalant allergens to reduce allergic rhinitis (Rinkle therapy). Another example is the administration of small doses of food extracts (sublingual food drops or subcutaneous neutralization) to treat symptoms caused by food allergy.

Finally, several widely practiced therapeutic approaches are simply irrational. These include injection of the patient's urine to reduce symptoms, enzyme-potentiated transepidermal desensitization, extreme and arbitrary dietary manipulation including rotational diets, the use of nystatin to eliminate intestinal *Candida*, and confinement to aluminum foil lined rooms.

## Selected Readings

California Medical Association Scientific Board Task Force on Clinical Ecology. Clinical ecology: a critical appraisal. West J Med 1986;144:239.

Galli SJ, Lichtenstein LM. Biology of mast cells and basophils. Middleton E Jr, Reed CE, Ellis EF, Adkinson NF, Yunginger JW, eds. Allergy: principles and practice, ed 3. St. Louis: CV Mosby, 1988:106.

Gleich GJ. The late phase of the immunoglobulin E-mediated reaction: a link between anaphylaxis and common allergic disease. J Allergy Clin Immunol 1983;70:160.

Kaliner M, Eggleston PA, Mathews KP. Rhinitis and asthma. JAMA 1987;258:2851.

Platts-Mills TAE, Tovey ER, Mitchell EB, et al. Reversal of bronchial hyper-reactivity during prolonged allergen avoidance. Lancet 1982;2:675.

Sampson HA. Prospects for Control of the IgE Antibody Response. Pediatr Clin North Am 1983;30:773.

Sampson HA. Late-phase response to food in atopic dermatitis. Hosp Pract 1987;22(12):111.

Sporik R, Holgate ST, Platts-Mills TAE, Cogswell JJ. Exposure to house dust mite allergen (Der p I) in the development of asthma in childhood: a prospective study. N Engl J Med 1990;132:502.

Vercelli D, Geha RS. Regulation of IgE synthesis in humans: a tale of two signals. J Allergy Clin Immunol 1991;88:285.

*Principles and Practice of Pediatrics, Second Edition.*
edited by Frank A. Oski et al. J. B. Lippincott Company, Philadelphia © 1994.

## 14.2.2 *Asthma*

Peyton A. Eggleston

Asthma is a chronic disease characterized by increased responsiveness of the airways to various stimuli and manifested by widespread obstruction, which changes in severity either spontaneously or as a result of therapy.

A leading cause of morbidity among children throughout the world, asthma accounts for 2.2 million pediatrician visits per year and 28 million restricted activity days. Asthma is the most commonly cited reason for school absenteeism. In the United States, it accounts for one third of school days lost, and in most urban hospitals, it is the most frequent cause for hospitalization of chil-

dren. In most western countries, between 2% and 10% of children younger than age 16 years are affected; the prevalence in Scandinavian countries is somewhat lower, 2% to 3%. In tropical and third world countries, the prevalence is significantly lower.

Over the past 15 years, asthma's prevalence in the United States has increased. In children aged 6 to 11 years, the prevalence in 1963 to 1965 was 5.3%; it rose to 7.6% in 1976 to 1980. The frequency of hospitalization also is increasing. The reason for this increase is not clear, but it has been seen throughout the western world, and is likely related to increasing urbanization in these populations, increasing pollution, and more accurate diagnosis of asthma.

Death from asthma is uncommon in children and represents a small fraction of the total causes of death in children of all ages in the United States. In 1985, for instance, the rate was 0.2 per 100,000 children 5 to 14 years of age, compared to 12.5 per 100,000 for accidents in the same age group, 3.5 per 100,000 for malignant neoplasm, and 1.2 per 100,000 for homicides. Death rates attributable to asthma have been increasing steadily in the last 20 years. In children in the United States, the rate has increased by approximately 6.2% per year. Again, this trend is worldwide, and mortality rates in the United States are generally small compared to other western countries. For instance, general population mortality rates of 1.4 per 100,000 compare to 2.0 per 100,000 in Canada, 3.4 per 100,000 in Great Britain, 5.7 per 100,000 in Great Britain, and 6.5 per 100,000 in New Zealand.

Risk factors for general morbidity and mortality trends primarily relate to urbanization and poverty. When poverty is accounted for, hospitalization rate differences between black and white patients almost disappear. There are definite pockets of increased mortality in cities, especially among those in lower socioeconomic groups.

## NATURAL HISTORY

The median age of onset of asthma is 4 years; more than 20% of children develop symptoms within the first year of life. Risk factors include atopy, especially multiple positive skin tests or RAST tests. This risk factor is genetic, in that the parental history is almost as strong a risk factor as is an elevated level of IgE in cord blood. The association with parental smoking is less clear, and most studies have shown a weak or insignificant association with either the onset or severity of asthma. Other obvious risk factors for early onset include neonatal lung disease, especially infants with reduced lung volumes, and respiratory infections, especially with the respiratory syncytial virus (RSV). Between 40% and 50% of children with RSV bronchiolitis develop chronic asthma.

In 60% of cases, asthma beginning in childhood resolves by young adult life. Fifty percent of those who undergo remission in adolescence become symptomatic again as young adults, and tests of airway hyperactivity show that even in asymptomatic young adults, the airways have not returned to normal. In general, those who resolve have less severe, intermittent asthma, usually do not have multiple positive skin tests to inhalant allergens, and do not have persistent wheezing or rhonchi. Studies demonstrate that heavy exposure to pollution, allergens, or cigarette smoke makes resolution less likely.

## PATHOPHYSIOLOGY

### Inflammation

As shown in the pathologic specimen in Figure 14-10, asthma is an inflammatory disease. The infiltrate in the airway wall and

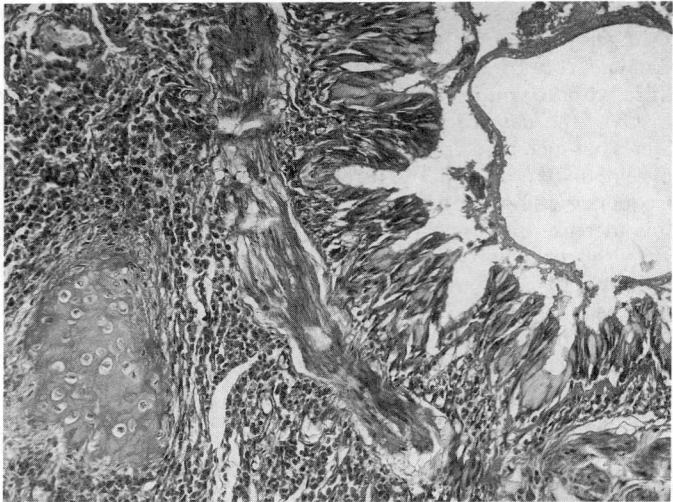

**Figure 14-10.** Pathology of asthma. Hematoxylin and eosin stained specimen of cross section of a small bronchus of an asthmatic patient.

the surrounding parenchyma is characteristically rich in eosinophils, but neutrophils, basophils, and mononuclear cells are common, without organized lymphoid nodules or granulomata. Large areas of respiratory epithelium are desquamated, and collagen is deposited in the area of the basement membrane. Bronchial smooth muscle is hypertrophied. Respiratory epithelium and inflammatory cells frequently fill large mucus plugs in the airway lumen.

This inflammatory process is thought to be caused by mast cell activation. Mast cells are a fixed tissue cell that may increase in areas of intense inflammation either through migration or proliferation. The cell is activated by either lymphokines or IgE-dependent mechanisms to produce a variety of proinflammatory substances. IgE-dependent inflammation requires antigen-specific IgE antibody. IgE antibody participates with other immunoglobulins in the normal immune response. It is produced from plasma cells that derive from B-lymphocytes influenced by T helper and suppressor cells. Characteristically, IgE binds with great avidity to mast cells and basophilic granulocytes and appears in the circulation in very small quantities. When it binds to mast cells, it confers on these cells the ability to respond to environmental allergens.

The nature of the antigen is an important component driving an IgE antibody response. Certain antigens such as penicillin, ovalbumin, ragweed pollen antigen, and parasitic proteins stimulate more IgE production than IgG. As a group, these allergens are 20,000- to 40,000-dalton molecular weight proteins that are constituent parts of such allergen vectors as plant pollens, foods, or animal dander. Although an IgE immune response occurs only after environmental exposure, modulation of IgE antibodies is genetically controlled. For example, certain inbred mouse strains preferentially produce IgE antibodies when immunized, while other strains produce IgG. The ability to respond to certain antigens has also been shown to be genetically controlled; for instance, the IgE response to certain pollen allergens is linked closely to the HLA-DW2 phenotype. Total serum IgE concentrations found in family and twin studies are inherited as a simple recessive trait.

On allergen exposure, the mast cell responds within seconds with an energy-dependent secretion of many pharmacologically active chemicals termed "mediators". These mediators result in an "immediate response," within 15 to 30 minutes, which includes vasodilation, increased vascular permeability, smooth muscle constriction, and mucus secretion in the respiratory and gastrointestinal tracts. This immediate response evolves into a late-phase reaction (LPR) within 2 to 4 hours after antigen exposure. Eosinophils and neutrophils begin to infiltrate the area, but by 48 hours, mononuclear cells predominate in the mixed cellular infiltrate. Symptoms associated with this LPR may include persistent tenderness or pain in the skin, persistent nasal congestion, or persistent asthma that responds poorly to beta-agonist treatment. Experimentally, it can be shown that the LPR is IgE-dependent. Recognizing LPR has been an important step in understanding asthma, because it provides a mechanism for the chronic inflammation seen in asthma. In addition, an important physiologic element of asthma, ie, airway hyperresponsiveness has been found to increase for days to weeks after LPR.

## Airway Hyperresponsiveness

Highly variable levels of airway obstruction are characteristic of asthma and are called airway hyperresponsiveness. This hyperresponsiveness is best illustrated in Figure 14-11, which shows the record of daily peak expiratory flow rate (PEFR) measurements on two patients with asthma. The patient with milder asthma usually has normal PEFR values, but these measures vary by more than 20% daily. The person with severe asthma has more abnormal PEFR measures together with daily variations of more than 60%. These variations in obstruction may be seen in response to many "precipitants" of bronchospasm. Typically, any patient responds to multiple precipitants, and the more severe the degree of airway hyperactivity, the greater the response to a stimulus. These multiple stimuli include irritants (cigarette smoke, odors, pollution, sulfite preservatives), weather changes, and emotions. Common colds (RSV, influenza, rhinovirus, parainfluenza) typically precipitate prolonged severe attacks. Certain drugs (beta-adrenergic antagonists, aspirin, and all nonsteroidal anti-inflammatory agents, except acetaminophen) cause brief, severe obstruction. Exercise causes brief obstruction by forcing the airway to adapt to hyperventilation and exposure to large volumes of cold dry air. Allergens cause attacks when specific IgE antibody is present.

Airway inflammation and airway hyperresponsiveness recently have been linked. In persons with a late-phase allergic response, airway hyperresponsiveness increases within a few hours and remains increased for 2 to 3 weeks, long after the late-phase obstructive response has subsided. During this period, the airway response to many stimuli including cold air, exercise, and allergens is increased. It is hypothesized that chronic and persis-

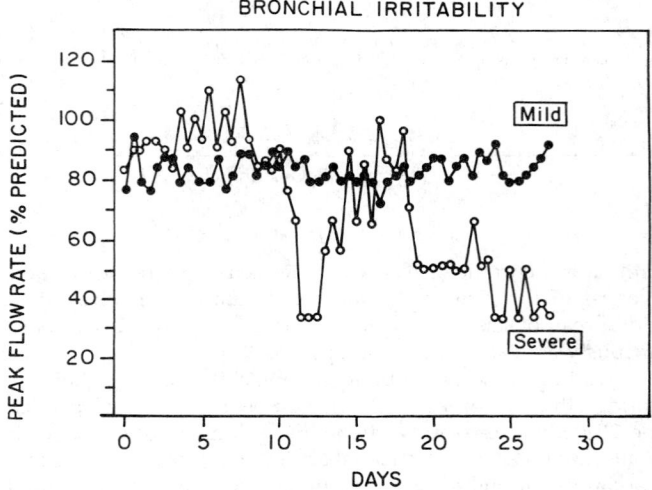

**Figure 14-11.** Daily PEFR measurement on 2 children with asthma.

tent allergen exposure causes not only immediate obstruction that can be noticed by a child, but also airway inflammation and physiologic abnormality that gradually increases and becomes more chronic and severe. This process can be reversed by removal from an allergic stimulus. Both in children and adults who are allergic to house dust mite allergen, avoidance for weeks to months will decrease airway symptoms, medication requirements, and response to environmental stimuli.

# PHARMACOTHERAPY FOR ASTHMA

## Beta-Adrenergic Agonists

The beta-adrenergic agonist group of drugs is the most important symptomatic therapy for asthma available. Airway obstruction

is reversed rapidly through their effects on the beta-2 receptor on bronchial smooth muscle. Available drugs and their doses are listed in Table 14-4. Because of its spectrum of effects and short duration, epinephrine is no longer the drug of choice for asthma, except as injectable preparations in infants when nebulized preparations cannot be given. The current drug of choice is either albuterol or terbutaline, which are beta-2 selective and longer acting. Newer drugs are being developed with much longer durations of action.

Whenever possible, beta-adrenergic agonists should be inhaled, because effective bronchodilation can be achieved with doses 10 to 20 times lower than with oral dosing. Toxicity includes tachycardia, palpitations, and central nervous system (CNS) excitement and muscular tremor. All these are dose-dependent and rarely are a problem with inhalation dosing. Nebulized drugs may be given with solutions from a nebulizer such as the De-

## TABLE 14-4. Available Drugs for Asthma

| | Preparations Available | | |
| --- | --- | --- | --- |
| | Tablets | Liquid | Dose |
| **Beta-Adrenergic Agonists** | | | |
| *Oral* | | | |
| Metaproterenol | 10, 20 mg | 10 mg/tsp | 1–2 mg/kg/d |
| Albuterol | 2, 4 mg | 2 mg/tsp | 0.4–0.6 mg/kg/d |
| Terbutaline | 2.5, 5 mg | NA | 0.4–0.6 mg/kg/d |
| *Metered Dose Inhaler* | | | |
| Metaproterenol | 0.625 mg/puff | | 1–2 puffs qid |
| Albuterol | 0.100 mg/puff | | 1–2 puffs qid |
| Terbutaline | 0.090 mg/puff | | 1–2 puffs qid |
| *Nebulized Solution* | | | |
| Metaproterenol | 50 mg/mL | | 0.2–0.5 mg/kg |
| Albuterol | 1, 5 mg/mL | | 0.1–0.15 mg/kg |
| Terbutaline | 1 mg/mL | | 0.1–0.15 mg/kg |
| **Theophylline** | | | |
| *Oral* | | | |
| Tablets | 50–300 mg | 50–80 mg/mL | 10–20 mg/kg/d to maintain peak serum concentration |
| Sustained release tablets, capsules (except Theodur sprinkles) | | | 5–15 $\mu$g/mL |
| *Aminophylline* (About 80% theophylline 100,200 mg/mL ampule) | | | 3–6 mg/kg bolus infusion 1 mg/kg/h to maintain serum concentration 10–20 $\mu$g/mL |
| **Cromolyn** | | | |
| Metered dose inhaler | 1 mg/puff | | 2 puffs/qid–bid |
| Powder | 20 mg/capsule | | 1 capsule qid–bid |
| Solution | 20 mg/ampule | | 1 ampule qid–bid |
| **Corticosteroids** | | | |
| *Oral* | | | |
| Prednisone | 1–50 mg | 5 mg/tsp | 1–2 mg/kg/d for 5·day acute course |
| Prednisolone | 5 mg | 5, 15 mg/tsp | |
| Methylprednisolone | | | |
| Dexamethasone | 4 mg | 0.5 mg/tsp | 0.75 mg/kg/d for 5 days *only* |
| *Inhaled* | | | |
| Beclomethasone | 0.042 mg/puff | | 2 puff qid–bid |
| Triamcinolone | 0.100 mg/puff | | 2 puff qid–bid |
| Flunisolide | 0.250 mg/puff | | 2 puff bid |
| *Injection* | | | |
| Prednisolone | 1 mg/mL | | 1–2 mg/kg then 1–2 mg/kg/d |
| Methylprednisolone | 20 mg/mL | | |

Vilbiss model 646 attached to a small compressor for home use or from a freon-powered inhaler. An inhaler is easier to administer when used with a reservoir device such as an Inspirease or Aerochamber; infants may be treated using an Aerochamber with a face mask. Adolescents must be cautioned against overuse of the inhaler and overreliance on its brief bronchodilatory effects.

In addition to being effective bronchodilators, beta-adrenergic agonists inhibit immediate asthmatic responses to allergens, exercise, and many inhaled irritants when given just before exposure. They have little effect on the LPR or on the resulting increase in reactivity.

Because beta-adrenergic agonists can not inhibit inflammation, their use as primary chronic therapy is questionable. Recently, a double-blind placebo controlled study suggested that chronic therapy could be detrimental. During the 1-year trial, asthmatic volunteers were treated regularly with inhalers containing beta-adrenergic agonists during one 6-month period and placebo during another 6 months. During the placebo period, the asthmatic volunteers had less acute medication requirements, fewer hospitalizations, more normal morning pulmonary function tests, and fewer chronic symptoms. The role of these drugs appears to be limited to controlling symptoms, and they should not be used as the only chronic therapy except in mild, episodic asthma.

## Theophylline

Theophylline was the most popular drug for the treatment of asthma in the 1980s, but is currently losing popularity to beta-adrenergic agonists because of toxicity and complex pharmacokinetics. The preparations available for current clinical use are listed in Table 14-4. Toxic effects include both mild (nausea, vomiting, stomach pain, diarrhea, headache, irritability, distractibility) and severe and life-threatening (intractable convulsion, tachyarrhythmia) reactions. Both therapeutic and toxic effects are related directly to plasma levels, with a therapeutic range of peak levels suggested from 5 to 20 $\mu g/mL$. Maximum levels of 15 $\mu g/mL$ are recommended for outpatient care because mild toxicity is seen in most patients with serum levels of 20 $\mu g/mL$. Distractibility, irritability, and poor school performance has been reported at all therapeutic levels; the consensus is that these effects are not significant when the effects of chronic illness are accounted for. Severe and life-threatening toxicity generally is not seen until plasma levels reach 30 $\mu g/mL$, but has been reported to occur at these levels without milder toxicity warnings.

Plasma theophylline levels depend on the amount of drug absorbed and the amount cleared by hepatic metabolism. Of the two, hepatic clearance is the most variable, with a range of difference as great as five-fold among individuals. Clearance is affected by many other factors (Table 14-5). Absorption also is quite variable. Fatty meals delay absorption, and absorption rate is lowest between 2 a.m. and 4 a.m. The absorption of certain time-released preparations (Theodur sprinkles) has been found to vary widely and unpredictably, although most are absorbed predictably. With the many variables described, it is imperative to measure serum theophylline concentrations when using the drug. In milder asthmatics treated with lower doses (10 mg/kg/d), a single level drawn at random may suffice. When the drug is used at higher doses, levels should be obtained whenever mild toxic symptoms occur, such as headache, stomachaches or vomiting, or when the child is exposed to conditions that may affect clearance, such as viral infections or erythromycin therapy.

Theophylline is an effective bronchodilator, although not as effective as beta-agonists. In acute emergency room use, theophylline is definitely inferior to beta-agonists and does not add to therapeutic effects while it does add side effects. Studies with hospitalized acute asthmatic children suggest that theophylline does contribute significantly to improvement. Theophylline is a

| TABLE 14-5. Factors Affecting Theophylline Clearance | |
|---|---|
| Factor | Approximate Multiple of Dose Needed to Produce Therapeutic Level |
| **Increased Clearance** | |
| Cigarette smoking | 2.0 |
| Phenytoin | 1.9 |
| Charcoal-broiled meats | 1.3 |
| **Decreased Clearance** | |
| Prematures, newborns | 0.1 |
| Cirrhosis | 0.4 |
| Congestive heart failure | 0.4 |
| Fever | 0.5 |
| Acute viral illness | 0.5 |
| Cimetidine | 0.6 |
| Erythromycin | 0.8 |

weak inhibitor of airway inflammation and of the LPR to allergens, but is unable to prevent the increased airway reactivity after allergen LPR. On the other hand, chronic therapy with theophylline or cromolyn have comparable effects on pulmonary symptoms and airway reactivity.

## Anticholinergics

Anticholinergic drugs are useful bronchodilators in acute asthma, but are not effective when used chronically. These muscarinic antagonists inhibit vagal reflex at smooth muscle and glands, but have no effect on CNS or neuromuscular transmission. Representative compounds in clinical use include atropine, ipratropium, and glycopyrrolate; only atropine is available for children younger than 12 years. Iprotropium bromide is a synthetic analog of atropine. It is poorly absorbed and has less systemic toxicity. These drugs are potent bronchodilators with peak effects that are delayed for 30 to 60 minutes. Treatment inhibits the response to irritants probably through interruption of vagal reflex, but exercise-induced and allergen-induced asthma is inhibited in only a fraction of patients. Toxic effects (xerostomia, mydriasis, tachycardia, and abdominal pain) are minor, but are annoying enough that the drug is not well accepted. The recommended dose of atropine for the treatment of acute asthma is 0.05 to 0.1 $\mu g/kg/$ dose.

## Cromolyn

Cromolyn was the first drug shown to prevent allergen-induced asthma in humans without having bronchodilator properties. Initially, it was thought to function by inhibiting mast cell activation, but recent information suggests that its effects can not be explained solely on mast cell activity. As shown in Table 14-4, it is available both as a solution for nebulization and as a metered dose inhaler. In single doses, cromolyn inhibits bronchospasm due to allergen, exercise, and sulfur dioxide. It is the only drug available that effectively inhibits both early and late-phase asthma caused by allergen exposure. In chronic use, airway reactivity is improved slightly, and disease activity is decreased. This effect requires approximately 2 to 4 weeks of chronic therapy, and approximately 25% of patients do not benefit. In trials directly comparing theophylline and cromolyn for chronic use in mildly to moderately asthmatic children (Furukawa, 1984), the two drugs are comparably effective, but theophylline is associated with a significantly higher rate of toxicity. Except for a rare allergic reaction, the cromolyn is nontoxic. A second drug, Nedocromil, with a very similar activity and has recently been approved for use in adults in the United States.

## Corticosteroids

Corticosteroids are the most potent drugs available for asthma. The mechanism of their effectiveness in asthma may relate to inactivation of various inflammatory cells including macrophages, monocytes, lymphocytes, basophils, and eosinophils. Acutely, their effectiveness may relate to increased numbers of beta-adrenergic receptors on bronchial smooth muscle and increased responsiveness to beta-agonists. With pretreatment for several days, inhaled and systemic steroids inhibit the allergen-induced LPR, but have little effect on immediate reaction. Chronically, airway hyperreactivity is significantly depressed.

Available preparations are listed in Table 14-4. For acute use, prednisone and methylprednisolone are equivalent. For chronic use, inhaled corticosteroids are an important new advance in asthmatic pharmacology. By modifying the glucocorticoid molecule, these compounds are about 100 times more potent than prednisone and methylprednisolone in anti-inflammatory activity. In addition, they are poorly absorbed from the respiratory tract and are rapidly cleared when absorbed from the gastrointestinal tract. This provides a wide therapeutic ratio and has led to recommendations for more widespread use in mild to moderate asthma. At the same time, studies show that signs of typical chronic toxicity may be seen with doses significantly higher than those shown in Table 14-4 and suggest the need for caution.

Corticosteroids have little serious acute toxicity except for hypokalemia. Eosinophil and mononuclear cells are reduced in peripheral blood, while neutrophils are increased and there is no demonstrable acute risk of infection. Chronic oral therapy with more than 5 mg/m$^2$ per day of prednisone or equivalent other drug produces growth suppression, adrenal suppression, decreased cortical bone mass, decreased oscalcin, and posterior subcapsular cataracts. These toxic effects are minimized by alternate day therapy or treatment with inhaled steroids.

## CHRONIC MANAGEMENT

Management of asthma in children is best considered in separate phases: chronic management and management of acute episodes. The goals of chronic management are to establish the diagnosis of asthma, to determine the most appropriate treatment program, and to educate the child and family to foster independent management of the disease. The National Asthma Education Program of the National Institutes of Health (NIH) recently published a monograph entitled "Guidelines for the Diagnosis and Management of Asthma," which is a consensus of a number of experts in the field. This section relies heavily on its organization and recommendations.

In most cases, little medical evaluation is needed to confirm the diagnosis of asthma, especially when there is a history of acute reaction to appropriate stimuli and quick relief by appropriate therapy. Other useful supporting evidence includes eosinophilia (greater than 400 eos/mm$^3$ in blood; greater than 10% in secretions), a personal or family history of atopic disease, and an elevated serum level of total IgE. Another screening test, the Phadeotope assay, has been shown to be both more specific and sensitive than the total IgE. To provide a basis for specific allergen control advice, allergy skin testing or RAST testing to common inhalant and food allergens should be performed on all children with moderate and severe asthma. At the same time, it is important not to equate asthma and atopy because 20% to 40% of children with asthma have no evidence of allergic disease.

The differential diagnosis in childhood is limited and should be considered only when atypical features are present. These are discussed in subsequent paragraphs that discuss the wheezing infant, because most of the conditions that can be confused with asthma present first in infancy.

## Allergic Aspects

Allergen avoidance is an essential first step in treating allergic asthma. The most common allergens associated with chronic asthma are house dust mites, cats, dogs, various molds, cockroaches, pollens, and various foods. House dust mite allergy is caused by pteroglyph mites that infest bedding, rugs, and other fabrics. The allergen is carried on fecal particles that are relatively large and settle quickly after disturbance; thus, close exposure (sleeping in an infested bed or lying on an infested rug) are important for sensitization and induction inflammation and symptoms. To avoid mite allergen, airtight covers must be installed to cover mattress and pillow completely. Bedding can be rendered mite-free by washing in hot water (55°C) or by dry cleaning; infestation usually recurs within a few weeks. Wall-to-wall carpeting in the child's bedroom should be eliminated as should excessive numbers of fuzzy toys if they are closely associated with the bed.

Pets contribute potent allergens, and about one third of patients with asthma have positive skin tests to cat or dog. The allergen originates in the animal's saliva. Pets should be eliminated from households with sensitized children. Because families often are unwilling to remove pets from the household, compromises may be employed. Keeping the pet out of the child's bedroom or in the yard is of questionable benefit. Washing the pet every 1 to 2 weeks does reduce concentrations in settled house dust, but cat antigen does not disappear from settled dust for more than 6 months after the animal has been removed. It is not clear whether compromise measures are adequate.

Mold antigens are ubiquitous in a home environment, and more than 25% of asthmatic children have positive skin tests. In general, the problem is worse in older houses or in moist environments. These sorts of environments are encountered with small room nebulizers, in basements, in homes in warm southern climates without air conditioning, or in rooms where vaporizers are used. The most effective way to remove mold and mildew is to remove contaminated materials and to reduce home moisture content.

Cockroaches recently have been found to contribute important allergens in urban environments, especially in the middle Atlantic and southeastern states. Elimination of the antigen usually requires pest control consultation and careful clean-up of the remaining insect parts and feces, which can be widespread and contain high concentrations of antigen.

Another approach to modifying the allergic response to environmental allergens is allergen immunotherapy, in which small amounts of aqueous extracts of source allergen vectors (pollens, dust mites, mold spores) are injected regularly over a period of months to years. Allergen immunotherapy reduces symptoms of allergic rhinitis, but it is less useful for asthma.

## Stepped Management of Medications

The first step in establishing stepped care is to establish the severity of asthma using a schema shown in Table 14-6. Symptoms of coughing and wheezing have the same significance in children. An episode occurs when an asthmatic child has more than two or three coughs or obvious wheezing. As asthma becomes more severe, intermittent episodes evolve to continuous symptoms.

In mild asthma, there are no symptoms or detectable signs of wheezing between episodes; they may, however, occasionally be

### TABLE 14-6. Assessment of Severity of Chronic Asthma

| Symptom | Mild | Moderate | Severe |
|---|---|---|---|
| Episodes of cough or wheeze | brief <2 per week | ≥2 per week | Almost daily, continuous |
| Symptoms or signs between episodes | no | Occasional | Present |
| Exercise tolerance | EIA with strenuous exercise | EIA with most exercise | Activity limited even with medication |
| Nocturnal cough or wheeze | <2 per month | Weekly | Frequent |
| School loss | None | >7 days | >21 days |
| ER, office visits for acute asthma | None | ≤3 per year | >3 per year |
| Hospitalization | None | None | 1 per year |
| PEFR % reference | ≥80% | 60–80% | <60% |
| PEFR variability | 20% | 20–30% | >30% episodes while medicated |
| Response to optimal medication | Symptoms controlled with prn inhaler | Regular medication required to control | Symptoms even with regular medication |

Adapted from NHLBI Expert Panel Report US Publication no. 91-3042.

seen in moderate asthma. Mild asthma never requires an emergency room or office visit for an episode, whereas moderate asthma may require up to three a year. During exercise, mild asthma may produce symptoms that last a few minutes but do not interfere with activity. Nocturnal cough may be present, but never more than two to three times a month in mild asthma.

Objective measurements of pulmonary functions are essential in managing asthma on a day-to-day basis. Symptoms and physical findings correlate poorly with objective measurements obtained in parallel. For chronic use, home peak expiratory flow meters should be used to educate patients about symptoms, to establish a baseline for measuring exacerbations, and to adjust medications. Acutely, peak flow meters should be used to establish the severity of obstruction. The PEFR is criticized as an inadequate measure of pulmonary function that provides little information compared to spirometry, but it is cheaper, more convenient, more easily performed by younger children, and correlates well with an $FEV_1$. Experience continues to confirm its usefulness. Equipment is cheap and includes the Assess and mini-Wright meters. Normal values are shown in Figure 14-12. Peak flows are within the normal range in mild asthma and never drop more than 20% during symptomatic episodes. Both figures escalate to more severe involvement in more severe asthma.

In general, children evolve from one stage of severity to another over long periods of time, usually months to years. Therefore, classification according to the categories described above can be used to plan therapy over extended periods of time.

### Mild Episodic Asthma

Mild episodic asthma is treated best with an inhaled beta-agonist as needed for symptoms. The drug should be used with a spacer device unless the child is demonstrably expert at inhaling it properly. It may also be used as a prophylactic before exercise or exposure to allergen. If use requires more than two doses a day (a new canister about every 6 weeks), the child should be considered for chronic therapy, and additional medications in different therapeutic classes should be added.

### Moderate Asthma

Moderate asthma should be treated with daily medications that induce long-term resolution. This may include cromolyn (two puffs taken two to four times a day) or theophylline taken at doses adequate to maintain levels of 5 to 15 mg/mL. Under these circumstances, the PRN use of beta-agonist may be increased

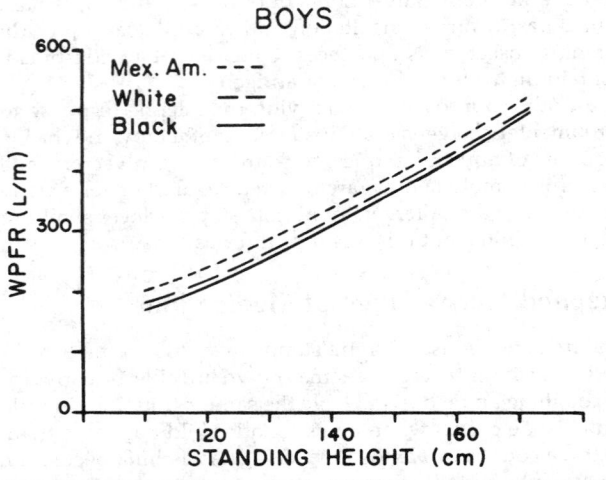
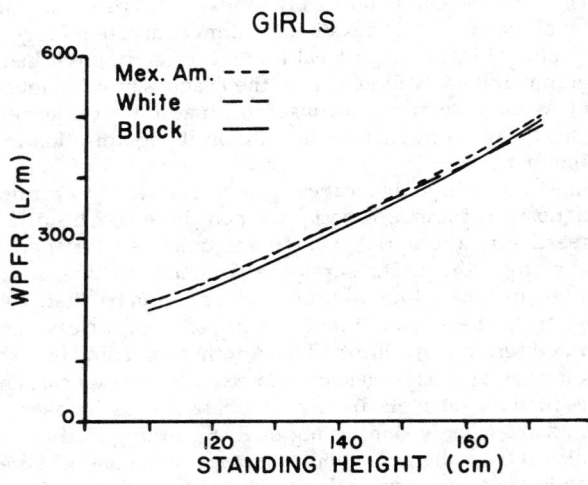

Figure 14-12.　Prediction curves for PEFR measurements in children (Hsu KHK, Jenkins DE, Hsi BP, et al. Ventilatory functions of normal children and young adults—Mexican American, white and black: II wright peak flow meter. J Pediatr 1979;95:192).

and may vary from zero to four times a day. Some authorities recommend inhaled steroids for children with moderately severe asthma.

## Severe Asthma

Severe asthma requires treatment with inhaled steroids in full doses (two puffs four times a day). In addition, a second drug for chronic use (eg, cromolyn, theophylline) is usually required. Inhaled beta-agonists are continued as PRN symptomatic therapy. If symptoms and pulmonary functions are not controlled with inhaled beta-agonists, oral steroids should be added in the range of 0.2 to 0.5 mg/kg every other day.

The goal of therapy is to normalize pulmonary function, decrease peak flow variability, and allow normal or near-normal activity with infrequent night symptoms and no absenteeism from school.

## TREATMENT OF ACUTE ASTHMA

The goal of treatment of acute asthma is to normalize pulmonary functions rapidly and to prevent progression of the attack. Essential to this process are early recognition of worsening lung function, prompt communication between patient and physician, removal from the allergen, irritant, or other trigger, and appropriate intensification of asthma medications.

A scheme to assess severity in acute asthma is shown in Table 14-7 and gives criteria for both home and hospital use. Generally, the most appropriate place to initiate treatment of an acute attack is in the home or at school. Certain patients are at risk for life-threatening severe attacks. These patients should be treated more aggressively than is outlined and sometimes can not be treated at home at all. High-risk patients include those with prior intubation for asthma, two or more hospitalizations for asthma in the last year, three or more emergency room visits for asthma in the last year, hospitalization or emergency room use within the last month, a requirement for oral steroid therapy, a past history of syncope or hypoxic seizures during an asthma attack, and a history of serious psychiatric or psychosocial problems.

Home management is recommended whenever possible so treatment begins immediately and families gain some control of the disease. Always, a written, brief plan of assessment and treatment should be provided by the physician. The first step is to assess severity using Table 14-7. In mild to moderate attacks, albuterol should be given by nebulization or metered-dose inhaler. A good response is indicated by a return to evidence of

mild obstruction. Routine medication should continue, albuterol should be given every 3 to 4 hours, and severity should be reassessed frequently. An incomplete response is indicated by persistent evidence of moderate obstruction. The physician should be contacted, oral prednisone 1 to 2 mg/kg per dose should be given and inhaled, and beta-agonist treatment should continue. If severity subsides to mild over the next 4 hours, continued home treatment is appropriate. If moderate asthma continues, the patient should be seen in the physician's office or a hospital-based emergency room. If a patient has severe asthma according to Table 14-7, albuterol treatment should begin. The patient should then go immediately to a physician's office or to a hospital-based emergency room.

The decision to treat in a physician's office or a hospital-based emergency room depends on many factors, including accessibility of the emergency room, the ability and interest of the physician to manage severe asthma in the office, and the physician's previous relationship with the patient.

In the office, a reassessment should determine severity and rule out complications such as atelectasis, pneumomediastinum, and pneumothorax. Oxygen should be administered together with nebulized albuterol every 20 minutes for 1 hour. Prednisone should be given unless the patient responds immediately to a nebulized dose. Epinephrine, 0.01 mg/kg, should be given if the patient does not generate a peak flow, has decreased consciousness, or cannot cooperate for treatment with nebulized drugs. If treatment is required past 4 hours, hospitalization should be considered, and if the response to treatment is poor, the patient should be admitted. Generally, a patient who has responded will be discharged on continued medication, which usually includes prednisone, and with a follow-up plan.

Hospital management offers little pharmacologically that can not be provided as an outpatient. The major indication for hospitalization is to observe for continued deterioration so more intensive treatment can be given, in an intensive care unit if necessary.

## THE WHEEZING INFANT

Because wheezy respiratory infections occur so commonly in infants and because chronic systemic illnesses present for the first time in infancy, the differential diagnosis of the wheezing infant is more extensive than that for older children. The most common cause of recurrent lower respiratory cough and wheeze in infants is simply recurrent colds, especially in day-care settings. Asthma is the second most common cause, but congenital anomalies

**TABLE 14-7. Estimation of Severity of Acute Exacerbations of Asthma**

| Indication | Mild | Moderate | Severe |
|---|---|---|---|
| Alertness | Normal | Normal | May be decreased |
| Dyspnea | Absent, speaks complete sentences | Moderate, speaks phrases | Severe, speaks short phrases, words |
| Pulsus paradoxicus (mm Hg) | <10 | 10–20 | 20–40 |
| Accessory muscle | None | Retractions sternocleido mastoid | Severe retractions, nasal flaring |
| Color | Good | Pale | Cyanotic |
| Auscultation | End-expiratory wheeze | Inspiratory, expiratory wheeze | Quiet breath sounds |
| O₂ saturation (%) | >95 | 90–95 | <90 |
| pCO₂ (mm Hg) | <35 | <40 | >40 |
| PEFR predicted or % best | 70–90 | 50–70 | <50 |

*Adapted from NHLBI Expert Panel Report US Publication no. 91-3042.*

(vascular ring, TE fistulae, congenital heart disease), metabolic abnormalities (cystic fibrosis), foreign body aspiration, immune deficiency syndromes, and gastroesophageal reflux must be considered. Any infant with significant steatorrhea, atypical wheezing with an inspiratory component or localization to one side, a history of aspiration or choking on food, or with failure to thrive or clubbing on physical examinations should receive further evaluation.

As a first step, any infant with recurrent wheezing should have a chest x-ray, a careful review of systems, and a careful physical examination. Laboratory evaluation and confirmation of an allergy history is more difficult because skin tests are generally smaller in infants and because RAST tests are more likely to be negative. In one study of 78 unselected asthmatic infants younger than 1 year of age, only 6 had positive skin tests. This contrasts with rates of 60% to 80% in older children and adults with asthma.

Treatment is more difficult in infants than in older children. Response to bronchodilator therapy is not striking, especially during an acute episode. Appropriate dosages for medication in infants are provided in Table 14-4. Specific problems with drug dosing include difficulty providing nebulized medications, differences in theophylline clearance, and a general concern that the chronic toxicity of all drugs may differ in rapidly growing infants than in older children. Aerosol medication usually must be given with a portable nebulizer. Some infants tolerate a face mask, whereas others only allow the nebulizer outlet to be held close to the face while sitting on the parent's lap; support for the parent and imaginative methods for increasing acceptance by the infant are required. A spacer device, the Aerochamber, is available with a face mask, allowing some infants to be treated with metered dose inhalers. Currently available drugs are not approved by the FDA for use in children younger than 6 years. Inhaled steroids, which have proven so important in the chronic therapy of older children, are not available for infants. In the United States, there is no available aerosol steroid preparation that can be used in a nebulizer; in Canada and Europe, however, budesonide has been used successfully.

## Selected Readings

Barnes PJ. A new approach to the treatment of asthma. N Engl J Med 1989;321: 1517.

Blair H. Natural history of childhood asthma: 20-year follow-up. Arch Dis Child 1977;52:613.

Buist AS. Asthma mortality: what have we learned? J Allergy Clin Immunol 1989;84: 275.

Charney E. The field of pediatrics. In: Oski FA, ed, principle and practice of pediatrics. Philadelphia: JB Lippincott, 1990:4.

Evans R III, Mullally DI, Wilson RW, et al. National trends in morbidity and mortality of asthma in the US: prevalence, hospitalization rate and death from asthma over two decades (1965–1984). Chest 1987;91:65S.

Gergen PJ, Weiss KB. Changing patterns of asthma hospitalization among children (1979–1987). JAMA 1990;264:1688.

Gregg I. Epidemiology of asthma. In: Clark TJH, Godfrey S, eds. Asthma. London: Chapman and Hall, 1977:214.

Murray AB, Ferguson AC. Dust-free bedrooms in the treatment of asthmatic children with house dust or house dust mite allergy: a controlled trial. Pediatrics 1983;71: 418.

Murray AB, Morrison BJ. The effect of cigarette smoke from the mother on bronchial responsiveness in severity of symptoms in children with asthma. J Allergy Clin Immunol 1986;77:575.

National Heart, Lung and Blood Institute. National Asthma Education Program Expert Panel Report: Guidelines for the diagnosis and management of asthma. US Publication no. 91–3042, US Department of Health and Human Services. National Institutes of Health, Bethesda.

Phelen PS. The natural history of childhood asthma into adult life. Immunology and Allergy Practice 1988;10:15.

Sly RM. Increase in deaths from asthma. Ann Allergy 1984;53:20.

Strunk RC. Asthma deaths in childhood: identification of patients at risk and intervention. J Allergy Clin Immunol 1987;80:472.

Tabachnik E, Levison H. Infantile bronchial asthma. J Allergy Clin Immunol 1981;67: 339.

Weinberger M, Lindgren S, Bender B, et al. Effects of theophylline on learning and behavior: reasons for concern or concern without reason. J Pediatr 1987;111: 471.

Weiss KB, Wagener DK. Changing patterns of asthma mortality: identifying target populations at high risk. JAMA 1990;264:1683.

*Principles and Practice of Pediatrics, Second Edition.*
edited by Frank A. Oski et al. J. B. Lippincott Company, Philadelphia © 1994.

## 14.2.3 *Urticaria and Angioedema*

Thomas B. Casale

Urticaria (hives) is characterized by erythematous, edematous wheals of the superficial layers of the skin or mucous membranes. The lesions blanch with pressure, are often pruritic, and usually are distributed symmetrically. Individual urticarial lesions are usually evanescent, commonly lasting less than 4 hours, but occasionally persisting for 24 to 48 hours. If the lesions persist, there may be underlying vasculitis. Angioedema is a similar process occurring in deeper layers of the skin and subcutaneous tissues. Angioedema is characterized by well-demarcated areas of nonpitting, nondependent, and not-hot swelling. Whereas urticaria may occur on any part of the body, angioedema often involves the extremities, face (especially the perioral and periorbital areas), or genitalia.

Pruritus or a chronic itch does not equal chronic urticaria. Pruritus without visible lesions can be caused by a number of different diseases unrelated to urticaria, such as renal failure and azotemia. These patients have severe pruritus and no evidence of urticaria. Although urticarial lesions are often pruritic, the presence of pruritus without urticaria is cause to formulate a distinct list of differential diagnoses.

Traditionally, the duration of urticaria has defined whether the disease is acute or chronic. Chronic urticaria is a disease in which the patient has urticarial lesions that are either continuous or frequent for 6 weeks or longer. Acute urticaria is a disease in which the lesions are present for less than that period of time. However, one must also include in any classification scheme the physical urticarias. Physical urticarias may last for several years, but are manifested by recurrent episodes of acute lesions in relation to a physical stimulus such as cold, exercise, or pressure. In addition, chronic urticaria as opposed to acute and physical urticarias may be distinguished pathologically. Biopsy samples of chronic urticarial lesions tend to show a non-necrotizing perivascular infiltrate that is generally not noted during acute episodes of urticaria or physical urticarias. In most studies, an etiologic agent in chronic urticaria is found in only 5% to 20% of patients. Thus, most cases of chronic urticaria are labeled "idiopathic." The success rates for identifying specific causes of acute urticaria are higher.

The incidence of urticaria and angioedema is extremely high. It is estimated that 15% to 20% of the population experience an episode of urticaria or angioedema at some time in life. Acute urticaria may occur at any age, and is the most common form seen in children. Chronic urticaria occurs more frequently in young adults (peak incidence in third and fourth decades) than in the pediatric population. Chronic urticaria may be persistent. In one long-term follow-up of pediatric and adult patients with chronic idiopathic urticaria or angioedema, the average duration of urticaria alone was 6 months, angioedema alone was 1 year, and urticaria with angioedema was 5 years (Champion et al, 1969).

Thus, it is readily apparent that all physicians can expect to see many patients with urticaria or angioedema. To facilitate the care of these patients, specific points about the pathophysiology, causes, diagnostic tests, and treatment of urticaria and angioedema are addressed in this chapter.

## PATHOPHYSIOLOGY OF URTICARIA AND ANGIOEDEMA

Urticarial lesions are caused by dilation of blood vessels in the superficial dermis (erythema or flare) and by increased vascular permeability with leakage of fluid into surrounding connective tissue (wheal). Histologically, urticaria is characterized by dilation of small blood vessels and by edema, which leads to flattened rete pegs, widened dermal papillae, and swollen collagen fibers. Angioedema shows similar changes but is confined to the deeper dermis and subcutaneous tissue.

Based on varied evidence, there are at least three pathogenic factors involved in the development of urticaria (Table 14-8). These include neuropeptides, mast cells and mast cell mediators, and inflammatory (especially mononuclear) cells other than mast cells.

### Neuropeptides

Intradermal injection of many neuropeptides results in erythema and a wheal or induration that closely resembles an urticarial lesion. These neuropeptides are present in skin and have direct effects on cutaneous vasculature including vasodilation and edema. In the physical urticarias, there is some evidence that neuropeptides might be important. The provocative stimuli in these conditions include such things as cold, heat, and pressure, which are expected to activate neuropeptide-containing sensory nerve fibers in the skin. The release of these neuropeptides can then cause vasodilation, edema, and possibly histamine release from cutaneous mast cells. Repeated topical application of capsaicin (a substance that depletes neuropeptides from afferent nerves) has prevented the urticarial response to thermal challenge in patients with cold- and heat-induced urticaria. The exact role of the neuropeptides in chronic urticaria and physical urticaria, however, is unclear.

### TABLE 14-8. Pathogenic Factors in Urticaria/Angioedema

**Neuropeptides of Unmyelinated Sensory Fibers**
Substance P
Calcitonin gene-related peptide
Vasoactive intestinal peptide
Others

**Mast Cells/Mast Cell Mediators**
Histamine
Bradykinin
Prostaglandins (eg, $PGD_2$)
Leukotrienes $C_4$, $D_4$, $E_4$
Platelet-activating factor

**Mononuclear Cells**
Monocytes
T-Lymphocytes

### Mast Cells

Mast cells and mast cell mediators have long been implicated in the pathogenesis of urticaria. Evidence for the roles of mast cells and mast cell mediators in the pathogenesis of urticaria includes morphologic and histologic definition of mast cell degranulation after specific physical stimuli in patients with physical urticarias; wheal and flare formation after intracutaneous injection of mast cell mediators; identification of mediators in biologic fluids collected during urticarial reactions; and the ability to suppress the urticarial tissue response with specific mediator antagonists (eg, antihistamines). Moreover, there is evidence of mast cell degranulation in chronic urticarial lesions and the skin of patients with chronic urticaria contains increased number of mast cells.

Overall, mast cells and mast cell-dependent mediators play a prominent role in the pathogenesis of urticaria and angioedema. A number of mediators other than histamine, however, are important in causing urticaria and angioedema (see Table 14-8). Therefore, selective $H_1$ antihistamines are seldom entirely effective in treating urticarial reactions. Studies on the role of mediators other than histamine in the pathogenesis of urticaria should aid in the development of new and better treatment modalities for this disorder.

Although mast cells and mast cell mediators are central to the pathogenesis of urticaria and angioedema, the presence of IgE antibodies to specific allergens is not necessary. A number of mechanisms other than "classic allergic reactions" may lead to mast cell degranulation. Activation of either the classic or alternative complement pathways may cause urticaria by producing anaphylatoxins (C3a, C4a, C5a), which can degranulate mast cells. A number of drugs including opioids, some antibiotics, and nonsteroidal anti-inflammatory agents may lead to nonimmunologic mast cell mediator release. Neuropeptides such as substance P and neurotensin can also cause mast cell degranulation. Inflammatory reactions resulting in the production of histamine-releasing factors from lymphocytes, macrophages, and neutrophils may cause mast cell mediator release as well. Finally, physical stimuli such as heat, cold, and pressure can cause mast cell mediator release and urticaria in susceptible individuals. Thus, there are many potential mechanisms leading to mast cell mediator release and urticaria.

### Mononuclear Cells

Numerous biopsy studies suggest that inflammatory cells other than mast cells play important roles in urticaria as well. Chronic urticarial lesions are characterized by a non-necrotizing perivascular infiltrate composed of T lymphocytes, monocytes, and mast cells. Because lymphocytes, monocytes, and other cells release histamine-releasing factors and mast cells may produce substances that activate T cells and monocytes, one might envision a cyclical propagation of an event initiated by mast cell degranulation. Corticosteroids work, in part, because T lymphocytes and monocytes likely play a role in the pathogenesis of chronic urticaria. Corticosteroids have not convincingly been shown to inhibit cutaneous mast cell degranulation, and, therefore, have not generally been shown to be effective in physical urticarias in which cellular infiltrates are generally not noted by biopsy sample (except delayed pressure urticaria/angioedema). In general, there is no evidence of complement or immunoglobulin deposition in chronic urticarial lesions.

## CAUSES OF URTICARIA AND ANGIOEDEMA

Because a number of mechanisms may lead to mast cell mediator release, a variety of etiologic factors have been found to cause urticaria and angioedema. The major etiologic factors producing acute and chronic forms of urticaria and angioedema are listed in Table 14-9. Acute urticaria is most frequently caused by a food or drug and usually dissipates within days to several weeks. As previously stated, the cause of chronic urticaria is usually not determined. The incidence of atopy in patients with chronic idiopathic urticaria does not appear to be higher than that found in the general population. The following paragraphs discuss many of the etiologic factors for urticaria and angioedema listed in Table 14-9.

## Drug Reactions

Drug reactions are one of the most common causes of urticaria and angioedema. The reactions are mediated by type I or type III immune mechanisms or by direct nonimmunologic mast cell mediator release. Depending on the mechanisms involved, the urticaria may occur immediately or days to weeks after drug exposure (eg, serum sickness syndrome with urticaria). Many drugs are associated with urticaria. Antibiotics, especially penicillin and related compounds, remain the leading causes of drug-induced urticaria. Aspirin and other nonsteroidal anti-inflammatory agents are common causes of urticaria. There is not convincing data to indicate, however, that patients who are not allergic to these drugs have an exacerbation of their disease when taking aspirin or nonsteroidals. Some drugs such as the opioids can directly cause mast cell degranulation. Other classes of drugs frequently associated with urticaria include diuretics, radiocontrast dyes, muscle relaxants, and sedatives or barbiturates. All drugs taken by the patient must be determined because any drug can be a potential cause of urticaria. Vitamins, lotions, contraceptives, laxatives, and various over-the-counter drugs represent possible offenders. When a drug reaction is suspected, all unnecessary

drugs should be eliminated, and an attempt should be made to switch to alternative, chemically distinct forms of necessary drugs.

## Foods

Foods are a common cause of acute urticaria, but may also cause chronic urticaria. Daily hives suggest foods eaten regularly, whereas sporadic, recurrent hives suggest foods eaten intermittently. The most common offenders include nuts, milk, eggs, chocolate, citrus fruits, tomatoes, and fish. Food dyes (tartrazine) and additives (benzoate derivatives, sulfates) may also infrequently cause urticaria. Patients with respiratory allergies to pollen may develop urticaria or angioedema after ingestion of certain foods with "cross-reactive" antigens. Reported examples include ragweed and banana and melons; birch and celery, nuts, and certain fruits; and grass and tomatoes.

## Infection

Many types of infections have been associated with urticaria. Viral infections are common causes of acute urticaria in children and adolescents. Although undetected infections have been considered a cause of chronic urticaria, the incidence is probably low. The most common infections known to be associated with urticaria include infectious hepatitis, infectious mononucleosis, coxsackievirus infection, mycoplasma infection, helminthic parasites, and acute beta hemolytic streptococcal infection. The association of urticaria with *Candida* or tinea infections is probably coincidental. If an infection is found it should be treated. However, extensive evaluation or empiric antimicrobial therapy for undetected infection is not warranted. Indeed, drugs used to treat suspected infections are more likely to cause hives.

## Inhalants

Inhalant allergens including pollen, animal dander, and spores are infrequently associated with urticaria. Allergic respiratory symptoms to the inhalant generally occur concomitantly.

## Insects

Children may get a hive-like reaction to biting insects such as fleas and mites, which is referred to as papular urticaria. These lesions are characterized by pruritic, papular lesions usually on exposed skin surfaces (especially the extremities). Acute urticaria and angioedema may also follow stings or bites from Hymenoptera in allergic individuals.

## Systemic Diseases

A number of systemic diseases are associated with urticaria and angioedema. If the urticarial lesions are accompanied by fever, arthralgia, or elevated sedimentation rate, an underlying connective tissue disorder and cutaneous vasculitis should be considered. Systemic lupus erythematosus, rheumatic fever, and rheumatoid arthritis may be accompanied by urticaria-like lesions. The rash associated with juvenile rheumatoid arthritis may appear before other signs of the disease. In patients with connective tissue disorders, lesional biopsy tests usually reveal vasculitis.

Urticaria also has been observed in adults and children with lymphoreticular malignancies, and in adults with carcinoma of the lung, rectum, or colon. Several studies suggest, however, there is not a higher incidence of malignancies in patients with chronic urticaria. Unless evidence suggest malignancy, an exhaustive search for cancer is not indicated.

Thyroid disease (especially Hashimoto's thyroiditis) and both

### TABLE 14-9. Major Causes of Urticaria and Angioedema

Drug reaction
Food
Infection
Inhalant
Systemic disease
  Collagen vascular diseases
  Malignancy
  Endocrine disorders
Urticaria pigmentosa and systemic mastocytosis
Hereditary disorder
  Familial cold urticaria
  Hereditary vibratory angioedema
  Urticaria with amyloidosis, deafness, and limb pain
  Hereditary angioedema (HAE)
Physical Urticaria
  Dermatographism
  Cholinergic urticaria
  Exercise-induced anaphylactic syndrome
  Familial and acquired cold urticaria
  Localized heat urticaria
  Aquagenic urticaria
  Delayed pressure urticaria/angioedema
  Solar urticaria
  Familial and acquired vibratory angioedema
Chronic idiopathic

hyperthyroidism and hypothyroidism are associated with urticaria. Exacerbations of chronic urticaria and cyclic urticaria have been noted during menses. These observations suggest a relationship between endocrine disorders, hormone levels, and urticaria.

## URTICARIA DISORDERS

### Urticaria Pigmentosa and Systemic Mastocytosis

Urticaria pigmentosa typically occurs during childhood and is characterized by persistent, pigmented, maculopapular lesions that urticate when stroked (Darier's sign). Biopsy of these lesions reveals mast cell infiltrations of the skin. Systemic mastocytosis is a generalized form of mast cell infiltration with involvement of the skin, bone marrow, long bones, liver, spleen, or lymph nodes.

### Hereditary Disorders

Several rare inherited disorders are associated with urticaria and angioedema. Familial cold urticaria and hereditary vibratory angioedema are discussed in subsequent paragraphs. Familial urticaria has been seen in combination with amyloidosis, nerve deafness, and limb pain. This syndrome appears to be inherited as an autosomal dominant condition.

Hereditary angioedema (HAE) is an autosomal dominant disorder caused by the absence of functional C1 esterase inhibitor. HAE is clinically characterized by recurrent episodes of angioedema (without urticaria) precipitated spontaneously and variably after trauma. Multiple parts of the body may be involved including, and especially, the face, extremities, and gastrointestinal tract. Edema of the bowel wall may result in crampy abdominal pain, obstipation, vomiting, and abdominal rigidity. The most severe complication is laryngeal edema, which may result in asphyxiation and death. Most cases of HAE manifest in childhood, but often worsen during adolescence. The severity and frequency of attacks vary greatly among patients. Only minor trauma is necessary to induce an attack with common triggers including contact sports and dental work. Sometimes an erythematous rash (erythema marginatum) may accompany attacks. The diagnosis of HAE is made by history and by evaluating complement levels (low C4, C2, and antigenic or functional C1 esterase inhibitor levels). Patients with HAE usually respond to androgen therapy.

### Physical Urticarias

The physical urticarias are a unique subgroup of chronic urticarias in which wheals can be reproducibly induced by a physical stimulus. Cold, heat, pressure, vibration, light, water, exercise, and increases in core body temperature are all provoking stimuli. Physical urticarias make up as much as 17% of chronic urticarias (Champion et al, 1969) and occur most frequently in young adults. The physical urticarias are distinguished by episodic lesions often limited to the areas of physical stimuli. In some patients, more than one type of physical urticaria may be present. The urticarial lesions are likely caused, in part, to mast cell activation and mediator release. Mast cell mediators, especially histamine, have been demonstrated in draining venous blood and in tissue fluids obtained from urticated areas in patients with various forms of physical urticarias. The mechanism by which a physical stimulus to the skin releases mast cell mediators is not fully understood, but may involve neuropeptides. In some forms of physical urticaria, a passive transfer factor (usually IgE) in the serum has been reported. Only the more common physical urticarias are discussed here.

### Symptomatic Dermatographism

Two percent to 5% of the general population may have dermatographism, but only a subgroup have symptomatic dermatographism. Dermatographism means "writing on the skin" and is manifest by transient wheal and erythematous responses occurring within minutes after stroking the skin with sufficient pressure (3600 g/cm$^2$). A transferable factor (probably IgE) has been identified in some patients. The disease usually can be treated with antihistamines.

### Cholinergic Urticaria

Cholinergic urticaria is fairly common, and occurs most frequently in teenagers and young adults. The skin lesions are often distinctive and appear as 2- to 4-mm pruritic wheals surrounded by extensive areas of macular erythema occurring most prominently on the upper trunk and arms. Systemic manifestations, including confluent urticaria, angioedema, hypotension, wheezing, and gastrointestinal complaints have been reported in patients with cholinergic urticaria after exercise. Furthermore, increases in blood histamine and neutrophil and eosinophil chemotactic factors have been demonstrated after provocative challenges. Cholinergic urticaria is a disease in which symptoms can be reproducibly induced by warming the body. It is postulated that the cholinergic nervous system effector mechanisms involved in the compensatory responses in thermoregulation may ultimately lead to mast cell degranulation. Elevation in core temperature induced by either exercise or passive heating (eg, hot bath), but not by endogenous pyrogen has elicited symptoms in susceptible subjects (Casale et al, 1986). Attacks can be aborted sometimes by prompt cooling of the patient (eg, cold bath). Some patients have a refractory period after a severe attack. This effect can be used to develop a program to induce tolerance by subjecting the patient to carefully graded increasing stimuli.

### Exercise-Induced Anaphylactic Syndrome

Exercise-induced anaphylactic syndrome (EIA) is clinically manifested by urticaria and the signs and symptoms of a classic anaphylactic reaction. Elevated plasma histamine levels have been demonstrated using provocative challenges. The disease appears to be more common among young adults. There have been reports of a family tendency in some subjects. Some subjects have symptoms only if exercise occurs postprandially. Celery, wheat, and shellfish are the foods most commonly implicated as precipitants, but any food may be associated with attacks. Subjects with postprandial EIA may avoid attacks by not eating for 4 to 6 hours before exercise. EIA and cholinergic urticaria are clinically similar in that both diseases may occur after exercise. EIA, however, is not related to core temperature and appears to be caused by either an abnormal release of a mast cell degranulating factor or an exaggerated response to a factor ordinarily released during exercise that is capable of inducing mast cell degranulation (eg, opioids). Because historical and clinical presentations of these two exercise-related syndromes are similar, diagnostic tests must be performed to distinguish those individuals having cholinergic urticaria/anaphylaxis from those with true exercise-induced anaphylaxis. Passive heat challenges are positive only in the subjects with cholinergic urticaria. A negative exercise challenge does not rule out the diagnosis of EIA because exercise does not always reproduce symptom development in these subjects.

### Cold Urticaria

Familial urticarias are autosomal dominant disorders characterized by burning erythematous papules with inflammatory cell infiltrates occurring after cold exposure. There are two forms of familial cold urticaria, an immediate form with onset of symptoms at ½ to 3 hours and a rare delayed form with onset of symptoms at 9 to 18 hours. The immediate familial form may be accompanied by a flu-like syndrome. Essential (acquired) cold urticaria is more common than the familial forms. Essential cold urticaria appears within minutes of cold contact and rewarming and is manifested by pruritic wheals. Syncope and anaphylaxis may occur after intensive cold exposure in the essential form. Indeed, swimming has resulted in massive mediator release and drowning. Provocative testing for the familial forms involves cold air exposure. The essential form, but not the familial forms, may be elicited by placing a plastic wrapped ice cube on the skin. Passive transfer has been accomplished only with the essential form. Connective tissue disorders, malignancies, or syphilis may be associated with acquired cold urticaria.

## Delayed Pressure Urticaria/Angioedema

Delayed pressure urticaria/angioedema is manifested by deep tender swelling with or without urticaria. The lesions are localized and occur 3 to 12 hours after exposure to sustained pressure. Flu-like symptoms may accompany these lesions. Common precipitating events include walking (foot swelling), clapping (hand swelling), sitting (buttock swelling), and swelling under belts or tight articles of clothing. This disease may respond to nonsteroidal anti-inflammatory drugs.

## Solar Urticaria

Solar urticaria can occur at all ages but is more common in the fourth and fifth decades. The disease is characterized by pruritic wheals or morbilliform erythema occurring within minutes on sun-exposed areas. Anaphylactic symptoms may occur when large body areas are exposed. If patients react only to the 400- to 500-nm wavelength, erythropoietic protoporphyria, and porphyria cutanea tarda should be excluded.

## Vibratory Angioedema

Vibratory angioedema is characterized by the rapid onset of localized angioedema proportional to the intensity and duration of the vibratory stimulus and body surface area involved. Common precipitators include vigorous towelling, lawn mowing, and motorcycling. A familial autosomal dominant form of this disease exists. Delayed pressure urticaria/angioedema and dermatographism should be excluded with appropriate tests.

## DIAGNOSTIC EVALUATION

As with most diseases, the history and physical examination are key to the evaluation of patients with urticaria and angioedema. A detailed history of drug and new food exposure is essential. Drugs that have been taken for several months or drugs that have just been added can cause urticaria. A diary containing information about urticarial outbreaks in relation to time of day, food ingestion, activity, and exposure to possible precipitants can be extremely helpful. A thorough physical examination should be performed. Signs and symptoms of systemic diseases and infections should be followed up with diagnostic tests. Provocative testing should be performed on patients thought to have a physical urticaria.

Because chronic urticaria in children is usually a benign disorder and most diagnostic tests are negative, extensive testing is indicated only when a systemic disease is suspected. Skin testing is generally not indicated for chronic urticaria and should be reserved for patients with histories suggestive of an allergen-induced disorder. If the cause is not obvious, I recommend a urinalysis, liver function tests, complete blood count, differential white blood cell count, and erythrocyte sedimentation rate or C-reactive protein to screen for hepatitis, infections, connective tissue diseases, eosinophilia, and leukemias. Stool for ova and parasites, complement assays, antinuclear antibodies, thyroid functions, and immunoglobulin levels are not routinely obtained unless a specific diagnosis is suspected.

Skin biopsy tests are generally not helpful. Skin biopsy tests should be performed, however, when individual urticarial lesions persist for more than 24 to 48 hours, or when the lesions are suggestive of cutaneous vasculitis or urticaria pigmentosa. Biopsy tests may be helpful if the lesions are hyperpigmented or leave a pigmented scar as they fade, or if the lesions have blisters. Another indication is refractoriness to therapy.

## TREATMENT

The general principles of treatment of urticaria or angioedema are outlined in Table 14-10. When a causative agent is identified, the treatment of choice, if feasible, is avoidance. This generally applies when a specific allergen is identified, or when the patient has a physical urticaria. If an associated systemic disease is found, treatment of the underlying condition is necessary. Patients should also be advised to avoid potentiating factors such as alcohol, opioids, and heat. Induction of tolerance may be attempted for some forms of physical urticaria (cholinergic, solar, cold, and localized heat urticaria and vibratory angioedema). Immunotherapy (allergy shots) is not indicated for urticaria without accompanying respiratory symptoms.

Drug therapy to relieve symptoms should be instituted while the cause is investigated. Therapy should be aimed at relieving most symptoms while keeping side effects from the drugs to a minimum. The patient may have some lesions despite therapy. To minimize side effects, additional drug therapy is not indicated when remaining lesions are not physically or emotionally disturbing to the patient.

In acute severe urticaria or angioedema, subcutaneous epinephrine is the treatment of choice (0.01 mL of 1:1000 epinephrine/kg body weight, up to 0.3 mL). Oral antihistamines of the $H_1$ class remain the drugs of choice for recurrent or chronic urticaria. Specific dosage recommendations are somewhat arbitrary. Therapy should begin with low doses and titrated upward to relieve symptoms without causing significant adverse side effects (usually drowsiness). Terfenadine and astemizole are the only nonsedating antihistamines available, but neither is currently approved for children younger than age 12 years. If symptoms con-

**TABLE 14-10.  Management of Chronic Urticaria or Angioedema**

Avoidance or treatment of underlying cause
Avoidance of potentiating factors (eg, alcohol)
$H_1$ antihistamines
   Classical (eg, hydroxyzine)
   Nonsedating (terfenadine or astemizole)
   Tricyclic antidepressants
Combinations of $H_1$ antihistamines
Combinations of $H_1$ and $H_2$ antihistamines
Addition of sympathomimetics (eg, ephedrine)
Corticosteroids (rarely)

tinue, the addition of a second, chemically distinct class of $H_1$ antihistamines, or the concomitant use of an $H_2$ antihistamine may be beneficial. Sympathomimetics such as ephedrine may also be useful adjuncts to $H_1$ antihistamine therapy. Tricyclic antidepressants such as doxepin and amitriptyline are potent antihistamines and are effective antiurticarial agents. For severe urticaria/angioedema unresponsive to these measures and disabling to the patient, corticosteroids may be tried. A short "burst" of corticosteroids usually relieves symptoms. Rarely, a patient requires low daily or alternate day corticosteroids for a longer time. Prolonged treatment with large doses of corticosteroids should be avoided because of the potential side effects. Antihistamines should not be discontinued during corticosteroid treatment. Newer drugs capable of antagonizing mediators other than histamine or inhibiting mast cell degranulation may prove more effective than traditional antihistamines.

## Selected Readings

Casale TB, Keahey TM, Kaliner M. Exercise-induced anaphylactic syndromes. JAMA 1986;255:2049.

Casale TB, Sampson HA, Hanifin J, et al. Guide to physical urticarias. J Allergy Clin Immunol 1988;82:758.

Champion RH, Roberts SDB, Carpenter RG, et al. Urticaria and angioedema: a review of 554 patients. Br J Dermatol 1969;81:588.

Fox RW, Russell DW. Drug therapy of chronic urticaria and angioedema. Immunology and Allergy Clinics of North America 1991;11:45.

Gorevic P, Kaplan AP. The physical urticarias. Int J Dermatol 1980;19:417.

Jorizzo JL, Smith EB. The physical urticarias: an update and review. Arch Dermatol 1982;118:194.

Kaplan AP. Urticaria and angioedema. In: Middleton E Jr, Reed CE, Ellis EF, Adkinson NF Jr, Yunginger JW, Busse WW, eds. Allergy: principles and practice, ed 4. St Louis: CV Mosby Company, 1993:1553.

Keahey TM. The pathogenesis of urticaria. Dermatol Clin 1985;3:13.

Kobza-Black A. The physical urticarias. In: Champion RH, Greaves MW, Kobza-Black A, Pye RJ, eds. The urticarias. Edinburgh: Churchill Livingstone, Inc., 1985:168.

Natbony SF, Phillips ME, Elias JM, et al. Histologic studies of chronic idiopathic urticaria. J Allergy Clin Immunol 1983;71:177.

Paul E, Greilich KD, Dominante G. Epidemiology of urticaria. Monogr Allergy 1987;21:87.

Soter NA. Urticaria: current therapy. J Allergy Clin Immunol 1990;86:1009.

Twarog FJ. Urticaria in childhood: pathogenesis and management. Pediatr Clin North Am 1983;30:887.

*Principles and Practice of Pediatrics, Second Edition.*
edited by Frank A. Oski et al. J. B. Lippincott Company, Philadelphia © 1994.

# 14.2.4 *Food Allergies*

Hugh A. Sampson

## FOOD ALLERGIES

Adverse food reactions are the result of food hypersensitivity (adverse immunologic responses) or food intolerance (adverse physiologic responses). Food intolerance makes up most adverse food reactions and is secondary to toxic or pharmacologic substances found in some foods, chemical or microbial contaminants, or metabolic disorders of the host (eg, lactose intolerance). Although an IgE-mediated mechanism is the most well-established form of hypersensitivity response, other less well-defined immunologic mechanisms are believed responsible for such disorders as celiac disease, milk- and soy-induced enterocolitis, and colitis syndromes.

## PREVALENCE

The term *food allergy* is frequently used to denote any adverse food reaction, a misnomer that leads to considerable confusion in this field. In addition, the perceived prevalence of food allergy is far greater than actual prevalence. Household surveys suggest that one third of American families alter their eating patterns in the belief that at least one family member suffers from a food allergy. In one survey of a general pediatric practice involving 480 babies followed from birth until their third birthday, 28% of the infants were reported to have experienced adverse food reactions. Only 8%, however, had symptoms confirmed by oral food challenge. In three large studies of infants followed through their third birthday, the prevalence of cow's milk allergy was found to be 2.2% to 2.5%. The majority of food allergies present in the first year of life, but only a minority (25%) persist beyond a child's third birthday. While comprehensive epidemiologic studies are not available, the prevalence of true food allergy is probably 3% to 4% in young children and 1% to 2% in adults.

## PATHOGENESIS

The pathogenesis of food allergy involves three areas: the food or allergen, the gastrointestinal barrier and its handling of food, and the individual's genetic predisposition to develop an allergic response. Despite a widely varied western diet, relatively few foods account for the majority of allergic responses. In children, egg, peanut, milk, soy, wheat, and fish account for about 90% of reactions. The allergenic fractions of these foods have several things in common: they are glycoproteins of about 20,000 to 60,000 daltons, they are largely heat- and acid-stable, and they are water-soluble.

The gastrointestinal tract utilizes both nonimmunologic and immunologic mechanisms to prevent intact foreign antigens from gaining access to the body while processing ingested food into forms that can be absorbed and used for energy and cell growth. IgA secreted into the gut lumen binds foreign antigens, such as food, and impedes their absorption. IgA-food antigen complexes become "hung up" in the glycocalyx, where enzymes in the mucosal cell brush border can break down these complex proteins. Food antigen-specific IgA and IgG in the blood may be involved in clearing antigens that enter the circulation. Although greater than 98% of ingested antigen is blocked by this gastrointestinal barrier, minute amounts of intact food antigens are absorbed and transported throughout the body. Factors such as decreased stomach acidity or the ingestion of alcohol increase antigen absorption. Antigenically intact food proteins entering the circulation, however, generally do not cause adverse reactions because most individuals develop tolerance to ingested food antigens.

Studies in mice provide some insight into the development of oral tolerance. After "gut closure" at 4 days of life, a single antigen feeding suppresses antigen-specific IgM, IgG, and IgE antibody responses and cell-mediated immune responses. Gut processing of food antigens to a "tolerogenic" form is essential in developing this oral tolerance. Lymphoid cells in the gastrointestinal tract are needed to generate the tolerogenic proteins; irradiation of mice abrogates their ability to form tolerogenic ovalbumin, while subsequent infusion of normal spleen cells restores their ability to form tolerogenic protein. Antigen presenting cells also appear to play a critical role in the development of oral tolerance. Agents that enhance antigen-presenting cell activity interfere with generation of $CD8^+$ (suppressor) cells and the development of oral tolerance.

Young infants are at increased risk for developing food allergic reactions because of immunologic immaturity, and to some extent, immaturity of the gut. Consequently, genetically predisposed infants ingesting food antigens may generate excessive food-specific IgE antibodies or other abnormal immune responses. Several prospective studies suggest that exclusive breast-feeding may promote the development of oral tolerance and prevent some food allergy and atopic dermatitis in infants and young children. This protective effect is speculated to be the result of decreased exposure to foreign proteins, passive immunologic protection provided by breast milk s-IgA, and soluble factors in breast milk that induce earlier maturation of the gastrointestinal barrier and the infant's immune response.

## CLINICAL SYMPTOMS

A variety of food-allergic reactions have been confirmed by controlled trials (Table 14-11).

## Gastrointestinal Food Hypersensitivity

There are a number of gastrointestinal syndromes associated with both IgE-mediated and non–IgE-mediated food allergy.

### Oral Allergy Syndrome

Pruritus and edema of the lips, tongue, palate, and throat may be the first symptoms of a generalized food allergic reaction or may be the sole manifestations of ingesting a food allergen. Symptoms isolated to the oropharynx constitute the oral allergy syndrome, which is analogous to contact urticaria of the oral mucosa and tongue. The oral allergy syndrome generally occurs in patients with allergic pollenosis and is associated with the ingestion of various fresh fruits and raw vegetables. Oral symptoms occurring after ingestion of raw potatoes, carrots, celery, apples, and hazelnuts are associated with birch pollen allergy; and symptoms secondary to bananas and melons (eg, watermelon, cantaloupe, honeydew) are associated with ragweed sensitivity.

### Gastrointestinal Anaphylaxis

Symptoms generally develop within minutes to 2 hours of ingesting a food allergen and consist of nausea, abdominal pain, cramps, vomiting, and less frequently, diarrhea. The frequent ingestion of a food allergen by an allergic individual frequently results in partial desensitization of gastrointestinal mast cells and subclinical symptoms such as poor appetite, periodic abdominal pain, and poor weight gain. Malabsorption has been demonstrated using various absorption markers (eg, lactulose, rhamnose, mannitol, polyethylene glycol). Elimination of the responsible food allergen may be followed by improved appetite and catch-up weight gain.

### Allergic Eosinophilic Gastroenteropathy

In a subset of patients with allergic eosinophilic gastroenteropathy syndrome, IgE-mediated food allergy is responsible for symptoms. Patients with this syndrome commonly present with post-prandial nausea and vomiting, abdominal pain, diarrhea, occasionally steatorrhea, and weight loss in adults or failure to thrive in young infants. Patients with food-induced symptoms generally have other atopic symptoms, elevated serum IgE levels, positive prick skin tests to a variety of foods and inhalants, peripheral blood eosinophilia, iron deficiency anemia, and hypoalbuminemia. In some infants, generalized edema occurs secondary to marked protein-losing enteropathy and hypoalbuminemia, often in the presence of minimal gastrointestinal symptoms. Rarely, allergic eosinophilic gastroenteropathy presents in infants as pyloric stenosis with outlet obstruction. Elimination of the responsible food allergen from the diet for 12 weeks may be necessary to bring about resolution of symptoms and normalization of intestinal histology.

### Infantile Colic

Double-blind crossover trials implicate food hypersensitivity as a pathogenic factor in about 15% of colicky infants.

### Food-Induced Enterocolitis Syndrome

Young infants between 1 week and 3 months of age with food hypersensitivity may present with protracted vomiting and diarrhea, resulting frequently in dehydration. Cow's milk or soy protein is most often responsible, but egg- and peanut-induced enterocolitis also has been reported. Stools generally contain occult blood, eosinophils, and polymorphonuclear neutrophils. IgE food-specific antibodies are absent. Jejunal biopsies reveal flattened villi, edema, and increased numbers of lymphocytes, eosinophils, and mast cells. Elimination of the responsible food generally leads to resolution of symptoms within 72 hours. The diagnosis is established by oral food challenge, which consists of administering up to 0.6 g/kg body weight of the suspected protein allergen. A positive challenge results in vomiting and diarrhea within 1 to 6 hours, and occasionally may be accompanied by shock. Monitoring the peripheral blood count reveals a rise in the absolute neutrophil count (more than 3500 cells/mm$^3$) 4 to 6 hours after symptoms develop. Neutrophils, eosinophils, and occasionally red blood cells may be found in the stools. Once diagnosed, children with cow's milk sensitivity should be placed on a hypoallergenic formula (Alimentum, Nutramigen, or Pregestimil) until about 9 to 12 months of age, because as many as 50% may develop a similar sensitivity to soy if placed on a soy-based formula. The majority of these children appear to "outgrow" their hypersensitivity in 1 to 2 years.

---

**TABLE 14-11.  Symptoms Substantiated by Controlled Food Challenges**

**Generalized Anaphylaxis With Cardiovascular Collapse** (sometimes associated with exercise)

**Respiratory**
  Upper airway—rhinoconjunctivitis, laryngeal edema
  Lower airway—wheezing (asthma)

**Cutaneous**
  Urticaria/angioedema
  Atopic dermatitis
  Urticaria associated with exericse
  Dermatitis herpetiformis

**Gastrointestinal**
  IgE-mediated—lip swelling, palatal itching, tongue swelling, nausea, abdominal pain, cramps, emesis, and diarrhea
  Coeliac disease and dermatitis herpetiformis
  Protein gastroenteropathy, especially to soy and milk—diarrhea, gross or occult blood loss, malabsorption, and failure to thrive (FTT)
  Milk-induced colitis—diarrhea and gross blood loss
  Heiner's syndrome—pulmonary infiltrates, iron deficiency, anemia, emesis, diarrhea, and FTT
  Colic—cow's milk-induced and allergen in breast milk
  Eosinophilic gastroenteritis

**Neurological**
  Migraine

## Food-Induced Colitis

As with the enterocolitis syndrome, food-induced colitis presents in the first few months of life and is generally secondary to cow's milk or soy protein hypersensitivity. However, these infants generally appear healthy and are discovered because of the presence of gross or occult blood in their stool. Bowel mucosal lesions are confined to the large intestine. Sigmoidoscopy findings are variable but range from areas of patchy mucosal injection to severe friability with small aphthoid ulcerations and bleeding. Biopsies reveal mucosal edema and a prominent eosinophilic infiltrate in the surface and crypt epithelium and lamina propria. Hematochezia generally resolves within 72 hours of appropriate food allergen elimination, but resolution of the mucosal lesions may take several weeks. Reintroduction of the responsible food leads to resumption of symptoms within several hours to days. Food-induced colitis often resolves after 6 months to 2 years of allergen avoidance.

## Malabsorption Syndromes

Excluding celiac disease, diarrhea (frequently steatorrhea) and poor weight gain in the first few months of life may be secondary to a variety of food proteins including cow's milk, soy, wheat and other cereal grains, and egg. Symptoms include protracted diarrhea, vomiting, and failure to thrive. Increased fecal fat and secondary carbohydrate malabsorption are frequently present. Cow's milk sensitivity appears to be the most frequent cause of this syndrome. Eliminating the responsible food from the diet brings about resolution of symptoms, but this may require several days to weeks. A patchy villous atrophy similar to celiac disease but generally less severe is seen on endoscopy, and biopsy tests reveal a prominent mononuclear round cell infiltrate of the epithelium and lamina propria with a small number of eosinophils. Complete resolution of the intestinal lesions may require 6 to 18 months of food allergen avoidance. The natural history of this disorder has not been well studied.

Celiac disease is a more extensive enteropathy leading to malabsorption. Total villous atrophy and extensive cellular infiltrate are associated with sensitivity to gliadin, a component of gluten found in wheat, oat, rye, and barley. Patients often present with diarrhea or frank steatorrhea, abdominal distention and flatulence, weight loss, and rarely nausea and vomiting. Oral ulcers and other extraintestinal symptoms secondary to malabsorption are common. Quantitation of IgA antigliadin and IgA antiendomysial antibodies appear promising as screening tests for celiac disease. The diagnosis, however, depends on demonstrating biopsy evidence of villous atrophy and inflammatory infiltrate while the patient is ingesting gluten, resolution of biopsy findings after 6 to 12 weeks of gluten elimination, and recurrence of biopsy changes after reinstitution of gluten. Although some patients tolerate small amounts of gluten as they get older, life-long elimination of gluten-containing foods is necessary to avoid increased risk of gastrointestinal malignancy and lymphoma.

## Respiratory Reactions

Both upper and lower respiratory reactions have been provoked during double-blind placebo-controlled oral food challenges (DBPCFC). Within minutes to 2 hours of ingestion, food allergens may induce typical signs and symptoms of rhinoconjunctivitis, although isolated upper airway symptoms are uncommon. These include periocular pruritus and erythema, and tearing; nasal congestion, pruritus, sneezing, and rhinorrhea. Nasal lavage fluid histamine levels rise significantly with the onset of nasal symptoms during DBPCFCs, strongly implicating a pathogenic role for nasal mast cell activation. Similarly, pulmonary function studies during DBPCFCs demonstrate significant drops in FVC, FEV$_1$, and MMEF in patients experiencing a positive food challenge.

Consumption of food allergens rarely are the main aggravating factor in chronic rhinoconjunctivitis and asthma, and recent studies suggest that ingesting food allergens leads to bronchial hyperreactivity. Two large series of asthmatic patients followed in pulmonary clinics were evaluated for food allergy. In one survey, 300 patients of all ages were evaluated for food allergy by history, prick skin tests, or RASTs. Findings suggestive of food-induced symptoms were evaluated by blinded food challenges. Six patients (2%) had wheezing provoked by the food challenge. In the second series of 140 children with asthma, 8 patients (6%) had wheezing induced by oral food challenge. All asthmatic children with food-induced wheezing either had atopic dermatitis or a history of eczema.

Food-induced pulmonary hemosiderosis is a syndrome of chronic or recurrent pulmonary disease (with hemosiderosis), chronic rhinitis, gastrointestinal blood loss, and iron deficiency anemia and failure to thrive secondary to milk ingestion; it was initially described by Heiner. Other foods rarely have been implicated.

## Cutaneous Reactions

The skin is the most common target organ in IgE-mediated food hypersensitivity. Ingestion of food allergens may provoke rapid onset of cutaneous symptoms or aggravate more chronic conditions.

### Urticaria/Angioedema

Acute urticaria and angioedema are among the most common symptoms of food allergic reactions. The exact prevalence of these reactions is unknown. In most cases, patients do not seek medical assistance (or even report the reaction) because the onset of hives or swelling occurs within minutes of ingesting the responsible food allergen making the cause-and-effect nature of the reaction obvious to the patient. The foods most commonly incriminated include eggs, milk, peanuts, and nuts in children and fish, shellfish, nuts, and peanuts in adults. Food hypersensitivity is occasionally incriminated in chronic urticaria and angioedema (symptoms lasting longer than 6 weeks). In one series of 163 children with chronic or recurrent urticaria, food allergy was implicated in only 10% of patients.

### Atopic Dermatitis

The pathogenic role of food hypersensitivity in atopic dermatitis has been debated since the turn of the century. In a series of children referred for evaluation of chronic, severe atopic dermatitis, IgE-mediated food allergy was demonstrated to be at least in part responsible for cutaneous symptoms in about 60% of children studied. In a more general population of patients seen by dermatologists and allergists, food hypersensitivity plays an etiologic role in about 30% of patients. As in the gastrointestinal tract, repeated ingestion of food allergens leads to a partial desensitization of skin mast cells, and a single ingestion of food allergen may not provoke obvious cutaneous symptoms. Repeated ingestion of food allergen leads to chronic inflammation and the typical eczematous lesions. (See discussion in Chapter 14.2.5.)

Dermatitis herpetiformis is a burning, erythematous, papulovesicular eruption sometimes mistaken for atopic dermatitis, which is associated with gluten-sensitive enteropathy in some patients.

Systemic anaphylaxis is an acute, occasionally fatal, immunologically mediated reaction involving many organ systems. Systemic symptoms include tongue swelling and itching, palatal itching, throat itching and tightness, nausea, abdominal pain, emesis, diarrhea, dyspnea, wheezing, cyanosis, chest pain, urticaria, angioedema, hypotension, and shock. In addition to direct induction of anaphylaxis, food ingestion is implicated as a cofactor in some cases of exercise-induced anaphylaxis.

A variety of symptoms are attributed to "food allergy," but the connection has not been substantiated in controlled trials. These include various behavioral disturbances, learning disorders, fatigue, sleep disorders, enuresis, myalgia, and arthralgia/arthritis. The Feingold Diet has been promoted by its supporters for children with hyperactivity and learning disorders. Several well-done controlled trials have failed to verify any consistent therapeutic effect from the diet.

## DIAGNOSIS

Symptoms secondary to food hypersensitivity that have been confirmed by appropriate controlled studies are listed in Table 14-11. Other symptoms often attributed to "food allergy" have not been substantiated in controlled trials. Some of these symptoms may be due to pharmacologic properties of certain foods such as sleep disturbances in children who drink caffeinated beverages. The differential diagnosis of food sensitivity is broad (Table 14-12), but careful history often suggests the appropriate diagnostic category to pursue.

Although history can be verified in only 30% to 40% of cases, it is important to the evaluation. History should reveal types of symptoms, when symptoms occurred after ingestion, severity of symptoms, whether symptoms occurred more than once, and whether co-factors (eg, exercise) are necessary to elicit symptoms. In general, symptoms occurring soon after ingestion are more likely to be due to food hypersensitivity than are those that take hours or days to develop. Physical examination may exclude some disorders in the differential diagnosis, but there is nothing in the physical examination that is unique for individuals with food hypersensitivity.

Various diagnostic studies (eg, x-rays, breath hydrogen, biopsy tests) exclude many anatomic and metabolic abnormalities. Laboratory studies such as prick skin tests and IgE-specific food an-

tibodies (eg, RAST, FAST, MAST) are of some value in discriminating among the foods responsible for immediate hypersensitivity reactions. There is no evidence to support the use of IgG-specific food antibodies or food antigen-antibody complexes in the diagnosis of food sensitivity.

In order to establish whether a patient has food hypersensitivity, a provocative oral food challenge is necessary. Food challenges may be performed openly, when both the patient and the physician know the contents of the challenge; single-blind, when only the physician is aware of the contents of the challenge; or double-blind, when neither the patient nor the physician knows the contents of the challenge. Placebo controls are necessary in the blinded challenges if they are to be truly blind. Only the double-blind procedure is free of psychological factors and inherent bias on the part of the patient and the physician. Several studies comparing results of single-blind and double-blind challenges in the same patient population have demonstrated the necessity of removing observer bias.

For research purposes, the DBPCFC should be the "gold standard" for diagnosing food allergy. In some cases, such as celiac disease, open challenge followed by intestinal biopsy is the diagnostic approach of choice. Although the DBPCFC provides a scientifically acceptable means of diagnosing food hypersensitivity, it is often not practical in the office practice setting. Table 14-13 outlines an approach that should be more useful to the pediatrician in the office setting. The initial evaluation consists of a careful history and physical examination, and laboratory studies suggested by the history or physical. If immediate hypersensitivity is suspected, results of prick skin testing to a battery of six to eight foods (egg, milk, peanut, fish, shellfish, nuts, soy, and wheat) or other foods suggested by history could be helpful. Negative prick skin tests, ie, a wheal diameter less than 3 mm larger than the negative control wheal, make immediate hypersensitivity extremely unlikely and preclude the further evaluation, unless the history highly suggests otherwise. Such skin testing is valuable only when an IgE-mediated mechanism is suspected.

Foods suspected by history should be eliminated from the patient's diet for 2 weeks. If symptoms have unequivocally improved, the diet may be continued unless it requires the elimination of more than one major food (egg, milk, soy, wheat) or two or more minor foods (any food other than major food). If symptoms persist unabated and food sensitivity is still contemplated, a brief trial (no longer than 2 weeks) of a severely restricted

### TABLE 14-12. Differential Diagnosis of Adverse Food Reactions

**Gastrointestinal Disorders**

Structural abnormalities—pyloric stenosis, hiatal hernia, tracheoesophageal fistula

Enzyme deficiencies—(primary versus secondary) lactase deficiency, sucrase deficiency, etc.

Malignancy—lymphoma

Other—cystic fibrosis, gallbladder disease

**Pharmacologic Agents**

Caffeine (coffee, tea, soft drinks, cocoa)

Theobromine (chocolate, tea)

Tyramine (cheese, banana, tomato)

Tryptamine (tomato, blue plum)

Histamine (fish, beer, wine)

Phenylethylamine (chocolate)

**Contaminants and Additives**

Flavorings and preservatives

Dyes

Toxins (bacterial, seafood-associated)

Infectious organisms

**Psychological Reactions**

### TABLE 14-13. Evaluating Food Sensitivity

**History and Physical Examination**

History—stress type of symptoms, timing, severity, and reproducibility

Physical examination—exclude many possibilities in differential

**Laboratory Test**

Studies suggested by history and physical examination (eg, x-rays, breath hydrogen, sweat test)

Skin tests—prick technique with commercial extract or fresh food

If negative (wheal <3 mm), immediate hypersensitivity very unlikely, further work-up probably unnecessary

If positive (wheal >3 mm), go to step 3

**Strict Allergen Avoidance Diet for 2 Weeks**

Include foods suggested by history for most sensitivities, also foods suggested by prick skin tests for immediate hypersensitivity

If unequivocal improvement and only 1 major or one or 2 minor foods involved, continue restricted diet

If equivocal improvement or more than 2 foods involved, refer to allergist or gastroenterologist for evaluation

diet may be warranted. The following diets may be used: for patients younger than 4 months old—milk substitute (Nutramigen, Pregestimil, or Vivonex); for patients aged 4 to 8 months—milk substitute, rice cereal (many infant cereals contain more than one grain), and pears; for patients aged 9 to 24 months—same as for 4- to 8-month-old patients plus rice, carrots, squash, and lamb; for patients older than 2 years—same as for 9- to 24-month-old patients plus fresh lettuce, potato, safflower oil, tea, and sugar.

If symptoms fail to improve, an adverse food reaction can be ruled out.

When improvement is not clear or several foods appear to be incriminated, a single-blind, or even an open, challenge should be performed in the office setting under observation. Because food challenges are time-consuming and may result in severe anaphylaxis, many pediatricians prefer to refer patients to a qualified allergist to perform these studies. When immediate hypersensitivity reactions are suspected, challenges should never be performed at home by parents. If challenges are performed in the office, appropriate equipment and personnel should be available in the office to deal with an emergency. If the office challenges reveal positive responses to only one major food or less than four foods in total, an appropriate elimination diet may be instituted. Such a diet would not be overly restrictive, and the results of such challenges would be acceptable.

Positive challenges to more than one major food or more than four foods in total should raise concern about the accuracy of the office challenges and suggest the need to refer the patient for DBPCFCs. Embarking on a diet restricted in a large number of foods without sound documentation subjects the patient to a diet that is extremely difficult to comply with and that may be nutritionally deficient.

If the clinician follows the protocol outlined in Table 14-13, it is likely that the DBPCFC is necessary in only a minority of patients. The need for sound documentation of food sensitivity by challenge procedures, however, cannot be overemphasized. Overly restricted diets in young children can lead to various eating disorders and create family conflict, especially around meal time. When various subjective complaints are ruled out (eg, vague abdominal complaints, behavioral problems), or when symptoms are reported to take several hours to days to develop, DBPCFCs may be conducted at home. Extreme caution should be exercised, however, when recommending that parents administer a food at home. Only foods that are felt to be unlikely to elicit an immediate-type allergic reaction should be tested at home.

Other procedures advocated as useful in making the diagnosis of food hypersensitivity are leukocyte cytotoxicity tests, sublingual provocation with drops of antigen extracts, subcutaneous provocation with varying concentrations of food extracts, and measurement of IgG- or IgG4-specific antibody. None of these procedures have been demonstrated to be useful in controlled studies.

## TREATMENT

Strict avoidance of the offending food allergen is the only proven therapy for food sensitivity. Drugs may modify symptoms in some cases, but such measures should only be considered palliative. Corticosteroids alleviate symptoms in some protein enteropathy syndromes and may be life-saving in some fulminant secretory diarrheas, but the side effects of long-term therapy generally are unacceptable. Antihistamines may modify symptoms of immediate hypersensitivity, but rarely, if ever, block them completely. Oral cromolyn sodium has been advocated, but carefully controlled trials in patients with challenge-confirmed food sensitivity failed to demonstrate efficacy. Rotational diets, immunotherapy, and sublingual or subcutaneous neutralization have never been shown to be efficacious in controlled trials.

Young infants sensitive to cow's milk generally can be managed adequately with hypoallergenic formulas such as Alimentum or Nutramigen. Infants with cow's milk protein enteropathy syndrome develop sensitivity to soy in as many as 50% of cases. Many infants develop diarrhea and localized skin rashes after ingesting various fruits and fruit juices (citrus, apple, grapes, tomato). These reactions appear to represent "intolerance" and are generally short-lived. Most infants with food sensitivity can have their diets expanded appropriately (ie, addition of fruits, vegetables, and meats) without difficulty. Adding only one new food every 3 to 5 days, however, is probably a useful practice.

Children older than 2 years of age rarely, if ever, require an elemental diet for treatment of food sensitivity. Appropriate oral challenge studies generally reveal only one or two specific food sensitivities in more than 90% of cases. The most practical method for implementing strict allergen avoidance diets is to teach parents (and older patients) to read food labels. Long lists of foods that patients "may" or "may not" eat are difficult to follow and are readily outdated. Educating patients to recognize key words, ingredient listings that indicate the presence of a specific food, allows the least restrictive diet and results in good dietary compliance. For example, the presence of milk may be indicated by any of the following key words: milk, dried milk solids, whey, casein, lactalbumin, caseinates, cheese, butter, or curds. A dietitian's assistance in suggesting alternative food preparation techniques and assuring a nutritionally sufficient diet is invaluable.

Implementation of strict allergen avoidance frequently leads to development of clinical tolerance to foods eliciting adverse responses. Virtually all young infants experiencing diarrhea in response to cow's milk or soy protein lose their sensitivity in 1 to 3 years. Several studies demonstrate the loss of immediate hypersensitivity reactions in about one third of patients after 1 year of antigen avoidance. Although young infants more consistently lose their food sensitivity, loss of hypersensitivity is not confined to the younger child. In addition, the clinical severity of the initial adverse reaction does not necessarily influence the longevity of the hypersensitivity. Infants younger than 2 years old with mild reactions may be rechallenged every 4 to 6 months to ascertain if symptoms persist. Older patients may be rechallenged every 1 to 2 years, depending on how difficult it is to avoid the food in question. Because loss of sensitivity varies with the antigen (eg, peanut, tree nuts, and fish appear to be persistent), rechallenging with some foods should be undertaken no sooner than every 4 to 5 years. In certain disorders, such as celiac disease or dermatitis herpetiformis, restricted diets should be continued indefinitely.

Clinical reactivity to a food appears to be highly specific, and rarely are children sensitive to more than one or two foods. Although results of skin tests and in vitro tests of specific IgE commonly demonstrate cross-reactivity among members of a botanical family or animal species, clinically relevant intrabotanical cross-reactivity and intraspecies cross-reactivity are rare. Consequently, it appears unwarranted to avoid all foods within a botanical family when one member is suspected of provoking allergic symptoms. By avoiding this practice, patient compliance with elimination diets is improved and a nutritionally deficient diet is less likely to be implemented.

Several contradictory reports discuss the role of breast-feeding in the prevention of food allergy. Several recent prospective studies suggest that exclusive breast-feeding for 6 months can reduce the infant's risk of developing food hypersensitivity and atopic dermatitis, but may only postpone development of other atopic disorders. Avoidance of highly allergenic foods (peanut, egg, milk) by the lactating mother may be beneficial, but dietary manipulation in the third trimester of pregnancy appears to offer no advantage and may compromise the pregnant mother's nutritional status.

## CONCLUSION

Food intolerance reactions probably represent the majority of food sensitivities in children, are more common in the young infant, and are short-lived. Both food intolerance and food hypersensitivity should be treated by strict avoidance of the inciting food. Repeated challenges should be conducted at varying intervals, depending on the age of the child, the type of reaction provoked, and the food involved to ascertain whether the sensitivity persists. Studies to accurately document the presence of food sensitivity will simplify the management of this disorder by reducing the number of foods that need to be eliminated from the patient's diet and the length of time they need to be avoided.

## Selected Readings

Anderson JA, Sogn DD, eds. Adverse reactions to foods. Bethesda, MD: US Department of Health and Human Services, July 1984; NIH publication no. 84–2442.

Bock SA. A critical evaluation of clinical trials in adverse reactions to foods in children. J Allergy Clin Immunol 1986;78:165.

Bock SA. Prospective appraisal of complaints of adverse reactions to foods in children during the first 3 years of life. Pediatrics 1987;79:683.

Leinhas JL, McCaskill CC, Sampson HA. Food allergy challenges: guidelines and implications. J Am Diet Assoc 1987;87:604.

Metcalfe DD, Sampson HA, Simon R, eds. Food allergy: adverse reactions to foods and food additives. Boston: Blackwell Scientific Publications, 1991.

Saarinen UM. Prophylaxis for atopic disease: role of infant feeding. Clin Rev Allergy 1984;2:151.

Sampson HA. Differential diagnosis in adverse reactions to foods. J Allergy Clin Immunol 1986;78:212.

Sampson HA. Immunologic mechanisms in adverse reactions to foods. Immunology and Allergy Clinics of North America 1991;11:701.

Sampson HA, McCaskill CM. Food hypersensitivity and atopic dermatitis: evaluation of 113 patients. J Pediatr 1985;107:669.

Sampson HA, Mendelson L, Rosen JP. Fatal and near-fatal food-induced anaphylaxis in children. New Engl J Med 1992;

Zeiger RS, Heller S, Mellon MH, et al. Effect of combined maternal and infant food-allergen avoidance on development of atopy in early infancy: a randomized study. J Allergy Clin Immunol 1989;84:72.

*Principles and Practice of Pediatrics, Second Edition.*
edited by Frank A. Oski et al. J. B. Lippincott Company, Philadelphia © 1994.

## 14.2.5 *Atopic Dermatitis*

Hugh A. Sampson

Besnier, a French physician, presented the first comprehensive description of atopic dermatitis a century ago. He emphasized its hereditary nature, its chronically recurring course, and its association with hay fever and asthma. Wise and Sulzberger later coined the term *atopic dermatitis* to further emphasize the relationship between atopic eczema, hay fever, and asthma (the allergic triad). Like asthmatics, patients with atopic dermatitis may be divided into those with extrinsic and intrinsic forms of the disorder. Patients with extrinsic atopic dermatitis are generally younger than 20 years old and flares of eczema are exacerbated by specific food or airborne allergens, whereas patients with intrinsic atopic dermatitis tend to be older and show no evidence of allergen-induced flares.

## INCIDENCE

Recent epidemiologic studies suggest that atopic dermatitis affects between 10% and 12% of the pediatric population and has been increasing in prevalence over the past 20 years. More than 20% of pediatric dermatology visits and about 1% of pediatric visits are related to atopic dermatitis. Earlier reports that atopic dermatitis is primarily a disease of industrialized societies have been refuted by more recent epidemiologic studies.

## DEFINITION AND CLINICAL FEATURES

Atopic dermatitis is a chronic cutaneous inflammatory disorder that generally begins in early infancy. About 60% of patients affected develop symptoms within the first year of life and 85% within the first 5 years. The skin symptoms generally present as an erythematous, papulovesicular eruption that progresses to a scaly, lichenified dermatitis over time. The distribution of the rash typically varies with age.

In infancy (3 to 6 months to 2 years), the cheeks, wrists, and extensor surfaces of the arms and legs typically develop papulovesicular, often weeping lesions that occasionally develop fine scaling or lichenification. The scalp and postauricular area frequently are affected with dermatitis. The eczematous dermatitis may involve the entire body, but generally the diaper area is spared. Frequent scratching results in obvious traumatic lesions and secondary infection.

Flexor surfaces, neck, wrists, and ankles generally are involved in the young child (2 to 12 years), with dry maculopapular lesions being a more prominent feature. Pruritus and scratching lead to excoriations, hyperpigmentation, and lichenification.

In the teenage patient and young adult, flexural surfaces, face (especially periorbital), hands, and feet frequently are involved. Extreme xerosis, marked papulation, and lichenification are characteristic of this stage. Older patients often have symptom-free periods that last for months, but even during remission, these patients retain a tendency toward dry, sensitive skin.

Unlike most dermatoses, atopic dermatitis has no primary skin lesion, but is identified by a constellation of symptoms. The classification system proposed by Hanifin and Rajka (Table 14-14) is the internationally accepted criterion for diagnosing atopic dermatitis. Modification of this criterion for the young infant is outlined in Table 14-15. Emphasis is placed on the extremely pruritic nature of the rash, its typical morphology and distribution, and its tendency toward a chronic or relapsing course. Some features, such as anterior subcapsular cataracts, nipple eczema, and upper lip cheilitis are uncommon but specific for diagnosing atopic dermatitis, whereas others such as orbital darkening, Dennie-Morgan infraorbital fold, and hyperlinearity of the palms are common but not specific.

There is no single, routine laboratory test that helps in diagnosing atopic dermatitis. Peripheral blood eosinophilia (5% to 20%) and elevated total serum IgE concentrations are present in as many as 80% of patients. Tests for specific IgE antibodies to foods and inhalants (eg, prick skin tests, radioallergosorbent tests) are positive in at least 80% of pediatric patients. Intracutaneous injection of acetylcholine (0.1 mL of 1:1000) leads to increased sweating and delayed blanching at the injection site (normal response—erythema, sweating, and piloerection).

## SKIN PATHOLOGY

Histologic changes in atopic dermatitis are not characteristic and may be similar to those of contact dermatitis, id reactions, acute photoallergic reaction, vesicular dermatophytosis, and others.

TABLE 14-14. Diagnostic Features of Atopic Dermatitis

**Major Features***

Pruritus
Typical morphology and distribution
   Flexural lichenification or hyperlinearity in adults
   Facial and extensor involvement in infants and children
Chronic or chronically relapsing course
Personal or family history of atopy (asthma, allergic rhinitis, or atopic dermatitis)

**Minor Features***

Xerosis
Ichthyosis/palmar hyperlinearity/keratosis pilaris
Immediate (type I) skin test reactivity
Elevated serum IgE
Early age of onset
Tendency toward cutaneous infections (especially S aureus and herpes simplex)/impaired cell-mediated immunity
Tendency toward nonspecific hand or foot dermatitis
Nipple eczema
Cheilitis
Recurrent conjunctivitis
Dennie-Morgan infraorbital fold
Keratoconus
Anterior subcapsular cataracts
Orbital darkening
Facial pallor/facial erythema
Pityriasis alba
Itch when sweating
Intolerance to wool and lipid solvents
Perifollicular accentuation
Food hypersensitivity
Course influenced by environmental/emotional factors
White dermographism/delayed blanch

   * Must have 3 or more

TABLE 14-15. Diagnostic Features of Atopic Dermatitis for Infants

**Major Features***

Family history of atopic disease
Typical facial or extensor eczematous or lichenified dermatitis
Evidence of pruritus

**Minor Features***

Xerosis, icthyosis, hyperlinear palms
Perifollicular accentuation
Postauricular fissures
Chronic scalp scaling

   * Must have 3 or more

Dermal pathology varies with the nature of the clinical lesion (Fig 14-13). The acute lesion is characterized by spongiosis (intercellular edema) and ballooning of the keratinocytes (intracellular edema) and by slight psoriasiform hyperplasia of the epidermis with hyperkeratosis. Normal numbers of mast cells are present and lymphocytes, rare monocytes, and macrophages infiltrate around venous plexes in the dermis. The chronic lesion is characterized by moderate to marked hyperplasia of the epidermis with elongation of the rete ridges and prominent hyperkeratosis. Varying degrees of intercellular edema are present. The inflammatory infiltrate consists of monocytes, macrophages, and lymphocytes (predominantly CD4 $TH_2^+$) in both the perivenular and intervascular areas. Mast cells and Langerhans cells (skin macrophage-like cell) are significantly increased in chronic lesions. Langerhans cells bear high-affinity receptors for IgE molecules on their surface and may be activated through allergen-IgE antibody interaction on their surface. Rarely, eosinophils are seen. Capillary number is often increased and capillary walls may be thickened. Demyelination and fibrosis of cutaneous nerves is seen at all levels of the dermis.

## PHYSIOLOGIC ABNORMALITIES

Physiologic abnormalities described in patients with atopic dermatitis are decreased itch threshold, increased transepidermal water loss, abnormal cutaneous vascular responses, and abnormal pharmacologic responses including "$\beta$-adrenergic blockade."

Itch is the dominant symptom in atopic dermatitis and the major cause of damaging excoriations, erosions, and lichenifications, which are characteristic of atopic dermatitis. The etiology of increased itching is unknown. Vasodilation precedes pruritus, suggesting that local release of mediators are responsible for increased pruritus. The increased number of mast cells and elevated tissue histamine in chronically involved areas support this hypothesis.

Increased transepidermal water loss is believed to be secondary to decreased sebum production. Sweating is abnormal in these patients. Studies evaluating amount of sweating are contradictory, but in general, sweating is believed to be increased. A variety of abnormal vascular responses include exaggerated constrictor response of cutaneous vessels and poor adaptability (vascular hyperactivity), white dermographism, delayed blanch to cholinergic stimuli, and paradoxical response to application of nicotinic acid. None of these responses are specific for atopic dermatitis.

Atopic dermatitis patients have several features suggesting the presence of $\beta$-blockade. Their skin lacks the expected inhibition of DNA synthesis after treatment with beta-adrenergic agonists, and their leukocytes show functional responses that correlate with subnormal cellular cyclic-AMP levels after beta-adrenergic stimulation. Some studies show a consistent increase in cyclic-AMP phosphodiesterase activity in untreated mononuclear leukocytes from patients with atopic dermatitis, but not in patients with contact dermatitis. This increased phosphodiesterase activity could account for the reduced cyclic-AMP levels seen in patients with atopic dermatitis.

## IMMUNOLOGIC ABNORMALITIES

Evidence suggests an underlying abnormality in some bone marrow-derived cells or factors. Patients with Wiskott-Aldrich syndrome experience clearing of eczematous rash after successful reconstitution by bone marrow transplantation, and latent atopy was transferred by successful bone marrow transplantation of a child from his atopic sibling.

Abnormalities of both humoral and cellular immunity have been described in atopic dermatitis patients. These are elevated serum IgE concentration in about 80% of patients; defective delayed-type skin responsiveness to various antigens; variably decreased lymphocyte response to mitogens, recall antigens, and alloantigens in vitro; defective generation of cytotoxic T-lymphocyte response in vitro; and variably decreased phagocytic capacity and chemotaxis of neutrophils and monocytes. These

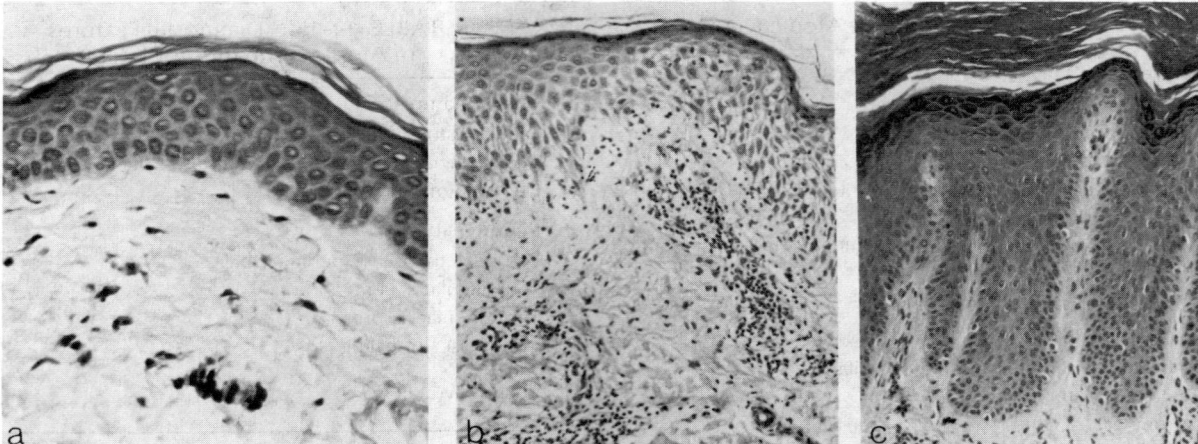

**Figure 14-13.** Skin biopsy sections from acute (*B*) and chronic (*C*) atopic dermatitis lesions compared to normal skin (*A*) at same magnification. Acute lesions are characterized by epidermal spongiosis and prominent mononuclear cell infiltrate. Chronic lesions have prominent hyperkeratosis, marked epidermal hyperplasia, and a mononuclear round cell infiltrate. (Courtesy of Dr. Antionette B. Hood, Department of Dermatology, Johns Hopkins University.)

defects generally fluctuate with disease activity and may revert to normal during long remissions.

Clinically, patients with atopic dermatitis experience increased numbers of skin infections. *Staphylococcus aureus* colonizes the skin of more than 90% of atopic dermatitis patients with high concentrations of the organism in areas of active dermatitis. The nearly constant presence of *S aureus* suggests a microbicidal dysfunction, perhaps due to abnormal fatty acid content of sebum or intermittently depressed neutrophil and monocyte chemotaxis. Superficial pustules, which are extremely pruritic and rapidly excoriated, usually are associated with active or flaring dermatitis. Septicemia generally is not a problem, and deep cutaneous infections are rare. The means by which *S aureus* causes flares of the dermatitis is unclear. Various enzymes and toxic products that can activate mast cells may be scratched into the skin, leading to further pruritus and inflammation. Some patients have been shown to have IgE antibodies specific to toxins excreted by *S aureus* (eg, *Staphylococcus* endotoxins A, B, C; TSST-1).

Both clinical and laboratory findings indicate depressed cell-mediated functions in atopic dermatitis patients. Cutaneous anergy is most striking with increased susceptibility to certain viral infections: herpes simplex (eczema herpeticum), verruca vulgaris (common warts), molluscum contagiosum, and rarely vaccinia. Dermatophyte infections also are reportedly more common in atopic dermatitis patients. Patients are less easily sensitized to *Rhus* (poison ivy) and dinitrochlorobenzene and show decreased delayed skin test reactivity to a variety of antigens.

## ETIOLOGY

The etiology of atopic dermatitis is unknown. Food and airborne allergens may reach cutaneous mast cells, lymphocytes, monocytes, and Langerhans cells by way of the circulation after entering at mucosal surfaces, or through breaks in the skin. The interaction of allergens with allergen-specific IgE on the surface of mast cells activates the cells to release histamine, $LTC_4$, platelet-activating factor, IL-4, and other cytokines that attract other cells (eg, eosinophils, lymphocytes, and monocytes) found in an IgE-mediated late-phase response. Release of IL-4 and IL-10 by infiltrating CD4 $TH_2$ lymphocytes inhibits local $CD4^+$ $TH_1$ cells and cell-mediated responses, and promotes up-regulation of IgE receptors on Lang-

erhans cells and monocytes leading to allergen-induced IL-1 release and the efficient presentation of allergens to T cells. Recent studies demonstrate the presence of allergen-specific CD4 $TH_2$ cells in the skin of atopic dermatitis patients. Repeated allergen exposure provokes chronic inflammation secondary to IgE-mediated mast cell and lymphocytic responses and contributes to the pathogenesis of atopic dermatitis.

Skin biopsies from chronic eczematous lesions of patients with atopic dermatitis reveal large quantities of major basic protein (MBP), excreted almost exclusively by eosinophils, in the superficial dermis, indicating that eosinophils were in the area, whereas actual eosinophils may be seen in more acute lesions. MBP is not seen in uninvolved skin sites in these same patients or in lesions of patients with contact dermatitis. In one series, some subjects developed a pruritic, erythematous, macular, or morbilliform rash, and plasma histamine levels rose after double-blind placebo-controlled food challenge. Skin biopsy specimens obtained 4 to 14 hours later revealed an infiltration of eosinophils and MBP deposition. This indicated that food allergen-induced mast cell activation triggered both an immediate and a late-phase response in the skin. Another eosinophil product, eosinophil-derived neurotoxin, may be responsible for the demyelination of nerves in the dermal layer seen in eczematous skin.

Inhalant allergens (pollens, molds, dust mites) may also play a role in IgE-induced pathology. Normal individuals passively sensitized to ragweed absorb sufficient pollen allergen via nasal challenge to produce a wheal and flare response at a distal skin site. In addition, eczematous skin changes are provoked by nasal challenge in some adult patients with *Alternaria* or ragweed allergy. Using a modified patch technique with dust mite antigen, eczematous changes and, later, increased mast cell numbers have been induced in patients with IgE antibodies to dust mite.

In addition to allergen-IgE initiated immediate and late-phase hypersensitivity responses, histamine-releasing factors (eg, lymphokines, monokines) have been discovered to bind surface-bound IgE molecules and activate mast cells and basophils to release various inflammatory mediators. IgE autoantibodies also have been found in 87% of patients with atopic disorders. Because low-affinity Fc ε receptors have been found on B cells, T cells, monocytes, macrophages, eosinophils, and platelets, histamine-releasing factors and IgE autoantibody immune complexes may affect a number of immunologic responses.

# DIAGNOSIS

The diagnosis of atopic dermatitis is based on the presence of sufficient major and minor features (see Tables 14-14 and 14-15). Absence of pruritus, typical morphology or distribution, and history of chronic or relapsing course should raise serious question as to the accuracy of the diagnosis. Seborrheic dermatitis and allergic contact dermatitis are confused most frequently with atopic dermatitis. Seborrheic dermatitis may be indistinguishable from atopic dermatitis in some cases, but often may be differentiated by its more frequent distribution in the axillae and diaper area, less prominent pruritus, and general absence of elevated serum total IgE and positive skin tests to foods and inhalants. Other less common disorders may be mistaken for atopic dermatitis: hyper-IgE syndrome, Wiskott-Aldrich syndrome, and a variety of genetic disorders such as phenylketonuria, biotinidase deficiency, and erythrokeratoderma variabilis, and histiocytosis X.

There are no consistent and distinctive laboratory abnormalities associated with atopic dermatitis. Skin biopsies are not specific, except for IgE-bearing Langerhans cells. Consequently, there are no routine tests to evaluate atopic dermatitis.

# THERAPY

Atopic dermatitis is characterized by intermittent inflammatory exacerbations superimposed on skin that is dry and easily irritated. The exacerbations may be infrequent with prompt resolution and healing, but more commonly, exacerbations occur regularly. A variety of trigger factors are known to exacerbate flares. These vary in patients and must be delineated in each patient for successful management.

Atopic dermatitis patients have a decreased itch threshold and are more sensitive to a variety of cutaneous irritants. Bathing in hot water and scrubbing vigorously with soap is one of the most frequent sources of irritation. Patients should be encouraged to bathe in tepid water (especially for hydration), avoid soap, and pat dry with soft absorbent towels. Clothing should be rinsed carefully after washing to remove all residual detergent.

Most patients recognize early that sweating causes pruritus. Whether sweating is induced by thermal change, exercise, or anxiety, it generally leads to cutaneous pruritus, scratching, and subsequent skin changes characteristic of atopic dermatitis. Avoiding excessive room temperature, wearing light, non-occlusive clothing (eg, cotton instead of polyester), keeping the bedroom cool, and avoiding excessive bedclothing helps reduce sweating.

Cutaneous infections are a frequent cause of acute flares in atopic dermatitis. *S aureus* is most frequently implicated, although streptococcal infections may be seen. Infection should be presumed in the presence of acute weeping or crusted lesions, small superficial pustules, or recalcitrant crusted patches. Staphylococcal organisms are generally resistant to penicillin (90% in the author's series of 120 patients) and many (31%) are resistant to erythromycin. Ideally, the physician is guided by results of culture and sensitivity tests. Antibiotic coverage generally can be started with erythromycin, but if there is a slow clinical response the presence of a resistant strain may be surmised. Oral dicloxacillin or cephalosporin may be substituted. Bactroban, a topical antibiotic effective for superficial *Staphylococcus* infections, may be used when infection is localized.

When lesions fail to respond to oral antibiotics, herpes simplex infection should be considered. A Giemsa stained Tzanck smear or culture indicates the presence of the viral infection. Patients at risk for ocular involvement or serious dissemination and systemic involvement of herpes simplex should be treated with intravenous Acyclovir. Others may be treated with povidone iodine compresses and ointment or topical Acyclovir. Occasionally, patients are flared from superimposed dermatophyte infections. These infections respond readily to either locally applied imidazole creams or oral Griseofulvin daily for 1 month.

Despite a long-standing debate on the significance of food allergens in the pathogenesis of atopic dermatitis, recent studies demonstrate a significant causative role in some patients. Eggs, milk, peanut, soy, and wheat are the most common offenders. Overall, about one third of children with atopic dermatitis have food hypersensitivity contributing to their symptoms. The role of inhalant allergens in the pathogenesis remains controversial. There is no evidence to support the use of immunotherapy in atopic dermatitis. In many cases, the dermatitis flares when allergy shots are initiated. Some attempt to reduce dust mite exposure appears warranted. Stuffed animals, stuffed furniture, and throw rugs may be removed, mattresses should be encased in plastic covers, and bedding should be laundered frequently.

Allergic contact dermatitis is uncommon in patients with atopic dermatitis. Occasionally, patients become sensitized, especially to topical medications or preservatives. Patch testing sometimes helps detect the offending contact allergen. Patients (or their parents) are generally aware that anxiety, anger, and frustration provoke pruritus and flares of atopic dermatitis. Patients should be encouraged to verbalize their emotional conflicts and occasionally psychological counseling sought. In children, potential stressful situations in the home or school should be assessed and discussed.

Several general measures may be taken to reduce pruritus and consequent skin damage secondary to scratching. Fingernails should be trimmed short and cotton gloves may be worn at night. Because dry skin is prone to itch, efforts to obtain maximal skin hydration are mandatory. Bathing for hydration, soaking in tepid water for 20 to 30 minutes, followed by immediate application of an emollient ointment or cream is the most effective form of therapy. Lubricant creams should be applied within 3 minutes of the child getting out of the tub so water absorbed into the stratum corneum does not evaporate. For patients with marked excoriation or weeping lesions, initial wet wraps with Burrow's solution (1:40) avoid the stinging or burning sensation sometimes seen with bathing. Adding oil to bath water is generally ineffective.

Topical corticosteroids are the mainstay of therapy for atopic dermatitis. For general management, midstrength corticosteroids such as 0.1% triamcinolone cream or ointment are optimal. Occasionally, more potent fluorinated steroids are required to suppress an acute flare. Use of these potent agents should be limited because of their accompanying side effects. In general, the least potent steroid that controls a patients symptoms should be employed. Systemic corticosteroids should be avoided in this chronic dermatitis because many patients experience a rebound flare after a short course, which only leads to further requests for systemic therapy. A course of antibiotics or hospitalization should be considered before utilizing systemic corticosteroids.

Most patients experience some symptomatic relief with antihistamines; whether this relief is due to an antipruritic or soporific effect is debated. Patient response to antihistamines varies, but hydroxyzine or doxepin appear most effective. Antihistamines are competitive antagonists and are best used on a regular basis. Single large doses of hydroxyzine (2 mg/kg up to 75 to 100 mg before bedtime) or doxepin before bedtime generally circumvents daytime sedation and facilitates nighttime sleep.

Tar preparations provide a useful nonsteroidal approach to therapy. However, gel preparations frequently irritate dry skin and the smell is unacceptable except to the most motivated patients. Ultraviolet light (UVA and UVB) therapy is beneficial in some recalcitrant cases but should be undertaken with extreme caution and careful professional supervision. PUVA (psoralen plus UVA) therapy has been beneficial in some severe cases. The dangers of squamous cell carcinomas and skin damage make these UV therapies unacceptable in most cases. Recent trials with immunomodulatory agents, thymopentin (TP-5) and interferon gamma, are promising in severe cases of atopic dermatitis.

Hospitalization, or a simulated hospitalization at home, should be considered as a therapeutic modality. Whether removal from daily stresses or environmental factors, a brief period of bed rest often leads to considerable symptomatic improvement.

## COURSE AND PROGNOSIS

The course of atopic dermatitis is capricious and marked by often unexplained exacerbations and remissions. A lack of distinct diagnostic criteria has interfered with epidemiologic studies of atopic dermatitis. Figures for persistent dermatitis vary from 10% to 83% of affected children, but recent studies indicate that the majority of patients retain some stigmata of the disorder throughout their life. Less favorable prognostic signs include late onset and reverse pattern (involvement of extensor surfaces instead of flexors), severe widespread dermatitis in childhood,

family history of atopic dermatitis, and associated allergic rhinitis or asthma. In general, the more severe the symptoms, the less likely is a permanent remission.

## Selected Readings

Hanifin JM. Epidemiology of atopic dermatitis. Monogr Allergy 1987;21:116.

Hanifin JM, Rajka G. Diagnostic features of atopic dermatitis. Acta Derm Venereol Suppl 1984;92:44.

Leiferman KM, Ackerman SJ, Sampson HA, et al. Dermal deposition of eosinophil granule major basic protein in atopic dermatitis: comparison with onchocerciasis. New Engl J Med 1985;313:282.

Leung DYM, Geha RS. Immunoregulatory abnormalities in atopic dermatitis. Clin Rev Allergy 1986;4:67.

Rajka G. Essential aspects of atopic dermatitis. Berlin: Springer-Verlag, 1989.

Ruzicka T, Ring J, Przybilla B. Handbook of atopic dermatitis. New York: Springer-Verlag, 1991.

Sampson HA. The role of "allergy" in atopic dermatitis. Clin Rev Allergy 1986;4: 125.

Sampson HA. Pathogenesis of eczema. Clin Exp Allergy 1990;20:459.

Sampson HA, Broadbent KR, Bernhisel-Broadbent J. Spontaneous release of histamine from basophils and histamine-releasing factor in patients with atopic dermatitis and food hyper-sensitivity. New Engl J Med 1989;321:228.

Soter NA. Morphology of atopic dermatitis. Allergy 1989;44 (Suppl 9):16.

Van der Heijden FL, Wierenga EA, Bos JD, et al. High frequency of IL-4 producing CD4+ allergen-specific T lymphocytes in atopic dermatitis lesional skin. J Invest Dermatol 1991;97:389.

Zeiger RS, Heller S, Mellon MH, et al. Genetic and environmental factors affecting the development of atopy through age 4 in children of atopic parents: a prospective randomized study of food allergen avoidance. Pediatric Allergy and Immunology 1992;3:110.

*Principles and Practice of Pediatrics, Second Edition.*
edited by Frank A. Oski et al. J. B. Lippincott Company, Philadelphia © 1994.

## *14.2.6 Allergic Rhinitis and Associated Disorders*

F. Estelle R. Simons

Allergic rhinitis, or inflammation of the nasal mucosa, is the most common chronic disorder of the respiratory tract, occurring in 10% of children and 15% of adolescents. Some patients with allergic rhinitis have associated disorders such as allergic conjunctivitis, chronic sinusitis, or otitis media with effusion. In allergic rhinitis and allergic conjunctivitis, severity of symptoms is clearly related to allergen exposure. In contrast, in chronic sinusitis and in otitis media with effusion, the allergic basis for symptoms may be much more subtle and controversial.

## ALLERGIC RHINITIS

### Anatomy

The nasal passages are separated by a cartilaginous and bony septum, which varies in thickness. The turbinates on the convoluted lateral wall of each nasal passage cause the incoming air stream to change direction and flow posteriorly and superiorly. The nasal cavities are lined anteriorly with nonkeratinizing squamous epithelium and posteriorly with ciliated pseudostratified columnar epithelium interspersed with goblet cells. The lamina propria is richly supplied with small seromucous glands, and

there are large serous glands scattered anteriorly. Air passing through the nose is humidified by exudate from these glands. Nasal secretions consist of mucous from the goblet cells, watery materials from the serous and seromucous glands, condensed water from expired air, tears, and transudate from serum.

The vasculature of the nasal mucosa is erectile tissue containing abundant arterial-venous anastomoses and venous sinusoids capable of intermittent engorgement. The smooth muscle of this vasculature is primarily under sympathetic (adrenergic) nervous control. Parasympathetic or cholinergic fibers are numerous around the glands, and stimulation of these fibers results in secretion. In allergic rhinitis, there is autonomic imbalance in the nasal mucosa with relative overactivity of the parasympathetic nervous system and hyperresponsiveness to nonspecific physical and chemical stimuli including changes in air temperature and humidity, irritants (eg, cigarette smoke, paint, perfume), and changes in the emotional state. This results in sneezes that expel foreign particles and in rhinorrhea that dilutes foreign water-soluble material.

The physiologic functions of the nose include olfaction, humidification, warming and filtration of the inspired air, provision of vocal resonance for speech, and defense of the lower airways. All foreign particles larger than 10 microns in diameter, and even some particles as small as 2 microns, are filtered as they traverse the nasal cavities.

### Pathophysiology

In allergic rhinitis, an immediate hypersensitivity response occurs in the nasal mucosa of a host who has become sensitized to inhaled allergens such as pollen. Specific immunoglobulin E (IgE) binds to high-affinity receptors on mast cells and basophils and to low-affinity receptors on other cells such as monocytes, eosinophils, and platelets. When the patient sensitized to an allergen is reexposed to it, an allergen-IgE antibody reaction occurs within minutes. The bridging of two or more mast cell or basophil-bound IgE molecules by allergen results in aggregation of IgE receptors on the cell surface, activation of membrane-associated proteolytic enzymes, and triggering of a cascade of enzymatic reactions within the cells. An energy-dependent, noncytolytic process then occurs, and the intracellular granules fuse with the cell membrane. Newly formed membrane-derived lipid mediators of inflammation such as arachidonic-acid metabolites and lipoxygenase products, as well as preformed mediators of inflammation such as histamine, eosinophilic chemotactic factor, and neutrophilic chemotactic factor, are released into the extracellular environment. The mediators cause increased permeability of the mucosa, facilitating entry of allergens and allergen contact with sensitized submucosal mast cells, thus amplifying the response. The mediators also directly produce smooth muscle contraction, vasodilation, mucosal edema, mucous secretion, stimulation of itch receptors, and reduction in the threshold for sneezing. Without additional exposure to antigen, many patients have a late-phase response 2 to 8 hours after exposure, characterized by infiltration with eosinophils and neutrophils, and by fibrin deposition. One to 2 days after exposure, infiltration of mononuclear cells such as macrophages and fibroblasts, and even tissue destruction may occur.

Seasonal allergic rhinitis is commonly caused by nonflowering, wind-pollinated plants. Tree pollens cause symptoms in the early spring, grass pollens cause symptoms in the late spring and early summer, and ragweed and other weed pollens cause symptoms in the late summer and autumn, until frost. A priming effect on the nasal mucosa occurs after continued daily allergen exposure in patients with allergic rhinitis; late in the pollen season, severe nasal symptoms may be caused by less antigen than the amount required to provoke symptoms at the beginning of the season.

Perennial allergic rhinitis is provoked by animal dander, house dust mites, and molds. In subtropical climates, pollens may cause perennial, rather than seasonal, rhinitis. Food antigens are seldom confirmed as etiologic agents in allergic rhinitis.

## Symptoms and Signs

The cardinal symptoms of allergic rhinitis are nasal congestion (stuffy nose), paroxysmal sneezing, itching, and watery, profuse rhinorrhea. Other symptoms that may be reported include noisy breathing, oronasal breathing, snoring, hyposmia or anosmia, itching of the palate or pharynx, and repeated throat clearing or cough secondary to drainage of nasal mucus into the pharynx. Ocular symptoms such as redness, itching, or tearing may also be present.

Children with allergic rhinitis may have "allergic shiners," a term used to describe the dark discoloration of the infraorbital regions secondary to obstruction of venous drainage. If they are chronic oronasal breathers, they may have hypertrophied gingival mucosa and halitosis. In contrast to children who breathe through unobstructed nasal passages, they are more likely to have a gaping expression, a long, retrognathic facies with a high, narrow palate, and orthodontic anomalies such as posterior dental crossbite. Pharyngeal lymphoid tissue, adenoids, tonsils, and the lymphoid tissue of the anterior cervical region may be hypertrophied. If hypertrophy of the adenoids is severe, obstructive sleep apnea, alveolar hypoventilation, and cor pulmonale may develop.

Examination of the nose of the child with chronic allergic rhinitis may reveal a transverse external wrinkle, secondary to rubbing and dorsal manipulation of the nose, also known as the "allergic salute." The nasal mucosa is a variable color in health and disease. In patients with allergic rhinitis, it usually appears edematous, but it is not necessarily pale or violaceous. Watery,

mucoid, or opaque material may be noted in the nasal cavity or the posterior pharyngeal wall. There may be evidence of recent epistaxis. Nasal polyps are rare in children and, if they are observed, cystic fibrosis must be ruled out. Ideally, the nasal mucosa should be inspected before and after application of a topical vasoconstrictor such as oxymetazoline. Examination using an otoscope is not always adequate, and examination using flexible fiberoptic rhinoscopy may be required for optimal diagnosis and management.

## Diagnostic Tests

Disorders that must be considered in the differential diagnosis of rhinitis are listed in Table 14-16. To confirm the diagnosis of allergic rhinitis, it is necessary to examine the nasal mucus or to obtain a specimen of nasal mucosa for cytologic examination using a disposable plastic Rhinoprobe scoop. The best method of collecting mucus is to have the child blow into a piece of nonporous paper, transfer the secretions to a glass slide, air-dry the specimen, and apply an eosin/methylene blue stain. In patients with allergic rhinitis, the percentage of eosinophils in specimens prepared in this manner will range from 10% to 100%. The total blood eosinophil count and the total serum IgE concentration may be elevated or normal in patients with allergic rhinitis.

Epicutaneous (prick) tests with common inhalant antigens may be helpful in patients with allergic rhinitis, especially those who have severe symptoms that do not respond to pharmacologic management and those who are curious about the etiology of their symptoms and are prepared to rid their environment of allergens to which they are sensitive. Skin tests cannot be interpreted accurately unless a positive control substance such as histamine and a negative control substance, preferably the antigen diluent, are tested concomitantly with the antigens. Measurement of allergen-specific IgE in serum by in vitro tests such as radioallergosorbent tests (RASTs) or enzyme allergosorbent tests (ELISAs) is also useful in patients with allergic rhinitis, particularly in those who cannot tolerate withdrawal of $H_1$-receptor antagonists before skin testing, or who have, in addition to their rhinitis, severe widespread atopic dermatitis that precludes skin testing. Skin tests and allergen-specific IgE measurement should not be

### TABLE 14-16. Differential Diagnosis of Rhinitis

Allergic rhinitis
Nonallergic eosinophilic rhinitis
Vasomotor rhinitis
Rhinitis medicamentosa from overuse of topical decongestants
Hormonal changes (pregnancy, oral contraceptives, hypothyroidism)
Infection: viral or bacterial
Acute or chronic sinusitis
Ciliary dyskinesia
Granulomatous disease, eg, Wegener's granulomatosis
Foreign body
Trauma (nasal septal deviation, septal hematoma, fracture of nasal bones, synechiae)
Adenoid hypertrophy
Nasal polyps
Choanal atresia
Cerebrospinal fluid leak
Congenital intranasal lesions (dermoid cysts, meningomyelocele, nasal glioma)
Neoplasm

used in place of a history and physical examination to "screen" patients for allergic rhinitis. The correlation among skin tests, allergen-specific IgE measurements, and nasal challenge tests is excellent for allergens such as pollens. Intranasal challenges with antigen, although not necessary for clinical diagnosis, have become a useful research tool, facilitating study of the pathophysiology of allergic rhinitis.

## Management of Allergic Rhinitis

The management of allergic rhinitis consists of avoidance of allergens, irritants, and other factors known to provoke symptoms; pharmacologic treatment to prevent or relieve symptoms; and, in selected patients, alteration of the immune response to allergens using immunotherapy (allergy shots).

The nasal mucosa of patients with allergic rhinitis is hyperreactive to many different environmental stimuli, including, in addition to allergens, irritants such as cigarette smoke or perfumes, and physical factors such as cold air or ingestion of hot liquids. The patient should avoid any environmental stimulus that is known to provoke symptoms. Well-maintained air-conditioning units are effective in reducing indoor pollen and mold counts and associated symptoms in patients allergic to pollens and molds. Similar beneficial effects are claimed for high-efficiency particulate air (HEPA) filter units.

Major advances in the pharmacologic treatment of allergic rhinitis have occurred. Treatment must be highly individualized. A patient's medication requirements may vary from season to season, or from year to year, and may range from occasional use of one medication for a few days to year-round use of several medications. Some of the newer $H_1$-receptor antagonists (antihistamines) such as terfenadine, astemizole, loratadine, and cetirizine do not cross the blood–brain barrier readily, and are associated with a lower incidence of sedation and other central nervous system adverse effects than older $H_1$-receptor antagonists such as chlorpheniramine. The newer medications also lack anticholinergic effects. Neither the new nor the older $H_1$-receptor antagonists relieve the symptom of nasal congestion as well as they relieve itching, sneezing, or rhinorrhea. Most of the new $H_1$-receptor antagonists are no more effective than chlorpheniramine.

Topically applied sympathomimetic medications such as xylometazoline and oxymetazoline should be used only in patients with severe nasal blockage, and only for brief periods. These medications increase nasal patency and facilitate examination of the nasal mucosa. They can be used to advantage during initiation of intranasal glucocorticoid treatment; to decrease blockage of the eustachian tube orifices during air travel; or to decrease obstruction of the sinus ostia and facilitate mucociliary clearance of the sinuses in patients with allergic rhinitis complicated by sinusitis. They may cause rebound congestion and, with long-term use, rhinitis medicamentosa. In infants and young children, they may even cause systemic symptoms, including central nervous depression and coma. Orally administered sympathomimetics such as phenylpropanolamine and pseudoephedrine are also best used for short-term relief of nasal congestion, rather than for long-term therapy, as they may exacerbate hypertension, and cause visual hallucinations, insomnia, and agitation in some patients.

Disodium cromoglycate (cromolyn sodium) 2% solution sprayed into the nasal cavity prophylactically four to six times daily is an antiallergic medication that prevents sneezing, rhinorrhea, and nasal itching in some patients with allergic rhinitis. It is not very effective in preventing nasal congestion. The chief advantage of cromolyn is its lack of toxicity. Nedocromil, which in vitro is more potent and has a broader spectrum of anti-allergic and anti-inflammatory effects than cromolyn, is being introduced.

Topically active, synthetic glucocorticoids such as beclomethasone, flunisolide, triamcinolone, or the newer agents budesonide and fluticasone, which are not yet available in the United States, are highly effective in the treatment of allergic rhinitis. In the nasal mucosa, these medications are rapidly degraded enzymatically to less active metabolites. Unchanged medication that is absorbed is metabolized in the first pass through the liver, and therefore the risk of hypothalamic/pituitary/adrenal axis suppression is small in patients receiving these medications intranasally in manufacturers' recommended doses. About 90% of patients with seasonal allergic rhinitis using an inhaled glucocorticoid regularly have excellent improvement of symptoms, and can reduce or eliminate the need for concomitant medications such as $H_1$-receptor antagonists and decongestants. Optimally, children should begin inhaling glucocorticoids 1 week before the pollen "season" begins. Regular monitoring of their technique of inhalation is essential. The spray should be directed away from the nasal septum.

Antibiotics are not required in the treatment of chronic rhinitis unless it is complicated by sinusitis or otitis media, or is associated with purulent nasal secretions, structural abnormalities of the upper respiratory tract, immunodeficiency disease, or ciliary dysfunction.

Immunotherapy for allergic rhinitis is time-consuming, inconvenient, and expensive, but it may reduce morbidity and medication requirements in patients whose symptoms are poorly controlled by optimal modification of the environment and by optimal pharmacologic management, including topical glucocorticoid treatment. Immunotherapy consists of a series of subcutaneous injections of increasing doses of specific antigens, identified on the basis of the patient's history, as well as on the basis of positive skin tests, RASTs or ELISAs performed and interpreted according to acceptable techniques. Placebo-controlled double-blind studies in patients with pollen-induced allergic rhinitis have shown that the response to immunotherapy is clearly antigen-specific and dose-related. Immunotherapy results in immunologic changes such as increase in antigen-specific IgG-blocking antibody, eventual decline in specific IgE antibody, reduction in sensitivity of basophils to antigen (as measured by their ability to release histamine), and decreased lymphocyte proliferation and lymphokine production in response to antigen, also an increase in blocking IgG and IgA antibodies in secretions.

The most common adverse effect of immunotherapy is a large local reaction at the injection site. Generalized systemic reactions, such as anaphylaxis or serum sickness, occur rarely. Standardized antigens for immunotherapy are now becoming available.

# DISORDERS ASSOCIATED WITH ALLERGIC RHINITIS

## Allergic Conjunctivitis

*Allergic conjunctivitis* is an IgE-mediated reaction to an airborne, antigenic stimulus. In temperate climates, it is usually a seasonal disorder. Symptoms include conjunctival erythema, tearing, lid edema, intense itching, and, occasionally, a mucopurulent discharge. Patients with allergic conjunctivitis often have associated allergic rhinitis, asthma, or eczema. Conjunctival scrapings show eosinophils, and skin tests with airborne antigens are positive.

Vernal conjunctivitis is a severe form of seasonal conjunctivitis in which patients have intense eyelid and conjunctival itching, as well as photophobia. In the palpebral form of vernal conjunctivitis, giant papillary reactions produce a cobblestone appearance in the everted tarsal conjunctivae, accompanied by a thick, white, ropy discharge. In the limbal form of vernal conjunctivitis, yellow-gray gelatinous limbal masses and white

Trantas' dots are observed. In both forms of vernal conjunctivitis, eosinophils are present in conjunctival scrapings. The IgE level is usually elevated in tears. Skin tests with airborne antigens are positive in most patients with this disorder. Patients with severe vernal conjunctivitis may develop secondary bacterial conjunctivitis, or corneal complications such as superficial keratitis and ulceration.

In management of allergic conjunctivitis, avoidance of airborne allergens, although ideal, is often impossible. Topical vasoconstrictors such as phenylephrine or naphthazoline can be helpful. Topical or oral $H_1$-receptor antagonists may contribute greatly to relief of itching and other symptoms. Cromolyn sodium in a 2% solution may be instilled in the conjunctivae four to six times daily. Topical glucocorticoids combined with a vasoconstrictor should be reversed for only severely affected patients, and monitoring of intraocular pressure before the start of treatment and every few weeks thereafter, by an ophthalmologist, is an important aspect of such therapy.

## Chronic Sinusitis

In children with allergic rhinitis and asthma, chronic sinusitis is remarkably common, causes considerable morbidity, and is easily overlooked. In this disorder, inflammation of one or more of the maxillary, ethmoidal, sphenoidal, or frontal sinuses is caused by partial or complete obstruction of the osteomeatal complex with subsequent hypooxygenation of the involved sinus, disturbance of ciliary function, and diminished local host resistance factors. In addition to allergic rhinitis and asthma, other conditions are predisposing to or associated with sinusitis: recurrent viral upper-respiratory infections, nasal obstruction due to foreign body, polyps, adenoid hypertrophy or tumor, cystic fibrosis, immotile cilia syndrome, hypogammaglobulinemia or other immunodeficiency disorders, nasal fracture, barotrauma, deviated septum, hypersensitivity to aspirin or other nonsteroidal anti-inflammatory agents, or damage to nasal and ostial mucosa from chronic use of topically applied drugs such as cocaine, oxymetazoline, and xylometazoline.

Symptoms of chronic sinusitis include nasal discharge, postnasal drip, frequent cough, nasal obstruction, and loss of smell or taste. Pharyngitis, headache, sore neck, malaise, nausea, irritability, fatigue, and low-grade fever may be reported. Pain over the sinuses is infrequent. The nasal mucosa is usually red and swollen. Mucopurulent material may be present in the nose and on the posterior pharyngeal wall. Adenoids may be enlarged.

Sinus radiographs reveal opacification, air fluid levels, or thickening of the sinus mucosa of greater than 6 mm. Occipitomental (Waters) views facilitate visualization of the maxillary sinuses, which are especially prone to chronic disease. Occipitofrontal (Caldwell) views for maximum visualization of ethmoid sinuses and lateral and submental vertical views may also be useful. Transillumination and ultrasonography generally are not helpful. Definitive methods used to diagnose chronic sinusitis are coronal computed tomography or nasal endoscopy. Polymorphonuclear cells, with or without intracellular bacteria, predominate in nasal secretions. There is poor correlation between organisms found in the nose and those found in the sinuses. Pathogens recovered from the sinuses of children with chronic sinusitis include *Streptococcus pneumoniae*, nontypable *Haemophilus influenzae*, and *Moraxella (Branhamella) catarrhalis* as well as *Bacteroides* species, *Fusobacterium* species, and anaerobic gram-positive cocci.

In the management of chronic sinusitis in children, an antimicrobial such as amoxicillin or trimethoprim/sulfamethoxazole should be administered for 21 days. If β-lactamase-producing *H influenzae* or *M catarrhalis* is implicated, amoxicillin/clavulanate or a second- or third-generation cephalosporin is recommended.

Sometimes a second course of antibiotic treatment is required. Topical or oral decongestants administered for 5 to 7 days may improve drainage. For noninfectious chronic sinusitis, intranasal glucocorticoids may reduce mucosal inflammation around the osteomeatal complex and facilitate drainage. Occasionally, surgical intervention is required.

Patients with chronic sinusitis may also have refractory asthma, said to be caused by "seeding" of the lungs with bacteria in the mucopurulent discharge from the sinuses, reflex bronchospasm via the parasympathetic nervous system, or enhancement of β-adrenergic blockade by infection. Although the association between sinusitis and asthma is not fully understood, relief of chronic sinusitis is often associated with marked improvement in asthma symptoms.

## Otitis Media With Effusion

*Otitis media with effusion* is a complex disorder in which allergy is only one of many potential etiologic factors. Other risk factors include young age, male sex, absence of breast feeding, chronic exposure to maternal cigarette smoking, frequent viral upper respiratory tract infections, adenoid hypertrophy, eustachian tube dysfunction, and congenital disorders such as cleft palate, Down syndrome, immotile cilia syndrome, and hypogammaglobulinemia.

Allergy can block the eustachian tubes and cause otitis media with effusion as the result of the following: (1) mucosal allergic reaction to antigen entering the middle ear via the nasal passages and eustachian tubes, (2) overgrowth of lymphoid tissue at the pharyngeal end of the eustachian tubes, or (3) the presence of allergic edema with peritubal swelling and obstruction of the drainage of the tube. If the eustachian tube is blocked, air cannot enter the middle ear. The air remaining in the middle ear is absorbed, and serous fluid collects because of the resulting negative pressure. In allergic patients, there is some correlation among intranasal provocative doses of antigen required, eustachian tube dysfunction, and elevation of serum IgE concentration to the specific antigen being tested.

Symptoms of otitis media with effusion may be subtle or inapparent. Some children present with school or behavior problems secondary to undetected hearing loss. Occasionally, children complain of hearing loss, "popping" of the ears, a dull earache, or a sense of "fullness" in the head. The tympanic membrane is often retracted, which may indicate negative middle-ear pressure, effusion, or both. The handle of the malleus may appear chalky white or acutely angled, and bony landmarks may be obliterated. In patients with middle-ear effusion, an air fluid level or bubbles of air mixed with liquid, and a bluish or yellowish hue to the drum may be noted. Signs of allergic rhinitis may be present.

*Impedance tympanometry*, in which the compliance of the tympanic membrane is measured at various positive and negative pressures, is widely used to screen for middle-ear functional abnormalities. Other aids in diagnosing otitis media with effusion include pneumatic otoscopy to detect decreased mobility of the tympanic membrane due to fluid or tympanic-membrane retraction, or both; the acoustic reflex threshold; and audiometry. A reliable audiogram can be obtained in most children older than age 5 years. Middle-ear effusions are associated with a hearing loss in the range of 25 to 50 dB. Younger children can be tested using behavioral audiometry or evoked potential tests.

The natural history of otitis media with effusion is favorable, with signs and symptoms resolving spontaneously over time in most children. Monitoring is essential, as a few patients will develop granulation tissue, tympanosclerosis, cholesteatoma, perforation, bone resorption, or sensorineural hearing loss. Nonspecific treatment of otitis media with effusion includes avoidance of smoke and other irritants and avoidance of known allergens.

It is not possible to predict the presence or absence of pathogenic bacteria from physical examination of the tympanic membrane. Fifty percent of chronic middle-ear effusions yield pathogenic bacteria, most commonly *S pneumoniae* and *H influenzae*, upon tympanocentesis and culture, so a 14-day course of an antimicrobial such as amoxicillin, trimethoprim/sulfamethoxazole, amoxicillin/clavulanate, or a second- or third-generation cephalosporin is usually appropriate. $H_1$-receptor-antagonist/decongestant preparations are often prescribed for patients with otitis media and effusion, although these medications may be no more effective than a placebo in this disorder. A short-term course of topical intranasal glucocorticoids may or may not improve the rate of resolution of middle-ear effusion. Indications for a myringotomy and aspiration of fluid with placement of ventilating tubes remain controversial. These procedures are usually reserved for children who have had otitis media with effusion for more than 90 days with no sign of improvement on otoscopic and tympanometric examinations, or those who have otitis media with effusion complicated by other major medical problems such as deafness, developmental delay, or speech disorders.

## CONCLUSION

Allergic rhinitis and associated disorders such as allergic conjunctivitis, chronic sinusitis, and otitis media with effusion are common in childhood, and cause considerable morbidity. Physicians providing primary care for children should be careful not to overlook these disorders, and should be aware of the relief that aggressive, modern management can provide for young patients who suffer from them.

### Selected Readings

Allansmith MR, Ross RN. Ocular allergy. Clinical Allergy 1988;18:1.
Fireman P. Otitis media and nasal disease: a role for allergy. J Allergy Clin Immunol 1988;82(Suppl):917.
Naclerio RM. Allergic rhinitis. N Engl J Med 1991;325:860.
Ott NL, O'Connell EJ, Hoffman AD, Beatty CW, Sachs MI. Childhood sinusitis. Mayo Clin Proc 1991;66:1238.
Pipkorn U, Proud D, Lichtenstein LM, Kagey-Sobotka A, Norman PS, Naclerio RM. Inhibition of mediator release in allergic rhinitis by pretreatment with topical glucocorticosteroids. N Engl J Med 1987;316:1506.
Simons FER. Allergic rhinitis: recent advances. Pediatr Clin North Am 1988;35:1053.
Simons FER, Simons KJ. Second-generation H₁-receptor antagonists. Ann Allergy 1991;66:5.
Varney VA, Gaga M, Frew AJ, Aber VR, Kay AB, Durham SR. Usefulness of immunotherapy in patients with severe summer hay fever uncontrolled by antiallergic drugs. BMJ 1991;302:265.

*Principles and Practice of Pediatrics, Second Edition.*
edited by Frank A. Oski et al. J. B. Lippincott Company, Philadelphia © 1994.

## 14.2.7 *Insect Sting Allergy*

Kenneth C. Schuberth

For most children, insect stings are common, painful, but not particularly hazardous. In about 1% of the general population, however, stings trigger systemic anaphylactic reactions that account for about 40 fatalities in the United States each year. Although the risk of a fatal reaction is lower in children than in adults, insect-allergic children cause anxiety in parents and pediatricians because children are more likely to be stung and young children can not handle emergencies and provide self-treatment.

During the past 15 years, major advances in understanding the biochemistry of insect venoms and the pathophysiology of the immune response have led to the development of safe and effective venom immunotherapy for highly allergic individuals. At the same time, long-term studies of the epidemiology and natural history of insect allergy have provided reassuring evidence that for most children the "allergic state" is a transient, self-limited process that may not require treatment.

## THE INSECTS

True "stinging insects" that account for the majority of allergic reactions belong to the order Hymenoptera (Table 14-17). The females of each species have a modified ovipositor stinger through which an injection of venom is delivered. Biting insects, such as mosquitoes, flies, and bugs, only rarely produce systemic reactions and are not considered in this discussion.

Honeybees are the most common members of the apid family. They are small, fuzzy, relatively docile insects that usually live in domestic hives and often are seen pollinating clover and flowering plants. They usually sting only when sat on or caught under foot, and leave their barbed stinger embedded in the victim. Bumblebees are large, slow-flying, yellow- and black-striped bees that are usually solitary and only rarely sting. Honeybees and bumblebees survive the winter and are present throughout the summer.

The vespid family includes yellow jackets, hornets, and wasps. In most areas of the United States, these insects account for the majority of stings. Yellow jackets are common in the Northeast, whereas wasps are dominant in the South and Southwest. Yellow jackets are small, black- and yellow-striped insects that usually nest in the ground or in decaying logs. They scavenge for food, are often seen around picnics and garbage, and become particularly aggressive late in the summer when their nests are crowded. White-faced hornets are large black insects with white faces that build teardrop-shaped paper nests suspended in trees. The thin-bodied brown- and yellow-striped Polistes wasp typically creates open-faced nests under the eaves of buildings.

The imported fire ants are less common members of the order. They inhabit the coastal areas of the Southeast and live in large dirt mounds. They attach themselves to the skin and deliver multiple stings that result in sterile pustules. Although they are a cause of systemic reaction, their venom has been less well-studied and is not commercially available for diagnosis and treatment.

## REACTION TYPES

After a sting, 90% of children experience transient redness, swelling, and pain localized to the sting site, usually less than 2 inches in diameter and lasting for less than 24 hours (Table 14-18). Hymenoptera venoms contain a variety of enzymes (phos-

| TABLE 14-17. Classification of Common Stinging Insects (Order Hymenoptera) |
| --- |
| Apid family |
|   Honeybee |
|   Bumble bee |
| Vespid family |
|   Yellow jacket |
|   White-faced hornet |
|   Yellow hornet |
|   *Polistes* wasp |
| Imported fire ant |

| TABLE 14-18.  Classification of Reactions to Insect Stings |
| --- |
| Reaction |
| **Normal**<br>Swelling <2 in in diameter<br>Duration <24 h |
| **Large Local**<br>Swelling >2 in in diameter<br>Duration 1 to 7 d |
| **Systemic**<br>Non-life-threatening<br>　Immediate-type generalized reaction confined to the skin<br>　(urticaria, angioedema, erythema, pruritus)<br>Life-threatening<br>　Immediate-type generalized reaction that may include<br>　cutaneous symptoms but also has respiratory (laryngeal<br>　edema or asthma) or cardiovascular (hypotension/shock)<br>　symptoms |

pholipase A, hyaluronidase), cytotoxic proteins (apamine, mellitin), and vasoactive compounds (histamine and kinins) which, in the normal individual, induces local vasodilatation, edema, and tissue damage.

In 10% of children, the sting results in a large local reaction that is extensively swollen and tender, is larger than several inches in diameter, and peaks in 3 to 7 days. Although the exact mechanism of this reaction is unknown, 75% of these individuals demonstrate venom-specific IgE, suggesting that immediate hypersensitivity plays some role in this exaggerated sting response.

True systemic anaphylactic reactions are less common. Estimates of their incidence in the general population range from 0.5% to 5%. Anaphylaxis is caused by the activation of mast cells sensitized by venom-specific IgE, with the release of large quantities of vasoactive mediators including histamine and kallikreins, leading to vasodilatation and increased vascular permeability. Most of these reactions (70% to 80%) are non–life-threatening. They begin several minutes to several hours after the sting and consist of simple urticaria, erythema, pruritus, and angioedema. The more serious life-threatening reactions begin within 5 to 10 minutes. Airway obstruction may occur secondary to laryngeal edema (tickle in the throat, gagging, difficulty in swallowing, or voice change) or bronchospasm (chest tightness or wheezing). Hypotension (dizziness or fainting) and frank cardiovascular collapse are accompanied by metabolic acidosis, clotting abnormalities (decreased Factor V, Factor VII, and fibrinogen), and evidence of complement activation. Although approximately 40 deaths per year are attributed to insect allergy, almost all of these occur in adults, particularly the elderly. Fatal outcome in children is extremely rare.

Several types of non–IgE-mediated reactions include serum sickness, renal disease, neurologic manifestation, and delayed hypersensitivity phenomenon. Their pathophysiology remains unknown. When a child is stung many times simultaneously, a "toxic," nonallergic reaction consisting of delayed fever, nausea, vomiting, and other systemic symptoms sometimes occurs. With an extremely large number of stings such as may occur with Africanized honeybees or "Killer Bees," this type of nonallergic reaction is occasionally fatal.

## ETIOLOGY AND NATURAL HISTORY

Systemic reactions are produced by venom-specific IgE directed against a variety of venom protein antigens. For honeybee, phospholipase A is the major antigen, while antigen 5, a protein of unknown function, is the most common in vespid sensitivity. Yellow-jacket, hornet, and wasp venoms share a variety of common antigens, and a sting by one species often results in sensitivity to all vespids. Crossreactivity is negligible between honeybee and vespid venoms. Nevertheless, almost 50% of children exhibit combined honeybee and vespid sensitivity, presumably as a result of previous stings from a variety of insects that did not result in unusual reactions. Although venom-specific IgE can be demonstrated in more than 90% of patients experiencing systemic reactions, it is also present in 75% of large local reactors and about 15% to 20% of the general population, especially in the 12 to 24 months after an acute sting. Exposure to venom proteins in the general atopic population may produce a transient period of subclinical sensitivity that usually disappears. In a small percentage of those patients, re-sting during that period of hypersensitivity results in systemic reactions.

Recent studies in the epidemiology and natural history of insect-sting allergy demonstrate several characteristics of the disease that were unrecognized. Children with a history of large local reactions only rarely go on to experience systemic reactions to subsequent stings (less than 3%). Children with a history of mild systemic reactions have only about a 10% chance of experiencing subsequent systemic reactions, almost all of which are less severe than the prior ones. These two pieces of information suggest that, for most children, insect allergy is not a progressive problem and is outgrown. Much of the anxiety and sense of panic relating to insect allergy in the past were the result of anecdotal reports and poorly controlled studies.

## DIAGNOSIS

The initial step in managing insect-sting allergy is an attempt, by careful history taking, to identify the insect culprit and clearly define the reaction by category, extent, and time course. The critical distinction to make is that between local and systemic reactions. If the reaction is systemic, particularly if life-threatening, referral for skin-test evaluation is necessary.

## VENOM SKIN TESTING

For children with a history of a prior systemic reaction, venom skin testing is the quickest and most sensitive way to determine the presence of venom-specific IgE and identify which insects are responsible. Testing may be done as soon as 1 week after the reaction and has been useful in children as young as 9 months old. A panel of purified processed venoms, including those of honeybee, yellow jacket, white-faced hornet, yellow hornet, and Polistes wasp, is available for intradermal testing at concentrations from 0.001 to 1.0 $\mu$g/mL. Although testing identifies the "sensitive state," there is no good correlation among the intensity of skin-test reactivity, the severity of the previous reaction, and the likelihood of reaction to subsequent stings. Positive skin tests must always be interpreted in light of clinical history. A negative skin test in a patient with a history of systemic reactions suggests non–IgE-mediated anaphylactoid mechanisms.

## RAST TESTING

Venom radioallergosorbent testing (RAST) detects the presence of venom-specific IgE in serum. Because it is less sensitive (15% false-negative) and more expensive than skin testing, it is not used routinely as a screening test but may be helpful in situations in which skin testing is equivocal.

| TABLE 14-19.    Treatment of Acute Anaphylactic Reaction |
| --- |
| Epinephrine—1:1000 aqueous 0.01 mL/kg subcutaneously up to 0.3 mL; may be repeated at 20-min intervals<br>Diphenhydramine—1 mg/kg up to 50 mg. IM or orally<br>Prednisone—1 mg/kg/day for 3 to 5 d<br>**In the event of a severe reaction:**<br>Oxygen/respiratory support<br>Intravenous volume expanders and vasopressor infusion |

## MANAGEMENT

### Treatment of the Acute Episode

Systemic reactions of immediate onset should be treated promptly with subcutaneous aqueous epinephrine in a dose of 0.01 mL/kg of a 1:1000 solution (Table 14-19). This dose may be repeated after 15 minutes if necessary. An injection of long-acting epinephrine (Sus-phrine 0.005 mL/kg) may be administered to prevent late recurrences. Oral and injectable antihistamines, such as diphenhydramine (1 to 2 mg/kg), are often administered, but their use should not delay the administration of epinephrine. Oral corticosteroids such as prednisone (0.5 to 1 mg/kg/d) may be given, but the delayed onset of action limits their effectiveness in the early stages of treatment. In any case, patients who are experiencing systemic reactions should be observed until all symptoms of the reaction are resolved.

The more severe anaphylactic reactions consist of hypotension or airway obstruction. The hypotension is secondary to a combination of loss of vascular tone and extravascular leakage of fluid. Initial treatment consists of intravascular volume support with as much as 50 mL/kg of normal saline over the first hour, followed, if necessary, by albumin or 5% plasma protein (Plasmanate) infusion. In prolonged or unresponsive cases, intravenous vasopressors such as epinephrine 1:10,000 (0.05 mL/kg/min) may be required. Respiratory obstruction is treated with supplemental oxygen in all cases. Upper-airway obstruction that does not respond to parenteral epinephrine should be treated with nebulized racemic epinephrine, and unresponsive bronchospasm may benefit from nebulized beta-agonists or cautious intravenous aminophylline.

Treatment of large local reactions consists of ice, elevation, antihistamines, and pain relievers. In persons with severe local reactions, a short course of corticosteroids has been advocated (prednisone 0.5 to 1 mg/kg/d for 5 days), but no controlled studies of their effectiveness have been performed.

### Emergency Self-Treatment

Patients who have experienced systemic reactions should be given an epinephrine-containing self-treatment kit to be carried when they are at risk for sting and medical care is not immediately available. The Epi-Pen device is an automatic self-injector that is available in two sizes (0.15 mg and 0.3 mg epinephrine) and is particularly useful in children.

### Avoidance Measures

Careful sanitation and extermination of vespid nests can significantly reduce the chance of yellow-jacket sting. For children especially, wearing shoes while walking in the grass eliminates the most common cause of honeybee sting. The usual insect repellents are not effective against Hymenoptera. In severely allergic children, wearing a Medic-Alert bracelet or necklace provides quick and useful information in case of accidental sting reaction.

### Venom Immunotherapy

In 1979, the Food and Drug Administration (FDA) licensed the use of purified extracts of insect venoms to prevent future systemic reactions in children and adults. The five venoms used in immunotherapy correspond to those used in skin testing. The selection of venoms for therapy is based on the demonstration of venom-specific IgE, either by skin testing or by RAST. The regimen consists of rapid advancement to maintenance doses at every 4- to 6-week interval for as long as 5 years of treatment. Children tolerate this regimen extremely well, although almost all of them sometime experience local redness or swelling at the injection site. About one fourth of them sometime experience a large local reaction at the injection site, and there is about a 5% risk of a systemic reaction at some time during the immunotherapy regimen. These are similar to risks encountered with other high-dose immunotherapy regimens using pollens or other inhalants. There is no evidence of any long-term adverse effects. Studies using in-hospital challenge stings after 15 weeks of venom immunotherapy, and at yearly intervals thereafter, demonstrate a 97% to 98% nonreaction rate in various groups of adults and children.

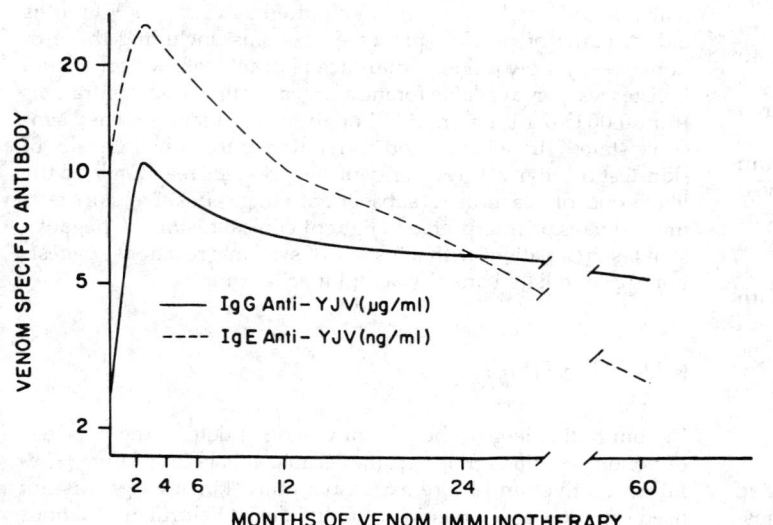

Figure 14-14. Antibody response to yellow-jacket venom immunotherapy.

TABLE 14-20.  Indications for Venom Immunotherapy

| | Venom Skin Test | |
|---|---|---|
| Prior Reaction | Positive | Negative |
| Life-threatening systemic | Yes | No |
| Non–life-threatening systemic | Yes | No |
| Adults | | |
| Children | No | No |
| Large local | Not indicated | |
| Normal local | Not indicated | |

During immunotherapy, a typical allergic patient responds initially by producing more venom-specific IgE at the same time that venom-specific IgG-blocking antibody increases. IgE peaks at about 8 weeks of therapy, then declines slowly over several years to a level lower than the initial baseline level (Fig 14-14). IgG antibody levels peak at about the same time and remain elevated for the duration of therapy. There is some correlation between the level of these antibodies and the certainty of protection conferred by immunotherapy so that in very high-risk patients, it is useful to monitor IgG titers to ensure protection. After 3 years, venom sensitivity, as measured by positive skin tests or RAST, disappears in approximately 20% of patients. For these patients, immunotherapy can be safely discontinued. The remainder should complete 5 years of treatment which confers long-term protection against stings regardless of skin test sensitivity at the time of discontinuation.

## Patient Selection for Venom Immunotherapy

Only those patients who have experienced a significant systemic reaction and who have positive skin tests or RAST are candidates for venom immunotherapy. The more severe the prior reaction, the more likely it is that the subsequent reaction will be serious. Although positive skin tests identify sensitive individuals, they do not predict the risk of future reactions. As many as 40% to 60% of adults who have had a systemic reaction and are skin-test positive do not experience any systemic reaction if they are stung again. Children have an even lower risk, as evidenced by the high frequency of mild cutaneous systemic reactions and the extreme rarity of fatalities. For children who have had mild systemic reactions and are skin-test positive, the risk of systemic reaction on re-sting is less than 10% and the risk of progression to more serious reactions is much less than that. For these children, observation and emergency precautions, without venom immunotherapy, appear to be sufficient. For children with life-threatening systemic reactions and positive skin or RAST tests, venom immunotherapy is mandatory, as it is in all adults regardless of severity of prior systemic reaction. Although the guidelines for treatment listed in Table 14-20 are specific, the decision for or against venom immunotherapy must be made for each patient after careful discussion between physician and family of risks, benefits, and individual concerns.

## Selected Readings

Freeman TM, Hylander R, Ortiz A, et al. Imported fire ant immunotherapy: effectiveness of whole body extracts. J Allergy Clin Immunol 1992;90:210.

Graft DF, Schuberth KC. Hymenoptera allergy in children. Pediatr Clin North Am 1983;30:873.

Hunt KJ, Valentine MD, Sobotka AK, et al. A controlled trial of immunotherapy in insect hypersensitivity. N Engl J Med 1978;299:157.

Levine MI, Lockey RF, eds. Monograph on insect allergy, ed 2. Committee on Insects. Milwaukee: American Academy of Allergy and Immunology, 1986: 107.

Reisman RE. Venom immunotherapy: when is it reasonable to stop? J Allergy Clin Immunol 1991;87:618.

Schuberth KC, Lichtenstein LM, Kagey-Sobotka A, et al. Epidemiologic study of insect allergy in children. II. Effect of accidental stings in allergic children. J Pediatr 1983;102:361.

Valentine MD, Schuberth KC, Kagey-Sobotka A, et al. The value of immunotherapy with venom in children with allergy to insect stings. N Engl J Med 1990;323: 1601.

*Principles and Practice of Pediatrics, Second Edition.*
edited by Frank A. Oski et al. J. B. Lippincott Company, Philadelphia © 1994.

CHAPTER 15
# Connective Tissue Diseases and Amyloidosis

## James T. Cassidy

The connective tissue diseases are a group of heterogeneous afflictions that commonly inflame the connective tissues of the body. A frequent manifestation of these diseases is arthritis—objective inflammation of a joint. Etiologies of these disorders are mostly unknown. Many have an immunogenetic background and are characterized by prominent autoimmune phenomena: circulating autoantibodies such as rheumatoid factors and antinuclear antibodies and, in some cases, deposition of gammaglobulins in the affected tissues. There is also tissue accumulation of lymphocytes and plasma cells. The connective tissue diseases are often chronic and self-perpetuating, although many respond to glucocorticoid and anti-inflammatory drugs or immunosuppressive agents.

Data on the prevalence of the connective tissue diseases in children are incomplete. Juvenile rheumatoid arthritis (JRA) is the most common disorder for which reasonable estimates of frequency are published. Our 1973 study in Michigan reported minimal incidence of referred cases of 9.2 per 100,000 children per year; a 1983 study from the Mayo Clinic cited an incidence of 13.9. A 1986 Finnish study estimated the annual incidence of JRA to be 16.8 cases per 100,000 children, and 108.5 per 100,000 for all forms of childhood arthritis.

The prevalence of other connective tissue diseases discussed in this chapter is estimated by noting their frequency among children in established pediatric rheumatology clinics. Table 15-1 includes composite data from three large clinics on the relative frequency of each of these diseases.

The combined prevalence of these disorders in the United States population in 1986 for children 15 years of age or younger would be about 70,000 for JRA and 17,500 for the other major connective tissue diseases. The total population of children with the various forms of juvenile arthritis would be about 175,000.

Table 15-2 is a condensed diagnostic classification for juvenile arthritis modified from a schema developed by the American College of Rheumatology. Each of the major types of rheumatic

TABLE 15-1. Frequency of Connective Tissue Diseases in Children in a Pediatric Rheumatology Clinic

| | |
|---|---|
| Juvenile rheumatoid arthritis | 75–80% |
| Systemic lupus erythematosus | 5–10% |
| Dermatomyositis | 5% |
| Juvenile anklosing spondylitis | 3% |
| Scleroderma | 3% |
| Vasculitis | 2% |

TABLE 15-2. Diagnostic Classification of Juvenile Arthritis

**Connective Tissue Diseases**
Juvenile rheumatoid arthritis
Systemic lupus erythematosus
Dermatomyositis
Vasculitis
Scleroderma

**Seronegative Spondyloarthropathies**
Juvenile ankylosing spondylitis
Psoriatic spondyloarthritis
Reiter's disease
Inflammatory bowel disease

**Infectious Arthritis**
Bacterial arthritis (including staphylococcal, gonorrhea, tuberculosis)
Viral arthritis
Fungal arthritis
Lyme disease

**Reactive Arthritis**
Rheumatic fever
Post-Yersinia arthritis

**Rheumatic Diseases Associated With Immunodeficiency**

**Congenital Anomalies and Genetically Determined Abnormalities of the Musculoskeletal System**
Constitutional diseases of bone
Lysosomal storage diseases
Heritable disorders of collagen and fibrous connective tissue
Amyloidosis

**Nonrheumatic Conditions of Bones and Joints**
Traumatic arthritis
Reflex neurovascular dystrophy
Legg–Calvé–Perthes disease
Slipped capital femoral epiphysis
Toxic synovitis of the hip
Osteochondritis dissecans
Chondromalacia patellae
Plant-thorn synovitis

**Hematologic Diseases**
Sickle-cell anemia
Hemophilia
Thalassemia
Leukemia and lymphoma

**Neoplastic Diseases**
Neuroblastoma
Malignant and benign tumors of cartilage, bone, and synovium
Histiocytosis

**Arthromyalgia**
Growing pains
Psychogenic rheumatism

disease is included, but only selected subtypes pertinent to pediatric practice are provided for each category. As in all other areas of medicine, correct diagnosis of a disease without a pathognomonic finding or known etiology requires careful exclusion of similar disorders that could afflict the patient. Most of the rheumatic diseases are more common in girls than in boys. Exceptions exist, however, such as for polyarteritis and ankylosing spondylitis.

In JRA, the primary focus of the clinical disease is on arthritis or synovitis. Arthritis should be distinguished from arthralgia, which is pain in a joint without objective findings on physical examination. Many more children have transient episodes of arthralgia or even of arthritis than can be categorized as JRA. One study estimated that only about 15% of children with unexplained arthralgia go on to develop chronic arthritis that meets classification criteria for JRA.

Although arthritis may be a characteristic of other connective tissue diseases, they often have more prominent manifestations in other systems. Table 15-3 compares signs and symptoms of major connective tissue diseases. In systemic lupus erythematosus (SLE), the primary focus is immune-complex vasculitis of the small arterioles that underlie the cutaneous, mucosal, and serosal surfaces of the body and involvement of internal organs such as the kidneys. In dermatomyositis, the shock organs are primarily the skin, skeletal muscles, and gastrointestinal tract. In scleroderma, the skin, gastrointestinal tract, and cardiopulmonary system are primarily involved. In vasculitis, the blood vessels are the predominant target organs with multisystem disease involving the central nervous system (CNS), cardiopulmonary tract, gastrointestinal and renal systems, and the skin, depending on the form that the vasculitis takes in a child.

## JUVENILE RHEUMATOID ARTHRITIS

Juvenile rheumatoid arthritis is the most common pediatric connective tissue disease with arthritis as the principal manifestation. It is one of the more frequent chronic childhood illnesses and a leading cause of disability and blindness.

The etiology of JRA is unknown. It likely does not represent a single disorder but a spectrum of diseases of diverse pathogenesis. Certain viral illnesses of childhood, especially rubella and mumps, have an associated arthritis. Immunodeficiency is associated with the occurrence of arthritis in children with selective IgA deficiency, agammaglobulinemia or hypogammaglobulinemia, and C2 complement component deficiency. An immunogenetic predisposition appears to be present in certain children. The HLA antigens DRw6, DRw8, DQw1, and DPw2.1 are associated with development of persistent oligoarthritis at early age in young girls with antinuclear antibody (ANA) seropositivity. Antibodies and cellular immune reactivity to Type II collagen have been demonstrated in children with JRA. Children with JRA may form antibodies to surface membrane antigens on T cells of the suppressor-inducer type. These cells are also low in number in the peripheral white cell population of these children.

## Pathology

The synovial membrane in JRA is characterized by villous hypertrophy and hyperplasia of the synovial lining layer. Edema

TABLE 15-3. Clinical Manifestations of Connective Tissue Diseases

| | Juvenile Rheumatoid Arthritis | Systemic Lupus Erythematosus | Dermatomyositis | Scleroderma | Vasculitis |
|---|---|---|---|---|---|
| Female-to-male ratio | 2:1 | 5:1 | 2:1 | 2:1 | 1:3 |
| Constitutional symptoms | +++ | +++ | +++ | + | +++ |
| Arthritis | +++ | ++ | + | + | + |
| Dermatitis | + | +++ | +++ | ++ | + |
| Photosensitivity | − | ++ | + | − | − |
| Mucocutaneous ulcerations | − | ++ | + | − | − |
| Subcutaneous nodules | + | + | − | + | + |
| Calcinosis | − | − | ++ | ++ | − |
| Alopecia | − | ++ | + | + | − |
| Raynaud phenomenon | − | ++ | + | +++ | + |
| Vasculitis | + | +++ | ++ | + | +++ |
| Myositis | + | + | +++ | ++ | + |
| Cardiac involvement | + | +++ | ± | ++ | ++ |
| Pleuritis | ++ | +++ | + | − | + |
| Pulmonary involvement | + | ++ | + | +++ | ++ |
| Gastrointestinal disease | − | ++ | ++ | +++ | +++ |
| Hepatomegaly | + | + | − | − | − |
| Splenomegaly | + | ++ | − | − | − |
| Lymphadenopathy | + | ++ | + | − | + |
| Renal disease | + | +++ | ± | ++ | +++ |
| Hypertension | − | ++ | − | ++ | +++ |
| Ocular involvement | ++ | ++ | + | − | ++ |
| Nervous system disease | − | +++ | − | − | +++ |
| Anemia | ++ | +++ | + | + | + |
| Leukocytosis | + | − | + | − | ++ |
| Leukopenia | − | ++ | − | − | − |
| Eosinophilia | − | − | + | − | ++ |
| Thrombocytopenia | − | ++ | − | − | − |
| Hypergammaglobulinemia | ++ | +++ | + | + | + |
| Rheumatoid factors | + | ++ | − | + | + |
| Antinuclear antibodies | ++ | +++ | + | ++ | + |

−, absent; ±, rare; +, minimal; ++, moderate; +++, severe.

and hyperemia are present along with vascular endothelial hyperplasia and infiltration of lymphocytes and plasma cells. Pannus formation eventually occurs in severely affected children and leads to destruction of articular cartilage and contiguous bone.

Infiltrates of inflammatory cells may be seen in parenchymal organs such as the liver. Rheumatoid nodules result from the small blood vessel vasculitis that occurs in JRA. The rash of JRA is characterized histologically by an infiltration of round cells surrounding capillaries and subdermal venules and a neutrophilic perivasculitis.

## Clinical Manifestations

Although onset of JRA before 6 months of age is unusual, the mean age at onset is characteristically young—1 to 3 years—with a substantial number of cases beginning throughout childhood and young adolescence. Girls are affected at least twice as frequently as boys.

Fatigue, low-grade fever, anorexia, weight loss, and failure to grow are common at onset of the disease in moderate to severely affected children. Morning stiffness, gelling after inactivity, and night pain are often encountered in uncontrolled disease. Children may not directly communicate these symptoms to their parents. The child may present, instead, with increased irritability, a posture of guarding the joints, or refusal to walk.

## Types of Onset

The classification of JRA is strengthened by recognition of three distinct types of onset of the disease Table 15-4: polyarthritis, oligoarthritis (pauciarticular disease), and systemic disease. These types of onset are characterized by specific signs and symptoms at presentation and during the first 6 months of the illness.

Polyarthritis is disease that begins in five or more joints. This onset occurs in nearly half the children and may be acute or insidious. Systemic manifestations are usually not severe or persistent. The arthritis generally involves large joints such as the knees, wrists, elbows, and ankles. The smaller joints of the hands or feet may be affected early or late. The pattern of arthritis is usually symmetric. The child may not complain of pain even though the joints are tender and painful on motion. The cervical spine is often involved in this type of onset, although onset of JRA solely in the cervical spine is rare. The neck may be painful or stiff with an alarmingly rapid loss over time of extension and

**TABLE 15-4. Classification of Types of Onset of Juvenile Rheumatoid Arthritis**

| Sign/Symptom of Onset | Polyarthritis | Oligoarthritis (Pauciarticular Disease) | Systemic Disease |
|---|---|---|---|
| Frequency of cases | 40–50% | 40–50% | 10–20% |
| Number of joints involved | ≥5 | ≤4 | Variable |
| Sex ratio (F:M) | 3:1 | 5:1 | 1:1 |
| Systemic involvement | Moderate involvement | Not present | Prominent |
| Occurence of chronic uveitis | 5% | 20% | Rare |
| Frequency of seropositivity | | | |
|   Rheumatoid factors | 10% (increases with age) | Rare | Rare |
|   Antinuclear antibodies | 40–50% | 75–85%* | 10% |
| Course | Systemic disease is generally mild; articular involvement may be unremitting | Systemic disease is absent; major cause of morbidity is uveitis | Systemic disease is often self-limited; arthritis is chronic and destructive in 50% |
| Prognosis | Guarded to moderately good | Excellent except for eyesight | Moderate to poor |

\* In girls with uveitis

rotation. Atlantoaxial subluxation may occur early and place a child at risk to injury of the cervical cord in an accident or with attempted intubation before general anesthesia. Temporomandibular joint disease is relatively common in children with polyarthritis and leads to limitation or asymmetry of bite and micrognathia.

The onset of JRA in half of the children involves four or fewer joints. Oligoarthritis or pauciarticular disease often is confined to the knees or ankles or may involve a single joint at onset and throughout the course of the disease. The hips are usually spared at onset. Extra-articular systemic disease except for chronic uveitis is distinctly unusual.

A small number of children have onset of JRA with severe constitutional and systemic disease. This systemic onset may precede the appearance of overt arthritis by weeks, months, or years. A hallmark of this type of disease is a high spiking fever, often combined with a rheumatoid rash. Temperature elevations occur once or twice a day, often in late afternoon or evening, to a level of 39°C or higher with a quick return to baseline temperature or lower. This quotidian pattern is highly suggestive of a diagnosis of JRA.

The rash of JRA develops with this fever and consists of 2- to 5-mm erythematous morbilliform macules (Fig 15-1). It is most commonly seen on the trunk and proximal extremities, and over pressure areas, but may occur on the face, palms, or soles. The rash is not generally pruritic; the most characteristic feature is its transient nature. Any single lesion generally does not persist for more than an hour. This rash may also be seen in some children with polyarthritis at onset but is never seen in children with oligoarthritis. The rash can sometimes be elicited in a child by rubbing or scratching the skin—the isomorphic response or Koebner phenomenon.

Children with systemic onset usually have hepatosplenomegaly and lymphadenopathy. Pericarditis, hepatitis, and other visceral disease may occur. Pulmonary involvement consists of a wide spectrum of abnormalities such as pleuritis and effusion, interstitial fibrosis, and hemosiderosis. The CNS may be affected, but encephalopathy may be difficult to distinguish from drug toxicity, viral infection, or other complications of the systemic illness and fever.

Tenosynovitis and myositis are also accompaniments of active disease. A stenosing synovitis of the flexor tendon sheaths may lead to loss of extension of the fingers or a trigger finger. Rheu-

matoid nodules may occur on the tendons or subcutaneously over pressure points. They are particularly found in children with widespread polyarthritis who are older at onset and who have prominent small joint disease, an unrelenting course with erosions, and rheumatoid factor seropositivity.

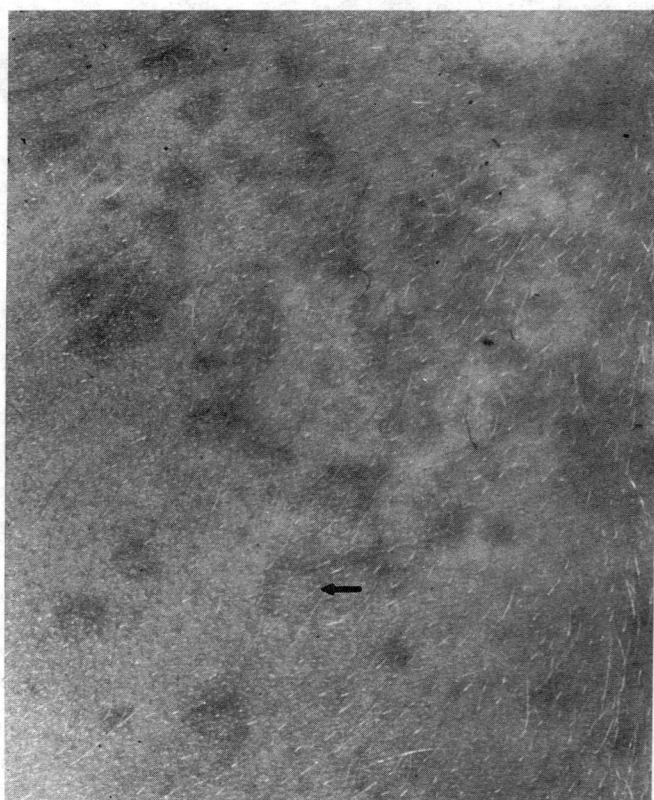

**Figure 15-1.** Rash of systemic onset JRA. This was a 4-year-old girl who presented with high spiking fever that occurred once a day accompanied by a transient nonpruritic rash. Shown is an area of active maculopapular rash on the back that was salmon pink in color. The arrow points to central clearing in a lesion. (Cassidy JT. Juvenile rheumatoid arthritis. In Kelley WN, Harris ED Jr, Ruddy S, Sledge CB (eds). Textbook of rheumatology. Philadelphia: WB Saunders, 1993:1193.)

## Chronic Uveitis

One of the most serious complications of JRA is the development of a chronic nongranulomatous uveitis involving the iris, ciliary body, and often the posterior choroid (Fig 15-2). This disease is usually bilateral and in 20% of children leads to blindness in the affected eye. Chronic uveitis characteristically has an insidious, asymptomatic onset and is only diagnosed by routine ophthalmologic and slit-lamp examinations at onset of the disease. These examinations should be repeated at frequent intervals during the first years after onset of JRA in all children. Chronic uveitis is confined to children with polyarthritis or oligoarthritis. It is particularly prone to occur in young girls of early age of onset with limited joint disease who are ANA seropositive. It is found in at least one fifth of these children.

## Growth Retardation

Disturbances of growth and normal development are complications of a chronic disease such as JRA. Linear growth is retarded during periods of active disease and during use of glucocorticoid drugs. There is often delayed development of secondary sexual characteristics. Psychological stunting is a frequent and potentially severe complication. Localized growth retardation may also occur in selective areas such as the jaw (micrognathia). Unequal leg or arm lengths develop with monarticular disease involving a single limb.

## Laboratory Examination

Most children with active disease develop a normocytic, hypochromic anemia characteristic of the chronic anemia of inflammation. This is often moderately severe with the hemoglobin in the range of 7 to 10 g/dL. Leukocytosis and thrombocytosis are common with active disease. These findings are not seen or are much less pronounced in children with oligoarthritis.

The acute-phase reactants are often positive at onset of the disease and are moderately useful in following the course of the disease. The Westergren erythrocyte sedimentation rate, C-reactive protein level, and immunoglobulin concentrations reflect the inflammatory activity. Serum complement components usually are elevated at onset and with exacerbations. The serum amyloid-like protein (SAA) is increased in concentration in children with JRA. Soluble immune complexes can be detected in the sera of some children, particularly those with systemic onset of the disease.

Tests for rheumatoid factors are positive in children with JRA less frequently than in adults with rheumatoid arthritis. Rheumatoid factors are IgM macroglobulins with antigenic specificity directed against the unfolded H-chains of IgG. About 20% of children with JRA eventually become seropositive, even though few children at onset of JRA are seropositive and a positive latex fixation test is seldom observed in a child younger than 7 years of age. Rheumatoid factors tend to be present in a child of later age of onset or in the older child, and in one who has prominent symmetric polyarthritis with involvement of the small joints, subcutaneous rheumatoid nodules, articular erosions, and a poor functional outcome.

ANA seropositivity is present in at least 40% of children with JRA. The pattern of fluorescent staining is usually homogeneous or speckled; the titer is generally low to moderate. The presence of these antibodies is significantly correlated with development of chronic uveitis. They are less commonly found in older boys and in children with systemic disease. A positive ANA determination is a valuable diagnostic measure in a child suspected of JRA because ANA are not frequently positive in other childhood illnesses except for SLE, scleroderma, and transient acute viral disease.

The synovial fluid white cell count in JRA is usually moderately elevated in the range of 10,000/mm³ to 20,000/mm³. Synovial glucose concentration is low. Complement levels may be depressed indicating intrasynovial complement activation.

Urinalysis generally is normal in children with JRA except for the few children who have a mild glomerulitis at onset. Proteinuria may occur with fever. Persistent proteinuria may be the first evidence of amyloidosis. Some children develop renal papillary necrosis during the course of the disease.

## Radiologic Examination

A wide range of distinctive radiologic findings are present in children with JRA. Early changes consist of soft-tissue swelling, juxta-articular osteoporosis, and periosteal new bone apposition. Development of the ossification centers may be accelerated or there may be premature epiphyseal closure leading to stunting of bone growth. In children with polyarthritis or systemic disease, especially late in the course, marginal erosions may develop along with narrowing of the cartilaginous spaces.

Cervical spine disease is characteristic of JRA. The upper cervical segments are principally affected with apophyseal joint fusion and atlantoaxial subluxation (Fig 15-3). The lower vertebrae may also be involved with failure to grow normally. Sacroiliac arthritis in children with JRA is not characterized by the degree of abnormality and reactive sclerosis that would be seen in ankylosing spondylitis. Fractures, particularly of the long bones and vertebrae, occur in children who develop generalized osteoporosis.

Routine radiographic studies generally are sufficient to delineate this progression of changes in evaluating a child's response to a management program. Newer methods of objectively evaluating joint disease can be employed, however, such as bone scans, computed tomography, and magnetic resonance imaging (MRI). MRI is more precise than routine x-ray examination in delineating soft tissue abnormalities in response to abnormal bone growth or fusion.

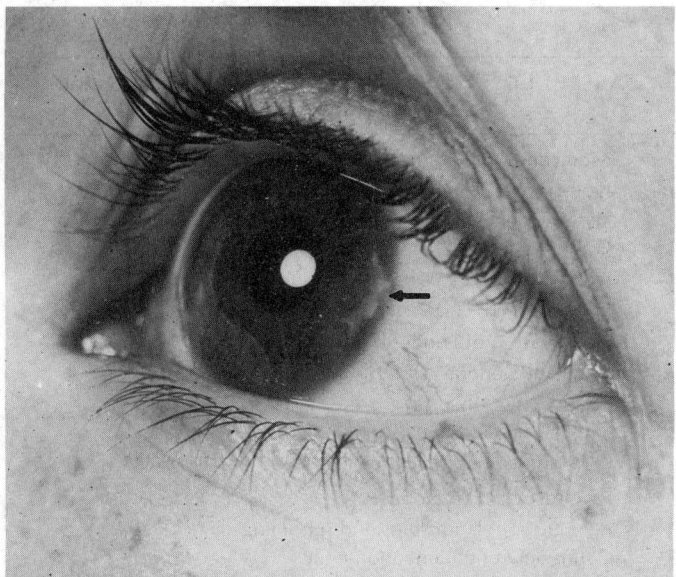

**Figure 15-2.** The arrow points to an area of band keratopathy just inside the limbus of the cornea in a girl who had ANA-positive oligoarticular JRA. Her chronic uveitis was bilateral and had resulted in a decrease in vision to 20/400 OD.

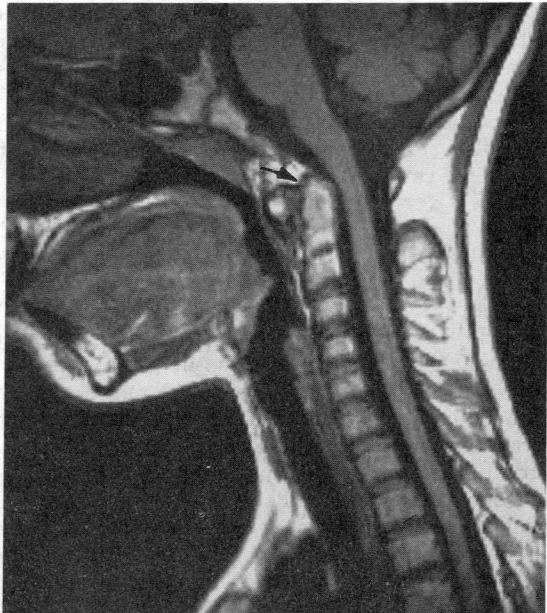

Figure 15-3. Magnetic resonance image of the cervical spine of a child with 7 mm of atlantoaxial subluxation. The arrow points to the odontoid, which is beginning to impinge on the upper cervical cord.

## Diagnosis

Classification criteria for JRA are listed in Table 15-5. JRA is defined as onset of idiopathic arthritis in a child younger than 16 years old. Arthritis is delimited objectively by the listed criteria. JRA is often a disease of exclusion and, therefore, similar diseases must be considered (see Table 15-2). The differential diagnosis generally includes other rheumatic and connective tissue diseases, especially rheumatic fever, SLE, and ankylosing spondylitis. Other forms of arthropathy such as Reiter's syndrome and psoriatic arthritis are uncommon in our experience. Particular attention must be accorded, however, to infectious arthritis, serum sickness, Henoch-Schönlein purpura, the enteropathies such as ulcerative colitis and regional enteritis, and the hematologic diseases such as leukemia, sickle-cell anemia, and hemophilia. The concurrence of arthritis and immunodeficiency has already been mentioned. Certain tumors may present as bone pain or arthritis in children, especially neuroblastoma in the young child. Onset of JRA in the hip is uncommon. In children with hip disease, transient synovitis, Legg-Calvé-Perthes disease, and slipped capital femoral epiphysis may mimic JRA, especially if the pain is referred to the knee.

---

**TABLE 15-5. Diagnostic Criteria for the Classification of Juvenile Rheumatoid Arthritis**

Age of onset <16 years

Arthritis in ≥1 joints defined as *swelling or effusion*, or the presence of two or more of the following signs: *limitation of range of motion, tenderness or pain on motion, or increased heat*

Duration of disease ≥ of 6 weeks

Type of onset of disease during the first 6 months

   Polyarthritis: ≥5 joints

   Oligoarthritis or pauciarticular disease: ≤4 joints

   Systemic disease: arthritis with intermittent fever

Exclusion of other forms of juvenile arthritis

*Cassidy JT, Levenson JE, Bass JC, et al. A study of classification criteria for a diagnosis of juvenile rheumatoid arthritis. Arthritis Rheum 1986;29:274.*

---

## Medical Treatment

Conservative management of JRA attempts to control clinical manifestations of the disease and prevent or minimize deformity. This approach ideally involves a multidisciplinary team that follows the child throughout the course of the illness. Management should be family-centered, community-based, and coordinated. The long therapeutic program must be accepted by the child and family and must be judged to have a favorable risk/benefit ratio by the pediatric rheumatologist.

Prognosis is excellent for most children with JRA, so philosophy of management should stress the simplest, safest, and most conservative measures. If this treatment proves inadequate, other therapeutic modalities should be chosen (Table 15-6).

Nonsteroidal anti-inflammatory drugs such as aspirin are effective in suppressing inflammation and fever. Aspirin has a long-term safety record and is generally started in a dose of about 75 to 90 mg/kg/d. Salicylate levels are occasionally useful as a guide to correct therapy. A child should not chew aspirin tablets because this results in gingival inflammation and erosion of the biting surfaces of the teeth. About 50% of children are treated satisfactorily with aspirin. The remainder should try another nonsteroidal anti-inflammatory drug.

A few children on the nonsteroidal drugs develop a "salicylate hepatitis" with elevation of the transaminase enzymes. Such an elevation indicates a need to lower the dose of the agent. The risk of Reye's syndrome is increased with salicylate administration according to recent Centers for Disease Control (CDC) data. Salicylates should be discontinued in children with JRA for about 2 weeks during outbreaks of influenza or varicella or with any illness characterized by vomiting. Because of this, some pediatric rheumatologists prefer other nonsteroidal drugs, such as tolmetin, ibuprofen, and naproxen. The latter two also can be prescribed as suspensions, which is particularly useful for younger children. All children with JRA should receive yearly influenza vaccines as a precaution.

Hydroxychloroquine is a useful adjunctive agent for treatment of the child with more progressive disease. Because of concern over retinopathy as a toxic reaction to this drug, a relatively low dose is chosen, eg, 5 mg/kg/d, and frequent ophthalmologic examinations are performed during its administration. Gold salts

---

**TABLE 15-6. Management of Children With Juvenile Rheumatoid Arthritis**

**Medication Program—Suppression of Inflammation**
Nonsteroidal antiinflammatory drugs
Hydroxychloroquine
Gold (IM and oral)
Glucocorticoid drugs
Immunosuppressive drugs

**Preservation of Function and Prevention of Deformities**
Local and general rest
Physical therapy
Occupational therapy
Orthopedic surgery—preventive and reconstructive

**Psychosocial Development**
Peer group relationships and schooling
Counseling of patient and family
Involvement of community agencies

**Maintenance of Adequate Nutrition**
Coordinated Care

either as intramuscular preparations or the oral compound are indicated in children whose polyarthritis is unresponsive to conservative management. Toxicities from these drug are primarily hematologic, renal, or hepatic, and those systems must be constantly monitored during treatment. D-penicillamine is not as widely employed as are gold salts. The expected response to treatment with D-penicillamine and its toxicities is similar to that for gold.

Glucocorticoid drugs should be reserved for treatment of the severely involved child who is recalcitrant to more conservative therapeutic regimens. Steroids have many toxicities associated with their use, eg, Cushing's syndrome, and severely retard normal growth and development. Steroids are indicated for resistant or life-threatening disease and its complications such as pericarditis. Ophthalmic administration is used for treatment of chronic uveitis. Occasionally intra-articular steroid is employed to achieve specific goals of a physical therapy program or for persistent monarticular involvement.

Methotrexate is the most successful and safe approach to advanced drug treatment of severe or resistant polyarthritis. In a large multinational, double-blind, randomized trial, a dose of 10 mg/M$^2$ once a week markedly reduced the articular severity index compared to placebo. This drug is attractive for pediatric use because it is taken only once a week orally as a pill or liquid, and has no proven oncogenic potential or untoward risk of sterility.

Other immunosuppressive agents seldom are used in the long-term approach to a child with JRA. There are children, however, who have failed on all other therapy, and are candidates for experimental protocols involving agents such as azathioprine or cyclophosphamide. Critical considerations are the oncogenic potential of these agents, along with potential sterility and bone marrow suppression. Alkylating agents are indicated in the treatment of amyloidosis as a complication of JRA.

## Physical and Occupational Therapy

Maintenance of function and prevention of deformity cannot be overemphasized in the total management of the child with JRA. Appropriate prescriptions for physical and occupational therapy, a balanced program of rest and activity, and selective splinting are usually employed. Normal play should be encouraged. Only unacceptable levels of stress on inflamed weight-bearing joints should be prohibited. Children with cervical spine disease should wear a padded plastic collar when traveling in an automobile or studying.

## Reconstructive Surgery

Synovectomy or tenosynovectomy is sometimes indicated in the course of management. Total joint replacement is generally delayed until after growth has ceased. Cosmetic surgery and orthodontic reconstruction for micrognathia or destruction of the temporomandibular joint are useful late approaches when indicated.

## Course of Disease and Prognosis

In general, 80% to 90% of children who develop JRA make a satisfactory recovery from their disease and enter adult life without serious functional disability. A small percentage of patients will have a recurrence of arthritis during the adult years. As many as 10% of children with JRA, however, enter adulthood with moderate to significant functional disability. The child most at risk is the one who has had polyarthritis of later age of onset, early symmetric involvement of the small joints of the hands or feet, the early appearance of erosions, unremitting activity of the joint disease, or prominent systemic manifestations, and the development of rheumatoid factor seropositivity and subcutaneous nodules. Progressive hip disease is also a major cause of long-term disability.

Serious functional disability is uncommon in children who have oligoarthritis and pursue a course of limited joint disease. About half of children with systemic onset will eventually recover completely; however, most deaths that occur in the United States are associated with systemic complications. Death occurs in less than 1% of children with JRA and often is a result of overwhelming infection. In Europe, renal failure secondary to amyloidosis is a leading cause of death. Amyloidosis is seldom seen as a complication of JRA in North America.

The prognosis for sight in children with chronic uveitis has dramatically improved, which is probably related to earlier detection and better management of this complication. Blindness still occurs in about 20% of affected eyes.

The prognosis for JRA is optimistic and in many children is excellent. It is important that both the child and parents understand the disease and share in its long-term management. The nature of JRA, the goals of therapy, and the course of the disease should be discussed in detail. A carefully selected program of coordinated care is initiated by the physician and needs constant reinforcement by the team nurse and social worker. Some families of children with JRA display psychiatrically important disruptions such as divorce, separation, death, and severe emotional disturbances. Thus, a priority in the management of a child with this chronic illness is to foster normal psychological and social development and peer group activities. Psychological regression to a more infantile pattern is present in most children who experience moderate to severe disease.

A child's unceasing potential for physical and psychological growth is a critical factor working in favor of the therapeutic program and team management. It is this natural endowment for future physical and psychological development that enables so much to be accomplished in the majority of children with JRA.

## LYME DISEASE

Lyme disease has emerged in the last 15 years as a clinical entity of near-epidemic proportions in the summer and autumn in endemic areas of the United States. Initially, an unusually large number of cases of arthritis were diagnosed as JRA in children from Old Lyme, Connecticut. In subsequent epidemiologic investigations, it was ascertained to be a tick-borne illness transmitted by Ixodes dammini and associated with widespread immune-complex disease. This arthropod vector multiplies in the white-footed deer mouse (adult ticks) and the white-tailed deer (larvae and nymphs). A spirochete, *Borrelia burgdorferi*, was isolated from adult ticks and proved to be a cause of this disease. The age of affected patients has been from 2 years to the ninth decade; the male-to-female ratio is equal. About half the patients are children. In endemic areas of the country, careful differentiation of Lyme disease from JRA (in particular the oligoarticular type) is essential.

A number of endemic areas are now recognized within the United States: the Northeast, the upper Midwest, the West Coast, and Texas. The spirochete has worldwide distribution; a similar disease is described in Europe and other countries. In the infected patient, the spirochete has been identified in the cutaneous lesions, blood, synovial fluid, and the cerebrospinal fluid. Related ticks (*Ixodes pacificus, Amblyomma americanum*) or other vectors (birds or feral animals) may be involved in the expanding distribution of the disease. The *Borrelia* organisms can be transmitted to the fetus and result in congenital anomalies, prematurity, developmental delay, and intrauterine death.

## Clinical Manifestations

Constitutional symptoms including lethargy and fatigue are often prominent (Table 15-7). Most patients complain of intermittent headache, fever and chills, and musculoskeletal aching. Lymphadenopathy and hepatosplenomegaly are frequent. The sedimentation rate is elevated along with the serum muscle enzymes. Hematuria and proteinuria are often present.

The cutaneous hallmark of the acute illness, erythema chronicum migrans (ECM), is an annular lesion measuring 3 to 70 cm in diameter that follows the tick bite by 3 to 21 days and precedes the onset of arthritis by weeks or months. The early cutaneous lesions may resemble urticaria and are often located in groin or axillae. They do not involve the palms, soles, or mucous membranes. Although the cutaneous manifestations of the disease may progress through a number of recurrences, initial signs and symptoms generally resolve within 1 month. Only about one third of the children give a history of a tick bite at the site of the initial lesion. Multiple secondary and migratory lesions develop within the first week in about half the patients. Often, these are smaller than the initial ECM, are not associated with tick bites, and are less likely to become vesicular, indurated, or necrotic. Other mucocutaneous lesions including a malar rash and conjunctivitis may develop. A late manifestation is acrodermatitis chronica atrophicans, which has been primarily described in Europe.

The spectrum of Lyme disease includes carditis, neurologic disease, and arthritis. Cardiovascular abnormalities occur within the initial 4 to 6 weeks after onset and include atrioventricular block, pericarditis, cardiomegaly, and left ventricular dysfunction. Cardiac disease usually runs a brief course of up to 6 weeks and seldom recurs.

The initial neurologic abnormalities generally resolve within 3 months. These consist primarily of meningitis, cranial neuropathy, and peripheral radiculopathy. Other variable signs and symptoms of central or peripheral nervous system disease may be present. The cerebrospinal fluid shows a mononuclear pleocytosis, slight elevation of the protein level, and a normal glucose concentration. The neurologic disease correlates with high antibody titers to the *Borrelia* spirochete. In 10% of patients, there is a late recurrence of CNS symptoms or peripheral neuritis including demyelinating disease or psychiatric illness years after onset.

Arthropathy follows the initial ECM by a few weeks to 2 years in about 80% of the children. Migratory arthralgia is characteristic initially. Recurrent attacks of asymmetric oligoarthritis occur months after onset of the illness and typically involve large joints such as the knees, although both large and small joints may be affected. A minority of children may have symmetric polyarthritis. The initial episodes of arthritis resolve in 2 to 4 weeks, but a child may experience exacerbations over several years. The synovial fluid white cell count is elevated to as high as 100,000/mm$^3$ with the polymorphonuclear leukocyte as the predominant cell. Synovial fluid protein concentration is increased and the complement level is decreased. In a small percentage of children (10%), arthritis involving the large joints becomes chronic with subsequent appearance of radiologic erosions of cartilage and bone. The severity of the musculoskeletal disease and the risk of erosive arthritis appear to be immunogenetically related to HLA-DR2. CNS and cardiovascular symptoms also may be more severe in children with this alloantigen.

## Antibody Titers

Specific IgM antibody titers against the spirochete reach a peak between the third and sixth week after the appearance of ECM. IgG antibody titers rise more slowly, are highest months after onset, and correspond to the time of the appearance of the arthropathy. The presence of an antibody titer in the diagnostic range is particularly important in differentiating Lyme disease from other rheumatic syndromes. Borderline results should be confirmed by Western blot analysis.

During the initial phases of illness, circulating immune complexes are present along with elevated IgM levels and IgM-containing cryoglobulins. There is a direct correlation between these observations and the severity and frequency of later CNS, cardiac, and joint involvement. The serum IgM concentration parallels disease activity in the neurologic and cardiac systems, but may return to near normal levels at the onset of the arthritis. At that point, immune complexes are present in the synovial fluid but often are not detectable in the serum. Complement levels in the synovial fluid are depressed although serum complement concentrations often are elevated as acute-phase reactants. Tests for rheumatoid factors and antinuclear antibodies are usually negative.

## Treatment

Oral tetracycline, 250 mg four times a day for 10 to 20 days, is the preferred treatment early in the illness for children older than 9 years. Doxycycline offers the advantage of twice-a-day administration and less concern over inactivation by food. In young children, phenoxymethyl penicillin 50 mg/kg/d in divided doses for 10 to 20 days or erythromycin 30 mg/kg/d are satisfactory alternatives. Established Lyme arthritis, a relapse, or major late complications such as meningitis or neuropathy may occur after early treatment. Intravenous penicillin-G, 20 million units a day in divided doses for 10 days, or ceftriaxone is the recommended therapy for those complications.

## SYSTEMIC LUPUS ERYTHEMATOSUS

Systemic lupus erythematosus (SLE) is a multisystemic disease in which widespread inflammatory involvement of the connective tissues and immune-complex vasculitis occur. It is a prototypic example of autoimmunity in humans that results from abnormal immunologic hyperreactivity and an immunogenetic predisposition to the disease.

### TABLE 15-7. Clinical Course of Lyme Disease

| Time from Onset | Organ System | Clinical Manifestation |
|---|---|---|
| Early (1 d to 1 mo) | Cutaneous | ECM |
| | | Lethargy/fatigue |
| | | Fever/chills |
| | | Headache |
| Intermediate (½ mo to 5 mo) | Cardiac | Syncope |
| | | Pericarditis |
| | | Congestive failure |
| | Neurologic | Meningoencephalitis |
| | | Cranial neuritis |
| | | Polyradiculitis |
| | Ophthalmologic | Uveitis |
| | Musculoskeletal | Arthalgia |
| | | Myalgia |
| Late (5 mo to 1 y) | Cutaneous | Acrodermatitis chronica atrophicans |
| | Neurologic | Demyelinating and psychiatric illness |
| | Musculoskeletal | Oligoarthritis |

## Pathogenesis

A number of environmental, hereditary, and immunogenetic factors are implicated in the pathogenesis of this autoimmune disorder. The F1 hybrid of New Zealand black and white mice develops an SLE-like disease with early onset of renal failure, more marked in females than males. Household dogs also develop an SLE-like illness, and, identical to their mouse counterparts, have circulating antibodies to native DNA and immune-complex deposition in tissues.

Environmental triggers such as excessive sun exposure, drug reaction, or an infection may precipitate the onset of SLE. The basic pathogenesis of SLE appears to be an immunologic abnormality of homeostatic control affecting nuclear and cytoplastic antigens. Antibodies found in children with SLE include those that are tissue-specific as well as those that are related to nuclear antigens. These antibodies result in some manifestations of the disease such as acute hemolytic anemia, thrombocytopenia, leukopenia, and bleeding diathesis, and in antigen-antibody complex deposition that results in systemic vasculitis and lupus nephritis. There are also impaired cell-mediated immunity and T-suppressor cell dysfunction.

Another connective tissue disease or an abnormal marker of immunologic function (eg, serum antinuclear antibody) is present in about 10% of family members of children with SLE. SLE has occurred in identical twins. It is associated with sporadic or familial immunodeficiency such as selective IgA deficiency and inherited disorders of complement components such as heterozygous C2 deficiency. A marked immunogenetic predisposition is evident in the extended haplotype present in many of these children: HLA-B8, DR3, and C4a null.

## Clinical Manifestations

Although SLE can develop at any age, onset in children is usually after 5 years of age and becomes increasingly more common during the adolescent years. The female-to-male ratio is about 8 to 1 except in the youngest children, when relatively more boys are affected.

The manifestations of SLE are variable and present with any degree of severity from an acute, rapidly fatal illness to insidious, chronic disability with multisystemic exacerbations. In more than three fourths of the children, SLE is diagnosed within the first 6 months after onset because of the acute nature of the early illness, but diagnosis is often delayed by 4 to 5 years in the rest of the patients.

Fever, malaise, and weight loss are common (Table 15-8). Each exacerbation of the disease tends to mimic previous episodes. If serious renal disease develops, it does so within 2 years after onset. The major exception to the predictability of SLE is in the occurrence of CNS illness; CNS disease may intervene at any time in about one third of the children.

A malar erythematous rash in a butterfly distribution across the bridge of the nose and over each cheek is characteristic of an acute onset or exacerbation (Fig 15-4). Other forms of cutaneous and mucocutaneous involvement are common and varied in character and distribution. Raynaud phenomenon is frequent in SLE. It may result in digital ulceration and gangrene in a few children. Osteonecrosis, particularly of the femoral heads, is common in SLE and made worse by glucocorticoid therapy.

Arthritis affects the majority of children and commonly involves the small joints of the hands, wrists, elbows, shoulders, knees, and ankles. This arthritis is characteristically transient and may be migratory. Pain may be more severe than is suggested by objective changes. The arthritis of SLE is almost never erosive nor does it result in permanent deformity in 95% of instances.

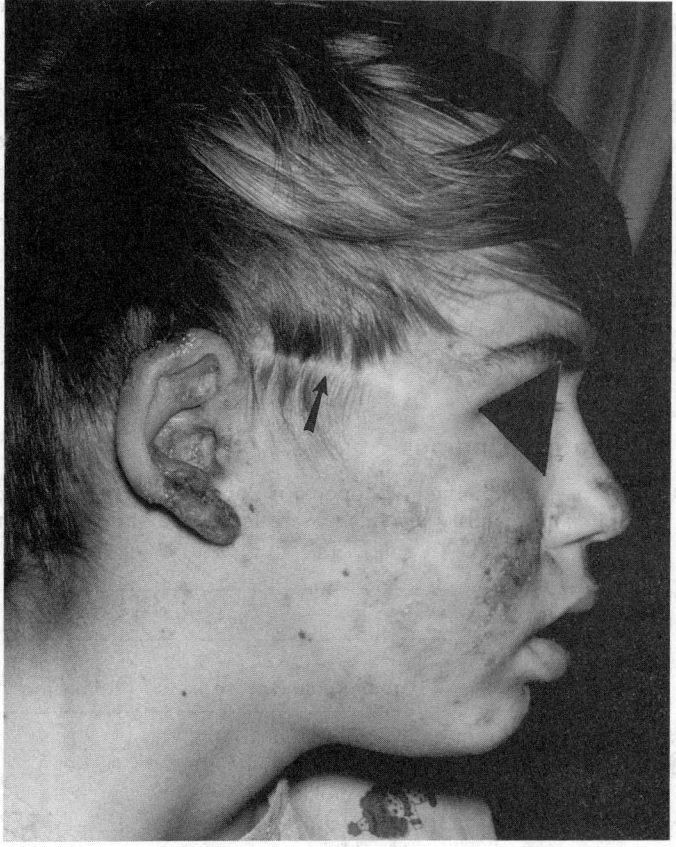

**Figure 15-4.** Excoriating erythematous facial rash of acute systemic lupus erythematosus in a 14-year-old boy. The crusting lesions are seen over the nose, malar areas, cheeks, and earlobes. The arrow points to a clear area corresponding to eyeglass frames, confirming the role of photosensitivity in the genesis of this lesion.

TABLE 15-8. Clinical Presentation and Course of SLE in Children

|  | At Onset (%) | During Course (%) |
|---|---|---|
| Nephritis | 84 | 86 |
| Hypertension | 10 | 28 |
| Arthritis | 72 | 76 |
| Dermatitis | 69 | 76 |
| Malar erythema | 51 | 56 |
| Photosensitivity | 16 | 16 |
| Alopecia | 16 | 20 |
| Oral or nasopharyngeal ulcerations | 12 | 16 |
| Pericarditis | 40 | 47 |
| Pleuritis | 31 | 36 |
| CNS disease | 9 | 31 |
| Raynaud phenomenon | 16 | 24 |
| Heptatomegaly | 43 | 47 |
| Splenomegaly | 20 | 20 |
| Positive LE cells | 86 | 100 |
| Anemia | 43 | 47 |
| Leukopenia | 60 | 71 |
| Thrombocytopenia | 22 | 24 |

*Modified from Cassidy JT, Sullivan DB, Petty RE, et al. Lupus nephritis and encephalopathy: prognosis in 58 children. Arthritis Rheum 1977;20:316*

Pericarditis is the most common manifestation of cardiac involvement. The child may also experience congestive heart failure, arrhythmias, or myocardial infarction. Valvular insufficiency develops in a few cases and a sterile verrucous endocarditis (Libman-Sacks) is particularly characteristic of SLE. Although previously reported from necropsy examinations, echocardiography has become a sensitive premortem method of confirming its presence. Pleuritis is also common and may involve the diaphragmatic pleurae along with a basilar pneumonitis. Pulmonary hemorrhage is rare but can be fatal.

Abdominal pain often presents a diagnostic dilemma in a child with SLE, especially when under treatment with glucocorticoids. Mesenteric thrombosis and acute pancreatitis are life-threatening events. Hepatomegaly and splenomegaly are common and splenic infarction may occur. Chronic active hepatitis is associated as an overlap syndrome with SLE.

Disease of the central and peripheral nervous systems are common causes of morbidity in these children. Pseudotumor cerebri may be a complication of SLE or the glucocorticoid therapy. Recurrent headaches, seizures, chorea, or frank psychosis are all encountered. Intracranial hemorrhage may result from hypertension, thrombocytopenia, or thrombosis associated with antiphospholipid antibodies. The so-called cytoid body of retinal vasculitis is often seen in disease involving the CNS or in lupus crisis. Systemic polyneuropathy, the Guillain-Barré syndrome, transverse myelopathy, or involvement of the cranial nerves have all been reported.

Some involvement of the kidneys is present in virtually all children with SLE. Even severe nephritis may not be detected early by the presence of an abnormal urinary sediment, proteinuria, or changes in the creatinine clearance. Evidence of active immune-complex disease such as increased levels of antinative DNA antibodies or hypocomplementemia correlate with active nephritis in most patients.

Lupus nephritis is categorized by the World Health Organization classification of Type I–normal, Type II–mesangial, Type III–focal proliferative, Type IV–diffuse proliferative, and Type V–membranous disease. The relation of these types of involvement to prognosis and eventual renal failure is shown in Table 15-9. Renal biopsy test is warranted in the majority of children with SLE unless there is no clinical evidence of significant involvement of the kidneys. The safest approach to long-term therapy is usually based on careful evaluation of the renal status. It is believed that serious renal lesions are more common in children with SLE than in adults, and prognosis for renal disease is more guarded.

## Laboratory Findings

Otherwise unexplained leukopenia is particularly characteristic of SLE. The majority of children are leukopenic at onset with neutrophils predominating in the peripheral count. During the course of the illness, the white blood cell count often does not become elevated to an appropriate degree even with bacteremia. Thrombocytopenia and acute hemolytic anemia may also be present. Coombs tests are often positive in these children. Other causes of anemia besides systemic disease include menorrhagia, septicemia, and gastrointestinal bleeding. SLE may present as thrombocytopenic purpura. The acute-phase indices are generally increased in active systemic disease.

Antinuclear antibodies are present in most children with SLE. They generally are found in high titer in a homogeneous pattern. A peripheral nuclear pattern is virtually synonomous with the presence of antinative DNA antibodies. Well-standardized assays for antinative DNA antibodies are critical to evaluating the degree of activity of the systemic immune-complex disease. Anti-Ro antibodies are characteristic of subacute cutaneous lupus and the neonatal lupus syndrome with congenital heart block. The LE-cell phenomenon is present in most children at onset of the disease and during acute exacerbations.

Rheumatoid factors and other antitissue antibodies such as antithyroglobulin are often positive in children with SLE. Cold agglutinins or cryoglobulins may result in peripheral anoxic phenomena. Antiphospholipid antibodies or circulating anticoagulants that cross-react with a phospholipid antigen of the Venereal Disease Research Laboratory (VDRL) test for syphilis predispose the child to repeated episodes of thrombosis. A young person with a biologic false-positive result for syphilis is at risk for development of SLE.

Components of both the classic and alternative complement pathways are consumed in the presence of active immune-complex vasculitis. The CH50 determination reflects the status of the total complement cascade; C3 concentration appears to be depressed less frequently, but a falling concentration of C4 is usually a reliable indicator of active disease. Occasionally, determination of circulating immune complexes, such as C1q binding or Raji cell assays, are useful in selected patients.

## Histopathology

An immune-complex vasculitis with fibrinoid necrosis is the basic inflammatory lesion of SLE. Vascular lesions are widespread throughout the parenchymal organs, in subdermal tissues, and on the mucosal and serosal surfaces. Soluble immune complexes are found beneath the vascular endothelium and along the dermal-epidermal junction (a positive lupus-band test).

Immune complexes are deposited in the kidney first in the mesangium, then in subendothelial areas beneath the basement membrane. This type of immunologic involvement is characteristic of focal proliferative glomerulitis, and when more extensive and severe, diffuse proliferative glomerulonephritis. In membranous disease, immune complexes are deposited along the epi-

| TABLE 15-9. Classification of Lupus Nephritis | | | | |
|---|---|---|---|---|
| Type of Renal Disease | Remission | Nephrotic Syndrome | Renal Failure | Uremic Deaths |
| Glomerular lesions | | | | |
| Mesangial | + | – | – | – |
| Focal proliferative | ++ | + | + | + |
| Diffuse proliferative | + | ++ | ++ | +++ |
| Membranous | + | +++ | ++ | + |
| Extraglomerular lesions | + | + | ++ | ++ |
| –, absent; +, minimal; ++, moderate; +++, severe. | | | | |

thelial side of the glomerular basement membrane, or, alternatively, circulating antibody forms immune complexes in situ with antigens that are fixed to that surface.

## Diagnosis

An early diagnostic suspicion that a child has SLE depends on recognizing an episodic, multisystemic constellation of clinical disease that is strongly associated with persistent ANA seropositivity. Eleven criteria have been tested by the American College of Rheumatology for the classification of SLE. These are listed in Table 15-10.

The differential diagnosis of SLE should consider JRA, other forms of acute glomerulonephritis, hemolytic anemia, leukemia, allergic or contact dermatitis, an idiopathic seizure disorder, mononucleosis, acute rheumatic fever with carditis, and septicemia. SLE remains today as the great masquerader!

## Treatment

Long-term supportive care of the child with SLE should include adequate nutrition, fluid and electrolyte balance, early recognition and treatment of infections, and control of hypertension. Fevers and potential infection should be attended promptly. Pneumonitis, septicemia and pyelonephritis are of particular concern.

Because SLE is a serious disease, a child with SLE benefits from contact with the same medical team over the course of the illness. The team should emphasize rationale supporting the treatment program and encourage prophylactic measures of avoiding excessive sunlight, unnecessary drug exposures, and transfusion. Appropriate clothing and sunscreens are prescribed. The child's general activities and interactions with peer groups should not be restrained unnecessarily.

Selected anti-inflammatory drugs are useful in treating minor manifestations of SLE such as arthralgia and myalgia. Hydroxychloroquine is an adjunctive medication that controls dermatitis

---

**TABLE 15-10. Criteria for Classification of Systemic Lupus Erythematosus***

Malar (butterfly) rash
Discoid-lupus rash
Photosensitivity
Oral or nasal mucocutaneous ulcerations
Nonerosive arthritis
Nephritis
    Proteinuria >0.5 g/d
    Cellular casts
Encephalopathy
    Seizures
    Psychosis
Pleuritis or pericarditis
Cytopenia
Positive immunoserology
    Antibodies to nDNA
    Antibodies to Sm nuclear antigen
    Positive LE-cell preparation
    Biologic false-positive test for syphilis
Positive antinuclear antibody test

\* Four of 11 criteria provide a sensitivity of 96% and a specificity of 96% for SLE.

*Adapted from Tan EM, Cohen AS, Fries JF, et al. The 1982 revised criteria for the classification of systemic lupus erythematosus. Arthritis Rheum 1982;25: 1271.*

---

or moderates glucocorticoid dosage. Glucocorticoid drugs are the mainstay of the basic regimen for children with this disease. Prednisone is the preferred analogue. A negative purified protein derivative (PPD) test for tuberculosis should be verified before a child is started on prednisone. The minimum prednisone dose possible is initiated at onset and maintained during the course of the disease to achieve the goals of the treatment program. Low-dose therapy, defined as 0.5 mg/kg/d in divided dosage, is used to treat noninfectious fever, dermatitis, arthritis, or serositis. These manifestations usually are suppressed promptly. Weeks are often required for improvement in anemia or the serologic tests reflecting active immune-complex disease. Low-dose glucocorticoid programs often control clinical disease in children with mesangial or focal glomerulonephritis.

High-dose prednisone therapy, defined as 1 to 2 mg/kg/d in divided doses, is employed for lupus crisis, CNS disease, acute hemolytic anemia, or the more severe forms of nephritis. Hypertension, azotemia, and preexisting psychosis are relative contraindications to prolonged high-dosage regimens. Results of treatment are monitored by the clinical course of the child and by periodic assessment of anti-native DNA antibodies and serum complement levels. Exacerbation of the disease during a steroid taper is signaled by a deterioration of the serologic indices. Although still a controversial matter, the precise glucocorticoid program and consideration of specific immunosuppressive drugs are often predicated on the classification of the renal disease determined by biopsy interpretation.

Intravenous pulse therapy with methylprednisolone may be used in an acute exacerbation of the disease to avoid increasing the daily steroid prescription. Immunosuppressive agents in addition to prednisone are necessary in some children. Although azathioprine has been employed extensively, recent data suggest that intravenous pulse cyclophosphamide is preferable, especially in children with severe nephritis. Dialysis and kidney transplantation have been successfully used in end-stage renal disease.

## Course and Prognosis

Prognosis in children with SLE has improved substantially during the past 25 years. Therefore, there is a guardedly optimistic attitude toward this disease. It is estimated that 85% to 90% of children with SLE will survive over a 10-year period. The most recent data from Minnesota indicate an overall outcome in this range with a survivorship in children with diffuse proliferative glomerulonephritis of 70% at 10 years. Infection has replaced severe nephritis and CNS disease as the leading cause of death in children with SLE. Malignant hypertension, gastrointestinal bleeding or perforation, acute pancreatitis, and pulmonary hemorrhage are also serious complications of the disease or its treatment.

SLE is characterized by repeated exacerbations and remissions; active disease is often prolonged over many years. Generalizations concerning prognosis for a specific child are especially unwise during the first 1 to 2 years after diagnosis. Later, a more reliable estimate can be offered the family based on the degree of systemic activity and its response to therapy and on the severity of nephritis, systemic vasculitis, and parenchymal organ involvement. Prognosis for life or function is poorest in diffuse proliferative nephritis or the organic brain syndrome and is best in minimal systemic disease, mesangial nephritis, and with a prompt sustained response to glucocorticoid therapy.

## DRUG-INDUCED SLE

In some children, acute SLE is precipitated or preceded by a drug reaction. Agents that are most frequently implicated are hydralazine, isoniazid, penicillin, sulfonamides, and the anticonvulsant medications. The most frequent clinical manifestations in drug-induced SLE are cutaneous and pleuropericardial. In most instances, drug-induced SLE is a self-limited illness that abates on withdrawal of the offending agent. Antibodies to native DNA are not present, but anti-DNA-histone reactivity is characteristic. The serum complement concentration remains normal, and CNS disease and nephritis are uncommon.

In children the anticonvulsant drugs, such as phenlhydantoin, mephenytoin, trimethadione, and ethosuximide have been the most frequently implicated in drug-induced SLE. Although the precise immunologic mechanisms have not been elucidated, some of these medications such as hydralazine may sensitize cutaneous DNA to degradation by ultraviolet light. A drug reaction may also precipitate SLE that is indistinguishable from idiopathic disease.

## LUPUS PHENOMENA IN THE NEWBORN PERIOD

A child born of a mother with active SLE may develop a neonatal lupus-like syndrome within the first few days of life from the transplacental passage of maternal IgG antinuclear antibodies. These infants have positive antinuclear antibody tests, LE-cell phenomena, and depressed complement levels. In the majority, there is no associated clinical disease and the serologic abnormalities abate within the first few months of life. In some infants, malar erythema or discoid lupus-like lesions develop. Thrombocytopenia may be present along with mild hemolytic anemia or leukopenia. SLE may recur in young adults who had transient manifestations of neonatal lupus.

Another neonatal lupus syndrome is the development of congenital heart block. Other cardiac abnormalities may be present including endomyocardial fibroelastosis. About one third of infants with congenital heart block are born of mothers who have SLE or who eventually develop SLE. The primary immunologic characteristic is the presence of anti-Ro (SS-A) antibody that is directed against a small cytoplasmic RNA-protein complex and binds to fetal cardiac epitopes. This antibody, and in some cases antibody to La (SS-B), has been found in every child and mother studied with this syndrome.

## MIXED CONNECTIVE TISSUE DISEASE

Mixed connective tissue disease (MCTD) was originally described in adults by Sharp and associates, but has been reported now in more than 75 children. This is an overlap syndrome that combines elements of JRA, dermatomyositis, scleroderma, and SLE with the presence of very high titers of antinuclear antibodies to an extractable nuclear antigen (ENA). This autoimmune reactivity is related to a ribonucleoprotein specificity (RNP) and specifically to antibodies to small nuclear $U_1RNP$.

MCTD was originally described as an autoimmune disease of unknown etiology with a consistently good prognosis. Rarely did life-threatening systemic disease involving the lungs, heart, gastrointestinal tract, or kidneys develop. An excellent response to low-dose glucocorticoid therapy was expected. A 10-year follow-up of adults, however, suggested that long-term prognosis was not so favorable. MCTD frequently progressed into a more scleroderma-like disease with sclerodactyly, gastrointestinal involvement, and pulmonary disease most prominent. Or, MCTD progressed into a course more typical of SLE. Even in the late stages of the disease, nephritis remained infrequent.

## SJÖGREN'S SYNDROME

The diagnosis of Sjögren's syndrome is based on a triad of findings: (1) the sicca syndrome (dry eyes and dry mouth), (2) a connective tissue disease, usually SLE or scleroderma, and (3) high titers of autoantibodies, usually rheumatoid factors or antinuclear antibodies.

Sjögren's syndrome (SS) can be divided into a primary disease in which a defined connective tissue disease is not present and a secondary disease in which a connective tissue disease is prominent. The secondary form of the disorder is far less common in children with a rheumatic disease such as JRA or SLE than in adults. The primary disorder has been reported in children as young as 5 years old. It is much more common in girls than boys.

The sicca component is the dominant symptomatic feature in SS and is directly related to lymphocytic infiltration of the lacrimal and salivary glands. There may be more widespread involvement of the entire upper respiratory tract, larynx, stomach, and genitourinary system. Even the primary syndrome is a multisystemic disorder that often involves many organ systems (Table 15-11). It is insidious in onset in many patients and slowly progressive. In children, although rare, it may present as recurrent bilateral parotid swelling.

Patients with SS may have achlorhydria or develop pancreatitis, hepatobiliary disease, chronic active hepatitis, or evidence of active vasculitis. Renal tubular abnormalities related to hypergammaglobulinemia or lymphocytic infiltration may be present and result in renal tubular acidosis. Hyposthenuria unresponsive to vasopressin occurs with decreased permeability of the distal convoluted tubules and collecting ducts to water. Other patients develop chronic interstitial nephritis.

**TABLE 15-11.  Associated Features of Sjögren's Syndrome**

**Sicca Complex**
Bilateral parotid enlargement
Hasimoto thyroiditis
Lymphoid myositis
Achlorhydria
Hyposthenuria and renal tubular acidosis
Hepatomegaly
Pancreatitis
Celiac syndrome

**Connective Tissue Disease**
Systemic lupus erythematosus
Vasculitis
Raynaud phenomenon
Nonthrombocytopenic purpura
Chronic active hepatitis

**Autoantibodies**
Rheumatoid factors
Antinuclear antibodies
LE-cell phenomenon
Antibodies to SS-A, SS-B, and RAP
Antisalivary duct antibodies
Antitissue antibodies

**Malignancy**
Pseudolymphoma
Lymphoma
Macroglobulinemia

## Laboratory Findings

Anemia and thrombocytopenia may be present but are usually not impressive. About one third of the patients have persistent leukopenia. A striking polyclonal hypergammaglobulinemia is almost always present. All patients have high titers of rheumatoid factors or other autoantibodies such as antinuclear antibodies. A speckled or nucleolar pattern frequently is found.

Most individuals with SS have circulating antibodies directed against small nuclear or cytoplasmic RNP antigens that are termed SS-A (Ro), and SS-B (La). These antigens can be extracted from continuously growing human lymphocytoid cell lines. Rheumatoid arthritis precipitin (RAP) is often present. About 15% of patients have positive LE cell preparations even in the absence of overt SLE. Other antitissue antibodies are found in 40% of patients including antiparietal cell and antithyroid antibodies.

Pathophysiologically, SS appears to be an extreme example of uncontrolled B-cell hyperactivity to a variety of antigens in conjunction with decreased T-cell responsiveness and suppression. Skin tests for delayed hypersensitivity are impaired and in vitro measures of lymphocyte transformation are decreased. The HLA antigens B8 and DR3 are strongly associated with development of this syndrome. Histopathologically, there is widespread infiltration in the parenchymal organs and the salivary and lacrimal glands by lymphocytes and mononuclear cells, and, to a lesser extent, plasma and reticulum cells. In some cases, germinal follicle formation is seen within the glands, and atrophy and obliteration of secretory acini develop. An important diagnostic feature of SS on salivary gland biopsy interpretation is the proliferation of ductal lining cells forming epimyoepithelial islands. It is often this feature that helps distinguish benign SS from malignant infiltration of these glands.

SS per se, however, is not always a benign disorder. At least in adults, pseudolymphoma and lymphoma may develop during its course and are particularly prone to occur in patients who do not have an overt connective tissue disease. In this regard, SS is remarkably similar to the spontaneous autoimmune disease observed in the New Zealand White/Black hybrid mouse.

## Diagnosis

Diagnosis is made by demonstrating the cardinal features of the sicca complex. A Schirmer test indicates decreased wetting of a filter paper strip placed in the conjunctival sac. Sialography with contrast media or scintigraphy of the salivary glands with $^{99m}Te$ are positive. Diagnosis may be confirmed by biopsy of the labial mucosa to demonstrate the characteristic round-cell infiltration in the minor salivary glands.

## Treatment

Treatment of the sicca complex is primarily symptomatic. The child may benefit from the use of artificial tears, saline nasal douches, or the use of sour lemon drops to provide relief from the xerostomia. Glucocorticoid and immunosuppressive agents can be considered if life-threatening complications occur. When SS is secondary to an established connective tissue disease, treatment is directed toward that disorder.

## DERMATOMYOSITIS

A classification of idiopathic inflammatory myositis is presented in Table 15-12. Dermatomyositis in children is characterized by nonsuppurative inflammation of striated muscle and skin. These multisystemic findings are accompanied early in its course by an immune-complex vasculitis and late by development of calcinosis.

TABLE 15-12. Classification of Inflammatory Myositis

Polymyositis
Dermatomyositis
Dermatomyositis or polymyositis with malignancy
Dermatomyositis with onset in childhood
Acute rhabdomyolysis
Polymyositis with Sjögren's or overlap syndrome

## Frequency and Age of Onset

Dermatomyositis occurs in about 5% of newly referred children to a pediatric rheumatology clinic. The disease is slightly more common in girls than boys at a ratio of about 1.6 to 1. The disease can present at any age, but onset is especially common from the 4th to 10th year.

## Etiology

Current investigations suggest that dermatomyositis is autoimmune in pathogenesis with both humoral and cell-mediated abnormalities. Immune-complex disease may be an initiating or perpetuating event. Immunoglobulins and complement are deposited in the walls of small blood vessels and in the skeletal muscles. There may be an immunogenetic predisposition to the development of dermatomyositis as HLA-B8 and DR3 may be increased in frequency in this disorder. Dermatomyositis has also occurred in patients with selective IgA deficiency and C2-complement component deficiency.

Dermatomyositis has developed after infections, vaccination, hypersensitivity reactions to drugs, and sunburn. A number of studies indicate that Coxsackie B-virus or toxoplasmosis may play a role in onset. An acute transient inflammatory myositis has been observed in otherwise normal children after certain viral infections, especially influenza A and B. A similar myositis has been described in a few children with agammaglobulinemia in association with ECHO-virus infection.

## Pathology

The initial lesion is an acute patchy inflammatory round-cell infiltration in striated muscle, skin, or gastrointestinal tract. Degeneration of striated muscle of all fiber types and accompanying regeneration follow with a moderate variation in fiber size observed on histologic specimens. Interstitial connective tissue and fat replace areas of focal necrosis during healing.

The nature and extent of immune-complex necrotizing vasculitis are important prognostic factors in the survival of children with dermatomyositis. Arterioles, capillaries, and venules are involved and lead to infarction, ulceration, and diffuse bleeding, especially in the gastrointestinal tract. Additional distinctive features associated with a noninflammatory, obliterative vasculopathy are related to a poorer prognosis associated with cutaneous ulcerations. Diffuse linear and occasionally granular deposits of IgM, C3d, and fibrin are found in the areas of noninflammatory vasculopathy.

Nail-fold capillary loop abnormalities are present in half the children with dermatomyositis and show simultaneous dilation of isolated loops, dropout of surrounding vessels, and an arborized cluster of peripheral capillary loops. These changes, like the noninflammatory vasculopathy, correlate prognostically with more severe, chronic, steroid-unresponsive disease.

Smooth muscle is not primarily affected in dermatomyositis. The heart is uncommonly involved. A few children have been described with focal myocardial fibrosis and contraction-band necrosis.

## Diagnostic Criteria

Dermatomyositis is diagnosed on the basis of an acute onset of proximal girdle muscle weakness accompanied by a characteristic dermatitis (Table 15-13). Polymyositis, or inflammatory myositis without dermatitis, is rarely encountered in children.

In the differential diagnosis of dermatomyositis, there is little confusion with the acute systemic onset of JRA or with SLE. Mild forms of dermatomyositis with a prominent degree of arthritis, however, may be confused with either of these two diseases. Scleroderma presents unique diagnostic problems in that about one fifth of the children present with a primary myositis not unlike that seen in dermatomyositis. An occasional child develops an overlap syndrome with varying features of the other connective tissue diseases. Eosinophilic fasciitis and mixed connective tissue disease are distinctive syndromes within this category.

The muscular dystrophies are diagnostic considerations in early disease. In these disorders, there should be an insidious onset, progressive or remitting disease, a positive family history, and a selective, predictable pattern of muscle involvement. Dermatitis and nail-fold capillary abnormalities are absent. The serum creatine kinase is increased in first degree relatives of children with muscular dystrophy and especially in the mothers of children with X-linked disorders. Other congenital myopathies, myotonias, and hypotonic syndromes, the metabolic and endocrine myopathies, paroxysmal myoglobulinuria, thyrotoxic myopathy, and myasthenia gravis must also be considered.

Poliomyelitis and the Guillain-Barré syndrome are other diagnostic possibilities in addition to influenza, Coxsackie, and ECHO-virus disease. Trichinosis and toxoplasmosis cause myositis of varying severity and severe pustular acne may be associated with inflammation of muscle. Rhabdomyolysis may follow an acute infection, trauma, or extreme muscular excretion. The acute onset is characterized by profound weakness, myoglobinuria, and, occasionally, oliguria and renal failure.

## Clinical Presentation and Course

Table 15-14 lists characteristic clinical features of dermatomyositis in children. Most patients have prominent constitutional symptoms of fatigue, malaise, weight loss, anorexia, and low-grade fever. Unexplained fever may be the circumstance that prompts referral to a physician. The proximal limb-girdle muscles of the lower extremities are affected initially. The shoulder girdle and proximal arm muscles are next most frequently involved. The child may be unable to hold the head upright or maintain a sitting posture because of weakness of the anterior neck flexors and back muscles. The distal muscles of the extremities may be involved later in the disease or in children with an acute onset. The affected child may stop walking, may be unable to dress or climb stairs, or may complain of muscle pain. The affected muscles

### TABLE 15-13.   Diagnostic Criteria for Dermatomyositis

Progressive symmetric weakness of proximal limb-girdle and anterior neck flexor muscles

Classic dermatitis of eyelids, metacarpophalangeal and proximal interphalangeal joints, elbows, knees, and medial malleoli

Elevation of serum muscle enzymes

EMG demonstration of myopathy and denervation

Muscle biopsy showing inflammatory myositis

### TABLE 15-14.   Clinical Features Associated With Dermatomyositis in Childhood

Muscle weakness
   Proximal pelvic girdle (95%)
   Proximal shoulder girdle (75%)
   Neck flexors (60%)
   Pharyngeal muscles (30%)
   Distal muscles of the extremities (30%)
   Facial and extraocular muscles (5%)
Muscle contractures and atophy (60%)
Muscle pain and tenderness (50%)
Skin lesions (85%)
   Heliotrope rash of eyelids
   Malar rash
   Subcutaneous and periorbital edema
   Periungual and articular rash (Gottron papules)
Raynaud phenomenon (20%)
Arthritis and arthralgia (25%)
Dysphagia, other GI symptoms (10%)
Calcinosis (40%)
Pulmonary fibrosis (5%)

are occasionally edematous and indurated. There is usually a pronounced inability to get up off the floor unaided or out of bed.

Ten percent of children with dermatomyositis develop involvement of the pharyngeal, hypopharyngeal, and palatal muscles. Dysphonia and difficulty swallowing may be related to this involvement and also to esophageal hypomotility. Palatal speech or regurgitation of liquids through the nose are early signs of impending respiratory difficulty. These children are at risk for aspiration. Profound involvement of the thoracic and respiratory muscles is seen in a few children and leads to increasing dyspnea at rest, aspiration, or death.

The classic rash of dermatomyositis is seen most of the children; in the remainder it is less characteristic but suggests the diagnosis (Fig 15-5). The severity of cutaneous involvement is

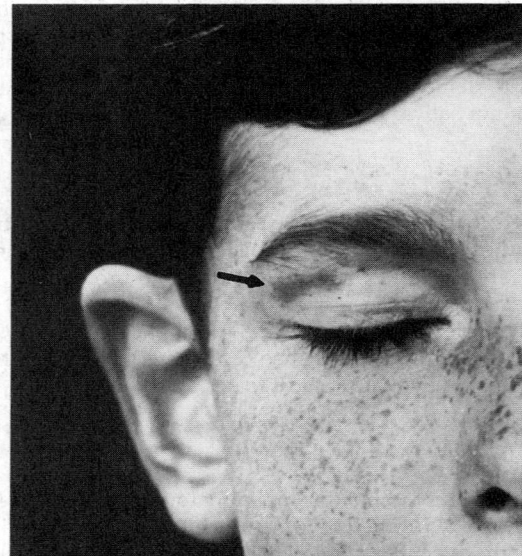

**Figure 15-5.**   The arrow points to the violaceous suffusion of the upper eyelid in a boy with active juvenile dermatomyositis.

variable and may be the first sign of the disease. It is most distinctive over the upper eyelids, malar areas, and the dorsal surfaces of the knuckles, elbows, and knees. Often at onset of the disease, there is indurative edema of the skin and subcutaneous tissues. Later, there is thinning and atrophy of the accessory epidermal structures with loss of hair and development of telangiectases. Vasculitic ulcers at the corners of the eyes, around the axillae, and over stretch marks may become serious.

The course of dermatomyositis often is divided into four characteristic clinical phases (Table 15-15). About 75% of children with dermatomyositis pursue a uniphasic course that lasts from 8 months to 2 years. The remaining 25% continue to have acute exacerbations and remissions; about half of these patients eventually develop a clinical disease more typical of systemic vasculitis. A small number of children late in the course assume more of the characteristics of scleroderma with profound sclerodactyly and cutaneous atrophy. Other children, even years after onset, have persistent elevations of serum muscle enzymes and demonstrate characteristic histopathologic features of the disease if muscle biopsies are performed.

## Laboratory Abnormalities

The acute-phase reactants such as the erythrocyte sedimentation rate (ESR) and C-reactive protein determination tend to correlate with the degree of clinical inflammation. Anemia is uncommon at onset except in the child with gastrointestinal bleeding. Urinalysis is generally normal except in the few children with microscopic hematuria. Serum antinuclear antibodies are variably present in these children, and specific antibodies such as to the PM antigen have been described. Half the affected children at onset have positive tests for circulating immune complexes.

The three most important diagnostic laboratory abnormalities are elevated serum muscle enzyme levels, which are present in 98% of the children, abnormal electromyographic changes in 96%, and specific histopathologic abnormalities on muscle biopsy in 79%. The levels of the serum muscle enzymes are important for diagnosis and in monitoring effective therapy. Generally, a panel of the creatine kinase, AST, and aldolase is followed. The amount of increase in serum concentrations ranges from 20 to 40 times normal for the creatine kinase (CK) or AST. The appearance of MB bands on the isozyme pattern of serum creatine kinase in children with dermatomyositis is usually interpreted as evidence of regenerative striated muscle and not of cardiac damage.

Electromyography (EMG) helps confirm the diagnosis of dermatomyositis in some children and helps determine the best site for a muscle biopsy. EMG changes are those of myopathy and denervation. MRI is also abnormal in those children and distinguishes between unaffected and affected muscles.

Although not often necessary for diagnosis, a muscle biopsy generally is indicated in the initial assessment of a child to support long-term glucocorticoid therapy or, eventually, immunosup-

pressive drugs. The muscle to be examined should be clinically involved but not atrophied. The best sites are generally a deltoid or quadriceps. The biopsy should be generous (2 cm) and usually is performed best by the open technique. Experience, however, is increasing with closed needle biopsy tests for diagnosis or at least for follow-up assessment.

## Treatment

General supportive care and a coordinated team approach are necessary to manage this serious disease in children. Treatment should include a program of graduated rest and positioning along with physical therapy to minimize contractures. Generally, it is necessary to use prednisone in a dosage of about 2 mg/kg/d in divided doses for at least the first month after diagnosis. If clinical response is acceptable and the serum muscle enzyme concentrations decrease, then a lower dosage in the range of 1 mg/kg/d is instituted. Thereafter, the prednisone is slowly tapered by frequent monitoring of improvement in the clinical status of the child, the degree of muscle weakness documented by objective testing, and the serum muscle enzyme concentrations. Myositis is not controlled satisfactorily until serum muscle enzymes return to normal (or nearly normal) levels and stay there while the steroid is tapered during an increase in the child's prescribed level of physical activity. Because long-term steroid administration is accompanied by significant toxicity in growing children, the glucocorticoid dose should be lowered as quickly as possible concomitant with continued improvement in indices of the disease.

Acute gastrointestinal complications are seen in a minority of children and may not be well controlled by glucocorticoid therapy. These complications have been an important cause of death. Respiratory insufficiency with or without aspiration is often a preterminal event. Cutaneous ulcerations are seen in a number of children and are likewise poor prognostic signs. During the course of the disease, progressive healing of the myositis and the extent of the rash may not correlate. These acute complications along with disease that is steroid-unresponsive are indications for the use of immunosuppressive agents. Methotrexate has been successful in resistant children. Intravenous cyclophosphamide and steroid-pulse therapy have also been used.

Long-term survival in dermatomyositis approaches 90%. If death occurs, it is often within the first years after onset. This observation suggests that the major factors to be assessed in estimating prognosis are the basic nature of the inflammatory disease, its early treatment and response, and whether vasculopathy is present, or if there is involvement of organ systems such as the gastrointestinal or pulmonary tracts.

The average child with dermatomyositis is expected to improve progressively to full functional recovery (Table 15-16). While the child heals, physical therapy is intensified to normalize function and minimize development of contractures secondary to muscle weakness or atrophy. Muscle strengthening exercises should be

---

| TABLE 15-15. Clinical Phases of Dermatomyositis in Childhood |
|---|
| Prodromal period with nonspecific symptoms (weeks to months) |
| Progressive muscle weakness and rash (days to weeks) |
| Persistent weakness, rash, and active myositis (up to 2 y) |
| Recovery with residual muscle atrophy and contractures with or without calcinosis |
| *Adapted from Hanson Clin Rheum Dis 1976;2:445* |

| TABLE 15-16. Prognosis for Dermatomyositis | |
|---|---|
| Recovery with no disability | 65% |
| Minimal atrophy or contractures | 25% |
| Calcinosis* | 20% |
| Wheelchair dependence | 5% |
| Death | 7% |
| *\* Children with calcinosis are also included in the other categories.* | |

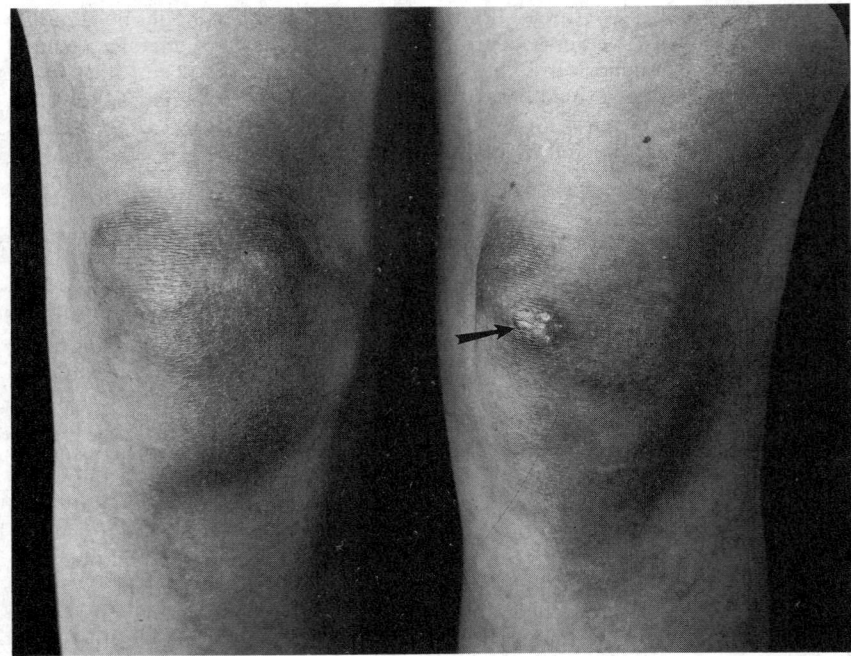

Figure 15-6. Knees of a girl with the erythematous prepatellar lesions of juvenile dermatomyosis. The arrow points to an area of calcinosis cutis.

added to the program only when acute inflammation subsides. Functional outcome appears best in children who have been seen early and treated vigorously. Most survivors function independently as adults, although some have residual atrophy of skin or muscle groups.

Late in the disease during the healing phase, about half the children develop calcinosis of the skin and subcutaneous tissues, about the joints, and within the interfascial planes of the muscles (Fig 15-6). The calcium salts have been identified as hydroxyapatite or fluorapatite. Many approaches to the therapy of calcinosis have been reported. None has been uniformly successful. Surgical excision of calcium tumors in areas of ulceration or pressure can be performed if necessary.

## SCLERODERMA

The sclerodermas are systemic or localized connective tissue diseases of unknown etiology. The development of scleroderma in a child is often unrecognized early because it is so rare. The localized forms of the disease such as morphea or linear scleroderma often are regarded as more dermatologic than rheumatologic. A classification of the sclerodermas is presented in Table 15-17. In all these disorders, girls are affected more often than boys and there is no peak age of onset during childhood.

### Systemic Disease

An idiopathic angiitis may be the basic lesion of scleroderma, and involves the lungs, heart, and kidneys in addition to the skin and gastrointestinal tract. The arterioles undergo eventual hyalinization and fibrosis. Perivascular infiltrates of mononuclear cells have been shown in some studies to be predominantly T lymphocytes. In systemic scleroderma, there is thinning of the epidermis and atrophy of the dermal appendages. There is an increased density and thickness of collagen deposition and a predominance of embryonal fibers.

Diagnostic abnormalities of the nail-fold capillaries are virtually universal at onset of the disease. Viewed through the +40 lens of an ophthalmoscope or the 100× objective of a microscope, there is a reduction in the number of vessels, thickening of vessel

walls, and a marked tortuousness and pebbling of the remaining vessels. Scattered fibrotic clear areas without capillaries are prominent. Telangiectases about the face, upper trunk, and over the hands appear during the early phases of the disease in these children as further evidence of vascular involvement.

### Clinical Manifestations

Often, there is a diagnostic delay of years in children with scleroderma because of the subtle nature of the onset. The presentation may be insidious and is characterized by the appearance of Raynaud phenomenon, thinning and atrophy of the skin of the hands or face, or the development of cutaneous telangiectases (Table 15-18). Dysphagia may be present early.

Tightening and thickening of the skin is virtually universal at onset and becomes more generalized. Acrosclerosis of the hands and feet and distal extremities is characteristic. Hypopigmentation and hyperpigmentation are present along with later development of subcutaneous calcification. Ulcerations may occur over the fingers, elbows, and malleoli. Raynaud phenomenon with a two- or three-color change occurs in most children and may antedate

| TABLE 15-17. Classification of Scleroderma |
|---|
| **Systemic Disease** |
| Scleroderma |
|    Classical |
|    CREST syndrome |
| Overlap syndromes |
|    Sclerodermatomyositis or other connective tissue diseases |
|    Mixed connective tissue disease, eosinophilic fasciitis |
| **Localized Disease** |
| Morphea |
|    Plaques |
|    Guttate disease |
|    Generalized skin involvement |
| Linear scleroderma |

TABLE 15-18. Clinical Manifestations in Children With Scleroderma

| Organ System | Frequency of Involvement (%) |
|---|---|
| Skin | |
| Ulceration | 30 |
| Subcutaneous calcification | 60 |
| Telangiectases | 30 |
| Pigmentation | 20 |
| Digital arteries (Raynaud phenomenon) | 75 |
| Musculoskeletal | |
| Contractures | 75 |
| Resorption of digital tufts | 60 |
| Muscle weakness | 40 |
| Muscle atophy | 40 |
| Gastrointestinal tract | |
| Abnormal esophageal motility | 75 |
| Colonic sacculations | 20 |
| Duodenal dilatation | 5 |
| Pulmonary tract | |
| Abnormal diffusion | 75 |
| Abnormal vital capacity | 70 |
| Heart | |
| Electrocardiographic abnormalities | 30 |
| Cardiomegaly | 15 |
| Congestive failure | 15 |

the onset of cutaneous abnormalities. Raynaud phenomenon is characterized by obstructive digital arterial disease and sympathetic hyperactivity that are often progressive. Digital gangrene may supervene with small atrophic pits on the soft surfaces of the fingertips. Radiographs of the hands or feet may show acroosteolysis of the digital tufts. This resorption is often accompanied by small areas of soft tissue calcification.

Many children have arthralgia and a few present with objective arthritis or contractures about joints. Muscle pain and tenderness are present in about 20% of patients. Elevation of the serum muscle enzyme levels, however, tends to be only mild to moderate. Cardiac involvement with arrhythmias may develop during the course of this disease and congestive heart failure is often a terminal event. Dyspnea on exertion may be related to skin tightness, intercostal muscle weakness, or intrinsic pulmonary disease. Symptomatic gastrointestinal disease is often confined to the esophagus with complaints of dysphagia or reflux esophagitis. Malabsorption may be minimal or become severe.

## Diagnosis

Diagnosis of systemic scleroderma is based on demonstration of the classic cutaneous findings of skin tightening of the face, hands, and feet, telangiectases, Raynaud phenomenon, and the presence of visceral disease, usually gastrointestinal or pulmonary. Plethysmography is abnormal in affected digits in children with Raynaud phenomenon and documents both the obstructive vascular disease and involvement of the sympathetic nervous system. Arteriography should not be performed as a diagnostic procedure because it may acutely exacerbate digital anoxia. Pulmonary diffusion and spirometry are sensitive measures of involvement of the respiratory tract. These studies are abnormal in many children at onset and progressive in a few additional patients. Upper gastrointestinal films usually document disordered motility of the

distal esophagus (Fig 15-7). Balloon esophageal motility and pH probe studies are more sensitive indicators of the degree of abnormality in these children.

The differential diagnosis includes dermatomyositis, SLE, the overlap syndromes, and, less frequently, JRA. Children with the CREST syndrome have prominent calcinosis, Raynaud phenomenon, esophageal abnormalities, sclerodactyly, and telangiectases. These patients were thought to have a more favorable prognosis; however, evidence for this judgment is not present in recent studies. Routine laboratory studies in scleroderma are often normal. Antinuclear antibodies are found in most children and on the HEp-2 cell substrate are characterized by high-titered speckled patterns. Distinct antigenic specificity may be present: anticentromere in the CREST syndrome, anti-Scl 70 (topoisomerase 1), or nucleolar antibodies.

A number of other entities mimic or duplicate abnormalities found in scleroderma. Scleroderma-like disease has developed as a toxic reaction to vinyl chloride, bleomycin, and pentazocine. It also has occurred in epidemic proportions, with many deaths in Spain secondary to contaminated cooking oil (rapeseed oil). It is occasionally encountered as a component of graft-versus-host disease in bone marrow transplant patients. Other forms of scleroderma-like changes may be seen in children with phenylketonuria and progeria.

## Treatment

Scleroderma is one of the most untreatable connective tissue diseases. Nonsteroidal anti-inflammatory drugs are useful to relieve the musculoskeletal components of this disease. Colchicine has also been tried. Children who present with gastrointestinal problems demand special consideration for esophageal stricture or obstruction, reflux esophagitis, or malabsorption.

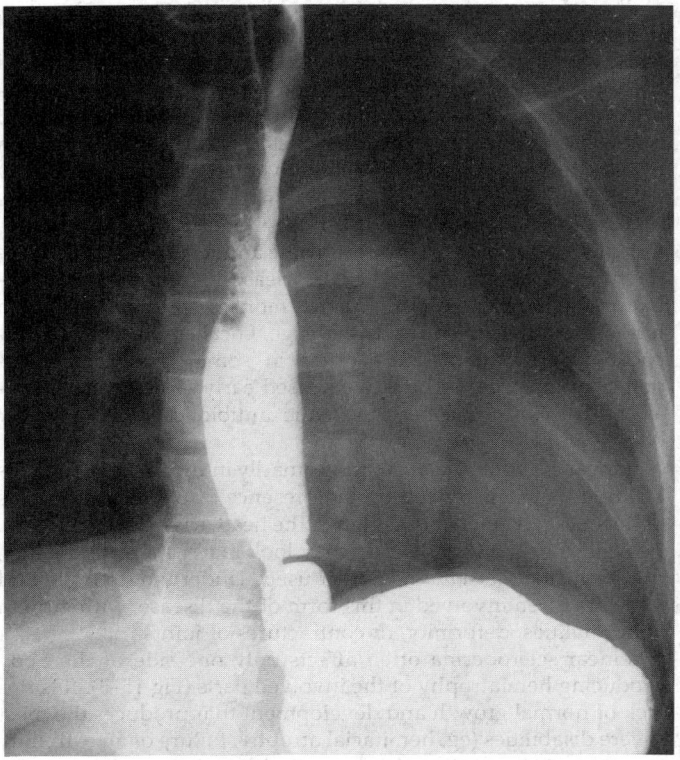

Figure 15-7. This is a barium swallow examination in the supine position of a 14-year-old girl who presented with severe dysphagia and scleroderma. The barium column collected in the patulous esophagus, which was virtually without peristaltic movement.

Raynaud phenomenon is managed with alpha-blocking agents such as phenoxybenzamine or with calcium-channel blockers such as nifedipine. Some investigators recommend early treatment of the angiitis of scleroderma by these drugs. Children with prominent Raynaud phenomenon need to dress seasonally and avoid cold liquids and objects that exacerbate not only the peripheral Raynaud disease but also vascular spasm within viscera. If prescribed early, D-penicillamine may be useful in managing cutaneous manifestations of the disease. Vigorous physical therapy to prevent contractures is important.

Glucocorticoid drugs are probably contraindicated in most of these children. They may exacerbate small blood vessel disease and renal involvement with hypertension. Renal failure and acute hypertensive encephalopathy may supervene as potentially fatal complications in a few children. As studied in adults, these events seems likely to occur early in the course of the disease. It merits emergency lowering of blood pressure to normal levels and expert intensive care management.

## Prognosis

The outcome of scleroderma is poor but has not been determined precisely because of the rarity of the disease in children. The prognosis is not judged to be any more favorable than in adults in whom survivorship at 7 years is only 35%. A child, however, may live decades after onset; therefore, an optimistic but realistic attitude should be taken in discussions with parents.

## Localized Scleroderma

Localized scleroderma is much more common than systemic disease. Fibrosis of connective tissues in morphea and linear scleroderma is limited to the dermis, subdermis, and superficial striated muscles. Morphea is subcategorized into single or multiple plaques, guttate morphea, consisting of small lesions in a generalized distribution, or extensive coalescent cutaneous involvement. In morphea, there are one or more circumscribed cutaneous lesions marked by hypopigmentation and induration surrounded by hyperpigmentation. Erythema and acute inflammatory edema are present especially at the margins. These lesions are located anywhere on the trunk or extremities. The child may complain of paresthesia or pain over the involved areas. Each lesion may enlarge centrifugally or coalesce and involve larger areas of skin.

Hide-binding from fibrosis of the involved skin and subcutaneous tissues may become extensive and result in marked contractures of an extremity. Active disease may undergo exacerbations and remissions for many months to years, although lesions tend to regress slowly with age. Local emollients and glucocorticoid ointments may result in some improvement. D-penicillamine may be effective if used early in the more generalized form of morphea. Systemic antibiotics are reportedly effective.

Linear scleroderma develops primarily in the first two decades of life. It is characterized by the presence of one or more areas of linear involvement of the skin of the head, trunk, or extremities. As lesions of the face or scalp may look like scars from dueling, the term *coup-de-sabre* has been used. Underlying muscle and bone are often involved in this form of the disease, with growth abnormalities, deformity, or contractures of joints.

Linear scleroderma often affects only one side of the body producing hemiatrophy of the involved parts (Fig 15-8). It is this lack of normal growth and development that produces the most severe disabilities (eg, hemifacial atrophy, failure of an extremity to grow in proportion to its opposite member, severe joint contractures).

There are few laboratory abnormalities in localized scleroderma. Serum antinuclear antibodies are positive in about 50%

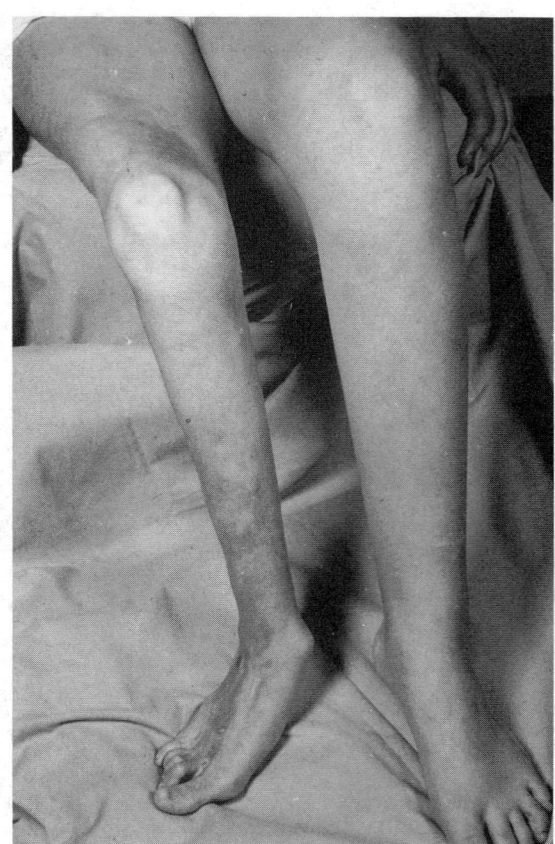

**Figure 15-8.** Severe linear scleroderma affecting the right leg of an adolescent girl. This lesion involves not just the skin but the deeper subcutaneous tissues, fascia, muscle, and bone. It had resulted in the deformity that is shown and a 7½-cm shortening of that limb. (Cassidy JT. SLE, juvenile dermatomyositis, scleroderma, and vasculitis. In Kelley WN, Harris ED Jr, Ruddy S, Sledge CB (eds). Textbook of rheumatology. Philadelphia: WB Saunders, 1993:1238.)

of the children. Antibodies to centromere or Scl-70 are generally not present in the localized forms of the disease.

Localized scleroderma may regress without treatment. Although linear lesions may improve with age, significant abnormalities of local growth persist particularly if deep tissues and bone are involved. Occasionally visceral disease or a seizure develops late in the course of the disease. A few children evolve into an overlap syndrome with another connective tissue disease such as SLE.

## EOSINOPHILIC FASCIITIS

Eosinophilic fasciitis was originally described in young adults who presented with painful inflammation and induration of cutaneous and subcutaneous tissues. This involvement occurred in upper and lower extremities, was often bilateral, and occasionally spread to the trunk or face. An acute onset of the disease was often preceded by unusual degrees of short-term physical exertion. Raynaud phenomenon, nail-fold capillary abnormalities, and visceral disease were absent.

Rare in children, the syndrome has been identified in fewer than 50 patients. These children present with marked induration of the cutaneous and subcutaneous tissues resembling that seen in scleroderma or dermatomyositis. There is controversy whether eosinophilic fasciitis is a distinct clinicopathologic entity or an unusual variant of scleroderma. Morphea may accompany or precede the disorder.

**TABLE 15-19. Classification of Primary Vasculitis**

Necrotizing vasculitis of medium and small arteries
  Polyarteritis nodosa
  Kawasaki disease
Necrotizing arteritis of small vessels
  Hypersensitivity angiitis
  Henoch-Schönlein purpura
Granulomatous vasculitis
  Allergic necrotizing granulomatosis
  Wegener's granulomatosis
Giant-cell arteritis
  Systemic giant-cell arteritis
  Takayasu arteritis
  Cranial arteritis

A remarkable eosinophilia and hypergammaglobulinemia occur in about half the children. The eosinophilia may reach the range of 40% to 60% of the peripheral white blood cell count. The ESR and other acute-phase reactants are also increased.

Diagnosis of eosinophilic fasciitis is established by a deep biopsy examination of skin, fascia, and muscle in an area of involvement. Inflammation is present in all layers, but the most characteristic feature is thickened fascia with round-cell infiltration of histiocytes and often eosinophils, and a prominent perivascular infiltrate of lymphocytes and plasma cells. IgG, IgM, and C3 may be deposited in these tissues.

Eosinophilic fasciitis originally appeared to be a self-limited disorder with spontaneous resolution after months to years, or a marked, satisfactory response to small doses of glucocorticoids. Occasionally, a more prolonged and steroid-resistant course was seen, or a more severe form of the disease evolved with hematologic abnormalities.

## VASCULITIS

Although vasculitis is a prominent component of the connective tissue diseases, this discussion describes distinct types of idiopathic vasculitis (Table 15-19). Several attempts have been made to classify the various forms of vasculitis. Table 15-20 presents a classification that accounts for the most significant features of histopathology and clinical findings. This schema is derived from the classification proposed by Zeek in 1953 and the reexamination of these diseases by a committee of the American College of Rheumatology in 1990. This classification is based on the size of the vessel involved, the distribution of the visceral involvement, and whether the predominant histopathology is necrosis of vessel wall or a granulomatous response.

In necrotizing arteritis, destruction of the vascular wall is often a direct consequence of immune-complex deposition. In most cases, the responsible antigen is unknown; however, in a few instances of classic polyarteritis nodosa, a causal relationship between hepatitis B infection and immune-complex formation has been proved. The predominant pathologic features of giant cell arteritis involve larger blood vessels and giant cells in the lesions. In Wegener's granulomatosis, the principal finding is a necrotizing granuloma.

All forms of vasculitis, except for Henoch-Schönlein purpura and Kawasaki disease, are rare in children. Hypersensitivity angiitis was more commonly encountered with the introduction of sulfonamides and penicillin.

### Necrotizing Vasculitis of Medium and Small Arteries

In necrotizing vasculitis of medium and small arteries, the medium-size muscular arteries are predominantly involved and the characteristic histologic abnormality is fibrinoid necrosis of the entire thickness of the vessel wall in all stages of development from acute to chronic. The inflammatory lesions are segmental with a predilection for vessel bifurcations. Angiography shows small aneurysms often in the celiac and renal vessels. Although each disease has characteristic features, it is not always possible clinically to distinguish among polyarteritis, hypersensitivity angiitis, and allergic granulomatosis.

#### Polyarteritis Nodosa

Early diagnosis and correct classification of polyarteritis nodosa (PAN) are often difficult. The classic form of PAN was initially described in 1866. Its course and progression are highly variable, and multisystemic disease leads to diagnostic confusion with other entities.

*Clinical Manifestations.* No single pattern of clinical presentation is characteristic, and the onset is frequently insidious.

**TABLE 15-20. Pathologic Classification of Necrotizing Vasculitis**

| | Size of Vessels | Location of Lesions and Organ Involvement | Histopathology |
|---|---|---|---|
| Polyarteritis | Small to medium-size muscular arteries, adjacent veins | Widespread near bifurcations; kidneys, gastrointestinal tract, mesentery, pancreas | Fibrinoid necrosis, aneurysms, lesions of various ages |
| Hypersensitivity angiitis | Arterioles, venules, and capillaries | Widespread; kidneys, heart, lungs, spleen, skin, serosa | Necrosis, lesions at same state of development, eosinophilic infiltration |
| Allergic granulomatosis | Small arteries and veins | Widespread; lungs, heart, spleen | Necrotizing granulomata, lesions of various ages, eosinophilic infiltration |
| Giant-cell arteritis | Large arteries | Aorta and major branches; temporal arteries | Granulomatous inflammation, no necrosis, multinucleated giant cells |
| Wegener's granulomatosis | Medium to small arteries and veins | Respiratory tract and kidneys | Necrotizing granulomata, giant cells |

*Modified from Zeek PM. N Engl J Med 1953;248:764.*

Constitutional symptoms of fever and weight loss may be the presenting complaints (Table 15-21). Renal, gastrointestinal, nervous system, and cardiac disease are often involved initially (Fig 15-9). Dermatitis, although characteristic, includes a spectrum of lesions of purpura, gangrene of the distal parts of the extremities, and erythematous, painful nodules. The initial clinical diagnosis in PAN may be renovascular hypertension or an acute abdomen. Severe, symmetric sensorimotor peripheral neuropathy (mononeuritis multiplex) is frequently observed.

*Laboratory Studies.* The level of anemia, leukocytosis, elevation of the ESR, concentration of the serum immunoglobulins, and urinary sediment changes often reflect the extent of multisystem involvement. Rheumatoid factors and antinuclear antibodies are unusual. A firm diagnosis is usually based on characteristic histological changes in a biopsy specimen or an angiogram showing multiple aneurysms.

*Treatment.* Glucocorticoid administration is the primary approach to the management of children with PAN. Prednisone is usually prescribed first in suppressive amounts in the range of 1 to 2 mg/kg/d in divided dose. The degree of cardiac or renal involvement or the presence of hypertension modulates therapeutic aggressiveness. Extensive systemic involvement, particularly of the intra-abdominal vessels with aneurysms or thrombosis, is generally an indication for the addition of cyclophosphamide.

*Prognosis.* Although the course of PAN is highly variable and fatalities do occur, death most commonly is secondary to renal failure, myocardial infarction, or hypertensive encephalopathy. Syndromes with more restricted organ involvement have a better prognosis. Cogan syndrome occurs in young adults and is characterized by ocular and inner-ear vasculitis. These patients present with interstitial keratitis, vertigo, tinnitus, and deafness. Serous otitis media may also be seen in children in association with PAN.

## Kawasaki Disease

Very young infants with a febrile illness that lasted from a few weeks to months were previously reported with a very rare syndrome referred to as *infantile polyarteritis nodosa*. This was probably the same disease as the acute febrile illness associated with systemic vasculitis affecting infants and young children that was noted by Kawasaki in 1961 in Japan. The first cases in the English literature appeared in 1974 under the designation *mucocutaneous lymph-node syndrome*. Since then, this form of vasculitis has become increasingly common in North America and Japan.

*Epidemiology.* Kawasaki disease (KD) occurs sporadically or in mini-epidemics every 2 to 3 years from fall to early spring.

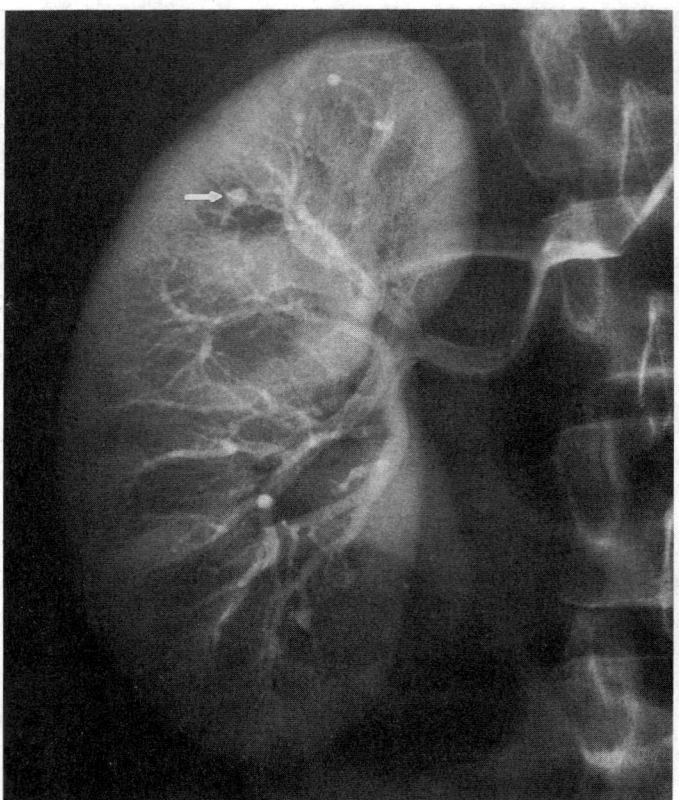

**Figure 15-9.** Renal angiogram of an adolescent boy with polyarteritis nodosa that presented with musculoskeletal aching, hypertension, and hematuria. The arrow points to an aneurysm that is characteristic of this disease.

These observations suggest that KD is incited by an infectious agent; however, secondary cases within a home are unusual. Although an immunogenetic predisposition has been suggested in Japanese studies, none has been identified in Caucasian children.

The mean age of onset is about 1½ years, and the male-to-female ratio is 1.5 to 1. The disease is more common in children of Japanese ancestry. In the United States, the risk factor for KD for those of Japanese descent is 17 times that of children of North European families. Risk for the single most important complication of KD, coronary vasculitis, is higher in boys with a very young age of onset. KD seldom occurs after the age of 7 years and rarely occurs after the age of 11 years. Adult cases have not been conclusively proven. Those that have been described may represent rare occurrences of this disease or other disorders such as toxic shock syndrome.

*Clinical Manifestations.* Clinical criteria for a diagnosis of KD established by the Japanese in 1974 are listed in Table 15-22. The disease course is divided into three phases: an acute febrile period of about 1 to 1½ weeks, a subacute phase of 2 to 4 weeks beginning with defervescence and a rise in the platelet count and ending with its return to near normal levels, and a recovery or convalescent period lasting months to years during which cardiac disease may first be noted.

Although the characteristic changes of KD may not all be present initially, fever is universal, and the correct diagnosis is often suggested at onset. The child may present with a febrile seizure, although other reasons for CNS involvement (eg, meningoencephalitis) must be carefully excluded. The fever is usually sustained and remittent, and elevations to 40°C are common; fever as high as 42°C may occur. The febrile phase lasts from 5 to 25 days with a mean of about 10 days.

| TABLE 15-21. Clinical Manifestations of Polyarteritis | |
|---|---|
| Constitutional signs and symptoms | 75% |
| Musculoskeletal involvement | 75% |
| Leukocytosis, eosinophilia | 75% |
| Dermatitis | 60% |
| Peripheral neuropathy | 40% |
| Mesenteric involvement | 40% |
| CNS disease | 30% |
| Pulmonary disease | 25% |
| Nephritis and hypertension | 25% |
| Myocardial infarction | 20% |

| TABLE 15-22. | Criteria for Diagnosis of Kawasaki Disease |
|---|---|

1. Fever lasting ≥5 d
2. Bilateral conjunctivitis
3. Changes of lips and oral cavity
    a. Dry, red, fissured lips
    b. Strawberry tongue
    c. Diffuse erythema of mucous membranes
4. Changes of peripheral extremities
    a. Erythema of palms and soles
    b. Indurative edema of hands and feet
    c. Membranous desquamation from fingertips
5. Polymorphous rash (primarily on trunk)
6. Acute nonpurulent swelling of cervical lymph node to >1.5 cm in diameter

Five criteria are required for diagnosis. One of the signs listed under 3 and 4 is sufficient to establish these criteria.
*Recommendations of the Japan MCLS Research Committee, 1974.*

A polymorphous rash accompanies the fever during the acute phase in most children and gradually resolves. Vesiculation does not occur, nor are petechiae or pruritus common. These cutaneous changes represent a vasculitis and perivasculitis of the dermis and subcutaneous tissues. Indurative edema of the hands, fingers, feet, and toes occurs within a few days of onset. Affected parts are often quite painful and the child may refuse to walk. During the subacute phase, desquamation of the skin of the extremities begins underneath and at the sides of the fingernails and toenails (Fig 15-10). These changes are most commonly seen during the third week after onset and persist for 1 to 2 weeks. Desquamation is also common elsewhere, including the perineal area and face.

Bilateral nonsuppurative conjunctivitis usually is present and persists for several weeks. Erythema of the lips with cracking and bleeding is observed in most children. Oropharyngeal erythema and a strawberry tongue (white to red) often accompany these changes and are similar to those seen in scarlet fever. Unilateral lymphadenopathy occurs in about half the children. A single, painful, enlarged cervical node is the most characteristic

finding. The lymphadenopathy disappears rapidly after the initial febrile period.

Involvement of almost any system can occur in KD. Relatively common at presentation are pneumonitis, tympanitis, meningitis, photophobia and uveitis, diarrhea, meatitis and sterile pyuria, and arthritis or arthralgia. Relatively uncommon are pleural effusion, severe abdominal colic, hydrops of the gallbladder, jaundice, or tonsillar exudate.

The extent and nature of involvement of the coronary arteries is the most important prognostic factor in KD. Early deaths and most of the long-term disability are usually related to cardiac disease. During the acute febrile phase of the disease, a universal myocarditis occurs. A variable number of children then develop coronary vasculitis, aortitis with necrosis of vessel wall, and aneurysm formation. Aneurysms of the coronary arteries may be present at onset of the disease or form as early as the second week of the illness. During the subacute period these aneurysms reach peak development, are usually multiple, and are found on average in 20% of children. In children with the risk factors for coronary aneurysms (male, age of onset less than 18 months, Japanese ancestry, and prolonged febrile course with early clinical myocarditis), frequency of aneurysms is increased to more than 50%.

Echocardiography is the most sensitive technique for delineating involvement of the proximal coronary arteries (Figs 15-11 and 15-12). Angiography in selected cases may demonstrate lesions of the peripheral cardiac vessels including narrowing or premature atherosclerotic changes. Aneurysms may be found in other arteries including the brachial, subclavian, and axillary.

The most common cause of early death in KD is myocardial infarction, which was originally described in about 2.5% of reported children and may be less frequent with early diagnosis and current therapy. This event occurs most commonly in the subacute phase of the disease. The child may die from coronary thrombosis, infarction, or rupture of an aneurysm. Giant aneurysms (more than 8mm) are especially serious prognostic developments. The extreme thrombocytosis that is observed during this phase of the illness (more than 550,000 to 1,000,000/mm$^3$) may contribute to thrombus formation on a damaged endothelium.

Close observation of the child in the hospital with cardiac monitoring is extremely important in the presence of developing,

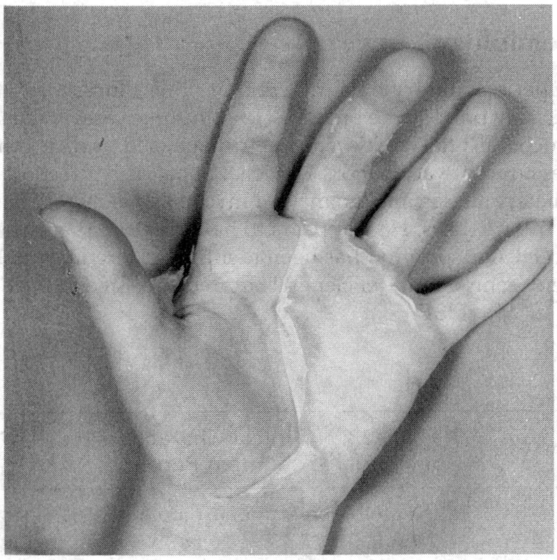

**Figure 15-10.** Hand of a 2-year-old boy in the subacute phase of Kawasaki disease. The skin of the hand is undergoing complete desquamation that started in the fingertip areas.

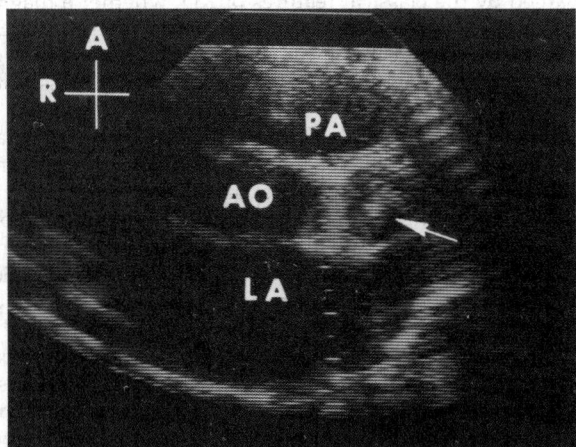

**Figure 15-11.** Echocardiogram showing pulmonary artery (PA), aorta (AO), and left atrium of the child with Kawasaki disease shown in Fig 15-10. The arrow points to increased echodensity corresponding to an aneurysm of the left coronary artery. (Cassidy JT. SLE, juvenile dermatomyositis, scleroderma, and vasculitis. In Kelley WN, Harris ED Jr, Ruddy S, Sledge CB (eds). Textbook of rheumatology. Philadelphia: WB Saunders, 1993:1241.)

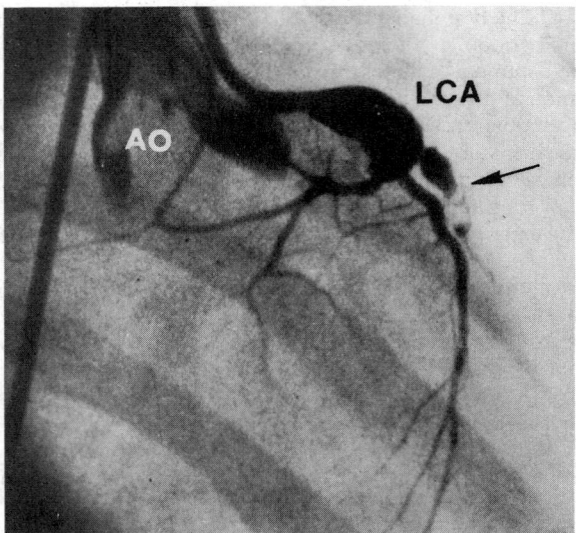

Figure 15-12.    Angiography of the child with Kawasaki disease shown in Figs 15-10 and 15-11 demonstrates a large aneurysm affecting the left coronary artery. (Cassidy JT. SLE, juvenile dermatomyositis, scleroderma, and vasculitis. In Kelley WN, Harris ED Jr, Ruddy S, Sledge CB (eds). Textbook of rheumatology. Philadelphia: WB Saunders, 1993: 1241.)

progressive, or unstable cardiac disease. Only by detecting early signs of congestive heart failure, infarction, or arrhythmia can appropriate critical measures be taken to save the life of a severely affected child. A child with established coronary artery disease may be a candidate for coronary bypass surgery.

Late death may occur in children who have had KD from coronary occlusive disease, rupture of an aneurysm several years after onset, or small blood vessel disease in the heart. Progressive myocardial dysfunction may develop secondary to these changes. Children who have survived an initial coronary insult may show extensive scar formation, arterial calcification, severe stenosis, or recanalization.

KD is now common enough that a careful history for previous KD is mandatory in all older children or young adolescents seen for pre-sport physical examinations. If a febrile illness was accompanied by the classical features of KD, whether a diagnosis of that disease was made or not, further investigation must include specific measures of cardiac function, which otherwise would not be indicated, including echocardiography and stress testing.

*Treatment.*    Treatment of KD is divided into two phases: administration of antiplatelet agents and the use of intravenous immunoglobulin. Aspirin at a level of 100 mg/kg/d in divided dose is started during the acute phase of the disease. With onset of the subacute period and thrombocytosis, lower antiplatelet doses of salicylate are substituted (eg, 5 mg/kg/d of acetylsalicylic acid). This dosage is continued for months or even years in children who have developed coronary disease or who were at risk for such involvement. Glucocorticoid drugs are contraindicated in KD because of early studies in Japan showing an increase in the frequency of coronary aneurysms in children treated with these agents compared to those receiving no therapy or treated with salicylate alone.

Intravenous immunoglobulin therapy of 400 mg/kg/d for 4 days was initially employed in controlled double-blind clinical studies and demonstrated to be effective in children with KD in reducing the incidence of giant aneurysms. In general, this therapy should be initiated within the first 10 days of the illness. The response to intravenous immunoglobulin is often dramatic with

a disappearance of fever and constitutional symptoms and a return of general well-being. Current recommendations include a single infusion of immunoglobulin of 2000 mg/kg.

## Necrotizing Vasculitis of Small Vessels

Leukocytoclastic vasculitis is a form of necrotizing vasculitis that involves the smaller blood vessels and post-capillary venules. Polymorphonuclear leukocytes infiltrate the entire vessel wall, and nuclear debris is present around the lesions. This form of vasculitis may be idiopathic or occur secondary to drug hypersensitivity, infectious endocarditis, or malignancy.

### Hypersensitivity Angiitis

Smaller blood vessels including arterioles, capillaries, and venules are the principal sites of involvement in hypersensitivity angiitis. The inflammatory lesions are at a similar stage of histologic development and eosinophiles are often prominent. The disease develops as a hypersensitivity reaction to administration of a therapeutic drug or after another systemic illness. Serum sickness is a form of this type of vasculitis. Experimental serum sickness in animals and soluble toxic immune-complex disease are laboratory counterparts of hypersensitivity angiitis. Immune complexes can be demonstrated in the circulation of many of the children and by fluorescent histopathology at the site of vascular inflammation.

Pulmonary and cutaneous disease are common in hypersensitivity vasculitis. Dermatologic lesions consist of palpable purpura or superficial hemorrhagic infarcts. The disease is characterized by a variable course often determined in large part by the presence of cardiac or renal abnormalities.

Glucocorticoids are usually effective in suppressing the clinical vasculitis and in preventing severe complications or death. Classically, this disease runs its course in about 6 weeks.

### Henoch-Schönlein Purpura

Henoch-Schönlein purpura (HSP) is the most common type of vasculitis of the small blood vessels that occurs in children and young adults and is an example of nonthrombocytopenic purpura. Table 15-23 lists the clinical characteristics of HSP. The classic purpuric rash consists of a maculopapular or purpuric eruption that affects the lower extremities and buttocks but may occur elsewhere.

## Epidemiology

An upper respiratory tract infection or other illness, often in the spring, may precede the onset of HSP. In some cases, β-hemolytic streptococcal pharyngitis has been diagnosed and in other instances a recent vaccination, varicella, hepatitis B infection, insect bite, dietary allergy, malignancy, or mycoplasmal disease has been cited. In rare cases, HSP appears to have familial predisposition, but no HLA association has been identified. Hereditary C2 complement-component deficiency is a predisposing factor in some children with HSP.

TABLE 15-23.    Clinical Characteristics of Henoch-Schönlein Purpura

Nonthrombocytopenic purpura
Arthritis
Abdominal pain
Nephritis

*Pathology.* A leukocytoclastic vasculitis is present in all affected organs with the skin, synovium, gastrointestinal tract, and renal glomeruli being most commonly involved. Arthritis may be symmetric or asymmetric and predominantly involves the large joints. Although usually painful at onset, it is always self-limited without residual damage. Submucosal hemorrhage, edema, and intramural hemorrhage are found in the gastrointestinal tract and occasionally lead to intussusception or perforation.

Clinical evidence of glomerulitis has been reported in about half of children in early studies of this disease. These patients develop microscopic hematuria within about 3 months of onset of the disease. The degree of renal involvement is from mild to severe crescentic disease and may occasionally be similar to that seen in rapidly progressive glomerulonephritis. Mesangial involvement is prominent at onset and is similar to that seen in Berger nephropathy of adults. IgA is uniformly identified in the cutaneous lesions of HSP and in the glomeruli in association with IgG and C3.

*Clinical Manifestations.* The extent of involvement of the necrotizing vasculitis determines the clinical manifestations of HSP in the skin, gastrointestinal tract, joints, and kidneys. An isolated CNS vasculitis has been described in a few children. Onset of HSP is usually acute with sequential manifestations appearing during the next few days to weeks. Purpura over the lower extremities is the first manifestation of the disease in more than half of the children. The trunk is often spared. Purpuric lesions appear in crops; some may go on to develop hemorrhage or ulceration and others mimic urticaria. The lesions may spread to form large areas of cutaneous involvement and may be interspersed with petechiae. Nonpitting edema occurs in 25% of the children and commonly affects the dorsal hands and feet, and, less commonly, the forehead, periorbital areas, scalp, perineum, and scrotum. Prominent edema is most common in the infant (younger than 2 years of age).

Involvement of the gastrointestinal tract occurs in more than 85% of children. Colicky abdominal pain, melena, ileus, vomiting, or hematemesis may be the initial presentation. Severe hemorrhage or intussusception with obstruction or perforation occurs in less than 5% of cases. These complications are more common in the older child (more than 4 years of age). Arthritis occurs at onset or shortly thereafter in about 75% of the children. Knees and ankles are most commonly affected, but wrists, elbows, and the small joints of the hands may also be involved. Periarticular swelling and tenderness, usually without erythema or warmth, are most characteristic. Large effusions are unusual. This arthritis is transient, generally not migratory, and usually resolves within a few days.

*Clinical Course.* Most children with HSP have self-limited disease that consists of a single exacerbation lasting about 4 weeks. The younger the child, the shorter the course and the fewer recurrences expected. Most exacerbations occur within the first 6 weeks. Generally, the disease is over in 3 months. An unusual child may experience exacerbations for as long as 2 years after onset.

*Laboratory Studies.* A moderate leukocytosis is seen in some children as is normochromic anemia, which may reflect gastrointestinal blood loss. The platelet count is normal to elevated, and coagulation studies are normal. Although this is an immune-complex disease, the total hemolytic complement is generally normal during the initial attack of HSP. Hemolytic and C3 complement levels are normal, but the concentration of properdin and factor B may be decreased in half the children during the acute illness. Serum IgA and IgM concentrations are elevated in half the patients. Split fibrin products may be present in blood and urine.

*Diagnosis.* Purpura and a normal platelet count must be present for a diagnosis of HSP. Abdominal pain, unexplained renal disease, or arthritis are additional diagnostic clues to the presence of HSP. This disease must be differentiated from a variety of other illnesses including acute poststreptococcal glomerulonephritis, rheumatic fever, SLE, septicemia, and disseminated intravascular coagulation. Other causes of an acute surgical abdomen or gastrointestinal bleeding must be considered as must be intussusception or pancreatitis.

A skin biopsy may be useful to confirm a diagnosis in some children. Characteristic features are a leukocytoclastic vasculitis with intravascular deposition of IgA and C3. A kidney biopsy is generally not indicated except to clarify the extent and nature of the renal disease in those children who are severely affected.

*Treatment.* General clinical support and meticulous observation for complications are critically important in the seriously ill child with HSP. Glucocorticoids are generally indicated only in gastrointestinal hemorrhage. The response to the use of these drugs may be dramatic. Generally, prednisone in the range of 1 to 2 mg/kg/d for at least 1 week is chosen, followed by a gradual reduction in the dose depending on response to therapy and extent of bleeding. Prednisone appears not to otherwise modify the extent of the disease, shorten its course, or affect the frequency or course of renal involvement. Clinical studies have not thoroughly evaluated the efficacy of glucocorticoid therapy administered early to children with nephritis. In progressive renal disease, consideration should be given to glucocorticoids and cytotoxic agents. Antiplatelet drugs should also be evaluated. Renal transplants have been successfully performed in children with irreversible renal failure related to HSP. Nephritis has recurred in the allografts of some of these cases.

*Prognosis.* Prognosis in HSP is generally excellent and depends on the extent of the disease and the age of the child; prognosis is better in the younger child. Morbidity and mortality are often related to the extent of involvement of the gastrointestinal tract or kidneys. Less than 5% of children who develop HSP progressed to end-stage renal disease in early studies of its course. Recent estimates of long-term prognosis are more optimistic. In children admitted to a hospital during the initial illness, however, careful follow-up shows increased evidence of renal disease.

## Other Types of Small Blood Vessel Vasculitis

A rare type of isolated cutaneous vasculitis presents with palpable purpura, painful nodules, or ridges that develop along the course of involved vessels. Otherwise, the child is well without systemic or constitutional symptoms. The clinical course is variable and is characterized by remissions and exacerbations, often over many years. Although each crop of lesions may respond to glucocorticoids or, occasionally, to acetylsalicylic acid, this disease is frequently of such long duration that it is difficult to treat the growing child with prednisone during the entire course of the problem. Alternate-day dosage may be acceptable therapy for such children.

Hypocomplementemic urticarial vasculitis has also been described in a rare child. Girls apparently are more at risk. The pathogenesis is unknown but an immune-complex process is suggested. The eruption affects principally the face, upper extremities, and trunk. The urticarial lesions last for only a few days with each exacerbation, then fade without scarring. Systemic features may accompany the cutaneous disease. The degree of hypocomplementemia parallels the severity of the illness. Some of these children warrant treatment with glucocorticoids.

Cryoglobulinemia, either essential or secondary to otherwise identified disease, causes an immune-complex vasculitis that can mimic any of the entities discussed above. Cryoglobulins can be demonstrated in plasma chilled to 4 to 22°C. Depending on the disease and the nature of the involvement, therapy consists of specific treatment of the underlying problem, the use of prednisone or immunosuppressive agents, or plasmapheresis.

## Granulomatous Vasculitis

### Allergic Necrotizing Granulomatosis

Allergic necrotizing granulomatosis is a rare systemic necrotizing vasculitis that occurs predominantly in young males with a history of chronic asthma. The histopathology is that of a necrotizing vasculitis with an eosinophilic infiltrate and extravascular necrotizing granulomata. Peripheral eosinophilia often is prominent. Other manifestations of this syndrome are identical to those seen in polyarteritis, especially in the gastrointestinal tract, CNS, and musculoskeletal system. Renal disease may be less frequent. Pulmonary disease is often the most important manifestation with prominent radiologic changes. Glucocorticoids are the main approach to treatment. Prognosis is variable; death often involves cardiopulmonary failure.

### Wegener's Granulomatosis

Wegener's granulomatosis is a rare syndrome in children, although it has been described as early as 3 months of age. It is characterized by a necrotizing granulomatous angiitis involving both the respiratory tract (sinuses, nasal passages, and lungs) and the kidneys. Characteristic granulomata may also be found in skin, heart, CNS, gastrointestinal tract, and synovia. Constitutional symptoms are almost always prominent.

Unexplained pain, rhinorrhea, mucosal ulceration, or bleeding of the upper respiratory tract may be the presenting sign. Nasal cartilage may be eroded. Hemoptysis and pleuritic pain are frequent. The pulmonary disease may progress to hemorrhage, obstruction, atelectasis, or repeated episodes of infection. Chest films demonstrate multiform pulmonary infiltrates and nodules. Most of the patients have moderate to severe renal disease that may progress progressive. Hypertension may be less common than in other types of nephritis.

The differential diagnosis includes the other forms of vasculitis, sarcoidosis, berylliosis, Loeffler syndrome, tuberculosis, disseminated fungal disease, syphilis, or lymphoma. Goodpasture's syndrome and other rare forms of granulomatous arteritis are easily confused clinically with Wegener's granulomatosis. Diagnosis is established by biopsy of an affected organ, usually the nasal mucosa, or an open-lung biopsy. Granulomata and a necrotizing vasculitis with leukocytic, lymphocytic, and giant cell infiltration are seen.

Historically, death from renal or pulmonary disease occurred with only rare long-term survivorship. Glucocorticoid treatment had some effect early in the disease, but recent trials support the use of cyclophosphamide in the managing these patients. A dramatic response to its use has altered the prognosis of this otherwise fatal disease to one of total remission, if not cure, in the adult series reported from the National Institutes of Health (NIH). More recent consideration is being given other immunosuppressive agents.

## Giant Cell Arteritis

Giant cell arteritis characteristically involves the aorta or its major branches. Histologically there is disruption of the internal elastic lamina, intimal proliferation, and infiltration of the wall with mononuclear cells and giant cells.

### Systemic Giant Cell Arteritis

Systemic giant cell arteritis involves major branches or segments of the thoracic or abdominal aorta at single or multiple locations. The child may present with constitutional symptoms such as weight loss, malaise and fatigue, fever of unknown origin, or hypertension. Vascular occlusion leads to the development of peripheral anoxia, cyanosis, and gangrene. Recanalization of involved vessels may occur spontaneously or during treatment with glucocorticoid drugs. Diagnosis is established by arteriography combined with biopsy test of a vessel if accessible.

### Takayasu Arteritis

Takayasu arteritis is a giant cell arteritis predominantly seen in teenage girls. Stenosis, occlusion, dilation, and aneurysm formation are confined to the aorta, its major branches, and the pulmonary arteries. This disease has been referred to as *pulseless disease* because of the obliteration of the radial pulses or reverse coarctation. Hypertension is frequent. The acute-phase reactants and the white blood cell count are usually elevated.

Takayasu arteritis appears to be more common in Asians, Latins, blacks, and Sephardic Jews. The female-to-male ratio is 8:1. Unidentified environmental or genetic factors may play a role in its pathogenesis. It is occasionally seen in families of children with other connective tissue diseases and has been reported in monozygotic twin sisters.

The course of Takayasu arteritis may be limited, lasting 3 to 6 months, or prolonged over many years. Early diagnosis is often difficult. Because of the insidious onset, an erroneous diagnosis (eg, systemic onset JRA, acute rheumatic fever) may be made. Eventually, signs of vascular insufficiency suggest the correct diagnosis, which can then be confirmed by angiography or MRI. On plain films, calcification may be identified in the affected vessels.

It is generally regarded that glucocorticoid drugs are indicated for early disease. Nonsteroidal anti-inflammatory drugs are useful in managing these patients during the acute early phases of the illness. Anticoagulants or antiplatelet agents may be indicated if there is widespread chronic occlusion of vessels. Vessel grafts have been successful late in the course of the disease.

### Cranial Arteritis

Cranial arteritis is generally found only in the older adult. However, it may rarely present in childhood. It is characterized by a severe, persistent headache and localized pain or tenderness directly over a cranial or temporal vessel. The ESR is very high. The threat of blindness (amaurosis fugax) from involvement of the ophthalmic and central retinal arteries is an important consideration in this disease and an indication for prompt initiation of glucocorticoid therapy. Diagnosis is established by biopsy of an involved superficial vessel.

## BEHÇET'S SYNDROME

Behçet's syndrome is uncommon in children in North America. It was originally described in the Near East and has been especially frequent in geographic areas characterized by Near-Eastern migration (eg, United Kingdom) and in Turkey, Cyprus, Greece, and Japan. This syndrome consists of a triad of recurrent uveitis, mucocutaneous ulcerations, and genital ulcerations. It is difficult to be certain of this diagnosis in a child without involvement of the CNS. Additional features include arthritis, gastrointestinal disease, and cardiovascular involvement.

No etiology has been identified. An infectious cause has been advanced because of the geographic foci of the disease. Inclusion bodies have been noted in exudative cells in some studies. The mucocutaneous lesions may represent lesions of delayed hypersensitivity. Superficial trauma such as a pin prick reproduces typical cutaneous lesions when active disease is present (pathergy).

## Histopathology

The basic pathologic lesion is a vasculitis of small- and medium-size arteries and veins with a mononuclear cell infiltrate, fibrinoid necrosis, and narrowing and obliteration of the vessel lumen. Venous thromboses of the terminal vascular beds or vena cava are especially common. Immunofluorescent microscopy demonstrates C3, C4, and the terminal components of the complement cascade in vessel walls along with IgG and fibrinogen. Circulating immune complexes are often present.

## Clinical Manifestations

Males are affected more frequently than females. The most common age at onset is 18 to 40 years. Occurrence of the disease in children as young as 2 years has been reported.

A nondestructive polyarthritis commonly occurs in about 75% of the children. The peripheral joint disease may be symmetric or asymmetric. Large joints such as the knees are most frequently affected, but small joints may be involved. Multiple recurrences of the synovitis develop during a period of several years, particularly in the knees and ankles, although bony erosions and functional disability are uncommon. Fever and erythema nodosum frequently accompany the arthritis.

Aphthous stomatitis is common as are ulcerative lesions of the mucous membranes of the upper and lower gastrointestinal tracts. The oral ulcerations are quite painful and interfere with swallowing and speech. Similar ulcerations occur in the genitourinary tract and are accompanied by a sterile pyuria. These ulcerations may resemble herpes simplex or the Stevens-Johnson syndrome. An incorrect diagnosis of regional enteritis or ulcerative colitis may also be made.

Involvement of the eye includes photophobia, pain, conjunctivitis, and blurred vision. Uveitis is most common. Scleritis, retinal vasculitis, and optic neuritis may also develop and lead to blindness.

CNS involvement in Behçet's syndrome ranges from trivial neurologic signs to confusion to papilledema and pseudotumor cerebri. These disorders occur in about one fourth of the patients and are divided into five syndromes: pseudotumor cerebri, meningoencephalitis, brain-stem involvement, dementia, and changes in personality and behavior. Cerebral spinal fluid abnormalities include pleocytosis and increased concentrations of protein.

The course of Behçet's syndrome is highly variable. It may span a period of a few weeks or extend to several years, and the pattern of involvement is characterized by frequent remissions and exacerbations. Prognosis is often directly related to the extent of CNS disease.

## Laboratory Findings

There are no specific laboratory findings. Hypergammaglobulinemia is characteristic. Autoantibodies reacting with mucosal cells have been demonstrated in some patients. HLA associations include B5 in North American studies and an increased prevalence of B27 in others, although the frequency of spondylitis does not appear to be increased. Behçet's syndrome can be confused clinically with the Reiter's syndrome.

## Treatment

Treatment is difficult and puzzling because the course is punctuated by frequent remissions. Reports suggest that immunosuppressive or alkylating agents may be indicated along with glucocorticoid drugs.

# AMYLOIDOSIS

Amyloidosis is characterized by the deposition of a homogeneous eosinophilic material in parenchymal organs and around blood vessels. Amyloidosis is divided into two types: primary amyloidosis in association with plasma cell disorders, on a familial basis, or occurring as an idiopathic disease; and amyloidosis found in conjunction with another disease such as JRA, familial Mediterranean fever, chronic pulmonary disease, or osteomyelitis. This classification is summarized in Table 15-24.

In primary amyloid deposition, principal sites of involvement are the skin and gastrointestinal tract. The patient may present with macroglossia, carpal tunnel syndrome or arthritis, congestive heart failure, malabsorption, or gastrointestinal bleeding. In secondary amyloidosis, the patient develops hepatomegaly, splenomegaly, and nephrotic syndrome. Secondary amyloidosis is rare in children but is seen in association with Hodgkin's disease or renal carcinoma. In young adults, it increases in frequency in chronic suppurative conditions, with the infectious complications of intravenous drug use, and in diseases such as leprosy or malaria. Amyloidosis has also been described in endocrine organs in association with endocrinologic disease and as localized cutaneous deposits.

## Immunopathology

All amyloid deposits display a green birefringence with Congo red dye under a polarizing microscope. These deposits appear microscopically homogeneous. The major component of amyloid deposits by electron microscopy is a 100 Å fibril that is thin, nonbranching, and rigid. Although the ultrastructural appearance of the fibrils in the various types of amyloidosis is nearly identical, their biochemical composition is distinct. In primary amyloidosis, these fibrils assume an antiparallel $\beta$-pleated sheet conformation by x-ray crystallography and their amino acid sequence is homologous with the variable region of immunoglobulin light chains.

In secondary amyloidosis, the major fibrillar protein is not homologous with light chains and the amino acid sequence is virtually identical in all patients who have been studied. A serum component that circulates normally in very low concentrations, SAA, cross-reacts immunologically with these amyloid fibrils. SAA is an acute-phase reactant, in part relating the occurrence of amyloidosis as a complication of inflammatory and infectious diseases. There is also a P component on electron microscopy that consists of an $\alpha$-1-glycoprotein that is absorbed onto the fibrillar structure. This pentagonal component is common to all types of amyloid but constitutes only about 5% of the deposits.

| TABLE 15-24. Classification of Amyloidosis | | |
|---|---|---|
| Terminology | Clinical Features | Probable Origin |
| AL | Primary, myeloma | L-Chains |
| AA | Secondary, FMF | SAA |
| AF | Familial | Prealbumin, etc |
| AS | Senile, heart, brain | Prealbumin, etc |
| AE | Endocrine | Thyrocalcitonin |
| AD | Dermal | ? |

It is a doughnut-shaped structure composed of five identical sub-units closely related in structure and function to C-reactive protein.

## Hereditary Amyloidosis

The most common type of amyloid deposition described on a hereditary basis is familial Mediterranean fever (FMF). This is a periodic disease inherited as an autosomal recessive trait. It is particularly common in Sephardic and Iraqi Jews, Turks, Armenians, and Levantine Arabs. Onset of disease occurs generally between the ages of 5 and 15 years. Each stereotypic exacerbation is characterized by fever, abdominal and pleuropericardial pain, arthritis, or ankle erythema. An attack begins acutely and may last 1 week before slowly subsiding.

Joint complaints include arthralgia, acute oligoarthritis, or chronic arthritis lasting for many years. Swelling and pain are predominant, erythema and increased heat are often absent, and the knees are most commonly affected. Residual damage is not characteristic except in the hips where secondary degenerative arthritis may develop. Radiographs are characterized by juxta-articular osteoporosis and occasional sacroiliac involvement.

Amyloidosis develops in some children with FMF and results in the nephrotic syndrome and eventual death from renal failure (FMF and amyloidosis may be inherited separately). Amyloidosis is not a common complication in North America. Other forms of periodic disease have been described with an unclear relationship with FMF.

Most of the other familial forms of amyloidosis are inherited as autosomal dominant disease. Each family presents characteristic clinical features and geographic distribution. These hereditary forms are quite rare and often have neuropathic elements in addition to visceral involvement. They have been especially well described in Portuguese and Japanese kindreds. Onset of the clinical disease is often not observed until the third decade of life.

## Treatment

There is no specific therapy for amyloidosis beyond appropriate treatment of the accompanying disease. In children with known malignant disease, treatment involves cytotoxic drugs. Amyloidosis seldom occurs in North America as a complication of JRA. It is a relatively common complication of JRA, however, in some Northern European countries (7%). Chlorambucil has been used in affected children as treatment for the nephrotic syndrome.

In FMF, no form of treatment is universally successful. Analgesics are useful for relief of symptoms. Colchicine has anti-inflammatory properties and may slow or prevent the development of renal failure.

## Selected Readings

Athreya B, ed. Pediatric rheumatology. Rheum Dis Clin North Am 1991;17(4).

Cassidy JT, Levinson JE, Bass JC, et al. A study of classification criteria for a diagnosis of juvenile rheumatoid arthritis. Arthritis Rheum 1986;29:274.

Cassidy JT, Petty RE. Textbook of pediatric rheumatology, ed 2. New York: Churchill Livingstone, 1990.

Cassidy JT, Sullivan DB, Dabich L, et al. Scleroderma in children. Arthritis Rheum 1977;20:351.

Cassidy JT, Sullivan DB, Petty RE, et al. Lupus nephritis and encephalopathy: prognosis in 58 children. Arthritis Rheum 1977;20:315.

Eichenfield AH, Goldsmith DP, Benach JL, et al. Childhood Lyme arthritis: experience in an endemic area. J Pediatr 1986;109:753.

Lovell D, White P, eds. Pediatric rheumatology into the 90's. J Rheumatol 1992;19 (Suppl 33).

Magilavy DB, Petty RE, Cassidy JT, et al. A syndrome of childhood polyarteritis. J Pediatr 1977;91:25.

Melish ME. Kawasaki syndrome: a 1986 perspective. Brewer EJ Jr, Cassidy JT, eds. In: Rheumatic diseases of childhood. Rheum Dis Clin North Am, 1987;7.

Sullivan DB, Cassidy JT, Petty RE. Dermatomyositis in the pediatric patient. Arthritis Rheum 1977;20:327.

# The Fetus and
# the Newborn

*Principles and Practice of Pediatrics, Second Edition.*
edited by Frank A. Oski et al. J. B. Lippincott Company, Philadelphia © 1994.

## CHAPTER 16
# *General Principles of Growth and Development*

## *16.1 Developmental Biology and Congenital Malformations*

### *16.1.1 Developmental Biology*

Merton Bernfield

The normal infant is the expected outcome of pregnancy, but fetal loss, preterm birth, and birth defects reduce this result to about one third of all conceptions. The perfectly structured and functioning infant that traverses the intrauterine to extrauterine environment normally is the product of a complex array of cellular and molecular interactions. The key to understanding both the normal adapting newborn and the abnormalities leading to adverse pregnancy outcome is developmental biology. Developmental biology is concerned with how a single-celled zygote undergoes programmed changes to emerge as a completely formed organism. The discipline encompasses information from a range of fields: molecular biology, genetics, cell structure and physiology, endocrinology, and anatomy. Because organs are diverse, the principles of human development would be overwhelmingly complex if each organ developed by distinct mechanisms. This is not the case. Instead, there are several major principles, each discovered by experimental manipulation of developing animals other than humans.

An understanding of developmental biology provides rational approaches to clinical problems. For example, knowledge of the preimplantation embryo led to the culturing of the early conceptus and to successful in vitro fertilization, as well as to the development of contraceptive agents. By identifying developmental genes and their regulatory mechanisms, birth defects can be screened for and prevented. Understanding the mechanisms of organ formation helps parents deal with both genetically and teratogenically induced malformations. The mechanisms of growth regulation of the embryo shed light on the control of growth of cancer cells. Knowledge of cell differentiation has led to novel therapies like the glucocorticoid stimulation of surfactant production in the prenatal lung. Understanding mechanisms of fetal growth gives insight into causes of low birth weight, a profound problem especially in disadvantaged populations in the United States. Finally, the intense application of technology in intensive care nurseries can result in iatrogenic diseases that are best understood in terms of the reparative response of developing tissues to injury.

## DEVELOPMENTAL BIOLOGY TRIES TO EXPLAIN HOW CELLS ORGANIZE AND SPECIALIZE

The human organism is constructed from hundreds of functionally distinct cell types, and the cells in each organ are organized in an exquisitely coordinated way. This intricate arrangement arises from a sequential developmental program of cellular behaviors. The zygote multiples into cells that organize spatially into a basic body plan. The cells at distinct sites coalesce into organ primordia and specialize by acquiring distinct functions. These cell populations then increase to generate the form and final relationships between organs. The information responsible for this development is encoded in the genome of each organism. Thus, genes control development by dictating behavior of cells.

Studies of invertebrate development indicate that the genes responsible for development are arranged in a hierarchy. Some genes control the expression of other genes. Activation of certain genes leads to a cascade of developmental programs, each involving activation of other genes. The various genes function at different times during development and have multiple functions. The action of these genes is then often modified by the consequences of interactions between cells, modifications which can either regulate gene activation or the function of their products. The concept of a gene hierarchy simplifies the understanding of cell differentiation, the process by which the cell specializes. Differentiation is understood by identifying the genes that control the expression of the other genes, then by assessing how these regulatory genes are controlled in time and in space.

Studies comparing vertebrate (including mammalian) and invertebrate development indicate that developmental genes are highly conserved in evolution. Although the precise developmental function of a conserved gene may differ between lower and higher forms, the genes can have similar protein products. Examples include the homeotic genes, a set of genes discovered originally in the fruit fly, *Drosophila melanogaster*, by mutations that affect where structures will develop in the fly. Structurally related genes are known in organisms as diverse as plants and humans. Indeed, mutations in the human homologues of *Drosophila* pair-rule genes can cause Waardenburg's syndrome and aniridia in humans (Table 16-1).

### Embryonic Cells Have the Same Properties as Cells From Mature Organisms

Although embryonic cells exhibit developmental cell behaviors, their fundamental structure and function are identical to those of cells in mature organisms. Their plasma membrane separates the cells from the external environment and is involved in cell interactions and the formation of cell junctions. The plasma membrane behaves as a highly selective sieve that allows either passive or active movement of molecules into the cell. The cells also bring materials into them by endocytosis. They secrete materials by exocytosis and produce substantial amounts of extracellular matrix, which they distribute around themselves. The cells contain a cytoskeleton, consisting of microtubules, microfilaments, and intermediate filaments that are responsible for changing cell shapes. The cells have the same kinds of membrane-bound organelles as those found in mature cells such as the endoplasmic reticulum, Golgi apparatus, and lysosomes. The mitochondria of these cells behave as they do in mature cells, producing adenosine triphosphate (ATP) and undergoing oxidative phosphorylation. The cell nuclei contain the chromosomal material where enzyme and protein-DNA interactions, many yet unknown, yield commitment of cell fate, specialization of cell function, and specific cell organization that are seen during embryogenesis.

**TABLE 16-1.    Mammalian Homologues of Developmental Genes in _Drosophila_**

| Type of Gene | _Drosophila_ gene | | Mammalian Gene | Homologues Syndrome |
|---|---|---|---|---|
| | Name | Action | | |
| Segmentation | | | | |
| Pair-rule | Fushi tarazu | Form alternate segments | pax 1 | Undulated (mouse) |
| | | | pax 3 | Waardenburg's (human) |
| | | | pax 6 | Aniridia (human) |
| Segment polarity | Wingless | Subdivide segments | wnt 1 | Swaying (mouse) |
| Homeotic | _Antennapedia_ | Specify fate of segments | Hox-1.1 to Hox-4.9 | — |

Moreover, the gene products that control cell behavior during development may not be distinct from those that maintain normal cellular physiology. The gene products with major developmental effects are in one of three classes of molecules. One, the DNA-binding proteins either regulate gene activation or control the rate of DNA synthesis and cell division. Two, the adhesion molecules cause cells to adhere together into groups of cells or as extracellular matrix components to segregate cell groups. Three, cytokines and growth factor peptides dictate developmental interactions between cells and tissues.

## Mouse Development Is a Useful Model for Human Development

Mammals, especially the mouse, have been used to provide information on the mechanisms of human development. Although there are clear differences between human and mouse development, the presumption is that the general mechanisms of development are similar. Indeed, genetically inbred mouse strains exhibit a variety of developmental mutants that share features with human malformations. Identifying the genes responsible for these abnormalities has been difficult. Technology, however, now enables identification of these genes, and in turn, provides greater understanding of both the gene products and processes that control development (Table 16-2).

New techniques of experimental embryology focused on the mouse include superovulation, culture of both preimplantation and postimplantation embryos, insertional mutagenesis, and introduction of transgenes into embryos by cell and DNA transfer. These techniques have led to construction of new mouse strains containing additional genes or genes that have been specifically deleted. These new mouse strains have yielded models of human diseases for use in studies of pathogenesis and treatment and of

prevention. The genes involved in development are ones in which abnormalities are most likely manifested early in life, and, therefore, are relevant to pediatrics.

Transgenic technology in the mouse is now used routinely to define genes involved in development. Retroviruses or cloned foreign genes are inserted into fertilized eggs or early embryos so the genes stably integrate into the mouse genome. These modified cells or tissues can be implanted into the oviduct of a pseudopregnant foster mother, enabling the development of the transgenic mouse. The resultant mice can be used to start a new colony. Integration of the retrovirus can disrupt a gene anywhere in the genome, leading to developmental abnormalities. The function of the added gene can often be assessed, especially if it contains genetic elements that enable it to be expressed as tissue-specific.

In a variation of this technique, a developmental gene can be mutated or deleted by targeting it specifically by homologous recombination in cultured embryonic stem cells. These stem cells are totipotent and can be inserted into a mouse blastocyst where they may be incorporated into the embryo. If the stem cells containing the mutated or deleted gene enter the germ line, a mouse is produced that can transmit the mutation to its offspring. Breeding these chimeric mice can yield mice strains containing the mutated or deleted gene. The abnormalities evident in the mice containing these gene "knockouts" give clues to the function of the gene. A large proportion of these newly constructed mouse strains either die at birth or in the newborn period, suggesting that the deleted genes function in the adaptation to extrauterine life. These results suggest hitherto unsuspected functions for several genes. Moreover, the results emphasize that the developmental functions of various genes are important to newborn medicine and that neonatology will play an increasingly important role in understanding the functions of these genes.

**TABLE 16-2.    Mouse Mutations Can Define Human Diseases**

| Mouse Mutant | Gene Defect | Human Abnormality |
|---|---|---|
| Spontaneous | | |
| _mdx_ | Dystrophin (cytoskeletal protein) | Duchenne's muscular dystrophy |
| _splotch_ | pax-3 (nuclear protein) | Waardenburg's syndrome |
| Induced | | |
| _hox 1.6_ deletion | Hox 1.6 (transcription factor) | DiGeorge syndrome |
| _c-fos_ deletion | c-fos (transcription factor) | Osteopetrosis |

Transgenic techniques complement the molecular genetic analysis of mouse mutants, most of which have been identified based on an abnormal developmental phenotype. Molecular analyses that identify mutant genes in these mice are now more feasible because of improvement in genetic and physical gene mapping techniques, including the vastly increased number of defined simple sequence repeat (microsatellite) loci in the mouse genome and the use of cloning vectors (eg, yeast artificial chromosomes) that enable manipulation of large DNA fragments. Polymorphisms of simple sequence repeat DNA are important in identifying genes potentially involved in human development because the most common human developmental abnormalities are polygenic traits. Both approaches—identification of potential developmental genes followed by analysis of the phenotypic consequences of inducing a mutation in these genes and identification of mutant genes responsible for an abnormal phenotype—are yielding information on human development.

# DEVELOPMENT RESULTS IN FORMATION OF HIGHLY SPECIALIZED CELLS ORGANIZED INTO DISTINCT STRUCTURES

Developmental biology attempts to answer two major questions. First, how does a single cell, the fertilized egg or zygote, generate all the highly specialized cells of the fully developed organism? This question asks how cells become specialized relative to each other. Developmental biologists cite two interrelated processes—cell determination and cell differentiation—for this specialization. Second, how do the cells organize at specific places and times to form tissues of specific shape? This question asks how the various cell behaviors are precisely integrated and controlled to yield organs. Developmental biologists term this process morphogenesis, which correlates in time during development with cell specialization.

## Cell Specialization Involves Commitment to a Restricted Developmental Fate

The zygote and early embryonic stem cells are totipotent; they can develop into all possible specialized cells of the body. After gastrulation and before actual specialization, however, the cells lose the ability to develop in alternative ways. Thus, they become restricted in their fate. During the developmental history of each

tissue, there is a time when the cells of that tissue could have become a different tissue or, earlier in development, even other tissues. The cells become increasingly committed or determined to a particular type of differentiation. Determination is the selection of a single developmental pathway from among several alternatives (Table 16-3).

The timetable for determination varies for different developmental pathways. Determination is often a gradual reduction in developmental options with the final restriction rendering the cells capable of producing only a single type of cell. Once a population of cells is determined, the restriction is permanent and stable, acquiring a genetic control in which the determined cells breed true. These stable phenotypes maintain differences between cells in mature organisms. The determination process also means that, after development, cell types that are lost cannot be replaced unless a preexisting parental cell type or an uncommitted stem cell exists. There is no organ regeneration in the mature human.

Although determination prevents certain genes from being activated, it does not involve elimination or permanent inactivation of any genetic material because all somatic, nongermline cells contain the same complement of genes. Rather, determination most likely involves the expression of one or a few regulatory genes that control the subsequent expression of many other genes in the hierarchy. These restrictions of gene expression can be considered to be developmental "decisions." These decisions can occur without any apparent change in the phenotype of the cells. Therefore, one can not establish when a cell has become committed until after the determination has occurred.

Nuclear transplantation experiments demonstrate that stability of the determined state depends on cytoplasm. In these studies, introduction of the nucleus from a determined cell into the cytoplasm of an uncommitted cell "de-programs" the transplanted nucleus in such a way that it expresses genes that had previously been restricted. This type of experiment approximates fertilization in which the nucleus of the determined sperm cell enters the egg cytoplasm and becomes able to express previously restricted genes. The cytoplasmic factors involved, however, are almost wholly unknown.

## Differentiation Involves Production of Specific Proteins

After determination, cells acquire distinct functional characteristics by differentiation. In this process, cells differentiate both

| TABLE 16-3. Growth Factor Peptides in Mammalian Development | | | |
|---|---|---|---|
| Family | Growth Factor (GF) | "Classical" Source | Developmental Action |
| Epidermal (5–6D) | EGF, TGF-$\alpha$ | Salivary gland Platelets | Mesenchymal mitogen, epithelial differentiation |
| Insulin-like (7.5D) | IGF-I, IGF-II, relaxin | Liver Amniotic fluid | Mesenchymal and epithelial differentiation |
| Fibroblast (16–17D) | a-FGF, b-FGF | Macrophages Brain | Mesenchymal mitogen, ECM production, angiogenesis |
| Transforming (25D [dimer]) | TGF-$\beta$, MIS Inhibin, activin | Platelets Bone | Mesenchymal mitogen and differentiation, epithelial growth inhibition, ECM production/ remodeling |
| Platelet-derived (30D [dimer]) | PDGF-A, PDGF-B | Platelets Macrophages Endothelia Smooth muscle | Mesenchymal mitogen and migration, ECM production/remodeling |

*EGF*, epidermal growth factor; *TGF*, transforming growth factor; *IGF*, insulin-like growth factor; *FGF*, fibroblast growth factor; *MIS*, Müllerian inhibitory substance; *PDGF*, platelet-derived growth factor; *ECM*, extracellular matrix.

from other cells and from their past. The differentiation of a cell is defined by the proteins that it synthesizes and by its shape. Both characteristics establish cell function. Cells produce a variety of proteins, and not all classes of proteins establish whether a cell is differentiated. Some proteins are for "housekeeping" use and are present in all cells (eg, mitochondrial proteins or glycolytic enzymes) or are common to a number of cell types (eg, collagens produced by fibroblasts or cytokeratins produced by epithelia). These proteins do not characterize the differentiated state. The proteins that establish differentiation of a cell type are those that enable the cell to carry out a unique function such as hemoglobin in red blood cells or IgG in plasma cells. Cell differentiation arises, in part, from controlling the synthesis of these "specialization" proteins.

There are many possible points at which the synthesis of specific proteins can be controlled. For example, various genes appear to be transcribed at different rates in different cell types. In oviduct cells, ovalbumin genes are transcribed but no globin gene transcripts are detectable, whereas in erythroid cells, there are abundant globin gene transcripts but no detectable ovalbumin mRNA. Genes that are transcriptionally active assume a different conformation on the chromatin, suggesting that not the gene but the proteins associated with the gene control rate of transcription. Nucleotide sequences known as promoters and enhancers initiate transcription of structural genes in a tissue-specific manner. These regions interact with proteins known as transcription factors, which are themselves products of differentiation. Other possible mechanisms of differentiation include selective posttranscriptional processing of mRNA. Cells could contain very similar or identical sets of RNAs as nuclear transcripts but produce different sets or different abundance of cytoplasmic mRNA by various mechanisms including alternative splicing of the primary RNA transcript or heightened/reduced metabolic stability of the mRNA. The efficiency of mRNA translation or various posttranslational modifications of the protein can also yield differences in the amount of specific proteins produced during differentiation.

During differentiation, cells also assume characteristic shapes that enable the cell to function effectively. The distinct shapes result from different arrangements of the various cytoskeletal components inside the cell: microfilaments, microtubules, and intermediate filaments. The shape of the cell may even control the production of specific proteins. For example, milk-producing mammary epithelial cells can synthesize milk proteins only when

allowed to assume a cuboidal shape, and chondrocytes can produce cartilage only when allowed to round up.

Some differentiated cells may no longer be able to undergo cell division. Some cells can synthesize their differentiated products in bulk only after they cease to divide, as in the production of cartilage by chondrocytes. Thus, there is often a reciprocal relationship between cell differentiation and proliferation. Tissues that contain cells in such a terminally differentiated state may also contain undifferentiated stem-cell populations that are able to divide. These stem cells subsequently differentiate, leading to the terminally differentiated cells (eg, red blood cells, plasma cells). Other tissues are not capable of producing new cells because they consist solely of terminally differentiated cells (eg, neurons, cardiac myocytes).

## Morphogenesis Involves a Limited Number of Cellular Behaviors

How do cells organize at specific places and times to form specific structures? That is, how is the one-dimensional array of genetic information in DNA transformed into the three-dimensional arrangements of cells and tissues in mature organisms? The precise organization of cell populations during development occurs by morphogenesis. Although the ultimate shape of each organ is distinct, the cellular behavior involved in the formation of these distinct organs is not. Morphogenesis involves a limited repertoire of cellular behavior: cell adhesion, change in cell shape (which accounts for both the motility of single cells and the movement of cell populations), localized cell proliferation, and localized cell death. Every developing cell, regardless of type, can perform these behaviors, but the distinct organ shapes arise from differences in the timing, extent, and location of these cellular behaviors.

The factors that integrate these cell behaviors into tissues and organs include the extracellular matrix and various growth factors, sometimes known as signalling peptides (see Table 16-3 and Fig 16-1). These integrating factors involved in embryonic inductions act on cells through receptors at their surfaces, which, when occupied, act transmembrane to influence intracellular events. Although these behaviors are listed as distinct processes in the table, this is an oversimplification that obscures their interrelationships. This simplification, however, allows apparently disparate mor-

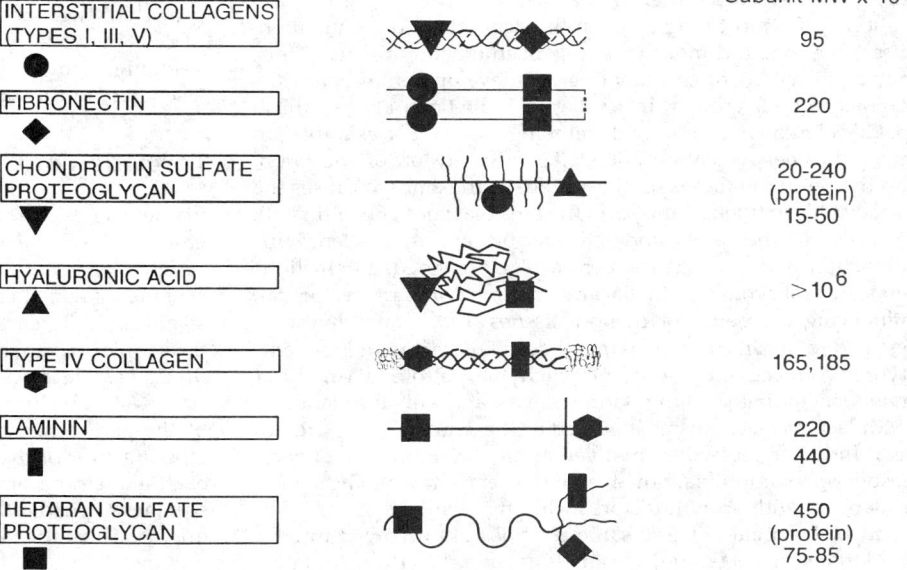

**Figure 16-1.** Major extracellular matrix components at tissue interfaces. Major components of the interstitial matrix include interstitial fluid and the interstitial collagens (types I, III, and V), fibronectin, chondroitin sulfate (includes dermatan sulfate) proteoglycan, and hyaluronic acid. Major components of the basal lamina include type IV collagen, laminin, and a specific heparan sulfate proteoglycan. Extensive binding interactions (represented by the symbols) cause these components to associate into cross-linked composites that are insoluble under physiologic conditions.

phogenetic events and their controls to be defined in molecular terms.

## STRATEGIES OF DEVELOPMENT

### Cell Lineages and Cell Interactions Regulate Developmental Processes

Determination, differentiation, and morphogenesis can account for the formation of organs, but how are these processes regulated? The aggregate behavior of cells leads to the formation of tissues that coordinate to form organs. But, how do the cells know where they are in a population? How is form controlled so that scale and proportion are achieved? There are two strategies for this regulation, cell lineage and cell interaction.

With cell lineage, the information dictating the developmental behavior of a cell is solely that which is encoded in its genome and is directly passed from parental cell to daughter cell. Events within the cell instruct it when to do something and what to do. In strict examples of this strategy, the developmental behavior of a cell is independent of the behavior or even the existence of neighboring cells. Such regulation leads to development in which the organism is assembled from more or less independent parts. Several invertebrates (eg, *Caenorhabditis elegans*, the well-studied nematode) develop predominantly, but not exclusively, in this manner.

With cell interactions, the parts of a developing organism influence the development of other parts. The information dictating the development of a cell is determined largely by interactions between it and its neighboring cells. For example, in the early mouse embryo, although each blastomere is totipotent, the actual variety of cell types that each will form depends on its position within the embryo. Mammalian development primarily involves such interactions. Such regulation leads to greater developmental plasticity. However, a cell's ability to respond to its neighbors depends on its lineage, and its response at any time increasingly depends on how it has been influenced. These constraints reduce the extent of plasticity with increasing developmental age.

### Embryonic Induction and Positional Information Integrate the Behavior of Cell Populations

Embryonic inductions are interactions between tissues of dissimilar origin that change the developmental behavior of the interacting tissues. These interactions, which occur during the formation of most organs, influence the determination, differentiation, and morphogenesis of interacting tissues. Thus, they are a means of coordinating the developmental behaviors of adjacent cell groups. In this way, inductions also establish spatial relationships among developing tissues. For example, an interaction between the optic stalk, an extension of the brain, and the ectodermal cells on the surface of the embryo causes the surface cells to thicken and form the lens placode. The optic stalk gives rise to the retina and the lens placode to the lens; this interaction ensures that these tissues are aligned. Interactions between embryonic epithelia and mesenchyme are reciprocal, influencing the behavior of both tissues. Embryonic epithelia, destined to become parenchymal tissues, interact with loose embryonic connective tissue, or mesenchyme, to form a variety of organs, including the lung, kidney, liver, and salivary glands. Molecular mechanisms involved in these interactions are not clear. Inducing molecules involved in the differentiation of early mesoderm in amphibia, however, have been shown to be similar or identical with growth factors including members of the TGF-$\beta$ and FGF families. These same peptides are involved in later developmental stages and as signals even in the adult. An inter-

action thought to lead to the formation of branched epithelial organs is remodeling by the mesenchyme of the basement membrane which lies beneath the epithelia. Here, the epithelium produces the basement membrane and stimulates the mesenchyme to produce matrix materials and various matrix-degrading enzymes, which in turn act on the basement membrane. Local alterations in the basement membrane cause the epithelial cells to arrange themselves into shapes that are characteristic of the tissue.

To produce organs of the correct shape, size, and pattern, cells must behave according to their position in the group. Moreover, the cells must act in coordination. The process proposed to account for these behaviors is positional information in which a cell "knows" its position in a population. This positional information is thought to result from the cell existing within a concentration gradient of some substance, often termed a morphogen. Retinoic acid, a vitamin A derivative, applied to developing chick limbs can mimic the behavior of a presumed morphogen. A gradient of retinoic acid presumably causes the limb bud cells to change positional information and to develop normal-appearing but misplaced digits. The evidence for retinoic acid being a morphogen is not unequivocal, and other signals or even mechanisms could specify positional information.

In both inductions and positional information, the signals appear to trigger cellular behaviors that are already within the repertoire of the responding cells. Thus, these signals do not appear to instruct the responding cells but to accelerate or select a developmental cell behavior.

## FIVE KEY MILESTONES OF HUMAN DEVELOPMENT

The complexity of human development begins with the formation of the gametes and includes five key sequential processes. These are fertilization, cleavage, implantation, gastrulation, and organogenesis. Fertilization is the formation of the fertilized zygote by union of the sperm with the egg. Cleavage is the rapid set of cell divisions that increase cell number without actual growth. Implantation is the invasion of the embryo into the maternal uterus. Gastrulation is the movement of cells that creates the basic body plan. And, organogenesis is the process by which individual organs arise, involving determination and differentiation and the cell behaviors involved in morphogenesis. These events occur early in human development. Organogenesis, for example, begins in the third week of development. The events are followed by growth of the embryo, due largely to an increase in the number of cells because of mitotic activity. The ultimate size of the developing embryo depends on many factors that are discussed elsewhere in this volume.

### Formation of Gametes

Gametogenesis produces highly differentiated male and female gametes that have undergone meiosis and thus contain a haploid number of genetically recombined chromosomes. The general scheme by which egg and sperm form is similar. The major and significant differences are the duration of meiosis and the amount of cytoplasm remaining. Meiosis consists of two sequential cell divisions, which result in reduction of the chromosomal number from 46 to 23. During the first meiotic division, the chromosomes of the gamete precursor cell recombine extensively because of crossing-over of the chromatids. At the end of the first division, each gamete becomes more distinct because the chromosomes sort into haploid cells independently of their maternal or paternal origins. Thus, the genetic complement of each human gamete is unique.

Spermatogenesis begins in the testis at puberty secondary to androgen stimulation and results in sperm bearing either an X or a Y chromosome. Meiosis lasts only a few days, and when complete, the cells differentiate. This process continues throughout life. Sperm are small, short-lived motile cells designed solely to reach and fertilize the egg. Their DNA is condensed and packaged in the nucleus of the sperm head, which is topped by the acrosome, a membrane-bound structure containing enzymes that assist in fertilization. The neck contains numerous mitochondria to provide energy for the motion generated by the flagellum tail.

Oogenesis is a slow and interrupted process that begins in the fetal ovary but pauses to be reinitiated after puberty. It periodically yields an egg that completes meiosis only after it has been fertilized. Many egg cell precursors begin meiosis in the human fetus, but most of these precursors die and no more will form. At about 5 months' gestation, meiosis arrests in the surviving cells. These cells lie dormant in the first meiotic division until puberty, when gonadotrophic hormones cause the ovarian follicle cells that surround the developing egg to differentiate into granulosa cells that assist in the maturation of the egg. The egg is large—the largest human cell. Eggs contain stores of RNA and ribosomes that enable protein synthesis to begin right after fertilization. Egg differentiation includes the production of a covering layer, the zona pellucida, which protects the egg during its early postfertilization passage through the fallopian tube.

A few developing eggs mature with each ovarian hormonal cycle. Early in the cycle, the meiotic process that began during fetal life reactivates, and the first meiotic division is completed. Near the midpoint of the cycle, with continued hormonal stimulation, ovulation occurs and usually a single egg with some adherent follicle cells, the corona radiata, is shed from the ovary. The egg then begins the second meiotic division, which is completed only after fertilization; if unfertilized, the egg dies in about 24 hours.

## Developmental Milestones

Developmental stages are illustrated in Figure 16-2.

### Fertilization

Fertilization restores the diploid number of chromosomes, determines gender, and initiates the developmental sequence. Fertilization of the egg occurs in the fallopian tube near the ovary by fusion of a recently ovulated egg with a sperm that has undergone capacitation induced by uterine fluids. Capacitation involves changes in the membrane covering the acrosome, allowing

release of the hydrolytic enzymes that enable the sperm to penetrate the corona radiata and the zona pellucida.

The sperm head attaches to the surface of the egg and the plasma membranes of the egg and sperm fuse. The egg reacts with depolarization of its plasma membrane, polymerization of the zona pellucida, and completion of the second meiotic division. These changes may be related to the release of calcium stores within the egg cytoplasm. The change in the plasma membrane and zona pellucida prevent the entry of other sperm. Once in the egg cytoplasm, the nucleus of the sperm enlarges. The male and female haploid nuclei fuse and their chromosomes intermingle, a process that forms the zygote, the fertilized egg.

### Cleavage

The zygote undergoes rapid cell divisions, called cleavages, forming a ball of cells, the morula, which develops an internal cavity, the blastocyst. The first division of the zygote occurs about 30 hours after fertilization, and repeated cleavages produce smaller cells, called blastomeres. This cell division occurs within the zona pellucida as the zygote is transported along the fallopian tube toward the uterus. At about 3 days after fertilization, the morula is a solid ball of 16 to 32 cells and enters the uterine cavity. The internal cells divide at a greater rate than do the outer cells and, on the fourth day after fertilization, a fluid-filled cavity develops within the morula, creating the blastocyst. The blastocyst is divided into two distinct cell populations—an outer trophoblast and an inner cell mass. The trophoblast cells form the extraembryonic structures such as the amnion and the chorion, and the inner cell mass cells produce the embryo proper.

### Implantation

The blastocyst implants into the endometrial lining of the uterus. On about day 5, the zona pellucida degenerates, exposing an adhesive region on the trophoblast cells overlying the inner cell mass. These cells adhere to the endometrial cells that have been suitably prepared during steroid hormone stimulation of the ovarian cycle. At about day 7, implantation begins by invasion of the trophoblast cells between these uterine lining cells. Thus, by the end of the first week, the blastocyst is superficially implanted within the uterus. The invading trophoblast differentiates into two layers, the syncytiotrophoblast—an outer layer lacking cell boundaries—and the cytotrophoblast—an inner cellular layer. The syncytiotrophoblast continues to invade while it produces chorionic gonadotropin, which converts the corpus luteum in the ovary into the corpus luteum of pregnancy. The steroid hormones produced by the corpus luteum maintain the lining of the uterus for development of the embryo.

During the second week of human development, the trophoblast cells of the blastocyst further differentiate and begin to form the rudiments of the placenta, the extra-embryonic membranes including the primitive yolk sac (contains no yolk), and the amniotic sac. The embryo grows into the cavity formed by the amniotic sac, which enlarges and obliterates the chorionic cavity formed by the surrounding chorion that is also derived from the trophoblast.

### Gastrulation

During the formation of the extra-embryonic membranes, the inner cell mass becomes "sandwiched" between the amniotic and the primary yolk-sac cavities. At this time, it consists of two sheets of epithelia that constitute the flat and circular embryonic disc. The lower of these two sheets is the roof of the primary yolk sac and is the embryonic endoderm. The upper sheet is the floor of the amniotic cavity and is the embryonic ectoderm. Thus, at the end of the second week of development, there are two layers of trophoblast, two sacs around the embryo, and two germ layers of the inner cell mass, which will become the embryo.

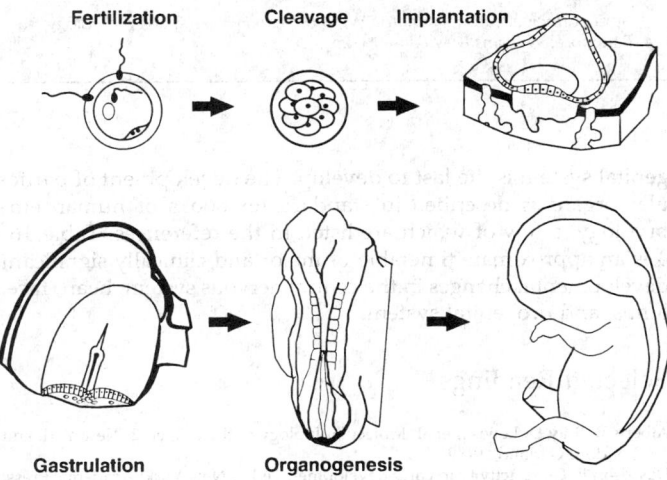

**Fertilization**  **Cleavage**  **Implantation**

**Gastrulation**  **Organogenesis**

Figure 16-2.  Milestones in development.

Beginning at about day 15, gastrulation converts the two germ layers into an embryo that has a basic body plan containing three axes: anterior-posterior, dorsal-ventral, and left-right. Gastrulation forms three distinct germ layers of the embryo: the ectoderm, the mesoderm, and the endoderm. The time of gastrulation coincides approximately with the first missed menstrual period.

Gastrulation occurs at a groove, the primitive streak, formed in the embryonic ectoderm at the midline of the embryonic disc near its posterior end. Embryonic ectoderm cells migrate into this groove and begin to fill the potential space between the sheets of embryonic ectoderm and endoderm. These cells, which migrate anteriorly and laterally, form the embryonic mesoderm or mesenchyme. A cord of these cells coalesces anterior to the primitive streak to form the midline notochord, which lengthens, causing the embryonic disc to become elongated. At the completion of gastrulation, which occurs by the end of the third week, the embryo is now in three layers, has each of the three body axes, and is spatially organized.

## Organogenesis

During organogenesis, the cells in the embryo undergo differentiation and morphogenesis to form specific tissues and organs. The ectoderm, the first layer to undergo organogenesis, begins to form the central nervous system on day 18 of gestation. The ectoderm will form the brain, its accessory organs, and neural crest, which forms the dorsal root and sympathetic ganglia, adrenal medulla, and melanocytes, as well as the epidermis and its derivatives, the sweat and mammary glands. Neurulation, formation of the central nervous system, begins by the thickening of the ectoderm in the dorsal midline. This thickened region then buckles, and folds appear at the margin of the buckle. The folds push toward each other, eventually meeting and fusing to form a continuous canal running from the head to the tail of the embryo, forming the neural tube. Because the neural tube grows faster than the rest of the embryo, the relatively flat embryonic disc begins to convex. This folding continues and ultimately repositions the germ layers so the originally dorsal ectoderm nearly surrounds the embryo.

The folding causes the originally ventral endoderm to be covered by the other two germ layers. This internalization enables the endoderm to form a tube that eventually becomes the gut lining and the numerous glands and outgrowths associated with the gut including the liver, pancreas, salivary glands, and lungs. By day 30, the folding process is completed and the future body regions are in their appropriate places within the embryo.

The mesoderm organizes into several regions, predominantly in the center of the embryo between the base of the head and the tail. The mesoderm consists of mesenchymal cells (the loose connective tissue of the embryo) that interact with epithelia of ectodermal and endodermal origin to form various organs. The somite (or paraxial) mesoderm adjacent to the notochord condenses into segments. Then, each somite splits into three—the dermatome, which forms the dermis, the myotome, which forms the muscles of the limbs and trunk, and the sclerotome, which forms the vertebrae. Lateral to the somites is the intermediate (or nephrogenic) mesoderm, which forms the urogenital system and its associated glands. Lateral to the intermediate mesoderm is the lateral plate mesoderm. This mesoderm forms serous linings and the blood and lymphatic vascular systems. Additionally, when associated with surface ectoderm, this mesoderm forms the bones and cartilage of the limbs; when associated with endoderm, these cells assist in the formation of the liver, pancreas, and intestines.

Different organs develop at different rates and involve the inductive tissue interactions discussed earlier. The earliest organ system to become functional is the cardiovascular system, which begins early in the fourth week of development to bring nutrients and oxygen from the mother to the developing embryo. The uro-

### TABLE 16-4.  Timetable of Human Organ Development

| Organogenesis Event | Approximate Embryonic Age (days) |
|---|---|
| Neural folds begin to fuse. | 21–22 |
| Heart tubes fuse. | |
| Optic evagination occurs. | 23–24 |
| Heart begins to beat. | |
| 1st and 2nd bronchial arches appear. | |
| Anterior neuropore closes. | 25–27 |
| Optic vesicle appears. | |
| Primitive atria fuse. | |
| Posterior neuropore closes. | 28–30 |
| Cardinal veins appear. | |
| 3rd bronchial arch appears. | |
| Arm bud appears. | |
| Ureteric bud appears. | |
| Lens placode invaginates. | 31–34 |
| Septum primum appears. | |
| Interventricular septum appears. | |
| Mandibular arches fuse. | |
| 4th bronchial arch appears. | |
| Leg bud appears. | |
| Urorectal septum forms. | |
| Cerebellum appears. | 35–38 |
| Lens separates. | |
| Atrioventricular canal fuses. | |
| Foramen secundum is present. | |
| Müllerian ducts appear. | |
| Hand plate forms. | |
| Aorta, pulmonary valves appear. | 39–44 |
| Upper lip fuses. | |
| Pinna appears. | |
| Adrenal cortex primordium forms. | |
| Finger rays appear. | |
| Cerebral commissurses appear. | 45–47 |
| Eyelids appear. | |
| Interventricular foramen closes. | |
| Palate fuses. | |
| Genital tubercle forms. | |
| Cornea develops. | 48–51 |
| Septum secundum appears. | |
| Anal membrane perforates. | |
| Urogenital membrane degenerates. | |
| Webbed fingers appear. | |

*Data principally from Hamilton WJ, Mossman HW. Human embryology, ed 4. Baltimore: Williams & Wilkins, 1972.*

genital system is the last to develop. The development of particular organs is described in standard textbooks of human embryology, a few of which are listed in the references. Table 16-4 is an approximate timetable of major and clinically significant developmental changes in the central nervous system, heart, face, limbs, and urogenital system.

## Selected Readings

Alberts B, Bray D, Lewis J, et al. Molecular biology of the cell, ed 2. New York and London: Garland, 1989.
Davidson E. Gene activity in early development, ed 3. New York: Academic Press, 1986.

Gilbert, Scott F. Developmental biology, ed 3. Sunderland, MA: Sinauer Assoc., 1991.

Moore KL. The developing human, ed 4. Philadelphia: WB Saunders, 1988.

Sadler T. Langman's medical embryology, ed 6. Baltimore: Williams & Wilkins, 1990.

Walbot V, Holder N. Developmental biology. New York: Random House, 1987.

Watson JD, Hopkins NH, Roberts JW, et al. Molecular biology of the gene, ed 4. Menlo Park, CA: Benjamin/Cummings, 1987.

*Principles and Practice of Pediatrics, Second Edition.*
edited by Frank A. Oski et al. J. B. Lippincott Company, Philadelphia © 1994.

## 16.1.2 Congenital Malformations

Lewis B. Holmes

### FREQUENCY OF MAJOR AND MINOR ANOMALIES

A major malformation is usually defined as a structural abnormality that has surgical, medical, or cosmetic importance. These are more common in spontaneously aborted fetuses than in term infants. About 2% to 3% of infants of at least 20 weeks' gestational age have a major malformation (Table 16-5). The frequency of malformations is higher among older children because "hidden" abnormalities, such as kidney malformations and heart defects, are detected when symptomatic or by accident during infancy. Having a single major malformation is much more common than having multiple malformations.

Minor anomalies, which are much more common than major malformations, are defined as having no surgical or cosmetic significance and as occurring in less than 4% of all newborns of the same race and sex. Minor abnormal physical features that occur in more than 4% of infants are considered normal variations.

The frequency of specific minor abnormal physical features varies among racial groups. For example, preauricular sinus and accessory nipples are more common among black than among white infants (Table 16-6). The pediatrician examining newborn infants should expect to find a few such minor abnormal physical features. Finding three or four minor anomalies should prompt a careful medical assessment for the presence of a major malformation, as such anomalies are present in about 20% of these infants. A few minor abnormal physical features are a significant physical finding that necessitates further diagnostic study. For example, an infant found to have a branchial sinus and a preauricular tag or sinus may have the branchio-oto-renal syndrome, a hereditary disorder in which serious kidney malformations occur. A capillary hemangioma and lipoma over the lumber spine can be a sign of a lipomeningocele in which tethering of the spinal cord can occur.

### RECOGNIZED ETIOLOGIES OF MALFORMATIONS

The cause of about 60% of major malformations can be predicted (see Table 16-4). The only etiology that can be proved is a chromosome abnormality, including trisomy, deletion, and unbalanced translocation. Attributions of malformations to autosomal-dominant and -recessive and X-linked genes are usually based on a comparison of the clinical findings in the affected individual with those of the recognized disorders. The presence of genetic abnormality will be established with more certainty as more mutations are identified in DNA studies, such as those now available to evaluate infants with the lethal (type-II) form of osteogenesis imperfecta.

### Malformations Due to Multifactorial Inheritance

The most common malformations (eg, heart defects and spina bifida) are attributed to multifactorial inheritance, a process in which mutant genes and environmental factors are involved. For all malformations attributed to multifactorial inheritance, the likelihood that a subsequent sibling (or the offspring of an affected parent) will be affected is 10 to 20 times greater than the risk in the general population (Table 16-7), but less than in instances

**TABLE 16-5. Congenital Malformations in Newborn Infants: Recognized Etiologies**

| | Number | % of Total | Example |
|---|---|---|---|
| **Genetic causes** | | | |
| Chromosome abnormalities | 157 (45) | 10.1 | Trisomies, deletions |
| Single mutant genes | 48 | 3.1 | Chondrodystrophies |
| Familial | 225 (3) | 14.5 | Renal agenesis |
| Multifactorial inheritance | 356 (23) | 23.0 | Anencephaly, some heart defects |
| Teratogens | 49 | 3.2 | IDM |
| Uterine factors | 39 (5) | 2.5 | Breech presentation |
| Twinning | 6 (2) | 0.4 | Acardia, conjoinings |
| Unknown cause | 669 (24) | 43.2 | Gastroschisis |
| Subtotals | 1549 (102) | 100.0 | |
| Overall total | 69,227 births | | |

Total frequency 2.2%.
( ) = therapeutic abortion.
*Nelson K, Holmes L. Malformations due to presumed spontaneous mutations in newborn infants. New Engl J Med 1989;320:19.*

**TABLE 16-6. Minor Abnormal Physical Features: Racial Differences**

| | Black Infants (%) (N = 871) | White Infants (%) (N = 4125) |
|---|---|---|
| Palpable metopic suture | 42.4 | 64.5 |
| Double hair whorl | 6.1 | 7.2 |
| Overfolded helix, left ear | 51.1 | 37.9 |
| Epicanthal fold, left | 1.3 | 2.5 |
| Anteverted nostrils | 2.0 | 2.6 |
| Preauricular sinus, left ear | 2.6 | 0.3 |
| Preauricular tag, left ear | 0.7 | 0.3 |
| Extra nipple, left or right side | 2.2 | 0.2 |
| Simian crease, left hand | 1.3 | 2.2 |
| Both hands | 0.7 | 0.5 |
| Sydney line, left hand | 8.5 | 14.0 |
| Clinodactyly, fifth finger, left hand | 7.2 | 8.1 |
| Syndactyly, toes 2–3 to first interphalangeal joint, left foot | 0.5 | 0.6 |

involving autosomal-recessive and -dominant genes with complete penetrance. For most conditions attributed to multifactorial inheritance, neither the genetic nor the environmental factors have been identified. However, progress is being made. Periconceptional supplementation with folic acid decreases significantly the occurrence of anencephaly or spina bifida. Recent studies show that parents of infants with anencephaly and spina bifida are more likely to share HLA alleles than are couples who have not had affected infants. Recent work suggests that a single autosomal-dominant gene is a more likely basis for cleft lip and palate than are multiple genes. The risk of heart defects shows a strong maternal influence with the offspring of affected mothers more likely to be affected than when the father is affected.

## Malformations Due to Teratogens

The teratogenic exposures during pregnancy that cause malformations include maternal conditions or diseases, maternal infections, drugs taken during pregnancy, exposures to heavy metals and the prenatal diagnostic procedure chorionic villus sampling (CVS) (Table 16-8). The first trimester of the pregnancy is the period of exposure that is most likely to produce malformations. Exposures in the second and third trimester are of equal concern, however, because these could be related to the occurrence of renal tubular dysplasia, microcephaly, growth retardation, and cognitive dysfunction. The risk that the exposed fetus will be damaged is typically expressed relative to the frequency of similar problems in the general population. It ranges from an increase of at least 20-fold for the drugs isotretinoin (retinoic acid) and valproic acid, to 2- to 3-fold for phenytoin and insulin-dependent diabetes mellitus. In general, one predicts that the higher the exposure, the greater the risk of damage. There is a pattern of major and minor anomalies in infants exposed to drugs such as thalidomide, diethylstilbestrol (DES), phenytoin, isotretinoin, and tetracycline and to maternal conditions such as alcoholism and systemic lupus erythematosus. Some maternal conditions, such as insulin-dependent diabetes mellitus, however, produce a variety of malformations involving several different organ systems but no consistent pattern of abnormalities. For some exposures, such as to alcohol and lead, there is a great need for more information on the risk, if any, from exposures to low levels, which are more common and more difficult to assess.

The mechanism of action is known for some teratogens. The hypothyroidism produced by iodides and propylthiouracil is caused by interference with the synthesis of thyroid hormone. The anticoagulant warfarin inhibits vitamin K reductase and interferes with the synthesis of the calcium-binding amino acid gamma-carboxyglutamic acid, thereby interfering with the function of growth factors that affect early chondrogenesis. It has been observed that parents with one child damaged by an exposure to the anticonvulsant phenytoin in utero have a greater risk of having a second affected child than do parents whose exposed children were unaffected. Recent studies suggest a genetic basis for this effect. Typically, one parent has a defect in ability

**TABLE 16-7. Malformations Attributed to Multifactorial Inheritance**

| Malformation | Race/Nationality | Prevalence in Newborn Infants (Rate/100) | Recurrence Risk Affected Sib, Normal Parents (%) | Recurrence Risk One Affected Parent No Affected Sibs (%) |
|---|---|---|---|---|
| Anencephaly, spina bifida | White | 0.1–0.2 / 0.2 | 2 to 3% | NA / 2 to 3% |
| Cleft palate | White | 0.03 | 4.3 | 6.2 |
| | Black | 0.01 | | |
| | Japanese | 0.05 | 2.3 | |
| Club foot (talipes equinovarus) | White | 0.08 | 2.9 | 1.4 |
| | Japanese | 0.08 | | |
| | Polynesian | 0.8 | | |
| Hypospadias | White | 0.08 | 7.0 | 7. |
| Intestinal agangliosis (Hirschsprung's disease) | White Short segment | 0.02 | 2.6, aff. brother 1.0, aff. sister | 2.0 |
| | Long segment | | 7.9, aff. brother 7.0, aff. sister | |
| Ventricular septal defect | White | 0.2 | 1.5–4.2 | 6–10, affected mother; 2, affected father |

## TABLE 16-8.  Recognized Human Teratogens

| Drugs | Radiation, therapeutic |
|---|---|
| Aminopterin/amethopterin | Cancer therapy |
| Androgenic hormones | **Maternal Conditions** |
| Angiotensin converting enzyme inhibitors | Alcoholism |
| Busulfan | Insulin-dependent diabetes mellitus |
| Carbamazepine | Maternal phenylketonuria |
| Chlorobiphenyls | Myasthenia gravis |
| Cocaine | Smoking (cigarettes and marijuana) |
| Cyclophosphamide | Systemic lupus erythematosus |
| Diethylstilbestrol | **Intrauterine Infections** |
| Etretinate | Cytomegalovirus |
| Heroin/methadone | Herpes simplex |
| Iodide | Parvovirus |
| Isotretinoin (13-cis-retinoic acid) | Rubella |
| | Syphilis |
| Lithium | Toxoplasmosis |
| Phenobarbital | Varicella |
| Phenytoin | Venezuelan equine encephalitis virus |
| Propylthiouracil | |
| Prostaglandin | **Other exposures** |
| Tetracycline | Chorionic villus sampling (CVS) |
| Thalidomide | Gasoline fumes |
| Trimethadione/paramethadione | Heat |
| | Hypoxia |
| Valproic acid | Methyl isocyanate |
| Warfarin | |
| **Heavy Metals** | |
| Lead | |
| Mercury | |

to detoxify phenytoin. The exposed fetus may inherit this metabolic abnormality and be damaged because of difficulty in metabolizing the drug that crosses the placenta into fetal circulation.

## Malformations Due to Uterine Factors

The presumed uterine factors that cause malformations are the effects of crowding, breech presentation, and entanglement. The amniotic band syndrome is attributed to entanglement of the fetal parts with strands of amnion. This pattern of abnormalities could also be due to factors such as hypoxia that are intrinsic to the fetus and produce the tissue damage. Breech presentation can produce hip dislocation and club-foot deformity because of continued fetal growth within the confines of the mother's pelvis. Crowding also occurs either in the septate uterus or in multiple gestations and produces positional deformities rather than true malformations. Monozygous twins are more likely to have major malformations than are singletons. Some of these abnormalities (eg, acardiac fetus, conjoined twins) occur only in monozygous twins. Other conditions such as cloacal exstrophy and sirenomelia are more common among twins and are attributed to the twinning process.

## Selected Readings

Leppig KA, Werler MM, Cann CI, et al. Predictive value of minor anomalies. I. Association with major malformations. J Pediatr 1987;110:531.

Mandell J, Blyth BR, Peters CA, et al. Structural genitourinary defects detected in utero. Radiology 1991;178:193.

McGimmis W, Krumlauf R. Homeobox genes and axial patterning. Cell 1992;68:283.

McKusick VA. Mendelian inheritance in man: catalog of autosomal-dominant, autosomal-recessive, and X-linked phenotypes, ed 9. Baltimore: Johns Hopkins University Press, 1990.

MRC Vitamin Study Research Group. Prevention of neural tube defects: results of the medical Research Council Vitamin Study. Lancet 1991;338:131.

Nora JJ, Nora AH. Maternal transmission of congenital heart diseases: new recurrence risk figures and the questions of cytoplasmic inheritance and vulnerability to teratogens. Am J Cardiol 1987;59:459.

Shepard TH. Catalog of teratogenic agents, ed 6. Baltimore: Johns Hopkins University Press, 1989.

Weitkamp LR, Schacter BZ. Transferrin and HLA: spontaneous abortion, neural tube defects, and natural selection. N Engl J Med 1985;313:925.

*Principles and Practice of Pediatrics, Second Edition.*
edited by Frank A. Oski et al. J. B. Lippincott Company, Philadelphia © 1994.

# 16.2 Growth and Metabolic Adaptation of the Fetus and Newborn

Ricardo Uauy, Patricia Mena, and Joseph B. Warshaw

## THE BASIS OF DEVELOPMENTAL PATHOLOGY

Many neonatal disease processes can be explained by preterm delivery, which determines unsuccessful adaptation and progressive compromise of specific organ function. The occurrence of hyaline membrane disease in babies born before 34 weeks gestation, that is, before surfactant production is adequate, is a good example of developmental pathology. The high prevalence of hypoglycemia in low–birth-weight (LBW) infants represents abnormalities in either storage or mobilization of glycogen. The patent ductus arteriosus (PDA) corresponds to an incomplete cardiovascular adaptation with failure of ductal closure.

Cardiovascular adaptations required by neonates include a drastic reduction in pulmonary vascular resistance needed to increase lung blood flow and reduce the right to left shunt through the ductus arteriosus. Subsequently, closure of the ductus arteriosus establishes separate right and left cardiac functions as two pumps in series. Pulmonary adaptations include the establishment of continuous rhythmic ventilatory movements to ensure oxygenation, the maturation of lung alveolar structure and a capillary network sufficient for gas exchange, and the biochemical development of the surfactant system including production, release, and recycling of disaturated phosphatydylcholine and phosphatydyl glycerol. Given the wide shifts in oxygenation, cellular metabolism must alternate between aerobic and anaerobic conditions for energy yielding processes.

Metabolic maturational events include the regulation of substrate flux and metabolism needed for maintenance and growth needs and the metabolism and excretion of waste products including acid, nitrogen, various electrolytes, and other minerals. As part of this successful adaptation to extrauterine life, the newborn must generate heat and maintain thermal balance independently. Heat production in the neonate depends on metabolic thermogenesis rather than muscular activity (shivering), which appears several months after birth. Successful metabolic adaptation requires that the neonate mobilize energy reserves (from glycogen and adipose tissue), generate glucose from amino acids and lactate, and regulate fuel supply to key organs by interaction of various hormones including insulin, glucagon, cortisol, and catecholamines. When continuous nutrient supply through the placenta is interrupted, the neonate must adapt to intermittent bolus feeds of nutrients that require processing before entry into circulation. The intestine during fetal life will recycle water ingested with the amniotic fluid; ex-utero, it must digest and absorb intact proteins, hydrolyze and reesterify fat, and convert lactose to dextrose and galactose. These maturational events are characterized structurally and biochemically and are dependent on systemic and gut hormonal mediators. Overall, these adaptive responses are integrated and mediated by the neuroendocrine system, which acts as a focal point to ensure successful adaptation (Table 16-9).

Many of the neonatal consequences of obstetrical problems can be avoided because of advances in prenatal and delivery room care. Thus, birth trauma and birth asphyxia are less frequent. Still, the consequences of preterm labor remain important because of poor understanding of the mechanisms responsible and of the interventions required to prevent premature deliveries. Even if premature labor and obstetrical complications associated with birth were eliminated, there would still be neonatal morbidity and mortality associated with genetic disorders and congenital malformations.

## GENETIC AND ENVIRONMENTAL INFLUENCES ON FETAL GROWTH

Fetal growth is regulated by and largely depends on the specific genetic endowment that defines normal range of growth. Envi-

---

### TABLE 16-9.   Immediate Neonatal Adaptations Necessary for Successful Extrauterine Life

**Cardiovascular**
Reduction in pulmonary vasculature resistance
Increased lung blood flow
Closure of ductus arteriosus
Separate right and left cardiac pumps

**Pulmonary**
Maturation of alveoli and capillary network
Development of the surfactant system (phosphatidylcholine and phosphatidylglycerol)
Rythmic respiration
Maturation of antioxidant enzyme systems

**Metabolic-Endocrine**
Thermogenesis and temperature regulation
Glucose homeostasis (glycogenolysis, gluconeogenesis)
Neuroendocrine responsiveness
Enzymatic maturation for detoxification, excretion, and metabolism of fuels and substrate

**Nutritional**
Intermittent rather than continuous feeds
Digestion and absorption of nutrients
Excretion of acid, nitrogen, and electrolytes
Maintenance of nutrient supply for growth and development

**Neurodevelopmental**
Integrated responses to environmental stimuli
Maintenance of autonomic regulation under new conditions
Activation of sensory input and processing necessary for learning
Operation of reflexes and behaviors needed for survival

---

ronmental factors modulate expression of genetic potential and may be important determinants of fetal growth. These nongenetic factors include the uterine and maternal environments and the external influences that may affect the mother and, thus, impact the fetus. Genetic influences on fetal growth play a significant role in the birth weight variability observed among different ethnic groups, ranging from a mean birth weight of 2400 grams among the pygmies to a mean of 3500 grams or greater in the affluent subpopulations of industrialized countries. Some of these differences may be explained by environmental factors, but in many cases, differences persist even after socioeconomic level and maternal nutritional status are controlled, suggesting intergeneration of genetic influences.

Another example of the effect of genotype is the increased birth weight among males, averaging 150 grams more than females at term. These differences are apparent only during the third trimester of gestation and may relate to increased androgens secreted by the male fetus. The effect of chromosomal alterations on fetal growth is another example of the influence of genetic factors. Turner's syndrome (45 XO) is associated with abnormal fetal growth. This has also been noted in infants with trisomy 21, Down syndrome, and with trisomies 13 and 18. LBW is also observed in infants with triploidy or polyploidy. Experimental studies show significant slowing of cell division in either trisomic or triploid cell lines. Genetic disorders not associated with specific chromosomal abnormalities may also be accompanied by decreased or increased fetal growth. Two extremes are hereditary gigantism (Sotos syndrome) and the genetic forms of dwarfism.

Environmental influences on fetal growth include the intra-uterine environment, which is determined largely by uterine blood flow, placental function, local uterine circulation, and placental and umbilical circulation. These factors determine the substrate and gas flux necessary to support fetal growth. In most cases, large babies are associated with large placentas and small babies associated with small placentas. The placenta usually weighs 20% of the baby's weight. Under some conditions, small babies may be associated with normal or large placentas. In extreme maternal nutritional deprivation, the placenta may actually continue to grow at the expense of the fetus, compromising its development. Intrauterine growth retardation, in most clinical conditions, is associated with diminished placental blood flow. This is true with maternal toxemia, severe diabetes, and long-standing hypertension and tobacco smoking. Doppler ultrasound evaluation of umbilical artery flow and resistance can be used to assess fetal well-being.

Other effects of placental function on fetal growth are mediated by several polypeptide or steroid hormones and growth factors produced by the placenta. These not only regulate substrate flow to the fetus but may be responsible for promoting and regulating cell replication and differentiation in the fetus. Abnormal uterine anatomy, ectopic placental insertion, placental abruptio or infarction, placental hemangioma or arteriovenous fistulae, congenital infections, and abnormal cord insertion all affect placental function and may adversely affect fetal growth.

The maternal environment is critical for optimal fetal growth. The mother usually acts as a buffer to ameliorate adverse environmental conditions, but a well-nourished, healthy mother can better provide the necessary substrates for fetal growth. Many studies show a positive correlation between maternal weight gain and fetal growth as measured by birth weight. The classic studies of the Dutch famine during the latter part of World War II showed a mean reduction in birth weight of 300 grams among infants whose mothers suffered severe caloric deprivation during the last trimester of gestation. The mean ration was 1300 kilocalories per day, barely enough to sustain the basal energy needs of the mother. In well-nourished mothers, caloric deprivation must be extreme before fetal growth is compromised. However, in women from developing countries where malnutrition may be entrenched over several generations, a moderate energy deficit adversely affects birth weight. Under such conditions, improving maternal nutrition during gestation is associated with small increases in birth weight. Several studies show that maternal height, which is determined by early nutritional influences, has an important influence on birth weight. Paternal size does not appear to influence birth weight. After 2 years of age, the growth of the infant correlates better with mean parental height rather than maternal height alone. This suggests that genetic factors contributed equally by both parents are important in determining final size, while early maternal nutrition, which is reflected in the maternal height, has a major influence on fetal growth. Moreover, there may be multigenerational influences on fetal growth. Mothers who were small for gestational age (SGA) are at a greater risk of having an SGA or preterm baby. Most likely, the effect of early maternal nutrition is mediated by the size of the uterus and its hypertrophic capacity in response to pregnancy.

Other maternal conditions that affect fetal growth include maternal age and parity. Mothers younger than 15 years and older than 35 years of age have a higher incidence of LBW babies. This effect is explained partly by parity and other socioeconomic risk factors. First-born infants usually weigh less than second- or third-born infants. Ideally, standards used to evaluate fetal growth should consider not only gestational age but also infant sex, maternal height, and birth order.

Maternal medical disease is an important determinant of diminished fetal growth. Maternal hypertension and preeclampsia have major impacts in determining low maternal weight gain and LBW. Chronic essential hypertension, collagen vascular disease, and renal disease all affect fetal growth either by compromising maternal nutritional status or by interfering with uterine perfusion. Severe maternal anemia caused by chronic blood loss or iron deficiency, diminished cardiac output secondary to heart disease or cyanotic congenital heart disease, and various autoimmune disorders may affect fetal growth by decreasing oxygen availability to the maternal uterine compartment. Recent in vitro and in vivo evidence suggests the perturbations in embryonic fuel metabolism caused by gestational diabetes may play a role in determining abnormal fetal growth and congenital anomalies. Mannose or other agents that inhibit glycolysis induce malformations in embryo cultures. The addition of glucose and oxygen to maintain fuel oxidation prevents the mannose-induced teratogenesis. Later in pregnancy, maternal hyperglycemia associated with gestational diabetes induces fetal hyperinsulinism and may cause macrosomia with enhanced growth of peripheral adipose tissue, muscle hypertrophy, and increased glycogen deposits in liver.

Intrauterine infections also are associated with growth failure. Rubella and cytomegalovirus infections have been implicated in SGA infants. Toxoplasmosis, syphilis, and herpes infections, although less frequent during the first trimester, may affect fetal growth by arresting cell replication during critical stages of development, causing typical patterns of malformations or severely compromised growth.

Other environmental factors that affect fetal growth include the effects of altitude, radiation, and environmental toxins, as well as drugs used for therapeutic purposes or because of maternal addiction. The effect of high altitude is to lower ambient oxygen tension, increasing the risk for fetal hypoxemia. At altitudes higher than 5000 meters, fertility may be compromised. Radiation exposure is associated with patterns of malformation including microcephaly and abnormal fetal growth. Other toxic substances include the heavy metals, especially mercury and cadmium, exposure to both of which are associated with malformation and compromised fetal growth.

There is an expanding list of drugs that may lead to intrauterine

growth retardation in humans. Many of these agents result in growth restriction or a spectrum of congenital malformations. Smoking, especially in the last trimester of pregnancy, has been shown to reduce birth weight and birth length. The effect is proportional to the number of cigarettes smoked by the mother. The fetal alcohol syndrome is characterized by prenatal and postnatal growth failure, microcephaly, mental delay, and characteristic craniofacial features including short palpebral fissures and midfacial hypoplasia. Infants born to heroin, cocaine, or methadone addicted mothers also show evidence of prenatal growth retardation; the effects of cocaine appear more severe. Other drugs with demonstrated adverse affects on fetal growth include anticonvulsants such as Dilantin, phenobarbital, and Tegretol, and antifolates such as methotrexate, Coumadin, and prednisone. Micronutrients such as vitamins and minerals are increasingly recognized as agents that ameliorate or, in some cases, enhance altered embryogenesis and congenital malformations. Folate intake before and during the early stages of embryogenesis has been suggested to be a factor in determining the prevalence of neural tube defects. Retinoic acid, derived from retinol (vitamin A), is a regulator of the expression of key genes and is a teratogen early in embryonic development. It also has been shown to enhance cell differentiation and decrease the risk of spina bifida in some animal models. Zinc deficit during gestation has been implicated in abnormal fetal growth and enhanced action of teratogens. Alcohol, valproic acid, arsenic, and other developmental toxins have been demonstrated to induce metallothionein synthesis by the maternal liver, thus sequestering zinc and enhancing the teratogenicity of these agents. The potential role of altered vitamin D metabolism in the skeletal abnormalities found in women receiving anticonvulsants has been recognized. In addition, the role of specific nutrients such as calcium and essential fatty acids in modulating pregnancy-induced hypertension have resulted in their present evaluation in the prevention of this condition. The balance of dietary essential $\omega$-3 and $\omega$-6 polyunsaturated fatty acids in cell membranes may affect the time of onset of labor because these fatty acids are precursors for prostanoids synthesis.

## INTERACTION OF NUTRIENTS, HORMONES, AND GROWTH FACTORS DURING PERINATAL GROWTH

Fetal growth is a complex process, and while fetal growth is ultimately controlled by genetic endowment, it is nonetheless influenced by diverse environmental factors. Fetal growth depends on adequate nutritional substrates; the action of a variety of hormones including insulin, thyroid hormones, and gonadal steroids; and the mediation of an array of growth factors such as IGF-I and IGF-II and epidermal growth factor. During fetal development, there are important interactions between nutritional state and hormonal and growth factor influences. Insulin, one of the principal hormones influencing fetal somatic growth, regulates fetal lipogenic activity and has a permissive role in hepatic glycogen deposition and protein synthesis. Fetuses with insulin deficiency secondary to pancreatic agenesis or with a defective insulin receptor as in "leprechaun" syndrome have marked intrauterine growth retardation (IUGR) with decreased adipose tissue and little weight gain during the last trimester of pregnancy. Conversely, fetal hyperinsulinism results in increased adiposity in human infants of diabetic mothers.

Protein feeding as well as several essential and nonessential amino acids stimulate insulin secretion in the fetus and neonate. Normal term infants fed cow's milk formula with a protein energy to total energy ratio (P:E) of 12% have higher levels of plasma insulin and urinary C-peptide than infants fed breast milk (P:E ratio 6%). Increasing arginine levels during parenteral infusion have been shown to increase serum insulin levels in newborn infants. Higher protein intakes in LBW infants are associated with a higher secretion of C-peptide. The significant correlation of urinary C-peptide excretion with weight gain suggests that insulin may be a growth promoting factor for infants on high protein diets. Preliminary evidence from a controlled clinical study in extremely small preterm infants shows increased tolerance to glucose and higher weight gain in infants infused with insulin during their initial postnatal days.

Other "classic" hormones including thyroxin, glucocorticosteroids, and sex hormones influence specific organ development and functional and metabolic adaptation, but have little influence on somatic growth. For example, thyroid hormones are important for central nervous system and skeletal maturation, glucocorticoids modulate lung maturation, and androgens are critical for sex differentiation. Pituitary growth hormone is not important in regulating fetal growth and does not appreciably influence size at birth. Males with growth hormone deficiency have a high incidence of micropenis. A growth hormone-like molecule, however, produced by the placenta—placental lactogen, or chorionic sommatomammotropin—may have a role in modulating fetal growth.

In the ovine fetus, maternal malnutrition reduces the number of placental lactogen receptors in fetal liver. The growth promoting role of placental lactogen in man is uncertain because pregnancies in which the gene for placental lactogen is missing result in normal birth weight.

Peptide growth factors that influence fetal growth and maturation include the insulin-like growth factors (IGF I and IGF II). In the fetus, these are independent of growth hormone regulation. IGF I influences terminal differentiation of a number of tissues, including brain astrocytes, neural outgrowth, and myogenesis. Even though the influences of IGF I appear to be local, serum concentrations of IGF I correlate with birth weight. Both IGF I and IGF II are complexed to binding proteins that modulate their biological activity. Growth retardation in fetal rats caused by maternal starvation has been associated with decreased expression of IGF I and IGF II and with increased expression of binding proteins in liver of the fetuses, suggesting that these factors have a role in regulating fetal growth. Epidermal growth factor and TGF-α, which may be its fetal form, influence growth and differentiation of epithelial cells including those in lung and gut. Receptors for EGF are present throughout development and are increased in number in placenta and lung in fetuses with growth restriction induced by uterine artery ligation, suggesting a role for EGF in fetal growth retardation. Additional evidence for an effect on EGF on somatic growth is the observation that exogenous EGF administered to rats less than 2 weeks of age decreases growth. This effect of EGF has been related to suppression of IGF-I concentrations in growth restricted fetuses.

It is likely that the changes in blood flow that characterize the hemodynamic response to fetal nutrient restriction are modulated by endocrine mechanisms. Stressed fetuses have increased circulating levels of arginine vasopressin, which may contribute to decreased splanchnic blood flow and increased blood flow to the brain that is associated with "brain sparing" during growth retardation. Vasoactive prostaglandins also are likely to be important in modulating blood flow to the fetus and the hemodynamic changes that result in "brain sparing."

Maternal constraint of fetal growth and fetal adaptations occur under conditions of decreased nutrient supply or when fetal growth is inappropriate for maternal size. The latter may involve changes in growth factor or hormonal signaling. Mice selected for high plasma IGF I concentrations were not only larger but produced litters with heavier fetuses than mice selected for low IGF I concentrations. Maternal constraints on fetal growth also are illustrated by the classic study of Walton and Hammond showing that foals born to shire horses bred with Shetland ponies (female) are small and, therefore, appropriate for maternal size. The adverse effect of maternal malnutrition on fetal growth may take several generations to correct after reinstitution of normal nutrition, which emphasizes the importance of maternal factors and the intrauterine milieu. Table 16-10 summarizes genetic, hormonal and environmental influences on fetal growth.

## PLACENTAL TRANSPORT AND METABOLISM

The placenta and fetal membranes facilitate the efficient transfer of substrates and other nutrients from the mother to the rapidly growing fetus. The placenta allows for the excretion of fetal waste products and performs metabolic and hormonal functions that may substitute for the corresponding immature fetal organ. The human placenta can be classified as hemochorial based on the number of layers separating the maternal and fetal circulations. In this type of placentation, the fetal villi are directly bathed by maternal blood; therefore, the fetal capillary circulation is separated from maternal blood by fetal connective tissue and the placental epithelium, which, in turn, is composed of the cytotrophoblast and the syncytiotrophoblast. Other mammalian species have "thick" placentas in which various layers of maternal tissues are interposed between the maternal circulation and the fetal tissues. An understanding of placental ultrastructure is necessary to discuss the functional correlates. As shown in Figure 16-3, the upmost layer of fetal tissues, the syncytiotrophoblast, directly contacts maternal blood. Microvilli increase the surface area necessary for transport. Syncytial vacuoles transport macromolecules and may be specifically targeted by cell surface receptors. The extensive endoplasmic reticulum network and the high density of mitochondria provide the anatomical basis for both synthetic activities and transport through the cytoplasm of the trophoblast.

---

**TABLE 16-10.    Genetic, Hormonal, and Environmental Influences on Fetal Growth**

**Genetic and Fetal Factors**
Species, racial, gender
Congenital anomalies
Chromosomal disorders
Fetal hormones (insulin, corticosteroids, thyroid hormone, androgens)
Growth factors (IGF I and IGF II, EGF and TGF-α)

**Maternal Uterine Environment**
Uterine and placental anatomy
Utero-placental function
Human placental lactogen
Substrate fluxes and transfer
Uterine blood flow
Maternal systemic disease

**Macroenvironment**
Infectious agents (STORCH)
Diet and nutrition
Social and emotional stress
Drugs and smoking
Teratogens and toxins
Altitude and temperature
Ionizing radiation

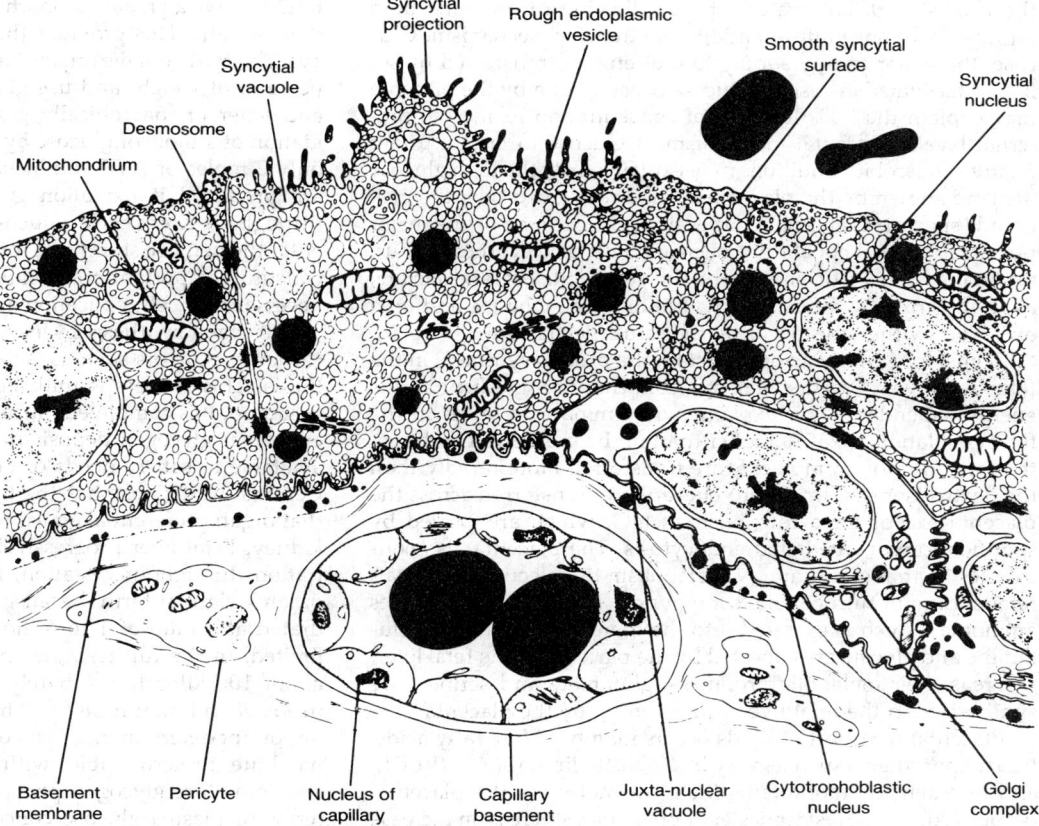

**Figure 16-3.** Diagram of structure of a placental membrane (seen by electron microscope). The syncytial trophoblast (upper portion of figure) is exposed to maternal blood. Microvilli increase the area for transfer. Syncytial vacuoles may be part of the pinocytotic process for protein transfer. The rich mitochondrial and endoplasmic systems provide the machinery for intense synthetic activity. The syncytiotrophoblast, which is incapable of cell division, derives from the cytotrophoblast. (Boyd JD, Hamilton WJ. The human placenta. Cambridge: Heffer & Sons, 1970.)

The multinucleated syncytiotrophoblast is incapable of cell division and derives from the actively replicating cytotrophoblast. The trophoblast represents the only uninterrupted cell layer interposed between the fetal capillary and maternal circulation. The trophoblast is also the basis for the immunologic barrier that protects the fetus from a host versus graft reaction. A homogeneous fibrin layer covering the trophoblast may also contribute in separating the mother and the fetus. Several experimental studies suggest there may be antigenic tolerance by the mother for the trophoblastic cells. This response may be facilitated by associated pregnancy endocrinologic changes that modify the maternal immune response.

The placenta grows rapidly during the initial stages of pregnancy. Placental growth is characterized by increased numbers of villi and microvilli and by proliferation of fetal capillary vessels. In this way, the surface area available for fetal–maternal exchange is greatly enhanced. The surface microvilli are bathed directly by maternal blood spurting into the intervillous space from the spiral arteries. Substrates circulating in maternal blood must cross the trophoblast cell layer and the basement membrane to reach the loose connective tissue surrounding the fetal capillaries.

Placental transfer can occur by diffusion in which the driving force is a concentration gradient across the placenta. The gradient is determined by the difference in concentration between fetal and maternal blood. Most small molecules appear to be transferred by simple diffusion; these include water, sodium, urea, oxygen, and carbon dioxide. A special case is the transport of glucose, the major energy substrate of the fetus. Fetal glucose uptake parallels maternal blood glucose concentration. There is evidence of a transport mechanism characterized by selective, facilitated diffusion with a high affinity for the substrate. Glucose transporter proteins have been described in the microvilli of the trophoblasts facing the maternal decidua and the fetal capillary.

The transporters are not responsive to insulin. They bind hexoses solely and have the highest affinity for glucose. Another mode of transfer is active transport. This is an energy-requiring transport mechanism that can occur against a concentration gradient. Such is the case for calcium, magnesium, and the specific transfer of L-amino acids. For many of these nutrients and for water soluble vitamins, specific transport proteins are identified within the lipid membrane of the placenta. The transfer of intact proteins or other hydrophobic macromolecules is probably mediated by pinocytosis or, more specifically, receptor-mediated endocytosis. The latter process requires a specific cell surface receptor with a binding site for the substrate or macromolecule that becomes internalized, processed, and released into the cytoplasm. This process initially described for the low-density lipoproteins is now characterized for iron, folate, vitamin $B_{12}$, insulin, and many other macromolecules. This mechanism probably accounts for the transfer of IgG, which occurs during the second half of pregnancy. Transplacental transfer of IgG is highly specific for this immunoglobulin and occurs faster than the transport of smaller circulating plasma proteins.

The major determinants affecting the placental transfer of small diffusible substances are related to maternal, placental, and fetal factors. The amount of substrate delivered to the placenta depends on blood substrate concentration and the blood flow to the intervillous space. Blood flow is regulated by both systemic and local factors. The placental surface area and the difference in concentration between the maternal intervillous space and the fetal villus capillary determines the driving force for diffusion. Resistance to diffusion depends on size, electrical charge, and polarity characteristics of the compound. Finally, the fetal perfusion pressure, flow to capillaries and blood concentration determines the extraction rate of diffused material.

The fetus totally depends on the intraplacental circulation for the provision of substrate. Fetal swallowing of amniotic fluid represents a nonsignificant additional transfer mechanism. Glucose, the major energy supply to the fetus, is transferred by selective facilitated diffusion. Glucose consumption by the placenta may explain the 20% lower fetal concentration relative to maternal levels. Placental metabolism of glucose to lactate under relative anaerobic conditions may explain partly the high glucose demand shown by the placenta. Evidence accrued over the past decade suggests that lactate rather than glucose may be the major precursor for fetal hepatic glycogen and fatty acid synthesis. Thus, the major sources of energy for the fetus, glucose and lactate, are transferred by diffusion. In addition, gas exchange and urea excretion by the fetus occur by the same mechanism.

Transfer of amino acids to sustain the protein synthesis in the fetus is active. It occurs against a concentration gradient and is energy dependent. This explains why amino acid levels in the fetal circulation are 30% higher than in the mother. In addition, the levo form of amino acids are transferred more rapidly than the dextro-isomers. Intact proteins are not transferred across the placenta except for a few, such as IgG, which are carried by specific receptor- mediated endocytosis. The placenta also contributes to amino acid and N metabolism by selective placental-fetal cycling of nitrogenous compounds. The placenta produces ammonia, which is excreted into the maternal circulation. Glutamine and glycine are exported by the placenta to the fetal liver, whereas their metabolic products—glutamate and serine—are synthesized in the fetal liver and taken up by the placenta.

Placental transport of lipids occurs mainly as free fatty acids. Intact lipoproteins such as very low-density lipoproteins (VLDL) and low-density lipoproteins (LDL) do not cross the placental barrier. During the last trimester of pregnancy, there is an increase in the fetal requirement for fatty acids, some of which is met by increased transport of fatty acids across the placenta. Most fatty acid accretion, however, is a product of fetal lipogenesis. Essential fatty acid needs of the fetus are met solely by transplacental transport and reflect maternal dietary supply. The placental transfer of fatty acids depends on lipid hydrolysis, maternal triglyceride hydrolysis, the transfer of fatty acids across fetal membranes, and reesterification with glycerol into triglycerides at the placental level. Experiment results suggest that short- and medium-chain fatty acids are transferred more easily than long-chain fatty acids. For essential fatty acids, a process of selective incorporation into fetal tissue has been described. The placenta may play an important role in the elongation and desaturation of the parent essential fatty acids forming the long-chain (greater than 18 carbon chain length) $\omega$-6 and $\omega$-3 fatty acids (ie, respectively, arachidonic acid, C20:4 $\omega$-6, and docosahexaenoic acid, C22:6 $\omega$-3) required as structural components of cell membranes. The chorion, the amnion, brain, and retina are particularly enriched with these essential polyunsaturated fatty acids.

## FETAL ENERGY METABOLISM

Glucose is the major energy substrate for the fetus and the newborn, although the fetus is capable of using lactate, free fatty acids, or ketone bodies under special conditions. Glucose transport across the placenta occurs down a concentration gradient with a maternal-to-fetal ratio for glucose concentration of 1.2- to 1.7-to-1. This transfer is stereospecific, exceeds the rate of transfer predicted from simple diffusion, and is linearly correlated with maternal glucose levels. These observations suggest that placental glucose transport occurs by facilitated diffusion. During the last trimester of pregnancy, it is estimated that 12 to 15 mg of glucose per kilogram of body weight per minute are transferred across the placenta. The placenta uses part of this glucose and may store part of it as placental glycogen. The liver, heart, and brain of the

fetus receive a greater proportion of cardiac output in relation to their weight. This provides these organs with greater substrate availability. The same organs have the highest energy expenditure per unit of weight and use glucose aerobically, producing $CO_2$ and water, or anaerobically, generating lactate. The complete oxidation of 1 mole of glucose by the anaerobic pathway generates only 2 moles of ATP and lactate. In contrast, 38 moles of ATP are produced if oxidation is completed in the mitochondria through the Krebs cycle. Glucose, by an alternative pathway, can enter the pentose shunt and form ribose. Ribose and deoxyribose constitute important precursors for the synthesis of nucleic acids necessary for cell replication and growth.

Glycogen synthesis in liver and muscle uses glucose and 3-carbon precursors such as lactate or pyruvate for glycogen synthesis. This process is initiated late in the second trimester of gestation. It is completed during the third trimester before delivery. Liver glycogen deposits represent stored glucose, which is available to satisfy needs of other organs, especially the brain. Cerebral hexokinase has the highest affinity for glucose, giving that organ preferential access to this fuel over liver, muscle, and kidney. Fetal liver progressively increases its glycogen concentration throughout gestation, reaching a maximum of 10% of organ weight at birth. Because glycogen within liver cells is hydrated at a ratio of 1 to 4, however, the total energy stored is limited. In the full-term newborn, glycogen stores account for about 100 kilocalories, barely enough to provide basal energy needs of an infant for 8 to 10 hours. Fetal glycogen stores are an important determinant of glucose homeostasis during early postnatal life. Preterm babies with diminished liver glycogen stores and immature glycogen phosphorylase, therefore, are labile in terms of plasma glucose concentrations. Some organs such as the liver, skeletal muscle, and heart can directly oxidize free fatty acids derived from lipolysis of triglycerides stored in adipose tissue. Adipose tissue represents the main energy reserve for the normal newborn, not only because the oxidation of 1 g of fat generates 9 kcal/g but also because triglycerides are stored within adipose tissue in a water-free environment, giving adipose tissue an energy density of 8 to 9 kcal/g as opposed to 1 kcal/g of wet liver. Table 16-11 lists energy stores at different gestational ages and birth weights. Only one third of the energy reserve from protein should be considered available because lean body mass losses of more than one third are associated with adverse functional consequences. This information allows for quantitative assessment of energy reserves for the fetus and clarifies survival potential under conditions of semistarvation. Thus, a full-term infant has an energy reserve that may support energy needs for several weeks, depending on catabolism, whereas the reserve for a 1000-g VLBW infant is spent within a couple of days.

**TABLE 16-11.  Energy Reserves of the Newborn at Various Birth Weights and Gestational Ages**

| Weight (g) | Gestational Age (weeks) | Energy Reserve (kcal) | | | |
|---|---|---|---|---|---|
| | | Glycogen | Protein | Fat | Total |
| 200 | 18 | 0 | 65 | 9 | 74 |
| 1000 | 27 | 4 | 416 | 90 | 510 |
| 2000 | 33 | 16 | 960 | 1080 | 2056 |
| 3500 | 40 | 70 | 1694 | 5040 | 6804 |
| 2200 | 40 | 26 | 871 | 1108 | 2005 |

*Adapted from Sharad DV, Ivengarm L. Composition of the human fetus. British Journal of Nutrition 1972;27:305 and Widdowson EM, Dickerson JWT. Composition of the body. In Diem K, Lentner C, eds. 1973 Scientific tables. Basle: Ciba-Geigy, p. 517.*

During the third trimester, the fetus forms triglycerides from glucose and lactate. There is also some transfer of free fatty acids across the placenta. Most fetal triglycerides are derived from direct lipogenic activity in the fetal liver and placenta because lipoprotein transfer from the mother as VLDL or chylomicrons is insignificant or nonexistent. The fetal brain and lung are also lipogenic organs in which lipids are components of structures with important functional roles. Triglycerides are transported in the fetal plasma as VLDL. In the periphery, triglycerides are hydrolyzed in the presence of lipoprotein lipase to free fatty acids which enter adipose tissue cells and are reesterified to triglycerides and stored. The adipose tissue exhibits dramatic hypertrophic growth during the last trimester of pregnancy. A 27-week fetus has only 1% of body weight as fat versus 16% in the full-term adequate for gestational age infant. Early in life, a significant amount of body fat is metabolically active, especially that located near major large vessels. This fat is rich in heme-containing cytochromes and in mitochondria and, hence, looks brown. Brown fat produces heat metabolically. The lipid vesicles provide fatty acids for oxidation, and the mitochondria possess a specific protein that functions as a proton channel in the inner mitochondrial membrane, thus dissipating the electrochemical potential generated by aerobic fuel oxidation without forming ATP. This mitochondrial protein is called uncoupling protein. Activation of thermogenesis is triggered by sympathetic stimulation of lipolysis. As the infant ages, shivering thermogenesis is established and most brown fat involutes or becomes white fat. The brain in early postnatal life can not oxidize free fatty acids directly; therefore, it usually relies on the availability of glucose. Ketone bodies produced by the liver from free fatty acids are the only significant alternative fuel for the brain. The fetal and neonatal brain can oxidize ketone bodies if a high enough concentration is present. The ketogenic response by the liver takes several days before it generates large numbers of ketone bodies because induction of necessary enzymes takes time. Maintenance of cerebral metabolism on an acute basis, then, depends on the adequacy of both liver glycogen stores and the glycogenolytic enzymes. Glucose cannot be formed from free fatty acids, but glucose can be formed from other substrates via the gluconeogenic pathway. The liver and the kidney are the main gluconeogenic organs in the fetus and neonate. Alanine and glutamine, generated from protein breakdown, as well as lactate and glycerol are the predominant gluconeogenic substrates. Thus, the newborn maintains glucose homeostasis while fasting or semistarved, typical conditions of early postnatal life. Early postnatal diets supplement and complement these metabolic responses by providing nutrients to obtain glucose and to supply free fatty acids. Human milk uniquely satisfies the needs of the newborn infant. It not only contains lactose but also significant amounts of easily absorbable medium-chain triglycerides. Even long-chain triglycerides in human milk have a special molecular configuration that makes them easier to digest and absorb. Palmitate is esterified predominantly to the sn-2 position of the glycerol, which improves its absorption because human milk lipase selectively hydrolyses this site. In addition, carnitine necessary for mitochondrial fatty acid transport facilitates fatty acid oxidation as shown by the higher levels of plasma ketone bodies observed in babies fed human milk.

Fetal growth not only depends on energy availability but also on an adequate supply of essential and nonessential amino acids. Protein synthesis in the fetus and in early postnatal life is estimated at 15 to 20 g/kg body weight/d. This is 5 to 8 times greater than that observed in adults. Based on amino acid transfer data from experimental studies and the fetal accretion of protein, it can be estimated that, during late gestation, placental transport of amino acid is 2.0 to 2.5 g/kg/d. The rapid anabolic rate of the fetus plus the presence of placental nitrogen exchange precludes the need for significant elimination of nitrogen waste by the fetus. The enzymes necessary for ammonia production and urea formation are all low in fetal life and exhibit significant rises in postnatal life as the protein load from both endogenous catabolism and dietary sources increases. Liver and kidney metabolism of nitrogen by-products is greatly activated postnatally. This is coupled to urea formation by the liver and ammonia genesis by the kidney that serves to excrete both nitrogenous waste products and acid equivalents.

## CARBOHYDRATE HOMEOSTASIS: ENDOCRINE RESPONSES AND INFLUENCES

Metabolic regulation in the newborn period is based on substrate availability and on the endocrine response induced by these substrates. During fetal life, after the 20th week of gestation, the fetal pancreas produces insulin in response to the normal flux of nutrients, especially glucose. This hormone regulates the accumulation of glycogen in liver, muscle, and lung. At the same time, it promotes lipogenesis and triglyceride storage within adipose tissue. Insulin also enhances protein synthesis in muscle and acts in general as a growth hormone-like substance. Insulin action is modulated by glucocorticoids, which regulate gene expression and induce activity of various enzymes related to glycogen and lipid synthesis. Steroid hormones are responsible for induction of glycogen synthetase type I, which is activated by insulin, and responsible for glycogen synthesis. Thus, despite detectable circulating insulin after 13 weeks' gestation, glycogen accumulation does not occur until the 27th week. The process of hormonal action requires the maturation of cell receptors and binding proteins, which are specific and necessary for adequate transcription and translation of genetic code at the cellular level. Insulin increases de novo fatty acid synthesis from acetyl-coA, which is derived from carbohydrate and lactate. Insulin also promotes the entry of amino acids into muscle and activates protein synthesis. High insulin levels inhibit lipolysis and glycogenolysis and are incompatible with adequate gluconeogenesis.

At the time of birth, the constant flux of glucose from the mother is interrupted, and there is an initial drop in the neonate's glucose level. This determines a lower insulin release and an increase in glucagon levels. The ratio between insulin and glucagon is essential in regulating gluconeogenesis and glycogenolysis. Glucagon activates adenylate cyclase in the hepatocyte membrane. This causes an increase in cyclic AMP within the cell, which activates the kinase system that is responsible for activating glycogen phosphorylase. This latter enzyme acts on hepatic glycogen to form glucose—6—phosphate, which forms glucose after phosphate cleavage by a specific phosphatase. The intracellular cascade triggered by cyclic AMP responds exponentially so small changes in glucagon induce large changes in glucose availability. The glycogenolytic response at birth depends on complete maturation of each step in this chain. Glycogen synthesis and degradation and gluconeogenesis are summarized in Figure 16-4.

Liver glycogen storage is limited. Despite the effective glycogenolytic response, this process ensures only short-lived glucose supply. Even for the full-term infant, glycogen as an exclusive fuel is estimated to provide energy substrate for only 10 hours of life. Glucagon and cortisol also are responsible for regulating gluconeogenesis. Formation of glucose from amino acids, lactate, or glycerol depends on an enzymatic system regulated by activity of the phosphoenolpyruvate carboxykinase and by glucose 1–6 diphosphatase. Glucagon determines an increase in the activity of these enzymes, generating glucose from 3-carbon precursors. This response requires enzymatic induction and availability of 3-carbon chain compounds derived from glycerol, lactate, or amino acids. Lactate is normally formed by anaerobic glycolysis

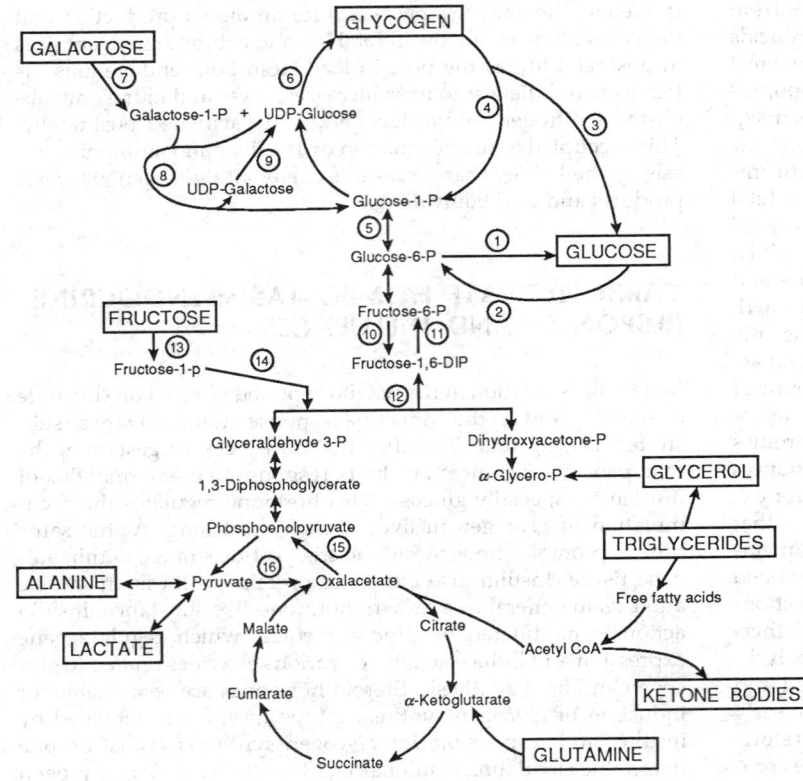

**Figure 16-4.** Metabolic pathways involved in glycogen synthesis and degradation and gluconeogenesis. Key enzymes are designated by number: *1*, glucose-6-phosphatase, *2*, glucokinase, *3*, amylo-1,6-glucosidase, *4*, phosphorylase, *5*, phosphoglucomutase, *6*, glycogen synthetase, *7*, galactokinase, *8*, galactose-1-phosphate uridyl transferase, *9*, uridine diphosphogalactose-4-epimerase, *10*, phosphofructokinase, *11*, fructose-1,6-diphosphatase, *12*, fructose-1,6-diphosphate aldolase, *13*, fructokinase, *14*, fructose-1-phosphate aldolase, *15*, phosphoenolpyruvate carboxykinase, *16*, pyruvate carboxylase.

of glucose. Gluconeogenesis from lactate is considered a recycling system rather than a net gain in glucose availability.

Glucagon and catecholamines, in addition to activating the glycogenolytic pathway, promote lipolysis, which generates glycerol and free fatty acids. High glucagon and cortisol and low insulin favor protein catabolism, especially skeletal muscle protein breakdown. This determines a net flux of alanine from muscle to liver. Muscle metabolism yields additional alanine from oxidation of branched chain amino acids such as leucine. Thus, the outflow of alanine from muscle is greater than the relative content of alanine in muscle protein. Free fatty acids are alternative fuels for the muscle, heart, kidney, and potentially the brain after ketone bodies are formed. Thus, free fatty acids are a major glucose sparing substrate for the newborn. Alanine from amino acid breakdown and glycerol from triglyceride breakdown, are the major gluconeogenic substrate that allow for normal glucose homeostasis after the first few hours of life and before adequate substrate are provided enterally or parenterally.

Postnatal changes in respiratory quotient, the ratio between carbon dioxide production and oxygen consumption, reflect the relative use of fuels early in postnatal life. Table 16-12 shows the respiratory quotient after birth. A value of 1.0 corresponds to predominant use of carbohydrates, specifically glucose, as a fuel for oxidation. A value of 0.7 corresponds to exclusive fatty acid oxidation. This information is validated by measurements of substrate flux using stable heavy isotopes labeled substrates such as $^{13}$C-glucose and $^{2}$H fatty acids to quantitate oxidation rates.

Other hormones that modulate glucose homeostasis include catecholamines, which act similarly to glucagon by increasing intracellular cyclic AMP to promote glycogen breakdown, lipolysis, and gluconeogenesis. Glucocorticoids potentiate the gluconeogenic action of glucagon and catecholamines. Steroids promote muscle protein breakdown and lipolysis and increase availability of gluconeogenic substrate. Thyroxine and growth

hormone promote lipolysis and further potentiate gluconeogenesis. Arginine vasopressin (AVP) also has been shown to induce a hyperglycemic response in the fetus. AVP is released during a variety of fetal stresses and may represent a major modulator of fetal metabolism in addition to regulating cardiovascular responses.

In summary, the goal of neonatal glucose homeostasis is to provide the brain and other vital organs with sufficient glucose as a key energy source. Virtually all hormones except insulin increase availability of glucose, which is taken up preferentially by the brain. The sequence described here is the basis for perinatal glucose adaptation and can be verified in virtually all mammalian species.

**TABLE 16-12. Respiratory Quotient (RQ) and Partition of Energy Used as a Fuel**

| | RQ | % Fat | % Carbohydrate |
|---|---|---|---|
| **Newborn** | | | |
| 15 min | 1.00 | — | 100 |
| 3 h | 0.90 | 33 | 67 |
| 48 h | 0.73 | 90 | 10 |
| 7 d | 0.82 | 40 | 60 |
| **Adult** | | | |
| Postprandial | 0.82 | 40 | 60 |
| Prolonged fast | 0.72 | 7 | 93 |

*Modified from Adams PAJ. Control of glucose metabolism in the human fetus and newborn infant. Advances in Metabolic Disorders 1971;5:183.*

# NUTRITION AND GROWTH OF PREMATURE INFANTS

Preterm infants are affected by significant illness usually associated with immaturity. They become malnourished because of intercurrent morbidity or because of iatrogenic practices leading to semistarvation. Eventually, when fed adequately they grow at a fast rate but usually do not fully catch up. Advances in neonatal clinical practices have allowed for survival of progressively smaller infants. The overall survival rate for VLBW infants (birth weight less than 1500 g) is 85% to 90%. For those less than 800 g, survival rate is close to 60%. The initial days or weeks of life for VLBW infants are characterized by significant weight loss due to catabolic illness and insufficient protein-energy supply. In most industrialized countries, VLBW infants constitute 1.0% to 1.5% of all births and account for a significant proportion of neonatal and infant mortality. The accepted practice of modern neonatal care is a 12% to 15% body weight loss period over the initial 10 days. After parenteral and enteral nutritional support is given, the infants take 15 to 20 days to regain birth weight. The catch-up growth phase observed in these infants may last 3 to 8 weeks. During this time, they grow at rates of 20 to 30 grams per kg body weight per day, which is nearly double the normal in-utero growth rate and three times that observed in the full-term newborn. Nutritional practices have helped significantly to shorten duration of hospital stay and may contribute to improved survival. The criteria for discharge includes not only attaining basic physiologic maturity but also reaching a critical weight, usually 1800 to 2200 g, depending on individual center practices. Thus, growth rate for VLBW infants has medical as well as practical implications. The duration of nutritional deprivation and the time to recover linear and head growth is correlated with subsequent developmental outcome. The study of nutrient needs for optimal catch-up growth of these infants and how to deliver nutrients to an immature gut have been the focus of extensive research for decades. Preterm human milk has a higher protein and sodium content relative to mature milk, thus is especially adapted to meet the needs of the LBW infant. Human milk fortifiers, which include nutrients (energy, protein, calcium, phosphorus, and trace elements) have been developed since human milk by itself is inadequate to fully meet the nutritional needs of very-low-birth-weight infants. Human milk also contains a variety of nutritional and nonnutritional factors that may modulate postnatal growth and development (Table 16-13).

Perinatal gastrointestinal development consists of sequential steps leading to successful digestion, absorption, and metabolism of nutrients needed for maintenance and growth. Early enteral feeding measurably affects maturational events; thus, postnatal semistarvation alone conspires against normal digestive functional development. Gastrin surges shortly after a feed, especially in a neutral pH environment (the pH of colostrum is 7.4). The likely stimuli for gastrin release are amines, decarboxylated amino acids products, which are taken up by G cells responsible for gastrin secretion. This gut hormone helps determine mucosal growth, smooth muscle contractions, and enzymatic maturation. Motilin and bombesin levels are also elevated after enteral feeds. Motilin modulates gut contractions and bombesin enhances gastrin release. Other gut hormones such as enteroglucagon, neurotensin, cholecystokinin, neuropeptide y, and gastric inhibitory peptide are liberated after a feed. Evidence suggests that even minimal enteral feedings (15 to 20 Kcal/kg/d) sufficiently maintain gut hormonal responses. Feeding tolerance and progression to full enteral feeding appears to be enhanced if minimal enteral feeding is established soon after birth. Nutrients supplied in excess of what can be tolerated at a given stage of functional development, however, increase the risk of acquiring necrotizing enterocolitis

---

**TABLE 16-13. Nutritional and Hormonal Factors Present in Human Milk That May Modulate Postnatal Growth and Development**

**Protein and Other Nitrogenous Compounds**

Casein
α-lactalbumin
Lactoferrin
Lysozyme
Serum albumin
IgA, IgG, and IgM
Urea
Creatine and creatinine
Uric acid
Ammonia
Choline and ethanolamine
Glucosamines
Polyamines
Nucleic acids and nucleotides
Cyclic nucleotides
Free amino acids (taurine, glutamine)
Carnitine

**Nonprotein Compounds**

Lactose
Oligosaccharides
Inositols
Phospholipids
Cholesterol
Triglycerides (medium- and long-chain fatty acids)
Polyunsaturated ω-3 and ω-6 fatty acids (arachidonate and docosahexaenoate).
Carotene and retinol
Folic acid

**Hormones and Growth Factors**

Epidermal growth factor
Insulin-like growth factor I and II
Insulin
Thyroxine
Cortisol
Prolactin

---

(NEC). Corticosteroids administered prenatally to mothers may enhance the biochemical, structural, and functional maturation of the gut and may help decrease the risk of NEC. Gastrointestinal motility measured manometrically in the duodenum normally becomes established, even in the absence of enteral feedings, by 28 to 30 weeks' gestation. The onset and strength of duodenal contractions is enhanced by maternal betamethasone administration. The rise in beta glucosidases is promoted by prenatal steroids, and lactase activity is particularly responsive to corticosteroids.

Multiple studies provide a wide range of recommended energy and protein intakes for LBW infants. They vary from 110 to 150 Kcal/kg for energy and from 2.5 to 4.2 g/kg/d for protein. The variability in the results on energy needs relates to differences in estimated fecal losses and the energy allowance for growth. The resting metabolic rate of preterm infants, including post-prandial thermogenesis, in most studies is 50 to 60 Kcal/kg/d. The energy expenditure related to minor thermal stress, despite a controlled environment, is 10 Kcal/kg. An additional 10 Kcal/kg are provided for activity. Fecal losses vary from 10 to 40 Kcal/kg depending on what is fed. Formulas with high saturated fats (butter fat) are less digestible than present formulas of unsaturated fats with some medium-chain triglycerides derived from vegetable sources. The allowance for synthesis and storage (growth) is 35 to 60 Kcal/kg the energy cost of weight gain is estimated at 4 to 5 kcal/g of weight gain. If the weight gain is predominantly lean, the cost is somewhat lower, 2 to 3 kcal/g. On the contrary, if adipose tissue is laid down, the cost may be as high as 8 to 9 kcal/g. The American Academy of Pediatrics (AAP) recommendations of 120 kcal/kg for energy and of 3.0 to 3.5 g/kg of protein for the nutrition of LBW infants remain essentially valid. Present efforts are directed at defining the needs of the extremely low–birth-weight (ELBW) infant (ie, birth weight less than 800 g).

Most studies have varied both the amount of calories and protein fed; therefore, it is difficult to evaluate the effect of protein or energy per se on weight gain and growth. Another key problem in evaluating these data is defining the goals for nutritional recovery of these infants. The present goal proposed by most national and international committees is a logical one: VLBW and LBW infants should attain as early as possible a body weight approximating that of a normal fetus of the same postconceptional age. A second, often nonspecified goal is that the quality of the tissue gain be similar to that accreted normally in utero at the equivalent gestation (ratio of lean to fat stored at 32 weeks is approximately 1 to 1). The first goal is clearly achievable with presently available commercial formulas specifically designed for preterm infants or by feeding fortified human milk. Most studies also show that the fat to lean ratio of tissue gained ex-utero is higher than what is normally accreted in utero. The higher fat to lean ratio of weight gain of VLBW infants during catch-up can be interpreted as an unavoidable consequence of postnatal nutrition and growth regulation. Alternatively, it may be interpreted as resulting from inadequate supply of key nutrients for optimal lean tissue accretion. Recent evidence suggests that this problem may be the result of the high energy supplied and the insufficient protein relative to energy in most commercial formulas. Others suggest that zinc or other micronutrients may be deficient relative to the needs for optimal lean tissue accretion.

Recent experimental observations in VLBW infants indicate that it is feasible ex-utero to attain in utero growth rates and to accrete sufficient lean tissue to reach normal body composition by 40 weeks' gestational age, that is, reaching the weight and composition equivalent to a term birth. To reach this goal requires not only a high energy intake (150 kcal/kg/d rather than 100 kcal/kg/d) but also an increased protein intake (4.5 g/kg/d rather than 3.3 g/kg/d). Thus, a high-energy intake may be required to optimize protein utilization for optimal catch-up. High-energy, high-protein infants in the experiment had significantly higher C-peptide excretion, suggesting that insulin response to feeding is greater. The accretion of fat was higher than in utero. Because the normal fetus increases fat gain during the last weeks of gestation, it was projected that the relative excess fat would decrease with advancing age.

The pending issue in improving growth of VLBW infants is how to enhance protein utilization without increasing energy stored as fat. The use of high-carbohydrate, low-fat energy sources can be proposed as the logical step based on the known effects of carbohydrates on insulin and IGF release. Another approach might be to add factors that enhance N retention. Growth hormone, IGF I, and insulin are likely candidates. Amino acid blends that induce anabolic hormones might be used. Arginine and the branched-chain amino acids may be considered because they promote N retention under catabolic conditions. High CHO diets may pose special problems for infants with cardiorespiratory problems. Carbohydrate relative to fat oxidation leads to higher carbon dioxide formation and may also increase energy expenditure, especially if the excess energy is converted to fat rather

than contributed to lean tissue synthesis. Results of investigations in progress may offer insight into how to optimize lean body mass accretion.

The use of whole body protein and nitrogen kinetic techniques allows a better understanding of protein metabolism in the neonate as well as in other groups. The preterm infant has been a preferred experimental subject for these studies because they are small and have high protein turnover rates. They require less isotope dose and attain steady state faster than older subjects. They are usually on controlled intakes, and because less is known on their true requirements, it is ethically permissible to evaluate ranges of intakes that may impact metabolic outcomes. Published information indicates that the LBW infant has an extraordinarily high rate of protein synthesis. When $^{13}C$ plasma leucine is used to assess synthesis, the reported rate is 5 to 10 g/kg/d, whereas using $^{15}N$ glycine and urinary urea enrichment, the values range from 13 to 26 g of protein per kilogram per day. The variance in these studies can be explained by clinical and experimental conditions under which the studies were conducted. These observations indicate that both synthesis and breakdown are extraordinarily active and that only a small proportion of what is synthesized is actually stored. Protein synthesis is an energy-demanding process. It has been suggested that nearly half the cost of lean body mass gain in the neonate can be explained by the energy cost of protein synthesis. Experimental studies demonstrate that for each 1 g of protein stored, 5 g are synthesized. Because 2 Kcal are required per gram of protein synthesis, the energy cost per gram of stored protein is 10 Kcal. This may be wasteful, but the system offers multiple sites for regulation and adaptation that would otherwise not be available. The high protein turnover rate favors tissue remodeling and appears to be a precondition for rapid growth. In the end, it is the balance between synthesis and catabolism that determines protein accretion. Dietary energy, protein, and hormonal regulators affected by maturation and nutrient supply affect rates of synthesis and breakdown. Two mechanisms may account for net protein accretion in response to diet: either protein synthesis increases or protein breakdown decreases. Both may also occur concomitantly. The evidence available from leucine oxidation kinetics studies indicates that in the full-term infant, the activation of synthesis after feeding determines protein accretion, but in the premature infant for whom synthetic rates are high, the inhibition of breakdown after feeding determines net accretion. The experimental data show a close relationship between protein synthesis, protein accretion, and energy expenditure, suggesting that these processes are closely linked.

This understanding of protein-to-energy and growth interactions may provide new ways to optimize growth of premature infants. These may include the following:

1. Use of different protein-to-energy ratios depending on developmental stage, degree of malnutrition, desirable weight gain, and target body composition. These regimens may be individually adjusted using growth rate, urinary N, and serum urea as simple markers of N metabolism. These laboratory measures are available in most settings.
2. Use of high-carbohydrate, high-protein, low-fat regimens during periods of rapid growth to induce higher insulin levels that may enhance N utilization and lean mass accretion.
3. Use of essential and nonessential N compounds such as glutamine, arginine, branched-chain amino acids, and nucleotides as potential growth modulators for specific organs. These compounds may induce hormonal or growth factor responses (ie, arginine and GH), provide fuels that favor growth of some organs (ie, glutamine and the gut) or spare amino acid oxidation (ie, branched-chain amino acids sparing of muscle protein breakdown), or serve as preformed precursors for tissue

synthesis (ie, nucleotide salvage for nucleic acid synthesis required by rapidly dividing cells).

4. Administration of growth hormone or insulin during periods of rapid growth or after lean tissue recovery slows to permit better recovery of linear growth or that of other tissues where hyperplastic growth is crucial. The potential use of these agents requires that safety considerations be fully addressed and that appropriate substrates be provided.

5. Use of organ-specific growth factors (eg, IGF I to promote muscle mass growth and recovery). The possibility of using other organ-specific growth factors may exist when more is learned about them (ie, epidermal growth factor, nerve growth factor, platelet growth factor, colony stimulating factor, osteogenic factor).

This is not a complete list of possibilities. The future of growth enhancement is yet to come.

## Selected Readings

Axelsson IEM, Ivarsson SA, and Raiha NCR. Protein intake in early infancy: effects on plasma aminoacid concentrations, insulin metabolism, and growth. Pediatr Res 1989;26:614.

Battaglia FC, Meschia G. Principal substrates of fetal metabolism. Physiol Rev 1978;58:499.

Bauer C, Bancalari E, eds. Perinatal nutrition and organ development. Seminars in Perinatology 1991;15:423.

Baumgart S. Reduction of oxygen consumption, insensible water loss, and radiant heat demand with use of a plastic blanket for low-birthweight infants under radiant warmers. Pediatrics 1984;74:1022.

Bier DM, Young VR. Assessment of whole-body protein—nitrogen—kinetics in the human infant. In: Fomon SJ, Heird WC, eds. Energy and protein needs during infancy. Orlando: Academic Press, 1986.

Brooke OG, Wood C, Barley J. Energy balance, nitrogen balance and growth in preterm infants fed expressed breast milk, a premature infant formula and two low solute adapted formulas. Arch Dis Child 1982;57:898.

Coleman RA. Placental metabolism and transport of lipid. Federation Proceedings 1986;45:2519.

Cornblath M, Schwartz R. Disorders of carbohydrate metabolism in infancy, ed 2. Philadelphia: WB Saunders, 1976.

Curry E, Warshaw JB. Higher serum carnitine levels and ketogenesis in breast fed as compared to formula fed infants. Pediatr Res 1978;12:504.

Dancis J. Placental transport of amino acids, fats and minerals. In: Placental transport. Mead Johnson Symposium on Perinatal and Developmental Medicine, 1981;18: 25.

D'Ercole AJ, Underwood LE. Growth factors in fetal growth and development. In: Novy MJ, Resko JA, eds. Fetal endocrinology. New York: Academic Press, 1981: 155.

Driscoll J, Driscoll Y, Steir M, et al. Mortality and morbidity in less than 1001 grams birthweight. Pediatrics 1982;69:21.

Ely JTA. Hyperglycemia and major congenital anomalies. N Engl J Med 1981;305: 833.

Fomon SJ, Heird WC, eds. Energy and protein needs during infancy. New York: Academic Press, 1986.

Gentz J, Kellum M, Persson B. The effect of feeding on oxygen consumption, RQ and plasma levels of glucose, FFA, and D-B-hydroxybutyrate in newborn infants of diabetic mothers and small for gestational age infants. Acta Paediatr Scand 1976;65:445.

Georgieff MK, Zempel CE, and Chang PN. Catch-up growth, muscle and fat accretion, and body proportionality of infants one year after newborn intensive care. J Pediatr 1989;114:288.

Gewolb IH, Warshaw JB. Influences on fetal growth. In: Warshaw JB, ed. The biological basis of reproduction and developmental medicine. New York: Elsevier, 1983;365.

Goodridge A. Regulation of the gene for fatty acid synthase. Federation Proceedings 1986;45:2399.

Gruenwald P, Funakawa H, Mitani S, et al. Influence of environmental factors on foetal growth in man. Lancet 1967;1:1026.

Haddad GG, Mellins RB. Hypoxia and respiratory control in early life. Annu Rev Physiol 1984;46:629.

Hack M, Horbar JD, Malloy MH, Tyson JE, Wright E, Wright L. Very low birth weight outcomes of the National Institute of Child Health and Human Development Neonatal Network. Pediatrics 1991;87:587.

Kimura RE, Warshaw JB. Metabolism during infancy. In: Warshaw JB, ed. The biological basis of reproduction and developmental medicine. New York: Elsevier, 1983;337.

Lechtig A, Habicht J-P, Delgado H, et al. Effect of food supplementation during pregnancy on birth weight. Pediatrics 1975;56:508.

Lucas A, Gore SM, Cole TJ, et al. Multicentre trial on feeding low birthweight infants: effects of diet on early growth. Arch Dis Child 1984;59:722.

Rigatto H. Control of ventilation in the newborn. Annu Rev Physiol 1984;46:661.

Silverman WA, Fertig JW, Berger AP: The influence of the thermal environment upon the survival of newly born premature infants. Pediatrics 22:876, 1958

Sparks JW. Augmentation of the glucose supply in the fetus and newborn. Semin Perinatol 1979;3:141.

Susser M. Prenatal nutrition, birthweight, and psychological development: an overview of experiments, quasi-experiments and natural experiments in the past decade. Am J Clin Nutr 1981;34:784.

Tanner JM. Physical growth from conception to maturity. In: Foetus into man, ed 2. Ware, UK: Castlemead Publications, 1989.

The Infant Health and Development Program. Enhancing the outcomes of low-birth-weight, premature infants: a multi-site, randomized trial. JAMA 1990;263: 3035.

Uauy R, ed. Current concepts in newborn nutrition: nutrition beyond growth. Seminars in Perinatology 1989;13:67.

Widdowson E. Chemical composition of newly born animals. Nature 1950;166: 626.

*Principles and Practice of Pediatrics, Second Edition.*
edited by Frank A. Oski et al. J. B. Lippincott Company, Philadelphia © 1994.

# CHAPTER 17
# *Obstetric Considerations*

## 17.1 *General Care*

Norman F. Gant

### PRENATAL CARE

Obstetric care always has been focused on recognizing and minimizing risks to mother and fetus. Initial prenatal care actually should begin before pregnancy. For example, all recreational drug use, including smoking and alcohol, but especially all hard-drug use, should cease before conception. The woman's general health should be at its peak before conception, and stringent efforts should be directed at the effective management of maternal disorders that place the gravida, or her fetus, at risk. For example, fewer congenital anomalies are seen in infants of diabetic women who have brought their diabetes under good glucose control before conception.

The pediatrician should have full access to relevant obstetric history and should be in close communication with the obstetric caregiver in any high-risk pregnancy. It is especially important for both of them to know accurate gestational age. The best estimate of gestational age is calculated from an accurate menstrual history. Failing this, after the first 6 to 8 weeks, gestational age can be established most reliably by the use of ultrasound to measure various diameters, lengths, and ratios of fetal size. After 14 weeks' gestation, a sonographic estimate of gestational age is accurate to plus or minus 10 days. Quickening usually occurs between 17 and 19 weeks' gestational age, and fetal heart tones can be identified by fetoscope between 17 and 20 weeks' gestation. Also, any past history of diabetes, cardiovascular disease,

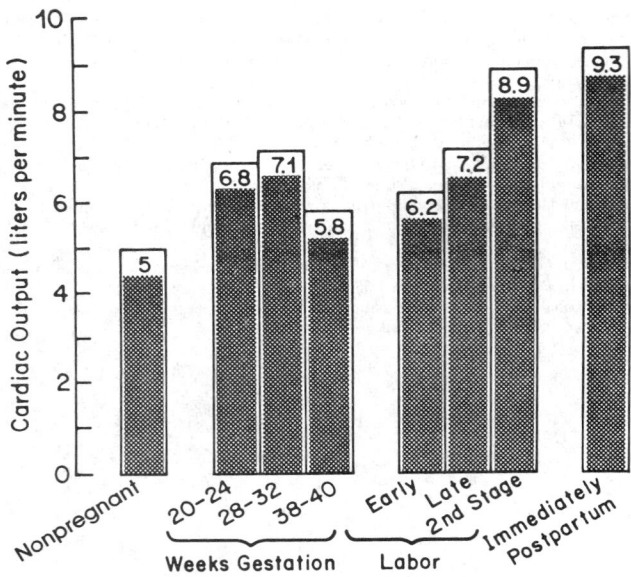

Figure 17-1.   Cardiac outputs during three stages of gestation, labor, and immediately postpartum are compared with values of nonpregnant women. All values were determined with women in the lateral recumbent position. (Adapted from Ueland and associates: Clin Obstet Gynecol 18:41, 1975 and presented by Hankins GDV, Cunningham FG, Pritchard JA: Cardiopulmonary consequences of hypertension during pregnancy and puerperium. *Williams Supplement No. 8*, 1986.)

renal disease, or other serious illnesses in the patient or in her immediate family should be identified.

## MATERNAL ADAPTATION TO PREGNANCY

Pregnancy is a normal physiologic condition; the pregnant woman is not an invalid. In fact, during pregnancy there are remarkable changes involving the cardiovascular system. Arterial blood pressure and vascular resistance decrease, while blood volume, maternal weight, and basal metabolic rate increase. These changes result in an appreciable increase in cardiac output, beginning during the first trimester and persisting throughout the pregnancy and the early puerperium (Fig 17-1).

With the fall in peripheral resistance, there is a rapid increase in blood volume that begins late in the first trimester and increases rapidly until about 34 weeks' gestation, when the rate of expansion slows appreciably. In the average-sized woman, blood volume expansion is about 1500 mL of whole blood. This results in a significantly increased requirement for iron, which can be met only by iron supplements.

Increased cardiac output and blood volume expansion are essential factors in providing the rapidly expanding uterus and its fetal occupant a sufficient uteroplacental perfusion. This blood flow is about 500 to 700 mL/minute at term and appears to be protected to some degree from the effects of several potent vasoconstrictors.

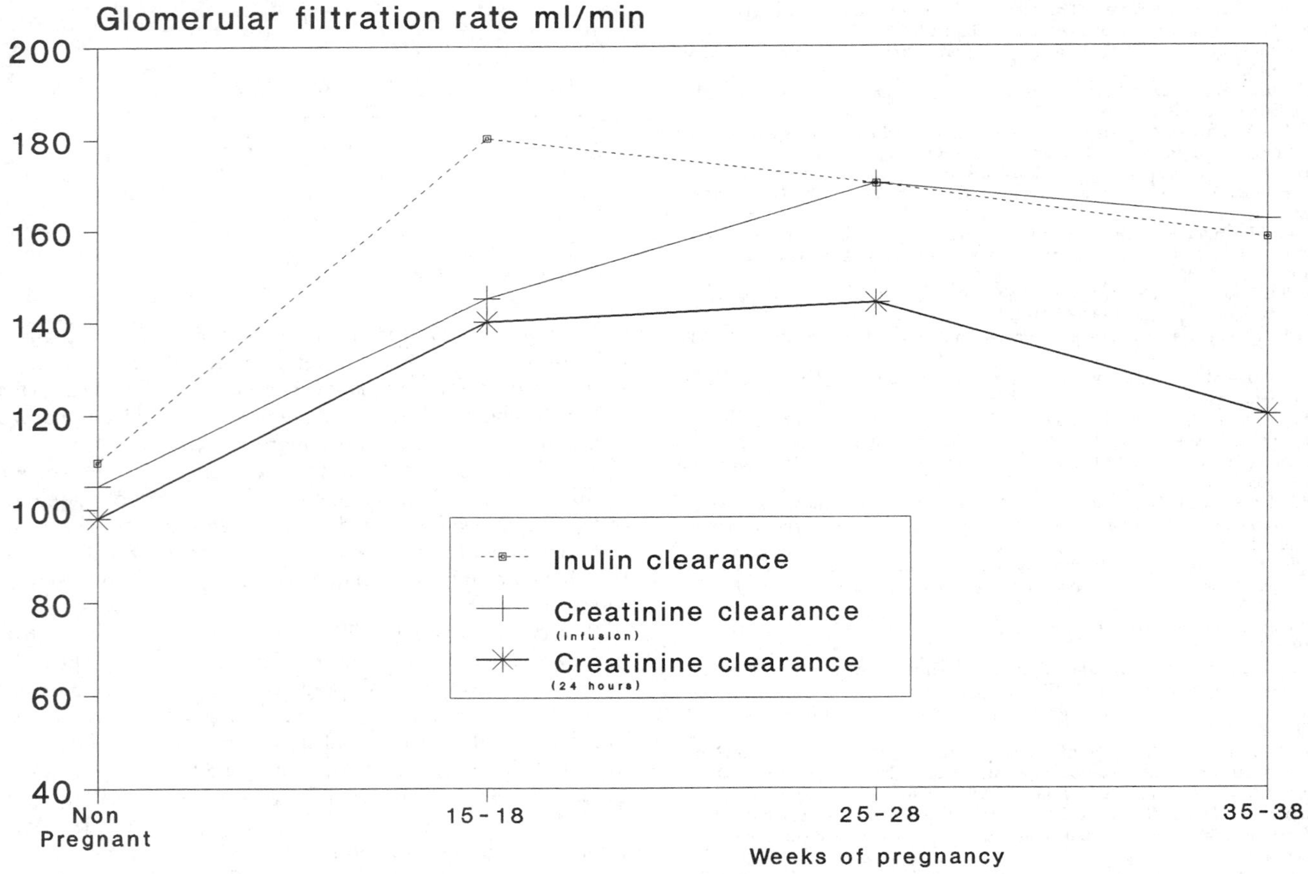

## Glomerular filtration rate ml/min

Figure 17-2.   Mean glomerular filtration rate in healthy women over a short period with infused inulin (*solid line*), simultaneously as creatinine clearance during the inulin infusion (*broken line*), and over 24 hours as endogenous creatinine clearance (*dotted line*). (From Davison and Hytten: J Obstet Gynaecol Brit Commonw 81:588, 1974).

Maternal renal function also is augmented as early as the first trimester. Specifically, glomerular filtration rate and renal plasma flow show significant increases early in pregnancy, and these changes roughly parallel those observed in cardiac output (Fig. 17-2). The augmented renal function results in a fall in normal nonpregnant values for plasma creatinine and urea nitrogen.

Finally, as might be expected, profound metabolic changes occur in pregnant women. Many of these are induced by the fetus to ensure an adequate and continuous source of nutrients. For example, human placental lactogen increases in parallel with the growth of the placenta, and the hormone is directed unilaterally into the maternal circulation, where it acts in a manner similar to growth hormone to increase lipolysis and the liberation of free fatty acids. These, in turn, serve as maternal energy sources to replace glucose, which is actively transferred to the fetus. Peak human placental lactogen concentrations correspond to the greatest insulin response by beta-cells of the pancreas. This response, as well as other possible mechanisms, results in maternal tissue resistance to insulin, which ensures a maternal glucose source for the fetus. Unfortunately, this also converts maternal metabolism into a state of "accelerated starvation" that renders a gravida diabetogenic, because each of these mechanisms requires an increased level and reserve of insulin.

## HIGH-RISK PREGNANCY AND ASSESSMENT

As many as 40% of all pregnancies may have risk factors identified at some time during the antepartum or intrapartum period. High-risk pregnancies include, but are not limited to, pregnancies with preexisting medical diseases such as connective tissue disorders or diabetes mellitus. Certainly, a history of previous pregnancy

problems, such as preterm delivery, fetal growth retardation, or recurrent perinatal mortality, places a woman in a high-risk category (Fig 17-3). Women who have experienced a placental accident, such as an abruptio, and those with evidence of vascular diseases or chronic hypertension also should be classified as high risk.

Biophysical tests of fetal well-being include the contraction stress test, the nonstress test, and the biophysical profile. A test frequently overlooked but equally important is the mother's own perception of fetal movement. The use of a fetal movement chart in high-risk patients is indicated whether or not any of the biophysical testing methods previously mentioned is used.

The *contraction stress test* consists of inducing uterine contractions in response either to parenteral oxytocin or to nipple stimulation. Fetal heart rate is monitored through three successive uterine contractions during a 10-minute window of time. A deceleration in fetal heart rate following a uterine contraction is considered to be a positive contraction stress test and usually indicates impaired uteroplacental perfusion (Fig 17-4). The *nonstress test* takes advantage of the fact that with fetal movement, fetal heart accelerations usually occur in excess of 15 beats per minute for more than 15 seconds. Failure of the fetal heart to accelerate with fetal movement is considered to be a positive nonstress test; it, too, may indicate a compromised fetus (Fig 17-5). Absence of heart-rate acceleration after fetal movement suggests that serious neurologic damage has occurred or is occurring. The *biophysical profile* usually consists of four to six biophysical assessments. These include the nonstress test and a real-time sonographic assessment of the adequacy of amniotic fluid volume, the presence of fetal movements and tone, the presence of fetal breathing movements, and occasionally the presence or absence of placental calcifications, indicating accelerated placental senescence. All of these tests of fetal well-being are considered to be

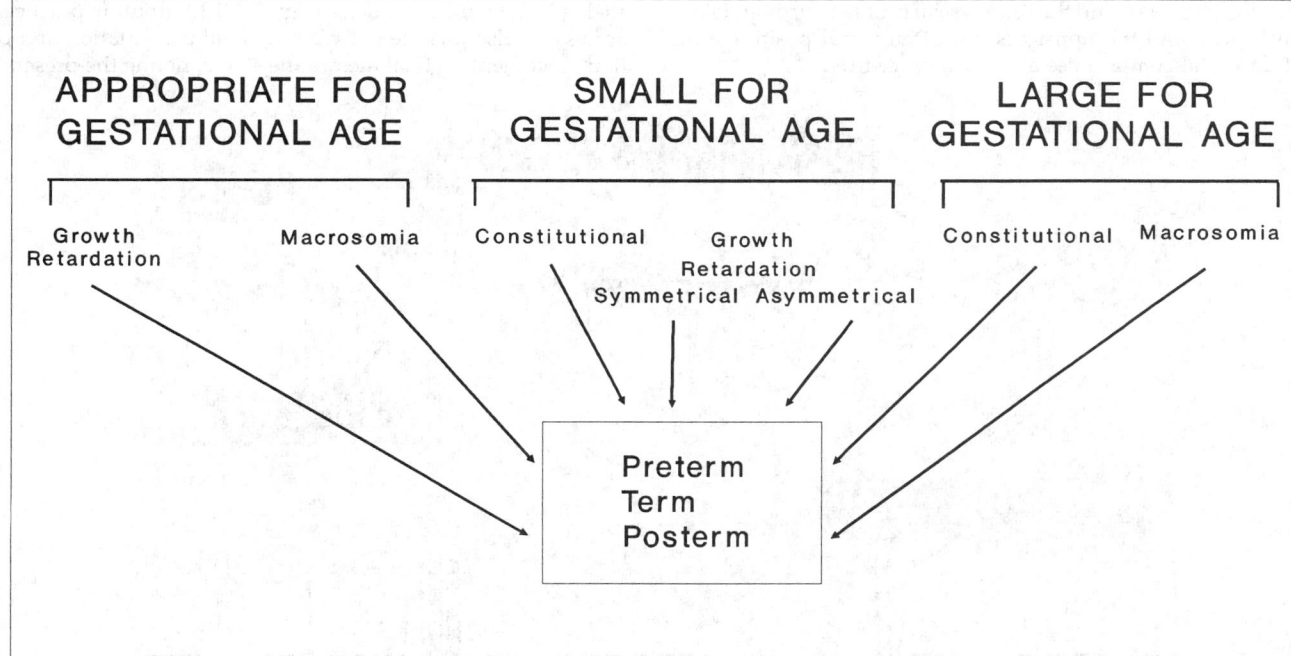

Figure 17-3.   Fetal-neonatal age compared to birth weight and functional growth. *Preterm* describes a neonate delivered before 38 weeks' gestation, and *postterm* after 42 weeks' gestation. A term neonate is one delivered between 38 and 42 weeks' gestation. A small-for-gestational-age fetus-neonate is below the 10th percentile for weight, whereas a large-for-gestational-age fetus-neonate is above the 90th percentile. An appropriate-for-gestational-age fetus-neonate is between the 10th and 90th percentiles. A fetus-neonate destined to be either large or small may be described as constitutionally large or small; that is, normal growth potential was reached for that infant. A pathologic process results in a growth-retarded or macrosomic fetus-neonate.

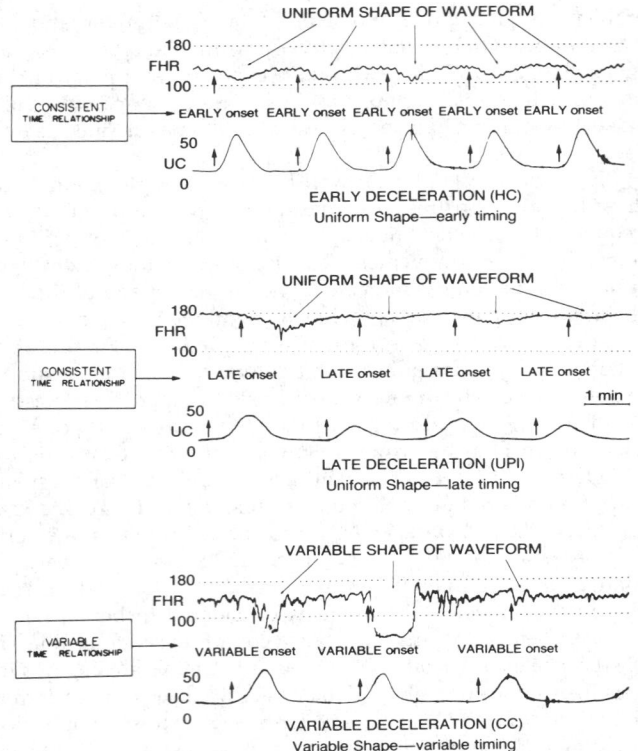

**Figure 17-4.** Fetal heart rate decelerations in relation to the time of onset of uterine contractions. *HC,* head compression; *UPI,* uteroplacental insufficiency; *CC,* cord compression. (From Hon. An atlas of fetal heart rate patterns. New Haven, CT: Harty, 1968.)

markers that identify current fetal health rather than absolute predictors of continuing fetal well-being. Unfortunately, the contraction stress test and the biophysical profile have high false-positive rates, and the nonstress test often is not positive until significant fetal compromise already has occurred.

# DIAGNOSIS OF LABOR

*Labor* is defined as the onset of regular uterine contractions accompanied by progressive cervical dilation and effacement with descent of the fetal presenting part.

## Stages of Labor

The intelligent management of labor depends on an understanding of its mechanism. Labor is divided into three stages: the first stage, from the onset of labor to full cervical dilation; the second stage, from full cervical dilatation to delivery; and the third stage, from delivery of the infant to placental delivery.

In North America, physicians traditionally divide the first stage of labor into latent and active phases (Fig 17-6). The *latent phase* is between the onset of regular uterine contractions until the beginning of the active phase, usually after the cervix is dilated 4 cm or more. Recorded graphically as cervical dilation against time, the *active phase* is seen as the period when the curve changes from the relatively flat portion or latent phase into a phase of maximal dilation. The average duration of the latent phase is 6.4 hours for nulliparas and 4.8 hours for multiparas.

## Conduct of Normal Labor

The woman admitted to the labor floor should have a thorough evaluation. A copy of the prenatal chart should be incorporated into the labor records so that those providing care get a full review of her past history and the events of her pregnancy. Certain historical data regarding the onset of labor, such as the nature of contractions, rupture of membranes, bleeding, and meals eaten, are essential. Usually, critical data such as the patient's blood type, serology, and rhesus factor already have been obtained and are present in the chart. A general physical examination on admission is routine, as are appropriate laboratory investigations, such as a hematocrit and serology (VDRL). Routine practices on admission also include determining fetal presentation and position, documenting fetal membrane status, noting the presence or

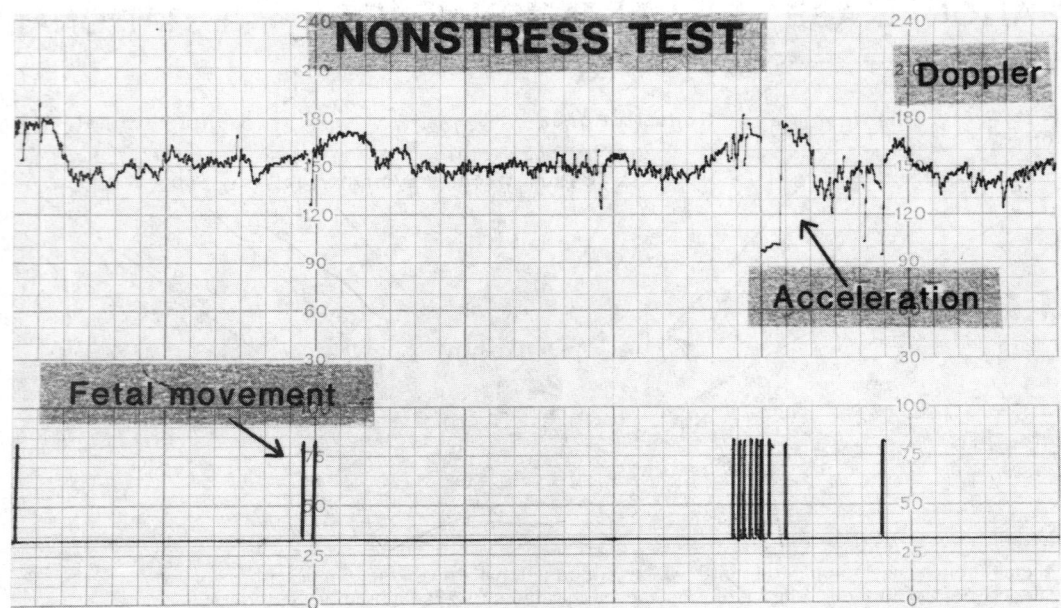

**Figure 17-5.** Reactive nonstress test. Notice increase of fetal heart rate to more than 15 beats per minute for longer than 15 seconds following fetal movements indicated by the vertical marks on the lower part of the recording. (Courtesy of Kenneth J. Leveno, MD, University of Texas Southwestern Medical Center at Dallas, and presented in Cunningham FG, Gant NF, MacDonald PC. Williams' obstetrics, ed 18. East Norwalk, CT: Appleton & Lange, 1989, with permission.)

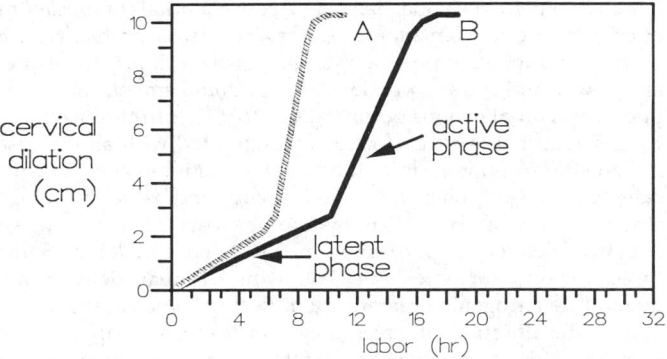

**Figure 17-6.** Normal labor during the first stage. A, average multipara; B, average primigravida.

absence of meconium staining, documenting cervical dilation and effacement, and noting the presenting part and the presence of fetal heart tones.

A graphic display of intrapartum data allows prompt visualization of the status and progress of cervical dilation and descent of the presenting part, and is used by many as an adjunct to intrapartum monitoring. This may be accomplished with a simple record of cervical dilation plotted against time on ruled graph paper, or by a more comprehensive recording of all intrapartum data related in graphic form to the progress of cervical dilation.

## Pain Relief In Labor

Pain relief during labor and delivery is important. Thoughtfully chosen analgesia probably improves labor, and it certainly improves the woman's memory of the experience. Proper anesthesia enhances the safety of difficult deliveries; conversely, poorly chosen analgesia may compromise labor, depress the fetus, and contribute to maternal or fetal morbidity and even mortality.

The choice of analgesic and anesthetic techniques depends on the experience and knowledge of the anesthesiologist or the personal preference of the obstetrician and patient, as well as the circumstances of labor and delivery. Choices include natural childbirth (ie, no analgesia or anesthesia), as well as narcotics, spinal and epidural regional blocks, pudendal block, and general anesthesia.

Narcotics ease the pain of contractions, are easy to administer, and cause little fetal depression if given in appropriate doses (eg, 25 to 50 mg meperidine intravenously) and repeated only if necessary. Larger doses given too close to delivery may depress the fetus.

Continuous lumbar epidural regional blocks provide safe, effective analgesia for the laboring patient. A pudendal block probably is the most popular form of obstetric analgesia used in North America. Administered vaginally by the obstetrician, it usually is adequate for spontaneous vaginal and outlet-forceps deliveries. In general, it is a very safe method for both mother and fetus. Its major complication is a local analgesic overdosage resulting from an inadvertent intravascular injection.

Spinal analgesia administered as a low spinal can provide optimum conditions for nearly any vaginal delivery, spontaneous or operative. With adequate precautions, the incidence of hypotension approaches zero. The main advantages of spinal and epidural analgesia are that the patient is awake and her infant has little if any risk of drug depression.

Although anesthetic agents do cross the placenta, when given by competent personnel it is unlikely that general anesthesia will depress the infant. General anesthesia usually is restricted to use when there is an absolute and relative contraindication to regional anesthesia.

## INTRAPARTUM FETAL MONITORING

Today, fetal monitoring is used widely throughout the world. Its increasing popularity prevails despite some controversy over its benefit. Advocates consider electronic fetal monitoring to be a routine technique potentially beneficial in all pregnancies. Critics believe that it is a meddlesome, cumbersome technique that offers no advantage over auscultation for low-risk patients. Electronic fetal monitoring allegedly identifies intrapartum fetal compromise with greater accuracy than other techniques or combination of techniques. It provides insights into the mechanisms that may cause asphyxia. Such monitoring may allow the obstetrician to correct some instances of fetal distress.

The major area of disagreement is the influence of monitoring on rates of perinatal mortality and on cesarean delivery. In a randomized trial of fetal monitoring conducted in Dublin, a higher incidence of cesarean delivery for fetal distress in monitored patients was not identified, and there was no difference in perinatal mortality between the group with continuous monitoring and the group with intermittent auscultation. There was, however, a higher incidence of neonatal morbidity in the nonmonitored group; neonatal seizures were used as the outcome marker.

One compromise is to use initial electronic fetal heart-rate monitoring for all patients admitted in labor. If there is any abnormality on this tracing, continuous electronic fetal monitoring is used throughout labor and delivery. If the fetal monitoring tracing is normal and the mother has no determinable maternal or fetal risk factors, intermittent auscultation may be used for the rest of labor and delivery.

## IDENTIFICATION OF RISK

In obstetrics, there are many different methods to identify or clarify risk. Hobel and colleagues used four major categories:

1. Those at low risk of either maternal or fetal problems throughout labor and delivery
2. Those with fetal or maternal risks identified only during the prenatal course but who have a normal labor and delivery (eg, a patient with premature rupture of membranes at 32 weeks' gestation)
3. Those who are normal prenatally but are at high risk during labor and delivery (eg, a baby who develops an abnormal heart-rate pattern during labor)
4. Those at high risk throughout the prenatal course, labor, and delivery (eg, a diabetic mother, who may have significant problems in the prenatal course or during labor and delivery)

Hobel demonstrated the relationship between these four categories and perinatal mortality. Category 1 had a perinatal mortality rate of 3/1000 live births; category 4 had a perinatal mortality rate of 145/1000 live births. In more than 40% of all pregnancies, some factor may be identified that places the woman or her fetus at risk.

Table 17-1 presents a convenient way to predict the high-risk neonate. It is beyond the scope of this review to consider all of these factors; instead, we have selected several specific maternal and fetal conditions for consideration.

## INDUCTION OF LABOR

Induction of labor is elective (ie, performed for the convenience of the professional staff or the patient) or is indicated for medical-obstetric or fetal indications. Elective induction of labor usually is not justified. Induction of labor is indicated if the prolongation of the pregnancy is dangerous for the mother or the fetus, and

TABLE 17-1.   Identification of Perinatal Risk Situations

**Maternal Conditions**
Maternal medical disease (hypertension, diabetes, cardiac disease)
Previous abnormal obstetric history (eg, stillbirth)
Antepartum hemorrhage
Postterm gestation—42 weeks
Prolonged rupture of membranes
Rhesus incompatibility
Low socioeconomic status
Maternal age <16 or >35
Maternal drug or alcohol abuse

**Conditions of Labor and Delivery**
Prolonged labor
Operative delivery (mid-forceps delivery, vacuum extraction, cesarean delivery, fetal distress)
Prolapsed umbilical cord
Maternal hypotension
Abnormal fetal presentation (eg, breech)

**Fetal Conditions**
Preterm labor and delivery
Fetal growth retardation
Multiple pregnancy
Polyhydramnios
Oligohydramnios
Malformation

if there are no contraindications to amniotomy or to uterine contractions.

Maternal indications for induction of labor include severe pregnancy-induced hypertension, fetal death, and chorioamnionitis. Fetal indications include any condition in which fetal jeopardy has been identified, such as diabetes mellitus, postterm pregnancy, hypertensive complications of pregnancy, fetal growth retardation, chorioamnionitis, or premature rupture of membranes with established fetal maturity. Contraindications for induction of labor in these situations are any condition in which spontaneous labor and delivery would be more dangerous for the mother or fetus than abdominal delivery; examples include fetal distress, shoulder presentation, placenta previa, and a previous uterine incision that would preclude a trial of labor.

## OPERATIVE DELIVERY

### Cesarean Delivery

Before 1960, cesarean deliveries constituted less than 5% of births in the United States. They were done primarily for maternal indications such as placenta previa, radiographically documented cephalopelvic disproportion, failure of induction, and severe preeclampsia. After 1960, more cesarean deliveries were done, primarily because of fetal indications. The cesarean birth rate in the United States increased nearly threefold, from 5.5% in 1970 to 15.2% in 1978. There is a trend toward increasing use of cesarean delivery in other countries, but the sharpest increase occurred in the United States. Four indications were found to account for 90% of the increase: dystocia (30%), repeat cesarean delivery (25% to 30%), breech presentation (10% to 15%), and fetal distress (10% to 15%).

Although cesarean delivery can be seen as a reasonably safe surgical procedure, it is associated with a higher risk of morbidity and mortality than vaginal delivery. Acute maternal complications of cesarean delivery include anesthesia accidents, problems with intubation, aspiration pneumonitis, hemorrhage, injury to bladder and bowel, and on rare occasions amniotic fluid embolism. Febrile puerperal complications occur in 20% to 30% of these women.

Cesarean delivery has long been associated with an increase in neonatal respiratory morbidity at all gestational ages. The incidence of this complication and its etiology and pathophysiology remain matters of dispute. The syndrome most often is seen when operative delivery is performed in the absence of labor. Some cases of respiratory morbidity following cesarean delivery are due to true iatrogenic prematurity; however, even careful attention to the duration of pregnancy and the use of appropriate amniotic fluid determination of fetal lung maturity have not eliminated the problem.

Reducing the incidence of maternal and neonatal complications of cesarean delivery begins with the proper respect for the dangers of the procedure, and careful patient selection. A straightforward generalization, although constituting a rational approach, does not do justice to the complexities of the decision in each case.

When cesarean delivery is necessary, the following measures help ensure the lowest morbidity and mortality risks for mother and fetus: preoperative administration of an antacid or hydrogen-ion blocker; administration of anesthesia by a skilled anesthesiologist; attention to maternal position and blood volume in the peripartum period; use of a transverse uterine incision whenever possible; awaiting the onset of labor whenever possible in cases of repeat cesarean delivery; and the presence of an individual skilled in newborn resuscitation.

### Obstetric Forceps Delivery

There are three types of forceps deliveries: outlet-forceps delivery, which usually is quite simple and uncomplicated for both mother and infant; low-forceps delivery, which is slightly more difficult technically but again usually is associated with good maternal and fetal outcomes; and mid-forceps deliveries, which may be associated with substantial trauma to either patient.

In an outlet-forceps delivery, the vertex is engaged and has reached the perineum. The vertex is visible between contractions, and the fetal sagittal suture is in the midline. Application of forceps in these situations usually is quite easy, and only limited traction is necessary to accomplish delivery.

In a low-forceps delivery, the same conditions generally apply, but the sagittal suture may be off the vertical by 45°.

A mid-forceps delivery is the application of forceps to the fetal head after it has entered the pelvis and the biparietal diameter has passed the inlet (engaged). In this case, however, the vertex is not visible between contractions. The debate about the indications and safety of mid-forceps delivery continues because it may be associated with increased morbidity and mortality. If a mid-forceps delivery is to be performed, an experienced obstetrician should be available and adequate general or regional anesthesia should be used. The procedure should be performed in an operating room, with personnel available to perform a cesarean delivery if needed. The attempt at vaginal delivery should be abandoned if the forceps cannot be applied easily. The attempt also should be abandoned if rotation does not occur with gentle pressure under moderate traction and does not result in immediate descent of the fetal head.

### PRETERM LABOR AND DELIVERY

Labor is considered preterm when it occurs in a woman who is less than 37 completed weeks from the first day of her last menstrual period. Among the problems arising from so simple a definition is the need to make a clinical decision about whether true labor has commenced. This frequently poses a problem because if pharmacologic inhibition of preterm labor is to be effective, it must be instituted early. *However, the efficacy of tocolytic therapy has not been established.* Therefore, unnecessary drug therapy with potentially harmful effects to mother or fetus is unwarranted if there is only marginal evidence of preterm labor or drug effectiveness. To avoid unnecessary treatment, the following criteria are helpful in making a diagnosis of preterm labor in patients who are 25 to 36 weeks' gestation:

Uterine contractions are occurring at a rate of four per 20 minutes or eight per 60 minutes.
The cervix is dilated to 2 cm and is effaced at least 80%.
Serial examinations, preferably by the same observer, reveal changes in the cervix.
The membranes are ruptured.

Preterm delivery continues to cause more neonatal deaths than any other single event except congenital malformations. All medical personnel responsible for the care of women at high risk for preterm labor and delivery must be expert in the management of these pregnancies. Only a fraction of women who present in labor remote from term are candidates for long-term tocolysis. If a decision for tocolytic therapy is made, the clinician must be familiar with the risks and benefits. Before any attempt is made to arrest labor, the clinician must ensure that prolonging the pregnancy is likely to benefit the fetus and not injure the mother.

General contraindications to tocolysis include but are not limited to:

Maternal conditions requiring delivery of the fetus (severe hypertension, preeclampsia, or eclampsia; uncontrollable diabetes, especially with ketoacidosis; chorioamnionitis; severe vaginal bleeding, such as abruptio placentae)
Fetal conditions (fetal death, fetal malformations incompatible with extrauterine survival, fetal distress, fetal growth retardation)
Gestational age. When the pregnancy has passed 34 completed weeks' gestation and the fetal weight is over 2500 g or pulmonary maturity is established, little is gained by prolonging pregnancy. With a special-care nursery, survival rates of preterm infants in these groups is excellent.
Imminent delivery. Cervical dilation of more than 4 to 5 cm renders attempts at tocolysis futile.

If delivery is imminent or indicated, intensive intrapartum monitoring of these fetuses, especially those weighing less than 1500 g, is mandatory. The mother should be transferred to a facility with expert obstetric care and a neonatal intensive care unit with staff experienced in the management of very-low-birth-weight infants. The aims of management of labor and delivery in the preterm infant include ensuring adequate fetal oxygenation throughout labor and delivery, and preventing traumatic delivery.

An episiotomy may be indicated to reduce pressure on the fetal head. Whenever possible, spontaneous delivery is preferable. It has been suggested that the use of outlet forceps will protect the preterm fetal head from vaginal compression and therefore improve outcome. This practice is questionable, as it is doubtful that less trauma results from the use of outlet forceps.

The preterm breech presentation poses special problems. For any infant in a breech presentation whose weight is estimated at less than 2000 g, delivery probably should be by cesarean section. The uterine incision, regardless of type, should be large enough to allow for nontraumatic delivery of the infant. If improvements in survival rates and outcomes of low–birth-weight infants are to continue, there must be close collaboration, not only between the obstetrician and the pediatrician, but also be-

tween all physicians and nursing staff who care for these high-risk patients.

# DIAGNOSIS AND MANAGEMENT OF FETAL DISTRESS

## Fetal Heart-Rate Deceleration

### Variable Decelerations

Variable decelerations reflect cord compression and are the most common form of deceleration seen in labor (Fig 17-7). There are two forms of variable decelerations: mild variable decelerations, which are very common, and severe variable decelerations, in which the heart rate drops to less than 60 beats/minute, lasts for more than 60 seconds, and demonstrates a slow recovery to baseline. Any variable deceleration indicates umbilical cord compromise, and even a mild variable deceleration rapidly may progress to a severe one and result in fetal death. Any variable deceleration is a sign for intense fetal vigilance; the umbilical cord is in jeopardy and with it the fetus's life.

### Late Decelerations

Late decelerations indicate fetal hypoxia. The most common situation in which late decelerations are seen in labor is during oxytocin infusion due to hypertonicity of the uterus.

## Fetal Heart-Rate Variability

Classifying the type of fetal heart rate deceleration (ie, late or variable) informs the clinician only of the mechanism of insult; the fetal response to that insult is reflected in fetal heart-rate variability. Most fetal heart-rate tracings show a jiggly, irregular line: this demonstrates the fetal heart-rate variability and represents a slight difference in calculated fetal heart rate from one heartbeat to the next (beat-to-beat variability) (Fig 17-8). Normal variability is classified as an amplitude range of 6 beats/minute. Absence of variability is less than 2 beats/minute, with a line that appears flat or smooth.

The most important aspect of variability is the fact that in the presence of normal fetal heart-rate variability, no matter what other fetal heart-rate patterns may be present, the fetus usually is not suffering asphyxia. The combination of an absence of fetal heart-rate variability and periodic decelerations, however, is ominous.

## Fetal Scalp Blood Sampling

In 1962, Saling introduced sampling of fetal scalp blood as a technique to evaluate fetal oxygenation during labor. Since that time, there has been great controversy about whether electronic fetal heart-rate monitoring or measurement of fetal scalp pH is the better means of evaluating the fetal condition during labor. Fetal scalp sampling affords only intermittent data and is technically more difficult to perform than fetal heart-rate monitoring; we do not use the technique.

## Management of Fetal Distress With Intrauterine Resuscitation

The interventions most commonly and successfully used in cases of fetal distress are those directed toward improving fetal oxygenation. If variable deceleration is a component of the distress, one or more changes in maternal position usually result in relief of the cord compression. Lateral positioning, cessation of any oxytocin administration, and correction of any hypotension gen-

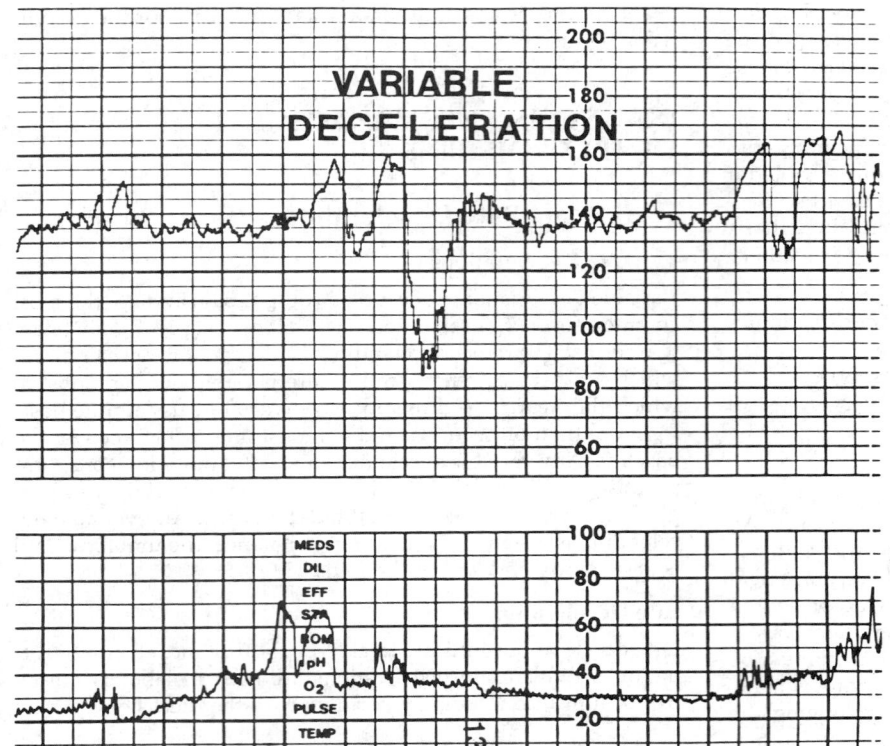

Figure 17-7. Variable deceleration, the most common form of deceleration during labor. The variable deceleration is reassuring because the heart rate does not drop to less than 60 beats per minute, does not last for 60 seconds, and returns quickly to the baseline fetal heart rate.

erally reverse a late deceleration pattern. Should intrauterine resuscitation efforts fail to resolve the distress pattern, expedient delivery often is warranted.

## Delivery of the Distressed Fetus

If fetal distress is irremediable, preparations should be made for immediate cesarean delivery. These preparations should begin when fetal distress is recognized and intrauterine resuscitation measures are being instituted. Precious minutes can be lost if operative preparations are delayed until it is obvious that resuscitative measures have failed; this is particularly important when extramural personnel must be called in for a cesarean delivery. Of course, if vaginal delivery is possible, this is the preferred method. Often, however, a difficult mid-forceps operation should be avoided when there already is evidence of severe fetal distress.

## MEANING AND MANAGEMENT OF MECONIUM

Meconium-stained amniotic fluid has been thought to represent fetal distress, but in many cases it probably is a normal function of the maturing fetal gastrointestinal tract. In the absence of signs of distress on a fetal monitor, expedient delivery usually is not indicated. If meconium-stained amniotic fluid is present, a combined obstetric and pediatric approach as described by Carson and associates should be used to prevent meconium aspiration syndrome. The obstetrician's responsibility is to perform vigorous suctioning of the nasopharynx and oropharynx after delivery of the head and before delivery of the shoulders. Once the infant is delivered, additional suctioning or stimulation should not be performed to prevent aspiration of the meconium left in the re-

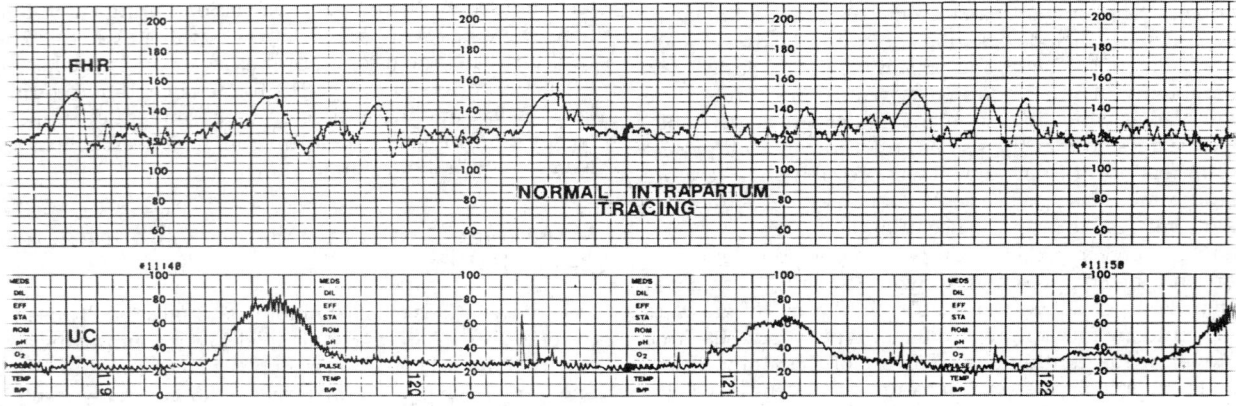

Figure 17-8.   A normal intrapartum fetal heart rate (FHR) tracing with uterine contractions (UC). No decelerations are seen. Variability and fetal heart rate accelerations are normal.

spiratory tract and mouth. The umbilical cord should be clamped immediately and the baby handed to the pediatric team. If laryngoscopy reveals meconium at the level of the larynx, tracheal intubation and suctioning should be done. Such combined obstetric and pediatric management almost always prevents meconium aspiration syndrome and its morbid consequences.

When meconium is associated with abnormalities in the fetal heart tracing, it portends a much more ominous outcome. In these situations, expedient delivery may be appropriate.

## MEDICAL COMPLICATIONS OF PREGNANCY

### Hypertension

Hypertension complicates about 10% of pregnancies and therefore is the most common medical problem requiring special attention in the intrapartum period. About 75% of hypertensive patients have pregnancy-induced hypertension (preeclampsia); the remaining 25% have chronic hypertension. Potential complications of intrapartum hypertension include placental insufficiency, abruptio placentae, and maternal seizures. Intrapartum management is aimed at preventing these complications by optimal timing and control of delivery.

Blood pressure levels above 170/110 mm Hg or mean arterial pressures above 130 mm Hg require urgent treatment. To stabilize blood pressure, treatment choices include but are not limited to the use of hydralazine, diazoxide, and methyldopa.

Hydralazine acts directly on the arterial wall; its major side effects are headaches, nausea, and reflex tachycardia. Marked hypotension may result in patients who are slow acetylators of hydralazine. Gradual lowering of blood pressure to moderate ranges is less dangerous to the fetus than a rapid fall in blood pressure. The aim of treatment is to achieve a diastolic blood pressure of about 100 mm Hg.

Diazoxide is a dangerous drug; we do not use it. A bolus dose of 300 mg IV may cause profound hypotension and fetal death. A titrated dose of 30 mg bolus every 60 seconds has been suggested as an alternative. Even so, intrapartum use of diazoxide should be reserved for those very few patients who do not respond to hydralazine.

Methyldopa, the most popular drug used in the treatment of hypertension in the antepartum period, has limited use in the intrapartum treatment of preeclampsia. The maximum antihypertensive effect may take 4 to 6 hours to achieve, an unacceptable length of time for the treatment of severe preeclampsia.

### Anticonvulsive Therapy

Prevention of eclampsia is one of the main goals of medical therapy. This goal is achieved by the use of parenteral magnesium sulfate, given in a loading dose of 4 g IV followed by an IV infusion of 2 g/hour or 5 g IM every 4 hours.

### Diabetes in Pregnancy

About one in 100 pregnancies is complicated by overt diabetes, and another 5% of pregnancies are complicated by gestational diabetes. Over the past 15 years, remarkable advances in perinatology and neonatology have reduced perinatal losses significantly in diabetic pregnancies. The goal of management in pregnant diabetics is to time delivery to ensure fetal maturity and avoid fetal death. With improved antenatal diabetic control and close obstetric monitoring, fetal death in the final weeks of pregnancy is now rare. Today, it is usual to continue a diabetic pregnancy until at least 37 weeks' gestation.

During labor and delivery, attempts should be made to main-

tain maternal normoglycemia. If induction of labor is planned, the morning subcutaneous insulin is omitted. An intravenous infusion is commenced, with 5% dextrose given via an infusion pump at 125 mL/hour. Regular insulin is added to the solution to achieve an initial rate of 1.25 units of insulin per hour. These levels should be monitored every 2 hours during labor and if possible kept within a range of 60 to 100 mg/dL. For elective repeat cesarean delivery, the morning insulin dose is omitted, and an infusion of normal saline is begun at about 7 a.m. At my institution, elective repeat cesarean deliveries in diabetic pregnancies are performed at 8 a.m. If the patient has run normal fasting levels, it is likely that plasma glucose will be normal at the time of surgery.

Vaginal delivery is planned for most diabetic pregnancies, and cesarean delivery is reserved for the usual obstetric indications. Diabetes in pregnancy need not mean an automatic cesarean delivery; however, evidence is mounting to suggest that cesarean delivery may be indicated for grossly macrosomic infants of diabetic mothers to prevent trauma, particularly shoulder dystocia.

## CONCLUSIONS

The challenge of modern obstetrics is to manage a pregnancy with the least interference and yet with the capability of recognizing and correcting any complications at the earliest possible moment. Early recognition of complications and identification of the at-risk mother and infant will allow transfer to the appropriate health-care center for optimum care. A high-risk situation can develop very quickly in an otherwise normal labor and delivery; therefore, every hospital that delivers babies must be equipped to give adequate intrapartum care and must be prepared to do a cesarean delivery within 30 minutes.

To deal with perinatal problems effectively, there must be full consideration of maternal, medical, and social factors that can affect the fetus and neonate. This can be achieved by cooperation among the mother, obstetrician, pediatrician, nurses, and social workers, and between regional centers and community hospitals. This collaboration affords the best opportunity for delivery of excellence in perinatal care.

### Selected Readings

Belizán JM, Villar J, Nardin JC, et al. Diagnosis of intrauterine growth retardation by a simple clinical method: measurement of uterine height. Am J Obstet Gynecol 1978;131:643.

Bowes WA, Bowes D. Current role of the mid-forceps operation. Clin Obstet Gynecol 1980;23:549.

Carson BS, Losey RW, Bowes WA, et al. Combined obstetric and pediatric approach to prevent meconium aspiration syndrome. Am J Obstet Gynecol 1976;126:712.

Consensus Task Force on Cesarean Childbirth. NIH Publication No. 82, 1981:2067.

Creasy RK. Prevention of preterm birth. In: Finely SC, Finely WH, Flowers CE, eds. Birth defects: clinical and ethical considerations. New York: Alan R. Liss, 1983

Freinkel N. Banting Lecture: Of pregnancy and progeny. Diabetes 1980;29:1023.

Freinkel N, Dooley SL, Metzger BE. Care of the pregnant woman with insulin-dependent diabetes mellitus. N Engl J Med 1985;313:96.

Friedman EA. Labor: clinical evaluation and management, ed 2. New York: Appleton-Century-Crofts, 1978.

Habicht J, Yarbrough C, Lechtig A, Klein RE. Relationships of birth weight, maternal nutrition, and infant mortality. Nutr Rep Int 1973;7:533.

Healy DL, Quinn WA, Pepperell RJ. Rotational delivery of the fetus: Kielland's forceps and two other methods compared. Br J Obstet Gynaecol 1982;89:501.

Hobel CV, Hyvarinen MD, Okader DM, et al. Prenatal and intrapartum high-risk screening. I. Prediction of the high-risk neonate. Am J Obstet Gynecol 1973;117:1.

Konte JM, Holbrook RH Jr, Laros RK Jr, Creasy RK. Short-term neonatal morbidity associated with prematurity and the effect of a prematurity prevention program on expected incidence of morbidity. Am J Perinatol 1986;3:283.

McDonald D, Grant A, Sheridan-Pereira M, et al. The Dublin randomized controlled trial of intrapartum fetal heart-rate monitoring. Am J Obstet Gynecol 1985;152:524.

Phelps RL, Metzger BE, Freinkel N. Carbohydrate metabolism in pregnancy. XVII.

Diurnal profiles of plasma glucose, insulin, free fatty acids, triglycerides, cholesterol, and individual amino acids in late normal pregnancy. Am J Obstet Gynecol 1981;140:730.

Pritchard JA, Scott DE. Iron demands during pregnancy. In: Hallberg L, Harwerth H-G, Vannotti A, eds. Iron deficiency: pathogenesis, clinical aspects, therapy. New York: Academic Press, 1970.

*Principles and Practice of Pediatrics, Second Edition.*
edited by Frank A. Oski et al. J. B. Lippincott Company, Philadelphia © 1994.

# 17.2 *Fetal Evaluation and Prenatal Diagnosis*

Mary E. D'Alton

Serious birth defects, often genetically determined, complicate and threaten the lives of 3% of newborn infants. These disorders account for 20% of deaths during the newborn period and contribute to an even higher percentage of serious morbidity in infancy and childhood. The cost of neonatal intensive care is staggering; higher still are the costs of rehabilitation programs for the severely handicapped. The family tragedy is perhaps unmeasurable. With growing recognition of the frequency and importance of congenital disorders and with social trends toward a smaller family size as well as delay in beginning a family, prenatal diagnosis plays an important role in the management of many pregnancies.

## INDICATIONS FOR PRENATAL DIAGNOSIS

The identification of a pregnancy with an increased chance of a diagnosable fetal disorder involves a search for general and specific risk factors. Counseling before prenatal diagnosis is important. The central issue is balancing the risk of an abnormal child against the risk of an investigative or interventional procedure. Prospective parents must understand the concept of excluding or establishing a specific diagnosis with a high reliability but without complete certainty. One of the most important goals in genetic counseling is to help patients understand the reproductive options available. A person's previous experience, ethnic and cultural background, and religious beliefs will affect the acceptability of prenatal diagnosis and the choices made following the diagnosis of an abnormality. Counseling should be nondirective and should concentrate on accurate presentation of all the facts and options available. Common indications for prenatal counseling and diagnosis are summarized in Table 17-2.

### General Factors

It is standard practice to offer prenatal cytogenetic diagnosis to all women who at their expected delivery date will be 35 years or older. Numeric chromosome abnormalities occur with increasing frequency with advancing maternal age (Table 17-3). Testing for biochemical markers in maternal serum identifies patients at risk for certain cytogenetic and structural abnormalities. Alphafetoprotein, the major protein of early fetal life, is synthesized

---

TABLE 17-2.   Indications for Prenatal Testing

**General Factors**

Maternal age ≥35 at time of delivery

Maternal serum alpha-fetoprotein concentration

Triple screening (maternal serum alpha-fetoprotein, human chorionic gonadotropin, and unconjugated estriol)

**Specific factors**

Previous child with structural defect or chromosomal abnormality

Stillbirths, neonatal deaths

Parent with structural abnormality

Parent with balanced translocation

Inherited disorders (cystic fibrosis, metabolic disorders, sex-linked recessive disorders)

Maternal medical disease (diabetes, phenylketonuria)

Teratogen exposure (ionizing radiation, anticonvulsant medicines, lithium, isotretinoin, alcohol)

Infections (rubella, toxoplasmosis, cytomegalovirus)

**Ethnic Factors**

| Disorder | Ethnic Group | Screening Test |
|---|---|---|
| Tay-Sachs disease | Ashkenazi Jews, French Canadians | Decreased serum hexosaminidase A |
| Sickle-cell anemia | Black Africans, Mediterraneans, Arabs, Indo-Pakistanis | Presence of sickling in hemolysate followed by confirmatory hemoglobin electrophoresis |
| Thalassemia (alpha and beta) | Mediterraneans, Southern and Southeast Asians, Chinese | Mean corpuscular volume <80 semtoliters followed by confirmatory hemoglobin electrophoresis |

| TABLE 17-3. Maternal Age and Estimated Rates of Chromosomal Abnormalities at Time of Expected Live Birth | | |
|---|---|---|
| Maternal Age | Risk of Down Syndrome | Total Risk for Chromosomal Abnormalities |
| 20 | 1/1667 | 1/526 |
| 25 | 1/1250 | 1/476 |
| 30 | 1/952 | 1/385 |
| 35 | 1/385 | 1/202 |
| 36 | 1/295 | 1/162 |
| 37 | 1/227 | 1/129 |
| 38 | 1/175 | 1/102 |
| 39 | 1/137 | 1/82 |
| 40 | 1/106 | 1/65 |
| 41 | 1/82 | 1/51 |
| 42 | 1/64 | 1/40 |
| 43 | 1/50 | 1/32 |
| 44 | 1/38 | 1/25 |
| 45 | 1/30 | 1/20 |
| 46 | 1/23 | 1/16 |
| 47 | 1/18 | 1/13 |
| 48 | 1/14 | 1/10 |
| 49 | 1/11 | 1/7 |

*Modified from Hook EB. Rates of chromosome abnormalities at different gestational ages. Obstet Gynecol 1981;58:282, and Hook EB, Cross PK, Schreinemacher MS. Chromosomal, abnormality rates at amniocentesis and in liveborn infants. JAMA 1983;249:2034.*

in the fetal liver and yolk sac. Open neural tube and ventral wall defects are associated with exposed fetal membrane and blood vessel surfaces, which increase the levels of alpha-fetoprotein in amniotic fluid and maternal serum. Low levels of maternal serum alpha-fetoprotein and unconjugated estriol are associated with trisomies 21 and 18.

The single marker that yields the highest detection rate for Down syndrome is human chorionic gonadotropin, which is significantly elevated in this syndrome. The combined use of the markers human chorionic gonadotropin, unconjugated estriol, maternal serum alpha-fetoprotein, and maternal age leads to detection of about 60% of cases of Down syndrome, with a false-positive rate of 6.6%; the use of ultrasonography to verify gestational age reduces the false-positive rate to 3.8%.

Maternal serum alpha-fetoprotein screening should be offered to women at 16 to 18 completed weeks of pregnancy. Careful evaluation of gestational age is of critical importance because maternal serum alpha-fetoprotein values increase steadily throughout the second trimester. Because of population differences of median maternal serum alpha-fetoprotein values, laboratories should provide interpretation of results that take into account the variables of race, multiple gestation, diabetes mellitus, and maternal weight. Most centers in the United States have chosen a cutoff of 2.0 to 2.5 times the median for the general population screened for neural tube defects. Invasive procedures such as amniocentesis may give rise to maternal alpha-fetoprotein elevations; therefore, blood samples for screening markers should be obtained before amniocentesis is performed.

### Specific Factors

After birth of one child with trisomy 21, the likelihood that a subsequent child will have a similar chromosomal abnormality is about 1%. The recurrence rate for neural tube defects is 2% to

5%, compared with a general population risk of one to two per 1000 births. The general recurrence risk of a cardiac defect is 2% to 4%, compared with the general population risk of four to eight per 1000 live births. If a parent has spina bifida, congenital heart disease, or a known chromosome translocation or inversion, there is as an increased chance that a child will have a related defect. Antenatal diagnosis is possible for many inborn errors of metabolism, almost all of which are transmitted in an autosomal recessive fashion. Maternal diabetes and maternal phenylketonuria are associated with an increased risk of fetal malformations. Other known teratogens include ionizing radiation, drugs, and maternal infections.

### Ethnic Factors

The gene frequencies of various genetic disorders differ among geographic population groups. Carrier detection programs can be applied to different ethnic groups at risk for specific diseases, for example for Tay-Sachs disease in Ashkenazi Jewish populations, hemoglobins in blacks, and thalassemia in people of Mediterranean origin. The populations involved and the methods of screening are listed in Table 17-2.

## PRENATAL DIAGNOSIS PROCEDURES

### Amniocentesis

Amniotic fluid contains viable cells of fetal origin plus dissolved proteins and other chemicals. The first diagnosis of a chromosomal abnormality by amniotic fluid analysis was reported in 1967, and by the mid-1970s the safety and accuracy of mid-trimester amniocentesis were well established. Mid-trimester amniocentesis created the field of prenatal diagnosis and has become established as the gold standard to which other procedures for prenatal diagnosis are compared.

Mid-trimester amniocentesis is usually performed under ultrasound guidance at 16 weeks' gestation in an outpatient setting. Chromosome studies can be done by culturing the few viable cells present in amniotic fluid, and the results are generally available in 10 to 14 days. Amniocentesis carries an estimated risk of fetal loss of 0.5% to 1%. Culture failure occurs in less than 1% of cases.

Chromosomal mosaicism is the presence of two or more cell lines with different karyotype in a single individual. This occurs as a result of postzygotic nondisjunction. The observation of multiple cell lines in a prenatal diagnosis sample does not necessarily mean that the fetus is a mosaic. The most common type of mosaicism detected in amniocentesis is pseudomosaicism. This should be suspected when an abnormality is seen in only one of several cultures from an amniotic fluid specimen. The abnormal cell lines arise during in vitro cultures; therefore, they are not present in the fetus and are not clinically significant. Maternal cell contamination can be minimized in amniocentesis by discarding the first few drops of aspirated amniotic fluid. True fetal mosaicism—the presence of the same abnormality on more than one cover slip—is rare (0.25%) but clinically significant. This is best resolved by karyotyping of fetal lymphocytes obtained by percutaneous fetal blood sampling, a method that provides results within 48 hours. Detailed ultrasound is also recommended to assess fetal growth and to rule out structural anomalies. If both the ultrasound and fetal blood sampling results are normal, this provides reassurance that the major chromosome abnormalities may be excluded.

### Chorionic Villus Sampling

The success of mid-trimester amniocentesis reduced the emphasis placed on first-trimester diagnosis, but because of the inherent advantages of first-trimester fetal diagnosis, a few investigators continued to explore this approach. Moreover, the development of molecular methods of gene analysis focused more attention on first-trimester fetal tissue sampling. Ultrasound guidance has been key to the success of the sampling procedure, and chorionic villus sampling is now done with a high success rate. By 1992, over 150,000 cases of chorionic villus sampling had been documented worldwide. Chorionic villi may be obtained by aspiration via a transcervical catheter or transabdominal needle using ultrasound guidance. The choice is based on placental location and operator preference and experience.

The main advantage of chorionic villus sampling over amniocentesis is the earlier availability of results, as the procedure is generally performed between 9 and 12 weeks' gestation. Results based on a direct preparation of spontaneously dividing cells are usually available in 24 to 48 hours, and final results from cultured cells in 10 to 14 days. An advantage of chorionic villus sampling is the increased amount of tissue obtained when compared to amniocentesis; this increased tissue mass is beneficial when DNA or enzymatic diagnosis is necessary. However, amniocentesis must be used for assays for which amniotic fluid is essential (for example, alpha-fetoprotein concentration).

Randomized trials comparing chorionic villus sampling with amniocentesis at 16 weeks' gestation have shown increased procedure-related fetal loss with chorionic villus sampling (about 2% to 3% of fetuses sampled). No difference has been found in the fetal loss rates between transcervical and transabdominal chorionic villus sampling.

Limb-reduction defects have been reported to occur with increased frequency in some series of chorionic villus sampling performed at 56 to 66 menstrual days. The proposed mechanism of the defects is a form of vascular insult leading to hypoperfusion of the fetus. This, however, has not been a consistent finding. Although a time-sensitive relationship for limb defects is possible, and operator experience may be a factor, a causal relationship between chorionic villus sampling and limb defects is not firmly established.

The increased observation of maternal cell contamination and mosaicism in chorionic villus samples contributes to reduced cytogenetic accuracy when compared to amniocentesis. Maternal cell contamination is uncommon in experienced cytogenetic laboratories; however, the reported incidence is about 2%. Villus specimens obtained must be meticulously separated from blood and decidual cells before undergoing cytogenetic analysis. Mosaicism occurs in less than 1% of cases, is more common with the direct preparations, and is usually due to confined placental mosaicism. This phenomenon occurs as a result of nondisjunction during embryogenesis and leads to the presence of aneuploid cells in the extra-embryonic tissues that are not present in the fetus itself. When mosaic results are reported, further testing with amniocentesis is warranted. Amniocentesis is necessary in about 1% of patients who undergo chorionic villus sampling.

These clinical disadvantages of increased risk and potential diagnostic error in chorionic villus sampling must be weighed against the disadvantage of the later timing of amniocentesis.

## Early Amniocentesis

Early amniocentesis (before 15 weeks) is technically easier to perform than chorionic villus sampling, and the success rates in obtaining samples are similar. On occasion, aspiration of fluid may be hampered due to tenting of membranes, as the amnion has not completely fused with the chorion at this early gestational age. The safety of early amniocentesis cannot be assumed to be the same as conventional amniocentesis. The volume of fluid removed constitutes a much greater proportion of the total fluid volume, which may have an effect on fetal loss and fetal lung function. An additional disadvantage is that standards are still being established for measuring and interpreting amniotic fluid alpha-fetoprotein before 14 to 15 weeks.

## Percutaneous Umbilical Blood Sampling

Fetal blood can be obtained from about 18 weeks' gestation with a 20- or 22-gauge spinal needle directed by ultrasound guidance into the umbilical cord. Access to the fetal circulation permits prenatal evaluation of many fetal hematologic abnormalities, including isoimmunization, hemoglobinopathy, thrombocytopenia, and coagulation factor abnormalities. Fetal blood can be used for the prenatal diagnosis of some inborn errors of metabolism and permits assessment of viral, bacterial, and parasitic infection by serology and culture. Fetal blood sampling may clarify chromosome mosaicism detected by cytogenetic analysis of amniotic fluid cells or chorionic villi.

Rapid karyotyping for congenital abnormalities is the most common indication for fetal blood sampling in the United States. Cytogenetic results are usually available from short-term fetal lymphocyte cultures within 48 to 72 hours.

The perinatal loss rate from percutaneous umbilical blood sampling is about 2% over the background risk to that fetus. Because many of the fetuses studied have severe congenital malformations, the background loss rate is high in comparison to the population undergoing amniocentesis or chorionic villus sampling. As percutaneous umbilical blood sampling carries a substantially greater risk of pregnancy loss than amniocentesis, it should be reserved for those situations in which a rapid diagnosis is essential or when needed diagnostic information cannot be achieved by safer means.

## Fetal Biopsy

Fetal biopsy was initially performed by fetoscopy but is now performed using ultrasound guidance. Certain genetic skin disorders such as epidermolysis bullosa that cannot at present be diagnosed by DNA analysis require fetal skin sampling. Fetal liver biopsy was in the past used to diagnose ornithine transcarbamylase deficiency. Fetal muscle biopsy has been reported to diagnose Duchenne muscular dystrophy in a family that was uninformative for DNA studies.

It is difficult to assess the safety and accuracy of fetal biopsy because experience is limited. Patients should be made aware of the investigational nature of the procedure. Rapid advances in DNA technology will delineate the molecular basis of many diseases that currently require fetal biopsy, and as this occurs the need for these procedures will decline.

## Ultrasound

Ultrasound is an important aid in assessing gestational age, monitoring fetal growth, confirming placental site, detecting multiple gestation, and diagnosing major fetal anomalies. Some teratogens and infections produce structural abnormalities that are potentially detectable via ultrasound but not via the other prenatal diagnostic approaches. Visualization of fetal anatomy is essential in diagnosing anatomical defects inherited in polygenic multifactorial fashion. Individual centers report excellent results in ultrasound diagnosis of renal and bladder anomalies, hydrocephaly, and neural tube and ventral wall defects. Ultrasound is also useful in Mendelian disorders characterized by anatomical defects such as skeletal dysplasia, and common chromosomal abnormalities can be identified by sonography (Table 17-4).

Opinions differ about the advantages of routine ultrasound screening. At a Consensus Development Conference sponsored by the National Institute of Child Health and Human Develop-

TABLE 17-4. Sonographic Findings
in Chromosomal Abnormalities

**Trisomy 21**
Duodenal atresia, tracheoesophageal fistula, esophageal atresia; polyhydramnios is usual if these gastrointestinal lesions present
Cardiac abnormalities (atrioventricular canal defects, ventricular septal defects, atrial septal defects)
Hypoplasia of middle quadrant of the fifth digit
Second trimester findings: thickened nuchal fold >6 mm; ratio of actual to expected femur length, 0.91

**Trisomy 18**
Intrauterine growth retardation
Polyhydramnios
Clenched hands with overlapping digits
Clubfeet, rocker-bottom feet
Cardiac abnormalities (ventricular septal defect)
Omphalocele, diaphragmatic hernia
Choroid plexus cysts

**Trisomy 13**
Holoprosencephaly
Cleft lip and palate
Cardiac abnormalities (ventricular septal defect)
Polydactyly
Omphalocele
Polycystic kidneys

ment the recommendation was made that ultrasound imaging be used only for specific indications. On the other hand, several countries, including Germany, France, and Britain, have adopted uniform screening ultrasound in all pregnancies. Most of the randomized trials evaluating the usefulness of routine ultrasound screening have not addressed the diagnostic accuracy for anatomical fetal defects. Trials conducted in the early 1980s did not demonstrate any benefit of routine ultrasound; furthermore, screened women had a significantly higher rate of hospital admission. The Helsinki randomized trial demonstrated that half of serious malformations were detected prenatally and that perinatal mortality was significantly lower in the screened group than in the control group (4.6/1000 versus 9.0/1000). This reduction was mainly due to improved early detection of major malformations, which led to induced abortion.

The most common congenital abnormalities are cardiovascular malformations, which are among the major malformations most frequently missed by prenatal ultrasound. A four-chamber view of the fetal heart is suggested for ultrasound examination in pregnancy. The use of a four-chamber view in obstetric sonography has resulted in a significant increase in referrals to perinatal centers, which permits the delivery to take place at a center capable of caring for the newborn with congenital heart disease. The reported sensitivity of the four-chamber view for detection of congenital heart defects was 92% in a referred high-risk population; however, the ultrasound at those centers was performed by experienced investigators.

When a fetal anomaly is diagnosed with ultrasound, echocardiography should be performed, as fetuses with an extracardiac anomaly have a 23% risk of having a cardiac defect. Conversely, fetuses with a cardiac defect have a 25% to 45% risk of having another anatomical defect. Karyotype analysis should be offered in most cases of cardiac and extracardiac malformations, as about one third will have a chromosomal disorder. Amniocentesis is the suggested technique; however, fetal blood sampling or pla-

cental biopsy may be performed if a rapid result is required. Knowledge of abnormal karyotype significantly affects perinatal management and may avoid unnecessary cesarean section. Several aneuploid chromosome defects exhibit characteristic ultrasonographic patterns (see Table 17-4). Karyotyping may not be necessary for all malformations detected with ultrasound (for example, congenital adenomatoid degeneration of the lung or isolated pyelectasis).

As a consequence of prenatal detection of fetal anatomical abnormalities, appropriate prenatal consultation can be obtained to make management decisions and determine the appropriate personnel and location and mode of delivery. Occasionally in utero treatment has been undertaken. Intrauterine shunts have been placed for bladder outlet obstruction and isolated pleural effusion. Open fetal surgery has been performed to manage congenital diaphragmatic hernia and complete bladder obstruction. All of these interventions are investigational and their effects on outcome unproven.

## Amniocentesis for Assessment of Fetal Lung Maturity

Iatrogenic preterm delivery still represents an important and preventable cause of prematurity and respiratory distress syndrome. Fetal pulmonary maturity should be documented by some method before elective delivery, and this applies equally to the low- and high-risk patient. Certain clinical situations such as diabetes mellitus are known to be associated with delayed pulmonary maturation. When the lecithin/sphingomyelin ratio exceeds 2:1 and phosphatidyl glycerol is present in normal amounts, the chances of respiratory distress syndrome in the newborn of a diabetic is remarkably low.

Other factors can affect the results of a lung profile. For example, blood or meconium in amniotic fluid can falsely lower the lecithin/sphingomyelin ratio. Subjecting amniotic fluid to a complete lung profile with analysis of phosphatidyl glycerol overcomes many of these problems. Neither blood nor meconium will cause false readings of phosphatidyl glycerol.

Various laboratories use different analytic techniques to perform a lung profile, so the clinician should discuss with the laboratory service the precise techniques used in lung maturity studies. Key steps in the assessment of lung maturity may include the cold acetone precipitation method and two-dimensional thin-layer chromatography. More expedient laboratory techniques are now available; they may have greater appeal to the clinical laboratory services but may be less accurate. The use of an inaccurate test may result in an increase in the incidence of respiratory distress syndrome in newborns despite laboratory evidence for lung maturity.

The assessment of fetal maturity is important in determining the timing of a repeat cesarean delivery. For patients being considered for elective repeat cesarean deliveries, if one of the following criteria is met, fetal maturity may be assumed and amniocenteses need not be performed:

Fetal heart tones have been documented for 20 weeks by fetoscope or for 30 weeks by Doppler.

It has been 36 weeks since a positive serum or urine human chorionic gonadotropin pregnancy test was performed by a reliable laboratory.

An ultrasound measurement of the fetal crown-rump length obtained at 6 to 11 weeks supports a gestational age of 39 weeks or more.

An ultrasound obtained at 12 to 20 weeks confirms the gestational age of greater than 39 weeks determined by clinical history and physical examination.

## Fetal Blood Sampling

Access to the fetal circulation provides a unique opportunity for direct evaluation of the fetal environment in at-risk pregnancies. Since cord blood pH is an accepted indicator of neonatal condition at delivery, antenatal demonstration of a low pH or low $PO_2$ may prompt early delivery; on the other hand, a normal acid–base balance would suggest that the pregnancy be allowed to continue.

While fetal blood sampling has a limited role in monitoring fetal well-being, acid–base determination does not predict perinatal outcome in growth-restricted fetuses. Studies of fetal–acid base status have demonstrated that while severe fetal antepartum hypoxia, acidemia, and acidosis are associated with poor perinatal outcome, it does not discriminate between fetuses who will die and those who will survive. Therefore, the place of fetal blood sampling in the evaluation of growth retardation has not been established other than for rapid karyotyping in the fetus with severe growth retardation to avoid unnecessary intervention if the fetus will be nonviable because of a chromosome abnormality.

## CURRENT EFFICACY OF SCREENING METHODS

Prenatal diagnosis for chromosomal analysis is currently offered to women who will be 35 years or older at the time of delivery. Nearly all genetic procedures performed in the United States are performed in the 5% of women who are over 35 years of age. This approach detects only 20% of cases of Down syndrome; the use of maternal serum alpha-fetoprotein screening in women of all ages will identify an additional 25% of cases. Use of maternal serum alpha-fetoprotein, human chorionic gonadotropin, unconjugated estriol, and maternal age will identify about 60% of cases of Down syndrome. Clinicians using a maternal serum alpha-fetoprotein screening program can expect to detect 80% to 90% percent of fetuses with neural tube defects, almost all cases of gastroschisis, and 70% to 80% of cases of omphalocele. The use of routine ultrasound screening, including a four-chamber view of the heart, potentially can diagnose about half of major cardiac, kidney, and bladder anomalies that would not be detected with maternal serum alpha-fetoprotein screening. When a targeted ultrasound examination is done to detect malformations suspected by history or screening ultrasonography in referral centers with skilled ultrasonologists, the sensitivity and specificity exceed 90%.

## THE FUTURE

The project of mapping the human genome is expected to be completed in the next 10 to 15 years, and as a result molecular genetic technology is likely to be available for detection of many additional common monogenic disorders. Cost-effective screening will be available for many disorders, including cystic fibrosis. Pre-implantation diagnosis is possible in certain circumstances and may allow fetal treatment before organogenesis.

A promising new technique for isolating fetal cells from maternal blood is under intensive study. The challenges of this technique include reliably separating fetal cells by identifying unique fetal cell surface antigens and modifying molecular genetic techniques such as the polymerase chain reaction so that small samples of fetal genetic material can be analyzed. It is likely that continued research into the fetal cell separation methods will make noninvasive prenatal diagnosis a reality.

## Selected Readings

American College of Obstetricians and Gynecologists. Antenatal diagnosis of genetic disorders. Technical Bulletin 108. Washington DC: ACOG, 1987.

American College of Obstetricians and Gynecologists. Ultrasound in pregnancy. Technical Bulletin 116. Washington DC: ACOG, 1988.

Bianchi DW, Flint AF, Pizzimenfi MF, et al. Isolation of fetal DNA from nucleated erythrocytes in maternal blood. Proc Natl Acad Sci USA 1990;87:3279.

Daffos F, Capella-Povlovsky M, Forestier F. Fetal blood sampling during pregnancy with use of a needle guided by ultrasound: a study of 606 consecutive cases. Am J Obstet Gynecol 1985;153:655.

Firth HV, Boyd PA, Chamberlain P, MacKenzie IZ, Lindenbaum RH, Huson SM. Severe limb abnormalities after chorion villus sampling at 56–66 days' gestation. Lancet 1991;337:762.

Froster UG, Baird PA. Limb-reduction defects and chorionic villus sampling. Lancet 1992;339:66.

Haddow J, Palomaki G, Knight G. Prospective prenatal screening for Down's syndrome using maternal serum markers. N Engl J Med 1992;327.

Hook EB. Rates of chromosome abnormalities at different gestational ages. Obstet Gynecol 1981;58:282.

Hook EB, Cross PK, Schreinemacher MS. Chromosomal abnormality rates at amniocentesis and in live-born infants. JAMA 1983;249:2034.

Merkatz IR, Nitowsky HM, Macri JN, Johnson WE. An association between low maternal serum alpha-fetoprotein and fetal chromosomal abnormalities. Am J Obstet Gynecol 1984;14:886.

National Institute of Child Health and Human Development National Registry for Amniocentesis Study Group. Mid-trimester amniocentesis for prenatal diagnosis: safety and accuracy. JAMA 1976;236:1471.

National Institutes of Health Development Conference Consensus Statement: The use of diagnostic ultrasound imaging in pregnancy. Washington DC: US Government Printing Office, 1984.

Rhoads GG, Jackson LG, Schlesseiman SE, et al. The safety and efficacy of chorionic villus sampling for early prenatal diagnosis of cytogenetic abnormalities. N Engl J Med 1989;320:609.

Saari-Kemppainen A, Karjalainen O, Ylostalo P, Heinonen OP. Ultrasound screening and perinatal mortality: controlled trial of systematic one-stage screening in pregnancy. Lancet 1990;336:387.

Wald NJ, Cuckle HS. Maternal serum alpha-fetoprotein measurement in antenatal screening for anencephaly and spina bifida in early pregnancy. Report of the U.K. Collaborative Study on alpha-fetoprotein in relation to neural-tube defects. Lancet 1977;1:1323.

Watson JD. The human genome project: past, present and future. Science 1990;249:44.

*Principles and Practice of Pediatrics, Second Edition.*
edited by Frank A. Oski et al. J. B. Lippincott Company, Philadelphia © 1994.

CHAPTER 18

# Management of the Normal Newborn

## William D. Cochran

Two hundred years from now, if we were asked what is clinically most the same now as 200 years before, we would probably be safe to answer, a newborn infant. Even so, newborns are, in reality, an extremely complex genetically engineered organism waiting to act and react with their environment. However, they are pretty consistently the same model, year after year. This chapter will deal with the usual medical care and evaluation of normal newborns and those with common variations.

## THE BIRTH AND NEWBORN ENVIRONMENT

Efforts are now made to create a natural and comfortable environment for childbirth in hospitals. A combination labor, delivery, and recovery room (occasionally even a postpartum room as well) has been incorporated into the construction of almost all new hospitals, and fathers and others close to the mother now can be present during the birthing process. Attempts to involve siblings of the new baby in the birthing process have mostly failed, but there is no inherent reason why they should not participate if the family so desires. The labor bed should be comfortable, chairs should be available, and typical delivery room equipment (for anesthesia and newborn resuscitation) should be as unobtrusive as possible. Mothers should be encouraged to hold the infant as soon after delivery as possible. This provides assurance of normalcy, and maternal attachment may also be enhanced during the hyperalert state that characterizes the newborn in the early minutes after delivery.

Since newborns are warmer than their mothers by about 0.5°C, they are born vasodilated and tend to lose heat rapidly. Also contributing to their heat loss is evaporative heat loss in the often too-cold environment. It is important to dry and wrap the newborn. A stocking cap placed immediately over the head while the rest of the infant is being dried helps to blunt this initial heat loss. Marked heat loss and consequent lowering of the infant's core temperature can cause an otherwise well infant to exhibit grunting respiration and cyanosis and to develop a measurable metabolic acidosis.

Apgar scores should be assigned (see Chap. 19), and a brief but essential examination of the baby should be done in the delivery room. This will determine whether the infant goes to the regular nursery or to a more acute care nursery. Major anomalies, labor- or drug-induced asphyxia or depression, and expected or unexpected prematurity should be recognized in the delivery room. It is also important for babies with malformations to be seen by the mother and father, with appropriate support and explanation.

## INITIAL PHYSICAL EXAMINATION

A thorough examination should be done within 24 hours of birth. Many pediatricians use warming lights during this exam, to keep the infant warm and hence less fussy. It is important to have an appropriate prenatal and delivery history available, as well as information provided by nurses concerning infant behavior and feeding patterns. Evaluations by nursery nurses are done at least every 8 hours and usually much more frequently close to admission or when deviations from normal such as hypothermia, grunting and retracting, questionable cyanosis, or hypotonia or jitteriness are noted. Febrile infants with rectal temperatures of 100°F or higher need especially careful observation and evaluation.

Three percent of all newborns have a major malformation, so unexpected anomalies such as those of the CNS, heart, skeleton, or gastrointestinal tract may be found. There may also be evidence of physical or hypoxic stress caused by the labor or the delivery process. The examiner should also be aware of risk factors for infection or hemolytic disease. The experienced examiner is alert for subtle signs related to newborn tone or level of arousal. An infant who becomes "alert" and stops moving or fretting in the presence of conversation can probably hear. Bright lights or a flashlight beam will almost always cause a blink, initially providing assurance of at least grossly intact vision.

Experienced examiners evaluate the neurologic system throughout the exam, using the infant's response to the general exam as an indicator of neurologic status. Painful components of the exam usually elicit an aversion response, the absence of which might indicate CNS pathology. Redressing or briefly holding and cuddling an infant will usually quiet a crying infant, although using a pacifier is often the most effective method. The infant's general patterns of response may provide clues to underlying pathology.

## Heart and Lungs

The heart and lungs are commonly examined first, while the infant is still quiet and unchilled. This part of the exam can be done with just the shirt pulled up and the diapers on, thus causing the least disturbance to and chilling of the baby. The infant should be examined for the presence of central cyanosis. *Acrocyanosis*—blue hands, blue feet, and occasionally even blue lips (but a pink tongue)—is normal, especially if the baby is cold. All the rest of the skin should be pink. Heart sounds loudest on the right suggest dextrocardia or possibly a left pneumothorax. Rate and rhythm should be noted; a rate between 90 and 160 is in the normal range. Some irregularity of rhythm, usually from premature ventricular contractions, is common, and if it is an isolated finding this is usually benign and transient. Systolic murmurs are common on the first day and usually reflect the closing ductus arteriosus or are simple flow murmurs. Persistent murmurs or murmurs accompanied by an overactive heart or in the presence of a fixed rate or tachycardia need careful evaluation (see Chap. 20.3.2). Femoral pulses may be difficult to palpate but should be sought in the presence of systolic murmurs to rule out coarctation of the aorta.

A pink, apparently well-oxygenated infant who is breathing quietly without retractions and grunting is immediately reassuring to the examiner. Most infants breathe rather irregularly in the first day or two of life, and the depth of each breath varies as well. Their abdomens often rise and fall because they use their diaphragms more than their intercostal muscles. Asymmetry, intercostal retractions, and tachypnea (a respiratory rate over 60) are worrisome if they are more than transient findings.

## Abdomen

Examination of the abdomen should be done with the infant naked. Again, observation is important. In the first day, the newborn abdomen is full and rounded, not asymmetric or scaphoid. *Diastasis recti*, nonunion of the two rectus muscles from the umbilicus to the xiphoid, often causes a mild herniation in the midline. Asymmetry, unless it is due to a big stomach bubble (often just after eating or crying), may be a clue to an abnormal abdominal mass. A scaphoid abdomen, usually with accompanying respiratory symptoms, might indicate a diaphragmatic hernia with some of the abdominal contents up in the chest. The veins in the skin over the upper abdomen often appear dilated. The cord and its three vessels will have been evaluated at delivery, but can be rechecked quickly. A two-vessel cord is accompanied by another major anomaly at least 10% of the time, so this should alert the examiner. The spleen is usually not palpable.

In the newborn, the liver edge can best be evaluated by approaching it from below with the thumb, held flattened on the abdomen and placed between the midline and axillary line, beginning the palpation at the level of the umbilicus and progressing upward. The pad of the thumb, with its greater sensitivity, will pick up the liver edge as the infant breathes. Generally, the liver edge will be felt 2 to 3 cm below the right costal margin. In infants with intrauterine growth retardation, the liver may not be palpable. In infants of diabetic mothers, the liver may be enlarged to as much as 4 cm below the costal margin.

Deep (and sometimes briefly painful) palpation is done to examine the bladder and the kidneys. With careful bimanual palpation, the left kidney can almost always be palpated, the examiner placing the third finger of one hand posteriorly in the lowest costovertebral angle and then trapping the left kidney against that finger with the index and third fingers of the other

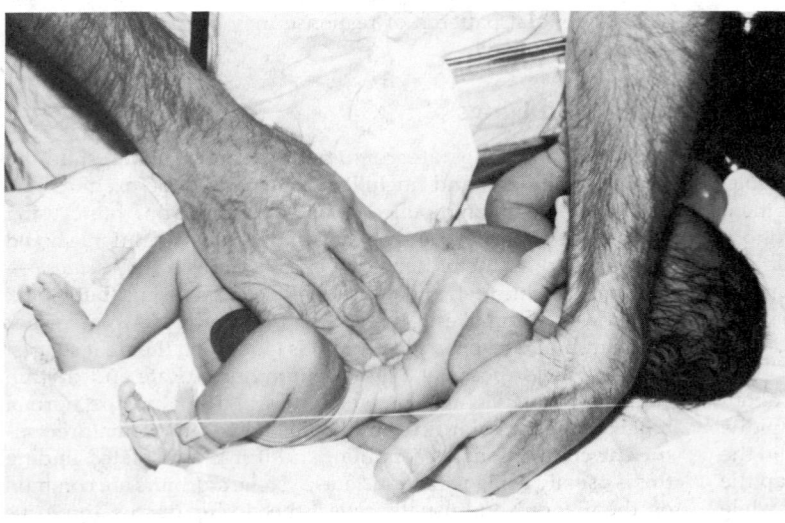

Figure 18-1.  Palpation of the left kidney.

hand (Fig 18-1). The lower pole of the normal right kidney is only occasionally palpated, but if the right kidney is enlarged it will thus be noted.

## Genitalia and Anus

The labia majora in the term female infant are enlarged and generally cover the labia minora, except in the clitoral region. The clitoris should be examined for size and palpated for diameter. Both labia should be spread, and the pink, glistening vaginal orifice should be examined for patency and discharge (usually creamy and white). An apparent imperforate hymen should be checked with a small soft catheter to see if it will slip by, because an enlarged Bartholin's gland often mimics imperforation. The fourchette should be checked for any fistula. The labia majora should be palpated briefly for masses (which when present are most commonly an ovary).

In the male, the penis and foreskin should be examined for hypospadias, with consideration given to the size of the penis. A hooded foreskin may be present in a first-degree hypospadias. The scrotum's rugation and size should be noted. Testes should be palpated bilaterally. Finding nonpalpable testes in any phenotypic male should raise a question of virilizing adrenal hyperplasia. Undescended testes are commonly found in males with less than 34 weeks of gestation.

The anus should be checked for patency and position. Occasionally, large fistulae are mistaken for a normal anus.

## Hips

Dislocated hips are the most common hidden and quiescent anomaly, and unfortunately, if not diagnosed until the infant (or even child) starts to walk, can result in permanent disability. The hips are examined by placing the legs in a frog-leg position, with the third fingertip on the greater trochanter and the thumb pressing laterally and down on the inside of the knee until the knee is pressed against the mattress; meanwhile, the third finger is pushing up toward the examiner. In other words, the femoral head most commonly has dislocated following a vector that has a posterior superior and a lateral component, so to relocate it the examiner is trying to bring the femoral head back upward. The knee abducted in the frog-leg position tightens the anterior segment of the hip capsule, thus creating a fulcrum that permits the head of the femur to move back into its socket. One sign of a dislocated hip is an asymmetric crease of skin folds under the buttock (Galeazzi's sign). This sign is not helpful if there is bilateral

dislocation. The possibility of undiagnosed dislocated hips should obviously be rechecked at follow-up physical examinations.

## Extremities and Joints

All long bones should be palpated briefly for unexpected fractures. Joints should be assessed for range of motion and evidence of uterine deformation. The most common deformation is tibial bowing and the next most common is forefoot adduction, with a clubfoot being the most extreme. Any foot that can be corrected passively to a neutral position will usually correct spontaneously over time. Counting the fingers and toes avoids the embarrassment of being asked later, "Why does my baby have six toes?" The clavicles should be palpated for fracture, which if present heals spontaneously. Thought should be given to the length of the limbs; the fingers should extend as far as the lower buttocks when stretched out. Infants presenting by breech often hold their legs in bizarre positions, yet in a matter of days all returns to normal.

## Head, Eyes, and Ears

Normal head circumference at term is between 33 and 38 cm. The head should be observed and palpated for the degree of molding and *caput succedaneum* (edema of the leading portion of the scalp in a vertex delivery). Occasionally, the degree of molding is marked but still benign (Fig 18-2). A caput occasionally obscures a developing cephalohematoma (the latter caused by bleeding under the outer periosteum of a parietal bone). Cephalohematomas usually do not mature until day 2 or 3 of life and, being subperiosteal, do not extend beyond the suture line as do caputs. The parietal and coronal sutures should be examined for patency and mobility. If the head circumference is within normal limits, the diameter of the anterior fontanelle can vary from 1 cm to 5 to 6 cm. Very large anterior fontanelles may be associated with hypothyroidism. *Craniotabes*, a ping-pong ball feel over the parietal bones with pressure, is a rare but normal variant.

The eyes may be difficult to visualize because the caput edema has migrated to the lids. In subdued light, while sucking on a pacifier or being held vertically, most infants will open their eyes. The eye exam is more easily done on the day of discharge, when the integrity of the iris, presence of a red reflex, and absence of cataracts can be evaluated. Hemorrhages in the conjunctivae are common, especially after strong labor. The ears should be examined for shape and the presence of an outer canal.

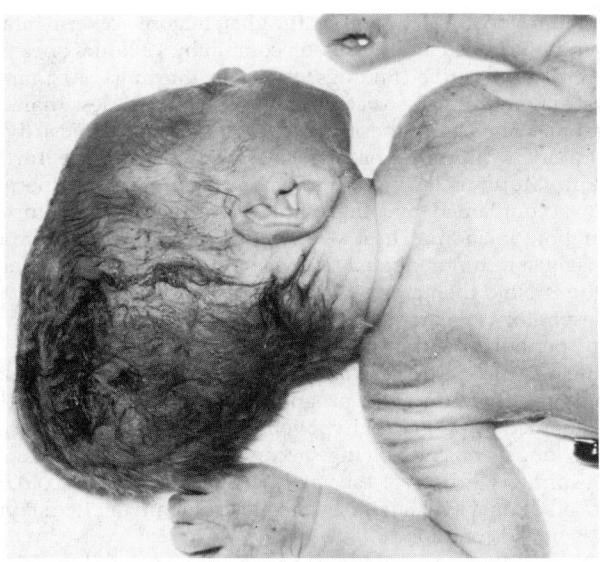

Figure 18-2.  Molding of the head.

## Neck and Mouth

Newborn infants may look like little football players because they have such short necks, so care must be exercised to rule out thyroid abnormalities or sinus tracts of the thyroid or of the second or third branchial arch. The tongue and gums should be checked carefully. The mouth should be examined, especially for palatal defects, which include bony clefts with an intact soft palate, a partial cleft, or a complete cleft of both the hard and soft palates. Visualization and palpation are usually necessary. *Ebstein's pearls* are small, white cysts often seen close to the midline at the junction of the hard and soft palates. They soon disappear with sucking. Abnormalities of the gums are less common, and sublingual cysts (ranulae) are unusual. If cysts are present, temporizing is worthwhile to see if vigorous sucking causes them to break spontaneously. *Asynclitism*, in which the maxillary gum line is not parallel to the mandibular gum line, is common, and extreme cases are associated with temporary feeding problems. It is often associated with arrest of descent during labor.

## Skin

Normal findings and variations on the first day include tiny milia (unbroken sweat glands), most commonly found on the nose, and petechiae, usually noted above the nipple line or on the head secondary to the pressure of labor. Occasionally, 0.5- to 1-cm vesicles or pustules, often broken, with no erythematous base are seen, usually clustered around the genitalia. Petechiae scattered more generally should prompt a more complete evaluation. Jaundice on the first day should always be considered abnormal. Mongoloid or blue spots up to 10 to 15 cm in size are often noted on the trunk or thighs of non-Caucasian infants. A nevus flammeus of the upper eyelids, at the nape of the neck, or occasionally extending down to the nose and upper lip is frequently seen but will soon fade.

As part of gestational age-dating, there are helpful variations to be recognized in the general appearance of a newborn's skin. The skin during late prematurity is still quite thin, and thus that infant's color is pinker (almost red) compared with that of a post-term infant, whose epidermis is thicker and, at least in repose, appears pale with a faint pink tinge. Although there is some racial variation, *lanugo* (fine hair found especially on shoulders) is more common as prematurity increases. *Vernix caseosa*, the greasy, white, often quite copious material produced in utero by the exocrine glands, is most common after 35 weeks of gestation, and is usually completely shed into the amniotic fluid after the 40th to 41st week. Postterm infants either have none left on their skin or have it only in creases in the skin.

## Neurologic Exam

The neurologic exam can be time-consuming, so the examiner should decide what is necessary and in what depth. Neurologic assessment of the newborn usually includes evaluation of cranial nerves, peripheral motor activity, general body tone, the quality of the cry, the level of alertness, the newborn reflexes, and occasionally some of the deep tendon reflexes (Table 18-1). The neurologic exam is often done concurrently with the rest of the physical exam. Movement of the facial muscles and movement and tone of the arms, legs, and trunk should be noted while handling the infant, with special attention to lack of movement of the arms and hands as a possible indicator of an Erb's palsy. When the mouth and palate are checked, the infant's gag reflex should be noted. Body tone is most easily evaluated with the infant held up off the mattress face-down, balanced over a hand on the chest. Held thus, the normal-term infant will generally hold the arms and legs flexed, and the head, although hanging down somewhat, will have some degree of extension. With the infant in this position, the spine can be examined for anomalies such as pilonidal sinus tracts and neural tube defects. Variations of the infant's cry can be assessed for strength and quality.

Most so-called "newborn reflexes," such as the Moro reflex, decrease with repetition. The sucking and rooting reflexes can be

| Reflex | Newborn | 2 Months | 4 Months | 6 Months | 8 Months |
|---|---|---|---|---|---|
| Moro | Present/Complete | Fading/Partial | | Absent | |
| Stepping | Present | Fading | | Absent | |
| Placing | Present | Fading | | Absent | |
| Tonic neck | Present | Fading | | | |
| Rooting | Excellent | Fading | | Absent | |
| Sucking | Present | Fading (replaced by purposeful activity) | | | |
| Head control | Poor but present | Improving | | Good | |
| Palmar grasp | Excellent | Fading | | Absent | |
| Plantar grasp | Excellent | Fading | | Absent | |
| Triceps | Present | | | | |
| Patellar | Present | | | | |

TABLE 18-1.  Common Reflexes of Newborns and Infants

assessed with a pacifier or a well-scrubbed finger. Lightly touching the upper lip laterally elicits the *rooting response*, with the mouth opening and the head turning toward the touch. The *Moro response* to being startled is characterized by extension of the arms with fingers extended, flexion of the thighs, grasping of the toes, and a strong cry, followed by folding of the arms and relaxation of the hands (Fig 18-3). The Moro reflex can be elicited by dropping the end of the crib 10° to 20° or by pulling the infant by the arms slightly off the bed, followed by a sudden release. The stepping and placing responses may be difficult to elicit. The *stepping reflex* is elicited by placing and pushing the infant's feet against the mattress and then leaning the infant far forward to flex the feet up toward the tibiae. With gentle rocking from side to side, the infant may take a few clumsy steps forward. (This is possibly a fetal reflex that may assist the fetus to the vertex position before delivery and may still be functioning in the early newborn period.) The *placing response* is brought out by holding the top of the infant's feet against the edge of the crib or a similar object. The infant will then lift that leg and place the foot on the object. Normal reflexes are indicators more of peripheral than central neurologic integrity at birth, and so cannot exclude occasional severe central nervous system pathology.

## Measurements and Gestational Dating

All infants should be weighed carefully on standardized scales. Length and head circumference should be measured accurately. The normal range for head circumference is between 33 and 38 cm. Body length is measured on a measuring trough or board and should be reproducible to within 1 cm. Measurement done with a tape while the infant lies in the crib is usually highly inaccurate. Accurate measurements are important for gestational age assessment, using standard grids.

Although parents are waiting to hear that their newborn has passed his or her first physical and therefore is "normal," in my opinion we should not put out such a verbal message. Rather, the verbal message should be, "I've just examined your baby and I didn't find anything wrong." Usually, but not always, these two messages are synonymous, but the latter message is the truth. We do a disservice to all of medicine when we posture unfairly (and occasionally untruthfully). We are constantly learning more, but there is so much to learn!

## Normal Variations

It is important for the examiner to decide whether particular variations of physical findings are within the normal range. For instance, most infants void within 24 hours and pass their first

meconium stool by 48 hours, yet the great majority of term infants have both urinated and passed meconium by 12 hours or earlier. Concern about cardiac findings, especially murmurs, is common. A first-day murmur associated with a heart rate of less than 160 at rest and an exam not associated with hyperdynamic activity, respiratory symptoms, or cyanosis may not require further workup. Murmurs lasting more than a day, however, especially when accompanied by other clinical symptoms, need further evaluation, including chest x-ray and ECG evaluation. Acrocyanosis must be differentiated from general cyanosis. If the infant's tongue is pink, then general cyanosis is not present.

Respiratory variations include transient tachypnea (a rate over 60) or periodic breathing. If the tachypnea changes minute by minute and there are intervals of minutes when the rate is below 60/minute, that is a good prognostic sign. Periodic breathing, accompanied by periods of hypoventilation, should be of no concern as long as no color change accompanies the finding. Persistent expiratory grunting, especially if the infant is not cold, requires additional evaluation. Cyanosis accompanying hard crying only is not uncommon.

CNS variations are common. For excessive irritability, the examiner must exclude problems such as previous hypoxia or trauma, hypoglycemia, drug withdrawal, or infection. If an irritable infant is easily soothed by a pacifier or by holding, the process is more likely benign. Infants may appear to be somnolent or stuporous after a long, hard labor. This behavior may wax and wane, with the infant "shutting down" for a brief period, but should generally resolve after an hour or two. A lack of motion or a decrease in motion of an arm or leg suggests nerve injury. Seizures are often difficult to diagnose and may be confused with the posturing and brief apnea some infants exhibit secondary to mucus or formula in the airway, but seizure activity usually involves the eyelids or hands and is usually clonic in nature. Also, when picked up, the infant with a seizure will usually continue such behavior. An infant's cry can be high and piercing, as might be seen with CNS involvement, or hoarse, as might be seen with vocal cord paralysis or hypothyroid, and yet be perfectly normal.

## BREAST-FEEDING AND FORMULAS

Breast-feeding of newborns has had a resurgence in the United States, and in many hospitals at least 75% of mothers breast-feed. Feeding schedules should ideally be adjusted to the infant's demand. This is more easily accomplished when infants room-in with the mother, so this should be encouraged whenever feasible. Breast-feeding should begin within the first hour after birth, even in the delivery or birthing room. During the first hour, the

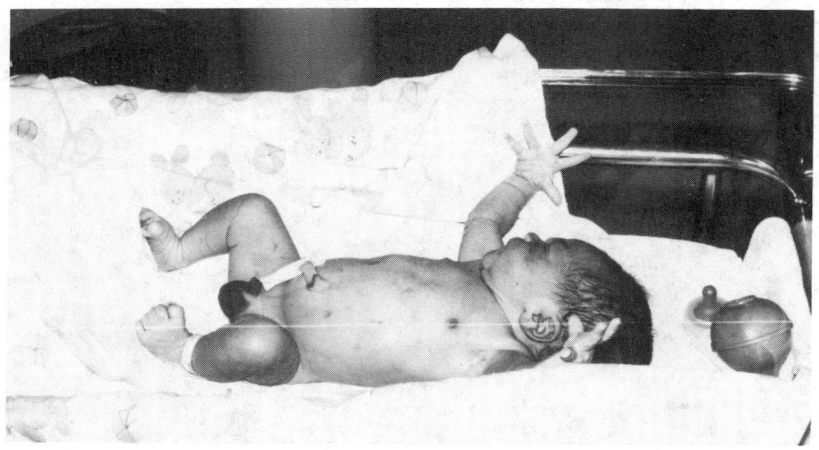

Figure 18-3.   The Moro reflex.

baby is often alert, awake, and anxious to suck. Infants less than 2 to 3 days old should be fed at least every 2 to 3 hours during the day and evening, and more frequently if awake and hungry. Newborns may awake frequently for a number of feeds before spacing out their next feeding to 2 to 3 hours. Within several days, they often can be so satiated by frequent day and evening feedings that they will begin to space their feedings as long as 5 to 6 hours apart at night. As the mother's milk supply builds up by day 3 or 4, more milk is taken per feeding, which lengthens the time between feedings. On the first day, the infant should nurse for only 5 to 10 minutes on a side, increasing to 15 to 20 minutes over the first 3 to 4 days and as the mother's nipples toughen. By a week of age, most breast-fed infants are on a fairly definite schedule of six to eight feedings per day.

Breast-feeding women need support and instruction by trained personnel. Women who have had cesarean deliveries may take an extra day or two to establish their milk supply. Breast-feeding and formulas are discussed in more detail in Chapter 24.1.

## MATERNAL-INFANT INTERACTION

Klaus and Kennell (see Selected Readings) argue strongly that mothers should hold their babies (and nurse if they plan to breast-feed) for much of the first hour after birth, because findings in their original and subsequent studies indicated that such mothers had a stronger attachment to and interest in their infants, observable for months later. Recent data suggest that the mother's voice (especially a repetitive sequence) becomes recognized by the fetus, who can identify it postnatally. A new mother should be especially encouraged to have her infant in the postpartum room with her most of the time, which allows her to feed the infant on demand. Rooming-in provides new mothers with an increased opportunity to interact with their infants and to anticipate questions about child care. The professional staff (especially the nurses) should be available 24 hours a day to answer questions about care, bathing, and breast-feeding while the mother is still in the hospital postpartum. Cesarean section or interventions such as phototherapy can interrupt mother-infant interactions. Rooming-in phototherapy can be used if necessary, permitting a nursing mother to nurse on demand more easily. It is useful for new mothers to meet as a group with a supervising nurse or other health professional to discuss common concerns.

## COMMON NEWBORN PROBLEMS

Many women these days have delayed having children until their late 20s or longer, and so have prolonged their anticipation as well as possibly heightened their expectations for a "perfect child." Conversely, mid-teenage pregnancies now make up 5% to 10% of all births, and these young mothers need to finish school as well as make the transition to adulthood and motherhood. Developing appropriate groupings of new mothers is an excellent educational technique. These groups can meet in the doctor's office at appropriate off-hour times or even in the home of one of the participants. Having the ongoing physician or nurse participating some or all of the time is helpful.

Excessive crying is one of the most common and exceedingly frustrating problems in the first 3 months of life, and can become the bane of the parents and often of their doctor. Hunger or illness must be eliminated as the cause of excessive crying, so appropriate signs and symptoms of illness or partial starvation must be elicited by history and examination. Pacifiers, formerly not recommended for fear they would never be discarded and also might misalign permanent teeth, are now widely accepted, and may offer relief. Thumb-sucking generates the same value

judgments; the thumb is always available but has the disadvantage of not being discardable. Generally, if the parents have no strong objection to either and feel that they will not be upset if the habit persists up to age 3 or 5 years, it is probably a very worthwhile approach. For persistent crying, mothers can also be told that picking their babies up and holding and rocking them will usually quiet them down. However, most infants enjoy this bodily contact and motion, and it soon becomes a fixed habit. The primary caregiver (usually the mother) should decide how much to let the baby cry, and those helping her should abide by her rules, thus helping to maintain consistency of care. Although crying is frustrating and worrisome, there is no evidence that it is physically or even psychologically harmful (at least to the baby!). Some professionals recommend letting the baby cry (especially at night) for up to an hour at a stretch, hoping that the infant will fall back asleep and soon learn to sleep through that feeding. If feasible, taking a crying infant for a car ride is often amazingly successful. It also permits the other parent or caretaker who is staying at home to get a rest.

Demand and scheduled feedings both have proponents. Certainly, for the mother planning on breast-feeding her infant, a demand schedule for at least the first 3 to 5 days is almost universally accepted and much more successful. Feeding on demand, the infant, when hungry and willing to suck the hardest yet not exhausted from crying, is put to the breast at the most appropriate time. After the first few days, many recommend a schedule of sorts, but this is almost always more easily carried out when bottle-feeding. Few people would dispute that a baby's parents are happier when the infant sleeps longer at night (and the longer the better, up to a point!). Instructing a parent to wake the infant during days and evenings as frequently as the infant woke the parent the previous night will soon swing the infant's longest sleep around to the night hours. Unfortunately, while it is possible to make the longest sleep occur during the night, that sleep will not necessarily last for 6 to 8 hours.

Jaundice (see Chap. 20.5), with its potential hyperbilirubinemia, is more of a concern at present because mothers are being discharged from the hospital so soon that the peak bilirubin level often occurs after discharge. Mothers should be alerted to this possibility, especially if they are breast-feeding.

Circumcision of newborn males continues, although recently there has been a slight decrease in the use of the procedure. In most instances, it is done for religious or cultural reasons. Although one or two recent reports have argued that there is less "urinary infection" found in circumcised males, variation in the method of documentation—clean-catch versus bladder taps—makes the evidence less conclusive. After circumcision, lathering the exposed raw glans with petroleum jelly at each diaper change for the next 3 days is all that is necessary. Superficial bleeding and minimal surface infection are normal.

Umbilical-cord care ranges from careful application of an antibiotic ointment 2 or 3 times per day, through alcohol wipes once a day, to no care at all other than observation until the cord falls off. All evidence seems to indicate that the more aseptic the care, the longer the cord hangs on, so some superficial colonization may speed the process. Certainly, quick bathing of that abdominal area even daily seems a benign process. The concern for doctor and parents is the development of an omphalitis, which appears as reddened, thickened periumbilical skin, sometimes (ominously) accompanied by a palpable thickened falciform ligament.

Sibling rivalry, particularly on the part of the next youngest sibling, is probably a universal phenomenon, whether overt or covert. Its clinical presentation can vary from overt hostility to compensated expressions of love and affection, or even to internalized changes such as a return of bed-wetting, thumb-sucking, or increased dependency. Parents should be informed of its myriad manifestations and counseled to be as consistent as possible in their planned response. Letting the older sibling participate as much as is reasonable in the care of the new infant seems to lessen his or her feelings of abandonment and neglect.

Exposing a newborn to other adults and especially to siblings with possible contagious diseases is a common concern. Although most newborns seem less prone to viral illnesses (probably because of passive immunity from their mother) than do older infants or young children, it is wise to minimize such exposure. If a mother is sure that she has had chicken pox, her infant is probably as protected as she is. Whether a newborn with that background should be allowed to stay at home with an infected sibling is controversial, but not prohibited by all. With no such maternal history, exposure should not be allowed until the older sibling has had the illness for at least 1 week.

The conflict and guilt that many mothers feel when they work outside the home have always been present, but now they are becoming problems for most mothers because more and more women work. Many women have no apparent guilt at all, and they seem to handle the double role best. When it is a matter of absolute economic necessity, mothers seem less ambivalent about their absence from home. Whatever the circumstances, the possible ambivalence should be addressed openly, at least as a question.

## Selected Readings

Anderson GH. Human milk feeding. Pediatr Clin North Am 1985;32:335.
DeCasper AJ, Spence MJ. Prenatal maternal speech influences newborns' perceptions of speech sounds. Infant Behav Dev 1986;9:133.
Klaus MH, Kennell JH. Maternal-infant bonding. St Louis: CV Mosby, 1976.
Wiswell TE, Roscelli JD. Corroborative evidence for the decreased incidence of urinary tract infections in circumcised male infants. Pediatrics 1986;78:96.

*Principles and Practice of Pediatrics, Second Edition.*
edited by Frank A. Oski et al. J. B. Lippincott Company, Philadelphia © 1994.

# CHAPTER 19
# Newborn Intensive Care

## 19.1 The Newborn Intensive Care Unit

Richard A. Ehrenkranz

## OVERVIEW

Newborn intensive care developed from the concept that a more intensive approach to neonates who require special care (both preterm infants and full-term infants with medical or surgical problems) would result in a significant decrease in neonatal morbidity and mortality. The first newborn special care unit was established at Yale-New Haven Hospital (YNHH) in 1960, and the subspecialty of neonatology evolved during the following years. Remarkable advances have been made in the care of neonates, and over 750 newborn special care units or newborn intensive care units (NICUs) have been built; each provides essentially everything necessary for the life support of a preterm or sick neonate. Many of the advances in neonatal care have been based on research in developmental physiology, biochemistry, pharmacology, and nutrition, which has increased manyfold the understanding of the uniqueness of neonates, particularly of the very-low-birth-weight infant. In addition, advances in medical technology have led to the development and neonatal application of life-support systems, monitors, equipment, and techniques such as ultrasound, CT, and MRI.

Today in many university and large community hospitals, newborn intensive care is just one component of a perinatal center. Such a center also includes facilities for prenatal evaluation, observation, and care of the fetus and mother both before and during labor; facilities for observation of neonates at risk of difficulties during their adaptation to the extrauterine environment; and facilities for continuing and rehabilitative care of growing preterm infants and of infants recovering from acute problems. In some perinatal centers, observation of high-risk neonates is done within the NICU, in others within a transitional nursery. In addition, the perinatal center has become a regional resource, accepting transfers of women in premature labor, with toxemia, or with other risk factors that indicate the probable need of maternal or neonatal special care or observation; and accepting transfers of neonates who are preterm or have other medical or surgical problems.

Finally, a NICU may exist in a hospital without an obstetric service (eg, a free-standing children's hospital) and will then provide care for only transferred neonates.

## Characteristics of NICU Patients

A large percentage of neonates admitted to NICUs are preterm infants. However, any infant who requires or may require the special attention available within a NICU is an appropriate admission. Since many neonatal problems can be anticipated before delivery, communication between the obstetric and pediatric members of the perinatal center (the perinatologists and the neonatologists respectively) is essential to optimize management plans.

Factors associated with high-risk pregnancies and infants are listed in Tables 19-1 and 19-2. High-risk pregnancy is associated with social and lifestyle characteristics of the pregnant woman, such as her socioeconomic status, and with her previous obstetric and medical history, such as a history of premature labor or delivery with a prior pregnancy or diabetes mellitus. Some of these factors have been shown to adversely affect maternal well-being with increasing gestation, and necessitate a premature delivery for maternal indications. Other factors develop during the pregnancy or are recognized during the process of labor and delivery, such as oligohydramnios, polyhydramnios, preeclampsia/eclampsia, or meconium staining of the amniotic fluid. Finally, unexpected medical or surgical problems will be recognized in the immediate neonatal period. Since these risk factors and problems correlate with an increased incidence of fetal and neonatal problems and account for a substantial percentage of perinatal mortality and morbidity, most of these high-risk infants are admitted to a NICU for observation, diagnosis, and management.

Table 19-3 correlates neonatal patient types with the level of perinatal services to be provided by a hospital. Such categorization has been useful in the development and organization of regional perinatal services. The staff at hospitals that provide only level I neonatal care would be expected to primarily manage uncom-

## TABLE 19-1. Factors Associated With High-Risk Pregnancies and Infants: Social and Historical

**Maternal Social and Lifestyle Characteristics**

Age <16, >40 years
Alcohol or substance abuse
Lower socioeconomic status
Noncompliance with health-care system(s)
Obesity
Poor diet
Poor physical fitness
Single parent
Smoking

**Obstetric History**

Infertility
Multiparity, especially grand multiparity (more than six pregnancies lasting beyond 20 weeks)
Rh or other blood group sensitization
Previous pregnancies with:
    Abnormal presentation
    Antepartum bleeding after first trimester
    Cephalopelvic disproportion
    Cesarean section delivery or instrumented delivery other than elective low forceps
    Gestational diabetes mellitus
    Poor pregnancy outcome, including multiple spontaneous abortions, fetal or neonatal death
    Postterm delivery
Preeclampsia/eclampsia
Premature labor or delivery
Premature rupture of fetal membranes
Prolonged labor
Previous infant with congenital malformation, genetic disorder, mental retardation, cerebral palsy
Primary or recurrent genital herpes simplex infection

**Medical History**

Anemia, nutritional (eg, iron, folate, or vitamin $B_{12}$ deficiency) or hemoglobinopathy
Cardiovascular disease, congenital or acquired
Collagen vascular disease
Diabetes mellitus, insulin-dependent or diet-controlled
Epilepsy
Hereditary disorders
Hypertension
Hyperthyroidism
Hyper- and hypoparathyroidism
Idiopathic thrombocytopenic purpura
Myasthenia gravis
Neoplasia
Pulmonary disorders, especially if associated with frequent episodes of hypoxemia or hypercapnia
Renal disease
Other chronic diseases or disorders requiring continued pharmacologic therapy

## TABLE 19-2. Factors Associated With High-Risk Pregnancies and Infants: Current Pregnancy, Labor and Delivery, Neonatal

**Current Pregnancy**

Abnormal biophysical profile
Abnormal fetal growth, intrauterine growth retardation or macrosomia
Age <16, >40 years
Alcohol or substance abuse
Decreased fetal movement
Exacerbation of preexisting medical disorder
Fetal arrhythmia or spontaneous decelerations
Infection, bacterial (gonorrhea, syphilis, tuberculosis), viral (rubella, cytomegalovirus, varicella zoster), parasitic (toxoplasmosis)
Intrauterine diagnosis or suspicion of anomaly or genetic disorder
Multiple gestation
Oligohydramnios
Polyhydramnios
Rh or other blood group sensitization
Smoking
Surgery and anesthesia
Vaginal bleeding from abruptio placentae or placenta previa
Vaginal colonization with chlamydia or Group B $\beta$-hemolytic streptococci

**Labor and Delivery**

Abnormal presentation
Acute blood loss at delivery
Amnionitis
Cesarean section delivery (especially if not elective repeat)
Fetal heart-rate abnormalities
Fetal pulmonic immaturity
Fetal scalp pH <7.2
Instrumented delivery other than elective low forceps
Meconium staining of amniotic fluid
Preeclampsia/eclampsia
Premature or prolonged rupture of the fetal membranes
Premature labor
Prolapsed umbilical cord
Prolonged labor

**Neonatal**

Apgar score at 5 minutes <3, or lack of spontaneous respiratory activity for longer than 5 minutes
Birth weight <2500 g (especially <1500 g) or >4000 g
Birth weight-gestational age discrepancy (SGA, LGA)
Hemodynamic instability
Major congenital malformations, such as abdominal wall defects, cardiac defects, CNS defects, diaphragmatic hernia, tracheoesophageal fistula with esophageal atreasia
Metabolic instability such as hypoglycemia, hypocalcemia
Nonimmune hydrops fetalis
Postterm birth, gestational age >42 wks
Preterm birth, gestational age <37 wks
Respiratory distress
Temperature instability

plicated deliveries, normal newborns, and larger, healthy preterm infants. However, they must be able to identify high-risk maternal, fetal, and neonatal conditions, to stabilize the patient until transfer to a level II or III center, and to successfully perform delivery room resuscitation. The staff at level II hospitals would be expected to provide level I services as well as the management of selected high-risk pregnancies and neonatal problems. Hos-

pitals with level III centers are usually perinatal centers that provide all types of obstetric and neonatal care. Many level III facilities are located at university medical centers and can therefore also provide the full range of medical, pediatric, and surgical subspecialty consultative services that level III obstetric and neo-

TABLE 19-3.   Neonatal Patient Types and Level
of Perinatal Services

**Level I**

Immediate resuscitation of depressed neonates

Management of high-risk infant until transfer to level II or III center

Nursery care of large premature neonates (>2000 g) without risk factors

Management of physiologic jaundice

Normal newborn care

**Level II**

Level I, plus management of selected neonatal problems, including:

Prematurity at ≥32 wks

Mild to moderate respiratory distress syndrome

Suspected neonatal sepsis

Hypoglycemia

Infants of diabetic mothers

Hypoxia/ischemia without life-threatening sequelae

**Level III**

Levels I and II, plus management of all neonatal problems, including:

Prematurity at <32 wks or with very low birth weight (<1500 g)

Severe respiratory distress syndrome

Persistent pulmonary hypertension

Sepsis

Severe postasphyxia sequelae

Major congenital malformations

Complex problems requiring subspecialty consultation

*Adapted from American Academy of Pediatrics, American College of Obstetrics and Gynecology. Guidelines for perinatal care, 1992, p. 236.*

natal patients might require. However, while the staff in some large community hospitals will provide most types of level III nursery care, infants who need cardiac catheterization or surgical subspecialty management must be transferred to centers that offer those services.

Newborn nursery services at YNHH are currently divided between the normal newborn nursery and the Newborn Special Care Unit (NBSCU), which includes a 20-bed intensive care nursery and a 24-bed continuing care nursery. Medical staff assigned to the NBSCU are called to be present at the delivery of

any infant believed to be at risk of developing neonatal problems due to the presence of factors associated with high-risk pregnancies (see Tables 19-1 and 19-2). Many of these infants, as well as other infants in whom high-risk clinical findings (see Table 19-2) are observed postnatally, are admitted to the NBSCU for observation, diagnosis, or management. Most of these infants are transferred to the normal nursery within 12 hours of birth or admission and are considered short-term admissions.

As shown in Table 19-4, between 1987 and 1991 about 50% of all NBSCU admissions (that is, about 15% of the live births at YNHH) were observed for periods up to 12 hours after delivery. Neonatal transfers represented about 8.5% of all NBSCU admissions. About 12% of YNHH deliveries accounted for the other NBSCU admissions, considered long-term admissions. Table 19-5 displays the birth weights of these infants between 1987 and 1991. About 57% of them had birth weights less than 2500 g, while about 22% had birth weights less than 1500 g and about 12% had birth weights less than 1000 g.

Survival of very-low-birth-weight infants has improved steadily. Figure 19-1 graphs survival data for infants born at YNHH in 1971, 1977, 1982, 1986, and 1991 with birth weights between 501 and 750 g, 751 and 1000 g, and 1001 and 1500 g. Although the percent survival increased within each birth weight group during these years, the greatest improvement is noted for infants born with birth weights 501 to 750 g. For infants with birth weights 501 to 1000 g, survival increased more than eightfold, from 8.0% in 1971 to 68.3% in 1991. Although the number of infants cared for at YNHH each year with birth weights between 500 and 750 g is small, the increased survival observed between 1986 and 1991 is most likely related to continued refinement in the management of extremely-low-birth-weight infants and possibly to the widespread use of surfactant replacement therapy during 1991. This observation is consistent with other reports of increased survival when the outcomes of infants managed before and after the introduction of surfactant replacement therapy are compared. Surfactant replacement therapy is discussed in Chapter 20.2.4.

Survival data for a 12-month period from eight centers participating in the National Institute of Child Health and Human Development Neonatal Intensive Care Network are presented in Table 19-6. This table also displays the intercenter differences in birth weight adjusted survival. This variation is most evident in the two lowest birth weight groups. Differences in the philosophy of care and management policies appeared to account for much of the intercenter variability in survival, and suggests that "the practice of neonatal medicine remains in part an art rather than an exact science" (Hack, 1991).

Surviving preterm infants with birth weights less than 1000 g

TABLE 19-4.   Admissions to the Newborn Special Care Unit, Yale-New Haven Hospital, 1987–1991

| | 1987 | 1988 | 1989 | 1990 | 1991 |
|---|---|---|---|---|---|
| Live births | 5551 | 5444 | 5544 | 5419 | 4938 |
| Total NBSCU admissions | 1584 | 1626 | 1595 | 1543 | 1614 |
| Short-term admissions | 738 | 818 | 769 | 759 | 842 |
| % NBSCU admissions | 46.6 | 50.3 | 48.2 | 49.2 | 52.2 |
| % YNHH live births | 13.3 | 15.0 | 13.9 | 14.0 | 17.0 |
| Neonatal transfer admissions | 111 | 144 | 134 | 154 | 132 |
| % NBSCU admissions | 7.0 | 8.9 | 8.4 | 10.0 | 8.2 |
| Long-term admissions, inborn | 707 | 638 | 684 | 616 | 619 |
| % NBSCU admissions | 44.6 | 39.2 | 42.9 | 39.9 | 38.4 |
| % YNHH live births | 12.7 | 11.7 | 12.3 | 11.4 | 12.5 |

| Birth Weight | 1987 | 1988 | 1989 | 1990 | 1991 | Total | (%)† |
|---|---|---|---|---|---|---|---|
| <600 g | 24 | 23 | 26 | 22 | 21 | 116 | (3.6) |
| 601–999 g | 49 | 52 | 50 | 65 | 54 | 270 | (8.3) |
| 1000-1499 g | 53 | 67 | 73 | 67 | 70 | 330 | (10.1) |
| 1500–1999 g | 117 | 132 | 136 | 103 | 103 | 591 | (18.1) |
| 2000–2499 g | 136 | 116 | 108 | 89 | 94 | 543 | (16.6) |
| ≥2500 g | 328 | 248 | 291 | 270 | 277 | 1414 | (43.3) |
| **Total** | 707 | 638 | 684 | 616 | 619 | 3264 | (100.0) |

TABLE 19-5. Admissions* by Birth Weight, Newborn Special Care Unit, Yale-New Haven Hospital, 1987–1991

\* Long-term admissions, live births
† % of long-term admissions.

remain patients within NICUs or intermediate care units for an average of 2 to 4 months. The length of hospitalization tends to be inversely related to birth weight and may be prolonged if complications develop. Therefore, while they may account for a minority of the admissions to a NICU, the majority of infants found on any day within an intensive care nursery may be very-low-birth-weight (VLBW, birth weight 1500 g or less) infants at various points in their hospitalization.

## NICU Staff

The size and composition of the medical staff varies according to the size of the NICU; the level of perinatal and neonatal services offered at the hospital (see Table 19-3); whether the NICU is part of a university medical center, a large community hospital, or a moderate-size community hospital; and the role that the NICU plays within the regional perinatal system. Most NICUs are directed by full-time physicians who are board-certified pediatricians with subspecialty training and usually certification in perinatal-neonatal medicine. NICUs at university medical centers and larger community hospitals usually have several additional full-time certified neonatologists sharing attending physician responsibilities, and provide 24-hour in-hospital coverage, usually with resident staff. At smaller community hospitals, a group of

community physicians, neonatal nurse practitioners, or physician assistants may assist one or two full-time neonatologists in managing NICU patients.

The size of the NICU nursing staff, particularly the number of nurses assigned per shift, is also a function of the size of the NICU, the level of neonatal care provided, and the case mix. Since large units require large nursing staffs, effective nursing management is essential. Most NICUs employ only registered nurses. Nurse-to-patient ratios of 1:1 for the sickest infants, 1:2 for intermediate care patients, and 1:4 for healthier infants who require little extra care have often been used to determine the number of nurses needed per shift. However, patient classification scoring systems that more accurately reflect the actual number of nursing care hours needed by the patients each shift have become more common.

For example, a neonate with persistent pulmonary hypertension who needs infusions of multiple vasoactive agents or one who has just returned from the operating room following repair of a diaphragmatic hernia would be classified at the highest level. Such an infant would require continual monitoring and assessment of vital signs, ventilatory parameters, and the response to infused medications. Infants classified at the lowest level would be stable and would require routine monitoring and assessment, and would include growing preterm infants who tolerate their

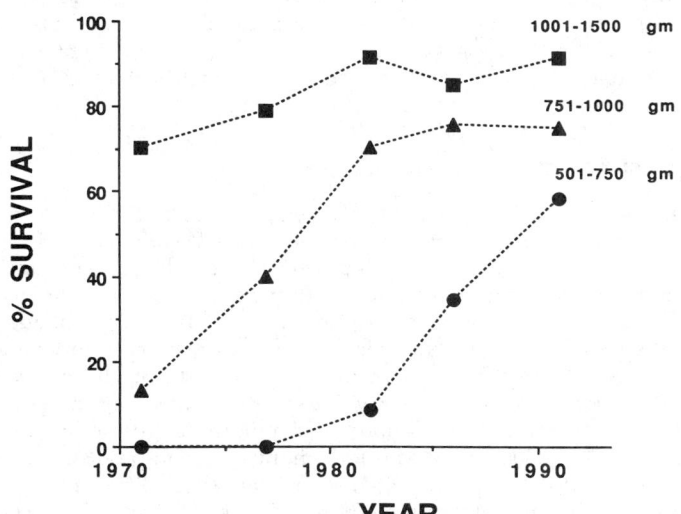

Figure 19-1. The percentage of survival for very-low-birth-weight preterm infants born at Yale-New Haven Hospital in 1971, 1977, 1982, 1986, and 1991.

| Birth Weight | Survivors/Total (%)† | Intercenter Range (%) |
|---|---|---|
| 501–750 g | 118/349 (33.8) | 20–55 |
| 751–1000 g | 252/382 (66.0) | 42–75 |
| 1001–1250 g | 419/480 (87.3) | 84–91 |
| 1251–1500 g | 514/554 (92.8) | 89–98 |
| **Totals** | 1303/1765 (73.8) | 69–77 |

TABLE 19-6. Survival Statistics, National Institute of Health and Human Development Neonatal Intensive Care Network*

\* University of Alabama at Birmingham, University of Vermont Medical Center, Case Western Reserve University, University of Texas Southwestern Medical Center at Dallas, Wayne State University School of Medicine, Dartmouth Hitchcock Medical Center, University of Tennessee at Memphis, University of Miami Jackson Memorial Medical Center
† Inborn survivors/live births (%) between 11/1/87 and 10/31/88
*Adapted from Hack M, Horbar JD, Malloy MH, Tyson JE, Wright E, Wright L. Very-low-birth-weight outcomes of the National Institute of Child Health and Human Development Neonatal Network. Pediatrics 1991;87:587.*

feedings but require monitoring for apnea and bradycardia, infants being treated for neonatal narcotic abstinence syndrome, infants receiving long-term central hyperalimentation, and infants completing a course of antibiotics. Intermediate classifications would apply to infants who require close monitoring and assessment and regular treatments and medications, including infants with resolving respiratory distress syndrome or ventilator-dependent bronchopulmonary dysplasia. The patient classification score is updated several times per day to account for changes in individual patient needs and patient census, and so that staffing needs can be anticipated and met. In addition, these systems also permit NICU nursing staffs to assess their ability to care for additional patients, and therefore often dictate the response to a request for transfer.

Expanded nursing roles are common in the NICU. Neonatal nurse transport teams have been trained at many centers. Using a packet of management protocols, they have assumed the responsibility of performing most neonatal transfers. To ensure ongoing ability to perform skills often needed on transport, education days on which the transport nurses perform all elective endotracheal intubations, umbilical vessel catheterization, and needle aspiration of pneumothoraces must be scheduled regularly. NICU nurses routinely perform most blood-drawing, obtain arterial blood gases via percutaneous radial artery sampling, and place most intravenous lines.

In addition to medical and nursing staffs, respiratory therapists and social workers play essential roles in the NICU. Since respiratory distress is one of the most common medical problems of NICU patients, a respiratory therapist is often assigned to the NICU full time. The respiratory therapist ensures that all respiratory equipment is functioning, assists in giving chest physiotherapy, and assists in monitoring the response to various respiratory treatments, such as bronchodilator therapy in infants with bronchopulmonary dysplasia. The respiratory therapist may also perform pulmonary function tests on intubated NICU patients, obtaining data about the infant's need for continued ventilatory assistance or response to medical therapies.

Having an infant admitted to a NICU, even for short-term observation, produces stress and anxiety in the parents. For parents whose infants are very small or very sick or have multiple problems, such stress is often overwhelming. Social workers assigned to NICUs work with parents during this emotionally and psychologically draining time. They ensure that the parents understand the information being told them by the medical team so that they can play an active role in selecting management options. If necessary, the social worker helps the parents to begin the grieving process. Often the social worker continues to counsel parents long after an infant's discharge or death.

## Neonatal Transport

Although the best transport isolette is the uterus, maternal transfer of a woman who develops a risk factor during labor (see Table 19-2) is not always possible. In addition, since many neonatal problems (see Table 19-2) are not predicted before delivery, regional neonatal transport systems have been developed. Maternal and neonatal transfers should be performed as soon as possible after a potential problem appears likely. For example, a woman who presents with premature labor should be transported to a hospital with a NICU before the cervix has dilated too much and transport becomes too risky. Also, infants with persistent respiratory distress should be transported within hours of birth, in anticipation that they might require long-term mechanical ventilatory assistance. If the medical and nursing staffs at referring hospitals can identify and stabilize high-risk neonates quickly while awaiting the transfer team, the birth weight adjusted mortality rate of outborn infants will be similar to that of inborn infants.

Equipment facilitating neonatal transport mirrors equipment available within the NICU, permitting treatment to begin at the referring hospital and continue during the transfer. The transport unit currently used by the NBSCU at YNHH includes a portable mechanical ventilator; an oxygen blender; an oxygen analyzer; small air and oxygen tanks; a monitor with channels for heart rate, ECG pattern, respiratory rate and pattern, and continuous intravascular blood pressure; a portable pulse oximeter; and portable syringe pumps. The YNHH transport ambulance is equipped with oxygen, air, and vacuum. A separate electric generator provides power for the isolette and the monitors when the patient is en route to the NBSCU. Transport systems using helicopters and fixed-wing aircraft have also been established to facilitate transport over highly congested areas or coverage of large referral areas.

Transport back to the referring hospital once an infant no longer requires the special services available at the NICU is an essential component of a regional perinatal system. Back-transfer helps to ensure the availability and efficient use of NICU beds for the care of critically ill neonates. Therefore, parents should be informed about this policy during discussions following maternal and neonatal transfer. They should be told that back-transfer facilitates increased family involvement in the infant's care in preparation for discharge home, and that it allows the primary-care pediatrician to become directly aware of the infant's health needs.

## Parents

The parents of a neonate admitted to a NICU must be encouraged to visit their infant regularly. Unlimited visiting privileges for parents are the rule in most NICUs. Provisions are usually made for visiting by grandparents, siblings, other family members, and friends. The NICU staff should explain to the parents the reason for admission, the initial management plan, expected hospital course with the more common difficulties, and standard NICU routines. The NICU staff should be prepared to repeat and augment this information so that each infant's parents understand it. Before an infant's discharge home, especially after a prolonged hospitalization, parents should be encouraged to become actively involved in daily care, such as feeding, diaper-changing, and bathing. If the infant will continue to receive medications after discharge, the parents must also learn to measure the dose and administer it. Finally, although the medical staff must direct medical care, parental input and guidance should be sought and considered when medical care becomes extraordinary and possibly futile.

## Cost-Effectiveness of NICU Care

In the United States and other developed countries, the use of life-support interventions (for example, assisted ventilation during the 1970s and now surfactant replacement therapy) has markedly improved the chance of survival and the quality of outcome for VLBW infants. As shown in Figure 19-1 and Table 19-6, about 50% of infants with birth weights of 750 g or less now survive. However, these infants, especially those with birth weights below 600 g, are at high risk for significant morbidities during their initial neonatal hospitalization, for significant long-term neurodevelopmental sequelae, and for continued health problems requiring ongoing care and often rehospitalization. Since charges for the initial hospitalization often average more than $1000 per day, the smallest, sickest infants commonly incur initial hospital charges well above $100,000. In addition, many incur significant post-hospitalization costs. Therefore, the cost-effectiveness of NICU care for infants with birth weights below 750 g has been questioned.

Neonatal intensive care is costly not only to the individual family, but also to society. These costs increase with decreasing birth weight and gestational age. However, any attempt to limit neonatal intensive care to those very-low-birth-weight infants most likely to benefit raises important ethical questions. In addition, neonatologists are usually unable to determine at birth which extremely-low-birth-weight preterm infant will survive intact and which one will survive with significant health or neurodevelopmental problems. Thus, as survival rates have steadily improved, the absolute number of handicapped survivors has increased with the number of normal survivors. It is essential, therefore, that neonatologists include parents in any discussion about whether to continue the extreme measures being provided to their extremely-low-birth-weight preterm infants.

## DELIVERY ROOM RESUSCITATION

Birth is a transition from the intrauterine to the extrauterine environment. It encompasses a series of complex events through which every infant must pass in order to successfully achieve an independent existence. Such adaptation demands major physiological changes in several organ systems as well as a reorganization of overall metabolic processes. For example, in utero the human fetus is totally dependent on the mother for respiratory gas exchange, nutrient supply, waste product removal, and thermoregulation. After delivery, the neonate's lungs must replace the placenta as the site of respiratory gas exchange; stored glycogen and absorption of nutrients by the gastrointestinal tract provide for metabolic homeostasis and growth; the task of waste elimination is taken over by the gastrointestinal tract and kidneys, with the latter also responsible for the maintenance of water and electrolyte balance; and the neonate must be prepared to supply energy to maintain body temperature. In most newborn infants (about 85% to 90%), these changes proceed smoothly, and the infants require little or no assistance after delivery. However, a few will require help and close observation until they complete the process of transition successfully, and the occasional infant will fail completely to adapt.

Resuscitation of an infant in the delivery room provides the assistance that newborn needs as he or she begins the transition from intrauterine to extrauterine existence. The main goals of delivery room resuscitation are the establishment of respiratory activity with gas exchange and the conversion from the fetal to the neonatal circulation.

Although most neonates do not require much assistance in the delivery room, several conditions have been identified that

increase the risk of perinatal asphyxia, including many of the factors listed in Tables 19-1 and 19-2. Early recognition of these conditions by obstetricians, midwives, and other delivery room attendants is one of the most important steps in ensuring prompt neonatal resuscitation. Many of these conditions are known before delivery, and a pediatrician or other appropriate person experienced in newborn resuscitation should be available to evaluate and resuscitate the infant. However, since many intrapartum problems cannot be anticipated, appropriate equipment and drugs must be available, all delivery room attendants must understand the principles of neonatal resuscitation, and at least one must be skilled at resuscitating a neonate.

### Apgar Score

In 1953, Dr. Virginia Apgar proposed a method of evaluating the newborn infant in the delivery room based on five easily determined signs. This evaluation, known as the Apgar score (Table 19-7), gives a rating of 0, 1, or 2 to each sign. A score of 10 indicates that the infant is in the best possible condition, whereas a score of less than 3 implies moderate to severe asphyxia. Currently a score is assigned at 1 and 5 minutes. The 1-minute score is a guide to the infant's well-being. It indicates the degree of asphyxia and previously had been used to suggest appropriate resuscitative measures. Although the 5-minute score had been thought to correlate with neonatal morbidity, it more accurately indicates the response to resuscitative efforts. If the Apgar score at 5 minutes is still less than 7, additional scores every 5 minutes for a total of 20 minutes have been recommended to assess response and the appropriateness of continued resuscitative measures.

In practice, the infant's respiratory activity, heart rate, and color are the best indicators of the need for resuscitation, not the 1-minute Apgar score. Bradycardia in a newborn is most often related to inadequate respiratory activity. Therefore, attention should be directed to ensuring airway patency and then to assisting breathing. Since cardiac output depends primarily on the heart rate, restoring the heart rate will improve circulation, resulting in improved color. In addition, it is important to remember that color, tone, and reflex irritability are partially related to the infant's gestational age and physiological maturity. The more preterm an infant is, the more likely that the completely pink body and the diminished tone and minimal reflex irritability are a function of immaturity and not asphyxia.

Furthermore, while the Apgar score at 5 minutes may indicate an infant's response to resuscitative efforts, it makes no clear distinction between the infant whose heart rate is greater than 100 beats/minute (bpm) after vigorous stimulation, the infant whose heart rate is greater than 100 bpm after initiation of positive-pressure ventilation, and the infant whose heart rate is

| TABLE 19-7. Apgar Score | | | |
|---|---|---|---|
| Sign | 0 | 1 | 2 |
| Heart rate | Absent | Slow (<100 beats/min) | >100 beats/min |
| Respiratory effort | Absent | Irregular, weak cry | Regular, strong cry |
| Muscle tone | Flaccid | Some flexion of upper extremities | Well-flexed active motion |
| Reflex irritability | No response | Grimace | Cough or sneeze |
| Color | Central cyanosis | Peripheral cyanosis | Completely pink |

Adapted from Apgar V. A proposal for a new method of evaluation of the newborn infant. Curr Res Anesth Analg 1953;32:260.

**TABLE 19-8.** Delivery Room Resuscitation Score

| Score | Resuscitation Effort |
|---|---|
| 0 | No intervention |
| 1 | O₂, tactile stimulation |
| 2 | Endotracheal suctioning only |
| 3 | Bag and mask positive-pressure ventilation |
| 4 | Endotracheal intubation and positive-pressure ventilation |
| 5 | Endotracheal intubation, positive-pressure ventilation, chest compressions, with or without drugs |

greater than 100 bpm in response to external cardiac massage and epinephrine administration. Therefore, the resuscitation effort score (Table 19-8) has been found to be helpful; it clarifies the Apgar score by defining the resuscitative measures used.

## Resuscitation in the Delivery Room

Figure 19-2 is an algorithm of the delivery room management and assessment recommended by the American Academy of Pediatrics and the American Heart Association. This overview will be briefly discussed; it is based not on the Apgar score, but on evaluation of respiratory activity, heart rate, and color. Table 19-9 lists equipment and drugs that should be available for delivery room resuscitation.

As soon as the infant's head is delivered, the mouth, nose, and pharynx are gently suctioned with a bulb syringe, DeLee trap, or suction catheter connected to mechanical suction. After the rest of the infant is delivered and the umbilical cord is clamped and cut, the infant is transferred in a head-down position and placed under a radiant heater on a resuscitation table. Most infants begin to cry between the time the body is delivered and the cord is cut.

On the radiant warmer, the infant's head should be in a slightly dependent position (20° to 30° below the horizontal), to aid in the drainage of secretions and amniotic fluid from the pharynx. The neonate should be quickly and thoroughly dried and not left in contact with or covered by wet towels or blankets. This should minimize evaporative heat loss, while placement under a pre-heated radiant warmer should minimize radiant and convective heat loss. Then the infant is positioned on the back with the neck slightly extended; elevating the infant's shoulders about 2 cm off the mattress with a rolled blanket or towel may help to maintain this position. Once correctly positioned, the mouth and nose are gently suctioned with a bulb syringe or a suction catheter. The mouth is suctioned first, so that there is nothing for the infant to aspirate. Blind deep and/or vigorous nasopharyngeal suctioning with a suction catheter can be hazardous if performed within the first minutes of life, since it can result in laryngeal spasm and increased vagal tone with apnea and bradycardia. For this reason, unless there is meconium staining of the amniotic fluid, deep suctioning of the oropharynx should be delayed for several minutes until normal ventilation has been established. The delivery room management of infants delivered with meconium staining of the amniotic fluid will be discussed separately.

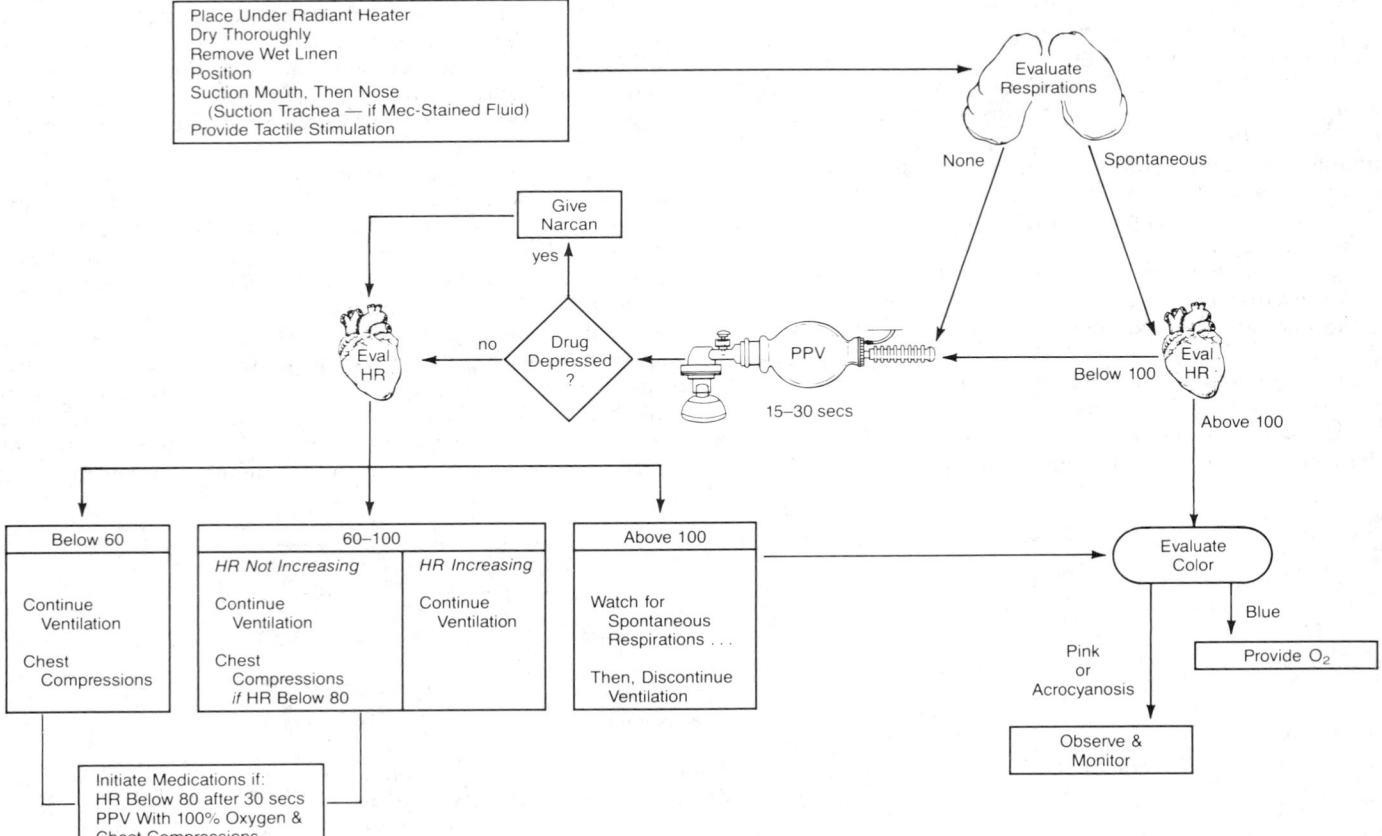

**Figure 19-2.** Overview of resuscitation in the delivery room. (Reproduced with permission from the American Academy of Pediatrics and the American Heart Association. Textbook of neonatal resuscitation. Elk Grove Village, IL: American Academy of Pediatrics, 1990.)

| TABLE 19-9. Equipment and Drugs Necessary for Delivery Room Resuscitation |
| --- |
| **Equipment** |
| Resuscitation table with radiant heat source |
| Oxygen with flow meter |
| Mechanical suction regulator |
| Ventilation bag with pressure manometer |
| Face masks with sizes for premature and term infants |
| Oral airways, sizes 0 and 00 |
| Endotracheal tubes and adaptors with stylets and without cuffs or shoulders (internal diameters of 2.5 mm, 3.0 mm, and 3.5 mm) |
| Laryngoscope with blade sizes for premature and term infants |
| Suction catheters, 6 Fr and 8 Fr, with thumb suction control |
| Meconium aspirators, with thumb suction control port |
| Bulb syringes |
| Syringes: 1 cc, 3 cc, 5 cc, 10 cc |
| Needles: 19- to 25-gauge, ⅝" to 1-½" long |
| Styletted small vein catheters, 16- to 24-gauge |
| Umbilical catheters: 3.5 Fr and 5 Fr vessel catheters; 5 Fr feeding tubes |
| Three-way stopcocks |
| Scissors |
| Adhesive tape |
| **Drugs and Fluids** |
| Albumin, 5% solution, 50-mL ampule |
| Atropine, 0.1 mg/mL preparation, 5-mL ampules |
| Epinephrine, 1:10,000 (0.1 mg/mL) preparation, 10-mL ampules |
| Naloxone, 1.0 mg/mL preparation, 2-mL ampules |
| Normal saline (or Ringer's lactate) |
| Sodium bicarbonate, 4.2% (0.5 mEq/mL) solution, 10-mL ampules |
| Sterile water, 10-mL ampules |

The neonate's respiratory activity is then evaluated. Both drying and suctioning provide stimulation that promote breathing. However, if respiratory activity is inadequate, additional tactile stimulation should be provided by flicking the heel or slapping the sole of the infant's foot or by rubbing the infant's back. The activities performed up to this point—drying the infant, suctioning the airway, and providing tactile stimulation—should be completed within 20 seconds.

If the infant has adequate spontaneous respiratory activity, then the heart rate is evaluated. Heart rate can be determined by auscultation or palpation of the umbilical cord or of the brachial artery. If the infant's heart rate is adequate (over 100 bpm), then color is evaluated. Free-flow oxygen should be given to the infant with central cyanosis who is breathing spontaneously and has a heart rate over 100 bpm. Free-flow oxygen is unnecessary for infants with only peripheral cyanosis (acrocyanosis). It is important to observe these infants and ensure that adaptation to extrauterine life is progressing satisfactorily.

If the infant is apneic or if the infant's respiratory effort is insufficient to maintain a heart rate over 100 bpm, positive-pressure bag and mask ventilation with oxygen should be initiated promptly. After a 15- to 30-second period of ventilation at a rate of 40 to 60 breaths/minute, the infant's heart rate should be evaluated. If the heart rate is over 100 bpm and if the infant displays spontaneous breathing activity, positive-pressure ventilation can be discontinued; free-flow oxygen should be provided until the infant remains pink. If the heart rate is between 60 and 100 bpm and increasing, positive-pressure bag and mask ventilation should be continued and the infant's heart rate should be reevaluated after another 30 seconds. If the heart rate is between

60 and 100 bpm and not increasing after the initial period of ventilation, positive-pressure ventilation should be continued and chest compressions should be initiated if the heart rate is less than 80 bpm. Also, positive-pressure ventilation should be continued and chest compressions should be initiated if the infant's heart rate is less than 60 bpm after the initial period of ventilation. Alternatively, if an individual skilled at endotracheal intubation is present in the delivery room, the infant can be intubated and the heart rate response to positive-pressure ventilation by bag and endotracheal tube can be used to determine the need for chest compressions.

Ventilation by bag and mask or by bag and endotracheal tube should be confirmed by movement of the chest and auscultatory evidence of equal, bilateral aeration. A ventilatory rate of 40 to 60 breaths/minute should be maintained. Chest compressions should be performed at a rate of 100 to 120 compressions/minute. Positive-pressure ventilation must always accompany chest compressions. Recommendations concerning the coordination of ventilation and chest compressions do not currently exist.

Chest compressions can be performed with either of two techniques. With one method, both thumbs are placed over the middle third of the sternum, and the other fingers encircle and support the back, while the sternum is compressed about 1 to 2 cm (Fig 19-3). The thumbs are positioned on the sternum just below the imaginary line drawn between the nipples; thumbs may have to be superimposed with VLBW infants. Alternatively, compressions could be administered with the ring and middle fingers of one hand placed on the sternum about one fingerbreadth below the nipple line; the other hand could be used to support the infant's back. The lower sternum should not be compressed, since abdominal organs might be injured.

If the heart rate improves and climbs above 80 bpm after about 30 seconds of chest compressions and ventilation, chest compressions can be discontinued. In most cases, positive-pres-

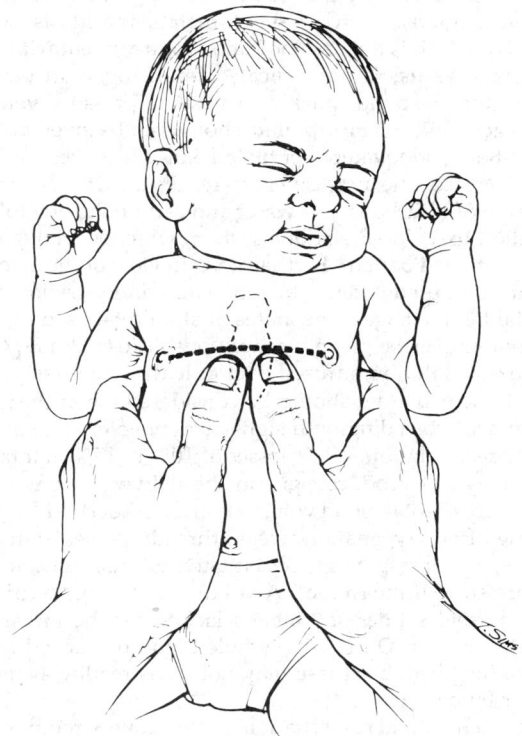

**Figure 19-3.** Side-by-side thumb placement for chest compressions in small neonates. (Standards and guidelines for cardiopulmonary resuscitation and emergency cardiac care. VI: Neonatal advanced life support. JAMA 1986;255:2969.)

sure ventilatory assistance should be continued until the infant has been transferred to the NICU, where blood pressure, perfusion, arterial blood gases, and acid–base status can be evaluated. If the infant's heart rate does not improve and remains less than 80 bpm after a 30- to 60-second period of adequate positive-pressure ventilation with oxygen and chest compressions, epinephrine should be given. Although epinephrine can be given intravenously, administration via the endotracheal tube is easier (dose: 0.1 to 0.3 mL/kg of a 1:10,000 solution, intravenously or endotracheally). Doses of epinephrine may be repeated every 5 minutes if required.

Recommendations for the use of other medications during delivery room resuscitation vary. Although there is little evidence to support the use of atropine and calcium during delivery room resuscitation, doctors at YNHH administer atropine (0.01 to 0.02 mg/kg/dose intravenously or via endotracheal tube) if there has been a minimal response to epinephrine. In addition to epinephrine, the neonatal resuscitation program developed jointly by the American Academy of Pediatrics and the American Heart Association recommends the use of naloxone hydrochloride (Narcan) to reverse respiratory depression associated with a history of maternal narcotic administration within the 4 hours immediately preceding delivery, sodium bicarbonate to restore acid–base balance, and volume expanders to improve tissue perfusion.

Infants who demonstrate respiratory depression secondary to maternal narcotic administration usually have adequate heart rates or respond readily to positive-pressure bag and mask ventilation. Naloxone, a competitive narcotic antagonist with a duration of action of 1 to 4 hours, can be administered (0.1 mg/kg/dose) intravenously, endotracheally, intramuscularly, or subcutaneously. Therefore, infants who are treated must be monitored closely for recurrent respiratory depression; repeated doses may be given. Administering naloxone to the infant of a narcotic-addicted mother may precipitate seizures.

Sodium bicarbonate should be given when a significant metabolic acidosis has been documented or is assumed to be present. Therefore, demonstration of a severe metabolic acidosis by arterial blood gas analysis is the best indication for treatment with sodium bicarbonate. Its use is not indicated following short periods of asphyxia that respond quickly to positive-pressure ventilation with oxygen. Sodium bicarbonate should not be given unless the infant is being adequately ventilated, since it causes the arterial $PCO_2$ to increase. The increased $PCO_2$ results from the spontaneous conversion of bicarbonate to water and carbon dioxide following its addition to a closed acidotic system, which is analogous to a poorly ventilated patient. Furthermore, in view of the association of rapid, undiluted sodium bicarbonate administration and intracranial hemorrhage in neonates, it should be used cautiously and should never be given by rapid push (dose: 2 mEq/kg of a 0.5 mEq/mL solution, infused over at least 2 minutes).

A volume expander should be considered when there is evidence of acute bleeding with signs of hypovolemia in an infant requiring resuscitation. While losses of 10% to 15% of total blood volume may not produce signs in the delivery room, a loss of 20% or more of total blood volume is often associated with pallor persisting after oxygenation, weak, thready pulses with a good heart rate, a poor response to resuscitative efforts, and a decreased blood pressure (if measured). A volume of 10 mL/kg of 5% albumin, normal saline, or Ringer's lactate can be infused over about 10 minutes; O-negative whole blood or packed red cells may also be given, but these may not be as readily available as the other fluids.

During a neonatal resuscitation in the delivery room, vascular access is most readily achieved by inserting a fluid-filled umbilical catheter (or feeding tube) into the umbilical vein. The tip of the catheter should lie just below the surface of the abdominal wall, at a location at which free flow of blood is present. Inserting the catheter farther into the umbilical vein might position the catheter tip within a branch of the portal vein; infusing resuscitative solutions into that vessel might result in liver damage. The catheter should be secured with a tape bridge. As described below, this catheter must be kept filled with fluid and closed to air at all times, because an air embolus might result if a large negative intrathoracic pressure were suddenly generated. Since emergency catheterization of the umbilical vein is usually not performed aseptically, the catheter should be removed after better vascular access has been established following transfer to the NICU. Consideration should also be given to the use of prophylactic antibiotic coverage. Umbilical vessel catheterization will be described later in this chapter.

In summary, delivery room resuscitation involves the same "ABCD" sequence used during any cardiopulmonary resuscitation: the airway is established, breathing is initiated, circulation is supported, and then if necessary drugs are given.

## Meconium Staining of the Amniotic Fluid

Meconium staining of the amniotic fluid occurs in 0.5% to 20% of all deliveries. Although the presence of meconium in the amniotic fluid may indicate fetal distress that might result in the birth of an asphyxiated or stillborn infant, there are numerous instances of fetal distress and asphyxia without meconium-stained amniotic fluid, and numerous instances of meconium staining without evidence of fetal distress. However, several studies have demonstrated increased rates of neonatal morbidity and mortality in association with meconium staining of the amniotic fluid, usually secondary to meconium aspiration pneumonia.

Since the development of meconium aspiration pneumonia requires the combination of meconium in the posterior pharynx and trachea and respiratory activity, the optimal management would be to remove any meconium from the trachea before the infant breathes, and thus prevent movement of meconium into the lower bronchial tree. Since several studies have demonstrated that this approach is effective in decreasing the incidence and severity of meconium aspiration pneumonia, management plans that have coordinated obstetric and pediatric efforts in the delivery room have been developed. First, the infant's mouth, pharynx, and nose are suctioned by the obstetrician with a suction catheter connected to mechanical suction as soon as the baby's head appears on the perineum, and before the delivery of the infant's shoulders and the onset of respirations. With a cesarean section, the infant is suctioned as soon as the head is delivered through the uterine incision and before the delivery of the thorax. Some obstetricians will also aspirate gastric contents before the delivery of the thorax. After delivery, additional suctioning or stimulation is not performed by the obstetrician. The infant is brought immediately to the resuscitation table, and additional suctioning of the airway is performed, if indicated, before the infant is dried.

The infant's respiratory status directs the pediatric management. Immediate tracheal suctioning is performed via an endotracheal tube connected to mechanical suction (maximum pressure of 120 mm Hg) if the infant does not cry and begin regular respiratory activity spontaneously, or cries and then demonstrates respiratory distress (for example, retractions or cyanosis). The duration of suction can be regulated via the thumb control port on the meconium aspirator. The endotracheal tube is slowly withdrawn as suction is applied. Suction catheters inserted through the tube may be inadequate to remove thick, tenacious meconium and therefore are not recommended. When possible, ventilatory stimulation or positive-pressure ventilation is not begun until meconium is no longer removed by tracheal suction. Although previous recommendations have suggested that suction could be applied to the endotracheal tube by mouth, current recommendations strongly encourage the use of mechanical suction so as to minimize the risk of exposure to potentially infectious body fluids. In addition, performing tracheobronchial lavage in the delivery room is not recommended and may increase morbidity.

However, the need for tracheal suctioning is controversial if the infant vigorously cries, spontaneously begins regular respiratory activity following delivery, and continues to show satisfactory adaptation to the extrauterine environment. Some clinicians argue that tracheal suctioning is unnecessary in these infants and have reported that such management has not increased the risk of meconium aspiration pneumonia. Other clinicians recommend that all infants delivered in the presence of meconium-stained amniotic fluid undergo tracheal suctioning under direct vision immediately after delivery. Still others suggest that the gastric contents be aspirated and evaluated first. Aspiration of the gastric contents is recommended in these infants because it demonstrates the consistency of the meconium-stained fluid present at the time of delivery, and because it alleviates the possibility that the infant might regurgitate and then aspirate meconium-stained gastric contents during direct laryngoscopy. As noted above, some obstetricians will have already aspirated gastric contents before the delivery of the thorax. If the amniotic fluid had been only thinly stained, and if the gastric contents are only thinly stained, then direct laryngoscopy and tracheal suctioning are not indicated. However, if they are thickly stained, then tracheal suctioning is performed at least once. Since meconium has been found in the trachea of some infants in the absence of meconium in the mouth or larynx during direct laryngoscopy, a decision to perform tracheal suctioning should not be solely based on the findings at direct laryngoscopy.

## Special Problems Interfering With Delivery Room Resuscitation

In addition to CNS damage or depression from intrauterine or intrapartum asphyxia, cervical spinal cord injury, and maternal analgesics and anesthetics, there are several other reasons why a neonate might experience difficulty in establishing and sustaining effective respiratory activity. Pediatricians and other delivery room personnel who manage delivery room resuscitation should always be alert to such possibilities.

VLBW preterm infants may lack the strength to maintain adequate respiratory effort and may require respiratory assistance in the delivery room to sustain gas exchange. Some of these infants may be further depressed by sepsis/pneumonia due to clinical amnionitis or by maternal therapies such as magnesium sulfate used to treat preeclampsia/eclampsia. Since the incidence of respiratory distress syndrome is substantial in infants at 30 weeks of gestation or younger, some clinicians prophylactically begin surfactant replacement therapy in the delivery room if the infants have been intubated.

As many as 3% of full-term infants develop a spontaneous pneumothorax or pneumomediastinum following a normal spontaneous vaginal delivery. This air leak appears to develop as a complication of the intrathoracic pressure generated by the infant during the initial respiratory efforts. While a pneumomediastinum may produce tachypnea, it rarely results in significant respiratory difficulty. A pneumothorax interferes with the establishment of respiratory activity only if it is large and under tension, producing mediastinal shift and compromising circulation and the contralateral lung. Breath sounds are diminished or absent on the side with the pneumothorax, but may also be decreased over the other side of the chest. Although some of these infants may require intubation and respiratory support, prompt aspiration of the free air is essential to permit the collapsed lung to reexpand. If a tension pneumothorax is suspected and the infant is deteri-

orating, with increasing cyanosis and worsening respiratory distress, aspiration of the chest should be performed in the delivery room. This technique is described below.

The presence of a scaphoid abdomen, immediate cyanosis, and respiratory distress suggests the presence of a diaphragmatic hernia. Diaphragmatic hernias usually occur on the left side of the thorax, inhibiting the normal growth and development of the left lung and often inhibiting the growth and development of the right lung because of displacement of the mediastinum and the heart to the right. Breath sounds are diminished or absent on the left, and the heart sounds are heard in the right chest. Endotracheal intubation should be performed quickly, since respiratory activity and cardiac function will be further compromised as the bowel fills with gas. An infant with a diaphragmatic hernia diagnosed by antenatal ultrasound should be delivered at a tertiary level hospital so that the delivery and immediate postnatal care can be coordinated by the obstetrician, neonatologist, and pediatric surgeon. The delivery room team must be prepared to intubate such an infant promptly if there is any evidence of respiratory distress after delivery; bag and mask ventilation is contraindicated. If the infant is breathing adequately by himself or herself, a nasogastric tube should be inserted so as to minimize distention of the bowel by swallowed air. The pathophysiology and management of diaphragmatic hernia are discussed in Chapter 20.2.11.

Congenital anomalies such as bilateral choanal atresia, laryngeal webs, and other obstructive malformations of the epiglottis, larynx, or trachea prevent air exchange. If respiratory movements are observed but there is no air movement when the infant's mouth is closed, the mouth and posterior pharynx should be cleared of secretions, an oral airway should be inserted, and the patency of each choana should be determined by attempting to pass a suction catheter through each nostril into the posterior oropharynx. If effective air exchange is not achieved, laryngoscopy and endotracheal intubation should be performed. The endotracheal tube should bypass any upper respiratory tract obstruction and permit air movement during respiratory activity. The management of these problems is discussed in Chapter 20.2.11.

Pulmonary hypoplasia may occur in association with renal agenesis or dysplasia and other congenital anomalies as part of Potter's syndrome. It may also occur secondary to prolonged rupture of the fetal membranes. These infants require immediate endotracheal intubation and very high peak inspiratory pressures to achieve chest expansion and air movement into the lungs. Multiple pneumothoraces may develop during these resuscitative efforts.

Nonimmune hydrops fetalis, a condition implying an excess of total body water that is not associated with a circulating antibody against a red blood cell, may hinder the establishment of effective respiratory activity. The excessive accumulation of extracellular fluid includes subcutaneous edema, pleural and pericardial effusions, ascites, polyhydramnios, and placental thickening. A pleural effusion interferes with expansion of the lungs by occupying intrathoracic volume; ascites interferes with expansion of the lungs by pushing the diaphragm up, disrupting its normal activity and decreasing effective intrathoracic volume. Therefore, once an airway has been established and positive-pressure ventilation initiated, it may be necessary to perform bilateral thoracentesis and abdominal paracentesis in the delivery room, so that pleural and ascitic fluid can be removed. Since polyhydramnios is often seen in conjunction with nonimmune hydrops, many affected infants are identified antenatally during a diagnostic obstetric ultrasound evaluation. Other infants may have been diagnosed prenatally during evaluation of a fetal tachyarrhythmia. Additional ultrasound examinations of these infants before delivery will alert the delivery room team about the presence, size, and location of pleural fluid and ascites, ensuring prompt action if necessary.

The pathophysiologic causes predisposing to the excessive extracellular fluid accumulation associated with nonimmune hydrops are unknown. Table 19-10 lists reported causes of nonimmune hydrops.

Occasionally an infant presents with pallor and shock at the time of delivery. This clinical picture results from an acute, significant intrapartum blood loss that may be associated with such problems as abruptio placenta; ruptured umbilical or placental vessels; fetal-placental, fetal-maternal, or fetal-fetal hemorrhage/transfusion; cesarean section incision through an anterior placenta; or intra-abdominal hemorrhage secondary to laceration of the liver or splenic rupture because of a difficult or breech delivery. As described above, volume should be administered if, after adequate ventilation with oxygen, there is a poor response to resuscitation, and the infant remains pale and tachycardiac, with weak pulses and poor capillary refill. In the delivery room, 10 mL/kg of estimated body weight of a 5% albumin solution, normal saline, or Ringer's lactate can be infused over about 10 minutes via a catheter (or feeding tube) inserted into the umbilical vein. After transfer to the NICU, 10 mL/kg of packed red blood cells can be given over about 30 minutes, and the need for additional volume expansion or pharmacologic support of blood pressure can be determined.

## Discontinuation of Resuscitative Measures

The decision to stop resuscitation remains a difficult one. It is based on personal experience with respect to the immediate and long-term success of the resuscitative efforts, consideration of the parents' feelings, understanding, and expectations, and the resources available for continued management and support of the infant. In most cases it is best to be as vigorous and aggressive as possible during a delivery room resuscitation. After transfer to the nursery, the status of the infant can then be evaluated and discussed with the parents. If continued care is futile, it is appropriate to discontinue extraordinary support.

## Transfer From the Delivery Room

As noted above, the aim of delivery room management of the newborn is to ensure the satisfactory transition from intrauterine to extrauterine existence. In addition to performing appropriate resuscitative efforts, personnel should also examine the infant for the presence of congenital malformations or other conditions that might require prompt medical or surgical intervention. If congenital malformations are noted, they should be shown and described to the parents in the delivery room. Heat loss should be minimized by drying infants with a warmed towel, caring for them beneath a radiant heat source, and wrapping them in a warm blanket.

Since most infants have 1-minute Apgar scores of greater than 7 and adapt well to the extrauterine environment, they should spend time with their mothers in the delivery or postpartum recovery room. If a mother intends to breast-feed, her child should be put to breast at that time. The infant should then be transferred to the nursery for routine admission procedures.

Most infants who require more than just tactile stimulation and facial oxygen in the delivery room should be transferred to a NICU or transitional nursery for observation, evaluation, and initial care. In addition, many infants who have a factor or prob-

TABLE 19-10.   Conditions Associated With Nonimmune Hydrops Fetalis

| Category | Conditions |
|---|---|
| Hematologic | Homozygous α-thalassemia, chronic fetomaternal transfusion, twin-to-twin transfusion, acardius, atrioventricular shunts, hemorrhage or thrombosis, maternal drugs (eg, chloramphenicol) |
| Cardiovascular | Severe congenital heart disease (eg, complex congenital heart defects, atrioventricular septal defects, premature closure of the foramen ovale, hypoplastic left and right heart), arrythmias or congenital heart block, myocardial and endocardial disease, cardiac tumors (eg, rhabdomyomas) |
| Respiratory | Cystic adenomatoid malformation of lung, diaphragmatic hernia, pulmonary lymphangiectasia, pulmonary sequestration, intrathoracic mass |
| Gastrointestinal | Bowel atresias, volvulus, duplications of the gut, peritonitis |
| Urinary/renal | Urethral and ureteral atresia, bladder neck obstruction, posterior urethral valves, cloacal malformation, congenital nephrosis |
| Chromosomal | Turner syndrome; trisomies 13, 18, 21; triploidy; miscellaneous aneuploidy |
| Placental | Umbilical vein thrombosis, torsion of cord, chorioangioma |
| Intrauterine infection (± hemolysis) | Cytomegalovirus, toxoplasmosis, syphilis, parvovirus, parasitic diseases |
| Recognized syndromes | Dwarfing syndromes (eg, thanatophoric, Jeune, hypophosphatasia, achondrogenesis), arthrogryposis, Neu-Laxova syndrome, Pena-Shokeir syndrome, Noonan syndrome, multiple pterygium syndromes, Meckel syndrome |
| Metabolic disorders | Lysosomal storage disorders (including mucopolysaccharidoses), Gaucher disease, gangliosidoses, sialidosis |
| Miscellaneous | Amniotic band syndrome, fetal tumors (eg, teratoma, neuroblastomas, Wilms', angiomas) |

Adapted from McGillivray BC, Hall JG. Nonimmune hydrops fetalis. Pediatr Rev 1987;9:197.

lem associated with high risk (see Table 19-2) should be transferred to a NICU for initial evaluation and care. Transfer from the delivery room should not occur until oxygenation, ventilation, and heart rate have been adequately established, but it is important to expedite transfer so that management can be continued and optimized.

## NICU ADMISSION ROUTINES, MONITORING, AND PROCEDURES

On admission to the NICU, every infant should be weighed; vital signs, including an apical pulse, respiratory rate, blood pressure, and rectal temperature, should be obtained; and a capillary hematocrit (or hemoglobin) and blood sugar (for example, with glucose oxidase-impregnated reagent strips) should be measured. Vitamin $K_1$ (1 mg) should be given intramuscularly and ophthalmic prophylaxis should be given (0.5% erythromycin ophthalmic ointment, 1% tetracycline ophthalmic ointment, or 1% silver nitrate). Surface electrodes should be placed and monitoring of cardiac function should be initiated, with simultaneous display of rate and ECG pattern. Proper placement of the surface electrodes permits some monitors to display a respiratory pattern based on thoracic impedance.

The normal heart rate and respiratory rate for neonates ranges from 120 to 160 bpm and 40 to 60 breaths/minute respectively. Arterial blood pressure is directly related to birth weight; Figure 19-4 displays the normal range for mean arterial blood pressure during the first 12 hours of life. After rectal temperature is determined on admission (occasionally leading to the diagnosis of an imperforate anus), body temperature can be monitored continuously with a skin temperature probe (or thermistor) or with serial axillary temperature measurements. Environmental temperature should be adjusted to maintain the skin or axillary temperature between 36.0°C and 36.5°C. Oxygen consumption has been shown to be minimized with such an environmental temperature (neutral thermal environment).

The hemoglobin concentration at birth is a function of the infant's gestational age, averaging 16.8 g% at term, 15 g% at 34 weeks, and 14.5 g% at 28 weeks. Infants with blood sugar measurements less than 45 mg/dL should receive intravenous glucose or if possible should be fed.

Any infant who has respiratory distress or who requires supplemental inspiratory oxygen after delivery should be monitored expectantly with a pulse oximeter or transcutaneous oxygen and carbon dioxide electrodes. Pulse oximeters measure oxygen saturation by detecting differences in the absorption of a red light and an infrared light signal by a pulsating arteriolar vascular bed. Transcutaneous oxygen and carbon dioxide electrodes estimate arterial oxygen and carbon dioxide levels by determining the partial pressure of these gases after diffusion across the skin. Depending on the severity of the respiratory distress, an arterial blood gas measurement should be considered, and the need for mechanical ventilatory assistance and placement of an umbilical (or peripheral) arterial catheter for serial arterial blood gas measurements evaluated. Although capillary blood gas measurements satisfactorily estimate arterial pH and $P_{CO_2}$ during the first 24 hours of life, estimates of arterial $P_{O_2}$ are inaccurate and unreliable. Fortunately, pulse oximetry provides an easily obtained, accurate assessment of inspiratory oxygen needs. The evaluation and management of infants with respiratory distress is discussed further in Chapter 20.2.

Serial blood pressure monitoring should be done on infants who are unstable (such as those with respiratory distress), who may have suffered some degree of intrapartum asphyxia, and who may have experienced an acute blood loss. Noninvasive blood pressure measurements can be performed by monitors that inflate a blood pressure cuff at preset intervals and then display systolic, diastolic, and mean blood pressure and heart rate. Continuous blood pressure monitoring can be performed from an arterial catheter with a pressure transducer. In addition, the hematocrit (or hemoglobin) should be rechecked 4 to 6 hours after admission in any infant who may have suffered an intrapartum blood loss. The need for blood transfusion, volume expansion, or pharmacologic support of blood pressure is made in response to the infant's evolving clinical status and the presence or absence of hypotension, poor capillary refill, a fall in hematocrit (or hemoglobin), metabolic acidosis, and decreased urine output.

These initial assessments, plus a physical examination and gestational age assessment, are often performed while the infant lies under a radiant warmer. If stable, the neonate is moved to a heated plexiglass isolette, which permits observation and easy maintenance of body temperature. If unstable, the neonate is often managed on the warmer to facilitate access by medical and nursing staff. For example, neonates requiring mechanical ventilatory assistance may be initially cared for on an open warmer, where such procedures as administration of surfactant replacement therapy, reintubation, placement of umbilical vessel catheters, chest tube placement, suctioning, and chest radiologic studies are more easily performed. However, as soon as possible that infant should be moved into an isolette, since an infant's insensible water loss is greater when cared for under a radiant warmer.

The age at which enteral feedings are initiated depends on such factors as the infant's birth weight and gestational age, a history of fetal distress, and the presence and severity of respiratory distress. Intravenous fluids and parenteral nutrition solutions should be provided until enteral feedings are well established so as to maintain normal fluid and electrolyte status and to approach nitrogen and caloric needs. At YNHH enteral feedings in infants weighing less than 1250 g at birth are delayed for at least 24 hours; then small volumes are offered by nasogastric tube if the infant's condition is stable. Enteral feedings are slowly increased in volume and caloric density as tolerated; intravenous fluids are maintained and slowly decreased as enteral feedings advance. Enteral feedings are delayed in infants with birth weights between 1250 and 1500 g for at least 12 hours. Then, if the infant is stable, feedings are advanced as described above, while intravenous fluids are tapered. Finally, with larger infants,

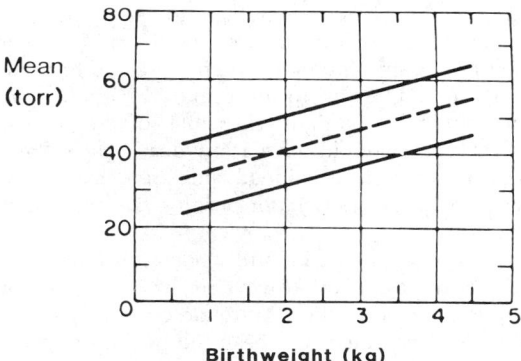

**Figure 19-4.** Linear regression (*broken line*) and 95% confidence limits (*solid lines*) of mean arterial blood pressure on birthweight in 61 healthy newborn infants during the first 12 hours after birth; y = 5.16 X +29.80, n = 443, r = 0.80; *p* < .001. (Versmold HT, Kitterman JA, Phibbs RH, Gregory GA, Tooley WH. Aortic blood pressure during the first 12 hours of life in infants with birth weight 610 to 4220 grams. Pediatrics 1981;67: 607.)

enteral feedings are initiated within 6 hours of birth if the infant is stable. However, feedings are delayed for at least 24 hours for any infant with a birth weight above 1250 g with a history of fetal distress or with respiratory distress.

## Initial Medical Management of Infants With Severe Perinatal Asphyxia

Infants who have suffered severe perinatal asphyxia may develop hypoxic-ischemic encephalopathy and may demonstrate a spectrum of multiorgan injury; therefore, they must be managed expectantly. Their level of consciousness and neurologic exam, including neurovital signs and level of arousal, must be followed carefully. If clinical signs of increased intracranial pressure develop, a cranial ultrasound should be performed to look for evidence of intraventricular or parenchymal hemorrhage, mass effect, generalized edema, or shift of the midline. A head CT scan should be done if subdural hemorrhage is suspected, or if the cranial ultrasound study produces questionable findings. Although it is not routine to perform a lumbar puncture to document increased intracranial pressure or to monitor intracranial pressure noninvasively (for example, with a pressure-activated device placed over the anterior fontanelle), many neonatologists take steps to minimize cerebral edema during the first 48 to 72 hours of life. These steps include hyperventilation of infants requiring ventilatory support and fluid restriction to maintain serum osmolality between 290 and 300 mOsm/L. A more detailed discussion of the neurologic evaluation and management of infants with hypoxic-ischemic encephalopathy is found in Chapter 20.1.4.

Severely asphyxiated infants usually require mechanical ventilatory assistance with correction and stabilization of arterial pH, $Po_2$, and $Pco_2$. As noted above, many neonatologists electively hyperventilate any severely asphyxiated infant who requires ventilatory support, aiming to maintain $Paco_2$ between 20 and 30 mm Hg for 40 to 72 hours. Since this practice may necessitate treatment of the infant with a muscle relaxant or a drug that will provide sedation, but which may interfere with the observation of seizure activity, serial EEG monitoring has been suggested. In addition, severely asphyxiated infants may require treatment for meconium aspiration pneumonia or persistent pulmonary hypertension; the management of these problems is discussed in Chapters 20.2.8 and 20.2.9.

Cardiac activity may be depressed by severe asphyxia, and ionotropic support may be required. Assessment of myocardial injury with echocardiography, ECG, and serial cardiac enzymes has been advocated. Central venous pressure monitoring may also be helpful in managing infants with severe myocardial dysfunction, impaired renal status, and uncertain volume status.

Acute renal failure is also commonly seen in severe asphyxia. Renal function should be monitored closely by determining urine output (oliguria is less than 0.5 mL/kg/hr) and performing serial laboratory measurements of BUN, serum creatinine, serum and urine electrolytes, and fractional excretion of sodium. Also, body weight should be measured at least once a day.

Asphyxia may predispose the gastrointestinal tract to the development of necrotizing enterocolitis due to intestinal ischemia. Therefore, these infants are usually observed without enteral feedings for the first several days of life, and then feedings are initiated and cautiously advanced when the infant has active bowel sounds and is considered stable.

In addition, severe asphyxia may produce hepatic damage and a coagulopathy. Hepatic injury is usually followed with serial serum bilirubin measurements; determination of liver enzyme (ie, ALT [SGPT], AST [SGOT]) activity would be performed if the direct (or conjugated) bilirubin level is elevated. Coagulation status is often evaluated clinically and by measuring the platelet count. If there is evidence of clinical bleeding or if there is thrombocytopenia, then coagulation studies should be performed.

## Ventilatory Equipment for Resuscitation

There are two standard types of ventilation bags, a self-inflating bag and an anesthesia bag. The self-inflating bag refills itself due to its elasticity, independently of gas flow. An intake valve or a series of valves at one end of the bag allows it to be rapidly reinflated. However, unless this type of bag is fitted with an oxygen reservoir that surrounds the intake valve(s), oxygen flowing into the bag is diluted by the air that is reinflating the bag, and high concentrations of oxygen cannot be delivered. Although the self-inflating feature makes this bag easier to use, some self-inflating bags will deliver oxygen only when they are compressed. Self-inflating bags that permit free-flow oxygen are preferable. Finally, even though many self-inflating bags are equipped with a pressure-limited pop-off valve that is preset at 30 to 40 cm of water, it is recommended that a pressure manometer be used during any positive-pressure ventilation. VLBW infants may require peak inspiratory pressures of only 15 to 20 cm of water to achieve adequate chest expansion, while asphyxiated term infants may initially require peak inspiratory pressures as high as 60 cm of water.

The anesthesia bag is reinflated by a continuous flow of air or oxygen from a compressed gas source. Delivery of an adequate ventilatory volume requires that the bag be sufficiently refilled between breaths. This is a function of the rate of air/oxygen gas flow into the intake port, adjustment of a flow control or exit valve, and the soundness of the seal between the infant and the face mask or endotracheal tube. If ventilation is interrupted and the mask is removed from the infant's face or the bag is disconnected from the endotracheal tube, the bag promptly deflates; it must be allowed to reinflate before positive-pressure ventilation can be restarted. However, this is a flow-through system, and facial oxygen can be provided by directing the ventilation port (with or without a mask) toward the infant's face. The anesthesia bag can deliver very high inspiratory pressures, so a pressure gauge must be included within the respiratory circuit so that peak inspiratory pressures can be monitored. In addition, the flow control or exit valve permits this type of ventilatory bag to maintain positive end-expiratory pressure during positive-pressure ventilation; in contrast, the end-expiratory pressure returns to zero after each breath with most types of self-inflating bags. Although the ability to deliver a high inspiratory pressure and to maintain a positive end-expiratory pressure are advantages of this ventilation bag, it is more difficult to use properly.

Face masks, oral airways, and endotracheal tubes should be available in sizes appropriate for premature and term neonates. Face masks should be able to conform to the infant's facial features and should form a tight seal while covering the nose and mouth. The masks should have a low dead space. Transparent masks and masks with cushioned rims are currently available. Such masks help the resuscitator position the mask and form a tight facial seal.

An oral airway may be helpful when an infant is ventilated with a bag and mask. Oral airways push the tongue down and forward into the floor of the mouth and ensure a patent airway.

Most of the endotracheal tubes used today are made of siliconized polyvinyl chloride, which is nonirritating and malleable and conforms to the trachea after being warmed to body temperature. The largest endotracheal tube that fits easily into the trachea should be used during intubation: the smaller the tube, the greater the airway resistance and the more difficulty in suctioning during pulmonary toilet. The tube should be noncuffed, and a small gas leak should be present around the tube during positive-pressure ventilation. Cuffed tubes have been associated with subglottic and tracheal necrosis. Appropriate endotracheal tube size (internal diameter) is a function of body weight; body weight less than 1000 g, 2.5 mm; 1000 to 2000 g, 3.0 mm; 2000 to 3500 g, 3.5 mm; and more than 3500 g, 4.0 mm. In addition, many endotracheal tubes have a black line above the tip of the tube, ranging from about 2 cm with 2.5-mm tubes to about 3.5 cm with 4.0-mm tubes. If this line is placed at the level of the vocal cords, the tip of the tube should be above the carina and in the mid-trachea.

The endotracheal tube should have a uniform internal diameter over its entire length. Tubes such as Cole-type tubes, which decrease their diameter at the tracheal end to produce a short, narrow segment that extends into the trachea while the tapered area or shoulder rests on the vocal cords, should not be used if positive-pressure ventilatory support will be continued. Although these tubes may be easier to insert during an emergency, they have been associated with significant damage to the glottis and they increase airway resistance and dead space.

## Laryngoscopy and Endotracheal Intubation (Fig 19-5)

To facilitate endotracheal intubation, the infant should be lying supine under the radiant warmer of the resuscitation table with a rolled or folded towel under the shoulders to produce slight neck extension. In this position, the infant's chin is slightly extended as if "sniffing." Hyperextending the infant's neck usually obstructs visualization of the glottic opening and the vocal cords.

The infant's head is steadied by the operator's right hand or by an assistant. The laryngoscope is held between the thumb and first finger of the operator's left hand and the infant's chin is grasped firmly with the second and third fingers of that hand. During intubation the infant's heart rate is monitored by auscultation or with a cardiac monitor. The appropriate-sized blade of a lighted laryngoscope is inserted near the right corner of the infant's mouth and advanced between the tongue and palate for about 2 cm. As the blade advances, it should be moved to the left side of the mouth. This maneuver moves the tongue to the left of the blade and permits visualization of the base of the tongue and epiglottis.

The blade is advanced into the vallecula, the space between the base of the tongue and the anterior surface of the epiglottis. Gentle elevation of the tip of the blade lifts the epiglottis anteriorly, revealing the glottic opening. In addition, the fourth or small finger of the left hand can press on the hyoid bone to move the larynx posteriorly and expose the glottis. Then, under direct visualization, the endotracheal tube is inserted along the right side of the blade into the trachea, about 2 to 3 cm below the level of the vocal cords (when applicable, the black line on the tube should be at the level of the vocal cords). The laryngoscope blade is then removed while the position of the tube is maintained by the right hand on the infant's face.

The laryngoscope blade should not be advanced below the epiglottis "to pick it up," since it is easily traumatized. Also, placing the blade below the epiglottis obscures visualization of the

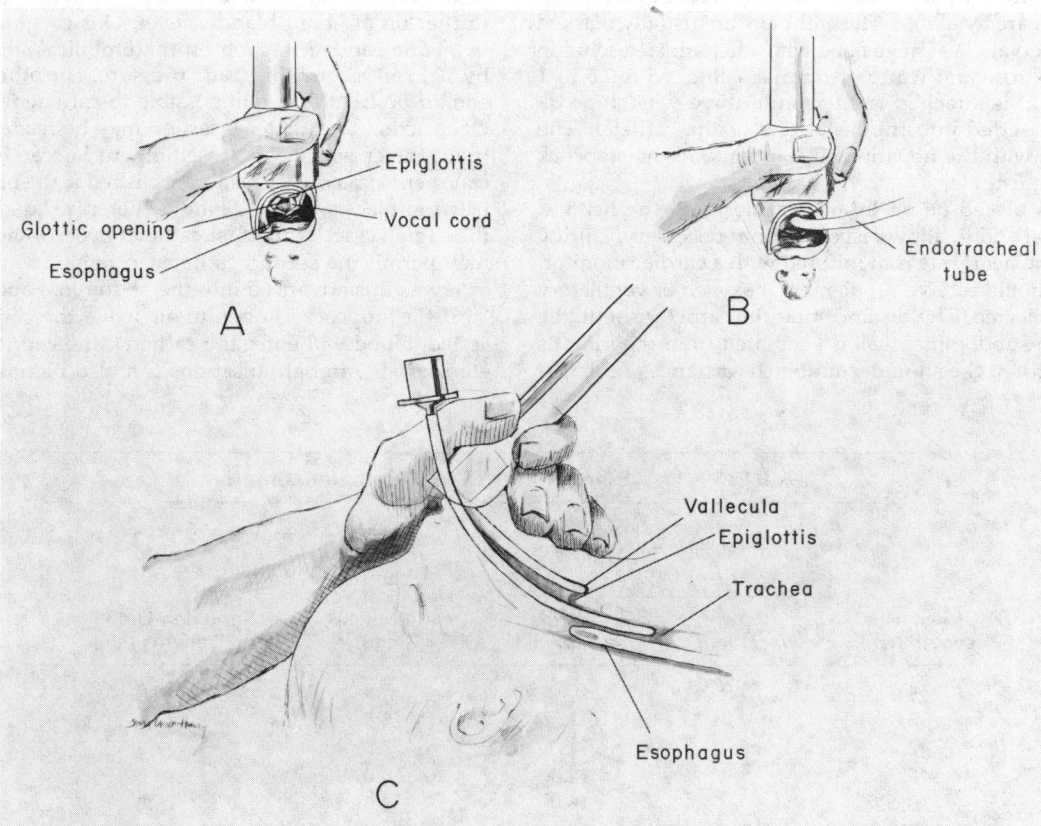

**Figure 19-5.**    Technique of endotracheal intubation. (**A**) Direct laryngoscopy. Note the glottic opening below the epiglottis and between the vocal cords. The esophagus is below the glottis. (**B**) Insertion of the endotracheal tube through the glottic opening from the right corner of the mouth. (**C**) The endotracheal tube is within the trachea. Note that the tip of the laryngoscope blade is in the vallecula, above the anterior surface of the epiglottis, and that the esophagus is below the trachea. (Ehrenkranz RA. Delivery room emergencies and resuscitation. In: Warshaw JB, Hobbins JC, eds. Principles and practice of perinatal medicine: Maternal-fetal and newborn care. Menlo Park, CA: Addison-Wesley, 1983:209.)

glottic opening. The endotracheal tube should not be passed through the grooved opening of the laryngoscope blade, since that will also obscure visualization.

When intubation is complete, the lungs should be expanded with a ventilation bag or by mouth. Tube placement should be confirmed by auscultatory evidence of equal, bilateral breath sounds over the axillary regions and symmetric chest movement. Unequal breath sounds and chest excursions suggest that the tube is probably in the mainstem bronchus of the lung producing the louder breath sounds. In that case, the tube should be withdrawn until breath sounds improve and become equal. Esophageal intubation results in poor breath sounds and chest movement, but loud sounds over the stomach. The tube should be immediately removed and then tracheal intubation reattempted after a brief period of bag and mask ventilation with oxygen. Once the tube is secured, a chest roentgenogram should be obtained to confirm tube position.

## Umbilical Vessel Catheterization

An umbilical arterial catheter is most often used for monitoring arterial blood gases and arterial blood pressure. An umbilical venous catheter is most often used for monitoring central venous pressure and performing exchange transfusions. Radiopaque, end-hole catheters should be used for umbilical arterial and central venous pressure monitoring; 3.5 Fr catheters are often used with infants under 1500 g and 5 Fr catheters for larger infants. A catheter with end and side holes may be used when the umbilical vein is being catheterized for an exchange transfusion; 5 Fr and 8 Fr sizes are available. The catheters are usually marked at centimeter intervals. A syringe filled with a heparinized solution (5% or 10% dextrose and water or normal saline, with 0.5 to 1 unit heparin/mL) is attached to the sterile three-way stopcock that has been inserted into the distal end of the catheter. The catheter is filled with the heparinized solution and the stopcock turned off to the catheter.

The infant is placed on an infant warmer with the head at the open or distal end to allow resuscitation if necessary. During the procedure the heart rate is monitored with a cardiac monitor, and the infant should receive supplemental oxygen or ventilatory assistance as indicated. The distance that the catheter should be inserted from the abdominal wall is estimated from the infant's crown-heel length or the shoulder-umbilicus distance (Table 19-

11). Umbilical vessel catheterization is done aseptically. Therefore, after adequately restraining the infant's extremities and grasping the end of the umbilical cord by the cord clamp or with a Kelly clamp, the umbilical cord, umbilicus, and periumbilical area are prepared with an iodine solution and then draped so that only the cord is exposed. Umbilical cord tape is tied loosely around the cord, as close to the abdomen as possible, and should be tightened if bleeding occurs. The umbilical cord is then cleanly cut about 1 to 1.5 cm from the umbilicus with a scalpel blade or large scissors. The length of cord remaining must be added to the estimated catheter length.

The side of the umbilical cord stump is then grasped with nontoothed forceps or a hemostat, the cut surface is blotted, and the umbilical vessels are isolated. The single large, thin-walled oval vein should be readily distinguished from the two smaller, thick-walled arteries, which are usually constricted and appear pin-point in size. With arterial catheterization, one of the arteries is gently dilated by placing the closed tips of a small nontoothed forceps into the lumen and allowing the spring of the forceps to spread the tips apart. A blunt probe may also be used to dilate the vessel lumen. Once dilated, the opposite walls of the artery can be grasped with small nontoothed forceps by an assistant. While the catheter is held about 1 cm from its tip with small curved forceps, the catheter is inserted in the lumen of the artery. If the artery is well dilated, an assistant may not be needed to hold the lumen walls apart. The catheter is then slowly advanced to the estimated length.

Obstruction to umbilical arterial catheter insertion may be encountered at either the level of the anterior abdominal wall or farther on at about bladder level. Obstruction may be relieved by gentle caudad traction on the umbilical stump accompanied by 30 to 60 seconds of steady pressure. The other umbilical artery should be tried if it is impossible to catheterize the first vessel. Obstruction to catheter insertion may be related to dissection of the catheter out of the vessel lumen. Successful catheterization can then occasionally be accomplished if the obstructed catheter is left in place while a second catheter is slid alongside it within the same vessel. If the first catheter is occupying a false track, it may permit the second catheter to remain within the umbilical artery as it is advanced into the abdominal aorta.

If the stopcock is open to air while the catheter is being inserted, blood will enter the catheter, indicating successful catheterization. Arterial pulsations can also be noted with blood in

| Crown–Heel Length (cm) | Length of Umbilical Artery Catheter (cm) | | Length of Umbilical Vein Catheter‡ (cm) | Shoulder–Umbilicus Length§ (cm) |
|---|---|---|---|---|
| | Low Placement* | High Placement† | | |
| 34 | 5.0 | 10.0 | 5.5 | 10.0 |
| 38 | 6.0 | 11.5 | 6.5 | 11.5 |
| 42 | 7.0 | 13.0 | 7.5 | 12.5 |
| 46 | 8.0 | 14.5 | 8.0 | 13.5 |
| 50 | 9.0 | 16.0 | 9.0 | 15.0 |
| 54 | 10.0 | 18.5 | 10.0 | 16.5 |

TABLE 19-11. Estimation of Vessel Catheter Length

* Length of catheter from abdominal wall to bifurcation of the aorta
† Length of catheter from abdominal wall to the diaphragm within the aorta
‡ Length of catheter from abdominal wall to reach the inferior vena cava just above the diaphragm
§ Length from above the lateral end of the clavicle to the umbilicus

Adapted from Dunn PM. Localization of the umbilical catheter by postmortem measurement. Arch Dis Child 1966;41:69.

the catheter and with the stopcock closed to the infant. However, if there is any question about whether the artery or vein is being catheterized, the stopcock should not be open to air during catheter insertion. If an umbilical venous catheter were opened to atmospheric pressure at a time when the infant generated a large negative intrathoracic pressure such as with crying, a large volume of air could be sucked in to the right heart and cause an air embolus.

Catheter placement should be confirmed by abdominal radiographs. Although an anteroposterior view of the abdomen is usually adequate for this purpose (Fig 19-6), if there is any question, a lateral view will demonstrate the location of the catheter tip and will confirm that an umbilical artery has been catheterized. There are two preferred locations for the tip of the umbilical artery catheter: lying within the lower abdominal aorta over the third or fourth lumbar vertebra, so that it is below the origin of the renal and inferior mesenteric arteries and above the aortic bifurcation (Fig 19-7); or lying just above the diaphragm in the thoracic aorta. However, little information exists to support a preference for low versus high catheter placement.

Once the catheter tip is in satisfactory position, it is secured to the Wharton's jelly of the umbilical stump with a suture or taped to the abdominal wall, and an intra-arterial infusion of a dextrose and electrolyte solution begun with an infusion pump. An arterial blood pressure transducer should also be attached to the catheter so that intravascular pressures can be continuously monitored. Infusion of a heparinized solution (0.5 to 1 unit heparin/mL) through an umbilical artery catheter is common but not standard practice. Furthermore, due to a report that administration of antibiotics through an umbilical arterial catheter was associated with an increased rate of complications (specifically, blanching or cyanosis of a lower extremity), many clinicians use these catheters primarily for monitoring blood pressure and for obtaining blood for arterial blood gas measurements and other laboratory studies. At YNHH antibiotics, medications, blood

products, or parenteral alimentation solutions are not routinely infused through an umbilical arterial catheter, but this practice varies among institutions.

Blanching or cyanosis of a lower extremity is commonly observed following placement of an umbilical arterial catheter. It is thought to represent vasospasm produced by the catheter's presence within the arterial system extending between the umbilical artery and the bifurcation of the aorta. This problem should be treated by warming the opposite leg; the warmth should increase blood flow to the affected leg due to reflex vasodilatation. It is contraindicated to warm the leg that is blanched or cyanotic, since the warmth will increase oxygen consumption in tissue that is already compromised, potentiating the problem. The catheter should be removed if there is no improvement. Infusion of lidocaine or tolazoline through an umbilical arterial catheter to diminish vasospasm is not recommended.

To monitor central venous pressure, a catheter may be placed via the umbilical vein into the inferior vena cava just above the diaphragm near the right atrium (see Fig 19-6). Before catheterizing the umbilical vein, any visible clot is removed with a forceps. Then, a catheter filled with a heparinized solution is introduced into the lumen of the vein. This catheter should always be closed to air, for the reasons noted above. The catheter is slowly advanced the estimated distance (see Table 19-11), from the abdominal wall through the ductus venosus into the inferior vena cava. Due to the orientation of the heart within the chest, it is common for an umbilical venous catheter to pass from the inferior vena cava through the right atrium and foramen ovale into the left atrium. In a well-oxygenated infant, this location can be easily discerned from the color of the blood within the catheter; in sicker patients, a blood gas or a chest radiograph is necessary. Leaving this catheter in the left atrium is not recommended.

Obstruction to umbilical venous catheter insertion indicates that it has entered the portal system and is probably wedged within a small vein in the liver. Reinserting the catheter after

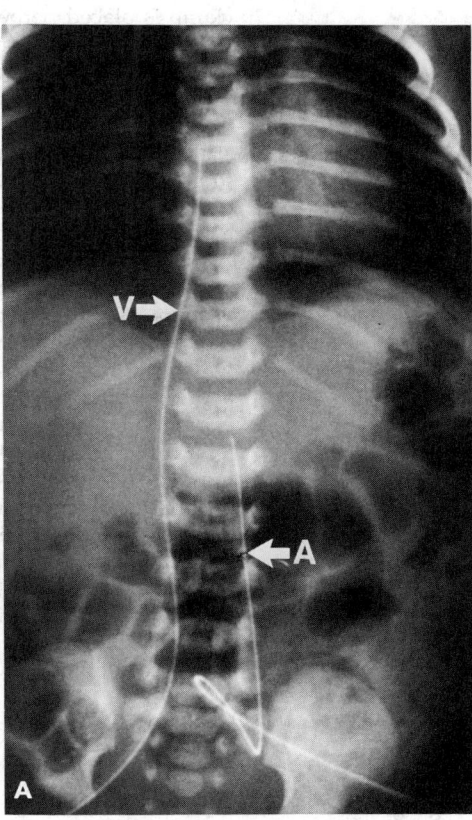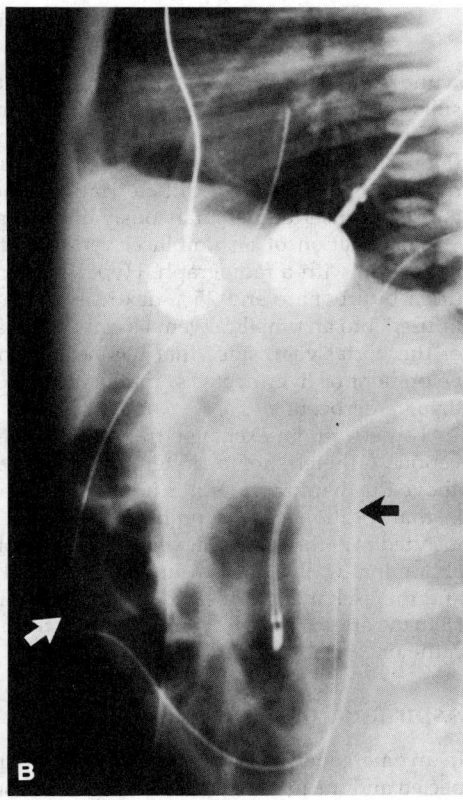

**Figure 19-6.** Umbilical vessel catheterization. (**A**) Anterior-posterior radiograph demonstrating an umbilical arterial catheter (*A*) in the abdominal aorta overlying the L1 and L2 interspace and an umbilical venous catheter (*V*) in the right atrium. Note the characteristic V-shaped appearance of the arterial catheter compared to the linear appearance of the venous catheter. (**B**) Lateral radiograph of the same neonate demonstrating catheters entering umbilical vessels at the abdominal wall (*white arrow*). The umbilical venous catheter proceeds cephalad as it passes via the ductus venosus into the inferior vena cava and then into the right atrium, while the umbilical arterial catheter (*black arrow*) initially proceeds caudally via the umbilical artery, then loops cephalad via the hypogastric artery and the common iliac artery into the abdominal aorta, lying over the spine.

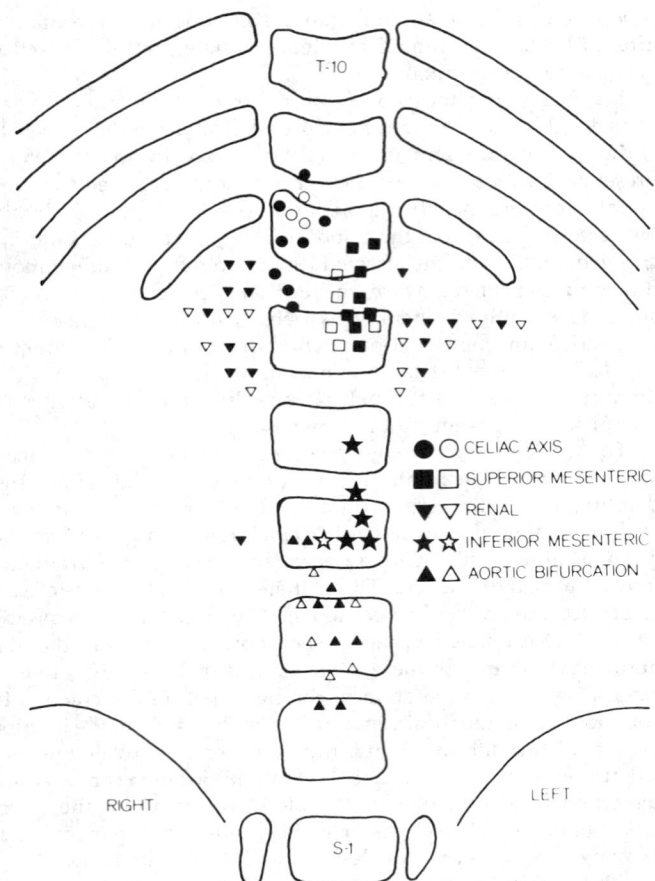

Figure 19-7. Distribution of the major aortic branches found in 15 infants. Filled symbols represent infants with, and open symbols without cardiac and/or renal anomalies. (Phelps DL, Lachman RS, Leake RD, Oh W. The radiologic localization of the major aortic tributaries in the newborn infant. J Pediatr 1972;81:336.)

withdrawing it several centimeters and rotating it frequently results in its passage through the ductus venosus. Occasionally it is impossible to insert the catheter into the inferior vena cava via the umbilical vein. If central venous pressure monitoring is required, another route of catheterization is necessary, such as by a catheter inserted percutaneously into a femoral vein.

The location of an umbilical venous catheter tip should be confirmed with a radiograph. Hypertonic solutions, such as sodium bicarbonate and 25% dextrose and water, should not be infused into an umbilical venous catheter located within a branch of the portal vein, since that has been associated with the development of liver necrosis, portal vein thrombosis, and necrotizing enterocolitis.

To perform an exchange transfusion, the tip of an umbilical venous catheter should preferably be in the inferior vena cava above the diaphragm. If it is impossible to place the catheter tip in that location via the umbilical vein, the catheter should be inserted into the umbilical vein to a depth of 2 to 3 cm from the abdominal wall. Then, an umbilical arterial catheter is inserted and the exchange performed by simultaneous removal of blood from the arterial catheter and infusion of the blood into the venous catheter.

## Aspiration of a Pneumothorax

In an emergency situation where a tension pneumothorax is suspected and the infant is deteriorating, a 16- or 18-gauge styletted,

small vein catheter can be used to evacuate the air from within the thorax. The appropriate anterior hemithorax is cleaned with an antiseptic preparation. The styletted cannula is inserted at a 45° angle to the skin between the anterior axillary and the mid-clavicular line, just above the fifth or sixth rib, but caudal to the breast. It is directed cephalad. When the stylet enters the pleural space, the cannula is advanced several centimeters at about a 15° angle to the skin as the stylet is withdrawn. A 20-cc syringe attached to a three-way stopcock is quickly connected to the adapter of the catheter. Air is aspirated into the syringe and then evacuated from the syringe when the stopcock is closed to the infant and open to air. If the infant is receiving positive-pressure ventilation, positive intrathoracic pressure is produced and air will not enter the pleural space if the cannula is left open. If possible, emergency aspiration of a pneumothorax should not be done with a needle that is left within the pleural space, since the needle point can penetrate and damage lung tissue after the air is evacuated and the lung reexpands. Furthermore, after emergency aspiration of a tension pneumothorax, a thoracostomy tube is often inserted to prevent reaccumulation of the air. The cannula may be left in place until insertion of the thoracostomy tube is completed.

Tube thoracostomy can be performed without prior aspiration of the pneumothorax if the infant is more stable and can withstand the extra time required for this procedure. Insertion of a tube thoracostomy is performed aseptically. The infant is positioned with the affected side of the chest raised about 60° off the bed and the arm on that side restrained, without external rotation over the head. The lateral aspect of the chest is prepared with an iodine solution and then draped. After administering a local anesthetic over the sixth or seventh intercostal space between the midaxillary and the anterior axillary line, a horizontal incision about 1 cm long is made. Then, with a curved mosquito hemostat, a subcutaneous tunnel is made by spreading the tissue from the incision site to the fourth intercostal space. If a thoracostomy tube with a trocar is used, the distal portion (about 2 to 3 cm from the tip) is bent to create about a 135° angle, and a straight clamp is placed perpendicularly across the tube, about 1.5 cm from the tip. The thoracostomy tube is directed through the subcutaneous tunnel toward the fourth intercostal space. Firm, steady pressure is applied to the tube so that it punctures the pleura just over the fifth rib in the fourth intercostal space. The perpendicular straight clamp should prevent the tip of the trocar from plunging too far into the chest and damaging the lung. After the straight clamp is removed, the trocar is withdrawn as the tube is advanced a predetermined distance toward the apex of the lung anteriorly. A rush of air indicates that the tube is in the pleural space. The proximal end of the tube is then connected to an underwater vacuum drainage system; bubbling in the water-seal chamber indicates evacuation of air. The tube is secured to the chest wall with a suture, the incision site is made airtight and dressed, and a chest radiograph is obtained to document tube position and evacuation of the pneumothorax.

If a thoracostomy tube without a trocar is used, the curved mosquito hemostat used to create the subcutaneous tunnel should be closed, directed into the tunnel, and used to puncture the pleura just above the fifth rib. The tube can then be inserted into the opening in the pleura by sliding it between the open tips of the hemostat. Alternatively, the tip of the tube can be grasped by the hemostat and directed through the tunnel into the thorax. Puncturing the pleura with the hemostat can also be done when a thoracostomy tube with a trocar is used.

## Selected Readings

American Academy of Pediatrics, American College of Obstetricians and Gynecologists. Guidelines for perinatal care, ed 3. Elk Grove Village, IL: American Academy of Pediatrics, 1992.

American Academy of Pediatrics, American Heart Association. Textbook of neonatal resuscitation. Elk Grove Village, IL: American Academy of Pediatrics, 1990.

Fanaroff AA, Graven SN. Perinatal services and resources. In: Fanaroff AA, Martin RJ, eds. Neonatal-perinatal medicine: diseases of the fetus and infant, ed. 5. St. Louis: Mosby/Year Book, 1992:12.

Fisher DE, Paton JB. Resuscitation of the newborn infant. In: Klaus MH, Fanaroff AA, eds. Care of the high-risk neonate, ed 3. Philadelphia: WB Saunders, 1986: 31.

Fletcher MA, MacDonald MG, Avery GB, eds. Atlas of procedures in neonatology. Philadelphia: JB Lippincott, 1983.

Gluck L. Design of a perinatal center. Pediatr Clin North Am 1970;17:777.

Gluck L. The newborn special care unit. Its role in a large medical center. Hosp Pract 1968;3:33.

Hack M, Horbar JD, Malloy MH, Tyson JE, Wright E, Wright L. Very-low-birth-weight outcomes of the National Institute of Child Health and Human Development Neonatal Network. Pediatrics 1991;87:587.

Hildebrand WL, Schreiner RL, Stevens DC. Endotracheal intubation of the newborn. Am Family Phys 1982;26:123.

Linder N, Aranda JV, Tsur M, et al. Need for endotracheal intubation and suction in meconium-stained neonates. J Pediatr 1988;112:613.

Swyer PR. The organization of perinatal care with particular reference to the newborn. In: Avery GB, ed. Neonatology: pathophysiology and management of the newborn, ed 3. Philadelphia: JB Lippincott, 1987:13.

U.S. Congress, Office of Technology Assessment. Neonatal intensive care for low-birth-weight infants: costs and effectiveness. Health Technology Case Study 38, OTA-HCS-38. Washington DC: US Congress, Office of Technology Assessment, 1987.

Wiswell TE, Henley MA. Intratracheal suctioning, systemic infection, and the meconium aspiration syndrome. Pediatrics 1992;89:203.

*Principles and Practice of Pediatrics, Second Edition.*
edited by Frank A. Oski et al. J. B. Lippincott Company, Philadelphia © 1994.

# 19.2 *The Premature Newborn*

Steven R. Mayfield, Ricardo Uauy,
and Joseph B. Warshaw

A *premature newborn* is defined as an infant born at an estimated gestational age of less than 37 weeks. This definition is distinct from low birth weight (LBW), which describes infants with a birth weight below 2500 g, and includes appropriate-for-gestational-age (AGA) premature infants and small-for-gestational-age (SGA) premature and term infants. AGA infants may be described as moderately-low-birth-weight (MLBW; birth weight 1501 to 2500 g), very-low-birth-weight (VLBW; birth weight 1001 to 1500 g) or extremely-low-birth weight (ELBW; birth weight 1000 g or less). Low birth weight occurs in about seven per 100 live births in the United States, of which 82% are MLBW infants, 12% are VLBW infants, and 6% are ELBW infants.

The risk of death among MLBW, VLBW, and ELBW infants is increased over that of infants of normal birth weight and gestational age by 40 times, 200 times, and 600 times respectively. Moreover, there may be significant morbidity among the survivors, particularly among VLBW and ELBW infants. The premature newborn infant presents the practitioner with a variety of problems that can be categorized broadly as those due to low birth weight and those due to functional immaturity.

The body composition of the LBW premature infant is characterized by low body fat, high total body water, and a large surface area to body mass ratio. These characteristics functionally translate to problems in extrauterine growth and thermoregulation.

## EXTRAUTERINE GROWTH

With the shift from intrauterine to extrauterine existence, the constant source of nutrition from the mother is interrupted and the infant's energy expenditure increases. Thus, achieving a positive energy balance adequate to promote growth depends on the level of nutritional support relative to energy expenditure. Moreover, the quality of nutritional support dictates the composition of weight gain. Ideally, the growth of the infant would approximate fetal growth. Ziegler and colleagues estimated the body composition of the fetus from 24 to 40 weeks of gestation from a retrospective compilation of cadaveric studies performed by different investigators. The reference fetus derived from this work has a body composition characterized by marked increases in body fat during the third trimester, and low glycogen stores (Table 19-12). For the VLBW infant born at the beginning of the third trimester, much of the body fat is in the form of structural lipids, which cannot be mobilized as an energy source. Thus, during early postnatal life, the LBW infant depends on exogenous sources of nutrition. In current practice, it is not uncommon to support infants with low fluid intakes (60 to 100 mL/kg/day) relative to their fluid losses during the first several days of life. Fluid restriction results in caloric deprivation as well, however, and VLBW infants often remain in negative energy balance for several days after birth. Thus, they must rely on available body fuel stores. Endogenous glycogen stores in LBW infants are low and are generally depleted within hours of the onset of negative energy balance. As mentioned, the body-fat stores that can be mobilized are also low. Thus, if inadequate calories are provided, energy must be generated from the body-fat free mass with loss of structural body protein, mainly skeletal muscle.

The energy expenditure of LBW infants depends on the basal metabolic rate, which reflects the minimum energy required for vital cellular processes such as the maintenance of transmembrane potentials, ion transport, and protein synthesis. Additional energy is expended with activity, with diet-induced thermogenesis, and in response to environmental cold stress. Typically the basal and other energy requirements can summarily be termed the *minimal energy expenditure*. Minimal energy expenditure for well LBW infants in a thermoneutral environment is 45 to 60 kcal/kg/day. Requirements for growth exceed the minimal energy expenditure: the *energy cost of growth* has been estimated at 4 to 5 kcal per gram of weight gain. Thus, the energy provision above minimal energy expenditure necessary to support a weight gain of 10 to 20 g/kg/day is 40 to 100 kcal/kg/day. While requirements vary, an adequate weight gain of 10 to 20 g/kg/day can usually be achieved by providing a total of 100 to 120 kcal/kg/day, and growth at a lesser rate can be achieved at caloric intakes of 80 to 100 kcal/kg/day.

Parenteral and/or enteral nutritional support is generally begun within the first week of life. The goals are to provide adequate calories to meet the energy requirements for growth and adequate

### TABLE 19-12. Body Composition of the Fetus

| Body Weight (g) | Body Composition (% body weight) | | | |
| --- | --- | --- | --- | --- |
| | *Water* | *Fat* | *Protein* | *Other\** |
| <1500 | 85 | 2 | 9 | 3 |
| 1501–2500 | 79 | 6 | 11 | 3 |
| >2500 | 72 | 12 | 12 | 3 |

\* Includes minerals, carbohydrate, and other body constituents.
*Adapted from Ziegler EE, O'Donnell AM, Nelson SE, Fomon SJ. Body composition of the reference fetus. Growth 1976;40:329.*

nitrogen for protein synthesis. Net protein accretion will not occur unless positive nitrogen and caloric balance are achieved. Generally, the protein needs of premature infants can be met by providing protein at 2 to 3.5 g/kg/day, with 50% to 70% of the nonprotein calories as carbohydrate. Essential fatty acid deficiency may occur as early as 7 to 10 days of age in premature infants receiving no fat intake. Essential fatty acid deficiency is associated with dry, scaly skin, which may desquamate. Exudation may occur in the body folds, particularly in the perianal area. Minimal essential fatty acid provision is generally achieved with 0.5 g/kg of intravenous lipid twice a week. Generally, lipid infusions are tolerated well without hyperlipidemia if the infusion rate is 150 mg/kg/hour or less for infants more than 1000 g of birth weight, and 50 to 100 mg/kg/hour for infants less than 1000 g of birth weight. Lipid infusions are typically not begun until after 48 to 72 hours of life and are better tolerated when prepared as 20% solutions.

The rate of weight gain can be related to postnatal growth curves (Fig 19-8) or to one of the intrauterine growth curves (Fig 19-9). The published intrauterine growth curves must be related to factors affecting fetal growth. These include maternal factors such as age, race, and socioeconomic status, environmental factors such as the ambient oxygen tension, and fetal-neonatal factors, which are a function of both intrinsic fetal maturation and the accelerated maturation associated with the transition from intrauterine to extrauterine life. Ideally, fetal and neonatal growth curves should relate gestational age to the composition of weight gain as well as to linear growth. However, such standards are not at present available, and an approximation of the Shaffer curves or one of the standard intrauterine growth curves is ac-ceptable. One must remember that the Shaffer postnatal growth curves include sick infants. Thus, these curves illustrate typical growth given current clinical standards of care, and do not necessarily reflect optimum growth as might be better defined by intrauterine growth curves.

## THERMOREGULATION

Fetal body temperature is 37.6°C to 37.8°C, and the fetus actually dissipates heat to the surrounding amniotic fluid. After delivery, the wet infant is exposed to delivery room air temperatures, which are 22°C to 25°C. As a result, significant heat losses can occur in the first few minutes after birth, resulting in a drop in body temperature of 1°C to 3°C. These losses can be diminished by drying and swaddling and placing the infant in a controlled, warm environment. In the nursery, environmental temperatures are rigorously regulated to a preset skin temperature of 36.5°C to 37.0°C. This is associated with extrauterine body temperatures, which range from 36.3°C to 37.1°C in premature infants and 36.5°C to 37.5°C in term infants.

The typical response of newborn infants to environmental cold stress is to increase total specific insulation and heat production. Total specific insulation depends on the ability to regulate vasomotor tone (peripheral vasoconstriction shunting blood away from the body surface and conserving heat), on the quantity of subcutaneous fat, which acts as an insulating medium, and on the skin surface area available for heat exchange with the environment. In the last case, surface area and heat exchange are reduced by postures of flexion and increased by postures of ex-

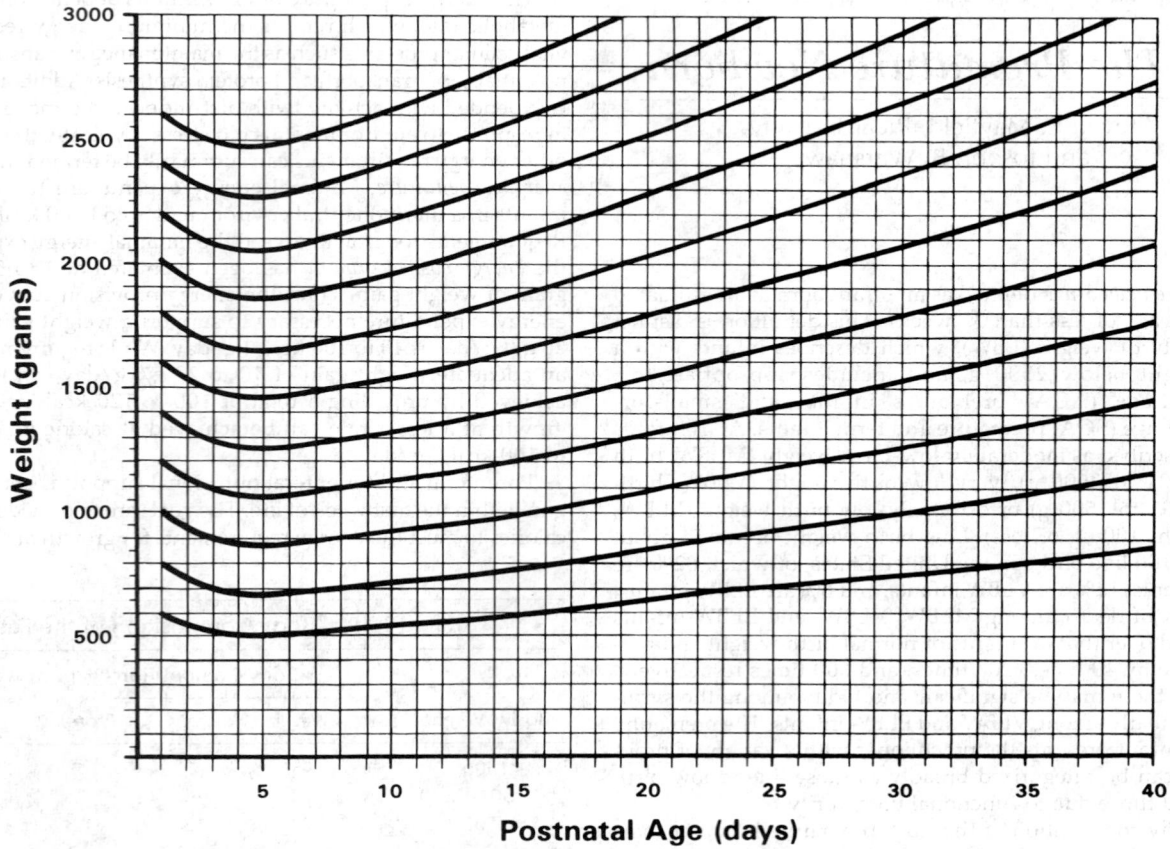

**Figure 19-8.** Postnatal growth grid, including growth curves for 100-g birth-weight groups. Derived from postnatal body weight changes in 385 surviving infants with birth weights of less than 2500 g. (Shaffer SG, Quimiro CL, Anderson JV, Hall RT. Postnatal weight changes in low-birth-weight infants. Pediatrics 1987;79:702.)

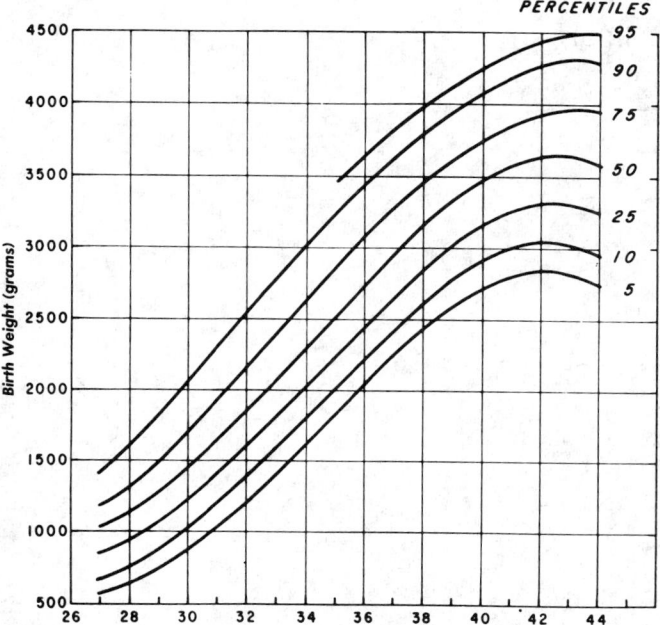

Figure 19-9.   Percentile curves of fetal growth in weight in relation to gestational age (calculated to the nearest week) for a white, middle-class population. (Babson SG, Behrman RE, Lessel R. Fetal growth: live-born birth weights for gestational age of white, middle-class infants. Pediatrics 1970;45:937.)

tension. Because premature infants do not shiver, heat production depends on the ability to generate heat by chemical thermogenesis in brown adipose tissue. Brown adipose tissue differentiates from reticular cells at around 26 weeks of gestational age. At term, it constitutes 6% of the body weight and 40% of the body fat stores. However, in the LBW premature infant, brown adipose tissue may be markedly diminished or even functionally absent. VLBW infants of less than 1000 g birth weight do not exhibit a thermogenic response to lowered skin temperatures until the third week of life. Thus, VLBW premature infants may be functionally poikilothermic for days after birth, dependent on the thermal environment for the maintenance of an optimum body temperature. The ability to thermoregulate improves with advancing postnatal age, and VLBW infants have been demonstrated to have increased subcutaneous body fat deposits and increased thermogenic potential at 3 weeks of age. Conversely, profoundly cold-stressed infants studied at autopsy have little or no residual brown fat stores.

Heat loss is a significant problem in LBW premature infants, especially during early postnatal life. Infants exchange heat via three routes: conduction, convection, and radiation. In addition, heat can be dissipated via evaporation. Modern nurseries use convection air incubators, radiant warmers, and heating mattresses to help stabilize body temperatures. In addition, attempts to decrease heat loss can be made by using a plexiglass radiant heat shield or polyethylene blanket.

In general, the goal of thermoregulation is to balance heat production and heat loss in such a way that the infant is maintained within the thermoneutral zone. The thermoneutral zone is defined as the environmental temperature at which the infant maintains a normal body temperature at the lowest level of energy expenditure. Energy expenditure increases at environmental temperatures higher or lower than the thermoneutral zone range of temperatures. Figure 19-10 demonstrates the effects of body size and postnatal age on the ranges of temperature defining the thermoneutral zone. Smaller, less mature infants have lower heat production, less subcutaneous fat, and a higher surface-area-to-mass ratio, with higher rates of heat loss. Thus, the range of temperatures defining the thermoneutral zone for those infants is higher and narrower. Body fat stores and thermoinsulation increase with postnatal age. In addition, advancing neurologic maturity allows the infant increasingly to assume a posture of flexion, which reduces the surface area available for heat exchange with the environment. Thus, as the infant gets older and grows, thermoregulatory capability improves and the range of temperatures defining the thermoneutral zone is lower and wider.

## PROBLEMS DUE TO FUNCTIONAL IMMATURITY

While the body organ systems are morphologically identifiable early in gestation, the function of the various body organs depends on the infant's stage of development. Although much attention is given to cardiopulmonary function in the early days of postnatal life, all organ systems are immature and undergo development with advancing postconceptional and postnatal ages. Different disease states and the quality of nutritional support further complicate the picture. Moreover, functional maturation of certain organ systems occurs with the transition from intrauterine to extrauterine life. Thus, there are both developmental and transitional changes to consider in the care of the premature infant, and the associated problems are both acute and chronic. In addition to being at risk because of lung immaturity and surfactant deficiency, premature newborn infants may have decreased central ventilatory drive, particularly if born before 30 to 32 weeks of gestational age, and asphyxia exacerbates this problem. Moreover, with decreasing gestational age, ventilatory muscle mass decreases and chest wall compliance increases. Thus, even with adequate central ventilatory drive, VLBW premature infants may not be able to perform the work necessary for effective ventilation. The fluid-filled alveoli and pulmonary interstitium result in a less compliant lung, exacerbating the problem. If ventilatory work is ineffective, alveolar surface area is diminished, with ensuing atelectasis and increased dead space ventilation. The net effect is poor respiratory gas exchange.

Most of the acute problems due to functional immaturity present in the first 72 hours of life. These are outlined in Table 19-13 and are discussed in greater detail in other sections. Chronic problems of the premature infant may be secondary to specific therapeutic interventions, as with bronchopulmonary dysplasia, or may be due to the long-term consequences of metabolic immaturity, as occurs in metabolic bone disease.

### Fluid and Electrolyte Balance

Infants born at less than 34 weeks of gestational age have a glomerulotubular imbalance that results in decreased free water clearance and increased urinary losses of sodium, bicarbonate, and glucose. In addition, there is a limited capacity to acidify the urine and excrete ammonia. Sodium losses may be as high as 8 to 10 mEq/kg/day, although the typical range is 2 to 3 mEq/kg/day. Bicarbonate loss may result in a metabolic acidosis unless adequate replacement is given. Most infants, term or premature, have a low urinary output in the first 24 to 36 hours of life. This may be due to increased plasma concentrations of arginine vasopressin or catecholamines resulting from the stress of labor. Generally, urine output averages at least 0.5 mL/kg/hour during the first 24 hours of life and more than 1 to 2 mL/kg/hour thereafter.

Fluid balance depends on the rates of sensible and insensible water losses relative to fluid intake. Thus, estimation of fluid needs requires measurement of ongoing urinary losses and es-

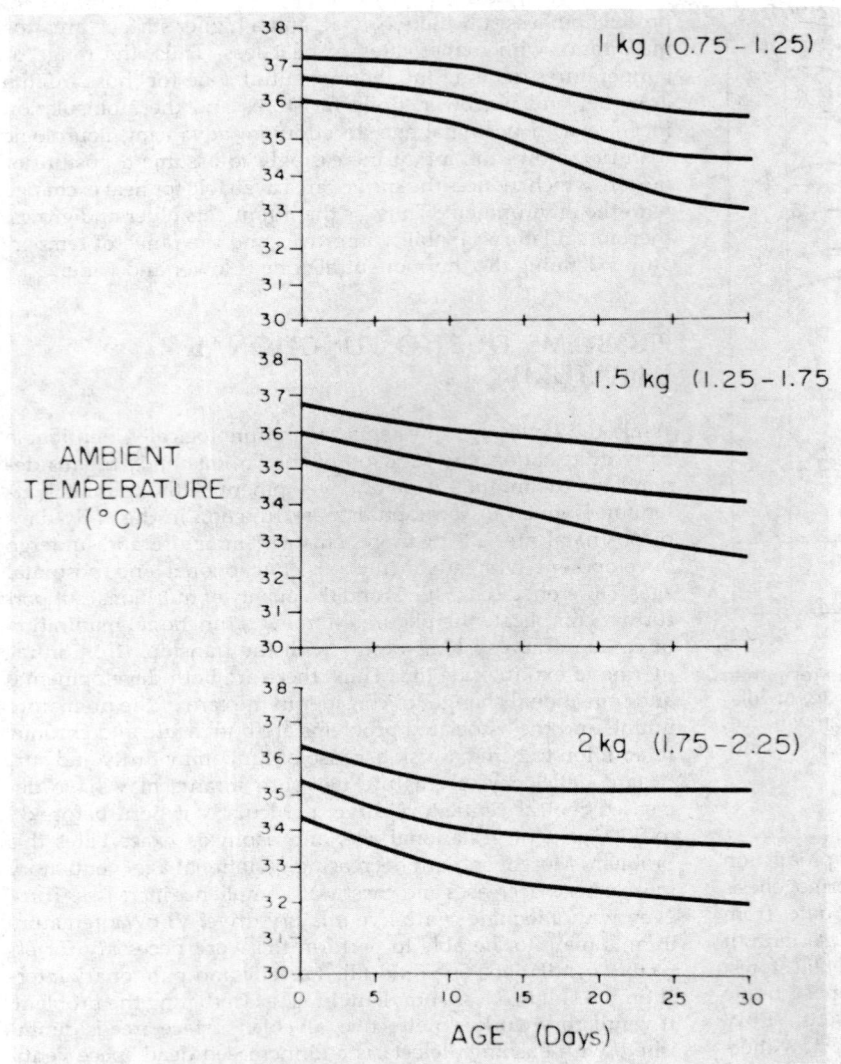

AMBIENT
TEMPERATURE
(°C)

1 kg (0.75 - 1.25)

1.5 kg (1.25 - 1.75

2 kg (1.75 - 2.25)

AGE (Days)

**Figure 19-10.**   Range of ambient temperatures defining a thermoneutral environment in infants with birth weights <1250 g (upper panel), 1250–1749 g (middle panel), and 1750–2250 g (lower panel). (From Bell EF et al. Pediatrics 1980;96:452.)

timation of insensible water losses, which consist primarily of evaporative water losses. Evaporative water loss consists of respiratory and transepidermal losses. Respiratory water loss generally accounts for about 33% of insensible water loss. This can be reduced to nearly zero for infants breathing humidified air from mechanical ventilators or oxygen hoods. Transepidermal water loss depends on body size, gestational age, and skin thickness. Smaller, less mature infants have higher transepidermal water losses due to their thin skin, low subcutaneous body fat

deposits, and high surface-area-to-mass ratios (Table 19-14). With increased postnatal age, the stratum corneum of the skin keratinizes and is less permeable. Accordingly, by the end of the first week of life, transepidermal water losses can be reduced by 50%. The thermal environment can affect transepidermal water losses. Higher environmental temperatures or the use of radiant heat increase transepidermal water losses. These losses can be reduced by using a thin plastic cover or conductive heating mattress.

Management of fluid and electrolyte balance is a critical feature

TABLE 19-13.   Problems of Premature Newborns

| Acute | Chronic |
|---|---|
| Respiratory disease | Necrotizing enterocolitis |
| Intracranial hemorrhage | Infection |
| Fluid and electrolyte imbalance | Bronchopulmonary dysplasia |
| Thermoregulation | Metabolic bone disease |
| Patent ductus arteriosus | Retinopathy of prematurity |
| Hyperbilirubinemia | Parental support |
| Hypoglycemia | |
| Hypocalcemia | |
| Apnea | |

TABLE 19-14.   Insensible Water Loss in an Incubator or Radiant Warmer

| Birth Weight (g) | Insensible Water Loss (mL/kg/day) | |
|---|---|---|
| | Incubator | Radiant Warmer |
| <1250 | 33–79 | 46–189 |
| 1251–1500 | 28–57 | 39–73 |
| 1501–1750 | 22–39 | 31–53 |
| 1751–2000 | 12–34 | 12–48 |

Adapted from Bell EF, et al, J Pediatr 1980;96(3):452, 460; Bell EF, Rios GR, Pediatr Res 1983;17:135; Marks KH, et al, Pediatrics 1980;66(2):228, and Baumgart S, Clin Perinatol 1982;9(3):483.

of premature newborn care and is also an area of considerable controversy. The controversy has arisen largely from the question of how fluid management relates to the development of patent ductus arteriosus (PDA). LBW infants given fluid at 160 mL/kg/day after the third day of life were found to have a higher incidence of PDA than infants given fluid at 120 mL/kg/day, while other investigators observed no difference in the incidence of PDA in LBW infants given 60 mL/kg/day versus 80 mL/kg/day. Animal studies have shown a vascular volume-dependent increase in circulating prostaglandins $E_1$ and $E_2$, which are associated with ductal patency. Based on the above studies, many nurseries have adopted the practice of providing fluids at 60 to 80 mL/kg/day, regardless of the infant's size and gestational age. For VLBW infants, in whom the risk of PDA is highest, this fluid intake may approximate or be considerably less than their ongoing evaporative water losses. Thus, the risk of dehydration and hypernatremia is increased.

At present there are two approaches to early fluid management of the ELBW premature infant. Both have three goals: maintaining an adequate vascular volume for effective cardiac output and renal plasma flow; avoiding vascular volume expansion; and preventing pathologic hypo- or hypernatremia. The first approach provides LBW infants with fluid intakes of 60 to 80 mL/kg/day; for ELBW infants nursed under radiant warmers, this may be less than their insensible water loss. Close surveillance is maintained, and fluids are increased as indicated to maintain urine flow and keep the serum sodium at 150 mEq/liter or less. The second approach is to provide infants with a fluid intake that approximates their estimated insensible water loss, resulting in a loss of body weight of 2% to 3% per day, up to 12% to 18% total body weight loss over the first week of life. This also results in a higher initial fluid intake per kilogram of body weight for ELBW infants than for other LBW or term infants. Again, close surveillance is maintained to ensure adequate urine flow and sodium balance. This approach must take into account the body size, gestational age, body posture, type of cradle (radiant versus convective heat source, with or without a conductive heat source), effects of postnatal age on skin thickness and transepidermal water loss, effects of radiant energy phototherapy, and other modifying factors. In practice, either approach is acceptable as long as close monitoring of body weight, urinary output, and serum electrolytes is maintained.

## Patent Ductus Arteriosus

In utero, the ductus arteriosus is patent, probably under the influence of circulating prostaglandins and the low oxygen tension of fetal blood. After birth, the plasma oxygen tension rises sharply, effecting a reactive vasoconstriction of the ductus arteriosus. In addition, the lung is a major site of prostaglandin catabolism, and the postnatal increase in pulmonary blood flow may result in a higher rate of prostaglandin degradation.

The ductus arteriosus remains patent in 15% to 35% of VLBW and ELBW infants. This may result in significant left-to-right shunting, with subsequent myocardial stress and pulmonary congestion. Progressive heart failure diminishes effective cardiac output and may reduce renal perfusion, glomerular filtration rate, and free water clearance. Typically, infants with a PDA have a systolic murmur and bounding pulses consistent with a wide pulse pressure. A precordial thrill may be palpable, and thoracic impulses are easily seen and are referred to as an active precordium. If heart failure ensues, tachypnea, tachycardia, and progressive respiratory distress occur, with cardiomegaly, hepatic congestion, and decreased urinary output due to poor renal perfusion.

The approach to a PDA depends on the severity of resultant symptoms. Some patients respond to fluid restriction. However, this approach should not be prolonged, as caloric deprivation may be an unavoidable complication. Pharmacologic closure may be attempted using indomethacin, an inhibitor of prostaglandin synthesis. Potential complications of indomethacin therapy include reduced glomerular filtration rate, impaired platelet aggregation, and reductions in both gastrointestinal and cerebral blood flow. Surgical closure is the final and only definitive option; however, the associated risks (transport to and from the surgical suite, effects of anesthesia, blood loss, and infection) must be considered.

## Intracranial Hemorrhage

Intracranial hemorrhage may occur at any time in the first several weeks of life, but the incidence is highest in the first 72 hours of life. The overall incidence of intracranial hemorrhage among LBW infants is 40% to 50%, so it is a major cause of mortality and morbidity of premature newborns (see Chap. 20.1.3).

## Hypoglycemia and Hyperglycemia

Regulation of blood glucose can be a problem for both the term and the premature newborn. Blood glucose in utero is typically about 20% lower than maternal levels. Except for the smallest premature infant, most neonates have glycogen stores adequate to maintain the blood glucose for the first several hours of life. However, infants of diabetic mothers who have become hyperinsulinemic secondary to chronic exposure to high glucose levels in utero may develop hypoglycemia within the first hour after birth, and fetal distress or neonatal stresses such as asphyxia or hypothermia may deplete glycogen stores and increase the risk for hypothermia. Moreover, SGA premature infants may not be able to use available glycogen stores, predisposing them to early hypoglycemia.

Hyperglycemia can occur in sick premature infants. While many ELBW infants can tolerate a glucose intake of 8 to 24 g/kg/day, sick ELBW infants may become hyperglycemic when receiving a glucose intake of more than 10 to 12 g/kg/day. If hyperglycemia results in severely restricted nutrient intake or in diuresis, then cautious insulin therapy should be considered.

## CHRONIC PROBLEMS

Many of the acute consequences of prematurity have presented by 3 days of age, and ongoing management of acute problems begins to blend with anticipatory management of chronic problems. Many of the chronic problems relate to the consequences of acute disease processes and to problems with nutritional support. These include such conditions as necrotizing enterocolitis, bronchopulmonary dysplasia, and retinopathy of prematurity, which are discussed in later sections.

## PARENTAL SUPPORT

Psychosocial issues and parental support are important in the care of any child. Premature delivery with or without intensive care nursing heightens the anxiety associated with childbirth. Even the ostensibly mundane circumstances associated with an uncomplicated premature infant may be the most unsettling, anxiety-provoking event that the infant's parents have ever faced. Moreover, the consequences may permanently affect the family's quality of life. Parents of sick children must contend with geographic displacement, disrupted sleep patterns, work conflicts or loss of income, fatigue, and the fright that accompanies an uncertain outcome for their child and their lack of control over the situation. These stresses should be recognized, and attempts should be made to remedy some or all of them.

The physician's goal should be to provide some structure and predictability in disordered, unpredictable circumstances. Thus, patience, honesty, and compassion are essential virtues. Providing a place to sleep, anticipating questions and concerns, willingness to offer the same messages repeatedly, defining the levels of care and supervision, and maintaining communication are responsibilities shared by physicians and nurses. Timely communication of both normal and abnormal findings is probably the most important factor in alleviating parental anxiety. Communicating with the mother in the delivery room and with both parents shortly after the infant is stabilized in the nursery is time well spent in alleviating parental anxiety regarding the infant's welfare, establishing a physician-parent relationship, and positively affecting parental attitudes toward visiting the intensive care nursery. Adolescent parents in particular may be fearful of their premature infant and of the busy intensive care nursery. If a good physician-parent relationship is not established in the early postnatal period, parents may avoid visiting after the mother is discharged, precluding an effective postdischarge transition to home for the infant and increasing the risk of child abuse and neglect.

## OUTCOME

Mortality among LBW infants, after declining sharply in the 1970s, has begun to level off. Current mortality and selective morbidity rates among LBW infants are shown in Table 19-15. As mortality has declined, morbidity among the survivors has increasingly distressed health-care providers. Nelson and Ellenberg associated a ten- to 33-fold increase in the risk of cerebral palsy with several factors, including birth weight of less than 2000 g, head circumference greater or less than three standard deviations from the mean, 5-minute Apgar score of less than 3, diminished activity or cry of greater than 1 day in duration, thermal instability, need for gavage feeding, hypotonia or hypertonia, apnea, or hematocrit of less than 40%. A 50-fold increase in cerebral palsy was associated with neonatal seizures or a 10-minute Apgar score of less than 3. Other studies have related LBW and the need for ventilator support to functional handicaps and an increased incidence of rehospitalization, most often related to chronic conditions that are consequences of prematurity (eg, bronchopulmonary dysplasia, posthemorrhagic hydrocephalus, failure to thrive), infections, and the need for herniorrhaphy.

However, infants of less than 1000 g of birth weight studied at 5 years of age were reported to have demonstrated an improvement in function, and in some cases appeared to have outgrown the developmental or neurologic disability. It is likely that such "improvements" reflect difficulties in early diagnosis of developmental or neurologic abnormalities. Moreover, low socio-economic status and decreased maternal age and experience can adversely affect motor and cognitive development. These environmental influences are not easily distinguished from the effects of premature delivery and its sequelae as causes of developmental delay.

In the final analysis, the outcome among LBW infants of more than 1000 g of birth weight is generally good in terms of both morbidity and mortality. However, the ethics and cost-effectiveness of intensive care for infants of less than 1000 g of birth weight, and particularly for those of less than 750 g of birth weight, continue to pose problems for health-care providers and society at large. Hack (1991) has described a 3-year experience with 98 infants of less than 700 g of birth weight. While overall mortality was 81%, resuscitation was attempted in only 45% of the infants. Survival among resuscitated infants was 43%. Morbidity among survivors was high and included bronchopulmonary dysplasia (70%), PDA (60%), septicemia (65%), necrotizing enterocolitis (10%), grade III or IV intraventricular hemorrhage (20%), and stage 3 or 4 retinopathy of prematurity (25%). Ninety-five percent of surviving infants demonstrated subnormal growth at term. Clearly, long-term follow-up is necessary, but these data illustrate that guidelines for resuscitation of extremely immature infants must be evaluated continually, particularly in the face of recent advances such as the use of artificial surfactant, which appears to reduce mortality while subsequent long-term neurologic morbidity among survivors is unknown.

The economic cost of providing tertiary care to the ELBW infant can be calculated, but it is not uniformly relevant to the perceived quality of life for the surviving infants and their parents. Moreover, in large public hospitals, distribution of personnel and services is severely affected, potentially affecting the care of more mature, more viable LBW infants.

## MANAGEMENT PRINCIPLES

The goal of intensive care medical practice is anticipatory management rather than crisis intervention. Each problem must be analyzed in terms of a history of illness, set of physical findings, differential diagnosis and assessment, and plan with contingencies for unexpected occurrences. Moreover, each problem must then be integrated into the sum of problems so that potentially conflicting assessments or interventions are avoided.

What causes an infant to be born prematurely? The origins of spontaneous premature labor are not well understood, and therapies designed to arrest premature labor have not been effective consistently. However, a number of infants are prematurely delivered for identifiable reasons. These include fetal factors such as uteroplacental insufficiency, fetal anemia, infection, or umbilical cord compression; and maternal factors such as preeclampsia, eclampsia, and placental separation.

TABLE 19-15.  Mortality and Major Neonatal Morbidity According to Birth Weight for the NICHD Neonatal Network

| | Weight (g) | | | |
|---|---|---|---|---|
| | *501–750* | *751–1000* | *1001–1250* | *1251–1500* |
| Survival (%) | 34 | 66 | 87 | 93 |
| Morbidity among survivors (%) | 56 | 39 | 25 | 15 |
| Chronic lung disease (%) | 26 | 14 | 7 | 3 |
| Intracranial hemorrhage (%) | 26 | 17 | 13 | 6 |
| Enterocolitis (%) | 3 | 8 | 6 | 4 |

*Adapted from Hack M, Horbar JD, Malloy MH, Tyson JE, Wright E, Wright L. Very-low-birth-weight outcomes of the National Institute of Child Health and Human Development Neonatal Network. Pediatrics 1991;87:585.*

A thorough maternal-fetal history may reveal preexisting conditions that will predict later pathophysiologic changes. These conditions must be identified, their logical outcomes predicted, and anticipatory surveillance or management instituted. The physical examination must include an assessment of gestational age in addition to the identification of abnormalities. The differential diagnosis and assessments should be complete and ranked according to the greatest likelihood of occurrence. Moreover, frequent follow-up assessments must be made and the priority ranking altered as indicated by new findings. The plan for intervention must focus on the primary cause of symptoms, the pathophysiology of the disease, and the risk-benefit ratio of each proposed intervention. Many therapies in the intensive care nursery are applied on presumptive grounds; only with appropriate surveillance can the physician be assured that the presumption was reasonable. Finally, the management plan must be flexible in such a manner that convenient dogma is not substituted for a more elusive but well-founded dialectic.

## Selected Readings

Bandstra ES, ed. Substance abuse in the perinatal period. Sem Perinatol 1991;15:263.

Bruck K. Neonatal thermal regulation. In: Polin RA, Fox WW, eds. Fetal and neonatal physiology, ed 1. Philadelphia: WB Saunders, 1992:488.
Butte NF. Energy requirements during infancy. In: Tsang RC, Nichols BL, eds. Nutrition during infancy, ed 1. Philadelphia: Hanley & Belfus, Inc., CV Mosby, 1988:86.
Cowett RM. Hypoglycemia and hyperglycemia in the newborn. In: Polin RA, Fox WW, eds. Fetal and neonatal physiology, ed 1. Philadelphia: WB Saunders, 1992:406.
Flynn JT. Retinopathy of prematurity. Pediatr Clin North Am 1987;34:1487.
Gerdes JS. Clinicopathologic approach to diagnosis of neonatal sepsis. Clin Perinatol 1992;18:361; Dis Child 1979;133:1119.
Green M. Parent care in the intensive care unit. Am J Dis Child 1979;133:1119.
Hack M, Fanaroff AA. Changes in the delivery-room care of the extremely small infant (<700 g). N Engl J Med 1986;314:660.
Hack M, Horbar JD, Malloy MH, Tyson JE, Wright E, Wright L. Very-low-birth-weight outcomes of the National Institute of Child Health and Human Development Neonatal Network. Pediatrics 1991;87:585.
Miller MJ, Marten RJ. Pathophysiology of apnea of prematurity. In: Polin RA, Fox WW, eds. Fetal and neonatal physiology, ed 1. Philadelphia: WB Saunders, 1992:872.
Nelson KB, Ellenberg JH. Neonatal signs as predictors of cerebral palsy. Pediatrics 1979;64:225.
Shaffer SG, Quimiro CL, Anderson JV, Hall RT. Postnatal weight changes in low-birth-weight infants. Pediatrics 1987;79:702.
Shaffer SG, Weisman DN. Fluid requirements in the preterm infant. Clin Perinatol 1992;19:233.
Ziegler EE, O'Donnell AM, Nelson SE, Fomon SJ. Body composition of the reference fetus. Growth 1976;40:329.

*Principles and Practice of Pediatrics, Second Edition.*
edited by Frank A. Oski et al. J. B. Lippincott Company, Philadelphia © 1994.

# 19.3 *Intrauterine Growth Retardation*

Joseph B. Warshaw

Intrauterine growth retardation (IUGR), or, preferably, intrauterine growth restriction, represents a final common pathway by which genetic and environmental influences result in low birth weight for gestational age. The diverse factors that influence fetal growth and may contribute to IUGR are reviewed in Chapter 16.2. IUGR has been defined most commonly in the United States as a birth weight of less than the 10th percentile for gestational age. This definition probably overestimates the incidence of IUGR, since it is unreasonable to consider 10% of all births as having pathologic restriction of growth. Small infants in whom there is no evidence that adverse genetic or environmental influences are limiting growth should be spared the IUGR label, which connotes pathology, and should be defined as small for gestational age (SGA). SGA should be applied to all infants less than the tenth percentile, and IUGR generally should be reserved for infants less than the third percentile, recognizing that some infants with growth restriction will fall out of this range if an insult occurs late in gestation. Thus, while all IUGR infants also are SGA, not all SGA infants are IUGR.

Confusion about definitions is amplified further by significant differences in the tenth percentile birth weights at each gestational age that have been published. Differences in published standards of growth have probably been influenced by racial composition, socioeconomic status of the population, and altitude above sea level when the standards were developed. The commonly used Lubchenco grids were developed in Denver, which is about 5000 feet above sea level, and may overestimate IUGR when these charts are used at sea level. What is necessary for an effective comparison between populations is the adoption of a single standard for fetal growth, for example the standards developed by Brenner from 30,772 deliveries from 21 to 44 weeks' gestational age in Cleveland. These standards include correction factors for poverty, race, and sex.

Recognition and treatment of IUGR requires an understanding of the diverse etiologies that result in restricted fetal growth. The pattern of growth of the infant with IUGR often reflects the underlying condition that has resulted in growth restriction. The terms *proportionate* and *disproportionate* have been used to distinguish newborns with decreased growth potential from those with restricted growth due to fetal malnutrition.

Newborns with decreased growth potential due to conditions such as chromosomal disorders, congenital infections, or exposure to environmental toxins characteristically have body proportions that are proportionate or symmetric; that is, the head, length, and weight generally occur within similar percentile grids, or the head is small relative to the body, as in microcephaly. Obstetric monitoring of the fetus with decreased growth potential characteristically demonstrates decreased body growth, including that of the head, from mid-gestation or earlier. Fetuses with decreased growth potential are at high risk for having major malformations or congenital infection.

Newborns with fetal malnutrition have weight reduced out of proportion to length or head circumference and may exhibit a sparing of head growth during late gestation. These infants are disproportionate, with the head circumference and length closer to the expected percentiles for gestational age than those for weight. Nutritional constraints on growth are unusual before 24 to 25 weeks of gestation; in most cases, only after that time will restriction in blood supply to the fetus result in IUGR. In mild to moderate degrees of IUGR, head growth may proceed along

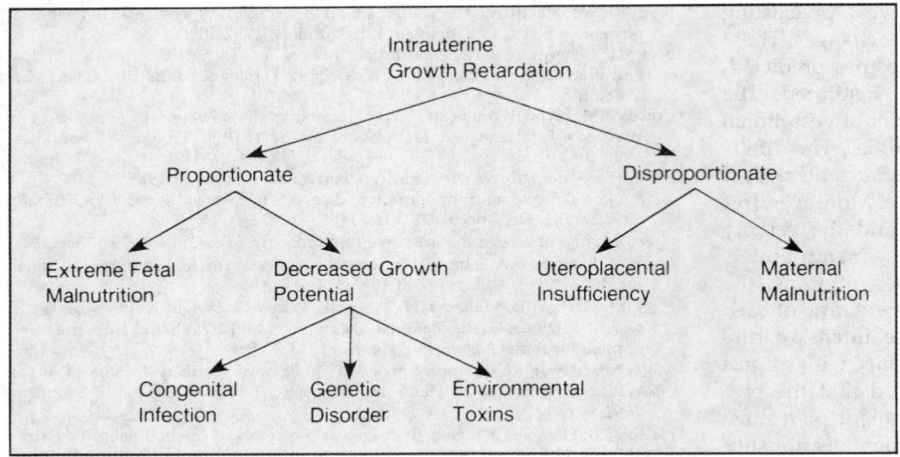

Figure 19-11. Classification of intrauterine growth retardation.

normal percentile grids, with a decrease in body fat and restriction in length and weight (disproportionate growth). This sparing of head growth is thought to result from circulatory changes in the fetus that favor a redistribution of blood flow to the heart and brain. There may be exceptions to this general pattern. In instances of extreme nutritional restriction in the fetus with class D diabetes or other conditions that result in severely compromised uterine blood flow, even head growth may be decreased.

Infants with either proportionate or disproportionate IUGR should be evaluated carefully for conditions causing hydrocephalus or microcephaly that may also confound the measurements. Figure 19-11 summarizes the etiology of IUGR. The importance of environmental exposures such as cigarette smoking can not be overestimated. In the developed countries of the world cigarette smoking is perhaps the single greatest determinant of low birth weight. It has been estimated that perinatal mortality would be reduced by 15% with elimination of all cigarette smoking in pregnancy.

The pattern of postnatal growth is also important to record and follow. As a consequence of decreased growth potential, infants with proportionate growth retardation may exhibit sluggish postnatal growth even with adequate nutrition. A slow rate of postnatal growth may be seen in genetic disorders, congenital infections, or the fetal alcohol syndrome. Infants with growth retardation secondary to fetal malnutrition often exhibit rapid growth when adequate nutrients are provided in the postnatal period; this is a good prognostic finding. About 30% of nutritionally induced IUGR newborns are still below the third percentile at 2 years of age.

## MANAGEMENT

Optimal management of IUGR should begin with recognition of the problem in utero so that informed decisions can be made concerning the appropriate time and method of delivery. This includes consideration of the options of cesarean section versus vaginal delivery. If biophysical data obtained during fetal monitoring show fetal distress, cesarean section may be the preferred mode of delivery. Decreased maternal weight gain and fundal growth should alert the obstetrician to the likelihood of fetal growth retardation. Ultrasonography can then confirm the diagnosis by monitoring such parameters of fetal growth as the biparietal diameter or the relationship of head size to body size.

Strategies to treat fetal growth retardation have included therapies to decrease the platelet aggregation and abnormalities in uteroplacental circulation seen in toxemia of pregnancy as well as maternal nutritional supplementation and oxygen therapy. In a promising study of 323 women at risk for fetal growth retardation, administration of 150 mg/day aspirin resulted in a 225-g newborn weight increase over the placebo group. The beneficial effect of low-dose aspirin probably related to inhibition of the synthesis of thromboxane $B_2$, which decreases the platelet aggregation and placental vasocclusion seen in the toxemic state.

Maternal parenteral nutritional supplementation is controversial. An adverse influence was observed when short-term administration of glucose to normal patients before delivery resulted in a significant increase in lactic acid and a fall in pH. When the fetus is "adapted" to a decreased nutrient supply, there may be a potential risk to increasing nutritional intake without a corresponding increase in fetal oxygenation. Indeed, several of the changes seen in IUGR can be considered adaptations to an adverse intrauterine nutritional environment: sparing of brain growth, increased red cell mass, and small size itself, in which the size of the fetus may be appropriate to the availability of nutrients. Even early lung maturation can be considered an adaptation that improves the opportunity for a good postnatal outcome.

Important problems of the infant with IUGR secondary to intrauterine malnutrition are summarized in Table 19-16. Appropriate management can prevent many of these problems (Table 19-17). If there is birth asphyxia, support measures should be instituted immediately, including the establishment of an effective airway and the management of meconium if present.

| TABLE 19-16.   Problems of the IUGR Newborn | |
| --- | --- |
| Birth asphyxia | Hypoglycemia |
| Meconium aspiration | Hypocalcemia |
| Persistent fetal circulation | Polycythemia |
| Hypothermia | Congenital malformation |

| TABLE 19-17.   Management of the IUGR Infant |
| --- |
| Gestational age assessment and careful history for drugs, etc |
| Prevent hypothermia |
| Check central hematocrit |
| Monitor blood sugar within first 45 min |
| Evaluate for congenital infections and congenital malformations |
| Chromosomal and genetic evaluation as indicated |
| Careful follow-up |

Suctioning and clearing the meconium from the airway before delivery of the thorax and establishing of the first breath, together with tracheal suction if meconium is present at the level of the cords, have greatly reduced problems associated with meconium aspiration. Meconium aspiration is rarely seen in infants of less than 35 weeks' gestation; therefore, in those infants, hypoxia per se is the major problem. An estimate of the degree of acidosis can be obtained from the cord blood pH. Hyaline membrane disease is generally less of a problem in infants with disproportionate IUGR because of the accelerated lung maturation commonly seen in these infants. Some asphyxiated newborns exhibit significant right-to-left cardiac shunting, making systemic oxygenation difficult to achieve. This is a consequence of chronic intrauterine hypoxia, which results in abnormal thickening of the smooth muscle of small pulmonary arterioles, thereby reducing pulmonary blood flow and increasing right-to-left blood flow at the atrial level or through the ductus arteriosus. Diagnosis is confirmed by measuring the disparity between preductal (right radial) and postductal (umbilical arterial) $PO_2$. Because acidosis and hypoxia modulate pulmonary arteriolar vasomotor tone, therapeutic efforts should be directed toward reversing these conditions. There is no clearly effective therapy, although some infants appear to improve with an induced respiratory alkalosis (pH 7.45 to 7.55). Tolazoline is often used to reduce pulmonary arterial pressure, but there is little evidence for its efficacy. Extracorporeal membrane oxygenation has had a surge in popularity in the treatment of this condition, but efficacy for this expensive and complex intervention has not been clearly established.

Apgar scores should be assigned in the delivery room, and the infant should be dried rapidly and warmed to prevent hypothermia. As soon as infant is stable, measurements should be taken and plotted on standard growth grids. As mentioned above, the Lubchenco charts are used in most institutions, although they may underestimate IUGR because the observations were made well above sea level and may have been influenced by racial and ethnic differences in the Denver population. Accurate measurements determine whether an IUGR newborn follows the disproportionate or proportionate pattern. Measurements include the standard growth parameters of weight, height, and head circumference. The *ponderal index* ([weight in grams × 100]/[length in cm³]) has also been used to identify infants with decreased weight relative to length; however, applications of standard measurements of length, weight, and head circumference to standard growth grids are generally more useful.

A careful assessment of gestational age should be done in all infants with IUGR. The examination most commonly used is a modification of a scale developed by Dubowitz that includes physical signs involving skin color and texture, hair, breast size, plantar creases, ear form and firmness, external genitalia, and neuromuscular assessment, which measures tone, posture, and reflexes. Scores are assigned for these measures, with a total score being used to assign gestational age. This examination can be completed in about 10 minutes and has a predictive error of plus or minus 2 weeks in infants weighing more than 1000 g. It is most accurate when performed within the first 6 hours of life and by two observers.

Newborns with IUGR secondary to fetal malnutrition (eg, those with decreased uteroplacental blood flow) are disproportionate, with the head and length generally in higher percentiles than the weight. These infants frequently appear scrawny as a result of their marked decrease in subcutaneous fat. They have an alert appearance and have higher Dubowitz ratings than do premature infants with similar weights.

Infants should be examined for genetic causes of IUGR, including the presence of congenital malformations. They should also be evaluated for any stigmata of congenital infection. The examination should include weighing and examining the placenta to determine whether there are structural or vascular abnormalities contributing to IUGR.

Many of the problems of IUGR newborns relate to their markedly decreased metabolic reserves. There is a risk of perinatal asphyxia when oxygen and metabolic demands exceed the oxygen provided by the uteroplacental circulation. This underscores the need for careful biophysical monitoring of the at-risk fetus to alert the obstetrician to the presence of uteroplacental insufficiency. Hypoglycemia is found frequently in the immediate postnatal period. Hypothermia may increase oxygen and glucose requirements. Blood glucose should be measured, and a central hematocrit test should be performed to detect polycythemia. Hyperviscosity and hypoglycemia are primarily problems of the nutritionally growth-retarded newborn. Those with IUGR secondary to congenital infection, genetic disorders, or environmental insults are less likely to experience these complications.

Hypoglycemia is best treated by early recognition and prevention. All infants with IUGR should be tested with Dextrostix within the first 30 to 45 minutes of life. These infants are at risk for hypoglycemia because of decreased fuel stores secondary to their fetal malnourished state, decreased gluconeogenesis, and an increase in the peripheral use of glucose due to polycythemia and cold stress. The best treatment for hypoglycemia is prevention by early feeding. Treatment of hypoglycemia is discussed in Chapter 20.8.

Hypocalcemia may also occur in the IUGR newborn, generally in association with neonatal stress. Only rarely do infants require a regimen of parenteral calcium, and this should be given with constant monitoring and with good venous access to avoid skin sloughing.

Hyperviscosity secondary to polycythemia in infants with IUGR can result in venous thrombosis and CNS injury and can also contribute to hypoglycemia. Polycythemia results from increased erythropoietin levels secondary to relative fetal hypoxia. Because blood viscosity sharply increases when the central hematocrit exceeds 65%, partial exchange transfusion should be considered in IUGR infants when the hematocrit exceeds that level.

There is some controversy concerning whether partial exchange transfusion should be done in asymptomatic polycythemic infants. Infants treated with partial exchange transfusion may have fewer neurologic problems than those not transfused. The symptoms of polycythemia include respiratory distress, plethora, cardiac failure, and neurologic signs, including jitteriness and seizures. Partial exchange transfusion is done using normal saline or 5% salt-poor albumin to replace blood that is removed. This is preferable to plasma because of the high viscosity due to adult fibrinogen in plasma. The formula used to calculate the amount of blood to be withdrawn (V) in a partial exchange transfusion is as follows: V = estimated blood volume × ([actual hematocrit − the desired hematocrit]/the actual hematocrit).

## NEWBORN OUTCOME

The most important aspect of IUGR is neurodevelopmental outcome, and this depends in large part on etiology. Infants with IUGR secondary to environmental insult or decreased growth potential generally have outcomes that are poor and reflect the underlying neuropathology of conditions caused by the environmental or genetic insult.

Generally, infants in whom brain growth has been spared have more favorable outcomes. Even those infants in whom there has been a decrease in intrauterine brain growth may show significant postnatal catch-up. The vast majority of full-term IUGR infants are of normal intelligence. Outcome is more difficult to predict in IUGR preterm infants, who appear to have a higher incidence of handicap than that of the general population. More extensive follow-up with these infants is required when they reach school age. The performance levels they achieve may be influenced by social class, with children from higher social classes scoring better on standard IQ tests and school achievement evaluations. The outlook for most infants with nutritional IUGR is favorable if the postnatal environment is adequate. Most IUGR infants, whether premature or full-term, achieve normal intelligence by 5 to 6 years of age, although there may be a risk for subtle deficits such as school problems and learning disability. Modern neonatal care has prevented death and much of the morbidity historically associated with IUGR.

Infants with IUGR with major genetic or chromosomal disorders—trisomy 18 or trisomy 13, for example—have virtually a 100% incidence of severe handicap and death, whereas outcome in those with congenital infection appears to be more variable. More than 75% of infants with congenital rubella infection will have a mental handicap requiring special education. They may also have learning deficits and disturbances associated with hearing loss or blindness. Infants with cytomegalovirus infection may have only minor or no sequelae, whereas those who present with microcephaly or significant growth retardation generally have poor outcomes, with handicap rates generally exceeding 50%. It is important to test for hearing loss in all infants diagnosed with cytomegalovirus disease.

When evaluating outcome of newborns exposed to pharmacologic agents, it may be difficult to dissociate the effect of the primary disease state from that of the medication. It is clear, however, that many drugs are associated with poor outcomes. The fetal alcohol syndrome, for example, is associated with slow postnatal growth and poor developmental outcome. Prenatal cocaine exposure has been associated with IUGR and microcephaly. Exposures to therapeutic agents such as phenytoin, warfarin sodium, and narcotics may result in IUGR, slow postnatal growth, and a spectrum of developmental disabilities. Infants with these conditions require thorough and thoughtful evaluation, including appropriate counseling with the family.

## Selected Readings

Allen MC. Developmental outcome and follow-up of the small-for-gestational-age infant. Semin Perinatol 1984;8:123.

Black VD, Lubchenco LO, Koops BL, et al. Neonatal hyperviscosity: randomized study of effect of partial plasma exchange transfusion on long-term outcome. Pediatrics 1985;75:1048.

Brenner WE, Edelman DA, Hendricks CH. A standard for fetal growth for the United States of America. Am J Obstet Gynecol 1976;126:555.

Dubowitz LM, Dubowitz V, Goldberg C. Clinical assessment of gestational age in the newborn infant. J Pediatr 1970;77:1.

Gewolb IH, Warshaw JB. Influences on fetal growth. In Warshaw JB, ed. The biological basis of reproductive and developmental medicine. New York: Elsevier, 1983:364.

Lubchenco LO, Hansman C, Dressler M, et al. Intrauterine growth as estimated from liveborn birth-weight data at 24 to 42 weeks of gestation. Pediatrics 1963;32:793.

Stein ZA, Susser M. Intrauterine growth retardation: epidemiological issues and public health significance. Semin Perinatol 1984;8:5.

Uzan S, Beaufils M, Breart G, Brazen B. Prevention of fetal growth retardation with low-dose aspirin: findings of the EPREDA trial. Lancet 1991;337:1427.

Warshaw JB. Intrauterine growth restriction revisited. Growth, Genetics and Hormones 1992;8:5.

*Principles and Practice of Pediatrics, Second Edition.*
edited by Frank A. Oski et al. J. B. Lippincott Company, Philadelphia © 1994.

# 19.4 *Follow-Up of Infants Discharged From Newborn Intensive Care*

David T. Scott and Jon E. Tyson

Some of the first newborn follow-up programs were questionnaire surveys undertaken in Europe in the second decade of this century. In these surveys, community physicians were asked to rate the growth and development of their low–birth-weight patients (Scott and Spiker, 1989). Not surprisingly, perhaps, these surveys did little to clarify the long-term prognosis of these infants (Benton, 1940). Fortunately, by the 1950s and 1960s, there had been significant advances in some of the methods available to investigators in this area; for instance, a few studies attempted to construct population-based samples, and more and more studies began to use some standardized assessments. With the advent of newborn intensive care units in the early 1960s, the population of low–birth-weight survivors began to grow, and follow-up programs began to be offered as a clinical service to address the special needs of such children.

The need for follow-up programs for high-risk newborns has now been widely accepted. However, there has been little discussion of the multiple (and sometimes competing) purposes of these programs, which have included providing comprehensive and specialized care for high-risk survivors, monitoring rates of handicap among infants discharged from intensive care units, and answering specific research questions.

In designing a follow-up program, a careful delineation of its specific purposes is central. Such a delineation will inform decisions about such issues as patient selection, the frequency of visits, the evaluation methods used, the interventions used, the communication with parents and community physicians, the duration of follow-up, and the funding of the program.

Two contrasting approaches to follow-up are outlined in Table 19-18. The *clinical service model* is designed to provide individualized medical care to high-risk survivors. This approach has the advantages of flexibility, efficiency, and orientation to patient needs. Although widely used, this approach is unlikely to provide unbiased estimates of the prevalence of health and development problems in surviving high-risk infants—information with considerable relevance for health policy. In contrast, the *epidemiologic model* is designed primarily to assess the effects of perinatal problems and therapies on various outcomes. However, this approach is labor-intensive and expensive because of the effort required to recruit, transport, and reimburse patients, to hire and train staff, and to maintain the calibration of the outcome assessments.

For most follow-up programs, some synthesis of the clinical service and epidemiologic approaches is needed to ensure that both follow-up care and outcome assessments are of high quality. Some of the outcome measures (eg, developmental assessments

## TABLE 19-18. Contrasting Approaches in Newborn Follow-up Programs

| Domain | Clinical Service Model | Epidemiologic Model |
|---|---|---|
| Initial identification of cases | "Convenience" samples (eg, all cases from one institution) | Population-based samples |
| Case selection | Composite clinical judgment of degree of risk | Fixed, objective criteria (eg, birth weight) |
| Recruitment | Samples often shaped by access factors (eg, distance from institution, access to telephone) | Great effort made to control differential loss of hard-to-follow patients in population |
| Frequency of visits | Often adjusted to fit severity of history/findings | Usually a fixed schedule of required visits with provision for extra visits if clinically indicated |
| Control/comparison groups | Only cases followed | Controls or some other comparison group also followed |
| Blinding of assessors | Assessor knowledgeable about neonatal course and prior follow-up findings | Assessor deliberately blinded to neonatal history and prior follow-up findings |
| Assessment reliability | Little attention to standardizing assessments and verifying reliability | Considerable attention to standardizing assessments and verifying reliability |
| Staffing | Clinician often serving as caregiver and evaluator; ideally, the same clinician for serial visits to facilitate rapport and familiarity | Ideally, a different evaluator at each visit to avoid examiner bias |
| Surveillance procedures | Procedures adapted to patient's clinical history and current clinical problems | Typically, a fixed battery of assessment procedures, focused on outcomes of greatest interest |
| Treatments/interventions | Variable treatments based on clinical judgment | Restricted treatment options to avoid altering phenomena under study |
| Communication with parents | Unrestricted and designed to increase understanding | Restricted to avoid self-fulfilling prophecies, "teaching to test," loss of blindness, etc. |
| Duration of follow-up | Patients often discharged when considered healthy or normal | Special efforts made to retain all patients throughout predefined evaluation period |
| Financial arrangements | Typically, fee-for-service; patient provides own transportation | Patients often reimbursed for expenses or paid for time; transportation often provided |

at specific age points) should be assessed by personnel carefully trained and blinded to previous findings. To reduce the likelihood that examiner expectations for high-risk infants would influence the evaluations, it is desirable for the examiners to know that some control infants (eg, healthy infants born at term) will be included for calibration purposes. At the same time, health care should be given on a schedule determined by patient needs, and it should be provided by personnel who are familiar with perinatal and follow-up findings and who have good rapport with the family. Whenever feasible, follow-up should be provided for infants with any of the neonatal problems listed in Table 19-19.

For infants followed by pediatricians skilled in the management of disorders such as bronchopulmonary dypslasia, short-gut syndrome, and the sequelae of intracranial hemorrhage and hypoxic-ischemic encephalopathy, follow-up clinics may need to provide no more than neurologic examinations and standardized developmental assessments. However, indigent populations have the most limited access to health care and the highest prevalence of neurodevelopmental morbidity; in such populations, the provision of primary medical care in the follow-up clinic may facilitate the management of health problems and help to reduce attrition. The prevalence of handicap becomes difficult to estimate if more than 10% to 20% of patients are lost to follow-up. The fact that traditional follow-up programs are not designed to provide comprehensive health care partly accounts for the uncertainty about the outcome of infants who are both medically at risk and socially disadvantaged.

## MEDICAL EVALUATION AND CARE

Routine medical care for high-risk infants includes administration of immunizations and evaluation of growth, vision, and hearing. Immunizations for preterm infants should be given at the same postnatal age as for term infants. Growth is assessed in much the same manner as for full-term infants, except that more stable growth trajectories—and better predictions of later growth status—are generally obtained by plotting growth measures on a postterm ("corrected") age scale. The American Academy of Pediatrics recommends that vision examinations be provided to all premature infants who receive oxygen therapy. If no retinopathy has been identified, periodic eye examinations should be done until the retina is mature (usually by 2 to 3 months after term); if retinopathy has been identified, eye examinations should continue until the disease process is stable or resolving. There are several indications for routine hearing screening in this population (Table 19-20). Screening for hearing loss may be based on behavioral or electrophysiologic responses to sound. Methods to assess behavioral responses to sound are relatively easy and inexpensive but are less accurate than assessment of auditory evoked electrophysiologic responses.

High-risk infants may be discharged from neonatal units with difficult unresolved medical problems. Methods of treatment or

## TABLE 19-19. Some Indications for Newborn Follow-Up Referral

Birth weight 1250 g or less
Treatment with mechanical ventilation for 12 hours or longer
Bronchopulmonary dysplasia
Recurrent apneic episodes at or beyond 38 weeks' postconceptional age
Grades 2 to 4 intraventricular hemorrhage, intracerebral lesions or ventriculomegaly by sonogram or CT
Seizures or persistent neurologic abnormality
Meningitis
Cystic white-matter disease
One or more major congenital anomalies
Any problem requiring major surgery in the neonatal period

TABLE 19-20.  Some Indications
for Audiologic Evaluation

Birth weight less than 1500 g
Potentially toxic levels of bilirubin
Congenital malformations involving the external ear, palate, face, or skull
Congenital nonbacterial infections
Meningitis
Prolonged administration of aminoglycosides or other ototoxic drugs
Family history of hearing loss

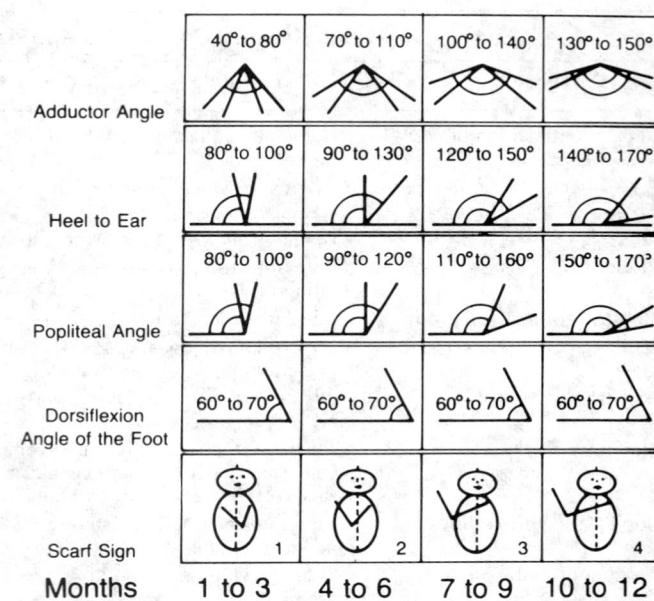

Figure 19-12.   Normal pattern of passive tone within first year of life. *Adductor angle:* the infant is supine. The legs are opened as far as possible by the examiner. The angle formed by the legs is measured. *Heel to ear:* the infant is supine. The buttocks are kept on the table. The legs are kept straight and the feet moved toward the ears. When there is resistance to the movement, the angle formed from the table surface to the legs is measured. *Popliteal angle:* the infant is supine. The buttocks are kept on the table. The legs are flexed to either side of the abdomen until there is resistance. Then the legs are extended. When there is resistance to this movement, the angle formed between the lower and the upper leg is measured. *Dorsiflexion angle of the foot:* the foot is flexed, and the angle between the foot and the leg is measured. *Scarf sign:* the infant is supine. The examiner takes one of the infant's hands and pulls the arm across the infant's chest until there is resistance. The position of the elbow is noted. (From Ellison P. Clin Perinatol 1984;11: 45. Adapted from Amiel-Tison C. Curr Probl Pediatr 1976;7:1.)

management that have been recommended for these problems include various anticonvulsant regimens for infants with recurrent seizures; a variety of specialized programs for infants with sensory or motor handicaps; bronchodilators, diuretics, physiotherapy, high-calorie feedings, and oxygen for infants with bronchopulmonary dysplasia; apnea monitors and theophylline for infants who have recurrent apneic episodes before nursery discharge; concentrated feedings or nutritional supplements for infants with growth failure; special formulas and parenteral nutrition at home for infants with severe short-gut syndrome; and bethanechol or fundal plication for infants with gastroesophageal reflux.

The pathophysiology and treatment of the difficult ongoing problems of high-risk survivors are complex, and a detailed discussion is beyond the scope of this chapter. The reader is referred to several reviews listed under Selected Readings (those by Hunt; Swanson and Berserth; Taeusch and Yogman; and Ballard). All the treatment methods noted above have potential hazards; only a few have been evaluated in controlled studies of discharged preterm infants. Thus, the indications for these treatments remain controversial. Whenever possible, their use should be carefully monitored by physicians with specialized experience.

## NEUROLOGIC ASSESSMENTS

Several methods of neurologic assessment have been described, both for the neonatal period (Volpe, 1987) and for the ensuing months (Ellison, 1984). The method most familiar to practicing physicians focuses on infant reflexes and posture. However, this method may not be adequate for early identification of subtle findings. The method of Milani-Comparetti and Gidoni emphasizes vestibular function and body posture. This method includes 27 assessments that are relatively time-consuming; many of these items are more familiar to physical therapists than to physicians. A method based on primitive reflexes has also been advocated.

Amiel-Tison has described a method for assessing neurologic status during the first year that is an extension of the neurologic items used in assessing gestational age in the neonatal period (eg, assessment of heel-to-ear maneuver, popliteal angle, dorsiflexion angle of the foot) (Fig 19-12). Ellison has recommended the Amiel-Tison method because of its familiarity to physicians, as well as its simplicity, reliability, and accuracy in distinguishing among normal, transiently abnormal, and abnormal children between 6 and 22 months of age. However, like other methods of neurologic assessment, this method has not been demonstrated to have high accuracy in predicting later handicap.

A low predictive accuracy for classic neurologic assessments in infancy was noted in the National Collaborative Perinatal Project (NCPP). The neurologic findings at 4 months were reported for children who had cerebral palsy at 7 years (Nelson and Ellenberg, 1982). At 4 months of age, only 33% of children with

cerebral palsy were classified as having an abnormal neurologic examination; 31% were regarded as neurologically suspect and 36% as normal at 4 months. Early neurologic examinations lack specificity as well as sensitivity. Many infants with suspect or mild neurologic findings (eg, mild hypotonia, mild hypertonia of the legs) subsequently become normal. This has led some follow-up investigators to describe a "transient dystonia" that appears and then resolves spontaneously during the first year (eg, Drillien and Drummond, 1977). However, in the NCPP sample, 84% of infants with moderate or severe quadriplegia at 1 year and 87% of those with moderate or severe hemiparesis at 1 year were classified as having cerebral palsy at 7 years.

A group of British investigators have developed a standard form for describing childhood motor deficits of central origin (Evans, 1989; Stewart, 1989). According to the former study, this record-keeping instrument was devised to "allow comparisons between areas and countries where registers of children with cerebral palsy are kept and to permit the grouping of children with similar deficits for research into aetiology and the effectiveness of interventions."

The causes of childhood handicapping conditions are often difficult to determine with certainty. There has been a tendency to attribute these conditions to perinatal complications. However, some investigators have reported an increased incidence of minor congenital anomalies and other dysmorphic features among handicapped children identified in population-based screening programs (Drillien, 1988). Such findings suggest that both perinatal complications and subsequent handicapping conditions may in some cases be consequences of antecedent biological abnormalities early in pregnancy.

## DEVELOPMENTAL ASSESSMENTS

The best-standardized infant development test is the Bayley Scales of Infant Development (Bayley, 1969). The Bayley Mental Scale includes 163 items, the Bayley Motor Scale 81 items. Both scales have items that nominally cover the age range from the first months of life up to about 2.5 years. The Bayley is the product of decades of refinement and restandardization. The current version includes norms based on a stratified national standardization sample of 1262 infants. A revision and restandardization of the Bayley is expected in 1993.

The Bayley scales each generate an age equivalent and a developmental index. The age equivalent is simply the age for which a given level of performance would be typical (ie, 50th percentile). The mental index and the motor index are standardized scores that are distributed in the same manner as scores for IQ, with a mean of 100 and a standard deviation of 16 in the general population. These indices permit comparison of a given infant with other infants of the same age. When evaluating a premature infant, many developmental clinicians now use the infant's "postterm" or "corrected" age (ie, the age computed from the child's due date), so that the comparison will be with other infants of the same biological (postconceptional) age.

Interpreting the Bayley index requires caution. In general, pairwise differences smaller than seven or eight points may arise from measurement error. In a high-risk sample, the product-moment correlation between the Bayley Mental Index and subsequent IQ (during the preschool years) is often about 0.5; this suggests that only about a quarter of the variance in preschool IQ is associated with variance in the Bayley Mental Index. Bayley indices obtained at either end of the test's age range (below about 4 months or above about 22 months) may be distorted to some degree by "basal" or "ceiling" constraints, respectively; that is, there may be too few items at the bottom and top of the test to document the full range of individual differences at those functional levels.

There is some variation among clinicians in the descriptive labels used to describe Bayley indices. An example of one set of such descriptive labels is provided in Table 19-21.

## ADDITIONAL METHODOLOGIC ISSUES

Several special methodologic issues should be considered in designing a follow-up protocol. Many of these issues affect outcome assessments in general, but they are especially salient for standardized assessments.

### TABLE 19-21. Example of Descriptive Labels for the Bayley Index

| Bayley Index | Descriptive Label |
|---|---|
| 110 or higher | Above average; ahead of schedule |
| 90 to 109 | Average; on schedule |
| 80 to 89 | Low normal |
| 70 to 79 | Borderline; gray zone |
| 60 to 69 | Developmental delay: mild to moderate |
| Below 60 | Developmental delay: moderate to severe |

## Demographic Issues

Follow-up studies have often been more careful in describing their samples' medical characteristics than their demographic characteristics. However, there is impressive heterogeneity in the environments into which high-risk children are discharged, and a vast literature documents the sensitivity of many of the commonly used outcome measures to environmental influences. There is some evidence that the sequelae of neonatal events are ordinarily more easily documented in the first or second year after discharge, after which time the effects of environmental factors often begin to obscure the effects of mild to moderate neonatal insults (Aylward, 1992).

## Blinded Assessments

Follow-up clinics based mainly on the clinical service model have often not used blinded assessments. However, there are many ambiguities inherent in the clinical assessment of children, particularly in the first year of life. The best way to ensure that outcome assessments have not been contaminated by self-fulfilling prophecies and other such biases is to keep certain follow-up personnel deliberately uninformed about the child's medical and social history.

## Calibration of Standardized Assessments

It has proven surprisingly difficult to compare follow-up data from different institutions, in part because of growing evidence that interexaminer calibration is more difficult to achieve and to maintain than has previously been acknowledged. There is recurring evidence that Bayley scores are often inflated, especially during the first year of life. In multisite studies that have taken a rigorous approach to reliability training, these inflated scores have often been associated with unwitting liberalizations of administration and scoring procedures. In some cases, Bayley scores have been inflated by half a standard deviation or more. In some clinical trials, the magnitude of the initial calibration error has been larger than the treatment effects that the trials were designed to detect.

## Developmental Instrumentation

Despite some recent additions to the array of neurodevelopmental instrumentation, the array of options remains relatively constrained for the first 3 years of life. Some of the methods that rely on visual attention or on habituation paradigms seem better suited for the laboratory than for the clinic, in that a substantial minority of infants may fail to meet the behavioral requirements of the procedure. On the other hand, several clinical assessment packages are now being used in "Birth to Three" programs developed in response to federal legislation. Some of these clinical instruments attempt to evaluate the child's developmental status in a dozen or more subdomains (eg, fine motor, social, speech). However, there is some psychometric evidence that early development may simply be too undifferentiated to permit reliable and valid assessment in numerous subdomains; scores purporting to represent such subdomains may in reality be only unreliable estimates of some broader common factor.

## Age Range

Some early newborn follow-up programs followed children until they were only 6 months or 1 year old. Conditions that are moderate to severe in degree can often be identified in the first year of life, but subtle and mild conditions often do not become apparent until later. We recommend that follow-up assessments continue until at least 18 months postterm age, in part to allow some opportunity to assess early language. Although sequelae such as learning disabilities cannot be identified with confidence until the early school years, it is often not feasible to extend routine follow-up to that extent.

## Choice of an Age Scale

Early follow-up studies often calculated the age of premature children from the date of their premature birth. Thus, premature children were compared to full-term children who were the same postnatal age but a more advanced postconceptional age. Not surprisingly, the full-term children were almost always taller, heavier, and further along developmentally. It was unclear whether the "delays" seen among the premature children were the genuine sequelae of prematurity and its complications or only the effects of the difference in postconceptional age. Other early studies attempted to put the premature children on the same biological footing as the full-term controls by calculating age from the child's due date. The age calculated from the due date has been called the real age, the postterm age, or the corrected age; the last of these terms is now the most common.

Although the use of the postterm age for premature children has gained ever-wider acceptance, there remains some controversy about the age range over which it should be used. In some early studies in which the degree of prematurity was modest and the samples were small, the use of the postterm age did not seem to make a significant difference after some age, and the investigators thus changed from the corrected-age scale to the chronologic-age scale after that point. However, as more survivors were studied with greater and greater degrees of prematurity, the effects of using the corrected versus the chronologic age could be seen at progressively later ages. Indeed, for a child born 3 months prematurely, the Wechsler IQ using the chronologic age is often five or six points lower than the Wechsler IQ using the corrected age; an effect of this size is not negligible. For this reason, some investigators now use the postterm age indefinitely.

## NEUROLOGIC AND DEVELOPMENTAL INTERVENTIONS

Therapies such as early physical therapy have been used in an attempt to prevent or ameliorate neurologic handicaps, but the few clinical trials in this area to date have not found much evidence to suggest that these interventions are effective (Piper, 1986; Palmer, 1988), at least not with respect to the limited range of outcome measures that have been used.

Since the early 1960s, several early intervention programs have been developed in an effort to facilitate normal development in socioeconomically disadvantaged children, in whom the incidence of developmental delays is often increased. A consolidated late follow-up of the children from several of these early intervention programs for the disadvantaged found evidence for "long-lasting effects in four areas: school competence, developed abilities, children's attitudes and values, and impact on the family" (Lazar and Darlington, 1982).

Unfortunately, there has been less evidence with which to assess the possible benefits of such interventions for children who are biologically at risk. Ferry (1981) found no persuasive evidence at that time that these programs were effective, largely because most of the early studies in this area were plagued by methodologic limitations (eg, nonrandomized designs).

A well-controlled multisite randomized clinical trial—the Infant Health and Development Program (IHDP)—has now been undertaken. At each of eight clinical sites, premature, low-birth-weight children were randomly assigned either to a follow-up group or to an intervention group. Children in the follow-up group received medical follow-up care and blinded developmental evaluations; children in the intervention group received these same follow-up services and a broad-spectrum early intervention program for the infants and their families.

At 3 years postterm age, there were differences in each of the three IHDP outcome domains. In the cognitive domain, there were large IQ effects: among children with birth weights between 2001 and 2500 g, intervention children exhibited a cognitive advantage of 13.2 IQ points; among children with birth weights of 2000 g or less, the IQ advantage was 6.6 points. Secondary analyses suggested that the IQ effects were largest for children from disadvantaged families. In the behavioral domain, there was a small but significant tendency for the mothers of intervention children to report fewer behavior problems than the mothers of follow-up children. In the health domain, mothers of children with birth weights of 2000 g or less reported more illnesses and health conditions for intervention children than for follow-up children; there were no differences on a measure of serious health conditions, however.

The IHDP sample has been followed beyond age 3, when the intervention ended. Additional findings from the early school years are expected in 1993 and 1994.

## RESULTS OF FOLLOW-UP STUDIES OF VERY-LOW-BIRTH-WEIGHT INFANTS

Parents, physicians, health economists, and others have worried that the increased survival of ever-smaller premature infants may increase the number of handicapped children. Many studies have compared recent survivors with those during the late 1940s to mid-1960s. However, neonatal outcome during these years was compromised by iatrogenic disease due to a variety of causes, such as misuse of oxygen, chloramphenicol, sulfonamide, and vitamin K (see Chapter 20.15.4). There is some evidence that before these years, low–birth-weight infants who did survive had a relatively low incidence of handicap that is unlikely to be equaled with the high survival rates in modern neonatal units. In the study of the 1946 British national cohort (all legitimate single births with a birth weight of less than 2000 g born in England during the first week of March 1946), the average IQ and the proportion of survivors who were handicapped at age 15 years were similar to those of matched children born at term (Douglas and Gear, 1976). However, no infants with birth weights below 1000 g had survived, compared with survival rates of 20% to 50% in recent population-based studies.

The incidence of handicap reported in recent years, although not so low as that noted for the 1946 cohort, has been lower than those reported in most follow-up studies before the introduction of intensive care. However, most of these studies have come from follow-up clinics based on a clinical service model, and their findings are thus difficult to interpret (Tyson and Swanson, 1987). The absence of blinded evaluations and control infants may allow the biases of even the most objective and careful examiners to influence the findings inadvertently. Moreover, most follow-up studies include small numbers of infants in the lowest birth weight categories. Studies from referral centers may be affected by a variety of selection biases that may influence the neonatal referrals (including death of the smallest and sickest infants before transfer can be arranged).

Two of the best follow-up studies evaluated whether the percentage of handicapped survivors in geographically defined areas changed as mortality diminished with increasing use of perinatal intensive care. The study of Shapiro and colleagues (1983) evaluated infants born in eight geographic areas during two periods (1976 and 1978–79) when neonatal mortality decreased by 18%.

A similar incidence of severe handicap at 1 year among infants of less than 1500 g (14.2% versus 12.3%) was observed. Saigal and colleagues (1984, 1989, 1990) evaluated the outcomes of infants of less than 1000 g birth weight in the same region during several time periods. Although the survival rate doubled, there was no increase in the proportion of functionally handicapped survivors.

In a population-based study in Australia, Kitchen and colleagues (1987) followed extremely-low-birth-weight children (birth weights 500 to 999 g) born in 1979 and 1980. Among those seen at 5.5 years corrected age, 72% were free of functional handicap; mild handicaps were found in 4%, moderate handicaps in 5%, and severe handicaps in 19%. Of the 89 survivors, 72 underwent standardized testing with the Wechsler Preschool and Primary Scale of Intelligence. (Of the 89 survivors, 17 children [19%] were not fully tested because of a sensory, motor, or marked mental handicap.) Among the nonhandicapped inborn children, the mean full scale IQ was 103.0; among nonhandicapped outborn children, the mean full scale IQ was 96.5. However, the authors acknowledged that these values would probably have been considerably lower if IQs had been available for the 17 handicapped children who were not fully evaluated.

Thus, at least during recent years, the increase in survival of small premature infants seems to have been accompanied by approximately the same percentage of survivors who are handicapped. While this finding is encouraging, it should be remembered that because there are more survivors, the absolute total number of handicapped survivors is likely to have increased. This conclusion is supported by the finding of a somewhat increased percentage of children with handicaps in large population studies that include children of any birth weight (Hagberg, 1982).

## Selected Readings

Aylward GP. The relationship between environmental risk and developmental outcome. J Dev Behav Pediatr 1992;13:222.

Ballard RA. Pediatric care of the ICN graduate. Philadelphia: WB Saunders, 1988.

Bayley N. Bayley scales of infant development. New York: The Psychological Corporation, 1969.

Benton A. Mental development of prematurely born children: a critical review of the literature. Am J Orthopsychiatry 1940;10:719.

Douglas J, Gear R. Children of low birth weight in the 1946 cohort. Arch Dis Child 1976;51:580.

Drillien CM. The growth and development of the prematurely born infant. Edinburgh: E & S Livingstone, 1964.

Drillien CM. Causes of handicap and impairment in a total population of Dundee (Scotland) children aged 8 weeks to 7 years. In: Kubli F, Patel N, Schmidt W, Linderkamp O, eds. Perinatal events and brain damage in surviving children. Berlin/Heidelberg: Springer-Verlag, 1988.

Drillien CM, Drummond MB. Neurodevelopmental problems in early childhood. Oxford: Blackwell Scientific Publications, 1977.

Ellison P. Neurologic development of the high-risk infant. Clin Perinatol 1984;11:41.

Evans P. A standard form for recording clinical findings in children with a motor deficit of central origin. Dev Med Child Neurol 1989;31:119.

Ferry PC. On growing new neurons: are early intervention programs effective? Pediatrics 1981;67:38.

Fitzhardinge PM, Flodmark O, Fitz CR, Ashby S. The prognostic value of computed tomography of the brain in asphyxiated premature infants. J Pediatr 1982;100:476.

Hagberg B, Hagberg H, Olow I. Gains and hazards of intensive neonatal care: an analysis from Swedish cerebral palsy epidemiology. Dev Med Child Neurol 1982;24:13.

Hunt H. Continuing care of the high-risk infant. Clin Perinatol 1984;11:3.

Infant Health and Development Program. Enhancing the outcomes of low-birth-weight, premature infants. JAMA 1990;263:3035.

Kitchen W, Ford G, Orgill A, et al. Outcome in infants with birth weights 500 to 999 grams: a continuing regional study of 5-year-old survivors. J Pediatr 1987;111:761.

Lazar I, Darlington R. Lasting effects of early education: a report from the Consortium for Longitudinal Studies. Monogr Soc Res Child Dev 1982;47 (2–3, Serial No. 195).

Nelson K, Ellenberg J. Children who "outgrew" cerebral palsy. Pediatrics 1982;69:536.

Palmer FB, et al. The effects of physical therapy on cerebral palsy: a controlled trial in infants with spastic diplegia. N Engl J Med 1988;319:796.

Piper MC, Kunos VI, et al. Early physical therapy effects on the high-risk infant: a randomized controlled trial. Pediatrics 1986;78:216.

Saigal S, Rosenbaum P, Stoskopf B, Sinclair J. Outcome in infants 501 to 1000 g birth weight delivered to residents of the McMaster Health Region. J Pediatr 1984;105:969.

Saigal S, Rosenbaum P, Hattersley B, Milner R. Decreased disability rate among 3-year-old survivors weighing 501 to 1000 grams at birth and born to residents of a geographically defined region from 1981 to 1984 compared with 1977 to 1980. J Pediatr 1989;114:839.

Saigal S, Szatmari P, Rosenbaum P, Campbell D. Intellectual and functional status at school entry of children who weighed 1000 grams or less at birth: a regional perspective of birth in the 1980s. J Pediatr 1990;116:409.

Scott DT, Spiker D. Research on the sequelae of prematurity: early learning, early interventions, and later outcomes. Semin Perinatol 1989;13:495.

Shapiro S, McCormick M, Starfield B, Crawley B. Changes in infant morbidity associated with decrease in neonatal mortality. Pediatrics 1983;72:408.

Stewart A. Standard recording of central motor deficit. Dev Med Child Neurol 1989;31:120.

Swanson J, Berserth C. Continuing care for the preterm infant after dismissal from the neonatal intensive care unit. Mayo Clin Proc 1987;62:613.

Taeusch HW, Yogman MW. Follow-up management of the high-risk infant. Boston: Little, Brown & Co, 1987.

Tyson J, Swanson M. Problems of neonatal follow-up programs in the United States. Proceedings of the Seventh Canadian Ross Conference in Pediatrics, 1987.

Volpe JJ. Neurology of the newborn, 2nd ed. Philadelphia: WB Saunders, 1987.

*Principles and Practice of Pediatrics, Second Edition,*
edited by Frank A. Oski et al. J. B. Lippincott Company, Philadelphia © 1994.

# 19.5 *Ethical Issues in Neonatology*

## Alan R. Fleischman

Dramatic changes in the technologic care available to newborn infants have resulted in the ability to save the lives of the majority of even the sickest and smallest neonates. Newborns as young as 25 weeks of gestational age and weighing 600 g survive at a rate of greater than 20% in most neonatal centers. Infants of 1000 g and 28 weeks of gestation, formerly thought to be at the threshold of viability in the 1960s and 1970s, have a greater than 90% survival rate in the 1990s. In addition, new surgical techniques have been developed over the past two decades to correct or ameliorate congenital anomalies of the heart, kidney, intestine, liver, and brain. Intravenous parenteral nutrition allows infants to grow and gain weight with normal development for weeks, months, or years without oral intake. These advances of neonatal medicine have enhanced the lives of countless children, yet at the same time they have also resulted in saving the lives of some children who are left with severely disabling and handicapping conditions.

Awareness of these ethical dilemmas or value conflicts is not new to those responsible for the care of infants. Historically, physicians felt obligated to make treatment decisions based on their personal beliefs about the future quality of life of their patient. At times, professionals shared this decision-making with the family, but often it was felt to be part of the job of the health-care provider to make such paternalistic decisions. These decisions were usually made within the privacy of the delivery room, the nursery, or the pediatric unit. There was little open discussion or even awareness by members of the society that value-laden ethical decisions were being made and rationalized as medical judgments. To a large extent, families and the society wished these decisions to be private matters because they were felt to be far too complex and personal for public involvement and debate.

However, concomitant with the evolution of the new technology of neonatal intensive care has been another sort of evolution. The physician in America has changed from the highly respected and rarely questioned paternalistic decision-maker into a collaborator who provides recommendations for health-care decisions that are made by the patient and family rather than solely by the physician. The changing expectation of the physician's role is consistent with an increasing desire for autonomy reflected in many parts of American society. Patients and families have become consumers of physician services, expecting to be fully informed and increasingly responsible for decisions about their own health care.

Respect for a person's fundamental right of self-determination, or autonomy, has resulted in the practice of allowing adults to make health-care decisions for themselves, even if at times the physician disagrees, and, more importantly, even if the physician perceives that the decision that is being made is not in the adult's best interests. This respect for a person's right of self-determination has been operationalized in medicine in the doctrine of informed consent. This doctrine assumes that the patient can understand the risks and benefits of alternative treatments and can make an informed choice. The process of informed consent when it relates to children or to any individuals who lack the capacity to decide for themselves invokes the use of a proxy or surrogate. Any proxy consent is not based on an individual's choice, but rather on another's perception of the appropriate choice.

Many have argued that the respect for a person's fundamental right of self-determination should be extended to respect the family as an autonomous unit making substituted judgments for its members who cannot participate in decision-making. This extension of the principle of respect for persons may occasionally be problematic when applied to neonates. The principle of informed consent for autonomous adults is extremely powerful in that it allows capable adults to refuse treatments despite negative consequences. However, parental refusals of treatments that are deemed to be beneficial for their infants do not hold the same weight as refusals by competent adults for treatments on themselves. Parental refusal of a needed therapy does not relieve the physician or other health-care provider from an ethical duty to the child, particularly if the refusal of such treatment puts the child at significant risk.

In a desire to preserve the child's future right to autonomous decision-making, the principle known as the "best interests of the child" has supplanted the "respect for persons" principle in regard to decision-making for infants. This principle supports making a decision solely for the benefit of the infant, sometimes, although rarely, even in conflict with parental beliefs. Thus, the "best interests" principle would preclude the right of a family to refuse a lifesaving blood transfusion for their newborn based on their strongly held religious or moral beliefs.

Often determinations of best interests are made in the presence of massive medical uncertainty as to the outcome of the proposed treatment. Physicians in general have a great deal of difficulty in admitting their lack of certainty as to the benefits of continued treatment or the initiation of new interventions. Jeff Lyon, in his book *Playing God in the Nursery*, graphically portrays the dilemma of uncertainty: "If it is hard to justify creating blind paraplegics to obtain a number of healthy survivors, it is equally hard to explain to the ghosts of the potentially healthy that they had to die in order to avoid creating blind paraplegics."

American neonatologists tend to deal with this uncertainty by considering it far worse to let an infant die who could have lived a reasonable life than to save an infant who becomes devastatingly disabled. Both outcomes are tragic, but is one truly worse than the other? It is clear that the value-laden decision about what is in the best interests of an individual infant is often uncertain. Many have argued that those who will bear the burden of the decision—namely, the family—ought to have the major role in making it. When faced with a lack of certainty as to what is in an infant's best interests, the physician's obligation is to share with the family a clear understanding of the various treatment options and make a recommendation consistent with what the treatment team believes is in the child's best interests. Ultimately, however, in these difficult cases, the family should decide. The physician's values should not be imposed inappropriately and force continued treatment when hope for benefit is uncertain.

Decisions, thus, should be collaborative, with the child's interests at the center of the analysis but with parents responsible for the choice, unless they are making a decision clearly against the best interests of the child. Prolonging an infant's life should not be viewed as an end in itself, but should be weighed against the probable quality of that future life.

At the core of all discussions concerning the appropriate process for making decisions for seriously ill neonates is the question of how much we value members of our society who have disabling and handicapping conditions. There remains a distinct tension between the ostensible societal valuing of the disabled, as represented by new legal initiatives and public policy, and the deeply held personal feelings of many individuals. In general, however, the last several decades have shown an increasing respect for the retarded and disabled in our society. Concomitantly, there has been an increasing public awareness that decisions are being made by physicians and parents in neonatal intensive care units to withhold or withdraw treatments from neonates who are at risk for disabilities and handicapping conditions. This resulted in the 1980s in several efforts by the U.S. Department of Health and Human Services to promulgate regulations concerning appropriate standards for foregoing of life-sustaining treatment for neonates. At the same time, the President's Commission for the Study of Ethical Problems in Medicine and Biomedical and Behavioral Research issued its report *Deciding to Forego Life-Sustaining Treatment*, and the Bioethics Committee of the American Academy of Pediatrics developed guidelines for the establishment and operation of bioethics committees, which would prospectively review cases where the foregoing of life-sustaining treatment was under consideration. It was hoped that these committees would provide consultation and decision review to assist families and health-care providers in the process of decision-making, as well as to protect the interests of the infants in neonatal intensive care units.

In 1984, the U.S. Congress amended the federal child abuse law, which added to the responsibility of each state's child protection agency oversight of the withholding of medically indicated treatments from neonates. The amendment and subsequent regulations state, "A new definition of withholding of medically indicated treatment is added in Section 3 of the Act to mean the failure to respond to an infant's life-threatening conditions by providing treatment (including appropriate nutrition, hydration and medication) which in the treating physician's reasonable medical judgment will be most likely to be effective in ameliorating or correcting all such conditions. Exceptions to the requirement to provide treatment may be made only in cases in which one of the following applies:

The infant is irreversibly comatose.

The provision of such treatment would merely prolong dying or not be effective in ameliorating or correcting all of the infant's life-threatening conditions or otherwise be futile in terms of the survival of the infant.

The provision of such treatment would be virtually futile in terms of the survival of the infant and the treatment itself under such circumstances would be inhumane.

These regulations, currently in effect, do not mandate unnecessary or inappropriate treatments. They allow physicians to use reasonable medical judgment in making treatment recommendations and allow physicians to involve parents in the decision-making process. The regulations give responsibility for protecting neonates with potentially handicapping conditions to the individual states; federal involvement is severely limited. Furthermore, the federal regulations strongly urge the formation of infant care review committees (which the American Academy of Pediatrics had called infant bioethical review committees) to facilitate decision review and to assist in the interaction among physicians, the family, the hospital, and the child protective services agency of the state.

Many fear that parental authority for decision-making for infants will be circumvented or supplanted by these regulations and by such a committee review process. Physicians have argued that these judgments are best made by the treating physician at the bedside, who is most knowledgeable of the medical facts as well as the infant's interests and the family's wishes. However, those who have used infant bioethics committees believe that they enhance the process of decision-making by reviewing the medical facts and protect the infant's interests by invoking ethical principles and not merely intuition in decision-making. Such committees can enhance the role of parents in decision-making and can increase the ethical comfort provided to both families and health-care professionals who are ultimately responsible for these difficult decisions.

Increasingly in the 1990s a new type of ethical dilemma is occurring in neonatal intensive care units. Physicians who have become comfortable with the concept of families having the discretion to choose to withhold or withdraw life-sustaining treatments from critically ill newborns are becoming increasingly concerned about families who insist on their infant's receiving life-sustaining treatments that are deemed by the professionals to have minimal if any benefit to the child. Physicians are invoking the concept of "futility" in an attempt to limit parental discretion to demand what is believed to be inappropriate treatment. One of the consequences of the development of an approach to decision-making for infants that respects the parents' role in that process is that the health-care professional will sometimes disagree with the parents' choice. Based on the physician's independent obligation to the child, we have elected to develop procedural mechanisms to override parental refusal of treatments felt to be in the child's best interests. This can be done through infant bioethics committee involvement or, ultimately, through the courts. Similarly, physicians have an obligation not to provide treatments to infants requested by parents that will only inflict pain and increase suffering and have no potential benefit for the child. However, when parents request a treatment that offers a low likelihood of benefit, even in the face of significant burden, health-care professionals ought not to arrogate to themselves the right to preclude treatment by calling the treatment futile. When caring, concerned parents request continued attempts to save the life of their child, if such treatments are possibly helpful, the physician should not use the language of futility in an attempt to impose his or her values over the values of the family.

Parental discretion should be given broad latitude in choices for children when there is honest uncertainty as to the ratio of benefits to burdens of continued treatment. However, parental discretion in demanding treatment ought not to be unlimited. Physicians and other health-care providers, based on their own strongly held personal beliefs, have the right to opt out of the care of an individual child for whom they believe the benefits of treatment do not outweigh the burdens. In addition, the society has the right through its laws, regulations, and institutions to limit individual resource allocation for patients unlikely or unable to benefit from continued treatment.

An ethical dilemma of a different variety is evident in the initiation of clinical interventions and experimentation in the neonatal intensive care unit. We need not discuss the therapeutic misadventures that are the hallmark of the early years of neonatology. These have included the excessive use of oxygen and resultant retrolental fibroplasia, the unexpected complications of the use of various antibiotics, and the use of rapid infusions of sodium bicarbonate to buffer metabolic acidosis, which caused intraventricular hemorrhage. All of these therapeutic modalities were instituted by well-intentioned clinicians whose motivation was based on a beneficent desire to help patients who would otherwise die or be severely impaired.

Physicians are often reluctant to subject innovative therapies to the discipline of a true experiment (ie, a randomized clinical trial) to ensure that the proposed therapy is not only effective but has few risks and negative consequences. Innovative clinicians are often self-deluding in an attempt to explain away a treatment failure or a complication of a new therapy that seems to have positive results. Galen, the famous physician of ancient Greece, reported the following analysis of his innovative therapeutic cocktail: "All who drink of this remedy recover in a short time, except those whom it does not help, who all die; therefore, it is obvious that it fails only in incurable cases." Neonatology has had too many clinical interventions that have not been subject to careful experimental scrutiny.

The clinical research scientist is certainly motivated by a desire to create new interventions that will ultimately benefit many patients. However, the motivating principle in clinical research, as distinct from clinical practice, is not beneficence but rather the seeking of truth. The subjects of a clinical research study should not believe that the experimental intervention is deemed effective by the clinician; rather, the clinician must maintain a healthy skepticism that allows the honest randomization of patients to an intervention or control group. Informed consent from the family is mandatory, and withdrawal from the research must be allowed at any time during the course of treatment. This experimental approach to innovative therapies, including such diverse treatments as extracorporeal membrane oxygenation, hypoplastic left-heart surgery, intestinal transplantation, and the initiation of a new antibiotic, is mandatory to protect the interests of present and future infants so that therapies become standard practice only after appropriate scrutiny.

Although the neonatal intensive care unit is a place for aggressive and innovative treatment as well as experimental clinical research, it is also the site of the death of many critically ill children. Each neonatal intensive care unit must develop an environment that allows for the humane care of the dying infant and the family. When a decision is made that continued therapeutic intervention is no longer in the child's interests or that the child is in the inexorable downhill spiral that will result in death, all technologic intervention should be withdrawn from the baby, and supportive care and caring should the treatment modalities used. Infants should not have to die attached to electronic machines and invasive technology. Neonatal intensive care units should have quiet, private areas where families can be together and relate to their child at the end of life. This enhancement of the dying process is an important step toward the resolution of this life crisis within the family. Appropriate counseling and bereavement services should be available both around the time of death and afterward.

Awareness of and concern for the value conflicts inherent in the field of neonatal intensive care is an important part of the practice of neonatology. Being sensitive to these issues and developing practices that are both in the best interests of infants and respectful of their parents will enhance the continued development of the field.

## Selected Readings

American Academy of Pediatrics. Guidelines for infant bioethics committees. Pediatrics 1984;74:306.

Department of Health and Human Services. Nondiscrimination on the basis of handicap. Federal Register 1983;48:9630.

Department of Health and Human Services. Child abuse and neglect prevention and treatment program and services and treatment for disabled infants: model guidelines for health-care providers to establish infant care review committees. Federal Register 1985;50:14878.

Fleischman AR. Bioethical review committees in perinatology. Clin Perinatol 1987;14:379.

Kliegman RM, Mahowald MB, Youngner SJ. In our best interests: experience and workings of an ethics review committee. J Pediatr 1986;108:178.

Kopelman LM, Irons TG, Kopelman AE. Neonatologists judge the "Baby Doe" regulation. N Engl J Med 1988;318:677.

Lyon J. Playing God in the nursery. New York: WW Norton, 1985.

McCormick RA. Ethics committees: promise or peril. Law Med Health Care 1984;11:150.

President's Commission for the Study of Ethical Problems in Medicine and Biomedical and Behavioral Research. Deciding to forego life-sustaining treatment. Washington DC: United States Government Printing Office, 1983.

Silverman WA. Human experimentation in perinatology. Clin Perinatol 1987;14:403.

Truog RD, Brett AS, Frader J. The problem with futility. New Engl J Med 1992;326:1560.

*Principles and Practice of Pediatrics, Second Edition.*
edited by Frank A. Oski et al. J. B. Lippincott Company, Philadelphia © 1994.

# CHAPTER 20
# *Diseases of the Newborn*

## 20.1 *Neonatal Neurology*

### 20.1.1 *Neuroembryology*

Laura R. Ment and Marvin A. Fishman

Congenital malformations of the central nervous system represent a major cause of infantile mortality and morbidity, and result in neuroanatomic abnormalities that range from the structural to the cellular levels. The basis for some of the well-described central nervous system malformations is discussed in this chapter within the context of development of the fetal neuraxis.

## NEURAL TUBE DEFECTS

The fetal nervous system begins development on the 18th day of gestation. The primordial neural tube is derived from the ecto-dermal layer, and the ectoderm on the dorsal portion of the embryo, along with the underlying notochord and chordal mesoderm, induce the formation of the neural plate. Closure of the neuroectoderm begins on the 22nd day of gestation and is accomplished by invagination of the lateral margins of the neural plate. Closure begins in the lower medullary and cervical regions, and it progresses in both directions. The anterior neuropore closes on the 25th to 26th day and the posterior neuropore closes 2 to 3 days later to form a closed, continuous cavity that constitutes the primitive ventricular system and central canal of the cord. Subsequent approximation of the cutaneous ectoderm occurs only when and if the converging edges of the neural groove come together to form this tube. Disturbances in neural tube closure range from anencephaly, to failure of rostral neural tube closure, to the dysraphic states, which represent disorders of caudal closure. Anencephaly, the presence of an exposed rostral mass of neural tissue, probably occurs before the 24th gestational day and has an incidence of 1:1000 births. About 75% of these infants are stillborn and the rest die shortly after birth.

Encephalocele, an insult thought to occur on about the 26th gestational day, is a less severe malformation involving defective closure of the rostral portion of the neural tube in association with a bony skull defect. Although 75% to 80% of these lesions occur in the occipital region, similar abnormalities have been noted in the frontal and parietal regions. Frontal and nasal encephaloceles are more common in infants of Asian ancestry and may be seen after the newborn period. In this condition, a soft sac of varying size protrudes through a bony defect and may contain only cranial meninges or meninges and neural tube. Communication usually is present between the ventricular cavity and the encephalocele, and hydrocephalus may be noted. The majority of cases of encephalocele are spontaneous events, and severe mental retardation, seizures, and motor deficits are commonly associated findings.

Further development of the caudal neural tube occurs by the processes of canalization and retrogressive differentiation, the latter continuing until sometime after birth. Myelomeningocele, a restricted failure of posterior caudal neural tube closure, is believed to occur before 26 days' gestation. The majority of these lesions occur in the the lumbar and lumbosacral regions, and the incidence is said to be between 1:1000 and 5:1000 live births, with the highest incidence found in the northern regions of the British Isles. Pathologically, the majority of lesions result in a dorsal displacement of neural tissue such that a sac or an open placode remains on the infant's back. Skeletal anomalies, including absence of the vertebral arches, lateral displacement of the pedicles, and a widened spinal canal, are present uniformly, and an incomplete, though variable, dermal covering is present. Clinical features relate to the region of the spinal cord that is involved and to the extent of the lesions. Generally, disturbances in lower-extremity motor function, sphincter function, and bladder function may be noted. Secondary orthopedic malformations of the lower extremities–congenital contractures known as arthrogryposis–occur in utero because of lack of fetal movement. Hydrocephalus is seen in almost 75% of cases and is associated nearly always with an Arnold-Chiari malformation, or kinking and elongation of brain stem structures. The morbidity and mortality seen in this disorder result from complications of meningitis (from the open sac), hydrocephalus, and renal involvement. Those infants who undergo the earliest closure of the meningeal sac appear to have the best neurodevelopmental outcome. Similarly, delivery by cesarean section has been advocated to preserve lower-extremity function to the fullest extent.

Other dysraphic states include meningocele, spina bifida occulta, and diastematomyelia. *Meningocele* is herniation of the meninges unaccompanied by neural tissue and covered by skin or a thin-walled membrane. Similar to myelomeningocele, these lesions are most common in the lumbosacral region, and defects in the vertebral arches may be present. Many patients have abnormalities of gait, particularly during periods of rapid growth, or loss of previously acquired bladder control. Meningoceles generally are not associated with hydrocephalus.

*Spina bifida occulta* usually refers to a vertebral defect without herniation of the contents of the spinal canal. This condition is found most commonly in the lumbosacral region. At birth, most patients are asymptomatic, although some may be identifiable by the presence of hairy tufts or birthmarks at the base of the spine. Occasionally, a sinus tract may lead into an intraspinal cyst or epidermoid structure. All infants with recurrent gram-negative bacterial meningitis should be examined carefully for sinus tracts, because these may provide a source of infection.

In *diastematomyelia*, the spinal cord is divided by a bony or cartilaginous spur extending from the dorsal surface of the vertebral body. This is associated with spina bifida occulta in more than 50% of cases and may cause neurologic deficits by producing traction on the cord. Lipomas are hamartomatous lesions associated with dysraphic states and are located most commonly in the region of the filum terminale.

Although the occult dysraphic states may go undetected in early childhood, 80% are associated with dermal lesions and vertebral defects. Later in childhood, as the spinal cord ascends to its position in adult life, patients may have gait disturbances, foot deformities, sphincter dysfunction, and scoliosis. The failure of the spinal cord to ascend, as a result of either primary malformation or secondary tumor, is known as *tethering of the cord*.

Prenatal diagnosis of defects in neural tube closure is widely available and is mandatory for mothers who are at high risk of having infants with these disorders. Maternal serum $\alpha$-fetoprotein tests performed during the 16th to 18th weeks of pregnancy will detect 88% to 100% of cases of anencephaly and 80% of cases of open spina bifida. False-positive test results are related to twin gestation, underestimation of gestational age, or threatened/missed abortion. When the serum $\alpha$-fetoprotein test is positive, a second test should be repeated in 1 week. If the second test result also is positive, an ultrasound examination to evaluate for twin pregnancy and a careful sonographic evaluation of the fetal spine to investigate spinal defects are necessary. In singleton pregnancies with normal vertebral arches, amniocentesis and amniotic $\alpha$-fetoprotein determination should be performed.

## DISORDERS OF VENTRAL INDUCTION

The concept of ventral induction refers to the developmental events that occur under the primary influence of the prechordal mesoderm during the fifth and sixth weeks of gestation. The major inductive relationship between the prechordal mesoderm and the developing cerebrum occurs ventrally at the rostral end of the fetus and influences the development of the forebrain and facial structures.

### Holoprosencephaly

Although malformations of the forebrain generally have been attributed to failure of normal segmentation and cleavage of the prosencephalon into paired cerebral hemispheres, more recent studies have suggested that holoprosencephaly should be considered a severe midline dysgenesis in a neuroembryologic spectrum that includes septo-optic dysplasia and agenesis of the corpus callosum (ACC). Thus, holoprosencephaly is the most severely involved malformation of this spectrum in which the cerebral hemispheres remain as a single-sphered structure with a large central ventricle and there are abnormalities of the basal ganglia, thalami, and hypothalamus. A computed tomographic

(CT) scan of a patient with holoprosencephaly is provided in Figure 20-1; note the presence of the large, single frontal ventricle in this young child with mental and motoric delay. Holoprosencephaly also frequently results in abnormalities of the optic and facial structures.

Holoprosencephaly has been reported to occur in 1:13,000 live births. Although its occurrence usually is sporadic and its etiology unknown, it has been associated with numerous chromosomal abnormalities, including trisomy 13 and various abnormalities at chromosome 18. Facial anomalies may range from a single median eye and rudimentary nasal structures to ocular hypotelorism or hypertelorism and median cleft lip and palate. Although many infants are reported to have severe neurologic impairment and to die shortly after birth, we have seen numerous children with holoprosencephaly become both ambulatory and sufficiently verbal to attend special schools.

### Agenesis of the Corpus Callosum

ACC, either partial or complete, may represent the opposite end of the spectrum of holoprosencephalies. This disorder principally is a migrational dysgenesis. Development of the corpus callosum is associated with migrational events in the divided cerebrum. The earliest fibers appear at 11 weeks of gestation and formation is complete at 20 weeks. The clinical features vary from the incidental finding of agenesis on CT scan or autopsy examination to developmental delay, seizures, and motor abnormalities. Although there are rare cases of X-linked ACC, most cases are believed to be sporadic in occurrence. A characteristic CT scan is shown in Figure 20-2.

## DISORDERS OF NERVE CELL PROLIFERATION

During the second through fourth gestational months, cells of the developing brain proliferate and migrate. Most of the devel-

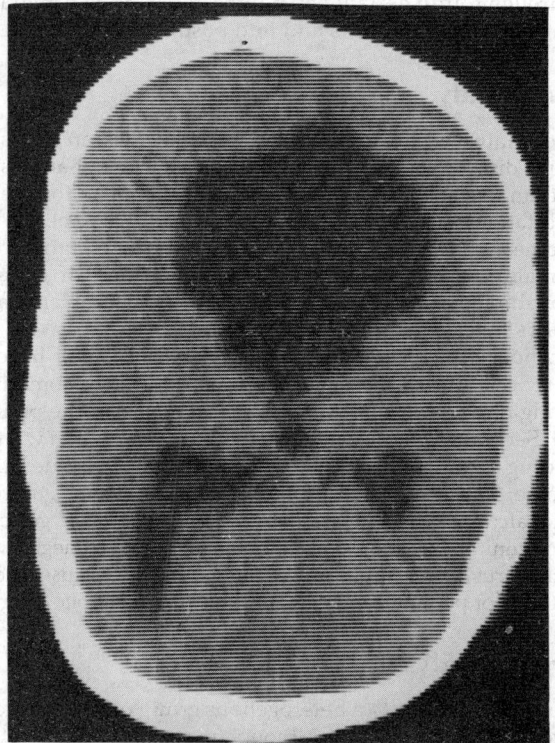

**Figure 20-1.** This CT scan of a young infant with a large head (>95% for age) demonstrates holoprosencephaly. Note the single large frontal ventricle with failure of division of the single frontal hemisphere.

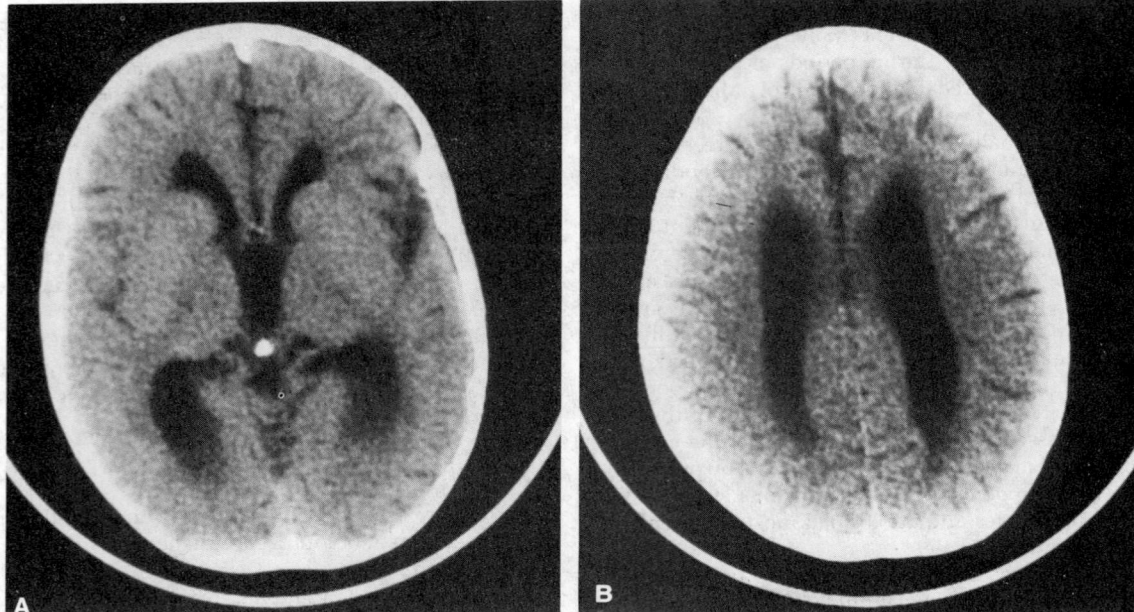

**Figure 20-2.** (**A** and **B**) In this CT scan of an infant with seizures and agenesis of the corpus callosum (ACC), the lateral ventricles appear parallel and closer in position than might be expected. The third ventricle is enlarged and occupies a relatively superior position in this study. Finally, the interhemispheric fissure can be traced dorsally to the third ventricle.

oping neurons and glial cells arise from the primordial cells found in the periventricular germinal matrix. Within this region, the cells migrate back and forth, dividing at the ventricular surface and alternately migrating outward toward the newly formed cortical plate. Although the primitive neuroblasts and glioblasts are indistinguishable, primary neuronal migrations occur in the second through fourth gestational months, whereas glial migrations continue through 40 weeks and into postnatal life.

## Microcephaly

Microcephaly vera, or primary microcephaly, is an autosomal recessive disorder characterized by severe microcephaly (usually more than two standard deviations below the mean for age, sex, and gestation), intellectual impairment, and poor speech. This syndrome is thought to derive from a neuronal cell proliferation abnormality that occurs before the fourth month of gestation. Neuropathologic defects in gyral pattern and cortical lamination, as well as heterotopias, have been reported.

Secondary microcephaly usually refers to a small head circumference and, thus, a small brain as a result of some insult occurring during the latter half of pregnancy or in the perinatal period. Secondary microcephaly is found in association with maternal drug ingestion; trisomies 21, 18, and 13; Cornelia de Lange's syndrome; Prader-Willi syndrome; Rubinstein-Taybi syndrome; the fetal alcohol syndrome; radiation before 20 weeks' gestation; and congenital infections, including rubella, cytomegalovirus, coxsackievirus, and toxoplasmosis. Suspected other causes include intrauterine or perinatal anoxia or trauma and metabolic disorders.

## Macrencephaly

Macrencephaly refers to a heterogenous group of disorders characterized by "heavy brains." Although macrencephaly is not well described neuropathologically, it is found in association with a number of genetic syndromes, including cerebral gigantism,

Beckwith's syndrome, achondroplasia, tuberous sclerosis, neurofibromatosis, multiple hemangiomatosis, and familial, isolated macrencephaly.

## DISORDERS OF NERVE CELL MIGRATION

### Lissencephaly

During the third to fifth months of gestation, abnormalities of the migrating neuroblasts and glioblasts may result in abnormal gyral development. Lissencephaly, or "smooth brain" with little or no gyral pattern, may represent a destructive premigrational lesion that occurs before the third month of gestation and results in a brain with a thickened cortical ribbon and a thin inner white matter region. The CT scans of infants with this condition are characterized by a paucity of periventricular white matter and a "squared" configuration of the lateral ventricles. Infants with lissencephaly have severe seizures, spasticity, and profound developmental delay. Although most cases are sporadic, familial cases have been reported. Similarly, the brains of infants with pachygyria demonstrate relatively few broad gyri with an abnormally thick cortical plate.

ACC, described previously, is seen in neuronal migration disorders, although it may occur alone. In the most common form, there is complete agenesis of the callosum and complete separation of the hemispheres except in the region of the anterior commissure and the lamina terminalis.

Polymicrogyria, a disorder characterized by the presence of multiple small gyri, seems to result from the fusion of molecular layers between gyri. Although one major variety of polymicrogyria includes those cases with evidence for cortical laminar neuronal necrosis after migration, a second major variety represents a disorder of neuronal migration throughout the developing cortex, cerebellum, and brain stem, as has been reported in Zellweger syndrome. Alternatively, polymicrogyria may be a localized dis-

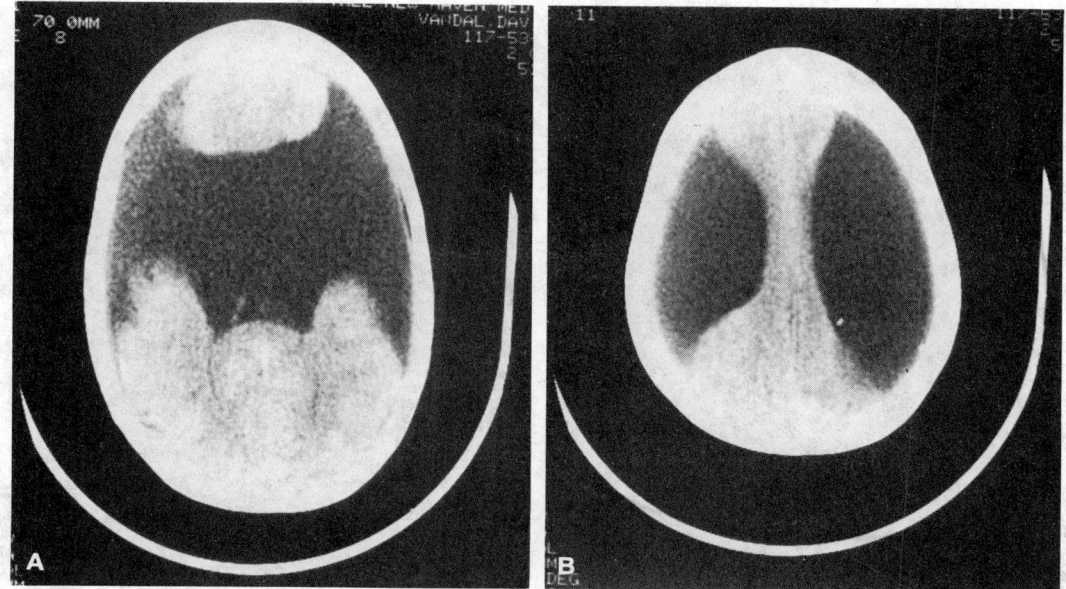

**Figure 20-3.** (**A** and **B**) This CT scan of a 2-year-old male with schizencephaly, seizures, and profound developmental delay is characterized by large bilaterally symmetric hemispheric clefts that communicate with the ventricular system.

turbance, found at autopsy and unassociated with neurologic impairment. In its most severe form, polymicrogyria has been associated with severe developmental delay, seizures, and hypotonia.

Schizencephaly similarly represents a severe form of migrational disturbance, probably also occurring before the third month of gestation. In this disorder, bilateral, symmetric congenital clefts are formed in the region of the sylvian fissures. Infolding of the cortical gray matter occurs, and a pial–ependymal seam extends from the surface of the brain into the ventricle. Clinically, most infants are delayed severely and have seizures and spasticity.

The CT scan of infants with schizencephaly (Fig 20-3) dramatically demonstrates the bilateral symmetric clefts.

Hemimegalencephaly, or unilateral megalencephaly (Fig 20-4), also is caused by abnormal neuronal proliferation and migration during the second trimester, and results in overgrowth and secondary polymicrogyria of one cerebral hemisphere. This condition may be diagnosed by prenatal ultrasonography and typically begins with a triad of clinical findings characterized by intractable seizures, profound developmental delay, and progressive hemiparesis. Patients with hemimegalencephaly may require epilepsy surgery to achieve adequate seizure control.

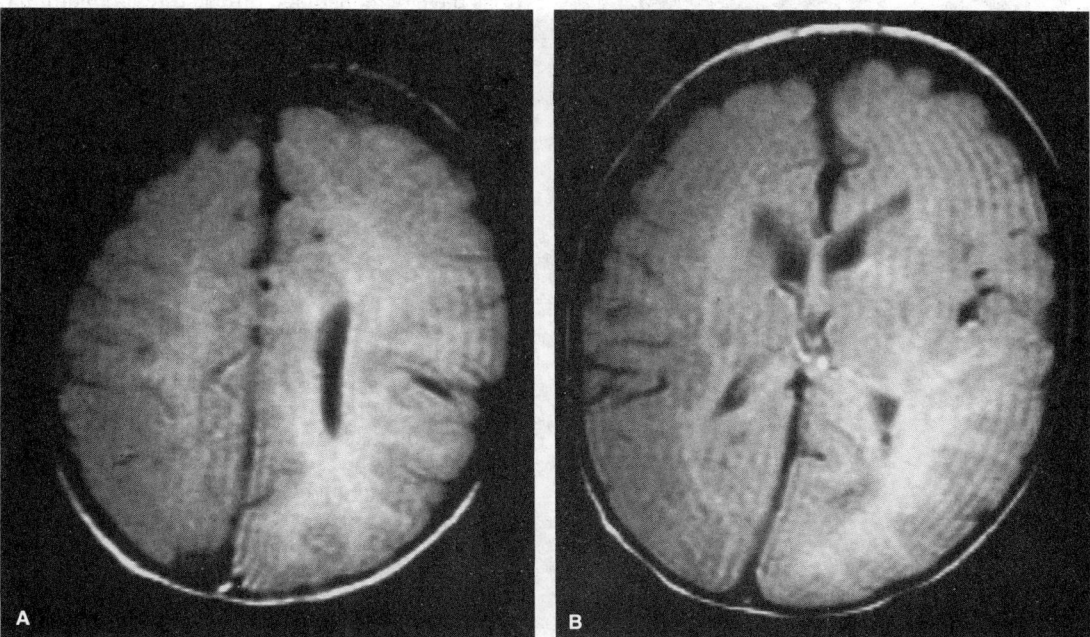

**Figure 20-4.** (**A** and **B**) Hemimegalencephaly, found in the hemisphere on the right in this cerebral MRI, is associated with the clinical triad of intractable seizures, profound developmental delay, and progressive hemiparesis.

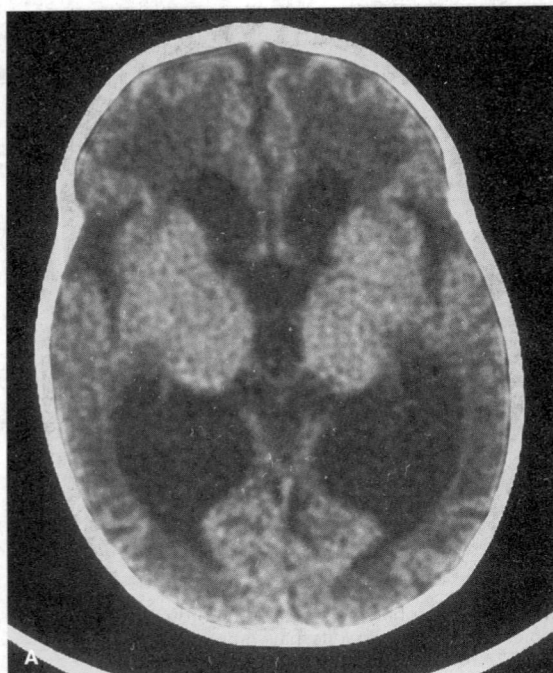
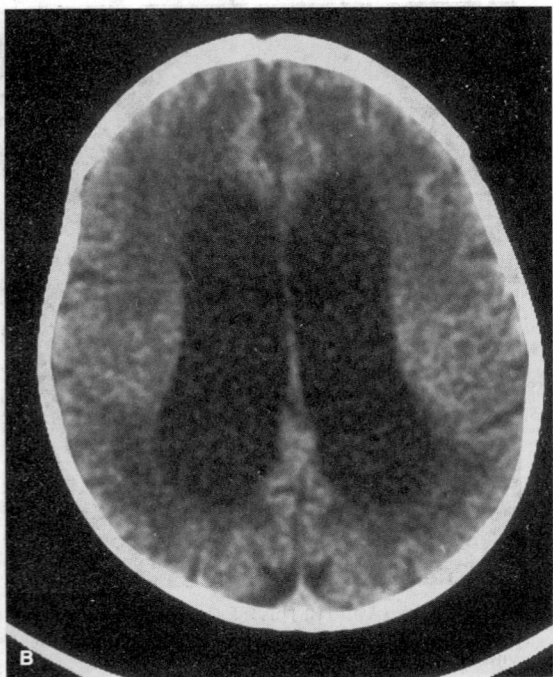

Figure 20-5. (**A** and **B**) A 6-week-old male was seen with hypotonia, lethargy, and seizures; his physical examination demonstrated microcephaly, central hypotonia, and hyperreflexia. A CT scan demonstrated ventriculomegaly and delayed areas of myelination in both frontal regions. Laboratory studies were consistent with the diagnosis of methylmalonic acidemia.

## DISORDERS OF NERVE CELL ORGANIZATION AND MATURATION

From the sixth month of gestation throughout several postnatal years, organizational events occur in the developing cerebrum. These events include proper layering of the cells, elaboration of

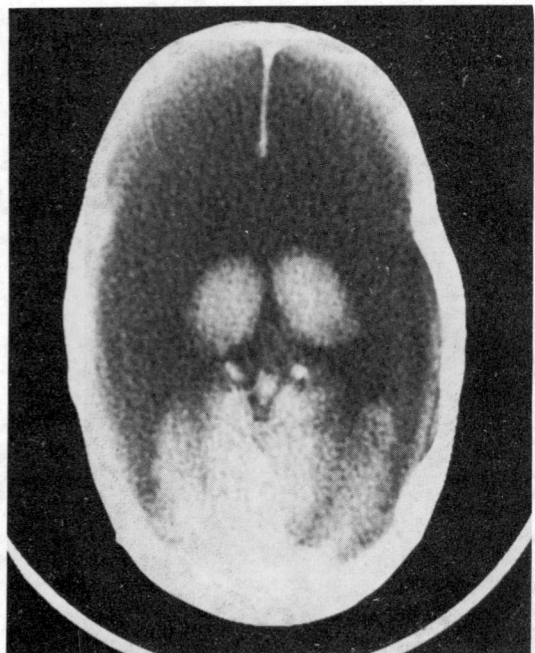

Figure 20-6. The CT scan of this 4-month-old female with a large head and bulging fontanelle was significant for the diagnosis of hydranencephaly—the presence within an intact cranium of deep gray, posterior fossa structures and brain stem, but nearly complete absence of hemispheric tissue.

dendritic and axonal ramifications, establishment of synaptic contacts, and glial proliferation and differentiation. Disturbances in any one or all of these events could have a major impact on the cortical connectivity and, thus, the neurologic function of an infant.

Although there are only limited studies available concerning developmental disturbances during this critical time, neuroanatomic and imaging studies of patients with untreated aminoacidurias have demonstrated diffuse cerebral maturational delay with decreased cell packing density, diminished cortical plate width, and myelination abnormalities (Fig 20-5). Neuronal studies of these patients also demonstrate poor development of dendritic arborizations and synaptic spines.

## DESTRUCTIVE LESIONS

### Hydranencephaly

Hydranencephaly, or the almost complete absence of the cerebral hemispheres with intact basal ganglia and brain stem structures (Fig 20-6), is postulated to be the result of a major vascular insult during the second trimester of gestation. Infants with hydranencephaly also experience abnormalities of the cerebellum, olfactory regions, and optic nerves. The normal-appearing cranium is filled with a meningeal sac that contains fluid with a high protein content, thought to be secondary to the primary destructive process. These infants frequently require ventriculoperitoneal shunts and, although many are seen in the newborn period with large heads, others are not detected until the third or fourth postnatal months when they fail to reach normal milestones. Finally, because of a persistent occipital cortical rim, some cortical visual behavior may be found.

### Porencephaly

Porencephaly refers to cavitary defects extending from the ventricular space into the cerebral hemisphere and it results from strokes in utero. Clinically, although affected infants may experience increased intracranial pressure from these lesions, the presentation generally depends upon the cortical location of the lesion.

## Selected Readings

Bauman ML. Neuroembryology–clinical aspects. In: Creasy RK, Warshaw JB, eds. Seminars in perinatology. Orlando: Grune & Stratton, 1987:74.

Gilles FH, Leviton A, Dooling EC. The developing human brain. Boston: Wright, 1983.

Grannum P, Pilu G. In utero neurosonography: The normal fetus and variations in cranial size. In: Creasy RK, Warshaw JB, eds. Seminars in perinatology. Orlando: Grune & Stratton, 1987:85.

Grannum P, Pilu G. In utero neurosonography: Neuroembryologic and encephaloclastic lesions. In: Creasy RK, Warshaw JB, eds. Seminars in perinatology. Orlando: Grune & Stratton, 1987:98.

Hicks SP. Developmental malformations produced by radiation. AJR Am J Roentgenol 1953;69:272.

Hobbins JC, Grannum PAT, Berkowitz RL, et al. Ultrasound in the diagnosis of congenital anomalies. Am J Obstet Gynecol 1979;134:331.

Lemire RJ, Loeser JD, Leech RW, et al. Normal and abnormal development of the human nervous system. Hagerstown, Md: Harper & Row, 1975.

Milunsky A, Alpert E, Neff RK, et al. Prenatal diagnosis of neural tube defects. IV. Maternal serum alpha-fetoprotein screening. Obstet Gynecol 1980;55:60.

Rakic P, Yakovlev PI. Development of the corpus callosum and cavum septi in man. J Comp Neurol 1968;132:45.

Volpe JJ. Neurology of the newborn. Philadelphia: Saunders, 1981.

Yakovlev PI, Wadsworth RC: Schizencephalies: A study of the congenital clefts in the cerebral mantle. I. Clefts with fused lips. J Neuropathol Exp Neurol 1946;5:116.

*Principles and Practice of Pediatrics, Second Edition.*
edited by Frank A. Oski et al. J. B. Lippincott Company, Philadelphia © 1994.

## 20.1.2 *Perinatal Cerebral Insults*

Laura R. Ment

Although the development of sophisticated perinatal intensive care techniques has brought about steady improvement in the survival rates of many critically ill and preterm neonates, the incidence of major neurodevelopmental handicaps in the graduates of newborn intensive care units has remained essentially unchanged over the past 10 to 20 years. Between 10% and 20% of the survivors of newborn special care have been reported to have serious abnormalities, including seizures, developmental delay, and motor problems. Those infants with parenchymal involvement of intraventricular hemorrhage (IVH) and perinatal cerebral infarct are believed to be at greatest risk for the development of such problems. These lesions are thought to be secondary to alterations in cerebral blood flow (CBF) to the developing brain.

## CONTROL OF CEREBRAL BLOOD FLOW

CBF in the newborn infant is felt to be largely independent of autonomic stimuli and controlled by local metabolic needs. Although "physiologic coupling" is the term frequently used to describe this relationship, the mechanism by which this coupling occurs is unknown. CBF is believed to be constant over a wide range of blood pressure, a phenomenon known as *autoregulation*. When blood pressure becomes too low, however, CBF falls and infarction may ensue. Similarly, a rapid increase in blood pressure

may increase CBF markedly, causing hemorrhage into damaged tissues. Hypercarbia, hypoxemia, rapid volume expansion, and seizures also produce marked increases in CBF.

Techniques to measure CBF in newborn infants have included [133]xenon injection or inhalation, venous plethysmography, near-infrared spectroscopy studies, and Doppler studies. Using these techniques, increases in CBF have been reported to occur in infants with hypercarbia, seizures, pneumothoraces, and volume expansion who subsequently developed germinal matrix hemorrhage (GMH) or intraventricular hemorrhage (IVH). A fluctuating pattern of CBF mirroring unstable systemic blood pressure also has been associated with GMH/IVH.

## Selected Readings

Armstrong D, Norman MG. Periventricular leucomalacia in neonates. Complications and sequelae. Arch Dis Child 1974;49:367.

Ashwal S, Majcher JS, Vain N, et al. Patterns of fetal lamb regional cerebral blood flow during and after prolonged hypoxia. Pediatr Res 1980;14:1104.

Cavazzuti M, Duffy TE. Regulation of local cerebral blood flow in normal and hypoxic newborn dogs. Ann Neurol 1981;11:247.

Duffy TE, Kohle SJ, Vannucci RC. Carbohydrate and energy metabolism in perinatal rat brain: Relation to survival in anoxia. J Neurochem 1975;24:271.

Goddard-Finegold J, Michael LH. Brain vasoactive effects of phenobarbital during hypertension and hypoxia in newborn pigs. Pediatr Res 1992;32:103.

Hernandez MJ, Brennan RW, Vannucci RC, et al. Cerebral blood flow and oxygen consumption in the newborn dog. Am J Physiol 1978;234:R209.

Kennedy C, Grave GD, Jehle JW, et al. Changes in blood flow in the component structures of the dog brain during postnatal maturation. J Neurochem 1972;19:2423.

Myers RE. Four patterns of perinatal brain damage and their conditions of occurrence in primates. In: Meldrum BS, Marsden DC, eds. Primate models of neurologic disorders. Adv Neurol 1975;10:223.

Rosenberg AA. Response of the cerebral circulation to hypocarbia in postasphyxia newborn lambs. Pediatr Res 1992;32:537.

Stewart WB. Blood flow and metabolism in the developing brain, In: Creasy RK, Warshaw JB, eds. Seminars in perinatology, vol 2. Orlando: Grune & Stratton, 1987:112.

Vannucci RC, Duffy TE. Cerebral metabolism in newborn dogs during reversible asphyxia. Ann Neurol 1977;1:528.

*Principles and Practice of Pediatrics, Second Edition.*
edited by Frank A. Oski et al. J. B. Lippincott Company, Philadelphia © 1994.

## 20.1.3 *Intraventricular Hemorrhage of the Preterm Infant*

Laura R. Ment

Intraventricular hemorrhage (IVH), or hemorrhage into the germinal matrix tissues with possible rupture into the ventricular system and parenchyma of the developing brain (Fig 20-7), remains a major problem of preterm neonates, and is believed to be the result of alterations in cerebral blood flow (CBF) to a damaged germinal matrix capillary bed. Because the germinal matrix begins to involute after 34 weeks of gestation, germinal matrix and intraventricular hemorrhages (GMH/IVH) are lesions of preterm infants, and a recent study of 2928 neonates of less than 1500 g birth weight demonstrated an incidence of GMH/IVH of greater than 45%. Seizures, hydrocephalus, periventricular leukomalacia (PVL), and neonatal death all are more frequent in infants with GMH/IVH than in those without hemorrhage, when matched for birth weight or gestational age. In addition, although the long-term neurodevelopmental outcome for those infants with

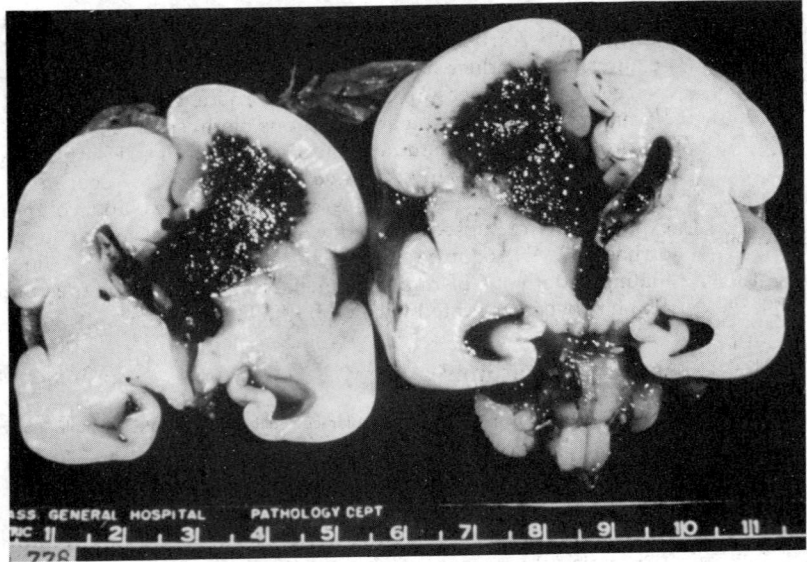

Figure 20-7.   Coronal sections of the brain of a 28-week preterm infant with a large intraventricular and frontoparietal parenchymal hemorrhage.

lower grades of hemorrhage remains unclear, most observers agree that infants with parenchymal involvement of hemorrhage are at higher risk for neurodevelopmental handicap.

Cranial ultrasound (Fig 20-8) is the method of choice for diagnosis of GMH/IVH in newborn special care units. A standard grading system (Papile, 1978), which originally was applied to the computed tomographic (CT) scan, has been adapted to cranial ultrasound examinations. Grade I, or GMH, describes blood in the germinal matrix only, grade II is blood filling the lateral ventricles without distention, grade III is blood filling and distending the ventricular system, and grade IV describes hemorrhages with parenchymal involvement (Table 20-1). The most common site for parenchymal involvement of hemorrhage is the frontal region; many hemorrhages occur bilaterally. Less commonly, the caudate nuclei and occipital periventricular white matter regions are involved.

In most newborn intensive care units, echoencephalography is performed on postnatal days 2 to 3 and then is repeated during the second postnatal week to screen preterm neonates of 1500 g or less or of 34 weeks' gestational age or less for GMH/IVH.

## PATHOPHYSIOLOGY

The germinal matrix is the site of proliferation of neuronal and glial precursors in the developing nervous system, and the capillary bed of the germinal matrix is composed of large, irregular vessels with little evidence for basement membrane proteins or glial supporting structures. These vessels represent the "watershed zone" of the ventriculofugal and ventriculopedal vessels of the developing brain (Fig 20-9) and are not readily distinguishable as arterioles, venules, or capillaries. These fragile vessels are unable to autoregulate the blood supply to this important region; thus, CBF to the germinal matrix is pressure passive. Neonates of less than 28 weeks' gestational age have been noted to have hemorrhage in the germinal matrix overlying the body of the caudate nucleus, whereas neonates of greater gestational ages are more likely to have hemorrhage in the germinal matrix at the head of the caudate nucleus at the level of the foramen of Monro. A small percentage of intraventricular hemorrhages in preterm infants also may originate from the choroid plexus, a second cerebral region that is believed to be unable to autoregulate blood flow; in contrast, the choroid plexus is the most common site of intraventricular hemorrhage in full-term neonates.

Despite the fact that the primitive cells of the germinal matrix are active through 34 weeks' gestational age and may be found in postmortem studies at least 1 year post-term, the risk period

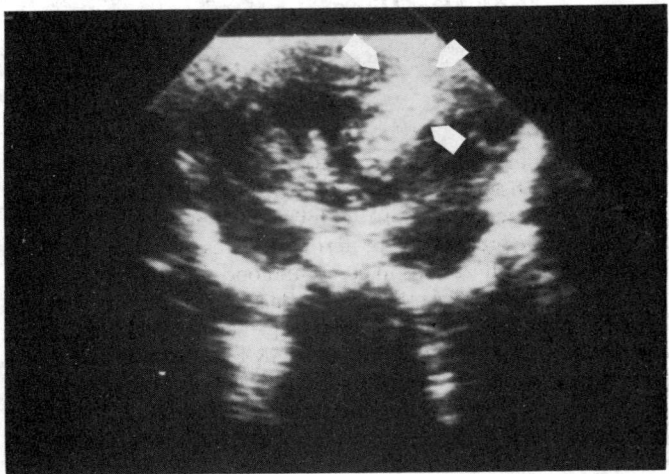

Figure 20-8.   Coronal ultrasound demonstrating a large right parenchymal hemorrhage in a 28-week preterm infant with bloody spinal fluid.

### TABLE 20-1.   Grading System for Neonatal Intraventricular Hemorrhage

| Grade | Description |
|-------|-------------|
| I | Germinal matrix hemorrhage |
| II | Blood within but not distending the lateral ventricular system |
| III | Blood filling and distending the ventricular system |
| IV | Parenchymal involvement of hemorrhage with or without any of the above |

*Adapted from Papile LS, Burstein J, Burstein R, et al. Incidence and evolution of the subependymal intraventricular hemorrhage; a study of infants with weights less than 1500 grams. J Pediatr 1978;92:529.*

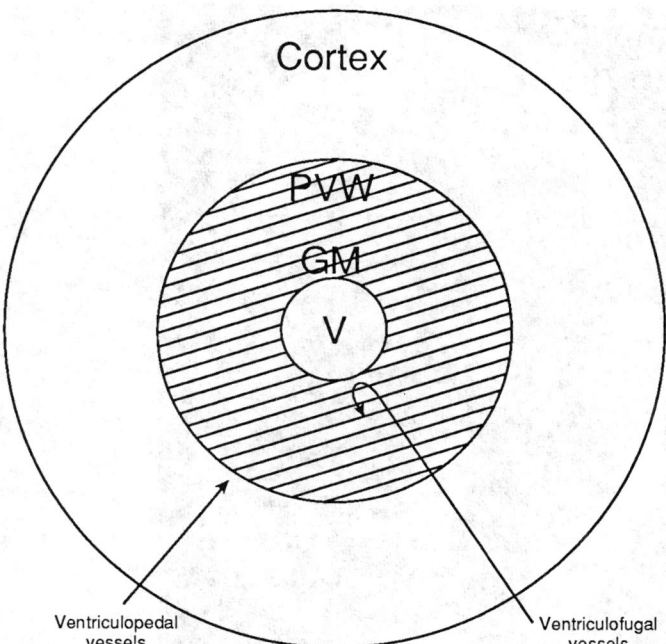

Figure 20-9. Model for cerebral blood flow patterns in the preterm brain. *GM,* germinal matrix; *PVW,* periventricular white matter; *V,* ventricle.

demonstrated prolonged ischemia for greater than the first postnatal week in preterm neonates with IVH.

A model for the development of neonatal GMH/IVH is found in Figure 20-10 and takes into account both the hypotensive/ischemic insults and those clinical events such as pneumothoraces, seizures, and rapid volume resuscitation to which many tiny and frequently critically ill preterm neonates are exposed.

The neuropathologic consequences of IVH include germinal matrix destruction, periventricular hemorrhagic infarction, and posthemorrhagic hydrocephalus (PHH). Germinal matrix destruction with secondary cystic formation is a common and expected feature of GMH.

In addition, 10% to 20% of patients with GMH/IVH have periventricular hemorrhagic infarction, also frequently called "hemorrhagic intracerebral involvement." Some investigators feel that the parenchymal involvement of insult that is readily visible by cranial ultrasonography (see Fig 20-8) represents a direct extension of hemorrhage from either the ventricular system or the germinal matrix; others believe that these lesions represent venous infarction of the periventricular white matter. Both proposed mechanisms are dependent on increased intracranial and, particularly, intraventricular pressure as a primary event. Distinguishing the two lesions in vivo is extremely difficult, and it is likely that parenchymal lesions occur secondary to both mechanisms.

The third consequence of IVH is PHH (Fig 20-11). PHH is more common in those infants with the highest grades of hemorrhage and is less common in those with the youngest gestational

for GMH/IVH appears to be the first 4 to 5 postnatal days and is independent of gestational age. Recent animal studies have suggested that these vessels are structurally different from those in both periventricular white and cortical gray regions, and that they may undergo the rapid perinatal induction of basement membrane deposition; for this reason, they may become more resistant to those insults that are associated with GMH/IVH after this 4- to 5-day interval.

The risk factors for GMH/IVH appear to include both perinatal and postnatal events, and several authors have speculated that the pathophysiology of early onset GMH/IVH (in the first 8 to 12 postnatal hours) may differ from that of postnatal onset GMH/IVH. The association between respiratory distress syndrome, vigorous resuscitation, hypoxemia, acidosis, and bicarbonate administration and hemorrhage have been well described, and the advent of bedside echoencephalography has permitted the demonstration of the relationship of such events as pneumothoraces and seizures and the acute onset of hemorrhage. All these factors have been shown to alter CBF in the preterm neonate. Perinatal risk factor studies for hemorrhage of very early onset (in the first hours of life) are less clear. Although some authors have suggested that vaginal delivery, labor, and intrapartum asphyxia may be related to the presence of early onset GMH/IVH, these studies require further investigation.

The relationship between surfactant, respiratory distress syndrome, and the development of GMH/IVH also must be mentioned. Although surfactant has been demonstrated to cause transient increases in CBF, most clinical studies have not noted an increase in GMH/IVH associated with its use. In addition, because surfactant may diminish the acute hypoxemia and hypercarbia that are associated with respiratory distress syndrome, it actually may contribute to the lower incidence of GMH/IVH that some centers are reporting.

Of equal concern, and perhaps more important for the neurodevelopmental outcome of these infants, is the observation of markedly diminished CBF following low-grade IVH. [133]Xenon inhalation CBF studies and positron emission tomography have

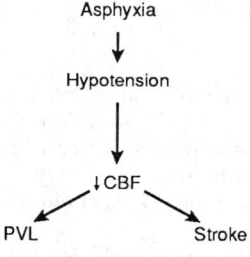

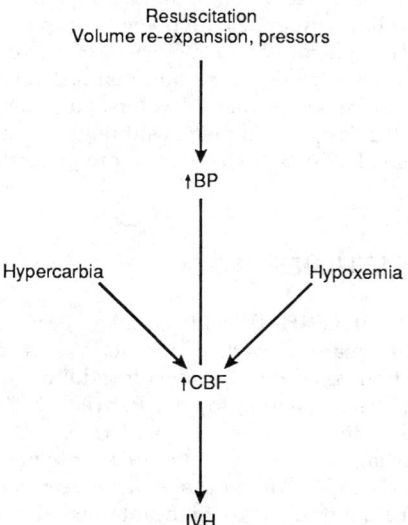

Figure 20-10. Model for the development of intraventricular hemorrhage in the preterm infant. *CBF,* cerebral blood flow; *IVH,* intraventricular hemorrhage; *PVL,* periventricular leukomalacia; *BP,* blood pressure.

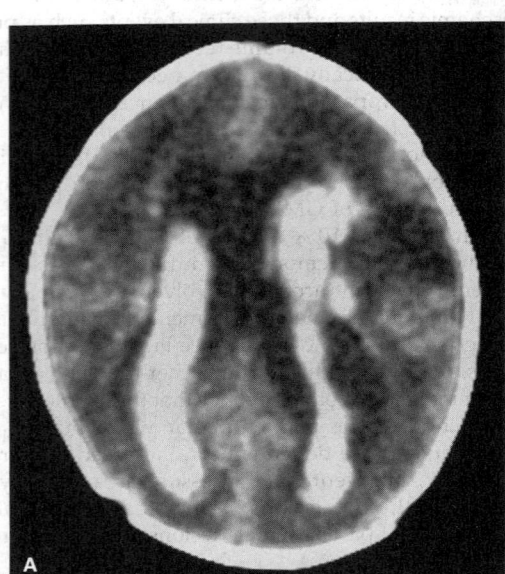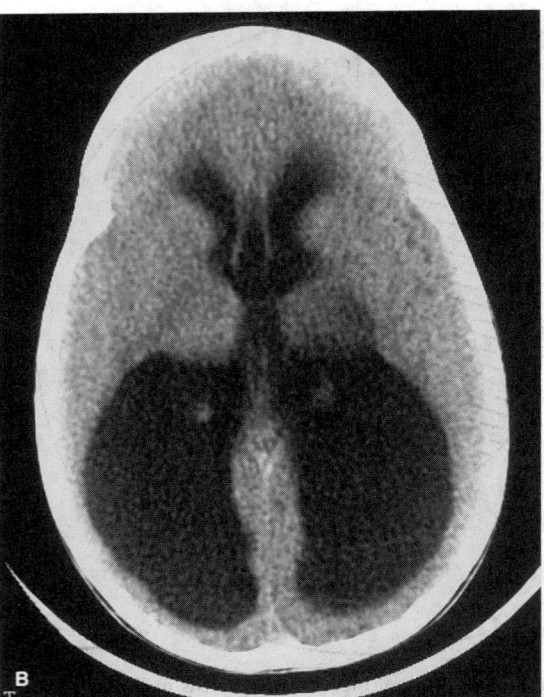

**Figure 20-11.** (**A**) CT scan of preterm infant of 28 weeks' gestational age with bilateral intraventricular hemorrhage. (**B**) Repeat CT, performed because of rapidly increasing occipitofrontal head circumference, lethargy, and increasing apneic spells, demonstrated ventriculomegaly. Lumbar puncture revealed an opening pressure of greater than 200 mm of water, consistent with the diagnosis of posthemorrhagic hydrocephalus.

ages. It is the result of obliterative arachnoiditis either over the hemispheric convexities with occlusion of the arachnoid villi or in the posterior fossa with obstruction of fourth ventricular outflow through the tentorial notch. Rarely, aqueductal obstruction is caused by an acute blood clot, ependymal disruption, or reactive gliosis.

PVL is a frequent neuropathologic accompaniment of GMH/IVH, but apparently is not caused by it. PVL is the generally symmetric injury of the periventricular white matter that is demonstrated readily as cystic lesions by cranial ultrasonography (Fig 20-12) and at postmortem examination. Frequently associated in risk factor studies with apneic, hypotensive, and other ischemic events, it has been reported in 25% to 50% of infants with GMH/IVH and is believed to represent non-hemorrhagic infarction of the periventricular white matter watershed zone. The clinical correlate of PVL is spastic diplegia, although some infants with extensive cystic PVL may experience more generalized changes in tone.

## CLINICAL STUDIES

The incidence of GMH/IVH increases as gestational age decreases, and as many as 50% of infants of less than 25 to 26 weeks' gestation have the disorder. In addition, although the incidence has been reported to vary between 20% and 40% in large cohorts of infants of less than 34 weeks' gestation, high-grade hemorrhages are found more commonly in neonates with very low birth weights. Hemorrhages have been reported within the first postnatal hour, and a significant number of hemorrhages occur by the sixth hour. About half of all preterm infants who will have GMH/IVH do so on the first postnatal day, and less than 5% have hemorrhage after the fourth to fifth postnatal days. This risk period for GMH/IVH appears to be independent of

gestational age. Finally, some infants, especially those with the earliest onset of GMH/IVH, will have extension of hemorrhage over the first several postnatal days; this progression has been linked to clinical events such as pneumothoraces and seizures that are known to increase CBF.

The presence of germinal matrix cysts at the time of birth in preterm infants, previously thought to be related only to congenital evidence, now also are believed to represent "in utero" GMHs.

The clinical manifestations of GMH/IVH are varied. In a significant percentage of cases, GMH/IVH is felt to be clinically silent, although infants with major hemorrhages may experience coma, seizures, abnormal eye findings (including dilated pupils and loss of eye movements), and changes in tone and reflexes. Persistent bradycardia and apneic spells may be secondary to increased intracranial pressure or alterations in CBF to brain stem respiratory centers. Infants may have significantly elevated values of blood glucose and evidence of inappropriate secretion of antidiuretic hormone. Finally, patients with large parenchymal hemorrhages frequently experience a persistent metabolic acidosis that is unresponsive to alkali therapy or pressor agents.

## OUTCOME STUDIES

Infants with GMH/IVH are at risk for the development of PHH and are known to have higher incidences of neonatal seizures and PVL than do infants with hemorrhage, as compared with normal infants matched for birth weight or gestational age. Finally, most investigators agree that those infants with parenchymal involvement of GMH/IVH are at high risk for neurodevelopmental handicap.

PHH (see Fig 20-11) is the combination of ventriculomegaly, diagnosed by serial echoencephalography studies, and increased

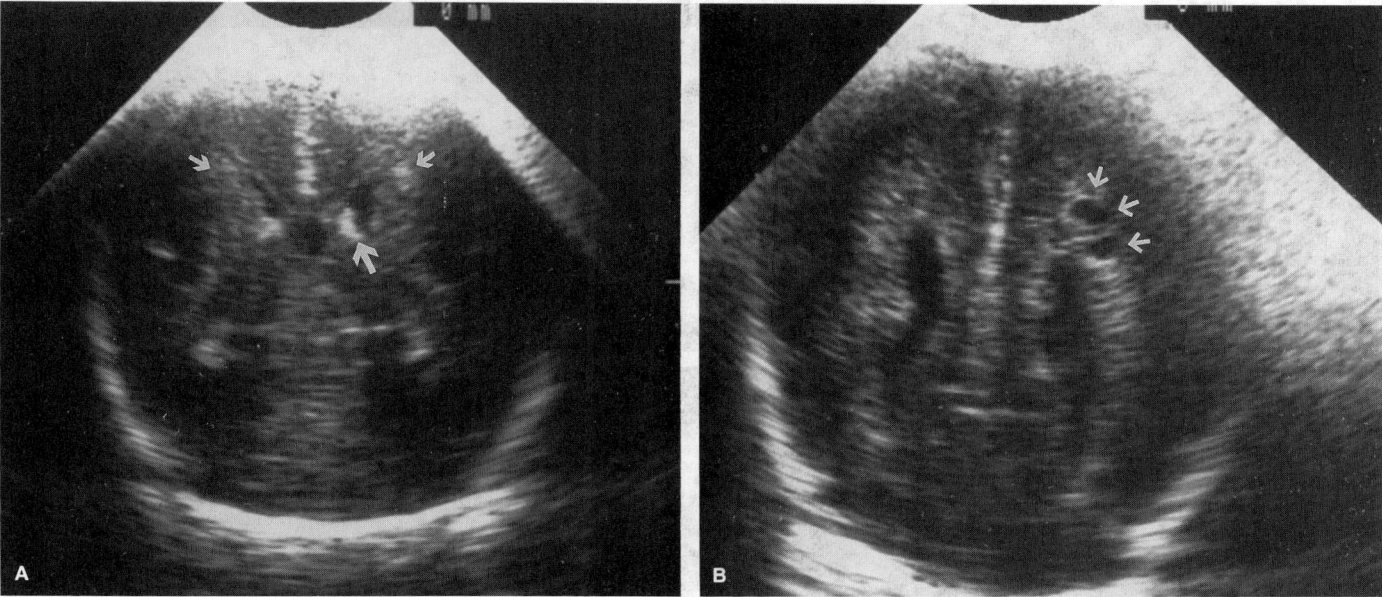

**Figure 20-12.** (**A**) Coronal cranial ultrasound studies of a 1000-g male of 29 weeks' gestation with bloody spinal fluid. Ultrasound on the second postnatal day demonstrated left-sided intraventricular hemorrhage (*large arrow*) and periventricular echodensities bilaterally (*small arrows*). (**B**) Follow-up study 1 week later revealed periventricular cystic lesions consistent with the diagnosis of periventricular leukomalacia (*arrow*).

intracranial pressure, defined as an opening pressure of greater than 140 mm $H_2O$ on either lumbar puncture or, if indicated, cerebral ventricular tap. PHH generally is a communicating hydrocephalus with a block at the level of the arachnoid villi or, less commonly, at the foramina of Luschka and Magendie in the posterior fossa. Hydrocephalus results when the blood and protein in the cerebrospinal fluid (CSF) produce a chemical arachnoiditis that may be transient or, less commonly, permanent. A small percentage of infants with IVH will have a noncommunicating hydrocephalus with a block at the level of the aqueduct secondary to an ependymal reaction similar to that of the arachnoid. Infants with the latter type of hydrocephalus will require neurosurgical intervention, whereas the treatment for neonates with communicating PHH, at least initially, is medical.

All infants with intraventricular blood require close ultrasound monitoring of ventricular size. These patients should undergo frequent head circumference measurements and cranial ultrasound examinations for determination of ventricular size. Because prolonged increased intracranial pressure may result in apnea, vomiting, lethargy, and, ultimately, optic atrophy, the intracranial pressure of infants with head circumferences crossing the expected growth curves and evidence for increasing ventricular size should be checked and, when the diagnosis is confirmed, treatment should be provided. Treatment protocols for infants with communicating hydrocephalus include lumbar punctures with removal of CSF to normalize intracranial pressure and frequent ultrasound checks of ventricular size. Alternatively, acetazolamide (25 to 100 mg/kg/d) and furosemide (1 mg/kg/d) may be used as a temporizing measure to decrease CSF production. The side effects of acetazolamide include vomiting, lethargy, and electrolyte abnormalities, and infants treated with this medication should undergo frequent assessment of their metabolic status with serum electrolyte and bicarbonate measurements. For those infants with evidence of noncommunicating hydrocephalus or intraparenchymal involvement of hemorrhage and shift of the cerebral midline, ventricular taps or the insertion of ventricular catheters with reservoirs performed by neurosurgical personnel are indicated, and the placement of a ventriculoperitoneal shunt ultimately may be necessary.

In many large series of preterm neonates, the incidence of motor handicaps appears to be low. These abnormalities include spastic diplegia, hemiparesis, and, rarely, spastic quadriparesis. Most infants with spastic diplegia have neuroimaging evidence for PVL, but in general have normal head circumferences, no evidence of seizures, and cognitive scores within the normal range. Although many investigators believe that there are no differences in the developmental outcome of infants with grades I, II, or III IVH when compared with infants with no known evidence of hemorrhage in the neonatal period, recent data suggest that the rate of cognitive deficits may increase with the grade of IVH in this patient population. Infants with parenchymal involvement of hemorrhage, or grade IV IVH, experience a wide range of outcomes; about 50% of all neonates with grade IV IVH will have motor and cognitive handicaps. For many of these children, the development of a porencephalic cyst follows resolution of the parenchymal blood, and this can be demonstrated easily both on CT scan (Fig 20-13) and with ultrasound.

## INTERVENTION STUDIES

A variety of measures have been suggested to prevent GMH/IVH. Clearly, the most important way to prevent GMH/IVH is to prevent preterm birth. When that is not possible, transport of the mother and fetus to a regional perinatal center specializing in high-risk obstetric care is preferred; "outborn" infants have consistently higher rates of GMH/IVH than do those who are "inborn."

Neonatal care should be based on an understanding of the pathogenesis of GMH/IVH. Abrupt increases in blood pressure and, thus, changes in CBF should be avoided. Blood pressure and transcutaneous $Po_2$ should be monitored continuously to avoid hypotension and hypoxemia. Hypercarbia should be avoided similarly. The role of the patent ductus arteriosus, and

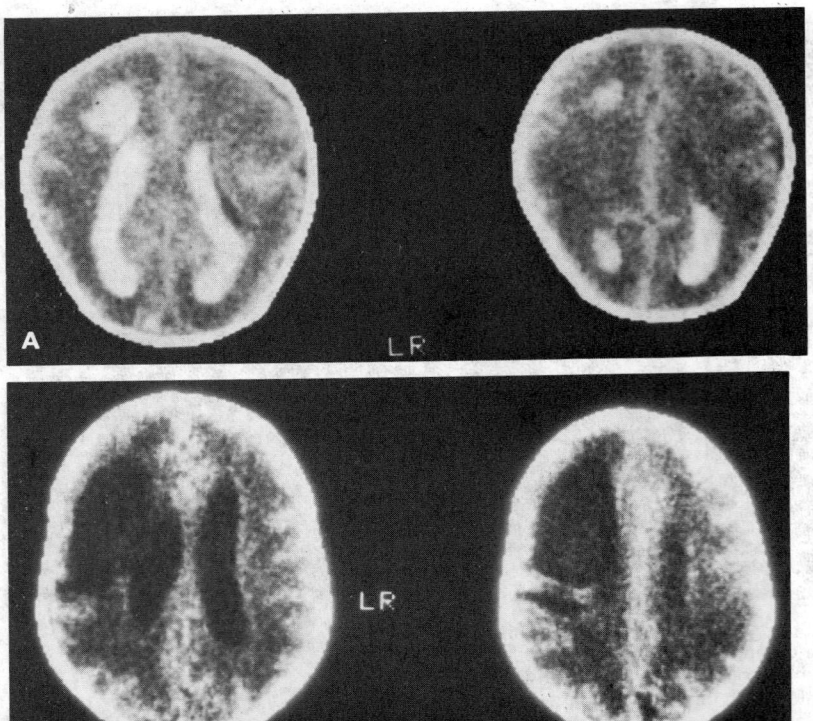

Figure 20-13.   This male of 27 weeks' gestation initially was found to have a bilateral intraventricular hemorrhage with a right frontal parenchymal component (**A**). Repeat CT 12 weeks later demonstrated a large right porencephalic cyst and moderate ventriculomegaly (**B**).

its abrupt closure, in the genesis of IVH long has been debated, and it appears that pharmacologic closure promotes smoother changes in blood flow than do surgical procedures.

Finally, multiple pharmacologic intervention trials have sought to prevent GMH/IVH. The drugs employed include phenobarbital, indomethacin, ethamsylate, vitamin E, and pancuronium bromide (Pavulon), among others. These agents lower CBF, alter the metabolic rate, scavenge free radicals, stabilize capillary membranes, and prevent fluctuations in CBF, respectively. Only phenobarbital has been given prenatally and, thus, none of the other drugs address the high incidence of GMH/IVH in the first 6 postnatal hours.

## Selected Readings

Del Toro J, Louis PT, Goddard-Finegold J. Cerebrovascular regulation and neonatal brain injury. Pediatr Neurol 1991;7:3.

Krishnamoorthy KS, Kuban KCK, Leviton A, et al. Periventricular-intraventricular hemorrhage. Sonographic localization, phenobarbital, and motor abnormalities in low birth weight infants. Pediatrics 1990;85:1027.

Leonard CH, Clyman RI, Piecuch RE, Juster RP, Ballard RA, Behle MB. Effect of medical and social risk factors on outcome of prematurity and very low birth weight. J Pediatr 1990;116:620.

Ment LR, Duncan CC, Ehrenkranz RA, et al. Intraventricular hemorrhage of the preterm neonate: Timing and cerebral blood flow changes. J Pediatr 1984;104:419.

Ment LR, Duncan CC, Scott DT, et al. Posthemorrhagic hydrocephalus. J Neurosurg 1983;50:343.

Papile LA, Burstein J, Burstein R, et al. Incidence and evolution of the subependymal intraventricular hemorrhage; a study of infants with weights less than 1500 grams. J Pediatr 1978;92:529.

Perlman JM, Rollins N, Burns D, Risser R. Relationship between periventricular intraparenchymal echodensities and germinal matrix-intraventricular hemorrhage in the very low birth weight neonate. Pediatrics 1993;91:474.

Szymonowicz W, Yu VHY, Walker A, Wilson F. Reduction in periventricular hemorrhage in preterm infants. Arch Dis Child 1986;61:661.

Volpe JJ. Intraventricular hemorrhage in the premature infant—current concepts. Part I. Ann Neurol 1989;25:3.

Volpe JJ. Intraventricular hemorrhage in the premature infant—current concepts. Part II. Ann Neurol 1989;25:109.

*Principles and Practice of Pediatrics, Second Edition.*
edited by Frank A. Oski et al. J. B. Lippincott Company, Philadelphia © 1994.

## 20.1.4 *Perinatal Asphyxia*

Bennett A. Shaywitz

Perinatal asphyxia, or hypoxic-ischemic encephalopathy (HIE), represents "the single most important perinatal cause of neurological morbidity" in the full-term as well as the low–birth-weight infant, occurring in 6:1000 full-term live births and in an even higher percentage of low–birth-weight infants. Follow-up studies indicate that 25% or more of infants who survive perinatal asphyxia demonstrate permanent neurologic sequelae, ranging from often subtle developmental disabilities such as learning disabilities and attention deficit disorder to more obvious problems such as cerebral palsy, mental retardation, pervasive developmental disorders, and seizures. Although the terms perinatal asphyxia and HIE often are used synonymously, more precisely, perinatal asphyxia refers to the disturbed exchange of oxygen and carbon dioxide, whereas HIE refers to the deprivation of oxygen to the brain by the combined effects of hypoxemia (the reduction in oxygen in the blood) and ischemia (decreased blood flow to the brain). In current usage in the fields of pediatrics and child neurology, the terms perinatal asphyxia, hypoxia, and HIE are interchangeable.

## PATHOGENESIS

The causes of perinatal asphyxia are considered most reasonably within a temporal framework as shown in Table 20-2. Thus, about 70% of the cases of perinatal asphyxia that are seen in

TABLE 20-2.  Etiology of Perinatal Asphyxia

| Time of Insult | Percent of Total |
|---|---|
| Antepartum | 20 |
| Intrapartum | 35 |
| Intrapartum ± antepartum | 35 |
| Postnatal | 10 |

*Volpe JJ. Neurology of the newborn, 2nd ed. Philadelphia: WB Saunders, 1987.*

TABLE 20-3.  Clinical Features of Perinatal Asphyxia

**Fetal**
Abnormal biophysical profile
Abnormal electronic fetal monitoring
  Bradycardia
  Late decelerations
  Variable decelerations leading to late decelerations
Abnormal fetal acid–base status

**Postnatal**
Evidence of asphyxia at birth
  Failure to initiate respiration
  Low Apgar scores
State of consciousness
  Ranges along a continuum from normal, to hyperalertness, through obtundation, lethargy, stupor, and coma
Evidence of damage to other organ systems
  Renal (oliguria)
  Cardiac (myocardiopathy)
  Liver (abnormal liver function test results)
Laboratory studies
  Neuroimaging abnormal
    Magnetic resonance imaging (MRI)
    Ultrasound
    Computed tomography
    Electroencephalography abnormal (eg, burst suppression)

full-term infants are related to events occurring during labor and delivery; these include fetal distress (eg, abnormal fetal heart rate patterns, meconium-stained amniotic fluid, or abnormalities in fetal acid–base values), abruptio placentae, cord prolapse, and traumatic delivery.

The onset of asphyxia is followed by metabolic changes and alterations in cerebral blood flow. Metabolic consequences include an acceleration of glycolysis with an increase in brain lactate levels and a reduction in high-energy phosphate concentrations. At the same time, failure of energy-dependent ionic pumps results in leakage from cells of the normally intracellular potassium and influx into cells of sodium, chloride, and calcium. As a consequence, membrane depolarization occurs, with concomitant release of the excitotoxic neurotransmitters, glutamate and aspartate; these, in turn, activate $N$-methyl-D-aspartate receptors, which are believed to play a critical role in neuronal damage. Alterations in cerebral blood flow accompany these metabolic changes and include an initial increase in cerebral blood flow, loss of vascular autoregulation, reduction in cardiac output, hypotension, and, finally, reduction in cerebral blood flow. The pathologic changes observed in the brain reflect the combined effects of the metabolic derangements that are occurring in the context of cerebral hypoperfusion. For example, selective neuronal necrosis, the most common pathologic finding noted in the brain, describes a process that affects some brain regions while sparing others. This selective vulnerability appears to reflect a combination of region-specific metabolic changes (including specific damage to areas known to exhibit high excitatory neurotoxic transmitter concentrations) and region-specific circulatory patterns. Circulatory changes are believed to play a more prominent role in the production of two other commonly observed pathologic changes after asphyxia: parasagittal cerebral injury and periventricular leukomalacia.

## CLINICAL FEATURES

Perinatal asphyxia may be recognized clinically both before delivery (antepartum and intrapartum) and after delivery (Table 20-3). Recent advances in technology such as ultrasonography, electronic fetal heart rate monitoring (EFM), and direct fetal blood sampling offer the opportunity to evaluate the status of the fetus before delivery. Perinatal asphyxia may be assessed in the antepartum period by two measures: the fetal heart acceleration test (nonstress test) and the biophysical profile. The former measures the increase in fetal heart rate after fetal movement. The latter combines the nonstress test with the ultrasonographic determination of fetal breathing, fetal movements, fetal tone, and amniotic fluid volume. During the intrapartum period, the evaluation of fetal heart rate and its relationship to uterine contractions has been used to assess fetal status. Investigations indicate that such findings as decelerations in fetal heart rate after a uterine

contraction (late decelerations) are related to uteroplacental insufficiency and are influenced considerably by fetal hypoxia. Similarly, decelerations in fetal heart rate beginning with or occurring shortly after the uterine contraction (variable decelerations) appear to be related to umbilical cord compression, which, if continued, can result in reduction in umbilical cord blood flow and fetal hypoxia. Finally, evaluation of fetal acid–base status by direct fetal blood sampling may provide another index reflecting the effects of perinatal asphyxia.

Recognition of perinatal asphyxia in the period immediately after birth reflects the continuous nature of the effects of this complication, a continuity that is reflected in the clinical appearance of an asphyxiated infant, which ranges from completely normal to stillborn. Although Apgar scores are by far the most widely used index of the condition of the infant at birth, pediatricians should recognize the difficulties inherent in attempting to relate hypoxia to the Apgar score. For example, a number of investigators have shown that Apgar scores are not well related to more direct measures of hypoxia such as umbilical cord pH, $P_{CO_2}$ and $P_{O_2}$ levels. Such studies indicate that, although "the Apgar score is an invaluable shorthand method of describing an infant's condition at birth," it reflects the infant's condition *only* at birth, which is "a narrow window in time through which the baby passes" (Editorial, Lancet 1982;1:1393). Another component of the evaluation of an infant who was subjected to perinatal asphyxia is assessment of the infant's state of consciousness, which ranges along a continuum from normal to hyperalertness, through obtundation, lethargy, stupor, and coma. Additional indicators of hypoxia include the involvement of other organ systems, specifically renal involvement (decreased urinary output), cardiac problems (cardiomyopathy), and liver abnormalities (abnormal liver enzyme levels). More specialized investigations also may be helpful in the assessment of perinatal asphyxia. Thus, imaging the brain may reveal evidence of those neuropathologic changes that are associated with perinatal asphyxia. Magnetic

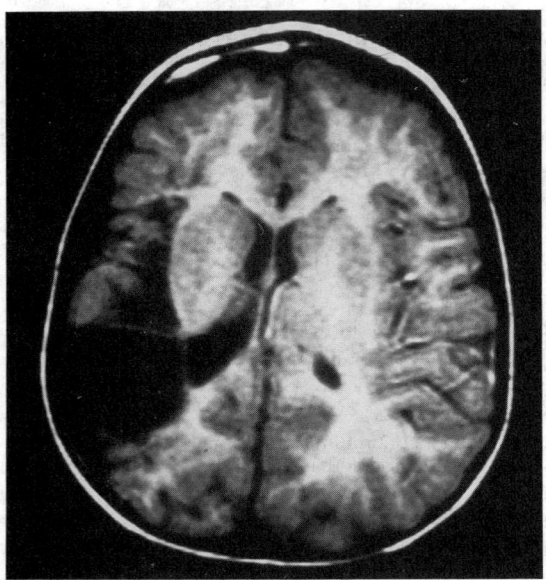

**Figure 20-14.** Magnetic resonance image of a full-term neonate with a right hemisphere porencephaly. In the perinatal period, the patient experienced a precipitous drop in fetal heart rate and low Apgar scores.

resonance imaging is most sensitive (Fig 20-14); ultrasonography is not quite as sensitive, but often is able to demonstrate periventricular echodensities. Magnetic resonance imaging and ultrasound both are considerably more sensitive than is computed tomographic imaging. The association of an abnormal electroencephalogram with perinatal asphyxia carries ominous prognostic implications. Whether newer studies, such as magnetic resonance spectroscopy (Fig 20-15), will offer an even finer-grained evaluation of the effects of perinatal asphyxia remains to be determined.

## MANAGEMENT AND OUTCOME

The management of perinatal asphyxia is focused on diagnosing the problem as early as possible and instituting interventions designed to eliminate or at least minimize the frequency, duration, and severity of the hypoxic insult. For example, when the diagnosis of fetal distress is suspected on the basis of EFM, immediate delivery by cesarean section often is indicated. Emergent care of the infant at birth includes respiratory support, correction of acid–base abnormalities, and treatment of any organ systems that were damaged by the asphyxia (eg, heart, kidney). If seizures complicate the neonatal course, these should be treated as well.

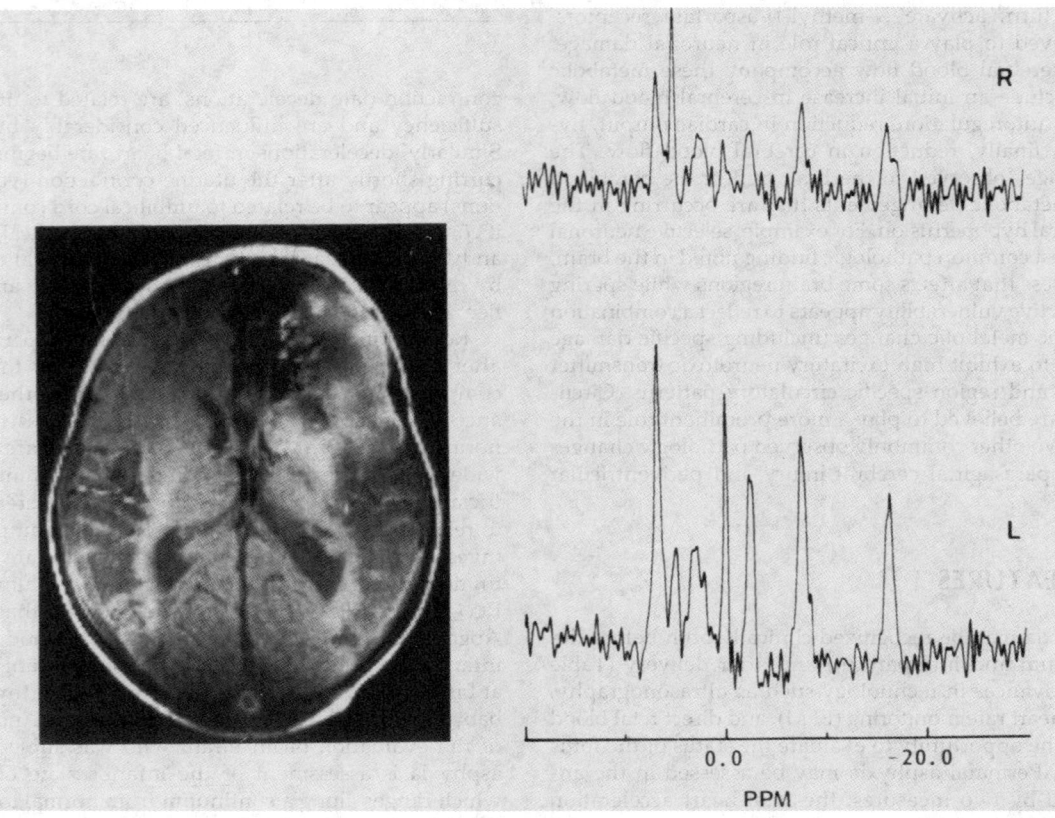

**Figure 20-15.** Magnetic resonance image and phosphorus magnetic resonance spectroscopy of a full-term infant with a cerebral infarct in the distribution of the right middle cerebral artery. On the left is a T$_2$-weighted axial image that shows the area of infarct in the right frontoparietal cortex. On the *right*, phosphorus magnetic resonance spectra were obtained in the same magnet. The spectrum on the *top* (R) is from the region of the infarct and the spectrum on the *bottom* (L) is from the homologous region of the normal left hemisphere. Note the decreased adenosine triphosphate (three peaks on the right side of the spectra) and phosphocreatine (peak at 0.0 ppm) levels when comparing the two sides. Also, note the increase in inorganic phosphorus (peak at 5 ppm).

Pharmacotherapy designed to minimize the central nervous system insult has been disappointing, although new medications directed at the presumed excitatory neurotoxic mechanisms are under development. The outcome of perinatal asphyxia ranges from normal, to subtle developmental disabilities such as learning disabilities and attention disorders, to more obvious and severe problems such as cerebral palsy, pervasive developmental disorder, mental retardation, and seizures, to death. Recognition of brain death in asphyxiated newborns often is difficult and, in contrast to the consensus criteria that exist for brain death in adults, no criteria have been agreed upon for either term or preterm infants. General guidelines are available to gauge outcome in infants who have been subjected to perinatal asphyxia. For example, those who exhibit very abnormal electroencephalographic patterns (such as burst suppression) and who evidence severe neuropathologic changes on neuroimaging studies (eg, multifocal cystic changes in cerebral cortex) will have very poor neurologic outcome. Prediction of long-term outcome in any given child remains problematic, however, and the pediatrician needs to tread cautiously in this area. Reasonable predictions of outcome may need to await follow-up evaluation at 6 months or even later.

## Selected Readings

Auer RN, Siesjo BK. Biological differences between ischemia, hypoglycemia and epilepsy. Ann Neurol 1988;24:699.

Cunningham FG, MacDonald PC, Gant NF. Williams obstetrics. Norwalk, Conn: Appleton & Lange, 1989:290.

Editorial. The value of the Apgar. Lancet 1982;1:1393.

Levene MI, Kornberg J, Williams THC. The incidence and severity of post-asphyxial encephalopathy in full-term infants. Early Hum Dev 1985;11:21.

Scheinberg P. The biologic basis for the treatment of acute stroke. Neurology 1991;41:1867.

Shaywitz BA. The sequelae of hypoxic-ischemic encephalopathy. Semin Perinatol 1987;11:180.

Vannucci R. Current and potentially new management strategies for perinatal hypoxic-ischemic encephalopathy. Pediatrics 1990;85:961.

Vannucci R. Experimental biology of cerebral hypoxic-ischemia: Relationship to perinatal brain damage. Pediatr Res 1990;27:317.

Volpe JJ. Neurology of the newborn, 2nd ed. Philadelphia: WB Saunders, 1987.

*Principles and Practice of Pediatrics, Second Edition.*
edited by Frank A. Oski et al. J. B. Lippincott Company, Philadelphia © 1994.

## 20.1.5 Perinatal Cerebral Infarction

Laura R. Ment

Perinatal cerebral infarction, or stroke, may be defined as a severe disorganization or even complete disruption of the gray and white matter architecture caused by embolic, thrombotic, or ischemic events. Infarcts in early fetal life result in cortical neuronal loss and architectural changes resembling polymicrogyria. Strokes later in gestation are characterized by cavitary changes, or porencephalies, and appear similar to well-defined adult cerebral infarctions. In full-term neonates with stroke caused by perinatal events, cortical necrosis and hemorrhage into gray and subcortical white matter structures may be apparent. In contrast, the periventricular white matter of the preterm neonate has shown a particular susceptibility to ischemic insult.

Strokes are a common finding in the survivors of newborn

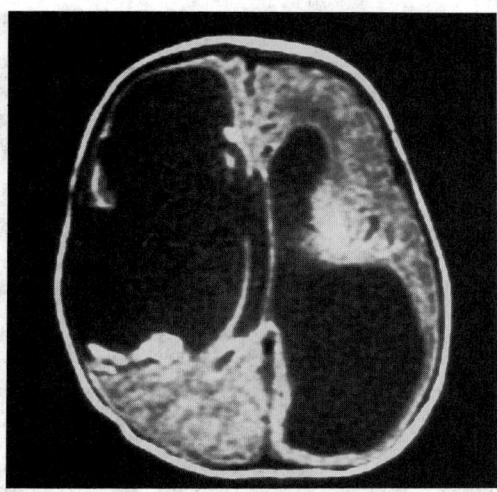

**Figure 20-16.**   This full-term infant with megalencephaly had petechiae at the time of birth. A cranial magnetic imaging study on the second postnatal day demonstrated cerebral infarcts of two different ages: an older left occipital infarct characterized by loss of occipital tissue, and a newer hemorrhagic stroke in the distribution of the right middle and anterior cerebral arteries. Laboratory study results were consistent with the diagnosis of isoimmune thrombocytopenia.

special care units, and their diagnosis must be entertained in those infants who have disorders ranging from congenital microcephaly to neonatal seizures or hemiparesis. Findings in an infant with perinatal cerebral infarction depend on both the timing of the insult in gestation and the mechanism of damage.

## IN UTERO STROKE

During the late second and entire third trimesters of gestation, three factors permit the development of cavitary lesions in response to cerebral insults. The high water content, relatively low myelin concentration, and paucity of active glial response in the developing brain make it susceptible to dissolution and to the secondary formation of such lesions as hydranencephaly, porencephaly, and schizencephaly (see Section 20.1.1). Less frequently,

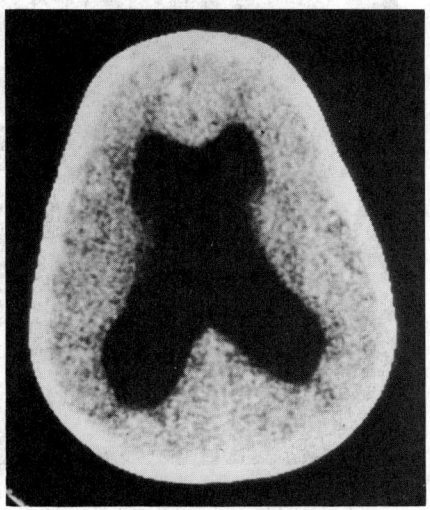

**Figure 20-17.**   Ventriculomegaly consistent with periventricular leukomalacia in a preterm infant with spastic diplegia.

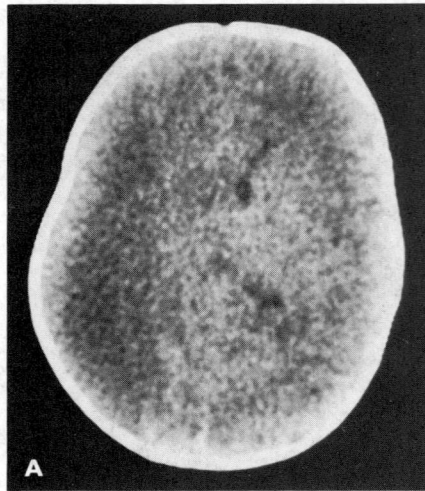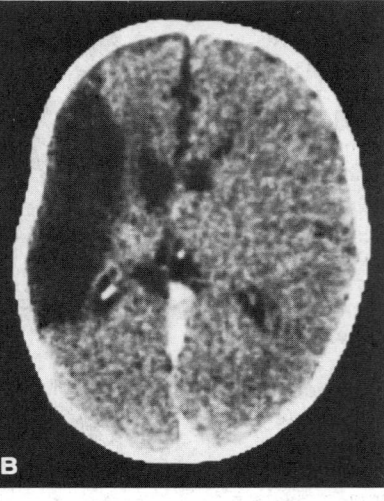

**Figure 20-18.**   CT scan demonstrating left hemispheric low density and effacement of the left lateral ventricle in a full-term infant with right-sided tonic-clonic seizures and meningitis (**A**). Follow-up scan (with contrast) at 1 year of age demonstrated focal tissue loss in the region of the left middle cerebral artery and corresponded to the patient's right spastic hemiparesis (**B**).

insults later in gestation result in regional neuronal cortical loss and areas of focal atrophy that may be accompanied by secondary ventricular system enlargement.

Recognized etiologies for in utero stroke include vascular maldevelopment, emboli, thrombus formation, isoimmune thrombocytopenia, disseminated intravascular coagulation, toxins, trauma, and intrauterine hypoxic-ischemic events. Focal vascular anomalies have been demonstrated in infants with focal porencephalies, and cerebral arteriography or neuropathologic examination of infants with hydranencephaly or schizencephaly (bilateral cyst-like clefts in the distribution of the middle cerebral

artery) have revealed attenuated vessels without recognizable occlusions. Emboli from placental infarcts and tumors, involuting fetal vessels, and punctured or catheterized fetal vessels may result in well-defined focal and multifocal parenchymal infarcts.

Thrombosis secondary to disseminated intravascular coagulation also may result in prenatal cerebral infarction. The finding of cavitary lesions in monozygotic twins or in the survivors of a twin fetal demise may be secondary to the development of disseminated intravascular coagulation, with the transfer of thromboplastic material or emboli from the deceased twin to the survivor through the monochorionic placenta. Similarly, isoimmune

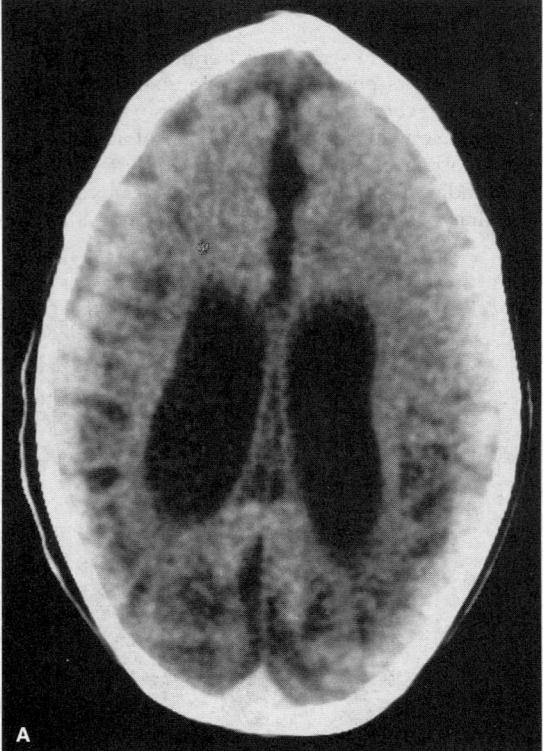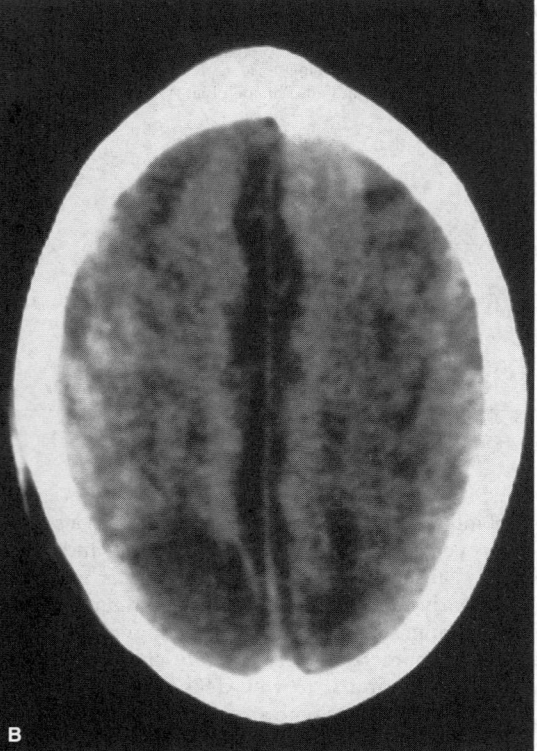

**Figure 20-19.**   (**A**) and (**B**) This 8-week-old female was evaluated for recurrent episodes of unresponsiveness beginning shortly after birth. Her neurologic examination was characterized by microcephaly, high-pitched cry, poor visual behavior, roving eye movements, and marked hypertonia. This CT scan performed at the time of admission demonstrated cortical and central volume loss, linear areas of low density in the periventricular white matter regions, and right occipital porencephaly. Metabolic study results were consistent with the diagnosis of molybdenum cofactor deficiency.

thrombocytopenia has been associated with multifocal hemorrhagic infarcts of varying ages in at-risk fetuses (Fig 20-16).

Other causes of in utero stroke include toxins such as maternal cocaine abuse, aspirin overdose, and carbon monoxide inhalation, and maternal illnesses such as seizures, asthma, or other conditions that are associated with single or recurrent episodes of hypoxemia or hypotension.

## PRETERM STROKE—PERIVENTRICULAR LEUKOMALACIA

Periventricular leukomalacia (PVL), the generally symmetric injury of the periventricular white matter that is readily demonstrable as cystic lesions by cranial ultrasonography, is a frequent neuropathologic accompaniment of germinal matrix and intraventricular hemorrhage, but apparently is not caused by it (Fig 20-17). The periventricular white matter is thought to represent the watershed zone for the developing preterm brain, and the cystic lesions of PVL are found more commonly in those infants with ischemic events such as prolonged perinatal hypotension, apnea, or pneumothoraces. Although rarely found on the first postnatal day, the cystic lesions of PVL may be demonstrated readily by cranial ultrasonography at the end of the first postnatal week. Later in the first year of life, computed tomographic studies may demonstrate ventricular dilatation without evidence of increased intracranial pressure. The clinical picture of spastic diplegia, normal head circumference, normal mental development, and no evidence of seizures is that most commonly associated with PVL, although quadriplegias, blindness, and severe handicaps may result from extensive cyst formation.

## FULL-TERM STROKE

Most strokes in full-term neonates occur in the distribution of the middle cerebral arteries, and more than 75% are found in the left hemisphere. Cerebral infarcts in full-term neonates may be the result of embolic, thrombotic, thrombocytopenic, infectious, iatrogenic, or ischemic events. Although perinatal asphyxia frequently is considered to represent the most common cause of stroke in full-term infants, many infants with stroke do not have the well-recognized risk factors for asphyxia, and other etiologies must be considered. Thus, infants with cyanotic congenital heart disease may be at risk for embolic phenomena. Similarly, those infants with thromboses secondary to meningitis (Fig 20-18), disseminated intravascular coagulation with or without sepsis, and indwelling catheters also are at risk for focal cerebral lesions. Thrombotic lesions also may be the cause of cerebral lesions in infants with polycythemia.

In contrast, deficiencies of coagulation factors may result in hemorrhagic infarction. These deficits include congenital deficiencies such as hemophilia A, severe liver disease, and vitamin K deficiency.

Other origins of stroke in the neonate include iatrogenic causes such as repeated cerebral ventricular taps, cardiac catheterization, and placement of catheters for extracorporeal membrane oxygenation therapy or hyperalimentation; metabolic defects including homocystinuria, molybdenum cofactor deficiency (Fig 20-19), and the mitochondrial encephalopathy lactic acidosis (or MELAS) syndrome; and autoimmune phenomena such as antiphospholipid antibodies.

## Selected Readings

Barmada MA, Moossy J, Shuman RM. Cerebral infarcts with arterial occlusion in neonates. Ann Neurol 1979;6:495.

Filipek PA, Krishnamoorthy KS, Davis KR, Kuehnle K. Focal cerebral infarction in the newborn: A distinct entity. Pediatr Neurol 1987;3:141.

Hofkosh D, Thompson AE, Nozza RJ, Kemp SS, Bowen A, Feldman HM. Ten years of extracorporeal membrane oxygenation: Neurodevelopmental outcome. Pediatrics 1991;87:549.

Mahoney BS, Petty CN, Nyberg DA, Luthy DA, Hickok DE, Hirsch JH. The "stuck twin" phenomenon: Ultrasonographic findings, pregnancy outcome, and management with serial amniocenteses. Am J Obstet Gynecol 1990;163:1513.

Ment LR, Duncan CC, Ehrenkranz RA. Perinatal cerebral infarction. Ann Neurol 1984;16:559.

Paneth N, Rudelli R, Monte W, et al. White matter necrosis in very low birth weight infants: Neuropathologic and ultrasonographic findings in infants surviving six days or longer. J Pediatr 1990;116:975.

Park YD, Belman AL, Kim T-S, et al. Stroke in pediatric acquired immondeficiency syndrome. Ann Neurol 1991;28:303.

Smith CD, Baumann RJ. Clinical features and magnetic resonance imaging in congenital and childhood stroke. J Child Neurol 1991;6:263.

Volpe JJ. Intraventricular hemorrhage in the premature infant—current concepts. Part I. Ann Neurol 1989;25:3.

*Principles and Practice of Pediatrics, Second Edition.*
edited by Frank A. Oski et al. J. B. Lippincott Company, Philadelphia © 1994.

## 20.1.6 *Neonatal Seizures*

Edward J. Novotny, Jr.

Seizures are an important sign of neurologic disease in the newborn. Their incidence varies between 1% and 20%, depending on the populations investigated and a variety of often imprecise clinical criteria. Over the last decade, studies using intensive bedside video/electroencephalographic (EEG)/polygraphic monitoring in neonates with suspected seizures have raised some important issues about the clinical diagnosis of seizures. Several studies have shown that less than half of the abnormal behaviors thought to represent seizures based on clinical criteria actually were epileptic seizures as defined by surface EEG recordings. Other investigators have shown that many epileptic seizures occur without any apparent clinical manifestations. This information suggests that past studies of neonatal seizures may have overestimated the incidence of certain types of neonatal seizures as well as underestimated the total number of seizures that occurred. These recent findings have resulted in alterations in the classification, diagnosis, and therapy of seizures in the newborn.

## CLASSIFICATION AND CLINICAL FEATURES

Neonates with neurologic dysfunction frequently are critically ill and may exhibit abnormal motor phenomena, autonomic instability, and alterations in consciousness. Abnormal motor activities, including posturing, clonus, choreoathetosis, dystonia, and seizures, are seen frequently in these newborns. Differentiation between seizures and other abnormal behaviors (nonepileptic seizure-like events [NESLEs]) traditionally is made on clinical grounds. Early neonatal seizure classifications were based on detailed clinical observations. These classifications were changed according to an improved understanding of the pathophysiology of seizures, movement disorders, and other abnormal phenomena observed in neurologically impaired newborns. The application of EEG to neonates in the 1960s began to clarify which clinical phenomena actually were epileptic seizures. An epileptic seizure

| TABLE 20-4. Classification of Neonatal Seizures | |
|---|---|
| Epileptic Seizures | Nonepileptic Seizure-Like Events |
| Focal clonic | Generalized tonic |
| Focal tonic | Myoclonic |
| Myoclonic |   Focal |
|   Generalized | Motor automatisms |
| |   Oral-buccal-lingual |
| |   Ocular |
| |   Complex movements |
| | Apnea |

is the result of an abnormal discharge of a population of neurons in the brain that may result in a clinical seizure. The use of video/EEG monitoring has allowed further distinction of epileptic seizures from NESLEs. A classification of neonatal seizures based on data from current studies is shown in Table 20-4.

Certain behavioral phenomena consistently show a high correlation with EEG seizure discharges. These include focal clonic, focal tonic, and generalized myoclonic seizures. Clonic seizures involving one limb, one side of the body, or axial structures such as the tongue and face reliably have accompanying synchronous EEG discharges. The EEG during the ictus has a characteristic progression of electrical changes in newborns with this type of seizure (Fig 20-20). The clonic movements are rhythmic and occur at a slow rate of 1 to 6 times per second. In neonates, the clonic activity often is multifocal or migratory and erroneously may be thought to be a generalized seizure. Focal tonic seizures in which the infant has sustained deviation of the eyes with or without head deviation and asymmetric posturing of the limbs or trunk frequently are associated with electrographic seizures. Generalized myoclonic seizures are another type that often have associated electrocortical discharges. The myoclonus occurs sporadically or in a few slow series of jerks. The EEG typically shows high-amplitude spike, sharp, and slow wave transients synchronized with the motor activity.

Other behavioral phenomena have an inconsistent association with EEG seizure discharges. These include generalized tonic, irregular focal myoclonic, and "subtle" neonatal seizures. The latter category also is called motor automatisms, and specific types may have a greater association with EEG seizures, depending on other clinical features. In several earlier studies, the subtle neonatal seizure was the most common type observed clinically. In current studies using EEG monitoring, the subtle neonatal seizure has been found to have a poor association with EEG seizure discharges in the full-term neonate. There is a greater association with electrographic seizures in the premature infant, however. There are other important EEG and clinical distinctions between term and preterm infants with subtle seizures. Premature neonates often have simple subtle seizures with eye, mouth, and tongue movements. Electrographic seizures in premature infants are very distinctive and often show characteristic progression and spread throughout multiple cortical regions with minimal accompanying

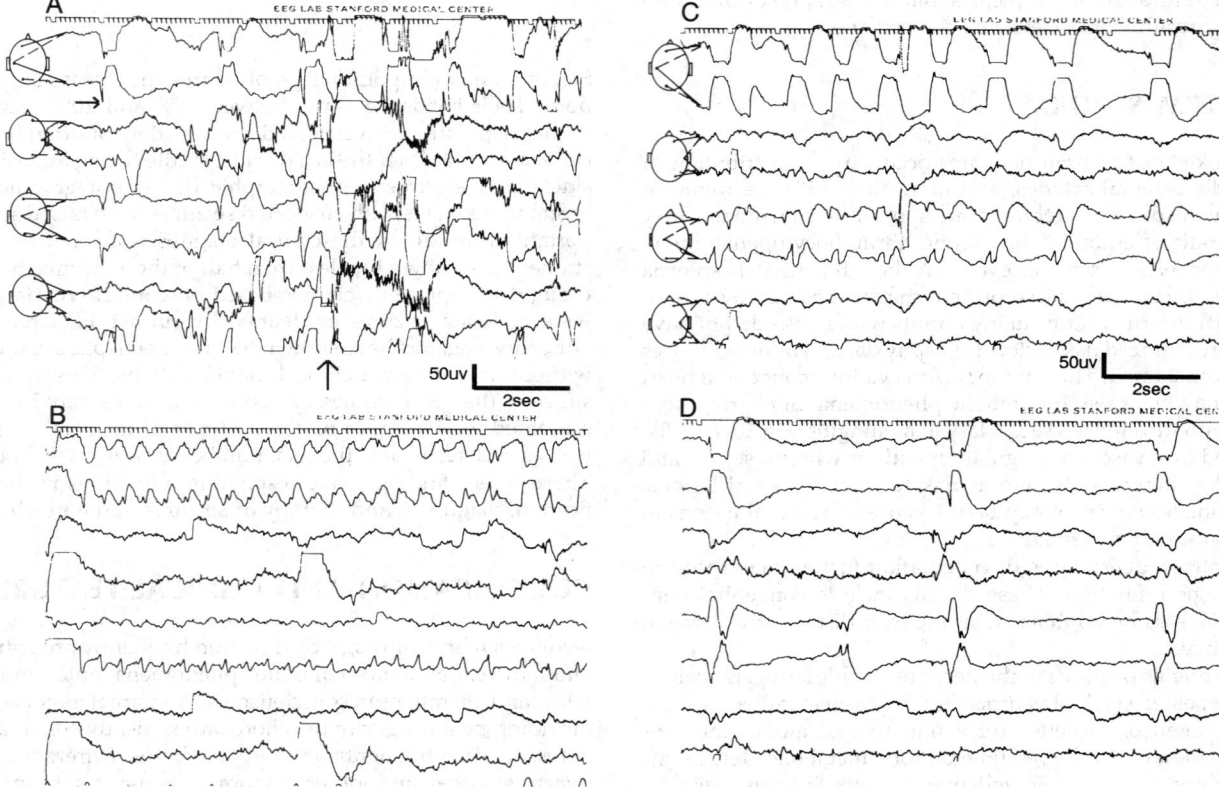

**Figure 20-20.** Electrographic seizure in a 9-day-old infant of 27 weeks' estimated gestational age with severe perinatal asphyxia. (**A**) Onset of the seizure arising from the left temporal region is indicated by the large vertical arrow. An interictal spike also is shown by the horizontal arrow. These spikes recurred erratically every 3 to 7 seconds immediately before the seizure. (**B**) No clinical signs were noted during this portion of the seizure (32 to 42 seconds into the ictus), while repetitive 2- to 3-Hz sharp-slow waves occurred in the left frontotemporal region. (**C**) During this period (76 to 86 seconds), rhythmic 1-Hz clonic activity of the right side of the face was noted. (**D**) Toward the end of the ictus (114 to 124 seconds), the sharp-slow wave complexes recurred every 4 seconds. They eventually stopped at 150 seconds.

clinical signs (Fig 20-21). In term infants, the subtle seizures often take on more complex motor automatisms such as peddling, swimming, and stepping behavior. Often, there are no associated EEG discharges in recordings of these infants.

Myoclonic activity that is irregular, multifocal, and stimulus-induced typically is not associated with any changes in electrocortical activity. These infants usually have markedly abnormal EEGs for gestational age, with suppressed and poorly differentiated background electrocortical activity. Neonates with episodes described as generalized tonic seizures rarely have them as a result of an epileptic seizure. In one study, less than 15% of infants with this clinical phenomenon had an epileptic seizure as a cause. Many of these episodes possibly represented decerebrate and decorticate posturing from acute intracranial pathology.

Several clinical attributes are helpful in differentiating NESLEs from epileptic seizures. Infants with clonic seizures have slower, more rhythmic motor activity that cannot be stopped by restraint, whereas infants with tremors and clonus have rapid, irregular motor activity that ceases with restraint and change in posture of the limb. Tremor, clonus, and other nonepileptic motor automatisms typically can be induced by various tactics such as touching the infant or making a sudden loud noise nearby. NESLEs also demonstrate properties of spatial and temporal summation by increasing in severity with increased intensity or frequency of the stimulus. These latter behaviors are abnormal and

usually indicate the existence of neurologic dysfunction, but they do not represent behaviors that warrant treatment with antiepileptic therapy. Another clinical characteristic that aids in distinguishing epileptic events from NESLEs is the fact that epileptic seizures typically are accompanied by changes in heart rate, respiratory pattern, pupil size, and blood pressure. Further video/EEG/polygraphic studies are required in the neonate to define the temporal and spatial relationships of these autonomic changes with the electroclinical seizure. An isolated episode of apnea also rarely is an epileptic seizure, though apnea is seen frequently in epileptic seizures in association with other clinical signs. Many other causes of apnea in term and preterm infants should be excluded before an epileptic seizure is considered as the etiology.

## ETIOLOGY AND DIAGNOSIS

Kellaway and Mizrahi suggest that conclusions derived from previous investigations regarding the etiology, treatment, and prognosis of neonatal seizures are of limited value. Past studies both overestimated and underestimated the incidence of neonatal seizures, and suffered from a lack of consensus about which phenomena in the newborn truly were epileptic seizures. These concerns have their greatest impact on treatment because prognosis and etiology are interdependent and the seizures are a symptom of an underlying neuropathologic process. Recent concerns about

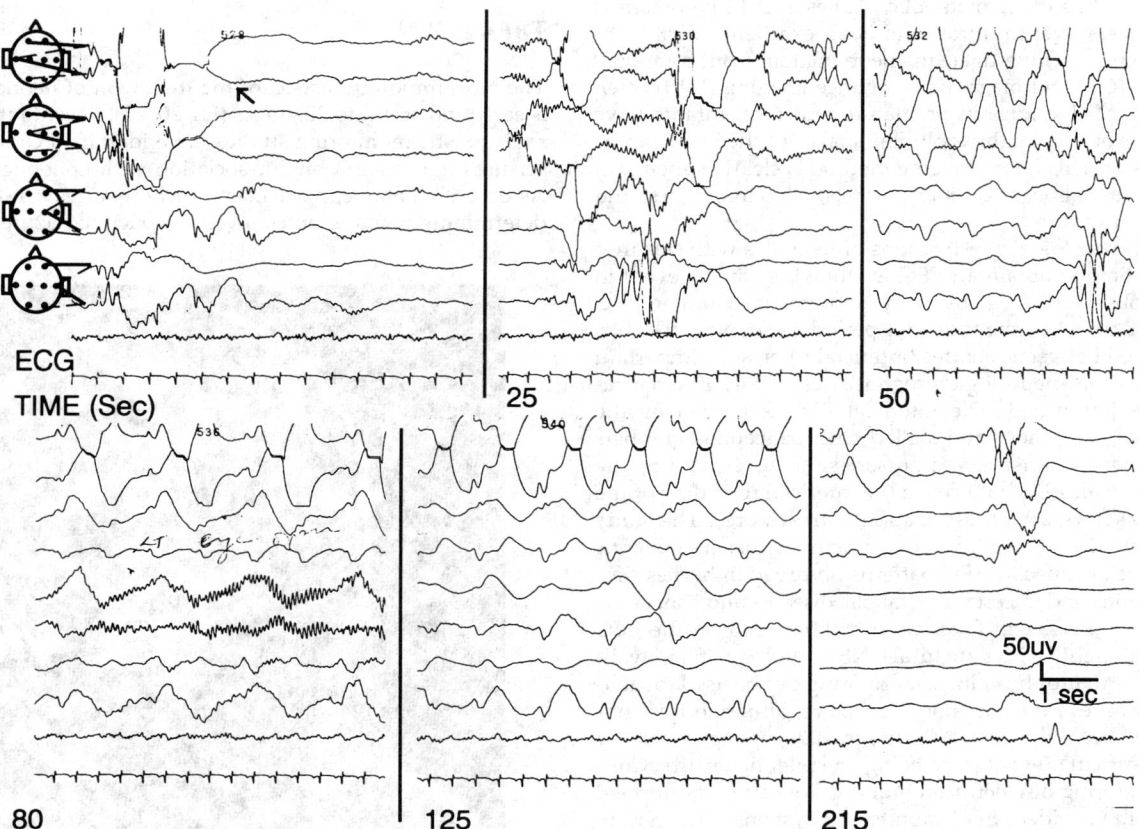

**Figure 20-21.** A subclinical electrographic seizure in a 2-day-old infant of 29 weeks' estimated gestational age with severe perinatal asphyxia. (**A**) The seizure begins with low-amplitude, rhythmic alpha activity in the left temporal region (*arrow*). This builds in amplitude and spreads to the left central region 25 seconds into the ictal event (**B**). Fifty seconds into the seizure, irregular, sharp-slow waves are observed over the entire left hemisphere, are higher in amplitude anteriorly, and spread to the right frontal region (**C**). Rhythmic alpha activity is observed to arise from the right central region 80 seconds into the seizure when the infant was noted to open the left eye (**D**). The sharp-slow wave activity is maximum over the left temporal region with spread over the entire cortex 125 seconds into the seizure (**E**), and it ends 215 seconds from its inception (**F**).

the effects of antiepileptic drug therapy on the developing nervous system have increased the importance of these issues in management.

In regard to etiology, perinatal asphyxia, central nervous system (CNS) infections, intracranial hemorrhages, and cerebral infarcts account for about 90% of the disorders that are responsible for neonatal seizures. Developmental anomalies, acute metabolic disorders, and rare inborn errors of metabolism are less common etiologies. Identification of the latter two etiologic categories is crucial because treatment is altered with respect to management of the underlying disease.

Initial evaluation of the newborn with seizures should begin with a thorough history, with emphasis on prenatal and perinatal drug exposure, details of labor and delivery, presence of maternal infection, maternal metabolic status, and family history of seizures. Early assessment of cardiorespiratory status and stabilization are critical. A careful general physical examination and a detailed neurologic examination are required. Funduscopic examination for retinal pathology indicating intracranial hemorrhage or CNS infection should be performed. Evaluation for hepatosplenomegaly and a thorough cardiovascular examination, including auscultation of the head for arteriovenous malformations, are necessary.

Initial investigations should include neuroimaging; cerebrospinal fluid examination; serum electrolyte determinations; calcium, magnesium, creatine, blood urea nitrogen, and glucose measurements; a complete blood count; and arterial blood gas determinations. Serum ammonia and hepatic enzyme concentrations, as well as other metabolic studies should be obtained in selected cases. Neuro-ultrasound is an excellent initial technique with which to investigate the neuroanatomy, but computed tomography (CT) and magnetic resonance imaging (MRI) often are required. MRI studies in premature and term infants have shown that exquisite, high-resolution images of the brain can be acquired easily. This neuroimaging method is clearly superior to CT for the illustration of cerebral infarcts, CNS anomalies, and certain CNS infections.

In neurophysiologic investigations of neonates with seizures, the optimal time to obtain an EEG is while the clinical event in question is observed. This obviously is impractical, and an EEG should be obtained in the interictal period as soon as possible. EEGs obtained between seizures (interictally) provide important information about neurologic prognosis, especially if serial recordings are performed. The interictal EEG is limited by the availability of equipment and skilled electroencephalographers in most neonatal intensive care nurseries, however, and by the absence of specific EEG patterns in the interictal recording of the newborn that have a high association with seizures. The study cannot verify whether a clinical event actually was an epileptic seizure. There are specific EEG patterns observed in herpes simplex encephalitis and in certain metabolic diseases and congenital malformations. Persistent focal abnormalities seen on the EEG are correlated highly with structural CNS pathology. If it is available, intensive neurophysiologic monitoring can be used to identify whether an event is an epileptic seizure, although it is controversial whether the lack of surface EEG epileptic activity excludes a particular event from being an epileptic seizure. Continuous monitoring of electrocerebral activity can be performed by cassette EEG, video/EEG monitoring systems, and certain commercially available physiology monitors that are present in newborn intensive care units. If a newborn continues to have persistent clinical seizures after careful clinical assessment and treatment with first-line antiepileptic agents, some form of neurophysiologic monitoring is indicated.

Certain types of seizures are seen in infants with specific disorders. For example, persistent partial motor seizures are noted typically in infants with strokes or congenital malformations. One

newborn with hemimegalencephaly of the left hemisphere (Fig 20-22) was reported to have persistent seizures primarily involving the right side of the body. Clonic seizures also are seen commonly in infants with hypocalcemia, although the incidence of this disorder has decreased dramatically over the last few decades. Both subtle and tonic seizures are seen more often in infants with hypoxic-ischemic encephalopathy.

Several specific epileptic syndromes are noted primarily in the neonatal period. These include benign neonatal convulsions, which occur in full-term infants, usually beginning on the fifth day of life. These seizures are self-limited and resolve spontaneously in a few weeks. Benign neonatal familial convulsions is a rare disorder with an autosomal dominant pattern of inheritance in which seizures begin during the first week of life and usually resolve in the first few months. Recent investigations have identified linkage to a specific region on the long arm of chromosome 20. Early myoclonic encephalopathy begins in the first few weeks of life with generalized and multifocal myoclonic seizures and depression of consciousness. Several metabolic disorders, including nonketotic hyperglycinemia and D-glyceric acidemia, have been identified in infants with this clinical syndrome. Finally, early infantile encephalopathy with burst suppression is observed in infants who have primarily tonic seizures and a progressive deterioration in neurologic function in the first month of life. This is associated with a burst suppression EEG pattern early during the disorder and the infants inevitably have a poor outcome.

## TREATMENT

The most important aspect of the treatment of neonatal seizures is early and accurate diagnosis (Fig 20-23). Recent intensive neurodiagnostic monitoring studies have identified certain types of seizures that have a high association with epileptic discharges. As described above, particular clinical features can be useful in determining whether an event is an epileptic seizure. Therefore,

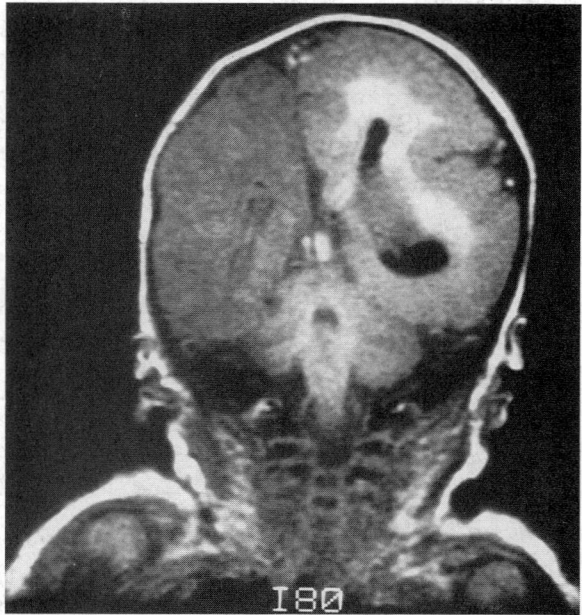

**Figure 20-22.** Head MRI of a 5-day-old, full-term male infant who began having seizures at a few hours of life. A coronal view of a T1-weighted image is shown. The left hemisphere is abnormal, with a dilated ventricle, increased signal intensity in the white matter, and abnormal architecture of the cortex. The neuroimaging changes are typical of infants with unilateral megalencephaly.

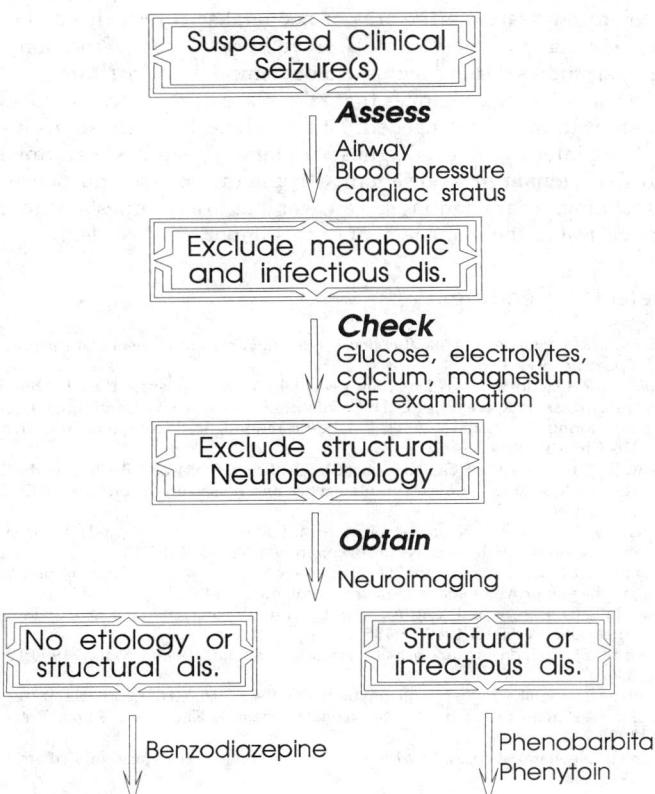

**Figure 20-23.** Flow chart of treatment and evaluation of neonatal seizures. *CSF,* cerebrospinal fluid; *dis,* disease.

**TABLE 20-5. Antiepileptic Drugs and Dosages**

| | Dose | |
|---|---|---|
| Antiepileptic Drug | Loading (mg/kg) | Maintenance |
| Phenobarbital | 15–40 | 3–5 mg/kg/d |
| Phenytoin | 15–20 | 8–10 mg/kg/d |
| Lorazepam | 0.05–0.10 | 0.1 every 6 h |
| Diazepam | 0.1–0.2 | — |
| Primidone | 10–20 | 10–20 mg/kg/d |
| Valproic acid | 20–50 | 15–50 mg/kg/d |
| Lidocaine | 2–3 | 3–10 mg/kg/h |

focal clonic, partial tonic, and generalized myoclonic seizures often can be treated based on clinical criteria alone. As recently recommended by Volpe, treatment with antiepileptic agents should be withheld in infants who have generalized tonic and subtle seizures, especially in the case of subtle seizures occurring in a full-term infant.

Initial management of the newborn with suspected seizures includes rapid assessment and stabilization of respiratory and cardiovascular status. This should be followed immediately by determination of glucose and electrolyte status, including measurement of the serum calcium level. Initial bedside measurement of the glucose level should be performed and, if it is abnormal, 2 to 4 mL/kg of $D_{25}W$ glucose should be given parenterally. Hypocalcemia should be treated by giving 1 mL/kg of 10% calcium gluconate parenterally. Next, evaluation for a CNS infection is indicated by examination of the cerebrospinal fluid. Neuroimaging should be performed to exclude any structural neuropathology, such as an intracranial hemorrhage, CNS anomaly, or cerebral infarct.

If the clinical seizures seen are definite epileptic seizures, treatment with either a benzodiazepine or phenobarbital is indicated (Table 20-5). Phenobarbital should be given at a dosage of 15 to 20 mg/kg intravenously. This dosage corresponds to a serum level of 20 to 30 mg/L. Additional 5-mg/kg doses of phenobarbital may be given to produce a serum level of 40 mg/L. A serum level greater than 40 mg/L does not produce an increase in the number of infants whose seizures will be controlled by this antiepileptic agent. If the seizures persist, 15 to 20 mg/kg of phenytoin should be administered intravenously at a rate of 1 mg/kg/min. Close monitoring of the blood pressure, electrocardiogram, and respiratory status is required with administration of this drug. If there is a question as to whether the events are epileptic seizures, treatment with a benzodiazepine should be

considered because these agents have a rapid onset of action and short half-lives. Cardiovascular instability and hyperbilirubinemia are relative contraindications to the use of these agents. Diazepam should be given at 0.1 mg/kg and lorazepam should be given at 0.05 to 0.1 mg/kg intravenously. Finally, primidone, valproic acid, lidocaine, and pentobarbital all have been used in the treatment of intractable seizures in the neonatal period. Use of these agents should not be considered unless the seizures are well documented both clinically and electrophysiologically. Infants with documented intractable epileptic seizures in the neonatal and infantile period should be given a trial of pyridoxine. This vitamin is an important cofactor for several enzyme systems, including the enzymes responsible for metabolism for the putative amino acid neurotransmitters. Fifty to 100 mg of pyridoxine should be given parenterally while the infant's EEG is being monitored. Infants with pyridoxine-dependent seizures will have a dramatic improvement in their EEG with the administration of pyridoxine.

Another significant issue regarding management that was brought about by neurophysiologic monitoring concerns the criteria that should be used for determining the adequacy of therapy. Should clinical or electrical criteria be used to judge therapeutic efficacy? Several studies have shown that the majority of electrical seizures in the newborn are of short duration and have no accompanying clinical signs. One investigator found that 79% of infants with electrographic seizures had electrical seizures without clinical manifestations. Most of these newborns already were being treated with antiepileptic agents. Other studies also have shown that electrical seizures persist even after treatment. Animal studies do not help with this question because most animal studies investigating neonatal seizures have shown significant biochemical changes only in animals that have prolonged seizures (those lasting longer than 30 minutes). Both clinical and electrical seizures in the human neonate typically last less than 3 minutes. Further information is needed to determine whether brief, subclinical electrical seizures are harmful to the immature nervous system. Until this has been defined, therapy should be guided by the response of clinical seizures that are determined to be epileptic.

The duration of therapy should be guided by the risk of recurrence of seizures and the possible toxicity induced by treatment. Infants with cerebral malformations and significant structural lesions are at high risk for continuing to have seizures, whereas those with hypoxic-ischemic encephalopathy or a metabolic cause have a much lower risk of recurrence. If the neurologic examination and the interictal EEG are normal, the chance of the infant having later seizures is small. Recent concerns regarding the effects of drugs on the developing nervous system also have dictated that the duration of therapy be kept to a minimum. Antiepileptic therapy is discontinued in most infants before they are discharged from neonatal intensive care and rarely is continued for more than 8 weeks after discharge. EEGs obtained after the acute illness and in the first weeks of life aid in deciding whether to continue antiepileptic therapy, in assessing the risk of the development of epilepsy, and in determining the long-term neurologic outcome.

## PROGNOSIS

The prognosis is associated closely with the etiology of the seizures. The presence of CNS anomalies or structural lesions on neuroimaging studies has a significant impact on the long-term outcome of the infant. For three decades, the EEG has been shown to be a valuable tool in determining prognosis in premature and full-term neonates with various pathologies, including seizures. If specific criteria are used to grade the severity of the background abnormality on the EEG, the degree of abnormality predicts long-term outcome better than does the clinical examination. Certain types of seizures determined both clinically and electrographically also permit further refinement of the ability to determine prognosis. Infants with tonic or subtle seizures often have diffuse, severe encephalopathies and a poorer outcome. A unique ictal EEG pattern characterized by bursts of rhythmic 8- to 12-Hz activity is seen commonly in newborns with severe encephalopathies (see Fig 20-21). These infants often have a poor prognosis. Further investigations combining both EEG and neuroimaging are required to refine our ability to determine prognosis.

Future research in the area of neonatal seizures is needed to address many of the issues discussed in this section. Additional animal studies dealing with the biochemical, ultrastructural, and molecular biologic changes that take place in repetitive seizures of short duration are needed. Finally, clinical investigations involving intensive neurodiagnostic monitoring studies performed on the neonate in association with pharmacologic and neuropsychologic examinations can answer many of the questions that are critical to the management of this important disorder.

## Selected Readings

Clancy RR, Legido A. Postnatal epilepsy after EEG-confirmed neonatal seizures. Epilepsia 1991;32:69.

Clancy RR, Legido A, Lewis D. Occult neonatal seizures. Epilepsia 1988;29:256.

Connell J, Oozeer R, De Vries L, Dubowitz LMS, Dubowitz V. Continuous EEG monitoring of neonatal seizures: Diagnostic and prognostic considerations. Arch Dis Child 1989;64:45.

Farwell JR, Lee YJ, Hirtz DG, Sulzbacher SI, Ellenberg JH, Nelson KB. Phenobarbital for febrile seizures—effects on intelligence and on seizure recurrence. N Engl J Med 1990;322:364.

Kellaway P, Mizrahi E. Neonatal seizures. In: Luders H, Lesser RP, eds. Epilepsy electroclinical syndromes. New York: Springer-Verlag, 1987:13.

Legido A, Clancy RR, Berman PH. Neurologic outcome after electroencephalographically proven neonatal seizures. Pediatrics 1991;88:583.

Mizrahi E. Consensus and controversy in the clinical management of neonatal seizures. Clin Perinatol 1989;16:485.

Novotny EJ. Epileptic syndromes and seizures in infants. Semin Neurol 1990;10:366.

Painter MJ, Alvin J. Choice of anticonvulsants in the treatment of neonatal seizures. In: Wasterlain CG, Vert P, eds. Neonatal seizures. New York: Raven Press, 1990:243.

Volpe JJ. Neonatal seizures: Current concepts and revised classification. Pediatrics 1989;84:422.

*Principles and Practice of Pediatrics, Second Edition.*
edited by Frank A. Oski et al. J. B. Lippincott Company, Philadelphia © 1994.

## 20.1.7 *The Floppy Infant and the Late Walker*

Richard S.K. Young

## HISTORY

In the diagnosis of neurologic disease, it is the history that furnishes clues to the nature of the disorder, and the physical examination and laboratory tests that provide confirmation. When the history of an infant with hypotonia is taken, information regarding any family history of neuromuscular disease, the quality of the fetal movements, and the presence of hydramnios should be obtained.

## PHYSICAL EXAMINATION

A general physical examination of any infant with suspected neurologic disease is essential to rule out motor delays caused by systemic disease. It should be determined whether congestive heart failure (dyspnea, edema, organomegaly) may be responsible for weakness or fatigue. The child should be examined for dysmorphic features (suggestive of a chromosomal abnormality) and

for signs of endocrinopathy (umbilical hernia, dull cry, brittle hair).

Weakness typically begins in the proximal large muscles of the neck and in the pectoral and pelvic girdles, producing poor head control in the infant and delay in walking in the older child. The muscles should be inspected for bulk, atrophy, fasciculations, and symmetry. The presence of fasciculations in the tongue muscle is evidence of denervation. The muscle stretch reflexes should be tested and it should be determined whether sensation is grossly intact.

## NEUROLOGIC EVALUATION

Based on the results of the history and physical examination, the physician first should determine whether a problem exists, or whether a child simply is at the lower limits of normal. If a neuromuscular disorder is suspected, it should be decided whether the lesion is central (spasticity correlates with upper motor neuron) or peripheral (hyporeflexia correlates with lower motor neuron arc). The pediatrician should think anatomically about each element of the motor system and determine whether it is involved, beginning with the cerebral cortex and proceeding along the corticospinal tract to the muscle fiber.

### Central Nervous System

Cerebral injuries are the most common cause of weakness ("central hypotonia"). Cerebral conditions that may cause an infant

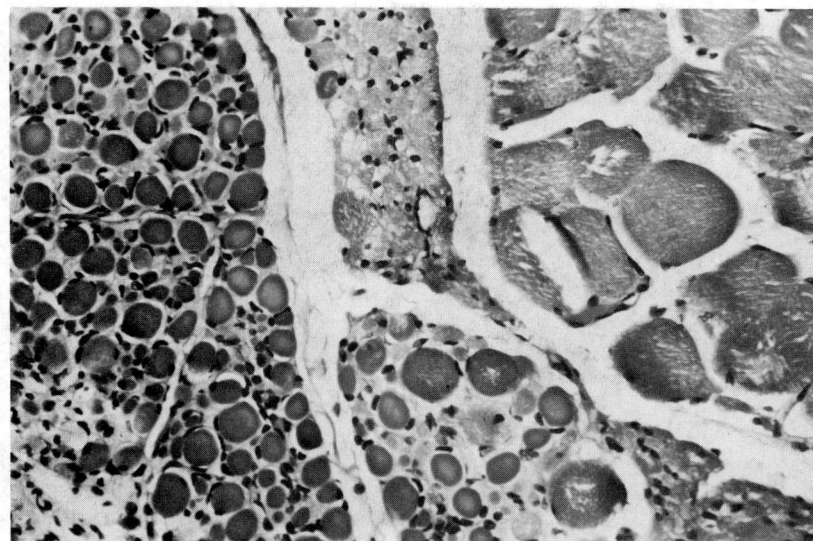

**Figure 20-24.** Muscle biopsy from a patient with Werdnig-Hoffmann disease. Muscle fibers are seen in the far left and right lower areas. They are round and markedly atrophic, whereas those seen in the upper right are either normal in size or hypertrophic. Hematoxylin-eosin stain. Magnification ×130. (Courtesy of J. Kim, MD, Yale University School of Medicine.)

to be floppy include hypoxic-ischemic encephalopathy, intracranial infection, cerebral hemorrhage, cerebral trauma, metabolic disorders, and cerebral malformations.

Children with these disorders may have seizures or other signs of cerebrocortical dysfunction. Central, as opposed to peripheral, causes of weakness result in spasticity, with ankle clonus, crossed adductor reflex, Babinski's sign, and fisting. Strabismus also may suggest central nervous system dysfunction causing floppiness in an infant.

## Spinal Cord

The most common causes of spinal cord disease producing a floppy infant are trauma, dysraphism (myelomeningocele), and degeneration of the anterior horn cells. Cervical spinal cord injury may result from tearing or shearing of the spinal cord during delivery of a large infant (Young et al, 1983). Tumors or infections of the spinal cord are relatively less common. Seesaw respirations are a sign of diaphragmatic breathing and indicate that the lesion is above the C4 level (emergence of the phrenic nerve). Widespread degeneration of anterior horn cells also may produce diaphragmatic breathing.

Selective loss of the anterior horn cells may occur during fetal life, in infancy, or during early childhood. If there is onset of paralysis in utero, the infant may exhibit widespread contractures (arthrogryposis multiplex congenita). Anterior horn cell disease also may be seen in the infant (Werdnig-Hoffman syndrome). Virtually all other sensory or association neurons in the nervous system are spared, leaving consciousness unimpaired. The diagnosis is confirmed by the presence of "group atrophy" on muscle biopsy samples (Fig 20-24).

The differential diagnosis of anterior horn cell disease also includes polio; this selectively affects the large motor neurons. In contrast to Werdnig-Hoffman syndrome, the pattern of involvement in polio is asymmetric, with prominent signs of inflammation in the cerebrospinal fluid (eg, elevated cerebrospinal fluid cell count, fever).

## Radiculopathies

Acute inflammatory polyneuropathy (Guillain-Barré syndrome) is an infrequent cause of weakness in the infant and young child. The disorder results from a postinfectious immune attack on the Schwann cell producing demyelination of peripheral nerves. Because of the interruption of the lower motor neuron arc, areflexia

is present. The diagnosis is established by the presence of elevated protein levels in the cerebrospinal fluid and delay in nerve conduction. Plasmapheresis and intravenous immunoglobulin have been advocated as therapies for Guillain-Barré syndrome.

## Disorders of the Peripheral Nerve

Peripheral nerve disease, other than Guillain-Barré syndrome, is an unusual cause of weakness in the neonatal period. Disorders of the peripheral nerve commonly are sporadic in occurrence (Leigh disease, Riley-Day syndrome or familial dysautonomia, and Möbius' syndrome), although Dejerine-Sottas disease is inherited in an autosomal recessive manner.

## Disorders Involving the Neuromuscular Junction

Disorders of the neuromuscular junction may cause an infant to be floppy or an older child to be a late walker (Table 20-6). Myasthenia gravis has a unique pattern of muscular involvement with predilection for the face and eyelids. Ptosis is prominent. Weakness of the bulbar musculature may produce dysarthria. Transient myasthenia gravis occurs in 10% to 15% of the infants born to mothers with myasthenia and results from an immune attack upon the postsynaptic receptor of the infant muscle. The diagnosis of neonatal myasthenia may be confirmed by the intramuscular administration of neostigmine, 0.1 mg/kg. Atropine (0.1 mg intramuscularly) should be kept on hand to counteract muscarinic effects such as diarrhea and tracheal secretions. Myasthenia in newborns also may be genetic and not mediated by antibodies to the acetylcholine receptor. Therapy for the infant with the transient form of neonatal myasthenia is largely supportive. Careful attention to feeding techniques and respiratory care is

| TABLE 20-6. Neonatal Diseases of the Neuromuscular Junction | |
|---|---|
| Myasthenia gravis | Transient, congenital |
| Metabolic disease | Hypermagnesemia |
| Toxins | Kanamycin, gentamycin, neomycin, streptomycin, polymixin |
| Infantile botulism | |

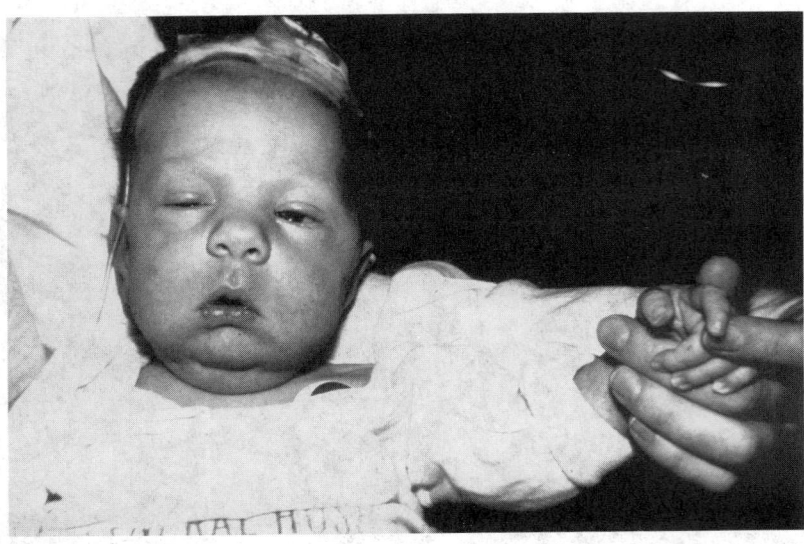

**Figure 20-25.** Myotonic dystrophy. Note the ptosis "fish-mouth" deformity in this infant.

needed; tube feedings may be required. Some authors advocate the use of anticholinesterases.

## Disorders of Muscle

Myotonic dystrophy is an autosomal dominant disorder and is determined by a genetic locus on chromosome 19. The mother with myotonic dystrophy may have a complicated obstetric course, with premature labor, uterine dystocia, and breech presentation. Polyhydramnios may result from inadequate swallowing by the fetus. Myotonic dystrophy should be suspected if the mother exhibits "hatchet" facies, upturned philtrum ("fish-mouth deformity"), ptosis, or percussion myotonia. Infants with myotonic dystrophy may have ptosis, apnea, or failure to thrive (Fig 20-25). Electromyography shows "dive-bomber" potentials, which consist of repetitive electrical potentials of up to 100 per second that wax and wane in frequency and amplitude. These infants may require ventilatory support, but, ultimately, should grow stronger and be able to breathe independently.

Metabolic myopathies are characterized by their histologic appearances. These disorders include central core disease, nemaline myopathy, myotubular myopathy, congenital fiber-type disproportion, (Fig 20-26), and mitochondrial myopathies. Although the specific metabolic defect still may not be clarified, the muscle biopsy sample may show a characteristic histopathologic picture. Patients with central core disease have cores that are central or somewhat eccentric, demonstrated well with histochemical stains for oxidative enzymes. The cores are more likely to be found in type 1 (oxidative) fibers. Central core disease is either slowly progressive or nonprogressive.

Nemaline (which is Greek for *rod*) myopathies have characteristic broad rods thought to represent abnormal deposition of Z bands of the sarcomere, possibly tropomyosin. There is predominance of type 1 fibers. Hence, the myopathy represents a defect in the cytoskeleton of the myocyte. Both a fatal infantile form and a more slowly progressive or nonprogressive form of the disease exist.

Muscle fibers in myotubular myopathy resemble fetal myotubes, suggesting maturational arrest. Muscle fibers contain one more central nuclei, surrounded by an area that is devoid of myofibrils. Facial weakness, ptosis, ophthalmoplegia, and generalized weakness are suggestive of myotubular myopathy. Mitochondrial myopathies are a group of disorders characterized by the presence of "ragged red fibers." Metabolic disturbances

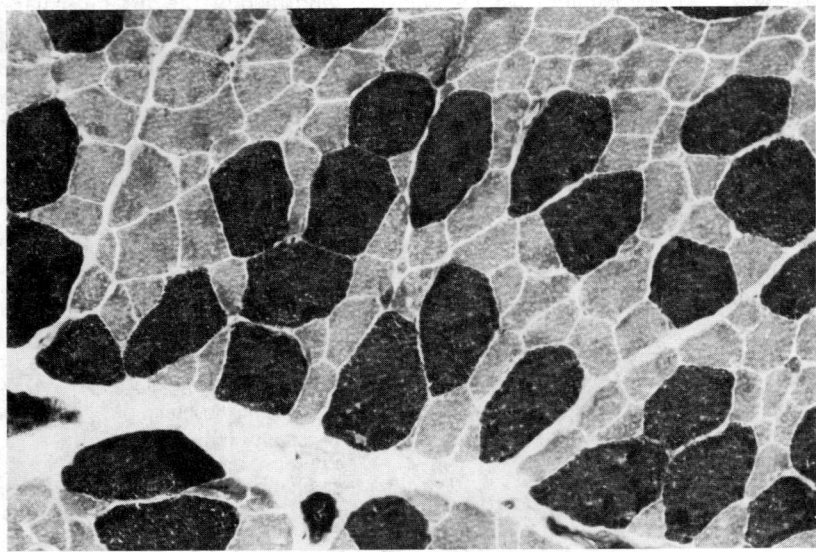

**Figure 20-26.** Muscle biopsy from a patient with congenital muscle-fiber-type disproportion. Lightly stained type I fibers are smaller than darkly stained type II fibers. Adenosine triphosphatase (pH 9.4) stain. Magnification ×160. (Courtesy of J. Kim, MD, Yale University School of Medicine.)

in mitochondrial myopathies include defects in substrate transport or utilization, the electron transport chain, or oxidative phosphorylation. For this reason, plasma lactate levels are elevated as in MELAS syndrome (myopathy, lactic acidosis, and stroke).

Further metabolic disorders that produce weakness involve the metabolism of carbohydrates (glycogen storage diseases such as Pompe's or McArdle's disease), and still others are mitochondrial in origin.

## Selected Readings

Bar-Joseph G, Etzioni A, Hemli J, Gershoni Baruch R. Guillain Barre syndrome in three siblings less than 2 years old. Arch Dis Child 1991;66:1078.
Byers RK. Spinal cord injuries during birth. Dev Med Child Neurol 1975;17:103.
Hoffman EP. Genetic aspects of myopathy. Curr Opin Rheumatol 1989;1:419.
Matthes JW, Kenna AP, Fawcett PR. Familial infantile myasthenia: A diagnostic problem. Dev Med Child Neurol 1991;33:924.
Shaw DJ, Harper PS. Myotonic dystrophy: Developments in molecular genetics. Br Med Bull 1989;45:745.
Storgion SA, Igarashi M, May WN, Stidham GL: Plasmapheresis for guillain barre syndrome. Pediatr Neurol 1989;5:389.
Towfighi J, Young RSK, Ward R: Is Werdnig-Hoffman disease a pure lower motor neuron disease? Acta Neuropathol (Berl) 1984;65:270.
Tzartos SJ, Efthimiadis A, Morel E, Eymard B, Bach JF. Neonatal myasthenia gravis: Antigenic specificities of antibodies in sera from mothers and their infants. Clin Exp Immunol 1990;80:376.
Young RSK, Gang DL, Zalneraitis EL, Krishnamoorthy KS. Dysmaturation in infants of mothers with myotonic dystrophy. Arch Neurol 1981;38:716.
Young RSK, Towfighi J, Marks K. Focal necrosis of cervical spinal cord in utero. Arch Neurol 1983;40:654.

*Principles and Practice of Pediatrics, Second Edition.*
edited by Frank A. Oski et al. J. B. Lippincott Company, Philadelphia © 1994.

# 20.2 *Respiratory Diseases*

## 20.2.1 *Developmental Considerations*

Ian Gross

## EMBRYOLOGY

The lung bud originates as an outpouching from the endodermal tube that will give rise to the gastrointestinal tract and grows out anteriorly into mesenchymal tissue, the forerunner of the interstitium and blood vessels of the lung. As the respiratory tract divides and branches, interstitial tissue and blood vessels surround the developing airways. The branching of the primitive respiratory tract gives rise to the lobes and lobules of the lung. At about 28 weeks of gestation in humans, alveolar formation begins. Although this process is active during fetal life, the major increase in the number of alveoli occurs after birth. There are about 1 million alveoli at birth, about 1 hundred million at 1 year, and about 300 million at 6 years, after which the number appears to stabilize. Thus, the capacity of the lung to generate new alveoli continues for a considerable time after birth.

Lung growth itself probably is regulated by hormonal and physical factors. It appears to be stimulated by the distending force of lung fluid in the airways and to be inhibited by the absence of this fluid, as occurs in oligohydramnios. Growth also can be inhibited by external compression, as occurs in diaphragmatic hernia, in which the bowel in the chest compresses the lung. The hormonal factors regulating growth are not well understood.

## ALVEOLAR MATURATION AND SURFACTANT SYNTHESIS

Because respiratory distress syndrome of the newborn is the result of immaturity of the lung, there has been considerable interest in the maturation of the fetal lung and the regulation of this process. At the microscopic level, development of the lung toward the end of fetal life is characterized by an increase in the number and size of the alveoli, and by thinning of the connective tissue septa between them. This reduces the distance between the alveolar lumen and the capillaries in the interstitium, thereby facilitating gas exchange. The alveolar lining cells also become flatter in late gestation, further reducing the barrier to gas exchange.

The onset of functional maturation is marked by the appearance of surfactant-filled lamellar bodies in the alveolar type II cells. The cuboidal type II cells are the sites of synthesis and secretion of pulmonary surfactant, the phospholipid protein mixture that lines the alveoli of the lung and prevents alveolar collapse caused by surface forces. Following synthesis, surfactant is stored in the lamellar bodies, which then are secreted onto the surface of the type II cell by a process of exocytosis. In the alveolar lumen, the lamellar body unravels to form a structure known as tubular myelin and, ultimately, the surfactant lines the surface of the alveolar cells.

The composition by weight of surfactant derived from lung lavage is as follows:

Phospholipids, 85%
  Phosphatidylcholine (80% of phospholipids)
  Phosphatidylglycerol (8% of phospholipids)
Neutral lipids and cholesterol, 5%
Proteins
  Serum proteins (contaminant), 9%
  Surfactant-specific proteins (SP), 1%
    SP-A, 28 to 36 kd
    SP-B, 4 to 5 kd
    SP-C, 7 to 8 kd
    SP-D, ± 40 kd

SP-A is a 28- to 36-kd glycosylated protein. It appears to play a role in regulation of the flow of surfactant in and out of the alveolar type II cell. In vitro studies have revealed that it acts to inhibit surfactant secretion and to enhance re-uptake of secreted surfactant into the type II cell (although this has not been confirmed by in vivo studies). Because SP-A is water soluble, it is not present in surfactant prepared by lipid extraction for clinical use. SP-B and SP-C (4 to 8 kd) are small lipophilic proteins that have been shown to be present in the clinically effective natural surfactant preparations. They are believed to be important for surface activity. SP-D (± 40 kd) is a collagenous carbohydrate-binding protein of unknown function.

Although the stimuli for the initiation of surfactant production are not defined clearly, it is known that this process may be accelerated by hormones. Glucocorticoids, thyroid hormone, cyclic adenosine monophosphate, and epidermal growth factor have been shown to enhance surfactant production in a variety of animal models, whereas the secretion of surfactant is stimulated by $\beta$-adrenergic agonists such as terbutaline, purinoceptor agonists such as adenosine and adenosine triphosphate, and leukotrienes. Fetuses in diabetic pregnancies have elevated glucose and insulin levels and delayed lung maturation. It is not clear whether it is the insulin, the hyperglycemia, or both that is responsible for inhibiting surfactant production in these infants.

Lung compliance and the ability of the lung to expand easily with inspiration are dependent on the development of the surfactant system, the maturation of the anatomic structure, and the development of tissue elasticity, which probably is related to the collagen and elastin components of lung tissue. Deficiencies in these components result in difficulty in breathing after birth.

*Principles and Practice of Pediatrics, Second Edition.*
edited by Frank A. Oski et al. J. B. Lippincott Company, Philadelphia © 1994.

## 20.2.2 *Physiologic Considerations*

Immanuela R. Moss

### THE ONSET OF AIR BREATHING AT BIRTH

Successful transition of the respiratory and pulmonary circulatory system from the fetal to the neonatal state determines the survival of the neonate. The fetal lung undergoes anatomic, physiologic, and biochemical development throughout gestation, so that, at term, the full complement of the airways (but not of the alveoli) is developed and the lungs are filled with fetal pulmonary fluid (30 mL/kg body weight), which includes surfactant. Whereas the fetus makes breathing movements (30% of the time in the near-term fetus), gas exchange is accomplished by the placenta. The resultant arterial oxygen tension of the fetus, although seemingly low (20 to 30 mm Hg), is functionally adequate because

the fetal hemoglobin dissociation curve is steep at this range, a property that permits facile oxygen delivery. Because of the low $PO_2$ levels, the fetal pulmonary circulation is constricted, pulmonary vascular resistance is high, and pulmonary blood flow is low. The recoil of the liquid-filled fetal lung at term is very low, and the fetal chest wall is highly compliant.

Thus, the following major changes must occur promptly at birth so as to render the lung suitable for its lifelong air-exchanging function: (1) the onset of continuous ventilation; (2) the absorption of fetal pulmonary fluid; (3) the establishment of an air-filled, compliant lung at functional residual capacity; (4) the establishment of an intra-alveolar film of surfactant-enriched material that lowers the surface tension of the lung; and (5) dilation of the pulmonary vasculature, as well as redirection of and increase in pulmonary blood flow to ensure adequate gas exchange across the alveolar-capillary barrier.

The first breath, which is crucial to the success of this transition, is brought about by a forceful contraction of the inspiratory muscles. The first inspiration is deep and is accompanied by large transpulmonary pressures that overcome surface and viscous forces; the first expiration is long and is accompanied by positive airway pressure brought about by laryngeal adduction and expiratory muscle activation. Some air already is retained in the lungs after the first breath—the beginning of the establishment of gaseous functional residual capacity.

After the first breath and over the next few hours, lung function changes progressively (Fig 20-27): functional residual capacity increases gradually as fetal pulmonary fluid is absorbed. This absorption is aided by positive airway pressure caused by partial closure of the upper airway during expiration. The fetal pulmonary fluid causes stimulation of J receptors, which, in turn, elicit by reflex a high breathing frequency. As the fluid is absorbed, breathing frequency decreases. After the initial deep breaths, tidal volume decreases. Lung compliance increases gradually, and total pulmonary resistance falls. Gas exchange adapts gradually to the postnatal state, as expressed by the decline in $PaCO_2$ and the rise in $PaO_2$. Although the time course of these changes varies depending on factors such as the mode of delivery, stable respiratory function usually is attained by the end of the first postnatal day (see Fig 20-27).

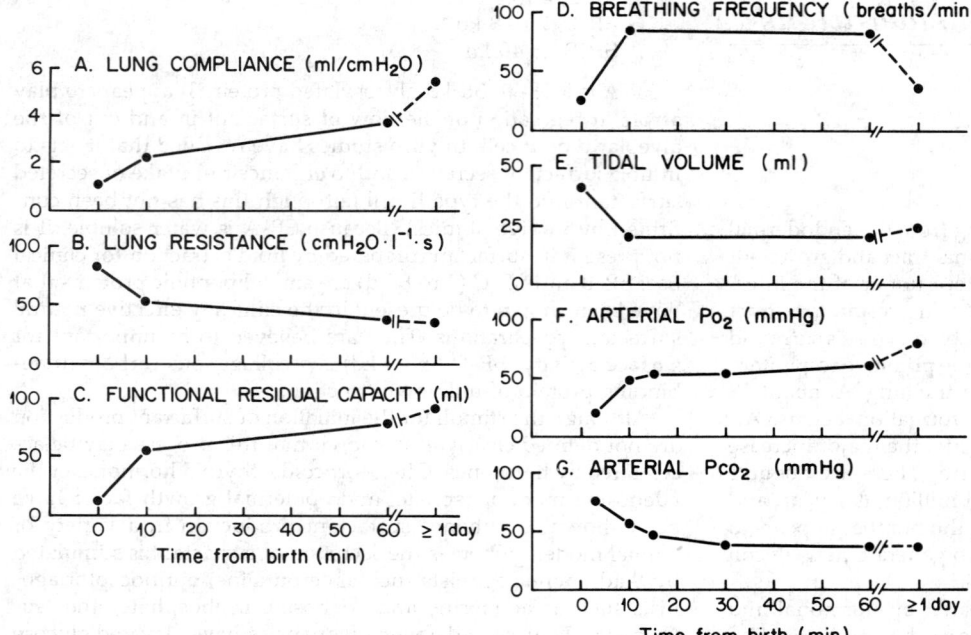

Figure 20-27. (**A** through **G**) Respiratory functions of term infants during the first hour after birth and at 1 day of age or greater. (Modified from Scarpelli EM, Moss IR [1983]; Mortola [1987]; and Nelson [1987].)

# RESPIRATORY MECHANICS, BREATHING DYNAMICS, AND GAS EXCHANGE IN THE NEONATE

Adequate gas exchange depends in part on the passive mechanical properties of the lung and the chest wall. Total respiratory compliance (ie, the change in lung volume per change in transpulmonary pressure) can be assessed in vivo from intraesophageal pressure and spirometric volume measurements. Newer, less invasive techniques for the assessment of respiratory mechanical parameters in the newborn are also under development. Lung compliance is measured in isolated lungs, and chest wall compliance is the difference between total respiratory compliance and lung compliance. As the chest wall of the neonate is very compliant, the relatively low total compliance in the newborn reflects largely the compliance of the lung itself. The latter (per unit of lung weight) tends to be smaller in the neonate than in the adult. The outward recoil of the newborn chest is relatively low. Inasmuch as the static resting volume of the respiratory system is determined by a balance between these two opposing forces, the transpulmonary pressure generated at that equilibrium and the resting volume are smaller in neonates than in adults.

Dynamic compliance, which is measured during normal breathing and is influenced by the frequency of breathing, is lower in infants than is static compliance. The reasons for the lowered dynamic compliance in the neonate are thought to be (1) the viscous properties of lung tissue, which have relatively greater importance in the newborn than in the adult; and (2) chest distortion, which is more typical of the newborn than of the adult and results in an imbalanced and unequal mechanical function of the chest wall.

During normal breathing, the dynamic functional residual capacity of the neonate is at a higher lung volume than the capacity that would result from the mere passive balance between the recoil of the lung and of the chest wall. This increased end-expiratory lung volume is caused by an insufficient time available to the neonate for full expiration. The longer time that would be required to bring about a complete expiration is caused in the neonate by continued inspiratory muscle activity (postinspiratory diaphragmatic contraction) and by increased upper airway resistance (laryngeal adduction) during the expiratory phase. The increased functional residual capacity during normal neonatal breathing is important, because it ensures the maintenance of an increased airway pressure throughout all respiratory phases. This pressure favors the reabsorption of intrapulmonary fluid and helps to keep the airways open, both of which enhance gas exchange. This situation changes in active sleep, during which laryngeal adductor muscle activity is reduced, so that the time required for complete expiration is shorter. The latter fact, in combination with decreased muscle tone and intercostal muscle activity, produces a lower end-expiratory lung volume and, thus, less optimal oxygenation during active sleep.

Airway resistance in neonates per unit of lung weight is greater than in adults, with the most peripheral airways contributing a relatively greater portion of this resistance. The upper airway of the neonate participates in the maintenance of airway patency by the action of dilatory muscles. When these are not operating, the neonatal upper airway is much more pliable than that of the adult, and can close at pressures of $-4$ cm $H_2O$. Neck extension in the neonate stiffens the upper airway, enhancing its patency, whereas neck flexion enhances its pliability and closure. The total nasal resistance of the neonate is proportionally smaller than that of the adult. Contrary to popular belief, neonates are not obligatory nose breathers, and can switch to oral breathing as needed. The more premature the infant is at birth, the more collapsible are the main airways and, therefore, the more uneven is the

distribution of air to various portions of the lung, and the greater is the chance for air trapping.

A striking characteristic of neonatal breathing is the paradoxic inward movement of the upper chest during inspiration, especially during active sleep. This movement can be explained in part by decreased intercostal muscle activity during active sleep, which allows the contracting and shortening diaphragm to pull the highly compliant chest wall inward. This mechanism might be enhanced further by an immaturity of the $\gamma$ and the intrafusal system, which would be activated by chest distortion in the adult and result in intercostal muscle contraction. Under circumstances such as crying or sighing, however, the intercostal muscles of the neonate function together with the diaphragm.

Similar to adults, neonates at rest breathe at an optimal frequency that requires minimal external work for a given alveolar ventilation. Whereas some energy required for the work of breathing is always lost during the shortening of the contracting muscles, in the case of the neonate, additional energy is lost because of chest distortion. Another possible cause for such wasted energy is the rounder skeletal contour of the neonatal chest, as contrasted with the flatter, more elongated contour of the adult chest. The rounded chest contour, with a spatial rib arrangement different from that of the adult, precludes an optimal length for the respiratory muscles at rest, thereby reducing the efficiency of their contraction during inspiration. The final contributor to the reduced efficiency of the neonatal respiratory muscles is their intrinsic mechanical properties during development. It seems that these muscles in the newborn, particularly in the preterm infant, have a relatively small mass, and are equipped poorly to sustain high work loads. The latter is because they contain relatively few fatigue-resistant, slow-twitching, highly oxidative fibers, have low glycogen and fat stores, and can easily become hypoxic. Thus, these muscles in the neonate may be vulnerable to fatigue. Although it is not easy to assess muscle fatigue noninvasively, attempts are under way with measurements of changes in spectra of diaphragmatic and intercostal electromyographic recordings.

Of the factors responsible for optimal gas exchange, a good match between ventilation and blood perfusion is of paramount importance. This match is less nearly ideal in neonatal than in adult lungs, partly because of the greater heterogeneity of air distribution throughout the lungs, resulting in increased venous admixture. The factors that contribute to the maldistribution of ventilation at birth include the pliable airways and the mechanical properties of the respiratory muscles at that time (see discussion above). As these mature with age, and as the alveoli continue to proliferate, air distribution improves. The pulmonary circulation also continues to develop postnatally, as exhibited by a change in the ratio of small arteries to alveoli from 20:1 at birth to 8:1 to 12:1 by 6 months of age (probably caused by the proliferation of alveoli); a gradual thinning of the vascular walls, including a reduction in their elastic tissue; a further decrease in pulmonary vascular resistance (perhaps related to a shift from the constrictive influence of lipoxygenase products during prenatal life to the dilatory effect of cyclooxygenase products postnatally) with an increase in pulmonary blood flow; and the ultimate establishment of a continuous film of capillary blood around the alveoli. These developmental improvements in both ventilatory distribution and pulmonary perfusion, and in the relationship between them, coupled with a change from fetal to adult hemoglobin, which is suited better for oxygen carriage and unloading ex utero, promote better gas exchange with postnatal maturation.

## RESPIRATORY REGULATION AND REFLEXES IN THE NEONATE

Inasmuch as neonatal respiration is a continuation of fetal breathing, consideration of the latter is important to the understanding of normal and abnormal respiratory control in the newborn.

The episodic breathing of the normal fetus is linked to its behavioral state: in the near-term human fetus (32 to 40 weeks' gestation), it has been shown by ultrasonographic techniques that breathing is least associated with the state of quiescence and most often associated with periods of body and eye movement as well as heart rate variability. Studies in animals, in which electrical assessment of states is possible, show that normal fetal breathing is not associated with a high-voltage, low-frequency electroencephalogram (typical of quiet sleep), but with a low-voltage, high-frequency electroencephalogram and eye movements (typical of active sleep and wakefulness). Of the respiratory reflexes that have been studied in the fetus, the breathing response to hypercapnia is excitatory and accompanied by arousal, but is blunted greatly compared with that in adults. In contrast to the $CO_2$ response, the fetal breathing response to hypoxia is inhibitory and associated with a change in state toward quiet sleep. Somatosensory stimuli also excite respiratory activity in the fetus. The most powerful of these is cooling, which produces vigorous fetal breathing and wakefulness.

Thus, it seems that some type of arousal is important for the sustenance of breathing activity. In fact, the "onset" of breathing at birth, which actually is the transition from discontinuous to continuous breathing, is associated with a barrage of stimuli that have an effect on arousal or a direct effect on respiratory reflexes. The former include cooling, light, sound, touch, and pressure. It also appears that the respiratory responses to the chemical stimuli $CO_2$ and $O_2$ change abruptly at birth; the response to $CO_2$, which involves carotid and aortic, but mainly ventral medullary chemoreception, is heightened, although it does not attain an adult-like sensitivity until several days postnatally. The response to hypoxia becomes biphasic, that is, an initial hyperventilation by peripheral chemosensory mechanisms is followed by respiratory attenuation or even apnea (Fig 20-28).

The causes of the differences in the chemical reflexes between perinatal and adult life are not understood as yet, although active research is ongoing in this field. Whereas some of the respiratory attenuation during severe hypoxia might be ascribed to hypometabolism, other prevalent explanations for the age differences in the chemical respiratory reflexes include the "immaturity" of respiratory-related receptors, neuronal structures, and synaptic connections. These age differences could also be explained by enhanced inhibition within the central nervous system during fetal life, which is either "lifted" or partly counteracted by excitatory reflexes around the time of birth. Such inhibition could emanate from cortical structures and could involve an activation of or an interaction among neurotransmitters and modulators, resulting in an inhibitory influence on respiration. Inhibitory neuromodulators under serious consideration for their possible role in perinatal respiratory control are adenosine and opioids (the antagonists to which are the xanthines and naloxone).

The behavior of other respiratory reflexes also differs in the perinatal period from that in later life. For example, the response of upper airway muscles to local changes in pressure, the coordination between the upper airway and the main respiratory muscles, and the intercostal–phrenic inhibitory reflex are all less developed in the newborn. Intrapulmonary reflexes are also less developed, including the slowly adapting (stretch), rapidly adapting (irritant), and C fiber (J receptor) vagal reflexes. A striking difference in behavior is shown by the laryngeal/pharyngeal chemoreflex: whereas stimulation of its chemoreceptors by materials perceived as foreign elicits a cough in the adult, it elicits apnea in the newborn. This apnea can be profound and irreversible in very young animals; its length is inversely proportional to postnatal age. Many of these differences can be explained by immaturity in the development of receptors, afferent nerves, and

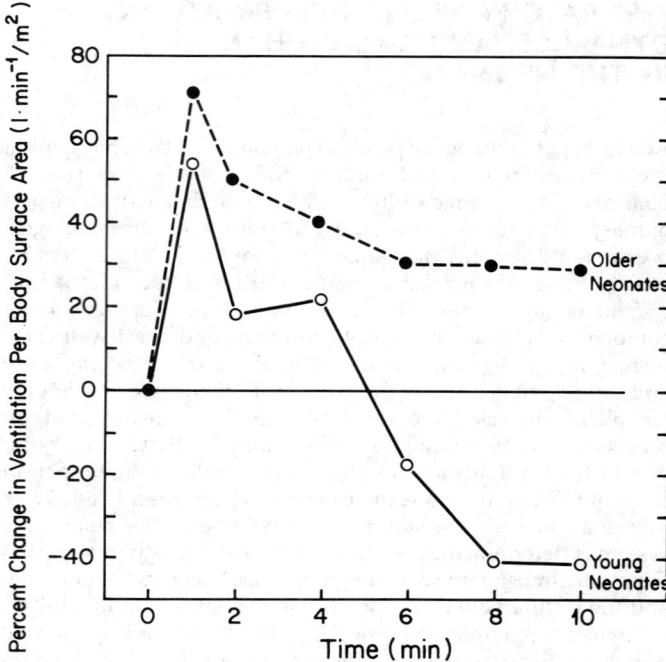

**Figure 20-28.** Percent change from control values in ventilatory response of young and older neonatal animals to 10 minutes of hypoxia ($F_{IO_2}$ = 0.06). The young, but not the older, neonates show a biphasic response to hypoxia (ie, transient hyperventilation followed by ventilatory depression). Neither metabolic nor sleep/wake state appeared to be involved in this response, as $P_{CO_2}$ and temperature were kept constant and all animals were studied at similar levels of anesthesia. (Modified from Moss IR, Runold M, Dahlen I, et al. Respiratory and neuroendocrine responses of piglets to hypoxia during postnatal development. Acta Physiol Scand 1987;133:533.)

central connections of the neuronal pathways participating in these reflexes.

Among the brain processes that undergo postnatal development, sleep/wake states have a special importance, as they reflect the maturation of neuronal networks that coordinate and integrate many somatic and autonomic systems and are linked tightly to respiration. The young neonate spends most of its time asleep, predominantly in active sleep. With time, the total time spent in sleep decreases, and quiet sleep becomes increasingly more pronounced. Furthermore, the length of sleep/wake cycles lengthens gradually, from 30 to 70 minutes in newborns to 75 to 90 minutes in children and adults. Even in normal neonates, and particularly in preterm infants, breathing pattern and respiratory reflexes depend on behavioral state. Periodic breathing and apnea are characteristic of premature infants during sleep, and are but a continuation into postnatal life of fetal patterns of breathing. The fact that these patterns exist during sleep and disappear with arousal (either natural or induced) underscores the importance of arousal in the maintenance of regular breathing. Sleep/wake states also play a role in the chemical respiratory reflexes, as these are relatively diminished in sleep, particularly in active sleep. Furthermore, the chemical respiratory stimuli, especially $CO_2$, produce wakefulness at the same time that they stimulate ventilation. Indeed, it is thought that deficient arousal mechanisms might account for a portion of near-miss sudden death or for crib death itself. The clinical aspects of these entities will be discussed in subsequent sections.

## Selected Readings

Bryan AC, Bowes G, Maloney JE. Control of breathing in the fetus and the newborn. In: Fishman AP, Cherniack NS, Widdicombe JG, eds. Handbook of physiology, vol II, section 3: The respiratory system. Baltimore: Williams & Wilkins, 1986: 621.

Davis GM, Coates AL. Pulmonary function testing in infants and neonates. Semin Respir Med 1990;2:185.

Fisher JT, Sant'Abmrogio G. Airway and lung receptors and their reflex effects in the newborn. Pediatr Pulmonol 1985;1:112.

Haddad GG, Farber JP, eds. Developmental biology of breathing. In: Lenfant C, exec ed. Lung biology in health and disease, vol 53. New York: Marcel Dekker, 1991.

Mortola JP. Dynamics of breathing in newborn mammals. Physiol Rev 1987;67: 187.

Moss IR, Inman JG. Neurochemicals and respiratory control during development. Brief review. J Appl Physiol 1989;67:1.

Nelson NM. The onset of respiration. In: Avery GB, ed. Neonatology: Pathophysiology and management of the newborn, ed 3. Philadelphia: JB Lippincott, 1987:176.

Scarpelli EM, ed. Pulmonary physiology: Fetus, newborn, child, adolescent, ed 2. Philadelphia: Lea & Febiger, 1990.

Scarpelli EM, Moss IR. Transition from fetal to neonatal breathing. In: Gootman N, Gootman PM, eds. Perinatal cardiovascular function. New York: Marcel Dekker, 1983:43.

*Principles and Practice of Pediatrics, Second Edition.*
edited by Frank A. Oski et al. J. B. Lippincott Company, Philadelphia © 1994.

## 20.2.3 *Causes of Respiratory Distress in the Newborn*

Ian Gross

Respiratory distress is a common presentation of disease in the newborn infant. The term is used to describe a constellation of easily observable physical signs, including rapid breathing (more than 60 breaths per minute), cyanosis, retractions (sucking in of the skin between the ribs, under the ribs, or above the sternum), flaring of the nostrils, and a grunting sound on expiration. There are many causes for these signs, and their presence is an indication that further observation or investigation is necessary. The causes of respiratory distress in the newborn include the following:

A. Airway obstruction
  1. Choanal atresia
  2. Congenital stridor (this may be caused by congenital defects such as laryngomalacia, tracheomalacia, laryngeal webs, or aberrant vessels compressing the airways)
B. Pulmonary disorders
  1. Respiratory distress syndrome (hyaline membrane disease)
  2. Transient tachypnea
  3. Pneumonia
  4. Aspiration syndromes
  5. Persistent pulmonary hypertension
  6. Air leak caused by interstitial emphysema, pneumothorax, or pneumomediastinum
  7. Congenital malformations caused by diaphragmatic hernia, pulmonary hypoplasia, tracheoesophageal fistula, or congenital lobar emphysema
  8. Atelectasis
  9. Chronic lung disease as a result of bronchopulmonary dysplasia or Mikity-Wilson syndrome
  10. Pulmonary hemorrhage
C. Nonpulmonary causes
  1. Cardiac disease
  2. Metabolic acidosis

  3. Central nervous system disorders
  4. Hypothermia or hyperthermia.

## APPROACH TO THE NEWBORN WITH RESPIRATORY DISTRESS

Babies may breathe rapidly during the first few hours after birth. This is related to the clearing of lung fluid from the airways and the cardiopulmonary adjustment to extrauterine life. Tachypnea also may be associated with transient conditions such as hypothermia. Isolated tachypnea, which is not associated with cyanosis, may be managed by observation only during the first few hours of life. If the tachypnea persists or is associated with other evidence of respiratory distress, however, further investigation is indicated. This usually includes a radiograph of the chest and determination of arterial blood gas levels or of blood oxygen saturation.

Because there are many causes of respiratory distress and they cannot be differentiated by clinical examination alone, a chest radiograph is indicated in any infant who has significant respiratory distress. A sudden deterioration in respiratory status also is an indication for obtaining a chest radiograph to rule out conditions that require urgent treatment, such as pneumothorax. Very early chest films (in the first 2 to 4 hours after birth) often are not helpful in differentiating the various forms of parenchymal lung disease because the presence of lung fluid tends to produce a hazy appearance or diffuse fine infiltrates. Early radiographs are useful, however, for excluding surgical conditions such as diaphragmatic hernia and air leaks.

If there is not a clear-cut pulmonary cause for the respiratory distress, it also will be necessary to exclude the presence of cardiac disease. This usually can be done by chest radiograph, electrocardiogram, and echocardiogram. The availability of echocardiography has diminished the need for cardiac catheterization and other potentially dangerous tests such as inspiration of 100% oxygen. In the presence of lung disease, the arterial $PO_2$ should increase after the inhalation of high concentrations of inspired oxygen, whereas with a fixed cardiac right-to-left shunt, there will be little increase in $PO_2$. This procedure carries the risk of causing closure of a patent ductus arteriosus in a ductal-dependent cardiac lesion. In some respiratory conditions (ie, persistent pulmonary hypertension), the echocardiogram not only is useful for excluding heart disease, but also plays a role in the diagnosis and management of the pulmonary disorder.

*Principles and Practice of Pediatrics, Second Edition.*
edited by Frank A. Oski et al. J. B. Lippincott Company, Philadelphia © 1994.

## 20.2.4 *Respiratory Distress Syndrome*

Ian Gross

Respiratory distress syndrome of the newborn (RDS, or hyaline membrane disease) is one of the most important causes of illness and death in the premature infant in developed countries. It is the result of immaturity of the lungs at birth and, therefore, with rare exceptions, is seen only in premature infants. Although alveoli first appear at 28 weeks' gestation, lung maturation usually is not adequate to sustain extrauterine life without some form of respiratory support until 32 to 34 weeks' gestation. Babies born earlier than this may have inadequate surfactant and decreased compliance of the lung. Other factors that contribute to lung compliance, such as tissue elasticity, also are believed to be abnormal in these infants. In addition, the anatomic structure of the lung is not suited as well to gas exchange as that of a full-term infant because there are smaller alveoli with larger amounts of interstitial tissue between them. The net result is a lung that is stiff and less well adapted for gas exchange.

## INCIDENCE

The incidence of RDS varies from institution to institution within the United States and from country to country throughout the world. It also depends on whether the infant's mother received antenatal glucocorticoid treatment. In general, the incidence of RDS in infants born before 30 weeks' gestation is about 60% in those who have not been exposed to antenatal glucocorticoids and about 35% in those who have received an adequate course of glucocorticoid therapy. Between 30 and 34 weeks' gestation, the incidence is about 25% in untreated or inadequately treated infants, and about 10% in those who have received full steroid treatment. In premature infants of greater than 34 weeks' gestational age, the incidence is about 5%. RDS is rare in full-term infants.

## FACTORS THAT MODIFY THE RISK OF RESPIRATORY DISTRESS SYNDROME OF THE NEWBORN

The factors associated with an increased risk of RDS include prematurity, maternal diabetes (classes A to C), delivery by cesarean section without antecedent labor, perinatal asphyxia, second twin, and history of a previous infant with RDS.

The increased incidence of RDS in infants of diabetic mothers may be related to the hyperglycemia or hyperinsulinemia that occurs during fetal life. Because labor enhances surfactant production, infants born by cesarean section that is not preceded by labor have an increased incidence of RDS. Acute asphyxia with hypoxia and acidosis appears to inhibit surfactant production. The incidence of RDS is higher in a second-born twin, as are a variety of other problems; whether this is related to asphyxia is not clear. Finally, there appears to be a familial tendency toward RDS, and a history of a sibling with RDS places a subsequent premature infant at higher risk.

There also are conditions that appear to decrease the incidence of RDS, such as long-term maternal stress (eg toxemia, hypertension), intrauterine growth retardation, maternal infection, maternal heroin exposure, and glucocorticoid treatment. Chronic low-grade maternal stress, as opposed to acute asphyxia, appears to accelerate lung maturation by a mechanism that is not entirely clear. It is possible that hormones such as glucocorticoids and catecholamines are involved.

## PATHOGENESIS

Current concepts of the pathogenesis of RDS are illustrated in Figure 20-29. The basic deficit is immaturity of surfactant production and lung structure. This results in a lung that is stiff and prone to atelectasis. Blood continues to perfuse the poorly ventilated areas, resulting in an intrapulmonary right-to-left shunt and hypoxemia. The hypoxemia in turn causes a metabolic acidosis as a result of poor tissue oxygenation. In the presence of hypoxemia and acidosis, the pulmonary arterioles tend to constrict, so that there is increased pressure in the pulmonary circulation. The pulmonary hypertension is reversible when normal

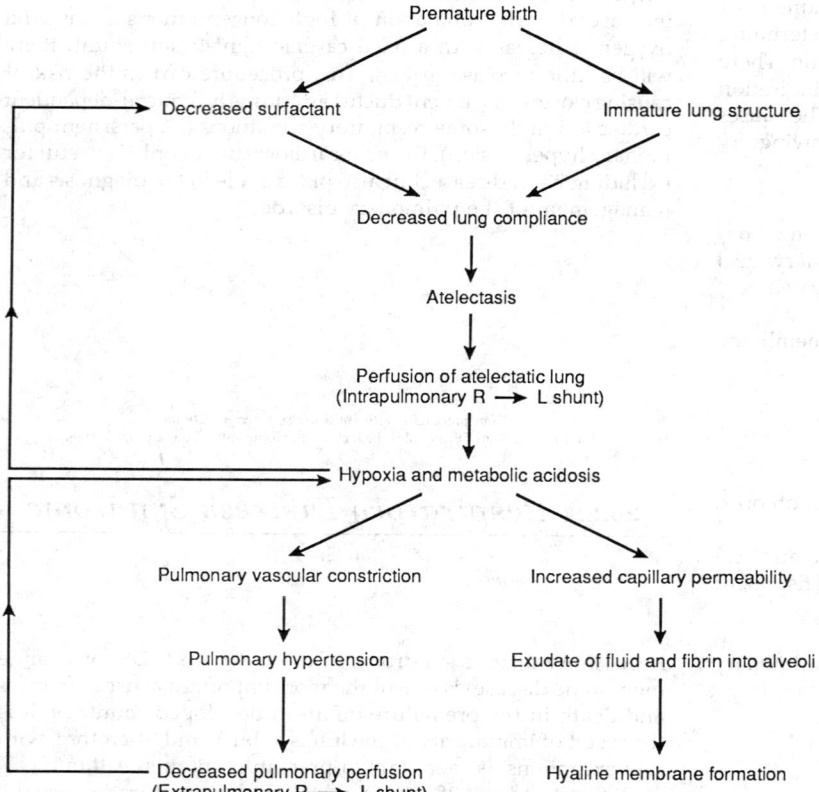

Figure 20-29. The pathogenesis of respiratory distress syndrome of the newborn.

blood gas levels are restored. With the increased pressure in the pulmonary circulation, shunting of blood from the right to the left atrium through the foramen ovale may occur, further aggravating the right-to-left shunt and hypoxemia. Depending on the relative pressures in the pulmonary and systemic circulations, there also may be right-to-left shunting through a patent ductus arteriosus.

Alveolar disruption and necrosis occurs, and there is leakage of fluid and fibrin from the pulmonary capillaries into the alveolar space. This fluid and fibrin exudate eventually coalesces to form intra-alveolar proteinaceous deposits that, at postmortem examination, are identified as the eosinophilic hyaline membranes that are characteristic of this disease. It is clear that hyaline membrane formation is a consequence and not a cause of RDS. Hyaline membranes never have been described in infants who are stillborn; they appear only in infants who have been alive and sick for at least a few hours.

The ductus arteriosus also plays a role in the development of this disorder. If it is patent, as it usually is during the first day after birth in premature infants, blood may flow from right to left, as discussed earlier. If aortic pressure exceeds pulmonary artery pressure, however, flow will be from left to right and flooding of the lungs and pulmonary edema may ensue. This will decrease lung compliance further.

Finally, because surfactant production is sensitive to hypoxia and acidosis, a vicious cycle may be initiated whereby the infant starts off with inadequate surfactant production and becomes hypoxic and acidotic, and this in turn further inhibits the production of surfactant.

## CLINICAL FEATURES

The clinical course of uncomplicated RDS usually follows a fairly consistent pattern. The infant demonstrates signs of respiratory distress that become worse during the first few hours after birth. In some infants, especially those who are extremely immature, the respiratory distress may be severe from the start. The disease then progresses for 48 to 72 hours, reaches a peak, and starts to improve. The onset of recovery often is associated with diuresis. This classic course may not occur, however, in infants with very low birth weights or those who are very sick. With the use of ventilators and high oxygen concentrations, oxidant or mechanical injury may induce secondary lung damage and a prolonged respiratory illness may ensue.

Infants with RDS initially have the classic features of respiratory distress in the newborn (ie, tachypnea, flaring of the nose, retractions of the chest, cyanosis, and grunting). Radiographs taken at about 6 hours after birth reveal evidence of diffuse atelectasis and loss of lung volume (Fig 20-30). The lung fields, which are relatively opaque, have been described as resembling "ground glass" or being "reticulogranular." Because the lung fields now are relatively radiodense, the heart border may be obscured. In addition, air within the bronchi stands out in contrast to the lung fields as "air bronchograms." The air bronchograms may extend down to the diaphragm. This radiographic picture, although characteristic of RDS, also may be seen in neonatal pneumonia in premature infants, and it may be impossible to distinguish RDS and pneumonia on radiographic grounds.

If the infant dies, the characteristic features at postmortem examination are disrupted alveoli and the presence of eosinophilic hyaline membranes within the alveolar spaces. Although these proteinaceous deposits give this syndrome its name, the presence of hyaline membranes is not pathognomonic of "hyaline membrane disease." They also are seen in pneumonia, cardiac failure, and other neonatal conditions that are characterized by lung injury.

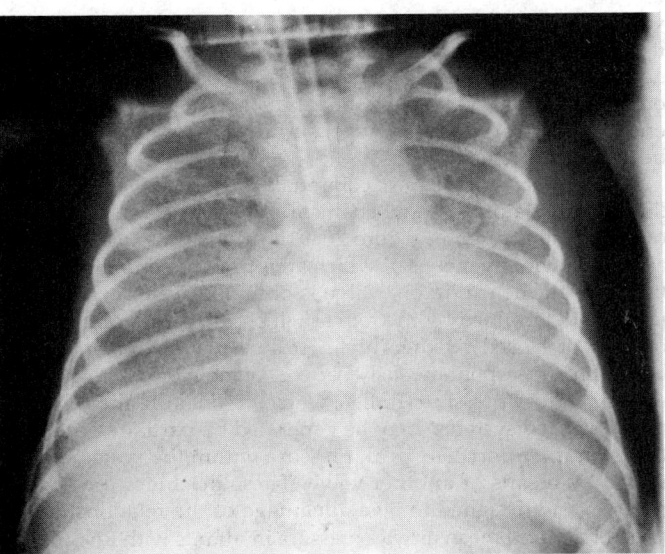

**Figure 20-30.** X-ray of the chest of an infant with respiratory distress syndrome. Note the diffusely opaque lung fields and the indistinct cardiac outline. Radiolucent "air bronchograms" also can be seen.

The differential diagnosis of RDS includes other causes of respiratory distress in the premature infant. The condition with which it is most likely to be confused is group B streptococcal pneumonia, which may mimic it in almost every respect. At times, it may be possible to differentiate these two disorders only retrospectively, by reviewing the course and pattern of the illness.

## MANAGEMENT OF RESPIRATORY DISTRESS SYNDROME OF THE NEWBORN

### Respiratory Care

Much of the work of neonatal intensive care units is concerned with providing respiratory care to infants with RDS. The level of intervention required depends on the severity of the respiratory distress. This is determined primarily by the arterial blood gas levels and by the amount of supplemental oxygen the infant needs to maintain an adequate arterial oxygen tension ($PaO_2$). The goal of therapy is to keep the $PaO_2$ in the range of 45 to 70 mm Hg, and the $PaCO_2$ between 35 and 45 mm Hg. Although these $PaO_2$ values are less than those observed in healthy full-term infants, they are used because premature infants are susceptible to oxygen injury to their eyes and it is felt that the range of 45 to 70 mm Hg is generally safe. $PaO_2$ levels lower than 35 mm Hg can result in tissue hypoxia and metabolic acidosis. Thus, the range used is a compromise designed to avoid hypoxia at the lower end and oxygen injury to the eyes at the high end.

The specific indications for, and methods of, respiratory support vary from center to center, but the following guidelines reflect common practice. If the $PO_2$ can be maintained in the range of 45 to 70 mm Hg by providing the infant with less than 30% to 40% oxygen, then the infant will be placed in a head box and oxygen will be delivered by this method. If a higher concentration of oxygen is required, assisted ventilation usually is initiated. The first step may be to attempt to deliver continuous positive airway pressure (CPAP) via nasal prongs, which are small catheters inserted into the nostrils and connected to a source of air and/or $O_2$. CPAP is generated by occluding expiration partially so that a distending pressure builds up within the airways. This promotes oxygenation by increasing the functional residual capacity and preventing alveolar collapse at the end of expiration. If the provision of positive airway pressure via nasal prongs is not adequate, if the infant is laboring to breathe, if the $P_{CO_2}$ is greater than about 60 mm Hg and rising, or if respiratory acidosis is developing, the infant will have to be intubated and ventilated via an endotracheal tube. At this stage, surfactant therapy also should be initiated (see below).

The ventilators used most commonly are time-cycled, pressure-limited ventilators. The mechanism by which these ventilators operate is illustrated in Figure 20-31. They can be thought of as a T tube device by means of which air is diverted into the infant's lungs when the expiratory valve is occluded. The rate of ventilation is determined by the rate at which the expiratory outlet is opened or closed by the valve. At slow ventilation rates, the infant breathes spontaneously between ventilator cycles. Positive end-expiratory pressure (PEEP), which is similar to the CPAP of nonventilated systems, may be generated by partially occluding the expiratory port. The peak pressure within the system is regulated by means of another valve. These machines are simple, reliable, and designed to take advantage of the relationship between $PaO_2$ and mean airway pressure in infants with RDS. Mean airway pressure is the integrated area under the inspiratory and expiratory portions of the curve that results when respirator pressure is plotted against time (Fig 20-32). It has been shown experimentally that, if oxygen concentration is kept constant, the $PaO_2$ in infants with RDS is dependent on mean airway pressure. As is shown in Figure 20-32, mean airway pressure may be increased during inspiration by increasing peak inspiratory pressure, or during expiration by increasing PEEP. It also may be increased by prolonging inspiration at the expense of expiration (inspiratory: expiratory ratio). Thus, if the $PaO_2$ is too low, it can be elevated by increasing the mean airway pressure or the inspired oxygen concentration. If the $PaCO_2$ is too high, more ventilation is required. This is accomplished by increasing the minute volume, that is, increasing the rate of respiration or the tidal volume (which is dependent on peak inspiratory pressure). On occasion, when

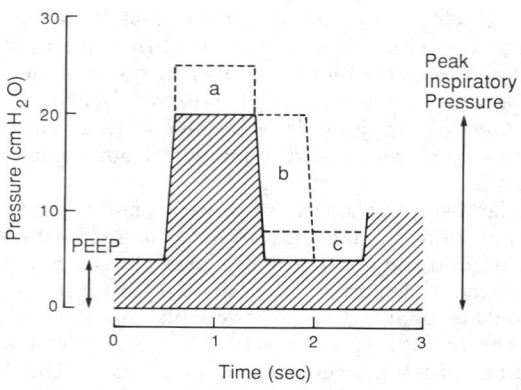

Figure 20-32.   Ventilator pressure curve. The shaded area represents the mean airway pressure. Mean airway pressure can be increased by (a) increasing peak inspiratory pressure, (b) prolonging inspiration, or (c) raising positive end-expiratory pressure (PEEP). (Modified from Reynolds O. Ventilator therapy. In: Thibeault DW, Gregory GA, eds. Neonatal pulmonary care. Menlo Park, Calif: Addison-Wesley, 1979: 217.)

the PEEP is very high, $PaCO_2$ may be lowered by decreasing PEEP and thereby increasing tidal volume.

Because the premature lung is extremely fragile and may be injured by the inspired oxygen or the pressure from the ventilator, the aim of therapy should be to provide adequate oxygenation by use of as gentle a mode of ventilation as possible. Many newborn units accordingly will accept a $PaCO_2$ in the range of 45 to 55 mm Hg, or even higher, rather than increase the peak inspiratory pressure to reduce the $PaCO_2$. There is an increasing tendency to accept blood gas levels that might not be considered optimal in the full-term infant or older child to prevent pressure injury to the lungs.

As the lungs start to recover and compliance improves, usually after 2 to 4 days, respiratory support can be reduced gradually and the infant can be weaned from the ventilator. Application of CPAP by nasal prongs after extubation often is helpful in the transition to unsupported breathing.

The role of high-frequency ventilators (oscillator and jet) in the management of RDS still is being evaluated. These machines provide an extremely high respiratory rate (eg, 600 to 1200 breaths per minute) with very low tidal volumes. They are believed to work by augmented diffusion rather than true ventilation. Although this type of ventilation is effective in animals with healthy lungs, multicenter studies have not revealed an advantage of high-frequency over conventional ventilation in infants with RDS, other than for the treatment of pulmonary interstitial emphysema. The indications for high-frequency ventilation in the management of RDS have yet to be defined.

## Monitoring

In addition to routine monitoring of temperature and heart rate, assessment of the respiratory status of infants with RDS by means of arterial blood gas determinations is essential. This usually is done by inserting a catheter through the umbilical artery into the aorta, or by radial artery catheterization. The catheter can be used to draw arterial samples to determine $PaO_2$, $PaCO_2$, and pH levels, and to record arterial blood pressure continuously via a transducer. Instruments for monitoring oxygenation by noninvasive methods also have been developed. The first such devices were transcutaneous oxygen sensors. Although these are useful for reflecting trends, they do not always report accurately the actual $PaO_2$ values. A more reliable instrument is the pulse oximeter, which records the oxygen saturation of the blood contin-

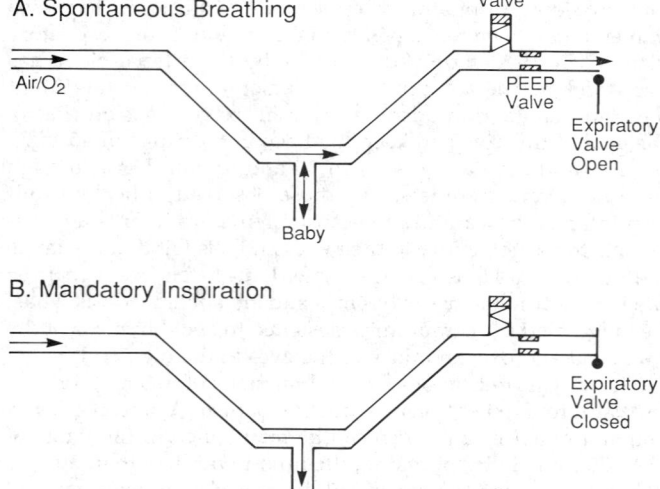

Figure 20-31.   Time-cycled, pressure-limited infant ventilator with intermittent mandatory ventilation. (A) When the expiratory valve is open, gas flows through the system. The baby can inhale and exhale spontaneously. Continuous gas flow clears the circuit of $CO_2$. The settings of the pressure and PEEP valves are variable. (B) When the expiratory valve closes, gas is forced into the baby's lungs, producing a mandatory inspiration. The inspiratory rate is determined by the rate at which the valve opens and closes. (Modified from Kirby RR. Design of mechanical ventilators. In: Thibeault DW, Gregory GA, eds. Neonatal pulmonary care. Menlo Park, Calif: Addison-Wesley, 1979:154.)

uously by means of a probe attached to an extremity, such as a fingertip. This device is easy to use and safe, and has found widespread application. In mild cases of RDS, it may be possible to follow oxygenation by means of a pulse oximeter alone and to avoid arterial catheterization. Capillary blood specimens (eg, a heelstick) can be used for determination of pH and $Pco_2$ levels; $Po_2$ values obtained in this manner will be unreliable, however.

## Surfactant Therapy

The successful use of pulmonary surfactant preparations for the prevention or amelioration of RDS represents one of the major advances made in neonatal care during the past decade. (The composition of surfactant is described in section 20.2.1.) Surfactant preparations generally are administered as liquid suspensions that are instilled into the lungs via an endotracheal tube. For this reason, surfactant therapy is confined to infants who are intubated and ventilated. Two approaches to surfactant therapy have evolved. "Prevention" therapy refers to the administration of surfactant to premature infants who are at risk for having RDS immediately after birth in the delivery area. "Rescue" therapy refers to the administration of surfactant to infants with diagnosed RDS, usually within 8 hours of birth.

Surfactant formulations for clinical use include the following:

Natural surfactant—surfactant recovered from bovine or porcine lung, or from human amniotic fluid

Modified natural surfactant—selected components, usually phospholipids added to lung extract. These preparations are used widely and are available commercially (eg, Survanta from Ross Laboratories).

Artificial surfactant—a mixture of synthetic compounds, usually including phosphatidylcholine, a spreading agent, and an emulsifier. Exosurf (Burroughs Wellcome) is an artificial surfactant that is available commercially in the United States.

Recombinant surfactants—surfactant proteins synthesized by recombinant DNA technology plus added lipid. These surfactants are in the research stage and are not available commercially.

Large, multicenter studies have confirmed the effectiveness of modified natural and artificial surfactants for the prevention or treatment of RDS. Initial studies, in which only one dose of surfactant was given, revealed an immediate short-term benefit (decreased need for ventilator support), but it was unclear whether there was a decrease in bronchopulmonary dysplasia or mortality. Further studies, in which up to four doses were administered during the first 48 hours after birth, have demonstrated a 33% to 50% reduction in mortality from all causes and an even greater decrease in the rate of death from RDS. This reduction in mortality was observed with both artificial and natural surfactants, whether they were given as prevention or as rescue therapy. Other benefits common to all therapies was a decrease in the amount of ventilator support needed and in the incidence of pulmonary air leaks (interstitial emphysema and pneumothorax). There also was a lower incidence of RDS in the prevention studies. (Rescue treatment is given only to infants with RDS.) A disappointing finding was the absence of a consistent decrease in bronchopulmonary dysplasia in surviving infants. This may be due in part to increased survival of sicker infants who would be at high risk for this complication.

Subsequent studies have compared the effectiveness of prevention versus rescue therapy. Potential advantages of prevention therapy include better distribution of surfactant in lung fluid that has not yet been absorbed, administration before lung injury from ventilation occurs, and the fact that some studies appear to demonstrate a greater reduction in mortality in the prevention component. Potential disadvantages include the fact that many pre-

mature infants do not have RDS and, therefore, would be treated unnecessarily with an expensive agent; treatment is given to a baby who is not yet stabilized; and endotracheal tube position cannot be checked carefully before therapy is initiated. Recent studies comparing the two modes of treatment directly have shown that prevention may be more effective than rescue for babies less than 26 weeks' gestation at birth. It is not clear whether prevention is the preferred therapy for infants over 26 weeks' gestation. In all cases treatment should be initiated as soon as it is safe and feasible. More mature infants should probably be stabilized, and endotracheal tube position and the diagnosis of RDS confirmed radiographically before surfactant therapy is initiated.

Surfactant therapy has been associated with few complications. There is no significant impact on the incidence of infection, patent ductus arteriosus, intraventricular hemorrhage, or necrotizing enterocolitis. In addition, there is no evidence of the development of antibodies to surfactant proteins in the serum of infants who have received natural surfactant therapy.

The dosing regimes used are derived from protocols developed for the clinical trials of the various preparations. In rescue mode, Survanta is given initially to intubated infants who require an $Fio_2$ of more than 0.4. Three more doses may be given at a minimum of 6-hour intervals if the $Fio_2$ is greater than 0.3. For rescue therapy with Exosurf, two doses are given 12 hours apart.

## Other Aspects of Treatment

Other components of treatment also are important. Body temperature should be maintained by caring for the infant on a radiant warmer or in an Isolette. Initially, fluids and calories will have to be provided intravenously, as infants who are breathing rapidly do not tolerate oral or nasogastric feedings. For the first few days after birth, the infant may be given intravenous glucose and electrolyte solutions. If it appears that gastrointestinal feedings will have to be deferred for any length of time, an intravenous amino acid and glucose solution usually is administered via a peripheral vein. Very immature infants or those with a prolonged and severe course may require total parenteral nutrition via a central vein. The fluid volume given will depend on the gestational age of the infant and on the type of environment in which the infant is being nursed. Very immature infants and those being managed on radiant warmers require more fluids. Antibiotics generally are administered, not because RDS is an infectious condition or to cover prophylactically invasive procedures such as catheters, but because, in many cases, pneumonia cannot be excluded.

Sodium bicarbonate should be used sparingly. Overuse carries the risk of inducing hypernatremia and may precipitate an intraventricular hemorrhage, particularly if it is given in bolus form. Acidosis should be treated initially by optimizing ventilation. A persistent metabolic acidosis with a pH level of less than 7.25 can be treated with a slow, dilute bicarbonate infusion of 1 to 2 mEq/kg. Persistent acidosis also is an indication to assess general perfusion and the presence of a significant patent ductus arteriosus. The latter should be treated by indomethacin therapy, or by surgical ligation if indomethacin is ineffective.

## COMPLICATIONS

The major complications of RDS are related to therapy and include the following:

1. Air leak caused by increased airway pressure from ventilation or CPAP. This complication is discussed in more detail later in this chapter.

2. Chronic lung disease (bronchopulmonary dysplasia). This is believed to result from injury to the lungs by oxygen and ventilator pressure. The fragile lung of the extremely premature infant is particularly susceptible to this injury and the incidence of bronchopulmonary dysplasia is increased greatly in infants with birth weights of less than 1250 g. Bronchopulmonary dysplasia is reviewed later in this chapter.

3. Catheter complications. The insertion of a catheter into the aorta can result in complications such as necrotizing enterocolitis, hypertension caused by renal arterial thrombosis, and infarction of other organs.

4. Intraventricular hemorrhage. There is an increased incidence of intraventricular hemorrhage in infants with RDS. The mechanism may be related to intravascular pressure swings.

5. Retinopathy of prematurity. Because RDS occurs in premature infants who are treated with oxygen, they are at particular risk for retinopathy of prematurity. Like bronchopulmonary dysplasia, this complication occurs mainly in infants with birth weights below 1500 g.

## PREVENTION OF RESPIRATORY DISTRESS SYNDROME OF THE NEWBORN

There are three approaches to the prevention of RDS in premature infants: antenatal prediction of fetal lung maturity, pharmacologic acceleration of fetal lung development, and prevention therapy with surfactant (see above). The best approach is prevention of prematurity itself.

### Antenatal Prediction of Fetal Lung Maturity

Before methods for assessing fetal lung maturity were developed, a significant number of infants born after elective induction of labor or elective cesarean section had RDS. In many cases, this was because of an inaccurate assessment of the duration of gestation.

The fetal lung secretes surfactant into the amniotic fluid. Examination of the amniotic fluid can reveal whether or not the lung is synthesizing surfactant-associated phospholipids in quantities sufficient to support respiration. This is done most commonly by measuring the lecithin:sphingomyelin (L:S) ratio and determining whether phosphatidylglycerol (PG), another surfactant-related phospholipid, is detectable. Lecithin (or phosphatidylcholine) is the most abundant component of surfactant, and the lecithin in amniotic fluid is derived from the fetal lung, whereas the sphingomyelin is derived from nonpulmonary sources. As the lung matures, the L:S ratio increases. When this ratio is greater than 2, the fetal lungs almost invariably are mature; a ratio of 1.5 to 2 is indeterminate; and a value below 1.5 predicts immaturity. The test errs on the side of overpredicting immaturity. If there is no PG in the amniotic fluid and the L:S ratio is below 1.5, an obstetrician considering an elective delivery may decide to delay this procedure until such time as the lung is mature.

Measurement of surfactant-specific proteins, particularly SP-A, in the amniotic fluid has been used experimentally to evaluate lung maturity and appears to be a good indicator. Rapid and relatively simple enzyme-linked immunosorbent assays may increase the clinical use of this test in the future. Determination of gestational age by measurements such as the biparietal diameter of the head on ultrasound examination also are useful for preventing inadvertent early elective delivery with the associated risk of RDS.

### Pharmacologic Acceleration of Fetal Lung Maturation

It is known that fetal lung development is under the control of multiple hormones. The agents that have been demonstrated clearly to enhance lung maturation are glucocorticoids, thyroid hormones, growth factors such as epidermal growth factor, and cyclic adenosine monophosphate. The role of estrogen and prolactin in this process still is controversial. Most of this information has come from animal studies, but there is a considerable body of evidence indicating that glucocorticoids accelerate lung maturation in humans, and these agents have been used clinically for more than 15 years for this purpose. Because glucocorticoids act by enhancing RNA transcription and protein synthesis, which is a process that takes time, they are effective only if the infant is delivered at least 24 hours after the initial dose of glucocorticoids is given. Their action also appears to subside after about 7 days and is not significant in infants of greater than 34 weeks' gestation. When they are administered appropriately, glucocorticoids have reduced the incidence of RDS by about 50% in most studies. The usual regimen is to administer betamethasone or dexamethasone, glucocorticoids that cross the placenta readily over a period of 48 hours. If the infant is not delivered within 7 days, another course of glucocorticoids may be necessary if threatened premature labor occurs again.

Attempts are being made to enhance the effectiveness of glucocorticoids by combining them with other agents. Recent studies suggest that a combination of TRH (thyrotropin-releasing hormone) with glucocorticoid is more effective than glucocorticoid alone in preventing both RDS and BPD.

It is recommended that antenatal steroids be used in cases of threatened premature labor before 33 weeks' gestation if pulmonary maturity is unknown, or whenever there is documented pulmonary immaturity and delivery is not anticipated for at least 12 hours.

### Synergy of Antenatal Hormone and Postnatal Surfactant Therapy

Both animal and clinical studies indicate that, although lung compliance and respiratory status are improved by either antenatal steroid therapy or postnatal surfactant, the effect of both therapies is greater than that of either alone. The use of antenatal steroids followed by postnatal surfactant if the infant has RDS appears to be the optimal approach to the management of this condition.

Although these new developments are exciting, it should be noted that one of the most effective means of preventing RDS remains good obstetric care, with the use of drugs such as β-adrenergic agonists to inhibit premature labor.

*Principles and Practice of Pediatrics, Second Edition.* edited by Frank A. Oski et al. J. B. Lippincott Company, Philadelphia © 1994.

## 20.2.5 Transient Tachypnea of the Newborn

Ian Gross

Transient tachypnea of the newborn (also called retained fetal lung fluid, wet lung, or respiratory distress syndrome type II) is a benign, self-limited condition seen primarily in full-term infants. It is believed to result from delay in the reabsorption of fetal pulmonary fluid. There is an association between delivery by cesarean section and the development of this condition, possibly because of the compression of the chest during vaginal delivery and the mechanical "wringing out" of fetal lung fluid. These infants have respiratory distress shortly after birth. The features are tachypnea, mild retractions, and, sometimes, cyanosis. The clinical course usually is transient and mild, with resolution of the problem in 24 to 48 hours. In some infants, the condition is more severe and may persist for 72 hours or longer.

The diagnosis is made by radiography. The classic appearance is that of a well-aerated lung with streaky markings radiating out from the hilum ("star-burst" appearance) and small amounts of fluid in the fissures, particularly the right middle fissure. The major condition from which transient tachypnea must be differentiated is pneumonia. Differentiation sometimes can be difficult in prolonged cases of transient tachypnea, although resolution usually is more rapid than with pneumonia.

Treatment essentially is symptomatic. Blood gas levels or oxygen saturation are monitored and oxygen is administered to maintain a $PaO_2$ of 60 to 90 mm Hg. Occasionally, a brief period of mechanical ventilation may be necessary and, if the diagnosis of pneumonia cannot be excluded, antibiotics are given, although transient tachypnea itself does not require antibacterial treatment. This condition is not associated with long-term sequelae such as bronchopulmonary dysplasia, and the prognosis is excellent.

*Principles and Practice of Pediatrics, Second Edition.*
edited by Frank A. Oski et al. J. B. Lippincott Company, Philadelphia © 1994.

## 20.2.6 *Pneumonia*

Ian Gross

Pneumonia in the newborn period may arise in the first 2 to 3 days after birth (early onset) or after the first week (late onset). It may occur as an isolated infection or in association with septicemia. Pneumonia that develops shortly after birth probably is acquired in utero or intrapartum by hematogenous spread from the mother, from ascending infection from the vagina and cervix, or by aspiration of contaminated secretions immediately after birth. Late-onset pneumonia, similar to other nosocomial infections in the newborn unit, can be transmitted by the infant's caretakers. The most common pathogens are the group B streptococci and gram-negative organisms such as *Escherichia coli* and *Klebsiella*, but a wide variety of organisms may be involved. During the 1970s, group B streptococci emerged as a major cause of pneumonia and septicemia in newborns. Although group B streptococcal infection still is prevalent, it occurs now with about the same frequency as does infection with gram-negative enteric organisms.

## CLINICAL FEATURES

Infants with early onset pneumonia usually have respiratory distress during the first few hours after birth. If they are premature, their symptoms may be indistinguishable from those of respiratory distress syndrome (RDS). Features that suggest pneumonia rather than RDS include prolonged rupture of the membranes, early onset of apnea, poor perfusion and shock, and other signs consistent with sepsis. The amniotic fluid lecithin:sphingomyelin ratio, if available, also is useful in differentiating pneumonia from RDS (a "mature" ratio rules out RDS).

The clinical course of neonatal pneumonia varies considerably. Some infants have fulminant disease with a rapid downhill course and early death. More commonly, moderate respiratory distress develops and assisted ventilation may be required for a few days, after which the baby recovers. The course is different from that of RDS, which tends to become progressively more severe and to peak at 48 to 72 hours, whereas pneumonia usually follows a more level course.

In addition to parenchymal lung disease, some infants also have severe pulmonary hypertension, presumably secondary to vasospasm, with right-to-left shunting of blood. These babies, who may be critically ill, tend to have a labile $PaO_2$ and a degree of hypoxia that is disproportionate to the severity of their lung disease as reflected by the chest radiograph. This complication is associated with significant morbidity and mortality.

## RADIOGRAPHIC APPEARANCE

Four different radiographic appearances have been described in newborn infants with pneumonia. The first is extensive infiltrates

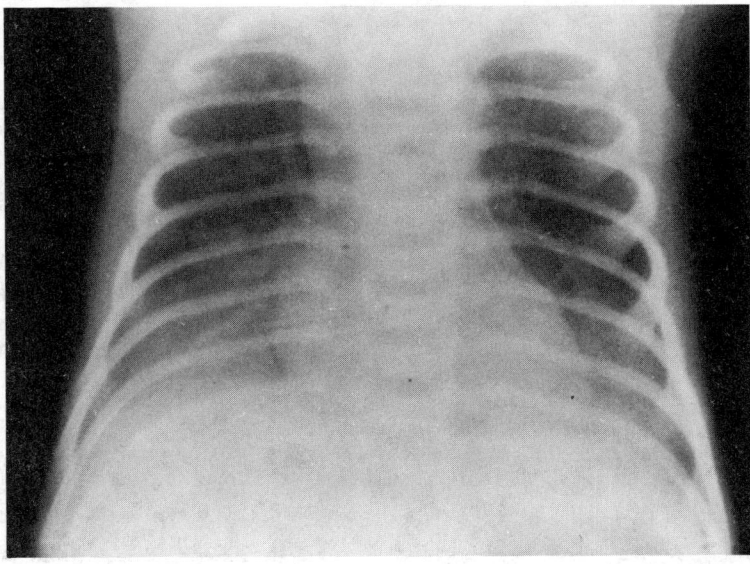

**Figure 20-33.** Bilateral lobar consolidation in an infant with pneumonia.

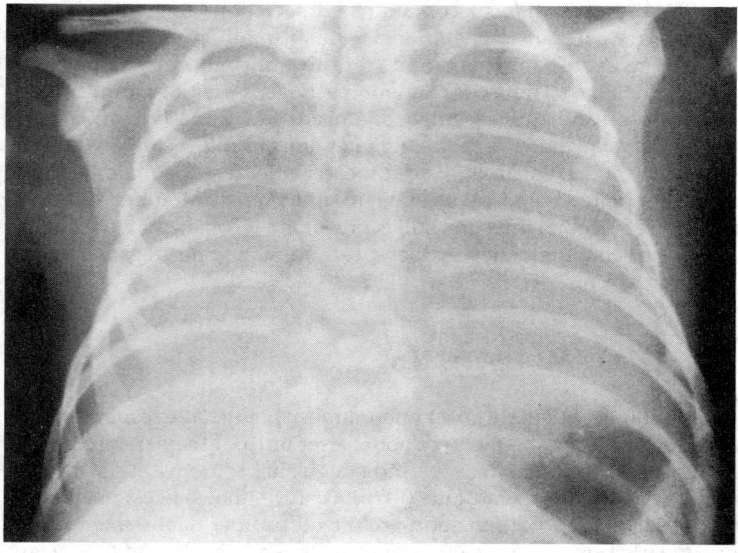

Figure 20-34. ''RDS-like'' pattern in a premature infant with pneumonia. The radiodensity of the lungs is greatly increased, resulting in an opacified appearance.

that appear as coarse infiltrates scattered throughout both lungs. Another radiographic appearance is that of lobar consolidation (Fig 20-33). Third, an RDS-like pattern (Fig 20-34) may be observed; the radiographic appearance of pneumonia in premature infants, particularly that caused by the group B streptococci, may be indistinguishable from that seen in RDS. It is possible that some of these infants have both RDS and pneumonia. Last, the chest radiograph of a newborn with pneumonia may reveal scattered small infiltrates in one or both lungs (this is more common in mature than in premature infants).

## DIFFERENTIAL DIAGNOSIS

In the full-term infant with a few scattered lung infiltrates on chest radiography, pneumonia must be differentiated from transient tachypnea of the newborn. Pneumonia usually persists for a few days, whereas transient tachypnea is more likely to resolve within 48 hours. In the premature infant with a radiographic appearance consistent with RDS, it may not be possible to distinguish the two conditions, at least in the early stages.

The use of cultures to identify the organism often is not helpful. Unless there is associated septicemia, the blood culture results will be negative. If the infant is intubated, tracheal cultures taken through the endotracheal tube can be misleading, particularly if the tube has been in place for some time, as the tube may be colonized with organisms that are not necessarily the same as those that are causing the pneumonia. A tracheal culture taken at the time of initial intubation may be of some value. Surface cultures are not helpful, as the organisms that colonize the skin may not be the pulmonary pathogens. In most cases, the bacteriology of the pneumonia is not established. If the infant dies, hyaline membrane formation may be noted in the lungs; Gram's stain of the lungs then may reveal gram-positive cocci enmeshed with the hyaline membranes in infants who die of group B streptococcal pneumonia (Fig 20-35).

## TREATMENT

The improvement that has occurred in the survival of infants with serious neonatal infections over the past 20 years is related to advances in supportive techniques as well as antibiotic therapy. Whereas milder cases may be treated with supplemental oxygen only, moderate and severe cases of pneumonia often require ventilator support. The infant's arterial blood gases, peripheral perfusion, blood pressure, and hematocrit should be monitored. If there is evidence of poor perfusion, this should be corrected

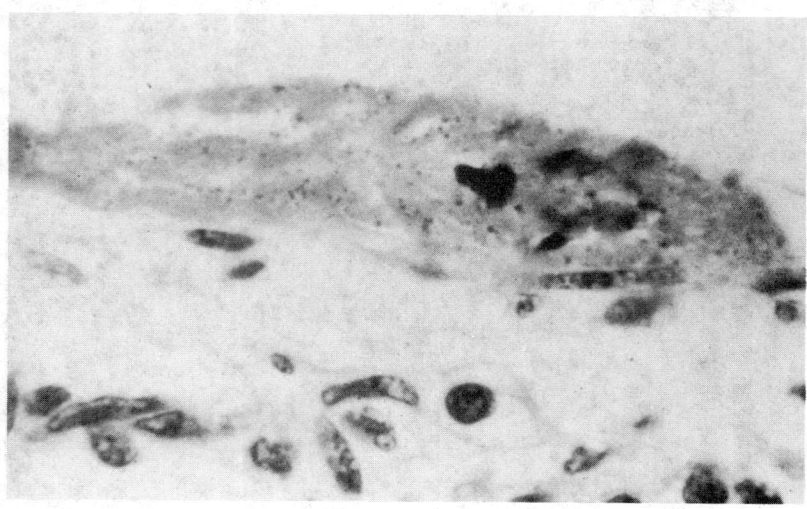

Figure 20-35. Gram's stain of hyaline membrane in group B streptococcal pneumonia. Enmeshed within the proteinaceous hyaline membrane are numerous gram-positive cocci.

with infusions of colloids such as albumin or inotropic drugs such as dopamine. If perfusion is a major problem, evaluation of central venous pressure and cardiac status will facilitate decisions related to the use of volume expanders or inotropic drugs.

Because a precise bacterial diagnosis usually is not available, broad-spectrum coverage, for example, with a penicillin and an aminoglycoside, usually is instituted for 7 to 10 days. If gentamicin is used, peak and trough levels of this antibiotic in the blood should be determined to ensure that the dose and frequency of administration are appropriate.

In those infants who demonstrate evidence of pulmonary hypertension and right-to-left shunting, a trial of tolazoline may be indicated, particularly if the PaO₂ is extremely low despite ventilation with high oxygen concentrations. If there is a favorable response to a test dose of tolazoline, a continuous infusion should be started and maintained as long as there is evidence of shunting. In some infants, the pulmonary hypertension is so severe and intractable that institution of extracorporeal membrane oxygenation (ECMO) is indicated. Tolazoline and ECMO therapy are discussed in the section on pulmonary hypertension (20.2.9).

Most infants with pneumonia do well and survive without long-term sequelae. Patients who require prolonged ventilation with high peak inspiratory pressures and high oxygen concentrations may have chronic lung disease.

*Principles and Practice of Pediatrics, Second Edition.*
edited by Frank A. Oski et al. J. B. Lippincott Company, Philadelphia © 1994.

## 20.2.7 *Pulmonary Air Leaks*

Ian Gross

Air leak is more common during the newborn period than at any other time of life. This probably relates to the facts that assisted ventilation is a relatively common mode of therapy in sick newborn infants, that premature infants have fragile lungs, and that high intrathoracic pressure gradients are generated during the first few breaths. It has been estimated that spontaneous air leak occurs in 1% of all live births, but many of these are asymptomatic. The sites of air leak in the newborn are the pleural cavities (pneumothorax), mediastinum (pneumomediastinum), interstitial tissue (interstitial emphysema), and, occasionally, pericardial sac (pneumopericardium) and peritoneal cavity (pneumoperitoneum).

Air leak begins with rupture of an overdistended alveolus. The air leaks into the interstitial space and tracks along the vascular sheaths into the mediastinum and then into the pleural cavity. Infrequently, air ruptures into the peritoneal or pericardial cavities. It is a significant problem in infants receiving assisted ventilation. The incidence of this complication varies between 15% and 40% in newborn infants on ventilators, depending in part on the nature of the underlying problem and its severity. The incidence of pneumothorax and interstitial emphysema in infants with respiratory distress syndrome (RDS) has been shown to be reduced by about 50% with the use of surfactant.

### PNEUMOTHORAX

Air leak, particularly pneumothorax, should be suspected in any infant receiving positive airway pressure who suddenly becomes cyanotic. The clinical features suggestive of a tension pneumothorax include shift of the apex beat, decreased breath sounds on the side of the pneumothorax, distention of the chest, and, occasionally, a readily palpable liver and spleen from downward displacement of the diaphragm. In addition, the infant may demonstrate poor circulation or shock.

Diagnosis and appropriate treatment of a tension pneumothorax is a matter of the greatest urgency. The differential diagnosis of an infant who deteriorates suddenly and becomes cyanotic while on a ventilator includes endotracheal tube or upper airway obstruction, pneumothorax, or massive intracranial bleed. Once it has been established that the airway is patent, the diagnosis of tension pneumothorax may be made on clinical grounds assisted by transillumination. This involves shining a bright, focused light on the chest wall after dimming the lights in the room. Often, the part of the chest into which air has leaked will become highly translucent. This test should be regarded as helpful rather than as absolutely diagnostic for the presence or absence of a pneumothorax. There usually is not time to obtain a radiograph of the chest if the infant is unstable; in this situation, the suspected pneumothorax will have to be managed without the benefit of radiographic confirmation. If the infant is stable and there is no acute interference with respiration or circulation, a chest radiograph may be obtained for confirmation of the diagnosis before proceeding to treatment.

The initial step is to insert a needle, preferably a plastic needle with a metal trochar such as is used for peripheral intravenous infusions, into the chest. The needle should be attached to a syringe by means of a three-way stopcock or, alternatively, to a short length of intravenous solution tubing, the end of which is placed under a water seal below the level of the chest. If the baby is lying supine, the air usually will collect in the anterior chest and a suitable site for needle insertion is the anterior axillary line in the fifth or sixth interspace. The diagnosis of pneumothorax is made when insertion of the needle results in the release of air under tension from the chest, with accompanying improvement in the infant's status. Once the diagnosis has been established, and preferably after radiographic confirmation has been obtained, a chest tube should be inserted. The chest tube should be connected to an underwater seal that is subjected to negative pressure. Drainage should be continued as long as air is evacuated from the chest. When it is clear that air drainage has stopped, the chest tube may be clamped. If the pneumothorax does not recur after clamping of the tube for a few hours, the tube may be removed.

A spontaneous pneumothorax that is not under tension and that is causing little distress may be treated by observation only. Some authors have recommended allowing the child to inspire 100% oxygen. This permits more rapid absorption of the pneumothorax because oxygen is absorbed more readily into the bloodstream than is the nitrogen in air. This condition usually is benign, however, and inspiration of 100% oxygen is unnecessary in most cases. Resolution usually occurs satisfactorily if the infant is allowed to breathe room air.

Pneumomediastinum generally is not treated surgically, and resolves spontaneously with time. A pneumopericardium that is causing significant cardiac tamponade will require drainage. This should be done by a physician who is skilled in this procedure.

### INTERSTITIAL EMPHYSEMA

If air tracks into the interstitial space and stays there, interstitial emphysema results. This problem has become increasingly more significant as more extremely premature infants survive after mechanical ventilation. Their fragile lungs seem to be particularly prone to interstitial emphysema, and air in the interstitial space may be seen early on when these infants are being ventilated for

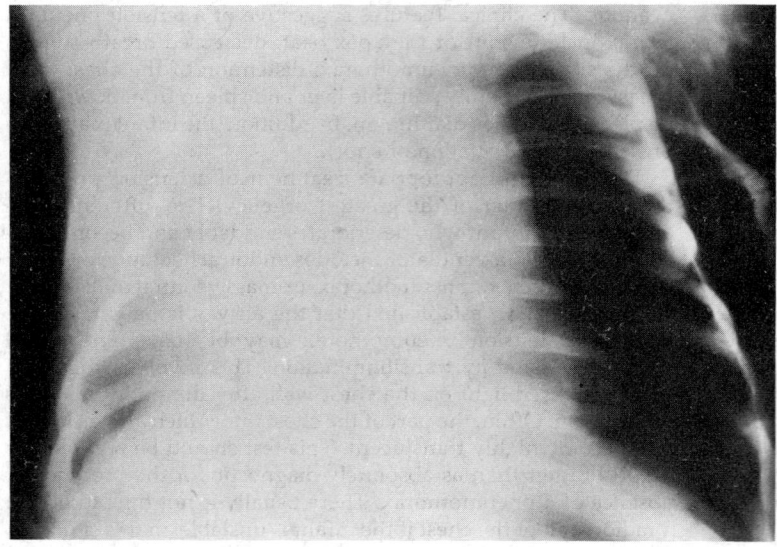

**Figure 20-36.**   Tension pneumothorax. Note the radiolucent air collection in the left chest, compression of the left lung, and shift of the mediastinum to the right.

*Principles and Practice of Pediatrics, Second Edition.*
edited by Frank A. Oski et al. J. B. Lippincott Company, Philadelphia © 1994.

RDS. The development of interstitial emphysema considerably complicates ventilatory management, as the lungs become even less compliant and higher ventilator pressures are required, which in turn further aggravates the interstitial emphysema. Very often, the pulmonary problem evolves into bronchopulmonary dysplasia.

Interstitial emphysema is difficult to treat. One approach, which sometimes is successful, is to position the infant so that the side of the chest that is most affected is dependent. The weight on this part of the chest may decrease the movement of the lungs there and assist resolution of the emphysema. Selective intubation may be useful in cases of unilateral interstitial emphysema. The endotracheal tube is inserted down the main stem bronchus of the unaffected lung, so that only that lung is ventilated. This procedure may result in resolution of the emphysema, but it often recurs when the endotracheal tube is pulled back and both lungs are inflated. Initial studies suggest that the use of high-frequency jet ventilation may be of value in infants with interstitial emphysema, and this condition may be an indication for this type of ventilation. High-frequency ventilation does not appear to prevent the development of this complication, however.

## RADIOGRAPHIC APPEARANCE

The definitive diagnosis of all these forms of air leak is made by radiography. A tension pneumothorax appears as a dark, radiolucent area in the pleural cavity (Fig 20-36). The compressed lung may be seen adjacent to the pleural air accumulation and the heart usually is shifted away from the pneumothorax. In an infant lying on his or her back, air tends to accumulate anteriorly, so that the free air is in the anterior medial portion of the chest. This may lead to confusion with pneumomediastinum. A lateral film always should be taken to localize further the site of air accumulation. In some cases of pneumomediastinum, the air compresses the thymus, resulting in the "sail" sign, which is caused by radiolucent air under a triangular thymic shadow. Pneumopericardium is characterized by air that surrounds the heart and adheres closely to its contour. The air crosses the midline underneath the heart as it follows the shape of the pericardial cavity. Interstitial emphysema is apparent as small, round, radiolucent blebs that track through the lung tissue. The air blebs sometimes follow a linear pattern.

## 20.2.8 *Meconium Aspiration Syndrome*

Ian Gross

Meconium is passed into the amniotic fluid in about 10% of all births. Although meconium passage may be associated with intrauterine fetal hypoxia, it also occurs in normal deliveries in the absence of asphyxia. Meconium aspiration is not seen in premature infants of less than 34 weeks' gestation, as these infants rarely demonstrate meconium-stained amniotic fluid. It is more common in postmature babies.

It is important that infants who are born covered with thick meconium and who have not yet cried vigorously have adequate aspiration of the meconium from their pharynx and trachea. It has been shown that tracheal suctioning in the delivery room before respiration is established is of benefit. The delivery room management of infants born with meconium staining is discussed in Chapter 17.1.

Meconium that has not been cleared from the trachea migrates peripherally and obstructs the smaller airways. Partial occlusion may result in a one-way valve effect, with distal hyperinflation. Alternatively, the small airways may be blocked completely, leading to atelectasis. In some infants, persistent pulmonary hypertension develops and this considerably complicates their management. The management of persistent pulmonary hypertension is discussed in the next section.

Infants with meconium aspiration present clinically with respiratory distress and an overdistended chest. Coarse rales may be heard. The chest radiograph reveals hyperinflation of the lungs with patchy infiltrates. Because of the air-trapping effect of meconium in the airways, pneumothorax is common, occurring in 20% to 50% of cases.

Management of these patients is symptomatic. They require oxygen supplementation and, frequently, ventilator therapy. The diffuse small-airway obstruction often necessitates the use of high peak inspiratory pressures to maintain adequate ventilation. The use of antibiotics is controversial; some neonatologists do not use antibiotics in uncomplicated cases of meconium aspiration, whereas others do because of concern for secondary infection.

*Principles and Practice of Pediatrics, Second Edition.*
edited by Frank A. Oski et al. J. B. Lippincott Company, Philadelphia © 1994.

## 20.2.9 *Persistent Pulmonary Hypertension*

Ian Gross

### PATHOGENESIS

During fetal life, there is increased tone in the pulmonary vasculature and the pressure on the right side of the heart is greater than that on the left. Consequently, blood is shunted from the right to the left side of the heart through the foramen ovale and the ductus arteriosus (Fig 20-37). The blood that enters the right atrium via the superior vena cava tends to flow into the right ventricle, whereas that which enters the right atrium from the inferior vena cava tends to be shunted across the foramen ovale to the left atrium. Much of the flow from the right ventricle then is shunted to the aorta through the ductus arteriosus. After birth, pressure in the pulmonary circulation decreases and there is functional closure of the foramen ovale, followed by anatomic closure of the ductus arteriosus. In some infants, pulmonary hypertension develops again after birth. This results in reestablishment of right-to-left shunting through the foramen ovale or ductus arteriosus; for this reason, this condition sometimes is referred to as "persistent fetal circulation."

The pulmonary vasculature is sensitive to hypoxia and acidosis, and responds to these stimuli by vasospasm. In infants with lung disease or other causes of hypoxia and acidosis, pulmonary hypertension may develop as a consequence of hypoxia resulting from the underlying disease. This secondary type of pulmonary hypertension usually reverses when the underlying problem has been resolved. There is, however, another group of infants in whom no obvious clinical cause for the pulmonary hypertension can be found. These usually are full-term infants with no lung or heart disease, but there may be a history of asphyxia. The underlying lesion in this primary form of persistent pulmonary hypertension (PPH) is believed to be premature muscularization of the small arterioles supplying the distal airways. At birth, the walls of the arterioles supplying the terminal and respiratory bronchioles normally are partially muscularized. Infants who die of this condition have been shown at autopsy to have extension of this muscularization into the arterioles that supply the alveolar ducts. The same abnormal arteriolar musculature also has been described in infants who die of meconium aspiration syndrome and PPH. It is possible that asphyxia or other insults after birth may trigger spasm of these thickened arterioles with resulting pulmonary hypertension.

Pulmonary hypertension also is associated with pulmonary hypoplasia, particularly that which results from diaphragmatic hernia. In this condition, there is not only pulmonary vasospasm, but also a smaller pulmonary vascular bed in association with the hypoplastic lung. The hypoxia in these infants may be particularly severe and resistant to therapy.

It has been suggested that the abnormal muscularization of the pulmonary vasculature is caused by intrauterine hypoxia during late fetal life. In utero, hypoxia also could account for the association of PPH with meconium aspiration and postmaturity. Infants who are stressed in utero, such as postmature infants, are less able to tolerate labor and have a greater tendency to experience intrapartum asphyxia and to pass meconium.

### DIAGNOSIS

The diagnosis of PPH is suggested by the triad of cyanosis, absence of heart disease, and clear lung fields or meconium aspiration. The usual presentation is that of a full-term or postmature infant who may have a history of asphyxia or meconium aspiration. The baby initially may appear to be well, but within the first 24 hours after birth, there is progressive cyanosis and tachypnea. A chest radiograph taken at this stage will reveal clear lungs or scattered infiltrates in the case of meconium aspiration. The lungs may have decreased vascular markings, consistent with diminished pulmonary blood flow. The cyanosis, if untreated, will continue to progress until, eventually, it becomes profound. Shock with decreased peripheral perfusion and hypotension also may become apparent.

The combination of severe cyanosis with clear lung fields or small infiltrates should raise the suspicion of PPH; the clue is cyanosis that is disproportionate to the underlying lung disease. The diagnosis cannot be made, however, and the infant should not be treated for pulmonary hypertension, until heart disease has been ruled out, preferably by an echocardiogram. Infants with transposition of the great vessels or other causes of cyanotic heart disease initially may exhibit very similar symptoms. The echocardiogram will exclude anatomic heart disease and confirm

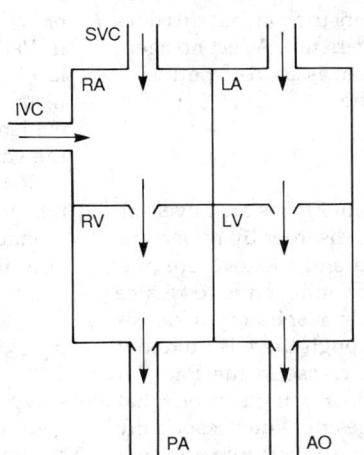

A. Mature Circulation  B. Fetal Circulation

**Figure 20-37.** (**A**) and (**B**) Comparison of mature and fetal circulations. In fetal life, blood is shunted from the right to the left side of the heart across the foramen ovale and the ductus arteriosus because of the increased pressure in the pulmonary circulation. If arterial pressure in the pulmonary circulation rises again after birth, the shunting recurs. *SVC,* superior vena cava; *RA,* right atrium; *LA,* left atrium; *RV,* right ventricle; *LV,* left ventricle; *IVC,* inferior vena cava; *PA,* pulmonary artery; *AO,* aorta; *FO,* foramen ovale; *DA,* ductus arteriosus.

the diagnosis of pulmonary hypertension and right-to-left shunting. It may reveal tricuspid regurgitation resulting from the high right-sided pressure. The echocardiogram also is useful for assessing right ventricular filling and myocardial contractility, and it can be used as a guide for determining intravenous fluid requirements.

Comparison of right radial (preductal) $PaO_2$ to umbilical artery (postductal) $PaO_2$ is useful in assessing shunting across the ductus arteriosus. The umbilical $PaO_2$ will be lower in the presence of right-to-left ductal shunting. The absence of such a difference does not rule out PPH and right-to-left shunting, because the shunt may occur at the atrial (foramen ovale) level only.

## MANAGEMENT

Infants with PPH present perhaps the most difficult medical management problem in the newborn intensive care unit and their care draws upon all the resources available to modern neonatology. They should be managed by physicians who are experienced with this problem and in an environment where the appropriate support is available.

### Monitoring

Careful monitoring is critical. An umbilical or radial artery catheter should be inserted so that blood gases and blood pressure can be determined. A central venous line may be inserted to monitor central venous pressure, although interpretation may be difficult if there is tricuspid regurgitation. Serial echocardiograms probably are more useful than is central venous pressure measurement for assessing intravascular fluid status. Two pulse oximeters or transcutaneous oxygen monitors, positioned so as to register preductal and postductal values (eg, on the right hand and left foot) also are extremely useful.

### Perfusion

These infants often have poor cardiovascular perfusion and may require large volumes of intravenous colloid or inotropic agents. If peripheral perfusion appears to be diminished, a determination of right-sided ventricular filling should be made. If the echocardiogram or the central venous pressure indicates that an intravenous fluid infusion is required, colloid such as albumin probably is the agent of choice. If intravascular fluid volume is adequate, but contractility is poor, an infusion of dopamine or another inotropic agent is indicated. Most infants with significant disease require both inotropic agent and albumin infusions. There is some concern that the infusion of dopamine at rates greater than 10 $\mu$g/kg/min may cause pulmonary vasoconstriction, but this does not appear to be borne out by clinical experience. A second agent such as dobutamine or epinephrine often is used if perfusion cannot be improved with dopamine alone.

### Ventilation

The ventilatory management of infants with PPH is controversial. Over the past 10 years, treatment of this disorder by hyperventilation has become common. Hyperoxia and alkalosis are pulmonary vasodilators. The goal of hyperventilation is to reduce the $PaCO_2$ to 20 to 25 mm Hg, so that a respiratory alkalosis develops, and to increase the $PaO_2$. Although there is no doubt that hyperventilation can produce an increase in the $PaO_2$, at least in the short term, there has been increasing concern that this form of therapy significantly damages the lungs, especially when it is prolonged. Pulmonary vasospasm and hypertension tend to resolve after a few days, and mortality in some cases

appears to be related to lung damage from barotrauma from the respirator rather than from the primary problem. For this reason, there has been a tendency recently to avoid hyperventilation and to use a more conservative approach to ventilator management. A number of centers now allow the $PaCO_2$ to remain at 45 to 55 mm Hg and will accept a $PaO_2$ in the range of 45 to 60 mm Hg. These blood gas levels can be achieved without having to hyperventilate the infant. The $PaO_2$ in many of these infants does respond favorably to an alkaline pH level, however, and some physicians maintain the pH in the range of 7.45 to 7.5 by the intravenous infusion of sodium bicarbonate.

Some infants are very labile and become hypoxic if they are touched or moved. They may become more stable with adequate sedation. Morphine or other opiates, alone or in combination with benzodiazepine derivatives, usually are effective for this purpose. The question of whether these infants also should be given muscle relaxants, such as pancuronium, to permit control of ventilation is controversial. Paralysis does facilitate ventilation if the infant is active and fighting the respirator, but the absence of muscular movement decreases venous return and results in significant edema. In addition, paralysis may mask seizures in asphyxiated infants. Muscle relaxants probably should be avoided, if possible.

The labile $PaO_2$ and right-to-left shunt usually persist for 2 to 5 days, after which recovery starts to occur. If the lungs have not been damaged by the respirator and oxygen therapy, the infant may be weaned slowly from the ventilator. Some infants become suddenly hypoxic when weaning is attempted ("flip-flop" effect), so this must be done slowly and cautiously.

### Pulmonary Vasodilators

Oxygen and alkalosis are potent pulmonary vasodilators, as discussed above. No specific pulmonary vasodilator drugs are available. A variety of agents with limited effectiveness are used for this purpose, however. The most widely used and probably the most effective agent is tolazoline, a histamine releaser and $\alpha$-adrenergic blocker. In about one third of infants with PPH, tolazoline is successful in dilating the pulmonary vasculature and improving the $PaO_2$. Tolazoline is a general vasodilator and does not act specifically on the pulmonary vasculature, so infusion of this drug may cause a drop in systemic blood pressure and aggravate the right-to-left shunt. Because of this systemic vasodilation, it often is advisable to infuse albumin before and during the administration of a test dose of tolazoline. The initial test dose is 1 mg/kg. If there is no response to this, a test dose of 2 mg/kg may be attempted. The blood pressure must be monitored while tolazoline is being infused and, if it drops significantly, this should be treated with an infusion of albumin, dopamine, or both. If the test dose of tolazoline produces a significant increase in $PaO_2$, a constant infusion of 2 mg/kg/h can be started. Tolazoline infusion can result in gastric bleeding, oliguria, and other histamine-like effects. It should be discontinued as soon as it is evident that the pulmonary vasculature no longer is labile and the vasospasm has resolved.

Recent preliminary reports suggest that endothelium-derived relaxing factor, which actually is nitric oxide, is a potent pulmonary vasodilator in adults and infants. Studies to evaluate the effectiveness of inhaled nitric oxide in the management of PPH are in progress.

### Extracorporeal Membrane Oxygenation (ECMO)

A type of pulmonary bypass, extracorporeal membrane oxygenation (ECMO) is being used increasingly for the treatment of severe cases of PPH. In this procedure, blood is diverted from the jugular vein, anticoagulated, pumped through a membrane oxygenator, and then returned to the baby via the carotid artery. The use of ECMO has been justified on the grounds that, if it were not used for the sickest infants, they would have a very high rate of mortality. Although the use of ECMO for infants with PPH has not been subjected to large-scale, randomized, controlled clinical trials, it does appear to be an effective rescue therapy for selected infants with severe irreversible hypoxia who are not responding to conventional medical therapy. Because the procedure involves ligating the carotid artery and heparinizing the blood, there have been concerns about bleeding and neurologic side effects, but follow-up studies of survivors have reported encouragingly good outcomes.

## PROGNOSIS

Although the rate of survival for infants with pulmonary hypertension was 50% or less in 1980, survival rates of 80% or better have been reported recently by a number of centers in association with advances in conventional supportive therapy. Similar survival rates also have been attained in severely ill infants with the use of ECMO. Those infants who survive appear to do fairly well. Some have residual lung disease resulting from prolonged ventilation and oxygen administration. Significant neurologic problems have been reported in about one fifth of the survivors, whether treated with conventional therapy or ECMO.

*Principles and Practice of Pediatrics, Second Edition.*
edited by Frank A. Oski et al. J. B. Lippincott Company, Philadelphia © 1994.

## 20.2.10 *Apnea*

Robert Herzlinger

Apnea is defined as a respiratory pause of 20 seconds or longer, or a shorter pause associated with cyanosis, abrupt pallor or hypotonia, or bradycardia. Apnea is an extremely common finding in premature infants. The incidence increases with decreasing gestational age. About 50% of infants weighing less than 1500 g at birth, and almost all infants weighing less than 1000 g, will require intervention for apnea. Because most cases of apnea are related to prematurity, the incidence of apnea decreases with increasing postconceptual age, and usually resolves by 35 to 36 weeks' postconceptual age. Infants with extremely low birth weights (less than 1000 g) may have persistent apnea beyond 40 weeks' postconceptual age.

Apnea can be categorized into three types. Central apnea is characterized by a total lack of chest wall movement and nasal airflow; obstructive apnea is associated with chest wall movement, without nasal airflow; and mixed apnea is obstructive followed by central apnea. The latter accounts for about 50% of apneic episodes in premature infants. In contrast to apnea, periodic breathing is defined as three or more respiratory pauses of more than 3 seconds with less than 20 seconds of breathing between pauses. Periodic breathing probably is a normal breathing pattern in premature and term infants.

## ETIOLOGY

Apnea is a symptom or sign of an underlying disorder; however, the most common cause of apnea in premature infants is related to immaturity of the ventilatory control mechanism. Anatomic correlates of impaired ventilatory control include decreased dendritic synapses and neural myelination. In addition, chemoreceptor function is impaired, resulting in a blunted ventilatory response to hypercarbia and paradoxic hypoventilation in response to hypoxemia. Functional obstruction of the upper airway results from uncoordinated brain stem control of posterior pharyngeal patency and diaphragmatic contractility. Active inhibitory respiratory reflexes also may contribute to apnea in premature neonates. In the face of an immature and unstable ventilatory control mechanism, a wide variety of conditions can induce apnea in premature infants. In contrast, a specific etiology is more likely to be found in term or near-term infants who have spells of apnea.

## MANAGEMENT

All infants at risk for apnea of prematurity (ie, those of less than 34 weeks' gestation) require cardiac or cardiac/thoracic impedance monitoring when they are admitted to the nursery. Apnea of prematurity is a diagnosis of exclusion, and before this diagnosis can be made, the other causes of apnea must be considered (Table 20-7). A careful history and physical examination will direct further evaluation. An investigation for sepsis/meningitis should be performed in infants who have other signs and symptoms of sepsis, in those with apnea beyond 34 weeks' gestation, in those with a sudden onset of apnea after being asymptomatic, and in those with severe apnea requiring bag mask ventilation. Management of apnea of prematurity is determined by the frequency and severity of the episodes. If these are mild and are not associated with cyanosis or bradycardia, they may be treated with gentle stimulation, clearance of secretions from the airway, and avoidance of neck flexion. If the infant continues to have significant apnea, the next step is to treat with methylxanthines.

**TABLE 20-7. Causes of Apnea**

Apnea of prematurity
Central nervous system disorders
  Intraventricular/periventricular hemorrhage
  Subarachnoid hemorrhage
  Infarction
Cardiorespiratory disorders
  Respiratory distress syndrome
  Bronchopulmonary dysplasia
  Patent ductus arteriosus
Metabolic disorders
  Hypoglycemia
  Hypocalcemia
  Electrolyte imbalance
Hematologic
  Anemia
Infection
  Sepsis/meningitis
Gastrointestinal
  Necrotizing enterocolitis
  Gastroesophageal reflux
Medications
  Phenobarbital
  General anesthesia
Temperature
  Rapid warming
Obstruction
  Secretions
  Neck flexion
  Congenital airway anomalies
Stimulation of inhibitory reflexes

These agents are effective against central and obstructive apnea. Proposed mechanisms of action of methylxanthines for apnea include increased sensitivity of the medullary respiratory center to $CO_2$, increased afferent nerve traffic to the brain stem, and improved skeletal and diaphragmatic muscle contraction. Theophylline is the most commonly used agent. It is given in a loading dose of 5 mg/kg, followed by a maintenance dosage of 1 to 2 mg/kg per dose every 8 hours. It is important to monitor blood levels, and to adjust the dosage accordingly. The therapeutic concentration is 8 to 12 $\mu$g/mL. Toxicity may occur with levels greater than 15 $\mu$g/mL, and usually presents as tachycardia, irritability, and vomiting. Caffeine, which is given orally and has a longer half-life and a wider therapeutic range, may be used as an alternative to theophylline. Theophylline is metabolized in part to caffeine in premature infants.

Persistent apnea despite methylxanthine therapy is an indication for nasal continuous positive airway pressure (CPAP), which is effective against obstructive and mixed apnea spells. The proposed mechanism of action for CPAP involves stabilization of the upper airway and chest wall, as well as reduction in inhibitory respiratory reflexes.

Intubation and mechanical ventilation are indicated if significant apnea persists despite the above measures. Severe apnea may be associated with a decrease in cerebral blood flow resulting in neurologic injury.

Infants with apnea of prematurity may be discharged home if they are more than 35 to 36 weeks' postconceptual age and remain free of apnea for 7 to 10 days. Although the incidence of sudden infant death syndrome (SIDS) increases with decreasing birth weight, parents should be reassured that apnea of prematurity is not an independent risk factor for SIDS. Pneumograms (recordings of heart rate and thoracic impedance) are not predictive of the risk for recurrent apnea or SIDS. Home monitoring may be used to shorten the hospitalization of premature infants with persistent apnea beyond 36 weeks' postconceptual age. The home monitor may be discontinued if the infant has no significant episodes for 2 or 3 months. No evidence exists, however, that home monitoring prevents SIDS. Apnea of prematurity that has resolved is not in itself an indication for home monitoring.

## Selected Readings

Ablow RA, Gross I, Effman EL, et al. The radiographic features of early onset group B streptococcal neonatal sepsis. Radiology 1977;124:771.

Abman SH, Wolfe RR, Accurso FJ, et al. Pulmonary vascular response to oxygen in infants with severe bronchopulmonary dysplasia. Pediatrics 1985;75:80.

Avery ME, Fletcher BA, Williams R. The lung and its disorders in the newborn infant, ed 4. Philadelphia: WB Saunders, 1981.

Avery ME, Tooley WH, Keller JB, et al. Is chronic lung disease in low birth weight infants preventable? A survey of eight centers. Pediatrics 1987;79:26.

Blanchard PW, Brown TM, Coates AL. Pharmacotherapy in bronchopulmonary dysplasia. Clin Perinatol 1987;14:881.

Bohn D, Tamura M, Perrin D, et al. Ventilatory predictors of pulmonary hypoplasia in congenital diaphragmatic hernia, confirmed by morphologic assessment. J Pediatr 1987;111:423.

Consensus Statement. National Institutes of Health Consensus Development Conference on Infantile Apnea and Home Monitoring, Sept. 29 to Oct. 1, 1986. Pediatrics 1987;79:292.

Escobedo MB, Gonzalez A. Bronchopulmonary dysplasia in the tiny infant. Clin Perinatol 1986;13:315.

Glass P, Miller M, Short B. Morbidity for survivors of extracorporeal membrane oxygenation: Neurodevelopmental outcome at 1 year of age. Pediatrics 1989;83:72.

HIFI Study Group. High frequency oscillatory ventilation compared with mechanical ventilation in the treatment of respiratory failure in preterm infants. N Engl J Med 1989;320:88.

Jobe A, Ikegami M. Surfactant for the treatment of respiratory distress syndrome. Am Rev Respir Dis 1987;136:1256.

Liechty EA, Donovan E, Purohit D, et al. Reduction of neonatal mortality after multiple doses of bovine surfactant in low birthweight infants with respiratory distress syndrome. Pediatrics 1991;88:19.

Monin P, Vert P. The management of bronchopulmonary dysplasia. Clin Perinatol 1987;14:531.

Thibeault DW, Gregory GA. Neonatal pulmonary care, 2nd ed. Norwalk, Conn: Appleton-Century-Crofts, 1986.

Wung J, James LS, Kilchevsky E, James E. Management of infants with severe respiratory failure and persistence of the fetal circulation without hyperventilation. Pediatrics 1985;76:488.

*Principles and Practice of Pediatrics, Second Edition.*
edited by Frank A. Oski et al. J. B. Lippincott Company, Philadelphia © 1994.

## 20.2.11 Surgical Considerations and Postoperative Care of the Newborn

Robert J. Touloukian

Major advances in the care of the newborn have improved survival and quality of life dramatically for a baby born with a major congenital anomaly or an acquired condition requiring emergency surgery during the first month of life. In most centers, the overall survival rate of these infants approaches 85% to 90%. The modern era of neonatal surgery can be traced to the early 1960s, with the establishment of tertiary care neonatal special care units, innovative surgical techniques, modern ventilatory management, intravenous nutrition, and the multimodal treatment of sepsis and shock. Perinatology, with its emphasis on the diagnosis and treatment of congenital anomalies in high-risk fetuses, has paralleled the development of the high-risk obstetric service, thereby reducing the need for infant transport from a community hospital to a tertiary care center. Improved radiologic modalities, including ultrasound, computed tomography, and magnetic resonance scanning, have revolutionized our ability to perform noninvasive evaluation of a sick newborn. Certain fetal intervention procedures have become safe, and even hysterotomy with open corrective operation has resulted in fetal salvage.

Most surgical procedures in the newborn are carried out by pediatric surgeons, who are general surgeons with an additional 2 years of training obtained in one of 28 approved training centers in the United States and Canada (as of 1993). This training encompasses the surgical fields of neonatal and general, head and neck, trauma, transplantation, burns, endoscopy, gynecology, and urology. Diaphragmatic hernia, esophageal atresia, Hirschsprung's disease, intestinal atresia, imperforate anus, omphalocele, and gastroschisis are certain "index" neonatal conditions for which exceptional technical skill and judgment must be learned by the pediatric surgical trainee. Because each condition occurs no more than once per 3000 live births, regionalization of care is required to achieve sufficient surgical expertise within the limited period of training. There are more than 500 board-certified pediatric surgeons in the United States and Canada, the majority of whom are affiliated with a tertiary care neonatal center.

The interface between neonatology and pediatric surgery begins at the time of initial evaluation of the infant and continues through the postoperative period. As in all other fields of pediatrics, good communication is needed. Because the infant's condition must be monitored closely, the neonatologist and primary nurse are essential partners of the surgeon. The surgeon, however, remains responsible for the overall care of the surgical patient, determining the timing of operation, the need for supplementary evaluations, the progression of feeding schedules, the use of antibiotics, and so on. It is essential that this relationship be both collaborative and collegial.

## PRENATAL DIAGNOSIS

Prenatal diagnosis has revolutionized the surgical care of the newborn with a correctable anomaly (Table 20-8). Screening ultrasound examination and determination of the maternal serum α-fetoprotein level provide the first level of evaluation by the obstetrician, who then refers the mother to a high-risk center for perinatology and pediatric surgical consultation. At this time, the surgeon and parents discuss the diagnosis and proposed treatment, further diagnostic testing such as amniocentesis for chromosome analysis, and the corrective surgery that is required, along with the risks and potential benefits. Furthermore, the family should have a clear understanding of the potential for long-term physical disability or neurologic impairment in their infant. Hand-drawn illustrations, the use of medical textbooks, and clinical examples taken from the surgeon's own experience may help to clarify many important questions about the fate of the fetus.

The advisability of terminating the pregnancy sometimes is raised if the diagnosis of an uncorrectable anomaly is made before the 24th week of gestation. Specific indications for termination include chromosome abnormalities that are incompatible with normal life (omphalocele with trisomy 13 or 18), severe neurologic impairment such as encephalocele or anencephaly, or hazards to maternal health, but the need for corrective surgery alone is not deemed an appropriate reason to terminate a pregnancy. Occasionally, the mother may wish to deliver at term in a community hospital if the anomaly is not life-threatening or does not require immediate surgical correction. My opinion, however, is that delivery in a tertiary care center obviates the need for infant transport and shortens the time from birth to surgical correction. This is mandatory for babies with congenital diaphragmatic hernia, abdominal wall defects, or intestinal obstruction, when emergency surgery is required within hours of birth. Recent reports have cautioned against unnecessary cesarean section when there is no evidence of fetal distress.

## INFANT TRANSPORT

Surgical conditions that are diagnosed postnatally require emergent transport of the neonate to a tertiary care center. Esophageal atresia, Hirschsprung's disease, and other forms of lower intestinal obstruction, including anorectal anomalies, are not detected routinely by prenatal ultrasound, but potentially are life-threatening within the first 12 to 24 hours of life. Although the number of babies with congenital diaphragmatic hernia diagnosed by routine prenatal screening is increasing gradually, some of these infants will not be detected until respiratory distress develops shortly after birth. The most frequently encountered indication for emergency transport (from a level 2 nursery) is the baby with "suspect" necrotizing enterocolitis in whom peritonitis develops after medical management is begun. For these reasons, a tertiary care center must provide the capability for prompt transport by ambulance, helicopter, or fixed-wing aircraft, depending on the distance of the referring hospital to the neonatal center.

The transport team consists of a cadre of neonatal nurses with advanced training in resuscitation, endotracheal intubation, institution of a peripheral intravenous line, umbilical artery catheterization, and insertion of a nasogastric or chest tube. The risks associated with specific anomalies and the means by which to prevent further injury or clinical deterioration should be understood. Babies born with a gastroschisis have rapid conductive heat and evaporative fluid loss. The exposed viscera must be covered in warm, moist saline sponges and plastic wrap to prevent additional fluid loss and inadvertent twisting of the mesentery or bowel. Early intervention with an intravenous glucose solution is lifesaving for a newborn with omphalocele and macroglossia (Beckwith's syndrome) who becomes hypoglycemic and potentially could have brain-damaging seizures.

## PREOPERATIVE PREPARATION

A number of special considerations make the surgical care of the neonate unique (Table 20-9).

### Temperature Regulation

The ratio of skin surface area to lean body mass of the premature neonate is higher than that of an older infant or child. With increased metabolic demands and the absence of a normal thermogenic shivering mechanism, peripheral vasodilatation results in rapid surface cooling and systemic hypothermia. This concern is particularly valid in the stressed preterm infant whose nutritional reserves are minimal, and when body cooling also leads to increased metabolism, thereby raising oxygen requirements. As heat loss continues, peripheral vasoconstriction occurs, with shunting of arterialized blood, increased lactic acid load, and, eventually, a profound metabolic acidosis.

Hypothermia is minimized by examining the infant under a radiant heat warmer, and by exposing him or her only for short periods when it is essential. Of particular concern is the infant with gastroschisis or omphalocele, because evaporative fluid loss compounds the hypothermia. Use of a warming mattress and supplementary radiant heating lamps are additional helpful measures to prevent hypothermia. Once the initial evaluation of

| | Incidence (live births) | Prenatal Detection Rate (%) | Diagnostic Markers | Overall Survival (%) |
|---|---|---|---|---|
| **TABLE 20-8. Prenatal Detection and Overall Survival of Common Neonatal Surgical Conditions** | | | | |
| Esophageal atresia | 1:2000 | 20 | Polyhydramnios | 90 |
| Intestinal atresia | 1:2500 | 75 | Polyhydramnios | 95 |
| Abdominal wall defects (with normal chromosomes) | 1:3000 | 90 | Elevated MSAFP | 95 |
| Cysts and tumors | 1:3000 | 25 | Elevated MSAFP | 95 |
| Neural tube defects | 1:400 | 95 | Elevated MSAFP | Variable |
| Diaphragmatic hernia | 1:2500 | 10 | Elevated MSAFP | 50 |
| Urinary tract obstruction | 1:3000 | 90 | Oligohydramnios | 90 |

**TABLE 20-9.   General Considerations in the Surgical Care of the Newborn**

Temperature regulation
Respiratory support
Cardiovascular status
Radiographic evaluation
Vascular access/fluid replacement
Antibiotic management
Catheters
Additional diagnostic tests
Informed consent

the infant is complete, the humidified and warmed Isolette provides the best substitute for the uterus.

## Respiratory Support

Careful attention must be given to the airway and lungs, as hypoxemia, hypercapnia, and oxygen desaturation often occur in the face of extrinsic compression of the airway or pulmonary aspiration of salivary or gastrointestinal secretions. This complication may develop rapidly in babies with cervical cystic hygroma involving the floor of the mouth and paratracheal tissues, those with thoracic problems such as congenital diaphragmatic hernia, or those with esophageal atresia with tracheoesophageal fistula. Abdominal distention and upward displacement of the diaphragm also may restrict ventilation in babies with neonatal intestinal obstruction. This problem is particularly common in association with more distal obstruction such as meconium ileus, or in babies with a large ovarian or duplication cyst or hydronephrotic kidney. Careful monitoring of respiratory status is essential to detect apneic spells. These risks are magnified in preterm infants because of their intrinsic tendency toward irregular respiratory patterns. Any tendency toward desaturation mandates continuous monitoring, use of supplementary oxygen, and, often, institution of nasal continuous positive airway pressure or placement of an endotracheal tube with intermittent mandatory ventilation. A primary example of the importance of careful respiratory monitoring is a newborn with congenital diaphragmatic hernia with adequate ventilation at birth. Because of the tendency toward accumulation of air in the herniated intrathoracic stomach or bowel, the contralateral lung rapidly becomes compromised. In these patients, a combination of peripheral oxygen saturation and arterial blood gas determinations is important to detect hypoxia or a rising carbon dioxide level. A mixed respiratory and metabolic acidosis is a common occurrence.

## Cardiovascular Status

Many infants with cyanotic congenital heart disease, such as aortic stenosis or hypoplastic left heart syndrome, will appear to be perfectly stable at birth and begin to show evidence of deoxygenation only after the ductus arteriosus closes 24 to 48 hours after birth. Increased resistance in the pulmonary vascular bed, such as occurs in infants with pulmonary hypoplasia and congenital diaphragmatic hernia, tends to keep the ductus patent and to cause right-to-left shunting of deoxygenated blood into the systemic circulation. The infant with a noncardiac anomaly also may have increased pulmonary vascular resistance secondary to hypoxia, acidosis, hypothermia, and hypovolemia. Unnecessary delays in treating newborns with intestinal obstruction predispose these infants to pulmonary aspiration, which will aggravate any underlying tendency toward increased pulmonary vascular resistance.

## Radiographic Evaluation

At least one set of radiographic studies should be obtained in any baby who needs an abdominal or thoracic operation. Additional studies, including ultrasound, computed tomography, and magnetic resonance imaging, also may be useful.

The plain chest radiograph is diagnostic of the great majority of surgically correctable thoracic problems, including diaphragmatic hernia, tension disturbances secondary to pneumothorax or hydrothorax, and even those lesions intrinsic to the lungs such as lobar emphysema and congenital adenomatoid malformation. Caution must be exercised in distinguishing suspected congenital pulmonary cysts from a diaphragmatic hernia by obtaining an ultrasound of the diaphragm or gastrointestinal contrast studies. Ventilation perfusion scans will provide valuable information about the possibility of pulmonary hypoplasia in patients with diaphragmatic eventration, a condition that may be either congenital or secondary to brachial plexus birth injury.

Plain abdominal radiographs obtained in multiple views (ie, supine, prone, decubitus, and cross-table lateral) remain the "gold standard" in evaluating babies for intestinal obstruction, perforation, or a mass lesion. Our choice for detecting free air with necrotizing enterocolitis is the cross-table lateral view. When this examination is repeated at 6-hour intervals, perforation with free air over the liver may be recognized before peritonitis is established and the baby becomes septic. Visualizing the number, distribution, and size of the dilated intestinal loops is very helpful in determining the site of obstruction. A diagnosis of duodenal stenosis can be facilitated by having the radiologist inject 30 or 40 cc of air through the nasogastric tube and obtaining a prone view of the abdomen to best visualize a "double bubble." When the etiology of duodenal obstruction remains uncertain, barium is introduced through the nasogastric tube to assess the location of the duodenum and rule out malrotation, which can be associated with with mid-gut volvulus. With more distal obstruction, the differential diagnosis between meconium ileus, ileal stenosis, meconium plug syndrome, and Hirschsprung's disease can be confusing. Because plain films are nondiagnostic, a barium (or water-soluble contrast) enema should be carried out on an emergent basis. In many instances, the enema is therapeutic, but a submucosal biopsy must be obtained if Hirschsprung's disease remains a diagnostic possibility.

Bulky external masses, such as cystic hygroma or sacrococcygeal teratoma, often are complex lesions in which vital structures, including major vessels or nerves, are involved. High-resolution ultrasound with color Doppler will clearly distinguish arterial and venous supply, and is helpful in guiding the surgeon at the time of excision. Intra-abdominal or thoracic tumors and cysts can be evaluated similarly and, in the case of a flank mass, ultrasound immediately distinguishes a cystic lesion, such as a hydronephrotic or multicystic kidney, from a solid mass such as a mesoblastic nephroma, for which prompt excision should be carried out. More complex lesions containing both solid and cystic components, such as a neuroblastoma, will require further evaluation by computed tomography or magnetic resonance imaging. Urinary catecholamine determinations and bone marrow aspiration and biopsy may be necessary before attempts are made at resection. Any paraspinal tumor is assessed best by magnetic resonance scanning.

## Vascular Access/Fluid Replacement

Prompt venous cannulation is essential and, often, a combination of venous and arterial access is required in a neonate who is undergoing surgery. A peripheral venous line in the hand or foot and an umbilical arterial catheter situated above the renal vessels provides access for both maintenance and replacement crystalloid fluids or blood, and the means to monitor arterial blood gas levels and systemic blood pressure. Arterial cannulation is important for the newborn with a congenital diaphragmatic hernia, or in similar circumstances when major fluctuations in oxygen or carbon dioxide concentrations are anticipated, but is needed less often in stable infants whose oxygen saturation is determined satisfactorily by a cutaneous oxygen saturation monitor. If the baby has an enlarged abdomen because of an intra-abdominal mass, obstructed intestine, or abdominal wall defect, venous cannulation in the upper extremity is preferred strongly to avoid impedance of antegrade flow in the inferior vena cava once corrective surgery has been carried out. Rarely, if ever, is a peripheral intravenous cutdown procedure required, but central venous catheter placement has become very useful, either by cannulation of the internal or external jugular vein under direct vision (Broviac 2.7-French catheter, Davol, Inc.), or by percutaneous insertion of the catheter in the upper or lower extremity and then passage to the cavo-atrial site. Percutaneous catheters and venous catheters may be inserted under fluoroscopic surveillance in the operating room, or in the unit after the primary operation has been carried out.

The composition and volume of maintenance and replacement crystalloid fluid will vary from case to case, depending principally on the estimate of dehydration. Although the normal fluid requirement during the first 24 to 48 hours of life is about half that of usual maintenance, both extrinsic and internal losses may occur that cause hypovolemia and increase the fluid requirement. The following formula, based on clinical assessment, has proven to be very useful in estimating the degree of dehydration or hypovolemia: 5%—just detectable, dry mucous membranes, poor skin turgor; 10%—skin tenting, sunken fontanelle, oliguria; 15%—shock, anuria.

Initially, salt-containing solutions may be given to reverse so-called "third space" loss in infants with intestinal obstruction or vomiting. Fluid deficits in excess of 5% of body weight can be corrected by giving 10 mL/kg normal saline fluid boluses until the urine specific gravity is less than 1.010. Infants with gastroschisis and omphalocele also have significant evaporative fluid loss that must be replaced before operation. Infants who are dehydrated severely, are unstable, or are hypotensive should be given bolus replacement equal to 1% to 3% of their body weight. Even babies with a large cystic hygroma or sacrococcygeal teratoma may sustain sudden internal hemorrhage or fluid retention that may cause clinical signs of hypovolemia.

Extensive preoperative laboratory evaluation of the newborn with an acute surgical problem usually is not needed. The necessity of obtaining certain basic studies, however, including a complete blood count with platelet determination, is obvious. Additional tests such as serum electrolyte, blood urea nitrogen, and creatinine determinations; liver function tests; and coagulation studies are required only under specific circumstances. Blood is sent routinely to the blood bank for typing and cross-matching at a time early enough for the results to be available in the operating room. A so-called "split" unit of 50 cc of packed red blood cells is sufficient for almost all neonatal procedures, except in unusual instances, such as in an infant with a large sacrococcygeal teratoma or abdominal neuroblastoma, or in similar situations when major blood loss might be encountered.

## Antibiotic Management

Unrecognized sepsis and inadequate antibiotic coverage are among the most common causes of morbidity and death in the surgical neonate. Both cellular and humoral immune mechanisms may be impaired or deficient, particularly in the preterm infant. IgG is passed transplacentally, whereas secretory IgA is acquired secondarily by absorption of the antibody-laden macrophage from the gastrointestinal tract. In most centers, the use of breast milk or fortified breast milk in the preterm infant is preferable to proprietary formulas because of the likelihood that some humoral immunity is transferable. Whether delayed acquisition of humoral antibodies plays a role in the pathogenesis of necrotizing enterocolitis remains conjectural. There is no evidence to substantiate the claim that a preterm infant who is fed fresh breast milk or colostrum-containing lymphocytes enriched with secretory IgA has a lower risk of having necrotizing enterocolitis.

Early signs of sepsis in the newborn are subtle and include the development of hypothermia, bradycardia, and lethargy; seizures or apneic respiratory arrest usually are later sequelae. For this reason, preoperative prophylactic antibiotics generally are administered to babies who are undergoing major surgery, or when sepsis is suspected after appropriate cultures are obtained. The standard is a triple combination of ampicillin, gentamicin, and clindamycin, which provides broad-spectrum coverage against the common gram-positive and gram-negative organisms, including the anaerobic flora. Gram-negative organisms usually are the cause of disseminated intravascular coagulation, which most commonly affects the preterm infant with necrotizing enterocolitis from peritonitis secondary to perforated bowel, or the full-term infant with meconium peritonitis, closed loop obstruction, or mid-gut volvulus. Deterioration of the vital signs and progressing thrombocytopenia are adjunctive indicators for early intervention when physical signs alone are confusing or misleading. Reversal of established sepsis requires a combination of prompt operation removing the source of infection, adequate antibiotic coverage, fluid resuscitation, and vasopressors such as dopamine or dobutamine, which improve cardiac output both by acting as inotropic agents and by stimulating the beta receptors of the heart. Dopamine and dobutamine may be used together when conventional measures have failed.

## Use of Catheters for Diagnosis and Treatment

The careful placement of a small catheter in the upper esophageal pouch, gastrointestinal or urinary tract, and pleural space may be appropriate for both diagnostic and therapeutic purposes, and may play an important role in the care of the surgical neonate.

A feeding tube (8-French) tests the patency of the choanae and upper esophagus. Passing the tube through each choana will rule out the possibility of membranous or bony choanal atresia in a baby with upper airway obstruction. Nasal discharge may be the only sign of unilateral choanal obstruction, but bilateral obstruction causes acute respiratory distress in the newborn, who is an obligate nasal breather. The diagnosis of esophageal atresia must be considered in babies with drooling or mucus-like oral secretions and episodes of coughing, choking, and cyanosis. This impression can be confirmed by gently passing a feeding catheter through the nose or mouth into the esophagus and meeting resistance in the upper thorax. It is important to use a tube that is firm enough to avoid coiling in the upper pouch. Confirmation of the diagnosis of esophageal atresia is made by obtaining a plain chest radiograph that reveals the air-filled upper pouch accompanied by air in the stomach of babies with an associated distal tracheoesophageal fistula. Continuous suction of the upper esophageal pouch with a sump suction catheter prevents pooling of secretions and minimizes the risk of pulmonary aspiration.

Emptying the stomach with a nasogastric tube is useful in determining whether a newborn who is vomiting at birth or is not tolerating feedings has partial or complete intestinal obstruction. Residual volumes that are bile-tinged or in excess of 25 mL strongly suggest intestinal obstruction or ileus, and nasogastric decompression and intermittent suction are required. The tube should be taped to the upper lip or, in the case of a preterm infant, passed through the mouth.

A 5- or 8-French feeding catheter also can be used to decompress the urinary tract in babies in whom it is obstructed by posterior urethral valves or in those with prune-belly syndrome, who have congenital absence of abdominal wall musculature. Intermittent catheterization of the enlarged bladder is essential to prevent reflux and urinary tract infection with eventual deterioration of the upper tracts and renal function. Careful placement of a catheter in a urogenital sinus or in the single orifice of a baby with a cloaca is done best under fluoroscopy to delineate the full anatomy. In some cases, the accessory orifices may be obstructed partially, and a full assessment of the underlying anatomy will require cystoscopy and, eventually, operative intervention.

The risk of a pneumothorax has decreased significantly with the advent of the pressure-limited, time-cycled ventilator, but any baby with unexplained oxygen desaturation or abnormal arterial blood gas levels requires prompt assessment for the presence of air in the pleural space or mediastinum. Transillumination of the thoracic cavity to confirm the clinical impression of a tension pneumothorax, followed by percutaneous aspiration of air with an Angiocath and subsequent insertion of a chest tube is a life-saving measure, because mediastinal shift and compression of the contralateral lung is a dramatic and possibly fatal event. Because the chest wall of a newborn is quite thin, a bronchopleurocutaneous fistula may develop, unless the chest tube is tunneled one or two interspaces above the insertion site, thereby preventing the tracking of air along the tube into the subcutaneous tissue and outside the baby. Connection of the chest tube to underwater suction is required until the air leak has sealed.

## Additional Diagnostic Tests

Evaluation of a newborn with one major life-threatening congenital anomaly for associated anomalies must be carried out within hours of birth. The incidence of an associated anomaly may be as high as 50% in babies with esophageal atresia or omphalocele, or quite low in babies with gastroschisis or jejunoileal atresia. Well known in the surgical neonate is the so-called VATER syndrome, which is an association of *v*ertebral, *c*ardiac, *a*norectal, *t*racheoesophageal, *r*enal, and limb anomalies. The cardiac anomalies in this condition may not be life-threatening (eg, a small ventricular septal defect), but they may be more complex, such as in a baby with multiple intracardiac defects, and they require preoperative echocardiography for full assessment. In general, this is carried out before the first operation in a baby with esophageal atresia or an anorectal anomaly, whereas urologic evaluation for associated renal abnormalities may be conducted by ultrasound in the early postoperative period. Some prioritization of the additional diagnostic tests is important to avoid delaying the operation. The importance of chromosome analysis as part of the prenatal diagnosis already has been discussed, but this rarely should interfere with the timing of surgery. In an emergency, rapid assessment of the chromosome status may be achieved by harvesting cells from the bone marrow. One instance in which operation may be delayed is to determine the chromosome status of a baby with an omphalocele and presumed trisomy 13 or 18. If this diagnosis is confirmed, we prefer nonoperative treatment by simply covering the omphalocele sac with allograft or amniotic membrane. The graft protects the sac and prevents rupture with evisceration, making surgery unnecessary in a patient with severe neurologic impairment and no hope for survival. On the other hand, an infant born with duodenal atresia and Down syndrome should undergo surgical correction. In unusual instances, a court order may be required to carry out the surgery at an opportune time.

## Informed Consent

Obtaining written operative consent simply is the final extension of preparation of the parents for their infant's surgery. Informed consent also should include a thorough understanding of the underlying condition, however, and the potential risks and benefits of the operation must be understood clearly by the parents before their signatures are obtained. Pertinent information should be given in each of the following categories: the diagnosis; the nature and purpose of the proposed treatment; the prognosis if the proposed treatment is carried out; the risks associated with the proposed treatment; the feasible treatment alternatives; and the prognosis if the treatment is refused. A written summary of what was told to the family by the surgeon also should be included on the operative consent and in the hospital record, both for further clarification and as an indication that these subjects were discussed if litigation ever is raised in the future.

## POSTOPERATIVE CARE

Certain general considerations and special issues regarding the postoperative care of the newborn should be emphasized (Table 20-10).

## General Considerations

The postoperative care of the newborn is largely a continuum of the many steps already described as part of the preoperative preparation. The surgeon summarizes these concerns in a list of steps known as the postoperative orders. Several important issues should be reemphasized.

Maintaining a normal core body temperature in the operating room is difficult because of the large skin surface area and the tendency for the viscera to be exposed to a cooler environment during an abdominal or thoracic operation. For that reason, it is imperative to return the infant to a servo-controlled Isolette or radiant warmer immediately after the procedure and to monitor core body temperature carefully. In most cases, a fluctuation of 1 to 2 °C can be reversed by rewarming within the first few hours after return to the newborn intensive care unit.

Some infants will require postoperative endotracheal ventilation until they are fully reactive and are sustaining a normal respiratory pattern. With appropriate weaning of the intermittent mandatory ventilation rate and inspired oxygen content, elective

---

**TABLE 20-10.   Postoperative Care of the Newborn**

**General Considerations**
Maintenance and replacement of intravenous fluids
Core body temperature
Ventilatory support
Vascular access
Antibiotic coverage
Nasogastric decompression
Pain control

**Special Issues**
Total parenteral nutrition
Extracorporeal membrane oxygenation
Stomal care
Family support
Discharge home

extubation is possible under controlled circumstances with the full staff available if the respiratory status falters. A preterm infant under 46 to 60 weeks' postconceptual age is at higher risk of having apnea and bradycardia after general anesthesia. This issue is particularly relevant after elective procedures such as inguinal herniorrhaphy in babies who have a history of previous mechanical ventilation, bronchopulmonary dysplasia, or a patent ductus arteriosus.

Adequate vascular access should be achieved before beginning the operative procedure. The position of the central venous line and the function of any peripheral line should be assessed again upon returning to the nursery. In most instances, a plain chest radiograph will provide information about the position of the tip of the endotracheal tube or a central venous catheter, the status of the lungs, and even the location of the nasogastric tube. If an umbilical venous or arterial catheter has been inserted, an abdominal film also should be obtained to ascertain the position of the tip of the catheter. Umbilical artery catheters should be positioned clearly above the level of the renal vessels superimposed on the T-11 and T-12 vertebrae, or just above the bifurcation of the aorta at the L2-3 level, but never at the presumed orifices of the renal or mesenteric arteries.

Appropriate antibiotic coverage should be continued for a minimum of 48 hours when any hollow viscus has been entered, or for as long as 2 weeks when established peritonitis or an intra-abdominal abscess is being treated. In high-risk patients, such as preterm infants requiring inguinal herniorrhaphy, our usual practice is to give a single dose of prophylactic antibiotics before commencing the operative procedure. In these patients, postoperative antibiotics are not required.

It is essential that adequate decompression of any hollow viscus that was entered during the course of the operative procedure be maintained. Paramount to this end is the use of nasogastric decompression for gastrointestinal surgery. The smallest catheter that is effective at preventing distention is an 8-French feeding tube. Smaller catheters are appropriate only for gavage feedings. Urinary tract drainage with a feeding catheter also may be indicated in selected instances, such as when hourly urinary output needs to be monitored or in cases in which bladder outlet obstruction is suspected. Bagging the perineum and performing a simple Credé's maneuver will enable the quantitation of total urinary output and determination of urine specific gravity.

Achieving adequate pain control has been a highly publicized, emotionally charged issue in the newborn. Pain-induced wincing and cries, splinted ventilation, and tachycardia all are recognized sequelae of inadequate pain control in babies who are undergoing major surgery. Morphine sulfate is, by far, the most effective analgesic and, given in small aliquots of .05 mg/kg in a carefully monitored patient, is both safe and desirable. Gradual weaning of the medication over 48 to 72 hours is possible.

## Special Issues

Achieving long-term venous access for the purpose of administering total parenteral nutrition, antibiotics, or blood and blood products has been a lifesaving measure in babies requiring major surgery. The majority of these patients have had multi-stage closure of omphalocele or gastroschisis, necrotizing enterocolitis with a proximal ileostomy, or short-gut syndrome after resection for mid-gut volvulus, intestinal atresia, or meconium ileus with meconium peritonitis. As indicated previously, a Broviac catheter can be placed in the operating room, or by the fourth or fifth postoperative day, when sepsis no longer is a contraindication. When parenteral nutrition is needed, the glucose concentration should be increased to provide a caloric intake over several days that is adequate to prevent glycosuria. In preterm infants with a low renal threshold for the tubular excretion of glucose, supplementary insulin may be required to prevent glycosuria. The success of total parenteral nutrition is judged by the observation of weight gain without catheter sepsis or metabolic complications.

Extracorporeal membrane oxygenation (ECMO) has progressed from a clinical research project to a recognized practice in the management of severe neonatal respiratory failure. By 1990, the Neonatal Extra-Corporeal Life Support Organization (ELSO) Registry (Ann Arbor, Michigan) reported a survival rate of more than 80% in 3000 babies treated in 64 centers. Indications included pulmonary immaturity, meconium aspiration syndrome, congenital diaphragmatic hernia, and persistent pulmonary hypertension, rather than pulmonary parenchymal disease. ECMO is achieved by cannulation of the carotid artery and jugular vein in the neck under local anesthesia in a specially dedicated area within the neonatal special care unit. A modified heart/lung machine (Fig 20-38) is used to take over part or all of cardiac and lung function for a period as long as 3 weeks, although the usual time on ECMO is 5 to 7 days. Vital to the success of this procedure is the experience and training of the ECMO team, which includes the pediatric surgeon, who supervises the procedure, with the assistance of the neonatologist, nurse, perfusionist, and respiratory therapist. Proper patient selection also increases the likelihood for success by excluding babies with severe bilateral pulmonary hypoplasia, intracranial hemorrhage, and structural cardiac defects; preterm infants below 34 weeks' gestation; and patients with irreversible lung disease, such as those with severe bronchopulmonary dysplasia.

Congenital diaphragmatic hernia in babies who have failed to respond to conventional mechanical ventilation and pharmacologic therapy for persistent fetal circulation remains the principal indication for ECMO in the postoperative patient. The potential for eventual survival after repair generally is heralded by a "honeymoon period," during which time reasonably normal oxygenation can be achieved. Extended use of hyperventilation and pulmonary arterial vasodilators, such as tolazoline, tends to aggravate underlying pulmonary disease by introducing an element of barotrauma. This factor is believed to be of such importance that trials of both preoperative and intraoperative ECMO are anticipated. Even the referral pattern of the baby with a congenital diaphragmatic hernia is being influenced by most perinatologists, who are reluctant to refer mothers for delivery to a hospital that does not have an experienced ECMO center.

Creation of an intestinal stoma is necessary in most babies with necrotizing enterocolitis or Hirschsprung's disease, and in selected patients with meconium ileus and anorectal anomalies. A centrally located, "matured" single stoma, to a large extent, will ease postoperative care. When the stoma begins to function by evacuating liquid meconium, effluent is captured with a collecting bag. Occasionally, the functional stoma will be accompanied by a second, more distal, stoma known as a mucus fistula. The stomas should be separated sufficiently to prevent spillover of intestinal contents. A Xeroform or petroleum jelly dressing of the second stoma is more than sufficient to prevent mucosal ulceration and bleeding. In almost all patients, except those with Hirschsprung's disease or anorectal malformations, intestinal tract continuity is restored before they are discharged from the unit. Several weeks may pass, however, during which time, adequate weight gain is achieved by a combination of parenteral and oral nutrition. Non-nutritive feedings of small aliquots of an elemental diet may minimize the risk of cholestatic jaundice and the subsequent development of sludge or calculi in the biliary tract. When a preterm baby reaches the approximate weight of 2.0 kg, contrast studies of the unused (distal) portion of the gastrointestinal tract are indicated, via either the rectum or the mucus fistula, to rule out the presence of an intrinsic obstruction or stricture. Then,

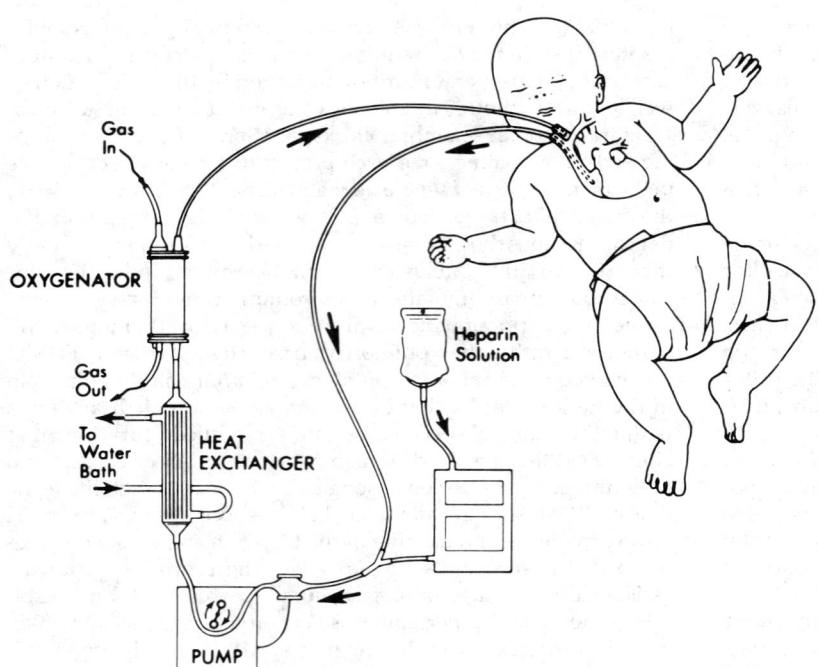

**Figure 20-38.** Extracorporeal membrane oxygenation (ECMO) perfusion system. (Krummel TM, Greenfield LJ, Kirkpatrick, BV, et al. J Pediatr Surg 1982;17:526.)

reconstitution of the gastrointestinal tract can be carried out and the risk of intercurrent salt and water imbalance from diarrheal illness largely will be avoided. Bile–acid diarrhea continues to be a problem in certain patients, even after the stomas have been closed. Cholestyramine, a bile salt resin that prevents choleretic enteropathy, and Pepto-Bismol both have been used successfully in our nursery to prevent this complication.

Perhaps the single most important role of the surgeon in the postoperative period lies in dealing with the family's anxiety and providing emotional support. Although much of this duty is shared naturally by the neonatologist, primary nurse, and social worker, the surgeon who performed the operative procedure needs to remain in close, even daily, contact with the family, and to explain clearly the steps and measures that are being employed in the recovery period. Because untimely events and even reoperation are common, early discussions of any trend are important to prepare the patient's family appropriately. The day of discharge home is one of great celebration for both the natural and the extended family of a baby who has required prolonged hospitalization in the newborn special care unit.

## Selected Readings

Barlow B, Santulli TV, Heird WC, Pitt J, Blanc WA, Schullinger JN. An experimental study of acute neonatal enterocolitis—the importance of breast milk. J Pediatr Surg 1974;9:587.

Bartlett RH, Toomasian J, Roloff D, et al. Extracorporeal membrane oxygenation (ECMO) in neonatal respiratory failure. Ann Surg 1986;204:236.

Bethel CAI, Seashore JH, Touloukian RJ. Cesarean section does not improve outcome in gastroschisis. J Pediatr Surg 1989;24:1.

Chervenak FA, Isaacson G, Touloukian RJ, Tortora M, Berkowitz RL, Hobbins JC. Diagnosis and management of fetal teratomas. Obstet Gynecol 1985;66:666.

Dudrick SJ, Wilmore DW, Vars HM, et al. Long-term parenteral nutrition with growth development and positive nitrogen balance. Surgery 1968;64:134.

Fonkalsrud EW. Pediatric surgery—a specialty come of age. J Pediatr Surg 1991;26:239.

Gertler JP, Seashore JH, Touloukian RJ. Early ileostomy closure in necrotizing enterocolitis. J Pediatr Surg 1987;22:140.

Gollin G, Bell C, Dubose R, et al. Predictors of postoperative respiratory complications in premature infants and inguinal herniorrhaphy. J Pediatr Surg, 1993;28:244.

Harrison MR, Golbus MS, Filly RA. The unborn patient. Management of the fetus with a correctable defect. San Diego: Grune & Stratton, 1984.

Pletcher BA, Friedes JS, Breg WR, Touloukian RJ. Familial occurrence of esophageal atresia with and without tracheoesophageal fistula; report of two unusual kindred. Am J Med Genet 1991;39:380.

Quan L, Smith DW. The VATER association. Vertebral defects, anal atresia, TE fistula with esophageal atresia, radial and renal dysplasia. J Pediatr 1973;83:104.

Touloukian RJ, Hobbins J. Maternal ultrasound in the antenatal diagnosis of surgically correctable fetal abnormalities. J Pediatr Surg 1980;15:373.

Touloukian RJ, Keller MS. High proximal pouch esophageal atresia with vertebral, rib, and sternal anomalies; an additional component of the VATER association. J Pediatr Surg 1988;23:76.

Touloukian RJ, Markowitz RI. A preoperative x-ray scoring system for risk assessment of newborns with congenital diaphragmatic hernia. J Pediatr Surg 1984;19:252.

Touloukian RJ, Weiss RM. The obstructed bladder syndrome in the neonate. Surg Gynecol Obstet 1976;143:965.

*Principles and Practice of Pediatrics, Second Edition.*
edited by Frank A. Oski et al. J. B. Lippincott Company, Philadelphia © 1994.

## 20.2.12 *Bronchopulmonary Dysplasia*

Kathleen A. Kennedy and Joseph B. Warshaw

Most neonates with acute lung disease recover completely within the first week of life. Some of these infants, however, have chronic respiratory disease characterized by tachypnea, dyspnea, hypoxemia, and hypercarbia. In 1967, Northway and colleagues first described the clinical, radiologic, and pathologic manifestations of chronic lung disease in survivors of hyaline membrane disease (HMD) and introduced the term *bronchopulmonary dysplasia* (BPD). These authors postulated that the disease was caused by oxygen toxicity and ventilator-induced barotrauma superimposed on the healing infant lung. In 1977, Edwards and associates reported a 21% incidence of BPD in infants ventilated for HMD. They identified an inverse relationship between gestational age and the incidence of BPD. As neonatal intensive care has become more sophisticated over the past 3 decades, the survival of infants with very low birth weights has increased dramatically. Although the birth-weight–specific incidence of BPD seems to have remained fairly stable with increasing survival rates, the result of this increased survival still is an increase in the absolute numbers of survivors with BPD. The impact of BPD is difficult to determine, because the incidence varies according to the definition used and the population studied. In a retrospective study of 1625 infants with birth weights between 700 and 1500 g who were treated in eight major medical centers from 1982 through 1984, chronic lung disease of prematurity was defined as an oxygen requirement greater than room air at 28 days of age, and the incidence of chronic lung disease in this population ranged from 6% to 33% in the different medical centers. Within the entire study population, lower birth weight, white race, and male sex were identified as risk factors for the development of chronic lung disease, but differences in patient populations did not account fully for the discrepancies in the incidence of chronic lung disease among the different medical centers. Although these observations suggest that certain aspects of patient management may alter the risk for chronic lung disease, no single cause or preventive measure is likely to be identified for this complex disease process.

## ETIOLOGY AND PATHOPHYSIOLOGY

Oxygen toxicity and barotrauma have been implicated frequently in the pathogenesis of BPD, but it is very difficult to isolate these factors from the pulmonary immaturity and acute lung injury for which these treatment modalities are used. Although BPD initially was described as a complication of HMD, chronic lung disease has become a significant problem in very premature infants with mild acute lung disease. Conversely, full-term infants who require aggressive oxygen and ventilator therapy for meconium aspiration, congenital pneumonia, or persistent pulmonary hypertension infrequently have chronic lung disease. Pulmonary air leak, pulmonary edema, patent ductus arteriosus, acquired pneumonia, and poor nutrition also are risk factors for the development of chronic lung disease, but these all are complications of acute lung injury in premature infants and their causal role in the pathogenesis of BPD is difficult to establish. For a variety of reasons, the premature lung seems to have an increased susceptibility to iatrogenic lung injury or a decreased capacity to undergo a normal healing process when lung injury occurs. Genetic factors predisposing BPD to develop in an infant are suggested by an increased incidence of asthma in first-degree relatives of infants with BPD.

Pulmonary edema and alveolar necrosis develop within 2 to 3 days in healthy mammals exposed to normobaric hyperoxia. This acute injury is followed by a chronic phase that is pathologically similar to BPD and is characterized by interstitial fibrosis with proliferation of alveolar type II cells and fibroblasts. The causal role of oxygen toxicity is supported best by the contribution of oxygen toxicity to BPD in the primate animal model of BPD. Term neonatal animals of some species are more resistant than are adults of the species to pulmonary oxygen toxicity. Protection from the toxic effects of oxygen seems to be related to the ability to prevent or repair cellular damage caused by oxygen free radicals. A variety of enzymatic and nonenzymatic antioxidants are involved in this protection, and the premature neonate may be relatively deficient in some of these antioxidants.

There is very little information available about antioxidant enzyme activity in the human neonatal lung. Several studies have suggested that the premature neonate with HMD may be deficient in superoxide dismutase, an enzyme that catalyzes the dismutation of the superoxide free radical. It is not known whether deficiencies of this and other antioxidant enzymes predispose an infant to the development of BPD, and there are no clinically feasible means by which to increase the intracellular levels of antioxidant enzymes in the human lung.

Vitamins A and E are nonenzymatic antioxidants that prevent free radical propagation in cell membranes. Although vitamin E deficiency exacerbates pulmonary oxygen toxicity in laboratory animals, pharmacologic doses of vitamin E do not afford additional protection in non-deficient animals or humans. Neonates have low vitamin E stores at birth and are at risk for deficiency if vitamin E is not provided enterally or parenterally. Premature neonates of less than 36 weeks' gestation also have low plasma concentrations and tissue stores of vitamin A. Vitamin A deficiency in laboratory animals results in necrosis of the tracheobronchial epithelium, with subsequent squamous metaplasia that is similar to the pathologic lesion seen in infants with BPD. Supplementation with intramuscular vitamin A to decrease the risk for the development of BPD has been studied in two groups of highly susceptible infants of very low birth weight. The results of these studies were conflicting; no conclusions can be drawn about the efficacy of vitamin A at this time. The intravenous administration of vitamin A is less efficient, and the optimal dosage and mode of administration have not been established.

Deficiencies of sulfur-containing amino acids and trace minerals such as selenium increase the susceptibility to oxygen-induced lung injury in animals. Such deficiencies are unlikely to occur in infants who are receiving formulas that are standard for preterm infants. Less is known about the optimal amounts of amino acids and trace minerals that should be supplied in parenteral nutrition solutions. Despite evidence from animal studies that pulmonary oxygen toxicity could be ameliorated by polyunsaturated fatty acid supplementation, preliminary studies in preterm human infants have shown no benefit.

A causal role of barotrauma in the pathogenesis of BPD is supported by the following observations. BPD was seen rarely before positive-pressure ventilators came into use, and some infants have BPD after receiving ventilator therapy with low oxygen concentrations. The acute manifestations of barotrauma, pulmonary interstitial emphysema, and pneumothorax are frequent precursors of chronic lung disease. Many investigators have attempted to reduce the severity of barotrauma by making alterations in the use of conventional mechanical ventilators to reduce peak airway pressure. There have been no large published trials in which a clear benefit was demonstrated for a particular style of conventional mechanical ventilation. In the national collaborative trial of high-frequency oscillatory ventilation compared with conventional ventilation for the treatment of respiratory failure in low–birth-weight infants, there was no difference between the study groups in the incidence of BPD.

A primary causal role for infection in the pathogenesis of BPD has not been established, but is suggested by the increased incidence of BPD in infants who are colonized with *Ureaplasma* at the time of birth. Whether early antibiotic treatment of this organism would be beneficial has yet to be established. Inflammation is a characteristic finding in the pathology of BPD, and inflammatory mediators have been implicated in the reactive airway disease and pulmonary hypertension that is associated with BPD. Inflammatory mediators, such as eicosanoids and platelet activating factor, have been found in high concentrations in lung lavage fluid from infants with BPD. Whether this inflammatory response results from infection, oxidant injury, or barotrauma as the primary insult, inflammation may exacerbate the primary lung injury and lead to more severe or prolonged lung damage.

## DIAGNOSIS

The diagnosis of BPD is suspected when a neonate with acute lung disease fails to follow the anticipated course of resolution or has a gradual increase in oxygen and ventilator requirements during the first month of life. In 1979, Bancalari characterized the disease as tachypnea, retractions, and supplemental oxygen requirement for more than 28 days in infants who had received positive-pressure ventilation for at least 3 days in the first week of life. Associated chest radiograph findings included strand-like densities in both lung fields alternating with areas of normal or increased lucency. The diagnosis must be made on the basis of both clinical and radiographic characteristics. There are no specific tests that can be used to confirm the diagnosis. The distinction between unresolved acute lung disease and chronic lung disease at 28 days of age is an arbitrary one, based in part on the likelihood that pulmonary dysfunction that persists for at least 4 weeks will be associated with increased long-term morbidity and mortality. The distinction can be problematic when considering therapeutic modalities begun at 1 to 3 weeks of age in infants with pulmonary dysfunction or when classifying deaths from respiratory failure at 1 to 4 weeks of age. More recently, a more stringent diagnostic criterion, oxygen therapy at 36 weeks' corrected postnatal gestational age, has been recommended. This recommendation was based on the observation that this definition is a more specific predictor of long-term pulmonary morbidity.

Two other forms of chronic lung disease in premature infants have been described. Wilson-Mikity syndrome and chronic pulmonary insufficiency of prematurity were described in 1960 and 1975, respectively, as consisting of progressive tachypnea, hypoxemia, and apnea in premature infants who have very mild or no lung disease in the first week of life. The radiographic findings of Wilson-Mikity syndrome are not unlike those of BPD. Neither of these syndromes has a specific etiology, and the clinical course in the first week of life is the main feature distinguishing infants with these syndromes from infants with BPD. This distinction may be somewhat arbitrary. These syndromes may represent different clinical presentations in a spectrum of chronic lung disease related to prematurity, with the clinical manifestations depending on the relative contributions of the various etiologic factors mentioned above.

Cystic fibrosis and $\alpha_1$-antitrypsin deficiency rarely cause pulmonary symptoms in the first weeks of life. Neonates with these genetic disorders who also have acute lung injury subsequently may experience slowly progressive chronic lung disease. Sweat chloride analysis, genetic screening, or determination of serum $\alpha_1$-antitrypsin levels is required to distinguish these disorders from BPD.

Patent ductus arteriosus commonly presents during the resolution stage of HMD in very premature infants. Similar to BPD, increased pulmonary blood flow from a patent ductus can cause prolonged oxygen and ventilator requirements during the healing phase of acute lung disease. The diagnosis and hemodynamic significance of a patent ductus arteriosus usually can be determined by physical examination and echocardiography.

Viral pneumonia acquired in the early neonatal period can cause progressive hypoxemia and respiratory failure. The diagnosis can be confirmed with nasopharyngeal viral cultures or urine culture for cytomegalovirus.

## COMPLICATIONS

Pulmonary hypertension and cor pulmonale can result from many forms of chronic lung disease, including BPD. Mortality is very high in infants with severe BPD and cor pulmonale, so therapeutic endeavors should be directed toward preventing the development of cor pulmonale. Pulmonary arterial pressure can be decreased by increased oxygen administration in infants with BPD.

Infants with BPD have an increased susceptibility to severe bacterial and viral pneumonia. In the first year after hospital

discharge, many infants with BPD are readmitted for pulmonary exacerbations. Respiratory syncytial virus and pertussis infections can be fatal in infants with BPD.

Congestive heart failure with pulmonary and systemic venous congestion frequently complicates the treatment of infants with BPD. The etiology of left heart failure in infants with BPD is uncertain. Fluid tolerance varies greatly and must be determined on an individual basis.

## PREVENTION

The management of acute lung disease in premature infants should be directed toward the prevention of BPD. As discussed above, BPD results from the complex interaction of many factors. Limited exposure to mechanical ventilation and oxygen therapy, judicious fluid administration, prompt management of the patent ductus arteriosus, and attention to optimal nutrition may reduce the risk of BPD in susceptible infants.

Because BPD originally was described as a complication of severe HMD, it was anticipated that surfactant replacement therapy to prevent or treat HMD would reduce dramatically the incidence of BPD. A number of large, multicenter, placebo-controlled surfactant trials have been published. Although most of the large trials have demonstrated a decrease in mortality with surfactant therapy, the incidence of BPD in the survivors generally has not been affected by the administration of surfactant. One explanation for this seemingly disappointing finding is that surfactant deficiency is only one of multiple factors involved in the pathogenesis of BPD, and it may be relatively less important in infants with extremely low birth weights than in the cohort with greater birth weights that was described in 1967. Another explanation is that the observed increase in survivors without BPD was matched by an increase in the number who would have succumbed, but survived with BPD as a result of surfactant treatment. This resulted in no change in the incidence of BPD among survivors, despite a significant increase in the number of infants who survived without BPD.

Short-term steroid treatment has been shown to be beneficial for ventilator-dependent infants at 3 to 6 weeks of age. Although there is evidence for short-term improvement in lung function resulting in reduced duration of assisted ventilation, the long-term benefits are less clear, and there are serious risks associated with steroid therapy. The optimal timing and duration of steroid therapy remain to be established. This form of therapy might be viewed as either prevention or treatment, depending on the accepted definition of BPD.

## MANAGEMENT

Although exposure to high concentrations of oxygen is thought to be a contributing factor in the pathogenesis of BPD, chronic administration of oxygen is one of the most important aspects in the management of chronic lung disease in infants. Maintaining a $PaO_2$ greater than 60 mm Hg or an $O_2$ saturation greater than 90% should reduce the risk of cor pulmonale from chronic hypoxemia. Many infants have decreased oxygenation during sleep and feedings, and may require additional oxygen therapy during these times.

Pulmonary and systemic edema develop in many infants with BPD when excessive parenteral fluid is administered, and chronic fluid restriction has become almost routine in the management of BPD in these patients. Because respiratory infection or hypoxemia predispose the infants to pulmonary edema, isolated episodes of pulmonary edema do not necessarily warrant chronic restriction of enteral fluid intake. Fluid given enterally generally is tolerated better than fluid given parenterally. This observation suggests that passive absorption of fluid from the gastrointestinal tract is controlled by osmotic forces. Modest fluid (140 to 160 mL/kg/d) and sodium (2 to 3 mEq/kg/d) restriction may decrease oxygen requirements and respiratory work in these infants. Severe fluid restriction at the expense of adequate nutrition is not indicated.

Although diuretic therapy is used commonly in infants with BPD, the diuretic and non-diuretic cardiopulmonary effects of chronic diuretic therapy in these infants have not been explored fully. Diuretic therapy may allow for increased fluid administration, and diuretic agents have been shown to improve pulmonary mechanics in infants with BPD. The efficacy of furosemide versus thiazide diuretics in infants with BPD is unknown, and careful attention must be given to electrolyte balance when diuretics are used in these infants. Replacement of potassium and chloride may be necessary to prevent metabolic alkalosis and hypoventilation during diuretic therapy. Sodium supplementation enhances fluid retention and defeats the purpose of diuretic therapy. Many infants with BPD also are at risk for osteopenia of prematurity, and thiazide diuretics may have the advantage of decreasing urinary calcium excretion.

Infants with BPD have increased airway resistance and increased work of breathing compared to age-matched control infants. Some of these infants have bronchial hyperreactivity that responds favorably to bronchodilator therapy with theophylline or β-adrenergic agonists. Response to bronchodilator therapy has been demonstrated in infants as young as 2 weeks' postnatal age.

Adequate nutrition is necessary for lung growth and repair, but meeting nutritional needs often is a challenge in infants with BPD. Infants with BPD have tachypnea and increased respiratory effort, and they may require more calories for adequate growth than do infants without respiratory disease. The caloric needs of an individual infant should be determined by the intake required to achieve a sustained weight gain of at least 10 g/kg/d. Some infants may require as much as 150 kcal/kg/d. If oral or nasogastric feedings are not tolerated, prolonged peripheral parenteral nutrition rarely provides adequate calories and central total parenteral nutrition should be considered. Supplemented formulas can be used to increase caloric intake in infants who cannot tolerate increased feeding volumes because of congestive heart failure or gastroesophageal reflux. If standard infant formulas or those for premature infants are supplemented with carbohydrate or fat to increase the caloric density, adequate intake of protein and trace minerals should not be compromised.

Respiratory infections should be prevented, if possible, by avoiding exposure of the infant to other patients, hospital personnel, and family members with viral symptoms. When viral respiratory infections occur in infants with BPD, requirements for oxygen, bronchodilator therapy, and diuretics often are increased for at least 1 week. If respiratory failure develops, requiring the reinstitution of ventilator therapy, the mortality is high and recovery may be very prolonged.

## PROGNOSIS

The mortality rate was very high (19 of 32 patients) in the initial cohort of infants with BPD described by Northway in 1967. Most deaths in infants with BPD are a consequence of cor pulmonale or respiratory infection, but these infants also have an increased incidence of sudden unexplained death after discharge from the hospital. There has been a reduction in the mortality over the past 20 years, but both morbidity and mortality remain high. In a study of 179 infants with BPD born between 1975 and 1982, the pre-discharge mortality rate was 14%. Those infants who survived until discharge from the hospital had a post-discharge

death rate of 11%. Survivors had an increased incidence of neurodevelopmental abnormalities, visual and hearing deficits, and rehospitalization for respiratory illness in the first year of life when compared to premature infants without BPD. Pulmonary function improves over the first several years of life in infants with BPD, and most survivors have normal exercise tolerance by school age. With formal pulmonary function testing, however, some evidence of increased airway reactivity persists into early adulthood.

With carefully monitored long-term oxygen therapy to reduce the risk of cor pulmonale and aggressive management of respiratory infections, the prognosis for infants with BPD may continue to improve. The long-term outlook for infants in whom BPD currently develops is impossible to determine. Encouraging information about 20-year-old survivors of HMD who had a different disease spectrum may not apply to the infants treated today.

## Selected Readings

Abman SH, Wolfe RR, Accurso FJ, Koops BL, Bowman M, Wiggins JW. Pulmonary vascular response to oxygen in infants with severe bronchopulmonary dysplasia. Pediatrics 1985;75:80.

Avery ME, Tooley WH, Keller JB, et al. Is chronic lung disease in low birth weight infants preventable? A survey of eight centers. Pediatrics 1987;79:26.

Bancalari E, Abdenour GE, Feller R, Gannon J. Bronchopulmonary dysplasia: clinical presentation. J Pediatr 1979;95:819.

Collaborative Dexamethasone Trial Group. Dexamethasone therapy in neonatal chronic lung disease: An international placebo-controlled trial. Pediatrics 1991;88:421.

Davis JM, Sinkin RA, Aranda JV. Drug therapy for bronchopulmonary dysplasia. Pediatr Pulmonol 1990;8:117.

DeLemos RA, Coalson JJ, Gerstmann DR, Kuehl TJ, Null DM. Oxygen toxicity in the premature baboon with hyaline membrane disease. Am Rev Respir Dis 1987;136:677.

Edwards DK, Dyer WM, Northway WH Jr. Twelve years' experience with bronchopulmonary dysplasia. Pediatrics 1977;59:839.

Ehrenkranz RA, Ablow R, Warshaw JB. Effect of vitamin E on the development of oxygen-induced lung injury in neonates. Ann N Y Acad Sci 1982;393:452.

Engelhardt B, Elliott S, Hazinski TA. Short- and long-term effects of furosemide on lung function in infants with bronchopulmonary dysplasia. J Pediatr 1986;109:1034.

Escobedo MB, Gonzalez A. Bronchopulmonary dysplasia in the tiny infant. Clin Perinatol 1986;13:315.

Frank L, Sosenko IRS. Prenatal development of lung antioxidant enzymes in four species. J Pediatr 1987;110:106.

The HiFi Study Group. High frequency oscillatory ventilation compared with conventional mechanical ventilation in the treatment of respiratory failure in preterm infants. N Engl J Med 1989;320:88.

Kao LC, Durand DJ, Phillips BL, Nickerson BG. Oral theophylline and diuretics improve pulmonary mechanics in infants with bronchopulmonary dysplasia. J Pediatr 1987;111:439.

Monin P, Vert P. The management of bronchopulmonary dysplasia. Clin Perinatol 1987;14:531.

Motoyama EK, Fort MD, Klesh KW, Mutich RL, Guthrie RD. Early onset of airway reactivity in premature infants with bronchopulmonary dysplasia. Am Rev Respir Dis 1987;136:50.

Nickerson BG, Taussig LM. Family history of asthma in infants with bronchopulmonary dysplasia. Pediatrics 1980;65:1140.

Northway WH, Moss RB, Carlisle KB, et al. Late pulmonary sequelae of bronchopulmonary dysplasia. N Engl J Med 1990;323:1793.

O'Brodovich HM, Mellins RB. Bronchopulmonary dysplasia: Unresolved neonatal acute lung injury. Am Rev Respir Dis 1985;132:694.

Rush MG, Hazinski TA. Current therapy of bronchopulmonary dysplasia. Clin Perinatol 1992;19:563.

Sanchez PJ, Regan JA. Ureaplasma urealyticum colonization and chronic lung disease in low birth weight infants. Pediatr Infect Dis J 1988;7:542.

Shenai JP, Kennedy KA, Chytil F, Stahlman MT. Clinical trial of vitamin A supplementation in infants susceptible to bronchopulmonary dysplasia. J Pediatr 1987;111:269.

Shennan AT, Dunn MS, Ohlsson A, Lennox K, Hoskins EM. Abnormal pulmonary outcomes in premature infants: Prediction from oxygen requirement in the neonatal period. Pediatrics 1988;82:527.

Sosenko IRS, Innis SM, Frank L. Polyunsaturated fatty acids and protection of newborn rats from oxygen toxicity. J Pediatr 1988;112:630.

Stenmark KR, Eyzaguirre M, Wescott JY, Henson PM, Murphy RC. Potential role of eicosanoids and PAF in the pathophysiology of bronchopulmonary dysplasia. Am Rev Respir Dis 1987;136:770.

Suave RS, Singhal N. Long-term morbidity of infants with bronchopulmonary dysplasia. Pediatrics 1985;76:725.

Weinstein MR, Oh W. Oxygen consumption in infants with bronchopulmonary dysplasia. J Pediatr 1981;99:958.

Yee WFH, Scarpelli EM. Surfactant replacement therapy. Pediatr Pulmonol 1991;11:65.

*Principles and Practice of Pediatrics, Second Edition.*
edited by Frank A. Oski et al. J. B. Lippincott Company, Philadelphia © 1994.

# 20.3 *Cardiovascular Diseases*

## 20.3.1 *Epidemiology of Congenital Heart Disease*

David E. Fixler and Norman S. Talner

Congenital heart disease (CHD) is a leading cause of death during the first year of life. Malformations of the heart occur in about 8:1000 liveborn infants, resulting in up to 36,000 cases per year in the United States. Children with CHD use between 25% and 30% of the beds in most pediatric intensive care units and, therefore, consume a large fraction of pediatric health care resources. Because the majority of severe cases now are being managed successfully by surgery, most of these patients are surviving into their reproductive years. Recent studies have shown that the off-spring of women with CHD are at much greater risk of having cardiac malformations. In the next decade, the prevalence of CHD may increase as a result of longer survival and the increase in incidence of heart defects in the offspring of survivors. Pediatric health care providers need to be informed of the incidence of CHD, the familial risk of CHD recurrence, and risk factors for CHD.

## INCIDENCE OF CONGENITAL HEART DISEASE

The incidence of CHD is the ratio of the number of cases to the number of births in a defined population. Estimating the incidence accurately requires precise diagnostic criteria for the identification of cases and complete ascertainment of all cases. Diagnostic criteria may include mild cases recognized solely by physical examination or be restricted to more severe forms diagnosed by cardiac catheterization, surgery, or autopsy. Many types of CHD are not diagnosed until after the neonatal period; therefore, the incidence rate is affected by the length of the period of observation. In the prospective study by Hoffman and Christianson, data are provided regarding the incidence of CHD at various age intervals (Table 20-11). These data indicate that fewer than half of the cases were identified during the first week of life.

The reported incidence of CHD in the United States varies

**TABLE 20-11. Cumulative Incidence of Congenital Heart Disease per 1000 Liveborn Children**

| Age Interval | Cumulative Incidence |
|---|---|
| Birth | 3.3/1000 |
| 1–6 d | 4.0/1000 |
| 7–31 d | 5.2/1000 |
| 1–5 mo | 7.3/1000 |
| 6–11 mo | 7.8/1000 |
| 1–2 y | 8.3/1000 |
| >2–3 y | 8.7/1000 |
| >3–6 y | 9.1/1000 |

from study to study because of differences in diagnostic criteria, methods of diagnosis, and completeness and length of follow-up (Table 20-12). Important discrepancies among these studies are noted that account for the large differences in reported incidence rates. The incidence of CHD among autopsied stillborn infants is 76.9:1000, which is nearly ten times higher than the rate found in liveborn infants. If stillbirths are included in the incidence figures, the rate increases by about 0.5:1000. The incidence figure also is influenced by the inclusion of infants born prematurely who have patent ductus arteriosus. Such patients were excluded in most of the recent studies listed in Table 20-12. Which incidence figure is most correct depends on how the data are to be used. For example, in estimating regional costs of inpatient services, use of the incidence rates for severe CHD might be most appropriate. In examining the association of heart disease with specific environmental exposures during pregnancy, however, the inclusion of mild cases might be more appropriate.

## PREVALENCE OF SPECIFIC TYPES OF CONGENITAL HEART DISEASE

The frequency of occurrence of various types of CHD among liveborn infants is shown in Table 20-13. This is a compilation of seven international studies, and is based on 3104 patients with CHD. These studies included both mild and severe forms of heart disease. Diagnoses of bicuspid aortic valve, patent ductus arteriosus in premature infants, and mitral valve prolapse were excluded, however. Isolated ventricular septal defects are by far the most common type of CHD noted, accounting for at least 30% of all congenital heart defects. Other lesions diagnosed frequently include patent ductus arteriosus, atrial septal defect, pulmonic and aortic stenosis, coarctation of the aorta, tetralogy of Fallot, and transposition of the great arteries. These eight lesions account for about 75% of the defects. Bicuspid aortic valve has been reported to occur in about 1% of adult hearts examined at autopsy. Although this is more common than any other type of congenital cardiac defect, it is diagnosed infrequently during life.

## FAMILIAL RISK OF RECURRENCE OF CONGENITAL HEART DISEASE

After the diagnosis of CHD has been made, parents want to know the chance of recurrence. In some cases, the affected offspring exhibits manifestations of a recognizable syndrome that has specific known genetic risks. CHD in about 8% of children may be explained on the basis of a primary genetic defect. In the majority of cases, however, a specific genetic defect is not recognized. It has been postulated that genetic predisposition interacting with an environmental trigger causes the cardiovascular malformation. In families having a child with CHD, the genetic predisposition already has been expressed, and subsequent pregnancies are associated with a higher risk of cardiac maldevelopment. The recurrence risk when one offspring has been born with CHD varies with the specific lesion, as shown in Table 20-14. Ranges of risk in the table are listed to indicate differences among studies. When a second case does occur, the infant frequently has a form of CHD that differs from that of the first child. It often is useful to present the information in a positive fashion; for example, in a family having a child with an atrial septal defect, the likelihood of the next infant having a normal heart is about 97%.

Over the past decade, more information has become available regarding the risk that a parent with a congenital heart defect will have a child with a heart defect (Table 20-15). The risk of recurrence is greater when the heart disease is in the mother.

TABLE 20-12.  Major U.S. Surveys of Congenital Heart Disease (CHD)

| Period | Population | Study Design | CHD Numbers | Incidence/1000 Liveborn |
|---|---|---|---|---|
| 1956–65 | 12 clinical* centers | Follow-up 1 mo to 9 y Mild and severe cases | 420 | 7.7 |
| 1959–66 | San Francisco† Kaiser Health Plan | Follow-up 5–13 y Mild and severe cases | 163 | 8.8 |
| 1969–77 | New England‡ | Follow-up 1 y Severe cases only, diagnosed by catheterization, surgery, or autopsy | 4065 | 2.4 |
| 1981–7 | Baltimore-Washington, DC§ | Follow-up 1 y Cases diagnosed by echocardiography, catheterization, surgery, or autopsy | 2659 | 4.3 |
| 1971–84 | Dallas County‖ | Follow-up 2–13 y Mild and severe cases | 2481 | 6.5 |

\* See Selected Readings: Mitchell et al, 1971.
† See Selected Readings: Hoffman and Christianson, 1978.
‡ See Selected Readings: Fyler, 1980.
§ See Selected Readings: Ferencz et al., 1991.
‖ See Selected Readings: Fixler et al, 1990.

Estimating the risk for mothers with cyanotic CHD is confounded by their higher rates of spontaneous abortion and interrupted pregnancy. Ranges of risk are shown in Table 20-15 because important discrepancies are found among different studies. Because it has not been feasible for any center to follow all patients with CHD through childbearing age, sampling biases may have occurred that result in underestimates or overestimates of risk. In addition, recent studies have reported higher risks of recurrence than those previously reported for families having left-heart obstructive lesions such as coarctation, aortic stenosis, and hypoplastic left-heart syndrome.

## PRENATAL RISK FACTORS FOR CONGENITAL HEART DISEASE

The embryo is most vulnerable to cardiopathic events during the developmental period from 20 to 45 days postconception. It is possible, however, for exposure before the 20th day to alter subsequent cardiac development. Likewise, it is possible for an agent introduced later in gestation to affect fetal or postnatal development—one example being rubella infection in the second or third trimester causing persistent patency of the ductus arteriosus. It has been difficult to establish associations between specific prenatal drug usage and particular cardiac defects. A major factor that interferes with the identification of specific cardiac teratogens is the low proportion of women taking any given drug and the low incidence of an individual cardiac defect (ie, the difficulty of detecting an increase in the risk of a rare occurrence). Several of the cardiac teratogens have been identified because exposure to them resulted in a high frequency of congenital heart malformations (Table 20-16).

In 1942, an ophthalmologist first reported clustering of anom-

TABLE 20-13.  Frequency of Specific Defects in Live Births With Congenital Heart Disease

| Lesion | Percent |
|---|---|
| Ventricular septal defect | 30.3 |
| Patent ductus arteriosus (full-term) | 8.6 |
| Pulmonary stenosis | 7.4 |
| Atrial septal defect (secundum) | 6.7 |
| Aortic coarctation | 5.7 |
| Aortic stenosis | 5.2 |
| Tetralogy of Fallot | 5.1 |
| Transposition | 4.7 |
| Endocardial cushion defects | 3.2 |
| Hypoplastic right heart | 2.2 |
| Hypoplastic left heart | 1.3 |
| Total anomalous pulmonary veins | 1.1 |
| Truncus arteriosus | 1.0 |

TABLE 20-14.  Estimated Risk of Congenital Heart Disease (CHD) Recurrence: One Offspring With CHD

| Lesion | Recurrence Risk (%) |
|---|---|
| Ventricular septal defect | 3–6 |
| Patent ductus arteriosus | 3–8 |
| Atrial septal defect | 3 |
| Tetralogy of Fallot | 3 |
| Pulmonic stenosis | 2–9 |
| Coarctation | 2–8 |
| Aortic stenosis | 2 |
| Transposition | 2 |
| Endocardial cushion defect | 2 |
| Endocardial fibroelastosis | 4 |
| Tricuspid atresia | 1 |
| Hypoplastic left heart | 2–10 |
| Truncus arteriosus | 1 |
| Ebstein's malformation | 1 |

TABLE 20-15. Estimated Risk of Occurrence in Offspring: Parent With Congenital Heart Disease (CHD)

| Lesion | CHD in Father (%) | CHD in Mother (%) |
|---|---|---|
| Aortic stenosis | 3–8 | 13–18 |
| Atrial septal defect | 1–7 | 4–14 |
| Atrioventricular canal | 1 | 14 |
| Coarctation | 2–8 | 4–6 |
| Patent ductus arteriosus | 2.5 | 4–9 |
| Pulmonic stenosis | 2 | 6–15 |
| Tetralogy of Fallot | 1.5 | 2.5 |
| Ventricular septal defect | 2 | 6–17 |

alies consisting of congenital cataracts, deafness, and heart disease associated with maternal rubella infection during pregnancy. Since then, the cardiac defects associated with the rubella syndrome have been described well, and consist of patent ductus arteriosus, pulmonary arterial stenosis, and myocarditis. In a study of 1275 infants with congenital rubella syndrome, the incidence of CHD was 48%. Since the initiation of rubella immunization in children in late infancy and in women of childbearing age, the impact of the rubella virus in causing CHD has been nearly eliminated. With public acceptance of vaccination being reduced in recent years, however, the rubella virus remains a potential public health risk.

Maternal alcohol ingestion during pregnancy has been associated with a cluster of cardiac anomalies, consisting primarily of ventricular septal defects and atrial septal defects. About 42% of children with the fetal alcohol syndrome have some form of CHD. From a compilation of 11 exposure studies, the risk of

CHD from maternal alcoholism was estimated to be 32%. Because the metabolism of alcohol varies from woman to woman and toxicity may vary from fetus to fetus, no safe range of maternal intake has been established.

Several anticonvulsive medications have been shown to be teratogenic. In 2148 treated epileptic mothers, 20% had offspring with CHD, the most frequent types being ventricular septal defect, tetralogy of Fallot, and transposition of the great arteries. The risk of CHD after prenatal exposure to barbiturates alone may be as high as 11%, and that after exposure to diphenylhydantoin alone may be as high as 29%. Other anticonvulsive medications, such as phenytoin, valproic acid, and carbamazepine, either alone or in combination, have been associated with a substantially increased risk of CHD.

Maternal diabetes and associated insulin therapy significantly increase the risk of CHD in an infant. It is difficult to ascertain whether this increased risk is the result of maternal diabetes itself or to its treatment with insulin. In the large Collaborative Perinatal Project, the risk of a congenital cardiac defect in offspring of diabetic mothers was found to be 2.5%. Maternal insulin dependence contributed significantly to the risk, as did poor control of the maternal diabetes.

The risk of CHD after prenatal exposure to exogenous female sex hormones remains controversial. Early exposure to these agents may result from the continuation of oral contraceptives or their intentional use for the diagnosis of pregnancy, prevention of implantation, and maintenance of pregnancy. Although there has been extensive investigation into the cardiopathic effects of these agents by epidemiologists, the estimated risk from early exposure probably is less than 2%. Prenatal exposure to several other agents, such as Bendectin (removed from the market in 1977), vitamin A congeners, amphetamines, tranquilizers, and mild analgesics, has been associated with an increased incidence of births involving CHD. Estimates of risk after these exposures have not been established clearly, however, because of the small

TABLE 20-16. Risk From Prenatal Teratogens

| Prenatal Exposure | Frequency of CHD (%) | Most Common Cardiac Defects |
|---|---|---|
| **Infections** | | |
| Rubella | 35 | Patent ductus arteriosus, pulmonary stenosis, septal defects |
| **Drugs/Substances** | | |
| Alcohol | 25–30 | Septal defects, patent ductus arteriosus |
| Hydantoin | 2–3 | Pulmonic/aortic stenosis, coarctation, patent ductus arteriosus |
| Trimethadione | 15–30 | Transposition of the great arteries, tetralogy of Fallot, hypoplastic left-heart syndrome |
| Lithium | 10 | Ebstein's anomaly, tricuspid atresia, atrial septal defect |
| Sex hormones | 2–4 | Ventricular septal defect, transposition of the great arteries, tetralogy of Fallot |
| Thalidomide | 5–10 | Tetralogy of Fallot, septal defects, truncus arteriosus |
| **Maternal Conditions** | | |
| Diabetes | 3–5 | Transposition of the great arteries, septal defects, coarctation |
| Phenylketonuria | 25–50 | Tetralogy of Fallot |
| Systemic lupus | 20–40 | Heart block |

CHD, congenital heart disease.

size of the studies and the very low rate of occurrence of the cardiac defects.

## Selected Readings

Boughman JA, Kate AB, Astemborski JA, et al. Familial risks of congenital heart defect assessed in a population-based epidemiological study. Am J Med Genet 1987;26:839.

Ferencz C, Neill CA. Cardiovascular malformations: Prevalence at live-birth. In: Freedom RM, Benson LN, Smallhorn JR, eds. Neonatal heart disease, chapter 2. New York: Springer-Verlag, 1991.

Fixler DE, Pastor P, Chamberlin M, et al. Trends in congenital heart disease in Dallas County births, 1971–1984. Circulation 1990;81:137.

Fyler DC. Report of the New England Regional Infant Cardiac Program. Pediatrics 1980;65(Suppl):375.

Hoffman JIE, Christianson R. Congenital heart disease in a cohort of 19,502 births with long-term followup. Am J Cardiol 1978;42:641.

Mitchell SC, Korones SB, Berendes HW. Congenital heart disease in 56,109 births: Incidence and natural history. Circulation 1971;43:323.

Nora JJ, Nora AH. Maternal transmission of congenital heart disease: New recurrence risk figures and the questions of cytoplasmic inheritance and vulnerability to teratogens. Am J Cardiol 1987;59:549.

Pexieder T. Teratogens. In: Pierpont MEM, Moller JE, eds. Genetics of cardiovascular disease. Boston: Martinus Nijhoff, 1987:55.

Rose V, Gold RJM, Lindsay G. A possible increase in the incidence of congenital heart defects among the offspring of affected parents. J Am Coll Cardiol 1985;6:376.

Whittemore R, Hobbins JC, Engle MA. Pregnancy and its outcome in women with and without surgical treatment of congenital heart disease. Am J Cardiol 1982;50:541.

Zierler S. Maternal drugs and congenital heart disease. Obstet Gynecol 1985;65:155.

*Principles and Practice of Pediatrics, Second Edition.*
edited by Frank A. Oski et al. J. B. Lippincott Company, Philadelphia © 1994.

## 20.3.2 *Cardiovascular Disease in the Newborn*

Norman S. Talner

The clinical approach to cardiovascular problems of the newborn must take into account the structural and functional basis of normal and abnormal cardiovascular development. This includes fundamental cardiac embryology; the transition from the fetal to the neonatal circulation (particularly the role of fetal flow pathways); basic differences between fetal, neonatal, and adult cardiac muscle; age-related responses to imposed circulatory loads; and the various types of functional impairment that may be encountered.

Within the above framework, this segment considers etiology, the essentials of the development of cardiac structure and function, elements of the fetal and neonatal circulations that may affect disease states, the clinical assessment of cardiovascular performance in the neonate, laboratory aids that permit recognition of a potential cardiac problem, and a functional approach to diagnosis and management that takes into account special clinical problems such as congestive heart failure, hypoxemia, and disturbances of cardiac rhythm.

## ETIOLOGY

Most cardiovascular diseases encountered in the newborn are congenital and, as such, they represent altered structural devel-

opment. This can be either abnormal development of a normal structure (aortic or pulmonary atresia, septal defects), failure of a structure(s) to progress beyond a particular embryonic stage (double-outlet right ventricle, truncus arteriosus), or modification of normal flow pathways (coarctation).

In addition to congenital heart lesions, cardiac function in the neonate may be compromised by serious rhythm disturbances (tachycardia, heart block), inflammatory diseases of the myocardium, metabolic defects (eg, glycogen storage disease, carnitine deficiency), defects of mitochondrial electron transport that interfere with the contractile process, and the adverse effects of intrauterine asphyxia on the myocardium, atrioventricular valve function, and pulmonary circulation.

Cardiovascular malformations often accompany chromosomal disorders such as trisomy 21, or are observed in the context of certain genetically determined syndromes, metabolic defects, abnormalities of cardiac rhythm, connective tissue disorders, and abnormal tissue growth. The prognosis in many of these syndromes is determined by the cardiovascular status; thus, detailed evaluation during the newborn period is required.

Because malformations result from an interaction between genetic and environmental systems, the etiology usually is multifactorial. In certain conditions, a specific etiology has been identified. Maternal rubella during early gestation produces a syndrome in which patent ductus arteriosus and pulmonary artery stenosis are common cardiovascular findings. Cardiac defects, particularly the ventricular septal defect, occur in almost 50% of infants with the fetal alcohol syndrome. The finding of complete heart block in a newborn has been linked to the presence of or subsequent development of lupus erythematosus in the mother.

Counseling on the incidence and recurrence rates for families of infants with congenital heart disease is extremely important. The availability of fetal cardiac ultrasound studies permits accurate determination of the presence or absence of significant structural heart disease in subsequent pregnancies and is recommended for families in which a previous child has been born with a congenital heart defect.

## NORMAL CARDIAC DEVELOPMENT

The heart develops from fusion of paired endothelial primordia during the first few weeks of gestation. Encapsulating the endocardium at this stage is the myoepicardium derived from mesoderm. The single cardiac tube has dilatations that constitute the sinus venosus, primitive atrium, primitive ventricle, bulbus cordis, and truncus regions. There is a constriction separating each of these regions, and these indentations define the sinoatrial segment, the atrioventricular canal, the bulboventricular foramen, and the bulbotruncal connection (Fig 20-39) (Anderson, 1978).

In early development, looping of the bulboventricular region occurs, which tends to move the bulbar component anteriorly and to the right of the primitive ventricle. This occurs because of differential cell growth. At the stage of "looping," the embryonic systemic venous return is to the sinus venosus, then to the primitive atrium and ventricle via the atrioventricular canal, and, finally, to the truncus through the bulbar region. The embryonic heart begins to beat concomitantly with the formation of the primitive heart tube and the onset of looping.

The looping process also confers two curvatures to the heart, with the outer curvature being more extensive than the inner. The inner curvature separates the atrioventricular canal, the locus for the developing atrioventricular valves, from the bulbar-truncal region where the semilunar valves will originate (Fig 20-40). The cardiac valves form from loose mesenchymal tissue that lines the cardiac tube distal to the atrioventricular junction. This en-

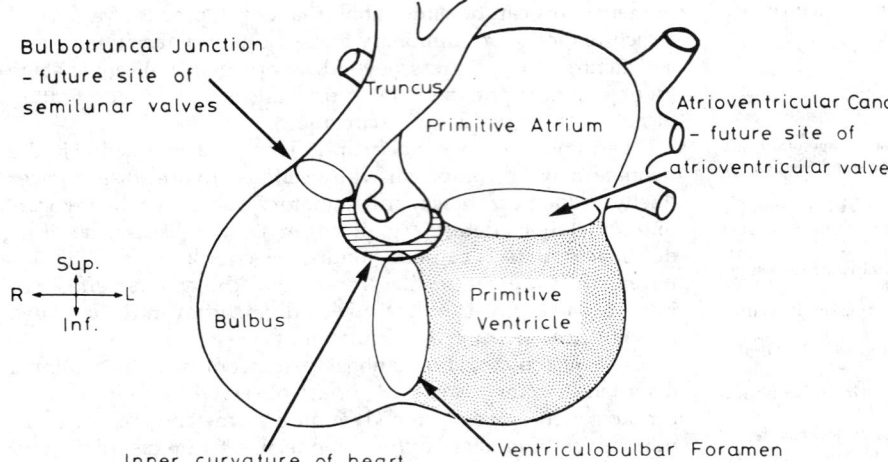

**Figure 20-39.**   The interrelations of the atrioventricular canal, ventricular bulbar foramen, and bulbotruncal junction following looping of the heart tube. The inner curvature of the tube, formed as a consequence of looping, separates the atrioventricular canal (potential site of the atrioventricular valves) from the bulbotruncal junction (site of the semilunar valves). (Anderson RH. Another look at cardiac embryology. In: Yu PN, Goodwin JF, eds. Progress in cardiology, vol 7. Philadelphia: Lea & Febiger, 1978:4.)

docardial cushion tissue will divide the heart into separate flow channels. The remainder of the early developmental process will result in partitioning of the atria, ventricles, and truncus, and establishment of the functioning fetal circulation by the sixth week of gestation (Fig 20-41).

## ABNORMAL CARDIAC DEVELOPMENT

Cardiovascular morphogenesis as described in the preceding section involves a number of important developmental mechanisms, including cell growth, migration, death, differentiation, and adhesion. Hemodynamic factors add another component to cardiovascular development. Based on pathogenetic mechanisms, structural defects may result from abnormalities in the migration of ectomesenchymal tissue (eg, conotruncal septal defects, abnormal conotruncal cushion position, aortic arch defects), abnormalities of intracardiac blood flow (eg, left and right heart obstructive defects, perimembranous ventricular septal defects),

cell death abnormalities (eg, Ebstein's malformation, muscular ventricular septal defects), extracellular matrix abnormalities (eg, endocardial cushion defects, dysplastic semilunar valves), abnormal targeted growth (eg, anomalous pulmonary venous return), and situs and looping defects (eg, heterotaxy, looping abnormalities).

The final form of the developing heart may be determined by extrinsic as well as intrinsic factors. Neural crest tissue has been shown to provide ectomesenchyme not only to the pharynx, but also to the outflow tract of the right ventricle and the postganglionic innervation of the heart. Ablation of neural crest primordia results in cardiac malformations, including double-outlet right ventricle and malalignment of the ventricular septum and aortic arches. Development of the parathyroid gland, thymus, and conotruncal region has been linked to neural crest function, and can account for the findings in DiGeorge syndrome.

The normal development of the great arteries involves the transformation from a paired six–aortic-arch system into a definitive vascular pattern, as shown in Figure 20-42. Anomalies of

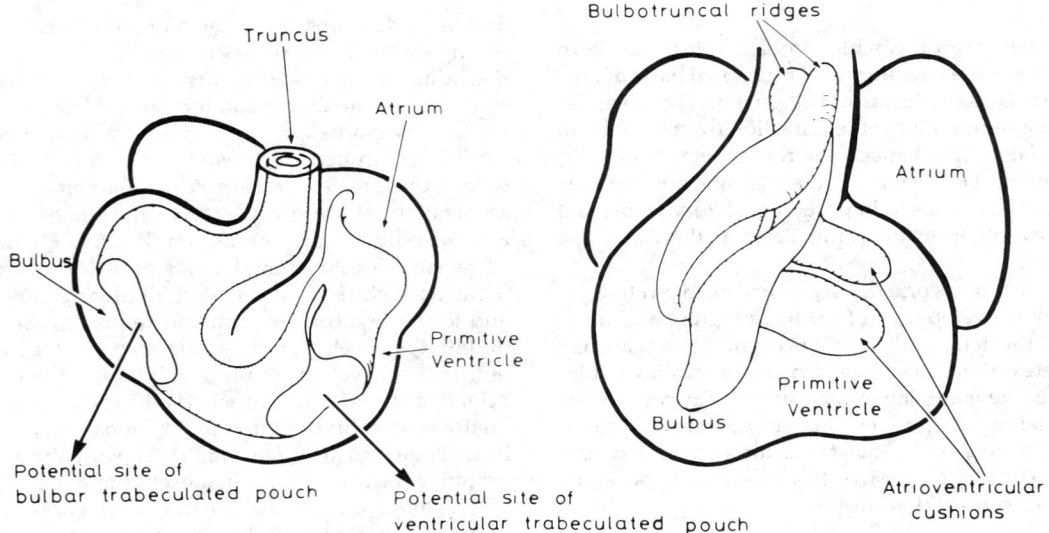

**Figure 20-40.**   Cardiac form just after the stage of looping, with endocardial "jelly" lining the ventricular bulbar loop except for areas destined to give rise to the trabeculated pouches (*left panel*). After further growth (*right panel*), the endocardial cushions are confined to the area of the atrioventricular canal and the bulbus truncus, where they form opposing masses that septate these parts of the cardiac tube. (Anderson RH. Another look at cardiac embryology. In: Yu PN, Goodwin JF, eds. Progress in cardiology, vol 7. Philadelphia: Lea & Febiger, 1978:5.)

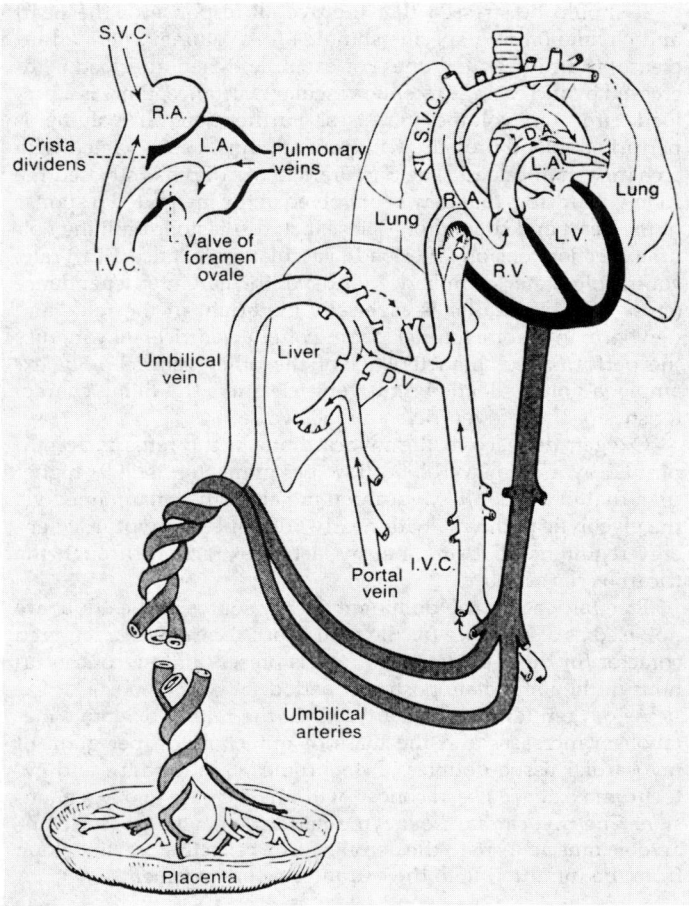

**Figure 20-41.** The fully developed fetal circulation, indicating the fetal flow pathways—foramen ovale, ductus arteriosus, and ductus venosus. The insert shows the direction of flow of the more highly oxygenated placental stream across the foramen ovale. *RA,* right atrium; *LA,* left atrium; *RV,* right ventricle; *LV,* left ventricle; *DA,* ductus arteriosus; *FO,* foramen ovale; *DV,* ductus venosus; *IVC,* inferior vena cava; *SVC,* superior vena cava. (Adams FH, Emmanouilides GC, eds. Heart disease in infants, children, and adolescents, ed 3. Baltimore: Williams & Wilkins, 1983: 12.)

clinical significance occur that can produce compromise of major conducting airways, such as the double aortic arch, right aortic arch with left ductus arteriosus (or ligamentum), and anomalous takeoff of the head vessels. Rarely, the left pulmonary artery takes its origin from the right and courses between the trachea and esophagus, producing tracheal and esophageal compression (pulmonary artery sling).

## THE DEVELOPMENT OF CARDIOVASCULAR FUNCTION

The primitive embryonic heart initially is a muscle-wrapped tube without valve function, partitions, or a coronary circulation. This system is capable of providing for the oxygen and nutrient needs of the embryo while at the same time removing end products of metabolism.

During fetal life, however, the placenta serves as the site for gas exchange, with blood almost fully oxygenated returning to the fetal body via the umbilical veins. The common umbilical vein enters the porta hepatis, where it is joined by the portal vein. Branches are provided to the left and right lobes of the liver, with the ductus venosus serving as a direct connection to the inferior vena cava, thus permitting umbilical venous blood to bypass the hepatic microcirculation. The well-oxygenated umbilical stream is directed across the foramen ovale, permitting blood of the highest $O_2$ concentration to perfuse the cerebral circulation. The third shunt channel, the ductus arteriosus, allows blood from the right ventricle to enter the descending aorta and essentially bypass the pulmonary circulation. The fetal circulation with functioning flow pathways is shown in Figure 20-41.

The patterns of blood flow in the fetal circulation have been studied in the fetal lamb model, using microsphere techniques. These studies have shown that about 20% of the total systemic venous return is derived from the superior vena caval stream, 3% is derived from the coronary circulation, and 7% is derived from the pulmonary vascular bed. Inferior caval flow accounts for 70% of the systemic venous return, of which 40% derives from umbilical veins, 5% derives from portal veins, and 25% derives from the lower fetal body. Fifty-five percent of umbilical venous flow passes through the ductus venosus, whereas 45% flows via the right and left lobes of the liver. Of interest, the left

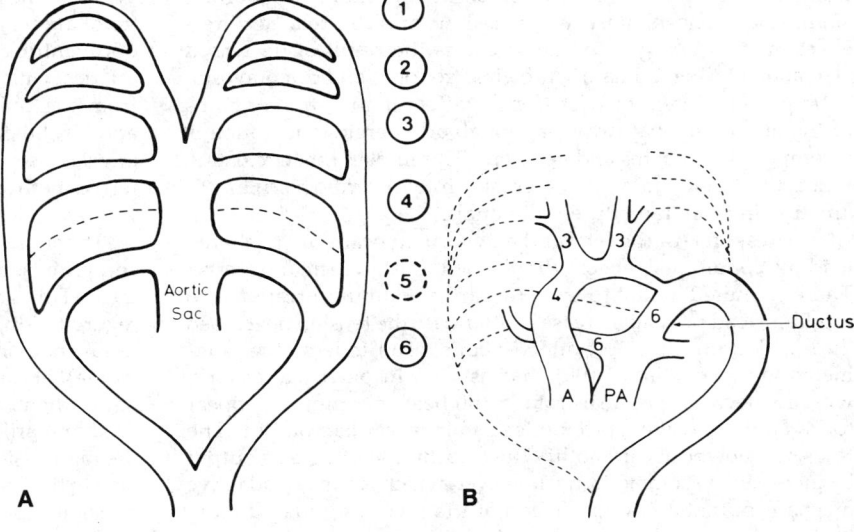

**Figure 20-42.** (**A**) The full aortic arch system. All arches do not exist at the same time during normal development, and the fifth arch probably is not functionally present. (**B**) The remnants of the aortic arch system with normal development. Shown are the definitive aorta (*A*), pulmonary artery (*PA*), and ductus arteriosus. (Anderson RH. Another look at cardiac embryology. In: Yu PN, Goodwin JF, eds. Progress in cardiology, vol 7. Philadelphia: Lea & Febiger, 1978: 40.)

lobe is supplied from the umbilical vein, whereas the majority of the right lobe is perfused with portal venous blood. Under conditions of hypoxemia and flow limitation, there is a redistribution of venous return favoring flow through the ductus venosus.

Thus, blood at the level of the entry of the inferior vena cava into the right atrium is derived from four sources: the ductus venosus (umbilical vein), the distal inferior cava, the right hepatic vein, and the left hepatic vein. The most highly oxygenated stream (ductus venosus) is directed preferentially across the foramen ovale, whereas distal caval blood with a much lower $O_2$ saturation passes across the tricuspid valve. The higher saturations of left ventricular blood ensure adequate oxygenation of the developing brain as well as provide vital substrates for brain metabolism.

The superior vena caval stream is directed across the tricuspid valve, with only 2% passing from right to left across the foramen ovale. The net effect of the fetal venous return pathways is a lower $O_2$ saturation on the right side compared to that on the left. The volume of blood in the right and left ventricles also favors the right side in the lamb. Ultrasound and Doppler-derived flow studies across the mitral and tricuspid valves in the developing human fetus, however, indicate that the volume flows on the right and left sides of the heart are almost equal, with only a slight dominance of right ventricular output.

The fetal cardiac output represents the combined output of both ventricles. Most of the right ventricular output of the fetus flows into the descending aorta via the ductus arteriosus, whereas the majority of the left ventricular output perfuses the upper body with the aortic isthmus (segment from the origin of the left subclavian artery to the ductus arteriosus) receiving only 30% of blood from the ascending aorta. The isthmus is the site of functional separation of the two circuits.

When compared to the adult heart, the fetal and newborn myocardium is unique with respect to its ultrastructure, mechanical and biochemical properties, metabolism, and autonomic innervation. The developing cardiac myocyte is smaller than the adult cardiac myocyte, and contains relatively more noncontractile mass with a reduction in cell density. Consequently, force generation and the extent and velocity of shortening are decreased, whereas water content and stiffness are increased. The process of excitation-contraction coupling also differs in the fetus and newborn when compared to that in the adult. There is less development of the sarcoplasmic reticulum and T tubule system in the fetus, which may interfere with the movement of calcium ions. Calcium ion increase in the cytosol appears to be provided by trans-sarcolemmal movement rather than by release of calcium from the sarcoplasmic reticulum, as in the adult. Myofibrillar adenosine triphosphatase levels are low, and age-related differences in contractility also may occur as the result of decreased activation of the modulatory proteins, troponin and tropomyosin.

Functional integrity exists for the afferent and efferent limbs of the autonomic pathways, although adrenergic innervation is incomplete in the fetus and newborn. This implies that circulating vasoactive agents may play a greater role in cardiovascular adaptation in more immature individuals.

The response of the fetal and newborn myocardium to altered loading conditions reflects diminished cardiovascular reserve. There is limited ability to increase cardiac output in response to a volume load or to an increase in afterload, the tension developed during ejection. Inotropic interventions result in less of an augmentation in cardiac output than is seen in older age groups, whereas decreases in heart rate (>100 beats per minute) appear to be associated with pronounced falls in cardiac output. The fetus and newborn can modify the distribution of cardiac output by increasing vasomotor tone, however, which is a major adaptive mechanism that allows perfusion of the myocardium and brain at the expense of the peripheral circulation.

It should be stressed that the overall response of the heart and circulation to a specific stimulus (eg, volume, afterload increase) is an integrated one. For example, when afterload is increased by increasing systemic vascular resistance, there is a preload effect as volume increases. Furthermore, if volume is perturbed, blood pressure will rise and, thus, be associated with a change in afterload. The San Francisco group has stressed the following factors that may be involved in the integrated response of the heart and circulation. These include diastolic or filling volume, ejection tension (afterload), vascular impedance, heart rate, contractile state, compliance, and ventricular interdependence (cross talk). The latter is especially important in the fetus and newborn, in whom volume loading of one ventricle may modify the performance characteristics of the other ventricle. For example, a volume-loaded right ventricle alters the filling characteristics of the left ventricle and vice versa.

Oxygen delivery to the myocardium in the fetus is accomplished by a coronary blood flow per gram that is 90% higher than that in the adult. Myocardial metabolism is maintained via the glycolytic pathway, with nearly 60% of fetal myocardial energy requirements being met by lactate extraction through the tricarboxylic acid cycle.

Free fatty acids, the dominant energy source in the adult, are not used as a substrate for the fetal heart. L-carnitine, a required cofactor for the $\beta$-oxidation of fats, is present in low concentrations in the immediate postnatal period.

As oxygen tension rises after birth, the rate of oxidative metabolism increases and the mass of mitochondria per gram of myocardial tissue doubles. Cytochromes $c_1$, a, and $a_3$, and cytochrome oxidase rise in concert with the increase in oxygen tension. The myocardial isoenzyme pattern changes from the anaerobic muscle form to the aerobic form, reflecting the transition from the intrauterine to the extrauterine environment.

## EFFECTS OF CARDIAC MALFORMATION ON FETAL CIRCULATORY FUNCTION

In most instances, cardiac malformations are tolerated well by the developing fetus because of the presence of the fetal flow pathways (which permit the bypass of obstructive lesions), the existence of the placenta for gas exchange, and the high pulmonary vascular resistance. On occasion, however, the presence of certain malformations interferes with the growth of chamber size, such as when a small foramen ovale compromises left heart development, or when incorporation of the common pulmonary vein into the left atrium fails, resulting in a hypoplastic left atrium (total anomalous pulmonary venous connection). Dominance of one ventricle over the other can modify the size of the great arteries, with the aortic isthmus becoming hypoplastic when flow from the pulmonary artery to the ductus into the descending aorta is the predominant flow pattern. When there is pulmonary atresia or severe obstruction of right ventricular outflow, the preferred pathway is via the aorta, which tends to be enlarged, whereas the pulmonary artery(s) is hypoplastic.

There are a few situations wherein fetal cardiac function is compromised, with cardiac failure arising in utero (hydrops fetalis). This occurs when there is massive atrioventricular valve regurgitation, semilunar valve insufficiency, a large systemic arteriovenous fistula (vein of Galen malformation, giant hemangioma), and severe anemia. These share the common hemodynamic theme of right-sided volume overloading, either primarily or secondarily, in the face of left-sided lesions. With the latter, the high-resistance pulmonary vascular bed shifts the circulatory load to the right heart. Hydrops fetalis with pericardial and pleural effusions, ascites, and generalized anasarca may occur in the face of the above-mentioned disturbances. This clinical picture also may develop with prolonged fetal tachyarrhythmias. These rhythm disturbances have been managed in some instances by the administration of antiarrhythmic pharmacologic agents (propranolol, digoxin, procainamide) to the mother, with transplacental passage of the agent to the fetus to enable control of the arrhythmia and resolution of the hydrops. Massive cardiomegaly that can be observed in association with fetal hydrops also may compromise lung development, an observation that is similar to that which takes place with diaphragmatic hernias.

## DEVELOPMENT OF THE PULMONARY CIRCULATION

The pulmonary arterial tree develops in conjunction with the airways. The periacinal, arterial, and airway branching pattern is completed by the 16th week of gestation. The intra-acinar vessels and alveoli develop during the latter part of gestation and postnatally. The multiplication of intra-acinar arteries keeps pace with alveolar ducts and alveolar development, and is particularly rapid during the first years of life. This progressive growth and remodeling of the pulmonary vascular bed provides a bed of sufficient capacity to ensure a low pulmonary vascular resistance.

During fetal life, the resistance vessels (precapillary) have a thicker wall than do those seen in a child or adult. This reflects the high pulmonary vascular resistance of the fetus (increased pressure drop across the bed and low pulmonary blood flow). In the remodeling process postnatally, there is a progressive decrease in muscularity as pulmonary vascular resistance falls. The important factors to be taken into consideration in the assessment of pulmonary vascular resistance are the pressure drop from the pulmonary arteries to the veins, pulmonary blood flow, surface area, muscularity and tone of the resistance vessels, and blood viscosity. The postnatal fall in hematocrit results in a decrease in blood viscosity and contributes to the lowering of pulmonary vascular resistance. The presence of pulmonary hypertension does not necessarily imply an increase in pulmonary vascular resistance if pulmonary blood flow is increased markedly, as occurs with large-volume left-to-right shunts.

In infants with persistent pulmonary hypertension of multiple etiologies, the pulmonary artery pressure is close to or at systemic levels, whereas pulmonary blood flow is decreased (high resistance state). It is imperative, therefore, in the assessment of cardiopulmonary disorders of the infant that the resistance of the pulmonary circulation be taken into consideration. Furthermore, persistent pulmonary hypertension is not in itself a definitive diagnosis. What is required is a precise diagnosis of the cause of pulmonary hypertension (eg, lung disease, cardiac problem, primary disorder of pulmonary resistance vessels) so that appropriate management can be carried out. Echocardiography occupies a key role in defining the specific nature of the problem in the pulmonary circulation.

## OXYGEN TRANSPORT IN THE FETUS AND NEWBORN

Oxygen transport (delivery) represents the product of the cardiac output and the arterial oxygen content. The arterial oxygen content is determined by the oxygen tension, the affinity of hemoglobin for oxygen, and the absolute hemoglobin level. The hemoglobin concentration is controlled by erythropoietin production. The liver is the site of erythropoietin production in the fetus, as contrasted with production by the kidney in the adult. Because the fetus is exposed to a lower oxygen saturation, the erythropoietin response differs qualitatively or has a different sensitivity to hypoxemia than does the response at later stages

of development. The affinity of hemoglobin to oxygen is greater in the fetus and newborn. This is accounted for by the fact that fetal hemoglobin has less affinity for 2,3-DPG (diphosphoglycerate), which competitively decreases hemoglobin–oxygen affinity. This is important for oxygen uptake in the fetus, because placental oxygen transfer occurs at much lower oxygen tension than does alveolar oxygen transfer. The $P_{50}$ ($PO_2$ at which hemoglobin is 50% saturated with oxygen) is 28 mm Hg for fetal blood and about 38 mm Hg for adult blood. Therefore, postnatally with an arterial $PO_2$ of 100 mm Hg and a venous $PO_2$ of 40 mm Hg, the amount of oxygen extracted from fetal blood is much less than that extracted from adult blood.

## THE TRANSITIONAL CIRCULATION

At birth, the critical event in the transition from the intrauterine to the extrauterine state is the establishment of lung inflation. This then initiates a series of events, culminating in a fall in pulmonary vascular resistance and functional closure of the fetal flow pathways. Contact of air containing oxygen with the pulmonary resistance vessels produces vasodilatation, which is accompanied by a marked increase in pulmonary blood flow as pulmonary vascular resistances fall acutely. A continued search has been conducted for the specific mediator of the pulmonary vasodilatation that occurs at birth. Initial focus was on bradykinin, then on prostaglandins, and, most recently, on the endothelial-derived relaxing factor, now thought to be nitric oxide. This very well may have clinical implications in the management of persistent pulmonary hypertension. Systemic vascular resistance rises consequent to obliteration of the low-resistance placental circuit. The ductus venosus flow channel also is eliminated at this time.

Left atrial pressure rises as pulmonary venous return increases, and this produces functional closure of the foramen ovale. The postnatal rise in arterial oxygen tension, together with local changes in prostaglandin metabolism, produces constriction of the ductus arteriosus, with functional obliteration complete in a full-term infant by 10 to 15 hours of life. In a preterm infant, however, the mechanisms responsible for ductal constriction are developed incompletely, and closure thereby is delayed.

Any interference with the establishment of ventilatory function (ie, birth asphyxia) tends to maintain the circulation in the fetal state, with a high pulmonary vascular resistance and right-to-left shunting via the ductus arteriosus and foramen ovale. This can produce the clinical picture associated with persistent pulmonary hypertension, as will be discussed later.

Final obliteration of the fetal flow pathways produces the adult-type circulation that is present in the term infant within a few weeks of birth. The two ventricles now operate in series, with a relatively high cardiac output resulting from the demands of growth. Pulmonary vascular resistance is almost at adult levels, with resistance vessels characterized by very little medial thickness and increased lumen diameter. Remodeling of the pulmonary vascular bed continues postnatally, however, in concert with airway development.

## KEY POINTS IN CLINICAL EVALUATION

Having established the fundamentals of the development of cardiovascular function, we can proceed to clinical assessment.

### History

The principal points in the history that aid in the clinical evaluation of the potentially critically ill infant with cardiovascular disease include the birth history, the presence of a chromosomal abnormality, a sibling with congenital heart disease, hydrops fetalis and ectopy, intrauterine infections, and other major-organ systemic malformations. A low Apgar score should raise the possibility of the deleterious effects of hypoxemia, hypercarbia, and acidemia on the myocardial, pulmonary, and systemic circulations. Chronic intrauterine hypoxia is associated with persistent pulmonary hypertension with right-to-left ductal and foraminal shunting. Almost all the chromosomal abnormalities are associated with a high incidence of congenital heart disease, with trisomies 21, 13, and 18 heading the list. Although defects involving the atrioventricular canal are observed commonly in infants with trisomy 21, other malformations such as tetralogy of Fallot and patent ductus arteriosus also can occur. Any infant born with a trisomy should undergo two-dimensional echocardiographic assessment to aid in the delineation of the total clinical problem.

Congenital heart disease in a previous child in the family should alert the clinician to possible involvement in a subsequent pregnancy. The use of fetal cardiac ultrasound studies to define the presence or absence of cardiac involvement has aided in the management of the pregnancy and the postnatal state when serious cardiac problems were discovered.

Intrauterine infections can be associated with life-threatening myocardial dysfunction. Therefore, myocardial structure and function should be assessed in all infants suspected of having a septicemic process.

The presence of malformations that affect multiple organ systems, such as tracheoesophageal fistula, imperforate anus, and cleft palate, should warrant a search for cardiac involvement. Abnormalities of cardiac position (dextrocardia, mesocardia) also demand a cardiac evaluation, whereas a midline liver with or without an abnormality of cardiac position should raise the possibility of atrial isomerism in association with absence of the spleen or polysplenia. Another important group consists of patients who have aortic arch anomalies with a strong association between absence of the parathyroid gland and thymus and conotruncal malformations (DiGeorge syndrome).

## Physical Examination

### Perfusion

The status of systemic perfusion must be evaluated carefully. A low output state with any one of a number of causes should be suspected when pulses are difficult to palpate, extremities are cold and pale, and capillary refill is slow. Although this could arise from overwhelming infection, it is common to encounter this clinical picture in newborn infants with critical left heart obstruction, tachyarrhythmia, or myocardial disease. It should be stressed that palpable femoral pulses in a newborn do not rule out coarctation if the ductus arteriosus is open (see the section on low perfusion states). Bounding peripheral pulses are observed with aortic runoff lesions, notably patent ductus, truncus arteriosus, and systemic arteriovenous fistulas, and in the face of severe anemia.

In regard to arteriovenous malformations, there have been reports of diminished femoral pulsations with large cerebral arteriovenous fistulas. In this situation, there is a steal from the peripheral circulation as blood flows through the low-resistance fistula.

### Heart Rate

The heart rate should be counted accurately. If it is higher than 250 beats per minute, an electrocardiogram (ECG) must be obtained to define the basis for the increase. Bradycardia (a heart rate of less than 100 beats per minute) may be encountered with hypoxic depression of the myocardium, possible central nervous system disease, or congenital heart block.

### Blood Pressure

Many new techniques permit the accurate determination of blood pressure in the newborn. This allows delineation of infants with serious hypertension and initiation of a search for the specific basis for the blood pressure elevation. On the other hand, if blood pressure is discovered to be low for developmental age, the causes of hypotension, such as hypovolemia, myopericardial disease, or left heart obstruction, must be defined quickly and corrected.

### Respiratory Pattern

The pattern of respirations may provide valuable clues to the presence of cardiovascular disease.

### Tachypnea

When lung water is increased, with the accumulation of fluid in the pulmonary interstitial space, tachypnea (rapid, shallow respirations) ensues in response to stimulation of juxtacapillary volume receptors. This response occurs under any circumstance in which there is a fluid leak into the pulmonary interstitial space (left-to-right shunting, left heart obstructive lesions, inflammatory diseases of the myocardium or lungs, delayed fluid reabsorption). Therefore, tachypnea is a nonspecific finding that demands a careful search for its underlying cause. The diagnosis of transient tachypnea, although descriptive of a breathing pattern, does not provide a precise delineation of etiology. Supporting studies are required to rule in or out cardiovascular or pulmonary problems associated with tachypnea.

### Hyperpnea

When the arterial oxygen tension is extremely low and pulmonary perfusion is decreased or normal, the ventilatory response is that of hyperpnea (rapid, deep respirations), in contrast to the congested lung in which tachypnea is observed. The hyperpneic response represents hypoxemic stimulation of the arterial chemoreceptors and results in the development of a respiratory alkalosis.

### Cyanosis

The presence of a generalized duskiness can arise from a number of causes. Diffuse cyanosis requires documentation of the level of arterial oxygen tension, along with determination of the pH level and the $PaCO_2$. Oxygen saturation levels can be derived from these measurements. Oxygen saturation levels also can be determined directly, in a noninvasive fashion, with pulse oximetry. Differential cyanosis, with the lower body being more cyanotic than the upper body, immediately should raise the suspicion of a high pulmonary vascular resistance with right-to-left shunting via the ductus arteriosus. This flow pattern can arise from a number of causes, including coarctation of the aorta, interruption of the aortic arch, and persistent pulmonary hypertension. In the rare situation in which the upper body is cyanotic while the lower body is pink, transposition of the great arteries in association with pulmonary-to-aortic shunting of oxygenated blood via the ductus arteriosus will produce this picture.

### Precordial Activity

The activity of the precordium, or lack thereof, provides valuable clinical information regarding cardiac performance. An active precordium is seen in the volume-loaded situation associated with increased ventricular contractility (left-to-right shunt, atrioventricular valve regurgitation, hypervolemia). A relatively inactive precordium with signs of compromised systemic perfusion is seen with myopericardial disease. Patients with the hypoplastic left-heart syndrome and coarctation characteristically have a hyperdynamic precordium along with decreased system perfusion. This reflects the volume-loaded right heart and pulmonary circulation, whereas systemic perfusion is impaired secondary to constriction of the ductus arteriosus. Precordial activity in the right chest suggests a cardiac malposition.

## Aortic and Pulmonary Valve Closure

The examiner should be able to detect normal splitting of the second heart sound, indicating the presence of aortic and pulmonary valve closure. A single second heart sound occurs if one semilunar valve is severely stenotic or atretic, or if the semilunar valves are closing in synchrony (transposition).

## Ejection Clicks

Aortic and pulmonary valve ejection clicks are heard just before the onset of turbulent flow. They represent the opening sounds of mobile but thickened semilunar valves. The aortic ejection click is heard at the cardiac apex or in the suprasternal notch. A pulmonary ejection click usually is heard at the left base. Ejection clicks also may be appreciated when there is an increased volume flowing into the pulmonary or systemic circulation, although they are heard most commonly when obstructive disease is present.

## Gallop Rhythm

A triple rhythm is encountered when there is increased flow across an atrioventricular valve or there is ventricular dilatation in association with decreased ventricular contractility or compliance.

## Murmurs

Auscultation of the heart should be performed in a fashion similar to ultrasound interrogation during echocardiography. This requires knowledge of specific anatomic positions, particularly those of the ventricular septum, great arteries, and atrioventricular valves. Stethoscopic probing of the cardiac base (second interspace on the right and left) will define outflow tract lesions. The ejection murmur of aortic stenosis is localized to the right base with transmission to the neck, whereas a similar ejection-type murmur, heard best at the second left intercostal space with transmission laterally and to the back, characterizes pulmonic stenosis. Murmurs localized along the lower left sternal border usually reflect defects of the ventricular septum. These murmurs are holosystolic, representing pansystolic flow from the left to the right ventricle. Holosystolic murmurs heard in a similar location occasionally may indicate the presence of tricuspid regurgitation, with some tendency to localize along the lower right sternal margins. An apical holosystolic murmur, usually heard well posteriorly, suggests the presence of mitral valve regurgitation.

The intensity of the murmur does not correlate with the severity of the lesion, and certainly can be influenced by cardiac output and changes in systemic and pulmonary vascular resistance. The total clinical picture must be taken into consideration when attempting to define the severity of a particular lesion.

Systolic ejection murmurs that localize to both axillae and are heard posteriorly are found with peripheral pulmonary artery stenosis. In the preterm and newborn infant, this may be a normal finding as a result of a discrepancy in size between the main pulmonary artery and its branches. Persistence of this type of murmur beyond 4 to 6 months of age should be considered abnormal, and indicates structural narrowing of the pulmonary arterial branches. Another murmur, one that is systolic ejection in timing, is associated with transient left-to-right shunting via the ductus arteriosus in the first 10 to 15 hours after birth, as the pulmonary vascular resistance falls and the ductus arteriosus is undergoing postnatal constriction. Echocardiographic studies in the preterm infant indicate that the ductus arteriosus may remain open for considerably longer periods of time.

Diastolic murmurs are heard rarely in the newborn. A decrescendo diastolic murmur after pulmonary closure is heard with pulmonary valve regurgitation, as might be encountered in the

absent pulmonary valve syndrome. In the latter instance, there may be significant airway problems caused by compression of major bronchi by a massively dilated main pulmonary artery and its branches. Low-pitched, diastolic rumbling murmurs heard along the lower left sternal border or at the cardiac apex, which time with rapid ventricular filling, are associated either with atrioventricular valve regurgitation or increased flow across normal tricuspid or mitral valves in the face of a left-to-right shunt lesion (relative stenosis).

The classic auscultatory finding of a patent ductus arteriosus is a continuous machinery-like murmur localized under the left clavicle. This represents systolic and diastolic flow into the pulmonary artery via the ductus arteriosus. Because a patent ductus arteriosus with left-to-right shunting may be a significant problem in the preterm infant, recognition of its presence is extremely important. The diagnosis should be suspected in any preterm infant with a hyperdynamic precordium and bounding arterial pulsations, even in the absence of significant murmurs. In infants with the respiratory distress syndrome, the ductus may be widely patent with no obvious clinical findings. Therefore, diagnosis is dependent on two-dimensional echocardiography with Doppler interrogation, which will demonstrate aortic-to-pulmonary artery shunting.

To-and-fro systolic and diastolic murmurs can be heard in the presence of semilunar valve regurgitation, with the systolic component arising from increased volume flow across a semilunar valve. With anemia, a number of murmurs may be appreciated, all arising from a high cardiac output state with increased flow across semilunar and atrioventricular valves.

## Hepatomegaly

The size and location of the liver edge provides valuable clinical clues related to cardiac disease and myocardial performance. A liver edge to the left is seen with situs inversus and dextrocardia (mirror-image type), whereas a midline liver raises the possibility of atrial isomerism and splenic abnormalities. Hepatic enlargement accompanies right-sided congestive heart failure. Systolic pulsations are seen with massive tricuspid regurgitation. Presystolic pulsations occur when there is tricuspid valve obstruction, and represent a prominent atrial contraction.

# IMPORTANT LABORATORY AIDS IN THE DIAGNOSIS OF CARDIAC DISEASE IN THE INFANT

## Chest Film

The chest film provides valuable structural and functional data relative to the underlying cardiac condition. Clinicians should discipline themselves to review the film carefully and to answer the following queries:

- What is the cardiac position (levocardia, mesocardia, or dextrocardia)?
- Where is the stomach bubble and liver (situs, solitus, inversus, midline liver)? Bronchi (right- or left-sidedness)?
- Is the heart enlarged (age-related normal, influence of thymic shadow)?
- What is the status of lung perfusion (increased pulmonary blood flow, pulmonary venous congestion, diminished pulmonary perfusion)?
- Is there associated lung disease (infection, hypoplasia, diaphragmatic hernia)?
- Is the airway compromised (vascular rings)?

Careful analysis of these points usually permits a physiologic and, sometimes, a correct anatomic diagnosis, although the presence of open fetal flow channels (ductus arteriosus, foramen ovale) may mask the eventual radiographic picture. Examples of rather typical chest radiographs encountered in critical cardiac disease in the infant are shown in Figure 20-43.

## Arterial Blood Gas and pH Levels

The data obtained from analysis of blood gas tensions and pH levels permit delineation of the severity of hypoxemia if it is present, the metabolic and respiratory consequences of the defect (metabolic and respiratory acidemia), and the degree of ventilatory compensation or decompensation (hypocarbia or hypercarbia). The response to the inhalation of high inspired oxygen concentrations (hyperoxia response) has not proven to be an accurate discriminator between heart, pulmonary vascular, and lung disease, and actually has been misleading on occasion. In situations in which there is ductal-dependent systemic blood flow (coarctation, aortic atresia), the $PaO_2$ may rise significantly, whereas systemic perfusion is compromised further, which re-

sults in severe metabolic acidemia. On the other hand, if there is ductal-dependent pulmonary blood flow (pulmonary atresia, tricuspid atresia), the arterial oxygen tension will rise only slightly as a result of the increment in dissolved oxygen. Oxygen saturation can be determined noninvasively with a pulse oximeter, which also is a valuable aid in assessing the response to medical or surgical interventions.

## Hemoglobin and Hematocrit

The packed cell volume and hemoglobin concentration provide clinical clues that aid in the assessment of cardiovascular disease. A hematocrit level elevated above 65% is associated with a high pulmonary vascular resistance (viscosity factor) and right-to-left shunting via fetal flow channels. With significant anemia (a hemoglobin level less than 12 g/dL), there may be a high output state. Infants with large left-to-right shunts evidence signs of congestive heart failure at a time when relative anemia is present (2 to 3 months). The decrease in blood viscosity and postnatal

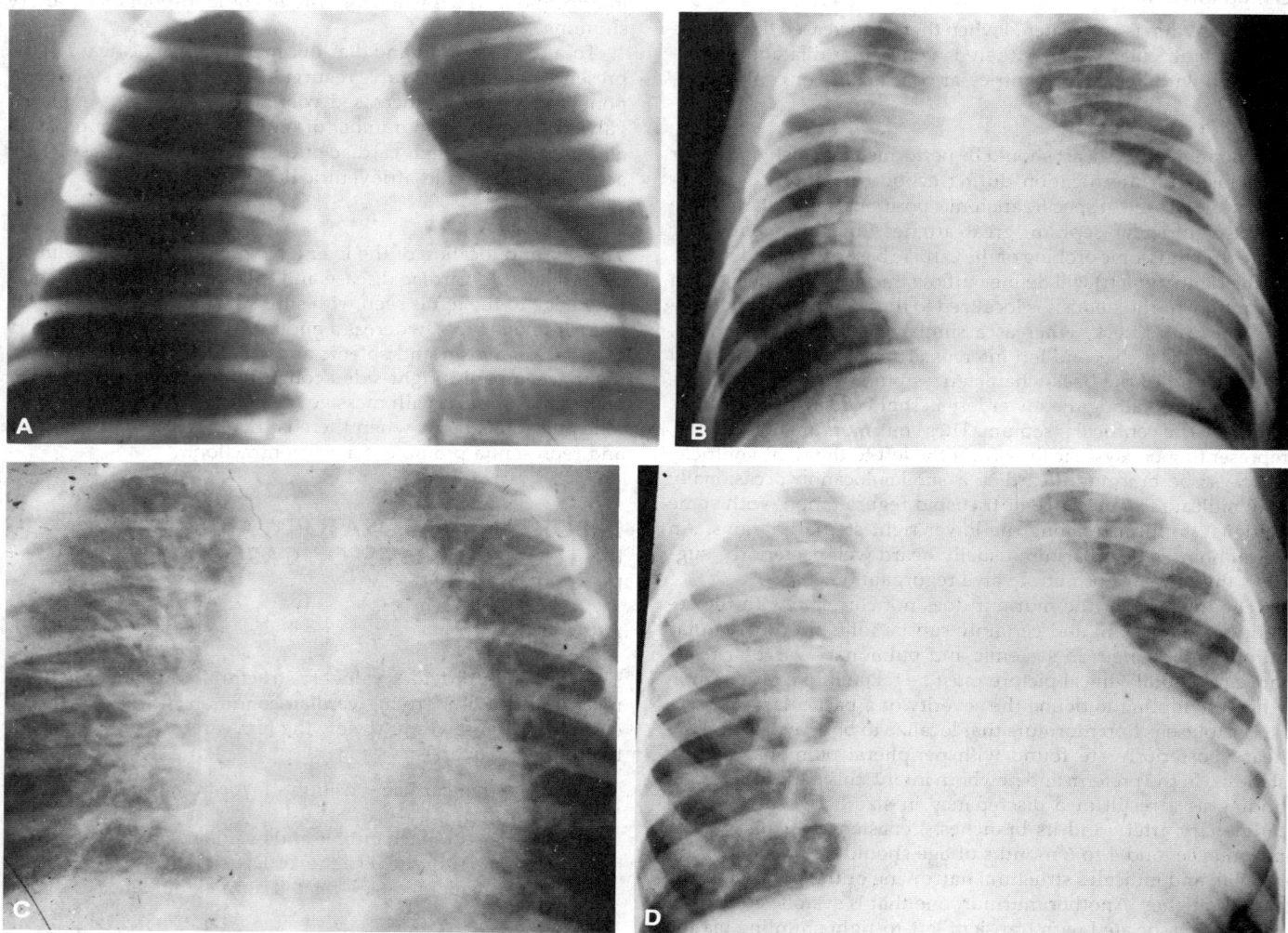

Figure 20-43.   Chest films illustrating various types of functional impairment observed with critical cardiac disease. (**A**) Striking decrease in pulmonary blood flow, as seen with tetralogy of Fallot or hypoplastic right heart syndrome. (**B**) Increased pulmonary vascularity in a newborn infant who also was severely cyanotic. This indication suggests the presence of transposition of the great arteries. (**C**) Marked pulmonary venous congestion of the type seen with severe obstruction to the left heart (coarctation, aortic stenosis) or compromise of pulmonary venous return. (**D**) Cardiomegaly and increased pulmonary vascular markings compatible with the finding of a large left-to-right shunt at the level of the ventricle or great artery. (Talner NS. Heart failure. In: Adams FH, Emmanouillides GC, eds. Heart disease in infants, children, and adolescents. Baltimore: Williams & Wilkins, 1989:899.)

remodeling of the pulmonary vascular bed both contribute to the fall in pulmonary vascular resistance and the resulting large left-to-right shunt.

## Blood Glucose and Calcium

Hypoglycemia and hypocalcemia have been implicated in clinical states characterized by low cardiac output. Therefore, these abnormalities should be corrected as part of any attempt to restore normal myocardial contractility.

## The Electrocardiogram of the Newborn

The ECG provides the clinician with valuable data relative to heart rate, potential rhythm disturbances, ventricular and atrial enlargement, myocardial ischemia, and possible electrolyte disturbances. During the newborn period, the ECG must be interpreted in terms of normative values for this age group.

The standard newborn ECG should consist of 12 leads and a rhythm strip as required. The lead system must be standardized to a known voltage so that proper interpretation can be made in terms of enlargement. The paper speed should be 25 mm/s so that rates and intervals can be calculated. Attention should be directed to proper lead placement, particularly of the precordial leads. If electrode paste is smeared, then a common lead usually is traced, which does not permit localization.

The following points should aid in evaluation. First, the ECG must be interpreted in conjunction with the history, physical examination, and other pertinent laboratory findings, electrolyte status, and medications. Second, a systematic approach should be used, paying attention to atrial rate, ventricular rate, and definition of the cardiac rhythm. Next, the PR interval should be

recorded, the QRS duration measured, and the QT interval derived. The QT interval, the period of electromechanical systole, should be corrected for heart rate ($QT_c$). Fourth, the P wave and QRS should be determined, and the ST-T wave segment assessed. Finally, atrial and ventricular enlargement should be looked for, comparing voltages and patterns to established normal values.

### Determination of Heart Rate

The pediatrician should calculate the heart rate and compare it to age-related normal values. Each major line represents 0.2 seconds when recorded at a paper speed of 25 mm/s. Thus, if one large line separates the RR interval, the rate is 300 beats per minute (one half beat every 0.2 seconds is equal to 300 beats per minute), which is abnormally rapid (Fig 20-44). On the other hand, if three large lines separate the R waves, the rate is 100 beats per minute, which is too slow for a newborn.

### Electrical Axis

As an approximation, the electrical axis will be perpendicular to the limb lead that adds up to zero (R + S), or parallel to the lead with the highest R wave voltage. The mean axis of the P wave can be determined in a similar fashion. In the newborn, the normal QRS axis is more to the right than in the older child and the adult. It should be stressed that, although the axis usually correlates with ventricular hypertrophy, this is not necessarily so. Hypertrophy must be assessed from the precordial leads.

### Right Ventricular Hypertrophy

At birth, the thickness of the right and the left ventricular walls is about equal and, thus, the infant has physiologic right ventricular hypertrophy. This results in increased rightward and anterior electrical forces, with tall R waves in the right chest and broad S waves over the left precordial leads (Fig 20-45). This makes the diagnosis of pathologic right ventricular hypertrophy difficult. Certain patterns are helpful in this regard. A pure R wave or qR pattern in the right precordial leads strongly suggests right ventricular hypertrophy at any age (Fig 20-46).

### Left Ventricular Hypertrophy

The diagnosis of left ventricular hypertrophy in the infant rests on an increase in posterior forces or a decrease in anterior forces for age. This is reflected by increased left precordial and decreased right precordial voltages (Fig 20-47). In the newborn, a decrease in anterior forces should suggest the possibility of underdevelopment of the right ventricle (tricuspid, pulmonary atresia). In the face of severe left ventricular hypertrophy, there may be accompanying ST-T wave changes, which indicate the presence of myocardial ischemia. The latter may be present with critical aortic stenosis.

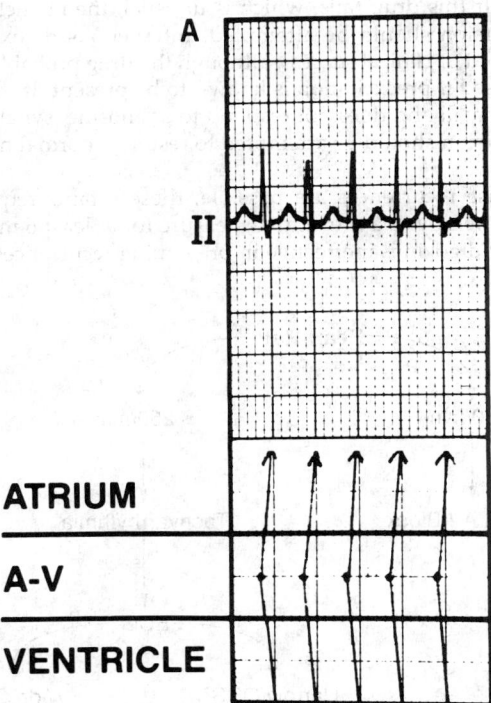

**Figure 20-44.** Supraventricular tachycardia at 290 beats per minute. There are no visible P waves. The P wave probably falls within the QRS complex. In the lower diagram, the *dot* indicates probable origin of the impulse from the atrioventricular (*A-V*) junction, with retrograde spread to the atrium and antegrade spread through the ventricles. The QRS morphology is normal. This is a reentry-type tachycardia. (Garson A Jr. The electrocardiogram in infants and children: A systematic approach. Philadelphia: Lea & Febiger, 1983:238.)

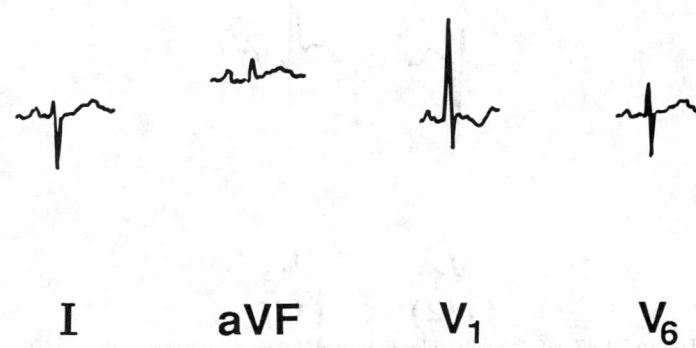

**I        aVF        V₁        V₆**

**Figure 20-45.** Selective electrocardiographic leads in a normal newborn infant, illustrating right axis deviation and right ventricular dominance.

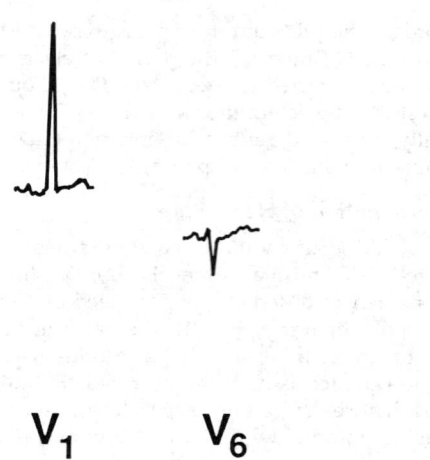

**V₁**     **V₆**

**Figure 20-46.** Significant right ventricular hypertrophy in a newborn infant with severe pulmonary valve stenosis (markedly increased R wave over right precordial lead V₁).

### Atrial Enlargement

Limb lead II usually is the optimal lead for use in assessing atrial size. Tall, peaked P waves (>3 mm) indicate right atrial enlargement, whereas bifid, broad P waves correlate with left atrial enlargement. Because the left atrium depolarizes after the right atrium, the latter part of the P wave may be deformed with any increase in left atrial volume.

### ST-T Wave Segment

Primary alterations in the ST-T waves occur with myocardial ischemia, electrolyte disturbances, and pericardial disease. Birth asphyxia has been associated with ECG abnormalities compatible with myocardial ischemia and, in rare instances, a true myocardial infarct pattern has been observed.

### Electrolyte Abnormalities

Hypocalcemia is associated with a prolonged QT interval that is heart-rate–dependent ($QT_c$ >0.45). The $QT_c$ is calculated by dividing the measured QT interval by the square root of the RR interval. A low serum magnesium level may intensify the findings in hypocalcemia. A prolonged QT interval also is seen in syndromes that are associated with life-threatening ventricular dysrhythmias. Hypercalcemia shortens the $QT_c$ interval.

An elevated serum potassium level is characterized electrocardiographically by peaked, elevated T waves, and indicates

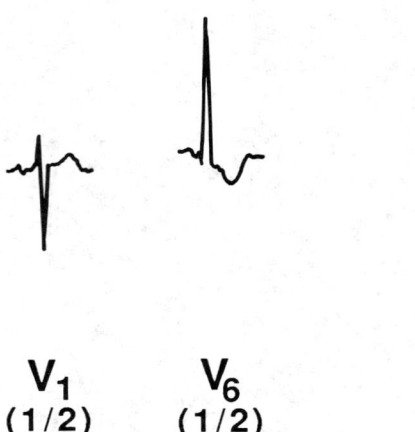

**V₁**     **V₆**
**(1/2)**     **(1/2)**

**Figure 20-47.** Left ventricular hypertrophy in a newborn with critical aortic stenosis (decreased forces over right precordial lead V₁ and increased R wave over lead V₆).

serum potassium valves of greater than 7.0 mEq/L. Higher values of serum potassium widen the QRS and decrease the amplitude of the complexes. Decreased serum potassium values lower the T waves and cause the appearance of U waves as serum values become less than 2.5 mEq/L.

## Life-Threatening Rhythm Disturbances

### Paroxysmal Supraventricular Tachycardia

Paroxysmal supraventricular tachycardia is a rhythm disturbance in the infant characterized by heart rates of between 250 and 300 beats per minute (see Fig 20-44). Although short bursts of tachyarrhythmia can be tolerated without clinical difficulty, episodes lasting for 24 hours or more can lead to low-output congestive heart failure. If the arrhythmia occurs in an infant with underlying structural heart disease, tolerance for the rapid heart action is decreased. The diagnosis is established by observing a rapid ventricular response with a normal QRS duration (Fig 20-48). Upon cessation of the tachycardia, one should look for evidence of preexcitation, involving bridges of muscle between the atria and the ventricles so that impulses can reach the ventricles via two pathways, the normal atrioventricular nodal tract and the aberrant pathway. There is early but slow excitation of the ventricles, producing a delta wave and the short PR interval. The QRS interval is prolonged as a result of a delay in ventricular activation via the normal and aberrant pathways.

Treatment of the supraventricular tachycardia requires conversion to a sinus rhythm and prevention of further attacks. The patient with a life-threatening tachyarrhythmia should have an indwelling venous line for the administration of drugs and fluids, and the ECG should be monitored continuously during interventions. Adenosine, administered intravenously, is the principal pharmacologic agent used to manage the tachyarrhythmia acutely. If this drug fails, which is unusual, then synchronized cardioversion should be attempted. Intravenous digoxin has a long record of clinical success, although the drug probably should not be used if preexcitation is known to be present. If the infant is seriously ill and does not respond to adenosine, synchronized cardioversion should be attempted to restore a normal heart rate quickly.

Because recurrences are possible, these infants require oral digoxin therapy as a preventive measure for at least 6 months to 1 year. If digoxin is ineffective in preventing recurrences, agents

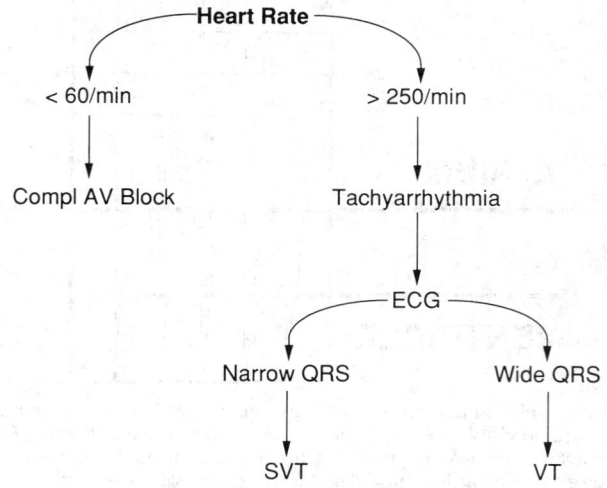

**Figure 20-48.** Decision tree in which heart rate is the entry point. See text for a detailed explanation of management options. *SVT,* supraventricular tachycardia; *VT,* ventricular tachycardia; *AV,* atrioventricular; *ECG,* electrocardiogram.

such as propranolol or quinidine should be considered. The latter agents also are useful if preexcitation is present.

## Ventricular Tachycardia

A tachycardia of ventricular origin is characterized by a wide QRS complex tachyarrhythmia (Fig 20-49). Although supraventricular tachycardia with aberrancy can produce a similar QRS picture, all wide-QRS tachycardias should be considered ventricular in origin until proven otherwise. This tachycardia usually is associated with serious underlying heart disease or overwhelming infection, and it demands prompt therapy. The infant should be placed on a lidocaine drip while the blood pressure is monitored. Cardioversion should be instituted immediately. Rarely, a benign form of ventricular tachycardia has been reported, with no compromise of circulatory performance.

The diagnosis and management of life-threatening arrhythmias requires prompt consultation with a pediatric cardiologist to provide for both acute and long-term management.

## Heart Block

Third-degree (complete) heart block with a heart rate of less than 60 beats per minute usually is congenital in origin (Fig 20-50). It may occur as an isolated event or in association with congenital cardiac disease. There is a strong association between isolated complete heart block and maternal lupus erythematosus. This should be searched for in the mother, even if she does not have manifest disease. Congenital heart block rarely requires a pacemaker or drug therapy, although there may be signs of congestive heart failure before compensatory adjustments to the slow heart rate are made.

## Ectopy in the Newborn

Premature supraventricular or ventricular beats are common. In the absence of underlying heart disease, they usually are benign, disappear during the first weeks of life, and require no therapy. Because there is a slight association with tachyarrhythmias, the infant should be monitored for 24 to 48 hours to determine that tachyarrhythmias or bradyarrhythmias are not occurring. All arrhythmias should have ECG documentation, with 24-hour ECG Holter monitoring usually required. Supraventricular premature beats are characterized by a QRS interval of normal duration,

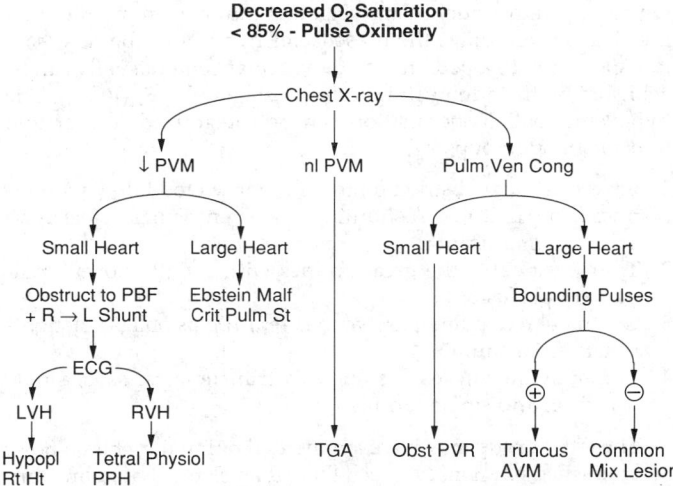

**Figure 20-50.**  Decision tree in which a low oxygen saturation as verified by pulse oximetry is the entry point. See text for a detailed explanation of management options. *PVM,* pulmonary vascular markings; *PBF,* pulmonary blood flow; *pulm ven cong,* pulmonary venous congestion; *Ebstein malf,* Ebstein malformation; *crit pulm st,* critical pulmonic stenosis; *hypopl rt ht,* hypoplastic right heart; *tetral physiol,* tetralogy physiology; *PPH,* persistent pulmonary hypertension; *TGA,* transposition of the great arteries; *obst PVR,* obstruction to pulmonary venous return; *AVM,* arteriovenous malformation; *nl,* normal; *ECG,* electrocardiogram; *R,* right; *L,* left.

with P waves that are distinctly different in shape from the normal P wave. Ventricular ectopy has a wide QRS interval and usually is unifocal. These beats, too, are of no consequence in the absence of underlying heart disease. Multifocal premature beats of ventricular origin are associated with underlying myocardial disease, and carry a guarded prognosis.

## CRITICAL CARDIAC DISEASE IN THE INFANT

Life-threatening cardiac disease in the newborn infant occurs in about 3:1000 live births. Of all cardiac conditions capable of producing cardiac failure or severe hypoxemia that were surveyed in New England, eight conditions accounted for about 75% of the total. These included ventricular septal defects, patent ductus arteriosus, transposition of the great arteries, tetralogy of Fallot, hypoplastic right-heart syndrome (tricuspid and pulmonary atresia), critical pulmonary stenosis with right-to-left atrial shunting, hypoplastic left-heart syndrome, and coarctation of the aorta. When these lesions are classified on the basis of their fundamental physiologic disturbance, they fall into three major categories, which constitute the bulk of the following discussion. These include hypoxemia (transposition, tetralogy, hypoplastic right-heart syndrome, and critical pulmonic stenosis), impaired systemic perfusion (hypoplastic left-heart syndrome and coarctation), and the large-volume left-to-right shunt (ventricular septal defect, patent ductus arteriosus). Additional life-threatening situations of importance in the differential diagnosis of these conditions will be discussed briefly. These include common mixing lesions (single ventricle, common atrium, truncus arteriosus), anomalies of pulmonary venous return, and persistent pulmonary hypertension.

## Hypoxemic States

Patients with severe hypoxemia represent an exceedingly important group with acute life-threatening cardiac disease. The clinical focus is on the degree of cyanosis, with arterial oxygen

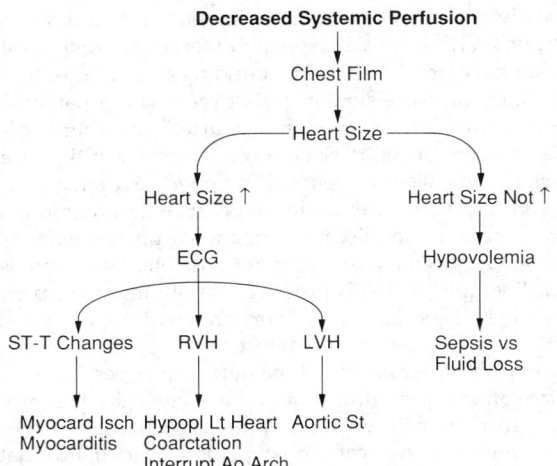

**Figure 20-49.**  Decision tree in which decreased systemic perfusion is the entry point. See text for details of management options. *ECG,* electrocardiogram; *RVH,* right ventricular hypertrophy; *LVH,* left ventricular hypertrophy; *myocard isch,* myocardial ischemia; *hypopl lt heart,* hypoplastic left heart; *interrupt ao arch,* interruption of the aortic arch; *aortic st,* aortic stenosis.

tensions usually under 35 mm Hg. It is extremely important that the clinician recognize the presence of hypoxemia, because safe transportation to a pediatric cardiovascular center usually can be achieved by the administration of prostaglandin E₁ (PGE₁). The hypoxemic patient population can be categorized further into four major subgroups:

1. Severe outflow obstruction to pulmonary blood flow with intracardiac right-to-left shunting (via a ventricular defect or an atrial communication)
2. Transposition of the great arteries with usually normal pulmonary perfusion
3. Obstruction to pulmonary venous return plus obligatory right-to-left atrial shunting
4. Common mixing lesions such as truncus arteriosus, single ventricle, and single atrium.

The latter group may have augmented pulmonary blood flow, or diminished pulmonary flow if there is an element of pulmonary stenosis. The chest film, along with the ECG, pulse oximetry, blood gas tensions, and pH level, provide vital data that usually permit physiologic definition of the patient's problem (Fig 20-51). Echocardiography and cardiac catheterization and selective angiography are required for precise delineation of the lesion(s).

Patients whose hypoxemia is the result of severe obstruction to pulmonary blood flow along with a right-to-left intracardiac shunt include those with tetralogy of Fallot, pulmonary atresia and an intact ventricular septum (right-to-left atrial communication), and tricuspid atresia. The latter two conditions constitute the hypoplastic right-heart syndrome, with the left ventricle being dominant. Lung perfusion is via the ductus arteriosus in the case of pulmonary atresia, and through a ventricular communication or ductus arteriosus with tricuspid atresia.

When pulmonary perfusion is reduced greatly and there is a marked reduction in arterial oxygen tension, the use of PGE₁ infusion to dilate the ductus arteriosus can produce striking improvement in the state of oxygenation in patients with hypoxemia. This can result in correction of metabolic acidemia and stabilization of the clinical state, which in turn will permit safe transportation of the infant to a pediatric cardiovascular center. Infants with severe hypoxemia caused by any of the conditions above require surgical intervention or balloon valvuloplasty to improve pulmonary blood flow (shunt operations, relief of outflow obstruction).

The diagnosis of transposition of the great arteries should be suspected in any infant with a low arterial oxygen tension and a radiographic picture showing normal to slightly increased pulmonary vascularity. With simple transposition, the fundamental problem is impaired intracardiac and extracardiac mixing of the systemic venous and pulmonary venous streams. The result is a systemic circulation of primarily systemic venous blood, while the pulmonary circuit carries the well-oxygenated pulmonary venous return. What limited mixing there is usually takes place at the level of the foramen ovale and ductus arteriosus, but is clearly inadequate. Suspicion of the diagnosis demands immediate echocardiographic confirmation. In the past, these infants were palliated by balloon atrial septostomy followed by an atrial switch operation (Mustard, Senning), usually at around 3 to 6 months of age. More recently, the arterial switch operation has become the operative procedure of choice. This approach is carried out in the first weeks of life, and relatively long-term follow-up indicates excellent results. The pathophysiologic features of the common hypoxemic lesions are shown in Figure 20-51.

Anomalies of pulmonary venous return, particularly if they are associated with pulmonary venous obstruction, must be considered in the differential diagnosis of hypoxemic infants with respiratory distress (lung infection, persistent pulmonary hyper-

tension, and transposition). These anomalies of pulmonary venous connection result developmentally from failure of incorporation of the common pulmonary vein into the left atrium, with persistence of primitive embryonic connections to system veins (cardinal system) or omphalomesenteric veins (portal system), or direct connections to the right atrium. The possibility of pulmonary venous obstruction exists when the abnormal connection is via a long pathway, as in connections to the portal circuit, where two microcirculations must be traversed (pulmonary and hepatic). There also is the possibility of venous obstruction when the connection is supradiaphragmatic as a result of intrinsic pulmonary venous obstruction (stenosis), or when the ascending vertical vein is caught in a hemodynamic vise between the pulmonary artery and the left bronchus.

The only access to the left heart in these conditions with anomalies of pulmonary venous return usually is via the foramen ovale or atrial septal defect. This results in hypoxemia of varying severity. If there is no pulmonary venous obstruction, pulmonary blood flow exceeds systemic flow and arterial desaturation is minimal. Signs of congestive heart failure dominate the clinical picture, and the clinical expression is similar to that encountered in a large-volume left-to-right shunt with a delay in clinical presentation. When pulmonary venous obstruction is present, however, presentation is earlier and hypoxemia is more pronounced. With pulmonary venous obstruction, pulmonary edema is severe because of the entrapment of blood in the pulmonary circuit. This produces the classic radiographic picture of hazy lung fields (lung edema) with a heart that is relatively normal in size (reflecting pulmonary venous entrapment outside the heart; see Fig 20-43).

A slight delay in clinical presentation may occur when the ductus arteriosus remains patent. This will mask the presence of pulmonary venous obstruction, but there will be significant hypoxemia. This condition can be confused with persistent pulmonary hypertension and transposition of the great arteries, and, therefore, demands early and careful echocardiographic assessment to define the pathway of pulmonary venous return and the position of the great arteries.

When a common mixing chamber exists, the clinical picture is dependent on the status of pulmonary and systemic perfusion. For example, if a single ventricle is the basic underlying lesion, the clinical picture will be dominated by hypoxemia if there is obstruction to pulmonary blood flow. Congestive heart failure will develop, however, if pulmonary vascular resistance falls postnatally and there is a large pulmonary blood flow. Infants with truncus arteriosus will have peripheral signs of a runoff into the pulmonary circulation, with bounding arterial pulsations and a wide pulse pressure similar to that seen with a patent ductus arteriosus. Unlike the patent ductus arteriosus, there will be a significant decrease in arterial oxygen tension resulting from the confluence of the well-oxygenated and poorly oxygenated streams at the ventricular and truncal level. Because the common mixing lesions represent complex malformations, precise diagnosis on purely clinical grounds usually is not possible. Two-dimensional echocardiography with Doppler color flow mapping permits a noninvasive diagnosis. Palliative or corrective surgery is in order, depending on the underlying defect.

Pulmonary hypertension of the newborn or persistence of the fetal circulation is a syndrome of multiple etiologies that produces hypoxemia in the first few days of life (see Chapter 20.2.9). This often is confused with certain congenital heart malformations, particularly transposition and anomalies of pulmonary venous return and right ventricular obstruction. It has been associated with neonatal asphyxia, meconium aspiration, diaphragmatic hernias and lung hypoplasia, hyperviscosity states, pneumonia, and lung hemorrhage. A primary disorder of the pulmonary vas-

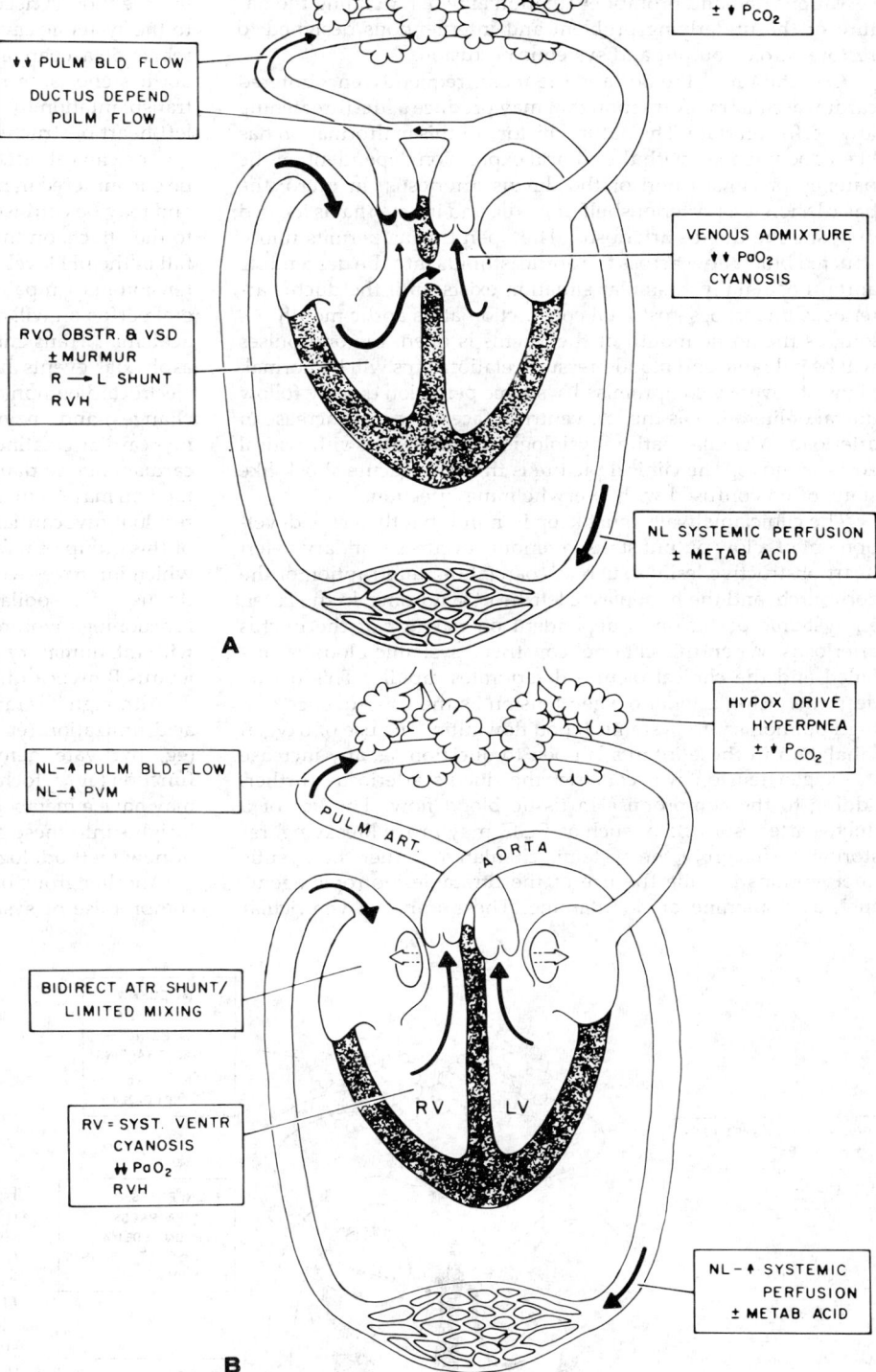

**Figure 20-51.** **(A)** Right-to-left shunt. This diagram shows an example of severe right ventricular outflow obstruction (*RVO obstr*) and a ventricular septal defect (*VSD*). There is limited pulmonary blood flow and mixing of oxygenated pulmonary venous blood with systemic venous blood (venous admixture), resulting in hypoxemia. In the newborn, as shown here, some or all of the effects of hypoxemia on respiratory function and systemic perfusion are shown. **(B)** Transposition of the great arteries. In the presence of transposed great arteries, most of the systemic venous blood returns to the aorta, resulting in an extremely low arterial oxygen tension. Similarly, most of the pulmonary venous blood flow returns to the pulmonary artery, and mixing of the two circulations is limited. In this example, what mixing there is occurs at the level of the atrium and great artery. The resultant effects of severe hypoxemia on ventilation and systemic perfusion are shown. *Hypox,* hypoxemic; *NL,* normal; *ventr,* ventricle; *LV,* left ventricle; *RV,* right ventricle; *art,* artery; *pulm,* pulmonary; *bld,* blood; *R,* right; *L,* left; *RVH,* right ventricular hypertrophy; *PVM,* pulmonary vascular markings. (Talner NS, Lister G. Recognition of critical cardiac disease in the infant. In: Warshaw JB, Hobbins JC, eds. Principles and practice of perinatal medicine—maternal, fetal, and newborn care. Menlo Park, Calif: Addison-Wesley, 1983:371.)

cular bed with increased muscularization of the distal pulmonary vessels has been described. The hypoxemia and pulmonary hypertension are linked closely, with right-to-left shunting via the ductus arteriosus, foramen ovale, or intrapulmonary vessels possible. Because multiple factors produce these physiologic alterations, a precise diagnosis is required. Therefore, an echocardiogram to define the status of the pulmonary venous connection and the position of the great arteries is mandatory.

## Low Perfusion States

Clinical signs of impaired systemic perfusion dominate in the face of critical obstruction of the left heart (coarctation, hypoplastic left-heart syndrome, aortic stenosis), disorders primarily affecting ventricular contractility (myocarditis, cardiomyopathies, birth asphyxia), and situations in which ventricular filling is impaired (tachyarrhythmias, pericardial disease). These signs include diminished pulses, cold extremities, poor capillary refill, and generalized pallor accompanied by a metabolic acidosis. Such observations demand prompt evaluation aimed at defining the nature of the underlying problem and interventions designed to restore cardiac output and systemic perfusion.

Coarctation of the aorta is the most frequently encountered cardiovascular malformation that may produce a life-threatening low perfusion state. The natural history of this malformation has been documented, with the clinical expression dependent on the patency or constriction of the ductus arteriosus. In utero, the basic lesion is a posterior shelf of media and intima that is located opposite the ductus arteriosus. The open ductus permits unobstructed blood flow across the aortic isthmus into the descending aorta. Postnatally, a similar situation exists until the ductus arteriosus undergoes postnatal constriction at its aortic mouth. As long as the aortic mouth of the ductus is open, femoral pulses will be palpable and blood pressure relationships will be normal. Signs of severely compromised systemic perfusion quickly follow ductal obliteration as the left ventricle faces an acute increase in afterload. A similar pathophysiologic picture exists with critical aortic stenosis. The clinical picture is that of an acute shock-like state, often confused with overwhelming infection.

The clinician always must keep in mind that the acute development of a low output state commonly occurs secondary to left heart obstructive lesions such as coarctation, interruption of the aortic arch, and the hypoplastic left-heart syndrome. In the latter, all systemic perfusion is dependent on patency of the ductus arteriosus. When this channel constricts, systemic blood is curtailed and the clinical picture deteriorates rapidly. This occurs despite a rising arterial oxygen tension as the consequence of a high pulmonary-to-systemic blood flow ratio. The use of oxygen inhalation in these infants is open to question, as any increase in oxygen tension will constrict the ductus arteriosus further, adding to the compromise in tissue blood flow. The use of a ductus arteriosus dilator such as $PGE_1$ may prove lifesaving, restoring perfusion of the systemic circulation. Other therapeutic interventions include the use of the titratable inotropic agents such as dopamine or dobutamine. These improve ventricular contractility, which usually is compromised severely, and provide peripheral vasodilatation as well. After the patient is stabilized, intervention is necessary to remove the mechanical obstruction to the systemic circulation. This may take the form of a surgical repair of a coarctation lesion, balloon valvuloplasty in critical aortic stenosis, or radical palliative surgical procedures or heart transplantation for aortic atresia. The pathophysiology of severe left heart obstructive disease is depicted in Figure 20-52.

The clinical picture of diminished systemic perfusion also may be encountered in neonatal states associated with birth asphyxia, and may be confused with the lesions just described. In addition to the effects on the pulmonary circulation (vasoconstriction), a fall in the pH level, elevation of $PaCO_2$, and a decrease in oxygen tension may impair myocardial contractility. As a result, peripheral perfusion will diminish with the development of a metabolic acidemia. Transient myocardial ischemia secondary to neonatal asphyxial events has been described. This is accompanied by electrocardiographic evidence of myocardial ischemia (ST-T wave changes) and enzymatic changes consisting of elevation of the myocardial creatine phosphokinase level that are indicative of cardiac muscle damage. On rare occasions, true myocardial infarction may occur, although usually these infants recover without residual myocardial impairment. Echocardiographic assessment of this group of infants has shown diminished systolic function, which improves with the administration of inotropic agents and the use of vasodilators to decrease the afterload on the poorly functioning myocardium. Similar physiologic abnormalities occur with inflammatory diseases of the myocardium such as coxsackievirus B myocarditis.

Although it is rare, newborns with inherited disorders of fatty acid utilization (eg, carnitine deficiency), pyruvate metabolism (eg, pyruvate dehydrogenase deficiency), and mitochondrial function (eg, cytochrome deficiencies, X-linked cardiomyopathy) may have a metabolic acidemia and low systemic perfusion. New insights into these diseases have been gained by the application of new methodologies in molecular and cellular biology.

Another group of conditions that may present with significant compromise of systemic blood flow are the tachyarrhythmias,

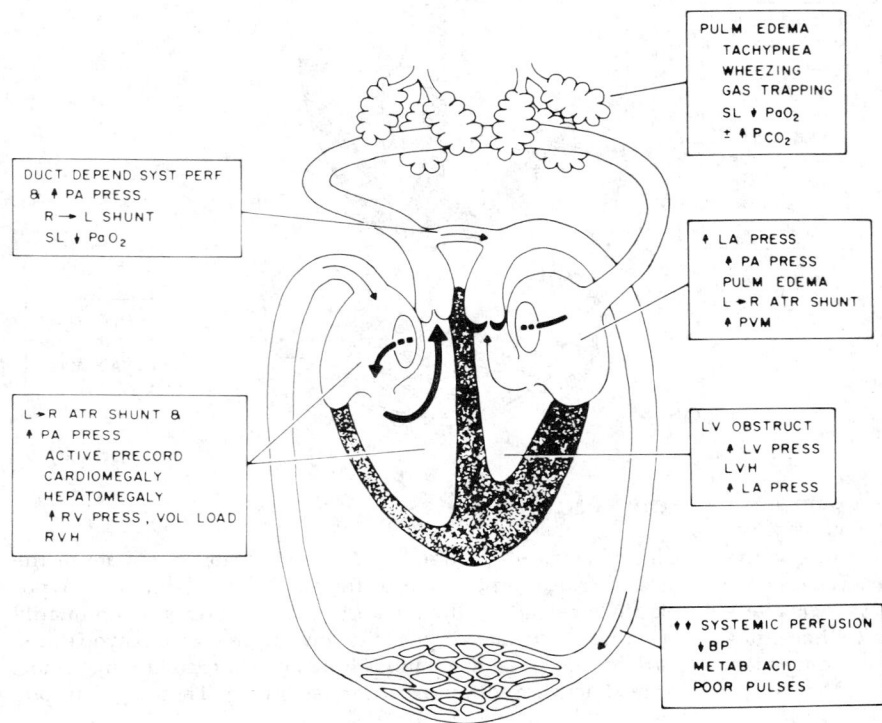

**Figure 20-52.** Left ventricular outflow obstruction (*LV obstruct*). This diagram shows an example of severe left ventricular outflow obstruction produced by critical aortic stenosis. The perfusion is decreased markedly and dependent on the right-to-left (*R → L*) ductus shunting for a portion of the systemic blood flow. The elevated left ventricular end-diastolic and left atrial pressures cause a left-to-right (*L → R*) atrial (foramen ovale) shunt and impaired respiratory function. *Duct depend syst perf,* ductus-dependent systemic perfusion; *atr,* atrial; *BP,* blood pressure; *metab acid,* metabolic acidosis; *Press,* pressure; *PA,* pulmonary artery; *precord,* precordial; *RV,* right ventricle; *LA,* left atrium; *vol,* volume; *RVH,* right ventricular hypertrophy; *pulm,* pulmonary; *LV,* left ventricle; *PVM,* pulmonary vascular markings; *LVH,* left ventricular hypertrophy; *SL,* slightly. (Talner NS, Lister G. Recognition of critical cardiac disease in the infant. In: Warshaw JB, Hobbins JC, eds. *Principles and practice of perinatal medicine—maternal, fetal, and newborn care.* Menlo Park, Calif: Addison-Wesley, 1983:368.)

either supraventricular or ventricular, as described in the section on electrocardiography. Without underlying heart disease, a heart rate of between 280 and 300 beats per minute can be tolerated for about 24 hours, after which systemic perfusion is impaired critically as a result of inadequate ventricular filling.

Pericardial disease, usually inflammatory or with tumors, also can produce signs of low perfusion secondary to the rapid accumulation of fluid in the pericardial sac that interferes with cardiac filling. Cardiac tamponade can be recognized by a decrease in, or loss of, peripheral pulses with inspiration, with a return of pulse volume on expiration. Diagnosis is confirmed by echocardiography, after which fluid must be evacuated from the pericardial space. The material should be gram-stained and cultured, and appropriate surgical drainage should be provided. Tumors of the pericardium may produce a similar picture.

## ALGORITHM FOR CRITICAL CARDIAC DISEASE IN THE NEWBORN

In an attempt to aid the clinician in detecting and stabilizing the newborn infant who may have critical cardiac disease, we have developed three algorithms, each of which focuses on a specific clinical problem previously discussed that may prove life-threatening to the infant. These include alterations in heart rate, the presence of cyanosis as verified by pulse oximetry, and decreased systemic perfusion. If the clinician will follow the decision tree pathway outlined in these algorithms, the key high-risk situations usually can be sorted out and appropriate management undertaken.

If the heart rate is less than 60 beats per minute or greater than 250 beats per minute, an ECG must be obtained. A rate under 50 beats per minute is associated most commonly with complete atrioventricular block and the presence of antiRo or antiLa immune responses. Although these infants rarely require pacing, they must be in a cardiovascular center where cardiologic evaluation can be pursued and, if necessary, a pacemaker inserted so that adequate perfusion can be obtained. If the heart rate is less than 40 beats per minute, an infusion of isoproterenol is required to provide a satisfactory output before pacemaker insertion.

With heart rates greater than 250 beats per minute, the most likely diagnosis is supraventricular tachycardia. The QRS is normal in this situation. As cited previously, intravenous adenosine is the treatment of choice, followed by digoxin as the agent for preventing recurrences. If there is a wide-complex tachycardia, this must be assumed to be ventricular tachycardia. Appropriate management in this situation is dependent on the infant's status. When perfusion is compromised acutely, direct-current cardioversion is necessary after placement of an intravenous line and infusion of lidocaine. The presence of ventricular tachycardia usually is associated with significant underlying heart disease such as myocarditis; therefore, management is complex and should be performed at a regional cardiovascular center. Rarely, the infant may have no change in circulatory dynamics, despite a persistent ventricular tachycardia. Nevertheless, these infants need precise electrophysiologic evaluation and possibly pharmacologic treatment.

When the presenting problem is cyanosis as verified by pulse oximetry, a chest film must be obtained primarily to assess pulmonary vascularity. If the pulmonary vascular markings are reduced, the fundamental physiologic abnormality is obstruction to pulmonary blood flow with a right-to-left shunt. An ECG permits delineation between the hypoplastic right heart, such as pulmonary or tricuspid atresia (left ventricular hypertrophy), and tetralogy physiology with right ventricular dominance. We recognize that some infants have persistent pulmonary hypertension

with right-to-left shunting via fetal flow channels. Nevertheless, these infants must be assessed at a regional center as well, and they need echocardiography to rule out a cardiac cause for the elevated pulmonary vascular resistance. If the pulmonary vascular markings are decreased in the face of massive cardiac enlargement, then Ebstein's malformation of the tricuspid valve or critical pulmonary valve stenosis should be considered.

When the pulmonary vascular markings are normal in association with a low $O_2$ saturation, transposition of the great arteries must be considered, particularly if the $O_2$ saturation is less than 65%. On the other hand, if the heart is small, but there is prominent pulmonary venous congestion, then the diagnosis of obstructed pulmonary venous return with right-to-left atrial shunting should be entertained.

With each of these hypoxemic states discussed above, an improvement in $O_2$ saturation can be improved by the intravenous administration of $PGE_1$. These infants usually require ventilation for transport and venous access by which to administer the pharmacologic agent and to provide volume if the systemic blood pressure falls. Irrespective of the diagnosis, the use of $PGE_1$ should stabilize the infant, as long as volume is provided as necessary to maintain systemic perfusion.

When there is cardiac enlargement and prominent pulmonary vascular markings in the face of an element of hypoxemia, a common mixing lesion such as truncus arteriosus or single ventricle, or a large arteriovenous malformation should be considered. If the pulses are prominent, truncus arteriosus or an arteriovenous malformation are distinct possibilities. Presentation within the first few hours with a large heart should encourage a search for a cranial or hepatic bruit. This latter group does not require $PGE_1$ for transport, but needs to be moved to a cardiac center for diagnosis and management.

The third high-risk situation concerns those infants with clinical signs of low systemic perfusion. For these patients, the differential diagnosis rests between a primary cardiovascular problem and hypovolemia, perhaps in association with septicemia. The chest film is an extremely helpful clinical aid. If there is cardiomegaly and lung congestion, then left heart obstructive lesions or myopericardial disease are likely to be present. When the heart size is normal, hypovolemia is likely, with sepsis being an important consideration.

The ECG provides additional data on which to base a specific diagnosis. Primary ST-T wave changes raise the possibility of myocardial ischemia, usually secondary to birth asphyxia. Myocardial enzymes should be determined as verification of myocardial damage. Right ventricular hypertrophy in association with low systemic perfusion is seen with hypoplastic left-heart syndrome, coarctation of the aorta, and interruption of the aortic arch. Left ventricular hypertrophy may be seen with critical aortic stenosis, as obstruction was taking place in utero and left ventricular hypertrophy ensued. With hypoplastic left heart, coarctation, and interruption of the aorta, no obstruction takes place until the ductus arteriosus constricts and, therefore, insufficient time has elapsed for ventricular hypertrophy to develop.

Stabilization and transport of this group of infants also requires venous access, withdrawal of blood for blood gas determinations and pH levels, and blood cultures to rule out a septic process. $PGE_1$ can be administered safely via an umbilical venous line to dilate the ductus arteriosus and improve systemic perfusion. Caution regarding the use of oxygen again is in order, because the ductus can be constricted as oxygen tension rises, which will compromise systemic perfusion further.

Ventilatory support is necessary in this group because apnea may occur with $PGE_1$ administration. We feel that antibiotic coverage with ampicillin and gentamicin is appropriate until a septic process has been ruled out. Myocardial support is provided best by an infusion of dopamine or dobutamine.

## The Large-Volume Left-to-Right Shunt

In contrast to the acute life-threatening situations just discussed, the clinical problems that are secondary to a large communication at the ventricular or great artery level develop gradually over the first months of life as a result of the postnatal fall in pulmonary vascular resistance, which permits a large increment in pulmonary blood flow. This occurs in response to remodeling of the pulmonary vascular bed, with an increase in lumen diameter and a decrease in blood viscosity as hemoglobin levels diminish. As pulmonary blood flow increases, the major clinical manifestations become apparent and reflect altered respiratory function. The accumulation of water in the pulmonary interstitial space, the site of the initial leak of fluid from the pulmonary capillary bed, is responsible for the pattern of respiration (tachypnea). At this point in the pathophysiologic process, there may be no fluid in the alveolar spaces and, thus, rales will be absent. Therefore, the only sign of interstitial pulmonary edema is an increase in respiratory frequency. This is thought to represent stimulation of juxtacapillary receptors in the pulmonary interstitial space. The clearance of lung water is via peribronchiolar and perivascular spaces into pulmonary lymphatics and finally into systemic veins. When fluid accumulation is excessive in terms of amount and rate of formation, the alveolar spaces are invaded and gas exchange is compromised, at first by an increase in the alveolar–arterial oxygen tension difference and later by a rise in carbon dioxide tension.

As clearance of lung water takes place, encroachment on the lumina of bronchioles can produce alterations in small airway resistance, manifested clinically by an increase in respiratory effort and wheezing. Large airways (bronchi) also may be involved in the face of a large left-to-right shunt. Significant bronchial compression by hypertensive, volume-distended pulmonary arteries and an enlarged left atrium and ventricle has been noted. The sites of predilection are the left main stem bronchus and the left upper and right middle lobe bronchi. Lobar atelectasis and obstructive emphysema secondary to these compressive effects can contribute to impairment of gas exchange, which then can effect an increase in pulmonary vascular resistance. In addition, secondary infection may occur at sites of compromised fluid drainage. The increase in the work of breathing raises oxygen requirements for these infants at the same time that the respiratory problems interfere with feeding. The result is a decrease in intake at a time when metabolic requirements are elevated. All these factors may contribute to the failure of these infants to grow.

Although respiratory signs tend to dominate the clinical picture, there are major alterations in the performance of the heart and systemic circulation as well. Systolic function of the myocardium usually is normal to supranormal. This is the result of increased adrenergic support, as evidenced by an increased heart rate and contractility, and by elevated levels of circulating catecholamines. A high cardiac output state exists, with most of the output flowing from the left to the right into the pulmonary circulation.

The systemic circulation also is altered by the left-to-right shunt. There is a redistribution of systemic blood flow, with perfusion of the skin, kidneys, and gastrointestinal tract potentially decreased by regional vasoconstriction. From the clinical standpoint, this is manifest as skin pallor and reduced urine formation. Compromise of mesenteric blood flow may result in ischemic gut necrosis, particularly in the preterm infant with a large patent ductus arteriosus. Peripheral vasoconstriction occurs as part of the increased adrenergic response that appears to redistribute cardiac output to the more vital organ systems (myocardium, brain).

The overall metabolic response to a large left-to-right shunt is variable. Initially, these infants may be hypermetabolic, creating a situation in which demands are increased in the face of limited supply. In the more chronic stages, oxygen consumption may fall, indicating severe compromise of oxygen supply.

There also are a number of compensatory mechanisms that operate in the face of the large-volume left-to-right shunt. These include the previously cited increase in adrenergic activity, the renin-angiotensin-aldosterone support mechanism, atrial natriuretic peptide, and alterations in the oxygen affinity of red blood cells. The adrenergic mechanisms result in tachycardia and enhanced contractility ($\beta_1$ effect), and the redistribution of cardiac output represents peripheral vasoconstriction ($\delta^1$ effect). The renin-angiotensin-aldosterone system triggered by a decrease in renal perfusion represents an attempt to preserve systemic volume. This decrease in renal perfusion leads to angiotensin formation, which, acting on the renal cortex, results in the production of aldosterone. Salt and water retention occurs in an attempt to preserve intravascular volume. The release of atrial natriuretic factor consequent to atrial distention in these patients may result in diuresis, but the exact function of this substance remains to be delineated. Oxygen delivery can be enhanced by alterations in red blood cell 2–3 DPG. This results in increased release of oxygen to the tissues at any given level of oxygen saturation.

Figure 20-53 depicts the pathophysiology of a large-volume left-to-right shunt at the ventricular level (a large patent ductus arteriosus would be similar), incorporating the material covered in this section.

## SPECIAL PROBLEMS IN MANAGEMENT

### Congestive Heart Failure

Treatment of congestive heart failure in the newborn must take into consideration the age-related differences in myocardial performance cited previously (which may influence the adaptation of the cardiovascular system), possible developmental differences in the response to pharmacologic agents, and the potential modulating influences of the fetal flow pathways and the pulmonary circulation. Appropriate management requires a precise anatomic and physiologic diagnosis, and may require support of lung as well as cardiac function; in many instances, reparative or palliative surgical procedures, or an interventional catheterization will be required to save the infant.

Congestive heart failure in the fetus is manifest as hydrops fetalis. As mentioned previously, this can arise from regurgitant lesions of the right-sided atrioventricular or semilunar valves, large systemic arteriovenous fistulas, myocardial disease, severe anemia, and prolonged tachyarrhythmias. Systemic venous congestion from the elevated right-sided filling pressures and volumes results in hepatomegaly and the accumulation of fluid in serous cavities, and may progress to generalized anasarca. Although the overall prognosis for survival when hydrops develops is poor, some infants have been salvaged by transplacental therapy of life-threatening cardiac arrhythmias with digoxin, propranolol, or procainamide. Intrauterine transfusions also have improved the hemodynamic status of fetuses with severe hemolytic disease.

In preterm infants, particularly those with birth weights less than 1500 g, patency of the ductus arteriosus can produce the clinical picture of congestive heart failure and complicate treatment of the respiratory distress syndrome. The classic clinical findings (bounding arterial pulsations, continuous murmur) may be absent in these infants, and diagnosis may rest on Doppler-derived flow-velocity determinations demonstrating left-to-right shunting via the ductus into the pulmonary artery. Management of the problem in these infants consists of the intravenous administration of indomethacin, which inhibits prostaglandin syn-

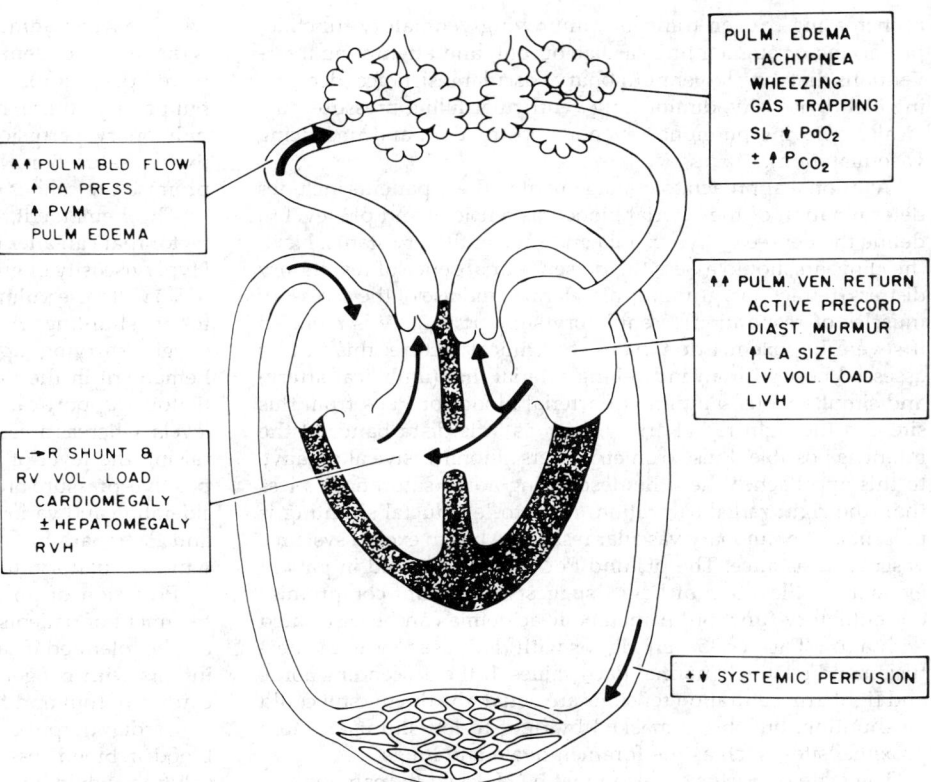

**Figure 20-53.** Large-volume left-to-right shunt. This figure shows the pathophysiologic consequences of cardiac malformations in the neonate. Flow of blood through the heart and the systemic and pulmonary circulations is shown by the *large arrows*, and the relative volume of flow is shown by the width of the arrows. This diagram is an example of a large left-to-right shunt at the ventricular level causing excessive pulmonary blood flow and pulmonary venous return. There is compromised respiratory function, along with extra demands on the ventricles and potentially inadequate systemic perfusion. ↑, increased; ↓, decreased; *pulm*, pulmonary; *bld*, blood; *PA*, pulmonary arterial; *press*, pressure; *PVM*, pulmonary vascular markings; *L → R*, left-to-right; *RV vol*, right ventricular volume; *RVH*, right ventricular hypertrophy; *SL*, slightly; ±, occasionally; *ven*, venous; *precord*, precordium; *diast*, diastolic; *LA*, left atrial; *LV vol*, left ventricular volume; *LVH*, left ventricular hypertrophy. (Talner NS, Lister G. The recognition of critical cardiac disease in the infant. In: Warshaw JB, Hobbins JC, eds. Pathophysiology of cardiac disease in the infant. Menlo Park, Calif: Addison-Wesley, 1983:366.)

thesis, if platelet counts are adequate and renal function is intact. In instances in which a course of indomethacin therapy does not produce ductal closure (<15%), surgical ligation is necessary.

When congestive failure accompanies a low perfusion state (coarctation, hypoplastic left heart), with systemic blood flow dependent on continued patency of the ductus arteriosus, the administration of $PGE_1$, which will dilate the ductus arteriosus, can restore tissue perfusion, as described previously. Restoration of systemic perfusion is the key.

Congestive heart failure is encountered most frequently in infants with large-volume left-to-right shunts (ventricular septal defects, atrioventricular canal defects, patent ductus arteriosus). Treatment of these infants requires interventions to lessen pulmonary and systemic venous congestion while attempts are made to improve systemic blood flow to allow for body growth. Furosemide is the diuretic agent used most widely to promote salt and water loss, and it may be required 2 to 3 times a day in the management of severe pulmonary edema. Spironolactone is a valuable adjunct to diuretic therapy, as it tends to reduce potassium loss. Serum electrolyte levels must be monitored when the loop diuretics are used on a frequent basis.

The use of cardiac glycosides in the treatment of the high-output congestive heart failure that accompanies a large-volume left-to-right shunt is somewhat controversial. Because myocardial contractility is not impaired, the need for an inotropic agent has been challenged. Nevertheless, more than 50% of these infants appear to improve clinically. This may be explained on the basis of withdrawal of adrenergic support, thus decreasing oxygen demands. Supporting this hypothesis is the fall in oxygen consumption that is seen in some patients with a favorable clinical response to cardiac glycosides, along with a decrease in the levels of circulating catecholamines.

Vasodilator therapy also has been introduced into the management schema for infants with large ventricular or atrioventricular septal defects and dilated congestive cardiomyopathies. With vasodilatation and a lessening of left ventricular afterload,

the left-to-right shunt, if present, may diminish, whereas systemic blood flow increases. Vasodilators in clinical use include sodium nitroprusside, hydralazine, and angiotensin converting enzyme inhibitors. Supportive measures for these infants include oxygen administration, maintenance of a semi-upright position, correction of relative anemia, intravenous hyperalimentation, and, possibly, the use of a ventilator if respiratory failure is present. A poor clinical response warrants early surgical repair of the defect.

Infants with a dilated cardiomyopathy should be evaluated for the presence of carnitine deficiency (serum, skeletal muscle), as replacement therapy with L-carnitine may be lifesaving by restoring myocardial oxidative function. In other situations, the ultimate management may be heart transplantation.

## Persistent Pulmonary Hypertension

Elevation of pulmonary artery pressures and an increase in pulmonary vascular resistance can complicate the management of some of the clinical problems encountered during the newborn period. Persistent pulmonary hypertension may occur rarely as a primary abnormality of the pulmonary vascular bed or be seen accompanying pulmonary disorders (infections, lung hypoplasia, respiratory distress syndrome), diaphragmatic hernias, and certain congenital and acquired cardiac diseases such as large-volume left-to-right shunts, anomalies of pulmonary venous return with pulmonary venous obstruction, and cardiomyopathies. It has become apparent that chronic intrauterine asphyxia can produce structural alterations in the pulmonary vascular bed, which may result in significant postnatal problems in oxygenation resulting from a restricted pulmonary circulation and persistent right-to-left shunting via fetal flow channels. Meconium aspiration at delivery may be only the terminal event in a more chronic intrauterine asphyxial state. This is discussed in detail in Chapter 20.2.8.

The treatment of these infants rests on establishing the underlying diagnosis and employing therapeutic strategies aimed at increasing oxygen transport, improving ventilatory function, preserving or augmenting cardiac output, and attempting interventions that may lower pulmonary vascular resistance (decreasing blood viscosity, diminishing ventricular filling pressure, surgically relieving pulmonary venous obstruction, and producing vasodilatation).

A rational approach to management in these patients includes determination of the arterial blood gas tensions and pH level to define the degree of hypoxemia and the ventilatory status. Next, the clinician should assess the presence or absence of respiratory distress (retractions, grunting, alar flaring, and use of the accessory muscles of respiration). Ventilatory support usually is required if severe hypoxemia dominates the clinical picture; this can be assessed best with an indwelling arterial line (umbilical artery) and simultaneous sampling of arterial blood for $PaO_2$ from this site and the right radial artery, with as little disturbance of the infant as possible. Pulse oximetry offers a noninvasive alternative to this approach. When the descending aortic saturation is less than the right radial saturation, right-to-left ductal shunting is present and pulmonary vascular resistance has to exceed systemic vascular resistance. The pH and $PCO_2$ values also aid in patient evaluation. Elevation of $PaCO_2$ suggests significant compromise of ventilatory function. A metabolic acidemia can be associated with a low $PaO_2$ (<35 mm Hg) or with decreased systemic perfusion and relatively normal $PaO_2$ values. If the descending aortic and right arm saturation tensions are equal, the ductus still could be shunting, but this is masked by right-to-left shunts at more proximal sites, such as the foramen ovale and lungs.

The state of perfusion also must be checked by palpation of the peripheral arterial pulses, capillary refill, and skin temperature. If perfusion is compromised, management must include provision of volume and inotropic support to restore perfusion of regional circulations. If perfusion and ventilation are not compromised, the clinician can proceed directly to determination of the site of right-to-left shunting.

The hyperoxia test (response to $FIO_2$ 1.0) has been touted as a way to separate a cardiac problem from one involving the lungs or pulmonary circulation. Interpretation of an increase in $O_2$ tension or saturation is fraught with error. Impressive increments have been observed in the face of cardiac disease, and little or no response in association with severe lung disease. Therefore, it is recommended that part of the assessment include an echocardiogram performed by a cardiologist who is experienced in the evaluation of critically ill newborns before vasodilator therapy is instituted.

A chest film focused on heart size, lung vascularity, and other malformations (eg, diaphragmatic hernia) is useful as part of the clinical evaluation. An ECG examined for evidence of myocardial ischemia (ST-T wave changes) and enzyme levels (myocardial creatine phosphokinase) also can aid in establishing a specific diagnosis.

Treatment of these patients is based on approaches aimed at raising arterial oxygen content and tension. The latter are functions of the following variables: pulmonary capillary oxygen content, cardiac output, the right-to-left shunt, and oxygen extraction. Each of these is capable of being manipulated, given that a change in one of these factors may influence one of the other variables. For example, increasing $PaO_2$ by positive-pressure ventilation may impede venous return and diminish cardiac output. On the other hand, raising cardiac output (eg, with inotropic agents) may increase metabolic demands and intrapulmonary right-to-left shunting.

Raising the inspired oxygen concentration may have a number of beneficial effects. An increase in dissolved oxygen permits about a 10% rise in oxygen saturation, even in the face of a fixed right-to-left shunt. Furthermore, oxygen is capable of dilating constricted pulmonary resistance vessels. The only situation in which oxygen administration may be deleterious is when there is ductal-dependent systemic blood flow (see the section on impaired perfusion). This will *not* take place in conditions such as pulmonary atresia, however, in which there is ductal-dependent pulmonary perfusion because pulmonary flow is limited, and oxygen saturation will rise only minimally—not enough to compromise the caliber of the ductus.

The hematocrit, by its effect on blood viscosity, is another factor that can alter the response of the pulmonary vascular bed. Hyperviscosity of greater than 65% (a hematocrit of greater than 65%) will raise pulmonary vascular resistance and increase right-to-left shunting. A low hematocrit, on the other hand, limits oxygen-carrying capacity. Therefore, it is appropriate to keep the hematocrit in the range of 40% to 50%. The provision of ventilatory support can lower an elevated $PaCO_2$ to normal or low levels, whereas areas of alveolar collapse may be inflated, thereby raising the level of $PaO_2$. If the potential deleterious effects of positive-pressure breathing on cardiac output are taken into consideration and various ventilatory maneuvers are tried while $PaO_2$ and $PaCO_2$ are monitored, an increase in $PaO_2$ can be achieved while circulatory function is maintained.

Provision of an adequate cardiac output is essential in the treatment of patients with severe hypoxemia. Hypoxemia usually can be tolerated if cardiac output is maintained, as in the case of infants with congenital heart disease. The combination of low cardiac output and hypoxemia, however, cannot be tolerated.

Cardiac output can be increased by volume infusions of whole blood if blood loss is a problem, or of electrolyte or albumin solutions when hemoglobin does not have to be replaced. If contractility is decreased, as assessed through echocardiographic evaluation, an inotropic agent such as dopamine or dobutamine should be administered. These have primarily $\beta_1$-receptor function (increased contractility and vasodilatation), and cause little change in heart rate.

The vasodilator tolazoline has had considerable use in the treatment of infants with persistent pulmonary hypertension, with varying degrees of success. The major risk of such therapy relates to the possibility of producing systemic hypotension, thereby worsening the clinical picture. Furthermore, its injudicious use in patients whose hypoxemia is on a cardiac basis (ductal-dependent pulmonary blood flow) can induce further right-to-left shunting and worsen the metabolic status.

Reduction in right-to-left shunt flow may be achieved by improving ventilation, particularly in those with impaired ventilation and stiff lungs. Oxygen extraction may be decreased by diminishing oxygen demands or by lessening the work of breathing and decreasing overall metabolic demands.

Conservative management consisting of some, but not a marked degree, of hyperventilation, provision of adequate volume, support of the myocardium, and increased inspired oxygen concentrations appears to result in reasonable survival data. Recent experience with extracorporeal membrane oxygenation also has yielded encouraging results, but that approach is expensive, requires specialized personnel, and has raised concern relative to the long-term central nervous system effects of ligation of a carotid artery, which is required for the procedure. The introduction of inhaled nitric oxide, a potent vasodilator, offers a novel approach to disorders of the pulmonary circulation, but large clinical trials are needed before this becomes the preferred approach.

## Other Cardiac Problems in the Infant

The infant of a diabetic mother may have cardiac involvement, particularly if the diabetes is under poor control. In addition to a higher than normal incidence of congenital heart disease, there may be the development in utero of a hypertrophic cardiomyopathy. This cardiac abnormality can be diagnosed by two-dimensional echocardiography. Of further interest is the fact that the pathologic process is reversible postnatally, usually within 6 months. Therapy with a $\beta$-receptor blocking agent rarely is required unless the infant has significant left ventricular outflow obstruction and compromised systemic perfusion.

## Endocrine Disorders With Cardiac Manifestations

Certain endocrinopathies are associated with cardiovascular manifestations. Hypothyroidism may be accompanied by cardiomegaly, decreased contractility, and bradycardia. Signs of cardiac involvement abate when replacement therapy with thyroid hormone is instituted. Tachycardia, increased contractility, bounding pulses, and tachyarrhythmias have been noted in infants of mothers being treated for hyperthyroidism because of high levels of long-acting thyroid-stimulating hormone.

Salt-losing adrenogenital syndrome with high serum potassium levels has been linked to cardiomegaly and decreased contractility. Myocardial function improves as the endocrine disorder is controlled. In addition, hypocalcemia accompanying parathyroid absence can impair cardiac performance, with contractility increasing as the level of ionized calcium is raised.

## Airway Obstruction With Vascular Malformations

Infants with certain vascular rings, slings, and dilated pulmonary arteries may have clinical signs of large airway obstruction, such as hoarseness, stridor, cough, and respiratory distress. These include double aortic arch, right aortic arch with left ductus arteriosus or ligamentum, and the pulmonary artery sling with the left pulmonary artery taking its origin from the right and crossing between the trachea and esophagus, thereby producing compromise of the tracheal lumen. Infants with the absent pulmonary valve syndrome or with marked pulmonary valve insufficiency have massively dilated pulmonary arteries, which results in tracheobronchial compression and a clinical picture dominated by manifestations of airway obstruction. When such manifestations are observed, diagnosis usually can be established by echocardiography with attention to great artery position and, more recently, by magnetic resonance imaging. Prompt surgical intervention is required to remove the obstructing vascular structure. It should be emphasized, however, that removal of the offending vascular structure will not eliminate immediately all signs of airway compromise; prolonged ventilatory support sometimes is required until the airway becomes more rigid.

## The Trivial Congenital Defect

The approach to the newborn infant who has a significant cardiac murmur but is entirely asymptomatic, with normal perfusion, respiratory pattern, and oxygenation, still requires additional noninvasive studies until the diagnosis (eg, a small ventricular defect or mild aortic or pulmonary stenosis) is established firmly. This usually involves obtaining an ECG and an echocardiographic and Doppler assessment of these infants so that the parents can be reassured as to the specific nature of their infant's defect. Further follow-up is necessary, however, to assess for spontaneous closure of ventricular defects and possible progression of any obstruction.

## SUMMARY

An approach to the newborn infant with heart disease has been developed that takes into consideration the potential influences of the fetal flow pathways, developmental changes in the pulmonary circulation, fundamental differences between developing and mature cardiac muscle, and possible deleterious effects on the transitional circulation of birth asphyxia, altered blood viscosity, and certain cardiovascular malformations. The common high-risk congenital cardiac defects have been classified on the basis of their primary functional abnormality (ie, hypoxemia, low perfusion state, and large-volume left-to-right shunt). Potential life-threatening disturbances in cardiac rhythm have been considered. Decision trees have been developed for the acute life-threatening situations.

The various laboratory aids to clinical diagnosis have been considered (eg, chest film, blood gas and pH levels, ECG). Finally, special problems that affect patient treatment, such as congestive heart failure and pulmonary hypertension, have been discussed.

This pathophysiologic approach on the part of the clinician should lead to prompt recognition of the at-risk infant, correct functional diagnosis, adequate stabilization, and appropriate medical and surgical interventions.

## Selected Readings

Anderson PAW. Physiology of the fetal, neonatal, and adult heart. In: Polin RA, Fox WW, eds. Fetal and neonatal physiology, vol I. Philadelphia: Saunders, 1992:722.

Anderson RH. Another look at cardiac embryology. In: Yu PN, Goodwin JF, eds. Progress in cardiology. Philadelphia: Lea & Febiger, 1978:1.

Friedman WF. Physiological properties of the developing heart. In: Marcelletti C, Anderson RH, Becker AE, et al. Pediatric cardiology, vol 6. Edinburgh: Churchill-Livingstone, 1986:3.

Garson A Jr. The electrocardiogram in infants and children—a systematic approach. Philadelphia: Lea & Febiger, 1983.

Kirby ML. Cardiac morphogenesis—recent research advances. Pediatr Res 1987;21:219.

Lister G. Persistent pulmonary hypertension of the newborn. In: Nelson NM, ed. Current therapy in neonatal-perinatal medicine. Philadelphia: BC Decker, 1985:278.

Rabinovitch M. Developmental biology of the pulmonary vascular bed. In: Freedom RM, Berson LN, Smallhorn JF, eds. Neonatal heart disease. London: Springer-Verlag, 1992:45.

Rose V, Clark E. Etiology of congenital heart disease. In: Freedom RM, Benson LN, Smallhorn JF, eds. Neonatal heart disease. London: Springer-Verlag, 1992:3.

Rudolph AM. Distribution and regulation of blood flow in the fetal and neonatal lamb. Circ Res 1985;57:811.

Talner NS, Lister G. The recognition of critical cardiac disease in the infant. In: Warshaw JB, Hobbins JC, eds. Principles and practice of perinatal medicine: Maternal-fetal and newborn care. Menlo Park, Calif: Addison-Wesley, 1983:363.

Teitel DW: Physiologic development of the cardiovascular system of the fetus. In: Polin RA, Fox WW, eds. Fetal and neonatal physiology, vol I. Philadelphia: Saunders, 1992:609.

*Principles and Practice of Pediatrics, Second Edition.*
edited by Frank A. Oski et al. J. B. Lippincott Company, Philadelphia © 1994.

# 20.4 *Gastrointestinal Diseases*

## 20.4.1 *Developmental Disorders of Gastrointestinal Function*

William M. Belknap and Colston McEvoy

## EMBRYOLOGY

Structural developmental anomalies are important causes of neonatal gastrointestinal disease. Several fundamental processes must occur during fetal development for normal intestinal structure to be present at birth (Table 20-17). Failure of these developmental events to occur may result in major defects in gut structure and function.

The primitive gut at 4 weeks' gestation is a hollow tube from mouth to cloaca and is subdivided into foregut, midgut, and hindgut. At 5 weeks' gestation, the cranial foregut separates longitudinally to become the trachea and the esophagus. During the fifth week of gestation, the stomach begins as a foregut dilatation just caudal to the lung buds. The duodenum forms by a fusion of the distal foregut and the first segment of the midgut just beyond the ampulla of Vater; it then rotates to the right and becomes fixed posteriorly in the retroperitoneum as a C-shaped loop. At this time, the duodenal lumen is obliterated temporarily by an overgrowth of lining cells. The remainder of fetal gut becomes the small and large intestines.

At 5 to 10 weeks' gestation, the intestinal loop grows faster than does the fetal body and must be projected outside of it through the umbilicus to achieve its normal length. A proper sequence of return of the gut to the abdomen with fixation of its mesentery to the fetal abdominal cavity is crucial. This is accomplished by fetal gut rotation counterclockwise through a 270° arc on its vascular axis; this process is completed by 20 weeks' gestation. During rotation, the gut returns to the fetal abdomen for positioning in the following sequence. First, the proximal jejunum fixes to the left upper quadrant. Second, subsequent loops enter and settle on the right side. The cecum enters last, and then descends to the right lower quadrant and fixes posteriorly to the abdominal wall. The descent of the cecum is associated with

completion of ascending and descending colons, and with the establishment of the small-intestine mesentery from the duodenojejunal junction to the ileocecal junction. At 4 weeks' gestation, the hindgut is joined to the allantois and the hindgut–allantois junction becomes the cloaca and cloacal membrane. In the sixth week of gestation, the cloaca divides with a septum in a process similar to the separation of esophagus and trachea. The dorsal compartment becomes the rectum and the ventral compartment becomes the urogenital sinus; by the ninth week of gestation, the definitive rectum and anus have been formed.

The solid parenchymal organs of the gastrointestinal tract, the liver and pancreas, begin as endodermal buds from the primitive foregut in the fourth week of gestation. The ducts of these secretory digestive glands are joined to the proximal gut very early in development. The liver bud will express three secondary buds: a cranial bud becomes the liver, a caudal bud becomes the gallbladder and extrahepatic biliary tree, and a more proximal segment becomes the ventral pancreas. The intrahepatic biliary tree forms at 6 weeks' gestation; the extrahepatic ductal system canalizes from solid epithelial cords by week 7. The pancreas develops from two buds, the aforementioned ventral pancreas and the dorsal pancreas. Both have central linear ducts; the dorsal pancreatic duct is connected to and opens into the duodenum, whereas the ventral duct remains associated with the common bile duct throughout development. As the two pancreatic anlage fuse, their ducts join to form the main pancreatic duct near the ampulla of Vater.

The maturation of a given digestive organ's function can be traced through development by identifying its differentiated cells and defining the times of expression of tissue-specific proteins during gestation (Tables 20-18, 20-19). The fetal gut begins as a hollow tube of endoderm, the epithelial cells of which become gastric cells, enterocytes, colonic cells, and all associated glands. An encasement of mesoderm supplies connective tissue, mesoderm, and peritoneum. At 5 to 6 weeks' gestation, the epithelium proliferates and forms villi; by 12 weeks, the entire gut is lined by fetal villi. Although villous growth and cell differentiation begin early in fetal life, the complete complement of villi and glands is not attained until childhood.

The digestive proteins of intestinal mucosal cells also are expressed during this time (see Table 20-19). Among the disaccharidases, sucrase appears first at 8 weeks' gestation; the remainder, with one exception, achieve adult levels by 10 to 11 weeks' gestation. Lactase, which is at a low level in the fetal gut before 24 weeks' gestation, increases to levels greater than those in the adult by 40 weeks' gestation. Innervation of this differentiating fetal gut occurs in a cranial–caudal progression that begins in week 6 and is completed by week 12. Neuroblasts, originating from the neural crest, migrate along the entire length

### TABLE 20-17. Principles of Normal Gut Development and Major Developmental Anomalies

| Principle | Developmental Mechanism | Developmental Anomaly |
|---|---|---|
| Growth | Gut elongation, rotation, and mesenteric fixation | Malrotation |
| Lumen formation | Recanalization from solid cell phase | Duodenal atresia, stenosis |
| Separation | Proximal: pulmonary tract | Tracheoesophageal fistula |
| | Distal: genitourinary tract (formation of rectum and anus) | Exstrophy, imperforate anus |
| Motility | Innervation for propulsion of fecal stream | Hirschsprung's disease |
| Regression | Closure of fetal remnant accessory intestine, the vitelline system | Meckel's diverticulum |

TABLE 20-18.    Development of the Gastrointestinal Tract in the Human Fetus: First Appearance of Development Markers

| Structure/Function | Developmental Markers | Weeks of Gestation |
|---|---|---|
| **Anatomic** | | |
| Esophagus | Superficial glands develop | 20 |
| | Squamous cells appear | 28 |
| Stomach | Gastric glands form | 14 |
| | Pylorus and fundus are defined | 14 |
| Pancreas | Endocrine and exocrine tissue are differentiated | 14 |
| Liver | Lobules form | 11 |
| Small intestine | Crypt and villi develop | 14 |
| | Lymph nodes appear | 14 |
| Colon | Diameter increases | 20 |
| | Villi disappear | 20 |
| **Functional** | | |
| Sucking and swallowing | Mouthing only | 28 |
| | Immature suck–swallow | 33–36 |
| Stomach | Gastric motility and secretion | 20 |
| Pancreas | Zymogen granules | 20 |
| Liver | Bile metabolism | 11 |
| | Bile secretion | 22 |
| Small intestine | Active transport of amino acids | 14 |
| | Glucose transport | 18 |
| | Fatty-acid absorption | 24 |
| Enzymes | $\alpha$-Glucosidases | 10 |
| | Dipeptidases | 10 |
| | Lactase | 10 |
| | Enterokinase | 26 |

Lebenthal E, Lee PC, Heitlinger LA. Impact of development of the gastrointestinal tract on infant feeding. J Pediatr 1983;102:1.

of the fetal gut and become identifiable as neuroenteric ganglia in week 9, when spontaneous rhythmic contractions of the gut first occur. Failure of neuroblast migration results in aganglionic bowel beyond the site of arrested migration.

Fetal swallowing and intestinal peristalsis are present at 16 to 20 weeks' gestation. At 16 weeks' gestation, the gut contains meconium, which consists of swallowed squamous cells, lanugo hairs, and sebaceous secretions. Colonic evacuation of meconium normally does not occur in utero; peristalsis in the fetal intestine, therefore, is only rudimentary.

Pancreatic acini, the functional exocrine units, are present first at 8 to 12 weeks' gestation. The fetal pancreas differs from that of the adult in morphology, enzyme content, and secretory capacity. Bile flow from fetal liver occurs in utero, as evidenced by the presence of fetal bile acids and pigment in meconium, but the rate of bile flow at birth is less than the adult rate.

## ADAPTATION

The newborn's ability to thrive is dependent upon successful adaptation from fetal to extrauterine life. In utero, the fetus receives maternal glucose and, to a lesser extent, fatty acids, both to satisfy energy needs and to provide essential substrate for tissue structural lipid. At birth, the focus of these same needs for energy and cell growth shifts to dietary triglyceride, the major nutrient of the infant diet. The infant's gastrointestinal tract must adapt to this change rapidly. Despite this necessity, many diges-

tive and absorptive functions at birth are not yet at adult levels of activity (see Table 20-19). The neonate, therefore, must adapt to and compensate for these circumstances.

The factors necessary for the appropriate neonatal intestinal response to extrauterine life are luminal nutrients, hormones, bile, and pancreatic secretions. Clearly, the first dietary challenge begins the process in the intestine that eventually will complete intestinal maturation. Conversely, neonatal starvation when feedings are withheld results in hypoplastic intestinal morphology and reduced gut function.

Some specific aspects of this process are as follows. Pancreatic secretion is not optimal at birth (see Table 20-19); fat digestion, therefore, requires compensatory support from alternative lipases, differing in chemical behavior from pancreatic lipase, to break down dietary triglyceride. Breast milk and lingual lipases are present in gastric aspirates of human infants; they originate, respectively, in breast milk and in the von Ebner's gland at the base of the newborn's tongue. Breast milk lipase requires bile salts for activation in the small intestine. Lingual lipase is uniquely active in the acidic environment of the stomach; from 30% to 50% of dietary triglyceride can be digested in the stomach of the neonate. Bile acids are key metabolites of cholesterol present in bile that are necessary for intestinal absorption of hydrolyzed dietary fat. The body bile acid pool size is diminished in newborns, particularly premature infants, compared to that in adults. As a consequence, fat digestion is more inefficient and stool fat is proportionately greater in newborns than in adults, resulting in "physiologic steatorrhea."

Lebenthal E, Lee PC, Heitlinger LA. Impact of development of the gastrointestinal tract on infant feeding. J Pediatr 1983;102:1.

TABLE 20-19. Digestion and Absorption

| Factors | First Detectable (week of gestation) | Term Neonate (% of adult) |
|---|---|---|
| **Protein** | | |
| H+ | At birth | <30 |
| Pepsin | 16 | <10 |
| Trypsinogen | 20 | 10–60 |
| Chymotrypsinogen | 20 | 10–60 |
| Procarboxypeptidase | 20 | 10–60 |
| Enterokinase | 26 | 10 |
| Peptidases (brush-border and cytosol) | <15 | >100 |
| Amino acid transport | ? | >100 |
| Macromolecular absorption | ? | >100 |
| **Fat** | | |
| Lingual lipase | 30 | >100 |
| Pancreatic lipase | 20 | 5–10 |
| Pancreatic colipase | ? | ? |
| Bile acids | 22 | 50 |
| Medium-chain triglyceride uptake | ? | 100 |
| Long-chain triglyceride uptake | ? | 10–90 |
| **Carbohydrate** | | |
| α-Amylases | | |
|   Pancreatic | 22 | 0 |
|   Salivary | 16 | 10 |
| Lactase | 10 | >100 |
| Sucrase-isomaltase | 10 | 100 |
| Glucoamylase | 10 | 50–100 |
| Monosaccharide absorption | 11–19 | <100(?) |

Two general classes of stimuli will produce growth in the intestine. First, thyroxine and growth hormone are necessary for intestinal mucosal growth. Second, the ingestion of nutrients both serves the nutrition of the intestine and evokes local and systemic hormone release that modulates growth. Other specific factors promoting the maturation of neonatal digestive organ function, such as growth factors or hormones, remain unknown. Several candidate compounds have been proposed, particularly those present in breast milk (eg, epidermal growth factor). The optimal diet for the adaptation of fetal digestive function to extrauterine life, therefore, appears to be breast milk.

## GASTROINTESTINAL OBSTRUCTION IN THE NEONATE

In this section, the disorders producing gastrointestinal obstruction in newborn infants are defined. The timing and severity of the clinical presentations of these disorders are variable. This variability is the result of both the level of obstruction and its pathophysiology. For example, high mechanical obstruction in neonates is apparent immediately at birth and requires urgent intervention and therapy. Disorders such as malrotation may be less abrupt in presentation, as clinical signs and symptoms may not be evident for days or weeks after birth.

The symptoms and signs suggesting obstruction are several. The immediate inability of the neonate to swallow secretions and saliva or his or her failure to tolerate the attempt at first feeding is the first manifestation of high esophageal mechanical obstruction. Alternatively, infants with intestinal obstruction may be seen acutely in a morbid state with either vomiting or abdominal distention, as obstruction may become apparent only several hours after the initiation of feedings. Bilious vomiting or obstipation in the neonate always demands immediate, careful, and comprehensive evaluation and care. As important, the infant who apparently tolerates early feedings but then fails to pass meconium in the first 48 hours of life must be investigated for distal bowel obstruction.

The pathophysiology of obstruction in the newborn may be functional or mechanical. Functional obstruction may be mediated by aberrant bowel innervation, inflammation, or a lumen impacted with abnormal meconium. Mechanical obstruction may be at any level of the gastrointestinal tract, from the esophagus to the anus. The latter may be intrinsic, as with an atretic or obliterated gut lumen, or extrinsic, as in the case of a constricting band. Obstruction, moreover, may be complicated; mechanical and functional obstruction may coexist.

Complete evaluation and intervention can be performed on an acute basis for all disorders producing gastrointestinal obstruction in the neonate. The benefits of a good history and a complete physical examination cannot be understated. Historically, polyhydramnios, a positive family history of other neonates with obstruction, and birth weight are helpful indicators. During the examination, it is essential that an attempt be made to pass a catheter into the stomach, that the presence of bowel sounds be sought, that the neonate's abdomen be palpated for the presence of a mass, and that the anus be examined carefully for patency. Documentation of extraintestinal anomalies may offer additional information to the clinician in the process of diagnosing the cause of gastrointestinal obstruction.

With the initial evaluation, acute supportive care is indicated uniformly. This includes providing circulatory support with intravenous fluids or colloid, checking for the possibility of sepsis with appropriate cultures and antibiotic therapy, and decompressing the obstruction through a nasogastric tube. The other general facets of neonatal intensive care are observed aggressively with these potentially very ill infants. A single radiograph of the abdomen and the chest will define the level of obstruction in a crude fashion, indicating the need for surgical therapy. Again, it is important to be prepared to identify sepsis or metabolic causes of ileus, which are the major functional causes of gastrointestinal obstruction in the neonate.

### Esophagus

Esophageal malformations that cause upper intestinal obstruction include tracheoesophageal fistula (TEF) and esophageal atresia. TEF is the failure of linear division of the trachea and esophagus during embryogenesis, and it occurs in three varieties (Fig 20-54). The most common type, occurring in 85% to 95% of patients with TEF, is a proximal blind pouch with a distal TEF. A second type is a proximal pouch containing a fistula to the trachea; a distal esophageal pouch communicates only with the stomach. In a third type, the esophagus is normal, with the exception of a single H-fistula connecting the mid-esophageal lumen to the trachea. Esophageal atresia as an isolated finding is second only to the first type of TEF as a cause for esophageal obstruction.

Clinically, all these patients may have aspiration at birth. Respiratory difficulty is apparent, with the inability to deal with swallowed secretions. Infants who cough and choke in the first hours after birth, such as during the first feeding, should be ex-

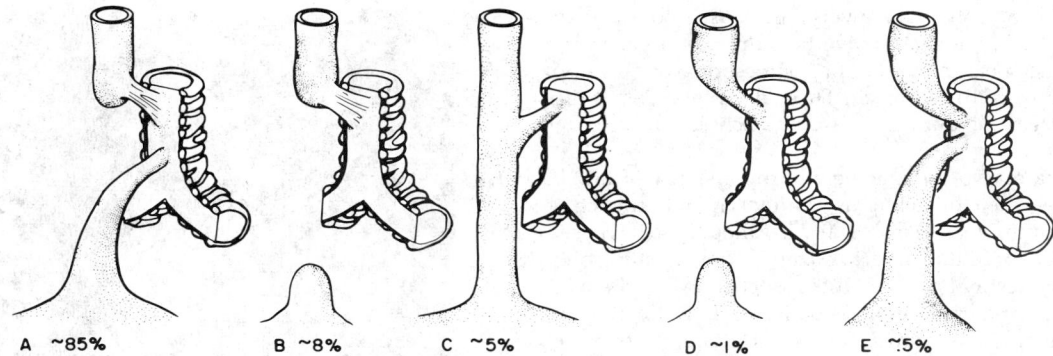

**Figure 20-54.** (**A**) through (**E**) Esophageal atresia and tracheoesophageal fistula. The most common type of these esophageal anomalies is a proximal atresia with a distal fistula to the trachea. Isolated esophageal atresia is the next most common esophageal anomaly; as indicated, the remaining types are far less common.

amined immediately for this disorder. Diagnosis can be made by attempting to pass a catheter into the stomach and encountering the obstruction (Fig 20-55A). A small amount of contrast material can be instilled through the catheter to demonstrate the blind proximal pouch on a chest radiograph; an abdominal radiograph will show bowel gas if a fistula is present. H-type fistulas commonly are seen later in infancy, and are more difficult to demonstrate (see Fig 20-55B). Surgical exploration confirms the diagnosis in each type; the fistula is ligated, and a gastrostomy is placed for nutrition. Later, the esophagus is anastomosed when the esophageal remnants are able to be brought together.

Mortality is 3% to 5% in stable infants, but can be as high as 41% when coexisting infection or anomalies are present. Poly-hydramnios and premature birth are two risk factors. TEF coexists with multiple anomalies in the VACTERL association (vertebral anomaly, imperforate anus, cardiac anomalies, TEF, renal defects,

and limb abnormalities [hypoplastic radii]). Complications distant from the neonatal period include uncoordinated esophageal peristalsis and gastroesophageal reflux resulting in stricture, aspiration, or a recurrent fistula. This occurs because the distal segment of the esophagus has abnormal motility and gastric acid clearance is impaired. Additional anomalies of the esophagus resulting in obstruction include a bronchopulmonary foregut malformation, extrinsic vascular compression, congenital esophageal stenosis, and an esophageal web in the upper or mid-esophagus.

## Stomach

The important malformations of the stomach resulting in neonatal obstruction are atresia, webs, microgastria, gastric duplication, gastric perforation, pyloric stenosis, gastric volvulus, and gastric

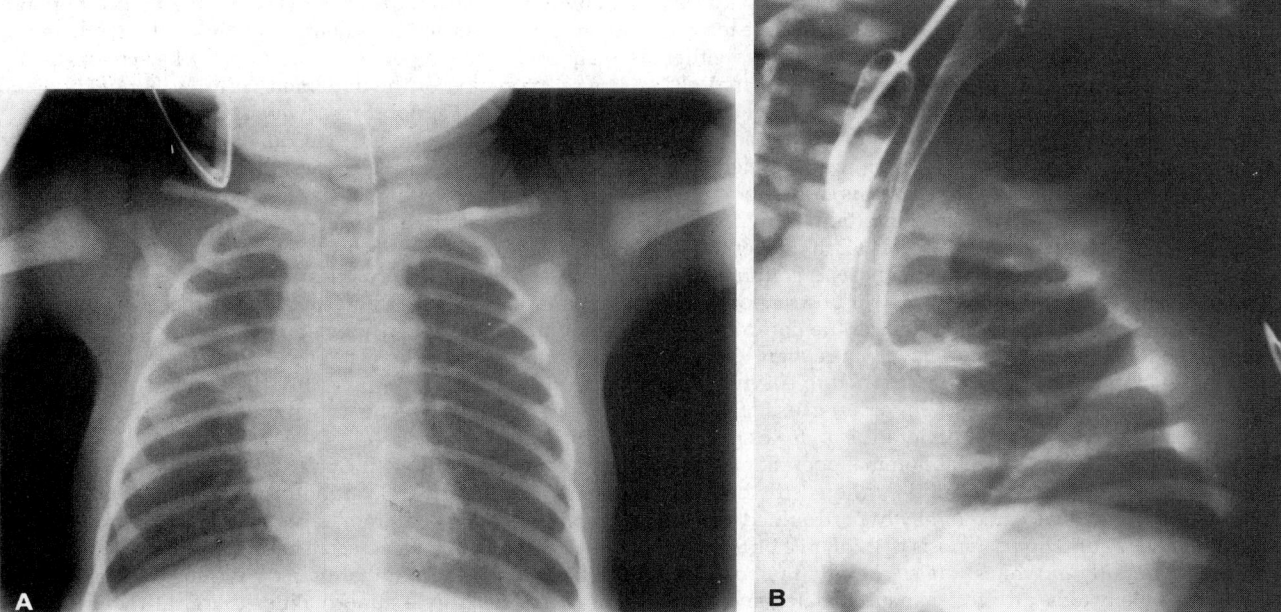

**Figure 20-55.** Radiographic appearance of esophageal atresia and tracheoesophageal fistula (TEF). (**A**) A radiopaque catheter that has been placed demonstrates the length of the proximal esophagus in an infant with the most common variety of TEF. (**B**) In another patient, contrast material is outlining an H-type tracheoesophageal fistula, a less common variety of TEF.

diverticulum. Gastric volvulus is a very rare cause of obstruction in the neonate. Rarely, a gastric diverticulum may occur in the area of the stomach near the cardiac or gastroesophageal junction, or near the pylorus of the stomach. These disorders are not discussed further; gastric duplications are discussed in another section.

Gastric atresia may present acutely in the first day of life; in this rare disorder, the stomach ends blindly. The inheritance of this condition is autosomal recessive, and it is thought to be caused by vascular factors or failure of recanalization. Representing only 1% of all gastrointestinal atresias, it is associated with the conditions trisomy 21 and epidermolysis bullosa. Clinically, the historic factors of maternal polyhydramnios, non-bilious vomiting, and a distended upper abdomen with a scaphoid lower abdomen and an abdominal radiograph that demonstrates a single gas bubble are suggestive of the diagnosis. Electrolyte disturbance, dehydration, and starvation are common features; surgical correction is necessary to establish a patent lumen.

Congenital webs, commonly found in the antrum of the stomach, also represent a failure of recanalization of the proliferating epithelial stage in fetal gut formation. These webs often are not noted in early infancy, but appear later in childhood or in adulthood; the web is mucosal and may have the morphology of a "wind sock" with a central opening. Symptoms include projectile vomiting, and barium studies of the stomach show a rounded, blunted pylorus and delayed gastric emptying. Some deformities are observed only at endoscopy; surgical treatment is necessary for membrane excision and pyloroplasty.

Microgastria or a hypoplastic stomach contrasts with gastric atresia in that there is patency of the stomach lumen. The foregut in this disorder, however, has failed both to differentiate into a reservoir "pouch" and to undergo epithelial cell differentiation, because acid secretion is absent. When these infants present with vomiting, the upper gastrointestinal series is diagnostic because there is failure of gastric rotation; the fundus, body, and pylorus are absent; and the esophagus may become dilated. No surgical therapy exists for this disorder, and its prognosis is quite poor.

An important gastrointestinal catastrophe in the neonate who has symptoms and signs of upper intestinal obstruction is gastric perforation. This disorder is rare, and 80% to 90% of cases occur in the first 5 days of life. It commonly occurs in premature infants who are hypoxic, require nasogastric suction, and have either peptic ulceration of the stomach or upper small-intestinal obstruction. These infants exhibit acute symptoms of refusal to feed, hematemesis, respiratory distress, and abdominal distention with tympany and tenderness. Gastric perforation must be identified very early in its clinical course, as peritonitis and shock may supervene shortly. Once the diagnosis is entertained, an abdominal radiograph is indicated immediately; free air in the peritoneal cavity will be evident (Fig 20-56). The diagnosis is confirmed by laparotomy; at the time, a distal small-bowel obstruction must be ruled out, and a gastrostomy is placed after the perforation is repaired. Infants whose treatment is delayed more than 12 hours after initial presentation should not be expected to survive.

The most frequently occurring and important cause of gastric obstruction in the neonate and young infant is pyloric stenosis; it is the most common reason for an abdominal operation during the first 6 months of life. In this condition, the gastric outlet is obstructed mechanically by a congenitally hypertrophied pyloric muscle. The incidence of pyloric stenosis is 1:250 live births, and it is seen predominantly in whites. Males, usually firstborn, are 3 to 4 times more likely to be affected than are females, and there is considerable aggregation of this disorder within families. When pyloric stenosis is recurrent in an extended family, a 5- to 50-times greater incidence among siblings of the patient is predicted. The average age at onset is 3 to 4 weeks, with a range of 1 to 12 weeks.

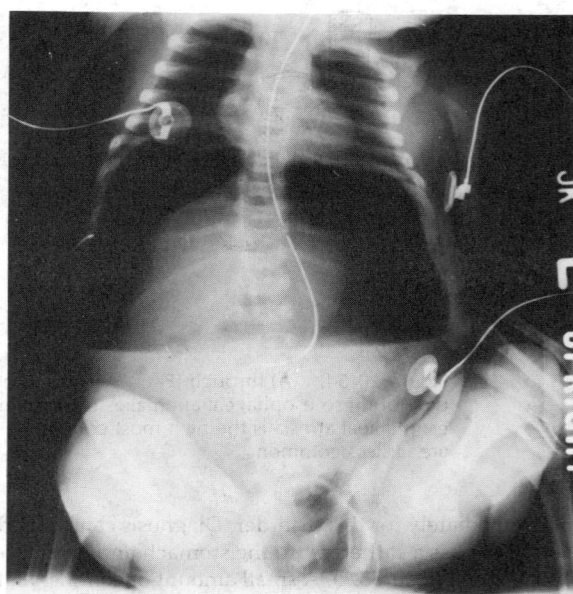

**Figure 20-56.** Acute gastric perforation. Free air is present in the peritoneal cavity and is displacing the abdominal viscera downward and toward the midline. The tip of a radiopaque catheter is within the lumen of the stomach, which is devoid of air.

The symptoms begin as regurgitation, particularly nasal, that progresses to the key sign, projectile vomiting. The emesis is non-bilious, but, in 20% of cases, contains blood in the form of "coffee grounds," a noteworthy and highly suggestive sign. Symptoms are present most commonly in the postprandial period, but they progress to occurring throughout the day if recognition is delayed. Initially, the appetite is retained, but weight loss, dehydration, a listless affect, constipation, markedly reduced urine output, and, occasionally, jaundice develop progressively in the infant. In extreme cases, the physical examination reveals cachexia, doughy skin, and sunken eyes and anterior fontanelle from profound dehydration. Fever, at times marked, may be present and raise suspicion of sepsis. Examination of the abdomen commonly is diagnostic. Visible peristaltic waves may be seen in the epigastrium; palpation of the abdomen with the flat of the hand will demonstrate an almond- to olive-sized tumor just to the right of the midline in the right upper quadrant. A test meal is given at times to help in eliciting these signs. The pyloric tumor is appreciated most easily, however, when the infant's stomach is empty. These confirmatory signs may not be apparent on initial examination, and a single negative examination should not preclude consideration of the diagnosis. These positive findings, when present, are sufficient data to confirm the diagnosis; an upper gastrointestinal series demonstrating a pyloric channel that is very narrow in a deformity known as the "tram-track sign" also is diagnostic (Fig 20-57). Recently, ultrasound has been used in some centers for patients in whom the disorder is more difficult to diagnose.

Complications are principally metabolic as a result of repetitive emesis of water and electrolytes typical of gastric secretion: hyponatremia, hypochloremia, hypokalemia, metabolic alkalosis, and azotemia. An elevated hematocrit at presentation indicates hemoconcentration. Initial therapy is aimed at correction of the fluid and electrolyte abnormalities. Surgical repair, the pyloromyotomy, is indicated; in the Ramstedt procedure, the pyloric muscle is incised on its anterior surface to the submucosa, and the operator can palpate a complete division. Persistent vomiting may occur after surgery secondary to continued delayed gastric emptying despite relief of obstruction. There is no evidence that

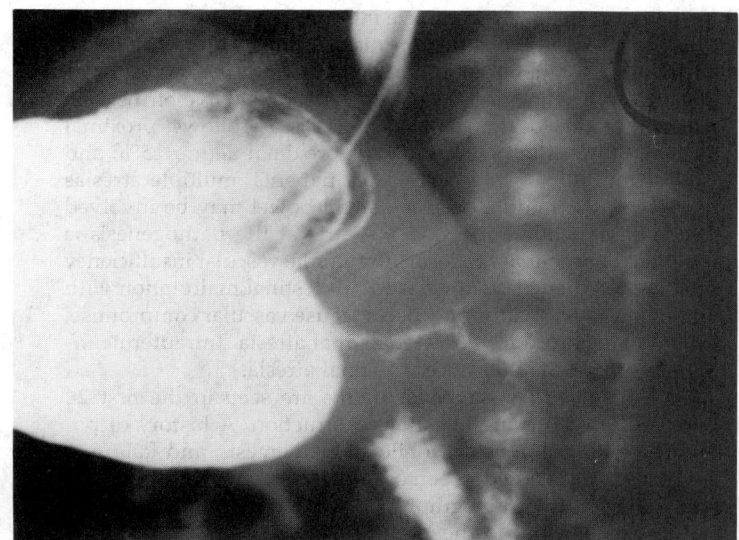

**Figure 20-57.** Pyloric stenosis. This radiograph is a lateral view from a barium study of the upper gastrointestinal tract performed on a vomiting infant. A thin stream of barium is seen exiting from the distended stomach through a markedly narrowed pyloric channel.

changing the infant's diet or dietary fat content will reduce the duration of this period of delayed gastric emptying. The overall prognosis is excellent; rarely, pyloric stenosis is associated with a genetic syndrome (Table 20-20).

## Duodenum

In the duodenum, the most common cause of obstruction in infancy and childhood is intestinal malrotation; in this disorder, a secondary extrinsic band across the upper abdomen mechanically obstructs the duodenum. In addition, the mobile redundant loops of small intestine that are fixed to a very narrow band of mesentery are prone to twist, or form a volvulus. This results in vascular obstruction of the most distal small intestine and in melena, with subsequent progression of intestinal ischemia resulting in bowel necrosis, sepsis, perforation, and peritonitis. Thus, there are two potential bases of intestinal obstruction: extrinsic duodenal obstruction and midgut volvulus. In 70% of these patients, the disorder will present in neonates; in half, it will present by 10 days of age; and in three fourths, it will present within the first month of life.

The presenting signs of prominent abdominal distention and bilious vomiting occur in the first 3 days of life. The diagnosis can be made based on the compatible clinical findings and a plain radiograph of the abdomen demonstrating intestinal obstruction, which demands surgical exploration. In less fulminant presentations, a barium study of the upper intestine reveals the absence of fixation of the duodenum and the fact that the duodenojejunal junction is freely mobile. A discrete level of obstruction resulting in a retrograde dilatation of the duodenum is present in symptomatic cases. Definitive therapy requires surgery, in which fibrous bands extrinsically obstructing the duodenum are lysed, the twists of the volvulus are taken down, and the cecum

| TABLE 20-20. Syndromes Associated With Pyloric Stenosis |
| --- |
| Trisomy 18 |
| Long-arm deletion 21 |
| Turner's syndrome |
| Smith-Lemli-Opitz syndrome |
| Cornelia de Lange's syndrome |

is stabilized. Intestinal resection of infarcted intestine is necessary; a critically shortened intestine may result, and many affected infants require prolonged total parenteral nutrition. Prognosis is dependent on identification and the timing of the operation after initial presentation; the overall mortality rate is 15% to 20%.

Less common causes of duodenal obstruction exist and are equally dramatic in their presentation. Duodenal atresia is defined as the complete obstruction of the duodenal lumen; in 80% of cases, the obstruction is distal to the ampulla of Vater. This disorder is rare, and occurs in 1:16,000 to 1:20,000 live births. The pathogenesis probably is failure of normal gut recanalization after the proliferative cell phase during early fetal life. Maternal polyhydramnios, premature birth, abdominal distention, and jaundice commonly are present. Although bilious vomiting occurs, meconium usually will be passed. The following occur in association with duodenal atresia: trisomy 21, intestinal malrotation, congenital heart disease, TEF, and renal anomalies. The prognosis is related primarily to early identification and therapy. In the compatible clinical situation, the diagnosis is suggested on an abdominal radiograph in which a distal bowel without gas coexists with two large gas bubbles in the stomach and proximal duodenum, the "double-bubble sign." The duodenum less commonly may be obstructed partially by congenital stenosis; in affected patients, this disorder may be noted at any time in infancy.

Duodenal obstruction also may be caused by annular pancreas, pre-duodenal portal vein, duodenal duplication, and incomplete rotation. Annular pancreas is obstruction in the second part of the duodenum caused by intrinsic bowel stenosis internal to an anomalous ring of pancreatic tissue. It occurs in 1:10,000 live births, and is associated with trisomy 21 in 20% to 30% of patients with annular pancreas, and with other anomalies in a further 40% to 50% of patients. The pathogenesis is unknown. Diagnosis may be suggested by an upper gastrointestinal series or ultrasound, but is confirmed by laparotomy. Surgery is required to construct a duodenostomy or duodenojejunostomy; however, there never is an intent to divide the pancreas. The prognosis after repair is good.

## Small Intestine

Atresias of the jejunum and ileum are the most common causes of intestinal obstruction in the first 2 weeks of life. As in duodenal atresia, the bowel lumen of jejunum or ileum ends abruptly in a blind pouch. Less commonly, incomplete obstruction of the lumen or stenosis with continuity of segments of bowel through a narrow lumen occurs. In atresia, complete intestinal obstruction is present at birth; in stenosis, obstruction may be mild, with little or no clinical manifestations, or it may approach the severity of complete atresia. The incidence of atresia is 1:20,000 live births. The incidence of the location of the atresia is as follows: proximal jejunum, 30%; distal jejunum, 20%; proximal ileum, 15%; and distal ileum, 30%. In 5% to 10% of patients, multiple atresias are present; the middle or entire small bowel may be involved in such cases. Unlike in duodenal atresia, the pathogenesis is thought to be secondary to focal intrauterine vascular insufficiency occurring relatively late in gestation. Intestinal malrotation with in utero midgut volvulus may occur, cause vascular compromise, and, ultimately, produce focal intestinal atresia. Intrauterine intussusception also may cause intestinal atresia.

Clinically, in all instances, patients are seen in the first 24 hours of life with acute intestinal obstruction. A history of polyhydramnios, vomiting with bile-stained emesis, and failure to pass meconium is noted; green or gray mucus may be passed per rectum. Abdominal radiography reveals intestinal luminal air–fluid levels proximal to the level of obstruction, with no distal bowel gas. Contrast studies are not necessary with these findings. At times, a water-contrast enema is performed to demonstrate the level of obstruction and the secondary findings of a congenital microcolon; a coincidental malrotation also may be suggested. Water-soluble contrast is necessary because the distal bowel segment may open directly into the peritoneal cavity.

Medical therapy is directed at acute support: fluid restoration, correction of electrolyte imbalance, and nasogastric suction for decompression of the proximal bowel. The diagnosis is confirmed by laparotomy, in which the atresia is localized; resection of the atretic area, plus a variable portion of the dilated proximal intestine, is undertaken and primary anastomosis commonly is performed. Whereas nearly 100% of infants with this disorder died of it in the middle of this century, less than one fifth do so today. Morbidity and mortality are minimized through early identification, aggressive supportive care, and the absence of complicating shock or sepsis.

Meconium ileus is an important cause of small-intestine obstruction in the neonatal period. This unique form of small-bowel obstruction is caused by occlusion of the intestinal lumen by an abnormally viscid meconium. Virtually all patients with meconium ileus have cystic fibrosis as an underlying primary diagnosis; meconium ileus is the presenting sign in 10% to 15% of infants with cystic fibrosis. The abnormal meconium is secondary to a reduced water content, a very high protein content, a high calcium concentration, and a reduction in other electrolytes.

The clinical features are those of intestinal obstruction within the first 48 hours of life. Contributing historic features are maternal polyhydramnios and a family history of cystic fibrosis; certain families afflicted with cystic fibrosis appear to be prone to this type of initial presentation. Affected infants have marked abdominal distention, bilious vomiting, and failure to pass meconium. Examination of the abdomen reveals palpable bowel loops, predominantly in the lower right quadrant. Rectal examination is difficult to perform, and will demonstrate either a paucity or a small plug of meconium. Abdominal radiography demonstrates bowel luminal air–fluid levels, small gas bubbles in meconium, or calcifications. Barium enema demonstrates a microcolon and a distal small-bowel luminal mass (Fig 20-58). The diagnosis is confirmed by laparotomy, in which the terminal ileum is of small caliber and appears focally beaded as a result of small collections of inspissated meconium. The distal colon also is of very small caliber; the intestine proximal to the terminal ileum is hypertrophied and grossly dilated, with massive distention caused by very viscous, green-black meconium.

In 50% of cases, meconium ileus is complicated by associated intestinal pathology; malrotation occurs with in utero midgut

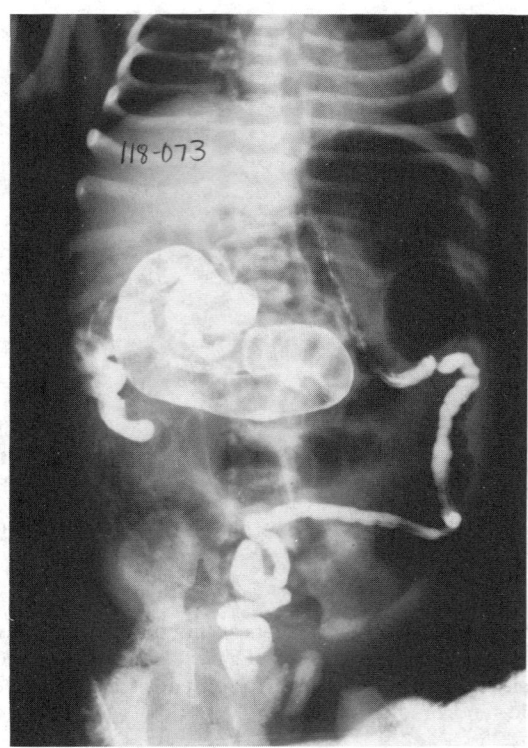

**Figure 20-58.** Meconium ileus. This is an anteroposterior view from a barium enema performed on an infant with intestinal obstruction in the neonatal period. Microcolon, which may occur in both meconium ileus and intestinal atresia, is evident. Unlike in ileal atresia, obstructing plugs of inspissated meconium are present within the lumen of this patient's terminal ileum, suggesting meconium ileus.

volvulus, at times leading to infarction and atresia of an intestinal segment. The most flagrant intrauterine complication of meconium ileus is intestinal perforation resulting in meconium peritonitis. As this usually occurs in utero, partial resolution may be evident by birth. Residual intraperitoneal pathology of varying clinical impact will be present: calcifications, adhesions, meconium, ascites, or a meconium pseudocyst. Intraperitoneal meconium may become infected and secondarily cause septic peritonitis after birth.

Therapy for meconium ileus can be individualized; uncomplicated cases can be treated with a water-soluble, hypertonic enema using diatrizoate meglumine or diatrizoate sodium (Gastrografin or Hypaque) to relieve the obstruction. Complicated cases require laparotomy and surgical correction, in which enterotomy is performed and the bowel is irrigated proximally and distally with either N-acetylcysteine (Mucomyst) or the detergent polysorbate 80 (Tween 80). Atretic segments of bowel are resected and peritoneal meconium deposits are evacuated. Although the prognosis depends on the presence or absence of complications, the overall survival rate is 50%, with an operative mortality rate of 30%. Long-term morbidity rates for such patients are no different than those for patients with cystic fibrosis past 6 months of age.

A rectal meconium plug does not imply the same morbidity or mortality rates as are given above. Upon relief of the temporary obstruction caused by the meconium plug, such patients should be evaluated carefully for cystic fibrosis and Hirschsprung's disease (see subsequent section).

## Colon, Rectum, and Anus

The principal disorders causing distal intestinal obstruction are either functional, resulting from a variable length of colonic aganglionosis, or mechanical, resulting from anorectal structural anomalies.

Colonic aganglionosis, or Hirschsprung's disease, is defined as functional obstruction of the rectum or colon. Aganglionosis is caused by an arrest in the cranial–caudal neuroblast migration in the gut during fetal life. Myenteric and submucosal ganglia, which are necessary for functional motility of the rectum and colon, are absent. The segment without innervation is of variable length proximal to the anus, is contracted permanently, and will not permit normal colorectal motility and fecal evacuation. This condition occurs in 1:5000 live births, and may be familial; there is a 3.6% incidence among siblings, and monozygotic twins are concordant for this disorder. Affected patients predominantly have intestinal obstruction and failure to pass meconium in the first week of life. Vomiting is present commonly within the first 48 to 72 hours after birth. Digital examination of the rectum usually will result in transient decompression of the obstruction. A barium enema in the neonatal period often will not show the transition of normal to abnormal bowel that is apparent at presentation in older infants and children (Fig 20-59). Infants may improve temporarily after the initial examination with evacuation of meconium or use of a suppository, with symptoms of obstipation recurring later. Thus, complete obstruction may be evident at birth or recurrent obstruction may occur during the neonatal period. A dramatic presentation as enterocolitis may occur with this disorder; symptoms of enterocolitis may simulate sepsis or necrotizing enterocolitis.

In the absence of colitis, suction rectal biopsy can be performed for diagnosis. A frozen-tissue section may be stained selectively for the neurotransmitter, acetylcholinesterase, to define abnormally large and undulant nerve trunks. Confirmation of the absence of submucosal ganglia on permanent hematoxylin and eosin–stained sections of the biopsy sample is required. Thereafter, full-thickness rectal biopsy and laparotomy are undertaken to establish the length of the involved colonic segment through

multiple biopsies of the colon in a retrograde fashion to determine where ganglia are located. Once this level of normally innervated colon is found, colostomy for decompression is performed, with subsequent colectomy and colonic or ileal pull-through performed at a later date. More than 80% of these patients have involvement of only the rectum and a small portion of the sigmoid colon. Less than 20% have long-segment aganglionosis; rarely, the entire colon is involved. The least common variety of the disorder involves the entire colon and a segment of ileum. There is a tenfold increase in the incidence of Hirschsprung's disease among patients with trisomy 21 compared with the normal population; 2% of patients with colonic aganglionosis have trisomy 21. In addition, Laurence-Moon-Biedl-Bardet and Waardenburg's syndromes have been associated; additional anomalies also may coexist (Table 20-21).

The second form of low intestinal obstruction in neonates is the anorectal anomaly, imperforate anus. This disorder is the result of a failure of anal development in which the bowel ends higher up in the pelvis, although a fistula coexists with an ectopic perineal or genitourinary opening. This lesion is associated with mechanical obstruction because the fistula is not completely effective for stool passage. Despite a failure to form part of the rectal and the entire anal segments of the bowel, the normal internal and external anal muscular sphincters are present. Complete separation of the developing rectum from the urogenital sinus is necessary during fetal development; this does not occur in this disorder, which explains the aberrant connection of the bowel to the urinary or genital tract. The incidence is 1:3500 to 1:9630 live births, and no familial pattern of inheritance is observed. The disorder is classified according to whether the terminal bowel or rectum migrates through the pelvic muscular floor (ie, through the puborectalis sling of the levator ani) during fetal life. Patients whose bowel does traverse the muscular pelvic floor (the infra-levator type of imperforate anus) have less morbidity, fewer associated anomalies, and a much better overall prognosis. In the supra-levator variety, in which the colon tip ends above the pelvic muscular floor, half of patients have lumbosacral spine defects that may include sacral agenesis, hemivertebrae, or lumbar segmentation defects. Seventy percent of such patients also have urologic anomalies such as hydronephrosis or a double collecting system. The ectopic opening of the distal bowel in affected females occurs in a defined order of incidence: perineum, vagina, and urinary tract. In contrast, three fourths of male patients have an ectopic opening into the urinary tract, whereas the opening is in the perineum in the remaining patients.

Either variety of imperforate anus may be associated with other anomalies, as one third of these patients will have one of the following: congenital heart disease, esophageal atresia, intestinal atresia, annular pancreas, intestinal malrotation or duplication, bicornuate uterus, vaginal atresia, septate vagina, ab-

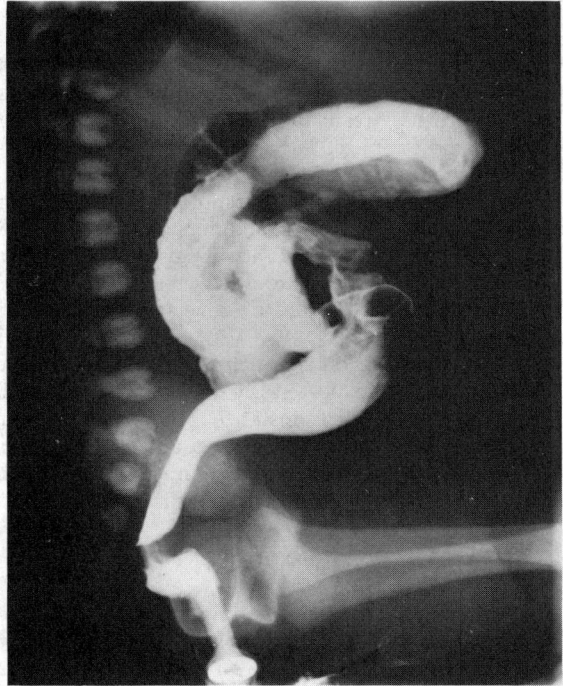

**Figure 20-59.** Hirschsprung's disease. This is a lateral view of a barium enema performed on an 8-day-old infant with constipation. The lumen of the rectum is contracted, suggesting congenital segmental aganglionosis; the diagnosis was confirmed later by suction rectal biopsy.

| TABLE 20-21. Anomalies Described as Associated With Hirschsprung's Disease |
| --- |
| Megacystis, megaureter |
| Hydrocephalus |
| Ventricular septal defect |
| Renal cystic disease |
| Cryptorchidism |
| Urinary bladder diverticulum |
| Meckel's diverticulum |
| Hypoplastic uterus |
| Colonic polyposis |
| Central hypoventilation |

sence of the rectus abdominis, trisomy 21, finger and hand anomalies, omphalocele, bladder exstrophy, and exstrophy of the ileocecal area. These patients usually have low intestinal obstruction, as described previously (Fig 20-60); they customarily have problems with defecation or urination and are noted to have unusual perineal anatomy. The extent of the disorder is defined by radiograph contrast studies. Temporary dilation of the ectopic opening to relieve destruction is possible if it is located in the perineum; otherwise, immediate surgical repair is indicated, involving an initial colostomy, eventually followed by an abdominal-to-perineal pull-through of bowel. After surgical repair, these patients are vulnerable to future episodes of fecal impaction, stricture formation, functional obstruction of the rectum, anal incontinence, and cryptic fistulas. The best surgical results are obtained in the infra-levator type of the disorder, whereas the worst are seen in patients with the supra-levator variety and concomitant sacral agenesis.

## Pseudo-Obstruction Syndromes

Disorders of the function of gastrointestinal motility often are seen in the newborn period. Although their overall occurrence is quite rare, their presentation often is dramatic. The spectrum of presentation is from simple constipation to apparent complete bowel obstruction. The etiologies include abnormalities of intestinal smooth muscle or innervation of the gut. Conditions involving smooth muscle also will manifest dysmotility in the gallbladder, ureter, and bladder. Radiographic, manometric, and radioisotope-labeled transit studies of the gastrointestinal tract are helpful in making the diagnosis. Exploratory laparotomy often is performed to rule out mechanical obstruction, and full-thickness intestinal biopsies can help distinguish between the neuropathic and myopathic forms.

The prune-belly or Eagle-Barrett syndrome is the abdominal muscle deficiency syndrome. Although renal and pulmonary anomalies and dysfunction predominate, these patients also have severe constipation.

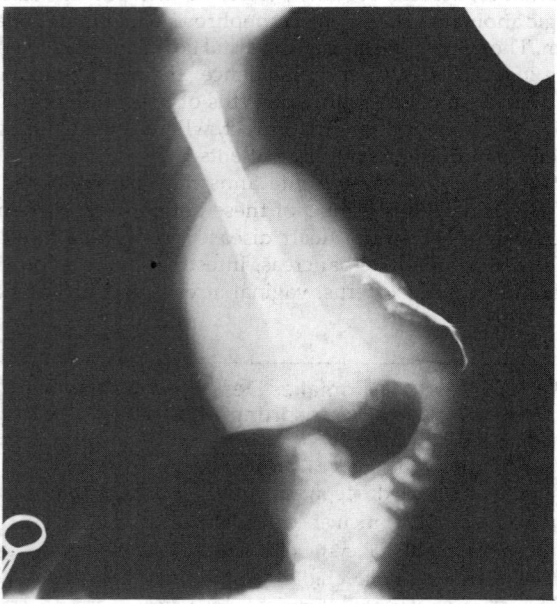

**Figure 20-60.**   Imperforate anus. This is a lateral radiograph of the sacrum with the patient upside down. Contrast is layered on the surface of the perineum; the level of obstruction in the rectum is outlined by bowel gas. The wide gap between the gas-filled distal rectum and the contrast-labeled perineum suggests the diagnosis of imperforate anus.

# GASTROINTESTINAL MALFORMATIONS

## Malrotation

The most important gastrointestinal malformation is malrotation of the small intestine. It has been stated previously that the process of rotation and fixation of the gut in the fetal abdomen is necessary to position the gut to ensure normal motility, normal passage of fluid through the intestine, an appropriate gut-to-mesentery ratio, and distribution of the gut's vascular supply. Malrotations are of several types; growth, rotation, and fixation of the small intestine in fetal life occurs in three stages, and a defect can occur at any stage.

A first-stage malrotation is associated with failure of the gut and, occasionally, the viscera to return to the abdominal cavity. The resulting anomaly, an omphalocele, consists of the midgut with or without viscera suspended outside of the abdominal wall within a bag of mesentery. Omphalocele is associated with several genetic syndromes, notably trisomies 13 and 18. Staged surgical reduction of the omphalocele is required for definitive repair.

Malrotation in the second stage of gut development may result in any of four possible anatomic malformations. The first is simple nonrotation, in which the small intestine remains entirely on the right side of the abdomen whereas the colon is on the left. This malformation does not result in intestinal obstruction or vascular insufficiency. In the second and most common form of malformation, discussed previously in the section on obstruction, the cecum remains on the left side during fetal life and does not complete its path of growth and fixation to the right lower quadrant. Therefore, it is never fixed within the abdomen and is quite mobile. Abnormal attachments are created through adhesions from the right side of the abdominal wall to the malpositioned cecum in the left upper quadrant. These fibrous or Ladd's bands are the extrinsic cause of mechanical obstruction, described previously in the section on the duodenum. This particular malformation within the second stage of rotation also is most likely to result in a very narrow mesentery serving the entire length of the mid-intestine. The major arterial supply, the superior mesenteric artery, proceeds from the base of this mesentery. The weight of the redundant loops of intestine with this narrow mesentery potentiates a twisting of mesentery around the axis of the superior mesenteric artery. This twist, or volvulus, may proceed through several turns to result ultimately in compromise of venous and arterial blood supplies. The gut mucosal lining, exquisitely sensitive to ischemia, is most affected; in extreme cases, total intestinal midgut ischemia and infarction occur. Bands extrinsically obstructing the duodenum in addition to concomitant midgut volvulus occur in half of patients with acute intestinal obstruction resulting from this type of malrotation. Less common types of malrotation in this second stage are reversed rotation and paraduodenal hernia.

A third-stage malrotation is principally a failure of the cecum and ascending colon to fix posteriorly to the abdominal wall. The small-bowel mesentery in this instance is long, but has a narrow base and abnormal fixation. The second and third parts of the duodenum also are mobile. Surgical therapy for correction of midgut malrotation and volvulus has been addressed previously.

## Duplications

Gastrointestinal duplications are defined as an anomalous secondary segments of bowel directly contiguous to normal bowel. Duplications contain a muscular wall and a mucosal lining of some variety of gastrointestinal mucosa, and may communicate with the true intestinal lumen. Duplications occur on the mesenteric side of the normal intestine, and may be either long and tubular or spherical. Enteric duplications may appear in the tongue, and are obvious at birth when they interfere with feeding; lingual duplications must be differentiated from cystic hygroma, hemangioma, lymphangioma, atopic thyroid, macroglossia, and rhabdomyoma. Duplications contiguous to the esophagus commonly are associated with hemivertebrae. Gastric duplications usually occur on the greater curvature; rarely, they may involve the pylorus, simulating true pyloric stenosis. Duodenal duplications may obstruct either the intestinal lumen or the pancreatic duct. Duplications are found frequently by the proximal jejunum or the proximal ileum, but occur most commonly adjacent to the distal ileum. Isolated ileocecal duplications may appear as cysts and obstruct the intestine at this level. Rarely, total colonic or rectal duplications occur; multiple duplications are found in 15% of patients with duplications. Patients may have a mediastinal or abdominal mass, intestinal obstruction, or gastrointestinal bleeding. The last instance is related to the presence of ectopic mucosa, usually gastric, which is found in one fifth of duplications. Ulceration can occur within the duplication, followed by bleeding, which may be occult. About two thirds of these cases are diagnosed before the patient is 1 year of age. Duplications must be distinguished from neurenteric cysts that are separate from the bowel; these lesions occur most commonly in the chest, and usually are in the posterior mediastinum. Lesions with gastric mucosa at any site can be identified by a technetium scan; diagnosis is made occasionally by barium studies or ultrasound. Based on clinical suspicion and the known distribution of duplications, laparotomy for confirmation and extirpation then is performed.

## Meckel's Diverticulum

Meckel's diverticulum, a 5- to 7.5-cm anomalous pouch projecting from the antimesenteric border of the ileum, results from persistence of a portion of the vitelline duct from the ileum. It usually lies within 100 cm of the ileocecal valve. Meckel's diverticulum is found incidentally in as many as 3% of autopsies; more than half of these reveal a mucosal lining other than ileal. In the vast majority of those cases, the ectopic mucosa is gastric epithelium. Unbuffered acid secretion from this source may result in ulceration of adjacent mucosa and cause the most common complication of this anomaly, intestinal bleeding. Hematochezia resulting from this lesion may appear as gross red blood or melena. Roughly two thirds of such cases present when the patient is less than 2 years of age; half present at less than 1 year of age. Patients with Meckel's diverticulum constitute about 50% of all cases of lower gastrointestinal bleeding in the pediatric population. This cause of intestinal bleeding usually is not accompanied by other symptoms. In rare cases, this lesion becomes inflamed and the patient's symptoms are quite similar to those associated with acute appendicitis: abdominal distention, ileus, low-grade fever, abdominal pain, signs of inflammation, and, possibly, peritonitis. Meckel's diverticulum also may be the lead point for intussusception. A band representing a fibrous remnant of the remainder of the vitelline duct also may persist, connecting the Meckel's diverticulum to the anterior abdominal wall, and may potentiate obstruction or twisting of the diverticulum. Diagnosis of those cases in which gastric mucosa is present can be made through labeled technetium scan. Surgical excision is curative.

## Heterotopia

In rare instances, rests of endoderm may differentiate in abnormal positions along the intestine, producing an ectopic focus of gastric or pancreatic tissue. The most common variety is gastric mucosa, which may be 3 to 12 cm in length, occurring in the small intestine as a mass or nodular lesion. Pancreatic rests may occur in similar fashion.

## Gastroschisis

Gastroschisis is a malformation of the anterior abdominal wall. It results in herniation of intestinal loops plus stomach from the right side. The umbilical cord and its insertion are normal in this disorder, in contrast to omphalocele. More important, there is no sac suspending the herniating bowel loops, which clearly differentiates this disorder from omphalocele at birth. Staged surgical reduction, as in omphalocele, is necessary. Mesenteric cysts, lymphangiomas, and tumors all will be seen in the neonatal period as abdominal masses and, therefore, will be discussed later in a specific subsection.

## Necrotizing Enterocolitis

Necrotizing enterocolitis is the most common and most dramatic cause of the septic abdomen in newborns and is the most common cause of acute intestinal obstruction in neonates. It is discussed in Chapter 20.4.5.

## Selected Readings

Bell MJ. Perforation of the gastrointestinal tract and peritonitis in the neonate. Surg Gynecol Obstet 1985;160:20.

Bower RJ, Sieber WK, Kiesewetter WB. Alimentary tract duplications in children. Ann Surg 1978;188:669.

Del Pin CA, Czyrko C, Ziegler MM, Scanlin TF, Bishop HC. Management and survival of meconium ileus. Ann Surg 1992;215:179.

Ford EG, Senac MO, Srikanth MS, Weitzman JJ. Malrotation of the intestine in children. Ann Surg 1992;215:172.

Ghory MJ, Sheldon CA. Newborn surgical emergencies of the gastrointestinal tract. Surg Clin North Am 1985;65:1083.

Lebenthal E, Lee PC, Heitlinger LA. Impact of development of the gastrointestinal tract on infant feeding. J Pediatr 1983;102:1.

Martin LW, Alexander F. Esophageal atresia. Surg Clin North Am 1985;65:1099.

Martin LW, Torres AM. Hirschsprung's disease. Surg Clin North Am 1985;65:1171.

Peña A. Current management of anorectal anomalies. Surg Clin North Am 1992;72:1393.

RyanET, Ecker JL, Christakis NA, Folkman J. Hirschsprung's disease: associated abnormalities and demography. J Pediatr Surg 1992;27:76.

Silverman A, Roy CC. Pediatric clinical gastroenterology, ed 3. St Louis: CV Mosby, 1983.

Sleisenger MH, Fordtran JS, eds. Gastrointestinal disease: Pathophysiology, diagnosis, management, ed 3. Philadelphia: WB Saunders, 1983.

Tanner MS, Stocks RJ. Neonatal gastroenterology—contemporary issues. Newcastle-Upon-Tyne: Intercept, 1984.

Van DW, West KW, Grosfeld JL. Vitelline duct anomalies: Experience with 217 childhood cases. Arch Surg 1987;122:542.

Vargas JH, Sachs P, Ament ME. Chronic intestinal pseudo-obstruction syndrome in pediatrics. J Pediatr Gastroenterol Nutr 1988;7:323.

Walker WA, Durie PR, Hamilton JR, Walker-Smith JA, Watkins JB, eds. Pediatric gastrointestinal disease: Pathophysiology, diagnosis, management. Philadelphia: BC Decker, 1991.

*Principles and Practice of Pediatrics, Second Edition.*
edited by Frank A. Oski et al. J. B. Lippincott Company, Philadelphia © 1994.

## 20.4.2 *Neonatal Cholestasis*

Donald A. Novak, Frederick J. Suchy, and William F. Balistreri

Neonatal cholestasis, defined as prolonged conjugated hyperbilirubinemia, is the end result of impaired bile flow and excretion. The cumulative incidence of neonatal cholestasis is about 1:2500 live births. Liver dysfunction in the neonate, regardless of the cause, commonly is associated with bile secretory failure and cholestatic jaundice. The potential mechanisms by which bile secretion may be impaired are many. Hepatocellular injury, such as that noted in neonatal hepatitis, may cause functional impairment of bile secretion. Mechanical obstruction to bile flow also may occur, as noted in extrahepatic biliary atresia. Although many disorders can present as neonatal cholestasis, neonatal hepatitis and biliary atresia are the most common syndromes, accounting for 70% to 80% of all cases of prolonged conjugated hyperbilirubinemia in infants (Fig. 20-61).

Identification of the infant with cholestasis begins with measurement of total and conjugated bilirubin fractions. The cholestatic infant will have an elevated conjugated fraction, generally at a level above 2 mg/dL and accounting for more than 15% to 20% of the total bilirubin. The possibility of liver or biliary tract disease must be considered in any neonate who is jaundiced beyond 2 weeks of age. Indeed, jaundice after 11 days in term infants and after 14 days in premature infants is unusual, occurring in only 0.5% of infants in one study. Subsequent efforts must be directed toward rapid diagnosis of and therapy for potentially treatable disorders, such as sepsis, galactosemia, and hypothyroidism or panhypopituitarism, in which delay of diagnosis may have catastrophic consequences; differentiation of biliary atresia from neonatal hepatitis, because the former will require surgical intervention; and effective management of the consequences of chronic cholestasis. Early in the workup of any cholestatic infant, vitamin K (2.5 mg) should be given in an effort to prevent life-threatening hemorrhage. Further description of specific diagnostic modalities is included with the discussion of each entity.

## INFECTIOUS CAUSES OF CHOLESTASIS

The fact that cholestasis may occur in patients with gram-negative bacterial infection long has been recognized. The incidence of jaundice during episodes of neonatal sepsis has been estimated at 20% to 60%. Urinary tract infections caused by *Escherichia coli* frequently have been associated with jaundice, particularly in male infants. The infants may appear clinically well and may have jaundice as their only symptom. Other bacteria, including gram-negative rods, staphylococci, and streptococci, have been implicated in causing cholestasis. Limited autopsy studies have shown centrilobular hepatic necrosis and canalicular bile stasis; this feature and direct experimental evidence suggest that bacterial toxins produce canalicular dysfunction. Jaundice is reversible with

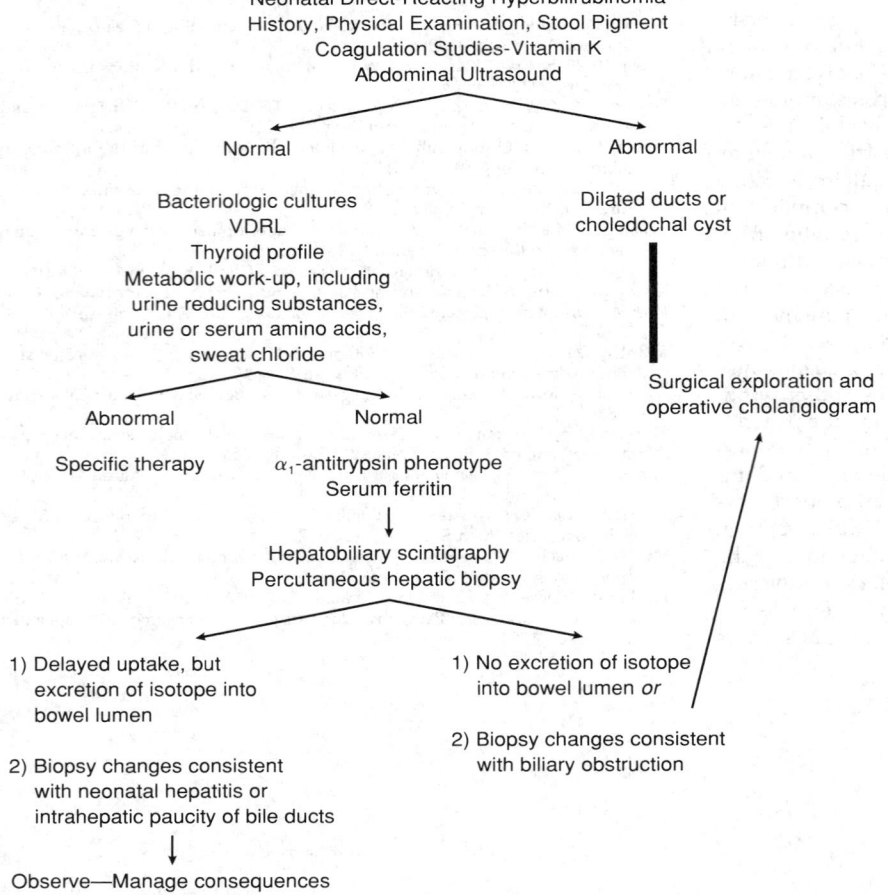

Figure 20-61.   Flow chart for the work up of neonatal cholestasis.

successful therapy for the underlying infection. Thus, cultures, of blood and urine in particular, are important components of the initial evaluation phase for neonates with cholestasis.

Other infectious causes of neonatal cholestasis include any of the so-called TORCH (toxoplasmosis, other [viruses], rubella, cytomegalovirus, herpes) agents, as well as coxsackieviruses and echoviruses. Parvovirus B19 and human herpesvirus type b recently have been associated with cholestatic liver disease. The infant with congenital toxoplasmosis may be noted at birth with hepatomegaly (60%) and hyperbilirubinemia (40%), or these features may develop later in the neonatal period. Although hepatic disease generally is mild, progressive hepatic dysfunction may occur. Hepatic pathology is nonspecific, and includes mononuclear periportal inflammation and canalicular bile stasis. Diagnosis may be made using the Sabin-Feldman dye test or through demonstration of the parasite in spinal fluid sediment. Antiparasitic therapy may arrest disease progression.

Congenital rubella may be associated with hepatomegaly in 65% of cases, and with jaundice in 15% of cases. The clinical presentation and hepatic pathology are nonspecific. Elevation of aminotransferase values may occur, as may acholic stools. The prognosis for the hepatic disease is good, with progression to hepatic fibrosis and failure uncommon. Diagnosis is through serology and viral isolation. No specific therapy is available.

Cytomegalovirus (CMV) infection may produce symptoms in the neonate of hepatosplenomegaly and, occasionally, hyperbilirubinemia, in addition to the other well-known stigmata of congenital CMV. In the jaundiced infant with abnormal serum aminotransferase levels, CMV infection is suggested by liver biopsy findings of focal areas of hepatocyte necrosis and portal inflammatory infiltrates composed of lymphocytes and neutrophils. Intranuclear viral inclusions may be noted in bile duct epithelial cells and, rarely, in hepatocytes. In addition, giant-cell transformation, bile stasis, and extramedullary hematopoiesis may be noted. Diagnosis is through culture of the organism from urine or tissue. The prognosis for CMV-related hepatic disease is generally good, with progression to severe chronic liver disease rare. Ganciclovir therapy may be indicated for severe congenital disease attributed to CMV.

Herpes simplex virus may cause jaundice and massive hepatic necrosis with liver failure in conjunction with the other clinical features of neonatal herpetic infection. Coxsackievirus and echovirus (types 11, 14, and 19) infection may present in similar fashion. Diagnosis in each case is through viral isolation and serology. Therapy for documented neonatal herpes simplex infection is with adenine arabinoside or with acyclovir.

Eighty percent of infants with congenital syphilis have hepatomegaly, whereas 40% are jaundiced. Hepatic biopsy may reveal extramedullary hematopoiesis, parenchymal or portal inflammatory infiltrates, and granulomatous lesions. Spirochetes may be seen; however, the diagnosis typically is made by serologic evaluation. Penicillin remains essential in the therapy of affected infants, but it may exacerbate hepatic disease resulting from syphilis.

## INTRAHEPATIC CHOLESTASIS

Intrahepatic cholestasis is a term that encompasses a diverse group of disorders, some associated with "paucity" of bile ducts, some associated with disordered bile acid metabolism, and others in which the underlying pathogenesis remains undefined. These disorders may present in the neonatal period with jaundice or later in life with chronic cholestasis. Paucity of the intrahepatic bile ducts, defined as less than 0.5 intralobular bile ducts per triad, in the presence of otherwise normal portal areas may represent either a congenital or an acquired disorder, with paucity being the end result of progressive bile duct injury. Some children with hepatic histology that demonstrates paucity have, in addition, unique features that suggest a syndrome. The best-studied example is Alagille syndrome (arteriohepatic dysplasia), which denotes a constellation of findings, including the following: abnormal facies (broad forehead, deep-set eyes, hypertelorism, long and straight nose with flat nasal bridge, and underdeveloped mandible), ocular abnormalities, cardiovascular abnormalities (typically peripheral pulmonic stenosis), vertebral arch defects ("butterfly" vertebrae, hemivertebrae, decreased interpediculate distance), and renal abnormalities.

Previously associated findings such as growth retardation, mental retardation, and hypogonadism may be secondary to nutritional deficiencies (eg, vitamin E). Patients with this disorder often are seen in the neonatal period with hepatomegaly and cholestasis. Liver histology early in life may be nonspecific, with portal inflammation, bile duct proliferation, and giant-cell infiltration. Biopsy findings later in life demonstrate the paucity of intrahepatic bile ducts and cholestasis. Although the etiology of this disorder remains unclear, bile secretory defects, perhaps in the Golgi apparatus, have been postulated. The prognosis for this disorder is generally good, provided careful attention is paid to management of the effects of chronic cholestasis, including fat-soluble vitamin deficiency. Inheritance appears to be autosomal dominant, and several patients with this disorder have been shown to have a partial deletion on the short arm of chromosome 20.

Paucity of the intrahepatic bile ducts that is unrelated to a specific syndrome most likely represents an eclectic variety of liver disease; the exact nature, however, is unknown. The prognosis for this form, which often recurs within a family, appears to be unfavorable, with progression to biliary cirrhosis and hepatic failure occurring frequently. Paucity of bile ducts may be seen on hepatic biopsy before 90 days of life, and bile duct destruction may be noted at that time.

Zellweger syndrome (cerebrohepatorenal syndrome) is a fatal autosomal recessive disorder that is associated with peroxisomal absence. Clinical characteristics include abnormal craniofacial development, severe hypotonia, hyporeflexia, eye abnormalities, hepatomegaly, failure to thrive, psychomotor retardation, calcific stippling of the patella, and renal cysts. Typically, jaundice is present in the first month of life. Death, often secondary to respiratory distress, sepsis, or liver disease, generally occurs within the first year of life. Histologic examination of the liver reveals cholestasis, focal necrosis, and, occasionally, paucity of the bile ducts. Electron-microscopic examination is significant for the apparent absence of peroxisomes. Lack of peroxisomal function causes the accumulation of very–long-chain fatty acids in the plasma, presumably because of deficient $\beta$-oxidation. Other abnormalities include low levels of plasmalogens, abnormal bile acid and cholesterol metabolism, and elevated levels of pipecolic acid. Apart from the fairly characteristic phenotypic features, diagnosis is aided by measurement of the C26/C22 fatty acid ratio and detection of abnormal bile acid intermediates. Prenatal diagnosis is possible. Other probable "peroxisomal" diseases include Refsum disease, neonatal-type adrenoleukodystrophy, X-linked adrenoleukodystrophy, and chondrodysplasia punctata, rhizomelic type.

Other forms of intrahepatic cholestasis include the following:

1. Benign recurrent intrahepatic cholestasis, with onset generally occurring during childhood. The clinical course includes recurrent episodes of cholestasis that resolve spontaneously. The etiology of this disorder is unknown; thus, diagnosis is by exclusion.
2. Hereditary cholestasis with lymphedema, which consists of episodes of recurrent jaundice, associated in later childhood

with lymphedema of the lower extremities. The etiology is unknown; inheritance may be autosomal recessive. Cirrhosis may occur later in life.

3. Byler's syndrome is a fatal familial disorder in which jaundice, at first episodic, becomes constant by 1 to 4 years of age. Liver pathology reveals progressive cholestasis and cirrhosis. Affected children have steatorrhea, failure to thrive, and rickets. Death occurs in childhood, and typically results from the consequences of hepatic failure and portal hypertension. Some patients with this disorder have benefited from partial cutaneous biliary diversion, which may promote the loss of potentially hepatotoxic bile acids.

## NEONATAL HEPATITIS

Idiopathic neonatal hepatitis is a descriptive term for neonatal cholestatic liver disease for which all other known causes, including metabolic and infectious diseases and extrahepatic obstruction, have been ruled out. The incidence of this disorder is about 1:5000 births, making it the most common cause of neonatal cholestasis, accounting for almost 50% of cases of prolonged neonatal jaundice. This category most likely represents a collection of multiple, as yet undescribed, disorders of hepatic function. There are a number of areas of overlap with the intrahepatic cholestasis category described above.

Clinically, 50% of infants with "idiopathic" neonatal hepatitis have jaundice in the first week of life. Hepatosplenomegaly is common, and about one third of these infants fail to thrive. Acholic stools may be present, making differentiation of this diagnosis from extrahepatic biliary atresia difficult. Liver histology is variable, but typically includes inflammation, hepatocellular unrest, multinucleated giant cells, and extramedullary hematopoiesis. Bile duct proliferation typically is not present. Diagnosis is through exclusion of other etiologies, including extrahepatic

---

**TABLE 20-22.   Differential Diagnosis of Conjugated Hyperbilirubinemia (Neonatal Cholestasis)**

| | |
|---|---|
| **Bile Duct Obstruction** | **Metabolic Diseases** |
| Cholangiopathies | Disorders of amino acid metabolism |
|    Extrahepatic biliary atresia |    Tyrosinemia |
|    Nonsyndromic paucity of intrahepatic bile ducts | Disorders of lipid metabolism |
|    Choledochal cyst |    Niemann-Pick Disease |
|    Neonatal sclerosing cholangitis |    Gaucher Disease |
|    Spontaneous perforation of common bile duct |    Wolman's Disease |
|    Bile duct stenosis | Disorders of the urea cycle |
|    Caroli's disease |    Arginase deficiency |
| Other | Disorders of carbohydrate metabolism |
|    Inspissated bile/mucous plug |    Galactosemia |
|    Cholelithiasis |    Fructosemia |
|    Tumors/masses (intrinsic and extrinsic) |    Type IV glycogenosis |
| | Disorders of bile acid synthesis |
| **Neonatal Hepatitis** | Peroxisomal disorders |
| Idiopathic |    Zellweger's syndrome |
| Viral | Disorders of oxidative phosphorylation |
| Cytomegalovirus | Other |
| Rubella |    Alpha-1-antitrypsin deficiency |
| Reovirus type 3 |    Cystic fibrosis |
| Herpesviruses |    Hypopituitarism [Septo-optic dysplasia] |
|    Simplex | Hypothyroidism |
|    Zoster | Neonatal hemochromatosis |
|    Human herpesvirus type 6 | |
| Adenovirus | **Toxic** |
| Enteroviruses | Drugs |
| Parvovirus B19 | Parenteral nutrition |
| Hepatitis B | |
| Hepatitis C | **Miscellaneous Associations** |
| ? Non A, non B, non C | Shock/hypoperfusion |
| Human immunodeficiency virus | Histiocytosis X |
| Bacterial and Parasitic | Intestinal obstruction |
| Bacterial sepsis | Erythrophagocytic lymphohistiocytosis |
| Syphilis | Neonatal lupus erythematosus |
| Listeriosis | Indian childhood cirrhosis |
| Tuberculosis | Extracorporeal membrane oxygenation |
| Toxoplasmosis | Autosomal trisomies |
| | Graft vs. host disease |
| **Idiopathic Cholestatic Syndromes** | Veno-occlusive disease |
| Arteriohepatic dysplasia [Alagille syndrome] | |
| Byler's syndrome | |
| Hereditary cholestasis with lymphedema [Aaqenaes] | |
| Benign recurrent cholestasis | |
| Familial cholestasis of North American Indians | |

biliary atresia (Table 20-22). Therapy is directed toward addressing the consequences of chronic cholestasis (Fig 20-62). The prognosis is variable, but about 80% to 85% of patients will recover, whereas 15% to 20% will have severe, progressive disease. The diseases that demonstrate a pattern of familial recurrence carry the worst prognosis.

## BILIARY ATRESIA

Extrahepatic biliary atresia, which occurs in about 1:8000 live births, consists of atresia or hypoplasia of any portion of the extrahepatic biliary system. The obstruction may occur as a discrete distal lesion, allowing surgical drainage of patent portions of bile duct proximal to the atresia. In the most common form, however, the atretic area extends to above the level of the porta hepatis and often affects intrahepatic bile ducts, making surgical drainage difficult.

The clinical presentation of this disorder is similar to that of neonatal hepatitis. Typically, infants are born at term and are of normal birth weight. Jaundice develops at 3 to 6 weeks of age in otherwise well-appearing, thriving infants, and the stool eventually becomes acholic. About 15% of infants may have associated defects, including polysplenia, cardiovascular anomalies, and malrotation of the intestine. There is no apparent genetic predisposition, and familial recurrence is rare. Hepatic pathology will vary with the age of the infant; early biopsy samples may feature the presence of multinucleated giant cells, which decrease in number with age. Classic features of biliary atresia include bile ductular proliferation, bile plugs, and portal or perilobular fibrosis and edema.

Biliary atresia appears to be an evolving lesion with progressive obliteration of bile ducts; this is supported by the fact that several

infants with previously documented patent extrahepatic biliary ducts have been found, on reexploration, to have biliary atresia. Thus, it is possible to speculate that neonatal hepatitis and extrahepatic biliary atresia represent different manifestations of hepatocyte or biliary tract injury by a single agent. However, the etiology of the disorder is unknown.

The diagnosis of biliary atresia involves the exclusion of other known causes of neonatal cholestasis. Differentiation of biliary atresia from neonatal hepatitis remains difficult. Clinical features aiding in discrimination include birth weight (biliary atresia is more common in term infants, whereas infants with neonatal hepatitis often are born prematurely or are small for gestational age); the presence of associated anomalies or an enlarged, firm liver (suggestive of biliary atresia); and the consistent absence of stool pigment (associated with biliary atresia). Duodenal fluid may be collected and assayed for the presence of bilirubin pigment or bile acids, the presence of which virtually excludes the diagnosis of biliary atresia. An abdominal ultrasound examination permits evaluation for the presence of a gallbladder, which often is absent in biliary atresia. Further studies should be directed at ruling out endocrine, metabolic, and other miscellaneous causes of cholestasis, as listed in Table 20-22.

Hepatobiliary imaging, using imidodiacetic acid derivatives, may be employed. The radionuclide is given intravenously. In patients with biliary atresia, uptake into the liver is rapid, but no excretion into the intestine occurs. Conversely, in patients with neonatal hepatitis, uptake is slow, but excretion does occur. This study typically is performed after phenobarbital, 5 mg/kg/d, has been given orally for 3 to 5 days to enhance biliary excretion of the isotope.

Percutaneous hepatic biopsy is of great value in the differentiation of neonatal hepatitis and extrahepatic biliary atresia. This procedure may be performed safely using the Menghini technique. Pathologic findings favoring the diagnosis of extrahepatic biliary atresia include bile duct proliferation, bile plugs, and portal and perilobular fibrosis.

If the diagnosis of extrahepatic biliary atresia cannot be ruled out definitively after the evaluation described above has been performed, operative exploration and cholangiography should be undertaken. This procedure enables recognition of biliary atresia as well as exclusion of other forms of extrahepatic bile duct disease (stenosis or perforation of the common bile duct). The surgeon should avoid transection of a biliary tree that is patent but small because of biliary hypoplasia or the diminished bile flow that is associated with intrahepatic cholestasis. Resection is *not* indicated in these cases. Correctable forms of atresia (distal obstruction), as mentioned previously, also may be found.

In about 80% of cases, however, a "non-correctable" atresia will be found. In these patients, further exploration is indicated and an attempt to establish biliary drainage should be made, using the hepatoportoenterostomy procedure of Kasai. This procedure consists of transection of the porta hepatis, with subsequent apposition of a Roux-en-Y loop of intestine. The rationale is to drain any small, persisting bile duct remnants. Prognosis after this procedure is affected by the age of the patient at the time of operation, with success rates of 90% in infants less than 2 months of age decreasing to less than 20% in patients greater than 90 days of age. Also important is the size of the lumina of the residual ducts that are encountered at surgery; those with diameters of less than 150 $\mu$m are associated with a poor prognosis. This operation rarely is definitive in patients with noncorrectable atresia, and most patients will have progressive hepatic disease as well as repeated episodes of bacterial cholangitis. Therapy of the patient after the hepatoportoenterostomy (Kasai) operation consists of prompt and vigorous treatment of the episodes of cholangitis and consistent attention to nutritional support. Patients in whom bile flow was attained initially after the

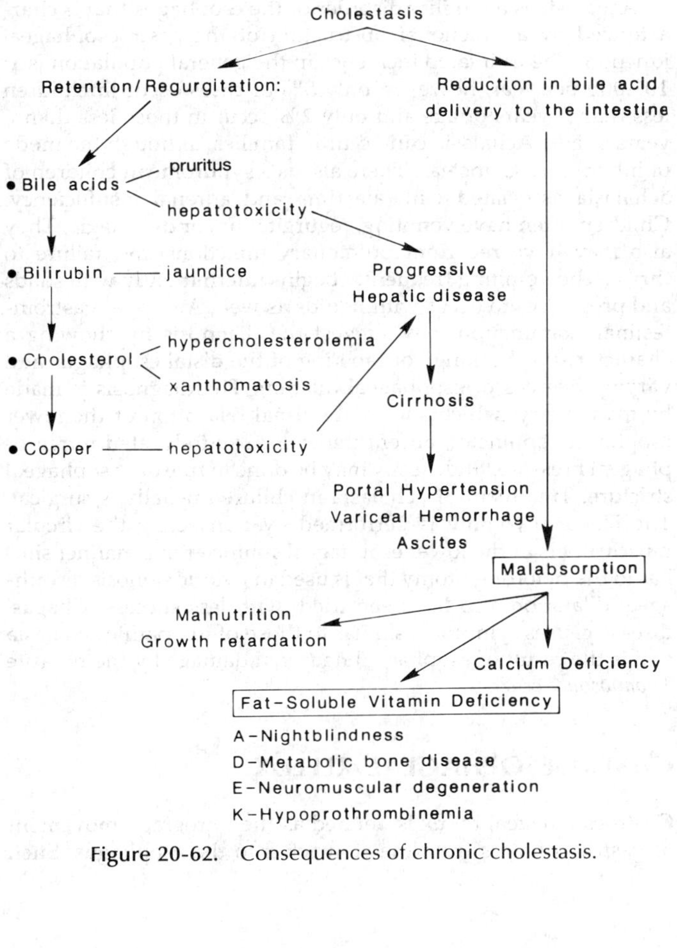

Figure 20-62. Consequences of chronic cholestasis.

Kasai operation, but who subsequently stop draining probably should undergo reoperation in an effort to establish bile flow again. Multiple attempts at reexploration and revision of a nonfunctional conduit should be avoided, however. Regardless of the eventual outcome, one beneficial effect of the Kasai procedure often is to provide adequate time for the patient to grow before hepatic transplantation becomes necessary. Biliary atresia without intervention is universally fatal, with the mean age of death being less than 1 year. Liver transplantation now is essential in the treatment of children whose operation is not successful in restoring bile flow, in those who are referred late (probably at 120 days of age or later), and in those in whom liver failure eventually develops despite some degree of bile drainage.

## Selected Readings

Allagille P, Estrada A, Hadchouel M, et al. Syndromic paucity of interlobular bile ducts (Alagille syndrome or arteriohepatic dysplasia): Review of 80 cases. J Pediatr 1987;110:195.

Balistreri WF. Neonatal cholestasis-medical progress. J Pediatr 1985;106:191.

Kahn E. Paucity of interlobular bile ducts: Arteriohepatic dysplasia and nonsyndromic duct paucity. In: Abramowsky CR, Berstein J, Rosenberg HS, eds. Transplantation pathology—hepatic morphogenesis. Perspect Pediatr Pathol 1991;14:168.

Kahn E, Daum F, Marowitz J, et al. Nonsyndromic paucity of interlobular bile ducts: Light- and electron- microscopic evaluation of sequential liver biopsies in early childhood. Hepatology 1986;6:890.

Karrer FM, Lilly JR, Stewart BA, Hall RJ. Biliary atresia registry, 1976-1989. J Pediatr Surg 1990;254:1076.

Kaufman SS, Murray ND, Wood P, et al. Nutrition support for the infant with extrahepatic biliary atresia. J Pediatr 1987;110:679.

Landing BH. Consideration of the pathogenesis of neonatal hepatitis, biliary atresia, and choledochal cyst: The concept of infantile obstructive cholangiopathy. Prog Pediatr Surg 1974;6:113.

Lilly JR, Karrer FM, Hall RJ, et al. The surgery of biliary atresia. Ann Surg 1989;210:289.

Mieli-Vergani G, Howard ER, Portman B, Mowat AP. Liver disease in infancy: A 20 year perspective. Gut 1991;32(Suppl):S123.

Mieli-Vergani G, Portman B, Howard ER, Mowat AP. Late referral for biliary atresia—missed opportunities for effective surgery. Lancet 1989;1:421.

Nelson R. Managing biliary atresia. Referral before 6 weeks is vital. BMJ 1989;298:1471.

Nietgen GW, Vacanti JP, Perez-Atayde AR. Intrahepatic bile duct loss in biliary atresia: A consequence of ongoing obstruction? Gastroenterology 1992;102:2126.

Rosenblum JC, Keating JP, Prensky AC, et al. Aggressive neurologic syndrome in children with chronic liver disease. N Engl J Med 1981;304:503.

Ryckman FC, Noseworthy J. Neonatal cholestatic conditions requiring surgical reconstruction. Semin Liver Dis 1987;7:134.

Schutzens RHB, Heymans HSA, Wanders RJA, et al. Peroxisomal disorders: A newly recognized group of genetic diseases. Eur J Pediatr 1986;144:430.

*Principles and Practice of Pediatrics, Second Edition.*
edited by Frank A. Oski et al. J. B. Lippincott Company, Philadelphia © 1994.

## *20.4.3 Sucking and Swallowing Disorders and Gastroesophageal Reflux*

William M. Belknap and Colston F. McEvoy

## SUCKING AND SWALLOWING

Normal sucking and swallowing are essential neurologic functions in the neonate. Primitive sucking and swallowing are present in the fetus by the 16th week of gestation. A completely mature suckling response usually is present by the gestational age of 34 to 35 weeks. The normal sequence of sucking and swallowing is as follows. At birth, the infant is capable of short bursts of suckling that fill the anterior chamber of the mouth. This chamber is created by the tongue, which fixes in a posterior position against the soft palate, occluding fluid entry into the pharynx during sucking. Next, swallowing is initiated when the liquid bolus is propelled from the mouth into the pharynx with a thrusting movement of the tongue. During this sequence, the tongue moves posteriorly and the larynx rises; as a consequence, the epiglottis closes and the airway is closed off to the pharynx. As the bolus enters the pharynx, the pharyngeal constrictor muscles relax to accommodate it; at the same time, the upper esophageal sphincter or cricopharyngeus muscle relaxes. The bolus then enters the upper esophagus and initiates a primary peristaltic wave within it, which propels the bolus to the distal esophagus. The gastroesophageal sphincter relaxes transiently, and the bolus enters the stomach.

Because the swallowing mechanism is a coordinated neuromuscular activity requiring intact neurologic and muscular functions, focal or global deficits will interfere with normal swallowing (Table 20-23). Structural anomalies of the mouth, pharynx, or larynx may interfere with the normal sequence of swallowing. Laryngeal anomalies such as laryngeal cleft may result in choking during swallowing. Birth asphyxia, congenital (Möbius' syndrome) or traumatic (birth injury) cranial nerve deficits, infantile botulism, congenital myopathies, myasthenia gravis, and Werdnig-Hoffmann disease are examples of neonatal diseases that cause sucking or swallowing dysfunction. As is apparent from the list of neurologic disorders, generalized hypotonia usually is present (see Chapter 20.1.6). Dysfunction of the muscle of the upper esophageal sphincter, the cricopharyngeus, also may result in these symptoms. More distally, swallowing dysfunction at the level of the esophagus may be caused by either intrinsic or extrinsic obstruction. Extrinsic compression of the esophagus or trachea by an anomalous course of a major thoracic blood vessel is addressed in another chapter.

Achalasia is a motility disorder of the esophagus that is characterized by a functional obstruction of the gastroesophageal junction. The estimated incidence in the general population is 1:100,000 per year; however, only 5% of cases occur in children less than 5 years of age and only 2% occur in those less than 6 years of age. Achalasia can occur in families, although the mode of inheritance is unclear. There also is a syndrome in children of achalasia associated with alacrima and adrenal insufficiency. Children often have vomiting, regurgitation, or dysphagia. They also may have recurrent pulmonary infections and failure to thrive. The vomiting frequently begins intermittently with solids and progresses to occur with liquids as well. An upper gastrointestinal examination may suggest the diagnosis by showing a characteristic "beaking" or tapering of the distal esophagus and varying degrees of esophageal dilation. The diagnosis is made by manometry, which shows abnormal relaxation of the lower esophageal sphincter, absent peristalsis, and elevated intraesophageal pressure. Endoscopy may be done to rule out esophageal stricture. Treatment of achalasia in children usually is surgical. The Heller myotomy is performed by transecting the circular muscle fibers of the lower esophageal sphincter in a manner similar to the pyloromyotomy that is used in pyloric stenosis. Esophageal dilatation also has been tried, with less success. Chagas' disease causes symptoms similar to those of idiopathic achalasia and is the result of esophageal neuronal damage by the parasite *Typanosoma cruzi.*

## GASTROESOPHAGEAL REFLUX

Gastroesophageal reflux is defined as the retrograde movement of gastric contents from the stomach into the esophagus. Such

TABLE 20-23. Causes of Abnormal Sucking and Swallowing
in the Newborn Period (Birth to 28 Days)

| Structural Anomalies | Neurologic | Muscular |
|---|---|---|
| **General** | **Congenital** | **Congenital** |
| Micrognathia | Möbius' syndrome | Benign congenital hypotonia |
| Cleft palate | Werdnig-Hoffmann disease | Myotonic dystrophy |
| Macroglossia | Neonatal myasthenia gravis | Muscular dystrophy |
| Ranula | Familial dysautonomia | Amyotonia congenita |
| Lingual hygroma | | |
| Lingual hemangioma | **Acquired** | **Acquired** |
| Lingual thyroid | Birth asphyxia | Hypocalcemia |
| Dermoid cyst (lingual) | Bulbar palsy | Hypomagnesemia |
| Choanal atresia or stenosis | Palatal paralysis | Hypokalemia |
| Pharyngeal cyst | Cricopharyngeal achalasia | Hypophosphatemia |
| Laryngeal cleft | Recurrent laryngeal nerve | |
| Esophageal anomalies | paralysis | |
| | Botulism | |
| **Syndromes** | Kernicterus | |
| Pierre Robin | Tetanus neonatorum | |
| Trisomy 21 | Sedation | |
| Trisomies 13–15 | | |
| Congenital hypothyroidism | | |
| Glycogen storage disease, type II | | |

*Modified from Gyboski J, Walker WA, eds. Gastrointestinal problems in the infant, ed 2. Philadelphia: WB Saunders, 1983.*

episodes frequently occur physiologically, and the event is brief, asymptomatic, and self-limited. It is well established that infants, particularly premature infants, have a greater frequency and duration of reflux episodes in both the sleeping and the awake states. The pathologic consequence of gastroesophageal reflux in the full-term and premature newborn usually is minimal.

The physiologic barriers for preventing reflux of gastric contents into the esophagus include the following. The first is a functional lower esophageal sphincter at the level of the gastroesophageal junction. It is most likely that the lower esophageal sphincter is the principal barrier against gastroesophageal reflux. The basal tone or pressure achieved at this specific anatomic site probably maintains gastric contents within the stomach. The second factor preventing gastroesophageal reflux is the ability to clear fluid actively from the distal esophagus by maintaining active motility. When normal distal esophageal motility is present, fluid entering the distal esophagus results in prompt clearance or return to the stomach. This prevents a peptic injury to the esophagus by the acidic contents of the stomach. This clearance is aided cooperatively by gravity, the ready flow of saliva from the mouth, and intact neuromuscular function of the distal esophagus. Thus, the ability of the distal esophagus to evoke local propulsive waves to clear its distal third is an essential reflux barrier. A third function important in maintaining normal upper gastrointestinal function is intrinsic gastric motility. Gastric emptying, the ability of the stomach to discharge efficiently and completely a milk feeding into the duodenum after it is emulsified and acidified, is a fundamental aspect of upper intestinal function and digestion. Failure of prompt and efficient emptying will overwhelm the reservoir capacity of the stomach and potentiate gastroesophageal reflux.

When examined closely, virtually all newborn infants are observed to have gastroesophageal reflux. This usually is manifested clinically at the time of feeding as the effortless regurgitation of a portion of the feeding. Dysfunction in or incoordination of the mechanisms of upper gastrointestinal motility cited above probably plays a role; this phenomenon is the result of a physiologic delay in the maturation of this function. Occasionally, unforced regurgitation of an entire feeding may occur, and should not occasion alarm. Rarely, either the overall frequency of reflux or the marked duration of single episodes may cause problems in a neonate, particularly a premature infant. Such reflux is problematic most often in infants with other diseases, such as chronic pulmonary disease or symptomatic congenital heart disease. In a minority of infants, reflux itself may occur excessively frequently or be of such duration as to create primary problems in the absence of a concomitant illness. Reflux may occasion reluctance to feed in the caretaker, and caloric deprivation may result, with failure of the infant to grow and thrive. In addition, the physical action of reflux of feedings itself may prevent the retention of sufficient intake to support normal growth. Reflux, by virtue of its frequency or duration, may result in peptic esophagitis. Infants with esophagitis will have frequent regurgitation, general irritability or colic, or reflux of small amounts of blood-tinged formula. The presence of esophagitis is a very important indicator for pathologic gastroesophageal reflux.

Much discussion has occurred about the role of gastroesophageal reflux in precipitating major respiratory events in neonates. Frequently, reflux events will result in coughing or choking. These commonly are associated with the feeding itself or occur in the immediate postprandial period. It is apparent that, on rare occasion, reflux itself may be a cause of obstructive apnea. The rarest and most serious complication of gastroesophageal reflux is tracheal aspiration.

Evaluation for the presence of esophageal reflux begins with excluding partial upper intestinal obstruction. Reflux never should be confused with such disorders as pyloric stenosis, gastric antral web, duodenal stenosis, annular pancreas, or malrotation. Vomiting secondary to increased intracranial pressure, metabolic disease manifesting acidosis or hyperammonemia, and drug toxicity, as well as the presence of infections such as pneumonia, otitis media, or urinary tract infection must be considered carefully and excluded. In general, the normal health of the infant, the absence of bloody or bilious vomiting, and a history of normal weight gain indicate that gastroesophageal reflux is physiologic and benign. If regurgitation of entire feedings has occurred and is of sufficient frequency, upper gastrointestinal obstruction or other causes of frank vomiting must be considered.

Barium contrast studies of the pharynx, esophagus, and upper gastrointestinal tract should be performed to confirm that anatomy and motility are normal. This study may demonstrate the occurrence of gastroesophageal reflux in roughly 50% of cases; unfortunately, reflux on barium swallow may be artifactual. This point is particularly relevant in small infants when the study is performed under stressful circumstances with an indwelling nasogastric tube. A very sensitive modality with which to define the actual frequency and duration of gastroesophageal reflux is the use of an indwelling pH monitor. Such a study may be performed in very small infants for as long as 12 to 24 hours. In addition, concomitant monitoring for cardiopulmonary dysfunction or recording of the cessation of active respiration occasionally is used in problem cases when reflux is thought to cause respiratory dysfunction in hospitalized infants. Last, in cases in which reflux is intractable and the possibility of gastrointestinal obstruction is eliminated, it may be necessary to investigate the infant specifically for a diagnosis of esophagitis. This may be accomplished either through a peroral suction biopsy of the distal esophagus or directly through visualization and biopsy by esophagoscopy. In many cases, the diagnosis of esophagitis is evident only histologically; the relevance of this finding must be individualized clinically. Pulmonary symptoms such as apnea can be ascribed to reflux only if a temporal association with apnea is documented carefully. Even in that event, causality is difficult to confirm.

Choking during feedings should not be attributed to gastroesophageal reflux; swallowing dysfunction may be present. Nasal–pharyngeal incoordination and other causes of swallowing dysfunction should be differentiated from gastroesophageal reflux in the infant who presents with feeding difficulties. The investigation for aspiration may include performing technetium–sulfur colloid scintiscanning of gastric emptying. In this case, the actual gastric emptying can be quantified, in addition to visualization and documentation of gastroesophageal reflux and actual aspiration.

Therapy for gastroesophageal reflux is individualized. In the uncomplicated patient with postprandial regurgitation of small amounts of the feeding, simple observation and reassurance are indicated. An upright, prone posture, taking advantage of gravity, is the next level of therapy. Formally placing the infant in a 30° posture after the time of feeding, or maintaining very difficult cases nearly continuously in this position, will minimize reflux. Frequent, small feedings are advantageous, in contrast with larger and less frequent feedings. Thickened feedings also have been advocated in some cases, but the utility of this practice recently has been brought into question. Documentation of esophagitis calls for prompt, aggressive therapy, including antacid administration after feedings; severe or unresponsive cases are treated pharmacologically with an $H_2$-receptor–blocking agent. Agents to enhance gastroduodenal motility and increase distal gastroesophageal sphincter pressure have been advocated. These drugs include bethanechol and metoclopramide; the latter agent has been associated with the undesirable side effects of restlessness and oculogyric crisis, particularly in newborn or premature infants. The routine use of these drugs in neonates cannot be advocated.

Because gastroesophageal reflux results from immaturity of the mechanisms necessary to maintain normal upper gastrointestinal motility, it will resolve rapidly in most infants. Indeed, most infants achieve normal function by 6 to 7 weeks of age; a minimum of 60% to 70% of infants with obvious gastroesoph-

ageal reflux achieve complete functional maturity without specific therapy. Because prolonged gastroesophageal reflux may occur during sleep as absent voluntary swallowing and salivation, resulting in prolonged episodes, placing the infant in a prone, upright position during sleep may be advantageous. In the remaining infants, continued reflux will improve or resolve by the time they are 6 months old; in 90% of them, it will resolve completely by the time they are 18 months old.

Intractable gastroesophageal reflux may occur in the neurologically impaired infant. In such cases, surgical fundoplication and gastrostomy tube placement may be indicated. Surgical therapy for gastroesophageal reflux also may be necessary in cases in which documented aspiration pneumonia has occurred on two occasions. Although surgical therapy may be of some benefit, it rarely is indicated. Surgical fundoplication is associated with postoperative complications in up to 10% to 20% of patients. In addition, a repeat surgical procedure may become necessary.

Patients who have undergone repair of a tracheoesophageal fistula very commonly have distal esophageal dysmotility and gastroesophageal reflux. Reflux may be very problematic in such cases.

## Selected Readings

Cucchiara S, Staiano A, DiLorenzo C, et al. Esophageal motor abnormalities in children with gastroesophageal reflux and peptic esophagitis. J Pediatr 1986;108:907.

Dedinsky GK, Vane DW, Black T, et al. Complications and reoperation after Nissen fundoplication in childhood. Am J Surg 1987;153:177.

Gyboski J, Walker WA, eds. Gastrointestinal problems in the infant, ed 2. Philadelphia: WB Saunders, 1983.

Hillemeier AC, Grill BB, McCallum R, et al. Esophageal and gastric motor abnormalities in gastroesophageal reflux during infancy. Gastroenterology 1983;84:741.

Nihoul-F'ek'e'e C, Bawab F, Lortat-Jacobs S, Arhan P, Pellnin D. Achalasia of the esophagus in childhood. J Pediatr Surg 1989;24:1060.

Orenstein SR. Controversies in pediatric gastroesophageal reflux. J Pediatr Gastroenterol Nutr 1992;14:338.

Orenstein SR, Orenstein DM. Gastroesophageal reflux and respiratory disease in children. J Pediatr 1988;112:847.

Weihrauch TR. Gastroesophageal reflux—pathogenesis and clinical implications. Eur J Pediatr 1985;144:215.

Werlin SL, Dodds WJ, Hogan WJ, et al. Mechanisms of gastroesophageal reflux in children. J Pediatr 1980;97:244.

*Principles and Practice of Pediatrics, Second Edition.*
edited by Frank A. Oski et al. J. B. Lippincott Company, Philadelphia © 1994.

## 20.4.4 *Distended Abdomen*

William M. Belknap

Abdominal distention in the newborn may result from several causes, including organomegaly, intestinal obstruction, pneumoperitoneum, hemoperitoneum, ascites, and an abdominal mass. The causes of hepatomegaly and hepatosplenomegaly in the newborn are discussed in the section regarding the liver. Intestinal obstruction, likewise, is discussed elsewhere.

## PNEUMOPERITONEUM AND HEMOPERITONEUM

Pneumoperitoneum, defined as free air within the peritoneal cavity, may result in massive abdominal distention. Pneumoperitoneum occurs most commonly as a result of perforation somewhere in the gastrointestinal tract, or because of an air leak in the pulmonary system with subsequent egress into the peritoneal cavity. In a large series of infants who were seen in the neonatal period with pneumoperitoneum, gestational ages varied from 22 to 43 weeks and birth weights were less than 1500 g in 75% of cases. Necrotizing enterocolitis complicated by bowel perforation was the leading cause of pneumoperitoneum in this group, occurring in 60% of the patients. Isolated gastrointestinal perforation was the next most common etiology. In the latter cases, the lesions occurred about equally often and were located at the following sites: stomach, duodenum, ileum, and colon. Spontaneous gastric perforation, acute duodenal ulceration, spontaneous ileal perforation or ileal atresia, and meconium plug or Hirschsprung's disease are the known causes for regional intestinal perforation. Roughly 10% of neonates with pneumoperitoneum have no gastrointestinal cause for this finding. In these infants, all of whom are critically ill with respiratory distress syndrome and are treated with mechanical ventilation, pneumoperitoneum develops after ventilator-induced pulmonary air leak occurs. In these cases, air dissects from the mediastinum to the peritoneal cavity. As implied above, all infants with pneumoperitoneum from gastrointestinal perforation are critically ill. Associated abnormalities are quite common and include premature birth, respiratory distress syndrome, sepsis, and congenital heart disease.

To determine the source of free air in the abdomen, radiographs should be taken in multiple views: flat-plate, upright, and cross-table lateral. A chest radiograph should be performed in ventilated infants to eliminate pneumomediastinum as the precipitating cause. Surgical co-management is indicated; infants with pneumoperitoneum of gastrointestinal etiology require abdominal exploration and surgical correction. Despite the fact that these infants are seriously ill, with early recognition and appropriate therapy, three fourths of them can be expected to survive.

Hemoperitoneum, or blood within the peritoneal space, occurs in the newborn as a result of active hemorrhage from the liver, spleen, or adrenal gland after birth trauma. Intraperitoneal hemorrhage commonly leads to shock and death unless it is recognized rapidly. Hemorrhage from the liver occurs as a result of a laceration sustained during birth trauma. These infants either are born prematurely or are large for their gestational age and present in the breech position. The mechanisms of hepatic injury are by compression to the chest with secondary pressure to the liver or by direct hepatic pressure. In both cases, the bleeding usually is self-contained in the liver as a subcapsular hematoma. Subcapsular hematomas are asymptomatic and may not be palpable; unfortunately, some hepatic lacerations continue to bleed, and the hematoma may rupture through the liver capsule after about 48 hours. Acute cardiovascular instability ensues as occult exsanguination occurs into the peritoneal space. In addition to tachycardia and acute hypotension, this event may be manifested by the clinical appearance of abdominal ecchymoses. Splenic laceration is the second, but much less common, cause of hemoperitoneum. This usually occurs as a result of rupture of the splenorenal ligament during birth; associated features may include difficult delivery, shoulder dystocia, fractured clavicle, brachial paralysis, or liver laceration. Hemorrhage from the disrupted splenic vessel is brisk, and cardiovascular collapse occurs earlier than with liver laceration. The third and least common cause of hemoperitoneum is adrenal hemorrhage; this entity more commonly presents as an abdominal mass, and is discussed below. Retroperitoneal hemorrhage from renal laceration is a much rarer consequence of birth trauma than are the lesions cited above. This lesion has a better prognosis, as hemorrhage in the retroperitoneum is more apt to be self-contained earlier.

The evaluation and treatment of all infants suspected of having

hemoperitoneum are the same. Diagnostic abdominal paracentesis confirms the presence of whole blood. A plain radiograph of the patient's abdomen demonstrates fluid densities bulging at both flanks, with the small intestine located centrally. If the infant is sufficiently stable, an abdominal ultrasound or computerized axial tomography scan may identify the specific organ of origin. Transfusion, correction of coagulopathy, and surgical exploration and repair are indicated in hemoperitoneum. Adrenal hemorrhage only rarely results in hemoperitoneum, as it often will remain self-contained in the retroperitoneal space; operative intervention, therefore, usually is not required. All patients with adrenal hemorrhage should be observed acutely and chronically for signs of adrenal insufficiency.

## NEONATAL ASCITES

Ascites, or fluid accumulation in the peritoneal space, occurs in the neonate either as a part of generalized body edema (hydrops fetalis) or as an isolated finding. Hydrops fetalis from Rh isoimmunization occurs as a result of low hematocrit, hypoproteinemia, and high-output cardiac failure, and is discussed elsewhere. Hydrops also occurs from nonimmunologic causes, and includes some of the disorders discussed below.

Ascites in the newborn may occur in the absence of generalized edema (Table 20-24). Urinary ascites resulting from perforation within a congenitally obstructed urinary tract is the most common cause of isolated ascites in the newborn. Idiopathic causes rank equally as causes of isolated neonatal ascites; cardiac arrhythmias and congenital heart failure are next in frequency. Congenital cirrhosis in hereditary tyrosinemia, acute metabolic injury to the liver in galactosemia, and extensive hepatic involvement in congenital infection are associated with neonatal ascites. In the biliary tract, spontaneous perforation of the common bile duct may result in biliary ascites. Whereas congenital infections may result in significant hepatic disease and ascites, idiopathic ascites also occurs in some infants who do not have significant liver disease. The most common congenital infections in which ascites occurs are syphilis, cytomegalovirus, toxoplasmosis, and parvovirus. Neonatal enterovirus, herpes simplex, and varicella infections all may cause serious systemic disease with multiple organ involvement; hepatic involvement and ascites frequently are present. These disorders have been discussed in detail in a previous section. A ruptured ovarian cyst in the neonate also will result in free intraperitoneal fluid. Patients with a history of maternal polyhydramnios who have ascites at birth are more likely to have

### TABLE 20-24.  Causes of Neonatal Ascites*

| Cause | Frequency (%) |
| --- | --- |
| Urinary | 30 |
| Idiopathic | 30 |
| Cardiac arrhythmia | 10 |
| Hepatobiliary | 5–10 |
| Congenital infection | 5–10 |
| Intestinal perforation | <5 |
| Ruptured ovarian cyst | <5 |
| Chylous ascites | <5 |
| Metabolic storage disease (see text) | <5 |

* Excluding hydrops fetalis from isoimmunization and nonimmunologic causes.

Griscom NT, Colodny AH, Rosenberg HK, et al. Diagnostic aspects of neonatal ascites: Report of 27 cases. AJR Am J Roentgenol 1977;128:961.

intestinal obstruction, with intrauterine bowel perforation causing ascites. In this case, the ascitic fluid may be either meconium or exudative fluid secondary to meconium-induced chemical peritonitis; peritoneal calcification also may be present. Chylous ascites is lymph in the peritoneal cavity; therefore, it has a high lipid content and is a consequence of lymphatic vessel leak or intestinal lymphangiectasia. The leak may be induced by intestinal malrotation and lymphatic perforation; a mesenteric lymphocele or cyst may distend massively and perforate into the peritoneal cavity. Chylous ascites may become apparent only after the baby is fed breast milk or a formula containing a long-chain triglyceride, which increases abdominal lymph production and flow. Neonatal ascites has been reported as a presenting sign of the following lysosomal storage diseases: Gaucher's disease, infantile sialidosis, Salla disease, and $GM_1$ gangliosidosis. The familial nature of these disorders and other manifestations, such as storage granules in peripheral blood leukocytes, suggest metabolic disease.

The strategy for evaluation of the newborn with abdominal distention and suspected ascites is as follows. The gestational history and preliminary physical examination are focused on precluding obvious and clinically serious conditions. Rh isoimmunization, other neonatal hemolytic diseases, congenital infection, and congestive heart failure resulting from tachyarrhythmia or structural heart disease are examples. The specific diagnosis of and therapy for these disorders are discussed elsewhere.

When the cause of ascites is not readily apparent, a careful sequence of studies should be performed. Abdominal radiographs of the infant in prone, upright, and lateral positions should be obtained. Pneumoperitoneum, diffuse abdominal calcification, and massive distention of bowel are indicative of intestinal obstruction and perforation. A pattern of laterally displaced bowel gas on the abdominal radiograph indicates, unlike in ascites, the presence of a regional abdominal cystic mass; the causes of this finding are discussed in detail below. Uncomplicated ascites is defined on the abdominal radiographs by fluid densities in the flanks that extend to a variable degree to the midline; loops of bowel are displaced to the center of the abdomen. In such cases, bilateral nephromegaly must be examined for carefully and excluded.

Investigation then is directed to the urinary tract. Ultrasound, a voiding cystourethrogram, and an excretory urogram are used to define a specific site of high-grade obstruction in the urinary tract that is complicated by perforation and urinary leak into the peritoneal cavity. If the infant has been voiding regularly and the abdominal ultrasound examination is normal, diagnostic paracentesis should be performed next. The fluid is inspected visually, and a microscopic cell count is made. Quantitative measurements of triglyceride, bilirubin, and protein are obtained. Hemorrhagic fluid may be indicative of hemoperitoneum and require immediate intervention; alternatively, a diagnosis of congenital toxoplasmosis infection or a ruptured ovarian cyst should be considered. Ascitic fluid that is white or has a high protein content and a large amount of triglyceride is chylous. Intestinal malrotation, mesenteric cyst, and a ruptured lymphangioma all should be excluded as causes of chylous ascites through barium studies of the gastrointestinal tract and abdominal ultrasound evaluation. If the ascitic fluid simply is a serous exudate, the following entities should be considered carefully: congenital infection, liver disease, and metabolic conditions, including the specific lysosomal storage diseases cited above. Despite careful investigation, nearly one third of infants with ascites as an isolated finding will show no discernible cause.

Therapy for ascites is aimed at surgical correction of specific urologic or gastrointestinal perforation. Treatment of specific congenital infection is indicated. In infants with documented chylous ascites, feeding with formula containing predominantly medium-chain triglycerides is instituted. This takes advantage of the alternate absorption pathway of medium-chain triglycerides, which are transported directly into the portal venous system after gastric or intestinal absorption. This maneuver will reduce the lipid load to the abdominal lymphatic system and allow time for the lymphatic leak to close. If chylous ascites persists and is symptomatic, surgical exploration for identification and repair of the leak is indicated. Unfortunately, neonatal chylous ascites on occasion is relentless, despite all treatment maneuvers, and eventually may be fatal. Specific diagnosis of lysosomal storage diseases causing neonatal ascites is discussed elsewhere.

## ABDOMINAL MASS IN THE NEWBORN

The lesions causing abdominal masses that present in the neonatal period usually are benign; only 10% to 15% represent malignant tumors (Table 20-25). Two thirds of abdominal masses in the neonate are retroperitoneal in location; the kidneys predominate as the most common origin of an abdominal mass presenting in the newborn period. Renal mass lesions, therefore, are the single most common diagnostic category of abdominal mass in the newborn, as well as the most common of the masses that arise specifically from the retroperitoneal space. The remainder of the regional abdominal masses detected in this age group originate in gastrointestinal, mesenteric, hepatobiliary, or genital tracts and are discussed individually below. Many of the specific aspects of these disorders in the newborn are discussed comprehensively elsewhere in this text.

### Renal System

Multicystic, dysplastic kidney is the single most common cause of abdominal mass seen in the newborn. This mass lesion presents, usually in the first day of life, as an asymptomatic, palpable, left flank mass. It is soft and irregular in contour because it is cystic and multilobar; on physical examination, these lesions will transilluminate. They are caused by developmental atresia of the ureteropelvic unit. Roughly 30% of afflicted infants have anomalies of the opposite kidney and collecting system. Nearly equal in frequency as a cause of abdominal mass in the newborn is hydronephrosis secondary to congenital anatomic obstruction to urine flow. This entity may not be apparent on the first day of life. Congenital ureteropelvic junction obstruction, posterior urethral valves, ectopic ureterocele, prune-belly syndrome, and ureteral or ureterovesical obstruction are the causes of hydronephrosis in the newborn, in decreasing order of frequency. Renal vein thrombosis with secondary renal enlargement resulting from venous occlusion and renal vascular engorgement and edema should be suspected in newborns younger than 3 days who are seen with abdominal distention and a palpable flank mass. These infants often have a history of hypernatremic dehydration secondary to vomiting, diarrhea, or sepsis, leading to a low urine output and shock. Afflicted infants also most commonly are male, are infants of diabetic mothers, and have a history of significant hypoglycemia, with or without a secondary seizure. A perinatal history of maternal dehydration or diuretic use may be elicited. The effect of the kidney enlargement resulting from renal vein thrombosis is a large mass that is firm, smooth in contour, and perhaps bilateral, and does not transilluminate. These infants may have systemic hypertension. Bilateral nephromegaly also may be a familial polycystic kidney disease, presenting as bilateral flank masses and associated with marked systemic hypertension; this entity is discussed more thoroughly in another section. Renal malignancy is very rare in the newborn. Nonetheless, Wilms' tumor (nephroblastoma) may be detected in the newborn as an

| TABLE 20-25. Causes of Abdominal Mass in the Newborn* | |
|---|---|
| **Renal (see section on the kidney)** | **Hepatic** |
| Unilateral cystic dysplastic kidney | Hepatomegaly (see section on the liver) |
| Hydronephrosis | Infantile hemangioendothelioma (calcification) |
| Renal vein thrombosis | Hepatoblastoma (calcification 40%) |
| Nephromegaly | Mesenchymal hamartoma |
| Renal polycystic disease | Subcapsular hematoma |
| Wilms' tumor | Epidermoid cyst |
| Mesoblastic nephroma | Benign teratoma |
| Neurogenic bladder | Focal nodular hyperplasia (rare) |
| | Angiosarcoma, undifferentiated sarcoma |
| **Adrenal** | Metastatic disease (neuroblastoma) |
| Adrenal hemorrhage | |
| Abscess | **Biliary** |
| Neuroblastoma (calcification 50%) | Hydropic gallbladder |
| Teratoma (calcification 75%) | Choledochal cyst |
| | Spontaneous perforation of the common bile duct |
| **Retroperitoneal** | |
| Lymphangioma | **Genital Tract** |
| Neuroblastoma | Hydrometrocolpos |
| Sacrococcygeal teratoma | Ovarian cyst |
| Ganglioneuroma | Ovarian teratoma |
| Leiomyosarcoma | Urachal cyst |
| Pancreatic cyst | Inguinal masses: hernia, hydrocele, calcified meconium |
| **Gastrointestinal** | |
| Intestinal duplication | |
| Segmental intestinal dilatation | |
| Mesenteric cyst (± intestinal malrotation) | |
| Lymphangioma | |
| Intraperitoneal meconium cyst | |

* See text for relative frequency and characteristics.

abdominal mass. A benign lesion, mesoblastic nephroma, also occurs in the newborn. Last, a pelvic mass representing a neurogenic bladder secondary to meningomyelocele or other pelvic neuropathy may occur; hydronephrosis may be present coincidentally.

The evaluation to define the cause of a regional abdominal mass in the renal system is primarily radiologic. Associated abnormalities in the blood or urine usually are present only in cases of renal vein thrombosis: hemoconcentration, hyperviscosity, thrombocytopenia, and gross or microscopic hematuria. Ultrasound is the principal mode of diagnosis. Multicystic dysplastic kidney will manifest multiple, variable-sized cysts that transmit echoes poorly on ultrasonography. A finding of one or several intrarenal or juxtarenal cystic masses on ultrasound suggests hydronephrosis; lower renal tract obstruction is diagnosed as the cause when concomitant ureteromegaly and bladder enlargement are present. Bilateral kidney enlargement with a uniform increase in echoes indicates the multiple small cysts of infantile polycystic kidney disease. Hepatic polycystic disease also may be present. Mesoblastic nephroma will manifest on ultrasound as an intrarenal solid mass, and an excretory urogram may be necessary to confirm this diagnosis. In renal vein thrombosis, ultrasound reveals uniform nephromegaly. Nephroblastoma, or early Wilms' tumor, is apparent on ultrasound as multiple, bilateral, subcortical masses. Occasionally, renal scintigraphy is required to differentiate between multicystic dysplastic kidney and hydronephrosis. With the exception of renal vein thrombosis, all the above lesions are treated surgically through nephrectomy or correction of the focus of obstruction.

## Other Retroperitoneal Masses

As stated previously, two thirds of abdominal masses in the neonate are retroperitoneal in location. Whereas the majority are renal in origin, 45% arise from a different location within the retroperitoneal space. A discussion of these other entities follows.

Hemorrhage into the adrenal gland is next in frequency to renal lesions as a cause of retroperitoneal abdominal mass in the newborn. Adrenal hemorrhage occurs on the right side in about 80% of cases; left-sided and bilateral hemorrhages are roughly equal in frequency. Injury to the adrenal gland during a difficult delivery is the usual cause. On the right side, this organ is quite vulnerable to compression trauma, as it lies between the liver and the bony surface of the vertebral column. The adrenal glands also are prone to injury via abrupt transient or sustained increases in caval venous pressure. Trauma or venous pressure changes in the presence of blood coagulopathy or hypoxia are particularly apt to promote adrenal hemorrhage. Fetal distress, maternal diabetes, septicemia, congenital syphilis, and hemorrhagic diseases presenting in the newborn are other predisposing conditions. Neonatal adrenal hemorrhage most commonly presents during the first through the fourth days of life. These patients may have a focal abdominal mass from a localized intra-adrenal hemorrhage, more extensive but self-contained retroperitoneal hemorrhage with associated intestinal ileus, or, in the most severe cases, hemoperitoneum. This diagnosis is confirmed through ultrasound and an excretory urogram demonstrating an adrenal mass compressing a normal adjacent kidney downward. The radiographic finding of circumferential calcification may be present by 2 weeks of age. The majority of these lesions may be followed clinically, and the infant occasionally may require blood transfusion. Rarely, surgical intervention for evacuation of blood clot, ligation of bleeding vessels, and possible adrenalectomy is required. If the lesion is bilateral but is followed clinically, the patient should be scrutinized prospectively for signs of adrenal insufficiency.

Neuroblastoma is an important, yet distinctly uncommon, cause of a retroperitoneal abdominal mass in the newborn. This entity is described in detail elsewhere. Briefly, congenital neuroblastoma may originate in the adrenal gland or elsewhere in the retroperitoneal area. Metastatic disease is common, with liver and skin lesions possible. Abdominal radiographs of neuroblastoma demonstrate diffuse, punctate calcifications in three fourths of the patients. Ultrasound will define the limits of the lesion further and will differentiate neuroblastoma from adrenal hemorrhage when it originates from that organ. A certain number of these lesions will regress spontaneously; a complete discussion of their therapy is contained in another section.

Abdominal teratoma is the most common tumor presenting in the newborn period; the site of origin is the retroperitoneal space anterior to the sacrococcygeal vertebrae. Although the lesion may be detected only through a digital rectal examination, a superficial mass may be evident extruding between the anus and coccygeus. Radiographic calcifications occur in two thirds of cases; occasionally, these are well-formed teeth and bone. Definition of the complete retroperitoneal extent of this tumor may require a combination of ultrasound and computerized axial tomography evaluation. Specific therapy through surgical extirpation is described elsewhere.

The remaining causes of abdominal masses arising from the retroperitoneal area occur infrequently. Ganglioneuroma, adrenal abscess, leiomyosarcoma, and pancreatic cyst are reported examples.

## Gastrointestinal System

Gastrointestinal and hepatobiliary lesions account for one fifth of abdominal masses in the neonatal period; 75% originate from the stomach or intestine. Intestinal duplication ranks as the most common gastrointestinal mass presenting in the neonatal period. The definition, distribution, diagnosis, and complications of this developmental anomaly have been discussed in a previous chapter.

Neonatal small-bowel obstruction may masquerade as a regional abdominal mass. In such cases, the characteristic finding during the newborn examination is a firm, mobile, middle abdominal mass. The mass represents a dilated segment of bowel. As discussed below, abdominal radiographs demonstrate a gas pattern consistent with intestinal obstruction. In some cases, in utero gut perforation occurs, and the leaking meconium may loculate as a uniform cystic mass in the peritoneal cavity.

Mass lesions may arise from the abdominal mesentery in the newborn. Such mesenteric cysts may be single or multilobar, and they may contain chyle or serous fluid. Intestinal malrotation may be associated. In contrast, the lesion may present as lymphangioma, a focal malformation of the mesenteric lymphatic system.

Diagnosis of the gastrointestinal mass lesion generally is made through prone and upright abdominal radiographs. Barium contrast studies of the bowel occasionally are necessary when complete luminal obstruction is not present. Ultrasound may be helpful in the more challenging cases of intramesenteric mass lesions.

The therapeutic approach to gastrointestinal or mesenteric mass lesions is complete surgical excision, and the overall prognosis is excellent.

## Liver and Biliary Tract

Abdominal mass lesions in the newborn rarely arise from the liver or biliary tract. All the lesions discussed below are seen far more commonly either later in infancy or early in childhood. The hepatobiliary disorders that present specifically as mass lesions in the newborn also are discussed in other sections of the text. The general causes of neonatal hepatomegaly are discussed elsewhere.

Vascular tumors are the most common cause of a mass lesion arising from or within the liver in the newborn. The specific lesions are hemangiomas, either as infantile hemangioendothelioma or as cavernous hemangioma; the majority are the former. Although they are histologically mesodermal in nature and benign, both conditions cause significant morbidity and have a high mortality rate. Affected patients usually are seen within the newborn period with marked hepatomegaly or a palpable hepatic mass. These tumors may be single or multifocal; they act physiologically as arteriovenous fistulas, with a secondary increase in the total blood volume, hyperdynamic circulation, and cardiomegaly. Congestive heart failure through eventual cardiac decompensation in this state of high cardiac output is the major cause of morbidity and mortality. In three fourths of patients, cutaneous hemangiomas also are present; the coincidence of cardiac failure without structural congenital heart disease, hepatomegaly with a hepatic bruit, and skin hemangiomas has been termed *multinodular hemangiomatosis of the liver*. Less commonly, hemangiomas of the liver may have the devastating complication of spontaneous rupture, producing hemoperitoneum. Anemia is present in most patients; cholestasis, portal hypertension, and other liver function abnormalities occur rarely. Diffuse cutaneous and visceral hemangiomatosis with thrombocytopenia and intravascular coagulation is known as the Kasabach-Merritt syndrome. The diagnosis of hepatic hemangioma can be suggested by filling defects observed on liver ultrasound examination; technetium liver scan confirms filling defects, and is diagnostic. Celiac angiography defines a large hepatic artery feeding the lesion(s). If the above complications are not present, the infant can be observed as even large hepatic hemangiomas resolve. If the patient has congestive heart failure in the neonatal period, hepatic artery ligation is indicated. Left untreated, half of such infants will die soon. If hemoperitoneum occurs, operative exploration and hepatic artery ligation are urgently necessary; if it is localized, the hemangioma is excised. Medical management of heart failure and the use of corticosteroids are reserved for patients who are older at the time of presentation, usually beyond 6 weeks of age.

The hepatic tumor that is next in frequency among benign lesions in the newborn is mesenchymal hamartoma. This benign tumor is rare, and usually presents as a mass in the right lobe of the liver; less commonly, the tumor hangs from the edge of the right lobe by a pedicle or involves both lobes. The tumor has both solid and cystic components. As a hamartoma, the tumor has both mesoderm and endoderm components. The major bulk of the tumor is composed of loose, nearly acellular connective tissue resembling mesenchyme. Tumor growth is progressive, often rapid, and expansive to the point of obliterating normal hepatic parenchyma. Tumor expansion occurs over a period of 3 to 22 months, although a period as short as a few days has been reported. The tumor eventually will achieve massive proportions, causing abdominal distention, respiratory distress, and vena caval obstruction. Because the tumor is highly vascular and may obstruct venous flow to the heart, cardiac failure may ensue. Ultrasound of the liver, computerized axial tomography, and, occasionally, selective celiac angiography are necessary to confirm the diagnosis. Mesenchymal hamartoma is very amenable to surgical extirpation, which always is indicated; preoperative radiation may facilitate resection. This tumor must be differentiated clinically from infantile hemangioendothelioma and hepatoblastoma.

Hepatoblastoma is a malignant liver-cell tumor of early life. The tumor may be purely epithelial in nature, or it also may contain mesenchymal tissue. The epithelial element is fetal, embryonal, or both. Congenital hepatoblastomas have been detected in the first day of life. Although they also are seen later in the neonatal period, the majority of hepatoblastomas occur in late infancy and early childhood. An abdominal mass arising from the right lobe of the liver is the usual clinical presentation. The infants usually are male, and the clinical findings of fever, irritability, and failure to thrive also may be present. Potential associated findings in the neonatal period include hemihypertrophy and hypoglycemia. The possible coincidence with Wilms' tumor is well established, as is isosexual precocity; these latter two associations are unusual and customarily are seen after the newborn period. The tumor itself is focal, and may have calcifications on abdominal radiography. As stated previously, the lesions must be differentiated clinically from those of infantile hemangioendothelioma and mesenchymal hamartoma. The serum $\alpha$-fetoprotein level is elevated in hepatoblastoma; computerized axial tomography and angiography will confirm the diagnosis. Therapy for hepatoblastoma is dependent principally on the ability to excise the total tumor surgically. Preoperative chemotherapy may permit better resection; cure is achieved in one third to one half of patients when surgical extirpation is successful. Overall mortality, however, may approach 75%.

Rarely, other benign and malignant tumors may be detected as a hepatic mass in the newborn. Solitary congenital epidermoid cysts of the right lobe of the liver occur rarely. These lesions are not calcified, do not progress, and are diagnosed noninvasively. Benign teratoma and focal nodular hyperplasia have been noted in the neonatal period. Massive hepatomegaly from metastatic neuroblastoma may occur in newborns; this clinical presentation is discussed in a previous section. The malignant tumors angiosarcoma and undifferentiated sarcoma (malignant mesenchymoma) occur rarely in the neonatal period. Specific delineation of these rare tumors is beyond the scope of this discussion.

Choledochal cyst and hydrops of the gallbladder both may present as right upper quadrant mass lesions in the newborn. These disorders are described in another section.

## Genital Tract

Anomalies of the female genital tract are presented in detail in another chapter. As these lesions may present as an abdominal mass in the neonate, they are described briefly here. The mucosal glands of the female genital tract have a maternal estrogen-responsive secretory function that is present in the fetus and newborn. The secreted fluid is discharged through a usually patent vaginal orifice, through the hymenal ring. This secretion ceases when maternal estrogen no longer is present. When the female genital tract is occluded congenitally at the level of the hymen, the middle of the vagina, or the cervix, this fluid accumulates and secondarily may distend massively the luminal space of the genital tract in utero above the level of the obstruction.

The most external of these conditions, imperforate hymen, results in complete obstruction and distention of the entire genital tract, known as hydrometrocolpos. Vaginal atresia or stenosis, or vaginal distention alone (hydrocolpos) may result in the same finding. Congenital uterine cervical stenosis results in isolated uterine distention, known as hydrometra. These conditions present as large, midline, lower abdominal masses. The mass is mobile, arises from the pelvis as appreciated by the digital rectal examination, and has an upper border that may reach the level of the umbilicus. In addition, the imperforate hymen is seen protruding

between the urethra and anus as a large hemisphere. Massive hydrometrocolpos may be complicated by secondary obstruction of the urinary tract. Alternatively, spontaneous decompression of fluid through the uterine tubes may result in peritonitis. Ultrasound of the pelvis and abdomen confirms the diagnosis of hydrometrocolpos and reveals patients who have secondary hydronephrosis. Complex anomalies may coexist with the lesions that obstruct the genital tract above the hymenal ring. In such cases, either the urethra or a ureter may be ectopic and enter directly into the vagina. Imperforate anus (see Chapter 20.4.1) may coexist with hydrometrocolpos, with a rectovaginal fistula entering the obstructed genital tract. In these complicated cases, a more complete evaluation is necessary, including an excretory urogram, cystography, a vaginohysterosalpingogram, and a barium enema. Surgical repair is indicated in all cases; this may be simple hymenal membrane excision or a complex abdominal-perineal repair. These lesions may remain occult through childhood and present later, at the time of menarche.

Ovarian cysts occurring in the neonatal period are of four varieties; all may present as an abdominal mass. The most common is a follicular cyst, the formation of which is the result of premature induction of ovarian follicles by maternal hormones. Ovarian follicular cysts may achieve remarkable dimensions in the newborn; torsion around the vascular pedicle may precipitate acute symptoms. The remaining causes of ovarian cyst in the newborn are far less common and include benign and malignant granulosa-cell tumors, benign cystic teratomas, and paraovarian cysts. Because these lesions achieve appreciable size and, consequently, are displaced from the pelvis into the abdomen in the newborn, their presentation usually is as a firm, smooth abdominal mass. Abdominal radiography shows a mass effect crossing the midline and displacing bowel; in the rare case of ovarian teratoma, calcification is present. Ultrasound confirms the cystic nature of the mass and demonstrates normal kidneys, ureter, and bladder. Surgical exploration and extirpation are indicated.

The inguinal area of the newborn is a common anatomic region for the clinical finding of a mass. The mass may represent a partially descended testicle; examination of the scrotum will confirm this impression. The processus vaginalis, the potential space of the inguinal canal from the peritoneal cavity to the scrotum, may fail to obliterate completely during development. Complete failure results in a potential space in which bowel may herniate and produce an inguinal mass. Partial obliteration with a narrow but patent residual lumen from the peritoneal cavity to the scrotum may result in a communicating scrotal cyst or hydrocele. Alternatively, partial, noncommunicating superior and inferior obliteration of the processus vaginalis may result in a mid-inguinal hydrocele. In the rare instance in which meconium peritonitis coexists in a patient with a patent processus vaginalis, a firm, calcified inguinal mass results. These lesions are diagnosed clinically; surgical repair and other specific aspects of these lesions are discussed elsewhere.

Complete patency or a cystic dilatation secondary to incomplete obliteration of the urachus, a midline fetal structure, may result in a midline, superficial, lower abdominal mass in the neonate. This lesion is discussed in detail elsewhere.

## Selected Readings

Case 1-1980. N Engl J Med 1980;302:104.
Effmann EL, Griscom NT, Colodny AH, et al. Neonatal gastrointestinal masses arising late in gestation. AJR Am J Roentgenol 1980;135:681.
Etches PC, Lemons JA. Nonimmune hydrops fetalis: Report of 22 cases, including three siblings. Pediatrics 1979;64:326.
Forouhar F. Meconium peritonitis: Pathology, evolution, and diagnosis. Am J Clin Pathol 1982;78:208.
Gillan JE, Lowden JA, Gaskin K, et al. Congenital ascites as a presenting sign of lysosomal storage disease. J Pediatr 1984;104:225.

Griscom NT, Colodny AH, Rosenberg HK, et al. Diagnostic aspects of neonatal ascites: Report of 27 cases. AJR Am J Roentgenol 1977;128:961.

Gryboski J, Walker WA, eds. Gastrointestinal problems in the infant, ed 2. Philadelphia: WB Saunders, 1983.

Hendren WH. Abdominal masses in newborn infants. Am J Surg 1964;107:502.

Hill LM, Breckle R, Gehrking WC. The prenatal detection of congenital malformations by ultrasonography. Mayo Clin Proc 1983;58:805.

Hutchinson AA, Drew JH, Yu VYH, et al. Nonimmunologic hydrops fetalis: A review of 61 cases. Obstet Gynecol 1982;59:347.

* Larcher VF, Howard ER, Mowat AP. Hepatic hemangiomata: Diagnosis and management. Arch Dis Child 1981;56:7.

Longino LA, Martin LW. Abdominal masses in the newborn infant. Pediatrics 1958;21:596.

* Merten DF, Kirks DR. Diagnostic imaging of pediatric abdominal masses. Pediatr Clin North Am 1985;32:1397.

Mollitt DL, Ballantine TVN, Grosfeld JL. Mesenteric cysts of infancy and childhood. Surg Gynecol Obstet 1978;147:182.

Raffensperger J, Abousleiman A. Abdominal masses in children under one year of age. Surgery 1968;63:514.

Srouji MN, Chatten J, Schulman WM. Mesenchymal hamartoma of the liver in infants. Cancer 1978;42:2483.

* Stevenson RJ. Abdominal masses. Surg Clin North Am 1985;65:1481.

Steves M, Ricketts RR. Pneumoperitoneum in the newborn infant. Am Surg 1987;53:226.

Wedge JJ, Grosfeld JL, Smith JP. Abdominal masses in the newborn: 63 cases. J Urol 1971;106:770.

* Weinberg AG, Finegold MJ. Primary hepatic tumors of childhood. Hum Pathol 1983;14:512.

* Key reference.

*Principles and Practice of Pediatrics, Second Edition.*
edited by Frank A. Oski et al. J. B. Lippincott Company, Philadelphia © 1994.

## 20.4.5 Necrotizing Enterocolitis

Kathleen J. Motil

Necrotizing enterocolitis is the most common gastrointestinal emergency in the infant. This disorder encompasses several distinct disease entities, which may be characterized according to their clinical presentation and course (Table 20-26). The most common form of the disease is idiopathic neonatal necrotizing enterocolitis. Although its etiology is unknown, specific precipitating factors may be implicated in many instances. The clinical manifestations of idiopathic neonatal necrotizing enterocolitis may mimic the symptoms and signs of various neonatal gastrointestinal disorders, and may be indistinguishable from those of sepsis neonatorum. Necrotizing enterocolitis has become the single most common surgical emergency among neonatal intensive care units. Early recognition and aggressive treatment of this disorder during the last 10 years have led to a markedly improved clinical outcome.

This work is a publication of the United States Department of Agriculture/Agricultural Research Service (ARS) Children's Nutrition Research Center, Department of Pediatrics, Baylor College of Medicine and Texas Children's Hospital in Houston, Texas. This project has been funded in part with federal funds from the Agricultural Research Service of the United States Department of Agriculture under Cooperative Agreement number 58-7MN1-6-100. The contents of this publication do not necessarily reflect the views or policies of the United States Department of Agriculture, nor does mention of trade names, commercial products, or organizations imply endorsement by the United States government.

**TABLE 20-26. Classification of Neonatal Necrotizing Enterocolitis**

Neonatal necrotizing enterocolitis (idiopathic)
  Sporadic
  Epidemic
Benign necrotizing enterocolitis (pneumatosis coli)
Neonatal necrotizing enterocolitis associated with precipitating factors
  Exchange transfusions
  Polycythemia
  Congenital heart disease
  Prolonged diarrhea
  Hypertonic agents (formulas, drugs, contrast media)
  Vitamin E therapy
Neonatal necrotizing enterocolitis associated with primary bowel pathology
  Intestinal obstruction
  Spontaneous bowel perforation
  Neonatal appendicitis
  Pseudomembranous colitis
  Hirschsprung's disease

## ETIOLOGY AND PATHOGENESIS

The precise etiology of neonatal necrotizing enterocolitis is unknown, but it probably is caused by multiple factors in a susceptible host. The features most commonly implicated in the pathogenesis of the disease are ischemic insult to the gut, the presence of bacterial or viral organisms in the intestinal tract, the availability of intraluminal substrate (usually formula or human milk) to promote bacterial proliferation or induce mucosal injury, and altered host defense (Table 20-27). The first three factors (ischemia, infectious agents, and milk feedings) are thought to be the predisposing variables that initiate the pathogenesis of necrotizing enterocolitis. Other factors, such as inflammatory mediators (cytokines), oxygen radicals, and bacterial fermentation products and toxins, are thought to propagate the disease process. Despite recent advances, the pathogenesis of necrotizing enterocolitis remains an enigma.

The regulation of mesenteric blood flow to the gut is understood poorly in the infant, but is thought to mimic the "diving reflex" in aquatic animals. During hypoxic conditions, this reflex is a defense mechanism that protects the brain and heart from ischemic damage by shunting blood away from the mesenteric, renal, and peripheral vascular beds. Comparable studies in asphyxiated neonatal piglets have demonstrated that blood flow to the stomach, ileum, and colon is reduced dramatically during a hypoxic episode. With resuscitation, perfusion rebounds, leading to vascular congestion and mucosal hemorrhages secondary to ischemic injury to the blood vessels. These studies support the hypothesis that ischemia contributes to the pathogenesis of necrotizing enterocolitis in the human infant.

Many perinatal events predispose the neonate to hypoxia. Birth asphyxia, respiratory distress syndrome, apnea, hypotension, hypothermia, patent ductus arteriosus, congestive heart failure, umbilical vessel catheterization, polycythemia, and exchange transfusion have been implicated as ischemic factors in the pathogenesis of neonatal necrotizing enterocolitis. Nevertheless, some infants with no evidence of these risk factors have the disorder. Moreover, in studies of multiple births in which risk factors such as perinatal asphyxia and respiratory distress are less common in the firstborn than in the second-born infant, necrotizing enterocolitis occurred in the firstborn twin in all cases, and

## TABLE 20-27. Pathophysiology of Necrotizing Enterocolitis

**Ischemia**

Hypoxia (birth asphyxia, respiratory distress syndrome, apnea, hypotension, hypothermia, patent ductus arteriosus)

Vascular congestion (congestive heart failure, exchange transfusion, polycythemia)

Thrombosis (umbilical vessel catheterization)

**Intestinal Microflora**

Bacterial organisms and toxins (*Escherichia coli, Klebsiella pneumoniae, Enterobacter cloacae, Pseudomonas, Salmonella, Clostridium difficile, Clostridium perfringens, Clostridium butyricum, Bacteroides fragilis*)

Viruses (coxsackie $B_2$, rotavirus, coronavirus)

Fungi (*Torulopsis glabrata*)

**Intraluminal Agents**

Human milk, commercial formulas (fermentation of fats and carbohydrates)

Hypertonic solutions (formulas, medications, contrast media)

**Altered Host Defense**

Developmental immaturity of the intestinal tract (corticosteroids)

Immaturity of neonatal immune system

Vitamin E therapy (scavenger of oxygen radicals)

---

in no case did only the second-born twin have necrotizing enterocolitis. Finally, when infants with necrotizing enterocolitis are compared with matched control infants, few, if any, ischemic risk factors are identified consistently.

The intestinal microflora provide an additional component in the development of ischemic necrosis of the intestinal tract. A number of bacterial, viral, and fungal organisms have been isolated in sporadic and epidemic outbreaks of necrotizing enterocolitis (see Table 20-27). Bacterial organisms normally found in the distal gastrointestinal tract, including *Escherichia coli* (56%), *Klebsiella pneumoniae* (28%), and *Pseudomonas* (11%), have been recovered from the blood and peritoneal cavities of about one third of all infants with necrotizing enterocolitis. Virus particles have been identified concurrently in the feces of infants with necrotizing enterocolitis and their mothers, the midwives, and the nursing staff involved in treatment of the infants. Fungi also have been isolated from infants born to immunocompromised mothers.

The role of gastrointestinal microorganisms in the pathophysiology of necrotizing enterocolitis remains unclear. Current hypotheses suggest that either bacterial invasion of tissue occurs after ischemic damage to the mucosal barrier of the gut in a passive manner or enteric bacteria and viruses cause the disease directly. Recently, several clostridial species have been implicated causally in the development of necrotizing enterocolitis because of their production of toxins, their association with pseudomembrane formation, and, most important, their ability to produce submucosal and subserosal gas blebs and intestinal gangrene. Nevertheless, in many epidemics of necrotizing enterocolitis, specific pathogens either cannot be identified or, when they are present, are isolated from healthy infants without the disease. Thus, cautious interpretation of the pathogenicity of specific microorganisms is warranted.

Recent evidence suggests that inflammatory mediators may aggravate further the injury induced by infectious agents. Bacterial endotoxin can initiate directly the production of tumor necrosis factor. This cytokine, in turn, stimulates the production of platelet activating factor. These inflammatory mediators act synergistically to produce intestinal injury similar to that found in necrotizing enterocolitis. Recent studies have demonstrated elevated levels of tumor necrosis factor and platelet activating factor in premature infants with necrotizing enterocolitis. Thus, these abnormalities may explain further the pathogenesis of this disorder.

Because bacterial involvement in necrotizing enterocolitis may be associated with usual intestinal flora, topical antibiotics are considered to be potentially useful in the prevention of this disease. The topical administration of aminoglycosides into the gastrointestinal tract either prophylactically or at the time of diagnosis decreases the total colony count of enteric flora. These antibiotics, however, do not provide protection from the development of necrotizing enterocolitis; do not alter its course, complications, or mortality rate; and may be associated with the emergence of resistant strains of enteric organisms and potentially ototoxic complications in the infant. Therefore, the use of topical aminoglycosides is not recommended for the routine prevention of necrotizing enterocolitis.

Milk feedings also have been implicated in the pathogenesis of neonatal necrotizing enterocolitis. About 93% of all infants in whom necrotizing enterocolitis develops have been fed enterally. Human milk and commercial formulas serve as substrates for bacterial proliferation in the gut. Because neonates partially malabsorb the carbohydrate and fat constituents in milk, reducing substances, organic acids, carbon dioxide, and hydrogen gas may be produced by the bacterial fermentation of these nutrients. When necrotizing enterocolitis develops, neonates have increased intestinal loss of carbohydrates, leading to reducing substances in the feces and hydrogen-filled cysts within the gut mucosa. Although these observations identify milk feedings as a contributory factor in the development of necrotizing enterocolitis, the disease may develop in some infants who have never been fed. Additional factors, such as the volume of milk and its rate of administration, were thought to be related causally to necrotizing enterocolitis. Nonetheless, recent studies suggest that early dilute feedings do not adversely affect the incidence of necrotizing enterocolitis.

Necrotizing enterocolitis may result from direct mucosal injury induced by hyperosmolar formulas. Although such formulas are used rarely in neonatal nurseries, medications that frequently are administered orally may contain hypertonic additives that irritate the intestinal mucosa and precipitate disease (Table 20-28). Other hyperosmolar agents instilled directly into the bowel for diagnostic studies, such as Renografin-76 (66% meglumine diatrizoate, 10% sodium diatrizoate), may precipitate necrotizing enterocolitis, presumably because of fluid shifts, bowel distention, and ischemia.

## TABLE 20-28. Osmolarity of Drugs Commonly Administered to Neonates

| Generic Drug | Osmolarity (mOsm/L) | Concentration (mg/mgL) |
|---|---|---|
| Ampicillin | 1843 | 50 |
| Nystatin | 3022 | 100,000* |
| Multivitamins | 6023 | — |
| Vitamin E | 605 | 36 |
| Ferrous chloride | 5079 | 157 |
| Calcium gluconate | 319 | 50 |
| Caffeine | 90 | 30 |
| Theophylline | 1012 | 193 |
| Methyl digoxin | 15250 | 0.6 |

* Concentration expressed as $\mu$/mL.

Altered host resistance as a result of immunologic and gastrointestinal immaturity in the neonate is believed to play a primary role in the development of necrotizing enterocolitis. At birth, the human intestinal mucosa has no secretory IgA, the major gastrointestinal immunoprotective antibody. Because human milk contains specific and nonspecific protective factors, such as immunocompetent cells, secretory IgA, lactoferrin, lysozyme, and the *Lactobacillus bifidus* growth factor, it has been fed to neonates to reduce the incidence and severity of necrotizing enterocolitis. Despite the presence of these presumed protective factors, necrotizing enterocolitis developed exclusively in neonates who were fed refrigerated, pasteurized, or frozen human milk. Recent studies, however, appear to support the protective role of human milk in the prevention of necrotizing enterocolitis.

Nonetheless, the issue of the developmental immaturity of the gastrointestinal tract itself may be central to the pathogenesis of necrotizing enterocolitis. Recent studies from a multicenter, randomized, blinded trial using antenatal corticosteroids demonstrated that the risk of development of necrotizing enterocolitis may be diminished significantly in infants whose mothers received antenatal corticosteroids. Although their mechanism of action is unclear, corticosteroids may function as nonspecific enzyme inducers, leading to accelerated maturation of the intestinal tract and enhanced protection from disease.

The use of vitamin E in the treatment of retinopathy of prematurity also has been associated with an increased incidence of necrotizing enterocolitis. This association was noted primarily in infants whose birth weights were less than 1500 g, and whose serum tocopherol levels were higher than 3.5 mg/dL. It was hypothesized that the mechanism of excessive scavenging of oxygen radicals, leading to diminished antimicrobial defenses, increased the risk of the development of necrotizing enterocolitis in these infants. Subsequent trials of vitamin E therapy for the prevention of neonatal intracranial hemorrhage failed to demonstrate an association with necrotizing enterocolitis, however, presumably because serum α-tocopherol levels were maintained in a range less than 3.5 mg/dL.

## PATHOLOGY

Neonatal necrotizing enterocolitis is a pathologic condition that may be characterized broadly as intestinal infarction. This disorder primarily affects the terminal ileum and colon, although, in severe cases, the entire gastrointestinal tract may be involved. The pathologic findings are variable and reflect the rapidity of disease progression and the presence of underlying pathogenic factors.

On gross examination, the bowel is distended and hemorrhagic (Table 20-29). Subserosal collections of gas may or may not be present along the mesenteric border. Gangrenous necrosis, with or without perforation, may be present on the antimesenteric border. Fibrinous adhesions, thickening of the bowel wall, and areas of stenosis are seen in the healing gut.

The histologic features of bowel ischemia include mucosal edema and hemorrhage, which may progress to transmural bland necrosis. Collections of gas, secondary bacterial infiltration, and acute inflammation may be present. Vascular thrombi are infrequent findings in necrotizing enterocolitis.

## EPIDEMIOLOGY

The overall incidence of necrotizing enterocolitis is 2.4:1000 live births (range, 0.0:1000 to 7.2:1000) or 2.1% (range, 1.0% to 4.1%) of all admissions to neonatal intensive care units (Table 20-30). The incidence of necrotizing enterocolitis averages 3% to 4% in infants whose birth weight is less than 2000 g, and decreases significantly to 1% in infants whose birth weight is greater than 2000 g. Males and females are affected equally. Black and white infants are affected more commonly than are those of Hispanic origin, but the racial patterns reflect the populations served by individual neonatal centers. Seasonal variation does not affect the incidence of necrotizing enterocolitis. Periodic clusters of cases or epidemics have been reported however.

## PREDISPOSING FACTORS

Risk factors that predispose the premature infant to necrotizing enterocolitis have been the subject of controversy. Because the disease affects predominantly low–birth-weight infants who require intensive care, "risk" factors for the development of necrotizing enterocolitis may be the same in low–birth-weight infants with or without the disease.

Several predisposing factors thought to be important in the development of this disorder in infants weighing less than 2000 g were identified in a prospective, multicenter investigation (Table 20-31). Prenatal risk factors included maternal age greater than 35 years, maternal infection requiring antibiotic administration, and premature rupture of membranes. Perinatal risk factors included maternal anesthesia at delivery and depressed Apgar scores at 5 minutes. Postnatal risk factors included patent ductus arteriosus, the use of total parenteral nutrition or gavage feedings, and the absence of prophylactic oral antibiotics before the onset of necrotizing enterocolitis. Factors not associated with the de-

---

**TABLE 20-29. Pathologic Features of Necrotizing Enterocolitis**

**Macroscopic**
Distended, hemorrhagic bowel
Subserosal collections of hydrogen gas (mesenteric border)
Gangrenous necrosis of the bowel wall
Perforation (antimesenteric border)
Fibrinous adhesions, thickened bowel wall, stenosis

**Microscopic**
Mucosal edema
Hemorrhage
Bland necrosis of the bowel wall
Collections of gas
Bacterial infiltration
Acute inflammation
Thrombus formation in blood vessels

---

**TABLE 20-30. Epidemiology of Neonatal Necrotizing Enterocolitis**

| Incidence | |
|---|---|
| Cases/1000 live births | 2.4 |
| Percent of NICU admissions | 2.1 |
| Percent of live births | |
| Birth weight < 1000 g | 3.4 |
| Birth weight 1000–2000 g | 3.9 |
| Birth weight > 2000 g | 1.0 |
| Sex (Male : Female) Ratio | 1:1 |
| Racial (White : Black : Hispanic : Other) Ratio | 14:18:1:1 |

## TABLE 20-31. Proposed Risk Factors Associated With Necrotizing Enterocolitis

**Group I: Preterm infants < 2000 g**

*Prenatal*
Maternal age > 35 y
Maternal infection treated with antibiotics
Premature rupture of membranes > 24 h before delivery

*Perinatal*
Maternal anesthesia at delivery
Normal Apgar score at 1 minute, low at 5 minutes

*Postnatal*
Patent ductus arteriosus
Administration of intravenous glucose or total parenteral nutrition before onset of disease
Gavage feeding
Absence of prophylactic oral antibiotics before the onset of disease
Transport to community hospital from regional neonatal intensive care unit
Cocaine exposure

**Group II: Older Infants > 2000 g**

*Perinatal*
Polycythemia
Respiratory Distress
Hypoglycemia
Postoperative Repair of Abdominal Wall Defects and Gut Lesions

## TABLE 20-32. Clinical Features of Necrotizing Enterocolitis: Incidence of Prematurity

| Prematurity Based on Age and Weight | Percent of Cases |
|---|---|
| **Gestational Age (wk)** | |
| <32 | 33 |
| 32–36 | 41 |
| 36–40 | 12 |
| >40 | 14 |
| **Birth Weight (g)** | |
| <1000 | 7 |
| 1000–1500 | 32 |
| 1500–2000 | 32 |
| 2000–3000 | 19 |
| >3000 | 10 |

velopment of the disease included catheterization of umbilical vessels, respiratory distress requiring oxygen support, mode of delivery, theophylline therapy, or feeding history (ie, feeding before diagnosis, age at first feeding, type of milk fed, method of feeding, rapidity with which feedings were advanced, and the presence of umbilical catheters during feedings).

More recently, the transport of stable premature infants from neonatal intensive care units to community hospitals for continued care and treatment of cocaine exposure has been suggested as a risk factor for the development of necrotizing enterocolitis. Despite these possibilities, the consensus is that prematurity is the only major risk factor that predisposes the neonate to this disorder.

Additional risk factors have been identified for infants who average more than 2000 g at birth. Polycythemia (peripheral venous hematocrit greater than 65%) is the most common condition associated with the development of necrotizing enterocolitis in this group of infants, particularly those who are small for their gestational age. Respiratory distress, defined by the need for supplemental oxygen for more than 24 hours, and hypoglycemia (serum glucose level less than 30 mg/dL) also occur more frequently in this group of infants. Therefore, larger infants with a history of perinatal stress or physiologic immaturity may be at greater potential risk for the development of necrotizing enterocolitis than are their otherwise normal counterparts.

Infants who have undergone major abdominal surgery within the first week of life may be at increased risk for the development of necrotizing enterocolitis. Late-onset necrotizing enterocolitis may develop in those with the diagnosis of gastroschisis, omphalocele, jejunal atresia, aganglionosis, and malrotation after surgical repair of the anatomic lesion. These infants have a relentless course, with substantial morbidity (67%) resulting from diarrhea, the short-gut syndrome, and sepsis, and with a mortality rate of 46%. Thus, the presence of abdominal wall defects and other intestinal lesions suggests a possible increased susceptibility

to necrotizing enterocolitis during the postoperative course in these infants.

## CLINICAL FEATURES

Nearly three fourths of all infants with necrotizing enterocolitis are born prematurely, with a gestational age of less than 37 weeks and a birth weight of less than 2000 g (Table 20-32). Full-term infants in whom necrotizing enterocolitis develops generally have congenital heart disease, congestive heart failure, or protracted diarrhea of unknown etiology that is complicated by malnutrition. The onset of symptoms occurs within the first 5 days of life in 44% of infants, although symptoms may occur as early as the first day and as late as the fourth week after birth (Table 20-33). Generally, the postnatal age at diagnosis is related inversely to the gestational age.

Significant maternal or perinatal risk factors may be present at the time of diagnosis; many of these factors, however, occur equally in premature infants in whom necrotizing enterocolitis does not develop. Most infants who are seen in the first week of life are recovering from their initial acute illness at the time of onset of this disorder, and many are considered to be "growing" premature infants.

Feedings with either human milk or commercial formulas have been instituted in 98% of infants in whom necrotizing enterocolitis develops. The feedings are tolerated poorly, however, and generate gastric retention, the earliest presenting symptom of the disease (Table 20-34). Other gastrointestinal symptoms and signs, including regurgitation, vomiting, abdominal distention, dimin-

## TABLE 20-33. Clinical Features of Necrotizing Enterocolitis: Age at Diagnosis

| Gestational Age (wk) | Age at Diagnosis* (d) | Postnatal Age at Diagnosis (d) | Frequency (%) |
|---|---|---|---|
| 26–30 | 20 ± 4 | 0–1 | 5 |
| 31–33 | 14 ± 2 | 1–3 | 18 |
| 34–37 | 5 ± 1 | 3–5 | 21 |
| | | 6–12 | 23 |
| | | >12 | 23 |

* Mean ± SEM.

TABLE 20-34.   Presenting Symptoms and Signs
of Necrotizing Enterocolitis

| Finding | Incidence (%) |
|---|---|
| **Gastrointestinal** | |
| Abdominal Distention | 89 |
| Hematochezia | |
| Guaiac-positive stools | 80 |
| Grossly bloody stools | 43 |
| Fecal Reducing Substances (3+, 4+) | 71 |
| Gastric Residual | 73 |
| Vomiting | 37 |
| Diarrhea | 25 |
| **Systemic** | |
| Lethargy | 84 |
| Temperature Instability | 81 |
| Apnea | 66 |
| Respiratory Failure | 40 |
| Hypotension | 37 |

ished bowel sounds, reducing substances in the stools, and hematochezia (with either guaiac-positive stools or frank blood), follow rapidly. Diarrhea is an infrequent finding. Systemic manifestations of necrotizing enterocolitis, including temperature instability, lethargy, apnea, respiratory failure, and hypotension, also may be apparent at the onset of the disease.

Subclinical necrotizing enterocolitis is suspected, but not confirmed, in about 25% of cases, and the symptoms resolve gradually. In 25% to 40% of cases, there is fulminant progression of the disease, with evidence of perforation and peritonitis that is characterized by abdominal tenderness on palpation, a feeling of fullness or a mass (particularly in the right lower quadrant), and erythema, ecchymosis, or necrosis of the abdominal wall. Lethargy, severe acidosis, sepsis, disseminated intravascular coagulation, and shock may supervene rapidly.

Premorbid risk factors associated with death from necrotizing enterocolitis have been proposed. Poor prognostic factors include premature rupture of membranes, low Apgar scores at 5 minutes, a prolonged oxygen requirement at birth, abdominal distention, portal vein gas on radiographic studies, *Klebsiella* septicemia, blood transfusion, and surgical intervention.

## LABORATORY AND RADIOGRAPHIC STUDIES

Laboratory studies of infants with necrotizing enterocolitis may demonstrate a decreased platelet count, increased prothrombin and partial thromboplastin times, and serum factor V concentrations of less than 40%, all of which are consistent with the diagnosis of disseminated intravascular coagulation. Platelet counts of less than 50,000/mm$^3$ have been found in 38% of infants with necrotizing enterocolitis and may lead to significant bleeding complications, such as intracranial hemorrhage. A serial decrease in platelets to levels less than 100,000/mm$^3$ is thought to correlate closely with gangrenous bowel and impending perforation. A complete blood count and differential are of little assistance in the diagnosis of necrotizing enterocolitis, but an absolute neutrophil count of less than 1500/mm$^3$ is associated with a poor prognosis.

The presence of 3+ or 4+ reducing substances, $\alpha_1$-antitrypsin, or blood in the stool may be an early, but nonspecific, presenting sign of necrotizing enterocolitis. Similarly, levels of C-reactive protein, $\alpha_1$-acid glycoprotein (orosomucoid), lysosomal acid hydrolase, and urinary D-lactate, a metabolite of carbohydrate fermentation produced by enteric microflora, are increased in infants with this disease and may serve as useful markers to discriminate between necrotizing enterocolitis and other intestinal insults. Elevated breath hydrogen levels may be useful to detect the onset of necrotizing enterocolitis 24 hours before symptoms appear in a premature infant who is at risk for the development of this disorder.

Serum biochemical abnormalities are nonspecific. Hyponatremia (serum sodium levels of less than 130 mEq/L) and persistent metabolic acidosis suggest the presence of sepsis or necrotic bowel.

Blood cultures may show bacterial growth in one third of all specimens obtained. Cerebrospinal fluid cultures may be warranted if sepsis or meningitis is suspected. Stool cultures generally show the presence of normal enteric flora. Additional cultures for *Clostridium difficile* and assays for its toxins may be indicated, however, when the history and physical findings support the clinical impression. When abdominal paracentesis is performed in infants with suspected peritonitis, Gram's stain and culture of the peritoneal fluid demonstrate enteric organisms in one third of the cases. Usually, these organisms are the same as those recovered from blood culture.

Radiographic features characteristic of necrotizing enterocolitis may be seen in 87% of patients before a definitive diagnosis is made (Table 20-35). An abdominal film in the supine, decubitus, or upright position may show the presence of pneumatosis intestinalis, edema of the bowel wall, dilatation of loops of bowel, ascites, portal vein gas, or free air in the peritoneum. Serial films may reveal the presence of fixed loops of bowel, which is an ominous feature suggesting the presence of intestinal perforation.

Barium contrast studies are contraindicated if the diagnosis of necrotizing enterocolitis and its complications are suspected. The metrizamide gastrointestinal series that has been introduced recently holds promise, however, as an aid in the diagnosis of necrotizing enterocolitis when clinical and radiographic information is inconclusive.

Abdominal ultrasonography also may prove useful to identify gangrenous bowel and impending perforation. The sonographic appearance of the pseudo-kidney sign (ie, bowel wall that is characterized by a hypoechoic rim with a central echogenic focus) may serve this purpose. Recently, this technique also has been used to demonstrate intermittent hepatic parenchymal and portal venous microbubbles of gas in the absence of the classic radiographic findings of necrotizing enterocolitis.

The diagnosis of necrotizing enterocolitis is confirmed when the following triad of clinical features is present: abdominal distention, hematochezia, and pneumatosis intestinalis. Pneumatosis intestinalis may not be identified, however, in nearly 15% of surgically or autopsy-confirmed cases. Similarly, portal vein gas, once thought to be a poor prognostic feature of necrotizing enterocolitis, may be a transient finding on radiographic exami-

TABLE 20-35.   Presenting Radiographic Features
of Necrotizing Enterocolitis

| Finding | Incidence (%) |
|---|---|
| Pneumatosis intestinalis | 91 |
| Dilatation of bowel loops | 83 |
| Persistent "fixed loop" | 33 |
| Peritoneal fluid (ascites) | 29 |
| Portal venous gas | 23 |
| Pneumoperitoneum | 17 |

---

**TABLE 20-36.    Differential Diagnosis
of Necrotizing Enterocolitis**

Anal Fissures

Pneumatosis coli

Infectious Enterocolitis
*Salmonella, Shigella, Campylobacter*
Pseudomembranous colitis (*Clostridium*)

Neonatal Appendicitis

Spontaneous Perforation

Intestinal Obstruction
Congenital (intussusception, meconium ileus, ileal atresia, volvulus)
Acquired (milk curds)

Hirschsprung's Disease

---

nation. Newer radionuclide scanning techniques that use technetium 99m diphosphonate may facilitate earlier detection of this disorder.

## DIFFERENTIAL DIAGNOSIS

The differential diagnosis of necrotizing enterocolitis includes anal fissures, pneumatosis coli, infectious enterocolitis, neonatal appendicitis, intestinal obstruction, spontaneous perforation, and Hirschsprung's disease (Table 20-36).

Anal fissures have been reported in conjunction with necrotizing enterocolitis, but the significance of the relationship is unknown. The fissures may have precipitated the development of the disease by creating a portal of entry for bacteria, or they may be secondary manifestations of the disease entity. A high index of suspicion when a premature infant has rectal bleeding or guaiac-positive stools should suggest no delay in diagnosis and treatment, despite the presence of anal fissures.

Pneumatosis coli is a benign form of necrotizing enterocolitis that is seen primarily in premature infants. Clinical features include gastric residua and vomiting (in some patients), transient episodes of lethargy and apnea, mild abdominal distention, and frank blood in the stools. Radiographic studies demonstrate intramural intestinal gas limited to the colon and the absence of small-bowel dilatation and pneumatosis. Recovery is complete within 3 days, and no sequelae are apparent. This entity can be differentiated from classic necrotizing enterocolitis by its clinical course.

Infectious enterocolitis may be attributed to a number of pathogenic organisms, including *Salmonella, Shigella, Campylobacter,* and *C difficile,* some of which also have been associated with necrotizing enterocolitis. Stool cultures should be obtained to identify the presence or absence of these organisms. The precise etiology of symptoms may be difficult to determine because of the association between necrotizing enterocolitis and intestinal organisms, and because of the similarities in the medical management of these enteric infections.

Neonatal appendicitis may masquerade as necrotizing enterocolitis. This entity is rare in newborn infants, however, presumably because of the persistence of the funnel-shaped configuration of the fetal appendix, which is less prone to obstruction. When it occurs, neonatal appendicitis has a predilection for premature male infants and is associated frequently with inguinal hernias. Radiographic features that may assist in the diagnosis of neonatal appendicitis include an abnormal gas pattern and peritoneal fluid in 85% of cases, psoas shadow obliteration in 56%, a thickened abdominal wall in 32%, a fecalith in 32%, and abscess formation in 20%. The findings at laparotomy will distinguish between neonatal appendicitis and necrotizing enterocolitis.

Gangrenous enterocolitis or perforation may be associated with intestinal obstruction resulting from intussusception, meconium ileus, ileal atresia, volvulus, or milk curds. Similarly, Hirschsprung's disease may present as fulminant enterocolitis with colonic obstruction, diarrhea, and sepsis. Infants with spontaneous perforation of the bowel often are more mature than are those with necrotizing enterocolitis. Perforations occur in the stomach, ileum, and colon. The lesion generally is localized, however, which differentiates this entity from necrotizing enterocolitis. Bilious vomiting, gastric aspirates, abdominal distention and tenderness, hematochezia, and pneumatosis intestinalis may be seen in any of these entities. A barium enema is of little use in distinguishing among these diagnoses, and generally is contraindicated because it may lead to perforation. Surgical intervention should clarify the dilemma introduced by these clinical conditions.

## TREATMENT

The treatment of infants with necrotizing enterocolitis is based on a method of clinical staging at the time of diagnosis (Table 20-37). Infants classified as having stage I or II disease require

---

**TABLE 20-37.    Staging Criteria for the Treatment of Necrotizing Enterocolitis**

| Stage | Systemic | Intestinal | Radiologic | Treatment |
|---|---|---|---|---|
| I. Suspect | Lethargy, temperature instability, apnea, bradycardia | Gastric residual, emesis, abdominal distention, hematochezia | Ileus, intestinal dilatation | Parenteral nutrition, nasogastric suction, antibiotics |
| II. Definite—same features as stage I plus: | | | | |
|   A. Mildly ill | — | Absent bowel sounds | Pneumatosis intestinalis | — |
|   B. Moderately ill | Metabolic acidosis, thrombocytopenia | Abdominal tenderness | Portal vein gas | NaHCO$_3$ |
| III. Advanced—same features as stage II plus: | | | | |
|   A. Shock | Respiratory arrest, hypotension, disseminated intravascular coagulation, combined respiratory metabolic acidosis | Peritonitis | Ascites | Intravenous fluids, isotropic agents, paracentesis |
|   B. Bowel perforation | — | — | Pneumoperitoneum | Surgery |

appropriate diagnostic studies and vigorous medical therapy, whereas those categorized as having stage III disease require surgical intervention.

The medical treatment of necrotizing enterocolitis primarily is supportive (Table 20-38). When the diagnosis is suspected, oral feedings should be withheld and nasogastric suction and intravenous fluid should be instituted. Initial laboratory studies should include a complete blood count and differential, a platelet count, prothrombin and partial thromboplastin time determinations, serum electrolyte measurements, and blood urea nitrogen, creatinine, and acid–base studies. Routine cultures of the blood, urine, stool, and cerebrospinal fluid should be obtained. Additional stool specimens should be sent for viral and fungal studies when appropriate. The stools should be checked routinely for pH, glucose, occult blood, and $\alpha_1$-antitrypsin. Total parenteral nutrition should be provided to maintain the nutritional status of the infant. Parenteral antibiotics that cover a broad spectrum of aerobic and anaerobic organisms should be administered for 10 to 14 days. Although the choice of antibiotic therapy will depend on the resistance patterns of individual institutions, the antibiotics currently recommended include ampicillin, aminoglycosides (eg, gentamicin and amikacin), clindamycin, and the newer cephalosporins (eg, cefotaxime). Although the administration of topical antibiotics such as gentamicin and colistin diminishes the bacterial flora of the gut, this therapy is not recommended in the treatment of necrotizing enterocolitis because of the development of resistant bacterial strains of significant virulence and the equivocal outcome of morbidity and mortality.

Serial abdominal films of the infant in the supine and decubitus positions are recommended every 6 to 8 hours as needed, and serve as the best guide in following the course of the disease. If there is no further progression of illness and the pneumatosis resolves, nasogastric suction may be discontinued. Oral feedings may be resumed gradually within 7 to 14 days after the acute illness.

Surgical intervention is necessary when the disease progresses clinically or when the complications of necrotizing enterocolitis become apparent (Table 20-39). The indications for surgery include rapid clinical deterioration manifested by thermal instability, bradycardia, persistent metabolic acidosis, progressive hypona-

---

**TABLE 20-39. Indications for Surgery in Necrotizing Enterocolitis**

Clinical deterioration
Peritonitis
Perforation
Abdominal mass
Obstruction

---

tremia, and thrombocytopenia; intestinal perforation manifested by pneumoperitoneum on abdominal flat plate; a palpable abdominal mass; intestinal obstruction; or peritonitis manifested as abdominal tenderness and rigidity, erythematous discoloration of the abdominal wall, or the radiographic appearance of a fixed and unchanging collection of intraluminal gas, usually in the right lower quadrant. Abdominal paracentesis and lavage have been recommended to identify infants with intestinal gangrene and impending perforation. The presence of brown, fecal-stained peritoneal fluid that contains bacteria on Gram's stain suggests intestinal gangrene and may be an indication for early operative intervention.

The operative procedures of choice include resection with primary anastomosis or a staged procedure involving resection and proximal enterostomy with distal mucous fistula formation, followed by closure 8 to 12 weeks later. The former procedure is favored in uncomplicated circumstances, because the problems of ileostomies, including wound dehiscence, stenosis at the enterostomy site, fluid and electrolyte imbalances, and delayed resumption of oral feedings, are not present. If an ileostomy or colostomy has been placed, however, a barium enema should be performed before reanastomosis is performed to exclude the presence of intestinal strictures. When the disease process is extensive, only unquestionably necrotic or frankly perforated bowel should be excised. When there is doubt about the viability of segments of the bowel wall, a second-look operation should be performed. In critically ill neonates with suspected perforation of the bowel, peritoneal drainage under local anesthesia may be warranted as a temporizing procedure. Operative mortality is significant, but has improved as a result of early aggressive medical and surgical intervention.

Preventive measures have been advocated to reduce the frequency or minimize the severity of necrotizing enterocolitis. These recommendations include delaying oral feedings for 1 week in low–birth-weight infants with a history of perinatal asphyxia; avoiding hypertonic formulas, medications, and diagnostic agents in sick newborn infants; performing a phlebotomy and exchange transfusion with plasma when polycythemia becomes critical (hematocrit greater than 70%); placement of arterial umbilical catheters in the aorta distal to the renal arteries; and avoidance of placement of venous umbilical catheters in the portal vein. More recent studies suggest that the administration of oral immunoglobulin (IgA-IgG) preparations may prevent the development of necrotizing enterocolitis in premature infants at risk for this disorder. Further studies that document the benefit of prophylactic immunoglobulin therapy are warranted.

## COMPLICATIONS

The complications of necrotizing enterocolitis may occur early or late in the course of the disease, and vary in the frequency of their appearance. The acute complications include sepsis (60%), peritonitis (20% to 30%), meningitis, abscess formation, thrombocytopenia, disseminated intravascular coagulation, and intestinal or extraintestinal bleeding. Antibiotic therapy provides cov-

---

**TABLE 20-38. Medical Treatment of Necrotizing Enterocolitis**

**Clinical**
Nothing by mouth
Intermittent nasogastric suction
Intravenous fluid replacement
Total parenteral nutrition
Broad-spectrum antibiotics
? Oral immunoglobulin therapy

**Laboratory**
*Hematology*
Complete blood count and differential
Serial (12-h) platelet counts, prothrombin and partial thromboplastin times
*Biochemistry*
Serum electrolytes, blood urea nitrogen, creatinine
Arterial blood gases
Fecal pH, glucose, occult blood, $\alpha_1$-antitrypsin
*Microbiology*
Routine blood, urine, stool, cerebrospinal fluid cultures
*Radiology*
Serial (6- to 8-h) abdominal films (supine, decubitus)

erage for the treatment of the infectious complications of necrotizing enterocolitis. Fresh-frozen plasma, platelet concentrates, or an exchange transfusion may be necessary for the hematologic complications. Shock, hypotension, respiratory arrest, hypoglycemia, and metabolic acidosis require aggressive resuscitative efforts in the early stages of advanced disease.

The late complications of necrotizing enterocolitis include stenosis, stricture formation, intestinal atresia, pericolic abscess, enterocele, enterocolic fistula, and short-gut syndrome. Intestinal stenoses and strictures are the most common complications of necrotizing enterocolitis, occurring in 11% to 36% of infants treated medically, and less frequently in those treated surgically. The interval during which a stricture may develop ranges from 1 to 20 months; the average abnormality is detectable by 2 months after the acute episode. About 80% of strictures occur in the colon, predominantly on the left side, but strictures also may be seen in the terminal ileum and jejunum. Multiple strictures may be seen in individual patients. Neither birth weight, gestational age, disease severity, nor the presence of pneumatosis intestinalis correlates with the likelihood of stenosis or stricture developing after an episode of necrotizing enterocolitis. Barium enema studies should be considered about 4 weeks after the acute episode of necrotizing enterocolitis, to avoid significant delays in the diagnosis of strictures. About 60% of infants have asymptomatic stenoses, of which half may progress to overt symptoms. However, about 20% resolve spontaneously.

Strictures are treated surgically. The procedures of choice are either resection and primary anastomosis or staged management (ie, resection and colostomy followed by closure). A short course of careful feedings may be justified in the treatment of symptomatic intestinal stenosis in the absence of frank intestinal obstruction. To implement nonsurgical management of stenoses, several criteria should be fulfilled, including the absence of symptoms associated with partial intestinal obstruction (ie, poor feeding, diarrhea, and abdominal distention), as well as the absence of radiographic findings consistent with intestinal obstruction (ie, minimal or no evidence of proximal dilatation of the bowel). The use of a balloon catheter to dilate focal colonic strictures located distal to an enterostomy has proven successful in the management of nonobstructive stenoses.

Significant malabsorption may occur postoperatively in about 8% of patients with necrotizing enterocolitis because the amount of small bowel remaining after surgery is insufficient. Prolonged parenteral or enteral nutrition may be required for survival. Vitamin $B_{12}$ malabsorption without megaloblastic anemia has been described in children after ileocecal valve and terminal ileal resection has been performed for neonatal necrotizing enterocolitis. Prolonged vitamin $B_{12}$ therapy may be necessary in these circumstances.

## PROGNOSIS

The prognosis for necrotizing enterocolitis has improved considerably in the last 10 years as a result of advances in the care of the critically ill infant, earlier diagnosis and treatment, and the institution of a standard aggressive approach in the treatment of this disorder. The overall survival rate currently is 70% to 80%. When classified on the basis of medical or surgical management, the survival rates are 71% and 65%, respectively. The prognosis is affected adversely by the degree of prematurity (Table 20-40) and the persistence of respiratory problems requiring ventilatory support. Late-onset necrotizing enterocolitis has a better prognosis than does the early onset form.

About 50% of the survivors of necrotizing enterocolitis become normal, healthy children. Fifteen percent have neurologic impairment. Neurologic morbidity probably is not related to the

**TABLE 20-40. Survival Rates of Infants With Necrotizing Enterocolitis**

| Birth Weight (g) | Survival Rate (%) |
|---|---|
| <1000 | 43 |
| 1000–1500 | 67 |
| 1500–2000 | 82 |
| 2000–2500 | 44 |
| >2500 | 80 |

occurrence of necrotizing enterocolitis itself, however, but rather is part of the spectrum of complications that is associated with prematurity and asphyxia. Late gastrointestinal morbidity is seen in about 10% of infants with necrotizing enterocolitis. Long-term follow-up (1 to 10 years) of these infants demonstrates that, in the absence of major intestinal resection (less than 25%), complete recovery of gastrointestinal function is expected. A small number of children with extensive resection may have the persistence of loose stools or increased frequency of bowel movements, however, as a result of lactose intolerance or the short-gut syndrome.

## Selected Readings

Bauer CR, Morrison JC, Poole WK, et al. A decreased incidence of necrotizing enterocolitis after prenatal glucocorticoid therapy. Pediatrics 1984;73:682.

Caplan MS, Sun X-M, Hsueh W, et al. Role of platelet activating factor and tumor necrosis factor-alpha in neonatal necrotizing enterocolitis. J Pediatr 1990;116:960.

Cheu HW, Brown DR, Rowe MI. Breath hydrogen excretion as a screening test for the early diagnosis of necrotizing enterocolitis. Am J Dis Child 1989;143:156.

Eibl MM, Wolf HM, Fürnkranz H, et al. Prevention of necrotizing enterocolitis in low-birth-weight infants by IgA-IgG feeding. N Engl J Med 1988;319:1.

Fish WH, Cohen M, Franzek D, et al. Effect of intramuscular vitamin E on mortality and intracranial hemorrhage in neonates of 1000 grams or less. Pediatrics 1990;85:578.

Gertler JP, Seashore JH, Touloukian RJ. Early ileostomy closure in necrotizing enterocolitis. J Pediatr Surg 1987;22:140.

Kanto WP, Wilson R, Breart GL, et al. Perinatal events and necrotizing enterocolitis in premature infants. Am J Dis Child 1987;141:167.

Kliegman RM. Neonatal necrotizing enterocolitis. Bridging the basic science with the clinical disease. J Pediatr 1990;117:833.

Lucas A, Cole TJ. Breast milk and neonatal necrotizing enterocolitis. Lancet 1990;336:1519.

McClead RE Jr. Neonatal necrotizing enterocolitis: Current concepts and controversies. J Pediatr 1990;117:S1.

*Principles and Practice of Pediatrics, Second Edition.*
edited by Frank A. Oski et al. J. B. Lippincott Company, Philadelphia © 1994.

## *20.4.6 Short-Bowel Syndrome*

Jon A. Vanderhoof

Short-bowel syndrome is perhaps the most common indication for the chronic use of parenteral nutrition in pediatrics. In the neonatal period, massive small-bowel resection often is necessary because of either congenital anomalies of the gastrointestinal tract or advanced ischemic injury from necrotizing enterocolitis. A smaller number of patients require resection later in life as a result of vascular injury of the small intestine, usually secondary to midgut volvulus, or they have short-bowel syndrome as a result of surgical management of advanced inflammatory bowel disease. Long-term survival without parenteral nutrition depends on the ability of the small intestine to increase its absorptive capacity so that the patient's nutritional needs can be provided through the enteral route.

Many patients with a surprisingly short segment of small intestine eventually develop the ability to live without parenteral nutrition as a result of a compensatory increase in mucosal surface area caused by the adaptive response to massive resection. This compensatory growth is dominated by villus hyperplasia, although some dilatation and lengthening of the remaining small intestine does occur.

As might be expected, increases in villus length and in the number of enterocytes available for absorption per centimeter of bowel are accompanied by a gradual increase in the absorption of nearly all nutrients.

Stimulation of the adaptation process becomes the primary goal of therapy in the treatment of patients with short-bowel syndrome. The importance of intraluminal nutrition in stimulating this process has been well documented in previous studies. The intraluminal nutrients not only are necessary to produce adaptation, but also are essential to maintain the structural and functional integrity of the small intestine.

Nutrients appear to stimulate mucosal adaptation through three independent, but possibly related, mechanisms:

1. Direct contact of concentrated nutrients with the mucosal surface appears to stimulate intestinal growth.
2. Trophic hormones produced in response to high concentrations of intraluminal nutrients are released both systemically through an endocrine mechanism and locally through a paracrine mechanism to stimulate the production of new enterocytes.
3. Release of trophic upper gastrointestinal secretions is stimulated by the presence of intraluminal nutrients.

The clinical management of short-bowel syndrome can be considered best in three phases. Phase I consists of nutritional repletion with total parenteral nutrition (TPN). Phase II includes the gradual introduction of enteral nutrition, usually by continuous infusion. During phase III, continuous enteral nutrition is reduced incrementally as the patient is weaned over gradually to bolus or solid feeding.

During phase I, achieving nutritional repletion and stabilizing fluid and electrolyte balance are the major goals of therapy. Home therapy also should be contemplated at this time and, if it is at all possible, organization of and instruction regarding home TPN should be initiated early.

Once it is apparent that the child will require long-term parenteral nutrition, a permanent indwelling central catheter, usually a Broviac or Hickman catheter, is placed in a large vein. The decision as to whether TPN will be necessary may be obvious in the case of massive small-bowel resection. In some patients, however, a trial of postoperative enteral nutrition after a brief period of central or peripheral parenteral nutrition will be required to make the decision. Parenteral nutrition usually is begun using a 10% dextrose, 2.5% crystalline acid solution infused at a rate about equal to 1.3 times the maintenance fluid rate for the patient. Incremental increases in dextrose concentration, to 15% and 20% each day, then follow to allow the patient to achieve total caloric requirements parenterally by the third day. Maintenance quantities of parenteral vitamins and trace metals are added to the parenteral nutrition solution, usually through the use of commercial preparations such as PTE4 trace element solution and MVI Pediatric multivitamin solution. In patients with high-output proximal fistulas, additional zinc supplementation may be re-

quired. Extra zinc also should be considered in small, preterm infants. Twenty percent intravenous lipid solution should be administered a minimum of twice weekly to provide at least 8% of the total caloric intake as fat if substantial enteral feedings are not administered concurrently. Although the primary purpose of intravenous lipid is to prevent deficiency of essential fatty acids, daily use of the lipid solution may allow additional calories to be provided, if they are needed.

With few exceptions, standard pediatric electrolyte concentrations can be administered with little variation. I routinely add 30 mEq of sodium chloride, 20 mEq of potassium phosphate, 10 mEq of calcium gluconate, and 5 mEq of magnesium sulfate to each liter of TPN solution. Depending on the amino acid solution used, some sodium may need to be administered in the form of acetate to buffer the solution. This will be readily apparent if the patient becomes acidotic while receiving parenteral nutrition.

The key to the use of standard solutions in patients with short-bowel syndrome is appropriate replacement of abnormal losses. Patients receiving long-term parenteral nutrition can be managed with infrequent changes in the composition of TPN, provided that abnormal losses are replaced. For example, if a patient has a jejunal fistula or high-volume stool losses, electrolyte concentrations can be measured in the fistula fluid or the stool, and a comparable mixture of fluid and electrolytes can be replaced on a volume-per-volume basis. This prevents excessive loss of fluid and electrolytes, and the patient then can be maintained on standard TPN solutions for prolonged periods. The additional cost of the second infusion pump is more than offset by minimized wastage of parenteral nutrition solution as well as by the relative stability of the patient, which results in a need for fewer serum electrolyte determinations.

During early phases of therapy, electrolyte, blood urea nitrogen, and glucose levels should be measured daily. After a short period, however, these determinations can be made less frequently. In patients receiving long-term therapy, monitoring is required as infrequently as every 1 to 3 months, once appropriate needs are established. Periodic determination of calcium, magnesium, phosphorus, liver enzymes, and, occasionally, trace element and vitamin levels is required.

Once the patient is stabilized on parenteral nutrition, fluid and electrolyte losses are under control, and gastrointestinal motility is returned, phase II begins with a gradual introduction to enteral nutrition, preferably by continuous infusion. This can be accomplished either by using a soft silicone rubber nasogastric tube or, if long-term infusion is planned, through a feeding gastrostomy. Initially, 3% to 5% of the total daily caloric intake is given in the form of an elemental diet such as Pregestimil. The stool volume, pH level, and reducing substances are monitored. A marked increase in stool volume or significant malabsorption, as indicated by a persistent stool pH level of less than 5.5 or stools that are positive for reducing substances, contraindicates further advancement of enteral nutrition. Otherwise, the rate of enteral nutrition should be increased gradually and that of TPN should be decreased isocalorically. The rapidity with which the increases can be made depends greatly upon the length of the remaining small intestine. The whole process may proceed so rapidly that it is completed in a few weeks. On the other hand, years of TPN may be necessary before total enteral nutrition is tolerated.

The selection of an appropriate liquid diet for continuous enteral feeding is controversial. Protein hydrolysates or crystalline amino acids typically are used for a protein source. Protein hydrolysates have the advantage of being absorbed more rapidly than nonhydrolyzed protein. As most protein is absorbed in the form of dipeptides and tripeptides, the use of amino acids may be unnecessary. Although complex diets sometimes are thought to be more trophic than elemental diets, there is no clear indication that an intact protein is better than a protein hydrolysate in inducing mucosal hyperplasia. Carbohydrate generally is provided in the form of either glucose polymers or sucrose. Glucose polymers are hydrolyzed readily by pancreatic and mucosal enzymes, and have the advantage of reducing the osmolality of the formula. Lactose generally is tolerated poorly and should be avoided. Many enteral formulations have a very low fat content. Those that do contain fats often contain a high percentage of medium-chain triglycerides. Contrary to popular belief, high-fat diets usually do not result in increased fluid loss in patients with short-bowel syndrome, and dietary fat may be important in stimulating intestinal adaptation.

During phase III, solid feedings are begun and the patient is weaned over gradually to bolus feedings of an elemental diet to supplement the solid feedings. Solids can be administered easily around the indwelling nasogastric catheter during continuous enteral infusion. During this phase, attention must be paid to potential nutrient-deficient states once the patient no longer is receiving parenteral nutrition. These nutrients specifically include vitamins, minerals, and trace metals. Carbohydrate, protein, and, to a lesser extent, fat are relatively well absorbed once parenteral nutrition is discontinued. Poor absorption of fat-soluble vitamins, calcium, magnesium, and zinc is common, however. Poor absorption of vitamin D and calcium may result in rickets or tetany, especially in preterm infants. After ileal resection, bile acid and vitamin $B_{12}$ malabsorption are major problems, and bile acid malabsorption may exacerbate further fat-soluble vitamin absorption. Additional vitamin D may be given as an aqueous suspension, as may vitamins A and D. Parenteral vitamin K is administered occasionally.

In addition to nutrient deficiency states, the clinician must consider the likelihood that medications administered orally will be absorbed at less-than-desired levels. This becomes important in the treatment of children with short-bowel syndrome who have otitis media or other common pediatric infections. From 10% to 90% of the antibiotics commonly used may be malabsorbed in these infants, resulting in unpredictable therapeutic outcomes in patients treated orally. In these instances, home intravenous antibiotic therapy often is required.

Chronic bacterial overgrowth is a frequent complication of short-bowel syndrome, further exacerbating malabsorption. Bacterial overgrowth is likely to occur when the ileocecal valve is absent, when a tight anastomosis or partial obstruction is present, or when a dilated segment of bowel with poor motility exists. Bacterial overgrowth exacerbates malabsorption because of injury of the intestinal mucosa and deconjugation of bile acids, facilitating their reabsorption and reducing bile acid availability for solubilization of long-chain fats. Such patients may respond to intermittent broad-spectrum antimicrobial therapy. I have found the combination of metronidazole with trimethoprim-sulfamethoxazole to be particularly helpful; clindamycin, because of its efficacy against anaerobic organisms, or oral gentamicin also may be useful. In some instances, continuous administration of cyclic antibiotics is required to control bacterial overgrowth. If possible, resecting a tight anastomosis or performing an intestinal tapering procedure is useful in alleviating bacterial overgrowth, and often results in marked improvement in absorption.

Metabolic acidoses have developed in some patients as a result of the production of excessive D-lactate by intestinal bacteria. Although both D-lactate and L-lactate are produced by intestinal bacteria, only the L form can be metabolized in humans. D-lactic acidosis is correctable by elimination of bacterial overgrowth, and should be considered in patients with short-bowel syndrome who have repeated attacks of dyspnea and drowsiness.

A colitis or ileitis picture similar to that associated with Crohn's disease has been described in patients with short-bowel syndrome and bacterial overgrowth. Frank ulceration may occur and, if it is unresponsive to antimicrobial therapy, the disorder may respond to anti-inflammatory agents such as sulfasalazine or even corticosteroids.

Gastric acid hypersecretion is common in infants with short-bowel syndrome. Cimetidine has been shown to decrease stool mass as well as fecal excretion of sodium and potassium in adults with short-bowel syndrome.

Cholestyramine, a bile acid–binding resin, is useful in reducing diarrhea in some patients with ileal resection. It is most effective when used in conjunction with medium-chain triglycerides or low-fat formulas, as cholestyramine may exacerbate fat malabsorption by reducing the functional bile acid pool.

A number of surgical procedures have been devised to improve absorption in patients with short-bowel syndrome. Most involve slowing intestinal transit. The most direct approach is construction of a valve or sphincter that functions in a manner similar to the ileocecal valve, causing constriction of the lumen and creating a partial mechanical obstruction. The intent also is to prevent retrograde reflux of bacterial contents into the small intestine. Clinical experience has been somewhat limited, and results usually are unsatisfactory. Antiperistaltic segments of small intestine also have been used.

Intestinal tapering or lengthening surgery occasionally may be helpful. A markedly dilated intestine often develops in patients with short-bowel syndrome secondary to both partial chronic obstruction and adaptation. Tapering dilated segments reduces stasis and bacterial content, improves intestinal function, and preserves intestinal length. In my experience and that of others, intestinal tapering procedures have proven to be a valuable adjunct in patients with dilated segments of bowel who respond poorly to antibiotic therapy for bacterial overgrowth.

The ultimate cure for short-bowel syndrome probably rests with intestinal transplantation. Recent improvements in immunosuppression with cyclosporine and, more recently, FK506 suggest that intestinal transplantation ultimately may be possible. Substantial experience has been gained in performing intestine transplants in experimental animals. Presently, in excess of 30 intestinal transplantations have been performed in children at a number of centers throughout North America and Europe. Most have been performed for short-bowel syndrome with severe TPN-induced liver disease and have included concurrent liver transplantation. Early reports are encouraging, but adequate early diagnosis of small-intestinal rejection remains a problem, and early reports of the development of intestinal lymphomas are worrisome. Although denervation of the small intestine and lymphatic disruption occur, these do not appear to major negative factors.

The prognosis for short-bowel syndrome has been altered markedly through the use of parenteral nutrition. Recent advances in parenteral therapy, including changes in catheter techniques, solutions, understanding of the importance of intraluminal nutrition, and, finally, use of parenteral nutrition in the home, have altered markedly the way in which patients with short-bowel syndrome are treated. In 1972, the classic paper by Wilmore defined the prognosis for short-bowel syndrome in infants. Of 20 infants with a jejunoileal segment length of 38 to 75 cm, 95% survived. Infants with 15 to 38 cm of jejunum and ileum survived 50% of the time, provided the ileocecal valve was intact. Those without an ileocecal valve died, as did infants with less that 15 cm of small intestine, including all those with intact ileocecal valves. This paper pointed out the importance of the ileocecal valve in determining the prognosis for short-bowel syndrome. Because this organ delays transit through the small intestine and reduces bacterial overgrowth at this site, it is the key to survival in many patients with short-bowel syndrome.

Recent data by Dorney and colleagues suggest that advances in parenteral nutrition have significantly changed the statistics regarding short-bowel syndrome in the 1980s. Thirteen children with less than 38 cm of jejunum and ileum were reported. Nine of the 13 survived, 5 successfully having discontinued parenteral nutrition therapy. The authors concluded that ultimate survival, including normal growth, without parenteral nutrition is possible with as little as 11 cm of jejunum and ileum and an intact ileocecal valve, and with as little as 25 cm of jejunum and ileum without an ileocecal valve. Patients with short-bowel syndrome now die of the complications of parenteral nutrition, such as severe TPN cholestasis or fulminant septicemia, rather than of malnutrition. The recent advent of intestinal transplantation likely will alter the prognosis further in the near future.

## Selected Readings

Cooper A, Floyd TF, Ross AJ, et al. Morbidity and mortality of short bowel syndrome acquired in infancy: An update. J Pediatr Surg 1984;19:711.

Dorney SFA, Ament ME, Berquist WE, et al. Improved survival in very short small bowel of infancy with use of long-term parenteral nutrition. J Pediatr 1985;107:521.

Dowling RH, Booth CC. Structural and functional changes following small intestinal resection in the rat. Clin Sci 1967;32:139.

Thompson JS, Rikker LF. Surgical alternatives for the short bowel syndrome. Am J Gastroenterol 1987;82:97.

Vanderhoof JA, Langnas AN, Pinch LW, Thompson JS, Kaufman SS. Short bowel syndrome: A review. J Pediatr Gastroenterol Nutr 1992;14:359.

Williamson RCN, Chir M. Intestinal adaptation (first of two parts): Structural, functional, and cytokinetic changes. N Engl J Med 1978;198:1393.

Williamson RCN, Chir M. Intestinal adaptation (second of two parts): Mechanisms of control. N Engl J Med 1978;298:1444.

Wilmore DW. Factors correlating with a successful outcome following extensive intestinal resection in newborn infants. J Pediatr 1972;80:88.

*Principles and Practice of Pediatrics, Second Edition.*
edited by Frank A. Oski et al. J. B. Lippincott Company, Philadelphia © 1994.

# 20.5 *Neonatal Hyperbilirubinemia*

William J. Cashore

Jaundice is one of the most common conditions found in the newborn infant, and measurement of the serum bilirubin concentration probably is the laboratory test performed most often in the newborn nursery. Although the cause of most neonatal jaundice is developmental and the clinical course nearly always is benign, physicians caring for newborn infants must be alert for the minority of cases in which the cause of hyperbilirubinemia is pathologic or the clinical course is atypical, with exaggerated and possibly harmful levels of hyperbilirubinemia. Observation and follow-up of the newborn infant must be diligent to identify such cases early enough in the clinical course to ensure prompt and adequate treatment.

## DEFINITION

The term *hyperbilirubinemia* implies an excessive level of serum bilirubin, potentially associated with a pathologic cause or outcome. In fact, during the first few days of postnatal life, most newborns have maximum serum bilirubin levels exceeding the upper limits of normal for adults, even when no disease is present. The reason for this "physiologic" hyperbilirubinemia is a developmental delay in the conjugation and excretion of bilirubin as the infant achieves a postnatal transition from dependence on maternal clearance of fetal bilirubin by re-excretion across the placenta and maternal conjugation of the unconjugated pigment, to a more mature and self-contained enzymatic and excretory pathway for bilirubin conjugation and elimination.

In the first 3 to 4 postnatal days, normal infants have a physiologic increase in serum bilirubin from cord bilirubin levels of 1.5 mg/dL or less at birth to a mean value of $6.5 \pm 2.5$ mg/dL (mean $\pm$ SD) on the third or fourth postnatal day. There is a difference in mean serum bilirubin levels even within the first 3 or 4 days between breast-fed infants ($7.3 \pm 3.9$ mg/dL) and formula-fed infants ($5.7 \pm 3.3$ mg/dL). This difference persists for the next several days, with clinically significant hyperbilirubinemia developing more frequently in breast-fed infants during the first week.

Although most newborns have hyperbilirubinemia by normal adult standards, physiologic jaundice is an event that is linked to normal development, is benign and self-limited, resolves by the end of the first week, and requires no treatment. Virtually all newborns manifest a phase of physiologic jaundice; during this time, the serum bilirubin level rises to between 6 and 8 mg/dL. This elevation, which results almost exclusively from an increase in the amount of unconjugated bilirubin (UCB), occurs in the absence of hemolytic disease and is more marked in premature infants. Classically, neonatal unconjugated hyperbilirubinemia has been attributed primarily to defective bilirubin conjugation and, indeed, low levels of glucuronyl transferase activity are detected in the human fetal and neonatal liver.

The role of inhibitors of glucuronyl transferase activity, such as maternal steroids, as well as postulated activators of enzyme expression, remains unclear. Other potentially important factors in the genesis of physiologic jaundice (unconjugated hyperbilirubinemia) include the following:

1. Persistent patency of the ductus venosus, which may divert blood flow away from the hepatic sinusoidal bed and, therefore, allow UCB to bypass the site of bilirubin metabolism—namely, the hepatocytes
2. Discontinuation of placental mechanisms for bilirubin removal and detoxification
3. A greater rate of bilirubin production in the infant (6 to 8 mg/kg every 24 hours) than in the adult, secondary to a larger red blood cell mass and shortened red blood cell survival time
4. Diminished binding of UCB to neonatal serum albumin
5. Diminished levels of intracellular bilirubin binding (Y) protein
6. Impaired canalicular excretion of organic anions in the developing human.

In addition, bilirubin appears to undergo a significant enterohepatic circulation in the newborn. Conjugated bilirubin in the intestinal tract of the adult is reduced by anaerobic intestinal flora to poorly absorbable urobilinogen. These flora are not present in the fetal and neonatal intestine. Instead, $\beta$-glucuronidase activity, present in the neonatal intestine, hydrolyzes bilirubin diglucuronide into UCB, which subsequently is reabsorbed into the portal circulation, contributing to the "bilirubin overload" and further taxing already stressed metabolic and excretory pathways. Thus, delayed passage of meconium can cause an elevation in the serum bilirubin level.

Some newborns show an unusually early onset, exaggerated and sustained levels, or an uncommonly long duration of hyperbilirubinemia, and these infants may require medical attention. Maisels and Gifford found that 6.1% of 2416 normal, asymptomatic, term infants had serum bilirubin concentrations greater than 12.9 mg/dL, or about twice the mean value of 6.5 mg/dL for healthy newborns. Nine percent of breast-fed infants had maximum serum bilirubin levels in excess of 12.9 mg/dL versus only 2.2% of formula-fed infants. A definite cause for this exaggerated hyperbilirubinemia was found in only 45% of the infants observed. Therefore, about 3% of term newborns may have exaggerated or sustained hyperbilirubinemia as part of the normal postnatal development of their ability to conjugate and excrete bilirubin, whereas another 3% to 5% of these infants may have clinically significant hyperbilirubinemia associated with some other identifiable cause. Even with exaggerated hyperbilirubinemia, about half of the cases encountered appear to be developmental, self-limited, and presumably benign. Hyperbilirubinemia, therefore, is a frequent observation in the nursery, and the term used by itself indicates only that the level of jaundice observed is greater than that expected for a healthy infant. Further observation and diagnostic studies may be necessary to arrive at a specific cause for the hyperbilirubinemia, or to alert the pediatrician that it is of pathologic origin and potentially is hazardous.

Because visible cutaneous and scleral jaundice in the newborn usually is noted only when the serum bilirubin level exceeds 7 to 8 mg/dL, most self-limited developmental jaundice with a maximum serum bilirubin level at or below the mean value for newborns remains undetected. There is no indication for routine serum bilirubin determination in newborns who are not clinically jaundiced. However, visible jaundice develops in about 15% of newborns with serum bilirubin levels in the range of 10 to 12 mg/dL or greater. The differential diagnosis of jaundice in these infants may be assisted by noting the rapidity of onset, the presence of major or minor blood group incompatibility between the mother and her newborn, the presence of associated findings such as hematomas or evidence of infection, the method of feeding being used, and the duration and clinical course of jaundice beyond the third day. If the presence of visible jaundice in the range of 13 to 15 mg/dL is accepted as a working definition of exaggerated hyperbilirubinemia, about 3% of the newborn population will have jaundice in this range as a result of a detectable cause potentially requiring treatment and follow-up, whereas about 3% will represent the statistical upper limits of normal. Strictly speaking, the term *hyperbilirubinemia* in the newborn should be reserved for cases that exceed the expected limits of normal or are associated with an unusual rapidity of onset, unexpected persistence beyond the first few days, or a recognized pathologic cause.

## CAUSES OF HYPERBILIRUBINEMIA

Bilirubin is the breakdown product of heme, derived via heme oxygenase and biliverdin reductase with liberation of 1 mole of carbon monoxide for each mole of heme metabolized. Circulating bilirubin is transported on serum albumin to specific receptor proteins in the liver, and then is conjugated by uridine diphosphate–glucuronyl transferase to its water-soluble form, also called "conjugated" or "direct-reacting" bilirubin. There is a somewhat complex family of bilirubin conjugates, but the two most important physiologic conjugation products are bilirubin monoglucuronide and bilirubin diglucuronide, the latter being the predominant conjugated form in the human infant. Bilirubin conjugates enter the small bowel via canalicular transport and bile excretion, and, in the course of normal metabolism, are oxidized further and excreted in the stool. Because the bowel does not function in fetal life, the hepatic conjugation and transport system is relatively inactive in the fetus, so that bilirubin produced from fetal red cells in utero mostly circulates in the unconjugated form. This unconjugated or "indirect-reacting" bilirubin is albumin-bound and relatively lipophilic, and can be transferred across the placenta again to the maternal circulation for conjugation and excretion by the maternal liver. At birth, this maternal excretory pathway is removed, and the development of normal conjugating capacity, canalicular transport, and metabolism and excretion of conjugated bilirubin in the small and large bowel require several days before this pathway becomes adequate for quantitative conjugation and excretion of bilirubin. Associated with the slow maturation of bilirubin conjugation and excretion is the accumulation of unconjugated or indirect-reacting bilirubin in the plasma until the conjugating system matures.

Infants of diabetic mothers often have polycythemia, with an increased red cell mass leading to an increased daily rate of bilirubin formation They may have some structural or metabolic instability of the red cell related to their glucose metabolism and, in general, they follow a less mature pattern of physiologic development than do term infants of similar birth weight whose mothers are not diabetic.

Delay in the conjugation and excretion of bilirubin appears to be highly individual, but some infants may have predisposing or contributing factors to delayed excretion. The most common underlying factor is immaturity. Otherwise healthy preterm infants (<37 weeks' gestation) tend to have maximum serum bilirubin levels 30% to 50% higher than those of their term counterparts, with increases in serum UCB continuing until as late as the sixth or seventh postnatal day and, sometimes, visible jaundice persisting into the second week.

Breast-fed infants may have combined inefficiency of bilirubin conjugation and excretion mediated by factors in breast milk that may suppress hepatic function, increase reabsorption of bilirubin from the small bowel, or both. As noted above, the mean bilirubin concentration is slightly higher, the duration of jaundice is somewhat longer, and the incidence of clinically detectable hyperbilirubinemia during the first week is more frequent in breast-fed than in formula-fed infants. In addition, about 2% of breast-fed infants have a prolonged (2- to 8-week) course of moderate unconjugated hyperbilirubinemia, usually in the range of 10 to 15 mg/dL, while they are feeding adequately on breast milk and have normal weight gain and no other abnormal clinical findings. Arias and colleagues showed that high levels of $3\alpha$-, $20\beta$-pregnanediol in their mothers' milk were associated with decreased hepatic conjugation of bilirubin and persistent hyperbilirubinemia in a group of infants with breast-milk jaundice, and proposed that the ingestion of pregnanediol in breast milk was the specific cause of this condition. In more recent investigations of breast-milk jaundice, however, not all infants exposed to high milk levels of pregnanediol have had hyperbilirubinemia, and not all cases of breast milk jaundice have been associated with high pregnanediol levels. Other possible contributing factors to breast-milk jaundice, proposed by some investigators but not confirmed by multiple independent studies, include high concentrations of lipase, $\beta$-glucuronidase, or polyunsaturated fatty acids in breast milk. Multiple hormonal or enzymatic factors may be involved in suppressing the conjugation of bilirubin or cleaving bilirubin conjugates in the small bowel in certain mother–baby pairs, thereby promoting the reabsorption and enterohepatic recirculation of UCB. Although the pathogenesis of breast-milk jaundice is controversial, most patients are asymptomatic and have only mild hyperbilirubinemia, and the majority respond to temporary cessation of breast-feeding for 36 to 48 hours with a prompt decrease in the serum bilirubin level.

The early onset of hyperbilirubinemia in breast-fed infants may be abetted by hospital feeding practices, which frequently call for an 8- to 12-hour period of postnatal observation without feeding, followed by a schedule of feeding every 4 hours. This type of scheduling may not allow sufficient nursing time during the first few days, resulting in the delayed onset of adequate lactation, suboptimal volume intake, and a delay in the normal bilirubin excretion that takes place as meconium is expelled, followed by normal neonatal stools that are rich in bile pigments.

Infants who are not fed or who have a high intestinal obstruction caused by conditions such as pyloric stenosis or intestinal obstruction or atresia may have exaggerated levels of jaundice as a result of the combined effects of lack of nutritional substrate for bilirubin conjugation, lack of peristalsis for the excretion of bilirubin in the stool, and consequent reabsorption of bilirubin from an obstructed or nonfunctioning bowel.

Crigler-Najjar syndrome (type I) is associated with extreme jaundice in the neonatal period; serum UCB concentrations may reach 15 to 35 mg/dL. Liver histology is normal, and no evidence of anemia or liver disease exists. This disorder is transmitted as an autosomal recessive trait, and is caused by an absence of hepatic glucuronyl transferase activity. Kernicterus occurs universally in patients with type I Crigler-Najjar syndrome. Phenobarbital does not increase bilirubin output or decrease serum bilirubin levels. This syndrome generally is fatal, and attempts at therapy, which have included consistent phototherapy and the use of bilirubin-binding agents, have been futile. Future prospects for therapy may include pharmacotherapeutic agents that selectively inhibit the conversion of heme to bilirubin, using agents such as Tin-protoporphyrin. In addition, hepatic transplantation, which provides the missing enzyme, is curative. This must be performed before irreversible neurologic damage occurs, however. Type II Crigler-Najjar syndrome is distinguished from type I by the fact that phenobarbital administration causes a prompt fall in the serum bilirubin level. Inheritance of this variety is thought to be autosomal dominant. The clinical course generally is milder than that in type I disease.

Gilbert's disease is characterized by a mild elevation in serum bilirubin levels, typically of 2 to 3 mg/dL. Liver function and histology are normal, except for minor changes noted on electron microscopy. The disorder appears to be inherited in an autosomal dominant fashion, with an estimated gene frequency of 2% to 6%. The cause of the increased UCB is uncertain; postulated mechanisms include diminished uptake or conjugation of bilirubin. Caloric deprivation often increases serum bilirubin levels twofold to threefold in patients with Gilbert's disease. No therapy is necessary.

Hypothyroidism is a cause of persistent unconjugated hyperbilirubinemia, and often is the presenting sign of thyroid hormone deficiency. Because diagnosis is through assay of thyroxine ($T_4$) and thyroid-stimulating hormone (TSH) levels, neonatal screening programs offer an early opportunity for detection of this disorder. Similarly, jaundice noted in infants with hypopituitarism presumably is secondary to hypothyroidism.

Lucey-Driscoll syndrome, which consists of severe neonatal hyperbilirubinemia and is capable of causing kernicterus, is thought to be caused by inhibition of glucuronyl transferase in the liver of the newborn by an unidentified factor present in maternal serum and urine. Infants with this disorder, which has been treated with exchange transfusions, subsequently have demonstrated normal development without further episodes of jaundice.

Many drugs presumably can inhibit glucuronyl transferase or hepatic bilirubin uptake and cause an elevation in the serum UCB level.

Circulating bilirubin levels in the newborn become abnormally high if the maturation of hepatic function is delayed or if new bilirubin is produced from heme at an abnormally high rate.

Bilirubin production is increased by hemolysis or, much more rarely, by inefficient erythropoiesis. The principal causes of hemolysis in the newborn are antibody-mediated hemolytic anemias (eg, Rh or ABO incompatibility); enclosed hemorrhage such as a cephalhematoma, skin bruising, or an intracranial hemorrhage; hemolysis resulting from bacterial endotoxin as in group B strep-tococcal or *Escherichia coli* septicemia; or an abnormality of red cell structure or metabolism such as hereditary spherocytosis or glucose-6-phosphate dehydrogenase deficiency (disorders that do not manifest often in the neonatal period, but may present with any degree of unconjugated hyperbilirubinemia, including hydrops fetalis). The increased bilirubin production associated with hemolysis can be detected as an increase in pulmonary carbon monoxide excretion using sensitive equipment to detect small amounts of carbon monoxide in expired air.

The most common causes of hemolysis in term infants are isoantibody-mediated hemolytic anemias resulting from maternal–fetal ABO or Rh incompatibility. Although not all susceptible infants are affected, 25% of normal pregnancies are ABO incompatible and about 12% are Rh incompatible.

Neonatal polycythemia, as seen in infants of diabetic mothers, infants with adrenal hyperplasia, twin-to-twin transfusion, or aggressive "stripping" of the umbilical cord, when combined with shortened fetal red blood cell survival time, may result in the accumulation of an increased bilirubin load that must be excreted postnatally. In these situations, hyperbilirubinemia becomes clinically evident after 48 hours of postnatal life and is treatable, in part, by partial exchange transfusion.

Extravasated blood, such as that found in the presence of a cephalhematoma, extensive cutaneous bruising, or swallowed maternal blood, also can present the neonatal liver with an increased bilirubin load. In small, premature infants, intracranial hemorrhage can contribute to increased bilirubin formation. Jaundice generally is evident by 3 to 5 days of postnatal life, because extravasated hemoglobin is metabolized slowly to bilirubin. Diagnosis is via inspection or, in the case of swallowed maternal blood, use of the Apt test.

Drugs, such as vitamin K given in excessive amounts, may cause hemolysis with a resultant increased bilirubin load. Augmentation of labor with oxytocin had been associated with neonatal hyperbilirubinemia, but this appears to be secondary to osmotic changes in the fetal/neonatal circulation.

The differential diagnosis of neonatal jaundice is summarized in Table 20-41.

# BILIRUBIN TOXICITY

High circulating concentrations of bilirubin are toxic to the central nervous system, with the basal ganglia being the most vulnerable areas and cortical damage occurring relatively infrequently. The reason for the susceptibility of the basal ganglia to bilirubin toxicity is not known and the metabolic abnormalities underlying bilirubin toxicity in the central nervous system are not understood. Clinical manifestations of bilirubin toxicity most frequently involve the basal ganglia and cranial nerve nuclei. The most characteristic findings are opisthotonos, extensor rigidity, tremors, ataxic gait, oculomotor paralysis, and hearing loss. Fatal cases in the newborn period often are characterized by loss of the suck response and lethargy, followed by hyperirritability, then seizures and death. The acute phases of bilirubin toxicity in severely affected infants often have been accompanied also by gastric and pulmonary hemorrhages. In fatal cases, the meninges and cortical surfaces may be stained lightly with bilirubin, but dense regional staining with bilirubin is found in the basal ganglia, globus pallidus, hippocampus, and, sometimes, cerebellum. In later deaths, scarring and gliosis may be found in these or adjacent areas that presumably were sites of bilirubin deposition. Neurologic damage in survivors corresponds to injury in the areas found to be stained in many autopsies. Intelligence and higher cortical functions are relatively spared, whereas ataxia, choreoathetosis, tremors, oculomotor palsy, and central hearing loss persist.

In general, the serum UCB concentrations that are associated

## TABLE 20-41. Differential Diagnosis of Neonatal Jaundice

| Cause | Associated Findings |
|---|---|
| **Unconjugated ("Indirect") Hyperbilirubinemia** | |
| *Hemolytic Disease (Isoimmune)* | |
| ABO incompatibility | Positive Coombs' antiglobulin test (anti-A or anti-B); microspherocytes |
| Rh incompatibility | Maternal anti-Rh titer; positive Coombs' test; nucleated RBCs |
| Other minor blood group incompatibility | Positive Coombs' test; RBC morphology variable |
| *Structural or Metabolic Abnormalities of RBCs** | |
| Hereditary spherocytosis | Family history; splenomegaly; microspherocytes |
| Glucose-6-phosphate dehydrogenase (G6PD) deficiency | Family history; recent exposure to an oxidant in food or drug; with or without splenomegaly |
| *Hereditary Defects in Bilirubin Conjugation* | |
| Crigler-Najjar syndrome | Complete lack of glucuronyl transferase; severe, lifelong unconjugated hyperbilirubinemia |
| Gilbert's disease (Arias syndrome) | Family history; partial defect of glucuronyl transferase; sometimes responds to phenobarbital |
| *Bacterial Sepsis* | History and findings compatible with neonatal infection; often an increase in direct bilirubin as well |
| *"Breast-Milk" Jaundice* | Mild to moderate, but persistent, hyperbilirubinemia; usually improves when breast milk is discontinued |
| *Physiologic Jaundice* | Usually mild to moderate; no predisposing factors; self-limited (duration <1 wk) |
| **Conjugated ("Direct") Hyperbilirubinemia** | |
| *Congenital Biliary Atresia* | Dilated intrahepatic ducts; no bile excretion |
| *Extrahepatic Biliary Obstruction* | Extrahepatic mass or cyst; dilated main or common bile ducts |
| *Neonatal Hepatitis* | |
| Bacterial | Findings compatible with neonatal sepsis |
| Viral | Inflammatory changes; other systemic signs of a specific viral infection |
| Nonspecific | Inflammatory changes without a specific viral etiology |
| *"Inspissated Bile Syndrome"* | Persistent direct hyperbilirubinemia associated with isoimmune hemolytic disease |
| *Post-Asphyxia* | Compatible history, plus increased hepatocellular enzyme concentrations |
| *$\alpha_1$-Antitrypsin Deficiency* | Decreased, $\alpha_1$-antitrypsin levels; recurrent or "chronic" lung disease |
| *Neonatal Hemosiderosis* | Hemosiderin-filled macrophages on biopsy |

* Only the two most common disorders are listed, as examples. *RBCs*, red blood cells.

with overt bilirubin encephalopathy (or kernicterus, the pathologic term for nuclear staining with bilirubin) are substantially higher than the indirect bilirubin levels normally seen among infants with hyperbilirubinemia in ordinary clinical practice. Bilirubin levels generally associated with clinical signs of kernicterus in term infants tend to be in the range of 25 to 30 mg/dL, or even higher. In epidemiologic surveys of bilirubin encephalopathy associated with Rh hemolytic disease, basal ganglion staining or clinical signs of bilirubin encephalopathy were encountered occasionally when the serum indirect bilirubin level reached or slightly exceeded 20 mg/dL. In most proven cases, however, the serum bilirubin level was considerably higher, often approaching 30 mg/dL. On the other hand, there are well-documented cases of patients with serum indirect bilirubin levels in the range of 30 to 35 mg/dL who did not experience serious long-term sequelae. Therefore, no precise bilirubin level has been established clearly at which either safety or permanent harm can be guaranteed.

Premature infants, especially those with a birth weight of less than 1500 g, and some infants with sepsis or metabolic complications of asphyxia or respiratory distress may be vulnerable to bilirubin toxicity at lower indirect bilirubin concentrations. During the 1960s and 1970s, numerous cases of basal ganglion staining at maximum serum bilirubin levels of 10 to 15 mg/dL, along with other, more perplexing, cases of generalized cortical and subcortical bilirubin staining, were reported in preterm infants or in larger infants with a complicated postnatal course often marked by sepsis or asphyxia. A few such patients had overt neurologic findings of bilirubin encephalopathy, but, in many cases, "low bilirubin kernicterus" was an incidental finding at autopsy, unsuspected from the clinical course. The clinical significance of low bilirubin kernicterus and its implication for follow-up of jaundiced preterm infants are uncertain, but the incidence of bilirubin staining in the central nervous system discovered at autopsy seems to have decreased in the 1980s. Moderate hyperbilirubinemia in the range of 15 to 20 mg/dL poses little or no acute or long-term developmental risk for otherwise normal infants. Term infants with hyperbilirubinemia in this range show, at most, only subtle and short-term behavioral changes, with no detectable long-term developmental or neurologic sequelae on follow-up. In the range of 20 to 25 mg/dL, some term infants become less active and responsive, and also show reversible increases in conduction time and occasional decreases in wave amplitude on determinations of auditory brain stem evoked potentials. The long-term significance of abnormalities in brain stem evoked potentials is not clear, but the study tracings return to normal as bilirubin concentrations fall back into the normal range or respond to treatment.

In summary, uncontrolled levels of severe hyperbilirubinemia produce a characteristic pattern of damage in the basal ganglia, manifested by basal ganglion staining at autopsy or by a subcortical neurologic deficit in survivors. In the range of 20 to 25 mg/dL of indirect bilirubin, some term infants show subtle but reversible sensory and behavioral changes of uncertain prognostic significance. Low bilirubin kernicterus in preterm infants remains a diagnostic and developmental puzzle, with a definitive solution becoming less likely as the incidence of low bilirubin kernicterus declines in this high-risk group.

The mechanism of bilirubin toxicity is not clear, but it probably is mediated by the entry of UCB into susceptible areas of the central nervous system. There are two possible mechanisms for bilirubin entry into the brain: diffusion of UCB, a somewhat lipophilic compound, across an intact blood–brain barrier, or damage to the blood–brain barrier with significant entry of plasma contents into the brain. Nearly all the bilirubin in the circulation is bound tightly to serum albumin, but at the very high bilirubin levels that usually are found in term infants with kernicterus, the total bilirubin concentration in the plasma may exceed the albumin concentration available to bind it, with increased diffusion of "free" bilirubin across the blood–brain barrier into the brain extravascular space. Because of the fact that, in most cell models of bilirubin toxicity, free bilirubin (ie, that which is not bound to plasma albumin) produces the abnormal metabolic or neurologic effect, whereas bilirubin bound to an equimolar concentration of albumin in the same system usually fails to produce the same effect, it is a plausible, but still unproven, hypothesis that the free fraction of UCB is the species responsible for the observed toxicity in patients with severe hyperbilirubinemia. In very immature or high-risk infants, however, especially those with kernicterus or cortical bilirubin staining as an incidental finding at autopsy, it also is plausible that injury to the blood–brain barrier allows quantitative entry of albumin-bound bilirubin, with incidental staining of susceptible structures, but without clinical evidence of bilirubin toxicity. The controversy regarding the relative contributions of "free" bilirubin and of underlying injury to the brain or blood–brain barrier in the finding of kernicterus at autopsy, or in the observation of neurologic abnormalities in the clinical setting, remains unresolved at this time.

## THE DIAGNOSIS OF HYPERBILIRUBINEMIA

Determination of the serum bilirubin concentration is indicated only for visible jaundice in healthy term infants, unless prenatal or delivery room screening procedures reveal the presence of a hemolytic anemia with a positive Coombs' test. Daily inspection of the baby, undressed and in adequate light, allows early recognition of cutaneous or scleral jaundice in most cases. For non-white infants, part of the examination can include brief compression with the examiner's thumb of the skin over a firm surface such as the forehead, sternum, or upper thigh; briefly blanching the skin may help to reveal an underlying yellow color. Skin

reflectance by means of a commercially available transcutaneous bilirubinometer is another aid to the evaluation of clinically evident jaundice in the nursery. The reflectance of jaundiced skin correlates well enough with serum bilirubin levels to be used as a screening test for hyperbilirubinemia with proper standardization of the technique and the instrument. Again, the correlation of skin reflectance with serum bilirubin levels is better in white than in non-white infants with jaundice.

Both clinical observation and skin reflectance document that cutaneous jaundice progresses from the face downward in term infants. Scleral and facial jaundice become visible at bilirubin levels of 6 to 8 mg/dL, jaundice of the shoulders and trunk becomes apparent at 8 to 10 mg/dL, jaundice of the lower body is noticeable at 10 to 12 mg/dL, and generally distributed jaundice can be seen at 12 to 15 mg/dL. Although this is only the roughest of guidelines, it serves to emphasize that daily observation of newborns for signs of jaundice often permits the timely recognition of developing hyperbilirubinemia, with the advantages that early detection may provide for timely diagnosis, intervention, and follow-up. Sometimes, the nurse is the first observer to note jaundice in the clinical record, and nurses' notes or messages should be followed up by reexamination of the infant and performance of appropriate laboratory studies when indicated. Visible jaundice on the first day is always abnormal, and requires prompt evaluation and follow-up. Faint jaundice, first appearing only on the third or fourth hospital day or on the day of discharge, usually is consistent with the average bilirubin levels expected in term infants who are otherwise well, and it may require no intervention.

In addition to a laboratory request for the measurement of total and direct (or conjugated) bilirubin, the clinical detection of hyperbilirubinemia should prompt a thorough examination of the infant's abdomen with palpation of the liver and spleen, and a review of the maternal and neonatal hospital records for evidence of blood group incompatibility, a positive antibody titer or Coombs' test, or a family history of neonatal or childhood jaundice in siblings or other relatives. All women who are receiving prenatal care or are admitted to a hospital for delivery should have their major (A,B,O) and minor (Rh) blood groups determined. If the mothers are Rh negative, they also should have a titer for anti-Rh antibodies determined during the course of prenatal care. At birth, a cord blood specimen for each infant should be sent to the hospital serology laboratory or blood bank. If the mother's blood type is group O, or if she is Rh negative (with any major group), the infant's major and minor blood groups should be determined and an antibody screen performed if the maternal and neonatal major or Rh blood groups are incompatible.

Although 25% of pregnancies potentially are ABO incompatible, only a minority (10% to 15%) have hemolytic anemia as documented by a positive Coombs' test. In the absence of a positive antibody test, it is not possible to confirm the diagnosis of hemolytic anemia in the newborn. If prenatal or postnatal screening tests reveal the presence of a Coombs'-positive hemolytic anemia, or if splenomegaly is present, then, in addition to serum bilirubin measurement, determination of hemoglobin, hematocrit, red cell indices, reticulocyte count, and red cell morphology should be undertaken. For the more common instance of benign, self-limited developmental hyperbilirubinemia, a complete blood count is not necessary unless there is strong reason to suspect hemolysis or infection as the source of hyperbilirubinemia. For known cases of Rh sensitization, hemoglobin, hematocrit, and bilirubin determinations should be performed on the cord blood as well as on subsequent postnatal specimens. For most cases of suspected ABO hemolytic disease, cord blood determinations are not needed because ABO incompatibility seldom causes significant jaundice or anemia at birth.

The age at first presentation of clinical jaundice and the subsequent rate of increase in serum bilirubin levels sometimes will allow the physician to infer the clinical course and probable outcome of an infant with hyperbilirubinemia. The rate of increase in the serum bilirubin level can be estimated simply by dividing the first serum bilirubin level by the patient's age at the time, and by dividing all subsequent changes in bilirubin level by the change in age between determinations. This will allow the physician to estimate whether the rate of increase is normal or abnormal, and whether the increase in bilirubin over time is sustained or declining. For example, the maximum rate of increase in bilirubin for otherwise normal infants with non-hemolytic hyperbilirubinemia is about 5 mg/dL/d, or 0.2 mg/dL/h. Visible jaundice on the first day or a bilirubin concentration greater than 10 mg/dL within the second 24 hours, therefore, is outside the normal range for rate of increase in bilirubin and potentially results from a pathologic cause. Estimating the rate of increase during the interval between bilirubin determinations also allows the physician to estimate the change in bilirubin level that is likely to occur over the next 12- to 24-hour interval, and to plan subsequent bilirubin determinations accordingly. In most cases, if an infant is jaundiced significantly (ie, serum indirect bilirubin level $\geq$10 mg/dL) at the first determination, and if the calculated rate of increase exceeds 0.2 mg/dL/h, repeat determinations are indicated about every 12 hours until the serum bilirubin levels stabilize or there is a clear indication for treatment. In the meantime, the clinician can use the initial rate of bilirubin accumulation in the plasma, and the subsequent rate of increase, as a guideline to further diagnostic efforts to determine the underlying cause of the jaundice, if it is not clearly physiologic.

Physiologic jaundice and hemolytic hyperbilirubinemia are always predominantly of the indirect-reacting variety. Because obstructive liver disease from various causes also may present with hyperbilirubinemia in the newborn period, the initial evaluation of a jaundiced infant always requires determination of the direct as well as the total serum bilirubin concentration. Direct bilirubin concentrations persistently above the range of 1.0 to 1.5 mg/dL should be regarded with suspicion and require a separate diagnostic evaluation, especially if the direct fraction continues to rise during subsequent postnatal days or weeks. Ideally, all neonatal bilirubin determinations should include measurement of direct as well as total bilirubin. Rapid methods that measure only total bilirubin are not acceptable for follow-up unless confirmatory measurements of direct bilirubin also can be performed at suitable intervals during follow-up.

# THE MANAGEMENT OF HYPERBILIRUBINEMIA

The clinical course in most cases of neonatal jaundice defines the problem as benign and self-limited. Unless the infant has clear evidence of a hemolytic anemia or some other significant perinatal or postnatal abnormality, most cases of "physiologic hyperbilirubinemia" can be managed with observation, serial bilirubin determinations, and reassurance. Despite an extensive differential diagnosis for neonatal jaundice, the vast majority of cases are attributable to a small number of causes that usually are detectable by serial bilirubin determinations, examination of the patient, and review of maternal and neonatal blood type and antibody studies. The benign and self-limited course of most cases of non-hemolytic hyperbilirubinemia makes it unnecessary to pursue further diagnostic studies in the first few days.

## Hemolytic Hyperbilirubinemia: Rh Disease

Until recently, Rh isoimmunization was a common cause of neonatal hemolytic anemia and hyperbilirubinemia, and was the un-

derlying cause for most cases of kernicterus in term infants. Sixteen percent of North American women are Rh negative, in most cases negative for the Rh "D" antigen. At delivery of her first Rh positive child, or sometimes because of a placental hemorrhage or spontaneous abortion of an Rh positive fetus, the Rh negative mother receives a small transfusion of Rh positive fetal cells. When these Rh positive cells enter the circulation of the Rh negative recipient, the maternal immune system develops an antibody response to the foreign Rh positive red cell antigen. Later exposure to Rh positive fetal cells, either during a subsequent Rh positive pregnancy or sometimes by later transplacental passage of fetal cells during the same pregnancy, increases the maternal IgG antibody titer against the cells of her fetus. Maternal anti-Rh IgG antibodies then re-cross the placenta to the fetal side, where they attack and destroy the Rh positive fetal cells. As the maternal production of antibody increases, fetal cells are attacked and hemolyzed extravascularly as well as intravascularly, as soon as they become sufficiently antigenic to be recognized by the circulating antibody. During the second half of a sensitized pregnancy, the fetus has a progressive hemolytic anemia and intrauterine hyperbilirubinemia. In the most severely sensitized cases, the intrauterine anemia becomes so profound that high-output cardiac failure, anasarca, and hydrops fetalis develop. Most infants with profound anemia and hydrops fetalis are stillborn or survive only a short time after birth. The course of an Rh-sensitized pregnancy may be monitored by measurement of maternal anti-Rh antibody titer; by serial ultrasound examinations to detect hepatomegaly, splenomegaly, or peripheral edema; and by transabdominal sampling of amniotic fluid for the presence of bilirubin pigments. An increase in the concentration of amniotic fluid bilirubin pigments, especially in combination with ultrasonographic evidence of developing hepatosplenomegaly or edema, indicates a worsening prognosis and a need for fetal rescue by transabdominal fetal red cell transfusion monitored by ultrasound or an emergency delivery if the fetus is near term.

Before effective prevention of Rh sensitization was possible, many of the most severe cases of hyperbilirubinemia and probably a majority of the neonatal cases of kernicterus were found among infants with Rh hemolytic disease. With proper maternal screening, all remaining cases of Rh sensitization should be detected prenatally and the pediatrician forewarned.

At birth, maternally crossmatched, packed, O negative red blood cells should be available. A specimen of cord blood should be sent to the laboratory for immediate determination of serum total and direct bilirubin levels, hemoglobin, hematocrit, red blood cell indices, and red blood cell morphology. The characteristic morphologic abnormality of the red cells in the newborn with Rh hemolytic disease is the presence of large numbers of nucleated red cells (erythroblasts), hence, the name *erythroblastosis fetalis*. The presence of these nucleated red cells represents the hyperactivity of the marrow and of foci of extramedullary hematopoiesis in an attempt to match the rate of destruction of maturing antigenic fetal red cells by the circulating antibody.

The immediate postnatal management of these infants may require replacement of red cell mass, diuresis, aggressive treatment of cardiac failure, and ventilatory support. Less severely affected infants are viable and even well at birth, but have a progressive course of postnatal anemia and hyperbilirubinemia. Without treatment, the hemoglobin concentration may fall by more than 1 g/dL/d to the level of a profound anemia, and serum bilirubin may progress from cord levels of 5 to 10 mg/dL to extremely high UCB levels at a rate of increase greater than 1 mg/dL/h.

Management of the newborn with Rh hemolytic disease may serve as a model for aggressive intervention in severe cases of neonatal hyperbilirubinemia. Immediate correction of the circulating hemoglobin level by the transfusion of packed red cells is indicated if the hemoglobin concentration at birth is 10 mg/

dL or less. The volume transfused, usually 25 to 50 mL/kg of packed red cells, is calculated to correct the newborn's hemoglobin level to the range of 11 to 13 g/dL. In addition, if the cord indirect bilirubin concentration exceeds 5 mg/dL, or if the immediate postnatal rate of increase is 1 mg/dL/h or faster, a double volume exchange transfusion with whole blood should be performed as quickly as possible. This procedure, outlined in Table 20-42, stabilizes the red cell mass by replacing most of the circulating red cells with Rh negative cells that are compatible with the major blood groups and cannot be hemolyzed by the circulating antibody. Replacement of the plasma decreases the circulating antibody level somewhat, although much of the antibody accumulated over the weeks before birth is outside the vascular system and is not immediately accessible. The exchange of plasma also replaces jaundiced with non-jaundiced plasma and allows re-equilibration of newly formed bilirubin into a non-jaundiced plasma compartment carrying fresh adult albumin that is not saturated yet with bilirubin.

After initial postnatal management, serial bilirubin determinations are performed as often as every 4 hours, but not less often than every 8 to 12 hours, depending on the rate of bilirubin increase after transfusion. The initial exchange transfusion reduces the serum bilirubin concentration to about 50% of its pre-exchange level. Extravascular bilirubin equilibrates rapidly with the plasma, causing a short-term 30% rebound increase in the plasma bilirubin level. For example, if the initial serum bilirubin concentration is 20 mg/dL and the exchange transfusion lowers it to 10 mg/dL, within an hour after the procedure, the serum bilirubin concentration will rebound to about 13 mg/dL. The rate of increase calculated after the initial exchange transfusion permits estimation of the bilirubin levels to be expected in the subsequent 12 to 24 hours. If the rate of increase persists at greater than 0.5 mg/dL/h over a 10- to 12-hour period and two or three successive bilirubin determinations, it is advisable to repeat the exchange transfusion before the serum bilirubin level reaches 20 mg/dL. A second exchange transfusion also may be needed if the postnatal anemia continues to progress and the hemoglobin again falls below 10 g/dL. After the first postnatal day, if the rate of increase in serum bilirubin is less than 0.5 mg/dL/h, and if the hemoglobin is stable, the infant should be observed closely and followed with serial bilirubin determinations, with a repeat exchange transfusion planned if the serum indirect bilirubin concentration reaches or exceeds 20 mg/dL. During the early, acute period of rapid hemolysis with progressive anemia and hyperbilirubinemia, auxiliary methods such as phototherapy and intravenous hydration have little measurable effect on the clinical course of anemia and jaundice in these cases.

Fortunately, the development of near-universal screening for Rh sensitization and the widespread use of anti-Rh immune globulin during the third trimester or in the period immediately after delivery have reduced the incidence of Rh hemolytic disease in the newborn until it now is comparatively rare. Continued screening and immunization will be necessary to maintain this therapeutic success, but there still may be occasional breakthrough cases related to undetected placental hemorrhage, missed spontaneous abortions, or other reproductive accidents.

## ABO Incompatibility

ABO hemolytic disease is more common than Rh hemolytic disease, but it is more benign. In nearly all cases, the mother's blood type is group O (the major blood type in 40% of the North American population) and the infant's blood type is group A or B. Prenatal detection of ABO incompatibility is not feasible and generally is not necessary. Instead of sensitization during pregnancy, preformed maternal anti-A or anti-B antibodies of the IgG class are transferred passively to the infant late in pregnancy or at parturition. Rapid early hemolysis of fetal red cells occurs, with splenic recognition and removal of antigen–antibody complexes. Because fetal red cells have only about 7500 to 8000 A or B antigen sites per cell (versus 15,000 to 20,000 in the adult), the fetal cells do not agglutinate, and they may not be destroyed completely. Splenic removal of the antibody may damage the cell membrane, which then repairs and reenters the circulation as a microspherocyte. Likewise, the decreased number of antigen–antibody sites on fetal cells may give a weakly positive or even a negative direct Coombs' reaction. The antibody may be identified correctly by incubation of the neonatal serum with incompatible adult red cells and performance of an *indirect* Coombs' test. Because not all ABO incompatible pregnancies result in neonatal hemolysis, a positive Coombs' test (direct or indirect) is necessary to confirm the diagnosis.

ABO incompatibility seldom presents with severe jaundice or severe anemia at birth, but the rate of increase in bilirubin on the first postnatal day may lead to preparations for an exchange transfusion in some cases. If the initial rate of increase exceeds 1 mg/dL/h, if the infant is significantly anemic (hemoglobin 10 g/dL or less), or if the serum bilirubin level reaches the range of 15 to 20 mg/dL within the first 24 hours, a double volume exchange transfusion is indicated after the indirect bilirubin level has exceeded 15 mg/dL and before it exceeds 20 mg/dL. After the first postnatal day, the rate of red cell degradation and the

---

### TABLE 20-42. Exchange Transfusion

**Criteria**

Cord indirect Br >5 mg/dL
Cord Hgb <10 g/dL
Postnatal increase in Br >1 mg/dL/h
Anemia (Hgb 10–12 g/dL) plus postnatal increase in Br >0.5 mg/dL/h
Postnatal increase in Br >20 mg/dL

**Technique**

Use citrate phosphate dextrose (CPD) blood, 160–170 mL/kg
Umbilical vein catheter (or continuous vein–artery technique)
Aliquots: withdraw/infuse 5 mL/kg/min
Operating time: 60–90 min
$Ca^{2+}$ replacement; monitor heart rate continuously
Hgb, Hcrit, and Br before and after exchange
No oral intake 1 h before and 5–6 h after procedure

**Results**

Decrease in plasma Br to 50% to 55% of pre-exchange value (30% rebound in 1 h)
Decrease in tissue Br: re-equilibration with plasma
Decrease in circulating antibody
Replacement of susceptible RBCs
Partial correction of blood volume and decreased RBC mass

**Complications**

Embolism
Unstable cardiac output and blood pressure
Ruptured spleen/liver
Hyperkalemia
Hypocalcemia
Hyperglycemia → hypoglycemia
Metabolic acidosis
Infection
Transfusion reaction

*Br,* bilirubin; *Hgb,* hemoglobin; *Hcrit,* hematocrit.

subsequent rate of increase in the serum bilirubin level begin to diminish as the antigen–antibody complexes are cleared and the rate of hemolysis slows. This often will be reflected in a rapid early increase in the serum bilirubin level to the range of 10 to 15 mg/dL or slightly higher, followed by a plateau level at 15 to 20 mg/dL on the second hospital day. In this case, blood may be crossmatched and preparations made for an exchange transfusion, but the transfusion need not be done unless the hemolytic anemia becomes more severe or the serum bilirubin concentration exceeds 20 mg/dL.

As a general policy, exchange transfusion should be considered for any newborn with an indirect serum bilirubin level in the range of 20 to 25 mg/dL from any cause. Sustained hyperbilirubinemia within this range is potentially hazardous, as evidenced by changes in brain stem conduction time, changes in feeding behavior and responsiveness as noted anecdotally by many observers, and occasional cases of overt kernicterus at these bilirubin levels. It also is significant that, after prolonged exposure to UCB at 25 mg/dL, the amount of extravascular bilirubin may represent 30% to 50% of the body's total bilirubin stores. After an initial double volume exchange transfusion at 25 mg/dL has been performed, the immediate decline in the serum bilirubin level to 12 to 13 mg/dL is followed rapidly by a rebound to the range of 16 to 17 mg/dL. If the source of hyperbilirubinemia remains untreated or if the failure of bilirubin excretion persists at these levels, within a few hours, the serum bilirubin level may rise again to its pre-exchange level, making a second exchange transfusion necessary. If the infant is treated with earlier exchange transfusions to maintain the post-exchange bilirubin concentration between 10 to 20 mg/dL, however, the risk of a second exchange transfusion becoming necessary is diminished somewhat, and the duration of exposure to extreme levels of hyperbilirubinemia is shortened.

## PHOTOTHERAPY

Just as bilirubin probably is the most common laboratory determination performed in the newborn nursery, phototherapy probably is the most common treatment performed. The systematic use of fluorescent light to lower serum bilirubin levels followed the observations of Cremer, Perryman, and Richards in 1958 that jaundice was less frequent in a well-lighted nursery in a new wing of their hospital than in a dimly lighted one in an older wing. The mechanism of phototherapy, once thought to be the degradation of bilirubin and excretion of its degradation products as smaller molecules, now is found to proceed through the light-induced formation of configurational and structural isomers of UCB. These isomeric forms of bilirubin are more water-soluble than the parent compound, bilirubin IX-$\alpha$; therefore, they are transported through the liver more rapidly than is the predominant form of UCB. The dose applied to the skin, ideally 5 to 10 $\mu$W/cm$^2$/nm in the spectral range of 400 to 500 nm, rapidly converts UCB to its isomers in a dose-dependent fashion at the level of the skin. Doses lower than 3 to 4 $\mu$W/cm$^2$/nm produce inefficient photoconversion, whereas the effectiveness of doses above 10 to 12 $\mu$W/cm$^2$/nm is limited by a plateau effect in the photoconversion response and by practical limits on achieving higher light doses in the nursery setting. The photoconversion to isomers is rapid, followed by slower distribution of the isomers from the skin into the circulation and subsequent excretion of the isomers by the liver.

Current studies of the photoconversion and excretion process point to the conclusion that the excretion step of photoisomers via the liver may be rate-limiting for the dose response in newborns. In addition, once isomerized bilirubin reaches the bowel, it may reconvert to the normal form of UCB, because it no longer

is exposed to light. Unless the photobilirubin that enters the small bowel is converted rapidly to other water-soluble products, or is excreted rapidly, some enterohepatic recirculation of photobilirubin via reconversion to bilirubin IX-$\alpha$ may occur. Therefore, even with rapid conversion of bilirubin to its photoproducts, a rapid decline in the serum bilirubin level may not always be seen. Rather, the bilirubin concentration in the plasma may be stabilized in equilibrium with its photoproducts, its rate of hepatic excretion, and its rate of recirculation from the bowel into the blood if, in the small bowel, it merely has entered a "third space" without being excreted. Perhaps, then, an apparent delay in serum bilirubin response to phototherapy is not surprising, given the balance that must be achieved between the rates of bilirubin production, excretion, and reabsorption in a complex system.

A potential advantage of phototherapy, however, even without a marked decline in the serum bilirubin level, is the conversion of 10% to 20% of the circulating bilirubin to water-soluble isomers, which, by definition, should be less likely to cross the blood–brain barrier than is the lipophilic parent compound, bilirubin IX-$\alpha$. Photoconversion of circulating bilirubin after the liberal early use of phototherapy in newborns at high risk may be part of the reason for a noted decline in low bilirubin kernicterus among such newborns, even though early phototherapy produces little or no change in eventual total serum bilirubin levels. Because the mechanism of phototherapy seems to proceed regardless of the underlying cause of jaundice, and because the photoconversion of bilirubin in the circulation may be somewhat protective, there is no strict contraindication to the follow-up use of phototherapy to control bilirubin levels in a newborn with hemolytic anemia, once the initial problems of hemolysis and rapid early onset of hyperbilirubinemia have been treated properly. Regardless of whether a newborn is receiving phototherapy, the criteria for an exchange transfusion should remain the same in these circumstances until the protective effect of bilirubin isomerization is proven clearly.

## OTHER THERAPEUTIC CONSIDERATIONS

Feeding promotes peristalsis and colonization of the bowel. Peristalsis increases the rate of bilirubin excretion as the stools change from meconium to transitional to the bilirubin-rich yellowish brown stools that are apparent at several days of life, whereas bowel colonization with normal flora promotes the enzymatic conversion of bilirubin to other bile products that cannot be reabsorbed or reconverted to UCB. Unfed or underfed newborns tend to have more persistent jaundice than do those who are fed adequately, so the underfed nursing infant may show improvement rather than worsening of jaundice with increased frequency of nursing and a rise in milk intake within the first few days. It is possible to reduce the enterohepatic circulation of bilirubin by feeding agar or charcoal to the newborn, but these approaches have not gained widespread popularity. On the other hand, phenobarbital in low doses stimulates the conjugating enzymes and the hepatic excretory system for bilirubin; thus, infants with a family history of significant neonatal hyperbilirubinemia or those with contraindications to exchange transfusion (eg, for religious reasons) may benefit from the maternal or early neonatal administration of phenobarbital in low doses—usually lower than would be required to achieve therapeutic levels for seizure control. This is an approach to hyperbilirubinemia that can be used selectively, but has not found widespread acceptance in North America.

Future therapy for unconjugated hyperbilirubinemia, both that seen in the neonate and that occurring in the older patient with Crigler-Najjar syndrome, may focus on the inhibition of bilirubin formation from its hemoglobin precursor. The synthetic heme analogue tin-protoporphyrin has been shown to inhibit competitively heme oxygenase, the rate-limiting enzyme in the degradation of hemoglobin to bilirubin. Experiments using animal models and some preliminary clinical studies have shown that administration of this agent results in decreased biliary excretion of bilirubin, with concomitant increases in the excretion of heme pigment into bile. In addition, when it is given to neonatal animals or human newborns shortly after delivery, hyperbilirubinemia is prevented. Thus, with further development and documentation of its safety and efficacy, this approach may offer a specific therapy for unconjugated hyperbilirubinemia.

## Management of Breast-Milk Jaundice

Most breast-fed infants have normal postnatal serum bilirubin levels that do not require any specific diagnostic or treatment measures. Early hyperbilirubinemia in breast-fed newborns may be associated with suboptimal feeding schedules and milk intake, resulting in excessive weight loss, infrequent stools, and inadequate excretion of bilirubin. No fixed interval between birth and the first breast-feeding should be necessary if the mother and baby are in good condition immediately after delivery. During the first several days postpartum, nursing on demand or at intervals more frequent than every 4 hours may help to stimulate lactation, avert excessive weight loss, and aid the transition from meconium to normal stools. Routine supplementation of breast-feeding with bottled water may be counterproductive, diminishing the thirst response between nursing periods while providing inadequate substrate for hepatic function and inadequate bulk for peristalsis. Water supplementation should be reserved for those few infants in whom milk intake and hydration are clearly inadequate and weight loss is obviously excessive.

Preterm infants of 35 to 37 weeks' gestation and weighing 2500 to 3000 g may appear healthy at birth, but may not nurse as well as term infants and still may have immature liver function. This group includes some infants delivered by elective cesarean section before term, with the smooth initiation of nursing complicated further by the mother's postoperative condition. Hepatic immaturity and inadequate intake may increase the likelihood of hyperbilirubinemia in such infants. Formula or water supplementation may be needed for adequate hydration and nutrition until lactation is well established, and phototherapy for hyperbilirubinemia in the range of 15 to 20 mg/dL may be used during the first several days, until hepatic function matures and adequate excretion of bilirubin begins.

The discontinuation of breast-feeding in a well baby with persistent hyperbilirubinemia is largely a matter of clinical judgment. Many cases of breast-milk jaundice are mild enough to require no intervention except for bilirubin determinations once or twice in the first several weeks after discharge, to follow the resolution of the problem. More severe cases, which often appear toward the end of the first week and then fail to resolve or progress to still higher levels of hyperbilirubinemia, may benefit from the therapeutic test of discontinuing breast-feeding for 36 to 48 hours. Discontinuation of nursing in the first few days, however, may not lower the bilirubin level or establish the probability of a breast milk inhibitor; the hormonal or enzymatic factors associated with persistent jaundice may not become operative until nursing is well established.

Hyperbilirubinemia caused by breast milk factors usually responds to the temporary cessation of nursing with a prompt decline of 2 to 4 mg/dL in the serum bilirubin level, after which nursing usually can be resumed with little or no further increase in bilirubin. In most cases, it appears that even temporary removal of the inhibiting factor allows an improvement in hepatic function and in the intestinal excretion of bilirubin. Only in rare cases is hyperbilirubinemia severe and persistent enough to require the complete discontinuation of breast-feeding. Phototherapy is indicated for a small minority only of breast-fed infants with hyperbilirubinemia that persists above 15 mg/dL and is unresponsive to the temporary discontinuation of breast-feeding.

Some authorities suggest that term breast-fed infants without other risk factors require no treatment until the serum indirect bilirubin exceeds 20 mg/dL, and that exchange transfusion is not indicated in these low-risk infants until the serum bilirubin level reaches or exceeds 25 mg/dL. Medical supervision and even daily follow-up of infants with "borderline," but still increasing, bilirubin levels is important. Undetected, unsupervised hyperbilirubinemia in breast-fed infants thought to be at no risk occasionally may progress to levels of 25 to 30 mg/dL or greater. Besides the uncertain risk of later neurologic damage from prolonged extremely high bilirubin levels, some unsupervised infants with extreme hyperbilirubinemia later are found to have risk factors that were not recognized at birth, and some of these are at risk for the development of clinically evident bilirubin encephalopathy.

## DIRECT (CONJUGATED) HYPERBILIRUBINEMIA

Obstructive hyperbilirubinemia resulting from intrinsic liver disease or a congenital hepatobiliary obstruction first may appear in the newborn. Early in the course, this condition may present with a predominantly indirect or unconjugated hyperbilirubinemia, but, in most cases, the direct or conjugated fraction of bilirubin quickly rises to levels in excess of 2 mg/dL and then remains elevated. Conjugated bilirubin appears not to be toxic to the central nervous system, but the persistence of conjugated hyperbilirubinemia indicates an urgent need for specific diagnostic evaluation of the infant to determine the nature of the hepatic abnormality. Underlying causes may include bacterial or viral infection, nonspecific neonatal hepatitis, persistence of direct hyperbilirubinemia with inspissation of bile after an episode of severe hemolysis (as sometimes is seen in Rh disease), or congenital intrahepatic or extrahepatic biliary obstruction. In general, mixed or obstructive hyperbilirubinemia represents a category of diseases that may present in the newborn period, but that persist well beyond neonatal life and have significantly different implications

---

**TABLE 20-43.   Anticipatory Management of Neonatal Jaundice**

1. Know maternal blood type
2. Know baby's blood type if mother is Rh-negative or Group O
3. Identify jaundice (especially if early onset)
4. Identify risk factors present by
     Serum bilirubin
               and/or
     Coomb's Test, Hgb, Hcrit, RBC indices
     and morphology
5. Observe, repeat, and discharge if jaundice is nonprogressive and no risk factor is present; or,
6. Start therapy as described below, if indicated by
   a. Approaching threshold
               or
   b. Risk factors present
7. Start phototherapy when unconjugated bilirubin is below expected exchange transfusion level
8. Exchange Transfusion
   a. Early, if conditions are met
   b. Later, if phototherapy fails to control serum BR

for the child's health and future development than do the usual causes of neonatal unconjugated hyperbilirubinemia. Therefore, specific details of the diagnosis and management of conjugated or mixed hyperbilirubinemia are beyond the scope of this chapter. Such infants, when they are detected in the newborn period, should be referred for diagnosis and treatment to a tertiary pediatric center where members of the pediatric staff have specific expertise in pediatric gastroenterology or liver disease.

## CONCLUSION

In summary, most cases of neonatal hyperbilirubinemia are developmental, benign, and self-limited. Significant hyperbilirubinemia may occur in a few normal infants, in a somewhat larger number of breast-fed infants, and in many infants with hemolytic anemia of prenatal or neonatal origin. The typical case of physiologic jaundice may be managed with serial bilirubin determinations, close observation, and reassurance. For more severe or more complicated cases, after initial neonatal stabilization and specific diagnosis, exchange transfusion is the treatment of choice for indirect hyperbilirubinemia with levels in excess of 20 mg/dL or levels that are rising rapidly in association with hemolysis. Phototherapy can be used to stabilize indirect hyperbilirubinemia resulting from any cause, and potentially may offer the brain additional protection by isomerization of UCB. Long-term follow-up of persistent hyperbilirubinemia is necessary for a minority of infants who have jaundice associated with breast-feeding. Table 20-43 outlines a suggested approach to the anticipatory management of neonatal jaundice.

## Selected Readings

Ahdab-Barmada M, Moosy J. The neuropathology of kernicterus in the premature neonate: Diagnostic problems. J Neuropathol Exp Neurol 1984;43:45.

Arias IM, Gartner LM, Seifter S, Furman M. Prolonged neonatal unconjugated hyperbilirubinemia associated with breast feeding and a steroid pregnane-3($\alpha$), 20 ($\beta$) - diol, in maternal milk which inhibits glucuronide formation in vitro. J Clin Invest 1964;43:2037.

Cremer RJ, Perryman PW, Richards DH. Influence of light on the hyperbilirubinemia of infants. Lancet 1958;1:1094.

Hegyi T, Hiatt IM, Indyk L. Transcutaneous bilirubinometry. I. Correlations in term infants. J Pediatr 1981;98:454.

Maisels MJ. Neonatal jaundice. In: Avery GB, ed. Neonatology: Pathophysiology and management of the newborn, ed 2. Philadelphia: JB Lippincott, 1981:473.

Maisels MJ, Gifford K. Normal serum bilirubin levels in the newborn and the effect of breast-feeding. Pediatrics 1986;78:837.

McDonagh AF, Lightner DA. "Like a shrivelled blood orange"—bilirubin, jaundice, and phototherapy. Pediatrics 1985;75:443.

Nakamura H, Takada S, Shimabuku R, et al. Auditory nerve and brainstem responses in newborn infants with hyperbilirubinemia. Pediatrics 1985;75:703.

Newman TB, Maisels MJ. Evaluation and treatment of jaundice in the term newborn. Pediatrics 1992;89:809.

Ritter DA, Kenny JD, Norton HJ, et al. A prospective study of free bilirubin and other risk factors in the development of kernicterus in premature infants. Pediatrics 1982;69:260.

Zipursky A. Isoimmune hemolytic diseases. In: Nathan DG, Oski FA, eds. Hematology of infancy and childhood, ed 2. Philadelphia: WB Saunders, 1981:50.

*Principles and Practice of Pediatrics, Second Edition.*
edited by Frank A. Oski et al. J. B. Lippincott Company, Philadelphia © 1994.

# 20.6 *Renal and Genitourinary Diseases*

Billy S. Arant, Jr.

## CONSIDERATIONS OF NORMAL DEVELOPMENT

### Embryogenesis and Morphology

Formation of the human metanephric kidney begins during the fifth week of gestation when the ureteric bud, an ectodermal outgrowth of the wolffian or mesonephric duct that will develop into the renal collecting system, makes direct contact with the caudal mesenchyma of the nephrogenic cord to induce the formation of glomeruli, proximal and distal tubules, and loops of Henle. Failure of these two distinctly different embryonic tissues to establish intimate contact will result in failure of the ipsilateral kidney to form normally. All glomeruli are located within the renal cortex, but the first ones formed will have their final position in the deep or juxtamedullary region, will contribute most to the function of the developing kidney until nephrogenesis is completed around 34 weeks' gestation, will be nearly equal in size to mature glomeruli at 40 weeks' gestation, and will have long loops of Henle and vasa rectae extending into the inner medulla and papilla—structures of the renal countercurrent multiplier mechanism. The last of the glomeruli formed will occupy the most superficial position of the subcapsular region of the cortex, will not exhibit filtration before 34 weeks' gestation, will be only about 25% of the size of juxtamedullary glomeruli at 40 weeks' gestation, will have short loops of Henle without vasa rectae that extend only into the outer medulla, and will contribute little or nothing to the urinary concentrating mechanism. Nephrogenesis follows a similar pattern after birth when the fetus is born prematurely—the infant born at 26 weeks' gestation exhibits continued nephrogenesis for about 8 weeks after birth. Differences in morphologic arrangement in the developing human renal cortex before and after the completion of nephrogenesis are illustrated in Figure 20-63.

Filtration by newly formed nephrons has been observed as early as 9 weeks after conception; however, the ureter is patent only from the 11th week. The transient hydronephrosis during this 2-week interval distends the proximal ureter to give the pelvicaliceal system its characteristic shape. Once the ureter is canalized, urine drains into the urogenital sinus that communicates with the amniotic sac. The urinary bladder is formed from the lower portion of the allantois and the urogenital sinus. The upper portion of the allantois closes by 32 weeks' gestation to form a fibrous cord unless the bladder outlet is obstructed, in which case the urachus may persist. The fetal ureter is composed mainly of connective tissue stroma lined by epithelium. The circumferential and longitudinal smooth muscle layers that allow the ureter to constrict and shorten during peristalsis, and the elastic fibers that permit the stretched, distended, or constricted ureter to resume its normal caliber and shape are formed between 36 and 48 weeks after conception—2 months postnatally in infants born at term.

The only role of the kidney that is essential to normal fetal

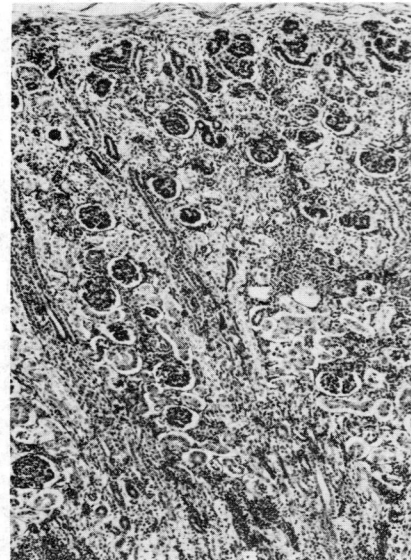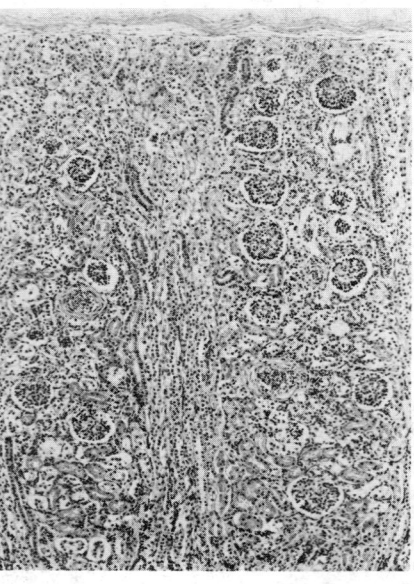

Figure 20-63. A comparison of morphology in the developing human renal cortex before and after nephrogenesis is completed. The larger glomeruli in the inner cortex are of similar size at 30 weeks (*left*) and at 40 weeks (*right*). In the superficial cortex, new glomeruli still are being formed at 30 weeks and have very little interposition of tubular structures, whereas at 40 weeks, glomerular size is more homogeneous throughout the cortex and tubular growth has separated the glomeruli and displaced the most superficial ones away from the capsule. Hematoxylin and eosin stain, ×100. (Photomicrographs courtesy of Dr. J. Bernstein, William Beaumont Hospital, Royal Oak, MI.)

development is its production of urine to increase the volume of amniotic fluid. Maintenance of a positive mineral and fluid balance and the excretory functions of the kidney required after birth are handled for the fetus by the placenta and maternal kidney. Failure of the fetal kidney to form urine or obstruction of the fetal urinary tract that prevents urine from reaching the amniotic space results in oligohydramnios and may cause fetal compression. In some fetuses with urinary tract abnormalities, oligohydramnios can be associated with pulmonary hypoplasia, although urinary volume is not considered to contribute significantly to the volume of amniotic fluid as early in gestation as pulmonary hypoplasia has been observed.

## Glomerular Filtration Rate

The glomerular filtration rate (GFR) has been measured at birth in healthy human neonates as early as 24 weeks' gestation and found to be about 0.2 mL/min, 0.5 mL/min/kg, or 5 mL/min/1.73 m$^2$. Such a low GFR in a child or adult would represent chronic renal insufficiency; therefore, it is not surprising that the neonatal kidney came to be mislabeled as functionally immature. Although growth and development of the fetus and its kidneys continue throughout gestation, the GFR changes little, if at all, before a conceptional (gestational plus postnatal) age of 34 weeks, the same stage of development at which nephrogenesis is completed. It is clinically relevant to understand that the neonate born at 26 weeks' gestation will not exhibit any appreciable change in GFR until nearly 8 weeks of age—34 weeks after conception. These changes have been demonstrated so consistently in recent developmental studies of human neonates that, when changes in the GFR are observed much before or after a conceptional age of 34 weeks, consideration should be given to the possibility that there has been an error either in estimating gestational age at birth or in measuring the GFR. In contrast, when birth occurs after 34 weeks' gestation, the GFR increases twofold to threefold during the first week of life, just as it does in full-term infants.

The developmental pattern of change in the GFR obtains whether infants are studied at birth and compared with gestational age or are studied during postnatal life and compared with conceptional age (Fig 20-64). A similar pattern of change in the GFR has been observed in all mammalian kidneys studied developmentally. The GFR remains relatively constant until nephrogenesis has been completed, which occurs antenatally in the

human and sheep born at term, and postnatally in the rat and dog. The biologic signal regulating the timing of these developmental changes is understood poorly, but, because the changes can occur abruptly, attributing them simply to a process of maturation seems inadequate. It is more likely that a vasoactive mechanism is responsible for the changes, because increments in renal blood flow are related inversely to changes in renal vascular resistance, in plasma renin activity, in circulating levels of angiotensin II, and in renal synthesis of vasodilator prostaglandins.

Further developmental increases in the GFR vary directly with postnatal age until the average normal adult GFR of 125 mL/min is attained during adolescence, when the kidney reaches its adult size at the approximate time that linear growth ceases and epiphyses close. When the GFR corrected for body surface area

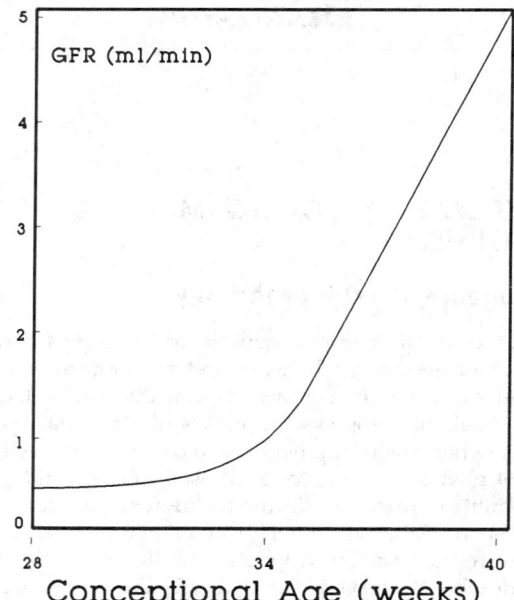

Figure 20-64. The pattern of change in glomerular filtration rate (*GFR*) compared with the conceptional (gestational + postnatal) age of healthy human neonates. The line represents the nonlinear relationship calculated from data obtained in healthy neonates during the first 8 weeks of life.

(mL/min/1.73 m²) is compared to chronologic age, the adult or mature value of 125 mL/min/1.73 m² is observed rarely before 6 months of age and sometimes at 12 months of age in infants born at term. During this period of early postnatal development, the rate of increase in the GFR exceeds the rate of body growth.

Measuring GFR in neonates is tedious and difficult when accurately timed and complete collections of urine are required; small errors in either can produce large errors in calculating the GFR. The expected developmental changes in GFR can be monitored satisfactorily in most neonates from serial measurements of serum creatinine concentration ($S_{Cr}$). Creatinine is a product of normal muscle metabolism and is a small molecule that crosses all membranes that are permeable to water, including the placenta; therefore, $S_{Cr}$ levels in the mother and her fetus are identical. There is no correlation at birth between $S_{Cr}$ and the gestational age of the infant. Hence, a single measurement of $S_{Cr}$ at birth or at any time during the neonatal period has no particular value for estimating GFR. When GFR increases rapidly after birth in infants born after 34 weeks' gestation, the excess creatinine of maternal origin in the neonate will be reduced by about 50% at the end of the first week of life, and usually will reach a stable normal value of 0.25 to 0.40 mg/dL during the second week. On the other hand, the GFR does not increase appreciably during the first week of life in infants born before 34 weeks' gestation, and $S_{Cr}$ actually may increase slightly during the first 48 hours after birth partially as a result of hemoconcentration and ongoing creatinine production of about 8 mg/kg/d, which is about equal to urinary creatinine excretion. Therefore, there is little net loss of creatinine from the body, and only minimal changes in $S_{Cr}$ can be expected during the first week of life in normal preterm infants. When a conceptional age of 34 weeks is reached, however, the GFR will increase rapidly, and $S_{Cr}$ will be reduced by about half within a few days, just as is observed in more mature neonates during the first week of life.

It also is possible to estimate the GFR corrected for body surface area from the formulas derived for premature infants (Brion and colleagues, 1986) or for full-term infants (Schwartz and colleagues, 1984). The formula for both is GFR (mL/min/1.73 m²) = k × body length (cm)/$S_{Cr}$(mg/dL); for preterm infants, k = 0.35, and for full-term infants after the first week of life, k = 0.45. Because GFR corrected for body surface area before 6 months of age is not comparable to the familiar normal adult value of 125 mL/min/1.73 m², the normal value for GFR must be recalled or referred to for neonates at every conceptional age. It is more convenient for clinical purposes, perhaps, to estimate changes in GFR from serial measurements of $S_{Cr}$. For neonates at high risk, it is advisable to measure $S_{Cr}$ on the first day of life for comparison, should the need arise, with subsequent measurements.

## Urinary Volume

Every normal neonate, as well as most with congenital renal abnormalities, will void some urine within 48 hours of birth. Urinary flow rate is, at best, only an indirect measurement of overall renal function. Because an exact measurement of GFR in neonates is impractical, however, clinicians have adopted urinary volume factored for time and body weight (mL/h/kg) as a convenient, although uninformed, indication of "renal function." The volume of urine formed in any given period depends not only on GFR, but also on tubular reabsorption of plasma ultrafiltrate that collects in Bowman's space. The final urinary volume may be minimal during hydropenic conditions when the kidney attempts to conserve or restore extracellular fluid volume (ECFV), or great when ECFV is excessive, when tubular dysfunction causes a greater fraction of glomerular filtrate to be rejected along the nephron, when arginine vasopressin (AVP) is not released from the hy-

pothalamus (central diabetes insipidus), or when the collecting duct epithelium is unresponsive even to high concentrations of circulating AVP (nephrogenic diabetes insipidus).

For example, GFR in the fetus is relatively low (<1 mL/h/kg), but urinary volume is high (10 mL/h/kg). Tubular reabsorption in the fetal kidney is inefficient; it is not necessary for it to be otherwise. The positive fluid balance or relative excess of ECFV that is normal for the fetus is assured by placental transfer from the expanded ECFV of the mother. Diuresis in utero is maintained, in part, by altered peritubular forces that reduce proximal tubular reabsorption, by the presence of minimal AVP in the circulation before parturition, and by increased renal synthesis of prostacyclin and prostaglandin $E_2$ (PGE₂) compared to that in the normal child or adult. The diuresis is interrupted briefly during labor with the normal release of AVP, but is resumed after birth as AVP levels decrease again. The duration of diuresis postnatally in a normal neonate is determined by the degree of ECFV excess, by hormonal interactions, and by hemodynamic changes. Because the ECFV in the preterm infant is greater relative to that in the full-term infant, the postnatal diuresis and relative weight loss after birth will be greater in the preterm infant. The normal pattern of changes in urine production begins with a rate of 10 mL/h/kg in the fetus, at least from 30 weeks' gestation; decreases to less than 0.5 mL/h/kg during parturition; and increases again spontaneously to 1 to 8 mL/h/kg, depending on the gestational age of the neonate, until the excess extracellular fluid for that infant is excreted. Thereafter, urinary volume in the neonate given appropriate fluid intake remains constant at between 0.3 and 2.0 mL/h/kg, with urinary osmolarity (specific gravity) at between 50 and 800 mOsm/L (1.001 to 1.024).

High-risk neonates of every gestational age usually are treated prospectively with parenteral fluid therapy. Clinical decisions for changing the volume of parenteral fluids given or for prescribing diuretic therapy are based usually on urinary volume and less often on change in body weight. Because hemodynamic and hormonal changes in the perinatal period may not be similar in every neonate, urine production will vary with factors other than GFR. For example, before 34 weeks' gestation, the premature neonate excretes about 10% of the volume of glomerular filtrate as urine. Although GFR increases after 34 weeks' gestation, tubular reabsorption increases as well, so that by 38 weeks, less than 3% of glomerular filtrate escapes the nephron. In general, the higher the urinary flow rate (mL/h/kg), the lower the fraction of glomerular filtrate reabsorbed—not only water, but also sodium chloride (NaCl), bicarbonate, amino acids, phosphate, calcium, and glucose. The fractional excretion of glomerular filtrate can be calculated as urinary flow rate (V) divided by GFR (V/GFR) when both are expressed in the same units. In other words, when urinary flow rate in a very preterm infant weighing 1.0 kg is 3 mL/h/kg, about 10% of glomerular filtrate is not reabsorbed along the nephron (V/GFR = 0.05 mL/min/0.5 mL/min = 0.10, or 10%). If this same infant were to excrete only 1% of glomerular filtrate in the urine, as does the normal adult, the urinary volume would be only 0.3 mL/h/kg. The physiologic basis for or clinical relevance of maintaining urinary volume at 1 mL/h/kg or greater in every infant has not been documented; however, there rarely is any delay in intervening with additional fluid therapy or diuretic agents in a neonate whose urinary volume falls below 1 mL/h/kg. The importance of maintaining urinary volume primarily is to assure that sufficient water is present in tubular fluid to permit excretion of the solute load imposed on the kidney. If there is no solute load in infants who are conserving NaCl and are given only dextrose in water to replace insensible water losses immediately after birth, no minimal volume of urine is required. When feedings were withheld routinely in the past from preterm infants to prevent aspiration, some infants made no urine for up to 5 days without evidence of renal injury. Moreover, acute renal injury was not obvious in neonates trapped during earthquakes, and they survived longer without fluid than did older victims.

It is important to identify other factors that may have caused the decrease in urinary volume, such as previously unrecognized heart failure, shunting of a greater fraction of cardiac output away from the renal circulation through a patent ductus arteriosus, changes in intrathoracic pressure from pneumothorax, or mechanical ventilation, which reduces cardiac output and stimulates baroreceptor-mediated release of AVP. In each case, the neonate's condition would be worsened by additional fluid therapy or furosemide administration.

## Renal Handling of Sodium Chloride

Although characterized previously as inadequate to maintain NaCl balance, it is known now that the developing kidney is limited only when extraordinary demands are imposed on it. Some very preterm infants, appropriate for gestational age, have survived (and more will survive in the future) with little or no clinical intervention, and they exhibit neither NaCl wasting nor any other tubular dysfunction. Renal tubular function in newborn infants is qualitatively similar to that in adults. When the function of the adult mammalian kidney is assessed during chronic saline expansion, hypotonic saline diuresis, increased glucosuria, hyperphosphaturia, hypercalciuria, hyperuricosuria, and increased bicarbonaturia are noted, just as in kidney function in the normal human fetus and preterm infant when ECFV is expanded. What is interpreted often as an inappropriate or immature response by the neonatal kidney can be attributed usually to the response by the normal mammalian kidney to changes in effective arterial blood volume (EABV), the blood volume/pressure force sensed by baroreceptors in the arterial circulation. When EABV falls because of decreased cardiac output or peripheral resistance, the normal neonatal kidney responds by conserving volume and exhibits functional oligoanuria, NaCl retention, and hypertonic urine. Because this response can follow a change in blood pressure, blood volume, or both, it may be observed when total body water is increased or decreased and when blood pressure is high, normal, or low. A schematic representation of the physiologic mechanisms that maintain or restore EABV is depicted in Figure 20-65.

During fetal development, body composition changes dramatically between conception and maturity. The content of body water decreases from 96% of body weight at 8 weeks' gestation to less than 80% at 40 weeks' gestation, as the NaCl content

decreases from 120 mEq/kg of body weight to 80 mEq/kg of body weight. This parallel reduction in total body water and NaCl accounts for the decrease noted in ECFV from 60% to 40% of fetal body weight during the last trimester of pregnancy. After birth, the ECFV is reduced further from 40% to less than 30% of body weight. This developmental decrease in relative ECFV occurs as body tissues expand and increase the demand for extracellular fluid, and as the constant hypotonic saline diuresis maintains amniotic fluid volume. When infants are born prematurely, a variable period of high urinary volume and negative NaCl balance occurs postnatally, in an apparent effort by the neonate to reduce its ECFV as would have occurred had the fetus remained in utero until term. Before the kidney of the preterm neonate can respond by conserving NaCl and water similar to the full-term infant, however, the relative differences in ECFV between the preterm infant and the full-term infant must be resolved.

Because neonates, regardless of their gestational age at birth, will vary somewhat in the exact timing of renal responses to reduced ECFV, each infant must be observed closely to determine when this important point in postnatal adaptation has been attained. The best clinical estimate of the timing for this event is made by observing changes in urinary volume and in the urinary excretion of NaCl. The fractional excretion of sodium ($FE_{Na}$) can be calculated from the sodium and creatinine concentrations in random samples of plasma and urine. These values are substituted in the formula $FE_{Na}$ (%) = urine sodium concentration × plasma creatinine concentration × 100/urine creatinine concentration × plasma sodium concentration. The relatively large volume of urine produced by the fetal kidney before birth and by the preterm neonate immediately after birth contains higher NaCl concentrations (>50 mEq/L) than does that of the full-term infant (<20 mEq/L); $FE_{Na}$ is 12% to 15% in the fetus, greater than 1% to 7% in the preterm infant, and less than 1% (usually <0.5%) in the full-term infant.

The continued hypotonic saline diuresis after birth results in a greater fractional loss of birth weight in preterm infants (10% to 30%) than in full-term infants (3% to 8%). When the excess ECFV has been excreted, further loss of body weight becomes more gradual and even may stabilize when insensible water losses are not unusual. This adaptational milestone is followed by a second period of normal oligoanuria after birth, when urinary volume becomes less than 1 mL/h/kg, urinary osmolarity increases to greater than 300 mOsm/L, and the tubules conserve NaCl ($FE_{Na}$ <1%). This observation may be made on the first day

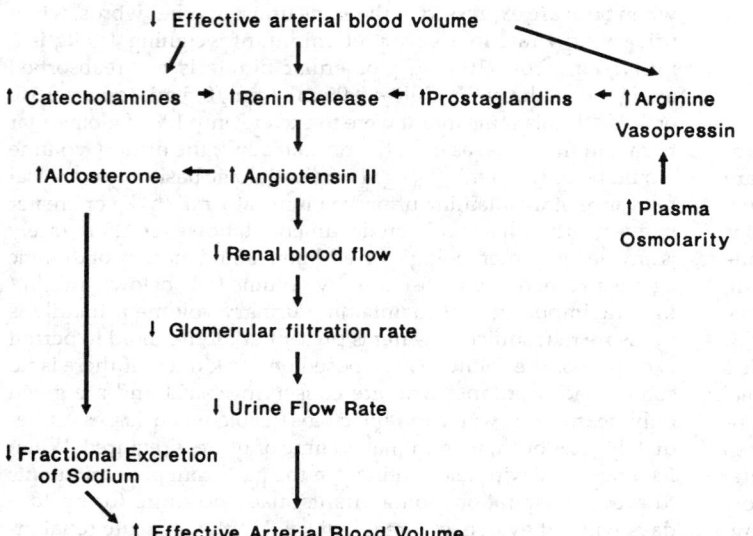

Figure 20-65. Schematic representation of the physiologic response to a decrease in effective arterial blood volume.

of life in infants born at term or may be delayed for 3 to 7 days after birth in those born prematurely. If only unusual insensible water losses, not urinary volume, are replaced with dextrose in water before this pivotal point in transitional physiology, subsequent oral or parenteral fluid therapy can be prescribed to replace urinary volume as well as insensible water losses. Then, body weight will be maintained and weight gain will be related to caloric intake and growth. Although urinary volume will increase and urinary osmolarity will decrease on such a regimen of "maintenance" fluid therapy, there should be no increase in urinary NaCl excretion. If, however, fluid therapy replaces both insensible water losses and urinary volume from birth (100 mL/ kg/d or greater), the relative excess ECFV of the fetus will be perpetuated postnatally in the neonate, and the hypotonic saline diuresis can continue almost indefinitely. When urinary volume, but not urinary NaCl, is replaced by 5% to 10% dextrose in water, hyponatremia will develop in the preterm neonate and clinical evaluation will suggest renal NaCl wasting, the so-called "immaturity" of neonatal renal tubular function.

The renal handling of NaCl in the neonate can be explained another way. The normal adult produces 180 L of glomerular filtrate daily, but excretes less than 1% of that volume as urine. The preterm infant, by comparison, produces about 750 mL of glomerular filtrate daily. For a 1000-g infant to excrete a urinary volume of 1 mL/h/kg (24 mL/24 h) or greater, 3.3% or more of the glomerular filtrate must be rejected along the nephron. If the urinary volume in the same infant actually were 5 mL/h/kg, which is not unusual in preterm infants given routine parenteral fluid therapy from birth, 16% of the glomerular filtrate would have been rejected by the tubule. And, if the sodium concentration of that urine were 75 mEq/L, which is usual in the fetus and in very premature neonates at birth, 9 mEq/kg/d of sodium would be lost in the urine. If the sodium added to the parenteral fluids provides only the maintenance requirements for older infants (2 to 3 mEq/kg/d), it is understandable that many preterm infants have a negative NaCl balance and hyponatremia. The provision of NaCl in excess of 2 mEq/kg to preterm infants when urine volume is high (V/GFR >3%) is associated with an increase in $FE_{Na}$ and a continued negative NaCl balance. On the other hand, when urinary volume is 1 mL/kg/h or less during periods of oligoanuria, urinary sodium concentration rarely is greater than 20 mEq/L; under these circumstances, in an infant of the same weight and maturity, less than 0.5 mEq/kg/d of sodium would be lost in urine. Moreover, the infant would exhibit the positive NaCl balance that is essential for growth when provided with only the maintenance requirements. Long-term management of negative NaCl balance, therefore, is not providing additional NaCl for the neonate, but rather restricting fluid volume from birth to replace insensible water losses only until the normally expected second period of oligoanuria and reduced $FE_{Na}$ is observed in the urine of the newborn infant.

## Renal Acid–Base Homeostasis

The neonatal kidney once was characterized as being unable to maintain acid–base balance because of its decreased ability to conserve bicarbonate, secrete hydrogen ion, or both. More recently, the kidneys of even premature infants have been demonstrated to excrete an acid load as well as does the adult kidney (about 80 mEq/1.73 $m^2$/d), which is more than adequate to dispose of a normal infant's daily hydrogen ion production. The relative metabolic acidosis commonly observed in preterm infants can be explained, in part, by the lowered renal threshold for bicarbonate, that is, the plasma level above which bicarbonate is wasted along the nephron and appears in the urine. Because the majority of filtered bicarbonate is reabsorbed in the proximal tubule, its renal conservation or wasting can be influenced by

extrarenal factors, especially changes in ECFV or EABV and regardless of the acid–base status of the infant. When the EABV is perceived by renal baroreceptors to be diminished, the fractional reabsorption of glomerular filtrate along the proximal nephron, including bicarbonate, increases, and the renal threshold for bicarbonate increases; consequently, plasma bicarbonate and arterial blood pH levels increase. Relative metabolic alkalosis will develop, but the urine will contain no bicarbonate and will have a pH level of less than 6.0, which constitutes renal tubular alkalosis. On the other hand, as EABV is restored or, in the euvolemic neonate, is expanded, tubular reabsorption of bicarbonate will decrease the renal threshold for bicarbonate, the plasma bicarbonate concentration will decrease both by dilution and by urinary excretion of bicarbonate, and the arterial blood pH level will return toward normal. If the process continues, relative metabolic acidosis will develop in the face of urinary bicarbonate excretion and a pH level greater than 6.0, which constitutes renal tubular acidosis. Because relative metabolic acidosis or alkalosis can be produced experimentally in normal animals by altering EABV, the relative metabolic acidosis of prematurity probably reflects the ECFV excess of the preterm infant compared to that of the full-term infant. The alkaline urinary pH of normal preterm infants during the first week of life becomes more acidic during the second week as the ECFV is reduced and tubular bicarbonate reabsorption is increased.

## Urinary Diluting and Concentrating Mechanisms

The ability of the neonatal kidney to dilute urine maximally to less than 50 mOsm/L in the absence of AVP is identical to that of the adult kidney. On the other hand, the inability of the neonatal kidney to concentrate the urine when the infant is deprived of fluid or loses fluid abnormally can be explained, not simply as immaturity of kidney function, but rather according to the gestational age and clinical management of the infant after birth. For instance, the fetal kidney has no need to form a concentrated urine because its only essential role is to replenish amniotic fluid volume. The fetal collecting tubule is relatively unresponsive even to very high circulating levels of AVP during normal labor or asphyxia. The physiologic basis for this observation is multifactorial. First, AVP-mediated water movement across the tubular epithelium is antagonized by $PGE_2$, the renal synthesis of which is increased in the fetus. In addition, $PGE_2$ inhibits tubular permeability to urea, which cannot contribute to the renal medullary osmotic gradient above that generated by NaCl. The maximum medullary osmotic gradient generated is limited further by $PGE_2$ inhibition of NaCl reabsorption in the ascending thick limb of Henle, in much the same way that furosemide effects a diuresis by stimulating renal synthesis of $PGE_2$. The greater synthesis of prostacyclin and $PGE_2$ by the renal vascular endothelium in the fetus maintains high renal medullary blood flow, which can wash out any gradient established by active NaCl transport.

Consequently, the maximum urinary concentration possible during adaptation by the fetus to postnatal life is only slightly hypertonic to plasma, or about 350 mOsm/L (specific gravity, 1.011). After birth, the renal synthesis of vasodilator prostaglandins decreases, NaCl reabsorption increases, and tubular permeability to urea increases. Then, the osmolarity of the medullary interstitium can be increased, the collecting duct epithelium can become more responsive to AVP, and urinary osmolarity can increase. The same stimuli responsible for the hypotonic saline diuresis that is considered to be physiologic in the fetus, if perpetuated after birth, become pathophysiologic for the neonatal kidney's capacity to concentrate the urine and conserve water. When these factors are diminished postnatally, the kidney of the very premature infant will become as capable as that of a full-term infant in maximally concentrating the urine to 600 to 800 mOsm/L when AVP is released from the hypothalamus. Comparing the maximum concentrating ability of the neonatal kidney to the greater ability of the adult kidney (1300 mOsm/L) is pointless, because it is rare for either the adult or the neonate to conserve water to such an extent.

In summary, the kidney of the newborn infant is able to maintain body fluid homeostasis within certain limits, but may be inadequate to support extraordinary demands placed upon it by disease, by the treatment of disease, or by the misinterpretation of its normal responses to extrarenal stimuli.

## STRUCTURAL ABNORMALITIES OF THE NEONATAL KIDNEY AND URINARY TRACT

### Failure in Morphogenesis

Developmental abnormalities of the kidney occur when metanephric induction fails, when it fails to permit normal differentiation and development after the metanephros is formed, or when the normal metanephros sustains an insult after nephrogenesis begins. When the ureteric bud does not establish contact with the mesenchyma of the nephrogenic cord, even minimal separation between the tissues of different embryonic origin will prevent induction of the metanephric blastema. Consequently, nephrogenesis does not occur, no urine is produced, and the proximal ureter is not distended to model the pelvicaliceal system. Radionuclide scanning for evidence of a kidney on that side would reveal no renal blood flow, an angiographic study would reveal no renal artery, and a retrograde urographic study would demonstrate that the ureter ends in a blind pouch. This condition is referred to as renal agenesis, and it can be unilateral or bilateral. If it is bilateral and associated with fetal compression, the criteria for Potter's syndrome are fulfilled. When the ureteric bud establishes contact with mesenchymal cells incompletely or only with certain regions, the metanephros will have neither a normal complement of nephrons nor a normal gross appearance. When the neonatal kidney is small, either in size or in weight, this is known as renal hypoplasia. If nephrogenesis is relatively uniform throughout the cortex, but does not result in the usual 1 million nephrons normal for a human kidney, existing nephrons will hypertrophy and be found subsequently to be quite large; this condition, referred to as oligomeganephronia, is recognized only by chance in the neonate because the complication responsible for determining the diagnosis when both kidneys are affected is chronic renal insufficiency, which develops toward the end of the first decade of life.

In some fetuses, the induction of metanephric formation may be either normal or abnormal, but further normal differentiation and development are interrupted by some insult to the fetus, such as exposure to teratogens or infection in the first trimester of pregnancy, or by uteroplacental dysfunction or urinary tract obstruction at any time during gestation. The term given to this kind of abnormal renal development is renal dysplasia, in which gross and microscopic findings may include hydronephrosis, parenchymal atrophy, broad or segmental scars, interstitial inflammatory cells in the absence of infection, aglomerular regions of the cortex, tubular atrophy or thyroidization, dilated tubules and collecting ducts (some of which are actual cystic structures), and aberrant structures that are formed also from mesoderm but normally are located elsewhere in the body, such as cartilage. Any one of these examples of abnormal renal development may be unilateral or bilateral. In addition, any two or more developmental abnormalities may coexist in kidneys of the same infant.

### Obstructive Uropathy

The most common abdominal mass in the neonate is a hydronephrotic kidney; however, every kidney that was obstructed in utero is not enlarged at birth. Hydronephrosis occurs only when hydrostatic pressure in the collecting system is increased, and it implies that urine formation continued at least until just before discovery of the enlarged kidney. If obstruction has been long-standing, glomerular filtration and urinary flow cease when the pressure within Bowman's space plus capillary oncotic pressure equals or exceeds glomerular capillary hydrostatic pressure. According to experimental studies of adult mammalian kidneys, normal renal function is not recovered when the complete obstruction persists for more than a week. Moreover, the longer the obstruction continues, the less is the expected return of renal function. When the fetal or neonatal ureter is obstructed, its smooth muscle layers are disorganized and it has few elastic fibers. The ureteral wall becomes a cylinder of connective tissue with ineffective peristalsis, which causes a relative obstruction to urinary flow and predisposes the infant to urinary tract infection. Eventually, the urine proximal to the obstruction is absorbed, leaving only a dilated and dysplastic cylinder of fibrous connective tissue. When the integrity of the collecting system is disrupted by increasing pressure within it, urine will be extravasated into the retroperitoneal space or, occasionally, into the peritoneal cavity. The resulting urinary ascites is a welcome sign in the fetus or neonate with obstructive uropathy, because the urinary tract has been decompressed and the kidney may be normal in spite of lower urinary tract obstruction. Another means of decompressing the obstructed fetal urinary tract occurs when the allantois does not close, but persists as a urachus or urachal cyst.

The clinical problem associated most often with renal dysplasia in the neonate is obstructive uropathy, which occurs in 1:1000 live births. Obstruction of the flow of urine can occur at any point along the urinary tract between the calyx and the urethral meatus; it can be partial or complete; and it can be transient, intermittent, or fixed. If, for example, the proximal ureter fails to canalize completely, ureteropelvic junction obstruction will result. This lesion is the most common form of obstructive uropathy; it may be partial or complete; and it is suggested or identified usually by routine ultrasonography in the fetus, during the evaluation of an abdominal mass or urinary tract infection in the neonate, and while investigating the complaint of intense flank pain after a large volume of fluid is ingested in the child or adult. If the diagnosis is unclear, an intravenous bolus of fluid given with furosemide will produce a brisk diuresis that will distend the urinary tract proximal to the obstructing lesion. Surgical correction is not always indicated because many uncomplicated lesions resolve spontaneously.

When mucosal folds obstruct the posterior urethra and limit the force or height of the urinary stream in male infants, the diagnosis of posterior urethral valves should be suspected and confirmed by voiding cystourethrography. Every male neonate should be screened for this obstructing lesion by having at least one experienced observer note the force or arc of the urinary stream during micturition. If this has not been recorded at the time of discharge from the nursery, parents should be instructed in how to make this observation and to report the finding to the pediatrician during the first week of life. Urethral or lower urinary tract obstruction affects both upper tracts similarly, resulting in bilateral renal and ureteral dysplasia, which is one of the most common causes of chronic renal insufficiency in male infants and children. For this reason, attempts have been made to intervene during pregnancy to relieve the obstruction as a means of salvaging some renal parenchyma for future function and increasing the volume of amniotic fluid in the hope of preventing pulmonary hypoplasia and fetal compression. Total destruction of both kidneys from cystic dysplasia, however, has been identified long before the fetus is large enough to undergo such surgery without significant risk. Furthermore, in spite of anecdotes to the contrary, no identifiable benefit to any fetus ever has been documented as being superior to immediate treatment at birth—irreversible damage usually has occurred by the time the obstruction has been identified. The best treatment still is considered to be early intervention by initiating a well-planned approach for definitive care of the neonate at birth.

## Prune-Belly Syndrome

Prune-belly syndrome is a condition in which the urinary tract findings are nearly identical to those for posterior urethral valves, but with one important exception—no obstructing lesion can be found. There is convincing evidence, however, that the developing prostate obstructs the fetal urethra transiently. Another similarity between the two conditions is that both can have a variable degree of muscle tone in the abdominal wall. The classic presentation of prune-belly syndrome is a male neonate who is found to have complete absence of abdominal wall musculature, so that the outlines of bowel loops can be seen and the abdominal cavity can be examined easily by palpation. In addition, there is a paucity of smooth muscle in the ureters, the urinary bladder, and, more rarely, the gastrointestinal tract. Clinical management of the neonate with prune-belly syndrome involves monitoring the urinary tract for relative obstruction to urinary flow and its major complication, infection; assessing GFR for subsequent comparison to identify change; establishing requirements for NaCl balance in an infant who will exhibit NaCl wasting and will fail to grow normally when replacement is inadequate; correcting the metabolic acidosis that develops because of decreased distal tubular secretion of hydrogen ion; and providing an activated form of vitamin D ($1,25(OH)_2$ vitamin D) because these infants, similar to those with other forms of primary uropathy, have hypocalcemia and renal osteodystrophy even when the GFR is nearly normal. Finally, appropriate counseling for the infant's parents is essential. Although renal function in the infant may seem normal at birth, end-stage renal disease develops in most patients before adolescence.

## Renal Cystic Disease

Renal cystic disease occurs in many different forms and nearly defies meaningful classification, at least any that would explain cystogenesis for each type. For instance, a unilateral, single cyst may be discovered incidentally in a neonate with normal renal function. This cyst may persist unchanged throughout life and cause no problem for the individual; it may disappear altogether, or it may be the first of many more cysts to form over the next 30 to 40 years in both kidneys. When this diagnostic dilemma is encountered in a neonate, the patient can be observed serially to document changes in the cyst, in kidney function, and in blood pressure, as has been the practice until very recently. In the absence of a family history of polycystic kidney disease, this option should be exercised only after both parents have had ultrasonographic examination of their kidneys for the presence of cysts. In a more aggressive diagnostic approach, which rarely is warranted, DNA probes can identify the gene that expresses autosomal dominant (adult) polycystic kidney disease when renal tissue is available. The finding of cysts in other organs, particularly liver, lung, or pancreas, supports the diagnosis of autosomal recessive (infantile) polycystic kidney disease. One further clue to the latter condition is the ability to identify early hepatic fibrosis in these patients by ultrasonography. Although this is not always present from birth, moderate to severe systemic hypertension develops in these patients within the first months of life, and they should be monitored prospectively for this problem. A multicystic kidney usually is unilateral, dysplastic, and nonfunctioning. Neonates who are found to have a multicystic kidney need only casual monitoring for the rare occurrence of enlargement or complicating infection; otherwise, these malformed kidneys should not be removed routinely. There once was concern that

malignancy might develop in these kidneys, but long-term follow-up of these patients has identified no such added risk. A voiding cystourethrogram will identify another genitourinary abnormality in 30% to 40% of these infants.

# ABNORMALITIES OF RENAL FUNCTION IN THE NEONATE

## Asphyxia Neonatorum

The kidney develops under conditions of relative hypoxia and is capable of considerable anaerobic metabolism. During the perinatal period, hypoxia alone probably has little, if any, well-defined effects on the kidney, but in combination with hypotension and either endogenous release of vasoactive substances or the administration of $\alpha$-adrenergic agonists, it can cause acute tubular necrosis, cortical necrosis, or medullary necrosis. On the other hand, asphyxia is a combination of severe hypoxia and intense pulmonary vasoconstriction, mediated in part through AVP release and, possibly, angiotensin II. Acute renal failure with oligoanuria is observed commonly in these infants, and recovery of renal function usually follows relief of pulmonary vasoconstriction with improvement in lung function. The kidney of an asphyxiated infant behaves as would a normal kidney when it is exposed to increased levels of circulating angiotensin II or to the infusion of angiotensin precursors into the renal circulation. A possible role for angiotensin II was dismissed after one study in an experimental animal model found no benefit to blocking angiotensin II; however, angiotensin II formation within the kidney is not overcome as easily as it is elsewhere in the body. It is possible, therefore, that intrarenal renin release stimulated by AVP and angiotensin II formation causes the intense renal vasoconstriction that is associated with asphyxia. One possible future treatment for this often devastating condition in the stressed neonate with meconium aspiration, respiratory insufficiency, and acute renal failure may be to inhibit AVP or angiotensin II formation, or to administer a precursor of nitric oxide.

## Nephrotoxic Drug Therapy

The neonatal kidney once was thought to be more tolerant of drug injury than is the kidney of the child or the adult. This assumption was based on a clinical study in which the assessment of renal function was made inaccurately and then was misinterpreted. The newborn kidney, like its adult counterpart, always is at risk of toxic injury when proximal tubular reabsorption is maximal, when EABV is decreased, during NaCl or potassium depletion, and during hypoxia. Oligoanuria does not always predispose the kidney to nephrotoxicity, because neonates are not dehydrated with inappropriate secretion of AVP; EABV is increased, total body NaCl and potassium levels are normal, proximal tubular reabsorption is decreased, GFR is normal, and the drug is diluted in the greater ECFV.

The nephrotoxic effects of antibiotics such as aminoglycosides, vancomycin, and amphotericin B occur with the same frequency in neonates as in older infants, children, and adults, even though they may not be recognized. For example, aminoglycoside therapy is prescribed for neonates in a higher dosage relative to body size than it is in adults. Moreover, therapy is adjusted according to arbitrarily chosen "effective" peak and trough plasma levels. Such levels can be misleading in the neonate because the drug is injected into the relatively larger volume of distribution, that is, the ECFV. Therefore, more drug must be given to achieve the same peak plasma levels in neonates compared to adults. Similarly, trough levels are determined by renal clearance of the circulating drug, and a much lower trough level will be observed in neonates than in adults. The decision to modify or discontinue nephrotoxic antibiotic therapy based only on an increase in plasma trough levels will come several days after GFR has decreased from the nephrotoxic effects of the drug. Such nephrotoxicity is manifested earlier by a serial rise in the $S_{Cr}$, which, in the adult, occurs almost predictably between 4 and 7 days after aminoglycoside therapy is initiated. A similar change in $S_{Cr}$ in the neonate may be masked before the excess maternal creatinine has been cleared from the neonatal circulation. Because neither $S_{Cr}$ nor plasma drug levels are ideal for monitoring the neonate for drug toxicity, therapy should be prescribed according to the drug's pharmacokinetics, which vary not with the infant's postnatal age, but with his or her conceptional age. For aminoglycosides and vancomycin, the drug dose interval is every 18 to 24 hours in neonates less than 34 weeks' conceptional age and every 12 hours in older infants. The same pattern of change in pharmacokinetics is characteristic of other drugs excreted by the kidney, such as furosemide and indomethacin.

## Urinary Tract Infection

Infections of the neonatal urinary tract are discovered most commonly when there is anatomic or functional obstruction to urine flow. Even in urinary tracts that are abnormal as a result of myelodysplasia or obstructive uropathy, the urine is sterile at birth. Urinary tract infection, therefore, is a disease that is acquired in the neonatal period and may be associated with, or the cause of, septicemia. Whether bacteria originate in the urinary tract or reach the urine as a consequence of bacteremia cannot be determined in every case. Consequently, significant bacteriuria in all neonates, regardless of the etiology, must be treated similarly by evaluating the urinary tract for evidence of obstruction once the urine is rendered sterile by effective antibiotic therapy. In the dilated urinary tract without anatomic obstruction, urinary stasis may occur along dysplastic or hypotonic ureters, and bacteria may grow in urine that fails to drain into the bladder. One characteristic of renal function in a urinary tract that is partially obstructed or one that becomes infected after obstruction is relieved is a clinical picture of pseudohypoaldosteronism: hyponatremia, hyperkalemia, and metabolic acidosis. Although it is rare in uninfected preterm and full-term infants, up to 65% of infants with first urinary tract infections have vesicoureteric reflux. The growing kidney of the infant is at greatest risk of injury from vesicoureteric reflux and urinary tract infection that, many years later, is the leading cause of hypertension and chronic renal insufficiency in adolescents and young adults.

## Diagnosis and Management of Renal Failure

Renal failure should be anticipated in any infant who is stressed unusually during the perinatal period. The diagnosis cannot be supported by a finding of oligoanuria alone. One infant at risk of acute renal failure may have a transient decrease in urinary volume ($<1$ mL/h/kg) after birth that is physiologic or functional oligoanuria when GFR is normal, whereas another infant with renal dysplasia or an obstructed urinary tract actually may have severely impaired renal function when the urinary volume is greater than 3 mL/h/kg. The immediate tendency to differentiate between acute renal failure and functional oligoanuria by bolus fluid administration or diuretic therapy cannot be acted on without some consideration being given to the risks inherent in such treatment. For instance, in a neonate whose body weight before significant caloric intake exceeds his or her birth weight, or in another with heart failure (both of whom already have excess ECFV), a fluid challenge would aggravate the clinical condition. In fact, the normal hemodynamic response to an acute increase in blood volume in the adult is an increase in cardiac output and a decrease in peripheral resistance, mediated in part by the

suppression of vasoconstrictor hormone release and the stimulation of endothelial synthesis of vasodilator prostaglandins, a cardiovascular response to stretch. Cardiac output in the neonate is nearly maximal, however, peripheral resistance is low, and both vascular and renal synthesis of prostaglandins is high. Additional volume put into the neonatal circulation can be accommodated only by shunting of blood through a previously closed ductus arteriosus or by increased flow through an already patent ductus arteriosus. Another mechanism for reducing circulating blood volume is to increase the movement of plasma into the interstitial space, which accounts for the frequent observation of edema in normal neonates, especially those who are allowed placental transfusion. When pulmonary interstitial water increases, respiratory distress develops or worsens, blood pressure decreases, renal perfusion pressure and GFR decrease, and, consequently, the urinary flow rate decreases even further.

The infant whose oligoanuria follows weight loss after birth and whose ECFV has been reduced will respond to a fluid challenge with an increase in blood pressure and urinary volume, a decrease in urinary osmolarity, and no appreciable change in $FE_{Na}$ if the infant has not been treated previously with a diuretic (the half-life of furosemide in preterm infants can be 24 hours or greater), if renal injury has not occurred already, and if EABV or blood pressure is not increased above normal. The diagnosis of renal failure in the newborn, therefore, should be made only after consideration is given, not only to urinary volume, but also to urinary osmolarity and $FE_{Na}$, to perinatal events, and to the clinical course of the infant after birth.

The causes of acute renal failure in the newborn are stated in Table 20-44 and can be considered under the broad categories of renal and non-renal causes. The renal causes of acute renal failure can be distinguished by morphologic criteria or as acute renal injury. When the kidneys are small or cannot be palpated, renal agenesis or hypoplasia/dysplasia should be considered. In contrast, large kidneys are associated with obstructive uropathy, prune-belly syndrome, and renal cystic disease. Acute renal injury that is unavoidable may be caused by asphyxia; significant blood loss at birth (from placental separation, twin transfusion, or cord accident); apnea or bradycardia with difficult or prolonged resuscitation; decreased cardiac output with acute tubular, cortical, or medullary necrosis; and renal vein thrombosis. Avoidable causes of acute renal injury include aortic and renal artery thrombosis as complications of umbilical artery catheter placement; nephrotoxic effects of contrast medium used for angiographic studies, such as cardiac catheterization and computerized axial tomography with contrast; combined drug therapy for pulmonary hypertension with tolazoline used as a generalized vasodilator and dopamine given to raise systemic blood pressure; and nephrotoxic drug therapy with aminoglycosides, vancomycin, or amphotericin B and indomethacin prescribed to prevent or close a patent ductus arteriosus.

Extrarenal causes of acute renal failure can be considered in two general categories, depending upon whether EABV is decreased or increased. EABV can be decreased when total body water is decreased, when cardiac output is decreased for any reason, when there is significant left-to-right shunting of blood through a patent ductus arteriosus, when low colloid oncotic pressure does not preserve the circulating blood volume but allows plasma to exit from the vascular space for the interstitium, and when furosemide therapy depletes blood volume and lowers peripheral vascular resistance by displacing angiotensin II from receptors and by stimulating vasodilator prostaglandin synthesis. Acute renal failure also can occur when EABV is increased by iatrogenic fluid overload or during inappropriate AVP secretion. Dopamine is a drug that often is given to raise blood pressure and increase cardiac output; contrary to a popular notion, it decreases renal cortical blood flow in the neonate—even at the

### TABLE 20-44.    Causes of Renal Failure in the Neonate

| Renal Causes | Extrarenal Causes |
|---|---|
| **Anatomical** | ↓ **Effective Arterial Blood Volume** |
| 1. Small kidneys | 1. ↓ Total body water |
|   a. Agenesis | 2. ↑ Left-right shunt |
|   b. Hypoplasia-dysplasia | 3. ↓ Cardiac output |
| 2. Large kidneys | 4. ↓ Colloid oncotic pressure |
|   a. Obstructive uropathy | 5. ↓ Peripheral resistance |
|   b. Prune-belly syndrome | 6. Furosemide therapy |
|   c. Cystic disease | ↑ **Effective Arterial Blood Volume** |
| **Acute Renal Injury** | 1. Inappropriate arginine vasopressin secretion |
| 1. Unavoidable |   a. ↑ Intracranial pressure |
|   a. Hypoxia-asphyxia |   b. CNS infection |
|   b. Blood loss |   c. ↑ Intrathoracic pressure (pneumothorax, positive-pressure ventilation) |
|   c. Apnea/bradycardia | |
|   d. Circulatory complications (acute tubular or cortical/medullary necrosis and renal vein thrombosis) | **Drug Effect** |
| 2. Avoidable | 1. Dopamine |
|   a. Renal artery thrombosis | 2. Pancuronium |
|   b. Radiographic contrast dye | |
|   c. Tolazoline/dopamine therapy | ↑ **Fluid Therapy** |
|   d. Aminoglycoside nephrotoxicity | |
|   e. Indomethacin | |

lowest recommended dose—and can cause acute renal failure. Any claim of benefit to renal function with dopamine infusion follows an improvement in EABV. Pancuronium or other paralyzing drugs given to mechanically ventilated infants can produce erratic sympathetic nervous system discharges, which cause the blood pressure to rise or fall unpredictably, accompanied by changes in EABV and renal function.

The mechanisms through which oligoanuria is mediated by a decrease in EABV are represented schematically in Figure 20-64. A decrease in EABV stimulates the release of catecholamines and AVP; both provoke renin release, which is followed by angiotensin II formation, renal arteriolar vasoconstriction, and a decrease in renal cortical blood flow, GFR, and urinary flow rate. Moreover, AVP release, stimulated either by a decrease in EABV or by a rise in plasma osmolarity, facilitates water reabsorption across the collecting duct epithelium, which reduces the urinary

flow rate. Angiotensin II stimulates aldosterone secretion, which promotes tubular Na/K adenosine triphosphatase activity to increase sodium reabsorption. In addition, angiotensin II can stimulate (at low or normal concentrations) or inhibit (at higher concentrations) proximal tubular Na reabsorption. The resulting NaCl and water conservation restores EABV, which then inhibits the compensating mechanisms.

Inappropriate AVP secretion should be suspected in any patient whose central nervous system has been exposed to infection, intracranial hemorrhage, change in intracranial pressure, or trauma (surgical or accidental). The pathophysiologic mechanisms involved in inappropriate AVP secretion are depicted in Figure 20-66. Moreover, any condition that reduces cardiac output or lowers EABV will stimulate baroreceptor-mediated AVP release, and an increase in plasma osmolarity will stimulate osmoreceptor-mediated AVP release. As urinary volume decreases, water being

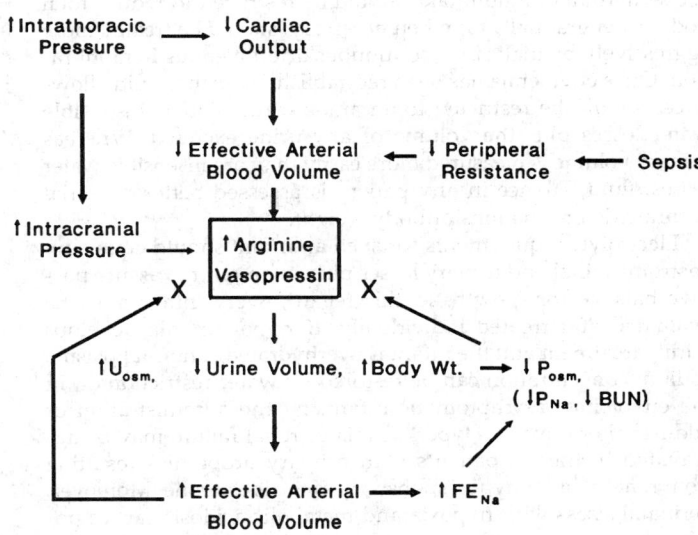

**Figure 20-66.** Pathophysiologic mechanisms that contribute to the consequences of inappropriate arginine vasopressin (AVP) secretion. The X indicates a failure of the normal feedback mechanism to reduce hypothalamic release of AVP. *Wt,* weight; *BUN,* blood urea nitrogen.

reabsorbed unnecessarily in the distal nephron and collecting duct is added back to body fluids, and plasma osmolarity decreases in proportion to the increase in body weight. Plasma sodium concentration and blood urea nitrogen decrease in proportion to plasma osmolarity. When AVP release is not inhibited (indicated by an X in Fig 20-65) either by an increase in EABV or by a fall in the tonicity of body fluids, and fluid intake is not restricted at the outset to urinary volume only, the dilution of body fluid and weight gain continue. Under normal circumstances, when AVP release is inhibited, urinary osmolarity should be the least or urinary dilution the maximum possible—30 to 50 mOsm/L (specific gravity, 1.001)—just as in diabetes insipidus. Urinary sodium concentration and $FE_{Na}$ may be either increased or decreased depending upon whether EABV is increased or decreased; therefore, urinary sodium excretion is irrelevant to the diagnosis of inappropriate AVP secretion. The most important treatment is anticipating the problem in patients who are at risk. When the diagnosis is suspected, fluid therapy should be limited to urinary volume plus an estimate of insensible water losses. Moreover, known stimuli to AVP release should be removed whenever possible. Although ventilator pressure settings cannot be changed just to facilitate diuresis, efforts should be made to decrease intrathoracic pressure in a stepwise fashion as quickly as the infant's condition permits. Administering hypertonic saline and furosemide simultaneously to reduce total body water and increase plasma sodium concentration is a naive approach to management. Because there is no deficit in total body sodium when AVP secretion is inappropriate, but only increased water, treatment appropriately is water restriction. Hypertonic saline infusion should be reserved for the infant whose condition develops unnoticed and is recognized after changes have taken place in the central nervous system.

The infant whose $S_{Cr}$ increases after birth rather than remains stable or decreases appropriately for his or her conceptional age should be considered to have acute or chronic renal failure. The onset of chronic renal failure may be more insidious, however, and may be discovered only after the neonatal period. Those whose kidneys fail to function at all after birth require dialysis therapy in the first week of life. It is possible to establish continuous ambulatory peritoneal dialysis, even in preterm infants, temporarily for those needing it while waiting for recovery from acute renal failure or longer for those who will become candidates for kidney transplantation.

Initial treatment of renal failure should include close attention to correcting and then preventing fluid and electrolyte derangements. If the infant is volume-depleted, euvolemic conditions should be restored by appropriate fluid replacement. If the infant is overhydrated, fluid intake should be restricted to reduce total body water gradually or, when necessary, should be treated more aggressively by dialysis or continuous arteriovenous hemofiltration. Once euvolemia has been reestablished, further fluid allowances should be restricted to an amount that equals insensible water losses plus the volume of any urine excreted. Whereas urinary volume is measured more easily than are insensible water losses, fluid balance in any patient is assessed better by serial accurate determinations of body weight.

Electrolyte requirements for such an infant should equal any gastrointestinal and urinary losses plus an amount to assure positive balance for growth. In this regard, every infant must be evaluated and treated individually. If hyponatremia develops during treatment and the infant is overhydrated, a normal plasma sodium concentration can be restored by water restriction or, in the euvolemic, asymptomatic infant, by the administration of additional oral NaCl. Hyperkalemia of renal failure may be aggravated further in patients with primary uropathies resulting from renal tubular hyporesponsiveness to aldosterone. Moreover, perinatal stress with hypoxia and metabolic acidosis causes po-

tassium to move out of cells and into the extracellular fluid. The clinical management of hyperkalemia in the neonate is no different than that in older patients.

Hypertension in the neonate is a problem encountered most often in association with circulatory or vascular causes of renal injury, such as renal artery or vein thrombosis and cortical or medullary necrosis. Hydronephrosis is a cause of hypertension less often in neonates than in older children and adults. The treatment objectives for hypertension should be to restore euvolemia by administering appropriate NaCl and fluid therapy, and to reduce peripheral vascular resistance by stimulating vascular endothelial synthesis of prostacyclin with hydralazine, diazoxide, or nitroglycerin, or by reducing vasoconstriction by inhibiting angiotensin converting enzyme activity or calcium channel blockade.

Systemic acidosis should be treated first with improved ventilation to reduce carbon dioxide tension and increase arterial blood pH, and then with alkali therapy (sodium bicarbonate or sodium citrate) to neutralize the excess hydrogen ion. *Hypocalcemia*, seen normally in the first week of life, especially in preterm infants, can become symptomatic in neonates who have renal failure. When renal function is impaired, the ability to excrete phosphate is limited and the hyperphosphatemia normally observed in the neonate will be exaggerated and result in further lowering of the serum calcium concentration. When fed, infants should be given a formula with reduced NaCl and phosphate compared to that in formulas given to normal neonates. However, NaCl may have to be added to the low-phosphate formula for neonates with primary uropathies. Calcium gluconate intravenously and calcium carbonate orally should be combined with activated vitamin-D therapy to maintain serum calcium concentrations at a high normal value.

All too often, adequate nutrition is achieved late in the treatment of neonates with acute renal failure. Attention is focused on the renal failure and its management. Providing appropriate caloric intake simultaneously makes fluid restriction and electrolyte adjustment more complex. This should not be the case in most neonates when the treatment of renal failure is appropriate and informed. Parenteral nutrition can be prescribed early in low volumes as essential amino acid preparations plus a hypertonic glucose solution. Intralipid can increase the caloric intake further. Whenever possible, consideration should be given to having vascular access lines always contain maximum caloric provision. Not only will the nutritional status of the infant be improved, but serum potassium and phosphate concentrations also will be controlled more easily.

Dialysis should be used to treat complications of renal failure, not during a crisis brought about by a complication of the neonate's previous treatment, but in a planned fashion whenever possible. Peritoneal dialysis can be initiated after percutaneous placement of a permanent or temporary catheter. Commercially available dialysis solutions with varying concentrations of glucose for altering ultrafiltration can be used; otherwise, special solutions can be formulated.

## Selected Readings

Aperia A, Herin P, Lundin S, et al. Regulation of renal water excretion in newborn full-term infants. Acta Paediatr Scand 1984;73:717.

Arant BS Jr. Developmental patterns of renal functional maturation compared in the human neonate. J Pediatr 1978;92:705.

Arant BS Jr. Neonatal adjustments of extrauterine life. In Edelmann CM Jr, ed. Pediatric kidney disease, ed 2. Boston: Little Brown, 1992:1043.

Arant BS Jr. Sodium, chloride and potassium. In Tsang RC, Lucas A, Uauy R, Zlotkin S, eds. Nutritional needs of the preterm infant. Baltimore: Williams & Wilkins, 1993:157.

Brion LP, Fleischman AR, McCarton C, et al. A simple estimate of glomerular filtration rate in low-birth-weight infants during the first year of life: Noninvasive assessment of body composition and growth. J Pediatr 1986;109:698.

Kleinman LI, Stewart CI, Kaskel FJ. Renal disease in the newborn. In Edelmann CM Jr, ed. Pediatric kidney disease, ed 2. Boston: Little Brown, 1992:1043.

Lorenz JM, Kleinman LI, Kotagal UR, et al. Water balance in very-low-birth-weight-infants: Relationship to water and sodium intake and effect on outcome. J Pediatr 1982;101:423.

Rees L, Brook CGD, Shaw JCL, et al. Hyponatraemia in the first week of life in preterm infants. Arch Dis Child 1984;59:414.

Schwartz GJ, Feld LG, Langford DJ. A simple estimate of glomerular filtration rate in full-term infants during the first year of life. J Pediatr 1984;104:489.

Seyberth HW, Wille L, Ulmer HE, et al. Renal pharmacology of the prostaglandin synthesis inhibitor indomethacin. In: Brodehl J, Ehrich JHH, eds. Paediatric nephrology. Berlin: Springer-Verlag, 1984:409.

Szefler SJ, Wynn RJ, Clarke DF, et al. Relationship of gentamicin serum concentrations to gestational age in preterm and term neonates. J Pediatr 1980;97:312.

Tulassay T, Machay T, Kiszel J, et al. Effects of continuous positive airway pressure on renal function in prematures. Biol Neonate 1983;43:152.

*Principles and Practice of Pediatrics, Second Edition.*
edited by Frank A. Oski et al. J. B. Lippincott Company, Philadelphia © 1994.

# 20.7 *Neonatal Endocrinology*

### Elizabeth A. Catlin and John D. Crawford

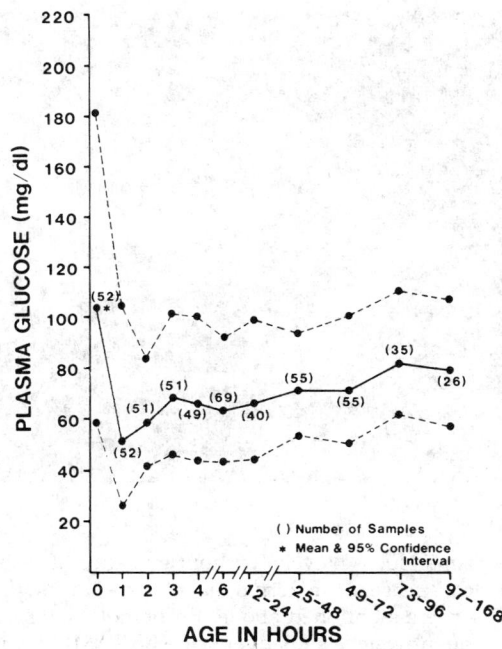

**Figure 20-67.** Predicted plasma glucose values during the first week of life in healthy term neonates with weights appropriate for their gestational age. (Srinivasan G, Pildes RS, Cattamanchi G, et al. Plasma glucose values in normal neonates: A new look. J Pediatr 1986;109:114.)

At the moment of birth, neonates face an intimidating list of requirements for independent living. Precise and appropriate hormonal regulation is one such key area for mastery by the newborn infant. Thus, it may not be surprising that the hormonal and metabolic responses of the neonate to stress, be it that of birth, surgery, or infection, are, if anything, even more vigorous than those of the adult. But neonates cannot talk; the very small ones seldom cry and move but little. The very vigor of the neonate's endocrine–metabolic response in the face of limited energy supplies in some situations may make it counterproductive; in circumstances in which it is defective, marked deviations of otherwise carefully protected body constituents develop rapidly. In either case, recognition must not be delayed because the manifestations characteristic of the older child or adult are absent. This chapter covers primarily the problems commonly encountered and several of the unusual imbalances and disorders of the newborn's endocrine system.

## GLUCOSE HOMEOSTASIS

Glucose transfer to the fetus by the placenta appears to be carrier-mediated. Whereas fetal growth and well-being depend on a maternally derived glucose supply, the fetus is not simply parasitic, but instead generates metabolic responses to nutritional states. At delivery, neonatal plasma glucose values normally are 70% to 80% of maternal values. In healthy term babies receiving enteral feedings by 3 hours of life, plasma glucose concentrations decline after delivery, reaching their lowest point at between 1 and 2 hours of life, with mean values (plus or minus the standard deviation) of 56±19 mg/dL (Fig 20-67).

Intermittent and unpredictable feeding in the early neonatal period stresses the newborn's carbohydrate homeostatic capacity. Glycogenolysis and gluconeogenesis (both stimulated by glucagon) actively contribute to neonatal glucose production, and high epinephrine levels stimulate glucagon release and lipolysis. In the first several hours after birth, 90% of hepatic glycogen is used. By 8 hours of age, 10% of plasma glucose in neonates with weights appropriate for their gestational age is derived from alanine via gluconeogenesis. Epinephrine-stimulated lipolysis results in a threefold rise in free fatty acid levels. The respiratory quotient immediately after birth is 0.9 to 1.0, but it drops to 0.7 as fat use increases. Animal data suggest that regulation of the glucose balance is less precise in the newborn than in the adult. Hepatic suppression of glucose production during glucose infusion, for example, is delayed in the newborn relative to that in the adult.

## Hypoglycemia

Hypoglycemia is defined as plasma glucose values of 40 mg/dL or less, and it is a common problem in newborn infants. Maintaining neonatal plasma glucose concentrations greater than 40 mg/dL is a sensible therapeutic goal, because fetal glucose levels are at least 40 mg/dL, and adults and older children may be compromised by glucose levels less than 40 mg/dL (as may neonates). Certain babies, including infants of diabetic mothers (IDMs), neonates with nesidioblastosis or Beckwith's syndrome, and neonates who are premature or growth-retarded are especially prone to the development of hypoglycemia. IDMs often exhibit hyperinsulinemic hypoglycemia (see Chap. 20.9).

Neonates with the Beckwith-Wiedemann syndrome (Fig 20-68) have macroglossia, visceromegaly, and omphalocele, and are large for their gestational age. Nearly 50% of reported cases exhibit hyperinsulinemic hypoglycemia caused by islet cell hyperplasia. Hypoglycemia in these infants may be severe and long-lasting, necessitating pharmacologic management of their hyperinsulinism in addition to glucose supplementation.

Nesidioblastosis, or primary hyperplasia of the islets of Langerhans, is an unusual cause of hyperinsulinemic hypoglycemia in the neonate; related pancreatic disorders producing hyperinsulinemia include islet cell adenomas and adenomatosis. Inappropriately high serum insulin levels (relative to simultaneously

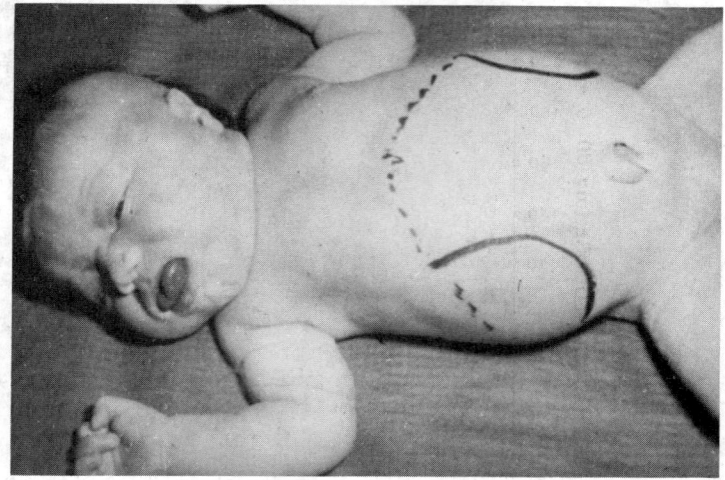

Figure 20-68.    Neonate with Beckwith-Wiedemann syndrome. This 38-week, 34-cm, 5.218-kg, plethoric infant was his mother's third child affected with the syndrome. Note, in addition to his large size and abundance of subcutaneous fat, the enlarged tongue and umbilical hernia. The enormously enlarged, multilobular kidneys have been outlined with a skin pencil. The vertical creases on the lobuli of the ears are not well shown. The infant required prolonged infusion of intravenous glucose to prevent hyperinsulinemic hypoglycemia as well as a partial glossectomy and repair of the umbilical hernia.

obtained plasma glucose levels) without evidence of Beckwith's syndrome, Rh disease, or maternal diabetes mellitus suggest the beta cell disorders mentioned above. Rh hemolytic disease (observed infrequently since the advent of RhoGAM) also is associated with hyperinsulinemic hypoglycemia; the cause of the islet cell hyperplasia in these babies is not known.

Small-for-gestational-age (SGA) neonates commonly are affected with hypoglycemia; 65% of premature and 25% of full-term SGA babies become hypoglycemic. Factors contributing to their low serum glucose levels include decreased glycogen and fat stores, large brain weight/body weight ratio, and functional delay in hepatic gluconeogenesis.

Hypoglycemia may develop in neonates with polycythemia/hyperviscosity. The reasons for this are not immediately apparent. Some glucose is lost by metabolism to the greater red cell mass, less glucose is carried in a given volume of blood as a result of the diminished plasma fraction, and sludging may leave tissues poorly oxygenated and, thus, more dependent on glucose for anaerobic metabolism. A venous hematocrit higher than 65% defines polycythemia; with increasing hematocrit levels, an exponential rise in blood viscosity occurs. The hypoglycemia in these instances resolves with partial exchange transfusion to reduce the hematocrit.

Premature neonates (<37 weeks' gestation) are at risk for the development of hypoglycemia. They often have inadequate dietary intake and lower total body energy stores. Premature neonates are affected more commonly with other conditions known to predispose to hypoglycemia: cold-stress, sepsis, hypoxia, or perinatal asphyxia. Each of these conditions results in hypoglycemia based on inadequate hepatic glucose production or inadequate substrate supply.

Very infrequently, hypoglycemia is caused by one of the inborn errors of metabolism such as galactosemia or type I glycogen storage disease (see Chap. 12.5).

### Diagnosis and Therapy

The clinician must have a low threshold for suspecting hypoglycemia in neonates. Affected infants may manifest signs such as tremors, apnea, seizures, poor feeding, or apathy, but they also may be essentially asymptomatic. A careful pregnancy history and physical examination may reveal evidence of growth retardation, visceromegaly, or other problems. A plasma glucose level should be obtained (if capillary sampling is used, care must be taken to warm the heel adequately); if the glucose concentration is 40 mg/dL or less, treatment should be instituted. Initial screening can be carried out using glucose oxidase strips (eg, Dextrostix,

Chemstrips) during the first 40 minutes of life. The strips should be fresh or packaged individually, because open bottles may lose activity and give erroneously low values. Stable and relatively mature babies may be treated safely with early enteral feedings and careful monitoring of subsequent plasma glucose values. If the Dextrostix reading is greater than 45 mg/dL, normal feeding can be started as soon as the infant's condition will permit; the capillary sugar level should be monitored by Dextrostix every 1 to 2 hours until there is clear evidence that the blood glucose level is stable. If the Dextrostix reading is between 25 and 45 mg/dL, the value is confirmed by obtaining a capillary blood sugar determination and the baby is given 10 to 15 mL of 10% glucose (orally or by gavage feeding), followed by normal milk feeding; the blood sugar should be monitored every 2 to 3 hours until the level is stable and above 40 mg/dL. If the blood sugar level is less than 25 mg/dL, parenteral glucose supplementation is required; it may be initiated with a "mini-bolus" of 2 to 3 mL/kg of 10% glucose intravenously in water, followed by a constant infusion of 10% glucose delivering 6 to 8 mg/kg/min of glucose, which approximates the normal rate of glucose utilization. Glucose values must be monitored closely, with titration of the infusate to maintain normoglycemia.

Infants with hyperinsulinemic hypoglycemia and SGA babies may require especially high glucose infusions (15 to 20 mg/kg/min), which usually must be delivered via a central venous catheter. Intravenous therapy should be maintained until the glucose level has stabilized. Rebound hypoglycemia in IDMs can be avoided by slow tapering of the intravenous glucose being administered. If nesidioblastosis or islet cell tumors are suspected, simultaneous plasma glucose and insulin concentrations should be obtained. Babies who require very high glucose infusions (>15 mg/kg/min) may need drug therapy to aid in the treatment of hypoglycemia. If there is difficulty in initiating intravenous glucose therapy for IDMs, glucagon (0.3 mg/kg to a maximum dose of 1 mg) can be given. Glucagon may override the inhibitory effect of insulin on glycogenolysis and raise the infant's blood sugar level within 10 to 15 minutes of the injection. It should be emphasized that glucagon benefits only the infant in whom there is a large glucose reservoir in the form of glycogen—it has no place in therapy for the hypoglycemia of low–birth-weight infants. Corticosteroids enhance gluconeogenesis, and hydrocortisone may be given at 5 mg/kg/d intravenously or orally. Diazoxide suppresses insulin secretion; the usual dosage is 10 to 15 mg/kg/d. Octreotide, a somatostatin analogue, is an effective suppressant of insulin release and has been useful in the long-term management of resistant hyperinsulinemia. Nesidioblastosis and islet cell adenomas usually require adenomectomy or subtotal (about 80%) pancreatectomy before glucose concentrations can be maintained at satisfactory levels.

## Hyperglycemia

Hyperglycemia in the neonate may be defined as plasma glucose concentrations higher than 145 to 150 mg/dL. The incidence of hyperglycemia appears to have increased in association with the increased survival of very premature and high-risk babies.

Some studies suggest that hyperglycemia contributes to increased morbidity and mortality in neonates. Although hepatic insulin insensitivity and, therefore, persistent glucose production are thought to be etiologic in the hyperglycemia that is observed so often in babies with very low birth weights, other conditions are associated with inappropriately high glucose concentrations in the newborn period. Sepsis, surgery, hypoxia, respiratory distress syndrome, and treatment with methylxanthines each is known to be associated with hyperglycemia. Stress-related hyperglycemia results, in part, from elevated catecholamine and cortisol levels. Pancreatic agenesis is a rare cause of neonatal glucose intolerance; these babies also exhibit significant intrauterine growth retardation. Transient diabetes mellitus may follow overwhelming sepsis, intracranial hemorrhage, and previous hypoglycemia; it is reported more often in growth-retarded neonates.

A rare, transient, insulinopenic type of diabetes mellitus may be seen in SGA neonates. The low birth weights of these infants, in contrast to the large size of IDMs, has been considered to reflect insulin's important role as an intrauterine growth hormone. These infants generally have severe hypertonic dehydration and require insulin treatment for 1 to 3 months.

### Diagnosis and Therapy

Plasma glucose levels of 150 mg/dL and greater are hyperglycemic. If the neonate is receiving intravenous glucose-containing fluids, the glucose infusion rate in milligrams per kilogram per minute should be calculated, and stepped decreases (by 1 to 2 mg/kg/min) every 3 to 4 hours should be implemented, monitored by glucose determinations every few hours; hypotonic infusates should be avoided. Fluid balance, glycosuria, blood pressure, oxygenation, and perfusion also should be checked carefully and, if sepsis is suspected, appropriate cultures should be obtained and antibiotics given. In infants with very low birth weights (1500 g or less), measures to minimize insensible fluid losses, such as transfer from radiant warmers to isolettes, should be considered. If, despite conservative measures, plasma glucose levels persist at greater than 200 to 250 mg/dL, insulin therapy may be required. Neonates may be treated initially with regular insulin, 0.10 to 0.25 U/kg given subcutaneously every 6 hours with frequent glucose monitoring, aiming to achieve euglycemia and taking care not to precipitate hypoglycemia. The larger requirement for insulin generally distinguishes the rare neonate with transient diabetes mellitus from the infant mounting a very vigorous stress response. In the latter, hyperglycemia lasts for a few days at most.

## CALCIUM HOMEOSTASIS

### Hypocalcemia

Hypocalcemia may be a significant metabolic problem in the neonatal period, and generally is subdivided into early and late categories (see Chap. 20.12). Early hypocalcemia is defined as a total serum calcium concentration of less than 8 mg/dL in the full-term neonate or less than 7 mg/dL in the premature neonate

during the first several days, with the nadir occurring at between 24 and 48 hours of life. Inasmuch as about 50% of the calcium in serum is bound loosely to protein and this inert fraction varies according to the protein concentration, pH level, and other factors, it may be more helpful, particularly where facilities are available for its measurement, to think in terms of the biologically active ionized calcium concentration. Thus, values for ionized calcium below 1.0 mmol/L are even more indicative of hypocalcemia. Premature and asphyxiated neonates and IDMs are particularly susceptible to early hypocalcemia; hypomagnesemia and hypocalcemia may coexist in the IDM. Late neonatal hypocalcemia (synonymous with infantile tetany) occurs at the end of or after the first week of life and is associated with hypoparathyroidism and high-phosphate formula consumption. Correction of the late hypocalcemia associated with hypomagnesemia requires magnesium repletion initially, with or without additional calcium supplementation. Hypomagnesemia may be seen in SGA babies, in neonates with hepatic disease or small-bowel resections, and, very rarely, in infants with magnesium malabsorption. It may result in late hypocalcemia because of decreased parathyroid hormone (PTH) production, relative end-organ insensitivity to PTH, decreased exchange of magnesium for calcium at the bone surface, and decreased calcium absorption via the intestine.

### Diagnosis and Therapy

Neonates with hypocalcemia may be completely asymptomatic. Physical findings in such neonates may include seizures, tremors, tetany or lethargy, and poor feeding. Seizures associated with hypocalcemia are treated with 1 to 2 mL/kg of 10% calcium gluconate given slowly intravenously over several minutes because of the possibility of bradycardia. Oral and intravenous calcium supplementation may be achieved with 40 to 75 mg/kg/d of elemental calcium, usually given for less than 3 days. Parathyroid agenesis requires lifelong therapy to prevent hypocalcemia. The subacute and chronic conditions of hypocalcemia are treated with calcitriol (1,25-dihydroxyvitamin D), starting with a dose of 0.25 μg once or twice daily (see Chap. 20.12).

When hypocalcemia and hypomagnesemia coexist, the magnesium deficit should be corrected first with intravenous or intramuscular magnesium sulfate, using 5 mg/kg of elemental magnesium given slowly over 10 minutes. Chronic therapy may be initiated with oral doses of 20 to 40 mg/kg/d of elemental magnesium (as magnesium sulfate, gluconate, lactate, citrate, or glycerophosphate).

## Hypercalcemia

Hypercalcemia in the neonate usually is the result of excessive calcium supplementation, especially in the very premature newborn. Babies with Williams syndrome (idiopathic infantile hypercalcemia syndrome with elfin facies and supravalvular aortic stenosis) occasionally may have hypercalcemia, possibly as the result of an increased sensitivity to vitamin D. Primary hyperparathyroidism also may be seen in the neonatal period, with potentially very severe hypercalcemia.

### Diagnosis and Therapy

Neonates with hypercalcemia may be asymptomatic or they may have vomiting, hypotonia, hypertension, or seizures. Hypercalcemia may develop in infants who are receiving calcium supplementation, particularly ill premature newborns who are being given parenteral nutrition only. These babies should have their serum calcium concentrations monitored daily and appropriate reductions made in their supplementation if there is evidence of developing hypercalcemia. In symptomatic term infants, total and ionized calcium levels, and total protein and phosphorus concentrations should be obtained to evaluate possible hypercalcemia. If elevated serum calcium levels are verified, maternal serum calcium as well as serum PTH concentrations in both the infant and the mother should be determined. Neonatal total calcium values between 10.5 and 11.0 mg/dL suggest hypercalcemia, and values greater than 11.0 mg/dL definitely are in the range of hypercalcemia. In the presence of such high calcium values, the serum concentration of PTH should be 10 pg/mL or less; primary hyperparathyroidism is indicated by PTH concentrations greater than 50 pg/mL.

Treatment of neonatal hypercalcemia should be prompt, and should include hydration at 1.5 to 2 times maintenance, using 5% dextrose with one half normal saline and 3 mEq of potassium chloride per deciliter; furosemide given at 1 mg/kg per dose intravenously twice or three times daily to inhibit renal tubular calcium resorption; and phosphate supplementation to maintain normal serum phosphorus values. Primary hyperparathyroidism may require surgical correction for definitive management.

## Magnesium Balance

Critically ill neonates and infants of insulin-dependent diabetics, drug abusers, and alcoholics appear to be at risk for hypomagnesemia. Perhaps maternal nutritional status contributes to the depressed total serum magnesium levels measured in some of their neonates, in that low amniotic fluid magnesium values have been found in diabetic women. A potential problem in interpretation of magnesium data is that of definition. Whereas magnesium exists in the extracellular compartment in ionized, protein-bound, and miscellaneously bound forms (similar to calcium), hypomagnesemia generally has been defined based on total magnesium levels. Because the ionized fraction of magnesium is considered to be physiologically more relevant, determinations of total magnesium may not represent a valid parameter for the assessment of neonatal magnesium balance. We evaluated the magnesium levels obtained by ultrafiltration (the protein-free fraction closely approximates the ionized fraction) in 84 critically ill and 33 normal neonates, and found 31% of critically ill newborns to have hypomagnesemia by ultrafiltration (<0.55 mmol/L) compared to normal neonates. Although low total serum magnesium levels (<0.6 mmol/L) correlated with levels obtained by ultrafiltration, they were neither sensitive nor specific in predicting hypomagnesemia by ultrafiltration. Clinically, neonates with hypomagnesemia by ultrafiltration required mechanical ventilation significantly more often than did patients with normal magnesium levels.

Neonatal hypomagnesemia may result from intestinal magnesium malabsorption, either caused by a rare X-linked defect presenting after the first few weeks of life and requiring lifelong magnesium replacement or associated with surgical short bowel with subsequent inadequate magnesium absorption. Hypomagnesemia caused by renal wasting may be seen as a result of aminoglycoside therapy or, rarely, as an autosomal dominant trait. Intrauterine growth retardation and hepatic disease predispose to neonatal hypomagnesemia. Hypoparathyroidism in the newborn infant results in hypocalcemia, sometimes with concomitant hypomagnesemia, because low magnesium concentrations reduce both the secretory response of the parathyroid gland to hypocalcemia and the end-organ responsiveness to PTH; refractory hypocalcemia may be the first clue to a primary magnesium deficit.

Hypermagnesemia (total serum magnesium levels >2.1 mEq/L or 1.05 mmol/L) is seen in babies of mothers being treated with magnesium sulfate or magnesium-containing antacids. A functional ileus often is present, and generalized central nervous system depression may result in lethargy, apnea, and diminished responsiveness. Parenteral alimentation may provide excessive

magnesium intake relative to excretion/utilization and result in elevated levels.

### Diagnosis and Therapy

Signs of neuromuscular irritability may be evident in neonates with hypomagnesemia. Studies of seizures in the first week revealed that as many as half of all neonates seizing with hypocalcemia had coexistent hypomagnesemia. Hypomagnesemia exists when total neonatal serum magnesium concentrations are less than 1.2 mEq/L (0.6 mmol/L). Therapy of hypomagnesemia coexisting with hypocalcemia is discussed above. No treatment recommendations for transient isolated asymptomatic hypomagnesemia exist, whereas lifelong oral replacement therapy is needed for magnesium malabsorption and hypoparathyroidism. Therapy of hypermagnesemia, on the other hand, is supportive, with intubation and mechanical ventilation as needed for apnea and airway control as well as parenteral fluid administration during the period of symptomatic ileus.

## WATER HOMEOSTASIS

Tonicity, the relationship between water and dissolved solutes, is protected jealously at all ages. Balance is accomplished by adjustments of both sides of the equation. Solutes, generally considered individually as glucose, sodium, urea, and the like, are regulated by familiar systems discussed elsewhere. Water is regulated by changes in intake, normally dictated by thirst, and by output in urine. Water losses in expired air or in the stool are not under facultative control. Losses via the skin are variable; while under facultative control, the amounts are mandated by the separate, almost equally jealously guarded need to maintain constancy of body temperature.

The neonate is at particular risk for disturbances of water homeostasis, both because turnover is so large relative to body stores and because of differences that affect both intake and output. Thirst is a far less discriminating sense than it will become with maturity; the neonate will accept hypertonic saline as readily as water. Furthermore, because of limited neuromuscular integration, the neonate is totally dependent on caretakers and can make needs known only by primitive behaviors such as sucking and crying.

Fortunately, the response generally provoked is the provision of breast milk, a fluid that is ideally suited for the maintenance of normal tonicity, with little call on the antidiuretic hormone system for modulation. This system ordinarily operates through the sensing of hypertonicity and the secretion of vasopressin, leading to renal water conservation.* Not surprisingly, this output limb of the regulatory system is not a great deal more effective in the neonate than is the intake arm; the term infant requires about 1 month's experience defending against hypertonicity before the losses of water in urine can be reduced to the small quantities characteristic of later life.

In this context, it must be recalled that urine is a solution, much as are the body fluids whose tonicity it serves to protect. Urinary water losses are regulated not as independent volumes, but relative to the osmotic activity of the solutes being excreted. Systemic hypotonicity is combated maximally when each osmotic solute particle in urine is accompanied by 10 mL of water (dilute urine); hypertonicity is combated when the water loss in urine is reduced to as little as 1 mL per milliosmole of solute. This wide range of facultative adjustment of urine tonicity makes possible

---

* A second stimulus to secretion is volume depletion. This operates through stretch receptors in the left atrium. It is reserved for emergencies but, when called upon suddenly, as by hemorrhage, it overrules tonicity, and this outpouring of vasopressin is so large that it has a pressor as well as an antidiuretic influence.

the protection of the very narrow range of normal systemic tonicity. The latter is expressed conventionally as 275 to 285 mOsm/kg, but it can be re-expressed to emphasize the water variable as 3.50 to 3.65 mL of water per milliosmole of solute.

Disturbances of systemic tonicity resulting from malfunction of the endocrine regulatory system are rare in the neonate relative to those resulting from other causes. These include inadequate or improper responses to thirst or to the extension of water losses by diarrhea, heat, or malfunction of the kidney, the endocrine effector organ. Nonetheless, diabetes insipidus—both the type caused by vasopressin deficiency and the receptor disorder—and examples of vasopressin overproduction are seen in the neonate. As indicated earlier, breast milk is ideally constituted to meet the needs of the particular species for which it has been formulated. Cow's milk is ideal for the calf, but not for the human neonate, tending, for example, to precipitate the late form of hypocalcemia known as tetany of the newborn. So perfect is the species match of milk to neonatal needs that diabetes insipidus is essentially asymptomatic in the breast-fed human neonate. With the introduction of solid foods, which yield solute in excess of needs for growth, the formation of concentrated urine begins to be required to prevent systemic hypertonicity. Very frequently, before diabetes insipidus is recognized, mother and pediatrician have been baffled by unexplained recurrent bouts of fever. Treatment in early life is continuance of breast milk or dilute formula and use of a thiazide diuretic rather than desmopressin, the long-acting vasopressin analogue. Desmopressin should be reserved for later use after a discriminating thirst mechanism and the ability to express preferences to parents or other caretakers has developed in the infant.

The causes of diabetes insipidus in the neonate are the same as those in later life (see Chap. 116.5). When there is no evidence of birth trauma or intracranial hemorrhage, the inherited forms should be considered; in boys, the X-linked nephrogenic type is particularly likely.

The syndrome of inappropriate antidiuretic hormone release (SIADH) may be seen transiently soon after intracranial hemorrhage, severe asphyxia, or trauma resulting in isolation of the neural lobe of the hypophysis. In these circumstances, there is loss of facultative control of vasopressin release. The transient excess of hormone may be followed by permanent diabetes insipidus. SIADH also is encountered in neonates with atelectasis or pneumothorax requiring positive-pressure ventilation. This presumably is the result of reduced pulmonary blood flow and decreased signals from the stretch receptors of the left atrium. SIADH is a frequent complication of infant botulism; venous pooling secondary to the generalized hypotonia similarly may reduce activation of the left atrial stretch receptors.

The treatment of SIADH is to reduce water intake relative to solutes. It should be recalled that, whereas metabolizable solutes such as glucose and lactate can be useful in affording intravenous infusates isotonicity with plasma, these solutes are degraded to $CO_2$, which is largely exhaled, and to more water. Hence, their residue is not useful in helping the kidney to correct the water excess of SIADH. If it is necessary because of seizures to return tonicity to normal abruptly, this should be done by the intravenous infusion of hypertonic saline.

## THE NEONATE WITH AMBIGUOUS GENITALIA

One of the most important decisions a clinician makes is the one announced in the delivery room: "It's a boy!" or "It's a girl!" This section deals with those rare situations in which this decision cannot be made with certainty. In this context, it is well to remember that the potential for development of the structures by which we recognize maleness and femaleness is common to all

zygotes, whether 46XX or 46XY. For example, should an accident rendering them functionless befall the gonads of an early embryo with a normal 46XY constitution, the neonate will be pronounced a girl without hesitation. On the other hand, female fetuses exposed to androgen, whether endogenous or environmental,[†] will undergo virilization to an extent dependent on the timing, duration, and severity of the exposure. Such infants are termed "female pseudohermaphrodites," whereas the term "male pseudohermaphrodite" is used for the "girl" described earlier. Not only is "she" an example of the testicular regression syndrome and correctly designated in scientific terms as a male pseudohermaphrodite, but such an infant is described correctly in social terms as a girl.

There are a number of different aspects of sexuality. Genetic sex refers to the sex chromosome constitution XX or XY, and gonadal sex refers to whether testes or ovaries are present. Phenotypic sex can be subdivided into the external components upon which that important "announcement" chiefly depends and the internal constituents, which may be quite disparate. Gender may differ from sex.

Once the announcement is made in the delivery room, a reaction that is reversible only in its earlier stages is set in motion. The parents are informed, and the way in which they and other caretakers treat the infant begins the process of gender identification in the child. Anything that occurs to threaten gender identification in the child's subsequent psychologic development can have serious consequences. Such events come early, and these experiences range from the child's sensing that the parents are troubled by his or her gender identity to discoveries in play group or nursery school that the child is not like others of the same sex. Later events are the doubts that develop at adolescence and in heterosexual relationships. The latter, whether the result of developmental delay, gynecomastia, hirsutism, or an inadequate introitus or penis, can have a disastrous emotional impact.

These are the reasons that examination of the genitalia in the delivery room should be done with care. Doubt, if any, as to the appropriate gender of rearing should result in an effort to restrain, at least briefly, initiation of the reaction leading to gender identification. It is well to bear in mind that even female infants who have undergone the most extensive virilization can be given a completely acceptable phenotype by the skilled modern plastic surgeon. The opposite cannot be accomplished. Accordingly, in instances in which phallic tissue is inadequate for the construction of a functional penis, the parents should be apprised of the facts and advised to rear the neonate in the female gender role. The success in societal roles of women with the classic syndrome of testicular feminization underscores the wisdom and correctness of this advice.

In male pseudohermaphroditism associated with testicular feminization, there generally is so little ambiguity that gender assignment is made without pause. Patients with a defect in testosterone biosynthesis, for example, $5\alpha$-reductase deficiency, may have significant ambiguity (Fig 20-69). When gender assignments cannot be made with assurance, the pediatrician immediately should call for a "time-out." The situation must be explained to the parents. They must understand that some time—a few days at most—will be required to determine whether the infant is a male who is incompletely developed or a female who has undergone virilization. The nursery staff must be instructed to avoid the personal pronoun in referring to the infant. The birth certificate should be put on hold and facilities should be mobilized to develop information as to genetic, gonadal, and internal body sex. Time is of the essence. Rapid karyotypes can be obtained on lymphocytes within 2 days. Smears of buccal mucosal cells to

---

† In this context, "environmental" may connote exposure to androgen arriving from a maternal endogenous source or from maternal ingestion.

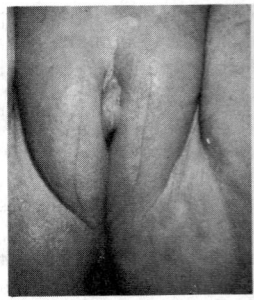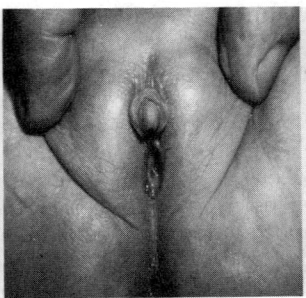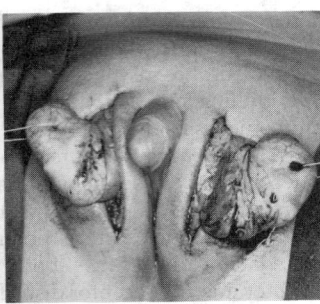

**Figure 20-69.** Male pseudohermaphroditism due to a defect in testosterone biosynthesis. This case serves to underscore the importance of careful examination of the genitalia in neonates. The infant was considered a normal female at birth. A nurse practitioner at 6 months questioned the nature of the symmetric masses in the labia majora. Spreading the labia (*middle panel*) discloses the obvious enlargement of the phallus and the foreshortened introitus. The latter is the result of partial embryonic fusion of the genital folds (labia minora). In the operating room (*right-hand panel*), the labial masses were shown to be testes, and were removed. The introitus ended blindly. Although secretion of adequate testosterone for full virilization was not possible, the secretion of müllerian-inhibiting hormone by the embryonic testes had caused regression of the uterus, tubes, and vagina. In addition to removing the testes, the surgeon carried out reduction of the phallus by resection of the corpora, taking care to preserve the dorsal and ventral neurovascular bundles. Throughout the diagnostic procedures, gonadectomy, and perineoplasty, every effort was made to maintain the parents' confidence that the gender role assigned at birth was correct.

look for Barr chromatin bodies or examination of leukocytes for Y chromosome fluorescence may provide helpful results within a few hours.

Ultimately, both the cytologic and the chromosomal information may be of importance. The functional connotations of the Y chromosome, in terms of both testosterone secretion and neoplastic degeneration of the gonads, mandate determination of whether a Y chromosome is present. The pediatric radiologist's help should be enlisted to ascertain with ultrasound or retrograde injection of contrast materials the nature of the pelvic organs and adrenals. The pediatric surgeon may need to be called upon for panendoscopy to confirm the radiologist's opinion, for gonad biopsy, and for consideration of the feasibility of reconstruction to give the infant an appearance consonant with the gender assignment being considered. Measurement of steroid and gonadotropin levels may be desirable, but is apt to be time-consuming, and time can be expended only when absolutely necessary. The decision as to gender assignment ultimately is made with the parents only after sharing with them all relevant information. This includes, in particular, the concept that the choice should be the gender in which the child can function happily; life can be miserable, indeed, with genitalia or secondary sexual characteristics inappropriate to the person's self-image.

## Clinical Considerations

Given the fact that every conceptus is endowed with the potential for either masculine or feminine phenotypic development, it follows that a diagnosis of genetic sex may be impossible on purely clinical grounds. A careful history may bring to light some valuable clues, such as androgen exposure in the mother or a pedigree in which there is an excess of females, many of whom are childless and amenorrheic. The latter is the usual finding in the classic androgen insensitivity syndrome (testicular feminization).

Physical examination should address such questions as whether the infant has a "chromosomal look" with multiple dysmorphisms. Such an appearance often is evident in the sex chromosome anomalies, especially the 45X (Turner's) and 45X/46XY (mixed gonadal dysgenesis) syndromes. It is even more pronounced in some of the anomalies of the autosomes, for example, in the genital hypoplasia (micropenis) of trisomy 21 or the chromosome 13 q syndrome. Ascertainment of the position of the

gonads is important. Mobile, oval masses felt in what apparently are normal labia majora almost certainly will prove to be testes in keeping with "Federman's rule" that a gonad felt below the inguinal ligament is a testis until proven otherwise. Asymmetry of the external (and internal) genitalia is the hallmark of mixed gonadal dysgenesis. Even if the vulva and introitus appear entirely normal, the vagina should be probed gently with a number 5 Hegar dilator to assess its depth. The vagina tends to be blind (ie, there is no cervix) and shallow (2 cm) in testicular feminization, and long (greater than 6 cm) and topped by a patulous cervix in mixed gonadal dysgenesis. In the female pseudohermaphrodite with congenital adrenocortical hyperplasia, there may be full masculine development of the phallus with no hypospadias and a roomy, rugated, and often deeply pigmented scrotum, but this always will be empty.

## Laboratory Data

The laboratory work required for the identification of sex and gender assignment already has been touched upon. In many instances, karyotyping is desirable for complete diagnosis. Thus, with the initial blood sample, an aliquot should be obtained to initiate this procedure. If subsequent findings indicate that the analysis is unnecessary, the culture can be discarded before harvesting and undertaking the tedious job of microscopic analysis, photographing, and karyotype preparation.

The importance of clear definition of the internal genital structures cannot be emphasized sufficiently. The whole class of female pseudohermaphrodites, and many of the infants with true hermaphroditism and mixed gonadal dysgenesis, will have vaginae and uteri that can be made functional. In females with adrenocortical hyperplasia, the ovaries will be normal and the affected child can look forward to fertility. In the true hermaphrodite, one gonad may be a normal ovary and the other a normal testis; more commonly, both are ovotestes, but the two types of tissue are functionally normal and are separated by a cleavage plane. Hence, surgical separation is feasible, with retention of the gonadal tissue appropriate to the gender assigned to the infant.

The best-known, if not the most common, of the disorders giving rise to ambiguous genital development are the congenital adrenocortical hyperplasia syndromes. The most common type, caused by deficient activity of the 21-hydroxylase enzyme, gives rise to female pseudohermaphroditism; in male neonates with this syndrome, there are no pathognomonic clinical findings until signs of adrenal insufficiency develop. The insufficiency of cortisol and aldosterone production in some infants with this and the other steroid biosynthetic deficiencies mandates that the clinician set up a watch in suspect infants for the rapidly developing hyponatremia and hyperkalemia that herald hypotensive collapse. On occasion, hypoglycemia may underlie the first clinical sign of cortisol deficiency. Hypocholesterolemia can provide an early clue to the excessive demand for substrate by the racing motors of the steroid biosynthetic machinery.

## Types of Genital Ambiguity

It is convenient to think of the common causes of genital ambiguity in the neonate in two major categories: the genetic and the environmental. The genetic causes can be subdivided into those resulting from major chromosomal anomalies, generally single events in a given family, and the single-gene disorders, which may affect more than one sibling. As already suggested, one subgroup of the chromosomal disorders involves aneuploidy, mosaicism, or deletion affecting the sex chromosomes, and another depends on similar morphologically evident abnormalities of the autosomes. These are thought to depend on accidents of disjunction at cell division, especially in meiosis, and generally are non-heritable. The other large category of genetic causes consists of heritable single gene disorders, a number of which already have been mentioned. Single gene disorders are responsible for the steroid biosynthetic defects in which the hormone products are either insufficient or abnormal and influence development of the fetus in a direction contrary to its genetic (chromosomal) sex. Similarly, single genes code for the receptor defects of the androgen insensitivity disorders.

Environmental accidents account for an equally diverse group of abnormalities of genital development. Just as the female fetus can undergo virilization by androgen deriving from her own adrenal glands, from an androgen-secreting tumor in the mother, or via maternal androgen ingestion, so, too, can the male fetus be prevented from full masculine development by inhibitors of androgen production or metabolism. Progesterone exposure has been proposed as having a role in hypospadias, an anomaly that also is a feature of the hydantoin embryopathy seen in the offspring of epileptic mothers taking this inhibitor of 5α-reductase activity.

A particularly instructive cause of genital ambiguity in the neonate is the syndrome of testicular regression. Intrapartum testicular infarction is developmentally the "latest" and probably the most familiar of the disorders constituting the spectrum of testicular regression. What might have been diagnosed as bilateral cryptorchidism had the infarction taken place a few weeks before birth constitutes the late end of a spectrum that extends from early fetal life to birth. The phenotype of the affected neonate depends on the timing of the functional demise of the testis. When this occurs before the time at which secretion of müllerian inhibiting hormone begins, the phenotype of the conceptus is female internally as well as externally. As Figure 20-70 illustrates, the phenotype undergoes an orderly transition from completely female (although anovarian) to completely male with bilateral anorchidism. Each example of the syndrome provides a structural array that differs from those in the others, depending on the moment in genital embryogenesis when testicular function ceased. This is not always the result of mechanical causes, such as twisting of the testicle on its pedicle and infarction. In certain families, it is programmed as a genetically determined event. It probably also occurs as a result of virus infection and as a manifestation of an immunologic disorder. Testicular regression syndrome illustrates, possibly better than any other of the multiple causes of genital ambiguity, that the outward appearance of the neonate

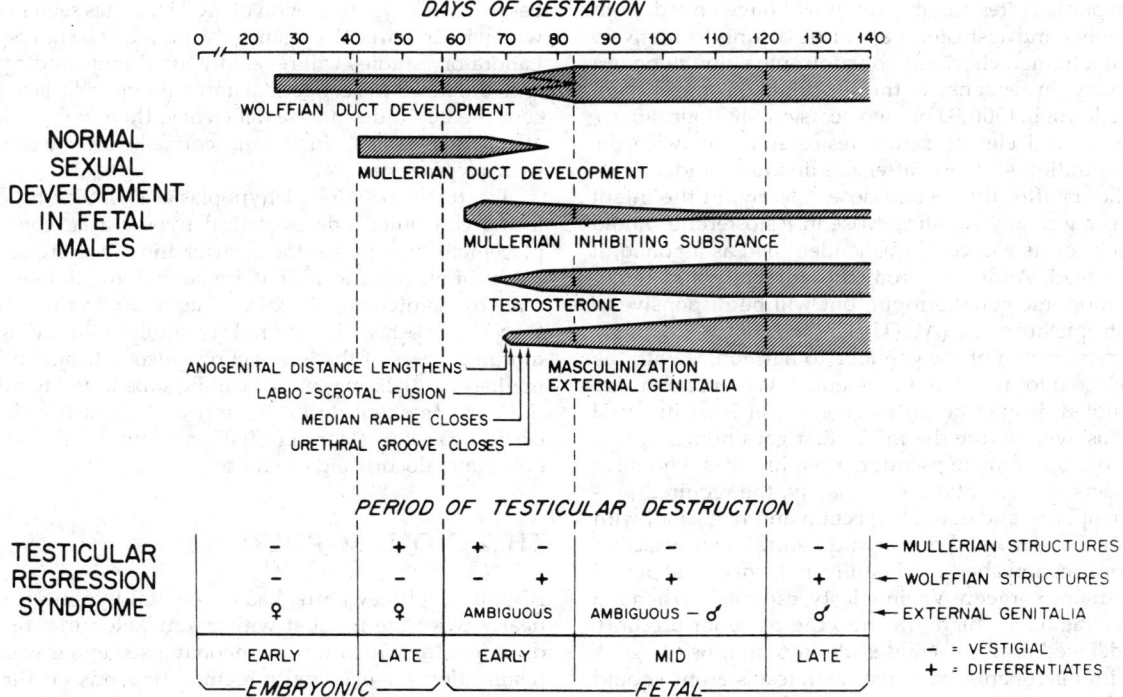

**Figure 20-70.** Timetable of normal genital development and dependence of neonatal appearance on timing in fetal life of loss of testicular function. (Welch WR, Robboy SJ. Abnormal sexual development: A classification with emphasis on pathology and neoplastic conditions. In: Kogan SJ, Hafez ESE, eds. Pediatric andrology. The Hague/Boston/London: Martinus Nijhoff, 1981:71.)

provides insufficient information to permit in every case a declaration of sex or even guidance for the parents in gender role selection.

## Management Considerations

The laboratory determinations required for gender assignment are different from those that ultimately may be needed for a final diagnosis. For gender role selection, one needs at least cytogenetics. One also needs definition of the internal genital structures by ultrasound, standard radiography using contrast materials, or endoscopy. All babies with ambiguity of the genitalia should be monitored for serum sodium, potassium, and glucose concentrations until the possibility of one of the adrenocortical hyperplasia syndromes with cortisol and aldosterone deficiency can be ruled out. In instances of mixed gonadal dysgenesis in which it is elected to rear the infant as a male, leaving the testis for its testosterone secretion (fertility is unreported in these persons), the parents and, later, the children must be taught to examine the gonad regularly to detect the tumors that arise so frequently in these gonads. Streaks, whether unilateral (the classic situation in mixed gonadal dysgenesis) or bilateral, always should be removed when the karyotype contains a Y chromosome or fragment. In mixed gonadal dysgenesis, streaks have the same high neoplastic potential that they do in more normal-appearing testes; the fact that the streak seems to be composed only of fibrous tissue is no indication that it should be left in place.

In an infant for whom the decision has been made to reconstruct and rear in the female gender role, any tissue should be removed that might begin to secrete androgen under pituitary gonadotropin stimulation at adolescence. It sometimes may be desirable in the neonate to address the question of whether there is any such tissue. High levels of gonadotropins (luteinizing hormone and follicle-stimulating hormone >20 mIU/mL) with negligible serum concentrations of testosterone (<20 ng/dL) indicate a negative answer. When this question has gone unaddressed in an infant of 6 months or older, the postnatal period of hypothalamic-pituitary-testicular activity will have ended. Both the gonadotropins and testosterone will be at uninformatively low levels, and a human chorionic gonadotropin stimulation test may be necessary. In response to the subcutaneous injection of chorionic gonadotropin (500 IU on two occasions 48 hours apart), the normal testis will elevate serum testosterone to twice the baseline concentration 48 hours after the first dose and will redouble it 72 hours after the second dose. Clearly, in the infant being raised as a girl, any significant rise in testosterone should lead to a search for its source; if this is identified as a gonad, it should be removed. Androgen from the adrenal gland is not increased by chorionic gonadotropin, but will be responsive to adrenocorticotropic hormone (ACTH).

Skillful reconstruction of the genitalia to harmonize with the gender role selected for the infant is essential. When parents are especially troubled, it may be an emergency, at least in social terms, to do this even before the infant first goes home. This is the case most often in female pseudohermaphrodites who have undergone extensive virilization. Fortunately, the required procedures (perineoplasty and clitoral resection and recession, with preservation of the glans and dorsal and ventral neurovascular bundles) can be accomplished successfully in the neonatal period by a skilled pediatric surgeon. Vaginoplasty, especially when the opening of the vagina is "high" (ie, into the posterior urethra), preferably is delayed until the child is about 6 months of age.

In males with micropenis, treatment with testosterone should not be delayed, because the responsiveness of the phallic tissues diminishes with age. Testosterone in one of the repository forms (testosterone cypionate or enanthate) can be given once a month,

at 15 to 25 mg per dose deep subcutaneously, until satisfactory growth has been achieved. The aim of the surgeon attending to the staged procedures, which may include relief of chordee, repair of hypospadias, and placement of small-sized testicular prostheses, should be to complete the work by the time the patient is 2 years of age, or shortly thereafter.

## ADRENAL DISORDERS

The most frequently occurring of the adrenal disorders of the neonate, the congenital adrenal hyperplasia syndromes, were considered in the previous section. Three other conditions deserve mention despite their rarity. These are bilateral adrenal hemorrhage as an accident of birth, leaving the neonate adrenally insufficient, and two genetic forms of adrenal hypoplasia. The cytomegalic type of congenital adrenal hypoplasia is an X-linked recessive trait in which the glands are composed of a fetal zone with large, vacuolated cells but no permanent adrenal cortex. In the other form, the miniature type, the adrenals resemble those seen in anencephaly and other disorders of hypothalamic and pituitary development, and may reflect either ACTH insufficiency or ACTH subresponsiveness. Surviving males with the cytomegalic form fail to undergo puberty in the years of normal adolescence. Their hypogonadism has been shown to be caused by deficiency of the hypothalamic gonadotropin-releasing hormone. It has been suggested that smallness of the genitalia may help in recognition of the syndrome in affected infants.

Adrenal insufficiency in the neonate seldom gives rise to symptoms in the first few days of life, when most newborns are in hospital nurseries being observed closely by trained personnel. Poor feeding and failure to gain weight often are recognized in retrospect after the sudden onset of vomiting, dehydration, and apathy at 1 week or 10 days of age. Questioning of the parents may bring to light the demise of a previously born sibling under similar circumstances. Clinical examination will be remarkable for signs of dehydration and prostration. Intense pigmentation bespeaks the hypersecretion of ACTH, and is seen in most infants with either adrenal cytomegaly or ACTH subresponsiveness. Laboratory studies will reveal hyponatremia and hyperkalemia, and, unlike all the congenital adrenal hyperplasia syndromes except the 20,22-desmolase deficiency, there will be low levels of all corticosteroids, including cortisol, testosterone, and 17-hydroxyprogesterone.

Treatment of adrenal hypoplasia is similar to that for salt-losing congenital adrenocortical hyperplasia, consisting of replacement therapy for the cortisol and aldosterone deficiencies. Doses of glucocorticoid that are large (5 to 10 times greater) relative to maintenance needs are necessary in the crisis situation. Once homeostasis is restored, carefully adjusted, single, daily, morning doses of the long-acting glucocorticoid analogue dexamethasone ($0.25 \text{ mg/m}^2/\text{d}$) can be substituted to advantage for the more frequent doses of short-acting glucocorticoid. Fludrocortisone acetate (Florinef), 0.05 mg daily for the neonate, is the oral mineralocorticoid of choice.

## THYROID DISORDERS

About 1:5000 newborns has congenital hypothyroidism; this is nearly twice the number with phenylketonuria, the first of the disorders for which routine neonatal screening was developed. Justification for neonatal screening depends on three principal factors other than the obvious criterion that clinical signs of the disorder are either absent or are overlooked easily. These factors include the cost of the test, the incidence of the condition being screened for, and the saving of life or improvement in its quality that can be achieved with treatment. Little argument is required for justification of screening programs for congenital hypothyroidism. With regard to subtlety of diagnosis, experienced pediatric endocrinologists have been amazed by the normalcy of affected infants brought to their attention by positive screening tests. The cost of the newborn thyroid screening test is modest; in comprehensive terms, it is about $3.00 per infant. Inasmuch as the incidence is 1:5000, the cost of each case found is roughly $15,000. The early proponents of screening argued that this was small when compared to the $30,000 quoted in the early 1970s as the annual cost of custodial care of a cretin at one of the state schools for the mentally retarded. The argument was brought home with the thought that the life expectancy of the hypothyroid infant was not 1 year, but the biblical 3 score and 10 years.

Most screening programs use the filter paper discs that are used for the Guthrie test for phenylketonuria. These are spotted with capillary blood in the neonatal nurseries, mailed to a central laboratory, and assayed per primum for thyroxine.[‡] In the specimens showing the lowest thyroxine values (ie, somewhere between 3% and 10% of the total), the thyrotropin value also is determined. If the serum thyroxine concentration is low and the thyrotropin level is elevated ($>20$ µU/mL), the primary pediatrician and family are notified by telephone. The turnaround time between obtaining the specimen from the infant and notifying the caretakers generally is no more than 10 days. Upon notification, it is incumbent upon the physician to obtain a fluid blood specimen promptly to confirm the results of screening and, without further ado, to start the use of levothyroxine (10 to 15 µg/kg/d).

Many feel that it is of value at this time to attempt to image any thyroid tissue and obtain an estimate of bone age. The thyroid tissue can be imaged by scintigraphy, using technetium or $^{123}$I. Imaging may indicate the complete absence of tissue (athyreosis, 15%), thyroid ectopia (43%, the most common anomaly in this group is intralingual or sublingual tissue), or a normally positioned gland that is either biosynthetically crippled (dyshormonogenesis, 22%) or is in the process of involution as the result of an autoimmune process (atrophic congenital hypothyroidism, 20%).

The only circumstance in the neonate in which the classic hand-and-wrist film for bone age may be of interest is in congenital hyperthyroidism. In infants with congenital hypothyroidism, much as in the normal neonate, none of the carpal centers or epiphyses of the wrist and hand will be calcified, so such a film has no value. The film that can be obtained expeditiously and provides the most information is the lateral view of a lower extremity from just above the knee to the foot. In this view, the bones of special interest are the calcaneus (which normally ossifies at between 24 and 26 weeks' gestation), the talus (which ossifies at 26 to 28 weeks), the cuboid (which ossifies at 35 to 40 weeks), the distal femoral epiphysis (which ossifies at 36 weeks), and the proximal femoral epiphysis (which ossifies at 38 weeks). It is believed that the duration and severity of the hypothyroidism are related to the retardation in bone maturation thus estimated. For example, in a term neonate brought to attention by screening, such a film showing ossification only of the calcaneus is both confirmatory of the diagnosis and suggestive of severe deficiency.

Neonates found to have low serum thyroxine and high thyrotropin values may not have permanent hypothyroidism. Five percent to 10% of neonates with these findings have them on the basis of transplacental transfer of maternal blocking antibodies against thyrotropin receptors of the thyroid gland. These antibodies are gamma globulins; with the gradual decline in all the maternally inherited gamma globulins that takes place during the first 3 months after birth, the block to normal pituitary–thyroid interrelationships is removed. Nevertheless, treatment for these infants is as essential as for those with athyreosis.

It is with these children particularly in mind that most pediatric endocrinologists advocate a review at 3 to 4 years of age of all patients designated as hypothyroid at birth. At this time, in contrast to during the first few months after birth, a brief period of hypothyroidism is not deleterious to the structural development of the central nervous system. Children in whom a misdiagnosis of permanent congenital hypothyroidism was made and who have been treated since birth with replacement doses of thyroxine react in a characteristic fashion when the previously employed levothyroxine dose is halved or discontinued altogether. They will show a slight decline in the thyroxine values, reaching a nadir at about 2 weeks, with a rise in thyrotropin, peaking at about 3 weeks; both values return to normal at 4 to 6 weeks in those with fully competent hypothalamic-pituitary-thyroid systems. Those in whom the diagnosis of permanent thyroid deficiency is upheld will show a much steeper drop in serum thyroxine concentration and rise in thyrotropin, so that there is little trouble at 2 weeks and almost none at 1 month in distinguishing between the two types of response.

Severe acute illness at any time of life is accompanied by a precipitous drop in serum thyroxine concentration unaccompanied by a rise in thyrotropin. Thus, neonates and preterm infants with respiratory distress syndrome or sepsis account for the majority of "positive" results noted in the neonatal screening programs, with subnormal values for serum thyroxine, but normal thyrotropin concentrations. Sometimes these findings seem to be attributable not to illness, but simply to immaturity. These findings also may be a manifestation of the common X-linked trait, deficiency of thyroxine-binding globulin; in male infants, the incidence may be as high as 1:5000 newborns. Such neonates should not be given thyroxine with the same alacrity as are those who show up in screening tests with both low thyroxine and elevated thyrotropin concentrations. About 1:30,000 neonates will turn out to have primary hypothalamic or pituitary disease and may need permanent replacement therapy. In the remainder of neonates with low values of thyroxine and normal thyrotropin levels, the thyroxine concentration will be restored to normal relatively rapidly. Most screening program directors, therefore, recommend that the primary pediatrician be notified promptly of the finding of a low value for thyroxine with a normal thyrotropin concentration, but that the pediatrician's reaction to the news be to consider the possibilities just discussed and to submit a second specimen to verify and extend the findings of the first screening test before beginning thyroxine treatment.

Just as there are false-positive screening test results, there also are false-negative results (ie, affected neonates may escape screening or positive results may be misinterpreted as being normal). Furthermore, even screening that is performed well is not infallible. About 1:150,000 newborns, or 3 of every 100 who ultimately will prove to have congenital hypothyroidism, on initial screening will have either a thyroxine level sufficiently high that the thyrotropin determination is not done, or low thyroxine but normal thyrotropin levels. These infants will escape detection until a second sample is analyzed or symptoms sufficient for clinical recognition develop. Thus, even in areas where screening is mandated, pediatricians caring for neonates still must be alert to the signs and symptoms of hypothyroidism, and must not dismiss the diagnosis as impossible because the program is in place.

Screening programs have enabled pediatricians to detect and initiate treatment within 30 days of birth in about 95% of all affected newborns in the program areas. The result has been an

---

[‡] The initial assay is for thyrotropin in European and Japanese programs; the relative merits of primary determination of thyroxine rather than thyrotropin in terms of case finding and cost still are being debated.

enormous improvement in the outlook for such infants. In the large patient cohort of the New England Hypothyroidism Collaborative Study, the affected, but quickly treated children have been compared, using a battery of neuropsychiatric tests, with their next-in-age siblings and have scored equally well.

Congenital hyperthyroidism is much less common than hypothyroidism. Nevertheless, it occurs with sufficient frequency to deserve mention. It usually is seen as a transient disturbance, the result of the transfer of maternal thyrotropin-stimulating immunoglobulins that act like thyrotropin to stimulate the pituitary thyrotropin receptors. It can be anticipated in infants born of mothers with Graves' disease, whether the disorder in the mother is active, is suppressed by propylthiouracil or another blocking agent, or is asymptomatic as a result of treatment, possibly years earlier, with radioiodine or by radical subtotal surgical thyroidectomy. Characteristics of the affected infant are excessive length for gestational age and less than normal weight for length. Clinically, these infants are scrawny in appearance, jittery in behavior, wide-eyed, and tachycardic, and they may not have an appreciable goiter until they are several days of age. Treatment is with propranolol (1 mg/kg/24 h in four divided doses, increasing daily as necessary to control tachycardia up to 5 mg/kg/24 h) either alone or in combination with propylthiouracil (5 mg/kg/24 h in four divided doses). This form of neonatal thyrotoxicosis may be severe, but usually runs its course in 3 months in keeping with the elimination of the maternal antibodies responsible for the condition. In rare instances, a dominantly inherited form of permanent Graves' disease is encountered, giving the same picture in the neonate, but persisting and requiring continuing thyroid-suppressive treatment or, ultimately, definitive therapy with either radioiodine or surgical subtotal thyroidectomy.

## Selected Readings

### Calcium and Magnesium

Demarini S, Tsang RC. Disorders of calcium and magnesium metabolism. In: Fanaroff A, Martin R, eds. Neonatal-perinatal medicine, 5th ed. St Louis: Mosby-Year Book, 1992:1181.

### Glucose

Cowett RM, Stern L. Carbohydrate homeostasis in the fetus and newborn. In: Avery GB, ed. Neonatology, pathophysiology and management of the newborn, ed 2. Philadelphia: JB Lippincott, 1987:691.
Srinivasan G, Pildes RS, Cattamanchi G, et al. Plasma glucose values in normal neonates: A new look. J Pediatr 1986;109:114.

### Thyroid

Naruse H, Irie M, eds. Neonatal screening. Amsterdam: Excerpta Medica, 1983:519.

### Stress

Anand KJS, Brown MJ, Carson RC, et al. Can the human neonate mount an endocrine and metabolic response to surgery? J Pediatr Surg 1985;20:41.

### Genital Ambiguities

Donahoe PK, Crawford JD. Ambiguous genitalia in the newborn. In: Welch KJ, Randolph JG, Ravitch MM, O'Neil JA, Rowe MI, eds. Pediatric surgery. St Louis: Mosby-Year Book, 1986:1363.
Griffin JE. Androgen resistance—the clinical and molecular spectrum. N Engl J Med 1992;326:611.
Josso N, ed. The intersex child. In: Pediatric and adolescent endocrinology, vol 8. Basel: S Karger, 1981:273.
Welch WR, Robboy SJ. Abnormal sexual development: A classification with emphasis on pathology and neoplastic conditions. In: Kogan SJ, Hafez ESE, eds. Pediatric andrology. The Hague/Boston/London: Martinus Nijhoff, 1981:71.

### Adrenal

New MI, Levine LS, eds. Adrenal diseases in childhood: Pediatric and adolescent endocrinology, vol 13. Basel: S Karger, 1984:235.

*Principles and Practice of Pediatrics, Second Edition.*
edited by Frank A. Oski et al. J. B. Lippincott Company, Philadelphia © 1994.

# 20.8 *Infant of the Diabetic Mother*

Joseph B. Warshaw

About 1 in 200 pregnancies is complicated by overt diabetes; gestational diabetes develops in an additional 2% to 3% of pregnancies. This statistic refers to a patient in whom diabetes develops during pregnancy and disappears after delivery. Despite advances in perinatal care over the past 20 years, infants of diabetic mothers (IDMs) remain a significant cause of perinatal morbidity and mortality. Diabetes in pregnancy is classified according to the Priscilla White classification (Table 20-45). The term *class A diabetic* often is used interchangeably with *gestational diabetic* or *chemical diabetic*, but this is not totally accurate because gestational diabetics may require insulin.

Overt diabetes in pregnancy should be managed in a perinatal center by a high-risk pregnancy health care group that is equipped to monitor the pregnancy and has a newborn facility capable of caring for the newborn in the event of an adverse outcome. All women should be screened for gestational diabetes between the 24th and 28th weeks of pregnancy. Those who have a plasma glucose level in excess of 150 mg/dL 1 hour after the oral administration of 50 g of glucose should be followed closely and have second evaluations. Insulin therapy may be required to treat gestational diabetics who have persistent hyperglycemia.

Fetal glucose levels reflect those of the mother. High levels of fetal glucose in response to maternal hyperglycemia stimulate the fetal islet to secrete insulin. Fetal islet cell volume has been shown to be proportional to maternal glucose concentrations, and macrosomia has been associated with increased insulin and C peptide levels in cord blood. Insulin functions as a fetal growth

**TABLE 20-45.   Priscilla White Classification**

| Class | Onset | | Duration |
|---|---|---|---|
| A | Any age | | Any length |
| B | > Age 20 y | and | <10 y |
| C | Age 10–20 y | or | 10–20 y |
| D | < Age 10 y | or | >20 y |
| F | Any (nephropathy) | | Any |
| R | Any (proliferative retinopathy) | | Any |

hormone, resulting in the characteristic macrosomia of IDMs. In utero, IDMs are not overgrown until some time after the 26th or 27th week; this staging may be related to the development of insulin receptors.

The risk for having a fetus with macrosomia is increased when the mean maternal glucose concentration exceeds 130 mg/dL. Measurement of glycosylated hemoglobin (HbA₁c) provides an important index of long-term diabetes control. Normal levels of HbA₁c generally are less than 8%. Many studies have demonstrated that increased perinatal morbidity is associated with elevated HbA₁c levels. The obstetric goal should be maintenance of fasting glucose levels below 100 mg/dL and other plasma glucose levels below 130 mg/dL.

IDMs have a characteristic appearance, with macrosomia, abundant adipose tissue, and a cherubic facial appearance; their head circumference, however, is similar to that of age-matched normal infants because insulin does not influence brain growth. A typical IDM is shown in Figure 20-71. The insulin-induced increase in glucose and amino acid transport into fetal tissues results in increased adipose tissue deposition and macrosomia. Adipose tissue of IDMs often exceeds the 16% of body weight that is fat in normal infants. The IDM has an increased glycogen content in the liver, kidney, skeletal muscle, and heart. The "growth hormone" effects of insulin result in increased linear growth.

Macrosomia may be associated with birth trauma and birth asphyxia. Perinatal asphyxia may occur in 25% of infants of insulin-dependent diabetics and correlates with maternal hyperglycemia before delivery and with maternal nephropathy. Maternal and fetal hyperglycemia during the intrapartum period may result in increased fetal oxygen requirements and place the fetus at greater risk during delivery. Nephropathy and hyperglycemia are associated with decreased placental blood flow, which may increase the risk of asphyxia further. Premature birth also is associated with birth asphyxia in IDMs.

Throughout early childhood, IDMs are large and may have increased adipose tissue. This tendency may have implications for the development of later obesity.

Problems of IDMs are summarized in Table 20-46. Despite their very large size, IDMs are functionally immature. The risk of hyaline membrane disease developing in these infants is six times that of normal infants until the 38th week of gestation. Fetal hyperglycemia and hyperinsulinism have been associated with pulmonary immaturity and decreased synthesis of surfactant phospholipids and their associated proteins. Hyperbilirubinemia also is an index of immaturity and occurs in about 20% of IDMs. Contributing factors include newborn polycythemia and hepatic immaturity.

At birth, the neonate is separated from the constant supply

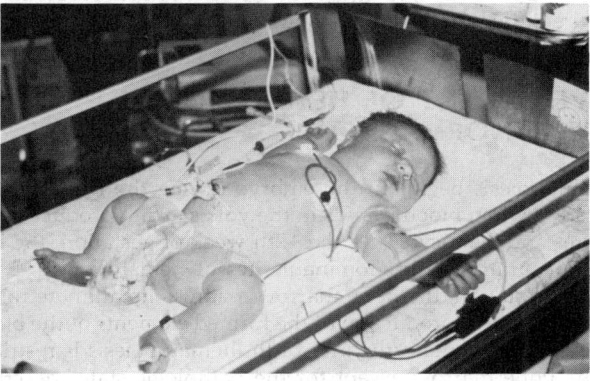

**Figure 20-71.** Infant of a diabetic mother.

### TABLE 20-46. Problems of the Infant of the Diabetic Mother

Birth trauma and asphyxia
Hypoglycemia
Hypocalcemia
Hyperbilirubinemia
Hyaline membrane disease
Polycythemia
Renal vein thrombosis
Septal hypertrophy and myocardiopathy
Congenital malformations

of glucose from the maternal circulation. Although IDMs have abundant adipose tissue and glycogen stores, they are less able than normal infants to use these substrate stores. These abnormalities largely are the result of the metabolic effects of insulin, which are summarized in Table 20-47. Insulin is an anabolic hormone that promotes growth and the movement of glucose and amino acids into tissues in the late stages of gestation and in the neonate. Normal neonates rapidly mobilize glycogen from the liver and other sites to maintain blood sugar; however, glycogenolysis is inhibited in the IDM. Fatty acid metabolism, ketone body oxidation, and gluconeogenesis also are important for the maintenance of normal glucose levels. These processes are impaired in the IDM. Newborn hyperinsulinism inhibits free fatty acid release from adipose tissue and limits the availability of fatty acids as an alternative substrate for glucose. Ketone body production from fatty acids also is decreased, making this important alternate energy source unavailable. These insulin-related influences result in increased glucose use, decreased glucose production, and decreased availability of alternate substrates. Factors responsible for hypoglycemia in IDMs are summarized in Table 20-48. Glucose should be monitored by Dextrostix within the first 45 minutes of life. Hypoglycemia is defined as a blood sugar level of less than 40 mg/dL. The best treatment is early feeding. A blood sugar level of less than 25 mg/dL requires intravenous glucose administration. All infants weighing more than 4 kg or with the physical characteristics of IDMs should be monitored carefully. The administration of a mini-bolus of glucose followed by continued intravenous glucose infusion is the preferred therapy when intravenous glucose is indicated. This regimen will minimize the risk of rebound hypoglycemia. Infants should receive 200 mg/kg of glucose (2 mL of 10% glucose per kilogram of body weight) over 1 minute followed by a constant infusion of 8 mg/kg/min (D₁₀/W at normal maintenance rates). Only rarely will more glucose be required.

Hypocalcemia occurs in a high percentage of IDMs. Hypocalcemia, defined as a calcium level of less than 7 mg/dL, may occur in about 50% of IDMs and contribute to agitation, irritability, and, in the occasional infant, decreased myocardial contractility. Treatment rarely is necessary, but, when indicated, consists of 1 to 2 mL/kg of 10% calcium gluconate given intravenously and 50 to 60 mg/kg/d given orally for maintenance.

### TABLE 20-47. Effects of Insulin on Metabolism

| Increase | Decrease |
|---|---|
| Glycogen synthesis | Glycogenolysis |
| Lipogenesis | Lipolysis |
| Protein synthesis | Gluconeogenesis |

| TABLE 20-48.   Causes of Hypoglycemia in Infants of Diabetic Mothers |
|---|
| Increased glucose utilization |
| Decreased glycogenolysis |
| Delayed onset of gluconeogenesis |
| Decreased fatty acids and ketone bodies |

Hypomagnesemia (<1.5 mg/dL) also can occur, but rarely is of clinical significance.

IDMs may have symptomatic polycythemia. Fetal hyperglycemia and hyperinsulinism result in increased oxygen consumption, which may lead to fetal hypoxia and increased levels of fetal erythropoietin. Polycythemia is treated by partial exchange transfusion using saline or salt-poor albumin to decrease the central hematocrit to below 65%.

The IDM also is at increased risk for the development of renal vein thrombosis. The pathogenesis may relate to polycythemia or to decreased cardiac output secondary to cardiomyopathy. Treatment is supportive. Cardiomegaly is common in IDMs, often associated with thickening of the intraventricular septum and subaortic stenosis. This complication may be a cause of the sudden late gestational deaths and stillbirths that occur occasionally. Septal hypertrophy is found by echocardiography in 30% to 40% of patients.

Congenital malformations are frequent in the diabetic pregnancy. The incidence of congenital heart disease and other major malformations is 2 to 3 times greater than that of the general population (3% to 5%) and has been related to poor maternal diabetes control during organogenesis. The incidence of all congenital malformations may be in excess of 10% in the poorly controlled diabetic pregnancy. The caudal regression syndrome, in which there is a general hypoplasia of the sacrum and lower extremities, is found almost exclusively in IDMs (Fig 20-72). These infants also may exhibit the small left colon syndrome. Most major congenital malformations occur very early in gestation and, therefore, cannot be attributed to fetal hyperinsulinemia. The fetal pancreas does not make insulin until after the 100th day of gestation, and the functional importance of insulin probably develops only after the 26th and 27th weeks of pregnancy. Malformations in the IDM probably relate to hyperglycemia during critical periods of organogenesis. There should be optimal control of maternal diabetes even before conception occurs to be certain of good control during the period of organogenesis, when congenital malformations occur.

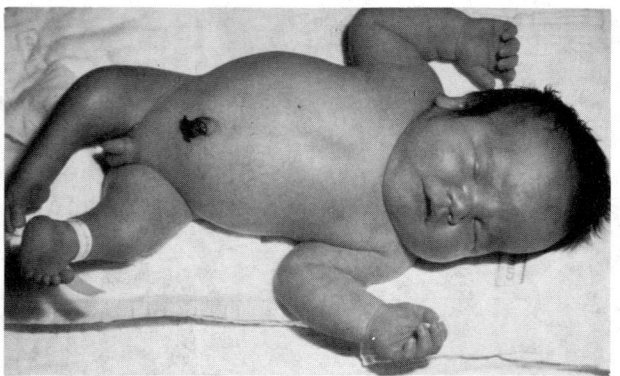

**Figure 20-72.**   The caudal regression syndrome.

Intrauterine growth retardation can occur if maternal diabetes is associated with severe vascular disease; these pregnancies should be monitored carefully and may require early delivery if fetal well-being is jeopardized.

## Selected Reading

Cowett RM, Schwartz R. The infant of the diabetic mother. Pediatr Clin North Am 1982;29:1213.

Freinkel N, Lews NJ, Akazawa S, et al. The honeybee syndrome: Implications of the teratogenicity of mannose in rat-embryo culture. N Engl J Med 1984;310:223.

Minouni F, Miodovnik M, Siddiqi T, et al. Perinatal asphyxia in infants of insulin-dependent diabetic mothers. J Pediatr 1988;113:345.

Morris MA, Grandis AS, Litton JC. Glycosylated hemoglobin concentration in early gestation associated with neonatal outcome. Am J Obstet Gynecol 1985;153:651.

Pedersen J. The pregnant diabetic and her newborn, ed 2. Baltimore: Williams & Wilkins, 1977:15.

Piper JM, Langer D. Does maternal diabetes delay fetal pulmonary maturity? Am J Obstet Gynecol 1993;168:783.

*Principles and Practice of Pediatrics, Second Edition.*
edited by Frank A. Oski et al. J. B. Lippincott Company, Philadelphia © 1994.

# 20.9 *Hematopoietic Diseases*

## George R. Buchanan

Hematologic problems are encountered daily by pediatricians caring for sick newborn infants. Alterations in the hematopoietic system are most often reactive, secondary, and even iatrogenic, but they are useful markers of underlying systemic diseases, including infection, asphyxia, and genetic and metabolic disorders. These secondary hematologic problems often have serious sequelae, so they must be recognized promptly and appropriately treated. Primary hematologic disorders, on the other hand, are rare during the newborn period. Yet, conditions such as hemophilia, immune-mediated thrombocytopenia resulting from transplacental maternal antibody, and inherited hemolytic anemia must be recognized by the pediatrician so that he or she can initiate appropriate management, both acutely and with regard to long-term therapy and genetic counseling.

This chapter reviews the hematopoietic system in the fetus and newborn infant, focusing on common clinical problems that require differential diagnosis and management.

## DEVELOPMENT OF HEMATOPOIESIS IN THE NORMAL FETUS

Hematopoiesis begins in the embryo during the third week of gestation when blood islands in the yolk sac first produce erythrocytes and leukocytes. By the 12th week of gestation, the liver and spleen are the predominant sites of hematopoiesis; by 30 weeks' gestation, the bone marrow assumes its ultimate role as the major site of production of the formed elements of the blood. At the time of or shortly after birth, hematopoiesis is restricted to the bone marrow except for the pathologic states described here.

## Production of Red Blood Cells

The predominant cellular element in the blood is the erythrocyte or red blood cell (RBC). The factors controlling erythropoiesis are similar in the fetus and newborn to those of older children. Pluripotent stem cells give rise to morphologically indistinct precursors committed to the erythroid lineage. Under the stimulus of erythropoietin and other humoral factors, these erythroid burst-forming units and colony-forming units give rise to identifiable erythroblasts, which proliferate, begin to synthesize hemoglobin, and mature into differentiated nucleated RBCs. In the final stages of maturation, the nucleus is extruded and the cell enters the circulation as a young erythrocyte. The major constituent of the erythrocyte is hemoglobin, which binds oxygen in the lungs and transports it to the tissues. Hemoglobin is composed of a tetramer consisting of two pairs of unlike polypeptide chains, each attached to a heme molecule of protoporphyrin and ferrous iron, the oxygen-binding site.

The major difference between erythropoiesis in the neonate and older child and adult is the dynamic but poorly understood "switch" from fetal to adult hemoglobin production. The primary hemoglobin in postnatal life is hemoglobin A, consisting of two $\alpha$ chains (whose genes are encoded on chromosome 16) and two $\beta$ chains (each of which derives from a 60-kilobase-long gene complex on chromosome 11). As shown in Figure 20-73, early in fetal life the hemoglobin tetramer contains several types of embryonic globin chains (eg, $\in$ and $\zeta$) whose synthesis soon declines. During the initial months of gestation, the embryonic $\in$ polypeptides are replaced by $\gamma$ chains, resulting in the predominant fetal hemoglobin or hemoglobin F ($\alpha_2\gamma_2$). Yet, as early as the 14th week of gestation, the $\beta$ globin genes are activated, $\beta$ chains are produced, and hemoglobin A ($\alpha_2\beta_2$) is detectable. Alpha-chain production is sustained at a high level throughout most of fetal life. At the time of birth, $\gamma$- and $\beta$-chain synthesis is about equal, and 60% to 80% of the total hemoglobin is hemoglobin F.

Gamma globin synthesis ceases during the initial months of life (see Fig 20-73). By 6 months of age, the percentage of hemoglobin F approximates that of the adult (less than 2%). An increased understanding of the $\gamma$-to-$\beta$ switch would have an impact on the treatment of a number of diseases (eg, sickle cell anemia and $\beta$-thalassemia) in which it is desirable to retain large quantities of hemoglobin F in the erythrocyte.

Fetal hemoglobin differs from hemoglobin A in a number of ways. Hemoglobin F is resistant to both alkali and dilute acid, forming the basis for two tests for its measurement (the Betke-Kleihauer stain for fetal hemoglobin in individual cells and

quantitative measurement of hemoglobin F in a hemolysate). Hemoglobin F can be differentiated from hemoglobin A by radioimmunoassay. It binds less avidly than hemoglobin A to 2,3-diphosphoglycerate, an organic phosphate in the erythrocyte important in modulating oxygen uptake and release by hemoglobin. Therefore, the affinity of hemoglobin F for oxygen is quite high.

The fetal RBC differs from its adult counterpart in a number of other characteristics. Fetal RBCs have higher levels of certain glycolytic enzymes, a relative deficiency of key defense mechanisms against excessive oxidation (eg, glutathione peroxidase, catalase, methemoglobin reductase), diminished deformability, and a shorter life span in the circulation.

## Leukocyte, Platelet, and Coagulation Protein Production

Like RBCs, granulocytes and platelets are derived from committed precursor cells in the yolk sac, liver, spleen, and then bone marrow. The developmental process and control mechanisms are similar to those noted in older children and adults. Blood coagulation factors and inhibitors, equal in importance to platelets in the fine balance of the hemostatic mechanism, are generally produced in diminished quantities during fetal life. The liver produces most blood coagulation factors as well as inhibitors such as antithrombin III and protein C; the physiologic immaturity of the liver in the fetus and neonate results in reduced levels of most of these factors.

## ANEMIA

### Normal Values

Because of intrauterine hypoxia and the high affinity of hemoglobin F for oxygen (resulting in a shift to the left of the oxygen-hemoglobin dissociation curve), erythropoietin secretion is enhanced during fetal life. Accordingly, during the final months of gestation and at birth, values for hemoglobin and hematocrit are higher than for older children. Representative values are shown in Table 20-49. The mean cord blood hemoglobin concentration in a term infant is 16.5 g/dL in a range of 14 to 22 g/dL. Premature infants have slightly lower values. Values depend on method of delivery, site of blood sampling, postnatal age, and other factors. Capillary specimens have a higher (by 1 to 2 g/dL) and generally wider range of hemoglobin values than samples obtained from the umbilical or peripheral vein. When performing

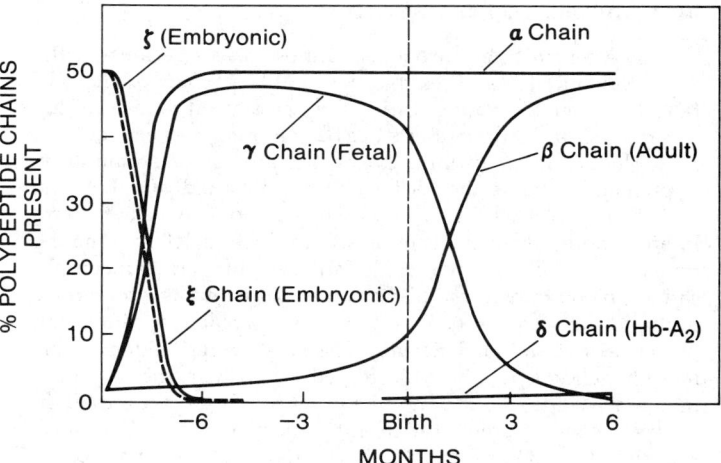

**Figure 20-73.** Changes in human globin synthesis during prenatal and neonatal development. (Bunn HF, Forget GB, Ranney HM. Human hemoglobins. Philadelphia: WB Saunders, 1977:107)

TABLE 20-49.  Normal Hemoglobin Values in the Newborn Infant

| Site and Time of Sampling | Hemoglobin Concentration (g/dL) | |
| --- | --- | --- |
| | Mean | Range |
| Cord blood | 16.5 | 14–22 |
| Venous specimen | | |
| 2 days of age | 18 | 14.5–23 |
| Capillary specimen | | |
| 2 days of age | 19 | 14.5–25 |
| 7 days of age | 16.5 | 14–22 |

serial hemoglobin measurements during the initial hours and days of life, such differences should be kept in mind; ideally, the same site of sampling is used consistently. Even though venous sampling is technically more difficult, it is preferred because neonatal blood is viscous (due to the high hematocrit and reduced deformability of individual cells) and peripheral circulation in sick neonates is frequently sluggish.

The blood volume in the newborn infant is 80 to 90 mL/kg at birth. During the initial hours of life, there is a decrease in plasma volume, resulting in an increase in the hematocrit compared to cord blood values (see Table 20-49). This alteration is followed by a progressive, slow decline termed the physiologic anemia of infancy. The life span of the fetal and neonatal RBC is about 80 days compared to 120 days in the mature adult RBC. Reasons for this shortened RBC survival are unclear; it is not due simply to the presence of fetal hemoglobin.

At birth, more RBCs are produced than in older patients, as shown by the elevated reticulocyte count and the appearance of nucleated RBCs on the peripheral smear. Erythropoiesis can be accelerated further by various causes of fetal hypoxia or anemia. The usual reticulocyte count in cord blood or during the first or second day of life is 2% to 8%, and 3 to 10 nucleated RBCs per 100 leukocytes are generally present. By 3 or 4 days of life, nucleated RBCs disappear, and the reticulocyte count falls (and remains low) until 3 months of age when recovery from physiologic anemia manifests. The erythrocytes of neonates are larger than those of older children. Mean cell volume is typically 100 to 115 femtoliters (fL) compared to 70 to 85 fL in children older than several months.

## Physiologic Anemia of Infancy and Anemia of Prematurity

Shortly after birth, erythropoiesis almost ceases because of the oxygen-rich milieu and relative excess of RBCs. The progressive fall in hemoglobin values during the first several months of life in term and premature infants has been termed, respectively, the physiologic anemia of infancy and the anemia of prematurity. In premature infants, the decline occurs more rapidly (with lowest values at 4 to 8 weeks as opposed to 10 to 12 weeks in term infants), and the anemia is more severe. Factors determining the time course and severity include birth weight, perinatal complications, blood transfusion history (premature infants who receive multiple transfusions generally exhibit a greater decline), and presence of vitamin E deficiency. Erythropoietin production during this period is relatively decreased. Nadir hemoglobin values may reach 9.5 g/dL at 3 months in term infants and 6 g/dL in 6- to 8-week-old premature infants. Recovery from physiologic anemia is heralded by a slight elevation in the reticulocyte count

and rise in hemoglobin value to levels seen throughout the remainder of infancy. To support erythropoiesis during the recovery stage of physiologic anemia, abundant iron must be available from existing stores, dietary sources, or exogenous supplements, particularly in rapidly growing premature infants, thus necessitating their daily iron requirement of 2 mg/kg/d.

The physiologic anemia of infancy does not respond to iron or folic acid. Healthy term infants and asymptomatic growing premature infants require no therapy. It has been demonstrated, however, that apneic episodes—as well as other signs and symptoms of hypoxia such as tachycardia, irritability, and poor feeding—may be eliminated by judicious use of packed RBC transfusions. Therefore, the anemia of prematurity may not always be physiologic or "normal."

## Differential Diagnosis of Anemia

Pathophysiologic mechanisms of anemia are similar to those of older patients. Hemoglobin concentration reduction can be due to diminished production, excessive blood loss (internal or external), or hemolysis (shortened RBC life span). Decreased production as a primary cause of anemia is uncommon during the newborn period. It is characterized by a relatively reduced reticulocyte response and paucity or absence of nucleated RBCs on the peripheral blood smear. Acute blood loss is common; it can be clinically obvious, occult, or iatrogenic. Hemolytic anemia during the newborn period may be due either to intrinsic inherited defects in the RBC or acquired causes. Hemolysis in the newborn infant is identified easily by the marked jaundice that usually results from hepatic immaturity.

Figure 20-74 is an algorithm of the differential diagnosis of anemia during the newborn period.

## Anemia Due to Blood Loss

Anemia due to blood loss is more common during the newborn period than at any other time in childhood. Signs and symptoms relate to the duration and amount of blood lost. Acute hemorrhage greater than 20% to 30% of the infant's blood volume results in signs and symptoms of shock (pallor, lethargy, tachycardia, hypotension). Jaundice is absent. External blood loss most commonly occurs from the gastrointestinal tract, sometimes from an identifiable anatomic lesion (eg, ulcer or duplication), but often without apparent cause. In instances of hematemesis or melena, whether the complication is swallowed maternal blood or blood from the baby is determined by the Apt test for fetal hemoglobin (Table 20-50). Hemorrhage may occur from one twin to another or into the umbilical cord, placenta (eg, abruption, placenta previa, or laceration during cesarean section), or maternal circulation (fetal–maternal hemorrhage). A Betke-Kleihauer stain for fetal hemoglobin-containing RBCs in the mother may allow for an estimate of the amount of transplacental hemorrhage. This complication is not uncommon; in 1 in 100 deliveries, blood lost can be more than 20% of the baby's blood volume, resulting in clinically significant anemia apparent at birth or manifesting later as iron deficiency. Occult blood loss of hemodynamic significance may also occur within the cranial vault of the neonate because of the relatively large head size and open sutures. Bleeding in the abdominal cavity, retroperitoneal space, subcutaneous tissues (eg, scalp), or other internal locations may result in jaundice (because of catabolism of hemoglobin from the resorbed hematomas) as well as anemia.

In sick premature infants, the most common cause of blood loss is the iatrogenic withdrawal of multiple specimens to monitor blood gases and other laboratory parameters. Such blood sampling can amount to more than 10% to 20% of the tiny infant's

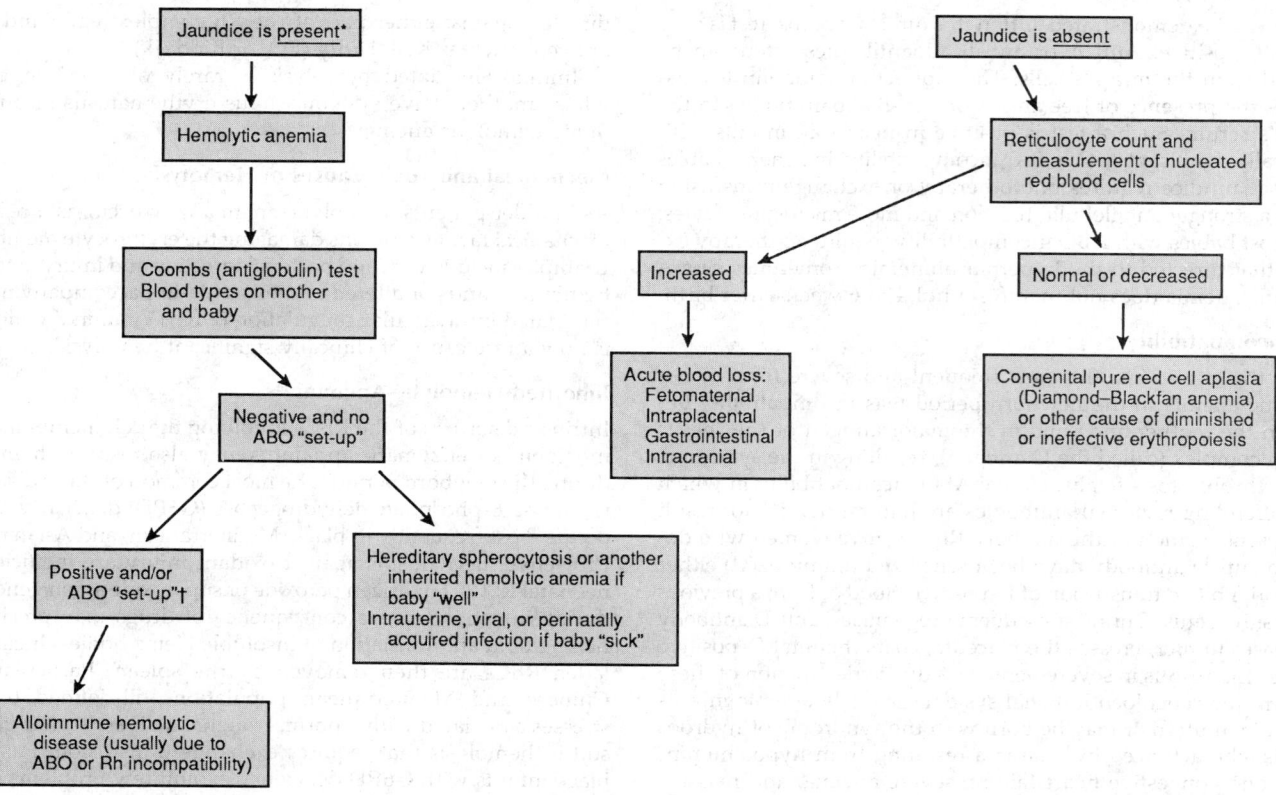

* In addition, reticulocyte count and number of circulating nucleated red blood cells are nearly always elevated.
† Mother group O and baby group A, B, or AB.

**Figure 20-74.** Diagnostic approach to anemia in the newborn infant (hemoglobin ≤ 14 g/dL with or without symptoms). The most likely diagnoses are provided in the boxes.

blood volume during each 24-hour period and represents the most frequent indication for blood transfusions in such babies.

The treatment of anemia due to acute blood loss depends on the amount and duration of blood loss. Infants with signs of hypovolemia should receive immediate volume replacement (crystalloid, plasma protein fraction, whole blood, or packed red blood cells). Packed RBC transfusions alone may be indicated for less acute degrees of anemia such as that resulting from repetitive blood sampling.

## Hemolytic Anemia During the Newborn Period

Destruction of RBCs intravascularly or by the mononuclear-phagocyte system (primarily spleen and liver) results in production of 32 mg of bilirubin from every 1 g of degraded hemoglobin.

---

**TABLE 20-50.   Apt Test for Differentiation of Fetal and Adult (Maternal) Hemoglobin in Stool or Vomitus**

Mix 1 volume of stool or vomitus with 5 volumes of water

Centrifuge mixture and remove clear-pink supernatant solution containing hemoglobin

Mix 1 mL of 1% sodium hydroxide with 4 mL of supernatant and observe color change after 2 min

   *Remains pink*—hemoglobin F

   *Turns yellow-brown*—hemoglobin A (maternal blood)

*Adapted from Apt KL, Downey WS. Melena neonatorum: the swallowed blood syndrome. J Pediatr 1955;47:6.*

---

The physiologically immature liver of the fetus and newborn is incapable of rapidly conjugating this excess pigment. Therefore, hyperbilirubinemia, usually with clinical jaundice, accompanies all severe hemolytic states during the initial days of life. Hemolysis in the neonate, as in older patients, is also accompanied by reticulocytosis, nucleated RBCs on the peripheral blood smear, and sometimes characteristic RBC morphologic changes.

### ABO Incompatibility

Usually, hemolysis during the newborn period is due to RBC injury resulting from antibody binding or mechanical effects. Immune-mediated hemolytic anemia results from maternally derived alloantibody directed against antigens on fetal and neonatal RBCs. In current practice, ABO incompatibility is seen most frequently. Generally, a blood group O mother exhibits IgG anti-A or anti-B alloantibody that crosses the placenta and binds to her infant's type A or B erythrocytes as well as to other tissues that contain blood group A or B. On the other hand, in women with blood groups A, B, or AB, anti-A or anti-B alloantibodies (also called isohemagglutinins) are generally of the IgM class and do not cross the placenta. Affected babies present with jaundice during the first several days of life. Anemia is usually absent or mild, but most patients exhibit an elevated reticulocyte count (usually 5% to 15%) and increased numbers of nucleated RBCs on the blood smear. Also characteristic on the peripheral smear are microspherocytes resulting from partial membrane loss.

Laboratory diagnosis of ABO incompatibility is confirmed by demonstrating the appropriate "ABO set-up" (ie, type O mother and type A or B baby) and a positive antiglobulin (Coombs') test. In the direct antiglobulin test, IgG antibody on the infant's washed

RBCs can be demonstrated. Often this direct Coombs' test is only weakly positive. Anti-A or anti-B alloantibodies often can be eluted from the infant's cells. The indirect antiglobulin test assesses the presence of free anti-A or anti-B alloantibodies in the baby's serum. Such a test is positive in nearly all infants with clinically significant A-O or B-O incompatibility. In general, babies whose jaundice requires phototherapy or exchange transfusion have a stronger antiglobulin reaction and more microspherocytes.

Most babies with ABO incompatibility require no therapy except that directed to the hyperbilirubinemia. Sometimes symptomatic anemia does not manifest until 4 to 6 weeks after birth.

## Rh Incompatibility

Until the late 1960s, the most frequent and severe form of hemolytic anemia in the newborn period was incompatibility between the mother and child in the major antigen of the rhesus or Rh complex (called the D antigen), resulting in the syndrome of erythroblastosis fetalis. Unlike ABO incompatibility in which the offending maternal antibodies are natural (ie, do not result from sensitization of the mother), Rh-negative women who develop anti-D antibody have been sensitized (immunized) either by a prior blood transfusion of D-positive blood or from a previous D-positive fetus. During subsequent pregnancies, anti-D antibody increases in titer, crosses the placenta, coats the fetal D-positive RBCs, and results in severe hemolysis due to destruction of these cells in the reticuloendothelial system. Severely anemic infants may die in utero or may be born with the syndrome of hydrops fetalis, characterized by anasarca resulting from hypoalbuminemia and congestive heart failure, severe anemia, and massive hepatosplenomegaly (resulting from cardiac failure and extramedullary erythropoiesis). The mortality rate is extremely high. Whether hydropic or not, a large percentage of these Rh-sensitized babies develop extreme jaundice, requiring multiple exchange transfusions.

The problem of Rh hemolytic disease has become less pronounced during the past two decades because of several key research advances. First, anti-D immune globulin is now administered routinely to all Rh-negative women immediately after delivery or after abortion; therefore, few women are now sensitized. Those women who do exhibit rising titers of anti-D antibody can be identified early in the pregnancy and monitored by amniocentesis, serial amniotic fluid optical density measurements, and estimation of the relative risk of fetal death. Intrauterine transfusions of packed RBCs can be administered to correct the anemia, and planned early induction of labor—followed by vigorous management of the jaundiced, anemic, and often premature infant—has resulted in a lower morbidity and mortality rate. Affected babies typically have a strongly positive direct antiglobulin test; the indirect test usually shows the presence of large amounts of free anti-D antibodies in the baby's and mother's serum. The degree of anemia is variable, but hyperbilirubinemia usually is present. An elevation of the direct fraction of bilirubin is seen in the most severely affected infants, probably resulting from intrahepatic cholestasis (inspissated bile syndrome). The peripheral blood smear shows polychromasia and nucleated RBCs (erythroblastosis) but no microspherocytes. Treatment consists of exchange transfusion for marked hyperbilirubinemia or anemia, simple packed RBC transfusions for less severe degrees of anemia, and careful follow-up during the first 2 or 3 months of life when delayed anemia resulting from persisting anti-D antibody may require additional transfusions.

With the diminished frequency and severity of anti-D antibody sensitization, fetal–maternal incompatibility due to minor blood group antigens has now become relatively more common. The pathophysiology and treatment are similar to those of ABO incompatibility and Rh incompatibility disease. The antibodies are directed against either part of the Rh complex (eg, c and E) or antigens such as Kell, Duffy (Fy), or Kidd (Jk).

Immune-mediated hemolysis is rarely observed in babies whose mothers have systemic lupus erythematosus or autoimmune hemolytic anemia.

### Mechanical and Toxic Causes of Hemolysis

As in older patients, hemolytic anemia may occur as a result of mechanical factors or toxins damaging the erythrocyte membrane. Examples include viral and bacterial infection and injury mediated by fibrin strands or altered microvasculature accompanying disseminated intravascular coagulation (DIC). Vitamin E deficiency is now a rare cause of clinically significant hemolysis.

### Inherited Hemolytic Anemias

Intrinsic disorders of the RBCs involving the cell membrane, hemoglobin, or enzymatic apparatus may also result in hemolysis during the newborn period. The most common of these disorders is glucose-6-phosphate dehydrogenase (G6PD) deficiency, which occurs most frequently in black, Mediterranean, and Asian males. Protective mechanisms against oxidant injury are inefficient in neonatal RBCs. Hydrogen peroxide or superoxide anion generated during infection or as a consequence of drugs may precipitate hemoglobin and formation of insoluble Heinz bodies. Inclusion-laden RBCs are then removed by the spleen. Particularly in Chinese and Mediterranean populations, ill-defined oxidant stresses associated with a normal vaginal delivery sometimes result in hemolysis that requires exchange transfusion. Full-term black infants with G6PD deficiency exhibit few problems in the absence of pathologic oxidant stress. Prematurely born black infants who are deficient in the enzyme, however, may exhibit marked hyperbilirubinemia. The diagnosis of G6PD deficiency is made by widely available screening tests and enzyme assays. False-negative results may occur in the affected black infant with reticulocytosis.

In whites of Northern European extraction, hereditary spherocytosis is the most common congenital hemolytic anemia presenting with jaundice and anemia during the newborn period. Although this condition is inherited as an autosomal dominant trait, the family history is negative for spherocytosis in nearly half of cases. Affected babies are jaundiced and have varying degrees of anemia. The blood smear typically contains numerous microspherocytes. Evidence of ABO incompatibility (a much more common cause of spherocytes on the neonatal blood smear) is absent.

Hemolytic anemia in neonates resulting from other RBC enzymopathies or membrane alterations occurs rarely. Because sickle cell anemia involves the β-globin chain, affected neonates have no apparent clinical or hematologic abnormalities. Special screening hemoglobin electrophoresis techniques are used for diagnosis of sickle cell disease, which is best made early in life to allow for education, counseling, and prompt initiation of prophylactic penicillin.

## Anemia Due to Decreased Production

Anemia resulting from diminished production of RBCs is uncommon at birth. The laboratory hallmark is a diminished or absent reticulocyte count. As in older patients, this deficiency may be due to a bone marrow replaced with malignant cells, absence of marrow precursors, nutritional deficiency, ineffective erythropoiesis, or diminished erythropoietin stimulation. Leukemia and aplastic anemia rarely occur this early in life. Iron deficiency resulting from chronic fetal–maternal hemorrhage is also uncommon. Hematologic features of iron deficiency (eg, microcytosis, reduced serum ferritin) are the same as those observed later in life. Relative bone marrow suppression occurs commonly during sepsis and may contribute to anemia seen in babies with diverse forms of infection.

The Diamond-Blackfan syndrome (congenital pure red cell aplasia) is an uncommon form of hypoproliferative anemia that usually presents at birth or soon thereafter. This disorder results from an absence of erythroid stem cells and is characterized by a macrocytic anemia and absence of reticulocytes, typically with normal values for leukocytes and platelets. These babies may be of low birth weight, and physical examination may show thumb anomalies or a phenotype similar to that of Turner's syndrome. The disorder occurs equally in males and females.

The major mechanism of anemia in thalassemia syndromes is ineffective erythropoiesis with diminished RBC production, although a hemolytic component exists also. Thalassemia results from quantitative reduction in the synthesis of one or more globin chains (usually $\alpha$ or $\beta$), resulting in microcytic anemia of variable severity. When there is diminished expression of the $\beta$-globin gene during fetal and neonatal life, $\beta$-thalassemia (like qualitative hemoglobinopathies such as sickle cell disease) does not express itself clinically during the newborn period. Babies with heterozygous forms of $\alpha$-thalassemia, however, do have microcytosis (ie, mean cell volume [MCV] less than 95 fL) and an abnormal hemoglobin electrophoresis with 2% to 6% hemoglobin Barts, a rapidly migrating, unstable tetramer of $\gamma$ chains. The $\alpha$-thalassemia trait, resulting from deletion of one or two of the four $\alpha$-globin genes, is common in black infants. The homozygous forms of $\alpha$-thalassemia result in the infant's being severely anemic, massively hydropic, or even stillborn. This syndrome is seen exclusively in Southeast Asians. In recent years, several such babies have survived as a result of vigorous resuscitation measures followed by chronic blood transfusions.

## NEONATAL POLYCYTHEMIA

Polycythemia, a pathologic increase in RBC mass, can cause multiple clinical problems that necessitate acute intervention and may have long-lasting effects. Polycythemia during the newborn period is defined as a venous hematocrit greater than 65%, ideally confirmed on two consecutive specimens. The etiology is usually ill-defined (Table 20-51). Maternal–fetal hemorrhage in utero is rarely documented, so the primary mechanisms are placental transfusion at birth (due to delayed clamping of the umbilical cord) or enhanced erythropoiesis associated with elevated erythropoietin production in utero. This condition presumably results from intrauterine hypoxia and is often seen in dysmature or postmature babies or infants of diabetic mothers.

The clinical features result from hyperviscosity in large vessels and in the microcirculation. The problem of excess RBCs can be compounded by their reduced deformability. Clinical features include plethora, tachypnea, irritability, jitteriness, and seizures. Laboratory abnormalities (in addition to high hemoglobin values) may include hypoglycemia, thrombocytopenia, and hyperbilirubinemia resulting from the breakdown of excess RBCs. Cerebral blood flow is reduced, and pulmonary artery pressure is usually increased.

Many infants are asymptomatic, and their management and outcome of treatment is controversial. There is little argument that symptomatic infants with polycythemia should be treated by partial-exchange transfusion consisting of isovolemic removal of the baby's blood and replacement with plasma protein fraction, saline, or lactated Ringer's solution. Fresh frozen plasma as replacement fluid should be avoided, and simple phlebotomy should never be undertaken without concomitant volume replacement. The amount of blood exchanged (in 10- to 20-mL increments) can be calculated by the following formula:

$$\text{Total volume removed (mL)} = \frac{\text{Baby's estimated blood volume (mL)} \times \text{Desired reduction in hematocrit (\%)}}{\text{Observed hematocrit (\%)}}$$

Reduction in the venous hematocrit to levels below 55% usually results in prompt disappearance of existing signs and symptoms. Most specialists would not recommend a partial exchange transfusion in asymptomatic infants incidentally found to have polycythemia. Yet, several studies demonstrate subtle long-term motor and psychological effects in young children who had polycythemia during the neonatal period; this subject warrants further investigation.

## BLOOD TRANSFUSIONS DURING THE NEONATAL PERIOD

The most common situation for blood transfusion in the newborn nursery is the sick premature infant in whom frequent blood sampling for monitoring requires replacement therapy. In this and in most other circumstances, packed RBCs (rather than whole blood) are recommended. Efforts must be undertaken to prevent the transmission of viral infection, especially cytomegalovirus (CMV), human immunodeficiency virus (HIV), and hepatitis C. To reduce exposure to multiple donors, many hospitals have instituted "walking donor" programs or other mechanisms to ensure availability of type O Rh-negative erythrocytes for multiple infants from limited numbers of regular volunteer blood donors. Reliance on CMV-antibody–negative donors or washed, previously frozen erythrocytes also enhances safety. Current blood bank screening practices have essentially eliminated HIV transmission in this setting, and hepatitis also occurs infrequently. Other complications of blood transfusion therapy are similar to those observed in older patients.

Currently under study is the use of recombinant human erythropoietin as treatment for the anemia of prematurity. A brisk erythropoietic response to parenterally administered hormone would obviate repetitive RBC transfusions to replace blood withdrawn for studies and to treat apnea of prematurity. There are no firm data regarding dose, efficacy, and toxicity, so this treatment must be viewed as investigational.

Platelet transfusions and granulocyte transfusions are discussed in subsequent paragraphs.

## ABNORMALITIES OF LEUKOCYTES

Neutrophils or granulocytes are the predominant form of leukocytes, or white blood cells (WBCs), important in the defense

---

**TABLE 20-51. Etiology of Polycythemia in the Newborn Infant**

| Etiology | Relative Frequency |
|---|---|
| Idiopathic | Most common |
| Delayed cord clamping | Common |
| Infant of diabetic mother* | Common |
| Intrauterine growth retardation* | Common |
| Down syndrome* | Less common |
| Maternal-to-fetal transfusion | Rare |
| Twin-to-twin transfusion | Rare |

* Demonstrated to be mediated by increased levels of erythropoietin

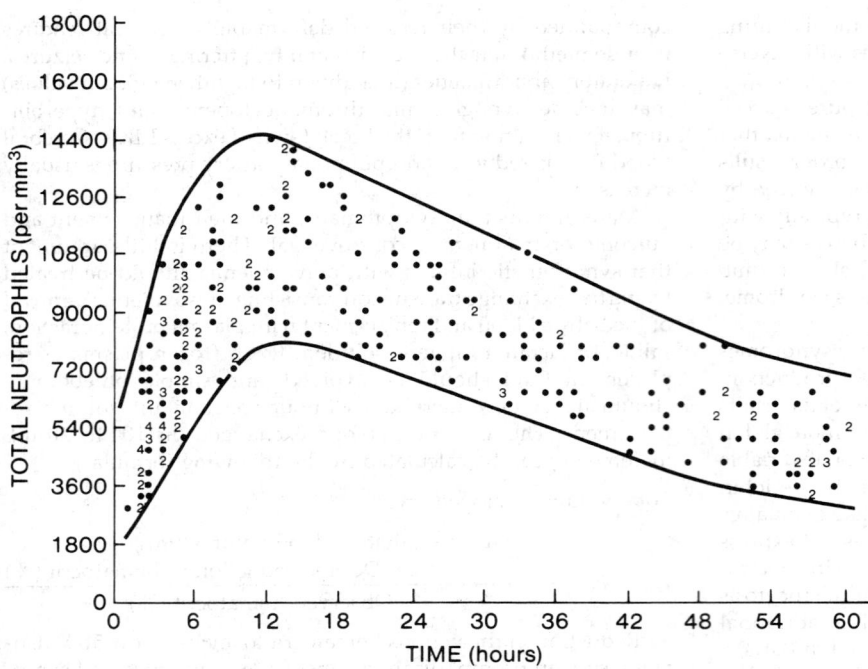

**Figure 20-75.** Total neutrophil count reference range in the first 60 hours of life. Points represent single values; numbers represent the number of values at the same point. (Manroe BL, et al. The neonatal blood count in health and disease. I. Reference values for neutrophilic cells. J Pediatr 1979;95:89)

against bacterial infection. The final stages of granulocyte maturation in the bone marrow result in condensation, folding, and segmentation of the nucleus. Normally, only the most differentiated segmented forms are released from the bone marrow. During periods of stress or infection, however, less mature, nonsegmented or band forms enter the circulation.

Varying neutrophil counts (best expressed in absolute terms, ie, number per mm³ of whole blood rather than as percentages of total WBC count) depend on postgestational age and other factors. Granulocytes are present early in fetal life and are the predominant form of circulating WBCs during the neonatal period. Numbers of segmented and band forms are normally higher during the first 2 days of life than at any other time during childhood (Fig 20-75).

The numerous factors affecting granulopoiesis and the circulation and distribution of neutrophils are similar in neonates and older patients. Evidence suggests, however, that the maturation and storage pool (ie, bone marrow reserves) of neutrophils are reduced in neonates, thus contributing to an impaired neutrophilic response during bacterial infection. Numerous alterations in neutrophil function have been described during the neonatal period, including reduced migration and impaired phagocytic capacity. The clinical relevance of these features with regard to risk of bacterial infection is not well understood.

Neutrophilic responses during bacterial infection are described below. Babies with bacterial infection, particularly septicemia, may have a normal total WBC count, but absolute neutropenia and a relative increase in immature band forms is often observed. This elevated band-to-segmented form ratio is useful in the diagnosis of bacterial septicemia.

## Neutropenia

Neutropenia (Table 20-52) during childhood is generally defined as an absolute neutrophil count of less than 1500 cells per mm³. Figure 20-75 shows a different definition applies during the first 3 days of life. The most common cause of severe neutropenia is bacterial sepsis; it is often accompanied by a relative increase in immature forms such as bands, metamyelocytes, or even myelocytes. Mild to moderate neutropenia is usually transient, resulting from intrauterine viral infection, maternal hypertension or preeclampsia, birth asphyxia, and certain drugs taken by the

**TABLE 20-52.** Differential Diagnosis of Neutropenia in the Newborn Infant

| Disorder | Relative Frequency | Associated Features |
|---|---|---|
| Severe bacterial infection* | Common | Relative increase in circulating band and other immature forms |
| Transient† neutropenia related to maternal factors | Common | Maternal hypertension or birth asphyxia |
| Congenital (intrinsic defect in myelopoiesis) | Uncommon | Sometimes familial; persists indefinitely |
| Alloimmune (isoimmune) neonatal neutropenia | Rare | Persists up to 3 months; due to maternal antibody against neutrophil antigen |

\* Especially septicemia due to group B streptococci and *Escherichia coli*
† Lasting hours to days

mother. Neutropenia may also be due to transplacental passage of an antineutrophil antibody due to neutrophil antigen incompatibility between the mother and fetus. This condition, termed alloimmune (isoimmune) neonatal neutropenia, results in profound neutropenia (usually less than 200 neutrophils per mm$^3$), with a corresponding increased risk of bacterial infection during the initial weeks of life. The disorder is self-limited. Antineutrophil antibodies, usually directed against the neutrophil-specific NA-1 antigen, can be demonstrated using specialized methods. Rarely, neutropenia is seen on a congenital basis because of inherited defects in myelopoiesis or accompanying some of the inherited organic acidurias. When neutropenia is a manifestation of hypersplenism, infiltrative disorders, or a bone marrow failure, other clinical and hematologic manifestations invariably coexist.

Management of neutropenia in the neonate is the same as that of older infants and children—treat the underlying disorder and vigorously manage infectious complications with antibiotics. Granulocyte transfusions may be useful in certain neonates with sepsis and severe neutropenia associated with neutrophil marrow depletion.

## Other Leukocyte Disorders

Leukocytosis, usually with a predominance of neutrophilic forms or their precursors, is seen in congenital leukemia, leukemoid reactions resulting from infection, and the unusual myeloproliferative syndrome observed in neonates with Down syndrome. Marked lymphocytosis is noted occasionally in intrauterine infection.

## BLEEDING DISORDERS IN THE NEONATE

Bleeding and thrombosis are common problems in sick newborn infants, and laboratory alterations in the hemostatic mechanism occur frequently even in the absence of hemorrhage. Because platelet and clotting-factor changes are sensitive measures of many disease processes, they may be thought of as acute-phase reactants.

## Pathophysiology and Normal Hemostatic Values

The hemostatic mechanism is a complex process by which blood vessels, platelets, and coagulation proteins interact to prevent excessive bleeding after tissue injury. Pathologic overactivity of this process may result in thrombosis. The initial component in the hemostatic mechanism is the blood vessel wall, which may be more fragile in the fetus and preterm infant than it is later in life. Blood platelets are produced in the bone marrow and interact with injured blood vessel walls to form primary hemostatic plugs, a process requiring a plasma cofactor (von Willebrand factor) and resulting in the generation of prostaglandin intermediates (primarily thromboxane A$_2$) and in secretion of the platelets' granular contents. The platelet count in the fetus and newborn infant is the same as in older patients with the lower limit of normal at 150,000/mm$^3$. Limited studies of platelet life span in neonates suggest a value similar to that in adults—9 days. In vitro studies reveal decreased platelet aggregation in neonates, but the clinical significance of these observations is unclear because the bleeding time, the most sensitive in vivo test of hemostasis, is similar to values in older subjects.

More than a dozen soluble blood coagulation proteins interact sequentially after tissue injury to produce an insoluble fibrin clot. This blood coagulation mechanism is the second line of defense after the initial formation of the platelet plug. Hepatic synthesis of blood coagulation factors begins early in fetal life. Plasma concentrations of nearly all such proteins are reduced in term infants as compared with that of older children and adults. Levels are lower still in premature infants; plasma concentrations of the vitamin K-dependent Factors (II, VII, IX, X) and the contact Factors (XI, XII, prekallikrein, and high-molecular-weight kininogen) may be only 10% to 40% of those in adults. In addition, there are concomitantly low plasma levels of antithrombin III and protein C, naturally occurring anticoagulants that guard against excessive thrombosis; their plasma concentrations are about half of those in adults. Moreover, the fibrinolytic mechanism is impaired in the fetus and neonate. Levels of both procoagulants and inhibitors rise toward adult values at a variable rate during the initial weeks of life.

## Laboratory Evaluation

As in older patients, the platelet count, prothrombin time (PT), and activated partial thromboplastin time (PTT) are the most useful screening tests of the hemostatic mechanism. Values for these tests in term infants are little different from those of older patients. In preterm infants, however, the PTT is variably prolonged, reflecting physiologic reductions in contact factors and vitamin K-dependent coagulation proteins and possibly heparin effects. Varying PTT values depend on sampling techniques and laboratory methods and reagents. Other tests useful in evaluating bleeding disorders in neonates are a fibrinogen determination (normal range 175 to 450 mg/dL) and quantitation of fibrin degradation (split) products (normal value less than 10 $\mu$g/mL) or D-dimer (normal value less than 0.5 ng/dL). Some laboratories also use the thrombin time as an indirect test of the final stages of coagulation. Measurement of each blood coagulation factor (other than fibrinogen) and assessment of platelet function are rarely necessary.

Obtaining blood specimens for coagulation tests can be difficult because of problems with venous access and the baby's small blood volume. In most hospitals, capillary specimens cannot be used for the PT and PTT. If test samples are drawn from a heparinized arterial catheter, spuriously prolonged PTT values may result, even if the catheter is first flushed with a saline solution. Also, the high hemoglobin value of newborn infants may result in an inappropriately increased anticoagulant-to-plasma ratio on the test specimen, resulting in artifactually abnormal values.

## General Diagnostic Approach to the Bleeding Neonate

As in older patients, the medical history and physical examination are more useful than myriad laboratory tests in the evaluation of a bleeding or thrombotic disorder. The differential diagnosis of altered hemostasis depends greatly on whether the infant is "sick" or "well" (Table 20-53). Ill infants, particularly those who are premature, generally have an underlying disorder such as respiratory distress syndrome, sepsis, birth asphyxia, or a metabolic disorder. The secondary bleeding signs and laboratory alterations generally result from mechanical consumptive thrombocytopenia or DIC. The bleeding infant who is well (ie, full-term, thriving, and exhibiting no underlying disorder) most frequently has immune-mediated thrombocytopenia, vitamin K deficiency, hemophilia, or a localized anatomic lesion responsible for hemorrhage. An algorithm for the differential diagnosis of thrombocytopenia is provided in Figure 20-76.

The history should include a family history of excessive bleeding with particular focus on the mother. Presence of an underlying disorder or maternal drug history may be important; for example, mothers taking anticonvulsants during pregnancy may give birth to babies with vitamin K deficiency. In addition to characterization of whether the baby is sick or well, physical findings of petechiae suggest a platelet deficiency or fragile vessels.

TABLE 20-53.   Bleeding Disorders in Newborn Infants: Differential Diagnosis Based on Characterization of the Baby as Well or Sick

| Well | Sick |
|---|---|
| Immune thrombocytopenia (maternal autoantibody or alloantibody) | Mechanical or immune-complex-mediated thrombocytopenia |
| Hemophilia | Disseminated intravascular coagulation |
| Vitamin K deficiency | Severe liver disease |
| Local vascular lesion (gastrointestinal tract, abdominal cavity, or retroperitoneal space) | Local vascular lesion (periventricular tissues in premature infant) |

Localized petechiae on the presenting part are usually of no concern. Diffuse petechiae, however, usually result from moderate to severe thrombocytopenia. Petechiae are not seen in primary coagulation disorders such as hemophilia or vitamin K deficiency.

Screening laboratory tests performed on all babies with hemorrhage should include a platelet count, PT, and PTT, with addition of fibrinogen and fibrin degradation product on D-dimer measurements in selected cases.

Treatment approaches are discussed below for each disorder. Because bleeding is so often a secondary phenomenon in sick neonates, treatment should be aimed primarily at the underlying condition. Because the prognosis is often poor, effective treatment of hemorrhage may not be possible. Blood products must be used judiciously. Focus should be on preventing or stopping hemorrhage rather than correcting abnormal laboratory tests.

## Consumption of Coagulation Factors or Platelets

The most common cause of impaired hemostasis and clinical hemorrhage in the neonate is DIC or mechanical consumptive thrombocytopenia. Nearly all sick neonates exhibit multiple

mechanisms that may trigger blood coagulation and accelerate platelet aggregation. DIC is observed often accompanying respiratory distress syndrome, birth asphyxia, and infection due to multiple pathogens. The problem is compounded by the physiologic diminution of protective anticoagulants such as antithrombin III and protein C.

Infants with DIC usually present clinically with oozing from multiple puncture sites or gastrointestinal bleeding; thrombotic manifestations are noted less frequently. Nearly all babies with clinically significant hemorrhage have striking prolongations of the PT and PTT. The majority also have thrombocytopenia of variable severity (see Fig 20-75). The PTT alone is not a reliable diagnostic test of DIC in the premature infant. Fibrinogen concentration is usually low, and FDP and D-dimer are elevated. Some babies with infection or respiratory distress show no laboratory evidence of depleted clotting factors but manifest only thrombocytopenia (see Fig 20-75), which is mediated by immune complexes, vasculitis, or endotoxin. Such consumptive thrombocytopenia is probably the most common hematologic abnormality in the newborn nursery. Mechanical injury to platelets is also encountered in babies with renal vein thrombosis, nec-

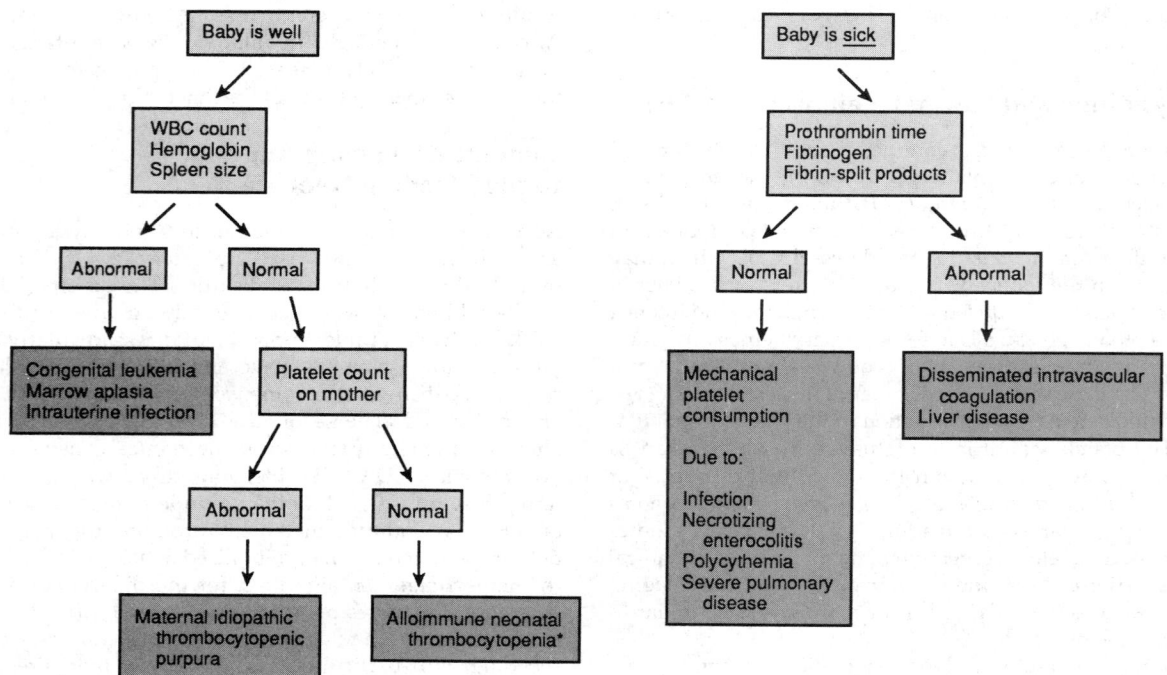

*WBC count may be low in alloimmune thrombocytopenia because of an anti-HLA antibody.

**Figure 20-76.**   Diagnostic approach to the newborn infant with thrombocytopenia (platelet count < 150,000/mm³ with or without symptoms). The most likely diagnoses are provided in the shaded boxes.

rotizing enterocolitis, and giant hemangiomas (Kasabach-Merritt syndrome).

Therapy for DIC or thrombocytopenia accompanying infection is directed primarily toward the underlying disorder. Fresh frozen plasma and platelet transfusions should be used sparingly and restricted to those babies with marked hemorrhage or grossly abnormal laboratory markers. One or two units of random donor platelets usually provide a temporary rise in platelet count. Repletion of coagulation proteins with fresh frozen plasma can be accomplished with a volume of 10 to 15 mL/kg every 12 to 24 hours. Exchange transfusion has not generally proved useful except for in those patients who have coexisting volume overload. At one time, heparin was advocated as treatment for DIC because it theoretically arrests the pathologic overactivity of coagulation; however, no data support its use except in cases of large vessel thrombosis.

## Immune-Mediated Thrombocytopenia

Well infants with petechiae, bruising, and moderate to marked thrombocytopenia, but no other abnormal laboratory or physical findings, usually have maternal antibody that has crossed the placenta, coated the platelets, and resulted in their destruction by the mononuclear-phagocyte system. Although bleeding usually is not severe, numerous deaths from intracranial bleeding have been reported. Immune-mediated thrombocytopenia during the newborn period includes two distinct conditions, which differ in the antigenic specificity of the offending antibody (Table 20-54).

Infants whose mothers have idiopathic thrombocytopenic purpura are usually known to be at risk before delivery. The extent of thrombocytopenia in the fetus and neonate that results from the maternal autoantibody is variable and does not necessarily correlate with the mother's platelet count. In alloimmune (isoimmune) neonatal thrombocytopenia, the mother's platelet count is normal. There is fetal–maternal platelet antigen incompatibility; the antiplatelet antibody is usually directed against the platelet-specific PLA-1 antigen that is present on the baby's platelets (as a result of inheritance from the father) but not on the mother's. Occasionally, the antibodies can be directed against other platelet membrane proteins. First-born infants may be affected because sensitization of the mother may occur early in gestation. A history of previously affected infants is sometimes obtained.

In both categories of infants affected by passive maternal antibody, the platelet count usually begins to rise by several weeks of age and invariably returns to normal by 3 to 4 months of age. Bleeding signs and symptoms are uncommon after the first 3 or 4 days of life.

Treatment of immune-mediated thrombocytopenia in the newborn infant is controversial. Therapeutic considerations begin with the pregnant mother, who is usually known to be at risk. Therefore, close cooperation between pediatrician and obstetrician is required in such cases. Administration of prednisone or intravenous gamma globulin to the mother during the pregnancy may cause a raise in the fetal platelet count, thereby lessening risks of internal hemorrhage especially during a vaginal delivery. Routine cesarean section is advocated by some, particularly if a platelet count taken from a fetal scalp specimen early in labor is less than 50,000/mm$^3$. Therapeutic intervention before delivery, however, is not usually necessary.

The existence of immune-mediated thrombocytopenia is often not appreciated until the 1- or 2-day-old baby exhibits petechiae and bruising. Mildly affected infants with platelet counts greater than 30,000/mm$^3$ need no therapy. More severely thrombocytopenic infants whose mothers have idiopathic thrombocytopenic purpura should receive a short course of prednisone or intravenous gamma globulin; platelet transfusions are usually of no value. Symptomatic babies with alloimmune thrombocytopenia should receive a transfusion of maternal platelets (because they lack the antigen to which the antibody is directed) or infusion of gamma globulin. Studies are needed to define further the most appropriate therapy for these infants. The overall prognosis is usually good.

### Vitamin K Deficiency

Newborn infants are at risk of vitamin K deficiency because of inadequate stores in the fetus, reduced bacterial synthesis of the vitamin in the colon (due to absence of endogenous microflora), and limited dietary intake. Human breast milk has relatively little vitamin K in contrast to cow milk-based formulas. Before the 1950s, hemorrhagic disease of the newborn, resulting from profound depletion of vitamin K-dependent coagulation factors, was a common cause of hemorrhagic death between the second and fifth day of life. Now, it is routine practice for 0.5 to 1 mg of vitamin K$_1$ (phytonadione) to be administered intramuscularly to all neonates. Administration of prophylactic vitamin K shortly after birth has nearly eliminated hemorrhagic disease of the newborn in the western world. Some studies show that oral dosing is as effective as an intramuscular injection; the less expensive oral route may be more feasible in underdeveloped countries where breast-fed babies frequently bleed because of vitamin K deficiency. Vitamin K deficiency may also occur in newborns whose mothers have taken anticonvulsants (particularly diphenylhydantoin) that have coumarin-like effects. Hemorrhagic disease resulting from vitamin K deficiency can sometimes be delayed until several months of life, particularly in breast-fed babies who have malabsorption syndromes or received broad-spectrum antibiotics.

Treatment, like prevention, is accomplished by oral or parenteral delivery of vitamin K, followed by prompt cessation of hemorrhage and correction of the prolonged PT and PTT within several hours.

### Hemophilia

Like vitamin K deficiency, hemophilia generally manifests in well neonates. Male infants at risk of Factor VIII or IX deficiency (hemophilia A or B) are often suspected on the basis of the family

| | Maternal Idiopathic Thrombocytopenic Purpura | Alloimmune Neonatal Thrombocytopenia |
|---|---|---|
| | **TABLE 20-54. Immune-Mediated Thrombocytopenia in the Newborn Infant: Differences in Pathophysiology, Diagnosis, and Management** | |
| Usual antigen specificity of offending antibody | "Public" antigens common to all platelets (eg, glycoprotein IIb-IIIa complex) | Platelet-specific antigen (usually PLA-1 or glycoprotein Ib) that is absent from the mother's platelets |
| Maternal platelet count | Usually reduced | Always normal |
| Therapy with maternal platelets | Not indicated | Treatment of choice for symptomatic infants |

history. The history may be negative, however, so any otherwise well newborn boy who exhibits excessive or prolonged bleeding from circumcision or heel puncture site, intracranial hemorrhage, or other unexplained bleeding should be investigated for hemophilia. In both Factor VIII and IX deficiency, the PTT is markedly prolonged but the PT is normal. Factor VIII and IX assays must then be performed to arrive at the specific diagnosis. Therapy consists of prompt administration of purified and viral inactivated concentrates containing the deficient factor.

During the newborn period, hemorrhage resulting from inherited deficiency of blood coagulation factors other than Factors VIII and IX is rare. Factor XIII deficiency usually presents with hemorrhage from the umbilical stump.

### Other Causes of Impaired Hemostasis in the Neonate

*Liver Disease.* As in older patients, hepatic injury resulting from viruses, metabolic disorders, or hypoxic insults may result in severe bleeding due to profound reduction in the synthesis of multiple clotting factors. DIC and excessive fibrinolysis may contribute to the hemorrhagic state. Other evidence of liver dysfunction is usually apparent; the PT and PTT are markedly prolonged. Treatment, which is often unsatisfactory, consists of administration of fresh frozen plasma.

*Platelet Dysfunction.* Although bleeding due to thrombocytopenia is common in neonates, it is uncertain how often qualitative platelet defects predispose to excessive hemorrhage. Infants of mothers who have taken aspirin during the final days of their pregnancies may have a mild bleeding tendency, resulting from impaired platelet aggregation. Also, clinically significant antiplatelet effects of indomethacin have been reported in premature infants receiving this agent to promote closure of the ductus arteriosus.

*Thrombocytopenia Due to Diminished Production.* Congenital leukemia and other infiltrative disorders, osteopetrosis (marble bone disease), congenital infection, and the thrombocytopenia absent radii syndrome may present with hemorrhage during the first days of life. Other clinical and laboratory features exist in all of these conditions.

*Local Vascular Lesions.* Bleeding from a single anatomic site is not always a consequence of generalized impairment in hemostasis. Most babies with intracranial or abdominal hemorrhage exhibit localized anatomic defects at the site of bleeding. For instance, a congenital malformation such as duplication may cause gastrointestinal hemorrhage; birth trauma may cause retroperitoneal or intraabdominal bleeding (eg, secondary to splenic rupture). In premature infants with respiratory distress syndrome, the most common cause of major morbidity and mortality is intraventricular hemorrhage. Although such babies may exhibit concomitant thrombocytopenia and the expected modest reduction in coagulation proteins, studies in which transfusions of plasma or platelets were administered to such premature infants show no convincing reduction in frequency or severity of intracranial hemorrhage. Therefore, localized anatomic defects predominate (see Chap. 20.1.3).

### Thrombosis in the Neonate

Despite the frequent occurrence of indwelling foreign bodies (eg, catheters) and the physiologic reductions in the anticoagulant proteins antithrombin III and protein C, large vessel venous or arterial thrombosis is relatively uncommon during the newborn period. It is occasionally encountered, however, in infants with severe dehydration, diabetic mothers, polycythemia, or DIC, especially at sites of catheter placement. Therapy consists of removal of foreign bodies and systemic heparinization. Thrombolytic

agents to dissolve existing clots (eg, streptokinase, urokinase, or recombinant tissue plasminogen activator) have been used successfully in a few cases.

Purpura fulminans, a syndrome of diffuse cutaneous thrombotic lesions associated with laboratory manifestations of DIC, is observed occasionally in babies with septicemia. It is also encountered in the rare infant with homozygous congenital protein C deficiency. Because protein C levels are markedly reduced or even undetectable in these babies, no defense mechanisms allow for the inactivation of Factors V and VIII; uncontrollable thrombosis therefore ensues. Treatment consists of administration of fresh frozen plasma, prothrombin complex concentrates, and coumadin.

## Selected Readings

Andrew M, Paes B, Milner R, et al. Development of the human coagulation system in the full-term infant. Blood 1987;70:165.

Andrew M. The hemostatic system in the infant. In: Nathan DG, Oski FA, eds. Hematology of infancy and childhood, ed 4. Philadelphia: WB Saunders Co, 1993;115.

Buchanan GR. Coagulation disorders in the neonate. Pediatr Clin North Am 1986;33:203.

Lane PA, Hathaway WE. Vitamin K in infancy. J Pediatr 1985;106:351.

O'Brien RT, Pearson HA. Physiologic anemia of the newborn infant. J Pediatr 1971;79:132.

Oski FA, Naiman JL, eds. Hematologic problems in the newborn, ed 3. Philadelphia: WB Saunders, 1982.

Shannon KM. Anemia of prematurity: progress and prospects. Am J Pediatr Hematol Oncol 1990;12:14.

*Principles and Practice of Pediatrics, Second Edition.*
edited by Frank A. Oski et al. J. B. Lippincott Company, Philadelphia © 1994.

# 20.10 *Dermatologic Diseases*

Lynne J. Roberts

## BIRTHMARKS

Birthmarks comprise a wide spectrum of common and uncommon congenital disorders, the recognition of which is crucial for predicting the natural course and potential for associated abnormalities. Jacobs and Walton (1976) determined the frequency of birthmarks in 1058 newborns under 72 hours of age (Table 20-55).

## Pigmented Lesions

Melanocytes are pigment- or melanin-producing cells that originate in the neural crest and migrate in utero to the skin, mucous membranes, eyes, and central nervous system (CNS). Tumors of melanocytes in the skin are composed of one of three types of cells: nevus cells, epidermal melanocytes, and dermal melanocytes (Table 20-56). All melanocytic tumors, except freckles, may be present at birth. Freckles are acquired later in childhood. Melanocytic nevi are further classified as junctional, intradermal, or compound when the location of the nevus cells is within the epidermis, the dermis, or both, respectively.

### TABLE 20-55. Frequency of Birthmarks

| Birthmark | Occurrence (%) |
| --- | --- |
| Salmon patch | 40.3 |
| Hemangioma | 2.6 |
| Port wine stain | 0.3 |
| Mongolian spot | 23.5 |
| Melanocytic nevus | 1.3 |

*Jacobs AH, Walton RG. The incidence of birthmarks in the neonate. Pediatrics 1976;58:218.*

### TABLE 20-57. Frequency of Mongolian Spots

| Race | Occurrence (%) |
| --- | --- |
| Black | 95.5 |
| Asian | 81.0 |
| Latin-American | 70.1 |
| White | 9.6 |

*Jacobs AH, Walton RG. The incidence of birthmarks in the neonate. Pediatrics 1976;58:218.*

## Congenital Melanocytic Nevus

Congenital melanocytic nevi (CMN) occur in up to 1% of all newborns and vary from a few millimeters to several centimeters or more in diameter. Giant CMN involving a major portion of the body have been referred to as "bathing trunk" or "garment" nevi. CMN may be flat or raised and range in color from pinkish tan to brown or black. They are significant because of their increased risk for development of malignant melanoma. Management of these lesions is controversial because data to predict which CMN will become malignant are lacking. The risk of malignancy in giant CMN is well documented and is at least 6.3% over a lifetime. Most investigators recommend excision of giant CMN during the first year of life because the incidence of melanoma is highest during the first 5 years. The precise risk for melanoma in the more common, smaller (less than 20 cm) CMN is not known, but may be as high as 1 in 20. Prophylactic removal of small CMN should be considered but probably can be delayed until the end of the first decade if the lesion appears benign and follow-up is ensured, because prepubertal melanoma in small CMN is rare. CMN grow with the child and are ultimately larger if excision is postponed. Features that suggest development of melanoma in a CMN include change in color, irregular or scalloped border, change in size or thickness, variation in color within the lesion, bleeding, or ulceration. CMN may have irregular borders and variation in color and thickness from the outset, making it difficult to follow these lesions for early malignant changes (Color Figure 1). All CMN with atypical or suspicious features should be excised regardless of size.

Midline CMN may signal the presence of spinal dysraphism and soft tissue tumors. Large CMN of the bathing trunk variety or those involving the head and neck may be associated with leptomeningeal melanocytosis in which benign melanocytic proliferation can result in seizures, hydrocephalus, or focal neurologic defects. There is a risk of developing a primary malignant melanoma in the leptomeningeal lesions as well as the cutaneous CMN.

### TABLE 20-56. Benign Melanocytic Tumors of Skin

Nevus cells
    Melanocytic/nevocellular nevus
Epidermal melanocytes
    Freckle (ephelide)
    Lentigo
    Cafe au lait spot
Dermal melanocytes
    Mongolian spot
    Blue nevus
    Nevus of Ota
    Nevus of Ito

## Mongolian Spot

Second to salmon patches as a cause of birthmarks, Mongolian spots are seen often in black infants (Table 20-57). These blue to blue-black macules occur anywhere on the body, but they are found mostly on the back and buttocks. When present in unusual locations, they have been mistaken for bruising as a sign of child abuse. Mongolian spots usually disappear with age but occasionally persist into adulthood.

## Blue Nevus

Blue nevi are uncommon benign tumors composed of dermal melanocytes that may be present at birth. The common blue nevus and the cellular blue nevus cannot be distinguished clinically but differ histologically. Blue nevi are well-circumscribed, slate blue or bluish black papules or nodules with a predilection for the buttocks, face, or dorsum of the hands and feet. Common blue nevi are usually less than 15 mm in diameter and are not at risk for the development of malignant melanoma. Cellular blue nevi are often larger and carry a small risk for malignant degeneration.

## Cafe au Lait Spot

Well-circumscribed, light brown macules, cafe au lait spots may be found on any part of the body. These lesions persist and may increase in number and size with age. Although cafe au lait spots occur in 10% of the normal population, the presence of six or more with a diameter of greater than 0.5 cm before puberty and 1.5 cm after puberty is highly suggestive, but not diagnostic, of neurofibromatosis. Cafe au lait spots are also seen in other disorders including tuberous sclerosis, Albright's syndrome, ataxia telangiectasia, and Bloom's syndrome.

## Mastocytosis

Mastocytosis should be considered in the differential diagnosis of pigmented lesions present at birth. Mast cell disease encompasses a spectrum from isolated cutaneous involvement to systemic disease (Table 20-58). Cutaneous lesions, produced by local

### TABLE 20-58. Classification of Mastocytosis

**Cutaneous Mastocytosis**
Isolated lesions
    Mastocytomas
Generalized lesions
    Urticaria pigmentosis

**Systemic Mastocytosis**
Organ infiltration
Mast cell leukemia

infiltration of the skin by mast cells, characteristically urticate with rubbing (Darier's sign) because of mast cell degranulation and histamine release resulting in increased vascular permeability, edema, and wheal formation. If the edema is marked, blistering may occur. Mastocytomas are present at birth or develop shortly thereafter and appear as reddish brown or brown plaques or nodules. Single lesions are the rule, although occasionally two or three will be present, typically involving the distal extremities, particularly the wrist. Most isolated mastocytomas resolve spontaneously after several years. The age of onset of the multiple red-brown, yellow, tan, or dark brown macules, papules, and plaques of generalized cutaneous mastocytosis (urticaria pigmentosa) ranges from birth to adulthood (Color Figure 2). Most affected children have significant clearing or complete resolution of the cutaneous lesions by early adulthood. Systemic symptoms may occur because of release of histamine and other mediators from cutaneous lesions including pruritus, flushing, hypotension, tachycardia, and less often, diarrhea, dyspnea, and syncope. Systemic mastocytosis with mast cell infiltration of bone, liver, spleen, lymph nodes, skin, and gastrointestinal tract is rare in children.

## Epidermal Nevus

Epidermal nevi are benign tumors in which the epidermis is hyperplastic. A variety of names has been given to this lesion, including linear epidermal nevus, nevus unius lateris, ichthyosis hystrix, and systematized epidermal nevus. Most epidermal nevi are present at birth and may become more extensive with age. The lesions are brown or black verrucous growths arranged in a linear, asymmetrical fashion and are more often unilateral than bilateral. Extensive epidermal nevi may be associated with congenital skeletal defects and CNS disease, including mental retardation, seizures, and focal neurologic defects (epidermal nevus syndrome).

## Nevus Sebaceous

Benign tumors of epidermis and epidermal appendages always present at birth, sebaceous nevi are characterized by a distinctive yellow-orange color because of the presence of a large number of sebaceous glands (Color Figure 3). Initially, they are well circumscribed, hairless, and flat or slightly raised with a finely cobblestoned texture. At puberty, enlargement occurs as the sebaceous glands become active under androgenic influence. Small, isolated lesions of sebaceous nevi are not associated with other defects and are most commonly located on the scalp or face. An extensive linear sebaceous nevus on the head, neck, or trunk may be associated with congenital skeletal defects and CNS disease including mental retardation and seizures much like those seen in the epidermal nevus syndrome. There is a 15% to 20% risk for the development of a basal cell carcinoma as well as other benign and malignant tumors within a sebaceous nevus, regardless of size; thus, excision before puberty is recommended.

## HYPOPIGMENTED LESIONS

## Ash Leaf Spot

Hypopigmented, oval, or leaf-shaped macules with smooth or jagged borders, ash leaf spots are the only cutaneous manifestation of tuberous sclerosis present at birth or in early infancy. Other skin lesions characteristic of this disorder develop later in childhood or in early adolescence including adenoma sebaceum, periungual fibromas, and shagreen patches. Ash leaf spots persist, and affected individuals may continue to develop new lesions during childhood. In fair-skinned infants, ash leaf spots are detected most easily with the aid of a Wood's light.

## Nevus Depigmentosus

Nevus depigmentosus (achromic nevus) is a single congenital hypopigmented macule that may appear to be in a dermatomal distribution and that does not change with age. This nevus is not associated with other defects.

## Piebaldism

Piebaldism is an autosomal dominant disorder in which depigmented patches of skin are present at birth. A distinctive feature is the presence of normally pigmented islands of skin within the leukoderma. Some affected individuals have been reported to have cerebellar ataxia, neurosensory deafness, or mental retardation. A white forelock or hypopigmented tuft of hair in the frontal region, heterochromic irides and fundi, hypertelorism, congenital deafness, premature graying of hair, confluence of the medial eyebrows, and a broad nasal root are manifestations of Waardenburg's syndrome. Also autosomal dominant, this disorder may be a variant of piebaldism.

## Hypomelanosis of Ito

Hypomelanosis of Ito (incontinentia pigmenti achromians) is a rare disorder of irregular, linear, and whorled hypopigmentation on the trunk and extremities associated in up to 75% with one or more abnormalities of the CNS, eyes, teeth, nails, hair, and skeletal system. The pigmentary changes are present at birth or within the first year of life, in most cases, and may become more extensive.

## Nevus Anemicus

Nevus anemicus is a congenital developmental anomaly that appears to be a hypopigmented macule. The involved area is lighter than the normal skin, not because there is a loss of pigment, but because blood vessels are constricted, producing a permanent blanching of the area. This blanching is a functional rather than a structural abnormality, presumed to be caused by local increased sensitivity to vasoconstrictors, probably in association with unresponsiveness to vasodilators. The color difference between the nevus and the normal skin can be accentuated by brisk rubbing—the normal skin becomes red, while the nevus will not. A nevus anemicus is not generally associated with other defects and does not change with age.

## VASCULAR LESIONS

## Normal Variants

### Cutis Marmorata

Cutis marmorata is the normal, reticulated, cyanotic mottling of the skin that is a physiologic response to chilling. This change is not normal if it persists after the infant is warmed. Persistent mottling or livedo reticularis implies an obstruction to blood flow such as hyperviscosity or vasculitis.

### Harlequin Color Change

The harlequin color change is seen primarily in premature infants and is thought to be due to immature vasomotor control. When the infant lies on its side, the lower half of the body becomes reddened and the upper half blanches. An episode may last for several seconds or minutes and resolves spontaneously when the infant is placed in a supine position.

# Congenital Vascular Malformations

Congenital vascular malformations may be classified as telangiectasias (nevus flammeus) or hemangiomas (Table 20-59). A telangiectasia consists of normal numbers of blood vessels that are dilated. A true hemangioma is produced by proliferation of endothelial cells.

## Telangiectasia

The most common of all birthmarks, salmon patches are pink macules located over the glabella, eyelids, nasolabial folds, or nape of the neck. Some refer to salmon patches on the face as "angel kisses" and those on the nape of the neck as "stork bites" because the former resolve but the latter do not.

Port wine stains (PWSs) are pink to red vascular malformations present at birth, usually on the face. They are frequently unilateral. PWSs do not resolve, tend to darken and thicken with age, and many develop nodular angiomas. Soft tissue hypertrophy may produce deformity and dysfunction of the involved area. In addition to these medical indications for treatment, the psychological trauma of a large or disfiguring PWS should not be underestimated. Tunable dye laser surgery has been shown to be a safe and effective method for removing PWS with minimal risk for scarring. Several treatments of the entire PWS are necessary for optimal fading or resolution. Beginning laser surgery early in life reduces the number of treatments required for clearing and prevents progression of the PWS. By definition, the Sturge-Weber syndrome includes a facial PWS in the distribution of the ophthalmic branch of the trigeminal nerve, angiomatosis of the ipsilateral leptomeninges, and gyriform intracerebral calcifications. If the PWS occurs exclusively below the ophthalmic division, there is no CNS involvement. The PWS may involve the trunk and extremities in addition to the face, but there is no correlation between the extent of the cutaneous involvement and the severity of the CNS vascular malformation. Other features of the Sturge-Weber syndrome include seizures (80%), mental retardation (60%), hemiplegia (30%), and glaucoma (45%). The highest risk for glaucoma is seen in those individuals with PWS involvement of both the ophthalmic and maxillary divisions of the trigeminal nerve. Studies suggest that all patients with a facial PWS in this distribution are at risk for glaucoma, regardless of the presence of Sturge-Weber syndrome. Therefore, any infant with a PWS involving the V-1 or V-2 divisions of the trigeminal nerve should be followed closely for evidence of glaucoma.

## Hemangiomas

Two types of congenital hemangiomas are recognized—capillary and cavernous. Both components may be present in one lesion. Capillary hemangiomas are characterized by proliferation of endothelial cells with relatively few capillary lumina. Cavernous hemangiomas are composed primarily of large, irregular vascular spaces without as much endothelial cell proliferation. Strawberry hemangiomas are of the capillary type but frequently have a cavernous component as well (Color Figure 4). The fully developed, bright red, pebbly strawberry hemangioma may be present at birth or may be preceded by a flat or slightly raised area composed of telangiectatic vessels surrounded by an area of pallor (Color Figure 5) or a solid red macule that begins to proliferate within a few weeks to produce the typical strawberry appearance. These early lesions are often mistaken for PWSs. The deeper location and less compact structure of cavernous hemangiomas give them a soft, compressible texture and a less distinct outline. The overlying skin may be normal or may have a bluish hue.

Parents frequently become alarmed when a hemangioma begins to grow, particularly if it becomes eroded or develops bleeding. It is important to stress the natural history of these lesions, because more than 90% resolve spontaneously. Hemangiomas grow rapidly during the first 6 months of life with most reaching their maximal growth by 1 year. A general rule is that 50% will resolve by 5 years of age, 70% by 7 years, and 90% by 9 years. Involution is heralded by a fading of the bright redness and the appearance of gray or white areas within the lesion. Indications for aggressive treatment include compromise of a vital function (sight, respiration, nutrition), high output congestive heart failure, consumptive coagulopathy, and significant ulceration or deformity. Systemic corticosteroids is the treatment of choice with a starting dose of 2 to 4 mg/kg/d followed by a tapering course over 2 to 4 months. Preliminary data suggest that capillary hemangiomas are amenable to tunable dye laser surgery. Intervention is most successful when laser surgery is begun early, before significant proliferation has occurred. Dye laser surgery can reduce or eradicate some proliferating and mature capillary hemangiomas but is not effective for cavernous hemangiomas. Alpha-interferon is being investigated for treatment of capillary and cavernous hemangiomas. One potential complication of large cavernous hemangiomas, and rarely smaller lesions, is the Kasabach-Merritt syndrome in which platelets are trapped and coagulation factors are consumed locally within the hemangioma. This syndrome is manifested by an enlarging hemangioma with surrounding ecchymoses and may develop into a full-blown disseminated intravascular coagulation-like picture with thrombocytopenia and a hemorrhagic diathesis.

The Klippel-Trenaunay-Weber syndrome is characterized by a vascular malformation associated with localized overgrowth of bone and soft tissue of the involved extremity or portion of the trunk. The congenital vascular malformation may be of one or more types including a PWS, hemangioma, arteriovenous malformation, or lymphangioma. Hypertrophy of the limb or portion of the trunk may be present at birth or develop in infancy. In addition, superficial venous varicosities frequently develop within the affected area in childhood or adolescence. Treatment has been unsatisfactory.

The blue rubber bleb nevus syndrome is characterized by cutaneous and visceral cavernous hemangiomas. The cutaneous hemangiomas are present at birth but tend to increase in number with age and have a distinctive soft, blue, rubbery, wrinkled appearance. A diagnostic feature is the ability to express blood from the hemangioma, leaving an empty wrinkled sac that looks like a nipple. Spontaneous bleeding is rare with the cutaneous lesions but common with the visceral lesions. Most visceral hemangiomas are found in the small bowel, but they can occur anywhere in the gastrointestinal tract or in the liver, lungs, skeletal muscle, peritoneum, or mucous membranes. Affected infants are at significant risk for serious gastrointestinal bleeding.

Diffuse neonatal hemangiomatosis is a syndrome of multiple capillary hemangiomas of the skin with hemangiomas of the mucous membranes, liver, gastrointestinal tract, lung, and CNS. Affected infants are noted at birth to have small, red to bluish black,

| TABLE 20-59. Congenital Vascular Malformations |
|---|
| Telangiectasias |
| Nevus flammeus |
| Salmon patch |
| Port wine stain |
| Hemangiomas |
| Capillary |
| Cavernous |
| Mixed |

**TABLE 20-60.   Differential Diagnosis of Vesicles or Pustules in the Newborn**

| Noninfectious | Infectious |
|---|---|
| Miliaria | Candidiasis |
| Erythema toxicum | Staphylococcal folliculitis |
| Transient neonatal pustular melanosis | Herpes simplex |
| Infantile acropustulosis | Congenital syphilis |
| Incontinentia pigmenti | Varicella |
| Histiocytosis X | Bacterial sepsis |

papular hemangiomas 0.2 to 2.5 cm in diameter, and they may develop hundreds of similar lesions in infancy (Color Figure 6). Prognosis is guarded because significant gastrointestinal bleeding or high-output congestive heart failure due to hepatic arteriovenous malformations may develop. Treatment with prednisone, 2 to 4 mg/kg/d, may result in involution of the cutaneous and visceral hemangiomas. There have been several recent reports of infants with cutaneous lesions without apparent symptomatic visceral involvement. If the infants survive, the hemangiomas tend to regress with time, much like typical strawberry nevi.

### Cutis Marmorata Telangiectatica Congenita

Cutis marmorata telangiectatica congenita is a rare congenital vascular malformation characterized by red-purple, reticulated mottling (livedo reticularis) and telangiectasia, with or without ulceration and atrophy of the skin (Color Figure 7). One extremity is most commonly affected, but lesions may be bilateral and the trunk may be involved. A variety of associated defects has been reported in up to 50% of cases. The cutaneous lesions tend to improve with age and may disappear completely.

### Angiokeratoma

Angiokeratomas are characterized by dilation of superficial blood vessels of the dermis with hypertrophy of the overlying epidermis. At least six types are recognized, but only one, the angiokeratoma circumscriptum, is present at birth. Lesions are composed of papules and nodules with a warty surface and a deep red to blue-black color, often arranged in a grouped or linear pattern. Although the lesions remain localized, they do not resolve spontaneously.

### Lymphangioma

Lymphangiomas are tumors of lymphatic origin classified much like hemangiomas into capillary or cavernous types. A lymphangioma circumscriptum is a capillary lymphangioma, present at birth or early childhood, made up of thick-walled, deep-seated vesicles. If purely lymphatic, the vesicles appear clear or translucent, but a hemangiomatous component will give them a red or bluish hue (Color Figure 8). Cavernous lymphangiomas or cystic hygromas are deeper tumors commonly involving the neck that can be extensive, difficult to remove, and life threatening.

## VESICULOPUSTULAR AND BULLOUS DISORDERS

### Vesicles and Pustules

Table 20-60 and Figure 20-77 present the differential diagnosis of vesicles and pustules in the newborn.

### Miliaria

Resulting from the occlusion and rupture of sweat ducts in the skin, miliaria (heat rash) occurs in two forms—miliaria crystallina

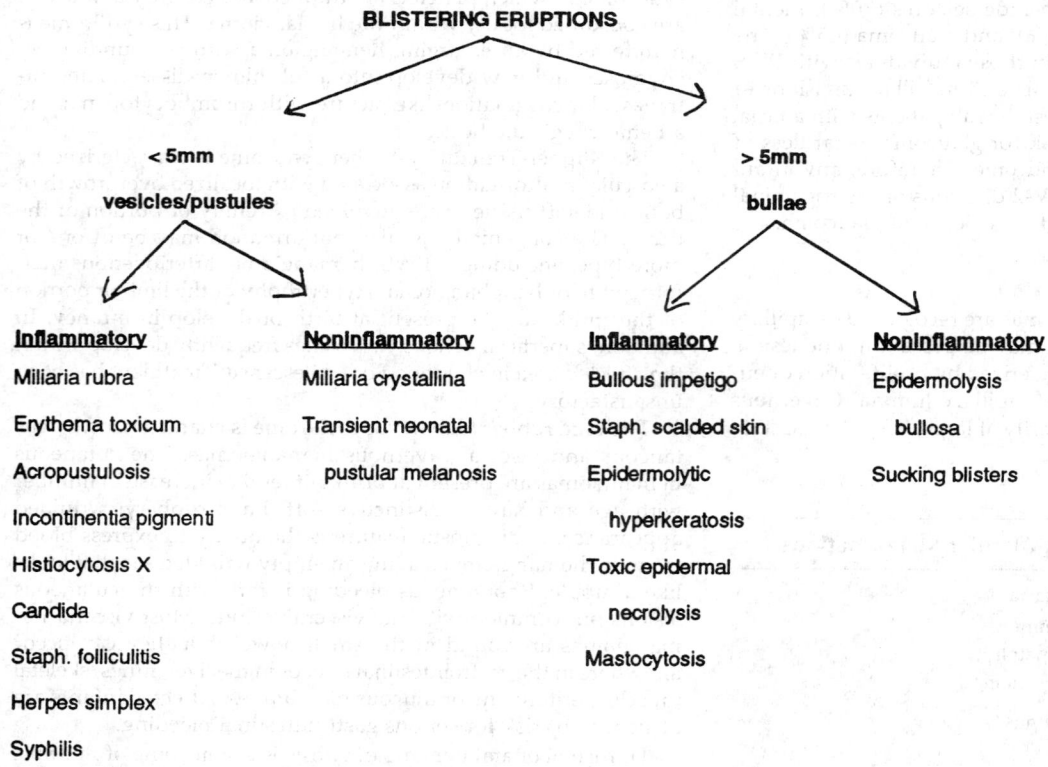

**BLISTERING ERUPTIONS**

**< 5mm** — **vesicles/pustules**

**Inflammatory**
Miliaria rubra
Erythema toxicum
Acropustulosis
Incontinentia pigmenti
Histiocytosis X
Candida
Staph. folliculitis
Herpes simplex
Syphilis
Varicella
Sepsis

**Noninflammatory**
Miliaria crystallina
Transient neonatal
   pustular melanosis

**> 5mm** — **bullae**

**Inflammatory**
Bullous impetigo
Staph. scalded skin
Epidermolytic
   hyperkeratosis
Toxic epidermal
   necrolysis
Mastocytosis

**Noninflammatory**
Epidermolysis
   bullosa
Sucking blisters

**Figure 20-77.**   Approach to blistering eruptions.

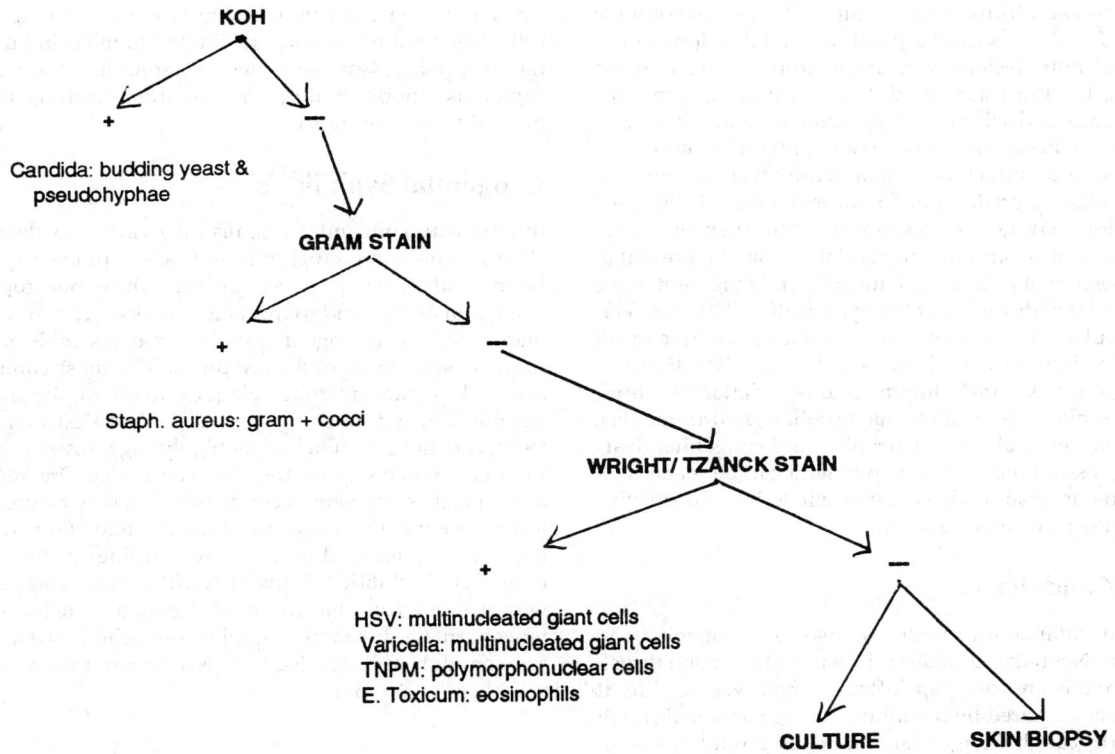

**Figure 20-78.** Diagnostic procedures for blistering eruptions.

and miliaria rubra. If the ducts rupture superficially in the skin, small, clear vesicles, miliaria crystallina, form; they are not associated with inflammation. These tiny, fragile, noninflammatory vesicles appear like dew drops on the skin. In miliaria rubra, sweat ducts rupture more deeply within the skin and provoke an inflammatory response resulting in erythematous papules that may evolve into vesicles and pustules. Both types are seen most often on the face, upper trunk, neck, and other body-fold areas but may become widespread. Miliaria resolves spontaneously if the infant is kept cool and dry and if topical creams or lotions, which aggravate the condition, are avoided.

## Erythema Toxicum

Erythema toxicum is a common eruption occurring in up to 50% of normal newborn infants. It may be present at birth but usually develops on day 2 or 3 of life and is characterized by large, splotchy areas of erythema studded with urticarial papules, vesicles, and pustules (Color Figure 9). Lesions are found in greatest numbers on the trunk, with fewer on the face and extremities. The palms and soles are not involved. The eruption lasts 7 to 14 days and resolves spontaneously without pigmentary change or scarring. The diagnosis can be confirmed with a Wright-stained smear of the pustule, which will reveal eosinophils with few or no polymorphonuclear cells and no organisms (Fig 20-78).

## Transient Neonatal Pustular Melanosis

An eruption always present at the time of delivery, transient neonatal pustular melanosis is characterized by noninflammatory pustules. The pustules are fragile and rupture quickly, often resolving within 24 hours, leaving a hyperpigmented macule surrounded by a collarette scale (Color Figure 10). Rarely, pigmented spots without pustules are noted at birth. The pigmented macules resemble freckles and may last for several weeks before resolving. The most common areas of involvement are the lower face, chin,

neck, and extremities, although lesions may occur anywhere, including the palms and soles. The incidence is much higher in blacks than whites. A Wright-stained smear of a pustule reveals polymorphonuclear cells with few or no eosinophils and no organisms (Fig 20-77).

## Infantile Acropustulosis

Infantile acropustulosis is a recently described syndrome of intensely pruritic 1- to 3-mm vesicles and pustules distributed primarily on the palms, soles, wrists, ankles, and backs of the hands and feet. The trunk and buttocks are less commonly affected. Onset is from birth to 1 year of age with spontaneous resolution within 2 or 3 years. Response to topical corticosteroids and antihistamines is poor, and intractable cases may be treated successfully with dapsone or sulfapyridine.

## Incontinentia Pigmenti

Incontinentia pigmenti is an X-linked dominant disorder with a 50% spontaneous mutation rate. Ninety-seven percent of the affected individuals are female, suggesting that the disorder may be lethal to male fetuses. The cutaneous manifestations occur in three distinct stages, not all of which are present in every patient (Table 20-61). The first stage begins at birth or shortly thereafter and is characterized by crops of vesicles in linear streaks or bands

| TABLE 20-61.  Cutaneous Stages of Incontinentia Pigmenti |
| --- |
| Vesicular stage: birth to 3 weeks |
| Hyperkeratotic/verrucous stage: 2 to 6 weeks |
| Pigmentary stage: 12 to 26 weeks |

on the extremities and trunk (Color Figure 11). Vesicles continue to develop for 2 to 3 weeks and are followed by development of warty, hyperkeratotic lesions in a linear array, particularly on the extremities. The third stage tends to begin after age 3 months with linear streaks and whorls of hyperpigmentation. This pigmentation does not necessarily occur in areas preceded by vesicles or warty lesions and, in fact, is predominantly truncal, whereas the early lesions have a predilection for the extremities. Ultimately, the pigmentation may fade or disappear. More than one stage may be present at once, and the pigmentation may be present at birth. Eighty percent of infants with incontinentia pigmenti have significant associated disorders of the eyes, teeth, CNS, and skeletal system. Ocular involvement may be serious enough to result in visual loss or blindness in 20% of patients. CNS disorders occur in 30% of infants, including mental retardation, seizures, spastic paralysis, motor retardation, microcephaly, hydrocephalus, cerebellar ataxia, cerebral cortical atrophy, and congenital deafness. The diagnosis of incontinentia pigmenti can be made with a biopsy of a characteristic early vesicular skin lesion. No effective treatment is known for this disorder.

## Cutaneous Candidiasis

In the newborn, cutaneous candidiasis exists as a congenital and a neonatal form. Neonatal candidiasis is manifested as oral thrush or diaper dermatitis and develops after the first week of life. It is presumed to be acquired by the infant during passage through an infected birth canal. Congenital cutaneous candidiasis is an ascending, intrauterine infection. The eruption is noted at birth or within 12 hours after delivery and is characterized by erythematous macules and papules that evolve into vesicles and pustules scattered widely over the body, including the palms and soles. Oral lesions are rare, and the diaper area is relatively spared. After several days, the eruption resolves with desquamation. The diagnosis is established by demonstrating pseudohyphae and budding yeast in a direct smear of the pustules. Most infants with congenital cutaneous candidiasis do not have systemic involvement and therefore do well with topical treatment alone. Conversely, systemic congenital candidiasis does not usually present with skin lesions and can lead to death in utero or in the immediate neonatal period. The most reliable indicators for predicting the outcome of congenital cutaneous candidiasis are the infant's birth weight and the presence of respiratory distress. Infants with birth weights of less than 1.5 kg or with early onset of respiratory distress are at risk for systemic disease, including candida sepsis or pneumonia.

## Staphylococcal Folliculitis

Staphylococcal folliculitis should be considered in the differential diagnosis of pustular eruptions in the newborn. Initial lesions are erythematous, follicular papules that evolve into pustules. Lesions remain discrete and do not coalesce. The diagnosis may be confirmed with a Gram stain or culture of a pustule.

## Herpes Simplex Virus

Herpes simplex virus may result in congenital infection but more commonly produces neonatal infection acquired as a result of passage through an infected birth canal or from an ascending infection associated with prolonged rupture of membranes. Cutaneous vesicles may be the first clue to the diagnosis but they are absent in 20% of affected infants. Although occasionally present at birth, skin lesions usually develop between 4 and 14 days of age and, when few in number, are often on the presenting part of the infant. Typical lesions are grouped vesicles on an erythematous base. A rapid diagnosis can be made with a Tzanck smear of the base of a vesicle, which reveals multinucleated giant cells. Neonatal herpes may be limited to the skin but more commonly produces disseminated systemic involvement with encephalitis, chorioretinitis, and hepatitis resulting in significant morbidity and mortality.

## Congenital Syphilis

Infants with congenital syphilis may vary considerably in their clinical expression, ranging from few symptoms to an acutely ill infant with fever, jaundice, anemia, thrombocytopenia, hepatosplenomegaly, and lymphadenopathy. The mucocutaneous manifestations of congenital syphilis may resemble or be identical to those seen in secondary syphilis. The most common lesions are oval, papulosquamous plaques involving the trunk and extremities, including the palms and soles. Vesicular or pustular lesions are not common but are highly suggestive of the diagnosis, especially when seen on the palms and soles. Oral mucous membrane patches and genital condyloma lata may be present. Similar lesions occur at the mucocutaneous junction of the mouth, which may become fissured and scarred, leading to the formation of rhagades. Syphilitic rhinitis or snuffles usually appear at 2 to 6 weeks of age from ulceration of the nasal mucosa with profuse mucopurulent discharge. Syphilitic osteochondritis and periostitis are common and can lead to pseudoparalysis, which may be mistaken for trauma.

## BULLAE

Differential diagnosis of bullae in the newborn is presented in Table 20-62 and Figure 20-77.

## Staphylococcal Toxin Syndromes

Three distinctive Staphylococcal toxin syndromes are produced by group II *Staphylococcus aureus:* bullous impetigo, staphylococcal scalded skin syndrome, and staphylococcal scarlet fever. All three syndromes represent varying cutaneous responses to an exfoliative toxin produced by this group of staphylococci. Bullous impetigo occurs primarily in newborns and older children and is characterized by initially clear bullae that rapidly become purulent. These superficial bullae rupture easily, forming thin crusts or erosions. The organism can be grown in cultures from the blister fluid.

Staphylococcal scalded skin syndrome (Ritter's disease) is preceded by a localized staphylococcal infection, usually a purulent conjunctivitis, omphalitis, rhinitis, pharyngitis, or infected circumcision site (Color Figure 12). Within a few days of the initial infection, diffuse erythema of the skin develops abruptly with marked skin tenderness and fever. Large, flaccid bullae develop and rupture almost immediately. Large sheets of skin separate and exfoliate, leaving a moist, red surface. Healing is usually

TABLE 20-62.    Differential Diagnosis of Bullae in the Newborn

Bullous impetigo
Staphylococcal scalded skin syndrome
Epidermolytic hyperkeratosis
Epidermolysis bullosa
Mastocytosis
Sucking blisters
Toxic epidermal necrolysis

TABLE 20-63. Differentiation of Staphylococcal Scalded Skin Syndrome (SSSS) and Toxic Epidermal Necrolysis (TEN)

| | SSSS | TEN |
|---|---|---|
| Etiology | Infectious; group II Staphylococci | Immunologic; usually drug related |
| Morbidity/mortality | Low | High |
| Mucous membrane involvement | Rare | Frequent |
| Nikolsky's sign | Present | Absent |
| Target lesions | Absent | Often present |
| Level of blister | Subcorneal | Subepidermal |

complete in 5 to 7 days, and mucosal involvement is rare. In contrast to bullous impetigo, organisms cannot be grown in cultures from the flaccid bullae but can be recovered from the initial site of infection. The widespread blistering is the result of a circulating exfoliative toxin produced by the staphylococcal organisms in the original site of infection. The blister forms high within the epidermis, just under the stratum corneum. Antistaphylococcal antibiotics are the treatment of choice.

## Toxic Epidermal Necrolysis

Staphylococcal scalded skin syndrome must be differentiated from toxic epidermal necrolysis (TEN) because their etiologies, courses, treatments, and ultimate prognoses differ (Table 20-63). TEN is presumed to be a hypersensitivity reaction and is a serious disorder with a high morbidity and mortality rate. It shares clinical and histologic features with, and is thought by many to be the most severe form of, erythema multiforme. Drugs are usually implicated in the etiology of TEN, although it may also be precipitated by viral or bacterial infections. TEN begins abruptly with fever and widespread macular or papular erythema that quickly becomes bullous (Color Figure 13). Target lesions may be present. As blisters rupture, large areas become denuded. Mucous membranes are severely affected, including the oral, conjunctival, and genital mucosa, as well as the lips. Less commonly, the respiratory and gastrointestinal mucosa is involved. Histologically, the entire epidermis is necrotic, and blisters form subepidermally.

## Epidermolytic Hyperkeratosis

An autosomal dominant form of ichthyosis with a 50% spontaneous mutation rate, epidermolytic hyperkeratosis is also referred to as congenital bullous ichthyosiform erythroderma because affected infants are born with widespread blistering and red, moist, denuded skin (Color Figure 14). Within 1 to 2 weeks, generalized blistering resolves and the skin becomes dry, thick, and scaly. During infancy and childhood, crops of localized blisters may occur and heal without scarring. Ultimately, blisters are replaced by dark, foul-smelling, verrucous, hypertrophic lesions that are most pronounced in body-fold areas.

## Epidermolysis Bullosa

Epidermolysis bullosa (EB) is a group of disorders whose primary feature is the formation of blisters following minor trauma to the skin. The inherited forms of EB are generally categorized according to the level of blister formation in the skin (Table 20-64). More than 16 variants of EB have been described. All types except localized EB simplex begin at birth or early infancy. Bullae arise on normal-appearing skin of the cheeks, chin, elbows, knees,

hands, feet, and other easily traumatized sites (Color Figure 15). Distinguishing among the types of EB clinically may be impossible in early infancy. Specific diagnosis requires light and electron microscopic histopathologic studies.

## Mastocytosis

Isolated mastocytomas or generalized cutaneous lesions of mastocytosis may present as blisters in the newborn. When blisters predominate, they are frequently mistaken for other disorders such as neonatal herpes or bullous impetigo. Mast cell degranulation with release of histamine may result in enough edema to produce grossly visible blisters.

## Sucking Blisters

Vigorous sucking by the fetus in utero may produce isolated bullae 5 to 15 mm in diameter on the forearm, wrist, hand, fingers, and, rarely, the toes. No treatment is necessary for these blisters because spontaneous resolution is the rule.

## SCALING DISORDERS

### Ichthyosis

Ichthyosis is classified into four major groups: autosomal-dominant ichthyosis vulgaris, autosomal-recessive lamellar ichthyosis/congenital ichthyosiform erythroderma, X-linked recessive ichthyosis, and autosomal-dominant epidermolytic hyperkeratosis. Recent data suggest that lamellar ichthyosis and nonbullous congenital ichthyosiform erythroderma are separate and distinct disorders. Onset in the neonatal period may occur in all but ichthyosis vulgaris in which symptoms develop later in childhood. Infants with epidermolytic hyperkeratosis are born

TABLE 20-64. Classification of Epidermolysis Bullosa (EB)

**Blister formation in the epidermis**
Autosomal-dominant generalized EB simplex
Autsomal-dominant localized EB simplex

**Blister formation in the basement membrane zone**
Autosomal-recessive junctional EB/EB letalis

**Blister formation in the dermis**
Autosomal-recessive dystrophic EB
Autosomal-dominant dystrophic EB

with widespread blistering. The collodion baby may be the first manifestation of more than one type of ichthyosis, but most infants subsequently develop lamellar ichthyosis. Rarely, the skin remains normal in appearance after the collodion membrane is shed. Collodion babies are encased in a tight, shiny membrane that restricts movement and results in ectropion (Color Figure 16). Fissuring and peeling begin shortly after birth, although complete shedding of the membrane may take weeks to months. Infants should be managed in an isolation incubator with careful temperature control and high humidity, which maximizes flexibility of the skin. Occlusive emollients should be avoided. The harlequin fetus is a severe form of congenital ichthyosis that probably represents a heterogeneous group of disorders. Affected infants are born with thick yellow skin that rapidly becomes crisscrossed by deep fissures with moist red bases (Color Figure 17). Marked ectropion and eclabium are common, as are malformed hands, feet, and ears from restriction of normal development in utero by the inflexible skin. Survival beyond infancy is rare.

## Seborrheic Dermatitis and Atopic Dermatitis

Classically, it has been said that seborrheic dermatitis begins shortly after birth and that atopic dermatitis has its onset at 2 or 3 months of age or later. Recent information suggests that the age of onset in infancy is similar for both disorders, ranging from 2 to several weeks. The morphologic characteristics and distribution of lesions may be alike with erythema, papules, and scale involving the scalp, face, diaper area, and trunk. Infants with seborrheic dermatitis are more likely to have axillary involvement, while lesions on the extremities are more common in atopic dermatitis. Both disorders may be treated with a low-potency topical corticosteroid such as 1% hydrocortisone cream once or twice daily.

## Psoriasis

Infantile psoriasis is uncommon. The diaper area is the most frequent site of involvement, thus making it difficult to differentiate from other causes of diaper dermatitis. Typical psoriatic lesions are sharply demarcated, beefy red plaques with thick, silvery scale (Color Figure 18). In infants, the scale may be less prominent and may be absent in the diaper area because of the moist environment.

## Neonatal Lupus Erythematosus

Round-to-oval, erythematous, scaling plaques with varying degrees of atrophy, telangiectasia, and scarring are the hallmarks of neonatal lupus erythematosus. The face is nearly always involved (Color Figure 19), and lesions may develop on the trunk and extremities. Affected infants may have systemic disease with congenital heart block, hepatosplenomegaly, pulmonary disease, anemia, neutropenia, or thrombocytopenia. Infants and their mothers have a high incidence of circulating anti-Ro/SS-A antibodies, but up to 35% of mothers have no overt signs or symptoms of connective tissue disease. Resolution of the skin lesions corresponds with the disappearance of transplacentally acquired maternal Ro/SS-A antibody between 6 and 12 months of age. Evaluation should include a thorough physical examination, biopsy of a characteristic skin lesion, complete blood count, platelet count, antinuclear antibody and Ro/SS-A antibody screen, and electrocardiogram. Because photosensitivity has been reported, protection from the sun, including the use of sunscreens, is advisable.

## Histiocytosis X

Histiocytosis X may mimic seborrheic dermatitis, with an erythematous scaling eruption on the face, scalp, axillae, and diaper area. Discrete, red-brown scaling papules with petechiae or purpura and failure to respond to topical corticosteroids are features that distinguish histiocytosis X from other similar-appearing disorders. Affected infants may have mucosal erosions or ulcerations, hepatosplenomegaly, and chronically draining ears. The diagnosis can be confirmed with a skin biopsy of a characteristic lesion.

## Diaper Dermatitis

A number of disorders may present with or include involvement of the diaper area. Regardless of the cause, diaper dermatitis persisting longer than 2 or 3 days is usually complicated by a *Candida albicans* infection that should be treated with topical antiyeast preparations. Irritant contact dermatitis tends to spare the body folds, with accentuation on the convex surfaces exposed to urine and stool. Keeping the skin as dry as possible with frequent diaper changes as well as emollient protection such as petrolatum will speed resolution.

## Selected Readings

### Birthmarks

Altman AR, Tschen JA, Wolf JE Jr. Cutis marmorata telangiectatica congenita: a case report. Pediatr Dermatol 1984;1:223.
Ashinoff R, Geronemus RG. Flashlamp-pumped pulsed dye laser for port-wine stains in infancy: Earlier versus later treatment. J Am Acad Dermatol 1991;24:467.
DiBacco RS, DeLeo VA. Mastocytosis and the mast cell. J Am Acad Dermatol 1982;7:709.
Enjolras O, Riche MC, Merland JJ. Facial port-wine stains and Sturge-Weber syndrome. Pediatrics 1985;76:48.
Esterly NB, Margileth AM, Kahn G, et al. Special symposium: the management of disseminated eruptive hemangiomata in infants. Pediatr Dermatol 1984;1:312.
Fost NC, Esterly NB. Successful treatment of juvenile hemangiomas with prednisone. J Pediatr 1968;72:351.
Hurwitz S. Epidermal nevi and tumors of epidermal origin. Pediatr Clin North Am 1983;30:483.
Jacobs AH, Walton RG. The incidence of birthmarks in the neonate. Pediatrics 1976;58:218.
Margileth AM, Museles M. Cutaneous hemangiomas in children: diagnosis and conservative management. JAMA 1965;194:523.
Rhodes AR. Pigmented birthmarks and precursor melanocytic lesions of cutaneous melanoma identifiable in childhood. Pediatr Clin North Am 1983;30:435.
Scheibner A, Wheeland RG. Use of the argon-pumped tunable dye laser for port-wine stains in children. J Dermatol Surg Oncol 1991;17:735.
Stevenson RF, Thomson HG, Morin JD. Unrecognized ocular problems associated with port-wine stain of the face in children. Can Med Assoc J 1974;111:953.
Tallman B, Tan OT, Morelli JG, et al. Location of port-wine stains and the likelihood of ophthalmic and/or central nervous system complications. Pediatrics 1991;87:323.
Tan OT, Sherwood K, Gilchrest BA. Treatment of children with port-wine stains using the flashlamp-pulsed tunable dye laser. N Engl J Med 1989;320:416.

### Vesiculopustular and Bullous Disorders

Carney RG. Incontinentia pigmenti. A world statistical analysis. Arch Dermatol 1976;112:535.
Crissey JT, Denenholz DA. Congenital syphilis. Clin Dermatol 1984;2:143.
Fine J-D. Epidermolysis bullosa: Clinical aspects, pathology, and recent advances in research. Intl J Dermatol 1986;25:143.
Johnson DE, Thompson TR, Ferrieri P. Congenital candidiasis. Am J Dis Child 1981;135:273.
Melish ME, Glasgow LA. Staphylococcal scalded skin syndrome: the expanded clinical syndrome. J Pediatr 1971;78:958.
Ramamurthy RS, Reveri M, Esterly NB, et al. Transient neonatal pustular melanosis. J Pediatr 1976;88:831.
Vignon-Pennamen M-D, Wallach D. Infantile acropustulosis: a clinicopathologic study of six cases. Arch Dermatol 1986;122:1155.
Whitley RJ, Nahmias AJ, Visintine AM, et al. The natural history of herpes simplex virus infection of mother and newborn. Pediatrics 1980;66:489.

### Scaling Disorders

Farber EM, Jacobs AH. Infantile psoriasis. Am J Dis Child 1977;131:1266.
Roper SS, Spraker MK. Cutaneous histiocytosis syndromes. Pediatr Dermatol 1985;3:19.
Siegel MD, Deng J-S, Sontheimer RD. Ro/SS-A antibody-associated cutaneous lupus erythematosus: neonatal and subacute cutaneous lupus. Sem Dermatol 1985;4:69.
Weston WL, Lane AT, Weston JA. Diaper dermatitis: current concepts. Pediatrics 1980;66:532.

Williams ML, Elias PM. Genetically transmitted, generalized disorders of cornification: The ichthyoses. Dermatol Clin 1987;5:155.

Yates VM, Kerr REI, MacKie RM. Early diagnosis of infantile seborrhoeic dermatitis and atopic dermatitis—clinical features. Br J Dermatol 1983;108:633.

*Principles and Practice of Pediatrics, Second Edition.*
edited by Frank A. Oski et al. J. B. Lippincott Company, Philadelphia © 1994.

# 20.11 *Mineral Metabolism in the Newborn*

### Joseph M. Gertner

## DEVELOPMENTAL CONSIDERATIONS

### Histogenesis and Organogenesis of the Skeleton

At the end of a 40-week term of gestation, the neonatal skeleton has reached an organization close to that familiar in the adult. The skeleton and the homeostatic control systems for the skeletal minerals, calcium and phosphate, develop in the protected intrauterine environment. Most of the functions of the skeleton— protection of vulnerable organs, anchoring of muscles, maintenance of the body's shape against gravity, and provision of a metabolic buffer of calcium and phosphate—are not needed until delivery. Development of the skeleton depends on integration of events directing cells derived from primitive mesenchyme to produce bone matrix, to mineralize that matrix, then to remodel the resulting bone. This process is under complex genetic control and can be distorted by disordered formation of fibrous and nonfibrous matrix proteins, by faulty migration of bone forming cells, by failure to recruit appropriate cells for bone remodelling, and by abnormalities of the hormonal and ionic milieu needed to promote mineralization.

Precursors of bone cells begin to form at about 5 weeks' gestation from membranes or rods of mesenchymal cells. Intramembranous bone forms the sides and vault of the skull and the clavicles while endochondral ossification accounts for most of the remaining bones, particularly those of developing limbs. In both forms of ossification, osteoprogenitor cells condense, mature into alkaline phosphatase-positive osteoblasts, secrete an extracellular ground substance, and begin to mineralize. A network of collagen fibers forms the framework upon which the first bony trabeculae mineralize to form "primary spongiosa." Secondary foci of ossification that eventually become epiphyseal centers differentiate from mesenchyme in an analogous manner. Remodelling of the skeleton begins as soon as the primary spongiosa is formed; osteoclasts resorb existing bone while osteoblasts form new bone.

## Ionic and Hormonal Effects on the Fetal Skeleton

The mineralization process depends on controlled delivery of calcium and phosphate to sites of ossification and on local effects of the calcitropic hormones, parathyroid hormone (PTH), calcitriol (1,25-dihydroxyvitamin D), and calcitonin. Calcium and phosphorus are transported across the placenta against a concentration gradient that appears as early as 12 weeks. The quantity of mineral transported increases sharply until late in the last trimester of pregnancy when the fetus accumulates up to 85 mg/kg/d of phosphorus and 150 mg/kg/d of calcium (Fig 20-79). Evidence shows placental calcium transport depends on availability of calcitriol, but there are no known intrinsic disorders of the placenta that specifically limit fetal calcium and phosphorus accumulation. Mineral deficiency may accompany the general fetal malnutrition characteristic of placental insufficiency. Pathologic consequences can arise from disordered transplacental calcium transport when calcium concentrations in the maternal serum are too high or too low. These disorders are discussed in the following paragraphs.

The parathyroid glands are formed from cells of the 3rd and 4th pharyngeal pouches at the 6th to 7th week of gestation and stain positively for PTH by the 12th week. The parathyroid glands are the principal regulators of extracellular ionized calcium concentration. The chief cells serve both as calcium sensors and effectors, detecting ionized calcium concentration in the extracellular fluid and secreting PTH, an 84-amino acid peptide that elevates ionized calcium by promoting bone resorption. Hypoparathyroidism does not affect the fetus because maternal calcium regulation prevails in utero and PTH does not seem necessary for skeleton development. Intrauterine hyperparathyroidism, on the other hand, can lead to pathologic resorption of the fetal skeleton.

The C-cells of the thyroid are derived from ultimobranchial (5th pharyngeal pouch) tissue and begin to secrete their 22-amino acid peptide hormone, calcitonin, at an early stage of gestation. Acutely, calcitonin lowers the extracellular ionized calcium concentration by inhibiting bone resorption. Humans of all ages,

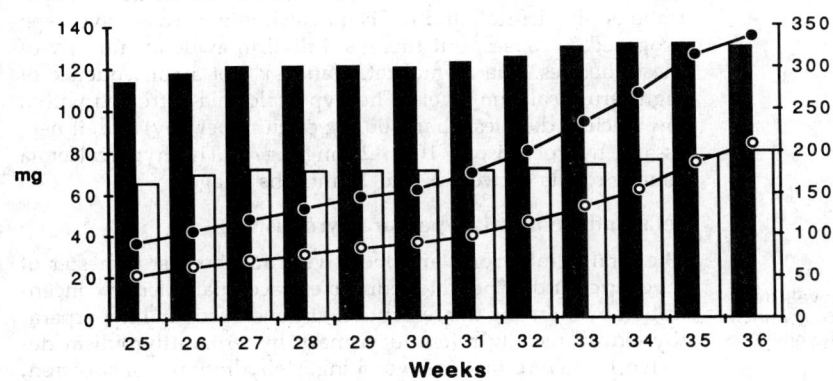

Figure 20-79.   Interuterine accumulation of phosphorus and calcium during late pregnancy.

however, maintain normal calcium homeostasis and bone turnover in the absence of calcitonin (athyreosis) and in the presence of large excesses of the hormone (medullary carcinoma of the thyroid). Thus, the physiologic function of calcitonin, both in utero and in the neonatal period, is obscure. Neonatal hypercalcitoninemia may contribute to neonatal hypocalcemia.

The third calcitropic hormone, calcitriol, is a lipid-soluble sterol that, unlike the two peptide hormones, can be transported across the placenta. Both the fetal kidneys and the placenta can make calcitriol. It is unknown how much of this hormone is transported from the maternal circulation and how much is synthesized in the fetus or placenta. It is known that the precursor sterol, calcidiol (25-hydroxyvitamin D), is transported across the placenta. Calcidiol concentration level in fetal blood correlates with the maternal level, and it is needed for fetal synthesis of calcitriol. The major biologic action of calcitriol, the promotion of intestinal calcium absorption, is unnecessary during fetal life. The role of fetal vitamin D metabolites in bone development is unclear, but the existence of congenital rickets as a pathologic entity suggests that vitamin D sterols directly affect mineralization.

In recent years, the role of another substance that may affect prenatal and perinatal bone mineral physiology has come under investigation. Parathyroid-hormone related peptide (PTHrP) is a 141 amino-acid peptide first characterized in malignant cells derived from patients with the syndrome of humeral hypercalcemia of malignancy. PTHrP shares a region of homology with PTH encompassing the 13 N-terminal amino acids and it shares with PTH the power to bind to PTH receptors, activating bone resorption and renal tubular phosphate reabsorption. Once the gene for PTHrP had been cloned, a search for mammalian tissues expressing the RNA message for the peptide was conducted. Active peptide was discovered in the placenta and in the lactating breast with considerable quantities secreted into the milk. It is not known what role is served by PTHrP to which the fetus might be exposed from the placenta and which the infant ingests orally from breast milk.

## Perinatal Mineral Homeostasis

After delivery, the fetus must adapt to the sudden withdrawal of an abundant placental supply of calcium and phosphate. Mean fetal calcium levels fall from around 11 mg/dL at birth to a nadir of around 8.5 mg/dL in full-term and 7.0 mg/dL in premature infants. Corresponding data for ionized calcium levels in preterm infants are shown in Figure 20-80.

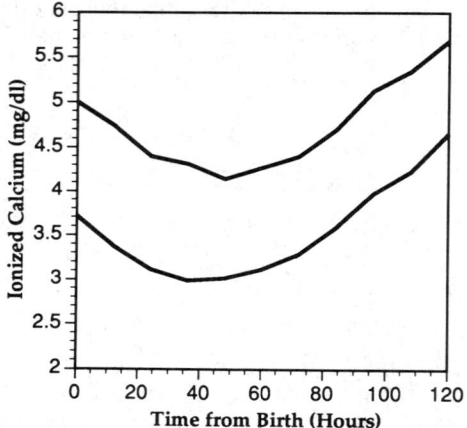

Figure 20-80. Fall and rise in mean serum ionized calcium levels over 120 hours after birth. (After Mayne PD, Kovar IZ. Calcium and phosphorus metabolism in the premature infant. Ann Clin Biochem 1991;28:131.)

These minimum levels of serum calcium occur 1 to 2 days after delivery and give rise to hormonal adjustments that promote the infant's metabolic adaptation to postnatal mineral homeostasis. PTH levels appear to increase postnatally, which is an appropriate response to the fall in serum calcium. Literature on this topic is contradictory, perhaps because of inconsistencies in PTH immunoassays. Serum calcitonin levels are said to be high in the perinatal period, but there is little information concerning changes during the first few days of postnatal life.

Mean serum calcidiol and calcitriol concentrations are lower in neonates than in mothers, but do not differ between full term and premature babies. In full term and premature infants, serum calcitriol increases from birth to day 5 and decreases again by day 30; in preterm infants, calcitriol levels are higher than in full term infants on day 30. The role of calcitriol in calcium homeostasis largely depends on promotion of gastrointestinal calcium absorption. Thus, the postnatal rise in calcitriol is less effective in infants whose oral calcium intake is inadequate or who have disordered intestinal function. Disorders of calcium control in the neonate can arise because of failures of the PTH-vitamin D homeostatic system or because that system is overwhelmed by unfavorable circumstances. These disorders are discussed as hypercalcemia and hypocalcemia in subsequent paragraphs.

## HORMONAL AND METABOLIC DISORDERS

### Congenital Rickets

Congenital rickets is a rare condition in modern times, but of theoretical interest in view of the importance of rickets as a component of metabolic bone disease of prematurity. The appearance in the term neonate of frayed and cupped epiphyses with general skeletal rarefaction and sometimes with deformities is well described in older literature.

The condition accompanies severe maternal vitamin D deficiency and is attributed to the same deficiency in the fetus. Some cases may be due to fetal hyperparathyroidism secondary to maternal and fetal hypocalcemia, but some may result directly from deficiency of vitamin D metabolites supplied to the fetus.

### Neonatal Hypercalcemia

#### Idiopathic Infantile Hypercalcemia (IIH) or Williams' Syndrome

Congenital facial and cardiovascular anomalies (supravalvular aortic stenosis and peripheral pulmonary stenosis) and mental retardation are often accompanied by transient infantile hypercalcemia. The hypercalcemia may not be recognized until many weeks of age but retrospective evidence may be obtained from a history of poor feeding or constipation in the neonatal period. The cause of the hypercalcemia is unknown and familial cases are rare. Elevations in calcidiol, elevated and subnormal concentrations of calcitriol, and deficient calcitonin release have been proposed as causes, but there is little firm evidence for any of these theories. The mental retardation is not a consequence of high serum calcium levels. The hypercalcemia is treated with a low calcium diet (less than 100 mg calcium per day) and, if necessary, hydrocortisone 10 to 25 mg/kg/d. The hypercalcemia usually remits between 9 and 18 months of age.

#### Fetal and Neonatal Hyperparathyroidism

The fetal parathyroids are operative from the first trimester of pregnancy and respond to reduced extracellular calcium concentration by inducing the resorption of bone. Neonatal hyperparathyroidism usually refers to primary hyperparathyroidism detected by severe malaise (vomiting, dehydration, constipation) during the first few days of life. These infants are always hypercalcemic, and soon after delivery they become hypophosphatemic. Immunoreactive PTH levels are high. Aminoaciduria is common, probably due to a direct effect of PTH on the renal tubule. The condition is most often due to parathyroid hyperplasia occurring either spontaneously or as part of a familial syndrome, in which, cases may be homozygous for a trait represented by benign hypocalciuric hypercalcemia in the heterozygous persons. Emergency treatment for dehydration and hypercalcemia is often needed. The most effective therapy is rehydration with 0.9% saline which corrects the dehydration of hypercalcemia and induces a calciuresis. Urinary calcium losses can be further increased by administration of furosemide 6 mg/kg/d (in divided doses). Calcitonin given subcutaneously may be effective for a few days but tolerance to its action soon develops. Corticosteroids are not beneficial in hypercalcemia due to hyperparathyroidism. These children have been treated by emergency parathyroidectomy with, in some cases, autotransplantation of some of the parathyroid tissue into an accessible site such as the forearm.

In secondary hyperparathyroidism the fetal glands are stimulated by fetal hypocalcemia caused by maternal hypocalcemia. These circumstances can occur when there is maternal vitamin D deficiency and when the mother has untreated hypoparathyroidism. As in primary hyperparathyroidism, the bones are rarefied and spontaneous fractures may occur. Biochemically, the condition evolves from hypocalcemia (present prenatally and responsible for the condition) through normocalcemia to hypercalcemia due to an autonomous release of PTH even when the neonate receives adequate oral calcium intake. There is hypophosphatemia due to PTH-induced phosphaturia. During the first few months of life, skeletal lesions tend to heal rapidly, and the parathyroid glands regress and resume normal function.

## Hypocalcemia

Neonatal hypocalcemia is generally divided into early and late forms according to the age (in days) of onset. The early form generally begins on the first to third day of life, while the late form becomes evident after about a week.

### Early Neonatal Hypocalcemia

Hypocalcemia occurs in low–birth-weight and sick infants 1 to 4 days old. Hypocalcemia may present with jittery movements, convulsions, apnea, or myocardial dysfunction. It may be considered an exaggeration of the physiologic drop in ionized calcium seen at this age. Causes of this hypocalcemia, which is more marked in preterm infants, are unknown. Parathyroid underactivity secondary to the normally high serum calcium of the fetus, diminished bone resorption associated with high calcitonin levels, and poor dietary calcium intake and absorption have all been proposed as causes. Direct measurement of ionized calcium is often more useful than measuring total serum calcium level because no correction need be made for protein concentration or blood pH. An ionized calcium concentration less than 2.5 mg/dL can lead to clinical symptoms. The electrocardiogram (long QT interval) may also provide a useful clue.

### Late Neonatal Hypocalcemia

Late neonatal hypocalcemia presents clinically at 5 to 10 days of age in full-term, and apparently healthy, neonates. Hypocalcemia is associated with elevated serum phosphate levels. The causes are summarized in Table 20-65.

*Permanent Hypoparathyroidism.*    Primary hypoparathyroidism may be due to inherited or sporadic isolated absence of the parathyroid glands. In some cases, hypoparathyroidism is combined with some or all of the other features of the DiGeorge

**TABLE 20-65.    Causes of Late Neonatal Hypocalcemia**

Hypoparathyroidism
  Permanent
  Transient (secondary to maternal hypercalcemia)
Excessive phosphorus intake (unmodified or inadequately modified cow's milk diet)
Renal glomerular failure

syndrome (thymic aplasia, various forms of congenital heart disease, and some facial abnormalities). Some cases of the DiGeorge syndrome appear to be dominantly inherited. Cause of the syndrome is not known, but an association with structural abnormalities of the 22nd chromosomes has been described in several cases. Hypoparathyroidism reduces the capacity of affected babies to regulate serum calcium and to excrete phosphate. Symptomatic hypocalcemia may occur within the first day or two after delivery. More commonly, it appears as serum phosphate levels rise at 6 to 9 days of age. PTH levels are low. The treatment is to restore extracellular fluid ionized calcium with oral or intravenous calcium and to restrain the accumulation of phosphate by feeding a low phosphorus formula such as PM 60-40. If hypocalcemia is severe or if it tends to recur when calcium supplements are reduced, a vitamin D metabolite can be added. Permanent therapy is needed in most cases of primary hypoparathyroidism, but some cases, even with DiGeorge syndrome, recover enough PTH secretory capacity to come off treatment after a few months.

*Transient (Secondary) Hypoparathyroidism.*    The parathyroid glands can be suppressed by prolonged intrauterine hypercalcemia, itself secondary to maternal hypercalcemia. Usually, mothers of these babies have primary hyperparathyroidism. The clinical picture is virtually identical to that of primary hypoparathyroidism, but cases due to maternal hypercalcemia remit spontaneously within the first few weeks of life. Maternal serum calcium must be checked as part neonatal hypoparathyroidism evaluation.

*Phosphorus Overload.*    Ingestion of unmodified cow's milk is no longer a practical problem in developed countries. Cow's milk contains six times as much phosphorus as human milk (950 mg/L versus 162 mg/L). Ingestion of a calorically adequate volume of cow's milk overwhelms the capacity of the neonatal kidney to excrete phosphate, causing hyperphosphatemia, which shifts the equilibrium in calcium flow between bone and the extracellular fluid toward bone. It also diminishes calcitriol synthesis. Both of these changes operate to reduce the plasma calcium level. Phosphate accumulation is also a feature of chronic glomerular renal failure with hypocalcemic tetany as a presenting feature in severely affected babies.

### Treatment of Hypocalcemia

Mild hypocalcemia may not require therapy. A neonate with a serum calcium level below 7.0 to 7.5 mg/dL (ionized calcium less than 2.8 mg/dL) should be treated to prevent tetany and other symptoms. In severe symptomatic hypocalcemia, intravenous therapy is required. Slow parenteral infusions of 20 to 50 mg/kg/d of elemental calcium as the gluconate may be diluted with saline or dextrose infusion fluids and given intravenously. Alternatively, 10 to 20 mg/kg of elemental calcium can be given every 4 to 6 hours. Occasionally, higher doses are needed. Intravenous calcium should be given carefully because over-rapid administration can cause cardiac arrhythmias, while extravasation of calcium salts can lead to local tissue inflammation and even necrosis. Serum calcium should be monitored frequently and the infusion adjusted accordingly. Chronic hypocalcemia is treated by administration of vitamin D or its metabolites. Calcitriol has largely replaced dihydrotachysterol, an analog of vitamin D, as the treatment of choice for chronic hypocalcemia. Circulating calcitriol has a half-life of less than 1 day, greatly enhancing therapeutic safety. Based on weight adjustment, calcitriol dosage in small children (0.125 to 2.0 µg/d, occasionally higher) is generally higher than adult dosage.

# METABOLIC BONE DISEASE OF PREMATURITY

## Definition, Nomenclature, and Prevalence

Metabolic bone disease of prematurity (MBDP) encompasses a spectrum of disturbances in preterm infants, which results in rickets, osteomalacia, and osteoporosis. Milder cases may show only biochemical changes. Rickets and osteomalacia describe undermineralization of normal organic bone matrix (osteoid), while in osteoporosis there is reduced bone mass with a normal ratio of mineral to matrix. Osteopenia describes decreased bone density on imaging. The term does not distinguish between decreased mineralization of quantitatively normal matrix and normal mineralization of diminished quantities of matrix. Little histologic information is available, and it is difficult to assess the relative importance of rickets versus osteoporosis in MBDP.

The reported frequency of MBDP varies depending on diagnostic criteria. The condition mainly affects premature infants, but also affects those close to term but small for gestational age. In one prospective radiologic survey, fractures were detected in 20% of newborns with birth weight less than 1500 g and gestational age less than 34 weeks. Subclinical disease may be more common as suggested by the prevalence of elevated serum alkaline phosphatase and decreased bone mineral content.

## Etiology

The primary cause of MBDP seems to be a deficiency of phosphate and calcium due to decreased intake. Initial reports of MBDP involved infants fed human milk and sick neonates (usually with respiratory disease). Human milk is relatively low in calcium and phosphate. Infants with respiratory disease are at risk because of the low mineral concentration in hyperalimentation fluid, fluid restriction when on oral feedings, and increased urinary mineral losses secondary to furosemide therapy. From prospective studies, however, it appears MBDP also affects "well" preterm infants fed standard formulas.

Although phosphate deficiency is usually associated with osteomalacia, it can also lead to osteoporosis. Phosphate deficient rats show a modest increase in osteoid and a marked decrease in trabecular bone volume, indicating osteoporosis. Calcium deficiency also can cause metabolic bone disease. Calcium deficiency is implicated in some cases of childhood rickets and in postmenopausal osteoporosis.

Eighty percent of calcium and phosphate accretion for the fetal skeleton occurs by active transport across the placenta during the third trimester of pregnancy (see Fig 20-78). To maintain an intrauterine growth rate postnatally, comparable quantities of calcium and phosphate must be provided from external sources to premature infants at an equivalent stage of gestation. There are inadequate quantities of these minerals in human milk and standard formulas. Assuming an intake of 150 to 200 mL/kg/d, human milk provides only 25% to 50% of the phosphorus and 35% to 70% of the calcium accumulated in the third trimester of pregnancy. A standard formula provides only 55% to 90% of the phosphorus and 45% to 100% of the calcium. Only some of

the minerals absorbed are retained. Retention of phosphorus and calcium depends on the balance between net intestinal absorption and renal excretion. Preterm infants satisfactorily absorb phosphorus and calcium from the intestine and reabsorb the minerals in the renal tubule. However, the following dietary factors may influence mineral retention:

1. Calcium to phosphorus ratio in the diet affects the intestinal and renal handling of both these minerals.
2. Quantity and quality of dietary fat influence calcium absorption.
3. Soy formulas, which contain phytates, bind phosphorus and calcium in the gut and decreases their absorption.
4. Relatively large volumes of intestinal secretions in preterm infants, a consequence of the large food volume needed to satisfy their caloric requirements, affect mineral retention.

Adequate mineral delivery via total parenteral nutrition (TPN) is confounded by the difficulty of maintaining the solubility of concentrated mixtures of calcium and phosphorus. Thus, the amounts of phosphorus and calcium that can be delivered by TPN provide less than 50% of the supply of these minerals delivered to the fetus in utero. It is not known whether "TPN bone disease" or TPN-associated skeletal aluminum toxicity, both described in older children and adults, also plays a part in the osteopathy of low–birth-weight infants receiving TPN.

It has been suggested that calcidiol levels are low in these infants and that levels of this metabolite do not respond to supplementation with 400 IU/d of vitamin D. Most preterm infants, including those with bone disease, however, appear to have normal levels of calcidiol and calcitriol and absorb calcium and phosphorus from the intestine efficiently. In some cases with MBDP, calcitriol levels are elevated, probably because of stimulation by hypophosphatemia. Such elevated calcitriol levels may contribute to MBDP by stimulating bone resorption. Despite high levels of calcitriol, such infants are not hypercalcemic, possibly because of concomitant dietary calcium deficiency. There is no evidence that abnormalities of PTH or calcitonin production or secretion contribute to bone disease in preterm infants. The role of possible insufficiencies of factors such as trace elements, other nutrients, and growth factors has yet to be excluded.

## Diagnosis: Clinical, Imaging, and Biochemical

MBDP covers a spectrum extending from overt bone disease (rickets and fractures) (Fig 20-81) to mild biochemical disturbances. Fractures usually are located where the infant may be physically manipulated during diagnostic or therapeutic maneuvers (ie, extremities, ribs). If one fracture is noted, other fractures are likely. Limb fractures may cause pain, loss of movement, or deformity, while rib fractures can exacerbate respiratory distress syndrome (RDS). Several methods are used to diagnose MBDP before it manifests clinically. Radiography is unsatisfactory because conditions under which films are taken are not standardized. In addition, there must be considerable bone loss for osteopenia to be detectable by routine x-ray. Despite this, the classification given in Table 20-66 has been proposed. Photon absorptiometry quantifies bone mineral content rather than total bone mass. A photon beam (photon source of $^{125}$I) is passed through the bone. The attenuation of detectable counts is proportional to the mineral content (g) per bone length (cm). With this technique preterm infants show decreased BMC compared to that of fetuses of similar postconceptional age. The methods used and correlations with clinical bone disease have yet to be fully validated.

Biochemical tests may detect early MBDP. Alkaline phosphatase values in subjects with and without radiologic evidence of bone disease overlap. An alkaline phosphatase level that is more

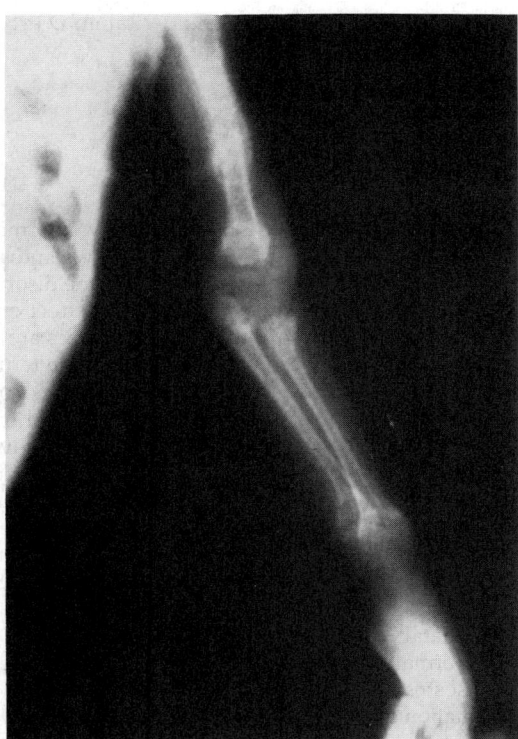

**Figure 20-81.** Osteopenia, rickets, and a healing humeral fracture characteristic of the metabolic bone disease of prematurity. (Courtesy of Dr. D.E. Carey, Schneider Children's Hospital, New Hyde Park, NY.)

| TABLE 20-66. Radiologic Classification of Metabolic Bone Disease of Prematurity |
| --- |
| Grade 0: Normal bone |
| Grade I: Bone rarefaction only |
| Grade II: Metaphyseal changes (fraying, cupping) with subperiosteal new bone formation |
| Grade III: The above changes with fractures |

but to a lesser degree than in classical vitamin D deficient controls. Osteoporosis, which was not a feature in the vitamin D deficient controls, was pronounced in the infants with MBDP.

## Course and Prognosis

The age at which the bony changes manifest may depend on growth rate. According to one study, infants who were later to develop rickets had a low serum phosphate by age 2 weeks and an elevated alkaline phosphatase at 4 weeks. Decreased mineralization is evident on photon absorptiometry as early as age 2 weeks. Radiographic changes have been found at 4 to 20 weeks. In one prospective study, 75% of abnormal x-rays were noted by 3 months and all abnormalities by 6 months.

Although some infants with MBDP may develop fractures and acute biochemical disturbances, little morbidity is noted in most infants with biochemical and radiologic evidence of MBDP. Increasing evidence shows the condition as self-limiting with recovery of bone mineral content during the first few weeks and months of postnatal life.

## Prevention and Treatment

A growth rate similar to that in utero is a sensible goal and has been endorsed by the American Academy of Pediatrics Committee on Nutrition. Therefore, the amount of phosphorus and calcium retained by the preterm infant must approximate that of the fetus in utero. Supplementation of feeds with phosphorus and calcium is difficult because of the formation of insoluble salts when these ions are combined. Some formulas that contain increased quantities of these salts have to be shaken well before use, which can be a problem with continuous naso-gastrointestinal feeds. Alternating administration of phosphorus or calcium is complicated by high urinary losses of the supplemented mineral. Nevertheless, fortified human milk and some of the special formulas for preterm infants (Similac Special Care, Enfamil Pre-

than five times the maximum adult level, however, may suggest MBDP in a patient who is not on TPN and has no bone disease. Table 20-67 summarizes laboratory tests used to evaluate infants at risk of MBDP and indicates findings expected in "pure" calcium or phosphate deficiency. The mixed picture found in clinical practice leads to correspondingly intermediate results. Other types of metabolic bone disease are unlikely to present in the newborn period and rarely pose a problem of differential diagnosis. Vitamin D deficiency, however, produces radiologic rickets and a biochemical picture similar to that of calcium deficiency, except for low calcidiol value (less than 5 to 8 ng/mL).

## Histology

There are few reports on bone histology in MBDP. The ribs from three preterm infants who died of RDS showed osteomalacia,

| TABLE 20-67. Evaluation of Infants at Risk of MBDP | | | |
| --- | --- | --- | --- |
| | Phosphate Deficiency | Calcium Deficiency | Value for Premature Infant |
| Serum phosphate | ↓ | ↓ | 5.0–8.5 mg/dL |
| Serum calcium | Normal or ↑ | Normal or ↓ | 8.0–11.0 mg/dL* |
| TRP | ↑ | ↓ | 85%–95% |
| Alkaline phosphatase | ↑ | | <5 times adult upper limit; varies with assay |
| Urinary calcium | ↑ | ↓ | <4–6 mg/kg/d |
| Parathyroid hormone | ↓ | ↑ | Varies with assay |
| Calcidiol (25-OH Vitamin D) | | | 3.6–10.8 ng/mL† |
| Calcitriol (1,25-OH₂ Vitamin D) | ↑ | ↑ | 40–80 pg/mL† |

\* Value for premature infant at 1 week of age
† Fifth day of life

mature) do permit an increase in absorption and retention of phosphorus and calcium approaching the fetal accretion rate. For example, volumes of 140 to 200 mL/kg/d provide 185 to 200 mg/kg/d calcium, 65% of which is retained (ie, 120 to 130 mg/kg/d), thus approximating the accretion rate of a fetus over 28 weeks. As for phosphorus, an intake of 100 to 113 mg/kg/d, 71% of which is retained (ie, 71 to 80 mg/kg/d), approximates the accretion rate of a fetus over 28 weeks.

Increasing phosphorus and calcium retention does not necessarily translate into improved bone structure. There are case reports of preterm infants with severe MBDP that resolved after supplementation with phosphorus or in combination with calcium. The natural course of this condition, however, suggests that resolution was spontaneous. Several prospective studies investigated whether MBDP could be prevented by increasing the intake (and presumably retention) of phosphorus and calcium. The results and conclusions of these studies vary, perhaps because mineral retention depends on factors other than the total calcium and phosphorus content of the formula and because different densitometric criteria were used to evaluate response.

In one study, the BMC of the radius in preterm infants fed calcium- and phosphorus-supplemented breast milk was greater than that of babies fed only breast milk. BMC was even higher in infants fed a premature formula with a calcium content of 94 mg/dL and a phosphorus content of 47.5 mg/dL. However, in another study, the use of fortified human milk failed to increase BMC in the humerus above values seen in control infants.

Most available prospective studies pertain to enterally fed preterm infants. Recently, however, Pelegano and colleagues published the results of a short-term (48 h) study of mineral retention in parenterally fed sick preterm infants. The calcium-to-phosphorus ratio of 1.7:1 led to a grater degree of calcium and phosphorus retention than parenteral feeds formulated with greater or lesser calcium-to-phosphorus ratios.

Despite inconclusive evidence from the supplementation studies, the consensus is that unfortified human milk is not adequate for preterm infants. On the other hand, little overt MBDP is reported in "healthy" preterm infants fed standard milk formulas. Therefore, it is recommended that all low–birth-weight infants receive phosphorus and calcium in excess of what is present in breast milk. Such supplementation is suggested to be continued until the infant's weight reaches 2 kg, depending on circumstances.

Commercial premature formulas given in quantities mentioned above contain maximal allowable intakes for preterm infants of gestational age over 28 weeks. The American Academy of Pediatrics Committee on Nutrition advises a calcium intake of 210 mg/kg/d for preterm infants weighing 800 to 1200 g. The Committee on Nutrition makes no recommendation for infants outside this range and does not make its own recommendation on phosphorus requirements.

The minimal requirement of phosphorus and calcium for preterm infants on TPN is 30 to 40 mg/kg/d of each element (American Academy of Pediatrics). It may be possible to circumvent the problem of low solubility of ionic mixtures of calcium and phosphorus by lowering the pH of the solution or providing a soluble source of both minerals such as calcium glycerophosphate. This compound has improved bone mineralization in piglets. Regarding vitamin D, a daily intake of at least 400 IU is recommended in addition to the vitamin D in the feeds. Higher intake of vitamin D may be necessary when there is maternal vitamin D deficiency.

Potential adverse effects of excessive calcium administration are hypercalcemia, hypercalciuria (with potential for nephrocalcinosis), hypophosphatemia, and decreased fat and phosphorus absorption. Calcium preparations such as calcium lactate may result in metabolic acidosis. A potential adverse effect of phosphorus supplementation is hypocalcemia. Vitamin D excess can lead to hypercalcemia and hypercalciuria.

## DISORDERS OF BONE FORMATION

### Disorders of Shape

Because the internal structure of a bone critically determines its shape, it is somewhat artificial to distinguish between disorders of morphogenesis and histogenesis. There are some disorders of matrix formation, however, that have a striking effect on bone morphology. Many disorders of limb morphogenesis are genetically determined, but, except in the most descriptive terms, the genetic error is unknown. Such disorders may involve all or most of the skeleton diffusely, in which case a generalized error of histogenesis is likely to be responsible or may specifically affect one bone or a defined group of bones. International efforts to devise a rational nomenclature for these disorders has led to their classification as dyschondroplasias, which are subdivided into five groups (Table 20-68). Achondroplasia is one of the more common representatives of the osteochondrodysplasias. Severe forms of this dominantly inherited condition may be recognized at birth or prenatally by ultrasound or radiology.

Defective formation of specific groups of bones is seen in a variety of dysostoses such as the Klippel-Feil syndrome, a vertebral segmentation defect, and in numerous syndromes involving syndactyly and polydactyly.

Congenital defects of bone may be limited to the skeleton, or they may be part of wider syndromes of congenital malformation. In the latter case, the bony malformation may be a consequence of a non-osseous defect (eg, spina bifida that accompanies the Arnold-Chiari malformation), or it may bear no logical link to other features of the syndrome (eg, femoral shortening seen in Down syndrome and radial hypoplasia of Fanconi's anemia) (Fig 20-82).

Acquired disorders of skeletal morphogenesis may be due to unfavorable circumstances in the external environment. The best-known examples are the phocomelia of thalidomide ingestion and limb reductions caused by constricting bands in utero. Other skeletal defects are ascribed to chemical toxins and irradiation.

While molecular pathogenesis of most osteochondrodysplasias remains unknown, genetic linkage analysis attempts to assign responsible mutations to specific regions of the genome. In at least one case (spondyloepiphyseal dysplasia), a developmental dysplasia of bone was traced to a mutation in one of the genes coding for proteins of connective tissue, in this case, type II collagen.

### Disorders of Structure

Disorders of structure may be due to abnormal bone matrix synthesis or to abnormalities of the ionic or hormonal milieu in which the skeleton develops. In the mucopolysaccharidoses, the bio-

---

### TABLE 20-68. Classification of Chondrodysplasia

I. Osteochondrodysplasias in which cartilage or bone formation is disordered

II. Dysostoses in which individual bones or combinations of bones are malformed

III. Idiopathic osteolyses

IV. Skeletal disorders associated with chromosomal anomalies

V. Primary (systemic) metabolic disorders

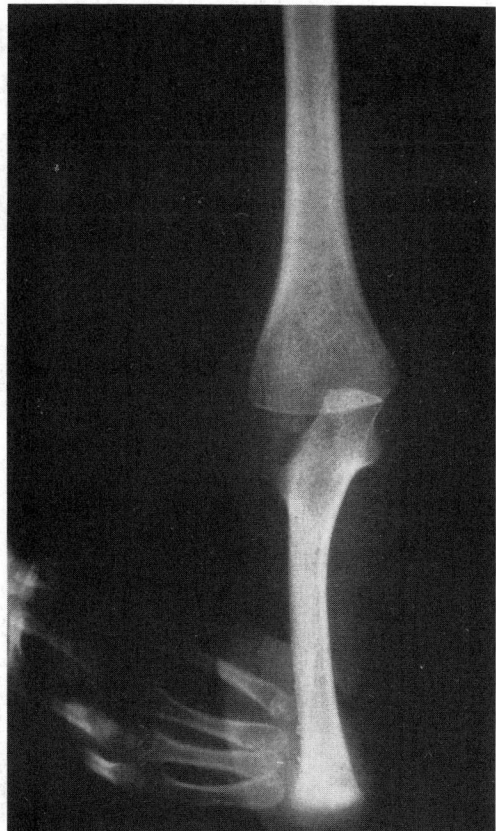

**Figure 20-82.** Absence of the radius in a young child with Fanconi's anemia.

chemical defect in the synthesis of cartilaginous matrix is relatively clearly defined. The resulting skeletal dysmorphia is usually mild and is rarely recognized at birth.

## Osteogenesis Imperfecta

Osteogenesis imperfecta (OI) is a group of inherited diseases in which the bones are unusually brittle and liable to fracture. Division into tarda and congenital forms of the disorder has been abandoned in light of more detailed studies of nosology and inheritance and the advent of our first insights at a molecular level into the etiologies of the various forms. The best clinical classification of osteogenesis imperfecta is that due to Sillence (Table 20-69).

Babies with type II disease generally have suffered many fractures in utero. They are obviously malformed with femoral

shortening and often upper limb deformities at birth. The radiologic appearances of the widened, shortened femora, which are due to repetitive fracture and healing with callous formation, are characteristic. The disorder was thought to be recessively inherited because more than one affected infant may be born to unaffected parents. New evidence, however, shows that this type of OI is dominantly inherited with new mutations affecting a parental germ line and being capable of transmission to a number of affected offspring arising from fertilization of affected germ cells. Infants with Sillence type I disease pose a greater diagnostic dilemma. They may not fracture until during or after birth, raising the possibility that their fractures are the response of a normal skeleton-to-perinatal or -postnatal trauma or the effects of nutritional disturbances. In some cases, a positive family history of OI in a parent or sibling leads to correct diagnosis. In general, OI is due to any one of a number of mutations of the genes coding for type I collagen. However, there remain clearly affected infants in whom mutations cannot be detected by current techniques. In addition, biochemical studies of collagen structure may also be normal in some such infants, so precise laboratory diagnosis of all such infants is not yet possible. The diagnosis is currently one of exclusion and retrospective evaluation combined with an increasing frequency of confirmatory laboratory data. Prenatal diagnosis can be performed when the propositus is a parent or sibling provided an abnormality in collagen structure or the coding sequence of the COL1 gene can be characterized in the propositus. In such cases, the diagnosis can be made from cells obtained at chorionic villus biopsy sample. In fetuses of more advanced gestational age, a prenatal diagnosis of severe OI can be obtained by ultrasound examination. No manifestly effective nonsurgical therapy is available for any form of OI.

## Osteopetrosis

Osteopetrosis is a disorder of bone composition attributable to a dysfunction of the cells that resorb bone. In the most common, recessively inherited form of the condition, the bones consist at birth of dense primary spongiosa because the resorption and remodelling that normally proceed during intrauterine development cannot take place. The resistance of the bone to resorption "crowds out" the hematopoietic marrow with consequent anemia and extramedullary hematopoiesis leading to hepatosplenomegaly (Fig 20-83). There is failure also of bone resorption needed to accommodate structures that must pass through bone, particularly the neural foramina of the skull. The consequent compression of cranial nerves leads to blindness and deafness at an early age. Affected infants are recognized by their cranial bossing, or by any of the clinical signs mentioned above, most of which become apparent in the first few weeks of life. Diagnosis is confirmed radiologically by the opaque density of the bones and by the "bone within bone" appearance of some limb bones. Serum

| OI Type | Fragility | Sclerae | Dental Involvement | Inheritance | Comments |
|---------|-----------|---------|--------------------|-------------|----------|
| IA | Present | Blue | Yes | Aut Dom | Relatively common |
| IB | Present | Blue | No | Aut Dom | Variable severity |
| II | Extreme | Blue† | — | ? Dom (Germ cell) | Perinatal |
| III | Severe | Normal | No | ? Dom (Germ cell) | Skeletal deformity |
| IVA | Present | Normal | Yes | Aut Dom | Uncommon |
| IVB | Present | Normal | No | Aut Dom | Variable severity |

**TABLE 20-69.** Sillence's Classification of Osteogenesis Imperfecta*

* Forms presenting at birth or the neonatal period are II and III of the Sillence classification.
† Blue sclerae are frequently seen in healthy neonates.

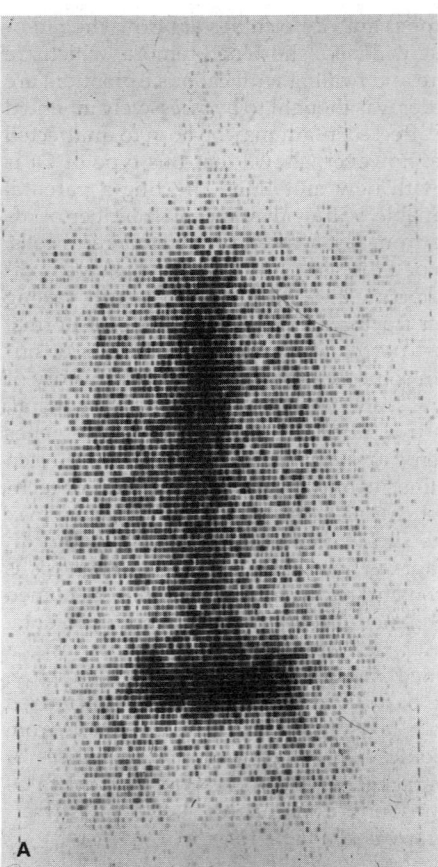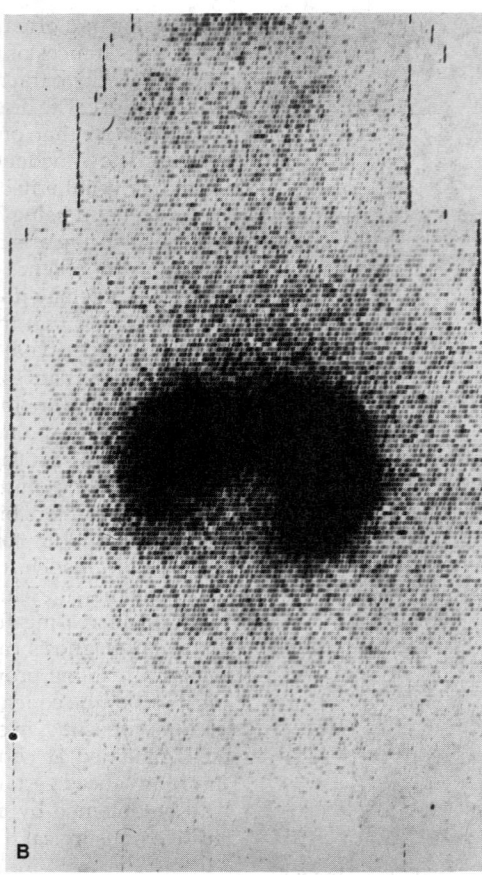

**Figure 20-83.** Radioactive iron scans in a normal infant (**A**) and an infant with osteopetrosis (**B**) indicate the predominance of extramedullary hematopoiesis in the latter.

biochemistry may be normal, but the failure of bone resorption may negate the skeleton's role as a calcium buffer, leading to intermittent hypocalcemia and consequent secondary hyperparathyroidism and hypophosphatemia.

The treatment of infantile osteopetrosis, formerly a uniformly fatal disease, is unsatisfactory. An important theoretic advance is the discovery by Walker that, in an animal model of the disease, defective cells were of lymphoreticular origin and that bone resorption could be restored by transplantation of spleen or marrow cells from isogeneic unaffected animals. Excellent results have been obtained using human bone marrow transplantation in affected infants. When this approach is not possible, there has been some success with use of large doses of calcitriol. Recently, in the osteopetrotic rat, dysfunction in both the immune and osteoclastic systems have been shown to be reversible on treatment with interferon gamma. This line of therapy is being pursued in human infants.

## TRAUMA

The majority of fractures noted at birth are due to trauma at the time of delivery. When more than one fracture is present, one should suspect underlying bone disease such as OI. Multiple birth fractures may also occur in arthrogryposis due to the rigid extension of joints. Fractures of the fetal skeleton are infrequent but may also occur as part of a systemic disorder such as OI.

Postnatally, fractures also tend to be due to generalized bone disease such as OI or Menkes' kinky hair syndrome (an abnormality in copper metabolism). The possibility of child abuse should be kept in mind, too.

Fractures associated with delivery are usually either midshaft

fractures of the clavicle, humerus, or femur or epiphyseal separations of the humerus or femur. Fractures distal to the elbow and knee are unusual. Fractures, mostly of the clavicle and often unrecognized, occur in less than 1% of newborns. In contrast, midshaft fractures of other long bones generally are recognized immediately, often by the obstetrician, when they occur. Epiphyseal separations may be only slightly displaced and remain undetected. Bony injuries occur more often when there is difficult labor, abnormal fetal position, a large infant, or rapid extraction because of fetal distress.

Clinically, the infant with a fracture has a tender red swollen extremity, often noted the day after delivery. The fractured extremity hangs limply and the infant avoids voluntary movement of the limb (pseudoparalysis). There may be a low-grade fever.

Radiographically, if the fracture is midshaft, often the fracture line can be seen. An epiphyseal separation may not be initially visible; conversely, displacement of the shaft may be so marked as to suggest a dislocation, especially because some epiphyseal ossification centers are not visible at birth. Dislocation of the major joints, however, is rare at this age. Comparison views of the uninjured extremity and arthrography may help distinguish between an epiphyseal separation and a dislocation of the joint. If the differential includes infection, the joint may be aspirated during arthrography. Usually by the third day, a faint callus is discernible and the fractures may achieve clinical union by the 10th to 13th day.

Clavicular fracture usually occurs during vertex delivery and is often of the "greenstick" type at the junction of the middle and lateral thirds. Most fractures are unrecognized. Occasionally, crepitations are felt or an asymmetric Moro reflex is noted. Pseudoparalysis of the ipsilateral arm, requiring exclusion of brachial plexus or humeral injury, may follow completely dislocated fractures. In the week after birth, callus formation is palpable. With greenstick fractures, usually care in handling is the only necessary treatment. With complete fractures, the ipsilateral limb and shoulder are immobilized. Prognosis is excellent with solid union in 7 to 10 days.

In the case of epiphyseal separation of the proximal humerus, the fractured limb is limp and the condition can be confused with Erb's palsy. Moderate displacement warrants a closed reduction. Avascular necrosis of the proximal epiphysis has not been reported. With midshaft humeral fractures, there is motion at the center of the shaft. There may be associated radial nerve paralysis and resultant wrist drop, which resolves. Splinting of the limb to the chest is usually sufficient. Injury of the distal humeral epiphysis is uncommon.

With a fracture of the proximal femoral epiphysis, the injured extremity appears shorter. When displacement occurs, this may be confused clinically and radiographically with a congenital dislocated hip. In the latter, however, there are acetabular changes and less displacement. This injury is often associated with an abnormal presentation, usually footling breech, which necessitates manipulation during extraction. Treatment consists of reduction and immobilization. Long-term results have been satisfactory. Avascular necrosis has not been reported. With midshaft femoral fractures, the extremity also appears shortened. Early professional intervention is needed because serious vascular problems can occur during management of this fracture. Injury to the distal femoral epiphysis is rare.

## Selected Readings

### Developmental Considerations

Barlet JP, Davicco MJ, Coxam V. Synthetic parathyroid hormone-related peptide (1–34) fragment stimulates placental calcium transfer in ewes. J Endocrinol 1990;127:33.
Budayr AA, Halloran BP, King JC, Diep D, Nissenson RA, Strewler GJ. High levels of a parathyroid hormone-like protein in milk. Proc Natl Acad Sci U S A 1989;86:7183.

### Hormonal and Metabolic Disorders

Colletti RB, Pan MW, Smith EWP, Genel M. Detection of hypocalcemia in susceptible neonates: the Q-oTc interval. New Engl J Med 1974;290:931.
Jones KL. Williams syndrome: an historical perspective of its evolution, natural history, and etiology. Am J Med Genet Suppl 1990;6:89.
Marx SJ, Attie MF, Levine MA, Spiegel AM, Downs RW, Lasker RD. The hypocalciuric or benign variant of familial hypercalcemia: clinical and biochemical features in 15 kindreds. Medicine 1981;60:397.
Mascarello JT; Bastian JF; Jones MC. Interstitial deletion of chromosome 22 in a patient with the DiGeorge malformation sequence. Am J Med Genet 1989;32:112.
Salle BL, Delvin E, Glorieux F, David L. Human neonatal hypocalcemia. Biol Neonate 1990;58(suppl 1):22.

### Metabolic Bone Disease of Prematurity

American Academy of Pediatrics Committee on Nutrition. Nutritional needs of low-birth-weight infants. Pediatrics 1985;75:976.
Congdon PJ, Horsman A, Ryan SW, Truscott JG, Durward H. Spontaneous resolution of bone mineral depletion in preterm infants. Arch Dis Child 1990;65:1038.
Ehrenkrantz RA, Gettner PA, Nelli CM. Nutrient balance studies in premature infants fed premature formula or fortified preterm human milk. J Pediatr Gastroenterol Nutr 1989;8:58.
Hillman LS, Rojanasathit S, Slatopolsky E, Haddad JG. Serial measurements of serum calcium, magnesium, parathyroid hormone, calcitonin, and 25-dihydroxy-vitamin D during the first week of life. Pediatr Res 1977;11:739.
Koo WW, Sherman R, Succop P, Ho M, Buckley D, Tsang RC. Serum vitamin D metabolites in very low birth weight infants with and without rickets and fractures. J Pediatr 1989;114:1017.
Pelegano JF, Rowe JC, Carey DE, et al. Effect of calcium/phosphorus ratio on mineral retention in parenterally fed premature infants. J Pediatr Gastroenterol Nutr 1991;12:351.
Rowe JC, Wood DH, Rowe DW, Raisz LG. Nutritional hypophosphatemic rickets in a premature infant fed breast milk. N Engl J Med 1979;300:293.
Venkataraman PS, Blick KE. Effect of mineral supplementation of human milk on bone mineral content and trace element metabolism. J Pediatr 1992;113:220.

### Disorders of Bone Formation

Cohn DH, Starman BJ, Blumberg B, Byers PH. Recurrence of lethal osteogenesis imperfecta due to parental mosaicism for a dominant mutation in a human type I collagen gene (COL1A1). Am J Hum Genet 1990;46:591.
Hochman N, Hojo H, Hojo S, et al. Reversal of immune dysfunction in osteopetrotic rats by interferon-gamma: augmentation of macrophage Ia expression and lymphocyte interleukin-2 production and proliferation. Cell Immunol 1991;137:14.
Lee B, Vissing H, Ramirez F, Rogers D, Rimoin D. Identification of the molecular defect in a family with spondyloepiphyseal dysplasia. Science 1989;244:978.
Lenarsky C, Kohn DB, Weinberg KI, Parkman R. Bone marrow transplantation for genetic diseases. Hematol Oncol Clin North Am 1990;4:589.
Lynch JR, Ogilvie D, Priestley L, et al. Prenatal diagnosis of osteogenesis imperfecta by identification of the concordant collagen 1 allele. J Med Genet 1991;28:145.
Rimoin DL, Lachman RS. The chondrodysplasias. In: Rimoin DL, Emery AEH, eds. Principles and practice of medical genetics, ed 2. II. Edinburgh: Churchill Livingstone, 1990:895.
Sillence DO. Osteogenesis imperfecta: nosology and genetics. Ann N Y Acad Sci 1988;543:1.

*Principles and Practice of Pediatrics, Second Edition.*
edited by Frank A. Oski et al. J. B. Lippincott Company, Philadelphia © 1994.

## 20.12 *Craniofacial Defects*

### Robert J. Gorlin

## EMBRYOLOGY OF THE PRIMARY AND SECONDARY PALATES

Neural crest plays an integral part in facial morphology. When the neural folds fuse to form the neural tube around the fourth week of gestation, ectomesenchymal cells adjacent to the neural plate migrate into the underlying regions. Those in the head and face form essentially all the skeletal and connective tissues of the face: bone, cartilage, fibrous connective tissue, and all dental tissues except enamel. This transformation is effected by induction of these ectomesenchymal cells by the adjacent oral ectoderm and pharyngeal endoderm. Langman (1985) and Hall (1988) report that neural crest cells also migrate into the visceral arches where they surround mesodermal cores.

By the end of the fourth week, the anterior neuropore has closed. What is to be the face consists of a large frontal prominence overlying the first or mandibular arch. If one manually elevates the frontal prominence, one can see into the primary mouth or stomodeum. The primary mouth is separated from the foregut by the buccopharyngeal membrane, which undergoes programmed cell death and ruptures at about this time in development. On both sides of the frontal prominence, the nasal placodes are forming. These bilateral structures, located just above the primitive mouth, are represented by local thickening of the surface ectoderm. Rapid proliferation of tissue known as nasal swelling occurs both lateral and medial to the nasal placodes. By means of selective cell death and proliferation of tissues, nasal or olfactory pits that extend into the primitive mouth are formed; these are the primitive nostrils.

Extremely active growth occurs during the fifth and sixth weeks (Fig 20-84). The maxillary swellings, which represent the

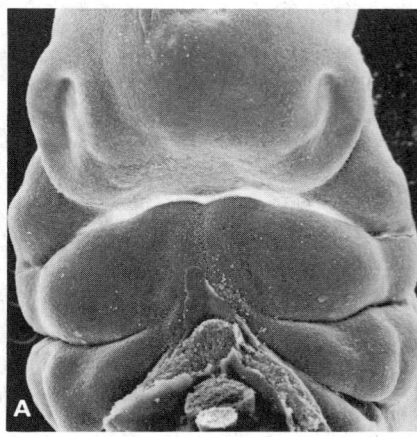 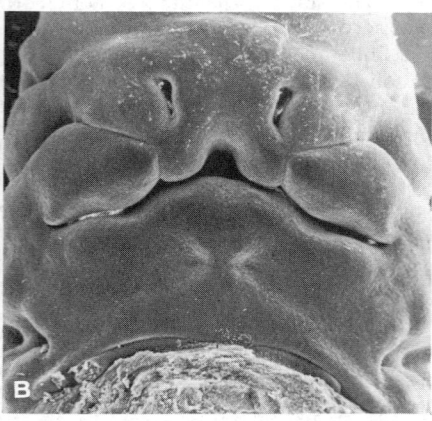

Figure 20-84. Embryology of the primary and secondary palates. Scanning electron microscopy of human embryos. (**A**) Early fifth week after fertilization. (**B**) Sixth week after fertilization. Median nasal process is not yet fused with maxillary process of first arch. (Courtesy of K. Sulik, Chapel Hill, North Carolina.)

upper portion of the first pharyngeal arch, enlarge considerably, and by pushing the nasal swellings or prominences medially, cause them to approach each other in the midline. When the two prominences meet, the median nasal prominences and the maxillary swellings merge. Thus, the upper lip is formed laterally by the maxillary prominences and medially by the fused median nasal prominences. This development occurs around the seventh week. The lateral nasal prominences play no role in formation of the upper lip but form the alae or wings of the nose.

The primary palate consists of the two merged medial nasal processes that form the intermaxillary segment. The intermaxillary segment consists of two portions: (1) a labial component that forms the philtrum of the upper lip, that is, the indented area flanked by roughly parallel ridges that run from the columella of the nose to the middle of the upper lip; and (2) the triangular palatal component of bone that includes the four maxillary incisor teeth. The primary palate extends posteriorly to the incisive foramen or, clinically, to the incisive papilla.

The so-called secondary palate comprises at least 90% of the hard and soft palates, that is, all except the anterior portion that holds the incisor teeth. Its development appears to be somewhat more complicated than originally thought. The palatal shelves originate as swellings or shelf-like burgeonings of the medial surfaces of the maxillary prominences. They appear in the sixth week and grow downward, lateral to and somewhat beneath the tongue. Elevation of the palatal processes to a horizontal plane is more "rigorous" anteriorly, nearer the primary palate. Elevation begins during the seventh week (Ferguson, 1987).

What promotes the elevation has been called intrinsic shelf force but has a complex biochemical and physiochemical basis. When the shelves are elevated to the horizontal plane, there is programmed cell death of the overlying epithelium, permitting flow of ectomesenchyme from each side to close the gap. Com-

plete fusion is effected by the tenth week (Fig 20-85). In some infants, cystic degeneration of the epithelial remnants occurs, producing evanescent midline palatal microcysts.

## CLEFT LIP AND CLEFT PALATE

### Epidemiology and Genetics

The degree of cleft formation varies greatly. Minimal degrees of involvement include bifid uvula, linear lip indentations (so-called intrauterine-healed clefts), and submucous palatal cleft. Clefts may involve only the upper lip or may extend to the nostril and may be combined with defects of the hard or soft palate. Isolated palatal clefts may be limited to the uvula or they may be more extensive, cleaving the soft palate or both the soft and hard palates to just behind the incisor teeth.

A combination of cleft lip and cleft palate is more common than isolated occurrence of either. Cleft lip with cleft palate composes about 50% of the cases, with cleft lip and isolated cleft palate each constituting about 25%, generally irrespective of race. Vanderas (1987) reported that cleft lip with or without cleft palate occurs in about 1 per 1000 white births (range 0.8 to 1.6 per 1000). Frequency is higher in Native Americans (3.5 per 1000), Japanese (2.1 per 1000), and Chinese (1.7 per 1000); it is lower among blacks (0.3 per 1000).

Isolated cleft lip may be unilateral (80%) or bilateral (20%). When unilateral, the cleft is more commonly on the left side (about 70%), but it is no more extensive. Lips are somewhat more frequently clefted bilaterally (about 25%) when combined with cleft palate. The cleft lip and palate combination is more common in men than women. About 85% of cases of bilateral cleft lip and 70% of cases of unilateral cleft lip are associated with cleft

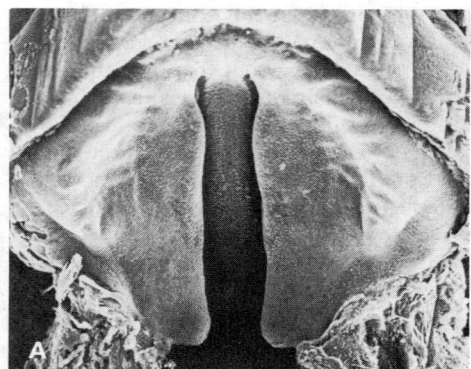 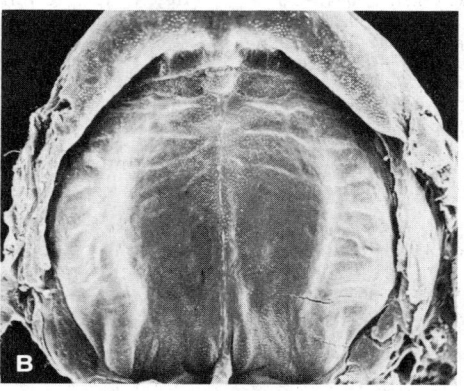

Figure 20-85. Scanning electron microscopy. (**A**) View of secondary palate at 8 weeks. (**B**) At 10 weeks. (Courtesy of K. Sulik, Chapel Hill, North Carolina.)

palate. Cleft lip is not always complete, that is, extending into the nostril. In about 10% of the cases, the cleft is associated with skin bridges or Simonart's bands.

Isolated cleft palate appears to be an entity separate from cleft lip with or without cleft palate. Numerous investigators have determined that siblings of patients with cleft lip with or without cleft palate have an increased frequency of the same anomaly but not of isolated cleft palate, and vice versa. The incidence of isolated cleft palate among both whites and blacks appears to be 1 per 2000 to 2500 births. It occurs somewhat more often in girls, comprising about 60% of the cases. While there is a 2:1 female-to-male predilection for complete clefts of the hard and soft palate, the ratio approaches 1:1 for clefts of the soft palate only.

Cleft uvula varies in degree of completeness. Incomplete clefts are more common. The frequency of cleft uvula (1:80 white persons) is much higher than that for cleft palate with no sex predilection. The frequency in parents and siblings of probands ranges from 7% to 15%. Cleft uvula among Native American groups is high, occurring in 1 per 9 to 14 births depending on tribal group. In blacks, it is extremely rare. Estimates are 1 per 350 to 400 births.

Congenital pharyngeal incompetence, characterized by cleft palate speech (50%) without an overt cleft, is due to a short soft palate (60%), an imperfect muscular union across the soft palate (submucous palatal cleft), or increased depth of the nasal pharynx. Submucous palatal cleft is relatively uncommon, occurring in 1 in 1200 children. There appears to be no sex predilection. About 30% of those with submucous palatal cleft have bifid uvula with poor mobility demonstrated in 20%. There is a median deficiency or notch in the bone at the posterior edge of the hard palate. It can be detected digitally or by a light probe placed within the nose.

Recurrence data do not suggest a simple pattern of inheritance. This finding is bolstered by twin studies indicating the relative roles played by genetic and nongenetic influences. Among twins with cleft lip with or without cleft palate, concordance is far greater in monozygotic (35.0%) than in dizygotic (4.5%) twins. In twins with isolated cleft palate, concordance is not quite as great between the two groups (monozygotic, 26.0%; dizygotic, 5.8%). This finding suggests a stronger genetic basis for cleft lip with or without cleft palate than for isolated cleft palate. Both cleft lip with or without cleft palate and isolated cleft palate consist of three groups, sporadic (75% to 80%), familial (10% to 15%), and syndromal (1% to 5%). Melnick and colleagues (1980) report that clefting is heterogeneous, its variation and liability probably being determined by major genes, minor genes, environmental insults, and a developmental threshold.

## Mechanisms of Cleft Production

By definition, cleft lip involves the failure of closure of the primary palate, and cleft palate involves failure of closure of the secondary palate.

Knowledge regarding mechanisms involved in regulation of embryonic growth is sparse at best. Growth patterns can also be affected by environmental factors. A long list of teratogenic substances (eg, corticosteroids, vitamin A, phenytoin, various folic acid antagonists) can produce clefting in rodents. Little evidence, however, suggests that any of these agents play even a minor role in cleft palate production in humans (Jones, 1988).

Various genetic and environmental factors may inhibit the flow of neural crest cells or may affect their volume or mass so that contact between prominence is impossible or inadequate. The epithelium covering the ectomesenchyme may not undergo programmed cell death, so fusion cannot take place. Exact timing and exact positioning play critical roles.

Clefts of the primary and secondary palates occur in associ-

ation in about one half of cases. A common mechanism of production has been sought. Reduction in size of both the labial maxillary prominence and the palatine process of the maxillary prominences appears to be a reasonable explanation.

Clefts of the secondary palate probably result from either hypoplasia of the shelves or delay in timing of shelf elevation. Experiments carried out on susceptible strains of mice suggest that both mechanisms are operative but at different times in gestation. For example, Johnston and Bronsby (1991) report that large doses of vitamin A given early in gestation inhibit palatal shelf growth and that cortisone given later in gestation inhibits palatal shelf elevation.

## Risk of Recurrence

In most cases, the cleft is either isolated or associated with a constellation of anomalies that do not form a recognizable syndrome. Although more than 300 cleft syndromes or associations are recognized, Gorlin and coworkers (1990) report that they constitute a low percentage of cases. Efforts must be made to recognize a cleft syndrome, because the pattern of inheritance may be simple and the genetic risk for future affected children may then be more precise. For example, a parent with or without a cleft who has paramedian pits of the lower lip has a 50% chance of having a child with cleft lip or palate.

In the case of isolated clefts, the risk to a first degree relative of an affected individual is 2% to 4%. This information applies only to risks for similar anomalies (ie, a parent with isolated cleft palate has no greater risk of having a child with cleft lip with or without cleft palate than anyone else, and vice versa). The risks increase as more individuals are affected. For example, if a parent and a child have clefts, the risk for a future affected sibling increases to about 10% to 12%. These and other situations are presented in detail in Table 20-70.

The severity of a facial cleft also affects recurrence risk in the offspring. For example, it has been found that if a parent has isolated unilateral cleft lip, the recurrence risk is 2.5%. If there is unilateral cleft lip and palate, the risk increases to 4%; if there is bilateral cleft lip with cleft palate, the risk is more than 5.5%.

## Associated Anomalies

Cleft lip and palate often occur as isolated anomalies; that is, thorough examinations conducted over several years have revealed no other primary abnormalities. This statement would

| | Siblings | | Cleft Lip | Cleft |
|---|---|---|---|---|
| Parents | Normal | Affected | (Palate) % | Palate % |
| Normal | 0 | 1 | 4.0 | 3.5 |
| | 1 | 1 | 4.0 | 3.0 |
| | 0 | 2 | 14.0 | 13.0 |
| One affected | 0 | 0 | 4.0 | 3.5 |
| | 0 | 1 | 12.0 | 10.0 |
| | 1 | 1 | 10.0 | 9.0 |
| | 0 | 2 | 25.0 | 24.0 |
| Both affected | 0 | 0 | 35.0 | 25.0 |
| | 0 | 1 | 45.0 | 35.0 |
| | 1 | 1 | 40.0 | 35.0 |
| | 0 | 2 | 50.0 | 45.0 |

TABLE 20-70.  Facial Clefts—Risk of Recurrence

Adapted from Tolarová M. Empirical recurrence risk figures for genetic counseling of clefts. Acta Chir Plast (Praha) 1972;14:234.

exclude, for example, the middle ear infections that occur so frequently secondary to cleft palate.

When data are broken down according to subtype, general agreement exists that isolated cleft palate (20% to 50%) is more often associated with other congenital anomalies than either isolated cleft lip (7% to 13%) or cleft lip with cleft palate (2% to 11%). The frequency with which one or more malformations accompanies clefts of all types is almost 28%.

More malformations are found in infants with bilateral cleft lip with or without cleft palate than in those with unilateral cleft lip. The more malformations a child has, the lighter the birth weight (Shprintzen et al, 1985). Congenital palatopharyngeal incompetence has been found to be frequently associated with cervical anomalies. As noted earlier, some of these associated findings form recognizable syndromes. Cohen (1978) listed 133 such disorders. In 1980, there were an estimated 204 cleft conditions: 47 autosomal-dominant, 55 autosomal-recessive, 6 X-linked, 32 chromosomal, and 64 disorders of unknown nature associated with facial clefting. The current number of "cleft syndromes" is more than 300, according to Melnick and colleagues (1980) and Gorlin and colleagues (1990). Only the Robin malformation sequence, oculoauriculovertebral malformation, and mandibulofacial dysostosis are discussed here.

### Care of Infant With Cleft Lip or Cleft Palate

A cleft palate team—usually composed of a maxillofacial surgeon, audiologist, speech pathologist, prosthodontist, otolaryngologist, pedodontist, and geneticist—is extremely important in helping parents understand the sequential approach to therapy for the many attendant problems. The desirability of a team approach is discussed by Bardach and Morris (1990). A recommended handbook for parents is that of Moller and colleagues (1989).

Feeding usually requires considerable patience. Those with more severe clefts of the lip or palate should be fed by placing the infant in a sitting position to minimize fluid loss through the nose. Various techniques and equipment are used to feed infants with clefts, but Clarren and coworkers (1987) report that no one method is optimal for all infants. Infants with cleft lip or cleft palate swallow normally but suck abnormally. A cleft in the lip or palate generally does not allow sufficient negative pressure. In the case of cleft lip only, breast-feeding or an artificial nipple with a large, soft base works well. For infants with cleft lip or palate, regular breast-feeding or normal bottle feeding is often not successful because they are unable to seal either their lips or their velopharynx. With cleft of the palate only, breast-feeding or normal bottle feeding usually can be carried out if the cleft is narrow or involves only the soft palate. Soft artificial nipples with large openings are more effective.

Regular bottle nipples do not work well for infants with wider

palatal clefts or the Robin malformation sequence. Enlarging the nipple opening in association with a softer nipple with a large base and a long shaft often enables tongue movement to express a greater quantity of milk. One can also deliver milk directly into the mouth with a soft plastic bottle.

Children with cleft palate are prone to repeated infections of the middle ear and paranasal sinuses. The tonsils and adenoids enlarge and chronic nasopharyngitis may lead to recurrent otitis media with resultant conductive hearing loss. Nasopharyngeal infection should be treated promptly with antibiotics. The tonsils and adenoids may play a vital role in allowing normal speech. Thus, tonsillectomy and adenoidectomy, especially in those with velopharyngeal insufficiency, may result in postoperative nasal speech.

Fria and colleagues (1987) stress the importance of assessing auditory function in infants with cleft palates. Assessment may be more accurately carried out in the infant or young child by auditory specialists.

### Surgical Repair of Clefts

Closure of the lip is usually carried out between the 2nd and 10th week after birth, depending on the infant's weight and state of health. The primary purpose is to create a seal to allow normal sucking. Various techniques have been employed for repair of the lip, depending on the degree and extent of defect. In those cases in which tissue in the two lip segments is insufficient to create an acceptable lip and nostril, the surgeon may have to move small flaps of tissue from other places in the upper or, occasionally, the lower lip. For bilateral cleft lip, surgery is more difficult. The primary palate may not be attached to the secondary palate and requires repositioning. Subsequent surgery is usually required to correct nasal alar form, to compensate for uneven growth of tissue on the two sides of the lip, or to match evenly the vermilion line on both sides. This secondary surgery is best done during the teen years (Cronin and Denkler, 1988).

Surgical closure of the hard and soft palate is often done at about 18 to 24 months of age, but some surgeons prefer to wait longer. The object is to create airtight and fluid-tight closure of the cleft and to preserve the length and mobility of the soft palate, which often involves multiple surgical operations. If insufficient tissue is available for closure by any of the many techniques available, an obturator or speech bulb is made by the prosthodontist.

### Robin Malformation Sequence

The Robin malformation sequence consists of micrognathia, glossoptosis, and cleft palate (Fig 20-86). About 30% of the cases

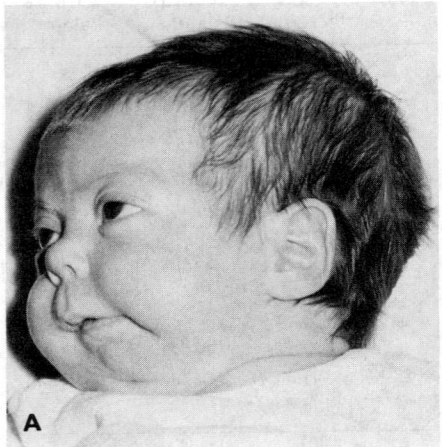
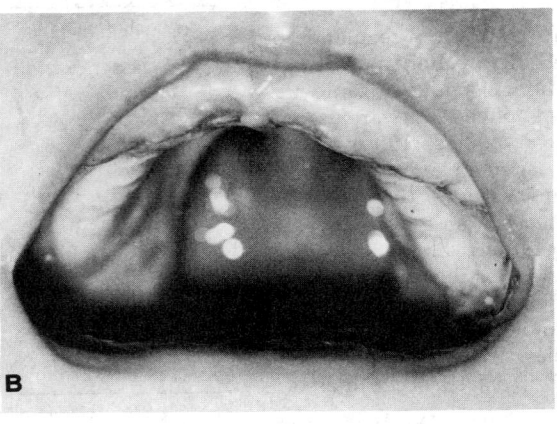

**Figure 20-86.** Robin malformation sequence. (**A**) Small retruded lower jaw. (**B**) U-shaped palatal cleft.

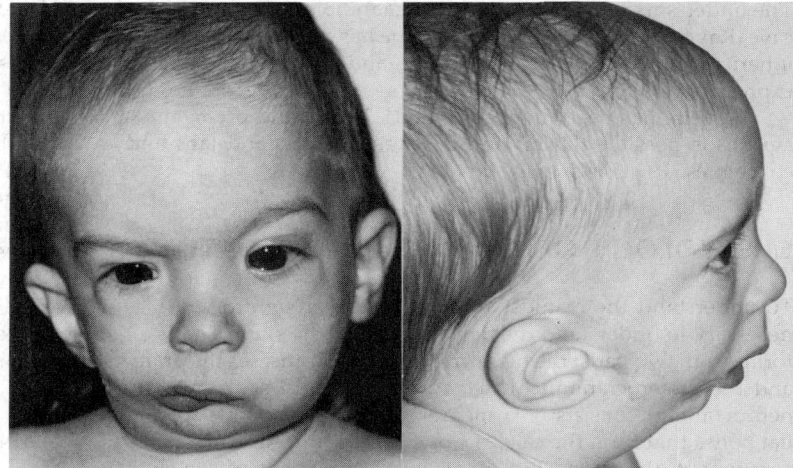

Figure 20-87. Oculoauriculovertebral malformation. Note hemifacial microsomia, repaired macrostomia, and low-set, somewhat dysmorphic pinna. Ear tags have been removed. (Courtesy of M. M. Cohen Jr., Halifax, Nova Scotia, Canada.)

represent Stickler's syndrome (Sheffield and colleagues, 1987). The mandible is small and symmetrically receded. Congenital murmurs or heart anomalies (eg, ASD, PDA, VSD) have been observed in 15% to 20% of those who have died in early infancy. Esotropia and congenital glaucoma are relatively common. About 20% exhibit severe mental retardation, but it is not known whether this condition is primary or secondary to asphyxia. The palatal defect may vary widely from cleft uvula to clefting that involves two thirds of the hard palate and is horseshoe shaped. The small mandible often achieves catchup growth by 4 to 6 years of age, but the angle is always somewhat abnormal. Difficulty in the inspiratory phase of respiration is apparent, with periodic cyanotic attacks, labored breathing, and recession of the sternum and ribs, especially apparent when the child is supine. The respiratory difficulty is usually evident at birth, but it may not be severe for the first week. Immediate airway maintenance is critical. In mild cases, it may be accomplished by keeping the individual prone with the head suspended by a pulley in a stockinette cap. In more severe cases, the tongue tip may be temporarily sutured to the lower lip or anterior mandible. Tracheotomy is rarely required.

## Oculoauriculovertebral Malformation

Facial asymmetry due to hypoplasia or displacement of the pinna is common in oculoauriculovertebral malformation (hemifacial microsomia, Goldenhar's syndrome, Fig 20-87). The maxillary, temporal, and malar bones on the involved side are reduced in size and flattened, and the ipsilateral eye is set low. Bilateral involvement occurs in about 10% of cases. Malformation of the external ear varies from complete aplasia to a crumpled, distorted pinna displaced anteriorly and inferiorly. Supernumerary ear tags may occur anywhere from the tragus to the angle of the mouth. When epibulbar dermoids are present, ear tags tend to be bilateral. Conductive hearing loss, due to middle ear abnormalities or absence or deficiency of the external auditory meatus and canal, is found in 40% of cases. Epibulbar dermoid is variable, white to yellow, flattened, ellipsoid, solid, and usually located in the lower, outer quadrant at the limbus. Coloboma of the upper lateral eyelid is common in patients with epibulbar dermoids. When unilateral microphthalmia or anophthalmia is present, mental retardation is increased. About 5% of cases have cleft lip or palate. Radiographically, vertebral anomalies, found in about 50% of cases, include complete or partial synostosis of two or more vertebrae and hemivertebrae. There is aplasia or hypoplasia of the mandibular ramus on the ipsilateral side. A small percentage of cases have agenesis of one lung and various renal anomalies (eg, absent kidney, double ureter). The frequency of the condition is about

1 in 3000 live births. Almost all cases appear to have multifactorial inheritance with a recurrence risk of about 1% (Cohen and colleagues, 1989). However, Gorlin and colleagues' (1990) research shows that, in a few families, the disorder appears to be autosomal dominant.

Surgical correction ranges from lengthening the mandible to construction of a new temporomandibular joint and ramus with rib grafts and costochondral junction (Kaban and colleagues, 1988).

## Mandibulofacial Dysostosis

Mandibulofacial dysostosis, or Treacher Collins syndrome, is characterized by downward-slanting palpebral fissures and coloboma of the outer third of the lower lid with deficient cilia medial to the coloboma (Fig 20-88). The nose appears large because of lack of malar development. A nasofrontal angle is commonly obliterated. Micrognathia is a constant feature. Cleft palate is found in 30%. The external ear is frequently deformed, crumpled forward, or misplaced, with some patients having absence of the external auditory canal or an ossicular defect with conductive hearing loss (Phelps and colleagues, 1981). Extra ear tags and blind fistulas may be found between the tragus and angle of the mouth. Radiographs show defects in the zygomatic arches.

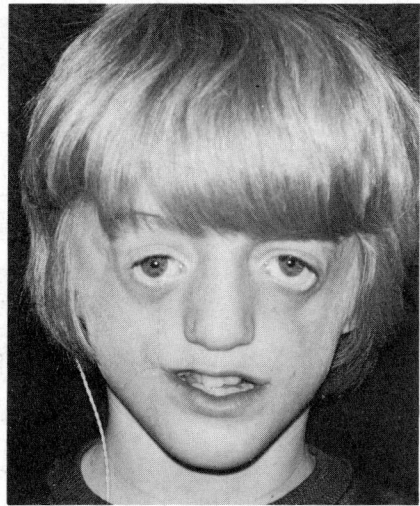

Figure 20-88. Mandibulofacial dysostosis. Boy with malar hypoplasia with downward slanting palpebral fissures. Colobomas of outer third of lower lids. Note hearing aid cord.

The under-surface of the body of the mandible is markedly concave (Kay and Kay, 1989). The syndrome has autosomal dominant inheritance with high penetrance and markedly variable expressivity.

The gene has been mapped to 5q31.3–33.3 and prenatal diagnosis is possible (Dixon and colleagues, 1991, and Jabs and colleagues, 1991).

## EMBRYOLOGY OF CRANIOFACIAL SKELETON

To understand the craniosynostoses and their syndromes, it is necessary to understand the development of the skull. The skull forms from two parts: the neurocranium, which encases the brain, and the viscerocranium, which forms the facial skeleton. The neurocranium consists of a membranous portion composed of flat bones that form the calvaria, or cranial vault. A cartilaginous component, the chondrocranium, forms the bones of the skull base. The flat bones of the calvaria develop by membranous ossification. Langman (1990) reports that several primary ossification centers, consisting of needle-like bone spicules, progressively enlarge and radiate peripherally, forming the frontal, parietal, and occipital bones.

In the newborn, the flat bones of the calvaria are separated by sutures, that is, narrow bands of connective tissue. At points where more than two bones meet, there are wide sutural openings known as fontanelles. The largest of these is the anterior fontanelle, where the two parietal bones and two frontal bones meet. The posterior fontanelle is situated at the junction between the two parietal bones and the occipital bone. A third fontanelle is occasionally present in the sagittal suture about 1 cm anterior to the posterior fontanelle. There are two other embryonal fontanelles: the anterolateral or sphenoidal fontanelle and the posterolateral or mastoid fontanelle. The sutures and fontanelles permit skull bones to overlap during passage of the head through the vaginal canal. After birth, the bones resume their position. The anterior fontanelle is usually clinically closed by 13 months of age (range 7 to 19 months). The posterior fontanelle, usually clinically inapparent at birth, closes anatomically at about 3 months of age. The sutures and fontanelles remain membranous to allow growth of the cranial vault in response to expansion of the brain. Many sutures remain open until adult life.

In contrast to the membranous neurocranium, the base of the skull, or chondrocranium, initially consists of several cartilages that fuse and undergo endochondral ossification.

The viscerocranium or facial skeleton is mainly formed from the cartilages of the first two pharyngeal arches. The first pharyngeal arch is divided into a dorsal maxillary process and a ventral mandibular process. The former gives rise to the maxilla, the zygomatic bone, and part of the temporal bone. The cartilage of the first pharyngeal arch is known as Meckel's cartilage. The ectomesenchyme surrounding the cartilage condenses and ossifies, giving rise to the mandible by membranous ossification. Meckel's cartilage actually acts only as a template, except for its most dorsal portion, which gives rise to the malleus and incus. Remnants may be found in the sphenomandibular ligament.

## CRANIOSYNOSTOSIS

If obliteration of sutures takes place before or soon after birth, it inhibits the growth of adjacent bones perpendicular to the course of the obliterated suture. Consequently, skull diameter is reduced in this direction. Compensatory and abnormal growth, however, proceeds in directions permitted by open sutures and fontanelles (Fig 20-89). If a single suture is involved, it is termed simple craniosynostosis; if multiple sutures, compound craniosynostosis. Early obliteration of the sagittal suture results in scaphocephaly (dolichocephaly, Fig 20-90). The skull is long and narrow and the parietal protuberances are absent. As the brain expands, the coronal and lambdoidal sutures are widened and fronto-occipital elongation takes place. In some cases, a bony crest is seen in place of the sagittal suture. In brachycephaly, the coronal sutures are prematurely fused, resulting in a short, squarish cranial configuration (Fig 20-91). Plagiocephaly refers to skewing of the skull due to premature unilateral fusion of a coronal or lambdoidal suture. Trigonocephaly describes a keel-shaped forehead due to premature fusion of the metopic suture. Acrocephaly (turricephaly) results from multiple suture closures. The highest point on the calvaria is usually near the anterior fontanelle, head form being short, high, and broad. The coronal suture is chiefly affected, although the sagittal and lambdoid sutures are frequently involved. If the anterior fontanelle and metopic suture remain open, the skull expands in abnormal directions, resulting in steep

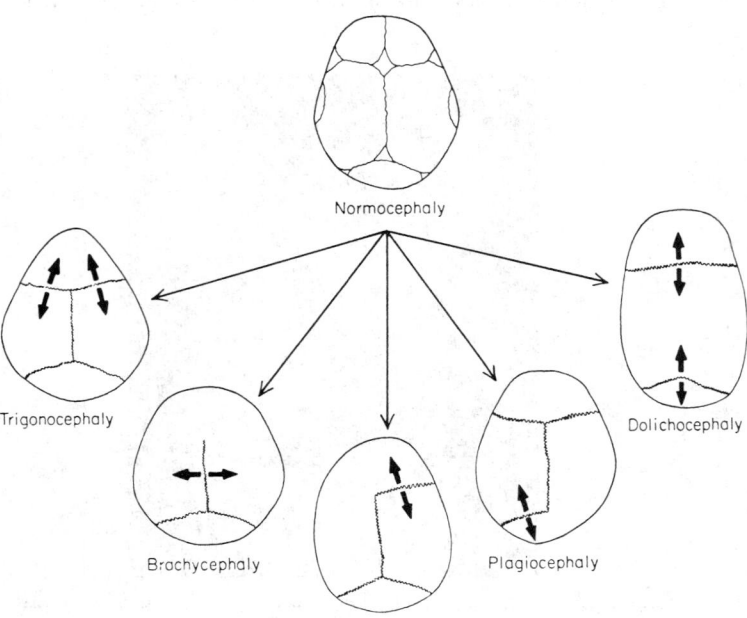

**Figure 20-89.**   Craniosynostosis. Various skull shapes resulting from premature fusion of individual sutures or groups of sutures. (Courtesy of M. M. Cohen Jr., Halifax, Nova Scotia, Canada.)

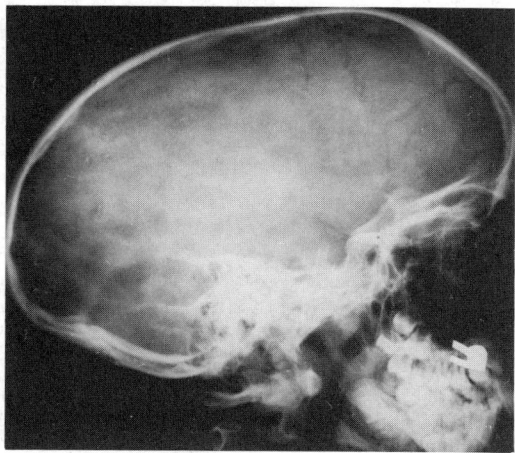

Figure 20-90. Scaphocephaly (dolichocephaly).

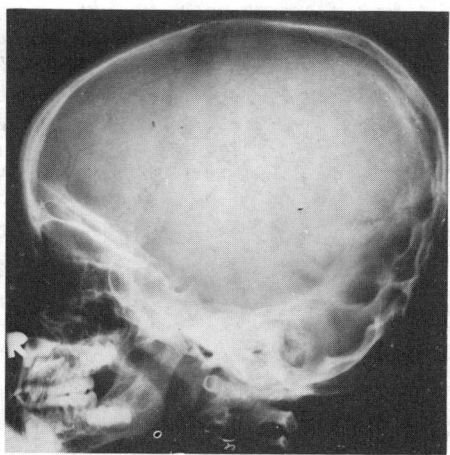

Figure 20-91. Brachycephaly.

frontal, parietal, and occipital bones and a high, broad, short skull. There often are digital impressions.

Craniosynostosis may be primary, as in simple or compound premature fusion described earlier, or it may be secondary to a known disorder (eg, thalassemia, hyperthyroidism, microcephaly, mucopolysaccharidoses, rickets).

Finally, craniosynostosis may be isolated or syndromic. In 1987, Cohen listed 64 syndromes of craniosynostosis (monogenic 31, chromosomal 14, environmentally induced 3, unknown genesis 10, miscellaneous 6). A few more common ones are discussed in this chapter. They are Crouzon's disease, Apert's syndrome, Saethre-Chotzen syndrome, Pfeiffer's syndrome, and Carpenter's syndrome.

## Epidemiology and Genetics

The frequency of simple or nonsyndromal craniosynostosis is approximately 0.4 per 1000 newborns. There appears to be no racial predilection. Premature fusion of the sagittal suture is the most common type of simple synostosis, constituting approximately 55% of cases. Boys are more commonly affected 4:1 over girls. Unilateral or bilateral coronal synostosis comprises approximately 20% to 25% of cases with a slight predilection for female infants. Metopic synostosis and lambdoidal synostosis each constitute a few percent. Two or more sutures comprise 15%.

Simple craniosynostosis is usually sporadic. Of patients with coronal synostosis, about 10% are familial; of patients with sagittal synostosis, about 2% are familial. In those with familial occurrence, autosomal dominant inheritance is far more common than autosomal recessive inheritance. In some kindreds, the same suture is synostosed in affected individuals, and in others, different sutures are fused. Hunter and Rudd (1976) found that sagittal synostosis appeared to be most consistent with multifactorial inheritance, the frequency in the general population being approximately 1 in 4200, with a recurrence risk of approximately 1 in 64 siblings. Twin studies clearly indicate that single-gene inheritance does not play a large role in craniosynostosis because discordance is more frequent than concordance in monozygotic twins.

## Treatment in Infancy

Treatment of craniosynostosis in infancy is controversial. The craniosynostoses represent not only diverse groups, but also extreme variables if found within each group. Opinions regarding treatment vary from conservative observation until completion of facial growth to radical extensive surgical correction in the first months of life. Complications such as increasing intracranial pressure or progressive corneal exposure secondary to exorbitism often mandate early treatment.

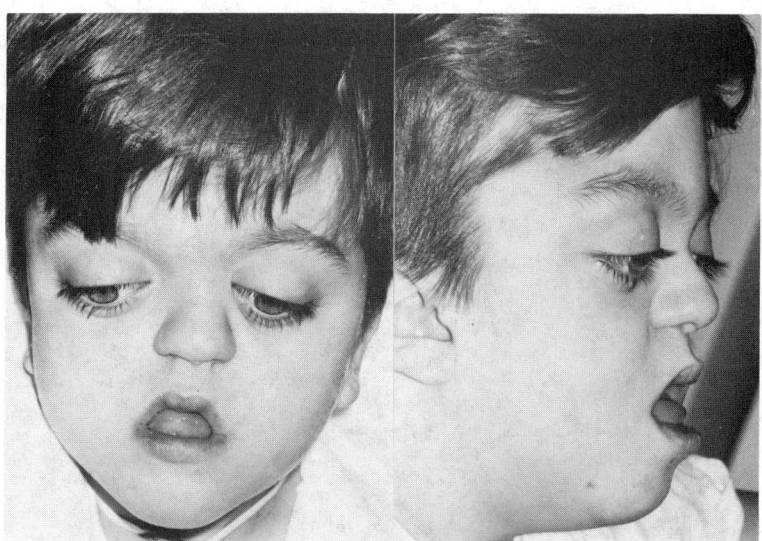

Figure 20-92. Crouzon's disease. Downward slanting palpebral fissures, facial asymmetry, hypoplastic midface, exorbitism, relative mandibular prognathism. (Courtesy of M. M. Cohen Jr., Halifax, Nova Scotia, Canada.)

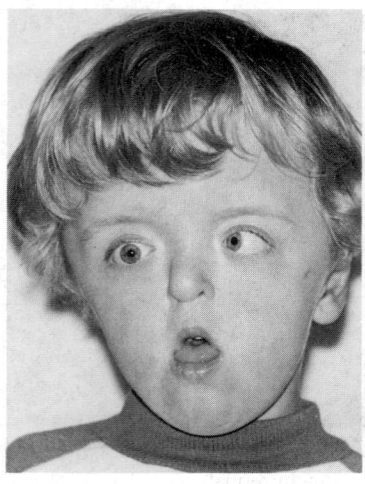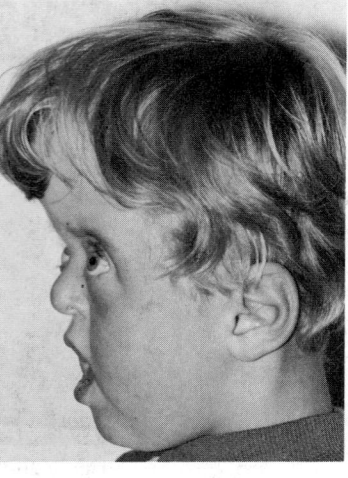

Figure 20-93. Apert's syndrome. Frontal bossing, brachycephaly, hypertelorism, strabismus, exorbitism, depressed midface. (Courtesy of M. M. Cohen Jr., Halifax, Nova Scotia, Canada.)

Albin and colleagues (1985) suggest that patients with premature closure of cranial sutures be surgically treated under the age of 2 years and those patients with metopic suture closure under the age of 6 months. The operation most frequently performed for simple craniosynostosis is linear craniectomy parallel to the prematurely fused suture. Polyethylene film is inserted over the bony margins to delay secondary closure. Bilateral, premature closure of the coronal sutures is frequently accompanied by anomalies of the facial, orbital, and sphenoid bones with downward displacement of the orbital roof and overgrowth of the lesser wing of the sphenoid, the orbits being markedly reduced in size, thus causing exophthalmos. Maximum decompression of the cranial vault rather than orbital decompression is carried out. Canthorrhaphy is performed to avoid dryness of the cornea and prolapse of the globe. Complex plastic surgical treatment of severe facial deformities of craniofacial dysostoses has been described in detail by Tessier (1986). The optimal time for such operations is at 10 to 12 years of age. Bartlett and colleagues (1990) and Bruneteau and Mulliken (1992) extensively discuss surgical treatment of unilateral suture closure and plagiocephaly.

Surgical techniques are reviewed by Whitaker and colleagues (1987). In general, they conclude that asymmetric synostosis treated at younger than 1 year of age by unilateral orbital repositioning and forehead remodeling gave excellent results. No further surgery was needed in greater than 90% of patients. For bilateral or symmetric synostoses and mild upper face deformity,

orbital advancement and forehead reshaping carried out within the first year of life was less satisfactory, with about 50% of patients needing another major osteotomy. For those with moderate to severe symmetric synostoses (Crouzon's disease and Apert's syndrome), extensive facial reconstruction is carried out between 7 and 14 years of age. Despite delayed and aggressive treatment, surgical outcome is less satisfactory (David and Sheen, 1990.)

## Crouzon's Disease

Crouzon's disease is characterized by premature craniosynostosis, midface hypoplasia with shallow orbits, and ocular proptosis (Fig 20-92). Premature and progressive craniosynostosis usually begins during the first year of life and is usually complete by 2 or 3 years of age. About 30% of patients complain of headache; seizures have been documented in 10%. The hypoplasia of the midface is associated with relative mandibular prognathism, drooping of the lower lip, and short upper lip. The nasal bridge is often flat, and the nasal tip may appear beaklike. Narrow, high-arched palate due to lateral palatal swellings, crowding of upper teeth due to hypoplastic maxilla, and open bite are characteristic. About 35% of patients are obligate mouth breathers. Cleft palate is observed in about 30% and bifid uvula in 10% of cases.

Exophthalmos, secondary to shallow orbits, is a constant finding. Exotropia (75%), exposure conjunctivitis (50%) or keratitis

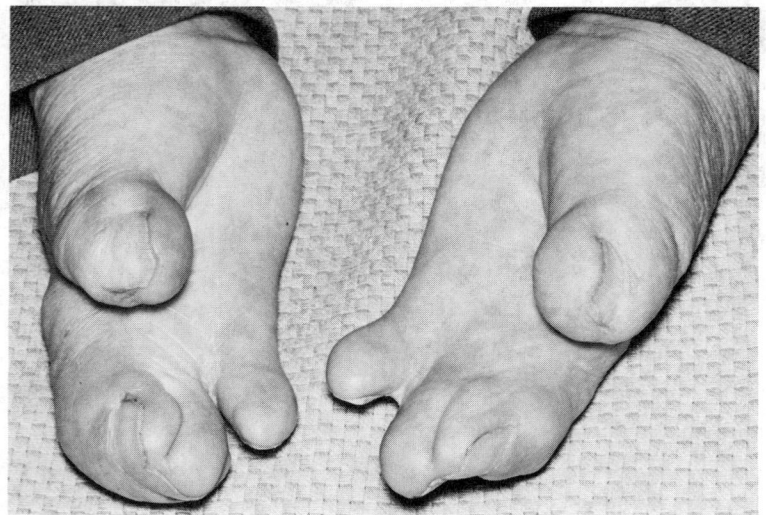

Figure 20-94. Apert's syndrome. Extensive soft tissue syndactyly of hands. Note middigital hand mass composed of digits 2 through 4 and separate thumb and little finger. (Courtesy of L. Bergstrom, Los Angeles, California.)

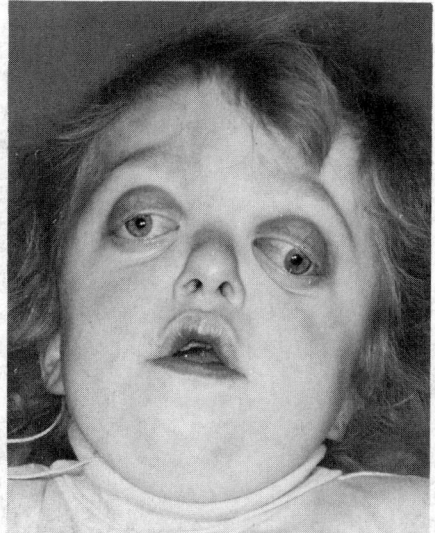

**Figure 20-95.** Pfeiffer's syndrome. Exorbitism, downward slanting palpebral fissures. Note hearing aid cord.

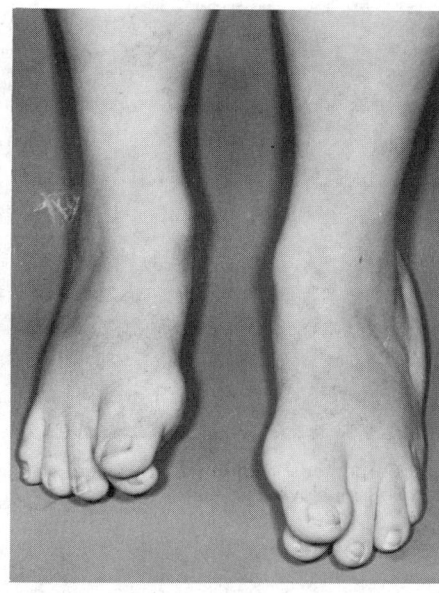

**Figure 20-97.** Wide halluces of Pfeiffer's syndrome.

(10%), poor vision (45%), optic atrophy (25%), hypertelorism, and nystagmus are noted. There is rare spontaneous luxation of the globes. Atretic auditory canals (15%) and malformed ossicles are associated with conductive hearing loss in more than 50% of patients. Stiffness of joints, especially the elbows, has been reported in about 15%. Head circumference and body height are generally smaller than normal.

Radiographically, the coronal and sagittal sutures are nearly always fused, the lambdoidal in 80% of patients. Other findings include digital markings (90%), calcification of stylohyoid ligament (85%), deviation of nasal septum (35%), obstruction of nasal pharynx (30%), and cervical spine anomalies (30%). Cephalometric studies have shown the calvaria to be short, the forehead steep, the occiput flattened, and the cranial base shortened and narrowed with the clivus especially abbreviated. Inheritance is autosomal dominant, with sporadic cases constituting approximately 50% of cases.

## Apert's Syndrome

Apert's syndrome is characterized by congenital craniosynostosis leading to turribrachycephaly, syndactyly of hands and feet, various ankyloses, and progressive synostoses of the hands, feet, and cervical spine (Figs 20-93, 20-94). Most patients are mentally

retarded. There is marked facial variability; the orbits are markedly hyperteloric with the midface usually underdeveloped, lending prominence to the mandible. The skull is malformed with the frontal and occipital bones flattened and the apex of the cranium located near or anterior to the bregma. Cleft of the soft palate has been observed in approximately 35% of cases. Malocclusion is common because of midface hypoplasia. The hands and feet are symmetrically deformed. A middigital hand mass with bony and soft tissue syndactyly of digits 2, 3, and 4 is often found. Digits 1 and 5 are often completely attached to the middigital hand mass. The hallux is frequently partially separated from the rest of the toes, which have complete soft tissue syndactyly and often a common nail. Six metatarsals have been noted in several cases. The upper extremities are shortened, and there may be ankylosis of joints, especially those of the elbow, shoulder, and hip. Acne vulgaris is commonly noted, with extension to the forearms. Apert's syndrome occurs in about 1 of 160,000 births. Inheritance is autosomal dominant, but the number of cases of transmission from parent to child is few because of the mental retardation and physical appearance.

## Pfeiffer's Syndrome

Pfeiffer's syndrome consists of craniosynostosis resulting in turribrachycephaly. Broad thumbs and great toes and partial soft

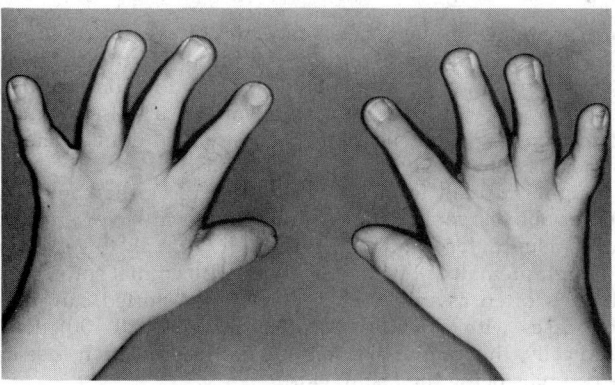

**Figure 20-96.** Wide thumbs of Pfeiffer's syndrome.

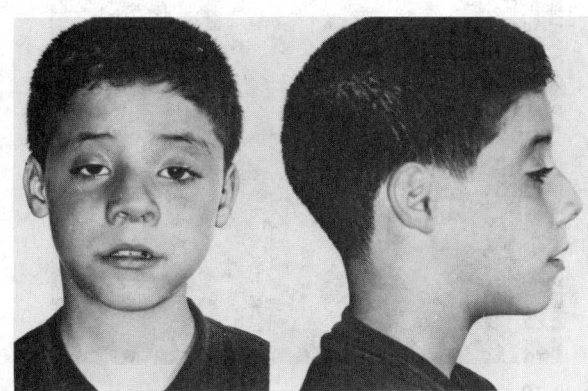

**Figure 20-98.** Saethre-Chotzen syndrome. Note facial asymmetry and ptosis of eyelid.

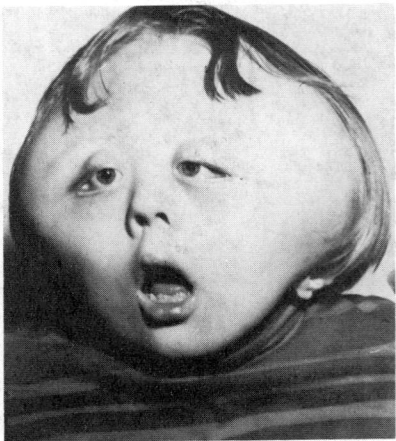

Figure 20-99.   Carpenter's syndrome. Downward slanting palpebral fissures, hypertelorism, cloverleaf skull.

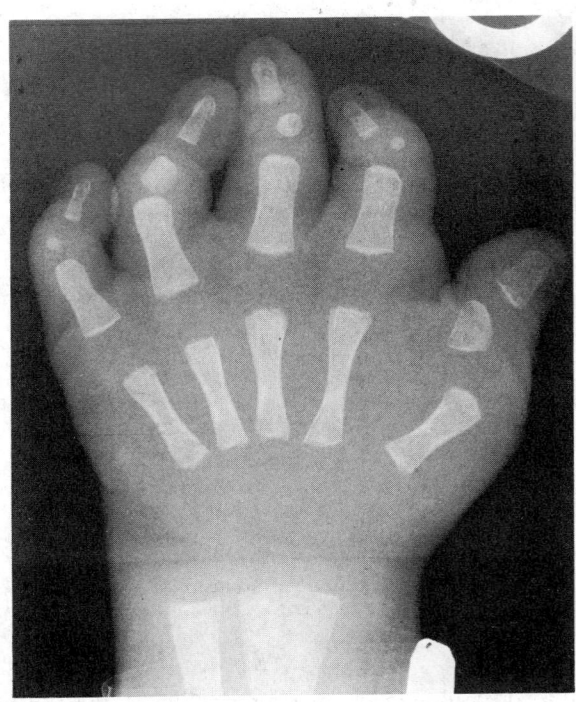

Figure 20-101.   Hypoplasia of middle phalanges in Carpenter's syndrome. (Courtesy of A. Poznanski, Chicago, Illinois.)

tissue syndactyly of the hands and feet are common. There is autosomal dominant inheritance with complete penetrance and variable expressivity.

Craniosynostosis, especially involving the coronal suture, results in turribrachycephaly; increased digital markings may be observed with age. Maxillary hypoplasia, shallow orbits, and depressed nasal bridge are also seen. Orbital hypertelorism, downslanting palpebral fissures, proptosis, and strabismus have been reported (Fig 20-95). Perhaps 5% of cases are associated with cloverleaf-skull malformation. Intelligence is usually normal, but severe retardation and various central nervous system defects are observed in those with the cloverleaf-skull anomaly.

The thumbs and great toes are broad, usually with varus deformity (Figs 20-96, 20-97). Mild soft tissue syndactyly especially involves the second and third digits. Middle phalanges are occasionally absent. The proximal phalanges of both thumbs are trapezoidal but may be triangular. Pollux varus is commonly found. The proximal phalanges of both great toes are trapezoidal, and hallux varus is common. The first metatarsals are broad, with partial reduplication in some cases. Symphalangism of both hands and feet has been reported. Fusion of carpals, tarsals, and the proximal ends of the metatarsals has been noted. Radiohumeral and radioulnar synostoses have been described.

## Saethre-Chotzen Syndrome

Asymmetric craniosynostosis produces plagiocephaly and facial asymmetry (Fig 20-98). Acrocephaly and occasionally scaphocephaly have been noted. Head circumference is frequently reduced, and often there is a low frontal hairline. Strabismus, myopia, hyperopia, ptosis, and hypertelorism are frequent. The ears may be dysplastic with folded helices, prominent antihelices, and posterior rotation. Some degree of hearing loss is common. The nose tends to be beaked, with deviation of the nasal septum. The nasofrontal angle is flattened. There is occasional partial cutaneous syndactyly of the second and third fingers. Intelligence is usually normal, but mild to moderate mental retardation has been found occasionally. Inheritance is autosomal dominant, with complete penetrance and variable expressivity. The gene has been mapped to chromosome 7p21.2 (Brueton, et al, 1992). Roentgenographically, there is usually coronal synostosis, reduced length of posterior cranial base, low position of the sella turcica, reduced facial depth, steep mandibular plane angle, and absence or reduced size of paranasal sinuses.

## Carpenter's Syndrome

Carpenter's syndrome consists of acrocephaly, soft tissue syndactyly, especially involving the third and fourth fingers, brachymesophalangy, preaxial polydactyly and syndactyly of the toes, coxa valga and pes varus, congenital heart disease, mental retardation, hypogenitalism, mild obesity, and hernia. The syndrome has autosomal recessive inheritance.

Height is usually in the low 25% range of normal, but weight is often above average. The obesity mainly involves the trunk, proximal limbs, face, and nape. The skull is usually tower shaped. Although premature fusion may involve all cranial sutures, synostosis is often asymmetric, producing a distorted calvaria, in some cases with cloverleaf skull (Figs 20-99, 20-100). Radiographically, the sagittal and lambdoidal sutures often fuse first, the coronals being the last to close.

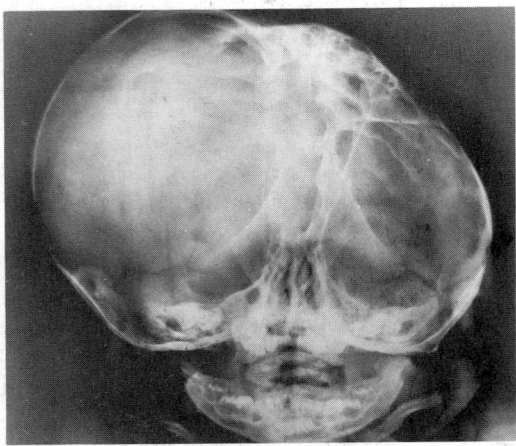

Figure 20-100.   Asymmetric cloverleaf skull of Carpenter's syndrome. (Courtesy of H. Schönenberg, Aachen, Germany.)

The hands are short and the fingers somewhat stubby, with a simple flexion crease (Fig 20-101). Soft tissue syndactyly often occurs between the third and fourth fingers, with less pronounced syndactyly between other fingers. Radiographically, there is brachymesophalangy of all digits or agenesis of some middle phalanges of the second to fifth digits. There usually are bilateral varus deformities of the feet and preaxial polydactyly with duplication of the first or second toe. The toes usually exhibit soft tissue syndactyly. Metatarsus varus and replication of the second toe are frequent. The first metatarsal is short and remarkably broad with only two phalanges present in each toe. In nearly all cases, there has been genu valgum with lateral displacement of the patellae. Congenital heart disease of various types (eg, VSD, ASD, PDA, pulmonary stenosis, tetralogy of Fallot) have been reported. Most patients are mildly retarded, but some have normal intelligence.

## Suggested Readings

Albin RE, Hendee RW, O'Donnell RS, Majure JA. Trigonocephaly: refinements in reconstruction. Experience with 33 patients. Plast Reconstr Surg 1985;76:202.

Bardach J, Morris HL. Multidisciplinary management of cleft lip and palate. Philadelphia: WB Saunders, 1990.

Bartlett SP, Whitaker LA, Marshac D. The operative treatment of isolated craniofacial dysostosis (plagiocephaly): a comparison of the unilateral and bilateral techniques. Plast Reconstr Surg 1990;85:677.

Bonaiti-Pellie C, Smith C. Risk tables for genetic counselling in some congenital malformations. J Med Genet 1974;11:374.

Brueton LA, von Herwerdon L, Chotai KA, Winter RM. The mapping of a gene for cramosynostosis: evidence for linkage to the Saethre-Chotzen syndrome to distal chromosome 7p. J Med Genet 1992;29:681.

Bruneteau RJ, Mulliken JB. Frontal plagiocephaly: synostotic, compensational, or deformational. Plast Reconstr Surg 1992;89:21.

Clarren SK, Anderson B, Wolf LS. Feeding infants with cleft lip, cleft palate, or cleft lip and palate. Cleft Palate Journal 1987;24:244.

Cohen MM Jr. The Robin anomaly—its nonspecificity in associated syndromes. J Oral Surg 1976;34:587.

Cohen MM Jr. Syndromes with cleft lip and cleft palate. Cleft Palate Journal 1978;15:306.

Cohen MM Jr. Craniosynostosis: diagnosis, evaluation and management. New York: Raven Press, 1986.

Cohen MM Jr, Rollnick BR, Kaye CI. Oculoauriculovertebral spectrum: an updated critique. Cleft Palate Journal 1989;26:276.

Cronin TD, Denkler KA. Correction of the unilateral cleft lip nose. Plast Reconstr Surg 1988;82:419.

David DJ, Sheen R. Surgical correction of Crouzon syndrome. Plast Reconstr Surg 1990;85:344.

Dixon MJ, Read AP, Donnai D, Calley A, Dixon J, Williamson R. The gene for Treacher Collins maps to the long arm of chromosome 5. Am J Hum Genet 1991;49:17.

Ferguson MWJ. Palate development. Development 1988;104(Suppl):41.

Fria TJ, Paradise JL, Sabo DL, Elster BA. Conductive hearing loss—in infants and young children with cleft palate. J Pediatr 1987;111:84.

Friedman JM, Hanson JW, Graham CB, et al. Saethre-Chotzen syndrome: a broad and variable pattern of skeletal malformations. J Pediatr 1977;91:929.

Gorlin RJ, Cohen MM Jr, Levin S. Syndromes of the head and neck, ed 3. New York: Oxford University Press, 1990.

Hall BK. The neural crest. Oxford: Oxford University Press, 1988.

Hunter AGW, Rudd NL. Cramosynostosis. I. Sagittal synostosis: its genetics and associated clinical findings in 214 patients who lacked involvement of the coronal suture(s). Teratology 1976;14:185.

Jabs EW, Li X, Coss CA, Taylor EW, Meyers DA, Weber JL. Mapping the Treacher Collins syndrome locus to 5q31.3->q33.3. Genomics 1991;11:193.

Johnston MC, Bronsky PT. Animal models for human craniofacial malformations. J Craniofac Genet Dev Biol 1991;11:277.

Jones JC. Etiology of facial clefts: prospective evaluation of 428 patients. Cleft Palate Journal 1988;25:16.

Kaban LB, Moses MH, Mulliken JB. Surgical correction of hemifacial microsomia in the growing child. Plast Reconstr Surg 1988;82:9.

Kay ED, Kay CN. Dysmorphogenesis of the mandible, zygoma and middle ear ossicles in hemifacial microsomia and mandibulofacial dysostosis. Am J Med Genet 1989;32:27.

Kreiborg S. Crouzon syndrome: a clinical and roentgencephalometric study. Scand J Plast Reconstr Surg 1981;18 (Suppl):1.

Langman, J. Head and neck. In: Thomas W. Sadler, ed. Langman's medical embryology, ed 6. Baltimore: Williams and Wilkins, 1990.

Marchac D, Renier D. Craniofacial surgery for craniosynostosis. Boston: Little Brown, 1982.

Melnick M, Bixler D, Shields ED, eds. The etiology of cleft lip and cleft palate. New York: Alan R. Liss, 1980.

Moller KT, Starr CD, Johnson SA. A parent's guide to cleft lip and palate. Minneapolis: University of Minnesota Press, 1989.

Pashayan H, McNab M. Simplified method of feeding infants with cleft palate with or without cleft lip. Am J Dis Child 1979;133:145.

Phelps PD, Poswillo D, Lloyd GAS. The ear deformities in mandibulofacial dysostosis. Clin Otorhinolaryngol 1981;6:15.

Shah CP, Wong D. Management of children with cleft lip and palate. Can Med Assoc J 1980;122:19.

Sheffield JA, Reiss K, Strom CJ. A genetic follow-up study of 64 patients with Pierre Robin complex. Am J Med Genet 1987;28:25.

Shprintzen RJ, Siegel-Sadewitz YL, Amato J. Anomalies associated with cleft lip, cleft palate, or both. Am J Med Genet 1985;20:585.

Spence MA, Westlake J, Lange K, Gold DP. Estimation of polygenic recurrence risk for cleft lip and palate. Hum Hered 1976;26:327.

Tessier P. Craniofacial surgery in syndromic craniosynostosis. In: MM Cohen Jr, ed. Craniosynostosis: diagnosis, evaluation and management. New York: Raven Press, 1986:321.

Turvey TA, Long RE Jr, Hall JD. Multidisciplinary management of Crouzon syndrome. J Am Dent Assoc 1979;99:205.

Vanderas AP. Incidence of cleft lip, cleft palate, and cleft lip and palate among races: a review. Cleft Palate Journal 1987;24:216.

Whitaker LA, Bartlett SP, Schut L, Bruce D. Craniosynostosis: an analysis of the timing, treatment, and complications in 164 consecutive patients. Plast Reconstr Surg 1987;80:195.

*Principles and Practice of Pediatrics, Second Edition.* edited by Frank A. Oski et al. J. B. Lippincott Company, Philadelphia © 1994.

# 20.13 *Eye Evaluation in the Newborn*

David S. Walton

Understanding the normal ocular system is essential preparation for evaluation of the normal newborn. Personnel caring for infants must be sensitive to the possibility of and have familiarity with common neonatal ocular abnormalities. Skillful eye examination allows early recognition of abnormalities.

When an ocular abnormality is recognized or when parents repeatedly question some aspect of the visual system, prompt referral to an ophthalmologist with experience with children is indicated. Generally, the medical and surgical management of any ocular abnormality should not be undertaken or continued without consultation. Some conditions are more emergent than others.

## EXAMINATION

Careful and complete ocular examination of the newborn is an essential component of any neonatal physical examination. This examination can be carried out relatively quickly. It is important to examine the eyes of all newborns to rule out unsuspected ocular defects.

To perform this examination, the infant should be comfortable and warm. The examination can be performed in the nursery bassinet while the baby is being fed. Only a penlight and ophthalmoscope are needed. A 2× magnification loupe can be helpful for observing anterior segment structures. The examination should be done systematically with the least upsetting maneuvers performed first. Results should be carefully recorded.

The newborn eye examination should include appraisal of the following structures and functions: vision and pupillary responses; eyelids and tears; eye position and movements; conjunctiva; corneal size and transparency; iris appearance and symmetry; pupil size, position, and shape; lens transparency; funduscopy and red reflex.

Vision testing of the newborn requires clinical acumen and lacks precision. Laboratory methods reveal that a term newborn possesses a visual acuity of approximately 20/200 and begins to focus (accommodate) by 3 months of age. This adjustment represents a high level of visual function. When presented with an object or light, the normal newborn may stare, halt movement of the extremities, and follow the object briefly. Blinking or blepharospasm is expected in response to bright light, but its presence should not be interpreted as evidence of cortical function. Pupillary response to light is the most reliable sign of sensory ocular function in the newborn. It is best performed in a somewhat darkened room; the direct pupillary responses should be compared and consensual responses judged. Nystagmus is always a significant finding and may be caused by decreased vision.

The eyelids and tears often can be appraised by momentary observation. The examination may, however, be made uncertain by postpartum lid swelling or by silver nitrate irritation of the eyes. A good blink is the appropriate response to a puff of air. The superior lid crease should be similar in each lid. A slight asymmetry in palpebral fissure width is usually not significant. The presence of turning out (ectropion) or turning in (entropion) of the lashes toward the cornea should be ruled out. An excess of tears makes the newborn eye look excessively wet.

Extraocular movements and position should be examined. The eye position in the straight-ahead position (primary position) should be observed. A deviation especially with sleep is common. A persistent deviation is always significant and deserves careful reexamination. Vertical and horizontal eye movements can be stimulated by head rotation. The presence of abduction (sixth nerve function) in each eye should be established. Vestibular nystagmus with both fast and slow phases is expected in the term newborn and is also best seen by rotation, holding the infant facing the examiner.

Inspection of the conjunctiva of the newborn requires careful assessment. Look for increased redness (injection) and discharge. Persistent discharge would suggest conjunctivitis. Familiarity with the usual response to and course after silver nitrate application is helpful.

Careful inspection of the anterior segment of each eye consists of inspection of the corneal size and transparency, the clarity of the anterior chamber as indicated by the view of the iris, the appearance of the irides, and the shape and size of the pupils. With practice, this examination can be done confidently and quickly. A 2× magnification loupe can be used for this phase of the eye examination.

Each lens should be examined for evidence of opacification (cataracts). This inspection is done best and most reliably by focusing an ophthalmoscope on the pupillary border, then moving it slightly closer and studying the red reflex. Even a small central opacity is revealed as a dark defect. Diffuse cataracts cause the red reflex to be of poor quality and inhibit a clear view of the ocular fundi.

The fundus examination should include inspection of the disks, retinal vessels, and macular regions, but it is not a necessary part of the normal newborn examination. The small pupils of the newborn make this examination difficult, so it is enough to be assured by the presence of an equal red reflex from each fundus. Darker pigmented people reveal a darker reflex (nearly gray in blacks). This variation is in proportion to the amount of pigment in the choroid.

## DISORDERS OF THE EYE IN THE NEWBORN

Disorders of vision are rarely detectable in the newborn period. Even anencephalic infants have pupillary responses and blepharospasm in response to light. Visual behavior, however, develops rapidly and often becomes a cause for parental concern by 1 month of age. Parents concerned that their child "does not see" should not be disregarded.

A common abnormality of the eyelid consists of ptosis (drooped eyelid), which is caused by weakness of muscles attached to the lid. This abnormality is usually an isolated defect, but it may be bilateral. Weakness of the levator palpebralis muscle is usually associated with an absent superior lid crease. Slight ptosis may be evidence of Horner's syndrome and associated with pupillary miosis along with possible homolateral upper extremity paralysis. Widening of the palpebral fissure may be the first evidence of a congenital facial nerve palsy or may be caused by proptosis. Proptosis in the newborn may be caused by a retrobulbar tumor or by hemorrhage associated with birth trauma. The eyelid position relative to the eye should be observed for evidence of an entropion that might put the lashes in harmful approximation to the cornea.

Normal tears for lubrication of the eye are present at birth. Excessive tears may suggest a common tear duct obstruction. This condition is usually noticed by parents promptly and becomes complicated by a discharge early in its course. There should be careful assessment of the eyelids after facial trauma associated with difficult birth because of the possibility of injury to the tear drainage system.

An intermittent eye deviation in early life is common and is seen usually only with sleep or fatigue. Deviation in this setting is normal. A congenital esotropia is seen in approximately 1% of infants. Usually the deviation is large and may be associated with impaired abduction of both eyes. A sixth nerve palsy may occur with birth, is usually unilateral, and often resolves spontaneously. A congenital fourth nerve paralysis also can occur but is less frequently recognized early in life. Congenital third nerve palsies are rare, cause ptosis, pupillary abnormalities, and external ophthalmoplegia often associated with an exotropia, and are frequently associated with other evidence of central nervous defects such as hemiplegia.

Nystagmus is always a sign of ocular disease. Tonic defects of eye position of supranuclear origin occur, are usually associated with tonic down gaze, and are often transient.

Disorders of the conjunctiva other than from infection are unusual in the newborn period. Ophthalmic neonatorum (conjunctivitis of the newborn) is described in Chapter 34. Other defects include hemorrhage, cysts, and choristomas including dermoid and lipodermoid cysts.

Failure to carry out a careful assessment of the anterior segment of the newborn may result in delayed diagnosis of significant ocular disease of the newborn. Corneal opacification may be an early sign of glaucoma or may be caused by a congenital defect of the cornea. The possibility of birth trauma to the cornea must also be considered, particularly after a history of difficult delivery and use of forceps. A small cornea may indicate microphthalmos and the presence of serious, more posterior defects such as a coloboma of the choroid, chorioretinitis, or cataract.

The irides are ordinarily similar in appearance. The pupils should be round and similar in size. Congenital defects to be ruled out include a coloboma of the iris, which gives the pupil a keyhole appearance; vascular congestion of the iris; poor view of the iris suggestive of a hyphema (blood in the anterior chamber); and abnormal iris pigmentation (albinism, congenital melanosis).

The most common lens defect in the neonate is cataracts. This opacification of the lens may be unilateral or bilateral and is detectable with use of an ophthalmoscope or a hand-held slit beam and a magnification loupe. Cataracts may be unilateral or bilateral, anterior or posterior in the lens, and partial or total. They may occur as an isolated defect or be associated with other ocular or systemic abnormalities. They may be inherited or sporadic and have hereditary significance, or they may represent a noninheritable, sporadic defect.

The diverse etiologies of congenital cataracts dictate the need for a careful and complete ocular and general examination of the young cataract patient to determine the significance of the cataract abnormality. Table 20-71 lists causes of congenital cataracts.

The presence of a cataract in infancy may represent a significant impediment to the development of vision. Increased opacification, irregularity, posterior location, and greater size are features of a potentially more significant defect. Vision develops

---

**TABLE 20-71.  Cataracts in Childhood—Etiologic Classification**

I. Congenital (0–1 y)
  A. Hereditary (Isolated Cataracts)
    1. Anterior polar
    2. Lamellar nuclear cataracts (D)
    3. Bilateral posterior lenticonus
    4. Discoloration anterior capsule (green)
    5. Star and nugget cataracts (D) (personal observation)
    6. Cataracts with microcornea or microphthalmia (D or XR)
    7. Cataracts, microcornea, and dental anomalies (Nance-Horan syndrome) (XR)
    8. Sutural opacities (carrier of Nance-Horan trait) (XR)
    9. Carrier of chondrodysplasia punctata (Clin Genet 1981;19:64)
    10. Ectopia lentis et pupillae
  B. Idiopathic
    1. Unilateral/bilateral cortical cataracts
    2. Unilateral posterior lenticonus
    3. Isolated lens capsule pigmentation
    4. Residual anterior capsule pupillary membrane plaque
  C. Embryopathic
    1. Maternal rubella syndrome
    2. Severe toxoplasmosis
    3. Herpes simplex infection (Arch Ophthalmol 1971;85:220)
    4. Maternal varicella (J Pediatr 1974;84:239)
  D. Trauma
    1. Birth
    2. Trauma X
  E. Cataracts or Prematurity
    1. Transient cataracts (J Pediatr 1973;82:314)
  F. Chromosomal Disorders
    1. 21 Trisomy
    2. 13 Trisomy
    3. 18 Trisomy
    4. 13 Long arm deletion
    5. Group G monosomy
    6. 18 Short arm deletion
    7. Autosomal dominant cataracts with [t(3;4) (p26.2;p15)] (Arch Ophthalmol 1987;105:1382)
    8. Cri Du Chat 5q⁻
    9. Aniridia 11p⁻
  G. Primary Systemic Disease
    1. Galactosemia–transferase deficiency
    2. Hallermann-Strieff syndrome
    3. Chondrodysplasia punctata (Rhizomelic) (R)
    4. Lowe's syndrome
    5. Marinesco-Sjögren's syndrome (mental retardation, hypotonia, dwarfism, ataxia, and cataracts)
    6. Syndromes of mental retardation, microcephaly, microphthalmia, and cataracts
    7. Kniest syndrome (skeletal dysplasia) (D)
    8. Incontinenti pigmenti
    9. Atopic dermatitis
    10. Smith-Lemli-Opitz syndrome
    11. Infantile hypopglycemia
    12. Congenital cataracts associated with skeletal and caradiac myopathy (J Pediatr 1975;86:873)
    13. Turner's syndrome
    14. Rubinstein-Taybi syndrome
    15. Blepharophimosis with somato facial dysmorphism (Schwartz-Aberfeld's Disease) (Arch ophthalmol 1969;82:1)
    16. Congenital cataract with renal necrosis and encephalopathy (Arch Dis Child 1963;38:505)
    17. Phenylketonuria (1 case)
    18. Hereditary spherocytosis
    19. Trichomegaly, spherocytosis, and bilateral cataracts (Am J Ophthalmol 1972;73:333)
    20. Oxycephaly (Am J Ophthalmol 1961;52:207)
    21. Schafer's syndrome (mental retardation, dwarfism, hyperkeratosis, nail abnormality)
    22. Seimen's syndrome (cataracts and skin hypoplasia)
    23. Oculocerebral syndrome with amino aciduria and keratosis follicularis (Arch Dis Child 1967;42:435)
    24. Maple syrup urine disease (J Ped Ophthalmol Strabismus 1973;10:70)
    25. Cataracts, microcephaly, kyphosis, and limited joint movement (Am J Dis Child 1973;125:553)
    26. Metaphyseal and epiphyseal dysplasia, unusual facies, and cataracts (Am J Dis Child 1973;125:553)
    27. A syndrome of hypohidrotic ectodermal dysplasia and cataracts (Frene-Maia. NJ Med Genet 1975;12:308)
    28. Familial organic aciduria with cardiomyopathy
    29. Mevalonic aciduria (N Engl J Med 1986;314:1610)
    30. Warburg syndrome
  H. Cataracts Associated With Primary Ocular Anomalies
    1. Persistent primary hyperplastic vitreous
    2. Congenital aniridia
    3. Peter's anomaly
    4. Ectopia lentis et pupillae (R)
    5. Unilateral microphthalmia
    6. Associated with ocular coloboma
    7. Congenital retinal disinsertion syndrome (Trans 1975;79:827; Ophthalmol 1968;80:325)
    8. Microphthalmos and cataracts with or without other ocular defects
    9. Bhaduri syndrome of congenital cataracts, blepharophimosis, cataracts, and iris anomalies (D) (personal observation)

rapidly early in life, and if this process is impeded beyond a critical period of approximately 4 months after birth, the potential for development of as high a level of vision as possible is lost. Thus, recognizing cataracts early in life is important. After cataracts are detected, prompt ophthalmologic evaluation is done, during which the infant is considered for cataract removal. Both the associated eye health and general health of the infant is considered when determining his or her potential for improved vision by way of cataract extraction.

Neonatal retinal hemorrhages frequently are present in the newborn and are seen less frequently when delivery is by cesarean section. Vitreous hemorrhage is far less common than retinal hemorrhage. Visualization of retinal hemorrhages requires focusing the ophthalmoscope on the ocular fundus. Such hemorrhages are usually numerous, occupy the inner layers of the retina, and subside rapidly. When seen, it is important to document their disappearance. Correspondingly, retinal hemorrhages seen later in the newborn (eg, after 3 weeks of age) should be interpreted as secondary to birth trauma with great reservation. The probability of more recent trauma, possibly caused by accident or by child abuse (whiplash-shaken infant) must be seriously considered, even in the absence of other immediate evidence of injury.

Infants born prematurely must be considered at risk for retinopathy of prematurity (ROP). Well cared for infants with a birth weight of 1500 g or less are at risk. Those infants below 1200 g may be considered at high risk and show an incidence of ROP of about 50%.

Parents should be informed of the risks of ROP early in the infant's hospitalization. The considerable efforts that are made to monitor oxygen dose, light exposure, occurrence of apnea, need for transfusions, and other treatments should be repeatedly reviewed as the infant's progress is reported to his or her parents.

Ophthalmic assessment should begin when the infant is clinically stable and 4 to 6 weeks of age. More premature babies tend to be examined later in life, eg, 6 to 7 weeks of age versus 1 month for those less premature. This examination is done by indirect ophthalmoscopy and requires pupillary dilation. For pupillary dilation tropicamide or cyclopentolate 0.5% to 1.0% and Neo-Synephrine 1.0% to 2.5% is recommended, with the application of a single drop of each to each eye. Overflow onto the skin should be avoided because further systemic absorption can occur is also helpful. The eyes may be examined individually on different days to lessen the burden on the patient.

On examination, the ophthalmologist looks for retinal abnormalities characteristic of ROP. If found, the defects should be classified in respect to their stage, using the international classi-

fication of retinopathy of prematurity (Table 20-72). This system permits definition of the retinal defect in respect to location, extent, and severity. Depending on location and severity of the defect, reexamination should be carried out regularly. Each affected infant is evaluated in respect to his or her candidacy for cryotherapy or laser treatment, which may be helpful for progressive disease. ROP is also associated with a high incidence of spontaneous regression of the abnormality, especially when retinal vascularization has prenatally achieved a position anterior to the equator. The indication, efficacy, and safety of prophylactic vitamin E therapy has not been established. Its use to prevent vitamin E deficiency is indicated.

A "normal" newborn examination report must include that the eyes have also been examined and found healthy without disease or congenital anomalies. The ocular examination of the newborn with suspected abnormalities requires skill that can best be acquired by the careful repeated examination of normal neonates. An ophthalmologist should be consulted frequently so that normal variations are learned and disease managed promptly. Like neonatology, pediatric ophthalmology has come far in the past decade.

## Selected Readings

Crawford JS, Morin JD. The eye in childhood. New York: Grune and Stratton, 1983.
Flynn JT, et al. A cohort study of transcutaneous oxygen tension and the incidence and severity of retinopathy of prematurity. New Engl J Med 1992;326:1050.
Isenberg SJ. The eye in infancy. Chicago: Year Book Medical Publishers, 1987.
Nelson LB, Calhoun JH, Harley RD. Pediatric ophthalmology. Philadelphia: WB Saunders, ed 3, 1991. An international classification of retinopathy of prematurity. Pediatrics 1988;82:37.
Robb R. Ophthalmology for the pediatric practitioner. Boston: Little, Brown & Co, 1981.
Sira IB, Nissenkorn I, Kremer I. Retinopathy of prematurity (major review). Surv Ophthalmol 1988;33:1.

*Principles and Practice of Pediatrics, Second Edition.*
edited by Frank A. Oski et al. J. B. Lippincott Company, Philadelphia © 1994.

# 20.14 *Bacterial and Viral Infections of the Newborn*

## 20.14.1 *Sepsis Neonatorum*

Jane D. Siegel

The terms *neonatal sepsis* and *sepsis neonatorum* refer to invasive bacterial infections that involve primarily the bloodstream in infants during the first month of life. As a "compromised host," the neonate does not localize infection well, and invasion of the meninges occurs in about 10% to 25% of bacteremic infants. The incidence of neonatal sepsis in the United States varies from 1 to 10 per 1000 live births, with an average of 2 or 3 per 1000. Although these infections are relatively uncommon, they may be associated with case fatality rates of 15% to 30% and sub-

| TABLE 20-72. Stage of Retinopathy of Prematurity | |
|---|---|
| Stage No. | Characteristic |
| 1 | Demarcation line |
| 2 | Ridge |
| 3 | Ridge with extraretinal fibrovascular proliferation |
| 4 | Subtotal retinal detachment |
| | Extrafoveal |
| | Retinal detachment including fovea |
| 5 | Total retinal detachment |

| Funnel: | Anterior | Posterior |
|---|---|---|
| | Open | Open |
| | Narrow | Narrow |
| | Open | Narrow |
| | Narrow | Open |

stantial morbidity in surviving infants. The pediatrician must be familiar with the etiologic agents, pathogenesis, and clinical manifestations of neonatal sepsis so appropriate cultures may be obtained and effective antimicrobial therapy may be initiated promptly.

## ETIOLOGY

Although the incidence of neonatal sepsis has varied little over the years, the predominant pathogens have varied considerably from one decade to the next (Table 20-73). In the 1970s, group B streptococcus emerged and has persisted into the 1990s as the predominant pathogen in most United States nurseries. The virulence of the group B streptococcus, however, has decreased in recent years. Within the United States, there has been an unexplained year-to-year as well as geographic variation in the reported rates of group B streptococcal infections. Yearly incidence of neonatal group B streptococcus infection may vary in the presence of stable maternal colonization rates for unknown reasons. Replacement of the gram-negative enteric bacilli and *Pseudomonas* spp by the group B streptococcus as the predominant pathogen in Latin American and Asian nurseries has lagged behind the pattern observed in North American nurseries by several years.

Although group B streptococcus and *Escherichia coli* account for 60% to 70% of all infections, several other pathogens are noteworthy. *Staphylococcus aureus, Klebsiella-Enterobacter, Serratia, Salmonella,* and *Pseudomonas* spp are most frequently isolated from infants with late-onset infections, especially during nosocomial outbreaks. Aminoglycoside-resistant strains of gram-negative bacilli and methicillin-resistant *S aureus* (MRSA) are particularly difficult to eradicate from nurseries for low–birth-weight infants. The incidence of *Listeria monocytogenes* is highly variable with temporal clustering related to maternal infection associated with food-borne outbreaks.

Several other pathogens have come to the forefront during the past decade. In a study by Broughton and colleagues (1981), the non-group D, α-hemolytic streptococcus was cited as second only to the group B streptococcus as an etiology of neonatal sepsis. This organism is less virulent than most of the other neonatal pathogens. There is a low incidence of shock and meningitis, and a case fatality rate of only 9%. Group D streptococci, both enterococcal and nonenterococcal (*Streptococcus bovis*), have been associated with clinical illness indistinguishable from early-onset disease caused by the group B streptococcus as well as late-onset nosocomial infections. *Streptococcus pneumoniae, Neisseria meningitidis, Haemophilus influenzae,* and groups A, C, and G streptococci are respiratory tract pathogens that occasionally colonize the maternal genital tract and cause early-onset neonatal sepsis. Pneumonia associated with these pathogens may be clinically indistinguishable from uncomplicated hyaline membrane disease. Friesen and Cho (1986) report that, in contrast to *H influenzae* infections in infants beyond the first month of life, only 20% of such infections in the neonate are due to type B organisms. The remaining cases are associated with nontypable strains (56%), other types (D and C, 9%), or strains of unknown type (15%). The reported overall case-fatality rate for neonatal *H influenzae* infections is 55%. *S pneumoniae* is more likely to be associated with meningitis in the neonate than are other respiratory tract pathogens.

Coagulase-negative staphylococci and *Candida* spp have been isolated more often from septic, premature infants who have prolonged stays in the intensive care unit and who receive parenteral hyperalimentation through a central venous catheter and repeated courses of broad-spectrum antibiotics. *Candida* spp are associated with 5% to 10% of late-onset infections in low–birth-weight nurseries, whereas coagulase-negative staphylococci now account for more than 30% of late-onset infections. These two pathogens may cause right-sided endocarditis associated with catheter placement in the right atrium. The significance of anaerobes isolated from blood cultures of neonates remains unclear. Most anaerobic bacteremias are self-limited in the absence of a focal infection. *Bacteroides* and *Clostridium* spp may be associated with serious life-threatening disease, especially when peritonitis, fasciitis, or meningitis is present.

Overall case fatality rates have decreased from 90% in the 1930s to 15% to 25% in the 1980s and 1990s. This decrease is a result of earlier recognition of the nonspecific signs of sepsis and improved supportive care of the overwhelmed infant as well as development of more active antimicrobial agents.

## EPIDEMIOLOGY

Our knowledge of the epidemiology of perinatally acquired bacterial infections is based on extensive studies of the group B streptococcus performed during the 1970s and 1980s. The gastrointestinal tract is the major site of asymptomatic colonization with both the group B streptococcus and *E coli* for mother and infant. Several findings support the concept of a gastrointestinal reservoir for group B streptococcus: the rectum is the single most consistently colonized site; in the genital tract, group B streptococcus is more frequently isolated from vaginal than cervical cultures; and group B streptococci have been isolated from the prox-

**TABLE 20-73. Pathogens Most Frequently Associated with Sepsis Neonatorum**

| Years | Most Frequent | Other |
|---|---|---|
| 1928–1932 | β streptococcus | *Staphylococcus aureus, Escherichia coli* |
| 1933–1943 | Group A streptococcus | *E coli* |
| 1944–1957 | *E coli* | *Pseudomonas aeruginosa* |
| 1958–1965 | *E coli* (*S aureus**) | *Pseudomonas* spp., *Klebsiella-Enterobacter* |
| 1966–1978 | Group B streptococcus | *E coli, Klebsiella-Enterobacter* |
| 1979–1990 | Group B streptococcus, *E coli* | Coagulase-negative staphylococci, MRSA*†, gram negatives, enterococcus, *Candida* |

\* Nosocomial outbreaks in some nurseries
† Methicillin-resistant *S. aureus*
*Adapted from Freedman RM, Ingram DL, Gross E, et al. A half century of neonatal sepsis at Yale, 1928–1978. Am J Dis Child 1981;135:140*

imal small intestine in a small number of healthy adults who have been studied. Group B streptococcus may be isolated from the gastrointestinal or genitourinary tract in 5% to 30% of pregnant women. Younger, sexually experienced women from lower socioeconomic backgrounds have higher colonization rates. This organism is sexually transmitted. Of men who attend sexually transmitted diseases clinics, 2% to 24% harbor group B streptococci in either the urethra or the pharynx, and identical strains are carried by sexual partners of 45% to 60% of colonized women. Group B streptococcal colonization is persistent throughout pregnancy in 60% to 70% of women. Group B streptococci are suppressed but not eradicated from mucosal surfaces by treatment with antibiotics.

Between 40% and 70% of infants whose mothers are colonized at delivery (maternal infant concordance) become colonized themselves with group B streptococci by one of three mechanisms: transplacental transmission in the presence of maternal bacteremia, ascension from the vagina and cervix through microscopic leaks in the amniotic membranes or through frankly ruptured membranes, and surface contamination during passage through the birth canal. The risk of transmission increases when the density (inoculum) and number of sites of maternal colonization are increased; the risk is not influenced by route of delivery. Invasive disease develops in only 1 of every 50 to 75 colonized infants. Community acquisition of group B streptococci by the neonate after discharge from the nursery does not occur. A comparable relationship exists between colonization and disease rates for the pathogenic K1 strains of E coli that are associated with 75% of neonatal meningitis cases caused by E coli and 40% of sepsis cases caused by E coli.

*Listeria monocytogenes* is a worldwide soil organism with a large animal reservoir. A mechanism of transfer from animal to human has never been proved. However, the analysis by Schleck and colleagues (1983) of an outbreak of perinatal listeriosis associated with ingestion of contaminated coleslaw supports the hypothesis that vegetables contaminated by manure fertilizer obtained from infected animals are the source of human gastrointestinal tract colonization. Studies of pregnant women in epidemic areas have identified colonization rates of 5% to 8%, with the gastrointestinal tract rather than the genital tract being the site of carriage of L monocytogenes. In one Swedish study of 3000 human subjects, the asymptomatic fecal carriage varied from 1% in a group of hospitalized adults to 26% in a group of household contacts of patients with proven disease. Carriage did not persist beyond 2 to 4 weeks. Similarly, studies in association with a large food-borne outbreak of listeriosis in Los Angeles in 1985 revealed fecal carriage rates of 10.4% for employees of the cheese plant that processed the contaminated Mexican-style cheese and their household contacts and 8.3% for household contacts of pregnant women with listeriosis. More recently (1993), a carriage rate of 21% has been reported for asymptomatic household contacts of individuals with invasive listeriosis.

The epidemiology of late-onset disease is discussed in Chapter 20.14.4, Nosocomial Infection in the Neonate.

## PATHOGENESIS

Risk factors for the development of invasive bacterial infections may be generally categorized as obstetric, structural virulence factors of pathogenic strains of bacteria, and impaired host defenses (Table 20-74). The presence of any of these risk factors is associated with a 10-fold or greater increased risk of developing systemic infection. Most obstetric risk factors provide opportunities for prolonged exposure of the fetus to potential pathogens carried in the maternal gastrointestinal or genitourinary tract. Boyer and coworkers' 1983 epidemiologic studies of group B streptococcus revealed significantly increased attack rates (7.6 per 1000 live births) associated with the following conditions: birth weight of less than 2500 g, rupture of membranes for more than 18 hours, and maternal intrapartum fever higher than 37.5 °C. A rate of 26.2 per 1000 live births was observed in infants who weighed 1000 g or less. Similar associations have been observed with other neonatal pathogens. Twin pregnancy remains an independent risk factor for group B streptococcal infection after correction for low–birth-weight and is most likely related to genetic susceptibility factors and exposure to virulent strains common for both infants. Detection of group B streptococcal bacteriuria during pregnancy may be a means of identifying the heavily colonized woman whose infant is at increased risk of developing infection.

Inhalation of infected amniotic fluid or vaginal secretions containing pathogens may produce bronchopneumonia directly without primary bacteremia. Pathogens present in the maternal genitourinary tract or in the environment may adhere to epithelial cells on mucosal surfaces, then invade the infant's bloodstream. Common entry sites are the conjunctiva, nasopharynx, umbilical cord, and traumatized skin (eg, circumcision site). The infant occasionally is able to eliminate group B streptococci from the bloodstream without antibiotic therapy. Such transient bacteremias, however, are unpredictable. Delayed clearance from the bloodstream allows pathogens to multiply and cause either disseminated or focal disease. A critical level of 1000 colony-forming units per milliliter of blood must be produced for meningeal invasion to occur. Once pathogenic bacteria have invaded, pathophysiologic changes may be induced by the production and release of cell wall or outer membrane components such as endotoxin, extracellular bacterial products, or mediators of inflammation such as cachectin and interleukin 1. An endotoxin-like substance produced by group B streptococci can produce

| | Structural Virulence | |
|---|---|---|
| Obstetric | Factors | Impaired Host Defenses |
| Prematurity | Capsular polysaccharide | Specific humoral antibody |
| Prolonged rupture of membranes | Surface proteins | Complement |
| Internal monitoring devices | Cell wall components | Fibronectin |
| Twin pregnancy | Adhesins | Neutrophil supply |
| Maternal urinary tract infection | Protease | Opsonophagocytosis |
| Maternal fever | Neuraminidase | Chemotaxis |
| Maternal bacteremia | Endotoxin (lipid A) | |
| Chorioamnionitis | Extracellular toxin | |

TABLE 20-74. Risk Factors for the Development of Sepsis Neonatorum

effects on pulmonary hemodynamics and vascular permeability in sheep similar to changes observed in infected infants.

Of the various structural virulence factors, the polysaccharide capsule has been studied most extensively. For three neonatal pathogens, specific serotypes as determined by identification of the capsular polysaccharide have been associated with neonatal disease: group B streptococcus type III, *E coli* K1, and *L monocytogenes* IVb. The following evidence supports the pathogenicity of these strains. These serotypes account for 70% to 90% of cases of meningitis caused by these species of bacteria. Bacteria with these polysaccharide capsules have increased resistance to opsonophagocytosis by normal adult polymorphonuclear leukocytes. Monoclonal antibodies to specific antigenic determinants on the surface of these pathogens protect against disease in the infant rat and rhesus monkey models. The mothers of infants who are colonized with group B streptococcus type III and develop invasive disease are less likely to have protective levels (more than 2 µg/mL) of specific antibody when compared with mothers of those colonized infants who remain healthy. Poor outcome from meningitis is associated with larger concentrations of *E coli* K1 antigens measured in the cerebrospinal fluid.

Detailed studies of the type III group B streptococcus show that both the quantity of sialic acid residues in the capsular polysaccharide and the spatial conformation of the antigenic molecule determine the antiphagocytic properties of this pathogen. Rubens and colleagues (1988) identified and cloned a gene sequence that is specific for type III group B streptococci and is associated with virulence. Those strains with multiple copies of this gene sequence repeated within the chromosome have a lower lethal dose required to kill 50% of infected animals ($LD_{50}$) in the infant rat model of disease and are more resistant to opsonophagocytosis than strains that did not contain the gene sequence or had only one or two copies of the sequence.

Rabbit antibodies to the Ibc and R proteins of group B streptococcus are protective in animals and opsonic in vitro, and antibody to these proteins have been described in humans. Variations in these proteins may explain some strain difference in virulence. These proteins may be able to be linked to the capsular polysaccharide antigens to increase vaccine immunogenicity. The relative contribution of factors such as adhesins, proteases, and neuraminidase has not been clearly established, but these factors have been associated with virulence.

All arms of the defense system are deficient in the healthy neonate and are further impaired under conditions of prematurity, hypoxia, acidosis, and other metabolic derangements associated with bacterial infection. Treatment with specific antibody to group B streptococcus provides protection by improving several host defense mechanisms: opsonization via the alternative complement pathway, prevention of neutropenia and bone marrow depletion, release of neutrophils from bone marrow, and accumulation of neutrophils at the site of infection. Replacement of complement and fibronectin further improve opsonophagocytosis.

## CLINICAL MANIFESTATIONS

The clinical signs of bacterial infection in the neonate are presented in Table 20-75. These signs are distinctively nonspecific and may be associated with viral infections or with noninfectious disorders. Because the neonate is an impaired host, the clinical course is unpredictable and usually rapidly progressive. The presence of any of these signs alone or in combination is an indication for complete evaluation to rule out sepsis. The most commonly encountered clinical syndromes are described here.

**TABLE 20-75.    Nonspecific Signs of Sepsis**

| | |
|---|---|
| Temperature instability | Hypotension |
| Respiratory distress | Tachycardia |
| Feeding intolerance | Apnea and bradycardia |
| Vomiting | Irritability |
| Abdominal distention | High-pitched cry |
| Diarrhea | Lethargy |
| Jaundice | Weak suck |
| Pallor | Convulsions |
| Skin rash, petechiae | Bulging of full fontanelle |

### Early-Onset Syndrome

Clinical manifestations of the group B streptococcal early-onset syndrome may be present at birth or may appear at any time within the first 72 hours of life. Of the reported patients, 50% to 70% are term infants. Onset is usually sudden and follows a fulminant course, with the primary focus of inflammation in the lungs. In 60% of infected patients, the chest roentgenogram shows a reticulogranular pattern with air bronchograms indistinguishable from those seen with uncomplicated hyaline membrane disease. Gram-positive cocci may be seen within the hyaline membranes at postmortem examination. Persistent pulmonary hypertension may complicate the respiratory disease. In the most severe cases, apnea, hypotension, and disseminated intravascular coagulation cause rapid deterioration and result in death within 24 hours. Meningitis is present in 15% to 25% of infants with the early-onset syndrome. Even prompt administration of antibiotics and aggressive supportive therapy may be unsuccessful in these overwhelmed infants. The case-fatality rate has been as high as 40% to 80%, but it is now 15% to 25% because of early recognition and the availability of advanced intensive care facilities. Serotypes Ia and III are associated with most cases of group B streptococcal early-onset disease when meningitis is not present. Groups D and G streptococci and nontypable *H influenzae* are associated with a similar syndrome. Rarely, a transient group B streptococcus bacteremia may occur and produce mild, if any, clinical symptoms. If untreated, however, most bacteremia results in metastatic infection and fulminant disease.

The early-onset syndrome associated with *L monocytogenes* has several distinguishing features. There is often a flu-like illness in the mother just before delivery, and the maternal blood cultures may be positive. The lung is the primary focus of infection, but hepatosplenomegaly, purulent conjunctivitis, a skin rash consisting of irregular macules and papules or pustules in a truncal distribution, petechiae, and small granulomas on the posterior pharynx are characteristic of listeriosis. The chest roentgenogram shows a distinct reticulonodular pattern of bronchopneumonia that is pathognomonic for this infection. Case-fatality rate is 40% to 80%. Equal distributions of serotypes Ia, Ib, IVb are associated with early-onset sepsis when meningitis is not present.

### Late-Onset Syndrome

The late-onset syndrome associated with group B streptococci and *L monocytogenes* usually occurs in infants 10 to 30 days of age, but it may be seen as late as 12 to 16 weeks, especially in premature infants. The onset is most often insidious, and the affected infants present with the nonspecific signs of sepsis. Meningitis is the most characteristic finding. Group B streptococcus is known for its broad variety of foci, the most notable of which are osteomyelitis, septic arthritis, skin and soft tissue lesions, endocarditis, peritonitis, omphalitis, and pericarditis. Neonatal meningitis, osteomyelitis and septic arthritis, urinary tract infection, otitis media, skin and soft tissue infections, and nosocomial infections are discussed in detail in Chapter 20.14.2.

## DIAGNOSIS

Whenever bacterial infection of the neonate is suspected, cultures of blood, cerebrospinal fluid, urine, and infected body fluids that are normally sterile or an aspirate from an infected soft tissue site or bone should be obtained before initiating antimicrobial therapy. The optimal amount of blood for culture is 0.5 to 1.0 mL, but 0.2 mL may be adequate. Blood should be drawn from both a peripheral site and the central venous catheter when one is in place. Blood cultures should not be obtained from the umbilical cord at delivery or from umbilical catheters beyond the time of initial placement because of the high rates of contamination. Microorganisms isolated only from blood obtained through a catheter when peripheral venous blood cultures are sterile are more likely to represent colonization than septicemia. Bacteria such as coagulase-negative *Staphylococcus* or viridans streptococci that are common contaminants are more likely to be pathogens if isolated within 48 hours of incubation and if the same organism is isolated from blood cultures obtained from two separate sites. Cultures of mucosal surfaces are not helpful in distinguishing the infected from the colonized infant. Similarly, gastric aspirate cultures reflect the maternal environment and do not distinguish the infected from the colonized infant. The polymorphonuclear leukocytes present in the gastric aspirate are of maternal origin and may reflect fetal stress of noninfectious origin. In contrast, culture of the tracheal aspirate obtained at the time of intubation has been useful in identifying the etiologic agent of early-onset neonatal pneumonia.

Group B streptococcus is the only neonatal pathogen that can be detected reliably by commercially available latex particle-agglutination kits. The most useful body fluids for antigen detection are urine that has been concentrated 25- to 50-fold and cerebrospinal fluid. The sensitivity of this test for detecting culture-proven disease is reported to be 95% to 98%. The false-positive rates using urine range from 0% to 16% with an average of 3% to 6%. Perineal contamination may cause false-positive results in heavily colonized infants in the absence of invasive disease when the urine tested is obtained by bag collection. Therefore, group B streptococcal antigen detection tests should be performed on urine that has been obtained by suprapubic aspiration or in-and-out straight catheterization. Additionally, gastrointestinal absorption of swallowed amniotic fluid containing GBS may be associated with antigenuria in the first 24 hours of life in the absence of invasive disease. Negative antigen detection test results in a clinically ill infant do not rule out the possibility of systemic group B streptococcus infection. The *E coli* K1 capsular polysaccharide antigen is immunologically identical to the *N meningitidis* group B antigen and theoretically could be detectable by commercially available *N meningitidis* group B kits. The insensitivity of these kits and the frequent contamination of urine collected by bag with *E coli* K1 from gastrointestinal tract colonization decrease the usefulness of this test for diagnosis of invasive neonatal infection with *E coli* K1.

Several laboratory tests have been evaluated for their usefulness in rapid detection of the neonate with bacterial infection. Those evaluated either singly or in combination with a defined scoring system include the leukocyte count and differential count, platelet count, C-reactive protein level, erythrocyte sedimentation rate, haptoglobin level, IgM level, leukocyte alkaline phosphatase level, fibronectin level, nitroblue tetrazolium test, elastase-α-proteinase inhibitor level, and limulus lysate test for detection of

endotoxin. No single test alone or in combination with others is superior to the leukocyte count and differential count as a reliable indirect indicator of bacterial infection. After correction of the Coulter leukocyte count for the presence of nucleated red blood cells, the absolute total neutrophil count and the ratio of immature-to-total neutrophils (I:T) are compared with normal standards for age (Figs 20-102, 20-103). Neutropenia is more likely than neutrophilia to be associated with neonatal sepsis. Pregnancy-induced hypertension or asphyxia in the absence of infection, however, may produce neutropenia. The neutropenia of infection does not persist for more than 36 hours, whereas the neutropenia observed with noninfectious conditions may persist through the first 3 postnatal days. Similarly, neutrophilia may be associated with maternal fever before delivery or hemolytic disease of the newborn. Other noninfectious conditions that may affect the normal neutrophil values are presented in Table 20-76. The most useful indicator of bacterial infection is an I:T ratio of 0.16 or more. An I:T ratio of 0.8 or more indicates depletion of bone marrow reserves and a poor prognosis for survival. It is important to repeat the leukocyte count and I:T ratio determinations after 8 hours because studies in both animals and human

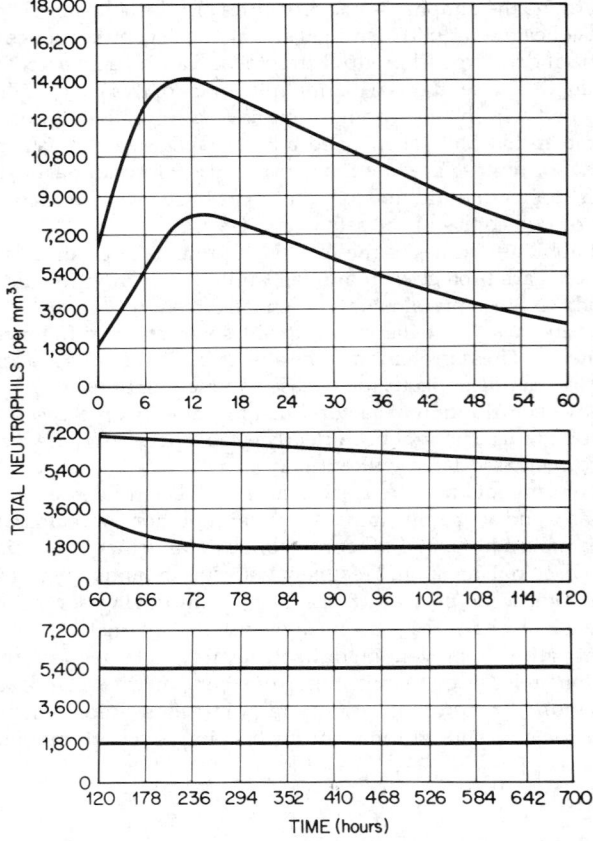

**Figure 20-102.** Normal total neutrophil counts after correction for nucleated red blood cells in neonates from birth to 700 hours of age. Formula for correction is as follows:

$$WBC = WBC_{cc} \times \frac{100}{NRBC + 100}$$

where WBC = corrected white blood cell count; $WBC_{cc}$ = Coulter counter white blood cell count; NRBC = nucleated red blood cells. (Adapted from Manroe BL, Rosenfeld CR, Weinberg AG, Browne R. The neonatal blood count in health and disease. I. Reference values for neutrophilic cells. J. Pediatr 1979;95:89. Reprinted from House Staff Nursery Manual, Division of Neonatal-Perinatal Medicine, Southwestern Medical School. Revised 1985.)

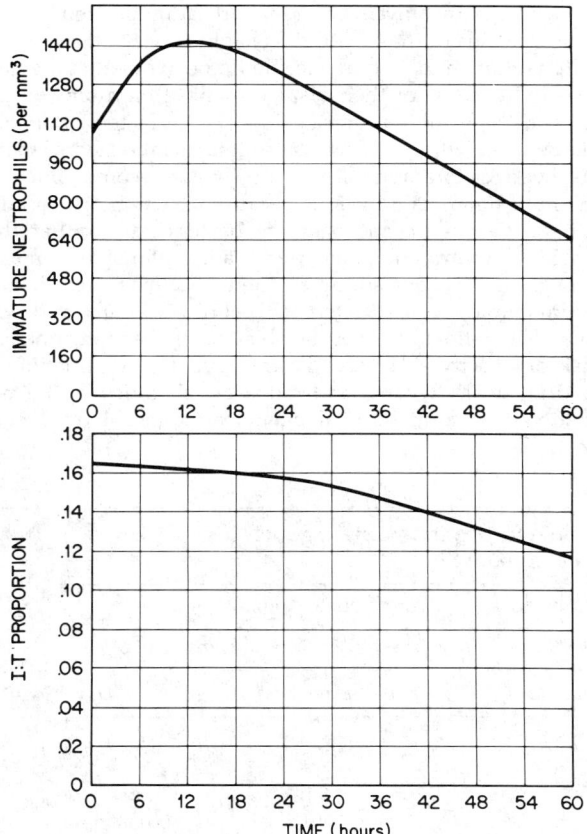

**Figure 20-103.** Normal total immature neutrophil counts and ratios of immature to total neutrophils (I:T) in neonates from birth to 60 hours of age. All bands and cell forms less mature than bands are classified together as immature neutrophils. (Adapted from Manroe BL, Rosenfeld CR, Weinberg AG, et al. The differential leukocyte count in the assessment and outcome of early onset group B streptococcal disease. J Pediatr 1977;91:632. Reprinted from House Staff Nursery Manual, Division of Neonatal-Perinatal Medicine, Southwestern Medical School. Revised 1985.)

### TABLE 20-76. Factors Affecting Neonatal Neutrophil Values

| Complication | ATN | ATI | ATI/ATN | Duration |
|---|---|---|---|---|
| Maternal hypertension | ↓ | | | 72h |
| Asphyxia | ↑↓ | | | 24h |
| Periventricular hemorrhage | ↓ | | | 120h |
| Hemolytic disease | ↑ | ↑ | ↑ | >28d |
| Maternal fever | ↑ | ↑ | ↑ | 24h |
| Stressful labor | ↑ | ↑ | ↑ | 24h |
| Pneumothorax | ↑ | ↑ | ↑ | 24h |
| Surgery | ↑ | ↑ | ↑ | 24h |
| >6-hour oxytocin induction | ↑ | ↑ | ↑ | 120h |

*ATN*, absolute total neutrophil count; *ATI*, absolute total immature neutrophil count

*House Staff Nursery Manual, Division of Neonatal-Perinatal Medicine, Southwestern Medical School, Dallas, TX, revised 1985*

infants demonstrate that the leukocyte count may be normal at the onset of group B streptococcal sepsis but becomes abnormal during the next 4 to 8 hours. No laboratory test result should ever negate a clinical impression of sepsis.

Chest roentgenogram should always be obtained as part of the diagnostic evaluation of the infant with suspected sepsis. Other radiographic studies may be indicated by the specific clinical condition. Sonography, computed tomography, and magnetic resonance imaging are the most useful imaging techniques in this age group. Technetium and gallium scans are rarely indicated in the neonate.

## THERAPY

The decision to initiate antimicrobial therapy in the neonate is based on the likelihood that an infant's clinical symptoms are a manifestation of infection or that the asymptomatic infant is at high risk for developing infection within the first few hours of life. Because of the increased risk of infection and the subtlety of clinical manifestations of infection in premature infants, antimicrobial therapy should be initiated in the premature infant with only a single obstetric or clinical risk factor. In contrast, the asymptomatic term infant with only obstetric risk factors presents more of a dilemma. An approach to the early management of

such infants is suggested in Figure 20-104. The goal of this scheme is to identify and treat all infected infants but to avoid excessive investigation and treatment of uninfected infants. It must be emphasized that such an approach is applicable only to asymptomatic term infants whose mothers do not have chorioamnionitis or sepsis in the peripartum period. Omission of a lumbar puncture in asymptomatic infants with only a single risk factor is unlikely to jeopardize the diagnosis of meningitis because term infants with in utero meningitis are symptomatic. If, however, the blood culture is positive, the lumbar puncture should be performed to be certain that meningitis has not developed. Furthermore, development of symptoms is an indication for immediate completion of the sepsis workup with lumbar puncture and initiation of antimicrobial therapy.

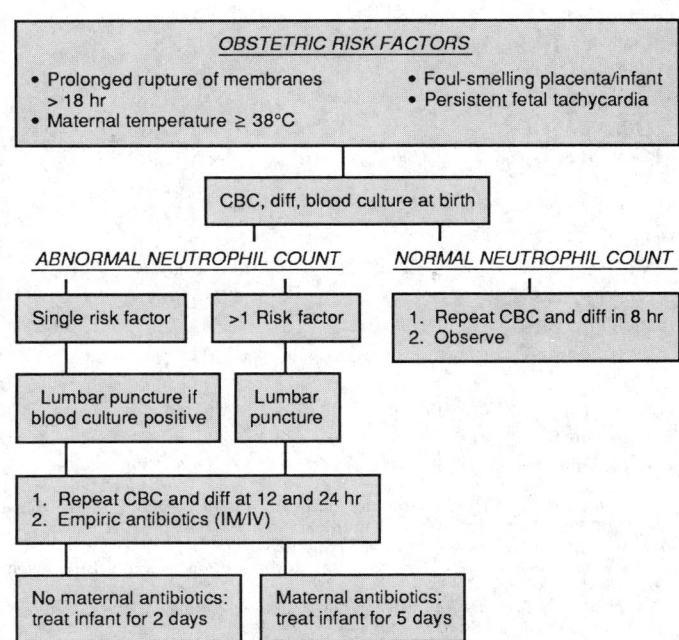

**Figure 20-104.** Recommended approach to diagnostic evaluation and treatment of the asymptomatic term (≥36 wk, 2200 g) infant with history of obstetric risk factors. *CBC*, complete blood count; *diff*, differential blood count; *IM*, intramuscularly; *IV*, intravenously. (Adapted from Engle WD, Sumner J, Lyttle B, Siegel JD. Abstract. Pediatr Res 1986;20:395A.)

The choice of antimicrobial agents is determined by several factors: the likely etiologic agent, susceptibility patterns within a specific nursery, central nervous system penetration, toxicity, and the infant's hepatic and renal function. Newly developed antimicrobial agents are not approved for use in the neonate until adequate clinical trials have been completed for determination of the pharmacokinetics, efficacy, and safety of each agent in this age group. The rapidly changing metabolic and physiologic processes as well as hepatic and renal immaturity of the neonate demand special considerations. For example, dosage schedules of antibiotics vary according to age and birth weight because of the improved renal function and clearance of drugs associated with increasing gestational and chronologic age. The half-life of vancomycin and the aminoglycosides is usually prolonged in low–birth-weight infants; therefore, serum levels of these drugs, as well as serum creatinine levels, must be monitored routinely to determine appropriate dosing interval in each patient. Amino-glycosides and vancomycin are frequently administered at 18- to 24-hour intervals in the low–birth-weight infant.

Sulfonamides and ceftriaxone should be avoided in the newborn period because of their displacement of bilirubin from albumin and the resulting increased risk of kernicterus. Nafcillin should be used with caution because it is metabolized primarily by the liver. Chloramphenicol is no longer recommended for treatment of neonatal infections because its action against most gram-negative enteric pathogens is bacteriostatic rather than bactericidal, in vitro antagonism with ampicillin against enteric gram-negative rods and group B streptococci has been demonstrated and may be associated with clinical failure, and wide individual variations in pharmacokinetics in neonates increase the risk of toxicity and necessitate frequent determinations of serum drug levels. Recommended dosage schedules for the most frequently used antimicrobial agents are presented in Table 20-77.

**TABLE 20-77. Recommended Dosage Schedule for Antimicrobial Agents Frequently Used for Treatment of Neonatal Sepsis***

| Antibiotics | Routes of Administration | Body Weight <2000 g | | Body Weight >2000 g | |
|---|---|---|---|---|---|
| | | 0–7 Days Old | >7 Days Old | 0–7 Days Old | >7 Days Old |
| Amikacin† | IV, IM | 15 div q 12 h | 22.5 div q 8 h | 20 div q 12 h | 30 div q 8 h |
| Ampicillin | IV, IM | | | | |
| Meningitis | | 200 div q 12 h | 300 div q 8 h | 200 div q 8 h | 300 div q 6 h |
| Other diseases | | 50 div q 12 h | 75 div q 8 h | 75 div q 8 h | 100 div q 6 h |
| Amphotericin B‡ | IV | 1 once daily | 1 once daily | 1 once daily | 1 once daily |
| Aztreonam | IV | 60 div q 12 h | 90 div q 8 h | 90 div q 8 h | 120 div q 6 h |
| Cefotaxime | IV, IM | 100 div q 12 h | 150 div q 8 h | 100 div q 12 h | 150 div q 8 h |
| Ceftazidime | IV, IM | 100 div q 12 h | 150 div q 8 h | 100 div q 8 h | 150 div q 8 h |
| Ceftriaxone | IV, IM | 50 once daily | 50 once daily | 50 once daily | 75 once daily |
| Clindamycin | IV, IM, PO | 10 div q 12 h | 15 div q 8 h | 15 div q 8 h | 20 div q 6 h |
| Erythromycin | PO | 20 div q 12 h | 30 div q 8 h | 20 div q 12 h | 30–40 div q 8 h |
| Flucytosine | PO§ | 100–150 div q 8 h | 100–150 div q 6 h | 100–150 div q 6 h | 100–150 div q 6 h |
| Gentamicin† | IM, IV | 5 div q 12 h | 7.5 div q 8 h | 5 div q 12 h | 7.5 div q 8 h |
| Methicillin | IV, IM | | | | |
| Meningitis | | 100 div q 12 h | 150 div q 8 h | 150 div q 8 h | 200 div q 6 h |
| Other diseases | | 50 div q 12 h | 75 div q 8 h | 75 div q 8 h | 100 div q 6 h |
| Metronidazole | IV, PO | 15 div q 12 h | 15 div q 12 h | 15 div q 12 h | 30 div q 12 h |
| Mezlocillin | IV, IM | 150 div q 12 h | 225 div q 8 h | 150 div q 12 h | 225 div q 8 h |
| Nafcillin | IV | 50 div q 12 h | 75 div q 8 h | 50 div q 8 h | 75 div q 6 h |
| Penicillin G | IV | | | | |
| Meningitis | | 100,000 U div q 12 h | 150,000 U div q 8 h | 150,000 U div q 8 h | 200,000 U div q 6 h |
| Other diseases | | 50,000 U div q 12 h | 75,000 U div q 8 h | 50,000 U div q 8 h | 100,000 U div q 6 h |
| Penicillin G | IM | | | | |
| Benzathine | | 50,000 U (one dose) | 50,000 U (one dose) | 50,000 U (one dose) | 50,000 U (one dose) |
| Procaine | | 50,000 U once daily | 50,000 U once daily | 50,000 U once daily | 50,000 U once daily |
| Ticarcillin | IV, IM | 150 div q 12 h | 225 div q 8 h | 225 div q 8 h | 300 div q 6 h |
| Tobramycin† | IV, IM | 4 div q 12 h | 6 div q 8 h | 4 div q 12 h | 6 div q 8 h |
| Vancomycin† | IV | 30 div q 12 h | 45 div q 8 h | 30 div q 12 h | 45 div q 8 h |

div, divided; h, hours; IM, intramuscularly; IV, intravenously; PO, orally; q, every.

* For detailed information about antibiotics in newborns, see McCracken HG, Nelson JD. Antimicrobial therapy for newborns, ed 2. New York: Grune & Stratton, 1983.

† For infants weighing <1200 g, smaller doses and longer intervals between doses may be advisable; monitor serum concentrations.

‡ Initial dose 0.25 mg/kg body wt/day × 2; then 0.5 mg/kg body wt/day × 2; then 0.75 mg/kg body wt/day × 2; then 1.0 mg/kg body wt/day. Maintenance dose 0.75 to 1.0 mg/kg body wt/day. Every-other-day dosing may be considered after good clinical response. IV infusions over 4 to 6 hours.

§ IV formulations available by special request for use when drug is not tolerated orally.

*Adapted from Nelson JD. Antibiotic therapy for newborns. In: 1993–1994 Pocket book of pediatric antimicrobial therapy, ed 10. Baltimore: Williams & Wilkins, 1993*

The regimen favored for empiric therapy of early-onset sepsis within the first 5 days of life is ampicillin and an aminoglycoside. Ampicillin is preferred over penicillin for its activity against *L monocytogenes* and enterococci. The choice of aminoglycoside (gentamicin, tobramycin, or amikacin) is guided by the prevalence of resistant strains within an individual nursery. Kanamycin is no longer used in most nurseries because of the resistance of many enteric gram-negative rods as well as *Pseudomonas* spp. Third-generation cephalosporins such as cefotaxime and ceftazidime should not be used routinely for empiric therapy of suspected sepsis because of the rapid emergence of resistance associated with heavy usage in a closed unit. Specific indications for usage of these newer drugs include prevalence of multiply resistant gram-negative rods, persistent gram-negative bacteremia, poor clinical response to aminoglycosides, extensive deep tissue infection or abscess, and gram-negative meningitis. The decreased activity of aminoglycosides under acidic and anaerobic conditions characteristic of abscesses and deep tissue infections makes this class of drugs less desirable for treatment of such infections. When a third-generation cephalosporin is administered before identification of the infecting pathogen, ampicillin should be administered additionally because cephalosporins are inactive against *L monocytogenes* and enterococci. The second-generation cephalosporin cefuroxime is inappropriate for empiric treatment of neonatal infections because of its limited spectrum of activity against the gram-negative enteric organisms and the lack of experience with treatment of the group B streptococcus. Beyond 5 days of age, staphylococci become more likely pathogens, requiring substitution of ampicillin with methicillin or with vancomycin if methicillin-resistant staphylococci are present within the nursery or if foreign bodies (eg, central venous catheters, shunts) are present and the risk of coagulase staphylococci is increased.

After the specific pathogen is identified, the therapeutic regimen may require adjustment according to susceptibility testing. Updated recommendations for antimicrobial therapy of specific neonatal infections and appropriate dosage schedules are published biannually (Nelson, 1993). Penicillin or ampicillin may be used for treatment of group B streptococcal infections. Minimal inhibitory concentration of penicillin is usually 0.125 µg/mL or less. Because of the occurrence of penicillin tolerance (ratio of minimum bactericidal concentration to minimum inhibitory concentration is greater than or equal to 32) in 4% of strains or less, Kim (1988) recommends that the minimum bactericidal concentration should be determined for patients with a slow or poor clinical or bacteriologic response. Rare tolerant strains are completely killed by the addition of an aminoglycoside to ampicillin or penicillin or by cefotaxime alone. Slow-to-respond or serious gram-negative infections are best treated by a third-generation cephalosporin combined with an aminoglycoside at least until sterilization has occurred. Ticarcillin or ceftazidime may be combined with an aminoglycoside for increased activity against *Pseudomonas* spp. Ticarcillin also provides moderate anaerobic coverage. However, clindamycin or metronidazole are preferred for treatment of serious anaerobic infections; only metronidazole is effective against anaerobic infections in the central nervous system. *Haemophilus* spp are best treated with ampicillin if β-lactamase-negative or with a third-generation cephalosporin if β-lactamase-positive. The newer agents, aztreonam and imipenem, require further evaluation before they can be recommended for routine use in the neonate.

Appropriate cultures should be repeated after 24 to 48 hours of effective antimicrobial therapy to document sterilization. Persistent bacteremia requires further diagnostic evaluation for identification of a focus of infection, removal of foreign bodies that may be the source of continued seeding of the blood stream,

and administration of a two-drug combination of antimicrobial agents with optimal activity against the specific pathogen.

The usual duration of treatment for most uncomplicated bacterial infections is 7 to 10 days. Longer courses of therapy are indicated for the treatment of meningitis and septic arthritis/osteomyelitis. The intravenous route of drug administration is preferred, but similar amounts of drug (area under the curve) may be delivered after intramuscular injections in infants with adequate muscle mass and stable cardiovascular function. Bacterial disease is documented by culture in approximately 10% of infants with suspected sepsis. Therefore, a 7- to 10-day course of antimicrobial therapy often is completed in infants whose bacterial cultures are negative at 48 hours when there is no other explanation for the infant's clinical condition and an apparent response to therapy has occurred.

Infants who are treated with vancomycin or aminoglycosides require initial determination of serum creatinine and peak and trough serum levels after 24 hours of therapy. Once a stable dosage schedule has been established and the infant has shown a good clinical response, trough levels only may be followed to monitor for toxicity. If renal function is changing, repeated peak and trough levels may be required. Optimal serum levels are as follows: vancomycin or amikacin, peak 20 to 30 µg/mL, trough less than 10 µg/mL; gentamicin or tobramycin, peak 6 to 8 µg/mL, trough less than 2 µg/mL.

Provision of general supportive care to the septic infant is of utmost importance in optimizing the outcome. The need for ventilatory support, volume expansion with fresh frozen plasma, replacement of blood or platelets, correction of electrolyte and other metabolic abnormalities, and early initiation of hyperalimentation must be determined. In recent years, attention has been directed toward enhancement of the neonate's deficient host responses. Exchange transfusion with fresh whole blood (less than 24 hours) may improve outcome by providing several different deficient components: granulocytes, specific antibody, complement, and fibronectin. Granulocyte transfusion has been beneficial for treatment of a small number of infants with bone marrow depletion of the neutrophil storage pool. The logistical problems associated with identification of infants with bone marrow depletion and collection of granulocytes from volunteers when needed makes this modality impractical for routine use. Furthermore, neutropenia resulting from increased margination of neutrophils by endotoxin is not improved by granulocyte transfusion. Administration of intravenous immunoglobulin preparations may improve neutrophil use and prevent bone marrow depletion as well as provide specific deficient antibodies and improved opsonophagocytosis. Redd and coworkers (1988) reported a beneficial effect only if immunoglobulin is given early in the course of disease in animal models. Very large doses, however, may cause a blockade of neutrophil receptors that are necessary for opsonization and phagocytosis of group B streptococci. The optimal immunoglobulin preparation (IgM versus IgG or specific high-titer monoclonal antibody versus lower-titer broad-spectrum antibody) has not yet been determined. Further studies are required to demonstrate efficacy and safety before such immunologic enhancement measures become routine.

An approach to the evaluation and treatment of neonates with suspected sepsis is shown in Figure 20-105.

## PREVENTION

Studies of prevention of neonatal infections have focused on group B streptococcus because of its greater prevalence and immunogenicity than the other common pathogen, *E coli* K1. Both chemoprophylaxis and immunoprophylaxis measures have been

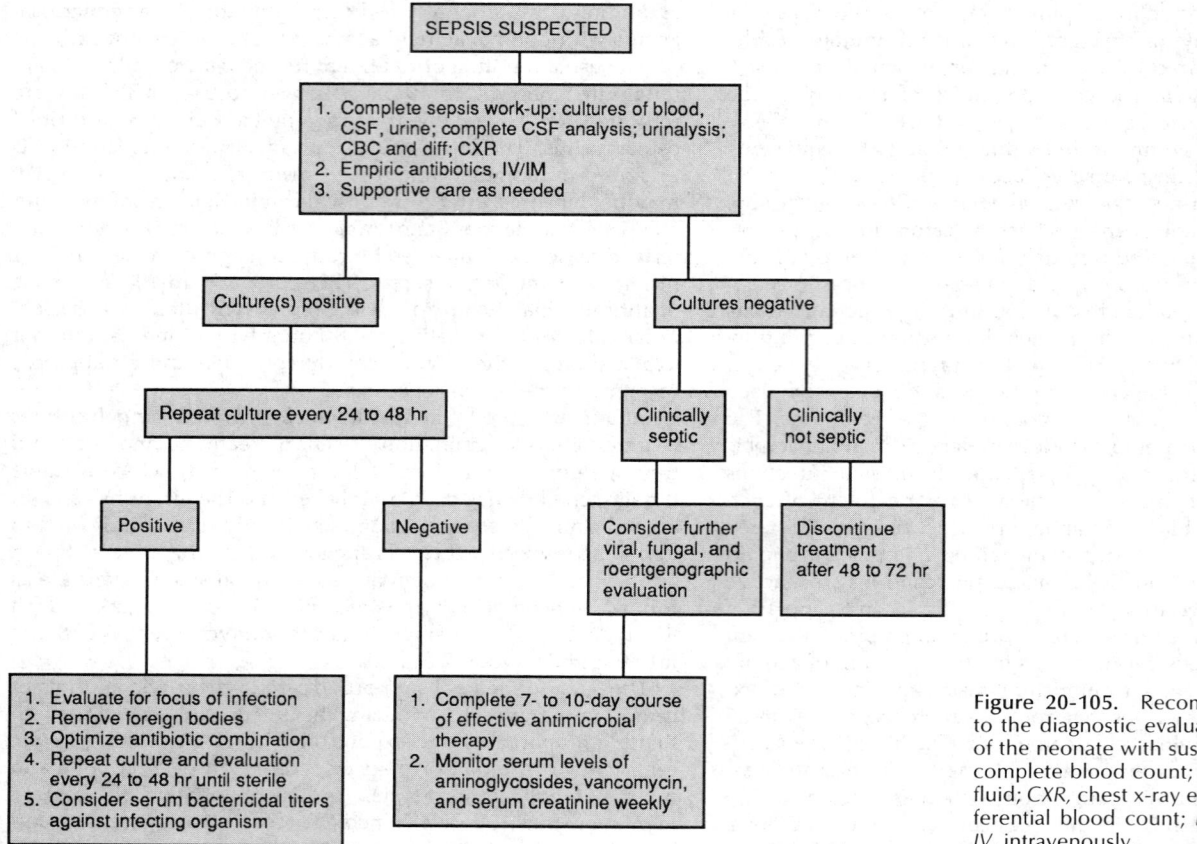

Figure 20-105. Recommended approach to the diagnostic evaluation and treatment of the neonate with suspected sepsis. *CBC*, complete blood count; *CSF*, cerebral spinal fluid; *CXR*, chest x-ray examination; *diff*, differential blood count; *IM*, intramuscularly; *IV*, intravenously.

under investigation. The efficacy of administration of ampicillin or penicillin antepartum, intrapartum, or postpartum has been discussed by Noya and Baker (1992) and universal screening of pregnant women at 26 to 28 weeks gestation for group B streptococcus carriage with selective intrapartum prophylaxis is now recommended by the American Academy of Pediatrics (1992), and no ideal regimen suitable for routine use has been identified. Several clinical trials have demonstrated that group B streptococcus cannot be eradicated from mucosal surfaces of colonized pregnant women by the administration of oral therapy during pregnancy. Animal studies demonstrate efficacy of penicillin combined with rifampin; however, rifampin is contraindicated during pregnancy because of its potential teratogenicity.

In contrast, two groups of investigators have reported that administration of 1 g of ampicillin intravenously to colonized women every 6 hours from the onset of labor to the time of delivery nearly eliminated group B streptococcal colonization of their infants. The incidence of group B streptococcal invasive disease was significantly decreased in one study. According to the protocol for the latter study, pregnant women colonized with group B streptococcus were identified at 26 to 28 weeks' gestation and randomized to receive intrapartum ampicillin or placebo if they had either premature labor (less than 37 weeks' gestation) or prolonged rupture of membranes (more than 12 hours). While this is the most promising approach that has been identified, the problems of universal colonization screening and accurate identification of women colonized at the time of delivery combined with the risk of serious reactions to penicillin or ampicillin present logistical problems for routine management. Development of a sensitive and specific rapid antigen detection test for group B streptococcus would facilitate identification of the colonized woman at the onset of labor and make this protocol more readily

applicable to the general population. Current recommendations are discussed in detail in Chapter 20.14.2.

The findings that specific antibody to group B streptococcus is protective in both human infants and in infant rat and rhesus monkey models of infection provided the impetus for development of effective active and passive immunoprophylaxis measures. Group B streptococcus-specific polysaccharide vaccines have been developed and tested in a small number of women, but they are not commercially available. Preliminary results of research by Baker and Kasper (1985) suggest the type III polysaccharide vaccine is immunogenic in only 60% of antibody-deficient women. It is likely that a second-generation vaccine consisting of the polysaccharide antigen linked to a protein carrier will be more immunogenic as observed with *H influenzae* vaccines in young infants. Other problems with reliance on immunization of pregnant women for prevention of neonatal infection include unreliable transplacental transfer of protective antibody before 32 to 34 weeks' gestation, noncompliance of the target population with prenatal care of any type, and difficulties encountered in conducting efficacy and safety vaccine trials in pregnant women.

Preliminary observations of the efficacy of administration of intravenous immunoglobulin preparations to low–birth-weight infants during their nursery stay for the prevention of nosocomial infections have not been confirmed in recently completed multicenter trials (Fanaroff et al, 1992; Baker et al, 1992). A decrease in late-onset bacterial sepsis in infants weighing less than 2000 g at birth was reported by Clapp and coworkers (1989) in infants who received 0.5 to 1.3 g/kg of intravenous immunoglobulin adjusted to maintain a level of IgG of 700 mg/dL or greater. There was no significant reduction in infections, however, when this regimen was studied in a multicenter randomized trial of 2416 infants (Fanaroff et al, 1992). In another multicenter randomized study of 588 neonates (Baker et al, 1992), the number of first infections was reduced in the recipients of IVIG. No relation between levels of IgG and susceptibility to infection was demonstrated nor was there a significant reduction for overall morbidity or mortality. Additional concerns about lot-to-lot variability in antibody content and absence of antibody to coagulase-negative staphylococci in IVIG preparations suggest that we must await the completion of adequate studies of efficacy and safety, and the determination of the most appropriate immunoglobulin preparation before such preventive measures can be recommended for routine use.

## Selected Readings

Baker CJ, Melish ME, Hall RT, et al. Intravenous immune globulin for the prevention of nosocomial infection in low–birth-weight neonates. N Engl J Med 1992;327:213.

Baker CJ, Rench MA, Edwards MS, et al. Immunization of pregnant woman with a polysaccharide vaccine of group B streptococcus. N Engl J Med 1988;319:1180.

Boyer KM, Gadzala CA, Burd LI, et al. Selective intrapartum chemoprophylaxis of neonatal group B streptococcal early onset disease. I. Epidemiologic rationale. J Infect Dis 1983;148:795.

Broughton RA, Krafka R, Baker CJ. Non-group D alpha-hemolytic streptococci: new neonatal pathogens. J Pediatr 1981;99:450.

Christensen RD, Brown MS, Hall DC, Lassiter HA, Hill HR. Effect on neutrophil kinetics and serum opsonic capacity of intravenous administration of immune globulin to neonates with clinical signs of early-onset sepsis. J Pediatr 1991;118:606.

Clapp DW, Kliegman RM, Baley JE, et al. Use of intravenously administered immunoglobulin to prevent nosocomial sepsis in low birth weight infants: report of a pilot study. J Pediatr 1989;115:973.

Committee on Infectious Diseases and Committee on Fetus and Newborn. Guidelines for prevention of group B streptococcal (GBS) infection by chemoprophylaxis. Pediatrics 1992;90:775.

Fanaroff A, Wright E, Korones S, Wright L for NICHD Neonatal Research Network. A controlled trial of prophylactic intravenous immunoglobulin (IVIG) to reduce nosocomial infections in very low birth-weight infants (abstr). Pediatr Res 1992;31:202A.

Friesen CA, Cho CT. Characteristic features of neonatal sepsis due to *Haemophilus influenzae*. Reviews of Infectious Diseases 1986;8:777.

Kim KS. Clinical perspectives on penicillin tolerance. J Pediatr 1988;112:509.

Manroe BL, Rosenfeld CR, Weinberg AG, et al. The differential leukocyte count in the assessment and outcome of early onset group B streptococcal disease. J Pediatr 1977;91:632.

Manroe L, Weinberg AG, Browne R. The neonatal blood count in health and disease. I. Reference values for neutrophilic cells. J Pediatr 1979;95:89.

Nelson JD. Antibiotic therapy for newborns. In: 1993–1994 pocketbook of pediatric antimicrobial therapy, ed 10. Baltimore: Williams and Wilkins, 1993.

Noya FJD, Baker CJ. Prevention of group B streptococcal infection. Infect Dis Clin North Am 1992;6:41.

Redd H, Christensen RD, Fischer GW. Circulating and storage neutrophils in septic neonatal rats treated with immune globulin. J Infect Dis 1988;157:705.

Rubens CE, Heggen L, Wessels M. A genetic marker for virulence of the type III group B streptococci (abstr). Pediatr Res 1988;23:380A.

Schleck WF, Lavigne PM, Bortolussi RA, et al. Epidemic listeriosis—evidence for transmission by food. N Engl J Med 1983;308:203.

Schuchat A, Deaver K, Hayes PS, et al. Gastrointestinal carriage of *Listeria monocytogenes* in household contacts of patients with listeriosis. Clin Infect Dis 1993;167:1261.

*Principles and Practice of Pediatrics, Second Edition.*
edited by Frank A. Oski et al. J. B. Lippincott Company, Philadelphia © 1994.

## 20.14.2 *Clinical Syndromes*

# MENINGITIS
*Marc H. Lebel*

## EPIDEMIOLOGY

The incidence of neonatal bacterial meningitis is about 0.5 cases per 1000 live births. The rates vary according to nursery and predisposing maternal and infant risk factors. There is a preponderance of male infants with meningitis caused by gram-negative enteric bacilli, but the ratio of male-to-female cases is comparable to that for group B streptococcus. The incidence of meningitis in low–birth-weight infants is about three times that of infants with birth weight greater than 2500 g. The other risk factors associated with an increased incidence of neonatal septicemia and meningitis include premature or prolonged rupture of membranes, maternal fever or chorioamnionitis, and traumatic delivery.

## MICROBIOLOGY

Group B streptococci and *Escherichia coli* are the two most frequent pathogens causing meningitis. *Listeria monocytogenes* is also an important but less frequently encountered pathogen. In some institutions, neonenterococcal group D streptococci cause a substantial proportion of meningitis cases. *Enterobacter* spp, *Salmonellae* spp, and other gram-negative bacilli are infrequently encountered. *Citrobacter diversus* can cause sporadic or epidemic meningitis in the neonate. *Staphylococcus* and *Candida* spp occasionally cause meningitis in the sick premature infant who is subjected to invasive supportive management and monitoring devices. Common pathogenic organisms (*Haemophilus influenzae* type b, *Neisseria meningitidis*, and *Streptococcus pneumoniae*) of meningitis in older infants and children are infrequent causes of meningitis in the neonate.

## PATHOGENESIS

Most cases of meningitis result from hematogenous dissemination. Factors that predispose to septicemia predispose also to meningitis; about one third of infants with septicemia develop meningitis. Rarely, meningitis is secondary to extension from infected skin or a skin structure site through the soft tissues and skull (eg, infected cephalhematoma). Infants with congenital malformations of the neural tube such as meningomyeloceles can be infected by direct spread from skin surfaces.

The choroid plexus may be the portal of entry to the cerebrospinal fluid (CSF) because ventriculitis is present in at least 70% of cases of neonatal gram-negative enteric meningitis; ventricles probably are the initial site of infection and serve as a reservoir for spread of infection throughout the subarachnoid space.

Many organisms causing meningitis in the newborn possess specific surface antigens. The K1 polysaccharide of *E coli* is present in 75% to 85% of strains isolated from neonates with meningitis. The BIII polysaccharide of group B streptococci is recovered from 30% of early-onset and 90% of late-onset strains causing neonatal meningitis. Type IVb strains of *L monocytogenes* account for most meningitis cases.

The K1 antigen of *E coli* confers resistance to phagocytosis and does not activate the alternate complement pathway. Immunochemical similarities between glycopeptides of the brain containing sialic acid and the capsular polysaccharide of *E coli* have been reported. It is possible that immunologic tolerance plays a role in the pathogenesis of meningitis caused by *E coli* K1 strains. Specific antibodies to the K1 antigen, however, appear to be highly protective against sepsis and meningitis. Delayed clearance of *E coli* because of decreased phagocytosis may allow replication of the organism in the blood to a concentration of 1000 or more organisms per milliliter, a concentration associated with an increased incidence of meningitis.

The capsular polysaccharide of serotype III of the group B streptococci seems to mediate resistance to phagocytosis; strains expressing this antigen adhere to buccal epithelial cells of neonates better than to those of adults. The presence of type-specific antibodies are necessary for opsonization of type Ia, II, and III strains, and high concentrations appear to confer resistance to the newborn infant. Phagocytosis of the organism is normal in presence of type III polysaccharide, but chemiluminescence of neutrophils is decreased when exposed to this antigen; however, this decrease in chemiluminescence has also been found with other pathogens.

The pathogenesis of late-onset disease caused by group B streptococci is unclear. In most instances, serotype III is the infecting pathogen. Predisposing risk factors are usually absent. A history of preceding respiratory tract infection is present in many patients. This infection may alter the nasopharyngeal epithelium and facilitate invasion by the streptococci.

Interleukin 1-β and tumor necrosis factors are detectable in the CSF of almost all infants with bacterial meningitis and are considered important mediators of the inflammation within the central nervous system. High levels of interleukin-1β or prolonged persistence of detectable levels of this mediator are associated with a poorer outcome.

Brain abscesses occur in 70% of cases of *C diversus* meningitis, whereas other gram-negative enteric bacilli cause abscesses in less than 10% of infants. Hematogenous spread is the most likely source of dissemination.

## PATHOLOGY

The pathologic findings of meningitis in neonates are similar to those found in older children. A diffuse purulent leptomeningitis is almost always found and is more pronounced at the base of the brain. In the acute phase of the illness, brain edema is fre-quently present, but cerebral herniation is uncommon. Vasculitis is common with resultant thrombosis and possibly infarct of brain tissue. Brain abscesses can develop in these areas and can involve multiple lobes. Ventriculitis is present in three fourths of infants, and hydrocephalus develops in about one third. Subdural effusions occur rarely in the neonate. Leukomalacia with porencephaly can develop as a result of tissue anoxia.

## CLINICAL MANIFESTATIONS

The clinical manifestations of meningitis in the newborn infant are often nonspecific and indistinguishable from those of septicemia. Meningitis should always be considered when the diagnosis of septicemia is suspected. The cardinal signs of meningitis in older children, such as stiff neck, Kernig's and Brudzinski's signs, are absent in most infants.

The most frequent signs are temperature instability, respiratory distress, irritability, lethargy, and poor feeding or vomiting. Seizures occur in 40% of newborn infants. Other signs include a bulging fontanelle, hyperactivity or hypoactivity, alteration of the level of consciousness, tremor, twitching, apnea, stiff neck of opisthotonos, hemiparesis, and cranial nerve palsy. Some patients will present with a severe protracted state of shock. Group B streptococcal infection also may present as hydrocephalus without other signs of infection.

## DIAGNOSIS

The diagnosis of meningitis is based on examination and culture of the CSF. In most instances, a lumbar puncture should be performed at the time of the sepsis workup. In a critically ill child, however, the lumbar puncture can be postponed until the cardiorespiratory condition is stable. Although CSF cultures may be sterile in the infant who has received antibiotics before diagnosis, examination of CSF for cellular and biochemistry values and for antigen detection is almost always indicative of the diagnosis of meningitis.

A Gram-stained smear of CSF should be made for all infants, because grossly clear fluid with only a few cells can contain many bacteria. Gram-stain or acridine orange smear of CSF reveals bacteria in at least 80% of infants with culture-proven meningitis. Because of the low concentrations of organisms (ie, $10^3$ CFU/mL of CSF), most Gram-stain smears of CSF from infants with *L monocytogenes* meningitis do not reveal bacteria.

The CSF laboratory findings in the neonate differ from those in older children (Table 20-78); this difference may be a result

| TABLE 20-78. | Normal Values for Cerebrospinal Fluid (CSF) Examination in Neonates | | | |
|---|---|---|---|---|
| | | Term | | Preterm* |
| Leukocyte count/μL | 7 | (0–32)† | | 8 (0–29) |
| Percent of polymorphonuclear leukocytes | | 61% | | 57% |
| Protein (mg/dL) | 90 | (20–170) | | 115 (65–150) |
| Glucose (mg/dL) | 52 | (34–119) | | 50 (24–63) |
| CSF: blood glucose ratio | 51% | (44%–248%) | | 75 (55%–105%) |

\* Preterm: less than 38 weeks' gestation.
† Mean (range)

*Adapted from Sarff LD, Platt LH, McCracken GH Jr. Cerebrospinal fluid evaluation in neonates: comparison of high-risk infants with and without meningitis. J Pediatr 1976;88:273.*

of an increase in the permeability of the blood-brain barrier (ie, cerebral capillary endothelial cells). By 1 month of age, an infant's leukocyte count should be in the range of 0 to 5 cells/mL. An overlap exists in the different cellular and biochemical characteristics between the infants with and without meningitis. Fewer than 1% of infants with proven meningitis, however, have an initial CSF examination that is completely normal. It is important to determine simultaneously obtained blood and CSF glucose concentrations because low CSF glucose can reflect concurrent hypoglycemia, and a CSF-to-blood glucose ratio of less than 0.6 (60%) should be considered abnormal. The CSF leukocyte count is elevated in most newborns with meningitis, and polymorphonuclear leukocytes are preponderant except in some patients with listerial meningitis. The protein concentration may not be elevated at the time of diagnosis. CSF changes characteristic of bacterial meningitis associated with sterile cultures may occur in association with anaerobic infection, most commonly *Bacteroides fragilis, C diversus* brain abscesses, or subarachnoid hemorrhage.

Blood culture specimens should be obtained in every patient; 85% of neonates with bacterial meningitis have positive blood culture results at the time of presentation. Counterimmunoelectrophoresis or latex agglutination for group B streptococci and *E coli* K1 antigens in CSF and concentrated urine can be performed to facilitate a rapid diagnosis of infection. The sensitivity of these tests can be increased by evaluating specimens from more than one source with detection of the antigen in 65% to 95% of patients with culture-proven infection.

## THERAPY

After CSF and blood cultures are obtained, antibiotic therapy should be initiated promptly with ampicillin plus cefotaxime or with a combination of ampicillin and an aminoglycoside such as gentamicin or amikacin in meningitis dosages. Therapy should be adjusted depending on results of cultures and of susceptibility testing. For group B streptococcal or *L monocytogenes* infection, 14 days of ampicillin therapy is adequate in the uncomplicated patient. The addition of an aminoglycoside to ampicillin has been suggested by some authors because of synergistic activity against group B streptococci and *Listeria* spp, especially if the strain demonstrates in vitro tolerance (ie, a 32-fold difference between the minimal inhibitory concentration and minimal bactericidal concentration). However, no clinical studies have proven superiority of one regimen over another.

For gram-negative enteric meningitis, ampicillin and gentamicin have been used extensively in the past 20 years. Delayed sterilization for 3 or more days occurs in half of infants with meningitis caused by gram-negative pathogens. Because the outcome of meningitis is correlated directly with duration of positive CSF culture results with a poor prognosis in those with culture results positive for more than 3 days, many therapeutic regimens have been evaluated in an effort to improve the rate of bacteriologic response.

In the first study from the Neonatal Meningitis Cooperative Study Group, systemic therapy with ampicillin and gentamicin alone was compared with systemic therapy with the same drugs combined with intrathecally administered gentamicin 1 mg/d for at least 3 days. The peak CSF concentrations in the lumbar area were considerably higher 2 to 4 hours after administration of intrathecal gentamicin than after systemic therapy alone, but the concentrations were similar for the two groups at 18 to 24 hours after a dose (mean, 1.6 µg/mL). No differences were seen between the two treatment groups in duration of positive CSF culture results, mortality rates, and incidence of neurologic sequelae. Lack of beneficial effect was thought to be secondary to the poor distribution of the aminoglycoside in the CSF space,

specifically in the ventricular system. Because ventriculitis is present in most infants with gram-negative enteric meningitis, failure to achieve ventricular concentrations of the aminoglycoside that were many times greater than the minimal inhibitory concentration of the gram-negative enteric pathogen could possibly allow persistence of the infection and continuous seeding of the subarachnoidal space.

On the supposition that larger concentrations of antibiotic resulting from direct inoculation in the ventricular space would result in earlier sterilization and better outcome, the Neonatal Meningitis Cooperative Study Group conducted a second study evaluating systemic ampicillin and gentamicin therapy versus systemic therapy with the same drugs combined with intraventricular administration of 2.5 mg/d gentamicin for a minimum of 3 days. The mean concentrations of gentamicin 1 to 6 hours after a dose were 48 and 32 µg/mL in the ventricular and lumbar spaces, respectively. Despite the higher concentrations of aminoglycoside achieved in the CSF compared with those after systemic therapy alone, no differences were noted between the two treatment groups in the duration of positive CSF culture results and morbidity. Furthermore, the mortality rates were 12.5% in the systemic therapy group and 42.9% in the intraventricular therapy group. Three children developed porencephaly along the needle track associated with repeated ventricular taps. From these data, intraventricular administration of aminoglycosides cannot be recommended for routine therapy of neonatal meningitis.

The third-generation cephalosporins offer potential advantages for therapy of meningitis in the neonatal period. They possess extraordinary in vitro activity against gram-negative enteric bacilli (including most of the causative pathogens of neonatal meningitis), achieve high serum concentrations, and penetrate well into the CSF. They appear to be safe and well tolerated and lack the nephrotoxicity and ototoxicity associated with use of aminoglycosides. Except for moxalactam, the third-generation cephalosporins are active against most streptococci but are inactive against *L monocytogenes* and enterococci. Only ceftazidime provides adequate activity against *Pseudomonas aeruginosa*.

In the third study from the Neonatal Meningitis Cooperative Study Group, moxalactam and ampicillin therapy was compared with amikacin and ampicillin therapy in 63 infants with meningitis caused by gram-negative enteric bacilli. Moxalactam was comparably effective to the conventional regimen. The duration of positive CSF culture results was approximately 3 days in each group; no significant differences were noted in the case-fatality rates and subsequent neurologic sequelae. The reasons for the delayed CSF sterilization in some patients in presence of excellent CSF bactericidal activity (greater than or equal to 1:8) is not fully understood. The CSF space may be considered an area of impaired host resistance. Polymorphonuclear leukocytes have an altered phagocytosis in the subarachnoidal space; there is reduced opsonic and bactericidal activity, and the concentrations of immunoglobulins and complement are low in that space. Also, it is possible that an inoculum effect exists that results in decreased activity of the antibiotics in presence of a high bacterial colony count at initiation of therapy. Such an effect can be demonstrated in vitro for some antibiotics versus specific pathogens.

Cefotaxime is preferred for therapy of neonatal meningitis over other new-generation cephalosporins because of more extensive experience with this drug in the neonatal period and because it does not alter substantially the bowel flora. Extensive or exclusive use of a cephalosporin in a closed newborn unit, however, invariably leads to rapid emergence of resistance. Outbreaks of cefotaxime-resistant *Enterobacter cloacae* infections have been described shortly after beginning routine therapy with cefotaxime for suspected sepsis in two neonatal intensive care units. These agents should be used selectively and as alternatives to the conventional regimen. Because of high biliary excretion and marked alteration of the normal intestinal flora and because of the potential concern for displacement of bilirubin, ceftriaxone should not be used frequently in the newborn infant. Moxalactam has been associated with prolongation of prothrombin time and is no longer prescribed for treatment of neonatal infections.

Dexamethasone adjunctive therapy is currently being evaluated in neonatal meningitis to determine whether or not this adjunctive treatment can improve the neurological and audiological outcome.

For gram-negative enteric meningitis, the duration of therapy should be 21 days or longer and should continue for at least 14 days after the first sterile CSF culture.

For premature infants hospitalized in the nursery for prolonged periods, staphylococci, enterococci, and gentamicin-resistant gram-negative organisms are potential pathogens. An alternative antimicrobial regimen should be considered. A combination of ampicillin and cefotaxime or ceftazidime could be used as initial empiric therapy. When there is an indwelling vascular catheter or a ventriculoperitoneal shunt or when staphylococci are frequent causes of infection, vancomycin and amikacin or cefotaxime can be used initially. Metronidazole is indicated for treatment of central nervous system infection caused by *B fragilis*.

Another CSF culture should be made after 48 to 72 hours of therapy to ensure sterility of the CSF. If culture results are positive after 48 hours for group B streptococci and 72 hours for coliform organisms, the susceptibilities of the pathogen should be reviewed. Cranial sonography, computed tomography (CT), or magnetic resonance imaging (MRI) should be considered. In all cases of meningitis caused by *C diversus*, cranial CT or MRI scans should be obtained early because of the frequent association with brain abscesses. In patients with an uncomplicated course of gram-negative meningitis, cranial CT or MRI scans should be obtained before discharge. The duration of antibiotic therapy for brain abscess should be at least 4 to 6 weeks depending on clinical evolution and resolution of the lesion based on repeated tomograms. Neurosurgery should be considered early for needle aspiration of the abscess to identify the etiologic agent and to provide drainage or for excision of the abscesses. Aminoglycosides are not very effective because of decreased activity in abscess cavities that have a low pH and anaerobic conditions.

Supportive care of the newborn is similar to that of the septic infant. Careful neurologic examination should be performed daily and the head circumference measured. Seizures should be controlled with intravenously administered phenobarbital or dilantin. The serum electrolytes should be followed for detection of hyponatremia as a result of inappropriate secretion of antidiuretic hormone; fluid restriction is instituted if this condition develops. Some newborns with group B streptococcal meningitis develop diabetes insipidus during the course of the illness. Serum concentrations of aminoglycosides in the newborn period are unpredictable, especially for the low–birth-weight premature infant, and should be routinely determined to achieve therapeutic concentrations and avoid toxicity. Every infant should have a brain-stem-evoked response audiogram at discharge or within 6 weeks after discharge from the hospital to detect hearing impairment.

# PROGNOSIS

Despite improvement in intensive care facilities and excellent in vitro activity of the third generation cephalosporins, meningitis in the neonatal period is still a devastating disease. The case-fatality rate remains about 15% to 30%, depending on causative pathogen, predisposing risk factors, and availability of intensive care facilities.

A poor outcome is associated with presence of coma at admission, persistent seizures, low–birth-weight, ventriculitis, duration of positive CSF culture results, very low or very high CSF leukocyte count, protein concentration higher than 500 mg/dL, and presence of brain abscess. High concentrations of the K1 antigen of *E coli*, of interleukin 1-$\beta$, and of the polysaccharide of group B streptococci in the initial CSF specimen have been inversely correlated with clinical outcome and with severity of the disease.

For group B streptococcus, about 15% to 20% of survivors have major sequelae including spastic quadriplegia, profound mental retardation, hemiparesis, deafness, or blindness. Hydrocephalus develops in 11% of cases, and 13% have a seizure disorder. Survivors without major sequelae on physical examination, however, seem to function within normal limits and comparably with their siblings.

Sequelae are found in 35% to 50% of survivors of gram-negative meningitis. Ten percent have severe sequelae as defined by failure to develop beyond the age at which the disease occurred or required custodial care. About 25% to 35% have mild to moderate sequelae, which many times do not interfere with adequate, albeit delayed, development. Hydrocephalus develops in one third of patients. The prognosis of infants with brain abscesses is generally poor.

## Selected Readings

Berman PH, Banker BQ. Neonatal meningitis: a clinical and pathological study of 29 cases. Pediatrics 1969;38:6.

Gandy G, Renie J. Antibiotic treatment of suspected neonatal meningitis. Arch Dis Child 1990;65:1.

Heusser MF, Patterson JE, Kuritza AP, et al. Emergence of resistance to multiple beta-lactams in *Enterobacter cloacae* during treatment for neonatal meningitis with cefotaxime. Pediatr Infect Dis J 1990;9:509.

Kaplan SL, Patrick CC. Cefotaxime and aminoglycoside treatment of meningitis caused by gram-negative enteric organism. Pediatr Infect Dis J 1990;9:810.

Kline MW. *Citrobacter* meningitis and brain abcess in infancy: epidemiology, pathogenesis and treatment. J Pediatr 1988;113:430.

McCracken GH Jr, Mize SB, Threlkeld N. Intraventricular gentamicin therapy in gram-negative bacillary meningitis of infancy. Report of the Second Neonatal Meningitis Cooperative Study Group. Lancet 1980;1:787.

McCracken GH Jr, Mustafa MM, Ramilo O, et al. Cerebrospinal fluid interleukin 1-beta and tumor necrosis factor concentration and outcome from neonatal gram-negative enteric bacillary meningitis. Pediatr Infect Dis J 1989;8:155.

McCracken GH Jr, Threlkeld N, Baker CJ, et al. Moxalactam therapy for neonatal meningitis due to gram-negative enteric bacilli: a prospective controlled evaluation. JAMA 1984;252:1427.

Shattuck KE, Chonmaitree T. The changing spectrum of neonatal meningitis over a fifteen-year period. Clin Pediatr 1992;31:130.

Wald ER, Bergman I, Taylor HG, et al. Long-term follow-up of group B streptococcal meningitis. Pediatrics 1986;77:217.

*Principles and Practice of Pediatrics, Second Edition.*
edited by Frank A. Oski et al. J. B. Lippincott Company, Philadelphia © 1994.

# OSTEOMYELITIS AND SEPTIC ARTHRITIS
*Marc H. Lebel*

## EPIDEMIOLOGY AND PREDISPOSING FACTORS

Osteomyelitis and septic arthritis are uncommon diseases in the neonate. When they occur, however, they can cause significant morbidity and permanent disability. The exact incidence of these two diseases is difficult to determine because most centers see only a few cases per year. A preponderance of male infants is affected, and debilitated newborns subjected to invasive monitoring are at increased risk.

In most cases, no precipitating factors are noted. Osteomyelitis of the newborn has been reported, however, after heel punctures, umbilical vessel catheterization, exchange transfusion, total parenteral nutrition, fetal monitoring, femoral venipuncture, suprapubic aspiration, and other needle punctures. Osteomyelitis has also been described as a complication of infected cephalhematoma. Broad spectrum antibiotic therapy, prematurity, central venous catheters, and total parenteral nutrition are risk factors for fungal bone and joint infections.

## PATHOGENESIS

Hematogenous dissemination is the most frequent source of suppurative bone and joint infections in the newborn period, but skeletal infection can occur after direct inoculation or as an extension from a contiguous site. The long bones are most commonly affected. Ogden and Lister (1975) reported that the pathogenesis of osteomyelitis differs in the neonate compared with the older child. In the neonatal period, there is a communication between epiphyseal and metaphyseal vessels by sinusoidal vessels that transverse the growth plate. The sluggish flow in the sinusoidal loops of the metaphysis near the growth plate predispose to bacterial sequestration and development of hematogenous osteomyelitis. The infection can spread through the transphyseal vessels and extend to the epiphysis. Infection of the epiphysis may rupture through the periosteum and enter the joint space with secondary suppurative arthritis, especially for such joints as the hip and shoulder where the epiphysis is intraarticular. Another unique feature of neonatal osteomyelitis is the frequency of multiple-bone involvement and contiguous joint involvement. This is particularly true for skeletal infections caused by *Staphylococcus aureus*. Destruction of the hyaline cartilage and of the growth plate can lead to long-term sequelae.

The mechanisms of infection secondary to umbilical vessel catheterization may be related to multiple septic embolization through an infected umbilical stump and catheter and to decreased blood flow that might predispose to infection by altering the host defense mechanisms. The infection is generally in the ipsilateral inferior limb, distal to the tip of the catheter.

In group B streptococcal osteomyelitis, the right proximal humerus tends to be more frequently affected. The predilection for this site seems related to minor trauma to the shoulder while passing beneath the pubic bone during delivery.

Osteomyelitis of the os calci may result from direct introduction of bacteria at the time of heel puncture for blood sampling; im-

proper site and techniques have been reported as causative events. Osteomyelitis of the skull is associated with use of fetal scalp monitoring and rarely as a result of extension from an infected cephalhematoma.

Yousefzadeh and Jackson (1980) stress the importance of *Candida* spp in causing neonatal osteomyelitis and suppurative arthritis in the debilitated newborn. Bones and joints are frequent secondary foci of infection in infants with disseminated candidiasis.

## MICROBIOLOGY

The leading pathogen causing osteomyelitis is *S aureus*, and the group B streptococci, especially serotype III, have been reported with an increased frequency in the last decade. In certain centers, group B *Streptococcus* is the most frequently isolated pathogen in neonatal osteoarticular infections. *Neisseria gonorrhoeae* as well as gram-negative bacilli such as *Klebsiella pneumoniae*, *Haemophilus influenzae* (type b and nontypable), *Proteus* spp, and *Escherichia coli* are infrequent pathogens.

The pathogens causing suppurative arthritis in the neonate are the same as those causing osteomyelitis; differences in etiology are influenced principally by whether the infection is hospital-acquired. In a review of 92 cases, Dan reports that the pathogens involved for hospital-acquired infections were *Staphylococcus* spp (62%), *Candida* spp (17%), gram-negative enteric bacilli (13%), *Streptococcus* spp, and *H influenzae* (4%). For community-acquired infections, the pathogenic organisms were streptococci (mainly group B) (52%), *Staphylococcus* spp (26%), gonococci (17%), and gram-negative bacilli (4%).

## CLINICAL MANIFESTATIONS

Skeletal infections in the neonate are difficult to diagnose because of their indolent presentation. Osteomyelitis and suppurative arthritis coexist in many neonates; signs and symptoms can be similar.

Failure to move an extremity spontaneously or apparent pain on movement (when picking up the baby or changing the diaper) may be the first manifestation. Osteomyelitis of the upper extremity may occasionally be misdiagnosed as an Erb's palsy. Fever and signs of systemic toxicity are absent in most patients. This lack may cause a delay in diagnosis because parents do not seek medical advice. Irritability and crying at the time of the diaper change can signify involvement of the femur or hip. In the more severe form of osteomyelitis, the initial signs and symptoms can be those of a septic process with lethargy, fever, and irritability.

On physical examination, decreased range of motion of the affected extremity may be the only objective sign, but redness and warmth are occasionally seen. Pittard and coworkers (1976) report that suppurative arthritis of the hip presents with decreased range of motion of the articulation and tendency to maintain the joint in an abducted, flexed, externally rotated position.

Edwards and colleagues note that osteomyelitis and septic arthritis caused by group B streptococci occur most often in otherwise normal neonates with no predisposing risk factors. These infants have fewer signs of systemic toxicity and frequently are afebrile. Single-bone involvement, particularly of the right proximal humerus, is the most frequent presentation.

Osteomyelitis of the superior maxilla produces a rare but specific syndrome in early infancy that is often misdiagnosed for orbital cellulitis or dacryocystitis. The infant presents with fever, redness and swelling of the cheek, unilateral purulent rhinorrhea, and proptosis if the orbital contents are involved. *S aureus* is the usual pathogen.

## DIAGNOSIS

When the diagnosis of suppurative arthritis and osteomyelitis is suspected, roentgenograms of the affected part and the contralateral extremity should be obtained. These examinations are frequently abnormal, showing edema of the deep soft tissues, joint space widening, subperiosteal elevation, or lytic lesions. Many patients have multifocal osteomyelitis with other sites found on roentgenograms that do not seem clinically apparent. Technetium pertechnetate bone scans are frequently normal in infants with osteomyelitis. False-negative results in the presence of abnormal roentgenograms have been reported in many infants, but sensitivity of the newer high-resolution camera seems to have improved diagnostic accuracy significantly. False-positive bone scans may result from calcium extravasation in the soft tissues. Gallium scans should be used with caution because of the high dose of radiation.

The peripheral leukocyte count is usually not helpful, but the erythrocyte sedimentation rate is generally elevated and is useful in determining duration of therapy. Aspiration of the material from the joint space or from the affected bone should be performed, and the contents should be examined for organisms by Gram-stained smears and culture. Blood cultures yield the causative pathogen in about half of patients and should always be obtained. Urine can be tested for presence of group B streptococcal antigen by latex agglutination.

The differential diagnosis includes Erb's palsy, pseudoparalysis of congenital syphilis, and deep cellulitis. Some cases of congenital neuroblastoma or leukemia can produce roentgenographic changes similar to those seen in osteomyelitis.

## THERAPY

After specimens have been obtained for culture, an initial empiric therapeutic regimen consisting of a penicillinase-resistant penicillin such as methicillin and an aminoglycoside should be initiated, unless the results of the Gram-stained specimens suggest a more specific etiology. The antibiotic therapy is adjusted depending on results of the cultures and susceptibilities. There is no indication for intraarticular administration of antibiotics, because the penetration of parenterally administered antibiotics in the joint space is adequate.

For hip and shoulder joints, open drainage is an essential part of therapy to prevent vascular compromise and possibly subsequent necrosis of the head of the femur or humerus. For other joints, repeated aspirations generally suffice; if there is persistent reaccumulation of pus, open drainage should be performed. For cases of suspected osteomyelitis, aspiration of the site of maximum tenderness or of a positive result of a bone scan should be performed. There is no consensus on the utility of surgical decompression of the subperiosteal space and metaphysis when pus is obtained at the subperiosteal or bone aspiration.

The duration of therapy should be at least 3 to 4 weeks. The treatment must be individualized and based on the resolution of the clinical signs and symptoms and the return of the sedimentation rate to normal. For streptococcal infections, the therapy consists of ampicillin or penicillin, sometimes combined with an aminoglycoside. For staphylococcal infections, methicillin, nafcillin, or vancomycin (when the strain is methicillin-resistant) should be administered. *Candida* spp infections are treated with amphotericin B for at least 4 weeks. There are insufficient data on the efficacy and safety of fluconazole in the neonatal period to recommend its use. Physical therapy should be instituted to prevent joint contractures. Although the combination of parenteral and oral regimens is acceptable therapy for older children, there is insufficient experience to recommend that regimen for most neonates with suppurative bone and joint infections.

## PROGNOSIS

Effective antimicrobial agents have contributed to the significant decrease in mortality rate, and death results only occasionally. The degree of residual damage depends on the presence of joint involvement and the duration of illness before diagnosis. As many as 30% to 40% of infants have moderate to severe sequelae, mainly impairment of growth with joint deformation or shortening of limbs. Osteomyelitis or osteoarthritis of the femur with hip or knee joint involvement is most frequently associated with sequelae. In contrast, skeletal infections caused by group B streptococci rarely cause long-term sequelae.

Careful clinical and roentgenographic follow-up is essential, because growth retardation with resultant discrepancy in the limb length can occur and joint dysfunction may not be apparent until many months later. Chronic osteomyelitis is a rare complication of neonatal infections.

### Selected Readings

Bergdahl S, Ekengren K, Eriksson M. Neonatal hematogenous osteomyelitis: risk factors for long-term sequelae. J Pediatr Orthop 1985;5;564.
Dan M. Septic arthritis in young infants: clinical and microbiological correlation and therapeutic implications. Rev Infect Dis 1984;6:147.
Edwards MS, Baker CJ, Wagner ML, et al. An etiologic shift in infantile osteomyelitis: the emergence of group B *Streptococcus*. J Pediatr 1978;93:578.
Fox L, Sprunt K. Neonatal osteomyelitis. Pediatrics 1978;62:535.
Ish-Horowicz MR, McIntyre P, Nade S. Bone and joint infections caused by multiply resistant *Staphylococcus aureus* in a neonatal intensive care unit. Pediatr Infect Dis J 1992;11:82.
Ogden JA, Lister G. The pathology of neonatal osteomyelitis. Pediatrics 1975;55:474.
Pittard WB, Thullen JD, Fanaroff AA. Neonatal septic arthritis. J Pediatr 1976;88:621.
Williamson JB, Galasko CS, Robinson MJ. Outcome after acute osteomyelitis in preterm infants. Arch Dis Child 1990;65:1060.
Wopperer JM, White JJ, Gillespie R, et al. Long-term follow-up of infantile hip sepsis. J Pediatr Orthop 1988;8:322.
Yousefzadeh DK, Jackson JH. Neonatal and infantile candida arthritis with or without osteomyelitis: a clinical and radiographical review of 21 cases. Skeletal Radiol 1980;5:77.

*Principles and Practice of Pediatrics, Second Edition.*
edited by Frank A. Oski et al. J. B. Lippincott Company, Philadelphia © 1994.

## SKIN AND SOFT TISSUE INFECTIONS
*Jane D. Siegel*

The most common manifestations of skin and soft tissue bacterial infections are presented in Table 20-79. Most of these conditions occur beyond the first 3 days of life. Most frequently observed are pustular lesions (impetigo neonatorum) that cluster around the umbilicus and diaper area and usually are not associated with fever or systemic illness. Gram-positive cocci present on Gram-

## TABLE 20-79. Infections of the Skin and Soft Tissues

Pustules
Impetigo
Scalded skin syndrome (Ritter's disease)
Abscess: skin, scalp, breast
Omphalitis
Cellulitis
Adenitis
Necrotizing fasciitis
Ecthyma gangrenosum

stained smear examination may help distinguish pustules from erythema toxicum. If only a few lesions are present, they are treated effectively by cleansing alone or cleansing followed by application of a topical antibiotic ointment. More extensive lesions may be treated with oral cloxacillin for 5 days. Bullous impetigo is more likely to spread and should be treated with systemic antibiotics in the absence of a prompt response to local or oral therapy.

Staphylococcal scalded skin syndrome, or Ritter's disease, is a much more extensive, exfoliative disease caused by phage group II staphylococci. These organisms elaborate an exotoxin that causes intraepidermal cleavage at the stratum granulosum. Infants first present with a tender, sunburn-like erythematous rash, then bullae develop with desquamation of large areas of skin. The presence of a Nikolsky's sign (desquamation of the superficial layer of skin after light pressure over areas that appear to be uninvolved) is pathognomonic. The site of toxin production is distal from the area of involvement and is usually the conjunctiva, nasopharynx, umbilicus, or circumcision site. Staphylococcal bacteremia and superinfection are absent. These infants require intravenous antibiotic therapy to eliminate the toxin-producing staphylococci.

Toxic shock syndrome (TSS) is associated with a unique toxin produced by certain strains of *Staphylococcus aureus*. The focus of infection may not always be apparent. Clinical manifestations in neonates are similar to those seen in older children and adults: sunburn-like rash with mild desquamation occurring in the second week of illness and multiorgan system involvement with cardiovascular instability. Blood cultures are usually sterile, and the toxin-producing staphylococci may be recovered from mucosal surfaces or sites of tissue infection. Intravenous antibiotics and aggressive supportive care are required. Fluid requirements are greater than estimated due to severe capillary leak.

Scalp abscess is a complication of fetal monitoring with scalp electrodes. Any of the microorganisms present in the birth canal may be implicated. Superficial abscesses are treated locally with incision and drainage. The presence of cellulitis requires systemic antibiotics. An infected cephalohematoma should be distinguished from a large superficial scalp abscess because an infected cephalohematoma may be complicated by an underlying osteomyelitis.

Breast abscess is a well-localized lesion that is usually unilateral and presents more commonly in female infants. There are few if any systemic signs. The only clinical findings are swelling with erythema and warmth. Although group B streptococcus and *S aureus* are the most common agents, gram-negative enteric bacilli have been isolated by Rudoy and Nelson (1975). Rarely, bacteremia may be present. A diagnostic aspiration of the abscess should be performed and the infant should be treated with parenteral antibiotics. Incision and drainage, when required, should be carried out by a skilled pediatric surgeon to avoid damage to normal breast tissue in female infants.

A wet, malodorous umbilical cord with minimal inflammation is usually associated with group A streptococcus or *S aureus* and may be treated with a 5- to 7-day course of methicillin. More severe infection with bacteremia, cellulitis, necrotizing fasciitis, or peritonitis may, however, be associated with any of the neonatal pathogens and therefore requires treatment with broad-spectrum antibiotics for 10 to 14 days. Anaerobes, especially *Clostridium* sp., may be important pathogens in severe necrotizing omphalitis; therefore, clindamycin or metronidazole should be included in the antibiotic regimen.

A characteristic syndrome of submandibular cellulitis or lymphadenitis was first described by Patamasucon and associates (1981) in infants with group B streptococcal bacteremia. These infants present at 2 to 10 weeks of age with the nonspecific signs of sepsis, fever, and a characteristic swelling with overlying erythema in the submandibular or submental area. Occasionally, the focal cellulitis appears during the first few hours after the patient is admitted to the hospital for treatment of suspected sepsis without a focus. Group B streptococcus is isolated from blood and tissue aspirate, and meningitis is usually not present. Response to parenteral antibiotic therapy is prompt.

Overwhelming sepsis and shock are associated with necrotizing fasciitis and ecthyma gangrenosum. An indurated area of skin with violaceous discoloration, overlying bullae, and rapid progression to necrosis is characteristic of necrotizing fasciitis (Color Figures 20 and 21). Group B streptococcus alone or mixed bacteria are associated with this process. Extensive debridement and broad-spectrum antimicrobials are required to control the systemic toxicity. This is the most serious infectious complication of circumcision. Ecthyma gangrenosum is a manifestation of vasculitis of the cutaneous blood vessels associated with *Pseudomonas aeruginosa* bacteremia or, less commonly, other gram-negative bacilli such as *Serratia* spp. The lesion first appears as a vesicle on an erythematous base, then forms a well-demarcated area of induration with a necrotic center. The infecting organisms may be isolated from the skin lesion. Treatment of the septicemia with parenteral therapy is required.

## Selected Readings

Adamkiewicz TV, Goodman D, Burke B, et al. Neonatal *Clostridium sordellii* toxic omphalitis. Pediatr Inf Dis J 1993;12:253.

Florman AL, Holzman RS. Nosocomial scalded skin syndrome. Am J Dis Child 1980;134:1043.

Patamasucon P, Siegel JD, McCracken GH. Streptococcal submandibular cellulitis in infants. Pediatrics 1981;67:378.

Rudoy AC, Nelson JD. Breast abscess during the neonatal period. Am J Dis Child 1975;129:1031.

*Principles and Practice of Pediatrics, Second Edition.*
edited by Frank A. Oski et al. J. B. Lippincott Company, Philadelphia © 1994.

# URINARY TRACT INFECTIONS
*Marc H. Lebel*

## EPIDEMIOLOGY

The incidence of bacteriuria in the neonate is low, ranging from 0.1% to 1.9% in full-term infants and up to 10% in low–birth-weight newborns. In the neonatal period there is a preponderance of infection in male infants. In infants less than 2 months of age presenting with fever, urinary tract infection is found in 7.5% of patients. Recent studies report an increased susceptibility to urinary tract infections in uncircumcised male infants. Other reports suggest that breast-feeding is associated with a lower incidence of infection.

## PATHOGENESIS

Urinary tract infections can be acquired by hematogenous infection of the kidney in association with neonatal septicemia or by the ascending route via the urethra. It is thought that the short female urethra allows for ascending infection and explains the higher frequency of infection in girls older than 3 months of age. In the uncircumcised male infant, accumulation of bacteria in preputial folds with meatal contamination is likely. Specific fimbrial receptors on the foreskin and along the urethra may allow for ascending infection. Malformations of the urinary tract may predispose to infection. Between 4% and 20% of infants presenting with urinary tract infection have an underlying malformation of the urinary tract.

Bergström and colleagues (1972) reported that in infants, 50% to 70% of *Escherichia coli* strains causing urinary infection belong to one of the eight common pyelonephritogenic O serotypes found in older patients; data conflict concerning frequency of specific polysaccharide K antigens on the surface of *E coli*. Furthermore, *E coli* can attach to specific receptors on uroepithelial cells. *E coli* strains isolated from infants with urinary tract infection show a higher percentage of P and X fimbriation and more type 1 pili than found in matched control patients. Concentration of Tamm-Horsfall protein in the urine of infected infants appears to be lower, but the role of this protein in the pathogenesis of urinary tract infection is uncertain.

## MICROBIOLOGY

*E coli* is the most frequent pathogen, causing 75% to 85% of infections. Other gram-negative organisms such as *Klebsiella pneumoniae*, *Enterobacter* spp, *Proteus vulgaris*, and *Pseudomonas aeruginosa* are encountered less often. Gram-positive bacteria (including enterococci, group B streptococci, and *Staphylococcus* spp) are uncommon pathogens in neonates. Candidal infections are seen in debilitated newborns as part of disseminated candidiasis or in the presence of an indwelling urinary catheter. A few patients have been reported with mixed bacterial infections.

## CLINICAL MANIFESTATIONS

Few specific symptoms or signs of urinary tract infection are recognizable in the newborn period. Conversely, clinical manifes-

tations vary widely, and many infants are completely asymptomatic. When symptoms are present, they often consist of fever, irritability, decreased feeding, and lethargy. Some patients present with diarrhea, vomiting, or weight loss. Jaundice is seen in approximately 7% of cases and can be accompanied by hepatomegaly and splenomegaly. The genitalia should be carefully inspected and the abdomen palpated gently to detect malformations or enlargement of the kidneys and bladder. Occasionally, an alert caretaker notices crying on urination (ie, dysuria) or an increased occurrence of wet diapers (ie, frequency).

## DIAGNOSIS

The diagnosis of urinary tract infection is based on examination and culture of an appropriately collected urine specimen. A urine culture should be included in the sepsis workup of all infants older than 72 hours of age. Within the first 3 days of life, urinary tract infection occurs secondary to bacteremia; therefore, such infants are identified by blood culture. The most reliable test is when urine is obtained by suprapubic bladder puncture. This technique is safe and easy; bleeding or perforation of the bowel occurs rarely. Dehydration, abdominal distension, and a bleeding diathesis are contraindications for suprapubic aspiration. To optimize the yield of a successful tap, it is recommended that aspiration be done 30 to 60 minutes after the infant has voided. Any bacterial growth in cultures obtained by a suprapubic puncture is considered significant. In Slosky and Todd's 1977 report of urine cultures obtained by suprapubic aspiration, 55% of children had fewer than the traditional 100,000 colonies/mL and 9% had fewer than 10,000 colonies/mL. Furthermore, mixed cultures and unusual organisms such as *Staphylococcus epidermidis* were occasionally seen. Catheterization of the bladder is a valuable and safe procedure when suprapubic aspiration is unsuccessful.

The simplest method of collecting a urine culture is by application of a sterile plastic bag after careful disinfection of the perineum; the bag is removed shortly after the child has voided. If more than 30 to 60 minutes elapses after the bag is applied or if stool is passed, the procedure must be repeated. Results of urine cultures obtained by bagged specimens are helpful when they are sterile, but a positive result is not necessarily indicative of infection because of frequent contamination during the collection process. False-positive rates of 33% and 15% have been reported after obtaining one and two bagged urine specimens, respectively. It is preferable to obtain a urine specimen for culture by suprapubic aspiration or catheterization before initiation of antibiotics in infants evaluated for possible sepsis.

Pyuria (more than 10 leukocytes/high-power field) occurs in 75% of infants with proven urinary tract infection. Hematuria and proteinuria may be present. Gram-stained smear of urine sediment reveals bacteria in 80% of cases (including patients without pyuria). Some infants with proven infection, however, have completely normal urinalysis. An elevation of blood urea nitrogen and creatinine concentrations and electrolyte abnormalities can be secondary to dehydration or underlying renal abnormalities.

The peripheral leukocyte count is variable, and about one third of patients have a preponderance of polymorphonuclear leukocytes and immature forms. Hemolytic anemia is seen in some patients presenting with jaundice. Ginsburg and McCracken (1982) found bacteremia in 20% to 30% of infants, depending on postnatal age. Concurrent meningitis is rare but must be ruled out in the septic-appearing newborn. Sterile pleocytosis is seen occasionally.

In the young infant presenting with jaundice, hepatomegaly and poor weight gain, biliary atresia or neonatal hepatitis must be ruled out. Both conjugated and unconjugated bilirubin concentrations are elevated, while other liver function tests such as alanine aminotransferase (ALT) or aspartate aminotransferase (AST) are often only mildly elevated. Urinary tract infection should be included in the differential diagnosis of gastroenteritis in the young infant because both can have similar clinical presentations.

## THERAPY

The initial therapy should be given parenterally because of the frequent association with bacteremia in the newborn period. Ampicillin and an aminoglycoside are appropriate before results of cultures and of in vitro susceptibilities are available. If an infection with S aureus such as a renal abscess is suspected, a penicillinase-resistant penicillin (methicillin, oxacillin, nafcillin) should be started. When blood and cerebrospinal fluid (CSF) (if obtained) cultures are shown to be sterile, the usual doses of antibiotics can be reduced. Repeat urine cultures should be done after 48 hours of therapy to document sterilization. Most patients respond promptly to antimicrobial therapy, becoming afebrile in 1 to 2 days. If clinical response or urine sterilization is delayed, an immediate evaluation for urologic obstruction or abscess must be made and the pathogen's in vitro susceptibilities reviewed. Therapy should be continued for 10 to 14 days in the uncomplicated patient and a repeat urine culture is performed 1 week after discontinuation of antibiotic therapy.

Aminoglycoside drug concentrations should be determined if they are used for more than 3 days or if blood urea nitrogen and creatinine concentrations are elevated.

Radiologic evaluation of the urinary tract is essential for all infants with their first episode of infection to detect underlying anatomical lesions. A renal ultrasound scan is used as an early screening procedure because the imaging does not depend on a good renal function and it is a safe and noninvasive procedure. A voiding cystourethrogram is performed within 4 to 6 weeks after treatment. About 50% of infants with urinary tract infection have some abnormalities seen on radiologic evaluation, vesicoureteral reflux being the most common abnormality encountered.

## PROGNOSIS

The goal of management is to prevent progressive renal damage and its consequences. Children should have regular follow-up, including repeated urine cultures. For infants with reflux, sonography and a voiding cystourethrogram or radionuclide scan should be repeated 6 to 12 months later, regardless of whether infection occurs in the interim. Chemoprophylaxis with trimethoprim-sulfamethoxazole is provided to all infants with grade II or greater reflux and to those with frequent urinary tract infections, regardless of the urologic status. The incidence of recurrent infection is 20% to 30%, and almost all recurrences happen during the first year. Minimal or moderate (not involving calyceal system) reflux eventually disappears in most infants. Medical management, however, should be coordinated with a pediatric urologist for infants with more severe reflux. The place of circumcision for prevention of urinary tract infection in male children should be individualized.

## Selected Readings

Abbott GD. Neonatal bacteriuria: a prospective study in 1,460 infants. BMJ 1972;1: 267.

Bergström T, Larson H, Lincoln K, et al. Studies of urinary tract infections in infancy and childhood. XII. Eighty consecutive patients with neonatal infections. J Pediatr 1972;80:858.

Crain EF, Gershel JC. Urinary tract infections in febrile infants younger than 8 weeks of age. Pediatrics 1990;86:363.

Ginsburg CM, McCracken GH Jr. Urinary tract infections in young infants. Pediatrics 1982;69:409.

Majd M, Rusthon HG, Jan Tausch B, et al. Relationship among vesicoureteral reflux, P-fimbriated *Escherichia coli* and acute pyelonephritis in children with febrile urinary tract infection. J Pediatr 1991;119:578.

Pisarcane A, Graziano L, Mazzarella G, et al. Breast feeding and urinary tract infection. J Pediatr 1992;120:87.

Ring E, Zobel G. Urinary infection and malformations of urinary tract in infancy. Arch Dis Child 1988;63:818.

Schoen E. The status of circumcision of newborns. N Engl J Med 1990;322:1308.

Slosky DA, Todd JK. Diagnosis of urinary tract infection: the interpretation of colony counts. Clin Pediatr 1977;16:698.

Wisswell TE, Roscelli JD. Corroborative evidence for the decreased incidence of urinary tract infections in circumcised male infants. Pediatrics 1986;78:96.

*Principles and Practice of Pediatrics, Second Edition.*
edited by Frank A. Oski et al. J. B. Lippincott Company, Philadelphia © 1994.

# GROUP B STREPTOCOCCAL DISEASE
*Carol J. Baker*

Until two decades ago, Lancefield group B streptococci were recognized infrequently as human pathogens. This organism was better known as a cause of epidemics of bovine mastitis. Sporadic reports of puerperal sepsis and occasional neonatal infection with group B streptococcus in humans surfaced during the 1930s and 1940s but remained largely academic until the early 1970s, when reviews documented a dramatic increase in the incidence of neonatal sepsis caused by group B streptococcus. Since then, it has emerged as the single most common bacterial pathogen responsible for neonatal sepsis and meningitis. The reasons for this shift in patterns of neonatal infection are unclear despite considerable advances in our understanding of bacteriologic and immunologic properties of the organism and the pathophysiology, treatment, and prevention of the infections it causes.

## BACTERIOLOGY AND EPIDEMIOLOGY

*Streptococcus agalactiae*, or group B streptococcus, is a facultative, encapsulated, gram-positive diplococcus that produces a narrow zone of $\beta$-hemolysis on sheep blood agar surrounding flat, grayish white, mucoid colonies. Nonhemolytic and $\alpha$-hemolytic strains have been isolated infrequently from humans but rarely cause systemic infection.

All strains of group B streptococcus share the group B-specific cell wall carbohydrate antigen originally defined by Lancefield. The strains may be classified into seven serotypes based on capsular polysaccharides (type-specific antigens) and a surface protein, c. The polysaccharide antigens are designated Ia, Ib, II, III, IV, and V. Strains possessing both the Ia polysaccharide antigen and c protein antigen are designated Ia/c. The c protein is found on all type Ib and some type II, III, IV, and V strains. Surface proteins identified as R and X antigens are found on some strains but do not seem to be associated with virulence. Nontypable strains are quite uncommon.

Group B streptococci may be recovered frequently from the lower genital tract of pregnant women, but their presence is rarely associated with symptoms before delivery. Recent studies indicate that the lower gastrointestinal tract may be the true reservoir for the microorganism and that genital colonization may represent contamination from this site. Reported carriage rates of group B streptococci in parturients vary from 4% to 40%. Variations are due not only to differences in age, socioeconomic status, and geographic location, but also to the site and number of culture specimens taken and to differences in bacteriologic method for growth and isolation. Some factors not influencing colonization rates include marital status, number and frequency of sexual partners, use of oral contraceptives, presence of vaginal discharge, and active gonococcal infection. Some controversy concerns the effect of ethnic background, but Hispanic women may have lower carriage rates than white and black women when other factors influencing colonization are controlled.

Transmission of group B streptococci to the neonate can occur whenever a delivering mother harbors the organism. Exposure may occur by ascending infection through ruptured or sometimes intact amniotic membranes or by surface contamination as the infant descends through the birth canal. Vertical transmission accounts for asymptomatic infection (or colonization) in 42% to 72% (mean, 58%) of infants born to mothers carrying group B streptococci at delivery. Mothers with "heavy" colonization documented by semiquantitative culture techniques are more likely to transmit the organism to their infants. Similarly, their infants are more likely to develop group B streptococcal disease. Of infants born to women whose culture results are negative at delivery, about 8% become colonized with group B streptococci. The rate of asymptomatic neonatal infection is increased by prolonged (more than 18 hours) rupture of membranes, maternal fever during the early (12 to 48 hours) postpartum period, and preterm delivery. Despite the high rate of transmission and colonization in newborns, overall only 1% to 2% of infants born to colonized mothers develop serious infection. Initial colonization may persist for weeks to months at various mucous membrane sites, but acquisition of the organism by neonates after hospital discharge is uncommon.

Clinically and epidemiologically, neonatal group B streptococcal infection can be divided into two distinct syndromes based on age of onset. Early-onset disease appears within the first 7 days of life, and occurs in 1.3 to 3.7 of 1000 live births. Maternal factors increasing risk for early-onset disease are similar to those for neonatal colonization: prolonged rupture of membranes, preterm delivery, multiple births, intrapartum infection, and, perhaps, black race and age less than 20 years. Late-onset disease,

that which occurs after 7 days of age, is documented in several studies to affect 0.6 to 1.7 of 1000 live births. The obstetric complications commonly accompanying early-onset disease are not factors associated with the later presentation of infant group B streptococcal infection. In both subsets of neonates, however, deficiency of maternally derived IgG antibody directed against group B streptococcal capsular polysaccharide increases the risk for invasive disease.

The distribution of serotypes has both epidemiologic and clinical significance. In surveys of large numbers of colonized adults, children, and neonates, the major serotypes are represented equally. Colonized neonates reflect the serotype of their mothers in all but the rare infant who acquires group B streptococci from nursery personnel or the community. Serotypes I (including Ia, Ib/c, and Ia/c), II, and III each account for approximately one third of the cases of early-onset disease not involving the central nervous system. Types IV and V account for only a few cases. Serotype III causes 80% to 90% of cases of group B streptococcal meningitis, regardless of age, and 90% of late-onset disease, irrespective of clinical presentation. In all, serotype III is responsible for two thirds of cases of group B streptococcal disease.

## CLINICAL PRESENTATIONS

The frequency of neonatal group B streptococcal infection in the 1970s led to the recognition of two distinct clinical presentations based on age at onset of symptoms (Table 20-80). Early-onset infection usually appears at or within a few hours of birth. The highest attack rate is observed in preterm infants born to women with known obstetric factors posing risk for neonatal sepsis. Clinical syndromes include bacteremia without a focus, pneumonia, and meningitis. Pneumonia and meningitis typically are accompanied by bacteremia. It has been estimated that blood cultures are sterile, however, in about 10% of cases of these focal infections. Respiratory signs such as tachypnea, grunting, retractions, and cyanosis or an unexpected apneic episode in a previously well neonate, especially at term, are the first clues of illness in most infants, regardless of the primary focus of infection. Poor perfusion or "cold shock" is a presenting finding in about one fourth of cases and may be found at birth in infants with in utero onset of infection. Nonspecific symptoms such as lethargy, poor feeding, tachycardia, jaundice, and temperature instability most often occurs in the term infant without respiratory symptoms.

Forty to fifty percent of neonates with early-onset group B streptococcal infection have pulmonary involvement. One third

| TABLE 20-80. Comparison of Early and Late Onset Group B Streptococcal Infection in Neonates | | |
|---|---|---|
| | **Early Onset** | **Late Onset** |
| Mean age at onset of symptoms | 8 h | 27 d |
| Incidence | 1.3–3.7/1000 live births | 0.6–1.7/1000 live births |
| Maternal obstetric risks for sepsis | Common | Uncommon |
| Common clinical presentations | Pneumonia (40%); meningitis (12%); bacteremia without focus (45%) | Bacteremia without focus (50%); meningitis (35%); osteomyelitis arthritis (5%) |
| Common serotypes | I (Ia, Ib/c, Ia/c) II III | III (85%) |
| Case-fatality rate | 8%–16% | 2%–10% |

of these infants demonstrate radiographic evidence of congenital pneumonia with distinct infiltrates, and about one half have findings typical of hyaline membrane disease. Among remaining infants, some have increased vascular markings compatible with the radiographic diagnosis of transient tachypnea of the newborn, a few exhibit small pleural effusions or pulmonary edema, and occasionally the initial chest radiograph is normal. Recent reports describe neonates with early-onset group B streptococcal sepsis manifested by respiratory distress, persistent fetal circulation (or persistent pulmonary hypertension), and a normal radiograph.

Group B streptococcal meningitis is clinically indistinguishable from bacteremia with or without pulmonary involvement. For this reason, lumbar puncture for cerebrospinal fluid (CSF) studies is always required for accurate diagnosis and appropriate therapy. Recent reports indicate that this focus of infection has decreased frequency from about 25% to 12% of cases. While seizure activity may develop in half of neonates with group B streptococcal meningitis, it is rarely the presenting symptom. Prolonged seizure activity or coma is associated with poor outcome, as is the occurrence of shock, neutropenia, or a CSF protein level greater than 300 mg/dL.

Late-onset group B streptococcal infection is observed in infants from 8 days to 12 weeks of age and has diverse clinical manifestations. The mean age at onset is 24 days. The obstetric and early neonatal course is usually uneventful. While some infants exhibit only fever and mild irritability, others have a few hours of illness culminated by septic shock and death. As with early-onset infection, infants may present with bacteremia without a focus or may have localization to the central nervous system, skeletal system, soft tissues, or a variety of other foci.

When first described, the most frequent clinical manifestation of late-onset group B streptococcal infection was meningitis, which accounted for 85% of cases. Recently, however, bacteremia without a focus is an increasingly common presentation, perhaps reflecting earlier diagnosis and therapy as familiarity with this disease increases. Infants with late-onset group B streptococcal syndrome have comparatively fewer respiratory symptoms than their early-onset counterparts, but a preceding or concurrent upper respiratory infection is noted in 20% to 30%. Subdural effusions occur in almost one fourth of infants, but these are rarely symptomatic. More serious intracranial complications such as obstructive ventriculitis, subdural empyema, and brain abscess are rare.

Infants with nonmeningeal focal late-onset infections regularly have accompanying bacteremia. The exception is osteomyelitis. The somewhat older age at onset (mean, 31 days) and the finding of a lytic bone lesion at presentation suggest that this form of infection may be acquired during a self-limited early-onset group B streptococcal bacteremia. Group B streptococcal osteomyelitis follows an indolent course with few systemic symptoms. Decreased use of the involved extremity and pain with passive movement are typical findings. Infants often have a relatively long history before diagnosis (mean, 9 days). Unlike other pathogens causing neonatal osteomyelitis, group B streptococcus has a predilection for the proximal humerus; the femur is the second most common site involved. Rarely is more than a single bone involved. Up to 70% of infants have accompanying pyarthrosis of the adjacent joint. Group B streptococcal septic arthritis without osteomyelitis occurs exclusively in the lower extremities and usually involves the hip joint. Onset of illness is acute (mean duration of symptoms before diagnosis, 1.5 days) and concurrent bacteremia is usual. Functional impairment after antimicrobial and surgical therapy is uncommon.

A variety of foci of late-onset group B streptococcal infection have been reported, but these are uncommon when compared to bacteremia without a focus, meningitis, and bone and joint infection. Infants with facial or submandibular cellulitis due to group B streptococci have been described, as have other soft tissue infections including necrotizing fasciitis, omphalitis, and scalp and breast abscesses. Otitis media alone or in association with facial cellulitis or meningitis also occurs. Endocarditis, pericarditis, myocarditis, endophthalmitis, urinary tract infection, pleural empyema, pneumonia, and peritonitis are rare.

## PATHOPHYSIOLOGY

Genital colonization in the mother is the primary determinant of early-onset infant group B streptococcal infection, and the risk for sepsis correlates directly with the number of genital organisms to which the infant is exposed. Also, a direct relationship exists between length of membrane rupture before delivery and risk of invasive infant disease. Both risk correlates suggest the mode of acquisition by the infant is by the ascending route. Amniotic fluid contains undetectable levels of type-specific group B streptococcal antibodies and readily supports the growth of these organisms. Several case series indicate that 36% to 65% of infants are symptomatic at birth, indicating that infection often begins in utero.

In experimentally induced group B streptococcal bacteremia, decreased mesenteric blood flow and myocardial dysfunction have been noted and are thought to contribute to the occurrence of fulminant sepsis. Further, in one animal model of early-onset group B streptococcal infection, an initial phase of pulmonary hypertension and fever was ablated by the prostaglandin inhibitor, indomethacin. A later phase characterized by granulocytopenia, granulocyte trapping in the lungs, and increased pulmonary vascular permeability was unresponsive to this intervention but seemed to be inhibited by steroids. These findings, however, are not specific for group B streptococcus and have been observed with other etiologic agents.

Human immunity is important in considering pathogenesis of group B streptococcal infections. One of the earliest observations was that neonates at greatest risk for infection with type III strains were those with low levels of maternally derived type-specific antibody to the capsular polysaccharide of this serotype in their sera. In vitro assays of the functional capacity of this type III-specific group B streptococcal antibody correlate a serum antibody concentration of more than 2 $\mu$g/mL with opsonization, ingestion by polymorphonuclear leukocytes, and killing of type III group B streptococcus. Similar observations have been reported for group B streptococcal serotypes Ia, Ib, and II. Antibody to the group B polysaccharide is immunogenic and appears to cross the placenta, but it is not protective. The relative deficiency of type-specific group B streptococcal antibody in infant sera may be related to either maternal deficiency common in women of childbearing age or failure of placental transport in the preterm infant born before 34 weeks' gestation.

While the pathogenesis of late-onset group B streptococcal infection is not as well understood, it appears that type III strains are uniquely virulent for the healthy term infant more than 1 week of age. As in early-onset infection, infants with late-onset disease exhibit low levels of type-specific antibody in their sera, as do their mothers. The common association of upper respiratory infection with late-onset group B streptococcal meningitis leads to speculation that alteration of the respiratory epithelium by a viral agent favors penetration of group B streptococci into the bloodstream. Type III strains, the cause of 90% of late-onset disease, elaborate high levels of type-specific polysaccharide into the blood as they multiply, and this contributes to their virulence. The relationship between the terminal sialic acid determinant to the tertiary structure of the type III polysaccharide also allows these organisms to escape several host immune mechanisms.

Infants with group B streptococcal osteomyelitis exhibit a somewhat different immune response to infection than either infants with early-onset sepsis or those with other foci of late-onset infection. Serotype III strains are isolated most frequently from these infants; however, in contrast to infants with other clinical types of group B streptococcal infection, these infants often develop type-specific IgM class antibody in their sera in convalescence. The levels persist for a few weeks, then wane. Infants with group B streptococcal osteomyelitis usually have an uncomplicated neonatal course and they have not had manipulative procedures so often found among neonates with osteomyelitis caused by other bacteria. In addition, they infrequently have bacteremia at presentation, have single rather than multiple bone involvement, and have few systemic symptoms. The minimal trauma of the shoulder passing under the symphysis pubis may provide a nidus for infection during a transient group B streptococcal bacteremia at birth, which would explain the frequency with which the proximal humerus is involved.

Many other factors have been related to the pathogenesis of early- and late-onset infection. Presumably, the first step in acquisition of infection involves adherence of the bacterium to mucosal cells. In vitro studies show that type III strains adhere better to both adult vaginal and neonatal buccal epithelial cells than do the other serotypes. Interactions between type-specific antibodies and serum complement components are important in the opsonization and phagocytosis of type III group B streptococcus, and presumably bloodstream clearance. The role of surface receptors and functional abnormalities in neonatal polymorphonuclear leukocytes appears important in the pathogenesis and outcome of invasive infection. It is known that the development of profound neutropenia in fulminant early-onset sepsis relates to an exhaustion of neutrophil reserves in the bone marrow and that this development occurs rapidly in some infants. Immaturity of a variety of host defense mechanisms undoubtedly contributes to the age-limited susceptibility of infants to invasive group B streptococcal infection.

The pathologic findings in infants with fatal group B streptococcal infection depend on age at onset and clinical syndrome. Histologic findings of congenital pneumonia and atypical hyaline membranes containing these bacteria are characteristic of infants with early-onset group B streptococcal sepsis with pulmonary involvement. In early-onset meningitis, evidence of meningeal inflammation is present in few infants. Perivascular inflammation with small vessel thrombosis and parenchymal hemorrhage are found frequently. Some premature infants surviving group B streptococcal sepsis complicated by hypotension develop periventricular leukomalacia, indicating infarction of the white matter around the lateral ventricles. Older infants with group B streptococcal meningitis usually have purulent leptomeningitis and a large number of organisms in the CSF.

## DIFFERENTIAL DIAGNOSIS

The clinical manifestations of early-onset group B streptococcal infection resemble those of neonatal sepsis due to other pathogens. In the preterm infant, the clinical and radiographic distinction between group B streptococcal pneumonia and hyaline membrane disease at onset of illness is impossible. Helpful features suggesting group B streptococcal pneumonia in this kind of patient are maternal risk factors for sepsis, apnea, and shock within the first 24 hours of life, an Apgar score of less than 5 at 1 minute, neutropenia, and cardiomegaly or pleural effusion by chest radiograph. None of these features, however, is specific for group B streptococci, and each may be observed with other etiologic agents causing early-onset neonatal pneumonia. Because clinical findings alone cannot identify the 10% to 15% of infants

with meningeal involvement, each infant with suspected or proven group B streptococcal sepsis requires a lumbar puncture.

The differential diagnosis for late-onset group B streptococcal infection somewhat depends on the focus of infection. Infants who have bacteremia without a focus may present with nonspecific symptoms and fever, and they may be thought to have a viral illness. Only a high index of suspicion and collection of a blood culture specimen provides a specific diagnosis. In infants with meningitis, a presumptive diagnosis may be made if CSF is abnormal or the Gram-stained smear reveals gram-positive cocci in pairs or short chains. If the CSF Gram-stained smear is negative, other etiologic agents causing meningitis in early infancy must be considered including *Listeria monocytogenes, Escherichia coli,* and viral agents as well as agents affecting older infants (*Haemophilus influenzae* type b, *Streptococcus pneumoniae,* and *Neisseria meningitidis*). The relative lack of systemic symptoms in an infant with a metaphyseal lytic bone lesion, especially of the humerus, strongly suggests group B streptococcal osteomyelitis. Until group B streptococci are isolated from a bone aspirate or biopsy sample of the affected area, however, other etiologic agents such as *Staphylococcus aureus* and gram-negative enterics must be contemplated. The diversity of clinical presentations of late-onset group B streptococcal infection requires that it be appreciated as a possible etiologic agent in unknown infection at any site in infants 1 to 12 weeks of age.

Isolation of group B streptococci from a normally sterile body site (blood, CSF, bone, synovial fluid, urine) is the only way to prove invasive group B streptococcal infection. The long wait for culture results, however, led to development of rapid diagnostic tests based on detection of the group B polysaccharide antigen in body fluids by latex particle agglutination (LPA). Although group B antigen can be detected in a variety of body fluids (CSF, serum, urine, joint fluid), concentrated urine is the most likely specimen to be positive. In infants with group B streptococcal meningitis, CSF also is often positive for group B antigen. LPA may be useful in diagnosis after the initiation of antimicrobial therapy because antigenuria persists for a few days in about half of infants with proven group B streptococcal sepsis and for weeks in patients with meningitis. The persistence of group B antigen in a body fluid specimen after therapy is begun is of unknown clinical significance. LPA false-positive results occur in up to 5% to 10% of specimens. Thus, a positive LPA result for group B streptococcal antigen does not prove invasive disease. The clinician should use judgment when interpreting this result in a patient whose culture results are negative. Enzyme immunoassay employing a monoclonal antibody is a sensitive technique for detecting group B polysaccharide antigen, but its primary clinical usefulness may be its rapid detection of group B streptococcal genital colonization of women in labor, so selective intrapartum antibiotic prophylaxis may be given in high-risk situations.

## COMPLICATIONS AND SEQUELAE

Complications of infant group B streptococcal infection range from negligible functional deficits in infants with septic arthritis to profound neurologic consequences of severe meningitis. The mortality rate for early-onset infection ranges from 8% to 16% and for late-onset disease from 2% to 6%. Factors associated with a fatal outcome in early-onset infection include prematurity, shock, neutropenia, apnea, a 5-minute Apgar score of less than 6, pleural effusion, and an initial blood pH of less than 7.25. Those factors related to death or permanent neurologic sequelae following meningitis are hypotension, a peripheral leukocyte count less than 4000/mm$^3$, coma, status epilepticus, and a CSF protein greater than 300 mg/dL. Three series report sequelae in survivors of group B streptococcal meningitis up to 8 years after illness. Major neurologic sequelae including global mental retardation, spastic quadriplegia, uncontrolled seizures, cortical blindness, deafness, hydrocephalus, and hypothalamic dysfunction occurred in 17% to 21%. Less severe sequelae such as spastic or flaccid paresis of one limb, speech and language delay, controlled seizure disorders, unilateral deafness, and mild cortical atrophy seen by computed tomography of the head were found in about 20%. The decreasing mortality rate found in many centers may result in a somewhat higher sequelae rate. Despite this significant mortality and morbidity, nearly 70% of the survivors of group B streptococcal meningitis function at or near their age-expected level.

One unusual complication of group B streptococcal sepsis is the unexplained association of early-onset infection with acquired right-sided diaphragmatic hernia. It has been hypothesized that insufficient diaphragmatic motion predisposes infected infants to the development of pneumonia and that subsequent respiratory effort leads to herniation.

Relapse or recurrence of infection of both the early- and late-onset type have been reported in a few infants. Inadequate dose or duration of antimicrobial therapy is one explanation for relapse. In a few cases, however, circumstances (maternal mastitis, undrained brain abscess, or congenital heart disease in an infant with endocarditis) may predispose infants to recurrence. In the majority, the reason for recurrence is inapparent. The opportunity for recurrent infection with optimal therapy exists in most patients, because intravenous antibiotics do not eliminate mucous membrane infection with group B streptococci nor do most infants develop protective immunity after recovery from sepsis or meningitis.

## TREATMENT AND PREVENTION

Group B streptococcal isolates remain uniformly susceptible to penicillin G. They also are susceptible in vitro to first-, second-, and third-generation cephalosporins, semisynthetic penicillins, and vancomycin. Resistance of group B streptococci to the aminoglycosides, colistin, bacitracin, trimethoprim-sulfamethoxazole, and metronidazole is uniform. Despite universal susceptibility to penicillin G, the minimal inhibitory concentration is 4- to 10-fold greater than that for group A streptococci. In vitro, susceptibility of group B streptococci to penicillin G is related directly to the inoculum size. Concentrations of $10^{-7}$ to $10^{-8}$ organisms/mL, often found in the CSF of infants with meningitis, require significantly higher antibiotic concentrations to inhibit growth. The combination of an aminoglycoside (usually gentamicin) with penicillin G or ampicillin is synergistic in killing group B streptococci in vitro. Ampicillin and gentamicin produce rapid killing of group B streptococci and are recommended for initial treatment of group B streptococcal infection and for maternally acquired sepsis of unknown etiology in the infant younger than 1 month of age. Once group B streptococci are identified in cultures from septic infants, therapy may be modified to penicillin G alone. Group B streptococcal isolates from CSF should have minimal inhibitory concentrations and minimal bactericidal concentrations determined before changing from two drugs to penicillin G alone. Delay in sterilizing CSF (achieved in 95% of patients within 36 hours) may be related to inadequate antibiotic dose or an unexpected suppurative focus. Ampicillin and gentamicin should be continued until sterilization of the CSF has been documented by repeat lumbar puncture, at which time the regimen may be changed to penicillin G alone. In cases when gentamicin is used for synergy, serum levels usually considered therapeutic may not be necessary, but levels should be monitored to avoid potential drug toxicity.

The optimal dose of penicillin G for treatment of group B streptococcal meningitis has not been investigated, but several facts argue for the use of high-dose therapy. Group B streptococcus has a relatively high minimal inhibitory concentration to penicillin G, especially when considering levels achievable in the CSF. Infants with group B streptococcal meningitis often have a high group B streptococcal inoculum in the CSF that would increase the minimal bactericidal concentration. Reported cases of relapse primarily have been associated with doses of penicillin G of less than 200,000 U/kg/d. Finally, penicillin G is safe in neonates in doses up to 600,000 U/kg/d. For these reasons, penicillin G at a dose of 400,000 to 500,000 U/kg/d or ampicillin 300 to 400 mg/kg/d are recommended for treatment of group B streptococcal meningitis. Doses of about half these amounts are suggested for treatment of noncentral nervous system infections. Therapy for 10 days is adequate for pneumonia, bacteremia without a focus, and most soft tissue infections. About 2 to 3 weeks of treatment are suggested for meningitis and septic arthritis, and 3 to 4 weeks for osteomyelitis, endocarditis, and ventriculitis (Table 20-81). These recommendations, however, must be tailored to each case. In rare cases of recurrent infection, prolonged therapy with penicillin should be followed by an attempt to eradicate mucosal colonization with oral rifampin given once daily for 5 days (10 mg/kg/d). The safety and efficacy of oral rifampin for this indication has not been investigated.

**TABLE 20-81. Recommended Treatment Regimens for Group B Streptococcal Infections in Infants**

| Clinical Presentation | Antibiotic | Dose (kg body wt/d) | Duration (d) |
|---|---|---|---|
| Meningitis | Ampicillin plus gentamicin, then penicillin G | 300–400 mg plus 7.5 mg,* then 400,000–500,000 U | Until cerebrospinal fluid is sterile and strain is known to be susceptible to penicillin G; to complete 14–21† |
| Bacteremia, soft tissue infection, pneumonia | Penicillin G | 150,000–200,000 U | 10 |
| Septic arthritis | Penicillin G | 200,000 U | 14–21 |
| Osteomyelitis | Penicillin G | 200,000 U | 21–28 |
| Endocarditis | Penicillin G | 300,000–400,000 U‡ | ≥28 |

\* Antibiotic levels should be monitored to avoid toxicity.
† If ventriculitis, extend therapy for 21 to 28 days.
‡ Plus gentamicin for the first 14 days.

Aggressive supportive measures are responsible for much of the increased survival in infants with invasive group B streptococcal infection. Improved ventilatory care has eased management of respiratory distress secondary to group B streptococcal pneumonia. Evidence of poor perfusion and metabolic acidosis can be treated with both volume expansion and infusion of pressor agents, and seizure activity can be controlled with anticonvulsants. Modern monitoring equipment makes anticipation of these consequences of group B streptococcal infection less problematic. Less conventional adjunctive therapies have been explored in many centers. Granulocyte transfusions in neutropenic infants, infusion of human intravenous immunoglobulin, and ECMO are among the therapeutic modalities being investigated. So far, none shows clear therapeutic advantages, and all are investigational.

Efforts to prevent neonatal group B streptococcal infection have aimed either to decrease frequency of group B streptococcal exposure of infants at birth or to alter the infant's immune status. Most widely investigated are attempts to eradicate maternal genital colonization. Courses of oral ampicillin or penicillin in colonized women (with or without concurrent treatment of sexual partners) during the third trimester of pregnancy have been ineffective in decreasing colonization at delivery. Further, this approach is impractical because to ensure "prophylaxis" for the infants at highest risk for sepsis, antibiotics would have to be initiated at the beginning of the third trimester and continued until delivery. Use of intravenous ampicillin during labor in women known to carry group B streptococci eliminates infant colonization without disturbing maternal genital flora. Because a large number of women are colonized with group B streptococci during pregnancy, the risk of anaphylactic reactions is significant compared to the number of infant cases that might be prevented. Treatment of high-risk infants in the delivery room with intramuscular penicillin G has not been shown to be effective either, because so many of these infants are already bacteremic when prophylaxis is given. An analysis of maternal risk factors for infant group B streptococcal sepsis was performed at one urban hospital to determine which obstetric groups were most likely to benefit from intrapartum chemoprophylaxis. Seventy-four percent of neonates who developed early-onset infection had at least one of these risk factors: birth weight less than 2500 g, rupture of mother's membranes more than 18 hours before delivery, and maternal intrapartum fever. In this group, the attack rate for group B streptococcal sepsis was estimated at 45.5 per 1000 live births. Additional maternal risk factors identified by other investigators include multiple pregnancy, preterm (less than 37 weeks) labor, group B streptococcal bacteria, and perhaps black race and age less than 20 years.

The first study to document the efficacy of maternal intrapartum prophylaxis in preventing group B streptococcus-associated early-onset disease and maternal morbidity was reported in 1986. Women at 26 to 28 weeks gestation had lower vaginal and anorectal cultures for group B streptococcus. Group B streptococcus-positive women who had preterm labor or rupture of membranes more than 12 hours before delivery were randomized to receive routine care or intravenous ampicillin until delivery. Women with intrapartum fever also received ampicillin. Five of 79 infants born to untreated women but none of 85 born to am-picillin-treated women developed group B streptococcal sepsis (p = 0.02). A similar study from Madrid confirmed the efficacy of this approach. Others have restricted intrapartum maternal prophylaxis to group B streptococcus-colonized women who present with preterm labor. Excellent outcome for mother and infant were reported. Additional studies provide evidence that when selective prophylaxis is indicated, ampicillin should be administered at least 4 hours before delivery (if possible) to achieve sufficient concentrations in the placental circulation and the amniotic fluid to kill group B streptococcus. Screening for group B streptococcus during pregnancy by culture of lower vagina and anorectum appears to be an effective method to identify women who, if they develop risk factors associated with neonatal sepsis, could be given intrapartum prophylaxis. Although some controversy regards selection of high-risk women, previous delivery of a sibling with invasive group B streptococcus disease always warrants intrapartum maternal chemoprophylaxis in subsequent pregnancy. Management of newborns born to mothers receiving chemoprophylaxis should be based on the infant's clinical findings and gestational age; routine treatment is not always necessary in healthy-appearing, term neonates.

Immunoprophylaxis is the optimal "permanent" method for prophylaxis against early-onset disease, and it is the only proposed method for prevention of late-onset infection. Type-specific IgG serum antibody directed against the capsular polysaccharides of group B streptococcus in excess of 2 to 3 $\mu$g/mL appears to correlate with protective immunity. Purified native group B streptococcal polysaccharides have been shown to be safe and variably immunogenic as vaccines in nonimmune adults. These antigens induce antibodies primarily of the IgG class that readily cross the placenta. Vaccine nonresponders do exist and their numbers vary by serotype. Thus, protein-polysaccharide conjugates may be better candidates for widespread use as vaccines. Clinical studies in progress must be followed by multicenter efficacy trials before immunoprophylaxis can be recommended.

## Selected Readings

Baker CJ, Edwards MS. Group B streptococcal infections. In: Remington JS, Klein JO, eds. Infectious diseases of the fetus and newborn infant, ed 3. Philadelphia: WB Saunders, 1988.

Baker CJ, Kasper DL. Group B streptococcal vaccines. Rev Infect Dis 1985;17(4): 458.

Boyer KM, Gadzala CA, Burd LI, et al. Selective intrapartum chemoprophylaxis of neonatal group B streptococcal early-onset disease. I. Epidemiologic rationale. J Infect Dis 1983;148(5):795.

Boyer KM, Gotoff SP. Prevention of early-onset neonatal group B streptococcal disease with selective intrapartum chemoprophylaxis. N Engl J Med 1986;314: 1665.

Dillon HC Jr, Khare S, Gray BM. Group B streptococcal carriage and disease: a 6-year prospective study. J Pediatr 1987;110:31.

Edwards MS, Rench MA, Haffar AAM, et al. Long-term sequelae of group B streptococcal meningitis in infants. J Pediatr 1985;106:717.

Payne NR, Burke BA, Day DL, et al. Correlation of clinical and pathologic findings in early-onset neonatal group B streptococcal infection with disease severity and prediction of outcome. Pediatr Infect Dis J 1988;7:836.

Schuchat A, Oxtoby M, Cochi S, et al. Population-based risk factors for neonatal group B streptococcal disease: results of a cohort study in metropolitan Atlanta. J Infect Dis 1990;162:672.

Yagupsky P, Menegus M, Powell KR. The changing spectrum of group B streptococcal disease in infants: an eleven-year experience in a tertiary care hospital. Pediatr Infect Dis J 1991;10:801.

*Principles and Practice of Pediatrics, Second Edition.*
edited by Frank A. Oski et al. J. B. Lippincott Company, Philadelphia © 1994.

# ENTEROVIRUSES
*Marc H. Lebel*

## MICROBIOLOGY

Enteroviruses are small RNA viruses that are a subgroup of the picornaviruses. Four major classes are described: polioviruses (serotypes 1 to 3), coxsackieviruses group A (serotypes 1 to 24) and group B (serotypes 1 to 6), and echoviruses (serotypes 1 to 34). These originally were classified according to their different effects in tissue cultures and animals; however, some strains possess in vitro characteristics belonging to more than one class. Furthermore, newer strains have been assigned only an enterovirus number (68 to 72); hepatitis A virus has been reclassified as enterovirus 72. After viral isolation, type-specific antisera are used to identify the different enteroviruses by in vitro neutralization.

## EPIDEMIOLOGY AND PATHOGENESIS

Enteroviruses have a worldwide distribution and tend to produce seasonal outbreaks during summer and fall in the temperate climates. Sporadic infections can occur at any time. There is a geographical and year-to-year variation of the serotypes producing infections. For isolates reported to the Centers for Disease Control in infants younger than 2 months of age in 1972 through 1975, echoviruses caused 51% of all nonpolio enteroviral diseases, coxsackie B viruses 45%, and coxsackie A viruses 4%. Viral isolates in the neonatal period parallel isolates circulating in the community at that time. Male infants are more often affected than female infants, with a male-to-female ration of 1.4 to 1.0.

Perinatal infections can be acquired by transplacental transmission (during maternal viremia and from the infected placenta), but this seems to occur rarely. Most often, infants are infected at the time of delivery, or from human-to-human contact (maternal or nonmaternal sources) after birth. Outbreaks of echoviruses and coxsackieviruses in special-care and well-baby nurseries have occurred; the source of infection was either an infected baby or the nursing personnel. The incidence of congenital infection is rare, but during the peak season of enterovirus activity, the incidence of infection in the first month of life can be as high as 13%. Most of these infections probably are acquired after birth. An increased risk of infection has been associated with lower socioeconomic status, lack of breast-feeding, and absence of passively transferred maternal antibodies. Gauntt and coworkers have reported a possible association between coxsackievirus B infections and severe congenital anatomic defects of the central nervous system.

After initial replication of the virus in the gastrointestinal or respiratory tract, the infection spreads to the lymphoid tissue. From there, a primary viremia occurs with dissemination to other lymphoreticular tissues such as liver, spleen, and bone marrow. In congenital infection, this viremia corresponds to the initiation of the infection. The virus can multiply in these secondary sites, with production of a secondary viremia and appearance of clinical signs and symptoms; the central nervous system, heart, and striated muscle can be seeded during this phase of the illness. With mounting antibody response, the viremia ceases.

Enteroviruses can produce inflammation and tissue necrosis in different organs, depending on the strain involved and the inoculum of the virus. There seems to be an age-related difference in the severity of illness, with very young neonates more severely affected than older infants and children, especially if there has been vertical transmission from the mother to the fetus before or at the time of delivery.

## CLINICAL MANIFESTATIONS

The spectrum of infection is wide, ranging from asymptomatic colonization to fulminant disease with myocarditis and death. The percentage of neonates asymptomatically infected is variable according to different studies, strain involved, presence of transplacentally acquired specific antibody and time of the year. Many children with enterovirus infections will be asymptomatic; some heavily infected children manifest only mild clinical symptoms.

Some infants will present with only fever and irritability. The temperature can be as high as 39°C and last an average of 3 days (maximum, 8 days). The most severe manifestation is a sepsis-like illness manifested by fever, lethargy, irritability, abdominal distension, decreased feedings, rash, and hypotonia. Disseminated intravascular coagulation, hypotension, hepatitis, and jaundice may also be present.

Viral myocarditis in the newborn period is most often caused by coxsackievirus B infections. The onset is acute with fever, anorexia, listlessness, tachycardia, tachypnea, and cyanosis. Cardiac arrythmias have been reported, and heart failure can occur. In many instances, there is a biphasic pattern of fever and symptomatology. The mortality rate is elevated for these children, and the recovery, if they survive, is slow. Many infants have concomitant involvement of the central nervous system and liver.

Meningoencephalitis is common as part of disseminated disease. The clinical presentation is frequently that of a nonspecific febrile illness, but other symptoms can include lethargy, seizures, vomiting, diarrhea, poor feeding, and tremor. The CSF findings are variable and sometimes can be comparable to those found in bacterial disease. The CSF leukocyte count can vary from few to several thousand cells with a predominance of lymphocytes; however, polymorphonuclear leukocytes can be seen early in the disease. The CSF protein and glucose concentrations are usually within normal limits, but the protein concentration can be elevated; hypoglycorrhachia and a CSF/blood glucose ratio of less than 0.5 is not uncommon.

Gastrointestinal infections can be manifested by vomiting and diarrhea; some children have heme-positive stools. Hepatitis with fulminant hepatic failure, jaundice, hepatomegaly, and disseminated intravascular coagulation has been reported with certain echoviruses. Pancreatitis is rare.

Respiratory symptoms are frequently present with other signs or symptoms. Pharyngitis, rhinitis, laryngitis, and interstitial pneumonitis have been associated with enterovirus infections. Cutaneous manifestations include macular, maculopapular, or petechial rashes.

Polioviruses can lead to spontaneous abortion, and poliomyelitis has a high rate of paralysis and mortality in the infant, especially if maternal infection occurs late in pregnancy.

Outbreaks of enterovirus infections in newborn nurseries have been described in many institutions and tend to occur during the peak incidence of enteroviral activity in the community. An increased risk of infection has been associated with mouth care and gavage feeding. This finding is consistent with a fecal-oral or oral-oral mode of transmission of the virus. The spectrum of disease depends on the infecting serotype.

## DIAGNOSIS

A specific etiologic diagnosis of enterovirus infection is based on recovery of the infecting strain and rarely from serology. No rapid diagnostic techniques are readily available, but the use of polymerase chain reaction and in situ hybridization may prove usefull in the future. With sterile bacterial cultures in the presence of myocarditis and meningoencephalitis, an enteroviral infection should be suspected. Viral culture results of the nasopharynx, CSF, and stool may be positive in 50% to 70% of patients. Some strains of enteroviruses produce a cytopathic effect cell line culture in 3 to 7 days; therefore, viral culture can help in the clinical management of some patients by allowing discontinuation of antibiotic therapy and earlier discharge from the hospital.

The excretion of enteroviruses in the stool can last for as long as 6 to 8 weeks after onset of infection. Isolation of a virus from the stool does not necessarily imply that this agent is the infecting strain of the present illness. Isolation of enterovirus from other sites, especially from CSF and tissue specimens, is the best proof of causality. Because of the vast number of serotypes and the absence of a common group antigen for enteroviruses, serologic diagnosis is impractical except when evaluating paired sera for an antibody rise (fourfold or greater rise in neutralizing antibody titer) for coxsackieviruses B in cases of myocarditis, or if a specific serotype is suspected or when an enterovirus has been isolated in tissue culture.

Differentiating between viral and bacterial etiologies can be difficult, but epidemiologic circumstances are helpful. In enteroviral infections, the mother frequently has a history of a febrile illness or gastrointestinal symptoms in the days preceding the delivery. Season of the year and geographic location are two other important considerations. Prolonged rupture of the membranes, prematurity, and low Apgar scores occur less often in enteroviral rather than in bacterial infections. *Herpes simplex* infections can present a fulminant course with multisystemic involvement and should be included in the differential diagnosis.

## THERAPY

No specific antiviral drugs are available for therapy of enteroviral infections, and treatment is supportive. After appropriate bacterial cultures have been obtained, the decision to give or withhold antibiotic therapy is based on history, clinical status of the patient, and experience of the physician. Supportive care is important, with particular attention to the fluid balance and cardiac and hepatic functions. No evidence suggests that corticosteroids are beneficial in cases of myocarditis, and data from experimental carditis in animals suggest a detrimental effect.

Human immunoglobulins do not alter the course of established enteroviral infections, and data are contradictory regarding their efficacy for prevention of clinical disease in exposed newborns in the setting of an outbreak of enteroviral infection in the nursery. Isolation measures, cohorting of patients, and emphasis on handwashing techniques are still the most important measures for limiting spread of infection.

## PROGNOSIS

Although most infants with enteroviral infections have a self-limited illness, some develop a fulminant disease with multisystemic involvement. Virulence of the strain and the presence or absence of passively acquired maternal antibodies are thought to alter the outcome. Modlin reports that about 80% of children with severe hepatic necrosis die. For myocarditis, a case fatality rate as high as 53% has been reported. A recent follow-up study of enteroviral meningoencephalitis by Bergman and coworkers showed no neurologic or cognitive defects, but another study by Farmer and colleagues has shown impairment in language and speech skills in some survivors if twitching or seizures occurred

during the time of the acute illness. Long-term neurologic follow-up is advisable for those children.

## Selected Readings

Amsley MS, Miller RK, Menegus MA, et al. Enterovirus in pregnant women and the perfused placenta. Am J Obstet Gynecol 1988;158:755.
Bergman I, Painter MJ, Wald ER, et al. Outcome in children with enteroviral meningitis during the first year of life. J Pediatr 1987;110:705.
Farmer K, MacArthur BA, Clay MM. A follow-up study of 15 cases of neonatal meningoencephalitis due to coxsackievirus B5. J Pediatr 1975;87:568.
Gauntt CJ, Gudvangen RJ, Brans YM, et al. Coxsackievirus group B antibodies in the ventricular fluid of infants with severe anatomic defects in the central nervous system. Pediatrics 1985;76:64.
Jenista JA, Powell KR, Menegus MA. Epidemiology of neonatal enterovirus infection. J Pediatr 1984;104:685.
Modlin JF, Polk BF, Horton P, et al. Perinatal echovirus infection: risk of transmission during a community outbreak. N Engl J Med 1981;305:368.
Modlin JF. Perinatal echovirus infections: insights from a literature review of 61 cases of serious infections and 16 outbreaks in nurseries. Rev Infect Dis 1986;8:918.
Modlin JF. Echovirus infection of newborn infants. Pediatr Infect Dis J 1988;7:311.
Morens DM. Enteroviral disease in early infancy. J Pediatr 1978;92:374.
Nagington J, Gandy G, Walker J, et al. Use of normal immunoglobulin in an echovirus 11 outbreak in a special-care baby unit. Lancet 1983;2:443.

*Principles and Practice of Pediatrics, Second Edition.*
edited by Frank A. Oski et al. J. B. Lippincott Company, Philadelphia © 1994.

## 20.14.3 *Congenital and Perinatal Infections*

## HERPES GROUP

### CYTOMEGALOVIRUS
*Pablo J. Sánchez and Jane D. Siegel*

Cytomegalovirus (CMV) has worldwide distribution and is the most common cause of congenital infections. CMV occurs in 0.4% to 2.4% of all live births. Acquisition of CMV is nearly always asymptomatic in the immunocompetent host. Seroprevalence studies indicate that an inverse relationship exists between socioeconomic status and development of infection. CMV seropositivity in women of childbearing age varies in the United States from 45% in higher socioeconomic groups to 70% in crowded areas with substandard living conditions; this figure increases to nearly 100% in developing countries. Two likely sources of primary CMV infection for pregnant women are infected sexual partners and young children in day-care centers. High rates of infection have been observed among young children in Israeli kibbutzim and in day-care centers in Sweden and the United States, where the rate of viruria may be as high as 70% among children aged 2 to 3 years. Serologic studies demonstrate a 30% seroconversion rate among parents whose children shed CMV as compared with no seroconversions among parents whose children do not excrete the virus (Adler, 1988).

### Transmission

Stagno and colleagues (1983) note that perinatal transmission of CMV can occur in utero, at delivery, or after delivery. In utero infection occurs transplacentally during maternal viremia. Primary CMV infection acquired during pregnancy is associated with a 30% to 40% risk of congenital infection with more severe fetal effects when maternal infection occurs in the first half of pregnancy. However, symptomatic disease is present in only 10% to 15% of these infants. CMV can also be transmitted to the fetus after reactivation of latent infection in the mother. About 1% to 3% of infants born to women who are seropositive before becoming pregnant are infected in utero, but they do not have clinically apparent disease at birth. Transmission of CMV to the newborn infant also occurs at the time of delivery from contact with infected cervical secretions. In the postpartum period, maternal-infant transmission of CMV occurs during breast-feeding because 20% to 40% of seropositive women shed CMV into their breast milk. Asymptomatic infection occurs in 60% of infants fed infected breast milk. Breast-feeding is, therefore, an effective means of providing passive-active immunization of the young infant.

An important iatrogenic source of CMV infection is transfusion of blood from a seropositive donor to a seronegative infant. The incidence is 10% to 30% and usually occurs in infants who weigh less than 1300 g. The risk of infection is related to the volume of transfused blood, the number of donors, and elevated complement fixation titers to CMV in donor blood. Horizontal transmission of CMV in a neonatal intensive care unit has been documented, but is rare.

## Clinical Manifestations

Cytomegalic inclusion disease (CID) is the most serious but least common manifestation of congenital CMV infection. This syndrome is characterized by multiorgan involvement with the reticuloendothelial and central nervous systems most frequently affected. Typical clinical features of cytomegalic inclusion disease include intrauterine growth retardation, hepatosplenomegaly, jaundice, petechiae or purpura, microcephaly, chorioretinitis, and cerebral calcifications (Table 20-82). These features may also occur singly or in combinations.

Hepatomegaly with direct hyperbilirubinemia and mild elevation of serum transaminase levels are the most common abnormalities noted in the newborn period. Giant cell transformation with associated extramedullary hematopoiesis or large inclusion-bearing hepatocytes characteristic of CMV infection are present on pathologic examination of the liver. Hepatitis usually resolves in the first year of life, and development of cirrhosis is rare. Splenomegaly is common and may be the only abnormality present at birth.

Thrombocytopenia with petechiae is usually transient but may persist through the first year of life. "Blueberry muffin spots" are discrete, well-circumscribed lesions often mistaken for purpura; they represent dermal erythropoiesis in the more severely affected infants (Color Figure 22).

Central nervous system infection with CMV can result in en-

### TABLE 20-82. Frequency of Clinical Findings in Infants with Congenital Infections

| Clinical Findings | Congenital Infection | | | | |
|---|---|---|---|---|---|
| | *Rubella* | *Toxoplasma* | *CMV* | *Syphilis* | *HSV* |
| Intrauterine growth retardation | +++ | ± | ++ | ++ | + |
| Reticuloendothelial system | | | | | |
|   Jaundice | + | ++ | +++ | +++ | |
|   Hepatitis | ± | + | +++ | +++ | + |
|   Hepatosplenomegaly | +++ | ++ | +++ | +++ | + |
|   Anemia | + | +++ | ++ | +++ | |
|   Thrombocytopenia | ++ | ± | +++ | ++ | |
|   Disseminated intravascular coagulation | − | − | ± | | |
|   Adenopathy | ++ | ++ | | ++ | |
|   Dermal erythropoiesis | + | − | + | − | − |
| Skin rash | − | + | − | ++ | +++ |
| Bone abnormalities | ++ | − | ± | ++ | |
| Eye | | | | | |
|   Cataracts | ++ | ± | − | − | |
|   Retinopathy | ++ | +++ | + | ± | +++ |
|   Microphthalmia | + | ± | − | − | + |
| Central nervous system | | | | | |
|   Microcephaly | + | ± | ++ | − | +++ |
|   Meningoencephalitis | ++ | +++ | +++ | ++ | +++ |
|   Brain calcification | ± | ++ | ++ | − | + |
|   Hydrocephalus | − | ++ | ± | ± | ++ |
|   Hearing defect | ++ | + | ++ | + | − |
| Pneumonitis | ++ | + | + | + | − |
| Cardiovascular | | | | | |
|   Myocarditis | + | − | ± | ± | − |
|   Congenital defect | +++ | − | − | − | − |

±, rare; +, 5% to 20%; ++, 20% to 50%; +++, more than 50%; □, prominent feature of particular infection; *CMV*, cytomegalovirus; *HSV*, herpes simplex virus.

cephalitis with seizures and an elevated protein content in the cerebrospinal fluid (CSF). Cerebral calcifications occur in less than 10% of infected infants and date the maternal infection to the first trimester of pregnancy. The calcifications usually occur in the periventricular areas (Fig 20-106) and are best visualized by ultrasonography. Arrested brain growth results in microcephaly, and obstruction of the fourth ventricle may result in hydrocephalus. Ocular defects include chorioretinitis (Color Figure 23), strabismus, optic atrophy, microphthalmia, and cataracts.

The most common manifestation of congenital CMV infection is sensorineural hearing loss resulting from direct viral invasion of the inner ear. It occurs in 15% of infants with symptomatic congenital infection and in about 5% of those with otherwise asymptomatic infection at birth. The hearing loss may be unilateral and unsuspected until the second year of life. All infants with congenital CMV require evaluation of hearing with brain stem auditory-evoked responses.

A diffuse interstitial pneumonitis occurs in less than 1% of newborns with CID. Bone abnormalities in CMV infection consist of longitudinal radiolucent streaks in the metaphysis of long bones ("celery stalk" appearance), particularly the distal femur and proximal tibia (Fig 20-107). Generalized osteopenia with irregular metaphyseal fragmentation has also been described. Defective enamelization of the deciduous teeth occurs in 40% of symptomatic newborns and in 5% of infants with asymptomatic infection at birth.

Attempts have been made to implicate CMV in cardiovascular, genitourinary, gastrointestinal, musculoskeletal anomalies, and particularly inguinal hernias in males, but the teratogenicity of CMV remains in doubt.

Of infants with asymptomatic congenital CMV infection, more than 90% have no apparent sequelae and only rarely manifest severe neurologic impairment. In contrast, severe intellectual and sensory deficits are consistently observed in infants and children with chorioretinitis, microcephaly, and intracranial calcifications. Symptomatic infants without central nervous system abnormal-ities at birth are at less risk for development of neurologic and developmental abnormalities.

CMV infection acquired at delivery is manifested by an afebrile pneumonia in 50% of exposed infants or, rarely, hepatitis or encephalitis after an incubation period of 4 to 12 weeks (mean, 8 weeks). In premature infants, CMV pneumonitis is associated with development of chronic lung disease. Late neurologic sequelae are not associated with perinatally acquired infection.

Transfusion-acquired CMV infection in low–birth-weight infants may be severe and is characterized by a gray ashen pallor, respiratory distress, pneumonia, hepatosplenomegaly, hepatitis, atypical lymphocytosis, thrombocytopenia, and hemolytic anemia; it has a 10% mortality rate.

## Diagnosis

All infants with congenital CMV infection have high titers of virus in their urine and pharynx at birth. Viruria and pharyngeal shedding appear after an incubation period of 4 to 12 weeks in infants infected with CMV perinatally. Viral excretion in the urine may persist for years, but the titer decreases markedly after 3 months. Pharyngeal shedding is not as prolonged. The diagnosis of congenital and perinatal CMV infection is best confirmed by isolation of the virus from the urine (Table 20-83). Recently, culture of saliva was as sensitive as urine for detection of congenital CMV infection. Characteristic cytopathologic developments occur within 2 weeks of inoculation of the specimen onto a human fibroblast monolayer. CMV may be identified in tissue culture after 24 to 48 hours of incubation by the shell-vial technique, which uses a monoclonal antibody to detect early CMV antigen. To diagnose congenital CMV infection accurately, cultures should be obtained within the first 2 weeks of life. After 3 weeks, viral shedding can occur from either congenital or postnatally acquired infection. CMV has been detected in the urine by electron microscopic study using the pseudoreplica method, which permits detection of herpesvirus particles within 15 to 30 minutes. This

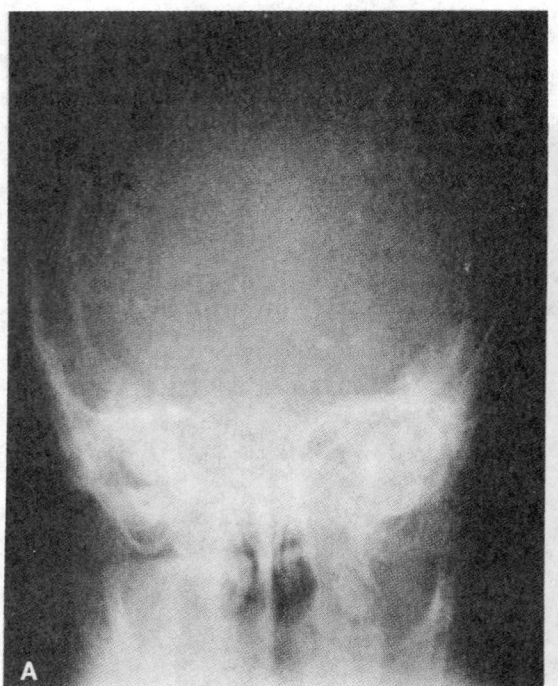
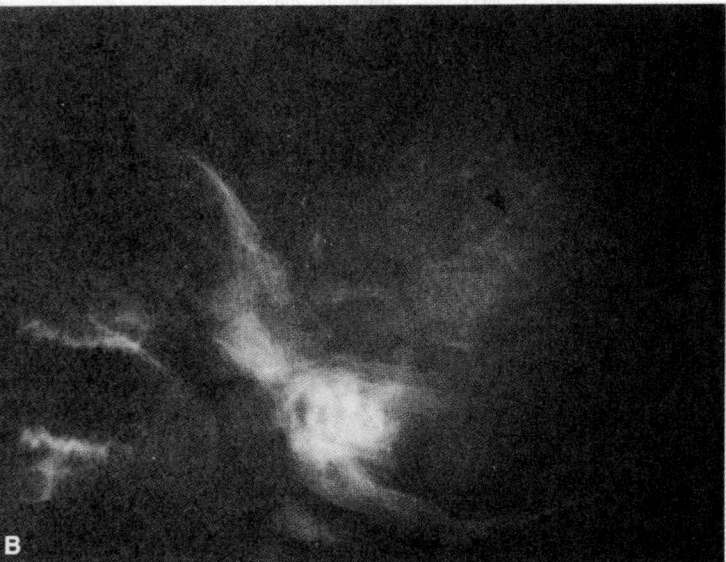

**Figure 20-106.** Anteroposterior (**A**) and lateral (**B**) skull roentgenograms demonstrating cerebral calcifications (*arrows*) lining the ventricles in a neonate with congenital cytomegalovirus infection. (Courtesy of Guido Currarino, MD, Dallas, Texas.)

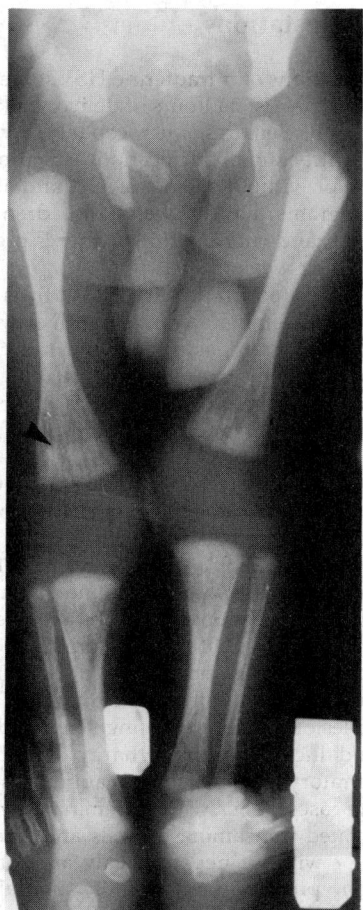

**Figure 20-107.** "Celery stalk" appearance of the femur (*arrow*) and tibia associated with congenital rubella, cytomegalovirus, and syphilis. Alternating bands of longitudinal translucency and relative density represent a disturbance of normal bone metabolism. (Courtesy of Guido Currarino, MD, Dallas, Texas.)

**TABLE 20-83. Methods of Diagnosis of Congenital and Perinatal Infection**

| | Isolation of Organism | Antigen Detection | Measurement of Antibody |
|---|---|---|---|
| Cytomegalovirus | ++ | − | + |
| Herpes simplex virus | ++ | + | + |
| Varicella-zoster | ± | − | ++ |
| Epstein-Barr virus | ± | − | ++ |
| Rubella | ± | − | ++ |
| Toxoplasmosis | ± | − | ++ |
| Syphilis | ±* | ± | ++ |
| Human immunodeficiency virus | ± | + | ++ |
| Hepatitis | | | |
|   A | ± | − | ++ |
|   B | − | ++ | ++ |
|   Delta | − | ++ | ++ |
|   C | − | − | ++ |
| *Neisseria gonorrhoeae* | ++ | − | − |
| *Chlamydia trachomatis* | ± | ++† | ++‡ |
| Mycoplasmas | ++ | − | ± |

+, alternative method but usually less helpful; ++, preferred method; ±, possible, but may not be performed routinely by clinical laboratories; −, not available
* Spirochetes visualized by dark-field examination of suspected lesions
† Preferred for conjunctivitis
‡ Preferred for pneumonia

technique detects virus in 95% of specimens with high infectivity titers (greater than or equal to $10^4$/mL); sensitivity is decreased when specimens are stored at 4 °C.

Alpert and Plotkin (1986) report that serologic studies have a limited role in diagnosis of congenital CMV infection. The presence of CMV-specific IgG antibody denotes passively transferred maternal antibodies. On serial determinations, antibody titers to CMV in most congenitally infected infants show either a rapid or gradual decline to low levels between 4 months and 2 years of age. A minimum of infected infants demonstrate persistence of the high initial titer. An increase in titer has not been demonstrated in these infants despite continued shedding of the virus. False-negative antibody levels determined by the complement fixation method have been seen in infected infants. Although the CMV-IgM immunofluorescent test detects 76% of congenitally infected infants, a false-positive rate of 21% is documented. Enzyme-linked immunosorbent assays (ELISAs) that are commercially available for measurement of CMV-IgG and CMV-IgM have improved sensitivity and specificity. To interpret test results, the accuracy of the specific kit used must be known.

At present, no effective antiviral agents are available for treatment of congenital CMV infection. There is an ongoing clinical trial with ganciclovir for treatment of congenital CMV infection; preliminary results have noted an exacerbation of chorioretinitis in some infants treated with ganciclovir.

## Prevention

Hand washing after exposure to urine or saliva from young infants is the most effective means of preventing primary CMV infection in pregnant women. Transfusion-acquired CMV infection is eliminated by administration of CMV antibody-negative blood products to infants less that 1500 g in birth weight. Frozen deglycerolized red blood cells are a suitable alternative because they lack viable leukocytes. CMV vaccine ultimately may be the best preventive strategy, but vaccine development remains investigational.

## Selected Readings

Adler SP. Nosocomial transmission of cytomegalovirus. Pediatr Infect Dis J 1986;5: 239.

Adler SP. Cytomegalovirus transmission among children in day care, their mothers and caretakers. Pediatr Infect Dis J 1988;7:279.

Alpert G, Plotkin SA. A practical guide to the diagnosis of congenital infections in the newborn infant. Pediatr Clin North Am 1986;33:465.

Fowler KB, Stagno S, Pass RF, Britt WJ, Boll TJ, Alford CA. The outcome of congenital cytomegalovirus infection in relation to maternal antibody status. N Engl J Med 1992;326:663.

Stagno S, Pass RF, Dworsky ME, et al. Congenital and perinatal cytomegalovirus infections. Semin Perinatol 1983;7:31.

Principles and Practice of Pediatrics, Second Edition.
edited by Frank A. Oski et al. J. B. Lippincott Company, Philadelphia © 1994.

# HERPES SIMPLEX VIRUS

*Pablo J. Sánchez and Jane D. Siegel*

The estimated rate of occurrence of neonatal herpes simplex virus (HSV) infection in the United States is about 1 per 5000 to 7500 deliveries per year. Most neonatal infections are due to HSV-2 with some 25% to 30% due to HSV-1. More than 50% of infants who develop HSV infection are born to women who are asymptomatic for genital infection with HSV at the time of delivery and have neither a history of genital herpes nor a sexual partner with genital HSV infection. The frequency of asymptomatic shedding of HSV at the time of delivery varies from 0.2% to 1%.

## Transmission

Acquisition of HSV by the infant can occur in utero, during delivery, or after birth. In utero infection with HSV accounts for about 10% of cases. Transmission occurs either transplacentally during a maternal viremia or by an ascending route from an infected maternal genital tract. The virus may pass through microscopic tears in the amniotic membranes to produce infection in infants delivered by cesarean section with intact membranes. HSV has been isolated from the blood of a pregnant woman with primary HSV infection, as well as from amniotic fluid, placenta, cord blood, and fetal tissue obtained at the time of spontaneous abortion. In utero acquisition of HSV is also suggested by reports of congenital malformations in infants born to women with genital herpes infection during pregnancy.

Transmission of HSV to the newborn infant usually occurs at delivery. Risk of neonatal infection is higher with primary maternal HSV infection than with recurrent infection (50% versus 4%) because of the infant's prolonged exposure to large quantities of virus in the absence of protective neutralizing antibody (Table 20-84). Prematurity, duration of rupture of amniotic membranes greater than 4 hours, and use of a scalp electrode for fetal heart rate monitoring also increase risk of HSV infection. Infants are at risk for developing disease after exposure to HSV infection in the first month of life.

Postpartum transmission of HSV to the newborn infant may occur after contact with a maternal breast lesion during breastfeeding, after endotracheal suctioning for meconium aspiration by a physician with herpes labialis, and from contact with other family members with active herpes labialis lesions. Nosocomial transmission of HSV in newborn nurseries has been documented by restriction endonuclease analysis of viral isolates, but it is rare.

TABLE 20-84. Maternal Genital Herpes Infection and Risk of Perinatal Transmission

|  | Genital Herpes Simplex Virus Infection | |
| --- | --- | --- |
|  | *Primary* | *Recurrent* |
| Risk of perinatal transmission | 50% | 3% to 5% |
| Site of viral shedding | Cervix | Labia |
| Duration of viral shedding | 3 wk | 2–5 d |
| Quantity of virus shed | Large | Small |
| Neutralizing antibody | Absent | Present |

## Clinical Manifestations

Clinical manifestations of intrauterine HSV infection are present at birth or within the first 24 hours of delivery. Skin vesicles with scars are common. Seizures, microcephaly, hydranencephaly, porencephaly, intracranial calcifications, microphthalmia, hepatomegaly with or without splenomegaly, and abnormalities on bone roentgenograms may be seen. The adrenal gland is frequently involved, and chorioretinitis either is present at birth or develops in the first week of life.

Neonatal HSV infection acquired at birth is categorized by extent of disease: disseminated disease with or without evidence of central nervous system, skin, eye, and mouth involvement; central nervous system disease (encephalitis) with or without skin, eye, and mouth involvement; and localized infection of the skin, eye, and mouth without visceral organ or central nervous system involvement (Table 20-83).

Disseminated disease accounts for 20% to 50% of neonatal HSV infection. Whitley and coworkers (1988) observed a 50.5% frequency of disseminated disease from 1982 to 1987 which significantly decreased to 22.9% from 1973 to 1981. This decrease is probably a result of prompt diagnosis and treatment of localized infection before dissemination occurs. The average onset of illness is between 9 and 11 days of life and the principal organs involved are the liver and adrenal glands. About 50% of infants manifest central nervous system involvement and 90% manifest skin, mouth, or eye lesions. The presenting signs and symptoms are nonspecific and include fever, lethargy, irritability, anorexia, vomiting, respiratory distress, apnea, jaundice, seizures, and, in the most severe cases, shock with disseminated intravascular coagulation. Elevated transaminase levels and direct hyperbilirubinemia with or without hepatomegaly are common. Splenomegaly is often present. Pneumonitis, pleural effusion, and roentgenographic lesions in long bones occur rarely. Without therapy, case-fatality rate exceeds 80%; pneumonitis and disseminated intravascular coagulopathy are associated with an increased risk of death among infants with disseminated infection. Most survivors develop psychomotor retardation and ocular defects.

Central nervous system disease accounts for about 30% of neonatal HSV infections. Clinical manifestations typically occur at 11 to 17 days of life and include lethargy, irritability, bulging fontanelle, focal or generalized seizures, opisthotonos, decerebrate posturing, and coma. Examination of the CSF reveals an elevated leukocyte count with a predominance of lymphocytes and an elevated protein content. Red blood cells are occasionally present, indicating hemorrhagic brain involvement. A normal cell count and protein concentration, however, may be found on the initial lumbar puncture. Mortality in untreated infants with localized central nervous system disease is 40% to 50%. Most survivors have neurologic sequelae consisting of seizures, spastic quadriplegia, chorioretinitis, microcephaly, hydrocephaly, porencephalic cyst, and psychomotor retardation.

Localized diseases of skin, eye, and mouth occur in 20% to 40% of infants with HSV infection. The hallmark of neonatal HSV infection is the discrete vesicular lesions that occur in 90% of infants with localized infection (Color Figures 24 and 25). The vesicles usually appear first on the presenting part of the body that was in direct contact with the virus during delivery. About 70% of untreated infants who present with skin vesicles develop disseminated infection or have progression of disease to involve the eyes or central nervous system. Although infants with skin lesions suffer recurrences during the first 6 months of life, recurrences after 1 month of age are generally not associated with further clinical progression of disease. Ulcerative lesions of the mouth, tongue, or palate occur less commonly. Ocular involvement with HSV is manifested by keratoconjunctivitis, uveitis, chorioretinitis, cataracts, and retinal dysplasia. Sequelae of ocular HSV infection include corneal ulceration, microphthalmia, optic atrophy, and blindness. Some 10% of infants with localized infection of the skin, eyes, or oral cavity have subclinical involvement of the central nervous system as manifested by the development of severe neurologic impairment. Three or more skin recurrences in the first 6 months of life are associated with an increased risk of abnormal development.

## Diagnosis

The preferred diagnostic method is isolation of HSV from skin vesicles, buffy coat, brain tissue, CSF, stool, urine, throat, nares, or conjunctivae (Table 20-82). HSV can also be isolated from duodenal aspirate in infants with hepatitis. Typing of HSV is not routinely performed, although recent evidence suggests that neurologic outcome may be better with neonatal encephalitis due to HSV-1 as compared with that due to HSV-2. When mucocutaneous lesions are present, scraping from the base of a vesicle may reveal intranuclear inclusions and multinucleated giant cells by Tzanck test or Wright's stain in 60% to 70% of cases; specific HSV antigen may be detected by immunofluorescence in 70% to 80% of cases.

Traditionally, diagnosis of HSV encephalitis in the absence of mucocutaneous lesions is confirmed by biopsy test of brain tissue because HSV is isolated from the CSF in only 30% to 50% of cases. Recent experience demonstrates usefulness of the electroencephalogram, technetium brain scan, computed tomography (CT), and magnetic resonance imaging (MRI) for identification of infants with HSV encephalitis. The characteristic electroencephalographic abnormality is a periodic slow and sharp wave discharge; more commonly, multiple independent foci of periodic activity are present. Technetium brain scan may demonstrate increased perfusion to the involved brain area. CT scan may be normal early in the course of the disease with characteristic abnormalities appearing 3 to 5 days later. The most frequently observed findings in the acute phase are patchy areas of low attenuation in both cerebral hemispheres, or hemorrhage or calcification in the thalamus, insular cortex, periventricular white matter, and along the corticomedullary junction. Late findings include multicystic encephalomalacia and ventriculomegaly as a result of brain atrophy and destruction. MRI is more sensitive in detecting early abnormalities in the periventricular white matter and in defining the extent of parenchymal lesions. Positive findings in any neurodiagnostic study provides enough evidence to initiate antiviral therapy. Recently, HSV DNA in CSF of patients with HSV encephalitis has been detected by polymerase chain reaction; this technique holds promise for identification of infected infants.

Serology is not helpful acutely because antibody may not yet be present with primary maternal infection, and, when present, antibody to HSV in neonates may be maternal. Increase in antibody titers in the convalescent phase indicates neonatal infection. Routine serologic methods do not distinguish reliably between antibodies to HSV-1 and HSV-2.

## Treatment

Two antiviral agents, acyclovir and vidarabine, have decreased the mortality rate and improved the outcome of neonatal HSV infection. Antiviral therapy is initiated when the characteristic clinical features are present or when neonate with overwhelming sepsis and negative bacterial cultures does not respond to broad-spectrum antibiotics. HSV may be recovered from brain biopsy specimens even after 24 to 48 hours of antiviral therapy. Acyclovir (10 mg/kg body wt every 8 h) or vidarabine (15 to 30 mg/kg body wt over 12 h) is administered intravenously for 10 to 14 days. A 21-day course may be required for treatment of encephalitis; there is increasing recognition of early relapse after shorter duration of therapy. Moreover, acyclovir at doses as high as 60 mg/kg/d may be more effective for treatment of encephalitis. Although there is no difference in mortality rates in infants who receive either the 15 or 30 mg/kg body wt/day dosage of vidarabine, a significantly lower percentage of infants who receive the higher dosage have progression of disease while on therapy. Ocular HSV infection requires topical antiviral medication with either 1% trifluridine or 3% vidarabine in addition to parenteral therapy. Treatment with acyclovir may prevent development of neutralizing antibody with relapse of disease after therapy is stopped. Acyclovir is the preferred drug, however, because of the insolubility of vidarabine and the large fluid volume required for vidarabine infusion. The mortality rate with disseminated disease has been reduced from 75% in untreated infants to 57% in infants treated with either acyclovir or vidarabine; 40% of these infants are normal at 1 year of age. Among infants with central nervous system disease, mortality is about 15%, and 35% are normal on follow-up examination at 1 year of age. No deaths have occurred among treated infants with localized infection of the skin, eye, or oral cavity, and 90% of infants are normal at 1 year follow-up examination. About 2% of infants treated with antiviral therapy for 10 to 14 days have recurrence of infection leading to central nervous system disease. Relapse of HSV encephalitis also has been reported after a 10-day course of vidarabine or acyclovir therapy.

A beneficial effect of human immunoglobulin that contains a large concentration of anti-HSV antibody has been observed in animal models when administered early in the course of disease. Clinical efficacy in humans has not been demonstrated.

## Prevention

Delivery of the infants of pregnant women with active genital herpes by cesarean section within 4 to 6 hours of rupture of amniotic membranes is the only intervention shown to prevent neonatal HSV infection. Results of antepartum genital HSV cultures from pregnant women with a history of genital herpes do not predict the infant's risk of exposure to HSV at delivery. Even if asymptomatic, infants born by vaginal delivery or cesarean section after prolonged rupture of membranes in the presence of active genital herpes lesions should have appropriate cultures for HSV taken 24 to 36 hours after delivery. Virus present at this time represents active replication and invasive infection, whereas virus isolated from mucous membrane cultures obtained at birth merely reflects surface contamination. If the mother has primary genital herpes and the infant is premature or has had invasive instrumentation or skin laceration during delivery, prophylactic or "anticipatory" antiviral therapy is recommended. If the mother has recurrent genital herpes and no other risk factors are present, antiviral therapy is withheld until culture results are known or clinical signs of disease develop. Antiviral therapy is initiated if HSV is isolated from any infant culture. This approach is widely recommended, but its efficacy is unproved. Infants born to women with active genital herpes should be in contact isolation in the nursery or should room with the mother. Careful hand washing before handling the infant should be stressed to the mother to prevent postpartum transmission. Breast-feeding is contraindicated only if the mother has vesicular lesions on the breast. Delay of circumcision for approximately 1 month for infants at highest risk of disease may be warranted.

Nursery personnel with oral and genital HSV lesions are at low risk of transmitting infection to infants as long as their lesions are covered. They must practice strict hand washing when handling infants. Personnel with herpetic whitlow should not have direct patient-care responsibilities until the lesions have healed.

## Selected Readings

Arvin AM, Johnson RT, Whitley RT, et al. Consensus: management of the patient with herpes simplex encephalitis. Pediatr Infect Dis J 1987;6:2.

Jenkins M, Kohl S. New aspects of neonatal herpes. Infect Dis Clin North Am 1992;6:57.

Overall JC, Whitley RJ, Yeager AS, et al. Prophylactic or anticipatory antiviral therapy for newborns exposed to herpes simplex infection. Pediatr Infect Dis J 1984;3: 193.

Prober CG, Sullender WM, Yasukawa LL, et al. Low risk of herpes simplex virus infection in neonates exposed to the virus at the time of vaginal delivery to mothers with recurrent genital herpes simplex virus infections. N Engl J Med 1987;316:240.

Whitley RJ, Corey L, Arvin A, et al. Changing presentation of herpes simplex virus infection in neonates. Journal of Infectious Diseases 1988;158:109.

Whitley R, Arvin A, Prober C, et al. Predictors of morbidity and mortality in neonates with herpes simplex virus infections. N Engl J Med 1991;324:450.

*Principles and Practice of Pediatrics, Second Edition.*
edited by Frank A. Oski et al. J. B. Lippincott Company, Philadelphia © 1994.

# VARICELLA-ZOSTER VIRUS
*Jane D. Siegel*

Varicella-zoster virus (VZV) is a member of the herpesvirus family and is the etiology of two clinical syndromes—chickenpox (varicella) and shingles (zoster). Primary infection usually occurs in childhood. It is rare for healthy adults to develop chickenpox; 90% of adults with no history of clinical chickenpox have evidence of previous infection when tested serologically. An increased risk exists, however, for development of pneumonia in adults with chickenpox. The incidence of maternal varicella is reported to be 0.7 per 1000 pregnancies. Zoster is a result of reactivation of the latent VZV and does not have a viremic phase in normal hosts.

## PATHOGENESIS

The neonate whose mother has never had VZV infection is at risk of acquiring varicella either transplacentally during the viremic phase of maternal chickenpox or postnatally by airborne transmission or direct contact with an acutely infected person in the neonatal nursery or at home. Transplacental transmission occurs in 25% of cases. Maternal varicella infection occurring between weeks 8 and 20 of gestation may be associated with a characteristic fetal varicella syndrome (Table 20-85). Varicella in the second and third trimester rarely is associated with birth defects. In a prospective study by Paryani and Arvin (1986) of 43 pregnancies complicated by varicella and 14 pregnancies complicated by herpes zoster, the congenital varicella syndrome occurred in 1 (9.1%) of 11 infants of women with first trimester varicella and in none of the infants whose mothers were infected in the second and third trimesters. According to the review of Alkaly and colleagues (1987), the most frequently observed features of fetal varicella syndrome are cutaneous scars in a dermatomal distribution, limb hypoplasia and paresis, and eye lesions. The characteristic segmental distribution suggests that these lesions result from fetal zoster after in utero varicella infection. No evidence supports an association between maternal varicella and chromosomal damage, spontaneous abortion, or prematurity. Some infants with congenital VZV infection are normal at birth

**TABLE 20-85. Characteristic Features of Fetal Varicella Syndrome**

Skin lesions: unilateral cicatricial lesions that correspond to dermatome distribution

Neurologic: limb paresis/paralysis, hydrocephalus/cortical atrophy, seizures, delayed development, sphincter dysfunction

Eye: chorioretinitis, anisocoria, nystagmus, microphthalmia, cataract

Skeletal: hypoplasia of extremities, digits

Gastrointestinal and genitourinary anomalies

Failure to thrive

but develop zoster during the first few years of life without an episode of postnatal varicella. The usual latency of several decades is, therefore, not maintained after intrauterine exposure to VZV. Fetal infection rarely occurs in association with an episode of maternal zoster during pregnancy because of the presence of large concentrations of antibody and the absence of maternal viremia.

Infants whose mothers develop chickenpox within the 21 days before delivery have a 25% chance of developing chickenpox in the early neonatal period. Because a large inoculum of virus is transmitted directly to the fetus during maternal viremia, the usual incubation period of 10 to 21 days in older children is decreased to 9 to 15 days in the neonate. When the maternal rash develops 6 to 21 days before delivery, sufficient quantities of maternal antibody are produced and delivered to the fetus to protect against postnatal development of severe chickenpox. Those infants whose mothers develop chickenpox fewer than 5 days before delivery or within 2 days after delivery are at risk of increased morbidity and mortality.

Development of chickenpox after exposure during the neonatal period is unusual in the infant whose mother is immune because of the placental transfer of antibody. Wang and coworkers (1983) report that VZV antibody levels are low or undetectable in infants of birth weights less than 1000 g or less than 25 weeks' gestation; therefore, such infants should be considered unprotected until antibody titers are determined. Rarely, infection occurs despite the presence of maternal antibody, but clinical disease is mild. Infants of susceptible mothers are not protected, but they generally do not develop serious disease after postnatal exposure.

## DIAGNOSIS

The diagnosis of VZV infections is based on characteristic clinical findings. Several methods of laboratory confirmation are available. Multinucleated giant cells or cells containing eosinophilic intranuclear inclusions identified in scrapings from the base of a vesicle indicate the presence of a herpesvirus. Virus is present in vesicular fluid during the first 3 days of illness, but VZV is difficult to isolate in the viral diagnostic laboratory; therefore, cultures are not routinely performed. IgG and IgM antibodies may be detected in serum by the fluorescent antibody to membrane antigen (FAMA) or by enzyme-linked immunosorbent assay (ELISA) methods. The ELISA test is preferred for its increased sensitivity. Congenital VZV infection may be diagnosed during gestation by detecting IgM antibody to VZV in fetal blood obtained by percutaneous umbilical blood sampling. After birth, the diagnosis is confirmed by presence of IgM antibody to VZV at birth or persistence of VZV-specific IgG antibody after 1 year of age.

## TREATMENT AND PREVENTION

Acyclovir 45 mg/kg body wt/d intravenously in three divided doses is administered for 5 to 7 days for treatment of severe disease in the neonate. Vidarabine 10 mg/kg body wt/d is an alternative agent, but an increased fluid load is required because of its relative insolubility.

Varicella-zoster immunoglobulin (VZIG) is recommended for susceptible pregnant women who have significant exposure to chickenpox. The recommended dose is 125 U/10 kg body wt (maximum 625 U). It is advisable first to confirm maternal susceptibility by measuring antibody to VZV. If antibody is not present, VZIG should be administered as soon as possible but not longer than 96 hours after exposure. It is uncertain whether prevention of clinical disease in the mother protects the fetus. A decision concerning termination of pregnancy must be made by the woman and her physician, taking into consideration the risk of having a malformed infant. The live, attenuated VZV vaccine administered to susceptible women before pregnancy may prove to be the most effective method for prevention of congenital varicella syndrome.

VZIG (125 U) is administered to neonates whose mothers develop chickenpox within 5 days before or 2 days after delivery because of the increased morbidity and mortality observed when infants develop chickenpox within the first 10 days of life. Although VZIG is not completely protective against infection, clinical disease is generally less severe. These infants must still be considered potentially infective and are maintained in strict isolation until 21 days of age if hospitalization is required. VZIG is not routinely administered to full-term infants exposed to chickenpox postnatally because the risk of complications is not increased. VZIG is recommended after exposure of neonates of less than 28 weeks' gestation or other premature infants who are seronegative.

## Selected Readings

Alkaly AL, Pomerance JJ, Rimoin DL. Fetal varicella syndrome. J Pediatr 1987;111: 320.

Paryani SG, Arvin AM. Intrauterine infection with varicella-zoster virus after maternal varicella. N Engl J Med 1986;314:1542.

Wang EEL, Prober CG, Arvin AM. Varicella-zoster virus antibody titers before and after administration of zoster immune globulin to neonates in an intensive care nursery. J Pediatr 1983;103:113.

*Principles and Practice of Pediatrics, Second Edition.*
edited by Frank A. Oski et al. J. B. Lippincott Company, Philadelphia © 1994.

## EPSTEIN-BARR VIRUS
*Jane D. Siegel*

Sporadic case reports suggest an association of Epstein-Barr virus (EBV) with congenital infection. EBV is the most prevalent herpesvirus worldwide, and seroconversion usually occurs by 3 years of age in primitive societies or in crowded living conditions. In the United States, acquisition of antibody may be delayed until age 15 years in women from lower socioeconomic backgrounds and until late in the third decade in women from middle to upper socioeconomic backgrounds. Primary EBV infections rarely occur during pregnancy because of nearly universal seropositivity of women of childbearing age. Large prospective studies of more than 12,000 pregnant women in France, Canada, and the United States demonstrate seronegativity rates of less than 5%. Most studies demonstrate no seroconversions during pregnancy. Seroconversion during pregnancy is not associated with intrauterine infection. Nearly universal presence of maternal antibody is probably protective against transmission by blood transfusion during the neonatal period.

Reactivation of a primary EBV infection in association with the relative immunodeficiency of pregnancy could provide another opportunity for intrauterine infection. Because the titers of antibodies to the EBV early antigen (anti-EA) increase as additional amounts of EBV-associated antigens are released during reactivation, a prospective study by Fleisher and Bolognese (1983) compared the incidence of anti-EA in 200 pregnant women to that in 200 control patients. Anti-EA was present in significantly more pregnant women than control participants, 55% versus 22% to 32%, P less than .005. In this study, however, no difference was noted in the incidence of low–birth-weight, congenital anomalies, or jaundice in infants whose mothers had EBV reactivation during pregnancy compared with those who did not. No evidence of intrauterine infection was found in those infants born to women with reactivation and available for testing. Another study of 719 women in France, however, demonstrated a lower incidence of anti-EA (16%), but there was a significant association between reactivation and pathologic outcome.

Several case reports have attempted to associate intrauterine EBV infection with congenital anomalies. Most are inconclusive because of absence of complete serologic studies or because of simultaneous infection with another viral agent known for association with a congenital infection syndrome. The manifestations of EBV infection in one case well documented by Goldberg and colleagues (1981) are micrognathia, cryptorchidism, central cataracts, hypotonia, thrombocytopenia, persistent monocytosis, proteinuria, and multiple areas of metaphysitis present at birth. Serologic and virologic studies failed to detect any other infectious agents. EBV-specific serologic studies were performed at 22 days of age with the following evidence of intrauterine infection: IgM antiviral capsid antigen (anti-VCA) 1:40; IgG anti-VCA 1:640 (maternal 1:80); anti-EA 1:10; and anti-Epstein-Barr nuclear antigen (anti-EBNA) less than 2. At 5 months of age, the EBNA was detected in 18% of lymphocytes that spontaneously persisted in culture for 3 months. A case report by Weaver and coworkers (1984) describes an infant with extrahepatic biliary atresia and onset of jaundice at 5 days of age and who at 3 weeks of age demonstrated IgM-VCA greater than 1:10 and IgG-VCA 1:640; IgG-VCA was 1:320 at 1 year of age.

When a clinical diagnosis of infectious mononucleosis is made in a pregnant woman, serologic confirmation should be obtained with acute and convalescent determinations of IgM-anti-VCA, IgG-anti-VCA, anti-EA, and anti-EBNA. Acutely, IgM-anti-VCA, IgG-anti-VCA, and anti-EA are elevated; anti-EBNA is absent and does not appear for 3 to 6 months. At birth, the infant should be carefully evaluated; most infants are unaffected. If in utero infection with EBV is suspected, acute and convalescent serologic measurements as well as spontaneous lymphocyte transformation studies should be obtained.

## Selected Readings

Fleisher G, Bolognese R. Persistent Epstein-Barr virus infection and pregnancy. J Infect Dis 1983;147:982.

Goldberg GN, Fulginiti VA, Ray G, et al. In utero Epstein-Barr virus (infectious mononucleosis) infection. JAMA 1981;246:1579.

Weaver LT, Nelson R, Bell TM. The association of extrahepatic bile duct atresia and neonatal Epstein-Barr virus infection. Acta Paediatr Scand 1984;73:155.

*Principles and Practice of Pediatrics, Second Edition.*
edited by Frank A. Oski et al. J. B. Lippincott Company, Philadelphia © 1994.

# SYPHILIS

*Pablo J. Sánchez and Jane D. Siegel*

Congenital syphilis, a result of fetal infection with *Treponema pallidum*, is a major public health problem in the United States. From 1977 through 1990, there was a steady increase in the incidence of primary and secondary syphilis among women in the United States (Fig 20-108). Subsequently, the number of cases of early congenital syphilis reported to the Centers for Disease Control and Prevention (CDC) increased from 108 in 1978 to more than 4000 cases in 1991 (see Fig 20-110). The majority of reported cases are from large urban areas such as Detroit, Houston, Los Angeles, Miami, and New York City. At Parkland Memorial Hospital in Dallas, the incidence of congenital syphilis also has increased steadily from 1980 through 1989; 0.2 cases per 1000 live births were reported in 1980, 0.6 cases per 1000 live births in 1982, 1.3 cases per 1000 live births in each of the years 1984 through 1987, and 1.7 cases per 1000 live births in 1989.

A major contributor to the increase of syphilis is the exchange of illegal drugs (notably crack cocaine) for sex with multiple partners whose identities are not known. Partner notification, a traditional syphilis-control strategy, is impossible to implement. The recent decrease in early syphilis (Fig 20-108) has been attributed to novel intervention programs aimed at identification and treatment of these high risk individuals. The dramatic increase in the number of cases of congenital syphilis is due to both an increase in actual cases and the use of revised reporting guidelines. Beginning in 1989, the surveillance definition for congenital syphilis was broadened. The new definition includes not only all infants with clinical evidence of active syphilis, but also asymptomatic infants and stillbirths born to women with untreated or inadequately treated syphilis. Use of the new surveillance case definition increases the number of confirmed/presumptive cases of congenital syphilis by almost four times.

## TRANSMISSION

Pregnant women with primary or secondary syphilis are at highest risk of delivering infected infants. Transmission of infection to the fetus usually occurs transplacentally from maternal spirochetemia, but the neonate also can be infected through contact with a genital lesion at the time of delivery. Although congenital infection can occur anytime during gestation, the risk of fetal infection increases as the stage of pregnancy advances. The theory that the Langhans' cell layer of the cytotrophoblast forms a placental barrier against fetal infection before the 18th week of pregnancy was disproved by demonstration of spirochetes in fetal tissue from spontaneous abortion at 9 and 10 weeks' gestation. Also, electron microscopy demonstrates the persistence of the Langhans' cell layer throughout pregnancy.

## CLINICAL MANIFESTATIONS

Syphilis during pregnancy is associated with premature delivery, spontaneous abortion, stillbirth, nonimmune hydrops, perinatal death, and two characteristic syndromes of clinical disease, early and late congenital syphilis. Early congenital syphilis refers to those clinical manifestations that appear within the first 2 years of life. Those features that occur after 2 years are designated as late congenital syphilis. The clinical manifestations and laboratory findings of early congenital syphilis may be present at birth or may be delayed for several months if the infant remains untreated (see Table 20-83). The physical signs are a direct result of active infection and inflammation.

Infants with congenital syphilis may be growth-retarded at delivery. Hepatitis with hepatosplenomegaly occurs in 50% to 90% of affected infants. Splenomegaly does not occur without liver enlargement. Extramedullary hematopoiesis is seen in both the liver and spleen. About one third of infants have direct and indirect hyperbilirubinemia and elevated transaminase levels. Liver abnormalities may require more than a year to resolve, but they rarely lead to cirrhosis. Generalized nontender lymphadenopathy occurs in 20% to 50% of cases, with characteristic involvement of the epitrochlear nodes. A Coombs' test-negative

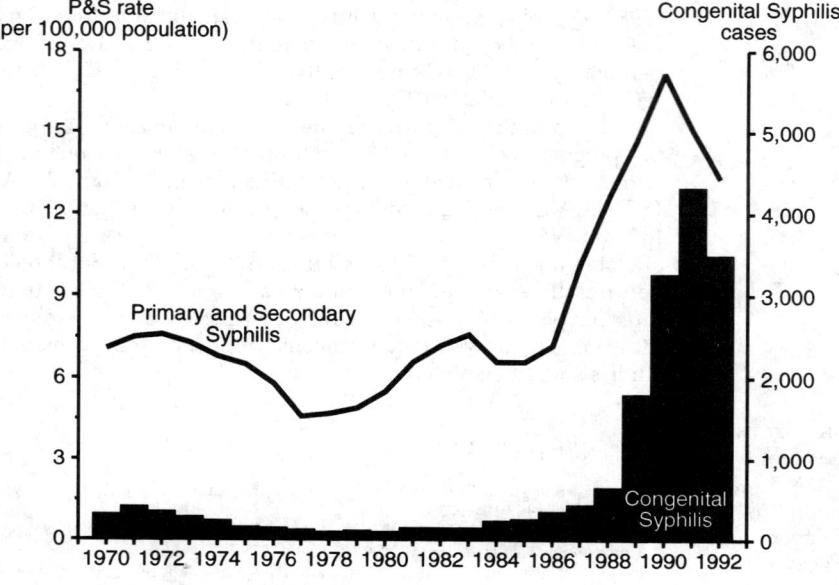

**Figure 20-108.** Case rates of primary and secondary syphilis among women and congenital syphilis cases in the United States, 1970 to 1992. The rate of congenital syphilis has steadily increased since 1983. The surveillance case definition for congenital syphilis changed in 1989; 1992 cases are projections based on reporting through June 1992. (Centers for Disease Control, Atlanta, Georgia, Public Health Service, 1991.)

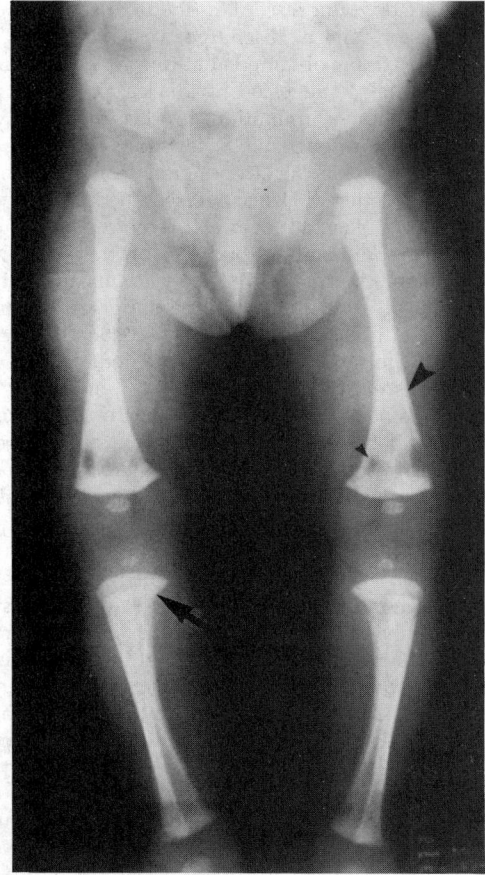

**Figure 20-109.** Bony lesions of early congenital syphilis: symmetric periostitis (*large arrow*); radiolucent metaphyseal area of osteochondritis (*small arrowhead*); bilateral metaphyseal defects on the upper medial aspect of the tibia, Wimberger's sign (*arrow*). Similar changes may occur at the upper ends of the humeri. (Courtesy of Guido Currarino, MD, Dallas, Texas.)

hemolytic anemia is common. The peripheral leukocyte count can show either leukopenia or leukemoid reaction. Thrombocytopenia with petechiae and purpura occurs in about 30% of infants and may be the sole manifestation of congenital infection.

Mucocutaneous lesions are specific for congenital syphilis and occur in 40% to 60% of affected infants. The rash of congenital syphilis is usually maculopapular and located on the extremities.

The lesions are initially oval and pink but then turn coppery brown and desquamate. Desquamation occurs mainly on the palms and soles. A characteristic vesicular bullous eruption known as pemphigus syphiliticus may develop with erythema, blister formation and eventual crusting as healing occurs (Color Figure 26). Nasal discharge associated with rhinitis or snuffles is initially watery, but it becomes thick, purulent, and even blood-tinged (Color Figure 27). Nasal discharge and vesicular fluid containing large concentrations of spirochetes are highly infectious. Rarely, mucous patches of the lips, tongue and palate, and condyloma lata in the perioral and perianal areas may occur.

Bone roentgenograms show skeletal abnormalities consisting of osteochondritis, periostitis, and osteitis in 80% to 90% of infants (Figs 20-109, 20-110). These abnormalities tend to be multiple and symmetric, with the lower extremities involved more often than the upper extremities. The long bones (tibia, humerus, femur), the ribs, and the cranium are principally affected. Rarely, bone lesions may be painful or have superimposed fractures resulting in pseudoparalysis of the affected limb (pseudoparalysis of Parrot). Osteochondritis involves the metaphysis and is evident roentgenographically about 5 weeks after fetal infection. Typical findings are metaphyseal demineralization and a radiodense band below the epiphyseal plate that represents a widened and enhanced zone of provisional calcification. An underlying zone of osteoporosis is evident as a radiolucent band. Bilateral demineralization and osseous destruction of the proximal medial tibial metaphysis is referred to as Wimberger's sign (see Fig 20-109). The classic transverse saw-toothed appearance of the metaphysis (see Fig 20-110) is often not seen on the plain roentgenogram but is evident on xeroradiography of long bones of stillborn infants with congenital syphilis. Periostitis requires 16 weeks for roentgenographic demonstration and consists of multiple layers of periosteal new bone formation in response to diaphyseal inflammation. Osteitis is the "celery stalk" appearance of long bones (see Fig 20-107) resulting from involvement of the medullary canal with resultant diaphysitis. After several months, complete healing of the affected bones occurs even without antibiotic therapy.

Neurosyphilis occurs in 40% to 60% of infants with congenital syphilis. Two types of central nervous system involvement are described. Acute syphilitic leptomeningitis occurs in early infancy. Chronic meningovascular syphilis with progressive hydrocephalus, cranial nerve palsies, and cerebral infarction secondary to endarteritis usually presents toward the end of the first year of life. Cerebrospinal fluid (CSF) examination reveals pleocytosis with an elevated protein content and positive serologic test results for syphilis.

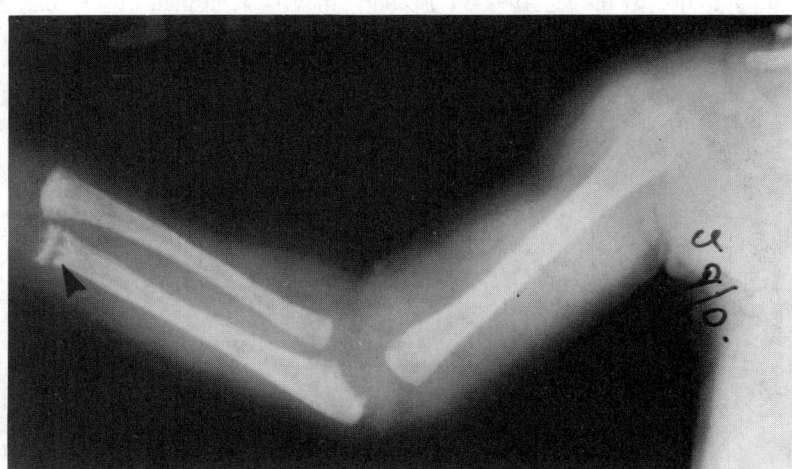

**Figure 20-110.** Saw-toothed appearance of the metaphysis of the distal radius (*arrow*) of an infant with early congenital syphilis. The lucent area represents syphilitic granulation tissue. (Courtesy of Guido Currarino, MD, Dallas, Texas.)

Ocular findings include chorioretinitis, cataract, glaucoma, and uveitis. Nephrosis with generalized edema, ascites, and proteinuria usually occurs at 2 to 3 months of age as a result of immune complex deposition in the renal glomeruli. Other uncommon manifestations include pneumonia alba, myocarditis, pancreatitis, and inflammation and fibrosis of the gastrointestinal tract leading to malabsorption and diarrhea.

The clinical manifestations of late congenital syphilis result from ongoing inflammation or from scars caused by infection of early congenital syphilis. Development of the characteristic lesions is prevented by treatment during pregnancy or within the first 3 months of life. Infants with late congenital syphilis are not infective.

Dental stigmata result from the inflammatory response to *T pallidum* infection in the developing permanent teeth during late gestation. The affected permanent upper central incisors (Hutchinson's teeth) are small, widely spaced, barrel shaped, and notched, with thinning and discoloration of the enamel (Fig 20-111). The first 6-year lower molars (mulberry or Moon's molars) may also be affected. The top surface has many small cusps instead of the usual four. Enamelization is defective. Infection before the 18th week of gestation may result in involvement of deciduous teeth, which then are misshapen, hypoplastic, and prone to dental caries.

The sequela of periostitis of the skull is frontal bossing, of the tibia is saber shins, and of the clavicle is Higoumenakis' sign with sternoclavicular thickening. Clutton's joints, or painless synovitis and hydrarthrosis without involvement of the adjacent bones, is rare. Osteochondritis affecting the otic capsule may lead to cochlear degeneration and fibrous adhesions resulting in eighth-nerve deafness, for which steroid treatment may be beneficial.

The sequelae of syphilitic rhinitis include rhagades and short maxilla with a high palatal arch. If the inflammation of the nasal mucosa extends to the underlying cartilage and bone, perforation of the palate and nasal septum occurs, resulting in a "saddle nose" deformity.

Late ocular manifestations include uveitis and interstitial keratitis. Interstitial keratitis usually appears at puberty and is not affected by penicillin therapy. Although steroid treatment may be beneficial, keratitis resolves spontaneously after 18 to 24 months. Possible sequelae of central nervous system infection include mental retardation, hydrocephalus, seizure disorder, cranial nerve palsies, paralysis, and optic nerve atrophy.

## DIAGNOSIS

The diagnosis of congenital syphilis is established by the observation of spirochetes in body fluids or tissue or by serologic testing (Ingall and coworkers, 1994). *T pallidum* may be identified by darkfield microscopy, fluorescent antibody or silver stain of mucocutaneous lesions, nasal discharge, vesicular fluid, amniotic fluid, placenta, or tissue obtained at autopsy. A diagnosis of congenital syphilis is also suggested by a large, pale, firm placenta, which on microscopic examination, reveals immature villi, vasculitis, and diffuse fibrosis. Serologic tests for syphilis are classified into nontreponemal tests and treponemal tests. Nontreponemal tests include the Venereal Disease Research Laboratory (VDRL) tests and the rapid plasma reagin test. Treponemal tests include the fluorescent treponemal antibody-absorption (FTA-ABS) test and microhemagglutination assay for *T pallidum* antibody (MHA-TP). A diagnosis of congenital syphilis is supported by an infant's nontreponemal antibody level that is at least four times greater than that of the mother's serum. Measurement of total cord IgM levels and results of specific fluorescent treponemal IgM (FTA-ABS-IgM) tests have not proved useful in the diagnosis of congenital syphilis. Elevated cord IgM levels can result from other congenital infections as well as from noninfectious abnormalities. Rheumatoid factor, which occurs frequently in congenital syphilis, interferes with the interpretation of FTA-ABS-IgM test results by producing as many as 35% false-positive results. A 10% false-negative rate also is reported with the use of this test. Recent studies by Sánchez and colleagues (1989) using Western blot analyses of highly purified IgM fractions of sera from infants with congenital syphilis suggest that fetal IgM reactivity with a membrane lipoprotein of *T pallidum* having an apparent molecular mass of 47 kd may accurately identify both symptomatic and asymptomatic infants with congenital syphilis. Similar IgM reactivity to the 47-kd antigen also has been found in the CSF of infants with congenital syphilis.

Recently, a polymerase chain reaction (PCR) technique was developed to detect specific *T pallidum* DNA in tissues and body fluids. Preliminary studies with PCR on amniotic fluid, neonatal serum, and CSF yielded sensitivities of 100%, 80%, and 71%, respectively, with a specificity of 100%. Combined use of IgM immunoblotting and PCR ultimately will aid in early identification of infected infants, regardless of clinical status.

A practical approach to the evaluation of infants born to mothers with reactive serologic tests for syphilis is presented in Figure 20-112. Testing of all pregnant women with reactive serologic tests for syphilis for antibody to the human immunodeficiency virus (HIV) is strongly recommended. Any infant with clinical findings suggestive of congenital syphilis requires a complete diagnostic evaluation, including serum VDRL test, bone roentgenograms, and CSF examination for cell count protein content and VDRL test. The diagnosis of congenital neurosyphilis is difficult to establish. Diagnosis is based on CSF examination that shows a reactive result to the VDRL test, pleocytosis (greater than or equal to 25 leukocytes/mm$^3$), and an elevated protein

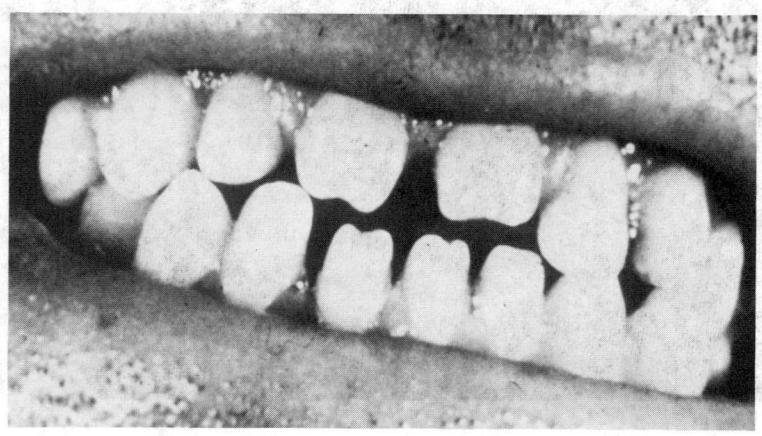

**Figure 20-111.** "Hutchinson's teeth" in a child with late congenital syphilis. The small, widely spaced, notched upper central incisors may be detected by radiography while deciduous teeth are in place. (Courtesy of George H. McCracken, Jr., MD, Dallas, Texas.)

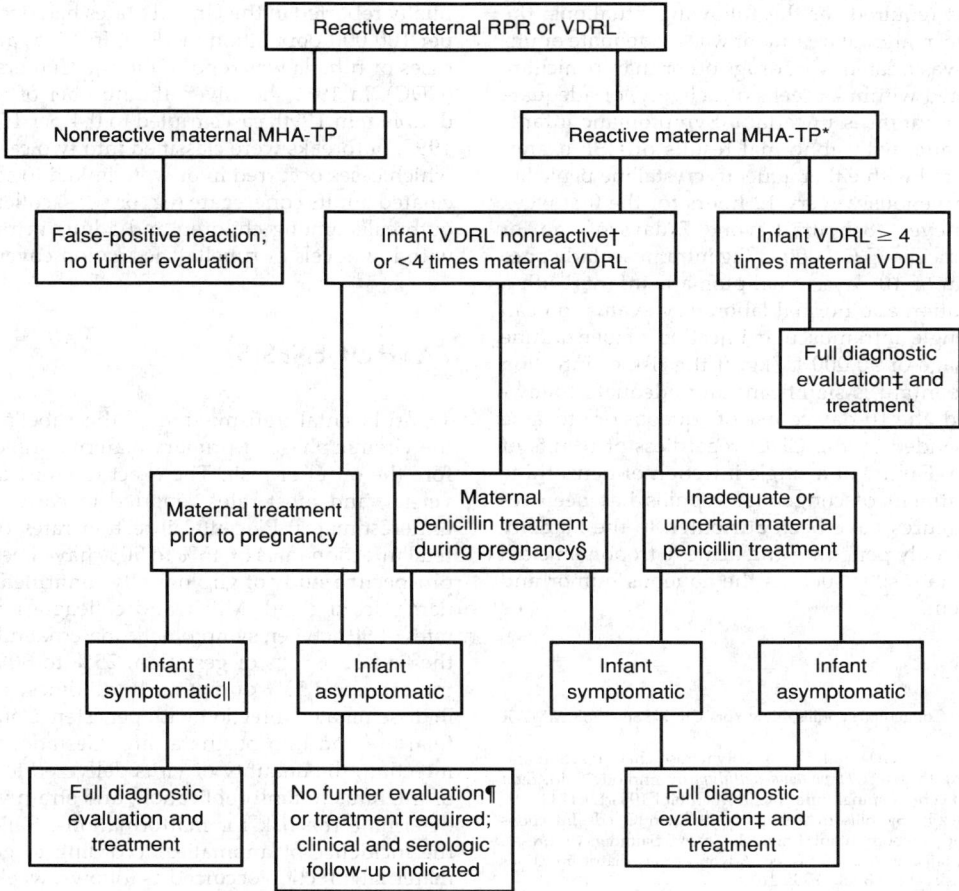

* Testing for HIV antibody recommended.

† Infant's VDRL may be nonreactive due to low maternal VDRL titer, prematurity, or recent maternal infection.

‡ Includes CBC, platelets, retic, LFT (ALT, AST, Bili T&D), long bone x-rays, and CSF examination for cell count, protein, and quantitative VDRL; eye exam if symptomatic.

§ Maternal treatment within 4 weeks of delivery is considered inadequate treatment of the infant.

‖ Women who maintain a VDRL titer ≤ 1:2 beyond 1 year after successful treatment are considered serofast. Symptomatic infants born to women believed to be serofast represent aternal reinfection.

¶ Full diagnostic evaluation of infants if maternal titers have not declined fourfold after appropriate therapy in a mother with early syphilis; no treatment is required if work-up is negative and follow-up is certain.

**Figure 20-112.** An approach to the evaluation of infants born to mothers with reactive serologic tests for syphilis. MHA-TP, microhemagglutination assay for *Treponema pallidum* antibody; RPR, rapid plasma reagin test; VDRL, Venereal Disease Research Laboratory test.

content (more than 150 mg/dL). The presence of red blood cells in the CSF as a result of a traumatic lumbar puncture can produce a false-positive serologic reaction. Also, a reactive CSF VDRL test may be due to passive transfer of nontreponemal IgG antibodies from serum into the CSF. Examination of the CSF for IgM reactivities to specific *T pallidum* antigens and *T pallidum* DNA by PCR may prove more useful for diagnosis of congenital neurosyphilis.

Infants with reactive serology at delivery should have serial quantitative nontreponemal tests performed until the test results show nonreactivity. Similarly, infants who are seronegative but whose mothers acquired syphilis late in gestation should be followed with serial testing after penicillin therapy is instituted. Follow-up for these infants can be incorporated into routine pediatric care at 2, 4, 6, 12, and 15 months. In infants with congenital syphilis, nontreponemal serologic tests become nonreactive within 12 months after appropriate treatment. Uninfected infants usually

become seronegative by 6 months of age. Infants with persistently low, stable titers of nontreponemal tests require retreatment. A reactive treponemal test at 12 to 15 months of age when the infant has lost all maternal antibody confirms the diagnosis of congenital syphilis. Infants with abnormal CSF findings should have a repeat lumbar puncture performed at 6 months after therapy. A reactive CSF VDRL test result or an abnormal protein content or cell count at that time is an indication for retreatment.

## TREATMENT AND PREVENTION

Congenital syphilis is effectively prevented by prenatal screening and penicillin treatment of infected women, their sexual partners, and their newborn infants. The decision to treat an infant for congenital syphilis is based on the clinical presentation, previous serologic test results and treatment of the mother, and the results of serologic testing of the infant and mother at the time of delivery.

Treatment at birth is required for the following situations: the infant is symptomatic, maternal treatment was inadequate or unknown, the mother was treated with drugs other than penicillin, the mother was treated within 4 weeks of delivery, or adequate follow-up care of the infant is uncertain. Symptomatic infants or asymptomatic infants with abnormal results of CSF examination should be treated with either aqueous crystalline penicillin G (50,000 U/kg intravenously every 12 hours for the first week of life, followed by every 8 hours beyond 7 days of age) or aqueous procaine penicillin G (50,000 U/kg intramuscularly once daily) for a minimum of 10 days. Asymptomatic infants with a normal CSF examination and normal laboratory evaluation can be treated with a single intramuscular injection of benzathine penicillin G at a dosage of 50,000 U/kg. If the risk of infection in the asymptomatic infant is significant and adequate follow-up cannot be ensured, the 10-day course of aqueous or procaine penicillin is recommended by the CDC, regardless of results of the CSF examination. Failure of a single injection of benzathine penicillin in the treatment of congenital syphilis has been reported. Treatment failures have been attributed to the inability of penicillin to adequately penetrate and achieve treponemicidal concentrations in certain sites such as the aqueous humor and central nervous system.

## Selected Readings

Centers for Disease Control. Congenital syphilis, New York City, 1986–1988. MMWR 1989;38:825.

Grimprel E, Sánchez PJ, Wendel GD, et al. Use of polymerase chain reaction and rabbit infectivity testing to detect *Treponema pallidum* in amniotic fluid, fetal and neonatal sera, and cerebrospinal fluid. J Clin Microbiol 1991;29:1711.

Ingall D, Musher D, Sánchez PJ. Syphilis. In: Remington JS, Klein JO, eds. Infectious diseases of the fetus and newborn infant. Philadelphia: WB Saunders (in press).

Sánchez PJ. Congenital syphilis. In: Aronoff SC, ed. Advances in pediatric infectious diseases. St. Louis: Mosby-Year Book, 1992:161.

Sánchez PJ, McCracken GH, Wendel GD, et al. Molecular analysis of the fetal IgM response to *Treponema pallidum* antigens: implications for improved serodiagnosis of congenital syphilis. J Infect Dis 1989;159:508.

Sánchez PJ, Wendel GD, Grimprel E, et al. Evaluation of molecular methodologies and rabbit infectivity testing for the diagnosis of congenital syphilis and neonatal central nervous system invasion by *Treponema pallidum*. J Infect Dis 1993;167:148.

Sánchez PJ. Syphilis. In: Burg FD, Ingelfinger JR, Wald ER, eds. Gellis & Kagan's Current Pediatric Therapy. Philadelphia: WB Saunders 1993:590.

Stoll BJ, Lee FK, Larsen S, et al. Clinical and serologic evaluation of neonates for congenital syphilis: A continuing diagnostic dilemma. J Infect Dis 1993;167:1093.

*Principles and Practice of Pediatrics, Second Edition.*
edited by Frank A. Oski et al. J. B. Lippincott Company, Philadelphia © 1994.

# RUBELLA
*Jane D. Siegel*

Rubella first was recognized in 1814 as a mild exanthematous disease distinct from scarlatina, roseola, and urticaria and responsible for large epidemics. In 1941, an Australian ophthalmologist, Norman McAlister Gregg, made the association between congenital cataracts and a history of rubella early in pregnancy. His was the first description of the variety of defects now known as the congenital rubella syndrome. Isolation of the rubella virus in tissue culture in 1962 was soon followed by the development of live, attenuated vaccines. Since licensure of the vaccine in the United States in 1969, the total number of cases of rubella annually reported in the United States had declined by 99% to 0.23 per 100,000 population in 1986. In 1988, an all-time low of 225 cases of rubella was reported to the Centers for Disease Control (CDC). In 1989, however, the number of reported cases nearly doubled. In 1990, cases tripled to 0.4 per 100,000 population. In 1990, outbreaks were classified into two categories: outbreaks in which cases occurred in or were linked to settings where unvaccinated adults congregate (eg, prisons, colleges, workplaces) and outbreaks among children and adults in religious communities with low levels of rubella vaccination coverage (eg, Amish).

## PATHOGENESIS

Transplacental transmission of the rubella virus occurs during the viremic phase of primary maternal infection in the week before the onset of rash. The exact rate of transmission is controversial, and most rates reported in early studies are probably underestimates. Placental infection rates of 85% to 91% with fetal infection rates of 45% to 50% have been reported. In a 1982 prospective study of virologically confirmed rubella during pregnancy in England, Miller and colleagues found fetal infection rates of 90% when symptomatic maternal rubella occurred during the first 12 weeks of gestation, 25% to 30% during the second trimester, and 53% during the third trimester. Fetal viremia results in disseminated infection with persistence of the virus throughout fetal life and into postnatal life. Gestational age at the time of infection, the quantity of virus delivered to the fetus, the ability of the fetus to limit replication, and strain variation in virulence determine the risk for malformations. Sallomi (1966) reported the incidence of anomalies according to gestational age when maternal infection occurred as follows: weeks 1 to 4, 61%; weeks 5 to 8, 26%; weeks 9 to 12, 8%; weeks 13 to 16, 1% to 4%; weeks 17 to 20, 0.5% to 2%; weeks 21 to 40, less than 1%. Most studies report no defects after maternal infection later than 18 to 20 weeks' gestation. Congenital infection after maternal reinfection is rare, but both congenital rubella syndrome and late-onset rubella syndrome are reported. Rubella virus may be transmitted to the susceptible newborn in breast milk or by the respiratory route, but postnatal disease is usually not severe.

Several mechanisms of fetal damage have been proposed. The rubella virus has both a mitotic inhibitory and cytolytic action on fetal cells that is selective for cells from different tissues. Depressed mitotic activity results in intrauterine growth retardation, a diminished number of cells per organ, and specific malformations of organs. Cytolytic action on cells resulting in necrosis may occur in organs with normal architecture and development, but the virus persists within cells. Examples of this mechanism of action are damage to the organ of Corti associated with deafness, myocarditis, hepatitis, and interstitial pneumonitis. Vasculitis of the placenta decreases the fetal blood supply, resulting in intrauterine growth retardation; vasculitis of the fetus results in vascular anomalies. Circulating immune complexes containing rubella viral antigens have been identified in the acute phase of the late-onset rubella syndrome.

## CLINICAL MANIFESTATIONS

Spontaneous abortion, stillbirths, and major organ defects are associated with congenital rubella infection. Maternal disease prior to implantation (just before and 3 weeks after the last menstrual period) may result in fetal infection. Although some investigators report no adverse effects associated with infection this early, an increased incidence of spontaneous abortion during this period is likely. Multiple-organ defects are most likely to result from maternal infection before completion of organogenesis in the first 12 weeks of gestation. The most commonly observed intrauterine defects are as follows:

1. Auditory. Sensorineural hearing loss of varying degrees is present in nearly all patients. Deafness occurs in 50% of patients as one of several defects or as an isolated defect associated with infection beyond 12 weeks' gestation. All infants with congenital rubella require evaluation of hearing with brain stem auditory-evoked responses.
2. Cardiac. Patent ductus arteriosus with or without pulmonary artery or pulmonic valvular stenosis, aortic stenosis, and ventricular septal defect.
3. Ophthalmologic. Cataract, pigmentary retinopathy, and microphthalmia.
4. Neurologic. Central auditory imperception, delayed development, microcephaly, and hypotonia.
5. Growth. Intrauterine and postnatal growth retardation.

Clinical manifestations related to persistent infection that may be present at birth include thrombocytopenia, hepatitis, jaundice, dermal erythropoiesis or "blueberry muffin spots" (see Color Figure 22), osteopathy with the characteristic "celery stalk" lesions (see Fig 20-107), meningoencephalitis, interstitial pneumonitis, and myocarditis. These lesions may resolve, but when present in combination with severe malformations, the risk for mortality is increased.

Some infants with intrauterine infection have few or no symptoms at birth but develop severe multisystem disease after a latent period of several months. The most notable manifestations of this late-onset rubella syndrome are a generalized interstitial pneumonitis associated with cough, tachypnea, and cyanosis, chronic rubelliform rash, chronic diarrhea, recurrent infections associated with defects of both the humoral and cell-mediated immune system, and progressive neurologic deterioration. Finally, endocrine abnormalities associated with an increase in autoantibodies may be observed. Insulin-dependent diabetes mellitus, hypothyroidism, and thyrotoxicosis manifest at several years of age in children with congenital rubella infection.

## DIAGNOSIS

The diagnosis of congenital rubella infection is confirmed by isolation of the virus from the nasopharynx, urine, buffy coat, stool, cerebrospinal fluid (CSF), or cataract. Eighty percent of infected infants excrete the virus at birth and for as long as 1 or 2 years. Viral isolation is often impractical because the tissue culture cells required for isolation of the rubella virus are not usually available in routine virology laboratories. Demonstration of rubella-specific IgM antibody at birth and an increase in the infant's IgG titer over 3 to 6 months with stable or decreasing maternal IgG titers provides serologic confirmation of the diagnosis. Not all infants with congenital rubella infection have IgM present at birth; therefore, absent rubella-specific IgM does not exclude the diagnosis. The traditional hemagglutination inhibition and fluorescence immunoassay tests have been replaced by kits that use latex agglutination and enzyme-linked immunosorbent assay (ELISA) techniques. Sensitivity and specificity of the method employed by the individual laboratory should be verified before interpreting the results of serologic testing.

## PREVENTION

Active immunization with live, attenuated rubella virus vaccine is the most effective means of prevention of congenital rubella syndrome. The only vaccine available for use in the United States—the RA 27/3, a strain grown in human embryonic lung tissue culture—is immunogenic in more than 89% of recipients and provides long-term protective immunity that is probably lifelong. The strategy of immunizing all infants at 15 months of age is more efficacious for decreasing the incidence of congenital rubella syndrome than a selective strategy that calls for routine immunization of prepubescent girls and women of childbearing age only. Women who are identified during pregnancy as nonimmune should be immunized in the postpartum period. Vaccine virus shed by the mother does not cause disease in the neonate. Postpartum immunization is not a contraindication for breastfeeding.

Immunization with rubella vaccine is contraindicated during pregnancy, and it is recommended that a woman not conceive during the 3-month period after immunization. Since 1971, the CDC has maintained a register to monitor the risks to the fetus of exposure to live, attenuated rubella virus vaccine within the 3 months before or the 3 months after conception. Data collected from more than 500 infants whose mothers received a rubella vaccine during this high-risk period show that vaccine viruses can cross the placenta and infect the fetus but do not produce the defects of congenital rubella syndrome (MMWR, 1987). The rate of isolation of vaccine virus from the products of conception is only 3% for the currently used RA 27/3 vaccine as compared with 20% for the Cendehill and HPV-77 vaccines used before 1979. Serologic evidence exists for subclinical intrauterine infection in 1% to 3% of infants born to susceptible vaccinees for all vaccines used. The theoretical maximum risk for the occurrence of congenital rubella syndrome after immunization is 1.2%. This is considerably less than the 20% to 50% risk associated with maternal infection with wild-type rubella virus during the first trimester of pregnancy and no greater than the 2% or 3% risk of major birth defects occurring by chance alone. Thus, while pregnancy remains a contraindication to rubella immunization, inadvertent administration of rubella vaccine during the first trimester of pregnancy should not be considered an indication to interrupt the pregnancy.

If a nonimmune pregnant woman is exposed to rubella during the first trimester of pregnancy, serial IgM and IgG rubella antibody studies should be performed to determine if infection has occurred. Termination of pregnancy is considered if infection occurred during the first 12 weeks of pregnancy. If termination of pregnancy is not an option, immune globulin 0.55 mL/kg administered within 72 hours of exposure may prevent or modify infection in an exposed, susceptible person. Protection is not complete even in the absence of clinical disease in the mother because infants with congenital rubella have been delivered by women who received immune globulin shortly after exposure.

Infants with congenital rubella are considered contagious and are maintained in blood and body fluid isolation. Only healthcare workers known to be seropositive should be permitted to care for such infants. Pregnant personnel and visitors who are not known to be immune should be restricted from contact with infants with congenital rubella.

## Selected Readings

Burke JP, Hinman AR, Krugman S, eds. International Symposium on Prevention of Congenital Rubella Infection. Reviews of Infectious Diseases 1985;7(Suppl 1):S1.

Centers for Disease Control and Prevention. Rubella vaccination during pregnancy—United States, 1971–1988. MMWR 1989;38:289.

Centers for Disease Control and Prevention. Rubella prevention: recommendations of the Immunization Practices Advisory Committee. MMWR 1990;39:RR-15.

Centers for Disease Control and Prevention. Increase in rubella and congenital rubella syndrome—United States, 1988–1990. MMWR 1991;40:93.

Miller E, Cradock-Watson JE, Pollock TM. Consequences of confirmed maternal rubella at successive stages of pregnancy. Lancet 1982;2:781.

Sallomi SJ. Rubella in pregnancy. Obstet Gynecol 1966;26:252.

*Principles and Practice of Pediatrics, Second Edition.*
edited by Frank A. Oski et al. J. B. Lippincott Company, Philadelphia © 1994.

# TOXOPLASMOSIS

*Jane D. Siegel*

*Toxoplasma gondii* is an intracellular parasite with a worldwide distribution. The cat family is the definitive host for this organism. Nonfeline mammals or birds ingest infective oocysts from contaminated soil. Tissue cysts then accumulate in the organs and skeletal muscle of these animals. The possible routes of transmission from animal to human are direct contact with cat feces, ingestion of undercooked meat containing infective cysts, and ingestion of fruits or vegetables that have been in contaminated soil. Infection may be passed from human to human by the transplacental route and rarely by transfusion of infected leukocytes or transplantation of infected organs or bone marrow. Most human infections are asymptomatic, and significant disease develops when reactivation occurs in association with suppression of the immune system. Toxoplasmosis is now an important opportunistic infection in patients with the acquired immune deficiency syndrome (AIDS). Encephalitis develops in 30% of previously infected AIDS patients.

The prevalence of chronic or latent infection with *T gondii* varies widely among different adult populations throughout the world. Seropositivity increases with age. In the United States, overall seropositivity of pregnant women is 32%, with variation from 16% for the 15- to 19-year age group to 50% for women 35 years of age or older. In contrast, the overall seropositivity rate for women in France is 87% with variation only from 80% at age 15 to 19 years to 96% at 35 years of age and older. The incidence of congenital toxoplasmosis in the United States is estimated to be 1.3 of 1000 live births as compared with a rate of 3 to 10 of 1000 live births in Paris, Vienna, and the Netherlands.

## PATHOGENESIS

Congenital *Toxoplasma* infection occurs only during maternal parasitemia associated with primary infection. Clinical signs are present in 10% of infected adults, but transplacental transmission results from asymptomatic as well as symptomatic maternal infection. No cases have been reported to occur in subsequent pregnancies of women who gave birth to congenitally infected children. Chronic infection is not associated with infertility or spontaneous abortion. Although the actual rate of fetal infection increases as pregnancy advances, the severity of clinical manifestations is greatest when maternal infection is acquired during the first trimester. Overall, the risk of transmission without treatment is 30% to 50% with variations of 25% in the first trimester, 54% in the second trimester, and 65% in the third trimester. Desmonts and Couvreur (1974) report the risk of severe manifestations of infection decreases from 75% in the first trimester to 0% in the third trimester.

## CLINICAL MANIFESTATIONS

Stillbirth and death in the early neonatal period are the most severe results of congenital infection. Most infants born with congenital *Toxoplasma* infection are asymptomatic in the neonatal period with severe disease at birth in only 10% of infants. Long-term follow-up of asymptomatic infants reveals chorioretinitis in as many as 85% and severe neurologic sequelae in 10% to 20%. At birth, these infants are indistinguishable from those who are asymptomatic. Infants with generalized congenital toxoplasmosis may have clinical syndromes indistinguishable from those associated with other agents of congenital infection. The central nervous system is always involved in symptomatic infants. The prominence of neurologic abnormalities is indicative of toxoplasmosis. The classic triad of hydrocephalus, chorioretinitis, and intracranial calcifications can be accompanied by fever, maculopapular or petechial rash, hepatosplenomegaly, jaundice, convulsions, and abnormal cerebrospinal fluid (CSF) (xanthochromia and mononuclear pleocytosis). Markedly elevated protein concentrations (more than 1 g per 100 mL) in ventricular fluid and hydrocephalus may be explained by periaqueductal and periventricular vasculitis with necrosis that are specifically associated with toxoplasmosis. Intracranial calcifications are distributed diffusely throughout the brain (Fig 20-113) in contrast to the periventricular pattern associated with cytomegalovirus. Severely affected infants may also have myocarditis, pneumonitis, thrombocytopenia, and nephrotic syndrome.

## DIAGNOSIS

*T gondii* may be isolated from the placenta, amniotic fluid, CSF, or blood by inoculation into mice or tissue culture using human fibroblasts. Because these techniques are available only in research laboratories, routine diagnosis is made serologically. The Sabin-Feldman dye test is considered the gold standard to which all newer tests are compared. This test is performed only in reference laboratories because of the requirement for viable *Toxoplasma* organisms. Commercially available methods for measuring specific IgG and IgM antibodies to *T gondii* include indirect immunofluorescent antibody, direct agglutination tests, and enzyme-linked immunosorbent assays (ELISAs). Immunoblot techniques are being evaluated. ELISAs are preferred over the previously used immunofluorescent antibody tests for their improved sensitivity and specificity. It is important to know what test method is used for antibody determination, because there is considerable variation in reliability of commercially available kits. For example, the "double-sandwich" or antibody-capture ELISA technique for detection of IgM antibodies has substantially greater sensitivity and specificity than the conventional IgM ELISA technique.

The presence of IgM antibodies or rising titers of IgG antibodies in a pregnant woman is indicative of acute infection. Serial determinations are needed because IgG antibodies may remain elevated at high titer for long periods with chronic infection. Daffos and coworkers (1988) demonstrated the ability to diagnose infection during gestation in 39 (93%) of 42 fetuses studied in France using a combination of the following studies: culture specimens of amniotic fluid and fetal blood obtained from the umbilical cord under ultrasound guidance, presence of *Toxoplasma*-specific IgM and nonspecific measures of infection (leukocyte count and differential, platelet count, total IgM level, lactic dehydrogenase level, and Γ-glutamyltransferase level) in fetal blood, and ultrasound examination of the fetal brain. Absence of IgM in fetal blood does not exclude the diagnosis of congenital infection because production of IgM may be delayed until after birth due to the immaturity of the immune system and possible inhibition of synthesis by maternal IgG. This extensive prenatal evaluation may be helpful in making decisions concerning interruption of pregnancy and prenatal therapy.

Postnatally, the diagnosis of congenital toxoplasmosis may be proved by isolation of the organism from the placenta or by serial determinations of specific IgM and IgG antibody levels in the infant and mother. Initially, low IgG titers and absent IgM antibody in mother and baby suggest infection before pregnancy and do not require continued follow-up. The presence of IgM antibody in the first 3 months of life and increasing IgG in the infant during the first year of life support a diagnosis of congenital toxoplasmosis. Specific IgM antibody in the CSF is diagnostic of congenital *Toxoplasma* infection.

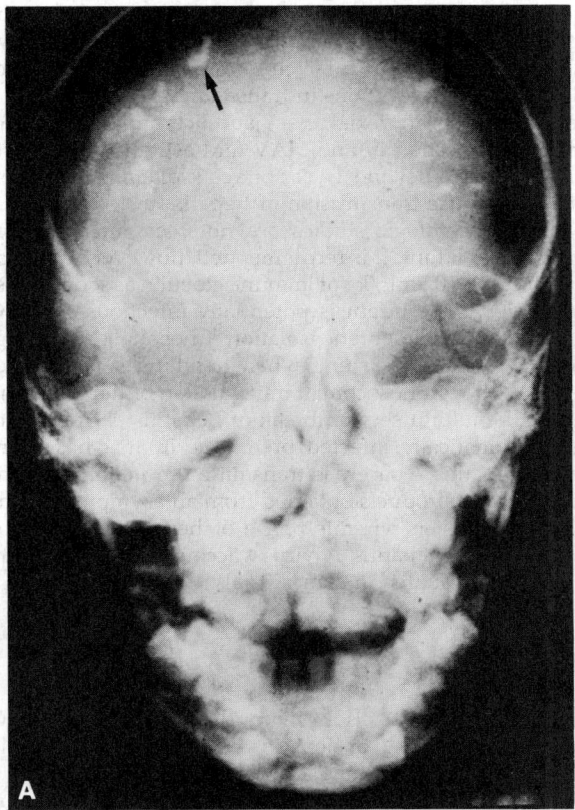
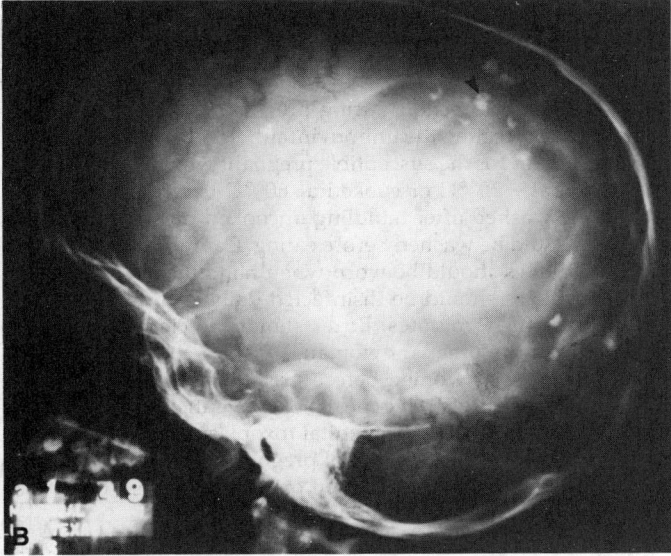

**Figure 20-113.** Anteroposterior (**A**) and lateral (**B**) skull roentgenogram demonstrating diffuse cerebral calcifications (*arrows*) in an infant with congenital toxoplasmosis. (Courtesy of Guido Currarino, MD, Dallas, Texas.)

## TREATMENT

In large studies of several hundred women with well-documented acute toxoplasmosis acquired during pregnancy, Desmonts and Couvreur (1974) and Daffos and coworkers (1988) have demonstrated the efficacy of treatment with spiramycin during pregnancy for the prevention of severe fetal abnormalities. Spiramycin is a macrolide antibiotic that is active against *T gondii* in animal experiments. It does not consistently cross the placenta; therefore, therapeutic benefits are attributed to its action within the placenta. Spiramycin is readily available in most countries, but in the United States, it must be obtained from the Food and Drug Administration by special request. A 3-week course of spiramycin (2 to 3 g/d in four divided doses) repeated at 2-week intervals until delivery resulted in significantly more normal children: 76% versus 44%, P less than .001 (Desmonts and Couvreur, 1974). The addition of pyramethamine and a sulfonamide to the treatment regimen of a mother with a prenatal diagnosis of congenital infection may have a beneficial effect on fetal outcome, but additional data are needed before a recommendation for routine addition of these drugs can be made.

Evaluation of postnatal treatment of congenitally infected infants is difficult because of the variations in outcome of infection and disease associated with *Toxoplasma* infection. Postnatal treatment has no effect on the severe damage that has occurred before delivery, but it may prevent progression of disease and allow healing of tissues that are not irreversibly damaged. Long-term follow-up care is necessary because sequelae of congenital infection such as chorioretinitis may not appear for several years.

The organism is never completely eradicated, and tissue cysts persist for life, especially in the eye and central nervous system. Because Wilson and coworkers (1980) report that the incidence of late adverse sequelae may be reduced significantly in treated children, treatment is recommended for both asymptomatic as well as symptomatic children with a confirmed diagnosis of congenital *Toxoplasma* infection. The combination of pyramethamine and sulfadiazine is the preferred regimen because of synergism against *Toxoplasma* organisms. The usual dose of pyramethamine is 1 mg/kg/d in two divided doses administered daily initially but decreased to 3-day intervals because the half-life of the drug is 4 or 5 days. For infants with severe disease, a daily loading dose of 2 mg/kg/d for the first 2 or 3 days may be beneficial. Sulfadiazine or trisulfapyrimidines, 50 to 100 mg/kg/day, are given in two divided doses. Sulfisoxazole should not be used because it is less effective in in vitro studies. Folinic acid, 5 mg twice a week, is also administered because pyramethamine is a potent folic acid antagonist.

The optimal duration of therapy has not been established. Infants with proven congenital infection should receive an initial 21-day course of pyramethamine, sulfadiazine, and folinic acid followed by a 4- to 6-week course of spiramycin, 100 mg/kg/d in 2 to 3 divided doses. No additional therapy is given for infants whose mothers acquired primary *Toxoplasma* infection during pregnancy but do not have serologic evidence of congenital infection. Infants with confirmed congenital infection should receive alternating courses of these two regimens for the remainder of the first year of life. In the presence of active inflammation (eg, chorioretinitis, CSF protein ≥100 mg/dL), the addition of prednisone, 1 to 2 mg/kg/d may be beneficial. The prednisone is tapered after the active inflammation has resolved. Spiramycin alone may be considered as initial therapy for infants whose mothers have serologic evidence of infection but the date of infection is unknown; therapy is discontinued when congenital infection is ruled out serologically.

Infants with congenital toxoplasmosis must be followed for several years to detect reactivation and evaluate the extent of neurologic and developmental sequelae.

## PREVENTION

Prevention of primary infection during pregnancy is the most effective means of protecting the unborn infant. Several practices are effective measures for the susceptible pregnant woman. Meat should be frozen at −20 °C or cooked at 60 °C before eating. Hands should be washed after handling uncooked meat. Fruits and vegetables should be washed before eating. Cat feces should be avoided and gloves should be worn when handling cat litter boxes. Cat litter boxes should be disinfected daily with boiling water left in place for 5 minutes. Boxes should be cleaned by someone other than the pregnant woman.

Serologic screening of women before pregnancy or early in pregnancy may be a cost-effective means of prevention in areas of the world with high rates of congenital toxoplasmosis. When primary infection occurs, interruption of pregnancy or treatment of the pregnant women with spiramycin or the combination of pyramethamine and sulfadiazine should be considered.

### Selected Readings

Alpert G, Plotkin SA. A practical guide to the diagnosis of congenital infections in the newborn infant. Pediatr Clin North Am 1986;33:465.
Carter AO, Frank JW. Congenital toxoplasmosis: epidemiologic features and control. Can Med Assoc J 1986;135:618.
Daffos F, Forestier F, Capella-Pavlovsky M, et al. Prenatal management of 746 pregnancies at risk for congenital toxoplasmosis. N Engl J Med 1988;318:271.
Desmonts G, Couvreur J. Congenital toxoplasmosis. N Engl J Med 1974;290:1110.
Wilson CB, Remington JS, Stagno S, Reynolds DW. Development of adverse sequelae in children born with subclinical congenital *Toxoplasma* infection. Pediatrics 1980;66:767.

*Principles and Practice of Pediatrics, Second Edition.*
edited by Frank A. Oski et al. J. B. Lippincott Company, Philadelphia © 1994.

## HEPATITIS VIRUSES
*Pablo J. Sánchez and Jane D. Siegel*

### HEPATITIS A

Maternal infection with hepatitis A virus (HAV) in early pregnancy may result, on rare occasions, in prematurity and spontaneous abortion. It has not been associated with increased rates of congenital malformation or intrauterine growth retardation. Pregnant women with HAV hepatitis generally do not transmit the infection to their offspring because the associated viremia is transient and low grade.

These infants, however, are at risk of acquiring infection during delivery if the mother has jaundice or had acute hepatitis within the prior 2 weeks. Most infected infants are asymptomatic and exhibit only mild elevations in transaminase levels. Rarely does nausea, vomiting, anorexia, fever, jaundice, and dark urine occur in infancy. Detection of anti-HAV IgM acutely and persistence of anti-HAV IgG beyond 1 year of age is diagnostic of neonatal infection. Because transmission of hepatitis A to the neonate is rare, routine serologic studies are not recommended for the asymptomatic infant. It is recommended, however, that exposed infants receive 0.02 mL/kg of immune globulin as soon as possible after delivery. The infant is potentially infectious for 6 weeks and is maintained in enteric isolation if hospitalized during this period. Strict hand washing when handling soiled diapers is stressed. Although nosocomial transmission of hepatitis A is not common, a multinursery outbreak of hepatitis A from exposure to asymptomatically infected premature infants has been described. Hepatitis A rarely is transmitted to neonates by transfusion of blood products obtained from an asymptomatic donor during the transient viremic phase of hepatitis A infection. A live, attenuated hepatitis A virus vaccine has been developed and is being evaluated in clinical trials.

### HEPATITIS B

Hepatitis B virus (HBV) is a 42-nm, double-shelled DNA virus. The inner core consists of hepatitis B core antigen, hepatitis B e antigen (HBeAg), DNA, and DNA polymerase. The outer shell is composed of hepatitis B surface antigen (HBsAg). In about 5% to 10% of adults with acute HBV hepatitis, a chronic HBsAg carrier state develops. HBeAg is found in the serum of some individuals who are HBsAg-positive. Ninety percent of infants delivered of women who are positive for both HBsAg and HBeAg become infected. If the HBsAg-positive mother is HBeAg-negative or has antibody to HBeAg, only 25% or 12% of infants, respectively, become infected.

Vertical transmission of HBV occurs when the mother has acute hepatitis B during the third trimester or within the first 2 postpartum months, or if the mother is a chronic HBsAg carrier. About 5% of neonatal hepatitis B infection is transmitted transplacentally, presumably as a result of leakage of infected maternal blood into fetal circulation. HBV infection is not associated with congenital defects or fetal malformations. Ninety-five percent of neonatal infections occur at the time of delivery from the infant's exposure to infected maternal blood or cervical and vaginal secretions. If perinatal infection does not occur, the infant may be at risk for subsequent infection from close contact with household members who are infected or are chronic carriers.

Neonatal infection usually is asymptomatic with only mild elevation of transaminase levels, although chronic active hepatitis B with or without cirrhosis, chronic persistent hepatitis, and fatal fulminant hepatitis can occur. Infected infants usually do not become HBsAg-positive until several weeks after birth. About 90% of infants infected perinatally become chronic HBV carriers, and one in four infants who become chronic carriers develops cirrhosis or hepatocellular carcinoma. There is a 275-fold increase in the risk of developing hepatocellular carcinoma during the third and fourth decades in chronic carriers. This risk is greatest for carriers who acquired the infection perinatally.

Effective prophylaxis of HBV infection has been possible since licensure of the first hepatitis B virus vaccine in 1982. Both the highly purified vaccine prepared from human plasma (Heptavax B, licensed but no longer produced in the United States) and the recombinant DNA vaccines (Recombivax-HB, Engerix-B) are safe, are highly immunogenic in neonates, and have an efficacy of about 90%. The Centers for Disease Control and Prevention

(CDC) suggests that universal screening of all pregnant women for HBsAg is cost-effective and is the most suitable strategy for control of perinatal HBV transmission. Prenatal questioning designed to identify women in high-risk groups in urban populations fails to detect about 50% of those who are HB$_s$ Ag-positive. Moreover, prenatal screening allows prompt institution of neonatal prophylaxis after delivery and minimizes risk of delivery room attendants' exposure to the mother's infective blood and body fluids.

The CDC recommends a combination of passive immunization with hepatitis B immune globulin (HBIG) and active immunization with hepatitis B virus vaccine for all newborns whose mothers are HBsAg-positive, regardless of the HBeAg or anti-HBe status. HBIG (0.5 mL) is administered intramuscularly as soon as possible after delivery, preferably within 12 hours. HBIG efficacy decreases markedly if treatment is delayed beyond 48 hours. Hepatitis B virus vaccine is administered intramuscularly at a separate site at birth or within 7 days, and administration is repeated at 1 and 6 months after the first dose. HBsAg may be detected for 24 hours after a dose of vaccine. An HBsAg-positive result at any other time indicates a vaccine failure, and the infant should not receive additional doses of HBIG or vaccine. Testing for HBsAg and measurement of anti-HBs is recommended at 9 months of age or later to determine the efficacy of therapy. The presence of anti-HBs indicates successful prophylaxis and immunization. Although the efficacy of booster doses in infants is not yet known, infants who are negative for anti-HBs and HBsAg should receive another dose of vaccine and be retested. Protection from immunization persists for at least 5 years. Household members and sexual contacts of HBsAg-positive mothers should be screened, and if no evidence exists of previous HBV infection, they should also be immunized.

Infants delivered by HBsAg-positive women are bathed as soon as possible after delivery to remove all maternal blood and secretions. Intramuscular injections should be delayed until bathing is completed. These infants are placed on blood and body fluid precautions. Those infants who remain in the hospital and later require surgical procedures should be tested for HBsAg. Infants who have received both active and passive prophylaxis may be breast-fed.

Recently, both the American Academy of Pediatrics and the CDC have recommended universal immunization of all infants with hepatitis B virus vaccine in an effort to control hepatitis B virus infections. The first dose of hepatitis B virus vaccine should be administered to newborns before hospital discharge, the second dose at 1 to 2 months of age, and the third dose at 6 to 18 months of age. An alternative schedule of the three doses administered at 2, 4, and 6 to 18 months concurrently with other routine vaccines, may be used for HBsAg-negative infants not vaccinated at birth. For premature infants and ill infants in the first few days of life, hepatitis B virus vaccine may be delayed until hospital discharge, if the mother is not HBsAg-positive.

## DELTA HEPATITIS

Hepatitis D virus (delta virus) is a 35- to 37-nm RNA virus with an internal protein antigen (delta antigen) coated with HBsAg. Because it requires HBV for replication, hepatitis D may occur as a coinfection with acute HBV hepatitis or as a superinfection of an HBsAg carrier. The route of transmission is similar to HBV. It is diagnosed by detection of delta antigen in serum during acute infection and by the appearance of delta antibody. Vertical transmission has been reported, but the risks to the infant are undefined. Infants who become HBsAg carriers as a result of perinatal infection are also at risk of delta infection. No product is available to prevent delta infection in HBsAg carriers either before or after exposure.

## HEPATITIS C

Most cases of non-A, non-B (NANB) hepatitis recently have been attributed to hepatitis C virus (HCV) infection. HCV is a single-stranded RNA virus closely linked to the family of *Flaviviridae*, which includes the arboviruses of yellow fever and Dengue fever. Seroepidemiologic studies show that approximately 1% of volunteer blood donors screen positive for anti-HCV antibody. Transmission of HCV occurs after transfusion of infected blood products, intravenous drug use, sexual intercourse, occupational injury with blood-contaminated needles, and human bites. Intrafamilial transmission also has been documented. Because about half of all cases of HCV infection have no identifiable risk factor, other modes of transmission seem to exist. Perinatal transmission has been documented; although its frequency is not yet fully known, it may play a role in sustaining a reservoir of HCV infection in the general population. Recent studies also suggest that vertical transmission from an HCV-antibody positive mother to her newborn infant may be enhanced by the presence of maternal and infant coinfection with the human immunodeficiency virus.

Infants born to HCV-antibody positive mothers should have serial measurements of serum alanine aminotransferase levels and HCV antibody for at least the first 15 months of age. Tests for HCV antibody include an enzyme-linked immunosorbent assay (ELISA) and a recombinant immunoblot assay (RIBA), both of which measure IgG antibody to recombinant HCV antigens. Recently, a polymerase chain reaction assay was developed for detection of viral RNA. Infected infants can develop a chronic hepatitis. In adults, half of all HCV infections appears to be chronic; in 20% of patients, the disease progresses to cirrhosis. Moreover, HCV is implicated as a cause of hepatocellular carcinoma. HCV infection may benefit from use of interferon alpha.

No preventive strategy is available. Immune serum globulin (0.06 mL/kg) may be useful in preventing HCV infection after accidental exposure to blood from a patient with hepatitis C, but efficacy has not been established, and its use for prevention of vertical transmission is not routinely recommended.

Transmission of NANB hepatitis by blood transfusion may be prevented by screening donors for antibody to HCV, elevated serum alanine aminotransferase levels, and antibody to the hepatitis B core antigen.

## Hepatitis E (Epidemic or Enterically Transmitted Non-A, Non-B Hepatitis)

Another agent has been described in water-borne epidemics of NANB hepatitis in several areas of Southeast Asia, North Africa, and Mexico. The viral agent appears to be a small RNA virus of the family caliviridae with similar characteristics of the picornaviridae, which include enterovirus type 72, the hepatitis A virus. Transmission occurs by the fecal-oral route similarly to that of hepatitis A. Epidemic NANB hepatitis occurs more frequently during pregnancy, particularly in the second and third trimester according to research by Khuroo and coworkers (1981). The attack rate in the first, second, and third trimesters is reported to be 9%, 19%, and 19%, respectively, with an overall rate of 17% during pregnancy. This statistic compares to a rate of only 2% in similarly exposed men and nonpregnant women of childbearing age. Pregnant women with acute epidemic NANB hepatitis in the third trimester are also at higher risk for developing fulminant hepatic failure, which is associated with a case-fatality rate as high as 75%.

No serologic test has been developed. Prophylactic therapy with immune serum globulin has not been shown to be effective. The only preventive measures available are good sanitation and avoiding ingestion of potentially contaminated food and water.

## Selected Readings

Bohman VR, Stettler W, Little BB, Wendel GD, Sutor LJ, Cunningham FG. Seroprevalence and risk factors for hepatitis C virus antibody in pregnant women. Obstet Gynecol 1992;80:609.

Centers for Disease Control. Prevention of perinatal transmission of hepatitis B virus: prenatal screening of all pregnant women for hepatitis B surface antigen. MMWR 1988;37:341.

Centers for Disease Control. Hepatitis B virus: a comprehensive strategy for eliminating transmission in the United States through universal childhood vaccination: recommendations of the Immunization Practices Advisory Committee (ACIP). MMWR 1991;40(No. RR-13):1.

Committee on Infectious Diseases, American Academy of Pediatrics. Universal hepatitis B immunization. Pediatr 1992;89:795.

Khuroo MS, Teli MR, Skidmore S, et al. Incidence and severity of viral hepatitis in pregnancy. Am J Med 1981;70:252.

Lan Y-L, Tam AYC, Ng KW, et al. Response of preterm infants to hepatitis B vaccine. J Pediatr 1992;121:962.

Snydman DR. Hepatitis in pregnancy. N Engl J Med 1985;313:1398.

Watson JC, Fleming DW, Borella AJ, Olcott ES, Conrad RE, Baron RC. Vertical transmission of hepatitis A resulting in an outbreak in a neonatal intensive care unit. J Infect Dis 1993;167:567.

Weintrub PS, Veereman-Wauters G, Cowan MJ, Thaler MM. Hepatitis C virus infection in infants whose mothers took street drugs intravenously. J Pediatr 1991;119:869.

*Principles and Practice of Pediatrics, Second Edition.*
edited by Frank A. Oski et al. J. B. Lippincott Company, Philadelphia © 1994.

# NEISSERIA GONORRHOEAE
*Pablo J. Sánchez and Jane D. Siegel*

The prevalence of gonococcal infection during pregnancy varies from 0.6% to 7.6%. The highest rates are found in single, low-income, nonwhite women younger than 30 years old. Gonococcal infection during pregnancy has been associated with septic abortion, chorioamnionitis, premature rupture of membranes, delayed delivery after rupture of membranes, and premature delivery.

## TRANSMISSION

Transmission of *Neisseria gonorrhoeae* to the newborn infant can occur in utero, during delivery, or after birth. In utero acquisition occurs via an ascending route after rupture of amniotic membranes. More commonly, neonatal infection occurs at delivery from passage through an infected birth canal. About 30% of infants born vaginally to infected mothers become colonized with *N gonorrhoeae*. Horizontal transmission via fomites and by nursery personnel also is documented.

## CLINICAL MANIFESTATIONS AND DIAGNOSIS

Conjunctivitis is the most frequently observed clinical manifestation of gonococcal infection in newborns. Although *Chlamydia trachomatis* is the most common cause of ophthalmia neonatorum, *N gonorrhoeae* is important because it can cause severe eye damage. Gonococcal conjunctivitis typically appears 2 to 5 days after birth and produces an acute, purulent, bilateral conjunctivitis with lid edema and chemosis. If treatment is delayed, the cornea may ulcerate and scar with loss of visual acuity. Ultimately, the eye may perforate, resulting in panophthalmitis and loss of the eye. Presumptive diagnosis of gonococcal conjunctivitis may be made by Gram stain of the conjunctival exudate, which demonstrates gram-negative intracellular diplococci. The diagnosis must be confirmed by isolation of the organism on selective media, especially because *Moraxella catarrhalis* has a similar appearance on Gram stain. Sandstrom and colleagues (1984) report that other bacterial pathogens associated with conjunctivitis in the neonate that may be visualized on Gram stain are *Haemophilus* spp, *Staphylococcus aureus*, enterococcus, and *Streptococcus pneumoniae*. *Pseudomonas aeruginosa* may cause conjunctivitis with severe complications in debilitated neonates.

Not only the conjunctiva but also the pharynx, umbilicus, urethra, vagina, and rectum can serve as a focus of local or disseminated disease. Disseminated infection is usually manifested by septicemia, meningitis, or septic arthritis that typically involves multiple joints. Cutaneous gonococcal lesions in infants are rare, but gonococcal scalp abscess at the site of previous placement of a scalp electrode has been described.

## TREATMENT

Infants with gonococcal ophthalmia should be hospitalized and placed in contact isolation for 24 hours after initiation of parenteral antibiotic therapy. Because of the increased incidence of both penicillinase-producing and chromosomally mediated resistant strains of *N gonorrhoeae*, for empiric therapy the Centers for Disease Control and Prevention recommends ceftriaxone administered intravenously or intramuscularly at a dosage of 50 mg/kg/d (maximum 125 mg). Laga and colleagues claim that a single dose of ceftriaxone may be sufficient, but therapy is usually continued for 5 to 7 days. Alternatively, cefotaxime can be used. Hourly irrigation of the infected eye with saline until the purulent discharge resolves is an important part of effective therapy. If the organism is susceptible to penicillin, aqueous crystalline penicillin G administered intravenously at a dosage of 100,000 U/kg/d in two to four divided doses also is effective. Duration of therapy is at least 7 days for disseminated infection and at least 10 days for meningitis.

All *N gonorrhoeae* isolates should be tested for β-lactamase production and for chromosomally mediated resistance, which occurs to penicillin, tetracycline, erythromycin, cephalosporins, spectinomycin, and other aminoglycosides. Identification of plasmid-mediated high-level tetracycline resistance (minimal inhibitory concentration greater than or equal to 16 μg/mL) is of epidemiologic importance because of the propensity of these resistant strains to acquire other resistance determinants. The prevalence of these strains in a community influences the choice of agent used for topical prophylaxis as well as for treatment of disease.

## PREVENTION

Ophthalmic prophylaxis in the immediate postpartum period with either 1% silver nitrate, 0.5% erythromycin ointment, or 1% tetracycline ointment is effective in preventing gonococcal ophthalmia. Even with topical prophylaxis, some infants born to mothers with untreated gonococcal infection may develop gonococcal ophthalmia or disseminated disease. These infants should, therefore, receive a single intramuscular injection of ceftriaxone. If the isolate is known to be susceptible to penicillin, a single intramuscular injection of penicillin G (50,000 U for a full-term infant and 20,000 U for a low–birth-weight infant) may be administered. The optimal preventive measure is diagnosis and treatment of maternal gonococcal infection before delivery.

## Selected Readings

Centers for Disease Control. Antibiotic-resistant strains of *Neisseria gonorrhoeae*. MMWR 1987;36(Suppl 5):1.

Laga M, Naamara W, Brunham RC, et al. Single-dose therapy of gonococcal ophthalmia neonatorum with ceftriaxone. N Engl J Med 1986;315:1382.

Sandstrom KI, Bell TA, Chandler JW, et al. Microbial causes of neonatal conjunctivitis. J Pediatr 1984;5:706.

*Principles and Practice of Pediatrics, Second Edition.*
edited by Frank A. Oski et al. J. B. Lippincott Company, Philadelphia © 1994.

# CHLAMYDIA TRACHOMATIS

*Pablo J. Sánchez and Jane D. Siegel*

Chlamydiae are bacteria that possess both RNA and DNA but are incapable of producing adenosine triphosphate outside of cells. Therefore, these organisms are obligate intracellular pathogens that require tissue culture cells for growth in the laboratory. Of the two species, *Chlamydia psittaci* and *Chlamydia trachomatis*, only the latter is a genital pathogen associated with neonatal infection. *C trachomatis* has 15 serotypes divided into 2 groups: oculogenital serovars A to K and lymphogranuloma serovars L-1 to L-3. Oculogenital serovars are divided into trachoma serovars A to C, which cause hyperendemic blinding trachoma in the Far East, and genital serovars D to K, which result in genital neonatal infections.

The rate of cervical colonization with *C trachomatis* during pregnancy varies from 2% to 37%. The highest rates are found in young, unmarried, nonwhite women of lower socioeconomic status. Chlamydial infection during pregnancy is usually asymptomatic. Pregnant women with cervical chlamydial infection who have IgM antibody against *C trachomatis*, however, may be at increased risk for premature rupture of amniotic membranes and delivery of low–birth-weight infants.

## TRANSMISSION

Chlamydial infection of the newborn infant occurs most often at delivery, secondary to passage through an infected cervix. Neonatal infection after delivery by cesarean section reflects an ascending route of infection. Transplacental transmission is doubtful because *C trachomatis* is not associated with abnormalities present at birth that are characteristic of other congenital infections, and IgM antibody directed against *C trachomatis* has not been detected in umbilical cord blood.

Schachter and colleagues report that about two thirds of infants delivered vaginally by mothers colonized with *C trachomatis* develop IgM antibody or exhibit a persistence or rise in IgG antibodies to *C trachomatis* beyond 9 to 12 months of age. About 28% to 66% of exposed infants are colonized in the conjunctivae, 15% to 20% in the nasopharynx or throat, 8% to 14% in the vagina, and 14% to 20% in the rectum. Initial colonization with *C trachomatis* occurs in the conjunctiva and pharynx, and the rectum and vagina usually become colonized in the second through sixth months of life. Of infants colonized with *C trachomatis*, 50% to 75% develop conjunctivitis, and 11% to 29% develop pneumonia.

## CLINICAL MANIFESTATIONS

### Conjunctivitis

*C trachomatis* is the most common cause of ophthalmia neonatorum in developed countries where it causes 13% to 74% (mean, 29%) of neonatal conjunctivitis. Onset is usually 5 to 14 days after birth. Clinical illness ranges from a mild mucoid discharge in the medial canthus without significant conjunctival erythema to a profuse, purulent bilateral discharge with lid edema, severe chemosis, and edematous, friable conjunctivae. In the most severe cases, the clinical findings are indistinguishable from those associated with *Neisseria gonorrhoeae*. Subconjunctival lymphoid hypertrophy and follicular conjunctivitis rarely occur in the neonatal period. Some 19% to 83% of infants with conjunctivitis have nasopharyngeal carriage of *C trachomatis* when first examined.

Gram stain examination of the ocular discharge reveals both polymorphonuclear leukocytes and mononuclear cells. A Giemsa stain examination of a conjunctival scraping that contains a large number of epithelial cells detects chlamydial inclusions in the cytoplasm of the epithelia cells in 50% to 90% of cases.

Untreated chlamydial conjunctivitis resolves spontaneously after several weeks to months. Ocular carriage of the organism may persist for 2½ years. Occasionally, chlamydial conjunctivitis results in mild conjunctival scars with punctate keratitis and micropannus. Normal visual acuity is preserved in most cases.

### Pneumonia

*C trachomatis* accounts for 15% to 73% of afebrile pneumonia in infants 3 to 11 weeks of age. There is often a history of conjunctivitis or mucoid rhinorrhea, followed by gradually worsening tachypnea and a characteristic staccato cough. Most infants are afebrile or have mild temperature elevations. Infants may present with apnea in the absence of other signs of respiratory involvement, or they may develop apnea during the course of the pneumonia. Auscultation of the chest reveals diffuse rales with few wheezes. Hyperexpansion and diffuse bilateral interstitial or alveolar infiltrates are present on chest roentgenogram. Lobar consolidation and pleural effusion are unusual. Blood gas values typically show mild hypoxia but not $CO_2$ retention. Total leukocyte count is usually normal, but 50% to 70% of infants have eosinophil counts greater than $300/mm^3$. Serum levels of IgM, IgG, and IgA are usually elevated. Untreated infants gradually improve after 5 to 7 weeks of illness. About half of affected infants will have middle ear abnormalities, with *C trachomatis* isolated from some middle ear aspirates.

Chlamydial pneumonia in premature infants may be severe and require mechanical ventilatory support resulting in chronic lung disease. Children hospitalized for chlamydial pneumonia in early infancy have an increased risk of developing long-term pulmonary sequelae such as asthma, chronic cough, and abnormal pulmonary function tests.

The clinical significance of vaginal and rectal colonization with *C trachomatis* in infancy remains unknown. Nasopharyngeal colonization is associated with rhinitis and nasopharyngitis with nasal congestion without rhinorrhea lasting for weeks or months. Chlamydia is an uncommon cause of myocarditis and otitis media.

## DIAGNOSIS

Diagnosis of chlamydial infection is confirmed by inoculation of McCoy cells in tissue culture with conjunctival or nasopharyngeal scrapings and by demonstration of the characteristic intracytoplasmic inclusions after several days of incubation. Conjunctivitis is diagnosed by sampling the inflamed lower conjunctiva, not the purulent drainage, because the organism resides within the epithelial cells of the conjunctiva. Diagnosis of chlamydial pneumonia is based on a typical clinical syndrome and demonstration of *C trachomatis* in specimens obtained from the nasopharynx or endotracheal aspiration. Chlamydia also may be identified in lung tissue and pleural fluid.

Rapid detection tests of chlamydial antigen in clinical specimens are available for routine use. A monoclonal antibody directed against chlamydial elementary bodies in a direct immunofluorescent stain of clinical specimens has shown a sensitivity and specificity of 100% in chlamydial conjunctivitis. In nasopharyngeal specimens, however, the sensitivity is only 85% and the specificity, 75%. A second method is an enzyme-linked immunoassay that is semiautomatic and demonstrates sensitivity of 93% and specificity of 97% in examination of conjunctival smears.

Serologic evaluation is not useful in the diagnosis of chlamydial conjunctivitis because most infants do not develop IgM antibodies, and their antichlamydia IgG is of maternal origin. When pneumonia is present, however, measurement of antichlamydia IgM titer is preferred over nasopharyngeal culture for the diagnosis of chlamydial pneumonia because it is always elevated when clinical disease is apparent.

## TREATMENT

The recommended treatment for both chlamydial conjunctivitis and pneumonia is a 2-week course of either erythromycin estolate (10 mg/kg every 8 hours) or erythromycin ethylsuccinate (10 mg/kg every 6 hours) administered orally. The advantage of orally administered erythromycin over topical antibiotic containing ophthalmic solutions or ointments is the eradication of *C trachomatis* from the nasopharynx in infants. A shorter clinical course with lower relapse rates after oral therapy for conjunctivitis has been observed. Topical therapy in addition to oral erythromycin is not necessary because therapeutic levels of the drug are achieved in tears after oral administration. Treatment of the mother and her sexual partner with erythromycin, tetracycline, or doxycycline for 7 days is recommended at the time of diagnosis of the infant's infection. Recently, 1 g of azithromycin as a single oral dose was found effective for treatment of chlamydial infection in adults.

## PREVENTION

Hammerschlag reports that ophthalmic prophylaxis at birth with 1% silver nitrate, 0.5% erythromycin ointment, or 1% tetracycline ointment does not prevent chlamydial conjunctivitis. Identification and treatment of pregnant women colonized with *C trachomatis* and their sexual partners with erythromycin (tetracycline or doxycycline for the partner) is currently the most efficacious method of preventing infection and disease in neonates.

## Selected Readings

Hammerschlag MR. Efficacy of neonatal ocular prophylaxis for the prevention of chlamydial and gonococcal conjunctivitis. N Engl J Med 1989;320:769.
Rettig PJ. Chlamydial infections in pediatrics: diagnostic and therapeutic considerations. Pediatr Infect Dis 1986;5:158.
Rettig PJ. Infections due to *Chlamydia trachomatis* from infancy to adolescence. Pediatr Infect Dis 1986;5:449.
Schachter J, Grossman M, Sweet RL, et al. Prospective study of perinatal transmission of *Chlamydia trachomatis*. JAMA 1986;255:3374.

*Principles and Practice of Pediatrics, Second Edition.*
edited by Frank A. Oski et al. J. B. Lippincott Company, Philadelphia © 1994.

# GENITAL MYCOPLASMAS
*Pablo J. Sánchez and Jane D. Siegel*

The genital mycoplasmas consist of *Mycoplasma hominis, Mycoplasma fermentans, Mycoplasma genitalium,* and *Ureaplasma urealyticum* (T-strain mycoplasma). Only *M hominis* and *U urealyticum* are clinically significant. Mycoplasmas are pleomorphic organisms that lack a cell wall. Serologic studies demonstrate 7 serotypes of *M hominis* and at least 14 serotypes of *U urealyticum. M hominis* and *U urealyticum* are sexually transmitted organisms accounting for female urogenital colonization rates of 20% to 30% and 60% to 80%, respectively. Although both organisms are associated with a variety of adverse pregnancy outcomes, convincing evidence exists only for their association with histologic chorioamnionitis and with postpartum fever and endometritis.

## TRANSMISSION

The rate of vertical transmission of *U urealyticum* is 45% to 65% in full-term and 59% in preterm infants. Similar data are lacking for *M hominis.* Vertical transmission of mycoplasmas occurs in utero or during delivery. In utero transmission occurs either transplacentally or by an ascending route from a colonized maternal genital tract. Mycoplasmas have been isolated from maternal blood at the time of delivery and from amniotic fluid, endometrium, placenta, and aborted fetal tissue. Mycoplasmas also have been isolated from mucosal surfaces of newborn infants delivered by cesarean section performed before the onset of labor and rupture of amniotic membranes. More commonly, however, acquisition of mycoplasmas by newborn infants occurs at delivery through contact with a colonized birth canal. Colonization of newborn infants increases with decreasing gestational age and birth weight. Postpartum or nosocomial transmission in neonates is not well documented, but probably occurs.

## CLINICAL MANIFESTATIONS

The role of these organisms in neonatal disease is being defined. *M hominis* and *U urealyticum* have been recovered from the lungs, brain, heart, and viscera of aborted fetuses and stillborn infants with histologic finding of bronchopneumonia present in the lungs of these fetuses. The genital mycoplasmas also have been isolated from blood, urine, cerebrospinal fluid (CSF), and lung tissue of newborn infants with clinical signs of infection. The following clinical associations with *U urealyticum* have been made: fatal neonatal pneumonia in a term infant documented by isolation of the organism from lung at autopsy and demonstration of elevated serum IgG and IgM titers to *U urealyticum* in the infant; pneumonia and persistent pulmonary hypertension in five infants from whom *U urealyticum* was isolated from blood, endotracheal aspirate, pleural fluid, or lung at autopsy; afebrile pneumonitis in infants younger than 3 months of age; development of chronic lung disease in low–birth-weight infants whose respiratory tracts are colonized with *U urealyticum* in the first week of life; isolation of *U urealyticum* from lung biopsy tissue of four infants with chronic lung disease; and isolation of *U urealyticum* from CSF of both preterm and full-term infants.

Isolation of *U urealyticum* and *M hominis* from the CSF of predominantly preterm infants with suspected meningitis is associated by Waites and coworkers with CSF pleocytosis consisting of a polymorphonuclear or mononuclear cellular response, hypoglycorrhachia, and elevated protein content. Sequelae of meningitis due to *U urealyticum* and *M hominis* include hemiplegia, hydrocephalus, and developmental delay. The isolation of *U urealyticum* from CSF in preterm infants is associated with severe intraventricular hemorrhage. Among full-term infants, isolation of *U urealyticum* and *M hominis* is associated with minimal, if any, CSF abnormalities.

Other manifestations of infection with *M hominis* are brain and scalp abscess, ventriculitis, submandibular adenitis, conjunctivitis, and pericardial effusion. Clinical significance of the isolation of genital mycoplasmas from urine obtained by suprapubic bladder aspiration in infants is undetermined.

## DIAGNOSIS

Genital mycoplasmas may be isolated on special broth and solid media that are commercially available. *M hominis*, but not *U urealyticum*, may be presumptively identified on blood agar as tiny pinpoint colonies.

The diagnosis of mycoplasmal infection is made by isolation of the organism from a normally sterile body fluid or suppurative focus. Because colonization of newborn infants with mycoplasmas occurs frequently, an etiologic role for these agents cannot be supported by isolation from mucosal surfaces only. Serologic tests used to measure antibody to genital mycoplasmas include modified metabolic inhibition test, mycoplasmacidal test, indirect hemagglutination, indirect immunofluorescent test, enzyme-linked immunosorbent assay; and Immuno blotting. Use of these tests for diagnosis of mycoplasmal infection in infants is problematic and not well established.

## TREATMENT

Mycoplasmas are not susceptible to antimicrobial agents routinely used to treat neonatal infections. Because mycoplasmas lack a cell wall, they are insensitive to penicillins, cephalosporins, polymyxins, and vancomycin. Although they may have moderate sensitivity to aminoglycosides, the minimum inhibitory concentrations of these agents for the genital mycoplasmas are usually too high for therapeutic use. The drugs of choice for treatment of infection due to *M hominis* are chloramphenicol, clindamycin, doxycycline, and tetracycline; for treatment of ureaplasmal infections, erythromycin, doxycycline, tetracycline, and chloramphenicol. *M hominis* is resistant to erythromycin. Antibiotic susceptibility testing should be performed on all clinically significant isolates because multiple-drug resistance occurs.

### Selected Readings

Cassell GH, Crouse DT, Waites KB, et al. Does *Ureaplasma urealyticum* cause respiratory disease in newborns? Pediatr Infect Dis J 1988;7:535.

Cassell GH, Waites KB, Crouse DT. Perinatal mycoplasmal infections. Clin Perinatol 1991;18:241.
Cassell GH, Waites KB, Watson HL, Crouse DT, Harasalua R. *Ureaplasma urealyticum* intrauterine infection: Role in prematurity and disease in newborns. Clin Microbiol Rev 1993;6:69.
Sánchez PJ. Perinatal transmission of *Ureaplasma urealyticum*: current concepts based on review of the literature. Clin Infect Dis (In press).
Sánchez PJ, Regan JA. *Ureaplasma urealyticum* colonization and chronic lung disease in low birth weight infants. Pediatr Infect Dis J 1988;7:542.
Waites KB, Rudd PT, Crouse DT, et al. Chronic *Ureaplasma urealyticum* and *Mycoplasma hominis* infections of central nervous system in preterm infants. Lancet 1988;2:17.

*Principles and Practice of Pediatrics, Second Edition.*
edited by Frank A. Oski et al. J. B. Lippincott Company, Philadelphia © 1994.

## 20.14.4 *Nosocomial Infection in the Newborn*

John D. Nelson

## BACKGROUND

The fetus who has not been infected in utero is first exposed to microorganisms during vaginal passage. Subsequently, normal skin and mucous membrane microflora are established from environmental sources. This normal process is referred to as nosocomial infection only when a microbe has pathogenic potential. It is often difficult to ascertain whether an infection is nosocomially acquired. The time of onset of disease does not help differentiate among congenital, perinatal, and nosocomial sources because there can be a lag of many days between infection and clinical expression of that infection. For these reasons, the National Nosocomial Infections Study conducted by the Centers for Disease Control (CDC) designates all infectious diseases in the first 28 days of life as nosocomial, regardless of the actual source of those diseases.

Horan and colleagues (1984) note that hospitals participating in the National Nosocomial Infections Study reported a mean nosocomial infection rate in newborn nurseries of 1.4%, ranging from 0.9% in community hospitals to 1.7% in large university hospitals. Rates of infection depend on the prevalence of risk factors discussed below. Rates as high as 25% in neonatal intensive care units have been reported by Jarvis (1987). In contrast, primary care community hospital nurseries populated mainly by healthy, term infants had a nosocomial infection rate of only 0.86%.

Skin infections, diarrhea, respiratory infections, and septicemia are the most common nosocomial infections encountered in a nursery. Epidemic situations are particularly characteristic of organisms that colonize skin and mucous membranes frequently but cause disease infrequently. In this situation, the organism perpetuates itself in the environment over a prolonged time. Because it causes invasive disease only periodically, it can be difficult to recognize that a nosocomial infection problem exists.

Historically, shifts in nosocomial etiologic agents occurred about every 10 years in the United States. A severe problem with invasive strains of *Staphylococcus aureus* emerged in nurseries during the 1950s; its disappearance in the 1960s was largely unrelated to the many attempts made to control the problem. Since then, the strains of *S aureus* causing periodic outbreaks of skin lesions have not been invasive, virulent organisms. In the 1960s, *Pseudomonas aeruginosa* was a serious nosocomial pathogen in many nurseries because of contamination of water in incubators and of respiratory therapy equipment. The 1970s were the decade of group B streptococcal infections. In the 1980s, methicillin-resistant strains of S aureus and Staphylococcus epidermidis emerged as difficult nosocomial problems in neonatal intensive care units. Group B streptococci remain important pathogens in vertical transmission from mother to baby, but their role as nosocomial agents, which was documented in some nurseries by Boyer and colleagues (1980), has diminished.

Occasionally, clusters of cases suggesting nosocomial transmission turn out to be unrelated coincidences when strain markers such as bacteriophage types, restriction endonuclease digestion analysis, or antimicrobial susceptibility patterns are investigated.

Neonatal nosocomial infections are significant determinants of mortality, especially in low–birth-weight infants, as reported by LaGamma and coworkers (1983). Prevention, recognition, and appropriate management of nosocomial infections is an important goal.

## RISK FACTORS

All newborn infants are immunologically deficient. The degree of immunologic deficiency relates principally to immature gestational age, but it is further compromised by invasive intensive care measures.

The skin and mucous membranes are barriers to microbial invasion. By 37 weeks' gestation, the skin is an effective barrier, but in premature infants with scant stratum corneum, the skin is quite permeable. This defect allows easy entry of bacteria, especially in the preterm infant of less than 32 weeks' gestation. After about 2 weeks of age, the stratum corneum is well developed, regardless of gestational age.

The normal microflora of the skin and mucous membranes play a major role in defense against pathogens, but these tissues are sterile at birth unless there is intrauterine infection.

Polymorphonuclear leukocytes and monocytes of newborns exhibit sluggish migration toward exogenous antigens. Chemotactic activity is only one fourth to one half that of adult leukocytes. Phagocytosis is also decreased; however, intracellular bactericidal activity of neonatal polymorphonuclear cells is normal. Reticuloendothelial activity is decreased in the term neonate and essentially absent in the preterm infant. The classic and the alternate pathways of the complement system have decreased activity, and fibronectin is deficient.

Maternal IgG begins passing transplacentally to the fetus at about 15 weeks' gestation, and the fetus begins synthesizing IgM at about 30 weeks' gestation. The preterm infant at 32 weeks' gestation has a serum IgG concentration that is less than half that of a term infant. Preterm infants commonly have a large portion of their blood volume withdrawn for diagnostic laboratory tests, which further depletes humoral factors. Replenishing the infant with packed red blood cells rather than whole blood aggravates the situation. Consequently, many sick preterm infants have severely depleted immunoglobulin stores.

## SOURCES OF INFECTION AND MODES OF TRANSMISSION

Both routine and invasive procedures in a nursery provide opportunities for neonates to acquire infection and for infection to be transmitted from infant to infant.

Intrapartum scalp electrodes have caused infection by both bacteria and viruses. The umbilical stump can be colonized by virulent nosocomial organisms. All types of intravascular catheters carry risk of infection. Nelson (1988) reports that outbreaks of

infection in nurseries have been caused by contaminated eye wash, resuscitation equipment, scrub brushes, hand lotions, various disinfectants, topical ointments, and intravenous fluids. Although these and other fomites are potential risks for spreading infections in nurseries, Jarvis (1987) notes that transmission on the hands of nursery personnel is the most common cause of outbreaks of infections in neonates.

Nasal carriage of staphylococci in personnel can be responsible for outbreaks of skin infections in newborns. Group A streptococcal infections can occur in nurseries as can outbreaks of diarrheal illness caused by enteropathogenic bacteria and viruses. In most such outbreaks, fecal-oral spread via hands of personnel is the mode of transmission. Coxsackie virus and toxigenic Clostridium difficile infections are also spread by the fecal-oral route, but the mode of transmission of rotavirus infection is not entirely clear; Rodriguez and colleagues (1982) report that it may involve fecal-oral, respiratory, or vertical routes of spread.

Echovirus 11 and respiratory syncytial virus are spread both by airborne droplets and by hands of personnel touching contaminated objects; the viruses survive well on hard surfaces in the nursery environment.

Banked breast milk for preterm infants that becomes contaminated during collection or storage has caused Salmonella and Klebsiella infections.

Numerous possibilities exist for nosocomial infection in newborn nurseries and intensive care units. The examples cited here are merely representative of the problem.

A unique feature of nurseries compared with other areas of hospitals is that most infants enter it without an established microflora of the skin and mucous membranes. An aim of infection control is to allow the infant to establish a microflora consisting of nonpathogenic organisms, rather than the potentially pathogenic organisms common in the hospital environment.

The infant's first exposure to microorganisms is the maternal vaginal flora. In Thadepalli and colleagues' study (1978) of the endocervical flora during labor, 75% of women had a mixture of aerobic and anaerobic bacteria and 25% had only aerobes. The major organisms were S epidermidis, diphtheroids, Gardnerella vaginale, and various Bacteroides spp. Potential pathogens in the vagina or cervix are group B streptococci, gonococci, chlamydia, Listeria monocytogenes, cytomegalovirus (CMV), and herpes simplex virus, among others.

The newborn's nares commonly become colonized with S epidermidis and nonhemolytic streptococci. Those organisms, Klebsiella spp, and Enterobacter spp colonize the umbilical stump. Escherichia coli colonization increases in summer, and increased humidity favors E coli and P aeruginosa.

An anaerobic fecal flora develops rapidly in neonates. By 1 week of age, the frequency of colonization with Bacteroides fragilis and other anaerobes in infants born vaginally and fed formula approaches that of adults. Breast-feeding or delivery by cesarean section decreases substantially the rate of Bacteroides colonization but not that of C difficile.

Infants in intensive care nurseries become colonized with Klebsiella, Enterobacter, and Citrobacter spp. Antibiotic therapy suppresses anaerobic bacteria and increases the likelihood of colonization with gram-negative aerobes, especially those resistant to commonly used antibiotics. Nasotracheal tubes lead to colonization of the trachea and bronchi with organisms that normally colonize the nasopharynx. Nasojejunal feeding tubes result in colonization of the proximal small bowel with coliform bacilli.

## RECOGNITION

When a cluster of similar cases occurs within a short time, it is an easy matter to recognize the situation. This is the pattern with organisms that have a high disease-to-colonization ratio such as several infectious diarrheal agents and group A streptococci.

More commonly, nosocomial infections are caused by diseases with low disease-to-colonization ratios such as group B streptococci and *S. aureus.* There may be only 1 or 2 cases of overt disease for every 100 infants colonized with the microorganism. Infants colonized with a potential pathogen may not develop disease until after discharge from the nursery.

Bacterial, fungal, and viral cultures; rapid antigen detection methods; and acute and convalescent serum specimens for antibody studies are variously needed to establish the pathogens involved in nosocomial infections, depending on the circumstances.

## SURVEILLANCE

The nursery staff must be alert to occurrences of possible nosocomial infection and must report them to personnel responsible for infection control. Periodic inpatient education of nursing and technical personnel about infection control practices helps maintain awareness.

Monitoring events in the nursery is easier than monitoring for diseases acquired in the nursery but manifested after discharge. Infants are usually followed by several physicians and communication is not good.

Snydman and colleagues report that routine surveillance cultures from neonates, personnel, and environmental sources in the nursery are not useful, recommended, or cost-effective. Most nosocomial infections are spread from infant to infant by the hands or clothing of personnel. Transmission of infection from infant to personnel or from personnel to infant is unusual, and environmental surfaces and fomites are seldom the source of infection in a modern nursery. The organism causing infection and the anatomic site of the infection can provide clues to the possible sources of contamination. If the nosocomial pathogen is an enteric gram-negative bacillus typically transmitted by the fecal-oral route, it is likely that hands of personnel are responsible for transmission and that environmental cultures are not worthwhile. If the site of infection is the lower respiratory tract of intubated infants, however, procedures for suctioning and possible contamination of suctioning equipment should be suspected. Careful thought about procedures and close scrutiny of their implementation are usually more productive than taking indiscriminate culture specimens of the inanimate and animate environment.

Whenever new procedures are introduced in the nursery, the potential for nosocomial infection should be considered, particularly in the case of invasive procedures. Depending on the nature of the procedure, it may be desirable to do prospective surveillance cultures to monitor for nosocomial infection.

## MANAGEMENT

Recommended isolation practices based on guidelines developed by the CDC are presented in Table 20-86. These guidelines are in addition to universal precautions for blood and body fluids. Universal precautions suffice for CMV, human immunodeficiency virus, syphilis, and hepatitis B and C infections.

Congenital infection usually connotes syphilis, rubella, toxoplasmosis, herpes simplex, listeriosis, CMV infection, hepatitis, and varicella, even though most infections with herpes simplex, CMV, and hepatitis are acquired at or shortly after birth rather than congenitally.

Nosocomial infection with *Toxoplasma gondii* does not occur, so no isolation precautions are necessary for a congenitally infected infant.

**TABLE 20-86.    Isolation Procedures**

| Category | Conditions |
|---|---|
| Strict | Varicella in mother |
| Contact | Gonorrhea |
| | Herpes simplex infection |
| | Pneumonia |
| | Respiratory viruses infection |
| | Rubella |
| | Staphylococcal or streptococcal skin infection |
| Drainage/secretions | *Chlamydia* infections |
| | Syphilitic mucosal or skin lesions |
| Enteric | Diarrhea |
| | Hepatitis A in mother |
| | Meningitis, aseptic |
| | Necrotizing enterocolitis |

Categories are Centers for Disease Control definitions.
*Garner JS, Simmons BP. Guideline for isolation precautions in hospitals. Infect Control 1983;4:245*

Skin and mucous membrane lesions of an untreated infant with congenital syphilis contain many spirochetes, and the infant may have spirochetemia. Blood precautions are necessary, and gloves should be worn when handling the infant. *Treponema pallidum* in the environment is rapidly killed by drying, heat, and soap. Once treatment with penicillin is started, the organisms are eliminated rapidly, and isolation precautions can be discontinued after 24 hours.

On rare occasions, intrauterine infection of the fetus with herpes simplex virus occurs. In most cases, the infection is acquired during vaginal delivery. Nosocomial transmission of herpes simplex infection is rare, but it has been transmitted during endotracheal suctioning, by fetal scalp electrodes, from a maternal breast lesion, and from oral lesions of nursery personnel. Contact isolation precautions should be used with an infant born to a mother with a history of genital herpes whether lesions are present or not. Maternal vaginal cultures and cultures of the eyes and mouth of the infant can guide future management. If an infant who has been treated for active herpes simplex infection must remain in the nursery for other medical reasons, isolation precautions should be maintained because recurrence of skin lesions is common. Personnel with genital herpes can work in the nursery as long as strict hand-washing technique is used, but personnel with herpes labialis should not have direct contact with infants until lesions are crusted.

Several reports have been made of clusters of cases of neonatal listeriosis and of protracted outbreaks in nurseries. In general, investigations have failed to uncover the source of infection; specifically, nosocomial sources have not been implicated.

Transmission of hepatitis A from mother to newborn is rare; nevertheless, if the mother had onset of jaundice within a week of delivery, the infant should be considered possibly contaminated by hepatitis virus in the mother's feces, and enteric precautions should be used with the infant. The infant is given human immune globulin for prophylaxis.

With hepatitis B infection in the mother, the risk of infection of her newborn is great, particularly if she carries the e antigen. Vertical transmission is effectively prevented by combined use of hepatitis B immune globulin and hepatitis vaccine. The infant should be considered potentially infected. Gloves should be worn when cleansing the infant's skin after birth. Blood and body fluid precautions are used until the immune status of the infant is verified at 1 year of age.

Infants whose mothers have varicella at the time of delivery typically develop disease between the 5th and 10th day of life unless effective prophylaxis is used. Severe infection is most likely if the mother's illness began between 4 days before delivery and 48 hours after delivery. Passive immunization with varicella-zoster immune globulin should be given immediately after birth. Prophylaxis is not uniformly effective, so strict isolation technique should be used until the infant is 10 days old. If infants are exposed to nursery personnel with varicella, a serologic test for V-Z antibody is done in infants whose mothers do not have verifiable histories of chickenpox or in any infant who has had multiple blood drawings and transfusions that could make interpretation of the infant's antibody status difficult. Varicella-zoster immune globulin is given to infants who lack antibody.

Chronic infection is characteristic of congenital rubella. The virus can be recovered from pharyngeal secretions, urine, conjunctival fluid, and feces for many months and occasionally years. Contact isolation precautions are used in the infant with congenital rubella for at least 1 year.

CMV infection is the most common congenital infection. Many additional babies acquire the virus during delivery or after birth. The neonate can also acquire infection from breast milk or from blood transfusions. CMV can survive on paper diapers for as long as 48 hours, posing a potential hazard to nursery personnel who handle diapers. Transmission of CMV infection among neonates in an intensive care unit has been documented using restriction endonuclease digestion analysis. Garner and Simmons (1983) show that apparent nosocomial infections in nurseries were actually caused by different strains. Despite the frequency of CMV in a nursery setting, transmission between babies and personnel is rare. The virus is present in saliva and urine of infected infants, but routine hand washing appears to be an effective preventive measure.

The risk of horizontal transmission of sepsis or meningitis in a nursery is virtually nonexistent, so routine precautions are sufficient. A possible exception is the case of *Citrobacter diversus*, an organism with unusual tropism for the central nervous system and a proclivity to cause brain abscesses. Outbreaks related to horizontal transmission of *C diversus* have occurred and been documented by Lin and colleagues (1987). Because the reservoir of that organism is the gastrointestinal tract, enteric precautions are recommended.

Aseptic meningitis in the neonate is commonly caused by enteroviruses, and outbreaks are common. Enteric precautions are important in preventing transmission of enteroviruses.

*S aureus* is the most common cause of nosocomial skin infections in a nursery. Daily bathing of infants with hexachlorophene-containing soap decreases skin colonization rates but does not reliably control outbreaks. Rates of skin and mucous membrane colonization do not always correlate with rates of disease.

Coagulase-negative strains of staphylococci are a major nosocomial infection problem in neonates with central venous catheters. Such strains are usually resistant to antistaphylococcal β-lactam antibiotics and are treated with vancomycin.

In recent years, methicillin-resistant strains of *S. aureus* have caused nosocomial infections in many tertiary care nurseries.

When multiple cases of staphylococcal disease occur within a limited time in a nursery and it is determined by laboratory testing that a single strain is involved, cohorting of neonates by day of birth may help contain the outbreak. Strict adherence to hand-washing technique is necessary.

Group A streptococcal nosocomial infection usually involves the umbilical cord stump. Funisitis is mild with little inflammation and minimal secretions, which are characteristically sticky and have a musty odor. Local measures such as applying triple dye

or bacitracin ointment to the umbilical stump may stop the outbreak, but sometimes it is necessary to give an injection of benzathine penicillin G to all newborns until the epidemic is stopped. Contact precautions are recommended for group A streptococcal and staphylococcal skin or mucous membrane infections.

Nosocomial chlamydial infection has not been reported but drainage and secretion precautions are recommended. In preantibiotic days, gonococcal infection in a nursery was exceedingly difficult to control, but with present day therapy, gonococcal ophthalmia is not a nosocomial problem. Nevertheless, the CDC recommends that full contact precautions instead of drainage and secretion precautions be used.

Most outbreaks of respiratory infections are caused by viruses, especially respiratory syncytial virus (RSV). RSV infection in infants with underlying cardiopulmonary disease is often lethal. Evans and colleagues report that gowning and use of masks alone are ineffectual in preventing transmission of respiratory infections among infants and personnel because RSV survives on hard surfaces such as the incubator or bassinet and is transmitted by hands of personnel. Again, hand washing is important. Infants with respiratory symptoms should be housed in nurseries separate from asymptomatic babies. In the intensive care unit, separate isolation facilities should be available. Aerosolized ribavirin therapy shortens the period of shedding of RSV.

The syndrome of necrotizing enterocolitis (NEC) is probably multifactorial in origin, but clusters of cases associated with intestinal pathogens suggest an important role for infection in pathogenesis. Outbreaks of NEC have been temporally associated with *Enterobacter cloacae*, rotavirus, and enteric coronavirus; however, in most outbreaks of NEC, no enteric pathogen is found. In isolated cases of diarrhea or when outbreaks occur, all infants with diarrhea should be housed separately from other infants. Strict enteric precautions for handling soiled diapers and washing hands should be stressed. When a bacterial pathogen is responsible for the outbreak, appropriate antibiotic therapy is instituted.

Candidal infection of the oral mucous membranes and diaper area is common in neonates who have received broad-spectrum antibiotics, but nosocomial transmission is not obvious in such cases. Therefore, no special precautions are necessary. No special precautions are needed for infants with urinary tract infection or for those born to mothers with tuberculosis. Infants exposed to nursery personnel with tuberculosis have a small risk of acquiring the infection; nevertheless, it is prudent to test them intradermally for tuberculin reactivity 2 to 3 months later and to ensure that the physician who gives continuing care to the infant is aware of the exposure.

Antibiotic usage is not great in a nursery for term infants, but in NICUs, more than half the infants receive antibiotic therapy at least once. Antibiotics alter the normal respiratory and gut flora, so resistant bacteria often replace the antibiotic-susceptible flora. By monitoring antibiotic susceptibilities, problems with multiply-resistant organisms are detected. The source should be sought, although it generally is not found because the infections are usually endogenous from altered flora. Colonized infants should be placed in a cohort, and scrupulous aseptic technique should be used in handling them. Ill infants are treated with an appropriate antibiotic, but it is not possible to eliminate asymptomatic colonization with use of antibiotics. Periodic surveillance culture specimens are made and new cohorts of colonized and uncolonized infants are formed until the epidemic is controlled.

## PREVENTION

Detailed guidelines for design of nurseries and for routine perinatal care are available and should be consulted when planning a new nursery and when setting policies for routine care in any nursery. Deviations from those guidelines are sometimes necessary because of peculiar local situations, but the principles remain constant. The modern trend in routine care policies has been to abandon restrictive and excessive precautionary procedures of unproven worth and to adopt simpler measures of proven benefit in the hope of increasing compliance with those procedures.

## Selected Readings

Adler SP. Nosocomial transmission of cytomegalovirus. Pediatr Infect Dis J 1986;5: 239.

American Academy of Pediatrics and American College of Obstetricians and Gynecologists. Guidelines for perinatal care, ed 2. Evanston, IL: American Academy of Pediatrics, 1988.

Boyer KM, Vogel LC, Gotoff SP, et al. Nosocomial transmission of bacteriophage type 7/11/12 group B streptococci in a special care nursery. Am J Dis Child 1980;134:964.

Evans ME, Schaffner W, Federspiel CF, et al. Sensitivity, specificity, and predictive value of body surface cultures in a neonatal intensive care unit. JAMA 1988;259: 248.

Garner JS, Simmons BP. Guideline for isolation precautions in hospitals. Infect Control 1983;4:245.

Horan TC, White JW, Jarvis WR, et al. Nosocomial infection surveillance, 1984. MMWR 1984;35(1SS):17SS.

Jarvis WR. The epidemiology of nosocomial infections in pediatric patients. Pediatr Infect Dis J 1987;61:344.

LaGamma EF, Drusin LM, Mackles AW, et al. Neonatal infections: an important determinant of late NICU mortality in infants less than 1,000 g at birth. Am J Dis Child 1983;137:838.

Lin F-Y, Devoe WF, Morrison C, et al. Outbreak of neonatal *Citrobacter diversus* meningitis in a suburban hospital. Pediatr Infect Dis J 1987;6:50.

Nelson JD. Neonatal nosocomial infection. In: Donowitz LG, ed. Hospital acquired infection in the pediatric patient. Baltimore: Williams & Wilkins, 1988.

Planning and design for perinatal and pediatric facilities. Columbus, OH: Ross Laboratories, 1977.

Rodriguez WJ, Kim HW, Brandt CD, Fletcher AB, Parrott RH: Rotavirus: a cause of nosocomial infection in the nursery. J Pediatr 1982;101:274.

Snydman DR, Greer C, Meissner HC, McIntosh K. Prevention of nosocomial transmission of respiratory syncytial virus in a newborn nursery. Infect Control Hosp Epidemiol 1988;9:105.

Thadepalli H, Chan WH, Maidman JE, Davidson ED Jr. Microflora of the cervix during normal labor and the puerperium. J Infect Dis 1978;137:568.

*Principles and Practice of Pediatrics, Second Edition.*
edited by Frank A. Oski et al. J. B. Lippincott Company, Philadelphia © 1994.

# 20.15 *Cardiovascular Surgery in the Newborn*

Gary S. Kopf and Michael L. Dewar

With significant progress in neonatal cardiovascular surgery, cardiology, intensive care, and anesthesia over the last few decades, definitive primary repair in the neonatal period is now feasible for a variety of life-threatening congenital heart defects. Risks and complications associated with palliation and additional surgical procedures are avoided. When primary repair is not feasible, effective palliation ensures continued survival and growth until a more corrective procedure is possible. Neonates with the most complex lesions, hitherto considered untreatable, are undergoing successful palliation or, if no other treatment option seems worthwhile, organ replacement.

## GENERAL CONSIDERATIONS

### Preoperative Management

Resuscitation and stabilization of cardiac, renal, and respiratory function are critical in optimizing surgical outcome. Diagnosis is expedited by using echocardiography and color flow Doppler, often without cardiac catheterization. Preoperative shock or renal failure is strongly associated with poor surgical outcome and must be corrected. Neonates dependent on a patent ductus arteriosus (PDA) for pulmonary blood flow (as for pulmonary atresia) or on systemic blood flow (as for hypoplastic left heart syndrome or interrupted aortic arch) are treated with infusion of prostaglandin E1 to reverse severe cyanosis or low output states. Inotropic agents, particularly dopamine and dobutamine, increase cardiac output and renal blood flow. Mechanical ventilation ensures adequate gas exchange and oxygenation. To avoid secondary complications, surgery should be done as soon as the infant's condition is optimized and stable.

### Intraoperative Management

#### Monitoring

Arterial blood pressure is monitored via umbilical artery, radial, or posterior tibial cannulation. An internal jugular venous line as well as peripheral venous lines is placed. A bladder catheter monitors urine output. Several electrocardiographic leads are continuously monitored. Temperature monitoring is a critical part of the operative management and is accomplished with tympanic, esophageal, and either bladder or rectal temperature probes.

Median sternotomy is the standard incision for virtually all open heart procedures and many palliative procedures in the neonate. The sternum is incised vertically using a heavy scissors. Often, the thymus gland is partially resected to facilitate exposure, but effort is made to spare some thymus tissue for regeneration. The pericardium is harvested for use as a vascular patch when necessary, and may be treated with a glutaraldehyde solution to increase its strength. Isolated coarctation repair, systemic-pulmonary artery shunts, pulmonary artery banding, and PDA ligation usually are done through a left or right lateral thoracotomy. The chest cavity is entered through the fourth intercostal space. The lung is retracted gently to expose the mediastinum.

#### Cannulation for Cardiopulmonary Bypass

Venous blood is siphoned into the venous reservoir of the heart-lung apparatus via a single cannula placed in the right atrium or two smaller cannula inserted into each vena cava. After traversing a membrane oxygenator, heat exchanger, filter, and roller pump, blood is returned to the patient in the ascending aorta via an aortic cannula. Each component of the system is designed to minimize priming volume and blood trauma and to increase efficiency of gas exchange and heat transfer to provide for the special needs of the neonate. Bypass is initiated by removing clamps from the venous line, which opens the siphon to the pump. Simultaneously, the roller pump is started to reinfuse blood into the patient. Pump flows of 100 mL/kg/min are adequate to maintain tissue oxygenation. The time during which blood is continuously exchanged between the heart-lung apparatus and the patient is referred to as the total bypass time.

Cardiopulmonary bypass results in a whole body inflammatory response, producing generalized edema and increase in total body water. The pump's priming volume is several times the neonate's blood volume. This severe hemodilution decreases oncotic pressure and tends to increase the loss of intravascular fluid. Diuretics, and rarely dialysis or hemoconcentration, are needed after bypass. Dilution of clotting factors may result in severe coagulopathy. Pump priming with fresh blood and administration of blood components help prevent severe bleeding complications. With current methods and technology, less than 3 hours of total bypass time is usually well tolerated by the neonate.

Successful repair of complex lesions requires meticulous attention to every detail of surgical technique. A bloodless, motionless field with a relaxed heart greatly aids the surgeon. This is often accomplished on bypass by clamping the ascending aorta between the root of the aorta and the aortic cannula. The heart is thereby isolated from the rest of the circulation, and cardioplegia solution can be infused selectively into the root of the aorta and the coronary arteries. Cardioplegia is a cold crystalloid-blood solution containing glucose, buffer, electrolytes, and, in particular, a high potassium concentration. With coronary cardioplegia infusion, the heart becomes flaccid, and a bloodless, motionless surgical field is produced. The time during which the ascending aorta is clamped and the heart is ischemic is called the aortic cross-clamp time. Current techniques of myocardial protection with cardioplegia and with topical and systemic cooling allows for cross-clamp times up to 2 hours with almost complete preservation of myocardial function. The most complex repairs usually can be accomplished within this time frame.

On bypass, body temperature is lowered to 20 °C or lower to protect the heart and other organs using a heat exchanger. Body temperatures of 20 °C or lower are referred to as deep hypothermia. At this temperature, pump flow can be temporarily reduced to as low as 25 to 50 mL/kg/min as metabolic demands decrease with hypothermia. This is known as the low flow technique.

Another way to create ideal surgical conditions is to turn the pump off for a time once deep hypothermia levels are achieved throughout the body. This condition is called deep hypothermia with circulatory arrest. The time during which the pump is turned off and there is no circulation is the circulatory arrest time. Arrest times less than 45 minutes are considered safe, but the incidence of neurologic sequelae increases significantly with longer periods. Most surgeons use a combination of low flow and circulatory arrest techniques to perform complex neonatal heart surgery. With these methods, most neonatal procedures can be carried out with incision and exposure through the atria or great vessels. Ventriculotomy size in the pulmonary ventricle is kept to a minimum. Incision in the systemic ventricle is poorly tolerated in the neonate and is avoided if possible.

## Postoperative Care

Neonates are closely monitored for at least 48 hours in the intensive care unit. Pulmonary compliance may be temporarily decreased and total lung water increased after bypass in the neonate. Several days of ventilatory support using positive end expiratory pressure may be necessary. Post-pump coagulopathy is treated with platelets, cryoprecipitate, and fresh blood. Echocardiography is an important tool for postoperative evaluation to check ventricular function, residual shunts, atrioventricular valve regurgitation, or obstruction to blood flow. A deteriorating neonate in the postoperative period must be aggressively evaluated with echocardiography or recatheterization. Prompt reoperation for residual defects may be lifesaving, but must be accomplished early before severe organ dysfunction produces an irreversible downhill spiral.

## SPECIFIC LESIONS

## Ventricular Septal Defect

Ventricular septal defect (VSD) is the most common congenital heart anomaly. Congestive heart failure may manifest within the first few weeks of life as pulmonary vascular resistance falls with consequent increase in left-to-right shunting. Surgery is indicated in those infants with large VSD, congestive heart failure, and failure to thrive. Primary closure is the procedure of choice in most infants with VSD. The VSD can be closed through the right atrium in most cases. Defects larger than a few millimeters are closed with a prosthetic patch. Operative mortality is low and complications few for simple VSD closure. Heart block is avoided by keeping sutures on the right side of the septum in the area of the conduction system. Palliation consisting of pulmonary artery banding (PAB) is done for those infants with extreme low–birth-weight, poor preoperative condition, severe coexisting anomalies, or multiple VSDs not amenable to primary closure.

### Pulmonary Artery Banding

PAB is carried out through a left anterior or lateral thoracotomy. The pericardium is opened longitudinally anterior to the phrenic nerve, and Teflon banding tape is placed around the base of the main pulmonary artery. The band is tightened to lower the distal pulmonary artery pressure to one fourth to one third of systemic pressure. This should result in a simultaneous increase in systemic pressure to 10 to 20 mm Hg. A prominent thrill is felt on the distal pulmonary artery, and systemic saturation on 50% oxygen should not fall below approximately 90%. Complications of banding include narrowing of the takeoff of the main pulmonary artery branches, particularly the right branch. This can be repaired easily, however, with patch arterioplasty at the time of VSD closure.

## Transposition of Great Arteries

The arterial switch operation for transposition of the great arteries (TGA) is the most common open heart procedure performed in the neonatal period at many institutions. Over the past decade, it has replaced atrial switch operations (ie, Mustard procedure, Senning procedure) as the operation of choice for TGA. Although the results of atrial switch procedures had been satisfactory with low initial mortality, long-term follow-up revealed a significant rise in the incidence of right (systemic) ventricular failure and arrhythmias. Jatene (1976) reported the first clinical success with arterial switching for TGA with VSD. Initially, operative mortality was high. Over the next decade, technical modifications and improvements in surgical technique resulted in low operative mortality similar to that reported for atrial switch operations. The arterial switch operation restores normal anatomy and physiologic function. Intermediate long-term follow-up studies show a low incidence of arrhythmias, normal ventricular function, and excellent overall results.

### Management

Operation is performed within the first few weeks of life before the left ventricle loses significant muscle mass, rendering it unable to support the systemic circulation. Diagnosis is made by echocardiography and associated lesions such as VSD are noted. Cardiac catheterization may be performed to elucidate details of coronary or other unusual anatomic details. Balloon atrial septostomy is done to improve oxygenation in most patients, which allows for a more elective operation on a stable patient. If echocardiographic examination is satisfactory and cyanosis not too severe, catheterization and balloon septostomy may be unnecessary if surgery can be carried out within a few days. Left ventricle thickness should appear adequate by echocardiography, and fixed left ventricular outflow obstruction should be ruled out.

About 25% of patients have a large VSD. High left ventricular pressures are sustained. Operation usually can be done electively within the first 6 weeks of life before the onset of severe congestive heart failure.

## Operative Technique

The aorta and the pulmonary arteries are extensively mobilized out to the hilum of the lung. The PDA is ligated and divided. Cardiopulmonary bypass is established. Operation is facilitated with the aid of deep hypothermia and low flow or with periods of circulatory arrest. The aorta and pulmonary artery are divided (Fig 20-114A and B). Buttons of aortic tissue containing the left and right coronary ostia are mobilized to allow for coronary transfer posteriorly to the neo-aorta (Fig 20-114C). The coronary buttons are sewn into place, creating the new aortic root (Fig 20-114D). The ascending aorta is then transposed underneath the pulmonary arteries, the "LeCompte maneuver" (Fig 20-114B and F). Anastomosis is carried out between the neo-aortic root and the distal aorta (Fig 20-114F). The base of the new pulmonary artery is reconstructed with a pericardial patch (Fig 20-114E), and the distal pulmonary artery is anastomosed to the new proximal pulmonary artery (Fig 20-114G). The atrial septal defect is closed through the right atrium. If necessary, a VSD can be closed via the right atrium or through the aorta. The result is a total physiologic and anatomic correction (Fig 20-114H).

Operative mortality is between 2% and 10% and is primarily related to technical problems associated with the coronary transfer. It is more common with unusual coronary variants, particularly an intramural coronary or a coronary artery traversing the space between the aorta and pulmonary artery. The most common postoperative complication is supravalvar pulmonic stenosis. The pulmonary artery may be stretched over the neo-aorta, resulting in stricture or compression. Adequate reconstruction of the new pulmonary artery base with a generous pantaloon-shaped patch of autologous pericardium (Fig 20-114E) helps prevent this.

Potential long-term problems include coronary artery stenosis or occlusion, supravalvar pulmonary or aortic stenosis, and aortic insufficiency. To date, intermediate follow-up studies show a very low incidence of coronary or aortic valve problems.

## Right-Sided Obstructed Lesions

Complete or partial obstruction of pulmonary blood flow in the neonate is caused by a variety of conditions including tetralogy of Fallot (TOF), pulmonary stenosis, and pulmonary atresia with

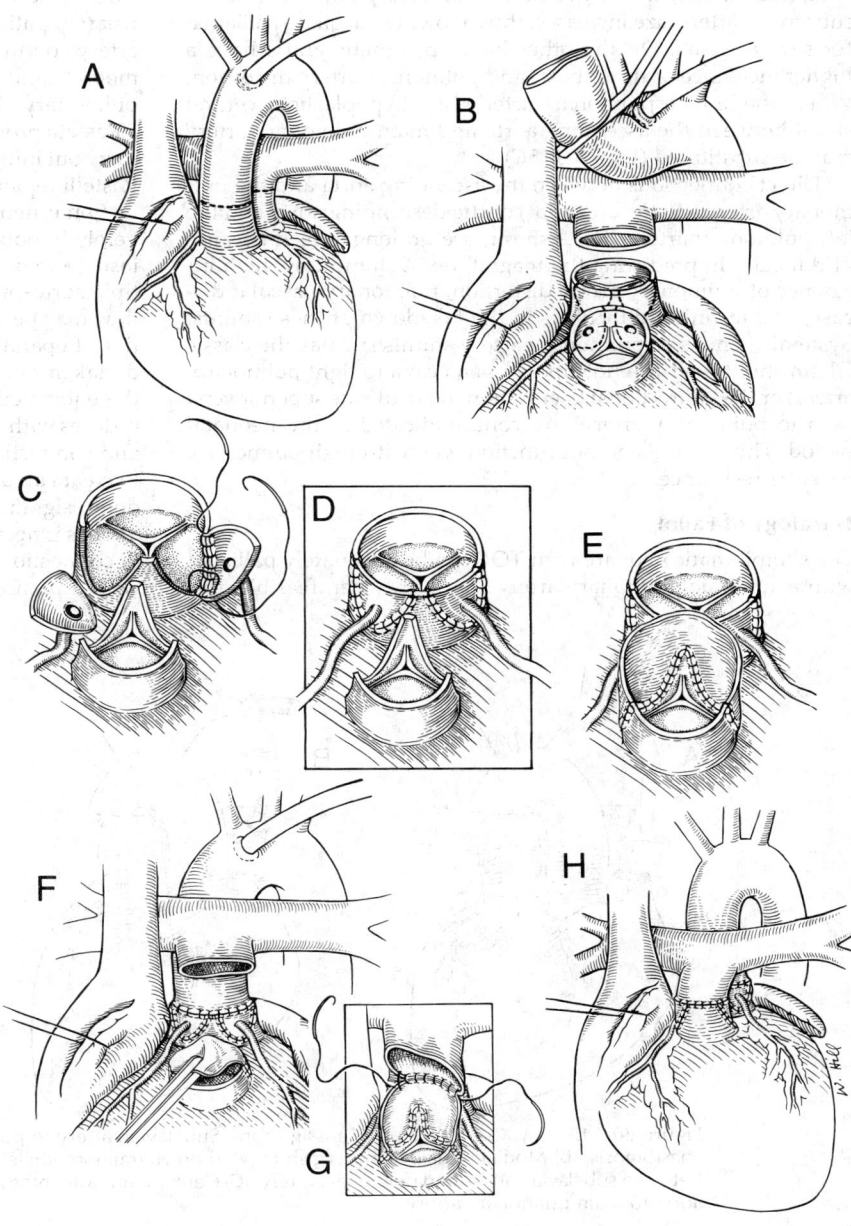

**Figure 20-114.** The arterial switch operation for transposition of the great arteries.

or without VSD. When pulmonary blood flow is dependent on a PDA, severe cyanosis and acidosis usually develop in the first few days of life, and prompt onset of prostaglandins infusion is imperative. If reparative surgery is not feasible, the first palliative step is to create a systemic to pulmonary artery shunt or right ventricle-pulmonary artery connection to provide pulmonary blood flow.

### Palliative Shunts in the Neonate

Stabilization with prostaglandins infusion is essential to reverse acidosis and severe cyanosis before the patient is taken to the operating room. The classic Blalock-Taussig (BT) shunt, first performed in 1945, consists of transection of the subclavian artery on the side opposite the aortic arch with end-to-side anastomosis to the pulmonary artery (Fig 20-115A). Most surgeons now use the "modified Blalock-Taussig" shunt. A 4- or 5-mm tubular interposition graft of polytetrafluoroethylene (PTFE) is placed between the subclavian and pulmonary artery (Fig 20-115B). This has several advantages over the classic BT shunt. The subclavian artery need not be sacrificed, graft length can be readily adjusted, and the operation can be performed on either side. Shunt flow is limited by the size of the subclavian artery and increases as subclavian artery size increases, thus allowing adequate palliation for several years. On the other hand, prosthetic grafts have a higher incidence of thrombosis and pulmonary artery distortion. Where the branch pulmonary arteries are hypoplastic, a central shunt between the ascending aorta and main pulmonary artery may be substituted (Fig 20-115C).

Direct connections between the ascending aorta and the pulmonary artery (Waterson shunt) or the descending aorta and the left pulmonary artery (Potts shunt) are no longer used because of difficulty in predicting the magnitude of shunt flow, high incidence of pulmonary artery distortion, pulmonary vascular disease, and technical difficulties in the takedown of these shunts. Systemic venous to pulmonary artery shunts such as the classic Glenn shunt (end-to-end superior vena cava to right pulmonary artery) or the bidirectional Glenn shunt (end-to-side superior vena cava to pulmonary artery) are contraindicated in the neonatal period. These shunts do not function well with high pulmonary vascular resistance.

### Tetralogy of Fallot

The symptomatic neonate with TOF can be adequately palliated with a systemic-pulmonary artery shunt or, when feasible, undergo primary corrective surgery. Primary repair carries an acceptably low risk for the neonate who is in otherwise good condition and has favorable anatomy for repair, that is, acceptable pulmonary artery size, single rather than multiple VSDs, and no major coexisting anomalies. Primary repair consists of patch closure of the large malalignment VSD through the right ventricle or right atrium. Right ventricular outflow tract obstruction (RVOTO) is relieved by any or all of the following: pulmonary valvotomy, infundibular incision and resection, and pericardial patch reconstruction. If the pulmonary annulus is severely hypoplastic, it is enlarged with a transannular pericardial patch that extends across the pulmonary annulus. Most symptomatic neonates require this type of reconstruction.

### Pulmonary Atresia With VSD

Pulmonary atresia with VSD is characterized by absence of continuity between the right ventricle and pulmonary artery. Palliation consists of a systemic-pulmonary artery shunt to ensure adequate pulmonary artery blood flow and pulmonary artery growth. Definitive repair with transannular patch or homograft connection between right ventricle and pulmonary artery, and VSD closure is possible in some patients with reasonably low risk (eg, patients with TOF). When right ventricular-pulmonary artery continuity is established with a prosthetic conduit or homograft and the VSD is closed so as to separate systemic and pulmonary blood flow, the procedure generally is referred to as a Rastelli procedure. To lower the risk to the patient, most centers carry out initial palliation with a shunt, followed by the definitive Rastelli repair within the first few years of life.

Some neonates with pulmonary atresia with VSD have severely hypoplastic pulmonary arteries with absent ductus arteriosus, and derive most of their pulmonary blood flow from multiple aorto-pulmonary collaterals (MAPCAS). Pulmonary blood flow may be increased if the collaterals are large with no obstruction. Reparative reconstruction of the Rastelli type can be undertaken only if an adequate pulmonary arterial tree supplying the equivalent of at least one lung is established. Multiple procedures with detachment of MAPCAS from the descending aorta and connection to central pulmonary arteries may be necessary to create an adequate pulmonary arterial tree. Before this can be done, significant growth of the native hypoplastic pulmonary arteries is necessary. A central shunt to the main pulmonary artery or connection of the right ventricle to the main pulmonary artery with a homograft or transannular patch stimulates pulmonary

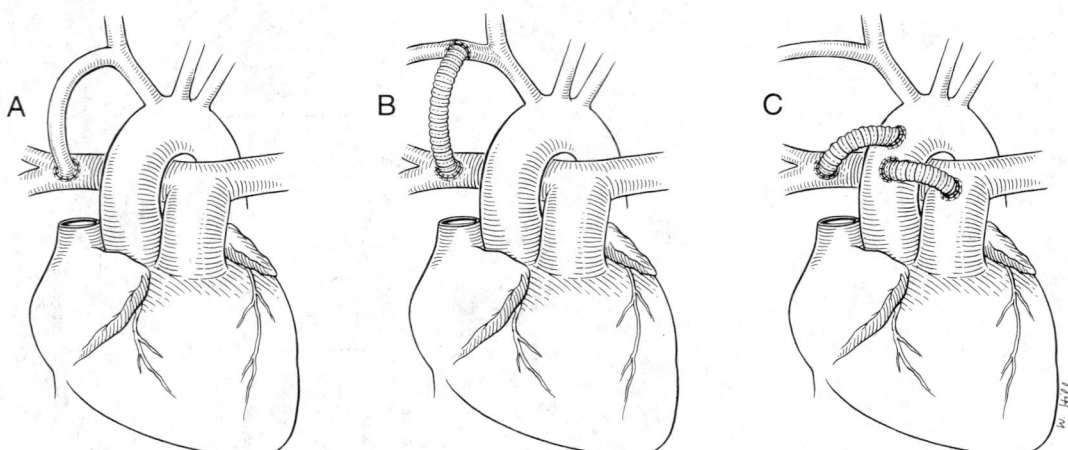

**Figure 20-115.** (**A**) Classic Blalock-Taussig shunt. Subclavian artery to pulmonary artery end to side anastomosis. (**B**) Modified Blalock-Taussig shunt with polytetrafluoroethylene (PTFE) interposition graft between subclavian artery and pulmonary artery. (**C**) Cental shunt with interposition graft from ascending aorta to main pulmonary artery.

artery growth. Banding or takedown of some of the unobstructed large aorto-pulmonary collaterals may be necessary to prevent congestive heart failure and development of vascular disease in those lung segments.

### Pulmonary Atresia and Intact Ventricular Septum

In neonates with intact ventricular septum as well as pulmonary atresia, the right ventricle is hypoplastic and hypertensive to varying degrees. Ventriculocoronary fistulas are present in a significant proportion of such patients. Surgical strategy depends on the degree of the right ventricular hypoplasia. The pulmonary arteries usually are well developed with ductal-dependent pulmonary blood flow. Patients with severely hypoplastic right ventricle and tricuspid annular hypoplasia are staged toward a univentricular repair (Fontan operation). A systemic-pulmonary artery shunt is the initial palliation to maintain pulmonary blood flow. In patients whose right ventricular size is at least two thirds normal, palliation encourages right ventricular growth by establishing a right ventricular-pulmonary artery connection by using valvotomy, a transannular patch, or a homograft. In addition, a systemic-pulmonary artery shunt is usually necessary because the hypoplastic right ventricle may not supply adequate pulmonary blood flow. Patients with coronary fistula formation may have significant obstruction of the native coronary circulation. Neonatal heart transplantation may be the only way to salvage these patients.

## Left-Sided Obstructive Lesions

### Aortic Stenosis

Critical aortic stenosis in the neonate is a surgical emergency. Patients often present severely hypoperfused with acidosis. Usual supportive measures of inotropic agents and mechanical ventilation are only partially and temporarily effective in improving their condition. Prompt relief of aortic obstruction is critical.

Aortic valvotomy is performed by a variety of techniques including open valvotomy with cardiopulmonary bypass or with inflow occlusion. Transventricular dilation can be done without bypass by introducing a dilating balloon catheter through the left ventricular apex and passing it across the aortic valve. A variable degree of left ventricular hypoplasia is present. Survival correlates closely with left ventricular size. Left ventricular size less than two thirds normal is rarely compatible with survival. Such patients are really variants of hypoplastic left heart syndrome (HLHS) and are treated with either heart transplantation or a Norwood procedure.

### Coarctation of the Aorta

Neonatal coarctation is a narrowing of the aorta, usually in the periductal area, but a variable length of hypoplastic aortic isthmus and arch may be present. Though coarctation of the aorta may exist as an isolated congenital defect, it is frequently associated

with other forms of congenital heart disease, most commonly, persistent ductus arteriosus, ventricular septal defects, and anomalies of the aortic valve. Fifty percent of infants with coarctation of the aorta have symptoms in the first month of life. The most prominent symptom is congestive heart failure. In the neonatal variety, a severe preductal coarctation becomes more obstructive as the ductus closes, resulting in severe hypoperfusion of the descending aorta. Such infants can present with fulminant congestive heart failure and shock. Immediate medical treatment requires infusion of prostaglandin E to open and dilate the ductus arteriosus, thus improving both hemodynamic and metabolic state of the patient. Surgery is indicated in all symptomatic infants but requires preoperative stabilization including treatment of metabolic acidosis, poor renal output, and often mechanical ventilation to ensure adequate gas exchange. Attention to preoperative stabilization has improved surgical results remarkably.

*Surgery.* Operation is performed through a left lateral thoracotomy and the chest cavity is entered through the fourth intercostal space. The extended resection with end-to-end anastomosis is the procedure of choice in the neonate. Operative repair entails closure of the persistent ductus arteriosus, excision of the coarctation, and end-to-end anastomosis between the aortic arch and isthmus and the descending aorta (Fig 20-116). The aorta is dissected from the transverse aortic arch starting from the innominate artery down to the descending aorta, four or five intercostal arteries below the coarctation. The aorta is completely mobilized and the persistent ductus isolated. The patient's blood pressure is controlled using nitroprusside and by altering mechanical ventilation. Vascular clamps are then placed proximally on the aortic arch occluding the left subclavian artery but permitting the innominate artery to provide cerebral profusion. The distal clamp is placed below the level of the coarctation. The persistent ductus is ligated and the coarctation is sharply excised. The medial border of the aortic arch is opened (Fig 20-116*B*). The two vascular clamps are approximated, and the anastomosis is carried out with 6-0 Prolene or absorbable PDS suture (Fig 20-116*C*). With an uncomplicated procedure, the total clamp ischemic time for the distal extremities and viscera should be less than 25 minutes.

Those infants who also have large isolated VSD can undergo concomitant pulmonary artery banding through the same incision. In most patients, primary VSD closure later in the neonatal period without preliminary banding carries an acceptable low risk. Neonates with associated complex anomalies have a poorer prognosis. Coarctation may be repaired through a median sternotomy used to repair other intracardiac anomalies.

Recurrent coarctation may occur in 10% to 25% of neonates and usually can be treated with balloon dilation. The radical end-to-end anastomosis technique is particularly useful in infants who have hypoplastic aortic isthmus and small transverse aortic arches.

An alternative surgical technique is the subclavian arterial flap

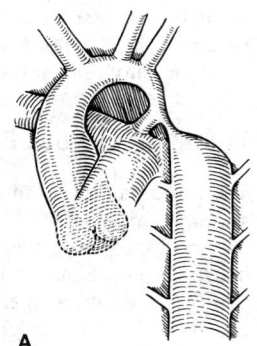
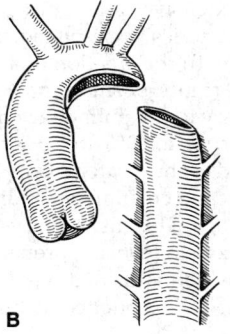
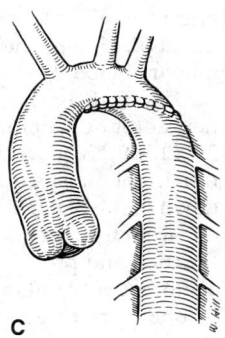

**Figure 20-116.** (**A**) Severe coarctation of the aorta with hypoplastic isthmus. (**B**) Resection of coarctation. (**C**) Extended end-to-end anastomosis.

**A**          **B**          **C**

in which the left subclavian artery is sacrificed and used as a pedicled flap to augment the coarctation. Another alternative is the use of prosthetic patch material to enlarge the area of coarctation, although a disturbingly high incidence of late aneurysm formation is reported with this particular technique.

Complications include chylothorax, recurrent laryngeal nerve injuries, and phrenic nerve damage. The incidence of paraplegia in neonates and infants is extremely low.

### Interrupted Aortic Arch

Interrupted aortic arch (IAA) can be considered an extreme variation of coarctation of the aorta. It is distinctly less common than coarctation. There is an 80% mortality within the first month of life with untreated IAA, and it is rare that infants are not profoundly symptomatic. IAA is classified into three types: type A, in which the interruption is distal to the left subclavian artery (42%); Type B, in which the interruption is between the left carotid and left subclavian arteries (50%); and Type C, an uncommon form in which the interruption is between the innominate and the left carotid artery. Neonates may present in profound congestive heart failure with systemic hypoperfusion and profound metabolic acidosis as a result of PDA closure and descending aortic hypoperfusion. Diagnosis is made with echocardiography and cardiac catheterization. Preoperative stabilization includes use of prostaglandin E1 and inotropes. If renal failure is present, peritoneal dialysis is also begun preoperatively.

Operation consists of a left lateral thoracotomy for Type A. Repair is essentially the same as a coarctation repair using the extended end-to-end anastomotic technique. Type B and Type C require the use of cardiopulmonary bypass, systemic hypothermia, and total circulatory arrest. Repair requires closure of the persistent ductus arteriosus, dissection of the proximal and distal segments of the interrupted aorta, and end-to-end anastomosis of the two segments. During total circulatory arrest, other intracardiac anomalies, including VSD which usually is present, are also repaired. Mortality in most reported series is high, but has improved in recent years due to increasing experience with total circulatory arrest and with careful attention to preoperative stabilization.

### Hypoplastic Left Heart Syndrome

HLHS is a common form of single ventricle, characterized by aortic and mitral valve atresia and a severely hypoplastic or absent left ventricle (Fig 20-117A). Systemic blood flow arises via a PDA from the pulmonary artery trunk with coronary perfusion retrograde through a severely hypoplastic ascending aorta. Until recently, this common form of univentricular heart was deemed inoperable. Over the past decade, a treatment strategy consisting of neonatal palliation followed by a Fontan procedure in infancy has been developed by Norwood. Commonly referred to as a Norwood operation, neonatal palliation consists of reconstructing the ascending aorta and aortic arch using the main pulmonary artery, ascending aorta, and an extensive homograft patch (Fig 20-117B, C, D). The pulmonary arteries are isolated, and pulmonary blood flow is established with the creation of a modified Blalock-Taussig shunt using a short interposition graft from the new aortic arch or innominate artery to the pulmonary trunk (Fig 20-117E). Neonatal palliation carries a 10% to 30% mortality rate in the most experienced hands. The strategy calls for takedown of the Blalock-Taussig shunt and creation of a bidirectional Glenn shunt at about 6 months of age. This maintains ventricular function and provides adequate oxygen levels in preparation for a subsequent Fontan procedure, which is carried out during the second or third year of life. Using this sequence of operations,

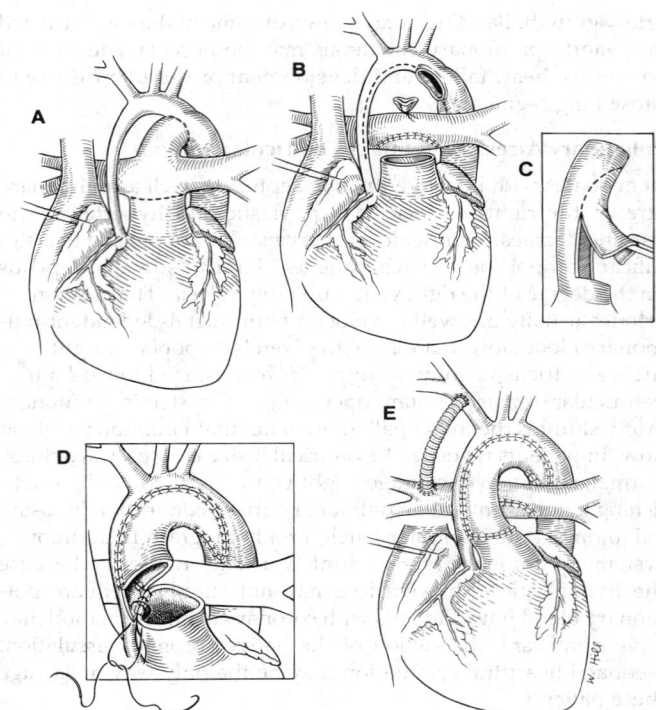

**Figure 20-117.** The Norwood procedure for hypoplastic-left-heart syndrome.

Norwood's group produced good long-term palliation in a significant proportion of these patients.

### Neonatal Heart Transplantation

Bailey's group at Loma Linda report a large series of neonatal heart transplantations for hypoplastic left heart syndrome (77%) or other complex neonatal heart disease. Ninety percent survived operation, and actuarial survival at 1 and 5 years was 86% and 84%. These results compare favorably to those in adult patients. The belief that transplantation in the neonatal period may allow for good long-term results with minimum chronic immunosuppression due to "extension of the fetal immune state" is supported by their data. Severe rejection was uncommon, and episodes occurring after 1 year were infrequent on a modest immunosuppression regimen. Initial immunosuppression consisted of cyclosporine and azathioprine with steroids reserved for acute rejection episodes. Of the patients followed for more than a year, 92% were on cyclosporine monotherapy. Few other groups have been as successful, but these results are encouraging, and continued trials of neonatal heart transplantation appear justified.

The shortage of suitable donors, however, is a major problem because 20% to 30% of infants succumb while awaiting transplantation. A combined treatment strategy for infants with HLHS using both transplantation and palliation may yield better overall results. With further progress in immunosuppression, use of xenografts may help solve the donor shortage.

### Total Anomalous Pulmonary Venous Return

Total anomalous pulmonary venous drainage is an uncommon anomaly in which all pulmonary venous blood drains into a common collecting vein, which drains to the right side of the heart. Different anatomic subgroups are established according to whether pulmonary venous blood drains into the superior vena cava (supracardiac), right atrium (intracardiac), or portal system (infracardiac). All pulmonary and systemic venous return mixes in the right side of the heart. Blood flow to the left side of the heart is via an atrial septal defect. Diagnosis is made in infants who are suffering from congestive heart failure but are cyanotic and have plethoric lungs with a small heart shadow on chest x-rays. Diagnosis is confirmed with cardiac catheterization and echocardiography. Poor clinical conditions correlate with the degree of pulmonary venous obstruction. Severe obstruction leads to hypoperfusion and consequent oliguria, subendocardial ischemia, and metabolic acidosis in the neonate. Preoperative preparation requires stabilization with inotropic support and prostaglandin E1 infusion to improve systemic flow and correct metabolic acidosis.

### Surgical Technique

All repairs are done with cardiopulmonary bypass using deep hypothermia with or without total circulatory arrest. The heart is protected with cold crystalloid or blood cardioplegia. The repair depends on the anatomic type of anomalous pulmonary venous drainage.

*Supracardiac Repair.* The heart is approached from the right side and a transverse bi-atrial incision is made. This allows opening of the foramen ovale and the left atrium, and pulmonary veins can be seen. Direct anastomosis is performed between the open pulmonary veins which lie in the retrocardiac space behind the pericardium and the posterior wall of the left atrium. The foramen ovale is closed with a generous pericardial patch, ensuring that the usually small left atrium is enlarged. The ascending vein is ligated carefully so as not to damage the phrenic nerve that runs near its lateral surface.

*Intracardiac Type.* Cardiac type, in which pulmonary veins drain into the right atrium via the coronary sinus or via direct connection, is approached through the right atrium. The coronary sinus is unroofed, and the atrial septal defect is enlarged to allow free drainage of pulmonary venous return into the left atrium. The atrial septal defect is then closed with a pericardial patch.

*Infracardiac Type.* Infracardiac is the most technically challenging surgery in that the collecting vein lies posterior and inferior to the heart in the extrapericardial space. Infants present with the most severe metabolic acidosis and hypoperfusion because pulmonary venous return is almost always severely obstructed. Patients are difficult to stabilize, and surgery is undertaken as an emergency. The heart is retracted upwards and to the right, allowing dissection of the veins in the retrocardiac space. Once the veins are dissected, a direct anastomosis is made to the back of the left atrium. This requires particular attention to each pulmonary vein orifice to avoid obstruction.

*Complications.* Complications associated with repair of total anomalous pulmonary drainage include the anastomotic strictures or stenosis of the ostiae of the pulmonary veins due to a hypertrophic growth of the vascular media. Hepatic failure has been reported to occur with the infracardiac type, secondary to ligation of the inferior collecting vein. Mortality rates in the neonate are 10% to 30% in most series, with the infracardiac group having the worst prognosis.

## Truncus Arteriosus

### Anatomy and Pathology

Truncus arteriosus is a ventriculoarterial abnormality characterized by a single arterial trunk overriding both ventricles (Fig 20-118A). A VSD is almost always present. Pulmonary blood flow arises from the single arterial trunk, and a main pulmonary artery may be absent or present to a variable degree. The underlying pathophysiology relates to unrestricted pulmonary blood flow. Infants with truncus develop congestive heart failure when pulmonary vascular resistance starts to drop within the first few months of life. If untreated, 85% of infants die in the first year of life.

Infants are treated vigorously for congestive heart failure with fluid restriction, diuretics, digitalization, and afterload reduction. Previous attempts at palliation of truncus, including pulmonary artery banding, have been unsuccessful; therefore, definitive surgical repair consisting of a Rastelli operation is carried out electively within the first few months of life or sooner for severe congestive heart failure and growth failure.

### Surgical Technique

Surgical repair consists of septating the single truncus into two separate pulmonary and systemic vascular trunks receiving blood

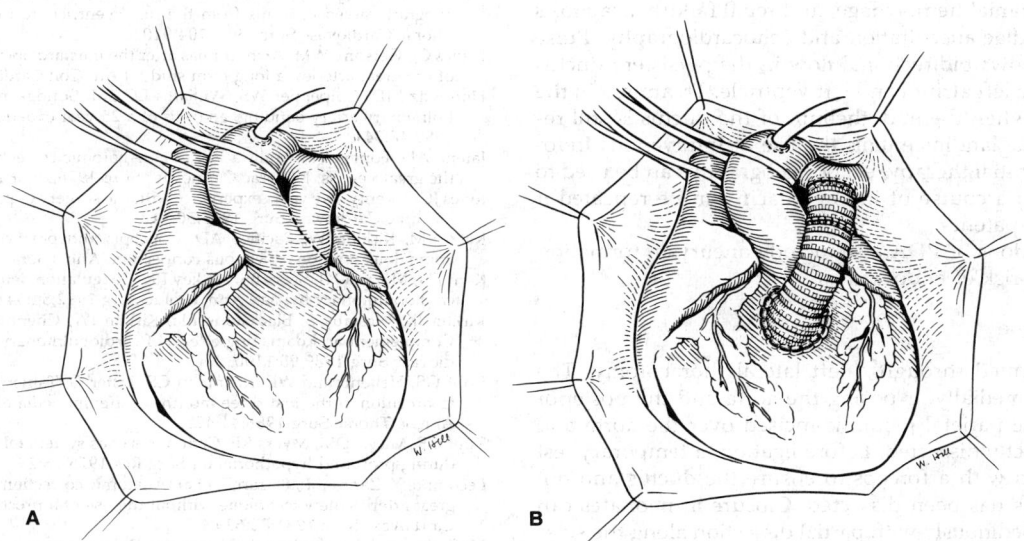

**Figure 20-118.** Rastelli type repair for truncus arteriosus. (**A**) Anatomy of type 1 truncus arteriosus. (**B**) Conduit from right ventricle to pulmonary artery. The VSD has been closed through the right ventricular incision to rout left ventricular blood out the aorta.

from their corresponding ventricles, another form of Rastelli repair (see Fig 20-118). The operation is performed with deep hypothermia and usually requires a period of total circulatory arrest. The heart is protected with cold cardioplegic solution and topical hypothermia. After aortic cross-clamping, the pulmonary arteries are separated from the aorta, and the aortic wall is reconstructed with a patch. The VSD is patched closed through a right ventriculotomy so as to direct left ventricular blood out the aorta. Finally, the right ventricular outflow tract is reconstructed with a 10- or 12-mm diameter homograft or porcine valved Dacron conduit between the right ventricle and pulmonary arteries. When available, homografts are preferred to Dacron conduits. Homograft tissue handles easier, and anastomosis to the thin neonatal pulmonary artery is facilitated, which results in less distortion and bleeding. Postoperatively, infants are subject to pulmonary hypertensive crises marked by sudden pulmonary vasoconstriction and severe right ventricular failure. This must be managed aggressively with sedation, paralysis, hyperventilation, and vasodilators including prostaglandins, if needed. Operative mortality rate in most institutions is 15% to 30%. Operation on infants younger than 6 months of age has improved surgical results over children operated on after that time. All infants require reoperation for conduit replacement usually within 3 to 5 years.

## Persistent Ductus Arteriosus

The ductus arteriosus is a normal fetal structure connecting the main pulmonary artery to the descending aorta. It arises from the superior portion of the bifurcation of the pulmonary artery and connects directly to the descending aorta just distal and medial to the left subclavian artery. Its length and diameter vary, whereas an increased amount of smooth muscle is always present in the wall of the vessel. In the fetal circulation, more than 60% of the blood flow from both ventricles is directed through the ductus. After birth, when the pulmonary vascular resistance falls and oxygenation increases, the ductus normally constricts. Spontaneous complete closure occurs in most infants during the first weeks of life.

Persistent PDA causes left to right shunt, which may result in congestive heart failure. These symptoms, though minimal at birth, may increase over the first month of life as pulmonary vascular resistance falls. The premature infant with large ductus and pulmonary disease is particularly prone to necrotizing enterocolitis, intracranial hemorrhage, and renal failure. Diagnosis is made with cardiac auscultation and echocardiography. Pulse wave Doppler shows bidirectional flow in the persistent ductus along with a large left atrium and left ventricle. Treatment in the neonatal period when the endothelium of the ductus is still responsive to prostaglandins entails the use of intravenous Indomethacin. After initial therapy, echocardiography can be used to assess results and a course of indomethacin can be repeated if the ductus is still patent.

Late complications of PDA also include aneurysm formation and an increased risk of endocarditis.

### Surgical Technique

Surgery is performed through a left lateral thoracotomy. The lung is retracted medially, exposing the aorta and the posterior mediastinum. The parietal pleura is incised over the aorta and the ductus is directly dissected. Before ligation, a temporary test closure is affected with a forceps to ensure the ductus and not the aortic isthmus has been dissected. Closure in neonates can be carried out expeditiously with partial dissection along the sides of the ductus and placement of a metal clip. In full-term infants with a short, large ductus, vascular clamps may be used to divide

and oversew both ends of the ductus. One pleural chest tube is left to be removed the following morning.

Complications include uncontrolled hemorrhage from a friable ductus, injury to the recurrent laryngeal nerve that loops around the ductus near the area of dissection, and disruption of significant lymphatics, resulting in chylothorax. The latter usually responds to conservative treatment consisting of drainage, dietary therapy, and nutritional support.

## Selected Readings

Albanese SB, Carotti A, DiDonato RM, et al. Bidirectional cavopulmonary anastomosis in patients under 2 years of age. J Thorac Cardiovasc Surg 1992;104:904.

Amato JJ, Galdieri RJ, Cotroneo JV. Role of extended aortoplasty related to the definition of coarctation of the aorta. Ann Thorac Surg 1991;52:615.

Bailey LL, Nehlsen-Cannarella SL, Concepcion W, Jolley WB. Baboon-to-human cardiac xenotransplantation in a neonate. JAMA 1985;254:3321.

Bove EL, Beckman RH, Snider AR, et al. Repair of truncus arteriosus in the neonate and young infant. Ann Thorac Surg 1989;47:499.

Castaneda A, Mayer J, Jonas R, Lock J, Wessel D, Hickey P. The neonate with critical congenital heart disease: repair–a surgical challenge. J Thorac Cardiovasc Surg 1989;98:869.

Castaneda AR, Trusler GA, Paul MH, Blackstone EH, Kirklin JW. The early results of treatment of transposition in the current era. J Thorac Cardiovasc Surg 1988;95:14.

Chiavarelli M, Boucek MM, Nehlsen-Cannarella SL, Gundry SR, Razzouk AJ, Bailey LL. Neonatal cardiac transplantation: intermediate term results and incidence of rejection. Arch Surg 1992;127:1072.

Corno AF, Bethencourt DM, Laks H, et al. Myocardial protection in the neonatal heart: a comparison of topical hypothermia and crystalloid and blood cardioplegic solutions. J Thorac Cardiovasc Surg 1987;93:163.

Danford DA, Huhta JC, Gutgesell HP. Left ventricular wall stress and thickness in complete transposition of the great arteries: inplications for surgical intervention. J Thorac Cardiovasc Surg 1985;89:610.

Dewar ML, Stark J. Complications of correction of total anomalous pulmonary venous connection. In: Waldhausen J, ed. Complications in cardiac surgery. New York: Mosby Inc. 1992:159.

DiDonato R, Jonas R, Lang P, Rome J, Mayer J, Castaneda AR. Neonatal repair of tetralogy of Fallot with and without pulmonary atresia. J Thorac Cardiovasc Surg 1991;101:126.

Farrell P, Chang A, Murdison K, Baffa J, Norwood W, Murphy J. Outcome and assessment after the modified Fontan procedure for hypoplastic left heart syndrome. Circulation 1992;85(1):116.

Greeley WJ, Kern FH, Ungerleider RM, et al. The effect of hypothermic cardiopulmonary bypass and total circulatory arrest on cerebral metabolism in neonates, infants, and children. J Thorac Cardiovasc Surg 1991;101:783.

Hardin JT, Muskett AD, Canter CE, Martin TC, Spray TL. Primary surgical closure of large ventricular septal defects in small infants. Ann Thorac Surg 1992;53:397.

Hawkins JA, Bailey WW, Dillon T, Schwartz DC. Midterm results with cryopreserved allograft valved conduits from the right ventricle to the pulmonary artery. J Thorac Cardiovasc Surg 1992;104:910.

Hayes CJ, Gersony WM. Arrhythmias after the mustard operation for transposition of the great arteries: a long term study. J Am Coll Cardiol 1986;7:133.

Horowitz MD, Culpepper WS, Williams LC 3rd, Sundgaard-Riise K, Ochsner JL. Pulmonary artery banding: analysis of a 25 year experience. Ann Thorac Surg 1989;48:344.

Jatene AD, Fontes VF, Paulista PP, et al. Anatomic correction of transposition of the great vessels. J Thorac Cardiovasc Surg 1976;72:364.

Jones JC. Twenty-five years experience with the surgery of patent ductus arteriosus. J Thorac Cardiovasc Surg 1965;50:149.

Katz NM, Kirklin JW, Pacifico AD. Concepts and practices in surgery for total anomalous pulmonary venous connection. Ann Thorac Surg 1978 25:479.

Kern FH, Morana NJ, Sears BS, Hickey PR. Coagulation defects in neonates during cardiopulmonary bypass. Ann Thorac Surg 1992;54:541.

Kirklin JK, Westaby S, Blackstone EH, Kirklin JW, Chenoweth DE, Pacifico AD. Complement and damaging effects of cardiopulmonary bypass. J Thorac Cardiovasc Surg 1989;98:1100.

Kopf GS, Hellenbrand WE, Kleinman CS, Lister G, Talner NS, Laks H. Repair of Coarctation in the first three months of life: immediate and long term results. Annals Thorac Surg 1986;41:425.

Kopf GS, Mirvis DM, Myers RE. Central nervous system tolerance to cardiac arrest during profound hypothermia. J Surg Res 1975;18:29.

Lecompte Y, Zannini L, Hazan E, et al. Anatomic correction of transposition of the great arteries: new technique without the use of a prosthetic conduit. J Thorac Cardiovasc Surg 1981;82:629.

McCaffrey FM, Leatherbury L, Moore HV. Pulmonary atresia and intact ventricular septum: definitive repair in the neonatal period. J Thorac Cardiovasc Surg 1991;102:617.

Moulton AL, Brenner JI, Roberts G, et al. Subclavian flap repair of coarctation of the aorta in neonates. Realization of growth potential. J Thorac Cardiovasc Surg 1984;87:220.

Norwood W, Lang P, Hansen D. Physiological repair of aortic atresia-hypoplastic left heart syndrome. N Engl J Med 1983;308:23.

Pigott J, Murphy J, Barber G, Norwood W. Palliative reconstructive surgery for hypoplastic left heart syndrome. Ann Thorac Surg 1988;45:122.

Puga FJ, Leoni FE, Julsrud PR, Mair DD. Complete repair of pulmonary atresia, ventricular septal defect, and severe peripheral arborization abnormalities of the central pulmonary arteries. Experience with preliminary unifocalization procedure in 38 patients. J Thorac Cardiovasc Surg 1989;98:1018.

Quaegebeur JM, Rohmer J, Ottemkamp J, et al. The arterial switch operation: an eight year experience. J Thorac Cardiovasc Surg 1986;92:361.

Ridley PD, Ratcliffe JM, Alberti KGMM, Elliott MJ. The metabolic consequences of a washed cardiopulmonary bypass pump-priming fluid in children undergoing cardiac operations. J Thorac Cardiovasc Surg 1990;100:528.

Sade RM, Crawford FA, Hohn AR, Riopel DA, Taylor AB. Growth of the aorta after prosthetic patch aortoplasty for coarctation in infants. Ann Thorac Surg 1984;38:21.

Sell Je, Jonas RA, Mayer JE, Blackstone EH, Kirklin JW, Castaneda AR. The results of a surgical program for interrupted aortic arch. J Thorac Cardiovasc Surg 1988;96:864.

Siebenmann R, Von Segesser L, Schneider K, Schneider J, Senning, Turina M. Late failure of systemic ventricle after atrial correction for transposition of great arteries. Eur J Cardiothorac Surg 1989;3:119.

Smith VC, Caggiano AV, Knauf DG, Alexander JA. The Blalock-Taussig shunt in the newborn infant. J Thorac Cardiovasc Surg 1991;102:602.

Starnes VA, Griffin ML, Pitlick PT, et al. Current approach to hypoplastic left heart syndrome: palliation, transplantation or both? J Thorac Cardiovasc Surg 1992;104:189.

Tamisier D, Vouh'e PR, Vernant F, Lec'a F, Massot C, Neveux JY. Modified Blalock-Taussig shunts: results in infants less than 3 months of age. Ann Thorac Surg 1990;49:797.

Turley K, Bove E, Amato J, et al. Neonatal aortic stenosis. J Thorac Cardiovasc Surg 1990;99:679.

Ungerleider RM, Greeley WJ, Sheikh KH, et al. Routine use of intraoperative epicardial echocardiography and Doppler color flow imaging to guide and evaluate repair of congenital heart lesions. J Thorac Cardiovasc Surg 1990;100:297.

Vernovsky G, Hougen TJ, Walsh EP, et al. Mid-term results after the arterial switch operation for transposition of the great arteries with intact ventricular septum: clinical, hemodynamic electrocardiographic and electrophysiologic data. Circulation 1988;77(6):1333.

Watterson KG, Wilkinson JL, Karl TR, Mee RB. Very small pulmonary arteries: central end to side shunt. Ann Thorac Surg 1991;52:1132.

Zeimer G, Jonas R, Perry S, Freed M, Castaneda A. Surgery for coarctation of the aorta in the neonate. Circulation 1986;74(suppl I):1.

*Principles and Practice of Pediatrics, Second Edition.*
edited by Frank A. Oski et al. J. B. Lippincott Company, Philadelphia © 1994.

# 20.16 *Malignancy in the Newborn*

Jack van Hoff

Cancer in neonates is an uncommon problem and one that presents unique challenges to pediatricians regarding both diagnosis and therapy. Many neoplasms discovered at birth or within the first month of life are benign, and others with apparent malignant histology may behave as benign. While this has important implications regarding the possible role of oncogene expression and modulation in embryonal and fetal cells, it complicates the clinician's decisions regarding therapy. Neonates are particularly susceptible to many of the adverse effects of both chemotherapy and radiation therapy, and they may have coexistent problems of prematurity or congenital malformations. Because of these issues, great care must be taken in deciding whether and how to treat neonatal tumors.

## INCIDENCE, PRESENTATION, AND SURVIVAL

Few population-based estimates of incidence exist; most reports represent the experience of a single institution. These results are subject to selection bias because of referral patterns and can rarely be used to estimate incidence. One of the best population-based sources in the United States is the Third National Cancer Survey, in which the incidence of cancer in infants less than 29 days of age is 36.5 per million live births. This number includes cancers that begin in the last few months of prenatal life, but are not diagnosed until birth. Therefore, the number is probably not significantly different from the incidence of cancer during the rest of childhood, which in the United States is 130 per million per year or 11 per million per month. Neonates account for about 2% of all cases of childhood cancer in institutional reports, a number proportional to their "time at risk." Based on this information, it is concluded that although cancer is uncommon during the newborn period, it is probably no less common than it is during later childhood.

The mortality from cancer in the first month of life—6 to 8 per million per year—is substantially lower than the incidence. The majority of newborns with cancer survive the neonatal period.

Types of tumors seen in the neonatal period are listed in Tables 20-87 and 20-88. Table 20-87 presents all neonatal tumors, both benign and malignant, seen at the Children's Hospital of Los Angeles from 1958 to 1985. Hemangiomas, the most common benign lesion of infancy, are generally excluded from discussions of neonatal tumors and are not included here. While teratomas and other soft tissue tumors constitute the majority of all tumors, neuroblastomas, leukemias, and sarcomas account for the majority of cancers.

Table 20-88 presents data compiled from the four largest series of neonatal cancer in North America. Neuroblastoma is the most common, accounting for 41% of all cancers. Leukemias (16%), sarcomas (12%), and retinoblastoma (12%) are the next most common cancers. Melanoma and carcinomas, which are uncommon during the rest of childhood and more common in adults, are present in several of the series. Overall, the cancers seen in neonates differ substantially from those seen during the rest of childhood when leukemias (31%), brain tumors (19%), and lymphomas (13%) predominate.

Half of neonatal malignancies and an even larger percentage of benign tumors are diagnosed on the first day of life. The re-

### TABLE 20-87. Neonatal Tumors, Children's Hospital of Los Angeles

|  | Total (%) | Malignant (%) |
|---|---|---|
| Teratoma | 46 (38) | 2 (4) |
| Soft tissue | 25 (20) | 8 (16) |
| Neuroblastoma | 17 (14) | 17 (33) |
| Leukemia | 13 (11) | 13 (25) |
| Renal | 7 (6) | 3 (6) |
| Brain tumor | 5 (4) | 2 (4) |
| Hepatic | 4 (3) | 1 (2) |
| Retinoblastoma | 3 (2) | 3 (6) |
| Carcinoma | 2 (2) | 2 (4) |
| Total | 122 (100) | 51 (100) |

*Adapted with permission from Isaacs H. Congenital and neonatal malignant tumors. Am J Pediatr Hematol Oncol 1987;9:121.*

### TABLE 20-88. Neonatal Malignancies, Relative Frequency and Long-Term (>5 Year) Survival

|  | Number | (%) | Long-term Survivors | (%) |
|---|---|---|---|---|
| Neuroblastoma* | 79 | (41) | 50 | (63) |
| Leukemia | 30 | (16) | 2 | (7) |
| Sarcoma | 23 | (12) | 10 | (43) |
| Retinoblastoma | 23 | (12) | 17 | (74) |
| Brain tumor | 11 | (5.5) | 1 | (9) |
| Renal | 10 | (5) | 6 | (60) |
| Germ cell | 9 | (4.5) | 7 | (78) |
| Carcinoma | 3 | (1.5) | 1 | (33) |
| Hepatoblastoma | 2 | (1) | 1 | (50) |
| Melanoma | 2 | (1) | 2 | (100) |
| Malignant schwannoma | 1 | (0.5) | 1 | (100) |
| Total | 193 | (100) | 98 | (51) |

\* Excludes neuroblastoma in situ discovered incidentally at autopsy.

*Adapted from Isaacs H. Congenital and neonatal malignant tumors. Am J Pediatr Hematol Oncol 1987;9:121; Crom DB, Williams JA, Green AA, Pratt CB, Jenkins JJ, Behm FG. Malignancy in the neonate. Med Pediatr Oncol 1989;17:101; Gale GB, D'angio GJ, Uri A, Chatten J, Koop CE. Cancer in neonates; the experience at Children's Hospital of Philadelphia. Pediatrics 1982;70:409; and Becker LE. Malignant tumors in the neonate. Arch Dis Child 1987;62:19.*

mainder present over the next month. Numerous lesions have been diagnosed prenatally by ultrasonography, and this is likely to occur more often in the future. Neonatal tumors usually present as visible or palpable masses whether they are malignant or benign (Table 20-89). Visible masses include hemangiomas, teratomas, benign soft tissue tumors or sarcomas, and skin nodules from leukemia, neuroblastoma, or congenital viral infection. Hemangiomas are the most common of all neonatal "tumors." Hemangiomas occur in as many as 2% of all newborns and almost always resolve without therapy. When subcutaneous, hemangiomas are differentiated from solid tumors by their characteristic appearance. Deeper hemangiomas can often be differentiated from solid tumors by their blood flow characteristics on magnetic resonance imaging. Neonatal teratomas occur most commonly in the sacrococcygeal region. Other relatively common locations include the neck and midline of the face. They are usually benign but may contain malignant elements. Sarcomas may present as masses on almost any part of the body including the head, neck, trunk, and extremities. Sarcomas are often clinically indistinguishable from benign soft tissue tumors.

Neonatal solid tumors also may present as palpable abdominal masses. Solid tumors in the upper abdomen are usually neuroblastomas or are renal or hepatic in origin. Common solid tumors in the lower abdomen and pelvis include teratomas, rhabdomyosarcomas of the genitourinary system, and neuroblastomas. They usually are differentiated from cystic urinary or gastrointestinal malformations by ultrasonography. Solid lesions must be biopsied or resected to differentiate malignancies from benign hamartomas.

Neonatal brain tumors may present with an abnormally large head circumference or bulging fontanelle in addition to the more typical symptoms of increased intracranial pressure such as irritability, decreased responsiveness, or vomiting. Leukemia in newborns usually presents with pallor, petechiae, or purpura.

### TABLE 20-89. Benign and Malignant Tumors in the Neonate (by Location)

| Location of Mass | Benign Lesion | Malignancy |
|---|---|---|
| Subcutaneous or soft tissue, visible | Hemangioma | Sarcoma |
|  | Teratoma | Teratoma |
|  | Fibroma | Neuroblastoma |
|  | Congenital viral infection | Leukemia |
|  | Branchial or thyroglossal duct cyst |  |
|  | Cystic hygroma |  |
| Abdominal or pelvic, palpable | Teratoma | Neuroblastoma |
|  | Polycystic kidneys | Wilms' tumor |
|  | Urinary tract obstruction | Teratoma |
|  | Hepatic hamartoma or hemangioma | Hepatoblastoma |
|  | Gastrointestinal duplication | Rhabdomyosarcoma |
|  | Hepatosplenomegaly | Leukemia (hepatosplenomegaly) |
| Intracranial | Hemorrhage | Brain tumor |
|  | Hydrocephalus |  |
|  | Teratoma |  |
|  | Vascular malformation |  |

*Adapted with permission from Reaman GH. Special considerations for the infant with cancer. In: Pizzo PA, Poplack DG, eds. Principles and practice of pediatric oncology. Philadelphia: JB Lippincott 1989:265.*

Occasionally, subcutaneous leukemic nodules are seen as dark blue spots on the skin. Retinoblastoma usually presents as leukocoria or strabismus. More advanced lesions may demonstrate signs of local inflammation or heterochromia iridis.

Long-term survival after neonatal cancer is not uncommon (see Table 20-88). Neuroblastoma, retinoblastoma, germ cell tumor, and kidney tumor all have long-term survival rates better than 50%, whereas long-term survival rates after leukemia or brain tumor are very poor.

## MANAGEMENT OF SPECIFIC TUMORS

### Solid Tumors

#### Teratoma

Teratomas are the most frequent perinatal neoplasm, occurring more commonly in females with a female-to-male ratio of 1.5:1. By definition, teratomas contain tissue from more than one of the three main germ layers (ectoderm, mesoderm, endoderm). They are classified as mature (containing only adult-type tissue), immature (containing embryonic type tissue), or malignant (containing embryonal carcinoma, endodermal sinus tumor, choriocarcinoma, or germinoma).

In the newborn, teratomas are found primarily in the sacrococcygeal region with a large external and relatively small internal or presacral component. Less than 10% of neonatal teratomas contain malignant elements, usually embryonal carcinoma or endodermal sinus tumor. In contrast, more than 50% of sacrococcygeal teratomas presenting after 2 months of age are malignant. About 30% of neonatal teratomas contain immature elements. These should be managed the same way as mature tumors, by complete surgical resection including coccygectomy for sacrococcygeal primaries. Mature tumors rarely recur. The incidence of recurrence for immature tumors may be as high as 15%. These tumors should be followed closely postoperatively with ultrasonography or computed tomography scans. Malignant teratomas, or germ cell tumors, in newborns are best treated with aggressive resection. The role of adjuvant chemotherapy is less clear. It appears warranted in light of the beneficial effects of cisplatin-based regimens on germ cell tumors occurring at older ages. The survival of newborns with extragonadal germ cell tumors appears better (see Table 20-88) than it is in older children for whom long-term survival is uncommon.

#### Neuroblastoma

Neuroblastoma is the most common form of neonatal cancer, accounting for 30% to 50% of all malignancies in most series. Congenital neuroblastoma is unique in that it may spontaneously regress. Routine postmortem examinations show neuroblastoma in situ in the adrenal glands of 1 in 200 to 1 in 500 newborns. This is more than 10 times higher than the lifetime incidence of neuroblastoma estimated at 1 in 7000, implying that the majority of these cases regress without ever being identified. A correlate to this is seen clinically in infants with a unique form of metastatic neuroblastoma—stage IV-S (consisting of a localized primary lesion plus liver, bone marrow, or cutaneous involvement)—which often spontaneously regresses. In a recent study, about one fourth of all newly diagnosed cases of IV-S neuroblastoma regressed without any tumor-directed therapy. Half required immediate treatment with either radiation or chemotherapy because of severe abdominal distention causing respiratory distress or inferior vena cava compression. The remaining one fourth required delayed therapy. The extended survival rate in that study, which included patients diagnosed beyond the neonatal period, was 75%. Localized neuroblastoma without metastases also has an excellent prognosis; 89% of stage I, II, and III neonates are long-term survivors. Only stage IV newborns with unresectable primary tumors

and bony or distant lymph node metastases do very poorly. Recommendations are surgical resection and observation for neonates with localized disease, aggressive chemotherapy for stage IV patients, and observation without therapy for stage IV-S patients, if possible. Stage IV-S patients who require therapy should be treated with either low dose radiation or chemotherapy.

Although the stage at presentation is a good indicator of the prognosis, the behavior of neuroblastoma can be more accurately predicted by biologic factors such as hyperdiploidy and oncogene (N-myc) amplification. These are currently used to help determine therapy. Routine screening for all newborns to detect early neuroblastoma by measuring urinary catecholamine levels is feasible; however, it is not yet recommended. To date, no large controlled trial has documented a decrease in neuroblastoma mortality related to screening. Current recommendation is to wait for evidence before instituting widespread screening programs.

#### Retinoblastoma

Although rare at older ages, retinoblastoma is a relatively common cause of cancer in neonates. Retinoblastoma has played an important role in the understanding of oncogenesis. Its familial predisposition attracted attention early and placed it in the center of research on the molecular biology of cancer. Retinoblastoma studies led to recognition of an entire new class of oncogenes, the tumor suppressor genes, and identification of the mutant protein product is providing new information on cell cycle regulation. About 40% of all retinoblastomas are familial, related to a germ line mutation on chromosome 13q. Laboratory DNA studies of affected families can identify individuals at risk for developing retinoblastoma.

Familial tumors are almost always bilateral or, if unilateral, multifocal, indicating an extreme predisposition to the development of retinoblastoma. Nonfamilial tumors are always unilateral and unifocal. Familial tumors present at an earlier age than nonfamilial tumors, and they are, therefore, overrepresented in neonatal series. In the largest reported neonatal series, 13 of 17 cases were bilateral indicating a familial predisposition.

Retinoblastoma can be treated successfully by enucleation or by radiation therapy. Radiation therapy is used more often in bilateral (ie, familial) cases to preserve vision. Radiation therapy increases an already elevated risk of second cancers in these children with a defective tumor suppression mechanism. As a result, children with familial retinoblastoma are more likely to die of a second cancer than of retinoblastoma, which is highly curable. Neonates with retinoblastoma, therefore, represent a complex problem that extends beyond their initial therapy and that requires careful, lifelong follow-up.

### Soft Tissue

Benign and malignant soft tissue tumors are second in frequency only to teratomas in the neonate. Malignant sarcomas are among the most common forms of neonatal cancer (see Tables 20-87, 20-88). Rhabdomyosarcoma is the most common malignant soft tissue tumor in the newborn, as it is later in childhood. A variety of other sarcomas also occur. Infantile or congenital fibrosarcoma has an excellent prognosis despite its aggressive appearance histologically. Although local recurrence may follow initial resection, congenital fibrosarcomas usually are curable with more extensive surgery, and fewer than 10% metastasize. Unresectable primaries appear to be treatable by chemotherapy. Rhabdomyosarcoma in newborns has a much less favorable prognosis, even when treated aggressively. Only 1 of 11 patients treated with surgery and radiation or chemotherapy was a long-term survivor. Recommendations are for multimodal therapy for rhabdomyosarcoma, similar to treatment at older ages, despite the poor prognosis. In general, other sarcomas in newborns should be managed with surgery and followed closely for local relapse.

## Renal

Solid tumors are a less frequent cause of renal enlargement in the neonate than is hydronephrosis or cystic kidneys. Furthermore, a majority of the solid lesions are mesoblastic nephromas. These are renal hamartomas that may progress to Wilms' tumor but generally are considered benign and curable by surgery alone. The remaining solid lesions are malignant, primarily Wilms' tumors with occasional rhabdoid tumors. While infants with rhabdoid tumors do very poorly, the prognosis for neonatal Wilms' tumor is quite good. Wilms' tumors should be managed with surgery and adjuvant chemotherapy, much the same as in older patients.

## Leukemia

Congenital leukemia is one of the most serious neonatal malignancies, accounting for less than 15% of cancers but 30% of all deaths (see Table 20-88). Acute myelogenous leukemia is more common than acute lymphoblastic leukemia (ALL) in newborns. During the rest of childhood, 75% of all leukemias are ALL.

Decisions regarding therapy are difficult with neonatal leukemia for two reasons. First, long-term survivors are rare; only 2 of 30 infants counted in Table 20-88 were long-term survivors and one of those was never treated, remitting spontaneously. Second, a benign entity known as the transient myeloproliferative or myelodysplastic disorder (TMD) occurs in newborns and can mimic acute leukemia. Unlike leukemia, TMD requires no therapy and resolves spontaneously over weeks to months. TMD is seen mostly in infants with Down syndrome and appears to depend on and be unique to trisomy 21. TMD has also been described in phenotypically normal infants. In virtually every case, however, the affected child was either a trisomy 21 mosaic or had trisomy 21 in the proliferative bone marrow cells alone. TMD usually can be distinguished from acute leukemia on clinical and laboratory grounds, even though both can present with high white blood cell counts and myeloblasts on the peripheral smear (Table 20-90). Therefore, it is recommended that careful evaluation, including bone marrow aspirate and cytogenetic analysis of both bone marrow and skin fibroblasts, precede any decision to treat a newborn with leukemia. Infants with Down syndrome or isolated trisomy 21 on bone marrow cytogenetics should be observed without treatment. Treatment with chemotherapy should be reserved for infants with other cytogenetic abnormalities in their bone marrow cells and either organ involvement such as skin nodules or clear progression of disease. Most hematologists offer supportive care only in uncertain cases, including exchange transfusion to lower a markedly elevated white blood cell count, while studies are being obtained.

---

**TABLE 20-90. Characteristics of the Transient Myeloproliferative Disorder (TMD) Compared to Acute Leukemia**

| TMD | Acute Leukemia |
|---|---|
| Well infant | Sick infant with skin nodules or organomegaly |
| High WBC, rest of CBC normal | Pancytopenia or high WBC with low hemoglobin and platelets |
| Blasts on peripheral smear | Blasts on peripheral smear |
| <15% blasts in bone marrow | >40% blasts in bone marrow |
| Trisomy 21 in marrow cells | Other cytogenetic abnormalities in marrow cells |
| Bone marrow cells mature in culture | Persistent growth of abnormal cells in culture |

## Brain Tumors

Neonatal brain tumors differ from brain tumors in later childhood in histology, location, and prognosis. Teratomas are the most common neonatal brain tumor, accounting for almost 50% of all lesions. Other relatively common types include gliomas (15%), medulloblastomas (10%), and craniopharyngiomas (8%). The majority of these lesions are supratentorial. Unlike many solid tumors, congenital and neonatal brain tumors have a much poorer prognosis than those occurring at older ages (see Table 20-88). A 1984 review of the world's literature identified 115 infants with congenital brain tumors, only 8 of whom had prolonged survival. Many of these tumors are very large at diagnosis and the poor survival may be partly due to the degree of loss of normal brain tissue secondary to the tumor itself or to tumor-related hydrocephalus. The most common mode of presentation is macrocephaly with or without a bulging fontanelle, and 32% of affected neonates suffer dystocia secondary to the large fetal skull size. This may account for the high incidence of stillbirths and tumor-related hemorrhage seen in these patients. The prognosis is so poor that some have discouraged an aggressive surgical approach to any of these lesions. Nonetheless, individual cases must be considered because long-term, disease-free survival has been reported after surgical resection of both low- and high-grade lesions.

## Selected Readings

Abramson DH, Notterman RB, Ellsworth RM, Kitchin FD. Retinoblastoma treated in infants in the first six months of life. Arch Ophthalmol 1983;101:1362.

Abramson DH. Retinoblastoma 1990: diagnosis, treatment, and implications. Pediatr Ann 1990;19:387.

Altman RP, Randolph JG, Lilly TR. Sacrococcygeal teratoma: American Academy of Pediatrics Surgical Section Survey—1973. J Pediatr Surg 1974;9:389.

Bader JL, Miller RW. US cancer incidence and mortality in the first year of life. Am J Dis Child 1979;133:157.

Barnett PL, Clark AC, Garson OM. Acute nonlymphocytic leukemia after transient myeloproliferative disorder in a patient with Down syndrome. Med Pediatr Oncol 1990;18:347.

Campbell AN, Chan HS, O'Brien A, Smith CR, Becker LE. Malignant tumors in the neonate. Arch Dis Child 1987;62:19.

Crom DB, Williams JA, Green AA, Pratt CB, Jenkins JJ, Behm FG. Malignancy in the neonate. Med Pediatr Oncol 1989;17:101.

Gale GB, D'Angio GJ, Uri A, Chatten J, Koop CE. Cancer in neonates: the experience at the Children's Hospital of Philadelphia. Pediatr 1982;70:409.

Gallie BL, Dunn JM, Chan HS, Hamel PA, Phillips RA. The genetics of retinoblastoma. Pediatr Clin North Am 1991;38:299.

Howell CG, Othersen HB, Kiviat NE, Norkool P, Beckwith JB, D'Angio GJ. Therapy and outcome in 51 children with nesoblastic nephroma: a report of the National Wilms' Tumor Study. J Pediatr Surg 1982;17:826.

Hrabovsky EE, Othersen HB, deLorimier A, Kelalis P, Beckwith JB, Takashima J. Wilms' tumor in the neonate: a report from the National Wilms' Tumor Study. J Pediatr Surg 1986;21:385.

Isaacs H. Congenital and neonatal malignant tumors. Am J. Pediatr Hematol Oncol 1987;9:121.

Jooma R, Kendall BE, Hayward RD. Intracranial tumors in neonates: a report of seventeen cases. Surg Neurol 1984;21:165.

Kalousek DK, Chan KW. Transient myeloproliferative disorder in chromosomally normal newborn infant. Med Pediatr Oncol 1987;15:38.

Koscielniak E, Harms D, Schmidt D, et al. Soft tissue sarcomas in infants younger than 1 year of age: a report of the German soft tissue sarcoma study group. Med Pediatr Oncol 1989;17:105.

Reaman GH. Special considerations for the infant with cancer. In: Pizzo PA, Poplack DG, eds. Principles and practice of pediatric oncology. Philadelphia: JB Lippincott Co, 1989:263.

Silverman RA. Hemangiomas and vascular malformations. Pediatr Clin North Am 1991;38:811.

Soule EH, Pritchard DJ. Fibrosarcoma in infants and children. Cancer 1977;40:1711.

Suarez A, Hartman O, Vassal G, et al. Treatment of stage IV-S neuroblastoma: a study of 34 cases treated between 1982 and 1987. Med Pediatr Oncol 1991;19:473.

Tuchman M, Woods WG. Neuroblastoma screening. Am J Pediatr Hematol Oncol 1992;14:95.

Wakai S, Toshimoto A, Nagai M. Congenital brain tumors. Surg Neurol 1984;21:597.

Whalen TV, Mahour GH, Landing BH, Woolley MM. Sacrococcygeal teratomas in infants and children. Am J Surg 1985;150:373.

Wienk MA, van Geijn HP, Copray FJ, Brons JT. Prenatal diagnosis of fetal tumors by ultrasonography. Obstet Gynecol Surv 1990;45:639.

# PART III

## Ambulatory Pediatrics

Catherine D. DeAngelis, Editor

*Principles and Practice of Pediatrics, Second Edition.*
edited by Frank A. Oski et al. J. B. Lippincott Company, Philadelphia © 1994.

# CHAPTER 21
# *Ambulatory Care: Present and Future*

## Morris Green

The purpose of ambulatory pediatric visits is to diagnose and treat acute disease, provide continuing care to children with long-term illnesses or handicaps, promote health, and offer consultation for biomedical, developmental, educational, or behavioral problems. Approximately one third of the visits made to the pediatrician's office are for acute illnesses, usually viral and respiratory. Health supervision and promotion take about 50% of the practitioner's time, and the care of children with chronic illness accounts for an additional 3% to 10%.

Except for those living in poverty, in whom illness continues to be proportionally overrepresented, children in the United States are physically healthier than ever before. The infectious and nutritional problems that once occupied so much of the pediatrician's time are now often supplanted by problems of a developmental, behavioral, social, or educational nature.

The American family has changed because of a dramatic increase in the number of mothers who work outside the home, one-parent families, separations, desertions, divorces, remarriages, and aggregate families. In a highly migratory society, grandparents and other relatives are less available to provide emotional and other types of support for their children and grandchildren. Pediatric patients come from more diverse ethnic and cultural backgrounds than they did just a few years ago. With the trend toward fewer children, parents are heavily invested in learning more about how they may be more active and better informed in the service of each child's optimal growth, development, adaptation, and function.

The delivery of pediatric care is changing, with a trend toward group settings, rather than solo practices. Only about one quarter of pediatricians remain in solo practice, and an increasing number of young pediatricians elect to practice in small or rural rather than urban or suburban communities. There is a significant amount of hospital care given in ambulatory and day hospital settings, and there is an increase in managed care through health maintenance organizations, independent practice associations, and preferred provider organizations.

Most children in the United States do not have insurance coverage for ambulatory visits. Although financial incentives may promote efficiency, there is widespread concern that misdirected cost-containment efforts may limit access to care and impair its quality. The fact that a disproportionately high use of ambulatory health services is made by a relatively few families should be explored to ensure that the real needs of the family are being met and that parents are counseled on how to use services more appropriately and parsimoniously.

The average pediatrician cares for about 2000 patients (range, 100 to 4000) each year, including about 100 newborns. Three quarters of pediatricians practice in areas with over 100,000 persons. With the decline in the birth rate, fewer episodic illnesses among children in economically secure families, and the recent increase in pediatric personnel, many practitioners have time to devote to the management of adolescents, children with chronic disease, and patients with psychosocial, developmental, genetic, or school problems. Pediatricians are involved in sports medicine and health promotion, including prenatal visits.

Most pediatricians prefer to practice both general and special-interest pediatrics and to see more patients with complex diagnostic and management problems. Except in the small town where there are not enough patients for more than one pediatrician or for the individualistic physician, there are compelling reasons for pediatricians to practice together. A group practice provides the opportunity to share knowledge and concerns, have easy access to consultation, avoid fatigue, secure time for continuing education, develop a special interest area, participate in a community child health program, pursue research in practice, or teach students and residents.

## STAGES OF PEDIATRIC AMBULATORY CARE

The staging of primary care is an idea whose time has come because of the growing dimensions and complexity of ambulatory care, the importance of cognitive and procedural services, changes in the organization of health-care delivery, and the regionalization and progressive hierarchy of office and clinic services. It seems timely and appropriate to reconceptualize pediatric ambulatory services into three levels of service. This staging of ambulatory care recognizes the importance of compensation based on the time required, the complexity of the specific problem, and the number of professional disciplines required for management. Current methods of reimbursement usually do not provide adequately for the time that cognitive services require.

Analogous to hospital-based practice with its traditional division into primary, secondary, and tertiary care, the three progressive or hierarchic levels of ambulatory care are defined by the length of time required for a specific service, whether the services are procedural or cognitive; the special training, experience, and competence required to provide that care; the complexity of the problem; and whether the pediatrician works alone or in an interdisciplinary or multidisciplinary team. Just as there is an occasional need to consult subspecialists or refer patients with biomedical disorders, the general pediatrician must have access to community professionals, facilities, and services for children with psychosocial, developmental, or educational problems.

The allocation of time by practitioners to the three levels of care depends on their special competence, the needs of the population served, and their practice organization. As special areas of interest and further specialization evolve among general pediatricians, those with the appropriate postresidency training are likely to devote a larger percentage of their time to level II and III care.

### Level I Care

Level I care is delivered in the office or similar setting by the general pediatrician and pediatric nurse. It includes health supervision visits, the management of acute episodes of illness, and the treatment of minor trauma. Telephone advice, acute illness follow-up visits, and maintenance immunotherapy are briefer level I services.

Level I or primary care is often offered in sites other than the pediatric office. Primary and secondary schools are being explored as opportune sites, especially in medically underserved areas, for medical care and for screening and health promotion. Provided by nurse practitioners or part-time physicians with backup by community medical and other consultants, these health services are capacity building, readily accessible to the target population, and well used. The professional staff available in some school-based health services include social workers, mental health counselors, and psychologists. Although secondary school health services generally include care for episodic illnesses, their major attraction lies in prevention and early intervention in relation to sexually transmitted diseases, alcohol and drug abuse, risk-taking behaviors, trauma, depression, violence, eating disorders, and pregnancy.

Some practice groups have initiated early morning, evening, and weekend hours to meet the needs of working parents, but much primary care is given (at considerable expense and with little continuity) in hospital emergency rooms or freestanding "urgent care" centers. Some community hospitals and private practice groups have established primary care satellite units to increase geographic access and enlarge their patient populations. In rural areas, a pediatrician from a nearby community may hold office hours a few times a week, and in less medically populated areas, the satellite unit may be staffed by nurse practitioners with pediatric consultation available by phone.

## Level II Care

Level II pediatric ambulatory care is provided by general pediatricians for children with chronic illnesses or long-term handicaps or provided by those with a special interest or expertise in child development, learning problems, developmental disabilities, behavior, allergy, adolescent health, sports medicine, neurology, or endocrinology. This level of care may be delivered by the pediatrician and the pediatric nurse solely; by the pediatrician and nurse complemented by a part- or full-time psychologist or social worker in the physician's office; or through collaboration with these and other professionals in the community, including the child psychiatrist, special educator, occupational therapist, physical therapist, audiologist, nutritionist, speech pathologist, family therapist, and vocational counselor. Community resources may include schools, special education programs, family service agencies, marriage counselors, community mental health centers, developmental day-care centers, early-intervention programs, respite centers, parent education programs, and self-help groups.

The 1986 amendments to the Education for All Handicapped Children Act authorized each state to develop comprehensive, multidisciplinary programs for infants and toddlers up to the age of 3. The pediatrician provides a level II or III definition of the child's problems; delineates the specific services needed by the child and parents; determines which intervention program best provides the needed service; communicates the findings and suggestions to the staff of the recommended program; and monitors the child's and family's response or lack of progress through periodic program reports and regularly scheduled health supervision visits.

## Level III Care

Children with complex problems that require level III services usually are referred to academic health centers, regional diagnostic and treatment centers, or large group practices to be seen by subspecialist pediatricians who have completed a fellowship or equivalent training. Level III services include multidisciplinary or interdisciplinary clinic teams for children with disorders such as myelodysplasia, cerebral palsy, craniofacial anomalies, birth defects, cystic fibrosis, developmental disabilities, learning problems, and genetic disorders.

## Level II and III Master Pediatric Clinicians

As staging and regionalization of ambulatory care evolves and academic health centers seek to preserve or enlarge their referral bases, level II and III master general pediatric clinicians may increasingly serve as consultation clinic directors. Pediatricians trained in the biomedical and psychobiological aspects of pedi-

atrics are important resources for excellent patient care, resident education, and clinical investigation. These exemplary physicians have a continuing commitment to patients and their families, recognize and respond to feelings, are aware of their own reactions, have effective coping strategies for dealing with personal discomfort, tolerate uncertainty, promote parental participation, identify the parents' and child's strengths and their vulnerabilities and problems, are expert observers of behavior, give parents and children the feeling that they are understood, and establish productive physician–patient relationships.

Caring for children with long-term problems requires an effective plan for continuity of care, including regularly scheduled visits for reevaluation, the development of a trusting relationship, and the patient's identification with the physician's attitude toward child health. The pediatrician who cares for patients with long-term disorders serves as the child's advocate, enlists the best help available, communicates closely with other professionals, assesses the patient's and family's adaptation to the handicap or illness, is aware of family interactions, is available when needed, and coordinates or is aware of the comprehensive management plan. The pediatrician helps the child understand his or her illness, enhances the child's sense of competence and active role in the management of the illness, prepares the child for what is going to happen, is experienced as a long-time friend and physician, promotes the child's positive identity, and maintains an optimistic, supportive outlook.

Parents of children with special health care needs are encouraged to participate actively in the child's care and communicate with each other and with the child. They should avoid social isolation, develop effective coping strategies, and master feelings of guilt and inadequacy. The parents are encouraged to focus on the child as a person rather than an extension of the handicap and to recognize the child's strengths and potentialities rather than dwell on weaknesses and vulnerabilities. They should feel comfortable in asking for advice and in sharing their problems, worries, and questions with the pediatrician.

## Facilitating Level II and III Care

Because of the low prevalence of chronic pediatric disorders, a general pediatrician is less likely to deliver subspecialty care for problems other than those of a behavioral, developmental, allergic, neurologic, or dermatologic nature. If referral is made to a subspecialist, the consultant may be requested to attend only to the specific problem or to give total care. These roles should be defined early in the course of treatment for each family.

Community hospitals may greatly facilitate the practice of level II and III pediatric care by providing ready access to hospital-based allied health professionals for collaboration in the care of children whose management requires a team approach. The team may include a psychologist, social worker, nutritionist, occupational therapist, physical therapist, audiologist, or speech therapist.

The delivery of level II care by the general pediatrician may be facilitated by traveling teams of consultants from academic health centers. Level II or III ambulatory care services may also be used for preadmission evaluations of children with problems that require hospitalization. This preparatory process, which may include an admission history and physical examination, subspecialty consultations, and diagnostic procedures, can significantly shorten the subsequent hospital stay.

## HEALTH SUPERVISION AND PROMOTION

The model of pediatric health supervision that has evolved over the years must be reevaluated and renewed periodically. Although the current preoccupation with cost containment may suggest otherwise, the question is not how to do less in health promotion but how to do more and with better effectiveness, especially in relation to behavior and development. The American Academy of Pediatrics and other child advocacy groups are seeking to make health supervision and promotion a covered benefit in all health insurance programs.

Linked to other community resources, the pediatric office can represent a parent and child resource center with the following potential roles:

- Promotion of health and the prevention of illness
- Management of pediatric biomedical, developmental, behavioral, educational, and social problems
- Care for patients with chronic illnesses or long-term handicaps; case management
- Promotion of adaptation to family crises and other transitions
- Advocacy for the benefit of children and families
- Patient education

The pediatrician may have a role in school health education, in associated environmental programs, and in the continuing professional education of the teacher. In addition to the pediatric office, the practitioner may provide care in community health clinics, adoption agencies, day-care centers, Head Start programs, migrant labor camps, juvenile detention centers, and other institutions for dependent or developmentally disabled children. The pediatrician may also be asked by a community agency to serve as a consultant for an individual child or to help evaluate programs and plan new services.

Health supervision and promotion include appraisal of the psychosocial status of the child and family, physical and developmental assessment, and identification, monitoring, and containment of biomedical and psychosocial vulnerabilities. Health promotion also encompasses anticipatory guidance and assessment of the adaptation of a child and parents to a recent developmental change or family crisis. Parent education and support includes reassurance and relief of anxiety, promotion of constructive parent–child interactions, acceptance by parents and children of self-responsibility, enhancement of family communication, early intervention for problems, and identification of the need for consultation or referral.

Excellent clinical care is always highly personal, with attention to the patient as a person the hallmark of any thoughtful pediatric encounter. In health supervision, this goal can be approached by familiarity with the questions, concerns, and problems and anticipatory guidance that apply to all children of the same developmental age. Although such "routine" packages of care ensure that the basic needs of the patient will be met, personalized interventions are likely to be more effective. These require a more extensive database, particularly of the family and the community, consistent with the practice of contextual pediatrics. Family data include the composition of the household, parental health, parental work, family discontinuities, and other risk factors balanced by the family's strengths and resilience. Community data include child care centers, preschools, schools, religious affiliations, and support systems.

The database can be developed by having new patients complete a personal data sheet that can be updated during subsequent visits or supplemented with key words identified informally during sessions (eg, sports activities, school projects, hobbies, trips planned). Unless the pediatrician sees a family frequently, it is difficult to remember all these bits of information.

Many families do not think contextually and do not consider that the child, the parents, and the community constitute a system in which what happens to one affects the others. Many do not relate stressful family events, such as maternal depression, divorce, alcoholism, a disruptive move, or other discontinuities, to the symptoms or problems of the child. Just as parents have insufficient knowledge about the causes of biomedical disease to be able to report spontaneously all the relevant facts that physicians need to know and must be queried for elaboration, they are often unaware of the pertinence of the historic data the physician needs to understand and manage psychosocial problems.

Health promotion has as its goal the identification, validation, and enhancement of the strengths of parents, including their sense of efficacy and confirmation of their personal contribution to the child's health and development. Honest compliments, given in the form of a "sound bite" that the mother can later share (ie, "What did the doctor say?") with her spouse or others, are highly supportive (ie, "The doctor said that Benjamin is progressing wonderfully and that you and I are doing just a super job!").

Parents value the reassurance of the physician's examination, answers to their questions, suggestions for managing perceived problems, and anticipatory guidance. Most parents find it relatively easy to ask for help, but others do not. Some are hesitant to disclose their concerns because it may indicate their inadequacy. Others tend to be passive and expect the doctor to tell them what they need to know. Because the success of the visit is largely determined by the extent to which their agenda is addressed, an important goal of the interview is to help parents express their questions rather than leave the session with them unasked and unanswered. One advantage of an occasional group session is that one parent in the group may raise a question that others would have been be too shy to ask in an individual visit.

Some topics are difficult for any parent to mention, such as the worry that their child may be mentally handicapped, a secret fear that their child is highly vulnerable to illness and likely to die prematurely, or parental problems, including alcoholism or depression, family violence, marital discord, intrusive grandparents, anger, and financial stress.

## Office Visits

Health supervision visits are commonly scheduled for 10 to 15 minutes, although they may be shorter or much longer. By intensively using the time available during several visits, supplemented by occasionally longer but less frequent appraisals and some group sessions, many observations and much cogent advice can be squeezed into the time available. However, 10 to 15 minutes may be insufficient time for a detailed appraisal or response in some encounters, such as dysfunctional, troubled, or high-risk families.

In health supervision visits, the interview is largely nondirective, with open-ended questions cued to the parent's or child's cues and concerns. The effectiveness and efficiency of such visits may be increased by a home curriculum for the parent and the older child or adolescent, consisting of pamphlets, books, newsletters, information sheets, and audio- or videotapes. If the study is complemented by self-administered developmental and behavioral screening instruments, the time available for the health promotion visit can be used mostly for personalized teaching and to answer the family's questions.

It is not possible to remember all of the relevant personal and demographic data about a patient or family, especially if the same pediatrician does not see them on each visit, the family is relatively new to the practice, or the child is seen infrequently. For selected patients, the visit may be more personalized if a cue card is attached to the patient's record to enable the pediatrician, before walking into the examination room, to review at a glance the previous biomedical, psychosocial, or developmental complaints, recent major family changes, past family crises, employment, special vulnerabilities, names and relationship of persons living in the home, school performance, previous questions or concerns, and prior advice given.

Health promotion visits also provide opportunities to enhance the parent–child relationship, teaching parents how to interact more positively with their children and how to understand and meet their developmental needs. Parents who are identified during health promotion visits as not doing well need special help promptly. Infants and children who are not progressing adequately or who are apathetic, highly irritable, or at risk of abuse and neglect also require urgent intervention. Families with poor communication should be identified, including those who have a child with a major handicap, parents who are away from home much of the time because of work or community activities, families in which there is parental depression or alcoholism, and families of divorce.

Well-functioning families usually require only level I health promotion care, but dysfunctional families require lengthier level II or III visits. Because of time constraints, level I health promotion visits are an inappropriate way to attempt to solve complex behavioral and developmental problems. The pediatrician cannot expect to change patient behavior in any major way in such a brief session. If problems are identified during a health supervision visit, a return level II or III appointment may be offered or the patient can be referred to a mental health professional for further care.

Level II pediatric counseling services for behavioral or developmental problems include help in adaptation to family crises and transitions such as death, separation, divorce, or remarriage; the care of children with long-term illness or disability; developmental delay; learning disabilities; and school failure. Counseling is needed for behavioral problems and physical symptoms, such as failure to thrive, toddler out of control behavior, persistent sleep problems, separation anxiety, hyperactivity, chronic headaches, recurrent abdominal pain, and chest pain.

Although most health supervision services are appropriately delivered to the individual patient, others should be population based to achieve desired health outcomes. If the environment is unhealthy, the effectiveness of preventive and health-promoting interventions is predictably limited. The trend in health promotion is toward developing and enhancing supportive environments rather than attempting only to change lifestyles directly. Brief interventions, especially those attempting behavior modification, do not work if families are preoccupied with obtaining food, clothing, and shelter.

## Alternatives to Office Visits

Group sessions may be a highly effective way to transmit information and offer shared experiences, mutual support, and social reinforcement. Parents gain a greater appreciation of the wide range of developmental and behavioral differences among children and learn what has worked for others. Group visits can be substituted for or held in conjunction with an individual visit prenatally, quarterly during the first year of life, twice in the second year, annually during childhood (especially before puberty), and twice during adolescence. Separate sessions could be held for groups of older children and adolescents, including teenage single parents.

Home visits, usually by a nurse or home visitor, represent another alternative to an office visit to be used selectively, especially for the young, single parent who has no evident social supports, the family whose infant was born prematurely or with a handicap, the early-discharged mother who hopes to breast-feed, and the mother with underdeveloped nurturing resources.

Organized home care programs increasingly include visits by physicians, occupational therapists, physical therapists, social workers, child development specialists, and nurses. Many hospitals have programs to facilitate and support the care of terminally ill children whose parents choose to have them die at home rather than in the hospital. There are also services for ven-

tilator-dependent children and for those receiving intravenous hyperalimentation or antibiotics.

Day surgery and day hospitals have experienced rapid growth in recent years. Day hospitals and short-stay units are being used increasingly for the regulation of diabetes, the treatment of cystic fibrosis, the infusion of blood and chemotherapeutic agents, and the management of acute asthmatic episodes.

Collaboration with health education programs offered in schools or sponsored by community hospitals, churches, civic organizations, social agencies, or other groups may complement the pediatrician's efforts to help children and adolescents acquire and maintain good health habits such as physical activity, good nutrition, and dental health; avoidance of smoking, obesity, and alcohol or other substance abuse, adolescent pregnancy and risk-taking behaviors; coping with stressors; enhancement of social skills; help in developing a social support network; and education in conflict resolution.

## Promotion of Adaptation

An important role of the pediatrician is to help parents and children successfully adapt to the changing circumstances of their lives. Positive parental outcomes include self-confidence, self-esteem, and autonomy; enjoyment of parenthood; adequate family communication; maintenance of social linkages; understanding of child development; nurturing parent–child interactions; a good marital relationship; and comfort in seeking help for current problems and major stressors. Maladaptive parental behaviors include inadequate parent–child interaction, child abuse, excessive use of health services, and under- or overstimulation of the child. Positive adaptive outcomes in children include the ability to communicate well, express feelings, relate positively to others, and develop trusting relationships. Other strengths of children are physical fitness, personal achievement, a constructive assessment of personal capacities, good grooming, self-responsibility for health, high self-esteem, and the security of being cared for and loved.

The promotion of adaptation is a long-established pediatric tradition. It has been the pediatrician's job to enhance a child's capacity to adapt to a variety of biologic stressors. Pediatricians have the opportunity to facilitate mastery of expected and unexpected transitions, events and crises that test the coping repertoires of parents and children. Pediatricians may help children and parents identify their strengths and resources, suggest protective strategies, intervene early, or initiate treatment of maladaptive symptoms or problems.

Adaptation to change and stressors may be prospective or anticipatory, such as preparation for an adoption, for a toddler's autonomy, for hospitalization, for surgery, for the changes initiated by puberty, or for the remarriage of a parent. Adaptation can be concurrent, as in coping with an infant with a difficult temperament, the birth of a baby with a handicap, separation, divorce, death, unemployment, suicide, homicide, accidents, sexual assault, serious illness, or the mother's return to work. Adaptation can also be rehabilitative, as in providing care for the disorders and symptoms that result from maladaptation.

Ambulatory services must continue to adapt to remain responsive to rapidly changing needs and circumstances. Financial constraints, consumer decisions, and the control increasingly exercised by managed care systems and third-party payors make this a challenging time.

## Selected Readings

Green M. Coming of age in general pediatrics. Pediatrics 1983;72:275.
Green M. The role of the pediatrician in the delivery of behavioral services. Dev Behav Pediatr 1985;6:190.

Green M. Behavioral and developmental components of child health promotion: how can they be accomplished? Pediatr Rev 1986;8:133.

Green M. On making a difference. Pediatrics 1991;87:712.

Green M, Haggerty RJ, eds. Ambulatory pediatrics, ed 4. Philadelphia: WB Saunders, 1990.

Horwitz SM, Leaf PJ, Leventhal JM, Forsyth B, Speechley KN. Identification and management of psychosocial and developmental problems in community-based, primary care pediatric practices. Pediatrics 1992;89:480.

*Principles and Practice of Pediatrics, Second Edition.*
edited by Frank A. Oski et al. J. B. Lippincott Company, Philadelphia © 1994.

# CHAPTER 22
# *Outpatient Versus Inpatient Management*

## Catherine D. DeAngelis

One of life's absolutes is change, and health care provision for children in the United States has changed dramatically during the past few decades. Some of these changes have resulted in better health; some of them have not. All of these changes have been expensive, whether or not they have been effective. Consequently, cost containment has received much more attention recently than ever before. These circumstances have placed the onus on pediatricians to ensure the highest quality care possible for children with the lowest risk for morbidity and for the lowest cost. This is not an easy task.

Much of the improvement in children's health has not been the direct result of costly alterations in medical care. For example, health indices such as infant mortality and life expectancy have improved dramatically since the turn of the century. However, close scrutiny of the data reveals that better nutrition, shelter, and sanitation have had at least as strong an impact as costly technology on improving these health indices. Unlike the relatively unexciting evolutionary changes brought about by improved nutrition and sanitation, modern medical technology has proven dramatically effective in many cases. Everyone wants the full benefit of all possibilities when his own child's health is involved, and because pediatricians are trained to be advocates for each child entrusted to their care, it is difficult to deny any diagnostic test or treatment, no matter what the cost to society.

Another cost of modern technology not usually considered is iatrogenesis—the problems that result from medical management. In general, advanced technology and medications have greater risks than simpler diagnostic and treatment modalities. Each new medical advance brings greater likelihood of undesired side effects in addition to higher financial cost, and much more of the high-cost technology and therapy occurs in hospitals than in ambulatory facilities.

Fear of malpractice also has generated higher costs, because physicians often feel compelled to order unwarranted, expensive diagnostic tests to be sure of not missing a diagnosis. They are reluctant not to hospitalize children even when close observation

may be all that is indicated. Both of these practices increase financial and iatrogenic costs. It should be no surprise that hospitalizations are the most financially and iatrogenically expensive contributors to the cost of health care.

Physicians should have taken the lead in reserving hospitalizations for only very ill patients or those with chronic illnesses who could not receive care in an outpatient setting. Unfortunately, the shift to outpatient care has been implemented by nonmedical professionals because organized medicine failed to make the necessary alterations even when it became obvious that curtailment of spending was essential. The enforcement of payment for hospitalizations by diagnostically related groups (DRGs), which is discussed in Chapter 4, has shown positive and negative effects. It has forced physicians to think carefully about admitting patients to the hospital and about discharging them as soon as possible. However, the DRGs often do not fit the medical needs of patients. This is especially true for children, because their special needs were not considered in the original DRG plan.

Too often DRG appears to say "Da Revenue's Gone," so do the best you can. It is essential for pediatricians to consider the positive aspects of the movement from hospitalizations to ambulatory management and use them to ensure quality medical care for children. It is probably easier for pediatricians than other specialists to adapt to this change, because pediatrics always has been primarily an ambulatory specialty, and it will become even more so in the near future.

This shifting of care has a significant impact on the resources needed in inpatient and outpatient settings. Hospital units are beginning to function more like intensive care units, requiring different types of resources and support for children and their families in these high-stress areas. The ambulatory settings, which traditionally had relatively fewer support staff and resources, require increased input to care for patients who previously would have been hospitalized. An 8- to 10-hour experience in an outpatient setting can be as intense and stressful to a child and his family as a 24- to 36-hour overnight stay for the same therapy. The advantages are that the child can be returned to his home sooner, there is much less risk for possible nosocomial infections and iatrogenic problems, and the financial costs are diminished.

A realistic expectation is that only a small proportion of all health care in the twenty-first century will occur in hospitals, and this will usually be intensive and expensive. Most care will occur in ambulatory settings and in the home. This change will be a challenge for physicians educated in traditional settings.

## OUTPATIENT MANAGEMENT

The approach to evaluating and treating a child or teenager in the outpatient clinic is quite different from that of a hospitalized patient. The timing, goals, and follow-up are distinctly different. Outpatient care is well described by Howell, Lurie, and Wolliscroft (1987).

One goal of outpatient medical management of children is to keep them from being admitted to the hospital. Although this may initially appear simplistic, further analysis shows that it is an important goal. Only sick children, whose problems cannot be managed outside the hospital, should be admitted. Preventing illness is one of the hallmarks of pediatric care. If pediatricians were completely successful in managing all preventable illnesses and problems in children, the number of children's hospitals needed would be few. Hospitals would admit children with significant congenital anomalies, inborn errors, immunologic defects, infectious diseases for which there are no vaccines or effective antibiotics, and certain neoplastic diseases, and most beds currently occupied by children with injuries, poisonings, and certain infectious diseases would be empty.

Many of the diseases that cannot be prevented can be managed effectively in the outpatient setting. For example, some emergency rooms now have 24-hour holding rooms for children with asthma or dehydration and those requiring further studies to rule out infectious diseases that would require hospitalizations.

In the past, children with neoplastic diseases or those with immunologic problems that required infusions of chemotherapy or immunoglobulin over a 6- to 8-hour period had to be admitted to the hospital. These children can now be scheduled in outpatient day units. These units have had a significant impact on lowering hospitalization rates.

Providing children with continuity of care can decrease the need for hospitalizations by early diagnosis and treatment before complications or severity dictate admission. This type of care, with one pediatrician coordinating the child's health care, ensures quicker discharge from the hospital and follow-up provided by someone who is familiar with the child and his family.

The three key points in ambulatory care that reduce costs while maintaining quality are use of health supervision standards as suggested by the American Academy of Pediatrics, monitoring and approval of all referrals to specialty services by the primary pediatrician, and careful monitoring and managing of all admissions, length of stay, and diagnostic procedures by a pediatrician familiar with the child. These criteria could reduce unnecessary emergency room visits, which seem to increase the likelihood for admissions because the emergency room pediatrician is not familiar with the child and his family. Close follow-up also becomes difficult. It is less expensive for a child to be seen in a private office or clinic than in an emergency room.

## HOSPITALIZATIONS

Some children require hospitalization to receive the kinds of care they need. These include children with infections requiring intravenous antibiotics, severe trauma, and other life-threatening diseases and disorders. In the past, all children requiring surgery were admitted to the hospital. Most medical centers and community hospitals now have less-expensive, same-day surgical centers, which are in the hospital and from which the child is discharged within 12 hours of admission. Unfortunately, some children require postoperative management that requires the resources of the hospital and must remain.

All of these factors have led to the increased acuity of care required for the "average" patient. The pediatric intensive care units (PICUs) are often full. Less-intensive care or intermediate units that relieve the burden on PICU while not stressing the management capabilities of the regular hospital units are becoming more popular. These are laudable and necessary changes that should decrease the risk for iatrogenic morbidity or mortality, but the hospital remains a not very safe place for children.

Children who require hospitalization should be prepared for the admission to help them with the associated stresses. In general, hospitalized children who understand what is happening to them and who have the emotional support of their parents and the hospital staff do better than those children without this understanding and support.

Several factors affect how a child reacts to hospitalization. Misconceptions about the staff and the hospital can lead to undue stress. Remember that children must use their relatively immature cognitive ability to process what they hear about hospitals. For example, watching television or having family conversations about seriously ill or dying hospitalized persons may cause them to expect the same treatment and outcome.

The child's life is centered on familiar persons, places, and routines. The hospital can abruptly break this familiarity by preventing access to some loved family members or friends. The

separation is rarely deliberate, but it may be impossible for those persons to come to the hospital. The hard-won developmental achievements, such as urinating or defecating into a toilet, can be altered in the bedridden child who must use a urinal or bed pan. This can be a devastating loss if the child or parents are not prepared for it.

Unfamiliar persons may perform procedures on the child that are uncomfortable and frightening. His parents probably spent much time and energy teaching him not to touch wires and sharp objects, but in the hospital, he can be connected to a monitor or electrocardiogram wires, receive injections, or have sutures removed with scissors. Preparation for such procedures can prevent short- and long-term problems.

The child's parents or another special person should be encouraged to stay with him and assist the staff in alleviating apprehension and pain. Studies have shown that parents who stay with their hospitalized children and prepare them simply, briefly, and recurrently help them to be more cooperative.

Many children's hospitals employ or have volunteer child-life specialists who augment the role of parents or provide the main support for some children whose parents cannot be with them. These specialists provide the support and organize the materials that contribute to the child's understanding of medical procedures. These materials include special dolls, hand puppets, stuffed animals, picture books, paper and pencils or crayons for drawing, and in some cases, special closed-circuit television programs. Play as a teaching method works wonderfully for children.

Although there is unanimous support for play teaching a child who must be hospitalized, there is some controversy about preparing well children for possible future hospitalization. Much of the controversy centers on the appropriateness of routine, short, group tours of hospitals for young school children. Frequently, these routine tours do not consider sufficiently the cognitive and emotional development of the children. It is probably unrealistic to expect young children to understand and integrate the information and stimuli from a 1-hour hospital tour. Some hospitals are now sending their staff to give presentations in the schools, which eliminates many of the unfamiliar visual, auditory, and olfactory stimuli of the hospital from the learning experience.

According to Azarnoff (1985), programs to prepare well children for possible future hospitalizations should include the following steps:

1. Identify parent's views about health care.
2. Explore the children's recent health care experiences.
3. Allow sufficient time for preparation.
4. Use multisensory experiences.
5. Provide real medical equipment that can be safely touched and used on dolls.
6. Plan ways to listen, observe, and respond to children's reactions to the program.
7. Systematically document the efforts and the children's later responses if they are hospitalized.

The last step is essential for monitoring the effects of the previous six steps, because few well-planned, correctly implemented, and properly analyzed studies on this subject exist.

## HOSPICE CARE

The concept of hospice care for children is relatively new, but it is an idea that fits nicely into the spectrum of pediatric medical care. According to the National Hospice Organization, "A Hospice is a program of palliative and supportive services which provides physical, psychological, social, and spiritual care for dying persons and their families. Services are provided by a medically supervised interdisciplinary team of professionals and volunteers. Hospice services are available in the home and an inpatient setting. Home care is provided on part-time, intermittent, regularly scheduled, and around-the-clock on-call bases. Bereavement services are available to the family. Admission to a Hospice program of care is on the basis of patient and family need."

Hunter (1984) and Seale (1991) have written extensively on the subject of hospice care.

## IATROGENESIS

Adverse drug reactions are a significant cause of morbidity and mortality and have been blamed for prolonging hospitalization and adding significantly to annual health care costs. Although adverse drug reactions can occur in outpatient and inpatient settings, at least one study has shown that they do not occur commonly among pediatric outpatients and that most of these are mild and self-limited (Kramer, 1985). Unfortunately, this is not the case for inpatient adverse drug reactions.

Many iatrogenic problems occur in hospitalized children, including intravenous infiltrates resulting in sloughing of skin, fluid overloading, nosocomial diarrhea and thrush, unnecessary intensive and noninvasive diagnostic procedures, and undetermined long-term problems, such as behavior problems. Many of these problems are preventable, and these are the ones that require the efforts of the entire hospital health team. For example, not every child who is admitted to the hospital requires intravenous infusion; fluid overloading and sloughing of skin can be prevented in these children. Frequent hand washing by hospital staff can eliminate much of the hospital-acquired diarrhea found especially in infant units.

Medicine is not an exact science; medical practice has its foundation in basic sciences integrated with clinical experience. Diagnostic and therapeutic procedures, instituted supposedly to benefit patients, may involve concomitant risk for harm. A guideline exists that is somewhat crude but difficult to forget, and it holds a valuable lesson: Ordering a diagnostic test is like picking your nose in public; first think of what you're going to do if you find something. This guideline is pertinent in all medical settings, but its impact is possibly greatest in hospitalized children, because so much opportunity exists to order tests.

Ordering unnecessary tests can lead to diagnostic misadventures that can be harmful and expensive. For example, contaminated cultures can lead to unnecessary antibiotic use and extended hospitalization, and repeated lumbar punctures of infants with bacteremia can increase the risk of meningitis, epidermal spinal cord tumors, and intramedullary spinal abscesses. Unnecessary radiographs expose patients to irradiation that may have long-term ill effects.

Iatrogenesis is directly related to the primary principle of ethics for the medical profession: *primum non nocere* (first do no harm). This tenet designates the practice of medicine as a moral enterprise and implies that the physician will render care while taking into account the risks and benefits and the iatrogenic and financial effectiveness of the care. Procedures instituted to benefit patients may involve concomitant risk for harm. It is possible to determine for large groups of patients an approximation of the risk–benefit ratio using statistical and epidemiologic methods. Pediatricians should be aware of the limitations of applying these ratios to the care of individual patients to avoid ineffective or dangerous practices.

Traditionally, the quality of medical care has been determined by the ethics and peer review of physicians. Recent changes in the health delivery system in the United States have allowed businesses and legal interests to have increasing influence on medical practice. A pediatrician or any physician should not be guided by fear of litigation in making decisions about his or her patients. Decisions about diagnostic tests, therapeutic procedures, hospital admissions, and every other aspect of medical care should be based on sound medical judgment. This is the best way to prevent litigation, and it is the only way for a physician to provide the best care for the patient.

## Selected Readings

Azarnoff P. Preparing well children for possible hospitalization. Pediatr Nurs 1985;1: 53.

Brennan TA, Leape LL, Laird NM, et al. Incidence of adverse events and negligence in hospitalized patients. N Engl J Med 1991;324:370.

DeAngelis C. Medical malpractice: does it augment or impede quality care? J Pediatr 1987;110:8780.

DeAngelis C, Joffe A, Willis E, et al. Hospitalization and outpatient treatment of young, febrile infants. Am J Dis Child 1983;137:1150.

DeAngelis C, Joffe A, Wilson M, Willis E. Iatrogenic risks and financial costs of hospitalizing febrile infants. Am J Dis Child 1983;137:1146.

Gordon T, DeAngelis C, Peterson R. Capitation reimbursement for pediatric primary care. Pediatrics 1986;77:29.

Howell J, Lurie N, Wolliscroft J. Worlds apart: Some thoughts to be delivered to house officers on the first day of clinic. JAMA 1987;258:502.

Hunter M, ed. Children's hospice advisory panel conference report. Washington, DC: Division of Maternal and Child Health, Health and Human Services, 1984.

Kregar BE, Restuccia JD. Assessing the need to hospitalize children: Pediatric appropriateness evaluation protocol. Pediatrics 1989;84:242.

Seale C. A comparison of hospice and conventional care. Soc Sci Med 1991;32:147.

*Principles and Practice of Pediatrics, Second Edition.*
edited by Frank A. Oski et al. J. B. Lippincott Company, Philadelphia © 1994.

CHAPTER 23
# *Getting Started in the Real World: How to Set Up Your Private Practice*

Lawrence K. Epple, Jr.

As the Lord Chancellor has said of good judges, so we may say of good child-health experts—they must have impartiality, the gift of wise silence, wide knowledge of human and natural laws, a quick grasp of fact, and vast experience of human nature.

A. V. Neale

Medicine is not only a science; it is also an art. It does not consist of compounding pills and plasters; it deals with the very processes of life, which must be understood before they may be guided.

Paracelsus

The end of pediatric residency or fellowship marks the beginning of a pediatrician's career. The resident has completed three or more years of intense training during which he or she has been exposed to the basic and esoteric points of pediatric health, illness, disease, and treatment. If the resident was lucky, emphasis was also placed on developmental, psychosocial, and environmental factors. The brand new pediatrician emerges from this intense period armed with all that modern medicine has to offer: the textbook knowledge, batteries of available tests, hi-tech wizardry to match any George Lucas movie, and an eagerness to use these tools. She or he is prepared and eager to begin life in a solo or group practice, emergency room, health maintenance organization, or clinic.

In American medical education, little or no time is devoted to teaching the medical student or pediatric resident about the practicalities and day-to-day operation of a medical office. This seems ludicrous, because residencies last only 3 years but a pediatric practice continues for 30 or 40 years.

This chapter attempts to fill in some of the gaps left after residency training is completed and to make the transition period less stressful. This information can help the newly graduated resident achieve satisfaction in his or her career in clinical practice.

## OBTAINING PROPER DOCUMENTATION

After the location of the practice has been decided, the next step is to obtain proper licensure, controlled substances forms, and hospital privileges. This should be done at least 6 months before starting practice. Write to the Department of Health in the state where the practice will be located, and ask for a state medical license application and state controlled substances application. These forms allow a physician to practice and prescribe drugs in a particular state. The forms should be filled out quickly and returned with the appropriate fees. Maintain copies of the forms and the accompanying check for your records. Send the applications by registered mail.

After receiving state licensure and state controlled substances approval, write to the Drug Enforcement Administration (1405 I Street NW, Washington, DC 20537) to request a Drug Enforcement Administration (DEA) number. A physician's DEA number is required on all prescriptions written for controlled substances.

The next step is to apply for staff privileges at the hospital(s) desired. Write to the medical staff secretary of each hospital to request an application. Allow plenty of time for this step, because many hospital committees are notoriously slow. Many hospitals require interviews during the application process. Sometimes sponsors are also required; these are physicians already on staff who recommend the new applicant. If time becomes a problem, temporary staff privileges can often be arranged while permanent privileges are being sought.

## FINANCIAL AND BUSINESS MATTERS

While proper medical licensure and hospital staff appointments are being obtained, financial matters must also be arranged. Most physicians do not leave residency training with pocketfuls of cash. Most are swamped by considerable debt. Many banks consider physicians preferred risks, however, and large amounts of collateral are rarely needed. Several months before beginning practice, make appointments with officers of the various local banks to discuss the sums needed, including start-up costs and living expenses. A newly graduated pediatrician needs money to live on during the first few months, because it is extremely difficult to pay debts, employees, and his or her own salary when the practice is just beginning. Many bankers are willing to arrange a mortgage on a home as well.

This is an excellent time to hire a reputable and aggressive accountant, one who is willing to do more than just balance the books and prepare tax forms. He or she can estimate how much start-up money is needed and how much money to borrow from the bank. An accountant can assist in hiring employees, determining fair salaries for employees, deciding on whether to computerize the office, and give advice about many other matters. The accountant can help to obtain a pediatrician's Medicaid number, taxpayer identification number, insurance company notifications, and reliable malpractice insurance.

A specialist has emerged to assist new physicians in getting practices started—the management consultant. Many of these consultants are excellent and can provide valuable practical assistance. These consultants are usually expensive, but they often arrange acceptable payment plans for new physicians.

Obtaining a lawyer is also recommended. A lawyer can assist with rental agreements or the purchase of land or buildings if buying an office is contemplated. If partnership in a group or health maintenance organization is planned, a lawyer is a must to make sure that everything is legal and that all that is specified is actually delivered. The lawyer can also help with personal legal affairs.

## THE OFFICE

### Choosing a Location

The location of a pediatric office is an important decision. The office should be in a safe part of town, not in a declining part of town such as a rundown mall or a former main street being supplanted by new suburban malls. The office should be a relatively short distance (ie, 10–20 minutes of driving time) for most patients. The office preferably should not be located on a busy street, because ample parking might be a problem and many parents are reluctant to bring their children to an office where there is heavy traffic. Parking should be abundant and free. The office should be located on the street level if possible; if not, an elevator must be available. It is difficult for a parent to carry an infant, infant seat, diaper bag, and assorted toys up several flights of stairs. Many women are not allowed to climb stairs for several weeks after cesarean section. The office should not be located too far from the hospital if you spend a significant amount of time there.

### Office Design and Decor

Opinions about a pediatrician and staff are formulated from the moment the parent or patient enters the office. Consequently, the office design and comfort can be a real asset or drawback to a practice. Serious consideration must be given to the design and decor of the office. An excellent resource guide is the *Planning Guide for Physicians' Medical Facilities* published by the American Medical Association (Division of Medical Practice, 535 N. Dearborn Street, Chicago, IL 60603).

Several ideas about office decor should be considered. "No Smoking" signs should be prominently displayed. Surprisingly, many people will smoke around young children unless specifically told not to. The experts recommend using earth-tone colors. This gives the office a more subdued and relaxed effect. Strive for a feeling of accommodation and efficiency, and avoid an aloof, antiseptic, hospital-like decor. Resist the temptation to decorate the office with cartoon characters and other cute objects. Remember, pediatricians take care of children of all ages, including teenagers. Teenagers feel uncomfortable enough in the pediatrician's office without having the office decorated like a nursery school.

A coat rack or other place for umbrellas, boots, and coats located in the waiting area is helpful. Individual seating for patients and their families is preferred to couches. Chairs should have arms. To estimate the number of chairs needed in the waiting room, multiply the number of patients seen in an hour by a factor of 2.5. Carpeting should be placed in all patient areas because it helps lower the noise level and protect rambunctious children from injuring themselves.

A special area of the waiting room should be designated as a play area. A sturdy and safe table with chairs for reading, drawing, or puzzles helps children occupy the time while waiting. Toys, books, and puzzles should be sturdy and preferably made of washable material. These items should have no small parts or sharp corners that could be dangerous. A large aquarium or children-oriented videocassettes help keep children occupied, and appropriate and current reading material should be available for adults.

Patient and parent comfort is of the utmost concern in any successful practice. Office temperature is important. Heat lamps over examination tables and infant scales keep infants and young children warm during the examination and allow a more comfortable waiting and office area for those wearing clothing.

Relaxing music in the examination rooms and waiting room can increase patient comfort. The music volume should be controllable in each room. In addition to patient and parent relaxation, the music keeps the patient entertained while waiting for the pediatrician and prevents the patient and parent from hearing private discussions in adjoining rooms. When the pediatrician enters the room, the music can be turned down or off.

Other excellent patient comfort ideas include installing a telephone in the waiting room for patient use. This is most appreciated by parents. The telephone can be installed so that only local calls can be made. Having an infant seat located near where parents pay their bills and make their next appointments is a certain patient pleaser. It is difficult to juggle a crying infant, diaper bag, and coats while writing a check or making an appointment.

How the physical facilities appear often affects how the patient views the pediatrician. The office should be cleaned regularly (ie, two or three times a week for most offices), the carpets steamed regularly, and the wallpaper and paint kept in good repair. Commercial cleaning companies are available almost everywhere and are reasonably priced.

## Equipment

It is difficult to anticipate specific equipment needs for the average pediatric office because practice locales and styles are different. By no means are all items listed in Table 23-1 required for successful practice, but they can be helpful. A few items deserve special attention. Electric thermometers save several minutes per patient and are usually reliable. It is also good to have traditional thermometers on hand to demonstrate proper temperature taking to parents.

Emergency and resuscitation equipment must be in every pediatrician's office. This equipment should be located in a convenient and easily accessible location. Every office employee should know its location and use. Table 23-2 lists the drugs and equipment that should be in an emergency cabinet in the office.

The portable pulse oximeter can be especially helpful in the office setting. The size and price of oximeters have decreased significantly. The data garnered from this instrument can be vitally important in children with acute asthma, croup, or sepsis.

Almost every office needs laboratory equipment. Table 23-3 lists commonly needed items found in many pediatricians' offices. Many laboratory tests can be performed easily in the office with a modest amount of training of office staff. The convenience and speed with which results can be obtained is attractive to many pediatricians and parents. These tests are often performed inexpensively and provide additional revenue for the office. The testing and procedures done in the office must conform with the guidelines of the Clinical Laboratory Improvement Amendments, which were implemented in 1988. The American Academy of Pediatrics Division of Pediatric Practice can help decipher these regulations.

To manage a successful office, certain clerical and business equipment must be purchased. Table 23-4 lists the items that can

### TABLE 23-1.  Medical Equipment for a Pediatrician's Office

Vision screening apparatus (eg, Titmus test, Ishihara's test for color blindness)
Hearing screening equipment (eg, Audiometry, tympanometry)
Scales, adult and infant
Examining table (ie, pediatric, with extensions for adult-size patients)
Thermometers (ie, rectal and oral, preferably digital)
Blood pressure cuffs of various sizes and sphygmomanometers
Nebulizer for aerosol treatments, spirometer, and oxygen tank
ECG machine
GOMCO or other suction machine
Papoose board
X-ray view box, high-intensity light for viewing splinters and suturing
Ultraviolet light for fungus detection
Resuscitation and emergency equipment (eg, laryngoscopes, IV solutions, drugs)
Suture equipment and instruments
Pulse oximeter

### TABLE 23-2.  Suggested Contents of a Pediatrician's Emergency Cabinet*

**Intravenous Equipment**
Catheters
Liquids (D5½NS, NS) and infusion sets
Bone marrow needles for IO infusion
Lumbar puncture tray

**Airway Equipment**

| | |
|---|---|
| Bag/masks | D-stix |
| Oxygen | HCT tube |
| Suction | Dipsticks |
| Endotracheal tubes | (Lab tubes and BC bottles) |
| Laryngoscope | |
| Pulse oximeter | |

**Cardiac Monitor**

**Drugs**

| | |
|---|---|
| Ipecac/charcoal (nasogastric tubes/ Ewac tubes) | Phenobarbital |
| | Dilantin |
| 5% albumin | $D_{10}$ or $D_{25}$ |
| IV antibiotics du jour (Amp Gent Chloro) | Aminophylline |
| | Dexamethasone |
| Epinephrine 1:1000 | Succinylcholine (cold) |
| Epinephrine 1:10,000 | Benadryl |
| Bicarbonate | Methylene blue |
| Valium | |

* This is a complete list for physicians far removed from emergency rooms. It can be modified to meet individual needs.

| TABLE 23-3. Laboratory Equipment for a Pediatrician's Office |
| --- |
| Refrigerator with freezer area for drugs that require freezing (eg, polio vaccine) |
| Binocular microscope (10× through 100×) |
| Incubator |
| Centrifuge (blood, urine) |
| Complete blood count machine |
| Culture media (eg, blood, urine, strep screens vs. strep cultures) |
| Autoclave |
| Blood drawing apparatus |
| Cholesterol-testing machine |

| TABLE 23-4. Business Equipment for a Pediatrician's Office |
| --- |
| Copier with a stationary top, which makes it easier to make copies from books |
| Typewriter(s) |
| Dictation equipment |
| File cabinets of various sizes |
| Adding machines/calculators |
| Computer (type depending on extent of medical records, laboratory work, or billing) |
| Fax machine |

increase the efficiency and productivity of the office staff. The subject of computers deserves special attention. Computers have been demonstrated to be advantageous for many physicians and their staff. New software programs and hardware complements are flooding the medical marketplace. As of 1993, adequate systems cost $15,000 to $40,000 to start. The best advice for the fledgling pediatrician is to wait until the office is financially sound and its needs are known. A good source of information is other physicians with working computer systems in their offices. Many firms and individual professionals, including your accountant, can offer sound advice. Shop around for price and service. The financial commitment can vary greatly.

## Personnel

The hiring, training, monitoring, and firing of office personnel is one of the most time-consuming, ulcer-producing, and sometimes even rewarding parts of private practice. At the conclusion of residency, a pediatrician is well versed in antibiotic dosages, lumbar puncture techniques, and hyperbilirubinemia, but he or she is a veritable 28-week premature infant in the world of hiring, managing, and firing employees. Luckily, there are firms willing to teach. These firms host numerous 2-day seminars across the country cosponsored by many state medical societies for neophyte physicians. Their courses cover many areas of office management, their handouts are excellent, and the cost is reasonable at $100 to $300 per seminar.

The American Academy of Pediatrics (AAP) has an excellent resource for all areas of office management, the second edition of *Management of Pediatric Practice*. This booklet can be obtained for a nominal charge by writing to AAP headquarters (P.O. Box 927, 141 Northwest Point Blvd., Elk Grove, IL 60009-0927).

There is no right or wrong way to hire medical staff. Most employers learn best by trial and error. There are, however, definite *Don'ts* concerning employees:

- Don't hire relatives or spouses; this leads to favoritism or to stresses in close personal and social relationships. Ensconced family employees may present special concerns as new partners join the practice.
- Don't hire friends of present staff. This often leads to the formation of cliques, and if one employee must be fired, the friend may leave, resulting in a considerable gap in office staffing.
- Don't hire parents of patients unless you feel especially comfortable with them. Make it understood from the beginning that there will be no hard feelings on either side if the job does not work out.

When hiring staff, remember that these persons represent you. They are usually the patients' and parents' first glimpse of what your practice is like. They can be a valuable asset or a debilitating liability.

Consideration for your staff breeds loyalty. Being consistent is important; otherwise, the staff won't know what to do. Compliment and thank staff when appropriate. Everyone responds positively to praise. When reprimanding or correcting an employee, do it in private. The entire staff need not know unless it applies to all of them.

Job descriptions for each position, including nurse, medical assistant, bookkeeper, and receptionist, must be written. These written documents clarify what is required from each employee from the outset, and misunderstandings can be prevented. Regular evaluations of employee performance are important. During these evaluations, positive aspects of performance are applauded and recorded, problems corrected, and ideas and frustrations aired by both employer and employee. Raises should be decided on before these evaluations and announced during them.

Regular office meetings of the entire office staff keep everyone informed of changes in office procedures and provide a clearinghouse for problems that have arisen. Holding meetings every 1 to 2 months is a good guideline to follow; if meetings are held too frequently, they often degenerate into gripe sessions.

Staff should be designated to order medical and business supplies for the office. Supplies should be checked regularly, and shortages should not occur if this system works properly. One person should be designated to check the refrigerator and freezer regularly to ensure that correct temperatures are maintained to protect vaccine potency and maximize drug shelf life.

Many other aspects of the employee–employer relationship will emerge. Good advice can be obtained from firms dealing solely with this issue and from books, pamphlets, accountants, and other sources.

## Proper Use of the Office Telephone

The telephone is an integral part of any pediatric practice. Many hours each week are spent using it. All staff members must be taught how to use it correctly. Most staff can be trained to handle minor medical questions and problems. Several good references that can be used to help train staff are listed at the end of this chapter. If more than one pediatrician is in the practice, a special effort should be made to unify office philosophy on how to manage certain common problems (eg, uncomplicated colds, constipation, diarrhea, treatment of poison ivy). The office staff should be aware of the danger signs that herald more serious problems, such as a stiff neck, high fever, or unconsciousness.

Some pediatricians prefer a morning call-in hour, when their patients can talk to them directly. This is advantageous because the patients know they will talk directly with the pediatrician. It is important that the pediatrician be consistent with this time, although this is often hard to do. One potential drawback to the morning call hour is that it can limit the patients' or parents' access to the pediatrician at other times of the day. Some pediatricians prefer that their patients call at any time throughout the day. Nurses and medical staff can be used to screen the calls that require immediate physician attention.

A startling revelation from my own experience is the fact that many physicians do not return their patients' phone calls. As unbelievable as this may sound, it is often true. If a patient or parent is concerned enough about a problem to call, it is mandatory that the pediatrician respond in a reasonable amount of time. This is a common complaint from patients about physicians. When returning a call, try to do it in a quiet place and do not write or do other things while talking. Give the patient your undivided attention.

Messages from patients should be on a special color of paper so they can be recognized immediately and not get mixed up with other scraps of paper. They should be placed in a designated area where the pediatrician can readily review them.

Some pediatricians use a combination of answering machines and answering services. Check with established physicians in the area about the reliability of the different services available. Computer-assisted answering services are available in some areas. The physician is automatically beeped when a patient leaves a message. The physician then checks the computer-recorded message by dialing certain code numbers. Human backup is provided by these services in case the computer has problems.

The pediatrician should have several incoming lines to handle the influx of telephone calls. The more pediatricians in the practice, the more lines are needed. Too many lines, however, can unnerve even the best receptionist. A private line for personal calls is of great benefit, and a direct hospital extension can save many hours of dialing. Efficient use of the telephone is essential in the smooth running of a pediatric office.

## OPERATING A PRIVATE PRACTICE

### Medicolegal Considerations

Because of the rampant litigation and overabundance of lawsuits brought against physicians, proper documentation is imperative. Concise, pertinent, and legible documentation can prevent many problems. Every office visit by a patient must be recorded on a form, preferably a separate one for each visit. A line or two of "chicken scratch" is not acceptable. Some pediatricians use different forms for health maintenance visits and for acute visits. Phone messages, prescriptions, and treatment advice given over the telephone should be written in the chart. After being reviewed by the pediatrician, laboratory results should be entered promptly into the chart. When writing progress information about hospitalized patients, frequent and complete notes are important. If a diagnosis is uncertain or unknown, a brief discussion of differential diagnoses is crucial. This allows a person reading the chart to follow your logic.

Never write in any chart words or information that you would not want the patient to know. Personal opinions about a patient's social status, dress, or personality are rarely relevant to the medical problems at hand.

When a patient requests that his records be transferred, do so without delay. A signed form authorizing the transfer or release of records is recommended. Patients leave a practice for many reasons, including change of job, change of insurance, or personality conflict with the pediatrician. Do not take it personally; you cannot please everyone.

A patient's confidentiality must always be maintained. Office staff must never discuss patients while other patients are in the office. Office walls are notoriously thin. Information should never be given over the telephone to relatives, except to parents. In some cases, even a parent should not receive information. If unsure about who is on the other end of the telephone, do not give any information.

Office security is extremely important. Every pediatrician's office should have a security system with alarms and smoke detectors. Billing cards, charts, and computer disks, should be stored in fireproof containers. A locked cash box and locked drug box are also important. An ongoing log of narcotics kept in the office should be updated and changed as drugs are used. Well-lighted entryways are important for office security.

### Making Contacts and Publicity

On arrival at your place of practice, an important step is to make contact with colleagues and potential referral sources. Make appointments to meet with or have lunch with obstetricians, family practitioners, and emergency room physicians, all of whom are good potential sources of referrals. Let these physicians know your background and training and your willingness to assist them in any way possible. It is a good idea to meet your competition, your fellow pediatricians. You may be surprised at the warmth of your meeting. Some of them may be looking for someone to cover occasional night calls or someone to whom they can refer overflow patients.

When a patient is referred to you by another physician, send a note or thank him or her personally on the telephone. If a consultation is requested, let the referring physician know your findings and recommendations as soon as possible. Do not steal patients. Always insist that the patient return to the referring physician after a consultation. Never say anything derogatory about another physician. This only reflects negatively on you and often gets back to the person you least want to hear it.

Another important step is to locate qualified subspecialists in your area to whom you can confidently refer your patients. Talk with other pediatricians or family practitioners and ask them to whom they refer and if they are satisfied. Meet the specialists practicing dermatology, otolaryngology, neurology, surgery, and ophthalmology to whom you are considering referring patients. Your professional reference is looked on by the patient as an extension of you and your office. If the experience is positive, so are the patient's feelings about you. If the patient's experiences are negative, the referral reflects negatively on you.

When opening the practice, a prime objective is to let the community know that you are there. Several weeks before opening, put advertisements in the local papers announcing who you are, your office location, your hours (usually by appointment), and what type of patients you want to care for (eg, infants, children, adolescents). Announce whether you accept Medicaid and whether you are participating in any of the area's health maintenance organizations or managed care plans. Let the physicians in the area know you are opening your office by sending out announcements. Radio announcements of the opening may be feasible. Some pediatricians hold an open house for other physicians and potential patients to see the new facilities and meet the pediatrician and staff.

### Charges for Services

Deciding what your knowledge and services are worth is often a difficult task. No one is ever asked to do this during medical school or residency. Ask other pediatricians in the area what they charge for their services. Adjust your scale accordingly. Be competitive with the others in your area. Pediatricians tend to undervalue their services, perhaps because most of what a pediatrician uses in practice is knowledge, common sense, and reassurance and not the myriad instruments, machines, and exotic drugs used in other specialties. You should remember that it took at least 7 years to be able to recognize otitis media even though it takes only 1 to 2 minutes to diagnose it.

## Types of Services Offered

In all specialties of medicine, but especially in pediatrics, we are not selling a product in the usual sense of the word. We are not giving our patients a material object for their money, although good health certainly is a tangible product. We are providing knowledge and service. We are selling quality care, security, availability, comfort, personalized service, caring, and compassion.

Quality care means being up to date on the latest and best modes of diagnosis, laboratory analysis, and treatment and being willing to change as new information is discovered and old ideas are disproved. In private practice, there is little time to read after a hard day in the office, but many ways to keep updated are discussed later in the chapter.

Providing security and achieving the confidence of patients means being consistent with what you say and do to patients, even if it is not always easy. This may make you unpopular with some patients, but as long as you are practicing good medicine, you should not vacillate. Do not compromise your beliefs, as in giving antibiotics because you feel the parent is expecting to get a prescription even though you think the child has a viral illness. Once you have compromised, it is always easier to give in again and again. Do not be afraid to admit you are unsure of a diagnosis; tell the patient what it is not. This alone reassures many patients. If you have made a mistake, admit it. Most patients appreciate honesty. Lying or covering up mistakes may lead to the lawyer's office.

Comfort is important to your patients. The office visit and telephone conversations should be designed to put the patient or parent at ease and instill confidence. The encounter should be as pleasant as possible. Do not keep patients waiting, and do not overbook. Be prompt for office hours. Try to put yourself in your patient's position.

Personalized service is equally important. Parents or guardians are paying you for taking care of their children, and if your service is not good, they will go somewhere else. Always review the chart before entering the examination room. Know your patient's name and sex. Nothing is more embarrassing than calling Susie "Jimmy." Review special problems from the last visit. When you mention these items in the interview, the patient and parent know you are interested. Put a reminder page in each chart. This is used to make notations about special circumstances and events that are important in your patients' lives. Examples are adopting a new baby, winning the swimming meet, buying a new house, or a recent family vacation to Disneyland. Briefly mentioning some of these items during a visit shows the patient and parent that they are more than just a diagnosis or illness.

Call parents by Mr. and Mrs., not by their first names, unless you want them to call you by yours. While the parent or patient is telling you what has been happening or the history of the recent illness, try not to interrupt. This shows common courtesy. Answer the parents' questions first during the health maintenance visits, and then cover your topics. If you do this in reverse order, the parents may not hear a single word you have said because they are concerned about something else. When interviewing a patient, sit down. A pediatrician who is standing up leaning against an examination table gives a patient and parent the feeling that he cannot wait to leave the room. Maintain eye contact with parents and patients. Do not let your staff interrupt you for routine phone calls; your time with the patient is sacred except for emergencies.

Caring and compassion are of utmost importance for the pediatrician. Treat those you care for as if they are your own children or members of your own family. Think before you say things, and remember that medical jargon has little meaning to most families. There are many ways to show you care. Keep a sick list each day of the patients that you felt were sicker than average or the parents who seemed especially anxious. Call these families back after hours or the next day to see how the child is doing. Just knowing you are concerned will diminish the parents' concerns. Another good idea is to call all parents of newborns 1 or 2 days after discharge from the hospital to see how the baby and mother are doing. New parents are often too confused or too busy to remember to call you.

Sending thank you notes to patients who send new referrals to you shows your patients you appreciate their confidence in you. Most of a pediatrician's new patients come from the recommendations of patients and parents.

Try to make the office visit as enjoyable as possible for the children. Balloons and stickers have made many children forget an injection or blood test.

Although a pediatrician's hours are long and arduous, try to make them as much fun for yourself as possible. Even when situations seem impossible, try to look on the brighter side.

## Marketing the Practice

"Marketing" is considered a dirty word in many medical circles. This one word conjures up images of giant neon billboards which read, "Appendectomies Half Price—Two for One!" or "Have Your Second Inguinal Hernia Repaired for Free." In some areas of the United States, similar advertisements are being displayed or carried over television and radio. There are many more subtle and tasteful ways to market and augment a practice. Some of them have been discussed previously.

One easy way to become more visible in a community is to volunteer to speak to community groups. Timely subjects such as hypertension, pediatric immunizations, acquired immune deficiency syndrome, and behavior problems are just a few of numerous potential topics. High school classes, prenatal classes, Parent Teacher Associations, Boy and Girl Scout troops, and various service organizations are always looking for interesting speakers. You do not have to hand out business cards or give away balloons to recruit new patients. Your knowledge, appearance, and personality will attract potential patients.

Advertising can be accomplished discreetly and with taste. Many communities have groups or businesses that send out packets of brochures, coupons, and information to new home buyers. Some communities have plastic telephone book covers that list important medical information. For a nominal charge, the office number and address of your office can be included. This gives the practice higher visibility in the public eye, especially in smaller communities in which the number of available physicians is small.

Refrigerator magnets with the office name, address, and phone number are helpful to parents when they need to call the office. A supply of business cards should be kept in the patient waiting room in case a patient wants to take one home to a friend or relative. A supply should be kept in the local hospital's emergency department for the emergency physicians to hand to patients when appropriate.

Offering free prenatal visits to couples is good publicity. This gives the couple a chance to meet with you before selecting their child's pediatrician, and potential areas of misunderstanding can be dealt with before they become major problems.

An excellent resource in the area of marketing and advertising is the state Board of Medical Examiners. Most states have guidelines for physician marketing and advertising which must be followed. All of the methods described above can help the community know what you have to offer. The more exposure you have in the community, the greater the chance that parents will choose you to take care of their children.

## BALANCING PROFESSIONAL AND SOCIAL LIVES

A physician should strive to balance professional life with family and social lives. All too often a pediatrician becomes obsessed with the office, patients, and medical side of life only to watch family relationships disintegrate from lack of attention. On the other hand, too many extracurricular activities can be detrimental to even the best of practices.

Patients need care, as do pediatricians and their families. You should take frequent getaway weekends or day trips. A week off every 3 or 4 months prevents burnout and gives you something to look forward to throughout the year. Just getting out of town for a few hours or for a weekend can invigorate even the most harried practitioner.

Throughout the greater part of college, medical school, and residency, physicians are surrounded by fellow physicians and other medical professionals. This is not healthy! Actively seek out nonmedical people to associate with at times. This gives you a more realistic view of the world and allows you to see things from different perspectives. Joining organizations or clubs such as Rotary International, Kiwanis Club, Chamber of Commerce, or the Parent Teacher Association can open up new avenues of friendship.

Family should remain a priority at all times. Schedule trips or events when not on call. Try to foresee potential problems or schedule conflicts before they arise, and take appropriate actions to avoid them. All too often, physicians learn this lesson after their own children are grown.

## CONTINUING EDUCATION

It is astonishing with how little reading a doctor can practice medicine, but it is not astonishing how badly he may do it.
Sir William Osler

After the practice is established and a routine is in place, you may heave a sigh of relief. However, you cannot set your professional life on automatic pilot. Medical progress marches ever faster, and a pediatrician must work hard to stay current. New drugs, new procedures, and new information must be incorporated into practice so that high-quality care is continually provided. There are many ways for the private practitioner to do this.

One excellent way is to teach medical students or residents in the office. Even one session a week can keep you scrambling to textbooks and journals to look up the answers to a student's questions.

Reading pertinent literature on a regular basis is important. Because no one can read all the literature, choose those articles that are pertinent to your specific practice or areas of interest. There are innumerable Continuing Medical Education courses available to pediatricians, many of which are sponsored by the national and regional chapters of the AAP. The Academy's PREP series is also an excellent source of pertinent up-to-date clinical information for the practitioner.

The process of obtaining board certification and recertification, despite certain problems, does force a pediatrician to recall forgotten words of wisdom and to learn new ones. Skills must be updated and reviewed. Many teaching hospitals, and AAP workshops, offer courses on practical topics such as intubation,

infant resuscitation, umbilical vessel catheterization, and pelvic examination.

An extremely important source of information can be regional specialists at pediatric tertiary centers who are abreast of all current information in their particular specialty. These professionals are excellent information sources for the general pediatrician.

The choice of pediatrics as a career is a noble and enriching one. Pediatrics demands integrity, compassion, commitment, and diligence. The profession brings joy, challenge, and satisfaction. Pediatricians are in the unique position to watch the growth, development, and metamorphosis of an infant into an adult. It is a serious responsibility and a source of constant wonderment.

## Selected Readings

American Academy of Pediatrics. Management of pediatric practice, ed 2. Elk Grove, IL: American Academy of Pediatrics, 1991.

American Medical Association. Planning guide for physicians' medical facilities, ed 3. Chicago: American Medical Association, 1979.

Mallcin J. For office decor, fresh thinking beats free spending. Med Econ 1987;64: 178.

Schmitt BD. Pediatric telephone advice. Boston: Little, Brown, 1980.

*Principles and Practice of Pediatrics, Second Edition.*
edited by Frank A. Oski et al. J. B. Lippincott Company, Philadelphia © 1994.

## CHAPTER 24
# *Prevention of Diseases*

# *24.1 Feeding the Healthy Child*

### Modena Hoover Wilson

Providing nourishment that results in normal growth and development is the premier task of the parent. Parents judge their success in child rearing, and the pediatrician judges the child's overall well-being, by growth. Feeding and its results are central issues in pediatrics. Nourishment involves more than the simple offering of food, even if it is of adequate composition. Appropriate feeding is a metaphor for the nurturing relationship.

The body's handling of the more than 50 known required nutrients is complex. The growth of the child that depends on these nutrients and processes appears to the observer, if not the researcher, nothing short of miraculous. Although pages of guidelines exist, research findings fill volumes, and many parental questions and concerns focus on feeding and growth, most children thrive. Current generations in the United States and many other parts of the world achieve previously unmatched levels of growth. If food is available in abundance and variety, feeding the healthy child is easy.

## PRINCIPLES OF NUTRITION

For normal growth, a child's intake must include protein, fat, carbohydrates, water, vitamins, minerals, and trace elements in appropriate amounts. Clinically recognizable deficiency states are known for many of these nutrients, and for some, disease is associated with excess. However, desirable intake ranges are described for only about half.

In the United States, the Food and Nutrition Board of the National Academy of Sciences establishes and updates guidelines called the National Research Council Recommended Dietary Allowances (NRCRDAs) to which the dietary habits of populations can be compared and by which individual diets can be designed and monitored. The NRCRDAs are based on average need of healthy persons plus a 30% to 50% margin of excess to guarantee meeting needs at the high end of the range. For some nutrients, a "safe and adequate dietary intake" rather than a recommended daily allowance is described. These values represent a range considered adequate and subtoxic. The guidelines of the Food and Nutrition Board and the Committee on Nutrition of the American Academy of Pediatrics (CONAAP) inform the decisions of the Food and Drug Administration about formulas for infants. These guidelines help professionals provide nutritional advice for children and adolescents.

The nutritional needs of the normal term infant and the healthy child and adolescent are addressed in this chapter. Nutritional guidelines for prematurely born infants, sick infants, and children with health problems that jeopardize nutrition are covered in other chapters of this book. The NRCRDAs and estimates for other vitamins and minerals for pediatric populations are summarized in Tables 24-1 and 24-2.

### Energy Substrates

Energy is needed for the metabolic functions that sustain life, for growth, and for physical activity. The rapid growth rate of the infant creates energy needs that are not matched by the healthy organism during any other part of the life span. Energy intake is the prime mover of the diet, without which other nutrients cannot be appropriately used. In ways that are not completely understood, energy intake is closely regulated through appetite in most persons, leading them to eat enough to grow during childhood and to maintain weight during adulthood.

Energy needs are expressed in kilocalorie (kcal) units. A kilocalorie is the amount of energy required to raise the temperature of 1 kg of water from 15 °C to 16 °C. Caloric needs can be estimated by summing energy needed for growth, which averages about 5 kcal per gram of weight gain, and for activity, which varies with the work required, with experimentally measured baseline energy needs for the maintenance of life. Such maintenance needs are age and gender specific and are represented in calculations by basal metabolic rate (BMR), basal energy expenditure (BEE), or maintenance energy requirements (MER). BEE is 10% higher than BMR and takes into account some minimal activity during bed rest. MER approximates BMR plus 15% and is based on estimations of body surface area. Besides varying with age, gender, body size, and activity, caloric needs increase with abnormal losses of nutrients in stool or urine and with fever, illness, and injury. The average needs for male and female infants, children, and adolescents are presented in Table 24-3. "Average" needs cover considerable individual variation. Deficient intake is expressed in the individual child as inadequate growth or weight loss.

Protein, carbohydrates, and fats can be used to meet caloric needs, providing for each ingested gram 4 kcal, 4 kcal, and 9 kcal respectively. Essential nutrients, which are substances the body requires and cannot manufacture, are provided by the foods that supply these energy substrates, and the balance among them is crucial.

### Protein

Protein contributes to energy intake and supplies essential and nonessential amino acids needed for protein synthesis and tissue growth and replacement. Essential amino acids are those that must be present in the diet because they are not synthesized at all or in sufficient quantities. Amino acids that are dietary essentials for adults are isoleucine, leucine, lysine, methionine, phenylalanine, threonine tryptophan, valine, and probably histidine. Cystine and tyrosine are not synthesized by infants at rates adequate to meet their needs. Dietary sources of these amino acids can decrease, but not eliminate, the need for dietary methionine and phenylalanine. Infants may need taurine.

Current methods of estimating nitrogen and protein needs suggest that protein needs decrease with age from about 2 to 0.7 g/kg/day. Protein needs vary by gender because of differences in lean body mass and size, and they decline with age because of changes in growth rate (see Table 24-1). The quality of protein, especially in infant formulas, can be described by a calculated protein efficiency ratio (PER) that equals weight gain in grams divided by grams of protein consumed. Casein is used as a standard. If the protein considered has a PER that is less than 100% of the PER for casein, the amount in the diet must be increased. Proteins with a PER of less than 70% of that of casein are not used in formulas.

Good dietary sources of protein are legumes, fish, poultry, dairy products, meat, and eggs. Proteins of animal origin are of higher biologic value because they most closely match the amino acid distribution needed. Adequate protein can be derived from nonmeat sources, but more attention must be paid to variety and amount.

Too little protein intake results in kwashiorkor or, if caloric intake is also low, marasmus. The average American child consumes a larger percentage of calories in the form of protein than is recommended. The long-term results of this imbalance are unknown. No safe upper limit has been established.

### Carbohydrates

The need for carbohydrate as an essential nutrient exists but is small. The importance of carbohydrate to the diet is greatest as a contributor of energy calories, thereby minimizing the intake of protein and fat, both of which have deleterious effects when consumed in excess. Extreme deficiency of carbohydrate in the diet leads to ketosis.

Lactose is the primary carbohydrate in the diet of most infants, as is starch in the diet of most older children. Children also consume monosaccharides, disaccharides, and fiber, which is indigestible carbohydrate.

Many beneficial effects have been ascribed to high fiber content in the diet: eliminating constipation, lowering risk for diverticular disease and colonic cancer, and preventing obesity and cardiovascular disease. However, some of the supposed benefits are based on epidemiologic associations; a direct correlation is not proven. High fiber intake decreases intestinal transit time and increases stool bulk, softness, and number. Pectin has a serum cholesterol-lowering effect.

Concerns about very high fiber intake during childhood center on interference with mineral absorption and the large volume of high-fiber food needed to ensure adequate calories. Because current fiber intake in the average childhood diet is quite low, desirable increases can be instituted without approaching levels that interfere with caloric or mineral needs. CONAAP suggests that fiber emphasis begin after the first year and that appropriate

TABLE 24-1.  Recommended Daily Dietary Allowances for Healthy Children and Adolescents in the United States*

| Group | Protein (g) | Fat-Soluble Vitamins | | | | Water-Soluble Vitamins | | | | | | | | Minerals | | | | | | |
|---|---|---|---|---|---|---|---|---|---|---|---|---|---|---|---|---|---|---|---|---|
| | | Vitamin A (µg RE)† | Vitamin D (µg)‡ | Vitamin E (mg α-TE)§ | Vitamin K (µg) | Vitamin C (mg) | Thiamine (mg) | Riboflavin (mg) | Niacin (mg NE)‖ | Vitamin B₆ (mg) | Folate (µg) | Vitamin B₁₂ (µg) | Calcium (mg) | Phosphorus (mg) | Magnesium (mg) | Iron (mg) | Zinc (mg) | Iodine (µg) | Selenium (µg) |
| **Infants** | | | | | | | | | | | | | | | | | | | |
| 0–6 mo | 13 | 375 | 7.5 | 3 | 5 | 30 | 0.3 | 0.4 | 5 | 0.3 | 25 | 0.3 | 400 | 300 | 40 | 6 | 5 | 40 | 10 |
| 7–12 mo | 14 | 375 | 10 | 4 | 10 | 35 | 0.4 | 0.5 | 6 | 0.6 | 35 | 0.5 | 600 | 500 | 60 | 10 | 5 | 50 | 15 |
| **Children** | | | | | | | | | | | | | | | | | | | |
| 1–3 y | 16 | 400 | 10 | 6 | 15 | 40 | 0.7 | 0.8 | 9 | 1.0 | 50 | 0.7 | 800 | 800 | 80 | 10 | 10 | 70 | 20 |
| 4–6 y | 24 | 500 | 10 | 7 | 20 | 45 | 0.9 | 1.1 | 12 | 1.1 | 75 | 1.0 | 800 | 800 | 120 | 10 | 10 | 90 | 20 |
| 7–10 y | 28 | 700 | 10 | 7 | 30 | 45 | 1.0 | 1.2 | 13 | 14 | 100 | 1.4 | 800 | 800 | 170 | 10 | 10 | 120 | 30 |
| **Males** | | | | | | | | | | | | | | | | | | | |
| 11–14 y | 45 | 1000 | 10 | 10 | 45 | 50 | 1.3 | 1.5 | 17 | 1.7 | 150 | 2.0 | 1200 | 1200 | 270 | 12 | 15 | 150 | 40 |
| 15–18 yr | 59 | 1000 | 10 | 10 | 65 | 60 | 1.5 | 1.8 | 20 | 2.0 | 200 | 2.0 | 1200 | 1200 | 400 | 12 | 15 | 150 | 50 |
| **Females** | | | | | | | | | | | | | | | | | | | |
| 11–14 y | 46 | 800 | 10 | 8 | 45 | 50 | 1.1 | 1.3 | 15 | 1.4 | 150 | 2.0 | 1200 | 1200 | 280 | 15 | 12 | 150 | 45 |
| 15–18 y | 44 | 800 | 10 | 8 | 55 | 60 | 1.1 | 1.3 | 15 | 1.5 | 180 | 2.0 | 1200 | 1200 | 300 | 15 | 12 | 150 | 50 |
| Pregnant | 60 | 800 | 10 | 10 | 65 | 70 | 1.5 | 1.6 | 17 | 2.2 | 400 | 2.2 | 1200 | 1200 | 300 | 30 | 15 | 175 | 65 |
| Lactating | 65 | 1300 | 10 | 12 | 65 | 95 | 1.6 | 1.8 | 20 | 2.1 | 280 | 2.6 | 1200 | 1200 | 355 | 15 | 19 | 200 | 75 |

* The allowances, expressed as average daily intakes over time, are intended to provide for individual variations among most normal persons as they live in the United States under usual environmental stresses. Diets should be based on a variety of common foods to provide other nutrients for which human requirements have been less well defined.

† Retinol equivalents. 1 retinol equivalent = 1 µg retinol or 6 µg β carotene.

‡ As cholecalciferol. 10 µg cholecalciferol = 400 IU of vitamin D.

§ α-tocopherol equivalents. 1 mg D-α-tocopherol = 1 α-TE.

‖ 1 NE (niacin equivalent) is equal to 1 mg of niacin or 60 mg of dietary tryptophan.

*Subcommittee on the Tenth Education of the RDAs, Food and Nutrition Board, Commission on Life Sciences, National Research Council. Recommended dietary allowances, ed 10. Washington, DC: National Academy Press, 1989.*

TABLE 24-2.  Estimated Safe and Adequate Daily Dietary Intake
Selected Vitamins and Minerals

| Age Group | Vitamins | | Trace Elements* | | | | |
|---|---|---|---|---|---|---|---|
| | Biotin (μg) | Pantothenic Acid (mg) | Cu (mg) | Mn (mg) | F (mg) | Cr (μg) | Mo (μg) |
| **Infants** | | | | | | | |
| 0–6 mo | 10 | 2 | 0.4–0.6 | 0.3–0.6 | 0.1–0.5 | 10–40 | 15–30 |
| 7–12 mo | 15 | 3 | 0.6–0.7 | 0.6–1.0 | 0.2–1.0 | 20–60 | 20–40 |
| **Children** | | | | | | | |
| 1–3 y | 20 | 3 | 0.7–1.0 | 1.0–1.5 | 0.5–1.5 | 20–80 | 25–50 |
| 4–6 y | 25 | 3–4 | 1.0–1.5 | 1.5–2.0 | 1.0–2.5 | 30–120 | 30–75 |
| 7–10 y | 30 | 4–5 | 1.0–2.0 | 2.0–3.0 | 1.5–2.5 | 50–200 | 50–150 |
| **Adolescents** | | | | | | | |
| 11–18 y | 30–100 | 4–7 | 1.5–2.5 | 2.0–5.0 | 1.5–2.5 | 50–200 | 75–250 |

* Because toxic levels for many trace elements may be only several times the usual intakes, the upper levels for the trace elements given in this table should not be habitually exceeded.

Subcommittee on the Tenth Edition of the RDAs, Food and Nutrition Board, Commission on Life Sciences, National Research Council. Recommended dietary allowances, ed 10 Washington, DC: National Academy Press, 1989;284.

sources of fiber during childhood include whole grain bread, cereal, fruits, and vegetables.

## Fat

The most common dietary fats are triglycerides, consisting of glycerol plus three fatty acids. Fatty acids can be unsaturated, containing one or more double bonds, or saturated, containing no double bonds. Fats from most animal sources are saturated. Two fatty acids are essential dietary components. Linoleic acid, a component of cell membranes and a precursor in prostaglandin synthesis, cannot be synthesized by the body. From it, the body derives arachidonic acid. Linolenic acid, found in the nervous system, is also essential. Triglycerides containing the essential fatty acids should comprise at least 3% of the caloric content of the diet. Deficiency develops rapidly in newborn infants who do not receive dietary fat. After the newborn period, deficiencies are likely to develop only under the extreme situations of parenteral nutrition or fat malabsorption. Symptoms and signs reported clinically include a flaky dermatitis, diarrhea, poor hair growth, thrombocytopenia, failure to thrive, and susceptibility to infection (Hansen, 1958).

Fats contribute to energy needs substantially because of their high caloric density. The proportion of total energy intake to be derived from dietary fat provokes controversy, because a diet high in saturated fats may lead to an unfavorable serum lipid profile, a risk factor for the development of coronary heart disease. CONAAP recommends that no restriction should be placed on fat and cholesterol during the first 2 years of life (CONAAP, Statement on cholesterol, 1992). Thereafter, the fat and cholesterol content of the diet can be decreased gradually to achieve the goal of 30% of daily calories from fat, with fewer than 10% of total calories from saturated fats and fewer than 300 mg of cholesterol. This goal is achievable without sacrificing other important nutrients. It is feared that attempts at greater fat reduction may restrict the diet to the point of compromise.

If the diet is high in unsaturated fats, vitamin E (tocopherol) must be available in quantities sufficient to prevent their oxidation. At least 0.5 mg of tocopherol equivalent is recommended per gram of linolenic acid. If vitamin E is not sufficient, hemolysis may result, especially if extra iron, which generates free radicals, is added to the diet. This has clinical application in planning the diet of premature infants and other specialized diets.

## Water

Water is an essential nutrient. It is required for growth and to replace losses through the skin, from the respiratory tract, and in urine and stool. Daily water needs begin at 125 to 145 mL/kg at term and decrease on a unit basis as a child increases in size. After a weight of 3 kg is achieved, water requirements can be calculated as 100 mL/kg to 10 kg, 50 mL/kg for each additional kg up to 20 kg, and 20 mL/kg for each 1 kg thereafter (Kelts, 1984). More detailed discussion of water and electrolyte requirements can be found in Chapter 11.

TABLE 24-3.  Recommended Energy Intake for Children and Adolescents

| Age Group | Average Energy Allowance (kcal) | |
|---|---|---|
| | Per 1 kg of Weight | Per Day (Rounded) |
| **Infants** | | |
| 0–6 mo | 108 | 650 |
| 7–12 mo | 98 | 850 |
| **Children** | | |
| 1–3 y | 102 | 1300 |
| 4–6 y | 90 | 1800 |
| 7–10 y | 70 | 2000 |
| **Adolescents** | | |
| 11–14 y females* | 47 | 2200 |
| 11–14 y males | 55 | 2500 |
| 15–18 y females* | 40 | 2200 |
| 15–18 y males | 45 | 3000 |

* Add 300 kcal/day for pregnancy or 500 kcal/day for lactation.

Subcommittee on the Tenth Edition of the RDAs, Food and Nutrition Board, Commission on Life Sciences, National Research Council. Recommended dietary allowances, ed 10. Washington, DC: National Academy Press, 1989.

TABLE 24-4.   Vitamin Characteristics, Actions, Disease States, and Sources

| Name | Characteristics | Biochemical Action | Effects of Deficiency | Effects of Excess | Dietary Sources |
|---|---|---|---|---|---|
| Vitamin A (retinol) 1 IU = 0.3 μg retinol | Fat soluble, heat stable; bile necessary for absorption, specific binding protein in plasma; stored in liver | Component of visual purple; integrity of epithelial tissues; bone cell function | Night blindness, xerophthalmia, keratomalacia, poor growth, impaired resistance to infection | Hyperostosis, hepatomegaly, alopecia, increased cerebrospinal fluid pressure (also from 13-cis-retinoic acid) | Milk fat, egg, liver |
| Provitamin A (β-carotene; 1/6 activity of retinol) | Converted to retinol in liver, intestinal mucosa | | | Carotenemia | Dark green vegetables, yellow fruits and vegetables, tomato |
| Vitamin D (D₂-activated calciferol; D₃-activated dehydrocholesterol) 1 IU = 0.025 μg | D₂ from diet, D₃ from action of ultraviolet on skin; hydroxylated sequentially in liver and kidney to form 1,25-dihydroxycholecalciferol, the active compound; regulated by dietary calcium, parathyroid hormone; anticonvulsant drugs interfere with metabolism | Formation of calcium; transport protein in duodenal mucosa; facilitates bone resorption, phosphorus absorption; synthesis of Ca-binding protein in epithelial cells | Rickets, osteomalacia | Hypercalcemia, azotemia, poor growth, vomiting, nephrocalcinosis | Fortified milk, fish, liver, salmon, sardines, mackerel, egg yolk, sunlight |
| Vitamin E (1 IU = 1 mg α-tocopherol acetate) | Stored in adipose tissue; transported with β-lipoproteins; absorption depends on pancreatic juice and bile (iron may interfere); requirement increased by large amounts of polyunsaturated fats | Antioxidant, role in erythrocyte fragility; stabilizes biologic membranes, prevents peroxidation of unsaturated fatty acids | Hemolytic anemia in premature infants; otherwise, no clear-cut deficiency syndrome in humans | Unknown | Cereal seed oils, peanuts, soybeans, milk fat, turnip greens |
| Ascorbic acid (vitamin C) | Easily oxidized, especially in presence of copper, iron, high pH; absorption by simple diffusion | Exact mechanism unknown; functions in folacin metabolism, collagen biosynthesis, iron absorption and transport, tyrosin metabolism | Scurvy | Massive doses may lead to temporary increase in requirements and may predispose to kidney stones | Citrus fruits, tomatoes, cabbage, potatoes, human milk |
| Thiamine (vitamin B₁) | Heat labile; absorption impaired by alcohol, requirements a function of carbohydrate intake; synthesis by intestinal bacteria | Coenzyme for decarboxylation, other reactions as thiamine pyrophosphate | Beriberi: neuritis, edema, cardiac failure, hoarseness, anorexia, restlessness, aphonia | Unknown | Liver, meat, milk, whole grains, legumes |
| Riboflavin | Water soluble, light labile, heat stable; synthesis by intestinal bacteria (t) | Cofactor for many enzymes, synthesis FMN and FAD | Photophobia, cheilosis, glossitis, corneal vascularization, poor growth | Unknown | Meat, milk, egg, green vegetables, whole grains |

| Vitamin | Characteristics | Function | Deficiency | Toxicity | Sources |
|---|---|---|---|---|---|
| Niacin (nicotinic acid, amide) | Water soluble, heat and light stable; availability from corn enhanced by alkali; synthesized in the body from tryptophan (60:1), some by intestinal bacteria | Component of coenzymes I and II (NAD, NADP), many enzymatic reactions | Pellagra: dermatitis, diarrhea, dementia | Nicotinic acid (not the amide) causes flushing, pruritus | Meat, fish, whole grains, green vegetables |
| Pyridoxine (vitamin B$_6$) also pyridoxal, pyridoxamine | Water soluble, heat and light labile, interference from isoniazid; pyridoxal is the active form | Cofactor for many enzymes (eg, transaminases, decarboxylases) | Dermatitis, glossitis, cheilosis, peripheral neuritis; in infants, irritability, convulsions, anemia | Unknown | Liver, meat, whole grains, corn, soybeans |
| Folacin group of compounds containing pteridine ring, p-aminobenzoic, and glutamic acids | Slightly soluble in water, light sensitive, heat stable; some production by intestinal bacteria; ascorbic acid involved in interconversions; interference from oral contraceptives, anticonvulsants | Tetrahydrofolic acid the active form; synthesis of purines, pyrimidines, methylation reactions, one-carbon acceptor | Megaloblastic anemia, impaired cellular immunity | Only in patients with pernicious anemia not receiving cobalamin | Liver, green vegetables, cereals, oranges |
| Cobalamin (vitamin B$_{12}$) | Slightly soluble in water, heat stable only at neutral pH, light sensitivity; absorption (ileum) depends on gastric intrinsic factor; CoA part of the molecule | Coenzyme component; erythrocyte maturation, central nervous system metabolism, methylmalonyl CoA mutase | Pernicious anemia; neurologic deterioration, methylmalonic acidemia | Unknown | Animal foods only: meat, milk, egg |
| Pantothenic acid | Water soluble, heat stable; daily requirement unknown but estimated at 5–10 mg | Component only CoA; many enzymatic reactions | Observed only with use of antagonists: depression, hypotension, muscle weakness, abdominal pain | Unknown | Most foods |
| Biotin | Water soluble; synthesized by intestinal bacteria; deficiency only with large intake of egg whites, TPN | Coenzyme: acetyl CoA carboxylase | Dermatitis, anorexia, muscle pain, pallor, alopecia | Unknown | Liver, egg yolk, peanuts |
| Vitamin K (naphthoquinones) | Fat soluble; bile necessary for absorption; synthesis of intestinal bacteria | Blood coagulation: factors II, VII, IX, X | Hemorrhagic manifestations | Water-soluble analogues only: hyperbilirubinemia | Cow's milk, green leafy vegetables, pork, liver |

CoA, coenzyme A; FAD, flavin adenine dinucleotide; FMN, flavin mononucleotide (riboflavin 5'-phosphate); NAD, nicotinamide-adenine dinucleotide; NADP, nicotinamide-adenine dinucleotide phosphate.

From Committee on Nutrition, American Academy of Pediatrics. Pediatric Nutrition Handbook, ed 2. Elk Grove Village, IL: American Academy of Pediatrics, 1985:136.

## Vitamins, Minerals, and Trace Elements

Most vitamins, essential cofactors in metabolic processes, must be supplied by the diet. The characteristics of those vitamins most commonly given consideration in pediatric nutrition are described in Table 24-4 with suggested dietary sources.

The dietary need for some minerals is well established. Sodium, potassium, and chloride are discussed in Chapter 11. Calcium, phosphorus, and magnesium metabolism are discussed in Chapter 12.11; the deficiency states associated with iron and iodine are discussed in Chapter 90.1. Daily requirements are listed in Tables 24-1 and 24-2. For most American children, dairy products are the major dietary source of calcium, although other sources include greens, some seeds and nuts, soybean products, lentils, and raisins. Magnesium and phosphorus are contained in many foods and are rarely limiting. The small quantities of iodine needed are adequately provided by iodized salt. Dietary sources of iron are discussed later.

Additional elements are needed in small or minute quantities for normal growth and metabolism. Although more than 23 elements are recognized as essential, relatively few are thought to be limiting in the sense that deficiency states are of clinical importance (Table 24-5).

With few exceptions, American children fed a recommended diet throughout infancy and childhood receive adequate supplies of minerals, vitamins, and trace elements with their food. The relatively uncommon instances in which supplementation is routinely recommended are listed in Table 24-6. Predictable deficiencies based on the special requirements and dietary habits of children by age are discussed later.

## FEEDING THE INFANT

The establishment of a satisfying relationship between the infant and the parent during feedings is, in the usual situation, integral to parent–infant interactions. Through the feeding process, the parent provides adequate nutrition for growth and social interaction, without which growth and development do not proceed normally. The infant and the parent contribute to the emotional content of the feeding process, and feeding problems can develop even when the infant is apparently intact, the parent well intentioned, and the nutritional content of the presented food appropriate.

Healthy term infants obtain their nourishment by sucking. They do so in a pattern that appears to encourage social interaction. After a few minutes of vigorous sucking, they settle into a rhythm of bursts of sucking followed by pauses. The feeder's behavior during these pauses is usually to stimulate the infant, and a reciprocity develops. The feeding situation appears to be one barometer of overall satisfaction in the mother–infant rela-

### TABLE 24-5. Trace Elements Associated With Clinically Recognized Deficiency Diseases

| Element | Biochemical Action | Effects of Deficiency | Effects of Excess | Daily Requirement | Food Sources |
|---|---|---|---|---|---|
| Chromium (Cr) | Required for maintenance of normal glucose metabolism; potentiates the action of insulin | *Humans:* impairment of glucose use; *animals:* impaired growth, disturbances of carbohydrate, protein, and lipid metabolism | Relatively nontoxic; *humans:* not well documented; *animals:* growth retardation, liver and kidney damage | Safe and adequate range: infants, 0.0–0.04 mg; children, adolescents, 0.02–0.2 mg | Meat, cheese, whole grains, brewer's yeast |
| Cobalt (Co) | Component of $B_{12}$ | *Humans:* unknown; *animals:* anemia growth retardation | Relatively nontoxic; polycythemia, myocardial degeneration | Not established | Green leafy vegetables |
| Copper (Cu) | Constituent of ceruloplasmin; component of key metalloenzymes; role in connective tissue biosynthesis | Sideroblastic anemia, retarded growth, osteoporosis, neutropenia, decreased pigmentation | Relatively nontoxic; Wilson's disease, liver dysfunction | Safe and adequate range: infants, 0.5–1 mg; children, adolescents, 1–3 mg | Shellfish, meat, legumes |
| Manganese (Mn) | Activator of metal–enzyme complexes; important for synthesis of polysaccharides and glycoproteins; constituent of pyruvate carboxylase and certain superoxide dismutases | *Humans:* not documented; *animals:* growth retardation, ataxia of newborn, bone abnormalities, reduced fertility | Relatively nontoxic; neurologic manifestations from industrial contamination have occurred | Safe and adequate range: infants, 0.5–1 mg; children, adolescents, 1–5 mg | Nuts, whole grains, tea |
| Molybdenum (Mo) | Component of enzymes involved in production of uric acid (xanthine oxidase) and in oxidation of aldehydes and sulfides | *Humans:* unknown; *animals:* growth retardation, anorexia | *Humans:* goutlike syndrome, antagonist of copper | Safe and adequate range: infants, 0.03–0.08 mg; children, adolescents, 0.05–0.30 mg | Meats, grains, legumes |
| Selenium (Se) | Component of enzyme glutathione peroxidase | *Humans:* cardiomyopathy; *animals:* liver necrosis, muscular dystrophy, exudative diathesis, pancreatic fibrosis | Irritation of mucous membranes (eg, nose, eyes, upper respiratory tract), pallor, irritability, indigestion | Safe and adequate range: infants, 0.01–0.06 mg; children, adolescents, 0.02–0.2 mg | Seafood, meat, whole grains |

*From Committee on Nutrition, American Academy of Pediatrics. Pediatric Nutrition Handbook, ed 2. Elk Grove Village, IL: American Academy of Pediatrics, 1985:126.*

TABLE 24-6.   Guidelines for the Use of Vitamin and Mineral Supplements in Healthy Infants and Children

| Group | Multivitamin | Vitamins* | | | Minerals | |
|---|---|---|---|---|---|---|
| | | D | E | Folate | Iron | Fluoride† |
| Term infants (0–6 mo) | | | | | | |
|   Breast fed | 0 | + | 0 | 0 | 0 | ± |
|   Formula fed | 0 | 0 | 0 | 0 | 0 | ± |
| Preterm infants | | | | | | |
|   Breast fed‡ | + | + | ± | ± | + | ± |
|   Formula fed | + | + | ± | ± | + | ± |
| Older infants (>6 mo) | 0 | + | 0 | 0 | ±§ | ± |
| Children | 0 | 0 | 0 | 0 | 0 | ± |
| Pregnant women | ± | 0 | 0 | ± | + | 0 |
| Lactating women | ± | 0 | 0 | 0 | ± | 0 |

\* Vitamin K for newborn infants is not shown. Extract calcium for pregnant and lactating women is not shown.
† Depending on local drinking water supply.
‡ Sodium content of human milk is marginal for these infants.
§ Iron-foritified commercial infant formula and infant cereal are convenient and reliable sources.
*From Committee on Nutrition, American Academy of Pediatrics, Pediatric Nutrition Handbook, ed 2. Elk Grove Village, IL: American Academy of Pediatrics, 1985:40.*

tionship, with maternal behavior during feeding predicting her overall parenting behavior.

## Nutrient Requirements

The infant must rely completely on the caregiver. The ability to regulate the intake volume is limited for the young infant, whose signals must be interpreted by a caregiver. Adding to nutritional vulnerability is the fact that a rapid growth rate and a high surface-area-to-volume ratio make the infant's requirements for energy, protein, and water especially great. During the first 3 months, a normally growing infant gains between 25 and 39 g/day and, during the second 3 months, 15 to 21 g/day. Energy requirements are ordinarily calculated in the range of 115 kcal/kg/day during the first 6 months of life, but some studies of breast-feeding infants suggest good growth often is achieved with a more modest caloric intake. By the end of the first year, the requirement falls to about 105 kcal/kg/day (see Table 24-3). Water, calorie, and major nutrient requirements and those for most vitamins, minerals, and trace elements can be met during at least the first 6 months of life by human milk or by many commercially prepared formulas.

## Feeding Choice

Before the twentieth century, almost all infants were fed human milk. During this century, several factors made alternatives more attractive and acceptable. Industrialization and the emancipation of women decreased their availability for nursing. Technical advances made formulated alternatives to human milk ever more convenient. Breast-feeding fell to an all-time low in the United States around 1970, when fewer than 30% of infants were being fed human milk at 1 week of age. The practice of breast-feeding is enjoying a resurgence in popularity, and more than 50% of U.S. infants are taking human milk for at least some period. However, the return to breast-feeding has not affected all segments of the population equally. Although it is increasingly likely in all groups, the first infant of an older mother with higher education is most likely to be breast-fed. Employment remains a major barrier to the initiation and maintenance of breast-feeding. Mothers who plan to return to work within 2 months of their baby's birth are less likely to choose to breast-feed than are those who plan to stay home from work longer (Kurinij, 1989). Of mothers returning to work, those with professional or part-time positions breast-feed the longest.

Commercial formula is not a viable alternative if the parents' standard of living does not provide ample resources for obtaining, correctly preparing, and storing it. Unfortunately, the uncontrolled introduction of commercial formulas into developing countries has led to decreasing rates of breast-feeding and to increased infant mortality.

For a healthy, term infant and a healthy mother who wishes to breast-feed, there is no doubt that human milk is the best food. Its composition is assumed to most closely approximate the needs of the human infant. It contains nutrients and immunologic properties at least somewhat individualized to the infant's needs. Breast-fed infants are somewhat protected from gastroenteritis, otitis media, early wheezing illnesses, and allergic reactions. Although the mechanism is less apparent, breast-feeding appears to confer to the child small but consistent advantages in measures of mental development (Morley, 1988). Breast-feeding offers convenience: body temperature food stored aseptically and ready at a moment's notice in volumes determined by a feedback process partially controlled by the infant. Many persons believe that the act of breast-feeding offers a unique opportunity for mother–infant bonding that is difficult to replicate with other forms of feeding. However, if breast-feeding is contraindicated or not chosen, commercially prepared formulas offer an acceptable substitute.

Typically, a mother has deeply held beliefs about how her infant should be fed. These beliefs are influenced by other persons in her environment and her own plans for caring for the infant. Pediatricians have little influence on the decision because it is often made even before pregnancy and certainly before the birth of the child. Pediatricians can be influential in supporting the woman's decision to breast-feed by ensuring that newborn nursery policy does not subvert her chances of succeeding and that advice is readily available if problems arise. If a mother has decided to feed her infant formula exclusively, it is counterproductive to make her feel guilty. The mother's feeling of competence to provide adequate nutrition for her infant should be enhanced no matter which alternative she chooses.

# Human Milk Feeding

Human milk feeding as currently practiced in the United States is much more episodic and scheduled and is of shorter duration than is thought to be the "natural" state. Contemporary studies of hunter–gatherer societies reveal that children are breast-feed for about the first 3 years of life and that infants, carried by and sleeping with their mothers, nurse for 0.5 to 5 minutes every 10 to 20 minutes while awake.

## Lactation

Most women who wish to can breast-feed successfully. However, not every woman can. Failure to produce an adequate quantity of milk for the infant's needs most often results from failure to establish a suckling pattern that stimulates sufficient milk production, but primary lactation failure can occur. A few women have insufficient glandular tissue, prolactin deficiency, or some other neurohormonal disruption. If no breast enlargement occurs during pregnancy, there is cause for concern (Neifert and Seacat, 1986). Surgical procedures that interrupt the ducts or sever or damage nipple nerves may prevent successful breast-feeding.

Final breast development, indicated by the rapid growth of ducts and alveoli, is completed only during pregnancy. Relatively little is known about this phase, but animal studies suggest that estrogen and progesterone stimulation are probably necessary and operate in the presence of hormones from the pituitary and the adrenal glands.

Milk synthesis and secretion begins about the fifth month of pregnancy, but copious amounts are produced only after parturition when prolactin secretion by the anterior pituitary is triggered by the precipitous fall in maternal progesterone level after removal of the placenta. Prolactin stimulates milk production by the breast alveolar cells. An abrupt increase in milk production occurs about 3 days after delivery and is referred to as lactogenesis or, more colloquially, as the milk "coming in." By the time of lactogenesis, if breast-feeding is intended, suckling or, if that is not possible for some reason, pumping should be well established and frequent. Removing milk from the breast by suckling or by pumping stimulates prolactin. Suckling causes oxytocin release from the posterior pituitary. Oxytocin acts on mammary myoepithelial cells, which results in milk release or "letdown." Many women experience a tingling sensation in their breasts during letdown.

Lactogenesis occurs whether or not the mother initiates breast-feeding. If the breast is not emptied, maternal prolactin falls, d pressure atrophy of the glandular tissue ensues. The mammary gland rapidly involutes.

The quantity and quality of milk produced vary with time from delivery. Although the content does not change abruptly, the milk produced in the first 5 days is usually referred to as colostrum, in the next 5 days as transitional milk, and after that as mature milk. The volume of milk produced is affected by more than the infant's needs as they are translated through suckling time. In general, older mothers and malnourished mothers produce less than their counterparts; however, volume is in most cases sufficient. Milk secretion is decreased by conditions that decrease blood flow to the mammary gland, such as stress, catecholamine administration, and fasting. After other food is added to the infant's diet, human milk intake and production decrease.

## Human Milk Nutritional Content

Human milk would not meet industrial quality control standards for uniform consistency. There is considerable variation in content in the milk from different mothers and in samples from a given mother obtained at different times. Recognized changes in composition occur with time after birth, defining the stages of lactation described earlier. Changes can occur within a single feeding.

Colostrum, the milk produced during the first few days after birth, is yellowish and translucent, and the amount produced is quite small. The average weight gain when an infant suckles within the hour after birth is 2.2 g, and the average intake in the first 24 hours is about 37 g. By the third day, about 400 g of colostrum are suckled in 24 hours, and then milk production begins to increase dramatically, rising eventually to about 750 g/day.

Colostrum is more viscous than mature milk and richer in protein and many minerals. It contains cellular debris from flushed mammary glands and ducts. Colostrum is relatively rich in nonnutrient factors, such as immunoglobulins, but it is relatively poor in carbohydrate and fat (and therefore energy content) and in many vitamins. The exclusively breast-fed infant receives few calories in the first several days of life. In most cases, glycogen stores allow tolerance of this waiting period, and routine supplementation should be strongly discouraged because of its possible deleterious effect on the infant's suckling which promotes the mother's milk supply. However, if the risk of hypoglycemia is high, the infant should be carefully monitored and judicious use of glucose water after breast-feeding instituted temporarily, if needed.

As the initial days pass, the protein and mineral content of the milk falls, and the amount of fat, lactose, and B vitamins increases. Transitional milk, typical of days 6 through 10, is more milky looking and, except for having higher phosphorus content than either, has a composition that represents a progression between colostrum and mature milk. This progression continues throughout the first month of the infant's life.

Mature milk is a thin, somewhat oily, blue-white liquid higher in fat and lactose content than colostrum and lower in protein, most minerals, and in fat-soluble vitamins and immunologic elements. Mature human milk provides 65 to 75 kcal/100 mL, has a low electrolyte load, and is 85% to 90% water, 0.9% protein, 2.7% to 4.5% fat, and 6% to 7.6% carbohydrate. The source of calories is 50% to 55% fat, 40% to 50% carbohydrate, and 6% to 15% protein. In contrast to cow's milk, the major protein component of human milk is whey ($\alpha$-lactalbumin) with a whey-to-casein ($\beta$-lactoglobulin) ratio of 80:20. Human milk provides more cystine and taurine and less methionine and phenylalanine than does a cow's milk formula. Lactose is the major carbohydrate component, constituting 90% of the carbohydrate content. The fat in human milk is relatively high in oleic acid and low in short-chain fatty acids. Although the total fat content is not affected much by maternal diet, the composition is.

Human milk contains nonnutrient substances. Of these, the most important may be the soluble and cellular immunoprotective elements. Many are most prominent in colostrum, declining in the transition to mature milk. Human milk is rich in immunoglobulins, particularly secretory IgA. Lactoferrin, another soluble element, is an iron-binding protein that competes with bacteria for available iron. Milk contains lysozymes that aid in bacterial lysis; the bifidus factor, a nitrogen-containing polysaccharide that promotes the growth of *Lactobacillus bifidus* and consequently inhibits the growth of pathogens in the gut; an antistaphylococcal factor, a lactoperoxidase that retards bacterial growth; and the antiviral glycoprotein, interferon.

Cells in human milk include polymorphonuclear leukocytes, macrophages, and T and B lymphocytes. Freezing milk inactivates these white cells.

Several active enzymes are found in human milk, including lipase, which assists fat digestion in the infant's stomach. Practically all maternal hormones and several other proteins and peptides have been detected in milk, but their roles are largely unknown.

The milk produced by mothers who deliver their infants before term differs from that of mothers who deliver at term. Preterm milk is higher in protein, fat, sodium, chloride, and vitamins A and E and lower in lactose and vitamin C. By the end of the first month, the milk produced by the mother of a preterm infant is similar to that produced by a term infant's mother, but the immunoglobulin content remains higher.

Milk content varies from the beginning of a feeding to the end. The initial milk, called foremilk, is lower in fat and protein. These increase gradually during the feeding, and the hindmilk is three times richer in fat. Diurnal variations occur with fat, sodium, potassium, and iron, which are all higher at night.

## Vitamin and Mineral Supplementation

A breast-fed infant without sufficient exposure to sunlight may become deficient in vitamin D. A daily dose of 400 IU is recommended by CONAAP to provide optimal calcification of bone and prevention of rickets.

Iron in breast milk, although low in absolute terms, is highly bioavailable. Even so, the stores of the infant fed human milk exclusively are gone after the fourth or fifth month, and dietary sources of iron or iron supplementation should be provided. Dry infant cereal in the amounts ordinarily given probably satisfies about 20% of the daily iron requirement (CONAAP, The use of whole cow's milk in infancy, 1992).

Fluoride at 0.25 mg/day is recommended for infants who are breast-fed and who receive ready-to-feed commercial formula or formula made from concentrate with local water containing less than 0.3 ppm of fluoride to prevent dental caries. CONAAP suggests that supplementation begin shortly after birth, but acknowledges that the evidence that it is necessary before the child is 6 months old is weak. Concerns continue to be raised that fluoride intake excessive in dose or duration can lead to a discoloration of the teeth called fluorosis.

If a breast-feeding mother adheres to a narrow vegetarian diet, her deficiency in B vitamins may be reflected in the milk she produces. The mother should receive appropriate supplements.

## Breast-Feeding Techniques

*Prepartum Preparation.* Useful information is provided by examination of the breasts of a pregnant woman who intends to breast-feed. If she has experienced no increase in breast size during pregnancy, there may be insufficient glandular tissue. Surgical scars raise the question of whether ducts and nerves are intact. If nipples are inverted (ie, they retract toward the chest wall on stimulation), the woman can be advised to wear breast shells and to gently pull and roll the nipples, which may make them more projectile and easier for the infant to grasp. Although nipple preparation has been routinely advised, there are no data to document its effectiveness, and any procedure that may abrade the nipple should be discouraged. Prenatal breast-feeding classes should be encouraged.

*In-Hospital Procedures.* The mother who has just delivered should be allowed to breast-feed her healthy infant as soon as possible in the delivery or recovery room. If this is her first experience, a supportive person should be available to help her with technique. Thereafter, the infant should be put to breast as often as the baby is awake and will suckle. The infant should spend as much time as possible with the mother, with rooming in made the standard. Supplementation should be offered to the infant only if it is specifically indicated and should follow breast-feeding. When supplementation is necessary, the liquid can be delivered to the infant's mouth with a dropper or by small squirts from a needleless syringe so that the infant does not get accustomed to sucking on a bottle nipple. For the same reason, in-hospital use of a pacifier should be discouraged.

The hospital should not provide gift packs that contain formula

to nursing mothers, because these have been shown to reduce the likelihood that the mother will continue to breast-feed, as has supplementation. Because postpartum hospital stays are short, discharge probably precedes lactogenesis. Close follow-up, especially for the first-time breast-feeder, is crucial until feeding is well established. An early home visit by a health provider experienced in helping mothers breast-feed is highly desirable.

*Positioning.* Classic positioning requires that the mother hold her arm on the side of the breast she offers as if it were in a sling. She places the baby on its side on her arm with its head near her elbow and its buttocks supported by her hand. The infant is then facing her breast, and care should be taken to get its arms out of the way. The mother's free hand is used to grasp the breast, thumb above and first two fingers below.

Alternatives to this nursing position include the mother lying on her side facing the infant or sitting with the infant under her arm and supporting its head near her ipsilateral breast with her hand.

*Latching on and Breaking Suction.* Whatever position is chosen, when the infant's mouth is near the breast, the mother should touch the infant's cheek with her nipple. The infant then turns toward the nipple and opens its mouth (ie, rooting reflex). The mother inserts the nipple and areola into the infant's mouth as far as possible. The infant's mouth covers the nipple and areola when properly positioned, and much breast tissue is sucked into the mouth. This allows the infant to massage the milk out of the collecting system. Attachment that is too dainty does not allow efficient recovery of milk by the suckling infant and makes the nipples sore. After the infant has latched on, the mother need no longer hold on to her breast except to depress it away from the infant's nose as necessary.

After the infant latches on to the breast correctly and suckles for a few seconds, the letdown reflex occurs, accompanied often by a tingling sensation in both breasts and often, especially during early attempts, by spurting of milk from both. This letdown reflex may occur with other stimuli as well—a shower, an infant's cry, or sexual stimulation. Breast shields without plastic backs can be worn inside the bra, but they should be changed when wet so that skin breakdown does not occur.

Considerable suction is generated by the suckling infant. When the mother wishes to remove the infant from the breast, she can break that suction by inserting her fifth finger into the infant's mouth beside the nipple.

*Engorgement.* On about the third day, when the milk comes in, the breasts become swollen, firm, and often painful. This is a normal finding accompanying lactogenesis and is "cured" by allowing the baby to empty the breasts. If the firmness of the breast prevents the baby from latching on efficiently, enough milk can be hand expressed or pumped to make the breast more pliable.

## Patterns and Schedules

Suckling time should be limited to a few minutes per breast during the first few days of life to prevent nipple soreness, but most mothers soon become comfortable with a pattern of letting the baby suckle about 10 minutes on one breast, burping the baby, and then allowing it to suckle as long as it cares to on the second. The next feeding is started with the breast used second at the last feeding.

The young infant nurses 10 or more times in 24 hours, initiating feeding every 2 to 3 hours. Because each feed may take a half hour or more, the mother spends considerable time in breast-feeding. If all is going well, the breast-fed infant surpasses birth weight at about 2 weeks and gains at about 1 ounce (28 g) per day thereafter. As the infant ages, it gradually allows more time to elapse between feeds, particularly at night; but frequent feeds are the hallmark of the early weeks and help to stimulate adequate milk production. Demands for frequent feeds recur periodically (often at about 6 weeks and 3 months) as the infant's caloric needs for growth outstrip the milk supply. Such increases in feeding stimulate consonant increases in milk production after 2 or 3 days, and then the feeds space out again. At 4 months or more, when the infant becomes acutely aware of its environment, it typically goes through a period when it is easily distracted from the breast, making it seem uninterested in feeding. At that time, the mother may need to repair to a quiet, darkened room for morning and evening feeds to ensure satisfactory intake.

Breast-fed infants who are adequately nourished urinate eight or more times a day. The urine is colorless. In the early weeks, infants produce a soft, seedy, yellow stool after almost every feeding. Hard, dry stools are not expected in a breast-fed infant with adequate intake; infrequent stools are normal only after 1 or 2 months.

### Problems Specific to Breast Feeding

*Insufficient Lactation.* Risk factors that should alert the physician to the possibility of insufficient lactation are listed in Table 24-7. Most cases of poor weight gain are due to secondary causes of insufficient lactation, usually a poor feeding routine in which the infant is not being suckled often enough or efficiently enough to stimulate milk production. The infant's suckling ability may be impaired, or its temperament may be so placid it does not demand feeds.

Although the goal is to preserve breast-feeding whenever possible, restoration is the first priority if the infant's nutritional status is impaired. Formula supplements should be offered after each breast-feeding until the child's nutritional status is satisfactory. A well-fed, vigorous infant is more likely to be able to continue breast-feeding and the stress is lessened. If the baby is failing to latch on properly, a lactation-aiding device that presents pumped breast milk or formula at the mother's nipple helps to nourish the infant while training for breast-feeding continues. If the infant is not emptying the mother's breasts, an electric pump should be used so that milk production can be sustained.

*Sore Nipples.* If nipples are cracked and sore, the pain impairs the letdown reflex and makes feeding difficult. To avert nipple problems, mothers should keep them as dry as possible, avoid soaps, and vary the feeding position. If a sore nipple is interfering with feeding, the mother may be advised temporarily to initiate feeding on the breast that is least sore, because the infant sucks hardest initially. As a last resort, a nipple shield may be used briefly for a few feedings. After letdown has occurred, the pain decreases, and latching to the breast can be attempted.

*Maternal Mastitis.* Plugging of a mammary duct leads to milk stasis and sometimes to infection. Mastitis is accompanied by pain; local changes of redness, fullness, and tenderness; and systemic signs. Mastitis does not usually preclude breast-feeding, but it should be treated with antibiotic therapy and pain relievers that do not put the infant at risk. Continued breast-feeding helps to relieve the pressure.

*Breast Milk Jaundice.* Postnatal bilirubin levels rise more on average in breast-fed infants than in infants fed formula, and 1 or 2 in 100 breast-feeding infants suffer an exaggeration of physiologic jaundice produced by substances in breast milk that impair bilirubin degradation. If icterus in a breast-fed infant is prolonged without another explanation and the bilirubin level demands therapeutic intervention, breast-feeding can be temporarily suspended and the infant fed formula. The mother should pump her breasts to maintain lactation but discard the milk. The bilirubin level should fall. After it does and breast-feeding is reinstituted (usually after about 24 hours), the bilirubin may increase slightly again but should then stabilize and decrease.

*Maternal Diet.* The breast-feeding mother should eat a good, balanced diet. Milk production requires about 800 calories per 1 L, and an average of 700 mL are produced per day, requiring a modest increase in caloric intake. About one third of prenatal weight gain appears to be storage for lactation. No attempt to decrease maternal weight should be made at least until breast-feeding is well established.

Although intake of alcohol and caffeine should be modest at best, no other dietary exclusions need to be recommended from

| TABLE 24-7.    Risk Factors for Lactation Failure | |
|---|---|
| Inadequate Lactation | Inadequate Milk Intake |
| History of breast surgery with postoperative altered nipple sensation | Inability to latch onto maternal nipple well (may occur with routine use of a nipple shield) |
| Previously unsuccessful or close relative unsuccessful with breast feeding | Irregular or nonsustained sucking at breast |
| Marked asymmetry or abnormal appearance of breasts or nipples | Yellow urine in small amounts or failure to have a wet diaper with each feeding |
| Minimal or no breast enlargement with pregnancy | Fewer than five large, seedy, yellow stools each day in the first month |
| Minimal or no evidence of milk coming in or postpartum engorgement | Failure to demand to nurse at least eight times each day |
| Failure to initiate nursing or breast pumping during postpartum engorgement | Taking only one breast at each feeding |
| Nursing fewer than eight times each day in the first postpartum weeks | Minimal audible swallowing and gulping of milk while nursing |
| Breast not full before feedings or after 4-hour interval without nursing | Nursing fewer than 10 minutes per breast at each feeding |
| No sensations of letdown or leaking of milk from the contralateral breast during feedings | Crying, fussing, and appearing hungry after most feedings |
| Return of menses within the first 3 months postpartum | Gaining less than 1 oz/day |

*Neifert MR, Seacat JM. A guide to successful breast-feeding. Contemp Pediatr 1986;3:32.*

the start. Nursing mothers occasionally report a pattern that appears to be infant intolerance, most often expressed as vomiting or colic, of a certain food in the mother's diet. Cow's milk is most commonly implicated. It is reasonable to avoid that food for a few days and then retry it. If similar symptoms follow, the food may be omitted from the diet during lactation. If the mother reports many exclusions, the situation should be carefully assessed, because the need for restrictions is unusual.

*Substituting For and Storing Human Milk.* Many mothers return to work before weaning their infant and hope to continue to breast-feed. If the workplace is supportive and provides time and equipment for pumping, exclusive human milk feeding can be continued with the mother pumping her breasts for milk for the next day's feedings. For many reasons, including the decline in milk production that often accompanies interrupted feeding schedules, many mothers insert occasional or regular formula feeds into the schedule. Direct breast-feeding is often maintained before and after work, with additional feeds on days off to stimulate the milk supply. If formula or bottles of human milk are to be offered, it is best to introduce the artificial nipple after lactation is well established, usually at about 6 weeks.

Human milk can be safely stored in the refrigerator for 24 hours. It can be stored frozen in the refrigerator freezer for 30 days and in a deep-freeze for 6 months. The packages should be dated. It is best to freeze milk in small quantities, because it should be used immediately after thawing, which is accomplished by holding the bag under running water; it cannot be refrozen. Milk pumped during the work day can be stored in a disposable nurser bag kept on ice in a thermos.

*Weaning.* Between 4 and 6 months, most breast-fed infants outgrow their reliance on exclusive breast-feeding because of increasing caloric needs and because of the development of oral-motor mechanisms that allow drinking and eating. Liquids can be offered from a nursing (lidded) cup when the infant is sitting. Breast-feeding can be continued as long as desired. Offering foods in addition to human milk is not "unnatural." In hunter–gatherer societies, for example, premasticated foods are given to the infant at a early age.

When a mother is willing to continue breast-feeding as long as the child wants, a gradual weaning process takes place. The child takes a decreasing proportion of its calories from human milk, maintains suckling apparently for its comfort value for some time, and eventually loses interest in breast-feeding altogether. Weaning is accomplished in a way that is developmentally acceptable for the mother and the child.

*Toxicology.* Most medications ingested by or administered to the mother can be detected in breast milk. A nursing mother should avoid over-the-counter preparations and remind a prescribing physician that she is breast-feeding. Compendia of findings for drugs in human milk should be consulted if maternal medication is indicated. A partial listing is presented in Table 24-8. Recent publications should always be consulted if there is doubt.

Environmental pollutants appear in human milk, but so little is known about their impact in most cases that practical guidelines are not yet possible. A toxicologist should be consulted about individual concerns.

### Contraindications to Breast Feeding

There are relatively few circumstances for which a mother should be advised not to breast-feed although she wishes to do so. Infants with galactosemia may not be breast-fed, because galactose is contraindicated no matter what the source. Some other hereditary metabolic disorders require special formulas.

Some maternal medications may be dangerous for the infant and prohibit breast-feeding temporarily or permanently. In this category are some antibiotics, radiopharmaceuticals, anticancer drugs, some antithyroid drugs, and some anti-inflammatories. The safety of each drug for the infant should be checked. For some maternal conditions (eg, breast cancer, severe maternal malnutrition, systemic disease), the mother's health may be maximized by feeding the infant formula that provides an acceptable alternative to human milk.

Some maternal infections can be passed to the infant through breast milk or by the close contact breast-feeding requires. Breast-feeding should probably be temporarily suspended if the mother has group B streptococcal disease, herpes simplex or syphilitic lesions involving the breast, chickenpox, pertussis, or non-B hepatitis and while cultures remain positive if the mother is being treated for active tuberculosis. Some view maternal cytomegalovirus infection as a contraindication, because the virus has been cultured from human milk. Maternal hepatitis B and human immunodeficiency virus (HIV) infections are considered contraindications by many in developed countries where commercial formulas are readily available and easily used, because there is a risk (as yet unquantified in the case of HIV) of transmitting the virus through human milk.

## Formula Feeding

Commercially prepared formulas are available for healthy term infants and for some infants with special needs. They are designed to satisfy the needs of the infant as nearly as current research can define them and to resemble human milk as closely as possible with current technology and nutrient sources. The content of most are presented in Tables 24-9 through 24-12. The composition of whole cow's milk and its tendency to cause gastrointestinal bleeding make it unsuitable for infant feeding. Feedings that contain adequate energy and macronutrients and are somewhat less expensive than formula can be prepared from evaporated milk, but vitamin and mineral supplementation is necessary, and errors in mixing are possible. At least two recipes have been used. Mix a 13-ounce can of evaporated milk with 17 ounces of water and add 2 tablespoons of corn syrup, or mix a 13-ounce can of evaporated milk with one and one-half cans of water and 2 tablespoons of sugar. In general, for families with limited resources who choose not to breast-feed, access to commercial formula should be obtained.

Formula preparation is carefully regulated and monitored. Portions of the *Code of Federal Regulations* specifying procedures for the production of food for human consumption apply. The Food and Drug Administration regulates formula manufacture, and its legislative authority to do so was confirmed and expanded by the Infant Formula Act of 1980, PL 96-359. Nutrient composition specifications under the law are based largely on the recommendations of CONAAP. The formula manufacturers have developed voluntary guidelines. Freedom from microbial contamination is virtually assured, and expiration dates are clearly marked.

### Guidelines for Formula Composition

CONAAP (1985) has suggested to the Food and Drug Administration composition standards called "recommended ranges of nutrients" for formulas to be fed to healthy term infants from birth to 1 year of age. Guidelines for major nutrients include the following:

1. Caloric density should be 0.67 kcal/mL or 20 kcal/oz unless otherwise labeled.
2. Osmolality should be about 300 mOsm/L or at least less than 400 mOsm/L.

## TABLE 24-8.   Drugs and Human Milk

**Contraindicated for the Breast-Feeding Mother**

Amethopterin, bromocriptine, cimetidine,* clemastines, cyclophosphamide, ergotamine, gold salts, methimzaole, phenindione, thiouracil

**Cease Breast Feeding Until Drug is Excreted**

Radiopharmaceuticals: gallium 69 (2 wk), iodine 125 (12 d), iodine-131 (2–14 d), radioactive sodium (96 h), technetium 99m (15–72 h)

Chloramphenicol,† clindamycin,† clonidine,† zomepirac†

**Usually Compatible, but Adverse Effects Reported or Possible**

*Anesthetics, Sedatives*

   Alcohol, bromide, chloral hydrate, methyprylon, diazepam and flurazepam as single doses (avoid chronic use)

*Antiepileptics (avoid chronic use, if possible)*

   Carbamazepine, ethosuximide, phenobarbital, phenytoin, primidone, thiopental, valproic acid

*Antihistamines, Decongestants*

   Chlorpheniramine, cyproheptadine, dexbrompheniramine maleate with D-isoephedrine, diphenhydramine, brompheniramine, ephedrine, pseudoephedrine

*Antihypertensives, Cardiovascular Drugs*

   Quinidine, reserpine

*Anti-infective Drugs*

   Amantadine, ethambutol,† isoniazid,† methenamine, sulfas (avoid in immediate newborn period)

*Antithyroid Drugs*

   Carbimazole, methimazole, propylthiouracil

*Bronchodilators*

   Albuterol, isoproterenol, metaproterenol, terbutaline, prednisone in short-term use, theophylline

*Diuretics (may supress lactation)*

   Bendoflumethiazide, chlorothiazide, chlorthalidone, furosemide, hydrochlorothiazide, methyclothiazide, spironolactone

*Hormones*

   Estrogen/progesterone contraceptives

*Muscle Relaxants*

   Carisoprodol

*Pain Relievers*

   Indomethacin, salicylates†

*Psychotropic Agents*

   Antianxiety drugs: chlordiazepoxide, clorazepate, diazepam,* hydroxyzine, meprobamate,* oxazepam, prazepam*

   Antidepressants: lithium*

**Breast Feeding Need Not Be Interrupted**

*Anesthetics, Sedatives*

   Barbiturate, chloroform, diphenhydramine, halothane, hydroxyzine, magnesium sulfate, secobarbitol

*Anticoagulants*

   Bishydroxycoumarin, Coumadin, heparin

*Antihistamines, Decongestants, and Bronchodilators*

   Diphenhydramine, diphylline,* trimeprazine, tripelennamine

*Antihypertensives, Cardiovascular Drugs*

   Atenolol, captopril, digoxin, disopyramide, guanethidine, hydralazine, methyldopa, metoprolol,* nadolol,* propranolol

*Anti-infective Drugs*

   Cefadroxil, cefazolin, cefotaxmine, cefoxitin, cephalexin, cephalothin, chloroquine, dicloxacillin, erythromycin, gentamicin, nafcillin, nalidixic acid, nitrofurantoin, oxacillin, penicillin, tetracycline,† trimethoprim, vancomycin

*Muscle Relaxants*

   Baclofen, methocarbamol

*Pain Relievers*

   Acetaminophen, butorphanol, codeine, flufenamic acid, heroin, ibuprofen, mefenamid acid, meperidine, methadone, morphine, Naprosyn, oxycodone, phenylbutazone, prednisone, propoxyphene

*Psychotropic Agents*

   Antidepressants: amitriptyline, amoxapine, desipramine, dothiepin, imipramine, nortriptyline, tranylcypromine

   Antipsychotic drugs: chlorpromazine, haloperidol, mesoridazine, piperacetazine, prochlorperazine, thioridazine, trifluoperazine

* Accumulates in breast milk.
† Some consider these drugs contraindicated; others do not. Refer to original sources.

Information abstracted from Committee on Drugs, American Academy of Pediatrics. The transfer of drugs and other chemicals into human breast milk. Pediatrics 1983;72:375. Marx CM. Drugs excreted in breast milk. Nutrition and Feeding of Infants and Toddlers, Appendix 7. Boston: Little, Brown, 1984:433. See sources for reported side effects and monitoring suggestsions.

3. Protein should be at least 1.8 g/100 kcal, assuming a PER of 100%. Protein should not exceed 4.5 g/100 kcal.
4. Fat should supply at least 30% of calories or about 3.3 g/100 kcal with 2.7% of total kilocalories as essential fatty acid. No more than 6 g of fat/100 kcal or 57% of kilocalories as fat is recommended (Kelts and Jones, 1984).

Most formula-fed infants receive one of a limited number of modified cow's milk formulas intended for healthy term infants. Although parents may develop a strong brand-name preference, the formulas are basically interchangeable. The physician should be certain that the "with iron" alternative is chosen (CONAAP, Iron-fortified infant formulas, 1989). Controlled trials consistently show that formulas containing an adequate amount of iron do not cause gastrointestinal symptoms. Parents and physicians who continue to believe that they do and switch to a low-iron formula in an attempt to treat symptoms put infants at risk. Iron deficiency may cause irreversible developmental damage. For infants with cow's milk intolerance, there are several modified protein and lactose-free alternatives. Carnitine is now being added to some of these formulas after reports that it was lacking. Sucrose-free, corn-free, phenylalanine-free, protein-modified, and fat-modified formulas are commercially available for infants with special needs.

Infants fed one of the cow's milk or soy-based formulas fortified with iron and intended for healthy term infants need no routine vitamin, mineral, or water supplementation. Fluoride

TABLE 24-9.  Source of Macronutrients in Infant Formulas

| Formula | Manufacturer | Protein Source(s) | Fat Source(s) | Carbohydrate Source(s) |
|---|---|---|---|---|
| Alimentum | Ross | Casein hydrolysate | Fractionated coconut oil (median chain triglycerides), safflower oil, soy oil | Sucrose, modified tapioca starch |
| Carnation Follow-Up Formula | Carnation | Nonfat milk | Palm olein, soy, coconut, high oleic (safflower) oils | Corn syrup |
| Enfamil Infant Formula | Mead Johnson | Reduced-minerals whey, nonfat milk | Palm olein, soy, coconut, and high oleic sunflower oils | Lactose |
| Enfamil Premature Formula | Mead Johnson | Nonfat milk, whey protein concentrate | Medium-chain triglycerides (fractionated coconut oil), soy oil, coconut oil, mono- and diglycerides | Corn syrup solids, lactose |
| Gerber Baby Formula | Bristol-Myers Squibb | Nonfat milk | Palm olein, soy, coconut, and high oleic sunflower oils | Lactose |
| Gerber Soy Formula | Bristol-Myers Squibb | Soy protein isolate | Palm olein, soy, coconut and high oleic sunflower oils | Corn syrup, sucrose |
| Good Start | Carnation | Enzymatically hydrolyzed reduced minerals whey | Palm olein, soy, coconut, and high oleic safflower oils | Lactose and maltodextrin |
| Human milk, mature | | Whey (80%) and casein | Monounsaturated fat, saturated fat, and polyunsaturated fat | Lactose |
| Isomil | Ross | Soy protein isolate | Soy oil, coconut oil | Corn syrup, sucrose |
| Isomil SF | Ross | Soy protein isolate | Soy oil, coconut oil | Hydrolyzed cornstarch |
| I-Soyalac | Nutricia | Soy isolate | Soy oil | Sucrose, tapioca dextrin (liquid); potato malto-dextrin, sucrose (powder) |
| Nursoy | Wyeth-Ayerst | Soy protein isolate | Oleo, coconut, oleic (safflower or sunflower), and soybean oils | Sucrose (liquid), corn syrup solids (powder) |
| Nutramigen | Mead Johnson | Hydrolyzed casein | Corn and soy oils | Corn syrup solids and modified corn starch |
| Pregestimil | Mead Johnson | Hydrolyzed casein | Medium-chain triglycerides (fractionated coconut oils), corn oil, soy oil, high oleic safflower oil | Corn syrup solids, modified corn starch, dextrose |
| Portagen | Mead Johnson | Sodium caseinate | Medium-chain triglycerides (fractionated coconut oil), corn oil, lecithin | Corn syrup solids, sucrose |
| Preemie SMA | Wyeth-Ayerst | Demineralized whey, nonfat milk | Coconut, oleic, oleo, soybean and medium-chain triglyceride oils | Lactose and glucose polymers |
| ProSobee | Mead Johnson | Soy protein isolate | Coconut, soy, palm olein and high oleic sunflower oils | Corn syrup solids |
| Similac | Ross | Nonfat milk | Soy and coconut oils | Lactose |
| Similac Natural Care | Ross | Nonfat milk, whey | Medium chain triglycerides, soy and coconut oils | Hydrolyzed cornstarch and lactose |
| Similac PM 60/40 | Ross | Whey and casein | Corn and coconut oils (powder); soy and coconut oils (liquid) | Lactose |
| Similac Special Care | Ross | Whey and casein | Medium-chain triglycerides, soy and coconut oils | Hydrolyzed cornstarch and lactose |
| SMA | Wyeth-Ayerst | Reduced-minerals whey, nonfat milk | Oleo, coconut, oleic (safflower or sunflower) and soybean oils | Lactose |
| Soyalac | Nutricia | Soy bean | Soy oil | Sucrose, corn syrup, soy bean |

supplements should be provided to prevent dental caries if ready-to-feed formula is being used exclusively or if concentrate is being mixed with water containing less than 0.3 ppm well into infancy.

### Techniques

*Formula Preparation.*   Formulas come in three forms: powder to be mixed with water, liquid concentrate to be diluted in one-to-one volumes with water, and ready-to-feed liquids. The latter is the most expensive; the powder is generally least expensive, but it is hardest to prepare. The powder may be stored without refrigeration, but after it is mixed with water, the formula must be refrigerated. Liquid concentrate and ready-to-feed formulas must be refrigerated after opening.

Care must be taken not to introduce dirt and large numbers of bacteria during preparation, but strict sterilization procedures are no longer thought necessary if the water supply is known to

TABLE 24-10. Macronutrient Composition of Infant Formulas

| Formula | Manufacturer | Energy (kcal/oz)* | Composition Per 100 kcal | | | | | | |
|---|---|---|---|---|---|---|---|---|---|
| | | | Protein (g) | Fat (g) | Carbohydrates (g) | Water (g) | Linoleic Acid (mg) | Renal Solute Load (mOsm/L) | Osmolarity (mOsm/L) |
| Alimentum | Ross | 20 | 2.75 | 5.54 | 10.2 | 133 | 1600 | 123.2 | 330 |
| Carnation Follow-up | Carnation | 20 | 2.6 | 4.1 | 13.2 | 128 | 680 | 172 | 280 |
| Enfamil | Mead Johnson | 20 | 2.2 | 5.6 | 10.3 | 134 | 910 | 134 | 270 |
| Enfamil Premature 20/24† | Mead Johnson | 20/24 | 3 | 5.1 | 11.1 | 133/108 | 1060 | 176/210 | 230/270 |
| Gerber Baby Formula | Bristol-Myers Squibb | 20 | 2.2 | 5.4 | 10.7 | 134 | 880 | 138 | 290 |
| Gerber Soy Formula | Bristol-Myers Squibb | 20 | 3.0 | 5.3 | 10.0 | 134 | 860 | 181 | 210 |
| Good Start | Carnation | 20 | 2.4 | 5.1 | 11 | 134 | 850 | 135† | 241 |
| Human milk | | 21.9 | 1.5 | 5.4 | 10 | | 540 | 79 | 300 |
| Isomil | Ross | 20 | 2.45 | 5.46 | 10.3 | 133 | 1300 | 110 | 220 |
| Isomil SF | Ross | 20 | 2.66 | 5.46 | 10.1 | 133 | 1300 | 116 | 160 |
| I-Soyalac | Nutricia | 20 | 3.1 | 5.5 | 10.0 | 133 | 2810 | 132 | 246 |
| Nursoy | Wyeth-Ayerst | 20 | 2.7 | 5.3 | 10.2 | 134 | 500 | 109 | 266 |
| Nutramigen | Mead Johnson | 20 | 2.8 | 3.9 | 13.4 | 134 | 2000 | 172 | 290 |
| Pregestimil | Mead Johnson | 20 | 2.8 | 5.6 | 10.3 | 134 | 940 | 169 | 290 |
| Portagen | Mead Johnson | 20 | 3.5 | 4.8 | 11.5 | 134 | 350 | 200 | 210 |
| Preemie SMA 20/24† | Wyeth-Ayerst | 20/24 | 3.0/2.4 | 5.2/5.4 | 10.4/10.5 | 133/108 | 485/500 | 128 | 242/246 |
| ProSobee | Mead Johnson | 20 | 3 | 5.3 | 10 | 134 | 860 | 178 | 182 |
| Similac | Ross | 20 | 2.14 | 5.40 | 10.7 | 133 | 1300 | 96 | 270 |
| Similac Natural Care | Ross | 24 | 2.71 | 5.43 | 10.5 | 109 | 700 | 149 | 250 |
| Similac PM 60/40§ | Ross | 20 | 2.22 | 5.59 | 10.2 | 134 | 1300 | 93 | 250 |
| Similac Special Care 20/24† | Ross | 20/24 | 2.71 | 5.43 | 10.6 | 133/109 | 700 | 124/149 | 210/250 |
| SMA 20/24† | Wyeth-Ayerst | 20/24 | 2.2 | 5.3 | 10.6 | 134/109 | 500 | 91/110 | 271/322 |
| Soyalac | Nutricia | 20 | 3.1 | 5.5 | 10.0 | 133 | 2810 | 130 | 215 |

* For Ready-To-Feed product or when concentrated liquid or powder product is mixed according to preparation instructions for standard dilution.
† Calculation from Ziegler EE, Fomon SJ. Potential renal solute load of infant formulas. J Nutr 1989;119:1785.
‡ Available in two preparations (20 kcal/oz and 24 kcal/oz). Concentrations of some nutrients vary correspondingly.
§ Information given is for the powder consumer product. The Ready-to-Feed hospital product has 2.34 g protein and 5.56 g fat per 100 kcal and a renal solute load of 96 mOsm/L.

be safe. Although some continue to recommend sterilization of bottles for very young infants or under certain circumstances, it is unlikely that a parent will comply for many months with such a tedious procedure, particularly after the infant is obviously mouthing every object in reach. If sterilization is not used, it is best to prepare one bottle at a time immediately before feeding. Prepared formula should not be stored for more than 24 hours. No matter how a bottle is prepared, the formula remaining in the bottle after a feeding should be discarded to avoid bacterial contamination.

If sterilization is recommended, it can be accomplished by aseptic preparation or by terminal sterilization. Aseptic preparation involves boiling the washed bottles, nipples, and utensils used in preparation and, separately, the water to be used for dilution for 5 minutes and then filling the sterile bottles with the sterile formula, inverting the nipples into the bottle, capping them, and refrigerating. The second method involves mixing the formula with a clean technique, filling clean bottles, inserting nipples, capping the bottles, and boiling the filled bottles for 25 minutes, sterilizing formula and bottles together. These prepared bottles must be kept in the refrigerator.

*Feeding.* The infant should be held during feedings. Propping the bottle is dangerous during early infancy because the

baby may choke on the milk. Moreover, the social aspects of feeding are as important as the nutrients. As the infant ages, the milk from a propped bottle may pool around the teeth as he or she falls asleep and cause caries, or it may be sucked into the middle ear, predisposing to otitis media.

Several bottle and nipple styles are available. Most infants nurse adequately from any of them, but if feedings are not going well, experimenting with other nipples may provide a remedy. Infants tend to swallow air and to tire with feeds if the nipple hole is too small and to choke or to consume the feeding before sucking needs are met if it is too large. If the bottle is held upside down, the milk should come out in frequent drips, not a stream. While the infant is being fed, the bottle should be held so that formula fills the nipple.

*Warming.* Contrary to popular belief, formula does not need to be warmed before a feeding but can be used straight from the refrigerator. Warming may cause burns. Microwave ovens, for instance, do not warm liquids evenly, and hot spots may burn the infant's mouth. If warming is deemed desirable, the bottle may be put briefly in tepid, not hot, water.

*Burping.* The infant should be burped after every few ounces while held in a sitting position on the feeder's lap or with ab-

## TABLE 24-11.  Mineral Content of Infant Formulas

| Formula | Manufacturer | Composition Per 100 kcal | | | | | | | | | | |
|---|---|---|---|---|---|---|---|---|---|---|---|---|
| | | Ca (mg) | P (mg) | Mg (mg) | Fe (mg) | Zn (mg) | Mn (µg) | Cu (µg) | I (µg) | Na (mg) | K (mg) | Cl (mg) |
| Alimentum | Ross | 105 | 75 | 7.5 | 1.8 | 0.75 | 30 | 75 | 15 | 44 | 118 | 80 |
| Carnation Follow-up | Carnation | 135 | 90 | 8.4 | 1.9 | 0.63 | 7 | 76 | 5.7 | 39 | 135 | 90 |
| Enfamil* | Mead Johnson | 69 | 47 | 7.8 | 0.5/1.88 | 0.78 | 15.6 | 94 | 6 | 27 | 108 | 63 |
| Enfamil Premature* | Mead Johnson | 165 | 83 | 6.8 | 0.25/1.8 | 1.5 | 6.3 | 125 | 25 | 39 | 103 | 85 |
| Gerber Baby Formula* | Bristol-Myers Squibb | 75 | 58 | 6 | 0.5/1.88 | 0.75 | 5 | 90 | 8 | 33 | 108 | 70 |
| Gerber Soy Formula | Bristol-Myers Squibb | 94 | 74 | 7.5 | 1.8 | 0.75 | 30 | 75 | 15 | 47 | 115 | 88 |
| Good Start | Carnation | 64 | 36 | 6.7 | 1.5 | 0.75 | 7 | 80 | 8 | 24 | 98 | 59 |
| Human milk | | 39 | 19 | 4.9 | 0.04 | 0.17 | 0.08 | 35 | 15.3 | 25 | 73 | 58 |
| Isomil | Ross | 105 | 75 | 7.5 | 1.8 | 0.75 | 30 | 75 | 15 | 44 | 108 | 62 |
| Isomil SF | Ross | 105 | 75 | 7.5 | 1.8 | 0.75 | 30 | 75 | 15 | 44 | 108 | 62 |
| I-Soyalac | Nutricia | 102 | 63 | 11 | 1.9 | 0.78 | 30 | 117 | 7.8 | 42 | 117 | 78 |
| Nursoy | Wyeth-Ayerst | 90 | 63 | 10 | 1.8 | 0.8 | 30 | 70 | 9 | 30 | 105 | 56 |
| Nutramigen | Mead Johnson | 94 | 63 | 10.9 | 1.88 | 0.78 | 31 | 94 | 7 | 47 | 109 | 86 |
| Pregestimil | Mead Johnson | 94 | 63 | 10.9 | 1.88 | 0.94 | 31 | 94 | 7 | 39 | 109 | 86 |
| Portagen | Mead Johnson | 94 | 70 | 20 | 1.88 | 0.94 | 125 | 156 | 7 | 55 | 125 | 86 |
| Preemie SMA 20/24† | Wyeth-Ayerst | 110/90 | 55/50 | 10.5/8.6 | 0.45/0.38 | 1.2/1.0 | 30/25 | 105/86 | 12/10 | 47/40 | 110/90 | 80/66 |
| Pro SoBee | Mead Johnson | 94 | 74 | 10.9 | 1.88 | 0.78 | 25 | 94 | 10.2 | 36 | 122 | 83 |
| Similac* | Ross | 73 | 56 | 6 | 0.22/1.8 | 0.75 | 5 | 90 | 9 | 27 | 105 | 64 |
| Similac Natural Care | Ross | 210 | 105 | 12 | 0.37 | 1.5 | 12 | 250 | 6 | 43 | 129 | 81 |
| Similac PM 60/40 | Ross | 56 | 28 | 6 | 0.22 | 0.75 | 5 | 90 | 6 | 24 | 86 | 59 |
| Similac Special Care* | Ross | 180 | 90 | 12 | 0.37/1.8 | 1.5 | 12 | 250 | 6 | 43 | 129 | 81 |
| SMA* | Wyeth-Ayerst | 63 | 42 | 7 | 0.2/1.8 | 0.8 | 15 | 70 | 9 | 22 | 83 | 55.5 |
| Soyalac | Nutricia | 94 | 55 | 12 | 1.9 | 0.78 | 90 | 78 | 7.8 | 42 | 117 | 65 |

* Comes in both low iron and iron-supplemented formulations.
† Content of 20 kcal per oz preparation/content of 24 kcal per oz preparation.

domen against the feeder's chest and shoulder. The position should be one that allows air to escape up the esophagus. Burping is encouraged by rubbing or gently patting the infant's back.

### Patterns and Schedules

Although appropriate growth rate is the most salient marker of appropriate intake, ounces become the preoccupation in formula-fed infants. The stomach capacity at birth is between 1 and 3 ounces, increasing to 3 to 5 ounces at 1 month, and in the first few weeks, most infants do not consume a whole 4-ounce bottle. As the infant ages, fewer but larger feedings are demanded. Feedings usually take 15 to 20 minutes. Table 24-13 describes the usual ranges for number and volume of formula feedings by age. The rule of thumb is that an exclusively formula-fed infant needs 100 to 120 kcal/kg/day, which is provided by 150 to 180 mL of formula/kg/day.

### Problems Specific to Bottle Feeding

*Sensitivity.*  Some infants do not tolerate cow's milk protein. Prevalence figures for this problem vary with diagnostic criteria up to about 8% of infants. Symptoms attributed to cow's milk sensitivity include diarrhea, vomiting, abdominal pain, failure to thrive, asthma, eczema, and shock. A formula change is indicated if intolerance is suspected. About 30% of infants intolerant of cow's milk formula are also sensitive to soy protein formula. A casein hydrolysate formula or a meat-based formula can be tried. However, formulas are changed far more frequently than medically indicated; many changes are probably in response to frustration over infantile colic. Evidence has not supported a simple dietary basis for most cases of colic, but perhaps 10% or 15% do

improve on a "hypoallergenic" formula based on casein or whey hydrolysate.

*Improper Dilution.*  Many failures to gain weight at the expected rate and some electrolyte imbalances in young infants can be traced to misunderstandings about formula preparation. The problem may be too much or too little water added to the formula. Parents may dilute formula, because they cannot afford an adequate supply.

*Regurgitation.*  Although breast-fed infants spit up, bottle-fed infants seem especially prone to this, probably because they swallow more air when they feed. Some infants tolerate regurgitation well. When regurgitation is threatening appropriate caloric intake or blocking the airway and cannot be reversed by changes in feeding technique or volume, it is labeled reflux (see Chapter 20.4).

*Constipation.*  It is unusual for an infant who is being fed adequate amounts of formula and nothing else to become constipated because of dry, hard stools. If an infant who initially passed soft stools begins to pass dry, hard stools, a careful dietary history is in order. If diet corrections are not necessary and the child otherwise appears normal, 5 to 15 mL of infant prune juice or a small amount of sugar may be added to each bottle for a few days. Corn syrup was the recommended additive until questions were raised about it as a potential source of botulinum spores.

*Weaning.*  At about 5 months of age, an infant is capable of putting lips on the rim of a cup, and sometime in the last half of

TABLE 24-12.   Vitamin Content of Infant Formulas

| Formula | Manufacturer | Composition Per 100 kcal | | | | | | | | | | | | | | |
| --- | --- | --- | --- | --- | --- | --- | --- | --- | --- | --- | --- | --- | --- | --- | --- | --- |
| | | A (IU) | D (IU) | E (IU) | K (µg) | $B_1$ (µg) | $B_2$ (µg) | $B_6$ (µg) | $B_{12}$ (µg) | Niacin (µg) | Foliate (µg) | Pantothenic Acid (µg) | Biotin (µg) | C (mg) | Choline (mg) | Inositol (mg) |
| Alimentum | Ross | 300 | 45 | 3.0 | 15 | 50–60 | 90 | 60 | 0.45 | 1350 | 15 | 750 | 4.5 | 9 | 8 | 5 |
| Carnation Follow-up | Carnation | 250 | 65 | 2 | 8.1 | 80 | 96 | 66 | 0.32 | 1280 | 16 | 480 | 2 | 8 | 12 | 18 |
| Enfamil | Mead Johnson | 310 | 63 | 2 | 8 | 78 | 150 | 63 | 0.23 | 1250 | 15.6 | 470 | 2.3 | 8.1 | 15.6 | 4.7 |
| Enfamil Premature | Mead Johnson | 1250 | 270 | 6.3 | 8 | 200 | 300 | 150 | 0.25 | 4000 | 35 | 1200 | 4 | 20 | 12 | 17 |
| Gerber Baby Formula | Bristol-Myers Squibb | 300 | 60 | 2 | 8 | 100 | 150 | 60 | 0.25 | 1050 | 15 | 450 | 4.4 | 9 | 16 | 4.7 |
| Gerber Soy Formula* | Bristol-Myers Squibb | 300 | 60 | 3 | 15 | 60 | 90 | 60 | 0.45 | 1350 | 15 | 750 | 4.5 | 9 | 8 | 5.0 |
| Good Start | Carnation | 300 | 60 | 2.0 | 8.2 | 60 | 135 | 75 | 0.22 | 750 | 9 | 450 | 2.2 | 8 | 12 | 18 |
| Human milk | | 310 | 3.05 | 0.32 | 0.29 | 29 | 49 | 28.5 | 0.07 | 208 | 7 | 250 | 0.6 | 6 | 12.5 | 14.9 |
| Isomil | Ross | 300 | 60 | 3.0 | 15 | 60 | 90 | 60 | 0.45 | 1350 | 15 | 750 | 4.5 | 9 | 8 | 5 |
| Isomil SF | Ross | 300 | 60 | 3.0 | 15 | 60 | 90 | 60 | 0.45 | 1350 | 15 | 750 | 4.5 | 9 | 8 | 5 |
| I-Soyalac | Nutricia | 312 | 63 | 2.3 | 7.8 | 94 | 94 | 86 | 0.31 | 1250 | 15.6 | 469 | 7.8 | 12 | 12 | 10 |
| Nursoy | Wyeth-Ayerst | 300 | 60 | 1.4 | 15 | 100 | 150 | 62.5 | 0.3 | 750 | 7.5 | 450 | 5.5 | 8.3 | 13 | 4.1 |
| Nutramigen | Mead Johnson | 310 | 63 | 3.1 | 15.6 | 78 | 94 | 63 | 0.31 | 1250 | 15.6 | 470 | 7.8 | 8.1 | 13.3 | 4.7 |
| Pregestimil | Mead Johnson | 380 | 75 | 3.8 | 18.8 | 78 | 94 | 63 | 0.31 | 1250 | 15.6 | 470 | 7.8 | 11.7 | 13.3 | 4.7 |
| Portagen | Mead Johnson | 780 | 78 | 3.1 | 15.6 | 156 | 188 | 210 | 0.63 | 2100 | 15.6 | 1050 | 7.8 | 8.1 | 13.3 | 4.7 |
| Preemie SMA 20/24 | Wyeth-Ayerst | 475/300 | 75/60 | 2.2/1.9 | 10.5/8.6 | 120/100 | 190/160 | 75/60 | 0.3 | 980/750 | 15/12.5 | 530/450 | 2.5 | 10.5/8.6 | 19/16 | 4.4/4.0 |
| Pro SoBee | Mead Johnson | 310 | 63 | 2 | 8 | 78 | 94 | 63 | 0.31 | 1250 | 15.6 | 470 | 2.3 | 8.1 | 7.8 | 4.7 |
| Similac | Ross | 300 | 60 | 3.0 | 8 | 100 | 150 | 60 | 0.25 | 1050 | 15 | 450 | 4.4 | 9 | 16 | 4.7 |
| Similac Natural Care | Ross | 680 | 150 | 4.0 | 12 | 250 | 620 | 250 | 0.55 | 5000 | 37 | 1900 | 37 | 37 | 10 | 5.5 |
| Similac PM 60/40 | Ross | 300 | 60 | 2.5* | 8 | 100 | 150 | 60 | 0.25 | 1050 | 15 | 450 | 4.5 | 9 | 12 | 24 |
| Similac Special Care | Ross | 680 | 150 | 4.0 | 12 | 250 | 620 | 250 | 0.55 | 5000 | 37 | 1900 | 37 | 37 | 10 | 5.5 |
| SMA | Wyeth-Ayerst | 300 | 60 | 1.4 | 8 | 100 | 150 | 62.5 | 0.2 | 750 | 7.5 | 315 | 2.2 | 8.5 | 15 | 4.7 |
| Soyalac | Nutricia | 312 | 62 | 2.3 | 7.8 | 78 | 94 | 70 | 0.31 | 1250 | 15.6 | 469 | 9.4 | 12 | 12 | 10 |

* Information given is for the powder consumer product. The Ready-To-Feed hospital product has 3.0 IU vitamin E per 100 kcal.

**TABLE 24-13. Recommended Bottle Feedings for a Normal Infant by Age**

| Age | No. of Feedings | Volume (mL) |
|---|---|---|
| Birth– 1 wk | 6–10 | 30–90 |
| 1 wk–1 mo | 7–8 | 60–120 |
| 1 mo–3 mo | 5–7 | 120–180 |
| 3 mo–6 mo | 4–5 | 180–210 |
| 6 mo–9 mo | 3–4 | 210–240 |
| 10 mo–12 mo | 3 | 210–240 |

Kelts DG, Jones EG. *Manual of pediatric nutrition.* Boston: Little, Brown, 1984:38.

the first year, cup feeding of liquids can begin to replace bottle feeds. The bedtime bottle, often a source of comfort and nutrition, is usually the last to go, although the temptation to let the child take it to bed should be avoided. The child should be held during this feeding and the teeth cleaned after it. It is probably wise to be rid of this evening bottle by 2 years of age. Other bedtime rituals can be substituted. The toddler should not be given a bottle to carry about as a pacifier. Constant feeding can lead to caloric overload and perhaps to dental caries.

The "follow-up" formulas available for use during the weaning process are iron fortified and nutritionally sound (CONAAP, Follow-up or weaning formulas, 1989), but they are unnecessary. During the second half of the first year of life, the infant is better served when the diet consists of human milk or one of the standard infant formulas with iron and a variety of "solid" foods that make up an increasing proportion of the caloric intake.

By 1 year of age, a formula-fed child should be receiving a wide variety of other nutrients, and formula can be discontinued. Modest intake of whole cow's milk can begin at this time. Milks with reduced butterfat (eg, low-fat or skim milk) are not recommended until a child is about 2 years of age.

## Addition of Other Foods to the Diet

Nutrients are initially presented in liquid form because the infant cannot chew and swallow well. Other digestive processes, although still maturing during the first 3 months of life, are already quite good. Competence to handle food antigens matures with time, and the risk of inducing food allergies may be increased with early introduction of solids. The decision of when to begin to feed pureed and soft foods centers on the age at which they are nutritionally and developmentally appropriate. Customs have changed markedly through the years. Once not recommended until 1 year of age, nonliquid foods then came to be introduced as early as the first month. Currently, the recommended age is 4 to 6 months. Although widely resorted to, the addition of cereal to the bedtime feeding does not help a baby "sleep through the night."

### Readiness

At 4 to 6 months of age, the infant has the muscle control to close the mouth, to move the tongue back and forth, and to retain foods placed in the mouth with a spoon. By 5 to 7 months, these skills are more refined, with the child capable of moving the jaw up and down, forming the mouth around the spoon, and freely turning the head away. At about 8 months, the infant acquires the ability to pick up small pieces of soft food and bring them to the mouth. Food refusal skills increase steadily, and by 1 year of age, they are well developed.

The age at which additional food becomes a nutritional ne-

cessity is debated and is probably not uniform. Although there is no upper limit on formula volume that can be presented, many practitioners suggest rather arbitrarily that additional calories should come in the form of other foods after intake reaches 32 oz/day. Breast-fed infants do at some point outgrow their supply. This is heralded by a slow rate of growth and occurs as early as 4 months for some infants, but it may be as late as 9 months for others (Hijazi, 1989). Most baby foods are of lower caloric density and overall nutritional value than formula or human milk.

Although they may differ over the ideal timing, most parents and practitioners feel that infants benefit socially and developmentally from introduction of solids and that it is an enjoyable part of growing and maturing.

### Choice and Progression

Introduction of solids midway through the first year coincides with the time the child may have depleted iron stores and be outgrowing the iron dose available from formula or human milk. Because iron content is important, many suggest iron-fortified infant cereal as the first solid food, but only a small proportion of its iron is absorbed.

At the time of introduction of solids, most infants take five feedings a day, and nonliquid foods are introduced before the bottle or breast at one or more of these times, beginning with several spoonfuls. As a wider variety of foods are introduced and quantities increase, nonliquid foods satisfy a greater portion of the infant's hunger, and smaller volumes of formula or breast milk are taken after the meal, until they are omitted altogether at some and then all feeding times. By 2 years of age, most children are taking three small meals and two snacks a day.

Tradition, not scientific fact, underlies recommendations for the sequence of introduction of foods. The introduction of cereal is often followed by fruits, vegetables, and meats, but other sequences can be easily defended, particularly because meats are excellent sources of iron. Cow's milk and cow's milk formula is high in protein, and meat is not needed as a source of protein in a diet containing large quantities of either. High-carbohydrate foods are preferable.

Whatever sequence is chosen, it is recommended widely that only one new food be added during the span of several days, so that any adverse reactions can be easily attributed. Juices can be offered after the child drinks from a cup. They are not recommended from the bottle.

Most pediatricians reserve for last the foods they feel are most allergenic, including peanut butter, fish, eggs, and citrus. Tradition also undergirds these practices.

An important feature of first foods is their safety. They should be in a form that does not cause choking. Foods for infants are pureed or ground into tiny bits. Soft foods can be presented to toddlers, but hard, round items like nuts, grapes, popcorn, large pieces of raw vegetable, and hot dogs should be withheld until the child can chew and swallow effectively.

Guidance during the introduction of solid foods, an area about which many families seek counsel, can serve as an opportunity for nutritional teaching and for establishing sensible eating habits to last a lifetime.

### Preparation and Prohibitions

Canned or processed foods high in salt or sugar content should be avoided. Infants have not acquired a taste for salt, and none should be added to increase food intake. Commercially prepared baby foods are now low in or free from salt. Preservatives are not added; preservation is accomplished by sterilization. Home-prepared foods, especially those made from fresh or frozen ingredients, are equally desirable, if they are prepared without adding salt and are stored safely. Foods can be ground or pureed after cooking. Baby foods do not need to be sterilized. If large quantities are prepared at a time, meal-size portions can be frozen in small plastic bags or in ice cube trays.

During storage, nitrates in foods can convert to nitrites, which have precipitated methemoglobinemia in infants. For this reason, home preparation of beets, carrots, collard greens, spinach, and turnips has been discouraged. These are probably safe if they are prepared from fresh foods just before mealtime and then discarded. Commercial baby foods made with these vegetables do not have a dangerous nitrite level.

Honey is not recommended during the first year of life, because some cases of infantile botulism have been associated with it. *Clostridium botulinum* spores ingested with honey do not pose a hazard to older persons, but intestinal colonization with elaboration of toxin and subsequent symptoms may occur in infancy. Spores have been detected in commercial corn syrups.

Some foods, such as beans, onions, broccoli, and cabbage, may cause flatulence. These foods are reserved by some parents until the second year of life.

Small portions should be taken to the table, because after the feeding spoon has gone from the mouth back into the food, bacterial contamination is ensured, and the unfed remains should be discarded after the meal. Two to three tablespoons is a good first estimate.

## FEEDING THE OLDER CHILD

The onset of the desire and the skill to self-feed usually become apparent by 1 year of age, and ultimate control over intake shifts to the child. Although the transfer of complete dietary independence to the child takes place gradually over many years and at different rates in different families, the parental role increasingly becomes one of providing a balanced, healthy range of appropriately prepared foods from which the child can select and of discouraging inappropriate feeding behaviors. The latter must be done in ways that do not become counterproductive.

The conversion to self-feeding ordinarily begins at the same time growth velocity is slowing and separation–individuation is a prominent developmental theme. Parents are well advised to become as dispassionate as possible about the feeding process, to avoid assigning great meaning to the consumption of any particular food at any particular meal, to avoid using food as a reward or a punishment, and to avoid insisting that portions are finished. However, it must be acknowledged that food and feeding have immense cultural and social importance and that much of family life revolves around meals.

## Nutrient Requirements and Diet Planning

Recommended caloric and nutrient intakes for toddlers, preschoolers, and school-aged children are presented in Tables 24-1 and 24-2. By the time a child is 18 to 24 months of age, the meals are drawn almost exclusively from foods eaten by the rest of the family, although the foods must be specially cooled and chopped and may need to be set aside before spices are added. Portions are small, and the young child demands between-meal snacks, as most children do throughout childhood and adolescence.

CONAAP suggests that the fat content of the diet be restricted to about 30% of calories beginning at about 2 years of age (CONAAP, Statement on cholesterol, 1992). No more than 10% of total calories should come from saturated fatty acids, and the daily diet should contain no more than 300 mg of cholesterol. It is not unreasonable to encourage the whole family to decrease

---

TABLE 24-14. Daily Meal Planning for the Toddler, Older Child, and Adolescent

| Food Group | Examples and Serving Size | Minimum Number of Portions for Toddler per Day | Examples and Serving Size | Minimum Number of Portions per Day for Older Child | Adolescent |
|---|---|---|---|---|---|
| Meat or substitute | 1 oz meat<br>1 egg<br>2 Tbsp peanut butter<br>1 slice cold cut<br>½ cup cooked dried peas or beans | 2 | 2 oz cooked lean meat, fish, poultry<br>2 eggs<br>2 oz cheese<br>4 Tbsp peanut butter<br>1 cup dried peas or beans | 2 | 2–3 |
| Vegetables and fruits | 4 Tbsp yellow or green vegetable or fruit | 1 | ½ cup cooked* vegetable | | |
| | 2–3 Tbsp fresh, canned, or frozen fruit or ½ piece potato or fruit | 4 | 1 cup raw vegetable or fruit | 3 | 3 |
| | ½ cup tomato, orange, or grapefruit juice | 1 | ½ cup citrus juice or ½ grapefruit | 1 | 1 |
| Breads and cereals | ½ slice bread<br>½ cup dry cereal<br>2 Tbsp cooked cereal, rice, or pasta | 4 | 1 slice bread<br>1 oz dry cereal<br>½ cup cooked cereal, rice, or pasta | 4 | 4 |
| Milk or equivalent | ½ cup milk<br>1 oz cheese<br>½ cup cottage cheese<br>½ cup pudding<br>½ cup yogurt | 4 | 1 cup milk<br>1½ oz cheese<br>1 cup cottage cheese<br>1 cup pudding<br>1 cup yogurt | 3 | 3–4 |

* Three or four servings from this category each week should be dark green, leafy, or orange vegetables or fruits.
*Modified from Feeding Your Toddler. Boston: Department of Nutrition and Food Service, The Children's Hospital, 1987, and How to Eat for Good Health, National Dairy Council, 1985.*

the saturated fat content of the diet by choosing lean cuts of meat, trimming fat from meat, substituting fish and chicken for red meats, preparing foods by broiling or baking rather than frying, and cooking with polyunsaturated vegetable oil or margarine.

Protein needs are diminished between infancy and adolescence in tandem with the diminished growth velocity graphically represented by the more gentle slope of the growth chart at these interim ages (see growth charts in Chapter 6). Weight gain does not occur evenly throughout the year but rather comes in spurts.

Appropriate nutritional balance can be achieved by including daily in meal planning foods from the four food groups: dairy, meats or meat substitutes, grains, and fruits and vegetables. Salt, simple sugars, and saturated fats should be minimized, and good sources of fiber should be included. Overall daily meal planning can be predicated on a serving exchange system such as the one in Table 24-14.

## Vitamin and Mineral Supplementation

Healthy older children taking adequate calories from a well balanced, varied diet do not appear to develop deficiencies of vitamins and minerals. There are relatively few circumstances for which supplementation is indicated.

Iron deficiency is the most common nutritional deficiency in American children, manifested by behavioral changes before anemia is apparent. Some dietary sources of iron usually acceptable to children are presented in Table 24-15, and iron intake should be emphasized throughout childhood and adolescence. If deficiency is documented or suspected, iron may be given in

### TABLE 24-15.    Good Dietary Sources of Iron

| Food | Serving Size | Iron (mg) |
|---|---|---|
| **Sources of Heme Iron (Absorption Is 15%–30%)** | | |
| Pork chop | 3 oz | 3.3 |
| Lean steak | 3 oz | 3 |
| Hamburger | 3 oz | 2.7 |
| Sardines | 3 oz | 2.5 |
| Chicken, dark meat | 3 oz | 2 |
| Lamb | 3 oz | 1.7 |
| Tuna | 3 oz | 1.6 |
| Ham | 3 oz | 1.2 |
| Chicken, white meat | 3 oz | 1 |
| Salmon or white fish | 3 oz | 1 |
| **Sources of Nonheme Iron (Absorption Is About 5%)** | | |
| Dried apricots | 3 oz | 4 |
| Baked beans | ½ cup | 3 |
| Baked potato with skin | 1 medium | 2.8 |
| Almonds | 2 oz | 2.7 |
| Lima beans | ½ cup | 2.1 |
| Raisins | ½ cup | 2.1 |
| Macaroni, enriched | 1 cup | 1.6 |
| Bread, enriched white | 2 slices | 1.4 |
| Spaghetti, enriched | 1 cup | 1.4 |
| Peas | ½ cup | 1.2 |
| Peanut butter | 4 Tbsp | 1.2 |
| Egg | 1 | 1 |
| Breakfast cereal, enriched or fortified | 1 oz | 1–10 |

*Modified from University of California, Berkeley Wellness Letter, August 1987;5 and from Pipes PL. Selected food sources of iron. Nutrition in infancy and childhood. St. Louis: CV Mosby, 1981:81.*

supplemental form at a dosage of 3 mg/kg per day. Laboratory confirmation of a response should be sought after 1 month and supplementation continued for 3 or 4 months (see Chap. 90.1).

Children whose water supplies are not fluoridated should receive supplemental fluoride because of its well-documented anticariogenic effect. Optimal daily intake is thought to be about 0.05 mg/kg/day. The intake of fluoride from nonwater sources and even the intake of water are hard to quantitate and probably vary widely among people. CONAAP guidelines for fluoride supplementation are presented in Table 24-16. Excessive fluoride intake leads to discoloration of tooth enamel, which varies from dull white to brown mottling. At very high doses, the enamel may be hypoplastic.

The diets of children who are abused or neglected, who are trying to lose weight, who are on vegetarian diets without dairy products, or who are failing to thrive are to be scrutinized for possible caloric, vitamin, and mineral deficiencies. Strict vegetarian diets are likely to be deficient in vitamin $B_{12}$. They also lack the vitamin D supplementation many children obtain from milk. Recommended vitamin and mineral supplementation for healthy persons of all ages on nonrestricted diets is summarized in Table 24-6.

## Common Problems

### Bottle Dependence

If the infant is allowed prolonged access to the bottle as a pacifier, its use can become habitual. The result is a toddler who is never seen without one. Caloric intake may be inappropriately increased or the high fluid intake may cause the child to eschew other foods, with poor nutritional outcome. The developing teeth are almost constantly exposed to carbohydrates, which are cariogenic.

Weaning from the bottle during the "terrible twos" can be a turbulent task, and the necessity to do so should be avoided by making the transition to the cup before this age. If a toddler is still clinging to the bottle, at least two methods of intervention are available. All bottles can be literally thrown away, so there is no relenting when the toddler insists on a bottle. After a few days of unhappiness, demands for the bottle fade. A more gradual method is to make the bottle uninteresting by filling it with water only.

### Concern About Intake

Food intake of the older child waxes and wanes. Parents often express concern about its adequacy. As growth velocity slows, appetites become less voracious. Some parents, accustomed to the almost continuous feeding demands of infancy, find the toddler's and preschooler's lack of interest in meals nothing short

### TABLE 24-16.    Supplemental Fluoride Dosage Schedule*

| Age | Concentration of Fluoride in Drinking Water (ppm) | | |
|---|---|---|---|
| | *<0.3* | *0.3–0.7* | *>0.7* |
| 2 wk–2 y | 0.25 | 0 | 0† |
| 2–3 y | 0.50 | 0.25 | 0 |
| 3–16 y | 1 | 0.50 | 0 |

\* In mg/day; 2.2 mg of sodium fluoride contains 1 mg fluoride.
† 0.25 mg of fluoride should be given to infants at 6 months of age who are still being breast fed exclusively.

*Committee on Nutrition, American Academy of Pediatrics, Pediatric Nutrition Handbook. Elk Grove Village, IL: American Academy of Pediatrics, 1985:171.*

of shocking. They are prepared to increase intake by whatever techniques they can muster, and if not reassured, they may precipitate real problems with food refusal by insisting that the child eat.

Parental concern should be taken seriously and realistic dietary guidelines established. The best marker of adequacy is the continued normal growth of the child, and parents are often visibly relieved by the growth chart.

### Selection

Young children commonly express strong food preferences and may demand nothing but a particular food for several days. These fascinations pass and rarely jeopardize total nutritional goals. However, it does not appear to be true that children, given the chance, make wise and healthy food selections, and the parents should limit their access to foods high in salt, fats, and sugar by minimizing these foods in the home. Snacks of fresh fruit and vegetables and of baked products made from whole grains should be offered.

Although usually managed by the mother, family diet is traditionally most heavily influenced by the preferences of the father. The preferences of the child are usually given priority only for snacks and sometimes at breakfast when the menu is individualized. Dietary intervention is therefore a family affair.

### Television

American children spend many hours each day watching television. Viewing is often linked to eating, especially of high-calorie snack foods, and to obesity, probably by increasing intake and decreasing activity. Television advertising promotes cereals and other child-marketed foods high in sugar and low in other nutrients.

### Obesity

The overall nutritional status of American children is good. The most common nutritional problem is an excess of calories, leading to obesity. Restricting high-calorie snacks, limiting television viewing, not insisting that a child clean the plate, encouraging activity, and presenting a prudent diet help to prevent excessive weight gain. However, heredity contributes to obesity. The goal in the growing child who is obese is to maintain, rather than to lose, weight (see Chap. 30.8). The social stigma attached to obesity should not be condoned by the attitudes of the pediatrician.

### Failure to Thrive

Pockets of poverty so grave as to threaten food supply remain, and some children are growing poorly "simply" because their families do not have enough food to feed them. Undernutrition can occur if family dynamics or chronic disease prohibit the presentation, intake, or assimilation of adequate calories. Poor growth is a pediatric emergency and should be acted on expeditiously (see Chap. 39).

### Food and Behavior

Parents may attribute undesirable behavior, particularly hyperactivity, to dietary excesses, especially of refined sugars or additives. Controlled, masked trials have yet to confirm any general association.

Occasions of sugar excess, like holidays, are often excessive in many other ways. Restricted diets are often more trouble than they are worth, and if quite restricted, they may lead to dietary deficiencies. Restricted diets should be attempted only with medical supervision.

### Table Manners

Messiness is to be anticipated and should be tolerated as a young child develops self-feeding skills. An old bed sheet under the high chair can reduce parental anxiety over the consequences of the child's developmentally appropriate experimentation with food. As motor skills and social skills progress, table behavior can be molded gradually to fit the family's expectations; however, manners are somewhat family specific and are acquired more slowly than the ability to feed oneself. Teaching the child to say please and thank you should be orchestrated in a way that does not produce food refusal.

### Vegetarian Diets

It is important for the pediatrician to understand what food restrictions a family makes if they report a vegetarian diet. Most of these diets, especially those that include milk and eggs, are nutritionally adequate for the growing child. Table 24-17 describes the most common patterns and the deficiencies they may contain. Because a family following a vegetarian diet may become increasingly restrictive over time, information about the diet should be updated periodically.

## FEEDING THE ADOLESCENT

Behavioral issues in adolescence often dwarf nutritional issues, but it is a time of exceptional nutritional need. The rapid growth rate of early adolescence combined with rather sudden dietary independence and susceptibility to fads and peer influence put the adolescent in nutritional jeopardy. The careful attention paid to the nutritional needs of the young infant should be afforded the adolescent.

### Nutrient Requirements

Growth needs during the adolescent spurt demand a total nutrient intake that is unmatched throughout the male lifespan and is exceeded for the female only during pregnancy and lactation. Recommended calorie and nutrient intakes are displayed in Tables 24-1 and 24-2. Only the adolescent boy can routinely enjoy the coveted taste of "fast food" without exceeding caloric needs. The large volumes of food consumed and the usual teenage preferences for pizza and hamburgers ensure adequate iron intake for the large increase in muscle mass and erythrocyte volume adolescents experience. Additional iron needed by the menstruating adolescent presumes a high caloric intake and a high activity level to burn off the excess calories that bear the needed iron. The pregnant adolescent is at great nutritional risk, because her intake must meet the needs of her fetus and her own growth. Nutritional counseling is mandatory.

### Vitamin and Mineral Supplementation

The dieting adolescent may require supplemental iron, and the pregnant adolescent should be supplemented (see Table 24-6). Although adolescents may follow a diet fad for a few days, their tendency to change their minds frequently protects most of them from sustained dietary deficiencies. Fast food supplemented by a few home meals that contain sources of vitamin A can serve vitamin and mineral needs quite nicely, although this diet may contain excessive fat and salt.

### Common Problems

#### Sports-Related Dietary Manipulations

Activity expends calories, and the more strenuous and sustained the activity, the more calories are used (Table 24-18). Exercise is a good remedy for an adolescent who wishes to avoid excessive weight gain if caloric intake continues to be adequate for growth.

The diets of some adolescent athletes are manipulated in an attempt to achieve competitive advantage by increasing protein

## TABLE 24-17. Vegetarian Diets: Nutritional Implications and Recommendations

| Type | Nutritional Implications | Recommendations |
|---|---|---|
| Lacto-ovovegetarians (eat no flesh; milk and eggs acceptable) | Usually without deficiencies | Follow for growth and changes toward a more restrictive diet. |
| Lactovegetarians (eat no flesh or eggs; milk acceptable) | Usually without deficiencies | Follow for growth and changes toward a more restrictive diet. |
| Pure vegetarians (only foods of vegetable origin) | No problems while child is young and breast feeding, except possible $B_{12}$ and D deficiency | Mother or child should be supplemented with $B_{12}$; infant with vitamin D. Encourage use of commercial soy-based formula after weaning. |
| | Bulk, lower digestibility, and low-fat content of vegetarian diet make energy needs relatively more difficult to meet. | Supplement energy intake with vegetable oils and margarine. |
| | Protein completeness a potential problem | Cereals are good sources of methionine, legumes of lysine. Diets should have both. Protein should make up 11%–12% of total energy intake. Encourage use of refined or milled grains. Fruits should not make up a large part of the diet because they are low in energy and protein. |
| | $B_{12}$ and D requirements are not met by vegetarian diet. | Supplement diet with a vitamin preparation containing $B_{12}$ and D. |
| | Iron intake may be compromised by low energy intake and less bioavailable form. | Consider iron supplementation of 10–15 mg of elemental iron per day. |
| Zen macrobiotic diets (levels vary in their prohibitions) | At higher levels (most restrictive) diet is composed entirely or mostly of cereals and is not compatible with health. Weaning foods are often inadequate. At middle and lower levels, is similar to vegetarian and omnivorous diets, respectively. | Advise families against most restrictive levels. |

Tabulated from MacLean WC, Graham G. Pediatric Nutrition in Clinical Practice, chap 7. Menlo Park, CA: Addison-Wesley, 1982:134–147.

intake, by carbohydrate loading before events, or by rigorous fluid and food restriction to meet a weight standard. Such manipulations should be discouraged by the pediatrician, who should remain an advocate for the adolescent's long-term growth and development.

### Diets

Adolescents, especially girls, are forever dieting. Many believe they are too fat. If an adolescent is not overweight, every attempt should be made to reassure him or her and to advise a sound, balanced diet. If an adolescent is overweight and wishes to lose, he or she may be referred for group therapy as offered by Weight Watchers for teens. Vitamin and iron supplementation may be warranted. A diet that restricts calories modestly without jeopardizing balanced intake is always the best plan (see Chap. 30.8). The overall goal of achieving optimal growth and sound dietary habits that will last a lifetime should not be sacrificed to more immediate but ephemeral goals, but it is the rare adolescent who can be this forward looking.

### Anorexia and Bulimia

Many female adolescents believe they are too fat. Some develop complicated feeding disorders (eg, anorexia nervosa, bulimia) that, in their most blatant forms, carry a grievous long-term prognosis. The harbingers of these disorders should be recognized as early as possible by the pediatrician (see Chapter 30.8).

### Adolescent Pregnancy

The nutritional issues are likely to be submerged among the many unfortunate consequences of adolescent pregnancy. The pediatrician must remember, as the advocate for the teen who becomes pregnant, that the teen's own nutritional needs, in addition to the needs of the fetus, should be supplied. Although the practice of prescribing prenatal vitamins and iron to all pregnant females has been called into question, the case for vitamin and mineral supplementation (see Table 24-6) is rarely stronger than for the young pregnant adolescent.

### Alcoholism

Many adolescents drink alcoholic beverages regularly. Society, as advertising clearly documents, encourages the adolescent to view drinking as a part of becoming an adult. Alcohol, high in

## TABLE 24-18. Caloric Expenditure During Various Forms of Exercise

| Activity | Calories* |
|---|---|
| Bicycling, 6 mph | 240 |
| Bicycling, 12 mph | 410 |
| Cross-country skiing | 700 |
| Jogging, 5½ mph | 740 |
| Jogging, 7 mph | 920 |
| Jumping rope | 750 |
| Running in place | 650 |
| Running, 10 mph | 1280 |
| Swimming, 25 yd/min | 275 |
| Swimming, 50 yd/min | 500 |
| Tennis, singles | 400 |
| Walking, 2 mph | 240 |
| Walking, 3 mph | 320 |
| Walking, 4½ mph | 440 |

\* Average calories spent per hour by a 150-pound person.

American Heart Association. Courtesy of the Department of Nutrition, The Johns Hopkins Hospital, Baltimore.

caloric content at 7 kcal/g, contains no other nutrients. Although often lost among the many other ramifications of adolescent substance abuse, the calories obtained from alcohol are not a good nutritional investment, particularly for the growing body.

## Selected Readings

Committee on Nutrition, American Academy of Pediatrics. Follow-up or weaning formulas. Pediatrics 1989;83:1067.

Committee on Nutrition, American Academy of Pediatrics. Forbes GB, Woodruff CW, eds. Pediatric nutrition handbook. Elk Grove Village, Illinois: American Academy of Pediatrics, 1985:356.

Committee on Nutrition, American Academy of Pediatrics. Hypoallergenic infant formulas. Pediatrics 1989;83:1068.

Committee on Nutrition, American Academy of Pediatrics. Iron-fortified infant formulas. Pediatrics 1989;84:1114.

Committee on Nutrition, American Academy of Pediatrics. Statement on cholesterol. Pediatrics 1992;90:469.

Committee on Nutrition, American Academy of Pediatrics. The use of whole cow's milk in infancy. Pediatrics 1992;89:1105.

Hansen AE, Haggard ME, Boelsche AN, et al. Essential fatty acids in infant nutrition. III. Clinical manifestations of linoleic acid deficiency. J Nutr 1958;66:565.

Hijazi SS, Abulaban A, Waterlow JC. The duration for which exclusive breast feeding is adequate. Acta Paediatr Scand 1989;78:23.

Kelts DG, Jones EG, eds. Manual of pediatric nutrition. Boston: Little, Brown, 1984.

Kurinij N, Shiono PH, Ezrine SF, Rhoads GG. Does maternal employment affect breast-feeding? Am J Public Health 1989;79:1247.

Marx DM. Drugs excreted in breast milk. Appendix 7. In: Howard RB, Harland SW, eds. Nutrition and feeding of infants and toddlers. Boston: Little, Brown, 1984:433.

Mead Johnson Nutritionals. Dietary management of metabolic disorders. Evansville, IN: Mead Johnson & Company, 1991.

Morley R, Cole TJ, Powell R, Lucas A. Mother's choice to provide breast milk and developmental outcome. Arch Dis Child 1988;63:1382.

Neifert MR, Seacat JM. A guide to successful breast-feeding. Contemp Pediatr 1986;3:32.

*Principles and Practice of Pediatrics, Second Edition.*
edited by Frank A. Oski et al. J. B. Lippincott Company, Philadelphia © 1994.

## 24.2 *Immunization*

Modena Hoover Wilson

The virtual disappearance of many of the once common and dreaded infectious diseases of childhood since the introduction of immunoprophylaxis with vaccines is one of the most remarkable success stories of modern medicine. To sustain these gains and reach the ultimate goal of eradicating selected diseases requires constant vigilance and meticulous attention to immunization. Additional gains are possible by immunizing an even higher percentage of susceptible persons and by developing new and better vaccines. These challenges are being presented in developed countries to young clinicians and parents who have little or no personal experience with the diseases against which we immunize. It may take increased energy and resources to convey the lessons of history and to prevent a fall in immunization levels. Surveillance results and disease patterns suggest that a substantial proportion of inner-city preschoolers in the United States are inadequately immunized.

Although progress has been made in many developing countries, the breakdown of political systems, poverty, and inadequate infrastructure and resources continue to threaten immunization programs. Protecting children against vaccine-preventable diseases must remain a worldwide priority.

The late 1980s and early 1990s have seen broad changes in recommendations for childhood immunization. The health care community has been called on to examine its failure to immunize children. Documentation that many children who are inadequately immunized have had multiple contacts with health care providers demands that the immunization history become a high priority at every visit, that deferral of immunization be limited strictly to contraindications, and that access to immunization be improved and barriers removed.

Complicating the failure to immunize children with the vaccines long-recommended (eg, diphtheria, tetanus, pertussis, measles, mumps, rubella), new vaccines have been offered and schedules adjusted. There have been several vaccine-related changes in health care for children:

- A marked fall in the incidence of invasive *Haemophilus influenzae* type b (Hib) invasive disease has resulted from immunization of toddlers with polysaccharide vaccine and subsequently of infants with Hib conjugate vaccine.
- A limited immunization strategy failed to interrupt the transmission of hepatitis B virus (HBV) infection in the United States, prompting the recommendation of a more comprehensive strategy, including universal immunization against HBV in infancy.
- A second dose of measles vaccine, preferably given as measles, mumps, and rubella (MMR) vaccine, was added to the childhood immunization schedule as a reaction to the failure to eradicate measles disease and a resurgence in the number of reported cases.
- Acellular pertussis vaccine combined with diphtheria and tetanus toxoids (DTaP) is associated with fewer adverse reactions than whole-cell pertussis vaccine and has been made available for use after initial immunization with whole-cell vaccine.
- There has been progress toward a comprehensive strategy for the use of varicella vaccine.
- The need to combine immunizing agents in multiple-antigen vaccines to make the immunization process more efficient and acceptable has been recognized.

## THE IMMUNIZATION PROCESS

*Immunoprophylaxis*, the prevention of infectious disease with specific antibody, can be accomplished in two ways. *Active immunization* refers to delivering one or more antigens of an infectious agent to a person to stimulate the immune system to produce antibody before exposure to natural infection, thereby preventing disease. If live attenuated organisms are used as the active immunizing agent, a more complete and long-lasting response is expected than if killed organisms or their products are used. *Passive immunization* is accomplished by transferring to the person preformed antibody produced by another host. The protection persists a for limited period, disappearing as the antibody is degraded.

Active immunization can occur naturally, as when polio vaccine virus shed by an immunized person infects another host or when an adult immunized against pertussis as a child acquires a mild case of pertussis, which boosts his antibody level. Active immunization is usually deliberate, accomplished when killed or attenuated infectious organisms or selected antigens are injected, fed to, or sprayed into the nose of human hosts thought to be susceptible to the disease.

Passive immunization can occur naturally. The antibody passed transplacentally from mother to infant protects infants from many diseases in the first few months of life. It can interfere with attempts to actively immunize the child, governing the timing of successful vaccination. Passive immunization can be accomplished through serotherapy by injecting a person with antibody produced by other humans or an animal host. Serotherapy is used if disease risk is high but active immunization is not practical, such as if the recipient is not immunocompetent and will not respond in the expected manner to active immunization, if exposure has occurred and active immunization may not provide protection soon enough, or if no efficacious vaccine exists but serotherapy has shown to be efficacious.

Timing is a pivotal issue for active and passive immunization. Antibody must be present soon enough to prevent the agent from infecting the host or, in a few instances, soon enough to prevent spread of the infection in the host or the damage caused by a toxic product of infection.

## Sources of Information on Vaccines

After a period of relative stability in the field, vaccines and recommendations for who should receive them and at what age have been changing rapidly. The clinician needs a strategy for obtaining up-to-date information. Among the sources of vaccine information listed by the Committee on Infectious Diseases of the American Academy of Pediatrics, there are several likely to be consulted by pediatricians in routine practice situations.

The Red Book, also known as the *Report of the Committee on Infectious Diseases* of the American Academy of Pediatrics (AAP), is published every 2 or 3 years and can be purchased from the Academy. Information from the 1991 edition was used to prepare this chapter. In the interval between editions of the Red Book, new information and recommendations from the Committee on Infectious Diseases may appear first in the monthly *AAP News* and is published in *Pediatrics* as a "Statement from the Committee on Infectious Diseases."

A second influential body in regard to vaccines and immunization policy is the Advisory Committee on Immunization Practices (ACIP) of the Public Health Service. Recommendations from the ACIP appear in *Morbidity and Mortality Weekly Report*, which is published by the Centers for Disease Control (CDC), as are reports about the occurrence and prevalence of vaccine preventable diseases. The *Journal of the American Medical Association* carries updates from *Morbidity and Mortality Weekly Report*.

The *Physicians' Desk Reference* contains information provided by the manufacturers of vaccines and antisera on the constituents of the preparations, indications and contraindications, dosage and route of administration, and adverse reactions. The same kind of information is supplied in the circular inserted into each package. When a new or unfamiliar vaccine is being given, the package insert should always be consulted.

Other sources of information that may be consulted as the need arises include *Health Information for International Travel*, updated and published each year by the CDC, *Control of Communicable Diseases in Man* from the American Public Health Association, and the *Guide for Adult Immunization* from the American College of Physicians. The immunization recommendations of the American Academy of Family Practice are published in *American Family Physician*.

## Available Products for Immunization

Vaccines are suspensions of attenuated or killed microorganisms or their antigens, administered for the prevention or amelioration of infectious disease. Those widely available in the United States are listed in alphabetical order in Table 24-19. Recommendations for those in regular use are described in the sections below.

Antibody preparations available to provide passive immunization through serotherapy are listed in Table 24-20. Indications and recommendations for serotherapy for nonspecific immuno-

prophylaxis and for postexposure prophylaxis can be found in the disease-specific sections in this chapter and in the chapters of this book dedicated to the individual infectious diseases for which preparations are listed. Adverse reactions to antibody preparations should be anticipated and are occasionally severe. Sensitivity testing is required before administration of sera of nonhuman origin, and desensitization may be necessary. Serotherapy should be administered by experienced persons in a setting where emergencies can be handled. Guidelines for administration can be found in the product package insert, in the disease-specific chapters of this book, and in the Report of the Committee on Infectious Diseases of the American Academy of Pediatrics.

## Candidates for Active Immunization

Active immunization with a safe and effective vaccine, provided well before exposure to the infectious agent and at a time when the person is able to respond adequately, is the most desirable method of preventing common infectious diseases. The vaccine is designed to resemble the microorganism sufficiently to provoke an immunologic response by the host that prevents natural infection or damage from the toxic results of infection.

Some vaccines are recommended for all United States children without a specific contraindication. These include diphtheria and tetanus toxoids with pertussis (DTP); oral poliovirus vaccine (OPV); measles, mumps, and rubella vaccines (MMR); *Haemophilus* b conjugate vaccine (HbCV); and hepatitis B viral vaccine (HBVV).

Some vaccines are recommended only for children who are at special risk or live with someone at special risk. These vaccines include pneumococcal polysaccharide, meningococcal polysaccharide, inactivated influenza viral vaccine, and inactivated poliovirus vaccine. Varicella-zoster vaccine may soon be licensed and added to one of the lists.

Vaccines in a third group are administered at this time in the United States only under special circumstances of probable or accomplished exposure. Included in this category are bacillus Calmette-Guérin vaccine (BCG) for tuberculosis, cholera inactivated bacterial vaccine, plague inactivated bacterial vaccine, rabies inactivated viral vaccine, typhoid inactivated bacterial vaccine, and yellow fever live viral vaccine.

When considering delaying or omitting the administration of an age-appropriate vaccine dose, the provider must carefully weigh the risks and benefits. Although a few true contraindications to specific vaccines exist, and are listed in the vaccine sections that follow, there are not many general contraindications. In most cases a vaccine can be safely given and should not be delayed. Pregnant women are not usually given live viral vaccines, and immunocompromised children require special consideration. True hypersensitivity reactions to immunizing antigens or other vaccine components are rare, but if the history suggests specific allergy or reaction to a vaccine component (not a general allergic history), the vaccine should be omitted or administered after testing. Guidelines are provided by the Report of the Committee on Infectious Diseases of the AAP. Minor illness, such as an upper respiratory infection presumed to be viral in origin or a low-grade fever in a child who appears relatively well, should not delay immunization.

## Vaccines

There is variation among vaccines and preparations of the same kind of vaccine from different manufacturers in how the antigens are prepared and preserved. Vaccines actually consist of several components. Package inserts contain the specific constituents.

## TABLE 24-19.   Vaccines and Toxoids Commercially Available in the United States in 1992

**Cholera Vaccines**

Cholera vaccine, India strains (Lederle)

Cholera vaccine USP, Wyeth (Wyeth-Ayerst)

**Diphtheria and Tetanus Toxoids (Pediatric-DT)**

Diphtheria and Tetanus Toxoids Adsorbed Purogenated, aluminum phosphate-adsorbed, pediatric (Lederle)

Diphtheria and Tetanus Toxoids Adsorbed USP (DT), pediatric (Squibb/Connaught)

Diphtheria and Tetanus Toxoids Adsorbed, pediatric (Elkins-Sinn)

Diphtheria and Tetanus Toxoids Adsorbed Ultrafined, pediatric (Wyeth-Ayerst)

**Diphtheria and Tetanus Toxoids and Pertussis Vaccines (Pediatric)**

Acel-Imune, diphtheria and tetanus toxoids and acellular pertussis vaccine (Lederle)

Diphtheria and Tetanus Toxoids and Pertussis Vaccine Adsorbed USP, pediatric (Connaught)

Tri-Immunol, diphtheria and tetanus toxoids and pertussis vaccine adsorbed (Lederle)

*Haemophilus influenzae* b Conjugate Vaccines

HibTiter, *Haemophilus* b conjugate vaccine (Lederle); conjugate is diphtheria CRM197 protein

PedvaxHib, *Haemophilus* B conjugate vaccine, meningococcal protein conjugate (Merck Sharp & Dohme); conjugate is outer membrane protein complex (OMPC) of the B11 strain of *Neisseria meningitidis* group B

ProHibit, *Haemophilus* b conjugate vaccine, diphtheria toxoid-conjugate (Connaught); conjugate is diphtheria toxoid

**Hepatitis B Virus Recombinant Vaccines**

Energix-B, hepatitis B vaccine, recombinant (SmithKline Beecham)

Recombivax-HB, hepatitis B vaccine, recombinant (Merck Sharp & Dohme)

**Influenza Virus Vaccines**

Flu-Imune, influenza virus vaccine (Lederle)

Fluogen, influenza virus vaccine (Parke-Davis)

Influenza Virus Vaccine, purified subvirion (Elkins-Sinn)

Influenza Virus Vaccine, subvirion type (Wyeth-Ayerst)

**Measles Vaccine**

Attenuvax, measles virus vaccine live MSD USP, more attenuated Ender's strain (Merck Sharp & Dohme)

**Measles and Rubella Vaccine**

M-R-Vax, measles and rubella virus vaccine live MSD USP (Merck Sharp & Dohme)

**Measles, Mumps and Rubella Vaccine**

M-M-R, measles, mumps and rubella virus vaccine live MSD USP (Merck Sharp & Dohme)

**Meningococcal Vaccine**

Menomune A/C/Y/W-135, meningococcal polysaccharide vaccine, groups A, C, Y, and W-135 combined (Connaught)

**Mumps Vaccine**

Mumpsvax, mumps virus vaccine live MSD USP (Merck Sharp & Dohme)

**Plague Vaccine**

Plague Vaccine USP (Miles-Cutter)

**Poliovirus Vaccines, Trivalent**

Ipol, poliovirus vaccine inactivated (Connaught)

Orimune, poliovirus vaccine, live oral trivalent (Lederle)

**Pneumococcal Vaccines**

Pneumovax 23, pneumococcal vaccine polyvalent MSD (Merck Sharp & Dohme)

Pnu-Imune, pneumococcal vaccine, polyvalent (Lederle)

**Rabies Vaccine**

Imovax, rabies vaccine (Connaught)

**Rubella Vaccine**

Meruvax, rubella virus vaccine live MSD USP (Merck Sharp & Dohme)

**Rubella and Mumps Vaccine**

Biavax, rubella and mumps virus vaccine live MSD USP (Merck Sharp & Dohme)

**Staphylococcal Antigen**

Staphage Lysate (SPL), bacterial antigen made from *Staphylococcus* (Delmont)

**Tetanus and Diphtheria Toxoids (Adult Td)**

Tetanus and Diphtheria Toxoids Adsorbed, adult (Elkins-Sinn)

Tetanus and Diphtheria Toxoids Adsorbed, adult, aluminum phosphate-adsorbed, Ultrafined (Wyeth-Ayerst)

Tetanus and Diphtheria Toxoids Adsorbed Purogenated, adult, aluminum phosphate-adsorbed (Lederle)

Tetanus and Diphtheria Toxoids USP (Td), adult, (Connaught)

**Tetanus Toxoids**

Tetanus Toxoid Adsorbed (Elkins-Sinn)

Tetanus Toxoid Adsorbed, aluminum phosphate adsorbed, Ulltrafined (Wyeth-Ayerst)

Tetanus Toxoid Adsorbed Purogenated, tetanus toxoid aluminum phosphate-adsorbed (Lederle)

Tetanus Toxoid Fluid (Elkins-Sinn)

Tetanus Toxoid, fluid, purified, Ultrafined (Wyeth-Ayerst)

Tetanus Toxoid USP (Connaught)

**Tuberculosis Vaccine**

Tice BCG, BCG vaccine USP, (Organon)

**Typhoid Vaccine**

Typhoid Vaccine USP (Wyeth-Ayerst)

**Yellow Fever Vaccine**

YF-Vax, yellow fever vaccine (Connaught)

Compiled from Physicians' Desk Reference. Montvale, NJ: Medical Economics, 1992.

Each preparation contains the immunizing antigen or antigens, which may be one particular component of an organism (eg, protein, polysaccharide) or whole organisms (eg, attenuated viruses, killed bacteria). It may contain one or more of the following: preservatives, stabilizers, antibiotics, adjuvants such as an aluminum compound to increase and prolong antigenicity, and a suspending fluid. The recipient may be sensitive to one or more of these elements and develop an adverse reaction to the vaccine.

Vaccines should be administered in a setting where adverse reactions can be anticipated and treated.

Great care must be taken to store and handle the vaccines in accordance with the manufacturer's recommendations to preserve sterility and the integrity of the antigenic components. Some live viral vaccines are particularly vulnerable to heat, because the attenuation process may include cold adaptation. Under adverse conditions efficacy is lost or decreased.

TABLE 24-20. Antibody Preparations for Passive Immunization (Serotherapy) to Prevent Selected Infectious Disease

| Product Name | Description | Selected Indications |
|---|---|---|
| Immune globulin (IG) (intramuscular injection) | Immunoglobulin (mostly IgG) from pooled plasma of adult human donors. Specific immunity represents experience of donors. | Immunoglobulin-deficiency disorders except selective IgA deficiency; hepatitis A prophylaxis, before- and after-exposure; measles post exposure prophylaxis |
| Immune globulin, intravenous (IVIG) | IG modified for intravenous use | Immunoglobulin-deficiency disorders; Kawasaki disease IVIG to prevent a wide range of infections studied in low-birth-weight infants, pediatric AIDS, chronic lymphocytic leukemia, and bone marrow transplantation |
| Specific immune globulins: | | |
| Human origin | Immunoglobulin from donors known to have high titers of the desired antibody | Postexposure prophylaxis |
|    Cytomegalovirus (CMV IVIG) | | Prophylaxis in renal transplant recipients |
|   Hepatitis B (HBIG) | | |
|   Rabies (RIG) | | |
|   Tetanus (TIG | | |
|   Varicella-zoster (VZIG) | | |
| Animal Origin | | |
|   Botulism antitoxin | In U.S., derived from serum of horses by concentration of the serum globulin fraction with ammonium sulfate | Postexposure prophylaxis when specific immune globulin of human origin is not available |
|   Diphtheria antitoxin | | |
|   Tetanus antitoxin | | |
|   Antirabies serum | | |

*Adapted from Report on the Committee of Infectious Diseases of the American Academy of Pediatrics, 1991.*

## Vaccine Administration

Vaccines to be injected, which include all currently licensed products except oral polio viral vaccine, must be administered without damaging vital structures. Large muscle masses distant from large nerves and vessels are the ideal site for intramuscular injection, and the skin over these muscles is preferred for subcutaneous injection. The anterolateral thigh is the preferred area for vaccine administration in infants, and the anterolateral thigh or the deltoid area is preferred in older children. The gluteal region should be avoided, especially in infants. The sciatic nerve likely to be damaged if the injection is not carefully confined to the upper, outer quadrant of the buttock, and the muscle in this area is poorly developed in infants. HBVV vaccine should not be injected into the buttock at any age, because antibody response is inadequate.

Careful attention to site selection and technique may prevent the serious complications of intramuscular injection, which are nerve and muscle damage. Abscesses occur infrequently. Other uncommon complications of injection include inadvertent injection into a vascular or joint space; tissue necrosis, hemorrhage, atrophy, or infection; and residual pigmentation, cyst, or scar formation.

## Scheduling Vaccine Administration

Scheduling of vaccines involves consideration of the age of likely exposure and age at which antibody response is likely to be adequate. The latter depends on characteristics of the immunizing antigen, the host, and the likelihood of the presence of interfering maternal antibody. Recommended schedules are those found to provide protective antibody in most recipients before the age at which disease is likely to occur. A schedule used for routine immunization of infants and children is found in Table 24-21.

Vaccines routinely given to infants and children in the United States may be given simultaneously without sacrificing efficacy or producing untoward adverse reactions if recommended dosing schedules are followed. Because a recipient may not respond to all three strains of vaccine virus contained in oral polio vaccine

after a single dose, a schedule of multiple doses is provided. There are a limited number of known interferences that involve vaccines for special cases. Cholera and yellow fever vaccines should be spaced at an interval of at least 3 weeks for ideal antibody response. Reactions to some vaccines (eg, cholera, typhoid, influenza, DTP) may be accentuated if given together, and these vaccines should be given on separate occasions if possible.

TABLE 24-21. Immunization Schedule Conforming With Recommendations for Healthy U.S. Children With No Additional Risk Factors

| Age | Vaccine and Dose Number |
|---|---|
| Postpartum | HBVrV[1] |
| 1–2 mo | HBVrV[2] |
| 2 mo | DTP[1], OPV[1], PRP-OMP[1] or HbOC[1] or PRP-T[1] |
| 4 mo | DTP[2], OPV[2], PRP-OMP[2] or HbOC[2] or PRP-T[2]* |
| 6 mo | DTP[3], HbOC[3] or PRP-T[3] |
| 12 mo | HBVrV[3],† Any Hib† |
| 15 mo | MMR[1], DTaP[4], OPV[3], Any Hib (if not given at 12 mo) |
| 18 mo | DTaP[4] and OPV[3] (if not given at 15 mo) |
| 4–6 y | MMR[2],† DTaP[5], OPV[4]† |
| 11–12 y | MMR[2]* (of not given at 4–6 years) |
| 14–16 y | Td booster (to follow every 10 y) |

*DTaP*, diphtheria and tetanus toxoids with acellular pertussis vaccine; *DTP*, diphtheria and tetanus toxoids with whole-cell pertussis vaccine; *HBVrV*, hepatitis B virus recombinant vaccine; *OPV*, oral poliovirus vaccine; *MMR*, measles, mumps, and rubella vaccine; *Td*, tetanus and low-dose diphtheria toxoids.
\* One of the following vaccines is administered: PRP-OMP, *Haemophilus influenzae* b conjugate vaccine (polysaccharide plus outer membrane protein complex of *N meningitidis* B), or Oligo-CRM, *Haemophilus influenzae* b conjugate vaccine (oligosaccharide plus diptheria CRM197 protein).
† Final dose of the vaccine.

## Standards for Pediatric Immunization Practices

The National Vaccine Advisory Committee convened a working group from public and private sector organizations to develop standards for the provision of childhood immunization services. These standards have been approved by the U.S. Public Health Service as national standards and were distributed as such in 1992. They are intended for use by all health professionals administering vaccines and immunization services in the public or the private health care setting. They are presented in Table 24-22.

## Consent and Adverse Events Reporting

Immunization is the backbone of preventive pediatrics, with an efficacy that is perhaps unsurpassed by any other medical intervention. However, vaccination programs are threatened on several fronts, as illustrated by the acute shortage of DTP vaccine that developed in the United States in 1985. The particular crisis was precipitated by the fact that two of the three suppliers stopped producing the vaccine because of rising liability costs. The third suffered temporary technical production problems. As a result, many children had immunization delayed, and the delivery process was significantly disrupted.

A study committee of the Institute of Medicine published an analysis of vaccine supply and innovation in 1986, citing as major problems the decreased number of domestic vaccine manufacturers, which left production concentrated and competition limited; a highly fragmented system for the development and use of vaccines; a compensation system inadequate for providing predictable, timely, and equitable benefits for those few persons with vaccine-related injuries that created a liability situation unfavorable to vaccine producers and forced costs upward; and an underuse of vaccination in general.

The National Childhood Vaccine Injury Act (VICA) was promulgated to obviate some of the problems. With funds from a surcharge on each vaccine dose, a compensation pool was created to provide injury-related payments after adjudication to the parents or guardian of a child who experiences vaccine-related injury. The Act resolved some of the problems that threaten the immunization effort without making the cost of vaccines prohibitive in the short term. Mandated childhood vaccines covered under VICA, which became effective in 1988, include diphtheria, tetanus, pertussis, poliovirus, measles, mumps, and rubella. Under the specifications of the act, the providers of the vaccine are required to record in the patient's record the date of vaccine administration, the manufacturer and lot number of the vaccine, and the name, address, and title of the person administering the vaccine. The vaccine, date, and provider should also be recorded in a patient-held vaccination record.

Parents should be made aware of their right to request compensation for adverse events attributable to vaccine administration. Adverse events known to the health care provider should be reported to the Vaccine Adverse Event Reporting System (VAERS) on special forms. The toll-free number for VAERS is 1-800-822-7967. Reportable events include those listed in this chapter and any listed under the "contraindications" section of the manufacturer's vaccine package insert. VAERS accepts adverse event reports for vaccines other than those covered by VICA. Adverse events should be reported to the local health department as well.

The U.S. Public Health Service has prepared booklets for parents about each of the vaccines covered under VICA. The content of the booklets was specified by VICA and is quite comprehensive. The booklets should be provided to the parent and used as part of the informed consent procedure. Consent should be recorded in the patient's chart. Information about vaccines not covered under VICA may be available from the Academy of Pediatrics or from the CDC. Informed consent from the parent or guardian and assent from the older child should be obtained for the administration of all vaccines. Preventive pediatrics should be viewed by the pediatrician as a cooperative effort between the family and the health care provider.

In addition to supporting measures that continue vaccine innovation, production, and supply, pediatricians must continue to emphasize publicly and in their practices the importance of immunization of the nation's children.

| TABLE 24-22. Standards for Pediatric Immunization Practices From the National Vaccine Advisory Committee, 1992 | |
|---|---|
| Standard 1. | Immunization services are readily available. |
| Standard 2. | There are no barriers or unnecessary prerequisites to the receipt of vaccines. |
| Standard 3. | Immunization services are available free or for a minimal fee. |
| Standard 4. | Providers use all clinical encounters to screen and, if indicated, immunize children. |
| Standard 5. | Providers educate parents and guardians about immunization in general terms. |
| Standard 6. | Providers question parents or guardians about contraindications and, before immunizing a child, inform them in specific terms about the risks and benefits of the immunizations their child is to receive. |
| Standard 7. | Providers follow only true contraindications. |
| Standard 8. | Providers administer simultaneously all vaccine doses for which a child is eligible at the time of each visit. |
| Standard 9. | Providers use accurate and complete recording procedures. |
| Standard 10. | Providers co-schedule immunization appointments in conjunction with appointments for other child health services. |
| Standard 11. | Providers report adverse events following immunization promptly, accurately and completely. |
| Standard 12. | Providers operate a tracking system. |
| Standard 13. | Providers adhere to appropriate procedures for vaccine management. |
| Standard 14. | Providers conduct semiannual audits to assess immunization coverage levels and to review immunization records in the patient populations they serve. |
| Standard 15. | Providers maintain up-to-date, easily retrievable medical protocols at all locations where vaccines are administered. |
| Standard 16. | Providers operate with patient-oriented and community-based approaches. |
| Standard 17. | Vaccines are administered by properly trained individuals. |
| Standard 18. | Providers receive ongoing education and training on current immunization recommendations. |

## IMMUNIZATION FOR CHILDHOOD DISEASES

### Diphtheria

#### Susceptibility

Infants born of mothers immune to diphtheria are relatively immune, but this passive protection is usually lost in the first half year of life and does not prevent active immunization of 2-month-old children. Although long-lasting immunity can be induced by administering diphtheria toxoid, it is not lifelong. Natural infection is now uncommon and is an unlikely source of resistance. Serum antibody level surveys of United States adults suggest that at least 40% are susceptible. At particularly high risk are health workers, and their immunizations should not be allowed to lapse. Immunization protects against systemic disease that is caused by the exotoxin, but it does not prevent nasopharyngeal infection. Even the disease does not reliably confer immunity, and active immunization with toxoid should be initiated during convalescence.

## Active Immunization

Active immunization against the manifestations of diphtheria infection is usually achieved with diphtheria toxoid combined with tetanus toxoid and pertussis bacterial vaccine (DTP). A preparation combining the toxoids with acellular pertussis vaccine (DTaP) may be given as doses four and five. Also available are DT (ie, diphtheria and tetanus toxoid without pertussis) and Td (ie, tetanus toxoid and diphtheria toxoid at reduced concentration); Td is used in older children (after the seventh birthday in the United States) and adults. All preparations are injected intramuscularly because they contain adjuvant.

Although use of the triple vaccine is common, countries differ in the recommended age at which immunization is initiated, the interval between doses, the number of doses considered necessary for completing a primary series, and the age at which DTP is replaced by Td. In some countries, diphtheria and tetanus toxoids are combined with inactivated polio virus vaccine (IPV).

The initial three doses of DTP vaccine are given (unless pertussis vaccine is contraindicated) to infants in the United States at 2-month intervals, with the first dose given at about 2 months of age. Current evidence supports initiating the series at 2 months of age, even for infants born prematurely. A fourth dose is given at 15 or 18 months to complete the primary series. A fifth dose, considered a booster, is administered before the child starts kindergarten or first grade (ie, 4 to 6 years of age). Diphtheria toxoid is given in a reduced dose and combined with tetanus toxoid as Td after the seventh birthday. A booster dose of Td should be administered every 10 years throughout the life span to maintain adequate protection.

For a variety of reasons, immunization does not proceed on schedule for some persons. Additional guidelines are needed to govern diphtheria immunization in these cases (Table 24-23).

If a child older than 2 months but younger than 7 years has received no prior doses of DTP, immunization is initiated with three doses given at intervals of at least 4 weeks (usually 2 months); a fourth dose is given 6 to 12 months after the third and, if the child is not yet 4 years of age at the time of the fourth dose, a fifth or booster dose is given when the child is between 4 and 6 years of age. If the fourth dose of the primary series is given after the fourth birthday, no booster is needed. The next immunization is given 10 years later.

If an infant in the United States has a neurologic disorder that may preclude or delay pertussis immunization, diphtheria and tetanus toxoids may be deferred briefly, because it is extremely unlikely that an infant in this country will develop these diseases. However, the primary immunizing series should begin with DTP or DT as soon as the situation is clarified and not later than 12 months of age, when ambulation makes the risk of acquiring tetanus higher.

If pertussis vaccine is contraindicated, an infant should be immunized according to the same schedule, but with DT instead of DTP.

If an unimmunized child who should not receive pertussis vaccine is 1 year of age or older but younger than 7 years, two doses of DT are given approximately 2 months apart, a third is

TABLE 24-23.  Diphtheria, Pertussis, and Tetanus Immunization of U.S. Children

| Age at Presentation for the Initiation of the Series* | Candidacy for Pertussis Vaccine | Primary Series | Boosters |
|---|---|---|---|
| Early infancy | No contraindication | Initiate at age of 2 mo; give 3 doses of DTP at 2-mo intervals and a fourth dose as DTaP or DTP at 15 (or 18) mo | Give 1 dose of DTaP or DTP between ages 4 and 6 before child starts school. Follow with Td at 10-y intervals. |
| Older than 2 mo but younger than 7 y | No contraindication | Initiate at earliest convenience with 3 doses of DTP given at intervals of at least 4 wk and a fourth dose DTaP or DTP 6 to 12 mo later. | Give a fifth dose as dTaP or DTP between ages 4 and 6 unless the fourth dose was given after the fourth birthday. Follow the "preschool" dose with Td at 10-y intervals. |
| Early infancy | May have contraindication; situation likely to become clearer with passage of time | In areas where risk of tetanus in infancy is low, may delay initiation of primary series for a limited time. A decision should be made and a DTP or DT series initiated by about the first birthday. | |
| Early infancy | Contraindicated | Initiate at age 2 mo, give 3 doses of DT at 2-mo intervals and a fourth dose at 15 (or 18) mo | Give 1 dose of DT between ages 4 and 6 before child starts school. Follow with Td at 10-y intervals. |
| 1 y or more, but younger than 7 y | Contraindicated | Initiate series at earliest convenience with 2 doses of DT given 2 mo apart and give a third dose 6 to 12 mo later. | Give a fourth dose between ages 4 and 6 unless the third dose was given after the fourth birthday. Follow with Td at 10-y intervals. |
| 7 y or older | Persons 7 y or older not given pertussis vaccine | Initiate series at earliest convenience with 2 doses of Td given 1 to 2 mo apart and give a third dose 6 to 12 mo later. | Follow third dose with Td at 10-y intervals. |

* If interval between doses is extended, complete the series without beginning again. DTP, DT, and Td can each be given at the same visit as OPV, IPV, Hib conjugate, HBVV, and MMR. Total doses of D or T should not exceed 6 before the seventh birthday.

given 6 to 12 months later, and a fourth dose between 4 and 6 years of age, unless the third dose was given after the fourth birthday. Persons 7 years of age or older should not receive pertussis vaccine and receive a lower dose of diphtheria toxoid. Primary immunization against diphtheria and tetanus is accomplished with two doses of Td given 1 to 2 months apart and a third dose 6 to 12 months later.

All diphtheria toxoid preparations can be given concurrently with OPV, IPV, HbCV, HBVV, or MMR. After the seventh birthday, only Td is given if diphtheria or tetanus toxoid is indicated. Td contains fewer flocculating units of diphtheria toxoid per dose (not more than 2 Lf) than DT or DTP (7 to 25 Lf) and is less likely in older persons to cause adverse reactions.

Persons who require tetanus toxoid for wound management should be given the combined vaccine preparation appropriate for age to help ensure continued immunity to diphtheria.

Extra doses of DTP may be administered to a child whose series was begun with DT but who belatedly became a candidate for pertussis vaccine to ensure adequate protection against pertussis, because monovalent pertussis vaccine is not commercially available. However, in no event should a child receive more than six doses of diphtheria and tetanus toxoid before the fourth birthday.

### Adverse Reactions

Local reactions are common after immunization with preparations combining diphtheria and tetanus toxoids without and with pertussis vaccine. Systemic reactions are reported more rarely after DTP, DT, and Td doses. IgE antibodies against diphtheria and tetanus toxoids have been found in some patients with systemic reactions. Because pertussis vaccine is more commonly implicated, these reactions are discussed further in the pertussis section of this chapter.

Adverse reactions are diminished by the use of acetaminophen during the hours immediately after vaccination. The incidence of various reactions after DTP administration is summarized in Table 24-24. Certain serious adverse events occurring in an interval after, but not necessarily caused by, vaccination are to be reported under VICA. In the case of preparations containing diphtheria toxoid, reportable events include anaphylaxis or anaphylactic shock within 24 hours (DTP, DT, Td), encephalopathy within 3 days (DTP, DT, Td), shock–collapse or hypotonic-hyporesponsive collapse within 3 days (DTP), a residual seizure disorder (DTP, DT, Td), or any complication of one of these reactions, including death.

### Contraindication

The only absolute contraindication to the administration of diphtheria toxoid is a previous systemic hypersensitivity to the vaccine or a vaccine component. In addition to the toxoids (and pertussis vaccine in the case of DTP), the preparations may contain a small amount of a mercury preservative.

### Postexposure Prophylaxis

A person exposed to diphtheria by household or habitual close contact with a patient should, in addition to being cultured and receiving antibiotic prophylaxis, be given the age-appropriate preparation of toxoid (ie, DTP, DT, or Td) if a dose is due or 5 years or more have elapsed since the last dose. If unimmunized, a dose should be given to initiate active immunization.

### Passive Immunization

Diphtheria equine antitoxin can be obtained through the CDC Drug Service, and because of the severity of the disease, it is administered if diphtheria is strongly suspected without waiting for culture confirmation. No antitoxin of human origin is available in the United States. After tests to rule out hypersensitivity to

**TABLE 24-24.   Reaction Rates in the 48 Hours After Immunization with DTP**

| Reactions | Occurrence/Doses |
|---|---|
| **Local Reactions** | |
| Pain | 1/2 |
| Swelling | 1/2.5 |
| Redness | 1/2.8 |
| **Common Systemic Reactions** | |
| Fretfulness | 1/1.9 |
| Fever of 38.3°C or more | 1/2.2 |
| Drowsiness | 1/3.2 |
| Anorexia | 1/5 |
| **Less Common Systemic Reactions** | |
| Vomiting | 1/16 |
| Persistent crying | 1/32 |
| **Reactions Contraindicating Further Doses** | |
| Crying for 3 or more hours | 1/100 |
| Fever of 40.5°C or more | 1/330 |
| Convulsion | 1/1750 |
| Hypotonic-hyporesponsive episode | 1/1750 |
| Encephalopathy | 1/110,000 |
| Permanent brain damage* | 1/310,000 |

\* Based on the most recent analyses of available data, the Committee on Infectious Diseaes of the AAP has concluded that pertussis vaccine has not been shown to be a cause of brain damage.

(Occurrence estimates are from Cody CL, Baraff LJ, Cherry JD, Marcy SM, Manclark, CR. Nature and rates of adverse reactions associated with DPT and DT immunizations in infants and children. Pediatrics 1981;68:650 and Miller DL, Ross EM, Alderslade R, Bellman MH, Rawson NSB. Pertussis immunisation and serious neurological illness in children. Br Med J 1981;282:1595.)

equine serum, a single dose of the diphtheria antitoxin is administered intravenously or intramuscularly. The dose range is wide, from 20,000 to 100,000 U, and it must be estimated from the clinical situation. An infectious disease specialist should be consulted. The AAP Committee on Infectious Diseases makes the following suggestions:

Pharyngeal or laryngeal disease of 48 hours' duration: 20,000 to 40,000 U
Nasopharyngeal lesions: 40,000 to 60,000 U
Extensive disease of 3 or more days' duration or with brawny swelling of the neck: 80,000 to 100,000 U.

Administration of antitoxin does not preclude active immunization, which should begin during convalescence because disease does not always confer immunity.

## Tetanus

### Susceptibility

All unimmunized persons are susceptible, and all are candidates for active immunization with tetanus toxoid. Active immunization results in protection that persists for at least 10 years, and booster doses after complete immunization confer continued high levels of immunity. Transient immunity follows administration of human tetanus immune globulin (TIG) and of equine tetanus antitoxin (TAT). Persons who have recovered from the disease are not reliably immune and are candidates for active immunization.

### Active Immunization

Tetanus toxoid as a single immunizing agent (T) is available in fluid preparation and as an adsorbed aluminum salt that produces longer-lasting immunity. However, in most situations, tetanus toxoid should be presented in combination with other immunizing agents. Tetanus toxoid adsorbed is combined with diphtheria toxoid in high-dose (DT) or low-dose (Td) formulations, combined with tetanus toxoid in high-dose and whole-cell pertussis vaccine (DTP), and combined with diphtheria toxoid in high-dose and acellular pertussis vaccine (DTaP). The preparations that include pertussis vaccine are used for primary immunization and booster doses for children younger than 7 years of age who have no specific contraindications. All should be injected intramuscularly.

The recommended schedule for active immunization against tetanus in the United States is the same as that recommended for diphtheria (see Table 24-23). Infants receive three doses at 2-month intervals, usually at 2, 4, and 6 months of age. A fourth dose is administered 6 to 12 months after the third, usually at 15 or 18 months of age, and a fifth or first booster dose at school entry between the ages of 4 and 6 years. A booster should be given as Td every 10 years thereafter.

Neonatal tetanus can be prevented by immunizing the mother before the baby's birth. Tetanus toxoid is not contraindicated during pregnancy. A previously unimmunized pregnant woman should receive two doses of tetanus toxoid at least 1 month apart, with the second dose to be administered at least 2 weeks and preferably 1 month before delivery. Primary immunization should then be completed with a third dose 6 to 12 months later and should not be deferred even if the woman is pregnant again. Pregnant women who were immunized more than 10 years before pregnancy should receive a booster dose of tetanus toxoid. Women are often reluctant to be immunized during pregnancy, and not all women, particularly those whose babies are likely to be born at home, receive prenatal care. Increased efforts to ensure that all young women are adequately immunized before pregnancy may be required. The complete elimination of neonatal tetanus is a sound and achievable goal.

### Adverse Reactions

Local reactions are common and systemic reactions occur, but much more rarely after DTP, DTaP, DT, and Td doses. IgE antibodies against diphtheria and tetanus toxoids have been found in some patients with systemic reactions. Because pertussis vaccine is more commonly implicated, these reactions are discussed more fully in the pertussis section of this chapter. Adverse reactions are diminished by the use of acetaminophen during the hours immediately after vaccination. The incidence of various reactions after DTP administration is summarized in Table 24-24.

Certain serious adverse events occurring in an interval after, but not necessarily caused by, vaccination are to be reported under the VICA. In the case of preparations containing tetanus toxoid, reportable events include anaphylaxis or anaphylactic shock within 24 hours (DTP, DT, Td), encephalopathy within 3 days (DTP, DT, Td), shock–collapse or hypotonic-hyporesponsive collapse within 3 days (DTP), a residual seizure disorder (DTP, DT, Td), or any complication of these reactions, including death.

### Contraindications

The only absolute contraindication to the administration of tetanus toxoid is a previous systemic hypersensitivity response to a vaccine component. In addition to the toxoids (and pertussis vaccine in the case of DTP), the preparations may contain a small amount of a mercury preservative.

### Postexposure Prophylaxis

A dose of tetanus toxoid is not necessary as part of wound management for persons with clean, minor wounds who have completed a primary series of tetanus toxoid and for whom fewer than 10 years have elapsed since the last dose. If a person who has received fewer than three doses of tetanus toxoid sustains a wound, a dose of tetanus toxoid should be administered as DTP, DTaP, DT, or Td, depending on age and indications, and the series should be completed in a timely fashion.

If a more serious wound is sustained by a previously immunized person (eg, puncture wound, avulsion, burn, frostbite, missile wound, crush wound) or a wound is contaminated with dirt, soil, human or animal feces, or saliva, a booster dose of tetanus toxoid as DT or Td should be administered if 5 years have elapsed since the last dose. If a child younger than 7 years of age with a wound meets the 5-year criterion, she or he is by definition inadequately immunized and should, unless it is specifically contraindicated, receive tetanus toxoid in the form of DTP. Adequacy of immunization against other childhood diseases should be addressed.

### Passive Immunization

Passive immunization to prevent neonatal tetanus through immunization of the mother has been discussed. Serotherapy with TIG is also part of wound management.

Persons who have sustained clean, minor wounds should not receive tetanus antibody products whether or not they have been previously immunized. The only candidates for serotherapy are inadequately immunized persons with more serious wounds. Persons who have had three or more previous injections of tetanus toxoid do not need tetanus antitoxin, even for serious wounds.

Persons with serious wounds who have had fewer than three previous injections of tetanus toxoid should receive TIG at a dose of 250 to 500 U injected intramuscularly. If TIG is not available, after screening and testing for sensitivity, equine TAT is given intramuscularly at a dose of 3000 to 5000 U. It should rarely, if ever, be necessary to use TAT in the United States. With consultation from an infectious disease specialist, IVIG may be considered as an alternative (Lee, 1992). The administration of an antibody product does not eliminate the indication for immunization with toxoid. Both should be given, but in separate syringes into separate sites. Larger doses of TIG or TAT are given as part of treatment of established disease with antibiotics, wound management, and supportive care.

## Pertussis

### Susceptibility

Pertussis is highly communicable, and as many as 90% of nonimmune household contacts become infected. Unlike many other childhood diseases, there is no clear evidence that passive protection is conferred transplacentally.

Many cases are mild and undiagnosed. Infection results in prolonged immunity, but second cases occur, and cases in adolescents and adults suggest that many are incompletely immunized or that vaccine-induced immunity wanes. Because the pertussis syndrome is mimicked clinically by other infectious agents, only culture-proven disease, not a pertussis-like illness, obviates the need for immunization.

The pertussis components of vaccines available in the United States are of two types. Whole-cell pertussis vaccines (P) are prepared from disrupted or otherwise inactivated *Bordetella pertussis* bacteria. Acellular pertussis vaccines (aP) contain one or more bacterial components. Both are combined with diphtheria and tetanus toxoids as DTP or DTaP. The purpose for developing acellular pertussis vaccines was to decrease the rate of adverse reactions associated with immunization against pertussis while retaining immunogenicity and efficacy.

Whole-cell pertussis vaccine is associated with an efficacy of about 80% after three doses, and immunity lasts at least 3 years. Infection of the immunized person results in mild disease.

Acellular pertussis vaccines have been routinely administered in Japan since 1981 to children 2 years of age or older and to some children beginning at 3 months of age since 1989. Disease rates have declined, but questions remain about whether acellular vaccines are associated with acceptable efficacy if given during infancy and whether they confer immunity comparable to that associated with whole-cell vaccine at any age.

One acellular pertussis vaccine, Acel-Imune, was licensed in the United States in December 1991. The pertussis component is largely composed of filamentous hemagglutinin, but it also includes smaller amounts of inactivated pertussis toxin, the outer membrane protein pertactin, and an agglutinogen, fimbriae type 2. This DTaP is licensed only for use as a fourth or fifth dose of pertussis in children who are at least 15 months but younger than 7 years of age who have had at least three doses of whole-cell pertussis vaccine. It is preferred as the fourth and fifth doses because of its lower rate of adverse reactions. It cannot be substituted for whole-cell vaccine if whole-cell pertussis vaccine is considered contraindicated.

Five intramuscular doses of pertussis vaccine are recommended. Immunization should begin with DTP at about 2 months of age, with doses two and three following at 2-month intervals. Although diphtheria and tetanus are extremely unlikely in infants in the United States, pertussis is much more likely, making early initiation of immunization highly desirable. During outbreaks, pertussis immunization can begin as early as 2 to 4 weeks of age, and the first three doses can be given at 4-week intervals. Customary practice is to give the three doses (with other vaccines) at health supervision visits at 2, 4, and 6 months of age. A "reinforcing" dose is given at 15 to 18 months. It may be DTaP or DTP; DTaP is now preferred, because of the lower rate of adverse reactions. Unless the fourth dose was administered after 4 years of age, a fifth or booster dose of DTaP or DTP is administered at 4 to 6 years of age. Although complications of the disease are less likely at that age, maintaining immunity prevents the passage of pertussis from school-aged children to infant contacts. DTaP is preferred, and DTaP is strongly recommended for the fourth and fifth doses for children who have a personal or family history of seizures but have no contraindication for pertussis immunization.

The recommended immunization schedule in various circumstances is summarized in Table 24-18. If the schedule is for some reason interrupted, it is resumed where left off, not restarted. Pertussis vaccine is not usually administered to persons who are 7 or older, even if they have not received the recommended number of doses, because the risk of complications from the disease at that age is low and because adverse reactions to the vaccine are more common. The inadequately immunized older child's schedule is completed with Td.

Children initially immunized with DT who become eligible for pertussis immunization may have extra doses of pertussis vaccine combined with diphtheria and tetanus toxoids to complete the recommended number of pertussis doses. They should not, however, have more than six diphtheria or tetanus doses before the fourth birthday. Children who have recovered from culture-proven pertussis disease do not need to be immunized.

Before the administration of each dose of pertussis (and of all multidose vaccines), the parent should be asked if there were any adverse reactions after the previous dose or doses.

## Adverse Reactions

Local reactions at the site of injection (ie, redness, swelling, induration, tenderness, apparent pain) are common after pertussis vaccination (see Table 24-24). The frequency increases with increasing numbers of doses. Bacterial abscess indicates contamination of the preparation or inadequate procedure. Bacterial or sterile abscesses from the site of injection occur after six to ten of one million doses. Generalized symptoms, such as fever,

drowsiness, irritability, persistent crying, decreased appetite, and vomiting, are fairly commonly observed within hours of vaccination, but they resolve rapidly. Children who display these local or systemic symptoms with one dose are more likely to display them with subsequent doses.

Administration of acetaminophen (15 mg/kg/dose) at the time of DTP vaccination and at 4 and 8 hours afterward decreases the incidence of common local and systemic reactions, including fever. The ACIP recommends the use of acetaminophen at the time of vaccination and every 4 hours for 24 hours for children with a personal or family history of convulsions. Prophylaxis is recommended for children with a personal history of convulsions if the decision is made to administer DTP.

Local and mild generalized symptoms do not preclude additional doses. These appear to be less frequent with the acellular vaccines. Adverse reactions of children receiving the licensed DTaP as a fourth or fifth dose have been compared with those of children receiving a whole-cell vaccine for the same doses. Local reactions and common systemic reactions with DTaP appear to be 25% to 75% as frequent as with whole-cell vaccine, varying with the specific reaction. Although studies have not been large enough to fairly compare all serious systemic reactions, there is no evidence that they occur more frequently than with DTP. Most investigators expect them to occur somewhat less frequently. DTaP should not be administered if DTP is contraindicated; DT should be used.

Severe adverse events associated with pertussis vaccine are uncommon or rare (see Table 24-24). These include high fever, brief convulsions associated with fever, persistent ($\geq$ 3 hours) or unusual cry, and collapse with a shocklike (hypotonic-hyporesponsive) state. Other attributed associations, such as encephalopathy, "brain damage," onset of seizure disorder, infantile spasms, and sudden infant death syndrome, appear on close study to be temporally rather than etiologically associated. The risk of catastrophe in infancy from the disease, particularly if immunization rates wane, appears to be much greater than from the vaccine. Certain serious adverse events occurring in an interval after, but not necessarily caused by, vaccination are to be reported under the VICA. In the case of preparations containing pertussis vaccine, reportable events include anaphylaxis or anaphylactic shock within 24 hours, encephalopathy within 3 days, shock-collapse or hypotonic-hyporesponsive collapse within 3 days, residual seizure disorder, or any complication of these reactions, including death.

## Contraindications

Children who have a disorder characterized by progressive developmental or neurologic deterioration should not receive pertussis vaccine. Examples include infantile spasms, uncontrolled epilepsy, progressive encephalopathy, and tuberous sclerosis. After the child's condition has stabilized, pertussis immunization can be considered.

If the neurologic status of a child is uncertain, DTP immunization can be deferred several months until the situation is clarified. Included in this category are children who have recently had seizures, because they have an increased risk of seizures associated with fever after pertussis vaccination. Those whose seizures are well controlled or who are unlikely to seize again may be immunized. Antipyresis should be emphasized. The decision to undertake primary immunization with DTP or DT should be made by the first birthday when the risk of tetanus increases.

Children with cerebral palsy or developmental delay that is not progressive or associated with a predisposition to seizures should receive DTP. A family history of seizures, sudden infant death syndrome, or DTP reaction is not a contraindication.

Future doses of pertussis vaccine should not be administered if any of the following occurred after an administered dose:

Encephalopathy within 7 days

A convulsion with or without fever within 3 days

Persistent, unconsolable screaming or crying for 3 or more hours or an unusual, high-pitched cry within 48 hours

Collapse or shocklike state within 48 hours

Fever of 40.5 °C (104.9 °F) or greater, unexplained by another cause, within 48 hours

An immediate severe allergic or anaphylactic reaction to the vaccine.

### Postexposure Prophylaxis

Immunization and antibiotic prophylaxis should be considered for children younger than 7 years of age exposed to pertussis by close contact with a sick patient at home or in day care. Children who have had fewer than four doses of pertussis vaccine, who have not yet met usual age criteria for dose four but for whom 6 months or more have elapsed since dose three, or for whom 3 years or more have elapsed since dose four all should receive a dose of pertussis vaccine. If the child has already received at least three doses of whole-cell pertussis vaccine and is at least 15 months old, the postexposure dose can be DTP or DTaP.

## Polio

### Susceptibility

Unimmunized persons who have not had asymptomatic infections are susceptible to polio infection. Lifelong but type-specific immunity is conferred by recognized and asymptomatic infection. Second attacks are due to infection with a second of the three poliovirus types. Immune mothers pass transient passive immunity to the paralytic disease to their infants.

Although susceptibility to infection is universal, paralytic disease is rare. It is more common with increasing age at infection and during pregnancy, and it appears to develop where tissues have been recently damaged.

### Active Immunization

Two types of poliovirus vaccines are available: inactivated poliovirus vaccine (IPV) and oral poliovirus vaccine (OPV). Both are trivalent, immunizing against all three poliovirus types, and both prevent poliomyelitis.

IPV became available first, but is currently recommended only when OPV is contraindicated. It is prepared from poliovirus seed strains by formalin inactivation. Potency varied until 1968, when minimum potency requirements were established by the government for use in the United States. An enhanced-potency IPV, prepared in human diploid cell culture, is the product now in use. Seroconversion rates are comparable to those induced by OPV. Ninety percent or more of children have antibody to all three poliovirus types after three doses. Newer methods enabled the production of inactivated vaccines of even higher potency than those licensed in the United States. These IPVs are more immunogenic than OPV (McBean and Modlin, 1987), with more than 99% of children possessing antibody to all three types of poliovirus after two doses of vaccine.

Preparation of the oral vaccine involved multiple passages in monkey kidney cell culture and the selection of mutants of low virulence for primates. More than 90% of infants have antibody to all three poliovirus types after two OPV doses, and a third dose ensures antibody prevalence of at least 97% to type I, the type least immunogenic but most likely to cause outbreaks. OPV became available in the early 1960s and soon became the preferred vaccine, with touted advantages including superior protection, ease of administration, induction of gastrointestinal immunity, lower cost, and spread of the attenuated virus from the feces of the immunized to indirectly immunize others in the population.

Although considerable controversy has surrounded the decision, fueled by the fact that most cases of paralytic polio in the United States are now caused by the vaccine viruses, an Institute of Medicine study group in 1977 and 1988 recommended that OPV remain the vaccine of choice in the United States. The recommendation was approved by the ACIP and the Committee on Infectious Diseases of the AAP. However, when IPV in combination with DTP is licensed, decreasing the number of needed injections, new recommendations suggesting sequential use are expected. The recommendations may be for polio immunization to be accomplished with two or three doses of IPV/DTP followed by three or two doses of OPV. This combination would have the advantage of eliminating most cases of vaccine-related paralytic polio in recipients by producing humoral immunity before presenting live organisms while retaining the advantages of mucosal immunity and possibly improved herd immunity attributed to OPV.

Candidates for immunization with OPV include normal infants and children without immunodeficient or immunosuppressed household contacts who are undergoing the routine schedule of immunizations, inadequately immunized children at risk of exposure, adults at risk of exposure who have had one or more doses of OPV or IPV, and unimmunized adults who are at risk of exposure within 4 weeks. IPV should be offered to immunodeficient infants and children (including those with human immunodeficiency [HIV] antibodies or proven infection), infants and children with immunodeficient or immunosuppressed household contacts, infants and children whose parents have refused OPV, unimmunized adults at risk of exposure, beginning more than 4 weeks from the date of immunization, and adults known to be unimmunized who are in close contact with a child who receives OPV and may excrete polio vaccine virus.

The recommended schedule for immunizing a normal infant against polio in the United States is to administer two doses of OPV in early infancy, the first when the infant is 2 months old and the second after an interval of at least 6 weeks. Common practice is to administer the first two doses at the same visits as the first two doses of DTP at 2 and 4 months. A third dose of OPV is given between 12 and 24 months, usually concurrently with the fourth dose of DTP, at 15 months with MMR, or at 18 months. The primary series of three doses is then complete. A booster dose is given at the time of school entry, between the ages of 4 and 6. Multiple doses produce immunity to all three types of poliovirus.

If the risk of contracting wild-type virus is high, an additional dose is inserted into the primary series at least 6 weeks after the second dose, at about 6 months, usually concurrently with the third DTP. In endemic areas, an extra dose of OPV may be given at the time of newborn hospital discharge, with a complete primary series of three doses undertaken beginning at 2 months of age.

Children not immunized in the first year of life should receive two doses of OPV 6 to 8 weeks apart. A third dose should be given 6 to 12 months later, unless the risk of exposure is high, in which case the third dose may follow the second as closely as 6 weeks. A fourth dose is given at school entry, between 4 and 6 years of age, unless the third dose came after the fourth birthday. The schedule for administration of IPV is the same as for OPV. Doses are injected subcutaneously. Booster doses of IPV were recommended every 5 years, but are not considered necessary for recipients of IPV. Children who are found to be partially immunized should have the series completed. It does not need to be restarted. OPV and IPV may be administered at the same visit as any of the other vaccines.

Polio immunization is recommended for previously unvaccinated United States residents who are 18 or older only if they plan to travel to areas where polio is endemic or epidemic, are a member of a community or population that experiences wild-type poliovirus disease, handle laboratory specimens that may contain poliovirus, are in close contact with patients who may excrete poliovirus, or are in prolonged contact (eg, household, day care) with a child or children who may excrete OPV virus.

For unvaccinated adults who qualify for immunization, IPV is preferred to OPV, because adults have a very low but slightly higher risk of developing paralytic disease after OPV than do children. Two doses of IPV are administered at 1- to 2-month intervals, followed by a third dose in 6 to 12 months. If time does not permit giving the first three doses before protection is needed, the following modifications are recommended:

1. If 4 to 8 weeks exist before protection is needed, two doses of IPV are given 4 weeks apart.
2. If fewer than 4 weeks remain before protection is needed, a single dose of OPV is administered.

In both cases, the series should be completed with the initial vaccine if the person remains at risk or foresees future risk. For partially immunized immunocompetent adults at increased risk of exposure, the series is completed with either vaccine, regardless of the time elapsed since the most recent dose. Immunocompromised adults should receive only IPV.

Fully immunized adults who are at increased risk of exposure may be given a dose of OPV, if they have previously completed a primary course of OPV, or a dose of either vaccine, if they previously completed a primary course of IPV.

### Adverse Reactions

Live polio vaccine virus (OPV) rarely causes paralytic polio in a vaccine recipient or the contact of a vaccine recipient. Administration of OPV results in about one case of paralytic polio in a vaccine recipient or contact for every 2.64 million doses distributed. Most cases are among susceptible adult contacts. Beyond identifying households with an immunodeficient or immunocompromised member, no effort to screen for susceptibility (eg, adults who are inadequately immunized) is recommended, because such efforts are likely to delay adequate immunization of the infant. If susceptibility in adult contacts is recognized, they should be informed of the small risk involved. If complete immunization of the infant can be assured, it is acceptable to delay the infant's initial OPV dose until the susceptible adult is receiving the second of two monthly doses of IPV.

No serious side effects of the currently licensed IPV have been recognized. Cases of paralytic polio were attributed to a previous preparation that inadvertently contained infective particles. Current methods of vaccine production and testing are thought to eliminate this possibility completely. The IPV preparation may contain minute amounts of the antibiotics neomycin, streptomycin, and polymyxin B. Theoretically, persons with sensitivity to any one of these may exhibit adverse reactions to the vaccine.

Events reportable to the VAERS after immunization against polio with OPV include paralytic poliomyelitis occurring in an immunocompetent recipient within 30 days, in an immunodeficient recipient within 6 months, or a vaccine-related case in nonrecipient at any time. Also reportable are complications or death due to poliomyelitis. Anaphylaxis or anaphylactic shock within 24 hours of receipt of IPV is a reportable event, as are resulting complications or death.

### Contraindications

There is no convincing evidence that OPV or IPV is a risk during pregnancy for the mother or the fetus, but immunization of the pregnant woman is ordinarily avoided unless specifically indicated because of risk. If immediate protection against polio is needed, OPV may be administered.

Patients with immune states altered by immunodeficiency disease, by malignancy or its therapy, or by pharmacologic doses of corticosteroids should not receive OPV. IPV is safe in these patients, and although adequate protection may or may not ensue, it may be administered.

OPV should be avoided for children who have household contacts of any age with immunodeficiency disease or altered immune status, or who are immunosuppressed. IPV should be used instead, because live vaccine virus may be excreted by the vaccine recipient. OPV should not be given to any members of a family in which there has been a child with primary immunodeficiency disease until immunodeficiency has been excluded in the recipient and other members of the family.

## Measles

### Susceptibility

Infants whose mothers had measles are ordinarily immune for the first 6 to 9 months of life, and infants whose mothers were immunized against measles are protected, but probably for a shorter period. Other persons who have not experienced the disease or been immunized are almost universally susceptible. The disease usually confers lifelong immunity. Unless measles was diagnosed by a physician, an unimmunized young person should be considered susceptible, because lay persons often confuse measles with other rash-causing, febrile diseases. The period of immunity that follows active immunization with live measles vaccine is prolonged, but its exact duration is unknown.

### Active Immunization

Measles vaccines have changed through the years. Early immunization programs were undertaken with killed measles vaccine, which was available in the United States from 1963 through the end of 1967. These vaccines generated two problems. After exposure to natural measles, recipients of killed vaccine occasionally (but much more often than recipients of live measles vaccine) developed a severe and atypical form of measles. Recipients who were later vaccinated with live measles vaccine were prone to develop moderate or severe local reactions. Nevertheless, persons vaccinated before 1968 with killed vaccine or with an unknown vaccine should be revaccinated with live measles virus to prevent atypical measles.

Live measles vaccines made with the Edmonston B strain were available in the United States from 1963 through about 1970. These vaccines were apparently more likely than current vaccines to cause adverse reactions, among them leukopenia, mild thrombocytopenia, and suppression of tuberculin test response. Because the vaccine sometimes produced an illness nearly as severe as wild-type measles, it was originally used with immune serum globulin. The combination produced relatively frequent vaccine failure.

Since 1965, measles virus vaccines prepared in chick embryo cell culture and attenuated beyond the level of the Edmonston strain have been available and have been used exclusively since 1970. These are referred to as "further attenuated" or "more attenuated" (hence, Moraten). They typically produce no illness and rarely produce an illness resembling mild measles.

Live measles vaccines are injected subcutaneously. They are quite labile, with heat and light inactivating the virus. They must be refrigerated, used within hours after reconstitution, and shipped and stored frozen or freeze-dried and cold. These special handling requirements make effective immunization against measles in developing countries, where mortality from measles remains high, problematic.

The recommended age for administration of measles vaccine has changed through time. It has remained 15 months since 1977, but was 12 months from 1965 to 1977 and 9 months from 1963 to 1965. Far too few persons responded and were protected if the vaccine was given before 1 year of age. About 85% developed antibody if the vaccine was administered at 12 months, and 95% developed antibody if given the vaccine at 15 months. Age-specific attack rates after exposure appear higher among those vaccinated at 12 months. Patterns may be changing now that antibody passively transferred from the mother most often represents her response to vaccine rather than natural disease. In the United States, where exposure is relatively unlikely, vaccination at 15 months has been the rule, with vaccination at 12 months recommended in communities with recent measles outbreaks. (During an outbreak, infants as young as 6 months are immunized and then reimmunized at 15 months.) High-dose vaccines intended to produce a lasting protective response at a younger age of administration are being studied in developing countries.

Measles vaccine is available as a single agent (M), in combination with rubella vaccine (MR), and in combination with mumps and rubella (MMR). Unless disease or previous immunization has been documented, the combined vaccine should be used for measles immunization. MMR can be given at the same time as other vaccines without diminished protection or increased adverse reactions.

Measles vaccination is recommended for all susceptible persons 15 months of age or older unless a specific contraindication exists. Persons are considered susceptible unless they have had the disease documented by a physician, have laboratory evidence of immunity, have been immunized with live vaccine on or after the first birthday, or were born before 1957 and are therefore likely to have had natural infection. There exists no evidence to suggest that administration of MMR to a person already immune is harmful.

Recent measles outbreaks demonstrate that measles transmission can occur even among populations in which the vaccination rate is high. Cases during outbreaks can be classified in four categories: unvaccinated persons for whom vaccine was not indicated most often because of young age, unvaccinated persons for whom vaccine was indicated, vaccinated persons who failed to seroconvert, and vaccinated persons who seroconverted after the initial vaccination but did not maintain protective antibody. All four kinds have occurred, emphasizing the need to review the age at which the initial dose of measles vaccine is administered, particularly because antibody passively acquired from an immunized mother may not last as long (nor interfere with primary immunization as many months) as antibody acquired from a mother who had wild-type measles infection. Physicians must work harder to ensure that all children receive measles vaccine as soon as they are age eligible, and all children should receive a second dose of measles vaccine, preferably MMR.

The ACIP and the AAP currently recommend different timing of the second dose. The ACIP, placing their emphasis on early immunization and the practicality of ensuring immunization at school entry, have recommended the second dose at 4 to 6 years of age, before a child enters the primary school system. The AAP, concerned about outbreaks in middle and high school and college, recommends, if the local jurisdiction does not require a second dose at school entry, that it should be administered at 11 or 12 years of age, a strategy that may more quickly decrease outbreaks among older children. A reasonable compromise is to immunize persons at primary school entry and at entry to middle or junior high school until all 11- and 12-year-old children have had two doses because they belong to a cohort immunized at 4 to 6 years of age.

Vaccinating susceptible persons before international travel is especially important, because exposure to disease in other countries accounts for many cases. Finding and vaccinating susceptible adolescents and young adults is important, because outbreaks on campuses account for a significant proportion of remaining cases. Adequate immunity at the time of pregnancy is highly desirable so that passive immunity is conferred to protect the infant during the early months of life, when the risk of complications from the disease is greatest.

## Adverse Reactions

As many as 15% of persons who receive further attenuated measles vaccine develop fever, and about 5% develop a rash resembling mild measles, occurring 4 to 10 days after vaccination and lasting for 2 to 5 days. There is no evidence that reactions are age related. As with other febrile illnesses, seizures may occur. Reactions after the second dose are expected to be even less common, because many recipients are immune.

Encephalopathy associated with measles vaccine has been reported after fewer than one in one million doses. The fact that this is lower than the background incidence of encephalopathy permits the interpretation that at least some of the cases are merely temporally and not etiologically related to measles vaccine.

Subacute sclerosing panencephalitis (SSPE) has been reported in children who have no clinical history of measles but have been immunized, and a linkage between the vaccine and SSPE cannot be ruled out. However, the incidence of SSPE has fallen markedly with the incidence of measles, suggesting that immunization has had an overall protective effect.

Adverse events reportable to the VAERS after measles vaccine administration include anaphylaxis or anaphylactic shock within 24 hours, encephalopathy with onset within 15 days, a residual seizure disorder, or any complication of these reactions, including death.

## Contraindications

Measles vaccine as MR or MMR should not be given to women known to be pregnant or who intend to become pregnant within 3 months. This recommendation is based on theoretic risk of passage of one of the vaccine viruses to the fetus or of spontaneous abortion, not on direct evidence. Pregnancy should be delayed for 30 days after measles monovalent vaccine (M) administration.

Because the vaccine virus is grown in chick embryo cell culture, persons with hypersensitivity to chicken products may have adverse reactions to the vaccine. These usually consist of minor urticarial reactions at the injection site. Extremely rare, potentially life-threatening reactions to the vaccine have occurred in children with a history of anaphylactic reactions to egg ingestion. Persons with such a history should be immunized with extreme caution. Persons with nonanaphylactic reactions to eggs or with reactions to chickens or feathers are not at increased risk for severe reaction and should be vaccinated in the usual manner.

The vaccine contains small amounts of neomycin. A history of contact dermatitis-type reaction to neomycin does not contraindicate measles vaccination; a history of anaphylactic reaction to topically or systemically administered neomycin does.

Persons who recently have received immunoglobulin, whole blood, or another antibody-containing product may not adequately respond to immunization because of passively acquired antibody. Vaccination should be deferred for 3 to 10 months depending on the dose of IgG the product is estimated to have contained (Siber, 1993).

Tuberculosis may be exacerbated by natural measles infection but apparently not by the vaccine virus, and lack of knowledge of tuberculin status should not preclude vaccination. Measles vaccine may suppress reactivity to tuberculin tests placed during the next 4 to 6 weeks, and if tuberculin testing is indicated, it should be placed on the day of vaccination.

Immunocompromised persons, with the exception of those with HIV infection, should not receive measles vaccine. However, persons vaccinated with live measles vaccine do not transmit the vaccine virus to others, and the presence of immunocompromised household contacts should not prevent vaccination. Immunization is indicated to protect the recipient and to prevent the recipient from contracting natural infection and exposing the contact. Unimmunized children with HIV infection, even symptomatic infection, should receive measles vaccine (MMR) because fatal cases of measles have occurred in HIV patients, but no complications of MMR immunization have been reported.

The timing of immunization after the completion of immunosuppressive therapy must take into consideration the type of therapy, the disease for which it was given, and the likely interval over which immunocompetence is regained. The delay should not be shorter than 3 months.

After exposure, vaccination within 72 hours may be protective. Infants as young as 6 months may receive monovalent measles vaccine (M) or MMR if that is all that is available. Unimmunized exposed persons 12 months of age or older should receive MMR within 72 hours of exposure. Immunization plays a major role in outbreak control.

### Passive Immunization

If exposure is recognized within 72 hours, the exposed person should be vaccinated in most instances. However, if exposure occurred within 6 days but more than 72 hours before recognition, immunoglobulin must be used because the interval is too short to provide protection through active immunization. Immunoglobulin given within 6 days of exposure may prevent or modify the severity of the disease. The dose (0.25 mL/kg to a maximum of 15 mL for immunocompetent recipients and 0.5 mL/kg to a maximum of 15 mL for immunocompromised recipients) is administered intramuscularly. Particular consideration to providing passive antibody prophylaxis after exposure should be give to candidates who are household contacts younger than 1 year of age, household contacts who are young or pregnant and have asymptomatic HIV infection and are susceptible, and for children and adolescents with symptomatic HIV infection regardless of immunization history. Patients who regularly receive intravenous immunoglobulin should receive adequate postexposure prophylaxis from their usual dose of 100 to 400 mg/kg of intravenous immunoglobulin if it has been given in the prior 3 weeks. Active immunization should be delayed 3 months after administration of immunoglobulin, but it then should be administered promptly to HIV-infected and healthy children if they have reached the age of at least 12 months.

## Mumps

### Susceptibility

After infection, immunity is generally lifelong. Most adults can be considered immune through natural infection, even if they have no history of clinical disease, because the incidence of inapparent infection is high.

### Active Immunization

Immunization in the United States with live attenuated mumps vaccine began in 1967. No monovalent mumps vaccine is commercially available in the United States. The vaccine available is prepared from the Jeryl Lynn strain grown in chick embryo cell culture and is in combination with measles and rubella vaccines (MMR). Mumps vaccine is injected subcutaneously, producing protective, long-lasting immunity in more than 95% of recipients.

Mumps vaccine, delivered as MMR, is recommended for routine immunization of all children at 15 months unless there are specific contraindications. The timing is chosen to produce the best conversion rate to the measles component. Mumps vaccine itself can be administered any time after 1 year of age. Many children will receive a second dose of mumps vaccine if their second dose of measles vaccine is delivered as MMR.

MMR can be administered even if a patient is known to be immune to one of the three diseases. Adverse reactions because of existing immunity do not appear to take place. Special effort should be exerted to ensure immunization before the onset of puberty. Documentation of immunization after the first birthday or physician-diagnosed disease is required to ensure immunity. Immunization is not routinely advised for adults, because immunity from natural infection is likely. Studies suggest that about 90% of adults are immune.

MMR can be given at the same visit as DTP and OPV without compromising antibody response and without increasing adverse reactions. Separate injection sites should be used. Although administration at the same time as other vaccines has not been well studied, problems are not anticipated. Persons who recently have received immunoglobulin, whole blood, or another antibody-containing product may not adequately respond to immunization because of passively acquired antibody, and vaccination should be deferred for 3 months.

### Adverse Reactions

Fever occurs in about 5% of recipients of mumps vaccine, but other adverse reactions are rare. Because their incidence is below that expected for the age-specific population at large, central nervous system events that are temporally associated do not appear to be etiologically associated. Orchitis is reported rarely.

Adverse events reportable to the VAERS after mumps vaccine administration include anaphylaxis or anaphylactic shock within 24 hours, encephalopathy with onset within 15 days, a residual seizure disorder, or any complication of these reactions, including death.

### Contraindications

Patients with acute febrile illnesses should have mumps vaccine delayed until recovery.

Although mumps vaccine virus has not been isolated from fetal tissues, the virus can cross the placenta. Because of the theoretic risk, women should not be immunized during pregnancy and should be counseled to avoid pregnancy for 3 months after administration of the vaccine.

Allergic reactions have been reported rarely. Because the vaccine virus is grown in chick embryo cell culture, hypersensitivity reactions are possible in patients allergic to eggs. Live mumps vaccine (MMR) should be administered only with extreme caution to persons who have exhibited anaphylactic reactions to eggs. The contraindications are those discussed for measles vaccine.

Mumps vaccine and MMR contain trace amounts of neomycin. Persons with a previous history of anaphylactic reaction to neomycin should not receive them.

Patients who have immunodeficiency disease or are receiving or have recently received immunosuppressive therapy, except children with HIV infection (who should receive MMR), should not receive mumps or any other live viral vaccine. After immunosuppressive therapy is withdrawn, the vaccine is not administered for at least 3 months. Longer intervals may be indicated, depending on expected immunologic recovery from the specific disease or agent involved. Mumps vaccine or MMR need not be withheld if a household member other than the recipient is immunocompromised, because the vaccine viruses are not spread from the recipient to contacts.

### Postexposure Prophylaxis

Immunization after exposure does not protect contacts from infection resulting from that exposure, but it is not contraindicated because it offers future protection. Screening to identify susceptible persons is unnecessary before immunization. A negative history for clinical disease and for immunization is all that is required, because vaccinating a person who is immune has no known adverse consequences.

### Passive Immunization

Mumps immunoglobulin was not efficacious in preventing disease among contacts and is no longer produced. Standard immunoglobulin has no value as postexposure prophylaxis.

## Rubella

### Susceptibility

Unimmunized populations are susceptible to rubella infection. Contemporary serologic surveys in the United States suggest that 10% to 20% of young adults are susceptible, suggesting that congenital rubella syndrome should remain a topic of concern.

Efforts to eliminate congenital rubella syndrome can center on universal immunization for children of both sexes or on immunization of females before the childbearing years. Both strategies have advantages and proponents. Congenital rubella syndrome has decreased in areas using each method.

### Active Immunization

Live rubella virus vaccine in use in the United States contains the attenuated RA27/3 strain propagated in human diploid cell culture. One dose produces satisfactory antibody levels in more than 98% of recipients, who have lasting, probably lifelong, immunity. Rubella vaccine is available as a single agent, in combination with measles and mumps vaccines (MMR), and with measles or mumps vaccine. It is injected subcutaneously. Many children receive a second dose of rubella vaccine if their second dose of measles vaccine is delivered as MMR.

Rubella vaccine is recommended for all United States children given as MMR at 15 months of age, unless there is a specific contraindication. The timing of vaccination is chosen to obtain favorable response rates to measles vaccine. Adequate response to rubella vaccine is expected any time after the first birthday.

Every effort should be made to immunize susceptible girls before the onset of puberty, and immunization of susceptible males is recommended. Because it is difficult to diagnose rubella with certainty clinically and because many infections are asymptomatic, immunization or serologic confirmation of immunity is desirable unless a date of immunization is documented.

Susceptible postpubescent females should be immunized, but only if they are not pregnant. Pregnancy should be deferred for 3 months after immunization. The risk of congenital rubella syndrome from the vaccine virus administered during pregnancy appears to be low. Although vaccine virus has been cultured rarely from an infant or abortus, congenital rubella syndrome has not been observed, and inadvertent immunization during pregnancy, although it should be reported, is not an automatic indication for the recommendation of therapeutic abortion.

Rubella immunity is highly desirable before entry into educational institutions, military service, and professions in health care and day care because of the likelihood of acquiring and spreading the disease.

Women found to be serologically susceptible during pregnancy should be immunized in the immediate postpartum period. Neither breast feeding nor the concomitant administration of $Rh_o(D)$ immune globulin or blood products is a contraindication.

Rubella vaccine as a single agent or in combination with measles and mumps may be administered at the same visit as DTP and OPV without sacrificing efficacy or increasing adverse reactions.

### Adverse Reactions

Rash, fever, and lymphadenopathy follow vaccination in a few children. Less commonly, pain in peripheral joints is reported.

Frank arthritis is uncommon. Joint complications appear to be more common in postpubescent females, are transient, and usually begin 1 to 3 weeks after immunization. Transient paresthesias and limb pain have been reported, as have central nervous system complications and thrombocytopenia, but the etiologic association has not been established.

Adverse events reportable to the VAERS after rubella vaccine administration include anaphylaxis or anaphylactic shock within 24 hours, encephalopathy with onset within 15 days, a residual seizure disorder, or any complication of these reactions, including death.

### Contraindications

Pregnant women should not be given rubella vaccine. Immunocompromised persons, including those with immunodeficiency disease and those on immunosuppressive therapy except children with HIV infection (who should receive MMR), should not receive rubella vaccine. Immunization should be withheld at least 3 months after the discontinuation of therapy and may be withheld longer, depending on the timing of expected recovery of immunocompetence.

Rubella vaccine need not be withheld if household contacts are pregnant or immunocompromised, because there is no evidence that the vaccine virus, although shed in small amounts from the nasopharynx, is transmitted.

### Postexposure Prophylaxis

Active immunization after exposure does not prevent infection and illness from that exposure. However, exposure is not a contraindication to immunizing a person who is not pregnant for future protection. The reader is referred to the Report of the Committee on Infectious Diseases and the obstetrics literature for discussion of the care of the patient exposed during pregnancy.

## *Haemophilus influenzae* Type B

### Susceptibility

All persons who do not have the bactericidal or anticapsular antibody acquired passively through the placenta or by previous experience with infection are considered susceptible, but children younger than 4 years of age who are in close contact with another child who has developed invasive *Haemophilus influenzae* type b (Hib) disease are at highest risk. The highest incidence of invasive Hib disease is among children between the ages of 3 months and 3 years, with a peak at 9 months.

In the United States, Hib meningitis occurs disproportionately among boys, urban children, blacks, native Americans, the poor, children from large families, and those in day care centers. Children who have had one episode of Hib disease are at increased risk of incurring another, with a recurrence rate of approximately 1%.

Conditions that carry increased risk of Hib disease in early childhood and beyond include sickle cell disease, asplenia, antibody deficiency, and, perhaps, malignancy treated with chemotherapy.

### Active Immunization

Two types of Hib vaccine have been used in the United States: Hib polysaccharide vaccine (PRP), which is no longer recommended, and the newer conjugate vaccines in which Hib polysaccharide, or an oligosaccharide, is linked to a carrier protein. Disease incidence, especially well documented for Hib meningitis, has dropped markedly after introduction of immunization.

Hib polysaccharide vaccine PRP, first licensed in the United States in 1985, consists of purified capsular polysaccharide. PRP does not induce anticapsular antibody or provide protection against Hib disease reliably in children younger than 18 months of age. Antibody is produced by most children at 24 months, and efficacy of approximately 90% was demonstrated in an early study. Routine administration of this vaccine was initially recommended by the ACIP and by the Committee on Infectious Diseases of the AAP for all children at 24 months. The ACIP recommended selective use at 18 months for children in certain high-risk groups. Variable results and the recognized need for a vaccine that could be administered before the age of peak incidence stimulated continued research and development of conjugate vaccines that are immunogenic in younger recipients.

In 1988, when the first of the conjugate vaccines (PRP-D) was licensed, the Committee on Infectious Diseases of the AAP recommended it replace the use of PRP in most instances. PRP-D should be given to all children, especially those at high risk, at 18 months of age, and subsequently, the recommendation was lowered to 15 months of age. It is injected intramuscularly. Because other conjugate vaccines have been licensed for use beginning at 2 months of age, PRP-D is now reserved for use in the child who has escaped immunization or as a booster dose for a 12 to 15-month-old child initially given another preparation.

Active immunization against Hib disease should begin at about 2 months of age with one of the three vaccines licensed for use in infancy. PRP-OMP (PedvaxHib) is given in a three-dose regimen, ordinarily at 2, 4, and 12 to 15 months, or HbOC (HibTiter) and PRP-T (Act HIB) are given in a four-dose regimen, ordinarily at 2, 4, 6, and 12 to 15 months. HbOC is also available as a combination vaccine with DTP (Tetramune). The combination can be used at any visit where both HbOC and DTP are indicated. If the necessary information is available in a timely fashion, the initial 2 (PRP-OMP) or 3 (HbOC, PRP-T) doses should be the same vaccine. However, inadequate information should not delay immunization, because the peak risk of disease is at a very young age. The final dose at 12–15 months can be of any Hib conjugate vaccine. Summary information about the Hib conjugate vaccines is presented in Table 24-25 A child whose Hib immunization is delayed beyond 2 months should have the regimen initiated at the earliest possible age but need not receive a vaccine dose beyond one given at 15 months or older, because one dose given at that age is considered protective. Unimmunized children between the ages of 12 and 14 months should receive two doses of vaccine spaced two months apart. Unimmunized children between the ages of 15 and 60 months can be fully immunized with one dose of any of the conjugate vaccines. Immunization of children 60 months (5 years) of age or older is only indicated if they have a chronic condition associated with increased risk for invasive Hib infection.

Hib disease at a young age does not necessarily produce immunity, and children who have documented Hib infection before the age of 24 months should be immunized. Immunization status does not affect the recommendation for chemoprophylaxis with rifampin after exposure.

### Adverse Reactions

Local reactions, including tenderness, erythema, and induration at the injection site, have been reported in about 25% of recipients, and systemic reactions defined as crying or fever have been reported in 10% to 15%. However, in neither category did these reactions exceed the rates in groups injected with placebo.

High fever and febrile seizures occur infrequently. Immunization is not protective immediately, and febrile illness occurring in the first few days after immunization should be evaluated. Extant PRP antibody levels decline in the 2 or 3 days after immunization, but early fears of immunization-precipitated Hib disease have not been substantiated with use of the conjugate vaccines in infancy.

### Contraindications

Except for serious acute febrile illness, there are no known contraindications to administration of Hib conjugate vaccines for the age groups for which they are considered indicated (2 to 59 months) and for older persons at high risk. Unvaccinated persons older than 12 months at high risk of invasive Hib disease should receive one or two doses, depending on their diagnosis, of Hib conjugate vaccine.

## Hepatitis B Virus

### Susceptibility

Most HBV infections occur among adults and adolescents. The virus is transmitted by contact with infected blood products and by sexual intercourse with infected persons, and the initial strategy was to immunize those from subpopulations with high rates of endemic infection and those with high-risk lifestyles, behaviors, or occupations. It proved difficult to immunize those known to be at high risk before infection, and infection continues to occur among persons who would not have been correctly classified as at risk and given the vaccine. The lifetime risk of HBV infection in the United States is 5%.

At particularly high risk of infection are children born to infected mothers. Depending on the mother's hepatitis B e antigen status, the risk of perinatal infection can be as high as 85%. Even if an infant escapes perinatal infection, the risk of acquiring infection during the first 5 years of life is high. Early infection is associated with an especially high rate of chronic infection and long-term mortality from liver disease. Persons with HBV infection are also at risk for co-infection or superinfection with the hepatitis delta virus (HDV) and consequent fulminant or chronic active hepatitis.

TABLE 24.25.  *Haemophilus Influenzae* b Conjugate Vaccines, 1992

| Vaccine Name | Manufacturer/ Distributer | Protein | Schedule |
|---|---|---|---|
| ProHibit PRP-D | Connaught | Diphtheria toxoid | 15 mo |
| HIBTITER HbOC | Lederle Praxis | Diphtheria CRM 197 | 2, 4, 6, 12–15 mo |
| PedvaxHib PRP-OMP Act HIB | Merck Sharp & Dohme | Outer membrane protein complex of *N meningitidis* B | 2, 4, 12–15 mo |
| PRP-T | Pasteur Merieux Vaccins | Tetanus toxoid | 2, 4, 6, 12–15 mo |

## Active Immunization

Currently targeted for active immunization are infants of hepatitis B surface antigen-positive (HBsAg-positive) mothers whose active immunization should begin immediately after birth and be combined with passive immunoprophylaxis (Table 24-26), infants of HBsAg-negative mothers, and adolescents and adults at high risk of infection. Vaccination is an essential component of postexposure prophylaxis (see Table 24-27). In each of these situations, the vaccine has been highly effective in preventing infection and its long-term sequelae.

The original vaccine prepared as a suspension of inactivated surface antigen particles purified from the plasma of chronic HBV carriers is no longer produced in the United States. The two licensed vaccines are both composed of HBsAg produced by baker's yeast into which the gene for HBsAg has been inserted with recombinant DNA technology. The vaccines (HBVrV) contain aluminum hydroxide as an absorptive and thimerosal as a preservative.

Three intramuscular doses of HBVrV are now recommended in most situations, administered into the anterolateral thigh in infants and in the deltoid of older children, adolescents, and adults. A variety of schedules are associated with high conversion rates and protective antibody levels. Dose and timing of the doses vary by product, age of recipient, and risk category. The recommended doses and schedules are displayed in Table 24-26. All pregnant women should be screened for the presence of HBsAg. The infants of HBsAg-positive women should receive postexposure prophylaxis with hepatitis B immune globulin (HBIG) and vaccine (Tables 24-26 and 24-27). Dosing schedules for immunizing infants of HBsAg-negative mothers are given in Table 24-26. To obtain reliable antibody response, prematurely born infants of HBsAg-negative mothers should begin the HBVrV series at 2 months or at a weight of 2000 grams. HBVrV can be administered at the same time as other vaccines. A vaccine recipient can receive either vaccine for subsequent doses with comparable results, and the vaccines, if given in the recommended doses, can be considered interchangeable. If the second dose of vaccine has been delayed for some reason, it should be administered as soon as possible. Increasing the interval between doses one and two has little effect on the final antibody titer. Because the third dose should be separated from the second by at least 2 months, there is less urgency if the third dose is delayed, but a missed third dose should be administered as early as is convenient so that full protection is afforded. Longer intervals (4 to 12 months) between doses two and three result in higher final antibody titers than shorter intervals (1 to 2 months).

Susceptibility testing, carried out by looking for antibody to the core antigen or to the surface antigen, is not recommended for children or for most adolescents before vaccination. The prevalence of infection and cost for vaccine are both low. If the risk of previous infection is high, the cost of vaccine is great compared with the cost of testing, and compliance with follow-up is expected, adolescents may have susceptibility testing before vaccination. Susceptibility testing before vaccination should be

**TABLE 24-26.** Recommended Dose and Immunization Schedule for Routine Use of the Currently Licensed Hepatitis B Vaccines by Age and Risk Status

| Immunization Groups | Energix-B* Dose (μg) | Energix-B* Dose (mL) | Recombivax-HB Dose (μg) | Recombivax-HB Dose (mL) | Immunization Schedule | HBIG† |
|---|---|---|---|---|---|---|
| Infant of HBsAg-positive mother | 10 | 0.5 | 5 | 0.5 | Birth (within 12 h), 1 mo, 6 mo‡ | Yes, within 12 h |
| Infant of mother whose HBsAg status is unknown | 10 | 0.5 | 5§ | 0.5 | Birth (within 12 h), 1–2 mo, 6 mo | Yes, if mother proves to be HBsAg positive‖ No, if mother proves to be HBsAg negative |
| Infant of HBsAg-negative mother▲ | 10 | 0.5 | 2.5 | 0.25 | Birth (before hospital discharge), 1–2 mo, 6–18 mo¶ or 1–2 mo, 4 mo, 6–18 mo | No |
| Children <11 y | 10 | 0.5 | 2.5 | 0.25 | 0, 1 mo, 6 mo | No |
| Adolescents 11–19 y | 20 | 1.0 | 5 | 0.5 | 0, 1 mo, 6 mo or 0, 2 mo, 4 mo# | No |
| Adults ≥20 y | 20 | 1.0 | 10 | 1.0 | 0, 1 mo, 6 mo | No |
| Dialysis patients** and immunocopromised persons§§ | 40 | 2.0†† | 40 | 1.0‡‡ | 0, 1 mo, 2 mo and 12 mo | No |

\* Also licensed for a four-dose series administered at 0, 1, 2, and 12 months. May be preferred when rapid response is sought; fourth dose cannot be omitted.

† HBIG, hepatitis B immunoglobulin. For infants, 0.5 mL is administered intramuscularly at a site different than the immunization.

‡ Serologic response (anti-HBs) should be measured 3 to 9 months after completion of the vaccination series, at 9 to 15 months of age.

§ Doses after the first can be 2.5 μg if mother proves to be HBsAg negative.

‖ Administer as soon as possible, ideally within 48 hours of birth and certainly within 7 days. If mother's antigen status will never be known, HBIG is probably indicated.

¶ Longer intervals between the last two does result in higher final anti-HBs titers.

# This shortened schedule can be used if compliance with follow-up is a concern.

** Annual antibody testing is recommended as is a booster dose when antibody levels decline to <10 mIU/mL.

†† Dose given as two 1-mL injections at different sites; four-dose schedule (0, 1, 2 and 6 months).

‡‡ Special high-dose formulation.

§§ Postvaccination testing should be performed at 1 to 6 months if results may affect subsequent clinical management.

▲ Infants prematurely born of an HBsAg-negative mother should begin the HBVrV series at 2 months or a weight of 2000 grams.

TABLE 24-27. Postexposure Immunoprophylaxis Against Hepatitis B Virus

| Type of Exposure | Immunoprophylaxis |
| --- | --- |
| Perinatal, HBsAg-positive mother) | HBIG × 1 within 12 h of birth; doses of HBVrV within 12 h of birth, at 1 and 6 mo; antibody testing 3 to 9 mo later |
| Infant (<12 mo) whose primary caregiver has acute infection | HBIG × 1 as soon as possible; HBVrV vaccine beginning at time of HBIG and at 1 and 6 mo |
| Household contact with person who has acute infection | |
|   has no known exposure | No immunoprophylaxis indicated |
|   has known exposure to blood | Treat like sexual exposure |
|   is a chronic carrier | HBVrV by usual schedule for age |
| Sexual contact with person who | |
|   has acute infection | Test exposed person for anti-HBc. If susceptible and within 14 d of exposure or if exposure is ongoing, give HBIG × 1 and initiate HBVrV series |
|   is a chronic carrier | Vaccination with HBVrV by usual schedule |
| Inadvertent percutaneous or permucosal exposure to blood | See guidelines from the ACIP |

*HBsAg*, hepatitis surface antigen; *HBIG*, hepatitis B immunoglobulin (for infants <12 mo, dose is 0.5 mL and thereafter is 0.06 mL/kg to a maximum of 5 mL, delivered intramuscularly at a site different than the vaccine); *HBVrV*, hepatitis B viral recombinant vaccine.

Adapted from the Advisory Committee on Immunization Practices. Hepatitis B virus: A comprehensive strategy for eliminating transmission in the United States through universal childhood vaccination. MMWR 1991;127:337, and from Peter G, ed. Report of the Committee of Infectious Diseases, American Academy of Pediatrics. Elk Grove Village, IL: American Academy of Pediatrics, 1991;238.

considered in certain cases if postexposure prophylaxis is under consideration (see Table 24-27).

Although universal immunization in infancy against HBV infection is recommended, it is prudent to continue to try to immunize older persons who may be at special risk, including hemophiliac patients (at the time of diagnosis), patients with recently acquired sexually transmitted diseases, prostitutes or those who have had multiple sexual partners in the previous 6 months, sexually active homosexual males, household and sexual contacts of HBV carriers (see Table 24-27), household members of adopted children who are HBsAg positive, children from populations with a high rate of endemic HBV infection (eg, Alaskan natives and refugees from Africa and eastern Asia), staff and residents of institutions for the developmentally disabled, staff and perhaps attenders of nonresidential programs for developmentally disabled persons where one or more HBV carriers attend, patients with renal disease who are likely to require dialysis in the future, health care workers and others with occupational exposure to blood, and persons who plan international travel that includes living 6 months or more in an area with highly endemic HBV infection. Particular consideration should be given to immunizing adolescents at the time of health supervision, ideally before sexual activity is initiated.

Testing for serologic response is not necessary after the routine immunization of infants whose mothers are HBsAg negative, of children, or of adolescents. If knowledge of the status affects subsequent management, postvaccination serology should be measured 1 to 6 months after the series is completed or 3 to 9 months for infants born to HBsAg-positive mothers. One or more additional doses should be considered for those who did not respond, because seroconversion follows in as many as 25% to 50%. Clinical trials estimate effectiveness to be in the range of 80% to 95%. As with other vaccines, some recipients fail to seroconvert, but if antibody response is adequate after immunization, protection against disease appears assured.

Immunity appears to be long lasting. Although HBV vaccines have not been available long, protection has been shown to last at least 9 years. Booster doses are not recommended in routine settings, but the need for additional doses may be reconsidered as clinical experience through time dictates.

### Adverse Reactions

Although pain at the injection site and fever are reported by a small proportion of vaccine recipients, these reactions appear to be just as common in placebo recipients. When HBVV is administered at the same time as DTP, there is no increase in local or febrile reactions. A possible rare association between the first dose of plasma-derived HBVV and Guillain-Barré syndrome was reported (Shaw, 1988). No association has been observed between HBVrV and Guillain-Barré syndrome. HBVVs are safe for infants, children, adolescents, and adults.

### Contraindications

Pregnant and lactating women can be vaccinated, because there has been no apparent risk to developing fetuses with vaccine use. No risk is anticipated, because the vaccine does not contain live virus.

### Postexposure Prophylaxis

HBIG is prepared from plasma with high titer of antibody against HBsAg but no antibodies to HIV. The preparation process excludes viable HIV. HBIG protection lasts for 3 to 6 months and is recommended only in some situations for postexposure protection (see Table 24-27). If exposure has occurred or is imminent, HBIG protection is essential in the interval between vaccination and adequate antibody response.

## Varicella

### Susceptibility

Susceptibility to infection with the varicella-zoster virus (VZV) is high among persons who have not had known previous infection. Studies of household exposure suggest that 80% of those without a history of chickenpox develop disease. Natural infection is thought to confer long-lasting immunity for most persons, but it may not be complete for all. Second infections occur. Zoster represents reactivation of virus latent in dorsal root ganglia and may be associated with an inadequate cell-mediated immune response or to VZV infection.

Considerations that have delayed the adoption of routine vaccination against varicella have included the widespread opinion that there is little urgency because the disease is more benign than the others for which healthy children are traditionally immunized, questions about duration of immunity, and concern about how immunization would affect the incidence of zoster.

It has been estimated that the complications of varicella lead to more than 50 deaths in otherwise healthy children each year. About the same number develop encephalitis associated with chickenpox. VZV infection is responsible for many physician and pharmacy visits, with the accompanying costs, and with many missed work days for parents and school days for child patients. VZV infection can cause severe disease in susceptible leukemia patients and other immunocompromised persons, in adults, and in the newborns of mothers infected late in pregnancy. Many researchers suggest that the weight of this combined burden argues in favor of active immunization. The vaccine has been in investigative use long enough to assert that immunity appears to be long lasting. "Breakthrough" is more likely in persons with low initial antibody response to the vaccine, and clinical cases occur at the relatively low rate of about 2% a year. Adding further impetus for immunization is the accumulating evidence that the rate of zoster after immunization is no greater and may be lower than the rate after infection with wild-type VZV.

### Active Immunization

A live attenuated varicella vaccine has been derived from the Oka varicella strain isolated and first attenuated in Japan in the early 1970s, where it is now licensed and in widespread use. The vaccine has been studied in the United States since 1981 and is expected to be licensed soon. It has been tested in leukemic children and in healthy children and adults. One dose of vaccine leads to seroconversion in 95% of healthy children but in fewer than 90% of adults or leukemic children, for whom two doses have been used.

Placebo-controlled, double-blind studies with follow-up and studies of protection after household exposure have led investigators to estimate that the efficacy of varicella vaccine in healthy children to be approximately 95%. Most cases that occur in previously immunized persons are mild and are associated with few skin lesions. Antibody levels decrease in some vaccine recipients and may fall below detectable levels. It is not yet apparent that there will be an increase in disease incidence with time. If long-term experience suggests there is, a booster dose of the vaccine may be recommended.

After the Oka vaccine is licensed for use among healthy children in the United States, it is expected that the relevant vaccine committees will issue statements suggesting that its use be left up to parents and providers. After a preparation is available combining varicella with measles, mumps, and rubella (MMRV), a recommendation for universal immunization against varicella by giving MMRV at the time of initial measles immunization (12 or 15 months) may be forthcoming.

Although licensure for use in leukemic children is not anticipated, compassionate use may be considered. Although the likelihood of vaccine-related rash is as high as 50% and may be severe enough to prompt antiviral therapy with oral acyclovir, studies have shown that disseminated infection does not develop, and the vaccine can be used safely. Vaccination of children with leukemia who are susceptible decreases the likelihood of wild-type VZV infection after exposure markedly, and cases that occur are almost always milder than unmodified disease would be. Se-

vere morbidity and death are prevented. Routine vaccination of toddlers would provide protection against VZV infection before the onset of most leukemia cases.

### Adverse Reactions

Reactions after vaccination include fever and other mild nonspecific symptoms, rash at the site of injection ($\approx$12%), and mild, generalized, varicella-like rash. Between 5% and 10% of healthy children develop a few papulovesicular lesions about 1 month after immunization. Vaccine virus can be cultured from vesicular lesions. No recipient, including no leukemic vaccinee, has developed disseminated infection with the vaccine virus.

### Contraindications

As is the case with other systemically administered live viral vaccines, varicella vaccine use is not recommended during pregnancy. It is not anticipated that varicella vaccine will be licensed for use in persons who are immunosuppressed, although compassionate use in leukemic patients may continue to be the practice. Because preparation of the vaccine involves sterilization with neomycin, persons with documented allergic reactions to neomycin should not receive varicella vaccine.

## IMMUNIZATIONS FOR SPECIAL SITUATIONS

### Pneumococcus

The available pneumococcal vaccine contains the purified capsular polysaccharide antigens of 23 pneumococcal serotypes, including those that cause most episodes of bacteremia and meningitis in children. The vaccine may be injected subcutaneously or intramuscularly. As with Hib PRP, another polysaccharide vaccine, the antigenicity of pneumococcal vaccine in children younger than age 2 is poor.

Side effects from the vaccine are soreness at the injection site and low-grade fever. Anaphylaxis is rare.

Pneumococcal vaccine is recommended at 2 years of age (or at any subsequent age, if not previously administered) for children who are at increased risk of acquiring pneumococcal infection, including children with sickle cell disease, functional or anatomic asplenia, or nephrotic syndrome or congenital or acquired immunodeficiency. The vaccine should be administered 2 weeks or more before elective splenectomy or planned immunosuppressive therapy. Vaccination during chemotherapy or radiation therapy is not likely to be effective. Vaccination should follow chemotherapy by 3 months.

Pneumococcal vaccine should be considered for children at increased risk of serious disease if they contract pneumococcal infection, such as children with diabetes, an organ transplant, congestive heart failure, chronic pulmonary disease, or renal failure. The need to repeat doses has not been established, but revaccination should be considered every 3 to 5 years.

Pneumococcal vaccine is contraindicated during febrile illness and has no proven efficacy in preventing recurrent respiratory infections or otitis media in healthy children.

### Meningococcus

Quadrivalent polysaccharide meningococcal vaccine is available for serogroups A, C, Y, and W-135. Meningococcal C vaccine has been administered to United States military recruits for a number of years and has decreased type C disease within that population. The quadrivalent vaccine is now used. The immunogenicity of group C polysaccharide is poor for children younger than 2 years of age, and duration of immunity in those older than 2 years may be short. Monovalent group A polysaccharide vaccine did produce immunity with a duration of less than 3 years in younger children and can be given when indicated and available to children as young as 3 months of age. Two doses given 3 months apart are recommended for children younger than 18 months, and only one dose is used for older children. Meningococcal vaccines are injected subcutaneously.

Adverse reactions to the meningococcal vaccine are not common and consist of mild reactions at the injection site.

Routine immunization of children with meningococcal vaccine is not recommended by the Committee on Infectious Diseases of the AAP. However, the quadrivalent vaccine is recommended at 2 years of age or later if not previously administered for children in certain high-risk groups, including those with functional or anatomic asplenia or with terminal complement component deficiencies.

The vaccine is recommended along with rifampin chemoprophylaxis for close contacts of cases with disease caused by one of the included groups, because secondary cases can continue to occur for several weeks. The vaccine is effective in outbreak control.

Travelers to epidemic areas may benefit from the vaccine.

## Influenza

The antigenic characteristics of influenza strains cultured from cases inform the selection of virus strains to be used in vaccines that are developed annually. In 1987, the vaccine was trivalent, comprising an A(H1N1), an A(H3N2), and a B organism. Current vaccines are made from highly purified viruses grown in egg culture that are then inactivated. Children receive a "split-virus" preparation that is associated less often with febrile reactions. Vaccine efficacy, defined as protection against clinical disease, is lower than for other vaccines given in childhood, peaking at about 70% in young adults. However, protection against death from influenza conferred by the vaccine is probably somewhat higher in younger and older age groups. Inactivated influenza vaccine is injected intramuscularly. Live attenuated vaccines with the prevalent antigen subtypes are being developed for intranasal administration.

The goal of influenza immunization is to protect persons who are at high risk of acquiring disease and its complications and to prevent transmission of influenza to high-risk susceptibles.

Children who are at high risk for influenza complications or for decompensation with an ordinary case of influenza and who are 6 months of age or older should be immunized annually in the fall, before the influenza season. High-risk groups probably include children with chronic pulmonary diseases like moderate or severe asthma, cystic fibrosis, or bronchopulmonary dysplasia; children with hemodynamically significant cardiac disease; children receiving immunosuppressive therapy; and children with hemoglobinopathies. Consideration should be given to immunizing children with conditions such as chronic renal or metabolic disease, those with diabetes, or those requiring long-term aspirin therapy, because they may be at increased risk of developing Reye's syndrome as a complication of influenza.

During the first year influenza vaccine is administered, a child younger than 9 years should receive two doses, which should be given 4 or more weeks apart in the fall preceding the influenza season. Children between the ages of 6 and 35 months receive split-virus vaccine in a dose of 0.25 mL. Children between 3 and 12 years receive 0.5 mL of split-virus vaccine. Those older than 12 may receive 0.5 mL of split- or whole-virus vaccine. In subsequent years, children who remain at high risk should receive one dose of the vaccine type and volume appropriate for age. Influenza vaccine is not recommended for normal children, but it is safe and not contraindicated. Administration can be condoned if requested.

Influenza vaccine may be administered at the same time as MMR, OPV, or polysaccharide vaccines, but it should not be administered within 3 days of immunization with DTP to permit attribution of adverse reactions to either vaccine.

Information is not available about the reactivity, immunogenicity, and efficacy of inactivated influenza vaccine in infants younger than 6 months, and immunization is not recommended, although those with chronic disease are probably a high-risk group. There is little experience with chemoprophylaxis with amantadine among infants, and protection of high-risk infants from influenza may be accomplished best by immunizing caretakers and other close contacts and by universal immunization of the health care workers, who are likely to be exposed and with whom high-risk infants have frequent contact.

Adverse reactions to the current influenza vaccines, especially split virus, are infrequent. Systemic reactions, including fever, do not appear causally related to vaccine given according to current recommendations. Local reactions are infrequent in young children, but they occur in about 10% of those over age 13.

Neurologic complications, particularly the Guillain-Barré syndrome experienced after the administration of A/New Jersey/ 76 swine influenza vaccine, have not been associated with current vaccines for which surveillance has been rigorous. It is extremely unlikely that current vaccines are associated with serious adverse reactions of any type. The memory of the previous isolated experience has resulted in apparent reluctance to use influenza vaccine, but that reaction must be overcome to benefit high-risk persons.

Influenza vaccine should not be administered to children with a history of anaphylactic reactions to eggs. Amantadine prophylaxis during the influenza season may be used as an alternative.

## Human Immunodeficiency Virus

Because of the increasing numbers of infected children, the progressive immunodeficiency characteristic of the disease, and increased susceptibility to infectious diseases, the immunization needs of children with HIV infection demands special attention. There has been concern that because of immunocompromise, protection may not follow immunization, and that live vaccines may cause disease in HIV patients. Experience is still accumulating on both subjects. Vaccine-related disease is reported only for BCG, which is not administered to HIV-infected patients in the United States, but continues to be recommended for HIV-infected asymptomatic children in parts of the world where tuberculosis in highly endemic and BCG is routinely offered.

The immunization schedule for children with HIV infection is modified compared with healthy children only in the following ways: eIVP is administered instead of OPV, and influenza and pneumococcal vaccine are administered. In all other ways, the routine immunization schedule is honored. DTP, Hib vaccine, HBVV, and MMR are administered according the usual schedule for infants and toddlers.

MMR vaccine consists of live attenuated organisms and represents a theoretic risk, but no serious consequences have been reported after vaccine administration. Serious cases of measles, including fatalities, have occurred in children with HIV infection. A dose of MMR at 15 months or at 12 months in communities with increased risk of measles exposure is recommended. The decision about whether a second dose should be administered before elementary or middle school entry as is recommended for healthy children awaits further clinical experience and may depend on the clinical status of the patient at that time.

Vertical transmission of HIV infection may imply a high risk for transmission of HBV as well, and that HBIG and HBVV may be indicated after birth. The hepatitis B status of the mother should be established immediately.

## Hepatitis A Virus

Field studies have repeatedly shown that immunoglobulin given before exposure or early in the incubation period (15 to 50 days) protects against clinical hepatitis A virus (HAV) disease. It is 80% to 90% protective if given early, after which its value declines. Several recommendations have been made by the Committee on Infectious Diseases of the AAP for pediatric patients.

Household contacts of persons with serologically confirmed HAV should receive 0.02 mL/kg of immunoglobulin as soon as possible after exposure without waiting for serologic confirmation of the recipient's susceptibility, which unnecessarily delays administration. If more than 2 weeks have elapsed since last exposure, immunoglobulin is not indicated.

The infant of a mother with jaundice due to HAV at the time of delivery should be given immunoglobulin at the 0.02 mL/kg dose, although efficacy has not been confirmed. If the mother is not jaundiced, immunoglobulin is not recommended.

The spread of HAV infection in day-care facilities is high. An infectious disease or public health consultant may be needed to assist in outbreak control. In centers with an index case among enrollees or staff and only children more than 2 years of age or toilet trained, immunoglobulin is recommended only for all employees and children who share the room with the index case. In day-care centers with younger children and children not toilet trained and an index case among employees or enrollees, immunoglobulin is recommended for all employees and enrollees. New employees and children entering during the 6 weeks after the last case should receive immunoglobulin. If recognition of the case is delayed by 3 or more weeks from onset of the illness or illness has already spread to three or more families, immunoglobulin should be considered for all employees, enrollees, and the household contacts of enrollees who are 3 years of age or younger.

Schoolroom exposure of older children does not generally carry risk, and immunoglobulin is not indicated under ordinary circumstances. As in day care, HAV infection is readily transmitted in institutions for custodial care, and after an outbreak occurs, all residents and staff who have had close personal contact with the patient should be treated with immunoglobulin.

The source of infection during food- or water-borne outbreaks of HAV is usually recognized too late for prophylaxis. If possible, immunoglobulin should be administered to exposed persons before 2 weeks have elapsed. Travelers who spend extended time outside of the usual tourist spots in underdeveloped countries, including children, should receive an initial dose of 0.02 mL/kg of immunoglobulin. If the stay is extended beyond 3 months, additional injections of 0.06 mL/kg should be administered every 5 months.

## Rabies

The decision about providing postexposure prophylaxis against rabies must be made frequently by physicians for patients with animal bites, scratches, or other contact. Important factors in the decision are the species of the animal involved and its regional history of positivity for rabies, whether the animal was captured and can be observed and then sacrificed, whether the animal was provoked, and the type and anatomic location of the exposure. Although bites from domestic animals are much more common, more wild animals are proved rabid, with seven species accounting for most cases: skunks, bats, raccoons, cattle, dogs, cats, and foxes, in descending order of importance. Rodents and rabbits are rarely rabid. Transmission is probably by way of infected secretions passed by a bite. Licks, scratches, and aerosolization may rarely transfer the virus.

Decision-making trees have been provided to aid the physician (McCracken, 1984); when in doubt, the advice of local public health experts should be sought. A treatment guide from the Committee on Infectious Diseases of the AAP is adapted as Table 24-28 Cleansing of the wound and evaluation of the need for tetanus prophylaxis should not be neglected in the process of making decisions about rabies prophylaxis.

When the decision is made to provide postexposure prophylaxis, it should always include human rabies immune globulin (HRIG) and rabies vaccine, regardless of the interval from ex-

### TABLE 24-28. Postexposure Antirabies Treatment Guide*

| Species of Animal | Condition of Animal at Time of Attack | Treatment of Exposed Human |
|---|---|---|
| Wild<br>  Skunk<br>  Coyote<br>  Raccoon<br>  Bat<br>  Other carnivores | Regard as rabid unless proven negative by laboratory test. | HRIG† and HDCV‡ |
| Domestic dog and cat | Healthy, under surveillance | None§ |
| | Unknown (escaped) | Call public health official for advice |
| | Rabid or suspected rabid | HRIG and HDCV |
| Livestock | | Consider individually |
| Rodents and lagomorphs (rabbits and hares) | | Consider individually |

\* These recommendations are only a guide. They should be applied in conjunction with knowledge of the animal species involved, circumstances of the bite or other exposure, vaccination status of the animal, and prevalence of rabies in the region.
† HRIG, human rabies immunoglobulin.
‡ HDCV, human diploid cell vaccine, given intramuscularly. Discontinue vaccine if fluorescent antibody stains of tissues from the animal killed at the time of attack are negative for rabies antigen.
§ Begin HRIG and HDCV at the first sign of rabies in a biting dog or cat during a holding period (10 days).
*From Report of the Committee of Infectious Diseases of the American Academy of Pediatrics, 1991.*

posure. The exception is persons who were previously immunized with an inactivated human diploid cell rabies vaccine (HDCV) or with another vaccine who had documented antibody response; this group should receive vaccine only and only two doses, the second on day 3. The only vaccine now available in the United States is HDCV. It is far less reactogenic than the immediately previous vaccine prepared in duck embryo culture, but local reactions occur in as many as 25% of patients and mild systemic reactions in slightly fewer. Rarely, serious adverse reactions have been associated temporally with HDCV.

Persons receiving booster doses as part of a preexposure immunization regimen may experience immune complex-like reactions. If a patient has any allergic reaction to HDCV, a report should be made to the CDC and advice sought about possible continuation of the regimen with an investigational vaccine prepared in other cell lines.

At initiation of prophylaxis, HRIG is administered in a dose of 20 IU/kg. Up to half is infiltrated at the site of the wound, if possible. The rest is given intramuscularly. On the same day, the first of five 1-mL doses of HDCV is injected intramuscularly. Continuing from the first day of treatment, additional doses are given on days 3, 7, 14, and 28. The regimen may be discontinued only if 10-day observation by a veterinarian of a domestic animal or examination of the brain of a wild animal proves the animal to be rabies free.

Pregnancy should not be considered a contraindication to postexposure prophylaxis if it is indicated, because the disease rabies is almost always fatal.

## Bacillus Calmette-Guérin

Few indications for BCG vaccine are thought to exist in the United States and other countries where the prevalence of tuberculosis is low. The efficacy of the vaccination is controversial and appears to be inferior to chemoprophylaxis with isoniazid. The BCG available in the United States is derived through many years of culture from the original live attenuated strain of *Mycobacterium bovis*, but no test of potency is available, and no recent field trials have been carried out.

BCG may be indicated for an infant or child who is tuberculin skin test negative and is being raised in a household with repeated exposure to persons who remain persistently sputum positive because they are not treated or are ineffectively treated or have drug-resistant strains or indicated for persons in population subgroups in which the rate of new infection remains excessive (>1%/year) and the usual surveillance and treatment techniques have failed or cannot be carried out.

If use is considered, the guidelines for tuberculin testing of candidates and recipients should be reviewed and the instructions on the package insert followed. BCG can cause ulceration at the vaccination site, regional lymphadenitis, osteomyelitis, and rare lupoid reactions. Disseminated BCG infection has been associated with fatality.

Contraindications to BCG administration include burns, skin infections, immunosuppression, and immunodeficiency disease, including HIV infection. Malnutrition is not a contraindication, but pregnancy is, although no fetal problems have been reported.

BCG is used widely in some areas with a high prevalence of tuberculosis. Vaccination with BCG is not a contraindication to tuberculin testing. A positive result in a vaccine recipient may need to be clarified with a chest roentgenogram.

## Immunizations for Travelers

Infants and children who travel to other countries should have up-to-date immunizations. Recommendations for additional vaccines are dictated by exposures likely in the country of des-

tination and by what vaccination requirements are placed on persons who enter and return from that country. The most complete source of information for use in the United States is *Health Information for International Travel*, which is available from the Superintendent of Documents of the United States Government Printing Office and which is updated annually. The country's embassy is a good source of information for those who plan a long stay. In addition to the vaccines used routinely for healthy children in the United States, yellow fever, cholera, typhoid, and rabies vaccine may be indicated by the circumstances of travel, and immunoglobulin may be indicated for the prevention of HAV infection. Chemoprophylaxis against malaria may be indicated (see Chap. 62.1.5).

## CONCLUSION

A schedule for healthy children beginning immunization in infancy and consistent with current recommendations is presented in Table 24-21. Because more than one Hib conjugate vaccine is available for use in infancy, each with its own schedule, because the hepatitis virus vaccine can be presented on a variety of schedules to unexposed infants, and because no consensus has developed about the timing of the second dose of measles vaccine, no one schedule should be considered absolute. The schedule for a child who is presenting for immunizations at an advanced age should be individualized.

The introduction of new vaccines, changes in recommendations, and abrupt changes in immunization strategy can be perplexing for parents and for the health care provider, but these changes should produce a healthier future for our children through one of the most trustworthy of health care modalities—prevention of infectious diseases through childhood immunization.

## Selected Readings

Advisory Committee on Immunization Practices. Hepatitis B virus: a comprehensive strategy for eliminating transmission in the United States through universal childhood vaccination. MMWR 1991;40:1.

Advisory Committee on Immunization Practices. Immunization of children infected with human T-lymphotrophic virus type III/lymphadenopathy-associated virus. MMWR 1986;35:595.

Advisory Committee on Immunization Practices. New recommended schedule for active immunization of normal infants and children. MMWR 1986;35:577.

Advisory Committee on Immunization Practices. Pertussis immunization; family history of convulsions and use of antipyretics—supplementary ACIP statement. MMWR 1987;36:281.

Advisory Committee on Immunization Practices. Pertussis vaccination: Acellular pertussis vaccine for reinforcing and booster use—supplementary ACIP Statement. MMWR 1992;41:1.

Advisory Committee on Immunization Practices. Prevention of *Haemophilus influenzae* type b disease. MMWR 1985;34:201, 1986;35:170, 1987;36:529.

Advisory Committee on Immunization Practices. Recommendations for protection against viral hepatitis. MMWR 1985;34:313.

Benenson AS, ed. Control of communicable diseases in man, ed 15. Washington, DC: American Public Health Association, 1990.

Bergeson PS, Singer SA, Kaplan AM. Intramuscular injections in children. Pediatrics 1982;70:944.

Committee on Issues and Priorities for New Vaccine Development, Division of Health Promotion and Disease Prevention, Institute of Medicine. New vaccine development: Establishing priorities, vols 1 and 2. Washington, DC: National Academy Press, 1985.

Gershon AA. Varicella vaccine: Still at the crossroads. Pediatrics 1992;90:144.

Institute of Medicine. Vaccine supply and innovation. Washington, DC: National Academy Press, 1986.

Ipp MM, Gold R, Greenbert S, et al. Acetaminophen prophylaxis of adverse reactions following vaccination of infants with diphtheria-pertussis-tetanus toxoids-polio vaccine. Pediatr Infect Dis J 1987;6:721.

Katz SL. Controversies in immunization. Pediatr Infect Dis 1987;6:607.

Lee DC, Lederman HM. Anti-tetanus antibodies in intravenous gamma globulin: An alternative to tetanus immune globulin. J Infect Dis 1992;166-642.

McBean AM, Modlin JF. Rationale for the sequential use of inactivated poliovirus vaccine and live attenuated poliovirus vaccine for routine poliomyelitis immunization in the United States. Pediatr Infect Dis 1987;6:881.

McCracken GH. Post-exposure rabies prophylaxis. Pediatr Infect Dis 1984⁴1.

Peter G, ed. Report of the committee on infectious diseases, American Academy of Pediatrics. Elk Grove Village, IL: American Academy of Pediatrics, 1991.

Shaw FE Jr, Graham DJ, Guess HA, et al. Postmarketing surveillance for neurologic adverse events reported after hepatitis B vaccination: experience of the first three years. Am J Epidemiol 1988;127:337.

Siber GR, Werner BG, Halsey NA, Reid R, Almeido-Hill J, Garrett SC, Thompson C, Santosham M. Interference of immune globulin with measles and rubella immunization. J Pediatr 1993;122:204.

*Principles and Practice of Pediatrics, Second Edition.*
edited by Frank A. Oski et al. J. B. Lippincott Company, Philadelphia © 1994.

# 24.3 Injury Control

### Modena Hoover Wilson

In industrialized countries, injury is the leading cause of death for pediatric patients who survive the perils of the first few days and months of life. Injury is also a prominent cause of morbidity and disability. It precipitates numerous emergency room visits and hospitalizations and adds substantially to health care costs. It is not an exaggeration to say that injury is now the most important health problem of childhood.

Injury is a disease that is neither inherited nor congenital. An agent outside of the child is always involved, and injury therefore can be prevented. After injury occurs, prompt and appropriate medical care is needed to minimize the consequences.

Injury control includes preventing events that may cause injury, commonly referred to as accidents; preventing or modifying the transfer of energy, which eliminates or minimizes the injury if the event occurs; and ensuring timely and age-appropriate field care, transport, treatment, and rehabilitation for the injured person after injury occurs.

## EPIDEMIOLOGY OF INJURY IN CHILDHOOD AND ADOLESCENCE

Injury causes about half of all childhood and three quarters of adolescent deaths in the United States (Table 24-29). Although during early infancy injury is numerically exceeded by other causes of death, the importance of injury should not be overlooked. Injury death rates during the first year of life are high when compared with injury death rates in other preadolescent age groups (Table 24-30). Moreover, many of the deaths due to perinatal problems and congenital anomalies are not preventable with current knowledge. Injury deaths are.

The events leading to injury death vary by age, because children differ in vulnerability, ability, and exposure to hazards by age. Contrast the infant who inadvertently hangs in the drapery cord with the intoxicated adolescent driver who crashes into a tree after the graduation party.

Death from injury is tragic and all too common, but it is only a portion of the injury problem. An intensive study of children up to the age of 19 years in several Massachusetts communities revealed that for every death due to injury, there were almost 50 injury-related hospitalizations and almost 800 emergency room visits (Gallagher, 1982). The data combined suggest that injury causes a serious problem for about 1 in 5 children every year.

## PRINCIPLES OF INJURY CONTROL

The enormous number of injuries has prompted an increasingly organized effort to understand and control the problem. Several key principles have emerged.

Injury control is more than accident prevention. An injury is not the same as an accident. The focus for the health professional should be on controlling the disease or injury.

The word *accident* conveys a sense of surprise and bad luck. Although unintended, most events and the injuries they produce are predictable. For example, it is easy to foresee that a child riding a walker may fall down an unguarded stairway and be injured on the concrete floor below. These injury-producing events can be predicted and avoided, and injuries can be prevented even though accidents occur. To illustrate, seat belts do not prevent car crashes (ie, predictable events we call accidents), but they do decrease injuries during a car crash.

Injury can be viewed in the same epidemiologic framework as infectious disease. Energy is the agent of injury. Although the full list includes chemical, radiation, and electrical energy, most pediatric injury is caused by mechanical or thermal energy. The injury occurs when energy impinges on the host at a level the host cannot resist. Like the microbial agents of infectious diseases, the agents of injury can be conveyed to the host by an inanimate object (eg, vehicle) or an animal (eg, vector). The agent and host interact in an environment that is subject to biological, social, and economic influences, all of which may influence the result. Injury can be controlled by influencing one or more of these factors: agent, vehicle, vector, host, or environment.

| TABLE 24-29. Causes of Death of Children in the United States, 1984 | | | | | | | | |
|---|---|---|---|---|---|---|---|---|
| | <1 y | | 1–4 y | | 5–14 y | | 15–24 y | |
| Cause of Death | No. | % | No. | % | No. | % | No. | % |
| All causes | 39,580 | 100 | 7372 | 100 | 9076 | 100 | 38,817 | 100 |
| Infections | 1732 | 4 | 660 | 9 | 408 | 4 | 746 | 2 |
| Cancer | 192 | <1 | 612 | 8 | 1287 | 14 | 2293 | 6 |
| Cardiovascular disease | 1084 | 3 | 411 | 6 | 470 | 5 | 1507 | 4 |
| Congenital anomalies | 8548 | 22 | 946 | 13 | 484 | 5 | 516 | 1 |
| Perinatal problems | 18,682 | 47 | 144 | 2 | 26 | <1 | 9 | <1 |
| Injuries | 1075 | 3 | 3155 | 43 | 4859 | 54 | 29,646 | 76 |

*Advance Report of Final Mortality Statistics, 1984. NCHS Monthly Vital Statistics Report 1986;35(Suppl 2):6.*

TABLE 24-30. U.S. Injury Death Rates per 100,000 Population by Age and Cause

| Category of Injury* | <1 | 1–4 | 5–9 | 10–14 | 15–20 |
|---|---|---|---|---|---|
| Motor vehicle occupant | **4.78*** | **3.34** | **2.35** | **3.48** | **29.00** |
| Bicyclist | 0.00 | 0.11 | 0.77 | 1.24 | 0.75 |
| Pedestrian | 0.34 | 2.73 | **3.12** | **1.83** | 3.05 |
| Pedestrian, nontraffic | 0.21 | 1.18 | 0.13 | 0.04 | 0.07 |
| Drowning | 2.34 | **4.70** | **1.99** | **2.01** | 4.07 |
| Poisoning | 0.57 | 0.53 | 0.14 | 0.19 | 1.13 |
| Falls | 1.23 | 0.68 | 0.20 | 0.24 | 0.82 |
| Fires/burns | 3.81 | **4.85** | 1.82 | 0.90 | 0.84 |
| Firearm, unintentional | 0.05 | 0.29 | 0.39 | 0.97 | 1.43 |
| Aspiration | **5.35** | 0.87 | 0.17 | 0.16 | 0.21 |
| Suffocation | 4.72 | 0.57 | 0.24 | 0.46 | 0.34 |
| Suicide | 0.00 | 0.00 | 0.03 | 1.17 | **9.08** |
| Homicide | **6.16** | 2.51 | 0.93 | 1.42 | **9.33** |
| Total injury deaths | 34.27 | 24.94 | 13.80 | 16.52 | 68.05 |

* The three highest injury death rates for each age are in boldface type. Data are for the years 1980 through 1986.

Excerpted from Baker SP, O'Neill B, Ginsburg MJ, Li G. The injury fact book, ed 2. New York: Oxford, 1992.

Reducing injury requires preventing or reducing the interaction between the agent and host. Although there are numerous ways of accomplishing this goal, Haddon (1980) has provided an organizing framework. These generic strategies are listed in Table 24-31 with illustrations for three injury events. This framework clarifies injury causation, and it is useful in generating ideas for new ways to approach an injury problem.

Injury control strategies can be grouped by their temporal relation to the injury event. Some strategies are pre-event phase; they reduce the likelihood that an event with injury-producing

TABLE 24-31. Injury Control Strategies

| Strategy | Examples | | |
|---|---|---|---|
| | *Injury to Motor Vehicle Occupants* | *Injury to Football Players* | *Injury by Handguns* |
| Reducing potentially injurious agents | Alternative travel modes; reduction in speed limits and speed capabilities of cars | Fewer games; shorter quarters; speed restrictions in tackling drills | Reduced production of handguns and bullets |
| Preventing inappropriate release of the agent | Vehicles and road designs that simplify driver's task | Playing surfaces that reduce likelihood of falls | Locking up guns; eliminating motive for shooting (eg, no cash) |
| Modifying release of the agent | Use of seat belts to decelerate occupant with vehicle | Short cleats on shoes allowing foot to rotate, rather than transmit sudden force to knee | Single-shot guns that require reloading between firings |
| Separating in time or space | Restricting transport of hazardous materials to certain times and places | Limited-contact practice drills; placing fixed structures farther from field | |
| Separating with physical barriers | Highway medians | Face masks | Bulletproof vests; bulletproof glass |
| Modifying surfaces and basic structures | Air bags to spread forces over wide area of body; removing projections in car | Padding outside of helmets | Soft, doughnut-shaped bullets for target shooting |
| Increasing resistance to injury | Therapy for osteoporosis | Musculoskeletal conditioning | |
| Emergency response | Systems that route patients to appropriately trained physicians | Personnel trained to recognize serious injuries and physicians on call | |
| Medical care and rehabilitation | | | Occupational rehabilitation for paraplegics |

Baker S, Dietsz P. Injury prevention in healthy people: The Surgeon General's report on health promotion and disease prevention., Background papers. Washington, DC: US Government Printing Office, 1979.

**TABLE 24-32.   Three Basic Injury Control Strategies**

| Stages of Prevention | Phase of Prevention | Example |
| --- | --- | --- |
| Prevention of events that may cause injury | Before event | Bicycle paths separate from roads used by motorized vehicles |
| Prevention of injury when the event occurs | During event | Helmets for bicyclists |
| Prevention of unnecessary severity or disability after an injury occurs | After event | Neuroresuscitation in a pediatric trauma center |

*Adapted from Wilson MH. Childhood injury control. Pediatrician 1985;12:20. Used by permission of S Karger AG, Basel.*

potential will occur. Some are event phase in that they reduce injury during the event. Post-event phase strategies reduce the resulting damage even after the injury has occurred. Table 24-32 lists examples of these strategies. A complete approach to injury control requires attention to all three phases.

To be effective, a strategy must decrease injury if it is used, and it must be used. These are separate considerations. Many strategies have never been adequately evaluated for efficacy. Some strategies can be supported before the evidence is conclusive, because they make scientific sense or because they are similar to other successful strategies. If strategies are retained despite demonstrated lack of efficacy, resources are diverted from developing or promoting alternatives.

Efficacious strategies may fail because people fail to use them. Unfastened seat belts do not reduce injury. A prime role for health professionals is to help to educate and motivate families to use strategies known to prevent or reduce injury.

The most effective injury control strategies are automatic. Strategies that require frequent individual action, such as buckling a seat belt, are called active. These strategies are likely to be omitted by at least some persons at least some of the time. Achieving widespread use of new active strategies appears to require the addition of incentives and removal of disincentives and may only occur after a gradual change in cultural attitudes. Some persons, often those at highest risk, are unprotected because they fail to comply.

Automatic or passive strategies are those that protect persons without individual action, or they are "built in." For example, if all passenger cars were factory equipped with driver-side air bags, male adolescent drivers, a group at extremely high risk for car-crash injuries and death, would benefit without any change in their knowledge or behavior.

Many strategies fall between the two extremes of active or passive. For example, a parent may take action once to protect family members through time by turning down the water heater to prevent scald burns or by installing an automatic sprinkler system to reduce the possibility of fire. Purchasing, installing, and maintaining a smoke alarm powered by batteries requires periodic action.

Passive strategies are usually preferable to active strategies, because they avoid the issue of compliance and are therefore more effective. Unfortunately, passive strategies are not available for all injury events. Health care providers must continue to encourage with the best techniques available the use of active strategies that are known to be efficacious.

Strategies that prevent unintentional injuries may also prevent some inflicted injuries: abuse, homicide, and suicide. For instance, if water heaters do not heat water to a temperature that will burn skin, tap water scalding is prevented no matter what the intent of the caregiver. Reduction in the availability of handguns can be expected to prevent unintentional childhood and adolescent firearm deaths and many homicides and suicides.

## AVENUES OF INJURY CONTROL

### Education and Health Promotion

Health professionals traditionally try to change behaviors that affect health by counseling patients and their families. An increasing number of injury issues are being added to the list of recommended topics for health supervision. However, rarely is traditional health education sufficient to prevent injury. It is possible to increase knowledge about an injury problem and about prevention strategies, but increased knowledge does not lead reliably to action.

Gains have been made with a health promotion approach that delivers the message from many respected sources and provides rewards for demonstrating the desirable behavior. Schools, community groups, agencies, and the popular media can all have roles in modifying beliefs and behaviors that affect injury and injury prevention. Informed health care providers can stimulate and advise on these efforts by providing leadership or consultation.

Educating persons in power may produce the best results. These are key persons whose decisions determine the risk of injury for many. Included in this group are architects, engineers, manufacturers, designers, law enforcement specialists, lawyers, school personnel, agency heads, legislators, and health personnel.

### Regulation and Legislation

Agencies that control personal practices and the environment (eg, boards of parks and recreation, health departments, schools, athletic associations, traffic authorities, regulators of consumer products) can promulgate within their authority regulations that decrease the likelihood of childhood and adolescent injury. Fire extinguisher and smoke alarm requirements can be set for rental housing, specific pool fencing requirements can be mandated, children transported in private cars on school trips can be required to wear seat belts, and fireworks can be prohibited within city limits. Legislative authority or specific legislation must precede agency action in many cases. The success of well-designed regulations depends on enforcement or the perception of enforcement. Unenforced regulations and legislation, like knowledge without behavior change, cannot prevent injury.

Legislative and regulatory efforts to bring about injury control can occur at the local, state, or federal level. There is little uniformity among local jurisdictions or states in regard to measures affecting injury. Illustrating this is motor vehicle occupant safety. Although an increasing number of states require seat belt use by front seat car occupants and all require car safety seat use for particular categories of young passengers, the specific legislation varies widely. Some states allow "primary enforcement," which means that noncompliance is sufficient reason to stop the driver. Others allow only "secondary enforcement, " meaning that the citation can be made only if another offense has prompted action. Passenger ages and positions, vehicle types, and penalties under the law also vary, leaving many persons unprotected even by full compliance with the law. The level of enforcement is not uniform and often is so spotty that it negates the intention of the measure. Nevertheless, the impact of such legislation on injury can be documented. States with long-standing car seat laws have experienced decreased infant motor vehicle occupant death rates. Specifically designed legislation has been shown to be an effective strategy for injury control. Health professionals should be advocates for children in the legislative arena.

Legislation enacted for other reasons may also have injury reduction potential. The Emergency Highway Energy Conservation Act (1974) reduced the speed limit to 55 to conserve gasoline. The highway death rate fell. When several states later revoked this conservative limit, deaths increased with speeds. A bill requiring a deposit on glass bottles, promulgated for environmental reasons, resulted in fewer pediatric emergency room treatments of lacerations.

The activity of the Consumer Product Safety Commission (CPSC), created by the Consumer Product Safety Act of 1972, is the centerpiece of federal efforts to eliminate unreasonable hazards associated with consumer products. In this role and as administrator of several earlier acts—the Flammable Fabrics Act (1953), the Refrigerator Safety Act (1956), and the Federal Hazardous Substances Act (1960), and Poison Prevention Packaging Act (1970)—the CPSC has had a special role in injury control for children. The CPSC can negotiate voluntary product changes, and it can regulate sales and force product recalls. It reacts to petitions complaints or clues from its surveillance systems, including the National Electronic Injury Surveillance System (NEISS). Health professionals should bring product-related injuries to the attention of the CPSC and CPSC findings to the attention of their patients and communities.

## Litigation

If educational, regulatory, and legislative options have failed to bring about injury control, litigation may succeed. Pertinent to the protection of adolescent drivers, for instance, is the facilitating role litigation against automobile makers has played in expediting the provision of air bags in automobiles. Air bags are a proven technology that can automatically protect motor vehicle drivers and front seat passengers in head-on crashes. Despite demonstrated effectiveness, automobile makers were slow to install them until the financial penalty for failing to do so became prohibitive.

## INJURY CONTROL AND PERSONAL FREEDOM

Objections to the implementation of injury control strategies are often framed as arguments against interference with personal freedom. For younger children, the assumption is sometimes made that injuries are a part of the trial and error learning process of growing up and that protection may restrict their education. However, automatic strategies—those that protect the child without constant action—can be viewed as freeing the child to explore with less restriction in an inherently safer environment.

Protection of the young child is generally accepted with less tension than measures addressing any other segment of the population. There are many precedents for societal intrusion to ensure the health and welfare of children.

The argument against restricting adolescents to protect them from injury is one made also on behalf of adults: the informed person has a right to take risks. Unfortunately, the injuries and the psychologic and financial burden are not always confined to the person taking the risk.

## INJURY RISK

Injury is a common problem. No child or adolescent can be considered free from risk. However, some patterns may be helpful in designing programs or counseling individual patients.

## Demographic Issues

Throughout the life span, males have higher injury death rates than females. This increased risk is apparent even before the age of 1 year; the total injury death rates for infant boys is about 1.2 times the rate for girls. In adolescence, the differential is even more striking, with a male-to-female ratio of about 3.2:1 (Baker, 1992). Higher risk for males is recorded for almost every cause of injury, although the degree of increased risk differs and appears to reflect differences in likelihood of involvement in hazardous activities. It is not clear whether these differences in male behavior are entirely due to socialization (ie, role expectations) or reflect innate behavioral characteristics specific to the male. Gender differences are greatest for fatal and other severe injuries. Because the total number of nonfatal injuries for males is only slightly greater than for females, the exaggerated differential in death rates suggests that injuries sustained by males are on average more serious.

If the full spectrum of injury is considered, rates are highest for both sexes during adolescence. The adolescent injury death rate is exceeded only by that for the most elderly segments of the population.

Injury death rates vary with ethnicity and economic status. Native Americans have the highest injury rates of all population groups. African-Americans are a second group at particularly high risk. Asian-Americans have the lowest rates. Part of the differences by race can be explained by differences in socioeconomic status. There is considerable evidence that unintentional injury rates are highest in the lowest income areas. Unintentional injury death rates fall markedly as the per capita income increases. Whites and blacks of the same income level have about the same death rates from unintentional injury (Baker, 1992).

Although homicide rates are highest where the population is most dense, unintentional injury rates are highest in the most remote rural areas. Unlike differences in injury rates by race, disparities by population density do not narrow when adjustments are made for differences in per capita income (Baker et al, 1992).

Demographic associations, although they provide interesting clues to the complexity of injury causation and are helpful in program development, do not significantly narrow the task for health care providers. Persons who belong to the higher-risk demographic categories may require extended counseling time and effort, but patients who do not fall into the demographic categories of highest risk cannot be excluded from counseling, because no group is free from all injury risk. Although the concept of the "accident-prone" person has been popular, evidence has provided no easy rubric for limiting injury control counseling to a small subset of patients. Injury appears to be far too evenly spread across the population to allow any narrow definition of the subpopulation at risk.

## Developmental Issues

The type of injuries to which a child is most vulnerable varies with personal circumstance and with age. Age is a rough correlate of size, developmental ability, and lifestyle, which influences exposure.

### Infants

The small size of infants may be the first of their developmental disadvantages predisposing to injury. With small body size comes a small airway that is easily occluded. A small body slips through small spaces that do not always permit the relatively large head to follow, resulting in entrapment injury. Infants, completely dependent on their caregivers, are handled on elevated surfaces for the caregiver's convenience, precipitating falls.

The motor skills of infants are primitive, not allowing them to escape danger easily, causing a relatively high rate of drownings, suffocations, and deaths from fires and burns. The combination of complete dependence, small size, and primitive motor and language skills may make the infant an easy target for inflicted injury.

Infants spend most of their time in their own homes or in the homes of substitute caregivers, and most injuries in infancy occur in the home. It is worthwhile making the home a safe (ie, child-proof) environment.

An additional worry in infancy is motor vehicle occupant injury. Infants not properly restrained in a safety seat are at exceptional risk in a crash. Tests with anthropomorphic dummies suggest that unrestrained infants become missiles during crashes or are crushed between the car interior and the body of the adult who was holding them. Small size is a disadvantage.

After adolescents, infants are the pediatric age group with the highest injury death rate.

### Toddlers

After babies develop motor skills that allow them to get around on their own, by creeping or crawling and especially by walking, their injury profile changes. Toddlers are busy pushing, pulling, finding, poking, mouthing, climbing, and exploring all day long. An active toddler can exhaust even the most vigilant parent. The explosive toddler is likely to run into the street, to tumble down stairs, and to disappear in crowds. Even the most passive toddler occasionally escapes a distracted parent. Toddlers have no impulse control. They do not understand cause and effect. Making the indoor environment a safe area for exploration is worthwhile. Although the injury death rate for the toddler does not stand out, the rate of nonlethal injuries is quite high.

### Preschoolers

Increasingly sophisticated motor and intellectual skills combined with the desire to imitate the behavior of older children and adults bring the preschooler in contact with a whole new group of injury risks. For example, the child in this age group becomes a tricyclist and then a tentative bicyclist. Curiosity about matches and fires burgeons. Although skills are becoming sophisticated, judgment is not. The child of this age cannot be relied on to recognize danger. Thinking is magical. "If superheroes can fly, why not I?"

### Elementary School-Age Children

The grammar school age group is quite healthy. Persons of this age boast the lowest injury death rate of the life span. Perhaps this is because these children spend so much of their total time sitting at a desk! About half of deaths that occur are due to injury, as are many urgent medical visits and hospitalizations.

Often for the first time, the child is coping independently with the traffic environment. More children this age die as pedestrians than as motor vehicle occupants, and bicycling injuries begin to take their toll. Children of this age are still not capable of making accurate judgments about speed and distance. Their decisions begin to be heavily influenced by the actions and opinions of their peers. Their motor skills and knowledge (eg, how to light a fire, how to fire a gun, how to start a lawn mower or car) far outstrip their judgment.

### Early Adolescents

As they approach adolescence, children are given more freedom, spend more time without adult supervision, and range farther from home. Peer pressure exerts its most profound influence. Helmets and seat belts may be eschewed by the group. Risk taking becomes more conscious. The traffic environment poses the biggest hazard, particularly for those who ride with older adolescent friends who drive, who operate any kind of motorized vehicle themselves, or who ride a bicycle in traffic.

### Older Adolescents

Adult privileges and practices are attained by older adolescents without adult experience, ability, and responsibility. The assumption of the adult behaviors of drug and alcohol use and use of weapons play an important but incompletely understood role in this age group, in which injury accounts for about 75% of all deaths. The older adolescent has the highest risk of any age group for motor vehicle occupant death and for drowning. Intentional injuries (ie, suicide, homicide) also take a striking toll.

## MAJOR INJURIES

More than 22,000 persons younger than 20 years of age lost their lives in injury events in the United States in 1986 (Baker, 1992). As a category, unintentional injuries claimed the largest share, about 17,000 or 80%. Transportation injuries alone were responsible for about 10,500 deaths in this age group, about half of all injury deaths. Other unintentional injuries claimed about 6500 of the lives, 30% of the injury total. The remaining 5000, still a significant number, were classified as homicide (13%) or suicide (10%). Selected sources of data on childhood and adolescent injury are listed in the bibliography at the end of this chapter.

Not all potential causes of serious injury can be presented in this chapter. The rest of this section concentrates on the most severe unintentional injury events as reflected in mortality statistics. Injury events are grouped in the broad categories of transportation injuries and other unintentional injury events. Homicide and suicide are covered in more depth in other chapters of this text.

### Transportation Injuries

Most children and adolescents who die of transportation-related injuries were motor vehicle occupants, and pedestrians struck by motor vehicles in traffic situations make up the second largest group. A significant number of deaths also is attributed to motorcycle and bicycle incidents. The number of deaths secondary to transportation injuries in 1986 for persons younger than 20 years of age is shown in Table 24-33. Because of their impressive numbers and severity, preventing transportation-related injuries should be a high priority. Transportation injuries are also an important area because much is known about how to prevent them. The prevention of motor vehicle occupant deaths has served as the flagship effort of the field of injury control, and the efforts to protect child passengers need continuing attention. Specific suggestions are given by topic for major transportation injury issues. Additional areas for injury control related to transportation

TABLE 24-33. Number of U.S. Transportation-Related Injury Deaths, 1986

| Category of Injury | Deaths by Age Groups in Years | | | | |
|---|---|---|---|---|---|
| | 0–4 | 5–9 | 10–14 | 15–19 | 0–19 |
| Motor vehicle occupant | 640 | 380 | 614 | 5664 | 7298 |
| Pedestrian | | | | | |
| Traffic* | 368 | 471 | 275 | 494 | 1608 |
| Nontraffic | 129 | 28 | 9 | 4 | 170 |
| Motorcycle | 2 | 11 | 73 | 583 | 669 |
| Bicycle | 17 | 126 | 230 | 152 | 525 |

\* On public roads.

*Data compiled from Baker SP, O'Neill B, Ginsburg M, Li G. The injury fact book, ed. 2. New York: Oxford University Press, 1992:308.*

or to motor vehicles not explored in this chapter but included in the selected readings include trains, aircraft, school buses, farm machinery, and riding lawn mowers.

For the United States population as a whole, motor vehicle crashes cause about half of the annual 100,000 unintentional injury deaths. Injuries from motor vehicle crashes are a leading cause of death well into adulthood, and they are an important cause of permanent disability. For every death, there are at least 10 hospitalizations and 100 injuries. Motor vehicle injuries account for a large proportion of brain and spinal cord injuries and of disfiguring facial injuries.

The pediatric age group at highest risk is the adolescent. For older adolescents and young adults, motor vehicle crashes cause about 40% of all deaths. The male-to-female ratio, which portrays an increased risk for males at every age after 1 year, is especially high during the highest-risk years. Although the risk of being involved in a crash is lower for the younger pediatric age groups, the case-fatality rate for motor vehicle injury is particularly high for the youngest children; if an unrestrained infant is involved in a crash, injuries are more likely to be fatal. The preadolescent age groups are almost unique in that the number of pedestrian deaths comes close to, and for children 5 through 9 actually exceeds, the number of motor vehicle occupant deaths. For all other age groups except the very elderly, motor vehicle occupant injuries far outstrip pedestrian injuries as a cause of death.

Although motor vehicle travel increases with income, motor vehicle injury and death rates decrease, for several likely reasons: differences in urbanization, local road conditions, vehicle types, driving behavior, seat belt use, and quality of medical care. In the United States, Native Americans have the highest motor vehicle-related death rates—twice that of whites, who have the next highest rate, followed by blacks and Asian-Americans. The motor vehicle death rate in rural areas is twice that in urban areas, a difference accounted for almost entirely by motor vehicle occupant deaths. Motor vehicle occupant death rates are highest in western and southern states, a fact not explained by variations in miles traveled. Pedestrian deaths are highest in the Southeast and Southwest, and motorcycle deaths are highest in the West. Bicycle deaths show no clear geographic pattern.

## Motor Vehicle Occupants

*Incidence.* Motor vehicle occupant fatalities are more common during warm months, at night, and on weekends. Direct frontal impacts account for 46% of the fatal crashes; side impacts initiate the second largest group. Single-vehicle crashes produce a higher death rate than do multiple-vehicle crashes. Occupants

who are ejected from a vehicle in a crash or at the time of a sudden stop are particularly likely to sustain severe or fatal injury. Occupants of smaller, lighter vehicles are at increased risk in both single- and multiple-vehicle crashes, even in crashes with other vehicles of the same size. Urban roads are associated with lower death rates per passenger mile than are rural roads and limited-access roads with lower death rates than uncontrolled-access roads. Probably because of superior engineering and the separation of opposing traffic, the crash rate per passenger mile is low on the interstate system. However, when crashes do occur, they tend to be severe because of high vehicle speed.

In about half of all crashes with fatalities, a driver's blood alcohol is found to be elevated. Night crashes and young and middle-aged male drivers are factors associated with an increased likelihood of intoxication. Elevated blood alcohol is more often found with night-time crashes and with young and middle-aged male drivers.

Motor vehicle occupant death rates have been declining during the last 30 years, a fortunate fact attributed to changes in roads and vehicles and with the propitious effect of lowering the speed limit to 55 mph promulgated in the mid-1970s as an energy-saving measure.

More than 7000 children and adolescents younger than 20 years of age are killed as motor vehicle occupants in the United States annually. Motor vehicle occupant death rates for pediatric age groups are shown in Table 24-30. Unrestrained infants have excessive rates and are at particular risk if riding on an adult's lap. The child's effective weight is markedly increased during the rapid deceleration of a crash and far exceeds the adult's ability to hold on. The weight of the adult, also exaggerated during deceleration, may crush the child against the car's interior. Adolescents are also at increased risk. Injury and death rates peak during adolescence for both girls and boys, although adolescents travel fewer car miles than adults. Male teenage drivers have higher fatal crash rates than any other group.

*Prevention.* Motor vehicle occupant injuries can be reduced by preventing crashes or by reducing the forces that impinge on the body during crashes. In addition to modifying vehicles and reducing speed, forces can be reduced by spreading them over a wider area of the body and by increasing the distance over which the body decelerates. This is accomplished by restraint systems and by air bags. Measures of specific interest to health professionals caring for children include counseling and advocacy issues.

*Counseling Points.* Injury can be prevented by the use of appropriate restraint systems for age and size. Parents of very small premature infants, of children with severe developmental disabilities, and of children in casts that preclude using a standard safety seat need special guidance. Counseling should include information about the correct use of car safety seats. The AAP publishes a "Family Guide to Car Seats" each year with support from the National Highway Traffic Safety Administration.

Parents should be encouraged to make the transition from safety seats to the three-point seat belt system, to continue use of seat belts through adolescence and adulthood, and to set the standard by using their own seat belts. Stress the advantage of air bags plus seat belts. Discourage drinking and driving, and encourage parents to provide adolescents a safe ride home.

*Advocacy Issues.* Advocacy issues include the provision of restraint devices for children with special needs, extending persons and vehicles covered under state car safety seat and seat belt laws, enforcement of safety seat and seat belt laws, increasing the minimum licensing age or the provisional licensing period or extending the curfew (ie, limitation on nighttime driving) associated with provisional licenses, and maintaining lower speed limits.

## Pedestrians

*Incidence.* The second largest category of vehicle-related deaths is that of persons on foot struck and killed by motor vehicles. In such crashes, the pedestrian is completely unshielded and is at great disadvantage. The severity of the injuries that result from a motor vehicle striking a pedestrian is well illustrated by the high death-to-injury ratio. Of every 1000 pedestrians injured, 52 die. There are "only" 27 deaths for every 1000 motorcyclists injured in crashes with other motor vehicles and 12 deaths for every 1000 injured as motor vehicle occupants. The overall trend in pedestrian death rates has been downward. About 1800 children and adolescents younger than 20 years of age are killed each year as pedestrians in the United States.

The highest pedestrian death rates are experienced by the elderly, but there are also peaks in childhood and adolescence. During the pediatric years, the death rates are highest for those between 5 and 14, and boys are more likely to die, with the sex differential appearing by the second year of life. During the high-risk years, children—especially city children—are more likely to be killed as pedestrians than as motor vehicle occupants. Pedestrian deaths are an urban disease, with two thirds of the deaths and even more of the injuries occurring in urban areas. Although less frequent than urban pedestrian injury events, rural events are much more likely to result in death, probably because of increased vehicle speeds.

Only 20% of adult pedestrian deaths occur at intersections, and even fewer pediatric deaths occur there. Most occur when children run into the street or attempt to cross between intersections. Some occur when the motor vehicle invades the pedestrian's space on a sidewalk or median strip. Allowing motorists to make a right turn after stopping at a red light has increased pedestrian injuries in urban areas, because as drivers look left for oncoming traffic, they do not always see approaching pedestrians. Although most pedestrian injuries and deaths do occur in traffic, during the first few years of life a sizable proportion of pedestrian deaths occur in nontraffic areas (eg, driveways, lanes). Nontraffic pedestrian deaths are particularly high in rural areas.

Pedestrian injuries peak at about 4 p.m., but the peak time of fatal injury is about 1 hour after sunset, with the time changing with the season. Adult pedestrians believe that motorists can see them from a much greater distance than is possible. Children probably are even more likely to misjudge the ability of the driver to see and to stop, and they may not consider the possibility at all.

Most often, the front of a motor vehicle strikes the pedestrian, but children are also killed when they run into the side of the moving vehicle, are struck by the vehicle's protruding hardware (eg, mirror), or are run over by the rear wheels of a truck or bus. More pedestrians are killed walking along a roadway in the same direction as traffic than against traffic.

The weight of the vehicle and the speed at which it is traveling are important determinants of the severity of injury. The death to injury ratio is about three times higher for heavy trucks than for cars, and it increases as the posted speed limit increases.

*Prevention.* Wherever and whenever possible, motor vehicle traffic and pedestrians should be physically separated with barriers or space, or they should not be using the same space at the same time. Young children cannot be trusted near traffic. They must have fixed barriers between them and traffic or continuous supervision from an adult. Children younger than 7 years of age should cross streets only with assistance. Even during the next few years, children are still too young to cross unassisted where traffic volume is high. They have difficulty judging speed and distance. Ideally, incursions into the street should only be made at intersections and in accordance with traffic rules. Adults must set a good example. Children playing and in groups often forget all about traffic, and yet many children must cope with traffic and street crossings as they make their way to school. They should demonstrate their knowledge of and adherence to safe pedestrian practices before they make that journey unassisted. The parent should plan a route that avoids heavy, high-speed traffic and walking in the street.

*Counseling Points.* Counseling should include advice on street-crossing timing and training, using barriers between play area and traffic, planning the route to school, and avoiding walking in or along streets or roads, especially at night.

*Advocacy Issues.* Advocacy issues include the development of safe, attractive off-street play areas, diverting traffic from residential areas and around schools, loading and unloading school buses and cars bringing children to school away from traffic, making convenient walks where pedestrian traffic is heavy or making other modifications of high-risk sites, using and constructing sidewalks, slowing motor vehicle speeds in residential areas, and prohibiting parking where children are likely to cross.

### Motorcycles and Other Motorized Vehicles

*Incidence.* The rate of injuries associated with high-speed vehicles that provide no external protection for riders is high. Although children and adolescents may be physically capable of operating vehicles such as motorcycles, minibikes, mopeds, trail bikes, all-terrain vehicles, and snowmobiles, the risk under many conditions, including off-road driving, is excessive. Use by children and young adolescents should be strongly discouraged.

Motorcyclists account for one tenth of all traffic deaths. For teenagers and young adults, the proportion is even higher. More than half of all motorcycle-related deaths occur during these years. A peak in motorcycle deaths occurred in the early 1980s. Subsequently, the number of registered motorcycles and the number of motorcyclist deaths declined. In 1986, just over 650 persons younger than 20 years of age were killed while motorcycling. Most were adolescents.

Compared even with passenger cars, motorcycles are extremely dangerous: the per mile death rate is fifteen times higher, the number of deaths per registered vehicle is three times higher, and the death to injury ratio is twice as high. The disparity between death rates by gender is extreme, with rates for young males ten times those of female riders. Fifteen male motorcycle drivers die for every female driver, but more females than males die as motorcycle passengers. Collisions with other motor vehicles account for slightly more than one half of the deaths. Crashes and injuries increase with increasing vehicle power. Alcohol abuse plays a part, particularly in nighttime, single-vehicle crashes. Helmets clearly decrease severe injury and death rates among motorcyclists. Deaths decrease when laws requiring riders to wear helmets are in place, although there is not perfect compliance with the laws.

Minibikes, minicycles, and trail bikes are all motorized two-wheeled cycles that range from little more than a bicycle to almost a motorcycle. They vary in speed and other capabilities. Because they are marketed for off-road use, they do not fall under federal safety standards for road vehicles or the usual licensing procedures for vehicle and driver. The size and marketing of many are clearly targeted at children and adolescents.

Although minibikes may be considered the most benign because of their low horsepower, they carry an injury per vehicle rate four times that of bicycles. Trail bikes, which are more powerful, account for 33,000 injuries a year, more than a third of them to children younger than 14 years of age. Although trail bikes are not intended for the roadway, many injury-producing crashes occur there and involve other motor vehicles.

In 1986, almost 30,000 children between 5 and 14 years of age were injured riding all-terrain vehicles (ATVs). ATVs come in three- or four-wheel versions and are marketed for use on rugged terrain. The three-wheeled version is notably unstable, with overturn on slopes leading to catastrophic injury. A ban on the sale of three-wheeled ATVs in the United States went into effect in December of 1987, but many are still in use. Manufacturers have agreed that high-powered ATVs should not be marketed to children younger than 16, but dealer compliance is thought to be less than perfect. High speeds, lack of differential on the rear wheels making turning difficult, especially for children, and vehicle weight all contribute to the high risk.

Snowmobiles, capable of reaching high speeds, also take a heavy toll among the pediatric age groups. Of the 12,000 to 13,000 injuries in 1 year, almost 20% were to children 14 or younger, with persons between 15 and 24 years of age incurring almost half of all injuries. Given the seasonal and regional limitations on snowmobile use, the injury rate appears quite high. Although some states require registration of snowmobiles, few put restrictions on driver age. Head injuries from crashes and rollovers cause most of the deaths, but drowning is also important, because snowmobiles are often operated over frozen bodies of water. The low profile of the snowmobile may make it especially difficult for motorists to see when operated on or near the roadway.

*Prevention.*   The vehicles discussed in this section, especially the heavy and powerful ones, carry a very high injury risk. They are not toys. Operation of motorized vehicles by persons under the legal driving age should be strongly discouraged. At whatever age operation is undertaken, careful instruction by an experienced and mature operator should precede it, and helmets and protective clothing should be worn. Adults should be discouraged from carrying children as passengers on these vehicles, but if they do, they should be experienced, sober, and willing to drive slowly.

*Counseling Points.*   Counseling should include information about avoiding motorcycles and off-road vehicles for children younger than driving age, discouraging the use of motorcycles and off-road vehicles by adolescents because of the high rate of serious injuries, using helmets and other protective clothing for operators and passengers, and avoiding use of motorcycles on public roads because other motor vehicles may be encountered.

*Advocacy Issues.*   Advocacy issues include regulating the marketing and sales of the products to children, licensing of operators and minimum age requirements, prohibiting the use of off-road vehicles on public roads, and enforcement of helmet laws.

### Bicycles

*Incidence.*   Children and adolescents are disproportionately represented among the 900 bicyclists killed in the United States annually. The death rate is highest for children between the ages of 10 and 14. Bicyclist deaths account for about 20% of all transportation-related deaths during those years. Nine of 10 bicycling deaths involve collision of the bicyclist with a motor vehicle, and most involve head or neck injury. Male riders have higher injury rates and much higher death rates than females.

Most injuries and deaths occur during warm months and in the afternoon or early evening. The weekend is not a particularly vulnerable time, as it is for other motor vehicle deaths, probably because alcohol abuse does not play as large a part. Rates also vary less with urbanization, socioeconomic status, and region.

Children are often seriously injured when they ride out of a driveway, side street, or alley into the path of a motor vehicle. Cyclist error can be identified as a precipitating factor in many crashes, although this is unlikely to be the most fruitful area for prevention. Collisions during street riding occur most often at intersections or when the cyclist is riding on the wrong side of the street against traffic.

Although collisions with motor vehicles are more likely to result in severe injury or death, falls from bicycles are much more common, with some resulting in serious head injuries or fractures of the extremities. The quality of the riding surface affects the likelihood of a fall. Also contributing to injury are mechanical failure, clothing entanglement, stunt riding, and double riding. Infants and young children carried on the back of an adult's bicycle are a special case of double riding. The extra weight of the passenger makes the bicycle more difficult to maneuver and to stop. Without a special carrier that shields and restrains the child, the child may fall from the bicycle or get feet or legs caught in bicycle spokes. The infant passenger is vulnerable during any crash.

The pressure of the handlebars or seat can cause neuropathy or perineal irritation. Falls on the top bar of the boy's-style bike cause straddle injuries, and abdominal injuries result from falls on the handlebars.

*Prevention.*   Whenever and wherever possible, bicyclists, especially child bicyclists, should be separated from motor vehicle traffic. All cyclists should wear helmets, because most serious injuries and deaths are due to head injury. Helmets can reduce the likelihood of brain injury in a crash or fall by as much as 88%.

*Counseling Points.*   Counseling should include advice about always wearing a helmet, carrying infants in a special protective seat, avoiding riding in the street or on the road (ie, children), obeying traffic rules when riding on the road (ie, older children and adolescents), avoiding riding after dark, adding lights for bikes and reflective clothing for riders, and buying a bike of the correct size.

*Advocacy Issues.*   Advocacy issues include bicycle helmet laws, separating bicycle and motor vehicle traffic, decreasing the speed of motor vehicles on shared roadways, and improving the riding surface.

## Injuries Not Involving Transportation

Injuries occur wherever children are—at home, at school, in places of recreation. Causes and kinds of injury are so numerous that no discussion can be exhaustive. The clinician and parent must be alert for injury potential when viewing the child's whole lifestyle and milieu. Demanding particular attention are the injury risks children and adolescents may face during recreation (eg, sports-related injuries) or occupation (eg, farm injuries, burns and lacerations in fast-food jobs). The principles of prevention are sufficiently generic to permit wise choices when hazards are identified. The most common unintentional injury events resulting in death (Table 24-34) are discussed in the following sections.

### Drowning

*Incidence.*   Drowning (ie, death from submersion) is second only to transportation injuries as a cause of unintentional injury death for children and adolescents, accounting for about 2000 deaths each year. Drowning death rates peak at 1 to 2 years of age and again in older adolescence. The increased drowning risk experienced by boys is apparent at a very early age, but it becomes even more exaggerated in adolescence when male drowning death rates are the highest of the life span and almost ten times higher than rates for girls of the same age.

Most toddler and preschooler drownings occur when a briefly unattended child falls into a body of water. One third of these drownings, about 250 each year, take place in swimming pools, often at home. The increasing popularity of home whirlpools, hot tubs, and spas is providing a new place for young children

## TABLE 24-34. Number of U.S. Nontransportation-Related Injury Deaths, 1986

| Category of Injury | Deaths by Age Groups in Years | | | | |
|---|---|---|---|---|---|
| | *0–4* | *5–9* | *10–14* | *15–19* | *0–19* |
| Drowning | 754 | 326 | 323 | 659 | 2062 |
| Fires/burns | 793 | 292 | 144 | 153 | 1382 |
| Asphyxiation | | | | | |
|   Suffocation | 250 | 31 | 66 | 64 | 411 |
|   Choking/ aspiration | 280 | 21 | 28 | 28 | 357 |
| Unintentional shootings | 34 | 57 | 143 | 238 | 472* |
| Poisoning† | 93 | 24 | 30 | 219 | 366 |
| Falls | 117 | 22 | 33 | 150 | 322 |

  * Total firearm deaths far exceed this number because firearms are responsible for many homicides and suicides.

  † About 60% are due to solid or liquids, the rest to gases or vapors. Many in the 10–19 ages groups are classified as suicides.

  *Data compiled from Baker SP, O'Neill B, Ginsburg M, Li G. The injury fact book, ed. 2. New York: Oxford University Press, 1992:308.*

to drown. Toddlers can drown in any amount of water that is sufficiently deep to cover the nose and mouth; diaper pail, toilet bowl, large bucket, and bathtub drownings occur. Older children, adolescents, and adults also inadvertently fall into water and drown, and about one third of unintentional drowning deaths occur that way. Only one quarter of the drowning victims were swimming before death. Of those, most were not swimming in designated areas but in unsupervised rivers, creeks, or quarries. Drowning while scuba diving, skin diving, or surfing contributes only a small proportion of all cases. Most boating-related drownings are associated with small recreational boats. Drowning follows a capsize or a fall overboard. Personal flotation devices often were not available or were not in use.

Drownings are more likely to occur on the weekend and during the warm months. Alcohol is involved in many adolescent drownings. The number of boating drownings has decreased modestly and other drownings more dramatically in recent years, with the largest decrease for those between 5 and 19 years of age.

Water is associated with additional injury hazards. For instance, diving where the water depth is inadequate accounts for about 700 spinal cord injuries a year, a significant proportion of all such injuries. Body surfing is also associated with spinal cord injuries. Hair can become trapped or body parts affixed by the suction developed by improperly grated pool and spa drains, resulting in submersion injury.

*Prevention.* Home water hazards should be eliminated. Children should not play in or near water without supervision. Wherever possible, fixed physical barriers should prevent young children access to water hazards. Particularly important is the requirement for unbreechable fencing around all four sides of home and public swimming pools. Swimming and boating should be permitted only in designated areas, after adequate training, and with supervision by an adult who has not been drinking alcohol. All persons in boats should wear personal flotation devices.

*Counseling Points.* Counseling includes advice on maintaining constant visual contact by an adult of young children in and around water, four-sided fencing of back yard pools, decreasing

water hazards in a young child's environment, discouraging swimming lessons for infants because of the risk of water intoxication and hypothermia, swimming and boating in designated areas only, wearing personal flotation devices, avoiding use of alcohol during water-related recreation, and cardiopulmonary resuscitation training for pool owners.

*Advocacy Issues.* Advocacy issues include requiring four-sided pool fencing, draining or fencing quarries and other such sites where water may pool over hidden hazards, decreasing the drinking of alcohol during water-related activities, and enforcing requirements for use of personal flotation devices.

### Fires and Burns

*Incidence.* Fires and burns cause about 1400 child and adolescent deaths each year. House fires cause most injuries. Most persons who die in house fires die of smoke inhalation and are dead before rescue and medical attention are provided. House fire death rates are highest for young children and for the elderly. Both groups are disadvantaged in at least two ways: They are less able to escape after fire breaks out, and they have high fatality rates with burn injury. Although males have higher fire and burn death rates, the disparity between the sexes is not so great as for some other kinds of injury.

Only about 10% of house fires are attributed to children playing with matches or other ignition sources. Cigarettes are a much more common cause. Typically, a cigarette falls onto upholstery or a bed during the evening hours and smolders there until conflagration breaks out in the early morning hours while the residents sleep. Heating equipment (eg, portable heaters, chimney fires, wood sparks) is the next most prominent cause of residential fires. Improperly installed or maintained heaters also cause deaths from carbon monoxide poisoning. About 5% of fire fatalities occur in fires attributed to arson.

Racial differences in death rates are particularly pronounced for young children, with black and Native American death rates at least twice as high as for whites. These rates are partially explained by socioeconomic differences, because the disparity decreases in high-income areas. Death rates are lower for blacks and whites in areas with higher per capita income. House fires occur more commonly in the winter and on the weekend, the latter perhaps reflecting a period of increased alcohol use.

Although house fire death rates had been increasing, that trend appears to have reversed in the early 1980s, and childhood deaths from other thermal injury have decreased even more. Clothing ignition burns, although second to house fires as a cause of death in the fires and burns category and once relatively common for young girls, account for only about 4% of all burn deaths and are now rare in children. Gasoline and automotive burns are important in adolescence. Although decreasing, fire and burn injury is still of marked significance because of the proportion of injury fatalities for which it is responsible and because of the terrible toll of pain, prolonged medical treatment, and permanent disfigurement it exacts.

Scald and contact burns are an important cause of injury morbidity in childhood. Hot liquids, often coffee or the liquid from a tipped-over cooking pot, cause most childhood burn hospitalizations. Another major source of scald burns is hot water from the tap. Burns from contact with a hot object, including the iron, the stove, the oven, the hot comb, the grill, charcoal, a cooking pot, a heater grate, a lighted cigarette, and fireworks, are common in childhood. Although occasionally severe or permanently damaging, these burns usually affect a more limited skin area and are therefore more easily treated than scalds. Burns to the face, eyes, hands, and genitals are particularly likely to result in long-term developmental problems. Burns are significant sources of injury because of their terrible toll of pain, prolonged medical treatment, and permanent disfigurement.

Some contact burns and hot water scalds are inflicted by the caregiver or result from willful neglect. Often, however, the circumstances of injury remain in doubt. Some prevention strategies may protect without regard to intent. If water from the tap was not hot enough to burn infant skin, the injury would be prevented no matter what the intent.

*Prevention.* The greatest gains in preventing fire and burn injuries can be made by the elimination and early detection of house fires. Working smoke detectors should be on every floor of every home. Although it would have a smaller impact on mortality statistics, decreasing hot water temperature can decrease morbidity, as can measures that reduce other sources of scald and contact burns.

The severity of burns can be decreased by immediately cooling the burned skin by immersing it in cool water or applying a cool wet pack.

*Counseling Points.* Counseling includes advice on having working smoke detectors on every floor of the home, turning down hot water heat so that water is not more than 120 °F to 125 °F, avoiding cigarette-initiated fires, planning escape routes in case of fire, placing home fire extinguishers near locations where fires are likely to start (eg, kitchen), keeping ignition sources away from children, using safe home heating, avoiding private use of fireworks, learning "drop and roll" in case of clothing ignition, and cooling a burn.

*Advocacy Issues.* Advocacy issues include smoke detector requirements, fire-safe cigarettes, childproof cigarette lighters, automatic sprinkler systems in new buildings, building codes that prevent house fire deaths, and fireworks bans except for community displays.

## Asphyxiation

*Incidence.* A major cause of injury death during childhood is asphyxiation by choking ($\approx$350 deaths) or by mechanical suffocation ($\approx$400 deaths). The size of the asphyxiation problem is exaggerated by existing data, because the presence of regurgitated food in the respiratory tract, a common terminal finding, is included; it accounts for some of the cases coded as asphyxiation. The fact remains, however, that choking on food and on other items kills more than 200 children each year. Child fatalities are concentrated among children younger than 4 years of age, with the peak occurring in the first year. Round, firm food products (eg, pieces of hot dog, candy, nuts, raw vegetables, grapes) are the most common airway-blocking agents in early childhood. Also choked on are small objects like round or pliable toys (eg, small balls, uninflated balloons), pop tops, safety pins, coins, and pieces of makeshift pacifiers, bottle nipples, or plastic-lined disposable diapers. Older children and adults usually choke on meat.

Asphyxiation can occur when the child is trapped in an airtight space or when the child's airway is constricted from the outside, as in hanging. Crib strangulations occur when the baby's relatively small body slips between the bars and the head, too large to follow, is trapped. Current CPSC regulations for slat spacing for new cribs (2⅜ in or less) prevent such events, but old cribs must be checked.

Children are also asphyxiated in inadvertent hangings in drapery, pacifier, or toy cords; when lids fall on them as they peer inside a toy chest; when they are trapped between frame and mattress of a bed or in the folds of a mesh playpen; when nose and mouth are covered in a soft basket, pillow, beanbag, or waterbed; when, unattended, they slip out of a high chair; inside plastic bags; in old refrigerators; in excavations that collapse; or when inadvertently covered by materials such as grain in the farm environment. The likely events vary with age.

Part of the apparent decrease in asphyxiation deaths among babies in the past 30 years is an artifact of coding changes for sudden infant death syndrome, but a decrease has also been noted in the 1 to 4 age group, reflecting in part a decrease in refrigerator entrapments after design and disposal changes.

*Prevention.* Parents can be taught what to do if a child chokes and can be cautioned about the household choking and suffocation hazards, like foods that may block the airway of a young child and unsafe crib designs. However, the most promising prevention strategies are probably those that involve redesign and regulation of hazardous products.

*Counseling Points.* Counseling includes advice on avoiding foods and nonfood objects on which infants and toddlers are likely to choke, avoiding cords in children's environments in which they may hang, purchasing age-appropriate toys so that toys for young children do not have small parts, ensuring a safe sleeping environment for infants (eg, crib slat space no more than 2⅜ in, no soft enveloping surfaces), avoiding entrapment hazards, explaining danger of earthen caves, tunnels, and excavations, and knowing rescue techniques for choking. If the choking child is able to talk or breathe and is coughing, no maneuver should be attempted. If the child is unable to breath and cough, recommended maneuvers depend on the age of the child (Table 24-35).

*Advocacy Issues.* Advocacy issues include regulation of hazardous toys and children's furniture and fencing of construction sites and excavations.

## Unintentional Firearm Injuries

*Incidence.* Children in the United States have a uniquely high risk of being shot. As with burn injuries, intent is not always easy to judge. Guns in this culture are highly available and over all age groups are responsible for 2% of all unintentional injury deaths, about two thirds of homicides, and more than half of suicides. Children can be the victims of all three. Unintentional shootings kill about 500 and severely injure many additional children and adolescents each year. Even more children and adolescents are murdered with guns. Suicide, most often accomplished with a gun, is the third leading cause of death in male adolescents, exceeded only by unintentional injuries and homicide. Nonwhite adolescent boys are more likely to be murdered with a gun than to die in any other way.

No other type of injury shows such a strong inverse association with socioeconomic status. Rates for unintentional firearm deaths are 10 times higher in low-income areas than in high-income areas and are highest in rural and remote areas. Firearm homicide is more common in urban areas than in rural areas. Males are at highest risk, with a male-to-female ratio of 6:1 for unintentional shootings and 5:1 for homicide and suicide.

Boys between the ages of 13 and 17 have the highest rates of unintentional shooting death. The most common scenario for unintentional shootings is for one child to shoot another at home with a gun kept by the parents, ostensibly for the family's safety. Although unintentional firearm deaths have been decreasing, suicides and homicides have increased for adolescents and children, respectively. The presence of a gun in the home increases the risk of adolescent suicide.

Although some fiercely assert the right of the individual to keep a gun for protection, the fact remains that a gun in the home is much more likely to kill a family member than an intruder. Children cannot be trusted to handle a gun safely, even though they quickly acquire the mechanical skill and strength to fire one. No amount of exhortation is enough to ensure they will not make a deadly error. It is not clear what effect television or toy gun play has on the number of gun injuries in this country. It is clear that guns sold as toys, those that shoot nonbullet projectiles, and nonpowder firearms are associated with high injury rates.

## TABLE 24-35. Recommended First Aid for Children Who Are Choking

### Infant

1. Place the infant face down on the forearms in a 60°, head-down position with the head and neck stabilized. Brace the forearm against the body for additional support (or lay the infant face down over the lap with the head supported and lower than the trunk).
2. Administer four back blows rapidly with the heel of the hand high between the shoulder blades.
3. If the obstruction is not relieved, turn the infant over. Place him or her in a supine position on a firm surface and deliver four rapid chest thrusts (similar to external cardiac compressions) over the sternum using two fingers.
4. If breathing does not resume, open the airway using the tongue–jaw lift technique; this draws the tongue away from the back of the throat and may help relieve the obstruction. If the foreign body can be seen, it may be extracted by a finger sweep. No blind finger sweeps should be used. They may cause further obstruction.
5. If the infant does not begin to breathe spontaneously, attempt ventilation with two breaths by mouth-to-mouth or mouth-to-mouth-and-nose technique.
6. Repeat steps 1 to 5 and persist in performing the above techniques as needed, while rapidly seeking aid from emergency medical services.

### Small Child

1. Place the child on his or her back and kneel at the child's feet, placing the heel of one hand on the child's abdomen in the midline between the umbilicus and rib cage. Place the second hand on top of the first. Apply a series of 6 to 10 abdominal thrusts—Heimlich maneuver—until the foreign body is expelled. The maneuver should consist of rapid inward and upward thrusts.
2. If the obstruction is not relieved using the Heimlich maneuver, open the victim's mouth using the tongue–jaw lift. If the foreign body can be seen, it may be manually extracted by a finger sweep. However, blind sweeps may cause further obstruction and should not be used.
3. If the child does not begin to breathe spontaneously, attempt to ventilate him or her with mouth-to-mouth or mouth-to-mouth-and-nose technique. If unsuccessful, repeat a series of 6 to 10 abdominal thrusts.
4. Repeat steps 1 to 3 and persist in performing the above techniques as needed, while rapidly seeking aid from emergency medical services.

### Large Child or Adolescent

1. Perform the abdominal thrusts on a conscious child with the victim standing or sitting, as for an adult. Stand behind the victim and wrap the hands around the waist. Make one hand into a fist and grasp it with the other hand. Place the thumb side of the fist against the victim's abdomen between the umbilicus and rib cage. Repeat 6 to 10 quick inward and upward thrusts as needed until the foreign body is dislodged.
2. If the victim is unconscious, lay the victim on his or her back. Position yourself straddling the victim's hips or one thigh. Place the hands on top of each other against the victim's abdomen between the umbilicus and rib cage. This position allows the delivery of a greater inward and upward thrust.
3. If the obstruction is not relieved using the Heimlich maneuver, open the victim's mouth using the tongue–jaw lift. If the foreign body can be seen, it may be manually extracted by a finger sweep. Blind sweeps should not be used, as they may cause further obstruction.
4. If breathing does not resume, attempt ventilation with mouth-to-mouth technique. If unsuccessful, repeat abdominal thrusts alternating with mouth-to-mouth ventilation as needed, while rapidly seeking aid from emergency medical services.

Rapid transport to a medical facility is urgent if the above first-aid measures fail. An emergency tracheotomy or the insertion of a large-bore (14-gauge) needle through the cricothyroid membrane to secure a temporary airway can be performed by those with experience.

*Adapted from McIntire MS, ed. Injury control for children and youth, chap 18. Elk Grove Village, IL: Committee on Accident and Poison Prevention, American Academy of Pediatrics, 1987 and Committee on Accident and Poison Prevention, American Academy of Pediatrics. First aid for the choking child, 1988. Pediatrics, 1988;81:740.*

*Prevention.* Guns and children should be nowhere near each other. If parents choose to own guns, the guns should be locked away unloaded and separate from ammunition. If parents choose to allow older children to learn to shoot, it should be under the strictest training and supervision.

*Counseling Points.* Counseling includes advice about the danger of guns in the home, safe storage of firearms, removal of firearms from the homes of suicidal adolescents, and the danger of nonpowder firearms as toys.

*Advocacy Issues.* Advocacy issues include laws that prohibit access to firearms by minors and controlling the manufacture, sale, and use of handguns.

### Acute Poisoning

*Incidence.* Most deaths from acute poisoning are among adults. Two pediatric age groups incur most of the childhood poisoning events: children between the ages of 1 and 4 (<100 deaths/year) and adolescents between the ages of 13 and 19 ($\approx$250 deaths). For every death, there are more than 20 hospitalizations. Centers belonging to the American Association of Poison Control Centers, which cover 60% of the U.S. population, record more than 800,000 calls a year about children and adolescents. More than half of all calls to poison centers concern children, but children younger than 5 comprise only 1% of poisoning fatalities. Most fatalities among the young are secondary to ingested drugs—aspirin, antidepressants, and cardiovascular drugs. Petroleum products make up the second largest category in the youngest age group. Caustics, although much less frequently involved, remain a source of particularly damaging ingestions.

There has been a satisfying decrease in the number of early childhood poisoning deaths, due in part to the vigorous efforts of many health care professionals and a combination of strategies. The sharpest decline followed the introduction of child-resistant packaging in 1970, after legislation required that toxic substances accessible to children be sold in containers difficult for a young child to open and involving products covered by the packaging requirements. Effort is required to sustain and extend this success, and acute poisoning still results in many hospital admissions and emergency visits for children.

Adolescent intentional poisoning deaths (ie, suicides) have not decreased. In one state where hospitalizations of adolescents with drug ingestions were studied, aspirin and its alternatives, benzodiazepines, alcohol, and antidepressants, were the most common drugs used. More girls than boys were hospitalized. Female death rates from antidepressant overdose are higher than male rates throughout the life span, an association not found for any other kind of injury death.

Children and adolescents are not exempt from carbon monoxide poisoning from car exhaust and faulty heating systems. For all ages taken together, carbon monoxide from motor vehicle exhaust is the most common agent in poisoning deaths. There are many unintentional deaths from motor vehicle exhaust each year. Deaths peak in adolescence for females and early adulthood for males. Rates are higher in low-income and rural areas and during the coldest months. Suicidal deaths from carbon monoxide are much more common than unintentional deaths, with rates being highest for middle-aged females and in high-income areas of intermediate urbanization.

*Prevention.*   The key to preventing unintentional and intentional poisonings is to prevent access to lethal quantities of chemicals. This can be done in several ways, but the more automatic the approach (ie, the less it depends on the watchfulness of persons), the better.

*Counseling Points.*   Counseling includes advice on keeping medications in a locked cabinet, buying medications in child-resistant packages, safe storage of poisonous substances, knowing when and how to call the Poison Control Center, keeping syrup of ipecac in the home for use as a postingestion emetic when recommended by a physician or Poison Control Center, maintaining the home heating system and car exhaust system, and eliminating hazardous chemicals (eg, kerosene, caustics) from the home environment.

*Advocacy Issues.*   Advocacy issues include maintaining and extending requirements for child-resistant packaging, continuing the practice of packaging antipyretics for children in sublethal total doses, and supporting regionalized Poison Control Centers.

### Falls

*Incidence.*   About 13,000 deaths are attributed to falls each year, but most of these occur among adults and partly reflect the high injury rate and fatality rate in the elderly. In 1986, about 300 children and adolescents suffered fatal falls. The highest pediatric fall death rates are in the very early years and during adolescence.

Falls are the most common cause of nonfatal injury. Every year, 1 in 20 persons receives medical care for injuries suffered in a fall. Falls are the leading cause of unintentional injury emergency room visits for children and a prominent cause of hospitalization. Falls are an important cause of brain injury.

Falls are common at all ages, but the peak incidence of medically treated falls is 1 year of age. In contrast to the figure of 1 in 20 for the whole population, each year 1 in 10 children between the ages of 1 and 3 years receives emergency treatment for a fall. Of these, about one eighth fell down stairs, and stair-related falls constitute about one quarter of hospital series. Most of the other hospitalized children fell from one surface to another.

Little variation is seen between high- and low-income areas or between urban and rural areas in overall morbidity and mortality from falls, but the specific events vary. Illustrating the special risks of the environment and the success of intervention is the decrease in fatal falls of children from New York City high-rise

apartment windows after the Board of Health's program to install guards on the windows of apartments with young children.

Falls can occur on the same level (eg, slipping while walking on an icy sidewalk), from one surface to another (eg, off a bed or changing table to the floor, down stairs), from a vehicle (eg, a car, pickup, bike), or from a height (eg, out of an upper story window, off the slide).

Several risk situations have been implied by the examples used here, and no list can be exhaustive, but several additional common or severe types of falls should be mentioned. Most injuries that occur on playgrounds result from falls. Baby walkers appear to be associated with a very high risk, particularly because of their propensity for being ridden down unguarded stairways, and they cannot be recommended as safe. Falls from vehicles (eg, from the backs of pick-up trucks) and falls that occur while playing on roofs, in trees, on bridges, or other elevated structures affect older children and adolescents and are likely to be severe. Falls associated with recreation are common in childhood and adolescence—from the skateboard, bicycle, horse, or playground equipment, to name only a few. Work-related falls, such as from scaffolding or ladders, also occur in adolescence. It is important for the health provider to remember that many inflicted injuries are falsely attributed to falls.

The forces that cause injury in a fall depend on velocity at impact, which is determined by the height of the fall and the stopping distance. It is more serious to fall from greater heights. Perhaps not so intuitively obvious, it is better to stop slowly, that is, to decelerate over a greater distance. The compressibility of the surface and of the presenting body part are important. Contrast the head of a toddler landing on cement with the buttocks landing on a thick carpet; the laws of physics and clinical experience predict much less damage in the latter situation. Surfaces that allow increased distance for deceleration are referred to as "forgiving" and are greatly preferred where children are likely to fall.

*Prevention.*   Environmental redesign has much to offer in protecting all segments of the population from falls. Falls from a height should be prevented by barriers. Where falls are predictable, forgiving surfaces should be in place to greet the child who falls.

*Counseling Points.*   Counseling includes advice on choosing not to use a baby walker, timing of the move from crib to a low bed, guarding stairways with special gates in homes with toddlers, using restraining belts on baby furniture (eg, high chairs, changing tables) and constant attendance of babies on high surfaces, installing screens that cannot be pushed out or window guards on all open windows above the first story, choosing safe home playground equipment and installing it over a forgiving surface, using protective clothing and helmets where appropriate for recreational activities, using side rails on bunk beds, and not allowing children to ride in a vehicle where they cannot ride restrained (eg, back of a pick-up truck).

*Advocacy Issues.*   Advocacy issues include the design and regulation of baby walkers, the design and use of furniture for children, window guard regulations, guard rails small children cannot climb over or fall through, playground design and regulations, provision of forgiving surfaces where children are likely to fall, and building codes that reduce falls on steps.

## THE HEALTH CARE PROVIDER'S ROLE IN INJURY CONTROL

### Anticipatory Guidance

Health care providers cannot ignore in their professional encounters with children and adolescents the number one cause of

TABLE 24-36.   Age-Appropriate Injury Prevention Topics and Advice

| | Advice for Prevention |
|---|---|
| **0–Years** | |
| Car crashes, falls, choking, suffocation, fires, burns, drowning, poisoning | Use a safe car seat correctly.<br>Never leave infants alone on high places.<br>Avoid baby walkers.<br>Keep small objects, hard foods, and harmful substances out of reach.<br>Never leave a child alone in or near water, hot liquids, or any heat source.<br>Install a smoke detector.<br>Have syrup of ipecac in the home.<br>Write Poison Control Center number on the home phone.<br>Know how to save a choking child.<br>Lower hot water heater to 120°F–125°F. |
| **1–2 Years** | |
| Poisoning, falls, choking, fires, burns, drowning, car crashes | Use safety caps on medications.<br>Store all toxic household products and medicines out of reach.<br>Use window screens which cannot push out and gates.<br>Keep toddler in an enclosed space and closely supervised when outdoors.<br>Keep electrical cords and handles of pots and pans on stove out of reach, and keep hot foods away from edge of table.<br>Never leave child in a tub or pool.<br>Use toddler car seat.<br>Eliminate or safely store firearms. |
| **2–4 Years** | |
| Falls, fires, burns, poisoning, drowning, car crashes, pedestrian injury | Keep doors to dangerous areas locked.<br>Use screens, guards, and gates.<br>Teach children about watching for cars in driveways and streets and danger of following ball into street, but continue to supervise.<br>Keep firearms locked up.<br>Keep medicines, knives, electrical equipment, and matches out of reach.<br>Arrange group swimming lessons after 3 years of age.<br>Never leave child in a tub or pool.<br>Use toddler car seat and then belt-positioning booster seat.<br>Continue to keep syrup of ipecac in the home<br>Teach children to avoid unknown animals. |
| **5–9 Years** | |
| Car crashes, pedestrian injury, bicycle injury, drowning, firearms, burns | Teach pedestrian, motor vehicle, and bicycle safety.<br>Do not allow bicycling on roadway before 10 years of age.<br>Use seat belts and bicycle helmets.<br>Continue swimming classes.<br>Supervise around water.<br>Keep firearms locked up.<br>Avoid off-road motor vehicle use.<br>Supervise use of matches. |
| **10–15 Years** | |
| Car crashes, pedestrian injury, bicycle injury, firearms, drowning, burns, falls | Continue rules of bicycle, pedestrian, motor vehicle safety, with good examples set by adults.<br>Insist on seat belts and bicycle helmets.<br>Discourage night bicycle riding and riding of off-road and other motorized vehicles.<br>Discourage nonpowder firearms.<br>Provide safe facilities for recreation and social activities.<br>Stress the buddy system in all sports.<br>Prohibit unsupervised swimming or boating.<br>Discourage alcohol use.<br>Eliminate or safely store firearms. |
| **16–19 Years** | |
| Car crashes, drowning, pedestrian injury, other motorized vehicles, firearms, suicide, homicide | Provide appropriate driver's education.<br>Insist on seat belt use.<br>Insist on helmets for bicycling and for riding other motorized vehicles.<br>Prohibit driving or swimming when under the influence of alcohol or other drugs.<br>Prohibit firearms except under the most stringent safety and training conditions. |

*Adapted from McIntire MS, ed. Injury control for children and youth. Elk Grove Village, IL: American Academy of Pediatrics, 1987.*

morbidity and mortality. However, discussion of every possible event and safety measure would overwhelm both practitioner and patient. Issues must be chosen for emphasis. When the practitioner follows a child through time, advice can be staged in an age-appropriate schedule. Topics can be chosen for a particular child because they meet one or more of the following criteria:

- The injuries are severe, ie, likely to result in death or permanent disability.
- The injuries are quite common for the age group.
- Effective prevention strategies are known and practical.
- The child is at special risk because of developmental age, medical condition, or exposure.

If more than one of these criteria are met for a child during one visit, the invitation for anticipatory guidance is hard to ignore. The more a clinician knows about the patient and the patient's milieu, the more "on target" the anticipatory guidance can be.

To aid the practitioner, counseling schedules have been prepared that suggest the most important topics to be covered for most children of specific ages. A 1983 Injury Prevention policy statement by the American Academy of Pediatrics (AAP) suggests that, at the minimum, advice about car restraints and seat belts, smoke detectors, hot-water tap temperatures, window and stairway guards, syrup of ipecac, bicycle helmets, and pedestrian safety should be an integral part of pediatric medical care.

A specific list of precautions for parents and children that includes those in the safety counseling section of the Academy's *Injury Control for Children and Youth* (McIntire, 1987) is to be found in Table 24-36. The Statewide Comprehensive Injury Prevention Program of the Massachusetts Department of Public Health also provides an Injury Prevention Counseling Schedule. These and other organizations provide materials to assist in injury control counseling. The AAP provides an educational package called *The Injury Prevention Program*, which is composed of age-appropriate surveys and instructional sheets in Spanish and in English that outline the major causes of childhood injuries and their prevention, a schedule, and a physician's guide. The National Safe Kids Campaign, based at the Children's National Medical Center in Washington, D.C., provides materials for counseling and for community advocacy. Regional Injury Prevention Centers, funded by the Centers for Disease Control (CDC) and the Division of Injury Control at the CDC, are valuable resources.

Office-based anticipatory guidance as usually provided, no matter how well intentioned, falls short of accomplishing injury control. The word of the physician is not enough to protect children from injury. Clinicians must take the advice of the educational experts about how to maximize these limited moments with families. Group well-child care, for example, seems to be a more successful format for anticipatory guidance about injury prevention than individual counseling.

If all health providers do to prevent injury is to admonish patients and families during regularly scheduled health care visits, the injury disease will not go away. Clinicians can be very effective community advocates for injury control. When health care providers remain silent on injury issues, the community may mistakenly assume that injury is not a matter of health.

## Advocacy

Clinicians can be pivotal in the community approach to injury control by providing consultation, urging design changes, testifying for legislation, informing regulations, and ensuring that the trauma system serves children well. Many of the gains recorded in injury control have resulted from such open advocacy on the part of health care workers for their patients, our children and adolescents.

## Selected Readings

American Academy of Pediatrics, Committee on Accident and Poison Prevention. TIPP (the injury prevention program): A guide to safety counseling in office practice. Elk Grove Village, IL: American Academy of Pediatrics, 1989.

Baker SP. Childhood injuries: The community approach to prevention. J Public Health Policy 1981;2:235.

Baker SP, O'Neill B, Ginsburg M, Li G. The injury fact book, ed. 2. New York: Oxford University Press, 1992:308.

Baker SP, Waller AE. Childhood injury: State-by state mortality facts. Baltimore: Injury Prevention Center, The Johns Hopkins University, 1989.

Children's Safety Network. A data book of child and adolescent injury. Washington, DC: National Center for Education in Maternal and Child Health, 1991.

Committee on Trauma Research, Commission on Life Sciences, National Research Council, and the Institute of Medicine. Injury in America. Washington, DC: National Academy Press, 1985.

Division of Injury Control, Center for Environmental Health and Injury Control, Centers for Disease Control. Childhood injuries in the United States. Am J Dis Child 1990;144:627.

Gallagher SS, Guyer B, Kotelchuck M, et al. A strategy for the reduction of childhood injuries in Massachusetts: SCIPP. N Engl J Med 1982;307:1015.

Haddon W. Advances in the epidemiology of injuries as a basis for public policy. Public Health Rep 1980;95:411.

McIntire MS, ed. Injury control for children and youth. Elk Grove Village, IL: American Academy of Pediatrics, 1987.

National Committee for Injury Prevention and Control. Injury prevention: Meeting the challenge. New York: Oxford University Press, 1989.

Rice DP, MacKenzie EJ, et al. Cost of injury in the United States: A report to Congress. San Francisco: Institute for Health and Aging, University of California and Injury Prevention Center, Johns Hopkins University, 1989.

Rivara FP. Traumatic deaths of children in the United States: Currently available prevention strategies. Pediatrics 1985;75:456.

Runyan CW, Gerken EA. Epidemiology and prevention of adolescent injury: A review and research agenda. JAMA 1989;262:2273.

Widome MD. Pediatric injury prevention for the practitioner. Curr Probl Pediatr 1991;21:428.

Wilson MH, Baker SP, Teret SP, et al. Saving children: A guide to injury prevention. New York: Oxford University Press, 1991.

*Principles and Practice of Pediatrics, Second Edition.*
edited by Frank A. Oski et al. J. B. Lippincott Company, Philadelphia © 1994.

# CHAPTER 25
# *Special Needs of Children With Chronic Illnesses*

Nancy Hutton

Caring for children with chronic physical, emotional, and social problems accounts for a substantial amount of the practicing pediatrician's time and energy. The pediatrician in training sees more than the usual number of patients with chronic, complex, multisystem disorders. These facts make it easy to focus entirely on the problem and lose sight of the broad picture. It is important to step back and consider the needs of children with ongoing problems and identify those common to all children and those that are unique.

The fact that childhood chronic illness is becoming more common attests to the success of advances in medical care. The incidence of a particular problem may remain constant, but if survival is improved, the prevalence of that problem increases. For instance, major advances in neonatal care permit the survival of extremely-low-birth-weight infants. Even with no change in the annual number of premature births, increasing numbers of former premature infants are being cared for. There has also been a significant reduction in the incidence of certain acute diseases, such as measles, because of the success of immunizations. As the proportion of a pediatric practice committed to care for acute problems in normal children decreases, the proportion made up by children with chronic problems increases. Children with chronic problems make frequent health care visits and often have complex needs, but these needs are not always identified or met. The focus is usually on the specialized medical problem, eclipsing the rest of the child's needs.

Kanthor and colleagues (1974) surveyed mothers of children attending a birth defects clinic and found that most of them thought that no physician provided the overall direction of the child's health care. They reported receiving adequate services from the specialist for the evaluation, treatment, and education about the child's chronic illness. However, two thirds reported receiving no real help in the area of the child's need for special schooling, behavior problems, or adjustment to the handicap. Eighty percent of the mothers said no one discussed their child's future with them, including vocational possibilities, marriage, and sexual functioning. Almost one third had no offers of emotional support from someone who understood their problems. Those who did frequently sought this support outside the medical setting.

Although the children of these women had multiple needs, 18% received no help in coordinating the care of multiple specialists. Primary care physicians provided three quarters with well-child care and two thirds with acute-illness care. However, no one took responsibility for well-child care for 14% of patients or for acute illness care for 25%.

Stein and colleagues (1983) reported their survey of over 200 mothers whose children had a broad range of chronic health problems. They modified and consolidated the areas of need described by Kanthor and found that 80% to 90% received needed medical services (eg, health maintenance care, intercurrent illness care, explanation of child's illness, and an identified usual source of care), but almost half had no one who discussed whether the problem was hereditary, and two thirds had no one who offered general advice about schooling, behavior, handicaps, or what to expect in the future. Thirty percent of the mothers reported that health personnel listened to their concerns and understood the problems of raising a child with a chronic health problem. Another 30% looked to family and friends for this support, and almost 40% had no one to fill this need.

The researchers also asked mothers what other services they felt they needed. Three fourths wanted to learn more about the children's conditions. This was usually voiced as a desire to better control the child's illness at home and to fit the ongoing problem into the fabric of everyday home life.

During the past 20 years, children with chronic disorders have been progressively viewed as having many similar problems and needs that transcend specific diagnoses. Whether a child has asthma, diabetes, cerebral palsy, hemophilia, congenital heart disease, or leukemia, the child and the family face the challenges of a problem that will not go away quickly and without intense treatment. Their lives are affected by whether the problem is stable or unpredictable or life-threatening; by the frequency of home treatments, health care visits, and hospitalizations; by whether the condition is visible or invisible; and by whether the condition impairs the child's ability to develop into an independent person. The child and family must learn to negotiate the monolith of the health care system. They must learn how to incorporate the child's medical needs into the family's routine.

They need to make the child's life as normal and similar to that of peers as possible. They need to know how to set consistent limits and reasonable expectations for behavior of all family members. They need to have their fears for their child's life and health acknowledged and understood. They must learn to deal with nosy neighbors and strangers who stare. They need to learn how to work with the medical, educational, third-party payer, and governmental bureaucracies.

In essence, this approach is a return to the concept of treating the "whole child" in the context of his family and community, instead of focusing on a diseased organ system.

## MEDICAL NEEDS

All children, regardless of whether they have a chronic problem, deserve regular health maintenance care. It is just as important for the chronically ill child to be monitored for adequate physical growth, appropriate nutrition, and timely attainment of developmental milestones and to receive age-appropriate immunizations and health screening as it is for the healthy child. These assessments are often crucial pieces of information in determining how well controlled the chronic problem is. For instance, in the oxygen-dependent premature infant or the infant with congenital heart disease and congestive heart failure, inadequate weight gain signals the need for reassessment of the management plan. Does the infant need more oxygen? Does he need increased doses of medication or surgical intervention? Does the feeding regimen need to be revised to provide increased numbers of calories for growth? Very rapid weight gain may signal worsening fluid retention. Measuring length and head circumference as faithfully as weight fluctuations offers data for deciding what is "catch-up growth" and what is fluid retention. This approach is often neglected during prolonged hospitalizations because the focus is on acute care.

Children with chronic health problems need ongoing care for those problems. If, for instance, care is dictated by diabetes, the child needs periodic assessment of glucose control, insulin dosage, and overall compliance with the recommended protocol and needs monitoring for complications of the disease, such as renal disease, retinopathy, or hyperlipidemia. This type of care fits the classic model of the specialty clinic.

Some children have problems that do not fit a specific diagnostic category. For instance, a tracheostomy is a procedure that generates a list of problems and concerns unique to children with tracheostomies without regard to the primary diagnosis for which the tracheostomy was placed. The ongoing medical care of this problem does not always fall nicely into a particular specialty clinic because many specialists can care for children with diagnoses that require tracheostomies.

Some children carry multiple diagnoses and require the care of multiple specialists. They have the extra need for coordination among specialties in scheduling visits, tests, or procedures and in combining prescribed treatments.

All children have acute problems that may or may not be related to their special problem. Fever is exceedingly common in childhood and can be due to common conditions, although the cause is not always clear before medical evaluation. In a young child with meningomyelocele, hydrocephalus, a ventriculoperitoneal shunt, and a neurogenic bladder, a fever may be due to otitis media or the current respiratory virus spreading through the community, to a urinary tract infection, or to a shunt infection. Although this child may need the services of a neurosurgeon or a urologist in the course of evaluation or treatment of this problem, he or she first needs the services of a pediatric generalist to determine the likely diagnosis and which tests or consultations are necessary. This initial assessment is much more tailored to the individual child if the generalist has an ongoing knowledge of the child's medical history and patterns of illness.

## Nursing Care Needs

The range of nursing needs of children with chronic illnesses is broad. A child may require daily doses of oral medication, or the medication may need to be given by injection or by nebulizer. He may need regular chest physical therapy or range-of-motion exercises. A tracheostomy requires routine suctioning to maintain patency. Feeding by nasogastric or gastrostomy tube necessitates correct preparation of the liquid feeding, maintaining position and patency of the feeding tube, and monitoring for any untoward effects. A child with apnea requires close monitoring and may require emergency resuscitative efforts.

These needs exist regardless of the setting. We are most accustomed to these needs being met by health care professionals in the hospital setting, but the same needs exist in the child's home and often in the child's school. In all of these settings, family members often take on substantial portions of these nursing functions. They may do this with the support of a visiting nurse who comes to the home periodically to assess the child's status and how successfully the recommended regimen is accomplished in the home setting. The frequency of visits varies with the child's needs from several times per week to once every few months. A child who requires more constant attention, such as a ventilator-dependent child, often receives shifts of skilled nursing care in the home or school.

## Allied Health Care Needs

There are numerous health care professionals who specialize in the evaluation of particular problems, formulation of a treatment plan, and ongoing assessment of progress. They are usually based in a medical center or school, but they often make home visits as well.

Physical therapists assess gross motor function. This may begin early in life for the child with cerebral palsy who requires periodic evaluation and updating of passive and active movement protocols to maintain range of motion and maximize muscle strength and balance. They can assess the child's need for bracing, crutches, walker, or wheelchair. The physical therapist is active in rehabilitation of function after surgery or significant injury.

Occupational therapists assess fine motor and oromotor function. A young child with a cleft palate or neurologic impairment or who, due to prolonged illness, never learned to suck from a bottle, may have to be taught how to suck, chew, and swallow in a coordinated fashion or how to accept new textures and sensations in the mouth. Therapists can recommend splinting and passive exercises for children with hand deformities and develop activities that help maximize fine motor precision and eye–hand coordination.

Respiratory therapists assist in the assessment and care of children with pulmonary problems. They may assess oxygenation and pulmonary function. They can also set up and help maintain respiratory equipment. A respiratory therapist makes home visits to periodically assess a child on oxygen or a home ventilator.

Speech therapists work with children with language delay or language abnormalities. Their assessment is tied with that of the audiologist, who uses objective and behavioral measures to assess hearing. The audiologist recommends a hearing aid when necessary.

Psychologists are trained in the detailed testing of intelligence, problem solving, and projective testing. They assess learning disabilities and help determine the educational level for appropriate school placement.

## Equipment

There is a vast array of equipment used in the home care of children with chronic medical problems.

Monitors have become commonplace in the homes of premature infants and other children at risk because of pulmonary, cardiac, or neurologic disease. The machines require a wall outlet or battery and are attached to the child by wires or leads and a belt that wraps around the chest or small adhesive patches. The monitor is supposed to sound an alarm when the child is apneic or bradycardic; it should be set at sensitivities that pick up the normally small breaths taken by premature infants but not so sensitive that it incorrectly interprets nonbreathing movements. The physician must define what is apnea and bradycardia for each patient to determine at what respiratory and heart rates the machine should be set. These definitions should be reassessed as the child grows.

There are problems associated with monitors. There can be frequent false alarms that disturb the family's sleep and may make them less responsive to future alarms or even discontinue the monitor's use without medical advice. The machines depend on electrical current and do not work during a power outage without a backup system. Some children have been severely injured or killed when their leads were mistakenly plugged directly into the wall outlet. Some families and some physicians become dependent on the monitors and have difficulty discontinuing their use after they are no longer indicated.

Respiratory therapy needs include oxygen equipment, suctioning equipment, nebulized medication delivery systems, and mechanical ventilation equipment. Children can receive oxygen at various concentrations by nasal cannula, tracheostomy collar, or ventilator intermittently (eg, only during sleep) or continuously. Suctioning may involve the use of a bulb syringe to clear the mouth and nose or may require a suction machine with disposable suction catheters to clear the trachea. Home nebulizers greatly expand the drug therapy available to asthmatic children. They can be run using room air or oxygen. Mechanical ventilators are used at home intermittently or continuously for children with hypoventilation syndromes. Before the placement of a ventilator in the home, the child's ventilatory needs and adjustment to the proposed regimen should be completely assessed. Periodic reassessment helps determine whether the regimen needs to be changed.

Equipment used to assist in positioning and ambulation can be recommended by the occupational or physical therapist. This may include specific forms for use in bed or chair, splints or braces, crutches or walkers, and wheelchairs.

Intravenous therapy is becoming more common in the home setting. Children requiring long-term intravenous medications or parenteral alimentation may have central venous catheters in place. These usually require a daily protocol of flushing the line to maintain patency and periodic local care of the site of catheter entry. Newer catheters have subcutaneous ports, reducing the frequency of line manipulation.

Special feeding programs have equipment needs. Sucking problems may require special nipples or feeding syringes. A child with fine motor problems may need specially designed eating utensils to promote independent feeding. Tube feedings require special formula and a system for delivering it. A pump is often used for prolonged feedings, such as overnight.

## TRANSPORTATION NEEDS

Safe and available transportation is needed by all children with ongoing health problems to obtain necessary medical care, attend school, and participate in family activities. There may be financial barriers, as when a family has no car or cannot afford frequent trips using public transportation. There may be geographic barriers if the child lives a great distance from the medical center. There may be physical barriers; a child with contractures may not be safely positioned in a car safety seat or seat belt. A child who requires numerous pieces of supportive equipment needs to use a vehicle with ample storage space. A second adult is often needed to accompany the parent and child to help with all the paraphernalia or to monitor the child during the ride. Ambulance transport is sometimes the safest mode of transportation.

## EDUCATIONAL NEEDS

All children deserve the best education possible. In 1975, the United States Congress passed Public Law 94-142, the Education for All Handicapped Children Act. Its intent is to ensure access to free and appropriate education in the least restrictive environment for children with special needs. It states that these children should have a fair assessment of their learning needs, a formal written plan for the child called the *individualized educational program*, any needed supplementary aids and services, and due process procedures if the parent disagrees with school policy. For states to receive federal funds for education, they must comply with this law. States write their own regulations to meet these federal requirements. The federal law covers handicapped children from 3 to 21 years of age. Some states and school districts extend this coverage to include children from birth.

Because each child's medical and educational needs are unique, determining how best to meet these needs must be done by those who know the child best. This involves communication and teamwork among parents, teachers, physicians, and any other professionals with ongoing contact with the child. A child with asthma but with no learning problems needs to be on an appropriate medical regimen to minimize episodes of wheezing. This enables him or her to be in school and to concentrate on the day's work instead of remaining at home or in the hospital. Medication may need to be given during the school day, and the teacher or school nurse must know which activities or exposures trigger the child's wheezing and should be avoided. If the child's asthma is so severe that he must miss many days of school despite maximum therapy, arrangements for home or hospital teachers should be made.

A child with motor and intellectual deficits who also has a tracheostomy and is ventilator dependent needs special educational services, supplementary services such as physical or occupational therapy, and skilled nursing during the school day. Services may be home or center based; even children with this level of technologic dependence can often be accommodated in the public school. It requires willingness to be creative and flexible on the part of parents, school officials, and health care professionals.

## FINANCING HEALTH CARE

Caring for a child with chronic medical problems is a significant financial burden on families. No medical insurance program pays for everything that the child needs. A combination of private or government insurance and funds from family and charitable organizations is usually needed.

Private insurers offer a multitude of medical plans that vary in cost, eligibility, and coverage. Families are usually insured as part of a group plan through a parent's place of employment. This may give the family little flexibility in the company or type of policy available. Alternatively, families may purchase an individual policy directly from an insurer, but this is expensive.

Most policies have two main sections. There is a basic plan that pays for a defined list of tests, procedures, and some medications. It usually does not pay for physician visits. The major medical portion is intended to cover costs not covered by the basic plan. However, the amount that the family has to pay (ie, the deductible) before the policy reimburses them varies, as does the proportion of the bill that is covered after the deductible is met. There are types of service that may not be covered under the policy, and there is usually a lifetime limit to benefits paid. These limitations and exclusions usually make no difference to the average medical consumer, but they have substantial impact for the family of a chronically ill child who incurs medical bills totaling thousands of dollars year after year.

There are government programs that pay some or all the cost of medical care for eligible children. The Medicaid program is funded jointly by the federal and state governments, and the benefits and eligibility requirements vary from state to state. Its purpose is to ensure access to medical care for the medically needy. One segment of this population consists of low-income patients; without Medicaid, they would be unable to obtain needed medical services. Children with chronic conditions form another population of medically needy patients. Their medical expenses are completely out of line with the family's income, assets, and ability to pay. Although eligibility requirements vary, these children may be eligible for Medicaid even though their family's income does not fall below the poverty level. The Supplemental Security Income program revised its guidelines, expanding eligibility for children with chronic health impairments.

Several states have a Model Waiver for Disabled Children that enables coverage of certain children with special needs who would normally be ineligible for Medicaid benefits. It is often used to provide high-technology care in the home for a child who would otherwise remain hospitalized indefinitely. This legislation was a major step forward in providing cost-effective care and achieving unity of the family in their own home.

Crippled Children's Services is an assistance program for children with chronic or disabling conditions funded at the state and local levels. Benefits vary from state to state but may include physician visits, laboratory testing, medications, hospitalization, and equipment.

## BEHAVIORAL AND FAMILY ISSUES

Families have many concerns about dealing with behavior problems and discipline for their special child that frequently remain unaddressed. It is important that physicians realize how commonly parents are concerned about their children's behavior, how powerful an influence this has on family relationships and functioning, and the special risks involved for a family with a chronically ill child.

Although children vary in temperament and personality, they all seem to have stages or periods of time when their behavior causes their parents concern. Children with chronic illness go through the same periods. Because these children are considered special or vulnerable by their parents, these periods of behavioral concern may cause more crisis in the home. Teaching parents about developmentally normal behavior helps them define developmentally appropriate expectations for the special child. Consistent rules and appropriate responsibility within the family go a long way in helping any child learn to behave in a socially acceptable manner. Social competence promotes the child's sense of self-esteem.

Children who undergo painful procedures, are repeatedly hospitalized, or are physically restricted due to their chronic problem may act out or become withdrawn. It is important to differentiate expectations for family behavior in routine situations from those for difficult circumstances for which the special child bears most of the burden. For instance, a child undergoing a painful procedure normally cries and resists. Adults need to support the child's ability to tolerate the procedure. This same child should not be allowed to hit his siblings or throw food or refuse to go to school; no one in the family is allowed to do that. If the chronically ill child is allowed to be an exception, the behavior will continue to deteriorate, and he may feel that what he does is not as important to the parents as what his siblings do. Parents need to be reminded that much of their child is normal and needs to be treated as such.

Siblings may also be vulnerable. They may have less access to a parent's time and energy due to the chronically ill child's needs. They may feel they caused the sick child's problems or fear becoming sick, too. Parents can make great demands on them to behave perfectly, be quiet all the time, or help care for the chronically ill child. Although these expectations can be appropriate in small doses, parents should remember that the siblings are also children and have the usual needs to play and learn and spend time with their parents.

Vulnerable children are at increased risk for child abuse and neglect. Although it seems paradoxical that a parent who is concerned about a child's health could also do harm to the child, having a child with special needs can be quite stressful. For parents without successful coping strategies, anger and frustration may be vented on the perceived source, the special child.

Adult relationships, especially marriages, are stressed by a child's chronic illness. So much time and energy is consumed in caring for the child that little may be left for the spouse. Sometimes couples blame each other for the child's problems. Sometimes the illness is the last straw for a relationship that was not working well.

## ROLE OF THE PHYSICIAN

Many of the needs of the ill child or her parents can be filled by the child's physician. Primary care is supposed to be accessible first-contact care, which is vitally important for children with chronic illnesses that have exacerbations or crises. The child should be followed over time to assess changes in the child's illness and developmental level. Primary care should occur with a continuous provider. The same physician seeing the child over time for well and sick visits has a better perspective for evaluating the child when ill and develops a solid and supporting relationship with the family. This relationship, combined with the opportunity to meet with the family at times when the chronic problem is stable, permits the provider to begin to fill the needs for counseling and advice.

Primary care is comprehensive. It approaches the whole child within the context of the family and community. This is a crucial part of quality care for chronically ill children. The physician can function as the coordinator among medical specialties and liaison with schools and community agencies.

The physician should be responsible for the child's overall plan of care. It is too easy for multiply involved professionals to assume that someone else is taking care of a special need. Someone needs to assume the responsibility for seeing that the needs are recognized and met. In this kind of role, the pediatric generalist can find real satisfaction in knowing that he or she has been able to offer healing, even if there is no cure.

## Selected Readings

Chronic disease in children. Pediatr Clin North Am 1984;31:1.

Jones ML. Home care for the chronically ill or disabled child: A manual and source book for parents and professionals. New York: Harper & Row, 1985.

Kanthor H, Pless B, Satterwhite B, Myers G. Areas of responsibility in the health care of multiply handicapped children. Pediatrics 1974;54:779.

Stein REK. Pediatric home care: An ambulatory "special care unit." J Pediatr 1978;92:495.

Stein REK, Jessop DJ. A noncategorical approach to chronic childhood illness. Public Health Rep 1982;97:354.

Stein REK, Jessop DJ. Does pediatric home care make a difference for children with chronic illness? Findings from the pediatric ambulatory care treatment study. Pediatrics 1984;73:845.

Stein REK, Jessop DJ, Riessman CK. Health care services received by children with chronic illness. Am J Dis Child 1983;137:225.

*Principles and Practice of Pediatrics, Second Edition.*
edited by Frank A. Oski et al. J. B. Lippincott Company, Philadelphia © 1994.

# CHAPTER 26
# *Child Maltreatment*

## Lawrence S. Wissow

Infanticide and other forms of child maltreatment have been a part of human behavior since ancient times. Only toward the end of the 19th century was there a recognition that children might have rights and deserve the protection already offered to domestic animals against cruel treatment or neglect of basic needs. In the United States, it was not until the 1930s that federal legislation mandated a government role in child welfare. Laws mandating the report of suspected abuse cases were not in effect nationally until 1967.

Medical recognition of child maltreatment came even more slowly and with great skepticism. Radiologist John Caffey's studies of the association of subdural hematomas with long bone fractures in infants were first published in 1946, but the concept of the "battered child" was not widely accepted until the syndrome was more fully described by C. Henry Kempe and co-workers in 1962.

Child maltreatment is a problem of enormous proportions. Since national statistics were first collected in the 1970s, the number of suspected cases reported annually to child protective services in the United States has risen from about 700,000 to almost 2,000,000. In 1985, approximately three reports were made for each 100 children (American Humane Association, 1987). Although many of these reports cannot be substantiated, reporting is thought to greatly underrepresent the true incidence of maltreatment. Only about a third of the cases recognized by professionals are reported. Estimates from large-scale surveys suggest that as many as one third of children in the United States annually are "seriously assaulted" (eg, kicked, bitten, punched, hit with an object, assaulted with a weapon) by a caretaker and that as many as 10% of boys and 20% of girls are sexually abused at some time during childhood (Straus, 1980; Finkelhor, 1984).

Although for most pediatricians the battered infant represents the prototype case of child maltreatment, rates of maltreatment increase steadily among older groups of children and are highest in adolescence. The rate of maltreatment among children younger than 2 is estimated to be 6 per 1000, and the rate for those 15 to 17 years of age is estimated to be more than 14 per 1000.

## TYPES OF ABUSE

*Neglect* is thought to be the most common form of abuse, and it is probably the most lethal form of child maltreatment. It is found in about 60% of confirmed reports of maltreatment. Neglect may take many forms, but the common feature is the failure of a parent or other caretaker to provide a child with basic shelter, supervision, or support. This failure can be passive, such as not obtaining needed health care, or it can be active, such as knowingly exposing a child to some hazardous situation.

*Physical abuse* is found in about 25% of confirmed abuse reports. It is defined as inflicting of physical injury through malicious, cruel, or inhumane treatment. Vigorous debate still rages over the boundary between acceptable forms of corporal punishment and physical abuse. Although there is evidence that it is less effective than other forms of discipline and more likely to result in increased negative behavior, corporal punishment is still permitted and even institutionalized in many settings. In practice, punishments that result in injury (ie, leave marks, break the skin or bones, involve real or perceived threats to life or health) are regarded as abusive.

*Emotional abuse* is found in about 17% of confirmed abuse cases. It is one of the more difficult types of maltreatment to define or detect and has had relatively little recognition in child abuse reporting laws. Garbarino offered one working definition that may be useful to the clinician: "The willful destruction or significant impairment of a child's feeling of competence or security" by a parent or other caretaker.

*Sexual abuse* is found in about 6% of confirmed reports of maltreatment, although its actual prevalence may be much greater. The definition of sexual abuse includes inappropriate exposure to sexual acts or materials, passive use of children as sexual stimuli for adults (ie, child pornography), and actual sexual contact of children with older persons. A child's apparent "consent" to participate in sexual activity does not reduce the older person's responsibility or alter the diagnosis of abuse.

## CAUSES OF ABUSE

Child maltreatment takes many forms and has many causes, but as research into the cause of maltreatment has progressed, some common themes have begun to emerge.

### The Abuser's Childhood

Many abusive parents report having suffered what could be labeled emotional abuse during their own childhoods. This includes a consistent lack of empathy from their parents, a lack of support for their own development, and a chronic feeling of never having had their own needs met.

Physical and sexual abuse appear to be more common in the childhoods of abusers than of nonabusers. The American Humane Association, in its compilation of U.S. national abuse reports, found that 20% of abusing parents said that they had been abused as children. The reason for this connection is not certain. In the case of sexual abuse, several theories have been advanced, including the need to master the traumatic experience by becoming an aggressor, the "damaged goods" syndrome that leads victims to believe they cannot have normal relationships, and the possibility that the early abuse conditions an abnormal pattern of

sexual responses. Steele (1980) proposed that a person's experience as a child establishes what he then considers normal and acceptable for child rearing. Adults abused as children often believe that physical or sexual exploitation of children is implicitly accepted by society. They may unconsciously attempt to rationalize their own experiences by perpetuating abusive behavior and establishing its normality. Most abuse, however, is committed by persons who do not give a history of having been abused, and most persons abused as children do not grow up to become abusers.

### Family Stresses and Supports

Another theory of abuse causation is that excessive stress on the parent or family causes a breakdown of inhibitions and a release of frustration on a child. Straus, in the 1976 National Family Violence Survey, found that physical violence against a family's children increased as a function of the number of reported stresses. Frequently reported stresses included death or serious illness of a friend or family member, serious financial difficulties, and conflicts in the workplace. Most highly stressed parents, however, did not abuse their children.

Several factors were associated with families in which abuse did take place. Dissatisfaction with marriage and a frustrated expectation that the husband should be the dominant family decision maker were associated with a twofold increase in the rate of abuse. Abuse was also more likely to occur in families that approved of one spouse slapping another. Participation in social, business, or religious activity outside the family was associated with lower rates of abuse. These data support the theory that stresses alone do not cause abuse. Other forces, such as poverty or poor self-esteem, may make a person more susceptible to stress and more prone to abuse, and better social support or a more positive history of dealing with crises make maladaptive responses to stress less likely.

### Socioeconomic Status

In the Family Violence Survey, job status classification and educational level had little to do with the occurrence of violence toward children. Low income, however, was associated with a marked increase in violence, and in other studies, it was associated with increased rates of child neglect and sexual abuse.

### Maternal Age

Maternal age at the time of a child's birth appears to influence the likelihood of physical abuse but not of neglect. Mothers of abused children usually begin childbearing earlier than do nonabusing mothers; the explanation for this association is uncertain. Younger parents may have less knowledge of normal child behavior, and they may be more likely to be frustrated or disappointed by their child's activities. Pregnancy at a younger age may be a sign of other dysfunction within the parent's family and an indication that the parent has had less of a chance to experience appropriate care.

### Abusers as Adults

Although abusers as a group do not fall into any single psychiatric diagnosis, some patterns of mental illness have been associated with certain kinds of maltreatment. Neglectful mothers (fathers have been less well studied) may fall into one of several categories: victims of the "apathy–futility" syndrome, the overly impulsive, the mentally retarded, the extremely depressed, and those few who are actively psychotic. Apathetic mothers probably comprise the single largest identifiable group. These mothers are passive, withdrawn, and verbally inaccessible. They see much of life as a futile endeavor, and although their fund of knowledge may be good, they fail to carry out day-to-day tasks that others take for granted. They may be intensely lonely and clinging but react to helpful suggestions with passive aggression and resistance. A major weapon in their resistance to change is their ability to evoke feelings of futility in those who try to help them.

Physical abuse is more common in families in which the mother has made a suicide attempt. Parents who poison or otherwise create factitious illness in children may suffer from a form of delusional thinking that allows them to harm a child and convincingly deny having done so. These parents may also have abnormally close, symbiotic relationships with their children.

The symbiotic relationship of parent and child may be a general characteristic of abusing families. All human relationships are based to some degree on symbiosis, the mutual provision of support that makes life possible. Symbiosis goes too far when adults reverse roles and require children to supply them with self-esteem and self-determination. This transfer of power makes the child responsible for the parent's problems and the target for the parent's frustrations.

Pedophiles are another class of abusers that may have specific psychologic problems. As a group, pedophiles appear to develop physiologic sexual arousal to child stimuli. How these arousal responses develop or how they can be modified is unknown. Although there is little evidence that pedophiles have particularly immature or dependent personalities that cause them to prefer relationships with children over those with adults, some do display evidence of increased anxiety in relationships with other adults.

## Social Forces and the Promotion of Maltreatment

Many feel that the root causes of child abuse rest in wider social values, especially those that condone violent behavior and define the social position of children as parental property. These values may serve to disinhibit persons who would otherwise be kept from harming children by social pressures. Two main observations support disinhibition as an antecedent of abuse. One is the finding that the risk of sexual abuse by stepfathers appears to greatly exceed the risk from biological fathers. It is hypothesized that stepfathers, especially those who did not take on primary parenting relationships, may lack some of the attachments to their children that counter incestuous desires. Second, the high correlation of alcohol use and sexual offenses against children has also been considered evidence for disinhibition as a factor contributing to abuse. Several studies have found a high proportion of pedophiles to be chronic alcoholics or to have been drinking at the time of their assaults on children.

## Characteristics of Children at Risk for Abuse

Many clinicians feel strongly that the child is not a passive, random target for the abuser, but that certain children are more vulnerable or may act in ways that precipitate abuse. There is evidence for this viewpoint from studies of both physical abuse in early childhood and sexual abuse of older children. Sex differences, for example, play a role in how parents relate to their children. Parents have been found to be more likely to quarrel in front of boys than girls, and boys are more likely than girls to respond to family stresses with disruptive behaviors that can make them targets of abuse.

Infants perceived by their parents as being fussier or as being slow to develop or to be in poor health appear to be at a higher risk of abuse, as do children labeled by their parents as having undesirable characteristics reminiscent of disliked family members. These risk factors may be related to a lack of parental feeling of control and competency; parents may be more likely to feel frustrated and inadequate when they cannot comfort an inherently more irritable child. Alternatively, they may involve the parent's inability to overcome a past, appropriate concern about the child's health status. Although quite bonded to their children, they may never develop appropriate warmth and closeness, perhaps because they continue to fear that the child will die.

Increased rates of abuse have been reported among handicapped children. The families of handicapped children may need more emotional and logistical support to achieve feelings of satisfaction and competency in parenting. Particular points of stress may arise, as during school vacations when a sudden increase occurs in the family's need to provide care for the handicapped child. Work schedules may be disrupted, siblings may be conscripted against their wills into supervisory roles, and the handicapped child's behavior may change outside of a structured school environment.

Children who are socially, emotionally, and geographically isolated also appear to be at a higher risk for sexual abuse. These children may be more open to an abuser's advances, even if they perceive them to be wrong, as a substitute for other relationships. It may be harder for these children to reveal the abuse to others, or they may be less likely to get a supportive response to disclosure. Finkelhor speculated that abusers choose children who appear to be shy or less assertive in the belief that they will be less likely to reveal abuse.

## Early Parent–Child Interaction

Some workers consider the period immediately after birth to be a critical period for the formation of parent–child relationships. They theorize that if a bond between the two fails to form at this time, the mother will not be motivated to adequately protect and nurture her child. The existence of such a critical period has not been demonstrated in humans, but different effects on parent–child attachment have been observed with changes in early contact (ie, immediately after birth) and extended contact (ie, time spent together during the first few days of life). These observations have been made against a background of great individual variability. Some parents seem to desire close, immediate contact with their newborn, but others do not. In general, early contact between mother and child is associated with increased amounts of affectionate behavior toward the child in the first few days of life. After the infant is about 10 days of age, early-contact mothers are indistinguishable from those who did not interact with their children immediately after birth.

Extra contact during the first days of life may have more lasting effects on the parent–child relationship and on subsequent care of the child. Although not all studies agree, extra contact in the form of rooming-in has been associated with a reduced incidence in subsequent child abuse and placement with nonparent caretakers.

## EVALUATION OF CHILD MALTREATMENT

There are three main steps in the initial evaluation of a child suspected of having been abused:

1. Basic medical history and family assessment
2. Physical examination and diagnostic testing
3. Investigative interview of the child and family

The first two steps are usually performed by a physician, nurse practitioner, or physician's assistant. Investigative interviews are usually carried out by a social worker, psychiatrist, or other mental health professional.

## Medical History

The goals of the basic history are to establish immediate treatment needs and to begin formulating a level of suspicion of abuse. In many abuse cases, the history given is often misleading or false. Improbable or inconsistent stories are important elements of diagnosing abuse, but they do not help diagnose a child's immediate medical problems. A careful and complete physical examination is especially needed if the clinician suspects that the history is unreliable.

Any history must be carefully recorded. Those involved in the case later need to check what they have heard with what was said initially. Stories that change over time suggest abuse. Initial statements may also have importance as courtroom evidence. Most history related to a third party outside a courtroom is considered "hearsay" and cannot be admitted as direct evidence that something has happened. "Excited utterances," statements made in the crisis of initial disclosure, may be considered legal evidence if they are accurately recorded. In a similar manner, statements made to physicians in the course of treatment and duly recorded in the patient's chart can often also be admitted as evidence.

When a child is old enough to provide a history, he or she should always be spoken to separately from other family members. This may not be possible if the child is too fearful or if the parents refuse. If a family member must be present when the child is interviewed, seating should be arranged so that the parent and child do not have eye contact; a side-by-side arrangement facing the clinician is best. When interviewing children, physicians should remember that their goal is to elicit and record a spontaneous account of the abuse. Direct questions (eg, "Did anyone touch you on your penis?") should be avoided, because they risk raising the issue that the child was prompted or pushed to respond. In most cases, the child does not give an explicit history of abuse, and he or she should be referred to a social worker or mental health professional capable of performing a medicolegally correct interview.

When interviewing adults, carefully establish the source of the information provided. Is the informant a regular caretaker for the child? What is their relationship? If the evaluation involves a question of trauma, was the informant actually a witness, or is the information given second-hand? Be especially careful to ask for details of events, and do not volunteer or suggest answers. When inquiring about previous illnesses or treatments, try to obtain enough information so that the history can be verified if necessary. Include the name and location of hospitals, clinics, physicians, and schools, and approximate dates when the services were used.

Be alert for aspects of the history that do not make sense when compared with clinical experience. Does the story fit the child's developmental age and abilities? Is the proposed mechanism of injury plausible? Have you seen other children with similar histories that suffered the same degree of injury to the same part of the body? Do the symptoms fit with any fairly common condition, or do you find yourself having to imagine combinations of unlikely conditions to explain the child's illness?

It may be difficult to remain professional and nonaccusatory. It is usually not possible to hide the fact that abuse is being considered as part of the differential diagnosis. Assure the parent that your questions do not mean that you suspect him of being the abuser, and try to enlist his support in seeking the best and most timely care for his child.

## Social History

Depending on the resources available, a social worker ultimately may be called on to take a detailed family and social history.

However, the physician often must obtain this information to make a decision about referral or reporting. Several factors are thought to be related to the risk of abuse and the child's safety.

Information about the parents is important. What are the parents' ages, occupations, and extent of contact with the child? Do either of the parents have any major illnesses? If so, what medications may be in the home? Are the parents under any particular stresses, such as financial difficulties, job conflicts, or a recent death of someone close? Is there a history of spouse abuse or other violence in the family? Does either of the parents have an alcohol or substance abuse problem?

Information about child care in the home is valuable. Who is the child's primary caretaker, and who else (eg, sitters, relatives) has a caretaking role? What other children live in the home, and are there siblings who do not live in the home? What is the health status of these children? What type of home does the child live in? Do the parents describe it as adequate or does it have major safety or crowding problems? Does anyone else live there?

The physician also needs information about family functioning. What is the family's general level of functioning as a unit? How do members of the family communicate with each other? Are messages given clearly, or are there discrepancies between words a family member uses and the vocal tone or visual message that accompany the words? Are other family members able to understand these mixed messages or are they confused by them? How does the family seem to make decisions that affect more than one member? Is there extensive quarreling? Does anyone in the family seem to possess the ability to negotiate a solution rather than impose one? Is there difficulty in perceiving and assessing options or in seeing the problem from the perspective of other family members? Are the children always required to adapt to their parents' perspective, or is there evidence that the family's adults can appreciate the child's different point of view? Do the family members seem at all capable of sharing authority or taking turns and allowing various members to temporarily set the group's agenda?

## Developmental Review

Specific questions of interest in the evaluation of maltreatment cases include the child's usual source of medical care and past or present medical or behavioral problems. Were there difficulties with pregnancy, labor, and delivery or in the perinatal period that might have resulted in the child being labeled as bad or a problem? Have there been feeding difficulties such as colic, refusal of food, or difficulties in toilet training? Are the parents expecting too much from the child too soon? Do they feel that they are able to make the child happy? Do they feel that this is a difficult child to care for?

The examiner should document behavioral problems, especially of recent onset, such as running away, a marked decline in school work, an increase in disciplinary problems at home or at school, abusive or violent behavior toward other children, or recent change to excessively quiet and withdrawn behavior.

A history of previous trauma, ingestions, or frequent visits for vague complaints such as abdominal pain or genital discomfort may alert the physician to the possibility of abuse. Chronic health problems (eg, asthma, a learning disability, cerebral palsy) that require special medical attention or impair interaction with others or normal functioning may add to the prospect of abuse. Is there a history of secondary enuresis or encopresis?

## Physical Examination

The physical examination of a potentially abused child should be therapeutic and diagnostic. Abused children may have little sense of personal security and control over their life. One of the purposes in conducting the examination is to assure them that they are well, that someone respects them, and that they have some control over what happens to them. Accordingly, the physician should try to find the most quiet and unrushed setting consistent with the child's level of illness. Privacy and modesty are important even for young children, and it is important to keep the door closed or curtain drawn and to use appropriate drapes and gowns.

A complete head-to-toe examination is important for two reasons. First, the history may be misleading, and unexpected illnesses may be detected. Second, it gives the child a chance to experience the examiner's touch and presence before sensitive or embarrassing areas of the body are explored. A ruler or measuring tape, a good light, and anatomical diagrams to mark on should be available during the examination, although photographs may be deferred until the end. Major findings, especially skin lesions, should be documented while the patient is still available to confirm written descriptions and drawings.

Documenting present and past growth parameters is an essential part of any pediatric examination. In the setting of suspected child abuse, growth parameters serve as one indicator of the child's general level of care. A static low weight for height may indicate chronic undernutrition, and a decline in the growth rate may signal the onset of a period of neglect.

Lack of clean clothing and poor personal hygiene are frequently taken as signs of neglect, but they are poor predictors that a given child comes from an abusive home. The fact that a child is wearing clothing that is insufficient for the prevailing weather may be a sign of neglect, but it may also simply be a sign of poverty. Of more concern is a child with injuries, even minor, that show signs of inattention to simple home first aid or an unreasonable delay in seeking medical care.

The child's behavior in the examination room can provide clues about abuse or neglect. Does the child separate too easily from the parents? This would be especially worrisome for a toddler, for example, in whom clinging to a parent at all costs is usually the rule. Is the older child excessively fearful of separating or fearful of the examiner? Is the child withdrawn and unresponsive or angry and even destructive? These are nonspecific signs, but they indicate some degree of abnormality in the child's social environment and adjustment.

Infants who have been chronically neglected may have characteristic behavioral symptoms. They may seem watchful and constantly alert with minimal smiling; they may have decreased movement and prefer to remain in one place; and they may become distressed when approached by adults. Many seem initially to be more comfortable playing with inanimate objects than with people and appear to dislike touch and holding.

## Establishing the Plausibility of Injury

It is often difficult to assess a parent's story of how a child was injured. As has been described, one must be alert for a lack of detail or consistency in the story or for aspects that do not match the child's developmental abilities. Often a visit to the alleged accident scene is required. A knowledge of patterns of injury in known accidents can also help. Injuries of any kind to children under 2 or 3 months of age are unusual, mostly because these children have such limited mobility. Few children can roll over before 2 months of age, and some still cannot at 4 months. Falls from the height of most household furniture rarely result in serious injury. One of the most widely cited case series, by Helfer and coworkers (1977), examined the records of 85 children who had fallen to the floor of their hospital rooms from heights of about 3 feet. One child had an uncomplicated skull fracture and 57 of the 85 had no apparent injury at all. In general, the presence of intracranial injury (subdural or epidural bleeding) suggests greater force than generally occurs in household injuries. Falls to concrete floors or onto hard, pointed objects may be exceptions, but there may also be physical findings (eg, abrasions, bruises corresponding to the shape of the object) that corroborate the history.

## BRUISES, BITES, AND LACERATIONS

### Signs

Bruises and other skin lesions are the most common manifestations of physical abuse. Normal, active children may have many bruises and abrasions at any given time. These injuries are usually over bony areas such as the shins, knees, elbows, and forehead. Injuries in other areas, especially to soft tissues such as the abdomen, genitalia, buttocks, thighs, or mouth are more worrisome, because they are unusual in unintentional household trauma. Particularly worrisome are injuries to the inner aspects of the upper or lower arm. These surfaces may be injured when the arms are raised to protect the face from a blow. Bilateral injuries to the face raise the question of abuse. Because the prominence of the nose makes it difficult to accidentally strike both sides of the face at the same time, bilateral bruising may be a sign of multiple impacts, possibly of battering.

The color of a bruise is a rough indicator of its age. Bruises are caused when trauma ruptures blood vessels and blood escapes into the skin. The bruise is first dark red or violet, but as hemoglobin from the blood is broken down, the bruise changes color to blue-brown (ie, 1 to 3 days), yellow-green (ie, about 1 week), and finally to a light brown (>1 week). Two to 4 weeks from the time of injury, the bruise is usually gone, but this progression is variable. Deep bleeding may not be apparent immediately and may take longer to change colors. Its surface appearance may not correspond to the location of the injury, as in the case of raccoon eyes, in which bruising on the face is associated with a basilar skull fracture.

The shape of an injury may also be a clue to its cause. Some of the few lesions that are virtually diagnostic of abuse fall into this category. A looped cord leaves a characteristic mark in the shape of an oversized hairpin. The loop may have a double railroad track appearance if it was inflicted with an electrical cord or an abraded texture if it was made with a rope. Belt buckles leave characteristic marks, usually an erythematous band from the belt itself, terminating in a horseshoe-shaped mark from the buckle. A flat palm with spread fingers leaves a mark that the examiner can test by superimposing his own hand. Petechial lesions from the neck up, with or without bruising, or cordlike lesions on the neck may be a sign of strangulation.

Bites usually appear as a semicircular or crescent-shaped red area with or without breaking of the skin. It may be possible to differentiate between human and animal bites and between bites by adults or children. Human teeth are largely dull and produce mostly in crushing and bruising. Animal teeth are sharp and often cause punctures and even surgical-appearing lacerations. Human teeth are arrayed in a semicircle, and animal mouths are in more of an extended loop shape. The diameter and circumference of a bite may suggest that it was inflicted by an adult or a child. It is important to measure the bite or take a photograph with a ruler visible in the frame. If it seems that the bite will be important in trying to identify the abuser, a forensic dentist may be able to match the wound with a suspect's dentition. Serial photographs should be taken over several days. This is because most bite wounds are crush injuries that darken and become more visible with time.

If the bite has just occurred, as in many cases of sexual assault, the wound may be swabbed with a saline-moistened swab in an effort to collect saliva. Police laboratories may be able to detect blood group antigens that could help identify the abuser. An area of the victim's uninjured skin should also be separately swabbed as a control specimen.

## Differential Diagnosis

Trauma, intentional or accidental, is not the only cause of skin lesions. Alternative diagnoses must be carefully considered, because they may be signs of life-threatening illness and because the accusation of abuse, once made, is not easily retracted. Perhaps the most commonly occurring similar lesions are mongolian spots, areas of purplish or dark brown discoloration frequently seen on the buttocks and lower back of black or Asian infants. They may also appear on the trunk, upper extremities, or face. These spots are entirely benign and unrelated to trauma and usually have been observed since birth. The easiest way to differentiate them from bruises is to notice that they fail to change color over a period of days.

Thrombocytopenia from any cause, meningococcal disease, and Schönlein-Henoch purpura can cause bruise-like lesions. Especially if a child presents with altered mental status or seems to be acutely ill, these causes must be considered first or at least simultaneously with the diagnosis of trauma. A vasculitis associated with hypersensitivity can also produce streaky ecchymotic lesions on the extremities that look like welts. These patients often develop urticaria and other signs of systemic illness. Even if abuse is strongly suspected, it is usually reasonable to obtain a platelet count if bruising is the major sign pointing to the diagnosis. Although the clinician may not think that thrombocytopenia is likely, the platelet count may be useful in proving to a court that alternative diagnoses were carefully considered.

Hemophilia usually presents as joint or deep soft-tissue bleeding, often after minor trauma. Coagulation studies are usually abnormal, although patients who are only carriers of the condition may require determinations of individual clotting factor levels to make the diagnosis. Even if abuse is strongly suspected as the cause of a soft-tissue bleed, documenting normal coagulation studies may strengthen a case if it is brought to court.

Folk medicine practices from many cultures may leave cutaneous signs falsely suggestive of abuse. Cupping, the application of a heated cup to the skin to draw out an ailment, is practiced in some Middle Eastern, Latin American, Chinese, and Eastern European cultures. The procedure may leave circular red lesions, sometimes with petechiae, on the abdomen or other soft-tissue areas. The skin within the circle may have been abraded before the cupping. *Cao gio*, coin rubbing, is a Southeast Asian practice that may leave linear red marks on the back resembling whip or stick welts.

Patients who are critically ill or who have undergone cardiopulmonary resuscitation may have lesions suggesting abuse. It is often difficult to decide if these lesions represent the trauma that caused the child to become so ill or if they represent complications of treatment or agonal changes. Critically ill children with poor peripheral circulation may develop extreme friability of the skin. Frequent instrumentation, such as taking rectal temperatures, may then cause the skin to break down and resemble patterns seen in intentional injury. Bloody discharge from the nose and mouth, caused by hemorrhagic pulmonary edema and rupture of mucosal capillaries, may occur after shock or with death. Changes in the peripheral circulation that result in blotching and blanching can occur with the administration of drugs, such as epinephrine or dopamine, that are used to support blood pressure. After death, blood may pool in dependent areas and resemble antemortem bruising. Body orifices may begin to gape, and the female genitalia, for example, may assume dimensions suggestive of abuse that they did not have in life.

## BURNS

Burns are among the most serious forms of intentional injury. They may be inflicted by hot liquids or heated objects. In both cases, the shape of the injury and its depth (ie, first, second, or third degree) may offer a clue that the cause was not accidental. Most hot liquid burns are caused by tap water or hot drinks. Many homes have hot water heaters set above 130 °F to 140 °F; water at this temperature can cause a third-degree burn in less than 10 seconds. Immersion in hot liquids as a punishment for messiness or lack of bowel control results in a typical pattern of injury. The burn, which is usually second or third degree, is uniform in depth and has a smooth border corresponding to the liquid's surface. The burn may have a glove or stocking distribution when the child's extremities are immersed. If the child is forcibly seated in a tub of hot water, there may be sparing of thicker skin and skin that protruded from the water or was pressed against the cooler surface of the tub. The soles, knees, and buttocks may be spared while the rest of the legs, perineum, and lower back are burned. Clothing worn during immersion can prolong contact of the skin with hot water and result in unusual burn patterns; outlines of elastic waistbands or folds of cloth may be visible as deeper burns.

Spill or splash burns often show a pattern of flow of the hot liquid over the skin. Some areas may be burned more than others as the liquid cools on its way to and over the body. Splash burns often have satellite lesions from drops of liquid, unlike the large, smooth-bordered lesions of immersion burns.

Burns in the shape of hot solid objects often indicate abuse. Cigarettes, hair curlers, and heating devices are among the more common objects causing questionable burns. The physician is often asked to decide if these burns occurred by accident or if they were inflicted. Inflicted burns are rarely first degree (ie, only redness and pain). People seeking to harm children with hot objects usually hold the object in place long enough for it to cause a deeper injury. Children are no less sensitive to pain than adults and withdraw from hot objects if given the chance. Some household appliances, such as electric curling irons, attain surface temperatures in excess of 280 °F, hot enough to cause a second- or third-degree burn in a matter of seconds, and they may remain hot for many minutes after they are unplugged. It may be difficult to differentiate intentional from unintentional injuries attributed to such devices.

The child's size and developmental abilities must be consistent with the history. Immersion burns of the lower extremities are frequently explained by saying that the child fell into the bathtub, often after turning on the water himself. Most children cannot climb until 14 to 16 months of age, and at that stage, they would most likely go face-first over a high tub side, if they could get over it at all. It is only later that they learn to swing their legs up and have a chance to enter feet first. Ideally, a visit to the home can be made to see the bathtub and measure its height in relation to the child's height.

Cigarette burns may be difficult to differentiate from impetigo. The location may be helpful; both impetigo and accidental burns are rare on the palms or soles, although these may be prime places for punitively inflicted burns. Accidental brushing of a cigarette (and impetigo) produce injury only to the superficial layers of the skin. A deeper wound is more likely to represent an inflicted burn.

## HEAD INJURIES

The child's head is especially vulnerable to intentional injury. During infancy, the head is large and heavy in relation to the rest of the body. The neck muscles are weak and cannot control the head's movements. The infant skull is pliable and more readily transmits force to the brain itself. Head injury must be considered any time a child presents with a change in level of consciousness or with a focal neurologic finding. Care must be taken to keep an open mind about diagnosis until conditions such as meningitis, encephalitis, seizure disorders, diabetic ketoacidosis, and other acute toxic or metabolic conditions have been considered. Patients waiting for computed tomography (CT), usually the definitive procedure to detect head injury, should be closely monitored and sometimes receive treatment for other disorders that can not yet be ruled out.

Magnetic resonance imaging (MRI) may be useful if children are suspected of having head injuries but the result of CT scanning is negative. MRI, although less available and more expensive than CT, is better able to define small areas of subdural bleeding and subtle changes suggesting trauma to the brain parenchyma itself.

Initial inspection of the head may reveal some signs of injury. The anterior fontanelle may be used as a rough gauge of intracranial pressure. A tense or bulging fontanelle with the child in an upright position is an abnormal finding usually indicating increased intracranial pressure. If the pressure increase is longstanding, such as in the case of chronic subdural hematomas or hydrocephalus, palpable splitting of the cranial sutures may also be detected.

Patchy hair loss may be a result of pulling. There may be associated soft areas of the scalp, where traction on the hair has caused subgaleal bleeding. Hair loss may occur for other reasons; malnutrition may leave the hair brittle and easy to pull out. Occipital bald or thin spots, once considered a sign of neglect, are a fairly common finding in normal infants. Hair loss secondary to fungal infections is usually accompanied by scaling and oozing, and the condition is ultimately confirmed by positive cultures for the organism.

Battle's sign (ie, bruising over the mastoid process behind the ears), raccoon eyes, and blood behind the tympanic membranes may be signs of basilar skull fracture. Some depressed skull fractures can be palpated, although they are difficult to feel if the suspected fracture site is under an area of the scalp that is tender and swollen. Large, boggy areas of the scalp may be associated with blood escaping through a fracture line. However, serious intracranial injuries, even those caused by direct blows, may have few or no external signs of bruising or swelling.

An ophthalmologic examination is essential if head injury is suspected. Many physicians hesitate to undertake a funduscopic examination in an infant, fearing that it will be a time-consuming and frustrating procedure. It is true that little is usually visible through an infant's mobile, undilated pupil. With dilation, however, the fundus is usually easily visible. Physicians also hesitate to dilate the pupils of seriously injured patients, fearing that they will lose the ability to watch for changes in pupillary reactivity. To some extent this is true, but it is often of less importance in infants, in whom the flexibility of the skull and an open fontanelle make herniation and its resultant pupillary changes less likely.

Retinal hemorrhages may be caused by shaking of the head, direct blows, or violent compression of the chest. Their presence in the setting of minor head trauma suggests that the history given may be false. They are sometimes the only clue that a child suspected of having meningitis or metabolic disease was abused. Papilledema may be a sign of increased intracranial pressure, but it may not be present with an acute rise in pressure, such as that associated with a fresh intracranial bleed.

## ABDOMINAL INJURIES

Blunt trauma to the abdomen can cause serious injury that is difficult to detect with a physical examination alone. Duodenal hematoma is the lesion most associated with child abuse. Blunt force compresses the small bowel against the vertebral column, producing bleeding into the duodenal wall. In the absence of rupture and subsequent peritonitis, patients usually have a history of increasing abdominal pain and anorexia spanning a period of a few days. They are often thought to have a benign gastroenteritis until the hematoma becomes large enough to cause obstruction and bilious vomiting begins. Sometimes an upper abdominal mass is palpable, but the diagnosis is usually made radiographically. A flat plate of the abdomen may or may not show a mass effect, and the obstruction is high enough in the gastrointestinal tract that, with the stomach decompressed, there may be none of the usual signs of obstruction, such as air–fluid levels in dilated loops of bowel. Oral contrast studies are most often used to demonstrate the lesion, although ultrasound, abdominal CT scans, and MRI may also be used.

Ruptured bowel or stomach or laceration of the liver or spleen produces symptoms more rapidly than duodenal hematomas. They often present as shock from massive intracapsular or intraperitoneal bleeding and have a high mortality rate. Less extensive injuries may cause abdominal symptoms that mimic appendicitis or pelvic inflammatory disease. Unfortunately, cutaneous signs of intentional abdominal injury are more the exception than the rule. Urgent surgical consultation is required if one of these lesions is suspected.

## SEXUAL ABUSE

### Injuries to the Genitalia

Any injury to the genitalia raises the question of abuse, although this area of the body is also susceptible to unintentional injury. Most children who have been sexually abused have no detectable genital injury. A negative physical examination never rules out sexual abuse.

#### Female Genitalia

The examination of the prepubertal girl is usually restricted to an inspection of the external genitalia. Patients and parents should be reassured at the outset that an "internal" examination is not required and that the procedures used are basically the same as those involved in routine well-child care. Girls may be comfortable in the lithotomy position (without stirrups) or they may prefer the prone, knee–chest position. If an internal examination is indicated for a prepubertal child, the use of sedation or general anesthesia should be considered.

Prepubertal girls usually have a small amount of clear, nonodorous discharge. Exceptions to this occur in the first week after birth and in the 6 to 12 months preceding menarche. At these times, the discharge may be slightly thicker and gray-white, but even then, it occurs in modest amounts and is not foul smelling. The differential diagnosis of prepubertal vaginal discharge includes sexually transmitted diseases, foreign bodies, poor hygiene, and chemical irritants. Eliciting a habit of bubble baths, exploring for a history of occlusive clothing, inspection of the introitus, a digital rectal examination to feel anteriorly for a mass, and laboratory studies are usually helpful in establishing a working diagnosis.

Masturbation is often suggested as an explanation for excessive erythema of the external genitalia, frequent urinary tract infections, and foreign bodies in the vagina. Children do masturbate from the time that they can reach their genitalia, and this is a normal part of sexual development. Girls and boys (especially those who are circumcised) can irritate their genitals and develop some dysuria during normal self-stimulatory behavior. The insertion of toilet paper and small foreign bodies into the female genitalia is also considered to be part of normal exploratory behavior. Prepubertal girls, however, do not normally engage in autoerotic behavior that simulates intercourse. The insertion of objects that mimic a penis is reason to suspect abuse rather than self-stimulation.

The examination of the perineum can be organized with a "face of a clock" approach. With the child supine, tissues above an imaginary nine o'clock to three o'clock line evenly dividing the vaginal opening into anterior and posterior segments overlie the pubic bone and can easily be crushed, with resultant bruising, in a straddle injury. Tissues below this line are suspended on the perineal musculature; they retract with trauma and are more likely to be injured by anteroposterior penetrating forces, such as those encountered in intercourse. The first step in the examination is to inspect the external genitalia, with the labia majora slightly spread, and to document the location of any bruises, lacerations, irritation, or bleeding. Venereal warts, erythematous papules suggesting herpes infection, or chancres may be found.

The next step is to examine the anterior vagina and hymen. A good flashlight and a measuring tape are all that are required, although experienced practitioners are increasingly using a colposcope (ie, illuminated, binocular type of operating microscope) to obtain a magnified view and to have the capability of taking photographs. The colposcope does not come into contact with the child, although it may induce some anxiety simply because it is another piece of equipment. An otoscope (without the ear speculum) or a hand-held lens may also be used as a magnifying instrument.

The labia minora are retracted until the hymen is visible. The normal hymenal opening may be round, U shaped, slitlike, pinpoint, or irregular. Important observations include whether the hymen is irregular; the size of the opening; and whether there seems to be any bruising, bleeding, or scarring. Old scars may be visible to the naked eye as areas with a different coloration, as retracted areas or clefts in the hymen, or as adhesions of the hymen to the vaginal wall. Clefts in the lower quadrants of the hymen (from 3 to 9 o'clock) may be more significant for trauma than clefts in other locations. Friability or scars of the vaginal mucosa, especially in the posterior fourchette, should be observed. Increased vascularity of the mucosa may also be a sign of old trauma.

The horizontal diameter of the opening of the hymen should be measured by holding a millimeter ruler up to the perineum while the child is in the supine, frog-leg position. In general, children who have been subjected to abuse involving the genitalia have been found to have an opening that is larger than children who have not been abused, although in the limited data available, the range of normal and abnormal overlap. Emans and coworkers (1987) suggest that about 6 mm is the upper limit of normal for girls between the ages of 3 and 6 years. However, they found similar mucosal and hymenal variations in children with a history of abuse and children who complained only of genital problems such as vaginitis, vulvitis, or dysuria. Other workers have reported that the size of the opening of the hymen tends to decrease in the months after vaginal trauma and that children who had an abnormal examination at one point may appear normal when examined at a later date.

McCann and colleagues (1990) demonstrated that differences in technique alter the types of observations that can be made about the prepubertal genitalia and the apparent size of the structures observed. Time and patience are perhaps the most essential tools for examining small children's genitalia. Relaxation has a major impact on how much visualization can be obtained and on the appearance of the structures visualized. The effort to avoid any direct instrumentation, even with only a moistened swab, means that traction often must be applied, relaxed, or reapplied to free up moist, adherent tissues, and then observations can be made in another position. This is only possible if the child is cooperative and the parent supportive.

## Male Genitalia

Penile bruising, erythema, or discharge may suggest abuse. Papules or ulcers may be signs of sexually transmitted diseases. Phimosis, or a swelling of the foreskin, may be caused by trauma or infection. Small infants may develop phimosis from a piece of hair that accidentally becomes wrapped around the penis. Subsequent swelling and tenderness may make it difficult to find or remove the hair.

## Rectal Lesions

Visible injury to the rectum is rare in sexual abuse. Most pedophiles go to great lengths not to inflict trauma so that abuse remains undetected. The anus is expansive, and stools larger than the adult penis can be accommodated without injury. However, some signs may be present, especially after a violent rape.

The perirectal area should be examined for scars, warts, petechiae, bruising, and small skin tags. These tags develop as tears or hemorrhoidal bleeding resolve. Hemorrhoids are uncommon in children, and their presence or the existence of skin tags should be considered a possible indication of abuse. Many children, however, have midline skin tags immediately anterior or posterior to the anus. Parents typically notice that these have been present since birth.

Children who have been chronically sodomized may have thickening of the perianal skin. These observations may be difficult to make, because many children have some increase in pigmentation immediately around the rectum, and most have many folds of perirectal skin that may be difficult to examine and may resemble fissures or scars. Fissures can develop in children who pass very hard stools. Some observers think that scars from a stool moving out of the rectum can be differentiated from the scar resulting when an object is inserted into the rectum.

Rectal tone may be a clue to the presence of abuse. After forced penetration, the injured sphincter may remain lax for 2 to 4 hours and then go into spasm. Some children who have been chronically abused may develop reflex relaxation of the sphincter in response to a soft stroke on the adjacent buttocks, but this may also develop in children who have been examined repeatedly. Normal children may have an anal "wink," a reflex tightening of the sphincter, with the same stimulation. Few children, even those who have been repeatedly sodomized, have a patulous or lax rectum. An important exception is the child with a spinal cord lesion, such as meningomyelocele. Interruptions of the cord in the area of the third sacral vertebra may result in flaccid paralysis of the internal sphincter. A digital examination is not required unless a rectal foreign body or impaction is suspected. There is no indication for use of a test tube or other improvised anoscope. If internal lesions are suspected or if the suspicion of abuse is so great that internal hemorrhoids or trauma must be ruled out, the patient should be referred to a pediatric gastroenterologist or surgeon. Anoscopy can be performed with appropriate equipment, sedation, and photographic capabilities.

## Laboratory Evidence in Cases of Sexual Abuse

Of all the types of child maltreatment, sexual abuse requires the most meticulous collection of laboratory and forensic evidence. Most of this collection is aimed at detecting sexually transmitted diseases and other body fluids or tissues that may be transferred from the abuser to the victim during intimate sexual contact. Although this kind of evidence is found only in a minority of cases, it must be looked for carefully if sexual abuse is suspected, because it is compelling evidence that abuse has taken place and may help to identify a specific person as being the abuser.

A minority of sexually abused children are infected with a sexually transmitted disease (STD). Rimsza found that about a quarter of sexually abused children younger than 18 years of age had signs or symptoms of infection at the time of their initial physical examination.

## Genital Flora in Prepubertal and Postpubertal Girls

Before puberty, most infections of the female genitalia involve the vaginal mucosa. The prepubertal hormonal environment makes the vagina a hospitable site for organisms that after puberty are found instead in cervical infections. This is one of the major reasons why most prepubertal girls do not require a speculum examination when sexual abuse is suspected. The main purpose of using a speculum is to visualize the cervix and to obtain cervical cultures. Equivalent cultures can be readily obtained from the vagina of prepubertal patients.

Several organisms can cause vaginitis in prepubertal girls without being associated with sexual transmission. These include *Mycoplasma*, *Gardnerella vaginalis*, *Candida*, and several nongonorrheal species of *Neisseria*. These same organisms may be found in postpubertal vaginitis occurring without sexual contact, although they are found more frequently in postpubertal girls who are sexually active.

## Sexually Transmitted Diseases

Three organisms appear to be almost exclusively associated with sexual activity: *Chlamydia trachomatis*, *Neisseria gonorrhoeae*, and *Trichomonas vaginalis*.

*Gonorrhea.* The best studied and most commonly found STD in children who have been sexually abused is gonorrhea. Symptoms, if they occur, are present within 2 to 5 days of contact with the organism. The presence of symptoms seems to depend on the part of the body that becomes infected and on the age of the patient. Pharyngeal and rectal infections in children appear to more often be asymptomatic, and urethral or vaginal infections usually present with symptoms.

The laboratory identification of gonorrhea can be difficult. False-negative results are common if specimens are not promptly placed in culture or transport media. The major problem concerning child abuse investigations is that there are many other species of *Neisseria*, distinct from *N gonorrhoeae*, that are regularly found in children (especially in the conjunctiva and pharynx) and that are not thought to be sexually transmitted. Unless a laboratory rechecks using alternative procedures, some of the tests commonly used to identify *N gonorrhoeae* can falsely label the other species as being gonorrhea.

Because a mistake can lead to the false determination that sexual abuse has taken place, it is critical that clinicians clearly mark all specimens for gonorrheal testing with the body site from which the culture was taken. The risk of false-positive findings varies with the site cultured. They must make sure that the laboratory is aware of the problem of misidentification and take appropriate steps to check its results. They should never announce preliminary culture results to patients. The examiner must wait until the results are verified. Final determinations are usually made in a matter of days. It is impossible to undo the news of a positive gonorrheal culture, even if the laboratory later says that it was false. The physician must ask the laboratory to save positive specimens (at −70 °C or colder) for possible analysis at a reference laboratory. Confirmatory tests may be required if a perpetrator is ultimately charged and tried.

Parents and others may be reluctant to believe positive culture results for gonorrhea, especially if infections have been asymptomatic or there is no other evidence of abuse. The question is frequently raised about the possibility of nonsexual transmission of the organism. *N gonorrhoeae* can survive on exposed surfaces for prolonged periods, but no case has ever been documented in which contact with the organism on objects or on the skin was responsible for infection. The only two established means of nonsexual transmission are acquisition during birth (eg, neonatal ophthalmia) and laboratory accidents (eg, ingestion of culture-positive material).

*Chlamydia.* Infections with *C trachomatis*, an intracellular parasite, are increasingly recognized as perhaps the most common sexually transmitted disease in Western societies. *Chlamydia* has been difficult to detect, because it is not readily seen in stained preparations of clinical materials and because it is difficult to grow in laboratory cultures. However, rapid diagnostic techniques and improved culture methods have made it easier to diagnose. The poor specificity of rapid diagnostic tests makes culture preferable. Rapid diagnostic methods should never be used for nongenital specimens, except as a means of screening if culture is not readily available. Their use should usually be restricted to cases in which the likelihood of infection is high (eg, testing of genital specimens that are associated with symptoms).

Sexually transmitted chlamydial infections may occur in all of the sites listed for gonorrhea. There may be more of a tendency for *Chlamydia* infection to be asymptomatic, although conclusive evidence is not yet available.

As with gonorrhea, a perinatally acquired syndrome is also associated with chlamydial infection. Infection is presumed to be acquired during birth from an infected mother and presumably is avoided by cesarean delivery. Eye infection is usually diagnosed within the first 2 weeks of life, and many children develop pneumonia, which presents slowly over a period of weeks with increasing cough, tachypnea, and rales. The usual time of diagnosis is about the sixth week of life. Perinatal exposure may produce latent genital infection. Colonization may progress from original pharyngeal sites to rectal and genital areas. Asymptomatic colonization in these sites is thought to spontaneously clear between 1 and 2 years of age. Except for these perinatal syndromes, nonsexual transmission of chlamydial infection has not been reported. Positive genital cultures in older children are presumptive evidence of sexual contact.

*Trichomonas vaginalis.* *T vaginalis* is a protozoan that can cause vaginal and urethral infection in male and female patients. The organism can survive on wet surfaces, but nonsexual transmission has not been demonstrated, except in the case of perinatal infection. The incubation period of trichomonal infection is 5 to 28 days. It is rarely symptomatic in adult men, but over half of adult women have symptoms such as vaginal discomfort and discharge. Trichomonal infection is highly contagious: more than half the sexual contacts of an infected man are likely to contract the infection. It is best detected by microscopic examination of a "wet prep" of vaginal secretions (see Chap. 30.5).

*Other Infections.* Syphilis is not common in sexual abuse but is regularly found whenever a large enough group of abused children can be studied. Nonsexual transmission has been demonstrated through skin contact with contaminated materials. Chancres on the genitalia, however, suggest sexual transmission. Chancres may not appear until 2 to 3 weeks after exposure, and antibodies may not be detectable for 4 to 6 weeks. It is important that follow-up examinations and serology take place after a patient is seen immediately after an incident of sexual abuse or assault.

Condyloma acuminatum (ie, venereal warts) are caused by one or more types of papillomavirus, the family of viruses that also cause common skin warts. The different types of papillomavirus have different preferences for the skin on which they will grow; the types causing condylomata grow preferentially in the perirectal area or on the male or female external genitalia. The lesions they make range from small, velvety warts to large, disfiguring growths. Condylomata are usually diagnosed solely by their appearance. Because they may resemble condyloma lata caused by syphilis, a serologic test for that disease is indicated.

Genital warts in adults are highly contagious and are easily spread to sexual partners. Their incubation period is not well defined, but it may be as long as several months. Condylomata in children only recently have been recognized as being sexually transmitted. The presence of common warts on other parts of the body such as the fingers or soles of the feet does not seem to be related to the development of genital warts. Controversy still exists about whether all genital or anal warts in children are caused by the sexually transmitted types of papillomavirus. Experimental procedures are available to identify the type of virus in the lesions and to help make a more definitive diagnosis. At this time, however, it seems reasonable to presume that most condyloma are caused by genitally related types of virus.

Perinatal transmission of papillomavirus is well documented, although determination of its frequency is made difficult by the fact that genital infections in adult women are often asymptomatic or hidden within the vagina. Viral DNA can be recovered from apparently healthy tissue adjacent to obvious lesions, and the role of latent infection in perinatal transmission therefore remains uncertain.

As with gonorrheal and chlamydial infection, perinatal infection is thought to occur during passage through the birth canal. The only well-documented perinatal syndrome is that of laryngeal papillomatosis, in which genitally related virus types cause lesions in the infant's upper airway. In the case of genital lesions in infants, reports of small case series have found a high concordance between virus types isolated from maternal lesions and from the child. In the absence of other evidence suggesting abuse, it may be reasonable to attribute genital lesions in children younger than 1 or 2 years of age to perinatal exposure. This explanation would obviously be less likely if the child's mother did not have condyloma or if the child was not born vaginally.

No studies have documented nonsexual transmission of condyloma in older children. Although the virus itself is hardy and can survive for long periods of time on contaminated surfaces, infection appears to require skin or mucosal trauma and contact with the basal cell layer. At this time, it seems reasonable to consider genital or anal warts in children as strong grounds to conduct an investigation for sexual contact.

Herpes simplex virus infections are frequently found in children. The herpes simplex type 1 is commonly associated with stomatitis; type 2 is found in 85% of all genital herpes lesions. Both types can be spread sexually. Herpes infections can occur in many parts of the body. Genital infections are strong presumptive evidence of sexual contact. Inflamed or ulcerated mucosal lesions are often accompanied by tender regional lymph nodes.

Several other organisms are spread by sexual contact, although their importance in child sexual abuse is not well established. Hepatitis B virus can be transmitted sexually and by mucous membrane or broken skin contact with contaminated materials such as blood. Serology should be performed if the suspected abuser is known to be infected or is from a high-risk group such as a user of intravenous drugs. Preventive treatment can be given if the contact disclosed is recent.

The human immunodeficiency virus (HIV) is transmitted by sexual contact and has been involved in a few cases of sexual abuse. Many factors enter into the decision to test for HIV infection after abuse or assault. If the abuser is known to be a member of a high-risk group (eg, homosexual, bisexual, intravenous drug user), testing of the victim may be appropriate. Routine testing of sexual abuse victims may also be appropriate in areas where HIV exposure is prevalent among persons with other sexually transmitted diseases.

Molluscum contagiosum is a contagious viral condition that can be sexually transmitted but also is reportedly spread by other close contact and from contaminated surfaces. Molluscum is caused by a member of the poxvirus family and has an incubation period of 2 to 12 weeks. It is manifested by 2- to 5-mm, firm, umbilicated papules with pearly white centers. If the disease is sexually transmitted, lesions usually appear in the genital area, abdomen, and thighs, but nonsexual spread can reportedly cause disease most anywhere on the body.

### Diagnostic Protocol

It is important to have a fairly fixed protocol for diagnosis of STDs in sexual abuse cases. Although taking cultures and specimens must be tailored to the patient's psychologic condition, history, and symptoms, thorough evaluations often find infections that were previously unsuspected. Rimsza (1982) found that over half of the positive gonorrheal cultures obtained from a series of abused children came from sites that would not have been suspected from the child's account of what had happened. If one sexually transmitted disease is found, thorough testing for others is mandatory. The following protocol is based on these premises and is generally applicable to acute and chronic sexual abuse. Special procedures for acute abuse are also mentioned.

*Cultures.*    Cultures for gonorrheal and chlamydial infection should be obtained from the pharynx, anus, and genitals (ie, vagina in prepubertal girls, cervix in postpubertal girls if a speculum examination is indicated, urethra from boys). If there are no symptoms and the child is anxious, cultures may be deferred until a follow-up visit a few days later.

It often seems overly invasive to obtain urethral cultures from asymptomatic boys. Although its efficacy has not yet been fully documented, a first-part voided urine specimen may be an acceptable substitute as a screening test. The child should be given a sterile container and helped to collect the first few milliliters (no more than 10 to 15 mL) of urine produced. The presence of 10 or more leukocytes per high-powered microscope field (after centrifugation) is highly suggestive of urethritis, most likely due to gonorrheal or chlamydial infection. These children usually then undergo urethral cultures. Five to 10 leukocytes are considered borderline, and fewer than five cells are considered to be within the range of normal. The first-part urine itself can be sent for gonorrheal culture, although the sensitivity of this method is not documented. It cannot be used for chlamydial culture, because the organism only grows in epithelial cells and not in the leukocytes contained in the urine.

*Wet Preps and Gram Stains.*    Any obvious discharge should be put on a microscope slide, fixed, and Gram stained using standard procedures. If gonorrhea is found, the microscope slide should be labeled and kept as part of the permanent case records.

In prepubertal girls, fluid in the anterior vagina can be aspirated with a sterile dropper or the tubing from a butterfly intravenous set with the needle removed. If fluid is lacking, 1 or 2 mL of normal saline can be introduced with the dropper and then aspirated. Alternatively, a saline-moistened swab using nonbacteriostatic saline can be used to collect cells from the vaginal mucosa. In postpubertal girls, fluid or secretions may be obtained with a swab or wooden spatula from the posterior vaginal pool. In either case, a drop of the secretions, diluted with more saline if necessary, should be immediately examined under the microscope for the presence of motile organisms (eg, *Trichomonas* sp.) and for sperm. Another drop should be mixed with potassium hydroxide and examined for yeasts and hyphae. If any positive findings are made, another slide should be made and immediately placed in or sprayed with the fixative used for Papanicolaou (Pap) smears. This specimen should be sent to a cytopathology laboratory for official confirmation of the diagnosis. These tests should be coordinated with the other necessary examinations for cases of recent (ie, within 72 hours) sexual assault.

*Urinalysis.*  A urinalysis is always indicated in the evaluation of child abuse. It may reveal evidence of retroperitoneal trauma (eg, blood or heme) or urinary tract infection, or it may be contaminated with a vaginal discharge and help to diagnose a genital infection. Urine that shows signs of infection should be Gram stained and sent for culture.

*Serology.*  A Venereal Disease Research Laboratory (VDRL) test or some other screening test for syphilis should be performed, although it may be deferred for a few days if it would be traumatic to perform a venipuncture at the initial examination. If the suspected abuse is recent (ie, within the last few weeks), a follow-up titer should be drawn 1 to 2 months later.

*Forensic Procedures.*  If abuse or assault has occurred within the past 48 to 72 hours, it may be possible to detect secretions or tissues from the abuser on the victim's body. This may provide important evidence to demonstrate that abuse has taken place and may even help to identify the abuser. The procedures must be carefully followed to collect and preserve available evidence.

If the victim is still wearing clothing worn at the time of the assault, he or she should stand on a large, clean sheet and undress completely. The clothing should then be wrapped in the sheet, taking care not to spill any small objects that may have fallen onto it, and the bundle must be labeled and safely stored until it can be handed over to police.

An ultraviolet light can be used to examine skin and clothing for semen, which fluoresces. If positive areas are found, they can be swabbed with saline-moistened swabs that should be air dried and put into empty blood collecting tubes or a clean paper envelope. The swabs should be labeled with the patient's name and the place swabbed and handed to the police.

Slides should be made for STD evaluation. They should be examined immediately for sperm or other organisms. If the examination is taking place within 6 hours after the assault, preparations should be taken from the mouth (ie, a saline-moistened swab is moved around the gums, under the tongue, and in the posterior pharynx), the vaginal pool (ie, anterior or posterior, depending on the patient's development), and rectum. After 6 hours, only the rectum and vagina should be examined. Permanent smears should also be made from these sources, and an endocervical Pap smear should be obtained if appropriate for the child's age.

Acid phosphatase is an enzyme in semen that may be useful in documenting close contact of a male abuser with a victim. It can be measured in secretions or from dried swabs taken from exposed areas as already described. Analysis is usually conducted by police laboratories.

It is vital that a "chain of evidence" be maintained for STD and other laboratory specimens associated with a case of suspected child abuse or assault. The chain is a written record confirming that the specimen that arrived in the laboratory for analysis was the same specimen taken from the patient.

## Behavioral and Family Presentations of Sexual Abuse

Young sexually abused children may seem to be overly fearful and clinging, especially in situations in which they may be left alone with an abuser. Because most sexual abuse is committed by persons having some trusted family or child-care role, these fears are often discounted by parents or seen as attempts at ma-

nipulation. They should be taken seriously, especially if they represent a change from the child's previous attitude toward a person.

Children are frequently suspected of having been sexually abused after they report a dream or fear that seems to have sexual overtones. Children normally have many fears. Toddlers may develop fears of specific people, places, or objects, often without ever having had any negative experience that would explain the feeling. Preschool children often have dreams that involve monsters or fear of bodily injury. Children may also use an account of a dream as a way of telling something that they have consciously feared or experienced. It is uncommon for young children to dream or fantasize explicit adult sexual activities unless they have had some direct exposure to sexual material. Explicit dreams must be taken seriously and explored by a qualified therapist.

The development of enuresis or encopresis in a child who has previously been toilet trained may indicate sexual abuse. These behaviors may occur with other regressive behaviors as a sign of stress caused by the abuse, or they may represent organic problems, such as infection with a sexually transmitted disease or perineal trauma.

Changes in school performance and acting out behaviors such as fighting, fire setting, and running away are common among sexually abused children. Children may be too fearful or preoccupied to concentrate on their work, or they may avoid homework sessions that bring them into contact with an abusing parent. Antisocial behaviors represent a particular problem for the clinician because these children are often seen as victimizing their family rather than as victims themselves of some emotional difficulty.

Age-inappropriate sexual conduct is perhaps the most specific behavioral sign of sexual abuse. Although children have many opportunities to learn the motions of adult romantic behavior, the desire for others as sexual objects does not normally start until adolescence. Prepubertal children who attempt sexual acts with other children should be carefully assessed for a history of sexual abuse, although these activities must be carefully separated from normal, age-appropriate exploratory behavior. Even during the latency period, prepubertal children remain intensely interested in sexual topics.

## SKELETAL TRAUMA

### Signs

Bony injuries are most common in abused infants and toddlers, usually younger than 3 years of age, and it is in this age group that full skeletal surveys are recommended if there is other evidence suspicious of abuse or neglect. The age range may be extended for children with mental or physical handicaps that may make them more vulnerable to physical abuse. The x-ray skeletal survey consists of exploratory views of the entire body, usually including one or more views of the skull, a frontal view of the chest, lateral views of the spine, and frontal views of the upper and lower extremities, including the pelvis, hands, and feet. The smaller the child, the fewer images are needed to complete the series. Additional films are taken if abnormalities are found.

Radionuclide bone scans are also sometimes used in the evaluation of suspected abuse. Bone scans have some advantages over x-ray films, but they have some disadvantages as well. Scans are better than x-ray films for detecting recent trauma, because nondisplaced fractures may not be detectable on radiographs for 1 to 2 weeks, but they may be visible on a bone scan 24 to 48 hours after injury. Scans are also good for detecting injuries to the ribs, hands, feet, and skull that may be hidden or too subtle on x-ray survey films.

Scans have technical and logistical disadvantages. An area of bone is seen on a scan because of an increase in blood flow to the traumatized tissue, but some of the bony injuries most characteristic of child abuse occur in areas of bone that already have increased blood flow because of active bone growth. Unilateral injuries to these areas may be visible by comparing the injured with the normal extremity, but bilateral injuries may not be detected. Scans are also more costly than x-ray films, take longer to obtain, and may not be available outside of larger hospitals. Most practitioners start with x-ray bone surveys. If the survey is negative and the suspicion of abuse remains high or if the diagnosis must be made as quickly as possible, a bone scan can be obtained.

Two characteristics of children's bones make it difficult to see the kinds of fractures most related to abuse. The bones of young children are not as fully mineralized as they are later in life. Some areas of bone, particularly the epiphyses of long bones, may not be mineralized enough to be visible on x-ray films. Other bones, such as the ribs, are sufficiently flexible that they return to their original shape after injury. A fracture may not be visible by x-ray survey until 1 to 2 weeks later when minerals are removed or laid down as callus in the course of healing. If recent injury is suspected, x-ray films may need to be repeated at a later date. The healing of bone takes place over months. By 6 months, all but the most subtle radiologic evidence of injury is gone in children. This limits the usefulness of bone surveys, but it allows radiologists to give at least wide periods during which a fracture may have occurred. Fractures of differing ages suggest injury on more than one occasion, a finding that increases the suspicion of abuse.

## Bone Lesions Highly Suggestive of Abuse

### Metaphyseal Injuries

Injuries to the metaphyses of the long bones are among the lesions thought to be most diagnostic of intentional injury. They occur when the limbs are subjected to pulling and torsional forces as a child is shaken or pulled violently, causing fractures through newly forming bone just under (on the diaphysis side of) the growth plate (Kleinman, 1986). A thin disc of bone is formed just under the radiolucent growth plate and epiphysis. Projected onto radiographic film, the disc appears as tufts, arcs, or irregularities at the ends of the bone.

The most common place to see these injuries is in the distal humerus and femur or the proximal tibia. The metaphysis appears irregular and may have spurs or displaced chips. The results of periosteal bleeding may be visible as extensive calcification alongside the diaphysis and later as a thickening of the cortex of the bone. These lesions may be subtle; it is important for the radiologist to know that abuse is suspected. Changes may not be visible for days to weeks after injury, and films should be repeated if necessary.

### Rib Fractures

Rib fractures in young children are usually nondisplaced and visible only after healing has begun. They may occur posteriorly near the attachment to the spine, possibly as a result of a direct blow on the back or from squeezing the sides of the chest or occur laterally in the midaxillary line, possibly from anteroposterior forces. Lateral fractures are difficult to see on standard chest x-ray films because they are hidden by the overlapping shadows of the curving ribs. Oblique views of the chest should be obtained if there is any question of irregularity.

Rib fractures may occur in sick premature infants with osteoporotic bones, apparently caused in the course of urgent care. They occur rarely in cardiopulmonary resuscitation (CPR) of other children. Outside of these differential diagnoses, rib fractures should be considered as possible signs of abuse, especially if more than one fracture exists and if the fractures appear to be of different ages.

### Complex Skull Fractures

Simple, nondisplaced linear fractures of the parietal bone seem to occur from relatively minor trauma, although they can occur from abuse as well. Fractures that are wide (>3 mm), complex (eg, branching fracture lines, multiple fractures, involvement of skull suture lines), or occurring outside the parietal bone suggest significant force. These findings are consistent with an automobile accident, a fall from a considerable height, or a forceful blow to the head. A history of minor trauma or no known trauma at all, combined with the finding of a complex fracture, strongly suggests abuse. Unfortunately, skull fractures cannot be dated in the manner of long bone or rib fractures. They are more likely than long bone fractures to be seen acutely, but their appearance gives no clue about their age.

Children suspected of having suffered head injury often are taken for CT scans before conventional radiographs are performed. CT scans can easily miss fractures, and if abuse is suspected, conventional skull films should be obtained after it is medically safe to do so.

## Bone Lesions Less Suggestive of Abuse

Spiral or oblique fractures of the long bones are frequently cited as signs of abuse. However, they may occur in any setting in which there is rotational force on a bone. These forces frequently occur when the leg or arm is trapped under the rest of the body during a fall. Transverse fractures may actually be more common in abuse, because they imply a direct blow to the bone or the snapping of the bone over a fulcrumlike object. All of these fractures require careful attention to the details of the injury itself and an assessment of what other factors in the family may be grounds for suspecting abuse.

## Bone Lesions Rarely Suggestive of Abuse

Two common injuries rarely indicate abuse. The "nursemaid's elbow" (ie, subluxation of the head of the radius) occurs when force is applied to the already extended elbow joint. These injuries typically occur when toddlers are walking along with an adult and are being held by the hand. The toddler's arm is extended above his or her head. If the toddler trips and the adult holds on, pulling and twisting on the elbow can cause a dislocation. Some children appear to be congenitally susceptible to this injury and repeatedly dislocate the same elbow in the same fashion.

Similarly, toddlers may suffer nondisplaced, often spiral, fractures of the tibia. These are thought to represent injury in the normal course of learning to walk and are not considered evidence of abuse.

## Differential Diagnosis of Fractures

Several conditions may render the bones more susceptible to injury or have radiologic findings that mimic trauma. These include congenital syphilis, scurvy, infantile cortical hyperostosis, osteogenesis imperfecta, and Menkes' kinky hair syndrome. These are rare, and all have characteristic clinical or radiologic appearances that help to differentiate them from abuse. Extreme osteoporosis or rickets may affect sick premature infants or older children who are immobilized because of physical or mental handicaps. These children may suffer fractures from minor trauma or in the course of medical treatments such as CPR, chest percussion, or physical therapy. The underlying abnormality of the bones is usually readily apparent.

Osteomyelitis, septic arthritis, and malignancies such as leukemia or neuroblastoma may sometimes present radiographic or bone scan pictures that resemble trauma. These diagnoses are often considered when a child presents with a sudden onset of limp or unwillingness to bear weight on one leg. Only the course of the illness and subsequent laboratory tests may allow the diagnosis to be made. If suspicions of abuse exist or if the medical picture is atypical, the social evaluation for maltreatment should be undertaken with the medical evaluation.

Injury during traumatic delivery may produce fractures. Periosteal changes in the diaphyses of long bones may be visible, and fractures of the clavicle may occur, sometimes in conjunction with brachial plexus injuries. Skull fractures at the time of birth are mostly associated with forceps deliveries, abnormal position of the child in utero, and prolonged labor. These fractures are likely to be depressed and have a high incidence of accompanying intracranial injury.

## WHIPLASH OR SHAKEN BABY SYNDROME

Caffey (1974) was among the first to describe the so-called "shaken baby" syndrome of intracranial injury and long bone fractures occurring in children under a year of age. The syndrome represents an important masked presentation of abuse because these infants are often mistakenly thought to have meningitis, seizure disorders, or metabolic disease. The failure to diagnose their intracranial injury can be life threatening.

### Signs

The syndrome's major injuries are believed to occur when the infant is held by the chest and violently shaken. Flailing of the limbs causes metaphyseal lesions, and shaking of the head causes tears to bridging vessels and subdural bleeding. Variants of the syndrome may occur if the head strikes a solid object or if there is compression of the chest. Skull and rib fractures, and retinal and intracranial hemorrhages, may then result.

Symptoms of brain injury are what usually cause parents to bring the child for medical care. Seizures or respiratory arrest may occur immediately or may develop over a period of days as a subdural fluid collection increases in size. Alternatively, the child may present with developmental abnormalities, irritability, and an enlarged head or bulging fontanelle (again, secondary to subdural fluid or hydrocephalus). It is important for the clinician to keep trauma in mind as a possibility while considering other diagnoses.

Parents usually relate no history of trauma, or only that of a minor fall. There may be a history of colic or other infant temperament, feeding, or sleeping problem that stresses caretakers. There are usually no external findings of trauma. Often retinal hemorrhage is the only sign visible without radiologic studies.

Vital signs and laboratory studies may also be misleading. There may be instability of blood pressure and an elevation of the peripheral white blood cell count suggestive of infection. Bloody spinal taps may be ascribed to traumatic procedures, but the fluid should be centrifuged and the supernatant examined. A supernatant that is colored by broken-down red cells (ie, xanthochromic) suggests that the blood actually is coming from within the central nervous system. Chest films obtained in the course of evaluation for sepsis should be carefully examined for rib fractures.

### Differential Diagnosis

The most frequently raised alternative diagnosis to the shaken baby syndrome is that of birth trauma. Intracranial bleeding and the development of subdural hematomas or hydrocephalus are associated with precipitous vaginal deliveries of large babies, often to primiparous mothers. These injuries appear to be rare given current obstetrical practices, but when they do occur they usually present at 4 to 8 weeks of life with an enlarged head circumference and sometimes (especially if hydrocephalus is present) with neurologic findings. In contrast, the median age for presentation of the shaken baby syndrome is 6 months, and many of these children are acutely ill. Retinal hemorrhages may also occur during delivery, but they do not persist after the first weeks of life. The hemorrhages associated with trauma persist for long periods of time. Therefore, the most difficult cases are children in the first few months of life who have subdural effusions, normal development, and no history of precipitous or traumatic birth. At present there seems to be no way to say whether or not these children have suffered intentional injury.

Subdural fluid collections may also represent the late effects of bacterial meningitis. There may or may not be fresh bleeding associated with these lesions. Usually there is little question of whether or not a child has had meningitis in the past.

## SUDDEN INFANT DEATH SYNDROME

The sudden infant death syndrome (SIDS) is the most common cause of death of children between the ages of 1 and 12 months in the United States. Intentional injury, such as the shaken baby syndrome, is sometimes raised as a possibility when children die of SIDS or undergo what some clinicians call near-miss episodes. These cases call for close cooperation among the medical examiner, social services, and the child's health care provider.

Much controversy exists about the causes and manifestations of SIDS, but there have been consistent findings about the age at which the syndrome occurs in children who were normal newborns. The peak incidence is between 2 and 4 months of age, and cases are rare in children younger than 1 month of age and older than 12 months. Death usually occurs at night and usually occurs without warning. Only about 5% of those children who die from SIDS (with the exception of those who had demonstrated respiratory abnormalities related to prematurity) had apnea or a previous life-threatening event. These characteristics may help the clinician decide whether a death may have been caused by SIDS.

Deaths of very young or older infants may require more careful investigation. All SIDS deaths require intensive supportive efforts to help the stricken family. The medical examiner should be urged to conduct a thorough autopsy and, if possible, make a visit to the scene of the death. Even if intentional injury is not suspected, an accurate diagnosis is vital to the parents' ability to cope and plan future childbearing. The family requires continued social support, and through this contact may come a better understanding of the parents' functioning and any reason to suspect that SIDS was not the cause of death.

## MUNCHAUSEN SYNDROME BY PROXY

### Signs

In the classic version of the syndrome named for Baron Munchausen, adults injure themselves or falsify symptoms to appear ill. When carried out by proxy, adults inflict illness on a child or falsify symptoms so that a child requires medical evaluation. The spectrum of inflicted illness runs from death (eg, apparent SIDS) to fabrications of long and problematic medical histories. It is frequently difficult to convince law enforcement and child protective services workers that such kinds of child abuse exist.

There are many presentations of the syndrome. In some cases, long but vague histories of difficult-to-document medical complaints (eg, hyperactivity, somnolence, seizures, abdominal, chest or head pains) are accompanied by doctor shopping, erratic compliance with suggested treatment, and lack of satisfaction with negative findings on evaluation. Bleeding, hematuria, and hematemesis are also common signs. Parents have been known to put their own blood in the child's urine or stool samples during the course of a workup. Cases have been reported of blood removal from indwelling central venous catheters. Presenting central nervous system problems, including drowsiness, coma, seizures, and apnea, may be symptoms of ingestion, head trauma (including the shaken baby syndrome), or suffocation. In some cases, laboratory tests may be returned with values that do not have ready physiologic explanations or that suggest too many simultaneously occurring illnesses to be likely. If real, the findings may be the result of salt or fluid poisoning; if factitious, they may be the result of "doctored" laboratory specimens.

Children hospitalized for mysterious conditions often get better in the hospital, only to suddenly worsen when discharge is planned. In many cases of intentional poisonings, parents have continued administration of the toxic substance during the child's hospitalization.

## Common Family Findings

The child's mother is often the perpetrator in cases of Munchausen syndrome by proxy. She is often perceived by the hospital staff as a model mother during the child's hospitalization; she is always helpful on the ward and solicitous of the staff. It is not clear if this represents a conscious effort to deceive the staff or is a reflection of the mother's abnormally great need for affection and belonging. She may have a history of medical illness or complaints similar to that of the child and may have been prescribed drugs that are used to poison the child. She may have a history of medical training or extensive contact with medical care settings, giving her knowledge of symptoms that will elicit attention from the staff and allowing her to give convincing descriptions of these symptoms.

In some cases, the syndrome seems to have its origins in an abnormally symbiotic mother–child relationship in which the mother creates a special sick-role bond between herself and her child. The child may adopt the sick role as a means of staying close to the mother. In this way, the Munchausen syndrome by proxy has much in common with school avoidance and other parent–child separation problems. The father may take a distant or passive role in all of the child's illnesses. He may leave medical decisions about the child to the mother and may seem to have little regard for the apparently serious illness being experienced by the child.

## Diagnosis

Detection of the Munchausen syndrome by proxy requires a high index of suspicion. It should be considered if confronted with a medical history or constellation of symptoms that does not make sense or cannot be verified from previous records. Children with such problems are often hospitalized as a chance for further consultation and controlled observation of the symptoms. Hidden cameras are sometimes used to document the offense. During the hospitalization, the physician should inquire about illnesses in other family members, especially siblings. The occurrence of similar problems or the death of a sibling should be closely investigated. Independent confirmation of these facts and records from any previous source of medical care must be obtained.

Inquiries should be made about medications that may be in the home or illnesses of family members that may require toxic medications. Complete toxicology screens should be considered for patients with altered mental status, especially delirium. If the sensitivity of hospital testing is unknown, extra urine and serum samples should be obtained for freezing and further testing if required. If toxic drugs are known to be in the home, they should be mentioned specifically on the test requisition. This may help the laboratory to screen the samples more efficiently.

Ultimately, the diagnosis of Munchausen syndrome by proxy usually is made in one of two ways. The clinical team is able to confront the parent with incontrovertible evidence of induced or factitious illness (eg, adult blood in the child's urine, a toxic substance discovered in the child's blood), or the parent is actually observed tampering with a specimen or injuring the child. Many such abusers still deny having caused the child's illness, even if they acknowledge that somehow the child was poisoned. Unless the evidence specifically links the parent to the injury, observation and entrapment may be the only way to prove the identity of the perpetrator or to convince social service authorities to take action to protect the child.

## EMOTIONAL ABUSE

Emotional abuse is among the most difficult kinds of maltreatment to define and detect. As with child neglect, it raises difficult questions about what constitutes improper parenting and grounds for outside intervention and what is only unfortunate for the child and within the scope of private family functioning. One conceptualization of emotional abuse divides it into three general categories:

1. Verbal assault: scapegoating, inconsistent discipline, humiliation, and consistent unrealistic expectations with subsequent belittling
2. Psychologic unavailability of parent: preoccupation with adult problems, failure to provide nurturing, threats of removal or otherwise severing the parent–child relationship
3. Chronic role reversal: the child takes on the emotional parenting role and provides nurture to the adult, often then being assigned responsibility for the parent's problems (eg, child of an alcoholic).

The manifestations of emotional abuse are similar to the behavioral changes seen in other forms of maltreatment. Acute changes may include increased worry, fear, somatic complaints, and nightmares. In settings of chronic emotional abuse, parents may be observed in the medical clinic or office to have inappropriate expectations for the child's behavior, to use inappropriate discipline or language, or to belittle the child. Showing anger at the child's fears of the medical visit or belittling the child in front of siblings may represent standard parenting behaviors used at home. Infants may manifest emotional abuse by failing to thrive, and older children may have school avoidance or poor academic performance, poor peer relationships, and low self-esteem.

## CHILD NEGLECT

Clinicians rarely have a problem detecting neglect, but they often have difficulty deciding if the level of neglect warrants intervention on behalf of the child. There may be questions about whether events that have been labeled "accidental" or "chance" in some way involved negligence on the part of a parent or other caretaker. The following discussion outlines some of the more commonly recognized forms of neglect and presents possible guidelines for determining if neglect has taken place.

## Physical Neglect

Physical neglect may include the failure to provide basic food, shelter, and clothing. These requirements may be taken to mean food with calories and nutrients sufficient for normal growth, shelter that is safe, sanitary, and adequately ventilated or heated, and clothing that is in good repair and appropriate for the weather.

Assigning parents responsibility for unintentional trauma around the home is tempting but problematic. Most injuries to children happen in and around the home, and many can be traced to hazards that, at least in retrospect, were avoidable. These hazards include windows with loose screens enabling children to fall, tap water at scalding temperatures, and unprotected electrical sockets. Injuries involving these sorts of hazards are not generally considered neglectful unless prior serious injuries have occurred, and the parent already had been helped to remedy the problem. Steps should be taken to correct the hazards.

Children require adequate supervision for their safety and emotional well-being. Parents are given the responsibility of ensuring that this supervision is provided, by themselves or by someone they designate. Substitute caretakers should have sufficient information to care for the child and to contact the parent in the case of an emergency. Preadolescent children are usually not suitable caretakers for their younger siblings, even on a short-term basis.

## Medical Neglect

Failure to obtain recommended preventive care, lack of compliance with prescribed treatment, or delays in seeking care for acute illnesses may constitute medical neglect. The failure to obtain prenatal care or the use of harmful drugs or alcohol during pregnancy may also be considered medically abusive or neglectful. Making the determination of neglect in these situations may not be easy. The decision may be clouded by conflicts between the clinician and the parent or by judgments about the parent's lifestyle. In these or other types of neglect cases, several criteria can be useful in determining if intervention is justifiable.

Is there imminent danger to the child or the risk of some permanent damage? The purpose of this test is to keep the clinician focused on problems that are serious enough to warrant overriding the parents' freedom to raise their children as they see fit.

Is there reasonable evidence that the neglected action would have truly helped the child or that the neglectful act would or could have caused the child harm? The important part of this test is the clinician's certainty of the link between the neglect and its consequences. The child's problem may be serious (ie, cancer), but if the therapy the parent neglects cannot be said to have a reasonable chance of benefiting the child, a report of neglect may not be justified.

Has the parent or other caretaker disregarded timely and clear information (or what should be common knowledge among parents) that the child would be harmed by the action they have neglected? Parents should not be held accountable for retrospective determinations that a particular action would have been helpful, nor can they be asked to comply with treatments that they do not understand.

Is the neglect part of a more pervasive pattern of parental dysfunction? Is the episode of neglect an isolated event related to a misunderstanding or an oversight, or does it seem to be generally indicative of the way the child is perceived by the parent? Are other needs or aspects of care neglected? Does the parent seem willing to expend the material and emotional resources necessary to raise the child?

Affirmative answers to one or more of these questions may indicate reasonable grounds for making a report of suspected neglect. In some cases, the law does not require the examiner to consider a larger pattern of parental dysfunction. By law, parents are not permitted to neglect their children's education, and in many jurisdictions, immunizations are also compulsory aspects of medical care that parents must provide.

## Failure to Thrive

The failure to thrive syndrome is more fully discussed in Chapter 39. Children failing to thrive traditionally have been divided into those who had organic causes for their growth failure (eg, cystic fibrosis, cardiac disease, inborn errors of metabolism) or nonorganic causes (eg, failures of nurturing or feeding on the part of the parents). This dichotomous view has given way to a realization that almost all cases of failure to thrive involve both organic and nonorganic components and that the child's behavior and temperament must be considered, rather than just the parents' behavior.

Viewed in the context of child maltreatment, the clinician's job in the evaluation of a case of failure to thrive is to identify families in which gross neglect or abandonment have led to growth failure or in which the parent's perception of the child (eg, as sick, bad, or rejecting) is so distorted that short-term improvements in care giving are not probable. In some cases, public agency involvement may be required to obtain the myriad services required to treat failure to thrive, including nutrition support (eg, WIC), home health aides, therapeutic day care, and psychologic help for the parent.

# TREATMENT OF CHILD ABUSE

Medical personnel are often asked to take part in discussions about initial treatment and placement for newly discovered abuse victims. The following discussion briefly outlines issues in the determination of safe placement and referral to treatment resources.

## Characteristics of People in Crisis

The disclosure or suspicion of abuse is often a time of crisis for all members of a family, including the victim, the perpetrator, and others who are just becoming aware of the problem. Crises alter the way in which these persons function, and medical personnel must be careful in their evaluations and reactions. Specific problems include disorganized thinking, focusing on irrelevant or harmful courses of action, hostility or emotional distancing, and dependency. These reactions are sometimes misinterpreted as lack of cooperation and can provoke major confrontations between clinicians and parents. Rational discussions may be impossible until the crisis is past.

Staff members may have to do things for patients that they would otherwise be expected to do for themselves. It is important that this dependence not be automatically interpreted as unwillingness to help themselves, and it is equally important that providers not count on patients in crisis to take critical steps in their own care, such as arranging a follow-up appointment or finding adequate emergency shelter.

## Safe Placement of the Victim

A critical question is whether it is safe for an abuse victim to return home. If there are medical problems requiring hospitalization, an admission is indicated, and sometimes conditions that are otherwise treatable as an outpatient require admission for psychologic support or because reliable care at home cannot be guaranteed. It is important that hospital staff be informed of the medical indications for such admissions. Patients who are labeled as social admissions may not receive appropriate medical and emotional support.

When it is medically appropriate for the victim to be discharged, several factors can be considered. Has the perpetrator been identified, and if so, can he or she be kept from contact with the victim? Can the victim receive sufficient support and protection in the home? The home environment must be physically safe, but it must also be emotionally supportive. If other family members are sufficiently traumatized or angry about the disclosure, they may not be able to provide support for the victim. Particularly dangerous situations arise after a child has disclosed abuse, especially incest, and the nonabusing parent seems not to believe the child's story. In these cases, the victim fails to receive support and the nonabusing parent cannot be counted on to protect the child if the abuser attempts to return to the home.

How did the abusive crisis occur? Is it a general symptom of the family's level of stress or lack of resources? If abusing parents, for example, continue to show extreme anxiety and inability to cope and if the stresses that contributed to abuse continue to exist, the risk of repeat abuse may be high. Families that have a long history of dysfunction or that have no immediately available outside contacts may prove to be at risk for repeat abuse.

Is there evidence of serious mental illness in the abuser? This includes abuse without any apparent stressors or risk factors, injuries that seem premeditated or are characterized by torture or sadism, evidence of sociopathic behavior (eg, violent outbursts, frequent previous involvement with legal difficulties), and distorted views of reality (eg, seeing the child as evil or inherently sick). Injuries justified by unusual or rigid moral or religious beliefs also present a high risk of recurrence.

Safety issues involving pedophiles and incest offenders may be especially difficult to evaluate. These persons typically go through cycles of offense, remorse, and repeat offense. In their remorseful state, they may convincingly seem to be under control and fully motivated to not offend again. There is often a suppression effect at the time of disclosure, and in the short term, the offenders appear to lose interest in offending. However, pedophile or incest behavior can be seen as a habituated behavior, such as alcohol or drug abuse, over which the abuser initially has little control. For this reason, regardless of the abuser's initial appearance, many therapists consider separation of the sex offender and victim mandatory, at least until the victim is psychologically prepared and adequate safety can be guaranteed.

Child Protective Services (CPS) agencies are given the authority and responsibility to protect children suspected of being abused or neglected. Their initial approach is often to make a contract, sometimes written, with a family, and voluntary arrangements are made for the child's safety and the abuser's conduct. The abuser may agree to stay out of the home, and the nonabusing parent may promise to call the police if the abuser returns. The parents may agree to have the child live with a close relative or family friend with whom his or her safety will be assured. If the family is unwilling, the CPS agency may go before a family or juvenile court and get an order, enforceable by the police, granting authority over the child's whereabouts to CPS. The child may still be placed at home, with relatives, or in a foster home, but the agency is given formal legal authority, and the parents' consent is not required.

Whenever possible, the offender, not the victim, should be removed from the home. However, placement of the victim is sometimes unavoidable. In this case, several steps can be taken to ease the difficulty of separation. To the extent possible, parents and children should be involved in the decision to place the victim outside of the home. Everyone should understand the rationale for placement, why other alternatives are not appropriate, and that the separation is temporary. Care must be taken that removal is not seen by the parents or children as a punitive step, but rather viewed as a move that is therapeutic for the victim and the abuser. The best placements are with close family members or with a member of the extended family who can come and live with the child in his own home. The person caring for the child must be prepared to help overcome the guilt feelings that the child may have about causing the separation and must be careful not to vilify the offending parent. If possible, siblings should remain together, and familiar objects and toys should accompany the children. Preliminary plans for visitation should be discussed before the actual separation takes place.

## Treatment Resources

Treatment for families must address acute and chronic problems and the needs of parents and children. The variety of services prescribed require close coordination from a single provider serving as a case manager. This is often a task performed by a protective service worker or a primary health care provider.

### Therapy for Victims of Abuse

In the short term, the children need a chance to be relieved of any guilt or anxiety that they experience for seemingly being the cause of the family's problems. The child may simultaneously be fearful of the parents' anger and frightened of losing the parents' love. The child's condition determines which professional helps to meet these needs. In the hospital, it may be a nurse, social worker, or child therapist. If the child is at home or in foster care, the issues must be addressed in a follow-up visit to a medical or counseling facility. That visit should be scheduled within a few days of the initial disclosure of abuse. At times, a child's chronic medical problems (eg, asthma, learning disability, physical handicap) may put added stress on a family or serve as a trigger for abuse. Optimizing the medical care of these conditions may help to reduce the risk of future injury.

Victims of child sexual abuse are more likely than other abused children to be totally rejected by both parents. These children need continued support and reassurance that they have taken the right step in disclosing what has happened. Sexual abuse victims often undergo marked behavioral changes in the first weeks after disclosure. They may have an increase in fearfulness and nightmares, increased dependency on significant others, and regressive behavior, including enuresis in younger children. These problems require understanding and supportive care.

Although preschool children usually are not able verbally to work through their reactions to abuse, they may benefit from individual play sessions that allow them to experience a normal relationship with an adult and to develop better social skills. Children who have become extremely withdrawn or overly aggressive may benefit most from this sort of therapy. Group therapy may take place in therapeutic play or preschools specially dedicated to abused children or in mixed settings among other, nonabused children. These groups address several goals. First and foremost, they offer the child a place of total safety and acceptance. These qualities are often missing from the child's home environment. The child is helped to gain independence and self-confidence by separating from his parents and having a chance to try new skills without fear of being punished or ridiculed. The child can learn better communication skills and more normal ways of interacting with other children and adults. Head Start programs are a successful model of therapeutic preschools that allow abused children to contact other children from the community.

For older children, the first goal of therapy is to give a consistent message that the child is physically intact and will be able to have a normal life. Group treatment is especially important for older victims as a way of ensuring that abuse has not made the child different from others. Abused children are often afraid to tell their peers about what has happened and may feel marked or damaged, and groups provide a safe place to share experiences and the chance to see that abuse can happen to others, too.

Programs such as Big Brothers may help a child who has had little chance to build self-esteem and appropriate social skills by providing role models and individual support in the home. They also help the child's parent get time away from child-care responsibilities. It is important that volunteers commit themselves to work with a child for a fixed, extended period. Abused children are particularly vulnerable to feelings of loss and self-reproach when a meaningful relationship is unexpectedly ended.

Foster care is often considered as treatment for many kinds of abuse. Ideally it combines the assurance of safety with the provision of a nurturing and stable environment. Foster care may be provided by a relative or by families selected by public or private agencies. Unfortunately, it has many drawbacks. Although safety is often the primary concern of health care and social service workers, the child placed in foster care may be more concerned over losing the only love and consistency he has ever known. The child may see foster care more as punishment than as rescue. If foster care is used, it is important for the child to understand the necessity and to know that contact with the biological parents will not be cut off. Abuse has also been known to continue in foster care settings, and deaths of children in foster care have been reported.

After being placed in foster care, one of the most serious risks to the child is that he or she will be constantly shifted from one foster setting to another, never being returned to the family but never legally eligible for adoption or permanent placement. Children who remain in foster care for more than a short period are at a high risk for never being returned to their parents. Foster care is perhaps best seen as a treatment of last resort when no other alternatives are available and the risk to the child's safety is so great that it balances the risks of placement.

### Therapy for Abusing Parents

Treatment for abusing parents must be provided in a context of acceptance and approval; these persons have low self-esteem and fear rejection. They may not be sufficiently trusting or mature for insight-oriented therapy. A combination of emotionally supportive services with practical parenting aids often provides a basis on which to later explore more deep-seated issues.

Individual counseling or psychotherapy must ultimately involve both parents and later the entire family. The goal is to aid the parents in developing new responses to dilemmas that they currently find overwhelming. The therapy often has specific behavioral objectives, and sessions focus on replays of situations that cause the parent to become anxious or angry. Parents who are open to insight therapy may then be helped to explore issues that underlie their propensity to abuse. This treatment usually lasts for 6 months to 1 year.

Both supportive and explicitly psychotherapeutic groups can be effective means of helping parents to confront their tendency to abuse and to receive practical advice on the acquisition of new skills. In the United States, Parents Anonymous is one example of a successful group program that combines support and therapy in a community-based setting. Groups are available for acknowledged abusers and for parents who feel that they have the capacity to abuse.

A variety of services are available to help parents with the kinds of life stresses that seem to precipitate abuse. Lay therapists and parent aides often have the advantage of coming from a similar socioeconomic background as the parent. They may be able to model parenting and coping skills and provide a secure and uncritical friendship. They give the parent a chance to build skills without exacerbating his feelings of inadequacy. Hot lines and crisis nurseries may serve two functions: their very presence, even if not used, can help a parent feel more confident in facing stress, and in times of need, immediate support and concrete advice are available. Crisis nurseries—facilities that accept children for usually less than 72 hours—can provide a useful alternative to foster care for parents who suffer intermittent periods of dysfunction. Emergency funds for food or clothing or for decreasing isolation by paying for telephone service or transportation may be available from social service or community relief organizations. Transportation may be provided on a regular basis for medical visits or simply to allow parents the opportunity to go shopping or visit family members. The parents' own medical problems also need attention, ideally from a primary care provider with whom the parent can establish an ongoing relationship.

Treatment for neglect may prove much more difficult than for other forms of abuse. Neglectful parents are more likely to have serious character disorders, and those who are extremely apathetic or view life as futile may be especially hard to reach. Marital counseling may be especially important for intact couples to allow the parents to support and nurture each other. Group therapy may not be appropriate for many neglectful parents whose underlying problems make them extremely fearful of interactions with others. Home aides may be the best way to ensure that the child's basic needs are being met and to model for the parent an organized, pleasurable approach to day-to-day tasks.

Treatment for sexual offenders may take several paths using group and individual counseling. Initially, the offender must take full responsibility for the abuse and make a commitment to change his ways and repair the damage he has done. In cases of intrafamilial abuse, the abuser usually agrees to leave the home for an extended period while still upholding his responsibilities to financial support of the family. Subsequent steps in therapy involve addressing the abuser's learned sexual arousal to children and his ability to overcome forces that promote abuse. Treatment for alcoholism is often a part of this therapy. Offenders who are psychotic or sociopathic or who have never been capable of arousal to adult sexual stimuli have a poor prognosis. Therapists rarely speaks of cure; the goal is instead controlling the offender's behavior in the long term. The final step in the treatment of intrafamilial abuse involves family sessions during which the offender reacknowledges his responsibility for the abuse and the family members agree on rules of conduct that can protect the children and foster a better relationship between the parents after the offender returns to the home.

## PREVENTION OF ABUSE AND NEGLECT

Several studies have tested systematic interventions in the newborn period and in early childhood aimed at preventing later abuse and neglect. Although there have been mixed results, it does seem that rates of subsequent injury and neglect can be reduced using home visits (eg, by a public health nurse), programs of regular pediatric care, and rooming-in in the immediate postpartum period. Benefits may be greatest for young, disadvantaged mothers. An important part of these interventions has involved teaching parents to interpret and understand their children's behaviors, including an understanding of basic temperamental differences among infants and appropriate responses to normal infant behaviors. A second important element has involved attention to the parents' emotional needs and those of the child.

Attempts to prevent sexual abuse have taken several directions. Public awareness campaigns have been designed to facilitate recognition and reporting of abuse and to help parents cope with disclosures. Other programs have used theater and music to teach parenting skills and coping strategies. Dozens of programs, from school curricula to coloring books, have been developed for children. These programs have among their major messages that children may say "no" to adults, that adults should not ask children to keep secrets, and that telling someone trusted can get them out of uncomfortable situations. The programs have not been proven capable of preventing sexual abuse, although children over 5 years of age do seem capable of understanding and repeating the messages they contain. These programs have a great emotional impact, and if improperly used, they can make children fearful. Teachers using prevention curricula must be well trained and adhere closely to tested materials. They must also be prepared for children who, prompted by the program, disclose that they or someone they know has been abused. Such disclosures occur frequently and may be one of the most important functions of the program.

Parents may be counseled on the selection of day-care facilities for their children. Facilities should be licensed and staffed by persons with documented experience in child care. The facility should have a written policy that any suspected abuse is immediately reported to the authorities and to the parents of the child involved. There should be no restrictions on parental visitation, and parents should make an unannounced visit before enrolling their child. The physical layout of the center should be such that play areas are open and visible. The lesson plan should not include times during which individual work with a child takes place outside of the common areas.

Injuries from motor vehicle collisions, burns, poisonings, and falls from windows or household furniture cause over half of all deaths among children between 1 and 14 years of age. Most of these deaths are preventable, and some researchers (Wilson, 1983) have labeled them as "culturally condoned child abuse." In some cases, the burden of prevention falls on manufacturers or builders who design inherently unsafe products or dwellings, but in many cases, parents have control over home hazards that threaten their children. Health care workers can help to educate parents to recognize and correct hazards. Measures such as lowering hot water temperatures or removing firearms from the home may prevent accidents and impulsive, intentional injuries.

## Selected Readings

Altemeir WA, O'Connor S, Vietze PM, et al. Antecedents of child abuse. J Pediatr 1982;100:823.

American Humane Association. Highlights of official child neglect and abuse reporting, 1985. Denver: American Humane Association, 1987.

Araji S, Finkelhor D. Explanations of pedophilia: Review of empirical research. Bull Am Acad Psychiatry Law 1985;13:17.

Caffey J. Multiple fractures in the long bones of infants suffering from chronic subdural hematoma. Am J Roentgenol 1946;56:163.

Caffey J. The whiplash shaken infant syndrome: Manual shaking by the extremities with whiplash induced intracranial and intraocular bleeding, linked with residual permanent brain damage and mental retardation. Pediatrics 1974;54:396.

Dine MS, McGovern ME. Intentional poisoning of children—an overlooked category of child abuse: Report of seven cases and review of the literature. Pediatrics 1982;70:32.

Emans SJ, Woods ER, Flagg NT, Freeman A. Genital findings in sexually abused, symptomatic, and asymptomatic girls. Pediatrics 1987;79:778.

Finkelhor D. Child sexual abuse. New York: The Free Press, 1984.

Garbarino J. The elusive "crime" of emotional abuse. Child Abuse Negl 1978;2:89.

Green M, Solnit AJ. Reactions to the threatened loss of a child: A vulnerable child syndrome. Pediatrics 1964;34:58.

Helfer RE, Slovis TL, Black M. Injuries resulting when small children fall out of bed. Pediatrics 1977;60:533.

Hobbs CJ. Skull fracture and the diagnosis of abuse. Arch Dis Child 1984;59:246.

Kempe CH, Silverman FN, Steele BF, et al. The battered-child syndrome. JAMA 1962;181:17.

Kleinman PK, Marks SC, Blackbourne B. The metaphyseal lesion in abused infants: A radiologic-histopathologic study. Am J Radiol 1986;146:895.

McCann J, Voris J, Simon M, Wells R. Comparison of genital examination techniques in prepubertal girls. Pediatrics 1990;85:182.

Polansky NA, Chalmers MA, Buttenwieser E, Williams DP. Damaged parents: An anatomy of child neglect. Chicago: University of Chicago Press, 1981.

Rimsza ME, Niggemann EH. Medical evaluation of sexually abused children: A review of 311 cases. Pediatrics 1982;69:8.

Rosenn DW, Loeb LS, Jura MB. Differentiation of organic from nonorganic failure to thrive syndrome in infancy. Pediatrics 1980;66:698.

Rutter M. Psychosocial resilience and protective mechanisms. Am J Orthopsychiatry 1987;57:316.

Steele B. Psychodynamic factors in child abuse. In: Kempe CH, Helfer RE, eds. The battered child, ed 3. Chicago: University of Chicago Press, 1980.

Straus MA. Stress in child abuse. In: Kempe CH, Helfer RE, eds. The battered child, ed 3. Chicago: University of Chicago Press, 1980.

Waller DA. Obstacles to the treatment of Munchausen by proxy syndrome. J Am Acad Child Adolesc Psychiatry 1983;22:80.

Whittington WL, Rice RJ, Biddle JW, Knapp JS. Incorrect identification of *Neisseria gonorrhoeae* from infants and children. Pediatr Infect Dis 1988;7:3.

Wilson MH. Childhood injury control. Pediatrician 1983–85;12:20.

*Principles and Practice of Pediatrics, Second Edition.*
edited by Frank A. Oski et al. J. B. Lippincott Company, Philadelphia © 1994.

CHAPTER 27
# Developmental Disabilities

# 27.1 Streams of Development

### Frederick B. Palmer and Arnold J. Capute

The developmental disabilities are diverse but related clinical syndromes of chronic neurologic dysfunction. They can best be considered under the broad categories of cerebral palsy, mental retardation, and communicative disorders. The syndromes are grouped together because of similarities in presentation, natural history, and traditional treatments, not because of a common cause or pathology. The common thread is the existence of nonprogressive central neurologic dysfunction, which results in disruption of the otherwise expected normal sequences of infant and child development.

The pediatrician's role in managing developmental disabilities must include but transcend provision of general health care. This expanded role includes responsibilities for detection, developmental diagnosis, developmental monitoring, and coordination of developmental services.

Detection or recognition that the child is developmentally abnormal has been a traditional pediatric role because of the almost universal contact with the infant and the family during the first few years of life. This can be partially achieved by recognition of risk factors associated with concurrent or later development of developmental disability.

Few risk factors have an extremely high likelihood of poor developmental outcome. Most factors are unlikely to be associated with disability in an individual patient. Moreover, many infants who develop disabilities have no clear history of risk. In most cases, detection relies on the recognition of developmental abnormality, usually developmental delay in one or more developmental streams.

Developmental screening tests have been widely used in pediatric practice for years. They are not highly sensitive for developmental abnormality and at the same time highly specific, and they do not yield an acceptably small number of false positives. They have therefore been constructed so that a high number of infants with disability, mostly those with milder disabilities, are not detected. This is a major difficulty when the screening tests lead to pediatrician complacency and no further efforts at detection. It causes a significant proportion of disabled children, those with milder disabilities, to be missed. The pediatrician can avoid this by taking a broader clinical approach to developmental detection rather than solely relying on published screening measures.

Developmental diagnosis includes delineation of the specific developmental disability—cerebral palsy, mental retardation, or communication disorder—and quantitation of its severity. A complete developmental diagnosis must recognize the overlaps among these diagnoses. For example, mental retardation and cerebral palsy can coexist, and the moderately retarded child can have an additional expressive language disorder. Other associated deficits, such as neurobehavioral aberrations (eg, deficits in attention), seizures, orthopedic abnormalities, sensory dysfunctions, or growth abnormalities, must be identified. A complete developmental diagnosis usually requires information from other medical and nonmedical disciplines that is usually best compiled by and interpreted for the parents by the pediatrician.

Developmental monitoring and coordination of services often can be accomplished by the pediatrician because of his or her orientation as a generalist and experience in dealing with families, schools, and other community agencies. Particularly for younger infants and children, in whom all of the manifestations of a developmental disability may not yet be clear, it is important that the pediatrician abdicate this responsibility to other professionals, such as teachers or therapists.

For the pediatrician to fulfill these roles adequately, a general framework for developmental assessment is necessary. (The framework summarized in this chapter is expanded upon in Chapters 27.2 and 27.3.) For decades, pediatricians have separated the complex developmental processes into separate developmental streams for easier evaluation. These developmental streams, including language, visuomotor skills, gross and fine motor skills, social development, and self-help are best analyzed separately. Analysis of each should focus on detecting delay and deviancy.

Developmental delay is best quantitated by the developmental quotient: DQ = developmental age ÷ chronologic age × 100. In children with nonprogressive central nervous system (CNS) abnormalities (eg, static encephalopathies), it represents the rate of development in the measured stream. It provides a rough guideline for measuring progress. Because it implies a constant rate of development from birth, it should be used with caution after CNS injury acquired during infancy and childhood and if there may be a progressive neurologic process. A language or visuomotor quotient below 80 should be seen as frank delay, but a gross motor quotient below 50 is generally necessary before ultimate motor handicap is likely.

Developmental deviancy, a subtle sign of CNS abnormality, refers to atypical development within a single stream, such as developmental milestones occurring out of normal sequence (eg, infant who walks before crawling). Deviancy is useful in detecting mild abnormalities within a given stream if overt delay is not apparent. Recognition of dissociations between rates of development in different streams is essential for the early diagnosis of atypical development within a specific stream.

## COGNITIVE ASSESSMENT

### Language

The best single measure of cognitive development in infancy and in childhood is language development. Traditional psychologic testing relies heavily on language in its determination of an intelligence quotient, beginning in the preschool years and extending through school age and into adulthood. This is true as early as the third year of life, for which the Stanford-Binet Intelligence Test remains the most commonly used instrument. The Wechsler Scales, the most frequently used intelligence test in the school years and for adults, also have a dominant use of language. Infant development scales such as the Bayley Scales of Infant Development and the Cattell Infant Intelligence Test make little use of language items as measures of developmental progress. Infant language can be used as an objective tool for early assessment if professionals are familiar with language markers, their occurrence in the normal population, patterns of delay and deviance, and limitations in their use.

The pediatric assessment of early language relies almost entirely on milestones. These prelinguistic and linguistic milestones are related to later cognitive development, and recognition of early language delay is probably the most sensitive indicator of subsequent mental retardation. Subtle manifestations of language delay or deviancy indicate risk for school-age learning disability and general academic underachievement.

The assessment of infant expressive language development begins in the prelinguistic phase with the sequential occurrence of cooing, babbling, indiscriminate "dada" and "mama," and the discriminate "dada" and "mama," followed by the child's first true word at about 1 year of age. With the development of words used spontaneously and with clear meaning, the child enters the linguistic phase. Between 12 and 24 months, there is an accelerating increase in vocabulary size, which continues into and through the school years; it is easily measured up to about 2 years of age. Similarly, the increase in phrase length occurs with the sole use of single words to about 20 months of age, followed by development of two-word phrases, short sentences, and near-normal adult syntax by the late preschool years.

Receptive language development can be traced into the prelinguistic phase of the first several months of life. The earliest receptive language skills are neurosensory. They represent peripheral auditory functioning and the CNS response to sound. The normal newborn alerts to sound by crying, quieting, or otherwise changing state and by startling, blinking, or by other recognizable responses. By 4 months of age, the child orients to voice by turning to the source of the sound.

Delay in achieving this 4-month skill of auditory orienting may indicate hearing loss, but it may also indicate CNS dysfunction as seen in mental retardation or communication disorders. It may indicate that the child's receptive language abilities are not yet at the 4-month level. By 9 months of age, the child should indicate his understanding of interactive gesture games by participating in them. He should follow a single-step command accompanied by gesture at 12 months and without gesture by

15 months. A 15 months, he should begin to point to body parts on request, and by 2 to 2.5 years of age, the child should be able to follow a series of two independent commands.

The pediatrician should be able to detect language delay associated with mild mental retardation or moderate communication disorders in children by the age of 2.5 years. To detect milder communication disorders and subtle delays in language, further assessment by a speech pathologist or psychologist is required, although atypical or deviant language development may have been noticed in the early months of life.

Language delay is best identified by determining the child's level of consistent language performance by milestone criteria, expressing it as a language age, and dividing by the chronologic age to yield a language quotient. A language quotient below 80 is regarded as delayed. Previously attained milestones should be converted into language quotients to evaluate the consistency of the rate of development expressed as those quotients. Information can be recorded in graphic form, as in Figures 27-1 and 27-2. A "line of best fit" drawn through individual points on this graph represents a developmental rate expressed as the language quotient. This graphic approach allows easy recognition of changes in the developmental pattern, such as plateauing or loss of skills, which may indicate a neurodegenerative process.

Infants with milder degrees of language impairment may not have overt delay. Their language abnormalities may be reflected as deviant or atypical attainment of milestones. For example, there may be a dissociation between receptive language development and expressive language development, with language understanding at a significantly higher level than language expression, a rather common finding in preschoolers with communication disorders. Another common but less easily recognized phenomenon is a better single-word vocabulary than connected language ability. The child may have an age-appropriate expressive vocabulary, but she is unable to put these words together into phrases and sentences at the similar developmental level suggested by vocabulary size. This can be manifested as an "uncoupling" of the milestones that normally occur together, such as two-word phrases and a 25-word vocabulary or two- to three-word sentences and a 50-word vocabulary.

The same phenomenon is seen in receptive development. The preschooler has a large single-word receptive vocabulary (eg, names pictures), but he does not understand connected language (eg, follows commands) at the same developmental level. This phenomenon is especially important to recognize. If parents and educational personnel assume the relatively good vocabulary skills are representative of ability in connected language, they can overestimate the child's capacity and create unrealistic expectations and treatment goals for the child.

Echolalia, repetition of words and phrases without understanding, is normally seen in infants younger than 30 months of age. It may be seen in preschoolers with language disorders with good rote memory skills but poor language comprehension. If prominent, it suggests receptive language skills below the level of 30 months. Recognition of such deviancy is the key component in early detection of milder disorders. It should prompt a complete evaluation by a speech and language pathologist or psychologist.

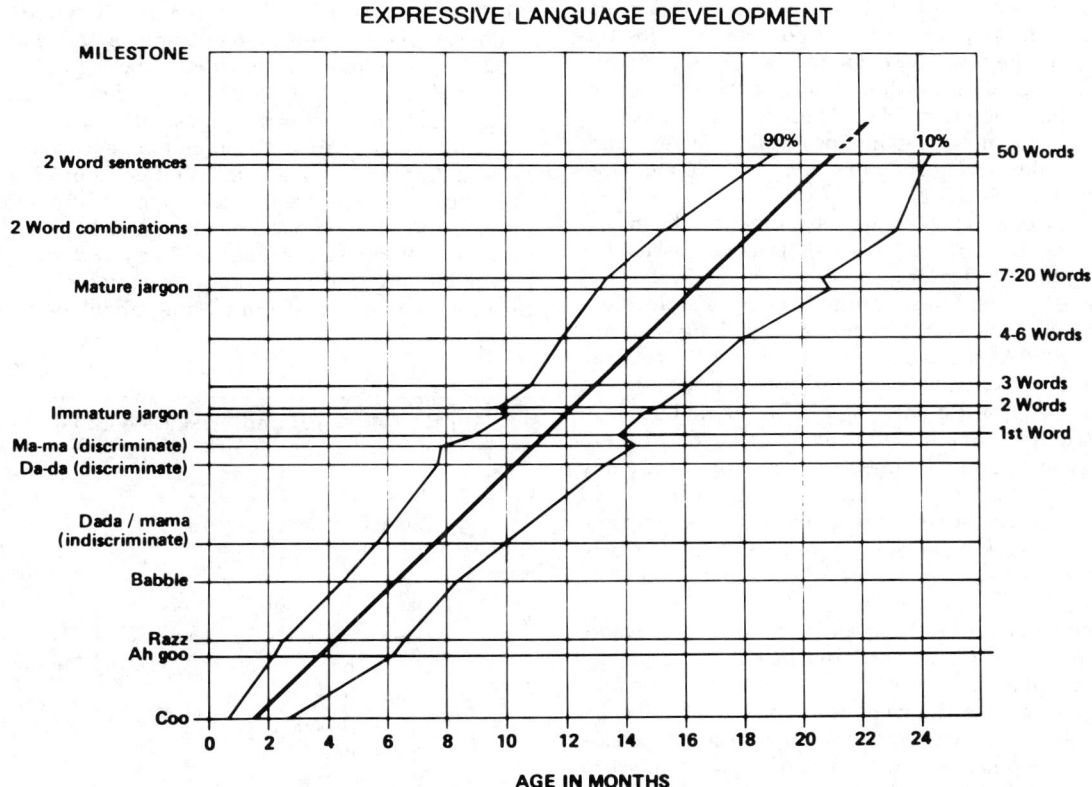

**Figure 27-1.** Expressive language milestones; 90th and 10th percentiles for normative population. Infants whose attainment of milestones is consistently later than the 10th percentile are at risk of language and cognitive delay. Slope of the line through the median of each milestone is 1.0 and corresponds to a developmental quotient of 100. Milestone attainment can be plotted on this figure to depict the rate of development, and the plateau or degeneration patterns. (Capute AJ, Palmer AJ, Shapiro BK, et al. Clinical linguistic and auditory milestone scale: Prediction of cognition in infancy. Dev Med Child Neurol 1986;28:762.)

## RECEPTIVE LANGUAGE DEVELOPMENT

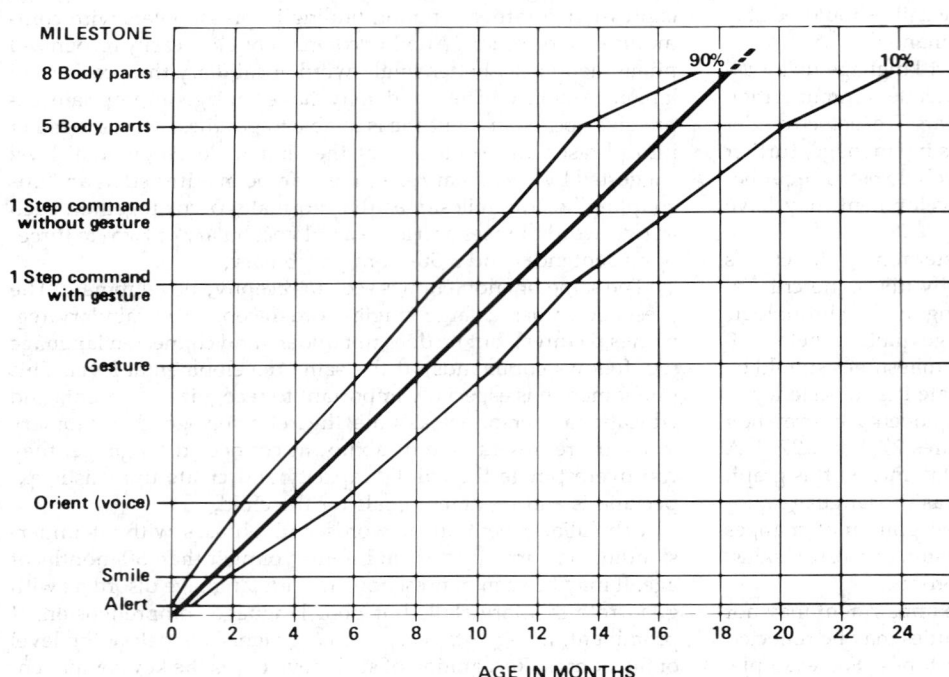

**Figure 27-2.** Receptive language milestones; 90th and 10th percentiles for a normative population (see legend for Fig. 27-1). (Capute AJ, Palmer AJ, Shapiro BK, et al. Clinical linguistic and auditory milestone scale: Prediction of cognition in infancy. Dev Med Child Neurol 1986;28:762.)

## Visuomotor Skills

Visuomotor or problem-solving skills comprise the other major cognitive stream of development. The purpose for assessing this stream is to quantify the cognitive components of visual and fine motor manipulative tasks. A task may not be achieved because of factors other than cognitive delay. These include visual impairment, gross or fine motor liability, or refusal. However, adequate cognitive abilities frequently overcome mild or moderate upper extremity motor limitations.

The earliest visuomotor tasks are assessable in the first 3 months of life. The visual neurosensory skills include visual fixation before 1 month of age and the developmental of visual tracking skills and the blink response to visual threat at 3 to 4 months. By this age, basic visual fixation and tracking skills approach full maturity. At the same time, the infant is gradually coming out of the neonatal flexor habitus (with suppression of primitive reflexes), and by 3 months of age, he should be able to bring his hands to midline and be relatively unfisted. With development of visual tracking abilities and early upper extremity control, eye, head, and upper extremity movements can be used in combination. This represents the beginning of assessable fine motor problem-solving skills, beginning with the ability to reach, attain, and transfer objects from hand to hand by 5 months of age.

During subsequent months, the infant's abilities become more sophisticated, and the examination draws heavily on tasks demanding the manipulation of blocks, peg boards, form boards, and pencil and paper. Like language development, as the child enters the preschool years, visuomotor abilities become increasingly complex and require the evaluation of a psychologist to describe and quantify the child's visuomotor abilities. Commonly used infant and preschool psychometric tests include the Bayley Scales of Infant Development, Cattell Infant Intelligence Scale, Stanford-Binet Intelligence Scale, McCarthy Scales of Children's Abilities, and the Wechsler Preschool and Primary Scale of Intelligence.

Although an infant or child may possess the motor ability to carry out certain visuomotor functions, these skills cannot be accomplished unless the necessary cognitive ability exists. This can be exemplified by the 9-month cognitive skill of examining a bell. If the infant is at the 9-month visuomotor level, examination of the bell and manipulation of the clapper is accomplished. If the infant is functioning below this cognitive level, this problem-solving activity is not carried out; the child ignores the bell, mouths it, or pushes it aside.

A valuable sequence of visuomotor pencil and paper tasks are listed in Table 27-1. These tasks range from 12-month random marking through the traditional copying of the Gesell figures and provide information up to a mental age of 12 years. This sequence of tasks should be a component of any visuomotor assessment.

Unlike language milestones, visuomotor tasks do not lend themselves to parental questioning about previously attained

**TABLE 27-1. Visuomotor Skills With Pencil and Paper**

| Skill | Age |
| --- | --- |
| Simple marks | 12 mo |
| Scribble in imitation | 15 mo |
| Scribble spontaneously | 18 mo |
| Stroke | 24 mo |
| Horizontal and vertical strokes | 27 mo |
| Circle in imitation | 30 mo |
| Copy circle | 36 mo |
| Copy cross | 42 mo |
| Copy square | 4 y |
| Copy triangle | 5 y |
| Copy Union Jack | 5–6 y |
| Copy horizontal diamond | 6 y |
| Copy vertical diamond | 7 y |
| Copy Greek cross | 8 y |
| Copy cylinder | 9 y |
| Copy cube | 12 y |

skills. The pediatrician is usually limited to determining a current visuomotor age and development quotient. Contrasting the rate of visuomotor development with the rate of language development allows the pediatrician to differentiate global mental retardation from a communication disorder. In the former, there is broad cognitive delay manifested in language and visuomotor skills. In language disorders, there is relative preservation of visuomotor abilities with significantly greater delay observed in language skills (ie, language—visuomotor dissociation). Before the developmental diagnosis of mental retardation can be made, assessment of language and problem-solving skills must be accomplished.

## MOTOR ASSESSMENT

Motor, particularly gross motor, development is the stream most familiar to parents and physicians. It is the key to early detection of many disabilities. Significant early motor delay and abnormalities of the neuromotor examination are the hallmarks of cerebral palsy. Most infants with moderate or severe cerebral palsy can be identified in the first 6 to 8 months of life by recognition of delay, abnormalities on examination, and perhaps accompanying risk factors.

There is no useful quantitative association between the rates of motor and language development. The degree of motor delay cannot be used to predict the degree of cognitive delay. However, there is a clear qualitative association; infants with motor delay are likely to have other nonmotor developmental abnormalities, including mental retardation and communicative disorders. Mild motor delay is often the first developmental concern expressed for an infant who ultimately is diagnosed as moderately mentally retarded.

Assessment of motor development begins with the determination of motor age by the best performance on milestone criteria, as outlined in Table 27-2 The motor quotient = motor age ÷ chronologic age × 100. A motor quotient less than 50 is likely to be associated with handicapping cerebral palsy (eg, child not sitting without support until after 12 months of age). Motor quotients above 70 are generally not associated with motor handicap. Infants and children with hemiplegia may represent exceptions to this basic rule, because their gross motor skills may be adequate, but they may have significant impairment of the affected upper extremity, a handicap that is not easily reflected in an overall gross motor quotient. After a complete motor history and neuromotor examination, it may be helpful to develop motor quotients for each of the four extremities to help establish the topography of the motor handicap.

The neuromotor examination offers considerable additional information in establishing topography and in contributing to the early detection of cerebral palsy before outright delay in motor milestones is apparent. The components of the traditional neuromotor examination, such as muscle tone, deep tendon reflexes, involuntary movements, and pathologic reflexes, must be seen in a developmental context. During the first year of life, changes in these parameters occur in normal infants. For example, ankle clonus and other manifestations of lower extremity hyperreflexia are common in infants younger than 4 months of age. Upper extremity synkinesias and other involuntary movements are frequent in infants younger than 8 months. The extensor plantar response should not be regarded as abnormal in infants younger than 12 months of age unless it is obviously asymmetric or associated with other abnormal neuromotor signs.

The evolution of primitive reflex activity during the first year of life offers a key to early recognition of CNS abnormality. Primitive reflexes are subcortical, whole-body motor responses, which develop during gestation, are elicitable at birth, and generally are suppressed during the first 6 months of life with CNS maturation. Abnormally intense primitive reflexes or reflexes that are not suppressed as expected during the first 6 months are signs of neurologic dysfunction. This finding combined with significant motor delay suggests cerebral palsy. With minimal or no delay, the primitive reflex abnormalities still reflect CNS dysfunction; abnormalities in other developmental streams should be pursued. Examples of clinically meaningful abnormalities in primitive reflexes are shown in Table 27-3. Asymmetries in primitive reflex activity, such as asymmetric grasps, toe standing, or shoulder retraction, are also clinical signs of abnormality.

Postural responses, unlike primitive reflexes, are maturational motor responses of righting and equilibrium that develop during the first year of life and are necessary antecedents of the more familiar motor milestones. Clinically elicitable postural responses are reflected in Table 27-4. These responses are helpful to the motor therapists in developing realistic short-term treatment goals for the child with cerebral palsy, and they also may be helpful to the pediatrician in recognition of early motor abnormality.

## ACTIVITIES OF DAILY LIVING

Assessment of self-help abilities or activities of daily living provides useful information. These skills of self-feeding, dressing, and related activities provide information on how the infant in-

### TABLE 27-2. Mean Age of Motor Milestone Attainment

| Milestone | Mean Age (months) | Standard Deviation |
|---|---|---|
| Roll prone to supine | 3.6 | 1.4 |
| Roll supine to prone | 4.8 | 1.4 |
| Sit tripod | 5.3 | 1.0 |
| Sit unsupported | 6.3 | 1.2 |
| Creep | 6.7 | 1.5 |
| Crawl | 7.8 | 1.7 |
| Pull to stand | 8.1 | 1.6 |
| Cruise | 8.8 | 1.7 |
| Walk | 11.7 | 1.9 |
| Walk backwards | 14.3 | 2.4 |
| Run | 14.8 | 2.7 |

### TABLE 27-3. Clinically Recognizable Abnormalities in Primitive Reflexes

| Primitive Reflex | Abnormality |
|---|---|
| Moro | Moro at any age associated with opisthotonos; visible Moro after 4 months |
| Asymmetric tonic neck reflex | An obligatory response from which the infant cannot free himself; visible reponse after 6 months of age. |
| Tonic labyrinthine in supine position | Persistent neck and trunk arching with the child in supine position at any age; visible arching or shoulder retraction after 6 months of age |

TABLE 27-4.  Selected Elicitable Postural Reponses

| Postural Response | Age of Appearance | Comment |
|---|---|---|
| Head righting in supported sitting | 6 wk–3 mo | Must be fully developed before adequate head control and sitting are attained |
| Landau response | 2 mo | Early measure of developing trunk control |
| Derotational righting | 4 mo | With Landau response, prerequisite to independent rolling from supine to prone positions |
| Upper extremity to protective extension in supported sitting | Anterior, 4 mo<br>Lateral, 6 mo | Prerequisite to sitting in the tripod position; prerequisite to sitting independently |

tegrates the developmental streams into basic daily functioning. Most activities of daily living require a minimal level of motor, language, problem-solving, and attentional maturity to be accomplished. Any problems with attaining these skills further clarify the level of competence in individual streams. For example, the mental age for toileting independently is usually about 18 months. A retarded child who is toilet trained by 36 months of age has a cognitive age of at least 18 months. However, failure to achieve toileting independence does not mean the child does not have the cognitive level of 18 months; it may suggest motor, problem-solving, attentional, or language deficiencies or a lack of opportunity.

## SOCIAL DEVELOPMENT

Social development, like activities of daily living, should be seen as an amalgamation of development in multiple streams, particularly cognition. Although environmental influences are important, social dysfunction may be a symptom of neurodevelopmental abnormality. For example, the child who prefers playing with younger children may do so because his communicative abilities are at that level. Certain traditional social milestones, such as play skills, domestic mimicry, and parallel play at 24 months and associative group play at 42 months, are best used as markers of language development.

## BEHAVIORAL ATTRIBUTES OF CENTRAL NERVOUS SYSTEM DEVELOPMENT

Neurologic dysfunction frequently presents as behavioral disturbance, sometimes independent of other obvious developmental abnormalities. Commonly recognized examples of behavioral manifestations of CNS dysfunction are listed in Table 27-5. A complete developmental evaluation, whether for the purpose of detection, diagnosis, or development monitoring, evaluates this behavioral stream. As with other streams, there may be nonneurologic factors contributing to a child's behavior, but the potential for a neurodevelopmental cause for these abnormalities should always be considered.

The child with more severe neurodevelopmental abnormalities, such as severe or profound mental retardation or severe communication disorder, may demonstrate exaggerated behavioral symptoms. These include markedly persevering or self-stimulatory behavior, self-injury, repeated violent temper tantrums, and dramatically short attention span. Management often requires a combination of pharmacologic means with strict behavioral modification techniques. Control of the symptoms often means the difference between institutionalization and supervised community living for the retarded child or adult.

## CONCLUSION

The expanding pediatric role in development disabilities requires a practical understanding of developmental assessment, including evaluation of individual developmental streams, recognition and quantification of delay and deviancy, and appreciation of the dissociated rates of development between different streams. The next two chapters extend these concepts in the context of cerebral palsy and mental retardation.

## Selected Readings

Accardo PJ. A neurodevelopmental perspective on specific learning disabilities. Baltimore: University Park Press, 1980.
Accardo PJ, Capute AJ. The pediatrician and the developmentally disabled child: A clinical textbook on mental retardation. Baltimore: University Press, 1979.

TABLE 27-5.  Behavioral Symptoms of Central Nervous System Dysfunction

| Common Age of Recognition | Behavioral Symptoms |
|---|---|
| Prenatal period | Increased, decreased, or late onset of fetal activity |
| Infancy | Poor feeding, need to awaken for feeding, sustained irritability, abnormal cry, excessive motor activity, excessive rocking or other self-stimulation |
| Late infancy through preschool years | Short attention span, distractibility, preservation, hyperactivity, impulsivity |
| School age | Hyperactivity, attentional aberrations, impulsivity, fire setting, excessive lying, stealing, cruelty to animals |
| Adolescence and adulthood | Above symptoms plus recurrent misdemeanors, substance abuse, accident proneness, and possibly sociopathy |

Capute AJ, Accardo PJ. Developmental disabilities in infancy and childhood. Baltimore: Paul H. Brookes Publishing, 1991.

Capute AJ, Palmer FB, Shapiro BK, Wachtel RC, Ross A, Accardo PJ. Primitive reflex profile: A quantitation of primitive reflexes in infancy. Dev Med Child Neurol 1984;26:375.

Capute AJ, Palmer FB, Shapiro BK, Wachtel RC, Schmidt S, Ross A. Clinical linguistic and auditory milestone scale: Prediction of cognition in infancy. Dev Med Child Neurol 1986;28:762.

Capute AJ, Shapiro BK. The motor quotient: A method for the early detection of motor delay. Am J Dis Child 1985;139:940.

Drillien CM, Drummond MB, ed. Neurodevelopmental problems in early childhood: Assessment and management. Oxford: Blackwell Scientific Publications, 1977.

Gesell AJ, Amatruda CS. Developmental diagnosis, ed 2. New York: Paul B. Hoeber, 1941.

Illingworth RS. The development of the infant and young child, ed 8. Edinburgh: Churchill Livingston, 1983.

Lyle JG. Certain antenatal, perinatal and developmental variables and reading retardation in middle-class boys. Child Dev 1970;41:481.

Nelson K, Ellenberg J. Antecedents of cerebral palsy, multivariate analysis of risk. N Engl J Med 1986;315:81.

Strauss AA, Lehtinen L. Psychopathology and education of the brain injured child. New York: Grune & Stratton, 1947.

*Principles and Practice of Pediatrics, Second Edition.*
edited by Frank A. Oski et al. J. B. Lippincott Company, Philadelphia © 1994.

# 27.2 *Mental Retardation*

Pasquale J. Accardo and Arnold J. Capute

Mental retardation represents a static encephalopathy with serious deficits in the cognitive realm. The term *mental retardation* is often criticized for reflecting a functional impairment rather than a medical diagnosis. Like cerebral palsy, it is best understood as a family of syndromes with sufficient theoretical analogies and practical similarities to make a separate consideration of individual clinical presentations more confusing to the pediatrician and less helpful to the medical management of the child with mental retardation. Despite much debate and disagreement among psychiatrists, psychologists, and educators about the ideal process model for mental retardation, the paradigm of the child with brain damage remains the best point of departure from which the pediatrician can pursue the necessary medical roles of diagnosis and counseling.

## HISTORY

Mental incapacity was recognized in the ancient and medieval worlds, but there was little incentive to pursue the problem beyond the bare minimum necessary to resolve questions of property rights. Radical conceptual changes in the philosophy of human nature and the legitimate goals of experimental science had to occur before the right questions were asked. The necessary social progress and the prerequisite scientific advances coincided at the time of the French Revolution. Victor, a "feral child" found in the woods at Aveyron, was pronounced an idiot by Pinel, one of the founders of modern psychiatry. Itard received one of the first government research grants of modern times to attempt to educate this significantly delayed boy. Over a 5-year period, Itard virtually invented the discipline of special education and pioneered much of behaviorist psychology. His student Seguin continued working on habilitation techniques and became an influential leader of the new residential treatment movement when he emigrated to the United States. With few changes, the special education methodologies these two physicians devised to help persons with mental retardation became the foundation for the early childhood education system popularized by a third physician, Maria Montessori in the first half of the 20th century.

In the early 19th century, Esquirol differentiated "imbeciles" from three classes of more severely limited "idiots" by their functional ability to use language. In 1877, William Ireland published *On Idiocy and Imbecility*, the first modern medical textbook on mental retardation, in which he delineated an etiologic classification that would remain valid for most of the next century. Ireland's book publicized the description in 1866 by Langdon Down of one of the first specific mental retardation syndromes. However, until Jerome Lejeune identified the specific trisomy chromosomal abnormality in 1959, difficulty in differentiating Down syndrome from cretinism and other disorders persisted. The pseudoscientific eugenics movement of the latter 19th and the early 20th centuries precipitated sterilization laws and distorted the initial idealism of the institutional movement. The flowering of the age of syndrome identification and molecular genetics in the latter half of the 20th century somewhat redeemed the contribution of scientific genetics to the study of mental retardation.

Major progress in the medical and behavioral areas depended heavily on the development of well-designed psychometric instruments for accurate classification. In 1905, the psychologist Alfred Binet and the physician Theodore Simon published the first standardized intelligence test. This technologic advance ushered in more than half a century of use and abuse of psychometric instrumentation that belied the authors' original intentions of introducing an objective and unbiased measurement device to replace the subjective and sometimes arbitrary opinion of the classroom teacher. The pediatrician and psychologist Arnold Gesell was the first to extend the quantification of development to the period of infancy and early childhood, and his assessment techniques succeeded in avoiding some of the major pitfalls of intelligence quotient (IQ) mismeasurement. Test scores did not stand alone but could acquire meaning only within the broader context of past history of biological risk and other factors and repeated detailed developmental assessments. The dissociation between the various streams of development was specifically used to more sharply focus the medical evaluation.

## DEFINITION AND CLASSIFICATION

The definition of mental retardation has three components: some degree of cognitive delay, impaired adaptive behavior, and onset before 18 years of age. Cognitive delay is delineated by the IQ, with the levels of mental retardation roughly correlating with the number of standard deviations below the mean (Fig 27-3). It is as imperative in mental retardation as in other developmental disabilities to remember that no child or adult can ever be reduced to a single number, such as IQ. Human behavior does not admit such simplistic reductionism. In addition to the IQ score as a first approximation to the level of retardation, neurobehavioral symptomatology, motor abnormalities, and other associated deficits should be considered to achieve an appropriate classification. The limited utility of IQ scores is further confused by such variables as chronic disease; sensory deficits; prematurity; environmental deprivation; intensive stimulation; the skill and experience of the examiner; the race, sex, and age of the child; the bias of the instruments used; and the interfering presence of behavioral and emotional disorders in the child and the family. These com-

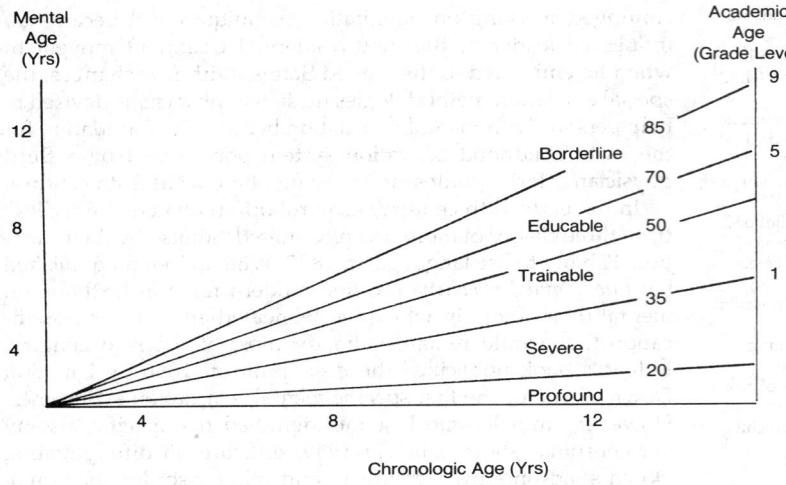

Figure 27-3. Levels of academic achievement to be expected with different degrees of mental retardation at successive ages. The difference between the two ordinal scales reflects the rule of five: mental age level (in years) = grade achievement level (as a grade level). This rule should be routinely used in the office practice of pediatrics. If a child's chronologic age and grade level differ by more than 5, after date of birth, age cut-off for entering school and current date have been allowed for, further investigation is warranted. Grade retention or failing a grade is almost never an acceptable treatment response for any developmental diagnosis. The neatness of the diagram is purely artifactual, and in real life, none of the lines is as clear, sharp, or straight as suggested in this first-order approximation. The diagram is itself a rule of thumb and not a presentation of statistical data.

plicating factors need not reduce the IQ score to complete insignificance; they should instead be viewed as the complex clinical circumstances in which children's cognitive behavior is routinely assessed. These difficulties also highlight the importance of special competence on the part of the pediatrician attempting to formulate a developmental diagnosis.

The fact remains that the single most important qualification for a diagnosis of mental retardation is a validly obtained IQ score of more than two standard deviations below the population mean for the test. Subject to various qualifications, the specific IQ score is the deciding basis for developmental diagnosis, biomedical assessment, parent counseling, educational habilitation, vocational rehabilitation, and disability determination. For using and interpreting the test instruments, the IQ cutoffs for the different levels of retardation (eg, 70, 50, 35, 20) are more accurately viewed as ranges (eg, 65 to 75, 45 to 55, 30 to 40, 15 to 25). For understanding adaptive behavior requirements, it allows a higher degree of correlation with cognitive level. In contrast to the more statistically defined field of psychometrics, the measurement of adaptive behavior does not yield precise quantification. Clinical judgment of self-help and socialization skills can be aided by the Vineland Adaptive Behavior Scales.

The third criterion, onset before 18 years, is least problematic because most cases of mental retardation are congenital, prenatal, or perinatal, and the onset and diagnosis are rarely delayed until after adolescence. The few cases of dementia (ie, degenerative central nervous system disease) and postnatally acquired brain damage are readily recognizable.

## PREVALENCE

Despite continued medical advances in prenatal maternal care and prenatal and perinatal treatment of the fetus and newborn, the overall incidence of mental retardation has remained remarkably stable at approximately 3% of the population. More than 80% of all persons with mental retardation are in the mildly retarded range, and there are twice as many male as female patients. Atypical children with the developmental pattern of borderline intelligence and superimposed language disorders or other deviance or dissociation can be misclassified as mentally retarded. Careful attention to the discrepancies between the different streams of development should allow the correct reclassification of these children and a lowering of the incidence of mild mental retardation.

The basic impact of technologic innovations that occur in neonatal intensive care units (NICU) is twofold. First, the mortality and morbidity curves retain the same shape and magnitude but are shifted horizontally, that is, babies who in the past would have died may now survive with handicaps, and babies who would have survived with handicaps now survive without them. Second, NICU follow-up and other epidemiologic surveys all suggest a marked increase in the newer morbidity of learning and behavior disorders in children. Most of this latter increase, however, is a product of increases in diagnostic skills, test sensitivity and methodologic refinement on the part of the examiners. The further extension of this improved ability to discriminate the finer shades of neurobehavioral dysfunction into the area of mental retardation represents a major future research direction for neurodevelopmental pediatrics.

## SCREENING AND EARLY DIAGNOSIS

Early diagnosis of mental retardation is the responsibility and prerogative of the pediatrician who provides well-child care. Existing screening instruments are far from ideal, and the pediatric practitioner must integrate the specific tests and milestones, neurobehavioral observations, and parental concerns into a larger pattern of specific disability categories and into existing community diagnostic and treatment referral sources. Adequate screening cannot be defined independently of how comfortable the physician feels in reaching specific developmental diagnostic formulations and how the particular pediatric practice has evolved its interactions with consulting subspecialists.

There is no accepted ideal screening or assessment methodology for the office pediatrician separate from a full range of multidisciplinary diagnostic services. In the past, when signs and symptoms of delay were noticed, they were considered to be temporary phases. Although this was often true, they were sometimes early markers for later mild neurodevelopmental dysfunction, such as the spontaneously resolving early articulation disorder, which later reappears as a reading problem. In some cases, they predicted more severe global mental retardation.

The first step in the pediatric assessment of mental retardation is to define the child at risk. Genetic, familial, prenatal, perinatal, and postnatal factors that can affect the developmental rate should be documented. However, the categorization "at risk" remains distinct from a developmental diagnosis. Most children at risk will progress normally, but many not at risk will exhibit severe delays. Many older children with confirmed developmental diagnoses were never at risk. Children at risk should have their development monitored more closely, with early signs and symptoms of brain dysfunction being weighted more heavily.

The treatment of undiagnosed children categorized as at risk remains problematic.

With few exceptions, motor development does not mirror cognitive development. Significant mental retardation is compatible with normal motor milestones. However, cerebral palsy is associated with mental retardation in 50% to 75% of patients, and severe mental retardation often exhibits some degree of motor dysfunction, such as transient hypotonia, visual motor organization problems, clumsiness, tremor, and ataxia. Some mental retardation syndromes exhibit motor deterioration over time, as occurs early in Rett syndrome and late in mental retardation with autistic features.

The most sensitive early marker for mental retardation is language development. Prelinguistic vocalizations in the first year of life show a clear pattern of delay even in mild mental retardation (Table 27-6). However, a significant disorder of language or a learning disability may also present with distortion of early language milestones, and these indications must be supplemented by an assessment of problem-solving skills. The evaluation can range from an observational description of type of play (ie, 0 to 3 months: visual tracking; 3 to 6 months: reach, grasp, mouthing; 6 to 9 months: grasp, transfer, bang; 9 to 12 months: voluntary casting and release) to the use of formal assessment instruments such as the Bayley Scales of Infant Development and the Cattell Infant Intelligence Scale. The pediatrician may also use formal (Table 27-7) or informal lists of developmental milestones or maturational sequences to arrive at one or more developmental quotients.

$$\frac{\text{Estimated Functional Age}}{\text{Corrected Chronological Age}} \times 100$$

$$= \text{Developmental Quotient}$$

A child with an overall developmental quotient (DQ) below 80 should be followed closely; persistence of a DQ below 80 should lead to formal evaluation. A child with a DQ below 60 should receive a comprehensive biomedical and psychologic assessment. This recommendation is a logical implication of the two-group theory of retardation in which organic brain pathology, identifiable causes, and other medical complications increase dramatically as the general cognitive level decreases below IQ 50 (Table 27-8). The milder the retardation, the later it comes to the pediatrician's attention. The preschool child with mental retardation often presents with language delay and the younger school-age child with grade retention.

Certain neurobehavioral symptoms and parental concerns can suggest severe cognitive impairment in infancy, especially if accompanied by CNS irritability and other signs of neurologic disorganization. To various degrees, these behaviors can be considered early nonspecific markers for mental retardation and other neurodevelopmental disorders: failure to thrive, prolonged colic, arching, standoffishness and lack of cuddliness, and suspected deafness or blindness. These markers are not to be interpreted in isolation but rather against the background of risk factors and the pattern of milestones yielded by the streams of development as discussed previously. Careful clinical analysis can often derive these behaviors from a preexisting substrate of delay, dissociation, and deviance.

Early diagnosis is important for a variety of reasons. Parental concerns about mentally retarded children often start in infancy and deserve accurate developmental feedback. The biomedical component of the developmental assessment may identify a hereditary or other recurrence risk about which young families should be informed. Supplementary disability income is available for significantly handicapped infants, and with appropriate

| Month of Age | Expressive Milestone | Receptive Milestone |
|---|---|---|
| 1 | | Alerts, soothes |
| 2 | | Social smile |
| 3 | Coos | |
| 4 | Laughs | Orients to voice |
| 5 | "Ah goo," raspberry | Orients (I) |
| 6 | Babbles | |
| 7 | | Orients (II) |
| 8 | "Dada" (inappropriately) "Mama" (inappropriately) | |
| 9 | Gesture | Orients (III) |
| 10 | "Dada" (appropriately) "Mama" (appropriately) | Understands "no" |
| 11 | 1 word | |
| 12 | 2 words | One-step command with gesture |
| 14 | 3 words, immature jargoning | |
| 16 | 4–6 words | One-step command without gesture |
| 18 | Mature jargoning, 7–10 words | Points to one picture, points to body parts |
| 21 | 20 words, 2-word phrases | Points to two pictures |
| 24 | 50 words, 2-word sentences | Two-step commands |
| 30 | Pronouns, repeats two digits | Concept of one, points to seven pictures |
| 36 | 250 words, 3-word sentence, repeats three digits, personal pronouns | Two prepositional commands |

**TABLE 27-6. Clinical Linguistic and Auditory Milestones Scale***

* The Clinical Linguistic and Auditory Milestones Scale (CLAMS) is an infant language assessment intended for office use by the practicing pediatrician.

## TABLE 27-7. CAT*

| Month of Age | Skills |
|---|---|
| 1 | Visually fixates momentarily, prone I |
| 2 | Visually follows horizontally/vertically, prone II |
| 3 | Visually follows in circle, prone III, visual threat |
| 4 | Unfisted, manipulates fingers, prone IV |
| 5 | Pulls down ring, transfers, regards pellet |
| 6 | Obtains cube, lifts cup, radial rake |
| 7 | Attempts pellet, pulls out peg, inspects ring |
| 8 | Pulls ring by string, secures pellet, inspects bell |
| 9 | Scissors grasp, rings bell, looks over the edge for toy |
| 10 | Combines cube in cup, uncovers bell, fingers pegboard |
| 11 | Mature overhand pincer movement, solves cube under cup |
| 12 | Releases one cube in cup, marks with crayon |
| 14 | Solves glass frustration, out–in with peg, solves pellet in bottle with demonstration |
| 16 | Spontaneously solves pellet in bottle, round block in form board, imitates scribble |
| 18 | Ten cubes in cup, round hole in reversed form board, spontaneous scribble with crayon, completes pegboard spontaneously |
| 21 | Obtains object with stick, square in form board, tower of three |
| 24 | Folds paper I, horizontal four-cube train, imitates pencil stroke, completes form board |
| 30 | Horizontal and vertical pencil strokes, reversed form board, folds paper II, train with chimney |
| 36 | Bridge, copies circle, names one color, draws a person with head and one other part |

* The CAT is a pediatric clinical observational instrument that measures fine motor, adaptive, and visual perceptual skills in the first 2 years of life and is intended to supplement the CLAMS in the diagnosis of mental retardation and other developmental disabilities in very young children.

medical documentation, private health insurance carriers may fund some part of the cost of habilitation programs. Public law (PL) 99-457 mandates early educational intervention for handicapped infants and preschoolers. The pediatric role in the implementation of this legislation should be as great as that for PL 101-47, the Individuals with Disabilities Education Act (IDEA), the most recent update of PL 94-142, Education for all Handicapped Children Act.

## MEDICAL EVALUATION

The pediatric assessment of the mentally retarded child consists of a careful history to obtain information about familial, genetic, prenatal, perinatal, and postnatal influences on development; a detailed listing of developmental milestones reinforced by records, baby books, photographs, and home movies or videotapes if appropriate; a neurodevelopmental assessment of the child's abilities that includes a formal psychometric evaluation by a competent child psychologist skilled in testing handicapped children; and a physical examination that focuses on neurologic correlates of organic brain dysfunction and the minor malformations associated with specific syndromes or that nonspecifically reflect prenatal causes (Table 27-9). The goals of this pediatric assessment are to measure functional level; determine the time of onset, duration, and impact of adverse biomedical influences on brain development; delineate associated dysfunctions or other organ system malformations needing treatment; and identify syndromes of genetic importance. Degenerative or progressive conditions can often be ruled out by a careful developmental milestone history.

Probably the single finding that most often confuses the question of developmental regression is the utterance from an otherwise globally retarded child of several words and perhaps even a rote phrase at about 1 year of age. This seemingly age-appropriate expressive language is lost before 18 months of age, giving rise to the suspicion of possible CNS deterioration. This benign regression pattern stands in striking contrast to that observed in Rett syndrome, which occurs only in girls and may account for as many as one third to one fourth of cases of female severe mental retardation. In this condition, girls who appear to be developing normally until 6 to 18 months of age undergo a fairly rapid dementia with a plateauing of head circumference and acquired microcephaly, a loss of purposeful hand movements replaced by stereotypies such as hand wringing reminiscent of those seen in autistic children, ataxia and marked loss of gross motor skills, and later development of seizures and scoliosis. Although the degenerative course is relatively short, the long-term prognosis is one of severe or profound handicap.

Parents should know whether their child is significantly delayed; how delayed their child is and what that level of delay implies for long-term function; why their child is delayed; with

## TABLE 27-8. The Two-Group Theory of Mental Retardation

| Level/% | Early Diagnosis | Long-term Predictability of IQ | Familial Occurrence | Genetic/ Metabolic Syndrome | Seizures and Other Neurologic Complications | Behavior Disorder/ Expanded Strauss | Positive Psychostimulant Response | Other Organ System Involvement |
|---|---|---|---|---|---|---|---|---|
| Sociocultural/Residual of Mild CNS Dysfunction* | | | | | | | | |
| Mild/80 | Difficult | Fair | Common | Very rare | Less frequent | Infrequent | Infrequent | Rare |
| Residual of Severe CNS Dysfunction | | | | | | | | |
| Moderate/12 | | | | | | | | |
| Severe/7 | | | | | | | | |
| Profound/1 | Easy | Very good | Rare | Common | Common | Frequent | Rare | Common |

* The terms used to describe the differences between the mildly retarded (IQ above 50) and the more organically impaired group are meant to indicate a trend that, with exceptions, varies continuously in the same direction as the IQ decreases.

## TABLE 27-9.  Minor Dysmorphic Features*

Electric hair
Hairwhorl abnormality
  Absent
  Poorly defined
  Multiple cowlicks
  Frontal upsweep
  Widow's peak
Head circumference (OFC) greater than 1.5 SD above or below the mean for age
Epicanthal folds
Hypertelorism or increased inner canthal distance
Low-set ears
Absent ear lobules or adherent ear lobes
Other pinnae abnormalities
  Malformed
  Protuberant ("jug handle")
  Flattened
  Rotated
High-arched or steepled palate
Geographic tongue
Clinodactyly of fifth fingers
Palmar crease abnormalities
  Simian—single four-finger transverse crease
  Sydney—proximal four-finger transverse crease
  Hockey stick crease
Sandal gap deformity of toes one and two
Syndactyly of toes two and three
Long middle toe

* Minor dysmorphic features may represent components of specific genetic or teratogenic syndromes, but they are also present in many other cases of mental retardation and the entire spectrum of neurodevelopmental disability, including learning disabilities and attention deficit hyperactivity disorder, and they then reflect the influence of a wide variety of factors that can affect the development of the fetal brain in the first trimester. They are nonspecific indicators for the prenatal cause of neurodevelopmental disorders. Conversely, infants with high dysmorphology scores (ie, weighted or unweighted scores >4) should have their development monitored more closely than usual and should probably be referred for more detailed developmental assessment at the earliest suspicion of delay or deviance.

## TABLE 27-10.  Sample Tests to be Considered in the Assessment of the Child With Mental Retardation*

Amino acids
Metabolic screening
Chromosome studies
  Karyotype
  Banding
  Fragile X (chromosome)
  Fragile X (DNA)
Skull x-ray films
Computed tomography scan of the head
Magnetic resonance image of the head
Electroencephalogram
Evoked potentials, auditory and visual
Thyroid function tests
Fibroblast cultures
Titers for infectious agents

* None of these procedures is routine. For specific indications, consultations with genetics, neurology, ophthalmology, and dermatology specialists may provide further diagnostic leads.

what degree of certainty the cause is known (eg, definite, probable, possible, unknown); what the recurrence risks are for all family members; what the parents should do in the immediate future to help their child; what the long-term goals are for which they should plan; and what further medical and behavioral tests can help answer these questions. A multidisciplinary approach is necessary to address all these issues.

As in other pediatric problem areas associated with many different causes, a shotgun approach to biomedical diagnosis is not warranted. Leads from the history and physical examination should be carefully followed, but there is no routine workup. Table 27-10 provides a list of diagnostic tests that can be considered. Appropriate consultations should be sought, but the family's energies and resources should not be squandered in pursuit of mythic comprehensiveness. In the earliest stages of the diagnostic process, the family is exquisitely vulnerable to overstated claims by physicians, psychologists, educators, and other involved professions. The eventual failure of implied promises can have serious long-term negative effects on the child with mental retardation, the parents' marriage, and the siblings.

It is especially important not to allow the biomedical data to overrule the most obvious clinical behavioral observations. Much of the data on expected developmental levels in rare and recently described genetic and metabolic disorders is seriously incomplete and potentially misleading. For example, short, dysmorphic, developmentally delayed females with three or four X chromosomes may exhibit significant language disorders instead of mental retardation. Profound microcephaly is compatible with normal, nonverbal intelligence.

## TREATMENT AND OUTCOME

The success of early diagnosis is predicated on a fundamental stability of the rate of intellectual growth. Unfortunately, long-term predictive validity improves only as the IQ drops and as the child's age increases. A careful assessment of and allowance for complicating factors increases the predictive validity of diagnoses made during infancy. Some children occasionally switch their developmental curves, which can be confusing. In the most common example, some perinatally stressed infants who appear to be developing at a consistently slow rate suddenly accelerate their developmental rate late in the first year of life and then continue to progress at a normal level. Alternatively, some children function at a mildly retarded rate through the first decade of life but then plateau in skills several years before or after the 16th birthday; this can lead to a change in their classification down to the moderately retarded or up to the borderline range. Such transitions appear to be genetically programmed and may be inherent in many of the less common genetic syndromes.

Something similar to this rate alteration occurs in children with the single most common genetic cause of mental retardation, Down syndrome. The younger child with Down syndrome in a preschool stimulation program can sometimes function in the borderline intellectual category. The school-age child with Down syndrome typically functions at the low-mild to high-moderate level of mental retardation. By late adolescence to young adulthood, IQ scores in the severely retarded range are not uncommon. Part of this decrement can be explained by the changing correlation between IQ test items at different age levels and the specific profile of skills in patients with Down syndrome. Part of this phenomenon may be related to the early onset of Alzheimer-type changes in 21 trisomy.

A large proportion of apparent change in IQ or functional ability may be secondary to the incomplete nature or poor quality of the initial assessment. The halo effect of striking dysmorphic features or marked neuromotor impairment may lead to underestimating a child's abilities. Most children with fetal alcohol syndrome are learning disabled rather than mentally retarded. Approximately two thirds of children with Prader-Willi syndrome are mentally retarded, but almost all have a superimposed learning disorder that makes an accurate estimate of their functional capacity difficult. Prader-Willi syndrome provides a dual object lesson: the possibility of the coexistence of diagnoses of mental retardation and learning disability in the same patient and the increasing irrelevance of IQ with age as the major determinant of the level of functioning or independence. Because of the severity of their food-related behavior disorder, many young nonretarded adults with Prader-Willi syndrome require group home or intermittent respite care placements.

The pediatric follow-up of the child with mental retardation depends on the nature of the underlying cause and the specific neurobehavioral pattern of cognitive deficits. For example, with an incidence of 14 in 10,000 live births, approximately 35% of children with Down syndrome have congenital heart disease, 20% develop thyroid dysfunction, 15% have cervical spine instability, and 80% have conductive hearing loss, with a higher-than-normal incidence of cataracts, strabismus, congenital duodenal atresia, Hirschsprung's disease, leukemia, and seizures. A complex, structured, multidisciplinary follow-up procedure is indicated, with the frequency of visits determined in part by the specific organ systems involved. In contrast, what may be the second most common (10 in 10,000 live births) genetic contribution to severe mental retardation, the fragile X syndrome, has fairly subtle phenotypic features without any commonly associated organ system malformations. As an X-linked disorder, it contributes to the marked excess of retarded boys over retarded girls.

In the absence of seizures and major organ system malformations, most of the treatment of mental retardation is carried out through the educational system, parent support groups, and other community-based resources. Progressing at a steady rate, the mildly retarded child eventually achieves a sixth grade academic level and is capable of economic independence (see Fig 27-3). The moderately retarded child does not attain a fourth grade academic level with its attendant functional literacy but is capable of sheltered workshop employment and group home living.

The education of severe and profoundly retarded children focuses on self-help skills; some can use group home settings, and others require more institutional residential placements. A few profoundly retarded adults do not speak and cannot be toilet trained (ie, functional age <18 months).

Regardless of the predicted long-term outcome and placement, the optimal environment for the young child with mental retardation is with his family. Parents of children with mental retardation should be advised early to specify guardianship arrangements in their wills and to finalize legal certification of permanent minority status by middle adolescence.

## BEHAVIOR DISORDERS

Any unexplained deviation from the slow but steady progress along the path predicted for the diagnosed level of mental retardation demands further investigation. In addition to medical complications to undiagnosed organ system involvement, there are three common syndromes that should be taken into account. First, despite an accurate overall IQ, the child with mental retar-

| TABLE 27-11. Psychotropic Medication | | |
|---|---|---|
| Class of Drugs | Generic Names | Trade Name |
| Neuroleptics (major tranquilizers) | | |
| | Chlorpromazine | Thorazine |
| Phenothiazines | Thioridazine | Mellaril |
| Butyrophenones | Haloperidol | Haldol |
| Sedatives/hypnotics | | |
| Anthihistamines | Diphenhydramine | Benadryl |
| Benzodiazepines (minor tranquilizers) | Diazepam | Valium |
| Miscellaneous | Chloral hydrate | Noctec |
| | Dextroamphetamine | Dexedrine |
| | Methylphenidate | Ritalin |
| Stimulants | Pemoline | Cylert |
| Tricyclic antidepressants | Amitriptyline | Elavil |
| | Desiprimine | Norpramine |
| | Imipramine | Tofranil |
| Anticonvulsants | Carbamazepine | Tegretol |
| | Clonazepam | Clonapin |
| | Diphenylhydantoin | Dilantin |
| | Phenobarbital | |
| | Primidone | Mysoline |
| | Valproate | Depakene |
| Miscellaneous | Clonidine | Catapres |
| | Naloxone | Narcan |
| | Propranolol | Inderal |
| | Benztropine mesylate | Cogentin |
| | Lithium | |

dation may have a superimposed learning disability or sensory-processing impairment that prevents his or her functioning at the predicted intellectual level. High expectations and undue pressures usually produce significant acting-out behavior. If behavior problems follow shortly after a trial of or an increase in mainstreaming, careful reevaluation of this placement decision is indicated.

Second, family stress and dysfunction are much more likely with a handicapped child and are much more likely to produce secondary behavioral symptoms in the immature child with mental retardation. Such stressors are fairly predictable occurrences at specific critical life stages. Family turmoil reflected in the retarded child's acting-out behavior or school underachievement can be expected at entrance into early childhood special education programs and into kindergarten, puberty or menarche, graduation, workshop or group home placement, and at similar critical events in the lives of other family members. Child abuse at home and sexual abuse in the community probably occur more frequently with retarded victims. The possibility of physical, sexual, and psychologic abuse should always be considered for a sudden or even a long-term behavior disorder unresponsive to routine interventions.

The third and probably most common reason for behavioral problems in persons with mental retardation is the expanded Strauss syndrome. In addition to the more typical hyperactivity, inaction, impulsivity, and perseveration, the more organically CNS impaired persons with mental retardation can exhibit greater degrees of aggressive, repetitive, self-stimulatory, self-injurious, and other bizarre and stereotypic behaviors. Although the incidence of these neurobehavioral symptoms does seem to correlate inversely with IQ, the syndrome complex can occur in persons with only mild degrees of mental retardation. The treatment of choice is behavior modification and environmental structuring.

Psychotropic medication can be a helpful treatment adjunct but should not be used alone (Table 27-11). Stimulant medication is occasionally helpful in persons with mild mental retardation, and its use should be given special consideration because the potential side effects of such medication are minimal compared with those of other drugs. Major tranquilizers may be effective, but their use runs the risk of sedation, dystonic reactions, tardive dyskinesia, and increased cognitive impairment. As a rule, such medications should only be used as part of a comprehensively designed behavioral intervention program after other contributing factors have been carefully addressed or excluded. Pharmacotherapy should be applied to specific target behaviors. Drug effects and potential side effects should be monitored closely. After these conditions have been met, the risk-benefit ratio might be acceptable. It is generally poor medical practice not to consider a trial of medication if family and school placements are at risk because of behavior.

A final word of caution is indicated on the use of medication that has direct or indirect effects on the CNS. Any such drug can be anticipated to have unpredictable effects, especially as the degree of mental retardation worsens. As the global percentage of normally functioning brain tissue decreases, fairly atypical responses become the rule. Paradoxic responses to stimulant and sedative drugs may occur; much higher dose of anesthetic may be needed for surgery, or homeopathic dose levels may prove fatal.

## CONCLUSION

In cerebral palsy, the presenting problem is motor abnormality, but the most handicapping aspect of the disorder is the cognitive dysfunction. In mental retardation, the presenting problem is the cognitive dysfunction, but the most handicapping aspect of the

disorder is society's inability to accept the limitations of the person with mental retardation. The expanded Strauss syndrome provides the greatest limitation on the ability of the adult with mental retardation to integrate successfully into the community. With appropriate educational habilitation, social competence can exceed the measured intellectual level. However, it is not uncommon to find neurobehavioral symptoms interfering with the achievement of social competence commensurate with mental age level. The issue of social competence assumes increasing importance as deinstitutionalization and normalization principles lead to the mainstreaming of persons into the community of persons with more severe degrees of mental retardation—with marriage and parenting as de facto choices currently being made. The children of parents with mental retardation promise to present to pediatricians a whole new set of challenges.

*Idiot* is ultimately derived from ancient Greek word indicating "a private person," a term with increasingly negative connotations for someone who did not involve himself in the active political life of the city-state. Pejorative terms such as idiot, imbecile, and moron have finally disappeared from the medical literature of the past 20 years, but the full integration of persons with mental retardation into modern community structures remains an advocacy objective for all professionals dealing with persons with handicaps.

## Selected Readings

Accardo PJ, Capute AJ. The pediatrician and the developmentally delayed child: A clinical textbook on mental retardation. Baltimore: University Park Press, 1979.

Accardo PJ, Whitman BY. Children of mentally retarded parents. Am J Dis Child 1990;144:69.

Brown FB III, Greer MK, Aylward EH, Hunt HH. Intellectual and adaptive functioning in individuals with Down syndrome in relation to age and environmental placement. Pediatrics 1990;85:450.

Capute AJ, Accardo PJ. Linguistic and auditory milestones in the first two years of life: A language inventory for the practicing pediatrician. Clin Pediatr 1978;17:847.

Capute AJ, Accardo PJ, eds. Developmental disabilities in infancy and childhood. Baltimore: Paul H. Brookes, 1991.

Cooley WC, Graham JM Jr. Down syndrome—An update and review for the primary pediatrician. Clin Pediatr 1991;30:233.

Coorsen EA, Msall ME, Duffy LC. Multiple minor malformations as a marker for prenatal etiology for cerebral palsy. Dev Med Child Neurol 1991;33:730.

Kanner L. A history of the care and study of the mentally retarded. Springfield, IL: Charles C Thomas, 1964.

Mehes K. Informative morphogenetic variants in the newborn infant. Budapest: Akademiai Kiado, 1988.

Ratey JJ, ed. Mental retardation: Developing pharmacotherapies. Washington, DC: American Psychiatric Press, 1991.

Shapiro BK, Accardo PJ, Capute AJ. Factors affecting walking in a profoundly retarded population. Dev Med Child Neurol 1979;21:369.

*Principles and Practice of Pediatrics, Second Edition.*
edited by Frank A. Oski et al. J. B. Lippincott Company, Philadelphia © 1994.

## *27.3 Cerebral Palsy*

Bruce K. Shapiro and Arnold J. Capute

Cerebral palsy is a disorder of movement and posture that results from an insult to or anomaly of the immature central nervous system (CNS). This definition recognizes the central origin of the dysfunction and differentiates cerebral palsy from neuropathies and myopathies. The definition implies that the cause is static in nature and excludes progressive neurologic disorders. The simplicity of the definition belies the diversity of the dysfunctions that result from diffuse neurologic damage.

Although a static encephalopathy, cerebral palsy is not unchanging. As the CNS matures, peripheral manifestations of the central lesions change. Some children improve, some require bracing and surgery, and others plateau.

## HISTORIC PERSPECTIVE

Just as the disorder changes with time, so too has the approach to cerebral palsy. Although known from ancient and biblical times, cerebral palsy was not differentiated from other crippling disorders until William John Little described spastic diplegia and related it to birth injury. Little treated the handicap that resulted from cerebral palsy, and others, including Sigmund Freud and William Osler, focused on classification and clinicopathologic associations.

At the turn of the 20th century, the emphasis shifted to the prevention of handicaps. Bronson Crothers and his coworkers are credited with the first programs of physiotherapy for cerebral palsy. Winthrop Phelps, an orthopedic surgeon, expanded the treatment of children with cerebral palsy and developed a comprehensive method of treatment that addressed nonmotor and motor dysfunctions. As scientific capabilities have increased, two major trends have emerged: reevaluating clinicopathologic correlations with noninvasive techniques to define anatomy and physiology and objective quantification of movement to more reliably define therapy. Early identification and intervention are mandated.

## EPIDEMIOLOGY

Cerebral palsy is the most common movement disorder of childhood. Estimates of its frequency vary from 1 to 6 per 1000, but most recent studies report a prevalence of 1 to 2 per 1000. The lower rate should be regarded as a minimal estimate because milder cases are not included; more severe cases may be obscured by other developmental disabilities, such as seizure disorders or mental retardation, and the most severe cases may die.

Traditionally spastic cerebral palsy has been the most frequent type, accounting for approximately 50% of cases. This is followed by athetosis ($\approx$20%), rigidity, ataxia tremor, and mixed forms ($\approx$25%). However, it is difficult to obtain good estimates of the frequency of cerebral palsy. Time trends have not been consistent, with some researchers reporting an increase and others a decrease. There is disagreement about whether to include children with acquired cerebral palsy (eg, neurotrauma, infection) and to what age cerebral palsy should be diagnosed, because the diagnosis is less stable in infants.

The causes of cerebral palsy have changed. Acute infantile hemiplegia, which was common during the late 19th century, has become rare. Modern obstetric techniques have markedly diminished major birth trauma. The understanding and successful prevention of hemolytic disease of the newborn have changed the spectrum of extrapyramidal cerebral palsy of the choreoathetoid type.

Most cerebral palsy is found in children who do not possess identifiable risk factors. Traditional risk factors are birth asphyxia, prematurity, and intrauterine growth retardation associated with cerebral palsy. When analyzed in a multivariate fashion, the strongest determinants of cerebral palsy are not related to events of labor or delivery. Data from the perinatal collaborative study more strongly support the hypothesis that abnormal antenatal events yield difficult pregnancies, labors, and deliveries and that perinatal difficulties are associated with, not the cause of, cerebral palsy.

The role of prematurity as a cause of cerebral palsy is not clear. As neonatal care has improved, the incidence of cerebral palsy in heavier-birth-weight groups has decreased. Very-low-birth-weight infants (<1500 g) may have a higher incidence of cerebral palsy, but the lower number of children at this birth weight should modify the contribution that these children make to the total pool of cerebral palsy.

## DIAGNOSIS

Some have challenged the classification of cerebral palsy as a static encephalopathy. Brains that have suffered an insult continue to develop in deviant fashions even if the insult is not ongoing. The results of the insult(s) may continue to unfold as the child ages. A person could appropriately ask, "What is static about cerebral palsy?" Two related clinical findings lend support to this dynamic view of cerebral palsy. The clinical picture changes in the first several years of life, and contractures and postural deformity may occur later in life.

The changing clinical picture of the first year of life has been noticed since the initial clinical descriptions of cerebral palsy. The younger the child, the less secure is the diagnosis of cerebral palsy. It was the inability to appreciate the manifestations of brain injury until late in the first year that led physicians to link cerebral palsy to teething. In the absence of signs of severe brain dysfunction, motor failure, or associated dysfunctions that interfere with physiologic homeostasis, the diagnosis of cerebral palsy is difficult. The early abundance of primitive reflexes, lack of inhibition of deep tendon reflexes until substantial myelination has taken place, and inability to predict the development of tone confound early diagnosis. Overidentification and underidentification are not uncommon in the first year of life, but the mandates for early intervention services have increased attempts at earlier diagnosis.

### Neonatal Period

It is not possible to diagnose cerebral palsy in the neonatal period by clinical methods. The relative immaturity of the full-term newborn limits the prognostic ability of the newborn examination. Although a normal neurologic examination may be reassuring, abnormal findings in the neonatal period do not usually prognosticate cerebral palsy.

Advances in noninvasive techniques of neuroimaging, particularly in ultrasound, have provided an alternative means of assessment that may better predict cerebral palsy than the clinical examination. Periventricular cysts, although uncommon, are specific for cerebral palsy. As the natural history of ultrasonic lesions is better appreciated and as techniques for assessing metabolism and blood flows (eg, emission tomography) are increasingly applied to neonates, the better is the chance of diagnosing cerebral palsy in the neonatal period.

### Birth to 6 Months

Attempts to identify cerebral palsy at an early age were hindered by a reticence to diagnose cerebral palsy until a handicap was clearly evident. This was based in part on the observation that some children evidenced early aberrations in their motor development that were associated with transitory abnormalities of tone. These abnormalities frequently did not result in a long-term motor handicap, and diagnosis was delayed to prevent misclassification. In recent years, the desire to ameliorate the effects of cerebral palsy has outweighed the potential adverse effects of misclassification.

The earliest presentations of cerebral palsy are subtle, because the infant has not yet developed a wide range of volitional movement. Feeding difficulties related to hypotonia or uncoordinated suck and swallow, difficulty with diapering because of adductor tightness, or behavioral disturbance, such as impaired periodicity, excessive colic, or cerebral irritability, are common manifestations of cerebral palsy.

The motor examination of the young infant is made difficult by the differential maturation of the underlying precursors of volitional movement. Flexor hypertonus occurs in term newborns and normalizes during the first half year. Primitive reflexes appear during the last trimester of pregnancy, are displayed at birth, and are suppressed during the first 6 months of life. Movement is undifferentiated and reciprocating initially but becomes more specific as the infant ages. Although rolling is usually considered the first motor milestone, predictable motor sequences that may assist early diagnosis occur before rolling.

Observing spontaneous movement is the most important aspect of the motor examination. Decreased amounts of the movement may be generalized or confined to specific limbs. The baby may not kick equally, exhibit fisting in one hand but not the other, transfer in only one direction, or show hand preference at too early an age. Such asymmetries are not normal.

Eliciting movements may yield information about axial abilities. In the prone position, the baby may clear his face at birth, lift his head by 1 month, lift his chest by 2 months, get up on his forearms by 3 months, and push up on his wrists by 4 months. By 5 months, he should be able to shift weight in a prone position while attempting to obtain a toy. In prone suspension, many infants are able to move their faces perpendicular to the plane of their bodies with vertebral extension by 3 months (ie, Landau reaction). The full-term baby should have only minimal overshoot when being pulled into the sitting position, and the 2-month-old infant can maintain his head in line with his body if gently displaced laterally from supported sitting; the 4-month-old infant flexes his neck from a supine position. The newborn can step and momentarily support his weight when held in vertical suspension (ie, neonatal positive support). By 2 to 3 months, the infant loses this stepping response and is able to support his weight (ie, a mature positive support response). Neuromotor signs indicating increased lower extremity tone, such as "scissoring" or assumption of an equinus position, are not normal.

The components of early movement may assist in delineating the nature of the dysfunction, but they are distant from the motor action and are not directly related. Passive tone assessment or measurement of deep tendon reflexes activity yields little in infants of this age. Primitive reflexes are difficult to interpret except if abnormally absent or in obligatory forms or if the most immature of the primitive reflexes persist, such as a Moro reflex beyond 6 months or stepping beyond 2 months.

If the pediatrician sees generalized decreases in movement, notices asymmetric findings, or elicits a neurodevelopmental examination that approximates that of an infant of half the child's chronologic age, the examination is abnormal. The examination is limited in prognostic ability because the situation is likely to change with maturation. However, early identification permits early intervention and monitoring. An abnormal motor examination requires delineation of other areas of neural functioning, because dysfunction usually is diffuse.

## 6 to 18 Months

Motor delay is the basis for the diagnosis of cerebral palsy. However, lesser motor delays may not be significant and resolve with maturation. One technique for qualifying the amount of motor delay is to compare the child's motor age with his chronologic age to develop a motor quotient. Motor quotients of less than 50 are associated with significant motor dysfunction and should be investigated further.

The examination of the infant who is motor delayed consists of assessing the degree and duration of primitive reflexes, assessing the child for postural responses that should be developing, noticing reactions that are never normal (eg, asymmetry), and searching for neurologic dysfunction in other areas, such as language.

As is true of the younger infant, direct observation of spontaneous movement is a sensitive method for detecting movement disorders. Watching the child's sitting; locomotion in prone posture, standing, and walking; and transitions between postures reveals important information about gross movement. Assessment of transferring, reaching, raking, finger isolation (eg, pincer use), and voluntary release reveals the status of the upper extremities.

The interweaving of the suppression of the primitive reflexes and the onset of postural responses serve as the basis for volitional movement. Persistence of significant primitive reflex activity beyond the first half year is abnormal. The Moro reflex (Fig 27-4), or "embrace" response, is elicited by sudden neck extension or by slapping the side of the pillow; extension, adduction, and abduction of the upper extremities occur, followed by semiflexion of fingers, wrists, and elbows. The asymmetric tonic neck reflex (Fig 27-5), or "fencer" response, is elicited by turning the child's head laterally with relative extension of the limbs on the chin side and relative flexion on the occiput side. The tonic labyrinthine reflex (Fig 27-6) is elicited by extending or flexing the neck. This alters the relation of the labyrinths and is associated with shoulder retraction and hip extension or shoulder protraction and hip flexion. If present to a substantial degree, these three reflexes interfere with midline activities, inhibit rolling, and preclude sitting.

A fourth reflex is the positive support (Fig 27-7) of the neonatal type, which gives some indication of neurologic integrity of the lower extremities. It is elicited by stimulating (ie, bouncing) the hallucal areas on a firm surface; the result is momentary lower

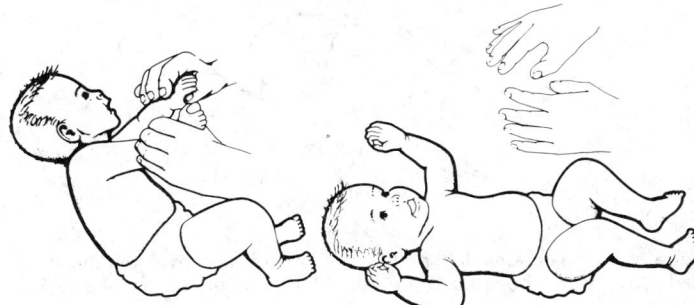

**Figure 27-4.** The Moro or "embrace" response is elicited by sudden neck extension or by slapping the side of the baby's pillow. The reflex is present at birth and disappears at 3 to 6 months.

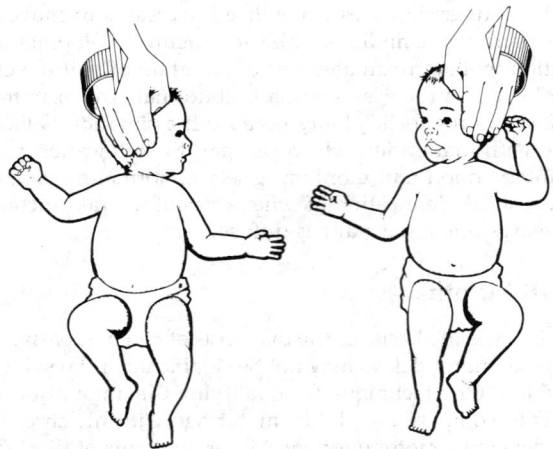

**Figure 27-5.** The asymmetric tonic neck reflex or "fencer" response. Limbs on the side the chin is turned toward extend, and limbs on the occiput side are flexed. The reflex is present at birth and disappears at 3 to 6 months.

extremity extension followed by flexion due to the co-contractions of the hip flexors and extensors. This neonatal or immature response is followed at about 2 to 3 months of age by the more mature one in which the extremities support the body weight for a longer period.

Just as important as the delineation of movement-inhibiting primitive reflexes is the evaluation of postural responses (eg, righting, equilibrium). Postural responses appear in the second half of the first year of life and coincide with volitional movement. Postural responses keep the head and neck in vertical alignment with the body. The 5-month derotative responses have the body following the turning of the head in a derotative fashion or the head following the body. Resistance to anterior displacement by extension of the arms (ie, anterior propping) occurs at 5 months, and lateral propping is seen at 7 months and posterior propping at 9 months. Anterior propping is associated with the ability to

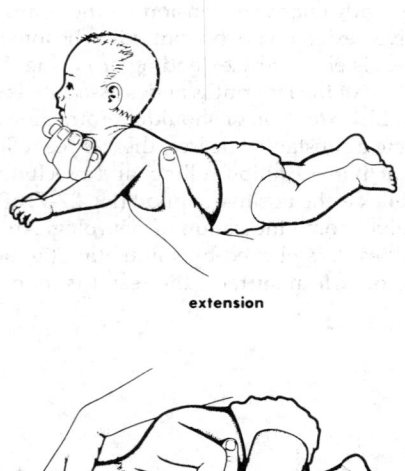

**extension**

**flexion**

**Figure 27-6.** The tonic labyrinthine reflex is elicited by extending or flexing the neck. The reflex is present at birth and disappears at 3 to 6 months.

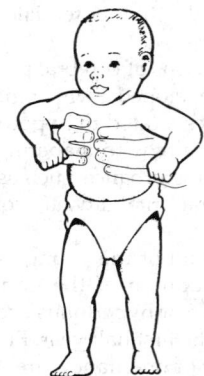

**Figure 27-7.** The positive support reflex is elicited by bouncing the hallucal areas on a firm surface. It is present at birth and disappears at 2 to 3 months.

sit in a tripod fashion, lateral propping correlates with independent sitting, and posterior propping permits pivoting in sitting. Propping responses without primitive reflex activity portends a good prognosis in the motor-delayed child.

## CLASSIFICATION

The classification of cerebral palsy is multiaxial and includes the type of dysfunction (eg, physiologic), site of dysfunction (eg, topographic), associated dysfunctions (eg, supplemental), and etiologic, neuroanatomic, functional, and therapeutic axes. Only the first three axes are used and are discussed here. The neuroanatomic axis awaits definition and the etiologic, functional, and therapeutic axes have been abandoned. The current classification is most useful for older infants and children. All cerebral palsy passes through a hypotonic phase, and attempts at early classification must be viewed as tentative until the evolution of the neurologic syndrome stabilizes. The changing peripheral manifestations also limit prognostication.

### Physiologic Classification

Cerebral palsy can be divided into two major groups, the pyramidal (spastic) and the extrapyramidal (nonspastic) types. Extrapyramidal cerebral palsy can be subdivided into choreoathetoid, ataxic, dystonic, and rigid forms. These groups are clinically useful but are not well correlated with neuropathologic findings.

The signs used to differentiate spastic from nonspastic types are listed in Table 27-12. The neurologic findings of the pyramidal type are consistent and persistent, varying little with movement, tension, emotion, or sleep. Variability is the main feature of extrapyramidal types, with findings increased with activity, tension, and emotions and decreased with sleep or relaxation.

The characteristic type of hypertonus seen in spasticity is clasp knife, similar to the opening and closing of a pen knife with a consistent "hitch." The tone in extrapyramidal types varies from hypotonic to hypertonic. Extrapyramidal hypertonus is of the lead pipe or candle wax type, but it is variable and can be diminished by repetitive movement (ie, "shaking it out"). The persistence of spastic hypertonus may be a factor in the development of contractures. The variability of extrapyramidal tone may protect against contractures.

Pathologic reflexes, such as Babinski or Chaddock, are readily elicited in spastic forms. A true Babinski reflex must be differentiated from the extensor plantar response that is seen as part of athetotic posturing. Primitive reflexes are more evident in the extrapyramidal forms.

| TABLE 27-12. Distinguishing Signs of Spastic and Nonspastic Types | | |
|---|---|---|
| Sign | Pyramidal (Spastic) Type | Extrapyramidal (Nonspastic) Type |
| Movement | Decreased | Disordered, but may be decreased in rigidity |
| Oral motor | Suprabulbar type (flat facies) | Athetotic (grimacing) or suprabulbar type. Common oral reflexes are root, palmomental, increased gag |
| Tone changes | Consistent and persistent; remain relatively constant when infant is asleep or challenged | Variable; changes with tension, challenge, or sleep (usually hypotonic when asleep or quiet) |
| Tone quality | Claps-knife spasticity; sudden give followed by resistance or vice versa (similar to the opening or closing of a penknife); more exaggerated with sudden increase in tendon stretching | Lead pipe or candle wax rigidity; sustained resistance throughout extension or flexion of a limb, brought out by slow movement |
| Primitive reflexes | Present (not noticeable as with choreoathetoid cerebral palsy) | Present; most evident in this type of cerebral palsy |
| Deep tendon reflexes | Hyperreflexia predominates, 3 or 4+ (frequently accompanied by overflow movement) | Normal or mildly increased, 1 to 3+ |
| Babinski, Chaddock, Oppenheim, or Gordon | Present | Absent, not to be confused with the athetotic positioning of the toes and foot (extensor plantar response) due to the posturing seen with choreoathetoid movement. |
| Ankle clonus | Sustained ankle clonus evident | Unsustained ankle clonus; possible to have some ankle clonus present |
| Contractures | Nonpositional contractures | Positional contractures such as hip and knee flexion contractures when child has been in a wheelchair for months or years |

Shapiro BK, Palmer FB, Capute AJ. Cerebral palsy: History and state of the art. In: Gottlieb M, Wilhams J, eds. Textbook of developmental pediatrics. New York: Plenum, 1987.

## Topographic Classification

The topographic classification is limited to the spastic types. It is not usually used with extrapyramidal types, because they have four-limb involvement and are classed by the nature of the movement disorder. The topographic axis includes hemiplegia, diplegia, quadriplegia, and bilateral hemiplegia.

Hemiplegia (ie, hemiparesis) describes involvement of either lateral side of the body. Upper extremities are more impaired than lower, and upper extremity dysfunction usually brings the child to attention.

Diplegia refers to four-limb involvement with the upper limbs only minimally involved although there is significant lower extremity impairment. The good upper extremity function seen in diplegia is of major assistance to habilitative efforts. Paraplegia is reserved for spinal and lower motor neuron dysfunctions, such as myelodysplasia.

Spastic quadriplegia is four-limb involvement with significant impairment of all extremities. Upper limbs may be less impaired than lower, but substantial functional limitations exist. Some researchers consider quadriplegia a furtherance of diplegia.

Bilateral hemiplegia has significant spasticity of both sides of the body, with upper extremities significantly more impaired. Monoplegia and triplegia are formes frustes or combinations of hemiplegia and quadriplegia.

The value of physiologic or topographic classification is that syndromes emerge that are related to patterns of neurologic deficit. For example, hemiplegia may be associated with growth arrest, a visual field defect (eg, homonymous hemianopia), sensory impairment (eg, astereognosis, deficiencies in two-point discrimination, position sense), and seizures. Cerebral palsy resulting from bilirubin encephalopathy has been associated with choreoathetoid movements that evolved into dystonia during adolescence, brown-green discoloration and dentin dysplasia of the deciduous teeth, upward gaze apraxia, and high-frequency hearing loss, frequently associated with central auditory processing dysfunction.

## Supplemental Classification

The child with cerebral palsy has an abnormally functioning CNS. The problem is expressed in many ways, all of which are associated with the primary problem. Cognitive, communicative, and behavioral disturbances are commonly seen. Seizures, sensory loss, and visual and auditory disturbances influence treatment programs.

Cerebral palsy rarely occurs without associated deficits. The diagnosis of cerebral palsy alone is not sufficient. In some cases, the cerebral palsy is not the most limiting condition. Associated dysfunctions alter treatment and affect long-term outcomes. An understanding of the interaction of the motor components and associated deficits is necessary for setting realistic goals. Evaluation and delineation of the associated deficits is part of the evaluation of cerebral palsy.

The presence of associated deficits, each with its own spectrum of severity, makes each case of cerebral palsy unique. It is necessary to completely describe the child's areas of strength and weakness because there is no "garden variety" of cerebral palsy. Failure to define a developmental profile usually results in incomplete habilitation, unrealistic goals, and therapeutic frustration.

Mental retardation coexists with cerebral palsy in approximately 60% of patients. In spastic forms of cerebral palsy, mental retardation is more frequent and more severe in proportion to the number of limbs involved. However, motor impairment does not always mean mental retardation.

Children who escape mental retardation are nevertheless brain damaged and have processing impairments. These may present as communicative disorders in the preschool child or learning disability in the older child. The communicative disorders are of central origin and must be differentiated from the speech disorders that result from oral motor dysfunction.

Deafness has been reported in approximately 10% of people with cerebral palsy, with the athetoid type having the highest incidence. Strabismus occurs in 50%, although it is less common in hemiplegics. However, visual field cuts occur in 25% of the hemiplegics. Refractive errors are also more common in cerebral palsy.

Abnormal neural control of oral motor mechanisms may result in speech and articulation problems, swallowing abnormalities, and repeated episodes of aspiration. Drooling, poor articulation, and difficulties in breath control are more evident in nonspastic forms of cerebral palsy. Most children are able to be successfully managed with oral motor treatment techniques and appropriate positioning. Swallowing abnormalities and aspiration are seen in children who have severe rigidity or dystonia. Severe oral motor dysfunction may be complicated by gastroesophageal reflux and may cause growth failure. In treating the child with severe oral motor dysfunction, the nutritional and motor aspects should be assessed separately. If the child is failing to grow appropriately, has repeated episodes of dehydration, or has gastroesophageal reflux, a feeding gastrostomy with or without an antireflux procedure should be considered.

Sensory impairments associated with hemiplegia are thought to be caused by parietal lobe dysfunction. A limb with sensory impairment (ie, a blind limb) is functionally useless. Fine testing of cortical sensory function is not possible in children younger than 7 years of age, and sensory impairment should be suspected in the child who uses the more motor-involved limb for function.

Seizures occur in one third of children with cerebral palsy. Most seizures are easily controlled with standard approaches. Recalcitrant seizure disorders, such as infantile spasms or Lennox-Gastaut syndrome, are more commonly associated with increased motor dysfunction. Hemiplegia is most commonly associated with seizures.

Behavioral disturbances occur in many children with cerebral palsy. Neurobehavioral disturbances, such as short attention span, impulsivity, distractibility, perseveration, and self-stimulation, may be seen. Emotional disturbances may intensify near adolescence, when issues of independence and peer-group interactions cannot be resolved successfully.

## Expanded Classification

The traditional definition of cerebral palsy does not specify that motor impairment is present to a handicapping degree, nor does it allow for temporal changes. If the physician concentrates only on the children with obvious motor handicap, a larger, more mildly dysfunctioning group of children will be overlooked. This is unfortunate, because many of these children have lasting developmental problems outside of the motor area and require surveillance and programming.

Children who have subclinical forms of cerebral palsy neither require motor therapy nor undergo orthopedic surgical procedures for their motor dysfunction. These children demonstrate clumsiness, awkwardness, transitory abnormalities of tone or postural responses, and other minor neuromotor signs. These signs are markers of central processing dysfunction and place the child at risk for a preschool learning disorder or specific learning disability. The term "cerebral palsy" should not be used with the parents, because it does not assist counseling and may cause the focus to be placed on the motor disturbance rather than the processing dysfunction.

The current definition of cerebral palsy is incomplete because it does not address the entire spectrum of motor dysfunction in children. Although the motor dysfunction may not be handicapping, deviations in motor development are markers for other de-

velopmental dysfunctions in cognitive and behavioral domains. Table 27-13 is a classification schema that expands the definition of cerebral palsy to include the entire spectrum of motor dysfunction of childhood.

## EVALUATION

The evaluation of the child with cerebral palsy seeks to determine the cause of the disorder and to delineate associated dysfunctions. The basis for the evaluation of the child with cerebral palsy is the same as that for any other condition—history, physical examination, and appropriate confirmatory tests. The main justifications for attempts to determine the cause of cerebral palsy are prevention and alleviation of parental guilt.

Prevention in this context refers to taking steps to diminish the likelihood of having a second affected child. This entails treating or preventing conditions that may result in cerebral palsy and excluding conditions that may present with motor dysfunction. These steps may be general, such as enrolling in a high-risk pregnancy clinic, or if the reason for the first child's cerebral palsy can be established, the steps may be specific, such as aggressive management of gestational diabetes. Determination of the cause of the cerebral palsy is often difficult. Many potentially damaging events may occur to the same child, or no risk factors may be present. The clinician must decide whether to go on a "fishing expedition" or follow the patient until signs are manifested. Taking an aggressive approach means many negative evaluations, but a less aggressive attitude may mean an affected sibling.

For children with substantial motor dysfunction a magnetic resonance scan permits the diagnosis of gross brain anomalies and allows an assessment of myelination. A complete blood count and measurement of electrolytes, glucose, kidney and liver functions, uric acid, pyruvate and lactate, ammonia, plasma amino acids, very-long-chain fatty acids, and urinary organic acids quantitated by gas chromatography may be warranted although the yield is low and indications are not clarified. Chromosomal analysis, when positive, rarely yields classic syndromes but more often shows deletions, insertions, or transpositions.

Evaluation of associated deficits is important for proper habilitation. To focus solely on the motor deficit and miss significant cognitive dysfunction may be harmful to the child and family. Specialists in audiology, dentistry, education, nursing, nutrition, neurology, occupational therapy, ophthalmology, orthopedics, otolaryngology, physical therapy, psychology, social work, and speech and language commonly have roles to play in assisting in the management of the child with cerebral palsy. Evaluations are necessary to define associated deficits, but it is possible to overdo it. It is up to the primary provider to direct the evaluation of the associated deficits.

As part of the process of accepting the diagnosis, parents frequently express a desire to know the cause of the cerebral palsy. Establishing an cause can reassure parents that they were not responsible for their child's cerebral palsy. If the cause cannot be established, questions about what could have taken to prevent the cerebral palsy may persist and lingering parental guilt results. This may negatively influence family function and attempts at treatment.

## TREATMENT

The treatment of cerebral palsy is directed toward maximizing function and preventing secondary handicaps. Normality is rarely achieved, although functional outcomes are not uncommon. Treatment objectives change as the child ages.

TABLE 27-13.  Expanded Classification of Cerebral Palsy

| Rate of Motor Development | Motor Signs | Associated Dysfunction |
|---|---|---|
| Minimal: normal<br>Motor quotient (MQ) 75–100<br>Qualitative abnormalities only | Subtle, transient abnormalities of tone<br>Persistence, exaggeration of some primitive reflexes to a mild degree<br>Deviant postural development<br>Soft signs reflected as clumsy or awkward motor performance | Communicative disorder<br>Specific learning disability<br>Strauss syndrome* |
| Mild: two thirds of normal<br>MQ 55–70<br>Walks by 24 mo | Transient abnormalities of tone<br>Occasional "hard" signs; more persistent, exaggerated primitive reflex development<br>Delayed postural responses<br>Exaggeration, persistence in soft signs; some may have functional importance (eg, tremor, synkinesis, poor coordination) | Communicative disorder<br>Specific learning disability<br>Mental retardation<br>Strauss syndrome* |
| Moderate: half of normal<br>MQ 40–55<br>Assisted ambulation<br>May need bracing<br>Usually does not require assistive devices or surgery | Traditional neurologic findings<br>Exaggeration, persistence of primitive reflexes with some obligates<br>Postural responses delayed or absent | Mental retardation<br>Communicative disorder<br>Specific learning disability<br>Seizures<br>Expanded Strauss syndrome† |
| Severe, profound: less than half of normal<br>Wheelchair ambulation<br>Usually need bracing, assistive devices, and orthopedic surgery | Traditional neurologic signs predominate<br>Obligatory primitive reflexes<br>Postural reactions absent | Mental retardation<br>Seizures<br>Expanded Strauss syndrome†<br>Nutritional disorders and others |

* Strauss syndrome: Hyperkinesis, attentional peculiarities (short attention span to perseveration), distractibility, easily frustrated, temper tantrums.

† Expanded Strauss syndrome: Components of Strauss to a greater degree and include repetitive stereotypic activities, such as rocking, head banging, flapping or spinning, and self-injurious behavior.

Shapiro BK, Palmer FB, Capute AJ. Cerebral palsy: History and state of the art. In: Gottlieb M, Wilhams J, eds. Textbook of developmental pediatrics. New York: Plenum, 1987.

The earliest treatments try to maximize motor function. Ambulation and performance of the activities of daily living are the major objectives. Handling techniques, positioning, pharmacologic approaches to tone reduction, bracing, and surgery may all be used to reach this goal. The child with cerebral palsy usually reaches his maximal level of motor function by the early years of school.

In the preschool years, enhancing communication becomes increasingly important. Communicative abilities are more closely related to long-term outcome than motor function. The most efficient means of communication is oral. However, this may not be possible for some children, and alternative methods may be used to circumvent oral motor dysfunction. Children whose motor dysfunction is severe enough to make intelligible speech unlikely but who possess the necessary cognition may be treated with augmentative methods of communication that circumvent oral communication. These methods may range from boards that require looking at the proper answer, to scanning systems, to pointing, to computer-synthesized speech.

As the child ages, concerns about communication evolve into concerns about school performance. Cognitive deficits, peer acceptance, and environmental issues are areas that commonly require intervention. Management of motor deficits focuses on the prevention of postural deformity and seeks to maintain gross motor function.

Focusing on the motor impairment alone may meet with early therapeutic success but will ultimately fail. Long-term outcomes are related more to associated deficits and motivation than to motor ability. Communication, ability to perform activities of daily living, and circumvention of transportation barriers are related more to societal integration than to the gross motor status.

## Motor Therapy

The motor deficit in cerebral palsy results from the combination of abnormal tone and abnormal control of movement. Normalizing tone may permit the expression of more functional abilities. Although conceptually simple, the application of specific techniques is complex because of the different patterns of tone that may be encountered. Hypertonus, hypotonus, mixed patterns of hypertonus and hypotonus, and shifting tone may be seen. Most techniques are designed to decrease hypertonus and its effects. Low tone in extreme forms is treated by positioning and support. Shifting tone is the most difficult to treat. No techniques have been consistently effective in achieving control of disordered movement.

Specific techniques of handling are the mainstay of physical therapy. The physical therapy of cerebral palsy is a diverse set of approaches. Neurodevelopmental physical therapy is the most commonly used physical therapy in the United States, but most therapists are eclectic and modify their programs by using other techniques to augment standard approaches. Motor therapy is tailored to the child and is determined empirically.

In young infants and in children with severe motor deficits, handling techniques are supplemented by positioning. Positioning seeks to diminish asymmetries, tonic influences of primitive reflexes, and to normalize tone. Proper positioning enhances the child's opportunity to interact with his environment. Benefits for oral motor function may be seen in improved feeding abilities and less difficulty in handling secretions. Modified seating devices ensure that most children can be in an upright position in addition to prone and side-lying positions.

Drugs may be used to decrease hypertonus. Diazepam is the

most commonly used agent, although baclofen and dantrolene are effective. Most of the experience with these agents is not derived from children with cerebral palsy, and only limited data exist for motor and nonmotor areas (eg, effects on learning with long-term use). Pharmacotherapy approaches must be coupled with targeted, measurable goals.

Nerve blocks with agents such as alcohol or phenol have been used to treat localized motor dysfunction due to spasticity (eg, heel cord tightness or adductor overactivity). Botulinum toxin has been used recently as well. These agents are more specific than other forms of pharmacotherapy but the effects are not permanent.

Bracing may be used to assist function, prevent deformity, or normalize tone. For example, in children who have spastic diplegia and obligatory positive supporting responses, such as marked equinus, bracing of the ankle and foot may be used to stretch tight muscles and prevent contracture or provide a more stable base for walking. By providing a fixed point to work against, bracing may improve the function of children with choreoathetosis. Bracing is most commonly used for foot and ankle problems, but splinting of the upper extremity may improve hand function.

Although surgery is the oldest intervention used in cerebral palsy, it is the approach that is in the greatest state of change. Surgical goals are similar to those of other motor therapies: improvement of function and prevention of deformity. Surgery may correct deformity. Surgery clearly changes the nature of the motor deficit, although the timing and appropriate procedure are frequently debated. Surgical approaches have moved away from consideration of static, single-joint function to more dynamic approaches. This has been facilitated by techniques that objectively quantify movement in great detail, such as gait analysis, and permit the delineation of individual muscle action during the course of a movement. As a result, lower extremity surgery is becoming more specific to the physiologic disturbance. Long-term study of these techniques is necessary to validate their efficacy.

Hand function is essential to the ultimate outcome in cerebral palsy. Good hand function may permit the person with cerebral palsy to circumvent other motor deficits. Surgical approaches to aid upper extremity function have traditionally been deferred until late adolescence to allow for full growth and maximal patient cooperation. Techniques for the surgical management of the upper extremity are evolving.

Neurosurgical approaches to cerebral palsy primarily seek to alter the abnormal control of movement. Some techniques also normalize tone. Ventrolateral thalamotomy, selective posterior rhizotomy, and cerebellar pacing are some of the more commonly applied neurosurgical techniques. Systematic study of these approaches is difficult, and criteria for their use are still being defined.

## Needs of Parents and Family

Parents of children with cerebral palsy are called on to perform many tasks. In addition to normal parenting roles, they act as therapists, case managers, and advocates. They are charged with selecting the best options from seemingly contradictory recommendations, with coordinating evaluations and treatment, and with ensuring that their child receives the services guaranteed by federal and state laws. They are required to provide skilled nursing care. At times, the amount of effort that the child requires seems endless. Sometimes this care is accomplished to the detriment of spouses and other children.

The continuing relationship with the family affords the pediatrician the opportunity to take the long-term view. Pediatricians can assist parents by providing health care to the child, reviewing treatment goals to ensure that they are attainable and

prioritized, periodically updating evaluations and imparting new information, and by providing a listening ear. The pediatrician's interactions with the family place him or her in a position to consider the needs of the entire family and see that those needs are considered in the development of a treatment program.

## Selected Readings

Capute AJ, Shapiro BK. The motor quotient: A method for the early detection of motor delay. Am J Dis Child 1985;139:940.

Capute AJ, Shapiro BK, Palmer FB. Spectrum of developmental disabilities: Continuum of motor dysfunction. Orthop Clin North Am 1981;12:3.

Crothers BS, Paine RS. The natural history of cerebral palsy. Cambridge: Harvard University Press, 1959.

Nelson KB, Ellenberg JH. Antecedents of cerebral palsy: Multivariate analysis of risk. N Engl J Med 1986;315:81.

Park TS, Owen JH. Current concepts: Surgical management of spastic diplegia. N Engl J Med 1992;326:745.

Penney JB Jr, Young AB. Movement disorders. In: Johnston MV, Macdonald RL, Young AB, eds. Principles of drug therapy in neurology. Philadelphia: F.A. Davis, 1992:50–74.Quzzetta F, Shackelford GD, Volpe S, et al. Periventricular intraparenchymal echodensities in the premature newborn: Critical determinant of neurologic outcome. Pediatrics 1986;78:996.

Scrutton D, ed. Management of the motor disorders of children with cerebral palsy. Clinics in Developmental Medicine, vol 90. Philadelphia: JB Lippincott, 1984.

Shapiro BK, Palmer FB, Capute AJ. Cerebral palsy: History and state of the art. In: Gottlieb M, Wilhams, J, eds. Textbook of developmental pediatrics. New York: Plenum, 1987.

Stanley F, Alberman E, eds. The epidemiology of the cerebral palsies. Clinics in Developmental Medicine, vol 87. Philadelphia: JB Lippincott, 1984.

Thompson G, Rubin IL, Bilinker RM, eds. Comprehensive management of cerebral palsy. New York: Grune & Stratton, 1982.

*Principles and Practice of Pediatrics, Second Edition.*
edited by Frank A. Oski et al. J. B. Lippincott Company, Philadelphia © 1994.

## CHAPTER 28
# Development and Disorders of Speech and Language

Beth M. Ansel, Rebecca M. Landa, and Rachel E. Stark-Selz

The pediatrician is often the first professional to see a child with a communication disorder. This is because parents are likely to seek the advice of a pediatrician if they believe their child is not hearing well or is not developing speech and language normally. Because it is important to take the concern seriously, pediatricians should become aware of the early landmarks of communication development, of the signs and symptoms of delayed or disordered development, and of the need for referral to appropriate professionals, such as audiologists and speech–language pathologists.

Although it is true that some children who show initial delays in speech and language development go on to develop quite normally, about 70% of language-impaired preschoolers continue to have problems during the school years. In 1979, the U.S. National Institute of Child Health and Human Development reported that communication disorders affect approximately 10% of the population (ie, 20 million persons in the United States). These figures represent the lowest defensible estimate of the rate of communication disorders. To improve the overall developmental status of children with handicapping conditions, early identification and intervention is critical. As Soboloff (1979) stated, "It can no longer be accepted that treatment for these children does not begin until 3 years of age. Early stimulation not only benefits the child, but the parents and the entire family." Federal law guarantees a free, appropriate public education for all handicapped children from 3 to 21 years of age. Services for children from birth to 3 years are provided under the 1991 reauthorization of the Individuals with Disabilities Education Act. Parents with concerns about their child's development have access to free assessment and intervention services through local public schools.

The term *communication disorder* is a global diagnostic label that indicates some abnormalities in speech, language behavior, or both, without consideration of cause. The diagnosis of communication disorder is established after examination of speech and language abilities relative to each other and to the child's chronologic age, cognitive abilities, physiologic capabilities, and cultural background.

A better understanding of communication development and disorders and of the decision process associated with establishing diagnosis and treatment recommendations is facilitated by considering a model of communication. The model presented in this text is based on cognitive-linguistic theory. This model may appear novel to pediatricians because it is dissimilar to the medical model they tend to use in the diagnostic and treatment process. In the medical model, the cause of presenting symptoms is sought, and the treatment associated with that cause is administered. However, the treatment of speech and language disorders is usually directed toward a set of behaviors that respond to complex intervention strategies, unlike the treatment of a disease that responds to a drug or surgery. Understanding the differences between the nature of communication disorders and of medical conditions and diseases requires that the knowledge and treatment of each be based on different models.

Communication is the result of a series of complex interactions between speaker and listener. The ability to receive, process, comprehend, formulate, and express messages are all indispensable to communication. Three dynamic, interactive phases are proposed for comprehension and production of spoken language. The input phases include the following:

*Sensation*—hearing or seeing the gestures in speech, sign, or other forms used to convey meanings
*Perception*—coding of auditory and visual input in relation to stored information about the sound and gesture system of a given language
*Comprehension*—decoding of words, grammatical structures, and meanings or concepts in relation to overall context

The output phases include the following:

*Formulation*—organizing concepts to be communicated and formulating them into linguistic structures (eg, words and sentences); organization of these structures within larger units (eg, conversations)
*Motor planning*—developing a motor plan for the concurrent actions of respiration, phonation, resonance, and articulation to express the formulated (intended) message
*Motor control*—executing motor plans in the volitional production of individual speech sounds or sign language gestures and their combinations into sequences to form words, phrases, and sentences

Impairment in any of these input or output phases may result in a distinctive communication disorder. Significant impairment of sensation leads to one of the most devastating forms of communication disorders. Severely or profoundly hearing impaired children have difficulty in understanding spoken language and may be unable to learn to speak intelligibly. They may learn a sign language system that allows them to communicate with others who use that system but that does not provide them with a good foundation for learning to read English or for academic progress in general.

Difficulty with speech perception, despite normal hearing, may give rise to impaired language comprehension. In its most severe form, the disorder may be referred to as *verbal auditory agnosia*. Failure to comprehend language may be related to a generalized cognitive deficit (ie, mental retardation). Some children, although they have normal intelligence and a good grasp of ideas and concepts presented nonverbally, may still fail to understand such ideas when they are presented in a spoken form. Some experts believe that this deficit is related to a difficulty in processing speech sounds, especially when rapid changes occur in these sounds. Because the movements made during speech take place quite rapidly, the cues to speech perception are brief and often rapidly changing. Others believe that comprehension problems are due to linguistic rather than perceptual deficits. Affected children may perform within normal limits on verbal and nonverbal portions of intelligence tests. Verbal items on intelligence tests do not assess grammatical knowledge, for example. These children may easily be misdiagnosed and may fail to receive appropriate services.

Many problems may affect formulation of output, including word-finding difficulties, difficulties in using any but the simplest grammatical constructions and in combining words to express meaning, difficulty in organizing ideas, problems in remembering the proper social forms to use, difficulties in considering the point of view of others, and problems in interacting socially. Impaired formulation may have a genetic or developmental basis or may result from central nervous system anomalies. It may be difficult to localize the anatomical basis of these disorders.

A child's difficulty may be primarily with speech production. Motor planning may be impaired, leading to a problem such as apraxia of speech. Alternatively, the child may lack the fine motor control needed to produce and to sequence gestures of tongue, lips, and jaw for the production of speech and to organize these movements within overall melodic and rhythmic patterns, according to the phonologic rules of the language governing permissible sequences of sounds in different sentence contexts (Fig. 28-1).

The more peripheral and observable functions of hearing and of speech motor control are addressed in this chapter before the more central functions of perception, comprehension, and formulation of spoken language.

## HEARING

The mechanism of hearing is designed to analyze sound according to changes in frequency and intensity over time. The speech signal is transmitted from the outer ear to the middle ear, where it is converted from pressure waves to mechanical vibrations by the three middle ear ossicles: the incus, malleus, and stapedius. These mechanical vibrations are transformed to vibrations in fluid in the inner ear. In the cochlea of the inner ear, nerve endings transform the vibrations of fluid into nerve impulses by means of electrochemical changes.

Hearing losses may be classified according to the portions of the auditory system that are affected or according to cause. Precise causes are frequently unknown. The classification of hearing loss

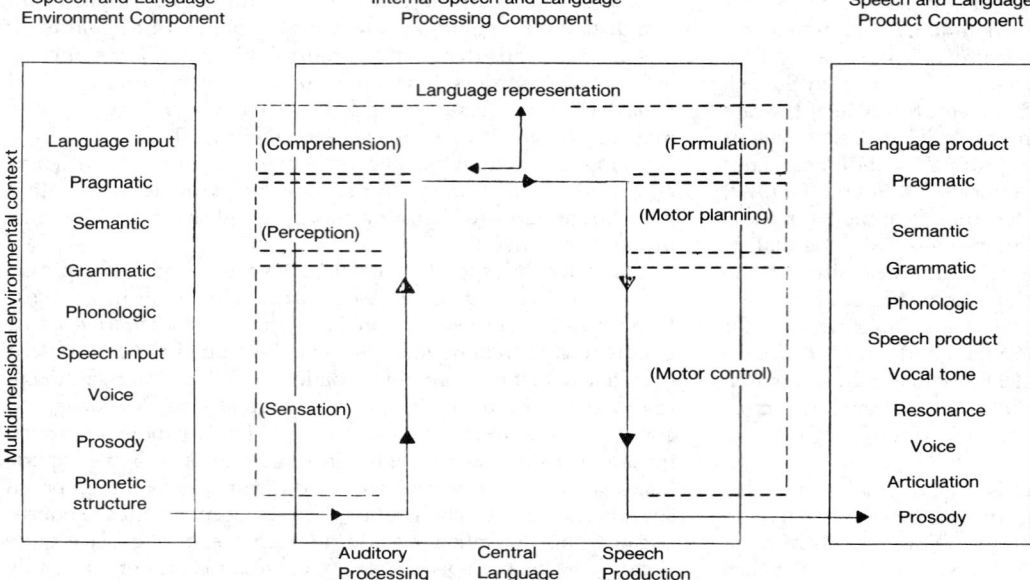

Figure 28-1. Speech and language processing model. (Adapted from Nation JE, Aram DM. Diagnosis of speech and language disorders. St Louis: CV Mosby, 1977.)

is usually based on the affected portion of the auditory system, and the three main classifications are conductive, sensorineural, and retrocochlear hearing loss. A *conductive loss* is related to infection, disease, or anomaly affecting a part of the conductive mechanism (the tympanic membrane and the ossicles of the middle ear). A *sensorineural loss* is associated with disease of the cochlea, such as viral infections, or with anomalies that may have a genetic basis. A *retrocochlear loss* is caused by damage to the auditory system at the eighth nerve, brain stem, or higher levels.

The symptoms associated with different types of hearing loss tend to differ, and the effects of each on speech and language acquisition may differ. Conductive losses are usually less severe than sensorineural losses, although both can be aided by the use of carefully selected amplification. It has been claimed that the relatively mild conductive losses, such as those related to otitis media commonly found in preschool children, may give rise to delays in language acquisition. This hypothesis remains unproved. However, it is likely that even mild language delays from other causes are compounded by the fluctuating hearing that accompanies chronic otitis media. This condition should receive prompt medical attention with close audiologic follow-up.

Mixed losses (ie, conductive and sensorineural) may occur. Only the conductive portion of a mixed loss is treated medically, but amplification may be indicated. Retrocochlear losses may be less common in children than in older adults but may give rise to difficulties in speech discrimination, a problem that can affect the acquisition of spoken language. Recent auditory brain stem studies suggest anomalies in brain stem functioning in certain language-impaired children. Auditory agnosia, a severe central disorder that may result from infections, injury, or seizures affecting cortical or subcortical nuclei, is particularly devastating for preschool children in whom language skills are not yet well established.

Hearing disorders in children vary in severity, but it is not meaningful to talk about percentage of hearing loss. The loss has to be measured in relation to a known standard of normal hearing. Thresholds of hearing are determined in terms of the intensity of a tone, measured in decibels (dB), at certain frequencies, measured in Hertz units. Hearing is usually measured across the frequencies 125 Hz through 8 kHz, which are important for everyday communication and for which hearing in normal humans is most acute. Hearing loss may then be discussed in terms of the slope

of the audiogram, which is the plot of frequencies by intensity that is used to represent hearing.

To determine the severity of a hearing loss, a child's average pure tone threshold is examined across the frequencies that carry the most important information about speech, which are 500 Hz through 2 kHz. It is widely believed that if the child's pure tone average level in the better ear is at least 90 dB, he may be successful in using amplification. If the loss is more profound, aided speech reception may not be achieved. However, some children with greater losses have been known to acquire spoken language comprehension and intelligible speech. Others with less severe losses have acquired only minimal spoken language, perhaps because they were not given amplification early enough or because of other factors influencing language learning, such as age at the onset of hearing loss.

Methods have been suggested for the classification of audiograms in terms of slope. An audiogram with a steep slope beginning from the lower frequencies and extending to only 1 kHz, such as type III in Figure 28-2, indicates a severe to profound loss. The child with this loss may have a more difficult time learning to understand and produce speech than one who has a flatter loss extending to 2 kHz or higher, such as type I in Figure 28-2.

Recent technologic advances in measuring hearing make it possible to diagnose hearing loss earlier in life than in previous decades. For example, acoustic immittance measurement, auditory brain stem response measurement, and behavioral measures to assess the hearing of infants as young as 2 weeks of age may be employed. Through these measures, information can be provided about middle ear status and possibly about other parts of the auditory system.

Philosophies about the education of severely to profoundly hearing-impaired children vary widely across different communities. Parents should be encouraged to consider all options, including the use of sign language, oral-aural training, and some combination of these approaches. The total communication approach employing sign and speech in the classroom has enjoyed popularity in recent years, but the advent of new devices, such as cochlear implants, wearable tactile aids, and other instruments designed to teach deaf children to speak intelligibly, are likely to redirect attention to oral-aural education, especially if the devices prove to be successful in long-term educational programs.

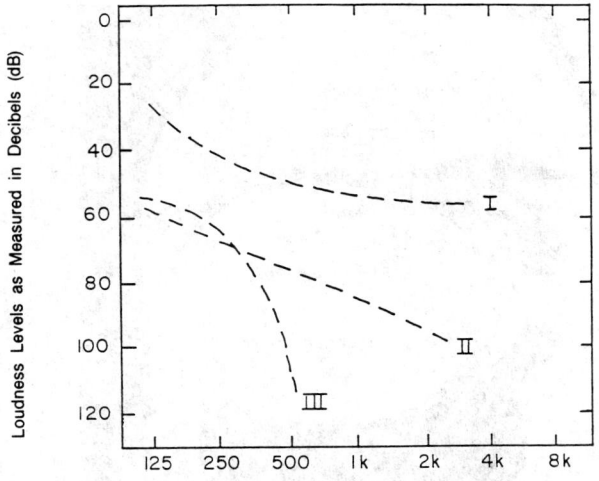

**Figure 28-2.** Sample audiograms of three groups of hearing-impaired children. (Levitt H, Pickett JM, Houde RA, eds. Sensory aids for the hearing impaired. New York: IEEE Press, 1980.)

# SPEECH

## Development of Speech Production

In one sense, the production of speech may be thought of as the entire chain of events occurring when a message is formulated by a speaker, encoded in terms of neuromotor sequences, and transformed by the movements of respiration, larynx, tongue, lips, and jaw into an acoustic pattern for transmission to a listener. No link in this chain is independent. However, the focus for this chapter is on the more familiar processes involving the peripheral movements of tongue, lips, jaw, and larynx, which create the desired acoustic patterns of speech.

The development of speech production in infancy and early childhood reflects increasing motor control. This control is exhibited in the ability to differentiate movements of the articulators (ie, tongue, lip, palate, jaw) and to coordinate these movements with respiratory and laryngeal action so that the prosodic features of rhythm, stress, intonation, and rate are conveyed to the listener. The sounds produced by infants are unlike those of adult speech in their temporal patterning, overall resonance, and acoustic characteristics.

The changes in vocalization during the first year of life cannot be understood without considering anatomical structural changes and the maturation of neuromotor control. These changes account for much of the speech behavior in infancy and early childhood. As the speech apparatus and its control are gradually reshaped by developmental processes, the acoustic signal generated by the motor system becomes more speechlike. The newborn infant's vocal tract is like that of the nonhuman primate, with the larynx high in the neck and the oral and pharyngeal cavities sloping gradually downward instead of showing a right angle as in the human adult. During the first year of life and more gradually thereafter, the larynx descends with the hyoid bone to which the tongue is attached. Downward and forward growth of the facial skeleton increases the size of the oral cavity in relation to the tongue, giving the tongue greater room within which to maneuver. From the standpoint of motor organization, the child must contend with a changing vocal tract anatomy and a maturing nervous system. Neuromotor control of the speech mechanism changes most rapidly during the first year of life, but it continues to develop into later childhood, perhaps to early adolescence.

Investigations by Stark suggested that the development of speech production in infancy takes place in a series of well-defined stages or levels. These levels, like the stages of cognitive development, are related to one another in a hierarchic fashion, with each new level building on preceding levels. New milestone behaviors emerge that are unrelated to previous activities. The levels are shown in Table 28-1.

At the reflexive level, crying and vegetative sounds such as burping and sneezing are produced. Infants are not able to produce open sounds or vowels until they can give up obligatory nasal breathing. They breathe through the mouth when they cry, and vowel-like sounds are heard in the cry. However, in pleasurable sound making or cooing, the mouth is often closed or partly closed. Vowel production in cooing or in neutral social contexts is a major achievement. At the expansion level, infants practice the sounds they have discovered they can make. Squeals, growls, "raspberries," and other sounds appear in different orders in different infants. In marginal babbling, infants begin to put consonant-like and vowel-like sounds together in longer utterances. However, the timing characteristics of these utterances are different from those of meaningful speech. In reduplicated babbling, infants produce recognizable syllables, usually "da" or "ba," in long strings. These utterances are much more speechlike in their timing and are considered to provide a foundation for meaningful speech. At the second expansion level, infants become able to produce different syllables within an utterance, not just the same or repeated syllables. They begin to use a variety of intonation contours and rhythmic patterns more like those found in speech.

Vocal development is cyclical in nature, with new behaviors elaborated and combined with old ones at each developmental level. The successive integration of features of speech appears to be related to increasing neurophysiologic maturity and to the experience of vocalizing in different situational contexts.

Immaturity of the speech motor control system in preschool and early school years is reflected in variability of control of vocal production or speech output. Increased control develops across the functional components of the speech mechanism, including respiratory, laryngeal, velopharyngeal, jaw, lip, and tongue motor milestones. Voluntary sensorimotor control of the muscles involved in speaking is usually well established between 3 and 4 years of age. Neurodevelopmental and acoustic studies by Kent showed that the variability of speech output progressively diminishes from 3 years of age until the age of 8 to 12 years, when adultlike stability is achieved. The order in which the sounds of speech are subsequently acquired by most normally developing children is shown in Figure 28-3. This order is related to increasing complexity of articulation of the sounds. As they acquire more complex sounds, children become increasingly accurate in their production of sound sequences. This process reflects increasing stability of anatomical structures and the automization of neu-

| TABLE 28-1. Level of Speech Motor Skill | | |
|---|---|---|
| Level | Descriptors | Age |
| 1 | Reflexive | 0–2 mo |
| 2 | Vowel production | 2–3 mo |
| 3 | Expansion 1 (consonant and vowel series, squeals) | 4–5 mo |
| 4 | Marginal babbling | 6–8 mo |
| 5 | Consonant—vowel syllables, reduplicated babbling, new vowel types | 9–12 mo |
| 6 | Expansion 2 (new syllable types, jargon, diphthongs) | 12–18 mo |

AGE LEVEL

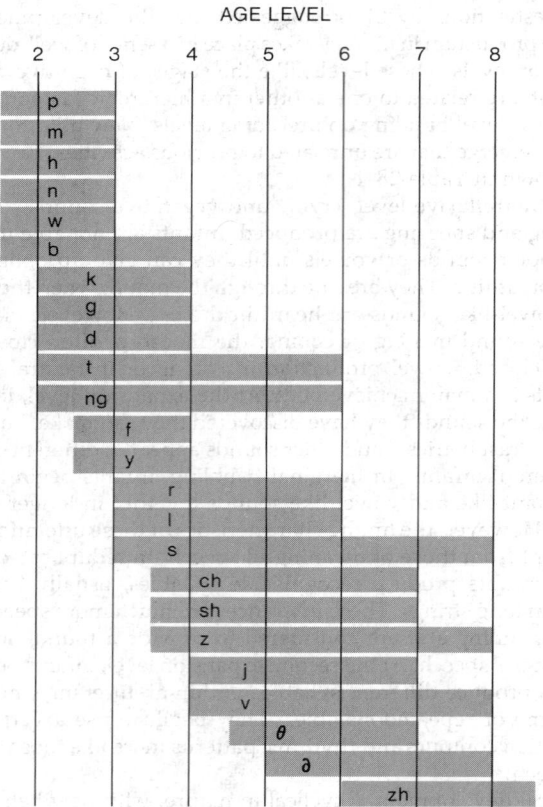

**Figure 28-3.** Speech sound development; average age estimates and upper age limits of customary consonant production. The solid bar corresponding to each sound starts at the median age of customary articulation; it stops at an age level at which 90% of all children customarily produce the sound. (Sander EK. When are speech sounds learned? J Speech Hear Dis 1972;37:55.)

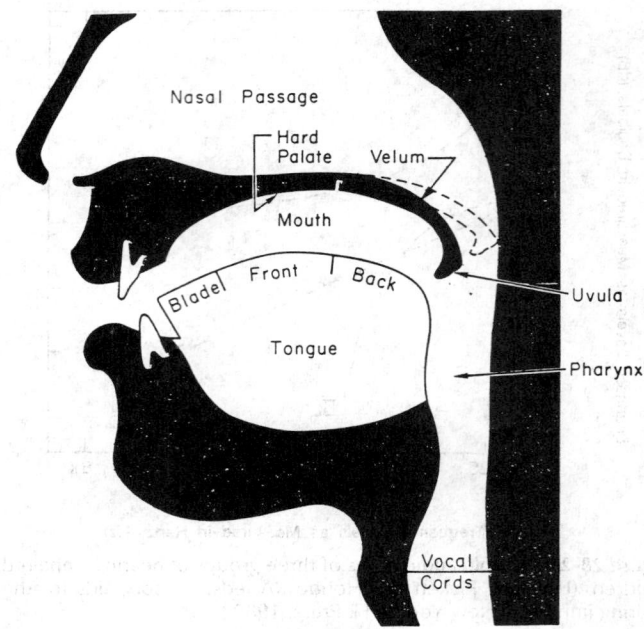

**Figure 28-4.** Schematic illustration of human vocal components. (Levitt H, Pickett JM, Houde RA, eds. Sensory aids for the hearing impaired. New York: IEEE Press, 1980.)

romotor processes. Measures of vocal fundamental frequency (ie, pitch), static formant patterns of vocalic sounds, and temporal properties of speech have shown consistent trends toward adult values and have highlighted the importance of development of timing and coordination of movement of the vocal tract.

It is useful to view the execution of speech output as the product of the interplay between a group of highly related interconnected mechanisms. There are several functional components: labial, lingual, velopharyngeal, mandibular, laryngeal, and respiratory (Fig. 28-4). Each of these components depends on the integrity of a structure or a combination of structures that generates or valves the airstream used for speech. The various valves interrupt, impede, and constrict the airstream in a variety of ways to produce the complete repertoire of phonation and the sounds of speech.

Energy, in the form of an unmodulated stream of air from the lungs, passes into the trachea and into the larynx. The larynx is the principal structure that produces a vibrating airstream, with the vocal folds constituting the vibrating elements. Rapid opening and closing of the vocal folds valve the airstream to produce a vocal or glottal tone within the pharyngeal, oral, and nasal cavities. Undifferentiated glottal pulses are transformed into meaningful speech by modification of the acoustic properties of these cavities. This modification is achieved by movements of the tongue, palate, lips, and jaw. These movements change the resonance properties of the oral, nasal, and pharyngeal cavities. Structural, neurophysiologic, or psychologic influences may impair the functioning of any of these mechanisms and give rise to a disorder of speech output or production (Table 28-2).

## Respiration and Phonation

The respiratory mechanism is the power source for phonation. Respiration for speech should provide an adequate supply of air with the least expenditure of energy or effort, allow for easy control of the expiratory air, and not interfere with speech production. A finely coordinated series of movements is needed to control or adjust the flow of air through the glottis or the vocal folds to produce phonation (Fig. 28-5).

Phonation is a specialized activity of the larynx and the muscles surrounding the larynx. Correct voice production requires that the respiratory and phonatory systems act in synchrony to produce appropriate intensity and pitch. As the vocal folds approximate, air pressure builds up in the trachea until it exceeds the resistance of the closed folds. The vocal folds are parted by the air pressure. As they open, air is expelled, decreasing the subglottal pressure. The elasticity of the laryngeal muscles causes the folds to close again. This cycle is repeated many times per second on a quasiperiodic basis. If there is aperiodicity in the glottal pulses, incomplete closure of the glottis, or asymmetry in the vocal fold motion, the normal characteristics of phonation change, and dysphonia results.

Respiratory support for speech is controlled by neurons in the anterior horns of the thoracic and cervical spinal cord, with some assistance from cranial nerve XI. This widespread anatomical arrangement has the potential for a great variety of clinical syndromes. Children may manifest abnormal breathing patterns as a result of inadequate or reduced respiratory support for speech secondary to muscle weakness, abnormal muscle tone, or incoordination. These motor problems may be encountered in children with dysarthria secondary to cerebral palsy, in severe dysarthria after cerebrovascular accident and trauma, and in the later stages of neurodegenerative diseases. Patients with these disorders may adopt a pattern of upper thoracic and clavicular breathing and extreme neck, laryngeal, and facial tension. The result is a harsh, high-pitched voice that is characterized by inadequate loudness and pitch variation.

Cerebral palsy is commonly characterized by anomalies of respiration and by consequent speech difficulties. Characteristic

## TABLE 28-2.  Possible Manifestations of Speech Disorders

**Disorders of Respiration**

Insufficient respiratory support for speech

Abnormal breath pattern: clavicular breathing, forced inspiration and expiration, audible inspiration

**Disorders of Phonation**

Abnormalities in loudness: monoloudness, excess loudness variation, inappropriate loudness

Abnormalities in pitch: pitch breaks, monopitch, inappropriate pitch

Abnormalities in voice quality: breathy, harsh, hoarse, strain-strangled, tremor, voice stoppages, aphonia

**Disorders of Resonance**

Hypernasality

Hyponasality

Nasal emission

Vowel distortion

**Disorders of Articulation**

Distortion of speech sound

Omission of speech sounds

Imprecision of speech sounds

Inconsistent speech errors

**Disorders of Prosody**

Abnormalities, in rate of speech: short rushes of speech, variable rate, increase in rate of sound segments, increase in overall rate

Abnormalities in rhythm of speech: excessive and equal stress, reduced stress, prolonged intervals, inappropriate silences

Prolongation of speech sounds (phonemes)

Repetition of speech sounds (phonemes)

respiratory difficulties may include too-rapid breathing, difficulty in deep inhalation, difficulty in controlling prolonged exhalatory movements, involuntary movements in the respiratory musculature, and antagonistic diaphragmatic-abdominal and thoracic movements. Certain neurodegenerative diseases, such as myasthenia gravis, may produce an isolated respiratory disorder. In

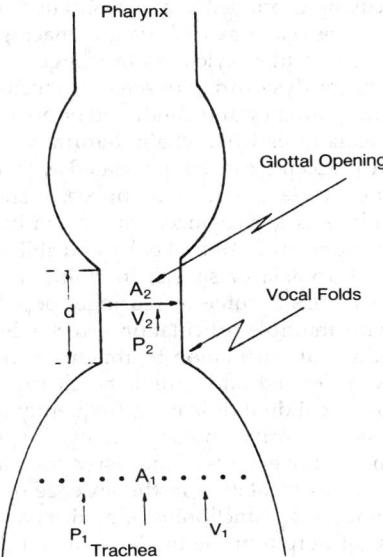

**Figure 28-5.**  Schematic diagram of the forces acting on the vocal fields: *d*, length of glottal constriction; $A_2$, cross-sectional area of glottal constriction; $V_2$ and $P_2$, particle velocity and air pressure at the glottal constriction; $A_1$, cross-sectional area of the trachea; $V_1$ and $P_1$, particle velocity and air pressure in the trachea. (Lieberman P. Vocal cord motion in man. NY Acad Sci 1968;155:28.)

patients with cranial nerve involvement, it may be difficult to differentiate respiratory disorders from those disorders resulting from ineffective laryngeal, palatopharyngeal, or articulatory valving of the airstream.

Disorders of phonation (ie, voice disorders) may be caused by structural abnormalities of the larynx and by neurologic and psychologic disorders. Most disorders of phonation are related to alterations in mass or size of the vocal folds or to approximation-adduction abnormalities of the vocal folds. Vocal fold mass abnormalities may have functional causes, such as speaking at an inappropriate pitch, or organic causes, such as enlarged vocal nodules or papillomas. Approximation-adduction abnormalities may be related to functional factors (eg, psychogenic), structural changes (eg, polyps), or neurologic insult yielding vocal fold paralysis.

Approximately 3% to 5% of all school-age children between the ages of 5 and 18 have phonatory disorders. The most common causes of phonatory disorders in children are vocal abuse or misuse yielding vocal nodules; allergy yielding edema of laryngeal tissue; nonmalignant growths such as juvenile papillomas; and neurologic conditions producing vocal fold paralysis.

There are three phonatory aspects of voice disorders: frequency, vocal intensity, and voice quality. The first two parameters are unidimensional and exist along a continuum. Voice quality is a multidimensional feature of voice production encompassing the characteristics of breathiness, harshness, hoarseness, and nasality. There are many physiologic and acoustic interactions that contribute to defining voice quality, and in cases in which abnormal voice quality exists, assessment by a speech–language pathologist and an otolaryngologist is necessary.

The diagnosis and treatment of voice disorders require a careful analysis of medical, neurologic, and psychologic factors, including a history of vocal use; careful delineation of alterations in quality, pitch, and loudness of the voice; and an examination of laryngeal anatomy and function through direct or indirect laryngoscopy. Psychologic factors can contribute to voice disorders and must be considered.

The primary purpose of the assessment of phonatory function is to identify the basis for deviant vocal behavior. This involves the evaluation of different aspects of laryngeal activity. The underlying basis for the phonatory disorder determines whether an aggressive or conservative management plan is indicated. If there is no laryngeal pathology, the speech pathologist may take complete charge of the voice rehabilitation process. Laryngeal pathology usually requires some combination of medical intervention and voice therapy. Conditions such as fractures of the larynx, cysts, congenital airway obstructions, growths on the vocal folds, laryngeal webbing, juvenile papilloma, and other structural abnormalities of the larynx require medical intervention. These abnormalities are usually treated by means of surgery followed by voice therapy or voice rehabilitation to prevent recurrence. For vocal polyps or nodules secondary to vocal abuse in children, vocal therapy should be implemented as a first step to reduce vocal abuse and the conditions leading to vocal abuse. Conservative management consists of medication alone and is the approach usually considered for disorders caused by edema associated with allergy.

## Resonance

The entire vocal tract is a resonating cavity. Normal speech production requires the coupling of the nasal and oral cavities, regulated by the velopharyngeal mechanism. The velopharyngeal seal results from elevation and posterior movement of the velum against the pharyngeal wall. Velopharyngeal closure allows for the effective separation of the oral and nasal cavities and the shaping of the intraoral airstream, permitting the production of all nonnasal consonants and vowels.

Resonance disorders include abnormalities in vocal tract shaping and disorders in oral-nasal coupling. Any specific resonance disorder, such as distorted vowels or hypernasality, may have an underlying anatomical or physiologic cause, which may be congenital or acquired. There may be compound problems, such as anatomical defects of the orofacial region and physiologic problems due to a central nervous system lesion.

Abnormal resonance can result from abnormal coupling or uncoupling of cavities caused by structural or physiologic dysfunction. Resonance disorders are usually thought of as involving deviations in nasal coupling. Resonance disorders include anatomical and physiologic defects of the orofacial region. Any defect that impairs normal positioning of the speech structures, including the tongue, lips, jaw, and teeth, has the potential for producing resonance disorders, regardless of whether there are orofacial defects, such as dysarthrias, acute myopathies, and peripheral neuropathies. Orofacial clefts are one of the most common craniofacial anomalies, occurring in 1 of 700 to 800 births in the United States and presenting with cleft lip, cleft palate, or both.

Perceptually, *hypernasality* refers to the resonance alteration of vowels and voiced consonants that results from abnormal coupling between the oral and nasal cavities or increased oral impedance relative to nasal impedance of the resonated airstream. Hypernasality is perceived when the velopharyngeal seal is incomplete. It is often accompanied by nasal air emission. The most obvious cause of hypernasality, with or without nasal emission of air, is inadequate function of the palatopharyngeal port. This disorder usually occurs in a person with complete or partial clefts of the velum and hard palate, submucosal clefts, or shortening of the velum.

*Hyponasality* is the resonance alteration resulting from decreased coupling of the nasal and oral tracts. Hyponasality is often attributable to underlying anatomical causes, such as significant obstruction of the nasal passageways or nasopharyngeal space, but it may result from improper velar timing, particularly in deaf persons. Because hyponasality is often associated with nasal or nasopharyngeal obstructions, significant enlargement of adenoid tissue, or edema of the nasal mucosal lining caused by allergy or chronic infection, referral to an otolaryngologist is indicated for medical or surgical intervention.

The study of resonance disorders and of articulatory problems due to structural defects has expanded beyond such relatively common problems as cleft palate to include craniofacial malformation syndromes and ablative surgery deficits. Patients in these two groups present with a variety of alterations in the anatomy and physiology of the speech mechanism and consequent aberrations of resonance that do not fit easily into the categories of hypernasality and hyponasality.

A characteristic quality that involves abnormal resonance patterns is often associated with the speech of deaf persons. Learning proper control of nasal coupling is difficult for deaf children for two reasons. First, raising and lowering the soft palate during speech is not visible and therefore not detectable by lip reading. Second, the activity of the soft palate (velum) provides little proprioceptive feedback. The deaf child has limited information on which to base monitoring of his own resonance patterns. Speech may be hyponasal or hypernasal depending on the degree of nasal coupling required and produced for particular sound combinations.

Dysfunction of the velopharyngeal port mechanism may cause articulatory, phonatory, and prosodic dysfunctions. An inadequate velopharyngeal valving mechanism places increased burden on the respiratory system, which could lead to production of short phrases and to phonatory abnormalities affecting the quality of vocal production, pitch, and loudness.

## Articulation

Articulation of speech is achieved by changing the size and shape of the vocal tract and its cavities. These changes are accomplished by movements of the larynx, pharynx, velum, jaw, tongue, cheeks, and lips.

Many articulation problems are associated with obvious structural anomalies, such as cleft palate, macroglossia, severe malocclusion, significant ankylosis of the tongue, neurologic impairment such as the dysarthrias, or sensory deficits as in hearing impairment during infancy and childhood or hearing loss due to serious otitis media or ossicular chain deformity.

Articulation problems can be associated with central motor disturbance, such as developmental apraxia of speech. Apraxia of speech in adults is a recognized clinical entity. It has been included in descriptions of cerebral palsy and childhood aphasia. The diagnosis of apraxia of speech in children without frank neurologic deficits has become increasingly popular, especially for children with multiple articulation errors who are slow to respond to traditional articulation treatment. Although the disorder is not well defined and cannot be clearly differentiated from dysarthria in children, it is most frequently described as a neurologically based deficit in motor planning for speech. It affects the coordination of movements of the respiratory, laryngeal, and oral musculature in articulation in the absence of impaired peripheral neuromuscular functioning. Impairment at the motor planning phase of output in the model shown in Figure 28-1 is implicated.

Many characteristics have been proposed as symptomatic of apraxia of speech in children, including a restricted repertoire of phonemes (ie, speech sounds) and inability to produce speech sounds requiring complex articulatory adjustments, such as *th, f,* and *sh*. Inconsistent sound production, vowel and consonant errors, and prosodic disturbances including an overall slow rate and monotony of stress patterns may characterize the disorder.

In some instances, no obvious etiologic factors account for an articulatory disturbance. Such articulation problems have been regarded as functional and are estimated to account for 75% to 80% of all speech problems in children.

Articulation problems occur more frequently among boys than girls and among younger than older children. Prevalence is estimated at 10% in children in kindergarten and first grade, with a gradual decline thereafter. However, the data on prevalence vary widely according to the source and method of detection. Approximately 4% of 11-year-olds and 1% of 17-year-olds continue to show articulation problems.

An articulation error traditionally has been defined as an omission, substitution, distortion, or addition of a sound or sounds. The degree of severity of the articulation disorder depends on the perceived interaction of these types of errors and the frequency with which an error is used in the language. The number of errors, frequency or consistency of errors, type or patterns of errors, stimulability (ie, difference in ability to imitate sounds and to produce the same sound spontaneously), contextual effects, and the relation between articulation and language function must be considered in evaluating the disorder.

Many changes have occurred since the 1960s in the way children with articulation disorders of unknown cause have been labeled, resulting primarily from shifts in the theoretical approaches applied to the disorder. For many years, articulation disorders were regarded as disorders of the speech motor system. Treatment was based on a motor-learning approach wherein speech behavior was viewed as a complicated skill that needed to be practiced at a conscious level until it became automatic.

More recently, the role of linguistics has been emphasized in the field of speech disorders, which has contributed information about phonologic systems, the rules by which sounds are combined in specific languages. Analyses are included in most phonologic examinations of children presenting with speech errors. The analyses examine the variability of a given speech error across phonetic contexts and allow the development of a systematic program of intervention. Articulation disorders characterized by faulty sound production rules are referred to as phonologic disorders.

Functional articulation disorders have been considered by many researchers to be the product of faulty phonetic learning. Because of the presumed importance of speech discrimination in early phonetic learning, deficient speech discrimination seems to be a potentially important factor in the development and perpetuation of functional articulation disorders. A somewhat more controversial extension of this notion is that the remediation of the perceptual dysfunction is an important preliminary step in alleviating the production deficit. The application of the term *functional articulation disorders* may be too broad. It fails to take into account the oral motor, auditory, and linguistic (ie, semantic and grammatical) deficits that may play a primary role.

Articulation disorders may be the result of impairment in one or more cognitive, social, linguistic, anatomical, or physiologic variables. For example, a child may have a cleft palate and mild mental retardation; another may have apraxia of speech and a concomitant language disorder. All of the relevant variables and their interactions must be examined. A thorough analysis of the child's articulation errors must be carried out before a diagnosis and plan of treatment is determined.

Current therapeutic methods afford a good prognosis for normal speech production. However, for the child with a severe communicative disorder related to a severe neuromotor speech disturbance, supplemental communication systems may be required. The selection of an optimal system is a complex matter requiring the cooperation of the speech–language pathologist, physical therapist, occupational therapist, special educator, and psychologist.

Oral speech communication may not be a viable or realistic option for persons with severe dysarthria or apraxia. It has been conservatively estimated that 1 to 2 million people in the United States are unable to communicate effectively through speech (ASHA, 1980; Blackstone, 1987). The inability to talk has been regarded as one of the greatest debilitative and socially stigmatizing of all disabling conditions.

Within the last decade, substantial progress has been made in the development of augmentative communication devices (eg, computers, nonelectronic devices) to facilitate the expressive communication of severely communicatively handicapped persons. Although most persons referred for augmentative communication evaluations have cerebral palsy or are otherwise obviously motorically handicapped, other populations (eg, autistic children) are reaping noteworthy benefits from augmentative communication devices. The evaluation process to determine the appropriateness of an augmentative communication system for a child and the type of system needed is complex and involves a multidisciplinary team. Augmentative communication devices are not viewed as a panacea for the motor-speech disabled. Many experts advocate using such devices at necessary points in the overall speech management plan for the dysarthric person, but if possible, they propose aiming for oral speech as a primary goal.

## Prosodic Aspects of Speech Production

The information in the speech signal can be imparted in one of two ways: through the words chosen or by the manner in which the words are produced. The second mode requires the speaker to make use of the suprasegmental or prosodic features of speech. The prosodic features of speech include rhythm, stress, intonation, and rate. They may be viewed as the vocal effects contributed by variations in the characteristics of pitch, loudness, articulation time, and pause time. Real-time physical events in the acoustic speech signal, such as fundamental frequency, intensity, and temporal spacing of acoustic events, serve as cues for the perception of prosodic features.

Prosodic features contribute information about the attitudes and intentions of the speaker. They contribute to referential meaning. The ability of a speaker to stress key words and syllables accurately in an utterance is critical in human communication. Stress patterning allows the speaker to mark specific locations within an utterance where the listener can decode significant semantic and grammatical information, improving the efficiency of communication. From a clinical perspective, optimizing stress patterning in a speaker is essential, because the patterns enhance the transfer of information, improve intelligibility, and contribute to the naturalness and acceptability of speech. Many categories of disordered speech are characterized by some degree of disturbed prosody. Although stuttering and cluttering have traditionally been described as prosodic disorders, abnormal or disturbed prosody is a primary, salient characteristic of the speech of the deaf, of all the dysarthrias, and of developmental apraxia of speech. Deficiencies in perception or production of prosodic features may be present in language-disordered children and adults, including persons categorized as mentally retarded, brain injured, or learning disabled.

Prosody was at one time viewed as something extra added onto the speech signal, which made it more aesthetically pleasing but was not crucial to its intelligibility. Prosodic aspects of a patient's speech used to be given some remedial consideration after the "more important" aspects such as segmental production, phonologic discrimination, syntax, grammar, and semantics had been rehabilitated. As a result, there was a lack of substantial research addressing problems related to perception or production of prosodic features. This view is changing with the recognition that prosody is intrinsic to perception and production of speech and that effective rehabilitation on other speech dimensions must incorporate an understanding of the functions of prosody. Researchers are beginning to document prosodic disruptions in speech production across the disorders with perceptual and acoustic methods of analysis. Current investigations have proposed that treatment of prosodic features should constitute a major focus of attention. Data support the hypothesis that prosodic features make a significant contribution to the intelligibility of speech and its communicative effectiveness.

## Fluency

Fluency disorders are a special case of disruption of prosody usually referred to as *stuttering*. In stuttering, the speaker experiences blocks that are significant disruptions in the flow of speech. The speaker may react to these blocks by struggling to overcome them, producing secondary reactions involving movements of other parts of the body, not just the articulators.

Many children exhibit periods of disrupted fluency, most commonly from 2 to 5 years of age. Because the disorder is frequently episodic in preschool years, the parent may be advised that the child will "outgrow it." Such advice runs the risk of overlooking an incipient problem and withholding treatment when it could be most successful. The longer the dysfluency exists, the more difficult it is to change, with secondary characteristics complicating the disorder. The earlier in the development of symptoms that intervention is begun, the greater is the likelihood that treatment will be successful. Concerned parents should not be counseled to ignore the child's dysfluent speech but should be referred to a speech and language pathologist for evaluation, counseling, and possible treatment.

When stuttering behaviors occur frequently and are severe, the family and physician may have little difficulty in recognizing that a disorder exists. More advanced stutterers, by their struggle or avoidance reactions and emotionality, show that they know they have a serious fluency problem. However, the differential diagnosis between stuttering and normal dysfluency is more difficult in young children. The following symptoms are guidelines to assist the physician in determining when a referral is appropriate:

The child is aware that a problem exists.

The child shows marked tension and audible or visible signs of struggle when speaking.

The child's speech pattern commands attention from listeners and interferes with communication.

The child's speech is characterized by sound prolongations, syllable or word repetitions, or silent pauses within word boundaries, before speech attempt, or after the dysfluency.

The child exhibits episodes of dysfluency of more than two sound repetitions per word or more than two word repetitions per 100 words.

The child avoids certain words or sounds.

The parent speaks for the child if a communicative difficulty is evident.

The child is frequently interrupted by a parent.

Parents are concerned about the way the child speaks and about the child's reaction to the dysfluencies.

According to one view of fluency disorders, there is a continuum of fluency that extends from highly fluent speech to severe breakdown of fluency in stuttering. Another view is that stutterers and normal speakers form two distinct groups. Many preschool children experience transitory periods of stuttering with complete remission in the school years. Persistent stuttering, sometimes with fluctuations in severity, occurs in less than 10% of the population.

Current research indicates that subject and environmental variables interact to bring about stuttering. One of the most important subject variables appears to be genetic predisposition. The incidence of stuttering is higher in the families of stutterers than in the families of nonstutterers. Stutterers tend to show speech motor, central auditory processing, and language impairment in childhood. As a group, they achieve developmental milestones in speech and language later than nonstuttering children, and they show a higher incidence of articulation problems. The incidence of stuttering is greater in boys than girls, but the severity of the disorder may be greater in girls who stutter than in boys.

Environmental variables that affect fluency are primarily social, interactive variables. Communicative stress is perhaps the most important. Stutterers can usually speak to animals or young children with relative ease. They may have most difficulty when they must compete with others to be heard or when they have to speak in front of a large group. The cause or causes of stuttering are unknown, but electrophysiologic and behavioral studies have the potential to increase our understanding of the disorder. Studies of intermittent stuttering as a sequel to neurologic insult should be taken into account. Although a number of approaches to treatment have proved quite successful, they are not based on a clear understanding of the nature of the disorder. It is agreed that the disorder is multifaceted and that an eclectic approach to treatment is more successful than one based on a narrow set of beliefs.

## LANGUAGE

Like speech, language is a multidimensional phenomenon. It may be conceptualized as four interdependent yet theoretically distinct subsystems: phonology, grammar (ie, morphology and syntax), semantics, and pragmatics. Phonology pertains to the sound system of the language and has been referred to in the section on speech production. The remaining three subsystems are described in this section. Each is discussed in terms of its development in the normal child and how it may be impaired in the child with a communication disorder (Table 28-3).

In the course of a child's acquisition of communication skills, a disruption may occur in the development of one or more of the language subsystems. This disruption may occur as delayed or deviant development of communication skills or result from an acquired neurologic insult, such as a closed head injury or stroke. In delayed development, a child exhibits communication behavior that is typical for a normally developing child of a younger chronologic age, and skills are acquired in a normal sequence at a slower-than-normal rate across all four major language subsystems. In deviant development, the child exhibits communication behaviors that are not observed in normal children, or the child acquires skills in an abnormal sequence. Children may exhibit delays that are more severe in some subsystems than in others. In these children, language subsystems are developing heterochronously, which is a deviant pattern of development.

Some causes of developmental language disorders include hearing impairment, mental retardation, infantile autism, and social and emotional disorders. In most cases, the cause is unknown, and no clear neuroanatomical or neurophysiologic basis can be identified. In these cases, behavioral analysis addressing the processes affected (eg, central auditory or motor planning processes) is informative.

TABLE 28-3.    Possible Manifestations of Language Disorders

**Disorders of Grammar**

Inconsistent, inappropriate, or no use of some grammatical markers (eg, past tense "ed")

Inappropriate arrangement of words in a sentence

Limited variety of grammatical forms in the sentences produced

Use of stereotyped phrases that result in limited flexibility of expression and may result in socially inappropriate message expression (eg, being too blunt)

Failure to produce or comprehend grammatically complex sentences

Difficulty recognizing grammatical errors produced by self or others

**Disorders of Semantics**

May have developed an inappropriate definition of a word, so may use words inappropriately

Difficulty comprehending words that have multiple meanings or abstract meanings and that require simultaneous consideration of multiple referents

May produce odd word combinations; failure to recognize inappropriate word combinations or to understand another's message

Difficulty integrating information in a conversation or story

Difficulty inferring information that is not explicitly expressed

Literal interpretation of expressions such as sarcasm, jokes, figures of speech

Word finding problems

Difficulty producing a well-organized story that portrays main events instead of insignificant details

Limited variety of meaningful relationships expressed (eg, possession, location)

**Disorders of Pragmatics**

Limited variety of communication intentions expressed

Difficulty expressing and understanding indirect messages

Monopolizing conversation

Reticence or unelaborated responses

Poor strategies for topic initiation, maintenance, elaboration, or termination

Abrupt topic changes or often gets on tangents

Difficulty assessing the informational needs of the listener (eg, provides insufficient background information)

Difficulty recognizing and repairing misunderstandings

---

Moderate to severe developmental language disorders are found in at least 6% of preschool children. As in the case of speech disorders, language disorders are more likely to occur in boys than in girls, and the incidence declines with age. Most children with psychiatric disorders have concomitant language disorders. Academic learning problems are likely to occur in children who are first identified as language impaired. It is important that language problems be identified as early as possible. Current knowledge permits identification of communication disorders as early as the first year of life.

In children with acquired language disorders, the cause is usually known. For example, language disorders are a common sequela to stroke, viral encephalitis, gunshot wounds, or closed head injury. The age of onset is thought to be a more important variable influencing recovery than the extent or site of the lesion. In younger children, the greater plasticity of the central nervous system may favor the reacquisition or recovery of speech and language. Recovery may take place over 2 years or even longer. Acquired language disorder (ie, aphasia) is frequently a concomitant of seizure disorder and may improve as seizures are brought under control. Aphasia may persist in children with focal lesions. In children with closed head injuries, speech and phonatory disturbances are almost always found in the early stages of recovery, and word finding and discourse (conversational storytelling) difficulties often persist.

Despite a relatively good prognosis for speech and language recovery in children sustaining neural insults, later academic difficulties are common. Poor academic records are typically found in longitudinal studies of these children. Academic failure in reading, spelling, and mathematics is often recorded after recovery of spoken language. These learning problems may be related to persistent generalized impairment in complex integrative linguistic processes that are necessary for acquisition of many academic skills.

In the following sections, the normal and abnormal developments of each language subsystem are discussed.

## Grammar

The grammatical rules of language that children learn are those that govern the arrangement of grammatical markers, such as verb tense markers and plural markers, and word sequences for sentence formation. To learn grammatical rules for sentence formulation, children must know that meaningful associations are conveyed by the way in which words are ordered and combined. Consider, for example, the sentences "Bob hit Sue" and "Sue hit Bob." Although they contain the same words, they clearly do not convey the same meaning. Children's knowledge of the grammatical rule system allows them to recognize that if Bob did the hitting, his name must precede the verb unless there are other grammatical markers present that indicate otherwise. For example, when the grammatical marker *was* precedes an uninflected verb and the verb is followed by the marker *by*, as in the sentence "Sue *was* hit *by* Bob," the listener knows that the first person mentioned was the recipient of the action, not the actor.

The use of grammatical rules becomes evident in children's

verbal output between 16 and 24 months of age, when they begin to combine words to express messages about relationships between people, events, and objects. The early grammatical structures employed by children are simple, usually taking the form of noun plus noun, such as *daddy car*; noun plus verb, such as *car go*; verb plus noun, such as *gimme cracker*; or adjective plus noun, such as *big boy*. During the early stages of grammatical development, children's sentence structure is sometimes described as "telegraphic" because their short, simple sentences resemble a telegram. These short sentences are primarily made of words such as nouns and verbs that are rich in semantic content or meaning. Consequently, function words, such as prepositions, conjunctions, and articles, tend to be lacking. The types of words children use in early sentences and the average length of these sentences may serve as indications of how normally the early grammatical system is developing.

Gradually, the grammatical rule system becomes more complex. Grammatical markers are added to sentences in a predictable order, first the "ing" verb marker, then the plural "s" marker, and so on. In addition, noun phrases and verb phrases are elaborated, enabling a child to express increasing amounts of information within a sentence. Rules are learned for embedding one sentence within another, resulting in an elaborate, complex sentence, such as "The boy who is sitting under the tree is eating apples." Rules are learned that enable a child to change one type of sentence structure into another type. For example, children learn the rules for changing a declarative sentence, such as "Bob hit Sue," into a negative sentence, such as "Bob did not hit Sue," or into an interrogative sentence, such as "Did Bob hit Sue?" This flexibility is critical if a child is to express his meaning accurately and in socially acceptable ways.

A common misconception about children's grammatical skill is that comprehension precedes production and that, if a child is able to produce a form, he must comprehend that form or type of sentence structure. Children sometimes produce complex forms or sentence structures for which they have not mastered the grammatical rules and which they may not understand. How is this possible? There are several means or strategies by which children may produce forms that they do not understand. One of these involves storing in memory multiword units that are perceived by the child as one giant word, such as "I wanna play." Another means involves repeating or building on an utterance that was produced earlier in the conversation by the child or his conversational partner. For example, the mother may say, "Does Johnny want his ball," and the child may say, "Johnny want ball." In such cases, the child may not really appreciate the complexity of the grammatical structure he has just produced. He does not realize how all the words in his sentence can be separated and combined with other words in his vocabulary. He cannot go on to say, "I want a cookie" or "I want a ride" in addition to "I want Mom." Misjudgment of children's grammatical comprehension and expression skills is likely if a child is credited with having acquired the underlying rules for all grammatical structures contained within his utterances. To determine whether the utterances produced by a child are rule based or strategy based, a careful grammatical analysis is necessary.

Knowledge of grammatical rules can enable a child to produce and comprehend an infinite number of novel sentences. Such knowledge affords the flexibility to express one particular message in several ways, permitting switching between formal and informal styles and tailoring sentence structure to express the child's specific communicative intention. By 5 years of age, a child can comprehend and produce many complex grammatical constructions. Grammatical knowledge is expanded and refined over time through individual encounters with infrequent and complex grammatical forms as in extended narratives.

## Grammatical Disorders

Grammatical development may be delayed, in which case a child's grammatical productions would be characteristic of those produced by a younger child. Such a delay may be observed only in the grammatical system, or it may be observed across communicative systems. Alternatively, a child may display disordered grammatical development, producing forms that are not commonly observed in normal children at any age, such as saying, "The baby is cry." In this case, the child displays a more specific disorder in the development of the grammatical rule system.

The way in which grammatical development is abnormal varies from child to child. Children may fail to learn the rules for using grammatical markers such as verb tense markers (eg, regular and irregular past tense forms), pronouns (eg, first person [I] versus second person [you]), or subjective case "I" versus objective case "me." Correct production of these markers may be inconsistent or lacking. Children may develop idiosyncratic ways of using grammatical markers to indicate time, person, number, or place. For example, language-disordered children may avoid the use of past tense markers (ie, irregular forms and the use of the "-ed" suffix) by frequent use of the form "did" with the uninflected form of the verb, as in "Sue did climb" rather than "Sue climbed." Grammatical errors may involve insertion of grammatical markers or forms where they are not called for, in addition to or instead of the correct form, as in "He done went," or they may involve the deletion of markers that are needed, as in "That Mommy hat."

Children with disorders of the grammatical system may display rigid or restricted rules for expressing their ideas. They may experience difficulty in altering a learned form to make the message simpler, more complex, and more or less formal or to communicate a slightly different type of intention, such as to inquire rather than to assert. Messages may be expressed through a limited variety of sentence forms. For example, a child who wishes to discuss events in a story book may talk about those events using only a "Noun is verb + ing noun phrase" sentence structure: "The girl is looking at the boy. A boy is sitting on a tree stump. A cat is washing the kitten. The kitten is sleeping." Contrast this story with one in which more varied and complex grammatical structures are used to express the same information: "The girl looks at the boy who is sitting on a tree stump. The cat is washing the kitten as it sleeps."

Although expressive grammatical problems may be noticeable, receptive (comprehension) problems may go unnoticed by parents. However, when presented with structured comprehension tasks involving complex sentence structures, language-disordered children often resort to immature grammatical processing strategies. They fail to recognize the significance of grammatical markers for interpretation of complex sentence structures. They may be able to handle conversations with highly predictable content quite well but have difficulty with a sudden change in topic or in understanding precise instructions of the kind that are frequently given in the classroom. Their scholastic progress is often severely affected by this kind of difficulty.

Children may have difficulty in recognizing grammatical errors. For example, language-disordered children may be less able than their peers to judge which of several sentences presented to them are agrammatical. Even when they can identify a sentence as agrammatical, they may be less than 50% successful in correcting the grammatical error.

## Semantics

Semantics, the knowledge of word meanings, may be divided into lexical and relational areas. *Lexical semantics* describes a child's acquisition of the lexicon, or vocabulary, of his language. The information about a word that is stored in the lexicon resembles that of a dictionary. It includes information about the phonetic shape of the word (ie, how it is pronounced), such as consonant-vowel-consonant; the grammatical class to which it belongs (eg, noun, verb); and the primary referential meaning and any alternative multiple meanings the word may carry. *Relational semantics* describes the way words are combined to express meaningful associations. A child's knowledge of relational semantics enables him to recognize that the grammatically correct sentence "Colorless green ideas sleep furiously" is semantically anomalous. Knowledge of the meanings of the words in the sentence enables the listener to recognize that this particular combination of words does not result in a meaningful relationship between words and therefore does not convey meaning. Knowledge of how the meanings of words interact enables a listener to recognize that the sentence "Flying planes can be dangerous" has two possible meanings.

Acquisition of semantic skill is closely tied to a child's conceptual growth. Children learn words to represent what they learn about people, events, objects, and relationships. If they cannot conceptualize a phenomenon, they do not use the word or words representing that phenomenon meaningfully. However, comprehension of a concept does not guarantee that a child is able to discuss the concept or even express it. The child's linguistic skills may be disordered in such a way as to interfere with learning the words that would be used to represent the concept. Verbal portions of intelligence tests may underestimate a language-impaired child's ability. In general, impaired conceptualization abilities lead to similarly limited semantic development.

The child acquires his first lexicon and begins to express meanings verbally at about 12 to 19 months of age. The child's mental dictionary in the early stages of semantic development does not contain the same type or amount of information found in the fully developed adult lexicon. Not all words are equal candidates for inclusion. The specific words that are acquired first vary from child to child but generally represent a person, object, or event that is salient to the child or a dynamic entity that directly affects the child. The word *ball*, an object on which the child may act and which has interesting motion patterns (eg, bouncing, rolling, flying through the air) is much more likely to be acquired early on than *wall*, which is static and has less relevance for the child in everyday life.

The meaning that a child attaches to a word differs from the adult meaning of the word, usually by being more general or more restricted than adult meanings. For example, the child who refers to all round objects (eg, moon, plate, ball, wheel) as "ball" is exhibiting a general, overinclusive definition of the word. Alternatively, the child who refers only to the red ball in his bedroom as "ball," and has no label for all other balls, is exhibiting an overly restricted definition. In a short time, children revise their incorrect definitions for words, and adultlike definitions are developed. However, they cannot verbally define words if presented with a task such as "Tell me what a ball is" until they are much older.

Vocabulary growth shows rapid acceleration in the second year of life, usually from 18 to 24 months. By the time they have at least 50 words in their lexicon, children should be expressing meaningful relationships between agents, actions, and objects by relating two words in an appropriate context. Examples of relationships expressed include *identity* ("this dog"), *recurrence* ("more cookie"), *nonexistence* ("no gum"), *location* ("sit chair"), and *possession* ("Heather coat"). As the child's conceptual and linguistic skills continue to advance, he begins to express multiple meanings within one utterance and to exhibit an even greater repertoire of increasingly complex relationships. Eventually, he is able to create lengthy, sequenced narratives with meaningful plots and characters.

Comprehension of spoken words begins toward the end of the first year. Children's ideas about a word's meaning may not be stable at this time, and the child often requires situational support to comprehend words spoken to him. For example, a child may comprehend "wave bye-bye" only if the phrase is spoken during the speaker's action of leaving the room or putting on a coat. From 12 to 18 months of age, children usually demonstrate their comprehension of a word or command within certain interaction routines but not in novel situations and not by pointing to one of two pictures presented by an examiner. A child may respond to "give mommy a kiss" or "show me your nose" within the context of interactive games in which the adult and child have prescribed roles. But he may not be able to retrieve his shoes from another room on command. During this period, children's responsiveness to spoken words varies with attention, interest, familiarity, context, and number of words spoken to them.

As their notion of word meaning and how meanings relate to each other becomes more stable, children's comprehension becomes less dependent on the environmental context. Between 16 and 24 months of age, children begin to comprehend novel combinations of familiar words such as "kiss the car." Gradually, they come to understand increasingly complex relationships, such as cause and effect, time, and kinship relationships. They are able to comprehend lengthy material, such as that presented in a narrative or conversation, to extract a main theme or topic, and to make inferences based on what they have heard. The ability to understand multiple word meanings and complex semantic relations enables children to appreciate verbal humor, idioms, and figurative language.

## Semantic Disorders

Many language-disordered children have problems processing and producing certain categories of lexical items, especially those that express spatial, temporal, and kinship relations. Words that refer to concrete objects, events, or actions usually pose no particular difficulty for these children unless they have specific word-finding difficulties. Relational terms, however, require that the child keep more than one referent in mind, and this places an extra burden on processing. For example, kinship terms such as "aunt" or "uncle" may pose a challenge to language-disordered children. In most listening situations, analysis of relational terms must occur instantaneously; otherwise, comprehension of the remainder of the incoming message is impaired.

Language-disordered children often have difficulty comprehending words that have multiple meanings, especially when those meanings represent more than one grammatical category, such as "run." "Run" functions as a verb and as a noun (ie, a run in a stocking or to run a particular route). In another case, run is a verb but is used figuratively, as in "Thoughts were running through my head." The difficulty that language-disordered children have in comprehending multiple meanings and complex relations plus their tendency toward literal interpretation of language compromises their ability to comprehend verbal humor and figurative language.

Language-disordered children have difficulty in compiling an overall theme or gestalt from a lengthy spoken or written story or dialogue. These children may find it difficult to understand the sequential relationship between events in a story, and they do not understand the plot. The ability to make inferences based on stated information may be impaired. Information and the relation between certain events may have to be spelled out for these children lest they fail to recognize the intended meaning of the speaker's utterance.

Language-disordered children may exhibit difficulty in retrieving words from their lexicons. This problem is seen when a child has learned a word but finds it difficult or impossible to think of the word under the stress of trying to express himself. In an attempt to produce the "forgotten" word (eg, sock), the child may produce a word that sounds similar (eg, shock) or that is perceptually or functionally similar (eg, shoe), a synonym, or a circumlocutory phrase (eg, you put it on your foot). When a child experiences word-finding difficulties, he may produce a word or series of words that are inappropriate for the context, appear to have trouble getting to the point, repeat parts of the previous utterance, or exhibit substantial midsentence pauses.

The formulation of stories or even of a sentence may be problematic for language-disordered children. Some appear to have difficulty organizing the content of their messages at an early stage of the expressive process. The result may be a sentence that contains many revisions and many relations that do not ultimately lead to one unified idea.

## Pragmatics

In addition to learning rules for how to express meaningful relationships in an appropriate form, children must learn the pragmatic rules that govern linguistic behavior in social contexts. They must learn the following:

To express a variety of communicative intentions (eg, protesting, requesting, persuading, informing) using appropriate sentence structures

To understand and produce intentions that are expressed directly (eg, "Get me a drink") and indirectly (eg, "I'm thirsty")

To take conversational turns

To keep the conversational ball rolling and to recognize when a turn should end

To change and maintain a topic

To consider the social context (eg, place of interaction, listener's social status, familiarity with listener, language conceptual skills of conversational partner) when deciding how to express an intention (eg, polite or colloquial language)

To judge the amount and type of information needed by the communicative partner and then to find a good way to communicate the information to meet the informational need

To recognize when a communication breakdown has occurred and how to repair the breakdown

Children begin to learn the rules for the social uses of language (ie, pragmatic rules) at a very early age. The precursors to the development of pragmatic skills are acquired during infancy, before a child learns to talk. The precursors include learning to establish eye contact, to engage in vocal turntaking, to smile socially, and to use anticipatory gestures. Failure to develop these precursors may indicate a pending communication disorder.

Before 8 or 9 months of age, children's unintentional behavior (eg, crying, facial expression, body position, tension) is interpreted by adults as meaningful. At 9 to 12 months of age, children begin to communicate intentionally. Through the use of gestures and nonspecific vocalizations, they begin to request actions and objects and to show things to others or to seem to make comments on actions and objects in their environment. The types of intentions they communicate gradually increase, and they learn to express their intentions in a variety of ways. By 4 years of age, children begin to express their intentions in less direct ways. This is an important ability, because certain social contexts require the use of such polite, indirect expressions. For example, while waiting for the school principal in the office, a child may be better off requesting a drink by saying "I'm thirsty" than "Give me a drink."

In the early stages of language development, young children are rather good conversational turntakers. The topic of their utterances is determined largely by objects, people, and events that catch their attention. As a result, young children do not tend to maintain another person's topic over a number of conversational turns unless their conversational partner presents them with a series of questions that obligate responses pertinent to that partner's topic. With increasing cognitive, social, and linguistic skill, a child becomes able to maintain a topic over many conversational turns, adding new information and relating the new to old, previously discussed information.

Young children do not fully recognize that listeners may not share their perspectives or background information. They may use pronouns without establishing their referents and may omit critical information in relating an event, and their listeners must make special efforts to understand them. By 4 years of age, children begin to demonstrate the ability to consider the informational needs of their partner. For example, they use simpler sentence structure, different types of verbs, and tend to be more directive when speaking to children younger and less linguistically mature than themselves than when speaking to peers or adults. Their ability to recognize the occurrence of communication breakdown increases. When a breakdown occurs, a child must rapidly assess how and why the initial utterance failed before he can correct it. A revision strategy is employed, and changes in the original message are performed. At about 3 years of age, children's strategies for revising their utterances include repetition of the original utterance, sometimes with clearer articulation and, less frequently, substituting new words or phrases for those that may have contributed to the communication breakdown in the first place. By the third grade, children are fairly adept at identifying how an utterance must be revised to make it comprehensible to the listener, and they employ rather extensive revision strategies.

## Pragmatic Disorders

Children with communication disorders sometimes evidence a deficit in one or more pragmatic skills. For example, they may inappropriately interpret indirect expressions of communicative intention. Although the context may indicate that an utterance such as "Is your mother there?" (spoken by someone on a telephone) should be interpreted one way (eg, as a request for an action), the communicatively disordered child may interpret the utterance incorrectly (eg, as a request for information) and answer the question "yes" rather than fetching his mother.

Language-disordered children may fail to communicate their intentions effectively because of poor implementation of their semantic and grammatical skills. They may tend to resort to simple, circumscribed behaviors (gestural or verbal) to communicate their intentions. Language-learning disabled children tend to have difficulty formulating requests with the range of linguistic strategies and devices used by normal children. Language-disordered children may also fail to develop the range of communicative intentions displayed by normal children. For example, autistic children characteristically fail to display communicative intentions such as commenting and informing, displaying a reduced inventory of communicative intentions.

The ability to maintain topics and elaborate them over multiple conversational turns is often deficient in language-disordered children. Abnormal topic maintenance is seen when children exhibit limited knowledge of a topic, attention deficits, reticence, perseveration, or echolalia. A child may fail to maintain a topic because he is unable to identify the information in an utterance that pertains to the main topic and may elaborate on insignificant details of his partner's message. This produces a qualitatively unusual conversation, placing a burden on the conversational partner, who must decide whether to concede to a shift in the intended topic or redirect the child to the original topic.

Poor topic maintenance skills may be characteristic of children who have difficulty with attention, memory, or integration of information. These children may have problems relating the information presented in current utterances to that presented in previous discourse. As a result, the partner's main conversational points may be missed. The language-disordered child may have trouble inferring the underlying message of an utterance presented to him if that message has not been overtly stated. He may have difficulty recognizing the implicit bridges that relate ideas to one another. A language-disordered child may fail to follow a conversational topic and may be subject to frequent communication breakdown.

The ability to recognize and repair a communication breakdown is often impaired in language-disordered children. Repair is accomplished, if at all, in a simplistic manner, such as repetition of the original message. The actual reason for the breakdown, such as failure to establish the referent of a pronoun, failure to supply sufficient background information, indistinct articulation, production of a word combination that conveys ambiguous messages, may not be recognized by the child.

## Treatment of Language Disorders

After the determination is made about which language subsystems are affected and how they are disordered, the speech–language pathologist must decide whether treatment is indicated and what methods should be used. One aspect of the disorder may be the focus of attention, or several aspects may be treated simultaneously. The main goal of treatment may be to facilitate rule acquisition and generalization of learned skills to new contexts. Typically, language skills are taught in such a way that the child's language behavior is communicatively relevant. Target behaviors are carefully selected, and children are systematically presented with opportunities to produce them in appropriate verbal and situational contexts. Prompts are employed as needed. Depending on the nature of the language disorder and the age of the child, the primary goal in treatment may be to teach the child strategies for comprehending and producing appropriate linguistic or communicative behaviors. Although most children benefit from language remediation, many continue to manifest some degree of language impairment in academic and social situations.

## MANAGEMENT OF COMMUNICATION DISORDERS IN CHILDREN

Communication is a complex process that involves the integration of many systems (eg, cognitive, affective, social, linguistic, motor). Effective management of communication disorders is based on careful assessment. Communication disorders may change and evolve over time, and management issues must be reevaluated at different points in the child's life when the interaction of handicapping conditions and new demands in school or home produce new problems.

Medical and nonmedical aspects of the problem should be addressed. Just as the pediatrician would not delegate the responsibility for diagnosis of medical aspects of a communication problem to a nonmedically trained professional, so the nonmedical diagnoses should remain the responsibility of the communication disorders specialist. The main responsibility of the pediatrician is to be aware of early signs that communication is not developing normally and to make early referrals to a speech–language pathologist. Referral to an audiologist should be made if there is any concern about hearing. As a guideline for determining when to refer, the child's history may be examined in relation to the High-Risk Register for Deafness, which was revised by the Joint Committee on Newborn Hearing. Children with chronic middle ear problems have fluctuating hearing losses of sufficient magnitude to place them at risk for speech and language delays that may affect academic performance in later years. Current audiologic assessment methods provide accurate estimates of hearing, even in infants. Identification of any hearing loss requires prompt attention. If a child requires hearing aids, it is critical that these be supplied at the youngest possible age.

If the complaint is one of failure to develop speech and language normally, the physician may elect to carry out screening procedures in his or her office. For example, the Clinical Linguistic and Auditory Milestones Scale (CLAMS) developed by Capute and Accardo and the Early Language Milestones (ELM) scale by Coplan may be used. Children failing these tests should be referred for audiologic evaluation and for evaluation by a speech–language pathologist. Alternatively, the physician may use a simple questionnaire or set of guidelines. The following indications can be considered in infancy and early childhood for this purpose:

Excessive crying in infancy after 3 months of age; failure to quiet to a familiar voice

Reduced crying by an infant or crying that is perceived as qualitatively abnormal

Lack of eye contact and smiling after 3 months of age

Lack of vocalization in response to smiling adults from 3 to 6 months of age (eg, when adults talk to the baby and wait for a reply)

Expressions of dislike of being held

Failure to produce consonant sounds in the first year of life

Delayed appearance of cooing, laughing, expansion sounds, reduplicated babbling, and other speech production milestones

Failure to express communicative intention nonverbally by 1 year of age

Failure to respond to environmental sounds

Difficulty in localizing a sound source correctly after 9 to 12 months

Failure to respond to voices of family members or other familiar person in the second 6 months of life

Failure to respond in interactive peek-a-boo and patty-cake games by 1 year of age

Failure to indicate one or two familiar objects when these are named by the beginning of the second year

Report that a child does not understand what is said to him, "takes no notice" of what is said to him, or takes "a long time to catch on" when he is spoken to by the end of the second year

Delayed appearance of single words, of the expected rapid increase in vocabulary some time thereafter, or of multiword utterances in the second and third years.

Parents are sometimes more likely to accept referral to speech and hearing professionals than to a psychologist, especially if they fear that their child may be mentally retarded. Nevertheless, referral to a psychologist should not be delayed if it is indicated. In a secondary or tertiary care facility, children must be evaluated by a team of professionals. The team should include a psychologist, an audiologist, a speech–language pathologist, a special educator, a physical therapist, and an occupational therapist. This staff has experience in evaluating and managing handicapping conditions in young children. Collaboration among a speech–language pathologist, audiologist, and physicians is particularly important for children with hearing loss, psychiatric disorders (including attentional deficit disorder and hyperactivity), vocal pathologies, structural anomalies of the oral-facial anatomy, and central nervous system dysfunction. In many cases, speech and language disorders are not associated with any definable medical condition. A social-linguistic analysis of the disorder is useful for designing speech, language, and academic management.

A careful assessment of a child's communication abilities is needed if a parent or pediatrician is concerned about unusual or delayed patterns of communication. The assessment will provide useful data for making informed decisions about how to maximize a child's strengths and compensate for weaknesses. This can best be carried out in an atmosphere of mutual respect of the physician and the communication disorders specialist.

## Selected Readings

Aronson A. Clinical voice disorders. New York: Thieme, 1990.

ASHA. Position statement on nonspeech communication. Am Speech Hear Assoc 1981;23:577.

Blackstone S. Augmentative communication: An introduction. Rockville: American Speech-Language-Hearing Association, 1987.

Coggins T, Carpenter R. Introduction to the area of language development. In: Cohen MA, Gross PJ, eds. The developmental resource: vol 2. New York: Grune & Stratton, 1979.

Coplan J. Evaluation of the child with delayed speech or language. Pediatr Ann 1984;14:203.

Darley FL, Aronson AE, Brown JR. Motor speech disorders. Philadelphia: WB Saunders, 1975.

Gerber SE. Prevention: The etiology of communicative disorders in children. Englewood Cliffs: Simon & Schuster, 1990.

Hardy J. Cerebral palsy. Englewood Cliffs: Prentice Hall, 1983.

Healey EC. Readings on research in stuttering. New York: Longman, 1991.

Hull F, Mielke PW, Willeford JA, Timmons RJ. National speech and hearing survey.

Final report. Project No. 50978. Grant No. OE-32-15-0050-5010 (607). Washington, DC: Office of Education, DHEW, 1976.

Jung JH. Genetic syndromes in communication disorders. Boston: Little, Brown, 1989.

Kent RD. Anatomical and neuromuscular maturation of the speech mechanism: Evidence from acoustic studies. J Speech Hear Res 1976;19:421.

Lahey M. Language disorders and language development. New York: Macmillan, 1988.

Love RJ. Childhood motor speech disability. New York: Macmillan, 1992.

McCarthy J. Early Intervention and school Programs for preschool handicapped children. In: Sell E, ed. Follow-up of the high risk newborn: A practical approach. Springfield, IL: Charles C. Thomas, 1980.

Netsell R, Lotz WK, Barlow SM. A speech physiology examination for individuals with dysarthria. In: Yorkston KM, Beukelman DR, eds. Recent advances in clinical dysarthria. Boston: Little, Brown, 1989:3–37.

Northern JC, Downs MP. Hearing in children, ed 2. Baltimore: Williams & Wilkins, 1978.

Peterson-Falzone SJ. Resonance disorders in structural defects. In: Lass NJ, McReynolds LV, Northern JL, Yoder DE, eds. Speech, language, and hearing, vol II. Pathologies of speech and language. Philadelphia: WB Saunders, 1982.

Rapin I, Mattis S, Rowan AJ. Verbal auditory agnosia in children. Dev Med Child Neurol 1977;19:197.

Speech and language development. Pediatr Ann 1985;14 (whole issue).

Stark RE. Stages of speech development in the first year of life. In: Yeni-Komshian GH, Ferguson CA, Kavanagh J, eds. Child phonology: Production, vol I. New York: Academic Press, 1980.

Rossetti L. High-risk infants: Identification, assessment, and intervention. Boston: Little, Brown, 1989.

Soboloff H. Developmental enrichment programs. Dev Med Child Neurol 1979;21:423.

Thompson CK. Articulation disorders in the child with neurogenic pathology. In: Lass NJ, McReynolds LV, Northern JL, Yoder DE, eds. Handbook of speech-language pathology and audiology. Toronto: BC Decker, 1988:548–591.

Yorkston KM, Beukelman DR, Bell KR. Clinical management of dysarthric speakers. Boston: Little, Brown, 1986.

*Principles and Practice of Pediatrics, Second Edition.* edited by Frank A. Oski et al. J. B. Lippincott Company, Philadelphia © 1994.

# CHAPTER 29
# *The Interface of Pediatrics with Psychiatry*

## *29.1 The Biopsychosocial Approach*

James C. Harris

When the parents and child come to the pediatrician, it is because they are concerned. Their "dis-ease" and disquietude must be appreciated as symptoms are elicited and signs are understood, so that a sense of confidence can be established. This then allows the parents confidently to carry out the recommendations made for the child's care and treatment. The approach to the patient

is developmental and biopsychosocial in nature (Engel, 1977). It is an interactional approach rather than an exclusively reductionist, biomedical one; it addresses current symptoms and physiologic changes, the meaning of the illness to both child and family, their current psychological state, their history of adaptation to past illnesses, the family genetic background, and their understanding of this particular illness.

To develop an appreciation for this approach, developmental models and the interaction of brain and behavior are reviewed in this chapter, followed by discussion of the stress response, resilience to stress, coping with stress, bereavement, and stress-related disorders. Finally, the epidemiology, assessment, diagnosis, and treatment of emotional, behavioral, and interpersonal conditions in childhood are reviewed from a biopsychosocial perspective. These include adjustment disorders, post-traumatic stress disorders, conduct disorder, oppositional defiant disorder, emotional disorders (phobic anxiety, separation anxiety, social anxiety, overanxious disorder), obsessive-compulsive disorder, depression, suicide, eating disorders (anorexia nervosa), pervasive developmental disorders, psychosis, and sleep disorders.

From a more personal developmental perspective, the child is viewed as active and fully engaged in life, using his or her individual genetic and temperamental endowment to master developmental tasks in relation to family, peers, and community, even when the child and the family are faced with illness. Psychological factors may assume importance in altering individual susceptibility to disease and recovery from illness.

In the psychiatric classification, the diagnosis "mental disorders due to general medical condition" is used when psychologically meaningful events relate to the initiation or exacerbation of a specific clinical condition. Considering children's behavior more generally, it may be quantitatively different from normal when developmentally appropriate symptoms persist, as in separation anxiety disorder, or qualitatively different from the average child's adaptation, as in major depression; both of these perspectives are addressed. The description of mental disorders used here is drawn from the *ICD-10 Classification of Mental and Behavioral Disorders: Clinical Descriptions and Diagnostic Guidelines* and the DSM-IV. The diagnoses are compatible in both systems, although DSM-IV maintains the numerical coding system of DSM-III-R. For specific, operationalized diagnostic criteria, DSM-IV should be consulted. For research purposes DSM-IV and the ICD-10 *Diagnostic Criteria for Research* should be considered.

## Selected Readings

Diagnostic and statistical manual of mental disorders, ed 4. Washington DC: American Psychiatric Association, 1993.

Engel GL. The need for a new medical model: a challenge for biomedicine. Science 1977;196:129.

Engel GL. Physician scientists and scientific physicians. Am J Med 1987;82:107.

Green WH. Child and adolescent psychopharmacology. Baltimore: Williams & Wilkins, 1991.

ICD-10 classification of mental and behavioral disorders: clinical descriptions and diagnostic guidelines. Geneva: World Health Organization: 1992.

Lewis M, ed. Child and adolescent psychiatry: a comprehensive textbook. Baltimore: Williams & Wilkins, 1991.

Rutter M. Child psychiatric disorders in ICD-10. J Child Psychol Psychiatry 1989;30:499.

Schab-Stone M, Towbin KE, Tarnoff MD. Systems of classification: ICD-10, DSM-III-R, and DSM-IV. In Lewis M, ed. Child and adolescent psychiatry: a comprehensive textbook. Baltimore: Williams & Wilkins, 1991.

Schetky D, Benedek E. Clinical handbook of psychiatry and the law. Baltimore: Williams & Wilkins, 1992.

Wiener J, ed. Textbook of child and adolescent psychiatry. Washington DC: American Psychiatric Press, 1991.

*Principles and Practice of Pediatrics, Second Edition.*
edited by Frank A. Oski et al. J. B. Lippincott Company, Philadelphia © 1994.

# 29.2 *Developmental Perspective*

## James C. Harris

The developmental perspective is basic to pediatrics. It emphasizes the capacity for change throughout life, an approach now referred to as the lifespan view of human development. The child is seen as an active, socially oriented, and developing person, rather than as either a passive respondent to the environment or an individual developing independently of the environment, with social experiences having only a limited impact. Development occurs in phases of progressive change as the individual child masters new development tasks. Early experiences are important in this process, but the child has a remarkable resilience to stress and as new abilities emerge the child often compensates for past difficulties.

*Growth* refers to changes in the size of the body as a whole, and *development* addresses the differentiation of form (ie, changes in function shaped by interaction with the external environment). Development is an interactive process and refers, particularly in psychiatry, to emotional and social development. The opportunity to develop one's full biological and psychological potential is a result of many interacting factors. Genetic factors are important in establishing the limits of potential, but they are interwoven with environmental experience. Physical trauma, particularly brain injury, affects growth, development, and behavior, and nutritional factors are important as well.

A developmental perspective has the following characteristics. It addresses changing contexts and patterns of behavior over time rather than behavioral stability. It recognizes that younger children have considerable developmental plasticity in the nervous system, but that with the pruning of neuronal synapses that occurs with maturation, the brain's capacity to adapt to injury becomes more circumscribed. It acknowledges discontinuity in development as well as connectedness and the persistence of temperamental traits over time. It asks why certain behaviors are present at one age and not another. It appreciates that there are vulnerabilities to some social experiences, but that as these experiences are mastered, they may be strengthening. It appreciates that stressors may have a different impact at one age than at another. It addresses the appearance of certain emotional and behavioral disorders that present first at one age but not at another. It suggests an opportunity for prevention by offering interventions within the developmental period. Finally, it studies how approaches to the interview, diagnosis, and treatment may be better informed by an appreciation of developmental processes, experience, and task mastery.

A developmental perspective is also applied to the study of major mental disorders when they occur during the developmental period. Through the study of developmental psychopathology, the natural history of a major mental illness is studied as it is manifested at different ages and influences developmental tasks.

From a developmental perspective, the pediatrician addresses all of the following: the full spectrum of behavior from the molecular level, as seen in enzyme activation in the course of differentiation; the interaction of metabolic and physical changes associated with the development of neurotransmitter and hormonal systems; the development of cognition, intelligence, and the emotions; and individual, reciprocal social relationships with family, peers, and community. The last category includes the quality of the interaction of the infant and child with parents, siblings, and others, the child's role in the family system, specific concerns for the child by the parents, and the type of child-rearing practices carried out. Child-rearing is influenced by the cultural and personal experiences of the parents.

## MATURATION OF THE BRAIN

The growth of the brain, in contrast to other organ systems, occurs primarily in the infant and toddler years. By 6 months of age the brain has reached half of its mature weight, and by 5 years, 90% of its adult weight. The rapid growth of the brain in contrast to the rest of the body has important implications from the developmental perspective. This rapid development has been linked to a maturational view of development that argues that abilities are little influenced by experience and that they gradually unfold as long as two primary conditions are met: adequate nutrition and an opportunity to interact in a normal, expected environment. Gesell argued that physical maturation occurs in an orderly sequence if there is not deprivation. One internal factor that apparently plays a part in brain growth is rapid eye movement sleep. Studies of infant sleep suggest that developmental changes in infancy do not indicate a unitary process but a change in the brain organization, or rather reorganization of the whole structure.

Some parts of the brain mature earlier than others; for example, the brain stem and limbic system mature before the cerebellum and higher cortical areas. Hearing and seeing are present early, but interpretation and understanding of what is heard takes place later. An understanding of the usual sequences of development is relevant in children with developmental delays, but there is considerable variability in development; for example, some children do not speak until age 3 or 4, suggesting a potential developmental delay. Delays are more common in boys than girls, suggesting gender differences in brain development. The association of developmental delay with maturation is hypothetical, and much more needs to be learned. However, in mental retardation the lack of maturation or interference with brain development is an important hypothesis.

The extent of brain growth determines the impact of specific training. This idea has been investigated through monozygotic twin studies in which one twin was given early training and the other was not; there was no difference in the twins' skills, demonstrating that the early training did not generally enhance skills. There are marked individual differences in brain development, so although there are average ages for maturational events, it is more appropriate to consider a range over months when development will occur (for instance, walking at 10 to 18 months).

Developing parts of the brain are more susceptible to damage from injury, infection, toxins, or malnutrition at times of their most rapid growth. However, the young brain is also more capable of adapting to damage, so that the practical consequences of damage may be less. This is probably because brain functions are not localized but instead involve connections that are present throughout the brain and involve multiple brain regions, as demonstrated by 2-deoxyglucose positron emission tomographic brain scan studies. Damage to regions vital to function in the adult (eg, the speech area in the left hemisphere) may be compensated for in the young child by the other hemisphere. Recovery in young children may be more complete than expected because of this neuronal plasticity.

## ENVIRONMENTAL INTERFACE

Development is not only a gradual unfolding, but a process in which experience plays an important role, and learning requires both brain growth and stimulation. The timing of development is not entirely genetically controlled, but external environmental stimulation may be needed to initiate it. The term *plasticity* is used to signify the fact that the organism can be modified by the environment. When behavior in response to a stimulus is measured, plasticity is being measured. For example, if infant kittens are raised with one eyelid sutured closed, vision is impaired in that eye; however, the loss is partially functional, and plasticity is demonstrated, because vision can be substantially restored by $\gamma$-amino butyric acid (GABA) agonists after the sutures are removed.

The chemistry of brain development is affected by deprivation, and in adults the lack of use of an extremity leads to some muscle wasting. Lack of stimulation may retard growth, but extra stimulation does not enhance it if adequate maturation has not occurred. Stimulation may influence particular behaviors as well; for example, babbling in infants is influenced by parents' talking to them and by accommodating the prosody or rhythm of their voice to that of the infant. Children who receive specific language training in a day-care center have enhanced abilities compared with those who are involved in free play. Stress may interfere with development, as demonstrated by the persistence of enuresis in children with severe burns and the return to bed-wetting in children who have been stressed.

## DEVELOPMENTAL TASKS

The development of the person, the personality, has been the focus of developmental theorists. Theoretic perspectives have addressed psychosexual development, cognitive development, the development of interpersonal relations, and identity. Psychotherapies have been suggested based on these approaches.

More recently, an emphasis has been placed on an ethological model of development that addresses behavior in reference to our biological background, patterns of behavior across species that serve the same purpose, the natural selection of behavioral traits, and behavior that is biologically based, such as infant attachment. Each of these frameworks for development makes assumptions about the capabilities of the infant and young child in regard to recognition and remembering of past experience, temperamental characteristics, and response to environmental uncertainty. Each of these perspectives suggests an emphasis on socially important features or goals; for instance, self-control, moral development, compassionate interpersonal behavior, and self-awareness are ideal goals. These goals are studied and represent developmental tasks to be mastered at different ages.

The child is an active person who has a series of developmental tasks to master through melding genetic and temperamental attributes with psychosocial support. For example, infants are actively involved, capable of interaction, and have individual responses. By their behavior they influence what goes on around them and what happens to them; parents respond to their preferences. This is in contrast to an older view that depicted the infant as passive, without individuality, and at the mercy of the environment. The parent–child interaction is one of social reciprocity as the parents adapt to the child in their individual personality, past experience with children, and family background. This interaction is particularly important to understand in the parents' response to a handicapped or premature child.

## DEVELOPMENTAL MODELS OF BEHAVIORAL AND EMOTIONAL DEVELOPMENT

To understand the complex interaction between children and the biological and environmental influences on them, the child's development can be approached from several perspectives. We will give an overview of each of these perspectives, emphasizing biological endowment, interpersonal experience, or environmental influences. The focus on biological endowment is emphasized through the maturational, ethological, and sociobiological approaches. The emphasis on the individual's interpersonal experience in mastering the environment is emphasized in the psychodynamic and systems theory approaches, whereas the emphasis on the environment as shaping the person is emphasized in behaviorism. References that offer a more detailed view of each approach are provided in the list of selected readings.

### Maturational Model

According to the maturational view, popularized by Gesell, development occurs through orderly, nonrandom, patterned sequences determined by our biological and evolutionary history. The rate of development, however, is influenced by the individual genetic family history. Although it may be altered by such things as illness, malnutrition, or stressful experiences, fundamental biological factors direct development. A favorable environment facilitates; an unfavorable one inhibits. Neither circumstance changes the basic biological potential. Gesell sought to describe the form of morphologic or structural growth and psychological growth. He argued that development has direction (eg, cephalocaudal and proximodistal); is organized through reciprocal relationships or interweavings (eg, flexors and extensors develop in a sequence that allows coordinated movement); and may demonstrate functional asymmetry or an unbalanced development that occurs to achieve mastery at a later stage of development (eg, development of "handedness").

In its basic form, development is not changed by the environment, suggesting that environmental influence is limited in this area. Finally, there is a self-regulatory fluctuation of development, with periods of instability followed by stability and consolidation, and cycles of development, with equilibrium following disequilibrium. Using this approach Gesell emphasized four areas of development: motor, adaptive, language, and personal/social.

Development is controlled by biologically predetermined patterns that are nonvarying, although the rate may vary from one child to another. Gesell's investigations focused on normal children from an average, expectable environment. In terms of motor development and individual differences in rate of growth and in personality pattern, his investigations have been often replicated. They show that pushing children excessively during the developmental period is futile, and they led to the concept of the child's "readiness" for intervention.

The normal expectable environment is active and stimulating. Gesell emphasized internal regulation, used age as a marker, provided guidelines for developmental level, noted the sensitivity of responsiveness at certain times in development, observed discontinuity in development, appreciated individual differences, and appreciated the impact of the environment as amplifying or reducing behavioral effects. His methods and the data-based approach he used continue to be models in approaching behavioral study.

## Ethological Model

The ethological view addresses the roots and mechanisms of behavior in both humans and animals. It addresses classes of behavior that are biologically based: reflexes, taxes, and fixed action patterns. Behaviors that are innate occur without learning (ie, without practicing) and are species-typical behaviors, such as imprinting in birds. A primitive reflex, like the tonic neck reflex, is an example in the infant. At least 25 such reflexes have been identified in the neonate, including the walking reflex.

The taxes are locomotor or orienting responses and include cuddling and other actions involving more than one reflex. The fixed action pattern is a sequence of coordinated motor actions. They are made up of innate releasing mechanisms associated with a signed stimulus; for instance, the mother leaves the room and that departure is associated with infant crying. The departure is a signed stimulus leading to an innate releasing mechanism followed by a fixed action pattern. Another example is the infantile appearance with large head, bulging cheeks, and large eyes, which acts as a signed stimulus for care-eliciting behavior toward the infant. Many parenting behaviors may have an ethological origin.

The ethologist develops an ethogram from the study of various categories of behavior as they are observed in their natural setting to establish links between behaviors. Bowlby, using the ethological approach in the study of infant attachment, has found four separate phases of attachment:

1. Pre-attachment, demonstrated by orienting behavior toward caregivers (eg, early following with the eyes, smiling, and vocalization)
2. Attachment in the making, as the parent responds to the infant's initiative
3. Clear-cut attachment, as the toddler walks away and then returns to the caregiver
4. Goal-corrected partnership.

This last phase occurs at the beginning of the third year of life, as the child begins to understand the adult's behavior and can take the parent's needs into account. The goal of attachment is to anticipate and increase physical proximity with the mother and to gain nurturance. As a consequence of these early experiences, a child increasingly develops internal working models of relationships. This approach includes an appreciation of genetic and environmental factors.

## Sociobiological Model

The sociobiological approach, unlike the ethological approach, places more emphasis on all aspects of development as related to and controlled by specific genes and gives less importance to the environment. Rather than potentials, the focus is on biological and psychological determinism. Sociobiology has been defined by Wilson, its prime proponent, as the "systematic study of the biological basis of all social behavior." Successful reproduction is emphasized. The theme of sacrifice or altruism is demonstrated in parents of all species in their efforts to preserve the next generation.

Sociobiologists posit several causes for the demonstration of social behavior. One cause is phylogenetic inertia, defined as the organism's tendency to remain unchanged under ecological pressures. Change is greatest if there is genetic variability in the species. An opportunity to increase the gene pool decreases phylogenetic inertia because as new material is introduced, the likelihood of change increases.

Antisocial factors that encourage individuals in that species to isolate themselves are also important considerations. Inbreeding of species increases recessive traits and minimizes genetic variability. Another important factor is complexity of behavior, which suggests that complex behaviors such as parenting would have higher phylogenetic inertia. The effect of change in behavior on other traits and characteristics is considered, in that the degree to which a change in one system affects another is related to the degree of phylogenetic inertia.

Ecological pressure represents that part of the environment that encourages the organism to change. This is the nurture side of the nature–nurture equation. The threat of predation is another aspect of ecological pressure in animals to adapt; for instance, ultrasonic separation calls in rodents protect them from predators and maintain social contact. Another pressure is the availability of food, leading to nomadic movement and increased demands to adapt in new environments. Wilson notes that "manipulation of the physical environment is the ultimate adaptation"; therefore, tool use is important in human adaptation.

Demographic characteristics, gene flow, and genetic similarity are important factors in sociobiology. Birth rates, death rates, and population size have important effects on behavior. For example, Calhoun has demonstrated that overcrowding in rats leads to an increase in aberrant social behaviors, increased death rates, and greater susceptibility to disease and stress. Gene flow results from interbreeding with other populations and introduces new genes into that population. Change is faster if new genes enter the population; however, the more genetic similarity in a population, the greater the stability of behavior and the more likely that genetically adaptive behaviors will be maintained. However, inbreeding may increase the risk of maintaining maladaptive traits in the community.

Sociobiologists argue that similar behaviors in humans and animals are genetically related. Research in this area that is pertinent to behavior may be relevant to parenting. An example is the separation cry, which has a similar sonographic frequency in various species of mammals and is a potential model for studies of separation anxiety in children.

## Sociocultural Model

The sociocultural approach emphasizes the importance of cultural transmission rather than genetic transmission for cognitive development. The major proponent of this approach is Lev Vygotsky, who focused on an interactional view of cognitive development and maintained that higher mental functions (cognitive processes) initially are experienced through interpersonal interaction and subsequently intrapsychically. The establishment of concrete logic is preceded by the internalization of representational language. Vygotsky emphasized the role of inner speech as a means of problem-solving. He discussed the interface of thought and language and emphasized how language originates and is established through social contact. For instance, a child loses a toy. His mother helps him mentally retrace his activities that day until he becomes aware of its location. Subsequently the child may use inner language to remember without relying on an adult.

Vygotsky referred to the distance between the actual developmental level, as determined by independent problem-solving, and the level of potential development, as determined through problem-solving under adult guidance or in collaboration with more capable peers as the zone of proximal development (Vygotsky, 1978). Self-talk becomes established in the zone of proximal development as an important process in cognitive development and as a means of self-monitoring and self-control. Both cognitive and interpersonal growth occur in the zone of proximal development. Vygotsky's approach has attracted more interest as developmental psychologists begin to study higher cortical functions, particularly regarding perspective taking and social cognition.

## Psychodynamic Model

The psychodynamic approach includes psychoanalysis, which was one of the first attempts to offer a systematic theory of development. Using energy models prevalent at the time, Sigmund Freud, the founder of psychoanalysis, described a hypothetic psychic energy, the libido, that was conserved in a closed biological system and was distributed to various psychological functions. His psychoanalytic theory addresses unconscious factors that influence development and includes this dynamic component, a structural system, and a series of progressive psychological stages. Originally based on studies of conversion symptoms that occurred without a demonstrable organic disorder, the distribution of this energy was said to depend on the organism's stage of development, experiential history, and current life setting. The primary source of psychic energy was initially suggested to be instinctually expressed through unlearned psychological drives whose tension was gratified through the infant's or child's behavior. Instincts were seen as psychological representations of biological processes. The bulk of psychic energy is unconscious in infants and is expressed in seeking pleasure and personal gratification. However, crying and increased motor activity serve to bring the infant into contact with the external world.

The most powerful of the unconscious instinctual drives are hunger, the sex drive, and the aggressive drive. For example, the hunger drive results in tension, which leads to crying, which is relieved by a parent. The child becomes gradually aware of the relationship to the parent and by adapting to these responses develops psychological structures to mediate future behavior. These psychological structures are described by Freud in his structural system under the hypothetical constructs of id, ego, and superego. The energy derived from original biological impulses is referred to as *id energy*, and its goal is to obtain instinctual gratification. Part of this id energy is adapted and transformed as conscious associations are made to psychosocial experiences. This complex of conscious associations is referred to as the *ego*. The ego facilitates adaptation by mediating new conscious behavior, and through the process of identification begins to discriminate a separate "self" and to obtain pleasure through adaptation to external reality. The third element, the *superego*, emerges as further psychic energy is transformed into conscious-

ness when the child becomes aware of and incorporates the parents' ethical standards. This ego ideal or conscience serves to modulate behavior in relation to parental standards, but it may conflict with the demands of the ego and superego.

The dynamic and structural components interact by a set of defense mechanisms to minimize experienced anxiety. These mechanisms distort reality in the face of potential danger that might threaten ego functioning. They are designed to alleviate the conflicts or stressors that give rise to the anxiety signal. They may be adaptive or maladaptive, depending on the context in which they occur. The most common defense mechanisms are denial, displacement, dissociation, idealization, intellectualization, isolation, passive-aggression, rejection, rationalization, reaction formation, repression, somatization, autistic fantasy, acting out, suppression, splitting, and undoing. Defense mechanisms aid in restructuring the personality as the child experiments with new experiences. They enable psychic energy to remain directed toward a goal rather than being expressed as excessive anxiety. With development, the ego acts as a more effective mediator in modulating anxiety, thereby reducing the need for defense mechanisms in dealing with reality.

## Psychosocial Model

The psychosocial perspective originated with Erik Erikson, who suggested that psychological development is the result of an interaction between maturational forces and social forces. This approach emphasizes socialization throughout the lifespan. Erikson suggested a series of eight stages of development that focus on the task of identity formation. In each stage a developmental crisis requires resolution, and so the importance of the ego is highlighted. Because Erikson said that an immature ego is present at birth, he is referred to as an ego psychologist. Erikson introduced the principle of epigenesis, based on an embryologic model with each psychosocial stage emerging from the previous one.

At each stage of development a different conflict has particular significance for the individual. These conflicts are expressed as polarities representing opposite tendencies that, when resolved, lead to a particular virtue. The first five stages deal with the tasks of children and adolescents, the next two address tasks of parents, and the final stages address tasks for older parents and grandparents. These are expressed as developmental tasks and are indicated most clearly as questions asked by the adolescent. Still, it is earlier experience that prepares the adolescent to ask these questions. The identity conflicts at each stage are as follows:

*Stage 1:* The polarity between trust and mistrust is experienced during the first year of life. If it is resolved with a predominance of trust, the outcome is hope. The question that must be answered is, can I trust?

*Stage 2:* The polarity between autonomy and shame or doubt is experienced in the second and third years of life. Resolution leads to confidence and a sense of self-control. The question that must be answered is, can I be free of self-doubt?

*Stage 3:* The polarity between initiative and guilt is introduced at 4 to 5 years of age, when the child is internalizing adult roles and standards. The resolution of the conflict leads to a sense of purposefulness. The question that must be answered is, can I act independently?

*Stage 4:* The polarity is between industry and inferiority, and its resolution leads to a sense of competence. This conflict presents itself between ages 6 and 11 years. The question that must be answered is, can I be successful in carrying out my goals?

*Stage 5:* The polarity relates to establishing a sense of identity and clarifying confusion of roles between ages 12 and 18 years. The questions that are asked are, who am I, what do I believe in, how do I feel about others, and what are my attitudes about myself? Successful resolution leads to fidelity or faithfulness, allegiance, and loyalty toward one's own beliefs.

*Stage 6:* With the establishment of fidelity, the young adult is prepared to consider marrying and starting a family. In this stage the polarity is between intimacy and isolation, and the resolution of this conflict is the experience of love in interpersonal relationships. The question that must be answered is, can I be intimate with another person?

*Stage 7:* Following the establishment of intimacy, the next stage presents the polarity between generativity and self-absorption. The resolution of this conflict is the ability to provide loving care to one's own children. The question that must be answered is, can I give of myself to the care of my children?

*Stage 8:* The final stage in the life cycle addresses the polarity of integrity and despair. It is the task of old age to reflect on having established contentment and satisfaction in one's life. That satisfactory outcome is wisdom. The question the older person asks is, have I found contentment and direction in my life?

Erikson's major contribution has been to stress the importance of the development of a strong ego identity. His formulations are widely used in medicine, psychology, and education.

## Behavioral Model

The behavioral perspective studies only observable behaviors; its theoretic framework emphasizes environmental factors in developmental outcome. The behaviorist suggests that development is a function of learning, that development is the consequence of different kinds of learning, that differences in individual development are the result of past experiences, that development is the result of the organization of current behavioral patterns, that general limits on behavior come from biological limitations but environmental factors determine the choice of behavior, and that the individual's behavior is not a direct consequence of biological stages. The behaviorist suggests that the behavior is neither biologically determined nor the result of internal biological processes.

Behaviorists emphasize classical conditioning and study conditioned reflexes (that is, the reinforcement and extinction of these conditioned responses). Having analyzed behavior, they study generalization of behavior by investigating factors in reinforcement. In the behavioral approach, learning is governed by the response to environmental stimuli, which are strengthened or weakened by environmental reinforcement. Behaviorists investigate how stimuli are discriminated. They assume that behavior is the function of its consequences; in particular, they study a type of learning called *operant conditioning*. Operant behaviors are controlled by their consequences and not what precedes them. The emphasis is on the behavior that is emitted and not on the preceding behavior. Factors that affect behavior are studied in terms of positive and negative reinforcers and punishment. Investigations of schedules of reinforcement that are broadly continuous or intermittent are used in behavioral analysis. Techniques of treatment include chaining and shaping of behavior and attempts to generalize behavior to appropriate environmental settings. A functional behavioral analysis should be completed and behavioral enhancement procedures should be emphasized in treatment.

## Selected Readings

Ainsworth MD. The development of mother-infant attachment. In: Caldwell B, Riccuiti N, eds. Review of child development research, vol 3. Chicago: University of Chicago Press, 1973.

Bowlby J. Attachment and loss. III. Loss, sadness and depression. New York: Basic Books, 1980.

Brenner C. An elementary textbook of psychoanalysis. New York: Doubleday, 1974.

Dare C. Psychoanalytic theories of development. In: Rutter M, Hersov L, eds. Child and adolescent psychiatry: modern approaches, ed 2. Oxford: Blackwell Scientific Publications, 1985:204.

Erikson EH. Identity and the life cycle. Psychological Issues 1959;1:1.

Gesell A, Amatuda CS. Developmental diagnosis. New York: Holber, 1947.

Rakic P. Development of the primate cerebral cortex. In: Lewis M, ed. Child and adolescent psychiatry: a comprehensive textbook. Baltimore: Williams & Wilkins, 1991.

Ross AO, Nelson RO. Behavior therapy. In: Quay HC, Werry JC, eds. Psychopathological disorders of childhood, ed 2. New York: John Wiley & Sons, 1979:303.

Rutter M. Child development. In: Rutter M, ed. Helping troubled children. New York: Penguin, 1975:54.

Salkind NJ. Theories of human development, ed 2. New York: John Wiley & Sons, 1985.

Smith P, Cowie H. Understanding children's development. Oxford: Basil Blackwell, 1991.

Vygotsky LS. Mind in society: the development of higher psychological processes. Cambridge. MA: Harvard University Press, 1978.

Wilson EO. Sociobiology: the new synthesis. Boston: Harvard University Press, 1975.

*Principles and Practice of Pediatrics, Second Edition.*
edited by Frank A. Oski et al. J. B. Lippincott Company, Philadelphia © 1994.

# 29.3 *Psychosocial Interview*

James C. Harris

After establishing demographic and other background information and determining the reliability of the informant, the pediatrician asks the parents about their specific concerns. The reason for referral is elicited, as well as the statement about the onset of the current difficulties and the family's life situation. Precipitating stressful events that may contribute to the behavioral difficulty are reviewed, and specific concerns are addressed; these include academic and school problems, antisocial behavior, emotional conflict, regressive behavior, and interpersonal difficulty. Previous treatment is reviewed, and the effects of the child's current behavior on family function are clarified. These questions are followed by asking the child and parents why they are seeking help at this time.

The family history is then reviewed, clarifying the child's status in regard to foster care, adoption, stepparenting, or other family issues. Questions include who has custody, who the child resembles in personality, and who the child is named after.

The family background of both parents is taken, including their own childhood, with particular emphasis on the family atmosphere in the parents' childhoods, stresses from emotional or economic cause, deaths, or separation from close relatives. Information on the grandparents and others closely affiliated with the child is gathered, along with a developmental family history of how the marriage evolved. The quality of relatedness in the current marriage, including frequency of disagreements and how they are expressed, coping mechanisms dealing with conflict in the family, and the relationship with the family of origin, is also covered. Siblings are described by age, school placement, history of significant illness, personality, and relationship with family members.

A history of familial diseases should include alcoholism, abnormal personality, suicide, homicide, manic-depressive disorder, and schizophrenia. When reviewing past and personal history, one should note the date and place of birth, birth weight, attitude of both parents toward the pregnancy, and whether it was planned or unplanned. If there were difficulties with the pregnancy or delivery, the psychological response by the parents to that event should be included.

Developmental milestones should emphasize social milestones, including eye contact, social smile, language communication, and interpersonal attachment. The quality of the parent–child (dyadic) relationship and the child–mother–father (triadic) relationship requires review. The interpersonal issues that relate to feeding and illness must be considered. The parents' attitudes toward child-rearing, particularly in regard to permissiveness and limit-setting, are assessed.

A behavioral review of symptoms, including information on temperament, early development, emotional responsiveness, antisocial behavior, attentional difficulties, self-stimulation, and play behavior, is obtained. Assessment of school includes the age of beginning school, the current grade, schools attended, type of class placement, and emotional adjustment to beginning school. Separation problems in initiating either preschool or school are reviewed. If there were prolonged absences from school or school years were repeated, this information, along with specific difficulties in reading, writing, spelling, and mathematics, is noted. Study habits and academic goals are reviewed, and the child's peer relationships are assessed. Whether the child is teased or is a bully is determined, and particular friendships are assessed. Attitudes toward teachers, peers, and schoolwork are also obtained.

Assessment is made of the child's awareness of sexual identity, which includes questions on curiosity about his or her own body and about reproduction, as well as sexual interests and activities.

For the adolescent, the interview includes information regarding the mastery of adolescent developmental tasks and the young person's attitude regarding entry into adolescence. One looks for mature versus pseudomature behavior and attitudes toward peers, family, and authority. Rebelliousness, drug-taking, periods of depression or withdrawal, and fantasy life are reviewed. How the young person has responded to puberty with its accompanying changes in body image (voice changes, hair growth, breast development, menarche) and masturbation and sexual concerns are assessed.

Previous mental health history is gathered, including details of disturbances for which treatment was received and how the treatment was done. This is followed by a description of life situation at present, which includes current housing, social situation, parents' work, and financial circumstances. The composition of the household, relationship with neighbors, recent stresses, bereavement, losses or disappointments, and how both parent and child have reacted to them are reviewed. A typical day in the child's life is described, which includes getting to school, activities during the school day, return home, and evening activities.

The physician should consider personality features that are pertinent to this particular child. These include habitual attitudes and patterns of behavior that distinguish him or her as an individual. Among personality characteristics are attitudes toward others, including the ability to trust others and to make and sustain relationships with them. Whether the child is secure or insecure in interpersonal relationships, a leader or a follower, is established. The attitude toward interpersonal relationships, whether it is friendly, warm, and demonstrative or reserved, cold, or indifferent, is considered. Other characteristics regarding aggressiveness, quarrelsomeness, sensitivity, and suspiciousness are noted. One also considers attitudes toward the self, including self-dramatizing behavior, egocentric behavior, self-consciousness, and ambition. Attitudes of the child toward his or her own health and bodily functions are included in the assessment of whether the child's self-appraisal is realistic or unrealistic.

An assessment of the personality also includes moral and religious attitudes and an assessment of whether the individual is easygoing, permissive, overconscientious, perfectionistic, or conforming. Mood is considered in regard to lability and whether the child is optimistic or pessimistic. Clarification about anxiety, irritability, excessive worrying, and apathy are noted. The ability to express and control feelings of anger, sadness, pleasure, and disappointment is reviewed.

Leisure activities and interests, including interest in books, pictures, music, sports, and creative activities, are noted. How the individual spends leisure time, either alone or with others, is assessed.

Finally, the physician asks about daydreams, nightmares, and reaction patterns to stress. This involves the ability to tolerate frustration, loss, and disappointment, and it includes a description of circumstances that arouse anger or anxiety and depression, and evidence of excessive use of particular psychological defenses, such as denial, rationalization, and projection.

## INTERVIEW WITH THE PARENT REGARDING ADJUSTMENT TO THE CHILD'S ILLNESS

The interview with the parent or parents should establish a sense of confidence in them in regard to carrying out medical and monitoring procedures and an acknowledgment of the nature of the child's illness. An effective interview facilitates appropriate care. Because the parent is an active participant in the child's care, it is essential to establish rapport with him or her and to remember that the parent is reassured not only by what is said, but also by *how* it is said. The parent is stressed by the child's illness and needs support.

To understand the parent's adaptation to illness, the psychological mechanisms normally present in a time of stress must be appreciated. The most common are denial, guilt or self-blame, projection or blaming others, and dependency by the parent on the caregiver or others. Self-awareness by the physician is critical in understanding the parent's adaptation. To determine the degree of the parent's acknowledgment of stress, the following questions are suggested:

1. *Whom do you talk to when you are concerned about your child?* This question helps establish the degree to which the parent is isolated and whether there is a confiding relationship with another person. It also helps to clarify if the parent is denying the seriousness of the child's illness, thereby putting the child at risk.
2. *Who or what do you feel is responsible for causing your child's illness?* This question asks about excessive guilt and self-blame. The self-blaming parent is at risk for developing symptoms of depression.
3. *Do you feel that the staff taking care of your child can be trusted?* This question deals with projection and excessive suspiciousness. Parents commonly criticize caregivers as an expression of their projected fear and anxiety.
4. *Do you feel adequate to take care of the child yourself, or do you automatically follow directions from others or feel increasingly dependent?* This question deals with dependency and passivity, which may be present in the overwhelmed parent. When this occurs, the physician experiences a sense of helplessness in the parent, often receives frequent telephone calls, and may be asked to make decisions unrelated to the child's medical care.

Difficulties in dealing with stress may relate to unresolved feelings that may be out of the parent's conscious awareness. To be effective in counseling, it is important to clarify the degree of stress and the psychological mechanisms used by the parent to adjust to the illness. An empathetic approach helps a parent to validate his or her responses and to act with greater confidence.

# INTERVIEW WITH CHILDREN FROM INFANCY TO ADOLESCENCE

In the interview with the child, one must take into account both the child's developmental level and level of communication. The purpose of the initial meeting is to establish confidence and co-operation as the examination progresses, to know the child, and to learn his or her response to illness and his or her ability to cooperate with treatment. No matter how benign the physician considers himself or herself to be, the child experiences anxiety in encountering a stranger. If the interview is one that deals with behavior and requires the assessment of emotional behavior and interpersonal issues, then a more extensive interview format is required.

In examining infants who have not established expressive language, initial observations focus on social milestones. In the first year the most important are the establishment of eye contact, attachment, stranger anxiety, and the use of language through babbling and jargon. One may communicate with the infant through nonverbal gestures and the form of language called "motherese," which involves extending vowel sounds and speaking more slowly. The infant responds to the adult's mood and gesture in an active and perceptive way but out of his or her own limited experience with familiar caregivers. The response to newness or change is more intense after 6 months, when selective attachments and stranger anxiety emerge as developmental milestones.

The approach to the infant, then, is an indirect, even casual one. The physician is still and quiet, but close enough to observe. He or she initially makes no direct gesture toward the child nor uses direct eye contact until the infant has looked him or her over from a safe distance. An outstretched hand may prove interesting and is offered to encourage the child to reach out. It is best if the infant makes the first move. Dramatic gestures such as facial contortions and staring may be threatening to an anxious child but not to a happy one, so in the examination the infant's psychological state must also be taken into account.

When holding an infant, it is best to observe the parent's preferred holding posture and imitate it. Infants tend to be most secure when they are held in an upright position facing but not directly face-to-face with a stranger. It helps if the infant can see the mother over the doctor's shoulder. After the doctor has established contact, the examination may proceed as the infant warms up to the examiner. During the examination, talking to the infant, particularly in a soothing tone, may be reassuring.

With toddlers, the physician should remember that although they may be too young to talk, they may understand what is said about them. Comprehension precedes verbal expression, and words can be misinterpreted. Also, an anxious tone of voice may have an adverse effect.

In children age 2 to 4 years who can talk and have a better understanding of what is said to them, the approach is somewhat different. Children at this age may continue to fear the unexpected. Strange procedures and new persons add to that fear, particularly if their earlier experiences have been negative. These fears must be dealt with, using the advantages of better language understanding. Children at this age are very literal in their understanding of the words they use and those they hear from others. Thinking is concrete and actions are understood in a concrete way; decisions are made based on literal word interpretations. Consequently, descriptions to young children should avoid the use of analogies and generally require that the child be asked to repeat what he or she has been told. For example, if the child overhears that someone has sticky fingers or that his head is in the clouds, he may expect to see clouds and resist being held by the people with "those fingers." Although the child gradually understands jokes and abstractions, they should be used cau-tiously when discussing an illness. Learning to speak the child's language is enjoyable, and time spent in this way facilitates future visits.

In addition to their literalness, children between 2 and 4 years also show a form of transductive reasoning that gives inanimate objects human attributes. The child attributes feelings and motives to household objects, or at least speaks as if they have them. The child may say that a machine that stopped has gone to sleep and frequently plays at putting toys to sleep and waking them up. In the office children may attribute characteristics of life to apparatus and instruments and may fear these things, worrying that they may harm them, cut them, or jump at them. It is therefore helpful for a child to play with instruments before they are used for an examination.

During this age, the child tends to be overactive and hard to please or satisfy. He or she may get into everything and act in a destructive and independent manner. Feelings such as sadness, anger, fearfulness, or jealousy are poorly modulated. The child may have difficulty controlling anger with a younger sibling. There is an unpredictability in the child's behavior, and things must be told over and over again, as stories are repeated and cartoons watched again and again.

Younger children frequently express fear of the doctor. Their fearfulness may represent what they have been told or what they have experienced from past examinations. Children also may be influenced by their parents' apprehension before coming for the visit. The parent who tricks the child into accepting medical treatment by saying painful procedures will not be painful or bad-tasting medications taste good makes the situation worse. The best approach is to describe the procedure to the child accurately, neither exaggerating nor minimizing it. This should be done even if the child says that he or she understands.

The examination should proceed even though a child continues to cry after routine precautions have been taken to prevent pain and relieve anxiety. Step-by-step explanations are important for the child who is anxious and also for the child who is crying and apparently does not seem to be listening. The child may be crying because he or she is frightened and in pain. This response may be age-appropriate or, if he or she is ill, appropriate for a child who is somewhat younger. If fearfulness or suffering are not expressed, there may be more cause for concern than if the child reacts strongly.

Fear of medical and surgical procedures is prominent between ages 4 and 7 years. This fear seems to be associated with anxiety about the integrity of the body. During this age, bodily awareness is enhanced and anxiety is heightened about potential threats of bodily harm. Concurrent with fear of injury is a sense of pride and a desire to be brave and strong. Valuing strength, children fear anything that might reduce their strength and force them to demonstrate weakness. Accompanying this increased bodily awareness is a new sense of self-esteem. Because of these concerns about the body, medical and surgical procedures should be delayed if possible in children whose concerns about bodily harm are heightened. If the procedure is necessary, the child's feelings must be discussed with him or her, and he or she must be carefully prepared in advance for the procedure. This is particularly true for genital surgery, because children in this age range are often particularly concerned with and aware of their genitals.

When talking to the child who does not admit to the presence of an illness, the physician looks for ways to reduce fear and anxiety. The child is helped to feel that he or she is safe and strong, despite the illness or the recommended treatment. During the examination, an initial period of warming up and talking to the child about his or her successes and interests can alleviate initial anxiety and can be a successful introduction to talking about treatment. By beginning the physical examination with body systems that are functioning well and then moving to the

## TABLE 29-1. Interview With an Older Child

### School

1. What grade are you in?
2. Where do you go to school?
3. What do you like best about school?
4. How are you doing in school?
5. Is your schoolwork as good as it used to be?
6. Do you have to push yourself to do your work?
7. At school, are you worried or sad about problems when you are trying to work?
8. Do you have trouble listening to the teacher?
9. Do you have trouble keeping your mind on your schoolwork?
10. How often are you absent from school?

### Friends

1. How many friends do you have in school?
2. How many friends in your neighborhood?
3. How many are good friends?
4. What do you like to do with your friends?
5. Do you wish you had more friends?
6. Do you ever feel shy or hopeless about getting friends?
7. Do you do favors for your friends and not expect to get something back from them?
8. Do you feel bad or guilty if you have done something wrong to a friend?

### Activities

1. What do you do when you are by yourself?
2. How do you feel when you are alone?
3. Do you like to spend time by yourself? (is it because it's fun, you are shy, you don't know how to make friends?)
4. What are your favorite hobbies?

### Family

1. Who lives in your house?
2. Who is the biggest troublemaker at your house?
3. Who are you closest to?
4. How do you get along with your mother?
5. How do you get along with your father?
6. What does your mother do that you like? don't like?
7. What does your father do that you like? don't like?
8. Do you have problems with your parents? (Who is usually to blame?)
9. If by magic you could change your family, what would you like to be different?
10. Are you happy in your family?
11. How are your parents getting along with each other?
12. How do you feel when you are away from home?
13. Have you ever thought about running away or leaving home?

### Fears and Anxieties

1. Most people are afraid of something; what are you afraid of?
2. Do you try to keep away and feel shy around strangers?
3. Do you feel worried or afraid about school?
4. Are there any specific people or situations that make you afraid?
5. Do you feel nervous or scared about the future?

### Worries and Concerns

1. Many children worry about different things; what do you worry about (bad things happening, being separated from your family)?
2. Do you worry about these things so much that it interferes with school, friends, or doing things that you like?
3. Do you worry that you make bad things happen?
4. Do you have thoughts that you can't get out of your mind?
5. Sometimes children check on things over and over again; do you do that?
6. Would you say that you worry a lot or just a little?

### Self-Image

(Request the child draw a picture of himself.)

1. Do you feel able to overcome your worries and/or fears?
2. Do you get embarrassed about what others think about you? (Do other people make fun of you?)
3. Do you think you're smart, good-looking, and popular?
4. What are you most proud of about yourself?
5. Is your family proud of you?
6. If by magic you could change yourself, how would you like to be different?

### Mood and Behavior

1. People have different feelings and moods; what kind of mood are you usually in?
2. How often do you feel sad (down, empty, like crying, unhappy, blue)?
3. Do you have less fun recently/have you lost interest in your usual activities?
4. What do you do when you have sad feelings?
5. Who do you talk to when you feel sad?
6. When sad, do you feel hopeless?
7. a) Do you ever think of hurting yourself?
   b) (If answer is yes) Or even killing yourself?
8. Do you ever think of a way to do it?
9. Do you feel things will work out for you?

### Physical Complaints

1. Sleep
   Do you have difficulty falling asleep at night?
   Do you have problems with waking up at night or waking up very early in the morning?
   Do you ever have nightmares? If you do, what are they about?
2. Eating
   During the past month, have you lost your appetite or have you been eating more than usual?
3. Aches and pains
   Do you have stomach aches, headaches or other aches or pains anywhere in your body (especially when you are upset about something)?
4. Bedwetting and fecal soiling
   Sometimes, do you wet the bed at night?
   When you are upset, have you ever lost control of your bowels and soiled yourself?

### Aggressive Behavior

1. What do you do when you feel mad or angry?
2. What kinds of things make you feel mad or angry?
3. Do you have trouble controlling your temper?
4. Do you have trouble following rules at school or at home?
5. Do you argue a lot?
6. Do other people think you are stubborn?
7. Do others think you are stubborn?
8. Have you had to see the principal at school for getting into trouble?

### Abnormal Mental Experiences

1. Do you ever feel things around you are strange or unusual?
2. Do you ever feel confused or unable to think?
3. Do you feel that people are after you?
4. Do you ever feel afraid of losing your mind or being crazy?
5. Do you ever feel you have special powers?
6. Do your eyes or ears ever play tricks on you (do you hear things or see things that other people don't see)?

*Adapted from The Children's Assessment Schedule, Kay Hodges et al, Duke University, Durham, NC, 1985.*

problem area, the examination can go more smoothly. The physician should not be misled by the child's apparent cooperativeness and bravery and should indicate that the procedure may be frightening. The desire to be brave and conceal fear is acknowledged, but at the same time the child is told it is all right to cry if he or she is frightened or if it hurts. Anticipating fearfulness and explaining that most children have fears about this procedure are a form of *psychological immunization*. Furthermore, allowing the child to play with the examining instruments or a syringe to be used for an injection may relieve anxiety as well as stimulate explanations about how healing occurs.

Younger children communicate their feelings through their behavior or through imaginary play. Children may demonstrate clearly through play their experience of office visits and their experiences at home or in school. During middle childhood, from age 7 on, children can more easily express feelings and fears verbally but may be unclear themselves about the nature of their concerns. Because they may present questions in a veiled fashion, it is important to understand the meaning of their questions. Frequent and persistent questioning ordinarily indicates a hidden concern.

When children reach middle childhood and adolescence, they can be interviewed more directly about their concerns and their life circumstances. An interview for an older child is outlined in Table 29-1. The interviewer should attempt to cover all the items listed. With some children a brief warm-up period for chatting or playing may be needed to make the child more comfortable before starting the formal interview. Sometimes, to preserve the spontaneity of the interview, it may be appropriate to ask the questions in a different order than listed. If one area seems more productive of feelings or pertinent fact, one should obviously spend more time and ask additional questions until the area seems exhausted, and then proceed to the next set of questions.

## Selected Readings

Bird B. Talking with patients, ed 2. Philadelphia: JB Lippincott, 1973:259.
Graham P. Assessment. In: Graham P. Child psychiatry: a developmental approach, ed 2. New York: Oxford University Press, 1991:17.

*Principles and Practice of Pediatrics, Second Edition.*
edited by Frank A. Oski et al. J. B. Lippincott Company, Philadelphia © 1994.

# 29.4 *Mental and Behavioral Disorders*

James C. Harris

The concept of mental disorder indicates an impairment in psychosocial adaptation occasioned by psychological distress and suffering or disability. It is not the expected response to a particular event but the expression of behavioral, psychological, or biological dysfunction. In assessing a child for a mental disorder, the physician must remember that the presenting symptoms may have multiple meanings to the child and family. Symptoms are signals that something is wrong with the child and might indicate that there is a biological syndrome or disease. On the other hand, they may point to a psychological disorder in the child or in the family, or the symptoms may be the child's only way to respond to an abnormal situation at home or school.

Physical or psychological symptoms may interfere with development by preventing a child from participating in age-appropriate activities and have secondary effects that must be addressed in a comprehensive treatment program. As with disinhibited behavior following head trauma, symptoms may be additionally disabling because of the negative response they elicit from others, and the potential effects of negative feedback on the child's self-esteem.

Assessment of symptoms leads to the diagnosis of problems or syndromes that may be dealt with in pediatric practice or referred for treatment to other professionals. To make this assessment, the current psychiatric classification follows a multiaxial system, sequentially addressing the clinical psychiatric syndrome, the presence of developmental disorders, the occurrence of physical disease, and the type and duration of stressors, which may be acute or chronic. It also provides for a global assessment rating of overall function. The DSM-IV system does not include mixed diagnostic categories (ie, mixed emotional and behavioral disorder), but the International Classification of Diseases does. Both classification systems should be consulted. The DSM-IV classification has a section on disorders usually first diagnosed during infancy, childhood, or adolescence.

## PSYCHOLOGICAL OR BEHAVIORAL FACTORS AFFECTING MEDICAL CONDITION

Psychological factors contribute to the maintenance, exacerbation, and sometimes the initiation of physical illness. The terms *psychosomatic* or *somatopsychic* have been used to emphasize this association in the past, but it is more useful to avoid these terms and to describe specifically the multiple, concurrent conditions or problems with which the child and family present. These might include a physiologic disorder with presenting signs and symptoms, the parent's and the child's response to symptoms based on individual temperament, the degree of anxiety, and the personal meanings of the illness, as well as associated psychosocial circumstances that may influence treatment compliance.

These are interacting circumstances and individual responses to "illness." They do not represent a unitary causality or a hypothetical entity called "psychosomatic." The parent's and child's interpretations and experiences of the illness make each case unique and add to the richness of the encounter between physician and patient. In this section, the term *psychological symptom* refers to the personal meaning the individual ascribes to the illness event. The psychological response to illness can affect the child's motivation to participate in a treatment program designed to facilitate recovery and can affect the parent's attitudes in supporting that recovery. Symptoms may be maintained if the "sick role" has become a comfortable one. However, even though the original personal meaning of a symptom may be lost, the interpersonal environment may continue to maintain the symptoms.

Clinical presentations are affected by general psychological factors related to being acutely ill and to factors related to chronic physical illness. The clinical presentation also is affected by life events, including chronic stress in the family, the parent's attitude and interpersonal behavior toward the child, attitudes toward hospitalization, and behavior following discharge. Finally, the motivation to recover must be considered. Among the specific disorders that have significant potential for psychological complications are asthma, heart disease, cystic fibrosis, epilepsy, gastrointestinal disease, diabetes mellitus, short stature, and malignancies.

As an example, a 7-year-old boy was seen in the emergency room for multiple visits because of asthma. His symptoms responded quickly to symptomatic treatment, yet his mother returned each week complaining about his asthma. When she was asked whether his symptoms reminded her of any past experience with illness in her life, she began to talk movingly about her father's death from emphysema that complicated black lung disease. She had nursed her father through his final illness while pregnant with this boy, who bore a striking physical resemblance to his grandfather and who was named after him. When her son wheezed she became terrified, remembering her father's terminal illness, and brought the child to the emergency room. The resolution of her bereavement was the essential ingredient in her appropriate support of the treatment of the boy's asthma.

Important considerations in treatment are the parents' concerns about the cause of the illness, their need for explanations, their understanding of the meaning of laboratory tests, their rejection of the child or overly protective attitudes toward him or her, and their understanding of the use of medication. Each illness has its own psychosocial context. Some issues that may require support are not being able to breathe in asthma, the experience of helplessness about when a seizure will occur, the frustration with encopresis, the fear of coma in diabetes, and the uncertainty about recovery in cystic fibrosis. For the child, excessive restrictions imposed by the parent during illness influence personality development. Developmentally, adaptation to the illness is an ongoing saga at home and at school, as the child's psychological experience and comments by others influence day-to-day activities. Yet most children with acute or chronic illnesses maintain their self-confidence and make full use of psychosocial support.

## STRESS AND ILLNESS

This section focuses on the factors that relate to the stress of illness and that facilitate recovery. The presence of psychosocial variables and the ways they might influence susceptibility, rather than cause disease, are an essential consideration. This approach requires evaluation of the circumstances that led to the consultation, as well as the specific presentation of symptoms. The child, in the unique context of his or her temperament, genetic background, family life, and community experience, is the patient. Both the symptom itself and how it is experienced must be appreciated. The physician should address the external environmental conditions at home and at school, along with the child's response to them, the risk factors that may lead to vulnerability to illness, nutrition and genetic predispositions, the family's and child's perception of the illness and how it affects their view of themselves, the child's temperament, the child's developmental level, the expected behavioral response to illness at that age, and the difficulty of relinquishing the dependence inherent in assuming the role of patient. All these factors are important in an initial assessment aimed at facilitating recovery.

## Resilience to Stress

Historically we have moved from a general emphasis on the effects of adverse life experience on behavior and symptoms to the specific kinds of life experiences that are most likely to lead to disorders. However, it is important to note that all children do not succumb to illness or become symptomatic when stressed. More than half of the children studied by Rutter were resilient to the effects of external circumstances on their behavior or somatic symptoms. Risk factors do interact with developmental stages; for example, an experience may be stressful and elicit a greater physiologic response in a younger child than an older one.

In the psychiatric classification system we not only describe the stressors as listed in Table 29-2, but we also consider protective factors. To understand vulnerability and resilience to stress, we must consider individual differences in how potential stresses are experienced, noting that what is initially stressful may have strengthened the patient for later exposure to similar events. Experiences may be sensitizing or strengthening depending on a variety of factors. Although the experience may be ultimately strengthening, it might not be initially experienced as positive by the child. The impact may be evident as protective only when new exposures to stress occur. For example, there are individual differences among separation experiences in younger children as compared to older ones. To be strengthening, early experience with stress must occur in the context of affectionate support and hopefulness, which may modify the effect of later stressors. On the other hand, early separation in primates may be sensitizing; instead of developing resilience, primates may show other symptoms when the stress of separation recurs.

An important preventive approach to separation and hospital stress is the hospital-based Child Life program, which provides anticipatory programming to prepare and strengthen the child for hospitalization and provides a normalized setting during the hospital stay. Social support is an important protective factor,

| Code | Term | Acute Events | Enduring Circumstances |
|---|---|---|---|
| | | **Examples of Stressors** | |
| 1 | None | No acute events that may be relevant to the disorder | No enduring circumstances that may be relevant to the disorder |
| 2 | Mild | Broke up with boyfriend or girlfriend; change of school | Overcrowded living quarters; family arguments |
| 3 | Moderate | Expelled from school; birth of sibling | Chronic disabling illness in parent; chronic parental discord |
| 4 | Severe | Divorce of parents; unwanted pregnancy; arrest | Harsh or rejecting parents; chronic life-threatening illness in parent; multiple foster home placements |
| 5 | Extreme | Sexual or physical abuse; death of a parent | Recurrent sexual or physical abuse |
| 6 | Catastrophic | Death of both parents | Chronic life-threatening illness |
| 0 | Inadequate information, or no change in condition | | |

TABLE 29-2. Severity of Psychosocial Stressors Scale: Children and Adolescents

Reprinted with permission from the Diagnostic and Statistical Manual of Mental Disorders, 3rd ed, revised. Copyright 1987 American Psychiatric Association.

and a particularly important element is a confiding relationship with one person, usually a parent. The parent's style of inter-action, psychological availability, and how, when, and to what degree he or she expresses emotion in the child's presence may be critical factors for the child's psychosocial development.

To understand the child's response to stress, several issues must be considered. The timing of the event, the child's devel-opmental level, and the degree of cognitive development all are important. Young children apparently are not as responsive to separation stress in the first months of life before developing selective parental attachment. After that time, an interpersonal bond is demonstrated by the child's response to reunion after separation from the parent.

To appraise events cognitively as stressful, the child must at-tribute personal meaning to them. The child's experience of self-efficacy also influences the response to the stress. The ability to develop strategies for controlling the environment is a psycho-logically protective element. Of importance are the kinds or pat-terns of stress that are experienced, individual differences in re-sponsiveness, previous interpersonal experiences outside the home, self-esteem and self-efficacy, opportunities to control the situation, availability of intimate relationships, and developmental strategies to cope. The ability to appraise a new situation is a cognitive landmark. Children's ability to act rather than react is important to gauge. They can respond with feelings of self-esteem and self-efficacy if they are secure in affection and achievement and have had positive experiences appropriate for their temper-ament. These interpersonal abilities are very important when the child is threatened or alarmed.

Usually a single stressor is not adequate to cause a disorder even if it persists; disorders ordinarily result from the experience of multiple stressors. Protective factors against stress include positive temperament, gender (school-age girls are less vulnerable than boys), parental warmth and affection, and the lack of per-sonal criticism. If only one parent is in the home and there is strife, supportive psychosocial measures at school can compensate for lack of support at home.

In a study by Werner and Smith on infants recovering from illness, those with a history of perinatal stress, poverty, family instability, and limited parental education had worse outcomes. Appropriate rule-setting and discipline led to skills in finding relevant models and sources of support from peers, older friends, teachers, and clergy. There may be other individual protective factors that are not fully appreciated. For example, in contrast to learned helplessness, the child's capacity to help others might be important to promote development and coping. The ability to show humor in adverse situations has recently been recognized as important and is associated with social competence in stressful situations.

## Reactions to Stress and Adjustment Disorders

When the child fails to master the physiologic consequences of stressful experience, the presence of severe or continued stresses may lead to impaired social functioning. The resulting disorders are referred to as acute stress reaction, post-traumatic stress dis-order, or adjustment disorder. The nature of the stress and its severity are designated as acute or enduring.

An *acute stress reaction* is immediate and subsides within hours or a few days. Typically the individual is dazed, has difficulty in comprehension, and may show initial signs of disorientation. Autonomic symptoms, including sweating, tachycardia, and flushing, are present. There may be partial or complete amnesia for the event. This period of initial disorientation is followed by a variety of symptoms such as anxiety, sadness, anger, or with-drawal. These symptoms ordinarily resolve within 2 to 3 days

with supportive management techniques, and if so do not spe-cifically constitute a disorder.

The *post-traumatic stress disorder* is a protracted or delayed response to a stressful event that is experienced with intense fear or terror and a sense of helplessness. Personal vulnerability may lower the threshold or affect the course but does not account for its occurrence. Characteristically, a traumatic event is reexperi-enced by the child through intrusive memories and dreams. The child avoids situations that are reminiscent of the trauma or shows a lessening of general emotional responsiveness to other persons and his or her surroundings. Increased arousal, an exaggerated startle, sleep disturbances, headache, and abdominal pain may occur. Younger children show post-traumatic play. Examples of trauma that can lead to this disorder include threats to life or physical integrity, destruction of the home or community, seeing another person who has been injured or killed in an accident or violent episode, or learning of severe loss or harm to another person. Directly witnessing an event is the most traumatic.

Symptoms ordinarily occur immediately after the trauma, but there may be a latency of several months. Avoidance of the sit-uation may occur, including phobic avoidance of similar situa-tions; this may interfere with developmental tasks such as inter-personal relationships or school. In some instances fluctuating moods, anxiety, sadness, and guilt may persist and require treatment.

In approaching the child with an acute post-traumatic stress syndrome, particularly following physical violence, the child may be numb or mute, and direct questioning may not be productive. A therapeutic interview that addresses the trauma indirectly through the imagination, using free drawings and story-telling, is often an effective approach that tends to alleviate traumatic anxiety. The family, police, or others involved can be consulted about the circumstances, the specific event itself, and the child's subsequent behavior. In the interview with the child, it is im-portant to keep in mind that after any stress or loss, a period of strategic emotional withdrawal may occur and should be re-spected (Caplan, 1981). However, with severely stressful events, intrusive memories of the trauma ordinarily are demonstrated in post-traumatic role play, stories, or pictures.

The focus of treatment is to provide sufficient support to help the child reenact the event until it is mastered. As the child plays, he or she is unaware of reliving the feelings associated with the events. After the events are reenacted in fantasy, the sequence of emotional release, the reconstruction of the experience, a review of the worst moment, and the direct revelation of the violent events to the therapist can be expected. To help the child cope with the experience, it is important to establish how it happened and what it meant to the child. Assigning responsibility for the traumatic event and clarifying a plan of action that might have rectified the situation are elements that ordinarily must be addressed.

A review of past trauma, current traumatic dreams, and current stresses also requires discussion. The child is helped to summarize what happened in his or her own words and to understand how anyone's responses would be similar in the same circumstances. It is important that the child not feel alone, learn to accept support from others, and appreciate that his or her own feelings are un-derstandable. The fact that the symptoms may return needs to be emphasized. At the end of an interview it often helps for the child to describe what was helpful or distressing about the in-terview itself. The goal is to relieve symptoms and reestablish trust in others and in the community environment.

Other family members also require support and ongoing pre-ventive interventions. This includes crisis management and availability of individual and group support networks. It is the physician's responsibility to convene a support group and give the family permission to ask for help (Caplan, 1981). The outcome depends on family support, affection, and the child's own efforts. The parents' ability to work through their concerns emotionally must be assessed, and the child's effort at mastery understood.

*Adjustment disorder* was previously called situation or adjustment reaction. It is a maladaptive response to a known stressor. In contrast to the post-traumatic stress disorder, the stressor is usually less severe, the precipitating event less overwhelming, and the characteristic reexperiencing of trauma not present. An adjustment disorder is characterized by the type of emotional and behavioral symptom (for example, adjustment disorder with physical complaints, anxious mood, depression, disturbance of conduct, or a combination of these). Symptoms are the result of the child's efforts to cope with stress.

Whether the child or adolescent develops a disorder depends on the stress-related factors that have been described previously. Younger children who lack mature coping strategies may be more vulnerable to a disorder; the impact of a stressor is related to the child's developmental level. Life changes such as the loss of a caregiver, abuse, divorce, moving, or school changes vary in their effects according to the child's age, temperament, and the extent of family support.

Adjustment disorder is more problematic to diagnose in adolescents because psychological turmoil may be an aspect of normal adolescent development. Still, psychological symptoms should be taken seriously. When adolescents are interviewed and asked specific diagnostic questions, they often reveal unexpected psychopathology. Although many symptoms prove to be transient, moods often fluctuate, with alternating withdrawal and good spirits. There is frequent concern about physical development, which is expressed differently in boys and girls.

Conflict over independence is a common concern in adolescence. Certain individuals undergo regression with external stressors and show aggressive behavior, delinquency, anxiety, depression, eating disorders, or physiologic disorders. In early adolescence, pubertal changes may be accompanied by rebelliousness and defiance against those in authority and may be manifested by guilt, moody withdrawal, or both. As the adolescent becomes older, heterosexual and homosexual concerns and occupational concerns become more apparent. In the late adolescent approaching the time of leaving home, long-term life goals and a philosophy of life become prominent concerns.

Since current terminology focuses more specifically on the phenomena of psychological experience and behavior, adjustment disorder is no longer the catch-all term it was in the past. Changes in definition mean that older studies are difficult to evaluate in regard to outcome. Adjustment disorders are characterized by their onset as a response to identifiable stressors during the previous 3 months and the absence of specific criteria for other syndromes. Each presents a primarily clinical picture that may suggest other syndromes or specific disorders. For example, the adjustment disorder with depressed mood is a partial depressive syndrome in response to psychosocial stress. The outcome of adjustment disorder with depressed mood has been shown to be substantially better than for a major affective disorder.

Adjustment disorders are common, affecting perhaps 5% to 15% of children. The incidence of the more severe forms is higher in adolescents. The disturbance begins within 3 months of a stressor and lasts no longer than 6 months following an acute stressor. If the stress or adverse circumstances endure, it will take longer to reach a more effective adaptation. If symptoms last more than 6 months, another disorder must be considered.

In an assessment, the type and severity of symptoms and the child's history and personality must be determined and the stressful event, situation, or life crisis must be clarified. The symptoms represent types of adjustment disorders and are described according to the clinical presentation as brief or prolonged depressive mood, predominant disturbance of other emotions,

predominant disturbance of conduct (eg, aggression toward others), mixed disturbances of emotion and conduct, physical complaints (eg, fatigue, headache), or academic inhibition.

In diagnosing an adjustment disorder, it is important to clarify whether there is impairment in functioning. Personality and temperamental traits may be exacerbated by stress. If psychological symptoms accompany physical illness, they are designated separately.

The etiology may be due to one or more stressors, with multiple events generally leading to more severe symptomatology. These may be recurrent, may occur in the family, or may accompany developmental changes.

Adjustment disorders may resolve without treatment if the stressor is removed. However, this may not be adequate, and symptoms may persist after removal. Certain problems, such as loud disagreement between parents before divorce or a death, may require continued coping. Short-term counseling or therapy may be indicated on an individual basis.

## Selected Readings

Berenbaum J, Hatcher J. Emotional distress of mothers of hospitalized children. J Pediatr Psychol 1992;17(3):59.

Caplan G. Mastery of stress: psychosocial aspects. Am J Psychiatry 1981;138:4.

Engel GL. The psychosomatic approach to individual susceptibility to disease. Gastroenterology 1974;67:1085.

Graham P. Psychosomatic relationships. In: Rutter M, Hersov L, eds. Child psychiatry: a developmental approach. Oxford: Oxford University Press, 1985:599.

Newcorn JH, Strain J. Adjustment disorder in children and adolescents. J Am Acad Child Adolesc Psychiatry 1992;31:318.

Richmond J. The family and the handicapped child. Clinical Proceedings, Children's Hospital National Medical Center, 1973;29:156.

Rutter M. Resilience in the face of adversity: protective factors and resistance to psychiatric disorder. Br J Psychiat 1985;136:598.

Werner EE, Smith RS. Vulnerable but invincible: a study of resilient children. New York: McGraw-Hill, 1982.

*Principles and Practice of Pediatrics, Second Edition.*
edited by Frank A. Oski et al. J. B. Lippincott Company, Philadelphia © 1994.

# *29.5 Disruptive Behavior Disorders*

## James C. Harris

"Disruptive behavior disorder" is the most recent designation for socially disruptive behavior that is generally more disturbing to others than to the person initiating the behavior. The impairment or disability is in the effects of the behavior on others rather than in distress experienced by the child. This section discusses conduct disorder and oppositional defiant disorder. Attention deficit hyperactivity disorder is often associated and is discussed in Chapter 29.15. The considerable overlap of these categories frequently leads to multiple diagnoses for a disruptive child in the DSM-IV system and to mixed diagnostic categories in the International Classification of Diseases, such as hyperkinetic conduct disorder and mixed disorder of conduct and emotions. In ICD-10, oppositional defiant disorder is categorized under conduct disorder. The categories *conduct disorder confined to the family context* and *depressive conduct disorder* also are included. The general terms "externalizing symptoms," such as activity and aggression, and "internalizing symptoms," such as anxiety and depression, have been introduced from factor analytic studies.

# CONDUCT DISORDERS

In both community and university clinics, the broad categories of *conduct and aggressive problem behavior* or of *emotional symptoms* constitute the primary reasons for referral for treatment. The distinction between emotional and conduct disorders is well validated. The conduct symptoms are externalizing symptoms and are of more concern to the parent than to the child. Furthermore, these are often chronic disorders that may, in a small but significant number of cases, be complicated by substance abuse, delinquency, and alcoholism or antisocial personality in adulthood. It is these future risks that involve the physician in the effort to intervene and to work with other nonmedical professionals to help prevent the frequently poor outcome of these conditions.

Disruptive behavior and delinquency have been a particular focus of attention since the initiation of the juvenile court system at the beginning of this century, when psychiatrists, psychologists, and social workers were drawn together in the legal assessment of behaviorally disordered children and adolescents. This early legal concern with prevention of antisocial behavior was a major factor in the initiation of the child guidance movement in the United States. Following these early efforts in intervention, Hewitt and Jenkins (1946) carried out the first systematic description of aggressive conduct disorder. Their early work suggested the usefulness of distinguishing socialized from unsocialized conduct disorders in children with disruptive behavior. Others investigators have suggested a useful distinction between aggressive and nonaggressive forms and between aggressive and delinquent or antisocial behavior.

In evaluating disruptive behavior, the child's age, sex, and life circumstances must be taken into account. The frequency and persistence of the problems are reviewed, as are specific or generalized situations in which they occur. Symptoms present in multiple settings have a poorer prognosis. For example, behavior may involve stealing, destructiveness, or fire-setting at home and in the community. Early intervention for conduct problems confined to the home (family context) may prevent subsequent difficulties in other settings.

The solitary aggressive or *unsocialized* form of conduct disorder is generally present in multiple settings and is associated with impairment in interpersonal relationship with other children and lack of close friendships. Lack of integration into a peer group is a key feature. It is evidenced by isolation or peer rejection, with unpopularity and lack of empathetic relationships with children of the same age group. Relationships with adults are marked by hostility, argument, and resentment. There is an absence of close, confiding relationships. Problems range from bullying and excessive fighting to frank destructiveness of property or violent assault. Ordinarily the problems are pervasive and occur in all situations, but they may occur predominantly at school or outside the home.

The group-type or *socialized* conduct disorder applies to conduct disorders occurring in children who are well integrated into their peer group. Often others participate in the antisocial behavior. Relationships tend to be poor with some adults, particularly those in authority, but they may be good with other adults. Stealing, truancy from school, running away from home, and criminal offenses occur with a group of companions.

Some children's behavior does not fit into these categories, but their behavior is severely enough disturbed to require treatment. Conduct disorder symptoms may occur in combination with emotional symptoms such as anxiety and depression. If the diagnostic criteria for depression are met, both diagnoses are made in DSM-IV and both are designated in ICD-10 (ie, depressive conduct disorder). The depressive symptoms must be addressed initially in treatment.

## Epidemiology

The Hewitt and Jenkins study noted that boys were referred more often than girls and that school-age boys were unsocialized and aggressive, whereas older adolescent boys more often presented with a socialized conduct problem. Others have made similar reports and noted a relationship to socioeconomic status. Frequently there is an association with adverse psychosocial environment, difficult family relations, and poor school performance. The onset may be as early as the preschool years, particularly for the solitary aggression occurring outside a social group, with temperamental traits that are associated with aggressive behavior identified in infancy (ie, the infant with a "difficult temperament"). Inflexibility reported by the mothers of preschoolers, negative parent–child interactions, and high family stress are highly associated with behavioral adjustment. Boys identified in first grade with the behavioral traits of aggression and social withdrawal were found on follow-up to be delinquents and substance abusers in adolescence. Associations with alcoholism, antisocial disorders, and somatization disorders in women occur in adult life. Antisocial personalities have been identified in fathers of affected boys. Affected girls reported more somatic complaints without diagnostic confirmation and more often injured themselves than boys. Postpubertal onset of solitary aggression was more common in girls. Early onset has been associated with attention deficit hyperactivity disorder, articulation problems, and in some studies perinatal hypoxia.

An estimated 9% of boys and 2% of girls under age 18 present with conduct disorder, making it the largest group of psychiatric disorders in older children and adolescents. In Rutter's Isle of Wight study, two thirds of 10- to 11-year-olds who were disturbed had conduct disorders. Population rates range from 2.5% to 12%, depending on the setting; they tend to be higher in socioeconomically deprived areas and more common in boys than in girls by a 4:1 ratio. Boys with conduct disorder make up at least one third of admissions to child psychiatry services.

## Natural History

The course depends on the number and severity of symptoms, their time of onset, the child's personality traits, and family and psychosocial circumstances. Milder cases may resolve; those with more risk factors may become chronic and may be associated with antisocial personality disorder in adulthood. The type of presentation also makes a difference: the solitary aggressive type may have a worse prognosis than the socialized but aggressive child or adolescent involved in group delinquency. About one third of those involved as preadolescents have difficulty in adulthood.

Symptoms may be severe enough to produce social impairment leading to removal from regular school classes or home placement, necessitating foster care or residential settings. Behavior problems often lead to school suspension, legal problems, unwanted pregnancy, and physical injury from accidents, fighting, and self-injury, including suicide and parasuicide. Aggressive and antisocial symptoms, fire-setting, and family deviance are associated with poor prognosis. Substance abuse is commonly associated. However, at least one study showed improvement at 2-year follow-up following intervention.

## Family Factors

Children who lack a permanent family are at particular risk. Frequent moves and impersonal home settings (eg, orphanages) lead to particular risks. Children placed outside the home early in life are at greatest risk. The failure of affectionate bonding is a major factor in the genesis of this disorder. Harsh discipline, rejection, lack of nurturing, inconsistent discipline, physical and sexual abuse, and exposure to loud arguments at home without support from either parent are common. Antisocial personality, especially in the father, and alcohol dependence and depressive symptoms in the mother are found more commonly than in the general population, resulting in poor parental models. Single-parent homes without fathers tend to affect boys adversely. Large family size is an issue, as are child-rearing patterns, including lack of self-confidence, which affects limit-setting by the mother. These risk factors are related to the severity of symptoms but do not specifically predict the behavior.

From the family systems viewpoint, antisocial behavior in one member may be the result of a failure in family relationships. If interpersonal communication, effective role modeling, appropriate family organization, and mutual nurturance are established and psychological disturbances in parents are treated, then the child's symptoms may diminish or resolve. The child's personality and temperament may make him or her more vulnerable to being the family scapegoat. The child's temperament interacts with that of the parent, and this interaction must be carefully considered.

## Psychological Features

Winnicott (1975) has suggested that when children are deprived of essential psychological support at home, antisocial behavior may result. The child may make demands on the personal and material environment—expressed as antisocial behavior—to elicit an interpersonal response. Winnicott termed this form of anti-social behavior, which draws attention to a child's legitimate emotional needs, the antisocial tendency. Having lost hope that others will provide for him or her, the child may demand a response from the environment. Such behavior includes stealing, lying, and a lack of concern for the rights and feelings of others. Bullying, abuse, and aggressive acts toward others may occur without apparent awareness of the hurt being caused to them. In some instances the parent may condone the behavior.

Stealing and associated lying, however, may be expressions of a child's hope that his or her needs will be satisfied. Those efforts and demands on the environment must be managed, because in some instances antisocial behavior may be a misguided attempt to demand the care that is a child's right, an aberrant form of reaching out. Another form of antisocial behavior is destructiveness, and this too may be meaningful if it is viewed as an attempt to test the environmental provision for care to see if it can withstand the strain. This formulation is most applicable to children whose stealing, lying, and destruction have a compulsive quality. The child often signals his or her intention to be disruptive.

If the demand for limits cannot be met at home, inpatient hospitalization or a residential setting may be required. The treatment for the antisocial tendency is to provide care despite the child's provocativeness, allowing the child to find again the personal care that was withdrawn. Because the failure of the family environment is perceived as a factor in the initiation of the antisocial tendency, reestablishing care is crucial to treatment.

## Biological Issues

Changes in social behavior have been documented following physical illness or injuries, particularly those involving the central nervous system. Many children presented with behavioral problems after the 1917 encephalitis epidemic. Head trauma, congenital brain dysfunction, and temporal lobe epilepsy are asso-

ciated with aggressive and antisocial behavior, but they account for only a small proportion of affected children. In children with early onset of severe conduct symptoms and family histories of aggressive behavior in first-degree relatives, genetic factors may increase vulnerability. There are ongoing efforts to identify biological markers for violent aggressive behavior, including EEG, endocrine, and neurotransmitter investigations.

## Assessment

Essential to the diagnosis of a conduct disorder is a repetitive and persistent pattern of conduct in which the basic rights and feelings of others, their person, or their property are violated. The duration of symptoms is at least 6 months. The patient is not responsive to the effect of his or her behavior on others. The behavior causes discomfort not to the perpetrator, but to others who must deal with him or her. The problem is a pervasive one, not a single occurrence.

Antisocial, aggressive, or defiant behavior presents in multiple settings and sometimes with peers. The most common referral symptoms are fighting, quarrelsomeness, stealing, lying, cruelty, fire-setting, sexual misconduct, and substance abuse severe enough to be distinguished from childhood mischief and adolescent rebellion.

The assessment takes into account the expected behavior for the child's developmental level; for instance, tantrums are common in 2- to 3-year-olds, and a child of 6 or 7 would rarely be involved in violent crime. Symptoms change with age. Younger children may be more oppositional and defiant, but older children are more directly confrontational with others. The disordered child ordinarily initiates the aggression in fighting with another person. Cruelty to people and animals is characteristic, and destructiveness extends to other's property. Stealing may be aggressive in older children and adolescents, and in severe cases it may involve confronting a victim physically with a weapon to demand money, take a purse, or initiate extortion. Rape, assault, or suicide may occur in the older individual. Stealing may range from taking without asking to burglary, shoplifting, or forgery. Lying and cheating in games or at school are common, as are school truancy and running away.

Robins suggests that the total number of symptoms and their early onset are of prognostic value, so it is important to clarify the age of onset of each symptom. Early and regular use of tobacco, liquor, or nonprescription psychoactive drugs is common. Of particular concern is the lack of interest in the welfare of others and absence of guilt or remorse after antisocial behavior. The blame for misconduct may be placed on others rather than accepted. Despite an apparent attitude of self-importance and power, self-esteem is generally low. Associated temperamental characteristics often include irritability, poor frustration tolerance, aggressive outbursts of temper, and recklessness, which may have a provocative quality.

## Differential Diagnosis

Isolated antisocial behavior does not justify this diagnosis but is designated as childhood or adolescent antisocial behavior, a problem that may require intervention but does not represent a persistent impairment in social and school functioning. There may be associated diagnoses of attention deficit disorder or symptoms of anxiety and depression that justify a second or underlying primary diagnosis of an emotional disorder. In the American diagnostic system, multiple diagnoses are often required, particularly when the child is seen in referral at a child psychiatry clinic, where concurrent attention deficit disorder, depression, or other disorders may be diagnosed. Poor academic achievement, particularly a history of language delay and reading retardation (ie, 2 years or more below expectation for age and intelligence), may require a second diagnosis.

## Treatment

Any child with a conduct disorder requires the care of a psychiatrist or psychologist working in conjunction with the pediatrician. Since family discord and difficult temperament are common, family treatment is needed for the child to change. The prognosis is related to the age of onset, number of symptoms, type of symptoms, family circumstances, and prior academic achievement. This condition has a poor prognosis, in contrast to the isolated antisocial symptoms that often occur in early adolescence and accompany a search for identity. The isolated symptom generally responds to a supportive psychosocial environment. The demands that the child or adolescent makes are ordinarily met by a caring and tolerant environment that withstands the demands for autonomy.

## OPPOSITIONAL DEFIANT DISORDER

Children who present with a pattern of hostile, negative, and defiant behavioral problems without serious violations of the basic rights of others are categorized as having oppositional defiant disorder. The common complaints are argumentativeness with adults, frequent loss of temper, swearing, defiance of adult requests, and deliberate acts that annoy others. They often blame others for their mistakes or difficulties rather than accepting blame. This disorder is ordinarily seen at home and may not be present at school. Symptoms are more apparent with adults or peers who know the child well; therefore, symptoms may be minimal during the clinical examination. The child shows lack of insight into his or her own behavior. Low self-esteem, poor frustration tolerance, mood lability, and temper outbursts are common. Older children and adolescents with this disorder have an increased use of alcohol and other drugs. Onset is usually by age 8 and no later than early adolescence. The disturbance may evolve into a conduct disorder or mood disorder when the child becomes older.

Oppositional behavior is common in children and adolescents. It may be part of normal adjustment, reactive, or a symptom of another disorder. Epidemiologic study shows negativism to be present in 16% to 22% of a nonreferral population at school age. Oppositional behavior is seen two to ten times more frequently in boys than in girls. The disorder may be diagnosed as early as age 3, but is more commonly seen in school-age children and adolescents.

The establishment of autonomy is a normal developmental task for children as they begin to develop self-awareness. Oppositional behavior is seen at the end of the first year of life as the child first assumes independence in feeding but more emphatically between 18 and 36 months. The behavior peaks between 18 and 24 months, when the need to separate and master the environment are strongest. If this developmental phase of oppositional behavior is interpreted by parents as a need to be in control, power struggles may ensue; excessive focusing on the behavior may reinforce it. A normal effort to become independent may become an attempt to be free of external control and perceived overprotection.

A second phase of normal oppositional behavior occurs in adolescence, when the developmental task has to do with becoming separate from the parent and establishing an independent, personal identity. If there is a perceived risk in expressing aggression overtly, it may be expressed in a passive oppositional manner. An appreciation for the need for autonomy is vital at this age, and effective support, although exhausting to provide, is essential for this age group.

Although the onset may be sudden following acute stress, it more commonly emerges as a prolongation and exaggeration of an earlier developmental stage, becoming increasingly maladaptive. Behavior that is seen as independent and "strong-willed" in the younger child may be viewed as oppositional and defiant in a school-age one. The prognosis is best for oppositional behavior that is the outcome of an acute event and poorest for temperamental traits of oppositionality. Without treatment, passive-aggressive personality may be the adult outcome of a non-accepting or controlling family environment.

Children with conduct disorder often have oppositional defiant symptoms, but because of the severity of their behavior the diagnosis of conduct disorder takes precedence. In psychotic disorders such as schizophrenia, oppositional defiant symptoms may be seen early in the course. Oppositional symptoms may also be present in major depression, dysthymia, and mania.

Treatment must address the individual child's need for autonomy and interpersonal relationship within the family. Individual psychotherapy and behavioral methods are commonly used. The child may be seen individually in therapy to develop more appropriate means of expressing autonomy. Family interventions often use treatment approaches based on social learning theory. This requires data-gathering by parents about their child's behavior, including both oppositional behavior and appropriate social interaction. Their cooperation is also necessary in providing appropriate consequences in behavior management. The child with less severe symptoms is often managed in collaboration with a psychologist; however, patients who meet the full criteria for the diagnosis may be referred for psychiatric assessment.

## Selected Readings

Ben-Amos B. Depression and conduct disorders in children and adolescents: a review of the literature. Bull Menninger Clin 1992;56:188.

Campbell M, Gonzalez NM, Silva RR. The pharmacologic treatment of conduct disorders and rage outbursts. Psychiatr Clin North Am 1992;15:69.

Gottlieb SE, Friedman SB. Conduct disorders in children and adolescents. Pediatr Rev 1991;12:218.

Hewitt L, Jenkins RL. Fundamental patterns of maladjustment: the dynamics of their origin. Springfield, Ill.: State of Illinois, 1946.

Keller MB, Lavori PW, Beardslee WR, et al. The disruptive behavioral disorder in children and adolescents: comorbidity and clinical course. J Am Acad Child Adolesc Psychiatry 1992;31:204.

Kelso J, Stewart MA. Factors which predict the persistence of aggressive conduct disorder. J Child Psychol Psychiatry 1985;27:77.

Lahey BB, Loeber R, Quay HC, Frick PJ, Grimm J. Oppositional defiant and conduct disorders: issues to be resolved for DSM-IV. J Am Acad Child Adolesc Psychiatry 1992;31:539.

Lavietes RL. Oppositional disorder. In: Kaplan HI, Sadock BJ, eds. Comprehensive textbook of psychiatry, vol. 2. Baltimore: Williams & Wilkins, 1985:1744.

Loeber R, Lahey BB, Thomas C. Diagnostic conundrum of oppositional defiant disorder and conduct disorder. J Abnorm Psychol 1991;100:379.

Robins LN. Conduct disorder. J Child Psychol Psychiatry 1991;32:193.

Spitzer RL, Davies M, Barkley RA. The DSM-III-R field trial of disruptive behavior disorders. J Am Acad Child Adolesc Psychiatry 1990;29:690.

Waldman ID, Lilienfeld SO. Diagnostic efficiency of symptoms for oppositional defiant disorder and attention-deficit hyperactivity disorder. J Consult Clin Psychol 1991;59:732.

Winnicott DW. The antisocial tendency. In: Winnicott DW, ed. Through pediatrics to psychoanalysis. New York: Basic Books, 1975:306.

*Principles and Practice of Pediatrics, Second Edition.*
edited by Frank A. Oski et al. J. B. Lippincott Company, Philadelphia © 1994.

# 29.6 *Emotional Disorders With Childhood Onset*

## James C. Harris

The term *emotional disorder* is used as a general term to designate symptoms that begin in childhood or adolescence. Childhood is a time of considerable developmental plasticity, and research findings have been consistent in demonstrating that most children with emotional disorders do not remain symptomatic and do not present as disordered adults. Although there is some continuity of symptoms into adulthood, the persistence of symptoms occurs more commonly with conduct disorders than with emotional disorders. Some emotional disorders in childhood appear as quantitative exaggerations of normal developmental trends rather than as qualitatively abnormal behavior. Symptom complexes beginning in early childhood form less clearly defined entities than adult disorders. From a developmental perspective the appropriateness of behavior must be gauged in terms of its intensity, frequency, age of onset, duration, and the setting in which it occurs.

Separation anxiety, phobic anxiety, social anxiety, obsessive-compulsive disorder, and overanxious disorder make up this category. The ICD-10 classification adds sibling rivalry disorder, and several forms of anxiety disorder may occur simultaneously. Panic attacks ordinarily begin in adolescence, although they may occur in preadolescence. This disorder is so rare, however, that it is not discussed here; interested readers are referred to the article by Alessi.

Children and adolescents may develop fears that are focused on a wide variety of objects or situations. Fears or phobias are not necessarily a part of normal development; some fears, however, do seem specific to a particular developmental phase and may arise in a majority of children (eg, fear of animals in preschool children). A distinction is made between fearfulness that is qualitatively different from normal behavior and fears that are exaggerations of normal behavior. The developmental age is considered along with the degree of anxiety. Some fears are specific to a particular situation, and others are part of a more generalized anxiety disorder.

In preschool children transient fears of insects, animals, monsters, and the dark are common. Fears of storms, heights, and bodily harm are common in school-age children, and fears of entering social situations and concerns about appearance (dysmorphobia) are common in adolescents. If these symptoms persist beyond the developmental period when they are common and are associated with sufficient anxiety to interfere with everyday activities, referral for treatment is recommended.

## SCHOOL REFUSAL/SEPARATION ANXIETY DISORDER

School-related problems, including school refusal due to separation anxiety disorder, are a rapidly growing part of pediatric practice. Excessive school absence is a problem of considerable importance nationwide, with both health and social implications. Patterns of absence are established early in the school career; thus, a small proportion of children make up a large percentage of the absences. Families at high risk for chronic organic and psychosocial problems could be identified by monitoring school absence patterns. School attendance has been suggested as one marker of how well a child is coping with chronic stress. Attending school is the first of many prolonged separations. Eighty percent of preschool children have difficulty adapting to school. By 6 to 8 years, symptoms are more common in only children and in those who have been overly dependent.

The child with anxiety related to school refusal was initially described by Broadwin in 1932 as having a variant of truancy, a term then used for all forms of persistent absence from school. Truancy was seen as an early indicator of delinquency, and the truant officer was a common character in the literature of that time. In Broadwin's description:

> The child is absent from school for periods varying from several months to a year. The absence is consistent. At all times the parents know where the child is. It is with the mother or near the home. The reason for the truancy is incomprehensible to the parents and the school. The child may say it is afraid to go to school, afraid of the teacher, or say that it does not know why it will not go to school. When at home the child is happy and apparently carefree. When dragged to school miserable, he is fearful and at the first opportunity runs home despite the certainty of corporal punishment. The onset is generally sudden. The previous school work and conduct has been fair.

Broadwin's observation that these children feared something terrible happening to their mother, which made them run home for reassurance and relief of anxiety, was repeated in many later clinical studies. It forms the basis for the observation that the apparent fear of school is really a fear of leaving home in many school refusers.

By 1941 the designation *school phobia* was used to distinguish it from the more common delinquent variety of nonattendance. Phobic tendencies and obsessional symptoms were described, and it was suggested that if cases were left untreated a more crippling adult disorder might develop. A family setting with maternal anxiety, marital disharmony, and parental inconsistency was associated. Early clinical presentations suggested that this form of school refusal was not one entity but might have more than one etiology.

Several initial distinctions must be made in diagnosing school refusal. Hersov emphasized the distinction between truancy and school refusal. In comparing 50 truants and 50 school refusers, the school refusers came from families with an increased incidence of emotional disorder; experienced less maternal absence in childhood; were passive, dependent, and overprotected; and showed a high standard of work and behavior at school. Anxiety and depressive symptoms also were noted in these children. The truant group came from larger families where discipline was inconsistent; maternal absence was greater in infancy and paternal absence in later childhood. School changes were frequent, and the standard of their work was poor. Truancy was one aspect of their antisocial conduct.

## Clinical Presentation

Separation symptoms are more common in girls than boys and present with the following:

1. Vague complaints before school or reluctance to attend, progressing to total refusal to go or remain in school despite entreaty, recrimination, and punishment
2. Overt signs of overanxiety and panic when the time comes to leave for school. The child often cannot set out for school or returns after going halfway. When the parent takes the child to school, the separation moment is a dramatic one.

3. Boys and girls are equally affected, although prepubertal separation symptoms occur more often in girls.
4. Average intelligence with school attainment equal to or better than expected is characteristic.
5. Average family size is common. Eldest and youngest children may be affected more frequently.
6. One fifth of the mothers suffer from psychiatric disorders, which are anxious or depressive in nature.
7. Acute onset occurs in younger children, but older children and adolescents often have a more insidious onset. Preadolescent children most often present with separation anxiety disorder. In the early adolescent group phobic disorders and major affective disorders are more common.
8. Precipitating factors may be a minor accident, illness or operation, leaving home for a new camp or school, the departure or loss of a school friend, or death or an illness in a relative to whom the child was attached. These events are experienced as threats to the child and elicit anxiety.
9. In adolescents and older children the onset may be more gradual, with a decline in peer group activities and activities outside the home. The child may cling to the mother and try to control her, may become stubborn and argumentative in contrast to earlier compliance, and often directs anger toward the mother. There may be no precipitating event other than a change to a more senior school. In this age group closer examination may demonstrate depressive symptoms or other behavior problems, or rarely a psychotic illness. Long-standing family pathology may be noted, with a personality history of anxiety when entering social situations. Lack of normal independence and poor sexual identification may be part of the young person's problems in coping with independence.
10. Symptoms may assume a somatic disguise with loss of appetite, nausea, vomiting, syncope, headache, abdominal pain, vague malaise, diarrhea, limb pains, and tachycardia. Complaints may be expressed in the morning before school or even in school without a clear expression of the fears, which are elicited only on careful inquiry. The child may anticipate the occurrence of symptoms, expecting to be ill, but becomes quickly asymptomatic when allowed to stay home. School refusal has also been reported in children with cancer who have been at home with continuous care over longer periods of time.

The prevalence of all forms of school refusal has been reported to be 17 per 1000 school-age children and represents 5% to 8% of referrals to child psychiatry clinics. In 10- to 11-year-olds the rate is lower, at 1% to 3%; in adolescents it is of greater severity. Children with separation anxiety disorder commonly have a second psychiatric diagnosis.

Rates are highest at three periods, including the time of school entry and soon after (ages 5 to 7), when separation anxiety is the most common presentation; at age 11, when symptoms are associated with school changes; and at 14 years and older, when symptoms begin to differ in type and severity and are associated with more severe psychiatric disorders such as depression.

Most often school refusal is part of an emotional disturbance; however, the term does not designate one etiology. Symptoms may develop in several ways according to the various theories:

*Psychodynamic theory:* Phobic symptoms arise from externalization of frightening impulses and displacement to a neutral object, which is then avoided.

*Learning theory:* Maladaptive responses are learned through operant conditioning by adult attention to symptoms.

*Interpersonal or family interaction difficulty:* An unduly dependent child is affected by maternal anxieties and conflicts and becomes symptomatic when he or she must leave home. There is often a mutual and hostile dependency in the parent–child

relationship. Symptoms result from a fear of leaving home. Sixty to eighty percent of younger children have this presentation.

*Fear of real situations at school* or concerns related to self-esteem make up 50% of cases in school-age children.

Multiple etiologies may be present, as when anxiety is related to some aspect of the school situation, and the child also has separation anxiety. A depressive mood must be distinguished from demoralization, especially in the older child and adolescent. A depressive subgroup of school refusers is important to identify, because depression with suicide has been reported in children and adolescents with school refusal.

Toddlers and preschool children normally show anxiety over real or potential separation from caregivers. A separation anxiety disorder is diagnosed when the fear over separation interferes with developmental tasks and persists, leading to impairment in peer and family relationships.

## Treatment

Treatment is based on a formulation of the individual case. From a psychodynamic view, the child's fears that harm will come to the parent may be based on hostile dependency; in other words, the child has a wish out of his or her awareness to harm a parent and fears this wish will come true. In attachment theory, the focus is on past experiences and specific threats and injury that are not imagined but are part of the child's actual life history. From a family therapy perspective, the father may not be strong and supportive but rather competes for a more maternal role, leading to sex-role confusion and ambivalence in parenting; more commonly, the father takes little role in family affairs.

Family therapy is recommended to reestablish parent–child boundaries and roles. An immediate goal is to assign family tasks, beginning with immediate return to school after clarifying the child's experience of the school situation.

In a 6-week double-blind, placebo-controlled study, Gittleman-Klein reported improvement with imipramine in 7- to 16-year-old boys and girls with separation anxiety disorder. The family and child were seen weekly, and individual support and desensitization were used along with drug or placebo. This finding was not replicated by Klein when contrasted with intensive behavior therapy. A subsequent study using fixed doses of clomipramine did not confirm these findings.

Tricyclic antidepressants may be considered for severe separation anxiety or depression leading to school refusal, but this should not be the only treatment. If pharmacotherapy is considered, psychiatric consultation should be sought and careful ECG monitoring carried out.

A specific treatment plan includes an early return to school, and the teacher and staff must be fully involved in treatment. The father or both parents should take the child to school in the morning. Regular support and praise for parents in their efforts is essential, and bringing in a school friend may help. Regular interviews, focusing on potential anxiety or stress at home and school, are needed to establish a regular pattern of attendance. A breakdown in attendance following a weekend, after an illness of a day or two, or at the beginning of a new term may be expected. Family illness or bereavement and changes to a new classroom increase the risk of recurrence. The parents must understand that being firm is supportive and not a rejection of the child's needs, because the child's pleas to stay home can be heartrending. Sometimes an outside person may have to be brought in to take the child to school. Regular office visits and telephone calls are required in the first weeks following the return to school. Family treatment and social work support may be needed, and parental disorders should be treated. The physician must establish a trusting relationship with the family, clarify situations causing anxiety at home, desensitize, confront, and persist. Hospitalization may be needed if the parent–child bond is strong and outpatient intervention fails.

In most series two thirds or more of patients improve. The prognosis is related to the severity of symptoms and psychosocial support.

## PHOBIC ANXIETY

A simple phobia is defined as a persistent fear of a specific object or situation. It is distinguished from a panic attack, in which the fear is of having another panic attack, or from a social phobia, in which the fear is of humiliation or embarrassment in a social situation. In a simple phobia, exposure to the phobic stimulus ordinarily provokes an immediate response of anxiety, which is associated with a panicky feeling, sweating, tachycardia, and problems breathing. The more physically distant the patient is from the phobic stimulus, the less the symptomatology. Anticipatory anxiety is generally noted when confrontation with the phobic stimulus is expected.

A diagnosis of simple phobia is made only if avoidance of the phobic stimulus interferes with normal activities or relationships. The anxiety is not relieved by knowing that other people do not regard the situation as threatening.

The age of onset of symptoms varies, but certain phobias such as animal phobias almost always start in childhood. These simple phobias beginning in childhood usually disappear without treatment. The degree of social impairment is related to how easily the child can avoid the phobic stimulus. Simple phobia may occur alone or along with another phobic condition. A recent study found a prevalence of 2.5% in a nonreferred population of 11-year-olds.

Phobias may be learned maladaptive responses. They may represent the persistence of age-related common fears, or they may have unrecognized personal psychological significance.

For simple phobias considered to be learned responses or developmental in nature, behavioral therapy is the appropriate treatment. Methods used include direct exposure to the feared situation with social support or desensitization through systematic presentation of the child's self-generated hierarchy of feared situations while the child is fully relaxed. Operant behavior methods also can be used by providing rewards to the child following planned entry into the feared situation. If the feared situation is a social one, role rehearsal before entering the situation or observing another child or adult deal with the feared situation is recommended. If the situation has a personal psychodynamic meaning for the child, individual or family treatment approaches may be necessary. Future phobic symptoms can be prevented by teaching the child coping strategies to deal with fearful and unexpected situations.

Specific fears ordinarily resolve over several months. The outcome is generally good for phobias, with remission in about two thirds of the cases over a 3- to 4-year period.

## SOCIAL ANXIETY DISORDER

Social anxiety disorder of childhood (avoidant disorder) is manifested by an avoidance of contact with unfamiliar people that is severe enough to interfere with social functioning in peer relationships and that has lasted at least 6 months. There is a desire for social contact with peers, family members, and friends. As a consequence of his or her behavior, the child is likely to seem socially withdrawn or timid when with unfamiliar people and may become anxious when minor requests are made to interact with strangers. The degree of anxiety may result in difficulty in speaking or muteness. Children with these problems are generally not assertive and lack confidence. The disorder is more apparent in adolescence, when increased socialization is expected. It ordinarily occurs along with another anxiety disorder.

The age of onset ordinarily is in the early school years, when children have their first opportunity for extensive social contact. However, sometimes it may represent a persistence or recurrence of stranger anxiety, which ordinarily would have disappeared developmentally. The course of symptoms is variable: some children have an episodic or even a chronic course and others remit spontaneously. Impairment in social functioning may be quite severe. Children with problems in language development may have an increased vulnerability and may avoid situations in which speech would be expected. As a result of this behavior, the child may not form age-appropriate social relationships and may feel isolated or sad. Social anxiety disorder of childhood is more common in girls than in boys and may be more common if the mother had similar symptoms. It should be distinguished, based on severity of symptoms, from children who are reticent or slow to warm up to new people.

Social anxiety may be part of an adjustment disorder; if so, adjustment disorder can be identified because of the presence of a recent psychosocial stressor. In the overanxious disorder, the anxiety is not limited to contact with strangers. In separation anxiety, the anxiety occurs at separation from the primary caretaker. An avoidant personality may be diagnosed if the personality traits persist over several years. In more serious personality disturbances, such as the schizoid personality, the child has difficulty with interpersonal relationships in all settings and is not specifically avoiding contact with strangers.

The initial treatment approach, following appropriate diagnosis and case formulation, addresses the child's individual needs. The focus is on increasing assertiveness in the psychotherapeutic setting and at school. Both child and parents are evaluated to clarify the family's response to the child's behavior and also to assess their ability to support treatment. In some instances, parents have similar personality traits. The parents must understand how the child is controlling interpersonal relationships by his or her shyness. Families are encouraged to introduce the child to experiences in which anxiety with strangers is manageable. Specific efforts are made to increase self-esteem by establishing new skills such as writing, music, or athletics.

An important issue in treatment is to restructure interpersonal relationships through supportive therapy that assists the child in facing new situations by mastering his anxiety. The parents need help in overcoming the child's excessive dependence on them. Tightly woven interpersonal relationships are often present that are difficult to modify. When the child leaves home and goes into a school setting or participates in recreational activities, the opportunity for change is greatest. Occasionally anxiolytic agents may be indicated on a short-term basis, but ordinarily they are not recommended.

The persistence of social anxiety symptoms may lead to avoidant personality structure in adulthood, when treatment outcome is less optimistic than with children. Parents and teachers must appreciate the child's needs and must work together to help the child develop greater autonomy.

## OBSESSIVE-COMPULSIVE DISORDER

An obsessive-compulsive disorder is characterized by recurrent obsessional thoughts or compulsive activity. Obsessional thoughts are ideas, images, or impulses that come to mind repeatedly in a stereotyped form. The disorder is indicated by the experience of anxiety and distress when the child or adolescent tries unsuccessfully to resist these mental experiences. Interference with the normal school routine or interpersonal relationships may result. The child attempts to ignore or suppress such thoughts and may try to neutralize them with another thought or action. Although they are not voluntarily produced, they are recognized as his own thoughts. They may be socially objectionable and associated with guilt. The most common obsessions have to do with repetitive thoughts of violence toward others, of doubt about one's own actions, or of becoming contaminated as a result of the compulsive behavior (eg, being infected by shaking another person's hand). Normal compulsive thoughts are common in middle childhood, as indicated by the familiar children's rhyme, "Step on a crack and you'll break your mother's back."

On the other hand, compulsions, acts, or rituals that are repetitive, purposeful, and intentional, and that occur in response to an obsession are expressed in a stereotyped fashion. This behavior is expected to neutralize or prevent discomfort related to a dreaded situation, which is objectively unlikely. The victims hope to prevent harm to themselves or harm they might cause to others. In older children, the behavior is generally recognized as pointless and ineffective, and attempts are made to resist carrying it out. However, younger children may not be as aware of the unreasonableness of their behavior. Despite its fruitlessness, there is some release of tension following the compulsive action, tension having mounted before the compulsive act.

Anxiety in obsessive-compulsive disorder is secondary rather than primary. Children and adolescents with obsessive symptoms, particularly those with repetitive thoughts, may also develop depressive symptoms as they become frustrated from repeated attempts to resist the thoughts. Individuals with a depressive disorder may develop obsessional thoughts during their episodes of depression. The severity of depressive symptoms and of obsessional symptoms may parallel each other.

Obsessional disorder usually begins in adolescence, but it may begin in childhood. This disorder makes up 1% of child psychiatric referrals. It is more common in boys than in girls by a ratio of 2:1 to 4:1. Recent data suggest that this disorder may be more common in children than previously expected. Early epidemiologic research suggested a prevalence of 0.3% in 11-year-olds. A report of 5000 unselected adolescents noted a prevalence of 2% in whom compulsive thoughts interfered with their daily activities. However, on follow-up interviews, 0.3% were affected. In reviewing adult cases of obsessional disorder, about 20% give a history of their first symptoms before age 10, and about a third experience symptoms by age 15.

Symptoms have been reported in children as young as age 3, but referral is most common in the early teens. In one study the average age of referral was 14.5 years. The symptom patterns in children are similar to those seen in adults. In one study cleaning rituals were most frequent, but counting and checking rituals and repetitive thoughts of violence or sex also were reported. Behavioral symptoms are qualitatively different, rather than an exaggeration of normal development. In adolescence a sudden onset has been reported. Obsessions have been noted following encephalitis, febrile seizures, and temporal lobe seizures.

The most common obsessional thoughts focus on fears of contamination (eg, dirt or feces) and fears of doing something wrong (eg, stealing or misbehaving). Although the child may try to resist them, these thoughts persist and lead to increased tension and anxiety, temporarily reduced by compulsive activity. Common compulsions are hand-washing rituals, having to touch objects in a particular sequence to avoid danger or trouble, and complex bedtime routines. Some children may become secondarily depressed by their perceived helplessness in dealing with obsessions. These symptoms may also be seen in individuals with severe depressive disorders and in anorexia nervosa. In those instances, the treatment is of the primary disorder.

Obsessive-compulsive disorder in children is treated most effectively by using behavioral methods and taking into account the child's appropriate developmental level. Efforts are also made to help the child find a meaningful context to express his or her symptoms. The alliance between the child and therapist is of considerable importance, as is the family's cooperation in planning treatment. Serotonin reuptake inhibiting drugs have been tested in adults, children, and adolescents; significant improvements were seen in a group of adolescents, and the effect was independent of an antidepressant action. The long-term effects of this drug treatment remain to be established. Resolution of obsessive symptoms leads to concurrent improvement in interpersonal difficulties.

The outcome is variable; however, symptoms tend to persist without treatment. Long-term outcome information is not available using newer treatment approaches.

## OVERANXIOUS DISORDER (GENERALIZED ANXIETY)

An overanxious disorder in childhood is characterized by excessive or unrealistic anxiety or worry that persists for 6 months or longer. Children with this condition are extremely self-conscious and worry about the future, particularly about their performance, possible injury, their relationships with peers, and how to meet peer group expectations. Concern may be expressed about tests, about completing tasks, and about their past behavior. Because of these concerns, the child may spend considerable amounts of time asking questions about the possible discomfort or the dangers of experiences that are anticipated. These children require considerable reassurance. Physical symptoms might include gastrointestinal distress, shortness of breath, nausea, dizziness, headache, or other somatic symptoms. The child may appear tense and may have difficulty falling asleep. Because of anxiety, he or she may refuse to attend school. His or her persistent questions may give a false impression of precocity. Perfectionism, self-doubt, excessive conformity, restlessness, and nervous habits may further complicate the course.

The onset of symptoms may be gradual or sudden, and worsening may occur with stress. In adult life, symptoms may persist as generalized anxiety disorder or in some instances as a social phobia. The age of onset is unknown, although symptoms are observed in school-age children.

The major impairment that may result from symptoms is an inability to work effectively in school or to relate appropriately at home. Unnecessary medical evaluations may be generated by the somatic symptoms.

The disorder is equally distributed among males and females, and it is more common in families in which the mother has an anxiety disorder or another mental disorder. It may be more common in the eldest child in small families, where there is considerable focus on achievement even when the child is apparently doing adequate work in school.

The differential diagnosis includes mixed anxiety disorders, which might commonly include separation anxiety and social anxiety in younger children. In separation anxiety, the focus is on the consequences of personal separation; the child with an overanxious disorder focuses on anticipated future problems. Attention deficit disorder should not be mistaken for this condition, since children with this diagnosis, although active, do not demonstrate the concurrent anxiety, nor are they overly concerned about the future. Both conditions may occasionally coexist. Adjustment disorder with anxious mood is demonstrated by the occurrence of a related psychosocial stressor during the past 6 months. If anxiety is related to a mood disorder or psychotic disorder, this would not be considered as a primary diagnosis.

The treatment of an overanxious disorder relies on the establishment of the diagnosis and an individual case formulation. The first issue is whether the anxiety has a symbolic meaning; if so, individual psychodynamic psychotherapy is indicated. Common conflicts that may be out of the child's awareness and need to be understood are sibling rivalry, aggressive or sexual feelings toward parents, and unrecognized conflicts about control. The therapist establishes a consistent setting, acknowledges the patient's emotional needs, establishes appropriate limits, and then initiates therapy. In this setting, a confiding relationship between adult and child may be established and specific target symptoms identified. Psychopharmacologic agents are ordinarily not prescribed for overanxious symptoms, although in adolescence the acute use of an anxiolytic agent may be indicated. Associated insomnia may require specific intervention. Family interviews clarify the parents' ability to support the individual therapeutic endeavor with the child and establish the need for concurrent family treatment.

## Selected Readings

Alessi NE, Magen J. Panic disorder in psychiatrically hospitalized children. Am J Psychiatry 1988;145:1450.

Beidel DC. Social phobia and overanxious disorder in school-age children. J Am Acad Child Adolesc Psychiatry 1991;30:545.

Bernstein GA, Borchardt CM. Anxiety disorders of childhood and adolescence: a critical review. J Am Acad Child Adolesc Psychiatry 1991;30:519.

Bowen RC, Offord DR, Boyle MH. The prevalence of overanxious disorder and separation anxiety disorder: results from the Ontario Child Health Study. J Am Acad Child Adolesc Psychiatry 1990;29:753.

Broadwin IT. A contribution to the study of truancy. Am J Orthopsychiatry 1932;2:253.

DeVeaugh-Geiss J, Moroz G, Biederman J et al. Clomipramine hydrochloride in childhood and adolescent obsessive-compulsive disorder—a multicenter trial. J Am Acad Child Adolesc Psychiatry 1992;31:45.

Eisenberg L. School phobia—a study in the communication of anxiety. Am J Orthopsychiatry 1958;114:712.

Gittleman-Klein R, Klein DF. Controlled imipramine treatment of school phobia. Arch Gen Psychiatry 1971;25:204.

Hersov L. School refusal. In: Rutter M, Hersov L, eds. Child and adolescent psychiatry: modern approaches, ed 2. Oxford: Blackwell Scientific Publications, 1985:382.

Johnson SB. Situational fears and phobias. In: Shaffer D, Ehrhardt AA, Greenhill LL, eds. The clinical guide to child psychiatry. New York: Macmillan, 1985:169.

Klein RG, Koplewicz HS, Kanner A. Imipramine treatment of children with separation anxiety disorder. J Am Acad Child Adolesc Psychiatry 1992;31:21.

Last CG, Hersen M, Kazdin A, Orvaschel H, Perrin S. Anxiety disorders in children and their families. Arch Gen Psychiatry 1991;48:928.

Last CG, Strauss CC, Francis G. Comorbidity among childhood anxiety disorders. J Nerv Mental Dis 1987;175:726.

Rapoport JL, ed. Obsessive-compulsive disorder in children and adolescents. Washington DC: American Psychiatric Association Press, 1989.

Rapoport JL, Swedo SE, Leonard HL. Childhood obsessive-compulsive disorder. J Clin Psychiatry 1992;53(suppl):11.

Reeve EA, Bernstein GA, Christenson GA. Clinical characteristics and psychiatric comorbidity in children with trichotillomania. J Am Acad Child Adolesc Psychiatry 1992;31:132.

Werry JS. Overanxious disorder: a review of its taxonomic properties. J Am Acad Child Adolesc Psychiatry 1991;30:533.

*Principles and Practice of Pediatrics, Second Edition.*
edited by Frank A. Oski et al. J. B. Lippincott Company, Philadelphia © 1994.

# 29.7 *Depression in Childhood and Adolescence*

James C. Harris

Depression is a pervasive emotional disorder manifested by a negative mood, an inability to obtain pleasure in everyday activities, poor concentration, cognitive complaints of self-blame and worthlessness, reduced personal motivation, and physiologic changes in sleep and appetite. As a symptom or syndrome, depression is not synonymous with sadness or unhappiness. The mood is referred to as dysphoric and is one of despair. Irritability, deterioration in school performance, difficulty in peer relationships, and problems in conduct may be the presenting symptoms; these were sometimes referred to in the past as masked depression. Without early recognition and effective treatment, depressive episodes can last for months and lead to continuing deterioration in school performance and a worsening in already poor peer and family relationships. Suicide as a consequence of depression has become a problem of increasing significance during adolescence.

Whether the preadolescent child could be depressed has been a subject of ongoing debate because of the child's level of psychological development and the lack of universally accepted diagnostic criteria for depression in children. In adolescence, depression often has been ignored and the symptoms attributed to "adolescent turmoil." However, diagnostic criteria originally developed for use with adults can be used to make the diagnosis in children and adolescents.

Although the same diagnostic criteria are used for adults and children, questions are asked of children based on their developmental level, and parent reports are also used. This approach has led to the recognition of major depressive disorder in children and adolescents. However, the diagnostic lower limit for other forms of depressive subtypes is not as clearly established.

A distinction must be made between the more common depressive moods seen in pediatric practice, which may be associated with somatic symptoms, unhappiness, bereavement, or demoralization, and a true major depressive disorder (ie, a constellation of symptoms with a characteristic prognosis). How the child's developmental level affects his or her presentation is ascertained through structured and semistructured interviews with the child and the parents, self-reports, and self-esteem inventories. Interview information from both child and parent is essential to make a diagnosis.

The earliest indication of depressive symptomatology can appear in a severely neglected infant. This nonorganic failure to thrive may represent a "reactive attachment disorder of infancy and early childhood" and is the result of a dysfunctional parent–child relationship. Information on prevalence is poorly documented, although failure to thrive with no specific etiology has been reported in up to 9% of infants in a rural area. For the preschool child, unhappy mood was reported in 4% to 8% of 3-year-olds in a behavioral survey; girls were affected more frequently than boys.

## EPIDEMIOLOGY

More than 40% of adolescents interviewed by a psychiatrist reported complaints of misery and depression. Furthermore, 20% had feelings of self-depreciation, and 7% to 8% had suicidal thoughts. In prepuberty, depressive feelings are much less common, with a rate of 9% to 12%. Symptoms were equally divided between boys and girls in prepuberty, but with the onset of puberty the prevalence increased in girls. In one study, major depressive disorder was found to be rare in 10- to 11-year-olds, with a ratio of three per 2000. However, when the same group was assessed 4 years later, the rate had increased threefold, suggesting a potential role of physiologic changes at puberty in the onset of major depression.

Other authors have identified a prevalence of 1.8% in major depressive illness and a 2.5% prevalence in dysthymic disorder in an epidemiologic population survey of 9-year-olds. In adolescence they found a prevalence of 4.7% in major depression and 3.3% in dysthymic disorder, which is similar to the adult prevalence.

Prevalence rates are substantially higher in referral populations either to pediatric hospitals or to child psychiatric inpatient and outpatient units. Consecutive admissions on a pediatric ward showed 7% depressive disorder and 38% dysphoric moods in children aged 7 to 12. A psychiatric outpatient study showed that one in nine prepubertal and one in four postpubertal young people seen for evaluation had depressive symptoms. Before puberty, symptoms were twice as frequent in boys, but after puberty they were twice as frequent in girls.

In recent years depression in children and youth has been more frequently recognized; the greatest prevalence is found in the postpubertal years. Planning based on epidemiologic studies requires agreement on diagnostic criteria for both major depression and less severe presentations. Achieving agreement is complicated by the recognition of subtypes of depression. There are ongoing efforts to validate assessment criteria and find biological markers that will help to improve recognition.

## PHYSICAL COMPLAINTS

Depression may be a biopsychosocial illness. It is a disorder of mood with symptoms related to neuroendocrine and autonomic dysfunction along with specific cognitive problems in self-perception. Problems in falling asleep and remaining asleep, anorexia and weight loss, abdominal pain, chest pain, headache, and constipation are associated somatic symptoms. Depression in the parent or child may lead to increased office visits and increased hospitalization for diagnostic evaluations for ill-defined complaints. How the child presents is influenced by the parent–child relationship and the words that the child has learned to use to describe emotional states. If the child does not recognize the bodily experience of feelings, his or her vague complaints of not feeling good may be misunderstood. An emotionally healthy child is active, feels good, and has fun.

The child also may have learned to use physical complaints to get attention when experiencing depressed feelings in a household where emotional expression is discouraged, or the child may have modeled his or her symptoms on a parent's complaints. These patterns may continue in adulthood, so they are best dealt with directly in childhood. Somatic symptoms and vague complaints may be the child's way of coping with the dysphoric feelings associated with grief and minor or major depression.

Complaints of sleep and eating problems are characteristic of depression. In addition, studies of hospitalized children have found headache, fatigue, muscle pain, recurrent vomiting, and abdominal pain to be physical symptoms associated with depression; gastrointestinal symptoms were found to be the most characteristic. Separation anxiety symptoms often accompany depressive symptoms and are classically associated with physical complaints on school mornings. Abdominal pain is often associated with separation anxiety, which may accompany depression. Chest pain is also associated with depression. In one study 13% of 100 children seen in a cardiac clinic had depressive symptoms; the chest pain had no associated cardiac diagnosis in any of this population.

Children with severe burns, trauma, or chronic illness are another group at risk for depressive symptoms. Restricted physical activity, sensory isolation, repeated treatment intervention, and sudden and severe loss of health may be factors in their apathy, regression, and withdrawal. Children with chronic handicaps also may be symptomatic. Twenty percent of 100 handicapped children coming for orthopedic hospitalization had depressive symptoms.

Although the focus is generally on the child's complaint, attention must also be paid to the parent's problems. In one study, children with recurrent abdominal pain were not different from a control group in degree of depressive symptomatology; however, 25% of the mothers were mildly to moderately depressed.

## ASSESSMENT

It is ordinarily the parents who request help for their distressed or dysfunctional child. Depression can present as a symptom, syndrome, or disorder. As a symptom it is the expected emotional response to stressful situations; as a syndrome or disorder it represents an abnormally persistent dysphoric mood. In clinical practice it is essential to differentiate between these transient mood changes, which may be normal reactions, and the despair, irritability, and loss of interest and pleasure that signify depression.

Depression involves not only dysphoria but also changes in self-perception. Those aspects of depression that involve self-blame and worthlessness become evident as the child matures. Thoughts of guilt, of helplessness, and of hopelessness about the future follow a developmental course, so diagnostic criteria for depression may need to be modified for younger children and for the mentally retarded. At age 4 or 5 children are aware of others being proud or ashamed of them, but it is not until around age 8 that they talk meaningfully about being proud or ashamed of themselves. By age 5 or 6 the child begins to distinguish accidental from intentional behavior, although earlier in life, bad outcomes are perceived as unintended. Similarly, 5- to 7-year-olds perceive that sadness comes from external events rather than internal feeling states. By about age 10, the child understands that a personal problem involves psychological distress as well as external stresses. Self-awareness with increased self-consciousness, as well as with anxiety about the future, develops in adolescence.

Age and sex are important factors in evaluation. In younger children, assessment is more difficult because of their difficulty in describing their emotions. Younger children do not divorce mood from the context of their experience. However, even in adolescence, parents and teachers often fail to recognize depression even though young people report it. An interview with both the child and parent is essential.

From a diagnostic perspective, the current classification of psychiatric diagnoses lists several emotional disturbances of increasing severity. These range from uncomplicated bereavement and adjustment reaction with depressed or anxious mood, to dysthymic disorder and major depression. An adjustment disorder with depressive symptoms following either acute or chronic stress is the most common diagnosis; the next most common is dysthymic disorder. In dysthymic disorder, symptoms have less intensity, are of shorter duration, and occur intermittently, in contrast to a major depression, which is accompanied by more severe physical symptoms, alterations in perception, and cognitive status. A description of symptom characteristics of a depressive disorder follows.

### Depressed Mood

Depressed mood can be expressed both verbally and nonverbally. Because young children vary in their ability to talk about their depressive symptoms, other informants are needed. For preschool children, teacher and parent reports are particularly important. Irritability and changes in activity, perhaps as a reaction to their dysphoric mood, are seen in preschool children. For these younger children symptoms vary more with the environmental setting than in older children. A parent report helps to distinguish changes in behavior but does not necessarily include the child's specific concerns. The child must be asked specifically about how he or she feels. The first step is to establish what words the child uses to describe the bad feeling inside (eg, down, bored, blue, empty, real sad). Nonverbally, a sad expression with downcast eyes and sagging lips is easily recognized; however, changes in facial expression are often more subtle. Adolescents can appropriately label feelings but they may be guarded in talking about them. They may distort their reports, perhaps because they lack the adult sense of time, and it seems to them that these feelings will never go away. Teenagers may try to hide their feelings from themselves and from adults.

## Loss of Interest and Pleasure

Characteristic of depression in children is the loss of a sense of pleasure or fun. The diagnosis of depression requires either this loss of interest or a persistent dysphoric mood. When children have difficulty using words to describe their mood, the demonstration of a loss of pleasure in their usual activities may suffice to make the diagnosis. For example, the child may have friends but loses interest in playing with them or stares at television but does not watch it and cannot remember or follow the story line. Typical adolescent boredom and apathy must be distinguished from a genuine loss of pleasure in activities. Depression may also occur in mentally retarded teenagers. For example, a depressed, moderately retarded young woman with Down syndrome manifested her depression by hiding in a closet at school, refusing to eat, and stopping her regular play with a coloring book after coming home from school.

## Preoccupation with Death

A depressed child may have preoccupations about death and persistently talk about the loss of a pet, a grandparent, or others who have died. Although the child's concerns may originate in real events, these may be exaggerated in fantasy or spontaneously and unexpectedly be revived.

Suicide, a topic children often know about from the media, should be directly addressed in every depressed child. It does not harm the child to ask about it, but rather offers an opportunity to discuss real concerns. Like adults, children and adolescents who deny their suicidal thoughts are at greater risk for impulsive self-injury. Although completed suicide is uncommon in preadolescents, children in this age group think about suicide and may make plans to carry it out. In adolescence, when suicide is more common, most completed suicides are associated with depression. Suicide attempts are more frequent than completed suicides and often follow arguments with parents or peers in homes where there is a family history of chronic interpersonal problems.

## Poor Self-Esteem

Low self-esteem may be difficult to explore in the interview, particularly in younger children. However, between age 8 and 10 the self-concept becomes more firmly established, making the interview more reliable. Younger children can talk about being liked by others, their appearance, and what they would want to have changed in their lives or about themselves. Children may

be particularly sensitive about self-concept and refer to themselves as "stupid"; they may reluctantly report derogatory names they are called by others. Their shifts in mood, irritability, and withdrawal adversely affect interpersonal relationships and may result in further reductions in self-approval. Alternatively, to compensate for poor self-image, older children and adolescents may brag unconvincingly about their presumed accomplishments.

## Excessive Guilt

Although children or adolescents may experience an overwhelming sense of guilt, it may be difficult to get reliable reports from them. The sensitive parent will say that the child assumes blame unnecessarily or feels overly responsible when things go wrong. A child under age 8 may not be able to describe guilty feelings or might deny them in an effort to make a good impression. However, guilt may be demonstrated indirectly through behavior (eg, when a punishment is deliberately sought, or toys are given away or destroyed because the child feels they are undeserved).

## Poor Concentration and School Failure

An abrupt change in school performance in a child who was doing well previously may herald the onset of depression. Unlike the learning-disabled child, previous school work would have been at least adequate. Performance may vary in different school subjects because of diurnal mood variability during the day, or may be worse in winter in the occasional child with a seasonal affective disorder. Both lack of interest and diminished ability to concentrate contribute to decreased performance. Unlike the hyperactive child, who is distracted by the environment, the depressed child is usually distracted by his or her internal emotional state. The teenager may continue to work hard for special teachers but derives little pleasure from learning and may spend considerable time in completing tasks to the detriment of participation in social activities.

## Social Withdrawal

Withdrawal from others commonly occurs with the onset of depression, but unlike the child with a conduct disorder, the depressed child ordinarily has previously demonstrated the capacity to make friends and socialize with them. The child may have talked about having been popular before but no longer does so, now saying that no one likes him or her; the child no longer socializes with peers. The child may set himself or herself up to be rejected by being unavailable, or may impose rules on others that they cannot meet. Chronically depressed children require considerable help with reestablishing peer relations as their depression improves.

## Psychomotor Activity

Psychomotor retardation is demonstrated by slowness in walking, speaking, eating, and general movement. Questions may be answered slowly and in short phrases with little imaginative elaboration. A depressed hospitalized child may remain relatively immobile during the day. When encouraged to go to the activity room he or she may be reluctant to go and may require considerable encouragement. On the other hand, the anxiety that frequently accompanies depression in children and adolescents may be demonstrated in increased psychomotor activity. This may be manifested as an agitated depression with excessive motor activity, or as restlessness.

## Fatigue

Increased fatigue as the day progresses is a frequent complaint of both children and parents. In contrast to previous exuberance, the child or adolescent may be too tired to go out with others or participate in family outings that he or she previously enjoyed. The parent may say the child is just lying around, and the child may want to take afternoon naps.

## Sleep Disturbances and Weight Loss

Difficulty falling asleep is the most usual sleep complaint, but nighttime walking and early-morning awakening also occur. The parent is often unaware of these symptoms and assumes that the child is sleeping. The child must be asked directly about sleep problems since often they are not spontaneously reported.

Weight loss is so characteristic of depression that this diagnosis should always be considered when unexplained weight loss occurs. In one study, depressed children were found to be 10 lbs lighter than a matched comparison group. Children and adolescents ordinarily do not complain about weight loss or changes in appetite. This symptom is often a sensitive topic with the parents, who have made considerable efforts to get the child to eat. In the hospital there may be food refusal or ambivalence about eating.

## Irritability, Crying Without Reason, Separation Anxiety

Irritability is commonly described by teachers and parents in depressed children and has been found at follow-up in preschool children. It may be a greater concern to adults than the depressed mood. Symptoms of irritability are best elicited from the teacher and parent rather than from the child. Crying for no reason or an unexpected urge to cry is a characteristic more often reported by parents than by children. Separation anxiety may be enhanced, particularly in the younger child.

## DIAGNOSTIC CRITERIA FOR DEPRESSIVE DISORDERS

To diagnose a major depressive disorder, the dysphoric mood or loss of interest or pleasure must have lasted at least 2 weeks.

### Dysthymic Disorder

A chronic disturbance of mood or loss of interest or pleasure is present but is not as severe or as long in duration as in a major depression. For children and adolescents the diagnosis requires that symptoms must be present for at least 1 year. The change in mood may be relatively persistent or intermittent and may be separated by periods of time when normal mood and interest or pleasure in routine activities last for several weeks. Anxiety disorders and conduct disorders may be present concurrently.

### Demoralization

Loss of self-confidence may result from frustration in being unable to accomplish developmental tasks, from inability to meet others' expectations, or as a consequence of negative feedback, negligence, or abuse. It is seen in both the learning-disabled and the behaviorally disordered child. These problems in self-esteem may respond to support in the mastery of specific tasks. Persistent failure in school or interpersonal relations may lead from demoralization to an adjustment disorder.

## Adjustment Disorder with Depressed Mood

In the past the most frequently used diagnosis in child psychiatry was adjustment reaction. The term *adjustment disorder* is now used, and specific symptoms are designated. In adjustment disorder, either psychological suffering and distress or an impairment in social functioning must be demonstrated. For example, a child with adjustment disorder might present with depressed mood, anxiety, or a conduct problem. A specific stressor is identifiable as leading to the symptoms, and the usual course is full recovery on removal of the stressor. Symptoms must be present for no longer than 3 months to make the diagnosis. Illness in the family, school changes, and parental separation are common stressors. An adjustment disorder with depressed mood is frequently accompanied by demoralization or loss in personal motivation; however, the symptoms are not of the same magnitude as a major depression or dysthymic disorder. Symptoms are of short duration and are responsive to environmental changes.

## Grief Response

Grief is a normal and expected consequence of personal loss. Immediate grief reactions are milder and of shorter duration in young children than in adolescents or adults. This is perhaps related to their developmental inability to conceptualize past relationships or view death as permanent. Following a loss, protest, searching, restlessness, and despair follow a rapid course in the younger child. The child experiences loss at his or her current level of maturation but may have to deal with the loss again when he or she is older and can reflect on the personal meaning of past experiences and to anticipate the future.

Unlike major depression, grief following bereavement is an adaptive process. Following the death of a loved one, the child may strategically withdraw until he or she can cope with or master life events. For example, a 5-year-old boy lost his parents in an automobile accident and went to live with his uncle and aunt. He was withdrawn and initially preoccupied, not talking to adults about the accident and speaking only to his cousins. His readjustment began gradually after he decided in church one Sunday that he now had two sets of parents watching over him, his real parents in heaven and his uncle and aunt in his new home.

Bowlby emphasized that the death of a parent may result in increased vulnerability to later depression, particularly when nurturant aftercare is not forthcoming following the loss. Unresolved bereavement may place the child at an increased risk for developing psychiatric disorders later in childhood or in adult life. Behavior problems may occur when feelings of grief are not fully expressed and experienced. Although bereaved children usually do cope and make the necessary major readjustments to develop normally, complicated bereavement may occur and may be associated with a depressive syndrome.

In a controlled follow-up study by Black of 105 children and adolescents who lost one parent, dysphoria (sadness, crying, and irritability), falling school performance, and social withdrawal were significantly increased in both sexes at a 13-month follow-up visit. Younger children demonstrated temper tantrums, bedwetting (particularly in girls), and loss of interest in their usual activities. A chronic mood disturbance was noted in 8.5% of the older children and adolescents but was seen most often in the older girls. The most severe depressive symptoms were found in the postpubertal age group, where changes in school performance were particularly noteworthy.

A major contributing factor in the child or adolescent's outcome is the surviving parent's adjustment to the loss. A poor outcome may relate to difficulty in the expression of grief, developmental factors associated with understanding the loss, and the surviving parent's difficulty in allowing the child to mourn and to share his or her own grief. Bereavement or other life events may precipitate depression in some vulnerable individuals, but most children do adapt.

## RISK FACTORS

The risk of having an affected family member with mood disorder is 50% for prepubertal children with major depression, 35% for adolescents, and 18% to 30% for adults. Affected children or adolescents are more likely to have a positive family history of depression than adults. Alcoholism and antisocial personality also occur more often in family members of children with major affective disorders.

Children who are at higher risk of developing depression may include those suffering from parental deprivation by separation or death before age 11, neglect, abuse, or parental physical or mental illness.

The most common risk factor is loss: of a person, an opportunity, hope about the future, or of potential following an accident or burn. However, most children with chronic illnesses do not become depressed. Temperament, acceptance by parents and others, and capacity to adapt all play a role in this adjustment. The loss of a parent is a major risk factor that may be modified by the substitution of another caregiver; the loss of the same-sex parent seems to be of special importance. The learned helplessness model of depression (Seligman) has been suggested to account for symptoms following unusual stress.

Genetic transmission, social transmission through identification with a depressed parent (in response to altered interpersonal relationships), or both increases the risk for the diagnosis. In a child under 18 with an affected parent, the risk is double that of someone having no parent with affective disorder; the risk increases fourfold if both parents are affected. There is an increased risk in monozygotic over dizygotic twins. Twin studies also suggest a concordance of 76% in monozygotic twins raised together, 67% for those raised apart, and 19% for dizygotic twins.

Ongoing studies of depression diagnosed in adolescence indicate continuity into adulthood. However, longitudinal studies have not yet been done to clarify the full implications of childhood onset. We do not know if there are childhood and adult forms of depression that require different approaches as, for example, may be the case in adult onset when compared to juvenile onset diabetes. Because of stronger family loading for the more severe form of depression, it is most likely related to the genetic form of the disorder.

The type of depression in the parent is important as well. Major depressive disorder or manic-depressive disorder in a parent has different consequences on a child's behavior. The child must deal with irritability, inconsistency, and erratic affection in a parent with manic-depressive disorder. Preschool children with a parent who is manic-depressive have been shown to have more difficulty regulating emotions, greater reactivity to stress, and difficulty sharing and socializing. On the other hand, if the parent has a major depression, children may show an increased tendency to suppress emotions and to be less persistent in their play with others.

## Biological Factors

Biological markers for depression in children and adolescents are being investigated, and such research includes neuroendocrine studies, biochemical investigations, and sleep studies. Studies showing the failure of a growth hormone response to insulin in psychosocial dwarfism have been extended to the study of major depression in prepubertal children. Reports of growth hormone

hyporesponsivity to insulin-induced hypoglycemia and increased growth hormone release during slow-wave (delta) sleep have been reported in children. In the older adolescent, the adult biological response to depression with a reduction in growth hormone release during sleep has been reported.

Although depressed children have multiple sleep complaints, including difficulty falling asleep and waking during the night, none of these sleep changes has been demonstrated to be characteristic of prepubertal depression in the sleep laboratory. Sleep changes in adult depression include decreased sleep efficiency, decreased deep (delta) sleep, early onset of dream sleep (shortened rapid eye movement [REM] latency), increased REM density in dream sleep, and abnormal distribution of REM sleep during the night. The failure to demonstrate these abnormalities in children may relate to maturational changes in both slow-wave and REM sleep with age. Some sleep continuity disturbance related to depression becomes evident on entry into adolescence, but REM latency becomes abnormal only in late adolescence. Future studies of sleep in children and adolescents, using more sensitive computerized methods, may help to clarify possible sleep abnormalities.

Biological markers may exist for major depression in prepuberty and adolescence, but they have not been convincingly demonstrated. Increased family prevalence and the growth hormone studies are the most similar to adult findings. Sleep EEG studies and abnormality in cortisol secretion have not been consistently demonstrated, which could relate to the degree of biological maturation. More sensitive methods to elucidate age-related changes in biological markers are needed.

## TREATMENT

Depression has no identifiable single cause; environmental, familial, and physical factors all contribute. Therefore, comprehensive treatment requires multiple therapeutic modalities. Preventive approaches include anticipatory guidance before hospitalization and in dealing with stressful life crises such as an impending death in the family. When the stress has occurred, preventive intervention programs using individual and family approaches to help deal with the impact of the loss have the goal of preventing complications and progression to a disorder. The convening of a support group is of considerable importance at the time of bereavement. One investigation found a preventive intervention program with three to six child-oriented bereavement counseling sessions led to fewer behavioral problems, fewer sleep problems, and less depressed mood in children at a 1-year follow-up. Children who received the intervention talked more about the deceased parent. Attending the funeral of the deceased also resulted in improvement in the child's behavior.

Early detection and referral for treatment of suspected cases of depression in children and adolescents is important. When a case is diagnosed, reducing disability and helping the child to achieve maximal function are the primary goals. There is an educational aspect to treatment that involves working with family members. There is also an interpersonal aspect to treatment that helps the child deal with the consequences of the depressive illness on his or her interpersonal relationships with others. Loss of peer relations and secondary family problems are common complications. Prevention or amelioration of poor performance at school, lack of social skills, social withdrawal, somatic concerns, and suicide are all targets for intervention and rehabilitation. Early diagnosis may prevent unnecessary medical evaluations. Psychotherapeutic modalities include crisis management, parental counseling, and individual, group, or family therapy.

In the major depressive disorder in which weight loss, sleep disturbance, and cognitive changes are severe, pharmacotherapy with antidepressants is frequently used; however, definitive studies on the effectiveness of these drugs are not yet available. This use requires routine monitoring of blood levels. Because there is a risk of self-poisoning, knowledge of drug overdose toxicity, especially for the most commonly used drug, imipramine, is essential. When a tricyclic antidepressant medication is used, a baseline ECG provides the most sensitive index for assessing later tricyclic toxicity. Imipramine dosage should not be increased if the resting heart rate exceeds 130 beats a minute, P-R interval greater than 0.21 msec, QRS interval greater than 130% of baseline, systolic blood pressure greater than 145, or diastolic blood pressure greater than 95 mm Hg. Tricyclic antidepressants should not be used in children with cardiac conduction defects. Because oral dosage is not well correlated with blood level, plasma levels must be routinely measured at least 8 hours following a dose.

The most convincing argument for pharmacotherapy is the chronicity and long duration of a major depressive disorder and the depth and extent of psychosocial impairment. However, pharmacotherapy alone does not ameliorate interpersonal problems with parents and peers; for these symptoms psychotherapy is indicated. A parent's depressive disorder must be considered and recognized, because the parent's symptoms may influence personality development and increase the likelihood of symptom expression in the child.

## PROGNOSIS

In one study of a high-risk group of children and adolescents with depressive symptoms, the average duration of a major depressive disorder was 7.5 months. Forty percent of the group went into remission within 6 months and 90% remitted in 18 months. The younger children had longer episodes than older ones. Within 5 years of the first episode there was a 70% risk of a second episode. The risk of recurrence of major depression was greater if there was an underlying dysthymic disorder. For dysthymic disorder the average duration was 3 years, but 6.5 years was the duration of symptom from diagnosis to recovery for 90% of this group, some of whom later developed major depression. Adjustment disorder with depressive mood was the most benign of the depressive disorders, usually occurring alone or with an anxiety-related disorder. The average case lasted 5.5 months, and 90% recovery was found within 9 months. None of the children in this group developed major depressive disorders. Prognosis has not been adequately evaluated in children from better psychosocial settings.

Although additional studies are critical to characterize further the natural history and to demonstrate appropriate treatment of depressive disorders in children and adolescents, the evidence to date demonstrates that current diagnostic criteria for depression can be meaningfully applied to children and adolescents. Furthermore, depressive disorders diagnosed using these criteria are not transient but may be acute or chronic conditions. Concurrent anxiety symptoms and conduct problems are often present and may complicate recognition of the depressive symptomatology. Efforts are underway to determine more effective treatments directed at more rapid recovery and prevention of future episodes.

## Selected Readings

Black D, Urbanowicz MA. Bereaved children—family intervention . In: Stevenson JE; ed. Recent research in developmental psychopathology. Supplement to J Child Psychology and Psychiatry. Elmsford, NY: Pergamon Press, 1985.

Bleiberg E. Mood disorders in children and adolescents. Bull Menninger Clin 1991;55: 182.

Bowlby J. Attachment and loss. III. Loss, sadness and depression. New York: Basic Books, 1980.

Harris JC. Don't overlook depression in children and adolescents. Contemp Pediatr 1987;4:70.

Hodges K, Kline JJ, Barbero G, Flanery R. Depressive symptoms in children with recurrent abdominal pain and in their families. J Pediatrics 1985;107:622.

Kashani JH, Barbero GJ, Boander FD. Depression in hospitalized pediatric patients. J Am Acad Child Psychiatry 1981;20:123.

Kashani JH, Lababidi Z, Jones RJ. Depression in children and adolescents with cardiovascular symptomatology: the significance of chest pain. J Am Acad Child Psychiatry 1982;21:187.

Kovacs M. A developmental perspective on methods and measures in the assessment of depressive disorders: the clinical interview. In: Rutter M, Izard C, Read, PB, eds. Depression in young people. New York: Guilford Press, 1986.

Kovacs M. Depressive disorders in childhood. IV. A longitudinal study of comorbidity with and risk for anxiety disorders. Arch Gen Psychiatry 1989;46:776.

Poznanski EO. The clinical characteristics of childhood depression. In: Grinspoon L, ed. Psychiatry 1982: The American Psychiatric Association annual review. Washington DC: American Psychiatric Press, 1982:296.

Puig-Antich J. Psychobiological markers: effects of age and puberty. In: Rutter M, Izard CE, Read PB, eds. Depression in young people. New York: Guilford Press, 1986.

Puig-Antich J, Goetz D, Davies M, et al. A controlled family history study of prepubertal major depressive disorder. Arch Gen Psychiatry 1989;46:406.

Puig-Antich J, Lukens E, Davies M, Goetz D, Brennan-Quattrock J, Todak G. Psychosocial functioning in prepubertal major depressive disorders. Arch Gen Psychiatry 1985;42:511.

Seligman MEP. Helplessness: on depression, development and death. San Francisco: WH Freeman, 1975.

Van Erdewegh MM, Beiri MD, Parilla RH, Clayton P. The bereaved child. Br J Psychiatry 1985;140:23.

*Principles and Practice of Pediatrics, Second Edition.*
edited by Frank A. Oski et al. J. B. Lippincott Company, Philadelphia © 1994.

# 29.8 *Suicide*

### James C. Harris

Suicide and parasuicide (suicide attempt) are common among adolescents and common enough among preadolescents to be an important concern. In a child psychiatry clinic, 10% of referrals are for this reason, and large numbers of adolescents are admitted to inpatient services. Suicide is the third leading cause of death in adolescents, exceeded only by motor-vehicle injuries and homicide. Of particular importance is the increase in completed suicides by more than 200% during the last 25 years. For each completed suicide there are 30 to 40 or more attempted suicides, depending on the age group. In preadolescents suicide may be overlooked as the cause of death when deaths are recorded as accidental.

## EPIDEMIOLOGY

Childhood suicide is described as a self-inflicted death occurring before the 15th birthday. It is the only psychiatric condition that is subject to documentation by age, sex, and method in all developed countries. At all ages the rate in whites is greater than in nonwhites. In males, completions are more common than in females. In 1978, 117 per 100,000 boys and 34 per 100,000 girls between ages 10 and 14 committed suicide, accounting for 2.4% of deaths in this age group. In the same year, 1367 per 100,000 adolescent males and 319 per 100,000 females between ages 15 and 19 committed suicide, accounting for 7.9% of deaths in that age group. The rate of suicide for the younger adolescent group was 9.81 per 100,000 and for the older adolescent group, 7.64 per 100,000. The rate in 10- to 14-year-olds has been stable for some years; the increases are found primarily in the 15- to 18-year-old age group.

It appears that suicide is related to maturation and that younger children may be protected, possibly because planning the event may require abstract reasoning, formulation of a plan, and the development of a poor self-concept. The child also must be able to understand the severity of the situation and understand the means to use to complete suicide. Certain psychiatric diagnoses, particularly major depression, occur most commonly for the first time in late adolescence and are important factors. Suicide may not be fully reported because of possible stigma, and such underreporting leads to difficulty in interpreting accident statistics that may include suicide in children. For example, if a child deliberately runs into the street, he may do so with suicidal intent. The specific means used for suicide is important to clarify.

It has been suggested that the increase in suicide in the United States for the 15- to 19-year-old group may be largely accounted for by the availability of firearms. In 1978, 59.5% of completed suicides were carried out with firearms, 20.5% by hanging or suffocation, 10% by poisoning, and 6.5% by the use of gas; other means were used in the rest. In England control of gas in the home led to a significant reduction of suicide, and it has often been suggested that the control of availability of firearms would have a similar effect in the United States.

Suicide attempts occur three times more often in girls than boys during the adolescent years. Young men often use firearms, jump from heights, or inhale carbon monoxide, and young women more often use self-poisoning; this has been the primary difference between sexes. The word "overdose" is often used in emergency-room settings to describe the behavior, but the more appropriate designation is self-poisoning.

## ETIOLOGY

Cognitive maturation is a factor in successful suicide. Children who have higher intellectual ability and higher standards of living may be more prone to deal with failure by blaming themselves. Pressure to admit antisocial behavior following a disciplinary crisis and other interpersonal disagreements may be followed by suicide attempts. The occurrence of psychiatric illness in families, particularly depression in siblings or parents, is another important consideration. The best predictor of a suicide attempt is a prior attempt; previous parasuicide has been noted to be as high as 40% in completed suicides. Suicide may occur in the context of psychiatric illness and may be the result of internal conflict. It varies in frequency and intensity with age, and is often related to interpersonal difficulties with parents and teachers.

An important etiology of suicide in adolescents is major affective disorder. This may be a primary condition or it may be secondary to another preexisting illness. It is the most significant event related to completed suicide, and risk occurs during the depressed phase or episode. When those with affective disorders are not depressed, the risk is not increased. The greatest risk is during the first years after the diagnosis of the depression.

Two other conditions are associated with completed suicide: drug abuse, particularly alcoholism, and schizophrenia. Suicide associated with schizophrenia is less common than in an affective disorder. With a schizophrenic individual, the history of a previous attempt, the presence of an associated depressive syndrome, or hallucinations that are self-destructive increase the risk.

In contrast to completed suicide, attempted suicide is more commonly associated with a hysterical personality style and antisocial personality traits. These personality traits, complicated by the use of drugs, increase the risk for an attempt. An additional risk factor is a family history of suicide. This may be related to the modeling that can occur from knowing that another family member has completed suicide. There also may be a small genetic contribution.

## CLINICAL PICTURE

Information about the clinical picture of completed suicide is gathered by techniques referred to as the psychological autopsy, a method initially developed for use with adults but more recently applied to adolescents. Interviews are conducted with those who knew the individual who has committed suicide. The completed suicide population has a dominance of depression as the primary diagnosis. Few individuals who complete suicide do not have psychiatric symptoms. Suicide assessment takes into account a history of behavioral change before the event; suicide does not just happen. The most common associated events are communication of suicidal thoughts, history of suicide attempts, and previous psychiatric contact. Most individuals have communicated their intent to others on several occasions, generally by indicating that they wish to die and that others would be better off without them, by comments about methods of suicide, and by predictions such as that others would find a dead person. Often these communications are not taken seriously by friends and family members, but it is extremely important to do so.

One should look for a family history of suicide, family and peer conflicts, isolation and withdrawal from contacts with others, the impact of recent disappointments, the presence of psychiatric illness, and particularly a sense of hopelessness.

The following background features are characteristic of the child and family where suicide or a suicide attempt occurs:

1. There is an increased prevalence of psychiatric conditions, especially depression and personality disorder in parents. There may be a family history of suicide. Difficulties in the parents' marriage are common.
2. Problems in discipline frequently occur. Discipline is often inconsistent; parents may alternate between being permissive and then restricting activity, which leads to conflict.
3. Problems in communication among family members, particularly in regard to confiding feelings, are evident.
4. A psychiatric disorder may be present in the child. This may represent a response of hopelessness on an acute basis or a chronic depressive disorder. For the suicide attempter, a history of antisocial behavior and drug and alcohol abuse are contributing factors.
5. The child or adolescent is socially isolated from peers and family members. A child who has had limited social support may report the loss of that support just before the attempt. In other instances there is a history of running away before the attempt.
6. Both pregnancy and chronic physical illness must be considered. The child with a chronic long-term physical illness may be at risk in adolescence, and the possibility of pregnancy must be considered as a potential precipitant in teenage girls.

## DIFFERENTIAL DIAGNOSIS

A completed suicide is a rare event in any individual pediatrician's practice. However, it is potentially preventable, so the danger signs must be kept in mind. Since depression most commonly is associated, an awareness of depressive symptoms is paramount. Depressed mood is often recognized, but clarifying whether or not there is a depressive syndrome present is more difficult. Suicidal talk must be taken seriously whether or not it makes sense that the person would be upset. Individuals who talk about committing suicide may do so, and finding out about their concerns is essential. Whenever the question of depression arises, the physician should ask about suicidal thoughts; doing so does not implant them into the patient's mind. If a patient remains depressed, one should ask about suicidal thoughts throughout the course of the illness, especially if a plan has been considered. Although most suicidal crises do not result in death, a miscalculation cannot be reversed. Consultation with a psychiatrist and hospital admission are the best choice when there is doubt.

## TREATMENT

Because there is no guarantee that suicidal intent can be reversed, it is essential to treat the underlying illness. If that illness is a major affective disorder, tricyclic antidepressants may be used, bearing in mind that there is a risk of overdose and self-poisoning with these agents. Because most individuals communicate their distress, attending to their distress is the most essential intervention.

Profiles of completed suicide and attempted suicide must be kept in mind. Completed suicides are associated with depressive disorder and schizophrenia. The act is carefully planned, and the method chosen is effective and is used in isolation, often with provisions to prevent the attempt from being interrupted. The plan is to die. In contrast, those who attempt are more often women than men, they are less likely to be suffering from a major psychiatric illness, and they act impulsively. The means chosen is often not carefully thought out nor rapidly effective. Caution is generally not taken to prevent rescue and the act may be carried out in the presence of others, or a means is available to notify others about the individual's despair. The plan is not to die, but to survive.

An attempted suicide should not be viewed as a failed suicide, because it might have led to death. The closer the individual's behavior to the pattern of completed suicide, the more concern is indicated. In the usual attempt, however, there is a wish to affect another person by the behavior. Consequently, the occurrence is in a social context, and it is a request for help. The distress is misdirected. These attempts are acts of desperation and are best considered in this way.

Assessment should be conducted as soon as the child or adolescent can participate in an interview after the appropriate emergency measures. This assessment should take place before discharge from the emergency room or hospital. Ideally the interview involves a psychiatrist, who can help in assessing the risk of recurrence and in other forms of intervention. Both the young person and family members are interviewed. If an adolescent is involved, it is preferable to interview him or her first, then the parents, and finally the family together. Table 29-3 lists the questions to be asked in assessing suicide.

The first issue to be addressed is whether treatment should occur on an inpatient or outpatient basis. Inpatient treatment is essential if major risk factors are present (ie, a serious life-threatening event planned and carried out in isolation by a child who is depressed) and if there are precipitating circumstances, an unsettled and poor support system, continuing suicidal thoughts, and an attitude of hopelessness. Each of these circumstances must be taken into account in developing a treatment plan, which includes treatment of the underlying psychiatric disorder, family intervention in regard to family treatment and psychosocial support, crisis intervention focusing on dealing with precipitating circumstances, and appropriate educational programming.

Hospital admission may be to a psychiatric unit for major psychiatric conditions or to a pediatric floor for observation and establishment of a treatment program. In some instances individual psychotherapy and in other instances family therapy is needed during admission. The impact of a suicide attempt on peers and the child's school is another important consideration in community treatment, because there have been several instances of multiple suicides in one school.

**TABLE 29-3.   Assessment for Suicide Risks**

1. Establish details of the attempt with specific emphasis on the means used, eg, self-poisoning, strangulation, self-inflicted wound.
2. What is the expressed intention about death in regard to the attempt?
3. Was anyone informed before or after initiating the attempt?
4. What were the circumstances that are said to have precipitated the attempt?
5. In what way has the attempt altered these circumstances?
6. Does the child or adolescent have current suicidal intentions and express an attitude of hopelessness?
7. What is the current mental status, with an emphasis on affective symptomatology?
8. Is there a history of emotional or behavioral difficulties in previous weeks or months?
9. Has there been involvement with a physician or a community agency?
10. What is the current support system: friends, family, teachers, religious groups, and other community contacts? How can a confiding relationship be established and a support system be convened?

## PROGNOSIS

The prognosis depends on the ability to alter the precipitating circumstances, effective treatment of underlying psychiatric conditions, and the availability of psychosocial support. Risk is greatest in those who have made previous attempts, when chronic stress persists, and if underlying psychiatric conditions are not resolved.

### Selected Readings

Mattison RE. Suicide and other consequences of childhood and adolescent anxiety disorders. J Clin Psychiatry 1988;49(suppl):9.

McKenry PC, Tishler CL, Kelley C. Adolescent suicide: a comparison of attempters and nonattempters in an emergency room population. Clin Pediatr 1982;21:266.

Murphy GE. Suicide and attempted suicide. In Winokur G, Clayton P, eds. The medical basis of psychiatry. Philadelphia: W.B. Saunders, 1986.

Pfeffer CR. Self-destructive behavior in children and adolescents. Psych Clin North Amer 1985;8:215.

Shaffer D, Fisher P. The epidemiology of suicide in children and young adolescents. J Amer Acad Child Psychiat 1981;20:545.

*Principles and Practice of Pediatrics, Second Edition.*
edited by Frank A. Oski et al. J. B. Lippincott Company, Philadelphia © 1994.

## 29.9 *Dissociative or Conversion Disorders*

### James C. Harris

Somatic symptoms are often associated with anxiety and depressive disorders. For example, abdominal pain may accompany separation anxiety and be used as a reason to stay home with the parent. Children with overanxious disorder may be preoccupied with medical illnesses or may present with headache or similar complaints. After bereavement, general pain complaints may be noted, and children with social anxiety disorders may feign illness to avoid social interaction. Children with mood disorders may be preoccupied with sickness and death. The most specific syndrome that presents with somatic complaints in children is dissociative or conversion disorder. Conversion disorders should be considered when there are no clear-cut medical reasons for somatic symptoms. This disorder may be present with or without an accompanying medical diagnosis.

## EPIDEMIOLOGY

The prevalence of conversion disorders depends on the clinical setting. Conversion symptoms are reported most often on the general pediatric service, the ophthalmology service, and the neurology service. Prevalence estimates range from 2% to 16%; the higher number is from a pediatric psychiatry inpatient consultation service. Rates are reported to be higher in children from rural poor populations than in urban children. The prevalence tends to be equal for males and females in the prepubertal years, but there is a greater prevalence in females in early adolescence. Many children with conversion symptoms have transient symptoms and can be treated as outpatients.

## CLINICAL DESCRIPTION

The most common presentations are neurologic or ocular. These include visual or hearing disturbances, localized pains, sensory disturbances such as paresthesias, problems in gait, weakness, seizures, and the loss of function of an extremity. Neurologic symptoms do not follow the expected anatomical localization. Emotional unconcern about symptoms may or may not be part of the clinical picture. Symptoms may be preceded by a traumatic life event or personal loss that the child cannot handle at his or her developmental level. Rapid remission is the rule; more than two thirds of patients improve within a 12-month period. A smaller percentage are subsequently found to have organic difficulties.

## ETIOLOGY

A variety of approaches have been taken to understanding conversion symptoms. The classic psychodynamic approach suggests that physical symptoms result from conflicts that are out of awareness. The symptom represents punishment for covert, unacceptable wishes. Other authors suggest that children with conversion symptoms find it difficult to put their feelings into words and need help in doing so. If symptoms persist, there may be secondary gain if the patient is allowed to avoid difficult situations and if developmentally appropriate demands are reduced. Learning theorists suggest that imitation of or identification with significant adults is related to symptom formation. For example, a boy who had difficulty dealing with his uncle's stroke could not use his arm.

Several authors have found symptoms of mood disorder in parents of children with conversion symptoms. In addition to specific symptoms in family members, stressful interpersonal family crises, threats to the child's dependency, or threatened losses of family members also may be related to etiology. The family may reinforce behavior that is passive, dependent, or even seductive. One must always ask, where did the child learn this symptom?

## DIFFERENTIAL DIAGNOSIS

Most children with conversion disorder do not have a histrionic personality. The diagnosis can occur in children with many psychiatric conditions. Symptoms may vary over time and from one situation to another. The child may or may not show emotional concern about the symptoms.

The physician must remember that some children with conversion disorders are later diagnosed with medical conditions, and that certain medical conditions, such as multiple sclerosis, may spontaneously remit. Children also present with undiagnosable conditions that are factitious, or a parent may falsify the medical history (Munchausen syndrome by proxy). These cases are more likely to be confused with other medical illnesses and not conversion disorder. As previously noted, separation anxiety disorder, overanxious disorder, and depressive disorders may have associated physical symptomatology. In addition, children with psychotic disorders may have somatic preoccupations or delusions.

## TREATMENT

If a conversion symptom is suspected, the pediatric medical evaluation should be done rapidly to avoid secondary gain from symptoms. As symptoms resolve, symptom removal generally does not result in the substitution of other symptoms. Interventions with parent and child include reassurance, enhanced expression of feelings verbally, behavioral treatments using suggestion, initiation of rehabilitation methods, relaxation techniques, and pharmacologic management. Basic to the assessment is an understanding of where the child may have learned the symptom and particularly what the child's symptom may mean to the child and to the family.

It is important to keep in mind that the symptoms are real to the child, although no specific physical disorder has been diagnosed. Efforts are made to find a way to allow the child honorably to give up the symptoms. For example, a child was referred for assessment of chest pain. He previously had several neurologic examinations and a hospitalization, all unrevealing. When his history was carefully reviewed, it was learned that symptoms began when a soccer ball hit him in the chest and knocked him to the ground. Concurrent with his recovery from the chest injury, his grandfather died of a myocardial infarction. The child slept in the same room with the grandfather, and during the terminal illness his grandfather had suffered severe angina pectoris. The boy was thought to be sleeping when his grandfather was taken out of the home to the hospital. The boy resembled his grandfather in appearance and did not grieve appropriately at the time of his grandfather's death; his mother also had a complicated bereavement. The chest pain was found to be associated with a complicated bereavement response by the child. After successful bereavement counseling, the chest pain resolved and the child could return to school.

Collaborative treatment between the pediatrician and child psychiatrist is recommended. The collaborative approach may be more effective than direct referral following assessment, because the family may not follow through on the referral. Interventions during the hospital stay that address the child's symptomatology and provide a comprehensive assessment of his or her psychopathology are integral to the treatment plan. The treatment plan develops mutually agreed-upon goals and defines carefully the role of each staff member in facilitating return to full functioning.

## Selected Readings

Anthony EJ. Hysteria in childhood. In Roy A, ed. Hysteria. Chichester: Wiley, 1982.

Dubowitz V, Hersov L. Management of children with nonorganic (hysterical) disorders of motor function. Dev Medicine Child Neurol 1976;18:358.

Goodyear I. Hysterical conversion reactions in childhood. J Child Psychol Psychiatry 1981;22:179.

Leslie SA. Diagnosis and treatment of hysterical conversion reactions. Arch Dis Child 1988;63:506.

Minuchin S, Baker L, Rosman BL, et al. A conceptual model of psychosomatic illness in children. Arch Gen Psychiatry 1975;32:1031.

*Principles and Practice of Pediatrics, Second Edition.*
edited by Frank A. Oski et al. J. B. Lippincott Company, Philadelphia © 1994.

# 29.10 *Eating Disorders*

### James C. Harris

Two important syndromes are recognized as eating disorders, anorexia nervosa and bulimia nervosa. Atypical forms occur with less severe symptom presentations. Overeating may be associated with other psychological disturbances. Anorexia nervosa, which we emphasize in this section, is a disorder characterized by deliberate weight loss induced or sustained by the patient, by unusual attitudes toward eating, by profound weight loss, and in females by persistent amenorrhea.

Probably the earliest report of anorexia is from 1659, when Richard Morton provided the following description:

> Mr. Duke's daughter in S. Mary Axe, in the year 1654, in the 18th year of her age, in the month of July, fell ill in a total suppression of her monthly courses from a multitude of cares and passions of her mind. From which time her appetite began to abate, and her digestion to be bad; her flesh also became flaccid and loose and her looks pale with other symptoms usual in universal consumption. I do not remember that I did ever in all my practice see one, that was conversant with the living, so much wasted with the greatest degree of consumption, yet there was no fever but on the contrary a coldness of the body; no cough or difficulty breathing nor an appearance of any other distemper of the lungs, or any other entrail; no looseness nor other signs of colliquation. Only her appetite was diminished and her digestion uneasy with fainting fits which did frequently return upon her.

The German term for the illness is *Pubertatesmagersucht*, which literally means "adolescent pursuit of thinness." It is this pursuit of thinness through dieting that distinguishes anorexia nervosa from other illnesses associated with weight loss. The term "anorexia" is incorrect, because loss of appetite is rarely seen until the patient becomes very emaciated. When continuous control over food intake is impossible, binge eating and vomiting may be used to lose weight. Laxatives and diuretics may be abused for similar reasons and may lead to medical complications if serum potassium levels are lowered, placing the patient at risk for cardiac arrhythmia. Chronic hypokalemia may produce renal tubular damage and persistent vomiting and may lead to dental problems. The presentation is commonly related to weight loss, although symptoms of hypothermia, dependent edema, bradycardia, and hypotension are common.

There is an intense fear of gaining weight and becoming obese, a fear that persists even in the face of increasing cachexia, which contributes to the characteristic disinterest and even resistance to treatment. Despite considerable weight loss, the patient describes a sensation of feeling fat after eating. Particularly in adolescents, there is a disturbance of body image and a lack of awareness of the degree of thinness. The degree of body image distortion is related to the outcome; the greater the distortion in body image, the more difficult it is to enlist the patient's cooperation in treatment.

The initial referral in girls may be for amenorrhea, which may occur before the onset of a major loss in weight. With extreme weight loss, there is a reversion to a prepubertal pattern of luteinizing hormone secretion. Physical and laboratory findings include lymphocytosis, hypocellular bone marrow, low fasting glucose, and elevated serum cholesterol.

## EPIDEMIOLOGY

Anorexia nervosa is primarily a disorder of females; the percentage of males in an anorexic population varies from 4% to 6%. One severe case in every 200 schoolgirls between the ages of 12 and 18 in English boarding schools has been reported. There is indirect evidence to suggest a familial pattern.

The onset of the disorder is ordinarily between ages 10 and 30 years, although younger patients have been reported. Eighty-five percent develop the illness between ages 13 and 20 years. Although rare in the retarded, there are occasional single case reports. There is indirect evidence of an increase in the prevalence of anorexia nervosa in the general population over the past few decades.

## CLINICAL COURSE

The presentation typically begins with concerns about mild obesity, which are followed by negative attitudes toward eating. Despite weight loss and in contrast to ordinary starvation, patients are usually alert and cheerful. They may also be overactive and engage in strenuous exercise, often in a specific effort to lose weight.

From the beginning of the illness, unusual behavior relating to food is seen. This includes gorging and induced vomiting and secretly hoarding food around the home. Amenorrhea may begin before, with, or after the disturbance in appetite.

The course varies from spontaneous recovery without treatment; to recovery after a single episode following a variety of treatments; to a fluctuating course of weight gain, with a series of relapses; and less commonly to a deteriorating course resulting in death due to complications of illness or starvation. The mortality rates at 4-year follow-up have been reported in the range of 5%; however, it is likely that mortality rates are decreasing with earlier diagnosis and referral. The best indicator of good outcome is an early age of onset. Poor prognostic factors are late age of onset and recurrent hospitalization. The primary impairments are the need for hospitalization and the effects of the disorder on peer relationships. An increased frequency of mood disorder has been reported among first-degree relatives of young people with anorexia nervosa.

## PREDISPOSING FACTORS

The illness may be associated with a stressful life situation. Children with anorexia nervosa are commonly described as being overly perfectionistic and model children before the onset of the illness.

The diagnostic criteria are as follows:

1. Refusal to maintain body weight over a minimum normal range for age and height (eg, weight loss leading to maintenance of body weight 15% below that expected), or failure to make expected weight gain during a period of growth, leading to a body weight 15% below that expected for age
2. intense fear of gaining weight or becoming fat, even though underweight
3. Disturbance in the way in which one's body weight, size, or shape is experienced (eg, the patient claims to feel fat even when emaciated and believes that one area of the body is "too fat" even when she is obviously underweight)
4. In females, the absence of at least three consecutive menstrual cycles at times when they are expected to occur (primary or secondary amenorrhea).

# DIFFERENTIAL DIAGNOSIS

In adolescence, this disorder must be differentiated from depressive disorders. Patients who are depressed do not become preoccupied with the caloric content of food, nor do they show food preoccupations, excessively collect recipes, or spend inordinate amounts of time preparing food. They do not deny the existence of a normal appetite but have a decreased appetite. Some patients may have both diagnoses; if so, both diagnoses should be made. In a somatization disorder, weight loss and vomiting can occur, but the weight loss tends not to be as severe, the patient is not preoccupied with losing weight, and amenorrhea is seldom a consistent finding. In schizophrenia there may be delusions about food, but the focus is not on the caloric content of food. Schizophrenic patients are not preoccupied with becoming obese and do not demonstrate the hyperactivity often seen in anorexia nervosa. Rarely, both of these diagnoses may occur.

*Bulimia* is a behavior present in about half of anorexia nervosa patients. It is differentiated diagnostically in that bulimic patients maintain their weight within a normal range despite large fluctuations in weight. Currently it is suggested that anorexic patients with bulimia are a subgroup among patients with this disorder (ie, anorexia nervosa, bulimic type). In this population self-induced vomiting, laxative abuse, and diuretic abuse are more prevalent. One may also see an increased evidence of impulsive behavior, alcohol and street drug abuse, suicide, and stealing. A separate diagnosis of bulimia nervosa is indicated for repeated bouts of overeating and preoccupation with the control of body weight that lead to behavior to mitigate the "fattening" effects of food. It may occur as a sequel to persistent anorexia nervosa (see ICD-10 criteria).

# ASSESSMENT

Interviews are conducted with both the patient and family members, because the anorexic patient may deny the characteristics of the disorder. In some instances, a diagnostic admission is necessary to make independent observations and clarify the diagnosis. Family history information should be gathered regarding eating disorders, depression, and alcoholism. During the assessment, how parents manage dieting and weight loss is assessed. The function of the symptom within family relationships is evaluated. Previous treatment must be considered, and a comprehensive physical examination must be conducted.

Psychological evaluation is carried out to determine both educational ability and intelligence level, since many affected young people are unrealistic in their own expectations of school performance and have been overachievers in the earlier years of school.

The mental status examination specifically addresses the questions regarding diagnostic criteria for the disorder. It should also address the patient's attitudes toward other family members and responses to siblings' and parents' behaviors and conflicts. It should identify social or sexual fears and review peer relationships. Specific questions about depressive symptoms and sleep disturbances are asked.

# TREATMENT

The treatment involves multiple therapeutic modalities, including the medical management of the weight loss and, depending on the case, individual, behavioral, or family treatment.

Patients tend to be unwilling and reluctant to be evaluated. Symptoms such as sleep disorder, depression, and the frustration about obsessive thoughts regarding food and body weight that interfere with ongoing life goals must be addressed. Reestablishing peer relationships may also be an important issue. Parental support for the treatment plan is essential.

The first step is to restore nutritional status. With weight gain, changes in mood, particularly decreased irritability and depression, less preoccupation with food, and an improvement in sleep may occur. Restoring weight generally requires a structured environment, often in a hospital. Outpatient treatment may be indicated in the following circumstances: early age of onset, symptoms present for less than 4 months, lack of vomiting or binging, and cooperative parents who can establish an appropriate structure at home and actively participate in family therapy.

Both outpatient and inpatient management are important to discuss with the family on initial visits because inpatient treatment may be needed. More severely ill patients require daily monitoring of their weight, fluid intake, caloric intake, and fluid output. The vomiting patient needs frequent assessment for serum electrolytes. In some instances, food supplements may be required to provide adequate calories. Refeeding edema may be noted if food intake is increased too rapidly. One approach is to provide a daily caloric intake to maintain admission weight and an additional 50% for increased activity. Daily caloric intake can be increased up to 50% every 5 days. Meals may also be divided into six equal feedings to avoid ingestions of large amounts of food at one time.

The whole family may participate in some cases; in others, marital therapy with both parents may be indicated. In still other instances, separate parent/patient or sibling/patient sessions may be required.

In a hospital milieu, nursing treatment programs can provide a regular feeding intervention by incorporating behavioral management principles in treatment. These include, for the overactive patient, making activity contingent on weight gain and requiring strict bed rest if weight is not gained. Some authors suggest that regular feedback be given about weight gain. Weighing should be done before breakfast in the same hospital gown each morning.

A baseline observation period of several days in the hospital is helpful in developing a behavioral management program to complement the medical rehabilitation and nutritional approach. Positive reinforcement, making physical activity contingent on weight gain, and participating in hospital programs should be encouraged. In addition to weight gain, behavioral approaches can be used to address vomiting by making the patient responsible for cleaning up after vomiting, and by using a commode in the room; regular bathroom privileges can subsequently be resumed. Other contingencies include remaining with other patients for 2 hours after eating.

During the initial hospitalization in which weight gain is facilitated, personal psychotherapy and family therapy are initiated to help maintain weight. Weight gain goals can be set in a 5-lb range, with the goal being to reach the middle of that range and then to maintain this weight at home. Of particular importance is the ongoing counseling of family members as an adjunct to behavioral treatments and individual or family therapy. Pharmacotherapy may include drugs such as amitriptyline and cyproheptadine.

Individual treatment approaches, rather than focusing on past life experiences, are initially centered on the present, addressing the patient's awareness of her behavior, the effect it has on maintaining her illness, and specifically emphasizing her responsibility for her own feelings and emotional states. Cognitive themes address fear of failure and anxieties about becoming independent from the family and acknowledging age-appropriate responsibilities. Considerable time is needed to deal with denial of the illness and to help the adolescent become aware of her need to control the environment through maladaptive behavior.

Anxiety and preoccupation with weight persist as weight is gained, requiring continued outpatient treatment. Outpatient management includes a behavioral contract, personal treatment for the child, and family treatment. Regular weekly weights are recorded. If weight falls below the agreed-upon level, removal from sports activities at school may be necessary.

Anorexia nervosa is a difficult, time-consuming condition to treat and is associated with a wide range of psychopathology. Early diagnosis and early vigorous intervention are effective in reducing its morbidity and mortality.

## Selected Readings

Bruch H. Eating disorders: obesity, anorexia nervosa and the person within. London: Routledge and Kegan Paul, 1974.

Fava M, Copeland PM, Schweiger U, Herzog DB. Neurochemical abnormalities of anorexia nervosa and bulimia nervosa. Am J Psychiatry 1989;146:963.

Goodwin DW, Guze SB. Anorexia nervosa. In Goodwin DW, Guze SB, eds. Psychiatric diagnosis, ed 3. Oxford: Oxford University Press, 1984.

Halmi KA. The diagnosis and treatment of anorexia nervosa. In Shaffer D, Ehrhardt, Greenhill LL, eds. The clinical guide to child psychiatry, New York: The Free Press, 1985.

Hodes M, Eisler I, Dare C. Family therapy for anorexia nervosa in adolescence: a review. J Roy Soc Med 1991;84:359.

Kennedy SH, Garfinkel PE. Advances in diagnosis and treatment of anorexia nervosa and bulimia nervosa. Can J Psychiatry 1992;37:309.

Nagel KL, Jones KH. Predisposition factors in anorexia nervosa. Adolescence 1992;27:381.

Steinhausen HC, Rauss-Mason C, Seidel R. Follow-up studies of anorexia nervosa: a review of four decades of outcome research. Psychol Med 1991;21:447.

*Principles and Practice of Pediatrics, Second Edition.*
edited by Frank A. Oski et al. J. B. Lippincott Company, Philadelphia © 1994.

# 29.11 *Pervasive Developmental Disorder/Autism*

James C. Harris

In 1980 the term *pervasive developmental disorder* (PDD) was introduced into the child psychiatric classification to describe children whose developmental difficulties cross multiple developmental lines. This category has been substantially expanded from one specific disorder, autistic disorder, to the inclusion of several other conditions in ICD-10. In DSM-IV these other conditions will be included as they are in ICD-10. The conditions described as PDD in ICD-10 are childhood autism, atypical autism, Rett syndrome (see Chap. 27.2), other childhood disintegrative disorder, overactivity associated with mental retardation and stereotypical movements, Asperger's syndrome, other and unspecified forms of PDD. Autistic disorder is described here; the ICD-10 and DSM-IV classifications should be consulted for the other conditions.

This category is particularly pertinent for the syndrome of autistic disorder, in which social, language, and cognitive deficits are apparent. The relationship between cognitive deficits and social abnormalities has been a focus of recent research. Diagnostic criteria have been introduced that focus on qualitative impairments in social interactions and in interpersonal communication, along with a stereotyped restricted pattern of interests and activities. These abnormalities affect functioning in all situations and in most instances are present from infancy onward. However, sometimes the onset is after the first year of life. The time of onset continues to be an area of research focus. The disorder is defined in terms of behavior that is deviant in relation to the child's mental age. The vast majority of children with this disorder have mental subnormality as a feature of their PDD. There are ongoing efforts to identify subgroups with this condition as described above. The relationship between cognitive deficits and social behavior is of particular interest.

Confusion sometimes exists about the language disorder in PDD, related to the dual nature and function of language. Language serves the purposes of being a mental tool in thinking and also the primary means of communication with others. Children with PDD have the most difficulty with the practical use of language as a communication tool (pragmatic language). The language disorder is in social communication, in sharing and discussing observations and thoughts. Sharing experiences with others is difficult regardless of the child's intellectual level. There are particular problems in communicating feelings because of the child's difficulty in interpreting the meaning of tone of voice, posture, and facial expression in others. Additionally, shared experience requires memories of one's own emotional experience in order to share the other person's frame of reference. Remembering and sharing affective experience is also a problem, particularly for the lower-functioning autistic person. There are deficits not only in initiating verbal social communication, but also in understanding the nonverbal communication of others.

## HISTORICAL BACKGROUND

The first description of a pervasive developmental disorder was by Kanner in 1943, when he described 11 children in his paper "Autistic Disturbances of Affective Contact." The emphasis was on the inability to develop relationships with other people, aloofness, delayed speech development, noncommunicative use of speech, lack of imagination, and efforts to maintain sameness in the environment. Rather than a withdrawal from previous social interests, these children from early life did not develop social communication. Subsequently there were differences of opinion regarding the term *autism*, the clinical features, and the role of psychosocial experience in the etiology.

It was not until 1980 that essentially the same criteria that Kanner introduced became formal parts of the psychiatric classification. By that time, autism had been distinguished from schizophrenia beginning in childhood, and it had become evident that it is a psychobiological condition whose course might be affected by psychosocial interventions but that was not caused by psychosocial circumstance. Most children with this disorder are mentally subnormal, and those who function at the lowest levels are the most symptomatic.

## DIAGNOSTIC ISSUES

Autism is seen as the most severe form of PDD. Impaired development is manifest before age 3 years, with characteristic abnormal functioning in social interactions, communication, and restricted, repetitive behavior. When the full autistic syndrome is not present, the term *atypical autism* is used in ICD-10. It may be atypical in regard to the age of onset or in not meeting the full diagnostic criteria. Asperger's syndrome should be considered in children with no general delay or retardation in language or in cognitive development who show qualitative abnormality in social interaction and demonstrate restricted, stereotyped interests. If the child has a period of normal development followed by a loss of previously acquired developmental skills (including social, communicative, and behavioral functions) that persists over time, the general diagnosis *childhood disintegrative disorder* may be used. Overall, the younger the child, the more severe the handicap and the more associated problems.

Associated with PDD are abnormalities in cognitive skills. The specific skill profile is usually uneven regardless of the level of intelligence. In most cases there is associated mental subnormality, most commonly in the moderate range (IQ 35 to 49). Abnormalities of posture and motor behavior may occur, such as stereotypes including repetitive jumping, grimacing, and arm flapping when excited, as well as walking on tiptoe and unusual hand or body postures. Motor coordination is variable. There may be unusual responses to sensory input; for example, insensitivity or excessive sensitivity to pain, cold, or heat, covering the ears in response to some sounds or resistance to being touched, and preoccupations with perceptual sensations, such as lights or odors. There also may be associated abnormalities in eating, drinking, or sleeping, with diet limited to a few foods, excessive fluid intake, or recurrent waking at night. It is difficult to identify feeling states in most of the younger children. Lack of fear of realistic dangers is of particular concern. One may see fluctuations in mood for no reason, but absence of emotional reactions is far more common. Self-injury may occur with head-banging or self-biting.

Other major mental disorders may also occur in autism, such as major depression or schizophrenia in adolescents. The simultaneity of these diagnoses is more easily recognized in higher-functioning individuals whose speech allows them to describe their symptoms accurately.

## ETIOLOGY

Autism has been associated with some genetic syndromes, such as phenylketonuria and the fragile X syndrome. The disorder occurs in boys three to four times more often than in girls. An increased prevalence has been shown in siblings of autistic children, of whom 2% are affected with the full syndrome. Because the general population risk is four per 10,000, this represents a 50-fold increase for siblings. The disorder has also been found more frequently (Folstein and Rutter, 1977) in same-sex twins: four of 11 twin pairs who were monozygotic were concordant for the disorder, but it occurred in none of ten dizygotic twin pairs. An increased association of organic brain dysfunction was noted in the affected twin, suggesting the possibility that genetic factors and postpartum stress may interact. However, it is unclear whether it is autism per se or a cognitive profile related to learning problems that is inherited, because the prevalence of learning difficulties is also increased in siblings.

## TREATMENT

The approach to treatment in autism requires clarification of the diagnosis and the development of an individual treatment plan. Autistic children have an abnormality in their development that involves socialization, language, and cognition. They are both delayed and deviant in each of these areas. Most autistic children (85%) are mentally retarded as well; they have a pattern of cognitive abilities that is uneven, with enhanced factual memory and visual-spatial and puzzle-solving abilities, but deficits in symbolic operations, conceptual understanding, and abstract abilities. Language is delayed, and some children do not acquire speech. When language does develop, it is abnormal in its development, particularly because the children fail to use language for the purpose of social communication in a normal socially reciprocal fashion characteristic for their age. Use of stereotyped phrases and echoing back words are common problems. Finally, socialization itself is deviant, and early milestones in initiating social interaction (eg, reaching to be picked up, developing selective attachments, shaking one's head no, recognizing the meaning of others' facial expressions, using the eyes to communicate needs, pointing with one finger, and developing social attachments) are abnormal. As the autistic child gets older, he or she wants to have friendships but often does not know how to go about establishing them.

Treatment is further complicated by the child's rigidity and inflexibility in learning new skills. Skills are often learned concretely, but generalizing to new situations is difficult. Applying knowledge to new situations is problematic, and a fear of change may be expressed with a preference for maintaining routines. Play is not imaginative, particularly at the younger ages. Objects are lined up and placed in patterns rather than used in an imaginative way. When imaginative activities do develop, they tend to be stereotyped, and specific rituals may be seen that have a strong compulsive or perseverative quality. Object attachment is deviant in that attachment is to inanimate objects such as stones, belts, or cans rather than to soft toys. Additionally, treatment of associated overactivity, behavioral disruption, tantrums, aggressiveness, and self-injury is required. Some children develop phobias and fears or have difficulty with sleep and with developing toileting routines. Each of these areas needs to be addressed in any treatment plan.

The overall goals of treatment are to foster normal development, to promote specific language development, to promote social interaction, and to promote learning. Treatment requires the establishment of active meaningful experiences. This involves planned periods of interaction, simplified communication, selection of specific learning tasks, and direct teaching. Individual therapy has a psychoeducational base to help the child understand and make appropriate adaptations. Family treatment is needed to help the family understand the nature of the disorder and to resolve guilt. Behavioral approaches are directed toward particular target symptoms such as self-injury.

## Selected Readings

Denckla MB, James LS, eds. An update on autism: a developmental disorder. Pediatrics 1991;87(part 2 suppl).

Folstein SE, Rutter M. Infantile autism: a genetic study of 21 twin pairs. J Child Psychology and Psychiatry 1977;18:297.

Frith U. Autism and Asperger syndrome. New York: Cambridge University Press, 1991.

Happe F, Frith U, Gillberg C, Volkmar FR, Cohen DJ. Is autism a pervasive developmental disorder? J Child Psychol Psychiatry 1991;7:1167.

Kanner L. Autistic disturbances of affective contact. Nerv Child 1943;2:217.

Prior M, Cummins R. Questions about facilitated communication and autism. J Autism Devel Disorders 1992;22:331.

Rogers SJ, Pennington BF. A theoretical approach to the deficits in infantile autism. Development and Psychopathology 1991;3:137.

Rutter M. The treatment of autistic children. J Child Psychol Psychiat 1985;26:193.

Szatmari P, Barttolucci G, Bremner R. Asperger's syndrome and autism: comparison of early history and outcome. Devel Med Child Neurol 1989;31:709.

Volkmar FR. Childhood disintegrative disorder: issues for DSM-IV. J Autism Devel Disorders 1992;22:625.

Volkmar FR, Cicchetti DV, Bregman J, Cohen DJ. Three diagnostic systems for autism. J Autism Devel Disorders 1992;22:483.

Whitehouse DW, Harris J. Hyperlexia in infantile autism. J Autism Devel Disorders 1984;11:31.

Wing L. Autism: a guide for parents and professionals. New York: Brunner/Mazel, 1985.

*Principles and Practice of Pediatrics, Second Edition.*
edited by Frank A. Oski et al. J. B. Lippincott Company, Philadelphia © 1994.

# 29.12 *Sleep Disorders*

## James C. Harris

Whereas disturbance in sleep is a common report in adults, children generally do not complain about sleep difficulties, although their parents might; more often, children's sleep problems go unrecognized and untreated. The usual concern presented by parents is of irregular sleep habits, insufficient or too much sleep, problems at bedtime, poor sleep, waking during the night, nightmares, night terrors, sleepwalking, bedwetting, and sleepiness during the day. Some disorders are more severe, such as narcolepsy, the sleep apnea syndrome, and sudden infant death syndrome associated with apnea. In addition, injuries may occur during sleepwalking. In other instances sleep problems may be related to other disorders, such as epilepsy with nighttime seizures or depression.

Sleep is one aspect of the 25-hour circadian sleep–wake cycle that is entrained to a 24-hour clock. Time cues related to bedtime and wake time, mealtime, and school schedules are all considerations in the daily cycle. The sleep cycle is accompanied by particular hormonal rhythms that occur during sleep, such as growth hormone, prolactin, and cortisol release, which is coupled with sleep. Growth hormone is released shortly after falling asleep during deep sleep, and prolactin reaches its peak between 5 and 7 o'clock in the morning. Corticosteroid secretion ordinarily is initiated during the night but becomes desynchronized in sleep with changes in the sleep–wake schedule. When the sleep schedule changes, cortisol is initially released at the same time as before, but it gradually adjusts to the new cycle.

Ordinarily, sleep problems are evaluated on an outpatient basis; more complicated cases, however, may require inpatient sleep laboratory assessment. Recent developments in classification of sleep problems have provided new information about when these assessments should be carried out.

## EPIDEMIOLOGY

The development of sleep is related to age. As children become older there are decreases in total amount of sleep, total amount of rapid eye movement (REM) sleep, and total amount of Stage 3-4 (deep) sleep. In premature infants, sleep is marked by more wakefulness than in full-term infants, with more irregularity and instability in the sleep–wake mechanism. In infancy, the amounts of REM sleep or active sleep are substantially greater than they are later in life, with almost half of the infant's time in the first week of life being spent in REM sleep. With time the REM sleep cycles are shifted to the second half of the night.

As children become older, separation anxiety becomes more of an issue for toddlers and young children; bedtime fears, nightmares, bedwetting, and night terrors emerge. The older group, particularly the adolescent, begins to show sleep patterns similar to those of adults. Difficulty falling asleep, waking during the night, difficulty getting up in the morning, and daytime sleepiness are commonly reported in adolescence. There are individual differences in sleep requirements and patterns among children, so rigid sleep schedules may complicate bedtime difficulties and sleep problems.

During the first year of life, following the establishment of a full-night sleep pattern, there is a period of wakefulness at approximately 9 to 11 months of age, followed by the reestablishment of a full night pattern. In toddlers, the major difficulties are in settling down to sleep and in nighttime waking. In the preschool child, problems around extensive bedtime routines and resisting falling asleep are common. One study found that two thirds of normal 5-year-olds require more than 30 minutes to fall asleep.

In the grade-school years, parents often note restless sleep. Sleep-related problems are increased in children with ear, nose, and throat symptoms. Children with emotional and behavioral difficulties have significantly higher numbers of sleep complaints than children who are not disordered. Achenbach found that clinically referred children had higher rates of nightmares, excessive tiredness, excessive sleep, difficulty with sleeping, and too little sleep compared to normal children. Simeon found, in a sample of 962 normal children and 103 child psychiatry patients, that sleep taking, difficulty falling asleep, night waking, and enuresis, as well as overtiredness, were three times higher among patients than in the normal group. Poor or restless sleep was six times as frequent.

Sex differences were not noted among normal children, but there were large differences between males and females in the psychiatric population, with boys having more sleep talking, enuresis, early morning waking, and daytime naps. Girls reported more restless sleep, night waking, and poor sleep. Therefore, both normal and behaviorally disturbed children have a variety of sleep problems. Furthermore, there is an association between frequency of sleep problems and psychological and behavioral disorders.

## CLASSIFICATION

The classification system for sleep disorders deals with chronic disorders, not transient disturbances that are part of everyday life. Sleep problems lasting a few nights following a psychosocial stressor are not diagnosed as sleep disorders. However, children who are chronically symptomatic for more than a month require further assessment for diagnosis and treatment.

Problems in sleep accompany both mental and physical disorders, particularly conditions involving changes in mood and those causing pain or discomfort. Sleep disturbances may occur at the beginning of an illness and can exacerbate other disorders. However, if the sleep disturbance is the predominant complaint, sleep disorder is the primary diagnosis.

The two major groups of sleep disorders are the dyssomnias and the parasomnias. In dyssomnia the primary difficulty and disturbance is in the quality, timing, or amount of sleep. In parasomnia, the primary disturbance is an abnormal event that occurs during sleep. Other conditions, such as sleep apnea, which is associated with increased daytime sleepiness, and narcolepsy, are classified as hypersomnias related to a known organic factor. Nocturnal enuresis occurring in the first third of the night and associated with sudden arousal from sleep may be regarded as a sleep disorder. A primary sleep condition independent of known mental or physical conditions would, for example, be considered a primary insomnia or hypersomnia.

Dyssomnias are manifested by disturbances in the quality, amount, or timing of sleep. Included are insomnias, hypersomnias, and sleep–wake schedule disorders. In insomnia, sleep is deficient in quality or in an amount necessary for normal active daytime functioning. In hypersomnia, the individual feels excessively sleepy during the daytime despite apparently normal sleep length. In the sleep–wake schedule disorders, the person's sleeping and daytime waking pattern is different and is not in keeping with an appropriate day–night routine for the environment. Insomnia includes a complaint of difficulty in both initiating and maintaining sleep or of not feeling rested after sleep that is apparently adequate.

To make the diagnosis, the sleep problem must occur at least three times a week for at least a month, and must lead to complaints of daytime fatigue or observations by others of symptoms related to sleep, such as irritability. It may be primarily related to a known organic factor or related to a nonorganic mental disorder.

There is considerable variation in the amount of time it takes for a person to fall asleep or in the amount of sleep that an individual feels is needed to be alert and rested. Ordinarily, sleep begins within 30 minutes after establishing a setting that is appropriate for sleep, although sleep length is variable depending on age. Insomnia may be complicated by treatment with pharmacologic agents such as sedatives or hypnotics. It occurs more often following periods of stress and is related to behavioral or emotional symptoms.

With childhood onset insomnia, it may take longer to fall asleep, and the sleep may be ill defined and associated with an atypical electroencephalographic (EEG) abnormality. In adolescents, the complaint may be difficulty in falling asleep or premature wakening. In other instances, there may be a delayed sleep phase syndrome in which sleep onset difficulties are associated with difficulty waking in the morning. However, if the individual is allowed to continue to sleep, he sleeps a normal number of hours. Price found that normal 11th- and 12th-grade students reported a 12.6% incidence of severe sleep disturbance. Those with the sleep problems also reported more tension, worries, moodiness, and difficulty with solving personal problems, as well as low self-esteem.

Insomnia may occur in conjunction with another mental disorder such as depressive disorder, anxiety disorder, and adjustment disorder with anxious mood or obsessive-compulsive personality. As noted, insomnia also may occur because of a known organic factor, such as a specific medical condition and the use of psychoactive drugs. These disorders are generally symptomatic when the patient is awake or asleep, as in the case of pain. However, some physical disorders seem symptomatic only during sleep, as seen in sleep apnea where waking respiration is normal. Drugs commonly influencing sleep are amphetamines or other stimulants, corticosteroids, and bronchodilators. However, psychoactive drugs and alcohol or amphetamine dependence may disturb sleep as well.

In primary insomnia, the individual frequently worries about not being able to fall asleep at night, and this may become a preoccupation. The individual's worries about possibly unsuccessful attempts to fall asleep increase arousal. However, he might be able to fall asleep when not trying to sleep, for example, while watching television or when away from the usual environment.

## HYPERSOMNIA DISORDERS

Children and adolescents with excessive daytime sleepiness (EDS) or somnolence may be thought to be inattentive and be labeled as lazy or poor learners. These symptoms may be a consequence of disrupted nighttime sleep in disorders such as sleep apnea and narcolepsy. However, these complaints sometimes are minimized by clinicians. The onset of excessive daytime sleepiness often first occurs during adolescence. A careful medical examination and sleep history, as well as physical examination, are important.

The primary features are excessive daytime sleepiness or sleep attacks (not accounted for by inadequate amount of sleep), or prolonged transition into a fully awake state when awakening (sleep drunkenness). The condition occurs every day for at least a month or episodically for longer periods of time and is severe enough to interfere with social activities, relationships, and school. Hypersomnia disorders may be primary or related to nonorganic mental factors, or organic conditions. Daytime sleepiness is defined as falling asleep easily, often in 5 minutes or less, anytime during the day, even after a normal prolonged amount of night sleep. Falling asleep is unintentional, making sleep attacks discrete periods of sudden irresistible sleep. Ordinarily, hypersomnia is present every day; it is most commonly related to sleep apnea or narcolepsy. It may be episodic in the Kleine/Levin syndrome and in some forms of atypical depression.

The course of this condition is related to the presence of other associated physical or mental disorders or to the primary condition. Social and occupational impairment may be mild or severe. Individuals with these problems may become demoralized, and the complications of accidental injury may ensue because of the excessive sleepiness.

Hypersomnia may be related to another mental disorder, particularly mood disorders such as depression. Hypersomnia associated with mental disorders occurs more often in adolescence; in contrast, older adults typically complain of insomnia. In other mental disorders such as somatoform disorder, personality disorder, or schizophrenia, hypersomnia is uncommon; daytime drowsiness is attributed to nonrestorative sleep.

The majority of cases of hypersomnia or excessive daytime somnolence are related to a known organic factor. About half of these are associated with sleep apnea, about 25% with narcolepsy, and 10% with sleep-related myoclonus.

If the hypersomnia is related to narcolepsy, cataplexy (episodic loss of muscle tone initiated by strong emotions) hypnagogic or hypnopompic hallucinations, and sleep paralysis (inability to move while falling asleep or upon sudden wakening) occur.

Narcolepsy ordinarily begins around the time of puberty. However, obstructive sleep apnea is seen primarily in infants and in older children with large tonsils and adenoids. Both of these conditions lead to impairment. In narcolepsy the person tries to exert control over his emotions, and this may lead to a lack of expressiveness that affects social relations. Individuals with sleep apnea may demonstrate mood changes or irritability, distractibility, and difficulty with attention and memory. On the other hand, primary hypersomnia is not related to another mental disorder or known organic factor.

## Sleep Apnea Hypersomnia Syndrome

Sleep apnea hypersomnia syndrome may occur in children of any age, but the incidence increases with age and involves males more often than females. Predisposing factors include enlarged tonsils or adenoids, upper airway or maxillofacial abnormalities, hyperthyroidism, and obesity. There is associated loud snoring followed by pauses in respiration and brief arousals that are often accompanied by restless movements. Associated symptoms include decreased school performance, excessive daytime sleepiness, recurrence of nocturnal enuresis, morning headaches, changes in mood and personality, changes in weight, and, if the condition is persistent and severe, development of pulmonary hypertension. Its effect on intellectual functioning may be greater than that of narcolepsy. Some children may be misdiagnosed as being intellectually limited. If symptoms are unrecognized at night, with time, symptoms may become more apparent during the day, particularly if cardiovascular or pulmonary abnormalities develop.

The sudden infant death syndrome (SIDS) is thought to relate to apnea in infants. It is responsible for the death of two to three infants per every thousand live births. Children at greater risk are those who have had prior intensive care and whose mothers are addicted to drugs. It occurs more often in males. Near-miss

SIDS is a disorder with various unrelated respiratory, cardiac, or sleep-stage difficulties. Siblings of children with this disorder may have a three- to fourfold increase of SIDS. Some studies have suggested longer intervals between active sleep in the newborn and a decreased tendency to enter short waking periods for 2 to 3 months, suggesting an increased tendency to remain asleep or a problem in arousal from sleep.

## Kleine-Levin Syndrome

In Kleine-Levin syndrome hypersomnia occurs in adolescent males and is associated with excessive eating and frequently with weight gain, abnormal sexuality, and mood disorders. It may represent hypothalamic and diencephalic dysfunction.

## Narcolepsy

Twenty percent of adult narcoleptics report that they had daytime sleepiness before age 11. Children with this disorder are usually referred when teachers complain about napping during class in school. Unrecognized microsleep may occur, and others may be unaware that naps are taking place. Children with this disorder have been viewed by teachers as poorly motivated and are thought to have attention deficits or learning problems. The child may become active or apparently overactive as he struggles with sleepiness. Hypnagogic, auditory, or visual hallucinations are vivid, often frightening, and may not be reported to parents. Children with this condition may be fearful of going to bed because of their hallucinatory experiences. Unlike those with seizure disorders, children who lose muscle tone with this condition remain aware of their surroundings.

## SLEEP–WAKE SCHEDULE DISORDERS

In sleep–wake schedule disorders there is a lack of synchronization between normal sleep–wake schedules demanded by the external environment and the individual's internal circadian rhythm. This results in complaints of either insomnia or hypersomnia, because the individual has difficulty in falling asleep until late at night and also has problems in waking the following day. Children with this condition may meet the criteria for either insomnia or hypersomnia disorder.

## DELAYED SLEEP PHASE OR ADVANCED SLEEP PHASE DISORDER

In this condition the onset of sleep is advanced or delayed in relation to sleep. If advanced cycles are evident, the individual falls asleep early in the evening and wakes for the day in the middle of the night. In the delayed type, sleep occurs later in the evening and waking occurs in the middle of the day. There is also a disorganized type in which sleep is generally random in pattern, and there is no major daily sleep period. Finally, the frequently changing type is the result of frequent changes in sleeping and waking times, eg, airline travel involving time zone changes.

Associated with sleep phase disorder are nonspecific symptoms such as lack of energy and irritability or malaise. Because the circadian rhythm normally lengthens during adolescence, there is an increased vulnerability to the delayed type during this age period. The disorganized type may occur at any age. Impairment in social function is primarily related to the time of day that the sleep disturbance occurs. The condition may be complicated by accidents because of lack of alertness. The DSM-IV diagnostic criteria for Circadian Rhythm Sleep Disorder are a mismatch between the normal sleep–wake schedule for a person's environment and his or her circadian sleep–wake pattern, resulting in complaints of either insomnia or hypersomnia.

## PARASOMNIAS

In this group of conditions an abnormal event occurs either during sleep or at the threshold between wakefulness and sleep. The primary complaint is this disturbance and not sleepiness or wakefulness, although symptoms such as sleep apnea, which occur during sleep, may lead to a complaint of daytime sleepiness. In a parasomnia such as night terror, the parent, not the child, complains about the event. From the perspective of the sleep disorder classification, enuresis occurring during sleep is a parasomnia. In some instances nocturnal seizure disorders may mimic the symptoms of parasomnia, thus requiring an overnight EEG to clarify whether or not the seizures are related to particular sleep stages.

## SLEEP TERROR DISORDER (PAVOR NOCTURNUS)

Pavor nocturnus is a condition marked by repeated episodes of abrupt wakening from sleep. It usually begins with a scream, and the episode ordinarily occurs during the first third of the night, in the first interval of nonrapid eye movement (NREM) sleep. Sleep terror is accompanied by EEG delta activity (sleep stages 3 and 4) and lasts 1 to 10 minutes.

In a typical episode, the child sits up abruptly in bed, appears frightened, and demonstrates signs of intense anxiety, including dilated pupils, excessive perspiration, piloerection, rapid breathing, and rapid pulse. The child is unresponsive to the efforts of others to comfort him or her until the agitation and confusion subside as the child gradually awakens. On the following morning there is no memory of the episode, and behavior may be entirely normal. Occasionally, the child recounts a sense of terror on being aroused from the night terror, but there are only fragmentary mental images unlike the recall of a dream. These episodes occur more often with fatigue and following stress.

Prior to a severe episode, EEG delta waves may be higher in amplitude than usual for that phase of sleep, and breathing and heart rate may be slower. The episode itself may be accompanied by a twofold or fourfold increase in heart rate. There is no consistently associated psychopathology with night terror in children. The age of onset is ordinarily between 4 and 12 years. The course is variable, usually occurring in intervals of days or weeks, but episodes may occur on consecutive nights. The disorder gradually resolves in children and often disappears by early adolescence.

The primary impairment related to sleep terror disorder is related to the avoidance of situations when others might become aware of the disturbance. The child must be protected if he gets up during the episode, to avoid accidental injury. Febrile illness has been reported as a predisposing factor. The prevalence is estimated to be 1% to 4% for the full disorder, although a larger percentage of children may have isolated symptoms. It is a condition more common in males than in females. The disorder is more common among first degree relatives of people with the disorder than in the general population (Table 29-4).

Treatment consists primarily of educating the family regarding the nature of the parasomnia. In those instances in which symptoms occur quite frequently and are disruptive to the family, pharmacologic treatment with diazepam (Valium) or alprazolam may be indicated.

TABLE 29-4.  Diagnostic Criteria
for Sleep Terror Disorder

A. Recurrent episodes of abrupt awakening from sleep, usually occurring during the first third of the major sleep episode and beginnng with a panicky scream.

B. Intense anxiety and signs of autonomic arousal during each episode, such as tachycardia, rapid breathing, and sweating.

C. No detailed dream is recalled, and there is amnesia for the episode.

D. Relative unresponsiveness to efforts of others to comfort the person during the episode.

E. Not due to the direct effects of substance (eg, drugs of abuse, medication) or a general medical condition.

*Reprinted with permission from the Diagnostic and Statistical Manual of Mental Disorders, 4th ed, draft criteria. American Psychiatric Association, in press.*

## SLEEPWALKING DISORDER

In sleepwalking there are repeated episodes of complex moments that lead to leaving bed and walking without the individual's being conscious of the episode or remembering it. It ordinarily occurs during the first third of the major sleep period, the period of NREM sleep that contains EEG delta activity, referred to as phases 3 and 4. Sleepwalking lasts for a few minutes to about half an hour. In a typical episode the child sits up, makes perseverative movements such as picking at a blanket, then proceeds to semipurposeful movements including walking, opening doors, eating, dressing, or going to the bathroom. The episode may terminate before sleepwalking is accomplished.

When observed, the sleepwalker has a blank face, appears to stare and is unresponsive to the efforts of others to communicate with him or efforts to influence the sleepwalking. Awakening is accomplished only with great difficulty. Coordination is poor during the episode; however, the individual may see and walk around objects. He may stumble or lose balance and be injured, particularly when taking a hazardous route. If walking terminates spontaneously, the child awakens but is disoriented. In other instances the child may return to bed without reaching con-

TABLE 29-5.  Specific Criteria for Sleepwalking

A. Repeated episodes of arising from bed during sleep and walking about, usually occurring during the first third of the major sleep episode.

B. While sleepwalking, the person has a blank, staring face, is relatively unresponsive to the efforts of others to communicate with him or her, and can be awakened only with great difficulty.

*Specify* type:

**Delayed sleep phase type:** A persistent pattern of late sleep onset and late awakening times, with an inability to fall asleep and awaken at a desired earlier time.

**Jet lag type:** Sleepiness and alertness that occur at an inappropriate time of day relative to local time, occurring after repeated travel across more than one time zone.

**Shift work type:** Insomnia during major sleep period or excessive sleepiness during major wake period associated with night-shift work or frequently changing shift work.

**Unspecified.**

*Reprinted with permission from the Diagnostic and Statistical Manual of Mental Disorders, 4th ed, draft criteria. American Psychiatric Association, in press.*

sciousness, or may fall asleep in another place away from the bed and be surprised at finding himself there on waking.

On the EEG, slow waves may increase in amplitude in stage 4 sleep just preceding the episode. There is a flattening of the EEG, indicating arousal before the episode itself. Ordinarily in sleepwalking, the high-amplitude slow wave pattern gives way to a mixture of NREM stages and lower-amplitude EEG activity. This condition is more likely to occur in children who are fatigued or have experienced stress the previous day.

During sleepwalking aggression toward other persons or toward objects in the environment is infrequent. The condition may be accompanied by sleep talking but, if so, articulation is poor. Sleepwalkers have an increased incidence of other episodic disorders associated with NREM sleep, such as sleep terrors. No specific psychopathology, however, has been observed in children with this condition. The onset is ordinarily between 6 and 12 years of age, and it lasts several years. Usually symptoms resolve by the end of the teens or in the early twenties. The primary impairment is the occurrence of injuries during an episode. Febrile illness may occasionally be associated.

Prevalence is estimated at 1% to 6%, but as many as 15% of children may have isolated episodes. It occurs more commonly in males than in females. It is also more common among first degree biological relatives than the general population (Table 29-5).

## Selected Readings

Achenbach TM, Edelbrock CS. Behavioral problems and competencies reported by parents of normal and disturbed children aged four through sixteen. Monogr Soc Res Child Dev 1981;46:1.

Ferber R. Solve your child's sleep problem. New York: Simon and Schuster, 1985.

Ferber R. Assessment procedures for diagnosis of sleep disorders in children. In: Noshpitz JD, ed. Basic handbook of child psychiatry (vol 5). New York: Basic Books, 1987:185.

Harris JC, DeAngelis-Harris C. Sleep and its disturbances in children. In: Moss AJ, ed. Pediatrics update reviews for physicians. New York: Elsevier, 1981:13.

Simeon JG. Treatment of sleep disturbances in children: recent advances. In: Noshpitz JD, ed. Basic handbook of child psychiatry (vol 5). New York: Basic Books, 1987:470.

*Principles and Practice of Pediatrics, Second Edition.*
edited by Frank A. Oski et al. J. B. Lippincott Company, Philadelphia © 1994.

# 29.13 *Psychotic Disorders*

James C. Harris

Psychotic disorders are major mental problems that involve abnormalities in thinking, belief systems, and perception. These are demonstrated clinically through incoherence in thinking, delusions, and hallucination. These symptoms are associated with major behavioral changes. The psychotic disorders are less common in preadolescence and primarily are evident for the first time in adolescence and adulthood. Assessment is more difficult in young children and the mentally retarded, because the major symptoms are identified through an interview assessment.

The conditions included are schizophrenia, affective and manic-depressive psychoses, organic psychotic states, and atypical psychoses. The last two conditions are not covered here. Pervasive developmental disorder/autism is categorized separately, because it is primarily a neuropsychiatric developmental disorder.

The underlying psychopathology has not been identified; however, there are both genetic and environmental risk factors.

The recent identification of a chromosomal disorder in two families with manic-depressive disease lends further credence to the eventual discovery of a genetic basis for some cases of this disorder. Ongoing investigations in brain imaging may provide additional information about brain dysfunction in each of these conditions.

## SCHIZOPHRENIA

Schizophrenia ordinarily presents for the first time in adolescence or young adulthood. It may occur in the prepubertal years, but the diagnostic criteria for adults are difficult to apply in children less than age 7. Whether the condition could be diagnosed before age 7 is a subject of disagreement. The characteristic features include the following:

1. A disorder in thinking. Thoughts are often incoherent, and the train of thought is lost. This difficulty in thinking is referred to as derailment or loosening of association.
2. Delusional beliefs. These are irrational beliefs and may take on a paranoid form in older children. The delusional beliefs arise out of ordinary consciousness and are not secondary to hallucinations or the result of a mood disturbance.
3. Hallucinatory experience. The hallucination is a false perception that occurs without external sensory stimulation. In schizophrenia, these are primarily auditory and are described as voices outside of the child's control that may speak with him or her directly or make reference to him or her in the third person.
4. Disturbance of mobility. In this instance, catatonic behavior may be present when the child assumes abnormal postures or refuses to change posture. Catatonia is present in both schizophrenia and in affective disorders.

The condition may have an abrupt or gradual onset. Particularly when onset is gradual, it may be more difficult for family members to recognize the seriousness of the condition. Children who develop schizophrenia often have a history of developmental delay, although their previous presentation may be normal. When developmental delay is present, language difficulties, clumsiness, social isolation, and muscular hypotonia may be noted. The condition may follow a remitting or a chronic course. There may be partial recovery with resolution of acute symptoms, but abnormal motivation and a decreased interest in routine events may follow the initial presentation as residual symptoms.

### Epidemiology

There is an increased risk in first-degree relatives. If a parent or a sibling is schizophrenic, the risk is about 12 times that of the general population. The rate of onset in adolescence is about three per 10,000, compared to 1% in the general population. Children of schizophrenic parents who are raised in foster or adoptive homes maintain the risk for the disorder. Concordance is greater in monozygotic twins.

A schizophrenic-like presentation may occur with stress in children who have organic brain dysfunction. These are more often brief reactive psychoses, but they may sometimes take on a more chronic picture. Family interactions may contribute to the course of the illness. Family difficulties in adapting to the disorder and strongly expressed, often hostile emotions may precipitate relapse.

### Assessment

Psychiatric assessment involves clarifying the major symptom picture. The diagnosis is generally straightforward in older adolescents, but in the rare instance that it occurs in a younger child, assessment may be more difficult; unless the specific diagnostic questions are asked, the child may be misdiagnosed as overactive or anxious. Whenever there is clouding of consciousness, an organic condition should be considered. Epilepsy is an important consideration, since confusion and sometimes unusual behavior may follow a seizure. Careful neurologic examination is essential in patient assessment.

Adolescents with a history of autism have a problem in language communication, which may be confused with schizophrenia. Brief psychotic episodes may occur following stress in this condition. Both delusions and hallucinations occur in affective psychosis; however, the classic manic symptoms—along with abnormal mental experiences that are congruent with mood, such as the belief that the body is decaying or that one has special powers—can usually differentiate the condition.

### Treatment

A comprehensive treatment program is essential in childhood. This takes into account the effect of the illness on the family, their response to it, and the need for an appropriate psychoeducational program. The family should be actively involved in the treatment, as families are involved in other chronic conditions. It is important to help the family understand that they are not to blame for this condition.

School programs must be carefully selected, because many programs for the emotionally disturbed inappropriately mix children who have schizophrenia with those who have antisocial behavior disorders. A program must be identified as one that is focused specifically on treating schizophrenia. During the acute phase of the illness, neuroleptic medication is indicated, and ordinarily this treatment is initiated on an inpatient unit. Following hospital discharge, careful psychiatric rehabilitation is required, particularly if there is a residual lack of motivation and difficulty in adaptation. Family counseling is ongoing to reduce excessive emotional involvement, and supportive psychotherapy is maintained for the child or adolescent. The outcome is variable, but the prognosis is better if a single acute episode occurs in a previously normal child or adolescent.

## DELIRIUM

Delirium is a syndrome with multiple etiologies. It is characterized by concurrent disturbances of consciousness and attention, perception, thinking, memory, psychomotor behavior, emotion, and the sleep–wake cycle. It is transient and of fluctuating intensity. Delirium occurs in young children with acute infections and after drug ingestion. Delirium is marked by clouding of consciousness with decreased response to environmental stimuli, misperception, often visual and tactile hallucinations, and disorientation. Treatment is that of the underlying disorder. The environment to be established is a supportive one that provides effective structure for the child.

## MANIC-DEPRESSIVE DISORDER

In manic-depressive disorder there is a severe disturbance of mood. Abnormalities in thought and perception emerge from the mood disorder. These conditions may occur as a single episode or as recurrent episodes; if there are recurrent episodes of both depression and hypomania, the term *bipolar disorder* is used.

During a manic or hypomanic episode, mood is elevated, and pressure in speech and irritability are observed. The young person is overly energetic, is disinhibited in his or her behavior, and sleeps less than usual. There are associated grandiose ideas about one's own capabilities. Hallucinations may occur but are not common.

## Epidemiology

The onset is rare before puberty, but the prevalence increases during the adolescent years. The disorder occurs with equal frequency in males and females. There is a genetic contribution: 12% of first-degree relatives have affective disorders. This is six times the frequency of affective disorder in the general population.

## Assessment and Diagnosis

If psychotic symptoms are present, a distinction must be made from schizophrenia. Organic mental disorders must be ruled out by examination, and associated suicidal behavior requires careful assessment. It is particularly important to clarify the family history for affective disorders.

## Treatment

The initial phase of treatment requires ensuring the safety of the patient and those around him or her, and it ordinarily requires hospital admission. Acute treatment with neuroleptic medications to deal with acute symptoms, and initiation of lithium carbonate in those with recurrent episodes, constitute the most effective pharmacologic management. Supportive psychotherapy for the child and family is needed to deal with the consequences of the irrational behavior and its effects on family and friends.

*Principles and Practice of Pediatrics, Second Edition.*
edited by Frank A. Oski et al. J. B. Lippincott Company, Philadelphia © 1994.

# *29.14 Child and Adolescent Psychiatric Referral*

James C. Harris

Pediatricians should identify a child and adolescent psychiatrist among their consultants. In considering referral, the pediatrician should remember that a mental disorder represents an impairment in social adaptation. It is accompanied by either painful psychological symptoms or disruptive behavior that is disabling as a result of its effects on others. Referral may be indicated in the following situations:

1. *Dysfunctional parent/child relationships*, particularly involving infants and toddlers, that have not responded to routine parenting strategies. Parent training is particularly important in an era when child abuse and sexual misuse occur far too frequently; these are preventable problems.
2. *Psychological and behavioral complications of medical illness.* This includes adjustment to the illness, as well as physiologic complications such as delirium. Warning signs for adjustment difficulties might be frequent office or emergency room visits, vague complaints that are difficult to ascribe to a physical condition, and continued difficulty adapting to a chronic disease.
3. *Persistent changes in behavior following stressful experiences.* An adjustment disorder or posttraumatic stress disorder may

occur following severe stress, such as an accident or loss of a significant family member. Changes in behavior may also accompany marital discord, family violence, psychiatric disorder in a parent, and drug or alcohol abuse by a family member.
4. *Disruptive behavior disorders and excessive risk-taking behavior.* Children with attention deficit disorder are vulnerable to both oppositional defiant and conduct disorders. Children with symptoms of stealing, lying, cruelty to animals or other children, drug or alcohol use, or inappropriate sexual behavior are at risk for subsequent delinquency and require early intervention. Risk-taking behavior is frequently seen in adolescents who are struggling with adjustment to a chronic illness or difficult family circumstances.
5. *Suicidal behavior (parasuicide) or threats.* These are among the most important reasons to seek consultation. Table 29-3 provides guidelines for establishing suicide risks.
6. *Somatic symptoms associated with a mental disorder.* Physical symptoms accompany many of the mental disorders of childhood and adolescence, including separation anxiety disorder, overanxious disorder, social anxiety disorder (avoidant disorder), depression, anorexia nervosa, schizophrenia, sleep–wake cycle disorder, and the dyssomnias.
7. *Problems related to psychotropic medications.* These include self-poisoning, the choice of medication, questions regarding side effects, and appropriate dosages. Children with attention deficit disorder who are receiving more than one medication for their behavior or are taking high doses of medication may require referral. When using psychotropic medications, it is essential to keep in mind that drug use is only one aspect of the treatment. All children who receive these medications need a multimodality approach to treatment. The modes of treatment include appropriate school placement and individual, family, or group therapy, in addition to the psychotropic agent.
8. *Treatment of major mental disorders.* The early recognition of affective disorder and schizophrenia in childhood is essential for the child and the family. Suicide is a major complication that may be avoided by early recognition and treatment of depression. Reluctance by the physician to make these diagnoses because of unrealistic fears about the stigma of having a major mental disorder is unwarranted. The Alliance for the Mentally Ill and other family support groups are effectively advocating to prevent the additional handicap of stigma in the life of the mentally ill.
9. *Mental disorder in a parent.* Psychiatric referral is indicated for personality disturbance and major mental illness, particularly depression and psychosis in parents. Substance abuse in parents is a particular concern.

*Principles and Practice of Pediatrics, Second Edition.*
edited by Frank A. Oski et al. J. B. Lippincott Company, Philadelphia © 1994.

# *29.15 School Failure*

Richard O. Carpenter

As trustees of children's health, pediatricians play an important role in the monitoring and prevention of childhood morbidity. For the school-age child, this monitoring role has become increasingly complicated as new research has highlighted complex interactions among genetics, biology, temperament, cognition, behavior, family factors, environment, and social factors in the genesis of childhood school failure. According to Freud, the school-age child enters the latency stage when triangular conflicts with parents abate, and the child's energies are focused on learning societal rules and technologies, exploring the world, and developing relationships with others outside the family. Erik Erikson described this period of childhood as the stage of "industry versus inferiority." The child's task is to build skills, gain confidence in innate abilities, and perform meaningful work.

Although the child's endeavors take place in many arenas, much energy and time are spent in school. Failure in school can have devastating consequences for the child. Failure leads to a child's deep sense of inadequacy, inferiority, and worthlessness. The cascading effects of school failure are far-reaching and can adversely affect self-esteem, future goals, peer and family relationships, and the child's ability to progress through subsequent developmental stages.

The pediatrician can play a crucial role in helping a child with school difficulties, using a comprehensive model of the range of variations in normal child development and an understanding of the multiple interacting factors influencing child development. Building on a child's strengths and helping family members and caregivers to prevent childhood experiences of failure must be a focus of preventive pediatric care. Comprehensive assessment of a child's abilities and appropriate matching of expectation to ability allow a child to grow and develop without experiencing the debilitating effect of school failure.

During this century, extraordinary achievements have resulted from the knowledge and technology generated under the tenets of the biomedical model of disease. The focus on the human body as a machine vulnerable to the consequences of faulty components and parts, inefficient engineering designs, poor maintenance, usage of improper fuel, contact with toxic substances, and the inevitable degeneration of physical material with time has allowed physician-scientists to construct powerful models for intervention and treatment of human disease. This reductionist approach, postulating that human disease can ultimately be understood in terms of genetic templates and molecular interactions, has advanced our understanding of child development and vulnerabilities during child development. We know that intelligence is heritable and can be adversely affected by exposure to toxins such as alcohol and lead. However, as George Engel and others have pointed out, there are significant limitations to the biomedical model. Learning and development are dynamic and interactive processes in which the child's cognitive and emotional functioning is shaped not only by genetic and physiologic events, but also by interactions with peers, family, culture, and society. By failing to take into account factors relating to psychosocial functioning in children, the biomedical model limits understanding of why a child in the violence-ridden inner city or the child of newly divorced parents might be failing in school.

Engel has proposed that physicians adopt a biopsychosocial model of human disease. The advances gleaned from the biomedical model are incorporated into the understanding of disease and dysfunction within the broader context of the child living and functioning in the world. Within this paradigm, the model of science as outlined by chemist Anna Harrison in her presidential address to the American Association for the Advancement of Science (investigation of the problem, identification of relevant phenomena, selection of study methodology, choice of instrumentation, delineation of protocol for data collection, execution of protocol, analysis of data, development of constructs, and assessment of certainty or uncertainty of results) becomes the method by which clinicians might understand the complex factors affecting a child with difficulties in development. The "physician scientist" is encouraged to become the "scientific physician" who investigates all relevant clues, carefully identifies

problematic issues, selects symptoms and signs to monitor, develops intervention strategies, and tracks the patient's progress over time.

This chapter will focus on the problem of childhood school failure. The biopsychosocial conceptual model will be used to highlight the interactions between genetics, behavior, environment, family, and society in its genesis. Syndromes associated with a high risk of school failure, including learning disabilities, school refusal, major depression, and attention deficit hyperactivity disorder, will be reviewed. Treatment strategies will be discussed and methods for prevention of school failure will be suggested (Table 29-6).

## PREVALENCE OF SCHOOL DIFFICULTIES

Over the last several decades, clinical researchers note that about one in ten children is at risk for significant school difficulties and failure. Interest in children at risk for school failure and our ability to identify them have risen. Pediatricians, educators, mental-health practitioners, and legislators have worked diligently to understand and address the educational problems in this group of children. In 1975, Public Law 94-142, the Education for All Handicapped Children Act, was passed. This law set forth procedures for identifying children with handicapping conditions and appropriate intervention services for these children in the public school system. The law listed categories that qualified children for special education services. Besides visual, hearing, and motor handicaps, other health-impaired, and mental retardation, learning disability and emotional disturbance were two other categories of educationally handicapping conditions identified under the law. These conditions have been recognized to impair a child's ability to learn and are a frequent cause of school difficulty and failure.

Data from the United States Department of Education that reviewed public school services for handicapped children in 1986–1987 as mandated under Public Law 94-142 identified over four million children with handicapping conditions, almost 11% of all children enrolled in public schools (Table 29-7). This figure undoubtedly underrepresents the total number of children in the United States suffering from handicapping conditions, because private school children are not included in these data. The breakdown of these data reveal that over one million children suffered from speech impairments, and close to one million children were classified as mentally retarded. Almost two million children were identified as having learning disabilities.

When compared to similar data from 1976, the 1986 data indicate that children with specific learning disabilities represent the largest and fastest-growing category of children receiving

---

### TABLE 29-6. Conditions Associated With Childhood School Failure

Neurologic disorders
Chronic medical illness
Medications that affect CNS function
Learning disabilities
School refusal
Major depression
Attention deficit hyperactivity disorder
Serious emotional disturbance
Lack of family involvement in their children's education
Diminished community educational resources

**TABLE 29-7.   Public School Services for Handicapped Children**

| Type of Handicap | 1976–1977 | Number of Children Served | 1986–1987 | Number of Children Served |
|---|---|---|---|---|
| All handicapping conditions | 8.33% | 3,692,000 | 10.97% | 4,374,000 |
| Learning-disabled | 1.80% | 796,000 | 4.80% | 1,914,000 |
| Speech-impaired | 2.94% | 1,302,000 | 2.85% | 1,136,000 |
| Mentally retarded | 2.16% | 959,000 | 1.61% | 643,000 |
| Seriously emotionally disturbed | 0.64% | 283,000 | 0.96% | 383,000 |

*Sikorski JB. Learning disorders and the juvenile justice system. Psychiatric Annals 1991;21:743.*

special education services. Curiously, these data identified fewer than 400,000 children as seriously emotionally disturbed. An alternate classification system of emotional disturbance used by mental-health practitioners, DSM-III-R, identifies considerably more children suffering from serious emotional disorders. Data from the United States Congress Office of Technology Assessment 1986 report on children's mental health estimates that over three million children and youths would be considered seriously emotionally disturbed by DSM-III-R criteria (Table 29-8). Both methods of ascertainment consistently agree with research demonstrating an increased prevalence of learning disabilities and serious emotional disorders in boys compared to girls, with ratios between 3:1 and 5:1.

Public Law 94-142 tends to be reductionistic in its definitions of handicapping conditions. The classification of subsets of handicapped children as either learning disabled or emotionally disturbed runs contrary to research and experience with this group of children. Epidemiologic studies such as Michael Rutter's work in the Isle of Wight demonstrate that learning disabilities, emotional disorders, and behavioral problems often occur as comorbid conditions in these children. The broader biopsychosocial perspective allows for the understanding of the interplay between reading difficulties, delinquent behavior, school dropout, and future entanglements with social and legal systems. Increasingly, common wisdom asserts that learning disabilities can predispose to emotional problems, and severe emotional disorders can impair attention and learning. Consequently, it is prudent for the office practitioner faced with a child floundering in school to consider that multiple factors, including medical illness, learning difficulties, and emotional problems, may play a combined role in the youngster's difficulties.

## EVALUATION

### Preschool Children

Risk factors for subsequent school difficulties in the preschool years include delayed motor, language, and social milestones. Office developmental screening procedures such as the Denver Developmental Screening Test (Denver II) help identify this group of children. If this brief screening procedure suggests developmental delays or abnormalities, more definitive evaluations should be undertaken to define more clearly the specific domains of developmental delay. Diagnoses including mental retardation, pervasive developmental disorder, autism, disabling cerebral palsy, severe speech and language delays, and visual and hearing impairments qualify these children for early intervention services.

Referral of these children to preschool intervention programs is crucial. Preschool intervention programs are mandated by fed-

**TABLE 29-8.   Diagnostic Criteria for Major Depressive Episode**

A. At least five of the following symptoms have been present during the same two-week period and represent a change from previous functioning; at least one of the symptoms is either (1) depressed mood, or (2) loss of interest or pleasure. (Do not include symptoms that are clearly due to a physical condition, mood-incongruent delusions or hallucinations, incoherence, or marked loosening of associations.)

1. Depressed mood (or can be irritable mood in children and adolescents) most of the day, nearly every day, as indicated either by subjective account or observation by others

2. Markedly diminished interest or pleasure in all, or almost all, activities most of the day, nearly every day (as indicated either by subjective account or observation by others of apathy most of the time)

3. Significant weight loss or weight gain when not dieting (eg, more than 5% of body weight in a month), or a decrease or increase in appetite nearly every day (in children, consider failure to make expected weight gains)

4. Insomnia or hypersomnia nearly every day

5. Psychomotor agitation or retardation nearly every day (observable by others, not merely subjective feelings of restlessness or being slowed down)

6. Fatigue or loss of energy nearly every day

7. Feelings of worthlessness or excessive or inappropriate guilt (which may be delusional) nearly every day (not merely self-reproach or guilt about being sick)

8. Diminished ability to think or concentrate, or indecisiveness, nearly every day (either by subjective account or as observed by others)

9. Recurrent thoughts of death (not just fear of dying), recurrent suicidal ideation without a specific plan, or a suicide attempt or a specific plan for committing suicide

*Note:* A "Major Depressive Syndrome" is defined as criterion A above.

B. 1. It cannot be established that an organic factor initiated and maintained the disturbance.

2. The disturbance is not a normal reaction to the death of a loved one (Uncomplicated Bereavement).

*Note:* Morbid preoccupation with worthlessness, suicidal ideation, marked functional impairment or psychomotor retardation, or prolonged duration suggested bereavement complicated by Major Depression.

C. At no time during the disturbance have there been delusions or hallucinations for as long as two weeks in the absence of prominent mood symptoms (ie, before the mood symptoms developed or after they have remitted).

D. Not superimposed on Schizophrenia, Schizophreniform Disorder, Delusional Disorder, or Psychotic Disorder NOS.

*Diagnostic and Statistical Manual of Mental Disorders, 3rd ed, revised. Copyright 1987, American Psychiatric Association.*

29.15: SCHOOL FAILURE    **741**

eral Public Law 99-457 (the Education of the Handicapped Act amendments of 1986) to provide free, appropriate, public education to all handicapped children between ages 3 and 5 years. Early intervention programs have demonstrated efficacy for this group of severely affected children. By matching educational expectations closely to the child's capabilities, self-esteem is maintained, and families are encouraged to participate in the special education process.

Children who pass initial early developmental screening procedures but who begin to develop academic problems in the school years will be the focus of the balance of this chapter.

## School-Age Children

Accurate assessment of a child's strengths and weaknesses in the cognitive, pragmatic, emotional, family, and social realms of day-to-day functioning is the first step in understanding factors related to school failure. The annual school physical provides the initial forum. A simple inquiry into how things are going at school may not suffice, because the child or family members may feel uncomfortable discussing concerns in a quick and superficial manner. Specific history from the child and family members about school attendance, homework management, favorite and least favorite subjects, interactions with the teacher, degree of comfort in relationships with classroom peers, popularity with peers, best friend at school, and visits to other friends' homes tends to be much more revealing and pertinent to the process of uncovering clues to the child's difficulty.

The clinician can assess the interactions between the child and parent or caregiver by interviewing them together. Excessive anger, anxiety, or distance in the relationship between child and adult requires further investigation. Separate meetings with the child and parent can be used to assess family function, potential economic or legal difficulties, or other traumatic stressors (death of a friend or relative, loss of a beloved pet, or significant parental illness).

During the physical examination, assessment of age-appropriate academic skills is instructive. By starting with easy tasks and progressing to more difficult tasks, the clinician can make the experience enjoyable for the child. A review of counting skills, reciting the alphabet, spelling first name forward and backward, testing math facts, and having the child tell a familiar fable or story may quickly highlight areas of concern such as problems with memory or language, articulation difficulties, calculation concerns, or problems with organizational skills. Drawing tasks such as writing the letters of the alphabet, drawing a picture of family members, and copying Gesell figures (Fig 29-1) may highlight potential fine motor or visual-perceptual difficulties. Assessing the child's attention to tasks, general level of impulsivity, and physical activity can provide further clues to areas that require more intensive investigation. Prudent diagnostic tests to confirm concerns about possible medical illness, medication toxicity, or toxin exposure may clarify the situation further.

The biopsychosocial model of disease focuses on the interplay of biological factors, cognitive/psychological factors, behavioral factors, family factors, and societal factors. Each of these areas will be examined more fully in the next section.

## BIOLOGICAL FACTORS

### Neurologic Impairments

At the extreme end of the spectrum of biological factors, neurological impairments and central nervous system damage or injury (chromosomal disorders, head trauma, birth anoxia, meningitis, seizure disorders, CNS malignancy) result in brain dysfunction and mental retardation syndromes that can adversely

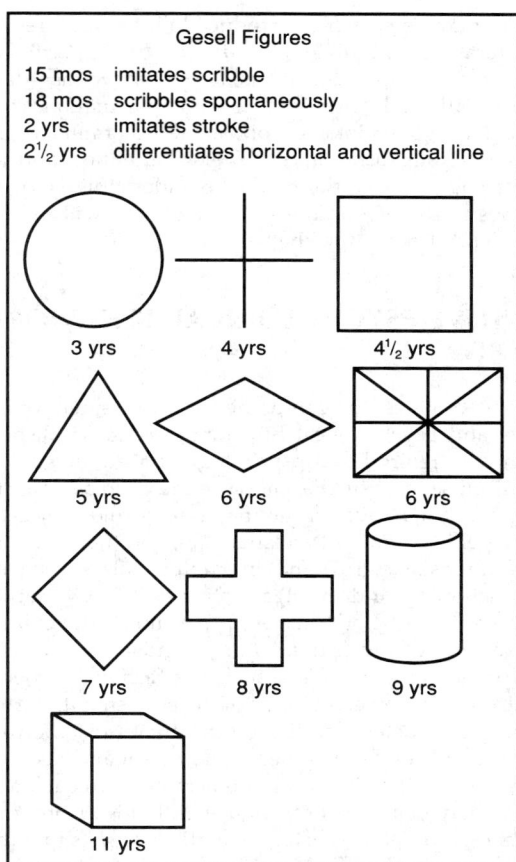

**Figure 29-1.**  The Gesell figures. (Illingsworth RS. The development of the infant and young child, normal and abnormal, ed 5. Baltimore: Williams & Wilkins, 1972:254.)

affect a child's school performance. These neurologic conditions require careful assessment, ongoing monitoring, and multidisciplinary habilitative efforts to maximize such a child's attainment in and adjustment to school.

### Nonneurologic Impairments

Nonneurologic, chronic medical problems such as asthma, diabetes, thyroid disease, inflammatory bowel disease, sickle-cell disease, and cancer can cause school difficulties because of chronic fatigue, anxiety, and physical discomfort. Chronic illness can divert a child's energy from school and compromise academic performance. Attention to these concerns by frequent monitoring of school issues during office visits, contact with teachers, and modifying or reducing schoolwork or homework can help ease the burdens carried by the child with chronic medical illness.

### Medication

Some pharmacologic treatments for chronic medical conditions (steroids, anticonvulsants, chemotherapeutic agents) alter and sometimes impair a child's cognitive and behavioral functioning, as well as cause depressed mood. Practitioners should be aware of the potentially deleterious CNS side effects of medication. Efforts should be made to use the lowest possible dose of required medications and to discontinue medications that impair optimal CNS functioning as quickly as possible.

### Brain and Neurophysiologic Alterations

Recent research using brain imaging (MRI and CT scans), positron emission tomography, and quantitative EEG techniques suggests that there may be specific, reproducible brain and neurophysiologic alterations in individuals suffering from specific learning disabilities, attentional difficulties, and affective disorders compared to unaffected controls. This new information, combined with previous epidemiologic work suggesting familial clustering of specific learning disorders, disorders of attention, and affective disorders, suggests that there may be underlying biological vulnerabilities to these conditions. These studies will be reviewed in more depth later in the chapter.

## COGNITIVE/PSYCHOLOGICAL/BEHAVIORAL FACTORS

In the United States, the comprehensive assessment of a child's cognitive and psychological functioning is accomplished most commonly by referral to a psychologist for administration of a standardized set of tests that measure the child's intellectual capacity, educational level in the major academic subjects (math, reading, spelling, and written language), and the developmental levels of other skills (gross and fine motor skills, speech and language functioning, and social/adaptive skills). A variety of projective tests might be administered to examine the child's emotional functioning and to assess for potential anxiety symptoms or signs of major mental illness such as affective disorder or psychotic disorder. Upon completion of the assessment, the test data are reviewed to determine if a discrepancy exists between the child's academic or developmental skill level and his or her intellectual potential. A significant problem in a particular academic area or a delay in a developmental skill that is disproportionate to the child's overall intellectual potential suggests that the child may have a specific learning disability. An emotional disturbance may occur as the primary reason for the child's school difficulties, or it may occur as a comorbid condition with specific learning disabilities.

### Brain Model For Learning

A current model for human learning postulates that new information is acquired in a series of brain operations that include inputting information, integrating newly input information with information previously learned, storing new information in memory, and outputting the processed information. Learning problems, in this model, are understood to occur when there is dysfunction in one or more of these brain operations. More specifically, each operation—input, integration, memory, and output—is viewed as a general category with component parts.

### Input

The input operation refers to the brain's ability to correctly perceive information from sensory end organs (visual, auditory, position sense, pressure). Dysfunction in the brain input operations can result in a child's misperception of written symbols (visual perceptual disabilities), spoken words (auditory perceptual difficulties), or body position in space (gross and fine motor disabilities).

### Integration

Integration or processing operations relate to the brain's ability to derive meaning from newly received information. Sequencing operations and the ability to integrate new information with past experience are important brain processing operations not only for correct understanding of language, but also for the correct interpretation of visual or multisensory information. A child with language processing problems may not understand a two- or three-step command given at one time; rather, the child may need requests that are given one step at a time with frequent prompts to ensure that information is understood.

At a higher level of information processing, disorders of the brain's active ability to organize incoming information (executive function) can occur. In this situation, a child appears confused and "out of it." Relevant information is not distinguished from background noise. Attention is not directed. Facts are muddled, and experiences are confused due to poor sequencing, organization, and integration.

### Memory

Memory operations refer to the brain's ability to store new information. Like a personal computer, the brain has two basic areas for memory storage. Short-term memory, akin to a PC's random access memory, stores information briefly while other areas of the brain process the information. Long-term memory functions like a floppy disk or a hard disk drive in a PC; this memory provides long-term storage of information in the brain. Children with memory impairments can have difficulty in either or both types of memory functioning. Also, the memory dysfunction may be limited to a specific sensory mode such as visual or auditory short-term memory functioning.

Long-term memory may be subdivided into procedural and declarative memory. According to neuroscientist Larry Squires, procedural memory refers to stored information about learned skills and how to go about the step-by-step execution of these skills. The information is analogous to computer software programs that direct the machine to perform certain tasks (word processing, database management, number crunching in a spreadsheet). Declarative memory refers to the storage of facts and "time-and-place" events. In a PC, this information would consist of documents generated by a word processor, data in a spreadsheet, or pictures generated in a graphics presentation software package. Children with difficulties in procedural memory might have difficulty learning rules to games, learning dance steps, or learning appropriate skills for social interaction. Children with difficulties in declarative memory might have difficulty remembering past events, vocabulary, math facts, or people's names.

### Output

Output operations refer to the brain's ability to organize the output of information either through words (expressive language) or through motor output (gross and fine motor skills). Children with expressive language disabilities may have difficulty using language to express their thoughts or demands. Gross motor disabilities may cause a child to be clumsy and awkward in team sports. Fine motor disabilities may be associated with slow written output and poor penmanship.

## FAMILY FACTORS

In the past decade, a national debate has focused on the decline in the quality of the United States educational system. Politicians and the news media have criticized the ability of some teachers to educate and some school systems to guide the educational agenda for the nation. The historical decline in our children's standardized test scores and the poor academic performance of our students compared with international competitors has focused discussion on issues such as high dropout rates, adolescent pregnancy, childhood drug abuse, and increasingly violent student behavior in and around school buildings. A national consensus has been building that proposes the educational system undertake primary responsibility for leadership in the nation's "war" to overcome its educational and social ills, but recent research suggests that this expectation is unrealistic and ill advised.

A study reported in the February 1992 issue of *Scientific American* examined the academic achievement of children of Indochinese refugee families who immigrated to the United States in the late 1970s and early 1980s. Despite tremendous physical and emotional hardships related to turbulent and destructive forces in their homelands, these children, like Jewish and Japanese immigrants before them, excelled academically in the inner-city schools of Orange County (California), Seattle, Houston, Chicago, and Boston. Despite poverty, economic disadvantage, and language and cultural barriers, these Indochinese students within 3 to 4 years of arriving in the United States were able to achieve overall grade-point averages of 3.05 (solid B average) and standardized test scores of academic achievement on the California Achievement Test with a mean score of 54%, placing them above the average for all students in the United States.

Careful analysis of the factors related to these students' academic success revealed the "pivotal role of the family." These Indochinese families were shown by the researchers to foster mutual honor and collective obligation between parents and children. Rather than focusing on personal or individual achievement, as is customary in American culture, these families emphasized respect, cooperation, equality, and interdependence. After dinner, parents cleared the dining-room table, finished household chores, and set up a family study period in which all family members were expected to teach and learn from each other. These homework sessions lasted 2.5 to 3 hours, compared to the 1.5 hours averaged by American high-school students. The Indochinese parents routinely read aloud to their younger children, and they placed a high value on the educational achievement of both male and female family members. In this environment, "a love of learning" was fostered, and learning became accepted as "normal, valuable, and fun." Older children were rewarded for teaching their younger siblings. In this way, the children developed a sense of accomplishment from their work and confidence in their academic abilities.

The remarkable academic success of the children of these Indochinese families highlights an important principle related to school success: families must play a role in their children's education. School personnel alone cannot instill a love of learning and a commitment to and respect for education in the nation's schoolchildren. Achieving these goals requires parental commitment and action.

## SOCIETAL FACTORS

In an era of massive federal and state budget deficits, services to children have been "streamlined" and "scaled back." Researchers have noted that more than 20% of American children live below the poverty line. The rise of violence, drug abuse, and family discord is matched only by the fall in mental-health services, educational initiatives, and funding for research solutions to these problems.

Educational cutbacks have increased regular public school class sizes from 20 students to 30 or 40 students. Special education classes have grown from about six students to 15 in many states. This doubling of teacher workload has changed the quality of education in the United States. School curriculums are less flexible and less able to be adapted to individual children's learning styles and needs. Children with problems are identified later in their struggles, when difficulties are more severe and when self-esteem and confidence have been significantly compromised. In general, intervention services are reserved for children who have faltered for several years rather than for several months. Efforts to provide "least restrictive" learning environments increasingly translate into "too little resources, too late."

Pediatricians and parents can play a vital role as child advocates in the educational system. Reforms and additional resources must be devoted to safeguarding our most valuable national resource, our children.

## SPECIFIC LEARNING DISABILITIES

In modern industrialized nations, there is a cultural expectation that children receive formal education and acquire basic literacy skills. These literacy skills enable children to record, share, and advance their culture's art and technology. Although the acquisition of these skills by children in the United States commonly is thought to occur as a part of normal human maturation and development, it is important to remember that the impetus for the attainment of literacy skills grew from sociocultural roots rather than from biological or evolutionary forces. The goal of universal adult literacy is a relatively recent expectation in human history and is not universally expected of children throughout the world. Our culture has come to accept that children naturally acquire academic skills at a rate commensurate with their overall cognitive abilities. Failure to meet these expectations is thought to suggest that a child suffers from a learning "disorder."

This model fails to highlight the tremendous diversity of human cognitive abilities. It posits that specific developmental delays in reading or math point to "disorder" and may not prompt the clinician to appreciate the child's genetically determined great artistic skill or musical ability. The clinician's task is to recognize that our school system expects all children to acquire specific academic skills at a predetermined rate. Most children can comply, but others have delays in the development of specific learning skills that may be transitory or lifelong. These children are conceptualized as having a specific learning disability. Remediation often is possible, but most importantly, intensive efforts should be made to preserve the child's self-esteem.

### Definition

Most public schools in the United States use the definition of specific learning disabilities established by Public Law 94-142:

> A disorder in one or more of the basic psychological processes involved in understanding or in using language, spoken or written, which may manifest itself in an imperfect ability to listen, think, speak, read, write, spell, or to do mathematical calculations. The term includes such conditions as perceptual handicaps, brain injury, minimal brain dysfunction, dyslexia, and developmental aphasia. The term does not apply to children who have learning problems which are primarily the result of visual, hearing or motor handicaps, of mental retardation, of emotional disturbance, or environmental, cultural, or economic disadvantage.

### Evaluation

To diagnose a specific learning disability, a psychologist uses standardized, individually administered tests to assess a child's performance in specific academic areas . Based on a child's overall cognitive ability, a delay in the expected developmental level of a specific academic, language, speech, or motor skill that is not the result of a physical or neurologic disorder, mental retardation, pervasive developmental disorder, or inadequate educational opportunity defines a specific learning disability. Historically, a delay in reading skills was called dyslexia, a delay in mathematics was called dyscalculia, and a delay in writing was called dysgraphia. Current nosology follows definitions set forth in DSM-III-R for a "specific developmental disorder." The subcategories of defined specific developmental disorders include academic skills disorders, language and speech disorders, and motor skills disorder.

Academic skills disorders focus on the three basic educational domains of reading, writing, and arithmetic. In practical terms, a child with a particular overall IQ can be expected to perform at predictable grade levels in each academic area. A child who is performing two grade levels below expectation in reading, writing, or math often qualifies for the diagnosis of an academic skills disorder and is eligible for special remediation services.

Language and speech disorders are subdivided into disorders of expressive and receptive language and articulation disorders. Rules of thumb that allow a clinician to suspect a developmental language disorder in a young child in the absence of mental retardation, neurologic or physical disorder (hearing loss, deafness), or pervasive developmental disorder include no use of single words by 18 months, no use of phrases by 24 months, reports of family members' inability to understand the child's speech by 24 months, or reports of the child communicating with unintelligible speech to people outside the family at 36 months of age. These difficulties should alert the clinician that the child may require a referral for a formal language assessment.

A child with a receptive language disorder has imperfect ability to "input" language information into auditory centers in the brain. This difficulty may arise from auditory perceptual problems such as the inability to distinguish *house* from *horse* or *red* from *read*, or it may be related to faulty language sound decoding. Once language information enters the child's brain, it needs to be comprehended and interpreted. Words and phrases are matched to stored meanings in the child's memory, then specific ideas can be assembled from the newly received language sequences. This cognitive operation, called central language processing, is complex and requires the simultaneous and cooperative operation of multiple cortical areas. Disorders of central language processing exist in children, although they are not coded in the DSM-III-R.

Expressive language skills require thoughts and intentions to be transformed into phonetic sequences that can be transmitted by speech through the coordination of motor neurons innervating the respiratory and oromotor centers. Children with disorders of expressive language or articulation can become quite frustrated by their inability to express their thoughts to other people, and this frustration commonly leads to behavioral problems. Early intervention strategies that use bypass techniques (sign language, communication boards) or speech and language therapy reduce frustration and can begin to remedy these problems.

Motor skills disorders can be divided into difficulties coordinating large muscle groups (gross motor disabilities) and problems with the coordination of small muscle groups (fine motor disabilities). A child with gross motor disabilities frequently is described by family members as accident-prone and clumsy. The child has difficulty participating in team sports. Not uncommonly, this child develops feelings of low self-esteem in middle childhood, when awkward physical abilities impede interactions with more physically agile peers. Fine motor disabilities come to light when a child begins to undertake longer writing assignments in school. The teacher will note that the child takes a long time to complete written assignments and applies unnecessary force to the pencil and paper. The child's work appears sloppy and difficult to decipher. The child often complains of hand and finger pain in the dominant hand, related to the pencil pressure that the child uses to obtain tactile feedback to compensate for the fine motor difficulties.

## Treatment

Public schools in the United States are mandated by federal law to identify children with learning disabilities. Thereafter, school authorities are required to provide each learning-disabled child with educational services appropriate to his or her learning needs. Public school systems in each community offer a continuum of alternative educational placements for learning-disabled students, ranging from several hours of extra tutoring per week to placement in a special residential school to work with severe emotional and learning handicaps. Efforts are made to place each student in the least restrictive educational environment.

Decisions regarding placement are formulated in a multidisciplinary meeting that includes the student's parents or legal guardian. At this meeting, an individual educational program (IEP) is written. The IEP is a legal agreement between the school and the child's parents that outlines educational goals and treatment strategies that will be used to help the child learn. If parents and school personnel disagree about school services, the IEP document should not be signed, and further negotiation between school officials and the parents must occur as mandated by federal law.

Data from the U.S. Department of Education in 1988 indicate that 21% of learning-disabled students are served in separate self-contained special education classrooms. Factors including lower teacher/student ratios, more individualized instruction with a special education teacher, and a supportive classroom milieu combine to make this type of self-contained class setting optimal for teaching severely learning-disabled children successfully. Sixty-two percent of learning-disabled students receive special education instruction for part of their school day in a resource room with four to eight other students. Flexible programming in the resource-room setting can combine with the student's regular class work to bolster weak skills and augment learning. Another 15% of learning-disabled students receive special education services in their regular classroom through consultation between their regular teacher and the special education teacher or via the use of special education materials to supplement learning materials in the regular class.

Clinicians can be most helpful to parents of learning-disabled students by encouraging these parents to become involved in and knowledgeable about the special education services available to their children. By advocating for their children within the educational system, parents help teachers and school administrators understand their child's special educational needs. By working collaboratively with special educators, pediatricians and parents can optimize each child's learning potential.

## School Refusal

Children with school refusal develop fearful feelings related to school attendance. Typically, these fears arise slowly over time and grow out of anxious concerns associated with physical separation from home or from parents. Some children develop fears of attending school due to concerns about a bullying peer at school or a "mean" teacher. Frequently, the condition occurs during points of school transition from a familiar setting to a new class situation (eg, starting kindergarten or first grade, moving to junior high school or high school). Age groups commonly affected include 5-, 10-, and 14-year-olds. Early age of presentation often correlates with less severe and more easily treated disorder. Boys and girls are equally affected. Severe school refusal is relatively uncommon, occurring in one to four children per 1000 students. Milder difficulties with anxiety symptoms associated with school attendance are much more common.

Unlike the truant child, who attempts to hide missed school attendance from teachers and parents, the child with school refusal openly communicates the desire not to be in school to family members. Another common presentation of school refusal symptoms includes somatic complaints (eg, chest pain, fatigue, headaches, sore throat, stomachaches) on school days that are not present in the late afternoon, on weekends, or on school vacations. Children who suffer from school refusal tend to be good students of average or better cognitive abilities.

### Evaluation

In many cases of school refusal, there is a common pattern of familial dysfunction. The central feature involves an overinvolved relationship between a parent and the child. One parent (usually the mother) is overprotective of the child; the other parent (usually the father) is peripherally involved with the child or openly disagrees with the spouse about the child's management. Occasionally, both parents may be overly concerned about their child's welfare. Usually these parents are unaware of the effects that their focused concern for the child has on the child's behavior. In these situations, the child receives considerable parental attention for not attending school, and the result is to reinforce child's anxiety symptoms associated with school attendance. The child's somatic complaints or anxiety symptoms associated with school attendance elicit parental attention and are powerfully reinforced by this parental attention. If unchecked by school officials or other concerned caregivers, the child and family become locked into an escalating pattern of behavioral and emotional dysfunction.

Although many children with school refusal have emotional symptoms only related to the process of getting to school, other children with this disorder experience significant emotional distress throughout the day that is heightened by their interactions with people outside the family. These children prefer to stay indoors. They withdraw from peer groups and over time can develop clinically significant psychiatric disorders, including separation anxiety disorder, overanxious disorder, phobic disorder, and mood disorder.

### Treatment

The treatment objective for the child with school refusal is to rapidly return the child to school. In most cases, the child's return to the regular classroom setting and the reestablishment of regular school and home routines causes the child's anxious symptoms to resolve. Family members benefit from an understanding of the interactive effects between their interpersonal behavior and the child's behavior. Supportive and empathetic counseling can facilitate parental understanding of these issues. Careful planning and coordination of services between school personnel, the clinician, and family members is important in bringing about the child's return to school.

The treatment of the child with school refusal and a serious psychiatric disorder requires the additional interventions of a mental-health provider. Concurrent mental-health evaluation should occur; thereafter, the pediatrician and the mental-health provider should work together with the family and school personnel to resolve the child's problem.

## Major Depression

Childhood major depression is not uncommon and can present either as school refusal or decreased performance in school. Epidemiologic studies in the United States have reported incidence figures of 0.9% in preschoolers, 1.9% in school-age children, and 4.7% in adolescents. The diagnosis of major depression is made using clinical data gathered from interviews with the child, family members, caretakers, and others involved with the child on a daily basis. Several rating scales have been developed over the past decade with concomitant refinements in the clinical criteria necessary for the diagnosis of depressive illness. The most commonly accepted set of criteria is contained in DSM-III-R; the specific features are summarized in Table 29-8.

### Evaluation

School problems associated with childhood depression can include diminished motivation, loss of interest in activities with peers, poor concentration, and a decline in school performance. Depressed children can be irritable, defiant, and emotionally labile. A child's demeanor may be either hostile and angry or quiet and withdrawn. Typically, children with depression appear unhappy, with downcast eyes and a sad facial expression. They may be excessively tearful, angry, or belligerent. Often their motor movements are slowed (psychomotor retardation), and if engaged in conversation, they respond slowly to questions and appear to have difficulty concentrating and staying on a topic. Speech content may reflect low self-esteem, guilt, and at times morbid or suicidal ideation. When directly questioned, these children report feeling sad and unable to enjoy interests and hobbies they pursued before becoming ill.

Research on childhood depression suggests that like major depression in adults, the illness has biological underpinnings reflecting changes in brain neurochemistry. Neurovegetative signs including changes in sleep, appetite, and energy are present to varying degrees. It is helpful to ask about weight changes over the past several months. Increases or decreases in appetite, sleep, and energy levels are relevant. Specific questions regarding length of time required to fall asleep (less than 30 minutes is normal), frequency of night awakenings, and early morning awakening are important. Detailed information about first- and second-degree family relatives suffering from depression, bipolar illness, or alcohol or drug abuse further highlights biological influences and contributes to the certainty of the diagnosis.

A variety of medical illnesses can mimic the signs and symptoms of childhood depression. Endocrine disorders (abnormalities in thyroid function, diabetes, hypoparathyroidism), infection (Epstein-Barr, tuberculosis, pneumonia, hepatitis, HIV), anemia, and electrolyte abnormalities may cause a child to appear depressed. Medication treatments with anticonvulsants (barbiturates), aminophylline, oral contraceptives, and corticosteroids can adversely affect mood. In older children, chronic alcohol or illicit substance abuse are major risk factors for subsequent mood disorder. These conditions should be investigated and ruled out before settling on the diagnosis of major depression.

### Treatment

Once the diagnosis of a major mood disorder is suspected, the child should be carefully assessed for possible suicidal risk and risk for aggressive behavior toward others. Depending on the severity of the child's condition, treatment options might vary from rapid inpatient psychiatric hospitalization for comprehensive evaluation and treatment to outpatient antidepressant medication treatment and psychotherapy.

## Attention Deficit Hyperactivity Disorder

Attention deficit hyperactivity disorder (ADHD) is a syndrome in which a child has difficulties with motor hyperactivity, impulsive behavior, and poor attention. The syndrome has been recognized by clinicians as the most common childhood neurobehavioral disorder, affecting 3% to 5% of school-age children. The literature on the subject comprises well over 2000 published articles. Over the past several decades, children with ADHD have been labeled with many different names including minimal brain damage, minimal brain dysfunction, hyperkinetic impulse disorder, and the hyperactive child syndrome, depending on which features of the syndrome clinicians determined were most salient.

Vigorous attempts have been made to discover an etiology for ADHD, but at present the cause remains unknown. Many clinical investigators support the hypothesis that ADHD comprises a heterogenous group of neurobehavioral difficulties. Analogous to the relationship of fever to its multiple possible etiologies, vulnerable individuals suffer from ADHD for a variety of reasons. Diverse factors including genetics, infection, metabolic abnormalities, exogenous toxins, and environmental, familial, and cultural influences have been associated with the symptoms and signs of the disorder. The severity of symptoms is modulated by the child's age, sex, developmental level, cognitive functioning, psychosocial and family setting, and comorbid conditions.

## Evaluation

As currently defined in the DSM-III-R, ADHD is a developmental disorder that affects attention span, activity level, impulse control, and rule-governed behavior (Table 29-9). It begins early in childhood and persists across developmental time and situations. The disorder becomes handicapping to the child when a poor match

---

**TABLE 29-9.   Diagnostic Criteria for Attention-Deficit Hyperactivity Disorder**

A. A disturbance of at least 6 months during which at least eight of the following are present:
   1. Often fidgets with hands or feet or squirms in seat (in adolescence, may be limited to subjective feelings of restlessness)
   2. Has difficulty remaining seated when required to do so
   3. Is easily distracted by extraneous stimuli
   4. Has difficulty awaiting turn in games or group situations
   5. Often blurts out answers to questions before they have been completed
   6. Has difficulty following through on instructions from others (not due to oppositional behavior or failure of comprehension), eg, fails to finish chores
   7. Has difficulty sustaining attention in tasks or play activities
   8. Often shifts from one uncompleted activity to another
   9. Has difficulty playing quietly
   10. Often talks excessively
   11. Often interrupts and intrudes upon others, eg, butts into other children's games
   12. Often does not seem to listen to what is being said to him or her
   13. Often loses things necessary for tasks or activities at school or at home (eg, toys, pencils, books, assignments)
   14. Often engages in physically dangerous activities without considering possible consequences (not for the purpose of thrill-seeking), eg, runs into the street without looking

*Note:* The above items are listed in descending order of discriminating power based on data from a national field trial of the *DSM-III-R* critieria for Disruptive Behavioral Disorders.

B. Onset before the age of 7
C. Does not meet the criteria for a Pervasive Developmental Disorder

Criteria for Severity of Attention-Deficit Hyperactivity Disorder

*Mild*: few, if any, symptoms in excess of those required to make the diagnosis and only minimal or no impairment in school and social functioning

*Moderate*: symptoms or functional impairment intermediate between "mild" and "severe"

*Severe*: many symptoms in excess of those required to make the diagnosis and significant and pervasive impairment at home and school and with peers

   *Note:* consider a criterion met only if the behavior is considerably more frequent than that of most people of the same mental age.

*Diagnostic and Statistical Manual of Mental Disorders, 3rd ed, revised. Copyright 1987, American Psychiatric Association.*

---

exists between environmental demands and his or her capabilities. It is helpful to view a child with ADHD from the biopsychosocial perspective. Biological factors interact with a child's cognitive and neuropsychological level of functioning. These factors are influenced in turn and to varying degrees by environmental, familial, social, economic, and political factors.

Researchers studying individuals with ADHD continue to uncover clues that suggest associations between the disorder and underlying disruptions in CNS function. Although ADHD is a heterogenous group of disorders, there is a suggestion that a final common brain pathology may exist. Genetic studies have shown that ADHD is a familial disorder. Joseph Biederman, a child psychiatrist at Harvard University, has demonstrated that ADHD is not uncommon in parents of probands with ADHD (morbidity risk 25% versus 5% in controls). Family studies show higher concordance rates of ADHD symptoms in monozygotic versus dizygotic twins. On an organ system level, researchers have suggested that the core features of ADHD may have their genesis in genetically determined differences in brain functioning. Recent studies of individuals with ADHD have demonstrated a variety of preliminary findings, including decreased regional cerebral blood flow to the caudate and frontal brain areas, decreased glucose metabolism in these brain areas on positron emission tomography scans, and frontal lobe deficits on neuropsychological tests. Studies of childhood exposure to neurotoxic agents or events that increase the risk for subsequent ADHD lend further weight to the concept of disordered CNS function in ADHD. Maternal tobacco and alcohol use during pregnancy, birth anoxia, and lead exposure are established risk factors for childhood ADHD.

Cognitive and psychological factors modulate the severity of the behavioral manifestations of ADHD. In general, children with higher intellectual capabilities are better able to capitalize on personal strengths and assets. Researchers have suggested that children with greater cognitive abilities generate and make use of compensatory strategies more fully than less cognitively able ADHD children. In a similar way, children with "easy" as opposed to "difficult" temperaments generally fare better with ADHD. These children are slow to anger, more adaptable, and generally cheerful in their dispositions. They tend to maximize the benefits of high energy, distractibility, and impulsivity, turning them into gains in imagination, creativity, and productivity.

It is important to be vigilant about the behavioral and environmental factors that affect a child with ADHD. Typically, the child with ADHD has difficulty taking turns and difficulty complying with the commonly accepted rules of social interaction. Interrupting in conversation, pushing to the front of lines, calling out in class, inappropriate laughter and comments about other people, and inability to censor thoughts and not say what is on his or her mind tends to alienate the child from family members and peers. The result often is poor self-esteem and further difficulties with social competence. Those caring for these children must fortify environmental supports (smaller class size, more individual attention, social skills training). Failure to recognize this aspect of a child's functioning inevitably contributes to the child's sense of disorganization and chaos.

The functioning of individual family members and the quality of familial interactions are other important areas to explore in the biopsychosocial realm. Since ADHD is often a familial disorder, parents may suffer from ADHD symptoms themselves. In adults, impulsivity may manifest itself as impatience and hyperexcitability. Inattention may continue with problems in task persistence, organization, and planning. These parents may have difficulty providing optimal support for the child suffering from ADHD. Recognizing these parental vulnerabilities and helping parents to obtain appropriate help and community support can add considerably to the positive outcome for the child with ADHD.

## Treatment

Management of children with ADHD is complicated by the fact that conditions other than ADHD can mimic the signs and symptoms of inattention, impulsivity, and hyperactivity. Medical and neurologic factors (eg, thyroid disorder, seizures, anticonvulsant or steroid treatment) must be identified and appropriately managed. Commonly associated learning difficulties may require special educational interventions or tutoring outside of school. Possible psychosocial factors (eg, parental divorce, child abuse, serious illness in a family member, overcrowded living quarters due to economic hardship in the family) should be investigated and appropriate counseling or social work interventions should be initiated.

Target symptoms of inattention, impulsivity, and hyperactivity that are manifestations of ADHD respond about 70% of the time to pharmacologic interventions. The short-acting stimulants methylphenidate hydrochloride and dextroamphetamine sulfate are the mainstays of medication treatment. Typically, stimulant medication is given 4 hours apart in divided doses of 0.3 to 1.0 mg/kg/day of methylphenidate or 0.15 to 0.5 mg/kg/day of dextroamphetamine.

Side effects of stimulant treatment can include increased pulse and blood pressure, decreased appetite, mood liability (particularly as the dose of stimulant wears off), and sleep disturbance. Psychotic symptoms including hallucinations and delusions can occur if stimulants are used at high doses. Children with preexisting major mental illness (affective, anxiety, or psychotic disorders) and ADHD may experience worsening of their psychiatric symptoms with stimulant treatment. Additionally, stimulants may aggravate an underlying tic disorder or may be associated with the emergence of a tic disorder in a child with a family history of Tourette's syndrome or motor tics.

Follow-up studies of children with ADHD have shown that they are at risk for having other psychiatric disorders, including conduct and antisocial disorders, drug and alcohol abuse, and affective disorders. Treatment, therefore, must be based on a comprehensive model that includes the careful assessment of a child's functioning at school, at home, and with peers. At various times, intervention strategies including combinations of individual or family counseling, behavioral modification, cognitive therapy, regular office monitoring, collaborative interactions with school personnel, and medication management may play important roles in the comprehensive treatment of a child with ADHD.

Long-term outcome studies of ADHD children demonstrate that between 30% and 50% of them continue to suffer from either the full or a significant part of the ADHD syndrome in adulthood. At present, data are not available to inform clinicians about which intervention strategies best protect these individuals from the long-term outcome risks of antisocial behavior, criminality, substance abuse, and school, job, or marriage failures. Clearly, interventions that preserve the individual's self-esteem and confidence and interventions that maximize his or her talents and skills offer the most hope for successful treatment.

## Serious Emotional Disturbance

Children with serious emotional disturbances can develop academic difficulties leading to school failure. Identifying these vulnerable children is challenging to clinicians because disorders associated with serious emotional disturbance (eg, psychosis, severe anxiety, obsessive-compulsive disorder, posttraumatic stress disorder, affective disorder) often occur along with other conditions such as attentional problems, behavioral problems, and learning disabilities. An understanding of the possible coexistence of learning and behavioral problems with an underlying serious emotional disturbance should prompt the clinician to refer a child failing in school for more intensive mental-health assessment, particularly when interventions for learning or behavioral problems have not been successful. A detailed discussion of serious emotional disturbances in childhood is presented in Chapter 29.6.

## Suggested Readings

Biederman J, Munir K, Knee D, et al. High rates of affective disorders in probands with attention deficit disorders and in their relatives: a controlled family study. Am J Psychiatry 1987;144:330.

Caplan N, Choy MH, Whitmore JK. Indochinese refugee families and academic achievement. Scientific American 1992; February:36.

Engel GL. The need for a new medical model. A challenge for biomedicine. Science 1977;196:129.

Engel GL. Physician-scientists and scientific physicians resolving the humanism-science dichotomy. Am J Med 1987;82:107.

Frankenburg WK, Dodds J, Archer P, Shapiro H, Bresnick B. The Denver II: a major revision and restandardization of the Denver Developmental Screening Test. Pediatrics 1992;89:91.

Gallico RP, Burns TJ, Grob CS. Emotional and behavioral problems in children with learning disabilities. Boston: College Hill Press, 1988.

Rutter M, Tizard J, Yule W, Graham P, Whitmore K: Research report: Isle of Wight studies, 1964-1974. Psychol Med 1976;6:313.

Silver LB. Learning disabilities: introduction. J Am Acad Child Adolesc Psychiatry 1989;28:309.

Sikorski JB. Learning disorders and the juvenile justice system. Psychiatric Ann 1991;21:742.

U.S. Department of Education: To assure the free appropriate public education of all handicapped children. Tenth Annual Report to Congress on the Implementation of the Handicapped Act. Washington DC: Government Printing Office, 1988.

*Principles and Practice of Pediatrics, Second Edition.*
edited by Frank A. Oski et al. J. B. Lippincott Company, Philadelphia © 1994.

# 29.16 *Disorders of Elimination*

### Richard O. Carpenter

The physiologic processes involved in the elimination of urine and fecal material from the human body are straightforward. Bladder and bowel structures designed to accumulate and temporarily store waste material send neural signals to the brain when these structures become filled near capacity. These brain signals, in concert with an individual's previous training and experience, prompt the individual to find an appropriate place to evacuate bodily waste products. Thereafter, the passage of urine and fecal material is accomplished through coordination of muscular activity. Sphincter muscles relax and muscles within the walls of the hollow organ structures contract.

Although the steps for elimination of waste products are readily accomplished by most children and adults, few of the requisite skills are present during infancy. Human infants eliminate waste products in a reflexive manner on a variable schedule. With neuromuscular maturation, socialization, proper nutrition and training, children develop voluntary control of urinary and fecal continence and the ability to eliminate waste products in a voluntary and socially permissible manner.

Complex interactions between the child's neuromuscular developmental maturity, genetic endowment, diet, prior training experiences, and parental and cultural expectations contribute to the difficulty inherent in correctly differentiating normal from abnormal functioning. Consensus about when a child's handling of urine or fecal material qualifies for a "disorder of elimination" remains elusive even among experts.

Scientific studies over the past thirty years have highlighted wide cultural variations in expectation and achievement of childhood continence. A study in 1965 by Hindley found median ages for the initiation of toilet training in London at 4.6 months, in Paris at 7.8 months, and in Stockholm at 12.4 months. Cohen reported in 1977 that early initiation of toilet training in China is customary and that many children achieve urinary and fecal continence by eighteen months of age. In the United States, Selma Fraiberg argued that children must master a series of developmental tasks and skills prior to successful attainment of continence. These steps include the ability to control sphincter muscles, the ability to postpone the urge to void or defecate, and the ability to signal the need to go to the bathroom. Charles Schaefer further suggests that the child should have an understanding of the social implications of evacuation of bodily waste in socially unacceptable places. The consensus among American pediatricians in the last ten to 20 years is that continence training probably should not be attempted before a child has reached cognitive and motor developmental age equivalents of 15 to 18 months. This principle has particular relevance for the toilet training of children who are developmentally delayed or mentally retarded.

Sociocultural expectations and a child's neuromaturational level are important factors in disorders of elimination. Likewise, the approach taken by parents or caregivers in toilet training plays an important role. Overly harsh, rigid, or punitive measures engender fearful, anxious, and occasionally hostile feelings in the child. Battles for control over the process can ensue, and the child's attainment of continence can be delayed. Permissive approaches with minimal expectations of continence may forestall the child's development of mastery of bowel and bladder control, leaving the child vulnerable to embarrassment when compared to the functioning of peers in school or day-care settings. A middle position between the overly restrictive and demanding approach and the indifferent approach is best tolerated by children and is most likely to lead to successful attainment of continence. Parental patience, gentle encouragement, and support are most likely to facilitate smooth acquisition of autonomous control of elimination.

This chapter focuses on the characterization, evaluation, and appropriate treatment of childhood disorders of elimination of urine and fecal material. The clinical disorders enuresis and encopresis are discussed individually. Understanding of the interactive influences of development and psychosocial and physiologic elements in the genesis and maintenance of these disorders is emphasized.

# ENURESIS

## Diagnosis

For years, health practitioners have had difficulty settling on a standard definition of enuresis. A classification system commonly used since 1987 is based on the definition of functional enuresis in the *Diagnostic and Statistical Manual* (DSM-III-R) of the American Psychiatric Association (Table 29-10). According to DSM-III-R criteria, functional enuresis occurs in a child aged at least 5 or 6 years (with a mental age of at least 4 years) who repeatedly voids urine during the day or night into bed or clothing. If a child is younger than 6 years, these events must occur more than once per month (if older, once per month) to make the diagnosis of functional enuresis. Primary functional enuresis refers to the situation in which the child has not been continent of urine in the past. Secondary functional enuresis occurs when the child becomes incontinent after a period of urinary continence lasting at least one year.

In children older than 5 or 6 years, functional enuresis is distinguished from other causes of enuresis by investigation and

| TABLE 29-10.   Diagnostic Criteria for Functional Enuresis |
|---|
| Repeated voiding of urine during the day or night into bed or clothes, whether involuntary or intentional. |
| At least two such events per month for children between the ages of 5 and 6, and at least one event per month for older children. |
| Chronologic age at least 5, and mental age at least 4. |
| Not due to a physical disorder, such as diabetes, urinary tract infection, or a seizure disorder. |
| Specify primary or secondary type. |
|    Primary type—the disturbance was not preceded by a period of urinary continence lasting at least one year. |
|    Secondary type—the disturbance was preceded by a period of urinary continence lasting at least one year. |
| Specify nocturnal only, diurnal only, or nocturnal and diurnal. |

*From Diagnostic and Statistical Manual of Mental Disorders, 3rd ed, revised. American Psychiatric Association, 1987.*

exclusion of organic causes of urinary incontinence such as disease, injury, or congenital malformation. Nocturnal enuresis refers to incontinence of urine during sleep time only. Diurnal enuresis refers to urinary incontinence during waking hours.

## Prevalence

Enuresis is a common childhood condition that has been estimated to occur in five to seven million children in the United States. The prevalence of the disorder decreases as the child's age increases. Studies by Michael Rutter in the Isle of Wight showed that at age 5, 13.4% of males and 13.7% of females wet their beds at night at least once per month; by 14 years, the prevalence of nighttime enuresis decreased to 3% among boys and 1.7% among girls. After 18 years, investigators report that approximately 1% of males have enuresis. Persistent enuresis in females after age 18 years is exceedingly rare.

Family studies show a strong genetic predisposition for enuresis. A study by Bakwin in 1973 showed that if both parents were enuretic as children, 77% of their children developed enuresis; 43% of children with one enuretic parent were enuretic. Concordance rates of enuresis among monozygotic twins were also greater compared to dizygotic twins (68% versus 36% respectively).

## Etiology

Investigations into various conditions predisposing to or maintaining enuresis in children have yielded a large body of literature indicating that the disorder has a multifactorial etiology. It is clear that physical and psychological factors play a role. Ideas that a child is enuretic as a means of expressing anger toward parents or to attract parental attention have been disproved. Instead, it is recognized that children with enuresis are emotionally sensitive to their condition and are likely to suffer loss of confidence, loss of self-esteem, and embarrassment if they are thought to be intentionally incontinent.

Physiologic and neuromaturational factors appear to be the most common etiologic factors predisposing to enuresis. Constitutional and genetic factors are suggested by the usual strong family history of childhood enuresis in other family members. Although not universal and comprehensive in scope, studies of age-matched enuretic and non-enuretic children suggest that some enuretic children suffer from a mild neuromuscular maturational delay in bladder function that results in a smaller functional bladder capacity compared to controls. These enuretic children have the same total bladder capacities as age-matched controls, yet they retain less urine in their bladders and are more prone to accidental incontinence.

Sleep arousal disorders have attracted much interest. Theories of bedwetting resulting from failure of arousal from deep sleep have been tempered by new understanding that urinary incontinence occurs in all phases of the sleep cycle, as documented by electroencephalogram. Frequency of incontinence is proportional to time spent in each sleep phase. Research has not ruled out that ''deep sleep'' and delayed arousal from sleep are factors in nighttime incontinence, but functional bladder capacity and time in each sleep phase are important.

Incontinence can be the result of organic causes, including anatomic defects of the genitourinary system (eg, epispadias, posterior urethral valves), constipation with a large fecal mass decreasing bladder capacity, urinary tract infections, or systemic illness such as diabetes mellitus or insipidus and seizure disorders. Although not as common as other conditions associated with childhood enuresis, these conditions are well understood; discoverable with a careful history, physical, and laboratory exam; and readily treated.

Psychological factors associated with enuresis are more difficult to categorize. Significant emotional disturbance occurs in a minority of enuretic children. The cause and effect relationship between emotional disturbance and enuresis often is unclear. A number of studies have shown that with effective treatment of the enuresis, the child's emotional disturbance resolves. On the other hand, studies of children during World War II indicated a relationship between high levels of fear and anxiety and higher prevalence rates of childhood enuresis. John Werry has pointed out that ''situational stress'' such as hospitalization of a young child, separation from the mother, birth of a sibling, or parental divorce is the most common cause of secondary enuresis. The association between anxiety and enuresis is of further interest in light of research by Yerkes and Dobson in 1908 that demonstrated that high levels of anxiety impede new learning. Charles Schaefer notes that parental toilet training procedures conducted in a high-stress and demeaning manner impede the child's ability to master the necessary skills for the maintenance of continence and set up a cycle of escalating anxiety and failure.

## Associated Features

Most children with functional enuresis do not have a comorbid emotional illness. The prevalence of functional encopresis, sleepwalking disorder, and sleep terror disorder, however, is somewhat greater in children with functional enuresis than in continent children in the general population.

## Course

Most children with functional enuresis become continent by adolescence, but approximately 1% of adolescents (almost exclusively males) continue to have the disorder in adulthood. The morbidity associated with the disorder is directly related to the adverse effects on the individual's self esteem. Anger, punishment and rejection by parents, caretakers and peers contribute to the individual's shame, embarrassment and damaged self-esteem.

## Assessment and Treatment

A wide range of treatment strategies for enuresis have been developed by health practitioners. Prevalence and etiologic information on childhood enuresis suggest that prevention of emotional difficulties in a child with enuresis may be possible by early education of parents and caregivers about the role of familial

inheritance, developmental maturational issues, the role of anxiety, and the importance of patient, supportive toilet training practices. For these interventions to be effective, such discussions should occur with the child's caregivers around the 12-month well-child visit and continue as needed through the early school years. The goal of preserving the child's self-esteem and confidence during the struggle to master continence is of paramount importance.

Although the high rate of spontaneous remission of enuresis with the child's advancing age (approximately 15% per year) prompts many practitioners to advocate an approach of reassurance and ''watchful waiting,'' this practice can lead to extended periods of suffering as the child is berated by frustrated parents and unsympathetic peers. Instead of the ''watchful waiting'' approach, health practitioners are well advised to use the combined methods of reassurance, careful physical examination, education, and behavioral treatment to address the concerns surrounding an enuretic child. This comprehensive approach will have the best chance of preserving the child's self-esteem, minimizing distress within the family, and resolving the incontinence.

### Organic Factors

A careful pediatric history that includes detailed information about the onset of difficulties with urinary incontinence (primary or secondary enuresis), frequency of accidents, precipitating circumstances, associated emotional or behavioral disturbance, and the motivation of child and caretakers to achieve change helps to guide the practitioner in ruling organic etiologies in or out. Physical examination and laboratory testing that checks electrolytes and serum glucose, urinalysis, and urine culture will alert the practitioner to possible difficulties with bladder infection, significant renal disease, or diabetes mellitus. Clinicians should be vigilant for children suffering from diabetes insipidus, seizure disorder, neurogenic bladder or structural anomalies of the genitourinary system, even though these are rarely the presenting cause of enuresis. Effective medical treatment of these conditions combined with education, reassurance, and behavioral training often leads to rapid resolution of the problem.

### Education and Behavioral Treatments

Frustrated parents and caregivers burdened by their child's repeated episodes of incontinence can develop the belief that their child's behavior stems from ''laziness'' or a desire to ''anger'' or ''get back'' at the caregiver. This frustration can lead to mutual resentment, higher levels of anxiety, and, occasionally, abusive situations. Clinicians are wise to intervene in these situations and to help the family and child understand that enuresis is a developmental condition that resolves with time and is amenable to treatment. Enuresis is *not* a product of ''willful misbehavior.''

The implementation of a behavioral reward system enhances toilet training procedures, structures parent and child interactions related to toileting, and effectively decreases episodes of urinary incontinence. A calendar can be hung in the child's room, with stickers or stars used to record successful voids in the toilet during the day or to record dry nights. This will emphasize and encourage the child's success. The calendar can be taken to visits with the treating clinician so that the child's progress can be monitored over time.

Another form of behavioral treatment involves bladder training. One method, ''retention-control training,'' advocates increasing the child's daily intake of fluid and encouraging him or her to hold urine in the bladder until the point of discomfort. As the bladder stretches to full capacity, the child may squirm and complain of discomfort. At this point, the child is helped by caregivers or teachers to link these feelings of bladder fullness to the need to go to the bathroom to void. Over time, this conditioning process allows the child to gain voluntary control over continence.

This method can be particularly helpful with children suffering from attention deficit hyperactivity disorder and enuresis because the method helps the child pay attention to bladder signals.

A second method of bladder training that is particularly helpful in developmentally delayed or mentally retarded individuals uses the behavioral approach of "clock training." In this treatment parents or caretakers place the child on the toilet at regular intervals throughout the day. The time intervals start at a point where the chances are maximized that the child will successfully void in the toilet—for example, an initial schedule consists of trips to the toilet every 30 minutes throughout the day with 10-minute sits on the toilet each time. Successful voids on the toilet are reinforced with praise or an opportunity to play with a favorite toy for several minutes. Once day-time continence is achieved and maintained on a particular clock interval schedule, intervals between trips to the toilet may be systematically lengthened by increments of half an hour to one hour. A goal of intervals of three to four hours between trips to the toilet may be reasonable in older children.

The most successful treatment for nocturnal enuresis involves the combination of behavioral rewards with the "urine alarm." As miniaturization technology has advanced, alarm devices have become smaller, lighter in weight, and more effective. The treatment involves the attachment of a moisture-sensing device to the pajama bottoms in the child's genital area and the placement of a buzzer alarm attached to a Velcro strip on the clothing over the child's shoulder. When the sensor device becomes wet, the alarm sounds. With the device, the child will be awakened from sleep quite quickly after the initiation of micturition. Once awake, the child should get out of bed and finish voiding in the toilet. Bed clothing should be changed and the child should return to sleep. Over time, the child is classically conditioned to awaken from sleep when the bladder is full prior to voiding. Numerous clinical studies have shown that approximately two thirds of children will respond favorably to this treatment. Subsequent relapse rates following this treatment are low.

### Medication Treatment

Two types of medication management have been used for the treatment of enuresis. In general, studies in the literature have demonstrated that these pharmacologic treatments are less effective than the behavioral treatments described above. Furthermore, after discontinuing the medication, relapse rates are quite high. Most clinical experience has been accumulated with the tricyclic antidepressant imipramine at a treatment dose of between 25 and 50 mg given by mouth as a single dose in the evening. Studies indicate that imipramine treatment stops enuresis in up to 80% of individuals within the first two weeks. Thereafter, however, continued treatment success may drop to below 50% of treated individuals. Long-lasting remission of nocturnal enuresis with imipramine treatment occurs in roughly 25% of patients. The mechanism of imipramine's therapeutic action is unknown. Proposed mechanisms include altered sleep rhythms or altered sleep architecture and anticholinergic effects on bladder musculature. The risk of death from accidental imipramine overdose, particularly with younger siblings in the household, is significant due to the degree of cardiac toxicity of high blood levels of this tricyclic compound. The potentially serious side effects of imipramine medication treatment for enuresis must be carefully weighed against the morbidity associated with this non–life-threatening condition.

A new pharmacologic treatment approach for nocturnal enuresis introduced in the United States in 1992 involves the intranasal administration of 1-deamino-8d-arginine vasopressin (DDAVP), the synthetic analog of the neurohypophyseal nonapeptide arginine vasopressin (antidiuretic hormone). Studies of DDAVP in humans have demonstrated enhanced antidiuretic potency, diminished pressor activity and a prolonged half-life and duration of action compared to treatment with antidiuretic hormone. The theoretic rationale for the use of DDAVP in children with nocturnal enuresis centers on the hypothesis that some children may not have the ability to concentrate urine and thereby decrease urine volume production at night due to dysregulation of the circadian release of antidiuretic hormone. Intranasal administration of DDAVP is postulated to restore urine concentrating ability, decrease nighttime production of urine, and reduce episodes of nocturnal enuresis. The medication is administered at night to the child via a nasal spray that delivers 10 $\mu$g of DDAVP to each nostril. Several studies with small numbers of children treated for periods up to four to eight weeks have demonstrated improvement in up to two thirds of treated patients. Adverse side effects have been limited to complaints of rhinitis and epistaxis. There have been no reports of significant difficulties with electrolyte imbalance or hypertension. Unfortunately, long-term data on treatment response or safety of continued use beyond eight weeks are not available. A study by Wille comparing pharmacologic treatment with DDAVP and behavioral treatment with the urine alarm demonstrated that there was improvement in 70% of individuals given DDAVP and 86% of individuals treated with the alarm. However, in follow-up, over 40% of individuals treated with DDAVP relapsed compared to a rate of relapse less than 5% among individuals treated with the alarm. The author felt that his study confirmed the role of conditioning treatment as preferable to the use of DDAVP in long-term treatment of nocturnal enuresis.

### Psychotherapy

Many authors in the field of child psychiatry acknowledge that monosymptomatic childhood enuresis is not an indication for interpretive psychotherapy. Studies have demonstrated that interpretive psychotherapy results in successful treatment of enuresis in approximately 20% of cases, but this rate may simply reflect the incidence of spontaneous remission of the disorder. Children, parents, and caretakers certainly benefit from education about the enuretic disorder conveyed by an empathetic clinician. In situations where there are clear environmental stresses, such as after a traumatic event or parental divorce, psychotherapy is appropriate and may be very useful in relieving fear and anxiety that contribute to the child's enuresis.

## ENCOPRESIS

### Diagnosis

The diagnosis of functional encopresis is made when a child is noted to have repeated bouts of involuntary passage of feces into places not appropriate for that purpose, such as in clothing or on the floor. Episodes must occur at least once a month for at least six months in a child with a mental and chronologic age of four years or older. Organic etiologies including inflammatory bowel disease, bacterial infection, and aganglionic megacolon (Hirschsprung's disease) must be ruled out. A child with functional encopresis might pass stool of consistencies varying from liquid to firm. Primary functional encopresis refers to the situation in which the child has not been continent of stool for a period of a year in the past. Secondary functional encopresis occurs when the child becomes incontinent of stool after a period of fecal continence lasting at least one year (Table 29-11).

### Prevalence

In a 1966 study by Bellman, a survey of 8863 children yielded a prevalence of 1.5% of encopresis among 7- and 8-year-old chil-

**TABLE 29-11.   Diagnostic Criteria
for Functional Encopresis**

Repeated passage of feces into places not appropriate for that
purpose (eg, clothing, floor), whether involuntary or intentional.
(The disorder may be overflow incontinence secondary to
functional fecal retention.)

At least one such event a month for at least 6 months.

Chronologic and mental age, at least 4 years.

Not due to a physical disorder, such as aganglionic megacolon.

Specify primary or secondary type.

   Primary type—the disturbance was not preceded by a period of
   fecal continence lasting at least 1 year.

   Secondary type—the disturbance was preceded by a period of
   fecal continence lasting at least 1 year.

*From Diagnostic and Statistical Manual of Mental Disorders, 3rd ed, revised.
American Psychiatric Association, 1987.*

dren. The male:female ratio was over 3:1. Other epidemiologic
data suggests that at 3 years of age, 16% of children will have
fecal incontinence once or more times per week. At 4 years, about
3% of children will be incontinent of feces. After 10 years of age
about 0.8% of children will continue to have difficulty with fecal
incontinence.

## Etiology

A variety of conceptual models have been proposed over the
years to explain why children develop encopresis. Like enuresis,
encopresis often has a multifactorial etiology.

A common scenario, which has been clearly conceptualized
by Melvin Levine, involves physiologic events related to stool
retention, bowel dilatation and stretching with subsequent overflow incontinence around an intraluminal fecal mass (Fig 29-2).
The genesis of the initial problem with severe constipation and
bowel dilatation might relate to either psychological or physiological factors. Psychological factors might include a child's anxiety about defecating in an unfamiliar place or simply relate to
an oppositional temperament. Physiologic factors might include
dehydration associated with a febrile illness, inadequate fiber or
bulk or fluid in the diet, or painful defecation associated with
previous injury to rectal mucosa (eg, perianal or rectal fissure)

following passage of a hard stool. Once the sequence of chronic
constipation and bowel dilatation is initiated, the child becomes
less able to exert voluntary control over fecal continence. Sensations of rectal fullness fade; muscular power within the bowel
wall to fully evacuate contents decreases, and external sphincter
control is lost. Support for the development of physiologic bowel
dysfunction in encopretic children has been found in the studies
of Loening-Baucke, who found that 56% of retentive encopretic
children were unable to defecate rectal balloons. Many of the
encopretic children also had abnormal contractions of the external
anal sphincter. These encopretic children with lower bowel
physiologic difficulties experience daily soiling accidents related
to overflow of liquid or semi-formed fecal material, which cir-
cumnavigates impacted fecal masses in the child's dilated lower
colon and rectum. The child is powerless to control these episodes
of fecal incontinence. Secretive behavior ensues in which the
child tries desperately to hide the evidence from parents, caregivers and friends. Levels of anxiety increase. Self-esteem is
eroded, and the child may become demoralized.

Fecal incontinence can be the result of organic causes, including anatomic defects of the gastrointestinal tract (eg, aganglionic
megacolon—Hirschsprung's disease, fistulas, stenosis of the rectum or anus); inflammatory bowel disease; viral, bacterial or parasitic diarrheal illness; or even systemic illnesses related to endocrine dysfunction or seizure disorder. These entities are readily
discovered by a careful pediatric history, physical examination,
and laboratory evaluation.

Children who are impulsive and hyperactive may have occasional episodes of encopresis simply because they do not attend
to the neural signals of rectal fullness until it is too late.

## Associated Features

Like children who suffer from urinary incontinence, children with
recurrent fecal incontinence experience profound negative effects
on self-esteem. Typically, these children try to avoid situations
that might lead to embarrassment, such as special family outings,
overnight visits to a friend's home, and even school. These children tend to hide their soiled underwear. They are shy and reluctant to socialize with peers and adults. Twenty-five percent
of children with functional encopresis also will suffer from functional enuresis.

On the other hand, children with deliberate fecal incontinence
or episodes of fecal smearing often suffer from comorbid severe
emotional disorders such as conduct disorder, major depression,

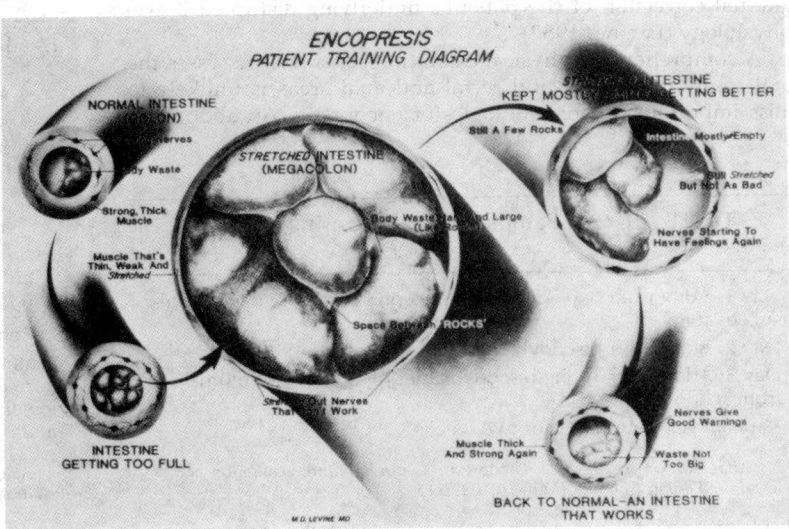

**Figure 29-2.**   Diagram developed by Mel Levine for de-
mystifying encopresis. (Levine MD. Encopresis: its potentiation, evaluation, and alleviation. Pediatr Clin North Am
1982;29:315.)

or psychotic disorder. Individuals with mental retardation can engage in fecal smearing as a self-stimulatory activity.

## Course

Childhood functional encopresis may develop after a period of fecal continence, or it may be continuous from birth. Most commonly, soiling occurs several times a day following the child's consumption of a meal, which initiates a sequence of peristaltic muscular contractions in the bowel via the gastro-colic reflex. The condition rarely lasts into adulthood, but it may continue for years unless appropriately identified and treated. The morbidity associated with functional encopresis is directly related to the adverse effects of peer and parental rejection and teasing (eg, complaints that the child "smells") on the child's self-esteem. Parental and caregiver anger, punishment, and rejection contribute to the encopretic child's shame, embarrassment, and damaged self attitude.

## Assessment and Treatment

As with each patient who comes to a clinician with a medical complaint, it is important when confronted with a child suffering from encopresis to take a thorough pediatric history that documents the frequency, nature, and circumstances of the child's soiling episodes in great detail. As a first step, it is useful to interview parents or caregivers separately from the child so that anger and hostility built up over time toward the child can be defused and vented without unduly embarrassing or distressing the patient. Thereafter, the child should be interviewed alone to further assess the situation.

In the absence of clear psychopathology in either the child or the caregiver, it is reasonable to approach the workup and treatment of encopresis from a comprehensive medical framework. Ordinarily, the child and family will be greatly relieved when the interviewer conceptualizes the encopretic disorder as a medical problem (ie, the disorder is not a willful act of defiance on the part of the child, and therefore the disorder is not the child's fault). Explanations of normal bowel functioning followed by descriptions of bowel physiology disrupted by chronic constipation, bowel distention, and ultimately overflow incontinence are sources of comfort and reassurance to a child and family who have struggled and suffered for long periods thinking that the problem was hopeless and unsolvable. This "demystification" process paves the way for an effective and trusting therapeutic alliance between patient, caregiver and clinician that will allow reversal of the emotional cycles of blame and shame as well as gradual correction of the patient's underlying disrupted bowel physiology (Levine, 1982).

A comprehensive physical exam that sensitively assesses the oral cavity, abdomen, and rectal and anal areas is unlikely to miss important organic etiologies of encopresis. An abdominal

flat plate radiograph provides visual evidence to the patient and family about the physiologic difficulties associated with chronic constipation and overflow incontinence.

Educational and supportive interventions with the child and family are followed by the establishment of a contract for ongoing treatment between the clinician and the family group. The discussion of treatment is best divided into two phases: a bowel "clean-out" phase and maintenance of a constipation-free phase. It is helpful to explain that the bowel clean-out is necessary to remove the fecal mass that chronically distends the bowel wall and interferes with normal nerve and muscle functioning. The cathartic regimen outline by Levine (Table 29-12) requires two weeks and can be done at home. In a clinic follow-up visit two weeks after the initial clean-out, it is expected that the child will have successfully removed the intraluminal fecal mass and will have been free from soiling. If this is not the case, the bowel clean-out procedure should be repeated.

Once the bowel lumen is clear, a maintenance contract should be established. Family members and the patient should be seen in regular follow-up clinic visits to ensure that the combination of daily doses of laxatives and mineral oil continue to facilitate daily bowel movements (Table 29-13). This regimen in combination with a behavioral reward system (eg, star charts or stickers on a calendar), regular toilet sits for five minutes following each meal, and a diet higher in fiber and fluid intake should facilitate return of the child's bowel physiology to normal functioning. The process takes patience, perseverance, and time. An analogy to a mother's abdominal musculature and skin returning to normal following normal childbirth often helps families and patients understand the bodily adjustment process once a distending force is removed.

Using this comprehensive approach, Levine and his coworkers have reported a 78% success rate for children suffering from encopresis. The treatment success is long-term without symptom substitution. A more intensive psychotherapeutic intervention might be necessary for children with intractable encopresis who also suffer from severe emotional disturbances.

## CONCLUSION

The childhood disorders of elimination are common. Often, a child's difficulties with enuresis or encopresis arise through the

---

**TABLE 29-12.  Sample Bowel Cleansing Program (3-day cycle)**

Day 1: Administer two adult hyperphosphate enemas (Fleet's) in succession.
Day 2: Administer biscodyl (Dulcolax) suppository.
Day 3: Administer 10 mg biscodyl tablet po after child returns from school.
Repeat cycle four times for two weeks.

*Adapted from Levine MD. Encopresis: its potentiation, evaluation and alleviation. Pediatr Clin North Am 1982;29:315.*

---

**TABLE 29-13.  Sample Constipation-Free Maintenance Regimen**

1. Administer 30 mL light mineral oil mixed in orange juice po bid.
   Adjust dose upward if child remains constipated.
   Adjust dose downward if child has orange mineral oil staining of underwear.
2. Administer multivitamin po qd.
   Minimizes possible effects of mineral oil-induced malabsorption of fat-soluble vitamins.
3. Administer Senna concentrate (Senokot) one tablet or 5 mL po bid.
4. Regular toilet sits for 5 minutes after each meal
5. Behavioral reward system

Continue for 3 to 6 months. As bowel physiology returns to normal, taper of medications will be possible, because daily bowel movements will occur with less need for assistance from medication.

*Adapted from Levine MD. Encopresis: its potentiation, evaluation and alleviation. Pediatr Clin North Am 1982;29:315.*

complex interactions of genetic, neuromaturational, physiologic, and sociocultural factors. Assessment and treatment using a multifaceted approach comprised of education, medical assessment, behavior modification and empathetic counseling are most successful in alleviating the child's symptoms and tempering parental anxiety and anger. For those clinicians treating children suffering from enuresis and encopresis, the wisdom of Patrick Friman should not be forgotten:

> . . . the treatment of enuresis can be a threat to the child's health, as can the parental, professional, and peer response to the wetting. Children cannot die from wetting the bed. They can die from the medicine given to them to stop bed wetting. Wet beds cannot cause contusions, abrasions, and concussions. Punishments administered for bed wetting can. Urine cannot cause emotional disturbance. Ridiculing, admonishing, or singling out a child for urinating can.

## Selected Readings

Bakwin H. The genetics of enuresis. In: Kolvin I, MacKeith RC, Meadows SP (eds): Bladder control and enuresis. Clinics in developmental medicine. Philadelphia: JB Lippincott, 1973:73.

Bellman M. Studies on encopresis. Acta Paediatrica Scandinavia [Suppl] 170, 1966.

Cohen TB. Observations on school children in the People's Republic of China. Journal of Child Psychiatry 16:165–173, 1977.

Fraiberg SH. The magic years. New York: Charles Scribner's Sons, 1959.

Freud A, Burlingham DT. War and children. New York, Medical War Books, 1943.

Friman PC. A preventative context for enuresis. Pediatr Clin North Am 1986;33: 871.

Hindley CB, Fillozat AM, Klackenberg G, Nicolet-Meister D, Sand EA. Some differences in infant feeding and elimination training in five European longitudinal samples. J Child Psychol Psychiatry 1965;6:179.

Levine MD. Encopresis: its potentiation, evaluation and alleviation. Pediatr Clin North Am 1982;29:315.

Levine MD, Bakow H. Children with encopresis: a study of treatment outcome. Pediatrics 1976;58:845.

Loening-Baucke VA, Cruikshank BM. Abnormal defecation dynamics in chronically constipated children with encopresis. J Pediatr 1986;108:562.

Rittig S, Knudsen UB, Norgaard JP, et al. Abnormal diurnal rhythm of plasma vasopressin and urinary output in patients with enuresis. Am J Physiol 1989;25: F664.

Rutter M, Yule W, Graham, P. Enuresis and behavioral deviance: Some epidemiological considerations. In: Kolvin I, MacKeith RC, Meadows SP (eds): Bladder control and enuresis. Clinics in developmental medicine. Philadelphia: JB Lippincott, 1973:137.

Schaefer CE. Childhood encopresis and enuresis: causes and therapy. New York: Van Nostrand Reinhold, 1979.

Wille S. Comparison of desmopressin and enuresis alarm for nocturnal enuresis. Arch Dis Child 1986;61:30.

*Principles and Practice of Pediatrics, Second Edition.*
edited by Frank A. Oski et al. J. B. Lippincott Company, Philadelphia © 1994.

# 29.17 *Psychometrics*

Leon A. Rosenberg

Psychometrics refers to a wide range of measurement techniques that provide data to assist in the diagnosis of cognitive and behavioral or emotional difficulties. There are several specific areas of measurement, each with a variety of tools that differ in the specific processes they measure and in their accuracy of measurement. The instruments also differ in their mode of interpretation. Some psychometric tools produce scores that have clearly defined meanings; others produce data that require much clinical expertise to allow accurate interpretation. Even those tools that provide relatively easily interpreted specific numbers also produce subtle issues of interpretation that require clinical expertise.

## COGNITIVE FUNCTIONING

### Measurement Process

The most commonly used measurement tools are listed in Table 29-14, along with the type of scores produced by each. These measures of cognitive development are crucial for the proper diagnosis both of intellectual development that is delayed or otherwise outside the range of normality, and of learning disabilities. The diagnosis of limited intelligence requires an objective assessment both of learning capacity and of overall social adaptation. The relationship between the two areas of measurement, the second of which is discussed in the next section, is not one of conflict. If the level of cognitive development is demonstrated to be significantly below normal, a measurement of social competence that scores higher does not indicate that the individual is not cognitively below normal limits, but only that he or she has received excellent social training from some source. If the measure of social competence scores significantly below the level of cognitive functioning indicated by an appropriate intelligence test, this does not indicate that the intelligence test is exaggerating the individual's level of functioning. Rather, the discrepancy indicates that the individual's level of independent social functioning is well below what one would expect from his or her level of cognitive functioning. When dealing with delays in cognitive development, this often indicates the absence of appropriate training toward independence. Both areas of measurement are essential to diagnosis and complement each other.

Several different types of instruments respond to the process of cognitive development and can provide insight into the child's developmental status. Not all of the instruments are equal in reliability and validity or scope of measurement. For example, the amount of detail presented in a human figure drawing directly correlates with the results from independent measures of cognitive functioning and with the chronologic age of normal subjects. As children get older the amount of detail they put in a drawing of a person increases. Hence, asking a child to "draw a person" has for many years been a rough estimate of the level of cognitive functioning. The fact that it is only a rough estimate is based on its relative weakness in predicting such things as levels of educational achievement when compared with other measures of cognitive functioning.

An individual's cognitive development must be sampled across a fairly broad range, touching on the many different ways in which complex reasoning is expressed in any individual. The most useful tools sample a range of intellectual functions providing a composite picture of the individual's capacity, with some additional information regarding specific areas of information processing.

The most well-known and well-validated instruments are the Wechsler series, the Wechsler Preschool and Primary Scale of Intelligence Revised (WPPSI-R), the Wechsler Intelligence Scale for Children, Third Edition (WISC-III), and the Wechsler Adult Intelligence Scale Revised. The WPPSI-R has replaced the 1967 Wechsler Preschool and Primary Scale of Intelligence for Children. The WISC-III is the result of an extensive revision of the 1974 Wechsler Intelligence Scale for Children Revised. Normative data was improved and the materials were extensively updated. These instruments produce a full-scale IQ score, separate verbal and performance IQ scores, and a series of subtest normalized standard scores within these two portions of the instrument.

Although the performance portion of a Wechsler instrument includes some perceptual-motor coordination skills, the instru-

## TABLE 29-14. A Descriptive Summary of Major Psychometric Instruments

### Tests of Cognitive Functioning

**Wechsler Preschool and Primary Scale of Intelligence-Revised**

Age range: 3 yrs to 7 yrs 3 mos

Scores produced: verbal I.Q., performance I.Q., full-scale I.Q.; 10 subtest normalized standard scores; 2 alternate subtests available. Average I.Q. = 100; standard deviation = 15

Year published: 1989

Publisher: The Psychological Corporation, New York, NY

**Wechsler Intelligence Scale for Children-third edition**

Age range: 6 yr 0 mo to 16 yr 11 mo

Scores produced: verbal I.Q., performance I.Q., full-scale I.Q.; 10 subtest normalized standard scores; 3 alternate subtests available, 4 index scores Average I.Q. = 100; standard deviation = 15

Year published: 1991

Publisher: The Psychological Corporation, New York, NY

**Wechsler Adult Intelligence Scale-Revised**

Age range: 16 yr 0 mo to 74 yr 0 mo

Scores produced: verbal I.Q., performance I.Q., full-scale I.Q.; 11 subtest normalized standard scores. Average I.Q. = 100; standard deviation = 15

Year published: 1981

Publisher: The Psychological Corporation, New York, NY

**McCarthy Scales of Children's Abilities**

Age range: 2 yr 4 mo to 8 yr 7 mo

Scores produced: general cognitive index (GCI); 5 subtest normalized standard scores. Average GCI = 100; standard deviation = 16

Year published: 1972

Publisher: The Psychological Corporation, New York, NY

**Kaufman Assessment Battery for Children**

Age range: 2 yr 6 mo to 12 yr 5 mo

Scores produced: sequential processing, simultaneous processing, mental processing composite, achievement; 7 to 13 subtest normalized standard scores, depending on child's age. Average score = 100; standard deviation = 15

Year published: 1983

Publisher: American Guidance Service, Inc, Circle Pines, MN

**Stanford-Binet Intelligence Scale—fourth edition**

Age range: 2 yr 0 mo to 23 yr 11 mo

Scores produced: verbal reasoning, abstract/visual reasoning, short-term memory, test composite; 8 to 13 subtest normalized standard scores, depending on child's age. Average score = 100; standard deviation = 16

Year published: 1986

Publisher: Riverside Publishing Co, Chicago, IL

**Bayley Scales of Infant Development**

Age range: 1 mo 24 d to 30 mo

Scores produced: Mental development index (MDI), psychomotor development index (PDI), infant behavior record (a descriptive rating). Average MDI and PDI = 100; standard deviation = 16

Year published: 1969

Publisher: The Psychological Corporation, New York, NY

### Tests of Social Adaptation

**Vineland Adaptive Behavior Scales**

Age range: birth to 18 yr 11 mo or "a low-functioning adult."

Scores produced: communication, daily living skills, socialization, motor skills, maladaptive behavior (optional), adaptive behavior composite. Average score = 100; standard deviation = 15.

Forms: *Survey*—for general assessment
      *Expanded*—for a more comprehensive assessment
      *Classroom*—for assessment of classroom behavior

Year published: 1984

Publisher: American Guidance Service, Inc, Circle Pines, MN

**AAMD Adaptive Behavior Scales**

Age range: 3 yr to 16 yr

Scores produced: percentile scores in 10 areas of independent functioning; scores are percentiles by age and sex.

Year published: 1974 revision

Publisher: American Association on Mental Deficiency, Washington, DC

### Tests of Educational Achievement

**Peabody Individual Achievement Test-Revised**

Age range: 5 yr 0 mo to 18 yr 11 mo

Educational range: kindergarten to 12th grade

Scores produced: mathematics, reading recognition, reading comprehension, spelling, general information, written expression; scores are grade equivalents, age equivalents, percentiles, and normalized standard scores.

Year published: 1989

Publisher: American Guidance Service, Inc, Circle Pines, MN

**Woodcock-Johnson Psychoeducational Battery-Revised**

Age range: 2.0 yr to adult

Educational range: preschool to 12th grade

Scores produced: reading cluster, mathematics cluster, written language cluster, knowledge cluster, skills cluster; scores are grade equivalents, instructional range, age equivalents, and percentiles.

Year published: 1990

Publisher: DLM Teaching Resources, Allen, TX

### Tests of Perceptual-Motor Functioning

**Developmental Test of Visual-Motor Integration**

Age range: 4 yr 0 mo to 13 yr+

Scores produced: age equivalents and normalized standard scores

Year published: 1982

Publisher: Follett Publishing Co, Chicago, IL

**Bender Visual Motor Gestalt Test**

Age range: approximately 4 yr to adult

Scores produced: several different scoring systems exist.

Years published: 1938–1979

Publisher: American Orthopsychiatric Association, New York, NY

**Motor-Free Visual Perceptual Test**

Age range: 4 yr to 8 yr

Scores produced: age equivalents and normalized standard scores

Publisher: Academic Therapy Publications, Novato, CA

---

ment was not designed for formal measurement of motor skills or visual-motor coordination. The performance portion of a Wechsler instrument measures complex verbal reasoning but does not require verbalization in the response system. For example, the child is shown a series of pictures in a mixed-up order; if he or she puts them together in the correct order, they show a person carrying out a fairly common problem-solving or social interaction activity. The child carries out very complex reasoning involving subvocal language, calling on his or her memory of practical life experiences and an appreciation of the sequence of behavior over time. The child presents the examiner with his or her solution by putting the cards in the "correct" order; the child says nothing. On the verbal portion of the instrument, similar problems are presented to the child in the form of verbal questions from the examiner. However, on the verbal portion of the instrument, the child responds in verbal form only.

Some subtests on the performance portion of a Wechsler test that clearly have a strong quality of visual-motor coordination also demand complex verbal reasoning for their solution, such as the block design and object assembly subtests. Obviously, if there is some type of significant perceptual or perceptual-motor integrative difficulty, the child will have difficulties with the co-ordination aspect of block design or the spatial orientation aspect of object assembly. However, those subtests were not specifically designed for that purpose. A child who scores in the retarded range on the verbal portion of the instrument and in the average range on the performance portion is not a cognitively delayed child with good mechanical skills, but rather a child of normal intelligence who has difficulty dealing with tasks requiring verbal expression.

The new WISC-III also provides the clinician with four index scores: verbal comprehension, perceptual organization, freedom from distractibility, and processing speed. These represent four structural factors in cognitive processing that contribute to our understanding of such special problems as retardation and learning disabilities.

Other measures of cognitive functioning also provide useful information. For example, the McCarthy Scales of Children's Abilities measure cognitive functioning by providing an overall score of cognitive development (general cognitive index [GCI]) and submeasures dealing with memory, verbal skills, quantitative reasoning, and perceptual-motor skills. The GCI of the McCarthy Scales is reasonably equivalent to the full-scale IQ of a Wechsler measure. The McCarthy Scales make a greater effort to measure areas of immediate or short-term memory than does the Wechsler series. This is important when examining learning-disabled youngsters, for whom interference in memory function is a major problem within the syndrome. However, clinicians have expressed some concern about the degree to which the measures of memory function overlap several portions of the McCarthy Scales, resulting in too sharp a drop in the GCI when the child does have a memory deficit. However, general clinical experience suggests that the McCarthy Scales of Children's Abilities can hold the attention of young children and can provide the examiner with a rich picture of the child's functioning.

The Kaufman Assessment Battery for Children (KABC), another instrument, also provides an overall measure of cognitive functioning but subdivides information processing into the two categories of simultaneous and sequential reasoning. The structural differences between the KABC and the Wechsler series are based on theoretic issues that are well presented in the KABC manual, which should be read along with Wechsler's presentations in the manuals for those instruments. There are no data to show that the Kaufman dichotomy of cognitive functioning is superior to the structure of the Wechsler series.

Nationally, the KABC has been used extensively, especially by school psychologists, who include it in an overall assessment of learning problems. Although the instrument certainly can provide useful information in many clinical situations, structural difficulties have led to a very serious caution regarding its use. Sattler in his 1988 review stated that the instrument may be useful when data are needed regarding nonverbal cognitive abilities, but "in most cases, however, the KABC should not be used as the primary instrument for identifying the intellectual abilities of normal or special children. . . . Neither should it be the primary instrument for measuring intelligence in clinical assessments."

A recent introduction to the scene is the fourth edition of the Stanford-Binet Intelligence Scale. The original instrument is one of the oldest measures of intellectual functioning. Although revised a few years ago, it maintained measurement limitations that clinicians found frustrating. It offered only an overall measure of level of cognitive functioning and did not permit analysis into subareas of cognitive processing. Various proposals for such

analyses have been in existence for some time, but the instrument itself was never designed nor validated for anything more than a single, global IQ score. The new Stanford-Binet provides an overall measure of developmental level along with measurements of subareas of significant clinical interest (verbal reasoning, abstract/visual reasoning, quantitative reasoning, and short-term memory).

Current validity studies indicate that the instrument is as valid as any other in accessing general ability level (Laurent et al, 1992). It can be especially useful in cases where there are concerns regarding short-term memory. The instrument measures a broad range of abilities. Although it can be used with children as young as age 2, it may not be the best procedure to use when examining very young children who are low functioning. It may be difficult to diagnose retardation in 2- and 3-year-old children because the items do not go low enough to adequately sample their functioning.

## What Instrument to Use

Deciding which instrument to use is first determined by the age of the child. Each instrument is valid only for children who fall into the specific age group on which that instrument was standardized. However, several of the instruments overlap in age ranges served. The Wechsler series overlap sequentially by a few months. The WPPSI-R has an upper age range that extends several months into the lower age range of the WISC-III, and the same relationship is seen between the WISC-III and the Wechsler Adult Intelligence Scale Revised.

The advantage of having such an overlap can be seen in the following example. If a child is within the age range for the WISC-III but is young enough also to be examined on the WPPSI-R, administering both instruments would result in very similar full-scale IQ scores regardless of whether the child is of average intelligence or below normal intelligence. However, a child of that age who has limited intellectual ability would tend to receive zero raw scores on several of the subtests of the WISC-III. Those zero raw scores would convert into standard scores that would then produce a valid full-scale IQ score. However, the test would have revealed what the child could *not* do, but not what he *could* do. If the same child were administered the WPPSI-R, he would receive a full-scale IQ score that would indicate the same degree of retardation, but the youngster would be able to respond positively to some of the items on all of the subtests. This is because the WPPSI-R has a lower age floor than the WISC-III. Choosing the WPPSI-R in this case would indicate the child's level of intelligence, but with the added advantage of obtaining a sample of his successes in a variety of areas of cognitive measurement.

Because of its wide age range, the new (fourth edition) Stanford-Binet Intelligence Scale provides a broader picture of functioning when examining retarded youngsters who are well into the age range appropriate for the WISC-III but of significantly lower-than-normal intelligence. The Stanford-Binet has a much lower age floor than the WISC-III. This type of reasoning is valid when comparing the Wechsler series, the Stanford-Binet, and the McCarthy Scales; those instruments have a great deal in common with one another.

Some measures of cognitive functioning are standardized on age groups much below that of the instruments discussed above. These "baby tests" can be used on infants as young as 2 months. However, any measure of cognitive functioning that purports to deal with such young children is very dependent on measures of motor development and is influenced by the normal variability of language development. Measures below age 6 years, and especially those below age 2.5 years, are negatively influenced by the variability of normal development. The best developed and validated measure of infant development is the Bayley Scales of

Infant Development, which starts at 2 months of age. Administering a complete Bayley gives an overall measure of development in both the cognitive (the mental development index) and the motor areas (the psychomotor development index). The motor scale is not expected to predict later cognitive development, although there are many items that overlap between the two measures. If a clear picture of the infant's developmental level relative to age peers is required, the Bayley Scales are at present the best instrument.

## Clinical Problems

The validity of the data from any measurement instrument is influenced by the level of cooperation and effort demonstrated by the child. The established instruments, such as the Wechsler and the Stanford-Binet, are fairly robust measures, meaning that they are not easily influenced by minor variations in cooperation or motivation. However, the child must put forth a reasonable effort and must be reasonably comfortable with the examiner, or the results can be affected negatively. Significant anxiety during test administration can also negatively influence results. Specific deficit areas can reduce the overall score and can falsely suggest retardation, but experienced examiners should identify this quickly. For example, the greater the degree of difference between verbal and performance IQ scores on a Wechsler, the less valid is the full-scale IQ score. Significant neurologic difficulties that influence language or affect perceptual-motor integrative processes may interfere with the subtests of any of the instruments. These difficulties can severely lower total scores; clinical expertise is needed to determine which scores can be interpreted and which cannot.

The patient does not have to know the examiner personally, and the examiner and the patient do not have to be from the same social class, the same religion, the same race, or the same sex. Well-trained examiners who know how to work well with children obtain good results regardless of the degree to which they are similar to or different from the child. Poor examiners who do not know the instrument well, are clumsy during its administration, are uncomfortable with children, or are in a hurry produce depressed scores regardless of the degree of similarity between themselves and the child. However, each child must be considered as an individual, and the child's response to the examiner must be considered when evaluating the validity of specific findings.

In recent years much emphasis has been placed on the issue of cultural bias in intelligence testing. When using older instruments, such as the original WISC, a 15-point difference has been found between the average scores obtained by the general population and those of extremely impoverished groups. At first, much was made of what appeared to be a racial difference in these data, but it appears that the bias was based on severe cultural impoverishment (Mercer, 1971). In addition, the problem was not in the clinical diagnosis of retardation, which starts at an IQ of 69 (DSM III-R, 1987). Children scoring below an IQ of 65 within the extremely impoverished population were significantly different from their own socioculturally matched peers. The bias occurred before the clinical range was reached (IQ scores below 70). Numerous impoverished youngsters scoring in the 75 to 80 range were not retarded, but the test could falsely suggest mild degrees of slow cognitive development as an answer to poor school performance.

All of the current instruments, the revisions of the Stanford-Binet, and the Wechsler and Kaufman instruments, have done a much better job of sampling racial groups and, more importantly, of sampling children of lower socioeconomic background, since the instruments were standardized.

Even though improved methods of test construction might

eliminate much of the cultural bias, intelligence testing remains a potentially controversial area because the data are sometimes used in a manner for which the instruments were not designed. Intelligence tests provide no information about why individuals score at whatever level they do. They simply provide the clearest picture currently possible regarding the child's current level of functioning. If those scores are to be related to genetic input, the role of sociocultural input, or the role of diet, race, and so on, appropriate research comparisons must be provided. For example, years of arguments about the use of intelligence test data for racial comparisons led to research indicating that extreme poverty was an influential factor but race per se was not. Obviously, when dealing with children of extremely impoverished backgrounds, accurate interpretation of test results requires experience with the effects of such impoverishment relative to the age of the child.

## Measurement of Social Adaptation

The Vineland Adaptive Behavior Scales measure several areas of social adaptation by considering that each of the areas of adaptation follows a developmental course from infancy onward. Reasonable estimates of the levels of independent functioning appropriate for each age have been determined through the standardization process in the construction of the instrument. An individual child's current level of independent functioning can be compared to his or her age mates by surveying the presence or absence of a wide variety of adaptive skills. In this manner, the Vineland Scales can provide the clinician with a reasonably objective measure of a child's rate of social development or, to be more specific, the rate at which the child is acquiring the ability to function independently.

The Vineland Scales are typically administered to the child's major caretaker. Hence, successful administration of the instrument requires the ability to interview parents who may be anxious about their child and who may deny problems and exaggerate skills, or, conversely, deny areas of achievement and exaggerate problem areas. The interviewer presents specific skills, such as whether or not the child can use a knife to cut food, and determines whether or not the skill is present and truly involves independent functioning by the child. If it is not present, the interviewer finds out whether the parents have not permitted the child to acquire this skill or the youngster has not acquired the skill despite the parents' efforts.

An expanded version of the instrument is available that breaks down each specific skill into smaller steps; thus, the instrument is sensitive to degrees of change that might be very small in the normal population but that would represent meaningful changes in the significantly retarded individual.

The American Association on Mental Deficiency has a similar survey instrument, the AAMD Adaptive Behavior Scales, that concentrates on behaviors specific to retardation and emotional maladjustment. Although providing a detailed survey of important skill areas, this instrument's norms are limited; this presents the clinician with some difficulty in generalization of findings and with limitations in the level of statistical analysis that can be used in research. However, when the instrument is used sequentially, it can serve to delineate clearly areas of positive or negative change in hospitalized mentally retarded patients.

## Measures of Educational Achievement

The field of special education has developed a variety of measurement tools primarily designed to aid in specific curriculum planning. The field of psychological measurement also has been strongly involved in the development of educational achievement measures, especially in delineating the child's specific level of current achievement and the measurement of variations in a child's method of learning or processing information.

The available tools differ from one another in what they specifically ask the child to do, and those differences can cause confusion in interpretation. For example, one measure of reading comprehension presents the child with a printed sentence that the youngster reads silently. Then the sentence is removed and the child is shown four pictures, one of which best matches the meaning of the sentence just read. The child demonstrates his or her level of reading comprehension by pointing to the picture he or she believes to be the correct one. The response system requires only pointing, because the child does not have to speak. The task involves a short-term memory factor because the youngster does not see the sentence while searching for the picture.

Another measure of reading comprehension presents the youngster with sentences he or she reads silently, each of which has a word missing. The child is to choose, from a list of presented words, the one that would complete the meaning of the sentence best if inserted in the missing space. While solving the problem the child has the sentence and the alternate words in front of him or her at all times. Again, the measure of reading comprehension does not involve the child's speaking. However, this time there is no memory factor, because all of the material remains in front of the child.

Hence, when both tests are given to the same child and a different score is obtained on "reading comprehension," there is a very good possibility that both scores are accurate even though different. One score demonstrates the child's level of reading comprehension when immediate or short-term memory is not involved, and the other measure indicates what level of skill is present when a demand on immediate recall is made. Differences seen between the two measures can be interpreted only by clinical experience and with caution. A lower score on the first instrument can suggest difficulty in immediate memory. A lower score on the second instrument is seen in children who have difficulty with an increased demand on visual tracking while maintaining an orderly left-to-right reading sequence. They must leave the sentence visually and examine a column or row of words, and then visually return to the sentence while maintaining a concept gleaned from the sequence of words they have read.

The Peabody Individual Achievement Test Revised (PIAT-R) provides two measures of reading, reading recognition and reading comprehension, which yield a total reading score. The instrument also includes measures of spelling, general information, and mathematics, which combine to yield a total test score describing the child's overall level of achievement. A separate subtest of written expression is combined with spelling to yield a measure of written language.

The Woodcock-Johnson Psycho-Educational Battery consists of two separate instruments: a series of tests of cognitive abilities and a series of achievement tests. The achievement battery is extensive. There is the standard battery consisting of letter-word identification and passage comprehension yielding an overall reading score, calculation and applied problems producing an overall mathematics score, measures of writing ability, and measures of knowledge in science, social studies, and humanities. The supplementary battery includes five more tests dealing with specific areas such as word attack and writing fluency.

Other instruments, which are all well-designed, high-quality measurement tools, are also available. The most valid interpretation of the findings obtained from any one of them requires an understanding of exactly what the child is being asked to do. Clinicians often find it worthwhile to measure academic areas with more than one instrument when they suspect that some type of disability is influencing the child's learning function.

## Learning Disabilities

A major demand on psychometrics is to assist in the diagnosis of learning disabilities and to contribute to an understanding of the processes that must be remediated. After years of confusion regarding the definition of learning disabilities, guidelines have been established that are extremely important to the educational field, but they leave psychologists and pediatricians with the need to differentiate carefully between diagnostic and legalistic definitions. Currently, a *learning disability* is defined as a condition that exists when there is a meaningful difference between the current level of academic functioning of a child and the level that would be expected from a child of that particular age and specific level of intelligence.

Several interrelated measurement issues must be considered. This is a discrepancy model that seeks differences between current levels of academic functioning and expected levels of functioning. Major issues to be considered are what size discrepancy is considered to be meaningful, what measures of intelligence are reliable and valid, and what measures of academic functioning are reliable and valid.

The model is based on the simple mental age concept, which can easily be computed from the old formula of IQ = mental age (MA) divided by chronological age (CA), multiplied by 100; or, solving for MA, MA = (IQ × CA)/100. If a child is 10 years of age and has an IQ of 100, mental age is 10. Five years are subtracted from mental age to obtain the expected educational level of fifth grade. Within rough limits, in the United States children start first grade at age 6, and normal progression results in a 10-year-old's being in fifth grade. That is the expectation for the average 10-year-old who would also have a mental age of 10 years. There is a lower expectation for children of less-than-normal cognitive ability. If the child is 10 years of age and has a mental age of 7, you subtract 5 and have an expected educational level of 2.

A 2-year discrepancy between actual and expected grade level has been required before a child could be considered as having a learning disability. This was due to economics: a smaller discrepancy would result in a larger number of children requiring expensive special education, whereas many of the youngsters are just demonstrating minor maturational delays that self-correct in time. A larger discrepancy would identify a much smaller number of youngsters, but that degree of difference was unacceptable to the professionals working in the field.

The psychometric issues, however, are much more complex than this. Educational achievement and intelligence are seen as being related in a linear fashion, because there is a statistically significant and highly meaningful correlation obtained between the two when the best measures are used. The actual relationship between the two variables, however, is affected by the mathematical artifact of regression to the mean.

The difference between the academic achievement levels of a 10-year-old person at the 60th percentile of intelligence and a 10-year-old at the 50th is not the same as that between 10-year-olds at the 90th and 80th percentiles, and the same is true at the other end of the spectrum. One cannot simply subtract 5 from their different mental ages to obtain a valid estimate of their expected achievement levels. Hence, techniques were developed that used the correlation between the measures of intelligence and achievement and the reliability coefficients of each separate measurement to specify the discrepancy level that would reach statistical significance ($p < .05$).

Tables are available that allow the clinician to make the necessary mathematical conversions quickly (Berk, 1984), and a simple computer program is available that provides a similar result (Reynolds and Stowe, 1985). The computer program already has built-in reliability coefficients for several intelligence and academic achievement measures, as well as the correlations among them. Different instruments can be used as long as the clinician can enter the reliability coefficients for both instruments, usually found in the test manuals, and the correlation between the two instruments, which may be present in one of the test manuals but may have to be obtained from the literature.

The previous discussion involves a legalistic definition of learning disability, and although the pediatrician must be aware of how these data will be interpreted by the local educational authority, the scientific and clinical aspects of the measurement of learning disability involve other concerns. After an appropriate intelligence examination determines the level of educational expectation, the next step is to identify the presence of cognitive processing difficulties that stress the child's ability to learn. This is true whether or not that stress results in a level of academic functioning that is significantly different from what is normally expected from that child. In other words, there may be a significant cognitive deficit that the child has struggled to overcome, and because of the level of success he or she has achieved, the youngster does not technically meet the definition of a learning disability.

Differentiation must be made between a *learning disability*, which has been formally defined as requiring a measurable discrepancy between expected achievement and actual achievement, and a *cognitive dysfunction*, which is a clinical problem of information-processing difficulties. The latter may not affect school learning to the point of meeting the criterion for a "learning disability." A child may show significant language-processing difficulties on cognitive (intelligence) tests and tests specific to language functioning, but he or she may read well despite the problem. A child may have significant directionality problems (ie, left-right disorientation) but may compensate well and read at an appropriate grade level. A 20-point discrepancy between verbal and performance IQ scores in either direction is often but not always associated with delayed learning. The "dysfunction" is present, but the "disability" may not be.

A more psychometrically accurate measurement would compare youngsters' intellectual functioning and current academic achievement with instruments that have been standardized on the same population. Hence, there was some interest in the KABC, because that instrument sampled both cognitive functioning and academic achievement, and the norms for both measures were derived from the same standardization group. However, there are procedures by which appropriate comparisons can be made between instruments not "normed" on the same population, as long as their intercorrelation and individual reliability coefficients are known.

Some evidence suggested that a combination of the Woodcock-Johnson Reading and Math Clusters and the Wechsler Intelligence Scale for Children identified learning-disabled children at a rate equal to, if not better than, the use of the two KABC measures (Heinfelden, 1986). In that study the "hit rate" improved when the assessment of intelligence was not limited to the full-scale Wechsler IQ score, but if there was a significant difference between the verbal and performance IQ scores, the higher of the two was used as the best estimate of the youngster's intelligence.

Further discussion of learning disabilities can be found in Chapter 29.2.

## Measures of Perceptual-Motor Functioning

The Bender Visual Motor Gestalt test requires the child to copy a series of designs, and the quality of the design reproductions is correlated with age. Hence, an estimate of the child's level of perceptual-motor integrative skills limited to a graphomotor task can be assessed. Rough guidelines of age norms are presented in the original monograph (Bender, 1979), and a scoring system is presented by Koppitz (1975). General clinical experience suggests that the instrument is sensitive to developmental differences in this area with children below age 10. With older children and adults, the instrument has a long history of being used in examinations of central nervous system dysfunction. Its current use with children, however, emphasizes the maturational process, examining for variability that might have an effect on learning skills, such as the negative influence of directionality errors on early reading and pencil-control difficulties that can negatively influence writing activities.

The Developmental Test of Visual Motor Integration includes many of the Bender items but has a wider range than the Bender Gestalt and may be more useful when dealing with older youngsters. Clinicians have found success in combining one of these two measures with other instruments such as the Motor-Free Visual Perceptual Test.

With a combination of tools, it may be possible to identify problems that are more perceptual than motor-output, versus those that encompass all aspects of visual-motor coordination. The use of any of these instruments requires a significant amount of clinical expertise, because the scoring procedures are still fairly general and require clinical interpretation. The same is generally true for most measures of perceptual-motor integration.

## Neuropsychological Batteries

Specific groups of psychometric measures have been presented as neuropsychological batteries based on their relevance to neurologic diagnosis and neurologic rehabilitation. Underlying neurologic processes obviously influence both overt and subtle aspects of motor dexterity, perceptual accuracy, visual-motor coordination skills, all aspects of memory functioning, language comprehension and language expression, and the complexities of reasoning or problem-solving. Comparing and contrasting the results of measurement in all of these areas can present a picture of the strengths and weaknesses in the individual's total functioning that can delineate specific functional losses. In turn, these may be indicative of some type of central nervous system dysfunction, may indicate areas of deterioration in functioning that might suggest an underlying neurologic process, and may point to problems in functioning that require remediation. Most neuropsychological approaches make heavy use of the Wechsler Intelligence Scale combined with a variety of other specific measures. There are two major batteries that relate to different theoretic positions regarding central nervous system organization and functioning, and they are somewhat in competition with each other: the Halstead Reitan battery (Reitan and Davison, 1974) and the Luria Nebraska battery (Golden, 1981).

At times, publications in the area suggest an almost cookbook approach through which score discrepancies can lead to a diagnostic or rehabilitation decision. However, in reality interpretation requires a good deal of sophistication regarding the clinical foundation of each of the measures, the statistical basis for intersubtest comparison, the neurologic basis of normal development, and the general clinical picture of the major neurologic issues presented. As a result, sophisticated neuropsychological assessment is often carried out by well-trained neuropsychologists who do not use either the Halstead Reitan or the Luria Nebraska batteries. These individuals select specific psychometric measures to examine areas of suspected weaknesses based on their clinical knowledge of the patient and their sensitivity to the meaning of neurologic symptoms. In their hands the neuropsychological examination follows a differential diagnostic decision tree within which the results of one psychological test indicate the need for the next area of measurement.

There is a good deal of interest in the use of these measures to aid neurologic diagnosis. One could debate what their future role will be in the face of continuing advances in the development of diagnostic procedures in neurology. At the same time, the sensitivity of the neuropsychological assessment to dysfunctional processes strongly suggests a tremendous potential in the area of rehabilitation or any aspect of treatment planning.

## Repeat Testing and Practice Effect

The evaluation of treatment effectiveness often requires repeated measurements. Diagnostic considerations also often require repeat measurements. For example, a child's response to a particular drug might have influenced WISC-III results, and his or her cognitive functioning must be reexamined when he or she is free of the effects of that drug.

How does repeat testing remain valid when just the act of taking the test the second time may produce a practice effect? When psychometric testing is done, it is assumed that the subject is naive and has no prior knowledge regarding the individual test items. Repeated administration of any intelligence test tends to result in a rise in IQ scores, and the increase is assumed to be caused by the effect of practice. The possibility of a practice effect decreases as a period of time elapses between the two test administrations. This is not simply due to a forgetting factor, but also is influenced by the basic structure of an intelligence test. For the IQ to remain the same over a period of time, for example, the youngster must be able to succeed on more items than he or she did before. In other words, the raw score must rise if the normalized score is to remain the same with an age-related instrument. As a result, if a year has elapsed, the child would be exposed to many items he or she has not seen before, and there would be no practice effect.

However, there are many clinical situations in which retesting is required within a short period of time. It is incorrect to believe that retesting, even within just a few days, automatically results in a practice effect and has an inflating impact on all aspects of measurement. It is very rare for a child to think about a verbal item that was administered, look up the item in a dictionary or talk about it with other people, and then do better on it when the test is readministered 3 or 4 days later. However, if the task was a timed one and required some planning before execution, the second administration could result in a higher score because the youngster does not have to go through a trial-and-error exploration process again. For example, on some of the more difficult puzzle items of object assembly, the child is not told what the object will make when he or she manages to put them together successfully. During the second administration, the youngster may remember what the puzzle will make; just the recall of that piece of information could result in his or her working faster and receiving a time bonus credit during the second administration, although he or she did not receive such credit during the first.

Practice effect occurs most frequently on timed tests, especially when there is a time bonus possibility, and on any test in which teaching by the examiner is permitted. For example, on the similarities subtest it is appropriate to give the child the correct answer if he or she fails some of the earlier items. The second time the child takes the test, he or she may receive full credit for those same items because he or she has gone through the training procedure before.

In general, practice effort can occur, but its presence can be recognized by the clinician, and practice effect is not a uniform problem common to the entire test protocol. Repeat testing, when needed for a clinical purpose, can be done despite the possibility that practice effect may influence some of the material, if the clinician has both test protocols available for an item-by-item analysis.

## BEHAVIORAL AND PERSONALITY MEASURES

### Behavioral Checklists

Several dozen instruments purport to provide clinical information based on behavioral reports made by a child's parents or teachers or those made directly by the child. An excellent example of development in this area of measurement is the Child Behavior Checklist of Achenbach and Edelbrock, which has a parent form, a teacher's form, and a youth self-report form. The norms that are presented allow one to determine whether or not the behavioral complaints indicated by the observer reach frequencies that fall into the clinical range or stay within the range of the general population. In addition, a comparison with the available norms may identify underreporting that makes the child look too perfect.

Such behavioral reporting systems are designed to aid clinical diagnosis, but they cannot stand alone. They are subject to the typical problems of reporting systems, such as the personal biases of those making the report or their variability in sensitivity to what is occurring even if there is no bias. However, such instruments allow an easily obtained survey of what parents and teachers feel they see in the child and, for the youngster old enough for the youth self-report form, what complaints the child has.

### Projective Measures of Personality

Projective tests sample the child's fantasy life by encouraging the youngster to tell stories in response to ambiguous pictures (Thematic Apperception Test) or to imagine what he or she might see in a series of vague inkblots (Rorschach). Projective testing has a dual foundation. First, normal personality functioning includes the use of fantasy as a release mechanism for areas of normal stress and conflict. When those areas of conflict become pathologic, fantasy expressions may reflect that pathology. Second, there is a long history of research in normal human perception that indicates that a subject's personal needs may influence his or her interpretation of ambiguous stimuli. True perceptions by normal subjects require stimulus clarity. Stimulus ambiguity produces variability among subjects in their interpretation of the stimulus, with their interpretations influenced by everything from different levels of hunger to different levels of anxiety.

Even though the history of perceptual research provides us with some clues to the mechanism by which projective testing operates, the primary factor is the role of fantasy in normal and abnormal personality functioning, whereby issues of conflict can be expressed despite the protective activity of unconscious defensive processes. For example, although unconscious mechanisms would prevent an individual from being able to be in touch with and report on sexual fears, these conflicts can be expressed in disguised form through fantasy. The individual is not talking about himself or herself but is referring to the make-believe figures in the story. The interpretation of projectives is, therefore, based on psychodynamic principles and is similar to the interpretation of dreams. The advantage of projectives is that we do not have to wait for the child to dream or to be able to recall and report a dream. Instead, the Thematic Apperception Test cards can bring the child into a game in which he or she makes up whatever story comes to mind about each card.

Projective material not only deals with areas of emotional conflict but also can provide the examiner with some insight into the child's strengths. However, projective test data are biased toward pathology. The data can present the experienced examiner with very significant information regarding unconscious emotional conflicts but may, at the same time, provide the same examiner with only limited information regarding how the individual deals with those conflicts. The projective data also provide the examiner with an impression of how the child perceives significant areas of life. However, the data relate to the child's perception and not to reality. It is extremely valuable to know, for example, that the child is struggling with fears of attack by maternal figures, because those feelings or fears motivate much of the child's behavior. However, a direct inference cannot be made about actual interaction between the mother and child from those data. The mother may actually be physically attacking the child, she may be using verbal threats, or she may act and speak only as a loving mother but in much more subtle ways communicate to the child an underlying quality of rejection. Hence, the results of projective testing add information to the overall evaluation of the child, but specific recommendations require the integration of the results of these measurements with the facts of history as well as an in-depth picture of the child's current functioning in all areas of life.

Attempts to develop specific scoring systems for projectives have been made. For example, with the Rorschach technique there are several competing scoring systems, with volumes written to support each approach. A great deal of overlap exists among these systems, as well as clinical approaches that make minimal use of scoring systems. Suffice it to say that with or without a scoring system, the interpretation of a projective test requires a great deal of clinical experience, not only with projective tests specifically but also with the psychological development of the child, childhood psychopathology, modern dynamic formulations of personality organization, and comparative experience with emotionally healthy children stressed by various problems such as physical illness. This last item provides the examiner with a sensitivity to the way in which children of different ages normally deal with stress, which greatly sharpens the examiner's ability to identify psychopathologic responses to different forms of stress.

## COMPUTERIZED PSYCHOMETRICS

Computer-produced psychometric assessments recently have become an important professional issue. There is an aura of greater scientific objectivity when a magical machine called a computer produces a written report. However, one must remember that a psychologist wrote a program calling for specific interpretations of the numbers achieved through whatever test measurement was being used. When a technician administers a test, scores it, and enters the numbers into the computer program, the resulting report is only as good as the qualifications of the psychologist who wrote the original program. Unfortunately, we very rarely have the opportunity to decide whether or not we value that person's qualifications. Furthermore, just as every pharynx does not look exactly like every other pharynx, and every beating heart does not sound precisely the same as every other heart, a myriad of subtle variations exist in psychometric data that require an alertness on the part of the examiner to warn us when the pattern being seen is not as uniform or predictable as one might like. We are still dependent on clinical expertise (Matarazzo, 1983 and 1986).

Another method of computer support that can be both very helpful and clearly not subject to errors of computer report-writing is the use of a computer-generated reminder to the clinician of what clinical and research information should be considered when dealing with a particular configuration of scores. For example, Quickscore and Scoring Assistant for the Wechsler Scales are personal computer programs that very quickly reviews Wechsler subtest scores and indicates whether any of the subtest deviations is statistically significant (Quickscore and Quickreport, 1985; Scoring Assistant for the Wechsler Scales, 1992). The clinician is left with the responsibility of integrating the psychometric data, determining their meaning, and delineating appropriate recommendations. The computerized system provides the clinician access to a wide range of data more rapidly than reaching for reference books or recent research articles would have done.

Unfortunately, what appear to be most marketable are programs that write full reports and allow the use of a technician to obtain the data. There does not appear to be a big market for computer systems that only support the more highly priced expert clinician.

This issue should not be confused with the long-standing discussion of clinical versus actuarial prediction. That is a totally separate scientific challenge, which has consumed years of research and is worthy of several more years. This involves determining the relationship between prediction of psychological status made by integrative clinical judgment and prediction produced only from the scores obtained from measures that do not require clinical decision-making.

Obviously, there are many psychometric tools that have not been discussed here, but the most prominent measurement areas have been touched on, and examples of instruments in each major area have been provided. When dealing with old or new tools of measurement, a clinician would be well served to seek additional data along specific lines. First, the American Psychological Association publishes a handbook specifying the level of information that should be available within any test manual before that instrument should be made available for clinical use (American Psychological Association, 1985). Using that publication as a guide, the clinician would next be well advised to read the manual of the psychometric measure in question. Third, published psychometric measures are frequently subject to critical review, not only available in published research literature but also compiled in book form (Weaver, 1984; Mitchell, 1985; Harrington, 1986).

## Selected Readings

Achenbach TM, Edelbrock C. Manual for the child behavior checklist and profile. Burlington: University of Vermont, 1983.

Achenbach TM, Edelbrock C. Manual for the teacher's report form and teacher version of the child behavior profile. Burlington: University of Vermont, 1986.

Achenbach TM, Edelbrock C. Manual for the youth self-report and profile. Burlington: University of Vermont, 1987.

Bender L. A visual motor gestalt test and its clinical use. New York: American Orthopsychiatric Association, 1979.

Berk RA. Screening and diagnosis of children with learning disabilities. Springfield, IL: Charles C Thomas, 1984.

Diagnostic and statistical manual of mental disorders, ed 3, rev. Washington DC: American Psychiatric Association, 1987.

Golden CJ. Diagnosis and rehabilitation in clinical neuropsychology. Springfield, IL: Charles C Thomas, 1981.

Harrington RG, ed. Testing adolescents; a reference guide for comprehensive psychological assessments. Kansas City: Test Corporation of America, 1986.

Heinfelden BB. A validity study of 15 discrepancy procedures for classifying children as learning disabled. Unpublished doctoral dissertation, The Johns Hopkins University Division of Education, Baltimore, 1986.

Koppitz EM. The Bender Gestalt Test for young children, Vol. II. New York: Grune & Stratton, 1975.

Laurent J, Swerdlik M, Ryburn M. Review of validity research on the Stanford-Binet Intelligence Scale, ed 4. Psychol Assess 1992;4:102.

Matarazzo JD. Computerized psychology testing. Science 1983;221:323.

Matarazzo JD. Computerized psychological test interpretations. Am Psychol 1986;41:14.

Mercer JR. Pluralistic diagnosis in the evaluation of black and Chicano children: a procedure for taking sociocultural variables into account in clinical assessment. Paper presented at the meeting of The American Psychological Association, Washington DC, September 1971.

Mitchell JV Jr, ed. The ninth mental measurements yearbook. Lincoln, NE: University of Nebraska Press, 1985.

Quickscore and Quickreport. Virginia Beach: Psytec Assoc, 1985.

Reitan RM, Davison LA. Clinical neuropsychology: current status and applications. New York: John Wiley & Sons, 1974.

Reynolds CR, Stowe ML. Severe discrepancy analysis. Bensalem: TRAIN Inc., 1985.

Sattler JN. Assessment of children, ed 3. San Francisco: Author, 1988.

Standards for educational and psychological testing. Washington DC: American Psychological Association, 1985.

Thorndike RL, Hagan EP, Sattler JN. The Stanford-Binet Intelligence Scale, ed 4: guide for administering and scoring. Chicago: Riverside, 1986.

Thorndike RL, Hagan EP, Sattler JN. The Stanford-Binet Intelligence Scale: technical manual. Chicago: Riverside, 1986.

Weaver SJ, ed. Testing children: a reference guide for effective clinical and psychoeducational assessments. Kansas City: Test Corporation of America, 1984.

*Principles and Practice of Pediatrics, Second Edition.*
edited by Frank A. Oski et al. J. B. Lippincott Company, Philadelphia © 1994.

# 29.18 *Crying in Infants*

### John D. Newman

Of all behavior patterns produced by preverbal infants, crying is the behavior most likely to attract attention to the infant. Crying is the primary means by which the infant can communicate, and it is a useful indicator of the infant's arousal state and level of neurologic development. Because parents frequently include an appraisal of their infant's crying behavior in reporting concerns about the infant's health status, it is important that the pediatrician understand both the value and the limitations of attending to the infant's cry sounds as part of a diagnostic procedure.

The pediatrician faced with diagnosing the status of the newborn infant will find attention to infant crying behavior to be of particular value, since it is during the earliest postnatal period that the clearest correlation exists between cry sound characteristics and the infant's developmental risk status. Diagnostic use of the infant cry falls into three broad areas: assessment of parental reports of infant crying behavior, clinical assessment of the infant's crying behavior during examination, and acoustic analysis of cry structure by specialized instruments.

Parents concerned about coping with an excessively fussy infant may benefit from the results of a study conducted in Canada (Hunziker and Barr, 1986). Infants who received supplemental carrying during weeks 4 to 12 (3.5 hours per day versus 2.7 hours in the control group) cried 43% less at 6 weeks and 23% less at 12 weeks of age. The greatest difference was observed in a drop in crying in the supplemented group during evening hours.

## PARENTAL IMPRESSIONS OF INFANT CRYING BEHAVIOR

The report by mothers that they can recognize the cry of their own infant in a nursery setting was confirmed by Formby under experimental conditions. Because mothers vary in the degree and the intensity with which they respond to their crying infants, the value of parental reports in evaluating the infant must be viewed with caution. Bell and Ainsworth documented the high degree of effectiveness in terminating crying by picking up the infant, and parents who succeed in comforting their infant after adopting this technique may perceive the crying behavior of their infant differently from those parents who cannot comfort their crying infant reliably.

The extent to which the cries of an infant signal different messages is a controversial topic. The most reliable differentiations for full-term, healthy infants are between pain-induced cries and cries arising in less stressful contexts. The identification of so-called "hunger" cries is not reliable. The cries of older infants may be more clearly differentiated according to the affective state of the infant and social conditions when the crying occurs, but this is a topic for which little specific information is currently available. Studies demonstrating the ability of adult listeners to identify cries produced by infants with neurologic pathologies reliably suggest that parents may first suspect a medical problem in their own infant by his or her crying behavior. Parental reports of an unusual cry from their infant may be the first indicator to the pediatrician that a detailed neurologic examination is required.

Good documentation exists for the differential perception of cry differences by parents and the resulting consequences on parental reactions to the infant. As Brazelton has reported, parents with infants who have regular, unconsolable crying bouts during their first 12 weeks become tense and anxious over their inability to quiet the infant, which may in turn lead to a feeling of inadequacy on the part of the parent, and even to the establishment of negative feelings by the parent toward the infant. Adult listeners clearly can discriminate the cries of high-risk infants and, in older infants, the cries of infants with difficult temperaments. In both cases, the cries of such infants are perceived to be more aversive by the listener. Cries of infants with high- and low-risk factors also produce different physiologic effects in the listener, as shown in a study by Bryan and Newman.

## CLINICAL ASSESSMENT OF CRYING BEHAVIOR

The clinical assessment of infant crying may begin in the immediate neonatal period, when both physicians and nursing staff can apply their auditory experience in evaluating the newborn. The extent and inducibility of crying during examination should be a routine part of the neonatal assessment. When the infant is in the neonatal nursery, audible differences in crying may be most useful. Techniques helpful in predicting recovery from insult to the central nervous system or in identifying marginally impaired or depressed newborns can include an acoustic evaluation of the infant's cry. Lester and Zeskind (1978) have shown that deviations in cry behavior correlate with behavioral responsiveness on the Neonatal Behavioral Assessment Scale.

Variations in crying may reflect a continuum of affective responses to distress. As Porter and colleagues have shown, infants undergoing circumcision exhibited longer bouts of crying with elevated peak frequency as the invasiveness of the procedure increased. Adult listeners trained in acoustics could judge accurately the degree of invasiveness by listening to tape recordings of the cries. In a Scandinavian study, experienced midwives were the most successful group of adult listeners in identifying birth cries correctly. Children's nurses recognized very few birth cries but could identify successfully pain cries recorded from healthy full-term newborns.

Wolff has described the basic pattern of crying in healthy infants as characteristically rhythmic, with each cry unit consisting of the cry proper followed by a brief inspiratory whistle. The natural cry unit perceived by the listener is the cry followed by the inspiration, rather than the other way around, because the interval between the cry and the inspiration is shorter than between the inspiration and the next cry. This rhythmic, continuous series of cries is observed within 30 minutes after birth and remains constant until the end of the second month, when the pattern becomes more variable. The cries of infants experiencing a painful stimulus, such as a heel prick, are distinguished by a sudden onset of loud crying without preliminary moaning. The perceived cry unit in this case consists of an inspiratory whistle immediately followed by a long expiratory cry. Clinical staff

TABLE 29-15. Pain Cry Measures Correlating with Patient Subtype

| Patient Subtype* | 1 | 2 | 3 | 4 | 5 |
|---|---|---|---|---|---|
| Duration (sec) | 2.6 | 3.7 | 1.7 | 2.7 | 3.9 |
| Maximum fundamental frequency (Hz) | 650 | 1320 | 1100 | 980 | 970 |
| Biphonation† | — | + | ++ | — | + |
| Glides† | — | + | — | — | + |

* 1, healthy full-term; 2, asphyxia neonatorium; 3, bacterial meningitis; 4, cri du chat (partial deletion of chromosome 5); 5, hydrocephalus

† *Biphonation* refers to the presence of two separate sets of voiced harmonics; *glides* are rapid changes in frequency over a limited part of the utterance. A "+" indicates occurrence in 13% to 25% of cases; a "++" indicates occurrence in about 50% of cases.

*Adapted from Michelsson and Wasz-Hockert (1980) and Michelsson et al. (1984).*

hearing cry patterns from newborns in the nursery or during examination that do not fall into one of these two acoustic patterns should be alerted to the possible need for further evaluation of the nonconforming infant.

To illustrate this point, Zeskind and Field (1982) found that among a group of healthy full-term infants, those requiring multiple applications of a rubber band snapped against the sole of the foot produced cries that were shorter in duration and had increased incidence of hyperphonation (perceived as an abrupt upward shift in pitch). Subsequent analysis of this group of infants showed greater instability of autonomic control than was found in the group of infants with more typical cry patterns.

The physiologic state of the mother during delivery influences the infant's condition at birth, and this influence may be detectable in abnormal crying. Blinick and associates found a high incidence of abnormal birth cries in the infants of drug-addicted mothers; the most characteristic perceived difference was a high-pitched, squealing quality to the cries.

## ACOUSTIC ANALYSIS OF CRY STRUCTURE

With ever-increasing sophistication, specialists in the analysis of the underlying acoustic structure of cry sounds are documenting differences that correlate with obvious neurologic pathologies, as well as with the subtle effects of suboptimal developmental and physiologic factors. The long-recognized stereotyped nature of infant crying during the first few weeks of life has, quite naturally, prompted efforts to describe in acoustic terms the nature of the cry in healthy full-term infants. These efforts have, in turn, served as a foundation for comparisons with cries from infants with a variety of disabilities stemming from abnormalities in fetal development or delivery. The conclusion from this work is that there are clear and consistent structural differences in the cries of certain infant patient populations that reflect disorders in neurologic organization and autonomic control.

The extent to which these differences in cry structure can be used in pediatric diagnosis is still under debate, but the pediatrician should be aware of their existence and of the resources available to provide this kind of information as warranted. Among the earliest investigators attempting to provide a diagnostically useful measure involving neonatal crying, Karelitz and Fisichelli in 1962 measured the stimulus threshold and latency to first cry of a group of infants, and found that normal infants generally respond more quickly and require less painful stimuli to begin crying than do infants with diffuse brain damage. A group of Scandinavian investigators has devoted more than 25 years to providing detailed documentation of these early findings and has developed a list of measurable acoustic characteristics that to-

gether have proved to correlate differentially with a variety of neurologic and chromosomal abnormalities. More recently, other research groups have used their own sets of acoustic parameters or attributes measured from graphic representations of infant cries in attempts to find acoustic correlates of neurologic or developmental abnormalities. Most of the findings from these studies must be viewed as preliminary, owing to small sample sizes and lack of standardized measurements or measurement techniques. Nevertheless, some generalities have emerged that should be of interest and possible clinical value to the practitioner.

Studies of the crying of full-term newborns have relied almost exclusively on the cries emitted during routine administration of brief, painful stimuli such as the heel prick during blood sampling. Although infants generally cry repeatedly following such a procedure, the first utterance has been the focus of quantitative study. This "pain cry" has a duration of about 2.5 seconds and a falling or rising then falling pitch; in about one third of the cries, the fundamental frequency shifts suddenly to a higher frequency at some point. These frequency shifts make computations of average frequency for the utterance problematic, and published values for mean fundamental frequency are difficult to interpret if it is not clear whether a shift occurred, and if the average frequency measurement included that portion of the utterance during which the upward frequency shift occurred. Comparisons of average frequency based on measurements of later utterances in a crying bout or of cries made under less stressful circumstances would be easier to make, because pitch shifts are very rare in these cases. However, information currently available from the crying of less stressed infants is inadequate to make general statements regarding differences correlated with neurologic or developmental abnormalities.

Table 29-15 is a guide to the pediatrician interested in knowing the most generally accepted pain cry measures that correlate with various clinical subtypes. Some of these measures may also be audibly detectable, and the pediatrician with access to expertise in acoustic analysis may wish to confirm an impression or judgment based on audible peculiarities in a particular patient's cry. However, accredited diagnostic facilities to which a pediatrician could send a tape-recorded cry sample for analysis are at present unavailable.

## Selected Readings

Bell SM, Ainsworth MDS. Infant crying and maternal responsiveness. Child Dev 1972;43:1171.

Blinick G, Tavolga WN, Antopol W. Variations in birth cries of newborn infants from narcotic-addicted and normal mothers. Am J Obstet Gynecol 1971;110: 948.

Brazelton TB. Application of cry research to clinical perspectives. In Lester BM, Boukydis CFZ, eds. Infant crying: theoretical and research perspectives. New York: Plenum Press, 1985:325.

Bryan YE, Newman JD. Influence of infant cry structure on the heart rate of the listener. In Newman JD, ed. The physiological control of mammalian vocalization. New York: Plenum Press, 1988:413.

Formby D. Maternal recognition of infant's cry. Dev Med Child Neurol 1967;9:293.

Green JA, Gustafson GE. Individual recognition of human infants on the basis of cries alone. Dev Psychol 1983;16:485.

Hunziker UA, Barr RG. Increased carrying reduces infant crying: a randomized controlled trial. Pediatrics 1986;77:641.

Karelitz S, Fisichelli VR. The cry thresholds of normal infants and those with brain damage. J Pediatr 1962;61:679.

Lester BM, Boukydis CFZ, eds. Infant crying: theoretical and research perspectives. New York: Plenum Press, 1985.

Lester BM, Zeskind PS. Brazelton scale and physical size correlates of neonatal cry features. Infant Behav Devel 1978;1:393.

Michelsson K, Wasz-Hockert O. The value of cry analysis in neonatology and early infancy. In Murry T, Murry J, eds. Infant communication: cry and early speech. Houston: College-Hill Press, 1980:152.

Michelsson K, Kaskinen H, Aulanko R, Rinne A. Sound spectrographic cry analysis of infants with hydrocephalus. Acta Paediatr Scand 1984;73:65.

Murry T, Murry J, eds. Infant communication: cry and early speech. Houston: College-Hill Press, 1980.

Porter FL, Miller RH, Marshall RE. Neonatal pain cries: effect of circumcision on acoustic features and perceived urgency. Child Dev 1986;57:790.

Wolff PH. The natural history of crying and other vocalizations in early infancy. In Foss BM, ed. Determinants of infant behaviour, vol 4. London: Metheun, 1969:81.

Zeskind PS, Field T. Neonatal cry threshold and heart rate variability. In Lipsitt L, Field T, eds. Infant behavior and development: perinatal risk and newborn behavior. Norwood: Ablex, 1982:51.

*Principles and Practice of Pediatrics, Second Edition.*
edited by Frank A. Oski et al. J. B. Lippincott Company, Philadelphia © 1994.

# CHAPTER 30
# *Adolescent Medicine*

*Principles and Practice of Pediatrics, Second Edition.*
edited by Frank A. Oski et al. J. B. Lippincott Company, Philadelphia © 1994.

## 30.1 Introduction

### Alain Joffe

Adolescence refers to the stage of human development encompassing the transition from childhood to adulthood. The term (derived from the Latin *adolescere,* to grow into maturity) is broader in scope than the word puberty, which usually refers to the biologic changes and sexual maturation that occur during this transition. Consequently, adolescence has not only physiologic but also psychological and sociocultural dimensions. An understanding of the significant events and processes occurring during this transition requires knowledge of each of these areas and of their interrelationships.

Statistics regarding adolescents are often difficult to interpret, because the age definitions used to compile data for this population group vary (eg, 10 to 14, 10 to 19, 15 to 19, 15 to 24). In 1980, there were approximately 39.4 million children and adolescents aged 10 to 19 years in the United States; by 1985, that number had dropped to 35.7 million. The adolescent population in the year 2000 is estimated at 38.3 million with slightly more than 50% being aged 10 to 14 years. Data regarding change among adolescents are expressed here as rates per 100,000 or as percentages. For example, despite a projected increase in the absolute number of adolescents in the United States as the year 2000 approaches, young people ages 10 to 19 years will constitute a smaller percentage of the total population (17.3% in 1980 versus 14.3% in 2000) than in prior decades.

Adolescence is viewed as both the healthiest period of life and the most problematic. For about half of teenagers, the former is true, and they make the complex transition into adulthood without significant difficulty. In doing so, they accomplish several critical developmental tasks: becoming accustomed to a new and markedly changed body, formulating a personal and sexual identity and developing the initial capacity for intimacy in relationships, and beginning to establish a social identity and preparing the groundwork for economic independence.

Many teenagers fail to achieve one or more of these goals and suffer significant morbidity and mortality during this developmental period. It is estimated that one fourth of 10- to 18-year-olds are at serious risk for school failure or of being injured or killed by various risky behaviors. An additional one fourth are at somewhat lower risk but are still confronted by significant threats to their health and optimal growth to adulthood. The mortality rate for 15- to 24-year-olds fell to a low of 95.9 per 100,000 in 1985 but has fluctuated above this level since then. The projected final death rate for 1990 is 99.2 per 100,000, an increase of 1.6% from 1989.

Age-specific death rates are listed in Table 30-1. Accidents, homicide, and suicide are the three leading causes of death for young people aged 15 to 19 years. Homicide is the chief cause of death for black males and exceeds even motor vehicle accidents as the single identifiable cause of death for black females. In 1988, 5718 youths aged 15 to 24 years died from homicide in the United States. In the same year, only 411 similarly aged youths died from homicide in all of Canada, France, Germany, Spain, the Netherlands, Switzerland, Finland, and the United Kingdom combined, despite a comparable total population of similarly aged youths.

Comparable data are not available for Hispanic youth. Table 30-2 lists the leading causes of death for 15- to 24-year-old Hispanic youths based on numbers (not rates). More than 75% of all deaths among this population are also attributable to accidents, suicide, and homicide.

Advance data for 1989 cite deaths from human immunodeficiency virus (HIV) as the sixth leading cause of death for 15- to 24-year-olds and the second leading cause, exceeding motor vehicle accidents, among 25- to 34-year-olds. If one assumes the average incubation period from infection to death is 7 to 10 years, then many individuals dying of acquired immune deficiency syndrome (AIDS) were infected during adolescence.

Morbidity associated with adolescence is associated also with risky behaviors and incorporates such problems as substance abuse (including alcohol and cigarette abuse), mental illness, school failure and dropout, delinquency (approximately 1.3 million 10- to 18-year-olds are arrested every year), sexually transmitted diseases and their sequelae (pelvic inflammatory disease, ectopic pregnancy, infertility), and adolescent pregnancy. Many of the risky behaviors leading to morbidity and mortality during adolescence co-occur; that is, individuals who engage in one behavior are more likely to engage in another.

Rates of substance abuse, although showing signs of diminishing somewhat in the last few years, continue to be highest in the adolescent and young adult age group when compared to

TABLE 30-1. Leading Causes of Death for Adolescents by Age, Race, and Sex
(Number of Deaths/100,000 Population)—1988

| All Races | | White | | All Nonwhite | | | |
|---|---|---|---|---|---|---|---|
| | | | | *Total* | | *Black* | |
| **10–14 Years (Males)** | | | | | | | |
| All causes | 34.1 | All causes | 32.8 | All causes | 39.5 | All causes | 42.3 |
| Accidents | 17.0 | Accidents | 12.3 | Accidents | 18.6 | Accidents | 19.8 |
| MVA | 9.0 | MVA | 9.8 | MVA | 8.0 | MVA | 8.5 |
| Malignancy | 3.4 | Malignancy | 3.6 | Homicide | 5.0 | Homicide | 5.7 |
| Suicide | 2.1 | Suicide | 2.1 | Malignancy | 2.9 | Malignancy | 2.9 |
| Homicide | 2.0 | Congenital anomalies | 1.6 | Cardiovascular | 2.0 | Cardiovascular | 2.3 |
| Cardiovascular | 1.7 | Cardiovascular | 1.6 | Suicide | 1.8 | Congenital anomalies | 1.3 |
| **10–14 Years (Females)** | | | | | | | |
| All causes | 20.5 | All causes | 18.7 | All causes | 27.8 | All causes | 30.0 |
| Accidents | 8.2 | Accidents | 7.8 | Accidents | 9.6 | Accidents | 9.6 |
| MVA | 5.5 | MVA | 5.6 | MVA | 4.9 | MVA | 4.6 |
| Malignancy | 2.7 | Malignancy | 2.6 | Homicide | 3.5 | Homicide | 4.4 |
| Homicide | 1.4 | Congenital anomalies | 1.1 | Malignancy | 2.9 | Malignancy | 3.0 |
| Congenital anomalies | 1.3 | Cardiovascular | 0.9 | Cardiovascular | 1.6 | Cardiovascular | 1.7 |
| Cardiovascular | 1.0 | Homicide | 0.8 | Congenital anomalies | 1.2 | Congenital anomalies | 1.3 |
| | | Suicide | 0.8 | | | | |
| **15–19 Years (Males)** | | | | | | | |
| All causes | 125.8 | All causes | 120.0 | All causes | 150.4 | All causes | 164.3 |
| Accidents | 67.1 | Accidents | 71.8 | Homicide | 64.4 | Homicide | 77.4 |
| MVA | 51.3 | MVA | 56.3 | Accidents | 46.9 | Accidents | 45.9 |
| Homicide | 18.8 | Suicide | 19.6 | MVA | 30.1 | MVA | 28.9 |
| Suicide | 18.0 | Homicide | 8.1 | Suicide | 11.0 | Suicide | 9.7 |
| Malignancy | 4.4 | Malignancy | 5.3 | Cardiovascular | 5.3 | Cardiovascular | 6.3 |
| Cardiovascular | 3.5 | Cardiovascular | 3.1 | Malignancy | 4.5 | Malignancy | 5.0 |
| **15–19 Years (Females)** | | | | | | | |
| All causes | 48.7 | All causes | 48.6 | All causes | 49.1 | All causes | 49.6 |
| Accidents | 25.4 | Accidents | 28.0 | Accidents | 14.6 | Accidents | 12.5 |
| MVA | 22.6 | MVA | 25.2 | MVA | 11.8 | MVA | 9.9 |
| Homicide | 4.4 | Suicide | 4.8 | Homicide | 10.2 | Homicide | 11.5 |
| Suicide | 4.4 | Malignancy | 3.7 | Malignancy | 3.6 | Cardiovascular | 4.4 |
| Malignancy | 3.6 | Homicide | 3.0 | Cardiovascular | 3.6 | Malignancy | 3.5 |
| Cardiovascular | 2.0 | Cardiovascular | 1.6 | Suicide | 2.6 | Suicide | 2.2 |

MVA, motor vehicle accidents; Malignancy, malignant neoplasms including neoplasms of lymphatic and hematopoietic tissues; Homicide, homicide and legal interventions; Cardiovascular, major cardiovascular diseases.
Data from National Center for Health Statistics. Vital statistics of the United States, 1988, vol II, mortality, part A. Washington: Public Health Service 1991.

other age groups. Furthermore, the age of initial use of these substances continues to decrease. The average age for first use of alcohol (excluding that associated with religious ceremonies) is 11 or 12 years.

Problems associated with adolescent sexuality also occur. Sexually transmitted diseases are most common in this population. The prevalence of gonorrhea increased 325% among 10- to 14-year-olds and 170% among 15- to 19-year-olds from 1960 to 1988. Women younger than 20 years accounted for 26% of reported abortions in the United States in 1987. Both the pregnancy rate and the abortion rate are higher for adolescents in the United States than for teenagers in any other industrialized nation. Ac-

cording to the Centers for Disease Control 1990 school-based Youth Risk Behavior Survey (involving a sample of 11,631 9th through 12th graders in all 50 states, the District of Columbia, Puerto Rico, and the Virgin Islands), one third of males and one fifth of females initiated intercourse before age 15. Nineteen percent of students (26% of males and 12% of females) had four or more lifetime sexual partners; less than half of all sexually active students used a condom at last intercourse.

Mental health problems are common during adolescence: about 600,000 suffer from mental disorders, and more than 115,000 adolescents were admitted to a psychiatric facility in 1986. According to the 1987 National Adolescent Student Health

TABLE 30-2. Leading Causes of Death for Hispanic Adolescents and Young Adults (Aged 15–24 Years)— 1988 (Numbers of Deaths)

| Males | | Females | |
|---|---|---|---|
| All causes | 2663 | All causes | 614 |
| Accidents | 1185 | Accidents | 232 |
| MVA | 854 | MVA | 192 |
| Homicide | 735 | Homicide | 90 |
| Suicide | 262 | Suicide | 41 |
| Malignancy | 88 | Malignancy | 41 |
| Cardiovascular | 76 | Cardiovascular | 35 |

*Data from National Center for Health Statistics. Vital statistics of the United States, 1988, vol II, mortality, part A. Washington: Public Health Service 1991.*

began smoking before age 18 years, and 80% to 90% began by age 21 years. Adolescents who eat a low-fat diet and exercise regularly promote cardiovascular health and can likely decrease their risk for developing coronary artery disease as adults.

Much of adolescent morbidity and mortality can be tied to risky behaviors. Research in the last several decades suggests that these behaviors are not distributed randomly among adolescents. Some behaviors fulfill various developmental needs. Others are adopted due to factors inherent within the adolescent or his or her social context (including family and community). Hence, some adolescents are at greater risk for adopting risky behaviors than others. Moreover, behaviors may coexist within an individual. That is, a young person who smokes cigarettes is more likely to engage in sexual intercourse at an earlier age. Many adolescents who appear to be at risk for initiating these behaviors, however, never do so. A burgeoning field of resiliency research has identified some factors that appear to protect adolescents from health-compromising outcomes. These include aspects of the adolescent's temperament and the presence of a warm, cohesive family that is caring despite poverty or other social ills. Support for an adolescent often is provided by a caring adult outside of the family. The interplay among these competing factors is shown in Figure 30-1.

The goal of adolescent medicine is twofold: to assist adolescents in making a healthy and successful transition into adulthood and to encourage healthy lifestyles that promote longevity.

Insight into the nature of the statistics that characterize the dimensions of adolescent health and the potential for improving

Survey, 34% of 8th and 10th graders had thought about suicide; 14% had attempted suicide at least once. Sixty-one percent of students reported feeling depressed and hopeless, and 45% indicated they had trouble coping with stressful situations at home and school.

Estimates are that 65% of diseases that figure prominently in adult morbidity and mortality, such as obesity, cardiovascular disease, and lung cancer are linked to behaviors that are adopted or rejected during adolescence. Almost 50% of adult smokers

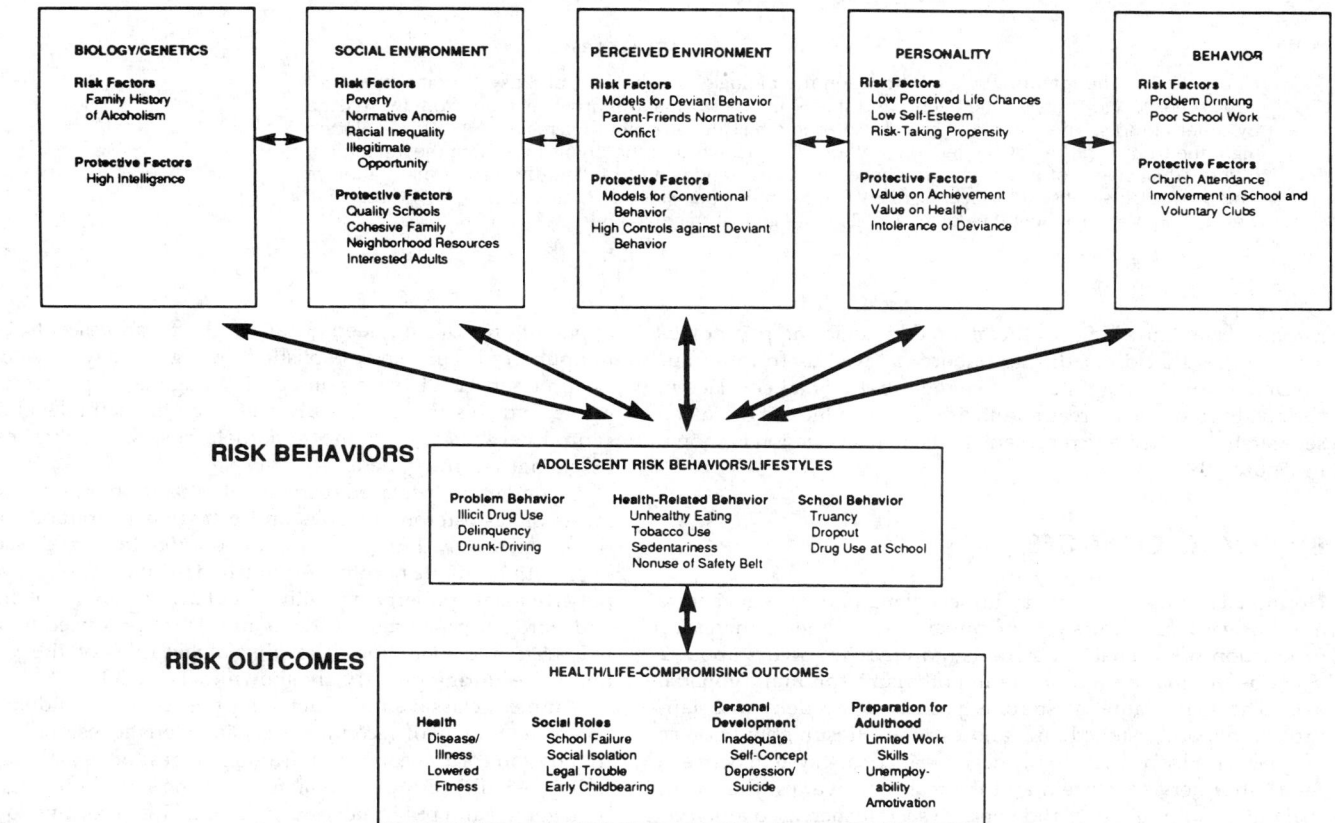

Figure 30-1. Interrelated conceptual domains of risk and protective factors.

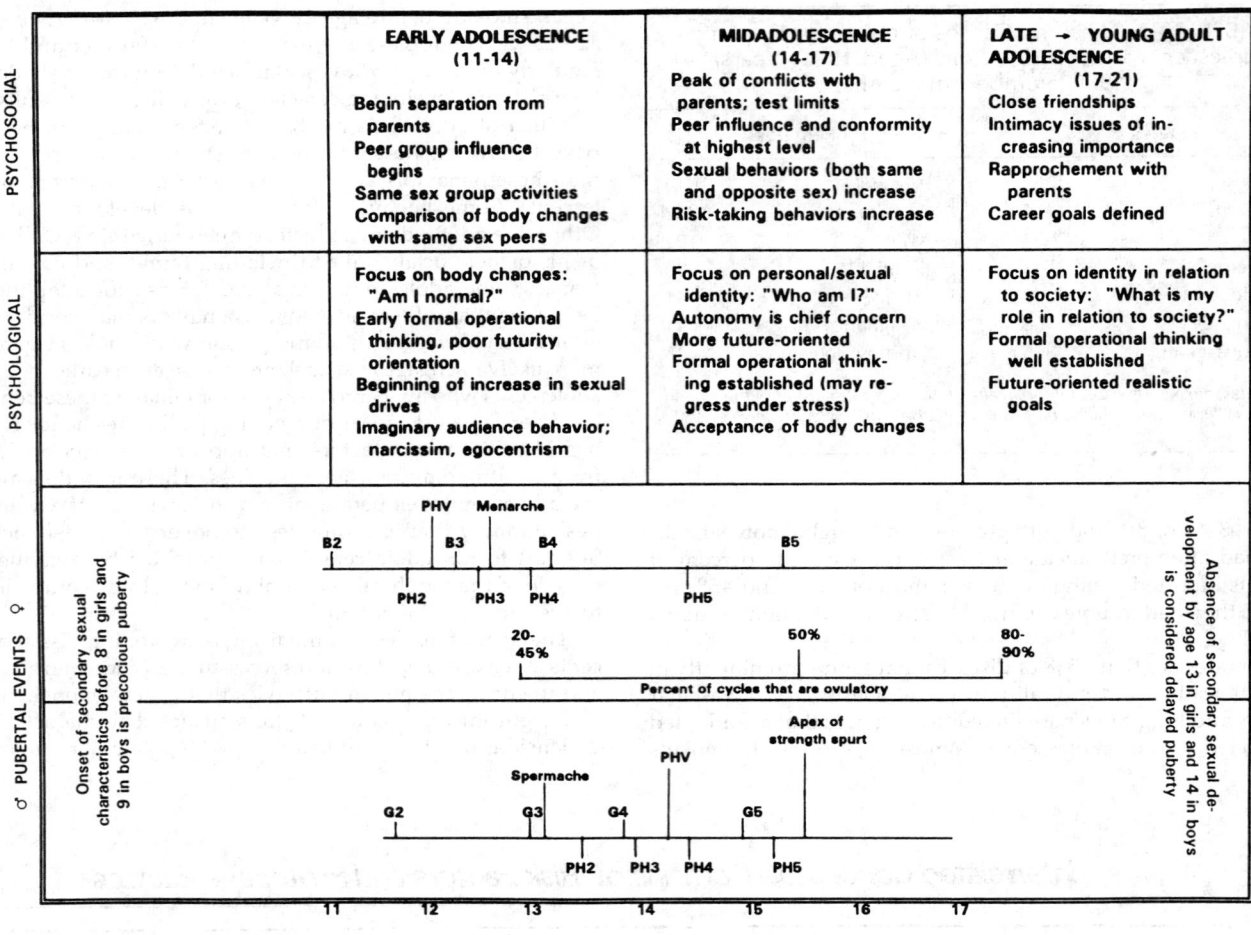

**Figure 30-2.** The temporal relation between the biologic, psychologic, and psychosocial events of adolescence. Age limits for the events and stages are approximations and may differ from those used by other authors. The mean age of onset of pubic hair development for males (=13.4) is likely too high due to bias in the data collection method. These limits and the points indicating the attainment of individual stages of puberty were chosen for consistency and to reflect the earlier maturation of American versus British adolescents. *PH2, 3, 4, 5*—pubic hair stage 2, 3, etc; *B2, 3, 4, 5*—breast stage 2, 3, etc; *PHV*—peak height velocity; *G2, 3, 4, 5*—genital stage 2, 3, etc.

it comes from knowledge of the marked biologic and psychological changes that occur during puberty as well as from an appreciation for the magnitude of change that has taken place in society. Each of these areas and their interrelatedness is discussed separately. A schematic representation of the discussion is shown in Figure 30-2.

## BIOLOGIC CHANGES

Hormonal changes associated with sexual maturation begin before any outward physical signs of puberty are evident. Increased production of adrenal sex steroids (adrenarche) occurs about 2 years before maturation of the hypothalamic-pituitary-gonadal axis. The major adrenal steroids produced are dehydroepiandrosterone, androstenedione, and estrone. Presumably because of a decreased sensitivity to the negative feedback system between the central nervous system and the testes or ovaries, the hypothalamus and pituitary gland begin to secrete increased amounts of gonadotropin releasing hormone (GnRH), follicle stimulating hormone (FSH), and luteinizing hormone (LH). This increase is

apparent only during sleep in early pubertal adolescents, but by midpuberty it becomes established during the day as well. The sleep-enhanced LH secretion occurs in agonadal patients, indicating that this process is truly maturational at the level of the central nervous system and hypothalamus, rather than caused by changes in the gonads.

Secondary to increased secretion of pituitary hormones, serum levels of testosterone in boys and estrogens (estradiol) in girls rise progressively during physical maturation. Increased secretion of growth hormone becomes established by midpuberty. By midpuberty to late puberty, a positive feedback system involving LH and estrogen production leads to an estrogen-induced midcycle LH surge and ovulation. The physiologic roles of the various hormones during puberty are shown in Table 30-3.

Tanner's classic studies detailing the growth of adolescents and development of secondary sex characteristics established the foundation for the concept of Tanner stages (or sexual maturity ratings—SMR). Boys are assigned a rating based on staging of both genital and pubic hair development, girls according to pubic hair and breast development. These various stages are shown in Figures 30-3 through 30-5. Most events occurring during ado-

TABLE 30-3.   Primary Action of Major Hormones of Puberty

| Hormone | Sex | Action |
|---|---|---|
| FSH (follicle-stimulating hormone) | Male | Stimulates gametogenesis |
| | Female | Stimulates development of primary ovarian follicles |
| | | Stimulates activation of enzymes in ovarian granulosa cells to increase estrogen production |
| LH (luteinizing hormone) | Male | Stimulates testicular Leydig cells to produce testosterone |
| | Female | Stimulates ovarian theca cells to produce androgens and the corpus luteum to synthesize progesterone. |
| | | Midcycle surge induces ovulation. |
| Estradiol ($E_2$) | Male | Increases rate of epiphyseal fusion |
| | Female | Stimulates breast development |
| | | Low level enhances linear growth; a high level increases the rate of epiphyseal fusion. |
| | | Triggers midcycle surge of LH. |
| | | Stimulates development of labia, vagina, uterus, and ducts of the breasts. |
| | | Stimulates development of a proliferative endometrium in the uterus. |
| | | Increases fat mass of the body. |
| Testosterone | Male | Accelerates linear growth |
| | | Increases rate of epiphyseal fusion |
| | | Stimulates development of the penis, scrotum, prostate, and seminal vesicles. |
| | | Stimulates growth of pubic, facial, and axillary hair |
| | | Increases larynx size and thus deepens the voice |
| | | Stimulates sebaceous gland secretion of oil |
| | | Increases libido |
| | | Increases muscle mass |
| | | Increases red blood cell mass |
| | Female | Accelerates linear growth |
| | | Stimulates growth of pubic and axillary hair |
| Progesterone | Female | Converts a proliferative uterine endometrium to a secretory endometrium. |
| | | Stimulates lobuloalveolar breast development |
| Adrenal androgens | Male and female | Stimulates pubic hair and linear growth |

*Reprinted with permission from Neinstein LS. Adolescent health care: a practical guide, ed 2. Baltimore: Urban & Schwarzenberg 1991:6.*

lescence correlate more closely with SMR or skeletal age than with chronologic age.

Studies indicate a definite sequence of pubertal events that most adolescents pass through as they mature. Although the sequence is the same, the age at onset of these events and the time interval between one event and the next vary. On average, puberty lasts approximately 3 to 4 years; the wide range of normal is shown in Tables 30-4 through 30-7. For girls, the average age of onset of breast budding, the first sign of pubertal development (especially for white girls), is approximately 10 years of age with a range from 8 to 13 years of age. Development of breast buds before age 8 years is considered premature, and absence of breast budding after age 13 years is indicative of delayed sexual development. Depending on the population studied, as many as 15% of girls develop pubic hair before or concurrently with breast development. Boys enter puberty approximately 1 year after girls, with enlargement of the testes occurring at about 11 years of age with a range of 9 to 14 years of age. Puberty is considered to be premature or delayed if it occurs outside this range. Because of the heterogeneity in the onset of these events, both boys and girls can be grouped into early, average, and late maturers, depending on whether an adolescent begins to mature before, along with, or after the majority of his or her age cohort. Considerable evidence shows these biologic differences correlate with a variety of psychological and sociocultural advantages and disadvantages, which contributes to a multiplicity of adolescent behaviors. Asynchrony between different aspects of development (eg between hormonal levels and age) appears to affect psychosocial adjustment of boys and girls.

A variety of other somatic changes occurs during puberty. Approximately 25% of adult height and 50% of adult weight accrues during puberty. During the year when adolescents grow fastest, their growth velocity (cm/yr) doubles from prepubertal levels. Males achieve a greater growth velocity than females. The peak growth spurt in girls occurs about 1 year after the onset of puberty, and growth is largely completed by the time women begin to menstruate. In boys, the growth spurt occurs 2 years after the onset of genital enlargement. Both the legs and trunk

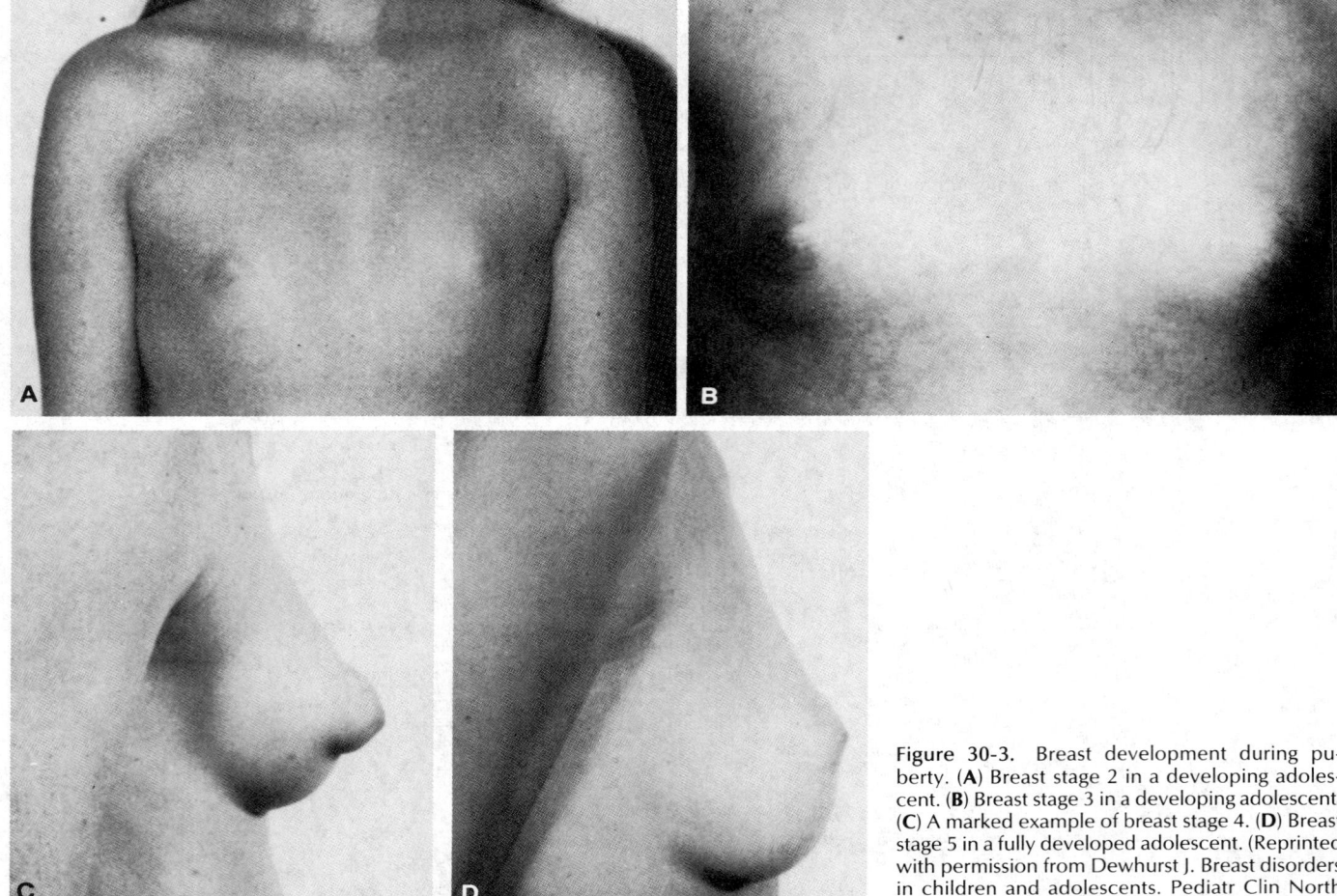

Figure 30-3. Breast development during puberty. (**A**) Breast stage 2 in a developing adolescent. (**B**) Breast stage 3 in a developing adolescent. (**C**) A marked example of breast stage 4. (**D**) Breast stage 5 in a fully developed adolescent. (Reprinted with permission from Dewhurst J. Breast disorders in children and adolescents. Pediatr Clin North Am 1981;28:288.)

grow rapidly, with final adult height due more to growth of the trunk. Influenced by circulating testosterone, lean body mass as a percentage of body weight increases from 80% or 85% to 90%. This increase is due to testosterone's effect on muscle development, giving rise to the concept of a strength spurt for boys occurring at Tanner Stage 5.

With maturation, girls have increased fat deposition, and their lean body mass decreases from 80% to 75%. The increase in body fat to a critical level of about 17% is postulated to trigger the onset of menses. This theory explains the trend for earlier onset of menarche observed in Western countries since 1840, based on improved nutrition among adolescents.

The size of the ovaries and uterus of an adolescent increases five to seven times during puberty. The penis doubles in size, and the volume of the testicles increases from approximately 2 mL to 18 mL.

These changes in sexual maturity, body size, and composition have significant implications for the health care of adolescents. Early adolescents become preoccupied with body changes and often seek assurances through their behaviors or from clinicians about the normalcy of their development. Gynecomastia, for example, occurs at Tanner Stage 2 or 3 and may prompt teenage boys to complain of chest pain in the hope that a visit to a clinician will bring reassurance that they are not, in fact, developing breasts. When breast budding is noted in females, they can be counseled that menarche will likely ensue in about 2 years. Certain illnesses or the risk for developing an illness is more likely to occur at one or another stage of development. For example,

scoliosis, if present, is likely to worsen at the time of rapid trunk growth. Other examples are provided in Table 30-8.

## STAGES OF ADOLESCENT DEVELOPMENT

Because adolescents vary over a wide range of chronologic ages in terms of their pubertal and cognitive development, it is useful to characterize an individual teenager as being in early, middle, or late adolescence.

Early adolescence incorporates the period of rapid body change and gives rise to a preoccupation with such changes and the need for reassurance regarding physical normalcy. Initial separation from parents begins during this stage but is still tentative. Adolescents are sporadically capable of formal operational thinking.

By middle adolescence, most bodily changes have occurred, and physiologic equanimity has been established. Separation from family, struggles concerning autonomy, and efforts at establishing an identity are at a peak level. Hence, testing of limits and a preference for peer activities are predominant behaviors during this stage. Interest in sexual activities increases substantially. Now able to engage in abstract thought, adolescents are more capable of considering the feelings of others, considering several options simultaneously, and viewing choices or situations within a future time perspective.

By late adolescence, major issues revolve around the relation of the individual to the surrounding society and the role one

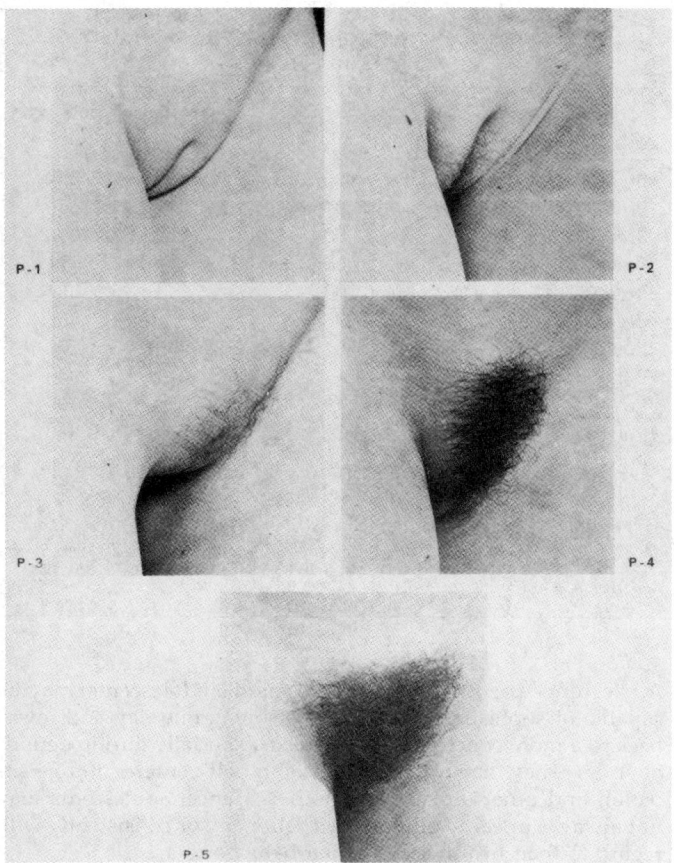

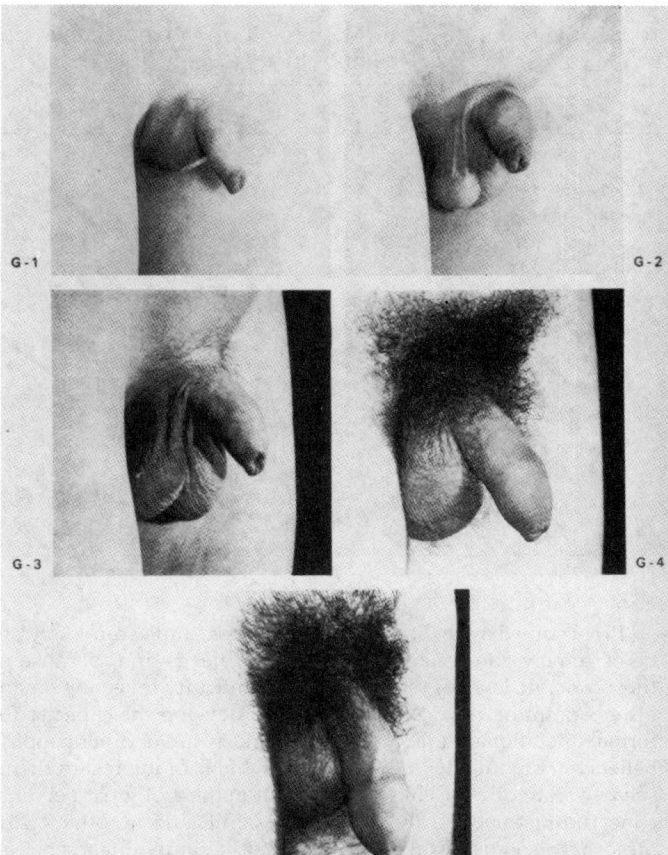

**Figure 30-4.** Stages of pubic hair development in girls.
Stage 1: Preadolescent; the vellus over the pubes is not further developed than that over the anterior abdominal wall, ie, no pubic hair.
Stage 2: Sparse growth of long, slightly pigmented, downy hair, straight or only slightly curled, appearing chiefly along the labia. This stage is difficult to see on photographs.
Stage 3: Hair is considerably darker, coarser, and curlier. The hair spreads sparsely over the junction of the pubes.
Stage 4: Hair is now adult in type, but the area covered is still considerably smaller than in most adults. There is no spread to the medial surface of the thighs.
Stage 5: Hair is adult in quantity and type, distributed as an inverse triangle of the classic feminine pattern. The spread is to the medial surface of the thighs but not up the linea alba or elsewhere above the base of the inverse triangle.
(Photographs by Van Wieringen, et al, Institute for Preventive Medicine, Groningen, Netherlands. © Wolters-Noordhoff, The Netherlands.)

**Figure 30-5.** Stages of pubic hair and genital development in boys.
*Genital*—Stage 1: Preadolescent. Testes, scrotum, and penis are about the same size and proportion as in early childhood.
Stage 2: The scrotum and testes have enlarged; there is a change in the texture and some reddening of the scrotal skin.
Stage 3: Growth of the penis has occurred, at first mainly in length but with some increase in breadth; there is further growth of testes and scrotum.
Stage 4: The penis is further enlarged in length and breadth with development of the glans. The testes and scrotum are further enlarged. The scrotal skin has further darkened.
Stage 5: Genitalia are adult in size and shape. No further enlargement takes place after Stage 5.
*Pubic Hair*—Stage 1: Preadolescent. The vellus over the pubes is no further developed than that over the abdominal wall, ie, no pubic hair.
Stage 2: Sparse growth of long, slightly pigmented, downy hair, straight or only slightly curled, appearing chiefly at the base of the penis.
Stage 3: Hair is considerably darker, coarser, and curlier and spreads sparsely over the junction of the pubes.
Stage 4: Hair is now adult in type, but the area covered is still considerably smaller than in most adults. There is no spread to the medial surface of the thighs.
Stage 5: Hair is adult in quantity and type, distributed as an inverse triangle. The spread is to the medial surface of the thighs but not up the linea alba or elsewhere above the base of the inverse triangle. Most men will have further spread of pubic hair.
(Photographs by Van Wieringen, et al, Institute for Preventive Medicine, Groningen, Netherlands. © Wolters-Noordhoff, The Netherlands).

desires to play within that society. Emotional intimacy and career planning become key concerns. For those lacking appropriate schooling or job opportunities, desiring of advanced education, or forced prematurely into adult status because of adolescent parenthood, it can be difficult to resolve these issues and the associated concerns regarding prolonged dependence on parents.

## PSYCHOLOGICAL CHANGES

A variety of psychological changes occur during adolescence. These are addressed by a variety of authors and theories. One major change is in cognition. Piaget characterized adolescent thought processes as increasingly sophisticated with movement from concrete to formal operational, abstract thinking. This maturation encompasses emerging abilities to reflect on concepts lacking concrete representation, to mentally arrange individual pieces into multiple combinations, and as a result, to construct ideals and situations distinct from or in contrast to those existing

in reality. Such changes allow increasingly sophisticated concepts and reasoning, making the teenager capable of exploring a broad range of possibilities or solutions when confronted with a new situation or problem. When combined with increased physical maturity, size, and strength, this new cognitive capacity affords the adolescent an increasing sense of mastery over the external world as well as a sense of invulnerability. Many risky behaviors among adolescents can be viewed as an attempt to test the limits and capabilities of newly developed physical and mental prowess.

TABLE 30-4. Age of Attainment of Pubertal Stages and Peak Height Velocity in Females

| Stage | Mean (yr) | Standard Deviation |
|---|---|---|
| Breast 2 | 11.15 | 1.10 |
| Pubic hair 2 | 11.69 | 1.21 |
| Peak height velocity | 12.14 | 0.88 |
| Breast 3 | 12.15 | 1.09 |
| Pubic hair 3 | 12.36 | 1.10 |
| Pubic hair 4 | 12.95 | 1.06 |
| Breast 4 | 13.11 | 1.15 |
| Menarche | 13.47 | 1.02 |
| Pubic hair 5 | 14.41 | 1.12 |
| Breast 5 | 15.33 | 1.74 |

Adapted from Marshall WA, Tanner JM. Variations in patterns of pubertal changes in girls. Arch Dis Child, 1969; 44:291. Reprinted with permission from Friedman IM, Goldberg E. Reference materials for the practice of adolescent medicine. Ped Clin North Am 1980;27:193

TABLE 30-6. Duration of Intervals Between Pubertal Stages in Females

| Interval | Mean (y) | Range From 5th to 95th Percentiles (y) |
|---|---|---|
| Breast 2 to 3 | 0.86 | 0.21–1.03 |
| Breast 2 to 4 | 1.80 | 0.69–3.63 |
| Breast 2 to 5 | 4.00 | 1.51–8.99 |
| Breast 3 to 4 | 0.89 | 0.13–2.19 |
| Breast 3 to 5 | 3.08 | 0.95–7.55 |
| Breast 4 to 5 | 1.96 | 0.12–6.82 |
| Pubic hair 2 to 3 | 0.62 | 0.16–1.27 |
| Pubic hair 2 to 4 | 1.13 | 0.50–2.04 |
| Pubic hair 2 to 5 | 2.49 | 1.39–3.10 |
| Pubic hair 3 to 4 | 0.51 | 0.18–0.93 |
| Pubic hair 3 to 5 | 1.85 | 0.94–3.85 |
| Pubic hair 4 to 5 | 1.30 | 0.57–2.37 |

Adapted from Marshall WA, Tanner JM. Variations in the pattern of pubertal changes in girls. Arch Dis Child 1969;44:291. Reprinted with permission from Friedman IM., Goldberg E. Reference materials for the practice of adolescent medicine. Ped Clin North Am 1980;27:198.

Preoccupied with bodily changes, early adolescents tend to be extremely concerned with their own needs and, because of their concrete level of reasoning, have difficulty reflecting on another's point of view. As they begin to develop the capacity for formal operational thinking, they become aware of other people's beliefs but are unable to differentiate what is of interest to themselves and to others. They assume that matters of great personal concern must necessarily be of equal significance to others. Adolescents also mistakenly assume that other individuals can read their thoughts. Hence, these young people sometimes act as if they are behaving for an imaginary audience. This notion that others are watching and thinking about them gives rise to the development of a sense of uniqueness and invulnerability (termed the "personal fable" by David Elkind). The adolescent believes that negative outcomes such as unintended pregnancy, drug addiction, HIV infection, or serious injury happen to others but not them. This personal fable helps explain why adolescents participate in behaviors adults view as risky.

With progression of the capacity for formal operational thought, adolescents become capable of considering perspectives other than their own, thereby becoming less egocentric. They also come to realize that other individuals have concerns of their own and are not focused exclusively on the adolescent's needs and desires. These changes do not occur in an all-or-none manner.

Adolescents, particularly early and middle adolescents, may be capable of sophisticated abstract reasoning one day and revert back to a more concrete level the next, especially during periods of stress. They may appear remarkably self-centered in one situation and other-directed in another. Hence, adolescents may not always appear to adults to act rationally or consistently with regard to their health care or their behavior.

As they mature in their ability to reason abstractly, adolescents also develop a more adult sense of time and the future. This involves the ability to project oneself forward in time to weigh future options or assess long-term consequences or benefits of various health decisions. It also presumes a belief that one has a future and the personal capability of influencing that future. Adolescents who have repeatedly failed at attempts to make decisions for themselves or have been given little opportunity to develop a sense of control are likely to be cynical or feel powerless when confronted with decisions in which time is critical.

Changes in sexual feelings and relationships during adolescence were key components of Freud's psychosexual theories. An upsurge in sexual feelings and impulses parallels hormonal and genital changes occurring during puberty. At first, such impulses are largely undifferentiated and directed toward persons

TABLE 30-5. Age of Attainment of Pubertal Stages and Peak Height Velocity in Males

| Stage | Mean (yr) | Standard Deviation |
|---|---|---|
| Genital 2 | 11.64 | 1.07 |
| Genital 3 | 12.85 | 1.04 |
| Pubic hair 2 | 13.44 | 1.09 |
| Genital 4 | 13.77 | 1.02 |
| Pubic hair 3 | 13.90 | 1.04 |
| Peak height velocity | 14.06 | 0.92 |
| Pubic hair 4 | 14.36 | 1.08 |
| Genital 5 | 14.92 | 1.10 |
| Pubic hair 5 | 15.18 | 1.07 |

Adapted from Marshall WA, Tanner JM. Variations in the pattern of pubertal changes in boys. Arch Dis Child 1970;45:13. Reprinted with permission from Friedman IM., Goldberg E. Reference materials for the practice of adolescent medicine. Ped Clin North Am 1980;27:199.

TABLE 30-7. Duration of Intervals Between Pubertal Stages in Males

| Interval | Median (y) | Range From 2.5 to 97.5 Percentiles (y) |
|---|---|---|
| Genital 2 to 3 | 1.12 | 0.41–2.18 |
| Genital 2 to 5 | 3.05 | 1.86–4.72 |
| Genital 3 to 4 | 0.81 | 0.24–1.64 |
| Genital 4 to 5 | 1.01 | 0.38–1.92 |
| Pubic hair 2 to 3 | 0.44 | 0.11–0.87 |
| Pubic hair 2 to 5 | 1.59 | 0.82–2.67 |
| Pubic hair 3 to 4 | 0.42 | 0.31–0.54 |
| Pubic hair 4 to 5 | 0.72 | 0.20–1.45 |

Adapted from Marshall WA, Tanner JM. Variations in the pattern of pubertal changes in boys. Arch Dis Child 1970;45:13. Reprinted with permission from Friedman IM., Goldberg E. Reference materials for the practice of adolescent medicine. Ped Clin North Am 1980;27:199.

TABLE 30-8. Factors Associated With Tanner Staging

| Process/Disorder | Tanner Stage |
|---|---|
| Hematocrit rise (male) | II–V |
| Alkaline phosphatase peak (male) | III |
| Alkaline phosphatase peak (female) | II |
| Adolescent hormonal levels (rise in estrogen for females and testosterone for males) | II–V |
| Peak height velocity (male) | III–IV |
| Peak height velocity (female) | II–III |
| Short male with growth potential | II |
| Short male with limited growth potential | IV–V |
| Usual timing of menarche | Late III or early IV |
| Appearance of menarche | 1–3.6 years post stage II |
| Slipped capital femoral epiphysis | (Obese) II or III |
| Acute worsening of idiopathic adolescent scoliosis (ie, time for close monitoring) | II–IV |
| Osgood-Schlatter's disease | III |
| Oral contraceptive prescription | IV |
| Diaphragm prescription | IV–V |
| Observe for worsening of straight-back syndrome | II–IV |
| Appearance of "normal" gynecomastia | II or III |
| Usual appearance of acne vulgaris | II or III |
| Gonococcal vaginitis | I |
| Gonococcal cerviticus (with or without pelvic inflammatory disease) | II+ |
| Timing of orchiopexy | I |
| Decreased incidence in serous otitis media | II or III |
| Mild regression in virginal hypertrophy | V |
| Timing of breast reduction | V |
| Timing of rhinoplasty | V |
| Strong suspicion for organic disease | II–V (abnormal progression or regression) |
| Counseling for further breast growth | II |
| Increased levels of serum uric acid in males | II–V |

Reprinted with permission from Greydanus DE, McAnarney ER. The value of Tanner staging. J Curr Adolesc Med 1980;February.

of the same sex but do not necessarily have implications for future sexual orientation. Group masturbation, especially among boys, is common. As the adolescent matures, these impulses generally become directed toward individuals of the opposite sex. As many as 10% of adolescents, however, continue to have sexual feelings directed predominantly or exclusively to members of the same sex.

An important component of the adolescent's maturing sexual identity is the realization that human sexuality involves more than the physical aspects of sex. The meaning of sexuality is influenced by parental beliefs and upbringing and by cultural, religious, and peer group norms. Given the importance of cultural and societal norms, those individuals who become aware of their persisting same-sex orientation usually must develop their sexual identity in secret without the needed support of parents, siblings, or peers. Hence support from a sympathetic pediatrician can be of great benefit.

Erik Erikson, another prominent theorist on human development, shifted from the Freudian emphasis on biologic drive states to highlight the critical issue of identity formation during adolescence. Building on skills achieved earlier in development, adolescents must achieve a sense of "who one is." This requires integration of both bodily and psychological changes, which, because of sexual awareness and maturity, result in a discontinuity with the past. Initial concerns focus on normalcy, then on characteristics of personal identity, and finally on the relationship between one's self and society. Developing a firm sense of identity is a prelude to resolving the young adult challenge of establishing the capacity for intimacy. Failure to do so leads to feelings of personal isolation. Erikson concluded that development of an individual identity depends on successful completion of previous developmental tasks. Adolescents who fail to achieve one or more of the preceding tasks during childhood or the various stages of adolescence (eg, as a consequence of heavy drug use) are at risk for failure to consolidate a sense of identity.

## SOCIOCULTURAL CHANGES

Adolescent development takes place within the context of a number of overlapping, interrelated spheres of influence. Parents, other family members, and peer groups are three primary social influences on adolescent development. These, in turn, are affected by other elements of the social web. Community (urban, suburban, rural), religion, cultural group (eg, Hispanic, Vietnamese), and school all have values, customs, and taboos that help shape the peer and family dynamics, which affect an adolescent's development. Families are in a rapid state of flux with many adolescents being raised by one parent, by a relative other than a parent, or in a household in which one or both parents have remarried.

The relationship between the adolescent and each of these socializing influences is complex. Adolescents derive many values from above-mentioned reference groups, and peer groups. These groups may also be influenced by personal characteristics of the adolescent. For example, teachers characterize late-maturing males as above average in intelligence less often than their early or average maturing classmates. Similarly, parents have lower expectations for these same individuals to complete college. Sexual activity, largely determined by peer norms, also appears to be influenced by an individual's physiologic maturity. Early maturing boys in one study engaged in various sexual behaviors earlier than age-matched counterparts who were normal or delayed in development (Westney, 1984). Early maturing girls initiate sexual intercourse at an earlier age than their less developed but same aged peers, perhaps because early maturing girls often have older friends and adopt the norms of that older peer group.

## Family

During early and middle adolescence, there is a gradual separation from parents and parental influence. This distancing occurs, in part, as a consequence of the more complex thought processes of the maturing adolescent who can now imagine a set of ideal parents to contrast with his or her real ones. The peer group becomes more important in an adolescent's life, particularly at middle adolescence. Family does not lose all its significance. Families, especially parents, are the primary socializing forces for infants and children up to early adolescence. The family continues to be the major source of nurturing and protection for adolescents who, as a result, enter puberty with values, goals, and beliefs instilled and modeled by parents. This value system is questioned, reanalyzed, and played down during the separation and individuation phase of early and middle adolescence, but it is not entirely abandoned. Rather, the adolescent shifts back and forth between seeking parental support at one moment and appearing to reject it the next. This seeming ambivalence can be frustrating for parents. By late adolescence, a rapprochement is reestablished, and the adolescent usually emerges with a belief system that incorporates, however modified, principles learned largely within the family context.

The challenge for parents, and perhaps other adult family members if they are present in the household, is to provide adolescents with an environment in which they can continue to develop and refine their emerging physical and cognitive skills. Such surroundings must constantly balance the adolescent's needs for adequate independence (which requires considerable parental flexibility) with legitimate parental expectations regarding respect for parental authority, for other members of the family, and for the orderly functioning of the household.

Such an environment can be best achieved if there is mutual respect among all family members and if there is effective communication. Effective communication is characterized by consistency, clarity, and completeness of expression and by a congruence between what family members say and do.

## Peer Group

Peer groups serve many important functions for adolescents. While adolescents try to determine who they are and whether they are normal, peer groups provide both social support and a safe way of trying alternative identities. Because they try to separate from parents, adolescents are unable to count on the ego support provided by the parents during the critical period when rapid body changes, increased drive states, and emerging cognitive abilities lead to a period of relative identity diffusion. The peer group provides an alternative support system.

The conformity required for peer group membership can have adverse developmental and health consequences if such behaviors as excessive drinking, cigarette use, or truancy are requirements for membership. As the adolescent becomes more secure in establishing his or her identity, the relationship with the peer group is restructured to a more equitable level.

Much has been written about peer group influence. Although adolescents look to peers for standards governing such things as dress, music, and hairstyles, they continue to respect and rely on parental values in many other areas. It is probably more accurate to say that decisions requiring choices about various aspects of lifestyle activate different referent groups.

## CHRONIC ILLNESS

Advances in medical care enable individuals with diseases that once resulted in childhood death to live into the adolescent and young adult age range. Still other adolescents develop chronic illness that persists into adulthood. Growing numbers, perhaps 10%, of adolescents and their families must confront the challenge of living with a chronic illness as they also confront the developmental tasks of adolescence.

The impact of chronic illness can be significant and complex. At a time when adolescents are concerned about bodily changes and desire to look like their peers, aspects of a disease or its treatment that result in altered body size or shape likely have an adverse affect on self-esteem and body image. Teenagers with chronic illnesses may be reluctant to take medications that produce visible changes in their bodies and set them apart from their peers. Part of the personal fable implies the need for medication no longer exists.

Chronic illness can interfere with normal adolescent development and create conflict between teenagers and parents. Anxious parents may be reluctant to grant age-appropriate independence or allow their teenager to make decisions about health care or other aspects of his or her personal life. Chronic illness gives parents justification for holding onto their teenager beyond the point when separation should occur.

Adolescents, in turn, may use their illness to manipulate their parents, avoid responsibility, or justify their unwillingness to meet the difficult challenges of growing to maturity. They also may shun social relationships out of fear of being perceived as different, or, having been excessively protected by parents, may be too immature to engage in appropriate peer activities. Alternatively, feeling the need to establish that they are like other adolescents, those with chronic illness may engage in health-risking behaviors. Such behaviors (eg, refusal to take insulin) can have serious deleterious effects on their health. Clinicians working with such adolescents and their families must be aware of these underlying dynamics.

## LEGAL AND ETHICAL CONSIDERATIONS

Providing health care for adolescents involves a variety of legal and ethical issues. In many health-care situations, there is a conflict among adolescents, their parents, physicians, and society about who makes decisions.

As with other areas of medicine, the framework for resolving such dilemmas is based on the patient's best interest from the patient's perspective and the principles of the doctor–patient relationship. The best interest standard recognizes the primacy of the adolescent's health and well-being and acknowledges that, in some circumstances in which lack of treatment poses a threat to health, adolescents do not seek care if they believe parents will be notified. Concerning the doctor–patient relationship, the physician should remember that the adolescent, not the adolescent's parents, is the patient. Hence, the adolescent should be afforded confidentiality, except when compelling evidence shows the adolescent is not competent to consent or is a threat to himself or herself (ie, suicidal or harmfully involved with drugs) or to others. In some situations, breach of confidentiality is mandated by law (eg, reporting sexual abuse or incest to social service agencies). Limits of confidentiality should be explained to the adolescent at the beginning of the visit.

There is no objective standard to determine at what age one is competent to give consent for health-care decisions. Recent evidence suggests that adolescents as young as 14-years-old have the same capacity as adults to give consent. Research by Kohlberg and Gilligan (1972) helps elucidate the manner in which adolescents make such decisions.

All 50 state courts recognize the doctrine of the "mature minor." This concept applies to those at the age of discretion, that is, age 15 years or older. For these youths, the doctrine applies if the following are true: the minor appears able to understand the procedure and its attendant risks and benefits sufficiently to give genuine informed consent, medical measures are taken for the patient's own benefit, measures are judged as necessary by conservative medical opinion, and there is good reason, including simple refusal by the minor to request it, why parental consent cannot be obtained (Holder, 1985).

Furthermore, competence need not be all-or-none. Given the adolescent's desire to be treated as an adult, competence can be presumed in situations in which there is little risk of harm to the adolescent from his or her decision. When situations involve considerable risk (eg, refusing life-saving treatment or when dealing with an extremely immature minor), the standard of competency should be more restrictive. Even with a stricter standard, it still may be concluded, as in the case of treatment for drug addiction or sexually transmitted diseases, that treatment without parental consent is warranted.

Rarely does the adolescent refuse any involvement of parents. Initially, out of fear or misunderstanding, adolescents may be reluctant to reveal information to their parents. With careful explanation of the issues involved and with adequate support by the physician, however, most adolescents eventually involve their parents.

By recognizing the competence of adolescents to give consent and based on concern that adolescents might avoid seeking care if confidentiality is not assured, most states have enacted legislation permitting physicians to treat adolescents in a variety of circumstances without parental consent. These include treatment for emergencies, sexually transmitted diseases, mental health problems, drug and alcohol abuse, pregnancy, and contraception. Abortion is a controversial topic, but the United States Supreme Court has ruled consistently that a minor may consent to an abortion without parental consent or notification, if she is willing to go to court to obtain a judge's consent in lieu of parental consent.

## HEALTH ASSESSMENT OF ADOLESCENTS

Health maintenance visits during adolescence are critical. Adolescents undergo a period of enormous physiologic and psychological change at the same time as they are confronted with a multitude of decisions about various behaviors that can enhance or threaten their well-being. The goals of the health maintenance visit are to reassure and support the adolescent about the normalcy of his or her development, to present information about how lifestyle choices affect health and help the adolescent assess the various choices, and to identify those youths at risk for, or having, adverse health problems as a means of preventing or treating such problems. The American Academy of Pediatrics

Committee on Practice and Ambulatory Medicine recommends a schedule of visits every other year. Such a schedule may be sufficient for those adolescents without significant illness who are fortunate enough to be raised in intact families with strong social support systems. More frequent visits (ie, at least once a year) may be warranted for many adolescents, especially those with chronic illness, who have dysfunctional families (eg, parental alcoholism) or who come from socially disadvantaged or impoverished backgrounds.

Adolescents have indicated the scope and range of services they would like to see provided by physicians caring for them. A classic study (Parcel et al, 1977) of a triethnic urban population of adolescents indicated that the majority wanted physicians to provide information about drugs, sex, sexually transmitted diseases, birth control, alcohol, and getting along with parents. Substantial numbers reported that they had personal concerns about one or more of those areas. At least 20% of the sample wanted help with acne, sexuality, depression, obesity, getting along with parents, miscellaneous health and dental problems, and nervousness. A similar study performed in Canada almost a decade later indicated almost the same range of problems and concerns.

In addition to the standard medical history usually obtained from patients and their families, certain aspects of the adolescent's level of functioning and lifestyle should be scrutinized. These are outlined in Table 30-9. A useful mnemonic to guide a clinician's systematic evaluation of these aspects of an adolescent's life is HEADSS: H–home, E–education, A–activities, D–drugs, S–sexuality, S–suicide/depression. Such information can be gathered from personal interview or from a combination of interview and questionnaire. Although some time will be spent with parents, most of the visit should occur alone with the adolescent, unless he or she specifically requests parental presence.

The direction and content of the interview depends on whether the patient is in early, middle, or late adolescence. Use of an open-ended, nonjudgmental style, interlaced with comments indicating that the intent of the questioning is for information gathering and that such areas are often of concern to adolescents, helps put the adolescent at ease. A good introductory clause is "Many young people your age are concerned about. . . ." In general, it is prudent to ask the adolescent the least threatening questions first. When asking about such things as illicit drug use or sexual activity, the physician may wish to inquire first about friends' behaviors.

Some time needs to be spent with parents to identify their concerns and to round out the picture of the adolescent's level of functioning. History appropriate to discuss with the adolescent and parents together includes immunization status, family history, history of chronic illness, previous hospitalizations, surgeries, and trauma. Medication, allergies, and diethylstilbestrol (DES) exposure in utero should also be reviewed.

Especially for early adolescents, the physical examination is exceptionally important. Concerned with changes in body size, shape, and function, adolescents often seek reassurance about the normalcy of their development. As the physician proceeds through the examination, it is worthwhile explaining the procedures and commenting about the results. For example, an adolescent may worry about his or her heart if the examiner listens for a long time without commenting that this is the usual manner of auscultation. See Table 30-8 for areas of the physical examination that should be highlighted.

There is no absolute consensus regarding the need for a pelvic examination in teenagers. In general, a nonsexually active teenager with normal menstrual function does not need a pelvic examination unless she specifically requests one. Examination of her external genitalia, however, should be part of the routine physical examination. Other than sexual activity, indications for a pelvic examination are severe dysmenorrhea unresponsive to

## TABLE 30-9.   Recommended Content for Routine Adolescent Health Visit

**Medical History**

Immunizations: DT, polio, measles (2 doses after first birthday), mumps, rubella, BCG

Chronic illness

Hospitalization

Surgery

Trauma: fractures, burns, head trauma; prior sports injuries

Medication: over the counter, prescribed (include oral contraceptives); food supplements

Diethylstilbestrol exposure

**Family History**

Cardiovascular: hypertension; diabetes; gout/hyperuricemia; obesity; elevated cholesterol/triglycerides; myocardial infarction or angina, peripheral vascular disease, or stroke in family members <60 years old

Alcoholism/substance abuse

Psychiatric disorders; suicide

Asthma, tuberculosis

**Review of Systems**

Dietary habits: typical foods consumed, special diets (eg, vegetarianism) types and frequency of meals skipped, use of laxatives or other weight loss methods

Recent weight gain or loss

Dental: last dental visit

Eye: last vision check

Female's gynecologic history: age of menarche; date of last menstrual period and previous menstrual period

  Characterization of menses: amount of bleeding; use of tampons/pads; dysmenorrhea (medications used for treatment); interval between menses; regularity of menses

Males: nocturnal emissions

**Psychosocial/Medicosocial History (HEADSS)**

**H(ome)**

  Household composition

  Relations with parents (including those not in home)

  Relations with siblings

  Living/sleeping arrangements

**E(ducation)**

  School attendance

  Ever failed a grade

  Grades

  Favorite, most difficult, best subjects

  Attitude towards school

  Special education needs

  Number of days missed

**A(ctivities)**

  Physical activity, regular exercise

  Sports participation, teams

  Work: type of job, hours, wages, satisfaction, safety hazards

  Special interests, hobbies, skills

  Peer relationships, best friend; activities with friends

**D(rugs)**

  Cigarettes/smokeless tobacco: age at first use, packs or cans per day

  Alcohol (beer, wine coolers): use at school or parties; use by friends, self

    If yes, CAGE: Have you ever felt the need to Cut down; have others Annoyed you by commenting on your use; have you ever felt Guilty about your use; have you ever needed an Eye-opener (alcohol first thing in morning)?

  Other drugs: CAGE can be modified; also age at first use, types of drugs used, routes of administration

**D(rugs) (Continued)**

  For any alcohol or other drug use: adverse consequences (driving while under the influence, accidents, truancy, vandalism; forced sex)

  Concerns about parental alcohol or drug use

**S(exuality)**

  Sexual feelings: opposite or same sex

  Sexual intercourse or types of sexual practices; age at first intercourse; gender of sex partner; number of lifetime partners

  Contraception/STD prevention: use of contraceptives, condoms, consistency of use; use at last intercourse

  History of STDs; last screen; history of PID (women)

  Prior pregnancies, abortions; ever gotten a girl pregnant?

  History of sexual abuse/date rape

  Females: vaginal discharge, dysuria

  Males: penile discharge, dysuria

**S(uicide)/depression**

  Feelings about self: positive and negative

  History of depression or other mental health problems, prior suicide attempts

  Sleep problems: difficulty getting to sleep, early waking, recurrent nightmares

  Suicidal thoughts

**Physical Examination (Most Pertinent Aspects)**

Height, weight, BP (with percentiles)

General appearance; affect

Skin: acne (type and distribution of lesions); scars; tattoos

Dentition

Spine (scoliosis)

Breasts: Tanner stage; masses

  Gynecomastia (males)

External genitalia (all)

  Pubic hair distribution—Tanner stage

  Testicular examination—Tanner stage, masses

Pelvic examination if indicated (see text)

**Laboratory Tests**

Tuberculosis skin test

Vision testing

Audiometry

Hemoglobin (indices and red cell distribution width if available)

  Hematocrit (if hemoglobin is unavailable)

Cholesterol, triglycerides, HDL-C, LDL-C if family history indicates

Sexually active adolescents

  Males: first part voided urinalysis (FPVU); gonorrhea and chlamydia cultures (or other detection tests) if FPVU positive; serologic test for syphilis

  Females: cultures (or other detection tests) for gonorrhea and chlamydia, serologic tests for syphilis, wet prep, KOH, cervical gram stain, PAP smear, midvaginal pH

  Homosexual males: same as above plus hepatitis B surface antigen and antibody

History of drug or alcohol abuse

  Hepatitis B surface antigen and antibody (IV drug users)

  Consider SGOT, SGPT, T-glutamyl transpeptidase (GGT)

  Consider HIV antibody testing (IV drug users)

HIV antibody testing should be considered for any sexually active adolescent. Informed consent is necessary and state laws vary as to specifics of consent procedure. Testing should occur if the patient requests it or if after a discussion of potential risk factors, benefits, and risks of testing, the patient determines it is in his or her best interest.

| TABLE 30-9. *(Continued)* | |
|---|---|
| **Immunizations**<br><br>Tetanus and diphtheria (update if ≥10 years since last dose)<br><br>Measles: Two doses of live attenuated vaccine are required after first birthday. Use MMR if not previously vaccinated for mumps or rubella. Do not administer rubella vaccine to woman anticipating pregnancy within 90 days<br><br>Hepatitis B vaccine: recommended for adolescents with multiple sexual partners (defined as more than one in 6 months) and for adolescents | **Immunizations** *(Continued)*<br><br>using intravenous drugs. Also recommended for adolescents living in areas where increased rates of parenteral drug abuse, teen pregnancy, and STDs occur. Also recommended for gay and bisexual males and for adolescents with a recent episode of an STD (Pediatrics 1992;89: 795). |

For a complete discussion of adolescent immunizations, see Report of the Committee on Infectious Diseases, ed 22. American Academy of Pediatrics, 1991.

*Modified from Marks A, Fisher M. Health assessment and screening during adolescence. Pediatrics 1987;80(suppl): 136.*

nonsteroidal anti-inflammatory agents, vaginal discharge, unexplained vaginal bleeding, amenorrhea or oligomenorrhea, in utero exposure to DES, and sexual assault. See Table 30-9 for recommended laboratory tests and immunization protocols.

## COUNSELING

As they mature, adolescents are faced with decisions regarding a myriad of lifestyle options. Pressures to perform a certain way are likely brought to bear by parents, peers, schools, and society (via television, radio, movies, and popular music). The adolescent should be provided with information concerning such areas as sexuality and contraception; safety (gun, seat belt, and bicycle helmet use); peer pressure; alcohol, cigarette, and illicit drug use; relationships with parents; and coronary artery disease prevention. The goal is not to lecture the adolescent but rather to assist him or her in understanding the ramifications of choosing a particular lifestyle. This dialogue signals the health-care provider's willingness to discuss such matters at future visits. Although the techniques are still of unproven efficacy, most physicians recommend teaching adolescents about self-breast and self-testicular examination.

Parents also should be able to discuss the development of the adolescent and to express concerns. Parents may need reassurance about the normalcy of the adolescent's development. Parents also may need guidance about setting limits, the role of peers, providing positive feedback to the adolescent, providing opportunities for independence and responsibility, and discipline. Because many teenagers model parental behavior, parents should be aware of the potential influence of such parental behavior as use of alcohol, cigarette smoking, driving while intoxicated, and use of seat belts. The visit should also be used to encourage parents to talk with their son or daughter about such topics as sexuality and drug use.

## Selected Readings

Cromer BA, McLean CS, Heald FP. A critical review of comprehensive screening in adolescents. J Adolesc Health 1992;13(supp).

Duke PM, Carlsmith JM, Jennings D, Martin JA, et al. Educational correlates of early and late sexual maturation in adolescence. J Pediatr 1982;100:633

Gilligan C. In a different voice: women's conceptions of self and morality. Harvard Educational Review 1977:481

Hechinger FM. Fateful choices: healthy youth for the 21st century. New York: Carnegie Corporation of New York, 1992.

Holder AR. Legal issues in pediatrics and adolescent medicine, ed 2. New Haven: Yale University Press, 1985:134.

Jessor R. Risk behavior in adolescence: a psychosocial framework for understanding and action. J Adolesc Health 1991;12:597.

Kohlberg L, Gilligan C. The adolescent as philosopher. In: Kagan J, Coles R, eds. Twelve to sixteen: early adolescence. New York: WW Norton and Co, 1972.

Lerner RM, Foch TT. Biological-psychosocial interactions in early adolescence. Hillsdale, NJ: Lawrence Erlbaum Associates, 1987.

Marks AM, Fisher M. Health assessment and screening during adolescence. Pediatrics 1987;80(suppl)136.

Muuss RE. Theories of Adolescence, ed 5. New York: Random House, 1988.

Parcel GS, Nader PR, Meyer MP. Adolescent health concerns, problems, and patterns of utilization in a triethnic urban population. Pediatrics 1977;60:157

Sebald H. Adolescents' shifting orientation toward parents and peers: a curvilinear trend over recent decades. Journal of Marriage and the Family 1986;48:4

Tanner JM. Growth at adolescence, ed 2. Oxford: Blackwell Scientific Publications Ltd, 1982.

Udry JR. Age at menarche, at first intercourse, and at first pregnancy. J Biosoc Sci 1979;11:433.

Westney OE, Jenkins RJ, Butts JD, Williams I. Sexual development and behavior in black preadolescents. Adolescence 1984;19:557.

*Principles and Practice of Pediatrics, Second Edition.*
edited by Frank A. Oski et al. J. B. Lippincott Company, Philadelphia © 1994.

# 30.2 *Breast Problems*

Michele Diane Wilson

During puberty, mammary tissue of the breast undergoes drastic alterations in response to the altered hormonal milieu. Many adolescents are uncomfortable with bodily transformations that occur as part of normal development. In American society, breasts are viewed as an essential component of female beauty and sexuality. Therefore, a young woman with a breast disorder may feel that her femininity is being threatened. Additionally, a breast mass is often feared to be cancer. In contradistinction, any breast enlargement in a young man may cause him to question his masculine identity. Breast problems are common during adolescence for both sexes.

In each situation, the individual may be extremely anxious regarding the implications of the breast disorder. Therefore, one should approach the individual with utmost sensitivity and provide adequate information and reassurances.

## BREAST MASSES IN FEMALES

Breast lumps frequently are encountered in adolescent women. A patient may find a lump by chance or as part of self-breast examination. Alternatively, the examiner may discover a lump during routine examination. It is useful to recognize the features of each type of lesion so a presumptive diagnosis can be made clinically.

## Fibrocystic Breast Disease

Fibrocystic disease, sometimes called proliferative breast changes, is characterized by diffuse bilateral breast thickening with non-discrete masses. Patients frequently complain of premenstrual tenderness. Fibrocystic breast disease is thought to result from mammary tissue stimulation by an estrogen-predominant and progesterone-deficient environment. Many therapies have been attempted with varying degrees of success. Vitamin E supplementation has been proposed as effective treatment but has not been adequately studied. The most well-known remedy, avoidance of methylxanthines (substances containing coffee, tea, and chocolate), is of uncertain benefit.

## Fibroadenoma

Fibroadenoma is the most common surgically excised breast lesion during adolescence, accounting for 64% to 72% of the diagnoses at pathology (Stone, 1977; Goldstein, 1982). Fibroadenoma is a benign neoplasm that occurs most often during late adolescence and early adulthood. Black women are affected disproportionately. On examination, the clinician finds one or multiple firm, easily mobile, painless masses. Recommended management of a suspected fibroadenoma is observation through two to three menstrual cycles because they will sometimes regress spontaneously. If the lesion persists, surgical excision is recommended. Rarely, the mass grows extremely large and is then called a giant fibroadenoma. Expedient surgical resection is required because the mass compresses normal breast tissue.

## Cystosarcoma Phylloides

Cystosarcoma phylloides accounts for less than 2% of all adolescent breast masses (Stone, 1977). The examiner detects a firm, smooth, mobile lesion similar in consistency to fibroadenomas. Appropriate management of this lesion is surgical excision because 10% to 15% of these tumors are malignant.

## Intraductal Papilloma

Intraductal papilloma is a rare tumor during adolescence. The patient presents with a bloody nipple discharge associated with discrete or multiple subareolar masses. When a discrete lump is present, surgical treatment is recommended because regression does not spontaneously occur. If a lump is not palpable, surgical exploration is unnecessary because of the uniformly benign prognosis.

## Breast Abscesses

A breast abscess manifests itself like an infectious process elsewhere; *Staphylococcus aureus* is the most common pathogen. Breast abscesses generally occur with predisposing conditions such as lactation, overlying skin infection, or local trauma. Application of warm compresses and antibiotics treat the condition. If infection is extensive and unresponsive to medical management, the abscess should be incised and drained.

## Breast Cancer

Breast cancer is rare in women younger than 20 years of age. Thus, a teenager with a breast lesion can be reassured that cancer is unlikely. Malignancies are characterized clinically by hard, irregular masses associated with overlying skin dimpling and nipple retraction. Surgical treatment is always indicated when malignancy is suspected.

## Patient Management

A careful history and physical examination can lead to a presumptive diagnosis. If the patient detects the lesion, it helps to know when it was first noted and whether it has changed in size. The clinician should ask whether it is painful or associated with signs of infection. If the lesion feels like a fluid filled mass, needle aspiration with resulting resolution confirms the diagnosis of an isolated cyst. If the lesion has qualities typical of a fibroadenoma, it can be followed clinically for 2 to 3 months before pathologic examination. Surgical intervention is indicated to obtain a definitive diagnosis and to allow for growth of surrounding healthy breast tissue when the mass persists for 2 to 3 months, the mass grows rapidly, or the mass has characteristics typical of cancer.

## Conclusions

Most breast masses in this age group are benign. Thus, the majority of lesions must be distinguished from the small number that represent serious disease. Careful physical examination, coupled with close follow-up, makes the distinction.

## ASYMMETRIC DEVELOPMENT

Breast asymmetry, commonly found in normal adult women, may cause anxiety for the teenager who is focused on her pubertal changes. Generally, the asymmetry is mild and the patient is satisfied by discussion regarding variations of normal development. More severe problems may be the result of a developmental anomaly known as amastia. This condition is manifested by the absence of chest wall structures, including muscles and ribs as well as mammary tissue. Management then entails surgical reconstruction when physical maturation occurs. In other circumstances, there is normal breast tissue bilaterally but marked difference in size, which is bothersome to the individual. Conservative management includes advocating a padded bra. If the young woman is fully mature and asymmetry persists, she may be referred to a plastic surgeon for reconstruction.

## GYNECOMASTIA

When a young man discovers breast growth, he is often extremely concerned and wants to know, "Am I normal?" His fear is shared by the majority of his peers entering puberty; 60% to 70% of male teenagers are affected. Gynecomastia, the presence of excessive breast tissue in males, has its peak prevalence between ages 12 and 15 years, which corresponds to Tanner stage II or III male genital development.

## Clinical Presentation

The young man often becomes aware of breast masses because they are exquisitely tender. The clinician finds unilateral or bilateral breast tissue localized under the areola or extending beyond it.

## Pathophysiology

Breast tissue grows whenever the ratio of estrogens to androgens is increased relative to normal adult male values. Thus, in early puberty during which increased estrogens are secreted before the surge in masculinizing hormones, ideal conditions exist for gynecomastia to develop.

## Differential Diagnosis

Most cases of adolescent gynecomastia are attributable to physiologic causes. Typically, breast enlargement begins in early puberty and regresses spontaneously within 6 to 24 months.

Nonphysiologic causes must be considered as well. Patients with Klinefelter's syndrome (47XXY) or hypogonadism produce deficient quantities of testosterone and therefore develop breast enlargement. Hepatic tumors or cirrhosis may result in breast masses as a result of altered steroid metabolism. Thyroid disease, starvation, testicular tumors, and adrenal tumors are associated with pathologic gynecomastia. Additionally, many medications induce male breast enlargement (Table 30-10). Substances of abuse, particularly marijuana and heroin, cause breast enlargement.

## Patient Evaluation

The evaluation of gynecomastia in an adolescent includes a complete history with particular attention to time of onset of breast growth in relation to initiation of puberty, its progression, as well as use of either prescription or illicit drugs. By examination, one should define the extent of gynecomastia. The presence of either hepatomegaly or a mass discovered on abdominal palpation suggests the possibility of liver or adrenal tumor. The genital exam is important for two reasons. First, the clinician should assess the individual's Tanner sexual maturity rating. Second, testicular palpation may reveal bilateral small testicles typical of Klinefelter's syndrome or a mass suggestive of testicular tumor. A more thorough laboratory evaluation for endocrine disorders and liver function assessment is indicated when the onset of gynecomastia precedes pubertal development or occurs after physical maturation or when the condition persists for more than 2 years. A careful history and physical examination can exclude nonphysiologic causes in most individuals.

## Management

If the evaluation is consistent with physiologic gynecomastia, the medical provider can reassure the patient and his family that the condition will spontaneously regress in less than 2 years. The clinician should examine the patient periodically until resolution occurs. Plastic surgery can be considered if the breast enlargement is disfiguring or causes emotional difficulties. Preliminary treatment trials with androgens and estrogen antagonists appear promising.

## Conclusions

Breast enlargement occurs in the majority of males during early adolescence but rarely is indicative of an underlying disease process. Reassurance of the patient and his family is the crucial element of treatment for physiologic gynecomastia. Rare pathologic etiologies are detected by careful history and physical examination. In these situations, treatment is directed toward the underlying disease process.

## Selected Readings

Beach RK. Routine breast exams: a chance to reassure, guide, and protect. Contemporary Pediatrics 1987;4:70.

Bower R, Bell MJ, Ternberg JL. Management of breast lesions in children and adolescents. J Pediatr Surg 1976;11:337.

Carlson HE. Gynecomastia. N Engl J Med 1980;303:795.

Diehl T, Kaplan DE. Breast masses in adolescent females. Journal of Adolescent Health Care 1985;5:353.

Dudgeon DL. Pediatric breast lesions: take the conservative approach. Contemporary Pediatrics 1985;61.

Goldstein DP, Miler V. Breast masses in adolescent females. Clinical Pediatrics 1982;21:17.

Lubin F, Ron E, Wax Y, et al. A case-control study of caffeine and methylxanthines in benign breast disease. JAMA 1985;253:2388.

Stone AM, Shenker IR, McCarthy K. Adolescent breast masses. Am J Surg 1977;134:275.

Vorherr H. Fibrocystic breast disease: pathophysiology, pathomorphology, clinical picture, and management. Am J Obstet Gynecol 1986;154:161.

Wilson JD, Aiman J, MacDonald PC. The pathogenesis of gynecomastia. Adv Intern Med 1980;25:1.

*Principles and Practice of Pediatrics, Second Edition.*
edited by Frank A. Oski et al. J. B. Lippincott Company, Philadelphia © 1994.

## 30.3 *Menstrual Disorders*

Michele Diane Wilson

Menstrual disorders are common concerns during adolescence. Certain problems such as dysmenorrhea are not unique to teenagers and may persist throughout adult life. By contrast, amenorrhea or dysfunctional vaginal bleeding are disorders for which the peak prevalence occurs during the second decade of life. Symptoms referable to the reproductive system often induce anxiety for patient and family. A sensitive and methodical approach allays unfounded fears and establishes appropriate diagnoses.

## DYSMENORRHEA

Dysmenorrhea is the most common gynecologic problem experienced during adolescence. Prevalence among the adolescent population approaches 60% (Klein, 1981). Dysmenorrhea is the leading cause of school absenteeism among young women.

| TABLE 30-10. Drugs That Cause Gynecomastia |
| --- |
| Hormonal medications |
| Corticosteroids |
| Tricyclic antidepressants |
| Phenothiazine |
| Diazepam |
| Ketoconazole |
| Isoniazid |
| Substances of abuse |
|    Heroin |
|    Methadone |
|    Amphetamines |
|    Marijuana |
| Insulin |
| Digitalis |
| Reserpine |
| Cimetidine |
| Spironolactone |
| Cytotoxic agents |

# Definition

The term dysmenorrhea is derived from the Greek and means "difficult monthly flow." Symptoms generally occur a few hours before or simultaneously with the appearance of menstrual bleeding. The pain is typically most severe on the first day of bleeding and usually resolves by the third day of menses. Women describe crampy, colicky, suprapubic pain that may be accompanied by other complaints. The most common associated symptoms include nausea, vomiting, diarrhea, and lower back pain. Less frequently, patients suffer from dizziness, syncope, and headaches.

## Differential Diagnosis of Dysmenorrhea

It is essential to distinguish primary and secondary causes of dysmenorrhea. Primary dysmenorrhea is more prevalent and refers to the occurrence of painful menses without pelvic pathology, whereas secondary dysmenorrhea indicates that an identifiable pelvic abnormality exists.

### Primary Dysmenorrhea

Primary dysmenorrhea has its peak onset 6 to 18 months after menarche, which corresponds to the transition to ovulatory menstrual cycles. The etiology of dysmenorrhea is the focus of recent research and debate. The association between dysmenorrhea and ovulation has been recognized for many years and is thought to explain the absence of pain during the first few menstrual cycles when ovulation is rare. Furthermore, therapies that suppress ovulation have been demonstrated to improve symptoms. Patients with severe dysmenorrhea have been shown to have abnormally high intrauterine pressure at the time of contractions during menses. Additional data demonstrate that prostaglandins act as pain mediators and as stimulators of uterine contractility, and patients suffering from dysmenorrhea have increased levels of prostaglandins in their menstrual fluid. Therapies with prostaglandin inhibitors have proved effective.

### Secondary Dysmenorrhea

Secondary dysmenorrhea indicates that an identifiable pathologic abnormality exists and is causing the pain. Congenital anomalies of the reproductive tract should be considered in the differential diagnosis of the young woman who presents with dysmenorrhea coincident with menarche. Uterine malformations such as a bicornuate uterus with unilateral outflow obstruction may be responsible. The pelvic examination may reveal a midline mass. Ultrasound confirms the diagnosis.

Pelvic tumors such as a cervical or uterine polyp or an endometrial fibroma may cause menstrual discomfort. Endometriosis, previously believed to occur only in older women, is increasingly recognized in adolescents. A surgical series of 282 teenage women who had laparoscopy because of chronic pelvic pain found endometriosis in 45% of the patients (Emans, 1990). The diagnosis should be considered in any patient whose symptoms are severe and unresponsive to conventional therapy. Additionally, nodularity of the cul-de-sac may be appreciated on pelvic exam.

### Infection

A young woman who is sexually active and experiences dysmenorrhea of recent onset may have a pelvic infection. The individual with acute salpingitis typically has a mucopurulent cervical discharge coupled with tenderness on bimanual palpation of the uterus and adnexa. A patient who has previously experienced a pelvic infection may suffer from dysmenorrhea as a consequence.

### Pregnancy and Its Complications

A sexually active individual may experience painful vaginal bleeding as the result of a complicated pregnancy including threatened, missed, or incomplete abortion. The classic triad of ectopic pregnancy includes lower abdominal pain, vaginal bleeding, and an abnormal menstrual history. Thus, diagnosis of pregnancy must be considered.

## Assessment of the Patient With Dysmenorrhea

The evaluation of dysmenorrhea must distinguish primary from secondary causes. The impact of the condition on the individual should also be assessed. It is important to determine how severe the symptoms are and the degree to which they affect the young woman's life. Questions to be asked include "How much school or work have you missed?" and "Does the pain interfere with participation in other activities?" The extent of the evaluation is dictated by the severity and impact of pain on daily life. A complete menstrual and sexual history should be obtained. Sexually active individuals must be considered at risk for pregnancy or for sexually transmitted diseases as etiologies for the problem. Age of onset and progression of dysmenorrhea should be assessed in relation to the time of menarche.

A complete physical examination with careful abdominal palpation should be performed. A pelvic examination is indicated at the initial evaluation if the patient is sexually active or the pain is severe. Any sexually active patient should have cervical cultures obtained for gonorrhea and chlamydia (if available) to aid in diagnosing endometritis or acute salpingitis. On bimanual palpation, it is important to note any uterine enlargement consistent with pregnancy. An adnexal mass suggests the possibility of an ectopic pregnancy. The cul-de-sac should be carefully palpated for the nodularity suggestive of endometriosis.

### Laboratory Data

The extent of laboratory evaluation is dictated by history and physical findings. When the diagnosis of a congenital anomaly is entertained, pelvic ultrasound may be obtained. If pain is severe and unresponsive to medical management, diagnostic laparoscopy to rule out endometriosis is indicated.

Treatment for secondary dysmenorrhea is directed toward correction of the responsible condition. Various treatment modalities are advocated for primary dysmenorrhea. Nonsteroidal anti-inflammatory agents (NSAIDs) inhibit prostaglandin synthesis. The ability of different NSAIDs to effect total symptom resolution ranges from 61% to 100%. For sexually active individuals, oral contraceptives protect against pregnancy and successfully treat primary dysmenorrhea in 80% to 90% of cases. Table 30-11 lists the response rate and appropriate dosages for various treatment modalities. Analgesics including aspirin are commonly used with results similar to those of placebo agents. The role of exercise and other nonpharmacologic agents is not clear.

Dysmenorrhea is common among adolescents. Evaluation of the patient with dysmenorrhea includes a careful search for pathologic etiologies. Most individuals with primary dysmenorrhea respond well to nonsteroidal anti-inflammatory agents or oral contraceptives.

## AMENORRHEA

Amenorrhea, the absence of menses, is a concerning symptom that generally brings teenagers in for evaluation. Sometimes, the patient is a young woman who has not experienced menarche—primary amenorrhea. Other times, the patient has previously

**TABLE 30-11. Pharmacologic Therapy for Dysmenorrhea**

| Medication | Dose |
| --- | --- |
| **Nonsteroidal Anti-inflammatory Agents** | |
| Ibuprofen | 400 mg every 4–6 h or 800 mg tid |
| Naproxen | 250–375 mg bid or tid |
| Naproxen sodium | 550 mg initial dose; then 275 mg qid |
| **Fenamates** | |
| Mefenamic acid | 500 mg initial dose; then 250 mg qid |
| **Oral Contraceptives** | As directed |

menstruated but experiences an interval without menses—secondary amenorrhea. The health-care provider should know what constitutes normal menstrual cycles and their variations before making an evaluation.

Primary amenorrhea is usually defined as the absence of menses by age 16 years in the presence of normal physical development, age 14 years without pubertal development, or 4 years after the onset of puberty. Secondary amenorrhea is defined as the absence of menses for at least 6 months or three cycle lengths after establishment of regular cycles. For both primary and secondary amenorrhea, the defined periods without menses are useful as guidelines and may be used with flexibility.

Control of female menstrual function is a complex and delicate process. Perturbations at any one of a number of levels can result in a common symptom: amenorrhea. The various levels of input include hypothalamus, pituitary, ovaries, uterus, and vagina. Other endocrine organs can impact menstrual function, particularly the thyroid and adrenal gland. Thus, the differential diagnosis of amenorrhea includes disorders of these organs. Primary and secondary amenorrhea are discussed together because many problems can cause either. Entities that are solely primary or secondary amenorrhea problems are noted.

## Differential Diagnosis of Amenorrhea

### Hypothalamus

Constitutional delay in puberty is a common reason for primary amenorrhea. Individuals who enter puberty at a late age typically progress normally. Family history of development often is similar. Kallman's syndrome, an isolated defect in GnRH production, is characterized by primary amenorrhea and anosmia.

### Pituitary

Hyperprolactinemic states caused by adenomas generally result in menstrual irregularities after initiation of menses. Patients often complain of headaches and galactorrhea. Visual field defects may be detectable by careful examination.

### Ovaries

Gonadal dysgenesis—Turner's syndrome (45XO) or mosaicism—is the most common reason for primary amenorrhea. Clues to the diagnosis include lymphedema at birth, webbed neck, short stature, shield chest, and wide-spaced nipples. Confirmation is made by karyotyping. Ovarian failure may occur after exposure to viral, toxic, radioactive, or chemotherapeutic agents. Polycystic ovary syndrome represents a spectrum of disorders variably manifested by amenorrhea or oligomenorrhea, hirsutism, obesity, and acne. Ovarian tumors are an unusual cause of menstrual disorders during adolescence.

### Uterus

If the uterus is unable to respond to circulating hormones, bleeding does not ensue. Congenital anomalies of the uterus that present with primary amenorrhea despite normal secondary sex characteristics include Rokitansky syndrome or müllerian agenesis, androgen insensitivity, cervical agenesis, and endometrial hypoplasia. Scar tissue in the uterus secondary to uterine instrumentation or trauma, Asherman syndrome, presents with secondary amenorrhea. Pregnancy is the most common cause of secondary amenorrhea and an infrequent cause of primary amenorrhea.

### Vagina

Congenital malformations of the vagina such as agenesis, septum formation, or imperforate hymen are manifested as outflow disorders. Women develop normally but do not have menses. An imperforate hymen causes cyclic pain because menstrual blood accumulates in the uterus.

### Thyroid

Overproduction or underproduction of thyroid hormone may result in amenorrhea. Symptoms of thyroid dysfunction for which inquiries should be made include change in energy, appetite, weight, skin texture, or bowel habits. Physical examination may demonstrate a goiter, exophthalmos, lid lag, and reflex changes.

### Adrenal Gland

The adrenal gland is the source of masculinizing hormones or androgens in females. Any process that increases steroid biosynthesis in the adrenal gland results in virilization. Deficiencies of 21-hydroxylase, 11-beta hydroxylase, and 3-beta-hydroxysteroid dehydrogenase may present with delayed menarche or oligomenorrhea as well as hirsutism.

### Chronic Illness

Any chronic illness, particularly those which interfere with normal growth and nutrition, may cause amenorrhea. Thus, patients with inflammatory bowel disease, cystic fibrosis, and chronic renal failure often suffer from amenorrhea.

Increasing evidence shows that a minimum amount of body fat is necessary to achieve menarche and to maintain menstrual function. Crash diets with loss of a significant percentage of body weight may precipitate amenorrhea.

Women who engage in competitive athletics are at risk for delayed menarche and secondary amenorrhea. The type of sport, extent of training, total body weight, percent body fat, stress, and genetic endowment are all factors.

Either physical or emotional stress may result in missed menses. Moving away to college or traveling may cause amenorrhea. Medications acting at the level of the central nervous system alter menstrual function. Post-pill amenorrhea occurs in a small percentage of women who discontinue use of oral contraceptives. Neuroleptic medications are commonly implicated.

## Evaluation of the Adolescent With Amenorrhea

A careful and complete history and physical examination direct the assessment and prevent unnecessary diagnostic testing. The clinician should inquire about the young woman's growth, onset of pubertal development and subsequent progression, lymphedema at birth, and family history of age of onset of puberty. Changes in weight or diet, participation in competitive athletics, and recent stress are possible causes of menstrual disorders. The clinician should ascertain whether any chronic illness exists and perform a complete review of symptoms. Specifically, one should ask about gastrointestinal symptoms suggestive of inflammatory bowel disease and symptoms of excessive or diminished thyroid activity. Severe headaches suggest the possibility of an intracranial tumor. The adolescent must be questioned privately regarding sexual activity, use of prescription medications, and use of illicit drugs. A young woman may not reliably provide information regarding sexual activity; therefore, a urine or serum pregnancy test must be obtained.

A complete physical examination is indicated. Because short stature is suggestive of Turner's syndrome and malnutrition is typical of anorexia nervosa, special attention should be paid to growth parameters. Excess body hair suggests a virilizing process. Careful ophthalmologic examination with attention to signs of papilledema and visual fields defects is indicated. The extent of breast, axillary hair, and pubic hair development should be assessed. The breast should be milked for discharge and the thyroid gland should be palpated. Pelvic examination is required. It is important to look for clitoromegaly (diameter greater than 5 mm). Although a speculum examination need not be performed on virgins, the patency of the vaginal orifice should be assessed by gently inserting one finger. Additionally, the cervix and uterus should be felt by either vaginal or rectal palpation. Enlargement of the uterus suggests pregnancy.

When the history and physical examination are completed, possible causes are identified. Figure 30-6 is a flow diagram useful in evaluating primary amenorrhea. If pubertal development has not started but the uterus is present and outflow tract is patent, there may be prepubertal levels of estrogen due to lack of hypothalamic or pituitary stimulation or there may be inability of the ovary to respond to stimulation. High levels of follicle stimulating hormone (FSH) implicate the ovary, and diagnostic possibilities are narrowed to gonadal dysgenesis from Turner's syndrome, mosaicism, or a nonfunctioning X chromosome. On the other hand, if puberty has begun and proceeded normally, men-

arche has not ensued because of an anatomic problem of the uterus or vagina. A karyotype is indicated because individuals with testicular feminization are 46XY, yet have normal female development. If the karyotype is 46XX, congenital absence of the uterus is diagnosed.

Figure 30-7 summarizes the evaluation of secondary amenorrhea. A pregnancy test should be performed before an extensive evaluation. If the young woman is not pregnant, the progesterone challenge test is a useful diagnostic tool. Uterine bleeding ensues from progesterone given either orally for 1 week or intramuscularly as one injection if the uterus is primed with endogenous estrogen and the anatomy of the lower reproductive tract is intact. Diagnostic possibilities, therefore, include stress, weight loss, medications, polycystic ovarian disease, and pituitary adenomas. If withdrawal bleeding does not occur, then serum FSH and luteinizing hormone should be obtained. High levels indicate ovarian failure, and low or normal levels implicate the hypothalamus or pituitary. It is appropriate to refer to a specialist in adolescent gynecology if the workup is inconclusive, a congenital anomaly is uncovered, or the physician feels uncomfortable with performing the evaluation.

Amenorrhea as a symptom suggests the need for a careful and thoughtful evaluation to discern the etiology for the problem. A complete history and physical examination provides direction for the evaluation.

# DYSFUNCTIONAL VAGINAL BLEEDING

## Introduction

Dysfunctional vaginal bleeding indicates the onset of abnormal vaginal bleeding secondary to anovulation. Commonly accepted definitions of excessive bleeding include bleeding that lasts 8 days

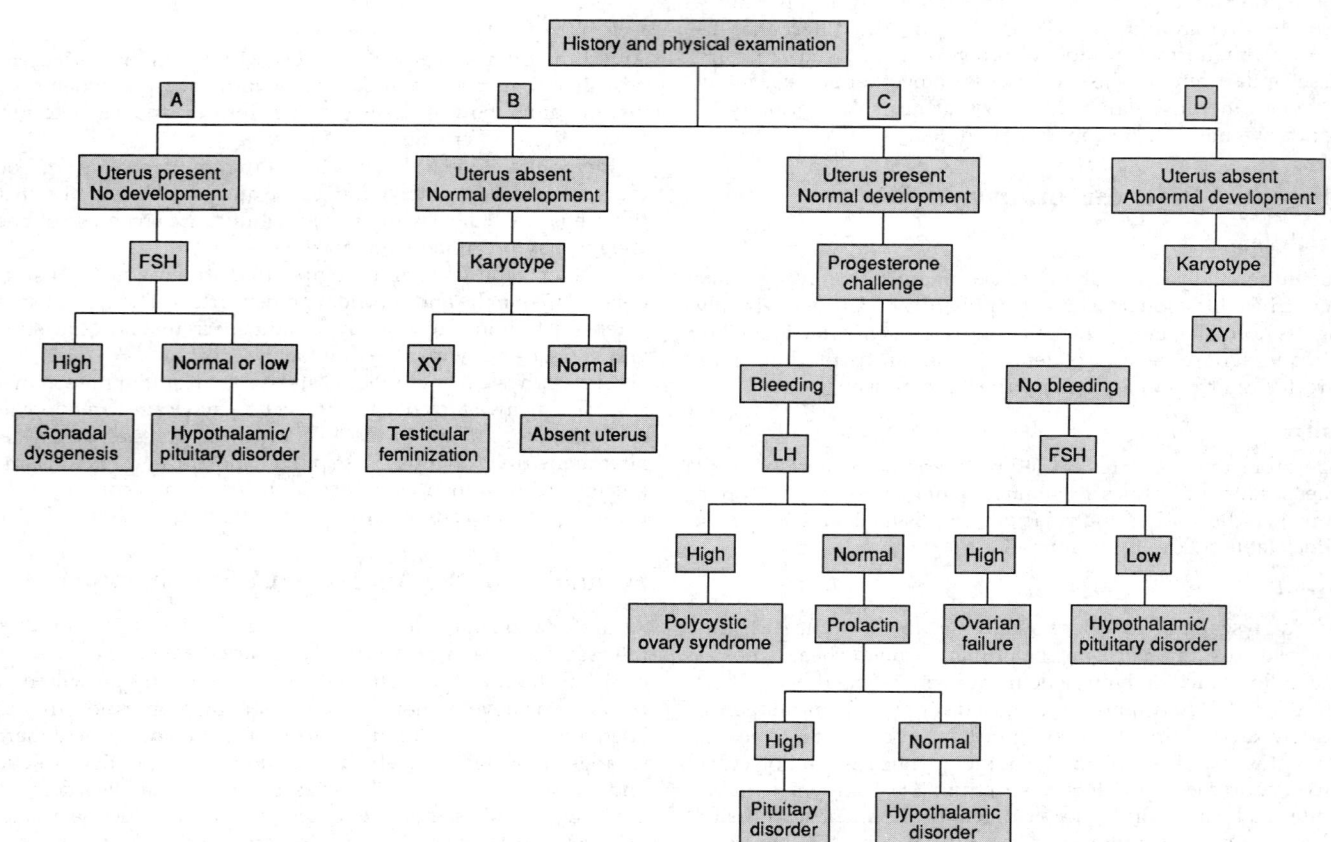

**Figure 30-6.** Evaluation of primary amenorrhea. Evaluation is indicated if menses are absent by age 16 with normal development, by age 14 without development, or 4 years after onset of puberty.

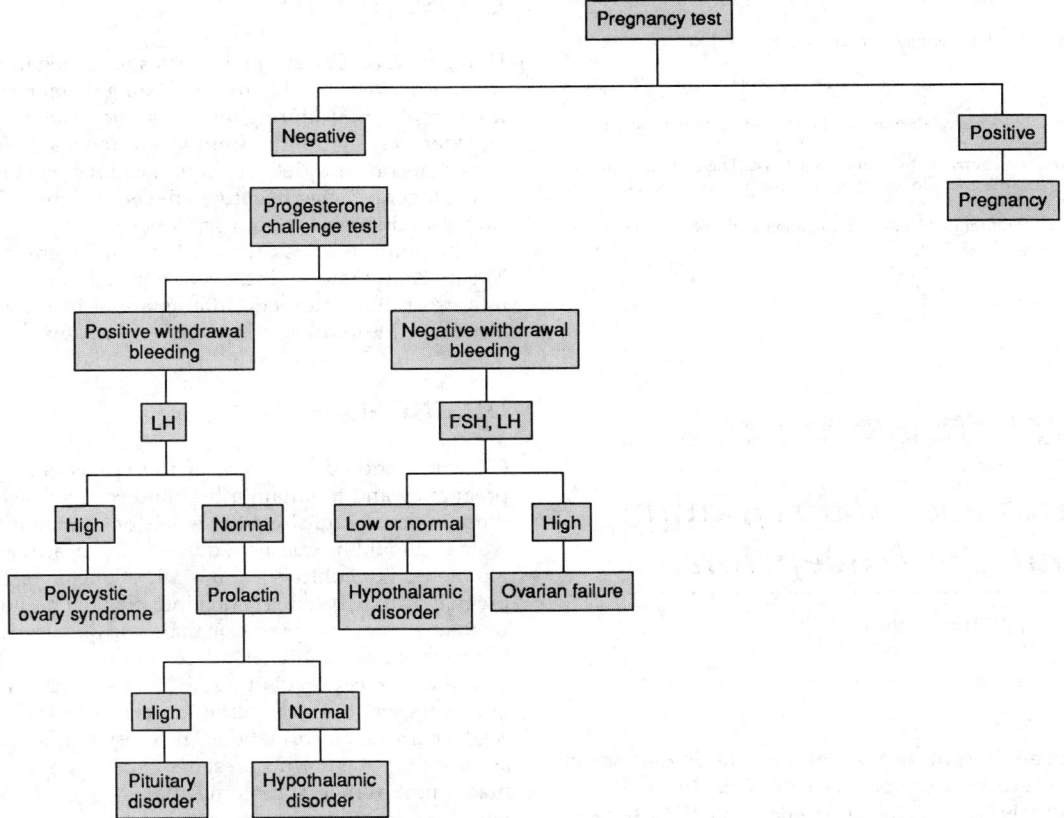

Figure 30-7.  Evaluation of secondary amenorrhea.

or longer, use of 10 sanitary pads per day, or frequency of bleeding more often than every 21 days. In the absence of one of the above criteria, abnormal bleeding exists if bleeding is associated with a drop in the hematocrit.

## Differential Diagnosis

The most common reason for abnormal bleeding in an early pubertal woman is anovulation. As a result, the endometrial lining is stimulated by unopposed estrogen, becomes thick, and sheds with heavy bleeding. Dysfunctional bleeding is a diagnosis of exclusion.

Pregnancy and its complications (eg, ectopic pregnancy; threatened, missed, or incomplete abortion) are causes for abnormal bleeding. Infectious processes such as endometritis or acute salpingitis may cause bleeding. Trauma from rape or coitus may result in bleeding. Foreign bodies, often a retained tampon, may present with bleeding. Blood dyscrasias accounted for 19% of hospitalized adolescents with bleeding. Tumors of the female reproductive system such as polyps, fibroids, and, rarely, malignancies must be in the differential diagnosis.

## Evaluation

The evaluation is important to assess the severity of the blood loss and to determine its cause. The history should indicate the amount of blood lost. A menstrual history including the age of menarche and the usual pattern of menses is important to obtain. Sexual activity should be discussed to assess risks of pregnancy and infection. The clinician also should ask about the possibility of trauma and should assess whether the patient shows evidence of a bleeding diathesis.

The physical examination provides evidence of severe blood loss if there are orthostatic changes in vital signs or pallor. The thyroid should be palpated. A full pelvic examination is indicated to localize the site of bleeding, to obtain cultures, to look for a foreign body or tumors, and to assess for pregnancy or tenderness as evidence of infection.

The extent of laboratory evaluation is determined by the extent of bleeding. A hematocrit confirms the degree of blood loss. Pregnancy should be excluded by the use of sensitive serum human chorionic gonadatropins (HCG). A white blood count and an erythrocyte sedimentation rate are increased with infection. Clotting studies should be obtained if bleeding disorder is being considered. Thyroid function tests should be drawn.

## Treatment

Therapy for most causes is directed toward the underlying condition. If the bleeding is anovulatory, therapy with progesterone supplementation stabilizes the endometrial lining and ends the bleeding. Various regimens include progesterone alone or oral contraceptives in high doses. Either treatment is effective. Therapy should continue for several months to build up the endometrial lining. Iron supplementation is recommended.

## Conclusion

Abnormal vaginal bleeding is common during adolescence. One must assess the extent of the bleeding, the reason for the condition, and provide treatment as indicated.

## Selected Readings

Alvin PE, Litt IF. Current status of the etiology and management of dysmenorrhea in adolescence. Pediatrics 1982;70:516.

Dawood MY. Dysmenorrhea. Clin Obstet Gynecol 1983;26:719.

Emans SJH, Goldstein DP. Pediatric and adolescent gynecology, ed 3. Boston: Little, Brown & Co, 1990.

Klein JR, Litt IF. Epidemiology of adolescent dysmenorrhea. Pediatrics 1981;68: 661.

Mansfield MJ, Emans SJ. Adolescent menstrual irregularities. J Reprod Med 1984: 29:399.

Marut EL, Dawood MY. Amenorrhea (excluding hyperprolactinemia). Clin Obstet Gynecol 1983;26:749.

Polaneczky MM, Slap GB. Menstrual disorders in the adolescent: amenorrhea. Pediatr Rev 1992;13:43.

Soules MR. Adolescent amenorrhea. In: Mahoney CP, ed. The pediatric clinics of North America: pediatric and adolescent endocrinology, vol 34. Philadelphia: WB Saunders, 1987:1083.

Vaughn TC. Dysfunctional uterine bleeding in the adolescent. Seminars in Reproductive Endocrinology 1984;2;359.

*Principles and Practice of Pediatrics, Second Edition.*
edited by Frank A. Oski et al. J. B. Lippincott Company, Philadelphia © 1994.

# 30.4 *Adolescent Pregnancy and Contraception*

Michele Diane Wilson

The age at which adolescents in the United States initiate sexual activity has decreased over the past few decades. In the United States, 79.8% of males and 53.2% of females ages 15 to 19 years of age had experienced sexual intercourse in 1988. Although adolescents experience an array of new sexual feelings and may be physically capable of engaging in sexual relations, frequently they are not emotionally prepared to make mature decisions regarding sexual activity and contraception.

Several factors cause difficulty for adolescents in their attempt to make responsible decisions regarding initiation of sexual activity and contraceptive behaviors. Young persons often lack adequate knowledge regarding fertility and contraception. Health services may be unavailable or difficult to access. Furthermore, adolescents may be unable to communicate with those individuals who can help them best in these decisions, ie, their parents, health professionals, and sexual partners. The psychological profile of an adolescent compounds the difficulty. Adolescence is characterized by risk-taking behaviors and impulsiveness. Young persons have difficulty with the future orientation required for effective contraception. Additionally, adolescents may be uncomfortable accepting their sexuality and fearful of discovery by parents. The end result is a large number of teenagers engaging in sexual activity without adequate protection against unwanted pregnancies.

## EPIDEMIOLOGY

The United States has the second highest pregnancy rate among all developed countries for which data are available. The higher rates of pregnancy in the United States versus other countries does not appear to reflect a greater rate of sexual intercourse but rather the lack of use or inadequate use of contraception by teenagers. On average, adolescent women delay 11.5 months from the time they initiate sexual intercourse until they go to a clinic for family planning. In 1988, women 19 years of age and younger gave birth to 488,940 infants in the United States. Overall, 1 in 10 adolescent women become pregnant during adolescence. Two thirds of these pregnancies are unplanned.

## CONSEQUENCES

Unplanned adolescent pregnancies have negative consequences for all involved individuals. The young woman is at risk for medical complications during her pregnancy. She is more likely than an older women to suffer from severe anemia, pregnancy-induced hypertension, and delivery complications. Furthermore, adolescent pregnancy has negative effects on future educational and career attainment for both parents.

The infant is at risk for mortality and significant morbidities. The mortality rate for infants of young mothers exceeds that for infants of older mothers. Infants are at increased risk for low–birth-weight, injuries, and learning problems.

## DIAGNOSIS

Clinicians should be aware of the epidemiology of adolescent pregnancy and maintain a high index of suspicion for the condition. After establishing the tenets of confidentiality, the young woman should be questioned in private regarding sexual activity. No method of contraception is 100% effective. The diagnosis of pregnancy may be entertained immediately because of the young woman's chief complaint or may not be suspected until much later in the evaluation. An adolescent may present with the concern that she is pregnant. Other times, pregnancy is uncovered only after lengthy evaluation, especially if the patient does not reveal pertinent information. The most common diagnosis in the adolescent patient who presents with secondary amenorrhea is pregnancy. Other symptoms that suggest pregnancy include nausea, fatigue, dizziness, syncope, urinary frequency, breast tenderness, and nipple sensitivity.

The physical examination can support the diagnosis of pregnancy. On abdominal exam, a midline lower abdominal mass may be palpable after the first trimester of pregnancy. On pelvic exam, the cervix acquires a cyanotic appearance and softens, and the cervico–uterine angle blurs. The uterine size should be assessed to estimate the length of gestation. At 12 weeks' gestation, the uterus is palpable at the symphysis pubis; at 20 weeks' gestation, the uterus is palpable at the umbilicus.

Laboratory confirmation of pregnancy can be made with either urine or blood measurement of human chorionic gonadotropins (HCG). Newer urine tests are extremely sensitive and can diagnose a pregnancy as early as within 7 days after conception, ie, 1 week before the missed menses.

## COUNSELING

Once a diagnosis of pregnancy is confirmed, the adolescent should be informed and counseled about her options. Ideally, the young woman should be counseled by an experienced professional who can present unbiased information to assist her in her choice. If personal reasons prevent the physician from doing so, it is appropriate to refer the patient elsewhere for services. Optimally, the parents should be involved to provide support. The options are to continue the pregnancy to term and keep the baby, continue the pregnancy to term and place the baby for adoption, or obtain an abortion.

There is no easy solution for the adolescent experiencing an unintended pregnancy. Supportive counseling should allow the patient to express her feelings so she can make the best decision.

In summary, early sexual activity and resultant pregnancy continue in epidemic proportions in the United States. Health care providers must anticipate unintended adolescent pregnancy, make a timely diagnosis, and provide or refer for choice counseling.

## ADOLESCENT CONTRACEPTION

There is a tremendous need for safe and effective methods of contraception that are acceptable to sexually active young persons. All counseling regarding contraception should include counseling regarding sexually transmitted disease (STD) and human immunodeficiency virus (HIV) infection risk reduction. An assessment made in confidence helps determine which adolescent plans to become or is sexually active. If contraception is needed, counseling regarding an appropriate method is indicated. In addition to obtaining a history and physical examination and determining which methods are contraindicated medically, it is important to elicit what method of contraception the patient desires. The choice must be acceptable to the young person and clinician. Ultimately, the patient must be comfortable with the method and be willing to use it correctly and consistently. The health-care provider needs to assess the patient's level of maturity as well as ability and willingness to use a given method of contraception.

Contraceptive counseling should include a discussion of the risks, benefits, side effects, and effectiveness for the methods being considered. Effectiveness is best described in terms of percentage of typical female users who become pregnant using the stated method for one year. It is important to recognize that the failure rate among adolescents using any contraceptive method is much higher than the rate among older individuals. Written materials generally augment verbal instructions. Table 30-12 summarizes the methods of contraception commonly used by adolescents.

## Oral Contraception

Oral contraception is one of the most frequently used methods of contraception used during adolescence. Birth control pills are prepared from a combination of estrogen and progestin, which is a synthetic progesterone. The three mechanisms of action of oral contraceptives are suppression of ovulation; alteration of cervical mucus, rendering it impermeable to sperm; and thinning of the endometrial lining, making it inhospitable to implantation.

Oral contraceptives offer many advantages that make them particularly well suited for teenagers. They are extremely effective, with 3.0 pregnancies occurring among 100 women in one year. Because a daily pill is ingested, use is not directly related to the act of coitus. Furthermore, many women experience noncontraceptive benefits from the pills. Specifically, dysmenorrhea, benign breast disease, rheumatoid arthritis, iron deficiency anemia, and

### TABLE 30-12. Methods of Contraception

| Method | Failure Rate in Typical User (%)* | Benefits | Risk/Disadvantages |
|---|---|---|---|
| Combined oral contraceptives | 3.0 | Use not related to coitus; decreased risk of dysmenorrhea, breast disorders, arthritis, iron deficiency anemia, ovarian and uterine cancers, ovarian cysts | Thromboembolic phenomena, cerebrovascular accident, coronary artery disease, hepatomas, gallbladder disease, hypertension, worsening of migraines, breakthrough bleeding, amenorrhea nausea, weight gain, acne, depression, glucose intolerance |
| Progestin-only pill (mini-pill) | † | Fewer metabolic complications, used for patients with hypertension, diabetes, sickle cell disease | Menstrual irregularities |
| Norplant | 0.04 | No demand after insertion, highly effective, long-lasting protection | Requires minor surgical procedure for insertion, removal; side effects—menstrual irregularities, headaches, nervousness, nausea, dizziness, dermatitis, acne, change in appetite, weight gain, breast tenderness, hirsutism, and hair loss |
| Condom | 12.0 | No major risks, low cost, nonprescription, male involvement, protects against STD, and cervical cancer | Allergy to materials (rare), loss of sensation, use with each act of coitus |
| Diaphragm with contraceptive cream or jelly | 18.0 | Protects against STDs, no major risks | Allergy (rare), toxic shock syndrome (rare), incidence of urinary tract infection, vaginal ulceration, requires motivation |
| Contraceptive sponge | 28.0 | Protects for multiple acts of coitus within 24 h, nonprescription, some STD protection | Cost, requires motivation, vaginal irritation, discharge, risk of toxic shock syndrome (rare) |
| Spermicide | 21.0 | Nonprescription, no major medical risks, some STD protection | Allergy (rare), use related to coitus |
| Intrauterine device | 3.0 | Minimal demands after insertion, secrecy | Pelvic inflammatory disease, ectopic pregnancy, infertility, dysmenorrhea, menorrhagia |
| Natural family planning | 20.0 | Natural, no risks, nonprescription | Not very effective with irregular menses, requires high motivation |
| Coitus interruptus | 18.0 | Useful when nothing else is available, no planning, no major medical risks | Less satisfying relationships |

* Percent of women who become pregnant during the first year using a specified contraceptive method.
† Lowest reported failure rate 1.1%
*From Hatcher RA, et al. Contraceptive technology 1990–1992, ed 15. New York: Irvington Publishers, 1990*

ovarian cysts are less common in pill users compared to nonpill users. Risk of ovarian and uterine cancer is significantly reduced in users. The relationship between oral contraception and cervical cancer is unclear.

Oral contraceptives do not provide protection against STDs or HIV infection. Thus, adolescents should be counseled to use oral contraceptives in conjunction with a barrier method, ideally condoms.

In general, oral contraceptives are extremely safe for teenagers. Physicians should be aware that mortality rates among women younger than age 20 years for using any method of contraception are significantly less than for carrying a pregnancy to term. Young, healthy women rarely have serious medical complications from oral contraceptive use.

Conditions that contraindicate prescribing oral contraceptives include thrombophlebitis, thromboembolic disease, cerebrovascular accident, and coronary artery disease. Because oral contraceptives alter hepatic metabolism and are associated with hepatomas (benign or malignant liver tumors), present impaired liver function or previous cholestasis during pregnancy contraindicate use of oral contraceptives. Known or suspected estrogen-dependent neoplasia and known or suspected carcinoma of the breast also are absolute contraindications. Individuals may have other medical problems that make oral contraceptive use more risky. Such conditions include severe headaches, particularly vascular or migraine headaches that begin after oral contraceptive use, hypertension, acute mononucleosis, elective major surgery, or immobilization planned in the next 4 weeks. Close follow-up is indicated if oral contraceptives are selected. Abnormal vaginal bleeding should be evaluated before initiating oral contraceptive use. Other conditions that make oral contraceptive use less than ideal include the following: diabetes mellitus, prediabetes or a strong family history of diabetes, sickle cell disease, active gallbladder disease, Gilbert's disease, or completion of a term pregnancy within the past 2 weeks. For any woman who wants oral contraceptives, counseling should encourage cessation of cigarette smoking because smoking increases the risk of pill-associated thromboembolic disorders.

Minor side effects include symptoms that, although not dangerous, may bother the patient and therefore result in her decision to discontinue use. A common complaint is gastrointestinal disturbance. Frequently, patients experience nausea and, occasionally, vomiting as their bodies adjust to an altered hormonal milieu. Taking the medication with meals, especially in the evening, alleviates this condition. The patient can be reassured that gastrointestinal problems generally resolve within the first few months of therapy.

Adolescents commonly experience either spotting or breakthrough bleeding in the first few months of oral contraceptive use. This problem often can be corrected by consistent time of intake. If irregular bleeding persists, selection of a pill with higher progestational activity usually corrects the condition. Expecting common problems and providing anticipatory guidance reassure patients and prevent unnecessary discontinuation of therapy.

Young women benefit from frequent medical follow-up after initiation of oral contraceptives. A suggested schedule includes a visit at 6 weeks and one every 3 months thereafter. At each visit, the physician should inquire about any of the following symptoms: chest pain, headaches, visual disturbances, leg or abdominal pains as possible indicators of thromboembolic disorders or hepatic neoplasm. It is helpful to review recent menstrual history and to inquire about minor side effects. The physical examination should include measurement of weight and blood pressure. Hypertension develops in a small percentage of individuals and necessitates cessation of therapy. Pelvic examination should be performed annually and more frequently if the patient has multiple or new sexual partners or if gynecologic symptoms supervene.

There are many preparations of combined oral contraceptives with varying compositions. All pills have 21 days worth of hormones followed by 7 days worth of an inert substance (or pill-free), during which time menses is expected. Fixed combination preparations contain a constant dose of estrogen and progestin for 21 days. Multiphasic pills have a slightly lower total dose of estrogen or progestin than fixed combination pills. Theoretically, any long-term complications of pill use would be less likely. Biphasic pills have two phases of hormonal treatment; triphasic pills have three phases of hormonal preparations. The ideal choice for an adolescent beginning therapy is a low dose combined oral contraceptive that has 35 $\mu$g or less of estrogen coupled with a low potency progestin. These pills offer excellent protection against pregnancy while minimizing significant side effects. Table 30-13 lists low dose oral contraceptives.

In contrast to the combined oral contraceptive, the mini-pill or progestin-only pill contains only synthetic progesterone. The mini-pill is less effective than the combined pill. It offers the advantage of inducing fewer metabolic alterations and thus is useful for women with diabetes mellitus, hypertension, or sickle cell disease for whom concerns about thromboembolic disorders are great. Menstrual irregularities occur in one third to one half of patients, however, and limit its usefulness in teenagers.

## Norplant Implants

Norplant is a long-acting, reversible method of contraception approved for use in the United States in 1991. It is implanted under the skin of the upper arm in a minor surgical procedure. Norplant is composed of six flexible Silastic capsules contain the progestin levonorgesterol.

Norplant is a long-lasting, highly effective contraceptive method that provides protection for up to 5 years. The failure rate in the first year of use is 0.04%. It is recommended that the capsules be removed after 5 years of use. The capsules may be removed earlier if the patient desires. Primary advantages of Norplant include its ease of use (once inserted, the patient does nothing more) and its high rate of effectiveness. Disadvantaged of Norplant are that a surgical procedure is required for insertion and removal and that many women experience bothersome menstrual irregularities. Contraindications to use include acute liver disease, unexplained vaginal bleeding, history of thrombophlebitis or thromboembolic disorder, coronary artery disease, or cerebrovascular accident. Other relative contraindications to Norplant use include diabetes mellitus, hyperlipidemia or hypercholesterolemia, hypertension, severe headaches, seizure disorder, depression, gallbladder, cardiac disorder, renal disorder, or breast disease suspicious for carcinoma. Common side effects

| TABLE 30-13. Low Dose Combined Oral Contraceptives | |
|---|---|
| Monophasic Preparations | Multiphasic Preparations |
| Loestrin 1/20 | Ortho-Novum 7/7/7 |
| Loestrin 1.5/30 | Tri-Norinyl |
| Ovcon 35 | Triphasil |
| Brevicon/Modicon | Ortho-Novum 10/11 |
| Ortho-Novum/Norinyl 1/35 | |
| Demulen 1/35 | |
| Lo/Ovral | |

include headache, nervousness, nausea, dizziness, dermatitis, acne, change in appetite, weight gain, breast tenderness, hirsutism, and hair loss.

Whether Norplant will be well accepted by young women is unclear. Because of its ease of use and low failure rate, some proponents tout Norplant as the answer to teenage pregnancy. Others are concerned that the high rate of menstrual irregularities will make it unacceptable for many teenagers. Studies are in progress to clarify the role of Norplant as a method of contraception for teenagers.

## Barrier Methods

The commonly recommended barrier devices include condoms, diaphragms, contraceptive sponges, and vaginal spermicide. Barrier methods, especially condoms, deserve increasing attention because of their role in preventing the spread of STDs including HIV infection.

### Condoms

The condom is the second most frequently used method of contraception during adolescence. Data from the 1988 Survey of Adolescent Males demonstrate that the rate of condom use has increased among 17- to 19-year-old males. Condoms have a failure rate in typical users of 12.0%. When used with spermicide, they are more effective. They are extraordinarily safe without any major medical risks. Condoms are easily available at low cost without prescription. Condoms provide a unique opportunity to involve male adolescents in contraceptive decision-making because they are the only available male-initiated, reversible method of birth control. In view of the current epidemic of STDs, particularly AIDS, all sexually active young people should receive instruction and encouragement for condom use even if they use another method of birth control. It is important to instruct adolescents to use latex condoms rather than animal skin condoms because only latex products have been shown to reduce the transmission of STDs. Additionally, condoms that have the spermicidal agent nonoxynol-9 provide additional protection against STDs. Patients may cite diminished sensation as a disadvantage to condom use. Occasionally, an allergy to the rubber or foam is encountered. Rarely, a condom tears with use. A great deal of motivation is required because the condom must be available and used consistently to be effective.

### Diaphragm

The diaphragm is chosen by only a small number of adolescents. It is a dome-shaped rubber cup that acts as a physical barrier to conception, while jelly or cream applied to it provides spermicidal properties. Like condoms, the diaphragm protects against STDs and has no major health risks. The clinician must perform a pelvic examination to fit a diaphragm. Additionally, the patient must feel comfortable with its insertion and removal. The individual must have her diaphragm available and insert it reliably before intercourse. The pregnancy rate among adult users is 18.0%. Allergies to materials and a few cases of toxic shock syndrome have occurred with diaphragm use. There is increased frequency of urinary tract infections.

### Contraceptive Sponge

The contraceptive sponge, unlike the diaphragm, is available without medical consultation. It is made of polyurethane imbedded with spermicide and is inserted into the vagina to cover the cervix. Failure rates are 18% in nulliparous women and 28% in parous women. The contraceptive sponge is expensive and, therefore, is most appropriate for individuals experiencing infre-

quent intercourse. The sponge provides protection for multiple episodes of coitus within a 24-hour period. Vaginal irritation, discharge, and an association with toxic shock syndrome are risks that accompany contraceptive sponge use.

## Vaginal Spermicide

Vaginal spermicide contains a spermicidal agent, either nonoxynol-9 or oxtoxinol-9, coupled with an inert substance, foam, cream, or suppository. Vaginal spermicide can be bought without prescription and must be inserted vaginally within 1 hour of intercourse. When used alone, vaginal spermicide has a failure rate of 21.0%. Therefore, it is recommended that spermicide be used with condoms. Nonoxynol-9 has antibacterial and antiviral properties that help protect against STDs.

## Intrauterine Device

The intrauterine device (IUD) is a plastic device inserted into the uterus. An IUD requires minimal patient motivation after insertion. Despite its low failure rate of 2.0%, it is no longer recommended for adolescents because of considerable risk of ascending pelvic infection, ectopic pregnancy, and infertility.

## Natural Family Planning

Natural family planning encompasses several techniques that require an awareness of the fertile period in the menstrual cycle and a willingness to practice abstinence during that time. Natural family planning methods include the calender method, Billings method (ie, recognition of symptoms of ovulation), and basal body temperature measurement. Pregnancy occurs in 20.0% of women. Natural family planning provides no STD protection. These methods require a regular menstrual cycle coupled with high motivation and body awareness. They are not generally recommended for teenagers.

## Coitus Interruptus

Coitus interruptus, or withdrawal prior to ejaculation, is used by many teenagers. It offers the advantage of easy availability without advance planning. Disadvantages include its poor use, effectiveness rates of 18%, potential interference with pleasurable relationships, and lack of STD protection.

## Noncoital Sex

Noncoital sex refers to sex without intercourse. Adolescents should know that if ejaculation occurs close to the vagina, pregnancy can ensue.

## Abstinence

Abstinence frequently is used without seeking medical advice. It offers the clear advantage of preventing pregnancy and STDs. Adolescents who practice abstinence should receive support and encouragement regarding their decision.

## EVALUATION FOR CONTRACEPTION

Before initiating contraception, it is important to obtain a careful history and physical examination to define medical and behavioral factors relevant to contraceptive choices. The physician must determine whether any condition exists that precludes use of a particular method. A complete gynecologic history should include age of menarche, recent menstrual pattern, and symptoms of dysmenorrhea. It is desirable for young women to experience regular menses for 1 to 2 years before initiating oral contraceptives. This allows for establishment of mature functioning of the hypothalamic-pituitary-ovarian axis. There is no evidence that long-term fertility is compromised by early oral contraceptive use. Thus, the desired establishment of regular menses is not absolute and may be waived if no other suitable method exists and the young woman is sexually active.

Any history of abortions or deliveries is important in defining a patient at risk for repeat pregnancy. Additionally, prior use of contraception and reason for discontinuation aids in future recommendations. Obtaining a sexual history is pertinent to the decision. A young woman or man who has not yet engaged in sexual intercourse but is feeling peer pressure might need reassurance regarding abstinence rather than contraception, whereas a young person who engages in infrequent intercourse may choose a barrier method. All individuals should be counseled regarding risks for STDs and desirability of condom use.

A complete physical examination is recommended. Particular attention is paid to blood pressure, cardiovascular system, thyroid, and breast. Skin should be inspected for xanthomas, chloasma, jaundice, or scleral icterus. Extent of pubertal development should be assessed because hormonal contraceptives are recommended only for those young women who are at Tanner sexual maturity rating stage IV or V. Abdominal examination checks for liver enlargement or tenderness. A pelvic examination should include a Papanicolaou smear as well as screening cultures for gonorrhea and chlamydia, if available. Syphilis serology should be obtained in the sexually active individual. When positive family history for hyperlipidemia or early cardiovascular disease is elicited, some clinicians recommend a serum lipid profile be obtained.

In summary, having identified an adolescent in need of contraceptive services, the medical assessment should include a comprehensive history, physical examination, and evaluation of the adolescent's level of maturity and needs. Ultimately, both the physician and the young patient must be satisfied with the selected method for safe and successful contraception.

## Selected Readings

Dickey RP. Managing contraceptive pill patients, ed 4. Durant, OK: Creative Informatics, 1985.
Edelman DA, McIntyre SL, Harper J. A comparative trial of the Today contraceptive sponge and diaphragm. Am J Obstet Gynecol 1984;150:869.
Forrest JD, Singh S. The sexual and reproductive behavior of American women, 1982–1988. Family Planning Perspectives 1990;22:206.
Greydanus DE, McAnarney ER. Contraception in the adolescent: current concepts for the pediatrician. Pediatrics 1980;65:1.
Hatcher RA, et al. Contraceptive technology 1986–1987, ed 13. New York: Irvington Publishers Inc, 1986.
National Center for Health Statistics: advance report of final natality statistics, 1984. Monthly Vital Statistics Report. Hyattsville, MD: United States Public Health Service 1990;39(4)(suppl).
Ory HW. Mortality associated with the control of fertility. Family Planning Prospectives 1983;15:57.
Ory HW, Forrest JD, Lincoln R. Making choices: evaluating the health risks and benefits of birth control methods. New York: Alan Guttmacher Institute, 1983.
Schirm A, Trussel J, Menken J, Grady W. Contraceptive failure in the United States: the impact of social, economic, and demographic factors. Family Planning Perspectives 1982;14:68.
Sonenstein FL, Pleck JH, Ku LC. Sexual activity, condom use and AIDS awareness among adolescent males. Family Planning Perspectives 1989;21:152.
Sonenstein FL, Pleck JH, Ku LC. Levels of sexual activity among adolescent males in the United States. Family Planning Perspectives 1991;23:162.
Stubblefield PG. Conception control: contraception, sterilization, and pregnancy termination. In: Kistner RW, ed. Gynecology: principle and practice, ed 4. Chicago: New York Medical Publishers Inc, 1986:583.
Tyrer LB. Oral contraception for the adolescent. J Reprod Med 1984;29(suppl):551.
Zabin L, Clark S. Institutional factors affecting teenagers choice and reasons for delay in attending a family planning clinic. Family Planning Perspectives 1983;15(1):25.

Principles and Practice of Pediatrics, Second Edition.
edited by Frank A. Oski et al. J. B. Lippincott Company, Philadelphia © 1994.

# 30.5 Sexually Transmitted Diseases

Hoover Adger

Sexually transmitted diseases (STDs) are generally defined as diseases that are transmitted primarily through sexual intercourse. The traditional list of STDs included syphilis and gonorrhea as the two major diseases of concern. Chancroid, lymphogranuloma venereum (LGV), and granuloma inguinale completed the list as the diseases of minor importance. Because of the increased attention given to clarifying disease processes in this area over the past two decades, substantially more is now known about sexually transmitted infections. The current expanded list of STDs also includes Chlamydia trachomatis infections, genital herpes, genital mycoplasmas, cytomegalovirus, hepatitis, bacterial vaginosis, human papillomavirus, and ectoparasitic diseases.

Adolescents are included in the population at risk for STD. The transmission of STDs among adolescents is now recognized as a major health problem. Sexual activity in the adolescent population has increased considerably over the past two decades. Current trends show adolescents in the United States begin sexual activity at an increasingly early age. Seventy percent of adolescent females and 80% of adolescent males are sexually activity before their 19th birthdays. With the increase in adolescent sexual activity, there is a concomitant increase in STDs.

When studies control for sexual experience, age-specific rates for many of the STDs are highest among sexually experienced adolescents. Prevalence rates for the two most common sexually transmitted organisms, C trachomatis and Neisseria gonorrhoeae, are highest in the young adult and adolescent age group, and the health habits and behaviors of these individuals puts them at an increased risk for adverse sequelae.

## GONOCOCCAL INFECTIONS

Gonorrhea is caused by the gram-negative diplococcus N gonorrhoeae. About 1 million cases are reported to the Centers for Disease Control each year. The true incidence of disease is estimated to be two to three times that which is actually reported. Of the total reported cases, approximately 25% occur in individuals between 15 and 19 years of age, and approximately two thirds of cases occur in those 15 to 24 years of age.

Trends for gonococcal infection from 1961 to 1975 showed a dramatic increase of incidence in the adolescent age group. There was an approximate fivefold increase for females 15 to 19 years of age and a threefold increase for males 15 to 19 years of age. Rates have stabilized since 1975; however, age-specific rates still show that adolescents and young adults have the highest risk of acquiring this infection. These rates mean that 1 in every 100 males and 1 in every 66 females aged 15 to 19 years acquire gonorrhea each year. Extrapolated to the estimated true incidence of disease, these figures translate into 1 in every 30 to 50 males and 1 in every 20 to 30 females acquiring a gonococcal infection each year.

The high number of acquired gonococcal infections occurs largely because of the high infectivity of the organism, the short incubation period of 2 to 5 days, and the lack of symptoms in many of those who are infected. The classic presentation of this infection in males is acute urethritis manifested by a purulent urethral discharge. As many as one third to one half of males infected by gonorrhea, however, may be asymptomatic. Likewise, it is estimated that as many as 80% of females with gonorrhea have few or no symptoms. This lack or scarcity of symptoms in those who are infected further complicates detection and treatment in the adolescent. When present, symptoms of genital gonorrhea in females may include abnormal vaginal discharge, dysuria, urinary frequency, and labial tenderness or swelling caused by infection of the Bartholin's gland. Abnormal vaginal bleeding, pelvic pain, and lower abdominal pain may indicate ascending infection and involvement of the upper genital tract.

## Clinical Presentation

The clinical spectrum of diseases associated with the *N gonorrhoeae* is broad. In males, gonorrhea is frequently a cause of urethritis. Complications due to direct extension to other sites is unusual in males; however, epididymitis, prostatitis, and seminal vesiculitis can occur. In females, in addition to localized infection of the cervix, urethra, and Bartholin's or Skene's glands, there is frequently an extension to the upper genital tract causing endometritis, salpingitis, parametritis, and perihepatitis (commonly known as FitzHugh-Curtis syndrome). Extragenital mucosal infections in males and females due to *N gonorrhoeae* are commonly manifested as proctitis and pharyngitis. Rare occurrences in both sexes include meningitis, endocarditis, arthritis, and dermatitis.

Anorectal infections due to gonorrhea are common in women and in men practicing anal intercourse. Even in the absence of rectal contact, it has been shown that 40% to 60% of women with cervical gonorrhea also have the organism isolated from the rectum. The majority of females with rectal gonorrhea are asymptomatic. Those males or females who have symptoms usually complain of perianal irritation, painful defecation, constipation, blood or mucus in the stool, or tenesmus. Frequently, other pathogens are associated with proctitis in males who engage in anal receptive intercourse including *C trachomatis*, herpesvirus, syphilis, *Campylobacter*, shigella, or other ectoparasites.

Disseminated gonorrhea, or the arthritis-dermatitis syndrome, occurs primarily in females and is present in less than 1% of all patients with gonorrhea. Dissemination occurs as a result of hematogenous extension of the gonococcus from the site of entry. It is seen frequently after menstruation. Patients may note the presence of myalgia, headache, malaise, fever, or anorexia initially, but the clinical manifestations noted most frequently are the characteristic hemorrhagic or necrotic appearing skin lesions, arthralgias, tenosynovitis, and monoarticular or oligoarticular arthritis. The joints most frequently affected include the knees, elbows, ankles, wrists, and small joints of the hands of feet.

Patients with disseminated gonococcal infection are frequently colonized with strains that cause asymptomatic mucosal infection. These strains have specific nutritional requirements, and they are usually exquisitely sensitive to penicillin. Often, it is difficult to recover the organism from nonmucosal sites such as blood, synovial fluid, or skin lesions. Blood cultures early in the course are positive in only 10% to 30% of cases. Gram stains of synovial fluid frequently contain an increased number of leukocytes but are positive for gram-negative diplococci in only 10% to 30% of cases, and fluid is culture positive in less than 30% of cases. Although the definitive diagnosis of disseminated gonococcal infection is made by recovery of the organism from the blood, synovial fluid, skin lesions, or cerebrospinal fluid in the case of meningitis, most often it is based on the typical clinical manifestations, the recovery of the organism from a mucosal site, and

the appropriate response to therapy. Hence, the cervix, urethra, pharynx, and rectum should be cultured before treatment.

## Diagnostic Tests

The in vitro isolation of *N gonorrhoeae* on selective media carried out in a 5% to 10% $CO_2$ environment is the gold standard by which all other methods are measured. There are several non-culture methods available for detecting *N gonorrhoeae*. Compared to culture, however, most are not low cost, timely, and accurate in both a high- and low-prevalence population. In addition, non-culture methods do not provide information on resistant strains, and some fail to differentiate among nonpathogenic strains. Culture-based detection can differentiate *N gonorrhoeae* from other species of *Neisseria* by specific growth characteristics, specific gram-negative morphology, oxidase-positive reaction, and its specific sugar fermentation pattern. Because of the increased demonstration of resistant strains, most culture isolates are routinely tested for antimicrobial susceptibility and $\beta$-lactamase production.

A Gram stain of a smear of urogenital secretions has been used to diagnose gonococcal infection of the male urethra and the female cervix for more than 70 years. In males with a urethral discharge, the Gram stain has a sensitivity and specificity almost equal to that of culture. Hence, in males with a urethral discharge, the demonstration of the typical gram-negative diplococci within polymorphonuclear leukocytes is sufficient for diagnosis. In males without a discharge, the Gram stain, although somewhat less sensitive, remains a specific test. A Gram stain of secretions from the cervix is less sensitive and not as reliable for diagnosing gonococcal infection in females. In experienced hands, however, it is a specific test and helps identify gonococcal or nongonococcal cervicitis.

## Treatment

The primary goal in treating gonococcal infections is to eliminate the infection as effectively, economically, and safely as possible. Important concerns are the treatment of coexisting chlamydial infection, which is documented in one third to one half of patients with gonorrhea, and the eradication of associated diseases such as incubating syphilis. To address these concerns, therapy is directed toward a single-dose regimen to treat gonorrhea followed by a 7-day course of treatment with doxycycline or tetracycline. The treatment regimen of choice for uncomplicated gonococcal infections is ceftriaxone 250 mg given intramuscularly. Alternatively, cefixime 400 mg given orally has be used with success. Most clinicians choose an oral regimen. Each of these regimens should be followed by doxycycline 100 mg b.i.d. or tetracycline hydrochloride 500 mg q.i.d. for 7 days.

For those patients in whom the use of tetracyclines is contraindicated, the appropriate single dose regimen may be followed by erythromycin base 500 mg q.i.d. for 7 days. Patients who are unable to take ceftriaxone can be treated with spectinomycin 2 g intramuscularly followed by doxycycline or erythromycin. Patients with incubating syphilis are likely to be cured by any of the regimens containing beta-lactams or tetracyclines.

Adolescents who have had recent exposure to gonorrhea should be cultured and treated as if they have infection. Follow-up test of cure cultures should include urethral and other appropriate specimens from men, and cervical, anal, and other appropriate cultures from women. These cultures should be obtained 7 to 14 days after completion of therapy. All teenagers with gonorrhea should have a serologic test for syphilis performed at the time of diagnosis. It is recommended that all patients with gonorrhea be offered confidential counseling and testing for HIV.

In cases with complicated gonococcal infections such as disseminated gonorrhea, the usual recommendation is for hospitalization and treatment with intramuscular or intravenous ceftriaxone or a substitute. Acceptable treatment regimens can be found in the frequently updated *Sexually Transmitted Disease Treatment Guidelines* published by the Centers for Disease Control.

## CHLAMYDIAL INFECTIONS

Chlamydiae are a group of obligatory intracellular microorganisms differentiated from other microbes by a unique developmental cycle. The chlamydiae have a restricted metabolic capability and multiply within the host cell by binary fission. They are similar to viruses in that they are obligate intracellular parasites, but they differ because they have both RNA and DNA, have a discrete cell wall, and are susceptible to antibiotics. *C trachomatis* includes the agents that cause trachoma, inclusion conjunctivitis, LGV, and genitourinary tract infections.

*C trachomatis* is the most commonly isolated sexually transmitted agent, causing an estimated 3 to 4 million sexually transmitted infections annually. It is most prevalent in the age group 15 to 19 years. *C trachomatis* infections are not reportable diseases; however, data from STD clinics suggest a sharp increase in incidence since 1975. *C trachomatis* has been isolated from 10% to 26% of adolescent females in teen clinics and is much more prevalent than gonococcal infection in most studies.

The most frequently noted risk factors for infection with *C trachomatis* include young age, history of multiple sexual partners, presence of other STDs, use of oral contraceptives, use of a non-barrier method or no method of contraception, and abnormal Papanicolaou smear. Young adolescents appear to be at particular risk for acquiring chlamydia. One explanation for this may be the presence of ectopy or ectopic columnar epithelium, which is often present on the exposed surface of the immature adolescent cervix and which is particularly susceptible to invasion by chlamydia.

### Clinical Presentation

The clinical presentation associated with chlamydial genital tract infections is similar to that of gonococcal infection. Infections commonly associated with *C trachomatis* include acute urethral syndrome, bartholinitis, cervicitis, salpingitis, nongonococcal urethritis, epididymitis, proctitis, conjunctivitis, and Reiter's syndrome.

Chlamydial infection in the female may be associated with mucopurulent cervicitis or urethritis, but frequently it is asymptomatic. Ascending infection may occur, leading to salpingitis and perihepatitis (FitzHugh-Curtis syndrome). Chlamydial salpingitis is frequently subclinical and is implicated as a significant cause of involuntary infertility.

Nongonococcal urethritis (NGU) is currently recognized as the most common form of urethritis in males. *C trachomatis* is the most common identifiable cause of NGU, being responsible for 30% to 60% of cases, depending on the population studied. In addition, *C trachomatis* is the most common cause of epididymitis and is a common cause of prostatitis in men younger than 35-years-old.

Infants born to women with cervical chlamydial infection are at significant risk for developing chlamydial infection. About 60% to 70% of infants exposed to chlamydiae during passage through an infected birth canal become infected. The approximate risk of developing conjunctivitis is 30% to 40%; pneumonia, 10% to 20%; and asymptomatic nasopharyngeal infection, 20%.

Because of the high prevalence and the potential for serious morbidity among infected individuals, all sexually active teenagers with genital tract symptoms should be evaluated for *C trachomatis* infection. Testing for chlamydia in sexually active females should be as routine as Papanicolaou smears and gonococcal cultures. Routine culture of adolescent males is impractical in most settings. Examination of a first voided urine specimen, however, may be a helpful adjunct in identifying the asymptomatic male with chlamydia urethritis.

### Diagnostic Tests

Several laboratory diagnostic methods are available to identify chlamydial infections including tissue culture isolation and serologic, cytologic, and immunodiagnostic techniques. Tissue culture techniques are the most sensitive and specific methods and are the preferred method of detection. Most hospital laboratories can isolate chlamydia by culture techniques, but in many clinical settings, culture capability is not feasible. Two rapid diagnostic nonculture methods—Microtrak, which depends on direct fluorescent staining of chlamydial elementary bodies, and Chlamydiazyme, an enzyme-linked immunosorbent assay (ELISA)—are helpful. The immunofluorescent antibody technique is quite sensitive for symptomatic patients but may be less sensitive in detecting infected asymptomatic patients. The ELISA appears to be relatively sensitive but may have more false positives associated with it. The technique used often depends on availability, cost, and laboratory experience of the laboratory. When possible, culture confirmation of positives is encouraged.

If detection methods for chlamydia are not available, presumptive treatment for this organism should be considered when genital symptoms suggest the possibility of infection. Anyone treated for gonorrhea should receive treatment for chlamydia as well.

### Treatment

Treatment regimens for chlamydial disease include doxycycline (100 mg b.i.d. for at least 7 days), tetracycline (500 mg q.i.d. for at least 7 days), or erythromycin (500 mg q.i.d. for at least 7 days or 250 mg q.i.d. for 14 days), as an alternative. Treatment of genital infections in individuals 8 years of age or younger is erythromycin 50 mg/kg/d for 7 to 10 days. The recommended therapy for chlamydial conjunctivitis or pneumonia is oral erythromycin 50 mg/kg/d for 2 to 3 weeks.

## SYPHILIS

Syphilis is caused by the spirochete *Treponema pallidum*. *T pallidum* is a pathogen only in humans and is transmitted from infected individuals through intimate contact. In 1991, there were more than 29,000 cases of primary and secondary syphilis reported in the United States.

### Clinical Presentation

The initial lesion of primary syphilis, the chancre, usually develops 14 to 21 days after the initial infection. The incubation period, however, varies from 10 to 90 days. The primary lesion usually appears as a small, solitary, round or elongated, indurated ulcer with a clean base. The chancre does not usually cause pain and, if located in an inconspicuous site, may go unnoticed. The lesions vary in size from 3 to 4 mm or 1 to 2 cm. Regional lymphadenopathy usually accompanies the chancre. The chancre usually remains stable in appearance for several weeks and, if untreated, slowly resolves.

Secondary syphilis is heralded by the presence of a generalized macular or maculopapular eruption which at times can also be nodulopapular in appearance and is usually not associated with pruritus. The rash of secondary syphilis is usually concentrated on the trunk, but the characteristic lesions frequently can be found on the face, palms, and soles. The rash may be accompanied by fever or malaise. Other clinical signs of secondary syphilis include the presence of flat moist papules in the anal or genital region referred to as condyloma lata, small patches of alopecia in the scalp, and loss of the lateral eyebrows.

When the symptoms and signs of secondary syphilis disappear, the disease is referred to as latent syphilis. Patients with latent syphilis have no signs or symptoms but may still be infectious, if untreated, for a period of several years. Approximately one third of those with latent syphilis progress to late syphilis if untreated; this condition may occur within 2 to 30 years after the original infection. The clinical manifestations are highly variable and take the form of benign late syphilis in about 50%, cardiovascular syphilis in about 30%, and neurosyphilis in about 20%.

## Diagnosis

The best method for verifying the diagnosis of primary syphilis is darkfield microscopic examination of a sample of material from the chancre. If positive, this is the only test required to establish the diagnosis of primary syphilis. When darkfield examination is not available, the diagnosis usually is based on the standard serologic tests, the VDRL (Venereal Disease Research Laboratory) and RPR (rapid protein reagin), which are used for screening. Because these two nontreponemal tests are nonspecific, a positive result should be confirmed by the highly specific fluorescent treponemal antibody (FTA) test. Approximately 90% of patients with primary syphilis have a positive FTA, while only 80% have a positive VDRL or RPR. The difficulty of using the FTA in the diagnosis of early syphilis is that, once positive, this test often remains positive over the life of the individual. Thus, it does not rule out a positive test as a result of prior infection. In contrast, although it may be negative in individuals early in the course of the disease, the VDRL test often has a titer that correlates well with activity of the disease and, therefore, can be used as a baseline for follow-up.

The diagnosis of secondary syphilis is easier, because the RPR or VDRL is positive in 99% of cases. False-positive results do occur, but they are found in only 2% of tests confirmed by FTA.

## Treatment

The choice of treatment for primary, secondary, or latent syphilis of less than 1 year's duration is benzathine penicillin G, 2.4 million units intramuscularly at one visit. Patients who are allergic to penicillin should be treated with tetracycline 500 mg q.i.d for 15 days. All patients should be encouraged to return for repeat VDRL tests at 3, 6, and 12 months after treatment. All patients with syphilis should be counseled concerning the risks of HIV and be encouraged to be tested for HIV antibody.

The optimal treatment regimen for syphilis of more than 1 year's duration is less well established. Except for neurosyphilis, the suggested treatment is benzathine penicillin G, 2.4 million units intramuscularly each week for 3 successive weeks or, for those allergic to penicillin, tetracycline 500 mg q.i.d. for 30 days.

## HERPES SIMPLEX VIRUS INFECTIONS

Infections due to herpes simplex virus (HSV) are increasingly common in the United States. The spectrum of clinical manifestations associated with this organism includes primary and re-

current genital herpes, pharyngitis, urethritis, cervicitis, proctitis, neonatal HSV infections, and possible association with cervical carcinoma.

Primary genital herpes may be caused by either type 1 (HSV-1) or type 2 (HSV-2) herpes simplex virus. In the United States, 70% to 90% of primary genital infections are caused by the HSV-2, although the two are clinically indistinguishable. Primary HSV infections may or may not produce clinically apparent symptoms. In general, first episodes of genital herpes are more likely than recurrent episodes to be associated with systemic signs and symptoms, more severe and prolonged symptoms, and increased and prolonged viral shedding. It is not uncommon for patients to experience central nervous system involvement during a primary HSV infection. Aseptic meningitis, autonomic dysfunction resulting in hyperesthesia or anesthesia, transverse myelitis, and encephalitis are frequently documented. Dissemination with viremia and widespread involvement can occur but is rare.

The clinical diagnosis of genital herpes is usually made by recognition of the characteristic lesions of grouped vesicles on an erythematous base. Both primary and recurrent HSV infections are accompanied by tender lymphadenopathy. The inguinal nodes, upon palpation, are usually mildly tender, nonfixed, and only slightly firm.

Several methods are available to document the organism including isolation by tissue culture, detection of viral antigen by direct fluorescent assay or ELISA, cytologic examination of clinical specimens, or serology. Diagnosis should be confirmed by culture if an alternative initial method of detection is used.

Symptomatic treatment for mild genital herpes usually includes good genital hygiene, topical anesthetics, cool compresses, and analgesia. Oral acyclovir is the preferred treatment in most episodes of symptomatic HSV disease. Topical therapy is substantially less effective than oral therapy. Systemic acyclovir provides partial control of the symptoms and signs of HSV infections; it accelerates healing but does not eradicate nor affect the subsequent risk, frequency, or severity of recurrences. Systemic therapy prevents new lesion formation, and because of the high incidence of urethral, cervical, and oral infections, oral acyclovir is preferred in first-episode infections. All patients with first-episode genital HSV who present with active lesions should be treated. The recommended dosage is 200 mg five times per day. Although intravenous acyclovir may be more effective, it is usually reserved for those with severe symptoms or complications that necessitate hospitalization.

## HUMAN PAPILLOMAVIRUS INFECTION

Genital warts are an STD caused by human papillomavirus (HPV). Genital wart virus infections appear to be increasing in prevalence and are rapidly becoming one of the most common STDs diagnosed. More than 50 HPV types have been characterized. Acute infections may be asymptomatic or produce exophytic or flat condylomas; chronic persistent infections may result in intraepithelial neoplasia or squamous cell carcinoma. HPV types 6 and 11 are the viral types most commonly associated with exophytic warts.

Genital warts are transmitted through intimate contact including sexual intercourse. It is unclear whether transmission rates differ for HPV types, and indirect transmission through fomites has never been demonstrated convincingly.

The association of HPV and genital malignancy is an area of study. HPV types 16 and 18 are the most frequent types found in malignancies, and types 10, 11, 33, and 35 are found in a small percentage of cases. HPV types 16 and 18, however, cause only a small percentage of genital warts; the most common cause of warts, type 6, is rarely found in genital malignancies. Hence, despite the strong association of HPV and genital malignancy, the precise role of HPV remains uncertain. Several methods for diagnosing HPV infection range from simple visual inspection to colposcopy, cytology, histology, antigen detection, and molecular DNA hybridization.

The standard treatment of genital warts traditionally is based on the ablation of grossly visible warty tissue. Recognition of subclinical disease and the association of cervical neoplasia, however, have caused this simple approach to be questioned. Methods used for ablation of tissue include the use of cytotoxic agents, laser vaporization, and cryotherapy.

Podophyllin is a cytotoxic agent that is applied to warts as a 20% solution in ethanol or tincture of benzoin and allowed to dry. It is washed off after 3 to 4 hours. Treatment is repeated once or twice a week. Treatment failures are common. Additionally, there are several reports of severe systemic side effects after generous application to large lesions including blood dyscrasias, hepatotoxicity, and neuropathy. Podophyllin may have oncogenic and teratogenic potential and should not be used during pregnancy. 5-Fluorouracil is a cytotoxic agent that has been used for the treatment of genital warts. Its effects are variable but it has been used successfully in treating intraurethral lesions. Another cytotoxic agent, trichloracetic acid, can be applied undiluted and washed off after 4 hours. It is sometimes effective against small lesions but has no advantage over other treatment modalities.

Routine screening with frequent Papanicolaou smears and close follow-up are important for those diagnosed with this infection. Examination and treatment of sexual partners is an important preventive strategy.

## SPECIFIC STD SYNDROMES

### Genital Ulcers

An ulcerated lesion on the genitals at any age should lead to a vigorous examination for STDs. Although it is often difficult to differentiate on visual inspection alone, several features help to distinguish those lesions which present as genital ulcers. The most common infections encountered in these circumstances include genital herpes, syphilis, chancroid, LGV, and granuloma inguinale or donovanosis (Table 30-14).

HSV is the most common cause of genital ulcers in the United States. The characteristic appearance is that of grouped vesicles that rupture to produce a painful, superficial ulcer on an erythematous base. The lesions are usually associated with tender inguinal adenopathy. If the vesicles have ruptured, the diagnosis of HSV may be suggested by a positive Tzanck smear prepared by scraping the base of the ulcer and staining the slide with Papanicolaou, Giemsa, or Wright stain. The diagnosis can easily be confirmed by viral culture.

The second most common cause of genital ulcers is syphilis. These ulcers are also superficial and sharply demarcated. The lesions are round or oval and are rarely painful. Painless inguinal adenopathy often is associated with the lesion unless there is secondary infection, in which case nodes are tender. The diagnosis may be established by darkfield microscopy of material collected from the suspected lesions. Material must be examined promptly.

Chancroid is the most common cause of genital ulcers in many developing countries. It occurs much less frequently in the United States where it is the third most common cause of genital ulcers. The etiologic agent of chancroid is *Haemophilus ducreyi*. The primary lesion in chancroid is multiple erythematous papules or pustules, which progress to a deep, commonly painful ulcer that may produce a purulent or hemorrhagic discharge. It is frequently accompanied by painful and often suppurative inguinal adenopathy. The definitive diagnosis requires isolation and identification of *H ducreyi*, which is a fastidious organism. Erythromycin or ceftriaxone offer effective treatment for most cases.

Although common in developing countries, LGV and granuloma inguinale (donovanosis) are uncommon in the United States as a cause of genital ulcers. LGV is caused by specific immunotypes of *C trachomatis*. In contrast to other ulcerating genital lesions, it is characterized best by only transient ulceration and the presence of marked regional adenopathy. Granuloma inguinale is caused by the gram-negative bacillus *Calymmatobacterium granulomatis* and is usually marked by the absence of adenopathy and occurrence of granulating ulcers. In both cases, tetracycline is the treatment of choice.

As a general approach, all patients with genital ulcers should have a serologic test for syphilis, even if an alternative diagnosis is established. The presence of grouped vesicles strongly suggests a diagnosis of HSV and should initiate the appropriate viral culture and treatment for such. If no vesicles are present, material from the ulcer should be examined by darkfield microscopy for spirochetes and, if positive, the patient should be treated for primary syphilis. The next diagnostic step is culture for *H ducreyi* and initiation of treatment for chancroid. If the ulcer persists, a repeat serologic test for syphilis and culture for HSV should be performed. Finally, consideration should be given to biopsy to establish the diagnosis of donovanosis or to rule out other causes.

**TABLE 30-14.   Clinical Features of Genital Ulcers**

| Infection | Appearance | Inguinal Adenopathy | Presumptive Diagnosis | Definitive Diagnosis |
|---|---|---|---|---|
| Genital herpes | Grouped vesicles, painful, shallow ulcers | Tender | Tzanck smear | Viral culture |
| Primary syphilis | Indurated, well defined, usually single ulcer | Nontender | Darkfield microscopy | Darkfield microscopy RPR/FTA |
| Chancroid | Multiple, ragged, painful, nonindurated ulcer | Painful, suppurative | Bipolar staining of gram-negative coccobacilli | Culture of *H ducreyi* |
| Lymphogranuloma venereum | Transient, small ulcers, often multiple | Most prominent feature | Complement fixation, Frie Test, serology | Culture of LGV-specific chlamydia |
| Granuloma inguinali (donovanosis) | Granulomatous ulceration with sharply defined border | Not present | Giemsa or Wright stain demonstrating Donovan's bodies | Biopsy of lesion |

## Vaginitis/Cervicitis

Lower genital tract infections in females, which can involve the urinary tract, cervix, vulva, and vagina, produce a variety of overlapping symptoms including pruritus, dyspareunia, dysuria, and alteration of vaginal discharge. Based on symptoms only, it is difficult to distinguish among the various lower genital tract infections. Physical examination and appropriate use of simple laboratory tests often can help clarify the presumptive diagnosis of vaginitis, cervicitis, or urethritis.

Normal vaginal secretions consist of a mixture of secretions from the vaginal wall, cervical mucus, exfoliated vaginal epithelial cells, and secretions from the sebaceous, sweat, Bartholin's, and Skene's glands. With the onset of menarche and under the influence of estrogen, the vaginal epithelium becomes thicker, and increased amounts of lactic acid are produced from the glycogen-rich cells, which causes the pH to fall. The low pH, which is normally less than 4.5, fosters the growth of *Lactobacillus* species, which are the most prevalent organisms in the normal vaginal flora.

Estrogen causes changes in the cervix as well. Typically, visual inspection of the adolescent cervix reveals the presence of an ectropion or ectopy (columnar epithelium on the outer surface of the cervix) with a well-demarcated squamocolumnar junction. Many adolescents have ectopy, which gradually is replaced by squamous epithelium through the process of squamous metaplasia as the cervix matures.

The three most common types of vaginitis are bacterial vaginosis (formerly called nonspecific or Gardnerella vaginalis vaginitis), *Trichomonas vaginalis* vaginitis, and Candida vaginitis. The adolescent complaining of a vaginal discharge often has a specific etiology for her symptoms (Fig 30-8). Careful evaluation should include measurement of vaginal fluid pH, examination of vaginal fluid saline and potassium hydroxide preparations, endocervical culture or antigen detection tests for *C trachomatis* and *N gonorrhoeae*, a Gram stained smear of endocervical secretions, and a Papanicolaou smear.

The characteristic findings of Candida vaginitis include vaginal and vulvar erythema, vulvar edema, pruritus, and the presence of a thick cottage cheese-like discharge. The diagnosis can be confirmed by the microscopic finding of yeast forms on a potassium hydroxide preparation or by culture. Predisposing factors include diabetes, recent use of antibiotics, immunosuppressive therapy, obesity, or use of oral contraceptives. Treatment with topical vaginal clotrimazole or miconazole usually results in relief of symptoms.

*Trichomonas vaginalis* vaginitis is characterized by a malodorous vaginal discharge that is homogenous and classically described as yellow-green and frothy and has a vaginal fluid pH greater than 4.5. The vagina and cervix may be erythematous, and occasionally punctate hemorrhages or strawberry spots are seen on the cervix. On examination of the saline wet preparation, flagellated organisms and polymorphonuclear leukocytes are seen. The only effective treatment for *Trichomonas vaginalis* vaginitis is metronidazole. A single 2-g dose appears to be as effective as the 7-day treatment regimen and is the preferred regimen for most adolescents.

Bacterial vaginosis is the most common cause of an abnormal vaginal discharge. Several anaerobic bacteria in addition to *Gardnerella vaginalis* are thought to be involved in this complex syndrome. This complex alteration of the vaginal flora appears to be closely linked to sexual activity, but no specific etiologic organism has been defined. The diagnosis is based on the finding of a gray homogenous discharge, a vaginal fluid pH greater than 4.5, a positive whiff test (fishy odor when KOH is added to vaginal fluid), and clue cells on the examination of a wet preparation of

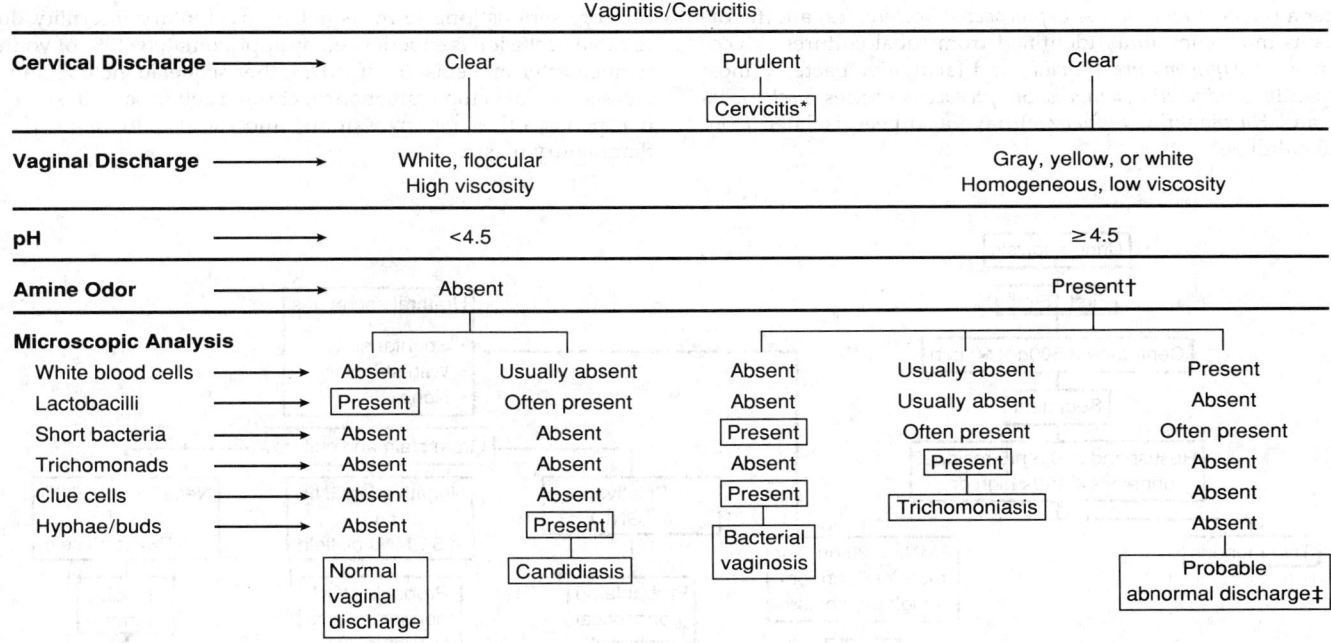

* Diagnosis supported by gram stain of endocervical secretion; confirm with culture and treat for *Chlamydia trachomatis* and *Neisseria gonorrhoeae*.

† An amine or "fishy" odor after addition of 10% KOH (the "whiff test") is a common feature of bacterial vaginosis

‡ Consider mixed infection

**Figure 30-8.** Vaginitis/cervicitis.

vaginal secretions. Metronidazole 500 mg b.i.d. for 7 days is the treatment of choice. Alternative treatment with ampicillin is less effective, and topical agents are no more effective than placebo.

Sexually active patients who present with dysuria or other urinary tract symptoms may have urethritis, cervicitis, cystitis, or vaginitis. Evaluation should include microscopic examination of a clean voided urine specimen. Women without evidence of vaginitis or cervicitis but with pyuria and bacteriuria usually have a bacterial urinary tract infection. Pyuria in the absence of bacteriuria may indicate urethral infection with *C trachomatis* or *N gonorrhoeae*.

Cervicitis is most frequently associated with infection due to *C trachomatis*, *N gonorrhoeae*, or HSV. The presence of a mucopurulent endocervical discharge and the presence of 30 or more polymorphonuclear leukocytes on a Gram stained smear of endocervical secretions correlate highly with infection caused by these three organisms. In addition, the observation of green or yellow mucopus on a white swab (positive swab test) helps to identify this disorder. Cultures should be performed for *C trachomatis* and *N gonorrhoeae*, and treatment should include a regimen that is active against both organisms.

## Pelvic Inflammatory Disease

Pelvic inflammatory disease (PID) is the syndrome resulting from the ascending spread of microorganisms from the vagina and cervix to the endometrium, fallopian tubes, and the contiguous upper genital tract structures. About 1 million women are treated each year for PID. It is a disease of young women, primarily, with adolescents 15 to 19 years of age constituting the group at highest risk when rates are adjusted for age. Although rates for women in other age groups show declines, rates for adolescents appear to be increasing.

Although the microbiologic etiology of PID is polymicrobial in nature, *C trachomatis*, *N gonorrhoeae*, and a variety of anaerobic bacteria (*Peptostreptococcus*, *Peptococcus*, *Bacteroides*) are the organisms most commonly identified from tubal cultures. Mycoplasmas, *Ureaplasma urealyticum*, and facultative bacteria (most frequently *Gardnerella vaginalis*, *Streptococcus* species, *Escherichia coli*, and *Haemophilus influenzae*) have also been isolated from tubal cultures.

PID frequently poses a difficult diagnostic problem and may be confused with appendicitis, pyelonephritis, and a host of gynecologic problems such as ruptured ovarian cyst, ectopic pregnancy, and septic abortion. The diagnosis is particularly difficult in adolescents with milder PID in whom chlamydia is more likely to be the causative agent. The suggested criteria for the diagnosis of PID include the presence of all three of the following: history of abdominal pain and presence of direct lower abdominal tenderness with or without rebound, cervical motion tenderness, and adnexal tenderness.

In addition, one or more supporting symptoms must be present. These include temperature of at least 38°C, leukocytosis (10,500 white blood cells per cubic millimeter), culdocentesis that yields peritoneal fluid containing white blood cells and bacteria, presence of an inflammatory mass noted on pelvic examination or sonography, elevated erythrocyte sedimentation rate, Gram stain of an endocervical smear revealing gram-negative intracellular diplococci suggestive of *N gonorrhoeae*, or a monoclonal directed smear from endocervical secretions revealing *C trachomatis*.

The goals of treatment are the prevention of infertility and the chronic residual of infection. To be effective, treatment should be instituted early and should cover the polymicrobial spectrum of the disease. Often the most difficult therapeutic decision for the physician is whether to hospitalize the adolescent with PID or to treat her as an outpatient. Current recommendations favor aggressive inpatient treatment of this disease in the hope of preserving fertility and minimizing complications caused by noncompliance or inaccuracy of diagnosis. Although several treatment regimens are suggested, intravenous cefoxitin and doxycycline is favored because of its excellent coverage for *N gonorrhoeae*, *C trachomatis*, and the anaerobic organisms.

If patients are treated as outpatients, it is important to ensure that there is adequate follow-up within 48 hours to evaluate the clinical course. Partner treatment should always be a part of the therapeutic approach.

At least one fourth of women with acute PID experience one or more serious long-term sequelae. Involuntary infertility due to tubal occlusion is experienced by approximately 20% of young women after one episode of PID. Other sequelae include an increased risk of ectopic pregnancy, chronic pelvic pain, dyspareunia, pelvic adhesions, pyosalpinx, and the development of inflammatory masses.

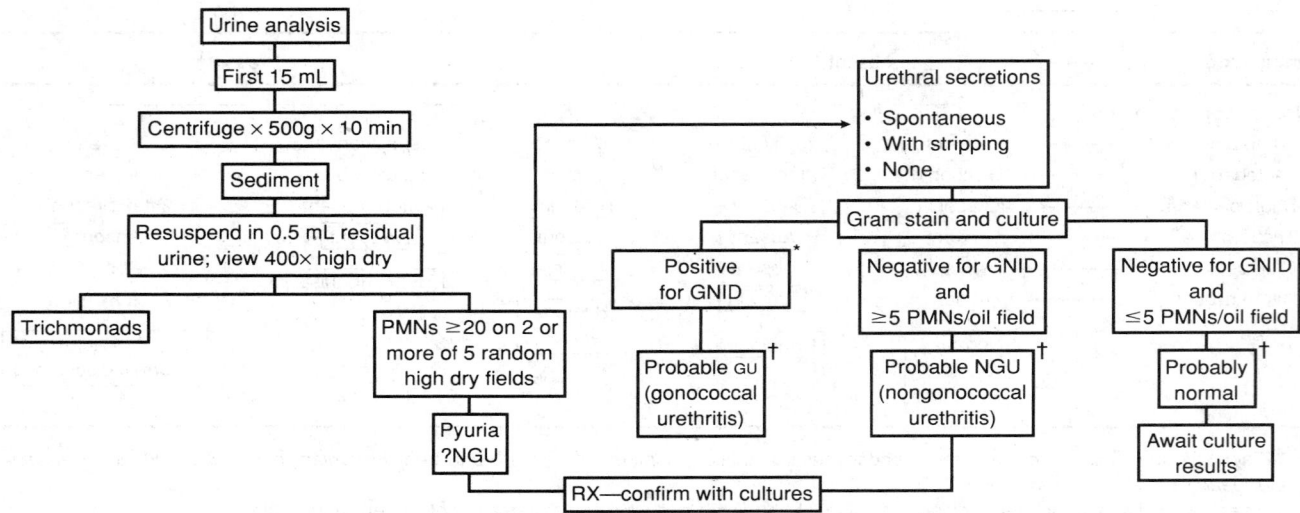

\* Gram-negative intracellular diplococci
† Confirm Rx with culture results

**Figure 30-9.** Diagnostic patterns to determine presence of urethritis in males.

The prevention of the sequelae through prompt and accurate diagnosis coupled with effective treatment should be a primary goal in the approach to adolescents with this disease.

## Urethritis

Urethritis is the response of the urethra to inflammation of any etiology. Urethritis is almost always sexually acquired and is classified as gonococcal or NGU depending on the presence or absence of *N gonorrhoeae*. Symptoms of urethritis may include urethral discharge, urinary frequency, burning on urination, and itching at the distal urethra or meatus; urethritis may also be present with no symptoms.

The incidence of urethritis is uncertain because it is not a reportable disease. It is generally appreciated that the incidence of NGU has increased despite the observed decrease in gonococcal urethritis.

*C trachomatis* is the most common cause of NGU. In addition, *U urealyticum* appears to be a common causative agent. Approximately 20% to 30% of patients with NGU have neither *C trachomatis* or *U urealyticum* identified. In this group, the etiologic agent may include other bacteria including genital mycoplasmas, *Haemophilus, Bacteroides*, or other anaerobes; herpes simplex virus; yeasts; or parasites such as *T vaginalis*.

Most males with symptoms of dysuria or urethral discharge, especially if the exudate is purulent, spontaneous, or easily expressed and either mucoid or yellow-green in color, have urethritis (Fig 30-9). On clinical grounds, however, it is impossible to distinguish gonococcal urethritis from NGU. Moreover, a clear discharge or a small amount of mucoid discharge does not always indicate urethritis. Procedures that provide information to support the diagnosis include the microscopic examination of a Gram stained smear of urethral secretions and the quantification of leukocytes in the centrifuged sediment from the first 10 to 15 mL of a first-voided urine specimen.

In most STD centers, the Gram stain is the procedure of choice. The presence of five or more leukocytes on a Gram stained smear is indicative of urethritis. The findings of gram-negative intracellular diplococci is a sensitive indicator of gonococcal urethritis and correlates well with culture positivity.

The presence of pyuria (20 or more polymorphonuclear leukocytes (PMN) in 2 or more of 5 random fields) in the sediment of a first-catch urine specimen is a valuable aid in the diagnosis of urethritis. This noninvasive test helps identify adolescents with asymptomatic urethral infection and, therefore, may be useful in screening patients with minimal or no symptoms. All individuals with urethritis should have appropriate cultures performed for *C trachomatis* and *N gonorrhoeae* and should be treated with an antibiotic regimen to cover both organisms.

## Selected Readings

Adger H, Shafer MA, Sweet RL, Schachter J. Screening for Chlamydia trachomatis and *Neisseria gonorrhoeae* in adolescent males: value of first-catch urine examination. Lancet 1984∞:994.
Bell TA. Major sexually transmitted disease in children and adolescents. Pediatr Infect Dis J 1983;2:153.
Centers for Disease Control. Chlamydia trachomatis infections—policy guidelines for prevention and control. MMWR 1985;34:35.
Centers for Disease Control. Sexually transmitted diseases treatment guidelines, 1989. MMWR 1989;38:S-8.
Emans SJ. Vulvovaginitis in the child and adolescent. Pediatr Rev 1986;8:12.
Eschenbach DH. Lower genital tract infections. In: Galask RP, Larsen B, eds. Infectious diseases in the female patient (clinical perspectives in obstetrics and gynecology). New York: Springer-Verlag, 1986.
Frau LM, Alexander ER. Public health implications of sexually transmitted diseases in pediatric practice. Pediatr Infect Dis J 1985;4:453.
Gilchrist MJR, Rauh JL. Office microscopic examination for sexually transmitted diseases. Journal of Adolescent Health Care 1985;6:311.
Holmes KK, Mardh PA, Sparling PF, et al. Sexually transmitted diseases. New York: McGraw-Hill, 1990.
Washington AE, Sweet RL, Shafer MA. Pelvic inflammatory disease and its sequelae in adolescents. Journal of Adolescent Health Care 1985;6:298.

*Principles and Practice of Pediatrics, Second Edition.*
edited by Frank A. Oski et al. J. B. Lippincott Company, Philadelphia © 1994.

# 30.6 *Hypertension*

### Michele Diane Wilson

Detection of hypertension during adolescence has important implications for optimal health in later life. Identification of the young person with persistent blood pressure elevations is important for two reasons. First, those studies in which blood pressure measurements are repeated serially suggest a relationship, albeit not always direct, between blood pressure in childhood and subsequent adult blood pressure. This phenomenon, known as blood pressure tracking, indicates that a young person who has a blood pressure reading that is above the 95th percentile for age is at increased risk for hypertension as an adult as compared to his normotensive peers. If hypertension is recognized and treated during childhood or adolescence, perhaps the long-term cardiovascular complications of hypertension, including stroke, heart disease, and premature death, can be prevented. Second, hypertension may be the presenting manifestation of serious disease. Recognition of elevated blood pressure may lead to a search for and identification of the causative process.

By contrast, an unwarranted diagnosis of hypertension has serious negative consequences. Giving an individual the diagnosis of hypertension commits him or her to frequent medical visits, an extensive evaluation, and the cost and potential side effects of medications.

## BLOOD PRESSURE MEASUREMENT

It is recommended that health care providers measure blood pressure in adolescent patients as part of routine health maintenance at least once a year. The technique for obtaining blood pressure readings is standardized to allow for meaningful interpretation of the values. Differences in patient position, arm selected, and cuff size may influence results. The patient should be calm because anxiety artificially increases blood pressure. The accepted technique is described as follows: the individual is seated and the blood pressure cuff is placed on the right upper arm. The arm rests on a table so that it remains at the level of the patient's heart. Either a mercury cuff or an aneroid cuff is used. An aneroid cuff is portable but needs frequent calibration to maintain accuracy. Cuff size must be carefully selected so that the internal bladder is long enough to completely encircle the arm and is wide enough to cover a minimum of three fourths of the length of the upper arm. After palpating the arterial pulse in the antecubital fossa, the stethoscope is lightly applied at that point. The cuff is then inflated to a pressure 20 mm Hg above the level at which the pulse is audible. Then, the cuff is deflated at a rate of 2 to 4 mm of mercury per second while the clinician listens for the first heart sound. This first heart sound or first Korotkoff sound is recorded as the systolic blood pressure. As the pressure continues to drop, the heart sounds become muffled. This point is called the fourth Korotkoff sound. Finally, the disappearance of all heart sounds is the fifth Korotkoff sound. If the fourth and fifth sounds are both heard, they should be recorded. In adolescents, the fourth Korotkoff sound is frequently not audible. Thus, the standards for diastolic blood pressures in this age group are based on the fifth Korotkoff sound.

# BLOOD PRESSURE STANDARDS

A clear definition of what constitutes hypertension is a key prelude to any discussion of hypertension. The standards for normal and abnormal blood pressures in the adolescent age group have long been debated. The Task Force for Blood Pressure Control in Children used results from nine large studies to establish the present standards for normal, high normal, and elevated blood pressures. These norms are defined for both age and sex. Normal blood pressure is defined as blood pressure that is less than the 90th percentile. High normal blood pressure is defined as a blood pressure between the 90th and 95th percentile. Hypertension implies that either the systolic or diastolic blood pressure is greater than or equal to the 95th percentile. Furthermore, weight and height are important determinants of blood pressure. Thus, the 90th percentile for height and weight should be taken into consideration in the individual with a blood pressure in the high normal range. Specifically, an individual who is either obese or unusually tall for age may have a blood pressure elevation. A patient without symptoms or any evidence of end-organ damage should not be labeled as hypertensive based on one abnormal blood pressure value. Only when the average of readings obtained on three different occasions is abnormal is the diagnosis of hypertension appropriate. Although 5% to 13% of adolescents are hypertensive on an initial blood pressure measure, only 1% remain persistently hypertensive on repeat evaluation.

# ESSENTIAL HYPERTENSION

Essential or primary hypertension indicates that significant hypertension exists for which an underlying etiology cannot be found. About 90% of adolescent hypertension fits in this category. Because essential hypertension appears to have a genetic component, a family history of hypertension or a history of cardiovascular disease makes the diagnosis more likely.

# SECONDARY HYPERTENSION

Secondary hypertension indicates that the blood pressure elevation has an identifiable cause. The more severe the degree of hypertension in an adolescent, the more likely it is that an etiology will be found. Oral contraceptives are frequently implicated in hypertension. If significant and persistent elevation occurs, treatment involves discontinuation of birth control pills. The common etiologies of hypertension are shown in Table 30-15.

# EVALUATION OF THE ADOLESCENT WITH HYPERTENSION

When it is determined that a young person is hypertensive, a complete medical evaluation is indicated. History may elucidate any complaints resulting from the blood pressure elevation, although symptoms are rare unless the blood pressure elevations are severe (ie, diastolic readings above 110). Symptoms may include occipital headaches, visual disturbance, chest pain, seizures, or epistaxis. History of kidney problems or trauma direct the investigation in the direction of renal disease. Symptoms of pheochromocytoma or hyperthyroidism should be sought. A careful drug history is important. Additionally, one should inquire about family history of hypertension, coronary artery disease, cerebrovascular infarct, renal failure, or virilization.

Physical examination should include a careful search for evidence of end-organ damage from longstanding or severe blood pressure elevation. Funduscopic examination may reveal hypertensive retinopathy (ie, arterial-venous nicking, hemorrhages, and exudates). Evidence of cardiac enlargement corroborates malignant disease. Elements of the physical examination may provide clues to the etiology of hypertension. Vital signs, growth parameters, body habitus, thyroid, cardiovascular system, and abdominal examination are important in the evaluation.

# LABORATORY EVALUATION

The extent of laboratory evaluation is determined by history and physical examination as well as by severity of hypertension. If essential hypertension is suspected based on positive family history coupled with an otherwise unremarkable history and physical examination, then laboratory assessment should not be extensive. A urinalysis is indicated to evaluate for signs of nephrosis, ne-

**TABLE 30-15. Differential Diagnosis of Hypertension in Adolescence**

Essential Hypertension
Renal Parenchymal Disorders
  Acute glomerulonephritis
  Chronic glomerulonephritis
  Hemolytic uremic syndrome
  Henoch-Schönlein purpura
  Systemic lupus erythematosus
  Nephrotic syndrome
  Pyelonephritis
  Polycystic kidney disease
Obstructive Lesions
  Hydronephrosis
Renal Vascular Lesions
  Neurofibromatosis
  Renal artery thrombosis
  Renal vein thrombosis
  Renal artery stenosis
Trauma
Endocrine Disorders
  Hyperthyroidism
  Congenital adrenal hyperplasia
  Hyperaldosteronism
  Pheochromocytoma
  Turner's syndrome
  Pregnancy-induced hypertension
Cardiovascular Disorders
  Coarctation of the aorta
  Takayasu arteritis
Drug/Toxin
  Oral contraceptives
  Corticosteroids
  Anabolic steroids
  Cocaine
  Phencyclidine
  Amphetamines
  Nonsteroidal anti-inflammatory drugs
  Heavy metal or lead poisoning
Central Nervous System
  Increased intracranial pressure
Miscellaneous
  Burns
  Leg traction

phritis, or urinary tract infection. Serum electrolytes including urea nitrogen and creatinine as measures of renal function are indicated. Routine complete blood count is recommended. Anemia may suggest the presence of undiagnosed chronic illness, and hemolysis directs the investigation to include hemolytic uremic syndrome. Lipid profile is obtained to assess for additional cardiovascular risk factors. Echocardiogram is optional to screen for left ventricular hypertrophy suggestive of longstanding hypertension. Renal ultrasound may show evidence of renal disease.

If secondary hypertension is suspected based on history, physical examination, or severity of blood pressure elevation, more extensive evaluation is suggested.

## TREATMENT

Treatment modalities include pharmacologic and nonpharmacologic methods. Patients with newly diagnosed mild hypertension (ie, between the 95th and 99th percentile) are initially treated with nonpharmacologic therapies. In those individuals who have more severe hypertension (ie, at the 99th percentile or higher), who are nonresponsive to nonpharmacologic measures over 6 to 12 months, or who develop evidence of target-organ damage, medications are indicated in addition to lifestyle changes. Nonpharmacologic methods are useful as either the primary therapy of patients with mild blood pressure elevation or as an adjunct to medication in cases of more severe hypertension. Weight reduction has a favorable effect on blood pressure in overweight individuals. A mean weight reduction of 9.2 kg in obese, hypertensive adults results in an average reduction in blood pressure of 6.3/3.1 mm Hg. The role of sodium is controversial, although some epidemiologic studies demonstrate that those cultures that consume a high sodium diet have an increased prevalence of hypertension. It appears that some hypertensive individuals are salt-sensitive and will respond to reduction in dietary sodium intake. Thus, moderate sodium restriction is advocated for hypertensive subjects. Exercise, particularly aerobic types, has a positive influence on blood pressure. Reduced intake of alcohol in adults improves blood pressure. The role of potassium, calcium, and magnesium supplementation on blood pressure is controversial. These nonpharmacologic therapies require lifestyle changes that may be difficult for adolescents to accomplish.

Pharmacologic treatment of hypertension has changed dramatically in the 1990s with the availability of new drugs that are easier to use and have fewer side effects. The initial therapy is a single medication, usually either an angiotensin converting enzyme (ACE) inhibitor, calcium-channel antagonist, or adrenergic blocking agent. The dose of the medication is gradually increased until the blood pressure responds, significant side effects occur, or the maximal dose is reached. If the initial medication does not adequately control blood pressure despite good compliance, another medication from a different class should be added or given as a replacement. Usually a diuretic is added as the second medication, and doses are again increased until there is adequate response, side effects occur, or the maximal dose is reached. If the diuretic fails, a direct vasodilator, either hydralazine or prazosin, is used. The fourth step is to use minoxidil as a vasodilator and a centrally acting agent rather than the ACE inhibitor or calcium-channel blocker.

## COMPLIANCE

Compliance problems are frequently encountered in hypertensive patients of all ages and may be more severe during adolescence. The disease is usually asymptomatic and therefore not bothersome to the patient. Thus, the young person may not fully comprehend the need for treatment. In addition, medications must be faithfully taken indefinitely. Finally, bothersome side effects often outweigh perceived benefits. The medical provider may enhance compliance by careful education about the disease process and the need for treatment. Counseling patients that different medications may be used if side effects occur may be helpful.

## CONCLUSION

A methodical approach to the diagnosis, evaluation, and treatment of hypertension results in optimal care for those in need of therapy and avoids unnecessary treatment for those who are healthy or have transient blood pressure evaluation.

## Selected Readings

The 1984 report of the Joint National Committee on Detection, Evaluation, and Treatment of High Blood Pressure. Arch Intern Med 1984;144:1045.

Freis ED. The effect of treatment on mortality in "mild" hypertension: results of the hypertension detection and follow-up program. N Engl J Med 1982;307:976.

Grobbee DE, Hofman A. Effect of calcium supplementation on diastolic blood pressure in young people with mild hypertension. Lancet 1986;703.

Hanna JD, Chan JCM, Gill JR. Hypertension and the kidney. J Pediatr 1991;118:327.

Kaplan NM. Non-drug treatment of hypertension. Ann Intern Med 1985;102:359.

Loggie JMH, Horan MJ, Hohn AR, et al. Juvenile hypertension: highlights of a workshop. J Pediatr 1984;104:657.

Report of the Second Task Force on Blood Pressure Control in Children-1987. Pediatrics 1987;79:1.

Rocchini AP, Key J, Bondie D, et al. The effect of weight loss on the sensitivity of blood pressure to sodium in obese adolescents. N Engl J Med 1989;321:580.

Shear CL, Burke GL, Freedman DS, et al. Value of childhood blood pressure measurements and family history in predicting future blood pressure status: results from 8 years of follow-up in the Bogalusa Heart Study. Pediatrics 1986;77:862.

The Trial of Hypertension Prevention Collaborative Research Group. The effect of nonpharmacologic interventions in blood pressure of persons with high normal levels. JAMA 1992;267:1213.

*Principles and Practice of Pediatrics, Second Edition.*
edited by Frank A. Oski et al. J. B. Lippincott Company, Philadelphia © 1994.

# 30.7 *Acne*

### Hoover Adger

Acne is one of the most common skin disorders and undoubtedly one of the most common problems of adolescence. Almost all adolescents are affected by acne. Although it is rarely a serious medical problem, the associated impact of this disorder is far-reaching. For most, it takes on at least a transient significance. For others, it can be emotionally crippling. Acne accounts for more than one fourth of all office visits to dermatologists and is responsible for a multitude of sales of over-the-counter products to combat this distressing skin disorder.

## ETIOLOGY AND PATHOGENESIS

Although much is known about the events resulting in the development of acne, there is yet to emerge a unifying hypothesis that clearly explains the sole etiologic agent responsible for the chain of events that results in this disorder. The lesions of acne develop in the sebaceous follicle. The sebaceous follicles consist of multi-lobulated sebaceous glands that empty into a wide infundibular canal, which often contains a hair follicle and terminates at the surface of the skin. The sebaceous glands are relatively inactive until early puberty when androgens, which are produced in greater amounts at this time, stimulate the sebaceous glands to enlarge markedly and to discharge sebum, the oily product that is produced by the glands. Many factors are thought to play a major role in the pathogenesis of acne, including obstruction of the pilosebaceous canal, excessive sebum production, bacteria, hormones, and genetic predisposition.

Androgens stimulate the growth of sebaceous glands and enhance the production of sebum. The increase in androgen levels at puberty is associated with an increased conversion of testosterone to dihydrotestosterone by sebaceous cells. Testosterone is converted in sebaceous glands by 5 alpha-reductase to dihydrotestosterone, which is a more potent metabolite. This compound directly stimulates sebaceous gland enlargement and apparently triggers the functional activity of the sebaceous cells. Measurements of sebum production are strikingly higher in individuals with severe acne.

Sebum produced by the sebaceous glands contains a mixture of lipids, wax esters, and squalene; the major component is triglyceride. Anaerobic bacteria that colonize the sebaceous gland (eg, *Propionibacterium acnes*) play a major role in the pathogenesis of acne by producing lipases that hydrolyze the triglycerides to free fatty acids in sebum, which then cause inflammation and aid in the formation of comedones. In conjunction with these changes is an abnormal keratinization pattern of cells lining the infundibular canal just below the surface of the skin; this leads to obstruction of the sebaceous follicle. Keratinized cells of normal follicles are loosely adherent and easily propelled to the surface of the skin. The abnormal keratinization of the epithelium of the pilosebaceous apparatus leads to obstruction of the follicle and impaction of the lumen with sebum, keratin, and bacteria. Accumulation of these products leads to cystic dilatation and disruption of the follicle. With the release of the follicular intraluminal contents, there is an associated inflammatory reaction and the genesis of the characteristic acne lesions.

## CLINICAL FEATURES

Acne is characterized by four basic types of lesions: open and closed comedones, papules, pustules, and nodulocystic lesions. One or more types of lesions may predominate, and there may be varying degrees of involvement. The primary lesions are comedones. Two types are recognized, the open comedone (blackhead) and the closed comedone (whitehead). Open comedones (blackheads) appear as 2- to 5-mm papules with dark centers. The dark centers result from the oxidation of various lipids and melanin and are not due to dirt in the pores as is commonly believed. The orifice of the follicular duct is widely dilated, allowing sebum, keratin, and other cellular debris to drain slowly to the surface. Hence, open comedones usually do not progress to inflammatory lesions. The closed comedones (whiteheads) are 1- to 3-mm, flesh colored papules with a pinpoint opening. These lesions are the precursors of the inflammatory acne lesions. The obstruction of the sebaceous follicle occurs just beneath the surface of the skin at the follicular opening, resulting in cystic swelling of the follicular duct. Rupture of the thin wall of the closed comedone results in an inflammatory response to the released contents.

If the process is superficial, a pustule forms. These raised, pus-filled, inflammatory lesions usually resolve in a few days without scarring. Papules represent a deeper inflammatory reaction. Papules appear as raised solid lesions, take longer to heal, and can be associated with scarring. Nodulocystic lesions are the most

severe category of acne lesions. These warm, tender, firm lesions are suppurative abscesses within the dermis that sometimes extend down to the intradermal fat. Over time, they become fluctuant. Because of the depth and extent of tissue reaction, these lesions often are associated with significant scarring.

Acne conglobata is a rare but severe and disfiguring form of acne that occurs predominantly in males. Papules, pustules, nodules, cysts, abscesses, sinus tracts, and severe scarring characterize this disorder, which usually requires specialized, aggressive management. Although the height of involvement occurs during adolescence, it frequently persists into early adulthood.

Acne fulminans is an acute, severe, explosive, and sometimes devastating variant of acne that affects primarily young males. Patients present with widespread, acute onset of comedones, inflammatory cysts, abscesses, and ulcerations of the chest and trunk. Systemic symptoms of fever, malaise, arthralgias, or arthritis commonly occur, and there is often an evident leukocytosis. Acne fulminans is distinct because of its abrupt onset, location (there is usually sparing of the face and neck), and presence of systemic manifestations. Patients are treated with the usual therapy for severe acne, but systemic corticosteroids are often recommended to control systemic manifestations.

## TREATMENT

Treatment is aimed at controlling the condition with the primary goal being improvement of appearance and prevention of permanent scarring. General cleansing of the face two to three times a day with a mild soap usually diminishes oiliness of affected areas. Vigorous scrubbing should be avoided, however, because it may lead to rupture of comedones. Adolescents should not squeeze comedones; this only increases tissue damage. Adolescents should avoid use of oil-based skin preparations, which can lead to plugging of the follicles and inflammation of comedones. Patients who must use makeup should be encouraged to use water-based products.

The majority of cases of simple acne can be controlled by a topical agent alone. The two most often prescribed topical agents are benzoyl peroxide and retinoic acid. Available as both prescription and nonprescription medication, benzoyl peroxide leads the list of the available armamentarium of treatment agents. The chief benefit of benzoyl peroxide is derived from its antibacterial effect. It also functions as an exfoliant, has comedolytic activity, and is sebostatic. Benzoyl peroxide is available in preparations with concentrations of 2.5%, 5%, and 10%. It comes as an alcohol- or water-based cream, lotion, or gel. Gel appears to be the most effective vehicle. Usually, therapy is initiated with the application of a 5% gel once daily. During early use, many patients complain of sensitivity marked by erythema and scaling. Some patients may prefer to initiate therapy on an every other day basis for the first 10 to 14 days, then progress to a daily or twice daily pattern of use. About 1% to 2% of patients manifest an allergic contact dermatitis to benzoyl peroxide (erythema, pruritus, or edema), which might preclude its use. Compliance is good, however, in most adolescents.

Retinoic acid (tretinoin) is another effective agent that can be applied topically. It is used to treat open and closed comedones of acne. Retinoic acid causes an increase in cell turnover and a decrease in the cohesiveness of the epithelial cells within the sebaceous follicle. This allows sloughing of the epithelium and inhibits the formation of comedones. Tretinoin is available as a cream, gel, or liquid in varying strengths. Although gel may offer the fastest response, often it is associated initially with more adverse effects than creams. Usually, treatment is started with a cream or a low-concentration gel (0.025% cream or 0.01% gel).

Side effects are common at the initiation of therapy and may be minimized by decreasing the frequency of application from daily to every other day during the first 2 weeks of therapy. Optimum therapy results are achieved after 3 to 5 months of continuous therapy. Limiting factors in the use of topical tretinoin include irritation, erythema, desquamation, and an initial worsening of acne in some. In patients with primary comedonal acne, topical retinoic acid may be used as the only agent. When there is only a small inflammatory component, the combination of a topical retinoic acid preparation in conjunction with benzoyl peroxide may be sufficient for treatment of most patients. In those with a moderate to severe inflammatory component, therapy can be maximized with the addition of a topical or systemic antibiotic.

Many dermatologists recommend that patients decrease exposure to sunlight during treatment with tretinoin because of reports of accelerated carcinogenic effects of sunlight caused by retinoids. Although this is not proved, it is prudent to advise patients to use sun screens during prolonged exposure to sunlight.

Systemic antibiotics commonly are used to treat acne that is unresponsive to topical therapy. Tetracycline or erythromycin in low doses appears to inhibit the growth of *P. acnes*. In inflammatory acne, these agents are effective for the treatment of comedonal, pustular, papular, and nodulocystic acne and are relatively free of side effects. Because of its low cost, tetracycline is usually the drug of choice. This antibiotic is usually administered in an initial dosage of 1 to 2 g/d. When inflammatory lesions clear after 2 to 3 weeks, the dosage may be tapered, frequently to a maintenance dosage as low as 250 mg/d.

Minocycline (Minocin), a second generation tetracycline, may be the most effective systemic antibiotic. It achieves a high intrafollicular concentration and is effective longer than tetracycline. The usual dosage is 100 mg or 50 mg twice daily. Although clinical efficacy of minocycline frequently surpasses that of tetracycline, its high cost makes it prohibitive. Hence, it is usually reserved for patients who do not respond to or cannot tolerate gastrointestinal side effects of tetracycline or erythromycin.

Erythromycin is an effective antibiotic in treating acne. The recommended initial dosage is 1 to 2 g/d in two to four divided doses. Nausea and diarrhea are major limiting factors. Trimethoprim sulfa is another effective but less frequently prescribed systemic antibiotic for acne therapy.

In addition to the systemic antibiotics, formulations of topical antibiotics including clindamycin, erythromycin, and tetracycline are available. As with systemic antibiotics, effectiveness of topical antibiotics is markedly enhanced when used in conjunction with benzoyl peroxide or topical retinoic acid. Although the exact mechanism of action is unclear, many studies report at least a 50% decrease in inflammatory lesions after 8 to 12 weeks of treatment with these topical agents.

The final group of therapeutic agents includes sebostatic compounds, of which 13-cis-retinoic acid (Accutane) is the most important addition. Accutane is recommended only for use in those patients who have cystic acne or acne conglobata. These severe forms of acne, which are usually refractory to conventional therapy, often respond to Accutane. The usual dosage of Accutane for treatment of acne is 1 mg/kg/d in two divided doses, preferably given with meals for 16 to 20 weeks. For some patients, a second course of therapy is given after a rest period of at least 8 weeks. The adverse effects of this medication include mucositis, cheilitis, conjunctivitis, pseudotumor cerebri, musculoskeletal pain, elevated plasma triglycerides, and abnormalities of liver function. Patients should have monitoring of liver function, triglycerides, and cholesterol levels. Because of the observed teratogenetic effects demonstrated in animal models, it is important to be sure that there is no risk of pregnancy.

In summary, most acne cases can be successfully treated with topical medications. Topical therapy in conjunction with systemic antibiotic therapy may be necessary and often proves to be ef-fective in patients with a marked inflammatory component to their acne. Severely disfiguring cystic acne or acne conglobata can often be effectively treated with aggressive management that includes 13-cis-retinoic acid. Management of these patients is probably most effective when performed in consultation with a dermatologic specialist.

## Selected Readings

Eichenfeld LF, Leyden JJ. Acne: current concepts of pathogenesis and approach to rational treatment. Pediatrician 1991;18:218.
Luckey AW. Endocrine aspects of acne. Pediatr Clin North Am 1983;30:495.
Luckey AW, Biro FM, Hustler GA, Morrison JA, Elder N. Acne vulgaris in early adolescent boys. Arch Dermatol 1991;127:210.
Martin RW, Klingler WG. Acne fulminans. American Family Practitioner 1989;40:135.
Matsuoka LY. Acne. J Pediatr 1983;103:849.
Schachner L. The treatment of acne: a contemporary review. Pediatr Clin North Am 1983;30:501.
Tunnessen WW Jr. Acne: an approach to therapy for the pediatrician. Curr Probl Pediatr 1984;15:1.
Weston WL. Practical pediatric dermatology, ed 2. Boston: Little Brown, 1985:23.
Wilson BB. Acne vulgaris. Prim Care 1989;16:695.
Winston MH, Shalita AR. Acne vulgaris. Pediatr Clin North Am 1991;38:889.

*Principles and Practice of Pediatrics, Second Edition.*
edited by Frank A. Oski et al. J. B. Lippincott Company, Philadelphia © 1994.

# 30.8 *Eating Disorders*

Alain Joffe

Anorexia nervosa and bulimia nervosa are the syndromes most often conceptualized as eating disorders, although obesity is more common than either. These disorders must be evaluated within the context of a culture that places such significance on thinness, body shape, and fitness that weight loss programs and health and fitness clubs are now a sizable and lucrative growth industry.

Thinness is so pursued, especially by women, that the quotation "You can never be too rich or too thin" has been taken literally by thousands of teenagers, especially girls. Even in the 1950s, according to a Roper poll, only 30% of women stated they did not make any attempts to control their weight. Another study of 446 senior high school girls in 1967 indicated that more than 60% had dieted some time in the past and 37% were dieting on the day of the survey. Of greater concern was that 53% of girls characterized as below average weight and 27% classified as lean in body fat (based on measurements of skinfold thickness) were dieting (Dwyer, 1967). In another study, girls expressed the desire to have smaller hips, thighs, and waists, whereas boys wanted larger biceps and chests (Huenemann and coworkers, 1966).

Given the prevalence of dieting behavior and concerns about body shape among adolescents, one of the major challenges associated with the study of eating disorders is to explain the process whereby some people limit their food intake sensibly while others progress to the full-scale disorder known as anorexia nervosa. Within the last decade or so, increasing numbers of adolescents, usually slightly older than those with anorexia but again predominantly women, have been identified as meeting criteria for diagnosis of bulimia nervosa. Again, although binge eating is common in the general population, only a small percentage of teenagers meet the specific criteria for bulimia nervosa.

About one half of women with anorexia nervosa manifest

some bulimic behavior. Similarly, 30% to 80% of patients with bulimia nervosa have a history of anorexia nervosa. Despite the overlap, these syndromes are discussed separately.

The terms "disorder" or "syndrome" are preferred to the term disease because evidence suggests both encompass a variety of distinct diseases with common manifestations.

## ANOREXIA NERVOSA

### Epidemiology

Most studies indicate an increase in the incidence of anorexia nervosa over the last four decades. Whether these observations are due to an absolute increase in the incidence of the disorder, better recognition and reporting, or both, is unclear. Statistics from Monroe County, New York, for 1960 to 1976 showed an increase from 0.49 to 1.16 cases per 100,000, almost entirely due to an increased incidence among females (Jones, 1980). This study probably detected only the moderately to severely affected patients. Lucas and colleagues detailed the incidence of anorexia nervosa in Rochester, Minnesota. In an initial study, there was a trend toward an increase in rates for 10- to 19-year-old girls from 1950 to 1979. However, the trend was not statistically significant. Subsequently (Lucas, 1991), these same investigators noted a highly significant increase from 7.0 per 100,000 10- to 19-year-olds in 1950 to 26.3 per 100,000 10- to 19-year-olds in 1984. On average, the rates increased by 36% every 5 years from 1950 to 1984. Studies from England suggest a prevalence rate of 1% among secondary school girls aged 16 years or older. The overwhelming majority, 90% to 95%, are females from middle or upper class families. Almost all are white, although reports of blacks, Asians, and Hispanics with the disorder exist. The association with race may be spurious, reflecting socioeconomic and cultural conditions rather than racial characteristics. Minority women seem to develop eating disorders as they move away from their traditional culture. One study found that scores on the Eating Attitudes Test (EAT) significantly correlated with acculturation. Age of onset is bimodal, with the first peak at about 13 to 14 years of age and another at 17 to 18 years of age. The

illness has been described in patients as young as 7 or 8. These characteristics hold true for most Western societies where the syndrome has been studied.

### Clinical Manifestations and Diagnosis

In terms of diagnosis, anorexia is a misnomer. During the early and middle stages of the illness, patients experience hunger but ignore it as a means of asserting self-control. It is not until the late stages of illness, after severe weight loss, that true loss of appetite develops.

An offhand remark by a parent or friend or the perception—whether real or imagined—that she is overweight triggers the adolescent to lose weight. The adolescent restricts calories, exercises, purges, or uses diuretics and laxatives. Some teenagers limit their weight loss. Those who achieve pathologic degrees of weight loss by limiting caloric intake and exercising are referred to as restrictive anorexics, whereas women who engage in purging behavior, laxative and diuretic use, or both are classified as having both anorexia and bulimia nervosa.

Amenorrhea is a prominent feature of the syndrome. In 20% of cases, however, the loss of menses precedes the onset of weight loss. Almost all of the physical and laboratory findings associated with anorexia nervosa are the result of the severe weight loss these women experience and the hypometabolic and hypopituitary status that ensues. Table 30-16 lists the more common physical findings and laboratory abnormalities. The decreased bone mineral density observed in these patients does not appear to completely reverse with treatment, leaving them at increased risk for fractures as they age.

The third revised edition of the *Diagnostic and Statistical Manual of Mental Disorders* (DSM-III-R, 1987) of the American Psychiatric Association criteria used to provide uniform and consistent diagnosis of anorexia is listed in Table 30-17. Adolescents who fail to gain the expected amount of weight associated with rapid body growth during puberty, resulting in a body weight that is 15% below normal, can still be diagnosed as anorexic if they meet the other three criteria listed in Table 30-17.

Bunnell and colleagues (1990) argue that the DSM-III-R criteria may exclude many adolescents, particularly younger ones, with

---

**TABLE 30-16. Physical Findings and Laboratory Abnormalities in Patients With Anorexia Nervosa**

| Physical Findings | Abnormal Laboratory Findings |
|---|---|
| Vital signs: bradycardia; hypothermia; hypotension | Neuroendocrine: decreased FSH and LH with immature secretory pattern; T3 low; "reverse" T3 elevated; growth hormone may be elevated; erratic vasopressin secretion; elevated serum cortisol; decreased estrogen and testosterone |
| Skin: lanugo hair; loss of subcutaneous fat; yellow, dry, or desquamating skin; scalp and genital hair loss; increased hair color pigmentation | Renal: elevated BUN if dehydrated; decreased glomerular filtration rate |
| Extremities: edema; cyanosis; mottling; cold temperature | Hematologic: Leukopenia; thrombocytopenia; anemia (late); decreased transferrin |
| Genital: dry, thin vaginal mucosa; small cervix and uterus | Metabolic: hypoglycemia; elevated cholesterol (early), decreased cholesterol (late); hypercarotenemia; elevated sweat chloride |
| Musculoskeletal: weakness; loss of muscle mass | Electrocardiogram: bradycardia; low voltage |
| | Radiographic: decreased cardiac silhouette; osteopenia |

If the patient is also vomiting or using laxatives or diuretics to maintain weight loss, physical findings and laboratory abnormalities seen in bulimia (see Table 30-18) may also be present.

**TABLE 30-17.** *DSM-III-R* Criteria for Diagnosis
of Anorexia Nervosa

Refusal to maintain body weight over a minimal normal weight for age and height (eg, weight loss leading to maintenance of body weight 15% below that expected) or failure to make expected weight gain during a period of growth, leading to body weight 15% below that expected.

Intense fear of gaining weight or becoming fat, even though underweight.

Disturbance in the way in which one's body weight, size, or shape is experienced (eg, the person claims to feel fat even when emaciated, believes that one area of the body is too fat even when obviously underweight).

In females, absence of at least three consecutive menstrual cycles when they are otherwise expected to occur (primary or secondary amenorrhea). (A women is considered to have amenorrhea if her periods occur only after hormone [eg, estrogen] administration.)

*Reprinted with permission from the Diagnostic and Statistical Manual of Mental Disorders, ed 3, revised. Copyright 1987 The American Psychiatric Association.*

significant eating disorder symptoms. They note that young adolescents in their clinic with many, but not all, of the DSM-III-R criteria were more similar psychologically to women who met the criteria than to normal controls.

Another controversial area is that of disturbed body image. Hsu (1991) points out that patients with bulimia nervosa also have disturbances in body image and that various measures used to identify body image disturbances yield differing, sometimes unreliable results.

The distinction between patients with anorexia who restrict caloric intake and those who also have bulimic behavior is significant. Impulsive behavior (such as stealing, suicide gestures, and alcohol and drug use) are more common among anorexic-bulimics than anorexic-restrictors. Family characteristics and premorbid weights are also different.

Although not specifically required for the diagnosis, several descriptive features of the adolescent and her family typically are seen. She is usually described as neat, even perfectionistic, and well-groomed, and she excels at schoolwork. Parents describe their daughter as a model child. She tends to be overly compliant with parental desires and lacks spontaneity. The family displays little emotion or evidence of intrafamilial conflict and is usually overprotective, enmeshed, and rigid. Members do not resolve

conflicts through direct confrontation; rather, issues are displaced onto the anorectic daughter. Although such characteristics are typical of these families, they are also found in other types of families, such as psychosomatic families.

When questioned, the adolescent tends to minimize the weight loss, appears unconcerned about her current weight, and may express the desire to lose a few additional pounds. Despite severe caloric restriction, she still participates in a vigorous exercise program.

A variety of psychological tests assist in the diagnosis of anorexia; these include the EAT and the Eating Disorders Inventory (EDI). Although they are useful for research studies or in helping confirm the diagnosis in someone suspected clinically of having an eating disorder, they should not be used in general practice or school settings as screening instruments to identify potential cases of eating disorders.

On a more practical basis, assessment of the adolescent suspected of having anorexia nervosa should cover a variety of areas. Included are the following key historical variables: weight history (highest and lowest weights achieved, method of losing weight, lowest adult weight, ideal weight); duration of weight loss; dietary history including diet recall, meals skipped, social context of eating, feelings accompanying eating, vomiting, and medications used to induce weight loss; menstrual history; perceived body image and concerns regarding weight gain; exercise patterns; and presence or absence of depressive symptoms or other physical symptoms (Comerci, 1985). Because other illnesses (such as inflammatory bowel disease) can produce anorexia and weight loss, a careful and thorough history and physical examination should be performed on all patients suspected of having an eating disorder.

## Etiology

A variety of hypotheses explains the characteristic manifestations of anorexia. The syndrome probably has a multifactorial origin with a reciprocal interplay between the forces outlined below. Anorexia then represents a final common pathway shown in Figure 30-10.

The sociocultural emphasis on thinness—both as an idealized body type and as an example of self-control—has accelerated in the last several decades and been directed at those in the upper socioeconomic strata, which explains some of the characteristic demographics associated with this syndrome. Similarly, women for whom thinness is a prerequisite for success (ballet dancers or models) or who serve as role models or ideals for other women, are at greater risk. Adolescents, who are normally preoccupied

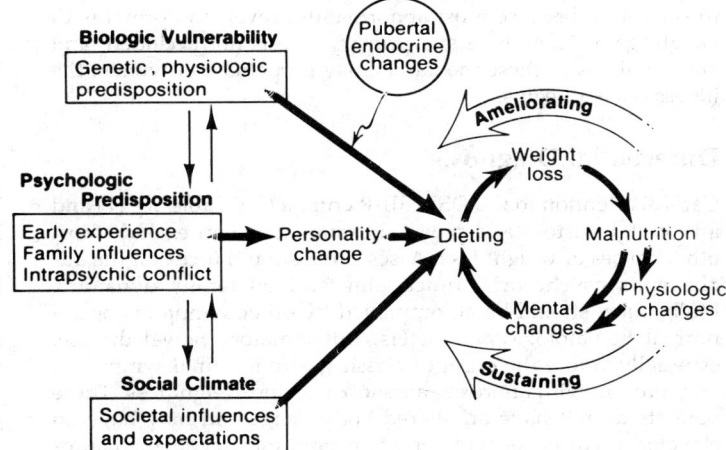

**Figure 30-10.** A theoretic model for understanding the multiple factors associated with anorexia nervosa. Such a model could be similarly constructed for bulimia. (Reprinted with permission from Lucas AR. Toward the understanding of anorexia nervosa as a disease entity. Mayo Clin Proc 1981;56:258.)

with their changing bodies, are particularly vulnerable to stereotypes about the idealized body shape.

Psychosocial factors center on the adolescent's normal developmental desire for independence within the context of a close-knit family that has trouble expressing emotion, denies family conflict, and is ambivalent about the separation of their daughter. The ability of the adolescent to separate from parents requires a sense of self-efficacy and personal autonomy, characteristics that are probably lacking in an adolescent who has grown up catering only to the needs and desires of others. Unable to express the desire for separation and ill-prepared to face the demands of the more complex social world of adolescence, the daughter expresses self-control and achieves a sense of identity by control over appetite and body weight.

The role of biology in the etiology of anorexia nervosa is uncertain. Most of the metabolic and laboratory abnormalities noted in these patients reverse with weight gain. Some abnormalities persist, however, and it is unclear whether these are primary or secondary phenomena. Twin studies indicate that the concordance rate for anorexia is higher among monozygotic twins than dizygotic twins. In one study, the concordance rate was 55% for monozygotic twins but only 7% for dizygotic pairs. This strongly suggests a genetic basis. An ascertainment bias is possible, however, in that twin pairs concordant for anorexia are more likely to come to medical attention. Anorexia nervosa also is noted to cluster in families, being approximately eight times more common in female first degree relatives of probands compared to the general population and absent among female relatives of probands with other types of psychiatric disorders.

Other reports demonstrate an increased risk for affective illness among first degree relatives of women with anorexia nervosa. The converse is not true: daughters in families in which one or more parents have an affective disorder do not have higher rates of anorexia. Not all investigators found an increased risk for affective illness in first degree relatives. If anorexia patients with depression are excluded from analysis, then parents of those remaining do not have a higher rate of affective illness.

A variety of neurotransmitters and hormones affect feeding behavior, appetite control, and mood. Increases in serotonin activity produce satiety; decreased serotonin activity increases food consumption and enhances weight gain. Norepinephrine also stimulates feeding behavior, even in animals who eat until full. Anorexic women have low cerebrospinal fluid (CSF) levels of both these neurotransmitters and have low plasma levels of tryptophan, a precursor of serotonin. Opioids normally increase food intake but, in animals with restricted access to food, they decrease appetite. Finally, peptide YY (PYY) is a highly potent stimulator of eating. These hormones and neurotransmitters affect each other's actions, further complicating study of their roles in anorexia. Alterations in CSF and plasma levels are likely secondary to starvation because most abnormalities revert to normal with weight gain. Nonetheless, a primary role is not excluded, and abnormalities of these mediators may perpetuate or worsen the illness once it begins.

## Differential Diagnosis

Careful attention to the DSM-III-R criteria (see Table 30-17) and a thorough history and physical examination can exclude most other causes of weight loss. Assessment should focus on the adolescent's psychosocial functioning and on family dynamics. Malignancy should be accompanied by other symptoms or abnormal hematologic parameters. Inflammatory bowel disease, especially before the onset of classic gastrointestinal symptoms, may present with anorexia, amenorrhea, and weight loss. These patients do not have an altered body image and may have an elevated erythrocyte sedimentation rate, microcytic anemia, or

stools positive for occult blood. Given that patients with anorexia become hypothyroid, hyperthyroidism as the cause of weight loss should easily be detected. Other metabolic diseases can be excluded by measurement of serum electrolytes, renal and liver functions, and blood glucose levels. Central nervous system pathology is suggested by the presence of severe headaches, papilledema, or visual field changes.

## Treatment and Prognosis

Rigorous long-term, double-blind studies of carefully defined patient populations and treatments for anorexia nervosa are scarce. Furthermore, outcome studies are based largely on clinical samples, which presumably represent more severely affected individuals. Hence, prognosis for patients is variable. Given the likely multifactorial etiology of the disorder, a multidisciplinary approach to treatment is prudent. These therapies involve attention to individual patient psychodynamics (insight-oriented therapy), family functioning (family therapy), and eating behavior and their meaning for the patient (cognitive-behavioral therapy). Further, nutritional therapy involves recognition and gradual reversal of biochemical, nutritional, and metabolic abnormalities. One important element of treatment is to reassure the patient that she will not gain an excessive amount of weight.

One critical aspect of therapy is the decision to manage the patient as an outpatient or an inpatient. Findings that indicate the need for hospitalization are evidence of hypovolemia (low systolic blood pressure), electrolyte imbalance (hypokalemia, hypomagnesemia, hypophosphatemia), hypothermia, uncompensated metabolic acidosis or alkalosis, weight loss to 30% to 40% below initial or expected levels, edema or congestive heart failure, suicidal ideation or severe depression, psychosis, or an uncertain diagnosis. Those who fail outpatient management or whose families do not participate in therapy should also be hospitalized.

A variety of pharmacologic agents are used in conjunction with individual, nutritional, and family therapy. Anxiolytic agents help briefly when given in low doses to lessen panic about gaining weight. Cyproheptadine is effective among restrictive anorexics but not among bulimic anorexics. Antidepressants occasionally are effective but often are accompanied by side effects. The role of such other medications as metoclopramide (to improve gastric emptying), lithium, and opioid blockers is uncertain.

Self-help groups, professionalized to varying degrees, also may play a role in treatment. These groups provide peer support as well as opportunity to interact with other patients in a nonprofessionally controlled environment.

Despite advances in the understanding of anorexia, the emergence of a multidisciplinary treatment modality, and research on optimum treatment strategies including drug treatment, this syndrome is still associated with significant long-term morbidity and mortality. Mortality figures range from 2% to 5%, to a high of 18%. Death may result from suicide, starvation, electrolyte imbalance, infection, gastrointestinal catastrophe, or cardiac insufficiency. Abuse of laxatives, diuretics, or other medications can also lead to fatal complications.

Statistics regarding long-term morbidity are more difficult to assess because the degree of morbidity is influenced by the number and types of outcomes measured (eg, weight gain, social adjustment, employment, persistence of abnormal eating behavior). Three reviews of outcome studies suggest that one third to one half of patients recover completely and that at least one third continue to have some difficulties with eating behavior. At least half of patients had difficulties in areas of social adjustment not related to eating or weight.

Factors that predict treatment outcome are elusive. Some suggest that early-onset disease and a short interval between diagnosis and treatment are favorable indicators, as are less denial of illness, admission of hunger, positive self-esteem, and a more supportive family environment. Unfavorable indicators are a combination of anorexia and bulimia, obesity before onset of illness, use of laxatives or vomiting to control weight, and psychiatric abnormality that precedes onset of anorexia.

## BULIMIA NERVOSA

### Epidemiology

Although anorexia nervosa has been well described for centuries, it is only in the last few decades that bulimia nervosa has gained attention and come under careful study as a distinct clinical syndrome. As with anorexia, bulimia appears to have increased in incidence recently. The DSM-III-R criteria for bulimia nervosa, however, are more conservative than the DSM-III criteria for bulimia. Hence, more recent prevalence data derived from surveys or interviews using DSM-III-R criteria are not readily comparable to earlier data using DSM-III criteria. Ten percent of female shoppers at a suburban mall revealed a history of bulimic behavior. One study among college students indicated an increase over a 3-year period from 1% to 3% of students. Several recent studies, using sophisticated interview studies, demonstrate a prevalence of 1%. An ongoing study of freshmen college students indicates bulimia nervosa may have declined in prevalence since the mid-1980s. Careful definition of binge eating is critical, because many adolescents view eating a single bowl of ice cream or several cookies as binge eating.

Bulimics are predominantly white and female. The relationship with social class is not nearly so clear as it is in anorexia. Most women with bulimia are normal weight or overweight; many of those who are underweight also fulfill the criteria for anorexia and as a group are distinct from bulimics. Bulimics tend to be slightly older than anorexics, with a peak age of onset of about 18 years.

### Clinical Manifestations and Diagnosis

Bulimics typically consume large quantities of food in a short time. Binges usually occur once a day, in the late afternoon or evening. Kaye and Weltzin (1991) noted that bulimic subjects ate the same number of meals over 24 hours as did controls and that 72% were of similar size. The other 28% of meals, however, contained from 1058 to 6728 Kcal. Invariably, binges occur when the adolescent is alone; secretiveness is a cardinal feature of the disorder. The sense of fullness, often painful, and the fear of weight gain leads the young woman to induce vomiting or to use laxatives or diuretics. Other feelings accompanying the binge include anxiety about not being able to stop, depression, guilt, shame, and self-deprecation. The episodes of binge eating may be followed by periods of fasting or rigorous exercise in attempts to control weight.

There may be few physical clues to the presence of bulimia. The most characteristic findings include dental enamel erosions and caries from repeated contact with stomach acid; callouses and abrasions on the dorsum of the hands from contact with the teeth; and salivary, especially parotid gland, hypertrophy. Other physical findings and laboratory abnormalities that suggest the diagnosis are shown in Table 30-18. The DSM-III-R criteria for bulimia are summarized in Table 30-19.

The evaluation of a patient suspected of having bulimia should include careful attention to details of binge episodes, the circumstances in which they occur, and the feelings accompanying them. Specific attention to the role of vomiting and the use of laxatives, diuretics, and emetics is critical.

### TABLE 30-18. Physical Findings and Laboratory Abnormalities in Patients With Bulimia

| Physical Findings | Laboratory Abnormalities |
|---|---|
| Oral: parotid gland hypertrophy; dental caries, pyorrhea; dental enamel erosion | Elevated serum bicarbonate (metabolic alkalosis secondary to vomiting) |
| Skin: ulcerations, calluses, scars on dorsum of hand | Hypokalemia, hypochloremia, hyponatremia |
| Neuromuscular: muscle weakness; hyporeflexia; peripheral neuropathy | Hyperamylasemia |
| Cardiac: arrhythmias | Metabolic acidosis (with laxative use) |
| GI: abdominal distention; ileus; acute gastric dilatation; esophageal tears | Hypo- or hypercalcemia; hypomagnesemia |
| Pulmonary: pneumomediastinum | |

### Etiology

There are probably multiple causes of bulimia. In one study, 9.6% of relatives of bulimic patients had bulimia compared to 3.5% of controls. First degree relatives of bulimics have a 7% to 22% prevalence of major depression. Alcoholism and obesity are also common among parents. Bulimics themselves are more likely to abuse alcohol or illicit drugs, to have personality and anxiety disorders, and to be depressed. Studies show a greater concordance for monozygotic twins as compared to dizygotic twins, although these studies are subject to the same ascertainment bias as studies analyzing the genetic role in anorexia nervosa. One study of twins identified the following as risk factors for bulimia: birth after 1960; low paternal care; history of wide weight fluctuations, dieting, or frequent exercise; slim ideal body image; low self-esteem; external locus of control; and high levels of neuroticism (Kendler, 1991).

The dynamics of interaction within bulimic families differ from those of anorexic families. Bulimic families tend to be more open in expressing emotions, and feelings of isolation and disillusionment within the marriage are often evident. Mothers of bulimic daughters are emotionally distant from their daughters. Interactions among family members are often negative and the family lacks cohesion and structure. Consequently, children raised in these families often feel disconnected and disorganized.

### TABLE 30-19. *DSM-III-R* Criteria for Diagnosis of Bulimia

Recurrent episodes of binge eating (rapid consumption of a large amount of food in a discrete period of time).

A feeling of lack of control over eating behavior during the binge eating.

The person regularly engages in self-induced vomiting, use of laxatives or diuretics, strict dieting or fasting, or vigorous exercise to prevent weight gain.

A minimum average of two binge eating episodes a week for at least 3 months

Persistent overconcern with body shape and weight.

*Reprinted with permission from the Diagnostic and Statistical Manual of Mental Disorders, ed 3, revised. Copyright 1987 The American Psychiatric Association.*

Enmeshment is characteristic of both anorexic and bulimic families. In anorexia the enmeshment is characterized by caring and deference, whereas in bulimia, families are trapped in a web of hostility, anger, and manipulation. The bulimic daughter often fears that the family would fall apart if she left home.

Sociocultural factors play a role in the pathogenesis of bulimia. It is intriguing to speculate how similar cultural cues can lead to starvation in one adolescent and to binge eating in another. Women with bulimia nervosa also demonstrate dissatisfaction with their body image, perhaps even more so than do patients with anorexia.

Several lines of investigation suggest a link between binge eating behavior and overactivity of the alpha-2 noradrenergic system, underactivity of the serotonergic system, or both. Administration of serotonin agonists to rats causes a decrease in meal size and number and in the percentage of carbohydrates consumed. Decreased serotonin activity among bulimics (documented in some but not all studies) could lead to binge eating behavior. Alternatively, binge eating with high carbohydrate foods could be an attempt to increase CSF serotonin levels. Alterations in cholecystokinin, opioid, and PYY levels have also been noted among bulimics; CSF norepinephrine concentrations are lower than normal. The significance of these findings is unclear. These abnormalities, however, cannot be explained by weight loss and may perpetuate abnormal feeding behavior once initiated.

## Treatment and Prognosis

Because bulimia has only recently come under systematic study, the long-term prognosis and optimal treatment regimens are not clearly defined. Complications resulting from repetitive vomiting can be severe and potentially lethal, including esophageal tears, acute gastric dilatation, and hypokalemia with resulting cardiac arrhythmias. Diuretic use can also lead to hypokalemia, and repeated self-administration of ipecac can result in myopathy and death.

A recent meta-analysis of 25 outcome studies comparing pharmacologic and nonpharmacologic therapy, including various combinations of psychotherapy or cognitive-behavioral therapy with or without dietary management, showed both to be effective although nonpharmacologic therapy appeared somewhat more effective. One effective nonpharmacologic approach is cognitive behavioral therapy, in which rigid food rules and distorted assessments of body shape and weight are corrected. Patients are taught to monitor themselves and to identify and avoid situations that lead to binge-eating. Also effective is interpersonal therapy, which focuses on such issues as dissatisfaction with social relationships and social impairments, low self-esteem, and anxiety and depression.

Only antidepressant medications have been shown to be effective in the treatment of bulimia nervosa. Virtually all antidepressants are effective, although their use does not entirely eliminate binge eating and purging behavior. Whether the patient is depressed at onset of treatment does not predict whether her binge eating or purging behavior will lessen with antidepressant use. Furthermore, the effect of the antidepressant appears short-lived. Several studies indicate a relapse rate of one third at 6-month follow-up, even for patients remaining on medication. Longer studies suggest that frequent switching of medication is necessary to control symptoms. Tricyclic antidepressants are not as effective in treating depression among adolescents as they are among older women; hence, their use in treating bulimic adolescents may be less favorable.

The long-term course of bulimia nervosa involves frequent relapses. Twelve-month follow-up studies of individuals treated as outpatients demonstrate recovery rates of 30% to 70%. Recovery rates for inpatients are substantially lower. Follow-up studies beyond 12 months are rare. One such study showed that almost 70% recovered by 3½ years, most within the first 12 months. Sixty-three percent relapsed within 8 months, however, and only one half of these recovered again. Ten to 85 weeks later, 50% of those making a second recovery relapsed yet again. Patients with less severe symptoms, a better self-image, and several close relationships did better. The significance of a concurrent depression as a predictor of outcome is uncertain, but alcohol abuse is negatively correlated with successful recovery.

## Selected Readings

Bunnell DW, Shenker IR, Nussbaum MR, et al. Subclinical versus formal eating disorders: differentiating psychological features. International Journal of Eating Disorders 1991;9:357.

Comerci GD, Williams R. Eating disorders in the young. Part 1: anorexia and bulimia. Curr Probl Pediatr 1985;15(8):7.

Dwyer JT, Feldman JJ, Mayer J. Adolescent dieters: who are they? Am J Clin Nutr 1967;10:1045.

Hsu LKG. Outcome of anorexia nervosa: a review of the literature. Arch Gen Psychiatry 1980;37:1041.

Hsu LKG, Sobkiewicz TA. Body image disturbance: time to abandon the concept for eating disorders? International Journal of Eating Disorders 1991;10:15.

Huenemann RI, Shapiro LR, Hampton MC, Mitchell BW. A longitudinal study of gross body composition and body conformation and their association with food and activity in a teen-age population. Am J Clin Nutr 1966;18:325.

Jones DJ, Fox MM, Babigian HM, Hutton HE. Epidemiology of anorexia nervosa in Monroe County, New York: 1960–1976. Psychosom Med 1980;42:551.

Kaplan AS. Biomedical variables in the eating disorders. Can J Psychiatry. 1990;35:745.

Kaye WH, Weltzin TE. Neurochemistry of bulimia nervosa. J Clin Psychiatry. 1991;52(suppl):21.

Kendler KS, MacLean C, Neale M, et al. The genetic epidemiology of bulimia nervosa. Am J Psychiatry. 1991;148:1627.

Laessle RG, Zoettl C, Pirke KM. Meta-analysis of treatment studies for bulimia. International Journal of Eating Disorders 1987;5:647.

Lucas AR, Beard CM, O'Fallon WM, et al. 50-year trends in the incidence of anorexia nervosa in Rochester, Minn: a population-based study. Am J Psychiatry. 1991;148:917.

Pyle RL, Halvorson PA, Newman PA, Mitchell JE. The increasing prevalence of bulimia in freshman college students. International Journal of Eating Disorders 1986;5:631.

Pyle RL, Neuman PA, Halvorson PA, Mitchell JE. An ongoing cross-sectional study of the prevalence of eating disorders in freshman college students. International Journal of Eating Disorders. 1991;10:667.

Steinhausen H-Ch, Rauss-Mason C, Seidel R. Follow up studies of anorexia nervosa: a review of four decades of outcome research. Psychol Med. 1991;21:447.

Swift WJ, Andrews D, Barkalge NE. The relationship between affective disorders and eating disorders: a review of the literature. Am J Psychiatry 1986;143:290.

Walsh BT, Devlin MJ. The pharmacologic treatment of eating disorders. Psychiatr Clin North Am. 1992;15:149.

Yates A. Current perspectives on the eating disorders: I. history, psychological and biological aspects. J Am Acad Child Adolesc Psychiatry. 1989;28:813.

Yates A. Current perspectives on the eating disorders: II. treatment, outcome and research directions. J Am Acad Child Adolesc Psychiatry. 1990;29:1.

*Principles and Practice of Pediatrics, Second Edition.*
edited by Frank A. Oski et al. J. B. Lippincott Company, Philadelphia © 1994.

# 30.9 *Adolescent Drug Abuse*

## Hoover Adger

Today's adolescent lives in a society in which use of alcohol and other drugs is prevalent and acceptable. Recent surveys outlining levels of use in youths support the notion that our children are growing up in a "do drug" society. Their use of alcohol and other drugs can no longer be seen as uncommon or restricted to small subgroups of problem youths. Prevalence patterns cut across gender, ethnic, cultural, and geographic lines. Young people have incorporated the use of alcohol, marijuana, and tobacco into their socialization to such an extent that those who abstain are in the minority. The consequences of such use are evident. Although individuals in all other age groups have experienced an improvement in overall health status and a prolonged life expectancy, young people aged 15 to 24 years constitute the only group to experience an increase in mortality rate over the past decade, with those aged 15 to 19 years experiencing the most acute increase. The major causes of mortality in this group are homicide, suicide, and unintentional injuries. A large proportion of these are associated with alcohol or other drugs. The increasing frequency and adverse consequences of drug use are critical issues for health care providers who care for youth.

## DEFINITIONS

Chemical dependence can be defined as a chronic and progressive disease process that includes both the physical and psychological reliance on a chemical. It encompasses both alcoholism and dependence on other psychoactive substances. Chemical dependence is characterized by loss of control over use, compulsion, and establishment of an altered state in which one requires continued administration of a psychoactive substance to feel good or avoid feeling bad. *Chemical dependence* replaces confusing terminology that placed substances into addicting and nonaddicting categories. Previous views concentrated on the addicting and nonaddicting properties of drugs and emphasized that the development of tolerance and evidence of physical withdrawal in discontinuing the drug were necessary components of dependence. Current definitions focus on loss of control over use and the interactive relationship between the individual and drug use.

In the *Diagnostic and Statistical Manual of Mental Disorders* (DSM-III-R), any person with a psychoactive substance abuse disorder is "dependent" if any three of the following criteria are met:

Frequent preoccupation with, seeking, or taking the substance
Frequent use in larger amounts or over a longer period than intended
Need for increased amounts of the substance to achieve intoxication or desired effect or diminished effect with continued use of the same amount
Display of characteristic withdrawal symptoms
Frequent use of the substance to relieve or avoid withdrawal symptoms
Persistent desire or repeated efforts to cut down or control substance use
Frequent intoxication or impairment from substance use when expected to fulfill social or occupational obligations, or when substance use is hazardous (eg, driving when drunk)
Relinquishment of some important social, occupational, or recreational activity to seek or take the substance
continuation of substance use despite a significant social, occupational, or legal problem, or a physical disorder that the person knows is exacerbated by use of substance.

*Substance abuse,* in contrast, is characterized by a maladaptive pattern of use, indicated by continued use despite consequences or recurrent use when such use may be physically hazardous.

## EPIDEMIOLOGY

Since 1975, the National Institute on Drug Abuse has conducted an annual nationwide survey of approximately 17,000 high school seniors on the use of alcohol, tobacco, and other drugs. Although surveys of drug use probably underestimate the magnitude of usage, they provide useful information about prevalence patterns and usage trends. Overall usage levels for many illicit drugs have declined from their peak levels during the late 1970s. Evidence continues to show, however, that the drug abuse problem among youth is a major dilemma.

Despite the decrease since the peak for reported illicit drug use in 1982, almost two thirds of young persons try an illicit drug before they finish high school, and 40% have used an illicit drug other than marijuana. Six percent of high school seniors in 1975 reported daily use of marijuana. By 1978, this figure increased to 11%, then dropped substantially by 1984 to 5%. Marijuana is the most widely used illicit drug with 37% of seniors in 1992 reporting some use in their lifetime, 24% reporting some use in the past year, and 12% reporting some use in the past month. Three percent reported actively smoking marijuana on a daily basis.

The use of some drugs has decreased dramatically from the peak levels in the late 1970s. Included in this group are tranquilizers, barbiturates, methaqualone, lysergic acid diethylamide (LSD), and phencyclidine (PCP). The use of stimulants, the most widely used class of illicit drugs outside of marijuana, started to decline in 1983. Despite declines in the reported levels of use for a number of drugs, the rate of decline has stabilized, suggesting that there may be a continuing level of drug use among youth. This trend continues to put this group at risk.

Not all drugs have declined in level of use. Substantial evidence suggests that cocaine is increasingly available throughout the United States. Since the advent of "crack," a powerful and easily marketable form of cocaine, reported use in youth has been a major concern. Almost 10% of high school seniors in 1976 reported ever using cocaine. By 1985, this figure had risen to 17%. This is the highest figure yet reported for this group, and it indicates the escalating impact of this drug. In addition, although only 10% of students reported cocaine use in 1976, nearly 40% of this same group, when questioned on follow-up 10 years later, reported having tried cocaine at some time. Hence, a large proportion of youth entering young adulthood shows evidence of placing themselves at risk for harmful effects of this dangerous drug.

While there has been a decrease in the reported prevalence for use of most illicit drugs, there has been relatively little change in the reported use of alcohol and tobacco, which are the major drugs of abuse. More than 90% of high school seniors in 1990 reported some experience with alcohol, 60% reported use in the past month, and 4% reported daily use. Additionally, problematic use among those who continue to use alcohol appears to be rising.

There has been a trend toward earlier initiation of use. There is also an inclination among today's youth to simultaneously use more than one drug. The earlier a person begins to drink or use other drugs, the greater the likelihood of later drug problems. Hence, potentially harmful effects are most serious in those who initiate use at a young age.

Nine classes of psychoactive substances are associated with both abuse and dependence: alcohol, amphetamines or similarly acting sympathomimetics, cannabis, cocaine, hallucinogens, volatile inhalants, opioids, PCP and similarly acting arylcyclohexamines, and sedative hypnotics. Despite their different physiologic effects, they all share one unique property: the ability to distort the sensory experience and produce euphoria. It is this easily induced euphoria that leads to the induction of behavior change, retardation of psychosocial maturation, and, at times, increasing levels and frequency of use.

### Etiology

Substance abuse is an excellent example of a condition reflecting a bio-psychosocial determination. There is no single cause. A number of biologic factors including genetic predisposition are well established. Psychological factors are less well understood. However, behaviors such as rebelliousness, poor school performance, delinquency, and criminal activity and personality traits such as low self-esteem, anxiety, and lack of self-control frequently are associated with or predate the onset of drug use. Environmental stressors, social pressures, and family attitudes and practices play important roles in shaping attitudes and behaviors of young people. The etiology, therefore, is multidimensional and multifactorial.

## Progression of Alcohol and Other Drug Use

Not all children and adolescents who use alcohol and other drugs (AOD) become problem users. Although risk factors may help identify those who are most vulnerable, it does not mean that any individual who exhibits them inevitably develops problems. For some, experimental or casual use progresses to heavy use and dependency. For others, even experimental or casual use leads to unfavorable outcomes. For this reason, it is helpful to look at AOD use and abuse on a continuum. Death can be an unfortunate outcome of use at any point on the continuum.

As is the case with other chronic and progressive processes, early treatment of chemical dependence leads to better outcomes. The key to early treatment is early recognition and intervention. A prerequisite for early recognition is a familiarity with and understanding of the natural history and progression of adolescent substance abuse from a stage of no use, to moderate use, to immoderate use, to dependency. MacDonald and others have popularized four successive stages of use that help characterize the progressive nature of substance abuse and chemical dependency: experimentation-learning the mood swing, seeking the mood swing, preoccupation with the mood swing, and doing drugs to feel normal or "burnout" (Table 30-20).

The use of a psychoactive substance such as beer or marijuana at the experimentation-learning stage generally occurs within the context of initial curiosity and is often in response to peer pressure. Hence, the experiential learning encompasses several facts. First is the knowledge that psychoactive substances result in a welcome or perhaps unwelcome mood swing. In addition, it may be ap-

| | Predisposition | Behavior | Family Reaction |
|---|---|---|---|
| **TABLE 30-20. Progression of Substance Abuse in Adolescents** | | | |
| **Stage 1: Experimentation—Learning the Mood Swing** | | | |
| Infrequent use | Curiosity | Learning the mood | Often unaware |
| Alcohol/marijuana | Peer pressure | Feels good | Denial |
| No consequences | Attempt to assume adult role | Positive reinforcement | |
| Some fear of use | | Can return to normal | |
| Low tolerance | | | |
| **Stage 2: Seeking the Mood Swing** | | | |
| Increasing frequency | Impress others | Use to get high | Attempts at elimination |
| Use of various drugs | Social function | Pride in amount consumed | Blaming others |
| Minimal defensiveness | Modeling adult behavior | Use to relieve feelings (eg, anxieties of dating) | |
| Tolerance | | Denial of problem | |
| **Stage 3: Preoccupation With the Mood Swing** | | | |
| Change in peer group | Using to get loaded—not just high | Begins to violate values and rules | Conspiracy of silence |
| Activities revolve around use | | Use before and during school | Confrontation |
| Steady supply | | Use despite consequences | Reorganization with or without affected individual |
| Possible dealing | | Solitary use | |
| Few or no "straight" friends | | Trouble with school | |
| Consequences frequent | | Overdoses, "bad trips," blackouts | |
| | | Promises to cut down or attempts to quit | |
| | | Protection of supply, hides use from peers | |
| | | Deterioration in physical condition | |
| **Stage 4: Using to Feel Normal** | | | |
| Continued use despite adverse outcomes | Use to feel normal | Daily use | Frustration |
| Loss of control | | Failure to meet expectations | Anger |
| Inability to stop | | Loss of control | May give up |
| Compulsion | | Paranoia | |
| | | Suicide gestures | |
| | | Physical deterioration | |
| | | Poor eating and sleep habits | |

Adapted from MacDonald DI. Marijuana and youth: clinical observation on motivation and learning. Department of Health and Human Services publication no (ADM) 1982;82:1186.

preciated that these mood swings or feelings can be reliably produced and even controlled to some extent by modulation of the amount, quality, or variations of the substance used. Often at this stage, there is little behavioral change and an absence of discernible consequences.

Through experience, some adolescents learn to anticipate and welcome the mood swing. For most, these experiences occur within the context of social functions in which it is perceived as fun, socially rewarding, and without untoward effects. For some at this stage, the euphoric feelings gained through the use of various substances seem to provide an answer by helping the adolescent to cope, relieving feelings of anxiety, or perhaps by providing a desired change in social or peer group status. At this point, there may be a change in peer group, new friends, and the beginning of deterioration in school and other life areas as substance use escalates.

Progression to the next stage involves a movement from anticipation to preoccupation. Drug use at this stage takes on a different relationship as the motivations and role of increasing substance use assume more of a primary role in the life of the individual. Often, problems with family, school, or the law become evident. Polydrug use becomes more frequent, and friends who do not also use drugs become scarce.

The final stage in the progression, dependence, is characterized by loss of control, compulsion, and evidence of dysfunction. The behavior of the chemically dependent adolescent shows a development of primary relationships with mood-altering drugs. Values, habits, and relationships that had been primary appear no longer to exist.

## RISK FACTORS

Individuals who have been identified as particularly at risk for development of alcohol and other drug problems include children from families in which alcoholism or drug abuse is present. In addition, the following adolescents are at increased risk: those who experience significant problems in behavior such as aggressiveness and rebellious deviancy; those with difficulties in cognition such as learning disabilities or attention deficit disorders; those with problems in psychological well-being such as depression, isolation, and low self-esteem; and those with impaired familial functioning such as neglect, abuse, loss, and lack of close relationships.

Genetics and environment play important roles in the risk profile of an individual. A family history of alcoholism or other chemical dependency is an important risk factor. Children of alcoholics are four to five times more likely to develop alcohol dependence than other children. Recent evidence indicates that there may be biologically measurable differences in such children that may be related to the metabolism of and tolerance to alcohol, in addition to the susceptibility to alcohol dependence. Further elucidation of these findings may have future applications to youth and risk counseling.

## Identification and Treatment

Diagnosing substance abuse rests on the realization that all children and adolescents are at risk but that some are at substantially more risk than others. Making the diagnosis must be part of a comprehensive diagnostic approach. Sources of diagnostic information might include: history and mental status examination, physical examination, self-report questionnaires, structured interview and standardized tests, and laboratory screening. While the ability to do an in-depth assessment and make an actual diagnosis may be beyond the time limitations and skills of most

practitioners, several approaches to office screening and assessment of adolescent substance abuse provide guidance for a meaningful role for the pediatrician.

Substance abuse should be included as a primary differential diagnosis whenever behavioral, familial, psychosocial, or related medical problems occur. As part of the routine health examination, all adolescents should be questioned about the use of cigarettes, alcohol, and other drugs. In addition, there should be an assessment of risk by reviewing risk factors and behaviors with adolescents and their parents.

The actual treatment of adolescents with chemical dependence is beyond the scope of most pediatricians. Even without special expertise in this area, however, most clinicians should be able to perform an initial assessment of an adolescent's use of drugs and to determine indications for further assessment and intervention. The primary tasks of the evaluation are to determine if the use of mood-altering chemicals is associated with identifiable consequences and if such use is causing behavioral impairment. A general assessment of psychosocial functioning is the most important part of the evaluation because it provides a basis for determining whether behavioral dysfunction exists. Information should be gathered specifically about family relationships, peer relationships, school performance and attendance, recreational and leisure activities, employment, vocational aspirations, frequency of conflicts with parents, and legal difficulties. Often, use patterns of peers and self-perceptions of the adolescent regarding his own use and whether or not it is a problem provide additional, useful information. Information gathered from the evaluation should help determine if substance abuse is a cause of behavioral dysfunction and the degree of patient involvement. It should also help in deciding whether there is need for further assessment or indication of need for treatment.

A number of treatment alternatives are available for the chemically dependent adolescent. Short-term inpatient treatment, residential care, and outpatient care span the spectrum from traditional office-based care to intensive and structured day programs. Most treatment programs share beliefs that treatment begins with the interruption of use, requires continued abstinence from drugs, and sets as a goal for the adolescent the development of a drug-free lifestyle. Because of the wide variety of settings and a number of different approaches to the treatment of adolescents, the clinician should be aware of resources in the community and become familiar with the philosophies of the agencies that render services. With this information, the physician can better assume a responsible role in terms of intervention and assisting the family in its search for appropriate treatment resources.

## Selected Readings

AAP Committee on Adolescence: The Role of the pediatrician in substance abuse counseling. Pediatrics 1983;72:251.

Adger H. Problems of alcohol and other drug use and abuse in adolescents. Journal Adolesc Health 1991;12:606.

Bailey GW. Current perspectives on substance abuse in youth. J Am Acad Child Adolesc Psychiatry 1989;2:151.

Comerci GD, MacDonald DI. Prevention of substance abuse in children and adolescents. Adolescent Medicine State of the Art Reviews 1990;1:127.

Duggan AK, Adger H, McDonald EM, Stokes EJ, Moore R. Detection of alcoholism in hospitalized children and their families. Am J Dis Child 1991;145:613.

Farrow JA, Deisher R. A practical guide to the office assessment of substance abuse. Pediatr Ann 1986;15:675.

MacDonald DI. Drugs, drinking and adolescents. Am J Dis Child 1984;138:117.

MacDonald DI, Blume SB. Children of alcoholics. Am J Dis Child 1986;140:750.

Schonberg SR, ed. Substance abuse: a guide for health professionals. American Academy of Pediatrics/Pacific Institute for Research and Evaluation, 1988.

Schwartz RH, Cohen PR, Bair GO. Identifying and coping with a drug using adolescent: guidelines for pediatricians and families. Pediatr Rev 1985;7:133.

Semlitz L, Gold MD. Adolescent drug abuse: diagnosis, treatment, and prevention. Psychiatr Clin North Am 1986;9:455.

Zarek D, Hawkins JD, Rogers PD. Risk factors for adolescent substance abuse: implications for pediatric practice. Pediatr Clin North Am 1987;34:481.

*Principles and Practice of Pediatrics, Second Edition.*
edited by Frank A. Oski et al. J. B. Lippincott Company, Philadelphia © 1994.

# CHAPTER 31
# *School Health*

## Catherine D. DeAngelis

The health of children directly affects their ability to learn, and the idea of providing some level of health services in schools is not new. The earliest school health programs emerged in response to the demographic, social, and economic conditions of the late 1800s and early 1900s. These programs often provided the only primary care received by immigrant children and those newly relocated into the nation's growing urban areas. Between 1891, when the first school health officer was appointed in Boston, and 1910, approximately 300 cities in the United States implemented school health programs. This was a remarkably swift adoption of a social innovation.

In most of these school programs, the key caregivers were nurses who provided a broad range of primary care and preventive services consistent with the state-of-the-art health care during this period. Despite the dedication of the nurses, many of these programs failed to prosper, and the provision of primary care health services in schools became rare. Over the years, school health became limited to screenings for vision, hearing, and general nutrition; recording of immunization histories; and overseeing children's return to school after illnesses.

The types of health care provided in the schools were curtailed because limited funds had to be used primarily for direct education resources and because of the increased supply of community providers. These community physicians provided little support for the direct provision of health services in schools because they could provide continuity of care to children in their private offices. Moreover, the idea that school children are healthy became a pervasive theme.

American school-aged children are remarkably healthy. Medical, social, and economic programs have contributed significantly to a decline in infectious and nutritional illnesses that formerly were the leading causes of morbidity and mortality in this age group. However, a significant number of acute and chronic physical and emotional illnesses still occur in children 5 to 18 years of age. For example, by the age of 15, about 10% of children have significant cardiac or renal problems; asthma and allergies occur in about 15% of children; about 40% have had surgical interventions; and more than half have been hospitalized at least twice.

The more subtle and perhaps more intractable developmental, behavioral, and emotional problems have become more evident in recent years. More than 4 million American school-aged children are enrolled in special education programs serving mentally or emotionally handicapped children and those with pronounced vision, hearing, orthopedic, or multiple special needs. According to federal law, states must provide appropriate public education to all handicapped children between the ages of 3 and 21 years, regardless of the severity of their disabilities or their families' abilities to pay for these services. At the local level, school districts must offer individualized instruction and related supporting services, including health services to these children.

Adolescents in middle and high schools have many health problems that affect their education, including substance abuse, sexually transmitted diseases, pregnancy, serious injuries, and poor nutrition. All of these topics are discussed in detail elsewhere in this book. Many of the behaviors leading to these problems can be affected by health education in the schools. Because of this and because realistic access to health care by school age children remains a problem in many areas, school health programs, especially for adolescents, have had a resurgence during the past decade.

## ROLE OF THE PEDIATRICIAN

Each state is responsible for enacting and enforcing regulations for school health. At the state level, 24 departments of education and 12 departments of health have the primary regulatory responsibility for school health services. In the remaining 14 states, more than one agency is involved. However, in 45 states, local boards of education have the primary responsibility for conducting health programs and in only 5 states does it rest with the local health departments.

There are about 16,000 school districts in the United States, and they spend more than 1 billion dollars annually on health services. They employ approximately 30,000 school nurses, and an unknown number of physicians participate in school health services.

The major role of the pediatrician in schools is to act as the child's advocate. The community-based or any available pediatrician can provide invaluable direct or indirect services to the school administrators, teachers, school nurses, and parents. School personnel can represent a wonderful resource for the pediatrician. Teachers and school nurses frequently identify problems and recommend medical intervention. Their insight to the child's behavior can be invaluable in determining the problem affecting the child. Their roles can extend far beyond routine screening and monitoring immunizations.

About 17% of the pediatricians in the United States are involved in some form of school health services. Many serve as the official athletic team physician, perform routine athletic physicals, consult with school nurses, assist in establishing health and safety guidelines for school personnel, or are members of the school board. Schools play a vital role in the lives of children, and health professionals can exert much influence on health curricula and attitudes by devoting a relatively small amount of time to this community service.

## SCHOOL HEALTH SERVICES

The types of school health services in which a pediatrician can and should exert influence and provide some intervention include physical, behavioral, or emotional educational and administrative issues.

### Physical Services

The traditional physical health services provided in schools are immunization monitoring and screening for problems that directly affect the child's ability to learn, including vision, hearing, and gross nutrition (usually weight and height); scoliosis and blood pressure screening have been added in some schools. The pros and cons of screenings are discussed elsewhere in this book. The pediatrician is often called on to intervene when a child scores abnormally on one of these screening tests. He or she must decide the appropriate management of the child and should use the school personnel to assist as much as possible. For example, if a child fails the vision screening, the pediatrician should first be sure the test results are accurate. If they are, the pediatrician should arrange for the child to receive corrective lenses or whatever treatment is appropriate. The school personnel should be aware that the child requires the lenses so they can assist by making sure the child wears them in classes.

Every state has a law prohibiting a child from attending school if he or she has not received certain immunizations, which usually include diphtheria, pertussis, tetanus, polio, rubeola, and rubella vaccines. Mumps immunization is required in a few states. Because by law a child must attend school until 16 years of age, the states indirectly mandate immunization for public health reasons. This law is an excellent way to assume control of certain communicable diseases that previously caused significant morbidity and mortality in children. A pediatrician assists in this process by ensuring that every child in his or her practice has received appropriate vaccines. The prekindergarten visit should be used to assess the child's readiness for school. A variety of developmental screening tests, discussed elsewhere in this text, can be used. Various investigators have identified specific signs associated with later school failure, including finger agnosia, poor impulse control and attention span, difficulty with using a pencil, inability to recognize letters and numbers, poorly established eye or hand dominance, and delayed laterality.

Attempts at early recognition of potential deviations raise the problem of labeling. If care is not taken to explain to the parents that no single test or sign can predict achievement and potential with certainty, the child may perform poorly because of the parents' expectations. If sufficiently concerned that the child is not ready for school, the pediatrician should seek the advice of a specialist in this area.

For many children, the significance of the ritual physical examination before entering school annually lies in reminding parents that the child has not seen the pediatrician in a year, except perhaps for an acute illness. The physician's examination of a child who has an ongoing source of care by one provider usually reveals little of significance beyond continuing growth. However, the visit should be used to address developmental and behavioral issues pertinent to the child's age.

Although routine school physical examinations may be considered repetitious for children who have continuity of medical care, they can uncover significant physical problems in children who have had poor access to medical care. In one study (De-Angelis, 1983), school physical examinations revealed 52 problems per 100 physical examination contacts. Moreover, 99% of these problems could not have been revealed by routine screenings, and 83% of the problems were previously unknown. These examinations were conducted in the schools on children who had had poor access to medical care, and they were performed as carefully as they could have been in a private office. No matter how healthy the child appears, a ritualistic, superficial examination before signing a school health report or sports permission record cannot be condoned.

In the best of all possible worlds, each child should have a pediatrician who provides high-quality care in a private office or clinic. Until this happens, the school may serve the health care needs.

## Emotional or Behavioral Services

A common reason for parents to seek the counsel of their physician is their child's underachievement or poor behavior in school. In many cases, parents have been encouraged by school personnel to have the child evaluated.

Reasons for a child's underachievement or poor behavior include unrealistic expectations by the parents or teachers, mis-

management of education, family problems causing stress, lack of motivation, chronic or acute physical illness, sensory deficits, subnormal intelligence or other handicapping problems, and psychologic problems. Some of these causes can be assessed by complete histories and physical examinations, including screening for hearing and vision. If results of these tests are normal, psychometric and psychologic evaluations may be indicated to evaluate the child's intellectual capacity and functioning. This aspect of the child's evaluation and management of these and other problems, including chronic truancy and school phobias, are discussed elsewhere in this text.

It is important for the pediatrician to retain the role of primary medical advocate for the child and to continue to assist the parents and teachers in the child's management, even though consultants or subspecialists may provide care for one specific problem.

## Educational and Administrative Services

If they make themselves available, physicians are frequently called on to provide education in the schools. Health education can take the form of speaking to the staff about common health issues that occur in schools, speaking to parent–teacher groups, or speaking directly to students. This commitment demands time, but much of it can occur over a few evenings each year. If the physician has children in school, it can be combined with a regularly scheduled parent–teacher meeting.

Some pediatricians assist teaching staffs in developing a health manual specific to the needs of the school. This assistance need not take much time, and it is a one-time commitment that usually requires only minimal annual updating. It is a nice way for the community physician to establish close communication with schools. It also can be invaluable in evaluating and managing children from the pediatrician's own practice.

Some pediatricians serve as paid or unpaid consultants to the school nurse in the community. This service has the potential for a significant time commitment and liability. However, if the service is needed because of difficulty in access to medical care—as occurs in some rural and densely populated, inner city areas—the school board or local health department should provide appropriate reimbursement.

Another role for pediatricians is to serve on school or Head Start boards. Much influence can be exerted on the general environment in which the school-aged child spends abundant time. For example, injuries, which account for much of the morbidity in school-aged children, can be prevented by careful inspection and repair or alteration of items in the playground, gymnasium, and other school areas.

Another aspect of potential influence is the emotional environment in the school. Many schools allow or condone corporal punishment, threats, insults, and condemnation of students. The pediatrician can encourage a more positive approach to foster learning in a peaceful environment. For example, some school systems have been able to reduce absenteeism from 33% to 2% by using praise or other rewards for perfect attendance. This praise and reward system in some schools has also resulted in decreased school vandalism, which costs school districts about 500 million dollars annually.

Pediatricians can influence the lives of school children in many ways besides providing for their medical needs in offices or clinics. The types of school health activities in which pediatricians can be involved include services to young athletes, consultations with school nurses, providing health education in the schools, serving on Head Start boards, serving as the designated school physician, and evaluating children with developmental disorders. These activities can be rewarding. They are the roles of a good pediatrician and a good citizen.

## Selected Readings

Committee on School Health. School health assessments. Pediatrics 1991;88:649.

DeAngelis C, Oda D, Berman B, et al. The comparative values of school physical examination and man screening tests. J Pediatr 1983;102:477.

Krugman R, Krugman M. Emotional abuse in the classroom: The pediatrician's role in diagnosis and treatment. Am J Dis Child 1984;138:284.

Meeker R, DeAngelis C, Berman B, et al. A comprehensive school health initiative. Image J Nurs Sch 1986;18:86.

Newton J, ed. School health: A guide for health professionals. Evanston, IL: American Academy of Pediatrics, 1987.

*Principles and Practice of Pediatrics, Second Edition.*
edited by Frank A. Oski et al. J. B. Lippincott Company, Philadelphia © 1994.

## CHAPTER 32
# Emergency Medicine

## 32.1 Emergency Medicine Except Poisoning

### Paula J. Schweich

Physicians in pediatric emergency departments or clinics care for children with a broad range of illnesses, from mild, nonurgent problems to life-threatening emergencies. The care of ill and injured children defines a new and growing pediatric specialty: pediatric emergency medicine. Physicians and nurses in this field provide resuscitation, stabilization, diagnosis, and initial treatment of children with the entire spectrum of pediatric illnesses and injuries. Most diagnoses are related to infection and trauma, and many visits are by children younger than 3 years of age. This chapter examines the common life-threatening pediatric emergencies.

## CARDIOPULMONARY RESUSCITATION IN CHILDREN

Most pediatric cardiopulmonary arrests occur in young, previously healthy children. Every attempt should be made to identify the cause of the arrest, because special considerations may affect treatment. The most common causes are listed in Table 32-1. Trauma is the leading cause of cardiopulmonary arrest in children 1 to 14 years of age.

In many patients, hypoxemia from respiratory obstruction or failure causes sinus bradycardia followed by cardiac arrest. In the case of an acutely ill or injured child, the rescuer may be able to prevent respiratory and circulatory arrest with the correction of hypoxia alone.

### TABLE 32-1. Common Causes of Cardiac Arrest

| Cause | Circumstances |
|---|---|
| Traumatic | Motor vehicle injuries, burns, child abuse, firearm wounds |
| Pulmonary | Foreign body aspiration, smoke inhalation, near drowning, respiratory failure |
| Infectious | Epiglottis, sepsis, meningitis |
| Central nervous system | Head trauma, seizures |
| Cardiac | Congenital heart disease, myocarditis |
| Other | Sudden infant death syndrome, poisoning, suicide, dehydration, congenital malformations |

Children who have delayed resuscitation or present in asystole have a poor prognosis, because hypoxemia has already caused extensive damage to the brain and other vital organs. Survival is more likely if cardiopulmonary resuscitation (CPR) is started immediately, there is respiratory arrest only, the arrest is witnessed in the hospital, there is extreme bradycardia rather than asystole, or oxygen is the only necessary drug.

Because many causes of arrest in children are preventable and because elapsed time until initial resuscitation is such an important factor in survival, special efforts should be made in prevention and prehospital care.

### Basic Life Support

The goals of life support are to optimize cardiac output and sustain tissue oxygen delivery; most important are the metabolic demands of the myocardium and brain. Basic life support should begin immediately after discovery of the arrest victim.

When first encountering a child who appears unresponsive, assess the adequacy of airway, breathing, and circulation. If the child is an accident victim who may have a neck injury, stabilize the neck with axial traction or a Philadelphia collar. Gently shake and call to the victim to determine if he or she is unresponsive or having respiratory difficulty. If conscious, allow the child to position his or her own airway; the child automatically assumes the best position. Position an unconscious child on a firm surface. When moving or turning the child, move the head and neck as a single unit. If a neck injury is not suspected, place a hand on the forehead and tilt the head back to a neutral position. Overextension of the neck obstructs the trachea. The fingers of the other hand are placed under the lower jaw at the chin to lift the chin off the airway. For further movement of the jaw, the rescuer's hands are placed on both sides of the victim's head, using the palms to tilt the head back, and two or three fingers are placed at each mandibular angle to lift the jaw upward (ie, jaw thrust). If a neck injury is suspected, use the jaw thrust without a head tilt.

After the airway is opened, the rescuer should simultaneously look at the chest wall and abdomen for movement, listen over the mouth and nose, and feel with his or her cheek for airflow. If the child is not breathing and the airway is in the correct position, the rescuer must breathe for the victim. The rescuer can cover the mouth and nose of an infant with his or her mouth or pinch closed the nose of an older child and breathe mouth to mouth. In successful mouth-to-mouth breathing, chest movement is visible. If unsuccessful, try to reposition the head and check for a foreign body in the mouth or pharynx.

TABLE 32-2.  Basic Life Support

| Patient | Respirations Per Minute | Compressions Per Minute | Depth (Inches) | Where to Compress |
|---------|------------------------|-------------------------|----------------|-------------------|
| Infant (<1 year) | 20 | 100 | 0.5–1.0 | Place index finger below intermammary line; press with middle and ring fingers |
| Child (>1 year) | 15 | 80 | 1.0–1.5 | Place middle and index fingers at base of sternum; place heel of hand above that and use for compression |

The airway of a child is easily obstructed by aspiration of small objects, such as removable parts of toys, hard candies, popcorn, peanuts, mucus, blood, vomitus, or the tongue. Initially, the child coughs and gags, but if the obstruction is complete and the airway cannot be cleared, the child loses consciousness. The rescuer should attempt to relieve the obstruction only if the child's cough is weak and ineffective and the respiratory difficulty is increasing.

If aspiration is witnessed or strongly suspected or if an unconscious victim has airway obstruction that cannot be relieved by head tilting and jaw thrust maneuvers, the rescuer should attempt to remove the object manually only if it is visible on careful inspection. Blind finger sweeps may push a foreign body further into the airway and should be avoided.

The Heimlich maneuver, a subdiaphragmatic abdominal thrust, produces an artificial cough and is considered safe for children older than 1 year of age. With the child supine, the heel of the hand is placed in the midline between the umbilicus and rib cage and pushed rapidly inward and upward. This maneuver can be repeated 6 to 10 times. It is not performed in a child younger than 1 year of age because of concern for intra-abdominal injury. Alternating back blows (ie, four blows between the scapulae) and chest thrusts (ie, four compressions as in CPR) is recommended.

As the rescuer is assessing and treating the airway and breathing, the adequacy of circulation is assessed by checking the pulse of a large artery, such as the carotid, brachial, or femoral. If no pulse is found, chest compressions are started immediately. In a small infant, the rescuer can encircle the baby's chest with both hands, support the back with the fingers, and compress the sternum with both thumbs. As in the adult, a child's heart lies under the lower third of the sternum, and compressions should be performed over this area. The compression phase should be 50% of the cycle.

Chest compressions and ventilation are coordinated at the rate of five compressions to one ventilation. The compressions are delayed for ventilation. Table 32-2 outlines breathing and circulation requirements for basic life support. The patient should be reassessed 1 minute after resuscitation begins and again every few minutes.

## Advanced Cardiac Life Support

When a child arrives in the emergency department, basic life support should be in progress. An initial assessment by the emergency physician includes state of consciousness, spontaneous respiratory effort, pulse, blood pressure, cardiac rhythm, temperature, perfusion and pupillary responses. In advanced life support, as in basic life support, start by assessing airway, breathing, and circulation.

### Airway and Breathing

Mouth-to-mouth resuscitation provides at most 17% of the fraction of inspired oxygen in advanced cardiac life support. Humidified 100% oxygen should be administered to the patient immediately on arrival at the hospital or sooner if possible. The bag, valve, and mask setup, later to be converted to bag, valve, and endotracheal tube, should deliver 100% oxygen and be equipped with a manometer and pressure-relief valve. Table 32-3 lists the differences between the two types of resuscitation bags. While equipment for intubation is being prepared, the bag and valve should be fitted to a clear plastic mask that allows for an airtight seal against the child's face and a small rebreathing volume. The soft circular masks seal well, and clear masks allow the physician to observe the color of the child and see any vomitus. An oropharyngeal airway in an unconscious child or a nasopharyngeal airway in a conscious child helps keep the tongue forward during mask ventilation. To determine the size of the oropharyngeal airway, place the airway next to the face. With the flange at central incisors, the tip of the airway should be at the angle of the mandible.

Intubation should be performed as soon as possible if the patient continues without spontaneous respirations or if prolonged ventilation is needed. Intubation provides better ventilation, higher oxygen concentration delivery, protection against aspiration, and the ability to give positive end expiratory pressure to the patient.

The pediatric airway is more flexible than the adult airway, the tongue is relatively larger, and there is an anatomical narrowing at the level of the cricoid cartilage, precluding the necessity of using a cuffed endotracheal tube. An endotracheal tube of

TABLE 32-3.  Resuscitation Bags

| Bag | Gas Filled | Oxygen Concentration | Pop-off Valve | Comments |
|-----|-----------|---------------------|---------------|----------|
| Self-inflating | Refill independent of gas flow | 50% to 60% (higher with reservoir) | Not necessary | Easy to use |
| Anesthesia | Refill depends on gas flow from source | Same as source | Necessary | Overfills easily; can transmit high pressure to lungs |

appropriate size is chosen, and one size larger and smaller should be available. If a stylet is used, its tip should be 1 to 2 cm proximal to the end of the endotracheal tube. Figure 32-1 outlines the formula for determining endotracheal tube sizes.

Before intubation, the patient should be preventilated with 100% oxygen by means of a bag, valve, and mask setup, and suction should be easily accessible. During use of the bag, valve, and mask and during intubation, an assistant should apply pressure to the cricoid cartilage, using the thumb and forefinger, to push the esophagus up against the cervical spine. This decreases inflation of the stomach and the risk of aspiration. The mouth and pharynx are suctioned immediately before intubation. The tip of a straight blade is placed under the epiglottis and lifted, or a curved blade is placed into the vallecula, the glottic opening is visualized, and the endotracheal tube is placed between the cords.

If ventilation is interrupted for more than 20 seconds or the heart rate drops below 60 beats per minute, mask ventilation should be resumed before another intubation attempt. As soon as the endotracheal tube has been placed, the bag and valve are attached for hand ventilation until a ventilator is available. After checking for symmetric chest movement and auscultation, the tube is secured at the mouth, and the position is confirmed by a chest radiograph.

### Circulation

While an airway is being secured, other members of the resuscitation team should be securing intravenous access and monitoring pulse and cardiac rhythm. The patient is placed on a hard surface, and chest compressions are performed if there is no pulse. Intravenous access is crucial for drug and fluid administration, but it is often difficult to achieve in a child with poor circulation. A peripheral intravenous line is usually difficult to place during an arrest, and placing a central line in the neck area interferes with resuscitation. The preferred methods for access are femoral vein catheterization, greater saphenous vein cutdown, or intraosseous vascular access. An intraosseous infusion is often the easiest and quickest method of access to the circulation, and it is recommended for children younger than 3 years of age. The method is outlined in Table 32-4.

Possible causes of the patient's arrest are considered before administering intravenous fluids. Patients with acute blood loss, shock, or dehydration may require vigorous volume replacement; those with head trauma or hypernatremic dehydration may be further harmed by overzealous fluid administration. Rapid volume expansion is best accomplished with isotonic crystalloid solutions, such as lactated Ringer's solution or normal saline until colloid such as blood, fresh frozen plasma, or human serum albumin is available.

### Drugs

A variety of drugs are used to correct hypoxemia, reverse acidemia or increase coronary and cerebral perfusion pressure. The goal is to restore spontaneous circulation and stabilize the child's cardiac rhythm.

Asystole and sinus bradycardia account for 90% of arrhythmias in pediatric patients in arrest. Because primary cardiac disease is a rare cause of cardiac arrest, other ventricular arrhythmias are uncommon.

$$\text{Inside diameter} = \frac{16 + age \text{ (years)}}{4}$$

Newborn, 3.0 to 3.5 Inside diameter (mm)

Figure 32-1.   Formula for determining the size of endotracheal tubes.

---

| TABLE 32-4.   Intraosseous Infusion |
| --- |
| Choose site: tibia, 1 to 2 cm below tibial tuberosity on flat anteromedial surface. |
| Clean site with an antiseptic. |
| If patient is awake, inject skin with 1% lidocaine. |
| Insert needle with stylet (18-gauge spinal needle or large-bore, 13-gauge, bone marrow needle) at 15° to 30° angle *away* from epiphyseal plate. Use screwing or boring motion until needle penetrates into marrow, noted by decreased resistance. |
| Remove stylet; aspirate into saline-filled syringe. |
| Flush with saline to check placement, even if there was no aspirate. Check for swelling around site. |
| Attach intravenous tubing. |

The preferred route of administration of drugs during resuscitation is intravenous bolus or infusion. If there is a delay in establishing intravenous access, epinephrine, lidocaine, or atropine may be given through the endotracheal tube. For endotracheal administration, the drug should be diluted to 5 to 10 mL, pushed in rapidly, and followed by five positive pressure breaths. All drugs and fluids may be given by intraosseous infusion. Intracardiac injection has serious risks and is used only as a last resort. Table 32-5 lists drugs, and Figure 32-2 displays protocols for cardiac arrest and arrhythmias. Recent research indicates that the use of a higher dose of epinephrine (0.2 mg/kg) may improve the resuscitation rate and long-term survival.

Ventricular arrhythmias may occur in patients with congenital heart disease, myocardial disease, chest trauma, or drug ingestions. Ventricular fibrillation is treated with electrical defibrillation, which causes asynchronous depolarization of the myocardium. If it is not possible to defibrillate immediately, the physician should try to correct hypoxemia and acidosis while setting up the defibrillator. If the rhythm is fine ventricular fibrillation, an intravenous dose of epinephrine and calcium is given to convert the rhythm to coarse ventricular fibrillation, which is more easily converted with defibrillation.

Pediatric paddles are available in 4.5- and 8.0-cm sizes. Use the largest paddle size that allows the entire paddle surface to contact the chest wall. One is placed to the right of the sternum under the clavicle, and the other is placed on the left anterior axillary line at the level of the xiphoid (ie, apex). The electrode–skin interface can be electrode paste or cream or saline-soaked pads; care is taken to apply interface only under the paddles. Bridging causes a short circuit. Alcohol pads can cause burns and should never be used as the interface.

The initial dose for defibrillation is 2 J/kg. Subsequent doses are doubled. Stop if the rhythm converts out of ventricular fibrillation. If three shocks do not correct the rhythm, CPR should be resumed with drugs, and the patient should be assessed again for acidosis, hypoxemia and hypothermia.

If the monitored rhythm is ventricular tachycardia and the patient is symptomatic, the patient undergoes cardioversion, which is a timed depolarization of myocardial cells and therefore different from defibrillation. The synchronizer circuit must be activated, and the dose is 0.25 to 2.0 J/kg. A lidocaine infusion is started.

Frequent reassessment, including body temperature, is mandatory during any resuscitation.

## PEDIATRIC TRAUMA

A serious pediatric health problem in the United States, trauma is the leading cause of mortality for children older than 1 year of age, accounting for approximately 25,000 deaths each year.

### TABLE 32-5.  Resuscitation Drugs

| Drug | Action | When Used | Route | Dose | Side Effects |
|------|--------|-----------|-------|------|--------------|
| Humidified oxygen | Improves arterial tension | Arrhythmias arrest | Mask ET tube | Highest FIo$_2$ possible 100% (adjust with Pao$_2$ later) | |
| Epinephrine | Vasoconstriction ($\alpha$) | Asystole | IV | 0.01 mg/kg (0.1 mL/kg of 1:10,000) | Tachycardia; VE; excessive vaso-constriction |
| | Inotropy ($\beta$) | Hypotension unresponsive | ET tube | 0.02 mg/kg (0.2 mL/kg of 1:10,000) | |
| | Chronotropy ($\beta$) | Convert fine to coarse, VF for DC defibrillation, bradycardia unresponsive to atropine | IV | start 0.1 $\mu$g/kg/minute¶ and titrate | |
| Sodium bicarbonate* | Reverse metabolic acidosis | Asystole (if acidotic); metabolic acidosis in arrhythmias | IV | 2 mEq/kg under 2 y (½ strength under 6 mo); can repeat every 10 min<br>1 mEq/kg over 2 y; further doses based on BD: mEq bicarbonate $= \dfrac{BD \times kg\ body\ wt \times 0.4}{2}$ | Hypersomolality; CSF acidosis; IVH in premature infants |
| Atropine sulfate | Accelerates sinus or atrial pacemaker | Asystole; symptomatic sinus bradycardia (hypotension, poor perfusion) | IV | 0.02 mg/kg (min, 0.16 mg/max, 2 mg) | |
| | Increases AV conduction | Vagally mediated bradycardia (intubation); sinus bradycardia with PVCs | ET tube | Same dose | |
| Calcium† | Increases myocardial contractile force | Hypocalcemia<br>Hyperkalemia<br>Hypermagnesemia<br>Calcium-channel blocker overdose | IV (peripheral) | Calcium gluconate, 30–60 mg/kg, IV (central) calcium chloride, 10–20 mg/kg | Bradycardia, toxicity; |
| Dextrose‡ | Increases blood glucose | Hypoglycemia | IV | 1 g/kg (25% solution) | |
| Dopamine§ | Low dose increases shock unresponsive to fluid resuscitation; increases renal and splanchnic blood flow<br>Intermediate dose stimulates cardiac $\beta$-adrenergic receptors<br>High dose stimulates $\alpha$-adrenergic receptors | Hypotension | IV | Start at 1 $\mu$g/kg/min# and titrate | Tachycardia; vasoconstriction; VE |
| Lidocaine | Decreases automaticity depressant | VF, VT<br>Sustained VA | IV<br>IV | 1 mg/kg<br>20–50 $\mu$g/kg/min** (with bolus) | Myocardial VT |
| Isuprel‖ | Increases HR, conduction velocity, and cardiac contractility | Symptomatic bradycardia | IV | 0.1–1.0 $\mu$g/kg/min¶ | Tachycardia |
| Bretylium tosylate | Prolongation of refractory period | VF, VT | IV | 5–10 mg/kg followed by defibrillation | Nausea, vomiting, postural hypotension |

*AV*, atrioventricular; *BD*, base deficit; *CSF*, cerebrospinal fluid; *DC*, direct current; *ET*, endotracheal; *HR*, heart rate; *IV*, intravenous; *IVH*, intraventricular hemorrhage; max, maximum; min, minimum; *PVC*, premature ventricular contraction; *VA*, ventricular arrhythmia; *VE*, ventricular entropy; *VF*, ventricular fibrillation; *VT*, ventricular tachycardia.

* Use sodium bicarbonate only after adequate ventilation has been established; otherwise, it causes a worsening respiratory acidosis.

† Calcium is no longer recommended for use during asystole. Calcium chloride is preferable (produces higher and more predictable calcium levels) to gluconate, but central line is needed for calcium chloride because it is sclerosing.

‡ Use glucose (dextrose) in any arrest situation. Poor glycogen stores and starvation predispose infants and children to hypoglycemia.

§ Low doses, 2–5 $\mu$g/kg/min; intermediate doses, 5–10 $\mu$g/kg/min; high doses; 15–20 $\mu$g/kg/min.

‖ Because of its $\alpha$-adrenergic activity, epinephrine is preferable to isuprel for patients in asystole.

¶ Preparation of infusion: 0.6 × kg body wt = mg added to 100 mL diluent; then 1 mL/h delivered 0.1 $\mu$g/kg/minute.

# Preparation of infusion: 6 × kg body wt = mg added to 100 mL diluent; then 1 mL/h delivered 1.0 $\mu$g/kg/min.

** Preparation of infusion: 120 mg added to 100 mL diluent; then 1 mL/kg/h delivered 20 $\mu$g/kg/min.

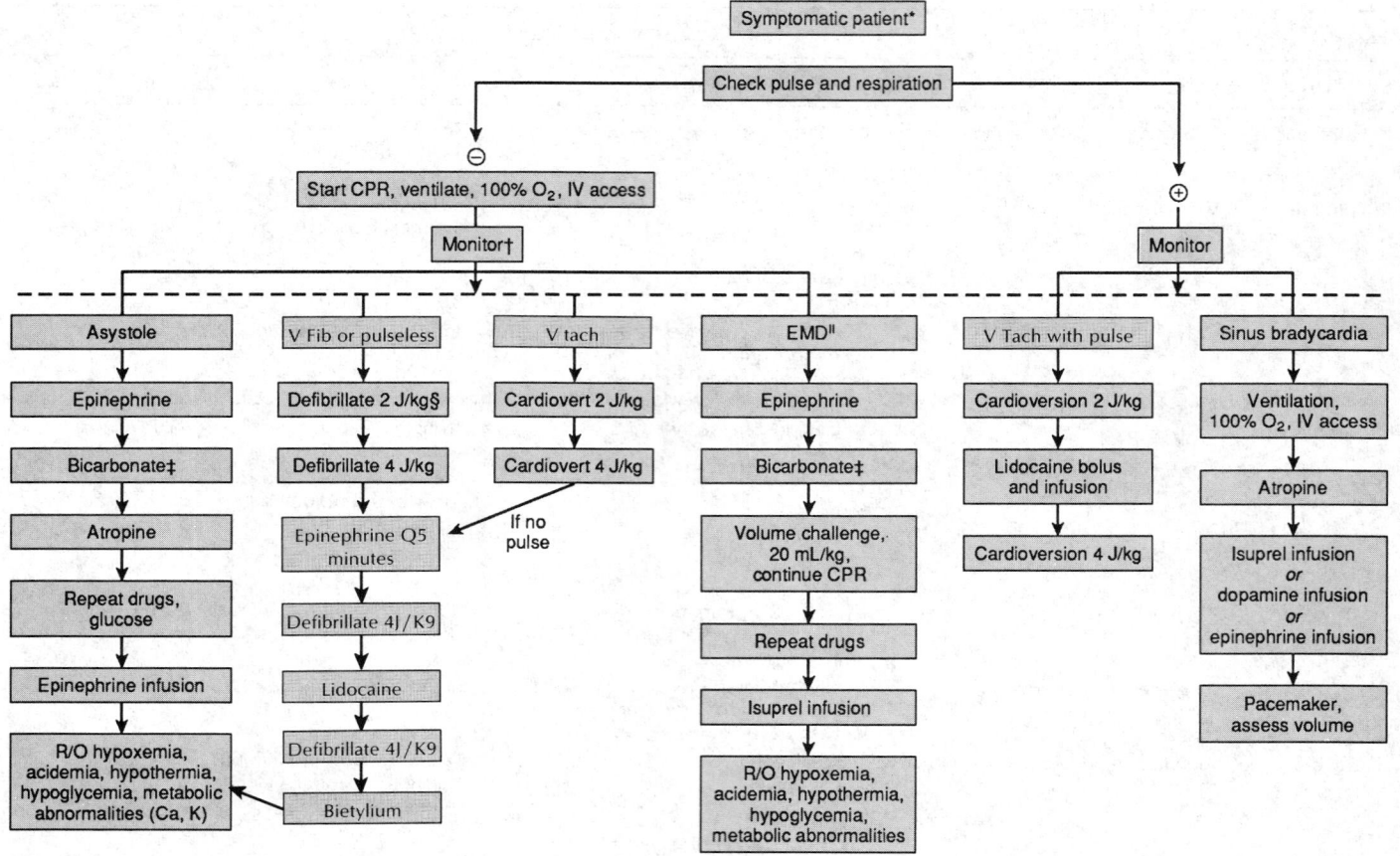

**Figure 32-2.**    Resuscitation protocols. *CPR,* cardiopulmonary resuscitation; *EMD,* electromechanical dissociation; *IV,* intravenously; *R/O,* rule out; *V fib,* ventricular fibrillation; *V tach,* ventricular tachycardia.

Motor vehicles are involved in more than half of pediatric trauma cases in which the child is a passenger or a pedestrian. As passengers, children are easily thrown; as pedestrians, they are vulnerable because of their smallness, quickness, and poor judgment. Other common causes of serious trauma are falls, drownings, and burns.

Trauma can be considered a disease that has host, agent, and environmental factors. The child host or victim is particularly vulnerable because of developmental limitations, curiosity paired with new motor skills, and a generally high level of activity. Each age group has its own set of common injuries. A child's world offers a constant supply of traumatic agents. In addition to motor vehicles, other common agents are bicycles, furniture, swimming pools, and household poisons. The most common environment is the child's own home, where he or she spends the most time. The danger of this environment correlates closely with parental factors, such as income, education, and psychologic stresses, and other stresses on the child.

Most childhood trauma is mild. Lacerations are the most common injury, followed by contusions, fractures and dislocations, ingestions, and bites. Approximately 90% of life-threatening injuries are from blunt trauma, in which multiple and occult organ injuries are common, and head trauma often is involved. These children often die of shock, respiratory obstruction, or brain stem damage. The child is occasionally a victim of penetrating trauma, such as a gunshot or stab wound.

When a child trauma victim is evaluated and treated, the unique anatomy and physiology should be considered, because they frequently create special problems. The head of a child is especially vulnerable in trauma, because it is proportionately larger relative to body mass than that of an adult and because it is not well supported by strong neck muscles. Head trauma occurs in more than 80% of severely injured children. Because of the elasticity of the child's chest wall, rib and sternal fractures are rare, and an intact chest wall can mask severe crush injuries to the heart and lungs. The liver and spleen are less well protected by the chest wall than other structures. The poorly developed abdominal muscles offer little protection for the viscera, including the kidneys and bladder. Because children with stress and screaming swallow a large amount of air, gastric distention is common and may impair diaphragmatic function.

The unique physiology of a child has advantages and disadvantages in trauma. Most injured children have been healthy and have large cardiac and pulmonary reserves. The brain and heart of a child can tolerate longer periods of hypoxia than those of an adult. Because of a reactive vascular system, the child can compensate for a 15% to 20% blood loss without a drop in systolic blood pressure. However, this apparently normal blood pressure can mask poor tissue perfusion. A child's metabolic status can change rapidly, requiring close observation of acid–base status and glucose level. The high ratio of body surface area to weight and small amount of subcutaneous fat greatly affect the child's ability to regulate core temperature. Hypothermic patients are more difficult to resuscitate.

## TABLE 32-6.  Trauma Surveys

| Primary Survey | Resuscitation | Secondary Survey |
|---|---|---|
| Airway maintenance with cervical spine control<br>Breathing<br>Circulation with hemorrhage control<br>Disability—alert, verbal, painful, unconscious<br>Expose—undress patient | Oxygenation<br>Shock therapy<br>Vital signs<br>Monitoring—electrocardiogram, nasogastric catheter,* urinary catheter* | Head and skull—pupils, fundi, vision, injury<br>Maxillofacial trauma<br>Neck—films, pulses, crepitation<br>Chest<br>Abdomen, perineum, rectum<br>Extremities—pulses, fractures<br>Neurologic examination—Glasgow Coma Scale<br>Radiographs, laboratory tests |

* If not contraindicated.

Committee on Trauma, American College of Surgeons. Advanced trauma life support course, instruction manual, 1989.

The key to decreasing morbidity and mortality from trauma is in prevention, particularly focusing on the environment. Because initial care is critical, improving emergency medical services and field treatment should improve the outcome for these unfortunate children.

## Multiple Trauma

When the injured child arrives in the emergency department, a quick initial assessment is performed to determine the level of care required. *Multiple trauma* is defined as injury to more than one organ system, major injury of one organ system from blunt trauma, multiple fractures, a deep penetrating wound of the trunk, or any trauma resulting in unstable vital signs. *Localized trauma* involves one region of the body. All trauma is multiple until proven otherwise. The nature of the injury, blunt or penetrating, and the severity of the injury are assessed in this initial triage. Various injury rating scales, including the Modified Injury Severity Scale, the Abbreviated Injury Scale, and the Injury Severity Scale, are designed to assess the clinical severity of injuries based on anatomical and physiologic measurements. They are useful in triage, treatment, planning, and prediction of morbidity and mortality.

### Initial Assessment and Treatment

The priorities in treating a patient with multiple trauma are to preserve or restore vital signs and to correct life-threatening injuries. Early, aggressive treatment in an organized fashion can greatly reduce morbidity and mortality. A systematized approach allows efficient diagnosis and treatment of life-threatening injuries without oversight of less serious injuries. To establish treatment priorities, the patient is assessed in a rapid primary survey. Any resuscitation that has begun during the primary survey is continued in the resuscitation phase. After resuscitation, the patient is thoroughly evaluated in the secondary survey, and plans are made for definitive care (ie, advanced trauma life support).

In the *primary survey* (Table 32-6), the airway is the first priority, with careful attention paid to possible cervical spine injury. The airway can be stabilized with in-line manual traction or a rigid Philadelphia cervical collar. After the airway is secured, breathing is assessed, and if necessary, mechanical ventilation is begun. Observe chest movement to assess any obvious abnormality impeding ventilation, such as a tension pneumothorax, open pneumothorax, or flail chest. Circulation is assessed by checking femoral or dorsalis pedis pulses, skin color, and capillary refill. Advanced cardiac life support should be initiated immediately for asystole. Blood pressure is not checked in the primary survey. Any obvious bleeding should be stopped with direct

pressure. Level of consciousness and pupillary responses indicate the neurologic status or disability. Using the AVPU mnemonic device, notice if the patient is *a*lert, responsive to *v*erbal stimuli, responsive to *p*ainful stimuli, or *u*nconscious. A full Glasgow Coma Scale (Table 32-7) assessment is done later. Life-saving measures are begun if a problem is identified during the primary survey. The patient is completely undressed, and the temperature is measured.

Treatment of life-threatening injuries is continued during the *resuscitation phase* (see Table 32-6). All multiple-trauma patients are given oxygen. Shock management is begun with the insertion of two large-bore intravenous lines. For shock, the pneumatic antishock garment (PASG) may be applied and used with intravenous fluid resuscitation. The child is monitored with electrocardiographic (ECG) leads.

A nasogastric tube is inserted unless a cribriform plate fracture is suspected in blunt head trauma. A midfacial fracture or cerebrospinal fluid (CSF) leaking from the ears, nose, or mouth may indicate this fracture. An orogastric tube can be inserted. A Foley catheter is inserted unless urethral transection is possible. In these

## TABLE 32-7.  Glasgow Coma Scale

| Observation | Response | Score |
|---|---|---|
| Eye opening | Spontaneous | 4 |
|  | To verbal command | 3 |
|  | To pain | 2 |
|  | None | 1 |
| Best verbal response | Oriented | 5 |
|  | Confused | 4 |
|  | Inappropriate words | 3 |
|  | Incomprehensible words | 2 |
|  | None | 1 |
| Best motor reponse | Obeys command | 6 |
|  | Localizes pain | 5 |
|  | Withdraws from pain | 4 |
|  | Flexion to pain (decorticate) | 3 |
|  | Extension to pain (decerebrate) | 2 |
|  | None | 1 |
| Total |  | 3–15 |

Modified from Mayer T, Matlak ME, Johnson DG, et al. The modified injury severity scale in pediatric multiple trauma patients; J Pediatr Surg 1980;15:719.

### TABLE 32-8.    Normal Vital Signs in Children

| Patient | Upper Pulse Limit | Lower Systolic BP Limit | Upper RR Limit |
|---------|-------------------|-------------------------|----------------|
| Infant | 160/min | 80 mm Hg | 40/min |
| Preschooler | 140/min | 90 mm Hg | 30/min |
| Adolescent | 120/min | 100 mm Hg | 20/min |

BP, blood pressure; RR, respiratory rate.

cases, a rectal examination must be performed before insertion of a catheter. If there is blood at the urethral meatus or a scrotal hematoma, a urinary catheter is not put into place before further diagnostic studies.

Success of resuscitation is repeatedly assessed by checking ventilation, pulse, blood pressure, urinary output, and arterial blood gases. Keep returning to the assessment of airway, breathing, and circulation.

A complete physical examination is performed in the *secondary survey* (see Table 32-6). Each area of the body should be completely visualized, palpated, and auscultated if appropriate. The cervical spine films are ordered, if not already done, with other appropriate radiographic and laboratory studies. After this examination is completed, the definitive care is begun.

### Definitive Care

*Airway and Breathing.*  Airway management is performed, always attempting to stabilize the neck. If any possibility exists of a cervical spine injury, the neck can be stabilized with in-line traction or a Philadelphia collar. If the child is breathing spontaneously but has signs of obstruction, open the airway with a chin lift or jaw thrust and suction it. An oral or nasopharyngeal airway may be all that is needed. Oxygen therapy is continued. If possible, cervical spine films are obtained before intubation. If not, orotracheal intubation is performed while another rescuer holds the neck stable. Intubation and ventilation are performed as described previously in the CPR section.

Emergency needle cricothyroidotomy is rarely necessary in children, but it may be needed if there is severe maxillofacial trauma or intubation proves impossible. A 14-gauge catheter-over-needle can be inserted through the cricothyroid membrane into the trachea.

If ventilation is compromised, examine the chest for tension pneumothorax, open pneumothorax, hemothorax, or flail chest. These conditions are often obvious on physical examination. Needle thoracostomy or chest tube placement may lead to immediate improvement in ventilation.

*Circulation.*  Because the early presentation of shock can be subtle in a child, the physician must be familiar with the normal vital signs of children at different ages (Table 32-8).

A child with major blood loss may present with only tachycardia but not be far from the more classic signs of shock, including cool extremities, poor capillary refill, altered sensorium, and low urinary output. Decreased systolic blood pressure and metabolic acidosis are late signs of shock.

Support of the circulation is easier in a child than in many adults, because children usually have normal cardiovascular systems before injury. Percutaneous lines are usually sufficient. A femoral venous percutaneous line or saphenous vein cutdown is useful when intravenous access is difficult, and central lines are of value in major trauma without reliable access or in an unstable patient. In a patient with abdominal trauma, an upper extremity vein is preferred in case abdominal vascular integrity is interrupted.

Patients in hemorrhagic shock require 300 mL of electrolyte solution for every 100 mL of blood loss. Blood loss can be estimated as shown in Table 32-9. Fluid resuscitation is initiated with an isotonic crystalloid solution, 5% dextrose in lactated Ringer's solution, or normal saline. The initial volume is 20 mL/kg given as a fluid bolus, which may be repeated. If the child does not respond to two fluid pushes, an ongoing serious blood loss is probably occurring, and blood or blood products should be administered as shown in Table 32-10.

Maintenance requirements must be added to the ongoing resuscitation fluids. The patient needs continual observation and reevaluation. Signs of improvement include clearing of the sensorium, decreased heart rate, warmth of extremities, faster capillary refill, increased urinary output, and increased blood pressure.

Resuscitation of a child in shock may be facilitated by the use of the PASG. Applied to the legs and abdomen and inflated, this garment translocates venous blood from the lower extremities and abdomen and increases peripheral venous resistance. It can be used to stabilize femoral or pelvic fractures and to tamponade intra-abdominal hemorrhage. The garment can be used for patients in shock with concomitant head trauma; the only absolute contraindication to the use of the PASG is pulmonary edema. These trousers are often applied in the field; if they are to be used, careful instruction in their application and removal is important. Sudden removal can produce a severe drop in blood pressure.

*Laboratory.*  If trauma is minimal and physical examination results are normal, a urinalysis is necessary to rule out injury to the genitourinary system. For multiple-trauma patients, the minimal laboratory studies include type and crossmatch of blood, complete blood count (CBC), electrolytes, amylase, blood urea

### TABLE 32-9.    Estimated Blood Loss

| Class | Blood Loss (%)* | Pulse | Blood Pressure | Perfusion Pressure | Capillary Blanch Test | Mental Status |
|-------|-----------------|-------|----------------|--------------------|-----------------------|---------------|
| I | 15 | Normal | Normal | Normal | Normal | Slightly anxious |
| II | 20–25 | Slightly ↑ | Normal | ↓ | + | Anxious |
| III | 30–40 | ↑ | ↓ | ↓ | + | Confused |
| IV | 40–50 | Nonpalpable | ↓↓ | ↓ | + | Lethargic |

\* Estimated blood volume is 80 mL/kg.

Adapted from Committee on Trauma, American College of Surgeons. Advanced trauma life support course, instruction manual, 1989.

**TABLE 32-10.    Blood Product Administration**

| Product | Volume (mL/kg) |
| --- | --- |
| Whole blood | 20 |
| Packed erythrocytes | 10 |
| Plasma | 20 |
| 5% human serum albumin | 20 |
| 25% human serum albumin | 4 |

*Adapted from Eichelberger MR, Randolph JG. Pediatric trauma: An algorithm for diagnosis and therapy. J Trauma 1983;23:91.*

nitrogen (BUN), creatinine, and urinalysis. Radiographs should include the lateral cervical spine, chest, abdomen, and pelvis. Other laboratory and radiologic studies are dictated by the history and physical examination. Commonly, special x-ray studies such as a liver–spleen scan, computed tomography (CT) scan, and arteriography are indicated.

## Head Trauma

### Initial Assessment and Treatment

Although central nervous system injury is the most common cause of pediatric traumatic death, most head trauma in children is blunt and mild. The initial evaluation includes a history of the force involved, any loss of consciousness and its duration, and a check of current vital signs and level of consciousness. Place a cervical collar if cervical spine injury is suspected.

As in any injured patient, the physical examination starts with the primary survey, including airway, breathing, and circulation evaluation and the beginning of necessary resuscitation. Particular attention should be paid to the blood pressure and pulse. A high blood pressure or low pulse may indicate increased intracranial pressure. If increased intracranial pressure is suspected, the patient should be immediately paralyzed with medications, intubated, and hyperventilated.

The Glasgow Coma Scale (see table 32-7), indicating the level of consciousness, is the most important part of the neurologic examination. The scale is useful in evaluating and following the child and in predicting immediate and future outcome. A Glasgow Coma Scale score less than 5 is associated with a high probability of mortality or permanent neurologic sequelae. Children with scores of at least 6 have a better prognosis.

After evaluation of level of consciousness, a complete neurologic examination is performed, including examination of pupils and cranial nerves. Pupillary inequality or eye deviation may herald impending herniation.

A more thorough physical examination includes palpation of all scalp wounds to determine depth of injury and possible depression of bone and signs of blood indicating a basilar skull fracture, including raccoon eyes, battle ears, and hemotympanum.

Skull films are rarely useful in the evaluation of head trauma in children because they are usually negative. They have a higher yield if restricted to children with at least one of the following criteria: age less than 1 year, a history of unconsciousness for at least 5 minutes, a penetrating wound, lethargy, a palpable depression, signs of a basilar skull fracture, or focal neurologic signs. Many of these children receive a CT scan, obviating the need for skull films.

### Definitive Care

If a child has a penetrating wound, radiologic evaluation and local exploration by a surgeon is necessary. If the inciting object is protruding from the wound, do not remove it because it may

be lodged near a critical area or tamponading a source of bleeding. These objects must be removed surgically.

If there is minor head trauma with a Glasgow Coma Score of 15 and a normal neurologic examination and cranial CT, the child may be observed at home for changes in mental status, vomiting, and gross motor ability.

A child with loss of consciousness for less than 5 minutes, indicating a concussion, may need hospital admission for close observation. If there is deterioration of the Glasgow Coma Scale score or focal neurologic abnormalities, a CT scan is obtained to look for an intracranial hemorrhage. Magnetic resonance imaging may be more sensitive than CT in detecting traumatic brain damage. Children with a longer period of unconsciousness, deteriorating examination results, or focal signs are at risk for major and sudden decompensation and need immediate treatment to reduce intracranial pressure. This treatment is outlined in Table 32-11.

A high intracranial pressure causes physical distortion of the brain and decreases cerebral perfusion pressure, preventing sufficient substrate from getting to the brain tissue. The three substances in the cranium—brain, blood, and CSF—normally are balanced, keeping intracranial pressure below 15 mm Hg. If the cause of increased intracranial pressure can be determined, therapy can be more specific. A CT scan helps determine whether there is a surgically treatable mass lesion, such as a hematoma, or diffuse cerebral swelling. This diffuse swelling is usually a result of increased cerebral blood volume and is best treated with hyperventilation. Barbiturate therapy and hypothermia can decrease cerebral blood flow by decreasing brain metabolism. If the primary problem is increased water content, mannitol is helpful, and if there is a high CSF volume, CSF can be drained.

If significant head injury and shock coexist, the shock is not due to the head injury and must be treated with vigorous fluid resuscitation, despite fears of increased intracranial pressure.

## Thoracic Trauma

Thoracic trauma can cause multiple threats to a child's life. More than 90% of thoracic trauma in children is blunt, resulting from motor vehicle injuries and falls. The injury from blunt trauma may be obvious, such as a tension pneumothorax, or more subtle, detected only during a careful physical examination. Penetrating trauma from a gunshot or stab wound usually causes significant damage, and penetrating wounds must be surgically explored.

### Initial Assessment and Treatment

The initial evaluation starts with a history of the force, an assessment of vital signs, and a primary survey. Air hunger, cyanosis, tachypnea, and anxiety are signs of ventilatory insufficiency. Retractions and stridor occur with partial upper airway obstruction. If the child is not moving air well, look for airway obstruction, open pneumothorax, tension pneumothorax, or flail

**TABLE 32-11.    Initial Treatment of Increased Intracranial Pressure**

Intubation with in-line traction of cervical spine*
Hyperventilation (Pco₂, 20–25 mm Hg) and oxygenation
Dexamethasone, 0.5–1.0 mg/kg IV
Mannitol, 0.25–0.5 g/kg IV†
Fluids, ⅔ maintenance‡
Computed tomography scan as soon as possible.

\* Obtain cervical spine films first, if possible.
† If herniation is suspected.
‡ If there is accompanying shock, start full fluid resuscitation.

chest. If shock exists, massive hemothorax, cardiac tamponade, and myocardial contusion must be considered. If evidence exists of a pneumothorax, a needle thoracostomy is performed, followed by placement of a chest tube. A chest tube is the initial treatment for a hemothorax. If respiratory distress continues, the patient is intubated.

If no immediate evidence exists of a major injury to the chest, a more careful physical examination, including inspection, palpation, and auscultation, is performed. Chest radiography, ECG, and arterial blood gas measurement may provide clues to other serious but less apparent injuries. For example, a widened mediastinum on x-ray film indicates the possibility of aortic rupture, necessitating an emergency aortogram. Mediastinal air may indicate tracheobronchial tree rupture. Arrhythmias are signs of myocardial contusion. Poor oxygenation and ventilation could be the result of significant ventilation–perfusion mismatch in a severe pulmonary contusion.

### Definitive Care

Patients with penetrating trauma that enters only the superficial tissues or with mild blunt trauma may be discharged from the emergency department if no other serious injuries are detected. Management of other injuries is summarized in Table 32-12.

## Abdominal Trauma

Like head and thoracic trauma, abdominal trauma in children is usually blunt and mild; most cases are due to motor vehicle injuries and falls. If the injury is penetrating, moderate or severe injuries are expected. Children with multiple trauma and severe neurologic impairment are at higher risk for intra-abdominal injury than those without coma.

### Initial Assessment

The history and primary survey precede the abdominal examination. If no resuscitation measures are necessary and the abdomen is an area of suspected injury, proceed with the abdominal examination. An accurate abdominal examination is often difficult to obtain because of an uncooperative child producing a falsely tight abdomen or because of an unconscious child producing falsely negative examination results. In a young, alert child, it is important to establish rapport before examining the abdomen and to examine the painful area last. As in a healthy child, look, listen, and lastly palpate. There may be injury to the genitourinary tract, spleen, gastrointestinal tract, liver, pancreas, or pelvis.

### Treatment

If the injury is mild, with only superficial tenderness or abrasions, the patient needs only a rectal examination and urinalysis. These patients can usually be discharged from the emergency department with reassurance.

In a more severe injury indicated by abdominal tenderness, guarding, and perhaps distention, the patient needs an intravenous line; diagnostic laboratory tests such as CBC, amylase, and type and crossmatch of blood; radiography; and observation. A child with a splenic or hepatic laceration may present with abdominal tenderness, guarding, and normal vital signs.

A severely ill child suffering from abdominal trauma may present in shock from bleeding, and the abdominal palpation may not be helpful. This patient needs surgery.

Patients with penetrating wounds to the abdomen need an intravenous line placed above the diaphragm, urinalysis, type and crossmatch of blood, CBC, BUN, amylase, and radiographs of the abdomen and chest. Patients with the possibility of free blood in the abdomen need peritoneal lavage, unless abdominal surgery is imminent. Other indications for lavage are lethargy or coma with abdominal injury, thoracic injury with suspected abdominal injury, or equivocal diagnostic findings. Before lavage is performed, an nasogastric tube and urinary catheter are placed unless contraindicated.

## Extremity Trauma

Care of the extremities is not part of the primary survey and resuscitation, except for control of major hemorrhage. During the secondary survey, the extremities are examined for perfusion,

### TABLE 32-12. Life-Threatening Thoracic Injuries

| Injury | Physical Examination Findings | Initial Treatment |
|---|---|---|
| Airway obstruction (eg, foreign body, secretions, severe maxillofacial trauma) | Decreased or no air movement (ventilatory insufficiency) | Suction, jaw thrust, chin lift, oropharyngeal/ nasopharyneal airway intubation |
| Open pneumothorax | Open wound in chest | Cover hole with occlusive dressing |
| | Ventilatory insufficiency (if large, air passes through hole with each respiration) | Chest tube through another site |
| Flail chest* (ie, multiple rib fractures) | Paradoxic motion of segment of chest wall | Turn patient onto affected side to stabilize flail |
| | | Intubate if ventilatory failure |
| Massive hemothorax | Decreased health sounds | Volume resuscitation |
| | Dull to percussion | Chest tube |
| | | Surgery |
| Tension pneumothorax | Decreased breath sounds | Needle aspiration |
| | Tracheal deviation | Chest tube |
| | Shift of point of maximum impulse | |
| | Hyperresonance | |
| Pericardial tamponade | Shock | Pericardiocentesis |
| | Distended neck veins | Surgery |
| | Decreased pulse pressure | |
| | Muffled heart tones | |

* Because the thoracic cage is very compliant in children, significant pulmonary contusion may be present without rib fractures. Flail chest is usually combined with lung contusion and ventilation–perfusion mismatch.

deformity and function. If not treated promptly, combined vascular and bone injuries can result in limb loss.

### Initial Assessment

The history indicates the severity of trauma and any prehospital care. The mechanism of injury, environment including possible contamination, and predisposing factors such as underlying illness and previous injuries should alert the physician to the severity of the injury. The person accompanying the patient should know if there was extensive bleeding, deformity, and spontaneous movement of the injured extremity. A history of tetanus prophylaxis can be obtained after the acute care.

After the limb is exposed, look for any angulation or shortening, swelling, bruising, or wounds. Feel gently for tenderness, crepitation, and signs of peripheral perfusion such as pulse, capillary refill, and warmth. Examine for sensation. A stable fracture, not evident on inspection, may have ecchymosis, crepitation, and point tenderness. Check for active and passive motion. If indicated, obtain appropriate radiographs. Neurovascular and musculoskeletal integrity may be compromised by penetrating trauma, by a compartment syndrome from blunt trauma, by dislocations, and by fractures.

### Treatment

Definitive care restores alignment and peripheral perfusion. All dislocations involving loss of pulse should be reduced immediately and arteriography performed if the pulse is not restored to prevent limb loss. All fractures are immobilized by splinting or traction. Immobilization is the best treatment for pain, but pain medication may be needed. As for any trauma patient, intravenous analgesics should be used sparingly. Open wounds should be debrided of gross contamination and covered with sterile dressings. Tetanus prophylaxis is administered if indicated.

## Wound Care

Wound care begins with a careful history of when, where, and how the injury occurred. The type of wound, the amount of contamination in the wound, and the delay until treatment determine the management. Other important history includes tetanus immunization status, allergies (especially to local anesthesia), bleeding disorders, and medications.

The initial examination determines the extent and severity of the visible lesion, where it is located, and the condition of the pulse and sensation distal to the injury. Check if there are any obvious associated injuries to nerves, muscles, tendons, vessels, or bones at the wound site or elsewhere.

**TABLE 32-13.  Sedatives and Analgesics**

| Drug | Dose | Route* |
|---|---|---|
| **Sedatives** | | |
| Midazolam | 0.1–0.2 mg/kg | IV, IM, PR |
| Diazepam | 0.05 mg/kg | IV |
| Chloral hydrate | 25–75 mg/kg | PO, PR |
| Pentobarbital | 2–4 mg/kg | IM, PO |
| **Analgesics** | | |
| Meperidine | 0.5–1.0 mg/kg | PO, IV, IM, SC |
| Morphine sulfate | 0.05–0.1 mg/kg | IV, SC, IM |
| Fentanyl | 1–2 µg/kg | IV |

*IM, intramuscularly; IV, intravenously; PO, orally; PR, per rectum; SC, subcutaneously.

**TABLE 32-14.  Local Anesthesia With Lidocaine**

| Approach | |
|---|---|
| Rule out allergy to lidocaine. | |
| Document sensation distal to injury. | |
| Topical anesthesia: ethyl chloride spray | |
| Inject 1 cm away from wound edge (if clean wound, can inject through wound margin). | |
| Lidocaine concentration | |
| Infants | 0.25–0.5% |
| Children | 0.5–1.0% |
| Lidocaine dose | 7 mg/kg (max) with epinephrine* |
| | 3–5 mg/kg without epinephrine |
| Onset | 5 min |
| Duration | 90–200 min |

* Do not use epinephrine for end organs, such as digits, ears, nose, or genitalia.

In young children, especially those younger than 3 years of age, restraint and sedation may be necessary for proper examination and repair of a wound. A papoose board is used to restrain a child. Sedatives, analgesics, and their doses are listed in Table 32-13. Combinations of a sedative, narcotic, and tranquilizer are not recommended, because they may cause oversedation and persist for an extended period.

Gently wash the wound and surrounding area with soap and water or dilute iodine solution and shave if necessary before injecting local anesthesia (Table 32-14). Lidocaine with epinephrine is used unless the wound is on the digits, nose, ears or genitalia. The liquid topical anesthetic TAC (ie, tetracaine, adrenaline [epinephrine], and cocaine) is a safe and effective method for anesthetizing minor lacerations of the skin (Table 32-15). Fingers and toes are most easily anesthetized with a digital block. When anesthetized, the wound can be properly washed and irrigated using a large needle and syringe, any devitalized tissue debrided, and irregular edges excised.

Explore the wound for injuries to deep tissues and structures, and remove any foreign bodies. If there is doubt about the presence of a foreign body, particularly glass, obtain appropriate radiographs.

Wounds should not be sutured if 12 hours have elapsed since injury. Face wounds may be sutured after a 12-hour delay. Other "dirty" wounds, such as animal bites and deep punctures, should not be immediately sutured; delayed primary closure may be possible after 4 or 5 days. If in doubt, leave the wound open. Surgical tape may be used in wounds partially through the dermis where there is no stress on the edges; this tape is not to be used

**TABLE 32-15.  TAC Solution***

To prepare:
  Cocaine, 6.0 g
  Adrenalin 1:1000, 25 mL
  Tetracaine, 250 mg
  Bring to 50-mL volume with sterile water, and put in 5-mL aliquots.
To use:
  Apply to sterile cotton ball, place on wound and tape for 10–15 minutes. Avoid eyes, mouth, and end organs.

* TAC = 0.5% tetracaine, 1:2000 adrenalin (epinephrine), 12% cocaine.

over joints or any area where the wound edges will be pulled apart. Extensive wounds to the face, hand, perineum, or genitals or a wound in combination with a fracture should be seen in consultation with a surgeon.

Absorbable suture material, such as Vicryl or chromic gut, is used to close the subcutaneous tissues in a deep wound and to avoid leaving dead space in the depth of the wound. The skin is closed with nonabsorbable suture, such as nylon, silk, or polypropylene. For suturing wounds, use the smallest suture needed to proximate the edges, use small stitches placed close together, approximate edges but allow room for edema, and evert the wound edges. A dressing is applied to absorb blood and to protect, compress, and immobilize the area. The first layer of the dressing should be nonadherent, with an absorbent material overlying it, wrapped with a bulky immobilizing dressing. Extremities should be elevated and ice applied during the first 24 hours.

Most patients with wounds do not need antibiotics. If the wound is more than 18 hours old before treatment or shows signs of infection, antibiotics should be prescribed for a short course. The patient is seen again in 24 to 48 hours to check the wound for healing and signs of infection. Sutures are removed from the face in 2 to 4 days, scalp in 5 days, extremities in 7 to 10 days, and joints in 10 to 14 days.

## BITES

Human and nonhuman animal bites are common among children. More than half of these bites are not serious, but certain initially innocuous-looking bites can lead to serious infectious complications. Dog bites account for about 90% of nonhuman bites that require medical attention, and cat bites account for almost 10%, with rodent and rabbit bites composing the remainder.

Most wounds are colonized by mixed aerobic and anaerobic organisms obtained from the skin of the victim and the oral cavity of the biter. An average infected wound yields three to five organisms on culture, with the highest estimate from human bites. The most common organisms in all bite wounds are *Staphylococcus aureus*, *Streptococcus* sp., anaerobic cocci, and *Bacteroides* sp. Dog and cat bite wounds commonly carry *Pasteurella multocida* and *Pseudomonas fluorescens*. Another coagulase-positive staphylococcal species, *Staphylococcus intermedius*, a common flora and pathogen of dogs, has recently been identified in dog bite wounds. *Eikenella corrodens* is frequently isolated from human bites. The *S aureus* and up to one half of the *Bacteroides* sp. have β-lactamase activity. Brook (1987) found that 40% of the wounds had at least one organism with β-lactamase activity.

### Assessment

The history and examination of the bite indicates how serious the injury and potential complications are. What bit the child? Most human bites in young children are inflicted by other children and are superficial. Adolescents may sustain hand bite injuries from striking another person on the teeth. Dogs have strong jaws and are capable of producing large crush injuries. Cats have small, sharp teeth that can penetrate into deeper tissues, increasing the chance of infection. The mechanism of injury, whether it is a puncture or crush, and the lapse of time from the injury to the examination are other factors influencing treatment. Wounds more than 12 to 24 hours old are more likely to become infected. On physical examination, notice carefully the location of the wound, the extent and depth, and whether there are any signs of infection.

### Management

After initial care, most children with bite wounds can be managed as outpatients with careful follow-up. Cleansing, irrigation, and careful debridement reduce the incidence of infection. The area around the wound should be cleansed with povidone iodine solution that has a wide antibacterial and antiviral spectrum. This treatment is followed by forceful irrigation with normal saline through a 19-gauge needle attached to a large syringe. This high-pressure irrigation is more effective in reducing bacterial counts than soaking. After local anesthesia, all visible devitalized tissue is debrided, and the wound is checked for foreign matter and injuries to tendons, joints, and bones. Irrigation is repeated.

Larger injured areas on extremities and wounds over joints are immobilized and elevated. Tetanus toxoid is given if indicated, and rabies prophylaxis is considered, depending on the animal species and area. In the United States, the animals most commonly infected with rabies are skunks, raccoons, and bats, but other animals, including dogs and cats, may be infected. A final decision about whether to treat a potentially exposed patient can be made in conjunction with the local health department. Treatment consists of thorough local wound care and passive and active immunoprophylaxis. Human rabies immune globulin is given as soon as possible to cover the time during which the patient has insufficient active antibody production. The dose of 20 IU/kg is given half into the wound and half as an intramuscular injection. At the same time, active immunization is begun with human diploid cell vaccine; 1 mL is given intramuscularly on days 1, 3, 7, 14, and 28. If the biting animal is found to be uninfected, treatment is stopped.

The patient is asked to return within 48 hours to check the wound, at which time any infection should be apparent by redness, swelling, tenderness, or drainage. Initial cultures of wounds do not predict subsequent infection.

Prophylactic antibiotics are probably useful for patients with wounds at a high risk for infection. High-risk wounds are identified by their location and nature and include all cat and nonsuperficial human bites, dog bites more than 8 hours after injury, hand wounds, deep puncture wounds, and wounds with the potential of delayed primary closure, as discussed in the section on wound care. Simple lacerations and face and scalp bites, unless sutured, have a low risk of infection and generally do not need prophylaxis.

Although penicillin and ampicillin provide the best coverage for *P multocida*, they do not cover *S aureus* and many *Bacteroides* isolates. Amoxicillin with clavulanic acid (Augmentin) covers all the common organisms. An alternative includes the use of penicillin in combination with a penicillinase-resistant penicillin or cephalosporin. Erythromycin can be used for patients with penicillin allergy. Additional therapy of infected wounds is guided by Gram stain and culture results.

If the wound is uninfected and seen within 8 hours of injury, it can be sutured or closed with wound tape. Primary closure does not increase the incidence of infection unless it is a hand wound, a human or cat wound, or a deep puncture wound. Human and cat wounds can be packed with gauze soaked in an antibacterial agent, and sutured in 4 to 7 days if there is no sign of infection.

All wounds that are infected or are more than 24 hours old are initially left open. Wound cultures for aerobic and anaerobic organisms should be obtained if the wound appears infected. If the bite is small and in a cosmetically acceptable area, it is left to heal by granulation and secondary intention. If it is a large wound or in a cosmetically important area, the wound can be packed with gauze and an antibacterial agent and can be seen again in 4 to 7 days for delayed primary closure if it is uninfected at that time. If this approach is planned, culture specimens should be taken and the child given antibiotics.

Facial wounds can be sutured up to 12 hours after injury if there is no sign of infection. The face is an area of rich vascularity with decreased risk of infection. Primary closure should be avoided on the hands, particularly in a clenched-fist injury. These wounds can heal by granulation or delayed primary closure.

Bite wounds that have a high incidence of complications and should be seen by a consultant include nonsuperficial or hand wounds older than 8 hours, wounds with extensive infections, severe disfigurement or tissue loss potentially requiring grafting, and wounds in which there is the possibility of tendon, joint, or cartilage injury. Most of these patients require hospital admission.

## BURNS

Burns are a common injury in children, exacting a large toll in terms of loss of function, deformity, pain, and psychologic strain. Burn injuries are classified as thermal (ie, flame, scald, contact, inhalation), electrical, or chemical, including battery burns. Most burned children are younger than 5 years old (average, 2.5 years). Eighty-five percent of these injuries are scalds from hot tap water or liquids spilled from cooking pots. Flame, electrical, and chemical burns are less common.

Burn injuries are responsible for 1300 deaths of children annually (McLoughlin and Crawford, 1985). Most of these deaths result from house fires, in which young children are at greatest risk. Death is usually caused by smoke inhalation rather than surface burns.

### Initial Emergency Treatment

The emergency management of a burn patient starts with removal of all clothing and assessment of airway, breathing, and circulation. Hot or smoldering clothes continue to burn the patient, and synthetic fabrics melt to become hot plastic and may extend the injury. Upper airway edema from smoke inhalation burns or soft-tissue edema of the neck and face may compromise airway patency and breathing. Respiratory status must be quickly evaluated and oxygen applied. Intravenous access is established if there is inhalation injury or if more than 10% to 15% of the body surface area is burned. If there is chemical injury, start copious irrigation with water as soon as possible.

### History

A detailed history of the burn injury (ie, environment of burn, materials burned, clothing worn) and the child's medical history are essential for care. For example, if the burn injury included a fall, explosion, or child abuse, there may be other serious injuries. If the child was in a fire in an enclosed space, smoke inhalation must be considered. If the burn was electrical, extensive damage may exist below the surface of the skin. The medical history, including history of tetanus immunization, guides care.

### Physical Examination

After any resuscitative or emergency management, a complete physical examination is necessary. The extent and depth of burns, hydration status, associated injuries, and neurologic examination determine the plan of management.

The extent of the burn can be roughly estimated using the "rule of nines" shown in Figure 32-3. Another helpful rule for estimating the extent of scattered, irregular burns is that one surface of the patient's hand represents approximately 1% of body surface area. Assessment of depth of burn injuries is illustrated in Table 32-16.

### Laboratory Studies

Laboratory and other studies to consider in the significantly burned patient are CBC, type and crossmatch of blood, carboxy-hemoglobin, electrolytes, BUN, creatinine, albumin and total protein, prothrombin time, arterial blood gas, chest radiograph, and radiographs of associated injuries.

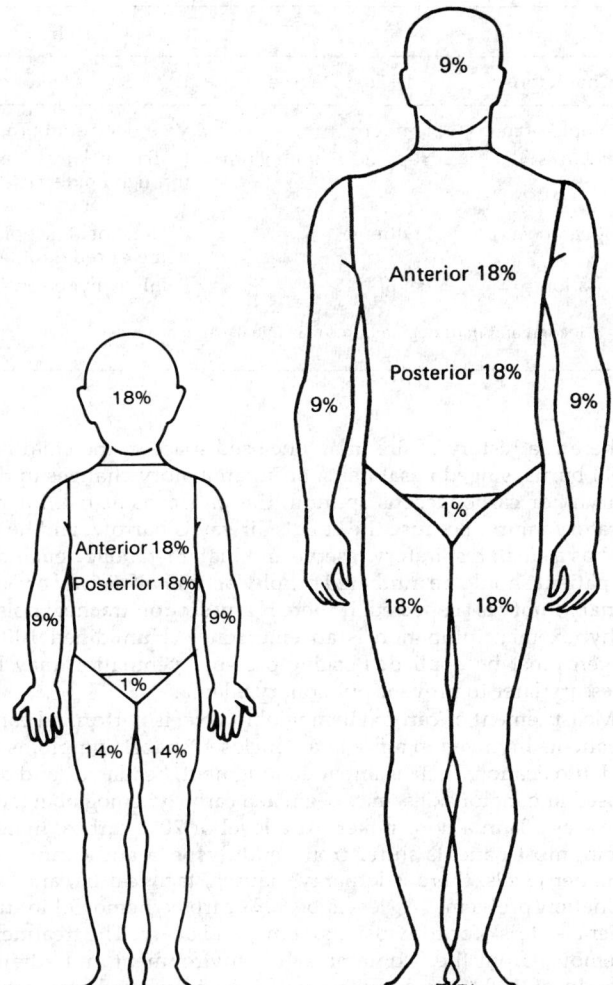

**Figure 32-3.** Rule of nines for child (*left*) and adult (*right*). (Adapted from Scherer JC. Introductory medical-surgical nursing, ed 4. Philadelphia: JB Lippincott, 1986:687.)

## Definitive Treatment

### Airway Management

Patients with inhalation injury have a marked increase in morbidity and mortality. The upper airway is extremely susceptible to swelling and obstruction from exposure to hot, moist air or toxic gases. Direct thermal injury from hot air is unlikely unless the heat is conveyed by steam. The subglottic airway is protected from direct injury by the larynx. Inhalation injury can damage the lower respiratory tract, resulting in pulmonary edema, aspiration pneumonia, and pneumonitis.

In the first 36 hours after an inhalation injury, acute pulmonary insufficiency can result from several different elements in a fire. Most of the damage is caused by toxic gases such as aldehydes, oxides of sulfur and nitrogen, and hydrochloric acid released from combustion. These agents cause atelectasis, pulmonary edema, and direct parenchymal damage. Acute asphyxia results when oxygen is consumed by the fire in an enclosed space. Inhalation of carbon monoxide seriously impairs oxygen delivery to the tissues, because carbon monoxide binds to hemoglobin with 200 to 300 times the affinity of oxygen and shifts the oxyhemoglobin dissociation curve to the left, causing more tissue hypoxia.

Diagnosis of airway or pulmonary injury is often difficult because the patient may initially show little or no respiratory distress.

TABLE 32-16. Depth of Burn

| Characteristic | First Degree | Second Degree | Third Degree |
|---|---|---|---|
| Example of injury | Sunburn | Very deep sunburn, scalds | Fire, prolonged exposure to hot liquids, electricity |
| Thickness | Superficial epithelium | Partial thickness: destruction into but not through epidermis | Full thickness: destruction of skin into hypodermis, death of all skin appendages, involves subcutaneous tissue |
| Appearance | Erythema | Blisters, peeling epidermis, swelling; white or red, mottled; weepy, wet* | Translucent, mottled, waxy white;* leathery, usually dry |
| Sensation | Painful | Painfully hypersensitive to air currents | Painless |

* Second and third degree burns may initially appear similar.

If there is a history of fire in an enclosed space or the child has facial burns, singed nasal hairs, or inflammatory changes in the pharynx or carbonaceous sputum, the patient is at risk for respiratory injury. Because the child's airway is narrow, and he or she has a small respiratory reserve and high metabolic demands, the patient should be intubated prophylactically if airway or pulmonary injury is suspected. If there is any stridor, tracheal noise, or hypoxemia, intubation is an emergency. Humidified 100% oxygen must be applied. Positive-pressure ventilation may be necessary later to prevent pulmonary edema.

Measurement of carboxyhemoglobin level is performed early in patients involved in a fire in an enclosed space. Symptoms of mild intoxication, such as impaired judgment, headache, and decreased fine motor skills, may begin at a carboxyhemoglobin level as low as 5% in a nonsmoker. At a level of 20% carboxyhemoglobin, most patients suffer from mild dyspnea and confusion; at higher levels, there is lethargy, nausea, tachycardia, and coordination problems. At levels of 60% carboxyhemoglobin, the patient is at risk for convulsions, coma, and death. The treatment is removal from the ''contaminated'' environment and administration of 100% oxygen. The half-life of carboxyhemoglobin decreases from approximately 4 hours in room air to less than 1 hour in 100% oxygen. Treatment with hyperbaric oxygen decreases the half-life even further, and it can be helpful in severely toxic patients. Arterial blood gas measurement is not helpful, because the $PO_2$ is not affected by carboxyhemoglobin.

A chest radiograph is always indicated if inhalation injury is suspected, but it may show no abnormalities in the first 12 to 24 hours after injury. After initial airway management, the patient is observed for pulmonary edema and later observed for bronchopneumonia. The care is generally supportive, because prophylactic antibiotics and steroids are not of proven benefit.

## Fluid Management

If the child is alert, has less than 10% full-thickness or 15% partial-thickness burns, and has no hypoxia or gastric distention, he or she can usually be hydrated orally. Otherwise, at least one large-bore intravenous line must be inserted. Upper extremity placement is preferable to the lower extremity because of a lower incidence of infection and phlebitis in the upper extremities. Careful aseptic technique is crucial, and although the intravenous line can be placed through burned skin, a nonburned area is preferable.

Shock associated with burn injuries is the result of loss of intravascular volume into the burn wound. Water, sodium, and protein are lost and should be replaced. Controversy exists about the volume and composition of fluids to be administered. Two formulas for volume replacement are shown in Table 32-17.

The problem encountered with a weight-related formula is that the ratio of body surface area (BSA) to weight changes with growth. A formula based on weight would tend to underestimate the fluid for a small child with a large BSA–weight ratio and overestimate the fluid for a larger child with a smaller BSA–weight ratio. Any formula, whether based on weight or body surface area, provides only an estimate of required fluids. It is essential to follow hydration status and adjust the fluids accordingly by following the general appearance and sensorium, vital signs, weight, urine output and specific gravity, capillary refill, serum osmolality, electrolytes, and acid–base status.

There are many theories on the proposed use of hypertonic and hypotonic fluids in burn resuscitation. It is easiest to start with an isotonic electrolyte solution, such as lactated Ringer's solution or 5% dextrose in normal saline. If there is more than a 20% BSA burn, it may help to add colloid to the rehydrating solution, because there is intravascular protein loss from increased vascular permeability. This protein loss is most marked in the first 6 to 8 hours after a burn, and 12.5 g of human serum albumin is added to each liter of fluid for the first 24 hours.

### Supportive Care

Because the burn patient has an elevated metabolic rate resulting in increased oxygen consumption, increased urinary nitrogen excretion, and fat breakdown, it is essential to minimize any extra metabolic work. Continuing care involves keeping the room temperature stable at 28 °C to 33 °C, minimizing pain, and supplying adequate calories.

All patients with significant burns should have a Foley catheter inserted to monitor urine output and a nasogastric tube to prevent acute gastric dilation. A physiologic ileus may last 1 or 2 days in a patient with burns over 20% of BSA.

### Wound Care

Full-thickness circumferential burns of the chest or extremities may compromise the child's ability to breathe or decrease peripheral perfusion. If there is decreased chest excursion because of a burn of the chest or decreased distal circulation due to an

TABLE 32-17. Fluid Requirements of Burn Patients During the First 24 Hours After a Burn*

| | |
|---|---|
| By weight† | 3–4 mL/kg body wt/% body surface area burn + maintenance (per weight per 24 hours) |
| By BSA‡ | 5000 mL/m² burned area + 2000 mL/m² body surface area per 24 hs (maintenance) |

* Half of the estimated fluid is given over the first 8 hours after injury, and the rest is administered over the next 16 hours.
† From the Committee on Trauma. American College of Surgeons. Advanced trauma life support course, instruction manual, 1989.
‡ From Carvajal HF. A physiologic approach to fluid therapy in severely burned children. Surg Gynecol Obstet. 1980;150:379.

**TABLE 32-18.  Criteria for Admission of Burn Victims**

Over 10% BSA of full-thickness burn
Over 15% BSA of partial-thickness burn
Serious burns of hands, feet, perineal area, face, joints
Inhalation injury
Other significant injuries or medical problems
Chemical or electrical burns
Suspected child abuse

*BSA*, body surface area.

extremity burn, an escharotomy should be performed immediately. An incision is made across the entire length of the eschar on the medial and lateral side of the limb or both sides of the chest until the sides of the wound separate. No anesthesia is necessary.

The burn surface is a warm, moist, protein-rich environment, and colonization with fungi and bacteria is a constant source of infection. Meticulous wound cleansing and dressing minimizes colonization and infection. With full-thickness burns, later skin grafts survive better on wounds with lower bacterial colony counts.

In initial treatment, cool, wet compresses can be applied to small burns, but they should be avoided on large areas to prevent hypothermia. The burn area is cleaned with a dilute antiseptic soap solution, and broken blisters are debrided. Intact blisters are left intact. Silver sulfadiazine (Silvadene) is the topical agent of choice, because it suppresses bacterial growth but does not prevent healing. It is not used on the face. Tetanus prophylaxis is given if indicated by the history.

If cared for as an outpatient, the child should be bathed twice each day and Silvadene then applied. A burned extremity should be elevated to avoid swelling. Oral penicillin for 3 to 5 days may be helpful in preventing infection of the wound. Broad-spectrum antibiotics are contraindicated. Daily follow-up care is necessary until clean healing is ensured.

### Pain Medications

If the child is anxious or restless and hypoxia is not a problem, analgesics or narcotics may be used sparingly. Morphine (0.1 mg/kg, given intravenously) or Demerol (1 mg/kg intravenously, orally, or intramuscularly) are effective analgesics.

### Criteria for Hospitalization

Table 32-18 lists criteria for admission of burn patients. If a specialized burn center is available, the child should be admitted there.

## Special Burns

Chemical burns are usually caused by acids or alkalis. Alkali burns penetrate deeply and are generally more serious than acid burns. The severity of a chemical burn is influenced by the amount of the agent, the concentration of the agent, and the duration of the contact. Treatment involves extensive irrigation for at least 20 minutes with large amounts of a neutral solution, such as water or normal saline. If the eyes are involved, irrigation should continue while an ophthalmologist is consulted.

Electrical burns range from a lip commissure wound from biting an electrical wire to electrocution from a lightning bolt. Lip commissure burns are frequently more serious than they appear and often involve deeper tissues. As current passes through the body, it may destroy muscles, nerves, and vessels. If an extensive burn is suspected, the patient must be observed with ECG monitoring, intravenous fluids, and general supportive care.

## Prevention

The key to decreasing morbidity and mortality from burn injuries, as in all accidents, is prevention. Burn deaths, caused mostly by house fires, can be prevented by extensive education of parents and children, increased adult supervision of children, and increased use of smoke detectors and sprinklers. Many hot water scald burns can be prevented if water heaters are turned down to 120 °F. Children can help themselves in fires if taught to drop and roll if they are on fire and to crawl under smoke. Many electrical injuries in the home can be prevented by plastic outlet protectors.

## RESPIRATORY DISTRESS

Respiratory distress may result from airway obstruction, pulmonary parenchymal disease, or from processes outside the respiratory system (Fig 32-4).

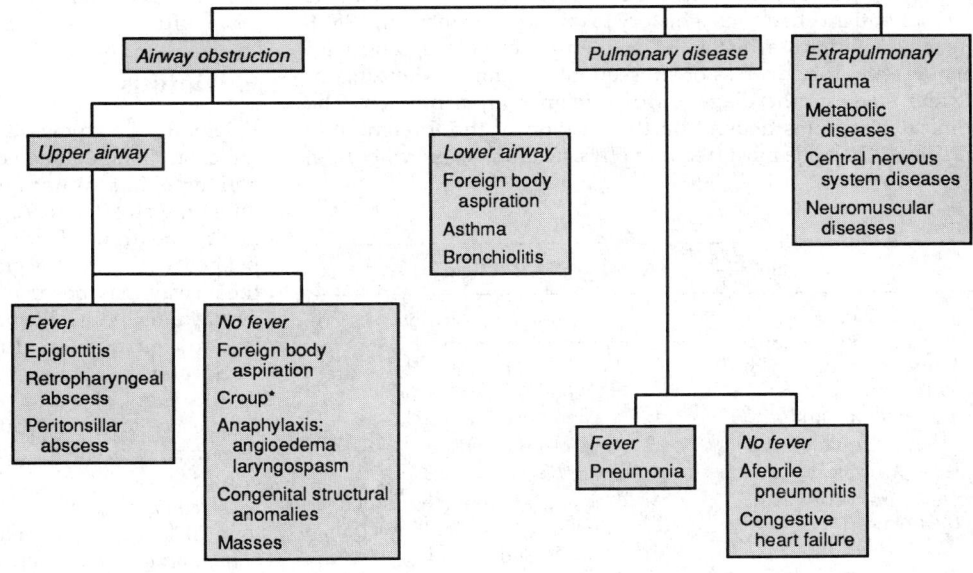

**Figure 32-4.**  Common causes of respiratory distress.

*May have low-grade fever.

Airway obstruction can be divided into upper and lower airway obstruction. The *upper airway* refers to the level above secondary bronchi, and the *lower airway* refers to the peripheral airways, which are usually less than 3 mm in diameter. Lower airway obstruction usually involves a diffuse distribution of obstruction. The differentiating characteristics are listed in Table 32-19.

Upper airway obstruction interferes primarily with inspiration. As upper airway obstruction progresses, a small increase occurs in respiratory rate, and a large increase occurs in respiratory effort, leading to dyspnea. The increased respiratory effort causes an increased negative intrathoracic pressure, manifested by retractions. Stridor, a low-pitched respiratory sound, increases. Complete obstruction above the bifurcation of the trachea causes asphyxia and death.

Lower airway obstruction interferes with expiration of air from the smaller airways, causing the expiratory phase to be prolonged. The turbulent airflow is heard as wheezing. As the obstruction increases, expiration is prolonged, and accessory muscles are used. Wheezing increases as the obstruction progresses, and then decreases as airflow becomes limited.

Foreign body aspiration, epiglottitis, croup, abscesses, asthma, and bronchiolitis are the more common causes of respiratory distress seen in a pediatric emergency department.

## Foreign Body Aspiration

Foreign body aspiration is a significant health hazard in young children, particularly between the ages of 6 months and 3 years. Most foreign bodies that children aspirate are small and, rather than lodging in the trachea and causing acute obstruction and death, pass through the trachea to lodge in a main stem bronchus. These small foreign bodies, usually composed of organic matter, are not immediately life threatening.

### Assessment

The child with foreign body aspiration may present with no history of aspiration and only subtle signs and symptoms, and the diagnosis is frequently missed. With delayed diagnosis, these children may present with recurrent attacks of wheezing diagnosed as asthma, pneumonia, or bronchiectasis. The diagnosis of foreign body aspiration requires a high index of suspicion and should be considered in any child with unexplained pulmonary complaints. A history of sudden onset of coughing while eating or playing with small objects is helpful but not always available; 70% of patients had such a history in one series (Moazam, 1983). In most children, a history of sudden onset of coughing with acute respiratory distress or subsequent coughing, wheezing, or stridor suggests the diagnosis of foreign body aspiration. The clinical symptoms depend on the location of the foreign body (Table 32-20). The most frequent physical findings are wheezing,

| TABLE 32-20. Foreign Body Aspiration | |
| --- | --- |
| Location of Foreign Body | Common Signs and Symptoms |
| Trachea | |
|   Total obstruction | Acute asphyxia, marked retractions |
|   High partial obstruction | Decreased air entry, inspiratory and expiratory stridor, retractions |
|   Low partial obstruction | Expiratory wheezing, inspiratory Stridor |
| Main stem bronchus | Cough, expiratory wheezing, Blood-tinged sputum* |
| Lobar/segmental bronchus | Decreased breath sounds†; wheezing, rhonchi |

\* Usually a later finding.
† Localized to area of lung related to affected bronchus.
*Adapted from Cotton E, Yasuda K. Foreign body aspiration. Pediatr Clin North Am 1984;31:937.*

decreased air movement, and rhonchi, all localized over the lung with the involved airway.

The most helpful supporting tests are inspiratory and expiratory or bilateral decubitus chest radiographs. Persistent air trapping on an expiratory or lateral decubitus radiograph is a common finding in foreign body aspiration. Persistent atelectasis or infiltration are other common findings. The foreign body itself is rarely opaque and therefore rarely visible on the radiograph. The chest film ranges from diagnostic to totally unremarkable. The diagnostic yield may be increased with fluoroscopy, which may show persistent lung inflation during inspiration and expiration.

### Management

If the child presents to the emergency room with no air movement, the Heimlich maneuver or back blows are administered (see CPR section at the beginning of this chapter). Most aspirations are not life threatening, and a thorough history and physical examination can be obtained. If suspicion of a foreign body aspiration is supported by physical examination or radiographs, bronchoscopy is the treatment of choice for its removal. The degree of urgency depends on the location of the foreign body. If the foreign body is in the distal airways, postural drainage and percussion may be helpful.

## Epiglottitis

Epiglottitis, or supraglottitis, is an acute, life-threatening bacterial infection. Cellulitis and edema of the epiglottis, aryepiglottic folds, and hypopharynx narrow the glottic opening. During inhalation, when the structures are sucked inward, there is stridor and difficulty breathing. During expiration, the airway structures are pushed away, and the glottis is opened. If the edema progresses, the airway may become completely obstructed, and an artificial airway must be established immediately. Pulmonary edema may lead to ventilation–perfusion mismatch and hypoxia.

Seventy-five percent of children with epiglottitis are younger than 5 years of age (average, 3.5 years). As many as 25% of affected children are younger than 2 years of age. Although infection may occur at any time, the incidence peaks during the winter.

*Haemophilus influenzae* type b is the etiologic agent in more than 90% of cases of epiglottitis. Other etiologic organisms include *Staphylococcus pneumoniae*, group A streptococci, and rarely, β-hemolytic group C streptococci.

| TABLE 32-19. Airway Obstruction | |
| --- | --- |
| Upper Airway | Lower Airway |
| Interferes primarily with inspiration | Interferes primarily with expiration |
|   Inspiratory stridor |   Expiratory wheeze |
|   Severe retractions |   Mild retractions |
|   Croupy or brassy cough |   Prolonged expiration |
|   Death from complete obstruction |   Hacking and repetitive cough |
| |   Patchy areas of atelectasis from areas of complete obstruction |

## Assessment

The child older than 2 years of age with epiglottitis typically presents with an acute febrile illness of less than 24 hours' duration. He or she may complain of a sore throat and show respiratory distress. On physical examination, the fever is often over 39 °C, and the child appears anxious and toxic. If the airway is compromised, he or she will sit forward with the neck extended and chin forward. The patient may have difficulty swallowing and may be drooling. Respiratory signs include a hoarse cough, tachypnea, inspiratory stridor, retractions, and late cyanosis. If epiglottitis is suspected, the throat should not be examined, and the child is left undisturbed. The clinical presentation of epiglottitis in children younger than 2 years of age is more variable and may mimic viral croup. These young children may have low-grade fever, a history of upper respiratory tract symptoms, and a croupy cough.

The laboratory and radiographs are helpful in the diagnosis of epiglottitis but are not essential early diagnostic tools. A lateral neck radiograph is necessary only if the clinical presentation is not straightforward and the patient is stable. If radiography is indicated, a physician experienced in difficult airway management should accompany the child. The lateral neck radiograph classically shows a thumb-shaped epiglottis and narrowing of the posterior airway. A CBC frequently reveals an increased leukocyte count with a shift to the left. Cultures of the blood and epiglottis, performed in the operating room, often reveal the causative organism, usually *H influenzae*.

## Management

Epiglottitis can be cured with few complications if there is early suspicion and rapid and smooth management. The physician who first sees the child needs to act quickly to prevent complete airway obstruction. If the child is seen at a tertiary care center, immediate involvement of emergency department physicians, an anesthesiologist, an otolaryngologist, and the pediatric intensive care staff is essential. If the child is first seen by a private pediatrician in an office or clinic, available support staff should be contacted and arrangements for transport made. The child should not be transferred without an accompanying doctor equipped to manage the airway.

The child should be allowed to assume the most comfortable position, and oxygen is supplied by mask or blown by the face. The physician or staff must not agitate the patient by restraining him or her, examining the throat, drawing blood, or starting an intravenous line. As soon as possible, the child is transported to the operating room, anesthetized, and intubated. The supraglottic structures are usually inflamed, and culture specimens are taken. Blood can be drawn for culture and CBC, and intravenous antibiotics are given for disease presumed to be caused by *H. influenzae*. If the airway is completely obstructed at any time and intubation is not possible, an emergency cricothyrotomy is performed.

Most cases of sudden death from epiglottitis can be avoided with rapid diagnosis and management. However, some deaths from epiglottitis occur in patients with a rapid course and respiratory obstruction before medical care can be obtained or in patients with secondary complications such as septic shock.

# Croup

Croup, or laryngotracheobronchitis, is a common syndrome involving inflammation or edema of the subglottic area and causing airway obstruction in the larynx, trachea, or bronchi. Croup usually affects children 6 months to 4 years old; the peak incidence is in 1- to 2-year-old children. It occurs all year, but the incidence increases in late fall and winter. There is a slight male predominance.

Most croup is viral, but it may also be spasmodic (ie, allergic) or bacterial. As many as 75% cases of viral croup are caused by parainfluenza viruses; other viruses include respiratory syncytial virus, influenza viruses, and adenovirus. *Mycoplasma pneumoniae* can cause croup.

## Assessment

Viral croup has an insidious onset after a few days of an upper respiratory tract infection. It progresses to hoarseness and the characteristic inspiratory stridor and barking cough. Symptoms wax and wane and are usually worse at night. Oral intake may be decreased.

Spasmodic croup appears as a sudden onset of severe stridor, usually at night, in a well child with no upper respiratory tract infection. The cause is thought to be allergic, but viruses may play a role.

Bacterial croup presents like viral croup but with higher fever and more severe respiratory distress. If the child is intubated, pus is found in the trachea. *Staphylococcus aureus* is the most common organism; *S pneumoniae*, *Streptococcus pyogenes*, and *H influenzae* type b are also isolated. Bacterial croup may be a bacterial superinfection of viral croup.

The child with croup is usually mildly or moderately ill; he or she rarely appears to be toxic. There are usually signs of an upper respiratory tract infection and a low-grade fever. The respiratory examination shows signs of upper respiratory obstruction: inspiratory stridor, suprasternal and intercostal retractions, and an increased respiratory rate. Children with croup have a characteristic barking cough and a hoarse voice.

There are no diagnostic laboratory tests for this illness. A lateral neck radiograph may be helpful to rule out other causes of upper respiratory obstruction, such as epiglottitis, foreign body aspiration, or retropharyngeal abscess. The lateral neck radiograph in croup usually shows a normal epiglottis, subglottic narrowing, and ballooning of the hypopharynx. On a posteroanterior neck view, there is narrowing of the air column at the top, known as the steeple sign.

## Management

Most children with croup can be managed as outpatients with a cool mist vaporizer or shower mist and careful observation of fluid intake. Children with spasmodic croup respond well to most therapeutic measures. If the child has moderate or severe respiratory distress, oxygen is given.

Racemic epinephrine, a local vasoconstrictor given by nebulization, temporarily relieves airway obstruction by decreasing edema, especially in spasmodic croup. Because the obstruction usually returns to pretreatment level or worse in 1 or 2 hours, the child must be carefully observed.

Steroids by intramuscular or oral routes may be helpful in patients with croup. A single intramuscular injection or oral dose of dexamethasone (0.6 mg/kg) may allow significant clinical improvement during the next 24 hours. Antibiotics are not indicated unless there is evidence of bacterial disease. Most patients with croup have excellent short- and long-term prognoses; artificial airway intervention is rarely necessary.

Croup and epiglottitis may occasionally be confused with each other. Table 32-21 shows the main differentiating characteristics of these two diseases. Croup is diagnosed approximately ten times as frequently as epiglottitis.

# Abscesses

## Retropharyngeal Abscess

A retropharyngeal abscess can cause significant upper respiratory obstruction. Usually a complication of bacterial pharyngitis, it is more rarely caused by contiguous spread of infection from ver-

| TABLE 32-21. | Differentiation Between Croup and Epiglottitis | |
|---|---|---|
| Characteristic | Croup | Epiglottitis |
| Age | 6 mo to 4 y | 2 to 8 y |
| Site | Subglottic | Supraglottic |
| Onset | Gradual history of upper respiratory infection | Rapid, usually less than 24 h |
| Presentation | Inspiratory stridor; hoarse, barky cough | Inspiratory stridor; high fever, toxic appearance; sits forward |
| Etiology | Viral | Bacterial |

tebral osteomyelitis. It occurs most commonly in children younger than 3 years of age, and the predominant organisms are *S. aureus*, group A β-hemolytic streptococci, and anaerobes. Children with retropharyngeal abscess usually have histories of pharyngitis or upper respiratory infection and a sudden onset of high fever. The patient may complain of throat pain or difficulty swallowing; a small child will refuse to eat. The child may be drooling and have a toxic appearance with the neck extended; meningism may be present. Breathing may be noisy, and if the abscess impinges on the larynx, the child will have stridor. On direct examination, there may be a bulge in the posterior pharyngeal wall, which can be palpated for fluctuance if the patient is placed in the Trendelenburg position and suction is ready in case of abscess rupture.

A lateral neck radiograph is helpful to rule out other diagnoses, such as epiglottitis, and to see an abscess that is not clinically visible. There may be thickening of the prevertebral soft tissues. If epiglottitis is suspected, do not examine the child further.

An untreated retropharyngeal abscess may rupture spontaneously and cause aspiration of pus or dissect laterally to the neck or medially to other structures. If the abscess is fluctuant, it should be incised and drained under controlled conditions and antibiotics begun. If the abscess is not fluctuant, parenteral penicillin G or a semisynthetic penicillin may prevent suppuration.

## Peritonsillar Abscess

A peritonsillar abscess, like a retropharyngeal abscess, can cause acute toxicity, high fever, and respiratory distress. This abscess is unusual in children younger than 10 years of age. The initial focus of infection is usually tonsillitis, and the most common organisms are group A β-hemolytic streptococcus, *S. aureus*, *H. influenzae*, and anaerobes such as *Bacteroides* species. The child or adolescent with a peritonsillar abscess usually complains of severe unilateral throat pain and has a history of a preceding or current pharyngitis. He or she may have difficulty speaking, swallowing, or opening the mouth. On physical examination, the teenager may appear toxic with a high fever and may be drooling because of difficulty swallowing; there may be torticollis or trismus. The tonsils are markedly inflamed and edematous, and one side protrudes farther than the other. The uvula may be pushed to the opposite side.

If there is respiratory compromise, the abscess can be drained in the emergency department with a needle and syringe.

If left untreated, a peritonsillar abscess will become fluctuant and eventually rupture spontaneously. If the abscess is fluctuant, drainage and culture are indicated. If it is prefluctuant or a cellulitis without abscess, parenteral penicillin G is given. If there is medical improvement, drainage is not necessary. If there is no improvement on intravenous antibiotic therapy, the area or abscess is aspirated. In younger adolescents, this drainage may not yield pus, and treatment is continued for cellulitis.

## Asthma

Children with asthma account for a large percentage of urgent emergency department visits. Smooth muscle spasm, mucosal edema, and mucus plugging all contribute to widespread airway narrowing and various degrees of airway obstruction in a child with asthma. The airway obstruction is diffuse but not evenly distributed, causing some alveoli to be overventilated while others are underventilated. This uneven distribution of ventilation creates ventilation–perfusion mismatch and subsequent hypoxemia. Because the child hyperventilates, the moderate asthmatic episode is also characterized by hypocapnia and respiratory alkalosis. If the attack becomes more severe and the patient cannot maintain adequate ventilation, the $PCO_2$ level rises and pH falls, resulting in respiratory acidosis. A normal or high $PCO_2$ level in the face of hyperventilation or fatigue indicates that the child's respiratory efforts are not able to overcome the airway obstruction. A child has status asthmaticus if he or she is unresponsive to initial treatment or has a significant chance of suffering from respiratory failure without vigorous further treatment. The course of an asthmatic episode may be unpredictable, and the patient must be carefully observed.

### Assessment

The assessment of a child with an asthmatic attack includes history, physical examination, pulmonary function tests, and laboratory tests.

The objective of the initial history is to obtain information important for the immediate treatment of the child in distress. The initial history should include the precipitating factors and duration of the attack, most recent times and doses of current asthma medications, the course of previous attacks, the last theophylline level, oral intake, vomiting, and other medical problems. A more detailed history can be obtained later in a more relaxed fashion.

The physical examination focuses on general appearance, mental status, respiratory status, and hydration. Moderate tachycardia is expected, but a value of over 150 beats/minute can indicate adrenergic stimulation and guide further treatment. The respiratory examination includes assessment of air movement, use of accessory muscles, wheezing, and cough. If the child has moderate or severe respiratory distress with wheezing, there is sufficient air movement to cause turbulence and at least some ventilation; if this patient is not wheezing, he or she is likely to be in respiratory failure.

Many scores have been devised to assess the severity of an asthmatic episode. Although a score may not be accurate in assessing the degree of hypoxemia, it is helpful for initial assessment of the severity of the episode and for continuing reassessment in a disease in which clinical status changes rapidly. An example of a scoring system is in Table 32-22. There is a statistically significant positive correlation between the score and the $PCO_2$.

The pulse oximeter and peak flow meter are helpful instruments when evaluating asthmatic patients. A decrease in oxygen saturation is an early sign of airway obstruction and alveolar hypoventilation, and the pulse oximeter gives an accurate and continuous reading of the oxygen saturation.

The pulmonary function test usually available in the emergency department is the peak expiratory flow rate using a handheld peak flow meter. This test is effort dependent and is not as accurate as a forced expiratory volume in 1 second (ie, $FEV_1$ measurement), but it is useful for assessing initial and posttreatment airway obstruction in a cooperative child.

The arterial blood gas is the single most useful laboratory test in asthmatic patients, because the ultimate test of respiratory function is the ability to maintain normal oxygenation and ventilation. An arterial blood gas test should be performed on every

TABLE 32-22. Asthma Score*

| Scored Items | 0 | 1 | 2 |
|---|---|---|---|
| PO$_2$ or cyanosis | 70–100 (RA) | <70 (RA) | ≤70 (40% FiO$_2$) |
| | None | In air | In 40% FiO$_2$ |
| Inspiratory breath sounds | Normal | Unequal | Decreased to absent |
| Accessory muscles used | None | Moderate | Maximal |
| Expiratory wheezing | None | Moderate | Marked |
| Cerebral function | Normal | Depressed/agitated | Coma |

* Score: ≥5 indicates impending respiratory failure; ≥7 and PcO$_2$ = 65 indicates respiratory failure.
RA, room air.
*Wood DW, et al. A clinical scoring system for the diagnosis of respiratory failure. Am J Dis Child 1972;123:227.*

child with status asthmaticus and repeated if the patient's clinical status remains steady or deteriorates. The PcO$_2$ level is interpreted in light of the physical examination. For example, a level of 40 is worrisome in a tired, lethargic patient, but it is acceptable in a relaxed child with an improving clinical picture. The changes in the arterial blood gas tensions are more meaningful than one isolated value. If repeated arterial sampling is anticipated, an arterial line should be inserted.

Other than arterial blood gas measurements, laboratory studies are of limited use in evaluating an asthmatic patient. Leukocytosis may be caused by asthma, adrenergic drugs, and steroids. A urinalysis may show ketones from poor oral intake and dehydration. The chest radiograph in an asthmatic patient typically shows hyperinflation, indicated by flattened diaphragms, increased anteroposterior diameter, hyperlucent lungs, peribronchial thickening, and areas of atelectasis that may be misinterpreted as pneumonia. Because the results of the chest radiograph rarely change the therapy, the study should be reserved for specific indications, such as an asthmatic patient with deteriorating clinical condition, chest pain, subcutaneous emphysema, suspected pneumothorax, or high fever. In rare instances, an entire lobe or lung collapses or pneumothorax exists.

## Management

Hypoxemia is an important and early component of asthma, and oxygen should be given to every patient. Further oxygen therapy is guided by the results of pulse oximetry and arterial blood gas measurement.

Initial management of an acute asthmatic episode consists of administration of β$_2$-adrenergic drugs. B$_2$-adrenergic receptors act on airway smooth muscle to produce bronchodilatation; stimulation of these receptors results in increased mucus clearance, vasodilation, and inhibition of mast cell degranulation.

Traditionally, adrenergic agents such as epinephrine have been administered by subcutaneous injection. Although epinephrine is a potent bronchodilator, its significant α- and β$_1$-activity limit its use because of serious side effects, including tachycardia and hypertension. Terbutaline is more β$_2$-receptor selective and has a longer duration of action. Injectable adrenergic drugs have been largely replaced by inhaled β$_2$-agonists as the mainstay in treatment of the acute asthmatic episode. The inhaled route of administration of β$_2$-adrenergic medications is equally as effective as the subcutaneous route, regardless of the severity of obstruction. The nebulized agents act faster, have a prolonged duration of action, and have fewer side effects than the subcutaneously administered drugs. Administration by nebulization delivers the agonist directly to the site of action, and a relatively small amount is needed. The margin of safety is wide, and there is no pain involved for the patient. These agents can be delivered with a hand-held mouthpiece. Respiratory cooperation is not necessary; a loose face mask can be used in infants and uncooperative children. Because the administration of inhaled β$_2$-adrenergic medications may cause a temporary decrease in oxygen saturation, these drugs should be delivered with oxygen. The three most effective agents are listed in Table 32-23. The newer agents, albuterol and terbutaline, are the preferred sympathomimetic agents because of their relatively complete β$_2$-receptor selectivity. A high dose of nebulized albuterol (0.03 mL/kg, maximum of 1 mL) every 20 minutes produces greater improvement in pulmonary function than a lower dose, is safe, and does not increase side effects (Schuh, 1989).

Steroids have long been useful in the long-term treatment of asthma. Because the patient with asthma progresses from the early bronchospastic phase to one with mucosal edema and mucus plugging, drugs directed at the inflammation are needed. Steroids are the drugs of choice for the inflammatory phase. There is con-

TABLE 32-23. Aerosolized β-Adrenergic Agents

| Drug | Activity* | How Supplied | Dose† |
|---|---|---|---|
| Metaproterenol (Alupent) | β2 > β1 | 5% inhalant solution | 0.1–0.3 mL/kg |
| Terbutaline (Brethine) | β2 ≫ β1 | 0.1% parenteral ampule | <2 y: 0.5 mL |
| | | | 2–9 y: 1.0 mL |
| | | | >9 y: 1.5 mL |
| Albuterol (Ventolin) | β2 ≫ β1 | 0.5% respirator solution | 0.01–0.03 mL/kg (max, 1 mL) |

* β$_1$, lipolysis and cardiostimulation; β$_2$, bronchodilation and vasodilation.
† May be administered every 20–30 min, depending on clinical response. Dilute each to total volume of 3 mL with normal saline. Deliver by nebulizer powered with oxygen at 6 L/min.

troversy about whether early administration of steroids in the emergency department affect the duration of the emergency visit and the rate of hospitalization. There may be a positive effect from steroid use within 3 to 4 hours. Intravenous methylprednisolone is the most commonly used steroid in the emergency treatment of asthma because of its limited mineralocorticoid effects (Table 32-24).

The role of theophylline in the acute management of asthma has been scrutinized in recent years. Its declining use can be attributed to its low potency as a bronchodilator, the lack of convincing trials concerning its efficacy, its narrow therapeutic index, and the question of increased morbidity when it is combined with certain beta agonists.

The bronchodilator response to theophylline is linearly related to serum drug levels. Its maximal bronchodilator effects occur when serum drug levels are high, at levels that are often associated with serious complications. There is controversy about whether theophylline adds bronchodilation to the regimen of $\beta_2$-sympathomimetic drugs and steroids. Further study should define whether theophylline has a role in the treatment of acute asthma in the 1990s.

Theophylline is most effectively given as a loading dose followed by a constant infusion with an infusion apparatus, which reliably delivers a steady rate of drug over time (see Table 32-24). If the patient is on a sustained-release theophylline preparation at home, obtain a theophylline level before beginning intravenous therapy, and adjust the loading dose. Drug levels must be monitored for maximal benefit and safety. A therapeutic level is considered to be 10 to 20 mg/100 mL, and toxic effects may occur in the high therapeutic range. The child should be observed for signs of theophylline toxicity, such as abdominal pain, nausea, vomiting, headache, tremors, tachycardia, seizures, and arrhythmias. Some of these same symptoms may be due to the asthma itself, adrenergic drugs, or viral illness.

The recognition of the parasympathetic nervous system's importance in the pathogenesis of asthma led to the use of anticholinergic drugs in the treatment of asthma. Atropine can be nebulized for delivery but has potential systemic side effects (see Table 32-24). Ipratropium bromide, not yet available in the United States, is a synthetic cholinergic antagonist with prolonged action of bronchodilation without the undesirable side effects of atropine.

Isoproterenol can be used for respiratory failure as a constant infusion to prevent the need for intubation. Other intravenous $\beta$-receptor agonists, such as albuterol or terbutaline, can be used

(see Table 32-23). Indications include faint or absent breath sounds, rising $PCO_2$ with respiratory distress or fatigue, and failure to respond to appropriate therapy. Other agents used in the asthmatic patient with impending or actual respiratory failure include continuous nebulization of $\beta_2$-receptor agonists or less conventional therapy such as magnesium sulfate and ketamine.

Other than drug therapy, general supportive measures are important in the care of an asthmatic child. Many children with asthma are at least mildly dehydrated, and hydration therapy proceeds as in any dehydrated child. No evidence suggests that large amounts of fluid have a beneficial effect in well-hydrated asthmatic children, and fluid administration may be contraindicated. Metabolic acidosis is treated with oxygen, hydration, and the drugs mentioned earlier. Rarely is there an indication for bicarbonate therapy. The child should be in as quiet and restful an environment as possible, a task often difficult to achieve in a busy emergency department.

Antibiotics are used in asthmatic patients only if there is good clinical evidence for pneumonia or other infection. A chest radiograph with atelectasis may be misinterpreted as pneumonia because the radiologic appearances are often indistinguishable. It is easier to assess the febrile asthmatic patient for pneumonia after the wheezing has cleared. There is no support for the use of expectorants, and sedatives are strongly contraindicated.

Many studies have looked at clinical variables such as peak flow rate, length of wheezing episode, and response to initial adrenergic treatment to try to predict the outcome of a particular asthmatic attack. No particular variable or set of variables accurately predicts outcome, and the degree of continued airway obstruction, inability to retain oral medications, and poor compliance with home therapy are used to determine the need for hospitalization.

## Bronchiolitis

Bronchiolitis is a common and acute viral infection of the lower respiratory tract that causes mild or severe respiratory distress. The organism invades the epithelial cells of the bronchioles, causing sloughing of cells, edema, and increased mucus secretion. The resultant narrowing of the small airways causes uneven air trapping and overdistention of the lungs; ventilation–perfusion mismatch can lead to hypoxia or hypercarbia.

Bronchiolitis most commonly affects infants 2 to 8 months of age but can be seen in children up to 2 years of age. Occurrence peaks in winter and spring. The organism in most cases is respiratory syncytial virus; others are parainfluenza viruses, adenovirus, influenza viruses, and *Mycoplasma pneumoniae*.

### Assessment

The diagnosis of bronchiolitis is made by clinical presentation, age of the child, and season. After a few days of an upper respiratory tract infection, the child has an acute onset of cough, expiratory wheezing, and rales. If there is moderate or severe respiratory distress, the child may eat poorly, be dehydrated from poor oral intake, and be irritable. The chest examination reveals wheezing and rales bilaterally; these findings may change on subsequent examinations. Increased respiratory rate and, in severe disease, nasal flaring and retractions are seen.

There are no routine laboratory tests for bronchiolitis. Viral culture results from the nasopharynx are positive for as many as 50% of cases but are not available in time for diagnosis. Some laboratories have immunofluorescent techniques for viral identification. A chest radiograph shows nonspecific changes; it may show diffuse hyperinflation with patchy areas of infiltration or atelectasis. An arterial blood gas determination may be necessary for more severely ill infants.

| Drug | Route | Dose |
|---|---|---|
| Methylprednisolone | IV | 2 mg/kg load, then 1 mg/kg q 6 h |
| Atropine | Nebulized | 0.05–0.1 mg/kg (min, 0.25 mg; max, 1.0 mg) |
| Aminophylline | IV | 6 mg/kg bolus |
| | | Drip 0.8 mg/kg/h |
| | | Adjust if on theophylline; 1 mg/kg raises level 2 µg/mL |
| Terbutaline | IV | Bolus 10 µg/kg over 5 min (max, 500 µg) |
| | | Drip 0.1 µg/kg/min |
| Isoproterenol | IV | Drip 0.1 µg/kg/min (titrate to heart rate) |

TABLE 32-24. Asthma Drug Doses

## Management

Traditional therapy for bronchiolitis is supportive and includes oral fluids, mist therapy, antipyretics, and oxygen if necessary.

Recent studies show that many children with bronchiolitis have a reversible component to their airway obstruction and benefit from a bronchodilator such as nebulized albuterol. If the child improves with a trial of a nebulized $\beta_2$-adrenergic agent or subcutaneous epinephrine, treatment with metaproterenol syrup (2 mg/kg/day, given in three divided doses each day) or albuterol syrup (0.1 mg/kg/dose, given three times each day) for 5 to 7 days may improve the symptoms.

The early use of steroids in bronchiolitis patients in the emergency department with $\beta_2$-adrenergic drugs may improve clinical status and allow a higher percentage of these patients to go home. Antibiotics have not been beneficial.

The only specific therapy for bronchiolitis involves the use of ribavirin for respiratory syncytial virus infection in very ill or high-risk infants.

The child with bronchiolitis should be hospitalized for severe respiratory distress or if aspiration, dehydration, and secondary bacterial pneumonia are concerns. If the child is an outpatient and is displaying high respiratory rate, fatigue, or poor oral intake, close follow-up care is necessary. The parent should be advised that the disease may worsen, especially at night, before it improves. Most children are completely well in 2 to 3 weeks.

When an infant presents with a first episode of wheezing with an upper respiratory tract infection, it is impossible to differentiate bronchiolitis from asthma triggered by a viral infection. If the patient has other signs of atopy or a family history of allergies or asthma or if the disease is reversible with bronchodilator treatment, the diagnosis of asthma is more likely.

The prognosis for a child with bronchiolitis is excellent, and the complications of persistent wheezing, apnea, or superimposed bacterial pneumonia are rare. Children with bronchiolitis are more likely to have reactive airway disease or asthma in the future.

## SEIZURES

Seizures are a common neurologic emergency; about 5% of children have at least one seizure by the age of 16 years. A *seizure* is a transient change in level of consciousness or an involuntary alteration of motor activity, sensation, or behavior indicating neurologic dysfunction. A *convulsion* is a seizure that manifests primarily as repetitive motor activity. *Epilepsy*, or seizure disorder, connotes recurrent seizures. Most seizures are brief, lasting less than 15 minutes; if the seizure is persistent or there are repetitive seizures without intercurrent regaining of consciousness for an hour or longer, the patient is in *status epilepticus*. Status epilepticus can cause significant morbidity and mortality; as the seizure continues, hypoxia, tachycardia, hypertension, and hyperthermia may occur.

The more common causes of seizures are listed in Table 32-25. A partial seizure from a localized focus in the brain can be motor, sensory, or psychomotor; it is simple, with no change of consciousness, or complex, with decreased level of consciousness. A generalized seizure involving both cerebral hemispheres initially or later during the seizure can be nonconvulsive (ie, petit mal) or convulsive. Generalized tonic clonic seizures (ie, grand mal) are the most common form of status epilepticus.

## Initial Management

The most common seizure emergency is generalized tonic clonic status epilepticus. If the level of consciousness is satisfactory,

**TABLE 32-25.    Common Causes of Seizures in Children**

Simple febrile seizures
Infections
    Intracranial infections—bacterial or aseptic meningitis, encephalitis
    Shigellosis
Head trauma
    Direct trauma
    Shaking injury
Metabolic abnormalities
    Hypoxia
    Hypoglycemia—insulin reaction in diabetics, alcohol ingestion
    Electrolyte disturbances or dehydration
    Hypocalcemia
    Pyridoxine deficiency
    Renal failure
    Hepatic failure
    Inherited metabolic disorders
Toxic ingestions (rule out suicide attempt)
    Alcohol
    Theophylline
Withdrawal of anticonvulsant medications
Miscellaneous
    Hypertensive encephalopathy
    Brain tumor
    Intracranial hemorrhage
    Idiopathic

most other seizures are not medical emergencies and can therefore be treated while an electroencephalogram (EEG) is being monitored.

Continuous generalized tonic clonic seizures need immediate treatment to prevent life-threatening complications. After advanced life support is established, the seizure is stopped with anticonvulsant medication and diagnostic studies are considered. Treatment starts with airway, breathing, and circulation assessment. Control of the airway is essential to prevent hypoxic brain damage and permanent neurologic sequelae. The airway is suctioned, an oropharyngeal or nasopharyngeal airway is inserted for bag and mask ventilation, and oxygen is applied to maintain cerebral oxygenation during this time of increased cerebral metabolic requirements. Be prepared to intubate if necessary. An intravenous line is started for administration of fluids and drugs. Blood is drawn at this time for diagnostic studies, and a Dextrostix is used to assess blood glucose quickly. A 25% solution of dextrose (2 mL/1 kg of body weight) is given in case the seizures are from hypoglycemia. Dextrose is necessary for the increased cerebral consumption of glucose. Isotonic fluids containing glucose are given at a slow rate so as not to exacerbate cerebral edema. A nasogastric tube is inserted to prevent vomiting and aspiration.

Intravenous anticonvulsants, as shown in Table 32-26, are used for the patient in status epilepticus; they allow prompt administration and produce quick therapeutic levels. The patient should be monitored while these drugs are given, because they have significant hemodynamic and respiratory-depressant side effects. The physician should be familiar with the potential problems and prepared to intubate or support the circulation if necessary.

There is no single best drug regimen for the patient in status epilepticus. Intravenous lorazepam is the drug of choice to rapidly stop a seizure; intravenous phenobarbital is an alternative in pa-

TABLE 32-26.　Drugs Used in Treating Status Epilepticus

| Drug | Dose and Route | Side Effects | Comments |
|---|---|---|---|
| Lorazepam* | 0.05–0.1 mg/min, IV, max 1 mL/min | Respiratory depression (unusual) | May have longer onset and longer duration then diazepam. |
| Diazepam† | 0.2–0.5 mg/kg, IV, slow push (1 mg/kg), max 10 mg per injection | Respiratory depression, hypotension, sedation (may be prolonged) | May push larger dose slowly until seizure stops. May repeat as necessary. |
| Phenobarbital† | 10–20 mg/kg, IV, over 5–10 min, max 120–150 mg | Respiratory depression, hypotension, sedation | Monitor serum level. |
| Phenytoin‡ | 10–20 mg/kg, IV, over 10–20 min (25 mg/min) | Arrhythmias, cardiovascular collapse, hypotension | Must be on cardiac monitor. No respiratory depression. Never use IM route. Monitor serum level. Must give directly into vein; may crystallize in solution. |
| Paraldehyde | 100–200 mg/kg over 5 min, followed by 20 mg/kg min (10% solution) | Pulmonary edema, metabolic acidosis | Monitor serum level. |

\* Lorazepam is the drug of choice for child with a known seizure disorder on maintenance doses of anticonvulsant drugs.
† Do not use intravenous diazepam and intravenous phenobarbital together, because of potentiated, cardio-respiratory side effects.
‡ Useful as second drug if diazepam or phenobarbital is ineffective.

tients who have not been on anticonvulsant medications. Diazepam is an effective initial anticonvulsant. It is best to give a full dose of one drug before beginning a second drug. Phenytoin is often used as the second drug. Intravenous diazepam and intravenous phenobarbital should not be used together because of their synergistic effect of respiratory depression. If the seizure cannot be stopped with these medications, other alternatives include paraldehyde, lidocaine, and general anesthesia. It may be difficult to terminate a seizure if there is an uncorrected underlying disorder such as hypoxemia, hypoglycemia, or an electrolyte disturbance. These conditions should be detected and treated as soon as possible. With cessation of the seizure, airway patency and adequate ventilation often return.

The patient having a seizure must be protected from physical harm. The child is placed on a soft surface and restrained as necessary. Fever control is part of supportive care. Body temperature may be elevated from infection or from the seizure itself, and the fever increases metabolic demands.

## Assessment

For diagnostic purposes, it is practical to divide seizure patients into four groups: febrile patients, patients with known seizure disorders, traumatized patients, and others. After the child is stable, a complete history and physical examination help to determine the cause of the seizure and guide ongoing management. It is essential to check for conditions that need immediate therapy. The history should include questions about the current seizure, including how it started, type, and duration; previous seizures and frequency; evidence of infection; abnormal behavior; development; pica; trauma; possible ingestion; birth history; and current medications, including anticonvulsants.

The physical examination includes assessment of vital signs, evidence of injury or infection, and the general medical condition. Abnormal neurologic signs, such as pupillary changes, increased or decreased muscle tone, or Babinski's sign, are common during and after a seizure. Serious neurologic abnormalities, such as asymmetric pupils, signs of increased intracranial pressure, focal deficits, and posturing may indicate a serious neurologic problem

that needs immediate further assessment and treatment by a neurologist.

The selection of laboratory studies is determined by the age of the patient, the history, and the physical examination. The traditional tests of electrolytes, calcium, and magnesium are rarely abnormal in children after infancy and are required only if there is suspicion of a relevant abnormality. A CBC with differential is obtained if there is suspicion of infection. Other studies, such as urinalysis, anticonvulsant drug levels, toxicology screens of serum and urine, blood cultures, liver function, ammonia, and lead levels may be indicated.

Skull radiographs are rarely indicated in a child with seizures, but they may be helpful if a skull fracture is suspected and CT scanning is not available. A CT scan is helpful if there is a focal deficit, history of trauma, evidence of increased intracranial pressure, or suspicion of a mass lesion. A lumbar puncture is indicated for a child with a febrile seizure and meningeal signs; seizures often occur in children with acute bacterial meningitis. If concern exists about increased intracranial pressure, a CT scan should be done before a lumbar puncture.

After a seizure has been stopped in the emergency department, any underlying conditions that may have caused the seizure must be treated. It is often advisable to treat the seizures themselves, and a neurologist should be consulted concerning ongoing seizure management.

If the seizure cannot be controlled, cardiovascular signs are unstable, or neurologic examination results are abnormal after the seizure and immediate postictal period, the patient should be hospitalized for further observation and management. The nonemergent care of children with seizures is discussed in Chapter 154.

## Management

### Simple Febrile Seizure

Children commonly have seizures as a consequence of an abrupt and steep rise in body temperature. For this simple febrile seizure, several criteria must be met: age 6 months to 6 years, generalized seizure of less then 20 minutes' duration, occurrence within 24 hours of onset of the fever, normal development and neurologic examination results, and no family history of afebrile seizures. If the child and seizure meet these criteria, the child is given an antipyretic and observed. If he looks fine, no further studies or treatment are indicated.

If the criteria are not met and the child does not look fine or is younger than 18 months, a lumbar puncture may be necessary to rule out meningitis. Central nervous system infections are rarely found, even in the children with "atypical" or complex febrile seizures. Other laboratory studies are performed as necessary. If the seizure is atypical, treatment may be started, usually with phenobarbital. The child with a simple febrile seizure has an approximately 30% risk of recurrence.

### Known Seizure Disorder

Many children presenting with seizures have chronic seizure disorders and are already on anticonvulsant medication. The seizures in these children often are due to inadequate anticonvulsant drug levels in the blood. It is important to ask whether this is a typical seizure for this patient (or does the child need further evaluation), how often the seizures usually occur (if at all), and whether he or she is taking the anticonvulsant medication. Often the patient has not been given the medication, has run out of medication, or is vomiting the medication. Management involves checking serum drug levels and loading the patient intravenously or orally. Follow-up care should be arranged with the patient's usual provider.

### Trauma and a Seizure

Seizures may be secondary to head trauma. This trauma may be obvious, with external bruising, or occult, as in a shaking injury. Post-traumatic seizures are classified by time after injury: immediate (<24 hours), early (during the first week), or late (after the first week). The sooner after the injury the seizure occurs, the better is the prognosis. Immediate seizures require no treatment, and the prognosis is excellent. Early seizures indicate a focal injury with a 25% incidence of further seizures. Late seizures indicate focal scarring and are associated with a high risk of additional seizures. Emergency studies to be considered include skull films, CT scan, subdural tap, and lumbar puncture. A neurologist should be consulted concerning treatment. If there is major head trauma and evidence of increased intracranial pressure, treatment for these problems should start immediately.

Certain conditions may easily be mistaken for seizures, including breath-holding spells, syncopal attacks, shaking chills, and hyperventilation.

## COMA

The child in coma or with an otherwise decreased level of consciousness is a common and perplexing problem for the emergency physician. Coma is a state of consciousness from which the patient cannot be aroused. Terms to describe other decreased levels of consciousness, such as obtundation and stupor, are confusing, and it is more efficient and exact to describe the particulars of the state of consciousness.

Processes causing coma can be divided into three groups: supratentorial mass lesions that compress or displace brain tissue, subtentorial mass or destructive lesions that directly affect the ascending reticular-activating system (ARAS), and systemic metabolic disorders that diffusely affect the brain. These processes depress the function of both cerebral hemispheres and can produce abnormal functioning of the ARAS in the brain stem, which arouses the cerebral hemispheres. The ARAS extends from the pons up to the diencephalon.

The more common causes of coma are listed in Table 32-27.

### Initial Management

Many causes of coma are reversible without long-term morbidity if they are properly diagnosed and managed. Certain conditions that are readily treatable can cause rapid deterioration if untreated.

After initial assessment, including blood pressure and temperature, all patients receive full resuscitation, because ultimate prognosis is unknown. One hundred percent oxygen and 2 mL of intravenous 25% dextrose per 1 kg of body weight are administered as substrates for brain metabolism. Naloxone (0.01 to 0.1 mg/1 kg of body weight) is given intravenously to reverse a possible narcotic overdose, and fluids are begun. The naloxone can be repeated in 2 or 3 minutes.

The patient should be undressed and checked for evidence of trauma, systemic illnesses, drug ingestion, and infection such as meningitis. After a thorough physical examination and a systematic consideration of etiologic factors, therapy is given for specific suspected causes, such as seizures, shock, infection, or increased intracranial pressure.

### Assessment and Further Treatment

After initial resuscitation, it is essential to assess the important historic and physical information that may indicate at what level the brain is impaired, to choose the most likely diagnoses, and to act quickly with further informative studies and treatment. Important historic information includes description and rapidity

---

TABLE 32-27. Common Causes of Coma in Children

| Cause | Circumstances |
| --- | --- |
| Trauma | Subdural and epidural hematomas, parenchymal bleeding |
| Poisoning/ingestions | Alcohol, barbiturates, opiates, aspirin, carbon monoxide, lead |
| Infectious disorders | Meningitis, encephalitis (eg, herpes simplex); severe systemic dysfunctions |
| Metabolic disorders | Hypoglycemia, diabetic ketoacidosis, uremia, electrolyte disturbances |
| Circulatory disorders | Shock, hypertensive encephalopathy |
| Respiratory failure | Airway obstruction, pulmonary disease, sudden infant death syndrome |
| Other | Tumors, seizures (postictal) |

Adapted from Kandt RS, D'Souza BJ, Kaplan RA, et al: Disorders of the central nervous system. In: Ehrlich FE, Heldrich SJ, Tepas JJ, et al, eds. Pediatric emergency medicine. Rockville MD: Aspen Publishers 1987; and Advanced pediatric life support course. The Johns Hopkins University School of Medicine, 1987.

of onset of coma, trauma, drug ingestion, medications, medical history, psychiatric history, and previous symptoms such as headache, vomiting, weakness, and seizures.

The neurologic examination starts with an assessment of level of consciousness. The Glasgow Coma Scale, based on eye opening and best motor and verbal responses, is used to standardize and communicate the level of consciousness (see Table 32-7). A modified scale, the Children's Coma Score, can be used in young children. These scales may predict future outcome.

The pattern and depth of respirations, pupillary reactions, ocular movements, funduscopic examination, and motor response to pain may help localize the level of the brain involved (Table 32-28). Cheyne-Stokes respirations (ie, alternating periods of breathing and apnea), central neurogenic hyperventilation (ie, deep, regular, and rapid respirations), and ataxic breathing (ie, respirations with irregular rate and depth) indicate a decreasing level of arousal, with ataxic breathing signaling an impending respiratory arrest. The size, reactivity, and comparison of the pupils provide information about the level of the lesion and possible lateralization. For example, if one pupil is fixed and dilated, there may be impending herniation of the temporal lobe and compression of the third cranial nerve on the side of the dilated pupil.

Intact oculocephalic and oculovestibular reflexes signify an intact brain stem. The oculocephalic reflex (ie, doll's eye reflex) is performed only if no possibility of a neck injury exists. When the head is turned in one direction, the eyes should move in the other direction before returning to mid position. If there is brain stem damage, the eyes turn with the head, as on a doll.

The oculovestibular reflex (ie, "cold water calorics") is performed after an ear examination ensures that the tympanic membranes are intact. The head is elevated 30°, and cold water is introduced into one ear canal. If the brain stem is intact, the eyes should have slow movement or tonic deviation toward the ear with the cold water. If one or both of these reflexes are preserved, the process causing coma is not in the brain stem but involves both cerebral hemispheres. The motor examination includes assessment of tone, movements, deep tendon reflexes, and gag reflex. In response to pain, the patient may have purposeful movement (ie, intact cerebral hemispheres), decorticate posturing (ie, hemispheric dysfunction), decerebrate posturing (ie, upper brain stem dysfunction), or flaccidity (ie, lower brain stem dysfunction). The arms are flexed in decorticate posturing (ie, point to the "core") and extended in decerebrate posturing; the legs are extended in both.

At the end of the neurologic examination, any focal findings should be evident. If there are findings such as unequal pupils, increased muscle tone, or brisk reflexes, the process is more likely

a primary central nervous system problem. If there are no focal neurologic signs, equal and reactive pupils, and decreased muscle tone and reflexes, the process is more likely systemic, such as metabolic or toxic encephalopathy. In end-stage disease of either origin, the pupils tend to be bilaterally fixed and dilated.

The laboratory investigation is guided by the most likely diagnoses, ascertained from the medical history and physical examination. A few initial studies are routine for any comatose patient: blood glucose, arterial blood gas, electrolytes, calcium, BUN, ammonia, liver function tests, CBC, urinalysis, toxicology screens of blood and urine, ECG, and a chest radiograph. A CT scan is the best way to detect a structural or mass lesion and is often indicated to determine the cause in a patient in coma or to evaluate the severity of a known process. A lumbar puncture is performed to rule out meningitis or encephalitis, but it is contraindicated if the physician suspects a mass lesion, head trauma, Reye's syndrome, or a bleeding diathesis. If there is any suspicion of increased intracranial pressure, with or without papilledema, a CT scan should precede a lumbar puncture. If meningitis is suspected but a lumbar puncture is contraindicated, empiric treatment should begin immediately. Other studies that may be helpful to determine the cause of coma or to localize the disease process include carboxyhemoglobin level determination, EEG, radionuclide brain scan, and cerebral arteriography.

The patient must be continually reassessed and treatment changed as indicated. With careful observation, the physician can gauge the progression of disease and the effectiveness of treatment.

# ANAPHYLAXIS

## Mechanism

Anaphylaxis is an extreme systemic allergic reaction. It is caused by hypersensitivity to a foreign substance and usually occurs within a few hours of oral or parenteral exposure to an antigen. Common causes of anaphylactic reactions include Hymenoptera stings, primarily bees and wasps; drugs, such as penicillins and local anesthetics; foods, such as nuts, seafood, and eggs; iodinated contrast media for radiologic studies; blood products; and hormones, such as insulin.

After exposure to a sensitizing antigen, IgE antibody is formed and binds to tissue mast cells. After a subsequent exposure, the antigen binds to the IgE–mast cell combinations and initiates degranulation of the mast cells, releasing preformed mediators, such as histamine, and subsequently releasing secondary mediators, such as slow-reacting substance of anaphylaxis.

TABLE 32-28.  Diagnosis of Level of Neurologic Lesion

| Level | Pupils | Ocular Movements | Breathing Pattern | Motor Response to Pain |
|---|---|---|---|---|
| Thalamus | Small, reactive | Intact oculocephalic and oculovestibular reflexes | Cheyne-Stokes respiration | Increased motor tone, decorticate |
| Midbrain | Midposition or dilated, nonreactive | Depressed oculocephalic and oculovestibular reflexes | Central neurogenic hyperventilation† | Decerebrate |
| Pons | Pinpoint, nonreactive | Absent* | Central neurogenic hyperventilation, apneustic or cluster breathing | Flaccid |
| Medulla | Dilated, nonreactive | Absent | Ataxic | Flaccid |

* Absent brain stem reflexes may also be due to metabolic encephalopathy or drug ingestion.
† Also may be present with acid–base disorders, hypoxia, sepsis.
Adapted from Pascoe DJ, Grossman M, eds. Quick reference to pediatric emergencies, ed 3. Philadelphia: JB Lippincott, 1984; and Plum F, Posner JB. The diagnosis of stupor and coma, ed 3. Philadelphia: FA Davis, 1980.

| TABLE 32-29.    Clinical Features of an Anaphylactic Reaction |
| --- |
| Cutaneous: pruritus, urticaria, angioedema<br>Respiratory: bronchospasm, laryngeal edema<br>Circulatory: hypotension, cardiac arrhythmias<br>Gastrointestinal: diarrhea, abdominal pain |

The most common clinical features of anaphylactic reactions are listed in Table 32-29. Urticaria may be localized to the exposed area or be generalized; it is often accompanied by angioedema, swelling of the lower dermis and subcutaneous tissues.

## Treatment

The history focuses on the time immediately preceding the reaction in an effort to determine exposure to an antigen.

The physical examination focuses on vital signs; airway, including swelling and bronchospasm; circulation, including heart rate and rhythm; skin changes such as urticaria and angioedema; and central nervous system changes. If there are clinical signs of respiratory distress, such as voice change or dyspnea, difficulty swallowing, or circulatory collapse, treatment must proceed immediately.

Treatment of a generalized reaction depends on the type and severity of the reaction. Treatment begins with support of the airway, circulation, and cardiac rhythm. Subcutaneous or intramuscular administration of a 1:1000 concentration of epinephrine in a dose of 0.01 mL/1 kg of body weight of (maximum, 0.4 mL) is the drug of choice in most systemic reactions. This drug should relieve laryngeal edema and severe bronchospasm and can be repeated every 15 to 20 minutes. Nebulized bronchodilators, such as salbutamol or Alupent, and intravenous aminophylline are helpful for reactive airway disease. If severe airway obstruction cannot be relieved, intubation or tracheotomy may be necessary.

Anaphylaxis may include a rapid decrease in plasma volume, requiring intravenous fluid boluses for support of blood pressure. Crystalloid infusion such as lactated Ringer's solution or normal saline can be given in 20 mL/1 kg of body weight boluses and repeated as often as necessary. If the patient remains hypotensive, the Trendelenburg position and a 1:10,000 epinephrine infusion starting at 0.1 $\mu$g/1 kg of body weight per minute may be used.

Generalized cutaneous reactions, such as urticaria or angioedema, may be treated with intravenous, intramuscular, or oral diphenhydramine at the dose of 1 mg/1 kg of body weight administered every 4 to 6 hours. The benefits of steroid therapy are controversial. In patients with persistent allergic urticaria, intravenous cimetidine may be of benefit.

## Selected Readings

Krauss BS, Harakal T, Flesher GR. The spectrum and frequency of illness presenting to a pediatric emergency department. Pediatr Emerg Care 1991;7:67.

### Cardiopulmonary Resuscitation

American Heart Association. Pediatric advanced life support. American Academy of Pediatrics, 1988.
Finholt DA, Kettrick RG, Wagner HR, et al. The heart is under the lower third of the sternum. Am J Dis Child 1986;140:646.
Goetting MG, Paradis NA. High-dose epinephrine improves outcome from pediatric cardiac arrest. Ann Emerg Med 1991;20:22.
Johnston C. Endotracheal drug delivery. Pediatr Emerg Care 1992;8:94.
Ludwig S, Fleisher G. Pediatric cardiopulmonary resuscitation: A review and a proposal. Pediatr Emerg Care 1985;1:40.
Nichols DG, Kettrick RG, Swedlow DB, et al. Factors influencing outcome of cardiopulmonary resuscitation in children. Pediatr Emerg Care 1986;2:1.
Zaritsky A. Selected concepts and controversies in pediatric cardiopulmonary resuscitation. Crit Care Clin 1988;4:735.

### Pediatric Trauma

Bruce DA. Manipulation of ICP. Pediatr Emerg Care 1985;2:139.
Committee on Trauma, American College of Surgeons. Advanced trauma life support course. , 1989.
Eichelberger MR, Randolph JG. Pediatric trauma: An algorithm for diagnosis and therapy. J Trauma 1983:23;91.
Gratz RR. Accidental injury in childhood: A literature review on pediatric trauma. J Trauma 1979;19:551.
Greenspan L, McLellan BA, Greig H. Abbreviated injury scale and injury severity score: A scoring chart. J Trauma 1985;25:60.
Leonidas JC, Ting W, Binkiewicz A, et al. Mild head trauma in children: When is a roentgenogram necessary? Pediatrics 1982;69:139.
Mayer T, Matlak ME, Johnson DG, et al. The modified injury severity scale in pediatric multiple patients. J Pediatr Surg 1980;15:719.
McCarthy J. Skeletal trauma in the multiple injury patient. Pediatr Emerg Care 1985;2:129.
Ros SP, Ros MA. Should patients with normal cranial CT scans following minor head injury be hospitalized for observation? Pediatr Emerg Care 1989;5:216.
Rutherford WH, Spence RAJ. Infection in wounds sutured in the accident and emergency department. Ann Emerg Med 1980;9:350.
Taylor GA, Eichelberger MR. Abdominal CT in children with neurologic impairment following blunt trauma. Abdominal CT in comatose children. Ann Surg 1989;210:229.
Tepas JJ, Discala C, Ramenofsky ML, et al. Mortality and head injury: The pediatric perspective. J Pediatr Surg 1990;25:92.
Trunkey DD. Blunt chest trauma. Pediatr Emerg Care 1985;2:133.
Yokota H, Kurokawa A, Otsuka T, et al. Significance of magnetic resonance imaging in acute head injury. J Trauma 1991;31:351.

### Bites

Brook I. Microbiology of human and animal bite wounds in children. Pediatr Infect Dis J 1987;6:29.
Callham M. Prophylactic antibiotics in common dog bite wounds: A controlled study. Ann Emerg Med 1980;9:410.
Talan DA, Goldstein EJC, Staatz D, et al. Staphylococcus intermedius: Clinical presentation of a new human dog bite pathogen. Ann Emerg Med 1989;18:410.
Trott A. Care of mammalian bites. Pediatr Infect Dis J 1987;6:8.
Wiley JF. Mammalian bites. Review of evaluation and management. Clin Pediatr 1990;29:283.

### Burns

Baxter CR, Waeckerle JF. Emergency treatment of burn injury. Ann Emerg Med 1988;17:1305.
Carvajal HF. A physiologic approach to fluid therapy in severely burned children. Surg Gynecol Obstet 1980;150:379.
Herndon DN, Thompson PB, Desai MH, et al. Treatment of burns in children. Pediatr Clin North Am 1985;32:1311.
McLoughlin E, Crawford JD. Burns. Pediatr Clin North Am 1985;32:61.
Thompson AE. Environmental emergencies. In: Fleisher GR, Ludwig S, eds. Textbook of pediatric emergency medicine, ed 2. Baltimore: Williams & Wilkins, 1988.

### Respiratory Distress

Anderson AB, Zwerdling RG, Dewitt TG. The clinical utility of pulse oximetry in the pediatric emergency department setting. Pediatr Emerg Care 1991;7:263.
Baker MD. Pitfalls in the use of clinical asthma scoring. Am J Dis Child 1988;142:183.
Bass JW, Fajardo JE, Brien JH, et al. Sudden death due to acute epiglottitis. Pediatr Infect Dis 1985;4:447.
Becker AB, Nelson NA, Simons FER. Inhaled salbutamol (albuterol) vs. injected epinephrine in the treatment of acute asthma in children. J Pediatr 1983;102:465.
Bentur L, Canny G, Shields MD, et al. Controlled trial of nebulized albuterol in children younger than 2 years of age with acute asthma. Pediatrics 1992;89:133.
Bolte, Robert G. Nebulized $\beta$-adrenergic agents in the treatment of acute pediatric asthma. Pediatr Emerg Care 1986;2:250.
Brilli RJ, Benzing G, Cotcamp DH. Epiglottitis in infants less than two years of age. Pediatr Emerg Care 1989;5:16.
Brook I, Frazier EH, Thompson DH. Aerobic and anaerobic microbiology of peritonsillar abscess. Laryngoscope 1991;101:289.
Conrad DA, Christenson JC, Warner JL, et al. Aerosolized ribavirin treatment of respiratory syncytial virus infection in infants hospitalized during an epidemic. Pediatr Infect Dis J 1987;6:152.
Costigan DC, Newth CJ. Respiratory status of children with epiglottitis with and without an artificial airway. Am J Dis Child 1983;137:139.
Cotton E, Yasuda K. Foreign body aspiration. Pediatr Clin North Am 1984;31:937.
Davis HW, Gartner JC, Galvis AG, et al. Acute upper airway obstruction: Croup and epiglottitis. Pediatr Clin North Am 1981;28:861.
Denny FW, Murphy TF, Clyde WA, et al. Croup: An 11-year study in a pediatric practice. Pediatrics 1983;71:871.
Faden HS. Treatment of Haemophilus influenzae type B epiglottitis. Pediatrics 1979;63:402.
Fleisher GR. Infectious disease emergencies. In: Fleisher GR, Ludwig S, eds. Textbook of pediatric emergency medicine, ed 2. Baltimore: Williams & Wilkins, 1988.

Kairys SW, Olmstead ED, O'Connor GT. Steroid treatment of laryngotracheitis: A meta-analysis of the evidence from randomized trials. Pediatrics 1989;83:683.

Koren G, Frand M, Barzilay Z, et al. Corticosteroid treatment of laryngotracheitis v spasmodic croup in children. Am J Dis Child 1983;137:941.

Kosloske AM. Bronchoscopic extraction of aspirated foreign bodies in children. Am J Dis Child 1982;136:924.

Littenberg B. Aminophylline treatment in severe, acute asthma. A meta-analysis. JAMA 1988;259:1678.

McConnochie KM. Bronchiolitis: What's in the name? [Marginal comment] Am J Dis Child 1983;137:11.

Moazam F, Talbert JL, Rodgers BM. Foreign bodies in the pediatric tracheobronchial tree. Clin Pediatr 1983;22:148.

Rapkin RH. The diagnosis of epiglottitis: Simplicity and reliability of radiographs of the neck in the differential diagnosis of the coup syndrome. J Pediatr 1972;80:96.

Schuh S, Canny G, Reisman JJ, et al. Nebulized albuterol in acute bronchiolitis. J Pediatr 1990;117:633.

Schuh S, Parkin P, Rajan A, et al. High- versus low-dose, frequently administered, nebulized albuterol in children with severe, acute asthma. Pediatrics 1989;83:513.

Schwartz RH, Knerr RJ, Hermansen K, et al. Acute epiglottitis caused by β-hemolytic group C streptococci. [Short report] Am J Dis Child 1982;136:558.

Schweich P. Lower respiratory tract infections. In: Schwartz MW, Charney EB, et al, eds. Principles and practice of clinical pediatrics, ed 1. Chicago: Year Book Medical Publishers, 1987.

Shoemaker M, Lampe RM, Weir MR. Peritonsillitis: Abscess or cellulitis? J Pediatr Infect Dis 1986;5:435.

Stecenko, Arlene A. Treatment of viral bronchiolitis: Do steroids make sense? Contemp Pediatr 1987;4:121.

Stein LM, Cole RP. Early administration of corticosteroids in emergency room treatment of acute asthma. Ann Intern Med 1990;112:822.

Super DM, Cartelli NA, Brooks LJ, et al. A prospective randomized double-blind study to evaluate the effect of dexamethasone in acute laryngotracheitis. J Pediatr 1989;115:323.

Welliver RC. Advances in the understanding of croup. Pediatr Virol 1987;2:1.

Wood DW, Downes JJ, Lecks HI. A clinical scoring system for the diagnosis of respiratory failure. Am J Dis Child 1972;123:227.

Wrenn K, Slovis CM, Murphy F, et al. Aminophylline therapy for acute bronchospastic disease in the emergency room. Ann Intern Med 1991;115: 241.

## Seizures

Lacey DJ, Singer WD, Horwitz SJ, et al. Lorazepam therapy of status epilepticus in children and adolescents. J Pediatr 1986;108:771.

Nypaver MM, Reynolds SL, Tanz RR, et al. Emergency department laboratory evaluation of children with seizures: Dogma or dilemma? Pediatr Emerg Care 1992;8:13.

Packer RJ, Berman PH. Neurologic Emergencies. In: Fleisher GR, Ludwig S, eds. Textbook of pediatric emergency medicine, ed 2. Baltimore: Williams & Wilkins, 1988.

Rothner AD. Status epilepticus. Pediatr Clin North Am 1980;27:593.

Selbst SM. Office management of status epilepticus. Pediatr Emerg Care 1991;7:106.

## Coma

Kandt RS, D'Souza BJ, Kaplan RA, et al. Disorders of the central nervous system. In: Eherlich FE, Heldrich SJ, Tepas, JJ et al, eds. Pediatric emergency medicine. Rockveille, MD: Aspen Publishers, 1987.

Pascoe DJ. Coma. In: Pascoe DJ, Grossman M, eds. Quick reference to pediatric emergencies, ed 3. Philadelphia: JB Lippincott, 1984.

Plum F, Posner JB. The diagnosis of stupor and coma, ed 3. Philadelphia: FA Davis, 1980.

Sacco RL, VanGool R, Mohr JP, et al. Nontraumatic coma. Glasgow Coma Score and coma etiology as predictors of 2-week outcome. Arch Neurol 1990;47:1181.

Yager JY, Johnston B, Seshia SS. Coma scales in pediatric practice. Am J Dis Child 1990;144:1088.

## Anaphylaxis

Kolski GB. Allergic emergencies. In: Fleisher GR, Ludwig S, eds. Textbook of pediatric emergency medicine, ed 2. Baltimore: Williams & Wilkins, 1988.

Rusli MR. Cimetidine treatment of recalcitrant acute allergic urticaria. Ann Emerg Med 1986;15:1363.

*Principles and Practice of Pediatrics, Second Edition.*
edited by Frank A. Oski et al. J. B. Lippincott Company, Philadelphia © 1994.

# 32.2 *Poisoning*

## 32.2.1 *General Principles*

J.D. Fortenberry and M. M. Mariscalco

Through intensive educational efforts by health care providers and the institution of childproof medication containers in the early 1970s, morbidity and mortality in children from poisoning have been reduced. Nevertheless, about 100 children younger than 5 years of age die from poisoning annually in the United States. Estimates of annual poisoning episodes in the United States range in the millions. Accidental poisonings make up 80% to 85% of all poisoning exposures, and intentional poisonings constitute the other 15% to 20%. Poisoning in a child older than 5 years is considered intentional and must be evaluated carefully. Accidental intoxication in young children is usually caused by ingestion of a single product, but multiple drugs often are ingested by the suicidal older child or adolescent.

## DIAGNOSIS

The diagnosis of poisoning may not be obvious. The diagnosis is difficult or often not considered because of purposeful falsification by an older patient or because the young or confused patient is unable to provide an adequate history. Poisoning should be considered particularly in children younger than 5 years of age who have acutely developed disturbed consciousness, abnormal behavior, seizures, coma, respiratory distress, shock, arrhythmias, metabolic acidosis, severe vomiting and diarrhea, or other puzzling multisystem disorders. Underlying drug or ethanol intoxication should be considered in adolescent and adult victims of accidental trauma.

During stabilization, information should be obtained from family members, friends, or paramedics who have transported the patient to the hospital about the possible agent, the mode of intoxication, the maximum potential dose, and the time since exposure. If poisoning is suspected but the history is not confirmatory, information regarding the different drugs in the home should be obtained by inquiring about illnesses of the patient and other family members.

The physical examination may be particularly helpful in the case of a questionable exposure to a toxic agent. Specific physical findings may suggest a diagnosis (Table 32-30). However, most children who arrive in the emergency department with a diagnosis of poisoning are asymptomatic. Of those who do present with clinical findings, gastrointestinal tract symptoms (eg, nausea, vomiting, diarrhea, cramps) and central nervous system depression (eg, drowsiness, coma) are most common. Other common findings are referable to the respiratory tract (eg, cough, dyspnea, respiratory depression), cerebellum (eg, ataxia, nystagmus), and central nervous system (eg, hyperactivity, tremor, convulsions). McGuigan (1983) has suggested that less common symptoms are due to alterations in cerebral function (eg, confusion, delirium, hallucinations) and to alterations of the cardiovascular system (eg, heart rate, cardiac arrest).

TABLE 32-30.    Toxidromes: Prominent Clinical Findings as an Aid to Diagnosis of the Unknown Ingestion

| Drug Involved | Clinical Manifestations |
| --- | --- |
| Anticholinergics (atropine, scopolamine, tricyclic antidepressants, phenothiazines, antihistamines, mushrooms) | Agitation, hallucinations, coma, extrapyramidal movements, mydriasis, dry mouth, tachycardia, arrhythmias, hypotension, decreased bowel sounds, urinary retention, flushed, warm, dry skin |
| Cholinergics (organophosphates and carbamate insecticides) | Salivation, lacrimation, urination, defecation, nausea and vomiting, sweating, meiosis, bronchorrhea, rales and wheezes, weakness, paralysis, confusion and coma, muscle fasciculations |
| Opiates | Slow respirations, bradycardia, hypotension, hypothermia, coma, meiosis, pulmonary edema, seizures |
| Sedatives and hypnotics | Coma, hypothermia, central nervous system depression, slow respirations, hypotension, tachycardia |
| Tricyclic antidepressants | Coma, convulsions, arrhythmias, anticholinergic manifestations |
| Salicylates | Vomiting, hyperpnea, fever, lethargy, coma |
| Phenothiazines | Hypotension, tachycardia, torsion of head and neck, oculogyric crisis, trismus, ataxia, anticholinergic manifestations |
| Sympathomimetics (amphetamines, phenylpropranolamine, ephedrine, caffeine, cocaine, aminophylline) | Tachycardia, arrhythmias, psychosis, hallucinations, delirium, nausea, vomiting, abdominal pain, piloerection |
| Alcohols, glycols (methanol, ethylene glycol; also salicylates, paraldehyde, toluene) | Elevated anion gap, metabolic acidosis |

*Mofenson NC, Greensher J. The unknown poison. Pediatrics 1974;54:337; reproduced by permission.*

Routine laboratory tests may play an important role in the diagnosis and management of the poisoned patient. Decreased hemoglobin saturation with a normal or increased $PaO_2$ is found in patients with carbon monoxide poisoning or in methemoglobinemia. An increased anion gap metabolic acidosis suggests metabolites of methanol, ethylene glycol, paraldehyde, and toluene. An elevated measured serum osmolarity compared with a calculated osmolarity indicates the presence of small-molecular-weight and osmotically active compounds such as methanol, ethanol, isopropyl alcohol, mannitol, and ethylene glycol. Hypoglycemia may affect patients intoxicated by ethanol, methanol, isopropyl alcohol, isoniazid, acetaminophen, salicylates, and oral hypoglycemic agents.

Toxicology testing may be helpful in confirming the clinical diagnosis of drug intoxication. Unfortunately, it is impossible to identify all available drugs with a high degree of specificity and sensitivity because of time limitations. Instead, a drug screen is performed. Because drug screens vary among institutions, it is important for the physician to know exactly which drugs can be detected. Toxicology screening tests generally detect a wide range of narcotics, analgesics, barbiturates, antidepressants, tranquilizers, sedative-hypnotics, and various other drugs and abused substances. Ethylene glycol, lithium, iron, cyanide, lead, and other heavy metals are agents that usually are not included in drug screening tests.

## TREATMENT

The three goals of treatment are preventing further drug absorption, providing antidotal therapy, and hastening the elimination of an absorbed poison. Several methods may be used to terminate the patient's exposure to a toxic substance or mitigate its effects.

For respiratory exposure, removal of the victim from the toxic environment is usually all that is necessary, with careful observation for latent effects of exposures to pulmonary irritants. Involved eyes should be washed for at least 10 to 15 minutes with water. For dermal exposure, the skin should be flushed immediately with water and then washed with copious amounts of water and soap. All contaminated clothing should be removed.

## Basic Life Support

Attention to basic life support and emergency cardiorespiratory support must precede any diagnostic studies in the poisoned child. Respiratory failure can result from upper airway obstruction, central nervous system depression, continuous convulsions, neuromuscular blockade, increased oral and airway secretions, aspiration, and pulmonary edema. An adequate airway is the first priority. It can be accomplished by jaw-thrust or chin-lift maneuvers or the placement of an oral or nasopharyngeal airway or an endotracheal tube. Only endotracheal intubation protects the airway of a comatose patient lacking a gag reflex from the hazards of aspiration.

Hypotension in the poisoned child usually is associated with hypovolemia from excessive volume losses or secondary to vasodilation or capillary leak with third-space losses. Guidelines for fluid resuscitation in the hypotensive patient that have been outlined in earlier chapters (see Chap. 42) can be applied. The insertion of a central venous line or pulmonary venous catheter to measure cardiac output and left ventricular filling pressure may be necessary if hypotension continues despite aggressive fluid administration.

Direct myocardial depression and arrhythmias are less frequent contributors to hypotension. Detection of arrhythmias depends on continuous electrocardiographic monitoring. All drugs used to treat arrhythmias can be dangerous and must be used with great care. It is best to use short-acting drugs. The frequency and recurrence of arrhythmias are increased by hypoxia, acidosis, and electrolyte abnormalities. Specific therapy of complicating arrhythmias is best accomplished after the intoxicating agent is known, but emergency therapy may be needed before a specific poison is diagnosed. The most common arrhythmias are frequent ventricular ectopic beats and ventricular tachycardia. These arrhythmias usually are treated with lidocaine or bretylium. However, in the case of membrane-depressant drugs such as tricyclic antidepressants, some conventional antiarrhythmic agents such as quinidine or procainamide are contraindicated. Lidocaine is the drug of choice. Sinus or junctional bradycardia may respond to intravenous atropine. Intravenous isoproterenol should be infused for unresponsive sinus, junctional, or ventricular bradycardia. Complete atrioventricular block should be treated with an isoproterenol infusion and possibly a transvenous pacemaker.

Control of convulsions is a common problem. Seizures can result from direct toxicity or indirectly from hypoxia, hypoglycemia, and electrolyte disturbances. Anticonvulsant drugs may be ineffective. The most useful are diazepam, lorazepam, phenobarbital, and paraldehyde.

Hyperthermia should be treated with cooling blankets or fans rather than antipyretic drugs. Hypothermia is treated or prevented with warming devices. Coagulopathies may occur, and blood or factor replacement therapy may be indicated.

## Gastrointestinal Decontamination

Traditional principles of gastrointestinal decontamination have undergone scrutiny in recent years. Dilution was previously recommended as an initial step in management of ingestions. Several studies demonstrated that dilution actually enhances absorption of ingested toxins, and therefore it should not be employed. Standard approaches to management have included gastric emptying by emesis or gastric lavage. Evidence suggests that these techniques may not significantly improve toxin retrieval when used in the emergency room and, in the case of ipecac, may delay the effective use of more beneficial agents such as activated charcoal and N-acetylcysteine.

Ipecac may effectively remove some toxins if given within 30 minutes after an ingestion, making it valuable for home use. However, its benefits after 30 minutes in the emergency room are uncertain. Recommended doses of syrup of ipecac are 10 mL for children 6 to 12 months of age, 15 mL for children 1 to 12 years of age, and 30 mL for adolescents and adults. Ipecac induces emesis within 30 minutes in more than 90% of children, although the contents returned may harbor minimal toxin. Absolute contraindications to the use of ipecac include the ingestion of caustic acids or alkalis, altered neurologic status or seizures, loss of airway protective reflexes, or hydrocarbon ingestions, unless the ingested distillate contains dangerous additives such as heavy metals or organophosphates.

Gastric lavage may be more effective than ipecac for removing toxins if gastric emptying is to be employed. Lavage is particularly beneficial within the first hour after ingestion and with drugs that delay gastric emptying, such as narcotics or tricyclic antidepressants. Lavage is contraindicated in alkali ingestions because of the increased risk for esophageal perforation. It should be employed cautiously in patients at risk for developing mental status changes, and endotracheal intubation should be performed first to protect the child with absent or compromised airway reflexes. Lavage should be performed with the patient in a left-side-down, head-down position and is best accomplished with use of a large orogastric hose. A 28-French (9-mm) Ewald tube is the smallest that can be used effectively, because pills and

fragments may not pass through smaller bores. This problem limits the benefits of lavage in small children. A 36-French (12-mm) tube is optimal for adolescents and adults. The most significant retrieval may result from aspirating gastric contents before instilling lavage fluid. Warm physiologic saline should be used in aliquots of 10 mL/kg in pediatric patients (200 to 400 mL in adolescents) and continued until the lavage return is clear. A total volume of at least 2 L is typically required.

Activated charcoal effectively minimizes gastrointestinal absorption of toxins by adsorbing them onto its large surface area. The use of activated charcoal has risen significantly as studies have demonstrated that activated charcoal produces better toxin recovery and fewer complications than emesis or gastric lavage techniques. It should be considered as the primary means of gastrointestinal decontamination in most ingestions, with the exception of a few compounds in which its use is not effective or recommended (Table 32-31). Activated charcoal is most effective if administered during the first several hours after ingestion. Approximately 5 to 10 g of charcoal is required for each gram of drug ingested. Treatment for ingestions of unknown amounts of toxin should be achieved by standard charcoal doses of 1 g/kg (50 to 100 g for adolescents) Initial doses of charcoal should be given with a cathartic such as sorbitol to minimize constipation. Commercial preparations containing both medications are available. Activated charcoal is odorless and tasteless, but its appearance often makes oral acceptance difficult. Nasogastric tube administration should be performed without delay if a child refuses oral intake. Charcoal aspiration can occur, causing bronchospasm and pneumonitis, emphasizing the need for adequate airway protection in the obtunded patient before administration.

Activated charcoal in multiple doses increases the serum clearance of certain toxins. Multiple-dose activated charcoal uses "gastrointestinal dialysis" to adsorb drugs across the gastrointestinal mucosa and take advantage of enterohepatic recirculation. This method has proven effective in oral and intravenous theophylline overdoses and is beneficial for other selected compounds (Table 32-32). A standard dose of activated charcoal should be given initially and then administered orally every 2 to 4 hours until serum drug levels are nontoxic or clinical symptoms of ingestion have resolved. Some patients tolerate repeated doses poorly. The $H_2$-receptor antagonists such as ranitidine may decrease vomiting, and administering charcoal as a continuous drip in saline through a syringe pump can be helpful.

Cathartics do not add significantly to decontamination achieved by other methods. They may be beneficial in ingestions with drugs that decrease gastrointestinal motility, such as tricyclic antidepressants and narcotics. A dose of sorbitol should be employed with the initial activated charcoal dose. Magnesium sulfate may be administered in a dose of 250 mg/kg (maximum dose, 30 g) in a 10% to 20% solution as a cathartic if desired.

**TABLE 32-31. Toxins Not Effectively Adsorbed by Activated Charcoal**

Ethanol
Methanol
Hydrocarbons
Cyanide
Iron
Ethylene glycol
Acids
Alkalis
Lithium

TABLE 32-32.    Toxins With Improved Clearance
by Multiple Dose Activated Charcoal

Theophylline or aminophylline
Phenobarbital
Carbemazepine
Benzodiazepines
Salicylates
Tricyclic antidepressants
Phenothiazines
Phenytoin

## Other Methods of Drug Elimination

The procedures available for enhancing the elimination of an absorbed poison that have the greatest value are diuresis, dialysis, and hemoperfusion. These methods should be used only if proved to be of value, in exceptional circumstances in which the danger of the persisting poison probably exceeds that of removing it, and if the physical and pharmacologic properties of the poison suggest the method would be effective.

For forced diuresis with pH alteration to be an effective therapeutic modality in hastening elimination, several criteria should be met. The drug must have a predominantly renal mode of excretion; drugs that are highly lipid soluble or primarily excreted by the liver are poorly removed with this method. If the drug is highly protein bound, adequate glomerular filtration does not take place. The pK of the drug (ie, the pH at which the proportion of the ionized and unionized forms of that drug are equal) must be such that by altering urinary pH, enough ionization can occur to ensure adequate trapping of the drug in the tubule lumen, which inhibits reabsorption. Alkaline diuresis enhances the excretion of drugs with pK values of 3.0 to 7.2 such as salicylate and barbiturates. Drugs with pK values in the range of 7.2 to 9.5 (eg, quinidine, PCP, fenfluramine, amphetamine) can be enhanced by acid diuresis.

Forced diuresis is achieved by the administration of intravenous fluids at two to five times maintenance requirements to establish urine output of 2 to 5 mL/kg/hour. Bladder catheterization allows the accurate measurement of urine output. Diuretics such as mannitol and furosemide can be used to maintain high urine output. Alkalinization of the urine (ie, pH 7.0 or greater) is accomplished by adding sodium bicarbonate in concentrations of 50 to 75 mEq/L to the intravenous fluids. Hypokalemia often complicates this therapy, and aggressive potassium supplementation may be required. Acetazolamide, a carbonic anhydrase inhibitor, achieves urinary alkalinization through its ability to enhance urinary bicarbonate excretion. However, systemic acidosis is induced and may worsen salicylate toxicity by increasing the proportion of unionized, lipid-soluble serum salicylate, enhancing its penetration into the central nervous system. Acidification of the urine to a pH of 4.0 to 5.0 with ammonium chloride or hydrochloric acid promotes excretion of poisons that are weak bases. Complications of forced diuresis include fluid overload with cerebral edema, pulmonary edema, hyponatremia, and water intoxication. Alkalemia and hypokalemia may complicate bicarbonate use. Hyperammonemia may complicate ammonium chloride use, particularly if there is underlying renal or liver disease.

There are guidelines for the use of hemoperfusion and hemodialysis to enhance actively the removal of intoxicating compounds in adults (indications for employing these techniques in children are not well defined): signs of severe or progressive clinical intoxication, particularly if unresponsive to aggressive medical therapy; ingestion and absorption of a potentially lethal dose of a toxin, even though the patient may not be symptomatic at that point; impaired normal route of excretion; and development of complications of coma.

Hemoperfusion over resins or charcoal has been shown in adults to be the most effective method of extracting some poisons, including barbiturates, methaqualone, glutethimide, tricyclic antidepressants, theophylline, and acetylsalicylic acid. Blood from a venovenous shunt is passed, with the help of a pump, over a ''bed'' of resin or activated charcoal, which binds the compound. The facilities and skills necessary are those that are needed to perform hemodialysis. With the use of smaller hemoperfusion devices, practice of this technique in children has become more common. Complications include thrombocytopenia, hypotension, hypothermia, and hypocalcemia.

Dialysis has been employed to remove toxic poisons. Drugs that are dialyzed effectively are poorly protein bound, are highly water soluble, have a low volume of distribution, and have molecular structures and physical characteristics that enable rapid diffusion across dialysis membranes. Molecules such as methanol, ethanol, ethylene glycol, and procainamide hydrochloride are removed by dialysis.

## MANAGEMENT OF SPECIFIC TOXINS

Although the preceding principles may be applied to most ingestions, an effective pharmacologic antagonist or chelating agent is available for fewer than 5% of poisonings (Table 32-33). These antidotes should be used in consultation with a local poison control center or person trained in the management of poisoning. The physician should be aware that many ingestions are nontoxic and do not require intervention.

Specific management of acetaminophen and salicylate ingestion are discussed in other chapters, but the management of several common toxins is reviewed here.

### Iron Ingestion

Iron ingestion is the most frequent cause of pediatric ingestion fatalities, accounting for 30.2% of deaths in the past 8 years re-

TABLE 32-33.    Systemic Antidotes and
Treatment Agents for Common Ingestions

| Ingested Chemical | Antidote or Treatment |
| --- | --- |
| Acetaminophen | N-acetylcysteine (Mucomyst) |
| Benzodiazepines | Flumazenil |
| Carbon monoxide | Hyperbaric oxygen |
| Cyanide | Sodium nitrite or sodium thiosulfate |
| Digoxin | Digibind (antidigoxin antibody) |
| Iron | Deferoxamine |
| Isoniazid | Pyridoxine |
| Methanol or ethylene glycol | Ethanol |
| Methemoglobinemic agents | Methylene blue |
| Opiates | Naloxone |
| Organophosphates | Atropine, pralidoxime |
| Phenothiazines | Diphenhydramine |
| Warfarin | Vitamin K |

ported by the American Association of Poison Control Centers. Overdoses in young children usually occur as accidental ingestions rather than intentional overdoses.

Ingested iron produces increased capillary permeability, intravascular permeability, and vasodilation on overwhelming the intestinal barrier and entering the circulation. When available free iron exceeds circulating transferrin-binding levels, toxicity of the liver and other parenchymal organs ensues. Iron intoxication usually follows four characteristic stages. The initial phase, occurring shortly after ingestion, is produced by direct effects on gastric and ileal mucosa to induce abdominal pain and vomiting. Gastrointestinal hemorrhage may occur. Fever, leukocytosis, and hyperglycemia are associated findings. In severe intoxications, shock and encephalopathy may ensue in this early stage. In the second phase, a deceptively stable period of ameliorated symptoms and subtle physical findings may follow for 6 to 72 hours. Some patients, however, advance to a third phase with return of gastrointestinal symptoms, metabolic acidosis, coagulopathy and overt shock, and liver dysfunction, rarely progressing to hepatic necrosis. Survivors may develop a fourth phase of gastrointestinal scarring and acute obstruction 4 to 6 weeks after ingestion.

Prediction of potential iron toxicity determines treatment. Estimation of the total dose ingested is helpful but often unreliable. A conservative estimate of 60 mg/kg elemental iron warrants physician evaluation. Serum iron levels should be obtained 2 to 4 hours after ingestion; after 6 hours, the liver has cleared most free iron and levels may be misleading. Mild toxicity may occur with iron levels of 100 to 300 $\mu$g/dL, and moderate toxicity occurs at levels of 300 to 500 $\mu$g/dL. Total iron-binding capacity lower than serum iron levels suggests risk for toxicity. Empiric deferoxamine challenge with 40 mg/kg (maximum dose 1 gram) administered intramuscularly can be used to demonstrate excess circulating free iron, which is chelated and excreted in the urine with a classic pink-orange "vin rose" color. Significant symptoms should encourage aggressive treatment, and abdominal radiographs should be obtained to look for tablet concretions.

Therapy for iron ingestion includes gastric lavage to remove fragments. The use of sodium bicarbonate in the lavage fluid may precipitate iron as insoluble ferrous bicarbonate and decrease absorption. Deferoxamine, an avid iron chelator, should be initiated in all cases of moderate or severe iron poisoning. Doses may be given intramuscularly or as an intravenous infusion. Deferoxamine should be continued until the urine color has normalized or serum iron levels are less than 100 $\mu$g/dL. Close monitoring and supportive therapy for shock are essential.

## Organophosphate Poisoning

Organophosphate poisoning is a leading cause of nonpharmaceutical ingestion fatality in children. Organophosphates such as parathion, malathion, and diazinon are common components of agricultural and domestic insecticides. They are absorbed across skin and mucous membranes by means of ingestion and inhalation, and they bind irreversibly to neuronal and erythrocyte cholinesterase and to liver pseudocholinesterase. This results in failure to terminate the effects of acetylcholine centrally at cortical, respiratory, and cardiac centers and peripherally at nicotinic and muscarinic receptor sites. Symptoms include muscle fasciculations, weakness, paralysis (ie, nicotinic effect), miosis, salivation, lacrimation, diarrhea, bradycardia (ie, muscarinic effect), obtundation, seizures, and apnea (ie, central effect). Symptoms are evidence for more than 50% reduction in enzyme activity. The onset of symptoms may be immediate or delayed for up to 24 hours.

Measurement of decreased serum pseudocholinesterase and erythrocyte cholinesterase confirms the diagnosis, but treatment should be based on elevated suspicion with these symptoms,

even without documented organophosphate exposure. Gastric emptying by lavage should be considered with adequate airway protection. Atropine given in high doses (0.05 mg/kg) antagonizes central and muscarinic effects, but it does not decrease muscle weakness and paralysis induced by nicotinic blockade. Repeated doses are given until cholinergic signs resolve. A continuous infusion may be necessary, because recrudescence can occur for at least 24 hours. The patient should be monitored for anticholinergic toxicity. Pralidoxime is a cholinesterase-reactivating oxime indicated for patients with significant muscle weakness, particularly those requiring mechanical ventilation for respiratory muscle dysfunction. Pralidoxime should be initiated early due to rapid development of resistance by organophosphate–cholinesterase complexes, and doses may need to be repeated over the first 24 hours of treatment.

## Hydrocarbon Ingestion

Hydrocarbon ingestion usually involves common household products, most commonly furniture polish or gasoline. Substances with low viscosity and high volatility such as gasoline and kerosene present the greatest risk for aspiration, which is the major danger from hydrocarbon ingestion. Determination of the exact formulation ingested is important, because some mixtures may include aromatic compounds such as benzene that produce central nervous system toxicity. Fluorinated hydrocarbons such as freon contained in aerosol propellants of various products can induce seizures and cardiac dysrhythmias if inhaled. Children rapidly develop coughing, gagging, choking, and vomiting, which limits the volume of ingestion but may increase the likelihood of aspiration. Dyspnea, cyanosis, and respiratory failure typically ensue over the first 24 hours. Roentgenographic changes are seen in most cases within 12 hours after exposure, and patients with these changes are almost always symptomatic on initial presentation.

Management of hydrocarbon ingestion is primarily symptomatic. Gastric emptying procedures should only be used in ingestions of aromatic substances, if the hydrocarbon is mixed with another toxin, or in very-high-volume ingestions; otherwise, the risk of aspiration may increase. Activated charcoal is ineffective in hydrocarbon ingestion. The patient with asymptomatic ingestion should be observed for approximately 6 hours and can be discharged if no symptoms or hypoxemia develop. Symptomatic patients should be hospitalized for observation, pulse oximetry monitoring, and serial roentgenograms. Neither prophylactic antibiotics or corticosteroids have proven beneficial and may increase risk for superinfection. Patients who develop respiratory failure require intubation and mechanical ventilation, often needing high levels of positive end-expiratory pressure for adequate oxygen delivery.

## Selected Readings

Banner W, Tong TG. Iron poisoning. Pediatr Clin North Am 1987;33:393.
Berkowitz ID, Rogers MC. Poisoning and the critically ill child. In: Roger MC, ed. Textbook of pediatric intensive care. Baltimore: Williams & Wilkins, 1987:1111.
Committee on Accident and Poison Prevention, American Academy of Pediatrics. The non-toxic ingestion. In: Aronow R, ed. Handbook of common poisonings in children, ed 2. Evanston, IL: American Academy of Pediatrics, 1983:16.
Henretig FM, Cupit GC, Temple AR, et al. Toxicologic emergencies. In: Fleisher GR, Ludwig S, eds. Textbook of pediatric emergency medicine, ed 2. Baltimore: Williams & Wilkins, 1988:548.
Kulig K. Initial management of ingestions of toxic substances. N Engl J Med 1992;326:1677.
Litovitz T, Manoguerra A. Comparison of pediatric poisoning hazards: An analysis of 3.8 million exposure incidents. Pediatrics 1992;89:999.
McGuinan MA. Poisoning in childhood. Emerg Med Clin North Am 1983;1:187.
Papadopoulou ZL, Novello AC. The use of hemoperfusion in children. Pediatr Clin North Am 1982;29:1039.

*Principles and Practice of Pediatrics, Second Edition.*
edited by Frank A. Oski et al. J. B. Lippincott Company, Philadelphia © 1994.

## 32.2.2 *Salicylism*

M. Michele Mariscalco

The frequency of aspirin ingestion in U.S. children peaked in the 1960s at 25% of all ingestions. Because of changes in product packaging and the introduction of child-resistant closures, a decline has been seen in the incidence of aspirin ingestion and the death rate associated with it. In recent years, more than 80% of fatal cases have occurred as the result of therapeutic overdose. Chronic salicylism produces greater morbidity than acute salicylate poisoning in the pediatric age group. Chronic salicylism can occur because of therapeutic errors, administration of several salicylate-containing preparations simultaneously, or normal dosing in a dehydrated child. The diagnosis of chronic salicylism may be delayed because its symptoms of fever, vomiting, and tachypnea resemble the disease process for which it is being used therapeutically.

In therapeutic doses, aspirin is absorbed rapidly from the upper small intestine, but absorption after overdose may occur more slowly, and blood salicylate concentrations can continue to rise for as long as 24 hours after ingestion. As higher doses of salicylate are ingested, biotransformation pathways become saturated, and elimination half-life increases from 2 or 3 hours to 15 to 30 hours. The time needed to eliminate a given fraction of a dose increases with increasing dose, and the steady-state plasma concentration of salicylate, particularly that of the pharmacologically active non–protein-bound fraction, increases more than proportionately with increasing dose. Renal excretion of salicylic acid becomes more important as the metabolic pathways of elimination become saturated.

## MANIFESTATIONS

The effects of toxic levels of salicylate include direct stimulation of the central nervous system respiratory center, uncoupling of oxidative phosphorylation, inhibition of Krebs cycle enzymes, inhibition of amino acid metabolism, interference with hemostatic processes, stimulation of gluconeogenesis, and increased tissue glycolysis. Secondary effects include fluid and electrolyte loss, respiratory alkalosis, metabolic acidosis, and impaired glucose metabolism.

The initial effect of respiratory stimulation is independent of increased oxygen consumption or carbon dioxide production. Metabolic acidosis is the result of the collective effects of elevated lactic acid and pyruvic acid secondary to Krebs cycle enzyme inhibition; increased ketone body formation from accelerated lipid metabolism; and aminoacidemia from inhibition of aminotransferases. In younger children, in chronic salicylate toxicity, and in large-dose poisoning in older children, metabolic acidosis appears early and is most prominent clinically with a concomitant respiratory alkalosis. Older children with moderate- or small-dose poisoning and most adults are able to compensate the metabolic acidosis by hyperventilation, resulting in respiratory alkalosis. Hypoglycemia is uncommon but quite severe when it occurs, and it usually occurs late. Hyperglycemia is more common. Significant central nervous system hypoglycemia can occur with normal blood glucose levels.

Severe fluid and electrolyte loss can occur with salicylate toxicity. Increased heat production due to uncoupling of oxidative phosphorylation, hyperpnea, and tachypnea all lead to an increase in insensible water loss. Decreased oral intake and vomiting and the increase in obligatory water and electrolyte loss necessitated by the enhanced renal solute load of organic acids further aggravate the water, sodium, and potassium loss. Renal excretion of bicarbonate is increased, contributing to the metabolic acidosis.

The clinical signs and symptoms of acute salicylate poisoning may be confused with diabetic ketoacidosis. Usual symptoms include disorientation, nausea, vomiting, dehydration, hyperpnea, hyperpyrexia, oliguria, tinnitus, coma, and convulsions. Unusual findings are bleeding, respiratory depression, pulmonary edema, acute tubular necrosis, inappropriate secretion of antidiuretic hormone, hepatotoxicity, nephropathy, bronchospasm, anaphylaxis, hemolysis, and electroencephalographic abnormalities.

The estimated amount of drug ingested may predict the severity of the clinical syndrome. Ingested doses of greater than 150 mg/kg of body weight are usually benign. Mild to moderate toxicity occurs with doses of 150 to 300 mg/kg. Ingestions of greater than 300 mg/kg generally cause more severe symptoms, and an overdose of more than 500 mg/kg may cause death. These guidelines do not apply to chronic salicylate intoxication. Observations show that chronic toxicity is likely if doses greater than 100 mg/kg/day have been ingested for 2 or more days. Clinical findings reflect the severity of the intoxication. Mild intoxication is characterized by mild hyperpnea, sometimes with lethargy. Severe hyperpnea with prominent neurologic disturbances (eg, marked lethargy, excitability) but not coma or convulsions suggests moderate poisoning. Coma, semicoma, and convulsions with severe hyperpnea mark severe intoxication.

The Done nomogram (Fig 32-5) is useful in acute poisonings

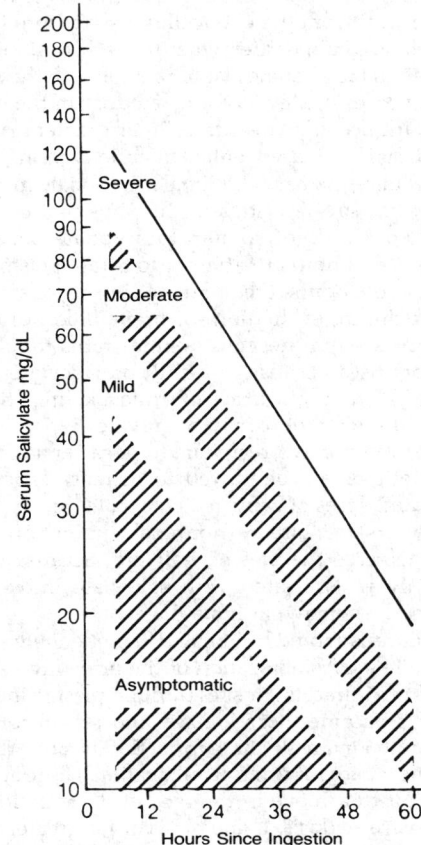

**Figure 32-5.** Done nomogram for estimating the severity of poisoning using serum salicylate levels. (Temple AR. Acute and chronic effects of aspirin toxicity and their treatment. Arch Intern Med 1981;141:364.)

for estimating the severity of toxicity based on the patient's serum salicylate level at 6 hours or more after the purported time of ingestion. The nomogram cannot be used for chronic aspirin intoxication. At each of three blood salicylate concentration ranges, studies have confirmed that severe symptoms occur with a much greater frequency in the chronically intoxicated group than in the acutely intoxicated group.

## TREATMENT

As with all ingestions, therapy initially is directed toward ensuring adequate ventilation, oxygenation, and cardiovascular stability. Gastric lavage or emesis should be performed even 12 to 24 hours after ingestion because salicylates delay gastric emptying. Activated charcoal then is administered. Salicylate levels should be obtained every 4 to 6 hours to determine that no further absorption is occurring.

Fluid therapy is aimed at promoting renal salicylate excretion and restoring hydration and electrolyte balance. Large volumes of isotonic solution such as lactated Ringer's solution may be necessary to restore the circulating blood volume, to correct hypotension, and to improve peripheral perfusion and urine flow. Subsequent fluid replacement depends on the degree of dehydration. The fluid should contain 5% dextrose with saline (0.45%), with 35 to 70 mEq of sodium bicarbonate per liter of solution. The addition of potassium is necessary to correct hypokalemia after the urine output is established. Vitamin K should be given, particularly in severe, chronic intoxication. Hyperpyrexia is managed by external cooling with a cooling blanket.

The therapy of acidosis is critical in the management of salicylate intoxication. Acidosis enhances the passage of salicylates (nonionized form) from the extracellular space into the cells, including the blood–brain barrier, where they disrupt mitochondrial function. Sodium bicarbonate alkalinizes solely in the extracellular space and increases the level of ionized drug in the extracellular plasma. The intracellular-to-extracellular gradient of diffusible, nonionized drug is increased, enhancing the trapping of salicylate in the extracellular plasma. Additional bicarbonate may be needed if the patient has severe acidosis. The physician can cautiously administer 1 to 2 mEq of sodium bicarbonate per kg of body weight every 1 to 2 hours to attempt to titrate plasma pH to 7.5 over the first 4 to 8 hours. Frequent monitoring of serum sodium and frequent clinical evaluation for brain–blood disequilibrium are mandatory. Central nervous system status may improve as the plasma pH rises because of a shift of salicylate equilibrium from brain to blood despite a lack of urine alkalinization. Sodium bicarbonate administration may aggravate hypernatremia and hypokalemia, and it may precipitate hypocalcemia and seizures.

Several methods are employed to increase salicylate elimination. Repeated doses of activated charcoal (1 g/kg immediately and every 4 hours) increase the nonrenal elimination of salicylate and greatly decrease the plasma half-life. Because of vomiting that commonly is associated with salicylate intoxication, this treatment may be somewhat limited.

Alkaline diuresis should be initiated in moderately and severely intoxicated patients. Alkalinization of the urine favors movement of salicylate from intracellular sites through plasma into the urine. The salicylates become more ionized and less absorbable from the tubular lumen in an alkaline urine. Sodium bicarbonate continues to be the choice for urine alkalinization. Urine alkalinization may be difficult to achieve in the face of dehydration, hypokalemia, and severe acidosis. Urine pH is of far greater importance than the volume of urine excreted. To achieve maximum excretion of salicylate, a urine pH above 7.5 and ideally between 8.0 and 8.5 is necessary. Diuretics should not be used until euvolemia is achieved. Clinical examinations and laboratory determinations must be repeated frequently to avoid cerebral and pulmonary edema from overhydration, hypernatremia, hyponatremia, hypokalemia, hypocalcemia, and severe alkalosis.

Dialysis or charcoal hemoperfusion should be considered for the severely ill patient with renal failure, severe central nervous system manifestations, pulmonary edema, or severe acidosis unresponsive to conventional therapy. Dialysis also should be considered for patients with elevated levels initially (ie, projected salicylate level at time of ingestion greater than 160 mg/dL) or a 6-hour level greater than 130 mg/dL. Peritoneal dialysis is less effective than alkaline diuresis, but it can be employed in the presence of oliguria. Hemodialysis is the treatment of choice. Charcoal hemoperfusion, although better than alkaline diuresis or peritoneal dialysis, is less effective than hemodialysis.

## Selected Readings

Berkowitz ID, Rogers MC. Poisoning and the critically ill child. In: Rogers MC, ed. Textbook of pediatric intensive care. Baltimore: Williams & Wilkins, 1988:1157.

Hentretig FM, Cupit GC, Temple AR. Toxicologic emergencies. In: Fleisher G, Ludwig S, eds. Textbook of pediatric emergency medicine. Baltimore: Williams & Wilkins, 1983:509.

Meredith TJ, Vale JA. Non-narcotic analgesics: Problems of overdosage. Drug 1986;32(S4):177.

Opheim KE, Raisys VA. Therapeutic drug monitoring in pediatric acute drug intoxications. Ther Drug Monit 1985;7:148.

Snodgrass WR. Salicylate toxicity. Pediatr Clin North Am 1986;33:381.

*Principles and Practice of Pediatrics, Second Edition.*
edited by Frank A. Oski et al. J. B. Lippincott Company, Philadelphia © 1994.

## 32.2.3 *Acetaminophen Overdose*

### M. Michele Mariscalco

Acetaminophen has been used increasingly for analgesia and antipyresis in children, partially because of studies linking the use of salicylates with the development of Reye's syndrome. Acetaminophen is widely available. Children younger than 6 years of age and adolescents are the two groups most often associated with acetaminophen overdoses. Overdose most commonly affects children younger than 6 years of age; it is usually accidental. The amount of acetaminophen consumed by this group of patients is less than that ingested by adolescents. In the adolescent group, the overdose is either a suicide attempt or a manipulative episode. Handfuls of tablets typically are consumed.

Children younger than 6 years of age and adolescents have different patterns of toxicity from acetaminophen overdose. Of the children younger than 6 years of age who ingested enough acetaminophen to have a level in the toxic range, only 5% developed hepatotoxicity, compared with the 30% of adults and adolescents with toxic acetaminophen levels. Adolescents and adults are twice as likely to develop plasma levels in the toxic range as children younger than 6 years of age. Adults and adolescents account for most serious and fatal cases of acetaminophen poisoning. The number of fatal cases has decreased since the addition of acetylcysteine to the treatment regimen. It is extremely rare for young children to ingest sufficient acetaminophen to cause more than minimal liver damage, but serious, even fatal, cases of overdose have been reported.

# PHARMACOLOGY

Acetaminophen is absorbed rapidly after an oral therapeutic dose, producing a peak plasma level between 30 and 60 minutes after ingestion. This absorption may be delayed in overdose so that peak plasma levels may not occur until 4 hours after ingestion. Approximately 94% of the drug is metabolized to the glucuronide or sulfate conjugate; 2% is excreted unchanged in the urine. Neither the conjugated forms nor the unchanged forms are hepatotoxic. The remaining 4% is metabolized through the cytochrome P-450 mixed-function oxidase system. It conjugates with glutathione to produce mercapturic acid, which is excreted in the urine. With a significant overdose, the P-450 mixed-function oxidase becomes the major system for metabolizing acetaminophen. When the liver glutathione stores are sufficiently depleted—usually to about 70% of normal—the highly reactive intermediate metabolite binds to hepatic macromolecules and produces hepatocellular necrosis.

The mechanism of acetylcysteine as an antidote for acetaminophen is not well defined. It is hypothesized that acetylcysteine is metabolized to cysteine, a glutathione precursor, and it protects by providing increased levels of glutathione. Hepatic toxicity is defined as a rise in serum glutamic-oxaloacetic transaminase (SGOT); significant toxicity occurs at SGOT levels of 1000 IU/L or greater. Other indicators of hepatotoxicity are a rise in bilirubin and prothrombin time. Hepatocellular necrosis may be severe enough to progress to acute fulminant hepatic failure.

Several mechanisms for decreased toxicity of acetaminophen in children have been postulated, including higher turnover rate of glutathione, which indicates more availability for detoxification and increased rates of sulfatization and spontaneous vomiting after ingestion. The co-ingestion of alcohol in children and adults appears to be hepatoprotective, probably due to the competition by alcohol at the P-450 site.

Chronic acetaminophen poisoning in a manner similar to chronic salicylate poisoning does not occur. Unlike salicylate, acetaminophen does not depend on renal excretory mechanisms. If the patient is receiving therapeutic doses of acetaminophen over a long period, he or she should safely manage the small load of toxic metabolites with the constantly regenerating glutathione stores in the liver. Studies performed in adults with chronic liver disease show no accumulation of therapeutic amounts of acetaminophen when administered for as long as 2 weeks. It is important to review carefully the history of a patient who was supposedly taking therapeutic doses of acetaminophen but has developed a high level.

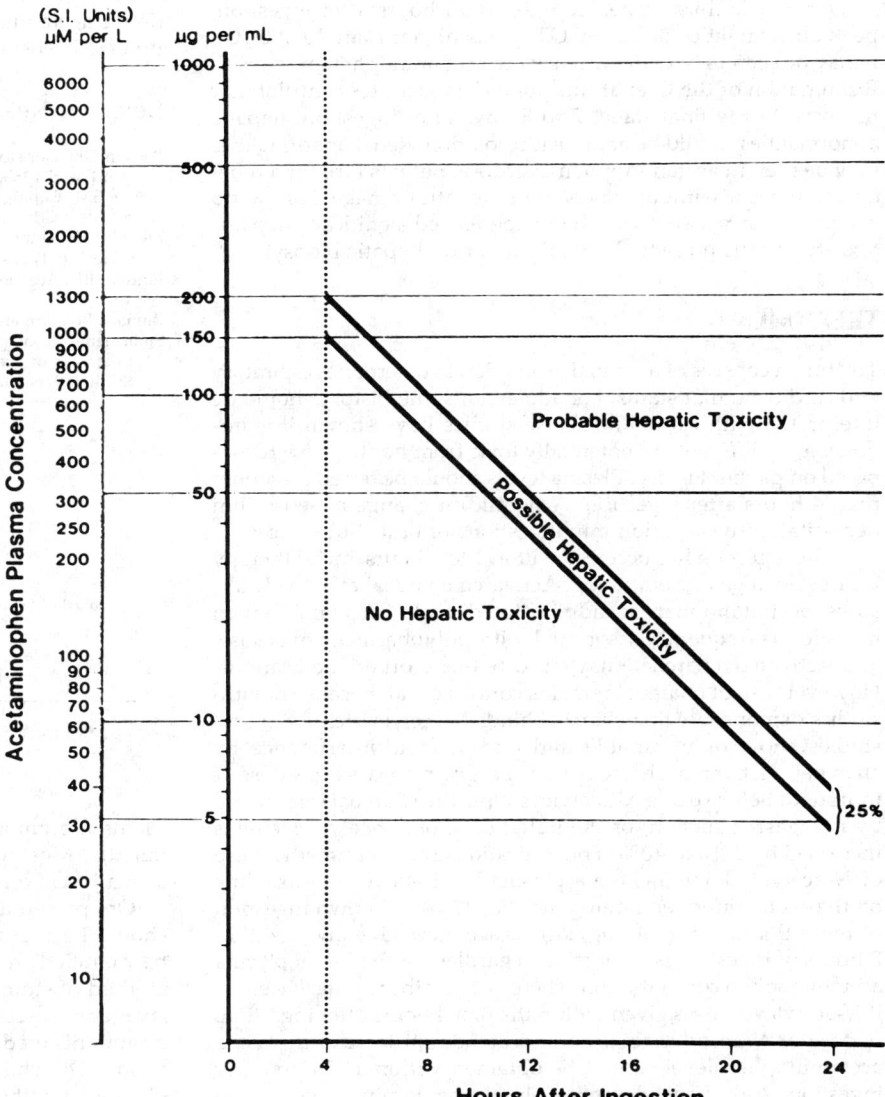

**Figure 32-6.** Semilogarithmic plot of plasma acetaminophen levels over time. Levels drawn less than 4 hours after ingestion may not represent peak levels. The lower solid line 25% below the standard nomogram is included to allow for possible errors in acetaminophen plasma assays and estimated time from ingestion of an overdose. (Rumack BH, Matthew H. Acetaminophen poisoning and toxicity. Pediatrics 1975;55:871; reproduced with permission.)

Clinical experience suggests that if an adult consumes more than 7.5 g of acetaminophen as a single dose or if a child ingests 150 mg/kg of body weight, hepatotoxicity may result. Plasma acetaminophen levels are not interpretable until at least 4 hours after ingestion. The overall mortality of unselected patients with untreated acetaminophen poisoning is 1% to 2%.

## CLINICAL COURSE

The clinical course of acetaminophen toxicity has four stages. In the first stage (ie, first 24 hours), adult and adolescent patients develop nausea, vomiting, diaphoresis, and general malaise. Children younger than 6 years of age show little diaphoresis and vomit earlier. They develop vomiting regardless of the acetaminophen level and have no symptoms unless the blood level is in the toxic range. Symptoms develop within 14 hours in patients with toxic levels of acetaminophen. Liver enzymes are normal during this period. Lethargy is rarely seen during this stage. If lethargy develops, some other agent should be considered in addition to or instead of the acetaminophen. During the second stage (ie, second 24 hours), most patients begin to feel better. If no treatment was received or treatment was unsuccessful, the SGOT, serum glutamic-pyruvic transaminase (SGPT), bilirubin level, and prothrombin time begin to become abnormal.

During the third stage, from 48 to 96 hours after ingestion, peak abnormalities occur. SGOT levels higher than 20,000 IU/L may be seen in patients with severe acetaminophen overdoses. Examination of the liver at this point demonstrates centrilobular necrosis. In the final stage, 7 to 8 days after ingestion, hepatic abnormalities should be at or near resolution. Renal abnormalities may be seen in acetaminophen overdose, but it is rare for a renal defect to occur without concomitant hepatic damage. Follow-up evaluation of patients who had experienced significant hepatotoxicity reveals no sequelae clinically or on hepatic biopsy.

## TREATMENT

Treatment consists of an initial evaluation to determine respiratory and cardiovascular status. For adolescents, the history should be interpreted with caution, because studies have shown it is impossible to differentiate potentially toxic from nontoxic overdoses based on patient history. Plasma levels should be tested no sooner than 4 hours after ingestion. A significant change in sensorium necessitates investigation into ingestions of other substances.

If the ingestion has occurred within 1 to 2 hours, initial therapy is directed at gastric emptying. Activated charcoal effectively absorbs acetaminophen if administered early. Acetaminophen ingestion is frequently associated with polypharmacy overdose, and activated charcoal may absorb these other medications. However, use of charcoal remains controversial, because in vitro studies demonstrate that charcoal binds N-acetylcysteine. Clinical studies show only variable and questionable interference by charcoal. Activated charcoal may be given in a single dose if indicated. Before using N-acetylcysteine, the charcoal is removed by nasogastric suction, or the initial dose of N-acetylcysteine is increased by 30% to 40%. The indications for the immediate use of N-acetylcysteine include a plasma level above the toxic line on the acetaminophen nomogram (Fig 32-6) or known ingestion of more than 7.5 g (150 mg/kg). N-acetylcysteine given within 8 hours of ingestion is protective, regardless of the initial plasma acetaminophen concentration. There is no further protective effect if N-acetylcysteine is given within the first 4 hours after ingestion. A dose of N-acetylcysteine should be administered if a plasma acetaminophen level cannot be obtained within 16 hours after ingestion, and N-acetylcysteine should be administered as late as 24 hours after ingestion.

In the patient with an unknown amount of acetaminophen ingestion (<7.5 g or <150 mg/kg), the plasma level is determined not earlier than 4 hours after ingestion, and the potential for toxicity is determined by the nomogram (see Fig 32-6).

Second and third levels are of interest, but they are not used to determine whether treatment should continue. Acetylcysteine is administered orally in a final concentration of 5% (weight/volume). The initial oral dose is 140 mg/kg, with subsequent doses at 4-hour intervals of 70 mg/kg for an additional 17 doses. The dose should be repeated if the patient vomits within 1 hour of administration. Antiemetic drugs are not recommended. Intravenous administration of acetylcysteine is by experimental protocol only. Intravenous acetylcysteine has been associated with the development of allergic reactions. If activated charcoal has been used, the stomach should be emptied before administration of oral acetylcysteine, because activated charcoal binds it. Baseline data should include SGOT, SGPT, bilirubin level, prothrombin time, and creatinine level. Another set of data should be drawn in at most 24-hour intervals after ingestion. Abnormalities become apparent 36 to 48 hours after ingestion, with the peak usually at 72 to 96 hours.

Although children younger than 6 years of age are unlikely to experience toxic effects, the recommendation is that any patient with a plasma acetaminophen level in the toxic range should be treated. A child accidentally consuming small amounts of children's acetaminophen can be managed safely at home if follow-up care is ensured.

## Selected Readings

Benson GD. Hepatotoxicity following the therapeutic use of antipyretic analgesic. Am J Med 1983;14:85.
Levine SM. Coping with drug overdose/poisoning, part 3: Analgesics and other agents. J Crit Illness 1991;6:995.
Meredith TJ, Vale JA. Non-narcotic analgesic problems of overdosage. Drugs 1986;32(S4):177.
Rumack BH. Acetaminophen overdose in young children. Am J Dis Child 1984;138: 428.
Rumack BH. Acetaminophen overdose. Pediatr Clin North Am 1986;33:691.
Smilkstein MJ, Knapp GG, Kulig KW, et al. Efficacy of oral N-acetylcysteine in the treatment of acetaminophen overdose. Analysis of the National Multicenter Study (1976–1985). N Engl J Med 1988;319:1557.

*Principles and Practice of Pediatrics, Second Edition.*
edited by Frank A. Oski et al. J. B. Lippincott Company, Philadelphia © 1994.

## 32.2.4 *Plant Poisoning*

M. Michele Mariscalco

Plants are among the accidental ingestions reported most frequently. Most ingestions involve house and garden plants, only a small fraction of which pose a serious toxic threat.

On presentation to the emergency department, the child should be evaluated and treatment begun unless the plant can be identified and is known to be nontoxic. Emesis is the preferred method of stomach evacuation, because it is more efficient than lavage in evacuating plant particles. Activated charcoal should be administered, because it is extremely useful in adsorbing plant toxins. The child should be observed for a short period. If the plant is identified and thought to be nontoxic or if it cannot be recognized and the child remains asymptomatic, the child may be discharged. If the child ingested a potentially toxic species or is symptomatic, he or she should be admitted for further observation and supportive treatment.

## PLANT TOXINS

Most of the symptomatic plant poisonings in the United States are from a large heterogenous group that cause gastrointestinal irritation. Philodendron and dieffenbachia leaves cause minor mouth and throat burning. Ingestion of the leaves from these plants can result occasionally in severe oropharyngeal injury with airway compromise. Severe vomiting, colicky abdominal pain, and diarrhea can result from ingestion of pokeweed roots and stems, wisteria seeds, buttercup leaves, daffodil bulbs, and seeds and pods from the bird of paradise. Twenty to 30 of the bright red or black berries of the holly tree are estimated to be a fatal dose for a small child. Holly contains ilicin and several unidentified toxins that cause diarrhea, vomiting, nausea, and abdominal pains. Boxwood contains a toxic alkaloid that can cause severe gastroenteritis if a moderate quantity of leaves is eaten.

The rosary pea (ie, jequirty bean or Indian bean) and castor beans are attractive seeds and are used extensively in inexpensive beadwork and jewelry. They contain a toxalbumin that is released when chewed, causing a violent hemorrhagic gastroenteritis, leading to profound dehydration and circulatory collapse. Therapy consists of fluid and electrolyte management. Alkalinization of the urine with sodium bicarbonate may prevent precipitation of hemoglobin and its products in the kidney tubules.

The leaves of common foxglove, oleander, and lily of the valley and the berries of mistletoe contain cardiac glycosides. Soon after ingestion, the child may complain of mouth irritation, vomiting, and diarrhea. As the digitalis is absorbed, acute digitalis effects ensue as evidenced by bradycardia with progressive heart block and hyperkalemia. Anecdotal reports indicate that digoxin-specific Fab antibody may be efficacious in reversing these acute effects. Mistletoe also contains sympathomimetics that may cause seizures and hypertension.

Nicotine or nicotinelike alkaloids are found in wild tobacco leaves, golden chain tree seeds, all parts of yellow jasmine, and poison hemlock seeds and leaves. Ingestion leads to spontaneous vomiting within 1 hour. Salivation, headache, fever, mental confusion, and muscular weakness may follow, and the child may deteriorate with convulsions, coma, and death due to respiratory failure.

Water hemlock frequently is labeled the most violent plant toxin known. Rapid-onset seizure activity has been reported after its ingestion. Ingestion is characterized also by tremors and muscle rigidity. Charcoal is especially useful in adsorbing these nicotinic alkaloids. Additional treatment consists of intensive supportive care with control of seizures and ventilatory assistance.

Other members of the nightshade family, such as the blue and black nightshade, Jerusalem cherry, and wild tomato, contain the toxic alkaloid solanine. Symptoms of solanine ingestion include vomiting, nausea, diarrhea, convulsions, and respiratory and central nervous system depression. Therapy consists of support of respiration and symptomatic treatment.

Jimsonweed, belladonna (ie, deadly nightshade), and angel's trumpet contain belladonna alkaloids, with atropine as a major constituent. Symptoms include visual blurring, dilated pupils, dryness of the mouth, hot and dry skin, fever, tachycardia, absent bowel sounds, urinary retention, delirium, or psychosis. Convulsions and coma may follow. Treatment consists of supportive care. Physostigmine may be used cautiously for severe sequelae.

A tea popular in Mexico and the southwestern and western United States called gordolobos (ie, tansy ragwort, fat wolf herb, groundsel, or mullein) has caused several deaths in children and adults. The alkaloids in the tea have been responsible for the acute and chronic liver disease that occurs.

Cyanide is an integral part of the chemical structure of amygdalin and prunasin, which are found in a surprising number of plants. Some examples of cyanide-containing plants include peach, apricot, plums, apples, chokeberries, lima beans, and hydrangea plant. Cyanide usually is concentrated in traditionally nonedible parts of commercial fruits, such as apricot kernels and apple seeds. There have been reports of serious illness and deaths among children who ate large amounts of raw apricot kernels. Gut hydrolysis is required for release of free cyanide, and intestinal decontamination using available cyanide kits may be lifesaving.

## MUSHROOM POISONING

Mushrooms cause an estimated 50% of all deaths from plant poisoning in the United States. Susceptibility to mushroom toxins varies greatly among species and persons. The severity of poisoning by a particular toxic mushroom also may depend on the season, the degree of maturity of the specimen, and the quantity of mushrooms consumed by the victim. Two main groups of mushrooms can be characterized on the basis of the interval between ingestion and symptom onset. Toxins that give rise to self-limited neurologic or gastrointestinal tract illness cause symptoms within 15 minutes to 2 hours after ingestion. More potent toxins capable of causing fatal poisonings do not produce symptoms until 6 to 18 hours after ingestion. Regardless of the type of mushroom, the initial management for all suspected mushroom poisonings includes emesis, charcoal, and catharsis.

Mushrooms with early-onset symptoms fall into three groups. Those with muscarinic effects produce cholinergic symptoms, such as sweating, lacrimation, blurred vision, miosis, watery diarrhea, abdominal cramps, and bradycardia, within 1 hour. Other mushrooms affect principally the central nervous system, causing dizziness, incoordination, ataxia, muscle twitching, hyperkinetic activity, and hallucinations within 2 to 3 hours of ingestion. Another group exerts its effect solely on the gastrointestinal tract, causing nausea, vomiting, diarrhea, and abdominal cramps. Management of patients who have ingested mushrooms with early-onset symptoms requires careful attention to fluid and electrolytes. The use of barbiturates and benzodiazepines should be avoided, because they may exacerbate symptoms.

Mushrooms causing symptoms that are delayed 6 to 24 hours after ingestion produce serious, potentially fatal poisoning. Two groups are recognized, both of which contain toxins causing cellular destruction. The first group produces nausea and vomiting followed by muscle cramps, abdominal pain, and severe watery or bloody diarrhea. In more serious poisonings, fever, liver failure, and central nervous system symptoms may supervene, sometimes followed by convulsions, coma, and death. The second group of poisonous mushrooms, *Amanita phalloides*, are responsible for 95% of fatal mushroom poisonings. The latent period of onset is 12 to 24 hours. The toxic effects are due to phallotoxins that act first, causing gastrointestinal symptoms including nausea, vomiting, abdominal pain, and diarrhea, and the amatoxins, which are responsible for cellular destruction, particularly renal and hepatic, through inhibition of protein synthesis.

The initial step in the treatment of any case of mushroom poisoning is rapid identification of the offending mushroom. A mycologist with experience in mushroom identification is essential for this task. Attention is paid to the latency period between consumption and symptom onset. Therapy should be geared to close monitoring of electrolyte and circulating volume status, hydration, and general supportive care. If more than 6 hours have elapsed between ingestion and onset of symptoms, potentially fatal poisoning from amatoxin should be anticipated. Gastric emptying often is delayed after ingestion, and attempts at gastric decontamination even many hours after ingestion may be beneficial. Charcoal appears to be helpful, even many hours after ingestion. Some toxins undergo enterohepatic circulation, making repeated doses of charcoal useful.

Patients may present with renal or hepatic failure. Appropriate laboratory tests such as blood urea nitrogen, creatinine, serum glutamic-oxaloacetic transaminase, serum glutamic-pyruvic transaminase, coagulation profiles, and bilirubin should be undertaken in any suspected amatoxin poisoning. Hypoglycemia, gastrointestinal hemorrhage, coagulopathy, and encephalopathy may occur in patients with liver failure. Therapies such as thioctic acid, pyridoxine, high-dose penicillin, and steroids have not been proved to be effective in controlled studies. In cases of potentially severe ingestions, contact should be made with toxicologists at a regional poison center to determine the current recommendations on management of these patients. Liver transplantation has been successful in patients with liver failure.

## Selected Readings

Arena JM. Poisonous plants, reptiles, arthropods, insects and fish. In: Arena JM, ed. Poisoning. Springfield, IL: Charles C Thomas, 1979:538.

Bivins HG, Lammers R, McMicken DB, Wolowodiuk O. Mushroom ingestion. Ann Emerg Med 1985;14:1099.

Committee on Accident and Poison Prevention, American Academy of Pediatrics. Plants. In: Aronow R, ed. Handbook of common poisonings in children, ed 2. Evanston, IL: American Academy of Pediatrics, 1983:120.

Hanrahan JP, Gordon MA. Mushroom poisoning. JAMA 1984;251:1057.

Henretig FM, Cupit GC, Temple AR, et al. Toxicologic emergencies. In: Fleisher G, Ludwig S, eds. Textbook of pediatric emergency medicine. Baltimore: Williams & Wilkins, 1988:548.

Kunkel DB. Plant poisoning in children. Pediatr Ann 1987;16:927.

*Principles and Practice of Pediatrics, Second Edition.*
edited by Frank A. Oski et al. J. B. Lippincott Company, Philadelphia © 1994.

## 32.2.5 *Lead Poisoning*

J. Julian Chisolm, Jr.

The Centers for Disease Control (CDC), in the 1991 Statement on Preventing Lead Poisoning in Young Children, identified lead poisoning as one of the most common and preventable pediatric health problems in the United States. It has been estimated that 3 to 4 million children between the ages of 6 months and 6 years had blood lead levels greater than 15 $\mu$g/dL of whole blood (0.72 $\mu$mol/L) in 1984. More comprehensive national figures for prevalence can be determined after data from the third National Health and Nutrition Examination Survey, conducted between 1988 and 1992, become available. It is estimated that the geometric mean blood lead concentration in the United States today among young children is 5 $\mu$g/dL of whole blood (0.25 $\mu$mol/L), with a long tail in the distribution on the high side of this mean. The CDC in its 1991 Statement reduced the level for concern from a blood lead level of 25 $\mu$g/dL to 10 $\mu$g/dL, based on evidence that children with a time-integrated mean blood lead level less than 25 $\mu$g/dL are at risk for adverse health effects. As sustained blood lead levels rise above 10 to 15 $\mu$g/dL (0.5 to 0.72 $\mu$mol/L), the children are at progressively increasing risk for future neurobehavioral and cognitive deficits, which are long lasting and can impede learning in school.

With the removal of lead from gasoline and its reduction in food, old paint, interior household dust, and possibly exterior soil are now the most significant sources of lead exposure for young children in the United States. Chronically increased lead absorption is most prevalent in young children who live in deteriorated dwellings built before 1950.

Most affected children are asymptomatic and are being identified through screening programs. Blood lead is the primary screening test, having replaced the less sensitive erythrocyte protoporphyrin (EP) test. Acute lead colic and lead encephalopathy, the most severe and potentially fatal form of this chronic disorder, are rare in the United States, but they may be more commonly encountered in some Third World countries. Current chelation therapy substantially reduces mortality. It is difficult to carry out successfully after the onset of severe symptoms but relatively simple to carry out before the onset of symptoms. In many areas of the United States, lead poisoning is a reportable disease. In some areas, under Child Wellness programs, screening is being mandated, particularly for children in public assistance programs.

## SOURCES OF EXPOSURE

The lead contents of food and air have decreased drastically during the past 15 years. After the almost complete removal of lead additives from gasoline, air lead levels decreased from 1.5 $\mu$g/m$^3$ to less than 0.2 $\mu$g/m$^3$, even in congested cities. This reduction and the systematic elimination of domestically produced food cans with lead-soldered seams diminished food lead in young children to 1 $\mu$g Pb/kg body weight/day. Lead in drinking water may be associated with significant overexposure in some areas of the country in which drinking water is acidic, plumbosolvent, and conveyed in lead pipes or in copper pipes with lead-soldered joints. This problem often can be managed in public water supplies by neutralizing the water. Uncontaminated drinking water contains less than 20 $\mu$g Pb/L. Such exposure are associated with a geometric mean blood lead level of 5 $\mu$g Pb/dL (range, 1 to 15 $\mu$g/dL). Although there appears to be no blood lead threshold for measurable adverse effects of lead, such exposure does not appear to be associated with clinically significant adverse effects.

After the substantial reductions in the lead content of food, drinking water, and air, lead in interior household dust and old residential paints constitute the major sources of overexposure to lead among children in the United States, and these will continue to be the major sources for the foreseeable future. Studies suggest that the exposure potential of lead in exterior soil may be highly variable, in part related to the chemical species of the lead. For example, exposure in the proximity of older lead smelting operations is quite hazardous, but exposure to lead in some types of mine tailings may not present much of a hazard. In the United States, 52% of the housing occupied in 1980 was built before 1950, when lead paints were widely used and basic lead carbonate was the almost universal white pigment. Interior dust in old housing may average 600 to 3000 $\mu$g Pb/g. Exterior surface soil in some areas may contain 2000 to 16,000 $\mu$g Pb/g. Multilayered chips of old lead pigment paints may contain 20,000 to 100,000 $\mu$g Pb/cm$^2$ of exposed surface area.

Increased absorption of lead is found among children living near lead processing smelters and among the children of workers who bring leaded dust into their homes on their work clothing.

In Third World countries, particularly in Northern Africa, the Middle East, China, southeast Asia and Mexico, ancient folk medicines and cosmetics (eg, azarcon, greta, paylooah, surma, al kohl, ghasard, liga, bali goli, bint, al dahab) and some infant tonics and teething powders containing lead (and sometimes arsenic and mercury) are still used and have caused fatal illness. These practices date back for millennia. Cases traceable to these sources have been found in the United States, because immigrants bring the practices with them. The physician must be familiar with immigrant ethnic groups and their practices.

Sporadic cases of clinical plumbism have been traced to other sources with very high concentrations of lead, including juices or cola drinks conveyed or stored in improperly lead-glazed earthenware; lead type sucked on; lead shot, fishing or curtain weights, and lead jewelry swallowed and retained in the stomach, where lead is dissolved and absorbed; "soft" drinking water conveyed in lead pipes or stored in lead-lined cisterns; lead-soldered vessels used in cooking; fumes from the burning of painted wood or casings of storage batteries; sanding and burning of paint containing lead. These exposures cause inorganic lead poisoning.

The sniffing of leaded gasoline by older children and adolescents causes organic lead poisoning, characterized by toxic encephalopathy. The organic solvents probably play a significant role in this type of poisoning.

## EPIDEMIOLOGY

The 1988 report of the Agency for Toxic Substances and Disease Registry on the nature and extent of lead poisoning in children in the United States, although based on data up to 1984, provides the most current estimates of environmental exposures to lead and its impact on infants, toddlers, and young children. In 1984, about 12 million children younger than 7 years of age were living in old housing with potentially toxic amounts of lead in the paint. About 1.8 to 2 million children lived in the oldest housing, which was also deteriorated, and were at the highest risk for toxic lead exposures. In 1983, according to the U.S. Census Bureau, 41.8 million (52%) dwelling units were built before 1950 but were still occupied and constituted the greatest hazard. The highest interior dust lead levels are found in and about such housing. Based on the small decline in the numbers of occupied, deteriorated housing between 1970 and 1980, it is not anticipated that the number of children at risk is much less in the early 1990s.

Exterior surface soil lead and interior paint contribute significantly to interior household dust lead. A major pathway of lead into the bodies of children is the hand-to-mouth route. When exposed to house dust containing greater than 1000 $\mu$g Pb/g of dust, the preschool child with extensive hand-to-mouth activity may sustain blood lead levels ranging from 16 to 60 $\mu$g/dL. More severe degrees of poisoning are generally associated with repetitive ingestion (ie, pica) of lead paint debris or some uncommon source.

## LEAD ABSORPTION

### Distribution, Retention, and Excretion

Lead is absorbed into the body through the respiratory and gastrointestinal tracts. It is also absorbed transplacentally by the fetus. The relative absorption through these different routes varies and is affected by age, nutritional status, and the particle size and chemical form of the lead. Absorption is inversely proportional to particle size, a factor that makes lead-bearing dust so important. From 30% to 50% of lead that is inhaled is deposited in the respiratory tract and absorbed. More than 75% of lead particles deposited in the upper respiratory tract that are too large to be absorbed in the lung are transported to the gastrointestinal tract for absorption. Adults absorb 5% to 10% of dietary lead and retain little of it, but young children absorb 40% to 50% and retain 20% to 25%. Spontaneous urinary excretion of lead in infants and young toddlers normally is about 1 $\mu$g/kg/24 hours. This may increase somewhat in acute poisonings.

Studies using animals show that diets high in fat, particularly those low in calcium, magnesium, iron, zinc, and copper, increase the absorption of lead. Diets suboptimal in calcium and iron are prevalent among young children in low-income groups. About 99% of the lead circulating in blood is in the erythrocyte, 50% of which is bound to hemoglobin $A_2$. Only 1% to 3% of circulating lead in blood is in serum, but this is the portion available for rapid distribution to target organs. Kinetic studies have been limited by the accuracy and precision of assays at normal serum lead concentrations of 1 to 3 $\mu$g Pb/dL of whole blood, and this determination is limited to a few research studies.

The body's lead burden is divided into three principle compartments: blood, soft tissue, and bone, with subcompartments in each of the principle compartments. The mean residence time of lead in blood is approximately 25 days, and most of this is excreted in the urine. In soft tissues such as the liver and kidney, lead has a mean residence time of about 40 days. Small amounts of lead are excreted in bile, hair, sweat, and nails. The mean residence time of lead in bone varies from about 3 years in trabecular bone to 30 years in cortical bone. There is also a subcompartment in periosteal bone that is more readily mobilized, as during chelation therapy. The periosteal bone is a factor in the rapid turnover of bone lead in growing infants. In view of the deep reservoir of lead in cortical bone, with a mean residence of 30 years, a woman who has absorbed much lead during childhood may transfer some of this lead to her fetus during the demineralization of bone that occurs during pregnancy. Bone lead may be rapidly released during extensive immobilization, such as with a hip and leg spica cast after serious fractures to the pelvis and femur.

### Toxicity

The main toxic effects of lead occur in the central and peripheral nervous systems, the erythroid cells, bone marrow, and the kidney. The developing nervous system is the system most sensitive to the toxic effects of lead in fetuses and young children. Reversible abnormal thyroid function and cardiac conduction have been reported in severe cases. Lead causes partial inhibition in the biosynthesis of heme at several enzymatic steps. Ferrochelatase and porphobilinogen synthase, sulfhydryl-dependent enzymes, are the enzymes most sensitive to inhibition by lead. Inhibition of ferrochelatase leads to increased zinc protoporphyrin in circulating erythrocytes. Compensatory erythroid hyperplasia and reticulocytosis result. Basophilic stippling is an inconstant finding in peripheral blood, but it is a relatively constant finding in bone marrow normoblasts in severe cases. Inhibition of 5-pyrimidine nucleotidase activity underlies the basophilic stippling of erythrocytes. As the concentration of lead in blood increases above 50 to 60 $\mu$g Pb/dL of whole blood, hemoglobin decreases. Lead causes a mild, well-compensated hemolytic normocytic anemia that can be differentiated morphologically from the hypochromic microcytic anemia of iron deficiency.

Lead interferes with normal cellular calcium metabolism, with a resulting intracellular build-up of calcium. Lead binds normally to some calcium-activated proteins with 100,000 times the affinity of calcium; once bound, it interferes with the normal actions of these proteins. Some lead-related disturbances, such as activation of protein kinase, show a dose-response relation with no evidence of a threshold, which may explain the apparent absence of a threshold for some of the adverse health effects of lead, particularly in the nervous system. Low-level lead exposure has subtle effects on growth rate, stature, and balance.

Severe acute lead poisoning (ie, blood lead level >150 $\mu$g Pb/dL of whole blood) can cause the Fanconi syndrome (ie, generalized renal aminoaciduria, melituria, hyperphosphaturia in the presence of hypophosphatemia) as a result of acute proximal renal tubular injury: this syndrome is reversible. Lead nephropathy, which is characterized by hyperuricemia with or without gout, has been reported as a late sequela of chronic plumbism in Australian children. Acute lead encephalopathy in the very young is characterized by massive cerebral edema, caused primarily by a generalized increase in vascular permeability. Neuronal destruction also occurs. In suckling animals, but not in mature animals, deficits in learning can be induced by doses of lead insufficient to cause histopathologic changes.

## Clinical Manifestations

The chronic course of unrecognized but moderately severe lead poisoning is characterized by recurrent symptomatic episodes, which may abate spontaneously. The earliest symptoms are anorexia, hyperirritability, decreased play activity, and a disturbed sleep pattern. Sporadic vomiting, intermittent abdominal pain, and constipation are manifestations of lead colic. Colic may occur at blood lead levels as low as 60 μg Pb/dL of whole blood, but children with levels up to 250 μg Pb/dL of whole blood may appear clinically well. Loss of recently acquired developmental skills may occur, and there may be delays in development, particularly of speech. Anemia may or may not exist.

The symptoms usually appear and slowly intensify over a period of 4 to 6 weeks before the clinical onset of acute encephalopathy, which is heralded by the sudden onset of persistent vomiting, ataxia, fluctuating state on consciousness, coma, and seizures. Younger children usually have massive cerebral edema, although the classic signs of increased intracranial pressure may not be found. In older children and adolescents, a toxic encephalopathy without massive cerebral edema is more common. Sudden premonitory behavioral changes may not be appreciated.

Blood lead concentration almost always exceeds 100 μg Pb/dL of whole blood and commonly exceeds 150 μg Pb/dL of whole blood in acute encephalopathy. The diagnosis can usually be made without lumbar puncture, which is dangerous. If examination of the cerebral spinal fluid is considered essential for differential diagnosis, the least amount of fluid required (several drops) should be obtained. The cerebrospinal fluid may show mild pleocytosis, mild or moderate increases in protein, and increased pressure in acute encephalopathy. The patient must be closely watched for inappropriate secretion of antidiuretic hormone, partial heart block, and profoundly impaired renal function. Peripheral neuropathy manifested by motor weakness in the distal muscles of the arms and legs is rare in children, but more than one half of the reported cases have occurred in children with sickle cell disease.

## PATIENT EVALUATION

## Clinical Diagnosis

Before the onset of acute encephalopathy, symptoms are subtle and nonspecific, and physical examination generally reveals little or nothing. Burton's lines are rare, seen only in severe cases in which there are dental caries. Plumbism should be included in the differential diagnosis of anemia, seizure disorders, severe behavioral disorders, mental retardation, colicky abdominal pain, and the arthralgia, bone pain, and cerebral and abdominal crises of sickle cell disease. Isolated seizures and self-limited episodes of vomiting during the recent past may represent episodes of unrecognized clinical plumbism, especially if the child lives in or visits and old house, if the parent is unavailable for much of the time, or if a history of excessive hand-to-mouth activity is ob-

tained. Recent changes of address, recent renovations in the home, and particularly time spent unsupervised or with baby-sitters and relatives should be ascertained. Persistent hand-to-mouth activity is associated with such histories. This information is essential in planning the appropriate management for each patient. Emphasis must be placed on environmental sampling for sources of lead and laboratory data. Whenever an index case is found, all housemates should have a blood lead test, and the possibility of uncommon sources should be ascertained.

## Screening

Under the 1991 CDC guidelines, the blood lead test replaced the EP test that was previously recommended as the primary screening test. The change was based on data showing that the developing nervous system is more sensitive than heme synthesis in the bone marrow to the adverse effects of lead; adverse effects in the developing nervous system are persistent, but effects on heme synthesis are reversible; and the EP test did not directly predict effects on the nervous system and did not uniformly predict an elevated blood lead concentration until it reached approximately 50 μg Pb/dL of whole blood.

Classification of children (Table 32-34) is based on a confirming venous blood lead concentration equal to or greater than 20 μg Pb/dL of whole blood. Although venous blood lead tests are preferable, capillary test results placing the child in classes I, IIA, and IIB need not be confirmed. Blood lead tests should be carried out by laboratories performing successfully in blind interlabo-

---

**TABLE 32-34. Classification of Children According to Blood Lead Concentration**

| Class | Blood Lead Concentration (μg/dL) | Comments |
|---|---|---|
| I | ≤9 | Acceptable; risk negligible, if any |
| IIA | 10–14 | Risk is minimal, particularly in class IIA. |
| IIB | 15–19 | Ensure good nutrition, particularly diets adequate in Ca and Fe. Use damp housecleaning practices to suppress dust. Rescreen more frequently, especially if child <24 mo of age to assess whether blood lead level is rising, stable, or decreasing. |
| III | 20–44* | Risk increases, particularly if blood lead level sustained in this or higher range. Provide more complete medical and environmental evaluation. Consider referring case to center specializing in management of childhood lead toxicity. Use pharmacologic therapy in selected cases. |
| IV | 45–69* | Treat as for class III and begin medical treatment and environmental assessment and remediation within 48 hours. |
| V | ≥70* | Begin medical treatment and environmental assessment and remediation immediately. |

* Based on confirmatory venous blood lead level.

*Adapted from Centers for Disease Control. Preventing lead poisoning in young children: A statement by the Centers for Disease Control. Atlanta, GA: Centers for Disease Control, October 1991.*

ratory proficiency testing programs. Such participation is required for licensing purposes in some states.

There is no unanimity of opinion regarding the use of chelating agents. In some programs, it is instituted at a blood lead level equal to or greater than 40 μg Pb/dL of whole blood and, in most programs, when blood lead level reaches a level equal to or greater than 45 μg Pb/dL of whole blood. It is generally agreed that chelation therapy should be instituted immediately if the blood lead level is equal to or greater than 70 μg Pb/dL of whole blood, because the onset of serious symptoms is unpredictable at these higher levels.

Among children residing in older housing with deteriorating lead-based paint, blood lead concentration increases most rapidly between 6 and 12 months of age and tends to reach a peak at 18 to 24 months. It is therefore recommended that the first screening test be given at 6 months of age. A detailed screening schedule is beyond the scope of this text. In general, testing should be more frequent in children younger than 24 months of age, in those with the higher blood lead levels, and in those with excessive hand-to-mouth activity living in older housing.

The 1991 CDC Statement proposes the use of a risk assessment questionnaire to be administered at every regularly scheduled health care visit (Table 32-35). When the physician is confident that highly reliable information can be obtained and the answers to all questions are negative, serial blood lead tests need not be done if the questionnaire is answered at each visit. In high-risk areas for childhood lead poisoning and when informants may not be able to answer all questions reliably, blood lead testing should be instituted starting at 6 months of age. Because lead-based paints have been found in some houses built after 1960 and because no questionnaire can cover all of the potential environmental sources of lead, it is considered prudent to do a blood lead test at least once at 12 months of age and, if possible, again at 24 months of age, even though the answers to all questions are "no." In some states, a blood lead screening test schedule is specified under the Early Periodic Screening, Diagnosis, and Treatment (EPSDT) or Healthy Kids programs. A blood lead test should be done whenever the answer to any of the questions in Table 32-35 is "yes."

## Laboratory Diagnosis

Because clinical diagnosis of lead poisoning in children is difficult before nervous system injury, early diagnosis depends on laboratory determinations. The basic test is a confirmed venous blood lead determination, which determines the level of toxicity, particularly to the nervous system. If blood lead concentration exceeds 40 to 45 μg Pb/dL of whole blood, measurement of δ-aminolevulinic acid in urine and zinc protoporphyrin in blood provide supporting evidence. Blood lead and zinc protoporphyrin (often determined as "free" erythrocyte protoporphyrin) can be determined in microliter blood samples and in venous blood obtained in hematology vacutainers containing EDTA as the anticoagulant. Special precautions are needed to prevent contamination of blood and urine samples by exogenous lead. Serial paired tests for lead and zinc protoporphyrin in blood are needed to determine trends. Iron deficiency may cause zinc protoporphyrin to be as high as 500 μg Pb/dL of packed erythrocytes if the blood lead level falls in classes I and IIA (see Table 32-34). Higher values usually indicate lead toxicity (ie, blood lead classes IV and V), with or without iron deficiency.

In emergencies, when these tests are not immediately available and acute lead encephalopathy is a diagnostic possibility, a strongly positive qualitative urinary coproporphyrin test, many stippled erythroblasts in bone marrow, glycosuria, and hypophosphatemia constitute presumptive evidence of plumbism. Studies have shown in chronically lead-poisoned rats that a single high dose of calcium disodium ethylenediaminetetraacetic acid (CaEDTA) is associated with an increase in brain levels of lead. Therefore, the diagnostic CaEDTA mobilization test for lead in urine is not recommended. Studies in children have shown that it is unnecessary if blood lead concentrations exceeds 40 μg Pb/dL of whole blood.

Radiopaque flecks in the intestinal tract indicating recent ingestion of foreign material containing lead are inconstantly found. The "lead lines" at the end of the growing long bone are generally associated with blood lead levels of 50 to 60 μg/dL of whole blood or higher and are of no use at the much lower blood lead levels likely to be encountered in screening programs.

Short-term responses to therapy are monitored by changes in blood lead levels. Blood lead values should always be obtained, because some local laws requiring the abatement of lead paint hazards in housing depend on the finding of an elevated blood lead concentration in the child. Such ordinances are invoked only after the child has been poisoned.

## THERAPY

The cornerstone of treatment is prompt separation of the child from the sources of lead, followed by careful reduction of lead hazards in the home. It is usually the local health agency's responsibility to identify and supervise the removal of lead hazards. Children and pregnant women, because of the sensitivity of the fetus to lead, must remain out of the home day and night until the abatement of lead paint hazards has been completed, the dwelling completely vacuumed with a high-efficiency particle accumulator (HEPA) vacuum, scrubbed with high-phosphate detergents two or three times, and vacuumed with a HEPA vacuum again to remove the fine particulate lead that is unavoidably generated by any deleading process. The deleaded areas should be repainted. Encapsulant paints have recently become available for this purpose.

Sanding, burning of paint with an open-flame torch, and heat guns should be prohibited. Abatement work should be performed only by those trained to do it safely. People who do abatement work should wear respirators (cloth or paper masks are grossly inadequate) and coveralls. These principles are briefly described in the 1991 CDC document. Thereafter, wet cleaning with high-phosphate detergents for dust control must be continued, particularly in old housing areas where the level of contamination

---

**TABLE 32-35. Assessing the Risk of High-Dose Exposure to Lead: a Sample Questionnaire**

| Does Your Child | Yes | No |
|---|---|---|
| 1. Live in or regularly visit a house with peeling or chipping paint built before 1960? This could include a day-care center, preschool, a babysitter's home, or a relative's home. | ☐ | ☐ |
| 2. Live in or regularly visit a house built before 1960 with recent, ongoing, or planned renovation or remodeling or repainting? | ☐ | ☐ |
| 3. Have a brother or sister, housemate, or playmate being followed or treated for lead poisoning (ie, blood lead ≥15 μg/dL)? | ☐ | ☐ |
| 4. Live with an adult whose job or hobby involves exposure to lead? | ☐ | ☐ |
| 5. Live near an active lead smelter, battery recycling plant, or other industry likely to release lead? | ☐ | ☐ |

*Adapted from Centers for Disease Control. Preventing lead poisoning in young children: A statement by the Centers for Disease Control. Atlanta, GA: Centers for Disease Control, October 1991.*

is likely to be high throughout the neighborhood. Play in dirt areas adjacent to such housing should be avoided. Preschoolage children should be tested periodically, according to the latest CDC and EPSDT guidelines.

Most children detected in current screening programs are asymptomatic and fall into groups I, IIA, IIB, and III (see Table 32-34). For those in groups I and II, the previously described measures and improved diet should suffice. Neither chelation therapy nor extensive removal of intact lead paint in good condition is likely to be of any benefit in group II. Chelation therapy may be of benefit in selected cases in group III.

## Chelation Therapy

Chelation therapy is advised for all children in groups IV and V, including the asymptomatic cases. Intramuscular therapy with CaEDTA is limited to 5 days at a daily dose of 1000 mg/m²/day, given in two divided portions when venous blood lead levels are greater than 40 but less than 90 to 100 $\mu$g/dL of whole blood. Chelation therapy before the onset of symptoms may simplify treatment and lessen the risk of cerebral injury. Repeat courses of CaEDTA with intervals of at least 4 days between courses may be indicated for children with higher body lead burdens. Treatment with oral CaEDTA is contraindicated. The use CaEDTA is regularly accompanied by transitory increases in serum transaminases and decreases in serum alkaline phosphatase.

CaEDTA may soon be largely replaced by meso-2,3-dimercaptosuccinic acid (DMSA, Succimer). DMSA has been approved by the Food and Drug Administration for the treatment of lead poisoning. It is given orally and has not been associated with serious adverse side effects. It does not induce acute zinc depletion as CaEDTA does. Nineteen-day courses are approved with a priming dose of 1050 mg/m²/day, given in 3 divided doses for the first 5 days, followed by a sustaining dose of 700 mg/m²/day, given in two divided doses, for the next fortnight. In animals, DMSA is more effective than CaEDTA in reducing the lead content of the brain, kidney, and blood. For those with higher body lead burdens, it is likely that multiple courses will be required. Under no circumstance should the drug be given on an outpatient basis to children concurrently overexposed to lead; an increase in blood lead during DMSA therapy has been observed.

Patients with symptomatic plumbism (eg, colic, seizures, acute encephalopathy) should be treated promptly with chelating agents on the basis of positive presumptive laboratory tests. Because the onset and clinical course of encephalopathy are unpredictable, the risk of delay far outweighs the risk of a few days of chelation therapy. If subsequent tests do not support the diagnosis of lead poisoning, treatment should be discontinued and the diagnosis reconsidered.

For acute encephalopathy or lead levels exceeding 90 to 100 $\mu$g/dL of whole blood, a regimen of 2,3-dimercaptopropanol (BAL) and CaEDTA is recommended. The dose for BAL is 500 mg/m²/24 hours, and the dose for CaEDTA is 1500 mg/m²/24 hours. The drugs are injected simultaneously at separate intramuscular sites in six divided doses each day for 5 days after an initial priming dose of BAL only. These patients usually need additional courses of chelation therapy and may be treated with either DMSA or CaEDTA alone after the blood lead concentration is less than 90 to 100 $\mu$g/dL of whole blood. If a symptomatic patient becomes anuric, administration of CaEDTA, but not BAL, should be temporarily withheld. CaEDTA is a nonmetabolizable drug that is excreted solely by the kidney; side effects include hypercalcemia, elevation of blood urea nitrogen, and renal injury. Side effects of BAL include vomiting, hypertension, and tachycardia. The side effects of each drug require careful evaluation because some of them are also features of acute lead encephalopathy. BAL may occasionally evoke intravascular hemolysis in patients with glucose-6-phosphate dehydrogenase deficiency. Adequate but not excessive hydration is particularly important for these patients.

## Fluid and Electrolyte Management

Proper fluid and electrolyte management is critical to survival in lead encephalopathy. After an initial infusion of 10% dextrose in water (and of mannitol if necessary to establish urine flow), continuous intravenous infusion should be restricted to basal requirements and a minimal estimate of the amounts required for correction of losses due to vomiting, dehydration, and activity associated with seizures. In mildly symptomatic patients with blood lead levels exceeding 90 to 100 $\mu$g/dL of whole blood, it is prudent to administer parenteral fluids initially in the same cautious manner until the trend of the clinical course becomes clear. Although enemas may be routinely given in asymptomatic patients to clear the bowel of lead before chelation therapy is started, the use of enemas to remove lead from the lower bowel should never be permitted to delay chelation therapy for symptomatic patients.

Seizures can be controlled initially with diazepam and thereafter with repeated doses of paraldehyde until the patient's state of consciousness has significantly improved. As the dose of paraldehyde is lowered, long-term anticonvulsant therapy with phenytoin or phenobarbital is phased in. If lead poisoning results from the ingestion of lead paint, as in most cases, effective longterm management requires the cooperative efforts of local health or environmental departments, the medical social worker, the psychologist or psychiatrist, the public health nurse, and the pediatrician. Control of pica is difficult to accomplish, although behavioral modification techniques may be helpful in selected cases.

## PROGNOSIS

Sequelae are related to the degree and duration of excessive tissue levels as indexed by serial blood lead measurements or the lead content of shed deciduous teeth. Recurrence of clinical manifestations increases the chance of permanent injury. Residual brain damage or dysfunction may not be evident until the early elementary school years. Sequelae of encephalopathy includes seizure disorders, impaired mentation, and rarely blindness and hemiparesis. Some survivors may require residential care. Seizures tend to abate before adolescence, but intellectual deficits persist.

There is general agreement that blood lead levels, if sustained during early childhood at levels greater than 10 to 15 $\mu$g/L of whole blood (0.5 to 0.72 $\mu$mol/L), carry an unacceptable risk for long-lasting but subtle injury to the nervous system, even if no clinical symptoms are detected. Follow-up of a cohort of children at 18 to 20 years of age has revealed that those with the higher dentin lead content at 6 to 8 years of age were seven times more likely to have dropped out of school and six times more likely to have a reading disability than those with the lower dentin lead content during the elementary school years. Some of these children had blood lead values during the preschool years averaging 35 $\mu$g/dL of whole blood. Attentional deficits and reading disabilities have been identified in other cohorts of younger children.

## PREVENTION

Actions by various federal agencies in the United States have substantially reduced air lead levels, reduced the lead content of foods, and reduced the lead content in public water supplies. Lead additives in automotive fuels were virtually eliminated in 1988. The use of lead additives in residential paint was banned in 1977. These steps constitute primary prevention, which is the only effective approach. However, until the large stock of older residential housing is renovated or replaced and substandard housing is brought up to code, screening programs are necessary for the early detection of lead toxicity in young children.

## Selected Readings

Aaseth J. Recent advances in the therapy of metal poisonings with chelating agents. Hum Toxicol 1983;2:257.

Agency for Toxic Substances and Disease Registry (ATSDR). The nature and extent of lead poisoning in children in the United States: A report to Congress. Atlanta, GA: Agency for Toxic Substances and Disease Registry, July 1988.

Aposhian HV, Aposhian MM: Meso-2,3-dimercaptosuccinic acid: Chemical, pharmacological and toxicological properties of an orally effective metal chelating agent. Ann Rev Pharmacol Toxicol 1990;30:279.

Baghurst PA, McMichael AJ, Wigg NR, Vimpani GV, Robertson EF, Roberts RJ, Tong SL. The Port-Pirie Cohort Study: Environmental exposure to lead and children's abilities at the age of seven years. N Engl J Med 1992;327:1279.

Baker EL Jr, Follard DS, Taylor TA, et al. Lead poisoning in children of lead workers: Home contamination with industrial dust. N Engl J Med 1977;296:260.

Bellinger DC, Stiles KM, Needleman HL. Low-level lead exposure, intelligence and academic achievement: A long-term follow-up study. Pediatrics 1992;90:857.

Bornschein RL, Succop PA, Krafft KM, et al. Exterior surface dust lead, interior house dust lead and childhood lead exposure in an urban environment. In: Hemphill DD, ed. Trace substances in environmental health—XX. Columbia, MO: University of Missouri, 1987:322.

Centers for Disease Control. Preventing lead poisoning in young children: A statement by the Centers for Disease Control. Atlanta, GA: Centers for Disease Control, October 1991.

Chisolm JJ Jr. Increased lead absorption and acute lead poisoning. In: Gellis SS, Kagan DM, eds. Current pediatric therapy. Philadelphia: WB Saunders, 1986:667.

Chisolm JJ Jr, Barltrop D. Recognition and management of increased lead absorption. Arch Dis Child 1979;54:249.

Cory-Slechta DA. Mobilization of lead over the course of DMSA chelation therapy and long-term efficacy. J Pharmacol Exp Ther 1988;246:84.

Cory-Slechta DA, Weiss B, Cox C. Mobilization and redistribution of lead over the course of CaEDTA chelation therapy. J Pharmacol Exp Ther 1987;243:804.

Dietrich KM, Berger, OG, Succop PA, et al. The developmental consequences of low to moderate prenatal and postnatal lead exposure: Intellectual attainment in the Cincinnati lead study cohort following school entry. Neurotoxical and Teratol 1993;15:37.

Farfel MR, Chisolm JJ. An evaluation of experimental practices for abatement of residential lead-based paint: Report on a pilot project. Environ Res 1991;55:199.

Fulton M, Raab G, Thomson G, et al. Influence of blood lead on the ability and attainment of children in Edinburgh. Lancet 1987;1:1221.

Graziano JH, Lolacono NJ, Moulton T, et al. Controlled study of meso-2,3-dimercaptosuccinic acid for the management of childhood lead intoxication. J Pediatr 1992;120:133.

Lyngbye T, Hansen ON, Trillingsgaard A, et al. Learning disabilities in children: Significance of low-level lead exposure and confounding factors. Acta Paediatr Scand 1990;79:352.

Mahaffey KR. Nutritional factors in lead poisoning. Nutr Rev 1981;39:353.

Markowitz ME, Rosen JF. Need for the lead mobilization test in children with lead poisoning. J Pediatr 1991;119:305.

Needleman HL, ed. Human lead exposure. Boca Raton: CRC Press, 1991:1–290.

Needleman HL, Gunnoe C, Leviton A, et al. Deficits in psychological and classroom performance of children with elevated dentine lead levels. N Engl J Med 1979;300:689.

Nriagu JO. Lead and lead poisoning in antiquity. New York: John Wiley & Sons, 1983.

Perlstein MA, Attala R. Neurologic sequelae of plumbism in children. Clin Pediatr 1966;5:292.

Rabinowitz MD, Wetherill GW, Kopple JD. Kinetic analysis of lead metabolism in healthy humans. J Clin Invest 1976;58:260.

Shukla R, Deitrich KN, Bornshein RL, et al. Lead exposure and growth in the early preschool child: A follow-up report from the Cincinnati Lead Study. Pediatrics 1991;88:886.

Wasserman G, Graziano JH, Factor-Litvak P, et al. Independent effects of lead exposure and iron deficiency anemia on developmental outcome at age 2 years. J Pediatr 1992;121:695.

Wolf DA. Etiology of acute lead encephalopathy in Omani infants. J Trop Pediatr 1990;36:328.

Ziegler EE, Edwards BB, Jensen RL, Mahaffey KR, Fomon SJ. Absorption and retention of lead by infants. Pediatr Res 1978;12:29.

*Principles and Practice of Pediatrics, Second Edition.*
edited by Frank A. Oski et al. J. B. Lippincott Company, Philadelphia © 1994.

# 32.3 *Minor Burns*

### Penelope Terhune Louis

Minor burns constitute approximately 95% of all burns treated in the United States. Minor burns are generally superficial and do not exceed 10% of the total body surface area. They have no significant involvement of the hands, feet, face, or perineum, and they rarely require hospitalization. No full-thickness component and no other complications exist. In the management of minor burns, survival is not the issue; most of these burns heal regardless of therapy. Undertreatment and overtreatment are common and may result in infection or delayed healing, with discomfort and prolonged morbidity. The goals of minor burn management include wound healing, patient comfort, and rapid rehabilitation.

## BURN ASSESSMENT

The seriousness of a burn injury can be defined by its depth, its location, the surface area involved, and patient age and general health. Even in minor burns, accurate estimation of the surface area is mandatory. The Lund and Browder chart (Solomon, 1985) should be used to adjust for the smaller surface area of the lower extremities of children.

The four-level burn classification is based on the depth of the injury: first-, second-, third-, and fourth-degree burns. In first-degree burns, the tissue destruction is superficial, involving only the epidermis. There is local pain and erythema without blistering or systemic response. First-degree burns are the result of contact with hot liquids, exposure to ultraviolet light, or flash burns. Except for the large burns of infants, first-degree burns generally require no treatment. However, various antiseptic and anesthetic ointments have been recommended for many years. Ointments and lotions may protect the burned area from the air and provide relief. Use of anesthetic agents in the ointment is not recommended, because large areas may be involved, and absorption of the anesthetic agent may cause toxic effects.

Second-degree burns can be divided into superficial and deep partial-thickness burns. Superficial partial-thickness injuries involve only the epidermis and dermis. The wounds appear red and moist, and blisters form. Tactile and pain sensors are intact. Caused by scalds, flash, and contact with hot objects, second-degree burns heal with minimal scarring.

The second-degree burns that are classified as deep partial-thickness burns involve the entire epidermis and dermis but leave the skin appendages intact. These deeper injuries have a mottled appearance, with areas of pale injury that are dry and anesthetic. These wounds usually heal spontaneously in 4 to 6 weeks. However, they may heal with late hypertrophic scarring and contracture formation. Deep partial-thickness burns may require excision and grafting.

Third-degree burns involve destruction of the epidermis, dermis, and subcutaneous tissue. The area appears white, red, or black and contains deep blisters or thrombosed blood vessels. The elasticity of the burned dermis is destroyed, resulting in a dry, leathery texture. These full-thickness burns require skin grafting if they are larger than 2 or 3 cm in diameter or are in an area of cosmetic importance.

Fourth-degree burns involve deep injury to bone, joint, or muscle, usually resulting from high-voltage electrical injury.

The location of the burn is important. Critical areas include the eyes, ears, face, hands, feet, and perineum. Other factors that are important are the age of the patient, associated trauma, inhalation injury, and preexisting health problems. Patients must be hospitalized for their injuries if they have severe burns; require fluid therapy; have involvement of the perineum, hands, feet, or joint surfaces; have circumferential extremity involvement, cellulitis, or infection at the burn site; or have associated trauma, facial burns, smoke inhalation, or carbon monoxide poisoning.

An important part of evaluating pediatric burn injuries is recognition of injury patterns suggesting child abuse. A detailed history is the most important element in establishing a diagnosis of child abuse. Characteristic patterns of nonaccidental burn injury seen on physical examination include the immersion burn caused by forcibly placing the child in a tub of hot water. Immersion injury is characterized by sharply demarcated burns of the hands, feet, buttocks, and perineum. The depth of the burn is uniform. Mirror-image or stocking-glove burn injuries are also associated with child abuse. Contact burns must be suspect when they appear on parts of the child not used in exploring his environment.

## MANAGEMENT

### Initial Treatment

Treatment of the burn begins at the scene of the accident, where the heat source is eliminated, and the areas of minor burn are placed in tepid rather than ice water. The burn area is wrapped in a clean towel, and the victim is taken to an emergency facility. The potential benefits of cooling the burned area are controversial. At best, these benefits last only through the first minutes after the injury. After this period, application of cold water may result in prolonged edema, impair healing, and convert a partial-thickness to a full-thickness injury.

Chemical burns should be irrigated with copious amounts of water. Adhered tar should be cooled with water, but the tar should not be removed at the scene of the accident.

An accurate history should be obtained, including when and where the accident occurred and the burn-causing agent. The history should help determine if smoke inhalation or associated injuries occurred. Pertinent medical history including drug allergies, medication record, and systemic illness must be obtained at this time.

Tetanus prophylaxis is the same for minor burns as it is for other injuries. In the management of clean wounds in patients who have completed the primary series of tetanus toxoid or received a booster within 5 years, a dose of tetanus toxoid is not required. In patients with burn wounds, a booster dose should be given if the primary series was not completed or if a booster has not been received in the past 5 years.

Burn wounds initially may be covered with saline-soaked sponges, which decrease the pain during patient evaluation. The wounds are then washed with mild soap and water, excess debris removed, and hair shaved from the margins of the burn.

Tar and asphalt are removed by a petroleum distillate with a hydrocarbon structure. Mineral oil and petroleum ointment, such as bacitracin or Neosporin, may also be used. Tar and asphalt should not be peeled off because of the additional damage to hair and skin that may result.

Chemical burns should be irrigated for 20 minutes. A neutralizing agent usually should not be administered because the resulting reaction may produce heat, causing a more severe injury.

Controversy exists about debriding blisters. Blisters may be left intact, fluid can be evacuated leaving the overlying skin intact, or the blister may be debrided. If the blister is left intact, the wound heals in the blister fluid environment. If the fluid is evacuated, the remaining skin acts as a protective layer covering the wound. The technique used depends on the burn's location and size and on the reliability of the patient's caretaker to care for the wound.

## Follow-Up Care

Minor burn injury is not associated with immunosuppression, hypermetabolism, or increased susceptibility to infection. Basic principles in wound care consist of keeping the wound clean and in a moist environment while it heals. Topical chemotherapeutic agents, such as mafenide acetate (Sulfamylon), silver sulfadiazine (Silvadene), silver nitrate, and providone-iodine (Betadine), are used in major burn injuries to prevent burn wound sepsis. These agents should not be used in minor burns, because they delay wound healing. Systemic antibiotics are not indicated in minor burns, because they may predispose the wound to infection with resistant organisms.

Follow-up wound care consists primarily of washing the wound with mild soap and water, drying the wound lightly, applying an ointment such as bacitracin or Neosporin, and covering the wound with nonstick porous gauze. Follow-up care may initially need to be performed daily if any question remains about the extent or depth of the wound or about patient reliability.

Each caretaker must be instructed in a program of range-of-motion exercises. Adequate physical therapy prevents prolonged edema that may impair wound healing.

The burn wound should have total epithelial coverage in 2 or 3 weeks. A patient with superficial partial-thickness injury must be followed until epithelial coverage occurs and then examined at 6 weeks for hypertrophic scarring. Recently healed partial-thickness burn wounds become dry. A mild lanolin lotion may be used until natural skin lubrication mechanisms return. The patient should avoid sun exposure during the period of wound healing. Sunscreen probably should be used even on healed areas when exposure to direct sunlight is expected. Pruritus is a common complaint in maturing burn wounds.

Multiple methods are available for managing outpatient burn wounds. Some physicians recommend bulky dressings for 2 weeks. Although bulky dressings prevent painful trauma to the burn area, they may encourage bacterial overgrowth in the warm, moist environment. Range-of-motion exercises are difficult with bulky dressings in place. Topical agents such as silver sulfadiazine often are used in the treatment of minor burns. Silver sulfadiazine must be readministered at least twice daily because it is inactivated by tissue fluids. A pseudomembrane may form with the use of this agent and result in painful, difficult removal. The use of prosthetic skin substitutes in the treatment of partial-thickness burns has become popular, but expertise in the use of this therapy is necessary.

Management of critical areas including the face, ears, eyes, hands, feet, and perineum often requires hospitalization. Superficial burns of the face are treated by exposure. The face is washed with mild soap and water. A thin layer of ointment may be applied to the open wounds to prevent drying. Superficial burns of the ears are treated with ointment. Deeper injuries are treated with topical chemotherapy and, to avoid chondritis, avoidance of excessive pressure to the area. Suspected corneal burns should be confirmed with fluorescein. Superficial corneal burns are treated with vigorous irrigation, ophthalmic antibiotic ointment, and eye patching. More serious injuries should be evaluated by an ophthalmologist.

To minimize swelling in superficial burns of the hands and feet, the extremity should be elevated. Range-of-motion exercises and instructions for the exercise program are an important part of initial management. Circumferential burns require patient hospitalization to observe for adequate circulation. Perineal burns require hospitalization for observation of urinary obstruction secondary to edema.

## COMPLICATIONS

Most complications in small burn injuries result from overtreatment, with too-vigorous dressing changes pulling off newly formed epithelium or the use of topical and systemic antibiotics resulting in infection with resistant organisms or pseudomembrane formation requiring debridement. Minor burns, which comprise most burns requiring treatment, are best managed with a simple protocol. These injuries are not associated with the severe complications of major burn injuries and do not require the same aggressive interventions in wound care.

## Selected Readings

Carvajal HF, Griffith JA. Burn and inhalation injuries. In: Fuhrman BP, Zimmerman JJ, eds. Pediatric critical care. St. Louis: Mosby Year Book, 1992:1209.
Carvajal HF. Management of severely burned patients: Sorting out the controversies. Emerg Med Rep 1985;6:89.
Cockington RA. Ambulatory management of burns in children. Burns 1989;15:271.
Goodwin CW. Current burn treatment. Adv Surg 1984;18:125.
Herndon DN, Thompson PB, Desai MH, et al. Treatment of burns in children. Pediatr Clin North Am 1985;32:1311.
La Ferla GA, Fyfe AH, Drainer IK. Minor burn injuries in children: Inpatient versus outpatient treatment? Ann R Coll Surg Engl 1983;65:394.
Meagher DP. Burns. In: Raffensperger JG, ed. Swenson's pediatric surgery, ed 5. Chicago: Appleton and Lange, 1990:317.
Solomon J. Pediatric burns. Crit Care Med 1985;1:161.
Spear RM, Munster AM. Burns, inhalation injury, and electrical injury. In: Rogers MC, ed. Textbook of pediatric intensive care. Baltimore: Williams & Wilkins, 1987:1323.
Swain AH, Azadian BS, Shakespeare PG. Management of blisters in minor burns. Br Med J 1987;295:181.
Warden GD. Outpatient care of thermal injuries. Surg Clin North Am 1987;67:147.

*Principles and Practice of Pediatrics, Second Edition.*
edited by Frank A. Oski et al. J. B. Lippincott Company, Philadelphia © 1994.

# *32.4 Oral Rehydration Therapy*

## Julius G. Goepp and Mathuram Santosham

Dehydration resulting from acute gastroenteritis (AGE) is the leading cause of child morbidity and mortality in the world. In the developing nations an estimated 4 million children die annually from dehydration, while approximately 1.5 billion episodes of AGE occur (Snyder and Marson, 1982). An estimated 16.5 million episodes occur annually in developing countries in children under 5 years of age (Glass et al, 1991). In the United States, dehydration still accounts for 300 to 500 deaths per year. Although most diarrheal episodes among children in the United States are mild, the resulting physicians' visits produce substantial health-care costs. In developing countries, where children are expected to have 7 to 10 episodes of AGE annually, and where significant malnutrition exists, the impact is still greater.

During the past 20 years, considerable progress has been made in the delineation of the etiologic agents of AGE and the pathophysiology of diarrheal dehydration. In particular, an improved understanding of the transport of fluids and electrolytes in the mammalian gut has led directly to the development of physiologically appropriate solutions for oral fluid therapy. Such therapy, in combination with appropriate dietary management of the child with AGE, has come to be known as oral rehydration therapy (ORT).

Restoration of circulating fluid volume was recognized as crucial to the treatment of dehydrating diarrhea in the early 19th century. Early attempts at parenteral fluid therapy were largely unsuccessful because of poor understanding of the nature of stool losses, the systemic effects of volume contraction, and inadequate aseptic technique and equipment. Even those patients who improved with this therapy worsened when therapy was discontinued, and more than 75% still died. By 1926, recognition of the importance of treating acidosis in dehydration led Powers to administer solutions of glucose, saline and bicarbonate, along with blood. Fasting was recommended. He reported a mortality among hospitalized patients of 33%. Over the ensuing two decades, the use of saline solutions with dextrose, accompanied by enforced fasting, was ineffective at reducing hospital mortality below 30%. In 1946, Darrow and Harrison, as a result of careful balance studies of salt and water losses, added potassium to rehydration fluids and reported mortality rates as low as 6%, still in fasting children.

Oral electrolyte solutions were pioneered in the 1940s by Harrison and Darrow. The first commercially available solution (Lytren, Mead, Johnson Co.) was developed in the 1950s, but simultaneous reports of hypernatremic dehydration and increased mortality led to a widespread distrust of ORT among pediatricians in the United States. In fact, the epidemic of hypernatremia was attributable to practices related to management of diarrhea and to the packaging of Lytren itself, not to problems intrinsic to ORT. Among those problems were the following:

Boiled skimmed milk was frequently recommended for use in diarrhea, and its high osmolality contributed to high serum sodium values.

Lytren was sold in bulk to be mixed at home, and parents often mixed the solution improperly.

Lytren contained 8% glucose, which made it excessively osmotic (see below for a discussion of the role of osmolarity in diarrhea).

The valuable lesson to be learned from the 1950s experience is that families must be taught how to use ORT and that proper feeding practices should be followed during diarrhea, not that ORT itself is a dangerous treatment.

Work throughout the 1950s and 1960s, including laboratory models of fluid and electrolyte transport in mammalian intestines, combined with improved measurements of stool electrolyte losses in cholera, led to the development of the first oral solutions to be truly tailored to the needs of patients with AGE, specifically those with cholera. Since then numerous studies have documented the effectiveness of ORT among children and adults with dehydration from AGE stemming from a wide range of causes.

The role of feeding in diarrhea has until recently been controversial. Park in 1924 and Chung in 1948 were among the first to challenge the established notion that feedings should be withheld during diarrhea. Chung found that duration of illness was unaffected and weight gain was improved in children who were fed during their illness. The demonstration of diminished volume and duration of diarrhea in infants receiving feedings has contributed to current recommendations that children be "fed through" diarrhea.

The decades-long evolution of the management of acute dehydration resulting from AGE has led to fundamental changes in the way dehydration is managed. ORT is a powerful, simple, and inexpensive approach that is credited with saving about a million lives annually. Paradoxically, ORT is used least in the industrialized countries where much of the original basic scientific research was done. Like any therapy, ORT relies on appropriate teaching and implementation for its ultimate effectiveness. In the balance of this chapter, we will describe the pathophysiology of AGE, the mechanisms of action of ORT, and practical aspects of delivery of ORT, particularly in an industrialized world setting.

# PATHOPHYSIOLOGY AND ETIOLOGY OF ACUTE DEHYDRATING GASTROENTERITIS

Although the terms "dehydration" and "rehydration" refer strictly to loss and replacement of water alone, they have become recognized as terms reflecting overall fluid and electrolyte status. More accurately, a patient suffering from AGE usually has sustained some degree of *volume depletion*, reflecting losses not only of water, but of sodium and other electrolytes as well. Initial losses of sodium during AGE are from the extracellular (and therefore intravascular) fluid compartment (ECF). With progressive loss of circulating volume and total body potassium depletion (see Intestinal Absorption, also Potassium, in section on Composition of Oral Rehydration Solutions), sodium also is lost from the ECF into the intracellular fluid (ICF) compartment. Thus, regardless of the measured serum sodium or potassium concentration, during dehydration from AGE total body sodium and potassium content is invariably diminished.

## Pathophysiologic Considerations

### Intestinal Absorption

A grasp of basic intestinal physiology is vital to understanding the concepts involved in fluid therapy of the volume-depleted patient. Here, we consider absorption of various substances in the bowel in the context of their physiologic roles in homeostasis.

Because of the tremendous rate of secretion of fluids and electrolytes in the healthy bowel (about 9 liters daily in adults), powerful mechanisms for reabsorption of secreted fluid must be present; otherwise rapid volume depletion would ensue. A circulatory pattern may thus be used to describe the normal flow of fluid into and out of the bowel lumen: secretions from salivary glands, pancreas, and gallbladder are added to the intrinsic bowel secretions to solubilize nutrients, and the vast bulk of fluid, as well as sodium and other electrolytes, is rapidly reabsorbed by mechanisms residing in the epithelial cells of the small and large bowel.

This complex system is modulated by the interactions of hormonal and intracellular mediators common to most tissues: the adenosine and guanosine nucleotide messenger systems, intracellular calcium, and metabolites of arachidonic acid (leukotrienes and prostaglandins).

The immediate driving force for active water absorption in the bowel is the movement of sodium. Uptake of sodium occurs by means of a two-step process, involving first active pumping of the ion out of intestinal epithelial cells at the basolateral membrane, then sodium entry down the resulting gradient from the bowel lumen into the cell. Sodium entry occurs passively as well as by several ion-coupled mechanisms: sodium–hydrogen exchange and coupled sodium chloride absorption. In addition, sodium cotransport with small organic molecules such as glucose and amino acids also occurs. A number of mechanisms and ratios of sodium to substrate have been proposed; the clinical relevance resides in the fact that uptake of sodium and, therefore, of water is dramatically increased when organic substrate is present at a molecular ratio of about 1:1 with sodium in the intact intestine. This observation is exploited in the design of orally administered rehydration solutions.

Sodium uptake and water absorption are modulated in part by the effects of aldosterone on sodium channels in enterocyte membranes. Elevated aldosterone levels result in increased sodium absorption. Antidiuretic hormone (ADH) and glucocorticoids also affect water and salt uptake from bowel. Catecholamines have profound acute stimulatory effects on sodium absorption.

Absorption of other electrolytes also is important, but these substances play a smaller direct role in movement of fluid, except as modulators of sodium uptake. Luminal potassium rapidly equilibrates with serum levels; even a severely potassium-depleted patient may continue to lose potassium in the stool. Additionally, elevated aldosterone in dehydration contributes to urinary potassium losses. Bicarbonate is secreted in substantial quantities by the pancreas and must be reabsorbed in order to maintain systemic pH. Luminal bicarbonate stimulates absorption of sodium as well.

### Features of Intestinal Secretion

As with water and electrolyte absorption, secretory processes in the mammalian intestine occur by numerous and varied mechanisms and are responsive to a host of modulators, both intrinsic and extrinsic. Because rates of secretion between small and large intestine vary greatly, we discuss each portion of the bowel individually and then describe the action of various substances on secretion in the intestine as a whole.

In the healthy gastrointestinal tract, net fluid absorption exceeds secretion, whereas in dehydrating diarrheal illness net intestinal losses exceed absorption. Such net loss may result from increased secretion in the proximal gut or from diminished absorption distally, or both. Each of the substances considered below may act on one or more of the secretory or absorptive processes to affect this balance. Their mechanisms of action are briefly discussed here.

### Secretion in the Small Intestine

Whereas most absorptive processes in small intestine occur in cells at the villous tip, secretion takes place chiefly in crypt cells. The secretion of chloride ion is a major determinant of ultimate fluid movement into the gut lumen. Chloride secretion appears to occur by means of energy-requiring, pump-mediated entry at the basal cell membrane, with subsequent conductive, channel-mediated exit at the apical membrane.

Control and modulation of chloride secretion in the small bowel depend on the interrelationship of a number of intracellular messenger systems, which appear to be fundamental signaling processes in most leukocytic cells. Known mediators of chloride secretion include free calcium ion ($Ca^{2+}$), cyclic adenosine monophosphate (cyclic AMP), cyclic guanosine monophosphate (cyclic GMP), and intracellular pH. Various endocrine and paracrine substances exert their ultimate effects on intestinal secretion by affecting one or more of these messenger systems.

Each of the intracellular messengers stimulates secretion, all by similar mechanisms. Neutral sodium chloride uptake is inhibited in apical cells, whereas chloride conductance is facilitated at the crypt cell membrane. In addition, calcium appears to increase the release of arachidonic acid, the metabolites of which themselves influence secretion (see below).

### Regulation of Absorption and Secretion in the Colon

The mammalian colon shares certain features of fluid and electrolyte transport with the small intestine but differs in a number of significant aspects. Rate and volume of electrolyte and water absorption are segmentally heterogeneous in the colon and may depend on volume, composition, and rate of flow of the luminal contents. Colonic sodium recovery occurs across a gradient three to four times greater than that found in the jejunum and responds to both mineralocorticoid and glucocorticoid effects.

Pathologically increased fecal water excretion in diarrhea may result from increased small or large intestinal fluid secretion, from diminished capacity of colon to absorb water and electrolytes, or from a combination of these factors. These effects may be mediated by a number of exogenous substances, which are discussed below, after a brief discussion of colonic mechanisms for normal absorption and secretion.

Under normal circumstances, the colon absorbs sodium and chloride by mechanisms similar to those in the small bowel and secretes potassium and bicarbonate in substantial quantities. Unlike the small bowel, the colon lacks significant mechanisms for the active co-transport of glucose, amino acids, and sodium beyond the neonatal period.

Intracellular mediators of secretion in the colon include those discussed above for the small intestine: calcium, cyclic AMP, and cyclic GMP. Cyclic AMP appears to increase colonic secretion of chloride and potassium, probably by increasing apical membrane conductances. Additionally, cyclic AMP reduces net sodium chloride absorption. The effects of increased intracellular calcium are also similar to those in small intestine, and there is evidence that increased cyclic AMP may result in elevation of intracellular concentrations of $Ca^{2+}$. Cyclic GMP may also play a role in colonic electrolyte modulation, but its effects are less well understood than those of calcium or cyclic AMP.

As is the case in the small bowel, the metabolites of arachidonic acid, prostaglandins (PGE), and leukotrienes play a role in the regulation of fluid and electrolyte movement in the colon, both as intermediaries that raise cyclic AMP levels and directly by some as yet unspecified intracellular mechanism independent of adenylate cyclase.

### Etiologic Agents of Diarrhea: Mechanisms of Action

A variety of intrinsic and extrinsic agents pathologically stimulate secretion in small or large intestine. These substances may be conveniently divided into three categories: (1) a single group of intrinsic biochemical signals (hormones, neurotransmitters, and mediators of inflammation); (2) extrinsic biologic pathogens (bacteria, viruses, and enterotoxins); and (3) extrinsic chemical secretagogues (laxatives). Each of the clinically important members of these categories appears to have its ultimate effect on one of the final common intracellular mediators discussed above—calcium, cyclic AMP, or cyclic GMP.

The effects of enterotoxins on secretory processes are most prominent in the small bowel. A number of these agents act by raising intracellular levels of cyclic AMP; they are all heat-labile multi-unit toxins that bind and activate cellular adenylate cyclase. The ultimate effects of these intracellular changes is that secretion in crypt cells is "switched on," whereas absorption in villous cells in "switched off." Toxins that act by this mechanism include the heat-labile *Vibrio cholerae* and *Escherichia coli* toxins, as well as those produced by certain strains of *Salmonella*, *Campylobacter*, and possibly *Shigella*.

A second group of toxins appears to function by stimulation of the guanylate cyclase pathway. This group comprises the heat-stable toxins of *E coli*, *Yersinia enterocolitica*, and *Klebsiella pneu-*

*moniae.* There is evidence that the effect of the toxins is mediated in part by calcium and by PGE, which in turn stimulate cyclic GMP production.

Effects of enterotoxin on fluid and electrolyte transport in the colon are less well understood and may be less important clinically in the production of water loss in diarrhea. Nonetheless, a reduction in neutral sodium chloride absorption in cholera has been suggested.

In addition to the effects of their enterotoxins, bacterial pathogens stimulate a host inflammatory response, resulting in release of mediators such as PGE and leukotrienes, which act both directly as stimulators of secretion and as modulators of intracellular second messengers.

Viral agents such as rotavirus appear to exert their pathologic effects by producing sloughing of intestinal villous (*i.e.*, absorptive) cells in excess of crypt (*i.e.*, secretory) cells. Because the damage to villous cells is patchy and absorption in the surviving cells is intact, oral fluid replacement in such cases is usually effective. Table 32-36 shows the etiologic agents of diarrhea and their mechanisms of action.

## ORAL REHYDRATION SOLUTIONS

It is the intestinal co-transport system of sodium on which oral rehydration therapy is based. In this system, sodium absorption from the small intestine is promoted by the passive co-transport of small organic molecules such as glucose. Water absorption follows that of sodium so that osmotic equilibrium is maintained. The co-transport system remains intact in surviving villous tip cells even in severe diarrhea. Thus, effective repletion of fluid and electrolytes can occur via the gut even when severe purging occurs.

### Composition of Standard Oral Rehydration Solutions

Oral rehydration solutions (ORS) have evolved over the past 2 decades. A single standard solution is currently recommended by WHO and is used in most countries in the developing world. Somewhat different solutions are available commercially in the United States, although currently there appears to be little difference in the ability of all of those solutions to produce adequate repletion of fluid. We will discuss the composition of the WHO recommended solution and examine the rationale for the presence of each constituent.

#### Glucose

Promotion of sodium absorption occurs over a range of glucose concentrations from 10 to 25 grams per liter (56–140 mmol/L). When glucose concentrations exceed 3% (30 g/L), the osmotic pressure exerted by glucose in the intestinal lumen produces passive fluid loss greater than absorption, and diarrhea may be exacerbated. Table 32-37 shows the concentrations of glucose in the physiologically appropriate oral solutions, as well as that of other fluids still commonly used during diarrhea. Soft drinks and juices all contain glucose in excess of 3%.

#### Sodium

ORS sodium concentrations have generated considerable research and controversy since the first solutions were evaluated. Patients with dehydration resulting from AGE may be isonatremic, hyponatremic, or hypernatremic. The earliest solutions to be used were developed to replete fluid losses in cholera patients, many of whom were poorly nourished; such patients tended to have a hyponatremic dehydration because stool losses of sodium in

TABLE 32-36. Classification of Etiologic Agents of AGE by Mechanism of Action*

| Toxin Producers† | Invasive Organisms‡ | Cytotoxic Organisms§ | Adherent Organisms‖ |
|---|---|---|---|
| Aeromonas | C jejuni | C difficile | E coli (Enteropathogenic Enterohemorrhagic) |
| E coli (Enterotoxigenic) | Salmonella | E coli (Enteropathogenic Enterohemorrhagic) | |
| | Shigella | | |
| | V parahemolyticus | | |
| lla | | Shigella | |
| V cholerae | Y enterocolitica | | |
| Y enterocolitica | | | |

* Some bacterial organisms exert pathogenic effects by more than one mechanism. Viruses such as rotavirus and Norwalk agent produce cell destruction of absorptive villous tip cells with resultant loss of absorptive surface area.
† Elaborate toxins that modulate ion and water transport in secretory cells.
‡ Cause mucosal injury, inflammation, and denudation of absorptive surface area.
§ Elaborate toxins that cause destruction of absorptive cells.
‖ Adhere to mucosal surface causing direct physical destruction of cells.

cholera are relatively high (Table 32-38) and hypokalemia, as we have seen above in the section on pathophysiology, tends to exacerbate hyponatremia because of the movement of sodium into ICF to replace potassium. In addition, high levels of antidiuretic hormone promote renal water resorption in excess of sodium. For these reasons, the early ORS had comparatively high sodium concentrations of 100–120 mEq/L.

In noncholera diarrheas, total body sodium losses are less severe, and concerns about producing hypernatremia have been raised. The use of hypertonic oral fluids such as juices and soft drinks may produce free water loss in excess of sodium loss and may worsen hypernatremia. It has been suggested that the common use of boiled skimmed milk as a feeding for children with diarrhea contributed to the epidemic of hypernatremic dehydration coincident with the use of Lytren in the 1950s. Because of these concerns, multiple solutions have been proposed for children with diarrhea of varying etiologies, and lower sodium concentrations have frequently been recommended. It must be recognized, however, that even patients with high serum sodium values have diminished total body sodium and that the effects of circulating volume depletion (acidosis, hypokalemia, and elevated aldosterone levels) tend to perpetuate hypernatremia. For these reasons, rapid restoration of circulating volume with a so-

lution similar in composition to ECF, which contains potassium and base and produces low osmotic forces in the gut, will best reverse these processes that perpetuate hypernatremia.

Both the physiologic considerations outlined above and practical ones related to production and distribution of solutions have led since 1975 to the acceptance by WHO and UNICEF of a single rehydration solution (WHO Packet, Table 32-37) for all children with diarrhea and dehydration. This solution contains 90 mEq/L of sodium and therefore provides a near 1:1 molar ratio to the glucose content of 111 mMol/L (20 grams/L).

### Potassium

Children with dehydrating AGE usually have diminished total body potassium levels. Potassium is lost in stool and, under the influence of elevated aldosterone levels, in urine as well. Acidosis contributes to the loss of intracellular potassium into the ECF, and thus additional potassium is renally filtered and excreted.

The clinical relevance of potassium losses is that hypokalemia may produce ileus, which in turn may reduce intestinal fluid absorption. Hypokalemia also may exacerbate hyponatremia as sodium leaves ECF to replace potassium in ICF. It may exacerbate hypernatremia as free water is lost into nonmotile segments of bowel during ileus. The partial repletion of potassium is thus an

TABLE 32-37. Compositions of Fluids Frequently Used in Oral Rehydration*

| Solution | Glucose/CHO g/L | Sodium mEq/L | HCO3 mEq/L | Potassium mEq/L | Osmolality mmol/L |
|---|---|---|---|---|---|
| Pedialyte | 25 | 45 | 30 | 20 | 250 |
| Ricelyte | 30† | 50 | 30 | 25 | 200 |
| Rehydralyte | 25 | 75 | 30 | 20 | 310 |
| WHO packet | 20 | 90 | 30 | 20 | 330 |
| Cola | 700 | 2 | 13 | 0.1 | 750 |
| Apple juice | 690 | 3 | — | 32 | 730 |
| Gatorade | 255 | 20 | 3 | 3 | 330 |

* Cola, juice and Gatorade are shown for comparison only; they are not recommended for use.
† Rice syrup solids.

TABLE 32-38. Initial Stool Sodium and Potassium
Concentrations (mmol/L) by Etiology of Illness

| | Cholera | Toxigenic E coli | Rotavirus |
|---|---|---|---|
| Sodium | 98 ± 23 | 67 ± 34 | 53 ± 26 |
| Potassium | 26 ± 11 | 37 ± 19 | 46 ± 21 |

Urinary potassium losses vary with degree of hypovolemia: as renin/
aldosterone system is increasingly active, obligate urinary potassium
losses increase. In severe dehydration, urinary potassium losses exceed stool potassium losses.

*Modified from Santosham M, Greenough WB. Oral rehydration therapy: A
global perspective. J Pediatr 1991;118:S44.*

important aspect of fluid therapy in AGE. Potassium is provided in the accepted oral solutions at 20 mEq/L. This quantity of potassium is insufficient to fully replete most children's potassium stores. Early restoration of normal dietary intake provides a good additional source of potassium repletion.

### Base

Latta recognized the role of acidosis in the hypovolemic state early in the 19th century, and decreased mortality among cholera patients followed the addition of alkali to replacement fluids in the early 20th century. Bicarbonate at 30 mEq/L has been a component of WHO recommended ORS since 1975. Trisodium citrate provides three bicarbonate ions per molecule, is more stable than sodium bicarbonate, and is currently the source of base in these solutions. Bicarbonate also stimulates intestinal sodium absorption independently of other organic substrates.

### Osmolality

The osmotic burden presented by oral solutions to the gut is of great importance. Fluids whose osmolality significantly exceeds that of serum (about 290 mOsm/L) exert forces resulting in retention of free water in the intestinal lumen. This effect not only reduces absorption of water but may result in free water losses from the intravascular space, contributing to or exacerbating hypernatremia. Most full-strength fruit juices, punches, and soft drinks have high osmolality contributed by their sugar content and are thus unacceptable as the sole source of fluid replacement in diarrhea. Although children with only mild diarrhea may tolerate such fluids, the potential for deterioration exists.

## Limitations of Oral Rehydration Therapy

Although ORT provides simple, safe, and effective therapy for the majority of children with dehydration, certain limitations exist. Physiologically, as indicated in the preceding section, ORSs are limited in the quantities of solute they can contain without becoming hyperosmolar and exacerbating fluid losses. Glucose-based ORSs, therefore, provide good rehydration but have no effect by themselves on stool output or duration of illness. Solutions that contain complex carbohydrate molecules (see below) may overcome this barrier and provide sufficient substrate to reverse fluid losses and decrease diarrhea.

In children presenting with severe dehydration who are in shock, oral solutions may be contraindicated because airway protective reflexes may be impaired. These patients should receive initial fluid repletion parenterally but are candidates for ORT once vital signs have stabilized.

Children with very high rates of stool output (> 10cc/kg/hr) may be unable to maintain positive fluid balance orally. Our experience, however, has been that most children do in fact retain

sufficient fluid for repletion to occur. We recommend that careful balance records be kept and that parenteral fluids be provided for the occasional child who remains in negative fluid balance after several hours of oral therapy.

A small proportion (about 1%) of children with AGE experience carbohydrate malabsorption, heralded by a dramatic increase in stool volume when ORS is given. These patients also have reducing substances present in stool following ORS administration. In infants with carbohydrate malabsorption, if ORS is discontinued and parenteral fluids are provided, a dramatic reduction in stool output occurs.

Vomiting is often (and inaccurately) cited as a contraindication to ORT. Most children with vomiting can be successfully rehydrated if fluids are provided in small frequent quantities. We recommend use of a 5-mL syringe or teaspoon, to prevent the thirsty child's rapid consumption of a large volume of fluid with subsequent vomiting related to gastric distention. Persistent gentle encouragement of parents is critical in this setting; many children "fail" oral therapy when parents give up in the face of vomiting. As tissue acidosis is corrected, vomiting generally ceases, although an occasional child may benefit from a few hours of parenteral fluids.

Other limitations of ORT in the clinical setting are behavioral, and many are perceived limitations in the minds of practitioners. These limitations include the notions that ORT is excessively time-consuming, that it is labor-intensive to staff, and that parents in the developed world are resistant to its use. We have found that each of these perceived barriers can be overcome. They are discussed more fully below in the section on delivery of ORT in the industrialized world.

## Clinical Studies

Oral rehydration solutions, although originally designed and field-tested for use in cholera patients, have subsequently been evaluated for use in dehydration resulting from diarrhea of all types. Early studies focused on children in the developing world, many of whom were poorly nourished. It was shown that ORS could be used safely for fluid repletion of children with hypo- and hypernatremia. Based on these findings, the WHO and UNICEF have recommended a single solution for use in diarrheal illness of all types, regardless of initial serum sodium values. Subsequent studies among well-nourished children on the U.S. Apache reservation also found ORS to be effective and safe.

Because of concerns that the WHO solution provided excessive amounts of sodium for children with noncholera diarrhea, we compared the WHO solution at 90 mEq/L of sodium with IV therapy and with a solution providing only 50 mEq/L of sodium. No difference in either stool output or in the ability of solutions to correct initial sodium abnormalities was found. Tamer has had similar results comparing IV with oral solutions. A study of well-nourished outpatients with mild diarrhea also showed successful rehydration with a variety of oral solutions with sodium contents of 30–90 mEq/L.

The current recommendations of the American Academy of Pediatrics reflect the findings of these studies (see Table 32-37), and commercially available solutions in the United States contain the recommended quantities of glucose and electrolytes.

### "Improved" Solutions

Although standard glucose-based ORSs are very effective at repletion of fluids and electrolytes, they have minimal effect on the volume and duration of stool output. In theory, by increasing the quantity of substrate available to the co-transport system, absorption of fluid could be promoted to the point of reversing water loss and actually reducing stool volume. In practice, because of the osmotic limitation alluded to above, the concentration of free glucose in ORS should not exceed 3%. Solutions that contain complex carbohydrates (starches) are able to supply a large number of glucose molecules in the intestinal lumen, while imposing a relatively low osmotic load. Starch molecules are broken down into their constituent glucose residues by intestinal amylase enzymes. The free glucose molecules then function as organic substrate to co-transport sodium ions. The glucose molecules liberated by amylase at the intestinal brush border are rapidly absorbed, so that high glucose concentrations do not develop. By providing large amounts of substrate for minimal osmotic penalty, starch-containing solutions may be capable of producing net fluid absorption in excess of losses.

A similar approach to improved solutions has been to provide other organic substrates such as amino acids, which function in cotransport systems independent of glucose. These solutions, however, have been found to provide little advantage over standard glucose-based solutions. They produce osmotic loads similar to that imposed by high glucose concentrations and are relatively expensive and unstable in solution. Glycine-based ORS have been shown to produce hypernatremia.

### Clinical Studies Using Cereal-Based Solutions

The use of fluids containing cereal starches for the treatment of diarrhea actually is among the oldest recorded medical therapies. It was not until the late 1970s and early 1980s, however, that systematic exploration of cereals as a carbohydrate source for ORS became widespread.

Rice has been most thoroughly studied as a carbohydrate source. Molla (1989) and Patra showed significant reduction in stool output in cholera patients given rice-based ORS (R-ORS) or puffed rice compared with those given glucose-based ORS. However, when R-ORS was compared with sucrose-based ORS in another study by Molla (1982), no difference in output was shown. Patra also showed a 40% reduction in duration of illness in the R-ORS group. In patients with noncholera diarrhea, minimal differences among groups have been shown. Similar findings (reduced stool output among cholera patients, no difference among noncholera patients) have been reported by investigators using a variety of other grains as the carbohydrate source.

Cereal-based ORSs have certain practical disadvantages. Primarily, they tend to be unstable without refrigeration. Fermentation of carbohydrate progresses rapidly at room temperatures, resulting in production of ethanol, which contributes an osmotic burden in addition to its obvious toxic properties. Cereal-based solutions settle rapidly and require frequent stirring. On the other hand, these solutions often are readily mixed from commonly available materials that are culturally acceptable. The risk of exacerbating diarrhea by using too much carbohydrate also is likely to be considerably lower with these solutions than it is with glucose or sucrose based fluids.

## DIETARY CONSIDERATIONS

Although Chung and Viscorova in 1948 reported good results among children who were fed during diarrhea, delayed feeding for most of the illness has remained the routine recommendation by most pediatricians until quite recently. Delayed feeding ("resting the gut") has the advantage of reducing the risk of osmotic diarrhea and usually does reduce stool output initially. The nutritional consequences of fasting, however, are profound. Children in the developing world may experience from 7 to 10 episodes of diarrhea annually, each one lasting for 7 to 10 days. Serious calorie deprivation and, ultimately, growth retardation may ensue. Fasting also has been demonstrated to inhibit enterocyte renewal, which along with increased susceptibility to new infection places the child at risk for prolonged or renewed diarrheal losses.

Enteral feeding, conversely, has been shown to increase cell renewal in the gut and to diminish intestinal permeability. In addition, the calories provided during feeding have been shown, in a careful balance study by Brown, to contribute to improved nutritional parameters among children who were fed during diarrhea.

The effects of feeding on severity of diarrhea also are marked. We have demonstrated reductions in both duration and volume of diarrhea among inpatient Apache infants fed a soy-based, lactose-free formula compared with those receiving only glucose-based ORS for the first 24 hours (Santosham et al, 1985). Duration of illness was reduced among outpatients with a similar regimen.

The effects of feeding during diarrhea have been directly compared with the use of cereal-based ORS. No difference in the duration of diarrhea was shown between infants who received only R-ORS during the first 24 hours of therapy compared with those receiving early feeding with soy formula or rice feeding or formula.

## Role of Lactose-Containing Feedings

Although the use of feedings early in the course of diarrheal illness is now widely recommended, the role of lactose-containing formulas or nonhuman milks remains controversial. A large number of studies have been devoted to attempts to identify the best formula for children with AGE by comparing lactose-containing to lactose-reduced or lactose-free diets. In a recent review, Brown (1991) evaluated these studies and analyzed differences between them. He found that those studies which suggested that lactose-containing feedings resulted in worse outcomes generally included children whose illness was more severe at the time of their entry into the studies. Also, one study of known lactose malabsorbers found differences between the two feeding regimens, whereas studies that excluded those patients did not. The studies in which control patients were given truly lactose-free feedings tended to show differences between groups; those providing reduced lactose feedings to controls were less likely to demonstrate differences.

Diminished absorption of lactose during diarrheal illness does occur, although the reported rates vary among studies and in different populations. On the basis of the analysis just discussed, it seems prudent to recommend reduction or elimination of lactose from the diets of children with severe AGE when such restriction is possible without compromising nutritional intake. Most children can safely tolerate lactose-containing feedings during diarrhea but should be carefully monitored, particularly during the initial hours of treatment. Those who develop increased stooling rates or abdominal distention should have lactose reduced or eliminated until they have recovered.

## Breast-Feeding During Diarrhea

Human breast milk contains more lactose than cow's milk or milk-based formulas, and breast-feeding has in the past been discouraged during diarrhea. Khin-Maung-U performed a controlled trial in hospitalized children and demonstrated reduced stool output among children who received continued breast-milk feedings compared with those whose feedings were interrupted.

A number of reasons have been proposed for the improved outcomes among breast-fed infants, although no completely satisfactory explanation has been demonstrated. Breast-milk has lower osmolality and contains secretory antibodies and enzymes that may reduce the severity of infections. Continued feedings may be superior to intermittent feedings, and breast-feeding may more closely resemble continuous feedings.

Mothers whose nursing patterns are interrupted may experience reduction or cessation of subsequent milk flow. Those mothers may then abandon breast-feeding entirely, to the nutritional detriment of the infant. For all of the above reasons, continuation of breast-feeding throughout diarrheal illness is always to be recommended.

## DELIVERY OF ORAL REHYDRATION THERAPY

### General Recommendations

Like any other form of treatment, ORT must be delivered in a controlled and reliable fashion to be effective. Because of its simplicity, many health care providers tend to offer ORS to patients without properly instructing them in its use and without adequate monitoring of its effects. The results are often discouraging both for parents and providers. We have found that when the following recommendations are observed, therapy is most likely to be successful.

### Clinical Assessment and Management

Patients presenting for therapy of AGE should initially be examined in light of their relevant history. In patients with abdominal pain, distension, and vomiting, acute abdominal processes such as appendicitis, volvulus, and intussusception should be clinically excluded. The physical examination should be directed at the assessment of dehydration. Table 32-39 shows the accepted system for such assessment. In children and infants with uncomplicated acute watery diarrhea, we discourage the routine use of laboratory diagnostic studies. Urine specific gravity, however, may provide a useful parameter for monitoring the progress of rehydration therapy.

The management of the dehydrated child is divided into two phases: rehydration and maintenance (see Table 32-39). Replacement of ongoing losses as well as maintenance fluids must also be provided throughout the treatment period.

### Rehydration Phase

In this phase, the total fluid deficit is intended to be replaced over a 4-hour period. This rapid restoration of circulating volume reverses systemic acidosis and improves tissue perfusion more successfully than the relatively slow repletion over 24 hours that has traditionally been recommended.

Children with mild or moderate dehydration should be given 60 to 80 mL/kg respectively over 4 hours. Patients with severe dehydration (frank or impending shock) should receive an initial bolus of normal saline or Ringer's lactate by the intravenous or intraosseous routes at 40 mL/kg/hr, until signs of shock resolve. The degree of dehydration should then be recalculated, and ORS should be continued as outlined above. While parenteral access is being sought, nasogastric infusion of fluid (using a small (5–7 French) soft catheter may be initiated at a rate of 30 mL/kg/hr, providing that the patient's airway protective reflexes remain intact.

At the end of each hour of rehydration, ongoing losses (stool and emesis) should be calculated and that volume added to the fluid remaining to be given. This fluid should consist of ORS (or isotonic IV fluid in children receiving initial parenteral therapy). Alternatively, parents may be instructed to provide 10 mL/kg or about 4 ounces of ORS for each diarrheal stool.

When the 4-hour rehydration phase is complete, clinical assessment should be repeated. If signs of dehydration persist, the rehydration phase should be repeated until fluid repletion has occurred. When rehydration is complete, the maintenance phase is begun (see Table 32-39).

### Maintenance Phase

The goal during this phase is to provide fluids for replacement of ongoing losses, as well as to meet requirements for maintenance fluids to meet baseline metabolic needs. Maintenance fluid replacements should be met with breast milk on demand in breast-fed infants. Formula-fed infants should receive approximately 150 mL/kg/day of lactose-free formula where available. If formula is unavailable, we generally recommend the use of cow's milk formula diluted 1:1 with water. Full-strength milk-based formula feedings may be offered in children with mild diarrhea who can be carefully monitored by their parents.

Ongoing stool losses should be replaced with ORS on a 1:1 basis. In hospitals and clinics, this can be accomplished using diaper weights. At home, 10 mL/kg or 4 ounces of ORS should be given for each watery stool. Parents should be instructed about

---

**TABLE 32-39.  Fluid Therapy Chart**

| Degree of Dehydration | Signs* | Rehydration Phase† (First 4 hours, repeat until no signs of dehydration remain) | Maintenance Phase (Until illness resolves) |
|---|---|---|---|
| Mild | Slightly dry mucous membranes, increased thirst | ORS 50–60 mL/kg | Breast feeding, undiluted lactose-free formula, ½ strength cow's milk or lactose-containing formula |
| Moderate | Sunken eyes, sunken fontanelle, loss of skin turgor, dry mucous membranes | ORS 80–100 mL/kg | Same as above |
| Severe | Signs of moderate dehydration plus one or more of the following: rapid thready pulse, cyanosis, rapid breathing, delayed capillary refill, lethargy, coma | IV or IO isotonic fluids (0.9% saline or Ringers lactate), 40 ml/kg h until pulse and state of consciousness return to normal, then 50–100 mL/kg of ORS based on remaining degree of dehydration‡ | Same as above |

* If no signs of dehydration are present, rehydration phase may be omitted. Proceed with maintenance therapy and replacement of ongoing losses.
† Replace ongoing stool losses and vomitus with ORS, 10 ml/kg for each diarrheal stool and 5 ml/kg for each episode of vomitus.
‡ While parenteral access is being sought, nasogastric infusion of ORS may be begun at 30 cc/kg/hour, provided airway protective reflexes remain intact.

the gastrocolic reflex that often results in a bowel movement immediately following a feeding and may result in poor compliance with ORT at home. Parents should be reassured that the fluid given by mouth is absorbed and is likely to exceed in quantity the amount lost in stool.

Because of their high osmotic load and low sodium content, fluids such as full-strength juices, punches, and soft drinks should *not* be recommended during AGE.

### The Older Child

Toddlers and school age children may present a special challenge for ORT, because they often refuse to drink physiologically appropriate solutions. Fortunately, such children are at lower risk for severe dehydration with noncholera diarrheas because of their smaller surface-area to volume ratio. We offer such children saltine crackers and half-strength apple juice, which provides a solution of acceptable osmolality and some sodium in a safe fashion (this regimen, however, has not undergone controlled clinical trials, and it should be recognized that it provides insufficient nutrition for prolonged use). These children should not be given soft drinks, teas, or full-strength fruit juices.

### The Vomiting Child

Infants and children with AGE often vomit. Vomiting is exacerbated by systemic acidosis, hypokalemia, and gastric distention. Most vomiting children can be successfully rehydrated orally, and vomiting generally resolves as systemic fluid repletion occurs. Patients should be instructed to provide ORS in small quantities (1 teaspoon, or 5 mL) frequently (every minute) and to persevere in spite of initially continued vomiting. As gastric distention is minimized and acidosis is corrected, frequency of vomiting is generally diminished and the rate of fluid administration can be increased. Children with truly intractable vomiting (as defined by an increasing or persisting negative fluid balance 4 hours after beginning therapy) should receive parenteral fluid therapy as outlined for severely dehydrated patients. Oral treatment usually can begin once vomiting ceases. Anti-emetic medications may have significant adverse effects and may mask serious underlying processes, and their use is contraindicated in infants and children with diarrhea.

## Diet

Once the rehydration phase has been completed and vomiting has diminished, children should be started back on regular feedings. When possible, foods high in lactose should be avoided. We have found that prescribing specific foods such as the standard BRAT (banana, rice, applesauce, toast) diet is less acceptable to families than is a careful description of foods high in complex carbohydrates and low in fats and simple sugars. Families then may make sensible choices from a wide variety of foods that are culturally acceptable.

## Delivery of ORT in the Developing World

Treatment and prevention of dehydration in children has been a priority of WHO for 20 years. Most developing countries currently have a diarrheal disease control program and provide centers for oral hydration as well as substantial promotional campaigns designed to be understood by both literate and illiterate parents. ORT centers may manage hundreds of children daily, usually as outpatients. Patients are rapidly assessed, deficits calculated, and fluids are provided as described above. The delivery of fluids is usually performed by parents, not by medical personnel. After rehydration, breast-feeding is encouraged and feeding instructions are provided.

## Use in Industrialized Nations

ORT centers in the developing world have contributed to the success of this simple therapy, making it truly one of the most important medical advances of this century. Health-care providers in the industrialized world, however, have been slow to take advantage of this therapy. The reasons for this underutilization have been elucidated by Snyder, and we have discovered some additional reasons during the development of an urban rehydration center in Baltimore (Katz).

### Perceived Obstacles to Implementation of ORT

Barriers to the successful use of ORT in the industrialized world generally involve perceptions on the part of health-care providers which are inaccurate or wholly mistaken. The following are examples of such misperceptions, along with recommended responses:

1. *The idea that parental involvement in medical care of children is impractical.* Parents often demand high technology care of their children by the health-care system. However, parents can be incorporated into the system so that they become active partners. Parents who have successfully provided ORS to their child and watched the child improve in their own hands often prefer the use of ORT to IV therapy.
2. *The time element.* Parenteral fluid delivery is usually seen as a more rapid, direct, and assured means of fluid repletion, whereas time spent teaching parents to provide oral solutions may be perceived as wasted. Several studies have compared ORT favorably with IV solutions. When 5 mL (1 teaspoon) of ORS is taken per minute, 300 mL (100) is delivered hourly, representing a rate of fluid administration sufficient to meet the needs of most children during the rehydration phase without inducing gastric distention.
3. *The notion that ORT can only be used in mild dehydration.* Providers are often concerned that moderately or severely ill children will not tolerate ORS or that electrolyte abnormalities or acidosis mandate intravenous therapy. In fact, standard ORS contain more base and potassium than standard IV solutions and are rapidly absorbed. As indicated above, rates of oral delivery can be quite high. Finally, the nasogastric route may be used in a child who is unable to drink (provided airway protective reflexes remain intact).
4. *The vomiting child.* Although children with truly intractable vomiting require parenteral fluids for a time, most can be rehydrated enterally when small volumes are presented to the stomach. The use of a 5-mL syringe or medicine cup can facilitate fluid delivery. The volume of emesis is usually overestimated by parents and staff. Generally, when careful measurements are made, children are found to maintain a net positive fluid balance.

### Real Obstacles

Certain genuine obstacles to the proper widespread use of ORT remain. One of these is cost: although ORT is cheaper than IV therapy, the cost of the former is often borne by the parent, because third-party insurers do not pay for ORT in hospitals. Currently, commercially available solutions cost from $3.00 to $7.00 per liter—a prohibitive expense for many families. Public assistance programs such as WIC provide solutions in only about half of the United States. One approach to the cost issue is to use the packaged dry salts, as WHO does. These packets (Oral Rehydration Salts, Jianis Bros, Kansas City, MO) provide salts for one liter of ORS at less than $0.75 per packet. The American Academy of Pediatrics currently recommends the use of these packets, when they are accompanied by an appropriately sized container for mixing to reduce the potential for misuse.

**Rehydration Orders**

**Mild Dehydration:**

60 cc ORS/Kg X _____ Kg = _____ ml ORS

**Moderate Dehydration:**

80 cc ORS/Kg X _____ Kg = _____ ml ORS

*Deliver calculated volume over 2-4 hours by administering 5cc/minute as tolerated*

**Treatment Record**

| Hours After Rx Starts | Time | T | P | R | BP | Volume ORS Calculated to be Given | ORS Ingested | Other Ingested | Volume IV given | Stool Loss (cc's) | Vomit (cc's) | Assessment of Dehydration | Init. |
|---|---|---|---|---|---|---|---|---|---|---|---|---|---|
| Start | | | | | | | – | – | – | – | – | | |
| 1 | | | | | | | | | | | | | |
| 2 | | | | | | | | | | | | | |
| 3 | | | | | | | | | | | | | |
| 4 | | | | | | | | | | | | | |

**Discharge instructions:**

_____

_____

_____

_____

**Figure 32-7.** Sample order sheet for rehydration fluids in an American Pediatric Emergency Department. This form is used for the *rehydration phase* only. After rehydration is complete, the patient is discharged to home with standard feeding and fluid recommendations.

## ORAL REHYDRATION PROTOCOL

A final obstacle to use of ORT is the lack of proper training in most medical centers. Health care providers must have a basic understanding of the pathophysiology of AGE and ORT and often must substantially change their existing practices to incorporate systematic protocols for delivery of ORT. A project recently was initiated at an urban teaching hospital to develop an educational program for physicians in training and for nurses. The following brief description of the protocol followed in that program may be modified to suit local needs:

1. All patients presenting to the triage desk with complaints of acute gastroenteritis (AGE), vomiting, poor intake, or dehydration, and/or those with clinical signs of dehydration excluding those exhibiting signs of circulatory collapse, are eligible for the ORT program. Of importance, patients with vomiting are eligible for the program, so long as they lack evidence of intestinal obstruction or acute abdomen.
2. Eligible patients are directed to the "walk-in" area of the Emergency Department, where staffing is provided by two or more pediatric house officers and a designated ORT nurse.
3. Patients are assessed by the physician. History and physical examination are performed. Patients with evidence of acute abdomen or serious underlying illness are excluded. Patients are then referred to the ORT nurse.
4. The ORT nurse evaluates the patient in the designated ORT room. Together with the physician, the degree of dehydration (mild or moderate) is estimated using standard criteria, and the fluid deficit is calculated (60 mL/kg for mild dehydration, 80 mL/kg for moderate).* Orders are then written for the replacement of the deficit over a 4-hour period. Initial data are recorded on the ORT data form (Fig 32-7).
5. The ORT nurse explains the principles of ORT and elicits parental participation. The parent is given the first hour's replacement volume in a container, and the ORT nurse demonstrates the technique of feeding small frequent volumes (we recommend giving 5 mL/minute; this provides a rate of 300 mL, or 10 ounces, per hour). A teaspoon, syringe, or graduated 60-mL bottle is used to deliver the fluid, depending on the age and preference of the child. More fluid is dispensed at the end of each hour.
6. Vomiting children are good candidates for ORT. In spite of their continued vomiting, patients are given fluids using the

* The current WHO standard for fluid replacement is 50 mL/kg for mild and 100 mL/kg for moderate diarrhea. In practice, children taking fluids as recommended in the text will consume 50 to 60 mL/kg or 80 to 100 mL/kg, respectively.

same technique of feeding small amounts with a spoon, syringe, or medicine cup. Both staff and parents must be taught that this approach provides continued absorption of fluid during vomiting.

7. The number of stools and emesis in each 1-hour period is recorded, as is the volume of fluid taken during that period. The fluid balance is calculated every hour by subtracting the volume taken from the calculated deficit, then adding 10 mL/kg for each stool during the period. Emesis volume is estimated and replaced as well. In practice, many children are found to consume their entire calculated deficit in the first 2 to 4 hours of treatment.

8. At the end of the first 4-hour period, or when the total calculated deficit has been replaced, whichever occurs sooner, the patient is clinically reassessed by the ORT nurse and physician. If signs of dehydration have resolved, further instructions on feeding and maintenance of hydration are given, and the patient is discharged to home with follow-up at the primary care physician's office. Discharge weight and vital signs are recorded. If the patient remains clinically dehydrated, the deficit calculation is repeated, and a second 4-hour rehydration phase is begun.

9. Patients who fail oral rehydration therapy are referred to the urgent care section of the ED for further evaluation and therapy. Criteria for treatment failure are as follows:

    An increasing deficit over the rehydration phase
    Intractable vomiting
    Clinical deterioration
    Failure to achieve clinical rehydration after 8 hours.

## Parent Education During the Emergency Department Encounter

Educational efforts are designed to take advantage of the time spent by family members in the Emergency Department during the rehydration period. In addition, a primary goal is to actively involve parents in the therapeutic process. The ORT nurse provides direct teaching to parents about how to use ORS in the hospital and at home, and how to detect and respond to the early signs of dehydration. A variety of printed material is provided to parents to reinforce instructions and provide some references at home for use during future episodes. Parents are actively solicited for their questions, comments, and feedback. Prior to discharge the children's maintenance fluid needs during AGE are calculated and presented to the parents in terms of a minimal number of 8-ounce bottles/glasses to be consumed daily. In addition, the nurse assists families in planning appropriate diets based on child and cultural preferences. Families also receive information about infection control, keeping their children comfortable during AGE, and general well-child care practices.

## CONCLUSION

Proper use of any therapy is critical to its success and depends on a thorough understanding of the pathophysiology of the disease process in question, the physiology of the therapeutic intervention itself, and the available systems for delivery of the treatment. In this chapter, we have endeavored to provide the clear physiologic basis for the use of ORT, as well as a practical framework to ensure its appropriate use and delivery. Although the last 3 decades have seen enormous progress in development and implementation of ORT programs, much remains to be accomplished. AGE and dehydration continue to be the leading causes of infant mortality globally. Only through the continued process of research, development, and education in this area will further progress be made. Technology and knowledge must be transferred not only from the research centers to the field, but from providers to parents, incorporating parents into the health care team. We must also continue efforts to effect the transfer of experience and skills from the less developed to the more developed nations. Our efforts to adapt ORT technology to the industrialized world represents the beginning of such an effort.

## Selected Readings

Alam AN, Sarker SA, Molla AM et al. Hydrolysed wheat based oral rehydration solution for acute diarrhea. Arch Dis Child 1987;62:440.

American Academy of Pediatrics Committee on Nutrition. Use of oral fluid therapy and posttreatment feeding following enteritis in children in a developed country. Pediatrics 1985;75:358.

Brown K: Dietary management of acute childhood diarrhea: Optimal timing of feeding and appropriate use of milks and mixed diets. J Pediatr 1991;118:592.

Brown KH, Black RE, Parry L. The effect of diarrhea on incidence of lactose malabsorption among Bangladeshi children. Am J Clin Nutr 1980;33:2226.

Brown KH, Gastanaduy AS, Saavedra JM et al. Effect of continued oral feeding on clinical and nutritional outcomes of acute diarrhea in children. J Pediatr 1988;112:191.

Chung AW. The effect of oral feeding at different levels on the absorption of foodstuffs in infantile diarrhea. J Pediatr 1948;33:1.

Darrow DC. The retention of electrolyte during recovery from severe dehydration due to diarrhea. J Pediatr 1946;28:515.

Darrow DC, Pratt EL, Flett J Jr et al. Disturbances of water and electrolytes in infantile diarrhea. Pediatrics 1949;3:129.

Flett J, Pratt EL, Darrow DC. Methods used in treatment of diarrhea with potassium and sodium salts. Pediatrics 1949;4:604.

Glass RI, Lew JF, Gangarosa RE et al. Estimates of morbidity and mortality rates for diarrheal diseases in American children. J Pediatr 1991;118:S27.

Govan CD Jr, Darrow DC. The use of potassium chloride in the treatment of the dehydration of diarrhea in infants. J Pediatr 1946;28:541.

Hirschhorn N, Cash RA, Woodward WE et al. Oral fluid therapy of Apache children with acute infectious diarrhoea. Lancet 1972;2:15.

Hirschhorn N, MmLarthy BJ, Ranney B et al. Ad libitum oral glucose–electrolyte therapy for acute diarrhea in Apache children. J Pediatr 1973;83:562.

Katz S, Goepp JG. The Johns Hopkins Oral Rehydration Project. In: Outpatient oral rehydration therapy protocol. Greer, Margolis, Mitchell, Grunwald and Associates, Inc., 1991.

Kenya PR, Odongo HW, Oundo G et al. Cereal-based oral rehydration solutions. Arch Dis Child 1989;64:1032.

Khin-Maung-U, Greenough WB III. Cereal-based oral rehydration therapy. I. Clinical studies. J Pediatr 1991;118:S72.

Khin-Maung-U, Nyunt-Nyunt-Wai, Myo-Khin et al. Effect on clinical outcome of breast-feeding during acute diarrhoea. Br Med J 1985;290:587.

Kinoti SN, Wasunna A, Turkish J et al. A comparison of the efficacy of maize-based ORS and standard WHO ORS in the treatment of acute childhood diarrhoea at Kenyatta National Hospital, Nairobi, Kenya: Results of a pilot study. East Afr Med J 1986;63:168.

Latta T. Malignant cholera: Documents communicated by the central board of Health, London, relative to the treatment of cholera by the copious injection of aqueous and saline fluids into the veins. Lancet 1832;2:274.

Lifshitz F, Coella-Ramirez P, Gutierrez-Topete G et al. Carbohydrate intolerance in infants with diarrhea. J Pediatr 1971;79:760.

Listernick R, Zieserl E, Davis AT. Outpatient oral rehydration in the United States. Am J Dis Child 1986;140:211.

Mehta MN, Subramaniam S. Comparison of rice water, rice electrolyte solution, and glucose electrolyte solution in the management of infantile diarrhea. Lancet 1986;1:843.

Mohan M, Sethi JS, Daral TS et al. Controlled trial of rice powder and glucose rehydration solutions as oral therapy for acute dehydrating diarrhea in infants. J Pediatr Gastroenterol Nutr 1986;5:423.

Molla AM, Ahmed SM, Greenough WB III. Rice-based oral rehydration solution decreases stool volume in acute diarrhea. Bull WORLD Health Organ 1985;63:751.

Molla AM, Molla A, Rohde J et al. Turning off the diarrhea: the role of food and oral rehydration solution. J Pediatr Gastroenterol Nutr 1989;8:81.

Molla AM, Molla A, Nath SK et al. Food-based oral rehydration salt solution for acute childhood diarrhoea. Lancet 1989;2:429.

Molla AM, Sarka SA, Hossain M et al. Rice powder electrolyte solution as oral therapy in cholera due to Vibro cholerae and Escherichia coli. Lancet 1982;1:1317.

Park EA. New viewpoints in infant feeding. Proc Conn State Med Soc 1924;20:190.

Patra FC, Mahalanabis D, Jalan KN et al. Is oral rice electrolyte solution superior to glucose electrolyte solution in infantile diarrhea? Arch Dis Child 1982;57:910.

Powell D. Intestinal water and electrolyte transport. In: Johnson LR (ed). Physiology of the gastrointestinal tract, 2nd ed. New York: Raven Press, 1987:1267.

Powers GF. A comprehensive plan of treatment for the so-called intestinal intoxication of children. Am J Dis Child 1926;32:232.

Santosham M, Burns B, Nadkarni V et al. Oral rehydration therapy for acute diarrhea in ambulatory children in the United States: a double-blind comparison of four different solutions. Pediatrics 1985;76:159.

Santosham M, Burns BA, Reid R et al. Glycine-based oral rehydration solution: Reassessment of safety and efficacy. J Pediatr 1986;109:795.

Santosham M, Daum RS, Dillman L et al. Oral rehydration therapy of infantile diarrhea: A controlled study of well-nourished children hospitalized in the United States and Panama. N Engl J Med 1982;306:1070.

Santosham M, Fayad I, Hashem M et al. A comparison of rice-based oral rehydration solution and "early feeding" for the treatment of acute diarrhea in infants. J Pediatr 1990;116:868.

Santosham M, Foster S, Reid R et al. Role of soy-based, lactose-free formula during treatment of acute diarrhea. Pediatrics 1985;76:292.

Santosham S, Duggan C. Management of acute diarrhea. MMWR 1992;41(RR16): 1.

Snyder JD. Use and misuse of oral therapy for diarrhea: comparison of U.S. practices with American Academy of Pediatrics recommendations. Pediatrics 1991;87: 28.

Snyder JD, Marson MH. The magnitude of the global problem of acute diarrhoeal disease: A review of active surveillance data. Bull WORLD Health Organ 1982;60: 605.

Tamer AM, Friedman LB, Maxwell SRW et al. Oral rehydration of infants in a large urban U.S. medical center. J Pediatr 1985;107:14.

Torres-Pinedo R, Lavastida M, Rivera CL et al. Studies on infant diarrhea. I. A comparison of the effects of milk feeding and intravenous therapy upon the composition and volume of stool of urine. J Clin Invest 1966;45:469.

*Principles and Practice of Pediatrics, Second Edition.*
edited by Frank A. Oski et al. J. B. Lippincott Company, Philadelphia © 1994.

# CHAPTER 33
# *Dental Problems*

## Katherine Kula

A multidisciplinary approach to pediatric health care is necessary to children's physical and emotional health. A physician, who examines a child earlier and more frequently than a dentist, can provide early education and dental referral to prevent or minimize oral problems. Although most problems in the oral cavity are traditionally considered to be in the realm of dentistry, the physician can diagnose oral problems that, left untreated, may contribute to systemic disturbances. The physician should examine the mouth for signs of physical or chemical insults. The prevention of dental problems reduces the cost and risk of dental care, particularly in medically or physically compromised patients.

Knowledge of the face and oral structures helps the physician diagnose various local and systemic problems. Some of the most common pediatric dental problems and their treatment are discussed in this chapter.

## NORMAL ORAL STRUCTURES

### Examination

Examination of the oral structures should be routinely performed at birth and at health maintenance visits. The newborn examination can reveal abnormalities and serves as a baseline against which to compare later development.

Knowledge of normal dental structures, processes, and timing and sequence of events helps a clinician recognize abnormalities.

The pediatrician performing an oral examination should remember that most children exhibit normal soft-tissue, hard-tissue, and dental symmetry and that accurate diagnosis and correct treatment of abnormalities usually requires dental referral for additional diagnostic tests.

Factors to be considered during an intraoral examination are support of the child's head, access, visibility, timing, systematic approach, and protection of the clinician's fingers. Extraoral and other portions of the examination may be accomplished while the parent is holding the child on his or her lap or against his or her shoulder. An intraoral examination can be conducted with the child in any one of a number of positions, depending on the child's age and willingness to cooperate. In most cases, a young child can be examined intraorally in a supine position, lying on the examination table. Alternatively, the parent and the clinician can sit knee to knee, with the child lying with his head on the clinician's lap and his arms and legs held on the parent's lap.

Extraoral structures are the easiest to observe. The proportions of the face, the profile, and the integrity of the lips should be evaluated. The physician can start the intraoral examination by using an index finger to palpate the hard and soft palate, ridges, and tongue. A sweeping palpation of the buccal vestibules can determine the presence of abnormal structures. The sucking reflex of an infant should be intact; she usually reacts to the examining finger as if it were a nipple. In examining older children, the physician should take care to avoid being bitten.

The next part of the intraoral examination is visual examination. Using the thumb and forefinger of each hand, the physician should slightly extend the lips in an apical direction for better visualization of the labial vestibules, anterior alveoli, and teeth. The cheeks should be slightly distended with a tongue blade or with a forefinger, preferably with the patient's mouth open, allowing the buccal vestibules, Stensen's duct, buccal mucosa, posterior alveoli, and teeth to be examined.

If the child is cooperative, she should be asked to open her mouth widely and extend the tongue so that the top of the tongue can be examined. She should then raise her tongue to the roof of the mouth so that the ventral surface of the tongue, floor of the mouth, and lower teeth can be viewed. The physician can hold the tip of the tongue with a piece of cotton gauze and then extend the tongue slightly to view its sides. If no small intraoral mirror is available for viewing the palate, the child's head, which may be rested on the examination table, in the crook of a parent's arm, or on the clinician's lap, can be tipped backward for viewing the palate and upper teeth. A pen light permits better visualization of the oral cavity.

If the child is uncooperative, the physician should use a mouth prop, constructed with several tongue blades stacked on top of each other and bound by a cushion of cotton gauze and then by tape. The physician can position the prop between opposing dentitions, inserting the narrow side first and then slowly rotating the prop to attain access between the arches. As long as the child's head is stabilized and the mouth prop held firmly, the child maintains an open mouth and cannot hurt herself. Alternatively, the physician can use a thimble with the end cut off, placed firmly over the examining finger.

### Primary Dentition

The dental stage in which only primary teeth are erupted is called primary dentition. Twenty primary teeth normally erupt between the ages of approximately 4 and 30 months (Table 33-1). The timing of eruption varies among ethnic and racial groups; for example, American blacks tend to have an earlier eruption and exfoliation pattern than American whites. Eruption is usually symmetric from side to side. Eruption tends to occur slightly earlier in the mandibular arch than in the maxillary arch. The sequence

### TABLE 33-1. Chronology of Human Dentition*

| Tooth | Hard Tissue Formation Begins | Amount of Enamel Formed at Birth | Enamel Completed | Eruption | Root Completed |
|---|---|---|---|---|---|
| **Deciduous Dentition** | | | | | |
| *Maxillary* | | | | | |
| Central incisor | 4 mo in utero | Five sixths | 1½ mo | 7½ mo | 1½ y |
| Lateral incisor | 4½ mo in utero | | 2½ mo | 9 mo | 2 y |
| Cuspid | 5 mo in utero | One third | 9 mo | 18 mo | 3¼ y |
| First molar | 5 mo in utero | Cusps united | 6 mo | 14 mo | 2½ y |
| Second molar | 6 mo in utero | Cusp tips still isolated | 11 mo | 24 mo | 3 y |
| *Mandibular* | | | | | |
| Central incisor | 4½ mo in utero | Three fifths | 2½ mo | 6 mo | 1½ y |
| Lateral incisor | 4½ mo in utero | Three fifths | 3 mo | 7 mo | 1½ y |
| Cuspid | 5 mo in utero | One third | 9 mo | 16 mo | 3¼ y |
| First molar | 5 mo in utero | Cusps united | 5½ mo | 12 mo | 2¼ y |
| Second molar | 6 mo in utero | Cusp tips still isolated | 10 mo | 20 mo | 3 y |
| **Permanent Dentition** | | | | | |
| *Maxillary* | | | | | |
| Central incisor | 3–4 mo | | 4–5 y | 7–8 y | 10 y |
| Lateral incisor | 10–12 mo | | 4–5 y | 8–9 y | 11 y |
| Cuspid | 4–5 mo | | 6–7 y | 11–12 y | 13–15 y |
| First bicuspid | 1½–1¾ y | | 5–6 y | 10–11 y | 12–13 y |
| Second bicuspid | 2–2¼ y | | 6–7 y | 10–12 y | 12–14 y |
| First molar | At birth | Sometimes a trace | 2½–3 y | 6–7 y | 9–10 y |
| Second molar | 2½–3 y | | 7–8 y | 12–13 y | 14–16 y |
| Third molar | 7–9 y | | 12–16 y | 17–21 y | 18–25 y |
| *Mandibular* | | | | | |
| Central incisor | 3–4 mo | | 4–5 y | 6–7 y | 9 y |
| Lateral incisor | 3–4 mo | | 4–5 y | 7–8 y | 10 y |
| Cuspid | 4–5 mo | | 6–7 y | 9–10 y | 12–14 y |
| First bicuspid | 1¾–2 y | | 5–6 y | 10–12 y | 12–13 y |
| Second bicuspid | 2¼–2½ y | | 6–7 y | 11–12 y | 13–14 y |
| First molar | At birth | Sometimes a trace | 2½–3 y | 6–7 y | 9–10 y |
| Second molar | 2½–3 y | | 7–8 y | 11–13 y | 14–15 y |
| Third molar | 8–10 y | | 12–16 y | 17–21 y | 18–25 y |

* Mean ages.

Logan WGH, Krenfeld R. Development of the human jaws and surrounding structures from birth to the age of fifteen years. JADA 1933;20:379. Slightly modified by McCall and Schour.

of eruption is usually the central incisor, lateral incisor, first molar, canine, and second molar. All primary teeth are usually into occlusion by the age of 3 years.

The upper and lower teeth are usually not held together but assume a physiologic rest position a few millimeters apart. They normally contact each other during swallowing and mastication. The gingiva surrounding the teeth is normally light pink and firm.

The dorsum of the tongue is occupied by numerous filiform and fungiform papillae. Circumvallate papillae separate the anterior portion of the tongue from the posterior portion. The lingual surface of the tongue and the floor of the mouth are well vascularized. Raised structures, which represent the salivary gland ducts, are usually visible in the floor of the mouth.

The oral tissues are moistened by saliva secreted from three major salivary glands and minor glands. The shape of the encapsulated parotid gland, the largest of the major glands, is irregular, and it extends within the cheek superiorly to the zygomatic bone and inferiorly to the angle of the mandible. The parotid may extend as far distally as between the external auditory meatus and the temporomandibular joint. A slight mass of tissue on the buccal mucosa approximately adjacent to the maxillary permanent molars usually surrounds the opening of the parotid duct (Stensen's duct), which extends from the anterior portion of the gland. The superior border of the submandibular gland lies in the floor of the mouth, and the inferior border extends to the hyoid bone. The submandibular ducts (Wharton's ducts) pass under the anterior portion of the tongue, where they appear as long, raised areas, and open into the sublingual caruncula, which lies at the midline of the tongue. The sublingual gland lies in the floor of the mouth. This gland may open directly under the tongue through multiple small excretory ducts or may unite with the submandibular duct through the sublingual Bartholin's duct. Minor salivary gland openings exist in the circumvallate papillae on the dorsum of the tongue, along the lingual frenum on the ventral surface of the tongue, and in the palate.

Salivary function is of utmost importance to the health of the oral cavity. Saliva is a multicomponent substance that serves numerous functions. It lubricates food and facilitates swallowing. Lubrication of the occluding surfaces of the teeth helps minimize tooth abrasion. The buffering of acidic, potentially destructive substances is primarily accomplished by bicarbonate ions, the concentration of which is increased with increased salivary flow. Various salivary proteins buffer acids. Salivary flow also clears oral debris. The greater the flow rate, the more frequently swallowing occurs, and the faster debris is cleared from the mouth. However, debris clears from various areas of the mouth at different rates because of the compartmentalization of the mouth. The differences in clearance rates makes teeth in some areas of the mouth more susceptible to caries than teeth in other areas.

Salivary amylase breaks down starch primarily in the mouth, because its action is inhibited in the acidic stomach. Immunoglobulin A and other proteins in the saliva are thought to prevent bacterial attachment. Numerous salivary proteins such as lysozyme, lactoferrin, and lactoperoxidase appear to be bacteriocidal or bacteriostatic. Fluid from the tissues around the teeth contributes antibodies, phagocytic cells, and antibacterial products. Multiple ions and other components in the saliva help maintain the oral tissues.

The flow rate of saliva from all areas of the mouth appears to increase with age up to 15 years, when it reaches that of an adult. Average stimulated salivary flow rate for 5-year-old children is approximately 0.5 mL/minute, slightly more than 1.0 mL/minute for 10-year-old children, and approximately 2.0 mL/minute for 15-year-old adolescents. Considerable variability in stimulated salivary flow rates exists. Unstimulated flow rates (eg, during sleep) are almost negligible and minimally clear food (eg, sugar in antibiotics or from the baby bottle) from the mouth. The increased time that these sugars and their acidic by-products spend in the mouth increases the susceptibility of teeth to caries.

In the lymphatic drainage of the oral structures, the submental nodes drain the mandibular anterior teeth, their surrounding labial gingiva, and the lower lip. The submandibular nodes receive lymphatic drainage from the submental nodes, the maxillary structures, the mandibular posterior teeth and surrounding structures, the tongue, and the nasal cavity. The parotid gland drains into the preauricular nodes. The cervical nodes receive lymphatic drainage from the base of the tongue, the sublingual area, and the posterior palate and from the preauricular, submandibular, and submental nodes.

## Newborn

The mouth of the newborn is similar to that of an older child but is characterized by toothless alveolar pads or ridges in the maxilla and mandible. The ridges vary considerably in shape and frequently have small bumps or protrusions under which lie the developing primary teeth. Teeth are normally lacking in the newborn. The maxillary alveolar ridge is usually demarcated from the rest of palate by a palatal alveolar groove that disappears with time.

The frenum may appear to extend over or through the alveolar ridge and may actually connect with the incisive papilla. With development, the frenum usually moves apically toward the vestibule.

## Mixed Dentition

Mixed dentition is a stage in which the roots of the primary teeth resorb, the primary teeth exfoliate and are replaced by the permanent teeth, and the first permanent molars erupt distal to the primary molars. Mixed dentition begins at approximately 6 years of age, when the first permanent molars or the permanent incisors erupt, and continues until approximately 13 years of age, when the last primary tooth is replaced by a permanent tooth. There is usually a 3- to 4-year span between the eruption of the permanent incisors and first molars and the eruption of the permanent canines and premolars. The sequence of eruption varies among children and between the dental arches, but in general, the first permanent molar or the mandibular central incisors erupt first.

Occasionally, a permanent tooth erupts before exfoliation of the primary tooth (Fig 33-1). This does not present a problem if the primary tooth is mobile; the permanent tooth usually moves into proper position within the arch. However, the child should be encouraged to extract the primary tooth as soon as possible. If the primary tooth is firmly attached, the child should be referred to a dentist for evaluation and potential extraction.

During the early stages of mixed dentition, the maxillary incisors may appear spaced and slightly splayed. This spacing frequently disappears as the permanent canines, which are developing against the roots of the lateral incisors, erupt, forcing the incisors together.

## Permanent Dentition

Permanent dentition is the stage that follows replacement of the last remaining primary tooth with a permanent tooth. Depending on the eruption sequence, the second and third permanent molars may not yet be erupted (see Table 33-1). However, the second molar should erupt within a year. The third molar varies in its eruption time but is not expected to erupt before the age of 17 years. The normal complement of permanent teeth is 32, with 16 in the maxilla and 16 in the mandible.

## DENTAL ANOMALIES

Various anomalies associated with developmental disturbances can be detected at birth, within a few weeks of birth, or at the time of tooth eruption. The categorization of dental anomalies into discrete entities is difficult. Some dental anomalies are manifestations of an entire tissue dysfunction, such as ectodermal dysplasia; others are nonspecific. Disorders involving mineralization, such as vitamin D-resistant rickets, affect bone and tooth formation. Although abnormalities of the teeth can be differentiated on the basis of tooth color, shape, number, position, and eruption, even this method of categorization has its pitfalls, and frequently overlaps exist.

The pediatrician should know that different tooth types undergo formation at different times and that crown formation starts at different times for the permanent teeth compared with the primary teeth. Knowledge of the effects of diseases (eg, ectodermal dysplasia), drugs (eg, tetracycline), and treatments (eg, head and

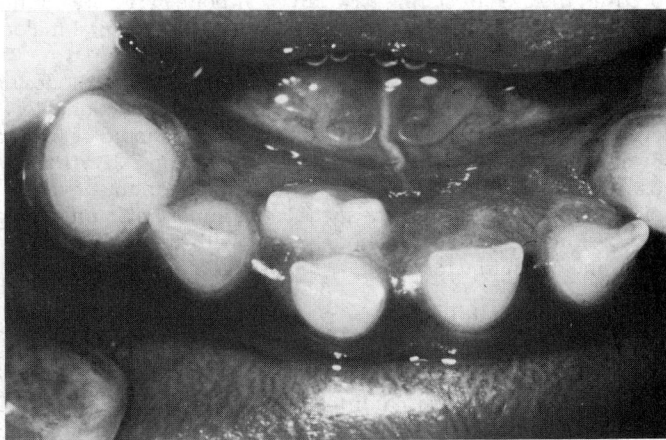

**Figure 33-1.** Double row of teeth in which a permanent incisor has erupted before primary tooth exfoliation. (Courtesy of Dr. Mark Wagner, University of Maryland Dental School.)

neck irradiation) on tooth formation allows the clinician to counsel parents about their children's future dental development and to assess the risks and benefits of treatment.

## Congenital Anomalies

### First Arch Syndromes

Examples of syndromes that result from numerous first arch malformations are the Treacher Collins and the Pierre Robin syndromes. The Treacher Collins syndrome, caused by an autosomal dominant gene, is characterized by malar hypoplasia, downslanting palpebral fissures, defects of the lower eyelid, and defects of the external, middle, and inner ear. The Pierre Robin syndrome is characterized by mandibular hypoplasia, cleft palate, and ear and eye defects. The abnormally small mandible may prevent vertical displacement of the tongue during palatal fusion, resulting in cleft palate.

### Clefts

Incomplete or total lack of fusion of the various processes can result in various types of clefting. Clefting of the lower lip or jaw is rarer than clefting in the maxillary area. Cleft lip can be unilateral or bilateral, resulting from failure of the maxillary prominences on the affected side(s) to unite with the merged medial nasal prominences. Clefting of the lip may vary from an incomplete cleft, with only a small notching in the vermilion border of the lip, to a complete cleft through the alveolar process to the distal portion of the incisive papillae. Boys are affected more frequently than girls.

Girls are more frequently affected by cleft palate with or without cleft lip. The severity of cleft palate can vary from a bifid uvula to a complete bilateral cleft of anterior and posterior palates. The severity depends on the extent of fusion between the median nasal process, the lateral palatine processes, and the median nasal septum. Cleft lip may occur with cleft palate.

Clefting can be manifested as part of a syndrome caused by single mutant genes or by chromosomal defects such as trisomy 13. Teratogenic agents such as anticonvulsant drugs are implicated in a few cases. The results of twin studies indicate that genetic factors are of greater importance in cleft lip with or without cleft palate than in cleft palate alone.

The patient with a palatal cleft may have numerous problems in addition to the cosmetic appearance. Palatal clefting may affect an infant's ability to feed because of interference with sucking. Later, it may affect the child's speech. A custom-made obturator minimizes some of these problems.

Abnormalities in tooth number, structure, and appearance may occur in the area of clefting. The alveolar bone in the area of the cleft is usually inadequate for the erupting teeth. Dental malocclusions are common and can become worse with age.

Surgical repair of the cleft lip and palate with orthodontic treatment can produce reasonable aesthetics and function. However, these patients have multiple problems and should be treated by a team consisting of a surgeon, speech pathologist, orthodontist, and pediatric dentist for maximum benefit. Timing of various procedures and the skill of the specialists is important in producing the best aesthetic and functional result with the least financial and time commitments.

### Natal and Neonatal Teeth

Premature eruption of primary teeth occurs in the United States in approximately 1 in 2000 to 3500 live births. Teeth present at birth are referred to as natal teeth; teeth that erupt within 30 days after birth are called neonatal teeth (Fig 33-2). Natal and neonatal teeth are usually part of the normal complement of primary teeth and may result from vertical displacement of the tooth follicle. In approximately 15% of reported cases, there is a

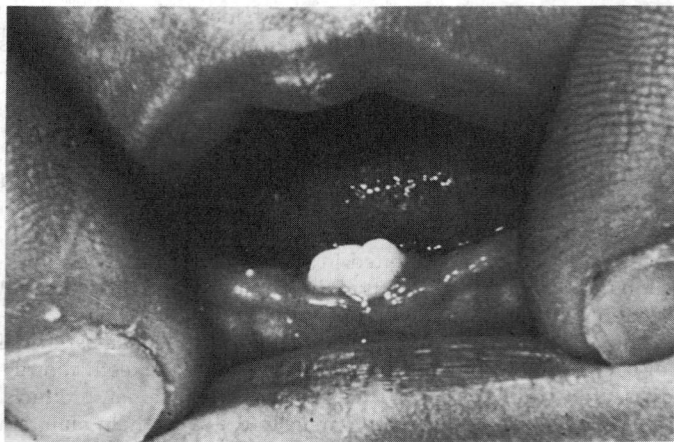

Figure 33-2. Neonatal teeth. (Courtesy of Dr. Mark Wagner, University of Maryland Dental School.)

family history of premature eruption, which may be associated with endocrine problems. Neonatal teeth erupt most frequently in the area of the mandibular central incisor. The crowns may appear well formed or yellow with an irregular surface. Although the gingival growth may eventually obscure them, the enamel portions that are clinically obvious do not continue to develop and remain hypoplastic. Crown and root formation is incomplete, and the teeth are frequently mobile, making aspiration of tooth shells a risk. Abrasion against these teeth can produce lesions called Riga-Frede on the tongue or the opposing ridge. Breastfeeding may produce maternal discomfort. Extraction is recommended if these teeth are mobile or cause lesions; otherwise, they can be allowed to remain.

### Cysts

Newborn infants may exhibit several types of dental cysts related to vestigial embryonic structures. The literature is confusing concerning some of their names and embryonic sources. Two cysts, Epstein's pearls and Bohn's nodules, occur in about 80% of newborns. Epstein's pearls are white-yellow cysts occurring along the median palatal raphes or at the junction of the hard and soft palates. They result from remnants of epithelial tissue entrapped during palatal fusion.

Bohn's nodules are white-yellow cysts occurring along the lateral aspects of the alveolar ridges and along the periphery of the palate. They may develop from heterotrophic salivary gland tissue or from remnants of the dental lamina.

Dental lamina cysts, named after their potential source, are fluid-filled cystic formations found on the crest of the alveolar ridges. In most cases, they are asymptomatic and regress spontaneously; however, if they interfere with eating, surgical intervention may be indicated.

Neonatal alveolar lymphangiomas are fluid-filled lesions occurring on the lingual alveolar process in the molar region of the mandible. Spontaneous regression is observed in some cases, but the progression of these lesions is unknown.

### Tumors

Congenital epulis, which consists of granular cells, is most often seen at birth in the anterior maxillary region. The epulis is usually pedunculated and varies from a few millimeters to several centimeters in diameter. Simple excision is the treatment of choice, and recurrence is rare. The origin of this tumor is unknown.

The neuroectodermal tumor of infancy is most often found in infants under the age of 6 months. Usually occurring in the maxilla, it is a smooth-surfaced, rapidly expanding lesion of the alveolus that may or may not be pigmented. Radiographs of the lesion show a radiolucency with displaced primary teeth. The treatment of choice is simple surgical excision. Recurrence has been reported.

## Tongue and Stoma

Microglossia, a rare anomaly, is manifested as a small or vestigial tongue and is most frequently associated with defects involving the limbs and digit reductions. Deformities of the arch and mandible are usually present and require correction. Speech is relatively unaffected.

Macroglossia, which is also rare, is enlargement of the tongue, resulting from lymphangiomas or muscle hypertrophy.

Ankyloglossia is abnormal restriction of the tongue caused by a tight lingual frenum. Surgical release is indicated if abnormal and destructive forces are placed on the gingival tissue or if speech problems exist. However, speech problems should first be evaluated by a speech pathologist. Most children adapt well to ankyloglossia and require no surgery. There are reports of ankyloglossia associated with deviation of the epiglottis and larynx. These patients develop dyspnea and other respiratory problems that are minimized with correction of the ankyloglossia and positions of the epiglottis and larynx. Other reports of ankyloglossia in the newborn relate to breast-feeding problems. Lactating mothers may develop sores because the nursing child's tongue does not cover the alveolus, which traumatizes the mother's nipple and areola.

A cleft tongue may result from incomplete fusion of the lateral embryologic swellings. A bifid tongue results from complete lack of fusion of the lateral embryologic swellings.

Microstomia, a small mouth opening, is a rare disorder associated with various syndromes, such as whistling face syndrome. Aesthetics, normal oral hygiene, and normal ambulatory dental care can be compromised by the restrictive oral opening.

## Tooth Anomalies

### Shape

Enamel hypoplasia, which can range from pits or furrows in the enamel surface to complete absence of enamel, results from disturbances in formation of the ameloblast layer, in matrix formation, or in mineralization. Factors such as excess fluoride supplementation, vitamin D deficiency, tetracycline therapy (Fig 33-3), hypothyroidism, head and neck irradiation, maternal infections while in utero, measles, and other infections (Fig 33-4) can cause temporary disturbances in enamel formation. As a result of the systemic nature of these disturbances, all teeth in which

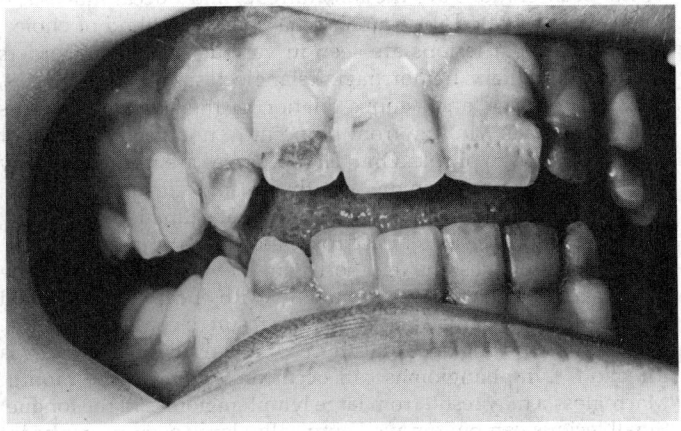

**Figure 33-3.** Linear hypoplasia resulting from tetracycline treatment of a child at approximately 2 to 3 years of age.

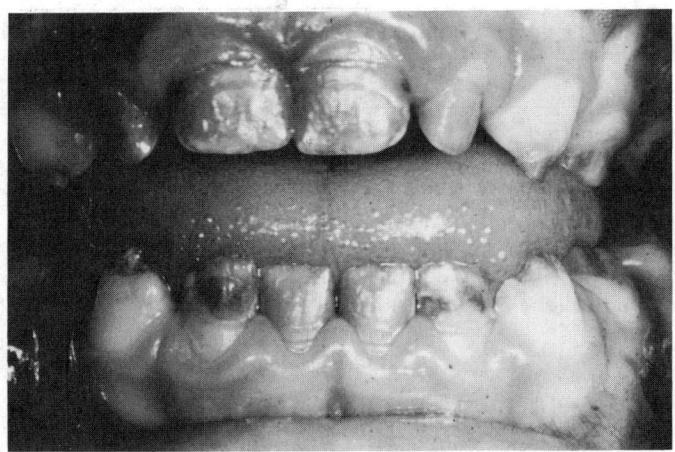

**Figure 33-4.** Linear hypoplasia and staining associated with repeated febrile episodes.

enamel was forming at the time of the insult may show permanent deformation in the particular segment of forming enamel. Localized hypoplasia affecting one or a few adjacent teeth is caused by factors such as trauma or a dental abscess. Generalized hypoplasia is obvious in hereditary forms of amelogenesis imperfecta. Congenital syphilis is manifested by permanent incisors that are shaped like screwdrivers and by first permanent molars that have irregular occlusal surfaces with multiple enamel blebs (ie, mulberry molars).

### Number

Congenital abnormalities such as absence or overproduction of teeth usually occur because of problems with initiation or proliferation. These abnormalities cause problems with function, dental arch spacing, and aesthetics.

Single supernumerary teeth occur most frequently in the area of the maxillary incisors; multiple supernumerary teeth are associated with various genetic syndromes, such as cleidocranial dysostosis and Gardner's syndrome.

The congenital absence of one or more teeth is called partial anodontia. Anodontia of premolars and lateral incisors occurs frequently in the general population and appears to be genetically controlled. Anodontia can be related to generalized defects of tissue involved in tooth formation, such as ectodermal dysplasia. Patients with ectodermal dysplasia may display partial or total anodontia.

### Size

Abnormalities of tooth size, shape, or number may occur separately or together. Many supernumerary teeth have abnormal shapes or sizes. Similarly, the teeth of patients with partial anodontia may be abnormally shaped.

Microdontia, smaller than normal tooth size, may be confined to a single tooth or may be generalized. Microdontia of the maxillary laterals is a frequent form of microdontia that appears to be genetically controlled. The contralateral incisor is often congenitally missing. Generalized microdontia, although rare, is exhibited in some cases of pituitary dwarfism.

Macrodontia, larger than normal tooth size, may be localized or generalized. Patients with hemifacial hypertrophy exhibit unilateral macrodontia; persons with pituitary gigantism may have generalized macrodontia.

### Color

Color can be used to diagnose tooth anomalies (Table 33-2). Bluish-brown or opalescent teeth that exhibit extreme wear and

TABLE 33-2.   Etiology of Common Tooth Discolorations

| Color | Cause |
| --- | --- |
| **Generalized** | |
| Bluish-brown | Dentinogenesis imperfecta |
| Yellow | Amelogenesis imperfecta |
| | Tetracycline ingestion |
| Reddish-brown | Porphyria |
| | Fluorosis |
| Blue/bluish-green | Rh incompatibility |
| Brown | Tetracycline ingestion |
| Gray | Tetracycline ingestion |
| **Localized** | |
| Yellow | Trauma |
| | Chromogenic bacteria |
| Gray | Trauma |
| Black/blackish-brown | Trauma |
| | Liquid iron supplements |
| | Tobacco |
| | Tea or other foods |
| | Chromogenic bacteria |
| Pink | Internal resorption |

fractures are usually caused by an autosomal dominant defect in dentin formation called dentinogenesis imperfecta. In this condition, dentin formation continues after eruption, obliterating the dental pulp and making the tooth susceptible to fracture. This abnormality may occur concurrently with osteogenesis imperfecta; both conditions may be related to collagen disorders.

A generalized yellow color may indicate a form of amelogenesis imperfecta, in which the enamel is defective.

In addition to causing enamel hypoplasia, tetracycline administration while teeth are forming can cause a generalized or linear pattern of yellow or brown, which may subsequently change to gray as a result of oxidation by sunlight (see Fig 33-3). The severity of discoloration varies with the type of tetracycline, the dosage, and the timing of administration during tooth formation. Doxycycline appears to cause little or no discoloration; oxytetracycline causes a light yellow color; and chlortetracycline, demethychlortetracycline, and tetracycline cause stronger yellow or gray-brown discolorations.

Generalized reddish-brown teeth are associated with porphyria. Teeth with a generalized blue or bluish-green tinge are associated with Rh incompatibility, in which hemosiderin is incorporated into the dentin. Symmetric reddish-brown discoloration of teeth superimposed onto white hypocalcified or hypoplastic areas is associated with moderate to severe fluorosis. A history of greater than optimal fluoride concentration in the water supply or improper fluoride supplementation dosage is necessary to substantiate the diagnosis.

Color localized to one or two teeth usually indicates trauma (eg, yellow, gray, or black) or internal resorption (eg, pink). Green, gold, or black generalized to the gingival borders of the tooth is usually caused by accumulations of chromogenic bacteria on the teeth or staining from liquid iron supplements, coffee, tea, or chewing tobacco.

## Eruption

The time of tooth eruption is highly variable between and within populations, making it difficult to diagnose some eruption problems until they are blatant. Generalized delayed eruption is as-

sociated with hormonal abnormalities (eg, hypothyroidism, hypopituitarism) and syndromes (eg, Gardner's syndrome, Down syndrome, progeria). Delayed eruption that is more localized is associated with syndromes such as cleidocranial dysostosis.

Generalized premature eruption of teeth can be associated with hyperthyroidism and precocious puberty.

Premature exfoliation of teeth can be attributed to disorders such as acrodynia, Papillon-Lefèvre syndrome, and Ehlers-Danlos syndrome. Localized problems of eruption (ie, eruption or exfoliation) may be caused by dental caries, periodontitis, trauma, cysts, and supernumerary teeth.

If problems with eruption are identified, the patients should be referred for a dental examination.

## ORAL LESIONS AND INFECTIONS

Soft or hard tissue lesions occurring in the areas of the face, neck, or mouth (Table 33-3) may be localized or may be manifestations of systemic disease. The physician should document the history, locality, lymph node involvement, number, texture, size, color, and pain or tenderness. Associative factors such as edentulous areas, caries, other lesions, and systemic diseases should be assessed to determine the potential source as localized or systemic.

## Lesions

### Pigmented Lesions

Oral freckles frequently occur on the lips of children exposed to sunlight. These are usually considered benign unless they are seen intraorally, in which case they should be biopsied.

Multiple pigmented lesions seen in the oral cavity and on the lips, the face, and possibly the fingers suggest Peutz-Jeghers syndrome. Dominantly inherited, this syndrome is characterized by intestinal polyps, which may cause abdominal cramping. Although skin spots fade with age, oral pigmentation remains throughout life.

A blue nevus may occur at any intraoral site but is most commonly found in the anterior region. It has a characteristic blue color and is usually flat or dome shaped in children. It should be biopsied because of a tendency for malignant transformation.

Racial or ethnic pigmentation is usually generalized over the gingiva and is considered normal. There is wide variation in intensity of color.

### Vascular Lesions

The most common intraoral locations of hemangiomas or blood vessel proliferations are the lips, tongue, and buccal mucosa. If removal is indicated, cryosurgery may be the method of choice.

Oral vascular lesions are seen in various systemic disorders such as hereditary hemorrhagic telangiectasia. Telangiectasias, multiple capillary and venous dilation of the skin and mucous membranes, vary in size from pinpoint to nodular and in color from bright red to purple. Oral telangiectasias are most frequently seen on the lips and tongue, but they also occur on the palate, gingiva, buccal mucosa, and mucocutaneous junctions. Bleeding occurs from oral lesions in approximately 20% of patients.

Angiomatous lesions (eg, port wine nevi) may occur on the gingiva and buccal mucosa of patients with encephalotrigeminal angiomatosis. Petechiae may occur as a result of continual trauma, such as digit sucking or sexual abuse, or as a result of *Streptococcus* infection. Lymphangiomas can occur anywhere in the mouth. Macroglossia may result from large lymphangiomas in the tongue. Small lesions can be removed surgically; large asymptomatic lesions are usually not removed.

## TABLE 33-3.    Oral Lesions

| Pigmented Lesions | Vascular Lesions | Raised Lesions | Ulcers | Swellings |
|---|---|---|---|---|
| Oral freckles | Hemangioma | Papilloma | Aphthae | Eruption cyst |
| Peutz-Jeghers syndrome | Telangiectasia | Pyogenic granuloma | Periadenitis mucosa necrotica recurrens | Eruption hematoma |
| Blue nevus | Angiomas | Fibroma | Behçet's syndrome | Dentigerous cyst |
|  | Petecchiae |  | Trauma | Primordial cyst |
|  | Lymphangioma |  | Mucositis | Odontogenic keratocyst |
|  |  |  |  | Branchial cleft cyst |
|  |  |  |  | Thyroglossal duct cyst |
|  |  |  |  | Periapical abscess |
|  |  |  |  | Fibrosarcoma |
|  |  |  |  | Ewing's sarcoma |
|  |  |  |  | Eosinophilia granuloma |
|  |  |  |  | Fibrous dysplasia |
|  |  |  |  | Cherubism |
|  |  |  |  | Central giant cell granuloma |
|  |  |  |  | Mucocele |
|  |  |  |  | Ranula |
|  |  |  |  | Torus |

## Raised Lesions

Papillomas are benign neoplasms that are usually pedunculated and have fingerlike projections. They occur anywhere on the soft tissue of the oral cavity and range in size from a few millimeters to more than 1 cm in diameter. The treatment of choice is simple excision at the base of the lesion.

Pyogenic granulomas usually occur on the gingiva in response to an irritant (eg, calculus, minor trauma). They are especially common in pregnant women. They are usually red, elevated, and ulcerated in their early stages; later they may become fibrotic, appearing similar to fibromas. The treatment of choice is removal of the irritant, simple excision of the lesion, and good oral hygiene.

Fibromas are sessile, smooth lesions up to 1 cm in diameter. They may become ulcerated or ossified. The treatment of choice is simple surgical excision.

## Ulcers

Aphthous ulcers are painful, yellowish depressions of necrotic tissue surrounded by erythema. There are usually fewer than six lesions during an outbreak. These ulcers range in size from a few millimeters to 1 cm in diameter and occur only on buccal or labial mucosa and other unbound oral tissue. Their onset may occur in childhood, and each recurrence may last as long as 14 days. Recurrent aphthous ulcers appear to be familial. Some investigators suggest that the causative factor is *Streptococcus sanguis;* others suggest autoimmune factors, deficiencies of vitamin B$_{12}$, folate, iron, and zinc, and gluten sensitivity. Cases of aphthous ulcers in which scarring occurs are called periadenitis mucosa necrotica recurrens. These lesions may persist for as long as 6 weeks and occur so frequently that the patient is rarely free of aphthae. Treatment for aphthous ulcers usually is empiric; however, for children older than 8 years of age, a tetracycline mouth rinse (125 mg/5 mL) used four times daily produces good results and prevents secondary infection.

Patients with ulcers similar to aphthae who have skin, ocular, and genital lesions may have Behçet's syndrome, which is discussed elsewhere in this text.

Traumatic ulcers, which occur relatively frequently, are associated with a history of trauma, such as tooth brushing, or with an obvious associative factor, such as a fractured tooth. Saltwater rinses or correction of the causative factor usually is adequate treatment. Viscous benzocaine should be used with caution because of the potential for seizures in patients who use it excessively.

Oral mucositis (Fig 33-5) is one of the major oral complications of cancer treatment and can be caused by head or neck irradiation or by chemotherapy. The mucositis produced by head or neck irradiation is painful at rest and particularly when eating hard foods. Chemotherapeutic treatment of leukemia produces stomatitis more frequently than chemotherapy for solid tumors because of the higher doses of drugs and greater immunologic suppression. Interference with DNA, RNA, or protein synthesis by the drugs results in a thinning of the oral mucosa, which may ulcerate and allow life-threatening bacterial, fungal, or viral infections to occur. Because indigenous oral flora are associated

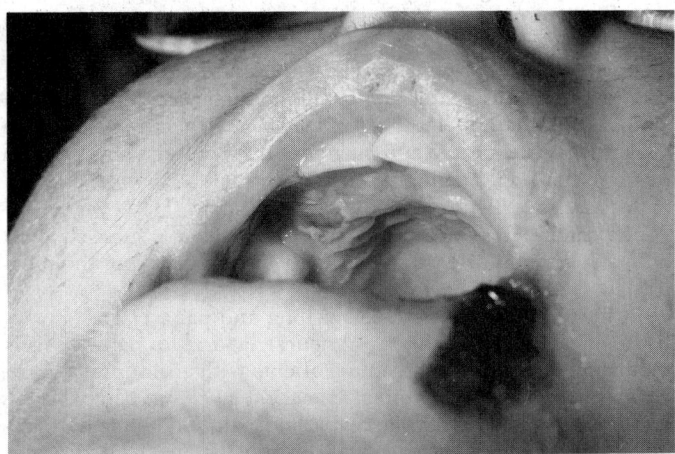

**Figure 33-5.** Extraoral lesion (*arrow*) and oral mucositis (*arrowhead*) in a patient receiving chemotherapy.

with many of these infections, it is important for cancer patients to establish and maintain good oral hygiene.

A high proportion of mucositis in immunologically suppressed patients is associated with herpes simplex virus (HSV). Diagnosis based on clinical impressions is inadequate and must be based on viral cultures or immunologic tests. Prophylactic regimens are suggested if a patient is seropositive for HSV. Mouthwashes such as chlorhexidine and allopurinol may reduce the severity of mucositis.

Before cancer treatment, all patients should have dental examinations to identify and remove or minimize potential sources of irritation and infection,. including orthodontic and prosthetic appliances and broken restorations and teeth.

## Swellings

A swelling on the gingiva of a young patient with an edentulous area where teeth are expected to erupt may be an eruption cyst. Occasionally, blood fills the cystic area, making the swelling appear bluish like a hematoma; this kind of cyst is called an eruption hematoma. Observation alone usually is the treatment of choice. However, simple incision into the crestal portion of the swelling may be necessary. This may cause bleeding, but it can be controlled easily.

The oral epithelial invaginations or ducts of epithelial processes (eg, palatine processes) are possible areas of cyst formation during fetal development. Whether all oral areas of embryonic fusion are involved in cyst formation is an unanswered question.

Hard-tissue swelling in the area of an unerupted tooth may be due to any number of cysts. For example, dentigerous cysts, which are associated with developing teeth, most commonly occur around third molars, maxillary canines, and mandibular premolars. The epithelial lining of a dentigerous cyst has a high probability of developing metaplasms and neoplasms. Alternatively, a primordial cyst may develop from a degenerated enamel organ that forms no tooth. Cyst formation in a person with the normal number of teeth suggests degeneration of a supernumerary tooth.

An odontogenic keratocyst is a particularly destructive cyst that is sometimes associated with multiple nevoid carcinoma syndrome. The peak incidence for the keratocyst alone is during the second decade of life, and the peak incidence for the syndrome is the first decade. Some patients with odontogenic keratocysts exhibit paresthesia of the mandibular teeth, gingiva, and lips.

Brachial cleft cysts may occur in the neck during late adolescence. They are usually fluctuant and unattached. The thyroglossal tract cyst forms between the foramen cecum of the tongue and the thyroid glands and is most commonly seen in young people. Its growth is usually slow and asymptomatic unless it is near the tongue.

Swelling and fever may occur with dental abscessing of teeth due to dental caries, trauma, or periodontal disease. Usually, a carious or fractured tooth is associated with this lesion. The swelling usually is rapid and may have been preceded by a parulis (ie, gum boil) on the gingiva. The teeth may be mobile, and the child may report spontaneous or elicited pain. However, many young children may not report pain. The gingiva of some children with periodontal disease may actually flap away from the roots if there is severe bone loss.

A fibrosarcoma may cause swelling and pain. Hard- or soft-tissue swelling with pain, facial neuralgia, and lip paresthesia is manifested in Ewing's sarcoma. Patients with eosinophilia granuloma, which also is manifested by oral swelling, usually have an inflamed gingiva, mobile teeth, and pain. Some of these patients may exhibit bone lesions, exophthalmos, and diabetes insipidus.

Fibrous dysplasia of the bone may occur in the jaws in monostotic form, in polyostotic form, or as a part of Albright's syndrome. The rate of expansion of a monostotic form, involving a single bone, is surprisingly rapid during the active growth phase. This form usually completes its active growth phase during childhood. The polyostotic form is associated with lesions in multiple bones. If endocrine disturbances are producing precocious growth, sexual development, and large café au lait spots, the clinician should consider the diagnosis of Albright's syndrome. Jaw lesions are hard, nonpainful, slowly enlarging masses that may interfere with tooth eruption and that usually produce facial asymmetry. Nasal obstruction and proptosis or exophthalmos may result if the lesions occur in the maxilla. Radiographically, lesions may look like ground glass.

Cherubism is a bilateral hard-tissue swelling affecting the maxilla and mandible. This fibro-osseous condition, inherited as an autosomal dominant disorder, becomes clinically apparent when the child is 2 to 4 years of age. Growth usually becomes static by 10 years of age. Tooth displacement and impaction are frequently observed.

Central giant cell granulomas occur in children. These lesions rarely involve pain, although they may aggressively expand and erode through the cortical bones of the mandible or maxilla.

Mucoceles (ie, mucous retention cysts) appear primarily on the lower lip but may occur elsewhere in the mouth. Superficial mucoceles are usually translucent and round, and deeper ones appear blue and manifest swelling, particularly if traumatized frequently. Mucoceles are generally painful and tend to recur even when ruptured. The treatment of choice is simple excision.

Ranulas are large mucoceles that occur under the tongue. They usually are unilateral, painless, and soft and may appear bluish. Continued growth of a ranula may cause respiratory distress. The treatment of choice is marsupialization. Recurrence requires excision of the lesion and the adjacent salivary gland.

Tori are benign, slowly expanding bone growths that frequently occur at the midline of the palate or along the lingual aspects of the mandible. Large growths may be traumatized during eating. They are rarely a problem in childhood.

## Infections

Oral candidiasis (ie, thrush) may appear anywhere on the soft tissue of the mouth. It ranges in appearance from mild erythema to small, white plaques to an extensively white mouth. The plaques are easily removed, leaving a raw-appearing surface. Severe ulcerative or necrotic lesions indicate invasive infection of underlying tissues and are therefore associated with a poorer prognosis than superficial lesions. Newborns can be infected during passage through the vagina of a mother with a *Candida albicans* infection, and infants can contract it from mothers with breast infections. Persons with angular cheilosis of the commissures of the mouth, which appears as a symmetric cracking of tissue, are susceptible to *Candida* infection. Immunosuppressed patients and patients on long-term, broad-spectrum antibiotics and oral contraceptives are susceptible to infection. Nystatin is used successfully in the treatment of infants. For older patients, removal of the primary problem in addition to nystatin rinses is necessary. Chlortrimazole troches are recommended.

Herpetic gingivostomatitis is a HSV infection in which the primary attack is characterized by fever, malaise, dysphagia, sialorrhea, pain, and lymphadenitis. Vesicles may occur on the lips and throughout the entire mouth. They usually rupture within 24 hours, leaving shallow yellow ulcers surrounded by erythema. Onset is usually in early childhood. Recurrent infections produce small vesicles or ulcers surrounded by erythema on tissue bound to bone (eg, attached gingiva and palate). Exfoliative cytology within 4 days of lesion formation is diagnostic. Treatment is primarily palliative and includes administration of nonacidic fluids. Prevention of dehydration is important. Lesions heal within 7 to 14 days.

Geographic tongue represents a benign reduction in the filiform papillae in patches that may migrate periodically. The cause is unknown, but psychosomatic factors have been suggested.

The effects of teething on infants remain in question. Although teething disturbances such as diarrhea, drooling, and fever have been reported, the association may not be causative. The 2-year period during which the primary teeth are erupting happens to be a period during which a child's immunologic capabilities are relatively low and infections are frequent. Hard or cold teething rings have variable effects, depending on the child. Acetaminophen liquid may help relieve an irritable child.

## DENTAL CARIES

Dental caries is exclusively a disease of the teeth. The average child between the age of 5 and 9 years has approximately three decayed, missing, or filled teeth as a result of dental caries. Approximately 60% of children in the United States between the ages of 5 and 17 years have one or more permanent teeth with dental caries. Approximately 20% of all children have eight or more permanent teeth with caries.

Caries increases with age as more permanent teeth erupt into the mouth. The rate of attack on permanent teeth appears to be the greatest during adolescence, when the posterior teeth with the most grooves and fissures erupt. In addition, the interproximal smooth surfaces of the teeth contact each other for long periods, making them more susceptible to caries.

Caries prevalence varies with geographic region in the United States and throughout the world. The northeastern and northwestern regions of the United States have the highest caries prevalence in the country; the southwestern region has the least. The incidence of caries has decreased in the United States and in various other areas of the world within the last 10 years, but it has increased in developing countries.

Dental caries results over time from a multifactorial interaction among a susceptible tooth (ie, host), microorganisms, and a cariogenic diet. A tenacious deposit of plaque, which is composed of salivary glycoproteins, bacteria, and bacterial products, forms on the teeth. Cariogenic bacteria metabolize dietary carbohydrates, particularly sucrose, and produce acids, such as lactic acid, which demineralize enamel and dentin. *Streptococcus mutans* and lactobacilli are the major bacteria in the caries process.

Frequent contacts with food, particularly food that is sticky and contains sucrose, expose teeth to prolonged drops in the pH of the plaque and potentially long demineralization times. Physical or chemical disruption of plaque, such as occurs with tooth brushing, flossing, or use of chlorhexidine rinses, minimizes the colonization of the cariogenic bacteria and the drop in plaque pH. Dental grooves and fissures, fluoride and carbonate ions, and salivary flow influence the susceptibility of teeth to dental caries.

Although caries may attack any surface of a tooth, the most susceptible surfaces appear to be those with pits or fissures in them. These areas may become carious within 6 to 12 months after eruption of the tooth. The smooth (ie, interproximal, buccal, lingual) surfaces of the teeth usually develop caries more slowly than the pits and fissures. A patient is considered to have rampant caries if the caries occurs in typically less susceptible areas, such as between the lower incisors and on the lingual surfaces of the mandibular molars. Although root caries are common in adults, developing as the periodontium recedes apically from the crown of the tooth, they may occur in children, in whom it may appear as an orange-brown softening below the bulge of the teeth. A child who exhibits root caries should be evaluated for periodontal disease or other systemic complications that allow the periodontium to recede.

The dynamic processes of demineralization and remineralization are continuously occurring on the enamel surfaces. The pellicle, or plaque, can act as a diffusion barrier to transient changes in salivary pH and to the by-products of enamel demineralization. If the rate of demineralization is slower or the same as the rate of remineralization, clinically apparent caries do not form. However, an area of remineralized by-products of demineralization may form what clinically appears to be an intact surface but microscopically is revealed to be porous. Approximately 5% of the mineral in this surface zone has been lost. As a result of the mineral loss and the changes of crystallization, the surface reflects light differently and appears to be whiter than the surrounding noncarious areas.

Internally, the white area is demineralized toward the pulp in what is described as zones. The innermost (ie, translucent) zone, which usually cannot be detected by radiography, has greater spaces between the hydroxyapatite crystals than sound enamel. External to the translucent zone is the dark zone, which can be detected by radiography. The spaces between the hydroxyapatite crystals are larger in the dark zone than in the translucent zone. However, these spaces may be narrowed by the deposition of mineral released during demineralization in the translucent zone. Between the dark zone and the surface zone is the body of the lesion, in which the area between the crystals may increase to 30% of the enamel.

Dental caries still in the white-spot stages with clinically intact surfaces can remain static or be remineralized by a decrease in the factors that contribute to demineralization or an increase in the factors that contribute to remineralization. This can be accomplished to varying degrees, depending on the extent of compliance by the patient, but it usually requires a multifactorial approach. Dental caries is best controlled through increased frequency of exposure to topical fluoride through fluoridated water, toothpastes, rinses, or gels; diet, with the emphasis on decreasing the number of sweets contacting the teeth throughout the day; and increased oral hygiene. Caries on the buccal and lingual surfaces is more easily controlled in this manner than interproximal caries or caries in the pits and fissures, because the former is detected visually at early, surface stages, when it is most accessible to fluorides and plaque removal. Caries in the pits and fissures is less accessible to such treatment and therefore not as easily controlled.

Dental caries in pits and fissures can be minimized by the placement of sealant materials that adhere to the surface of the enamel, by the creation of micropores in the enamel surface into which tags of sealant physically lock, or by chelation. These materials are most effective when introduced as soon as possible after eruption of a susceptible tooth. Sealants stop incipient caries and significantly reduce the number of vital bacteria in a groove. The effectiveness of sealants is related to their retention, which depends on patient cooperation, saliva control, and the eruptive status of the tooth.

In the case of carious lesions that have a broken surface, the tooth cannot be remineralized to the extent that the surface can be reconstructed. Although fluoride may allow remineralization of the outermost surfaces and slow demineralization processes interiorly, demineralization may continue into the pulp before it can be stopped, particularly if a cariogenic diet and poor oral hygiene are continued. Dental restoration is usually indicated to restore the surface and function of such a tooth, to prevent further deterioration of the tooth, to eliminate the foci of infection for caries or periodontal disease in the oral cavity, and to prevent loss of space within the dental arch. A child may be placed on a topical fluoride therapy to promote remineralization and inhibit demineralization throughout the mouth while dental restoration is being carried out.

Caries frequently progresses through the enamel as a wedge-shaped lesion that spreads laterally at the dentinoenamel interface when it reaches the dentin and undermines the enamel. By the time the enamel surface fractures under masticatory forces (eg, chewing on ice), the lesion is usually large and may have progressed as far as the pulp.

As caries progresses toward the pulp, inflammation may cause the pulp to form more dentin, which acts as a barrier to the carious process. However, if demineralization is taking place faster than dentin formation, caries may proceed into the pulp, causing more inflammation. The edema that occurs within the closed pulp chamber may cause dental pain.

A necrotic tooth may drain through the carious coronal tissue, causing the patient no pain. If coronal drainage is not available, necrosis may extend beyond the pulp chambers of the tooth to the root apices of the anterior primary teeth or to the furcation area between the roots of the primary molars, possibly affecting permanent tooth structure. Although the inflammation may localize around the tooth, it may cause bone expansion, which may produce pain. Fistulization through bone may occur, so that the tooth drains into the periodontal sulcus next to it or through the alveolus toward the tongue or the face. The alveolus may exhibit a fistula through the gingiva or mucosa or a parulis (ie, gum boil) that is not open to drainage. A fistula in the soft tissue usually is not associated with dental pain. The parulis can be chronic or acute, depending on the amount of drainage from it. Radiographically, the abscess may be diagnosed as a widening of the periodontal membrane or as a radiolucency in the alveolar bone at the root apices or in the furcation of the primary molars.

Cellulitis (Fig 33-6) is the most serious consequence of draining of the infection into the soft tissues. If the infection involves the submandibular, sublingual, and submental spaces, elevation of the tongue and floor of the mouth may obstruct the patient's airway. Trismus (ie, inability to open the mouth) may occur. The

child may not present with pain if the infection is in the primary dentition, even with cellulitis. High fever, malaise, and lethargy are frequently associated with acute dental infection. The patient may not eat properly as a result of pain on mastication or sensitivity to hot or cold.

If the patient exhibits pain and swelling due to a dental abscess, he or she should be referred immediately to a dentist for extraction or pulpal treatment to save the tooth. The patient should be placed on antibiotics for 7 to 10 days. The antibiotic of choice is penicillin; erythromycin is the second choice. Recalcitrant infections should be cultured for antibiotic sensitivity. Analgesics may be given for pain, but aspirin should be avoided in case tooth extraction is required.

Although numerous methods are used to detect caries for research projects and clinically, a clinician should be able to visualize white-spot lesions and cavitations on the exposed surfaces of the teeth. The clinician should keep in mind that incipient caries or even large cavitated lesions may exist on interproximal surfaces or other surfaces that cannot be seen.

Systemically compromised patients who are placed at increased risk by dental infections include those with immunosuppression, sickle cell disease, heart disease, liver disease, kidney disease, diabetes mellitus, and leukemia. Patients in whom systemic risk is increased by dental treatment include those with hemophilia, heart defects, connective tissue disorders, and osteogenesis imperfecta; in these patients, local anesthetic injections and other dental manipulations may increase the risk of bleeding or cause tissue sloughing, which may compromise airways or increase the chances of infection, scarring, or bone fracture. Dental treatment is not contraindicated in these patients, but special precautions must be taken, including antibiotic coverage, availability of plasma substitutes, and coagulation tests. Multidisciplinary cooperation is required in the treatment of such patients.

## Systemic Conditions Contributing to Dental Caries

Various systemic illnesses or conditions place children at increased risk for dental caries and, in some cases, may complicate dental treatment. A team approach to the prevention of caries and to necessary dental treatment is required for total patient care. At the time of diagnosis, a dental consultation should be obtained, with recommendations reinforced at each clinic visit.

In patients with the recessive, dystrophic form of epidermolysis bullosa, hypoplastic enamel and intraoral and circumoral bullae form at sites of pressure or trauma and result in severe and extensive scarring. The scarring can result in loss of oral vestibules, loss of mobility of the tongue, and microstomia. Tooth brushing can cause significant bullae formation, which contributes to scarring. The lack of oral hygiene, the formation of hypoplastic enamel, and these patients' soft diets probably contribute to their high caries rate. Routine dental treatment is complicated by the microstomia and by the potential for significant bullae formation as a result of oral manipulation.

Chlorhexidine and fluoride rinses are recommended. However, the chlorhexidine rinse may have to be applied with cotton-tip applicators to minimize the burning sensation about which some patients complain. Fluoride rinses that are nonflavored and contain low concentrations of alcohol are accepted better for the same reasons.

Patients with mental retardation are at increased risk for dental caries if they do not receive routine and thorough oral hygiene and a relatively noncariogenic diet. Patients who ruminate may exhibit generalized decalcification of their teeth as a result of prolonged contact with acid from the stomach. Other patients may require frequent feedings, which contribute to frequent acid exposure from plaque on their teeth. Ideally, a dental program for these patients should involve routine oral hygiene carried out

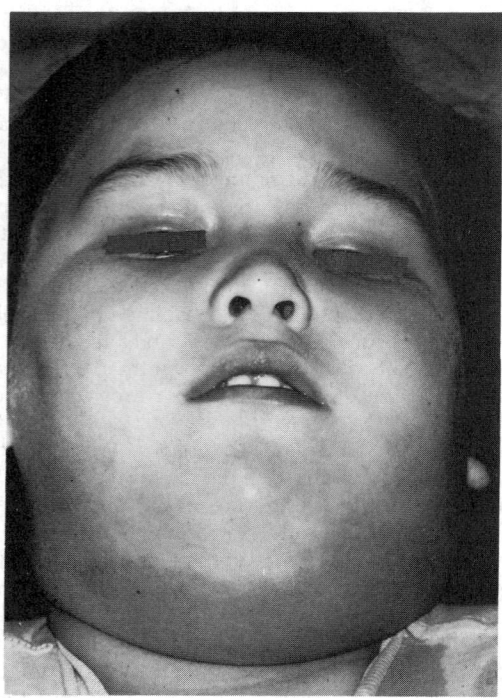

**Figure 33-6.** Cellulitis resulting from a dental abscess.

by a well-trained and motivated dental hygienist and a dental examination with preventive treatment at each routine checkup. Alternatively, the daily caregivers should be trained to provide oral hygiene care for the children. Training should include proper positioning of a child's head for access, visibility, and stability and comfort for the child and the care provider. It should include various methods of obtaining access to the mouth of an uncooperative child. Modified toothbrushes and flossing implements may be helpful for children who can handle some aspects of their oral hygiene themselves and for care providers.

In some patients with behavioral or muscle control problems, such as patients with spastic cerebral palsy or mental retardation, dental prostheses to replace extracted teeth may be contraindicated, and malocclusion may result. The key to maintaining health in these patients is the prevention of dental diseases such as caries.

Dental treatment can sometimes be accomplished only with behavioral management or sedation techniques. Physical restraints may be required to prevent patients from hurting themselves or the clinicians. General anesthesia is required for some children who have extensive dental needs, severe behavioral problems, or medical problems.

Gastrointestinal reflux and bulimia may cause decalcification of teeth due to frequent acid exposure. Repeated intake of various forms of medication, such as aspirin and antibiotics, is associated with high caries rates in some children, possibly as a result of a high sucrose content in the medication in conjunction with poor salivary clearance. Because of the dental problems seen in children who go to bed with sugary fluids in baby bottles, parents should be told not to administer oral medications with a high sugar content to a child just before bedtime unless the teeth are cleaned after ingestion.

Salivary gland dysfunction caused by head and neck irradiation, disease, or drugs may contribute significantly to the risk of caries. The buffering of acids and the oral clearance of sugar are related to salivary flow rate. Daily applications of a fluoride gel, scrupulous oral hygiene, and diet modifications to minimize the ingestion of cariogenic foods minimize the caries rate in children with this problem.

## Systemic Conditions Contributing to a Decrease in Caries

Children whose diets have been altered for systemic reasons (eg, fructose intolerance, diabetes) to exclude cariogenic foods appear to have a lower caries rate than other children their age.

## Nursing Caries

Dental caries can be particularly destructive in children older than 1 year of age who continue to nurse (Fig 33-7). Frequent contact with liquids from the bottle throughout the day and particularly during sleep, when the salivary flow rate is minimal, exposes the child to multiple and prolonged drops in salivary pH. Because the salivary flow rate is minimal during sleep, a child who nurses just before or periodically during sleep is particularly susceptible to caries. Decalcification is rapid in the newly erupting and partially mineralized primary teeth, and pulpal involvement occurs rapidly because the primary tooth enamel is relatively thin.

Continued and frequent breast-feeding is implicated as a causal factor in nursing caries. Mothers should be informed that nursing on demand past the age of 1 year can cause problems. Sweetened pacifiers are also sources of dental caries. The number of teeth and severity of caries involved in nursing caries probably depend on the eruption sequence of the primary teeth, the length of time nursing continues, the frequency of nursing throughout the day,

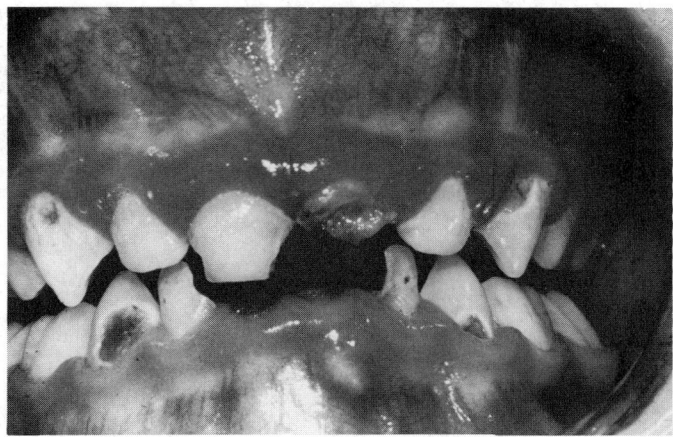

Figure 33-7.   Nursing caries.

the types of fluids given in the bottle, and whether nursing occurs just before or periodically during sleep.

Nursing caries begins as a white-spot lesion, usually on the buccal or lingual side of the tooth. The white-spot lesion is not likely to appear at the gingival border of the tooth, because primary teeth are continuously erupting. Depending on the rate of demineralization, the lesion cavitates and proceeds to the pulp. If the rate of demineralization is rapid, the root of the tooth may not develop fully before the tooth abscesses. If this occurs, the tooth usually must be extracted.

The maxillary incisors are most frequently and extensively involved, with the primary molars being the next most frequently and severely involved. The mandibular incisors are not as commonly involved, although they erupt at approximately the same time as the maxillary incisors. The position of the tongue during nursing and the saliva released from under the tongue may protect the mandibular incisors. Mandibular incisor involvement usually indicates frequent and probably continued nursing; in the case of patients who have continued to nurse until 4 years of age, the destruction can be devastating.

In particularly advanced cases, extraction of primary incisors has been necessary at 14 months of age. Early extraction of primary incisors before eruption of the canines (at approximately 18 months) may result in loss of arch space and create future orthodontic problems; extraction of primary incisors at a later age usually does not compromise arch space.

Water is the only safe fluid in a baby bottle for children past the age of 1 year. Sugar water, commercial sodas, sweetened tea, fruit juices, fruit drinks, and milk contribute to nursing caries.

If nursing caries is identified, the parent should be informed of the cause and of the potential results of lack of treatment and should be referred to a dentist who treats young children. Parents should be told to completely discontinue bottle feedings or, if necessary, to gradually dilute the contents with water until the child is taking only water in the bottle or discontinues use of the bottle completely.

A complete diet history should be obtained from the parents to determine whether the total diet is adequate. A child who is ingesting only the contents of the bottle may be malnourished. Extensive nutritional counseling may be required. Other members of the family should be involved if they provide care for the child.

Although most children with nursing caries do well with simple ambulatory dental care, some require sedation or general anesthesia, depending on the extent of disease, the extent of patient and parent cooperation, and the existence of compromising medical conditions.

Restorative procedures and tooth extraction for nursing caries are often carried out in same-day surgery units, although some patients may require overnight hospitalization because of medical problems. If the cost of same-day surgery or overnight hospital care is prohibitive for the parents, the procedures may be carried out in the dentist's office with sedation. Office extraction with sedation may be used in cases in which treatment is not extensive, the patient is amenable to ambulatory care, and parent cooperation is good.

## PERIODONTAL DISEASES

### Gingivitis

Gingivitis, the most common periodontal disease, is an inflammation of the gingival tissues usually caused by a bacterial infection. The amount of edema and the tendency for gingival bleeding increases with the severity of the gingivitis. The factor most commonly associated with gingivitis is poor oral hygiene, but other factors, such as mouth breathing, fractured or decayed teeth, and use of birth control pills, may contribute to an increasingly inflammatory response.

Bacterial colonization of the teeth and gingiva is normal. The pathogenicity of the organisms in the dental plaque is the key determinant in gingivitis. As gingivitis progresses, the bacterial population within dental plaque exhibits a characteristic shift from low to high numbers of organisms, from gram-positive cocci to rods and gram-negative anaerobes, filamentous organisms, and spirochetes. There is no conclusive evidence that gingivitis in children develops into periodontitis, a more progressive form of periodontal disease that involves loss of alveolar bone.

Calculus, which is calcified plaque, forms when plaque remains undisturbed on the teeth. This process is influenced by the ratio of calcium to phosphate in the saliva and by the pH of the saliva. Calculus can occur above or below the gingiva and is associated with varying degrees of gingivitis. Calculus is occasionally seen on the teeth of children with prepubertal periodontitis. Apparently heavy unilateral deposits of calculus may indicate that the child has pain on chewing as a result of a carious or periodontally involved tooth and therefore limits chewing to one side, allowing calculus formation on the other. Unilateral calculus deposits may indicate a unilateral salivary gland dysfunction.

Although an increased incidence of gingivitis has been associated with puberty, the relation between hormonal fluctuations and degree of gingivitis is unclear. Increased gingival metabolism of estrogen and increased prostaglandin production have been implicated in the increased severity of gingivitis during pregnancy. Gingivitis is associated with the eruption of primary and permanent teeth and appears to decrease in severity after the teeth erupt fully. Orthodontic and prosthetic appliances increase susceptibility to gingivitis as a result of the decreased accessibility for cleaning.

In most cases, a professional dental cleaning followed by good home care, including tooth brushing and flossing, decreases the incidence and severity of gingivitis. In some cases, restoration of fractured or carious teeth decreases the severity of localized inflammation.

A physician should recognize that the inflammation, bleeding, and openings through the epithelial layers around the tooth associated with gingivitis can contribute to profound systemic problems in compromised patients. In hemophiliacs who do not practice good oral hygiene, areas around the teeth may bleed spontaneously or with eating. Ulcerated gingiva is a source of bacterial infection in children who are susceptible to subacute bacterial endocarditis infection, children who are immunosuppressed, and children with uncontrolled diabetes mellitus, kidney disease, or transplanted organs. Children with leukemia who are undergoing chemotherapy are at risk for septicemia if they develop pericoronitis or periodontitis.

Fibrotic hyperplastic gingiva occurs in children receiving phenytoin (Dilantin) for seizure control. Careful titration of the dosage of Dilantin and excellent oral hygiene may control the severity of the gingival overgrowth. However, surgical removal of the overgrowth may be required in some cases.

### Mucogingival Problems

Recession of gingiva apically from the cementoenamel junction of the tooth can result in loss of support for the tooth, exposure of pulpal canals, and entrapment of bacteria in an area normally not cleaned by routine brushing. Recession can involve one or more teeth and could be the result of periodontal disease causing bone loss. Alternatively, a tooth may be abnormally positioned such that a thin layer of alveolar bone covers the root. Lack of adequate oral hygiene can cause inflammation, which destroys friable tissues covering the root, or vigorous scrubbing of the area can cause tissue destruction and root exposure.

Abnormal frenum placement can cause recession or clefting. A frenum may interfere with proper placement of a toothbrush, or muscle movement may pull the tissue from the root surface. Frenum problems may occur from the buccal or the lingual sides of the alveolus.

### Periodontitis

Periodontitis is the inflammatory destruction of the alveolar bone. Pain, abscessing, tooth loss, and loss of masticatory ability and aesthetics may result.

Juvenile periodontitis occurs around the permanent teeth of adolescents, especially the incisors and first molars. Bone loss is usually detected around or after puberty. Some children exhibit an apparent lack of dental plaque or calculus and mildness of gingivitis that masks severe bone loss. The bone loss may be localized to first permanent molars and incisors or may be generalized.

Reports are increasing of periodontitis around the primary teeth of apparently healthy children with nonsignificant medical histories or systemic findings. Little is known about this prepubertal periodontitis, but some children have a mild form of neutrophil chemotactic defect. Progression varies, with tooth exfoliation occurring close to the normal exfoliation time or so rapidly that almost all primary teeth are lost by 5 years of age. These patients have mild to severe gingivitis.

Periodontitis has been reported in children with various systemic diseases or syndromes associated with neutrophil dysfunction or neutropenia. Children with Down syndrome have greater than normal susceptibility to periodontal disease, which may be associated with impaired neutrophil function. Periodontitis has been reported in conjunction with various kinds of neutropenia. Significantly, not all patients with familial neutropenias exhibit periodontal bone loss. The differences have been attributed to various degrees of oral hygiene, suggesting that the susceptibility to periodontal disease is inherited but that bacteria may be the causative factor. Numerous bacteria are associated with juvenile periodontitis, but *Haemophilus actinomycetem comitans*, *Bacteroides gingivalis*, *B forsythus*, and spirochetes appear to be the most likely pathogenic organisms involved.

Periodontal disease and early exfoliation of primary teeth are associated with hypophosphatemia, diabetes mellitus, Papillon-Lefèvre syndrome, Chédiak-Higashi syndrome, scleroderma, leukemia, fibrous dysplasia, acrodynia, acatalasia, and histiocytosis X. Signs and symptoms of periodontitis include abnormal timing and sequencing of tooth exfoliation, recession, abnormal mobility of teeth, pain on occlusion, and gingival condition ranging from almost healthy to edematous with spontaneous bleeding.

Although there appears to be a genetic tendency toward periodontitis, the immediate causative factor seems to be dental plaque. This suggests that treatment should consist of antibiotic therapy, but bacteria that invade the gingiva are not very susceptible to antibiotics. The most successful treatment of juvenile periodontitis consists of scaling of the teeth, surgery, and tetracycline administration over a 3-week period. Although tetracycline is usually contraindicated for children younger than 8 years of age, it is the drug of choice if *Haemophilus* infection is confirmed. Little is known about effective treatment of prepubertal periodontitis; extraction of selected teeth with scaling and antibiotic coverage is suggested.

## Pericoronitis

An acute infection called pericoronitis may occur around erupting molar teeth as a result of the accumulation of bacteria under a flap of tissue called an operculum or as a result of abrasion from an opposing tooth. Pericoronitis is most commonly seen around third permanent molars but may occur around first or second permanent molars and primary molars. The tissue around the tooth becomes erythematous, edematous, and sensitive. Tissue swelling results in additional trauma from the opposing tooth. Cellulitis, fever, lymphadenopathy, pain (possibly radiating to the ear, throat, or floor of the mouth), trismus, and malaise may accompany the infection. The child may not be able to occlude properly if the swelling is extensive.

Treatment consists of irrigation under the tissue flap with a blunt-end needle and syringe and administration of antibiotics. Extraction of the opposing tooth in the case of third molars or excision of the operculum may be required. Incision and drainage are indicated in some cases.

## Acute Necrotizing Ulcerative Gingivitis

Acute necrotizing ulcerative gingivitis (ANUG) is a gingival infection caused by spirochetes. The disease is associated with stress, poor oral hygiene, and local tissue trauma. Severe bone loss and gingival recontouring may result.

The usual manifestations of ANUG are pain, a foul mouth odor, and craterlike destruction of the interdental papillae. The lesions may extend beyond the papillae and are covered by a pseudomembrane. Lymphadenopathy, fever, and malaise may occur.

Treatment consists of a professional dental cleaning and irrigation. Administration of antibiotics such as penicillin is suggested. Gingival surgery may be required after the acute phase of infection if significant tissue damage has occurred. Patients with ANUG should be checked for cyclic neutropenia.

## Hereditary Gingival Fibromatosis

Hereditary gingival fibromatosis is a nonpainful, generalized growth of firm, fibrotic gingival tissue. Onset is usually reported at the time of eruption of the primary teeth, and the condition usually ceases after all the permanent teeth have erupted. Proliferative gingival growth can cover the crowns of all the teeth, move teeth, and prevent eruption.

The cause of fibromatosis is unknown, although an autosomal dominant pattern of inheritance is seen in some cases. The condition has been reported in patients with mental retardation, epilepsy, and hypertrichosis.

The treatment of choice is surgical excision of the gingival tissue and increased oral hygiene, but recurrence is common even with meticulous hygiene. Tissue enlargement usually resolves after tooth extraction, a treatment alternative.

## TRAUMA

A child's attempts to walk initiate a traumatic period for child and parents. Falls due to lack of coordination and physical timing can result in numerous traumatic injuries to the face and oral structures. The incidence of these injuries peaks at approximately 2 to 4 years of age. Trauma to the permanent dentition tends to peak at about 8 to 10 years of age. Boys appear to be twice as prone to facial trauma as girls.

Falls, sports injuries, vehicular accidents, and physically handicapping conditions contribute to facial trauma, particularly in older children. Facial trauma is evident in approximately half of all children who are physically abused. Depending on the population, as many as 30% of 7-year-old children exhibit trauma to the primary dentition, and as many as 25% of 14-year-old adolescents exhibit trauma to the permanent dentition. Most injuries involve the anterior teeth, particularly the maxillary central incisors.

Examination of a child suffering from trauma should include several basic components: medical history; tetanus immunization history; description of cause, place, and time of accident; history of loss of consciousness; systemic conditions and symptoms; and extraoral and intraoral examinations. The priority of these components depends on factors such as acute bleeding and level of consciousness. Immediate referral to a dentist is required in almost all cases for additional evaluation and treatment. The success of treatment frequently depends on the rapidity with which it is provided.

Discussion of trauma in this chapter is limited to ambulatory patients, but the physician should realize that any child suffering from a blow to the head may have facial bone fractures, tooth injuries, and intraoral soft-tissue lacerations or contusions, all of which can contribute to blood loss, compromised airways, infection, pain, lack of healing, and future deformity. An intraoral examination should be performed as soon as possible, with the timing of dental treatment determined on an individual basis, depending on the severity of the child's condition and what other kinds of treatment are required.

Physical examination should include inspection of the ears for blood, which can indicate condylar fracture of the mandible. The nose should be checked for cerebrospinal fluid. The face, lips, and oral soft tissue should be examined for lacerations or ecchymosis. Acute bleeding should be controlled immediately. Lacerations should be gently cleansed and examined for extent of damage and presence of foreign bodies. Lacerated lips and tongues should be carefully inspected for pieces of teeth or other foreign bodies, particularly if teeth are fractured. Radiographs are required to check for foreign bodies before any suturing is done. Ecchymosis around the eye may indicate fracture of the nose or malar bone. Ecchymosis in the upper buccal vestibules may indicate fracture of the sinus, malar bone, or alveolar bone; ecchymosis in the lower buccal vestibules or floor of the mouth indicates possible mandibular fracture. The facial bones, alveoli, and jaws should be palpated for step fractures or point pain that would indicate fractures. Limitation or deviation on opening and closing of the mouth may indicate fracture of the mandible or other facial bones.

The occlusion should be examined for abnormalities, and if possible, the child's subjective evaluation of his occlusion should be elicited to determine whether alveolar fractures, jaw fractures, or tooth displacements have occurred. Parents can be asked to compare the child's occlusion before and after the trauma. Maxillary mobility should be determined as a screen for maxillary fracture. Teeth should be examined to detect fracture, mobility, displacement, gingival bleeding, pain, and loss.

Trauma may extend to more than one structure. More than one type of injury can occur as a result of one event, and injuries can be caused by a combination of numerous accidents. Although extensive classifications of trauma to the teeth and their supporting structures exist, a simplified classification is used for purposes of this discussion: crown fracture, root fracture, crown–root fracture, concussion, subluxation, displacement, avulsion, alveolar compression, and fracture of the supporting bones, including the alveolus, mandible, and maxilla.

## Crown Fracture

Crown fractures may be of various kinds and degrees of severity, as shown in Figure 33-8. Fracture of the enamel can be incomplete, such that no structure is lost but fine cracks, called crazings, are visible. Crazing alone usually requires no treatment, but if the fracture is complete but limited to the enamel only, smoothing of sharp tooth edges may be indicated as an emergency measure. Incomplete and complete enamel fractures have excellent prognoses.

Fractures extending into the dentin require immediate coverage to protect the exposed odontoblastic processes. The use of a calcium hydroxide dressing under the coverage may stimulate the pulp to produce more dentin as protection and acts as palliative treatment for the increased sensitivity to hot or cold. The prognosis is not as good as with crazings or enamel fractures; as many as 7% of teeth with dentin fractures become necrotic. If the teeth are treated within 24 hours, the prognosis is improved. The prognosis is worse as the amount of dentin exposure increases.

Fractures extending into the pulp require immediate pulpal therapy. Depending on the amount and time of pulpal exposure, a calcium hydroxide dressing and coverage should be placed on the tooth, or the pulp should be extirpated and a root canal started. Recently erupted permanent teeth with incomplete roots require additional treatment to stimulate root completion or closure before

definitive pulpal treatment. Primary teeth can be treated similar to permanent teeth. Cooperation of the patient and root length are two major factors in the decision to save primary teeth; extraction is often the treatment of choice. Lack of treatment inevitably results in necrosis, with possible abscessing and loss of the tooth. The prognosis for teeth with pulp exposure depends on the type of treatment and the amount of time elapsed before treatment.

Color is a good criterion for determining the extent of crown fracture. Enamel is relatively white, dentin is more yellow, and pulp is red. Therefore, an enamel fracture alone should be white, a fracture into dentin should exhibit yellow surrounded by white, and a fracture into the pulp should appear as red surrounded by yellow and white.

Approximately 20% to 65% of reported dental trauma is crown fracture without pulp exposure; approximately 5% to 8% is crown fracture with pulp exposure. Immediate dental referral is the treatment of choice.

## Root Fracture

Root fractures, which involve dentin, cementum, and pulp, constitute approximately 0.5% to 7% of traumatic injuries to the permanent dentition and approximately 2% to 4% of traumatic injuries to the primary dentition. Root fractures are relatively uncommon in primary or permanent incisors with incomplete root formation. They occur predominantly in the permanent maxillary central incisor area in persons between 11 and 20 years of age and in the primary dentition in those between 3 and 4 years of age.

Clinical findings include a slightly extruded tooth, frequently displaced in a lingual direction. Mobility depends on the site of the fracture. The child may express symptoms of sensitivity on occlusion. Radiographs are necessary for diagnosis. Other dental injuries (eg, alveolar fracture) frequently occur simultaneously.

Pulpal necrosis occurs in approximately 20% to 45% of teeth with root fractures. The type of dental treatment indicated depends on numerous factors. If the tooth can be retained, splinting is necessary. Dislocated permanent teeth that are not splinted are at the highest risk for necrosis. The patient should be referred to a dentist immediately.

## Crown–Root Fracture

Crown–root fractures extend from the crown into the root. The portions of the tooth may be visibly distinct, or a fragment may be missing. Depending on the direction of the fracture and soft tissue attachment, the extent of the fracture may not be visible. Crown–root fractures are reported in as many as 5% of trauma cases.

For primary teeth, extraction is usually the treatment of choice. It is possible to salvage permanent teeth if the fracture occurs less than one third of the root length from the crown.

## Concussion

The supporting structures of a tooth can be traumatized without clinically apparent mobility or displacement. The child may exhibit transient sensitivity to percussion or occlusion. The treatment of choice is relief of occlusion.

## Subluxation

Subluxation of a tooth may cause bleeding and mobility of the tooth as a result of injury to the periodontal fibers. Displacement of the tooth is not usually apparent. Approximately 15% to 20% of reported trauma cases exhibit concussion or subluxation. The treatment is similar to that for concussion.

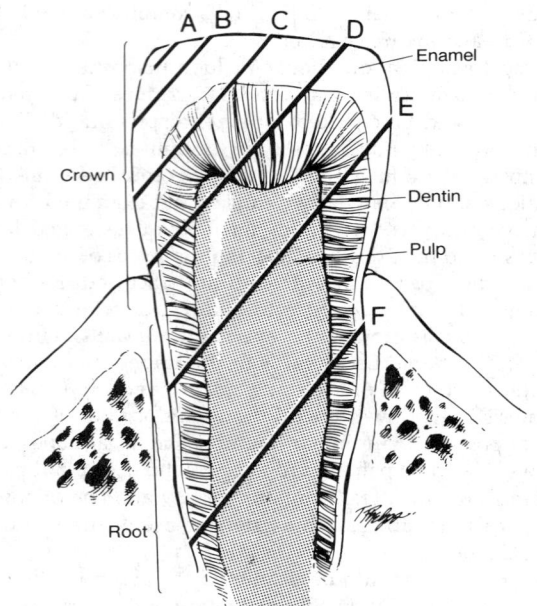

**Figure 33-8.** Diagram of various tooth fractures. **A,** crazing; **B,** enamel fracture; **C,** dentin and enamel fracture; **D,** fracture into pulp; **E,** crown-root fracture; **F,** root fracture.

## Displacement

Displacements with or without alveolar fractures include intrusive, extrusive, or lateral movement of the tooth. An injured tooth may undergo more than one movement, as may adjacent teeth.

Pulpal necrosis occurs with the highest frequency in cases of intrusion and extrusion, respectively. Obliteration of the pulp canal as a result of stimulation of dentin formation occurs in as many as 35% of displaced teeth. Pulp obliteration results in eventual pulp necrosis in 7% to 13% of these cases. External root resorption may be detected after trauma and occurs most commonly after intrusive luxation. It is not a problem unless it becomes progressive, in which case it can eventually result in loss of the tooth.

Intrusion forces the tooth apically into the alveolar bone. Clinically, the crown of the intruded tooth appears shorter than those of the adjacent teeth. Bleeding may be apparent.

Trauma to the primary teeth may cause injury to the underlying permanent teeth, which may be in various stages of development. The extent of injury to the permanent teeth may include one or all of the following: discoloration, malformation, hypomineralization, and eruption problems. The severity of each problem varies. Some of the problems may occur as an immediate result of the trauma; others may occur as a result of continued inflammation in the area of a traumatized tooth.

An intruded primary tooth may be allowed to reerupt by itself over a few months if it appears that it will cause no additional damage to the permanent tooth. A primary tooth with an exposed root should be extracted. Because inflammation occurs when primary teeth are allowed to erupt on their own, the medical history of the patient influences treatment. For example, in patients with susceptibility to subacute bacterial endocarditis or systemic immune deficiency, the affected primary teeth should probably be extracted if the prognosis is poor. If inflammation is severe when a tooth is allowed to reerupt, additional evaluation is necessary, and extraction may be indicated. Use of a relative benefits and problems list during treatment planning is recommended.

Intruded permanent teeth may require repositioning and splinting if it appears that the tooth will not erupt at all or will not erupt into an ideal position. Orthodontic repositioning of the teeth may be required if immediate ideal positioning is not possible.

An extruded tooth usually is longer than the crowns of the adjacent teeth. Treatment of extruded permanent teeth involves immediate intrusive force followed by splinting. The physician should force the tooth into the socket, have the child bite on gauze, and then immediately refer the child to a dentist. If the teeth cannot be repositioned fully into the sockets, the child should simply be referred immediately to a dentist. Local anesthesia may be required for the child to accept treatment.

Extruded primary teeth should be extracted. Injury to the permanent tooth follicles can occur if primary teeth are forced into the alveolus.

Teeth can be displaced laterally in any direction with or without alveolar bone fracture. Displaced segments of alveolar bone usually contain the teeth within them. The bone and teeth should be repositioned by application of opposite-finger pressure at the area of obvious fracture and at the incisal tips of the teeth. Splinting is required in many cases to retain the position of the fragment, and occlusal reduction may be required to avoid occlusal contacts. Occasionally, primary root tips project through the gingiva, and extraction is necessary.

## Avulsion

Avulsion is the total displacement of a tooth from its socket. The frequency of avulsion due to trauma ranges from 7% to 15% in the primary dentition and from 0.5% to 15% in the permanent dentition. The maxillary central incisors are most frequently avulsed because of their single conical tapering roots and their potential prominence.

A bleeding hole appears where a tooth should appear. However, the clinician should never assume that a tooth has been totally avulsed unless a radiograph shows no evidence of tooth structure or the child presents the entire tooth. Partial avulsion or total intrusion can occur.

In the case of avulsed permanent teeth, treatment should be instituted as soon as possible. The parent or guardian should quickly wash the tooth in saliva or saline solution and reinsert the tooth as closely as possible into the alveolus. If the tooth cannot be reimplanted by the parent or physician immediately, it could be stored in the buccal vestibule of an adult's or the child's mouth, depending on the child's age and cooperation. An alternate storage medium is saline solution. Keeping the tooth moist is of greatest concern. The child should be seen by a dentist immediately. Splinting and possibly root canal therapy is required.

The prognosis depends on the time elapsed between avulsion and treatment and the conditions under which the tooth has been stored. Root resorption is the most common complication after reimplantation. Root resorption increases in frequency from 10% when the tooth is implanted within 30 minutes of avulsion to 95% when reimplantation has not occurred within 2 hours.

Reimplantation of primary teeth is not indicated because of potential damage to the underlying permanent teeth.

## Fracture of the Supporting Bones

Discussion of treatment of fractures of the alveolus, mandible, or maxilla requires more detail than allowed in this chapter. However, the physician should be aware of the possibility of fracture of any of these structures. Fractures to these areas are infrequent, occurring most often in automobile injuries, fights, and bicycle accidents, but any fall or injury that involves a direct blow to the chin or the face can result in bony fractures.

Bruising, point tenderness, atypical occlusion, atypical mobility, percussion sounds, and step defects can be used to diagnose alveolar or jaw fractures. Radiographs must be taken that visualize these areas well. However, clinical or radiographic evidence of fracture may not be obvious at the time of the initial examination.

Alveolar fractures occur more frequently in permanent than in primary dentition, but the alveolus supporting newly erupted primary incisors without other erupted teeth is susceptible. Alveolar fractures are frequently associated with tooth dislocation.

Treatment of alveolar fractures of the permanent dentition involves reduction and splinting of the affected area with local anesthesia. Alveolar fractures of the primary dentition may not require splinting but do require a soft diet for several weeks.

The prognosis depends on the time elapsed between injury and treatment. Teeth splinted within 1 hour after alveolar fracture develop pulp necrosis less frequently than teeth splinted after longer intervals. Alveolar fractures involving permanent teeth usually heal. However, delayed complications of alveolar fractures, including pulpal necrosis, canal obliteration, root resorption, and loss of alveolar bone, are frequent. Root development of primary teeth may be arrested. Immediate and extended dental attention is required.

In the mandible, the region of the angle, the cuspid, and the neck of the condyle are the most common sites of fracture. The developing cuspid is positioned close to the mandibular border and provides a weak area for fracture to occur.

One frequent area of maxillary fracture involves separation of the palate from the body of the maxilla such that the fracture line occurs above the root apices and travels through the floor of the nose and the tuberosity. Another area of fracture involves the maxilla and frontal process and the nasal bones on both sides of the face but not the zygomatic bones, which remain intact. This fracture virtually separates the midface from the cranium. The third area involves complete separation of the entire facial skeleton from the cranial bones and passes through the sutures of the temporal and zygomatic bones, frontal and zygomatic bones, frontal bones and maxilla, and frontal and nasal bones.

Treatment of jaw fractures in children with developing teeth involves exact repositioning and usually intermaxillary fixation. The short bulbous primary dentition and the edentulous areas of mixed dentition may present problems of stabilization. Antibiotics are required if inflammation involves the fracture line. Fractures involving the follicles of developing teeth and fractures in which permanent erupted teeth are preserved require special attention to infection control. Swelling and abscess formation occur in 10% to 18% of children with developing permanent teeth. If possible, the developing or erupted permanent teeth should be preserved.

Fewer inflammatory complications of fractured jaws occur if the jaws are immobilized within 48 hours after injury than if immobilization is delayed. Delayed complications are similar to those of alveolar fractures and require dental follow-up.

## Prevention of Dental Trauma

The unexpected nature of injuries makes prevention of trauma difficult. The physician can identify high-risk children and make recommendations to minimize trauma. Dental factors such as increased overjet, flaring incisors, and insufficient lip closure contribute significantly to the risk of dental trauma. For example, children with overjets exceeding 6 mm have triple the number of traumatic dental injuries of children with normal occlusion. They should be referred to a dentist or orthodontist for orthodontic evaluation and treatment. Digit sucking, a significant contributing factor in the protrusion of anterior maxillary teeth, should be evaluated by a dentist and treated if indicated.

Sports injuries can be minimized by the use of intraoral mouth guards. In addition to protecting the teeth and soft tissue, mouth guards effectively minimize concussion, condylar fractures, and neck injuries and the complications ensuing from these injuries. Well-fitting mouth guards can be made by a dentist from a dental cast or can be mouth formed from stock guards that are purchased in a store, heated, and molded intraorally to the player. Commercial guards that are not molded to the individual player usually do not fit as well and are not as comfortable as custom-made guards. In general, custom-made guards provide better retention, comfort, speech pattern, and tear resistance than the other form of mouth guards; they are, however, more expensive than commercial guards, particularly if a child requires replacements as a result of loss or eruption of teeth. Mouth guards are mandatory in many organized football leagues. It is the responsibility of the team physician or a physician evaluating a player's fitness to recommend a mouth guard for any child participating in contact sports.

Players should be told to wear mouth guards into the shower after playing and to clean them, dry them thoroughly, and store them in a perforated tray. The guards should be rinsed with a mouthwash or antiseptic before use. Unfortunately, many sports injuries do not occur during organized sports, where the use of mouth guards can be controlled; many occur in yards, alleys, empty lots, and streets where children play informally.

Children with disorders such as epilepsy, cerebral palsy, chronic vertigo, self-mutilation, and other psychomotor conditions that contribute to loss of balance should be evaluated for protective headgear or a mouth guard to prevent orofacial trauma. Children with cerebral palsy, epilepsy, chorea, and other psychomotor disturbances who exhibit grinding of teeth may need a mouth guard to prevent severe abrasion to their teeth, but lack of patient compliance is a contraindication. Frequent reevaluation of the mouth guard may be necessary to determine its condition. The oral trauma or severe abrasion of teeth that results from grinding in some comatose and decerebrate patients can be minimized by use of mouth guards. Intraoral fixation may be required in some patients to prevent choking or removal of the guard.

The use of normal safety precautions, such as seat belts for children on child bicycle seats and car seats or safety belts in cars, minimizes injuries.

## BURNS

### Electrical Burns

Oral electrical burns occur most frequently in children between the ages of 3 and 6 years, usually when the children place the female portion of live extension or appliance cords into the mouth or bite into exposed or poorly insulated live wires. An electric arc is created when the electrolytic saliva forms a short circuit between the cord and the oral tissues.

The severity of injury ranges from superficial burns to extensive third-degree burns that may involve portions of the lips, the commissures of the mouth, the tongue, and other oral tissues. The extent of tissue destruction may not be immediately obvious, and the child may not experience pain, because nerves are frequently damaged.

The edema and drooling that may occur within a few hours usually subside within 1 week. The lesion generally consists of an erythematous band of tissue surrounding a mass of grayish or yellowish tissue. The necrotic tissue gradually forms an eschar, which is shed in 1 to 3 weeks. Although hemorrhage is not an immediate problem, it may occur from 3 days to 3 weeks after the burn, when the necrotic tissue sloughs, exposing granulation tissue, or when the weakened arterial walls rupture. As healing occurs during the next 2 to 3 months, fibrous tissue forms in the wound, causing it to become indurated. Within 6 months, the immature scar tissue that forms may cause defects ranging from minor scarring to significant unaesthetic and crippling deformations or microstomia. Potential contraction of the scar tissue is decreased within 1 year after trauma as the scar tissue softens.

Treatment depends on the severity of the burn and the physical status of the patient. The patient's tetanus immunization history should be updated if necessary. Conservative tissue debridement is suggested, and parents should be given instruction about cleansing and potential hemorrhage control. Antibiotics should be prescribed if there are signs of secondary infection. Small, superficial burns may require only observation, but extensive burns should be managed with an interdisciplinary approach. Within the first 10 days after the burn, the child should be seen by a dentist for construction of a burn appliance. Although required in some cases, surgery can be avoided or minimized by the appropriate selection, proper fit, and compliant use of a burn appliance. The purpose of the appliance is to limit scar contracture and prevent microstomia by applying pressure evenly to both commissures of the mouth. The design of the appliance depends on presence of teeth, the extent of the burn, and the extent of cooperation of the patient.

Parents should be taught to clean and replace the burn appliance after meals. Parents should be informed that the success of treatment depends on compliance with instructions. Repeat visits should be spaced frequently at the beginning of treatment (eg, 2 days, 1 week, and 3 weeks) and then once every 4 to 6 weeks for a year to determine patient compliance and to modify the appliance as necessary. At the end of 1 year, the patient should be reevaluated to determine the need for surgical intervention.

If surgical intervention is required, a burn appliance should be inserted when the sutures are removed. The appliance should be worn 24 hours a day until the clinician determines that it is no longer needed.

## Chemical Burns

Holding an aspirin over the area of a toothache to alleviate the pain is not recommended because the aspirin can cause oral chemical burns by the salicylic acid. The burn is an irregular, whitish lesion that usually approximates an abscess or carious tooth.

If a child complains of dental pain, parents should call a dentist, maintain proper oral hygiene, and administer acetaminophen systematically for pain. They should be informed of the potential tissue damage associated with improper use of aspirin. Parents should be informed that, if extraction is required, aspirin may contribute to bleeding.

## OCCLUSION

Occlusion refers to the manner in which the maxillary and mandibular teeth fit together in a typical bite and in the variety of contacts between teeth that occur during mastication, swallowing, clenching, grinding, and other normal and abnormal mandibular movements. Occlusion is affected by the relative positions of the skeletal bases, by the position of the alveolar bone on the base, and by the relative positions of the teeth within the alveolar bone.

In dentistry, every bite that differs from ideal occlusion is considered malocclusion. Malocclusion can be caused by skeletal or dental imbalance or by a combination of the two. There are various degrees of malocclusion. Some malocclusion is considered within the normal range and is compatible with good dental health and function. Between 75% and 90% of children younger than 18 years of age in the United States have some degree of malocclusion. Approximately 15% to 30% have a handicapping condition requiring orthodontic treatment.

The maxillary and mandibular teeth normally contact only during mastication and swallowing. During most of the day, they assume a rest position in which as much as 5 mm of interocclusal space exists between the two arches. However, some children clench or grind their teeth (ie, bruxism) as a result of dental or skeletal malocclusion or psychologic or physical stress for which they cannot compensate.

Malocclusion can interfere with mastication of coarse or tough foods. It may not be aesthetically appealing, an important factor that causes psychologic problems for some children. Certain types of malocclusion are associated with facial trauma.

Decisions concerning orthodontic treatment and possible surgical intervention are frequently based on evaluation of measurements of facial bony and dental landmarks on a lateral or an anteroposterior cephalogram. Numerous analyses are available to assist pediatric dentists, orthodontists, and oral surgeons in these decisions. Normal standards for several measurements may vary, depending on the patient's race.

The physician usually has no cephalograms to evaluate a child's orofacial growth or orthodontic needs. These bony landmarks are covered by soft tissue and are difficult to assess accurately. However, palpation and visual inspection allow general determinations about the need for further evaluation. The facial profile and proportions should be evaluated, because they have direct developmental and structural associations with occlusion.

## Evaluation of Occlusion

The occlusal form of each completed dental arch should be smooth, with continuous symmetry and without crowding or undesirable spacing. Lack of symmetry from the midline of the palate or mandibular arch may indicate skeletal growth discrepancy; lack of symmetry anteroposteriorly may indicate previous space loss, excessive rotation of teeth, a local skeletal growth problem, or a congenitally missing tooth.

Spacing in the primary dentition is generally ideal. The permanent teeth replacing the primary teeth are usually larger and require more space. Maxillary anterior spacing in the mixed dentition may be caused by pressure from the unerupted permanent canines on the incisor roots and may close on eruption of the canines. Crowding generally becomes worse with age, although slight crowding in the mixed dentition may be alleviated later. Spacing in the completed permanent dental arch generally does not close completely; the spacing can be caused by generalized or localized smaller tooth structure than arch space, hypodontia, supernumerary teeth, a large fibrous frenum, congenitally missing or extracted teeth, cysts, and abnormal and unbalanced forces on the dentition such as those seen with thumb sucking. In some cases, adjacent teeth drift into the spaces through rotation and tipping, contributing to malocclusion.

The dentition should be evaluated from the transverse view to determine that the cusps of the mandibular teeth occlude in the occlusal grooves of the maxillary teeth. Ideally, the maxillary teeth should extend approximately half a tooth buccally beyond the mandibular teeth. Extension of one or more of the maxillary teeth to the buccal of the mandibular teeth is called a buccal crossbite. Extension of one or more of the maxillary teeth to the lingual of the mandibular teeth is called a lingual crossbite. Crossbites can be the result of dental positioning or skeletal discrepancies in the maxilla or the mandible. Small dental or skeletal discrepancies can cause the cusps of the teeth of both arches to meet and deflect to one side, resulting in a functional crossbite. Small discrepancies are often difficult to detect and require more analysis than large discrepancies.

The midlines of the mandibular and maxillary arches should coincide with each other in occlusion and should coincide with the midline of the face. Midline discrepancies greater than 1 mm indicate skeletal or dental problems that require dental referral.

The vertical relation between the permanent front teeth (ie, overbite) is considered ideal when the maxillary incisors cover no more than 1 mm to 2 mm (approximately 20%) of the mandibular incisors. An overbite is considered deep if 50% of the mandibular incisors are covered; it is considered serious if more than 80% of the mandibular incisors are covered.

An open bite exists when the maxillary incisors do not touch the opposing incisors. The severity of the open bite can vary in the vertical height and in the number of teeth involved. Some children may have an open bite that extends to their molars. For these children mastication, such as biting through a sandwich, can be a problem.

The dentition should be evaluated from the side view to determine the relation of the posterior teeth and the anterior teeth. The lingual surfaces of the maxillary incisors should touch the labial surfaces of the mandibular incisors. The horizontal spacing between the maxillary and mandibular incisors is called overjet.

All posterior maxillary teeth should occlude with the mandibular teeth unless the patient is at a normal dental developmental stage in which primary teeth are exfoliating and permanent teeth are erupting. The lack of occlusion or the presence of vertical space may indicate a growth discrepancy in the area. Eruption proceeds at approximately 1 mm a month, and a space caused by a normal developmental process should be closed or almost closed within approximately 6 months. Occasionally, teeth are partially visible but impacted because of lack of arch space. If the physician is in doubt, the child should be referred to a dentist.

Determining the anteroposterior relation of the maxillary teeth to the mandibular teeth is difficult for the average nondental clinician. The key to screening a patient for gross malocclusion problems is that the profile frequently reflects the relation of the maxilla to the mandible. The maxilla and the mandible are the skeletal bases holding the teeth, but the teeth may not be ideally positioned on their bases, and the profile can be used to screen for gross malocclusion problems only.

A young child normally has a slightly convex facial profile that becomes straighter with growth of the mandible. If the maxilla and the mandible are in good relation to each other, the profile tends to be straight. A profile that is definitely convex indicates that the maxilla is too far forward compared with the mandible. This situation can be the result of growth problems in the maxilla only, the mandible only, or a combination of both. If the profile tends to be concave, the maxilla is not adequately forward, the mandible is too far forward, or a combination of both. Orthodontic referral is recommended for patients with convex or concave faces. Early intervention in the growth processes of the maxilla or mandible may prevent future surgical procedures to position the jaws better. However, mandibular growth can be difficult to predict. Mandibular growth can continue into adulthood, requiring surgery to correct the facial deformity and malocclusion it can cause.

## Habits

Habits such as digit sucking and lip sucking can contribute to malocclusions and, in the case of mouth breathing, to gingival inflammation. Other habits, such as bruxism and self-mutilation, cause destruction of oral tissues. However, most oral habits are little more than nuisances.

### Digit Sucking

Digit sucking, which usually begins during the first year of life or before weaning, is the most common oral habit. Although it usually diminishes in frequency with age, some adults retain the habit. There is a wide range in the reported prevalence, reaching a level as high as 86% of children between 1 and 10 years of age.

Possible explanations as to the cause of digit sucking include the rooting reflex, lack of sucking satisfaction during eating, peer modeling, and psychologic problems. Although the habit is considered normal during infancy, the older child who continues to suck may have an emotional problem. Peer pressure and highly critical parents often compound the problem.

Digit sucking is of dental and social concern, because it may detrimentally affect occlusion. Digit sucking does not always cause malocclusion, particularly in children who discontinue the habit early and have not sucked with considerable frequency and intensity. However, the habit is associated with malocclusions such as anterior open bite, flaring maxillary incisors, retruded and crowded mandibular incisors, increased overjet, posterior crossbite, anteriorly displaced maxilla, and retruded mandibles in the primary and permanent dentition. The greater the deformity, the better is the likelihood that the habit is frequent and intense.

The critical age at which digit sucking should be stopped to minimize the effect on the permanent dentition is controversial. Treatment is most often recommended at 4 or 5 years of age. However, some open bites self-correct if a child stops sucking before eruption of the maxillary permanent anterior teeth. Self-correction of the malocclusion depends on its severity, the perioral soft tissue, and the practice of other oral habits, such as tongue

thrust, mouth breathing, and lip habits. Severe oral changes require early intervention.

Digit sucking may involve the thumb or one or more fingers. A variety of positions for the digits are assumed during sucking and appear to cause varying occlusal changes. For example, a child who sucks only a digit on one side may exhibit a one-sided open bite on that side. In contrast, a two-thumb sucker usually exhibits a wide and more symmetric open bite.

Even if the clinician does not see the child sucking and the parents do not report the habit, digit sucking should be considered if an open bite or overjet is observed during oral examination. If the incisors involved in the overjet are spaced and have no lingual support from the mandibular incisors, the clinician should suspect a digit-sucking habit. Direct questioning of the child concerning the practice of digit sucking frequently results in lack of a response or an untruthful negative answer. Instead of asking directly, the hands of the child should be examined for extra clean, wrinkled, or red digits and calluses, which are diagnostic of frequent, intense sucking. The physician can then ask less threatening questions. "Are these the fingers that you suck the most?" "Do these fingers taste the best?" In the absence of signs on the hands, the examiner can ask "Which fingers do you like to suck the most?" to elicit more truthful answers.

If digit sucking is associated with an emotional problem, counseling should be encouraged. Counseling should be considered for parents or families who cannot cope with the child's habit. Negative reinforcement of the habit causes some children to become more adamant about sucking.

A simple explanation of the effects of the habit on the teeth may help some children. However, before deciding on any definitive treatment, the physician should determine the child's desire to stop. If the child is motivated, positive reinforcement programs with the parents' cooperation can be established. A reward system or a reminder such as an adhesive bandage on the digit can be used. If the habit is too deeply established to stop by positive reinforcement alone, the dentist can introduce an intraoral habit appliance to serve as a reminder. This is usually effective. Additional orthodontics may be required in some children.

If the child is not motivated to stop the habit, appliances should not be used. The child may continue to suck, embedding the appliance into the soft tissue or causing orthopedic movement of the maxilla or intrusion of abutment teeth. Alternatively, the child may cause tissue damage by removing the fixed appliance. Counseling should be suggested to determine the reason for the child's lack of motivation.

### Pacifier Sucking

Prolonged and intense sucking of a pacifier can cause malocclusions similar to those produced by digit sucking. The problems are usually minimal and tend to self-correct after the habit is discontinued.

Pacifiers are used to satisfy an infant's nonnutritive sucking needs and delay an infant's feeding time when nursing or bottle-feeding is inappropriate or inconvenient. Prevalence studies report that as many as 45% of infants use pacifiers. The habit is discontinued in most children by 3 years of age, but it should be discontinued by 1 year of age. The simplest form of treatment is to discard the pacifier so that the child cannot find it. Parents should be cautioned not to dip pacifiers in honey or other sweet liquids, a practice associated with rampant caries.

### Lip Habits

The two major lip habits involve wedging the lips between prominent upper incisors and the lower incisors and licking, sucking, or biting the lips.

Forcefully wedging the lower lip between the teeth can cause additional protrusion of the upper incisors. This is known as the mentalis habit, after the mentalis muscle, which is responsible for lifting the lower lip. Puckering of the skin over the chin occurs during this activity because the mentalis muscle inserts into the soft tissue of the chin. Because this habit is seen most frequently in patients with increased overjet, it is assumed that a malocclusion already existed before the habit was established. An intraoral appliance can be used to minimize the action, but it does not correct the malocclusion.

Licking, sucking, or biting the lips is not associated with malocclusion but may result in chapping or drying of the lips and surrounding skin. Lip balm, face cream, or other lubricating material is recommended for palliative treatment.

### Bruxism

Bruxism refers to the grinding together of the teeth. The clinical signs vary from small wear facets to extensive wear of the teeth. The abrasion appears to stimulate the odontoblasts within the pulp to form additional (sclerotic) dentin to protect the pulp. In some cases, the rate of abrasion is so great that the pulp can be seen through clear sclerotic dentin. In severe cases, the rate of abrasion exceeds the rate of dentin formation, exposing the pulp and resulting in a dental abscess. Bruxism can contribute to fracture of the teeth, muscle fatigue, and temporomandibular joint dysfunction and discomfort.

Bruxism is usually a subconscious activity and may occur during waking or sleeping periods. Parents usually report that the child "grits" his teeth together, particularly at night. Children with neurologic disorders are reported to brux with the same intensity day and night.

Bruxism has been attributed to numerous factors, including occlusal interferences, psychologic stress, iron-deficiency anemia, anal pruritus due to pinworms, and neurologic disorders. Identification of the underlying cause is the primary factor in managing bruxism. Eliminating occlusal problems by reshaping the teeth solves or minimizes some problems. Occasionally, crossbites are observed, in which case orthodontic treatment is indicated. If psychologic stress is discovered to be contributing to the bruxism, parental and child counseling and psychiatric referral may be necessary. Bite guards can provide palliative treatment when worn at night and, if necessary, during the day.

### Mouth Breathing

Mouth breathing is associated with excessive drying of the anterior gingiva with a concomitant increase in chronic gingivitis. This effect is seen in patients who cannot close their lips easily or whose normal rest position of the lips is open.

Mouth breathing is associated with a type of facial morphology characterized by a long, narrow face, a narrow nose and nasal passages, and flaccid lips. A person with this facial morphology, called adenoid facies, may exhibit a short upper lip and an apparently expressionless face. A malocclusion characterized by narrowing of the maxillary arch and palate, flaring of the incisors, and a decreased vertical overlap of the incisors is associated with adenoid facies.

The causal association between mouth breathing and adenoid facies is controversial. It would be logical to expect factors such as adenoidal hypertrophy and allergy to affect a child with narrow nasal passages more than a child with wide passages, but some children with open-mouth posture and a mouth breathing habit have no history of significant nasal obstruction. In addition, some children whose nasal obstruction is eliminated continue to mouth breathe.

Treatment consists of eliminating the malocclusion by orthodontics and stopping the habit. Evaluation by an otolaryngologist and an allergist may be necessary. If the mouth breathing continues despite a patent nasal airway, a program of positive reinforcement or the use of an oral shield over the lips may be effective.

### Tongue Thrust

Tongue thrust is an infantile pattern of swallowing in which the tongue flattens and moves forward between the anterior teeth. Approximately 97% of newborns exhibit tongue thrust. Tongue thrust decreases with age; 3% of 12-year-old children exhibit the habit.

Tongue thrust is associated with open bite, incisor protrusion, and mandibular retrusion. However, the relation is uncertain. Three fourths of children who exhibit malocclusion in the primary teeth do not develop malocclusion of the permanent teeth. The swallowing pattern appears to mature in most children by 8 or 9 years of age, the time in which the permanent incisors are completely erupted. The efficacy of intraoral appliances is documented, and such therapy is not recommended before 8 years of age. Treatment at this time is contraindicated if there is no malocclusion or speech problem.

The cause of tongue thrust is controversial. Functionally, it appears that the tongue compensates for a small jaw and large lymphoid tissue by anterior placement during swallowing. Growth of the mandible and reduction of lymphoid tissue appear to correspond with decreased thrust.

## PARENTAL COUNSELING AND REFERRAL

A physician should inform parents about the importance of good dental care to the overall health and future dentition of their children. Nursing by bottle should be stopped when the child is 12 months of age, and the child should never go to bed with a bottle filled with anything but water. A well-balanced diet containing few refined carbohydrates, particularly sticky sugars, should be emphasized. Between-meal snacks should consist of cheeses, fresh fruits and vegetables, and other nonsweet foods.

The importance of good oral hygiene should be stressed, and parents should be advised to clean their children's teeth at least once a day, preferably at night before they sleep. Tooth cleaning should be started with the eruption of the first primary tooth, when it can be accomplished with a soft gauze or cloth. A small, soft toothbrush can be used when the child is older and accepts it. Parents do not need to floss their children's teeth until tight contacts exist between adjacent teeth. The lack of fine motor skills prevents most children from learning to floss their own teeth adequately until approximately 8 to 10 years of age. Waxed and unwaxed floss are equally effective in removing plaque.

Children should be referred by 1 year of age to a dentist who is concerned about primary prevention. This is particularly important for children who have medical, physical, or mental handicaps. The focus should be on preventing dental disease. Physicians are strongly encouraged to find dentists willing to work with children.

The physician should inform parents of the importance of fluoride in controlling dental caries. Water fluoridation is the most effective and economic means of controlling caries and generally does not require patient compliance. In areas that have suboptimal fluoride concentrations in the drinking water (<0.7 ppm), fluoride supplements should be prescribed.

The current dosage schedule (see Chap. 24.1) for fluoride supplements is based on the age of the child and the fluoride concentration in the drinking water. Too great a dose of fluoride can result in dental fluorosis, a condition that may range in severity from thin, opaque areas on the teeth to large, discolored areas and hypoplasia. Fluoride supplementation should begin within a few months after birth, although a mild fluorosis may occur in low-weight children.

Prescribing fluoride supplements to breast-fed infants living in fluoridated areas requires caution. Mothers frequently supplement breast-feeding with tap water or liquids mixed with tap water and often discontinue breast-feeding earlier than they had originally expected. The infant can be exposed to higher than optimal doses of fluoride. Mothers living in an area with water fluoridation should be advised to discontinue fluoride supplements as soon as the infant is not exclusively breast-fed. Fluoride supplements ingested by a nursing mother result in little or no increase in the fluoride levels of her milk and are not recommended as a substitute for direct supplementation of the child.

The efficacy of prenatal fluoride supplementation is controversial. Clinical studies tend to support the efficacy of prenatal fluoride supplementation. However, many of these studies suffer from flaws of design and interpretation. The Food and Drug Administration does not currently approve the marketing of prenatal fluoride supplements, but physicians and dentists are not restricted from prescribing them. The reader is referred to Chan, Wyborny, and Kula (1990) for a more detailed review of fluoride metabolism and supplementation.

Children should use fluoride toothpastes that are approved by the American Dental Association. Toddlers should use no more than required to color the bristle tips of the toothbrush.

## Selected Readings

Abrams RG, Kula KS, Josell SD. Early childhood prevention programs. In: Hardin JF, ed. Clinical dentistry. Philadelphia: JB Lippincott, 1988.

American Academy of Periodontology. Perspectives on oral antimicrobial therapeutics. Chicago: KAP Graphics, 1987.

Andreasen JO. Traumatic injuries of the teeth. Philadelphia: WB Saunders, 1981.

Chan JT, Wyborny LE, Kula KS. Clinical applications of fluorides. In: Hardin JF, ed. Clinical dentistry. Philadelphia: JB Lippincott, 1990.

Josell SD, Abrams RG, eds. Pediatric oral health. Pediatr Clin North Am 1991;38;1049.

National Survey of Dental Caries in U.S. School Children: 1986–1987. Oral health of United States children: National and regional findings. NIH publication no. 89-2247. Bethesda: National Institutes of Health, 1989;379.

NIH Consensus Development Conference on Oral Complications of Cancer Therapies. Diagnosis, prevention, and treatment. USDHHS, PHS, NIH; Nat. Cancer Institute Monogr No. 9, 1990.

Proffit WR. Contemporary orthodontics. St. Louis: CV Mosby, 1986.

*Principles and Practice of Pediatrics, Second Edition.*
edited by Frank A. Oski et al. J. B. Lippincott Company, Philadelphia © 1994.

# CHAPTER 34
# *Eye Problems*

## Elias I. Traboulsi and Irene H. Maumenee

# NORMAL DEVELOPMENT OF THE EYE

Ocular and orbital structures are derived from two populations of cells: mesodermal and ectodermal. The vascular endothelium, extraocular muscles, and part of the temporal sclera are derived from mesoderm. The three types of ectodermal cells that contribute to the remaining ocular structures are neural ectoderm, neural crest cells, and surface ectoderm. Most mesenchymal tissues of the eye and orbit are derived from the neural crest.

At the end of the second week of gestation, through adjacent mesodermal induction, the ocular primordia arise from the neural plate. The optic vesicles form from neuroectoderm and approach surface ectoderm to induce the lenticular placode. At 4 weeks' gestation, the optic vesicle and lens placode invaginate, and vessels of the hyaloid system are incorporated into the globe through this formed embryonic fissure, located inferiorly in the developing globe. At the beginning of the fifth week, the embryonic fissure closes, and by the sixth week, the entire double-layered optic cup is formed. The inner neuroectodermal cell layer becomes the multilayered sensory retina, and the outer layer becomes the retinal pigment epithelium. The neuroectodermal layers induce the surrounding mesenchyme to produce the stroma of the choroid and the melanocytes of the uveal tract. The collagenous coats of the eye, the bones, and soft tissues of the orbit and the sheaths of the optic nerve are derived from the neural crest.

## Normal Milestones

Nonquantitative but clinically helpful techniques to assess visual function in children include examination of the pupillary light response, which normally indicates functioning afferent and efferent pathways. This response is usually present by 31 weeks' gestation. The blink response to light occurs by 30 weeks' gestation; in contrast, the blink response to threat is not observed until 5 months of age. Most examiners base their estimates of visual acuity and awareness in young infants on the ability to fixate and follow targets and on the absence of nystagmus and, in older infants, on the pattern of play behavior and interaction with parents. Human faces are used as visual targets by infants a few hours after birth. The mother's face is an even better target. Questioning the mother about her child's response to her face and smile is useful in assessing the child's ability to see in the absence of major neurologic and developmental impairment.

## Acuity Measurement in Infancy

Objective techniques of visual acuity assessment in infancy include optokinetic nystagmus (OKN), visual-evoked potentials (VEPs), and forced-choice preferential looking (FCPL) techniques. In the OKN technique, black and white stripes are moved in an arc across 180° of the infant's visual field. This results in a horizontal jerk nystagmus in the seeing infant, with a fast phase in the direction opposite that of the moving stripes. OKN response to a smaller stripe width reflects better visual acuity. The OKN drum is used routinely in the evaluation of children suspected of being blind.

Analysis of the latency and amplitude of VEPs elicited by variable sizes of phase-alternated checkerboards or square-wave gratings is used to determine visual acuity in infants. The level of visual acuity is directly proportional to the amplitude of the VEP and inversely proportional to the latency of the evoked response. VEPs are not affected by acoustic stimuli, movements of the observer's limbs, or some eye movements.

FCPL techniques are based on the observation that infants prefer to fixate on a pattern stimulus than on a homogeneous field. In this kind of test, the infant is presented simultaneously with a patterned stimulus consisting of black and white stripes and a gray screen of space-average luminance equal to the patterned stimulus. The observer, who sits behind a screen and is masked to the relative position of the striped or checkered stimulus and the gray screen, records the direction of the child's eyes and head as patterns with decreasing stripe widths are presented. Acuity is estimated from the smallest stripe width the child prefers over the homogeneous field. Although tedious, this is a useful behavioral technique for assessing visual acuity and diagnosing a variety of ocular diseases.

Table 34-1 summarizes estimates of normal visual acuity during the first year of life based on the three methods described. Each of these methods has its limitations and inconsistencies, but all have proved useful in the objective assessment of visual acuity in infants.

Some infants have a maturational delay in visual development in the absence of structural ocular abnormalities or nystagmus. These infants frequently have delays in motor skills as well. Normal or only slightly reduced electroretinograms differentiate these infants from those with Leber's congenital amaurosis, an autosomal recessive retinal dystrophy characterized by poor visual acuity, nystagmus, variable retinal pigmentary changes, and a markedly reduced electroretinogram.

## Acuity Measurement in Older Children

For a 2- or 3-year-old child who can recognize pictures with or without prior instruction by parents, the Allen picture cards or charts can be used to assess visual acuity. In another method, the Sheridan-Gardiner test, the child is shown geometric shapes, letters, or patterns in decreasing sizes and asked to point to identical patterns on a chart held at reading distance. For a child who is older than 3 years of age but cannot yet read letters, the E game can be used. In this game, the child is asked to point with his fingers or hand in the direction of the open end of the horizontal lines of Es of decreasing sizes on a chart or on cards. It may be necessary to teach the child to play the E game at home before the examination.

Caution must be used in interpreting visual acuity in children tested by a method involving letters. One potential problem is that the child may not know all the letters presented. Another potential problem with any of the described methods is "peeking" from the better eye by a child with uniocular decreased vision; the eye that is not being examined must be adequately occluded.

## OPHTHALMOLOGIC EXAMINATION

In consultation with the American Academy of Ophthalmology, the Committee on Practice and Ambulatory Medicine of the American Academy of Pediatrics has set up guidelines for vision screening and eye examination in children. Age-appropriate assessment for ocular problems should be performed in the newborn period and at subsequent health supervision visits. Examination by an ophthalmologist should be obtained in the nursery in infants at risk for ocular problems, such as those with retinopathy of prematurity or with a family history of congenital cataracts, retinoblastoma, or metabolic or genetic diseases. All infants should be examined by 6 months of age for fixation preference, ocular

alignment, and eye disease. Vision screening should begin by the age of 3 years.

Visual acuity can be assessed in the pediatrician's office with Allen cards or Sheridan-Gardiner cards for children 3 to 5 years of age and with Snellen acuity charts for older children who know the alphabet well. The E chart may also be used. In preverbal or retarded children, symmetry of visual acuity between the two eyes can be determined by the pattern of fixation. Vision is recorded as being central or eccentric, steady or interrupted by abnormal or involuntary movements, and maintained or preferred to one eye or the other.

The pediatrician can check ocular alignment using the cover test, the cover-uncover test, or the Hirschberg test, which determines whether the corneal light reflex is centrally and symmetrically located. The cover and cover-uncover tests are based on the finding that children with strabismus use one eye for fixation; the other eye is deviated. When the fixating eye is covered, the deviated eye moves in or out to pick up fixation. If the eye moves from the nasal side to the temporal side, it is esotropic; if it moves from the temporal side toward the nose, it is exotropic. Pupillary responses are checked with a bright light source, and the direct (ie, stimulated pupil constricts) and consensual (ie, other pupil constricts when light is shined in one eye) light reflexes are observed, as is the presence or absence of an afferent pupillary defect (ie, pupil dilates instead of constricting as light is moved from the other eye to the one with the dilating pupil).

Direct ophthalmoscopy can be used to check for the presence of cataracts. A plus-ten diopters lens is dialed into the ophthalmoscope, and examination is performed at a distance of about 1 m; cataracts appear as black shadows over a red background. Ophthalmoscopy allows examination of the disc, macula, and blood vessels in the posterior pole area. Children with strabismus or any obvious ocular problem should be immediately seen by an ophthalmologist, as should infants who are suspected to have impaired vision. Children with syndromes or diseases known to involve the eye, with a family history of early onset of ocular disease, or with developmental delay or suspicion of visual handicap should be examined immediately. Ocular handicaps need to be ruled out in the case of children with scholastic failure or learning disabilities.

To evaluate a child with an ocular problem, the ophthalmologist needs to obtain detailed pertinent ocular, developmental, and systemic histories; gestational, natal, and neonatal histories; and any family history of similar or other systemic and ocular diseases. The following examinations should be performed routinely: a test for estimated visual acuity in infants and toddlers and exact visual acuity in older children; an examination of ocular motility and determination of binocularity of vision; a good anterior segment examination, preferably using the slit lamp or biomicroscope; examination of pupillary responses; a dilated fundus inspection using the indirect ophthalmoscope; and a cycloplegic refraction test.

TABLE 34-1. Development of Visual Acuity in Infancy as Assessed by Various Techniques

| Method | Full-Term Newborn | 2 Months | 4 Months | 6 Months | 1 Year | Age at Which 20/20 Vision Is Detectable |
|---|---|---|---|---|---|---|
| OKN | 20/400 | 20/400 | 20/200 | 20/100 | 20/60 | |
| VEP | 20/100–20/200 | 20/80 | 20/80 | 20/20–20/40 | 20/20 | 6–12 mo |
| FCPL | 20/200–20/400 | | | 20/100 | 20/50 | 18–24 mo |

OKN, optokinetic nystagmus; VEP, visual-evoked potential; FCPL, forced-choice preferential looking

# CONGENITAL MALFORMATIONS

Congenital malformations may be observed at any age. The most common abnormalities and those requiring attention or screening for associated systemic abnormalities are discussed here. Children with any of these conditions should be referred to an ophthalmologist.

## Birth Trauma

Although birth trauma is not a congenital anomaly per se, it is discussed here because it is evident soon after birth. Forceps injuries to the eye are unilateral and most frequently involve the left eye, probably because the most common position of the infant's head is left occiput anterior. In these injuries, lid swelling and corneal opacification can be seen soon after birth. Characteristic vertical or oblique breaks in Descemet's membrane are observed on slit-lamp examination, in contrast to the horizontal breaks or Haab striae seen in congenital glaucoma. Myopia, astigmatism, and amblyopia may subsequently develop. More severe injuries can lead to intraocular hemorrhage or even rupture of the globe. Prolonged labor and anatomical crowding are predisposing factors.

## Adnexal Disorders

In cryptophthalmos, the upper and lower lids are completely fused, although the underlying eyeball may be completely normal. Surgical incision in the area of the palpebral fissure may open directly into the anterior segment of the eye. The cryptophthalmos syndrome includes lid fusion, hypertelorism, and cardiac and genital anomalies; it is inherited as an autosomal recessive disorder.

Upper lid colobomas (ie, full-thickness defects in lid tissue involving the lid margin) are seen in Goldenhar's syndrome, a variant of the oculoauriculovertebral sequence, in conjunction with epibulbar dermoids and preauricular skin tags. Lower lid colobomas are seen in Treacher Collins syndrome, a form of mandibulofacial dysostosis.

Distichiasis is the growth of true cilia in ectopic locations and in extra rows along the lid margin and out of the orifices of meibomian glands. The distichiasis-lymphedema syndrome is inherited in an autosomal dominant fashion.

Hypertelorism is a radiologic diagnosis that refers to an abnormally great distance between the two orbits. Telecanthus refers to an unusually long distance between the inner canthi; the ratio between the inter-inner canthal distance and the inter-outer canthal distance is normally about 1:3. Telecanthus and outer displacement of the inferior lacrimal puncti are seen in Waardenburg's syndrome, other features of which include heterochromia, deafness, and a white forelock; this syndrome is now classified with the neurocristopathies. Hypertelorism is seen in many dysmorphologic syndromes, discussed in Chapter 166.

## Anterior Segment Disorders

In microcornea, the corneal diameter is 10 mm or less. Microphthalmos may or may not be present.

In microphthalmos, the anteroposterior diameter of the eye is short (<18 mm at birth). High hyperopia or myopia is often present. Chorioretinal or iris colobomas and other eye anomalies may also exist. Microphthalmos may be unilateral, bilateral, isolated, or part of a multisystem dysmorphologic syndrome. Nanophthalmos (ie, pure microphthalmos) is an autosomal recessive disease involving high hyperopia and a predisposition to narrow-angle glaucoma and spontaneous choroidal effusion.

In megalocornea, the corneal diameter is increased to more than 12.5 mm. The intraocular pressure and endothelial cell count are normal. Megalocornea is usually X-linked recessive and may be rarely seen in Marfan syndrome. Congenital glaucoma should be ruled out in infants with enlarged corneal diameter, especially if there is no corneal clouding.

In sclerocornea, there is whitening of the cornea, with irregular arrangement of the collagen fibrils leading to loss of transparency and sclera-like appearance. Irreversible amblyopia and other ocular abnormalities usually coexist with sclerocornea.

Anterior segment dysgenesis (ie, anterior chamber cleavage syndrome) includes a gamut of developmental defects of the anterior chamber angle and iris. This syndrome is probably caused by a mesodermal defect involving the corneal endothelial cells, anterior chamber angle, and anterior iris. In the mildest form, called posterior embryotoxon, there is a prominent anteriorly displaced Schwalbe's line (ie, peripheral end of Descemet's membrane). In the Axenfeld anomaly, iris strands are attached to the anteriorly displaced Schwalbe's line. The Rieger anomaly involves hypoplasia of the anterior stroma of the iris in addition to the abnormalities already described.

Anterior segment dysgenesis is inherited in an autosomal dominant fashion. Developmental or adult open-angle glaucoma develops in 50% of these patients. The Rieger syndrome combines anterior segment dysgenesis, hypodontia, and loose umbilical skin and is inherited in an autosomal dominant fashion.

Peters' anomaly involves a central defect in Descemet's membrane, with various degrees of adhesion of the central iris and lens capsule to the central cornea. Cataracts are usually present. Combined cataract extraction and penetrating keratoplasty are required in severe cases. Most instances are sporadic, although autosomal recessive and autosomal dominant forms have been observed.

## Uveal Tract Disorders

In aniridia, a rim of rudimentary iris is always present at the iris root. The associated ocular features include cataracts, ectopia lentis, developmental glaucoma, corneal pannus, persistence of the retina over pars plana, and foveal hypoplasia leading to decreased visual acuity and nystagmus. Aniridia can be sporadic or hereditary with autosomal dominant transmission. Sporadically affected family members may have atypical iris defects and pseudopolycoria. Wilms' tumor has been associated only with sporadic aniridia, and the Wilms' tumor, aniridia, genitourinary abnormalities, and mental retardation (WAGR) syndrome has been associated with a deletion of the short arm of chromosome 11.

Ocular melanocytosis (ie, melanosis oculi) is a congenital condition involving hyperpigmentation of the uveal tract caused by increased numbers of normal melanocytes. This is a premalignant condition; uveal malignant melanoma develops in about 10% of patients. In oculodermal melanocytosis (ie, nevus of Ota), ocular melanocytosis is associated with congenital hyperpigmentation of the skin in the distribution of the trigeminal nerve. Oculodermal melanocytosis is more common in American blacks and Asians than in whites, but malignant melanoma is less frequent in these races than in whites.

Persistent strands of the pupillary membrane are a common condition resulting from failure of regression in the embryonal membrane that obliterates the pupil in utero. The strands seldom interfere with vision.

Colobomas are defects in the uveal tract caused by overlying defects in the retinal neuroectodermal layer. Various degrees of failure of the embryonic ocular fissure to close lead to the development of colobomas. Because the embryonic fissure closes inferonasally, typical colobomas are located inferiorly. The iris, ciliary body, and inferior choroid may be involved, as may the optic nerve head. Eyes with colobomas may be of normal size but are generally microphthalmic. Large colobomas may produce a white reflex from the pupil and have therefore been confused with retinoblastomas. Colobomas may be isolated, sporadic, or hereditary (most commonly autosomal irregular dominant with reduced penetrance), or they may be part of a complex malformation syndrome of known or unknown cause. Table 34-2 presents an etiologic classification of ocular colobomas.

## Vitreous Disorders

Persistence of hyaloid vessels and vascular loops at the optic disc results from incomplete regression of the hyaloid system of blood vessels. Vision is normal. Rarely, retinal vascular occlusive disease has resulted from twisted prepapillary loops.

Mittendorf's dot and Bergmeister's papilla are glial remnants of the regressed hyaloid system at the posterior lens capsule and optic disc, respectively. No patent blood vessels are found within these fibrous remnants.

Persistent hyperplastic primary vitreous (PHPV) is the most severe developmental anomaly involving the vitreous. The affected eye is microphthalmic, the ciliary processes are elongated,

---

**TABLE 34-2. Etiologic Classification of Ocular Coloboma**

**Genetic Disorders**
*Single-Gene Disorders With Isolated Coloboma*
Autosomal dominant
Autosomal recessive
Sporadic
*Single Gene Disorders With Multisystem Involvement*
Lenz microphthalmia syndrome
Goltz focal dermal hypoplasia
Basal cell nevus syndrome
CHARGE association
Meckel syndrome
Warburg syndrome
*Chromosomal Abnormalities*
Trisomy 13
Triploidy
Cat-eye syndrome (22)
4p-
11q-
13q-
18q-
18r
13r
Trisomy 18

**Teratogens**
Thalidomide
LSD

**Multisystem Disorders of Unknown Etiology**
Rubenstein-Taybi syndrome
Linear sebaceous nevus
Goldenhar syndrome
Other genetic or multisystem disorders with doubtful association with ocular coloboma

*After Pagon RA. Ocular coloboma. Surv Ophthalmol 1981;25:223.*

---

and there is some degree of anterior or posterior hyperplasia of the fibrous and glial tissue surrounding the hyaloid blood vessels. There may be an associated cataract. PHPV is a unilateral condition affecting male and female patients equally. Visual prognosis depends on the severity of the microphthalmia and the associated retinal traction and dysplasia. The younger the patient, the more likely it is that surgical intervention to remove the cataract and clear the visual pathways can improve visual potential. After a lensectomy and vitrectomy procedure, immediate aphakic correction and aggressive amblyopia therapy are necessary to produce useful vision. Surgery should be performed before 4 months of age, and parents should be informed about the guarded prognosis. Surgery prevents the later occurrence of angle-closure glaucoma, which otherwise develops in many patients with PHPV. Because it causes a white pupil, PHPV should be differentiated from retinoblastoma on the basis of clinical clues and ultrasonography or computed tomography.

## Retinal Disorders

Retinal cysts are discrete structures that have been described in various positions in the retina, including the macula. They vary in size and are usually nonprogressive.

Retinal dysplasia is a pathologic term describing abnormal, disorderly acinar, tubular, and rosette-like formations in the retina. It is a prominent feature in trisomy 13 and can be produced by intrauterine insults or infection. Retinal dysplasia can lead to the appearance of a white pupil and should therefore be differentiated from retinoblastoma.

Myelinated nerve fibers are found in about 1% of all autopsy eyes. These are present at birth, have a feathery appearance, and are usually found in the nerve fiber layer in contiguity with the optic nerve head, although they can be separate from it. Involvement can be minimal to extensive. In extensive cases a scotoma is produced. There exists a condition in which extensive myelinated nerve fibers are associated with high myopia and amblyopia.

There are several congenital vascular disorders of the retina. Retinal arteriovenous communications are large, dilated retinal vessels. Cavernous hemangiomas, composed of dilated saccular aneurysmal grapelike compartments, are associated with similar central nervous system and cutaneous hemangiomas. These vascular tumors may be inherited in a dominant fashion. Coats' disease (ie, congenital retinal telangiectasia) is discussed later in this chapter, in the section on retinoblastoma. Hippel-Lindau disease is an autosomal dominant condition characterized by retinal capillary hemangiomas; cerebellar, medullary, and spinal cord hemangioblastomas; and a variety of other cystic and neoplastic lesions throughout the body. The lesions include cysts of the pancreas, kidney, lungs, and ovaries; adenomas of the liver, epididymis, and adrenals; hypernephromas; pheochromocytomas; and familial islet cell tumors. Retinal lesions may be complicated by exudative retinopathy and retinal detachment and have been treated with various degrees of success by laser photocoagulation and cryotherapy.

## Optic Nerve Disorders

Optic nerve hypoplasia is a relatively common, nonprogressive developmental anomaly characterized by a subnormal number of axons in the affected nerve with normal mesodermal and glial supporting tissues. Subtle, segmental, and severe forms are seen. Classically, the nerve head is one half to one third of the normal size, pale to gray, and surrounded by a yellowish halo bordered on either side by a darker ring of pigment, the so-called double ring sign. The retinal vessels are frequently tortuous. Bilateral cases are more frequent than unilateral cases, with variable asymmetry. Visual acuity ranges from poor light perception to normal, and visual field defects are common. Severe bilateral cases are manifested in infancy with poor visual development and nystagmus; less severe and more subtle forms are detected only later in life.

Optic nerve hypoplasia has been reported with porencephaly, isolated cerebral atrophy, basal encephaloceles, congenital suprasellar tumors, colpocephaly, and anencephaly. Neuroradiologic abnormalities and hypopituitarism with growth retardation and hypothyroidism appear to be most common in patients with bilateral, severe involvement. Although most cases are sporadic, mother–daughter pairs have been reported. Maternal diabetes has been associated with an increased incidence of mild optic nerve hypoplasia and good visual acuity. Other rare associations include maternal viral infections and maternal ingestion of quinine and anticonvulsants. Optic nerve hypoplasia may be a common feature of the fetal alcohol syndrome. Other ocular features of the fetal alcohol syndrome are strabismus and a typical configuration of the lids with downslanting and horizontally shortened fissures.

In septo-optic dysplasia (ie, DeMorsier's syndrome), bilateral optic nerve hypoplasia is associated with lack of a septum pellucidum, partial or complete agenesis of the corpus callosum, and dysplasia of the anterior third ventricle. Hypopituitarism may be present.

The morning glory disc anomaly is a congenital malformation in which the optic nerve head is excavated, with white tissue at its center and a raised annulus of pigmentary chorioretinal change at its edge. Its appearance and the degree of dysplasia vary. Most cases are unilateral, and visual impairment varies greatly, with acuities ranging from 20/30 to light perception only. Several ocular anomalies may coexist with the disc anomaly. There have been no associated systemic abnormalities, except basal encephaloceles. Nonrhegmatogenous retinal detachment occurs in about one third of cases and is thought to be due to the accumulation of fluid from between the subarachnoid space into the subretinal space through the malformed optic papilla.

## Corneal Opacities

The five categories of disease leading to corneal opacification at birth or in the first few months of life are congenital anomalies, intrauterine and perinatal infections, birth trauma, glaucoma, and corneal dystrophies. Metabolic conditions such as the mucopolysaccharidoses and the mucolipidoses do not give rise to corneal opacification before 6 months of age. All children with corneal opacification should be referred to an ophthalmologist.

## Leukocoria

Leukocoria (ie, white pupil) is a white reflex in the normally black pupillary area. The reflex, which may be observed in certain ambient lighting conditions or only in certain directions of gaze, could theoretically result from opacification or tumefaction of any structure behind the iris (eg, lens, vitreous, retina, choroid). Table 34-3 lists conditions that may be associated with leukocoria. The exact cause of the white reflex should be determined as soon as possible so that treatment for the underlying disease can be started. Retinoblastoma, discussed elsewhere in this chapter and in Chapter 101, is a major concern for children with leukocoria.

## Retinopathy of Prematurity

Retinopathy of prematurity (ROP) is a vasoproliferative retinopathy seen in premature infants exposed to high concentrations of oxygen for prolonged periods. Two phases are seen: an acute proliferative phase and a cicatricial phase in which scarring and

### TABLE 34-3. Differential Diagnosis of a White Pupillary Reflex (Leukocoria)

**Hereditary Conditions**
Norrie disease
Congenital cataract
Coloboma
Congenital retinoschisis
Incontinentia pigmenti
Familial exudative vitreoretinopathy

**Developmental Anomalies**
Posterior hyperplastic primary vitreous
Cataract
Coloboma
Retinal dysplasia
Congenital retinal fold
Myelinated nerve fibers
Morning glory disc anomaly
Congenital corneal opacities

**Inflammatory Conditions**
Nematode endophthalmitis (toxocariasis)
Congenital toxoplasmosis
Congenital cytomegalovirus retinitis
Herpes simplex retinitis
Peripheral uveoretinitis
Metastatic endophthalmitis
Orbital cellulitis

**Tumors**
Retinoblastoma
Retinal astrocytoma
Medulloepithelioma
Glioneuroma
Choroidal hemangioma
Retinal capillary hemangioma
Combined retinal hamartoma

**Miscellaneous Conditions**
Retinal telangiectasia with exudation (Coats' disease)
Retinopathy of prematurity
Rhegmatogenous retinal detachment
Vitreous hemorrhage
Perforating ocular injuries
Battered child syndrome

*After Shields JA, Augsburger JJ. Current approaches to the diagnosis and management of retinoblastoma. Surv Ophthalmol 1981;25:347.*

tractional retinal detachment occur. More than 90% of patients with acute disease undergo spontaneous regression, and fewer than 10% of eyes develop significant cicatrization.

It is estimated that about 40,000 premature infants are born annually in the United States and that about 5% of these develop some degree of cicatricial ocular damage. Of the latter group, only 5% are totally blind or have severe permanent visual impairment. The most important risk factor in the development of ROP is low birth weight. The disease is rare in infants with a birth weight over 2000 g; it occurs in 2% to 20% of those weighing between 1000 g and 1500 g, and it occurs in 30% to 40% of those weighing less than 1000 g. Other risk factors include gestational age, duration and concentration of oxygen exposure, shift of the oxygen dissociation curve by transfused adult hemoglobin, sepsis, high light intensity, hypoxia, and hypothermia.

Retinal vessels start growing at the nerve head from hyaloid vessels at 4 months' gestation and progress centrifugally to reach the nasal retina by 8 months and the temporal retinal periphery by 9 months or shortly after birth. ROP results from incomplete vascularization and sprouting of new vessels from the demarcation line between vascularized and nonvascularized retina. The pathogenetic mechanisms of new vessel formation and the roles of the various agents implicated in ROP have not been fully elucidated; hypoxemia and hyperoxic damage to growing retinal vessels seem to be important factors. Fibrovascular proliferation results in traction on the normal retina, dragging of the macula and disc, and in partial or total retinal detachment in severe cases. In progressive ROP, the iris is involved, and dilated iris vessels can be seen on anterior segment examination.

An international committee developed a staging classification of ROP. In stage I, there is a demarcation line between vascular and avascular retina. In stage II, there is thickening of the demarcation line and formation of an intraretinal ridge. In stage III, new vessels arise from the ridge, and hemorrhages may be seen on or adjacent to the ridge. In stage IV, subtotal retinal detachment occurs posterior to the ridge, possibly involving one or more quadrants with tractional and/or exudative components; the detachment is extrafoveal in stage IV-A and involves the fovea in stage IV-B. In stage V, there is total funnel-shaped retinal detachment, the funnel taking on one of various configurations. Dilated posterior pole vessels are termed "plus disease," and the condition is associated with a greater chance of progression of disease. The various stages can be localized to one of three zones of anteroposterior involvement and quantified in clock hours of circumferential involvement.

Newborns at risk for ROP should be examined by an ophthalmologist after discontinuation of oxygen therapy and before hospital discharge. If ROP is discovered, examinations should be repeated frequently; significant changes may occur within days, and surgery may be indicated. If regression is documented, examinations may be done less frequently. The optimal time for examination is 6 to 10 weeks postpartum, when most cases are detected. Long-term complications of regressed ROP include high myopia and angle-closure glaucoma.

Treatment of ROP includes cryotherapy or laser surgery to the avascular retina to arrest progression of the disease. A large multicenter trial has documented the value of this therapy. Vitrectomy and scleral buckling are performed in stages IV and V of the disease; visual results are generally poor, with patients occasionally achieving ambulatory vision. Intravenous vitamin E supplementation is not helpful in the prevention of ROP in premature infants and may be associated with a higher than normal risk of intraventricular hemorrhage and other hemorrhagic complications of prematurity.

## COMMON EYE PROBLEMS

### Errors of Refraction

The most common cause of poor vision in childhood and adolescence is an error of refraction, the presence of which can be determined accurately by retinoscopy. Glasses should be prescribed if the resultant visual impairment is interfering with the child's activity, if the child is going to school, if the child shows symptoms of asthenopia (ie, ocular strain), or if the child has hyperopia, strabismus, anisometropia (ie, unequal error of refraction between the two eyes), or high astigmatism, which may presage bilateral sensory amblyopia.

### Visual Impairment

The pediatrician or ophthalmologist should handle the situation delicately when parents observe poor visual responsiveness in their baby; the situation is even more complex in the case of a concomitant developmental delay or associated systemic disease. On the basis of the normal visual milestones, the pediatrician can estimate what the infant should be able to see. However, before any statement is made about the infant's visual status or prognosis, a pediatric ophthalmologist should perform a thorough evaluation.

The clinical assessment includes observation of the infant's general responsiveness to the mother's face, to large and small objects, and to bright lights in the absence of auditory stimuli; recording of abnormal ocular movements; and documentation of wandering conjugate eye movements, which in blind children are usually horizontal and roving with or without tonic spasms and vertical jerky movements. Strabismus may or may not be present, and pupillary responses to a bright light stimulus may be reduced from normal levels. A careful search for organic eye disease and developmental anomalies is made, and refraction is tested. Optokinetic testing and cortical visual-evoked responses are helpful in documenting the presence of some vision. Electroretinography should be performed for children in whom blindness is strongly suspected but who have a normal ocular examination; this test determines the possibility of Leber's congenital amaurosis, in which fundus changes may be absent or minimal.

Unilateral vision loss is more difficult to detect. Affected infants or children usually present with strabismus or leukocoria, and the condition may be discovered on routine examination. Causes of unilateral blindness include retinoblastoma, various congenital abnormalities of the eye, and trauma. All efforts should be made to uncover the cause of severe visual impairment in infants and children so that appropriate therapy can be instituted early and that prognosis and genetic counseling for parents can be offered in cases of inherited diseases with ocular involvement.

Leber's congenital amaurosis is characterized by moderately to severely reduced vision before the age of 1 year, poor pupillary reaction, a tapetoretinal degeneration, and markedly reduced or extinguished results on electroretinography. In 90% of patients, the pattern of inheritance is autosomal recessive, but a few dominant cases have been described. The ophthalmoscopic appearance is variable, ranging from normal to a typical retinitis pigmentosa-like picture with bone spicule formation, attenuation of retinal vessels, and waxy optic atrophy. Associated retinal changes include a salt-and-pepper appearance, chorioretinal atrophy, macular colobomas, retinitis punctata albescens, disc edema, and a nummular pigmentary pattern with round to oval pigmented lesions. Affected eyes may develop cataracts or keratoconus when the affected person is in his teens or twenties. Congenital cataracts are rare. Infants with Leber's congenital amaurosis are usually seen in the first year of life because of poor vision, wandering eye movements, and oculodigital sign (ie, the infant rubs the blind eyes, probably in an attempt to elicit some visual images through mechanical excitation of the retina). Although ophthalmoscopic findings change with age, visual acuity remains stable except in a subgroup with macular "colobomas," in whom vision deteriorates. Associated systemic abnormalities include polycystic kidney disease, osteopetrosis, and skeletal anomalies. Neuropsychiatric disorders and mental retardation may coexist in patients with Leber's congenital amaurosis.

The electroretinogram is essential to the diagnosis of this condition. Other congenital conditions included in the differential diagnosis are achromatopsia, albinism, aniridia, congenital stationary night blindness, macular coloboma, and infectious chorioretinitis. Other syndromes with retinal findings similar to those in Leber's congenital amaurosis include Senior syndrome (ie, familial nephronophthisis and tapetoretinal degeneration), Saldino-Mainzer syndrome (ie, Senior syndrome plus cone-shaped epiphyses of the hands), Bassen-Kornzweig syndrome (ie, abetalipoproteinemia), infantile phytanic storage disease, and infantile neuronal ceroid lipofuscinosis. Peroxisomal disorders should be suspected in infants with pigmentary retinopathy, cataracts, hypotonia, and a Zellweger phenotype.

Retinitis pigmentosa is a group of hereditary diseases characterized by progressive degeneration of the retina, retinal pigment epithelium, and choroid, with resultant loss of visual field and acuity. Ophthalmoscopy characteristically shows thinning of retinal vessels, waxy pallor of the optic disc, and peripheral bone corpuscle pigmentary changes, first in the equatorial area. Choroidal sclerosis is a late feature of the disease. As the condition progresses, a peripheral scotoma appears, enlarges, and eventually reduces the visual field to a central area where acuity may be well preserved. Night blindness is a universal finding.

Diagnosis is made clinically and confirmed on electroretinography. The electroretinographic response is markedly subnormal or unrecordable, even in the absence of subjective visual symptoms. Other ocular findings include posterior subcapsular cataracts, myopia, keratoconus, and vitreous degeneration with a cellular response. About 25% of families with autosomal dominant retinitis pigmentosa have mutations in the rhodopsin gene. The Usher syndrome combines autosomal recessive retinitis pigmentosa with congenital deafness. Table 34-4 lists some conditions associated with a retinitis pigmentosa-like fundus picture and symptomatology.

Three modes of inheritance are recognized. X-linked recessive and autosomal recessive retinitis pigmentosa are more severe, start earlier, and result in earlier blindness than the autosomal dominant form. Nongenetic cases exist, confounding determination of the cause.

## Obstruction of the Lacrimal System

The majority (61%) of lacrimal drainage obstructions in children are developmental; others are caused by infections (24%), trauma (12%), and dysfunction (3%). Nasolacrimal duct (NLD) obstruction, most commonly caused by a failure of the distal membranous end of the NLD to open, occurs in 1.75% to 6.1% of infants and is bilateral in as many as one third of cases. NLD obstruction may be caused by blockage elsewhere in the lacrimal system or by a lack of some parts of the system, such as the puncti or canaliculi, interfering with the normal drainage of tears. Rarely, lacrimal obstruction is seen as part of the facial clefting syndromes and the Goldenhar syndrome.

---

**TABLE 34-4.   Syndromes and Metabolic Diseases Involving Retinal Dystrophy**

Usher syndrome
Alström syndrome
Kearns-Sayre syndrome
Bardet-Biedl syndrome
Cockayne's syndrome
Retinitis pigmentosa with nephronophthisis
Abetalipoproteinemia
Mucopolysaccharidosis I, II, III
Mucolipidosis IV
Neuronal ceroid lipofuscinosis
Cystinosis
Hyperornithinemia with gyrate atrophy of the choroid and retina
Methylmalonic aciduria with homocystinuria
Myotonic dystrophy
Olivopontocerebellar atrophy with macular degeneration
Sjögren-Larsson syndrome
Alagille syndrome

---

Infants with lacrimal obstruction present with a "wet-eyed" appearance, persistent or intermittent tearing, and various degrees of mucopurulent discharge over the medial canthal area and lids. Pressure over the lacrimal sac area expresses whitish material from the lacrimal puncti. Superimposed dacryocystitis may exist, and dacryocystoceles or fistulas may develop.

Most obstructions (90%) resolve spontaneously by 18 months of age, and lid hygiene alone is the indicated treatment in most cases. Fingertip or cotton-tip applicator massage over the lacrimal sac area, with massage directed inferiorly while the upper end of the lacrimal system is blocked, may be tried for a short period; this results in increased pressure inside the system, possibly causing the distal membrane to rupture into the nose. Chronic antibiotic therapy should be avoided. Some pediatric ophthalmologists prefer early probing after a short trial of conservative management for 2 to 4 weeks; this results in early patency of the system and avoids potential infections and continuous cosmetic annoyance. For young infants, probing can be performed in the office with topical anesthesia and restraint; older children are probed in the operating room under general anesthesia. Probing is successful in 90% of patients. If it fails, it may be repeated with or without silicone intubation of the lacrimal system; silicone stents are left in place for 3 to 6 months. If probing and silicone intubation fail, a dacryocystorhinostomy is performed. This provides direct drainage of tears from the lacrimal sac into the nose. Complex microsurgical procedures are performed for agenesis of the lacrimal puncti or canaliculi, lacrimal fistulas, and strictures of the lacrimal system. Dacryocystitis should be treated with systemic antibiotics and may resolve only after nasolacrimal probing.

## Infections

### Congenital Infections

The growing fetus acquires toxoplasmosis transplacentally in the third trimester of gestation from the often clinically healthy mother. At birth, affected infants have hydrocephalus, although intracranial calcifications may not yet be seen. Prematurity, low birth weight, microcephaly, and failure to thrive are frequent. The typical ocular lesions are large, healed chorioretinal scars with pigmented borders, usually in the macular area. Lesions may be unilateral or bilateral. Occasionally, a newborn exhibits active lesions; areas of active retinitis have a whitish, fluffy appearance and are associated with vitreous inflammatory cells. Strabismus and nystagmus may develop later. The diagnosis is made on clinical grounds and is confirmed serologically through complement fixation, indirect hemagglutination, and fluorescent-tagged antibody determinations.

Toxoplasma retinitis in older children, mostly around puberty, is usually due to reactivation of dormant disease at the edges of old congenital scarring. There is growing evidence that primary infection from the ingestion of organisms in raw meat can lead to retinitis. The condition may be associated with various degrees of vitreous and anterior segment inflammation.

Small peripheral lesions without vitreous inflammation can be observed. Larger lesions warrant antimicrobial therapy; sulfadiazine, pyrimethamine, clindamycin, and tetracycline have been used in various combinations. There is no strong evidence that antimicrobial therapy decreases the incidence of recurrences. Topical corticosteroids and cycloplegics should be given if ocular inflammation is mild. Severe inflammation and lesions impinging on the macula and optic nerve should be treated with systemic corticosteroids to minimize the damaging effects of necrotizing inflammation.

One of the main features of rubella embryopathy is the accompanying ophthalmopathy. Cataracts develop in more than half of patients with ocular rubella and are most likely to follow maternal infection between the second and eleventh weeks of gestation. The cataracts have a distinctive appearance, with a dense central opacity surrounded by a rim of more normal, although liquefied, cortex and a normal capsule. The lens may be swollen, and a total cataract may develop. Live virus in the lens may complicate surgical management, in which the lens has to be totally aspirated and preoperative steroids administered to minimize postoperative inflammation.

Because of associated ocular abnormalities, the visual outcome of cataract surgery in congenital rubella remains grim, despite early intervention and aggressive occlusion therapy. Corneal edema may exist at birth, and keratoconus and corneal decompensation may develop later. The developing iris and ciliary body may be affected by the viral infection, and iris atrophy, lack of a dilator muscle, and focal necrosis of the iris pigment epithelium may develop. The anterior chamber angle may fail to develop adequately, possibly causing cleavage abnormalities.

Rubella retinopathy, which gives the fundus a salt-and-pepper appearance, is most obvious in the posterior pole. The abnormal pigmentation is due to irregularities in distribution, hypoplasia, and hyperplasia of the retinal pigment epithelium. The retinopathy is progressive, and although vision is usually unaffected, visual acuities of 20/60 and less have been observed in the absence of cataracts or glaucoma. Ten percent of infants with congenital rubella have congenital glaucoma, which develops early in embryonic life and is therefore associated with a poor visual prognosis. Corneal clouding due to glaucoma should be differentiated from corneal clouding due to corneal involvement by the virus. Microphthalmos or microcornea may occur because of interference of the virus with normal ocular development. Oculomotor disorders such as strabismus, nystagmus, and ocular torticollis occur in 20% of children with congenital rubella syndrome. Strabismus is most often due to underlying amblyogenic factors such as cataracts, glaucoma, cortical blindness, optic atrophy, and high refractive errors.

Most cytomegalovirus infections at birth are clinically insignificant. Symptomatic babies are usually quite ill with hepatosplenomegaly, jaundice, petechiae, microcephaly, intracranial calcification, optic atrophy, and retinitis. Mortality is high. Long-term effects of congenital infection are deafness and slow development. The typical ocular feature is a retinitis similar to that seen in adults, with hemorrhages and exudates usually along blood vessels. Ocular disease is seen in 20% of symptomatic newborns who have other affected organs and occurs only if the infection is intrauterine. Associated ocular abnormalities include anophthalmia, optic nerve hypoplasia and colobomas, Peters' anomaly, and iridocyclitis. Cytomegalovirus retinitis has been observed in infants with acquired immunodeficiency syndrome and may lead to blindness if the macula is involved.

Congenital syphilis is rare in developed countries because of the widespread use of antibiotics, screening for the disease before marriage, and maternal screening at the onset of pregnancy. Infants with congenital syphilis have fever, skin rash, pneumonitis, and hepatosplenomegaly. Active choroiditis may be seen, but most affected babies have only peripheral pigmentary changes. Active keratitis is rare.

Neonatal herpes simplex virus (HSV) ocular infection is transmitted to the newborn in the mother's infected birth canal during delivery or shortly before though ruptured membranes. Twenty percent of neonates with HSV infection have ocular involvement, which can take the form, in order of decreasing frequency, of conjunctivitis keratitis, retinitis, cataracts, and microphthalmia. Most cases are associated with cutaneous herpetic vesicles. Neonatal HSV conjunctivitis and keratitis are seen in the first 2 weeks and must be differentiated from other causes of ophthalmia neonatorum. Cataracts associated with neonatal HSV infection may be unilateral or bilateral and develop secondary to uveitis or to direct viral invasion of the lens. Retinitis is usually diagnosed between 3 weeks and 3 months of age but may be seen earlier. Retinal findings range in severity from small peripheral chorioretinal scars to blinding necrotizing retinitis. Active retinitis is marked by patches of yellow-white intraretinal exudates, intraretinal hemorrhages, vascular sheathing, vitritis, and anterior chamber pleocytosis. Retinal detachment may occur in severe cases. Other causes of infantile retinitis include cytomegalovirus, syphilis, rubella, *Toxoplasma* infection, *Candida* infection, tuberculosis, and histoplasmosis.

## Ophthalmia Neonatorum

Conjunctivitis is the most common ocular disease of newborns, occurring in 1.6% to 12% of neonates. The cause and incidence of neonatal conjunctivitis have been altered by the routine use of silver nitrate prophylaxis. This treatment is effective in preventing gonococcal conjunctivitis, but it has no effect on *Chlamydia trachomatis*. The 1980s were marked by a dramatic increase in the prevalence of chlamydial neonatal conjunctivitis due to maternal genital chlamydial disease. The use of 1% tetracycline ointment and of erythromycin ointment, instead of silver nitrate drops, has reduced the incidence of gonococcal and chlamydial ophthalmia neonatorum.

Direct immunofluorescent monoclonal antibody staining has proved useful in the diagnosis of neonatal chlamydial conjunctivitis. Of 100 neonates with conjunctivitis in one study, 43 were found to have chlamydial disease; rates as high as 73% have been reported. Other causal agents in ophthalmia neonatorum include *Staphylococcus aureus*, *Haemophilus influenzae*, *Streptococcus pneumoniae*, *Escherichia coli*, *Proteus mirabilis*, *Klebsiella pneumoniae*, *Branhamella catarrhalis*, *Neisseria gonorrhoeae*, *Pseudomonas aeruginosa*, *Staphylococcus epidermidis*, *Streptococcus viridans*, and coxsackievirus A9.

The external appearance of the eye is the same regardless of the causal agent; in addition to swelling of the lids and conjunctiva, there is profuse and sometimes bloody discharge, especially if pseudomembranes are formed. The timing of the infection in relation to birth is helpful, although not diagnostic, in the determination of the causal agent. Chemical and mechanical conjunctivitis occur in the first day of life and are due to birth trauma and manipulation or to silver nitrate prophylaxis itself. Gonococcal conjunctivitis, which is acquired in the birth canal, usually manifests between days 2 and 4. The remaining organisms cause conjunctivitis at various times after birth. *Pseudomonas* conjunctivitis is particularly aggressive and may be complicated by corneal ulceration and blindness; it is acquired in the hospital and should be suspected in infants on mechanical ventilation with other foci of *Pseudomonas* infection. Treatment consists of frequent instillations of fortified topical aminoglycoside eye drops and systemic aminoglycosides if other foci of infection are present. Gonococcal conjunctivitis and chlamydial conjunctivitis require systemic and topical antibiotic therapy.

An infant suspected of having conjunctivitis should be immediately isolated. If the infant is in the nursery, strict handwashing precautions should be observed. If the mother is found to be free of gonorrhea, the nursery staff should be checked for the disease, which may be transmitted through the hands. Conjunctival scrapings for Gram and Giemsa stains and for a direct immunofluorescent monoclonal antibody stain for *Chlamydia* should be obtained. Aerobic, anaerobic, and chlamydial cultures should all be done. Therapy should be started based on staining, with definitive culture pending. Patients suspected of having chlamydial disease should be given oral erythromycin ethylsuccinate (50 mg/kg/day in four divided doses) for 2 weeks. If erythromycin fails to clear chlamydial conjunctivitis, a 2-week course of oral trimethoprim-sulfmethoxazole and a concurrent 1-week course of topical tetracycline usually result in clearing of infection.

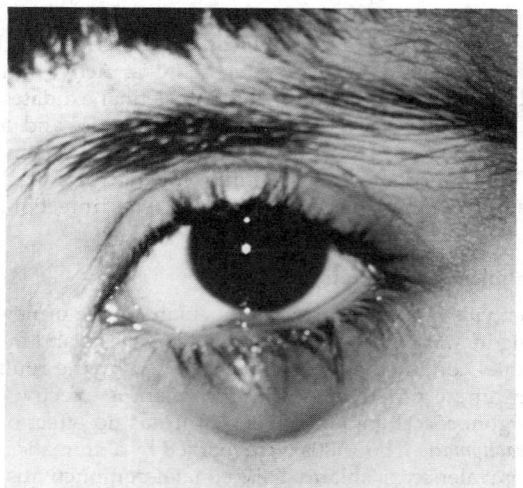

**Figure 34-1.** An unusually large chalazion of the lower lid. Chalazia are usually much smaller than hordeola and can be detected by palpation.

secrete the mucinous component of the tear film. It is characterized by localized swelling, redness, and pain near the lid margin. The inflammatory process leads to the formation of a small abscess that points and ruptures to the outside within a few days. Treatment consists of the frequent application of warm water compresses and the application of antibiotic ointment three to four times per day.

Granulomatous inflammation of the meibomian glands leads to the formation of chalazia, which appear as small bumps within the lid tissues over the tarsal plates (Fig 34-1). Treatment consisting of warm compresses and antibiotic–steroid ointment should be tried for 2 to 4 weeks. If the chalazion fails to resolve and is cosmetically blemishing, it can be excised through a conjunctival approach. Intralesional Celestone injections have been tried with some success.

## Conjunctivitis

Three major categories of conjunctivitis are recognized: infectious, allergic, and traumatic or chemical. Ocular conditions that should be differentiated from simple conjunctivitis include iritis (ie, inflammation of the iris, a form of anterior uveitis), acute glaucoma, traumatic corneal abrasions, and infectious corneal ulceration. Table 34-5 lists the differentiating features of these various conditions.

In bacterial conjunctivitis, conjunctival hyperemia is marked, and there is a moderate to copious purulent discharge. The patient is usually in pain and feels as if there is a foreign body in the eye. Vision, pupillary reflexes, intraocular pressure, and corneal clarity are all normal. Staphylococcal blepharitis (ie, chronic infection or inflammation at the lid margins) is a common associated finding. Cultures may be obtained, and bilateral antibiotic eye drops or ointment should be started. Ten percent sulfacetamide or erythromycin is a good initial choice; it may be changed later, depending on culture and antimicrobial sensitivity results. Antibiotics may prevent recurrences and shorten the course of the disease somewhat, but bacterial conjunctivitis usually improves within 4 to 5 days irrespective of treatment.

Viral conjunctivitis may involve a mild purulent discharge, but tearing and lid swelling, with or without preauricular lymphadenopathy, are the prominent features. Photophobia and blepharospasm (ie, squeezing of the lids, usually in response to light) occur if the cornea is involved. Adenoviruses are common causal agents. Primary herpetic conjunctivitis is not easily rec-

If gonococcal conjunctivitis is suspected, the infant is admitted to the hospital and started on intravenous aqueous penicillin G potassium (50,000 U/kg/day; [20,000 units/kg/day if the infant is premature] in four divided doses) and saline lavage of the eyes. Parents and their sexual partners should be treated for chlamydial and gonococcal infection in the usual manner. Gram-negative bacilli indicate treatment with gentamycin sulfate ophthalmic ointment, using one application four times per day for 1 week. If gram-positive cocci or inflammatory cells without organisms are found, erythromycin ophthalmic ointment should be given four times per day for 1 week.

Bacteria may be cultured from the conjunctivae of infants with chlamydial conjunctivitis. The child with recurrent conjunctivitis should be suspected of having nasolacrimal duct obstruction, and patency of the lacrimal system should be tested. The management of obstruction of the lacrimal system is discussed earlier in this chapter.

### Hordeolum and Chalazion

A hordeolum results from acute infection of the meibomian glands, which are located in the tarsal plates in the lid and which

| Finding | Acute Conjunctivitis | Allergy | Iritis | Acute Glaucoma | Corneal Abrasion/Ulcer |
|---|---|---|---|---|---|
| Pain | Mild | None | Moderate | Moderate | Severe |
| Tearing | Mild to moderate | Moderate | Moderate | None | Severe |
| Discharge | Moderate to copious | Moderate | None | None | Watery/purulent |
| Incidence | Very common | Very common | Uncommon | Uncommon | Common/uncommon |
| Vision | Normal | Normal | Mildly decreased | Decreased | Decreased |
| Injection | Diffuse | Diffuse | Perilimbal | Perilimbal | Diffuse |
| Cornea | Clear | Clear | Clear | Clear to cloudy | Clear/hazy |
| Intraocular pressure | Normal | Normal | Normal | Increased | Normal |
| Pupil size | Normal | Normal | Small | Mid-dilated | Normal |
| Pupillary reaction | Normal | Normal | Poor | Very poor | Normal |
| Culture | Causative organism | Normal | Normal | Normal | Normal/causative agent |

TABLE 34-5.   Differential Diagnosis of Conjunctivitis

*Modified from DeAngelis C. The eye. In: DeAngelis C, ed. Pediatric primary care, ed. 3. Boston: Little, Brown, 1984:221.*

ognized unless it is accompanied by herpetic lesions on the lids. Treatment of viral conjunctivitis (except for herpes simplex type 1) is nonspecific; mild steroid drops may be given if inflammation and swelling are severe.

The hallmark of allergic conjunctivitis is itching. There is usually a stringy mucoid discharge. Allergic conjunctivitis may be seasonal, associated with hay fever, and the patient frequently has a history of allergic disorders. Mild vasoconstricting, decongestant drops are usually sufficient to improve symptoms in mild cases; mild steroid drops may be necessary in more severe cases. In vernal conjunctivitis, a seasonal, rather severe allergic ocular condition characterized by large palpebral conjunctival papillae and perilimbal infiltrates, 4% cromolyn sodium drops have decreased recurrence rates and shortened the course of the disease if administered frequently and prophylactically.

The classic example of a chemical conjunctivitis is that induced by silver nitrate prophylaxis (ie, Crede procedure) in newborns. Any chemical that reaches the ocular surface is potentially toxic; the most serious of the chemical conjunctivitides are those caused by alkali. Many common household detergents are strong alkali that can cause serious ocular injuries if they come in contact with the eye. An ophthalmologist should be immediately consulted in case of suspected ocular alkali burns. Pending the ophthalmologist's arrival, topical anesthetic drops should be instilled and the eye copiously irrigated for as long as possible with at least 2 L of normal saline solution or until a litmus paper test reveals a normal pH. Any debris or foreign bodies should be washed out of the conjunctival fornices. Because the bulk of the ocular damage occurs within the first few minutes of exposure, irrigation should be done immediately. The ophthalmologist treats the patient for the ocular surface, cornea, and lid problems that follow these potentially severe injuries.

## Periorbital and Orbital Cellulitis

Periorbital cellulitis and orbital cellulitis are bacterial infections of the eyelids and orbital area. In preseptal or periorbital cellulitis, the infection remains anterior to the orbital septum, a fibrous structure located in the lids that separates the orbit proper from the subcutaneous lid structures. In orbital cellulitis, the infection involves the orbit proper and may affect all orbital structures, including extraocular muscles, sensory and motor nerves, and the optic nerve. The two types may coexist, and one may lead to the other.

Bacterial organisms may gain access through the lid skin secondary to insect bites, pustules, or trauma; they may gain access through adjacent infected paranasal sinuses, upper respiratory tract, or teeth. *Staphylococcus aureus* is the most common cause of disease acquired through the lids; other causal organisms are *Streptococcus pyogenes*, *Peptostreptococcus*, *Bacteroides*, and others. *Haemophilus influenzae*, which gains access to the orbit from upper respiratory tract infections, bacteremia, or sinusitis, is a leading cause of periorbital and orbital cellulitis in children. Children younger than 5 years of age are immunologically most susceptible to *H influenzae*, especially to the b serotype. Fungal orbital cellulitis (ie, phycomycosis, aspergillosis) is rare, usually occurring only in immunocompromised or ketoacidotic persons; the orbit is involved through extension of the disease from infected paranasal sinuses.

Proptosis and limitation of ocular motility differentiate preseptal from orbital cellulitis. Fever, lid swelling, redness, and hotness occur in orbital and periorbital infections. Computed tomography is helpful in documenting orbital involvement and delineating orbital and subperiosteal abscesses, and it is used to exclude the diagnosis of rhabdomyosarcoma.

Complications of orbital cellulitis include orbital abscess, subperiosteal abscess, cavernous sinus thrombosis, meningitis, brain abscess, and orbital apex syndrome.

Orbital cellulitis is a medical emergency, and early diagnosis and treatment are imperative. Children with this condition should be admitted, and a complete blood count and cultures of any skin lesion around the eye or nasopharynx, blood, cerebrospinal fluid, and subcutaneous aspirate should be obtained. Urine antigen studies for a variety of bacterial organisms may be helpful. Sinus x-ray films and computed tomographic films of the orbits should be obtained. An ophthalmologist should be consulted.

Periorbital cellulitis is treated with intravenous antibiotics until the periorbital induration and redness decrease. Oral antibiotics are then substituted for intravenous therapy for an additional 7 to 10 days. If a skin infection is documented in the etiology of the condition, a penicillinase-resistant penicillin (eg, methicillin, cloxacillin) should be administered. With the emergence of $\beta$-lactamase-producing strains of *H influenzae*, cephalosporins have become the mainstay of treatment. Cefuroxime (100 to 150 mg/kg/day in three divided doses) is preferred because of its relatively good penetration into the cerebrospinal fluid. For orbital cellulitis, intravenous antibiotics are given for 2 weeks, followed by oral antibiotics in the recovery phase. Surgical drainage of orbital abscesses may be necessary if these abscesses are localized. Surgery is necessary in the rare instance of mucormycosis.

## Keratitis and Corneal Ulcers

Bacterial keratitis and corneal ulceration are unusual in the absence of trauma or use of contact lenses. The conjunctiva is hyperemic, and there is a central or peripheral corneal epithelial defect with surrounding infiltration. There usually is an anterior chamber cellular reaction with or without hypopyon formation. When a bacterial ulcer is suspected, scrapings of the ulcer margins should be obtained for Gram stain and routine cultures should be taken.

Patients are started on hourly eye drops of fortified topical gentamycin (15 mg/mL) and cefazolin (50 mg/mL). The most common organisms to spread after trauma are staphylococci. For wearers of soft contact lenses with rapidly progressing central corneal ulceration and melting, *Pseudomonas aeruginosa* should be considered the causal agent until proved otherwise. Other organisms may cause bacterial ulcers in victims of trauma and contact-lens wearers. Antibiotic treatment should be modified according to results of cultures and antimicrobial sensitivities.

Fungal and amebic ulcers are rarely seen in the pediatric population but should be suspected in the case of chronic ulcers that are not responding to antibiotic therapy.

Herpes simplex keratitis is one of the leading causes of loss of vision in young adults. Primary infection occurs in childhood in the form of a conjunctivitis or keratoconjunctivitis with or without the formation of classic epithelial dendritic lesions. After primary infection, the virus remains latent in the trigeminal or other ganglia. In recurrences, the virus travels to the cornea by way of the sensory nerves, causing dendritic or geographic lesions. Treatment in such cases consists of debridement of the ulcer margin and frequent administration of topical antivirals (eg, idoxuridine, adenosine arabinoside, trifluorothymidine) until healing occurs. Stromal keratitis is characterized by stromal necrosis, thinning, and neovascularization. Because immunologic factors play a role in stromal disease, treatment involves use of steroids in conjunction with antivirals. Disciform keratitis develops in patients with previous dendritic disease owing to an immunologic stromal reaction to herpes antigens. Treatment consists of cautious use of mild steroids. Corneal transplantation may be necessary in patients with recurrent disease that has resulted in opaque vascularized corneas. Surgery is to be avoided during active disease, when chances of graft rejection are high because of host corneal vascularization and reactivation of the virus. Oral acyclovir has been used successfully to prevent recurrence of keratitis in grafted patients.

### Endophthalmitis

Nematode endophthalmitis (ie, ocular toxocariasis) results from invasion of the eye by the second- or third-stage larva of the dog roundworm. This systemic infection, known as visceral larva migrans, is characterized by fever, hepatosplenomegaly, pneumonitis, occasional encephalitis, and extreme eosinophilia. Transmission to humans occurs from ingestion of roundworm eggs in soil contaminated by feces from infected dogs or from contaminated hands or fomites. A history of geophagia or pica should be obtained in children suspected of having ocular toxocariasis.

In the United States, visceral larva migrans is most prevalent in the south-central and southeastern regions. Children with visceral larva migrans are most often boys between 6 months and 3 years of age at the onset of symptoms. There usually is a history of contact with puppies, and many children are reported by parents to be geophagic. Leukocyte counts range from 30,000 to 90,000 with 50% to 90% eosinophils, and the eosinophil count may remain elevated for months or years. Granulomas form in infected tissues after the acute stage of eosinophilic abscesses subsides.

Severe cases of nematode endophthalmitis are treated with steroids. Anthelmintics (ie, diethylcarbamazine, thiabendazole) relieve symptoms and shorten convalescence time. For most patients, prognosis is excellent, and in many, the disease is self-limited and subclinical. However, associated encephalitis and myocarditis may be lethal.

Ocular involvement may occur after a clear-cut episode of previous visceral larva migrans, concurrently with the systemic disease or without any previously manifested disease. It is usually manifested as endophthalmitis with a solitary chorioretinal granuloma with or without retinal traction. The granuloma may be in the posterior pole or in the fundus periphery.

The disease is most often unilateral in children, although bilateral occurrences have been reported in adults. There is no pathognomonic presentation; children are seen because of uveitis or endophthalmitis, strabismus, or poor vision. Ocular toxocariasis has commonly been confused with retinoblastoma, as a result of which the eyes of many children with toxocariasis have been unnecessarily enucleated in the past.

Ultrasonography differentiates the granulomas of ocular toxocariasis from retinoblastoma by the absence of high peaks due to calcifications in retinoblastoma. An enzyme-linked immunosorbent assay (ELISA) for *Toxocara canis* is positive at a 1:8 dilution in about 90% of patients with ocular toxocariasis, but it is uniformly negative in patients with retinoblastoma. Cytology of aqueous humor is likely to reveal eosinophils in toxocariasis and tumor cells in seeded retinoblastoma.

Severe ocular toxocariasis can lead to numerous complications and even loss of the eye. Systemic and topical steroids should be administered to reduce ocular inflammation and its sequelae, and anthelmintics should be given to destroy the larvae. Intraocular surgery and laser treatment are performed in selected cases.

Bacterial endophthalmitis is rare in the pediatric age group. It may occur after intraocular surgery (eg, cataract extraction, filtering surgery for glaucoma), after trauma, or secondary to bacterial embolization from endocarditis or disseminated infection. It can be a blinding condition if the intraocular contents are destroyed by necrotizing inflammation. Vitreous cultures and intravitreous injection of antibiotics should be performed early, and the patient should be started on systemic antibiotics and concentrated topical antibiotic eye drops. The visual prognosis is guarded.

### Pingueculae and Pterygia

Pingueculae are elevated conjunctival lesions that usually occur near the nasal or temporal corneoscleral limbus in the area of the interpalpebral fissure. When these growths impinge on the cornea, they are called pterygia (Fig 34-2). Histopathologically, the lesions consist of elastotically degenerated collagen, which is tissue that looks like elastin but is not digested by elastase. Ultraviolet radiation is thought to play an important role in the pathogenesis of pterygia. No treatment is required except in cases of recurrent inflammation of a pinguecula, for which mild steroid drops are given. If a pterygium grows toward the central corneal area, surgical excision may be indicated. There is a 30% to 40% rate of recurrence after excision.

### Strabismus and Amblyopia

The pediatrician often has reason to suspect ocular misalignment in an infant or child. Pseudostrabismus is a prominence of epicanthal folds or variations in orbital alignment in a young child producing a false impression of esotropia (ie, inward deviation of an eye) or, less frequently, of exotropia (ie, outward deviation of an eye). Good centration of the corneal light reflex in both eyes and normal fixation patterns are usually sufficient to rule out true strabismus. Parents can be reassured that epicanthal folds will decrease as the child grows and the nasal bridge becomes more prominent. A positive family history of strabismus should raise suspicion of true strabismus, in which case a detailed ophthalmologic assessment is always mandatory. Some common forms of strabismus are briefly described here.

Phoria is misalignment of the visual axes that is kept latent by fusional mechanisms and can be elicited by disruption of fusion, as produced by the monocular cover-uncover test. Phorias may become tropias when a child is ill or tired. Exophoria or esophoria is recognized, depending on the direction of drift of the covered eye.

An intermittent tropia (ie, deviation) exists if ocular misalignment occurs spontaneously, alternating with longer periods of good ocular alignment and fusion. Intermittent tropias occur when the deviation exceeds fusional capabilities, especially when the child is tired. In a tropia, one eye is constantly deviated while the other eye is used for fixation. In alternating tropias, vision is equal in the two eyes, and either one deviates when the other one is fixating. In constant tropias, one eye is always in the abnormal position, and there is a strong fixation preference for the

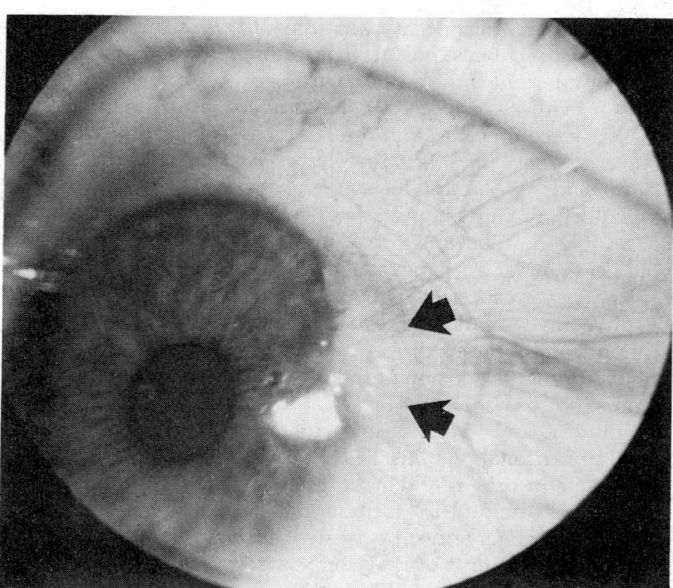

**Figure 34-2.**   Anterior-segment photograph showing a small pterygium (*arrows*).

other eye. Strabismic amblyopia develops with constant tropias in very young children.

Amblyopia is loss of vision caused not by an organic ocular or visual pathway lesion but rather by disuse of one eye and predominant use of the other. The mechanism of vision loss is thought to be of central nervous system origin. This is a reversible process in younger children, and a major aim of strabismus treatment is the prevention or reversal of amblyopia in addition to the restoration of good ocular alignment. Amblyopia therapy consists of patching of the better eye to allow stimulation of the central visual centers from the deviated eye. The younger the child, the faster and more dramatic is the response to short periods of occlusion therapy. Longer periods of patching are required in older children. There is some debate about the upper limit of age at which amblyopia is still reversible; it may be around 10 years of age. Continuous patching for several weeks may be needed for children older than 7 or 8 years of age.

Congenital or infantile esotropia is not present at birth but is diagnosed in the first 6 months of life. The angle of ocular deviation is usually large, and there is little refractive error. Associated conditions include overacting inferior oblique muscles and dissociated vertical deviations, which may manifest later in childhood despite the original therapy and apparently good ocular alignment (Fig 34-3). The mainstay of therapy is early surgical intervention and ocular patching for prevention of amblyopia.

Accommodative esotropia becomes evident in the first few years of life. It is due to accommodative efforts made in response to a relatively large degree of hyperopia. Therapy consists of use of corrective glasses and surgery for any residual deviation.

Exophoria is an intermittent outward deviation of either eye that may become evident when the affected child is tired or ill. Exophoric patients often squint in the sunlight. Treatment consists

of the correction of any error of refraction and close follow-up. There is no associated amblyopia. Surgery is indicated only if fusion breaks down and the deviation exists more than 50% of the time.

Duane's syndrome type I is characterized by esotropia, limited abduction of the eye, and retraction of the globe with palpebral fissure narrowing on attempted adduction. Two additional types are recognized. Several systemic congenital anomalies have been associated with the syndrome, especially radial ray skeletal defects. The condition involves abnormal innervation to the lateral rectus muscle from the oculomotor nerve and absence of the sixth nerve; this leads to co-contraction of the medial and lateral rectus muscles on attempted adduction.

Brown's superior oblique tendon sheath syndrome is characterized by an inability to elevate the eye in adduction. Most cases are congenital, although acquired cases have been documented.

Möbius' syndrome is characterized by unilateral or bilateral sixth and seventh nerve palsies. Affected persons usually demonstrate esotropia and an expressionless face. Associated anomalies include the Poland anomaly (ie, absence of the pectoral muscle and radial defects) and terminal limb defects.

Extraocular muscle palsies in children result in incomitant strabismus, in which different measurements are obtained from different directions of gaze; the most strabismus is found in the direction of gaze of the affected muscle. Children with acquired palsies may not verbalize a complaint of diplopia, but they may squint, cover one eye with a hand, or assume a compensatory head posture to avoid diplopia.

Third-nerve palsies are most commonly due to trauma or to increased intracranial pressure, and they may be complete or incomplete. Other causes include inflammation, infectious and parainfectious processes, vascular lesions, tumors, and degenerative and demyelinating disease involving the nerve. Diabetes is not a cause of third-nerve palsy in the pediatric population. Associated neurologic defects are good clues to the location of the lesion causing the nerve palsy. Like third-nerve palsies, fourth-nerve palsies are commonly due to trauma or tumor, but they may be idiopathic and present at birth.

Sixth-nerve palsies are common in children. They may indicate neurologic disease but are seen as a transitory benign postviral condition. Sixth-nerve palsy may be the result of increased intracranial pressure from hydrocephalus, tumor, intracranial hemorrhage, or cerebral edema. It may be due to trauma, inflammatory conditions such as meningitis, and degenerative or demyelinating conditions. Benign sixth-nerve palsy in children develops 1 to 3 weeks after a febrile illness and usually subsides within 6 months. A child with a cranial nerve palsy should undergo a complete neurologic evaluation, including computed tomography or magnetic resonance imaging of the head. A history of recent viral disease should be obtained, and the child should receive care from an ophthalmologist and a neurologist.

Nystagmus refers to rhythmic oscillations of the eyes that occur independently of normal movements. In pendular nystagmus, the velocity of movement is equal in the two directions. In contrast, jerk nystagmus has slow and fast components. The different kinds of nystagmus are named according to the refixation and the direction in which the nystagmus occurs (eg, in right-beating jerk nystagmus, the fast refixation component is to the right). In conjugate nystagmus, binocular oscillations are in phase, unlike disjugate or dissociated nystagmus, which can be monocular or binocular with a slow component that is out of phase. Latent nystagmus is elicited by interruption of binocular vision (eg, by occlusion of one eye). Congenital nystagmus is present at birth and may be associated with abnormal head movements and positions. Visual acuity is usually decreased.

Strabismus may be superimposed on congenital nystagmus,

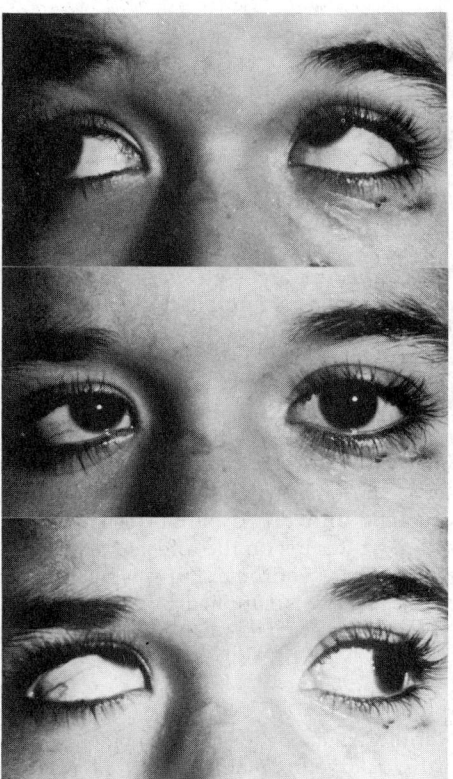

**Figure 34-3.** Right esotropia with overaction of the inferior oblique muscles. Notice the elevation of the adducted eye (toward the nose) in right and left gazes, indicating overaction of the inferior oblique muscles.

which can be inherited as an autosomal dominant, recessive, or X-linked recessive trait. Sensory defect nystagmus is due to defects in the afferent visual system. Any abnormality of the eye that interferes with good image formation and transmission from the retina can result in nystagmus. Motor defect nystagmus is due to a defect in the efferent motor system, possibly at the level of centers or pathways for conjugate motor control.

Spasmus nutans is characterized by small-amplitude and very-fast-velocity nystagmus accompanied by head nodding and sometimes torticollis. Spasmus nutans starts between 4 and 12 months of age and usually subsides spontaneously after 3 years of age. Intracranial tumors may be associated with nystagmus. Any child with abnormal eye movements should be promptly evaluated by an ophthalmologist.

## Cataracts

Developmental cataracts are unilateral or bilateral opacifications of the crystalline lens. Hereditary cataracts are most often inherited in an autosomal dominant fashion. Developmental cataracts may be associated with chromosomal abnormalities, intrauterine infections, and certain metabolic diseases. Cataracts may be associated with ocular diseases or abnormalities in the absence of systemic disease, as in the case of ROP, retinoblastoma, chronic uveitis, retinal detachment, microphthalmos, Peters' anomaly, and aniridia. Ocular trauma may result in the development of cataracts. Chronic steroid and other drug ingestion may lead to the development of cataracts, as may exposure to therapeutic irradiation for the treatment of orbital or ocular tumors. Table 34-6 lists various conditions associated with congenital or developmental cataracts.

Evaluation of the infant or child with cataracts includes a full ophthalmologic evaluation to exclude associated ocular disease and to assess visual status. Ocular ultrasonography should be performed in eyes with totally opaque lenses. The child should be evaluated by the pediatrician for associated systemic conditions as listed in Table 34-6. A family history of congenital cataracts in a parent or grandparent suggests dominant isolated cataracts.

Bilateral complete cataracts should be extracted early, and visual prognosis is generally good if there is no other ocular disease. Aggressive surgery as early as 1 month of age for unilateral cataracts is currently recommended. The infant is fitted with a contact lens soon after surgery, and the child's better eye is patched for an increasing number of hours each day through middle childhood to prevent the development of amblyopia. Frequent refractions and changes of contact lens power are needed, and parents should be aware of the importance of perseverance if good visual results are to be obtained. Conservative management of partial cataracts includes the use of mydriatics if the opacity is central and patching of the uninvolved eye for the treatment and prevention of amblyopia.

## Ptosis

Congenital ptosis, the most common cause of upper-lid drooping in children and young adults, is due to faulty development of the levator palpebrae muscle. Most cases are unilateral, and the degree of severity varies. Superior rectus palsy may exist. Familial cases are inherited as an autosomal dominant condition, and there is a dominant syndrome of congenital ptosis, phimosis, and epicanthus inversus. Infants with severe ptosis usually assume a chin-up head posture and look with both eyes in downgaze. Amblyopia is uncommon, and cosmetic surgery is usually delayed until the child attends school.

Acquired ptosis in childhood demands special attention because it usually indicates potentially serious neurologic disease. Paralytic ptosis is seen in third-nerve palsy, and the differential

| TABLE 34-6. | Chromosomal and Hereditary Conditions Associated With Cataracts |
|---|---|

**Chromosomal Disorders**
Trisomy 13
Trisomy 18
Trisomy 21

**Metabolic Disorders**
Galactosemia
Galactokinase deficiency
Albright pseudohypoparathyroidism
Wilson disease
Fabry disease
Refsum disease
Homocystinuria
Myotonic dystrophy

**Skin Diseases**
Incontinentia pigmenti
Ectodermal dysplasia
Rothmund-Thompson syndrome
Werner syndrome

**Mandibulofacial Syndromes**
Hallermann-Streiff syndrome
Stickler syndrome with Pierre Robin sequence
Rubenstein-Taybi syndrome

**Connective Tissue and Skeletal Syndromes**
Conradi syndrome
Marfan syndrome
All syndromes involving dislocated lenses
Other bone dysplasias

**Renal Diseases**
Lowe oculocerebrorenal syndrome
Alport syndrome

**Central Nervous System Diseases**
Marinesco-Sjögren syndrome
Sjögren syndrome

diagnosis of acquired paralytic ptosis is the same as that of acquired third-nerve palsy. Neuromuscular ptosis is seen in myasthenia gravis and in myopathies such as myotonic dystrophy and congenital myotonia. Lid trauma can result in transient or permanent ptosis. Inflammation, swelling, scar tissue, and tumors of the lids can lead to acquired ptosis.

Pseudoptosis may be due to hypotropia of the ipsilateral eye or to lid retraction or proptosis of the contralateral eye.

In Horner's syndrome, sympathetic denervation leads to mild ptosis, miosis, and anhydrosis of the ipsilateral face. Heterochromia, with a lighter iris on the affected side, may be present in congenital Horner's syndrome. Ptosis is due to denervation of Müller's muscle, which is supplied by the sympathetic nerves and inserts on the upper tarsal plate.

## Infantile Glaucoma

Primary infantile glaucoma, with an incidence of about 1 in 100,000 births, is due to maldevelopment of the trabecular meshwork (ie, trabeculodysgenesis), resulting in reduced outflow of aqueous humor from the developing eye and increased intraocular pressure. All ocular layers are stretched, leading to buphthalmos (ie, large, prominent eye) and optic nerve head damage with an abnormally large cup-to-disc ratio. Primary infantile glaucoma is inherited in an autosomal recessive fashion and is most common in populations with high rates of consanguineous marriages. About 80% of patients are detected by 6 months of age.

Symptoms and signs include corneal enlargement and clouding, tearing, photophobia, and blepharospasm. Thirty percent of cases are unilateral and the male-to-female ratio is 3:2, suggesting the existence of an X-linked variant. Intraocular pressure measurements vary from 20 to 50 mm Hg or more. Corneal diameter is usually enlarged but may be normal early. Corneal epithelial edema and stromal clouding result from failure of the endothelial cell pump, which normally dehydrates the cornea. Horizontal breaks in Descemet's membrane (ie, Haab's striae) are diagnostic. The corneal enlargement in congenital glaucoma should be differentiated from megalocornea, which is discussed in the section on anterior segment disorders in this chapter.

The treatment of infantile glaucoma is surgical. Goniotomy and trabeculotomy open Schlemm's canal to the anterior chamber. In trabeculotomy, the approach is through a sclerotomy site, but in goniotomy, it is through a directed incision at the opposite limbus by way of the anterior chamber. Multiple surgeries may be necessary to achieve optimal control of the intraocular pressure, but results appear to be equal for the two approaches. Oral acetazolamide (10 to 15 mg/kg/day) and topical timolol maleate (0.25%) may be given while the child is awaiting surgery, which should be performed as soon as possible. Optic nerve cupping is reversible in infants after normalization of intraocular pressure. High myopia and astigmatism are generally present because of ocular axial elongation and corneal deformity. Any error of refraction should be corrected postoperatively to prevent anisometropic amblyopia.

Infantile glaucoma is associated with several other conditions, including anterior segment dysgenesis, congenital rubella, neurofibromatosis, mucopolysaccharidosis I, Lowe oculocerebrorenal syndrome, Sturge-Weber syndrome, and several chromosomal abnormalities. In diseases manifested by microspherophakic or dislocated lenses, such as Weill-Marchesani syndrome, homocystinuria, and Marfan syndrome, pupillary block by the dislocated lens and secondary glaucoma may develop. Other causes of secondary glaucoma in children include trauma, inflammation, ROP with secondary angle-closure glaucoma, lens-induced glaucoma, steroid-induced glaucoma, and glaucoma secondary to intraocular tumors, such as retinoblastoma, juvenile xanthogranuloma, and medulloepithelioma.

## Uveitis

The uveal tract comprises the iris, ciliary body, and choroid. Iritis, cyclitis, iridocyclitis, choroiditis, and panuveitis refer to inflammation of the different parts of the uveal tract singly or in combination. Peripheral uveitis refers to inflammation of the extreme fundus periphery. Endogenous or nonpurulent uveitis is rare in children. As in the adult population, males are affected twice as frequently as females. About half of the cases have binocular involvement. The younger the affected child, the more diffuse is the inflammation. Uveitis can be classified as granulomatous or nongranulomatous, depending on the type of cellular reaction involved.

Iritis produces exudation of protein into the anterior chamber with the production of flare or diffraction of a light beam. Inflammatory cells, seen floating in the anterior chamber, can form keratic precipitates on the posterior surface of the cornea.

A hypopyon is the accumulation of inflammatory cells in the anterior chamber, forming a visible whitish fluid level inferiorly. Hypopyon may be seen in retinoblastoma, in which the malignant cells accumulate in the anterior chamber. Inflammation of the posterior uveal tract produces a cellular reaction in the anterior or posterior vitreous. Prolonged inflammation results in adhesions between the peripheral iris and cornea (ie, peripheral anterior synechiae) or between the iris and lens (ie, posterior synechiae). Cataracts may develop.

Choroiditis may spread to overlying retina, producing a chorioretinitis. Active chorioretinal lesions are white; inactive lesions or chorioretinal scars have black areas of hyperpigmentation and white areas of scarring. A particular complication of chronic uveitis in children is the deposition of calcium in a band-shaped pattern in the superficial layers of the cornea, mostly in the interpalpebral fissure area, producing band keratopathy. This complication is seen predominantly in conjunction with juvenile rheumatoid arthritis.

Children with uveitis may complain of pain, photophobia, lacrimation, and blepharospasm, and if they are old enough, they may notice disturbances in vision. Other children may be completely asymptomatic.

The most common cause of posterior uveitis in children is toxoplasmosis. Anterior uveitis is seen in Still's disease, herpes simplex, and sarcoidosis. Many cases are of undetermined cause. About 15% to 25% of cases of uveitis in children are of the peripheral variety, also called pars planitis. This disease is usually bilateral and can start as early as 7 years of age. Its onset is insidious; redness, photophobia, and tearing are usually absent. Progressive visual impairment occurs secondary to macular edema and posterior subcapsular cataracts. Characteristic "snowball" inflammatory deposits may be seen in the pars plana area, but they are not a universal finding. The cause of this disease is unknown. Therapy consists of administration of topical and systemic steroids. The disease runs a variable course, with exacerbations and remissions over several years. Other causes of uveitis in children include sarcoidosis, syphilis, tuberculosis, sympathetic ophthalmia, Behçet's disease, Vogt-Koyanagi-Harada disease, histoplasmosis, and ankylosing spondylitis.

Trauma can induce an iridocyclitis, with cells and flare in the anterior chamber and symptoms of pain, photophobia, lacrimation, and blepharospasm. Treatment consists of administration of cycloplegic drops with or without mild steroid drops for a few days.

## TUMORS

### Orbital Tumors

After inflammatory orbital infiltration, the two most common tumors in the pediatric population are dermoid cysts and capillary or infantile hemangiomas, which together make up more than 50% of all orbital tumors. Other orbital tumors, in order of decreasing frequency, are rhabdomyosarcoma, optic nerve glioma, neurofibroma, lymphangioma, metastatic neuroblastoma, inflammatory pseudotumor, lipoma, leukemia, lymphoma, meningioma, and other rarer tumors, including teratoma, orbital extension of retinoblastoma, schwannoma, and other even rarer conditions. Some of these tumors are discussed here.

#### Dermoid Cyst

Dermoid cysts account for about 40% of orbital tumors of childhood. They are choristomatous tumors due to the retention and proliferation of ectodermal derivatives along lines of fetal fissures within the lid, brow, or orbit. Deep orbital cysts arise within diploë of orbital bones and may have an hourglass appearance. Although these are congenital tumors, less than 25% are evident at birth; the delayed appearance in most cases is probably due to postnatal growth. The tumors are nontender, well circumscribed, and of a rubbery or doughy consistency. More than half are located in the upper outer orbital quadrant; less than 3% arise deep within the orbit. Diagnosis is made on the basis of clinical grounds, ultrasonography, and computed tomography. Orbital bony structures may be compressed by the tumor, and well-circumscribed defects may be seen.

Deeper tumors are harder to diagnose, and other orbital cystic tumors may be confused with dermoids. Anteriorly located tumors are easily excised, although care should be taken not to rupture the cyst wall, because the cyst contents may elicit a severe local inflammatory response. Deep orbital cysts are more difficult to excise.

## Capillary Hemangioma

Capillary hemangiomas of infancy are vascular orbital tumors composed of proliferating capillaries. The bulk of the tumor consists of proliferating plump endothelial cells. More than 90% of these tumors have a visible superficial component, allowing diagnosis on the basis of clinical inspection alone. There may be a bluish discoloration of the overlying skin, a tangled vascular mass, or the classic strawberry mark. The tumor swells when the child cries. One third of tumors are present at birth, and 95% are diagnosed by 6 months of age. The tumor continues to grow after birth but eventually regresses spontaneously; regression is complete in about 75% of patients by 7 or 8 years of age. Girls are affected more frequently than boys.

Local complications include ptosis, occlusion of the eye, ulceration and bleeding from the tumor surface, and infection. One rare complication in large hemangiomas is platelet sequestration. Amblyopia may result from occlusion of the eye by the tumor or from a high degree of astigmatism and resultant anisometropia because of pressure over the globe. One fourth of patients have one or more cutaneous capillary hemangiomas elsewhere on their bodies.

Treatment consists of observation if the visual axis is clear and there is no astigmatism. Systemic steroids and intralesional injections of Celestone are the mainstay of therapy in vision-threatening capillary hemangioma. One or more injections induce rapid regression of the tumors in most cases. Other modes of therapy include surgery and low-dose radiotherapy, but these are not commonly used.

## Idiopathic Inflammatory Pseudotumor

The diagnosis of idiopathic orbital psuedotumor requires exclusion of several inflammatory, tumorous, infectious, and traumatic orbital conditions that may have an inflammatory component; these include Graves' disease, systemic vasculitis, Wegener's granulomatosis, juvenile xanthogranuloma, sinus histiocytosis with massive lymphadenopathy, angioneurotic edema, bacterial orbital cellulitis, mucocele, orbital mucormycosis, parasitic infestations, trauma with retained foreign body, inflammatory reactions around primary benign tumors, and malignant orbital tumors. About 5% of patients with idiopathic inflammatory pseudotumor are in the pediatric age group, and only 2% of biopsied orbital masses in children fall in this disease category.

Pain differentiates this condition from other orbital mass lesions causing proptosis. Most cases are unilateral; bilateral cases are likely to be associated with a poorer prognosis or with the subsequent diagnosis of systemic disease, such as Wegener's granulomatosis. Iritis occurs in about 25% of cases. Erythrocyte sedimentation rates and eosinophil counts may be elevated.

Pathologically, there is a localized or diffuse aggregation of inflammatory cells that may form well-defined lymphoid follicles; there may be an aggregation of plasma cells, lymphocytes, or eosinophils, and a granulomatous inflammatory response. In some cases, proliferation of connective tissue predominates; in others, the inflammatory infiltrate is predominantly perivascular. Ultrasonography and computed tomography are helpful in diagnosing idiopathic inflammatory pseudotumor if components of inflammatory edema and an inflammatory mass lesion can be identified. A trial of systemic steroids is often used to confirm the diagnosis and initiate treatment. Response to treatment may be dramatic; about 75% of patients respond well to this modality. Low-dose irradiation has been used in refractory cases.

## Rhabdomyosarcoma

Rhabdomyosarcoma, the most common primary malignant orbital tumor, accounts for 9% of orbital tumors in children. Because it is lethal if untreated, it should always be suspected in the case of a child with acquired ptosis or with a lid, epibulbar, or orbital mass. This tumor arises from mesenchymal precursors of muscle cells and forms three pathologic types: embryonal (78%), alveolar (14%), and differentiated (8%). Over 90% of orbital rhabdomyosarcomas occur in children younger than 16 years of age.

The main presenting sign is unilateral, often fulminant proptosis. There may be ptosis or a palpable orbital or lid mass. Occasionally, the tumor presents as a lid or conjunctival mass. The two keys to diagnosis are a high index of suspicion and an early biopsy. Computed tomography is helpful in delineating the extent of the disease.

The major prognostic factor in this condition is the extent of disease at the time of institution of therapy. Metastases occur most frequently to lungs and bone marrow, and the tumor may extend locally to the intracranial cavity and paranasal sinuses. Excellent survival rates are obtained with combined supervoltage radiotherapy and chemotherapy, although many eyes are ultimately enucleated because of the complications of radiation therapy. Exenteration, once the mainstay of treatment, is reserved for cases in which medical treatment fails, cases of orbital recurrences, or cases in which megavoltage radiotherapy is not available.

## Metastatic Neuroblastoma

Neuroblastoma is a tumor of the embryonic sympathetic neuroblasts. It is the third most common malignant tumor in children after leukemia and brain tumors. Forty percent to 50% of neuroblastomas arise in the adrenal glands, 25% in other retroperitoneal sites, 10% in the mediastinum, and 2% to 5% in the neck. Primary intraspinous, intracranial, and soft-tissue tumors have been described. In some cases the primary site cannot be identified. Metastases spread by way of the bloodstream to distant sites, particularly the skull and orbit; by way of lymphatics to adjacent and distant lymph nodes; and by direct extension from the right adrenal gland into the liver. Metastatic neuroblastoma accounts for about 3% of orbital tumors in children. Orbital involvement may precede, concur with, or follow diagnosis of the primary tumor.

Patients most commonly present with proptosis and may have periorbital swelling and lid ecchymosis. Ptosis and miosis are seen in neck tumors because of the so-produced Horner's syndrome. Severe proptosis results in anterior segment complications, such as conjunctival necrosis and corneal exposure, and in restriction of ocular motility. Intracranial metastases produce papilledema and optic atrophy. Orbital metastases indicate stage IV neuroblastoma and are associated with an extremely poor prognosis; the 5-year survival is almost zero, regardless of therapy.

# Ocular Tumors

## Retinoblastoma

Retinoblastoma is discussed in Chapter 101, and the discussion here is restricted to some general diagnostic considerations. Retinoblastoma is the most common intraocular malignancy in childhood. It occurs in about 1 in 15,000 live births and is responsible for about 1% of deaths in the pediatric population. The hereditary and sporadic cases of retinoblastoma are caused by deletion or mutation of both alleles of the *RB1* gene on chromosome 13. Most cases are diagnosed before the age of 4 years. Boys and girls are equally affected. Mortality is low if treatment is instituted before metastases occur, with 5-year survival rates of 90% in unilateral and 80% in bilateral cases. It is vital that this condition be diagnosed and treated as early as possible.

The average age at diagnosis is about 1 year for bilateral disease and 2 years for unilateral disease. Disease in infants with a positive family history is discovered earlier because of examination shortly after birth. The most common manifestation of retinoblastoma is a white reflex from the pupil (ie, leukocoria), most often observed by parents when the child is looking in a direction that puts the tumor in the path of the incident light. Other manifestations include convergent or divergent strabismus, pseudohypopyon, hyphema, periorbital swelling, and red eye.

Accurate and prompt diagnosis is invaluable if adequate therapy is to be instituted and enucleation for simulating conditions is to be avoided. Pediatricians should suspect the tumor in any patient with leukocoria, especially if any other family member has had an eye enucleated in infancy or childhood. Strabismus is the next most common sign of retinoblastoma, and a search for retinal pathology or tumor should be routinely carried out in infants and children with ocular misalignment.

Age at presentation, sex, laterality of ocular involvement, and family history are good clues to the differential diagnosis of retinoblastoma, because the various simulating conditions appear in characteristic age groups and may show male predominance or predominantly uniocular or binocular involvement. More than 90% of retinoblastomas can be easily diagnosed by ophthalmologists using indirect ophthalmoscopy and ultrasonography or computed sonography. About 50% of patients referred to tertiary specialized ophthalmic oncology centers to rule out retinoblastoma turn out to have the tumor; the remainder have one of the several simulating conditions listed in Table 34-4.

Coats' disease (ie, idiopathic retinal telangiectasia) is usually a unilateral retinal disease of boys that is most often diagnosed in the first decade of life. However, bilateral cases, cases in girls, and cases with onset in adulthood can occur. Coats' disease is characterized by telangiectasia, aneurysms, and focal bulblike dilations of the retinal vessels. The dilated vessels leak fluid and exudates in the retinal and into the subretinal space, resulting in retinal edema, circinate exudates, and serous retinal detachment. The accumulation of mounds of yellow-white subretinal exudates leads this condition to be commonly confused with retinoblastoma. Patients may be completely asymptomatic or present with decreased vision, strabismus, or leukocoria. Fluorescein angiography and the demonstration of telangiectatic vascular abnormalities are diagnostic. Visual prognosis is poor in patients with diffuse retinal involvement; cryotherapy may be used in an attempt to obliterate leaky vessels. Patients with mild peripheral disease may be observed; laser photocoagulation is helpful in some cases of localized disease.

### Juvenile Xanthogranuloma

Juvenile xanthogranuloma affects the skin and eyes of children younger than 5 years of age; 85% of patients are younger than 1 year of age. The eyelid is most frequently affected, followed by the epibulbar area and orbit. Intraocular lesions are located in the iris and ciliary body and present as an iris tumor, spontaneous hyphema, unilateral glaucoma, or heterochromia iridis. Skin lesions, which appear suddenly on the upper part of the body, can be solitary or multiple; yellow, orange, or brown; and papular or nodular. They vary in size from a few millimeters to 1.5 cm in diameter and resolve spontaneously within 2 or 3 years.

Histopathologic sections of fibroxanthomatous tumor tissue reveal chronic inflammation and large multinucleated cells, called Touton giant cells, in which several nuclei are arranged in a circular fashion around a central area of foamy cytoplasm. The differential diagnosis of these iris tumors includes medulloepithelioma, primary iris cysts, melanoma, leiomyoma, and neurofibroma. The severity of ocular involvement varies, and if extensive or clinically aggressive tumors are left untreated, the eye may be lost from complications of glaucoma and recurrent intraocular hemorrhage. Surgical excision, systemic and topical steroids, acetazolamide, and external irradiation have been used with various degrees of success.

### Medulloepithelioma

Medulloepithelioma is a rare congenital tumor that arises from the nonpigmented ciliary epithelium. Cell type and arrangement are extremely variable because of the pluripotentiality of the cell of origin. If cartilage, brain, striated muscle, or other heterotopic cells are present, the tumor is called teratoid medulloepithelioma. Both simple and teratoid tumors may exhibit histologic evidence of malignancy. These tumors become evident in the first decade of life; the average age at enucleation is 5 years. The tumor is invariably unilateral, and the family history is negative for similar tumors.

Presenting signs include a visible iris tumor or iris distortion, secondary glaucoma, a white pupillary reflex, spontaneous and post-traumatic hyphema, and reduced visual acuity or strabismus. The differential diagnosis includes retinoblastoma, persistent hyperplastic primary vitreous, primary iris cyst, melanoma, leiomyoma, and neurofibroma of the ciliary body. Treatment is early enucleation, before the tumor extends orbitally. Prognosis after early enucleation is excellent. Excision of localized tumors is associated with good long-term survival. This tumor is not radiosensitive.

## OPHTHALMOLOGIC MANIFESTATIONS OF SYSTEMIC DISEASE

It is impossible to cover the ophthalmologic manifestations of all pediatric systemic diseases, and only selected common pediatric diseases with major ocular findings are discussed here.

### Marfan Syndrome

Marfan syndrome is an autosomal dominant condition characterized by skeletal abnormalities with excessive length of the distal limbs, loose jointedness, scoliosis, and anterior chest deformities. The affected person is usually taller than the rest of his family. Cardiovascular abnormalities in the form of aortic root dilation, dissecting aortic aneurysm, and mitral valve prolapse are commonly seen. Complications of aortic dilation have been the major cause of death, which occurs at an average age of 45 years.

Ocular abnormalities in Marfan syndrome include subluxation of the lens, usually but not invariably in an upward and outward direction (Fig 34-4); moderate to severe myopia; tremulousness of the iris (ie, iridodonesis); megalocornea; keratoconus; an unusually deep anterior chamber angle; and retinal detachment. Retinal detachment may occur spontaneously in eyes with axial myopia or after cataract extraction. Cataracts develop early in subluxated and nonsubluxated lenses. The lens does not usually subluxate into the anterior chamber in Marfan syndrome, and patients presenting with lenses in the anterior chambers and a marfanoid habitus should be considered to have homocystinuria until proven otherwise. Other diseases associated with lens subluxation include homocystinuria, the Weill-Marchesani syndrome, hyperlysinemia, sulfite oxidase deficiency, Kniest syndrome, and Stickler syndrome. Dislocated lenses can be an isolated finding in a hereditary condition called simple ectopia lentis, which is

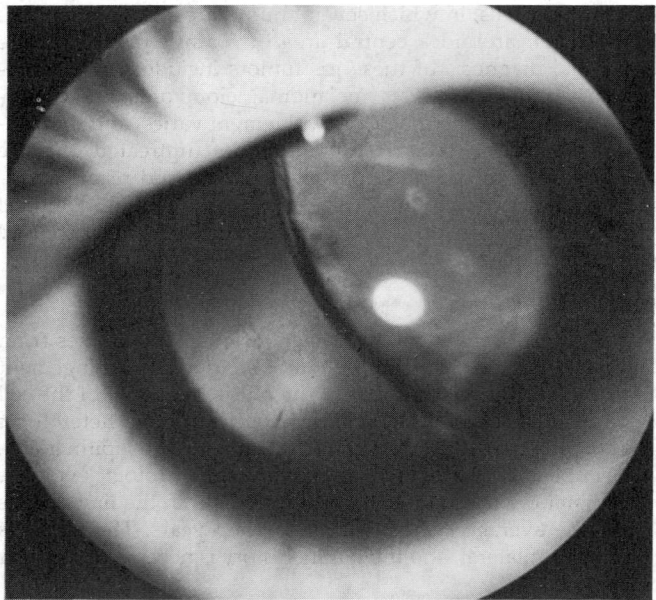

**Figure 34-4.** Subluxated lens in a patient with Marfan syndrome.

inherited as an autosomal recessive and occasionally as an autosomal dominant trait; they may be seen in combination with ectopia or abnormal position of the pupil in ectopia lentis et pupillae, which is inherited in a similar fashion.

## Albinism

Albinism refers to the absence or scarcity of melanin in the skin, eye, or both. All conditions featuring albinism are genetically determined and involve defects in the normal process of melanogenesis. There are nine forms of oculocutaneous albinism, three forms of ocular albinism, and 16 or more disorders involving dermal hypopigmentation without ocular albinism. The general aspects of albinism are discussed elsewhere in this textbook.

All types of oculocutaneous and ocular albinism are characterized by nystagmus, strabismus, decreased foveal reflex, absence of pigment in the retinal pigment epithelium and uveal tract with iris transillumination, prominence of choroidal vessels, and high astigmatic refractive errors. Although photophobia is generally believed to be a major symptom in albinism, it is not universal, and sunglasses may further compromise already decreased visual acuity. Abnormal decussation of temporal optic nerve fibers in the optic chiasm occurs in some forms of albinism.

In children with albinism, any error of refraction should be fully corrected to prevent additional amblyopia. Strabismus is corrected surgically, although patients never achieve binocular vision. Referrals for special education and low-vision aids are necessary. Monocular telescopes are prescribed at 5 or 6 years of age. Like all children with poor vision, albino children should be allowed to hold their reading material as close to their eyes as they like; they should be seated in the front row in class. Professional genetic counseling is advisable in families with an albino child. The genes for tyrosinase-positive and tyrosinase-negative oculocutaneous albinism are probably not allelic.

## Juvenile Diabetes Mellitus

Ocular complications of juvenile diabetes mellitus most often involve the retina but may affect the conjunctiva, cornea, iris, lens, optic nerve, and extraocular muscles. Transitory refractive changes causing transitory blurring of vision are due to swelling and detumescence of the lens secondary to changes in blood sugar levels. Diabetic cataracts are relatively rare in well-controlled juvenile diabetics. Transient lens opacities can be seen in poorly controlled patients. Cranial nerve palsy is occasionally seen in juvenile diabetics who have had the disease for more than 10 years.

Retinopathy in juvenile diabetes depends more on the duration than on the control of the disease. No retinopathy is detected by fluorescein angiography if the duration of the diabetes is less than 4 years, but the incidence rises to 25% after 5 to 9 years and to more than 70% after 10 years. One third of patients have proliferative retinopathy, and one third of those are legally blind. These figures can be expected to decrease with better blood sugar control, closer monitoring of retinal changes, and early institution of laser therapy, if indicated. Vitreoretinal microsurgical techniques have allowed salvage of the eyes of many patients who would have been doomed to blindness in the past.

Several syndromes combine diabetes and various ocular findings. Alström syndrome is characterized by diabetes, severe retinal degeneration with blindness and cataracts, obesity, and severe nerve deafness. Wolfram syndrome features diabetes mellitus, diabetes insipidus, optic atrophy, and sensorineural deafness. Other diseases with occasional diabetes mellitus and ocular manifestations include Bardet-Biedl syndrome, Cockayne's syndrome, Friedreich's ataxia, Prader-Willi syndrome, and Werner syndrome.

## Tuberous Sclerosis

Tuberous sclerosis (ie, Bourneville's disease) is characterized by multiple central nervous tumors, epilepsy, cutaneous lesions in the form of adenoma sebaceum of the face developing during puberty, subungual fibromas, shagreen patches, and sometimes café au lait spots and nevi. Mental deficiency is seen in 50% of patients. The major ocular abnormalities are hamartomas of the optic nerve and retina. Long-standing tumors have a refractile multinodular appearance that has been likened to mulberries, clumps of tapioca, and frog's eggs. Retinal tumors may have a flat contour and appear as spots in the fundus that range from smooth to fluffy and from milky white to yellowish. Central nervous system tumors may cause papilledema and optic atrophy, usually the main cause of visual loss. The size and location of the various tumors determine their effect on visual acuity. Secondary glaucoma, inflammation, and intraocular hemorrhage are rare complications.

## Neurofibromatosis

Neurofibromatosis (ie, von Recklinghausen's disease) has two types: central and peripheral. The peripheral type (*NF1* gene) is assigned to chromosome 17 and the central type (*NF2* gene) to chromosome 22. The central type is characterized by tumors of the pontine angle with no ocular involvement, except for the occurrence of combined hamartomas of the retina and retinal pigment epithelium in some patients and cataracts in late childhood and early adulthood. The peripheral type is characterized by neurofibromatous tumors in many parts of the body. The principal cutaneous lesions are café au lait spots and diffuse and plexiform neurofibromas (Fig 34-5). Neurofibromas, gliomas, and meningiomas occur in the central nervous system, and ependymomas of the spinal cord have been found. Patients may have neurofibromas of the peripheral and autonomic nervous systems. Pheochromocytomas occur in fewer than 1% of patients.

More than 90% of patients with peripheral neurofibromatosis who are older than 6 years have pigmented iris nodules, also known as Lisch nodules (Fig 34-6). These nodules are composed solely of cells of melanocytic origin and do not correlate with the extent or severity of other manifestations. Glaucoma, seen only

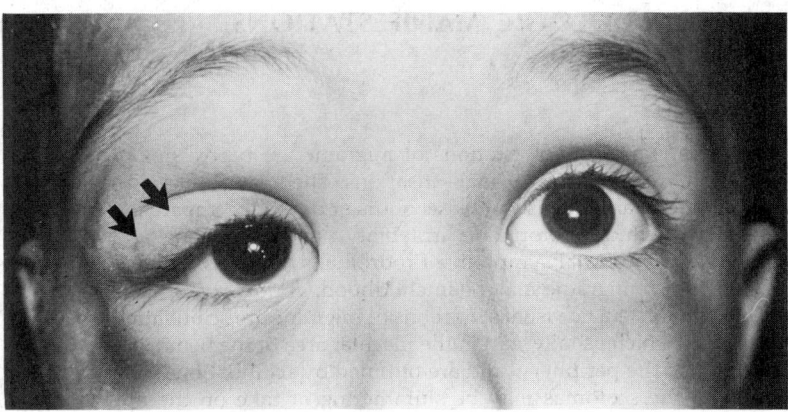

**Figure 34-5.** Plexiform neuroma of the lid (*arrows*) in a child with neurofibromatosis.

in eyes with lid involvement and only in conjunction with high myopia, may be the result of neurofibromatous involvement of the angle, incomplete development of the angle, overgrowth of melanocytic cells onto the trabecular meshwork, and peripheral anterior synechiae. Rubeosis iridis may or may not be present. Trabeculotomy is the procedure of choice for glaucoma in children with neurofibromatosis.

Patients with neurofibromatosis may develop gliomas of the optic pathways, most commonly in the orbital portion of the optic nerve with or without extension posteriorly into the optic chiasm. The clinical manifestations of optic nerve gliomas include proptosis, usually preceded by unilateral visual loss. An afferent pupillary defect and color vision defects usually exist, and there may be strabismus. Ophthalmoscopy may reveal disc pallor or papilledema; retinal striae and hyperopia may occur secondary to direct pressure from the tumor on the globe. Radiographic studies may reveal enlargement of the optic canal. Computed tomography of the orbits helps differentiate this tumor from optic nerve meningioma and delineates its posterior extension. Chiasmal gliomas may affect hypothalamic and pituitary function and may produce nystagmus and a variety of nonspecific visual field defects. If intracranial pressure is elevated, there may be bilateral papilledema. Bitemporal hemianopia may not develop.

Most optic nerve gliomas are diagnosed clinically on the basis of signs, symptoms, associated systemic findings of neurofibromatosis, and computed tomographic studies. Because these tumors are histologically benign, conservative management of lesions not extending intracranially is recommended. Tumor resection in blind, severely proptotic eyes is accepted.

## Leukemia

Ten percent of children with acute leukemia have clinically detectable ocular manifestations. Retinopathy is most common in patients with profound anemia and thrombocytopenia. Intraretinal blood in the form of nerve fiber layer hemorrhages, dot and blot hemorrhages, and white-centered hemorrhages is usually seen (Fig 34-7). Retinal and nerve head infiltration by leukemic cells is a sign of central nervous system involvement in more than 90% of the patients. Histopathologically, the uveal tract is the ocular structure that is most commonly infiltrated by leukemic cells. Choroidal infiltrates, which may appear as round, pale areas, are common, but they are difficult to detect clinically. Orbital involvement, which occurs less frequently, is manifested by the formation of chloromas, periorbital swelling, and exophthalmos.

The different types of leukemias are discussed in Chapter 96.

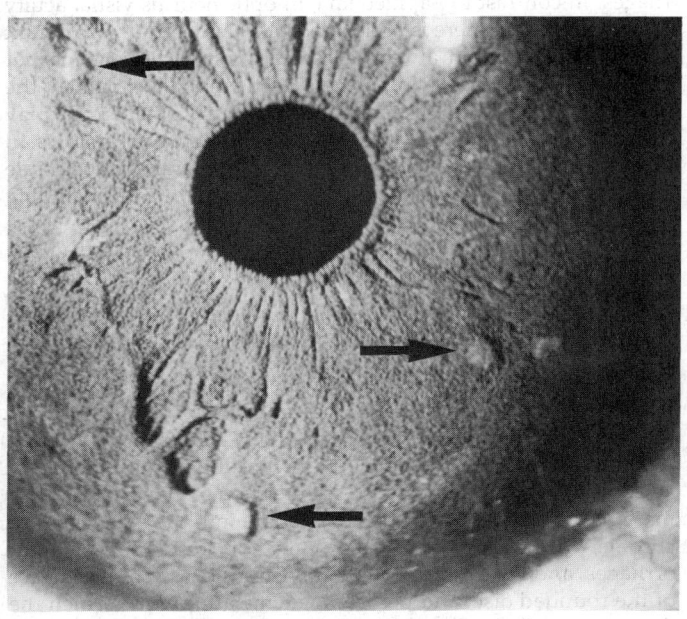

**Figure 34-6.** Hamartomas (ie, Lisch nodules) of the iris (*arrows*) in a patient with neurofibromatosis.

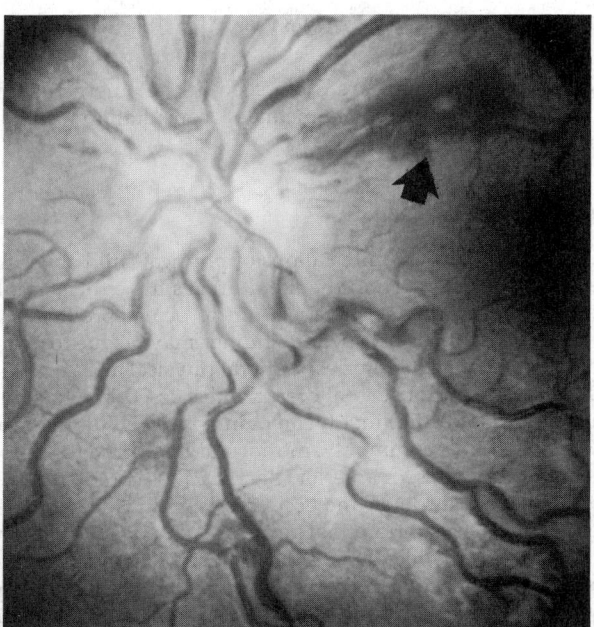

**Figure 34-7.** Retinal findings in a 7-year-old girl with acute lymphocytic leukemia. Notice the vascular tortuosity, optic nerve head swelling, blot hemorrhages, and white-centered hemorrhage (*arrow*).

# OPHTHALMOLOGIC MANIFESTATIONS OF HEADACHES

## Migraine

The main clinical manifestations of migraine are paroxysms of headache and abnormal visual sensations. The headache is usually unilateral and intense and lasts hours or days. Accompanying symptoms include photophobia, irritability, nausea, vomiting, and other gastrointestinal symptoms. Prodromal symptoms may occur. Onset of migraine may be in childhood, at puberty, or later in life. Characteristic visual sensations of migraine are scintillating scotomas, which usually start in the macular area of the hemifield, progress to the periphery, and are outlined by scintillations. The edges of the scotomas may be shimmering or take on the appearance of fortification figures. Scotomas may be transient, accompany or precede headaches, or be the only manifestation of migraine. They are caused by a focal disturbance in the occipital cortex.

Other sensory and motor disturbances can occur in migraine. Extracerebral ocular manifestations of migraine include unilateral visual loss, retinal arteriolar constriction, retinal and vitreous hemorrhage, and ischemic papillitis. Transient ophthalmoplegia is a well-recognized manifestation of migraine that usually has its onset before the age of 10 years. Most commonly, it takes the form of a third-nerve palsy with pupillary involvement; less commonly, the fourth and sixth nerves are involved. Treatment of migraine is discussed in Chapter 162.

## Errors of Refraction and Strabismus

Uncorrected astigmatism and hyperopia may give rise to headaches and ocular fatigue (ie, asthenopia) in children; corrective glasses should be prescribed in such cases. Myopia does not result in asthenopic symptoms. Phorias and intermittent tropias may result in headaches due to continued efforts to maintain ocular alignment and binocular vision.

Ocular problems are rare causes of headaches in children, and other possible causes should be investigated.

# EMERGENT EYE PROBLEMS

Emergent eye problems are often seen in the emergency room or clinic and require immediate consultation with an ophthalmologist.

## Battered Child

The ophthalmologic manifestations of physical child abuse have received much attention in the literature, as have the social and medical manifestations. The spectrum of ocular problems seen in battered children is broad, and findings may be due to delayed complications of acute injuries. General physical and social findings in physically abused children are discussed in Chapter 26. The incidence of ocular involvement in abused children is about 30% to 40%. Most commonly, intraocular hemorrhages are seen in the retina, vitreous, or anterior chamber. Less common findings include periorbital edema and ecchymosis, retinal detachment or dialysis, cataracts, chorioretinal atrophy, subluxated lenses, traumatic mydriasis, papilledema, subconjunctival hemorrhage, esotropia, corneal opacity, and optic atrophy. Bleeding into the optic nerve sheath may be the only finding in shaken babies. A detailed ophthalmologic examination should be part of the routine evaluation of children suspected of being physically abused.

## Trauma

Ophthalmologic trauma may be divided into blunt injuries, penetrating injuries, and injuries involving the globe, orbit, adnexae or any combination of these three. Nonpenetrating injuries to the globe include thermal, ultraviolet, electrical, and chemical burns, corneal abrasions, and contusions.

Contusions to the eyeball may result in subconjunctival hemorrhage, hyphema, iritis, iridodialysis and iris sphincter tears, subluxated lenses that may become cataractous, angle recession with delayed glaucoma, ghost cell glaucoma, vitreous hemorrhage, retinal and choroidal tears, detachment and rupture, and optic nerve injury with edema or avulsion.

Penetrating injuries to the globe may produce corneal lacerations, corneoscleral lacerations, scleral lacerations, or double-penetrating injuries. An intraocular foreign body may be retained. Lid lacerations may involve the lacrimal drainage system and may result in traumatic ptosis. Extraocular muscles may become entrapped in blow-out orbital fractures, leading to restrictive strabismus.

A detailed ophthalmologic examination by an ophthalmologist is mandatory in all cases of periocular and ocular injuries, and all of the described complications are looked for so the appropriate management plan can be instituted. Patients with suspected penetrating ocular injuries should have a protective metallic shield placed over their eyes, and no attempts should be made to open the lids forcefully; especially in the case of a young child, opening of the lids may need to be done with the patient under anesthesia. Tetanus immunization should be given, as in any penetrating injury.

Sports and work-related ocular injuries are receiving increased attention. The use of protective eyewear in athletic activities should be encouraged, especially in one-eyed children and children with compromised ocular function, a predisposition to retinal detachment, or subluxated lenses.

## Optic Neuritis

In children, optic neuritis is usually a manifestation of systemic or neurologic disease. Two forms are recognized: retrobulbar, in which the optic nerve head appears normal, and papillitis, in which the nerve head is swollen with nerve fiber layer hemorrhages. In contrast to papilledema, in optic neuritis visual acuity is decreased, and there is abnormal color perception, an afferent pupillary defect, and always a central scotoma. There may or may not be pain on moving the eye. If the retina is inflamed, the condition is called neuroretinitis. In children, optic neuritis may occur as a complication of the encephalomyelitis that follows an exanthem, or it may develop as part of acute meningitis. Multiple sclerosis may develop years later. A number of toxins, including lead, and drugs, including ethambutol and isoniazid, can cause optic neuritis. An ophthalmologist should be consulted in the case of any child with optic neuritis.

## Papilledema

Papilledema is optic disc swelling due to increased intracranial pressure (Fig 34-8). Several stages are differentiated ophthalmoscopically: early, with disc hyperemia, blurring of the disc margins, and mild disc swelling; fully developed, with more disc swelling, venous engorgement, splinter hemorrhages at the disc margins, and various amounts of exudate into the macular area; chronic, with persistence of disc elevation, resolution of hemorrhages, and the appearance of grayish exudates on the surface of the rounded disc; and postpapilledema atrophy, in which the disc becomes flat and atrophic and retinal vessels are attenuated.

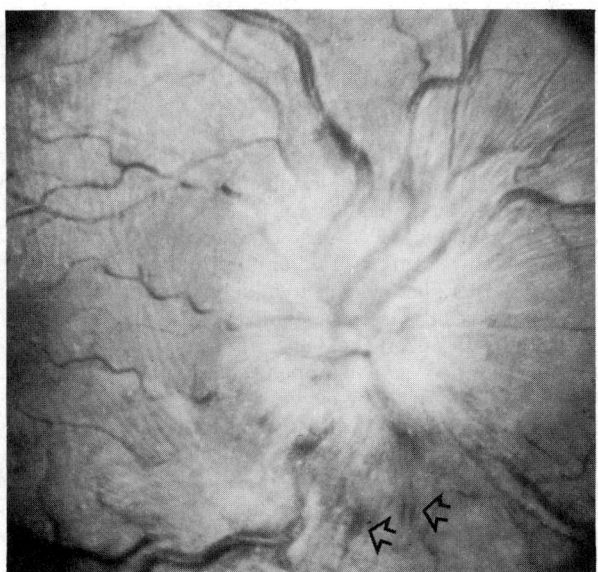

**Figure 34-8.** Papilledema. Notice the elevated disc, folds in the peripapillary retina, and the flame-shaped hemorrhages (*arrows*).

Papilledema may be simulated by several conditions, including high hyperopia, buried optic disc drusen, optic disc infiltration by tumor (eg, leukemia) or inflammation (eg, sarcoid), and primary optic disc tumors (eg, glioma, hamartoma, hemangioma). Neovascularization at the optic disc margin may be confused with papilledema.

Papilledema in children may be accompanied by headaches and nausea due to increased intracranial pressure. Vision is usually unimpaired, and visual fields show only an enlarged blind spot. There is no color vision defect and usually no afferent pupillary defect.

Chronic papilledema may be associated with visual field and acuity loss. Causes of papilledema include intracranial tumors, such as infratentorial lesions, subdural hematomas, brain abscesses, arteriovenous malformations, subarachnoid hemorrhage, and meningoencephalitis; rarely, papilledema is caused by a spinal cord tumor. Optic disc swelling is seen in the mucopolysaccharidoses, the craniostenoses, juvenile diabetes, and rarely, Guillain-Barré syndrome.

Papilledema in benign intracranial hypertension (ie, pseudotumor cerebri) is associated with increased intracranial pressure, normal or small ventricles, and normal cerebrospinal fluid. Symptoms of this condition include headache, disturbances of visual acuity, diplopia, nausea, dizziness, alterations of consciousness, and tinnitus. Pseudotumor cerebri is an isolated phenomenon in 50% of cases but may be associated with obstruction of cerebral venous drainage, endocrine and metabolic dysfunction, ingestion of certain drugs and toxins, and several systemic illnesses. Although this condition is thought of as benign, progressive visual field and acuity loss may result. Patients with intractable headaches or with evidence of optic neuropathy have been treated with various degrees of success by repeated lumbar punctures, dehydrating agents, steroids, shunting, and optic nerve sheath decompression.

## Retinal Detachment

Retinal detachment is rare in the pediatric population. Hereditary conditions featuring vitreoretinal degeneration and high myopia are associated with early onset of retinal detachment in some cases. These conditions include familial high myopia, the Stickler syndrome, Kniest dysplasia, spondyloepiphyseal dysplasia congenita, Ehlers-Danlos syndrome, and Marfan syndrome. Retinal detachment may complicate congenital ocular abnormalities, such as the morning glory disc anomaly, optic pits, and chorioretinal colobomas.

Symptoms of retinal detachment include sudden onset of floaters, flashes of light, and the appearance of a black veil in parts of the visual field. Early diagnosis and surgical correction are imperative, and patients with predisposing conditions should be examined at frequent intervals. Retinal breaks may be treated prophylactically. All children with signs or symptoms consistent with retinal detachment should be referred to an ophthalmologist.

## Selected Readings

Alfano JE. Ophthalmological aspects of neuroblastomatosis: a study of 53 verified cases. Trans Am Acad Ophthalmol Otolaryngol 1968;72:830.

Brown GC, Tasman WS. Congenital anomalies of the optic disc. New York: Grune & Stratton, 1983.

Committee for the Classification of Retinopathy of Prematurity. An international classification of retinopathy of prematurity. Arch Ophthalmol 1984;102:1130.

Committee on Practice and Ambulatory Medicine. Vision screening and eye examination in children. Pediatrics 1986;77:918.

Crawford JS. Pediatric ophthalmology and strabismus. Transactions of the New Orleans Academy of Ophthalmology. New York: Raven Press, 1986.

DeAngelis C. The eye. In: DeAngelis C, ed. Pediatric primary care, ed 3. Boston: Little, Brown, 1984:221.

DeLuise VP, Anderson DR. Primary infantile glaucoma (congenital glaucoma). Surv Ophthalmol 1983;28:1.

Dietz HC, Cutting GR, Pyeritz RE, et al. Marfan syndrome caused by a recurrent de novo missense mutation in the fibrillin gene. Nature 1991;352:337.

Drack AV, Traboulsi EI. Systemic associations of pigmentary retinopathy. Int Ophthalmol Clin 1991;:35.

Dryja TP, McGee TL, Hahn LB, et al. Mutations within the rhodopsin gene in patients with autosomal dominant retinitis pigmentosa. N Engl J Med 1990;323:1302.

Duane TD, ed. Clinical ophthalmology, vols 1–5. Hagerstown, MD: Harper & Row, 1985.

Fedukowicz HB. External infections of the eye, ed 3. New York: Appleton-Century-Crofts, 1985.

Font RL, Ferry AP. The phakomatoses. Int Ophthalmol Clin 1972;12:22.

Harley RD, ed. Pediatric ophthalmology, ed 2. Philadelphia: WB Saunders, 1983.

Heher K, Traboulsi EI, Maumenee IH. The natural history of Leber's congenital amaurosis. Age-related findings in 35 patients. Ophthalmology 1992;99:241.

Helveston EM. Atlas of strabismus surgery, ed 3. St. Louis: CV Mosby, 1983.

Hoskins HD, Shaffer RN, Hetherington J. Anatomical classification of the developmental glaucomas. Arch Ophthalmol 1984;102:1331.

International Committee for the Classification of the Late Stages of Retinopathy of Prematurity. An international classification of retinopathy of prematurity. II. The classification of retinal detachment. Arch Ophthalmol 1987;105:906.

Isenberg SJ. The eye in infancy. Chicago: Year Book Medical Publishers, 1989.

Kayser-Kupfer MI, Freidlin V, Datiles MB, et al. The association of posterior capsular lens opacities with bilateral acoustic neuromas in patients with neurofibromatosis type 2. Arch Ophthalmol 1989;107:541.

Kushner BJ. Congenital nasolacrimal system obstruction. Arch Ophthalmol 1982;100:597.

Lambert SR, Hoyt CS, Narahara MH. Optic nerve hypoplasia. Surv Ophthalmol 1987;32:1.

Lavery MA, O'Neill JF, Chu FC, et al. Acquired nystagmus in early childhood: a presenting sign of intracranial tumor. Ophthalmology 1984;91:425.

Lewis RA, Riccardi VM. Von Recklinghausen neurofibromatosis: incidence of iris hamartomata. Ophthalmology 1981;88:348.

Ludwig S, Warman M. Shaken baby syndrome: a review of 20 cases. Ann Emerg Med 1984;13:104.

Maumenee IH. The eye in the Marfan syndrome. Trans Am Ophthalmol Soc 1981;79:684.

Mottow LS, Jakobiec FA. Idiopathic inflammatory orbital pseudotumor in childhood. I. Clinical characteristics. Arch Ophthalmol 1978;96:1410.

Mottow-Lippa L, Jakobiec FA, Smith M. Idiopathic orbital pseudotumor in childhood. II. Results of diagnostic tests and biopsies. Ophthalmology 1981;88:565.

Nicholson DH. Cytomegalovirus infection of the retina. Int Ophthalmol Clin 1975;15:151.

Pagon RA. Ocular coloboma. Surv Ophthalmol 1981;25:223.

Palmberg P, Smith M, Watman S, et al. The natural history of retinopathy in insulin-dependent juvenile onset diabetes. Ophthalmology 1981;88:613.

Peterson RA, Robb RM. The natural history of congenital obstruction of the nasolacrimal duct. J Pediatr Ophthalmol Strabismus 1978;15:246.

Renie WA, ed. Goldberg's genetic and metabolic eye disease, ed 2. Boston: Little, Brown, 1986.

Ridgway E, Jaffe N, Walton DS. Leukemic ophthalmology in children. Cancer 1976;38:1744.

Ridley ME, Shields JA, Brown GC, et al. Coats' disease: evaluation and management. Ophthalmology 1982;89:1381.

Schlaegel TF. Ocular toxoplasmosis and pars planitis. New York: Grune & Stratton, 1978.

Shields JA. Diagnosis and management of intraocular tumors. St. Louis: CV Mosby, 1983.

Shields JA, Augsburger JJ. Current approaches to the diagnosis and management of retinoblastoma. Surv Ophthalmol 1981;25:347.

Spencer WH. Ophthalmic pathology: an atlas and textbook, ed 3. Philadelphia: WB Saunders, 1985.

Stern J, Jakobiec FA, Housepian EM. The architecture of optic nerve gliomas with and without neurofibromatosis. Arch Ophthalmol 1980;98:505.

Traboulsi EI, Maumenee IH. Peters' anomaly and associated congenital malformations. Arch Ophthalmol 1992; (in press).

Traboulsi EI, Shammas IV, Massad M, et al. Ophthalmological aspects of metastatic neuroblastoma: report of 22 consecutive cases. Orbit 1984;4:247.

von Noorden GK. Burian-von-Noorden binocular vision and ocular motility: theory and management of strabismus, ed 3. St. Louis: CV Mosby, 1985.

Walton DS. Primary congenital open angle glaucoma: a study of the anterior segment abnormalities. Trans Am Ophthalmol Soc 1979;77:746.

Wolff SM. The ocular manifestations of congenital rubella. J Pediatr Ophthalmol 1973;10:101.

Wright JE, McDonald WI, Call NB. Management of optic nerve gliomas. Br J Ophthalmol 1980;64:545.

*Principles and Practice of Pediatrics, Second Edition.*
edited by Frank A. Oski et al. J. B. Lippincott Company, Philadelphia © 1994.

# CHAPTER 35
# *Pediatric Dermatology*

## Walter W. Tunnessen, Jr.

Skin complaints are common reasons for children to visit physicians. A survey performed in a pediatric clinic setting indicated that 12.8% of primary and 11.2% of secondary concerns prompting clinic visits were related to the skin. Because of the volume of skin-related problems, it is incumbent on physicians who care for children to gain some facility in recognizing and managing the most common cutaneous disorders.

Dermatology is a visual specialty. With experience, most of the common problems affecting children's skin can be recognized, including the subtle variations in presentation. For uncommon cutaneous problems, atlases, texts, or other sources can be used to aid in identification. As in most medical specialties, an organized approach to the problem is most helpful in leading to the correct diagnosis.

This chapter is designed to assist the reader in the diagnosis of skin problems. The approach is based on morphologic appearance. If physicians can describe what they see, they already may have conquered a major obstacle to diagnosis. Physicians often rely simply on pattern recognition to make dermatologic diagnoses. Although that approach can be partially successful, a more comprehensive, descriptive evaluation of lesions is needed.

Describing cutaneous lesions is not as easy as it sounds. Practice in using descriptive terminology is the key to success. The sections of this chapter are based primarily on lesion morphology. The first step in an organized approach to skin lesions is to define the descriptors.

A *macule* is a circumscribed area of change in normal skin color without elevation or depression of the skin surface; macules generally are less than 1 cm in diameter. A *patch* is a large macule, greater than 1 cm in diameter. *Papules* are solid, elevated, palpable lesions less than 0.5 cm in diameter; *nodules* are larger papules that can lie in the epidermis or in the dermis or subcutaneous tissues. *Plaques* are elevated lesions, formed most frequently by the confluence of papules.

A *vesicle* is a fluid-filled blister less than 0.5 cm in diameter; a *bulla* is a blister that is greater than 0.5 cm in diameter. A *pustule* is a blister filled with cellular debris, generally white blood cells, which gives the lesion a white or yellowish color. A *wheal* is the result of localized edema in the skin. It is pink or pale and usually is rounded or flat-topped, sometimes with irregularly shaped margins. Wheals are evanescent, lasting less than 24 hours in any one place. They are associated almost invariably with pruritus.

*Telangiectases* are permanent superficial dilations of venules, capillaries, or arterioles that may or may not blanch with pressure. *Lichenification* is a thickening of the skin in which the normal skin markings usually are accentuated; prolonged rubbing or scratching of the skin is necessary to produce this change. *Crusts* are accumulations of dried serum, blood, pus, or other exudative materials on the surface of the skin. *Scales* are flakes of skin, either loose or adherent, that are composed of compact keratin. An area of *sclerosis* is one that feels indurated or thickened and has lost its normal elasticity. The surface coloration may show hyperpigmentation, hypopigmentation, or both. Normal skin appendages (ie, hair and sweat glands) are absent from the sclerotic area.

An *erosion* is a superficial loss of epidermis that has a moist base; an *ulcer* is a deeper lesion, extending into the dermis and sometimes below it. *Atrophy* of the skin produces a depression in the skin surface. If the epidermis is atrophic, the skin appears thin and translucent, and it wrinkles when the edges of the affected area are pinched.

In addition to the types of morphologic changes described above, the pattern the lesions form on the skin should be noted. Lesions may be arranged in lines, as are the linear vesicles seen in poison ivy dermatitis; they also may be grouped, as are the vesicles observed in herpes simplex, or dermatomal as in herpes zoster. The distribution of the lesions also should be noted. For instance, seborrheic dermatitis commonly involves not only the scalp, but the eyebrows and nasolabial folds as well. Psoriasis often affects areas that are traumatized, such as the elbows and knees. Pityriasis rosea presents as ovoid, slightly scaly lesions in a pine bough distribution, particularly over the back. Acne occurs almost exclusively on the face, shoulders, back, and chest.

The headings of most of the sections that follow are morphologic descriptors of cutaneous lesions. The most common dermatologic conditions are covered in these sections, with the emphasis placed on clinical appearance, differentiation from other lesions, and suggestions for management.

## SKIN LESIONS IN THE NEONATAL PERIOD

### Pigmented Macular Lesions

#### Mongolian Spots

Mongolian spots is an unfortunate name for this common, benign skin discoloration. Present at birth, mongolian spots are blue-gray or blue-green in color and represent areas of dermal melanocytosis. They occur most frequently in the lumbosacral area (Fig 35-1) and over the shoulders. Occasionally, they are found on the anterior trunk and extremities; only rarely are they seen on the face. The occurrence of mongolian spots is related to the

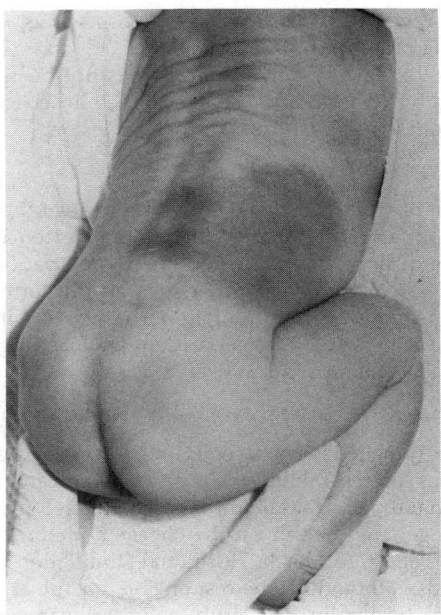

**Figure 35-1.** The blue-gray hyperpigmentation of mongolian spots is most common over the buttocks and back.

degree of natural pigment. The more pigment infants have, the more likely they are to have these spots. More than 90% of blacks and Asians have mongolian spots, whereas less than 10% of whites have them. Infants of Hispanic and Mediterranean heritage are more likely to have the spots than are infants of northern European ancestry.

Although these lesions tend to disappear with time, usually by the age of 4 to 5 years, the color change persists in 5% of children. Because mongolian spots have been mistaken for bruises associated with child abuse, it is important to educate parents and nursery or day-care workers regarding the congenital nature of the patches. The cause of these collections of melanocytes deep in the dermis is unknown. Because the spots are benign, no therapy is necessary. Malignant degeneration has not been reported.

### Nevi of Ota

A nevus of Ota is an uncommon, ill-defined, blue-gray to blue-black patch of pigmentation that occurs on the skin of the face, usually in the distribution of the second and third branches of the trigeminal nerve. About two thirds of affected infants have an associated bluish discoloration of the sclera of the eye on the same side. Although they are most common in Asians, the lesions may occur in blacks. About half are congenital; the rest appear later, often during the second decade of life. Histologically, this dermal patch is identical to the mongolian spot. Unlike the latter, however, it does not undergo spontaneous regression. Rare cases of glaucoma of the eye and malignant degeneration of the melanocytes have been reported.

### Nevi of Ito

A similar patch of hyperpigmentation occurring over the shoulders, in the supraclavicular areas, and on the sides of the neck, the upper arms, and the scapulae is known as the nevus of Ito. These patches also persist. Cosmetic cover-up is the recommended therapy.

### Café au Lait Spots

Café au lait spots are macules of various shapes and sizes. Their color ranges from light to dark brown, the pigmentation is even throughout, and the margins are defined sharply. In a cohort of 4641 newborns, 1.9% of black and 0.3% of white infants had at least one of these lesions. Black infants were more likely to have more than one lesion: 0.6% had two and 0.2% had three or more. None of the white infants had more than one lesion. Multiple café au lait spots are associated with neurofibromatosis; they also can be seen in other syndromes. (See the section on changes in pigmentation later in this chapter.)

## Macular Vascular Birthmarks

### Flame Nevi

Flame nevi are the most common vascular lesions in infancy, seen in almost half of all newborns. These dull pink macules composed of distended dermal capillaries are most prevalent over the eyelids and forehead. Almost all infants with lesions on the face also have lesions on the nape of the neck and on the occiput. Facial lesions tend to fade with time, generally within the first years of life. Neck lesions, however, are likely to persist. The macules often are called salmon patches, stork bites, or angel kisses. During crying, older infants and children may demonstrate flushing in areas of previous lesions that have faded.

### Port-Wine Stains

The benign flame nevus described above must be differentiated from the port-wine stain, which is a congenital vascular malformation composed of mature vessels. Port-wine stains are reddish or reddish purple, they are darker than flame nevi, and they may occur anywhere on the body, although they are seen most commonly on the face. If the skin corresponding to the first branch of the trigeminal nerve is involved, the stain may be associated with an angiomatosis of the leptomeninges on the same side, creating the Sturge-Weber syndrome (described later in this chapter). Treatment for port-wine stains during childhood consists simply of the use of cosmetic coverings. Tunable dye laser beam therapy performed early in childhood offers the most effective means of obliterating these lesions.

### Melanocytic Nevi

Histologically proven congenital melanocytic nevi are present in about 1% of newborns, although four times that many have lesions resembling melanocytic nevi (see Color Figure 1). Most of the nevi are small, well defined, and flat. Considerable controversy surrounds their management. Some specialists advocate removing all congenital nevi, regardless of their size, whereas others recommend removing only those greater than 20 cm in diameter. The risk of malignant melanoma developing in a large lesion is estimated to be between 6% and 7% over the child's lifetime. Unfortunately, not all the melanomas arise from cutaneous sites. Furthermore, the size and distribution of the nevus may make surgical removal difficult and disfiguring. The best means of managing large nevi must be decided on an individual basis. Unfortunately, there are no longitudinal data regarding the natural history of congenital nevi.

## Hypopigmented Macules

Macules or patches of depigmented skin in the newborn may signify the presence of underlying problems. Small hypopigmented macules are an early cutaneous sign of tuberous sclerosis, an autosomal dominantly inherited condition associated with seizures and mental retardation, among other things. Large patches or swirls of depigmentation may indicate the presence of Ito syndrome, a neurocutaneous disorder that affects various bodily systems, including the central nervous system and the bones. Infants with piebaldism, who usually have depigmentation of the skin of the forehead and other areas, also may have associated abnormalities, including deafness. Most hypopigmented lesions probably represent a simple absence of pigment, known as a nevus depigmentosus.

## Harlequin Color Change

Harlequin color change is a curious phenomenon usually noted in the first few days of life in low–birth-weight infants (see Color Figure 17). When they are placed on their sides, a sharp midline demarcation develops in the color of these infants' bodies, with the upper half turning pale and the lower half turning deep red. A change in position results in resolution of the color change. The phenomenon can last for a few weeks and is attributed to a temporary imbalance in the regulatory mechanisms of the autonomic nervous system.

## Papules and Vesicles

### Milia

Multiple 1- to 2-mm yellowish-white cystic lesions, known as milia, occur in about 40% of newborns. These lesions are found most commonly over the cheeks, forehead, nose, and nasolabial folds (Fig 35-2). Much less commonly, they may be found on the trunk or extremities. Histologically, the cysts are composed of keratin and are similar to Epstein's pearls, the whitish papules noted on the palates of many newborns. Treatment is unnecessary; the cysts disappear in the first few weeks of life.

### Erythema Toxicum

The erythematous macules, papules, and, sometimes, vesicles of erythema toxicum (see Color Figure 9) occur in at least half of full-term newborns; they are less common in premature infants. Generally, the lesions appear between the first 24 and 48 hours of life, and are described best as resembling flea bites. The individual lesions tend to last less than 24 hours, but new lesions can appear during the first 2 weeks of life and, occasionally, later. It may be difficult clinically to separate the lesions of erythema toxicum from those of more ominous conditions, such as staphylococcal pustulosis or herpes simplex. Identification of large patches of macular erythema surrounding the lesions is one way to recognize erythema toxicum; however, a more reliable method is to scrape the lesions and stain the contents with Wright's stain,

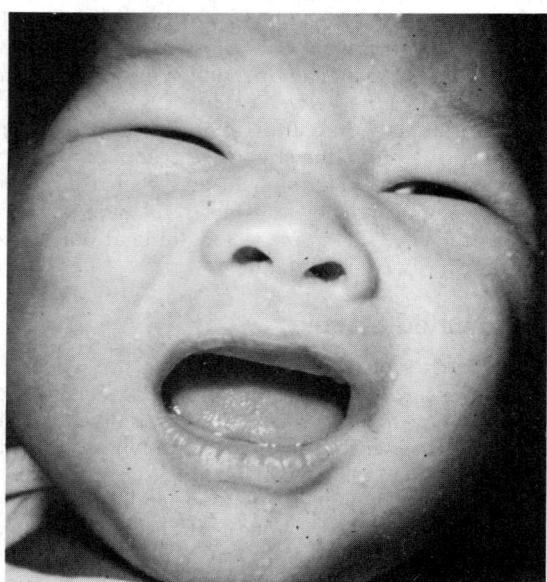

Figure 35-2.   Milia on the face of a newborn.

which will reveal the predominance of eosinophils. A peripheral eosinophilia often is present as well.

The etiology of erythema toxicum has not been elucidated. Histologically, the lesions are related to the pilosebaceous orifice. No treatment is necessary for this benign lesion.

### Sebaceous Gland Hypertrophy

Stimulation of the sebaceous glands, which lie at the base of the pilosebaceous units, by maternal hormones often leads to the appearance of tiny, yellowish to flesh-colored papules over the face and, less commonly, at other sites on full-term newborns. Because the source of the stimulation is removed with birth, the appearance of these papules is transient and clearing occurs in a few weeks. No therapy is necessary.

### Neonatal Acne

Comedones (plugged pilosebaceous units), erythematous papules, and pustules, all resembling the acne of adolescents, may occur in the neonatal period. Male infants are affected primarily, and the lesions generally occur on the cheeks and almost never are seen on the chest and back. Hormonal stimulation of the sebaceous glands is thought to be responsible for the appearance of the lesions. Generally, the eruption disappears in weeks or months, and no therapy is required. Occasionally, in severe or prolonged cases, a mild keratolytic agent, such as 2½% benzoyl peroxide, can be prescribed.

### Transient Neonatal Pustular Melanosis

Transient neonatal pustular melanosis is a relatively common neonatal dermatosis that was not described until 1976. The lesions, which consist of vesicopustules, ruptured vesicopustules with a collarette of scale, and small pigmented macules in the sites of previous lesions, occur in 4% to 5% of black infants and in less than 1% of white infants. The face, chin, neck, and shoulders are the most commonly affected sites. If vesicopustules are present, they disappear rapidly within 1 to 2 days. In contrast, the pigmented macules may take weeks or even months to fade. The pustules are 1 to 3 mm in diameter, usually are flaccid, and have no surrounding erythema (see Color Figure 10). Most have very little content on rupturing, including perhaps a few neutrophils. The cause of this disorder is unknown, but it appears to be an entirely benign condition. A simple Gram's stain of the contents of a pustular lesion should prove most helpful in differentiating transient neonatal pustular melanosis from bacterial pustulosis. No therapy is necessary.

### Miliaria

Miliaria crystallina are tiny, teardrop-like, clear, fragile vesicles caused by plugged sweat ducts. They may appear shortly after birth (particularly on the forehead), have no surrounding erythema, and disappear rapidly without intervention. Miliaria rubra, in contrast, are associated with surrounding erythema as a result of extravasation of sweat into the epidermis causing localized inflammation. Young infants seem particularly prone to miliaria, perhaps in part because of parental concern about keeping them warm. The face, neck, shoulders, and diaper area are most likely to be affected. Therapy consists of removing excessive clothing and lowering the level of humidity.

### Neonatal Impetigo

The appearance of pustules or pus-filled bullae suggestive of staphylococcal infection is cause for concern. Impetigo may occur after the first few days of life, but it generally begins to appear only in the second or third week. The individual lesions have a small rim of erythema. The bullae rupture easily, leaving a raw, moist base, which turns into dried lesions with rings of scale. Fresh lesions should be aspirated for culture and Gram's stain if impetigo is suspected or if there is difficulty in differentiating these lesions from some of the benign ones already discussed.

Impetigo requires treatment with systemic antibiotics to prevent secondary infections such as pneumonia or osteomyelitis. Affected infants must be observed carefully and should be hospitalized for treatment if there is any question about their health. The newborn nursery of origin should be notified of the problem, and the occurrence of more than one case in a single nursery should lead to a review of that nursery's procedures for handling infants.

Certain staphylococci produce exotoxins that may lead to the scalded skin syndrome, a generalized erythema that leads to separation of the skin, often in sheets. Fluid loss and thermal instability in affected infants can lead to serious complications and even death. Less commonly, streptococci may gain a foothold in the infant's skin and produce localized impetigo or cellulitis, including erysipelas, which is a rapidly spreading cellulitis with systemic toxicity.

### Congenital Cutaneous Candidiasis

Congenital cutaneous candidiasis is uncommon, despite the frequency of maternal vaginal candidiasis. The lesions are intensely erythematous macules, papules, and vesicles that rapidly become pustular and are present at birth or appear shortly thereafter. Examination of a scraping of the lesions should reveal the budding hyphae and pseudo-hyphae of *Candida*. To be present on the first day of life, the infection must have occurred in utero. More commonly, infants come into contact with *Candida* during passage through the birth canal and the typical intertriginous lesions develop a few weeks later. Interestingly, oral thrush usually is not present in congenital infections. Congenital cutaneous candidiasis dries quickly, and the skin undergoes desquamation within the first week of life with no therapy. *Candida* acquired on passage through the birth canal usually requires topical therapy for rapid resolution.

### Herpes Simplex

Vesicular lesions, whether they are grouped, as is typical in herpes infections, or scattered, as sometimes occurs in the neonatal period, always should suggest the possibility of acquired herpes simplex infection (see Color Figure 24). Because untreated neonatal infections with herpes can be devastating, surveillance for vesicular lesions should continue throughout the neonatal period. Unfortunately, the majority of infants in whom herpes infections develop are born to mothers who are unaware of their own infection with genital herpes. Infection usually is acquired during passage through the infected birth canal, although ascending infection, particularly in association with premature rupture of the amniotic membranes, also is recognized.

The mean age at onset of herpetic lesions is 6 days, although they can appear any time between birth and the age of 3 to 4 weeks. The initial lesion is an erythematous macule that develops into a vesicle. The presenting parts of the infant at delivery, as well as the scalp at the site where the monitoring electrodes were attached, are the most common sites at which the initial herpetic lesions appear (see Color Figure 25). The initial lesions occasionally resemble erosions.

The importance of immediate diagnosis of herpes simplex cannot be emphasized too strongly. Suspicious lesions should be cultured for herpesvirus, and the base of the lesions should be scraped and stained with Giemsa stain to reveal multinucleated giant cells indicative of the herpes group of viruses (Tzanck preparation). Parenteral antiviral therapy should be administered without delay. The risk of neonatal herpes is estimated to be 50% if the infant is delivered vaginally of a mother with a primary herpetic infection; it is less than 5% if the maternal lesions are recurrent.

### Congenital Varicella

Scattered vesicular lesions also may indicate the presence of varicella acquired in utero. Usually, the maternal history is positive for the disease. The lesions in neonates are similar to those seen in older infants and children, with crops of macules and papules developing into teardrop-like vesicles. A Tzanck preparation of the base of a vesicle will demonstrate the multinucleated giant cells that are characteristic of herpesvirus infections.

Infants in whom lesions develop between the fifth and tenth days of life have a 20% to 30% mortality rate. Those born with lesions and those in whom lesions develop before 5 days of age do much better.

### Incontinentia Pigmenti

Incontinentia pigmenti is a rare genodermatosis commonly manifested in the neonatal period by linear papules and vesicles (Fig 35-3; also see Color Figure 11). The presence of linear lesions in the newborn always should raise the suspicion of a neurocutaneous disorder. These lesions often are mistaken for infections, particularly because pustules and some crusting may occur. Wright's stain performed on the vesicular fluid will reveal eosinophils, and peripheral blood eosinophilia is present in the majority of affected infants. Ninety-seven percent of infants with this disorder are female. Because incontinentia pigmenti is X-linked dominant, the family history may reveal similar lesions. The vesicles disappear in weeks or months. Verrucous lesions often develop after the vesicles, or they may be the initial lesions. Eventually, the verrucous lesions disappear, followed by linear hyperpigmented streaks, bands, or swirls. A host of systemic defects can occur in this disorder, including seizures, bony abnormalities, and eye lesions.

## Bullous Lesions

### Sucking Blisters

Infants commonly suck their hands or fingers in utero. Occasionally, a thick-walled bullous lesion on the dorsum of the hand will result (Fig 35-4). The most helpful clue to this diagnosis is observation of the infant sucking the involved area of skin after birth.

### Epidermolysis Bullosa Congenita

Newborns affected by the group of hereditary disorders that cause fragile skin often have bullae or erosions as a result of the trauma associated with birth or minimal trauma induced by handling

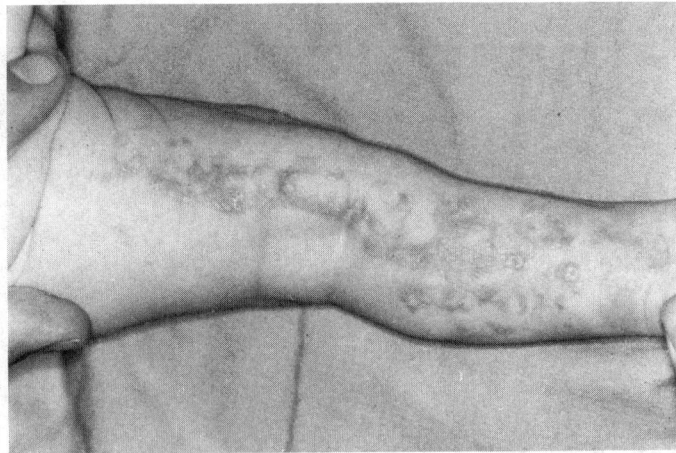

**Figure 35-3.** Papulovesicular lesions of incontinentia pigmenti in a linear distribution on the flexor surface of one leg.

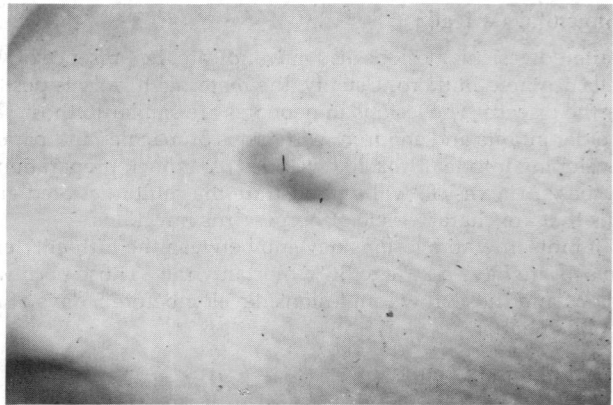

**Figure 35-4.** A solitary bullous lesion, due to sucking in utero, on the dorsum of a newborn's hand.

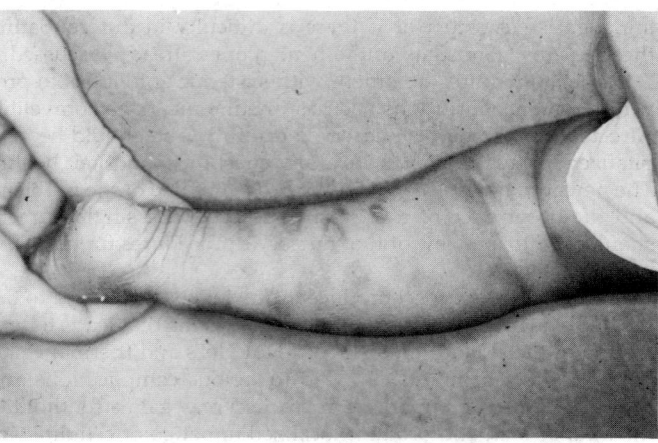

**Figure 35-5.** Ovoid, brownish lesions with a fine scale on the leg of a neonate with congenital syphilis.

and care after birth (see Color Figure 15). These disorders are discussed more completely later in this chapter.

### Congenital Syphilis

Bullae are an unusual presentation of congenital syphilis (see Color Figure 26). Most common on the extremities, they rupture rapidly, leaving a raw, oozing surface. Ovoid, macular, slightly scaly, salmon-colored lesions are much more common; they generally appear between the age of 2 and 6 weeks (Fig 35-5).

## Purpuric Lesions

Hemorrhagic lesions may occur on the skin of newborns for a variety of reasons. Infectious causes always should be considered, including bacteria and congenitally acquired infections.

### Congenital Rubella

Purpuric lesions of infants infected with rubella virus in utero are caused most commonly by thrombocytopenia. On occasion, the purpuric lesions take on an infiltrative or nodular quality, producing a "blueberry muffin" appearance (Fig 35-6). The lesions actually are areas of extramedullary hematopoiesis rather than true cutaneous hemorrhage.

### Congenital Cytomegalovirus Infection

Petechial lesions in conjunction with intrauterine growth retardation, hepatosplenomegaly, and hyperbilirubinemia always should raise the question of congenital infections. Cytomegalo-

virus is the most prevalent of these infections. Most of the purpuric lesions are the result of thrombocytopenia. Blueberry muffin-like lesions (see Color Figure 22) also have been documented.

## Lumps and Indurations

### Subcutaneous Fat Necrosis

Irregular lumps and bumps may occur in the subcutaneous tissue of neonates, probably as a result of pressure or trauma associated with the birth process. The areas most commonly affected are the cheeks, buttocks, back, arms, and thighs. The areas are irregular, hard, erythematous, or violaceous, and they seem nontender. The size of the lumps is variable. Occasionally, the lesions may become calcified, but generally they resolve spontaneously in 1 to 2 months without scarring. These lesions occur much less commonly later in life. No therapy is necessary.

### Sebaceous Nevi

The most common sebaceous nevus (nevus of Jadassohn) is found on the scalp of newborns (see Color Figure 3). The area is devoid of hair, slightly raised, smooth, and yellow to yellow-orange. The lesions vary in size and can be found on the face as well (Fig 35-7). Rarely, central nervous system lesions are associated with this nevus. The tissue is composed of an increased number of sebaceous glands. Removal before puberty is recommended, because the area becomes more verrucous with age and has a significant risk of neoplastic degeneration.

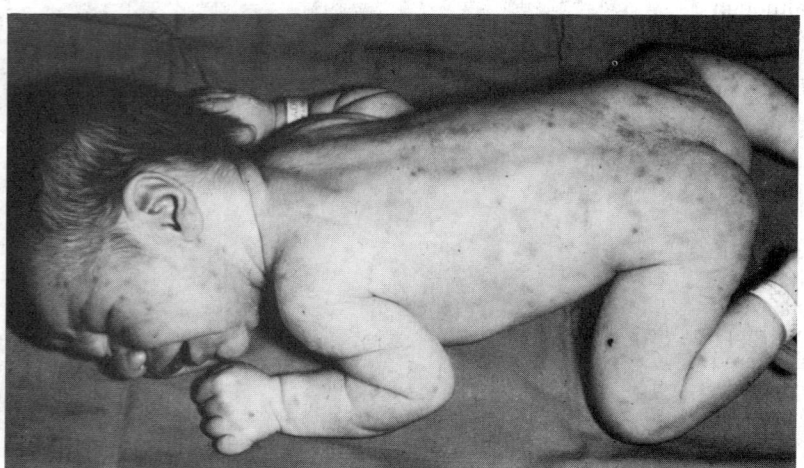

**Figure 35-6.** Diffuse, purplish papules and nodules create a "blueberry muffin" appearance in an infant with congenital rubella.

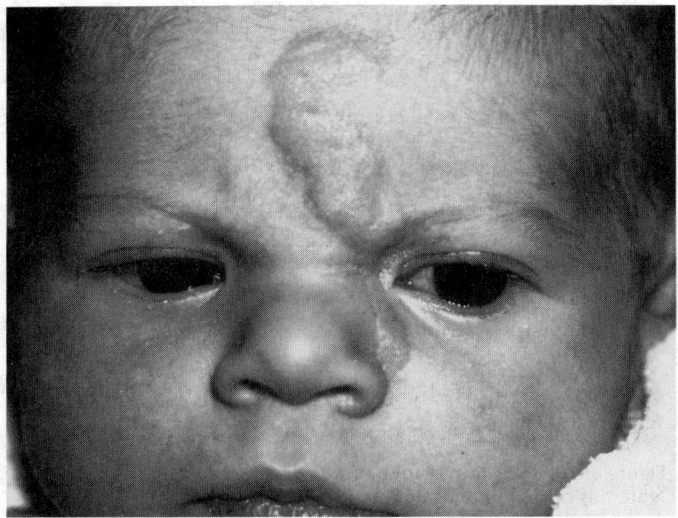

**Figure 35-7.** A tan-yellow plaque of nevus sebaceus on the forehead. (courtesy of P.J. Honig, M.D., The Children's Hospital of Philadelphia)

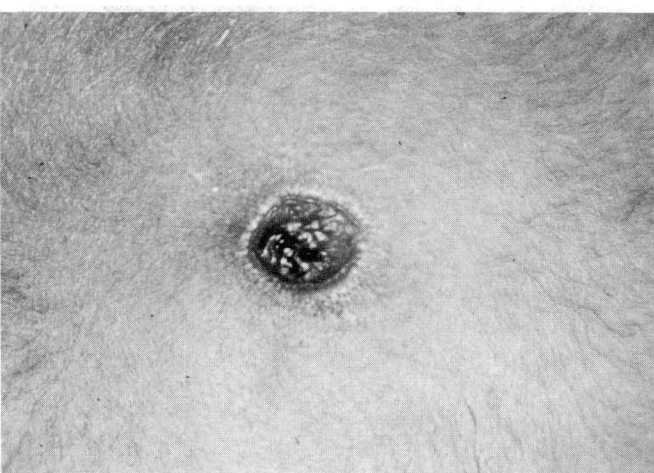

**Figure 35-8.** A discrete, punched-out lesion of aplasia cutis congenita on the scalp of a newborn.

### Epidermal Nevi

Verrucous-appearing, flesh-colored or pigmented lesions may occur in the neonatal period. Linear lesions may indicate a neurocutaneous disorder with central nervous system, eye, and skeletal abnormalities; this disorder is discussed in the section regarding linear lesions that appears later in this chapter.

### Sclerema Neonatorum

Sclerema neonatorum is an uncommon, rapidly spreading thickening of the subcutaneous tissue that occurs in preterm or ill infants during the first few weeks of life. The skin becomes tight-fitting, shiny, and non-pitting. Affected infants usually are seriously ill with other problems and rarely survive once this condition appears.

## Ulcers

Aplasia cutis congenita is a congenital condition characterized by punched-out, usually solitary ulcers that occur randomly and are not associated with malformation syndromes such as trisomy 13. The lesions may be deep or superficial, usually are 1 to 3 cm in diameter, and resemble ulcerated open wounds (Fig 35-8). Occasionally, they appear as well-healed atrophic scars. Hair will not grow in these lesions.

## PAPULAR DISORDERS

### Warts*

Warts are among the most common skin lesions affecting children; they also are among the most frustrating, because they often are difficult to treat and control. Warts are caused by infections with human papillomaviruses, DNA viruses of which at least 15 different types have been described. Each type of human papillomavirus usually can be related to a specific clinical presentation of the wart. The highest incidence of these infections occurs in the second decade of life. Untreated warts generally have a lifespan of a few months to 5 years or more. About two thirds disappear within 2 years, but self-inoculation and spread to other persons may occur.

* Gail Demmler, M.D., contributed to this section.

### Verrucae Vulgaris

The common wart is recognized by most laypersons without difficulty. The surface of the wart is rough, sometimes lumpy, and usually flesh-colored. Occasional lesions, particularly those on the face and scalp, may be linear or have finger-like projections. The lesions usually are round, and tiny dark specks frequently can be seen through the surface. These dots often are referred to as the seed of the wart, but they merely represent thrombosed capillaries in the warty tissue.

### Plantar Warts

When warts occur on the plantar surface, pressure forces their growth inward, resulting in deep, painful lesions. Plantar warts may be single, scattered, or grouped together in clusters. The black specks of thrombosed capillaries help distinguish warts from corns, which are localized areas of hyperkeratosis over pressure points.

### Flat Warts

Flat warts are tiny, flat-topped, flesh-colored papules that occur primarily on the face and dorsa of the hands and forearms. Their surface is smooth, and they may number in the hundreds. At times, they seem to form plaques as they coalesce.

### Condylomata Acuminata

Genital warts tend to be soft, flesh-colored to slightly pigmented, and papular or pedunculated (Fig 35-9). The occurrence of genital warts in children always should raise the suspicion of sexual abuse; viral typing by molecular hybridization examinations has revealed that these lesions are of the same type as those affecting adults. In children under 2 years of age, the condition may be the result simply of their having passed through a birth canal that is infected with papillomavirus. It is estimated that one third or fewer of the venereal warts seen in children are the result of sexual abuse.

### Treatment of Warts

When multiple therapies are recommended for a disorder, it is unlikely that treatment will yield excellent results. Such is the case with warts. Some clinicians use benign neglect, because warts have a finite lifespan. Parents and older children often desire treatment, so primary care physicians should be able to make some recommendations. For common warts, keratolytic agents such as salicylic and lactic acids in flexible collodion offer painless and effective, albeit slow-acting, therapy. It is extremely important

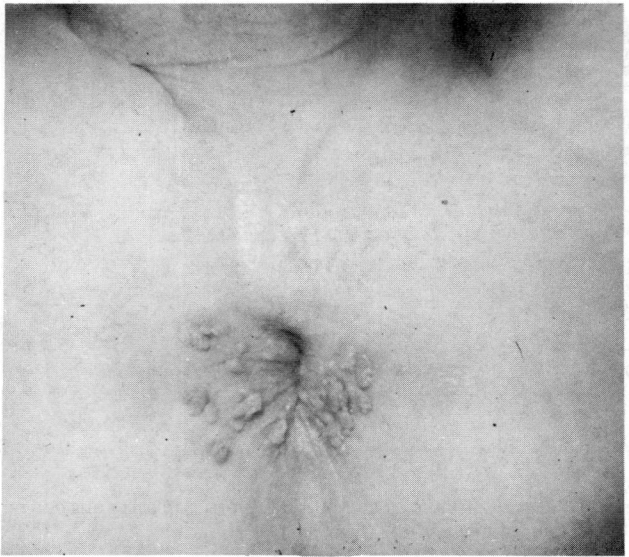

**Figure 35-9.** Flesh-colored papules of condylomata acuminata in the anal verge.

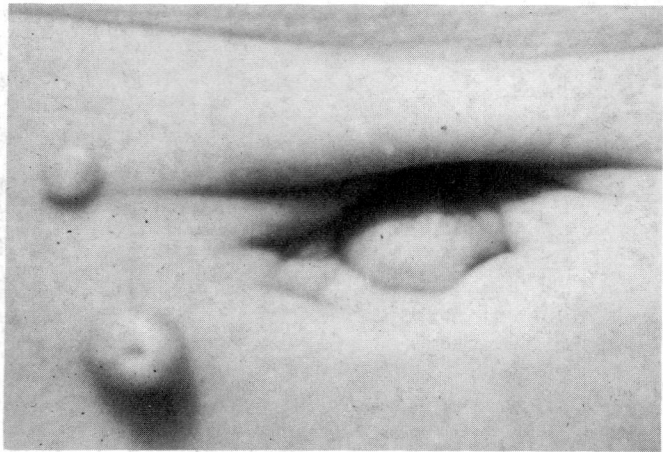

**Figure 35-10.** Pearly molluscum contagiosum papules on the abdomen. Note the central umbilication of the larger lesion.

to soak the warts in warm water for 10 to 20 minutes before "sanding" down the lesions with a pumice stone or an emery board and applying the keratolytic agent daily. Covering the wart with tape also seems to increase the effectiveness of the treatment. The application of liquid nitrogen and use of electrocautery are similarly effective, but these treatments are painful, particularly for small children. Plantar warts can be treated with higher-potency keratolytic agents that are applied after soaking and "sanding down." In resistant warts, cantharidin, a blistering agent, can be applied carefully to enhance removal.

Flat warts are tiny and are scattered over wider areas. Retinoic acid A or salicylic acid may be applied lightly on a daily basis over the areas involved. Genital warts often respond to the weekly application of podophyllin in a tincture of benzoin base, which is washed off after 3 to 4 hours, but referral for removal by laser therapy often is necessary.

The success of the various therapies is said to be 70%. Therefore, more than one therapeutic approach may be necessary for each wart.

## Molluscum Contagiosum*

Lesions of molluscum contagiosum, which are caused by a DNA pox virus, are described best as pearly papules. Their size may vary from that of a pinhead to more than 1 cm in diameter. The top of the lesion is almost translucent, often revealing a whitish core known as the molluscum body. Larger lesions may have a central umbilication (Fig 35-10). The number of papules present may vary from few to hundreds. Spread by autoinoculation is common; other members of the family also can become infected through contact with the affected person. The diagnosis may not be readily apparent on the basis of clinical examination alone; it may require opening of a lesion with a large-bore needle and extraction of the molluscum body.

Although some physicians recommend no treatment, the lesions have a lifespan of months to years, and parents frequently insist that something be done. If there are only a few lesions, they can be picked off or excised with a curet. Cantharidin, applied carefully in small amounts to each lesion, is effective in causing blistering and extrusion of the central core. This potent medication should be applied only by physicians or other trained personnel.

* Gail Demmler, M.D., contributed to this section.
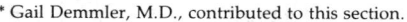

Liquid nitrogen and podophyllin also have been used. Individuals with atopic dermatitis are prone to the development of widespread lesions.

## Pityriasis Rosea

Although pityriasis rosea does not seem to fit neatly into the category of papular lesions, it is a papulosquamous disorder, consisting of oval lesions composed of tiny papules with a fine scale. At times, individual papular lesions may be prominent. The presence of a myriad of individual papules occasionally confuses the diagnosis by making the ovoid lesions less noticeable (Fig 35-11). The cause of pityriasis rosea is unknown, but is believed by many to be viral. The disorder occurs most commonly in teenagers and young adults, but has been described in infants. Recurrent episodes are not rare, and small epidemics have been reported among individuals in close contact.

The name *pityriasis rosea* means "rose-colored scale." The herald patch is a single, papular, erythematous lesion that enlarges over 1 to 2 days. It may precede the appearance of the more extensive rash, or it may not appear at all; its reported prevalence has varied in different series from 12% to 94%. At times, this raised lesion may be mistaken for tinea corporis. The interval between the appearance of the herald patch and the more generalized eruption is 1 to 2 weeks.

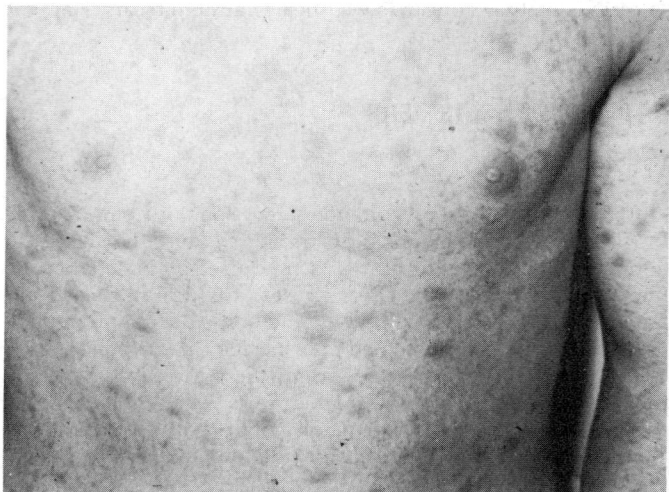

**Figure 35-11.** Pityriasis rosea. The diffuse erythematous papules may obscure the classic lesions, which are scattered, ovoid, pink plaques.

The typical ovoid lesions of pityriasis rosea have their longest axis along skin tension lines; thus, their distribution on the patient's back gives the appearance of the boughs of a pine tree. It often is helpful to view the child's rash from across the room to see the characteristic pattern. Individual lesions may have a pinkish to brownish color. Most lesions are covered by a fine, wrinkled scale (Fig 35-12).

The lengthy course of this disorder should be emphasized to the patient or the parents. The eruption itself develops over a 2-week period, persists for 2 weeks, and then fades over another 2 weeks. There is great variability in this pattern, however, and rashes lasting 3 to 4 months are not unusual. The lesions generally are distributed on the trunk, but a "reverse" distribution also can be seen, with lesions appearing primarily on the face and proximal extremities. Occasionally, the lesions may have urticarial, bullous, or even purpuric tendencies. Pruritus is one of the most annoying features of pityriasis rosea, occurring in up to half of the cases. Treatment with an emollient containing menthol and phenol is helpful. No therapy will shorten the course of the eruption.

The differential diagnosis includes dry nummular eczema and nummular dry skin. Because secondary syphilis can have a similar appearance, a serologic test for syphilis should be considered if the patient is in a sexually active age group. The histologic appearance of a skin biopsy specimen of pityriasis rosea lesions is nonspecific.

## Keratosis Pilaris

Keratosis pilaris is a common, benign skin condition that usually goes unnoticed, unless it involves the face. The scattered follicular papules with an adherent scale are distributed most commonly on the extensor surfaces of the upper arms and thighs. The lesions are not grouped, are occasionally erythematous, and give the appearance of gooseflesh. They appear most commonly in the second decade of life and, when present on the face, can be mistaken for early comedonal acne. The cause of the follicular keratinous plugs is unknown, but they are most prone to appear in individuals with atopic dermatitis or ichthyosis. For patients who are distressed by the appearance of the lesions, mild keratolytics, emollients with 3% to 6% lactic acid, can be used to reduce their prominence.

## Miliaria

Prickly heat, or miliaria, is a common papular condition caused by sweat retention. Eccrine ducts become plugged with keratin, resulting in the formation of vesicles and leakage of sweat below the level of obstruction, which in turn leads to an inflammatory response and erythema. Miliaria crystallina occur primarily in the first few weeks of life and are characterized by superficial vesicles without surrounding erythema. Miliaria rubra, as the name suggests, are associated with erythema, because the sweat obstruction is lower in the epidermis, causing an inflammatory response. The term *miliaria pustulosa* denotes the presence of white cell response.

Miliaria lesions are caused by exposure to high environmental temperatures, especially in areas where there is friction from clothing or the skin is subjected to occlusion from airtight material (eg, the back of a patient restricted to a bed with a plastic mattress cover). The forehead, neck, and body folds are common sites of involvement. The papules usually are discrete but close together and commonly are pruritic. Therapy consists of changing the environmental stimuli producing the rash (eg, no longer overdressing a young infant).

## Id Reaction

Dermatophyte infections, particularly tinea capitis, may be associated with the presence of a myriad of tiny flesh-colored papules, especially over the face, neck, and shoulders. The scalp infection may be subtle. The presence of papules, vesicles, and other lesions of the palms and fingers may suggest an id reaction caused by tinea pedis. Appropriate antifungal treatment of the site of infection will result in resolution of these papules.

## Milia

Tiny 1- to 2-mm whitish papules, similar to those that occur on the face of newborns, may appear at sites of traumatized skin. Milia are retention cysts composed of keratinous material in blocked pilosebaceous units. They may be seen in suture lines, in healed abrasions, at sites of chronic skin erosions in children with epidermolysis bullosa, and at damaged and then healed sites in children with porphyria.

## Frictional Lichenoid Eruption

Flesh-colored papules may appear on areas of the skin that are subject to repeated friction or rubbing. Groups of these papules are seen most frequently on the knees, elbows, knuckles, and dorsa of the hands. Lesions on the knees are prominent in young children, who play on wool carpeting or other rough surfaces;

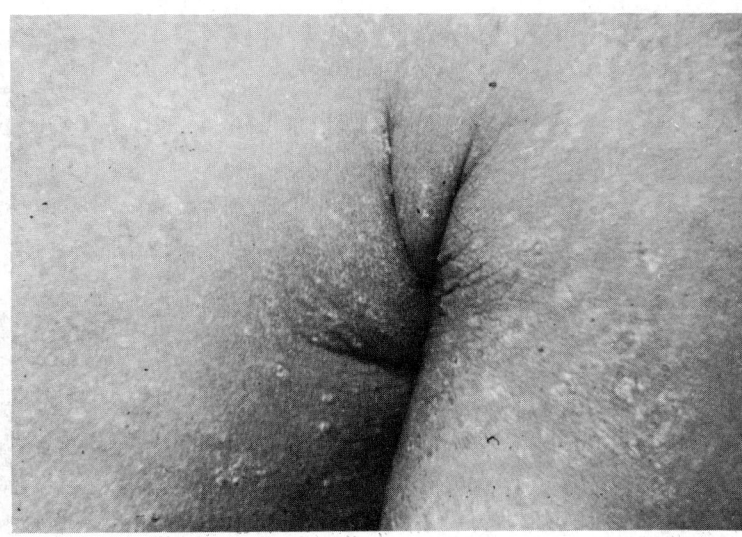

**Figure 35-12.** The fine scale on the ovoid plaques is characteristic of pityriasis rosea.

elbow lesions are seen more commonly in school-aged children, resulting from rubbing on desks. No therapy is necessary; simple avoidance of the rubbing will result in disappearance of the papules.

## Lichen Spinulosus

The key clinical feature of lichen spinulosus is patches of grouped, minute, spiny projections of various shapes and sizes. The lesions are flesh-colored, but usually stand out from unaffected skin. They generally are asymptomatic, but feel dry if rubbed. The lesions may appear in crops relatively rapidly and are found most commonly on the neck, abdomen, buttocks, lateral thighs, and extensor surfaces of the extremities.

The etiology of lichen spinulosus is unknown. The histologic picture is one of hair follicles dilated with a keratinous plug. Children with atopic dermatitis seem to be most prone to these lesions. The course is variable; the condition may last indefinitely, although affected sites can change over a period of months without therapy.

## Lichen Nitidus

The tiny papules in lichen nitidus also are flesh-colored, but their surface is smooth and shiny. They do not form the patterns seen in lichen spinulosus, although the areas of skin involved do have multiple lesions. The trunk, genitalia, abdomen, and forearms are affected most frequently. Linear lesions at sites of trauma, known as Koebner's phenomenon, are common. The etiology is unknown, and the pinhead- to pinpoint-sized lesions have a variable course, lasting months to years.

## Lichen Planus

The papules in lichen planus, a disorder found mostly in adults, are characteristically polygonal. When the lesions are examined closely, the flat-topped papules seem to form rectangles, squares, and other shapes (Fig 35-13). The classic lesions are violaceous and occur most frequently on the wrists and extensor surfaces of the forearms. They may coalesce to form plaques. Significant scaling of the lesions may occur on the lower extremities. Oral lesions, consisting of tiny white papules in lacy patterns, may occur on the buccal mucosa.

Lichen planus is intensely pruritic. Excoriations can lead to secondary infection and the occurrence of lesions in lines of

trauma. The cause of the eruption is unknown and the lesions persist for 8 to 18 months. Therapy is nonspecific, consisting of antihistamines for the pruritus and emollients for the associated dryness.

## Syringomas

Syringomas are firm, skin-colored to yellowish papules found most commonly on the lower eyelids and neck. They generally measure 1 to 3 mm, but can be as large as 1 cm in diameter. Females are affected twice as frequently as are males, and the lesions appear most often at puberty. Pathologically, the lesions are dilated cystic eccrine ducts. Syringomas persist and may increase in number over time. Although they are disturbing from a cosmetic standpoint, they are benign. The lesions seem to run in some families and tend to be most common in individuals with Down syndrome.

## Angiofibromas

Angiofibromas are hamartomatous papules and nodules composed of fibrous and vascular tissues. They are solid, are pink or flesh-colored, and generally appear after the age of 2 to 3 years, most commonly on the face. Their key significance is their association with tuberous sclerosis, a neurocutaneous, autosomal dominantly inherited disorder with central nervous system and systemic involvement. The lesions sometimes are mistaken for acne (Fig 35-14), but the age of the patient when the lesions begin to appear and the lack of comedones should eliminate this diagnosis rapidly. No effective therapy is available for this condition.

## Pityriasis Rubra Pilaris

Pityriasis rubra pilaris is an uncommon disorder characterized by the rapid spreading of erythematous, scaly papules and the subsequent formation of plaques. The papules are follicular, with tapered tips. A characteristic feature is the presence of islands of normal tissue between the joined plaques. Another clue is the development of thick, adherent scaling of the scalp, suggesting psoriasis, and thickening of the palms and soles, which may be marked. Some cases of pityriasis rubra pilaris seem to be hereditary; others are acquired. The disorder has been associated with vitamin A deficiency in some cases. The histologic picture of follicular plugs with hyperkeratosis is similar to that of vitamin A deficiency, further supporting a connection.

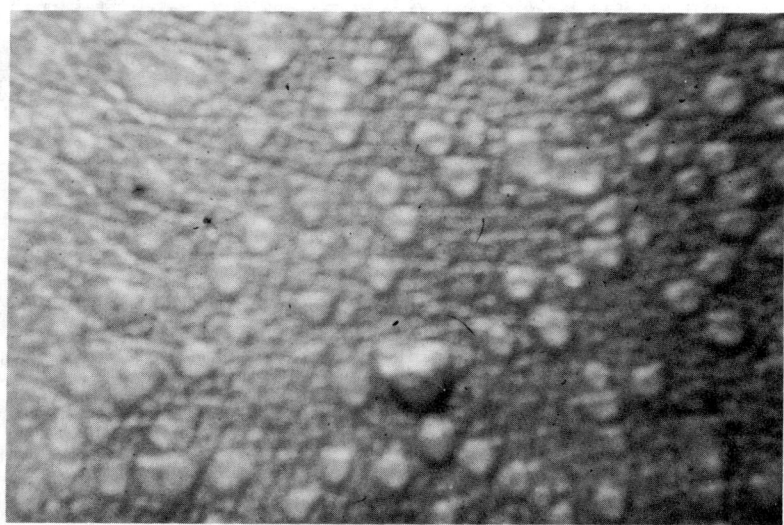

**Figure 35-13.**   The classic papules of lichen planus are not only flat-topped, but also polygonal in shape.

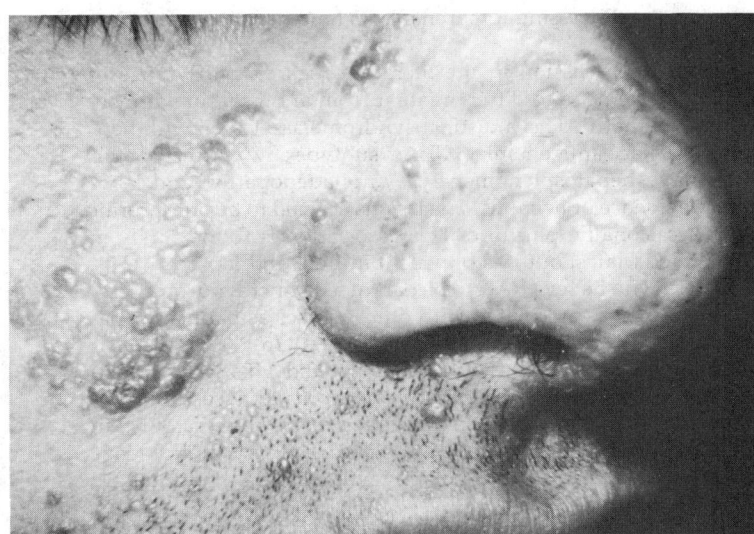

**Figure 35-14.**  Angiofibromas were mistaken for acne in this adult with tuberous sclerosis.

The course of pityriasis rubra pilaris usually is prolonged, interspersed by remissions and exacerbations. Some patients have responded to topical keratolytic therapy (organic acids in emollients), and etretinate, an oral retinoid, has been used successfully in a number of cases.

## Red Papules

### Papular Urticaria

Papular urticaria is a common, intensely pruritic disorder caused by hypersensitivity to insect bites. The fresh lesions are papules with an erythematous flare capped by a central punctum at the site of the bite (Fig 35-15). Lesions generally appear in crops, particularly on exposed skin surfaces. Most cases occur in the late spring and summer, but household exposure to fleas from animals can cause problems any time of year. Not all lesions have a central punctum. Linear or irregular clusters may be related to localized reactions caused by immunoglobulins and complement released into surrounding vessels.

Fleas are the most common cause of papular urticaria. Mos-

quitoes and other biting insects also may produce the lesions. Secondary infections from excoriations are extremely common and, in some children, the wheals may progress to bullae. Treatment success depends on eliminating the biting insects from the child's environment. Topical antipruritic agents may be of some help. Secondary infections also need to be treated. This severe reaction to the bites lasts 1 to 2 years.

### Gianotti-Crosti Syndrome

Gianotti-Crosti syndrome, also known as papular acrodermatitis of childhood (PAC), has a distinctive clinical picture because of the predominant location of the erythematous papules on the face and extremities (Fig 35-16). First described in Italy in 1955, it has received increasing attention throughout the world in association with a number of viruses. The papules generally are larger in infants (up to 5 mm) than in older children (2 to 3 mm); they tend to be of similar size, usually appear rapidly, and may be associated with pruritus. One of the features of this exanthem

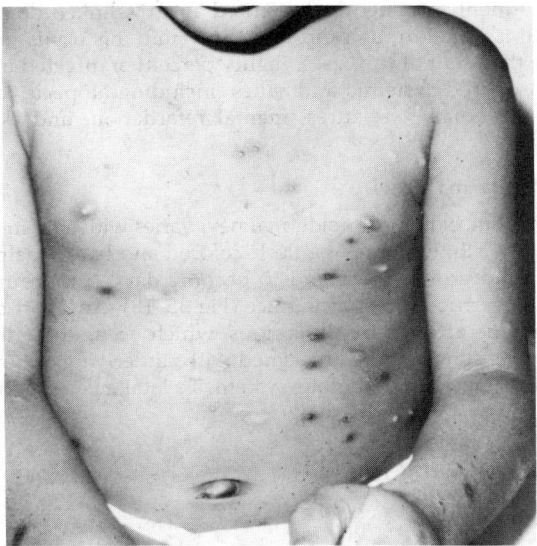

**Figure 35-15.**  Papular urticaria. Old, hyperpigmented lesions and recent, erythematous papules with central puncta from flea bites.

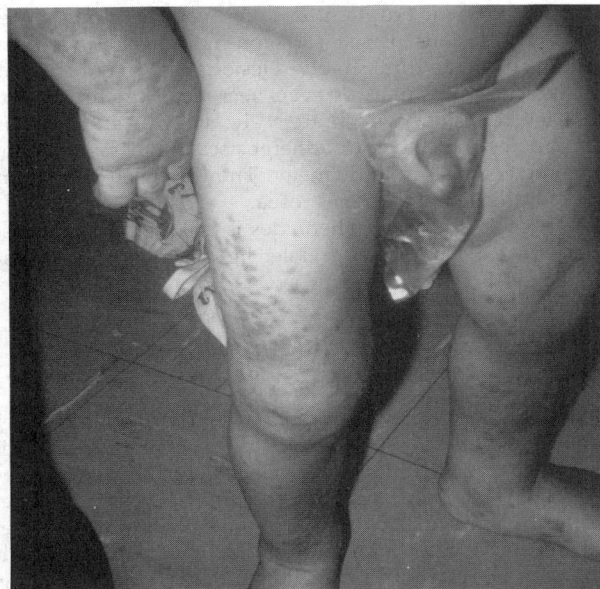

**Figure 35-16.**  Diffuse reddish papules are present over the arms and legs with sparing of the trunk in a patient with papular acrodermatitis of childhood.

that is most distressing to parents is its long duration, often 3 to 5 weeks.

There is discussion in the literature regarding the cause of PAC and the need to differentiate it from another, similar rash. Some feel that PAC is a distinct syndrome associated with hepatitis B surface antigenemia (HBsAg; subtype ayw). Affected children have hepatosplenomegaly, lymphadenopathy, and laboratory evidence of hepatitis. The lesions are said to be non-pruritic and, occasionally, purpuric. This association is found rarely in the United States, but it is prevalent in Italy and Japan.

Those who believe PAC to be part of a distinct syndrome refer to similar rashes associated with other viruses as papular or papulovesicular acrolocated syndromes (PASs). In PAS, pruritus is common, hepatomegaly is uncommon, and HBsAg always is lacking. Occasionally, juicy papules may have a vesicular appearance. PAS also has a prolonged course. Viruses found in association with PAS include Epstein-Barr virus, parainfluenza virus, coxsackievirus A16, poliomyelitis virus, and respiratory syncytial virus.

Regardless of whether PAC and PAS are classified singly or together, their association with HBsAg should be recognized, particularly in certain countries. The exanthem is much more common than generally recognized. The distinctive distribution and duration of the papules should help in making the clinical diagnosis. The rash is looked on best as a self-limited cutaneous response to a viral infection.

### Eruptive Vellus Hair Cysts

Eruptive vellus hair cysts, first described in 1977, are characterized by the presence of discrete, red-brown or brown-black, 1- to 4-mm, soft, smooth-surfaced papules. The lesions may be scattered or grouped, particularly over the anterior chest. The onset of lesions occurs in the first decade of life. The condition may resolve spontaneously or it may persist, and it usually is asymptomatic. An autosomal dominant mode of inheritance is suspected.

### Pityriasis Lichenoides

Pityriasis lichenoides is an uncommon disorder mentioned here only because it sometimes is confused with pityriasis rosea. There are two variants: an acute form, most commonly called Mucha-Habermann disease; and a chronic type, known as pityriasis lichenoides chronica. Both produce a generalized erythematous papular and macular eruption, usually over the trunk and extremities. The lesions persist for months or recur in periodic eruptions. The acute form involves lesions that may be hemorrhagic, vesicular, pustular, or even necrotic. The chronic form has less severe lesions, which are scaly. They begin as reddish brown papules that have an adherent scale and range from a few millimeters to 1 cm in diameter. The wafer-like plaques resemble old, thickened pityriasis rosea.

The cause of pityriasis lichenoides is unknown. Some cases resolve with exposure to ultraviolet light; others resolve with prolonged erythromycin therapy.

## Linear Papules

### Lichen Striatus

Lichen striatus, a self-limited eruption most common in children, is characterized by the rapid development of multiple tiny, discrete papules arranged in a linear, band-like pattern over an extremity (Fig 35-17). The bands may be 1 cm to several centimeters in width, irregular or fairly uniform, and continuous or interrupted; they occur most commonly on the upper extremities. The papules may be scaly and generally are flesh-colored, although in black individuals, a hypopigmented discoloration may be prominent. The cause of this distinctive lesion is unknown. It tends to have a duration of a few weeks to as long as a year. Topical steroids and keratolytics may hasten its resolution. Linear

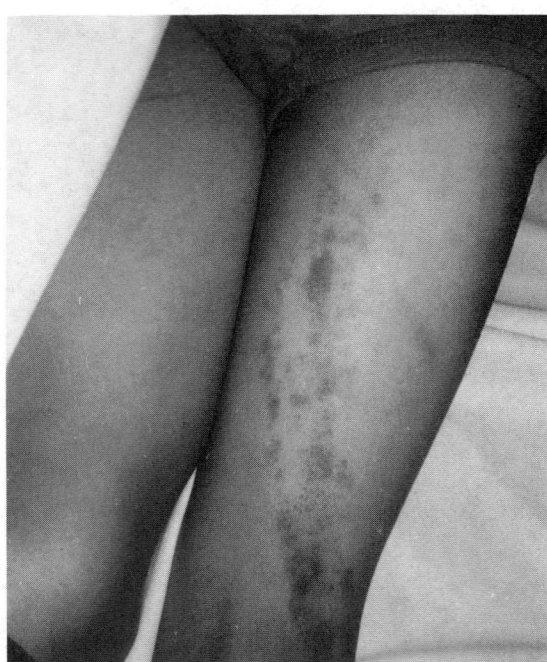

Figure 35-17. Linear arrangement of confluent papules in lichen striatus.

epidermal nevi, linear psoriasis, and linear lichen planus are included in the differential diagnosis.

### Incontinentia Pigmenti

Incontinentia pigmenti is a neurocutaneous disorder characterized by a rash that may progress through four distinct stages. The first, which usually is present at birth (and is discussed earlier in this chapter), consists of papules and vesicles distributed linearly. These lesions, which may fade in weeks or months, often are followed by the second stage, linear verrucous lesions. These wart-like lesions also fade gradually after several months. The pigmented stage follows, although not necessarily in skin affected by previous lesions. The pigment usually appears as large patches, bands, or swirls; eventually, it may disappear. The final stage is seen in some adult females and consists of subtle, hypopigmented, atrophic patches of skin, especially on the lower extremities.

Incontinentia pigmenti is inherited as an X-linked dominant trait that is lethal to males in utero. A family history is present in more than half of the cases. Eighty percent of affected infants have associated systemic anomalies, including alopecia, dental and eye anomalies, seizures, mental retardation, and skeletal deformities.

### Linear Epidermal Nevi

The appearance of linear epidermal nevi varies with age. Initially, usually at birth, they may be flesh-colored and barely palpable. As the child grows, they tend to become darker, more raised, and more verrucous on the surface (Fig 35-18). Any part of the body may be affected by the lesions, which occur sporadically. Extensive lesions may be associated with underlying abnormalities, including central nervous system, skeletal, eye, and kidney defects.

## NODULAR DISORDERS

### Red Nodules

#### Hemangiomas

Tumors composed of blood vessels come in various shapes, types, and sizes. They occur in 10% of all infants and generally are

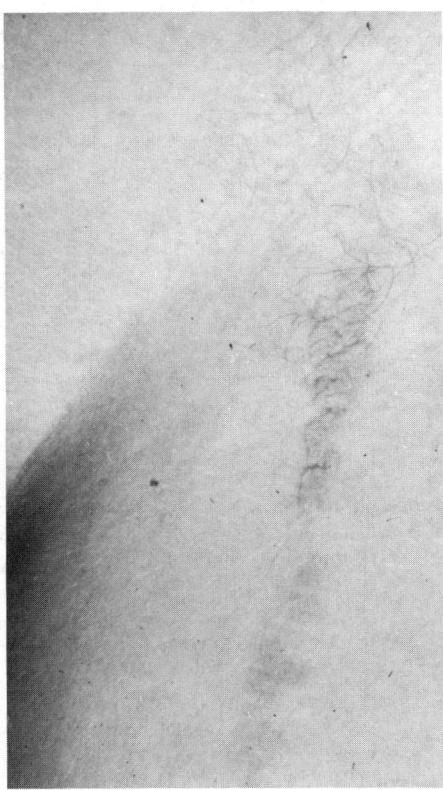

**Figure 35-18.** Grouping of linear epidermal nevi in the axillary area.

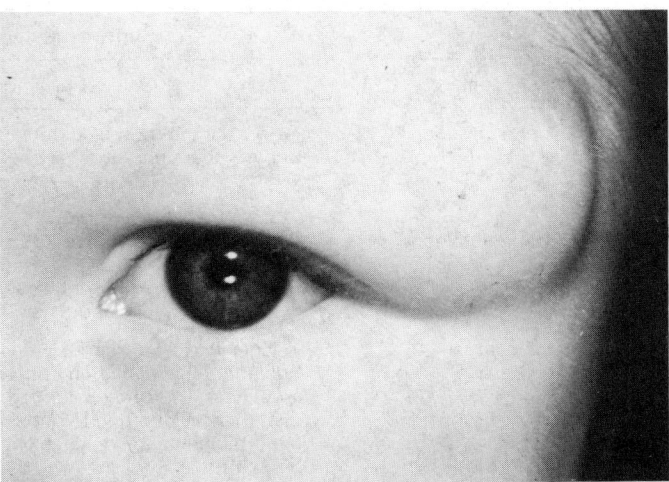

**Figure 35-20.** A soft, bluish cavernous hemangioma without epidermal involvement.

benign growths with an excellent prognosis. Capillary hemangiomas are tumors composed of a proliferation of endothelium-lined vascular spaces (see Color Figure 5). They generally project above the surface of the skin, are soft, and can be blanched with pressure. Cavernous hemangiomas are composed of large venous channels and they lie deeper in the skin, in the deep dermis and the subcutaneous tissues. The etiology of these vascular tumors is not known. Something stimulates angiogenesis; fortunately, something also turns it off, causing most of the tumors to regress over time.

Capillary, commonly referred to as strawberry, hemangiomas rarely are present at birth. Occasionally, a pink or hypopigmented

macule may be seen. The lesions grow rapidly during the first 6 months of life, reach a quiescent stage when the patient is 6 to 12 months old, and then begin to regress when the child is between 12 and 18 months old. The individual lesions may be pink, red, or a mixture of the two colors. Signs of regression include patches of white or gray on the surface of the lesion (Fig 35-19). By the time the patient is 5 years old, 50% of these lesions will show complete involution; by 7 years, 70% will have disappeared; and by 10 to 12 years, 95% will have regressed completely. Depending on the previous size of the lesion, a small scar or no blemish may remain. With large lesions, redundant skin may be the major cosmetic defect.

Cavernous hemangiomas may not show complete regression; these tumors impart a bluish tint to the overlying skin (Fig 35-20). Hemangiomas often are mixed, with superficial capillary and deep cavernous components (see Color Figure 4).

Complications of hemangiomas are infrequent. Superficial infections are the most common problem, because the surface of the lesion may become irritated or eroded (Fig 35-21). Bleeding occurs in less than 3% of cases, and bleeding lesions usually respond well to pressure. Platelet trapping may be a problem in some lesions, resulting in peripheral thrombocytopenia. Rapid enlargement of a hemangioma may signify platelet trapping, known as the Kasabach-Merritt syndrome. Rarely, arteriovenous shunts in large lesions may result in high-output congestive heart failure.

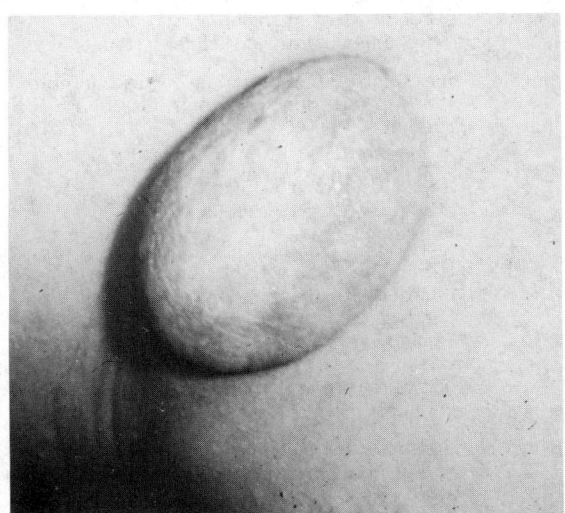

**Figure 35-19.** A large capillary hemangioma shows whitening of the surface, indicating the start of resolution.

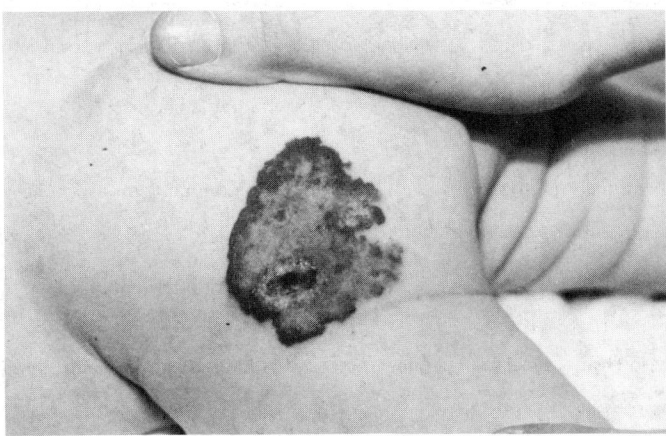

**Figure 35-21.** The surface of this capillary hemangioma has become ulcerated from continuous rubbing against a diaper.

TABLE 35-1.   Syndromes With Cutaneous Vascular Changes

| Syndrome | Cutaneous Findings | Associated Problems |
|---|---|---|
| Sturge-Weber (sporadic) | Nevus flammeus in first branch of the trigeminal nerve; other areas also may be involved | Seizures; mental retardation; angiomatosis of leptomeninges; glaucoma; hemiplegia; telangiectatic hypertrophy of oral mucous membranes |
| Klippel-Trenaunay-Weber (sporadic) | Port-wine stains; capillary or cavernous hemangiomas; varicose veins; telangiectasia; hyperpigmented nevi and streaks; lymphangiomatous anomalies | Hypertrophy of soft tissue and bone (present at birth or later); syndactyly, polydactyly, macrodactyly; dislocated hips; scoliosis; kyphosis; asymmetry; visceral hemangiomas |
| Ataxia-Telangiectasia (autosomal recessive) | Telangiectasia in progressive pattern, first on bulbar conjunctiva, then on ears, eyelids, malar area, neck, etc.; gray hair; pigmentary disturbances: mottled hypopigmentation and hyperpigmentation; café au lait spots; seborrheic dermatitis | Cerebellar ataxia; recurrent sinopulmonary infections; immunologic defects: reduced or absent IgA; reduced IgE; IgG2 deficiency; recurrent skin infections; insulin-resistant diabetes; increased incidence of malignancy; progeroid appearance |
| Hereditary Hemorrhagic Telangiectasia (Rendu- Osler- Weber; (autosomal dominant) | Telangiectatic mats—punctiform, 1–4 mm, macular, occasionally papular; mucosa of nose, lips, tongue and mouth involved | Recurrent epistaxis, starting as early as 8–10 years; mucocutaneous lesions rarely observed in children; gastrointestinal bleeding commonly results in anemia |
| Kasabach-Merritt | Hemangiomas—capillary or cavernous, usually large | Thrombocytopenia caused by sequestration in hemangiomas; microangiopathic hemolytic anemia; rapidly enlarging hemangiomas |
| Blue Rubber Bleb Nevus (sporadic) | Cavernous hemangiomas: multiple, soft, rubbery, compressible; size: 0.1–5 cm; number: 1->100; may be tender | Gastrointestinal bleeding from hemangiomas (most common in small intestine); iron deficiency in almost all; tumors may occur in liver, spleen, central nervous system; orthopedic abnormalities common—related to hemangiomas |
| **Marocephaly With Cutaneous Angiomatosis** | | |
| *Riley-Smith (autosomal dominant?)* | Hemangiomas usually appear in childhood | Macrocephaly; pseudopapilledema |
| *Bannayan (autosomal dominant)* | Multiple lipomas; hemangiomas | Macrocephaly; macrodactyly; visceral lymphangiomas; mental retardation; increased birth size |
| *Cutis Marmorata Telangectasia Congenita* | Persistent cutis marmorata phlebectasia; telangiectasia; areas of ulceration | Macrocephaly |
| Wyburn-Mason (Bonnet- Dechaume-Blanc) (sporadic) | Enlarged facial veins; facial angioma (nevus flammeus) | Unilateral cirsoid retinal vascular anomalies; intracranial arteriovenous anomaly involving the mesencephalon and base of the brain; unilateral exophthalmos; hemiparesis; ataxia, cranial nerve defects; mental retardation; seizures; subarachnoid hemorrhage |
| Gorham (sporadic) | Hemangiomas may or may not overlie affected bone; lymphangiomas | Massive osteolysis and complete or partial replacement of bone by extensive fibrosis secondary to hemangiomatosis and lymphangiomatosis of skeletal system |
| Cobb | Angiomas—port-wine stain most common, but angiolipomas to cavernous hemangiomas involved; characteristic dermatomal distribution on trunk and extremities | Intraspinal tumors (angioma) cause symptoms from compression and anoxia; may be gradual or sudden |
| Sacral Hemangiomas and Multiple Congenital Abnormalities | Sacral hemangiomas | Imperforate anus; fistulas; renal anomalies; abnormal genitalia; skin tags; lipomeningomyelocele; sacral bony defects |
| Maffucci's (sporadic) | Multiple hemangiomas: capillary, cavernous, and especially phlebectasia—often with grape-like appearance; lymphangiectasis occasional. Other: generalized nevi; vitiligo, cafè au lait spots; hyperpigmentation | Variable early bowing of long bones; asymmetric retarded growth; enchondromas primarily of hands, feet, and tubular long bones; hard, cauliflower-like growths of hands and feet; usually normal at birth, 25% of cases develop in first year; increased incidence of malignancy—chondrosarcoma; recurrent fractures |
| von Hippel-Lindau (irregular dominant) | Most have no abnormality; some have port-wine stain | Cerebellar hemangiomas—signs and symptoms of a posterior fossa mass; seizures; retinal angiomas with tortuous retinal artery and vein; renal cysts and tumors; pancreatic cysts; pheochromocytomas |

**TABLE 35-1.** *(Continued)*

| Syndrome | Cutaneous Findings | Associated Problems |
|---|---|---|
| Sternal Malformation/Vascular Dysplasia | Capillary/cavernous hemangiomas of face and anterior trunk | Sternal cleft of variable length; atrophic scar with abdominal raphe |
| Hemangiomatous Branchial Clefts, Unusual Facies (sporadic) | As per name | Four patients described; clefts in retroauricular areas extending down sternocleidomastoid muscle; retroverted auricles; nasolacrimal duct obstruction; epicanthal folds; flat nasal bridge; blunted alae nasi; microphthalmia |

Although these complications always must be kept in mind by any physician observing a child with a hemangioma, their infrequency speaks for a conservative management approach. In the past, surgical removal, irradiation, freezing, and other destructive measures were used to "treat" these tumors. The resulting scarring and complication rates were unacceptable; sane management consists of watchful waiting. A major task is convincing the parents that time is the best therapy. Before-and-after pictures of children with typical lesions are most helpful.

Nevertheless, therapy occasionally is indicated for hemangiomas and even can be lifesaving. Lesions that interfere with vision or impinge on an airway fall into this category. Large oral doses (2 to 4 mg/kg/day) of prednisone have proved beneficial in the treatment of some of these lesions. Infants with rapidly enlarging hemangiomas associated with thrombocytopenia, consumption coagulopathy, and hemolytic anemia from platelet trapping (Kasabach-Merritt syndrome) also may respond to such therapy. Infants with large arteriovenous fistulas in their hemangiomas who have intractable congestive heart failure and do not respond to prednisone may require embolization of the lesions. Recombinant interferon-alpha 2a, which appears to have antiproliferative effects on endothelial cells, may provide another alternative form of therapy. The tunable dye laser may obliterate the immature vascular channels when the lesion is still macular or minimally raised.

Eruptive hemangiomatosis refers to an uncommon condition characterized by the rapid proliferation of cutaneous hemangiomas. In many cases, visceral lesions are present, affecting the central nervous system, liver, gastrointestinal tract, and other organs. Reports of catastrophic complications secondary to these visceral lesions have promulgated a dismal prognosis for affected infants. Fortunately, the majority of infants do well, despite as many as 100 cutaneous lesions and the presence of multiple visceral lesions, all of which regress with time.

A number of syndromes involving cutaneous hemangiomas are listed in Table 35-1.

## Pyogenic Granulomas

Pyogenic granulomas are benign vascular proliferations arising from the connective tissue of skin or mucous membranes. They usually are precipitated by trauma and infection, although the mechanism for growth stimulation is not known. The lesions grow rapidly, may be papular or nodular, and often are pedunculated. They usually are solitary and dark red to purple, with a surface that generally is moist, crusted, or eroded and that may bleed easily when traumatized (Fig 35-22). The best known pyogenic granuloma is the fleshy tumor associated with ingrown toenails.

The differential diagnosis of pyogenic granuloma includes warts, molluscum contagiosum, and capillary hemangioma. The best treatment is excision and electrodesiccation of the base of the lesion to prevent recurrence.

## Erythema Nodosum

The lesions of erythema nodosum are fairly distinctive. The presentation usually is one of painful, erythematous, warm nodules on the pretibial surfaces. The number of nodules may vary from one to many. Their bright red color changes in a few days to brown-red or purple and later to yellow-green, as seen with a bruise. Lesions may occur on other body sites, including the arms and face. Erythema nodosum is a hypersensitivity reaction pattern triggered by a variety of different infections, drugs, and other conditions. It is not a disease entity in itself, but requires evaluation to uncover the underlying cause.

The most common precipitating agent in erythema nodosum in children in the United States is a preceding streptococcal infection. In the past, tuberculosis was the foremost cause. Other, less common precipitants include cat-scratch disease, histoplasmosis, coccidioidomycosis, and leptospirosis. An association with inflammatory bowel disease and sarcoidosis has been noted with increasing frequency. Drugs most frequently incriminated include sulfonamides, diphenylhydantoin, and contraceptive agents. Chronic or recurrent episodes suggest more serious systemic disorders, such as a collagen vascular disease, lymphoma, or inflammatory bowel disease.

The lesions of erythema nodosum initially may be confused with areas of cellulitis, insect bites, or bruises. Arthralgias occur in most cases, and arthritis is present in up to one third of cases, suggesting rheumatic disorders. Biopsy samples of lesions reveal intense inflammation deep in the dermis and subcutaneous tissues, with involvement of arteries and veins. Most patients re-

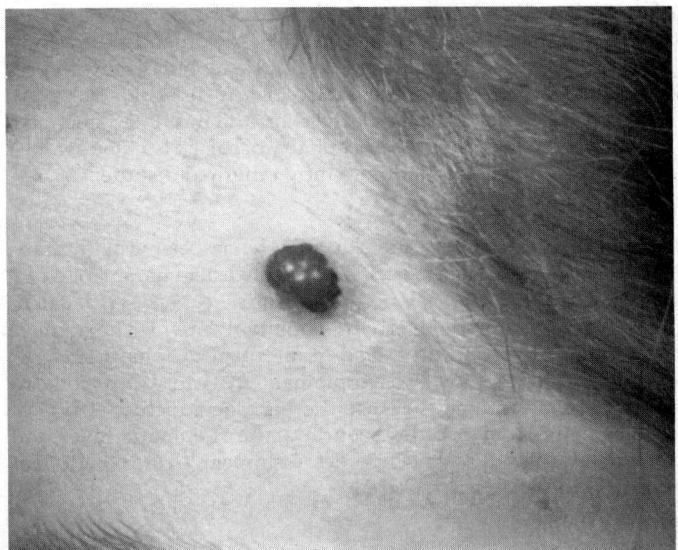

**Figure 35-22.** This pyogenic granuloma of the forehead is red, pedunculated, and moist.

spond to bed rest, and the episodes resolve in 2 to 3 weeks. The trigger for this delayed cell-mediated hypersensitivity reaction may not be found.

### Panniculitis

The name *panniculitis* denotes inflammatory nodules in the subcutaneous tissue. The blood vessels usually are affected also, with resultant fat necrosis. The clinical appearance commonly is one of erythematous, enlarging nodules that frequently are painful to palpation. The lesions may vary considerably in size, from less than 1 cm to many centimeters in diameter. As the lesions subside, the overlying skin becomes less erythematous, eventually leaving macular areas of hyperpigmentation. A depression in the overlying skin is common with resolution.

The causes of panniculitis are varied. Cold-exposure panniculitis is common on infants' cheeks. Some cases are associated with connective tissue diseases, particularly lupus erythematosus. Weber-Christian disease features recurring inflammatory subcutaneous nodules with systemic symptoms, particularly fever. The withdrawal of steroids also may result in the appearance of panniculitis.

## Skin-Colored Nodules

### Dermoid Cysts

The small, firm, smooth intracutaneous or subcutaneous nodules characteristic of dermoid cysts occur most frequently on the head and neck. Congenital lesions formed from embryonic ectoderm, they are lined by stratified squamous epithelium. Almost 40% are periorbital, and about 30% occur in the eyebrows. The lesions usually are solitary and asymptomatic, and they are managed by surgical excision.

### Epidermal Cysts

Most epidermal cysts occur after puberty. Clinically, they appear as discrete, enlarging, raised, somewhat compressible nodules of variable size. The margins may be irregular. The overlying skin is normal. Epidermal cysts occur most frequently on the face, scalp, and back, and they seem to be a result of the proliferation of surface epidermal cells within the dermis. Trauma may be responsible for some of these lesions.

### Lipomas

The subcutaneous tumors typical of lipomas are spongy and often lobulated. They occur most frequently in the subcutaneous tissue of the back and abdominal wall. The overlying skin is unaffected and not attached to these lesions, which are nontender and slow-growing, and may be solitary or multiple. Lipomas may be part of Gardner's syndrome (other features of which include polyposis of the colon, epidermal cysts of the skin, and multiple osteomas), have an accompanying macrocephaly, occur as isolated events, or occur as an autosomal dominantly inherited disorder.

### Pseudorheumatoid Nodules

Palpable nodules within the skin may be associated with granuloma annulare, a benign, self-limited disorder characterized by an enlarging ring-like lesion with a clearing center, an elevated, papular border, and no overlying skin involvement. The nodules most frequently occur on the scalp, pretibial regions, and dorsa of the feet. They are totally asymptomatic, but cause great concern if biopsy is performed, because the histologic picture is typical of the rheumatoid nodules seen in acute rheumatic fever and rheumatoid arthritis. The nodules disappear over a period of months; no therapy is required.

### Pilomatricomas

Pilomatricomas are firm to hard, slow-growing tumors. Most are flesh-colored, but some may be reddish or bluish. They occur most commonly on the head and neck, and almost always are solitary. When sectioning an excised nodule, a gritty sensation characteristic of calcification is noted. Pilomatricomas are benign, but should be removed for cosmetic reasons. They occur most commonly in the first 2 decades of life.

### Connective Tissue Nevi

Connective tissue nevi often are grouped together and tend to be elevated and firm. Mostly benign and hereditary, they represent localized collections of dermal collagen and elastic tissue. It is important to distinguish the isolated, benign lesions from those associated with tuberous sclerosis. The latter tend to form plaques and are associated with other skin lesions, including hypopigmented macules and angiofibromas of the face.

### Dermatofibromas

Dermatofibromas are solitary, hard, well-defined, dome-shaped nodules that occur occasionally in children. They are fixed firmly to the skin and vary in color from flesh-colored to red-brown to tan or black. They rarely exceed 2 cm in diameter. Some feel they occur as a reaction to insect bites.

### Neurofibromas

When they are associated with café au lait spots, neurofibromas are a major indicator of von Recklinghausen's disease. They also may occur as an isolated phenomenon, however. The shape and size of these lesions varies considerably; some are soft and well defined, whereas others are firm and interdigitate with the normal skin. Giant, grossly deforming lesions may occur. The neurofibromas of von Recklinghausen's disease generally do not begin to appear until after the first decade of life.

## Pigmented Nodules

### Mast Cell Disease

Lesions composed of infiltrates of mast cells may occur in a number of shapes and forms (see Color Figure 2). In infants and young children, solitary mastocytomas are most common. The typical picture is one of a raised brown or tan plaque, often with an orange-peel surface, that has recurrent flares of erythema or that develops vesicles, bullae, or, sometimes, crusting resembling an infectious process (Fig 35-23). Occasionally, the bullae take on a hemorrhagic appearance. Irritation of the lesion may cause

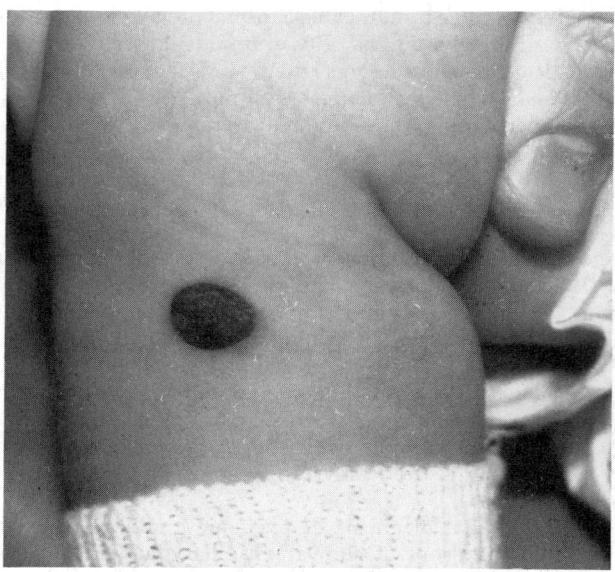

**Figure 35-23.**    A brownish mastocytoma on the lower leg of an infant.

the release of histamine, which in turn may stimulate facial flushing and colic.

The most common form of mast cell disease in childhood is urticaria pigmentosa. The lesions, which are macular or slightly elevated papules and nodules that occur primarily on the trunk, may number from a few to hundreds and often appear in the first few months of life, although they can occur at any time (Fig 35-24). The most helpful clue to diagnosis is the appearance of an erythematous or urticarial flare after vigorous rubbing of the lesion (Darier's sign). In some cases, systemic symptoms, including diarrhea and gastrointestinal bleeding, may be prominent.

Fortunately, mast cell disease in children generally is benign. The younger the child is when the lesions appear, the more likely it is that they will resolve. Isolated mastocytomas usually are gone by the time the child is 10 years of age, and half of all cases of urticaria pigmentosa that develop early in childhood are resolved by the late teenage years.

### Xanthogranuloma

Juvenile xanthogranulomas, or nevoxanthoendotheliomas, start to appear in the first few months of life. They begin as small, reddish papules and enlarge into 0.5- to 1.0-cm nodules (Fig 35-25). The lesions vary from yellow to brown to red and generally are firm and rubbery. Most commonly, multiple lesions are present, but only one or, conversely, hundreds of lesions may be present. Histologically, the nodules are composed of histiocytes and lymphocytes. There is no associated lipemia.

The cause of juvenile xanthogranuloma is unknown. No treatment is necessary, because about one third disappear within 6 months and another one third are gone within 12 months. Lesions may occur in the viscera. Iris xanthogranulomas may lead to hemorrhage into the eye, cause glaucoma, or be mistaken for an intraocular tumor. The most worrisome association is with juvenile chronic myeloid leukemia, which has been described with increasing frequency. Children with neurofibromatosis and juvenile xanthogranuloma seem to be at a much higher risk than normal for the development of this uncommon form of leukemia.

## VESICULAR AND BULLOUS ERUPTIONS

### Disorders With Grouped Vesicles

#### Herpes Simplex

Whenever a localized group of small vesicles is found anywhere on the skin, the most likely cause is infection with herpesvirus hominis, a DNA virus. Most primary infections are mild and almost inapparent. The vesicles rapidly become pustular, dry, and form crusts, or the tops are removed, leaving erosions or shallow ulcerations. The most common sites of infection are the lips and genital area. In young children, symptomatic primary infections most often involve the oral cavity, where multiple vesicles on the gums and buccal surfaces rapidly erode to form ulcers. The illness is accompanied by high fever, increased salivation, refusal to drink, and swollen, fragile gingiva. When affected children suck their fingers, vesicles may appear there as well (Fig 35-26).

Recurrent herpes simplex infections are very common. The vesicles appear at the sites of previous infections at various time intervals. Often, burning or itching of the area precedes the appearance of the vesicles. The virus appears to remain dormant in the regional nerve ganglion of the affected area until some event—often illness, stress, or sunburn—triggers the clinical infection. Although most laypersons recognize the "cold sore" or "fever blister" when it occurs on the lips, many fail to realize that this infection may occur on any surface of the body.

Some interesting labels have been applied to some of these

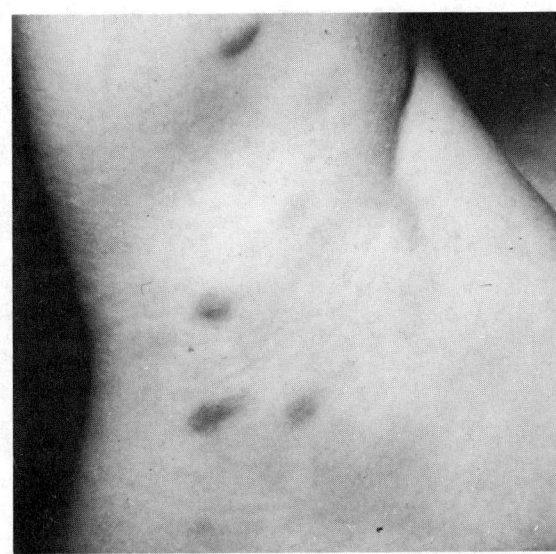

Figure 35-24.  Multiple pigmented nodules of urticaria pigmentosa in the axilla. Rubbing causes an erythematous flare and swelling.

infections. Herpes gladiatorum refers to herpes lesions occurring in wrestlers; abrasions of the skin on virus-laden mats promotes this association. Herpes rugbiformis refers to infection on the forehead, where rugby players most often are affected. Herpetic whitlow denotes the presence of vesicular lesions on a finger or fingers. Frequently, these pustular lesions are mistaken for recurrent bacterial infections. Because the lesions clear in a few days to a week in most cases, they may seem to respond to prescribed antibiotics. Eczema herpeticum, a potentially life-threatening herpes simplex infection, occurs in persons with atopic dermatitis. The viral infection spreads rapidly over the skin, producing widespread vesicles and pustules. Systemic toxic symptoms are common, and secondary bacterial infections may occur in herpes lesions. The clinical differentiation may be difficult.

Genital herpes in children always must be viewed with suspicion of possible sexual abuse. Neonatal herpes simplex infections have high rates of morbidity and mortality, and must be recognized and treated immediately (see Color Figure 24). Unfortunately, 60% to 80% of mothers being delivered of infected

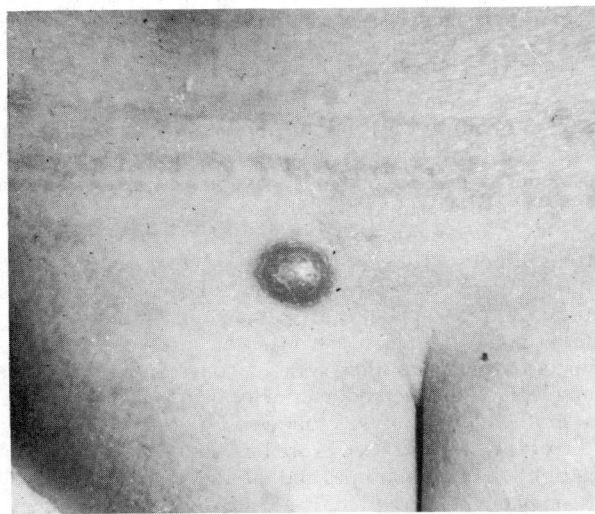

Figure 35-25.  A yellowish nodule of juvenile xanthogranuloma in the sacral area.

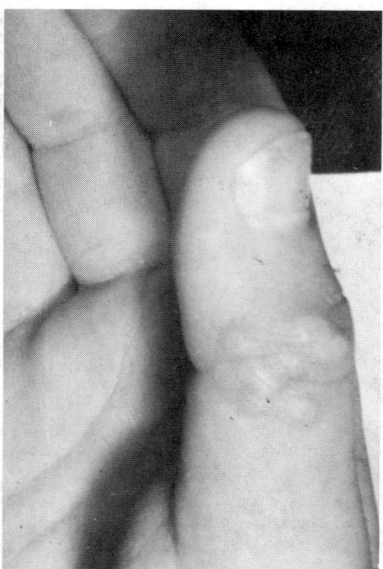

**Figure 35-26.** Herpes simplex infection always should be considered when grouped vesicles are present.

babies are asymptomatic, with no history of infections. Most of the infants are infected as they pass through the birth canal. If a mother's herpes infection is primary, her infant has a 40% to 50% chance of acquiring a herpesvirus infection if delivered vaginally; if the mother's lesion is recurrent, the risk is about 3%. The incubation period of natally acquired herpesvirus infections is 2 days to 3 weeks. Given that almost half of affected infants manifest no skin lesions, the absence of skin lesions does not indicate lack of infection. Neonatal herpes lesions may be localized at the site of trauma, particularly the scalp, where fetal monitors may have been applied (see Color Figure 25); they may be scattered over the skin; or they may be large areas of erosion, simulating epidermolysis bullosa. Whenever a suspicious vesicle appears on a neonate's skin, a Tzanck test should be done to reveal the multinucleated giant cells characteristic of the herpes group of viruses.

The use of acyclovir has led to a significant decrease in the morbidity and mortality associated with herpes simplex virus infections. This drug enters cells, where it is activated selectively by herpes simplex viral thymidine kinase and, in turn, specifically inhibits replication of the virus. The effectiveness of the drug depends on the timeliness of treatment initiation.

### Herpes Zoster

Herpes zoster, or shingles, is an acute vesicular eruption that occurs in dermatomal distribution and is caused by herpesvirus varicellae, the same virus that is responsible for varicella. For herpes zoster to develop, one must have had a previous infection with varicella virus. The varicella-zoster virus appears to remain dormant in the dorsal root ganglia until something triggers the cutaneous response. Triggers include trauma to the spinal column, radiation, immunosuppressive therapy, leukemia, and reexposure to varicella. Affected patients are contagious to others.

The lesions of herpes zoster often are preceded by painful stinging or burning sensations for a few days. Right lower quadrant involvement of the abdomen may be mistaken for appendicitis. Erythematous papules followed by vesicles then appear over the next week. The lesions are limited to band-like areas in the distribution of dermatomes and rarely cross the midline. The vesicles may not be continuous in a band and, on occasion, more than one dermatome is involved. The vesicles may coalesce to form bullae. Generally, the infection clears within 7 to 14 days,

but 10% of the cases may last longer. Persistent pain in the area previously affected by herpes zoster is unusual in young children, but may occur in adolescents.

Lesions that appear at the tip of the nose should be noted carefully; they may be associated with significant eye involvement. Most infections can be managed by the use of compresses to dry the lesions, keep them clean, and relieve the itching or pain. In extensive cases, or cases involving the eye, parenteral acyclovir may prove helpful. Although herpes zoster may be a presenting sign of malignancy in adults, it rarely is so in children.

### Dermatitis Herpetiformis

Dermatitis herpetiformis, the key clinical feature of which is the sudden appearance of symmetric areas of intense pruritus, is a very uncommon skin eruption in children. The areas most commonly affected in children differ from those in adults and include the face, torso, and genitals. The only cutaneous sign may be some erythema at the areas of itching, but papules and vesicles usually follow. The vesicles are most common and occur in groups, sometimes coalescing to form bullae. The lesions tend to come and go with exacerbations and remissions. Single eruptions may last for a few days to weeks.

Gluten-dependent enteropathy has been found in 85% to 95% of patients studied, but malabsorptive symptoms are rare. A jejunal biopsy sample will show the characteristics of celiac disease in almost all cases. Antigen HLA-B8 or -DR3 is found in 60% to 80% of affected patients. Treatment consists of a gluten-free diet and dapsone or sulfapyridine. Once the cutaneous lesions resolve, the drug therapy may be discontinued as long as the diet is followed.

### Lymphangiomas

Overgrowth of lymphoid tissue may be manifested in a number of different forms. In the simplex form, deep-seated, tense vesicles appear on the skin surface. Most are small (1 to 3 mm in diameter) and clear to hemorrhagic in color (see Color Figure 8). The surface of the lesions may be smooth or rough. Occasionally, a clear fluid may leak from traumatized lesions. Lymphangiomas are seen most commonly on the neck, upper trunk, tongue, and proximal extremities.

Cavernous lymphangiomas are ill-defined spongy growths that vary considerably in size. The overlying skin surface may be discolored. Secondary infections are common in these lesions, which may be difficult to remove surgically. Lymphangiomas, unlike hemangiomas, do not regress spontaneously.

## Disorders With Generalized Vesicles (Varicella)

Chickenpox is a highly contagious childhood disease caused by the same herpes group DNA virus that is responsible for herpes zoster. Infection usually follows contact with children infected with varicella, but zoster lesions are infectious also. The characteristic lesions occur in crops, with varying types present at the same time. The initial lesion is an erythematous macule/papule that becomes vesicular in a few hours. The vesicles then become pustular and umbilicated, and are covered with a crust in 1 to 2 days. Occasionally, the vesicles may appear teardrop-like on an erythematous base. Mucous membrane involvement is common. Lesions initially are scattered on the trunk, face, and scalp, with the extremities becoming involved within a short time.

The incubation period of varicella is 7 to 21 days, with most cases appearing 14 days after exposure. Pruritus often is marked, and fever is common. Generally, the disease is fairly mild, except in adults, immunocompromised children, and neonates. Secondary infections are common. When large, glistening erosive lesions or bullae appear, secondary staphylococcal infection is likely. Complaints of pain in lesions usually indicate a secondary infection. Treatment of uncomplicated varicella is symptomatic. Aspirin should be avoided because of its association with Reye's syndrome. Calamine lotion and cool compresses may reduce the itching and enhance drying of the lesions. In immunocompromised patients, acyclovir may be lifesaving. If the diagnosis is in question, a Tzanck test can be performed to demonstrate multinucleated giant cells. The Tzanck preparation will not differentiate varicella from herpes simplex or herpes zoster, however; all of these show the characteristic cells.

## Disorders With Linear Vesicles (Rhus Dermatitis)

Vesicles that occur in lines are characteristic of allergic contact dermatitis, which, in the United States, is caused most commonly by poison ivy or poison oak (Fig 35-27). The eruption is a delayed contact hypersensitivity reaction to a sap-like material known as urushiol that is present in the plants. Trauma to the leaves of the plants releases this material, which can be transferred to the skin. The rapidity of reaction to contact depends on the sensitivity of the individual and the amount of toxin deposited on the skin. Pruritic papules and vesicles may appear in a few hours in areas of heavy contamination, or over a few days on skin areas where contact was minimal. The development of new lesions over a few days' time has fueled the false tale that the vesicular fluid itself spreads the lesions.

Poison ivy most frequently occurs in the summer, but it can occur at any time of year. Dried leaves, stems, and roots may release the toxic material. Burning vines may release particles into the air that affect very sensitive individuals. Scrubbing areas that are known to have come in contact with these plants can prevent the development of lesions if it is done early enough. The urushiols are bound rapidly to the skin on contact, however.

The classic lesions of rhus dermatitis are vesicles arranged in lines, but linear and nonlinear erythematous papules can be found as well. Children's faces may be edematous and erythematous, resembling the manifestations of angioneurotic edema. The arms, legs, and neck should be examined carefully for the presence of linear lesions to establish the diagnosis.

The treatment of rhus dermatitis is symptomatic. Wet compresses and calamine lotion assist in drying the lesions, and antihistamines may help relieve the pruritus. Topical steroids prob-

ably are of little benefit in extensive cases. Oral steroids such as prednisone (1 to 2 mg/kg/day) in decreasing doses over a 2-week period are indicated. As in any other pruritic disorder, care must be taken to prevent or, if prevention is not possible, to recognize secondary skin infection.

## Other Vesicular Lesions With Typical Distributions

### Hand-Foot-and-Mouth Disease

The characteristic feature of hand-foot-and-mouth disease is the distribution of the vesicular eruption, as per the name. This viral exanthem occurs most often in the summer months, often in mini-epidemics. The most frequent site of lesions is the mouth, where the vesicular tops are eroded rapidly, leaving ulcers. The exanthem on the hands and feet is vesicular, but the vesicles often have a curious linear or arcuate shape (Fig 35-28). The rash may appear maculopapular at the outset. Occasionally, the buttocks may be involved. Coxsackievirus A16 is associated most frequently with this disease, with occasional coxsackievirus A5 and A10 infections.

The primary disorder to differentiate from hand-foot-and-mouth syndrome is primary herpes gingivostomatitis. Treatment is symptomatic, and the course of the illness usually is benign.

### Scabies

The characteristic feature of scabies is intense pruritus. Early lesions are vesicular before excoriation and lichenification of the skin. The head generally is spared, except in babies. Large vesicles and occasional bullae may appear on the palms and soles of infants and toddlers with scabies. The best means of documenting scabies infestation is to apply immersion oil, scrape the vesicles or papules with a scalpel blade, collect the oil, apply it to a glass slide, and examine the contents under a microscope for the presence of the mite or its eggs or feces. See the section on pruritic lesions later in this chapter for further discussion.

### Tinea Pedis

Athlete's foot is uncommon before puberty. The presence of erythema and scaling in the interdigital webs of the toes always

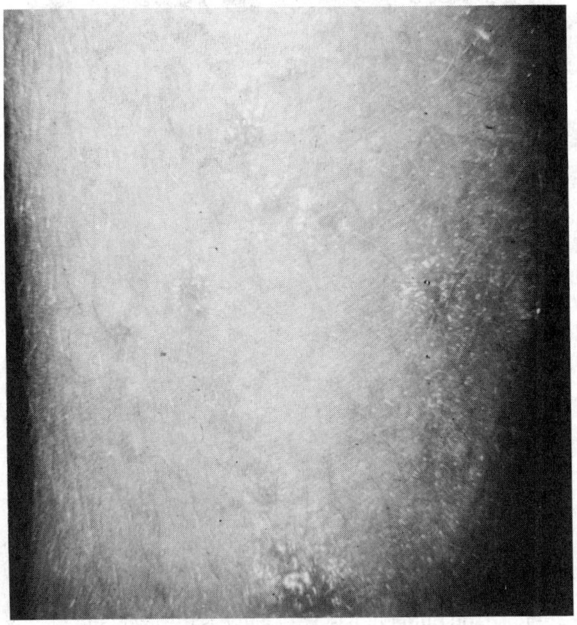

**Figure 35-27.** Rhus dermatitis caused by poison ivy is characterized by linear papules, vesicles, and bullae.

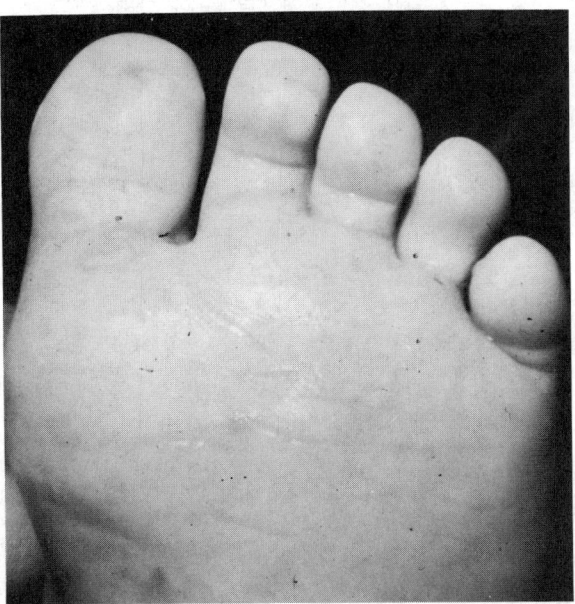

**Figure 35-28.** In hand-foot-and-mouth disease, vesicles are present on the hands and feet, as well as in the mouth. Note the linear configuration of these vesicles.

should suggest this diagnosis, particularly in adolescents and adults. The lesions may appear vesicular or bullous as well. An id reaction, resulting in lesions on the palms or fingers that vary from plaques to vesicles to other types of lesions, may be associated with tinea pedis. The presence of any lesion on the hands should prompt an examination of the feet for tinea pedis. Treatment usually can be accomplished with a topical antifungal agent. Following clearing, the feet should be washed and dried carefully and an antifungal powder applied daily.

### Dyshidrotic Eczema

Dyshidrotic eczema is a poorly understood, but relatively common vesicular eruption that appears most often on the hands and feet. The lesions are deep-seated vesicles that give the involved areas an appearance akin to that of tapioca. Pruritus associated with the vesicles usually is pronounced. If they are excoriated and ruptured, the lesions may be erythematous and crusted. Vesicles also may coalesce to form bullae. Despite the name of the condition, the eccrine apparatus is not affected.

Although its cause is not clear, dyshidrotic eczema tends to occur in individuals with a personal or family history of atopy. Contact dermatitis and id reactions of tinea pedis, as well as primary tinea infections, must be considered in the differential diagnosis. Treatment includes the application of compresses and a fluorinated topical steroid.

## Bullous Lesions

Many of the vesicular lesions mentioned above may result in the appearance of bullae secondary to the coalescence of vesicles.

### Burns

Bullae may be the result of thermal injury to the skin, either accidental or inflicted.

### Bullous Impetigo

The classic lesions of bullous impetigo, a staphylococcal infection, are bullae filled with cloudy fluid surrounded by a thin margin of erythema. Characteristically, many of the bullae have ruptured, leaving dried-up lesions scattered in contiguous areas (Fig 35-29). The most recently ruptured lesions have an erythematous, shiny base resembling lacquered paint, whereas older ones are

completely dry and nonerythematous, a collarette of scale being the only remnant. In infants and toddlers, the diaper area is affected most frequently. *Staphylococcus aureus* is the organism responsible for this infection, with the exfoliative toxin released locally by this bacteria causing production of the bullae.

Because the lesions are highly contagious and may spread cutaneously as well as systemically, parenteral rather than topical antibiotics are required for treatment.

### Staphylococcal Scalded Skin Syndrome

Some *Staphylococcus aureus* produce an exfoliative toxin, usually phage group II, type 70 or 71. Infections with these phage-producing strains often may be subtle, but they produce a striking picture befitting the name. The entire skin surface may be erythematous, and bullae may appear in areas of trauma or in areas that are rubbed or simply touched (see Color Figure 12). The separation of skin at sites of trauma is known as Nikolsky's sign. Affected children are in extreme pain. A characteristic feature is crusting in a radial pattern (sunburst) around the mouth, nose, and eyes (Fig 35-30). The mucous membranes are not involved, which may help distinguish this illness from Stevens-Johnson syndrome.

The skin separation in staphylococcal scalded skin syndrome is intraepidermal rather than deeper, at the epidermal basement membrane, as occurs in toxic epidermal necrolysis (TEN). In the latter disorder, there usually is mucous membrane involvement and no sunburst of crusting around the mouth and eyes. With or without antibiotic treatment, improvement occurs within 3 to 5 days. Antibiotic therapy should be used to prevent recurrences of the problem. Occasionally, dehydration is a major complication because of the loss of cutaneous covering.

### Blistering Distal Dactylitis

Blistering distal dactylitis usually is manifested by a single pus-filled bulla on the volar aspect of the distal phalanx of one finger. The cause is not clear, although insect bites have been known to precede the lesion. The bacterial cause commonly is group A β-hemolytic streptococci. Treatment may be accomplished by simple incision and drainage of the bulla or prescription of systemic antibiotics.

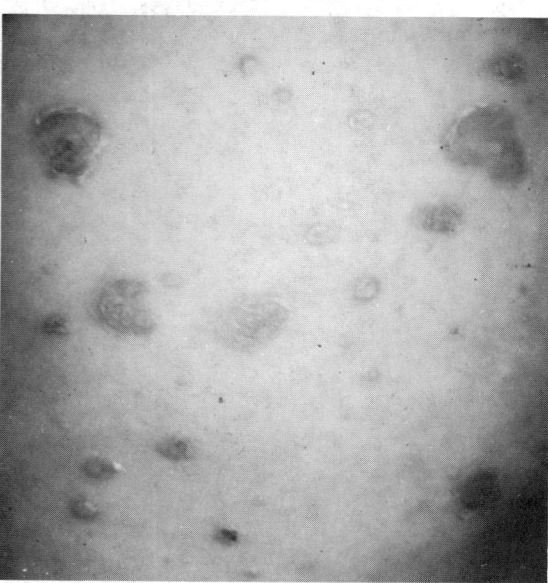

**Figure 35-29.** Fresh and ruptured bullous lesions of staphylococcal impetigo.

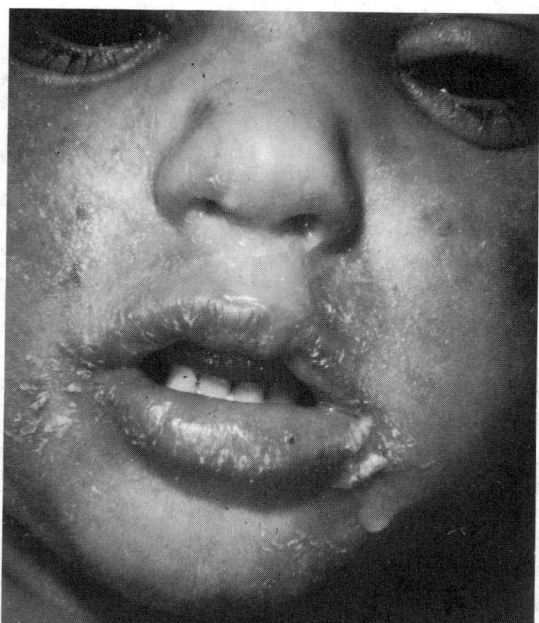

**Figure 35-30.** The purulent nasal discharge is the likely site of infection in this child with staphylococcal scalded skin syndrome. Note the early perioral scaling.

## Papular Urticaria

Although the characteristic lesions of papular urticaria are erythematous papules, impressive numbers of bullae may develop in involved areas in individuals who are highly sensitive to insect bites (see the earlier section regarding red papules).

## Urticaria Pigmentosa

Urticaria pigmentosa is manifested most frequently by the presence of small, pigmented macules and papules on the skin, varying in number from a few to hundreds. Vigorous rubbing of the lesions causes histamine to be released from the mast cells that are present in large numbers in the macules, which in turn causes the lesions to swell and develop an erythematous flare (Darier's sign). In early childhood, these lesions may form vesicles or bullae. In bullous mastocytosis, an unusual form of mast cell disease, recurrent bullae appear on normal-looking skin that is devoid of pigmented macules or nodules. The lesions generally are quite pruritic. Secondary skin infections are common. The disease usually remits by early adolescence.

## Erythema Multiforme Bullosum

Bullous lesions may appear in the target lesions of erythema multiforme (see the section regarding annular lesions later in this chapter).

## Chronic Bullous Disease of Childhood

Chronic bullous disease of childhood is the most common chronic bullous disease seen in children. It occurs sporadically, most commonly in the first decade of life (18 months to 8½ years), is characterized by spontaneous remissions and exacerbations, and has a duration of 2 to 4 years. The clinical spectrum of the disease often makes accurate diagnosis difficult, bullous impetigo being the most frequent misdiagnosis. The bullae may be large, tense, and clear or hemorrhagic, arising on normal or erythematous skin; alternatively, they may appear as large, rosette-like erythematous plaques with central clearing and annular borders marginated by vesicles and bullae. New lesions develop around older ones, creating a "cluster of jewels" picture. The lesions occur most frequently on the buttocks, genitals, thighs, and perioral areas. There are no mucosal lesions or herpetiform grouping.

Pathologically, the blisters are subepidermal and can be separated from similar-appearing blisters by immunofluorescent studies, which demonstrate linear IgA deposits at the basement membrane zone in uninvolved skin. It is thought that IgA deposits lead to complement activation and influx of inflammatory cells to produce skin lesions. Sulfapyridine seems to be effective therapy, especially when it is preceded by systemic steroids.

## Pemphigus Vulgaris and Pemphigus Foliaceus

Pemphigus vulgaris and pemphigus foliaceus are extremely rare in childhood. The cutaneous lesions of pemphigus vulgaris often are preceded by oral ulcerations. When blisters form, they progress rapidly to erosions. Childhood pemphigus foliaceus is confused most often with seborrhea or impetigo. The initial lesions are an erythema of the scalp with scaling, blistering, and oozing. The eruption then progresses to the trunk and extremities, producing erythematous, crusting plaques. The mucous membranes are not involved. Diagnosis of both forms of pemphigus requires immunofluorescent stains, and both forms are treated with systemic corticosteroids.

## Epidermolysis Bullosa

The skin disorders listed as epidermolysis bullosa are a mixed group of hereditary, mechanobullous diseases (Table 35-2). Their characteristic feature is the development, in response to trauma, of vesicles, bullae, or erosions. There is a wide spectrum of degree of skin fragility and involvement in this group.

The autosomal dominant form of non-scarring epidermolysis bullosa simplex may be present at birth and may involve the mucous membranes as well as the rest of the skin (see Color Figure 15). Although this form tends to be milder than some of the other types, it may be severe in newborns. Lesions develop over traumatized areas in most children, especially the hands, feet, extremities, and trunk. The disorder generally improves with time, although it worsens in warm weather.

An interesting form of epidermolysis bullosa simplex is the localized type (Weber-Cockayne syndrome), which is confined to the hands and feet. This also is inherited in an autosomal dominant fashion and may be confused with friction blisters unless a careful family history is obtained.

Junctional epidermolysis bullosa, an autosomal recessive disorder, may present at birth or shortly thereafter. Although this type may seem benign at first, it often is progressive. Death is common, although its timing varies; it may occur after weeks or

---

**TABLE 35-2. Major Types of Epidermolysis Bullosa**

| Type | Inheritance | Clinical Picture |
|---|---|---|
| I. Nonscarring generalized epidermolysis bullosa | Autosomal dominant | Present at birth; mucous membranes may be involved; feet and hand lesions most common, but may be generalized |
| Localized epidermolysis bullosa (Weber-Cockayne) | Autosomal dominant | Onset usually in first 2 years of life; lesions confined to hands and feet; merges with friction blisters |
| II. Junctional epidermolysis bullosa | Autosomal recessive | Present at birth or soon after; variable severity, usually progressive; large perioral granulomatous ulcers common; loss of nails, dysplastic teeth; complications: infection, growth failure, anemia |
| III. Scaring (dystrophic) Dominant dystrophic epidermolysis bullosa | Autosomal dominant | Hyperkeratotic lesions at sites of blistering; hypertrophic scars; nail loss; milia present; variable severity |
| Recessive dystrophic epidermolysis bullosa | Autosomal recessive | Onset at birth; progressive scarring and deformity; oral involvement; esophageal strictures; nail loss; mitten-like hands and feet; contactures of joints |

years. Large granulomatous ulcers usually appear in the perioral area (Fig 35-31). The nails are lost, and teeth are dysplastic. Mucous membranes frequently are involved early in the course of the disease, and strictures of the esophagus can develop. Scarring may be present. Complications include anemia from chronic blood loss and secondary infections.

The most severe and devastating form of epidermolysis bullosa is the autosomal recessive dystrophic type. The bullae and erosions usually are present at birth, and the entire skin surface may be affected at different times by minor trauma. Scarring, milia formation, and nail loss are prominent features. Oral involvement leads to scarring with the tongue bound down, and swallowing is affected by esophageal strictures. The hands and feet become mitten-like, and contractures develop in the large joints. The prognosis is poor, even with the best of care by parents. Secondary skin infections, anemia, growth retardation, amyloidosis, and skin cancer are complications.

The pathogenesis of these disorders seems to differ with each type, as does the depth of the blister formation. Treatment consists of careful attention to the skin to prevent friction, maintain cleanliness, treat secondary infection and anemia, and maintain adequate nutrition.

## VESICULOPUSTULAR LESIONS

### Impetigo

Bacterial infections of the skin are the most common dermatologic condition for which children are brought to physicians. Superficial infections account for the great majority of these infections, and impetigo is the most common pyoderma. The prevalence of impetigo varies with the season of the year, occurring most often in the warm summer months among individuals with poor hygiene and crowded living conditions. Impetigo previously was

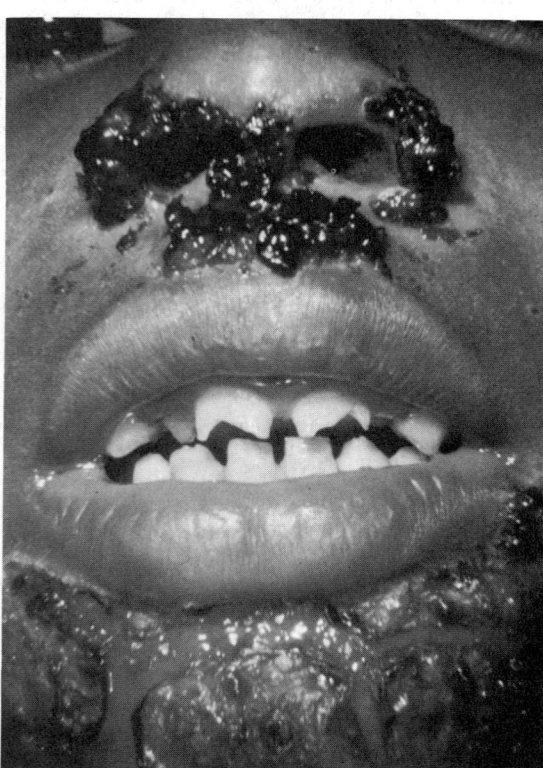

**Figure 35-31.**   In junctional epidermolysis bullosa, erosions with hemorrhagic crusting are typical in the perioral area.

divided into two types, each with a typical clinical picture and different bacterial etiology. An increasing number of studies have found that *Staphylococcus aureus* is the primary agent responsible for most impetigo, however, whether the lesion is golden crusted (which type used to be caused by group A β-hemolytic streptococcus) or bullous (which type always has been staphylococcal in origin).

The crusted lesions of impetigo have little surrounding erythema, but local lymphadenopathy is common (Fig 35-32). The lesions tend to spread locally, and scratching, particularly of insect bites, may result in widespread lesions. Family members often are infected as well. Any area of the body may be involved, and any break in the skin (eg, abrasions, excoriations, lacerations, burns) may provide access.

When group A β-hemolytic streptococci were the most common bacteria responsible for impetigo, secondary nonsuppurative complications, such as post-streptococcal glomerulonephritis, were common in some areas of the United States and other countries. Acute rheumatic fever, however, never has been reported to follow impetigo.

When impetigo is widespread, systemic therapy usually is indicated. Until reports of a change in the bacterial cause of impetigo appeared, crusted lesions were treated with penicillin and bullous impetigo was treated with an antistaphylococcic antibiotic. The trend at present is to treat all impetigo as if the infection were caused by *S aureus*. Mupirocin, a topical antibiotic cream, may be used effectively when the lesions are not widespread.

### Folliculitis and Furunculosis

Infections of the hair follicle unit are caused most frequently by *S aureus*. Folliculitis is a superficial infection; a small rim of erythema surrounds the hair follicle, which is topped by a small, yellowish pustule. Furuncles are deeper infections with a larger rim of erythema, more swelling, and, often, a cavity of pus in the center.

Common sites for these infections include the scalp in children who have their hair pulled tightly, the buttocks in infants wearing occlusive diapers, the beard area in some teenagers, and areas of the skin that are rubbed by padding in athletes. Folliculitis often can be treated successfully with topical antibiotics and washing, but furunculosis usually requires the addition of systemic antistaphylococcic antibiotics.

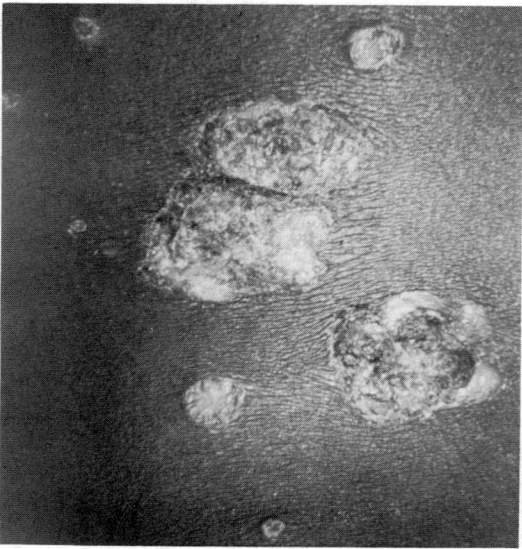

**Figure 35-32.**   Crusted lesions of superficial pyoderma in a perioral distribution.

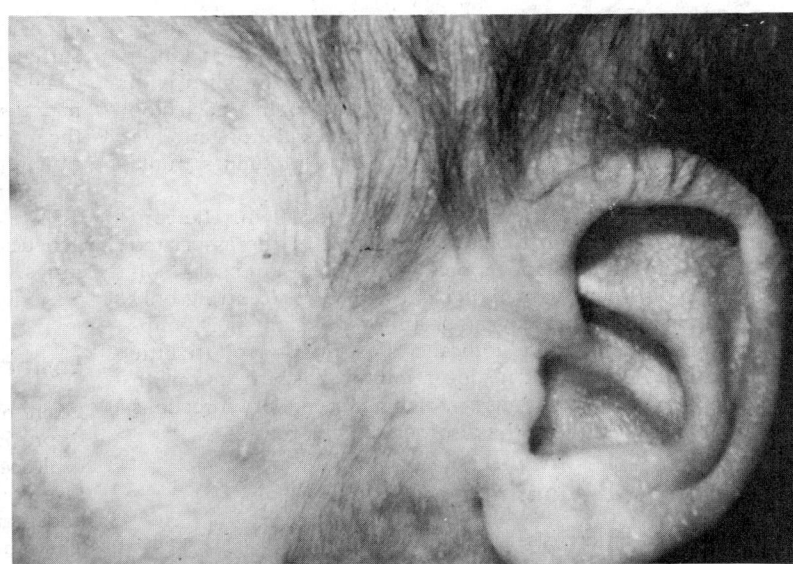

**Figure 35-33.** Diffuse, pinpoint papules and pustules of miliaria on the face of an infant.

A gram-negative folliculitis may occur in teenagers with acne who are treated with systemic antibiotics. Hot tub or whirlpool folliculitis is characterized by the appearance of erythematous macules, papules, or pustules 8 to 48 hours after immersion in these tubs. The lesions are most likely to occur under swimsuits. The bacterial agent responsible usually is *Pseudomonas aeruginosa;* because the infection is superficial, no treatment normally is required.

## Miliaria Pustulosa

Blocked sweat ducts may produce a folliculitis-like eruption. Although "prickly heat" generally is characterized by crops of small (1 to 4 mm) erythematous papules, pustules may be prominent (Fig 35-33). The lesions most commonly appear on areas subject to occlusion, particularly the neck, groin, and axilla, in warm weather or artificially produced warm environments. Treatment consists of the removal of excessive clothing and exposure to air.

## Candidiasis

Yeast infections are caused most commonly by *Candida albicans,* a dimorphic fungus that occurs in both budding and mycelial phases. *Candida* thrives in warm, moist places; the diaper area of infants, which can be likened to a tropical rain forest, is an ideal site for proliferation (Fig 35-34). Characteristically, the inguinal creases are involved in candidal infections, which produce a confluent erythema, often with maceration and fissuring. The earliest lesions of *Candida* are small vesicopustules on an erythematous base. The lesions enlarge and tend to become confluent. Their roofs then are lost rapidly, leaving the red base. Other common sites of candidal infection include the axillae, the neck in young infants, and the corners of the mouth.

Infants commonly have "thrush," which appears as adherent, cheesy plaques of candidal infection in the mouth. Infection of the nails and paronychia also may develop in young children who suck their fingers or in individuals who immerse their hands in water for extended periods on a regular basis. Outside the neonatal period, overt candidal infections are uncommon. The presence of *Candida* might suggest the presence of diabetes mellitus, hypoparathyroidism, Addison's disease, an altered immunologic response to infection, acquired immunodeficiency syndrome, or malignancy.

Cutaneous infection with *Candida* usually can be treated ef-

fectively with drying and the application of an anti-candidal agent, such as nystatin (Mycostatin).

## Dermatophyte Infections

Dermatophyte infections are common in children. The appearance of lesions varies with the site infected, but the basic lesion is a microvesicle that expands, creating an enlarging ring with clearing in the center (see the section regarding annular lesions later in this chapter).

## Scabies

Infestations with the scabies mite, *Sarcoptes scabiei,* may produce vesiculopustular lesions, particularly on the hands and feet of young children (see the section regarding pruritic lesions later in this chapter).

## Infantile Acropustulosis

Infantile acropustulosis is a highly pruritic skin disorder that was not described until the mid-1970s. The clinical picture is characteristic: the lesions are vesicles and pustules located primarily

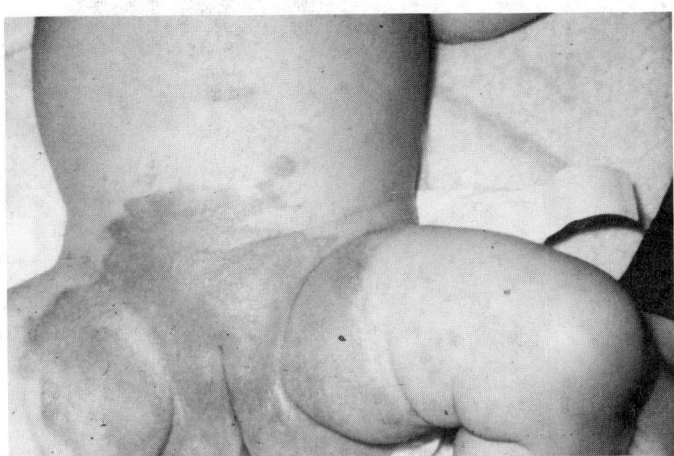

**Figure 35-34.** Candidal infection is characterized by involvement of the inguinal creases and satellite pustules.

on the palms and soles that occur in crops lasting 5 to 7 days and recur until the child is 2 to 3 years of age (Fig 35-35). Onset is between 2 to 10 months of age. The pustules are filled with polymorphonuclear cells and, occasionally, eosinophils. Each crop may be followed by a remission of a few weeks before another bout occurs. Lesions occasionally appear on the extremities, trunk, and face, as well as on the palms and soles.

The cause of infantile acropustulosis is unknown. The condition often is mistaken for scabies because of the associated intense pruritus and its appearance on the palms and soles. Although the disorder originally was described as occurring only in black individuals, all races can be affected. Treatment is symptomatic; antihistamines and topical corticosteroids produce little response. In severe cases, dapsone, a sulfone, has been used with success. Because of the intense scratching, secondary infections are common. Fortunately, the disorder abates with age.

## Hand-Foot-and-Mouth Disease

Hand-foot-and-mouth disease also is a highly characteristic vesiculopustular disorder. As the name denotes, the vesicles are distributed typically on the palms and soles, with ulcerations, or unroofed vesicles, present on the tongue, gums, and buccal mucosa (see Fig 35-28, and the earlier section regarding other vesicular lesions with typical distributions).

## Dyshidrotic Eczema

Dyshidrotic eczema is a poorly understood and often mislabeled disorder that is characterized by the appearance of pruritic deep vesicles and vesiculopustular lesions on the hands and feet. The sides of the fingers often are affected. Scratching leads to thickening of the skin and scaling, giving an eczematoid appearance. The eruptions generally are fairly symmetric. (See the earlier discussion of this disorder in the section regarding other vesicular lesions with typical distributions.)

## Pustular Psoriasis

Pustular psoriasis is a severe form of psoriasis that is uncommon in children. Innumerable pustules with an erythematous base

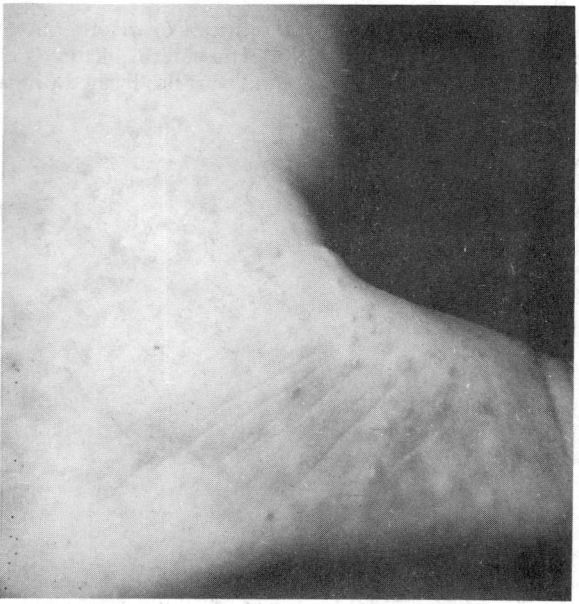

**Figure 35-35.** Intensely pruritic vesicles and pustules of the hands and feet are characteristic of infantile acropustulosis.

appear and spread on previously normal skin. The entire skin surface may become involved. The 2- to 3-mm pustules tend to coalesce, rupture, scale, and heal, often in waves. Healed areas may develop new waves of lesions. The mucous membranes of the mouth may be involved, and the tongue may appear to have a geographic pattern. The skin is tender, and systemic toxicity is common.

The cause of pustular psoriasis is unknown. There may be a genetic predisposition. Triggering factors include emotional stress, drugs, allergies, infection, and trauma. Treatment is supportive. Systemic and topical steroids seem to have no effect.

## Eosinophilic Pustular Folliculitis

Eosinophilic pustular folliculitis is characterized by recurrent crops of pruritic, follicular, papulopustular lesions. The lesions tend to coalesce into plaques and occur most commonly on the scalp, face, chest, and back. Smears from the pustules show eosinophils, and peripheral eosinophilia is common. The lesions are sterile. The cause of the lesions is not known and the course is variable. Treatment with topical steroids of moderate potency has met with modest success.

## SCALING AND DRY LESIONS

## Atopic Dermatitis

Atopic dermatitis, a common skin condition better known among laypersons as eczema, affects about 4% of the pediatric population. The cause is unknown, but seems to be multifactorial; heredity plays a role, modified by environmental factors. The basic problem seems to be a sensitivity of the skin to numerous stimuli, all of which produce pruritus. An apt description of atopic dermatitis is "an itch that rashes." If the itch can be controlled, the rash usually will not develop.

Atopic dermatitis is rare in infants less than 2 months of age, primarily because the "itch-scratch" mechanism does not mature until around 3 months of age. Onset of the rash occurs before the age of 1 year in 60% of affected children and before the age of 5 years in 85%. The rash of atopic dermatitis most often appears as dry patches, but sometimes it is eczematoid (weeping), particularly on the cheeks and the extensor surfaces of the arms and legs (Fig 35-36). Dry patches may occur on much of the body surface. Lesions may become hyperpigmented, especially in black individuals, from the scratching and rubbing. In toddlers, the rash characteristically appears in the popliteal and antecubital fossae, although other areas are involved as well. In adults, the periorbital and neck areas often are affected. The skin of most patients generally is dry, and the decreased humidity of the environment that is associated with heating in the winter commonly accentuates the problem.

In addition to appearing dry and somewhat scaly, the skin of individuals with atopic dermatitis is thickened or has undergone lichenification (Fig 35-37), and normal skin markings are accentuated (Fig 35-38). Scratching commonly results in secondary infections, particularly with staphylococci. The presence of infection, which may be occult, often leads to accentuation of the pruritus with a resultant flare in the rash.

The major and minor criteria used to diagnose atopic dermatitis are listed in Table 35-3. Because this disorder is chronic and relapsing, treatment involves a great deal of teaching and explaining to the parents and child, as well as prescribing of medications. Given that ichthyosis commonly accompanies atopic dermatitis, other medications may be necessary to give the skin a relatively normal texture and appearance.

Factors that may precipitate pruritus in atopic skin include

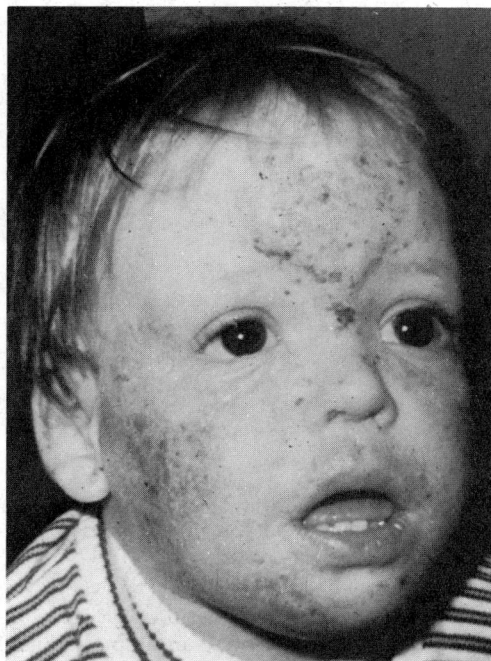

**Figure 35-36.** Typical morphology and facial distribution of infantile atopic dermatitis.

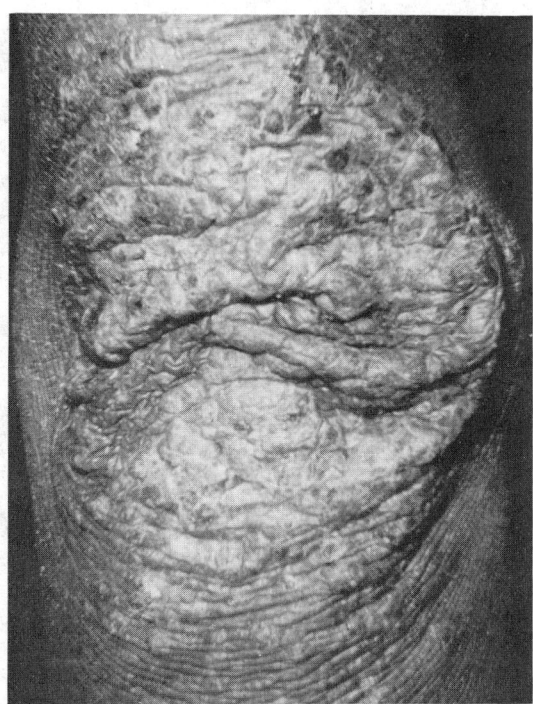

**Figure 35-38.** Dramatic lichenification from chronic scratching in atopic dermatitis.

soaps; sweating and, conversely, exposure to cool air; certain materials, especially wool and synthetic fibers; and stress. Well-controlled studies have demonstrated food sensitivity in as many as 5% of affected children. The foods most frequently implicated are eggs, milk, wheat, peanuts, soybeans, and chicken. The role of inhalants (pollen, mold, and dust mites) is not clear.

Atopic skin almost always is colonized by *Staphylococcus au-*

*reus,* and infections are common, often leading to exacerbation of the rash. The role of *S aureus* in exacerbation may be by direct biologic action or by indirect damage mediated by the immune and inflammatory systems.

Atopic skin also is prone to viral infections; herpes simplex may spread rapidly and extensively over the entire skin surface, resulting in severe disease and even death (Fig 35-39). Molluscum contagiosum also can be extensive on atopic skin. Interestingly,

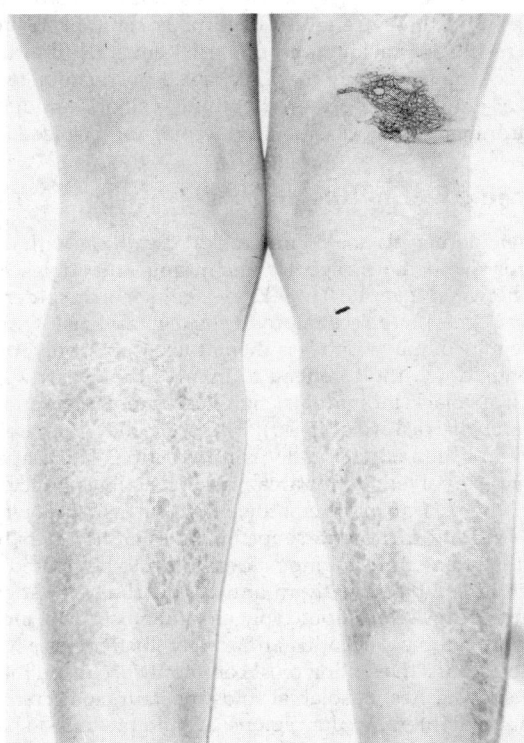

**Figure 35-37.** Lichenous plaques of atopic dermatitis involving both lower legs.

**TABLE 35-3. Diagnositic Criteria for Atopic Dermatitis**

I. All of the following
  A. Pruritus
  B. Typical morphology and distribution
    1. Facial and extensor involvement in infants
    2. Flexural lichenification in children
  C. Tendency toward chronic or chronically relapsing dermatitis
  D. II or III below
II. Two or more of the following
  A. Personal or family history of atopic disease (asthma, allergic rhinitis, atopic dermatitis)
  B. Immediate skin test reactivity
  C. White dermographism or delayed blanch to cholinergic agents
  D. Anterior subcapsular cataracts
III. Four or more of the following
  A. Xerosis/ichthyosis/hyperlinear palms
  B. Pityriasis alba
  C. Keratosis pilaris
  D. Facial pallor/infraorbital darkening
  E. Dennie-Morgan infraorbital fold
  F. Elevated serum IgE
  G. Keratoconus
  H. Tendency toward nonspecific hand dermatitis
  I. Tendency toward repeated cutaneous infections

*Hanifin JM, Lobitz WC Jr. Newer concepts of atopic dermatitis. Arch Dermatol 1977;113:663.*

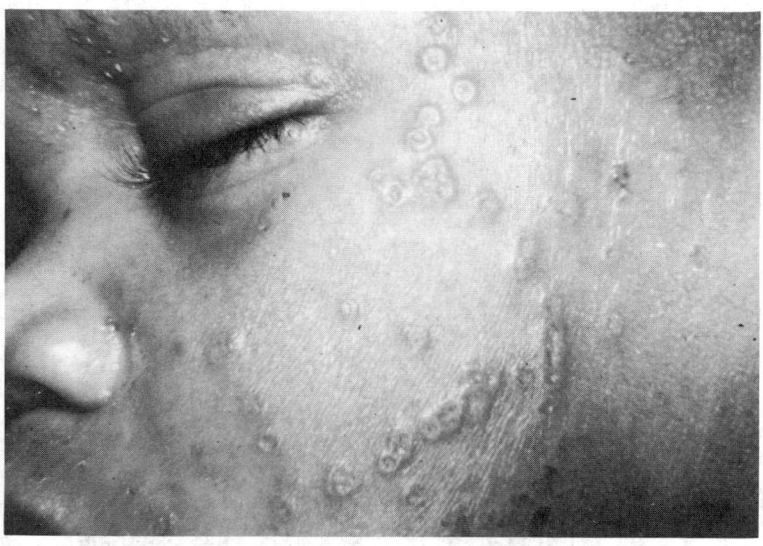

**Figure 35-39.** Children with atopic dermatitis are susceptible to the development of widespread cutaneous herpes simplex.

atopic children are less prone than are normal children to contact dermatitis.

Fifty percent to 80% of children with atopic dermatitis go on to have allergic rhinitis or asthma. Although the skin of the majority of children improves by adulthood, it tends to remain "sensitive," especially to winter dryness and soaps, throughout their lives.

The keys to treatment, in addition to education, are avoidance of precipitants (particularly drying soaps), use of emollients to keep the skin moist, and application of corticosteroids to reduce the inflammation and pruritus. Non-fluorinated steroids should be used to circumvent adrenal suppression and skin atrophy, which may occur with stronger medications. Topical fluorinated steroids should be applied only to the most severely affected areas for the shortest possible time, and they never should be used on the face or perineum. Hydrocortisone may be added to an emollient to produce a 1% concentration. A potent oral antipruritic agent such as hydroxyzine should be prescribed in doses large enough to reduce the pruritus, which results in the "itch-scratch-itch" cycle. A large dose at bedtime will help to reduce scratching during sleep.

If there is any suspicion of possible secondary bacterial infection, an antistaphylococcic antibiotic should be administered by mouth. In severe cases of recalcitrant atopic dermatitis, children may need to receive daily doses of antibiotics. As the rash improves, the frequency of application of steroid medications and the use of antipruritic agents may be reduced. Emollients, however, often need to be continued, particularly after bathing.

Atopic dermatitis may be confused with seborrheic dermatitis in young infants, or with "dandruff" in older children and adults. Scabies, which also is characterized by pruritus, should be differentiated easily from atopic dermatitis by the presence and distribution of the papulovesicular lesions and the short duration of the skin condition. Allergic or contact dermatitis also usually has a shorter course than does atopic dermatitis.

## Pityriasis Alba

Pityriasis alba is a common, asymptomatic skin condition that is characterized by a relatively distinct hypopigmented patch or patches with minimal to no fine scale. The lesions, which generally are round to oval, occur most commonly on the face and less often on the neck, upper trunk, and proximal extremities. Most cases seem to appear after sun exposure in children between the ages of 3 and 16 years. Individual lesions last 1 to 2 years. Although the lesions commonly occur in atopic individuals, the cause is unknown. The response to topical steroids and emollients is not good. The differential diagnosis includes tinea corporis, tinea versicolor, vitiligo, and psoriasis.

## Xerosis

Dry skin has many names, including winter eczema, eczema hiemalis, and eczema craquelé; whatever it is called, it is a common condition characterized by dryness and dehydration of the epidermis. Xerosis occurs most commonly during the winter months, when the indoor environment becomes dry from heating. Too frequent bathing and harsh soaps may contribute to the problem. The skin generally is dry and often has areas of scaly patches, particularly on the extremities. Pruritus is common. When the dryness results in cracking and fine erythematous fissuring, the appearance may resemble that of cracked porcelain. Treatment consists of emollients, decreased bathing, use of humidifiers for the environment and, occasionally, steroids for localized lesions.

## Seborrheic Dermatitis

Seborrheic dermatitis is a common skin condition with a predilection for two pediatric age groups, infants and adolescents. In infants between 2 and 10 weeks of age, seborrheic dermatitis generally begins on the scalp, producing a greasy, yellowish scale. The base may or may not be erythematous. Commonly, the scaling extends down the forehead to involve the eyebrows, nose, and ears. In black individuals, significant depigmentation may accompany the rash (Fig 35-40). The scale may be barely perceptible, and the rash generally is not pruritic. The diaper area also may be involved; in this area, which usually is infected with *Candida*, there is an erythematous, diffuse rash involving the creases. Without treatment, seborrheic dermatitis clears by 8 to 12 months of age. Intertriginous areas need to be treated with a mild steroid combined with an anti-candidal agent. Continued "dandruff" of the scalp should suggest other disorders, including tinea capitis, atopic dermatitis and, rarely, histiocytosis X.

In adolescents, the scaling most commonly occurs on the scalp, eyebrows, eyelashes, nasolabial folds, postauricular crease, and presternal and interscapular regions. A mild tar-based shampoo usually keeps the scalp involvement under control. Mild (0.5% to 1%) hydrocortisone will aid in clearing other areas of the skin.

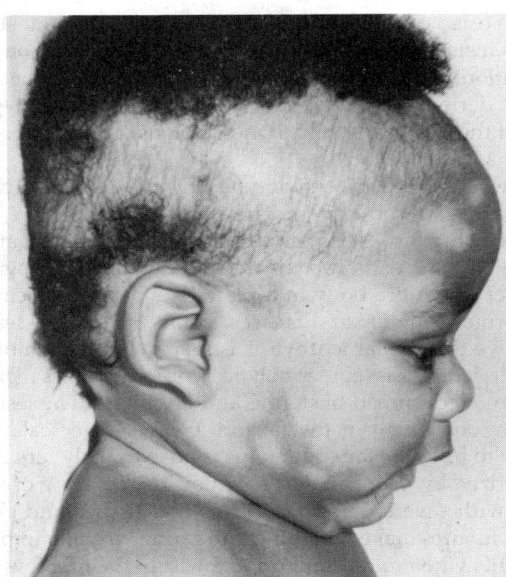

**Figure 35-40.** Note the facial depigmentation and scalp hair loss without prominent scaling in this child with seborrheic dermatitis.

The etiology of seborrheic dermatitis is not clear; the histopathology is nonspecific. The idea that the condition has something to do with sebaceous glands is supported by development of the dermatitis in areas with the highest density of these glands. The appearance of seborrheic dermatitis in infants probably reflects the effect of transmitted maternal sex hormones on these glands; reappearance of the condition during puberty occurs with the resurgence of sex hormones.

## Leiner's Disease

Leiner's disease is a rare disorder characterized by a generalized seborrheic dermatitis combined with severe diarrhea, failure to thrive, and recurrent infections. The disease usually has its onset in the first few months of life. The skin generally is erythematous, with pronounced desquamation of a fine scale. Dysfunction of the fifth component of complement has been demonstrated in some cases.

## Tinea Versicolor

The characteristic clinical presentation of tinea versicolor is the asymptomatic, gradual appearance and spread of hyperpigmented and hypopigmented areas on the neck, chest, and back. The lesions of this common fungal disorder are relatively discrete, are irregular in shape, and may be red, brown, or whitish. The macules may be ovoid or coin shaped and have a fine adherent scale. Pruritus is uncommon. Most cases occur after puberty, but facial lesions in infants have been described, probably resulting from contact with affected mothers.

The diagnosis may be confirmed by microscopic examination of the scale (to which potassium hydroxide has been added) for the presence of the budding cells and hyphae of *Pityrosporum orbiculare*, which give a spaghetti-and-meatball appearance. A Wood's light examination in a totally dark room should reveal a yellow to yellow-blue fluorescence, unless the patient has bathed in the previous 6 to 12 hours.

Treatment of tinea versicolor consists of selenium sulfide lotion applied in various therapeutic routines. Although this usually produces good results, relapses of the infection are common. Ketoconazole, 200 to 400 mg orally every month, also is effective.

## Psoriasis

The fact that psoriasis often has its onset in childhood is not commonly known. It is estimated that 10% of cases begin before the patient is 10 years of age and that 35% begin by 20 years of age. The cause of the condition is not known, although it is clear that hereditary factors play a role. Trauma to the skin is a common precipitant in susceptible individuals.

The clinical lesions usually are distinctive, with well-demarcated papules or maculopapular lesions covered with a scale (see Color Figure 18). Larger lesions form characteristic plaques with distinct borders, a silvery scale, and an erythematous base. The scale tends to build up in layers, and its removal may cause a bleeding point (Auspitz' sign). The papules enlarge to form plaques. The distribution usually is symmetric, with plaques commonly appearing over the knees and elbows because they are sites of repeated trauma. The Koebner phenomenon (ie, the appearance of rash at sites of physical, thermal, or mechanical trauma) often is evident. The scalp frequently shows a thick, adherent scale; the nails often demonstrate punctate stippling or pitting, or become discolored and crumbly; and the palms and soles may show scaling and fissuring.

A variety of inciting factors in addition to trauma have been associated with the appearance of psoriatic lesions. An interesting one in children is the development of guttate psoriasis, a condition that is characterized by multiple, small, teardrop-like lesions associated with group A β-hemolytic streptococcal infection (Fig 35-41). Other agents implicated are sunburn, drug eruptions, and viral infections. The histologic picture is one of hyperproliferation of the epidermis.

The course of psoriasis is unpredictable. Treatment consists of the application of a good lubricant. For small areas of involvement, fluorinated steroids may be successful; tars also may help. Exposure to sunlight, with care taken not to burn the skin, seems to be the best therapy. Oral psoralens combined with ultraviolet

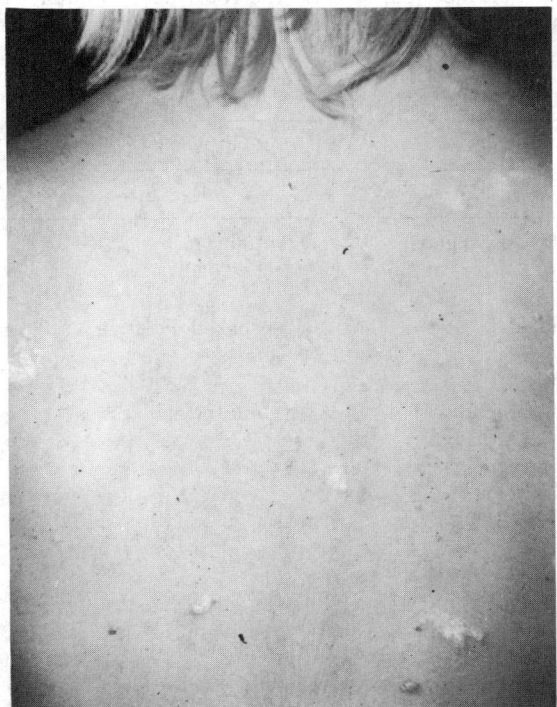

**Figure 35-41.** The sudden widespread appearance of small, scaly plaques is characteristic of guttate psoriasis.

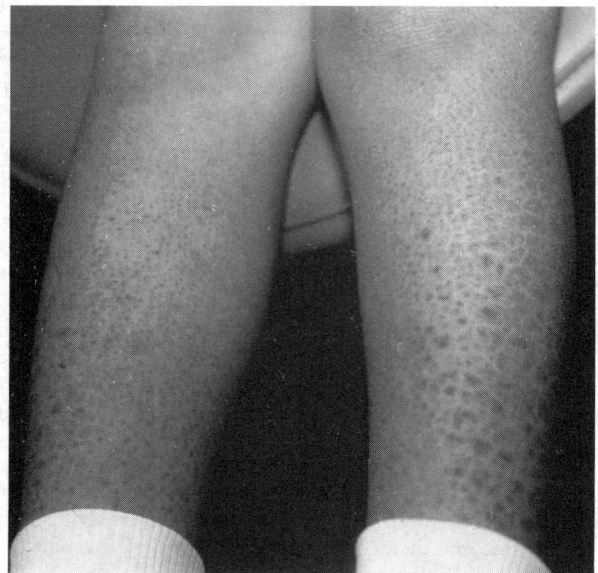

**Figure 35-42.** Large, plate-like scales of the lower legs in a patient with ichthyosis vulgaris.

light and methotrexate therapy rarely are indicated for use in children.

The differential diagnosis in childhood includes uncommon disorders such as pityriasis rubra pilaris, parapsoriasis, and lichen planus. Occasionally, atopic dermatitis may be confused with psoriasis, but psoriasis is not pruritic.

## Ichthyosis

Ichthyosis refers to a group of disorders that are characterized by the accumulation of visible scales and a general dryness of the skin surface (Fig 35-42). The four most common types of ichthyosis and some of their characteristic features are listed in Table 35-4.

Ichthyosis vulgaris is much more common than most people realize. Most cases are mild and are overlooked easily on routine examination. This type of ichthyosis commonly is misdiagnosed as atopic dermatitis, occasionally leading to confusion regarding failure of the skin to respond to medications prescribed for atopic dermatitis.

In the sex-linked, recessive type of ichthyosis, the scales are larger and yellowish-brown. The palms and soles are not involved, but the face, scalp, and neck characteristically are.

Lamellar ichthyosis is characterized by greasy, brown scales that cover the entire body in a plate-like fashion, resembling a suit of armor. The flexural creases, palms, soles, and scalp also are involved. Lamellar ichthyosis is relatively uncommon.

Bullous ichthyosis (epidermolytic hyperkeratosis) is manifested at birth by widespread blistering and erythema. The lesions are especially prominent in the flexural creases. The scale is thick and gray to brown. Harlequin fetus is an extremely rare disorder characterized by massive, dense, armor-like covering of the skin at birth with severe deformity of the soft tissues and skeleton. The skin fissures make breathing and eating virtually impossible, and infants who are not stillborn die within the first few days of life. Ichthyosis also is seen in numerous other syndromes, including Sjögren-Larsson, Refsum's, and Conradi's syndromes.

Considerable research into the pathogenesis of the ichthyoses has led to a better understanding of these disorders. Although the fundamental defect is unknown in most cases, it appears that disorders of lipid metabolism are somehow responsible. Steroid sulfatase deficiency has been found in X-linked ichthyosis.

The treatment of ichthyosis varies with the type. Generally, an emollient containing an organic acid, such as lactic or salicylic acid, applied once or twice a day will result in improvement in appearance.

## Nummular Eczema

As the name denotes, nummular eczema is characterized by the presence of coin-shaped plaques of eczema. The lesions of this poorly understood disorder may be "dry" (ie, covered with dry scales) or "wet" (ie, composed of papules and vesicles with a

**TABLE 35-4. The Primary Types of Ichthyosis**

| Type | Inheritance | Incidence | Onset | Clinical Features |
|---|---|---|---|---|
| Ichthyosis vulgaris | Autosomal dominant | 1:250 | >3 mo | Fine white scales; flexural creases spared; increased markings on palms and soles |
| X-linked | X-linked recessive | 1:6000 | Birth to 1 year | Dark scale; neck and trunk involved; face, palms, and soles spared |
| Lamellar ichthyosis | Autosomal recessive | <1:100,000 | Birth (collodion baby) | |
| ?Subtypes Classic lamellar ichthyosis | | | | Lemellar ichthyosis: large, dark, plate-like scale involving all surfaces |
| Nonbullous congenital ichthyosiform erythroderma (CIE) | | | | CIE: Finer, white scale erythroderma common |
| Bullous ichthyosis | Autosomal recessive | <1:100,000 | Birth (blistering and erythema) | Greasy brown scales; face less involved; flexures, palms, and soles involved |

*Williams ML. The ichthyoses—pathogenesis and prenatal diagnosis: A review of recent advances. Pediatr Dermatol 1983;1:1.*

scale that gives a wet appearance to the base). They are discrete, often on an erythematous base, and may be hyperpigmented or have undergone lichenification. Pruritus is variable. Lesions appear most commonly on the extensor surfaces of the arms and legs, and on the dorsa of the fingers and hands.

There seems to be an association between a dry environment and appearance of the lesions. Frequent bathing with drying soaps aggravates the rash. Other stimuli also may precipitate or contribute to the rash. Nummular eczema is not thought to be related to atopic dermatitis. Treatment consists of decreased bathing, frequent application of emollients, and, occasionally, for recalcitrant lesions, the use of corticosteroids. The differential diagnosis includes allergic contact dermatitis, atopic dermatitis, psoriasis, tinea corporis, and impetigo.

## Contact Dermatitis

In acute contact dermatitis, the skin usually is erythematous and features vesicles and oozing. In contrast, in chronic contact dermatitis, the skin is scaly and has undergone lichenification with or without crusting. (See the section regarding pruritic lesions later in this chapter.)

## Acrodermatitis Enteropathica

Although the early lesions of acrodermatitis enteropathica are vesicular/bullous and pustular, the primary clinical appearance usually is one of dry, scaly, or crusted lesions with sharply marginated borders (Fig 35-43). The lesions begin around the body orifices (ie, mouth, eyes, perianal areas). The vesicles rupture rapidly, revealing a moist, red base, and then they dry and become plaque-like. Lesions develop on the hands and feet as well and, with time, other areas of the body similarly may be involved.

Acrodermatitis enteropathica was a cruel and devastating illness until zinc deficiency was discovered to be the cause in the early 1970s. Affected children respond readily to oral zinc supplementation. The dermatitis has its onset between a few weeks and 20 months of age, and it often is accompanied by alopecia and diarrhea. Affected infants are irritable and listless, and fail to thrive. Secondary skin infections are common.

Patients receiving total parenteral nutrition are prone to zinc deficiency if they do not receive adequate zinc supplementation. In young infants receiving total parenteral nutrition, a recalcitrant diaper rash always should suggest this possibility (Fig 35-44). Zinc deficiency was thought to be rare in breast-fed infants; however, there has been an increase in cases associated with low levels of zinc in maternal milk.

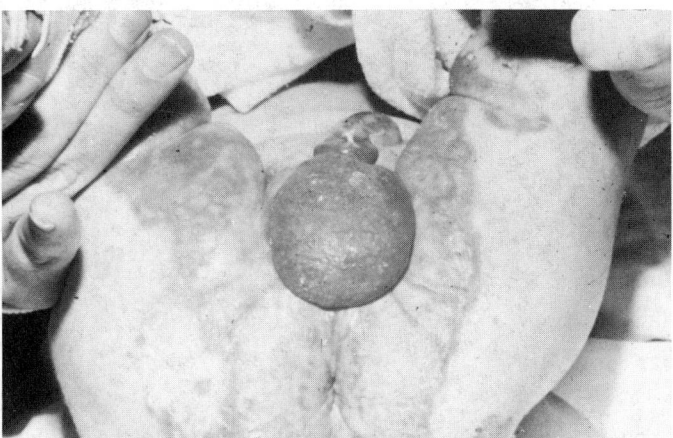

**Figure 35-43.** Erythematous, scaling, well-demarcated perianal dermatitis in an infant with acrodermatitis enteropathica.

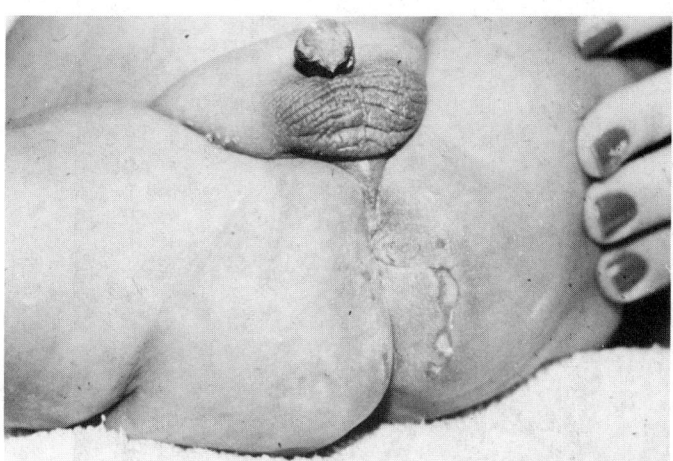

**Figure 35-44.** Ulcerative diaper dermatitis in a child on total parenteral nutrition with inadequate zinc supplementation.

## Dermatomyositis

Scaly, dry, papular lesions on an erythematous base are characteristic of dermatomyositis. The lesions, referred to as Gottron's papules, classically are found over the knuckles, elbows, and knees. At times, diffuse, fine, scaly lesions occur on the extensor surfaces of the arms and legs. A facial eruption, sometimes resembling a sunburn, frequently is present. In two thirds of cases in children, the onset is insidious, with gradually increasing muscle weakness.

## DISORDERS INVOLVING ABNORMAL SKIN TEXTURE

### Sclerosis

#### Morphea

Although most physicians have read about progressive systemic sclerosis, few seem to have heard of morphea, also known as localized scleroderma. Morphea is much more common than progressive systemic sclerosis, and its outcome generally is excellent. The lesions consist of well-demarcated patches of sclerosis of the skin. The patches may be singular, multiple, or linear, and they occur in various patterns and locations. The skin feels indurated to the touch and has lost its normal elasticity. The skin appendages also are lost. A slight depression of the area may be noted, with some loss of skin color. Areas of increased pigmentation occasionally are intermixed (Fig 35-45). Lesions may appear waxy, ivory to yellow, and plaque-like, and they may have violaceous borders.

Morphea comes in many varieties. Large patch, guttate (small, scattered lesions), and linear forms occur. The linear form may affect underlying subcutaneous tissue, muscle, and bone, resulting in significant shortening and deformity of an extremity. Facial lesions, known as coup de sabre, usually appear on the forehead and scalp just lateral to the midline and may cause significant cosmetic deformity.

The cause of morphea is unknown. The histologic picture is indistinguishable from that of progressive systemic sclerosis, but systemic involvement in the two disorders is quite different. Arthralgias are common and polyarthritis sometimes is found in morphea, but the progressive involvement of other organs does not occur. The relationship to progressive systemic sclerosis still is controversial. The lesions of morphea develop insidiously and remain for many years, although most show a tendency to resolve

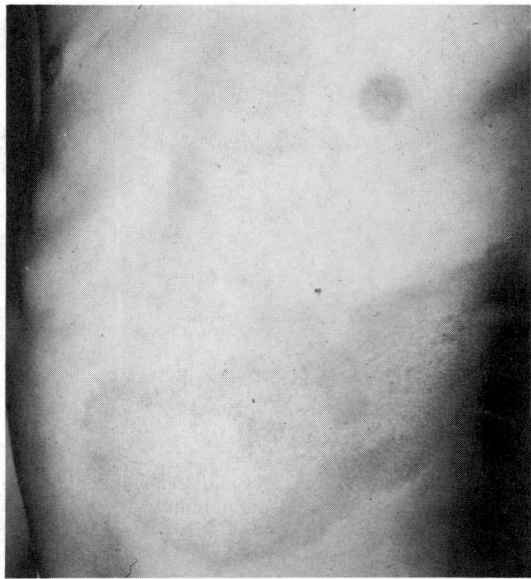

**Figure 35-45.** An irregularly pigmented patch of morphea on the abdomen. The skin has lost its elasticity and feels firm.

spontaneously within 3 to 5 years. There is no known effective therapy for the disorder. It is important not to confuse morphea with progressive systemic sclerosis.

## Progressive Systemic Sclerosis

Whereas morphea is localized, progressive systemic sclerosis is a generalized disorder of connective tissue that affects the lungs, heart, gastrointestinal tract, joints, and kidneys, as well as the skin. The initial lesions almost always develop on the distal extremities, with an insidious tightening and thickening of the involved areas. Raynaud's phenomenon is seen invariably. The involved skin may take on a shiny, blotchy appearance, and finger swelling and contractures are common. The tightness extends up the extremities and involves the face. Pits of the finger pulp are common, as are telangiectases of the nail cuticles. The fatal course may be as short as 1 year, but it often lasts for many years. There is no known effective therapy.

The CREST syndrome (subcutaneous *c*alcinosis, *R*aynaud's phenomenon, *e*sophageal dysfunction, *s*clerodactyly, and *t*elangiectasia) mimics progressive systemic sclerosis. Because major organ involvement is lacking, the course of this disorder is relatively benign. Mixed connective tissue disease may be difficult to differentiate from progressive systemic sclerosis in the early stages. The cause of all these disorders is unknown.

## Lichen Sclerosis et Atrophicus

The characteristic features of lichen sclerosis et atrophicus are patches of atrophy and whitening of the skin. The initial lesions begin as papules, which become white, enlarge, and, as dermal sclerosis occurs, appear to be depressed below the surface of normal skin. The surface is white and thin, almost resembling cigarette paper. The most common site of involvement in females is the perineum, where the lesions encircle the vulva and anus in an hourglass shape. Pain and pruritus of the area lead to excoriation and secondary infection. The lesions may be mistaken for sexual abuse. Vaginal discharges are a frequent accompaniment. In males, the foreskin may be involved, creating a phimosis.

The cause of lichen sclerosis et atrophicus is not known, although some believe that hormonal factors play a role. Females are affected 10 times as often as are males. Three fourths of

children have symptomatic improvement in 3 to 5 years. There appears to be no effective therapy for children; some success with testosterone cream has been reported in adults.

## Scleredema

Scleredema is a rare disorder of unknown cause characterized by the appearance of large areas of diffuse, brawny induration. The onset usually is sudden, often starting on the posterior neck and extending over the shoulders to the chest, face, upper extremities, and back. A strong association with a preceding streptococcal infection has been found in cases that have their onset within 6 weeks of a febrile illness.

The disease reaches its maximum extent in 2 to 6 weeks, and most cases improve spontaneously in 6 months to 2 years. About one quarter of affected children show only partial improvement. The induration and thickening of the skin may interfere with joint mobility and respiration. There is no known effective therapy. Histologically, the major change is in the reticular dermis, where the subcutaneous tissues are replaced by connective tissue with acid mucopolysaccharide deposition.

# Loose Skin

## Ehlers-Danlos Syndrome

Ehlers-Danlos syndrome has a number of variants, some with more skin hyperelasticity and others with more joint hyperextensibility (Fig 35-46). The basic problem is a hereditary disorder of collagen. The skin is fragile and hyperelastic, and feels velvety and soft to palpation. When stretched, it returns quickly to its previous position. Lacerations result in gaping wounds, which create scars resembling cigarette paper. The poor tensile strength of the skin does not allow it to hold sutures. Blood vessels also are fragile, with easy bruising being a common feature. Large vessels such as the aorta are prone to dissection, and massive bleeding may occur from major arteries. There is no effective therapy for Ehlers-Danlos syndrome. Management is supportive. Recognition is important, particularly if surgery is contemplated, because care must be taken in wound closure.

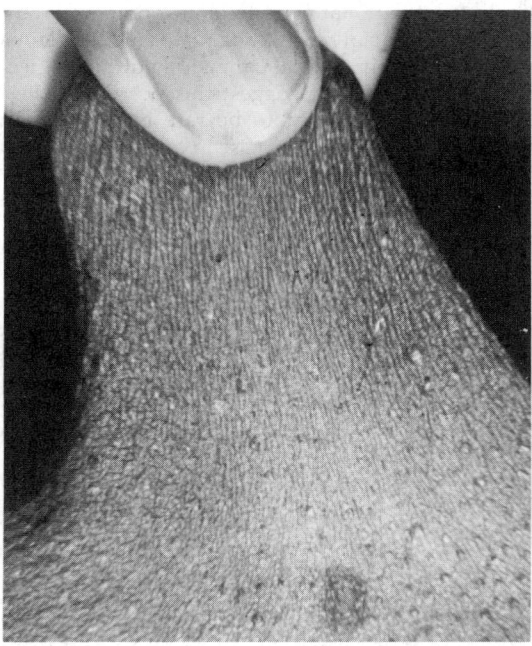

**Figure 35-46.** Striking hyperextensibility of the skin of the forearm in a patient with Ehlers-Danlos syndrome.

## Cutis Laxa

In cutis laxa, the skin hangs and sags, as a result of a loss of elastic fibers, and gives the affected individual an aged or hound-dog appearance. At least three heritable patterns exist: an autosomal recessive type, which is severe; a relatively benign autosomal dominant form; and a rare, sex-linked form. Systemic associations of this uncommon disorder include pulmonary emphysema, pneumothoraces, diverticula of the gastrointestinal tract, rectal prolapse, and hernias. There is no known treatment for this disorder.

## Pseudoxanthoma Elasticum

Pseudoxanthoma elasticum is a genetic disorder with both dominant and recessive forms. The characteristic feature is the development of soft, yellowish papules and plaques on the neck creating a cobblestone effect; the appearance resembles that of plucked chicken skin or orange peel. With age, the skin becomes inelastic and hangs in folds. The relatively benign skin changes belie the severity of ocular and cardiovascular problems. Angioid streaks—gray to brown linear bands—appear on the retina and, as fibrosis develops, central vision may be lost. In adults, significant vessel disease may occur, including coronary artery disease and gastrointestinal bleeding.

## Depressed Lesions

### Striae

Linear, shallow depressions of the skin commonly seen in adolescents, striae occur in areas where the skin has been subjected to stretching. Common sites include the shoulders, abdomen, hips, buttocks, thighs, and breasts. Initially, the lesions may appear red or red-blue, but they become white with time. The cause is not understood, but lesions are more likely to occur in individuals who are receiving systemic steroids. Topical steroids may cause similar lesions. Striae may appear after severe illness, such as infections or oncologic therapy, or after excessive weight loss or gain. No effective therapy is available for the lesions.

### Corticosteroid Atrophy

Depressions in the skin may develop at sites of intramuscular injections of steroids, particularly triamcinolone acetonide or diacetate. The dermis and subcutaneous fat demonstrate local atrophy. In most cases, the tissues regenerate. The overlying skin appears normal.

### Macular Atrophies

A number of types of anetoderma, or atrophy of the skin, may develop during childhood, although these conditions are uncommon. The characteristic feature is the appearance of white, pink, or bluish macules in which elastic tissue is lost. Most of these macules are round or ovoid. The skin may appear slightly depressed in the lesions, but outpouchings occur with time.

### Necrobiosis Lipoidica Diabeticorum

Necrobiosis lipoidica diabeticorum is a degenerative disorder of the skin that is characterized by the appearance of atrophic plaques on the anterior surface of the lower legs. The lesions begin as reddish papules or nodules that enlarge gradually to form oval yellowish plaques with purplish borders. The surface may appear waxy and depressed, with prominent telangiectasia. There is a strong association with diabetes mellitus; 90% of affected individuals have the disorder or a strong family history of it, or they will have diabetes eventually. The pathogenesis seems to involve microangiopathy, which alters dermal collagen. No satisfactory therapy is available.

## Discoid Lupus Erythematosus

The classic lesions of discoid lupus erythematosus are well-demarcated, slightly raised, indurated, red to purple plaques. The lesions appear most commonly over the face and scalp. An adherent scale is typical, as are telangiectases, and central atrophy is common. Changes in pigmentation occur with time. In young children, therapy might include the judicious use of fluorinated steroids along with sunscreens and avoidance of the sun. If this therapy fails, oral hydroxychloroquine may be used. Neonatal lesions of lupus frequently appear discoid. No therapy is necessary for these lesions; they resolve with time, although telangiectasia may remain at the sites of the lesions.

## CHANGES IN PIGMENTATION

### Dark Lesions

#### Mongolian Spots

It is important not to confuse mongolian spots, which are benign lesions, with bruises, particularly bruises caused by child abuse. (See the previous section regarding skin lesions in the neonatal period.)

#### Nevi

Lesions that represent collections of nevus cells, which are variants of normal melanocytes, are referred to as nevi or, by laypersons, as moles. They come in a number of varieties and often are cause for controversy and alarm.

*Congenital Nevocytic Nevi.* About 1% of newborns have histologically proven nevocytic nevi. These darkly pigmented, flat or slightly raised lesions can be huge or so small as to be barely perceptible (Fig 35-47). Debate regarding the management of these lesions is likely to continue, because prospective studies regarding the risk of the development of melanoma over a lifetime are almost impossible to carry out.

The risk of melanoma developing in a giant congenital nevus (ie, one greater than 20 cm in diameter) is estimated to be 6% over a lifetime. The risk in smaller lesions is not clear. Most authorities recommend that giant nevi be removed early in life. Difficulty arises when these lesions are extensive, creating major problems with skin grafting or resulting cosmetic appearance. Removal of the bulk of a lesion may decrease the risk of malignant change. Not all melanomas associated with these lesions develop from a cutaneous site; deep structures also may be involved. Some physicians recommend removal of all congenital nevi irrespective of their size, whereas others observe lesions carefully, watching for worrisome changes.

*Acquired Melanocytic Nevi.* The common mole may appear at any time after birth, with peaks in appearance occurring between the ages of 2 and 3 years and again between 11 and 18 years. The average number of nevi in white adults is somewhere in the vicinity of 40, but the range is large. Black individuals have many fewer lesions. Moles are divided into three clinical types, which may not be easy to differentiate. In the junctional nevus, which occurs predominantly in children, all the nevus cells are contained within the epidermis. The lesions are macular or only slightly raised and are smooth and hairless. Compound nevi have nevus cells both at the dermal–epidermal junction and lying free within the dermis. The lesions are raised and smooth bordered, and often contain hair. Intradermal nevi have their nevus cells entirely in the dermis. They are raised, dome shaped, smooth bordered, and even in pigmentation.

Nevi vary considerably in appearance and range from deeply

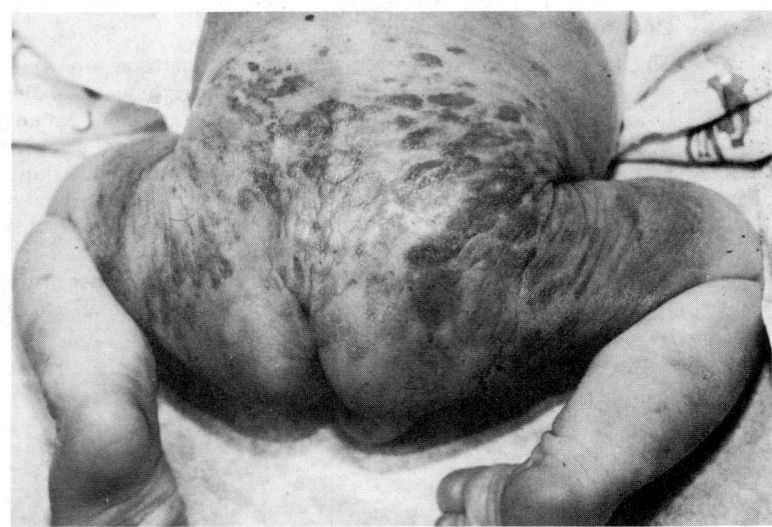

**Figure 35-47.** Extensive hyperpigmentation and nodular nevoid elements in a large congenital nevocytic nevus.

pigmented to colorless. Acquired nevi do not need to be removed routinely, unless worrisome signs of change suggestive of melanoma develop. Although malignant change is uncommon in children, melanomas may develop at any age. Features that should suggest further evaluation include rapid enlargement or darkening with the development of irregular borders; the appearance of whitish, fibrotic areas, or nevi with various shades of pink or blue; spontaneous bleeding or ulceration; and the development of satellite lesions or palpable regional lymph nodes. The lifetime risk of developing cutaneous melanoma is 0.6% in whites and about 0.06% in blacks.

*Dysplastic Nevi.* Attention has been drawn to the propensity of melanoma to develop in certain families. Members of these families seem to have an abnormally large number of acquired pigmented lesions, many of which are termed dysplastic. The dysplastic lesions are larger (5 to 12 mm) than common nevi, have macular and papular components, and are characterized by irregular and ill-defined borders. The color often is variegated, tan to dark brown, sometimes with a pink background. Dysplastic nevi begin in adolescence and continue to appear into adulthood. The risk for melanoma development among affected persons is 10% over their lifetime; the risk approaches 100% in melanoma-prone families.

*Halo Nevi.* Nevi occasionally develop a hypopigmented ring around them and, over time, disappear (Fig 35-48). Such halo nevi represent an apparent immunologic attack by the body against its own nevocytic cells. About one quarter of individuals with halo nevi also have areas of vitiligo. Halo nevi almost always are benign, although the associated color change frequently precipitates parental concern.

*Benign Juvenile Melanoma.* The name *benign juvenile melanoma* is unfortunate, because melanoma has a decidedly negative connotation, and these nevi are benign. This lesion best is called a Spitz nevus, for the person who first described it. Spitz nevi occur most commonly in young children around 3 years of age and in adolescents. They usually are solitary, occurring most commonly on the cheeks. The typical lesion is dome shaped, has a smooth surface and distinct border, is hairless, and is pinkish (Fig 35-49). Spitz nevi tend to grow rapidly over a 3- to 12-month period. They usually are removed because of concern about a true melanoma or for cosmetic reasons.

*Blue Nevi.* The blue nevus is a benign lesion that also may be mistaken for a melanoma. Blue nevi usually are solitary, blue to blue-black, and generally less than 15 mm in diameter. They tend to occur most frequently on the hands, feet, buttocks, and face. No malignant changes have been reported.

**Becker's Melanosis**

Becker's melanosis, a relatively common condition that occurs most frequently around the time of puberty, is characterized by acquired areas of pigmentation of the skin. The typical site is the shoulder, but lesions, which seem to develop fairly rapidly, have been described on any cutaneous surface. The borders often are irregular, the pigmentation is spotty, and there almost always is increased hair growth in the area (Fig 35-50). The lesions occur

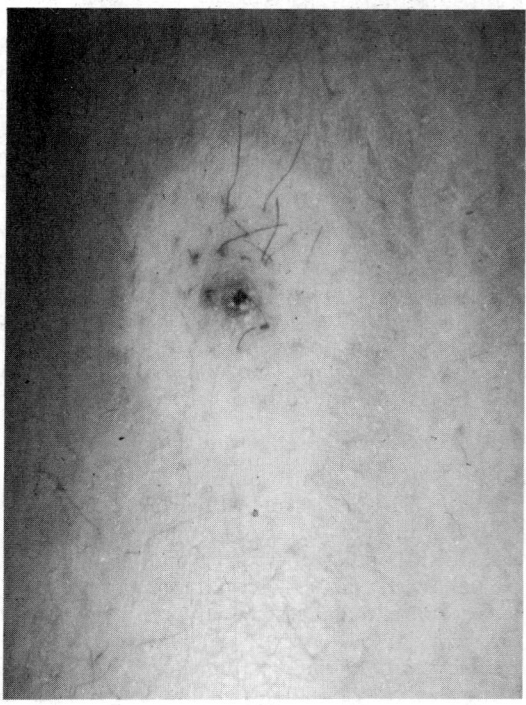

**Figure 35-48.** Depigmentation of the central nevus and surrounding skin in a halo nevus.

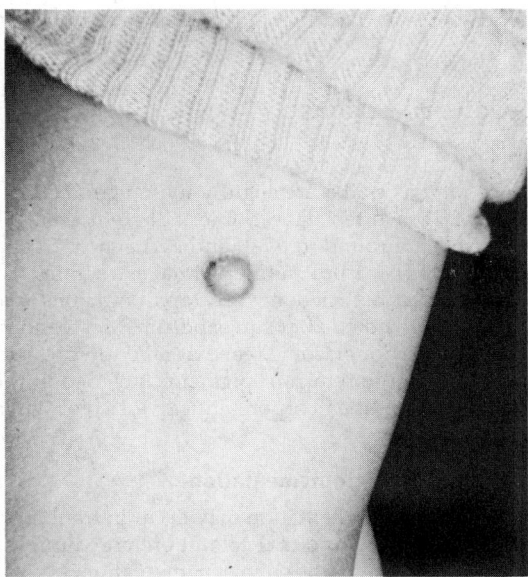

**Figure 35-49.** A well-circumscribed, pigmented spindle cell or Spitz nevus in a typical location, the upper arm.

more frequently in males than in females. The cause is unknown, although androgen stimulation is thought to play a role. On biopsy, it is difficult to differentiate this lesion from normal skin. Becker's melanosis is a benign lesion for which there is no treatment.

### Ephelides

Freckles is a much easier name to remember than is ephelides. These common, tan to brown, small macules usually develop around the age of 6 years in red-headed and fair-skinned children. Inherited as an autosomal dominant trait, the lesions develop only on sun-exposed areas and become more prominent in the summer months. After adolescence, they are less noticeable.

### Lentigines

Unlike freckles, lentigines develop not only on sun-exposed skin, but also on unexposed areas. They are small (0.2 to 1 cm), discrete, dark brown to black, round to oval macules. Lentigines may be present at birth, but they usually develop in early infancy and increase in number with age.

A number of different disorders have been associated with lentigines. The Peutz-Jeghers syndrome features multiple lentigines, usually in a perioral distribution, in association with intestinal polyposis. The LEOPARD syndrome is an acronym for the association of *l*entigines with *e*lectrocardiogram abnormalities, *o*cular hypertelorism, *p*ulmonic stenosis, *a*bnormalities of the genitalia, growth *r*etardation, and *d*eafness.

### Café au Lait Spots

Discrete macular areas of light brown pigmentation that are present at birth or develop shortly thereafter are common "birthmarks." They usually are seen as an isolated finding, especially among members of darkly pigmented races. The presence of multiple café au lait spots may provide an important cutaneous clue to von Recklinghausen's disease (neurofibromatosis). The presence of five or more café au lait spots greater than 0.5 cm in diameter in a child or six or more café au lait spots greater than 1 cm in diameter in an adult should prompt careful examination for other findings of this autosomal dominantly inherited disorder with protean features.

The presence of café au lait spots (rarely exceeding five or six in number) may be associated with other syndromes as well, including Russell-Silver syndrome, multiple lentigines, ataxia-telangiectasia, tuberous sclerosis, Fanconi's anemia, and Turner's syndrome.

### Postinflammatory Hyperpigmentation

Darkening of the skin at sites of preceding inflammation or irritation is a common phenomenon, especially in black individuals. The pathophysiology of the deposition of melanin is unclear. Varicella commonly produces macular, round remnants of previous infection, and children with atopic dermatitis often have significant pigmentation in the areas that have undergone lichenification. Generally, the pigmentation fades with time.

### Urticaria Pigmentosa

Collections of mast cells in the skin may create pigmented macular or slightly nodular lesions. (See the previous section regarding bullous lesions.)

### Phytophotodermatitis

A macular hyperpigmentation, phytophotodermatitis is caused by an increased sunburn response after contact with photosensitizers that are present in certain plants. Crushing of these plants releases furocoumarins, the photobiologically active portion of

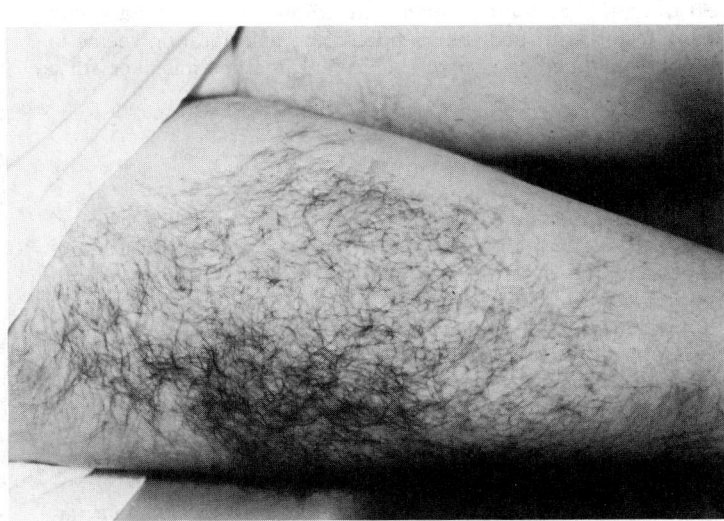

**Figure 35-50.** A large patch of irregular hyperpigmentation with hypertrichosis is characteristic of Becker's melanosis.

which, psoralen, induces cross-linking of DNA strands on exposure to ultraviolet light. Lime juice, particularly from lime skin, is a relatively common culprit. Other plants producing a similar effect include lemon, celery, parsnip, and fig. The hyperpigmented areas may assume unusual shapes, depending on the type of exposure. Rarely, the lesions may appear erythematous or vesicular. These lesions have been confused with bruises caused by child abuse.

### Fixed Drug Eruption

A fixed drug eruption is a localized drug reaction characterized by the appearance of a purple to red plaque with clearly demarcated borders. The plaque often is singular and occasionally is urticarial, nodular, or eczematous. Common drugs responsible for these lesions include salicylates, tetracyclines, barbiturates, and sulfonamides. The reason that systemically administered drugs cause such localized reactions is unknown. Each time the drug is given, the eruption recurs in the same spot.

### Acanthosis Nigricans

Acanthosis nigricans is manifested characteristically by the appearance of a hyperpigmented, somewhat velvety thickening of the skin. The most common sites of involvement are the nape and sides of the neck, the axillae, and the groin. Although acanthosis nigricans may be associated with an internal malignant tumor in adults, this association is extremely rare in children. The most common problem connected with the disorder is obesity. In some cases, in which the disease onset is early in life, a familial association may be found. Some individuals with endocrinopathies, particularly those associated with insulin resistance, have the hyperpigmentation. No effective therapy is available for the lesions.

### Blue Jean Coloration

Youngsters wearing new blue jeans may have their hands or other areas of the skin discolored by the dye used to color the blue jeans. The most common scenario is the appearance of bluish hands during the cold winter months. The children may be brought to their physicians because of concern about "circulatory problems." An alcohol swab rubbed on the affected areas usually removes the stain. The hands are affected predominantly because the children place them between their thighs to keep warm while sitting in class.

### Maculae Cerulae (Taches Bleuâtres)

Discrete, round, barely perceptible gray to bluish macules also known as taches bleuâtres, maculae cerulae occasionally are seen on the lower abdomen, thighs, and thorax of individuals who are infested with pediculosis pubis. The discoloration seems to occur at the feeding sites of the lice and may be mistaken for a bruise.

## Yellow Skin

### Carotenoderma

Carotenoderma is a common yellowish to orange skin discoloration caused by the ingestion of excessive amounts of carotene-containing foods. Carotenoderma occasionally is associated with hypothyroidism, diabetes mellitus, or nephrosis. Foods commonly connected with the disorder are carrots, squash, and other yellow vegetables. The areas most often involved are the face, palms, and soles. The disorder is asymptomatic and noninjurious; the main reason for concern is its possible confusion with jaundice. The sclerae are not yellow in carotenoderma.

### Lycopenemia

Less well recognized than carotenoderma is lycopenemia, an orange-yellow discoloration of the skin associated with high levels of lycopene, the red carotenoid of tomatoes. No therapy is necessary.

## Light-Colored Lesions

### Pityriasis Alba

Patches of pityriasis alba are slightly hypopigmented and fairly discrete, and they often have a fine, adherent scale. They are asymptomatic, are round to oval, and occur most frequently on the face, neck, upper trunk, and proximal extremities. The cause is unknown, but an association with atopic dermatitis is common, and most cases are noted after sun exposure. Most lesions resolve spontaneously, although some feel that mild topical steroids and emollients hasten the return of pigment. Included in the differential diagnosis are tinea corporis, tinea versicolor, vitiligo, and pityriasis rosea.

### Postinflammatory Hypopigmentation

Areas of decreased pigmentation may occur in traumatized skin. These areas regain their normal coloration more rapidly than do those with postinflammatory hyperpigmentation, because of the superficial nature of the problem.

### Tinea Versicolor

Hyperpigmented or hypopigmented macules and patches, often ovoid or round, with a fine scale, are typical of tinea versicolor (Fig 35-51). The lesions appear most commonly over the trunk and neck, most often in adolescents and young adults. The rash is asymptomatic; the cosmetic appearance prompts the medical visit. *Pityrosporum orbiculare*, a yeast-like organism, is responsible for the discoloration. The diagnosis can be confirmed easily by microscopic examination of the scale dissolved in potassium hydroxide for the classic spaghetti-and-meatball appearance of the hyphae and spores. Wood's light examination usually reveals a golden fluorescence, unless the patient has bathed in the previous 6 to 12 hours. The superficial infection tends to persist and is difficult to eradicate. Selenium sulfide lotion, 2½%, applied to generous areas of the skin for 10 to 15 minutes and then washed off in a regimen of nightly treatment for 3 to 4 nights, then weekly treatment for a month, then monthly treatment, usually is successful. Ketoconazole, 400 mg orally, in a single dose, also has proven effective.

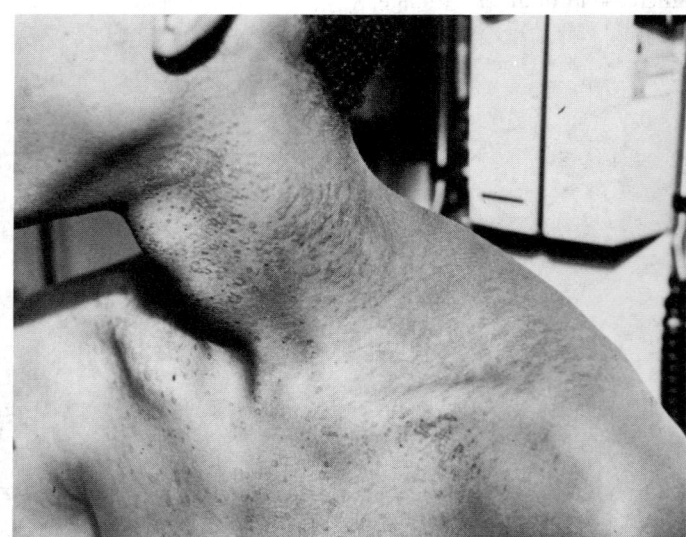

**Figure 35-51.** Hyper- and hypopigmented minimally raised tinea versicolor lesions on the neck, shoulders, and trunk.

## Seborrheic Dermatitis

Hypopigmented areas are common on the forehead, eyebrows, scalp, and other areas affected by seborrheic dermatitis. A greasy or fine scale usually is associated with the hypopigmentation. The darker the skin, the more visible are the lesions. Although the hypopigmentation is seen most commonly in infants, it may occur in any age group that is affected by seborrhea. A mild topical steroid will reduce the inflammation that causes the depigmentation. Seborrheic dermatitis occurs during the first year of life and not again until the onset of puberty.

## Vitiligo

The lesions of vitiligo are much lighter than those of the disorders listed above. Many or all of the pigment cells in the skin have been destroyed. The cause of vitiligo is unknown. It probably is not an autoimmune disorder, as once suspected, although individuals with autoimmune disorders are more prone than normal to this disorder. It is more common than most people suspect; as much as 2% of the general population may have vitiligo, and 50% of those have the problem before the age of 20 years.

The lesions usually are bilateral and symmetric, commonly appearing around body orifices (Fig 35-52). The most frequent sites of involvement are the face, backs of the hands and wrists, umbilicus, and genitalia. Halo nevi are common in individuals with vitiligo. Topical steroids result in the return of normal color to the skin in about 20% of treated patients. Treatment with PUVA (psoralens and ultraviolet A light) should be reserved for older children. Care must be taken to protect the depigmented skin from sunburn.

## Albinism

At least seven types of oculocutaneous albinism have been described. The hypopigmentation is present at birth. Melanocytes are present in the skin, but fail to produce melanin. In white individuals, the skin appears milk-white and the hair white to yellow. The pupils are pink, and severe photophobia is typical. Affected black individuals may have white or tan skin, blond to red hair, and blue to hazel irises. Most oculocutaneous albinism is inherited as an autosomal recessive disorder.

## Piebaldism

Piebaldism also is known as partial albinism, because the area of skin involved is limited. The most common sites affected by the congenital absence of pigment in this autosomal dominantly inherited disorder are the hair, which has a white forelock, and the forehead, which has a triangular area of hypopigmentation. Hyperpigmented macules are common in the white patches. Piebaldism may be associated with deafness, and some affected individuals have Hirschsprung's disease and cerebral ataxia.

Waardenburg's syndrome is an autosomal dominantly inherited disorder that is characterized by varying expressions of lateral displacement of the lacrimal puncta, a broad nasal root, partial or total heterochromia of the iris, piebaldism of the skin or hair, and congenital deafness. This syndrome accounts for as many as 1% of all deafness in children.

## Tuberous Sclerosis

Hypopigmented macules often are the initial clue to tuberous sclerosis, a neurocutaneous disorder that is inherited in an autosomal dominant manner. The hypopigmented lesions are small, ovoid, and scattered, and they vary in number. Larger lesions, known as ash leaf spots, may have jagged edges resembling a leaf. Any child with unexplained seizures should be examined carefully for cutaneous clues, particularly hypopigmented macules. Shagreen spots—connective tissue nevi resembling raised, leather-like lesions—generally appear later, as does adenoma sebaceum, manifested by angiofibromas on the face. Many normal individuals have isolated hypopigmented macules without underlying disorders.

## Hypomelanosis of Ito

Hypomelanosis of Ito is characterized by macular hypopigmented swirls, streaks, and other patterned patches that generally are present at birth (Fig 35-53). The syndrome is present if there are associated noncutaneous abnormalities. Central nervous system problems include seizures and mental retardation; eye abnor-

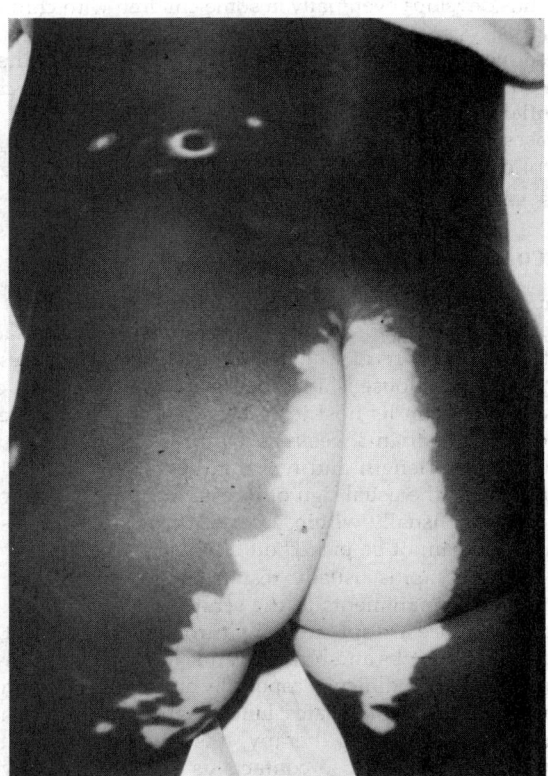

Figure 35-52. In vitiligo, depigmentation with distinct borders frequently involves the perineum.

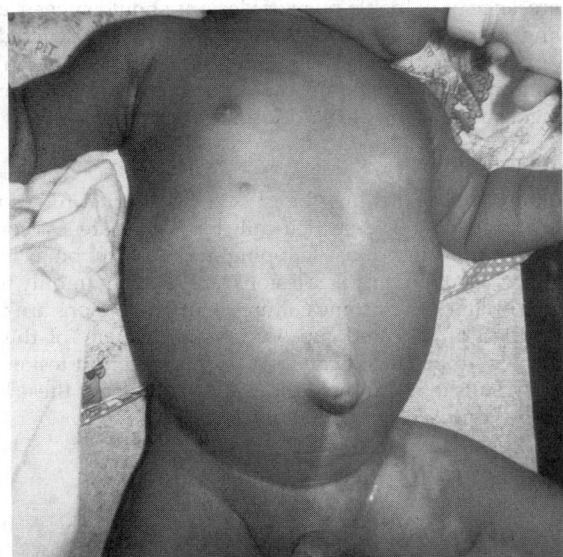

Figure 35-53. An irregular area of hypopigmentation in an infant with hypomelanosis of Ito.

malities, skeletal defects, dysplastic teeth, and alopecia, among other problems, also have been described. The mode of inheritance is not clear. Some cases seem to be sporadic. It is important not to diagnose cases of patches of hypopigmentation as Ito syndrome; the presence of such patches simply should alert the examiner to observe affected children carefully for anomalies. Nevus depigmentosus may have a similar appearance.

### Nevus Depigmentosus

Nevus depigmentosus, or achromic nevus, is much more common than is hypomelanosis of Ito. The hypopigmented areas are not completely devoid of pigmentation. They are poorly defined, often appear like splashes, sometimes in dermatomal patterns, and occur most frequently on the trunk and proximal extremities. Rare associations with neurologic defects have been reported.

## Purpuric Lesions

### Henoch-Schönlein Purpura

The rash of Henoch-Schönlein purpura is classically purpuric, but early on, it may appear urticarial or maculopapular. The characteristic distribution of the rash helps determine the diagnosis. The rash is located primarily from the buttocks on down the lower extremities. The upper extremities are involved less frequently, the face even less commonly, and the trunk only rarely. The characteristic lesion is that of a vasculitis (ie, palpable purpura), but the purpuric lesions may be macular and small or large, and, in severe cases, they may develop necrotic centers. Striking areas of edema involving the scalp, hands, feet, scrotum, or other areas may appear.

Individuals with Henoch-Schönlein purpura generally have associated disorders. A periarticular arthritis occurs in more than two thirds of the cases. Abdominal pain, gastrointestinal bleeding, and glomerulonephritis also are common. The purpuric lesions may appear in waves. One third of the cases resolve within 2 weeks, another third in 2 weeks to 2 months, and the remaining third in 2 to 6 months. It seems that the leukocytoclastic vasculitis of Henoch-Schönlein purpura may be precipitated by a variety of infections and exposures. Group A $\beta$-hemolytic streptococcal infections, *Mycoplasma*, varicella, hepatitis B, food allergens, insect bites, and exposure to cold have been implicated. Therapy is mainly supportive, although gastrointestinal bleeding and severe joint pain may respond to courses of systemic steroids.

### Vasculitis

The presence of palpable purpuric lesions should suggest an underlying vasculitis. The causes of vasculitis are discussed elsewhere in this textbook. The sudden development of purpuric lesions in an ill child should cause the pediatrician to consider meningococcemia and Rocky Mountain spotted fever.

### Factitious Lesions

Some purpuric lesions may be caused by external forces rather than by underlying disease. Self-inflicted lesions are less common in children than in adults. Cupping and coin rubbing, both of which may result in purpuric lesions, are used commonly to treat a variety of illnesses in some cultures. Cupping lesions are caused by inversion of a heated cup on the skin, usually of the back. The suction so produced causes a purpuric, round lesion. Coin rubbing results in linear purpuric lesions. Neither of these lesions should be confused with child abuse.

## PRURITIC LESIONS

## Contact Dermatitis

In allergic contact dermatitis, in contrast to primary irritant contact dermatitis, pruritus is a prominent feature. Rhus dermatitis, which includes poison ivy, is the most frequently recognized of the allergic contact group. The characteristic feature of this eruption is the appearance of vesicles and vesicular papules in a linear distribution. The rash may be localized with groups of erythematous papules and vesicles, have widely scattered lesions, or, on occasion, be limited to the face, which appears swollen. A history of contact with eruption-producing plants is helpful to the diagnosis. The linear vesicles, or papules if the lesions are early, may be subtle. Pruritus often is severe. Contrary to common belief, the vesicular fluid does not spread the rash. The rapidity of appearance of the rash depends on how sensitive the affected person is to the toxin and how much of the toxin has reached the skin. In sensitive individuals, areas of significant exposure may show a rash within hours, whereas areas of minimal toxin exposure may not show a rash for days. (Lesions might not develop in less sensitive individuals until several days or a week later.)

Rhus dermatitis should not be confused with atopic dermatitis, which is a chronic disorder. Atopic dermatitis usually begins in early childhood and has a morphology and distribution much different from those of poison ivy. In addition, individuals with atopic dermatitis usually do not react to exposure to poison ivy.

Other contact rashes may create problems in diagnosis. Some are localized to areas that indicate the underlying problem. Contact dermatitis from metal, for example, develops in areas where metal comes in contact with the skin (eg, on fingers with rings, wrists with watches, the neck with necklaces, earlobes with earrings). Cosmetics occasionally produce less obvious rashes. Eyelid dermatitis from fingernail polish is common.

Foot dermatitis in children often is mistaken for tinea pedis; however, prepubertal children rarely have tinea infections of their feet. If the rash involves the dorsum of the foot, an allergic contact dermatitis is likely. The reactions are caused primarily by rubber antioxidants and potassium dichromate leather-tanning agents. If the dermatitis is on the weight-bearing surface, the cause may be unclear, but contact dermatitis usually can be ruled out. Atopic dermatitis develops eventually in some children with chronic foot dermatitis.

Treatment of contact dermatitis involves removal of the cause of the outbreak. A topical steroid may aid in relieving the pruritus and inflammation. Oral antihistamines may be needed in extensive cases. Oral steroids, which sometimes are indicated in severe cases of contact dermatitis, should be given in decreasing doses over a 10- to 14-day course.

## Pediculosis

The human louse has a field day with children. Pediculosis capitis is an extremely common problem and a difficult one to eradicate, despite the best efforts of schools, health agencies, and physicians. The human head louse is an obligate human parasite; it cannot survive away from its host for more than 10 days in the adult form or for more than 3 weeks as a fertile egg. The insect, which is 2 to 4 mm in length and ivory, rarely is seen. Nits, the egg sacs of lice, are the usual sign of infestation. Firmly cemented to the hair shaft, usually within 1 cm of the scalp, they resemble dandruff but cannot be picked off easily.

Pediculosis capitis usually results in pruritus of the scalp. Common accompaniments to the scratching are folliculitis and impetigo. The lice are spread easily through close contact, toilet articles such as combs and brushes, and clothing, especially hats. Treatment may be difficult, especially in young children, who may be reinfested by playmates. Lindane and pyrethrin shampoos are the standard forms of therapy. It is important to treat other family members and close contacts as well. Black individuals rarely are infested with head lice; the reason for their resistance is not known.

Pediculosis corporis is a much less common problem in the United States. These lice live in the seams of clothing and feed on the skin, producing small, red papules and wheals. To rid the clothing of the lice, it must be sterilized or at least have a hot iron run over the seams.

Pubic lice usually are acquired through contact during sexual intercourse; thus, sexual abuse must be considered in the case of pubic lice in a child. Although the lice usually cling to pubic hair, in young children, they may attach to body hair. Nits may be found in the eyelashes as well. The primary symptom is pruritus, and excoriations are common in heavy infestations. The nits on hair shafts are seen more commonly than is the louse itself, which is broader and shorter than are head and body lice. Infestation sometimes is manifested by the appearance of bluish-gray, faint purpuric lesions. Known as maculae cerulae or taches bleuâtres, these spots are sites of feeding by the louse. Treatment consists of a 6- to 8-hour application of pyrethrin or lindane to affected areas.

## Scabies

Epidemics of scabies seem to occur in 30-year cycles. A peak in cases occurred in the United States in the 1970s, but the infestation still is prevalent. The culprit, *Sarcoptes scabiei*, is a 0.2- to 0.4-mm female mite that burrows into the stratum corneum, where it deposits eggs and excrement. The clinical picture, which usually develops 4 to 6 weeks after infestation, is thought to be the result of sensitization to the mite and its products. A person can have mites on the body and transmit them to others without having symptoms and signs of the disorder.

The pruritus of scabies usually is intense and unremitting. A characteristic feature is that it seems worse at night, perhaps as a result of a rise in skin surface temperature and increased activity of the scabies mites. The lesions of scabies are papules, tiny vesicles, and pustules. Most are excoriated and, in long-standing cases, lichenification may be extensive. Burrows (ie, linear tracks) are not seen commonly in children. The distribution of lesions usually is from the neck down, although young infants and children can have scalp and even facial lesions. Characteristically, the lesions are most intense on the hands, particularly the webs of the fingers in older children and adults, and the palms and soles in infants; on the wrists; in the axillae; on the belt line; on the gluteal cleft; and around the nipples and genitalia in adults and older children. Scabies in babies can produce nodular/vesicular lesions on the palms and soles that can mimic pyoderma. Secondary infections occur frequently.

Although the clinical picture may be typical of scabies, it always is prudent to try to identify the mite in a scraping from one of the lesions. A simple technique is to choose a non-excoriated, fresh vesicle or papule, place a drop of immersion oil on it, scrape it with a scalpel blade to open it, collect the oil from the skin, place the oil on a glass slide with a coverslip on top, and look for the mite, eggs, or feces.

Treatment of scabies usually can be accomplished effectively by the application of 5% pyrethrin cream to the entire body surface, including the head in infants. The pyrethrin cream should remain on for 8 to 12 hours and then be washed off. One treatment usually is effective, although some prefer a second application 10 to 14 days later. Lindane, applied as a 1% concentration, is also effective and should remain on the skin for 6 to 8 hours. The pruritus may take a week or more to resolve after treatment. All family members must be treated at the same time. Failure to treat close contacts, such as baby-sitters, grandparents, aunts, and uncles, often results in reinfection. Many contacts may be infested despite a seeming absence of lesions.

The use of lindane on children has been the subject of much concern and debate. A review of reported cases of toxicity, how-ever, has shown the preparation to be safe if it is not ingested or used inappropriately. Lindane is not recommended for use on pregnant women, however. Ten percent crotamiton is much less effective. Two applications, 24 hours apart, are recommended before the agent is washed off 48 hours later. Benzoyl benzoate, 12.5% to 25%, is effective, but difficult to obtain. A 6% to 10% precipitate of sulfur in petrolatum hardly ever is used because of its unpleasant odor. Clothing worn and bedding used by the family before treatment should be washed or stored for 72 hours before reuse to prevent reinfestation by mites.

Scabies can affect families at all socioeconomic levels. Its presence denotes contact with a source. Although the contact generally requires intimate exposure, epidemics can occur in hospital settings, where nurses and physicians care for children and adults with undiagnosed scabies. Simple hand washing after patient contact prevents infection of health care providers.

## Papular Urticaria

The red papules and wheals that are associated with papular urticaria, a reaction to insect bites, occur most commonly in the spring and summer. A more complete discussion of this topic is found in the previous section of this chapter regarding red papules.

## Neurotic Excoriations

Occasionally, a patient picks or scratches at the skin, creating erosions or ulcerations. The latter lesions may be confused with a primary skin problem; the real cause is emotional stress.

## Varicella

The vesicles of chickenpox are pruritic, sometimes intensely so. The lesions generally are present in a variety of stages, including erythematous papules, vesicles, pustules, and crusts. Calamine lotion may help relieve the pruritus. Varicella is discussed more fully in the previous section of this chapter regarding disorders with generalized vesicles.

## Fiberglass Dermatitis

An itchy, finely papular dermatitis may result from contact with glass fiber particles from insulation or fiberglass materials. Fiberglass drapes washed with clothing in the family washing machine also may be a source of the irritant.

## Swimmer's Itch

A pruritic, allergic response to schistosomes may occur in individuals who swim in freshwater lakes that are frequented by ducks, birds, and other carriers. Humans are accidental hosts of the schistosomes, which use snails as the intermediate host. The first exposure to the cercarial larvae produces no response; subsequent penetrations by this organism result in an allergic response. Tiny erythematous papules appear in the first hour after exposure and increase in size and pruritic effect over the next few days. The lesions appear most frequently on exposed body surfaces. Treatment is symptomatic with topical antipruritic agents.

## Creeping Eruption

The larvae of cutaneous larva migrans penetrate the skin and migrate through the superficial layers of the epidermis, creating characteristic serpentine patterns. A small, erythematous papule designates the entrance site of the hookworm larva. The tracks are a few millimeters in diameter and are pink or skin-colored. Pruritus is prominent. The lesions appear most frequently on the feet, the body part that most commonly is exposed to the soil that contains the larvae. Infection is most frequent in warm, humid regions with sandy soil. Secondary bacterial infection may result from scratching. Application of a topical thiabendazole suspension under an occlusive dressing seems to be effective in eradicating the organisms.

## GROUPED LESIONS

### Herpes Simplex

The appearance of erythematous papules that rapidly become vesicular and are clustered together should suggest the diagnosis of herpes simplex. (See the previous section in this chapter regarding disorders with grouped vesicles.)

### Insect Bites

The pruritic, erythematous papules of insect bites, particularly flea bites, commonly are grouped together. A central punctum on top of the papule or wheal is strong evidence that the papule is the result of a bite.

### Contact Dermatitis

The erythematous papules and vesicles of contact dermatitis may be grouped according to cause. Rhus dermatitis (poison ivy) is characterized by linear papules and vesicles. (See the previous section in this chapter dealing with pruritic lesions.)

### Lymphangioma Circumscriptum

Grouped, tense, small vesicles may indicate the presence of an underlying localized abnormality of the lymphatic system. The vesicles most commonly are deep seated, their surface may be rough, and the fluid may appear hemorrhagic rather than clear. The lesions are seen most frequently around the neck, the upper trunk, and the proximal extremities.

### Chronic Bullous Disease of Childhood

As the name implies, chronic bullous disease of childhood is a chronic disorder. The bullae or vesicles are grouped around the margins of an erythematous plaque, which represents an area of clearing. Multiple lesions usually are present. For more detail, see the previous discussion of this disorder in the section of this chapter dealing with bullous lesions.

## DIFFUSE ERYTHEMA

### Scarlet Fever

In the past, scarlet fever was manifested by a finely papular rash on an erythematous background that felt like sandpaper to the touch. Recently, however, the disease seems to have become much milder. Although still common, it frequently is not diagnosed because of a lack of typical features. The slapped cheek appearance is not common. Pastia's lines (ie, the erythematous accentuation of flexural creases), circumoral pallor, and even severe pharyngitis are seen infrequently. Most cases feature a fine, rough, papular rash predominantly over the bridge of the nose and face, shoulders, and upper chest. In fair-skinned individuals, the erythematous base may be present.

The rash of scarlet fever is produced by sensitization to those strains of group A β-hemolytic streptococci that produce an erythrogenic toxin. Because prior exposure to the toxin is required, it is rare to see this disorder in children less than 2 years of age. The incubation period is only 24 to 48 hours. It is important to warn parents that their child's hands and feet may show significant sheets of desquamation in 7 to 14 days.

### Staphylococcal Scalded Skin Syndrome

The diffuse erythema seen in staphylococcal scalded skin syndrome is, as implied by the name, strikingly suggestive of a scald or burn of the skin (see Color Figure 12). For a more detailed discussion of this syndrome, refer to the section earlier in this chapter regarding bullous lesions.

### Toxic Shock Syndrome

The typical skin eruption in toxic shock syndrome is a diffuse sunburn-like erythema. The other features of this serious illness, however, should separate it readily from scarlet fever and scalded skin syndrome. Early symptoms include a temperature higher than 38.9°C (102°F), bulbar conjunctival hyperemia, oropharyngeal and vaginal hyperemia, hypotension, a strawberry tongue, and striking palmar and plantar erythema and edema. There is evidence of multiple organ system involvement as well. The kidneys, muscles, central nervous system, gastrointestinal tract, and hematopoietic system all may be involved. Desquamation of the hands and feet develops 1 to 2 weeks after the illness.

The toxic shock syndrome is a medical emergency often requiring major medical life support. Hypotension leading to death is common. The toxin responsible for the disorder is produced by *S aureus* organisms. The disease occurs most frequently in young women using vaginal tampons during their menstrual period, but other infections also may be responsible, including osteomyelitis, cellulitis, and burns.

### Toxic Epidermal Necrolysis

At one time, the staphylococcal scalded skin syndrome was included under the category of TEN (see Color Figure 13). It became apparent, however, that the disorders were dissimilar in many respects. TEN usually is the result of a reaction to a medication, particularly penicillins, sulfonamides, or barbiturates. Early signs of this disorder include malaise, fever, inflammation of the eyelids and mucous membranes (including the genitalia), and a generalized painful erythema. Flaccid blisters may develop, areas of skin may become denuded, and a maculopapular morbilliform rash may be present. The site of skin separation on performance of a biopsy is subepidermal.

Children with TEN usually appear ill. Involvement of the mucous membranes may make oral intake difficult. Supportive care is the primary therapy available. TEN may be categorized with the group of disorders that includes erythema multiforme and Stevens-Johnson syndrome.

### *Corynebacterium haemolyticum*–Induced Rash

A rash similar to that of scarlet fever has been described in individuals infected with *Corynebacterium haemolyticum*. The infection, which produces a sore throat with pharyngeal erythema and exudate, occurs most frequently in teenagers and young adults. The rash is diffuse, erythematous, and macular, and it blanches when pressed. A fine, papular component occurs most frequently distally on the extensor surfaces of the extremities and then spreads centrally to the trunk within a few days. A mild desquamation may follow in 1 or 2 weeks.

## Acrodynia

Metallic mercury poisoning has become rare since calomel teething powder was found to be the source of this metal poisoning in England in the mid-1900s. Children's fascination with liquid-like metallic mercury still gives rise to occasional cases, however. Typical cases of acrodynia are unforgettable. Children are anorectic, irritable, and hypotonic. They sweat profusely and have a prominent rash similar to miliaria in addition to a background erythema of the skin. Their hands and feet are strikingly puffy, pink, perspiring, and painful, and they rub them together, causing desquamation. Hypertension is common.

## Miscellaneous Causes

Atropine intoxication, often caused by eye drops or similar substances containing atropine, should be suspected as the cause of erythema if fever, hallucinations, dilated pupils, and dry skin are present. The onset of symptoms is rapid.

Boric acid poisoning has become extremely rare since the toxicity of boric acid has been publicized. Anorexia, weight loss, and mild diarrhea are followed by a "boiled lobster" appearance, with desquamation occurring in a few days.

A diffuse, glowing, red discoloration of the skin associated with periorbital or facial edema and pruritus has been described in children receiving an overdose of rifampin.

A curious macular erythema, generally appearing on the head and neck or on the upper trunk, especially after stroking, is known as tache cérébrale. Originally, this phenomenon was described in association with tuberculous meningitis, but it may be seen with any central nervous system irritation.

## PHOTOSENSITIVITY DISORDERS

### Sunburn

The erythema resulting from damage to the skin by ultraviolet radiation is known as sunburn. Although, in our society, such damage to the skin is considered cosmetically pleasing and even a sign of good health, it actually is additive over the years, producing an appearance of premature aging and acting as a carcinogen. The relationship between the increasing incidence of malignant melanoma and sun exposure is conjectural, but concerning. Part of the role of physicians taking care of children should be early education of parents and children about care and protection of the skin.

Variations in skin types are recognized easily by laypersons. A classification system has been devised that grades the likelihood of irritation and resulting complications occurring from ultraviolet light exposure. Individuals with class I skin always burn and never tan; they generally have red hair and freckles, and are of Celtic origin. Those with class II skin always burn, tanning only minimally; they are fair-skinned, fair-haired, blue-eyed whites. Individuals with class III skin burn moderately and tan gradually; they generally are darker-skinned whites. Persons with class IV skin, who usually are of Mediterranean background, burn minimally and tan well. Individuals with class V skin rarely burn and tan profusely; examples are Middle Eastern whites and Mexicans. Finally, persons with class VI skin (ie, blacks) never burn and are deeply pigmented. This classification system can be used to counsel patients about the dangers of sun exposure and to advise them regarding the use of sun-protection agents such as sunscreens. Potent sunscreens contain active ingredients that absorb, reflect, or scatter light. Once sunburn has occurred, there is no effective therapy. For mild burns, an emollient and oral acetylsalicylic acid may provide relief. For moderate to severe burns, cold, wet compresses may be used to relieve the burning and tenderness. Simple sunburn needs to be separated from the disorders discussed below, which represent pathologic reactions to sunlight.

### Drug Photosensitivity

Drug reactions to light have been divided into two types, toxic and allergic. Toxicity reactions occur after a single exposure and appear to be an exaggerated sunburn. Immediate reactions may occur with sulfonamides, phenothiazines, griseofulvin, and some tetracyclines. Delayed phototoxicity may follow the systemic administration of furocoumarins or psoralens. Most photoallergic reactions occur after topical contact with chemical agents. Early signs are pruritus and eczema, which appear within 24 hours after the chemical and light exposure. Drugs in this category include sulfonamides, griseofulvin, hydrocortisone, benzocaine, coal tar, and phenothiazines. In reactions caused by the combination of drugs and light, the distribution of the rash, which is confined to sun-exposed areas, is an important diagnostic clue. Treatment consists primarily of removal of the offending agent and of the sun exposure.

### Plant Photosensitivity

Certain plants, particularly limes, contain natural furocoumarins, which may result in photosensitive reactions when present on the skin. (See the previous section of this chapter regarding changes in pigmentation.)

### Lupus Erythematosus

A wide variety of rashes have been associated with systemic lupus erythematosus. Many patients with this disease are photosensitive and have this type of rash as their initial manifestation. The "butterfly" rash, a slightly raised erythematous or violaceous rash over the malar areas and bridge of the nose, is the most frequently recognized lesion associated with lupus, but nonspecific maculopapular eruptions, erythema, and fine, scaling, annular lesions and urticarial reactions also are seen in this disorder. Patients with the Ro (SSA) antigen represent a subset of patients with lupus who seem to have photosensitivity as an early manifestation of their disease.

Individuals with discoid lupus lesions also are photosensitive and need to avoid sun exposure and to use protective sunscreens. The classic discoid lesion is a well-demarcated, indurated, red to violaceous plaque with fine telangiectasia, an adherent scale, and areas of atrophy. The lesions appear most commonly on the face and scalp and in the ears.

### Dermatomyositis

A butterfly distribution of erythema and swelling occurring after sun exposure or at least resembling a persistent sunburn may be the initial clue to or presentation of dermatomyositis.

### Polymorphous Light Eruption

As the name implies, polymorphous light eruption has a variable clinical presentation. The lesions, which represent a reaction to ultraviolet B light, range from small papules and papulovesicular lesions to plaques. They may appear eczematous and often are pruritic. At times, large nodules may appear in areas of light exposure. The eruption generally occurs within several hours to several days of exposure. Polymorphous light eruption may be confused with atopic dermatitis. A high incidence is found in North and Latin American Indians and in persons of Finnish descent; American Indians are most likely to have onset of the disease in childhood. Topical or systemic steroids may provide relief for acute lesions, but sun protection is the ultimate therapy. In some cases, prolonged treatment with antimalarial agents may be necessary.

## Hydroa Estivale

Hydroa estivale is a rare disorder that has its onset in childhood and shows some improvement in late teenage years. The lesions, which are pruritic, consist of erythema, edematous papules, and vesicles. Excoriations of sun-exposed areas may be a clue to the diagnosis. The rash generally appears in the summer months and occurs 1 to 2 days after sun exposure. Treatment consists of avoidance of sunlight.

## Porphyrias

The human porphyrias are an uncommon group of disorders caused by enzymatic defects in the metabolic pathway leading to the biosynthesis of porphyrins and heme.

### Erythropoietic Protoporphyria

Erythropoietic protoporphyria generally is a mild disease characterized by the burning, itching, and stinging of sun-exposed areas of skin. The skin may become erythematous, edematous, and thickened, but it rarely becomes blistered or scarred. Hepatic cirrhosis occurs in some of the individuals affected by erythropoietic protoporphyria, which has an autosomal dominant pattern of inheritance. Results of the free erythrocyte protoporphyrin test are unusually high in this disorder.

### Congenital Erythropoietic Porphyria

Congenital erythropoietic porphyria is a destructive, severe disorder that is inherited in an autosomal recessive manner. Symptoms occur early, with severe photosensitivity resulting in scarring and hypertrichosis. Hemolytic anemia and splenomegaly are common. The passage of red urine may be the first sign of the disease; progressive mutilation of the skin follows. There is speculation that ''werewolves'' may have been individuals affected with this terrible disorder, which is manifested by reddish teeth, hypertrichosis, disfigurement, and avoidance of sunlight. Free erythrocyte protoporphyrin levels are not elevated; urine levels of uroporphyrin I are increased greatly.

### Hepatoerythropoietic Porphyria

Hepatoerythropoietic porphyria is a rare autosomal recessive disorder characterized by photosensitivity beginning in infancy. Severe erythema and blistering occur, and scarring of sun-exposed areas is prominent. Affected individuals have more facial hair than normal, and their urine may be red. Levels of red blood cell free erythrocyte protoporphyrin are increased.

### Variegate Porphyria

Variegate porphyria rarely begins in childhood. The primary clinical manifestations are photosensitivity, episodes of bizarre neurologic symptoms, or both. Skin changes include fragility and blistering on sun-exposed areas.

### Porphyria Cutanea Tarda

Porphyria cutanea tarda, which is characterized by a photosensitive dermatosis, is extremely rare in children. The diagnosis is based on the finding of high levels of uroporphyrins in the urine.

## Syndromes With Photosensitivity

A number of uncommon syndromes feature photosensitivity as a major presenting clue. Brief descriptions of a few of these disorders conclude this section.

### Xeroderma Pigmentosum

Xeroderma pigmentosum is a rare, progressive, autosomal recessive, degenerative disease characterized by severe photosensitivity developing in the first few years of life. Erythema, bullae, pigmented macules, hypochromic spots, and telangiectasia develop rapidly. The skin becomes atrophic, dry, and wrinkled. A variety of benign and malignant growths appear early in life. The ability to repair DNA after exposure to ultraviolet radiation is defective.

### Cockayne's Syndrome

Individuals with Cockayne's syndrome appear normal at birth, but clearly demonstrate short stature, microcephaly, and developmental delay by late childhood. The eyes appear sunken, the ears large, and the limbs long. There is progressive neurologic degeneration, with deafness, loss of vision, dysarthria, gait disturbances, and ataxia. The skin is sensitive to light and develops erythema, blisters, and telangiectasia. The hands and feet are cool and often cyanotic. The mode of inheritance is autosomal recessive.

### Bloom Syndrome

The first clue to the diagnosis of Bloom syndrome, an autosomal recessive disorder, usually is the development of plaques of telangiectatic erythema over the butterfly area and dorsa of the hands after exposure to sunlight. The prenatal onset of growth deficiency continues after birth. Malar hypoplasia, a small nose, and a high-pitched voice are typical. The diagnosis is confirmed by the finding of chromosomal breakage and rearrangements with somatic exchange between sister chromatids. Malignancy accounts for the majority of deaths in individuals with this disorder.

### Hartnup Disease

A rare autosomal recessive disorder, Hartnup disease is caused by the malabsorption of tryptophan from the gastrointestinal tract. The skin changes resemble those of pellagra, with the development of an erythematous to vesicular eruption with scaling, lichenification, and hyperpigmentation over the sun-exposed areas of the body, particularly the face, back of the neck, and hands. Neurologic signs resemble those of cerebellar ataxia, and psychiatric disturbances are common. The diagnosis can be confirmed by the finding of large amounts of monoaminomonocarboxylic acids excreted in the urine.

### Rothmund-Thomson Syndrome

The striking cutaneous picture of Rothmund-Thomson syndrome develops within a few years of birth. The skin is pigmented in a reticulated or dappled pattern. Depigmentation, small areas of atrophy, telangiectasia, and vascular marmorization are other features. Half of the children are short in stature. Half develop cataracts and half have hypotrichosis. Photosensitivity occurs in one third.

# ANNULAR LESIONS

## Tinea Corporis

Superficial fungal infections probably are the most readily identified annular lesions of the skin. The ring-like lesions are recognized by most laypersons, although not all ringed lesions are tinea. Because the infection of non-hairy areas of the skin by dermatophytes is limited to the epidermis, only the most superficial layers of the skin are involved. The rings generally are erythematous. As the inflammation spreads, the active infection in the center of the lesions is destroyed, and this area clears, resulting frequently in the picture of an advancing border with central clearing. The border generally is scaly and slightly elevated, and, on close inspection, is seen to contain microvesicles and pustules (Fig 35-54). The lesions, which may be single or multiple, are not always round. Bizarre shapes and, occasionally, a coalescence of lesions may be noted, and borders may not be continuous. Target-like lesions may occur as a result of reinfection or failure of clearing of the central part of the lesion. Tinea corporis usually is asymptomatic, although pruritus may be present.

The organism responsible for most cases of tinea corporis is *Trichophyton tonsurans*. *Microsporum canis, Microsporum audouinii*, and *Trichophyton mentagrophytes* infections also are seen. Treatment consists of application of one of the topical antifungal agents, such as clotrimazole, haloprogin, or miconazole. Application twice a day for 2 to 3 weeks after the lesion clears usually is sufficient. The diagnosis may be confirmed by potassium hydroxide preparations. Because tinea corporis occurs on non-hairy skin, the lesions do not fluoresce with a Wood's lamp. The three lesions most frequently confused with tinea corporis are granuloma annulare, the herald spots of pityriasis rosea, and dry nummular eczema.

## Pityriasis Rosea

Pityriasis rosea is a disorder of unknown cause characterized by ovoid papulosquamous lesions that generally are distributed on the trunk. The herald patch, a large lesion that appears before development of the other, smaller ovoid lesions and papules, may be mistaken for tinea corporis. The full picture of pityriasis rosea, however, should not be confused with this diagnosis. The ovoid lesions are slightly elevated and papular, and they have a fine, wrinkled scale. The bases of the lesions are erythematous, although some may appear hypopigmented and others hyperpigmented, especially in black individuals. It is helpful to look at the patient from a distance of 90 to 180 cm (3 to 6 ft) to see the pattern of the lesions, which often resembles the boughs of a pine tree.

A marked papular component occasionally confuses the picture of pityriasis rosea. In some cases, involvement of the face and extremities is prominent. Pruritus occurs frequently. The duration of the eruption is long, often more than 1 month and

sometimes 2 or 3 months. The rash of secondary syphilis resembles pityriasis rosea so closely that a serologic test for syphilis may be in order for patients with pityriasis rosea who are in a sexually active age group. Additional discussion of pityriasis rosea can be found early in this chapter in the section dealing with papular disorders.

## Granuloma Annulare

The uninitiated almost always mistake granuloma annulare for tinea corporis. Granuloma annulare is an inflammatory disorder that is characterized by the eruption of papules, which may be superficial or subcutaneous, in a ringed arrangement. The initial papule enlarges outward and the center clears, sometimes seeming depressed (Fig 35-55). The key to differentiation from tinea corporis is close inspection of the borders. In granuloma annulare, the surface of the lesion is devoid of scale, vesicles, or pustules; skin markings are normal. In tinea, the border of the lesion is scaly, with microvesicles and pustules, and the color of the lesions varies from skin tone to erythematous. The lesions of granuloma annulare are asymptomatic, being neither pruritic nor tender.

The cause of granuloma annulare is unknown. Some believe that it represents a delayed type of hypersensitivity. Most lesions resolve spontaneously within 2 years, but some may last for decades. In adults, an association with diabetes mellitus has been reported, but this has not been noted in children. About half of all individuals with granuloma annulare have a single lesion. The lesions most frequently appear on the distal extremities. Deep-seated lesions can appear to be attached to the periosteum of bone, particularly the tibia. On biopsy samples, these lesions resemble rheumatoid nodules, but there is no association with connective tissue diseases. The nodules regress in 6 weeks to 6 months.

## Psoriasis

Annular lesions also may be seen in psoriasis. These lesions usually can be differentiated from other annular lesions by the pres-

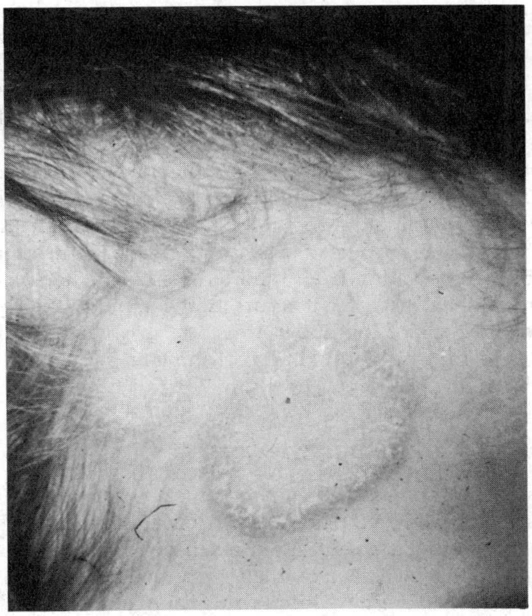

**Figure 35-54.** Annular lesion of tinea corporis with a raised border and scaling on the forehead.

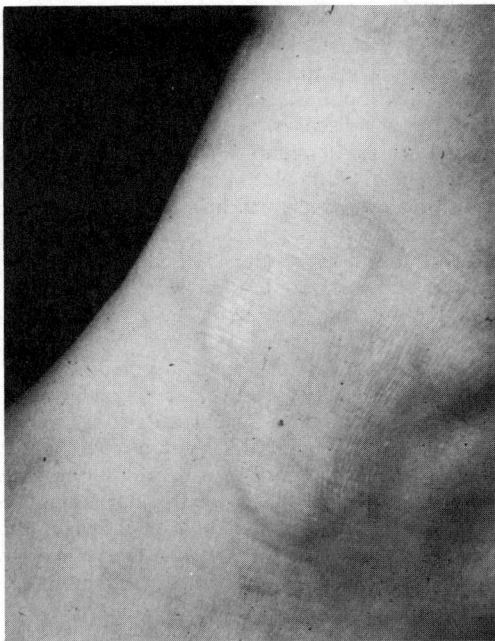

**Figure 35-55.** A granuloma annulare lesion on the ankle. Note the lack of epidermal involvement.

ence of a thick, adherent, silvery scale; clear demarcation of the erythematous borders; and symmetry of distribution of the lesions. See the previous section of this chapter regarding scaling and dry lesions for a more complete discussion of psoriasis.

## Nummular Eczema

As the name implies, lesions of nummular eczema are coin shaped. The surface generally is thickened and dry, and the borders are fairly discrete. Central clearing is not typical. The cause is not known, but seems to be related to dry skin. See the previous section in this chapter regarding scaling and dry lesions for further discussion.

## Lichen Spinulosus

The lesions of lichen spinulosus often are easier to feel than to see, except on black skin. Annular patches are common, although irregular patterns are more frequent. The lesion is composed of a base of tiny, spiny projections, which create the rough texture. The projections are grouped, giving rise to the lesions, which are flesh-colored to slightly hypopigmented and are asymptomatic. Patches may appear suddenly and have a tendency to clear and return. The back and extremities are common sites of occurrence.

The cause of lichen spinulosus is not known, but there is a definite association with atopic dermatitis. Treatment is not necessary unless there is concern about appearance. A good emollient, particularly one containing a small amount of lactic acid, often hastens resolution of the lesions.

## Urticaria

Hives, or wheals, are common in both children and adults. The lesions represent a localized vasodilation and transudation of fluid from capillaries and small blood vessels. Hives are transient, lasting less than 24 hours. They are lightly erythematous and may have central clearing, creating an annular pattern. Stasis of blood in the center of lesions frequently creates an appearance of purpura. Pruritus is a common feature.

Urticaria is a manifestation of the release of mediators from cutaneous mast cells, which increase vascular permeability. Histamine, kinins, and prostaglandins are among the mediators released. Urticaria may be caused by drugs, foods, inhalant allergies, infections, and arthropod bites and stings. Other agents include contactants, internal diseases, psychogenic factors, genetic abnormalities, and physical agents. Given the wide variety of possible agents, it often is difficult to pinpoint the cause of urticaria.

Infections that may cause urticaria include those with group A $\beta$-hemolytic streptococci, hepatitis virus, and Epstein-Barr virus. Physical agents that may result in urticaria include heat, cold, pressure, light, water, and vibration. Cholinergic urticaria is a fairly distinctive form manifested by the appearance of 2- to 3-mm papules surrounded by large erythematous flares. These flares are very pruritic and follow the onset of perspiration.

Uncovering the cause of chronic urticaria, defined as urticaria of at least 6 weeks' duration, is particularly difficult. In most series, the cause of the problem has been uncovered in less than 20% of the cases. The presence of urticarial lesions that persist for more than 24 hours should raise the suspicion of urticarial vasculitis. A skin biopsy of one of the lesions will be diagnostic.

Treatment of urticaria depends on the extent and severity of the condition. Acute episodes that threaten vital functions should be treated with epinephrine as well as with antihistamines. Systemic steroids are indicated occasionally. Usually, an antihistamine alone is satisfactory therapy until the problem resolves.

## Erythema Multiforme

The target-like lesions of erythema multiforme evolve over a period of 1 week and should not be confused with the lesions of urticaria, which occasionally resemble targets because of their bluish centers. The primary lesion of erythema multiforme is a dull red macule or wheal in the center of which is a papule or vesicle. The macule becomes papular and then plaque-like, and the center forms concentric rings of color. The center may blister and appear purpuric or even necrotic.

Erythema multiforme is a nonspecific hypersensitivity reaction that can be divided into two types, minor and major, depending on the extent and severity of the lesions. The minor form often is preceded by an upper respiratory infection. Herpes simplex recurrences are responsible most often for recurrent erythema multiforme. Other infections implicated include infectious mononucleosis, *Yersinia* infection, tuberculosis, and histoplasmosis. The underlying cause usually is not defined, however.

Erythema multiforme major is a much more serious disorder. Mucous membrane involvement is significant, and erosive lesions on mucous membrane surfaces may lead to dehydration from failure to take in enough fluids. Eye involvement may lead to blindness. Large areas of the cutaneous surface may become denuded. Affected children appear ill and have fever, prostration, and myalgias. Rarely, *Mycoplasma pneumoniae* infections have been implicated in erythema multiforme major. Usually, however, the condition is drug related. The drugs most frequently associated with this reaction are sulfonamides, penicillins, and phenytoin. The reaction follows drug therapy by 1 to 3 weeks, allowing time for the antigenic stimulus to cause the host immune response. The course of the illness is prolonged; Stevens-Johnson syndrome, which is the most severe form and which often has severe mucocutaneous involvement, lasts for weeks. Although therapy is mainly supportive, hospitalization is recommended. The skin is handled best as if it were burned, with the healing lesions being treated with wet compresses, whirlpool baths, and ointments. Ophthalmologic consultation is important because of the high incidence of corneal involvement with consequent scarring. The use of systemic steroids remains controversial.

## Erythema Marginatum

The clinical appearance of the skin lesions occasionally seen in acute rheumatic fever are not pathognomonic. Erythema marginatum begins as erythematous blotches or papules that spread peripherally. The borders may form annular lesions, sometimes polycyclic or serpiginous. The margins are sharp, and the lesions advance and change shape rapidly. Dull red, pink, or violaceous, the lesions may resemble urticaria, but they are not pruritic. Their rapid change distinguishes them from erythema multiforme.

Erythema marginatum occurs in about 10% of patients with acute rheumatic fever. The rash is not specific for acute rheumatic fever, however, having been reported also in patients with juvenile rheumatoid arthritis. It occurs most commonly on the trunk and inner aspects of the upper arms and thighs. A skin biopsy of the lesion may be helpful in establishing an early diagnosis of acute rheumatic fever.

## Erythema Chronicum Migrans

The rash of erythema chronicum migrans has two general forms. One is an expanding red patch with varying intensities of redness within it; the other is a central red patch surrounded by normal-appearing skin that is surrounded by an expanding red band, producing a target or ring-within-a-ring configuration. The lesions usually are flat or slightly elevated. The lesions tend to be asymptomatic, but burning, pruritus, or pain may be associated with the rash. The lesions are singular in three quarters of the patients and begin 1 to 3 weeks after a bite from a tick. The spirochete, *Borrelia burgdorferi*, which is responsible for the rash and its progression to Lyme disease, usually is transmitted by the deer tick, *Ixodes dammini*.

## Syphilis

The brownish to dull red macules and papules of secondary syphilis may appear annular and resemble pityriasis rosea. The lesions generally are discrete and follow lines of cleavage on the trunk, similar to pityriasis rosea. Reddish brown lesions on the palmar and plantar surfaces should be a clue to this diagnosis in sexually active patients. The rash appears 6 to 8 weeks after the primary syphilitic lesion, and it may last from a few hours to months.

## Lupus Erythematosus

A wide and confusing variety of cutaneous lesions may be seen in systemic lupus erythematosus. The butterfly rash is known best, but annular lesions, including erythema multiforme, may be early signs of the disorder. The antinuclear antibody test is helpful in diagnosing confusing cases. Lesions of discoid lupus erythematosus, which occur mainly on the face and sun-exposed areas, are indurated plaques that are violaceous and have an adherent scale. They occasionally appear annular in configuration.

## Sarcoidosis

Sarcoidosis is replacing syphilis as the great mimic of the second half of the 20th century. A rash develops in about 50% of children with this disorder of unknown cause. The most common cutaneous eruptions are soft, red to yellowish brown or violaceous, flat-topped papules, found most frequently on the face. Sometimes, these papules take on an annular configuration. Larger, violaceous, plaque-like lesions may be found on the trunk, extremities, and buttocks. Other cutaneous manifestations of sarcoidosis include nodules, ulcers, subcutaneous tumors, and erythema nodosum.

## LINEAR LESIONS

### Rhus Dermatitis

The most common linear eruption seen in children is caused by contact with the *Rhus* toxins produced by poison ivy and poison oak. (See the previous section of this chapter concerning disorders with linear vesicles.)

### Lichen Striatus

Lichen striatus is characterized by the sudden onset of rapidly spreading, discrete, tiny papules in a linear band 1 cm to several centimeters wide. The lesions occur most commonly on the extremities. The papules are not always continuous, sometimes appearing to jump over areas of normal skin. The papules usually are skin colored or pink and sometimes are topped by a fine, adherent scale. In black individuals, the bands may appear depigmented. If a finger or toe is involved, the nail may become irregular. The cause of this unusual phenomenon is unknown. Most cases reach their maximum extent within a few days or weeks and regress spontaneously over 6 to 12 months. The lesions flatten out during their involution. There is no effective therapy,

although topical steroids or steroids in a lactic acid emollient occasionally may hasten recovery.

## Linear Scleroderma

Morphea or localized scleroderma may take on a linear configuration. (See the section earlier in this chapter concerning disorders involving abnormal skin texture.)

## Nevus Depigmentosus

Nevus depigmentosus is a linear, whorled, or marbled area of depigmentation that is not associated with underlying systemic abnormalities. The cause of these lesions, some of which appear after birth, is not known. There is no treatment for the cutaneous changes. Children with such lesions should be examined carefully for underlying defects that might suggest Ito syndrome.

## Incontinentia Pigmenti

Incontinentia pigmenti, an unusual genodermatosis, is manifested by four stages of cutaneous abnormalities. The first is the presence of or development of linear papules and vesicles at or shortly after birth (see Color Figure 11). The lesions may take on a pustular or crusted appearance and resemble a cutaneous infection; they generally clear by the time the patient reaches 4 months of age. The next stage is the appearance of verrucous (wart-like) lesions, not necessarily in the same areas as the inflammatory lesions. The verrucous stage peaks at 12 to 26 weeks and resolves gradually, usually within 1 or 2 years. The third stage is one of hyperpigmentation. These lesions are tan to slate gray and may be arranged in irregular linear streaks, whorls, or speckles. Sometimes, a pattern reminiscent of a marble cake may be seen. This stage also resolves gradually over the years. The final stage is seen in adult women who have subtle, hypopigmented, atrophic patches of skin, especially on the legs.

The inheritance mode of incontinentia pigmenti is X-linked dominant. Only 3% of cases have been described in the male sex, suggesting that the disorder is lethal to males. Documentation of the condition in the mother of an affected infant is difficult unless a history of cutaneous lesions can be obtained or the mother manifests one of the many systemic anomalies that are associated with the disorder. Important defects include involvement of the central nervous system, with seizures, spastic paresis, microcephaly, or mental retardation; eye defects, including strabismus, blindness, cataracts, optic nerve atrophy, and retrolenticular masses; dental anomalies, particularly cone-shaped or irregularly spaced teeth; patchy alopecia; and skeletal defects, including hemivertebrae, extra ribs, clubfoot, and syndactyly. Curiously, a peripheral eosinophilia is common in the first few weeks of life. The prognosis seems to be poor for future normal development if seizures occur early in life.

## Linear Epidermal Nevus Syndrome

Epidermal nevi may take on a linear configuration. Generally present at birth, they usually are unilateral and singular, are flesh colored to yellowish brown, and become rougher and more wart-like with age. These lesions may become dark and rather raised as the years progress. The syndrome appellation is used when systemic abnormalities accompany the skin changes; these abnormalities include mental retardation, seizures, strabismus, hemihypertrophy, kyphoscoliosis, and eye and kidney lesions. Generally, the more extensive the cutaneous lesions, the more likely it is that there are underlying systemic alterations. Occurrence of the epidermal nevus seems to be sporadic, the result of overproduction of surface or adnexal epithelium. The nevus is removed most often for cosmetic reasons, although carcinomatous change in adulthood has been described.

# DISORDERS OF THE SCALP

## Scaling

### Tinea Capitis

Dermatophyte infections should be ruled out whenever scaling of the scalp is found (Fig 35-56). Over the past few decades, *Trichophyton tonsurans* has replaced *Microsporum* species as the most common fungus responsible for tinea capitis. With this change has come an alteration in the appearance of the scalp infection. *Trichophyton* infections are manifested by a variety of lesions; the most common of these, and the one that is mistaken frequently for other conditions, particularly seborrheic dermatitis, involves scalp scaling without significant hair loss. Patches of hair loss, pustules, and boggy masses are other types of presentation; they are discussed later in this section.

In the past, the Wood's lamp was used frequently as a reliable screen for tinea capitis. *Microsporum* species invaded the outside of the hair shaft (ectothrix), producing by-products of infection that fluoresced with ultraviolet light. In contrast, *Trichophyton* infections grow within the hair shaft itself (endothrix) and do not fluoresce. In addition, with *Trichophyton* infections, the hair becomes fragile and tends to break off near the scalp, resulting in the so-called black-dot alopecia.

Tinea capitis is transmitted easily among children and is the most common fungal infection occurring before puberty. After puberty, tinea capitis is much less common, for reasons that are not clear. The infection also can be transmitted by animals, although this mode of transmission has decreased in frequency.

A 10% potassium hydroxide preparation may be used to demonstrate the hyphae and spores causing the tinea capitis. The diagnosis is established most easily by the examination of plucked-out, broken hairs, which are most likely to be infected. If the diagnosis is in doubt, a culture of hair and scale may be placed on Sabouraud's medium to grow the fungus. Office culture

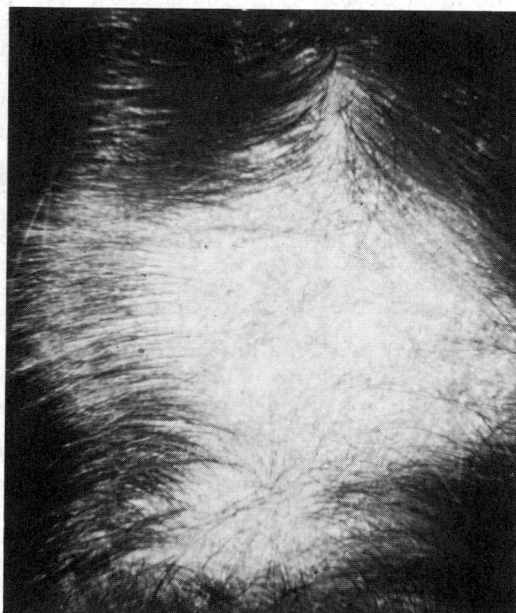

**Figure 35-56.**   Scaling and hair loss in the classic form of tinea capitis.

bottles that are inexpensive and easy to read are available for this test.

Given that the infection invades the hair shaft, topical antifungal therapy is not effective. Systemic antifungal agents, such as griseofulvin, 15 to 20 mg/kg/day, given once a day with a meal for 6 to 8 weeks, is effective in eradicating this infection. Care must be taken to examine other household members for similar infection. Selenium sulfide solution, 2½%, used as a shampoo twice a week will decrease the shedding of live fungi.

### Seborrheic Dermatitis

Most physicians generalize the adult experience with scaling of the scalp to children. Scaling of the scalp in children is diagnosed most commonly as seborrheic dermatitis, despite the fact that this condition generally is not found from about 12 months of age until puberty.

Infants commonly have the dry or greasy yellow scales of seborrhea, generally between 2 and 10 weeks of age. Some infants develop thick, brownish yellow scales over the anterior fontanelle because their parents are afraid to scrub or even touch this area. The dermatitis can cause erythema and hair loss, and the rash commonly spreads to the forehead, eyebrows, and retroauricular spaces. In black infants, depigmentation of the involved areas may be extensive. Candidal superinfection in moist areas is frequent.

Seborrheic dermatitis appears to be related to the presence of androgens. Infants receive maternal androgens transplacentally. When their effect dissipates, by 8 to 12 months of age, so does the rash. At puberty, with the swell of sex hormones, the sebaceous glands are stimulated again, and the typical changes of this dermatitis develop in predisposed individuals. That eunuchs do not seem to have seborrhea supports the idea that androgen is the underlying cause.

The scalp of infants usually can be treated with mild shampoo and fine combing or brushing to remove the scale. In recalcitrant cases, a mild hydrocortisone agent applied topically will suppress the dermatitis on the scalp, face, or other areas. In adolescent seborrhea, tar- or selenium-based shampoos are effective treatment.

### Atopic Dermatitis

Scaling of the scalp in children who have atopic dermatitis often is mistaken for seborrheic dermatitis. The scale generally is fine and white, and the scalp typically is pruritic. Excoriations of the scalp may be prominent, and secondary infections are common. Excessive hair washing may exacerbate the problem rather than helping it, as it does in seborrheic dermatitis. Clues to the presence of atopic dermatitis usually are found on other areas of the skin.

### Psoriasis

In most children with psoriasis of the scalp, other areas of the skin also are involved, showing the typical plaques set on an erythematous base (see Color Figure 18). Occasionally, however, only the scalp may be affected. The base of the scalp lesion always is inflammatory; thus, erythema underlies the whitish scale. The scale sometimes forms large plaques, resulting in hair loss with combing. The borders of the scalp often are involved. Topical steroids of moderate potency may be required to treat the scalp involvement. Thick, adherent scaling may require the use of a softening agent such as P and S Plus.

### Tinea Amiantacea

The massive, thick, adherent scaling of tinea amiantacea usually is mistaken for tinea capitis. The scales are silvery and tend to overlap, often trapping hair and thereby causing thinning of the scalp hair. Despite its name, tinea amiantacea is not caused by a fungal infection. The etiology is not clear, although some suspect a relationship to psoriasis. Aggressive applications of scale-softening agents, similar to those used in psoriasis of the scalp, often are helpful.

### Histiocytosis X

Histiocytosis X frequently is manifested by a scaly, erythematous dermatitis of the scalp and retroauricular areas. The scaling may be mistaken for seborrheic dermatitis until other systemic features appear. A clue to the diagnosis is the presence of petechiae underlying the scale (Fig 35-57). Other areas of the body may have a variety of lesions, including vesicular pustules, discrete erythematous papules, hemorrhagic crusted papules, and ulcerations in creases. This diagnosis always should be considered in any recalcitrant scaling eruption of the scalp.

## Pustules

### Tinea Capitis

As noted previously, tinea capitis can take on many disguises in the scalp. Scattered pustules are one of the various manifestations of dermatophyte infection. The most impressive, however, is the kerion, a boggy, indurated, raised mass on the scalp, the surface of which has no hair and is studded with pustules (Fig 35-58). On first glance, the kerion looks like a bacterial abscess. Incision and drainage of the mass, however, is unsuccessful; as implied by the name, which means "honeycomb," the kerion is made up of channels rather than a cavity.

A kerion is a hypersensitivity reaction to an infecting dermatophyte, usually *Trichophyton tonsurans*. The lesions may be single or multiple and often appear over a short period. Although a superficial culture frequently yields bacteria, often staphylococci, treatment need not include antibiotics. Most cases respond to a 6- to 8-week course of oral griseofulvin. Large lesions shrink rapidly with a tapering course of oral prednisone over a 2-week period. Although lost hair will not have grown back by the time the lesion resolves, it almost always regrows eventually.

### Traction Folliculitis

Prolonged or excessive traction on hair from tight braiding may result not only in hair breakage and loss, but also in the development of pustules at the borders of the areas of pulled hair. Resolution of the problem usually can be accomplished by removal of the traction. Occasionally, a secondary bacterial infec-

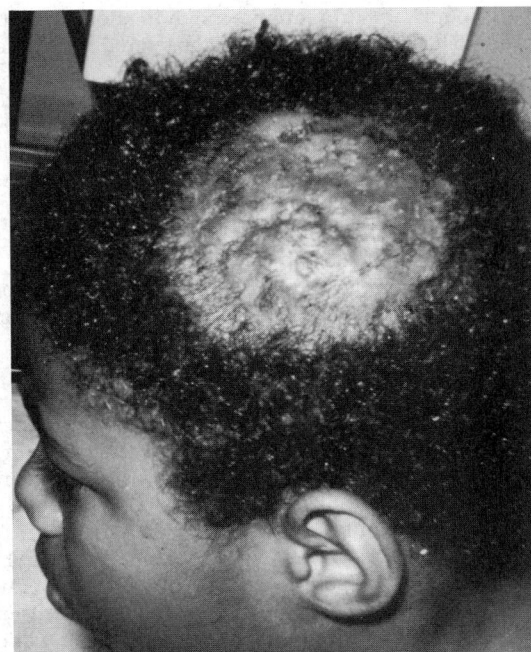

**Figure 35-58.** This boggy, oozing mass with pustules and hair loss is a kerion, one of the many varieties of tinea capitis.

tion, most commonly staphylococcal in origin, may become established in the hair follicles that were damaged by the pulling. Treatment with topical or systemic antibiotics may be indicated.

### Impetigo

Pustules and crusting of the scalp may be the result of secondary infection. A variety of stimuli may cause pruritus and subsequent excoriations of the scalp, preparing the way for bacterial infections. Precipitating causes include atopic dermatitis, occlusion from oils and greases, and head lice. The bacteria most frequently responsible are streptococci and staphylococci. Treatment with topical antibiotics may be effective, but with extensive lesions, systemic therapy may be required.

## Hair Loss

### Tinea Capitis

As mentioned previously, hair loss always should suggest the possibility of tinea capitis. The hair loss may be localized to one spot and be associated with scaling of the scalp or, less frequently, it may be associated with microvesicles at the advancing borders of the hair loss. More commonly, the scalp may look relatively unaffected except for the hair loss and the presence of black dots, which represent broken-off, infected hairs. There may be many patches of hair loss or a diffuse thinning of hair. If the cause of hair loss is not clear, a fungal culture is indicated.

### Alopecia Areata

The hallmark of alopecia areata is the appearance of well-circumscribed, round or oval patches of complete or relatively complete hair loss. The scalp appears normal, without scale or scarring. The lesions tend to appear rapidly, and may be single or multiple. Hair at the periphery of the lesions can be pulled out easily. Alopecia areata totalis is total loss of scalp hair; alopecia universalis is the complete loss of body hair.

Alopecia areata is much more common than most physicians realize. In reviews of dermatology clinics, as many as 2% of new patients have been found to have this disorder. The cause is not

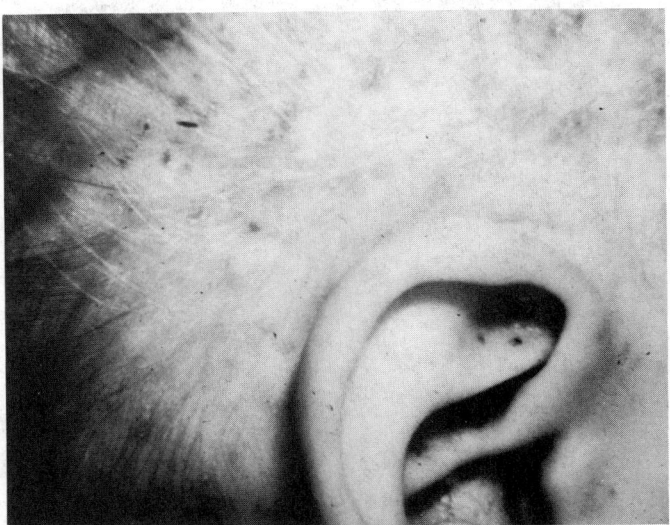

**Figure 35-57.** Seborrhea-like scaling of the scalp with underlying petechiae in a patient with histiocytosis X.

known, although an autoimmune phenomenon is suspected. Psychiatric disturbances used to be considered the underlying cause.

Alopecia areata rarely occurs in patients less than 4 years of age, but almost half of the cases appear in those less than 20 years of age. The course is totally unpredictable. Factors associated with a poor prognosis for eventual recovery include extensive alopecia in areas other than the scalp; occurrence in association with atopic dermatitis; the presence of nail changes, such as pitting; prepubertal onset; and ophiasis, the loss of hair in a swath above and behind the ears and across the occiput. The prognosis is good for most older children and adults. Hair may regrow in some places, however, only to be lost in others. Regrown hair often is light or even white.

The treatment of alopecia areata is disappointing. A wide variety of therapies have been tried with little sustained effect. Hair regrown during a course of systemic steroids is lost again when the steroids are discontinued. Local injections of triamcinolone into the scalp usually result in hair regrowth in injected areas, but the procedure is painful and the regrowth temporary. Topical irritants of various types were in vogue for some time, but rarely are effective. The key to treatment is careful, empathetic education of the patient and the parents. Support groups of similarly affected patients are increasingly common in large communities and offer a great deal of help for both patients and parents. Artificial hairpieces often help patients maintain a positive body image.

## Traction Alopecia

The hair loss in traction alopecia is secondary to prolonged tension on the hair shaft, usually from braiding of the hair. Traction most commonly produces hair loss at the margins of the scalp or as oval or linear areas in part lines (Fig 35-59). Permanent hair loss may result if pressure is maintained for a long time.

## Pressure Alopecia

Pressure alopecia is most common in young infants, who lie prone and rub their occiputs on the bedding. Such hair loss occasionally indicates a lack of stimulation by the parents. Persistent rubbing of the scalp by any means may result in hair breakage and loss.

## Trichotillomania

Hair loss as a result of trichotillomania, the pulling out of one's own hair, often assumes bizarre shapes and irregular patterns (Fig 35-60). The hair loss in this condition is never complete. A key feature distinguishing this from other forms of alopecia is the lack of scalp lesions and the presence of broken hairs of different lengths within the lesions. Body hair from other areas also may be lost, especially from the eyebrows or eyelashes. Rarely will a child admit to hair pulling, and rarely will the parents have noticed such behavior.

In young children, hair pulling usually represents a fairly benign reaction to stress. With time, most children discontinue the habit spontaneously. A short haircut and grease applied to the hair may help discourage the activity. In older children and adolescents, trichotillomania may reflect a more serious psychologic problem. An attempt should be made to uncover the cause of the stress. Open discussion with the child and the parents may lead to resolution of the problem.

## Telogen Effluvium

The hair loss in telogen effluvium is diffuse and rarely involves more than 50% of the scalp hair. Postnatal and postpartum alopecias affect almost all infants and many of their mothers. The hair loss actually is an acceleration of the normal physiologic process of aging of the hair. Eighty-five percent to 90% of hair on the scalp is in the anagen, or growing, phase, which generally lasts for 3 to 7 years. The remainder is primarily in the telogen, or resting, state, which lasts for 3 to 6 months and is followed by shedding. It is normal to shed 50 to 100 hairs from the scalp each day. In telogen effluvium, many of the hairs in the anagen phase are thrown suddenly into the telogen stage. Inciting factors include febrile illnesses, drug reactions, and severe stress. Hair loss begins 4 to 16 weeks after the inciting event; the hair returns to normal by 5 to 6 months. The diagnosis may be confirmed by pulling out a small patch of hair and examining the roots for the

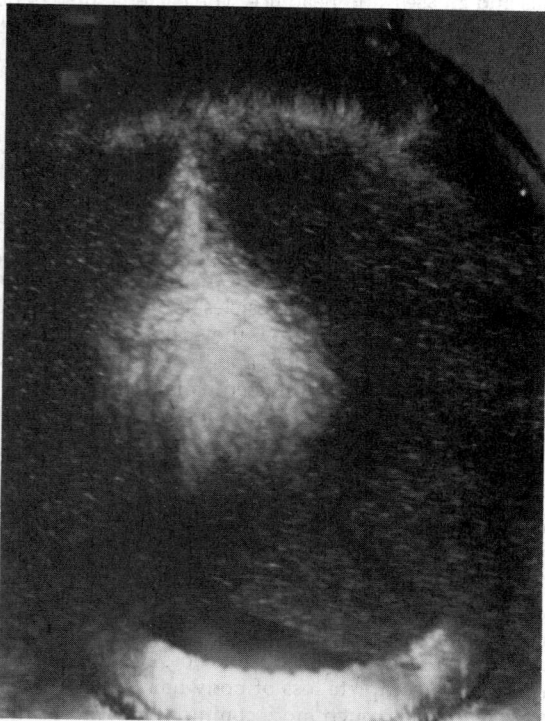

**Figure 35-59.**   Traction alopecia over the midline of the occiput as a result of braiding.

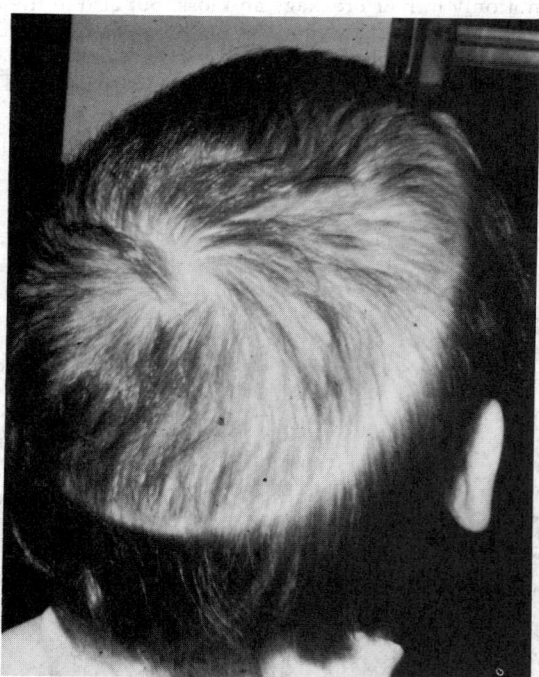

**Figure 35-60.**   Alopecia with various hair lengths in an unusual configuration is characteristic of trichotillomania.

appearance of hair in the anagen or telogen phase. In telogen effluvium, the number of hairs in the telogen phase is unusually high.

### Loose Anagen Syndrome

In the recently recognized disorder known as loose anagen syndrome, hairs in the anagen phase can be pulled easily from the scalp. Affected children have sparse, usually blond hair, with a history of rarely requiring cutting. On hair pulling, the normal anagen sheath over the root is missing and the root bulb is misshapen. The length and density of the hair tend to increase with age.

### Other Causes

Scalp hair may be absent, sparse, or abnormal for a wide variety of reasons, including reactions to drugs or chemicals, congenital defects in the hair shaft itself, and endocrine or systemic disorders. The list is too long and varied for this chapter. Table 35-5 presents a systematic classification of the causes of alopecia.

## DISORDERS OF THE NAILS

This section is limited to the description of only the most common and interesting nail disorders.

## Dystrophic Nails

### Psoriasis

As many as 50% of individuals with psoriasis have nail abnormalities. When the skin eruption is not diagnostic of psoriasis, the presence of nail abnormalities may help to establish the diagnosis. A variety of lesions may occur, including pits, discoloration, and separation of the nail plate from its bed. Subungual thickening, crumbling, and grooving of the nails also may be

found. Unfortunately, there is no effective therapy for nail involvement.

### Alopecia Areata

Fine stippling of the nails and, occasionally, ridging may occur in association with alopecia areata. The pitting is much finer than that associated with psoriasis.

### Nail-Patella Syndrome

The nail-patella syndrome is an inherited disease that is characterized by distorted or atrophic nails in association with absent or hypoplastic patellae. Some persons may have associated renal abnormalities, resulting in renal failure in adulthood. The condition is inherited as an autosomal dominant trait.

### Beau's Lines

Transverse grooves, the result of thinning of the nails, may be caused by trauma to the nail matrix or may follow a systemic disease. Given that the normal nail plate grows at a rate of about 1 mm/wk, the timing of the preceding insult may be determined by measuring the distance of the groove from the nail plate.

### Nail Dystrophy

Nail dystrophy is a condition with an autosomal dominant pattern of inheritance that begins in early childhood and is characterized by dystrophic involvement of many nails, usually all of them. The nail changes are variable, and different types may occur in the same child. Changes include thickening, thinning, pitting, ridging, opalescence, and spooning. Generally, there is gradual improvement with age.

## Nail Infections

### Tinea Unguium

Chronic fungal infections of the nail, also known as onychomycosis, are caused most often by *Trichophyton rubrum*, *Tricho-*

---

**TABLE 35-5.    Classification of Alopecia by Pattern and Time of Onset**

| Acquired Localized Alopecia | Acquired Diffuse Alopecia | Congenital Localized Alopecia | Congenital Diffuse Alopecia |
|---|---|---|---|
| Alopecia areata | Telogen effluvium | Sebaceous, epidermal nevi | Genetic syndromes |
|   Severe variants include alopecia totalis, alopecia universalis | Anagen effluvium | Melanocytic nevi |   Ectodermal dysplasias |
| |   Drug-induced | Hemangiomas |   Congenital hypothyroidism |
| Tinea capitis |   Endocrine-associated | Lymphangioma |   Marinesco-Sjögren syndrome |
| Traumatic alopecia |   Diet-associated | Aplasia cutis |   Atrichia-congenita |
|   Trichotillomania | Proximal trichorrhexis nodosa | Incontinentia pigmenti |   Cartilage hair hypoplasia |
|   Friction | Lamellar ichthyosis | Focal dermal hypoplasia | Hair shaft abnormalities |
|   Traction | Acrodermatitis enteropathica | Chondrodysplasia punctata |   Trichorrhexis nodosa |
|   Scars from accidents or burns | Multiple rare syndromes and disorders | Hallermann-Streiff syndrome (sutural alopecia) |     Proximal |
| Androgenic alopecia (male pattern baldness) | | Intrauterine trauma (eg, scalp electrodes) |     Distal |
| Seborrheic dermatitis | | |     Familial |
| | | |     Argininosuccinicacidura |
| | | |   Pili torti |
| | | |     Familial |
| | | |     Syndromal |
| | | |   Monilethrix |
| | | |   Trichorrhexis invaginata (Netherton's syndrome) |
| | | |   Trichoschisis (trichothiodystrophies) |

*Datloff J, Esterly NB. A system for sorting out pediatric alopecia. Contemp Pediatr 1986;3:53.*

*phyton mentagrophytes,* and *Epidermophyton floccosum.* These infections are not seen commonly in young children, but may appear in adolescents. The infection usually begins at the distal nail edge as an opaque white or silvery patch that later turns yellow or brown. Debris tends to accumulate underneath the nail plate. Treatment of this condition is frustrating and prolonged. Oral griseofulvin may need to be taken for 6 months, and the cure rate is only 50%.

### Candida

Infections with *Candida* are seen most often in young children who suck their fingers or in adults whose occupations require repeated immersion of the hands in water. The key to diagnosis is the appearance of a swollen, erythematous, and slightly tender area of skin adjacent to the involved nail. The nail itself is discolored, often greenish, and separates from the nail plate. The edges of the nail are eroded. Treatment consists of removal of the source of continued wetness as well as application of a topical anti-candidal agent to the infected nail.

### Pseudomonas

*Pseudomonas* infections of the nail often resemble *Candida* infections, with the nail bed taking on a greenish blue discoloration. Paronychial involvement, however, causes the skin surrounding the nail to be more tender in *Pseudomonas* than in *Candida* infections. Given that continuous immersion in water is an important contributing factor in this infection, keeping the nails dry is of utmost importance. A topical anti-pseudomonal antibiotic may be effective in clearing the infection.

## DISORDERS INVOLVING BLOOD VESSELS

Congenital vascular lesions come in a variety of shapes and sizes and account for the most common congenital malformation of the skin. The common macular erythematous lesion known as nevus flammeus is discussed at the beginning of this chapter in the section dealing with skin lesions in the neonatal period. The common hemangiomas, both capillary and cavernous, are discussed in the section on nodular disorders. This section describes a few of the less common cutaneous vascular lesions.

### Port-Wine Stain

The vessels composing the port-wine stain are mature capillaries. The lesion generally is macular, does not grow except in relation to the growth of the child, and tends to be pink to red. The stains may appear anywhere on the body surface, although they commonly involve the face. With age, they may darken and develop superficial or deep nodules. Hemangiomas and arteriovenous malformations occasionally may underlie the superficial lesion. These lesions do not regress with age. If the patient or parent desires treatment, cosmetic cover-up or more aggressive therapy with tunable dye laser offer the best results. It is important to recognize conditions that occasionally are associated with port-wine stains, such as Sturge-Weber syndrome and glaucoma.

The characteristic features of Sturge-Weber syndrome, which is an uncommon disorder, are a port-wine stain of the face and an ipsilateral angiomatosis of the leptomeninges, which commonly leads to seizures and mental retardation.

Experience with large numbers of children with port-wine stains has shown that distribution of the stain is of primary importance regarding development of the syndrome. Angiomatosis of the leptomeninges occurs only in association with stains in the distribution of the first branch of the trigeminal nerve (Fig 35-61). Not all children with a port-wine stain in this area develop the syndrome, however, and full coverage of the area with the

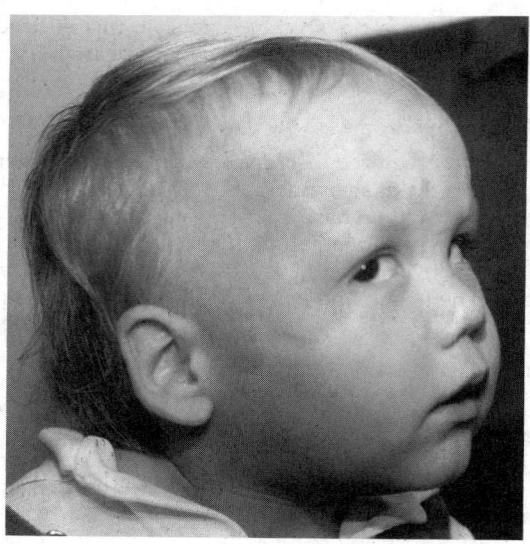

Figure 35-61.    A port wine stain involving the right frontotemporal area.

stain is more likely to be associated with the syndrome than is only partial involvement. The vascular malformation on the surface of the cortex eventually develops calcifications that take on an appearance similar to that of train tracks, but these changes may not be present in early life.

Glaucoma of the eye on the side of the stain is another important complication that needs to be checked closely. Involvement of both the upper and lower eyelids is associated with a high probability of glaucoma.

Hemiplegia, mental retardation, and hypertrophy of gingiva involved with the stain are other complications associated with the Sturge-Weber syndrome.

### Spider Angioma

Prepubertal children commonly have tiny, erythematous macular papules on the face, hands, and arms that blanch with pressure. These lesions generally represent benign telangiectases rather than those associated with liver disease, pregnancy, or estrogen therapy. Some of the lesions, particularly on the face, may develop thin branches radiating from the central punctum, resulting in the name *spider angioma*. Sometimes, the radiation of fine vessels produces a noticeable lesion.

Most spider angiomas do not regress with age. If it is cosmetically indicated or desired, careful microcoagulation of the central vessel with electrocautery, freezing, or the pulsed laser may result in eradication of the lesion.

### Ataxia-Telangiectasia

The appearance of fine telangiectasia, usually first on the bulbar conjuctivae, may be a clue to the cause of a child's ataxia, which usually has appeared much earlier. The telangiectasia generally develop between 3 to 5 years of age and become increasingly extensive over the years (Fig 35-62). This disorder is inherited as an autosomal recessive trait. Affected children face a relentless downhill course, with recurrent sinopulmonary infections and progressive central nervous system involvement. Death usually occurs during the second decade of life.

### Hereditary Hemorrhagic Telangiectasia

Rendu-Osler-Weber syndrome is an autosomal dominant disorder that is characterized by the appearance of numerous punctate,

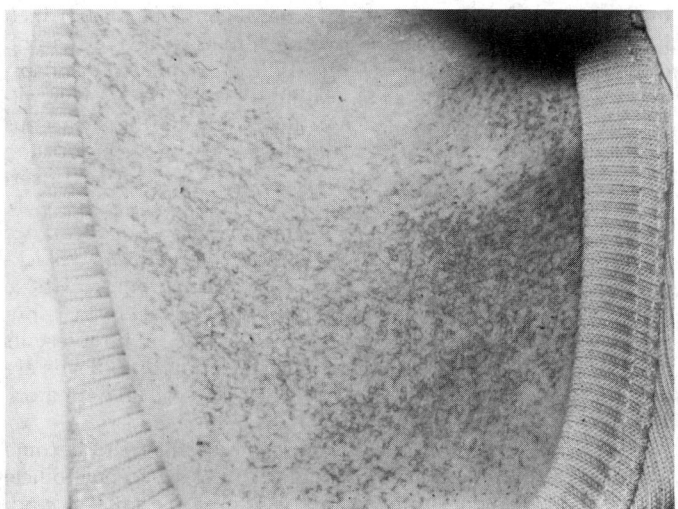

**Figure 35-62.** Diffuse telangiectasia on the upper chest of an adolescent with ataxia-telangiectasia.

slightly elevated telangiectasia of the skin. The lesions generally start to appear late in the first decade of life, primarily around the mouth and on the mucous membranes of the mouth and nose. The most common presenting complaint is epistaxis. Gastrointestinal blood loss with chronic anemia is another frequent complication.

## Other Vascular Disorders

Other cutaneous vascular syndromes are described in Table 35-1.

## DIAPER DERMATITIS

Almost all children in diapers have a rash in the covered area at some point during their diaper-wearing years. In most cases, the irritation is minimal and can be treated effectively with any of a host of available creams, ointments, and powders. As many as 10% of children, however, have a problem rash that leads to consultation with a physician. Diaper dermatitis is not a life-threatening condition, but it may produce discomfort for the infant and it certainly causes anxiety for the parents.

The etiology of diaper dermatitis is multifactorial. The rash itself may take on a number of forms and must be differentiated from a variety of other conditions. The basic problem is the diaper. If infants did not wear diapers, there would be no diaper rashes; in countries where diapers are not worn, diaper dermatitis is almost unheard of. Diapers protect us and the environment from the urine and stools of infants. As barriers, however, they also impede the evaporation of moisture from the skin. The stratum corneum becomes edematous and increasingly susceptible to friction from the diaper itself. Friction leads to maceration, which allows other irritants and bacteria (especially *Candida*) to gain a foothold and create even more inflammation.

Ammonia used to be thought to play a major role in diaper dermatitis. Bacteria that are capable of producing ammonia from urea are present in the perineal areas of most infants. Although ammonia itself will not initiate diaper dermatitis, it will aggravate the condition. In contrast, *Candida* may be able to initiate an inflammatory response in the skin and produce a diaper dermatitis.

Diaper dermatitis can be grouped into two major categories: primary irritant and candidal. Primary irritant diaper dermatitis, also called generic diaper dermatitis, is characterized by varying degrees of erythema and papules, often with a shiny, glazed surface. The creases tend to be spared; primarily involved are the convex surfaces, which are directly in contact with the diaper itself. *Tidemark dermatitis* is the name given to the form that features chafing from the recurrent wet-dry effect of urine contact. Nodules and ulcerations of the convex surfaces occur only rarely, usually as a result of prolonged contact of the skin with soiled diapers.

Candidal diaper dermatitis, caused by infection with the yeast *Candida albicans*, is characterized by the appearance of the rash in the inguinal and other creases, with erythema, superficial erosions, and numerous bright red satellite pustules and erosions. Infantile seborrheic dermatitis also may produce a diaper dermatitis involving the inguinal creases; however, although seborrhea may play a role, treatment should be aimed at eradicating the secondary *Candida* infection that usually is present.

The treatment of diaper dermatitis would be easier if diapers could be removed. Realities of daily life and societal pressures make such removal difficult for any length of time. Nevertheless, in recalcitrant cases, that may be the recommended treatment. Wet diapers always should be removed quickly. The perineum then should be washed gently with mild cleansing agents, these agents should be rinsed off thoroughly, and the whole area should be dried completely before a new diaper is put on. In primary irritant dermatitis, a number of soothing ointments, most of which contain zinc oxide, are available to protect the skin and decrease friction on it from diapers. Persistence of any diaper dermatitis for more than 48 to 72 hours indicates secondary infection with *Candida*; in such cases, an antifungal agent specific for this yeast should be used. Treatment of candidal diaper dermatitis requires use of the above measures, as well as application of an antifungal agent and a mild hydrocortisone cream to treat the inflammation. In some cases, it may be wise to use a separate antifungal agent and hydrocortisone product to be applied alternately every 2 hours with each diaper change.

Talcs and cornstarch may be used to protect the skin and absorb excess fluid. Parents must be warned that talc can be inhaled by the infant, however, resulting in respiratory problems. Cornstarch does not enhance candidal growth, contrary to common belief.

Whether cloth or disposable diapers are less likely to result in dermatitis is a moot concern. Some infants seem to react to the detergents used to clean cloth diapers; others react to certain types of disposable diapers. The plastic covering on disposable diapers may cause irritation of the skin. Elastic bands in disposable diapers and plastic covers for cloth ones may result in contact dermatitis in susceptible infants. Disposable diapers with absorbent gels will hold a greater amount of fluid and pull it away from the skin.

Although most diaper dermatitis is the result of primary irritant dermatitis or *Candida*, other disorders also may cause rashes in the diaper area. Impetigo, a bacterial infection, is common in the diaper area. Bullous impetigo, characterized by blisters that rupture rapidly and leave moist areas of erythema or dried lesions with collarettes of scale, is the most frequent bacterial infection found in the diaper region. This infection is caused by *Staphylococcus aureus* and, therefore, is treated best with oral antistaphylococcic antibiotics. Folliculitis and furunculosis may occur, particularly on the buttocks. Recurrent staphylococcal furuncles generally resolve once the child no longer wears diapers. Tinea corporis occasionally masquerades as diaper dermatitis. An advancing border of microvesicles, crusting, and erythema usually is present. The lesions may not be as clearly ring-like as they are on other body areas.

Psoriasis also may occur in the diaper area, because the skin at this site is subjected to repeated irritation. Because of the moisture produced by diapers, the thick, silvery, adherent scale typical of psoriasis may not be clearly evident. Allergic contact dermatitis also may mimic diaper dermatitis. Parents may apply a variety of ointments and creams that contain sensitizing agents to the skin of the perineum, only to create a worsening dermatitis. It is important to obtain a complete list of all medicaments used in this area.

Herpes simplex infections usually can be distinguished readily by the presence of grouped vesicles, but, occasionally, larger areas of erosion may simulate diaper dermatitis. Acrodermatitis enteropathica typically produces vesiculation and erosions around the mouth and nose, in the perineum, and on the acral surfaces (ie, hands and feet). Affected infants are irritable, usually have diarrhea and failure to thrive, and lose their hair. Infants with histiocytosis X may have an erythematous, papular/nodular, and, occasionally, ulcerative rash in the diaper area, particularly in the inguinal creases. The rash may mimic a candidal infection, but does not respond to appropriate treatment for such an infection. The scalp may be affected with a scaly rash, frequently with underlying petechiae. Scabies may result in a diaper dermatitis, but the infestation has signs of involvement in other areas as well and, therefore, is not difficult to diagnose. Finally, child abuse or neglect needs to be considered in cases of suspicious lesions of the perineum or severe, unattended diaper dermatitis.

A discussion of diaper dermatitis is not complete without mention of granuloma gluteale infantum. This is a rare, but worrisome-looking disorder characterized by red-purple nodules occurring in any portion of the diaper area, most commonly on the abdomen and upper thighs. The lesions are asymptomatic and are firm or soft and elastic. They usually develop in children who have had preceding irritant dermatitis. Although the cause is not known, many cases seem to occur in children who previously were treated with moderate- to intermediate-potency topical steroids. The lesions sometimes suggest lymphomatous nodules.

## ACNE

Acne undoubtedly is the most common skin problem of adolescents. Unfortunately, it often is relegated to a minor position in most medical school curricula. Acne is not a life-threatening illness, but its impact on adolescents in their formative years is significant. The scars on the face are only a superficial reflection of the psychologic scars, which may run much deeper. The magnitude of sales of over-the-counter medications for acne are an indication of the importance of this problem to adolescents.

### Pathogenesis

The pathogenesis of acne is not clearly understood. Many factors seem to contribute to development of the lesions. Development of acne starts in the sebaceous gland, a large, multilobular gland that empties into a relatively long canal containing a vellus hair, the follicle for which lies at its base. The concentration of sebaceous follicles is highest on the face, chest, and back, areas that commonly develop acneiform lesions. At puberty, the sebaceous glands are stimulated by androgens to increase in size and lipid production, resulting in an increase in the oiliness of the skin.

Dihydrotestosterone, a product of testosterone, is the most potent androgen end-organ effector. Dihydrotestosterone is formed primarily in cells located within the sebaceous glands. An important event along the path to acne is obstruction of the sebaceous follicle unit. For some reason, sebum and keratin from the shedding of cells lining the follicle stick together to form plugs. The plugs, called comedones, are invaded by bacteria, especially *Propionibacterium acnes*. The primary role of bacteria in the pathogenesis of acne may be the production of lipases, which hydrolyze the triglycerides of sebum into free fatty acids and other extracellular products, which in turn stimulate an inflammatory response (chemotaxis), leading to the rupture of the pilosebaceous unit. The presence of lipids outside the sebaceous follicle causes a further inflammatory response and the production of the papular pustules of acne. All these factors act in concert to produce the lesions of acne.

Acne vulgaris, or common acne, begins with the appearance of comedones, usually in early adolescence (Fig 35-63). Blackheads, or open comedones, represent sebaceous follicles whose orifices at the skin surface are patulous. The blackhead is not composed of dirt, contrary to popular belief; rather, it represents discoloration of the sebaceous plug by melanin. Blackheads are unsightly, but they are not typical precursors of inflammatory lesions.

The closed comedo, or whitehead, is more likely to become inflamed. In these lesions, the opening of the sebaceous follicle is tiny, and a plug of sebum pushes the skin up in a small mound. Rupture of the follicular wall is likely to cause the lesion to become inflammatory and to produce papulopustules in an attempt to clean up the "oil spill." Generally, the follicular wall re-forms; the neutrophils, macrophages, and other debris from the inflammation are expelled or cleared; and the lesion eventually recedes.

Deeper lesions, or nodules, may develop when the products of inflammation take longer to clear and fibrous tissue is laid down. Scars may result from the formation of this fibrous tissue. Nodules of inflammation may coalesce to form large lakes of pus, resulting in cystic lesions, which heal slowly, frequently become reinflamed, and may form sinus tracts. In acne conglobata, a severe, disfiguring form of acne generally occurring in adolescent males, a maze of channels may form in the dermis; the skin surface is distorted by large, purplish mounds as well as by a myriad of pustules and blackheads (Fig 35-64).

### Treatment

The treatment of acne begins with education. It is important that the adolescent understand as much as possible about the pathogenesis of the problem. Old myths should be discarded, particularly the relationship between "junk" food and acne. It must

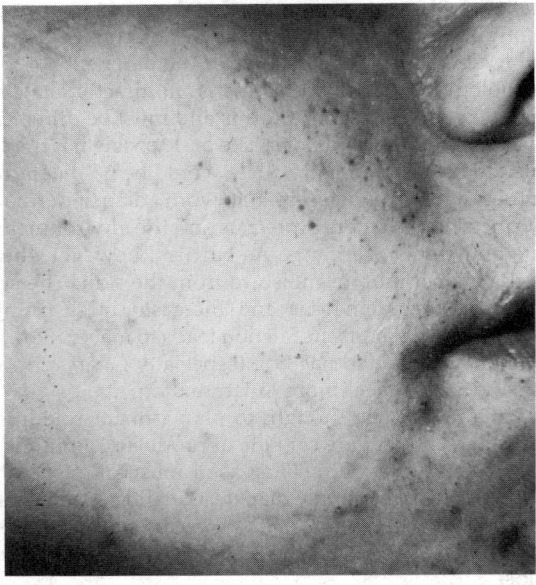

Figure 35-63. Comedones predominate in this teenager with acne.

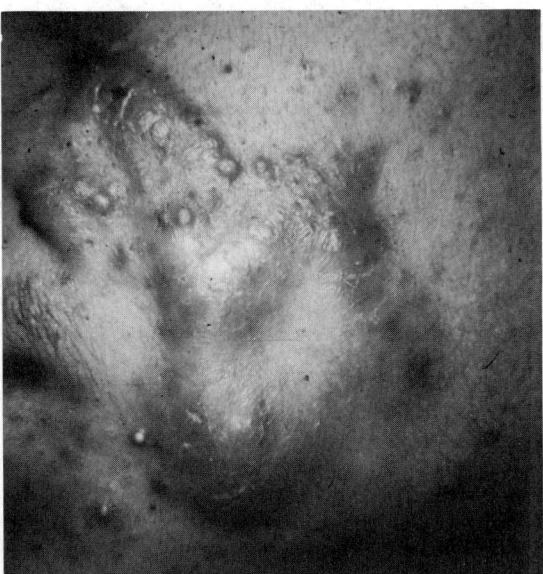

Figure 35-64.    Large cysts and pustules are characteristic of acne conglobata, a severe form of acne.

## Types

*Acne neonatorum* refers to the presence of small papulopustules, which may develop in the whitish yellow papules resulting from sebaceous gland hypertrophy that are present on the faces of some neonates. The glands of neonates are stimulated by maternal androgens in utero. The problem resolves within 1 to 2 months of birth and usually requires no treatment.

Infantile acne is a less well understood phenomenon; comedones and papulopustules may begin to appear in infants who are 3 to 4 months of age and may last until the infants are 12 to 18 months of age. Steroid acne is a result of the administration of oral or intravenous corticosteroids in large doses. The characteristic lesions—smooth, dome-shaped, erythematous papules of uniform size—appear suddenly in a crop (Fig 35-65). Comedones are absent, and pustules are uncommon initially, although they may appear later.

*Cosmetic acne* refers to the appearance of typical acne lesions after prolonged application of comedogenic cosmetics. Cocoa butter, a favorite moisturizer, is a proved comedogenic agent. The typical lesions of mechanical acne occur in areas subject to repeated trauma; examples are lesions of the forehead caused by brushing or combing of the hair, or lesions of the forehead and chin caused by helmet straps. Rubbing may result in rupture of the sebaceous follicle unit below the skin surface.

A number of lesions may mimic acne. Angiofibromas of tuberous sclerosis have been mistaken for acne, despite their onset at an age much too early for acne and the lack of associated comedones. Flat warts sometimes are extensive and appear acneiform. Again, comedones are absent, and pustules do not form.

## DRUG REACTIONS

One of the main difficulties in dermatologic differential diagnosis is deciding whether a rash is drug induced. Obviously, if the child is not taking a medication currently or has not received one recently, this is not a possibility. All too frequently, however, a febrile child is prescribed an antibiotic and later erupts in a rash. Is it an allergic reaction? Should the antibiotic be discontinued? The answers often are difficult to determine. The difficulty lies

be made clear that the medications used to treat acne take time to work and sometimes must be changed or combined.

The most commonly used medication is benzoyl peroxide, which appears to have three modes of activity: a sebostatic effect; mild comedolytic activity; and a strong inhibitory effect on bacteria. Most over-the-counter acne medications contain benzoyl peroxide. Unfortunately, the adolescent usually does not read the directions carefully, uses too much or too strong a concentration, and gives up after a short time because of irritation from the medication or lack of rapid response.

Retinoic acid A, a metabolite of vitamin A, is another excellent topical medication for acne. In addition to having a strong comedolytic effect, this medication increases superficial blood flow, enhancing clearing of existing lesions. Antibiotics long have played a role in acne therapy. Tetracycline and erythromycin reduce the surface concentration of bacteria and, equally importantly, decrease the surface content of free fatty acids. Their primary beneficial effect may be their ability to depress the chemotaxis of leukocytes, thereby reducing the pustular inflammatory response to follicular injury. Topical antibiotics are a more recent addition to the armamentarium of acne therapy.

A key to success in treating acne is development of a partnership with the patient. Most physicians should be able to treat the great majority of their patients with acne. Failure of therapy generally is the result of a lack of understanding of the disorder. Adolescents expect overnight cures and must be made to understand that it often will take 4 to 6 weeks before treatment effects much change.

Topical medications often are used only on papulopustules. They should be used on the entire surface involved in acne, however, to keep all sebaceous follicles open. Care should be taken not to apply too much of the topical medication. The fact that a little bit is good does not mean that a lot is better; excessive application leads to dryness and irritation of the skin, which often causes the patient to discontinue the medication.

In 1982, a derivative of vitamin A, isotretinoin, was approved by the United States Food and Drug Administration for oral use in cases of severe cystic acne. It has proved to be a highly effective agent. Unfortunately, it is expensive and has many annoying side effects, and its long-term effects are unknown. It also is a highly teratogenic agent.

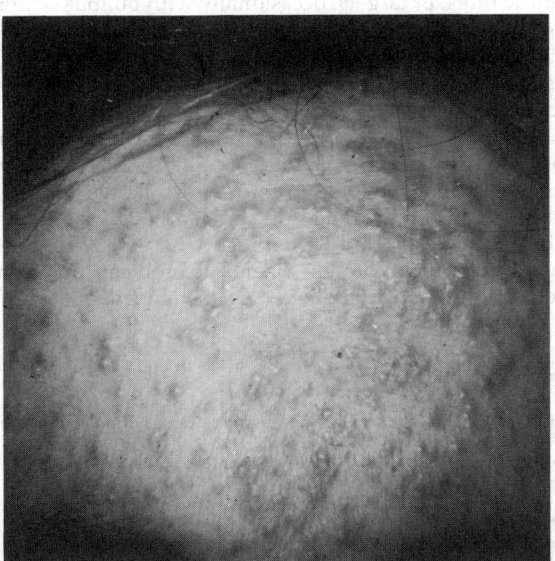

Figure 35-65.    Monomorphous papules appeared in this patient after steroid therapy.

in the fact that drug rashes can resemble almost any other kind of cutaneous eruption. Skin biopsies generally are nonspecific and provide no help in determining the cause of the problem.

In studies of types of drug reactions, four cutaneous types have been found to make up almost 90% of the rashes. About half of the rashes that are associated with drug reactions are similar to exanthems. These lesions may be maculopapular, morbilliform (similar to measles), macular, or scarlatiniform. They have no characteristic features that distinguish them easily from viral or bacterial exanthems. Penicillins, sulfonamides, trimethoprim sulfa, and erythromycin all are capable of producing this type of reaction.

The rash that is associated with ampicillin presents a special diagnostic problem. This rash may be allergic or, more commonly, nonallergic. The latter is not a true hypersensitivity reaction and is morbilliform and blotchy. It usually begins 5 to 10 days after ampicillin is initiated and resolves despite continuation of the drug. The difficulty lies in deciding which one of these reactions the rash represents. An extensive, erythematous, maculopapular rash develops in more than 80% of children and adults with infectious mononucleosis who receive ampicillin. This rash does not indicate penicillin allergy.

The difficulties associated with differentiating drug reactions from exanthems probably has resulted in a significant number of cases in which patients erroneously were designated as being allergic to a drug because they erupted with viral exanthems while receiving antibiotics.

Urticarial eruptions account for about 25% of drug eruptions. These reactions are IgE mediated, and their onset generally is sudden, usually occurring hours or days after drug exposure. The individual wheals are transient, but the entire process may last for 4 to 6 weeks. Penicillins, sulfonamides, barbiturates, and acetylsalicylic acid are drugs well known to cause this type of reaction.

Fixed drug reactions in children are less common than in adults; they are localized to a small area rather than being generalized, as usually is the case with drug reactions. The lesions are discrete, violaceous plaques that often are single or few in number and generally are asymptomatic. If the same drug is administered again, the rash will appear in the exact same spot. As many as 10% of drug reactions are of the fixed type.

Reactions resembling erythema multiforme, which feature concentric rings, or targets, occasionally with bullous or purpuric centers, account for 5% of drug reactions. Sulfonamides, penicillins, hydantoin, barbiturates, and griseofulvin have been implicated in this type of drug reaction. Infections and some systemic disorders can cause a similar eruption, however.

Other forms of drug reactions run the gamut of cutaneous lesions. Photosensitive dermatitis, vasculitic lesions with palpable purpura, vesicular/bullous eruptions, exfoliative lesions, erythema nodosum, and eczematous contact type reactions all have been described. The child with a rash who is receiving a medication will continue to present diagnostic problems until sensitive and reliable tests for drug allergy are developed.

## Selected Readings

Alper JC, Holmes LB. The incidence and significance of birthmarks in a cohort of 4,641 newborns. Pediatr Dermatol 1983;1:58.

Arvin AM, Prober CG. Herpes simplex virus infection: The genital tract and the newborn. Pediatr Rev 1992;13:107.

Cohen BA, Honig P, Androphy E. Anogenital warts in children. Arch Dermatol 1990;126:1575.

Ermacora E, Prampolini L, Tribbia G, et al. Long term followup of dermatitis herpetiformis in children. J Am Acad Dermatol 1986;15:24.

Esterly NB. Cutaneous hemangiomas, vascular stains and associated syndromes. Curr Probl Pediatr 1987;17:1.

Hanifin JM. Atopic dermatitis. J Am Acad Dermatol 1982;6:1.

Norton LA. Nail disorders: A review. J Am Acad Dermatol 1980;2:451.

Sampson HA, McCaskill CC. Food hypersensitivity and atopic dermatitis: Evaluation of 113 patients. J Pediatr 1985;107:669.

Tallman B, Tan OT, Morelli JG, et al. Location of portwine stains and the likelihood of ophthalmic and/or CNS complications. Pediatrics 1991;87:323.

Tunnessen WW Jr. A survey of skin disorders seen in pediatric general and dermatology clinics. Pediatr Dermatol 1984;1:219.

Van Arsdel PP Jr. Allergy and adverse reactions. J Am Acad Dermatol 1982;6:833.

Williams ML. The ichthyoses—pathogenesis and prenatal diagnosis: A review of recent advances. Pediatr Dermatol 1983;1:1.

Williams ML. Differential diagnosis of seborrheic dermatitis. Pediatr Rev 1986;7:204.

*Principles and Practice of Pediatrics, Second Edition.*
edited by Frank A. Oski et al. J. B. Lippincott Company, Philadelphia © 1994.

# CHAPTER 36
# Upper Airway Infections

## 36.1 The Common Cold

Sarah S. Long

Respiratory illness accounts for more than half of all acute disabling conditions in adults annually in the United States, and for an equal percentage of child outpatient visits to health care providers. The common cold, almost always caused by a virus, is the most common of the specific disorders. Most of the medical literature regarding the etiology, epidemiology, pathophysiology, and treatment of the common cold derives from studies performed in adults, with more occasional reports in children providing the bases for extrapolation to pediatrics. There is no specific association of any respiratory syndrome with a particular agent. Depending on the pathogen, the age of the patient, and the immunologic experience of the host, all respiratory pathogens can cause undifferentiated upper respiratory tract illness. Laboratory techniques are not available or cannot be applied practically for specific diagnosis in most instances of upper respiratory tract illnesses. A careful clinical history, including epidemiologic information, combined with physical examination can result in a reasonably accurate prediction of the cause of any particular episode.

## ETIOLOGIC AGENTS

Initially believed to be caused by either a single virus or a group of viruses, the common cold now is recognized to be associated with more than 200 viruses, occasional bacteria, protozoa, and *Mycoplasma*.

Table 36-1 gives an abbreviated list of the agents that cause the common cold and their relative prevalence in children. Rhinoviruses and coronaviruses have even more importance in

**TABLE 36-1. Etiologic Agents of the Common Cold in Children**

| Agent | Prevalence* |
|---|---|
| **Viruses** | |
| Rhinoviruses | +++ |
| Parainfluenza viruses | ++ |
| Respiratory syncytial virus | ++ |
| Coronaviruses | + |
| Adenoviruses | + |
| Enteroviruses | + |
| Influenza viruses | + |
| Reoviruses | + |
| **Other** | |
| *Mycoplasma pneumoniae* | + |
| *Bordetella pertussis* | + |

\* +++ Indicates most prevalent cause; ++ indicates prevalent cause; + indicates occasional cause.

overall, the role of other agents can be suggested by consideration of the information listed in Table 36-2. Season (Table 36-3), age, and prior immunologic experience have the most important influence on cause. For example, disease resulting from respiratory syncytial virus and parainfluenza viruses is most common and most severe in patients who are less than 3 years of age. Infection occurs less commonly and with milder symptoms (frequently those of the common cold) with increasing age.

Rhinoviruses belong to the family of picornavirus, included among enteroviruses. They are RNA viruses with a diameter of 15 to 50 nm. They are ether-stable, but, unlike other enteroviruses, are inactivated in 3 to 4 hours by a pH level of 3. More than 100 distinct serotypes are known and recent data suggest that new serotypes are not evolving; rather, a large pool of antigenically stable rhinoviruses exists.

Rhinoviruses are found in nasal secretions and are not found in stool specimens. Peculiar requirements for growth limit attempts at isolation in research laboratories. Most serotypes grow only in human cell lines, and some fastidious strains grow only in organ culture of human tracheal or nasal epithelium. No rapid antigen detection systems are available.

## EPIDEMIOLOGY

The common cold occurs frequently in childhood. The precise number of colds expected per child per year is difficult to glean from reported studies, as they vary with regard to the demography of the populations studied. Children normally experience 2 to 8 colds per year. The peak age of occurrence is the second 6 months of life. The incidence does not fall significantly until the child is

adults; symptoms of the common cold are the classic manifestations of these viruses.

Factors related to the host, pathogen, and environment that are gleaned from the child's history indicate the likelihood of causative agents in upper respiratory illness and provide an approach to the delineation of specific causes (Table 36-2). Although rhinoviruses are the most frequent cause of the common cold

**TABLE 36-2. Use of Historical Information to Differentiate Among Causes of Nonspecific Upper Respiratory Illnesses**

| Factor | Typical for Rhinovirus | Examples of Factors Typical for Other Etiologies | |
|---|---|---|---|
| Age | School age | Toddler | Parainfluenza viruses |
| | | School age | *Mycoplasma pneumoniae* |
| Season | Fall, spring | Winter | RSV, influenza |
| | | Summer | Adenoviruses |
| Immunization status | Any | Incomplete | *Bordetella pertussis* |
| | | Incomplete | Mumps |
| Sibling | School age | Infant | RSV |
| | | Adolescent | Adenoviruses |
| | | Toddler | Parainfluenza viruses |
| Illness in contacts | Common cold | Bronchiolitis | RSV |
| | | Croup | Parainfluenza viruses |
| | | Conjunctivitis | Adenoviruses |
| | | Exudative pharyngitis | Adenoviruses, Epstein-Barr virus |
| | | Ulcerative enanthem | Enteroviruses |
| Incubation period | 3–5 d | 2 wk | *Mycoplasma pneumoniae, Bordetella pertussis* |
| Acquisition | Home | Hospital | RSV, influenza viruses |
| | | Day care | All agents |
| Community epidemic | Common cold | Parotitis | Mumps |
| | | Hand-foot-and-mouth disease | Enteroviruses |
| | | Aseptic meningitis | Enteroviruses |
| | | Febrile upper respiratory tract infection | Influenza viruses, adenoviruses |

*RSV*, respiratory syncytial viruses.

## TABLE 36-3. Seasonal Peaks of Respiratory Tract Pathogens

| | |
|---|---|
| Fall | Rhinoviruses |
| | Parainfluenza viruses |
| | Group A *Streptococcus* |
| Winter | Respiratory syncytial virus |
| | Adenoviruses |
| | Influenza viruses |
| | Coronaviruses |
| Spring | Rhinoviruses |
| | Parainfluenza viruses |
| | Group A *Sterptococcus* |
| Summer | Adenoviruses |
| | *Bordetella pertussis* |
| | Enteroviruses |

well into school age. The number of respiratory illnesses is increased during day-care exposure in infancy. Exposure to viruses in day-care centers and schools serves to introduce viruses into the family. Boys have symptomatic respiratory illnesses more frequently than do girls. Adults usually are the victims rather than the sources of common cold viruses; primary caretakers and infants have the highest rates of secondary illness. Because there are more than 100 serotypes of rhinovirus alone, susceptibility to the common cold probably is lifelong.

Viruses causing the common cold spread from person to person by means of virus-contaminated respiratory secretions. Studies performed primarily with adult volunteers suggest that possible routes of spread of rhinovirus are by small airborne particles, by inhalation or impalement of large particles when transmitters and recipients are at very close range, and by direct contact with the transmitter's infected nasal secretions or contaminated objects. Accumulating evidence favors direct contact as the primary means for the spread of rhinovirus infections. Compared to adults, children with infection have relatively higher concentrations of virus in secretions and shed virus for longer periods of time. Secretions related to saliva (expressed by coughing, talking, drooling) are not very contagious. Kissing is an inefficient way to transmit rhinoviruses. They are transmitted by sneezing, by nose blowing and wiping, or from secretions that are on environmental surfaces. Recipients become infected by touching one of these sources and then inoculating their nose or conjunctiva.

## PATHOPHYSIOLOGY

Site of virus inoculation, cytopathic effects of multiplication, and degree and mode of spread vary with the many viruses that cause common cold symptoms. The events that occur after primary infection differ from those that take place after recurrent infection. Generally (and specifically for rhinoviruses), during primary infection, virus is inoculated or inhaled onto the nasal mucosa or the conjunctival mucosa. Replication follows and, within 2 days, cellular damage to respiratory epithelium leads to increased nasal secretions with elevated protein content. Local extension causes the symptoms of nasal stuffiness, sneezing, rhinitis, and throat irritation. Ciliary epithelium is denuded. Viral shedding peaks at 2 to 7 days in uncomplicated upper respiratory illness, but persists at lower quantities for as long as 3 weeks. Extension to the tracheobronchial area occurs frequently in adult volunteers after aerosol inoculation, but apparently occurs to a lesser extent in natural infection. Rhinovirus causes exacerbation of bronchitis

in adults and, alone or in consort with other viruses, occasionally causes pneumonia.

Mucociliary dysfunction is present maximally during the acute phase of illness and can persist for weeks after recovery. Studies of pulmonary function conducted during periods in which symptomatology is confined to the upper respiratory tract suggest that occult lower respiratory tract involvement occurs. Viremia is unusual during the common cold. Infection with rhinovirus and other common cold viruses predisposes to bacterial complications of otitis media, sinusitis, and pneumonia.

Host response to infection with rhinovirus is noted by day 2 after inoculation, when leukocytes with an increased percentage of neutrophils are recruited to the site of virus replication and cellular damage. Nasal discharge becomes mucopurulent. Interferon is produced locally by day 3 to 5, and plays an important role in halting viral replication for weeks after recovery. Specific serum neutralizing antibody peaks on day 14 to 21, and secretory antibody peaks 1 to 2 weeks later.

The roles of different immunologic factors in protecting against rhinovirus infections are not entirely clear. Concentrations of local nasal secretory antibody of the IgA fraction are related more closely to protection against subsequent infection than is the concentration of serum antibody. Infection with some serotypes of rhinovirus stimulates short-lived protection against other serotypes. Psychologic stress was associated with an increased risk of infection in adult research subjects who were exposed intentionally to respiratory viruses.

## CLINICAL MANIFESTATIONS

The common cold syndrome has been defined as that which most typically follows rhinovirus infection, its most frequently occurring cause. Throat irritation, sneezing, and nasal stuffiness are the primary complaints on the first and second days of illness; rhinitis, watering eyes, and, sometimes, hoarseness and cough follow on the second to fourth days of illness. Fever is absent or low grade. Chilliness, headache, and myalgia can be present early in the illness. Cough and nasal discharge are the most persistent complaints. Typically, illness caused by rhinoviruses lasts for 6 to 7 days. Nasal symptoms tend to be more prominent and throat and systemic symptoms less prominent in upper respiratory tract illness caused by rhinovirus compared to that caused by other viruses. The large number of rhinovirus types is associated predictably with variable symptoms and degrees of discomfort.

The symptoms described above are typical for older children and adults. Young infants are more likely to have a temperature of 38 °C or 39 °C, irritability, and restlessness. Nasal obstruction can interfere with sleeping and eating.

Complications of the common cold are those associated with extension of the virus to the lower respiratory tract and an increase in local susceptibility to bacterial infection by indigenous flora. Additionally, in children with hyperreactive airways, mild viral upper respiratory illnesses and their complications incite episodes of asthma.

## TREATMENT AND PREVENTION

Treatment of the common cold is supportive. No antiviral agent effective against rhinovirus is available. Although sales of proprietary cold remedies total more than $1 billion annually in the United States, these preparations have little benefit for children and may be harmful. The controversy of recent years regarding the efficacy of large doses of vitamin C for prophylaxis or treatment of the common cold has subsided. In placebo-controlled studies, both in volunteers artificially inoculated with rhinovirus and in research subjects infected naturally, vitamin C had no convincing benefit when provided either prophylactically or therapeutically. It should not be given to children in excess of normal daily requirements. Antibiotics have no place in the routine treatment of the common cold or other nonspecific upper respiratory illnesses. Antihistamines are not beneficial. The use of nasally applied or systemically administered decongestants has not been shown to be beneficial; they should be used infrequently in children and not at all in infants less than 6 months of age. Acetaminophen can be used occasionally to relieve fever or discomfort, but it should be used rarely for cold symptoms in infants less than 6 months of age. Aspirin should not be given, as it is implicated causally in influenza-associated Reye's syndrome, and assigning viral causes to nonspecific upper respiratory illnesses is difficult. In adults challenged intranasally with rhinovirus, aspirin and acetaminophen suppressed antibody response and increased nasal signs and symptoms compared to placebo.

The relief of nasal obstruction is the most important focus of supportive care. Comfortable environmental temperature and humidity should be maintained. Humidification provides comfort for irritated nasopharyngeal mucosa and helps to prevent drying of nasal secretions, thus promoting their elimination. In a placebo-controlled study in adults, there was no beneficial effect of steam inhalation on common cold symptoms. Use of isotonic saline nasal drops and gentle aspiration can provide temporary relief for young infants.

The transmission of respiratory viruses, documented especially well for rhinovirus and respiratory syncytial virus, depends mainly on hand contact with infected nasal secretions and then self-inoculation to nasal or conjunctival mucous membranes. Meticulous hand washing by staff should be practiced in hospitals and other facilities where small children are located. Personal hygiene should be taught to children. Phenol/alcohol solution (Lysol) is an effective disinfectant, as are tincture of iodine and povidone-iodine.

Interest in the development of a vaccine against the common cold viruses waned when continual antigenic drift of rhinoviruses was considered the best explanation for the multiple serotypes, conventional parenteral routes of vaccine administration did not provide protection against nasal challenge, and nasal inoculation provided only short-term benefit. The task of developing an attenuated nasal vaccine seems less formidable now that the serotypes of rhinovirus appear to be multiple but stable and the number of serotypes causing the majority of disease may be only 30.

Discovery of the role of interferon in halting viral replication in natural infection led to speculation that locally applied interferon could be used as therapy for the common cold. Successful production of interferon by recombinant DNA technology provided the hope of inexpensive, effective therapy. Unfortunately, in preparations used to date, side effects have followed the application of doses high enough to be effective. These effects, which include nasal stuffiness, bloody mucus, and nasal mucosal erosion, preclude the use of interferon for prophylaxis or treatment of the common cold.

## Selected Readings

Cherry JD. The common cold. In: Feigin RD, Cherry JD, eds. Textbook of pediatric infectious diseases, ed 3. Philadelphia: WB Saunders, 1992:137.

Cohen S, Tyrrell DAJ, Smith AP. Psychological stress and susceptibility to the common cold. N Engl J Med 1991;325:606.

Douglas RM, Moore BW, Miles HB, et al. Prophylactic efficacy of intranasal alpha$_2$-interferon against rhinovirus infections in the family setting. N Engl J Med 1986;314:65.

Graham NMH, Burrell CJ, Douglas RM, et al. Adverse effects of aspirin, acetamin-

ophen, and ibuprofen on immune function, viral shedding, and clinical status in rhinovirus-infected volunteers. J Infect Dis 1990;162:1277.

Hutton N, Wilson MH, Mellits ED, et al. Effectiveness of an antihistamine-decongestant combination for young children with the common cold: A randomized, controlled clinical trial. J Pediatr 1991;118:125.

Macknin ML, Mathews, Medendorp SVB. Effect of inhaling heated vapor on symptoms of the common cold. JAMA 1990;264:989.

Monto AS, Bryan ER, Ohmit S. Rhinovirus infections in Tecumseh, Michigan: Frequency of illness and number of serotypes. J Infect Dis 1987;156:43.

Wald ER. Purulent nasal discharge. Pediatr Infect Dis J 1991;10:329.

Wald ER, Guerra N, Byers C. Upper respiratory tract infections in young children: Duration of and frequency of complications. Pediatrics 1991;87:129.

*Principles and Practice of Pediatrics, Second Edition.*
edited by Frank A. Oski et al. J. B. Lippincott Company, Philadelphia © 1994.

# 36.2 *Paranasal Sinusitis*

### Ellen R. Wald

Acute infection of the paranasal sinuses is a common complication of allergic or infectious inflammation of the upper respiratory tract. About 1% to 5% of upper respiratory infections are complicated by acute sinusitis. As adults average 2 to 3 colds per year and children 6 to 8, sinusitis is a problem commonly seen in clinical practice.

The four paired paranasal sinuses are the ethmoid, maxillary, sphenoid, and frontal sinuses. All but the frontal sinuses are present at birth. The frontal sinuses develop from the anterior ethmoid sinuses, and become clinically important after the 10th birthday. The maxillary and ethmoid sinuses are the principal sites of sinus infection in young children.

## ANATOMY

The anatomic relationship between the nose and the paranasal sinuses is shown in Figure 36-1. The nose is divided in the midline by the nasal septum. From the lateral wall of the nose come three shelf-like structures, the inferior, middle, and superior turbinates. Beneath each turbinate is a natural meatus that drains one or more of the paranasal sinuses. The posterior ethmoid sinus and the sphenoid sinuses drain into the superior meatus, the anterior ethmoid sinuses, the frontal sinuses, and the maxillary sinuses drain into the middle meatus, and only the lacrimal duct drains into the inferior meatus. The position of the outflow tract of the maxillary sinus, high on the medial wall of the nasal cavity, impedes gravitational drainage of secretions and accounts for the frequency of involvement of the maxillary sinuses when upper respiratory tract inflammation becomes complicated by bacterial superinfection.

## PATHOPHYSIOLOGY/PATHOGENESIS

Three elements are important to the normal physiology of the paranasal sinuses: the patency of the ostia, the function of the ciliary apparatus, and, integral to the latter, the quality of secretions. Retention of secretions in the paranasal sinuses is caused by one or more of the following: obstruction of the ostia, reduction in number or impaired function of the cilia, or overproduction or change in viscosity of the secretions.

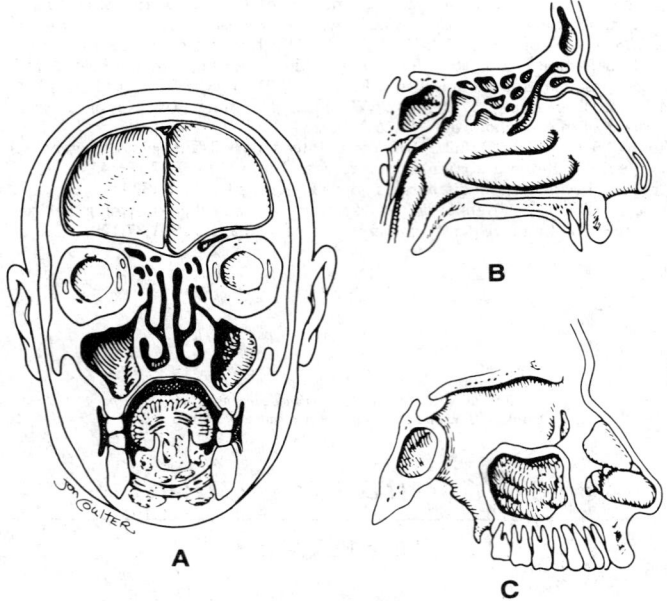

**Figure 36-1.** Anatomy of the paranasal sinuses.

The ostia of the paranasal sinuses are the key to pathology in the sinus area. The ostia are small, tubular structures with a diameter of 2.5 mm (cross-sectional area about 5 mm) and a length of 6 mm. The diameter of the ostium of each of the individual ethmoid air cells that drains independently into the middle meatus is even smaller, measuring 1 mm to 2 mm. The narrow caliber of these individual ostia sets the stage for obstruction to occur easily and often.

The factors predisposing to ostial obstruction can be divided into those that cause mucosal swelling and those that result from mechanical obstruction (Table 36-4). Although many conditions may lead to ostial closure, viral upper respiratory infection and allergic inflammation are by far the most common and most important.

In the posterior two thirds of the nasal cavity and within the sinuses, the epithelium is pseudostratified columnar, in which most of the cells are ciliated. The normal motility of the cilia and the adhesive properties of the mucous layer usually protect respiratory epithelium from bacterial invasion. Certain respiratory viruses (influenza, adenovirus), however, may have a direct cytotoxic effect on the cilia. The alteration of cilia number, morphology, and function may facilitate secondary bacterial invasion of the nose and the paranasal sinuses.

| TABLE 36-4. Factors Predisposing to Sinus Ostial Obstruction | |
|---|---|
| Mucosal Swelling | Mechanical Obstruction |
| Systemic disorder | Choanal atresia |
|   Viral upper respiratory infection | Deviated septum |
|   Allergic inflammation | Nasal polyps |
|   Cystic fibrosis | Foreign body |
|   Immune disorders | Tumor |
|   Immotile cilia | |
| Local insult | |
|   Facial trauma | |
|   Swimming, diving | |
|   Rhinitis medicamentosa | |

## CLINICAL PRESENTATION

In most children with acute or chronic sinusitis, the respiratory symptoms of nasal discharge, nasal congestion, and cough are prominent. During the course of an apparent viral upper respiratory tract infection, there are two common clinical presentations that suggest a diagnosis of acute sinusitis.

The first, most common, clinical situation in which sinusitis should be suspected is when the signs and symptoms of a cold are persistent. Nasal discharge and daytime cough that continue beyond 10 days and are not improving are the principal complaints. Most uncomplicated upper respiratory tract infections last for 5 to 7 days; although patients may not be asymptomatic by the 10th day, their condition usually has improved. The persistence of respiratory symptoms beyond the 10-day mark without appreciable improvement suggests that a complication has developed. The nasal discharge may be of any quality (thin or thick; clear, mucoid, or purulent) and the cough (which may be dry or wet) usually is present in the daytime, although it often is noted to be worse at night. Cough occurring only at night is a common residual symptom of an upper respiratory tract infection. When it is the only residual symptom, it usually is nonspecific and does not suggest a sinus infection; it is more likely to represent reactive airways disease. On the other hand, the persistence of daytime cough frequently is the symptom that brings a child to medical attention. The child may not appear ill and, usually, if fever is present, it will be low grade. Malodorous breath often is reported by parents of preschoolers. When the complaint of malodorous breath is accompanied by respiratory symptoms (in the absence of exudative pharyngitis, dental decay, or nasal foreign body), it is a clue to the presence of sinus infection. Facial pain rarely is present, although intermittent, painless, morning periorbital swelling may have been noted by the parents. In this case, it is not the severity of the clinical symptoms, but their persistence that calls for attention.

The second, less common presentation is a cold that seems more severe than usual: the fever is high (above 39 °C), the nasal discharge is purulent and copious, and associated periorbital swelling or facial pain may be present. The periorbital swelling may involve the upper or lower lid; it is gradual in onset (evolving over hours to days) and most obvious in the morning after awakening. The swelling may decrease and actually disappear during the day, only to reappear the following day. A less common complaint is headache (a feeling of fullness or a dull ache either behind or above the eyes), reported most often in children older than 5 years of age. Occasionally, there may be dental pain, either from infection originating in the teeth or referred from the sinus infection.

It is worth emphasizing that headache is not a common complaint in children with acute sinusitis. When headache is a symptom of acute sinusitis, it almost always is accompanied by prominent respiratory complaints. The headache usually is most severe on awakening, and is relieved partially when the patient is up and about. Chronic sinusitis is distinguished from acute sinusitis when respiratory symptoms (nasal discharge or cough, or both) persist beyond 4 to 6 weeks.

## DIAGNOSIS

### Physical Examination

On physical examination, the patient with acute sinusitis may have mucopurulent discharge present in the nose or posterior pharynx. The nasal mucosa is erythematous; the throat may show moderate injection. The cervical lymph nodes usually are not enlarged significantly or tender. None of these characteristics differentiates rhinitis from sinusitis. Occasionally, there will be either tenderness as the examiner palpates over or percusses the paranasal sinuses, appreciable periorbital edema (soft, nontender swelling of the upper and lower eyelid with discoloration of the overlying skin), or both. Malodorous breath in concert with nasal discharge or cough suggests bacterial sinusitis.

In general, for most children less than 10 years old, the physical examination is not very helpful in making a specific diagnosis of acute sinusitis. If the mucopurulent material can be removed from the nose and the nasal mucosa is treated with topical vasoconstrictors, however, pus may be seen coming from the middle meatus. The latter observation, or the presence of periorbital swelling or facial tenderness, probably is the most specific finding in acute sinusitis.

## Radiography

Radiography traditionally has been used to determine the presence or absence of sinus disease. Standard radiographic projections include an anteroposterior, a lateral, and an occipitomental view. The anteroposterior view is optimal for evaluation of the ethmoid sinuses, and the lateral view is best for viewing the frontal and sphenoid sinuses. The occipitomental view, taken after tilting the chin upward 45° from the horizontal, allows evaluation of the maxillary sinuses.

The radiographic findings most diagnostic of bacterial sinusitis are the presence of an air-fluid level in, or complete opacification of, the sinus cavities. An air-fluid level is an uncommon radiographic finding in children younger than 5 years of age who have acute sinusitis, however. In the absence of an air-fluid level or complete opacification of the sinuses, measuring the degree of mucosal swelling may be useful. If the width of the sinus mucosa is 5 mm or greater in adults or 4 mm or greater in children, it is likely that the sinus aspirate will contain pus or yield a positive bacterial culture. When clinical signs and symptoms suggesting acute sinusitis are accompanied by abnormal maxillary sinus radiographic findings, bacteria will be present in a sinus aspirate 70% of the time. A normal radiograph suggests, but does not prove, that a sinus is free of disease.

CT scans are superior to plain radiographs in the delineation of sinus abnormalities. However, they are not necessary in children with uncomplicated acute sinusitis and should be reserved for the evaluation of recurrent, chronic, or complicated sinus infections.

## Sinus Aspiration

Aspiration of the maxillary sinus (the most accessible of the sinuses) can be performed in children who are older than 2 years of age to establish the precise cause of a sinus infection. Puncture is performed best by the transnasal route, with the needle directed beneath the inferior turbinate through the lateral nasal wall. This route is preferred to avoid injury to the natural ostium and permanent dentition. Careful sterilization of the puncture site is essential to prevent contamination by nasal flora. Indications for sinus aspiration in patients with suspected sinusitis include clinical unresponsiveness to conventional therapy, sinus disease in an immunosuppressed patient, severe symptoms such as headache or facial pain, and life-threatening complications such as intraorbital or intracranial suppuration at the time of clinical presentation.

## MICROBIOLOGY

Maxillary sinus aspiration in children with acute sinusitis has shown the bacteriology of sinus secretions to be similar to that found in otitis media. The predominant organisms are *Streptococcus pneumoniae*, *Moraxella catarrhalis*, and non-typeable *Haemophilus influenzae*. Both *H influenzae* and *M catarrhalis* may produce β-lactamase and, consequently, may be ampicillin-resistant. Anaerobic isolates and staphylococci rarely are recovered. Several viruses, including adenoviruses, influenza viruses, parainfluenza viruses, and rhinoviruses, have been recovered from maxillary sinus aspirates. Summary figures for the prevalence of various bacterial species in children with acute sinusitis are shown in Table 36-5. The performance of nasal, throat, or nasopharyngeal cultures is of no value in patients with acute sinusitis, as the results are not predictive of the bacterial isolates within the maxillary sinus cavity.

The microbiology of chronic sinusitis differs slightly from that of acute sinusitis. Anaerobes of the respiratory tract, viridans streptococci, and, occasionally, *Staphylococcus aureus* are found in addition to the aerobes of acute sinusitis.

## DIFFERENTIAL DIAGNOSIS

The major symptoms that prompt consideration of the diagnosis of acute sinusitis are persistent or purulent nasal discharge and persistent cough. Alternative diagnoses to consider for patients with purulent nasal discharge are simple viral upper respiratory infection, group A streptococcal infection, adenoiditis, and nasal foreign body. In simple upper respiratory infection, the purulent nasal discharge usually is accompanied by low-grade fever and other elements of upper respiratory inflammation, such as pharyngitis and conjunctivitis. The symptoms commonly begin to improve after a few days. Streptococcal infection in children younger than 3 years, so-called streptococcosis, may present with persistent respiratory symptoms such as nasal discharge, low-grade fever, lassitude, and poor appetite. The diagnosis can be excluded by culturing the nasopharynx or throat for group A streptococci. Adenoiditis is suggested when purulent nasal discharge persists beyond 10 days without improvement in a patient with normal sinus radiographs. Nasal foreign body usually is characterized by unilateral nasal discharge, which is purulent and often bloody. Most strikingly, the nasal discharge is very foul-smelling—a fact that often can be noted from the doorway of the examining room.

Patients who have persistent cough as the most troublesome symptom prompt the consideration of several diagnoses, including reactive airways disease, *Mycoplasma pneumoniae* bronchitis, cystic fibrosis, and gastroesophageal reflux. Reactive airways disease triggered by upper respiratory infection may cause dramatic cough without accompanying wheezing. This occasionally occurs in conjunction with acute sinusitis, but more often is a residual symptom after an upper respiratory infection, and substantially prolongs the clinical course of the illness. *Mycoplasma* bronchitis usually occurs in children between 5 and 15 years of age. The illness begins with a prominent sore throat and fever. As the upper respiratory symptoms subside, cough begins and becomes prominent and persistent. Cystic fibrosis should be considered

| TABLE 36-5.  Bacteriology of Acute Sinusitis | |
|---|---|
| **Bacterial Species** | **Prevalence (%)** |
| *Streptococcus pneumoniae* | 25–30 |
| *Moraxella catarrhalis* | 15–20 |
| *Haemophilus influenzae* | 15–20 |
| *Streptococcus pyogenes* | 2–5 |
| Anaerobes | 2–5 |
| Sterile | 20–35 |

in children with persistent cough, although it is unlikely to explain the symptom in a previously thriving child who presents with an intercurrent illness. Gastroesophageal reflux may be responsible for pulmonary and neurologic symptoms as well as failure to thrive. It should be considered most seriously in children who have nighttime coughing only or in those who have had poorly controlled asthma or previous episodes of pneumonia.

## TREATMENT

The objectives of antimicrobial therapy for acute sinus infection are achievement of a rapid clinical cure, sterilization of the sinus secretions, prevention of suppurative orbital and intracranial complications, and prevention of chronic sinus disease.

## Antimicrobial Agents

The relative frequency of occurrence of the various bacterial agents suggests that amoxicillin is an appropriate drug for most uncomplicated cases of acute sinusitis (Table 36-6). Amoxicillin is safe, effective, and reasonably priced. Safety is an especially important consideration when one is treating an infection that has a 40% rate of spontaneous recovery. The prevalence of β-lactamase–positive, ampicillin-resistant *H influenzae* and *M catarrhalis* may vary geographically. In areas where ampicillin-resistant organisms are prevalent, in situations in which the patient is allergic to penicillin or has mild periorbital swelling, or in instances in which there has been an apparent antibiotic failure, several alternative regimens are available. The combination agent sulfamethoxazole/trimethoprim (Bactrim, Septra) has been shown to be efficacious in acute maxillary sinusitis in adults. This combination agent may be ineffective, however, in patients with group A streptococcal infections. Cefaclor (Ceclor) and the combination of erythromycin/sulfisoxazole (Pediazole) also are suitable. A combination of amoxicillin and potassium clavulanate (Augmentin) is another potential therapeutic agent for use in patients with β-lactamase–producing bacterial species in their maxillary sinus secretions. Potassium clavulanate irreversibly binds the β-lactamase, if it is present, and thereby restores amoxicillin to its original spectrum of activity. Cefuroxime axetil is a potent agent for treating most respiratory pathogens. It is available only in tablet formulation, however, and is bitter when crushed.

New antimicrobial agents that may be appropriate for use in children with sinusitis who do not respond to conventional therapy include cefprozil (Cefzil, a second generation cephalosporin), cefpodoxime (Vantin, a third generation cephalosporin), loracarbef (Lorabid, a carbacephem), and the new macrolides, clarithromycin (Biaxin) and azithromycin (Zithromax).

Patients with acute sinusitis may require hospitalization because of systemic toxicity or inability to take oral antimicrobial agents. These patients may be treated with cefuroxime at a dosage of 100 to 200 mg/kg/d, intravenously, in three divided doses.

Clinical improvement is prompt in nearly all children who are treated with an appropriate antimicrobial agent. Patients febrile at the initial encounter will become afebrile, and there is a remarkable reduction in nasal discharge and cough within 48 hours. If the patient does not improve, or worsens, in 48 hours, clinical reevaluation is appropriate. If the diagnosis is unchanged, sinus aspiration may be considered for precise bacteriologic information. Alternatively, an antimicrobial agent effective against β-lactamase–producing bacterial species should be prescribed.

The antimicrobial regimens recommended to treat acute sinusitis usually are prescribed for 10 to 14 days. If the patient is improved but not recovered completely by 10 or 14 days, it is reasonable to continue treatment for another week. In patients with chronic sinusitis, antimicrobial therapy should be maintained for 3 to 4 weeks.

The effectiveness of antihistamines or decongestants, or combinations thereof, applied topically (by inhalation) or administered by mouth in patients with acute or chronic sinus infection has not been studied adequately. Because appropriate antimicrobial therapy results in prompt clinical improvement within 48 to 72 hours, additional pharmacologic agents usually are not necessary.

## Irrigation and Drainage

Irrigation and drainage of the infected sinus may result in dramatic relief from pain for patients with acute sinusitis. Drainage procedures usually are reserved for those who fail to respond to medical therapy with antimicrobial agents or those who have a suppurative intraorbital or intracranial complication. If an episode of acute sinusitis cannot be treated effectively by medical therapy alone or by medical therapy and simple sinus puncture, more radical surgery may become necessary.

## Surgical Therapy

Surgical therapy in children with chronic sinusitis focused initially on creating a nasoantral window, or fistula, in the maxillary sinus to facilitate gravitational drainage. These fistulas proved to be relatively ineffective, however, in part because the cilia that line the maxillary sinus still transport secretions toward the natural meatus.

At present, the focus of surgical therapy is the osteomeatal unit. Most current surgical efforts involve using an endoscope to enlarge the natural meatus of the maxillary outflow tract by excising the uncinate process and the ethmoidal bullae and performing an anterior ethmoidectomy. A pilot study assessing the safety and efficacy of endoscopic sinus surgery in children with chronic sinusitis reported that 71 percent of the patients were considered normal by their parents one year after the operation. Endoscopic surgery in children is promising, but requires further study.

## COMPLICATIONS

Complications of sinus disease may cause both substantial morbidity and occasional mortality. Major complications result from either contiguous spread or hematogenous dissemination of infection. A complete list of the major complications of sinusitis is provided in Table 36-7.

## Orbital Complications

Orbital complications are the most common serious complication of acute sinusitis and, despite antimicrobial therapy, may lead to

| TABLE 36-6. Antimicrobial Agents for Sinusitis | |
|---|---|
| Antimicrobial Agent | Dosage |
| Amoxicillin | 40 mg/kg/d in 3 divided doses |
| Erythromycin/ sulfisoxazole | 50/150 mg/kg/d in 4 divided doses |
| Sulfamethoxazole/ trimethoprim | 40/8 mg/kg/d in 2 divided doses |
| Cefaclor | 40 mg/kg/d in 3 divided doses |
| Amoxicillin/K clavulanate | 40 mg/kg/d in 3 divided doses |
| Cefuroxime axetil | 250 or 500 mg/d in 2 divided doses |

### TABLE 36-7. Major Complications of Sinusitis

**Orbital**
Inflammatory edema (preseptal or periorbital cellulitis)
Subperiosteal abscess
Orbital abscess
Orbital cellulitis
Optic neuritis

**Osteomyelitis**
Frontal (Pott's puffy tumor)
Maxillary

**Intracranial**
Epidural abscess
Subdural empyema or abscess
Cavernous or sagittal sinus thrombosis
Meningitis
Brain abscess

by an abrupt onset, rapid progression, and severe systemic toxicity. The markedly swollen and tender periorbital tissue has a violaceous, almost hemorrhagic discoloration, the texture of the skin is altered, and the subcutaneous tissue is indurated. *H influenzae* type b is recovered frequently, and *S pneumoniae* less often, from blood cultures and tissue aspirate. Because most *H influenzae* organisms isolated from sinus aspirates are non-typeable, the relationship, if any, of these acute bacteremic *H influenzae* type b infections to sinusitis is unclear. Other entities to distinguish from inflammatory edema include an infected periorbital or blepharal laceration, insect bite, contact allergy, conjunctivitis, dacryocystitis, and eczematoid dermatitis.

When proptosis and ophthalmoplegia are present, stages II to V of orbital complications must be considered (see Table 36-7). When infection tracks backward into the cavernous sinus, the patient will have signs of meningitis, focal or generalized seizures, deterioration of consciousness, and, usually, involvement of the opposite eye by way of the circumfundibular communicating conduits between the two cavernous sinuses.

When eye swelling is the result of inflammatory edema, plain radiographs of the sinuses will disclose partial or complete opacification, mucous membrane thickening, or an air-fluid level. Most commonly, the ethmoid and maxillary sinuses are involved together, but, in patients with a history of chronic sinus disease, pansinusitis is the usual finding. In early and late stages, the orbit, the paranasal sinuses, and the intracranial dural venous sinuses all can be studied simultaneously with contrast-enhanced computed tomography (CT). Thin CT cuts of the orbit, using the multiplanar imaging technique, also are helpful in detecting and defining the extent of subperiosteal and orbital abscesses.

### Treatment and Outcome

Children with stage I disease occasionally can be treated carefully as outpatients by the usual regimen for acute sinusitis, provided the parents are cooperative and can return for reevaluation readily. The antimicrobial agent selected must provide an antibacterial spectrum that includes β-lactamase–producing *H influenzae* and *M catarrhalis*. Careful follow-up is essential to detect progression of infection and the need for hospitalization. If the infection has progressed beyond stage I, then hospitalization and intravenous antibiotics are mandatory. The choice of antibiotics is guided by knowledge of the usual bacteriology of acute sinusitis.

loss of vision and severe morbidity. The usual presenting feature of sinus-related orbital complications is a "swollen eye." A classification that is useful in establishing the severity of the orbital cellulitis is shown in Table 36-8. It is essential to establish the severity of the cellulitis clinically so that appropriate decisions can be made regarding specific therapy and the need for surgical drainage. With early involvement (stage I), the inflammatory edema is confined to the medial aspect of the upper or lower eyelid. There is gradual onset of lid swelling, minimal skin discoloration, and low-grade or no fever. No proptosis, visual impairment, or limitation of extraocular movement is observed. This is not an actual infection of the orbit, but, rather, swelling caused by impedance of the local venous drainage. As such, it must be distinguished from a much more virulent form of periorbital or so-called preseptal cellulitis caused by *H influenzae* type b. The septum is a connective tissue reflection of periosteum that inserts into the eyelid and provides an anatomic barrier protecting the orbit. Both "inflammatory edema" and *H influenzae* type b preseptal infection involve tissues anterior to the orbital contents. *H influenzae* type b periorbital cellulitis, however, is characterized

### TABLE 36-8. Clinical Staging of Orbital Cellulitis

| Stage | Clinical Features |
|---|---|
| I. Inflammatory edema | Inflammatory edema, beginning in medial aspect of upper or lower eyelid; nontender erythema may be prominent. No induration, visual impairment, or limitation of extraocular movement. |
| II. Subperiosteal abscess | Abscess beneath the periosteum of the ethmoid or frontal bone. Proptosis down and out, varying degrees of chemosis, and limitation of extraocular movement. |
| III. Orbital abscess | Abscess within the fat or muscle cone in the posterior orbit. Severe chemosis and proptosis; complete ophthalmoplegia and moderate to severe visual loss (globe displaced forward or down and out). |
| IV. Orbital cellulitis | Edema of orbital contents with varying degrees of proptosis, chemosis, limitation of extraocular movement, or visual loss. |
| V. Cavernous sinus thrombophlebitis | Proptosis, globe fixation, severe loss of visual acuity, prostration, signs of meningitis; progresses to proptosis, chemosis, and visual loss in contralateral eye. |

*Modified from Chandler JR, Langenbrunner DJ, Stevens ER. The pathogenesis of orbital complications in acute sinusitis. Laryngoscope 1970;80:1414.*

Cefuroxime at a dosage of 150 to 200 mg/kg/d, intravenously, in three divided doses, or cefotaxime at a dosage of 200 mg/kg/d in four divided doses is an appropriate selection. Ampicillin (200 mg/kg/d, intravenously, in four divided doses) and chloramphenicol (100 mg/kg/d, intravenously, in four divided doses) likewise is a reasonable combination. Blood and sinus aspirates should be obtained and cultured aerobically and anaerobically; appropriate antimicrobial agents should be added if unsuspected organisms are isolated or observed on Gram's stain of purulent material obtained from the sinus cavity or orbit. Surgical drainage is required if there is a subperiosteal or an orbital abscess, but orbital cellulitis may respond to antimicrobial agents without surgical intervention. The prognosis for patients with stage I and II disease usually is excellent if diagnosis and appropriate therapy are carried out promptly, but residual visual loss as a result of infection of the optic nerve may complicate orbital abscesses. Severe neurologic sequelae or death may follow cavernous sinus thrombophlebitis.

## Intracranial Complications

Intracranial extension of infection is the second most common complication of acute sinusitis. Although the incidence of suppurative intracranial disease in patients with sinusitis is unknown, paranasal sinusitis is the source of 35% to 65% of subdural empyemas.

### Clinical Features

Four groups of symptoms and signs may be recognized:

1. Signs of pansinusitis. About 50% to 60% of patients with subdural empyema secondary to sinusitis have symptoms of acute frontal sinusitis or an acute exacerbation of chronic pansinusitis. There is low-grade fever, malaise, frontal headache, and marked forehead and maxillary tenderness to digital pressure. Occasionally, subperiosteal pus overlying the anterior wall of the frontal sinus results in dramatic epicranial edema and a painful fluctuation called Pott's puffy tumor.
2. Signs of increased intracranial pressure. With increased intracranial pressure, an initial headache worsens despite repeated doses of analgesic and oral antibiotic agents. Vomiting becomes intractable, and the level of consciousness deteriorates gradually. High intracranial pressure results from local cerebral edema in the area adjacent to the subdural pus, and it may progress rapidly to cause stupor and coma. With an isolated extradural empyema, cortical involvement is less extensive and the patient generally remains alert.
3. Signs of meningeal irritation. During the stage of depressed sensorium, there usually is nuchal rigidity and photophobia. This reflects an intense inflammatory response in the leptomeninges in contact with a subdural abscess, rather than septic leptomeningitis.
4. Focal neurologic deficits. Focal neurologic deficits are caused by a combination of local brain compression (by the empyema), edema, and infarction. A frontoparietal convexity subdural empyema causes contralateral brachiofacial weakness, contralateral conjugate gaze palsy, and expressive dysphasia. Lower limb involvement usually occurs late. Focal seizures involving the arm and face occur in more than 60% of patients with dorsolateral lesions. With a parafalcine empyema, jacksonian seizures often begin in the foot and march upward to include the trunk, arm, and face. Weakness also primarily affects the leg, with sparing of speech and facial musculature. Bilateral parafalcine collections may present with paraplegia, simulating thoracic spinal cord compression. In the terminal stage, the patient is comatose and hemiplegic, has evidence of generalized and meningeal sepsis, and finally has signs of uncal or tonsillar herniation.

### Diagnosis

Intracranial infection should be suspected if signs of systemic toxicity and headache do not improve after an adequate course of oral antibiotics has been given for the original sinusitis. Diagnostic tests must be arranged immediately if the headache becomes excruciating, if systemic toxicity worsens, or if intractable vomiting or visual blurring develops. Whenever meningeal signs develop in a patient with sinusitis, the clinician may be tempted to obtain cerebrospinal fluid by lumbar puncture. It must be remembered, however, that pure meningitis rarely occurs with sinusitis, and all the other intracranial suppurative complications are mass lesions that are likely to cause brain herniation with lumbar puncture. This procedure should be deferred, therefore, until the CT scan has ruled out empyema and abscess.

CT scanning is recognized now as the most definitive test for the diagnosis of intracranial suppuration secondary to sinusitis, and virtually has eliminated the need for cerebral angiography, radionuclide scanning, and electroencephalography. This noninvasive procedure defines and localizes exactly even small purulent collections, delineates associated cerebral edema, assesses the amount of brain shift, and detects concomitant brain abscess or bilateral empyema that often was missed by angiography in the era before CT. The extent of sinus disease also can be evaluated concurrently by low axial cuts that include the ethmoid, sphenoid, and maxillary sinuses. A parenchymal abscess characteristically shows up as a low-density center with an intensely enhancing capsule and surrounding edema. An extracerebral empyema always possesses an enhancing inner membrane, and the underlying cerebral edema often causes an impressive midline brain shift that cannot be accounted for by the amount of pus present. This combination of a small extracerebral collection and a disproportionate degree of brain shift distinguishes a subdural empyema from a chronic subdural hematoma, in which the severity of brain shift is determined primarily by the size of the clot.

### Treatment and Outcome

The treatment of sinusitis-related intracranial suppuration requires antimicrobial agents, drainage, and excellent supportive care. Rarely, brain abscess or highly selected cases of subdural empyema may be treated nonoperatively. More commonly, aspiration rather than excision is the operative procedure performed. Because either acute sinusitis or an acute exacerbation of chronic sinusitis may precede intracranial complications, the antibiotics selected must be appropriate to include *S pneumoniae*, *H influenzae*, *M catarrhalis*, respiratory anaerobes, streptococci, and *S aureus*. A combination of aqueous penicillin G (200 to 300 U/kg/d, intravenously, in 4 to 6 divided doses) and chloramphenicol (100 mg/kg/d, intravenously, in four divided doses) is used frequently. If cultures or Gram's stain smears of purulent material reveal a predominance of gram-positive cocci in clusters, nafcillin (150 mg/kg/d, intravenously, in four divided doses) may be substituted for penicillin G. Additional drugs (cefotaxime for enteric gram-negative organisms or metronidazole for fastidious anaerobes) may be prescribed if unexpected bacterial flora are seen on Gram's stain or are recovered by culture.

Hyperosmolar agents should be given if high intracranial pressure threatens brain herniation. Systemic steroids should be prescribed with caution because of their theoretic suppressive effect on granulocytic and immune functions. Anticonvulsant agents should be given prophylactically to protect against a high incidence of associated seizures.

Extradural and subdural empyemas should be drained through a generous craniotomy. An underlying brain abscess is handled best by intracapsular evacuation and catheter drainage to avoid unnecessary brain damage associated with radical excision of deep-seated lesions within eloquent areas of the brain. In some cases of subdural empyema, the underlying brain is so swollen that the bone flap must be left out for external decompression.

Postoperatively, intravenous antibiotics should be maintained for a minimum of 2 to 3 weeks. The shrinking of the abscess or empyema can be observed accurately by serial CT scans. Despite modern diagnostic and surgical capabilities, the mortality associated with subdural empyema and brain abscess is more than 20%. Early diagnosis remains the most effective way of improving survival.

## Selected Readings

Chandler JR, Langenbrunner DJ, Stevens EF. The pathogenesis of orbital complications in acute sinusitis. Laryngoscope 1975;80:1414.

Evans RD Jr, Sydnor JB, Moore WEC, et al. Sinusitis of the maxillary antrum. N Engl J Med 1975;293:735.

Gwaltney JM Jr, Sydnor A Jr, Sande MA. Etiology and antimicrobial treatment of acute sinusitis. Ann Otol Rhinol Laryngol 1984;90(Suppl):68.

Hamory BH, Sande MA, Sydnor A Jr, et al. Etiology and antimicrobial therapy of acute maxillary sinusitis. J Infect Dis 1979;39:197.

Kovatch AL, Wald ER, Ledesma-Medena J, et al. Maxillary sinus radiographs in children with nonrespiratory complaints. Pediatrics 1986;73:306.

Rachelefsky GS, Katz RM, Siegel SC. Diseases of paranasal sinuses in children. Curr Probl Pediatr 1982;12:1.

Wald ER. Sinusitis in children. N Engl J Med 1992;326:319.

Wald ER, Chiponis D, Ledesma-Medina J. Comparative effectiveness of amoxicillin and amoxicillin-clavulanate potassium in acute paranasal sinus infections in children: A double-blind, placebo-controlled trial. Pediatrics 1986;77:795.

Wald ER, Milmoe GJ, Bowen A'd, et al. Acute maxillary sinusitis in children. N Engl J Med 1981;304:749.

Wald ER, Reilly JS, Casselbrant M, et al. Treatment of acute maxillary sinusitis in children: A comparative study of amoxicillin and cefaclor. J Pediatr 1984;104:297.

*Principles and Practice of Pediatrics, Second Edition.*
edited by Frank A. Oski et al. J. B. Lippincott Company, Philadelphia © 1994.

# 36.3 *Infections of the Oral Cavity*

Joseph F. Piecuch, Richard G. Topazian, and Thomas R. Flynn

Most infections of the oral cavity in children are odontogenic in origin and may be treated simply with local measures. Occasionally, spread to adjacent or distant fascial spaces or to the maxilla and mandible may result in life-threatening complications.

## MICROBIOLOGIC CONSIDERATIONS IN DENTAL INFECTIONS

### Normal Flora

The oral cavity provides an environment favorable to the growth of microorganisms. Bacterial counts in the range of $10^8$ to $10^{11}$ per milliliter of saliva have been reported. More than 30 species of bacteria normally can be identified in saliva, in varying proportions depending on a dynamic interaction of different micro-

bial ecosystems, including the tongue, the gingival crevice, and the presence of plaque. Age, anatomic relationships, eruption of teeth, presence of decayed teeth, diet, oral hygiene, antibiotic therapy, systemic disease, and hospitalization all can modify the microbial population. The estimated ratio of anaerobic to aerobic organisms in the oral cavity ranges from 3:1 to 10:1. Even the edentulous person may have a preponderance of anaerobes, because areas such as the buccal vestibule, when the cheek is approximated against the teeth or alveolar ridges, may have a greatly reduced oxygen tension.

The flora of children is quite similar to that of adults, with several exceptions. At birth, the oral cavity is sterile, but colonization with *Streptococcus salivarius* is rapid. This organism has been found in 80% of cultures taken from 1-day-old infants. The percentage of *Streptococcus* spp. decreases from 98% the day after birth to 70% at 4 months of age as other organisms become established. *Staphylococcus* spp., *Neisseria*, *Veillonella*, *Actinomyces*, *Nocardia*, *Fusobacterium*, *Bacteroides*, *Corynebacterium*, *Candida*, and a variety of coliforms gradually become established by 1 year of age. As eruption of the deciduous dentition occurs, anaerobic organisms become well established in the gingival crevice, yet spirochetes and *Bacteroides melaninogenicus*, which commonly are associated with the gingival crevice in adults, appear to be present in fewer numbers before 13 to 16 years of age.

## Pathogenic Organisms

Most odontogenic infections, whether they are periodontal or periapical, are polymicrobial, with a mixed aerobic-anaerobic flora averaging 4 to 6 isolates per case. A combination of an oral streptococcus and an anaerobe is involved in the majority of these infections. Early in the course of an infection, the streptococcus predominates, invading tissue and spreading infection by elaborating enzymes, such as hyaluronidases, that break down the ground substance of connective tissue. This process generates necrotic tissue and a reduced oxygen environment, and provides nutrients such as vitamin K, hemin, and succinate that favor the growth of oral anaerobes, including *B melaninogenicus*, *Fusobacterium*, and anaerobic streptococci. As the infection matures, the anaerobes cause tissue liquefaction via collagenases, producing an abscess with a mixed flora. Late infections, with chronic encapsulated abscesses, often yield a purely anaerobic culture. The primary pathogens in orofacial odontogenic infections are identified in Table 36-9.

**TABLE 36-9. Most Frequent Pathogens Isolated in Orofacial Infections In Two Recent Studies**

| Microorganism | Percent of Cases | |
| --- | --- | --- |
| | Lewis | Heimdahl |
| *Streptococcus milleri* | 50 | 31 |
| *Peptococcus* species | 64 | 31 |
| Other anaerobic streptococci | 8 | 38 |
| *Bacteroides oralis* | 40 | 9 |
| *Bacteroides gingivalis* | 28 | * |
| *Bacteroides melaninogenicus* | 24 | 26 |
| *Fusobacterium* species | 14 | 45 |

* This organism was not reported in this study.
*Flynn TR. Odontogenic infections. Oral Maxillofac Surg Clin North Am 1991;3: 311.*

More serious infections, in which spread to orofacial soft tissue has occurred, tend to have a mixture of anaerobic and aerobic organisms, with anaerobes predominating in some and aerobes in others. A possible explanation for this finding lies in the cause of these infections. Infections originating from non-odontogenic causes (eg, facial trauma, surgical manipulation, tonsillitis) in which contamination from the skin or oropharynx might occur, as well as odontogenic infections cultured only superficially with swabs over draining fistulas, may show aerobic organisms such as *Staphylococcus aureus* and aerobic streptococcus species. In contrast, infections originating solely from the dental periapical tissues that are cultured directly by needle aspiration are much more likely to reveal a predominance of anaerobic organisms.

The taxonomy of the oral flora is changing. Clinical isolates from orofacial infections still may be identified by the laboratory as *Streptococcus viridans* or *B melaninogenicus*; however, recent research involving genetic analysis of the various strains of these species has resulted in a rapidly changing classification and nomenclature for these organisms, with the acceptance of several new genera and species within these older classifications. Current classifications are summarized in Table 36-10.

## ANATOMIC CONSIDERATIONS

Most severe orofacial infections develop as a result of periapical, periodontal, or pericoronal dental infection, with spread occurring along the anatomic pathways of least resistance. Periodontal and pericoronal infections generally drain through the gingival sulcus into the oral cavity, and rarely have major sequelae, except for pericoronal infections involving erupting third molar teeth, which can spread into deeper anatomic spaces because of their posterior location in the oral cavity. On the other hand, infections associated with root apices usually are confined within the bony alveolar process. Should spontaneous intraoral drainage occur through either the periodontium or the pulp chamber, further spread through marrow spaces is unlikely. If such a drainage does not

occur, then spread through bone (osteomyelitis) or perforation of the cortical plate of the affected jaw may take place. Once penetration of the cortical plate occurs, infection will involve the adjacent soft tissues and may manifest either as a cellulitis or as a soft-tissue abscess that eventually may perforate mucous membrane or skin as a fistulous tract (Fig 36-2).

Perforation of periapical infections through bone usually follows a typical pattern that results from the position of the root apices in relation to the bony cortex and to muscle attachments (Fig 36-3). Abscesses that are associated with anterior teeth and the buccal roots of maxillary posterior teeth tend to perforate labially or buccally because the tooth roots are in close proximity to that cortical plate. Abscesses that are associated with mandibular posterior teeth may perforate either the buccal or the lingual cortical plate. When spread of a mandibular infection occurs lingually, the relationship of the tooth apex to the mylohyoid muscle origin is significant. If the roots are superior to the mylohyoid muscle, infections will localize intraorally in the floor of the mouth (sublingual space). Apices of the second and third molars usually are located inferior to the mylohyoid muscle and, consequently, the submandibular space will be involved, with extraoral localization.

In children, the maxillary and mandibular root apices often are located superior and inferior, respectively, to the attachment of the buccinator muscle. Consequently, dental infections in younger patients may have a greater tendency to spread into the facial soft tissues and localize extraorally.

Two fascial spaces commonly associated with odontogenic infections are the submandibular and masticator spaces. The submandibular space is formed within the superficial layer of deep cervical fascia, inferior to the mylohyoid muscle and inferomedial to the mandible. Anteriorly and posteriorly, it is limited by the digastric muscle. Within this space lie the submandibular gland and portions of the facial artery and anterior facial vein. This space is approximated closely to the sublingual and masticator spaces. Infections of the submandibular space may originate in these adjacent spaces as well as from the mandibular posterior teeth.

The masticator space also is formed with the superficial layer of deep cervical fascia. Its contents include the masseter muscle, the internal and external pterygoid muscles, and the temporal tendon, as well as the mandibular ramus and the inferior alveolar neurovascular bundle. The temporal and infratemporal spaces are considered to be superior extensions of the masticator space. Adjacent are the submandibular, lateral pharyngeal, and retropharyngeal spaces. Infections of the masticator space may originate in adjacent spaces or spread to it from periapical or pericoronal infections of the mandibular second and third molars and the maxillary third molar.

## TREATMENT OF ODONTOGENIC INFECTIONS

Patients with odontogenic infections may have symptoms ranging from minor to life-threatening. Too often, they receive thorough systemic and extraoral head and neck evaluations, but the intraoral examination is overlooked.

Thorough intraoral evaluation begins with assessing the degree of mandibular opening. Interincisal distance on wide opening may be 40 mm or more, even in young children. Painful limitation of opening, or trismus, is associated with inflammation of the muscles of mastication and indicates spread of the infection to the masticator space. If there is an associated high temperature, this can represent a serious turn of events because airway compromise may result. Teeth are inspected visually for caries, by percussion for tenderness, and by electrical sensitivity (Vitallometer) or hot and cold stimulation for pulpal involvement. Gin-

| TABLE 36-10. Recent Taxonomic Changes in Selected Oral Pathogens | |
| --- | --- |
| Older Terminology | Current Terminology |
| *Streptococcus viridans* | *Streptococcus anginosus* |
| | *Streptococcus intermedius* |
| | *Streptococcus constellatus* |
| | *Streptococcus mutans* |
| | *Streptococcus sanguis* |
| | *Streptococcus mitis* |
| | *Streptococcus salivarius* |
| | *Streptococcus vestibularis* |
| *Streptococcus milleri* | *Streptococcus anginosus* |
| | *Streptococcus intermedius* |
| | *Streptococcus constellatus* |
| *Bacteroides melaninogenicus* | *Prevotella melaninogenica* |
| | *Prevotella intermedia* |
| | *Porphyromonas asaccharolyticus* |
| | *Porphyromonas gingivalis* |
| | *Porphyromonas endodontalis* |
| | *Capnocytophaga* species |
| *Streptococcus faecalis* | *Enterococcus faecalis* |
| *Streptococcus faecium* | *Enterococcus faecium* |
| *Peptococcus* species | *Peptostreptococcus* species |

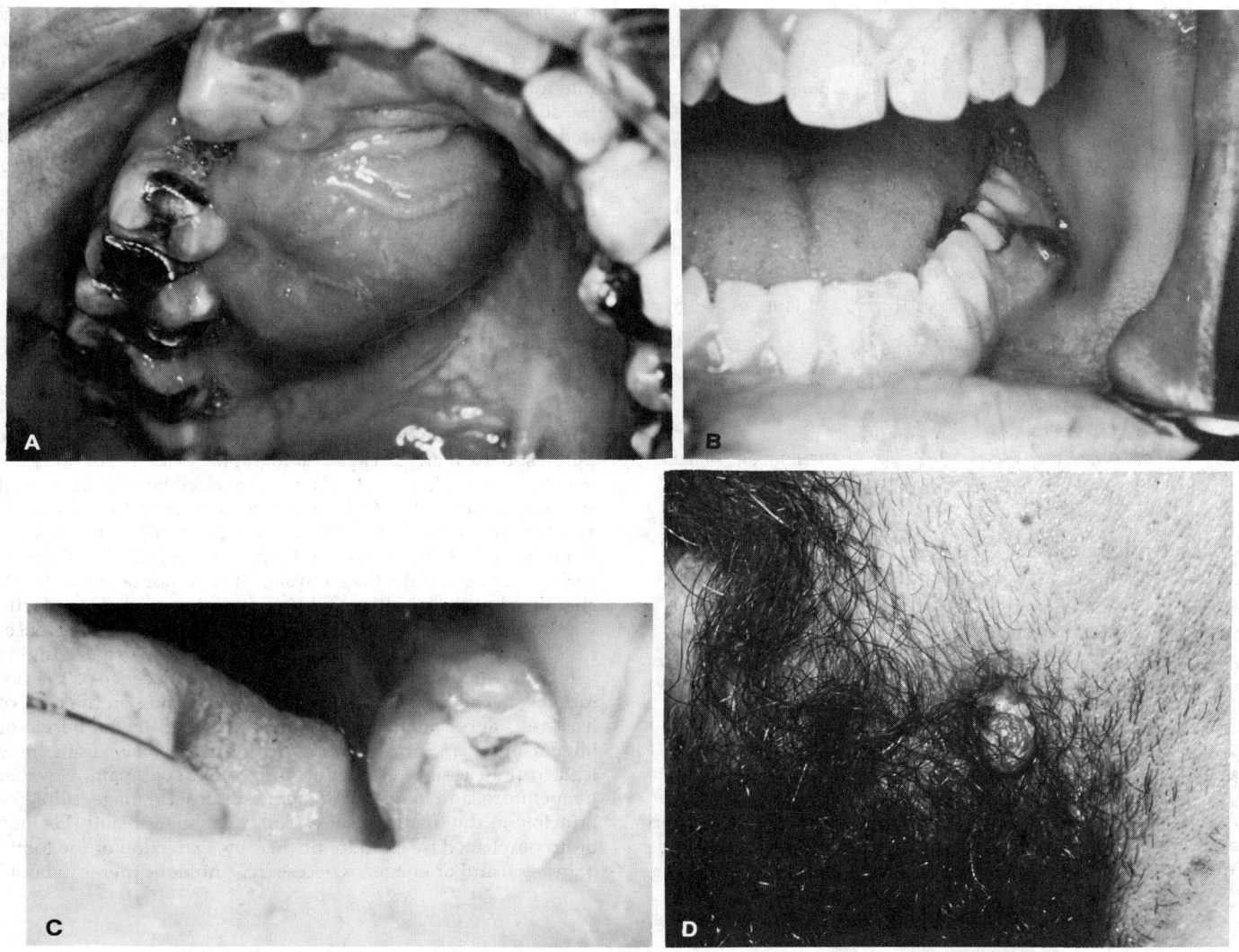

**Figure 36-2.** Spread of odontogenic infection. (**A**) Palatal abscess resulting from infected first premolar. (**B**) Intraoral mucosal fistula from periapical abscess of mandibular first molar. (**C**) Pericoronitis. (**D**) Extraoral fistula from mandibular second molar infection, adult patient. (Piecuch JF. Odontogenic infections. Dent Clin North Am 1982;26:135.)

gival tissues are probed for periodontal defects, and salivary glands are palpated for tenderness and are milked to be observed for purulent discharge from the duct orifices.

## General Therapeutic Principles

As with infections elsewhere in the body, the principles of treatment of oral infections involve surgical drainage and antibiotics. Surgical drainage may comprise standard incision and drainage of fluctuant abscesses or, in the case of localized periapical infection, it may involve endodontic drainage through the pulp or extraction of the offending tooth. Antibiotic therapy, although it is not necessary for minor, well-localized periapical lesions in non-compromised patients, is indicated if fluctuant abscesses, infections of adjacent bone (osteomyelitis), systemic signs (fatigue, anorexia, fever), trismus, or immunocompromise are present.

Antibiotic selection for odontogenic infections, although based ultimately on Gram's stain and aerobic and anaerobic cultures, generally is begun empirically, before culture results are available. Penicillin G or V is the logical first choice, based on its lack of toxicity, its bactericidal nature, and the sensitivity of most streptococci and oral anaerobes to this drug. If clinical signs or Gram's stain suggest the presence of *S aureus*, a penicillinase-resistant drug such as oxacillin or dicloxacillin may be added to the penicillin, pending the culture results. Alternatively, a cephalosporin, such as cephalexin, cephalothin, or cefazolin, may be used. Second-generation cephalosporins, such as cefoxitin and cefotetan, are useful if a β-lactamase–producing *B melaninogenicus* or *Bacteroides fragilis* is present; however, they rarely are indicated, partly because the latter bacteria are less likely to be involved in odontogenic infections and partly because of cost considerations. In the case of penicillin allergy, clindamycin may be substituted, but it remains the drug of second choice because of its greater toxicity. Erythromycin is less desirable because of its lesser activity against some anaerobes, its variable absorption after oral administration, its reversible binding to target sites, and the usually acidic nature of infected tissues. Tetracycline may result in severe staining of teeth in the young child and should be avoided, except when given specifically in cases of severe juvenile periodontitis. Similarly, the safety of using metronidazole in children has not been established, even though it is highly effective against obligate anaerobic bacteria.

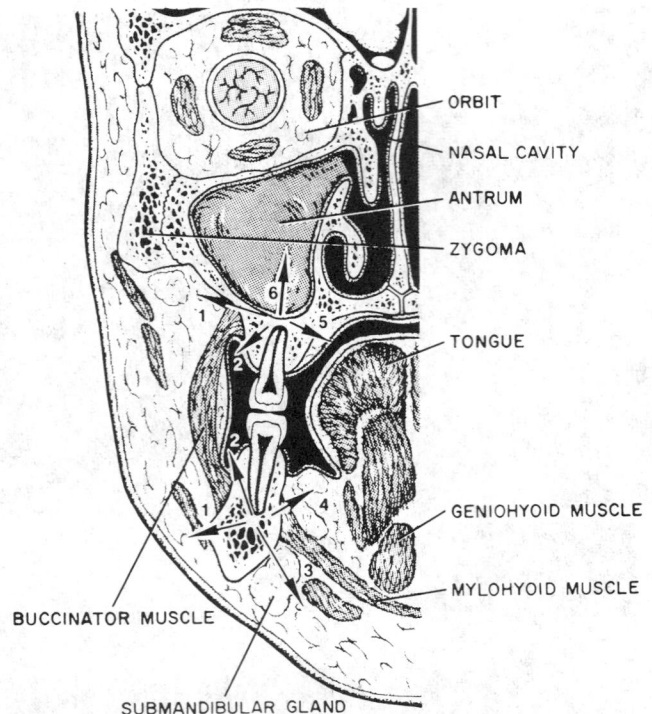

ORBIT
NASAL CAVITY
ANTRUM
ZYGOMA
TONGUE
GENIOHYOID MUSCLE
MYLOHYOID MUSCLE
BUCCINATOR MUSCLE
SUBMANDIBULAR GLAND

**Figure 36-3.** Possible pathways of spread of periapical infection. (Waite DE. Textbook of practical oral surgery. Philadelphia: Lea & Febiger, 1978.)

## Nursing Bottle Caries

A syndrome of tooth decay has been identified that affects primarily the deciduous upper incisors, and frequently the upper and lower deciduous molars, in children of bottle-feeding age

(Fig 36-4). It is caused by the practice of putting a child to bed with a nursing bottle filled with a sugar-containing drink, such as milk, fruit juices, or soft drinks. The child sucks on the bottle intermittently during sleep, when salivary secretion is low, and the sugar-containing liquids stay in the mouth for extended periods. This provides an excellent environment for the growth of caries-producing organisms. Nursing bottle caries can destroy virtually the entire primary dentition of a child as it erupts. It is incumbent on pediatric physicians and dentists, therefore, to instruct parents to avoid putting their child to bed with a nursing bottle or, if they must do so, to use only water in the bedtime drink.

## Periapical Abscess

Extension of microorganisms through the root apex will lead to the formation of an abscess. Early in this process, the acute abscess is indistinguishable clinically and radiographically from an acute pulpitis, particularly because radiographic evidence of bone destruction may take 7 to 14 days to develop. Sensitivity to heat stimulus (relieved by cold), exquisite sensitivity to percussion, and tenderness to finger pressure on the alveolar process are indications that the tooth has become abscessed. Vitallometer testing may be useful if the tooth shows no response to the electric stimulus, but the results may be equivocal in multirooted teeth. Chronic abscesses are diagnosed more easily by observing looseness of the tooth, the presence of suppuration from draining fistulas or from the gingival crevice, and the presence of a radiolucency on the radiograph (Fig 36-5). Depending on the path of least resistance, fluctuant areas may be noted in the buccal or lingual mucosa. Spread through the tissues, or cellulitis, may lead to the classic presentation of swollen face, pain, elevated temperature, and malaise. Adequate surgical drainage is the key principle in the treatment of periapical abscesses, and this may be accomplished by endodontic therapy, extraction of the tooth, or incision and drainage, as necessary. Antibiotic therapy should

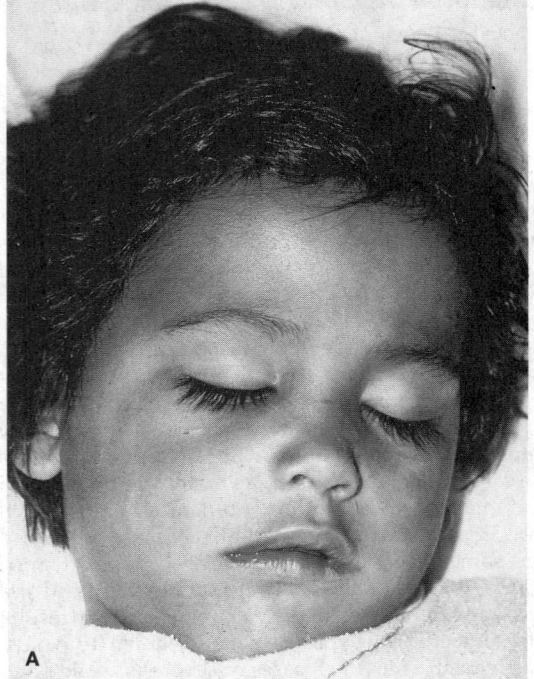
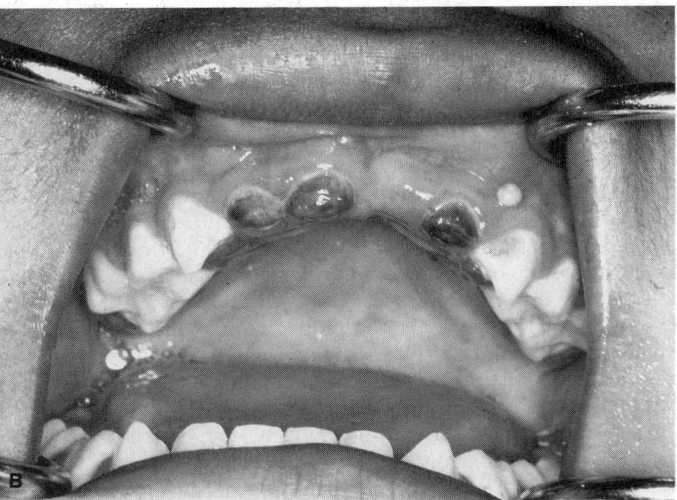

**Figure 36-4.** (**A**) Four-year-old boy with a right canine space infection resulting from nursing bottle caries. Note the swelling of the infraorbital region, elevating the ala of the nose and protruding the upper lip. (**B**) Intraoral view of the same patient. Note the darkened stumps of the carious upper primary incisors and the draining sinus tract (*white dot*) near the upper lateral incisor.

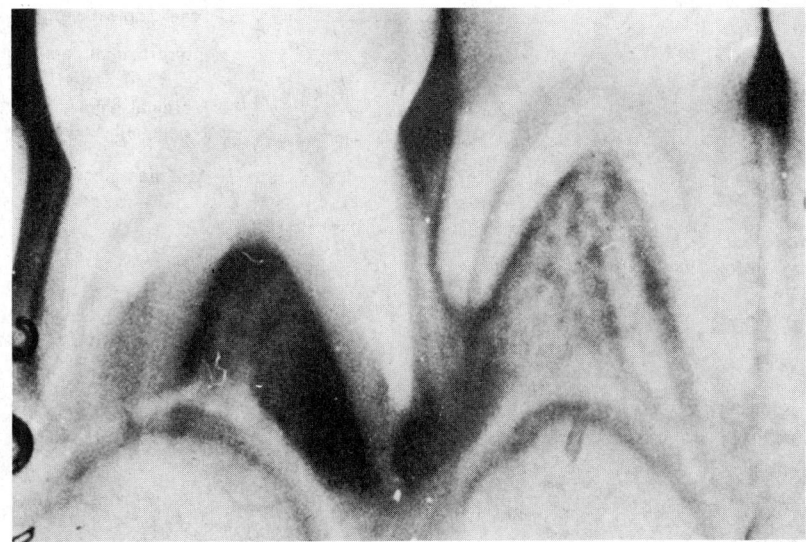

**Figure 36-5.** Radiolucency representing a chronic peri-apical abscess involving the mesial root of the deciduous second molar and the distal root of the deciduous first molar. The developing mandibular bicuspids are seen inferior to the deciduous roots. The cause of the abscess is the deep carious lesion in each tooth, which appears to have penetrated the pulp chambers.

be considered an adjunctive rather than a primary therapeutic modality, because antibiotics alone will not remove the cause of the infection.

Extraction of unsalvageable abscessed teeth soon after the diagnosis has been made has been found to be curative in about 97% of cases. Early extraction also has been shown to be associated with a decreased requirement for extraoral incision and drainage procedures, as compared to treatment only with antibiotics.

## Periodontal Infections

Surrounding the teeth is a distinctive, pink, keratinous mucosa known as the gingiva. Normal gingiva is attached firmly to the alveolar bone and extends between the teeth as the interdental papilla. A thin cup of free (unattached) gingiva surrounds each tooth, and the resulting crevice between the free gingiva and the tooth normally is about 2 mm in depth (Fig 36-6A).

The accumulation of food deposits and bacteria in the gingival crevice may result in gingivitis, a localized inflammation of the free gingiva that presents as an erythematous, painless swelling of the interdental papillae, accompanied by deepening of the gingival sulcus. In severe cases (see Fig 36-6B), the gingival architecture may become distorted and accumulations of plaque are evident. Gingivitis is prevalent at all ages and, in some studies, has been shown to affect more than 60% of children at 5 years of age and almost all adults. It often is most severe in compromised hosts, including diabetic individuals and immunosuppressed patients. Poor oral hygiene is the usual cause, however, and this condition generally responds well to gingival scaling and home care. Chlorhexidine gluconate mouth rinse (Peridex) has been shown to be effective in gingivitis, and is recommended for use in immunocompromised patients as an adjunct to good oral hygiene and regular professional care.

In adolescents as well as adults, gingivitis may progress to periodontitis, a progressively severe infection that is characterized by hypertrophied gingivae, tooth mobility caused by irreversible resorption of alveolar bone, and a purulent exudate. Unfortunately, this insidious condition generally is painless and may progress for years before being recognized. Localized periodontal treatment and meticulous oral hygiene may arrest the condition.

A rare variant, juvenile periodontitis, usually is localized to the molar and incisor regions of younger, otherwise healthy children. Deep gingival pocketing and severe bone resorption are characteristic of this disease, and may result in loss of the dentition

in these areas. The cause is thought to involve relative predominance of a gram-negative anaerobe, *Actinobacillus actinomycetemcomitans*, and localized bacterial inhibition of leukocyte function. Tetracycline has been shown to be useful, in combination with periodontal surgery and meticulous home care.

Acute necrotizing ulcerative gingivitis (ANUG), formerly referred to as trench mouth or Vincent's infection, is a specific disease caused by fusiform bacilli and spirochetes. Recent theories suggest a concomitant viral etiology. Erythema at the tips of the interdental papillae soon is supplanted by frank ulceration and fossae of spontaneous bleeding. A grayish, pseudomembranous, necrotic exudate forms along the marginal gingivae and the interdental papillae. The papillae later become blunted (see Fig 36-6C). ANUG is characterized by pain, foul breath and taste, thick saliva, malaise, and, occasionally, fever. Treatment consists of localized curettage and dental scaling, combined with oral rinses with 0.5% hydrogen peroxide or 0.12% chlorhexidine (Peridex). Systemic penicillin may be added to the regimen if fever is present. With treatment, resolution occurs within 3 to 5 days.

## Pericoronitis

Impaction of debris and microorganisms under the soft tissue overlying the crown of a tooth—often, a mandibular third molar—can lead to the development of inflammation. Drainage usually occurs spontaneously from under the flap, thus localizing the problem. Blockage of natural drainage may lead to spread of the infection to adjacent soft tissues and fascial spaces.

Pericoronitis may be classified into acute, subacute, and chronic forms. Acute pericoronitis characteristically has a sudden onset, with severe pain, trismus, swelling, and dysphagia. Fever is present, as well as tender enlargement of ipsilateral lymph nodes. Purulent material may be drained from beneath the erythematous, edematous flap. The subacute form generally is less severe, with only mild, if any, trismus. Pain is less severe and manifests only as a dull ache. Chronic pericoronitis presents as a recurrent discomfort of several days' duration. Radiographic changes, which generally are absent in acute and subacute forms of pericoronitis, may be seen as a crater-shaped defect posterior to the third molar.

A variety of treatment modalities are applicable to pericoronitis, including irrigation under the operculum, local incision and drainage, and extraction of the tooth. Penicillin is used if fever, lymphadenopathy, or trismus is present. After appropriate therapy is begun, resolution can be expected within 1 week.

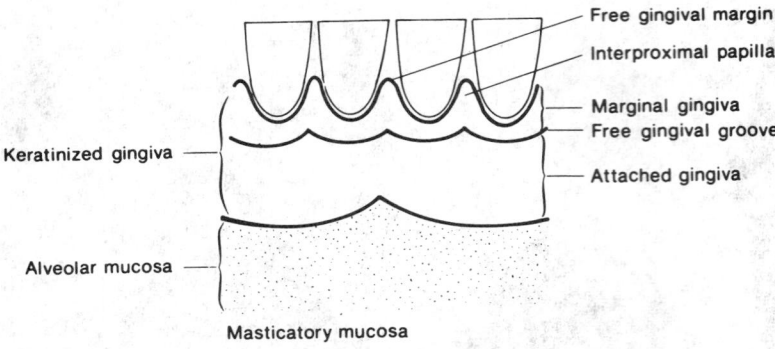

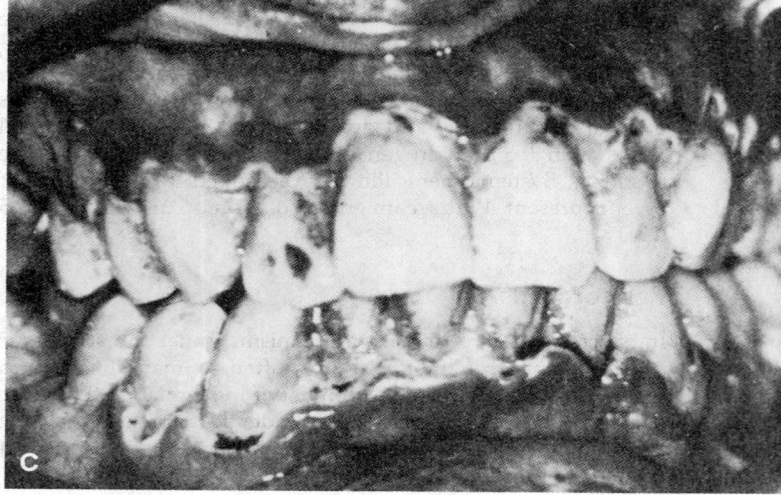

**Figure 36-6.** Normal and abnormal gingiva. (**A**) Normal gingiva. (**B**) Gingivitis: papillae are swollen and accumulations of white plaque are present on teeth. (**C**) Acute necrotizing ulcerative gingivitis. (Lesco B, Brownstein M. Recognition of periodontal disease in children. Pediatr Clin North Am 1982;29:457.)

## COMPLICATIONS OF ODONTOGENIC INFECTION

### Fascial Space Infections

Spread of infection to the fascial spaces may result in dramatic facial swelling, high temperature, and, if the infection is untreated, respiratory embarrassment. The characteristics of the more common fascial space infections related to odontogenic infections are described in the following paragraphs.

Canine space infections generally are connected with maxillary anterior teeth and are well localized to the canine fossa by the levator labii superioris and levator anguli oris muscles. Facial swelling lateral to the nose is prominent, as is weakness of the upper lip resulting from trismus of these muscles. If the infection is fluctuant, intraoral incision and drainage, with placement of a small Penrose drain for 1 to 2 days, generally is sufficient treatment. Antibiotics are indicated for *all* fascial space infections. Figure 36-4 illustrates a canine space infection in a 4-year-old boy caused by nursing bottle caries affecting the upper anterior teeth. It was treated by incision and drainage, and by extraction of the unsalvageable carious incisors.

Trismus is the classic sign of masticator space infection. Because this space is located both medial and lateral to the mandibular ramus, swelling may occur in either direction and resultant abscesses may point either extraorally or toward the lateral pharyngeal wall. Although an intraoral site for incision and drainage has been described, the classic extraoral Risdon incision made inferior and parallel to the inferior border of the mandible remains the technique of choice for incision and drainage.

Infections of the submandibular space (Fig 36-7) may be localized unilaterally or they may involve bilateral structures. Treatment of submandibular space infection is by means of extraoral incision and drainage.

First described in 1836, Ludwig's angina consists of infection of the sublingual and submandibular spaces bilaterally, and is characterized by hard, brawny swelling and a minimum of suppuration. The tongue often is edematous and raised to the roof of the mouth, with little mobility (Fig 36-8). Airway obstruction should be considered to be impending; indeed, the greatest cause of death with this affliction is asphyxiation, which occurred in more than 50% of patients before antibiotics were available. Today, death is rare, although the need for tracheostomy or prolonged endotracheal intubation is common. The cause of this infection often is odontogenic infection, but it also may result from laceration of the floor of the mouth and fracture of the mandible. Usually a disease of middle-aged individuals, it is rare in children, but may occur in greater frequency in those who are immunologically compromised. Surgical drainage of all four spaces is indicated, accompanied by vigorous antibiotic therapy.

## Odontogenic Sinusitis

Odontogenic sinusitis may result from infection of a tooth adjacent to the maxillary antrum or it may occur after extraction of a tooth that has roots in close proximity to the maxillary antrum. The diagnosis usually can be made on the basis of pain, tenderness to percussion over the sinus extraorally, purulent internasal discharge, and radiopacity of the sinus on a Waters' view radiograph. Initial treatment includes oral antibiotics and decongestants to combat microorganisms and promote drainage through the ostium. If an odontogenic infection is thought to be the cause of the sinusitis, penicillin remains the antibiotic of choice, rather than other agents that are used more commonly to treat nonodontogenic sinusitis. Occasionally, a nasal antrostomy or functional endonasal sinus surgery may be necessary to reestablish normal pathways of sinus drainage.

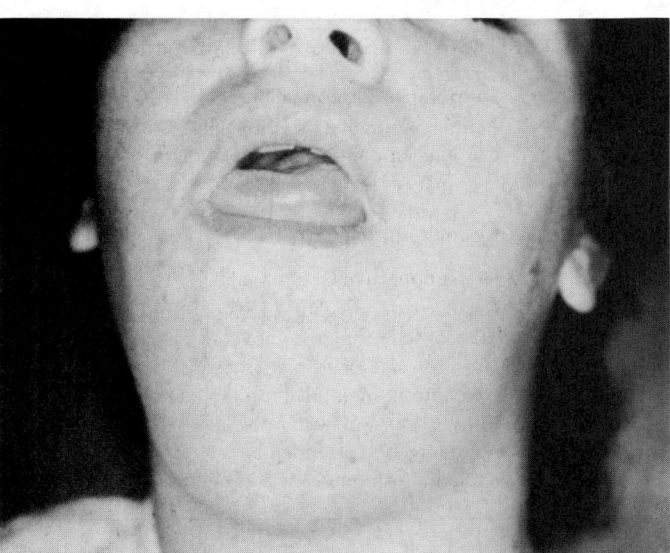

**Figure 36-8.** Ludwig's angina. (Feigin R, Cherry J. Textbook of pediatric infectious diseases, ed 2. Philadelphia: WB Saunders, 1987.)

## Orbital and Intracranial Complications

Orbital and intracranial complications of odontogenic infections are rare. They may occur by direct extension, through sinuses, and by hematogenous spread through the ophthalmic vein system. Probably no more than 5% to 10% of all cases of orbital cellulitis are odontogenic in origin. This infection generally is unilateral, and is characterized by proptosis, chemosis, lid edema, and restriction of extraocular movement secondary to the edema. No nerve palsies or visual changes are present. Treatment includes surgical drainage and antibiotics.

Cavernous sinus thrombosis, which may be difficult to differentiate clinically from orbital cellulitis, is considerably more serious because microorganisms proliferate intracranially. The risk of death is high. Characteristics include bilateral involvement, with rapid progression from one eye to the other, proptosis, chemosis, and lid edema. Extraocular movements are limited because of inflammation of the third, fourth, and sixth cranial nerves. Systemic signs of meningeal irritation and funduscopic evidence of obstruction of the retinal veins also are present. Treatment includes high doses of parenteral antibiotics.

Subdural empyema and brain abscess complicating odontogenic infection are exceedingly rare today compared to several decades ago. Computed tomography may be helpful in establishing the diagnosis, and intracranial drainage may be necessary.

## OSTEOMYELITIS OF THE JAWS IN CHILDREN

Osteomyelitis of the jaws in children usually results from the spread of odontogenic infection. Open fracture of the jaws with delayed treatment also is a significant cause of osteomyelitis. Extension from contiguous infections such as otitis, parotitis, and mastoiditis occurs much less often.

Osteomyelitis of the jaws occurring in children must be viewed with great concern, because it may result in the following problems: loss of primary and permanent teeth; sequestration of segments of the jaws; jaw deformities such as mandibular hypoplasia, asymmetry, and ankylosis of the temporomandibular joint; disfiguring facial scars and cutaneous fistulas; and lesions suggestive of malignancy, which require the performance of open biopsy.

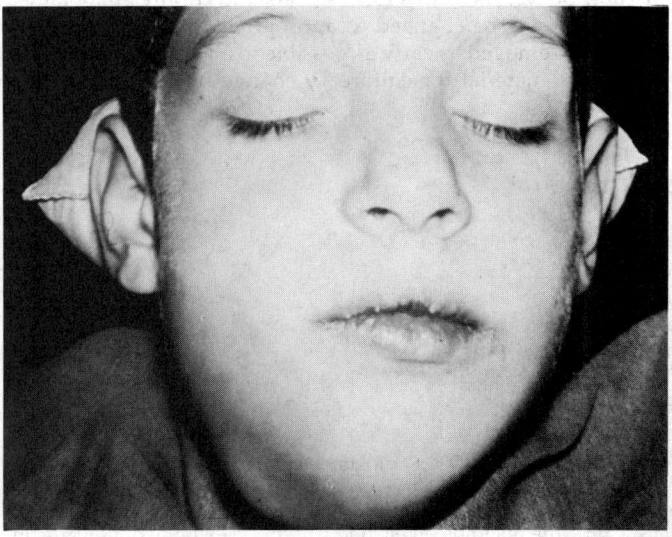

**Figure 36-7.** Submandibular space abscess.

| TABLE 36-11. Osteomyelitis of the Jaws |
| --- |
| **Suppurative Osteomyelitis** |
| Acute suppurative osteomyelitis |
| Chronic suppurative osteomyelitis |
|     Primary |
|     Secondary |
| Infantile osteomyelitis |
| **Nonsuppurative Osteomyelitis** |
| Chronic osteomyelitis |
|     Focal sclerosing osteomyelitis |
|     Diffuse sclerosing osteomyelitis |
|     Recurrent multifocal osteomyelitis |
| Garré's sclerosing osteomyelitis |
| Actinomycotic osteomyelitis |
| Radiation osteomyelitis and necrosis |

For these reasons, osteomyelitis of the jaws in children should be diagnosed rapidly and treated aggressively.

## Predisposing Factors

Preexisting systemic disease with accompanying alteration of host resistance plays a major role in the initiation of osteomyelitis of the jaws. This includes such conditions as diabetes, leukemia, sickle-cell disease, and febrile illnesses. Conditions that alter the vascularity of bone and, thus, the ability to combat infections, including bone tumors, fibrous dysplasia, Paget's disease, and radiation to the jaws, also are important predisposing conditions. Major maxillofacial injuries resulting in open fractures of the jaws, especially those that are not treated immediately, are an important cause of osteomyelitis. Osteomyelitis involves the mandible far more frequently than the maxilla because the relatively poor blood supply to the mandible comes primarily from one major vessel and the periosteum.

## Microbiology

Because the cause of osteomyelitis of the jaws is not always purely odontogenic infection, the bacterial spectrum is broad.

The majority of cases of osteomyelitis of the jaws are caused by those organisms that are found commonly in odontogenic infections. These include aerobic streptococci (*S viridans*), anaerobic streptococci, and other anaerobes, particularly *Peptostreptococcus*, *Fusobacterium*, and *Bacteroides*. Occasionally, anaerobic or micoaerophilic cocci, and gram-negative organisms such as *Klebsiella*, *Pseudomonas*, and *Proteus* are found. Specific forms of osteomyelitis are caused by *Actinomyces* spp., *Treponema pallidum*, and *Mycobacterium tuberculosis*. Unlike long-bone osteomyelitis, *Staphylococcus* rarely is a cause except when extraoral trauma involving soft tissues has been a contributing factor.

## Classification

A useful classification of osteomyelitis of the jaws is provided in Table 36-11. Four major forms of the disease may be distinguished clinically: (1) acute suppurative osteomyelitis; (2) secondary chronic osteomyelitis, the form that begins as an acute osteomyelitis and then becomes chronic; (3) primary chronic osteomyelitis, the form that has no acute phase and always has appeared to be a low-grade infection; and (4) nonsuppurative osteomyelitis. Those forms most often seen in children are the acute suppurative, the secondary chronic, and one nonsuppurative form known as Garré's sclerosing osteomyelitis.

### Suppurative Osteomyelitis

Suppurative osteomyelitis usually begins with deep, intense pain in the jaws, intermittent high fever, and an obvious etiology—most often, a deeply carious or discolored tooth. Occasionally, in the early stages, mental nerve paresthesia is present. Facial swelling develops over the course of several days and teeth begin to loosen, pus exudes around the gingival sulcus, and multiple mucosal or cutaneous fistulas form after 10 to 14 days. A firm cellulitis is present in the soft tissues, accompanied by trismus and cervical lymphadenopathy.

A leukocytosis occurs that typically ranges from 8000 to 15,000 cells per cubic millimeter, although it ordinarily does not reach the levels that are seen in acute osteomyelitis of the long bones. The erythrocyte sedimentation rate may be elevated, but, unlike in long-bone disease, this value rarely is a valid indicator of the extent or course of osteomyelitis of the jaws. After 10 days to 2 weeks, radiographs may show scattered areas of bone destruction with a "moth-eaten" appearance (Fig 36-9); periosteal reaction characterized by the laying down of new bone also is common. Smears of specimens and cultures should be taken whenever possible, including cultures of bone sequestra. Interpretation of cultures must be made with caution, because of the possibility of skin and oral contaminants in the specimen.

Initially, intravenous antibiotics (in dosages adjusted for weight) should be given empirically, using regimen I described in Table 36-12. As results from smears and culture are obtained, antibiotics may be changed as appropriate. The involved tooth should be removed as early as possible to allow for drainage and to provide material for culture. A change from intravenous to

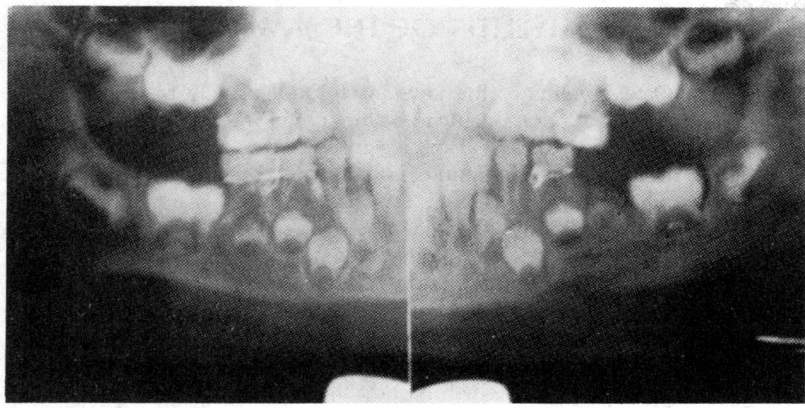

**Figure 36-9.** Radiograph of the jaws of a 4-year-old girl with suppurative osteomyelitis of the left mandible. The film shows marked destruction of the midbody and ramus of the mandible. (Feigin R, Cherry J. Textbook of pediatric infectious diseases, ed 2. Philadelphia: WB Saunders, 1987.)

be undertaken to prevent permanent optic damage, neurologic complications, loss of tooth buds in the bone, and extension to the dural sinuses. Initial antibiotic treatment includes intravenous penicillin and a penicillinase-resistant agent given simultaneously, pending results of Gram's stain and culture, and of sensitivity testing. Fluctuant areas must be drained. Antibiotics should be continued orally for 2 to 4 weeks after all signs of the infection have disappeared. If sequestra form, these should be removed conservatively. It should be noted that tooth buds may be lost, and that surviving teeth may be deformed or discolored after eruption.

### Chronic Recurrent Multifocal Osteomyelitis of Children

An uncommon form of osteomyelitis of the jaws has been described that affects children averaging 14 years of age and is characterized by unpredictable periods of exacerbation and remission. It is referred to as chronic recurrent multifocal osteomyelitis of children. Mandibular lesions are bilateral, irregular, mottled, and multilocular, and are located in the mandibular rami. Antibiotics and debridement appear to have little effect on the prolonged course of this disease.

### Garré's Sclerosing Osteomyelitis

Garré's sclerosing osteomyelitis, also known as chronic nonsuppurative sclerosing osteomyelitis and proliferative osteomyelitis

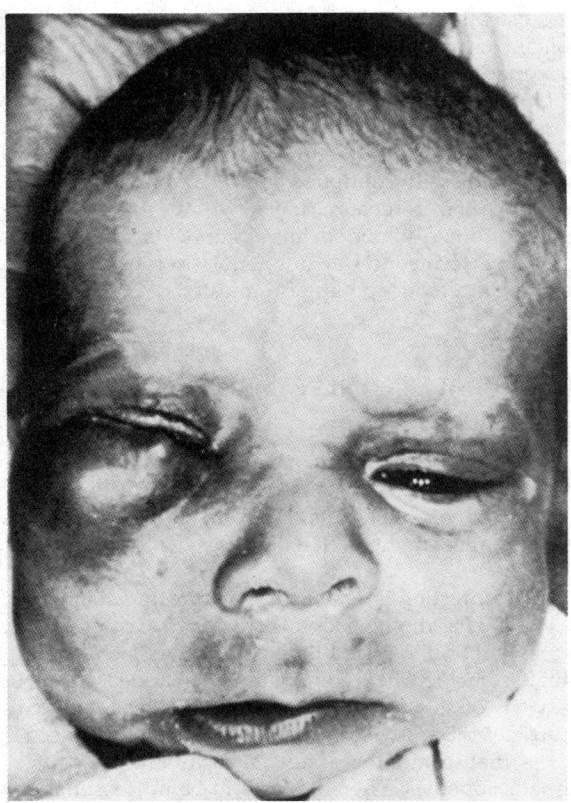

**Figure 36-10.** A 3-week-old child with infantile osteomyelitis. (Courtesy of M. Michael Cohen, Sr., D.D.S.)

oral antibiotics is permissible after the patient has been afebrile for 48 hours and all draining fistulas have closed.

Antibiotic therapy should be continued for at least 2 to 4 weeks after all symptoms subside. If the infection persists, repeated cultures should be obtained and the antibiotic changed, if necessary. Consideration should be given to sequestrectomy and saucerization, which involve removal of teeth in the immediate area and removal of the overlying buccal plate of bone, allowing access to the medullary portion and sequestra that may be present. Occasionally, it is necessary to place catheters via an extraoral approach for closed irrigation suction. This permits the instillation of antibiotics, allowing close contact with bone. Hyperbaric oxygen treatment may be considered in chronic cases that are refractory to antibiotic treatment.

### Infantile Osteomyelitis

Osteomyelitis of the jaws in the newborn is uncommon, but, because of its serious sequelae, it is worthy of special mention. This type of osteomyelitis occurs most often a few weeks after birth and usually involves the maxilla. It is not odontogenic in origin, but is thought to arise from neonatal trauma to oral tissues; from hematogenous spread from the skin, middle ear, mastoid process, or tonsils; or from an infected maternal nipple used in breast-feeding. Clinically, the patient has a facial cellulitis centered about the orbit (Fig 36-10). Irritability and malaise precede cellulitis and are followed by marked elevation in temperature, anorexia, and dehydration. Intercanthal swelling, palpebral edema with closure of the eye, conjunctivitis, and proptosis may be seen, along with a purulent discharge from the nose or inner canthus.

Oral examination reveals swelling of the maxilla on the infected side, extending to both the buccal and the palatal regions, with fluctuant areas often present with multiple fistulas. *S aureus* is the usual organism found. Aggressive, prompt treatment must

| TABLE 36-12. Antibiotic Regimen for Osteomyelitis of the Jaws | |
|---|---|
| Regimen I | *Empiric Therapy* |
| | Aqueous penicillin, 250,000 U/kg in 6 divided doses intravenously |
| | When asymptomatic for 48–72 h, switch to: |
| | Penicillin V, 500 mg orally every 4 h for an additional 2–4 wk |
| | *or* |
| Regimen II | *Initial Therapy With Gram's Stain Results* |
| | A. Smear suggestive of mixed infection: regimen I as above |
| | B. Smear suggestive of *Staphylococcus* infection: Penicillin as in regimen I |
| | *plus* |
| | Oxacillin, 200 mg/kg/24 h in 4 divided doses intravenously |
| | When asymptomatic for 48–72 h, switch to: |
| | Dicloxacillin, 75 mg/kg/24 h in divided doses orally for an additional 2–4 wk |
| | *or* |
| | Clindamycin, 30 mg/kg/24 h in 3 divided doses intravenously; then 30 mg/kg/24 h in 3 divided doses orally |
| | C. Smear suggestive of anaerobic infection: |
| | Aqueous penicillin, 250,000 U/kg in 6 divided doses intravenously |
| | When asymptomatic for 48–72 h, switch to: |
| | Penicillin V, 500 mg orally every 4 h for an additional 2–4 wk |
| | For patients allergic to penicillin, in order of preference: |
| | 1. Clindamycin, 30 mg/kg/24 h in 3 divided doses intravenously, then clindamycin 30 mg/kg/24 h in 3 divided doses orally |
| | 2. Cefazolin, 50 mg/kg/24 h in 3 divided doses, then cephalexin 40 mg/kg/24 h in 4 divided doses orally |

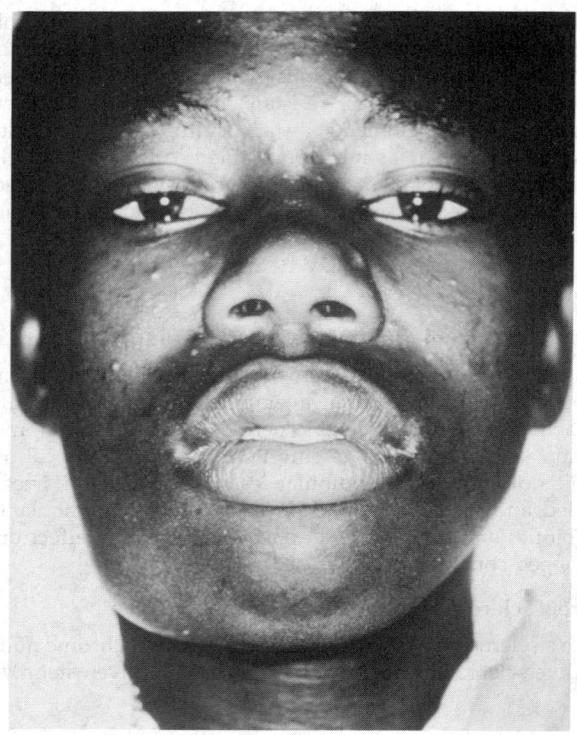

**Figure 36-11.** Enlargement of the right side of the mandible in a 12-year-old with Garré's sclerosing osteomyelitis. The swelling is hard and nontender.

of Garré, is notable because of the similarity of some of its characteristics to those of other neoperiostoses.

It is characterized by a localized, hard, nontender swelling of the mandible (Fig 36-11). Lymphadenopathy, hyperpyrexia, and leukocytosis are not present. It is associated commonly with a carious tooth, usually the lower first molar, with a history of a toothache that may have resolved. It also may be associated with a recent dental extraction or with an infected flap of tissue over an erupting tooth. Radiographs are quite impressive, showing a focal area of well-calcified bone proliferation that is smooth and often has a laminated or "onion-peel" appearance (Fig 36-12).

Garré's osteomyelitis is thought to be a response to a low-grade stimulus, such as a dental infection, that influences the potentially active periosteum of young individuals. Its appearance resembles that of infantile cortical hyperostosis, osteosarcoma, and Ewing's sarcoma, and must be distinguished from these conditions. Treatment consists of extraction of or endodontic therapy for the involved tooth, with continued clinical and radiographic follow-up of the patient to ensure that new bone formation does not progress. Ordinarily, remodeling occurs over time, but biopsies should be performed to rule out neoplasm if the lesion does not regress. No antibiotic therapy is indicated.

## HERPES SIMPLEX INFECTIONS

Herpes simplex type 1 infections are manifested commonly as a herpetic gingivostomatitis. Five stages of infection have been identified: primary mucocutaneous infection, acute infection of ganglia, establishment of latency, reactivation, and recurrent infection.

Primary infection is established by direct contact either with a person who has draining lesions or with an asymptomatic carrier who may continue to shed the virus despite lack of symptoms. The highest incidence of primary infection appears to occur from 2 to 4 years of age. In a series of 19,000 children with gingivostomatitis described by Juretic in 1966, no cases were seen in children less than 6 months of age; such infants are protected by maternal antibodies. There appears to be no seasonal variation or male–female difference in incidence.

The incubation period is thought to be about 6 days, followed by the development of small vesicles that may coalesce to form larger lesions or ulcers. In severe cases, the lips, gingivae, oral mucosa, and pharynx all may be involved (Fig 36-13).

Many patients with primary herpes labialis may be asymptomatic, however, and no symptoms may develop. Healing occurs in 1 to 2 weeks, with gradual crusting of the lesions followed by re-epithelialization.

Latency is thought to continue throughout life, with reactivation occurring at various times, possibly triggered by emotional and physical stress. Recurrent disease is manifested by vesicles at the mucocutaneous border that are painful for about 2 days, followed by crusting and complete healing in 7 to 8 days.

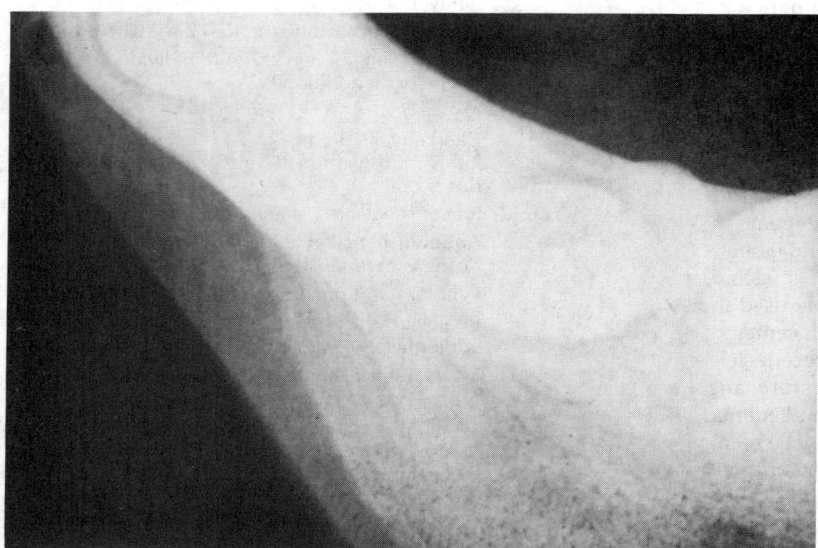

**Figure 36-12.** Characteristic radiograph of Garré's osteomyelitis, showing the laminated or onion-peel appearance of the mass.

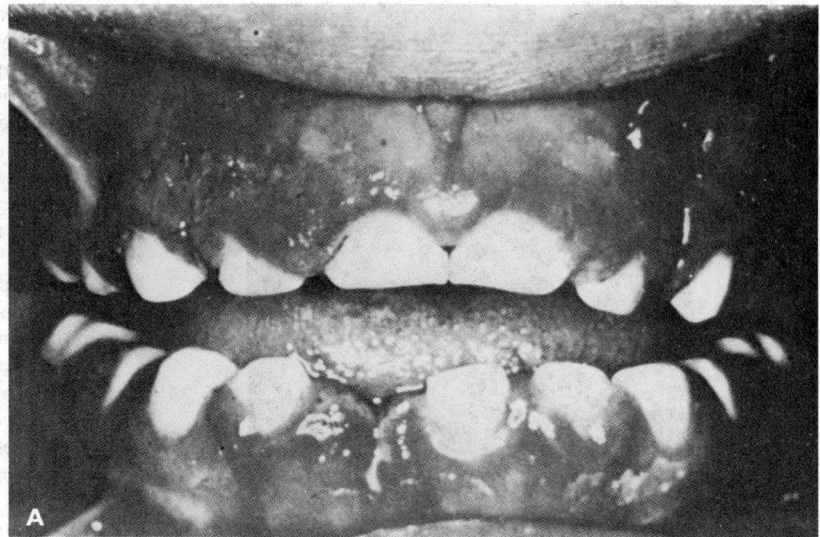

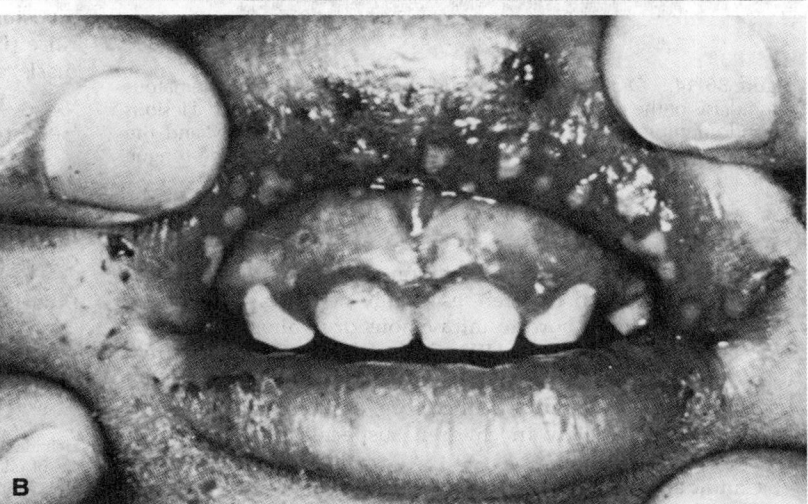

**Figure 36-13.** Herpetic gingivostomatitis. (**A**) Gingival lesions. (**B**) Lesions of labial mucosa. (From Sanders B. Textbook of pediatric oral and maxillofacial surgery. St Louis: CV Mosby, 1979.)

Although numerous confirmatory laboratory tests are available, including tissue culture, immunofluorescence, radioimmunoassay for antigen, and electron microscopy, there is no rapid, inexpensive, and sensitive test for herpes simplex. Consequently, the diagnosis often is made clinically.

Treatment of primary and recurrent lesions is palliative and supportive. Lesions should be kept clean and dry, and analgesic and antipyretic medications should be given as needed. Small children with severe primary gingivostomatitis may be subject to dehydration. Studies with acyclovir and other antiviral agents have not shown a reduction in duration of symptoms when the agents are used topically for recurrent lesions, but they may decrease the severity of the manifestations. Oral and intravenous therapy has shown some benefit in the compromised host for the reduction of pain and systemic symptoms.

As much as 50% of the adult population in industrialized countries, and a higher percentage in less-developed nations, may suffer from recurrent herpes labialis. Surprisingly, many, if not most, adults who suffer from recurrent "cold sores" are not aware that they can transmit the disease, and they should be counseled in this regard. Likewise, medical, dental, and nursing personnel also should be advised that the occurrence of cutaneous lesions (the herpetic whitlow) is not unknown after direct contact of the practitioners' fingers with lesions during the physical examination.

## ORAL LESIONS ASSOCIATED WITH THE HUMAN IMMUNODEFICIENCY VIRUS

Human immunodeficiency virus (HIV) infection first was recognized in children in 1983. Since then, it has become clear that the oral manifestations of this infection are frequent and protean, and that they are significantly different from those in adults.

Similarities between adults and children with HIV infection include failure to thrive, fever, lymphadenopathy, opportunistic infections with atypical pathogens, and persistent oral candidiasis. In contrast to adults, children infected with HIV have a greater susceptibility to bacterial infections, especially with encapsulated organisms, such as *Streptococcus pneumoniae* and *Haemophilus influenzae*. Septicemia from an oral focus of infection can become a life-threatening problem in the HIV-infected child; therefore, optimal oral health must be established and maintained vigorously in these children. Children with HIV also have a much greater incidence of persistent diffuse parotitis, in which the gland may become large and disfiguring. Parotid enlargement sometimes is caused by lymphocytic infiltration and intraparotid lymphadenopathy rather than by infection of the gland.

The oral lesions associated with HIV seropositivity can be classified as fungal, bacterial, viral, neoplastic, and idiopathic.

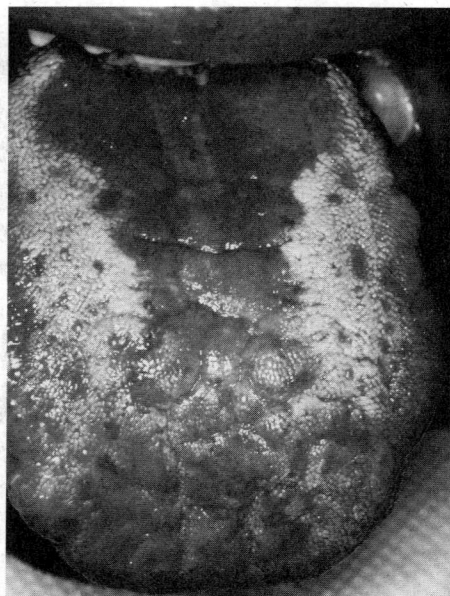

**Figure 36-14.** Oral candidiasis. Pseudomembranous and erythematous candidiasis of the dorsum of the tongue. Note the white candidal lesions (pseudomembranous type) on the filiform papillae laterally and the patchy red areas with loss of filiform papillae producing a bald tongue centrally (erythematous type).

The most common oral manifestation is persistent candidiasis, which is common in children, especially neonates. It has been reported in children born to intravenous drug-abusing mothers who are not infected with HIV. Oral candidiasis may progress to esophageal candidiasis, which is a marker for the acquired immunodeficiency syndrome; therefore, oral candidiasis should be treated aggressively in children suspected of having HIV infection.

Candidal lesions in the mouth may take four forms: pseudomembranous, erythematous, hyperplastic, and angular cheilitis. The pseudomembranous form is the classic manifestation, with white curd-like colonies on the mucosa that leave a raw, red underlying surface when the colonies are wiped off. The erythematous variant presents as reddened oral mucosa that may vary from fiery red to pink, without the presence of creamy white colonies. On the tongue, it causes loss of the filiform papillae, leaving bald patches resembling geographic tongue (Fig 36-14). The hyperplastic form is characterized by a papillary mucosal hyperplasia, especially in the palate. Angular cheilitis can be recognized by red, tender patches at the corners of the mouth, from which *Candida albicans* may be identified. Treatment is with antifungal agents, the preparation of which becomes very important in establishing compliance with therapy in children.

The most common oral bacterial infections seen in HIV-seropositive children are HIV gingivitis and acute necrotizing ulcerative gingivitis (ANUG). HIV gingivitis is characterized by linear erythema of the gingival margins surrounding the teeth, and it is unresponsive to improved oral hygiene. The progression of this lesion to the rapid destruction of periodontal bone and soft tissue that is seen in adults has not been reported in children. ANUG, recognized by necrotic loss of the interdental gingival

papillae, with pain and fetor oris, has not been reported in American HIV-positive children but is common in malnourished, immunosuppressed children from less well developed countries.

Herpes simplex virus infection, as described above, can be particularly severe in HIV-infected children, leaving large crater-like painful ulcers with a gray-white pseudomembrane. This infection is treated with acyclovir, orally or intravenously as necessary.

Oral neoplasms associated with HIV infection in adults, such as non-Hodgkin's lymphoma and Kaposi's sarcoma, have not been reported in children. Similarly, the persistent aphthous ulcerations that are common in HIV-positive adults are infrequent in children.

To prevent life-threatening infections and improve the quality of life in HIV-infected children, maintaining optimal oral health is of great significance. These children should have regular pediatric oral and dental examinations and care, consisting of excellent oral hygiene, frequent dental prophylaxis (cleanings) and fluoride treatments, and early and aggressive treatment of oral infections such as caries, gingivitis, candidiasis, and herpetic gingivostomatitis. Routine use of chlorhexidine gluconate mouth rinse (Peridex) may be helpful in minimizing gingivitis, candidiasis, and bacterial superinfections of the oral cavity.

## Selected Readings

Adekeye EO, Cornah J. Osteomyelitis of the jaws: A review of 141 cases. Br J Oral Maxillofac Surg 1985;23:24.

Benca PG, Mostofi R, Kuo P. Proliferative periostitis (Garré's osteomyelitis). Oral Surg 1987;63:258.

Coykendall AL. Classification and identification of the viridans streptococci. Clin Microbiol Rev 1989;2:315.

Dodson TB, Barton JA, Kaban LB. Predictors of outcome in children hospitalized with maxillofacial infections: A linear logistic model. J Oral Maxillofac Surg 1991;49:838.

Dodson TB, Perrott DH, Kaban LB. Pediatric maxillofacial infections: A retrospective study of 113 patients. J Oral Maxillofac Surg 1989;47:327.

Granite EL. Anatomic considerations in infections of the face and neck. J Oral Surg 1976;34:34.

Heimdahl A, VonKonow L, Satoh T, et al. Clinical appearance of orofacial infections of odontogenic origin in relation to microbiological findings. J Clin Microbiol 1985;22:299.

Kaban LB. Draining skin lesions of dental origin: The path of spread of chronic odontogenic infection. Plast Reconstr Surg 1980;66:711.

Leggott PJ. Oral manifestations of HIV infection in children. Oral Surg 1992;73:187.

Lewis MO, MacFarlane TW, McGowan DA. Quantitative bacteriology of acute dental alveolar abscesses. J Med Microbiol 1986;21:101.

Marx RE. Chronic osteomyelitis of the jaws. Oral Maxillofac Surg Clin North Am 1991;3:367.

Marx RE, Johnson RP, Kline SN. Prevention of osteoradio-necrosis: A randomized prospective clinical trial of hyperbaric oxygen vs penicillin. J Am Dent Assoc 1985;111:49.

Nyberg D, Jeffrey R, Brant-Zawadzki M, et al. Computer tomography of cervical infections. J Comput Assist Tomogr 1985;9:288.

Page RC. Gingivitis. J Clin Periodontol 1986;13:345.

Ranta H, Haapasalo M, Ranta K, et al. Bacteriology of odontogenic apical periodontitis and effect of penicillin treatment. Scand J Infect Dis 1988;20:187.

Scully C, McCarthy G. Management of oral health in persons with HIV infection. Oral Surg 1992;73:215.

Shah HN, Collins DM. Proposal for reclassification of Bacteroides asaccharolyticus, Bacteroides gingivalis, and Bacteroides endodontalis in a new genus Porphyromonas. Int J Syst Bacteriol 1988;38:128.

Shah HN, Collins DM. Prevotella, a new genus to include Bacteroides melaninogenicus and related spp. formerly classified in the genus Bacteroides. Int J Syst Bacteriol 1990;40:205.

Straus SE, moderator. NIH conference: Herpes simplex virus infection: Biology, treatment, prevention. Ann Intern Med 1985;103:404.

Whiley RA, Beighton D. Amended descriptions and recognition of Streptococcus constellatus, Streptococcus intermedius, and Streptococcus anginosus as distinct species. Int J Syst Bacteriol 1991;41:1.

Principles and Practice of Pediatrics, Second Edition.
edited by Frank A. Oski et al. J. B. Lippincott Company, Philadelphia © 1994.

# 36.4 *Pharyngitis*

## Margaret R. Hammerschlag

Children and young adults visit physicians more often for sore throats than for any other problem or symptom. Technically, pharyngitis is an inflammatory illness of the mucous membranes and underlying structures of the throat. Although the symptom of sore throat invariably is present with pharyngitis, it should not be used as the sole criterion for diagnosis. Sore throat can be a common complaint in children with colds in whom no evidence of pharyngeal inflammation is present.

Pharyngitis also can be subdivided into two categories: with and without nasal symptoms. This has important etiologic implications. Nasopharyngitis almost always has a viral cause, whereas illness without nasal symptoms (pharyngitis or tonsillopharyngitis) can have diverse causative agents, including bacteria, viruses, and fungi.

## ETIOLOGY

The etiologic agents involved in nasopharyngitis most often are viruses, with adenovirus types 7a, 9, 14, and 15 being the most common. Influenza and parainfluenza are the other major viral agents. Rhinovirus and respiratory syncytial virus infections are not associated often with objective pharyngeal findings.

Pharyngitis (including tonsillitis and tonsillopharyngitis) can be caused by a diversity of infectious agents, ranging from group A β-hemolytic streptococci to more obscure agents such as *Legionella pneumophila* and leptospires. As with other infections, the probability that any one agent is the cause of pharyngitis depends on the age and immune status of the patient, the season, and the environment. In normal, healthy children, more than 90% of all cases of pharyngitis are caused by the following organisms, listed in order of decreasing frequency of occurrence: group A β-hemolytic streptococci; adenoviruses; influenza viruses A and B; parainfluenza viruses 1, 2, and 3; Epstein-Barr virus; enteroviruses; *Mycoplasma pneumoniae*; and *Chlamydia pneumoniae*.

Other β-hemolytic streptococci, especially groups C and G, also have been isolated from children and young adults with pharyngitis. Other, less common bacterial sources of pharyngitis include *Archanobacterium haemolyticum*, formerly called *Corynebacterium haemolyticum*, an organism that is more likely to infect teenagers and young adults, and also can cause a scarlatiniform rash. Data are limited to only one report, however. *Neisseria gonorrhoeae* should be considered in adolescents who are sexually active or are known to have been exposed, and possibly in abused children. Most abused children who have had *N gonorrhoeae* isolated from the nasopharynx are asymptomatic, however.

Among viral causes, adenovirus is the most prevalent. A recent study has found viruses to be responsible for 42% of all cases of pharyngitis in a group of children, aged 6 months through 17.9 years, with acute exudative tonsillitis. Adenovirus was responsible for 19% of the cases, followed by Epstein-Barr virus. Two children (2%) had infections with herpes simplex virus, and five children had infection with *M pneumoniae*.

## CLINICAL PRESENTATION

Nasopharyngitis tends to be more common in younger children. The presentation can be variable, depending on the agent. Fever usually is present. Infection with adenovirus may be associated with conjunctivitis and exudative pharyngitis, whereas infection with influenza A or B frequently is associated with more severe systemic complaints. The onset of pharyngitis can be acute, with fever and the complaint of sore throat. The child also may have headache, nausea, vomiting, and, occasionally, abdominal pain. Physical examination usually reveals moderate to severe pharyngeal erythema and tonsillar enlargement, and varying degrees of cervical adenitis. The erythema can be associated with follicular, ulcerative, and petechial lesions, as well as areas of exudate. Follicular tonsillitis is fairly characteristic of adenoviral infections, and ulcerative lesions usually are observed with enteroviral infections. The presence of exudate has been thought in the past to be most common or characteristic of group A streptococcal infection or infectious mononucleosis. A recent, prospective, 1-year study of acute febrile exudative tonsillitis, however, found that 42% of the cases had a viral cause, predominantly adenovirus. The only clinical clues to the nature of the infecting agent were cough and rhinitis—both of which were observed in 45% of patients with viral disease and in only 10% of children with β-hemolytic streptococci. Pharyngitis in children is almost entirely acute and self-limited, lasting from 4 to 10 days, depending on the cause.

Streptococcal pharyngitis can have significant suppurative complications, including peritonsillar abscess and bacteremia. Post-anginal sepsis is a clinical syndrome that usually occurs in adolescents or young adults after an oronasopharyngeal infection, frequently infectious mononucleosis. After a latency period of several days, contiguous or lymphatic spread of local infection, septicemia, and septic metastases can be observed. Septicemia in these cases usually is attributed to thrombophlebitis in small and large vessels of the face and neck. The organisms most frequently involved in this syndrome are anaerobes, including *Fusobacterium* species and *Bacteroides* species

## DIFFERENTIAL DIAGNOSIS

Because of the numerous organisms that can cause pharyngitis and the significant overlap among them in clinical presentation and findings, it is difficult to make a specific diagnosis based on physical findings alone, such as the presence of exudate. The age and clinical status of the patient and the time of year should be taken into account. Age may be the most important factor in predicting the causative agent, with viral tonsillitis being most common in patients younger than 3 years of age and group A β-hemolytic streptococci found most often in children 6 years of age or older. The presence of rhinitis also is more suggestive of a viral infection. In adolescents and adults, viral infection with *M pneumoniae* and *C pneumoniae* is more likely.

## SPECIFIC DIAGNOSIS

Because infection with group A streptococci can have significant suppurative and nonsuppurative complications, streptococcal disease must be excluded in all instances of acute pharyngitis. If the child is young (less than 3 years of age) or has obvious viral infection such as pharyngoconjunctival fever (adenovirus) or herpangina, antibiotic therapy is not needed and, therefore, cultures are not indicated.

The only way to make a definite diagnosis of group A streptococcal infection is to identify the organism in the pharynx by culture. Recent confirmation that early treatment of severe streptococcal pharyngitis hastens recovery has made rapid diagnosis of this condition desirable. Even "routine" culture methods may have problems with sensitivity. The use of a single blood agar plate culture for the diagnosis of streptococcal pharyngitis has only 72% sensitivity compared to a two-plate culture method when the plate is read at 2 days. If the single plate is read only at 24 hours, the sensitivity drops to 58%. There are a number of rapid, non-culture antigen detection kits available for the diagnosis of streptococcal pharyngitis. Although these tests appear to be very specific, they often lack sensitivity. Even in several kits in which the sensitivities appear to be high (>90%), they actually are much lower because the kits were compared to less sensitive culture methods. The evaluation of any new technology is influenced by the choice of the reference method. An insensitive reference method causes a test to appear unjustifiably more sensitive. It may be postulated that those patients who have false-negative streptococcal antigen detection test results do not have significant pharyngeal infection. Several studies have demonstrated, however, that there is little correlation between the degree of positivity (number of colonies) and changes in streptococcal antibody titers. In one study, 45% of the children who had false-negative throat antigen test results using a rapid test kit had significant changes in their streptococcal antibody titers. If the prevalence of infection also is low (<50%) in a particular population, the positive predictive value of these tests may be 56% or less.

It has been suggested, on the basis of false-negative result rates that average around 15%, that the specimen be obtained using two swabs for the tonsillar sweep. If the rapid antigen detection test result is positive, the patient can be treated and the second swab discarded. If the test is negative, the second swab should be used for a standard culture on blood agar with a bacitracin disc. For identification of other bacteria, such as *A haemolyticum* or *N gonorrhoeae*, the laboratory must be informed specifically so that appropriate media are used. Examination of Gram's stains of the exudate does not appear to be an accurate way to identify group A streptococci, *N gonorrhoeae*, or *C haemolyticum*.

Rapid differentiation of infectious mononucleosis from streptococcal pharyngitis once was thought to be possible by demonstration of atypical lymphocytes in Wright-Giemsa–stained smears of the exudate. Newer tests using agglutination of red cells or latex particles to detect heterophil antibody responses are simpler, faster, and more accurate.

## TREATMENT

Because the majority of episodes of pharyngitis are viral and self-limited, specific therapy is not indicated except for a streptococcal pharyngitis. Generally, either intramuscular benzathine penicillin or a 10-day course of oral penicillin or another antibiotic such as erythromycin will be about 90% effective. Recent studies have suggested that some clinical and bacteriologic treatment failures after therapy with penicillins may have been caused by the presence of β-lactamase–producing bacteria, especially *Bacteroides fragilis* and *Bacteroides melaninogenicus*. Subsequent treatment with an antibiotic resistant to β-lactamase, such as clindamycin, or with a cephalosporin, frequently was effective.

The importance of accurate diagnosis and appropriate therapy of pharyngitis cannot be emphasized too strongly. Recently, there has been a resurgence of acute rheumatic fever in several parts of the United States, including Utah, Pennsylvania, and Ohio. In an outbreak in Akron, Ohio, the patients generally were not indigent and had good access to medical care. About 80% of the patients had had an illness suggestive of pharyngitis within 1

month of the onset of acute rheumatic fever; of these, 39% either had failed to receive a full 10-day course of antibiotics or had received no antibiotics at all.

## Selected Readings

Alpert JJ, Pickering MR, Warren RJ. Failure to isolate streptococci from children under the age of 3 years with exudative tonsillitis. Pediatrics 1966;38:663.

Bass JW. Antibiotic management of group A streptococcal tonsillopharyngitis. Pediatr Infect Dis J 1991;10:S43.

Brook I. Beta-lactamase-producing bacteria recovered after clinical failures with various penicillin therapies. Arch Otolaryngol 1984;110:228.

Brook I, Leyva F. Discrepancies in the recovery of group A beta-hemolytic streptococci from both tonsillar surfaces. Laryngoscope 1991;101:795.

Congeni B, Rizzo C, Congeni J, et al. Outbreak of acute rheumatic fever in northeast Ohio. J Pediatr 1987;111:176.

Houvonen P, Lahtonen R, Ziegler T, et al. Pharyngitis in adults: The presence and coexistence of viruses and bacterial organisms. Ann Intern Med 1989;110:612.

Kaplan EL, Hill HR. Return of rheumatic fever: Consequences, implications and needs. J Pediatr 1987;111:244.

Kellog JA. Suitability of throat culture procedures for detection of group A streptococci and as reference standards for evaluation of streptococcal antigen detection kits. J Clin Microbiol 1990;28:165.

Miller RA, Brancato F, Holmes KK. Corynebacterium hemolyticum as a cause of pharyngitis and scarlatiform rash in young adults. Am J Med 1986;105:867.

Pichichero ME. The rising incidence of penicillin treatment failures in group A streptococcal tonsillopharyngitis: An emerging role for the cephalosporins? Pediatr Infect Dis J 1991;10:S50.

Putto A. Febrile exudative tonsillitis: Viral or streptococcal. Pediatrics 1987;80:6.

Turner JC, Hayden GF, Kiscelica D, et al. Association of group C beta-hemolytic streptococci with endemic pharyngitis among college students. JAMA 1990;264:2644.

Van Cauwenberge PB, Vander Mijnsbrugge A-M. Pharyngitis: A survey of the microbiologic etiology. Pediatr Infect Dis J 1991;10:S39.

Wegner DL, Witte DL, Schrantz RD. Insensitivity of rapid antigen detection methods and single blood culture for diagnosing streptococcal pharyngitis. JAMA 1992;267:695.

*Principles and Practice of Pediatrics, Second Edition.* edited by Frank A. Oski et al. J. B. Lippincott Company, Philadelphia © 1994.

# 36.5 *Peritonsillar, Retropharyngeal, and Parapharyngeal Abscesses*

Paul E. Hammerschlag and Margaret R. Hammerschlag

A deep neck abscess is a collection of pus in a potential space bounded by fascia. These potential spaces are areas of least resistance to the spread of infection. An infection may begin with a minimal area of cellulitis and progress to a deep neck abscess, which then may extend to invade adjacent potential spaces; these frequently encompass vital structures in the neck. Destruction or dysfunction of these structures represent the major complications of deep neck infections.

## PERITONSILLAR ABSCESS (QUINSY)

A peritonsillar abscess is circumscribed medially by the fibrous wall of the tonsil capsule, and laterally by the superior constrictor muscle. The cause of peritonsillar abscesses is not constant; they may follow any "virulent" tonsillitis, with extension through the fibrous tonsil capsule. Peritonsillar abscesses are rare in young children. They are most common in late adolescence and in the early part of the third decade.

## Clinical Manifestations

The patient's recent history may include a sore throat with occasional unilateral pain, malaise, low-grade pyrexia, chills, diaphoresis, dysphagia, reduced oral intake, trismus, and a muffled "hot-potato voice." Trismus results from irritation and reflex spasm of the internal pterygoid muscle. Impaired palatal motion from edema contributes to the muffled voice.

On physical examination, there is minimal to moderate toxicity, dehydration, and drooling. Inspection of the oropharynx may be compromised by trismus. The soft palate is displaced toward the unaffected side, is swollen and red, and frequently contains a palpable fluctuant area. The edematous uvula is pushed across the midline. The displaced tonsil and its crypts rarely are coated with exudate. The breath is fetid, and there is ipsilateral, tender cervical adenopathy. Indirect laryngoscopy reveals supraglottic and lateral pharyngeal edema. The white blood cell count is elevated, with a predominance of polymorphonuclear leukocytes.

## Treatment

Aspiration of the fluctuant mass with an 18-gauge needle commonly confirms the diagnosis of peritonsillar abscess, especially if the pus is located in the superior pole. Aspiration along with intravenous antibiotics has been found to be very effective treatment. Some clinicians prefer the time-honored method of incision and drainage under local anesthesia, in which there is a slight risk of aspiration of the pus. Pus in locations other than the superior pole may not be accessible to aspiration intraorally or amenable to drainage by this route. An "acute quinsy tonsillectomy" with the medial wall of the abscess removed is the ideal procedure by which to provide adequate drainage. The length of the hospital stay for patients treated with immediate tonsillectomy has been found to be about half as long as that for those treated with incision and drainage. Although it is thought to be higher, the incidence of recurrent peritonsillar abscess was reported to be 10% in one study. Bilateral tonsillectomies often are advocated, although the incidence of abscess within the contralateral peritonsillar capsule varies from 2% to 24%.

Several recent studies have suggested that many patients with peritonsillar abscess can be treated with simple needle aspiration combined with antibiotic therapy on an outpatient basis. One prospective, randomized study found a cure rate of 92% with a single aspiration, compared to 93% in those patients who had standard treatment with incision and drainage. This approach should be considered with caution, however, as no data are available regarding the long-term follow-up of the patients who were treated with simple aspiration.

Preoperatively and postoperatively (in tonsillectomy, aspiration, or incision and drainage), patients should be treated with appropriate intravenous antibiotics until they are asymptomatic, then they should be switched to oral medications. Lavage with warm saline every 2 hours aids in debridement of the area, may reduce the peritonsillar edema, and provides some symptomatic relief.

Untreated peritonsillar abscess may point, with spontaneous rupture, or extend to the pterygomaxillary space, with potentially fatal complications.

## PARAPHARYNGEAL ABSCESS (PHARYNGOMAXILLARY, LATERAL, AND PHARYNGEAL SPACE ABSCESS)

The potential pterygomaxillary space is an inverted conical cavity lying along an oblique axis roughly parallel to the ramus of the mandible. The base of the skull at the jugular foramen forms the base of the "cone," and its apex is at the hyoid. The parapharyngeal space is contiguous with the peritonsillar, submandibular, and retropharyngeal spaces—all of which are potential avenues of extension of a parapharyngeal space abscess. The posterior portion of the cone contains the contents of the carotid sheath (the carotid artery and internal jugular vein, the cranial nerves IX through XIII, and the cervical sympathetic chain). The internal pterygoid muscle and fatty connective tissue are located anteriorly.

Involvement of these structures determines the clinical manifestations and complications of a parapharyngeal space abscess. An abscess in the posterior compartment may result in medial displacement of the lateral pharyngeal wall and parotid space induration and swelling, with variable overlying facial nerve weakness, carotid artery erosion and hemorrhage, internal jugular vein thrombosis, decreased gag reflex and dysphagia, ipsilateral vocal cord paralysis, weakness of the ipsilateral trapezius muscle, ipsilateral lingual deviation, and Horner's syndrome from cervical sympathetic chain involvement.

Extension of the abscess into the anterior compartment causes trismus as a result of irritation of the internal pterygoid muscle. Induration at the angle of the jaw and medial displacement of the tonsil and pharyngeal wall also occur with an anterior compartment abscess. By the time a patient with an abscess seeks medical attention, the source of the parapharyngeal space infection may be unclear. Reports indicate variable causes: incompletely or inadequately treated bacterial pharyngitis, tonsillitis, peritonsillar abscess, dental infection, bacterial parotitis, mastoiditis (Bezold's abscess from a mastoid tip infection traveling along the digastric muscles), petrositis, cervical adenitis with suppuration, cervical vertebral tubercular adenitis in the adult, or a foreign body. Local anesthetic infiltration for dental procedures and for management of post-tonsillectomy bleeding has been implicated in case reports.

## Clinical Manifestations

In addition to the preceding description, the patient may report tender cervical swelling, induration and erythema of the side of the neck, sore throat, dysphagia, trismus, hoarseness, malaise, chills, and diaphoresis. A variable low-grade fever is present with occasional temperature spikes. Examination discloses variable toxicity, respiratory distress, laryngeal edema, medial displacement of the lateral pharyngeal wall and inferior tonsil pole, trismus, and, infrequently, drooling. Indirect laryngoscopy may document ipsilateral vocal cord paralysis and obliteration of the piriform sinus. On palpation of the neck, a tender, high cervical mass is noted that initially is diffuse and later is fluctuant.

The complications of parapharyngeal abscess are related to the structures involved. Involvement of the carotid artery can produce hemiplegia from emboli. Internal jugular vein thrombosis with cephalad extension can lead to a cavernous sinus thrombosis, whereas inferior extension can lead to internal jugular vein thrombosis. Extension into the retropharyngeal region by a parapharyngeal abscess can lead to a posterior mediastinitis. Airway obstruction secondary to laryngeal edema and aspiration pneumonia from suppuration of the abscess into the pharynx have been reported.

Initially, a parapharyngeal abscess may be difficult to differentiate from a peritonsillar abscess, but the latter usually is less toxic and has a distinct, soft, fluctuant palatal mass. Parapharyngeal space abscesses are demonstrated well in axial computed tomographic (CT) scans of the neck. The CT scan has made the diagnosis and treatment of deep neck space infections more precise. In contrast to conventional radiologic studies, the CT scan distinguishes cellulitis of the neck, which usually does not require surgical treatment, from a deep neck abscess, which requires surgical drainage. With its ability to define differences in tissue density, CT scanning permits accurate determination of the extent of the abscess and its extension to and involvement of adjacent spaces. When there is more than one space involved, accurate assessment of these spaces may ensure sufficient surgical drainage. Vascular structures can be identified, as well as potential complications such as venous thrombosis. Gas also may be detected by CT scan.

## RETROPHARYNGEAL ABSCESS (POSTERIOR VISCERAL SPACE AND RETROVISCERAL SPACE ABSCESSES)

The anterior wall of the retropharyngeal space is the middle layer of the deep cervical fascia, which abuts the posterior esophageal wall (the superior pharyngeal constrictor muscle). The deep layer of the deep cervical fascia circumscribes the posterior wall of this potential space. Inferiorly, these two fasciae fuse to limit the depth of this pocket at a level between the first and second thoracic vertebrae. A retropharyngeal abscess can erode inferiorly through the junction of these fasciae to extend posteriorly into the prevertebral space. Subsequently, pus in the prevertebral space can descend inferiorly below the diaphragm to the psoas muscles.

The retropharyngeal space contains two paramedian chains of lymph nodes that receive drainage from the nasopharynx, adenoids, and posterior paranasal sinuses. These structures are prominent in early childhood and undergo atrophy at puberty. Retropharyngeal abscesses are most common in young children, and are thought to be secondary to suppurative adenitis of these retropharyngeal nodes. Other sources of infection are penetrating foreign bodies, endoscopy, trauma, pharyngitis, vertebral body osteomyelitis, petrositis, and dental procedures. In adults, tuberculosis and syphilis were common causes of retropharyngeal abscesses in the era before antibiotics.

### Clinical Manifestations

The symptoms of retropharyngeal abscess frequently begin insidiously after mild antecedent infection. Airway stridor from edema, cellulitis, or an obstructing mass is common. Laryngeal edema may cause dyspnea and tachypnea. Dysphagia, drooling, and odynophagia may occur. There is no trismus, but a stiff neck secondary to muscle tenderness may be present, along with an ipsilateral tender cervical adenopathy. In adults, the symptoms may be milder. Chest pain may reflect mediastinal extension. Early in the course, there is midline or unilateral swelling of the posterior pharynx. Later, gentle palpation may demonstrate a large fluctuant mass in the posterior pharynx. Vigorous palpation should be avoided, as the abscess may rupture into the upper airway.

### Treatment

The administration of intravenous antibiotics combined with incision and drainage is the treatment of choice for retropharyngeal abscess. If the mass is small, a peroral incision made with the patient in Rose's position (supine, with the neck hyperextended) may provide some drainage, but there is a slight risk of aspiration. If the mass is large or if there is persistent fever after peroral drainage, an external incision is preferred. A tracheostomy may be required if there is risk of compromising the airway.

Posterior mediastinitis can result from the spread of infection from the retropharyngeal area into the prevertebral space. Other complications may be seen when the abscess extends to the parapharyngeal space and involves the great vessels and cranial nerves.

## MICROBIOLOGY OF DEEP NECK ABSCESSES

Group A streptococci (Streptococcus pyogenes) and Staphylococcus aureus have been considered to be the organisms most frequently associated with pharyngeal space infections. Several recent studies, however, have demonstrated the presence of oral anaerobes in the majority of these infections. In recent studies of peritonsillar and retropharyngeal abscesses, anaerobes were isolated from all the patients and were the only isolates in about 20% of the patients. This is not surprising, because the main portals of entry for pharyngeal space infections are the nasopharynx, oropharynx, paranasal sinuses, mastoid, and lower molars—all of which are areas that are colonized with anaerobes. The predominant anaerobes isolated were Bacteroides species, peptostreptococci, and Fusobacterium species. The predominant aerobes were $\alpha$- and $\beta$-hemolytic streptococci, S aureus, Haemophilus species, and group A $\beta$-hemolytic streptococci. More than 70% of these isolates also were $\beta$-lactamase producers; these included all isolates of S aureus, 33% of Bacteroides melaninogenicus, and 67% of Bacteroides oralis. The data concerning the bacteriology of parapharyngeal abscesses are less complete. Many individual cases have been reported in which adequate cultures for both anaerobic and aerobic bacteria were performed. In general, the organisms isolated appear to follow the pattern seen with peritonsillar and retropharyngeal abscesses. One recent report of three parapharyngeal abscesses in children found, in addition to anaerobes, streptococci, and Haemophilus influenzae, one isolate each of Escherichia coli and Klebsiella pneumoniae.

One unusual cause of retropharyngeal abscess is Mycobacterium tuberculosis secondary to tuberculosis of the cervical spine eroding through the cervical vertebrae. Atypical mycobacteria and Coccidioides immitis have been isolated from retropharyngeal abscesses. These infections also were secondary to cervical vertebral osteomyelitis.

Because a large variety of organisms can be found in pharyngeal space infections, obtaining adequate cultures is of the greatest importance. The optimal material for culture is an aspirate of the pus obtained at operation. Throat swabs or swabs of the abscess obtained after drainage usually are inadequate because of contamination with normal oropharyngeal flora. The pus, when it is obtained, can be transported in a capped syringe if anaerobic transport media are not available. Most pathogenic obligate anaerobes can survive in a purulent exudate despite extended periods of air exposure. A Gram's stain of the exudate provides important clues to the bacterial cause. A Gram's stain showing a mixture of organisms suggests a mixed aerobic-anaerobic infection.

Because anaerobic bacteria are recovered frequently from deep neck abscesses, antimicrobial therapy should be directed at the eradication of these organisms. Antibiotic therapy is effective, however, only in conjunction with adequate surgical drainage. Resolution of some peritonsillar and retropharyngeal infections may occur without drainage when therapy is initiated at an early stage of infection, before suppuration occurs. Penicillin and ampicillin probably are adequate antibiotic therapy, but the frequent presence of penicillin-resistant bacteria such as S aureus and Bacteroides species may warrant the administration of antimicrobial agents that are effective against these organisms, such as clindamycin, amoxicillin/clavulanic acid, ticarcillin/clavulanic acid, ampicillin/sulbactam, or metronidazole in combination with an antistaphylococcic β-lactam. The newer, expanded-spectrum oral cephalosporins such as cefixime, quinolones, and new macrolides do not have adequate gram-positive or anaerobic coverage to enable them to be used alone for these infections.

## Selected Readings

Barratt GE, Koopmann CF, Couthard SW. Retropharyngeal abscess. A ten-year experience. Laryngoscope 1984;94:455.

Brook I. Aerobic and anaerobic bacteriology of peritonsillar abscesses in children. Acta Paediatr Scand 1981;70:831.

Brook I. Microbiology of retropharyngeal abscesses in children. Am J Dis Child 1987;141:202.

Dodds B, Manigila AJ. Peritonsillar and neck abscesses in the pediatric age group. Laryngoscope 1988;98:956.

Flodstrom A, Hallander HO. Microbiologic aspects of peritonsillar abscesses. Scand J Infect Dis 1976;8:157.

Kronenberg J, Wolf M, Leventon G. Peritonsillar abscess: Recurrence rate and the indication for tonsillectomy. Am J Otolaryngol 1987;8:82.

Morrison JE Jr, Pashley NR. Retropharyngeal abscess in children: A ten-year review. Pediatr Emerg Care 1988;4:9.

Ophir D, Bawnik J, Porat M, et al. Peritonsillar abscess. A prospective evaluation of outpatient management by needle aspiration. Arch Otolaryngol 1988;114:661.

Stringer SP, Schaefer SD, Close LG. A randomized trial for out-patient management of peritonsillar abscess. Arch Otolaryngol 1988;114:278.

*Principles and Practice of Pediatrics, Second Edition.*
edited by Frank A. Oski et al. J. B. Lippincott Company, Philadelphia © 1994.

# 36.6 *Otitis Externa*

## Mark W. Kline

Under normal circumstances, the external auditory canal is protected from infection by a physical barrier of squamous epithelium and a chemical barrier provided by the acidic pH of cerumen. Factors that disrupt these barriers, such as trauma, excessive cleansing or wetting, and high temperature and humidity, predispose to development of otitis externa.

## CLINICAL MANIFESTATIONS

A history of swimming or diving, or of repetitive ear cleansing with soapy water and cotton-tipped swabs often is elicited. Most patients are seen for evaluation of ear pain, itching, and fullness. Pain is exacerbated by manipulation of the pinna or tragus, a feature that is useful in differentiating between otitis externa and otitis media. Purulent discharge may be present in the external auditory canal. The canal walls are diffusely erythematous and edematous. Ipsilateral cervical lymph node enlargement may be noted, but fever usually is absent.

## DIAGNOSIS

Otitis externa is a clinical diagnosis. The historic features and physical findings are sufficiently characteristic that most patients present no real diagnostic dilemma. On the other hand, several other conditions mimic external otitis in some cases. Furunculosis is, in a sense, a focal form of otitis externa. Symptoms and signs resemble those of the diffuse condition, but otoscopy reveals a discrete furuncle or pustule with surrounding erythema in the outer portion of the external auditory canal. Otitis media causes ear pain that is not exacerbated by manipulation of the pinna. Perforation of the tympanic membrane usually results in symptomatic improvement, although the external canal may fill with purulent debris. Cleansing the canal permits otoscopic detection of the perforated tympanic membrane. A foreign body, usually visible in the external canal, may cause inflammation and discharge closely mimicking diffuse external otitis.

A microbiologic diagnosis helps to guide antibiotic therapy for otitis externa. A nasopharyngeal calcium alginate swab is used to obtain purulent material from the auditory canal for routine bacterial cultures and Gram's stain. Special stains and cultures for fungi, mycobacteria, or viruses may be indicated under unusual circumstances. The most common causative agents are *Staphylococcus aureus*, *Pseudomonas aeruginosa* and other gram-negative bacilli, and group A *Streptococcus*. Infections frequently are polymicrobial. Fungi, such as *Aspergillus niger* and *Candida albicans*, are isolated occasionally as the sole or predominant organisms. Varicella zoster virus may produce external otitis with ipsilateral oral vesicles and facial nerve paralysis.

## TREATMENT

After cultures are obtained, the auditory canal can be flushed with 3% saline or 2% acetic acid and dried with a cotton-tipped applicator. A suspension of polymyxin B-neomycin-hydrocortisone (Cortisporin) is instilled in the canal four times daily, generally for 10 to 14 days. Swelling may be so severe initially that drops will not enter the auditory canal. In these cases, Cortisporin cream may be placed in the canal on a wick and removed in about 24 hours when inflammation has subsided. Cutaneous sensitivity to neomycin, with local signs and symptoms mimicking those of otitis externa, is a potential complication of therapy with Cortisporin. Some authorities recommend initiating therapy with Cortisporin, then using an agent that does not contain neomycin (such as clindamycin or polymyxin B drops) once culture results are known. Prevention of recurrent otitis externa may be accomplished by use of 2% acetic acid ear drops after swimming.

Systemic antibiotic therapy for otitis externa is indicated if the patient is febrile or if there is associated cervical adenitis or cellulitis of adjacent tissues. Appropriate oral antibiotics for initial therapy include trimethoprim/sulfamethoxazole, cefuroxime axetil, or amoxicillin/clavulanate.

Malignant otitis externa, a particularly aggressive form of the disease, generally is diagnosed in elderly patients with diabetes. It occurs rarely in immunocompromised children, and is characterized by extensive destruction of soft tissues, cartilage, bone, and nerves around the external auditory canal. Granulation tissue may be seen in the canal itself. The causative organism is *P aeruginosa*. Effective therapy combines surgical debridement with intravenous antibiotics that are active against *Pseudomonas*.

## Suggested Readings

Bergstrom L. Diseases of the external ear. In: Bluestone CD, Stool SE, eds. Pediatric otolaryngology. Philadelphia: WB Saunders, 1983:347.

Feigin RD, Sheerin KA. Otitis externa. In: Feigin RD, Cherry JD, eds. Textbook of pediatric infectious diseases, ed 3. Philadelphia: WB Saunders, 1992:172.

Senturia BH, Marcus MD, Lucente FE. Diseases of the external ear. An otologic-dermatologic manual. New York: Grune & Stratton, 1980:31.

*Principles and Practice of Pediatrics, Second Edition.*
edited by Frank A. Oski et al. J. B. Lippincott Company, Philadelphia © 1994.

# 36.7 *Otitis Media*

Mark W. Kline

Otitis media is a general term denoting inflammation of the middle ear. Acute otitis media refers to suppurative middle ear infection of relatively sudden clinical onset. The term chronic otitis media encompasses several entities of insidious onset that are difficult to differentiate by clinical or pathologic criteria. Chronic suppurative conditions include tubotympanitis (eg, permanent perforation syndrome), atticoantral disease (eg, Shrapnell's disease or cholesteatoma), and end-stage disease (eg, atelectatic ear, adhesive otitis media, or tympanosclerosis). Otitis media with effusion (secretory otitis media) is a chronic condition that is characterized by the persistence of fluid in the middle ear. Temporally, otitis media with effusion usually follows an episode of acute otitis media. Extension of inflammation beyond the mucoperiosteal lining of the middle ear constitutes a complication of otitis media (eg, mastoiditis, epidural abscess).

## EPIDEMIOLOGY AND PATHOGENESIS

Otitis media is one of the most common infectious diseases of childhood. In one large study, 33% of pediatric office visits for illness of any kind were attributable to disease of the middle ear (acute otitis media or otitis media with effusion). Infants and young children are at highest risk for the development of otitis media, with a peak prevalence between 6 and 36 months of age. Two of every three children have at least one episode of otitis media before their first birthday. By 3 years of age, 80% of children have had at least one episode of acute otitis media, and nearly 50% have had three or more episodes. After an initial episode of acute otitis media, 40% of children have middle ear effusion that persists for at least 4 weeks, and 10% have persistent effusion after 3 months. Children in whom otitis media with effusion develops early in life are at increased risk of recurrent acute or chronic middle ear disease. The overall prevalence of otitis media with effusion in childhood is estimated to be 15% to 20%. The incidence and prevalence of otitis media decline after about 6 years of age.

Otitis media occurs more commonly in boys than in girls, and is particularly prevalent among Eskimos and Native Americans, and among children with cleft palate or other craniofacial defects. A familial predisposition to otitis media may exist in some cases. Other implicated predisposing factors include lower socioeconomic group status, bottle-feeding in the horizontal position, bottle-feeding versus breast-feeding, day-care center attendance, and atopy. In general, the highest rates of otitis media are observed in the winter months, coinciding with the peak incidence of respiratory viral infections.

Abnormal eustachian tube function underlies most cases of otitis media. The eustachian tube normally permits equilibration of middle ear pressure with atmospheric pressure, protects the middle ear from reflux of nasopharyngeal secretions, and drains secretions from the middle ear into the nasopharynx. Either obstruction or abnormal patency of the eustachian tube may lead to the development of otitis media. Intrinsic (eg, inflammation secondary to infection or allergy) and extrinsic (eg, tumor or adenoid enlargement) types of mechanical eustachian tube obstruction are recognized. Functional obstruction, caused by persistent collapse of an abnormally compliant eustachian tube, an abnormal active opening mechanism, or both, is common in young children and individuals with cleft palate. An abnormally patent, or patulous, eustachian tube, which is found commonly among Native American populations, permits reflux of nasopharyngeal secretions into the middle ear. Reflux, aspiration, or insufflation of nasopharyngeal bacteria into the middle ear on any basis leads to mucoperiosteal inflammation and otitis media.

## ACUTE OTITIS MEDIA

### Clinical Manifestations

The classic description of acute otitis media is of a child with upper respiratory tract infection who suddenly develops fever, otalgia, and hearing loss. A classic presentation, however, may be the exception rather than the rule. Fever and hearing loss are inconstant features of the disease, and otalgia may not be reported. In many young children in particular, otitis media must be inferred on the basis of nonspecific symptoms (eg, fretfulness or irritability, anorexia, loose stools) and subtle findings suggestive of middle ear disease (eg, scratching or tugging at the ear). Otitis media must be excluded before any child is labeled as having fever without localizing signs, or fever of undetermined origin.

The appearance of the tympanic membrane is key to the diagnosis of acute otitis media. All wax and debris must be removed from the external canal before examination. Otoscopy usually reveals a hyperemic, opaque tympanic membrane with distorted or absent light reflex and indistinct landmarks. A red appearance of the drum may be noted if the child is agitated or if inadequate illumination is provided; this is not evidence of otitis media in the absence of other findings. Adequate assessment of tympanic membrane mobility requires pneumatic otoscopy, using an ear speculum large enough to occlude the external canal completely. Decreased mobility of the drum results from either eustachian tube dysfunction or middle ear effusion.

The diagnosis of acute otitis media usually is made readily. Referred otalgia may be associated with infections and other conditions of the tonsils, adenoids, teeth, or pharynx, however. The tympanic membrane should appear normal in these conditions. Purulent otorrhea may indicate otitis media with tympanic membrane perforation, but otitis externa must be excluded. In diseases of the external canal, pain frequently is elicited by manipulation of the pinna.

### Specific Diagnosis

Bacteria may be isolated from middle ear fluid in about two thirds of patients with acute otitis media. The approximate prevalence rates of various bacterial agents of otitis media beyond the neonatal period are shown in Table 36-13. Several additional pieces of information are noteworthy. Eleven serotypes of *Streptococcus pneumoniae* account for about 85% of cases of otitis media caused by that organism, and all are included in the currently available pneumococcal vaccine. Most *Haemophilus influenzae* isolates from the middle ear are non-typeable; only a minority are type b. Many *H influenzae* strains and most strains of *Moraxella catarrhalis* produce β-lactamase and, therefore, are resistant to ampicillin and penicillin. Bacterial cultures of middle ear fluid are sterile in about one third of patients with acute otitis media. Studies assessing the role of viruses have found a low rate of isolation from middle ear fluid, with respiratory syncytial virus and influenza viruses being most common. *Chlamydia trachomatis* and *Mycoplasma pneumoniae* probably are infrequent causes of otitis media.

Other than the more frequent occurrence of disease caused by enteric gram-negative bacteria (about 20% of cases), and oc-

**TABLE 36-13. Bacterial Etiology of Acute Otitis Media in Children***

| Bacterial Isolate | Prevalence (%) |
|---|---|
| Streptococcus pneumoniae | 31 |
| Haemophilus influenzae | 22 |
| Moraxella catarrhalis | 7 |
| Group A Streptococcus | 2 |
| Enteric gram-negative bacteria | 1 |
| Staphylococcus aureus | 1 |
| Other | 3 |
| No bacterial isolate | 33 |

* Based on cultures obtained by needle tympanocentesis.

casional recovery of usual neonatal pathogens (eg, group B *Streptococcus*), the cause of otitis media in neonates is similar to that in older children.

Diagnosis of the specific causative agent is desirable in unusual or complicated cases of otitis media. Qualitative nasopharyngeal cultures correlate poorly with cultures obtained from middle ear fluid. Therefore, when the diagnosis of otitis media is in doubt or an unusual pathogen is suspected, aspiration of middle ear fluid should be performed. Specific indications for needle tympanocentesis or myringotomy include serious illness or toxicity; suppurative complications (eg, mastoiditis or meningitis); otitis media in the neonate or immunocompromised patient; otitis media in a patient receiving mechanical ventilation; and otitis media developing in spite of, or failing to respond to, antimicrobial therapy. Discordance in middle ear cultures may be found in 20% of cases of bilateral otitis media.

Pediatricians generally obtain middle ear fluid cultures by needle tympanocentesis. Rubber tubing can be attached to a plunger-free tuberculin syringe, leaving both hands free and per-

mitting the application of negative pressure orally to obtain specimens. The posterosuperior quadrant of the tympanic membrane should be avoided when performing tympanocentesis. Done incorrectly, the procedure may lead to bleeding, hearing loss, or other complications. Myringotomy, which is incision of the tympanic membrane, usually is performed by an otolaryngologist and is preferred when therapeutic drainage of the middle ear is desired.

## Treatment

In the era before antibiotics, otitis media frequently resolved spontaneously, but tympanic membrane perforation and suppurative sequelae were common. Antibiotic therapy has changed the clinical course of otitis media dramatically, arresting infection before complications develop. A number of agents that are active against the common bacterial pathogens of otitis media are available (Table 36-14). As a rule, children younger than 1 month who have otitis media should be admitted to the hospital. Cultures of blood, cerebrospinal fluid, and middle ear fluid should be obtained, and parenteral antibiotic therapy should be initiated. If blood and cerebrospinal fluid cultures are sterile after 72 hours and the infant appears well, with disease limited to the middle ear, therapy may be completed with an oral antibiotic that is active against the middle ear isolate.

The choice of an antibiotic for acute otitis media must take into account many factors, including the local antibiotic susceptibility patterns of common bacterial isolates, compliance of the patient population with various antibiotic regimens, and the cost of the various antibiotics under consideration. Oral amoxicillin is a reasonable first choice for the treatment of otitis media in older infants and children. An alternative agent may be needed if there is no response to therapy in 72 to 96 hours, or if a resistant organism is cultured from middle ear fluid. Cefuroxime axetil, cefixime, cefpodoxime proxetil, and amoxicillin/clavulanate are considerably more expensive than are other alternative antibiotics. Antibiotic ear drops are of no value in acute otitis media.

**TABLE 36-14. Antimicrobial Therapy for Acute Otitis Media**

| Age of Patient | Drug | Dosage* |
|---|---|---|
| Less than 1 mo | Ampicillin and | 200 mg/kg/d IM or IV in 4 divided doses |
| | Gentamicin | 7.5 mg/kg/d IM or IV in 3 divided doses |
| 1 mo to 15 y | Amoxicillin | 40 mg/kg/d po in 3 divided doses |
| | or Trimethoprim/sulfamethoxazole | 8–10 mg/kg/d trimethoprim po in 2 divided doses |
| | or Erythromycin/sulfisoxazole | 40 mg/kg/d erythromycin po in 3 divided doses |
| | or Cefuroxime axetil | 250–500 mg/d po in 2 divided doses |
| | or Cefixime | 8 mg/kg/d po in 1 dose |
| | or Cefpodoxime proxetil | 10 mg/kg/d po in 2 divided doses |
| | or Amoxicillin/clavulanate | 40 mg/kg/d po in 3 divided doses |

* *IM*, intramuscularly; *IV*, intravenously; *po*, orally.

Diverse opinions exist concerning indications for myringotomy in acute otitis media. Therapeutic myringotomy should be considered for relief of persistent severe pain or persistent conductive hearing loss. Nasal and oral decongestants, sometimes administered in combination with an oral antihistamine, have been advocated for relief of nasal and eustachian tube obstruction in children with otitis media. In clinical trials, these preparations have had equivocal, and sometimes contradictory, results in affecting rates of treatment failure, recurrence, or persistence of middle ear effusion. At present, the efficacy of these preparations is unproven, and their routine use cannot be recommended.

Supportive therapy, including acetaminophen and local heat, may be helpful in children with acute otitis media. Sedation should be avoided.

Ideally, children with acute otitis media should be reexamined after they have received 72 to 96 hours of antibiotic therapy. If symptoms and signs persist, needle tympanocentesis or myringotomy should be performed and subsequent antibiotic therapy determined by culture results. The usual duration of antibiotic therapy in uncomplicated cases of acute otitis media is 10 days. Every child should be examined at the end of therapy to document resolution of tympanic membrane inflammation. Complete resolution of middle ear effusion may require 2 to 3 months.

## RECURRENT ACUTE OTITIS MEDIA

Recurrent episodes of acute otitis media occur commonly. Underlying susceptibility to middle ear infection is important in the development of recurrent otitis media; recurrences represent reinfection more often than recrudescence or relapse. Early development of otitis media caused by *S pneumoniae* seems particularly likely to predispose to recurrent otitis media.

Several strategies have been employed for the prevention of recurrent acute otitis media. Antibiotic prophylaxis with amoxicillin (20 mg/kg once daily) or sulfisoxazole (75 mg/kg/d in two divided doses) is reasonable in the child who has at least three episodes of acute otitis media within 6 months or four episodes in 1 year. Prophylaxis generally is continued for 3 to 6 months, at which time the antibiotic is discontinued and the child is observed. Pneumococcal vaccine may benefit individual children, but it is least efficacious in infants, the group at highest risk for recurrent disease. Myringotomy with tympanostomy tube insertion is an option for patients who fail to respond to antibiotic prophylaxis. Adenoidectomy may be of benefit for selected patients. The relative efficacies of the various strategies for prophylaxis, alone and in combination, are unknown.

## OTITIS MEDIA WITH EFFUSION

After an episode of acute otitis media, 10% of children have middle ear effusion that persists for 3 months or longer (chronic otitis media with effusion). Clinically, otitis media with effusion is characterized by a sensation of fullness in the ears, muffled hearing, and tinnitus. Pneumatic otoscopy usually reveals an opaque tympanic membrane with decreased mobility. Frequent acute otitis media, catarrh, exposure to cigarette smoke, and atopy may increase the risk of persistent effusion. Language, behavioral, and learning deficits often result.

Bacteria are recovered from one third to one half of all middle ear fluid specimens obtained at myringotomy in cases of otitis media with effusion. The bacteriology closely mimics that of acute otitis media. It is not known whether the bacteria have a direct pathogenic role, but an initial course of antibiotic therapy similar to that used for acute otitis media seems warranted. Oral decongestant-antihistamine combinations and corticosteroids have not been found to be effective in the treatment of persistent middle ear effusion. Evaluation for respiratory allergy, obstructive adenoid enlargement, immune deficiency, or anatomic abnormalities such as submucous cleft palate may be necessary in patients whose disease does not respond to treatment.

For patients whose condition fails to respond to medical therapy, myringotomy with tympanostomy tube insertion may prevent subsequent accumulation of middle ear fluid and improve hearing. Tympanostomy tubes also are used to prevent structural middle ear damage and cholesteatoma in selected cases. Tonsillectomy is not efficacious in the treatment of otitis media with effusion.

## COMPLICATIONS

Serious complications of otitis media are uncommon when appropriate medical therapy is initiated promptly. Extracranial complications include serous or purulent labyrinthitis, mastoiditis, osteomyelitis of the temporal bone, and facial nerve paralysis. Intracranial complications are subdivided into meningeal and extrameningeal complications. Epidural and subdural abscess, meningitis, lateral sinus thrombosis, and otitic hydrocephalus are reported meningeal complications of otitis media. Lateral sinus thrombosis is characterized by high temperature, chills, signs and symptoms of increased intracranial pressure, and septicemia with embolization. The mortality rate is about 25%. Otitic hydrocephalus may follow acute otitis media by several weeks, and usually is associated with impaired intracranial venous drainage. Hydrocephalus commonly subsides spontaneously. Extrameningeal complications of otitis media include brain abscess and petrositis.

## Selected Readings

Bernard PAM, Stenstrom RJ, Feldman W, et al. Randomized, controlled trial comparing long-term sulfonamide therapy to ventilation tubes for otitis media with effusion. Pediatrics 1991;88:215.

Cantekin EI, Mandel EM, Bluestone CD, et al. Lack of efficacy of a decongestant-antihistamine combination for otitis media with effusion ("secretory" otitis media) in children. N Engl J Med 1983;308:297.

Carlin SA, Marchant CD, Shurin PA, et al. Early recurrences of otitis media: Reinfection or relapse? J Pediatr 1987;110:20.

Feigin RD, Kline MW, Hyatt SR, Ford KL III. Otitis media. In: Feigin RD, Cherry JD, eds. Textbook of pediatric infectious diseases, ed 3. Philadelphia: WB Saunders, 1992:174.

Giebink GS, Canafax DM, Kempthorne J. Antimicrobial treatment of acute otitis media. J Pediatr 1991;119:495.

Kaplan SL, Feigin RD. Simplified technique for tympanocentesis. Pediatrics 1978;62:418.

Macknin ML, Jones PK. Oral dexamethasone for treatment of persistent middle ear effusion. Pediatrics 1985;75:329.

Moran DM, Mutchie KD, Higbee MD, et al. The use of an antihistamine-decongestant in conjunction with an antiinfective drug in the treatment of acute otitis media. J Pediatr 1982;101:132.

Teele DW, Klein JO, Rosner B, et al. Epidemiology of otitis media during the first seven years of life in children in greater Boston: A prospective cohort study. J Infect Dis 1989;160:83.

Teele DW, Klein JO, Rosner EA, et al. Middle ear disease and the practice of pediatrics: Burden during the first five years of life. JAMA 1983;249:1026.

*Principles and Practice of Pediatrics, Second Edition.*
edited by Frank A. Oski et al. J. B. Lippincott Company, Philadelphia © 1994.

# 36.8 *Mastoiditis*

## Mark W. Kline

Inflammation of the mucoperiosteal lining of the mastoid air cells usually accompanies otitis media. Clinically evident suppurative infection, or mastoiditis, develops when inflammation causes progressive swelling and obstruction to drainage of exudative materials from the mastoid. Mastoiditis is uncommon in this era of effective antibiotic therapy for otitis media, but it remains a potentially life-threatening disease requiring prompt recognition and appropriate treatment.

## CLINICAL MANIFESTATIONS

Children with mastoiditis almost invariably have otitis media concomitantly. Classically, the child with acute mastoiditis presents with fever, otalgia, and postauricular swelling and redness. Swelling typically occurs over the mastoid process, pushing the earlobe superiorly and laterally, but in infancy, it may occur above the ear, displacing the pinna inferiorly and laterally. The clinical presentation of acute mastoiditis may be quite subtle, particularly in the child who has received oral antibiotic therapy for otitis media (so-called masked mastoiditis). Mastoiditis should be considered in a patient with otitis media that is unresponsive to antibiotic therapy.

Chronic mastoiditis generally develops in individuals with long-standing middle ear disease. The clinical course is indolent. Fever and local signs referable to the mastoid may or may not be present. Chronic purulent drainage from the ear and conductive hearing loss may occur.

## DIAGNOSIS

In some cases, the diagnosis of mastoiditis can be made with confidence on clinical grounds alone. Plain roentgenograms may show coalescence of mastoid air cells and loss of normal bony trabeculations. If osteomyelitis develops, sclerosis or destruction of adjacent bone sometimes is noted. Abnormalities on roentgenograms of the mastoid bone do not necessarily imply mastoiditis, however, and, conversely, normal study results do not exclude the diagnosis. Computed tomography sometimes is helpful in cases in which clinical findings and plain roentgenograms are equivocal or nonspecific.

A bacteriologic diagnosis is highly desirable in cases of mastoiditis. Tympanocentesis obtained through an intact tympanic membrane yields bacteriologic information that correlates well with specimens obtained from the mastoid bone itself. Common causative agents of acute mastoiditis include *Streptococcus pneumoniae*, group A *Streptococcus*, *Staphylococcus aureus*, and *Haemophilus influenzae*. In chronic mastoiditis, prevalent isolates include anaerobic bacteria, such as *Peptococcus* spp., *Actinomyces* spp., or *Bacteroides* spp., and aerobic gram-negative bacilli (including *Pseudomonas aeruginosa*). Chronic mastoiditis frequently is polymicrobial. *Mycobacterium tuberculosis* rarely causes chronic mastoiditis today, but it should be considered if there are suggestive epidemiologic or historic features in the case.

In all cases of mastoiditis, specimens from the middle ear or mastoid should be cultured aerobically and anaerobically, and a Gram's stain should be performed. Special fungal and mycobacterial stains and cultures may be indicated in some cases. A skin test for tuberculosis should be performed in all cases of chronic mastoiditis or if there is a history of exposure to tuberculosis.

## TREATMENT

Patients with acute onset of symptoms and no evidence of intracranial or local extracranial complications of mastoiditis usually are treated initially with myringotomy and parenteral antibiotics alone. Signs of increased intracranial pressure or meningeal irritation signal complications of mastoiditis, such as meningitis, brain abscess, epidural abscess, subdural empyema, or venous sinus thrombosis. A postauricular fluctuant area implies subperiosteal abscess formation. Because of proximity to the mastoid bone, other local structures may be involved by infection, producing facial nerve paralysis, jugular venous thrombosis, or internal carotid artery erosion and hemorrhage. Lack of appropriate response to medical therapy or development of complications necessitates mastoidectomy and possibly other surgical interventions.

The initial selection of specific antibiotic therapy is made empirically, with some guidance provided by Gram's stain of specimens from the middle ear or mastoid. In acute mastoiditis, a combination of a penicillinase-resistant penicillin (such as nafcillin or oxacillin) and one of the third-generation cephalosporins (such as cefotaxime or ceftriaxone) is reasonable. Alternatively, cefuroxime alone may be employed for initial coverage. In chronic mastoiditis, a penicillinase-resistant penicillin and an aminoglycoside with activity against *Pseudomonas* (such as amikacin or tobramycin) may be used initially. Clindamycin is a reasonable alternative to the semisynthetic penicillin if enhanced activity against anaerobic bacteria is desired. Eventual antibiotic therapy is determined by the bacteriology of the process. Provided complications have not occurred, and if it is feasible on the basis of the organisms' susceptibility to oral agents, the course of therapy can be completed orally once signs of acute inflammation have subsided. The minimum course of therapy for mastoiditis is 21 days, and it may be longer if complications of infection have occurred. For patients discharged on oral antibiotic therapy, careful monitoring of compliance and documentation of bactericidal activity in serum are desirable.

## Selected Readings

Holt GR, Gates GA. Masked mastoiditis. Laryngoscope 1983;93:1034.
Lewis K, Cherry JD. Mastoiditis. In: Feigin RD, Cherry JD, eds. Textbook of pediatric infectious diseases, ed 3. Philadelphia: WB Saunders, 1992:189.
Nadal D, Herrmann P, Baumann A, et al. Acute mastoiditis: Clinical, microbiological, and therapeutic aspects. Eur J Pediatr 1990;149:560.
Ogle JW, Lauer BA. Acute mastoiditis. Diagnosis and complications. Am J Dis Child 1986;140:1178.
Samuel J, Fernandes CM, Steinberg JL. Intracranial otogenic complications: A persisting problem. Laryngoscope 1986;96:272.
Venezio FR, Naidich TP, Shulman ST. Complications of mastoiditis with special emphasis on venous sinus thrombosis. J Pediatr 1982;101:509.

*Principles and Practice of Pediatrics, Second Edition.*
edited by Frank A. Oski et al. J. B. Lippincott Company, Philadelphia © 1994.

# 36.9 *Uvulitis*

### Ellen R. Wald

Infections of the uvula have been reported infrequently in the medical literature. When the uvula is the most inflamed structure in the posterior pharynx of a febrile child, acute infection should be suspected.

## ETIOLOGY

The bacterial agents that cause uvulitis in children include *Haemophilus influenzae* type b and *Streptococcus pyogenes*. Uvulitis caused by *H influenzae* may occur concurrently with epiglottitis or as an isolated site of infection. Two cases of uvulitis and associated epiglottitis caused by *Streptococcus pneumoniae* have been reported in adults. Uvulitis caused by *S pyogenes* appears always to occur in concert with pharyngitis. Other bacterial causes have not been reported; no search for viral agents has been conducted. Recently, two cases of uvulitis caused by *Candida albicans* were reported in immunocompetent infants.

## EPIDEMIOLOGY

The epidemiology of uvulitis is the epidemiology of its two etiologic agents: *S pyogenes* and *H influenzae* type b. As such, it can be seen in the school-age child between 5 and 15 years of age (the so-called streptococcal age group) in association with pharyngitis. Similarly, it can be seen in the "*H influenzae* age group" of 3 months to 5 years. Cases of uvulitis in association with epiglottitis have been reported in the United States as well as in England. The seasonality of infections caused by *S pyogenes* and *H influenzae* is primarily winter and spring, but both can occur throughout the year.

## PATHOPHYSIOLOGY

Uvulitis is an acute cellulitis characterized by dramatic swelling and erythema. Infection of the uvula probably arises from direct invasion by *S pyogenes* or *H influenzae* type b, both being recognized as normal nasopharyngeal flora. In the latter case, epiglottitis also may arise by direct extension, and the bacteremia may result secondarily from either the uvula or the epiglottis as a primary site of infection. Alternatively, the pathogenesis of most *H influenzae* type b infections is by hematogenous spread from the nasopharynx as a portal of entry.

## CLINICAL MANIFESTATIONS

In a review of five patients with streptococcal uvulitis, all had an associated pharyngitis. The patients had low-grade fever and sore throat. Three of the five patients experienced a choking or gagging sensation in the pharynx that induced coughing and spitting; one of these patients also had drooling. Although pharyngitis was noted on physical examination, the swelling and erythema of the uvula were most dramatic. None of the patients had evidence of respiratory distress.

In patients with uvulitis and epiglottitis, the presentation usually is typical for epiglottitis, with sudden onset of high temperature, dysphagia, and increasing respiratory distress. Rapkin, however, reported a case of uvulitis/epiglottitis in which the epiglottitis initially was unsuspected. The lateral neck radiograph (performed to evaluate the possibility of retropharyngeal abscess) belatedly alerted the clinicians to the correct diagnosis.

In patients with uvulitis and no epiglottitis, the presentation may be similar to that of epiglottitis (acute onset of fever, odynophagia, and drooling) or less specific (fever and irritability or decreased appetite). The diagnosis in the latter case is apparent on physical examination of the oropharynx, which shows a swollen and erythematous uvula.

## DIAGNOSIS

The diagnosis of streptococcal uvulitis is suspected when a school-age child is seen with low-grade fever, pharyngitis, and uvulitis. The diagnosis is confirmed by the recovery of *S pyogenes* from a surface culture of the throat, the uvula, or both. A lateral neck radiograph should be performed to eliminate the possibility of a concurrent epiglottitis.

The diagnosis of uvulitis caused by *H influenzae* is suspected in a highly febrile infant or preschool child who has uvular inflammation on physical examination. A lateral neck radiograph must be performed to evaluate the possibility of epiglottitis unless there are obvious signs of upper respiratory obstruction, in which case immediate endoscopy is warranted. If epiglottitis is discovered, the airway must be secured and appropriate parenteral antimicrobial agents initiated after blood and surface cultures are obtained. Any surface culture that is obtained to search for *H influenzae* must be plated onto chocolate agar. After appropriate cultures are obtained, parenteral antimicrobial agents should be initiated, as in other bacteremic *H influenzae* infections.

## DIFFERENTIAL DIAGNOSIS

The differential diagnosis of the patient with acute onset of fever, dysphagia, and drooling includes herpes simplex gingivostomatitis, uvulitis, epiglottitis, severe pharyngitis, and peritonsillar or retropharyngeal abscess. Although it is appropriate to be extremely cautious in examining the pharynx of any patient with suspected epiglottitis, some children tolerate attempted visualization of the oral cavity without undue upset. Instrumentation with a tongue blade should be avoided. If the examination does not show gingivostomatitis or peritonsillar abscess, a lateral neck radiograph should be performed. If epiglottitis or retropharyngeal abscess is confirmed, airway management and antimicrobial agents or incision and drainage combined with antimicrobial agents are indicated, respectively. If the lateral neck is normal and the uvula is inflamed, uvulitis with or without pharyngitis is confirmed.

Noninfectious inflammation of the uvula may be caused by allergy (as in angioedema) or irritants (as in marijuana abuse).

## TREATMENT

The treatment of uvulitis is guided primarily by the associated pharyngitis or epiglottitis, if either is present. In the case of streptococcal pharyngitis, penicillin therapy for 10 days is most appropriate; penicillin V, orally, 250 to 500 mg three times daily, will suffice. Clinical improvement of uvulitis and pharyngitis should occur within 24 to 48 hours after the initiation of treatment.

In the case of uvulitis/epiglottitis, management of the airway is most important. This can be accomplished by nasotracheal intubation or tracheotomy. Appropriate parenteral antibiotic therapy usually should be initiated.

In the case of uvulitis without epiglottitis, antimicrobial therapy appropriate for bacteremic *H influenzae* type b is necessary. In geographic areas where β-lactamase–producing *H influenzae* is prevalent, an advanced-generation cephalosporin is appropriate, such as cefuroxime, 150 mg/kg/d in three divided doses, or cefotaxime, 200 mg/kg/d in four divided doses. In a patient with serious penicillin hypersensitivity, chloramphenicol, 75 mg/kg/d in four divided doses, also is a satisfactory regimen. After the fever has subsided and the patient has improved clinically, an oral antimicrobial agent can be substituted. Clinical improvement can be expected within 24 to 48 hours. The results of blood and surface cultures then can be used to guide therapy. For an ampicillin-sensitive *H influenzae* organism, amoxicillin, 40 mg/kg/d in three divided doses, should be prescribed to complete a 7- to 10-day course of treatment. For β-lactamase–producing *H influenzae*, a variety of oral agents can be prescribed, including cefaclor, 40 mg/kg/d in three divided doses; sulfamethoxazole/trimethoprim, 40/8 mg/kg/d in two divided doses; erythromycin/sulfisoxazole, 50/150 mg/kg/d in four divided doses; or amoxicillin/potassium clavulanate, 40 mg/kg/d of the amoxicillin component in three divided doses.

## COMPLICATIONS

In extreme cases of uvulitis, obstruction of the oral airway may occur. When uvulitis is associated with epiglottitis, complete airway obstruction may result. The latter should be managed with nasotracheal intubation or tracheostomy. In isolated uvulitis, if obstruction is present, a nasopharyngeal airway will suffice until medical therapy results in clinical improvement.

### Selected Readings

Gorfinkel HJ, Brown R, Kabins SA. Acute infectious epiglottitis in adults. Ann Intern Med 1969;70:289.
Kotloff KL, Wald ER. Uvulitis in children. Pediatr Infect Dis J 1983;2:392.
Krober MS, Weir MR. Acute uvulitis apparently caused by Candida albicans. Pediatr Infect Dis J 1991;10:73.
Li KI, Kiernan S, Wald ER. Isolated uvulitis due to *Haemophilus influenzae* type b. Pediatrics 1984;74:1054.
Rapkin RH. Simultaneous uvulitis and epiglottitis. JAMA 1980;43:1843.
Westerman EL. Acute uvulitis associated with epiglottitis. Arch Otolaryngol Head Neck Surg 1986;112:448.

*Principles and Practice of Pediatrics, Second Edition.*
edited by Frank A. Oski et al. J. B. Lippincott Company, Philadelphia © 1994.

# 36.10 *Epiglottitis/ Supraglottitis*

Ellen R. Wald

Supraglottitis is an inflammation of the structures above the glottis, including the epiglottis, aryepiglottic folds, and arytenoids. The most common site of involvement is the epiglottis.

## ETIOLOGY

*Haemophilus influenzae* type b causes more than 90% of all supraglottitis involving the epiglottis. This undoubtedly will change, however, consequent to the increased use of *H influenzae* type b conjugate vaccines in infancy. Rarely, other organisms, including *Staphylococcus aureus*, *Streptococcus pyogenes*, and *Streptococcus pneumoniae*, have been documented. Several examples of supraglottitis involving mainly the aryepiglottic folds have been described and attributed to *S pyogenes*. Cases caused by *S pneumoniae* have occurred most often in adults.

Viral causes of supraglottitis have not been investigated extensively. Parainfluenza virus and herpesviruses have been reported to cause supraglottitis in individual cases.

## EPIDEMIOLOGY

Although supraglottitis resulting from infection with *H influenzae* type b can occur at any time from infancy to adulthood, it most often affects children between 2 and 7 years of age. Epiglottitis is unique among illnesses caused by *H influenzae* type b in that it characteristically develops in older children; infection with this bacterial species usually is seen in those aged 3 months to 3 years. Cases occur year-round and boys and girls are affected equally. The illness has been observed in virtually all geographic areas, but it is rare in those populations in which the peak age incidence of meningitis caused by *H influenzae* type b is shifted toward infancy (ie, in Alaskan Eskimos and Native Americans). Occasionally, associated cases of invasive disease caused by *H influenzae* type b may precede or follow a case of *H influenzae* epiglottitis within a household or day-care center. When *S pyogenes* causes supraglottitis, the children most often are of early school age and their illness occurs during the winter and early spring.

## PATHOPHYSIOLOGY

Epiglottitis is the second most common expression of invasive disease caused by *H influenzae* type b. This bacterial species may be part of the normal pharyngeal flora or it may be acquired by respiratory transmission from an intimate contact. In the absence of serum antibody to the polysaccharide capsule of *H influenzae* type b (which is protective), these bacteria may become blood-borne and subsequently seed the meninges, epiglottis, facial skin, lungs, or joints.

Supraglottitis is an acute cellulitis of the structure of the upper airway, characterized clinically by dramatic swelling and erythema. In cases of epiglottitis, as the edema increases, the epiglottis curls posteriorly and inferiorly to produce a horseshoe appearance on cross-section (Fig 36-15). The aperture of the airway is reduced considerably. If the epiglottis has any remaining mobility, an inspiratory effort will draw it down to occlude the airway further. With the airway partially obstructed, a bolus of mucus easily can complete the obstruction of the glottic orifice. Histologically, there is a diffuse infiltration with immature polymorphonuclear leukocytes and inflammatory edema. Neither membranes nor severe ulceration of the mucosa is seen, although slight ulceration on the surface of the epiglottis may be observed.

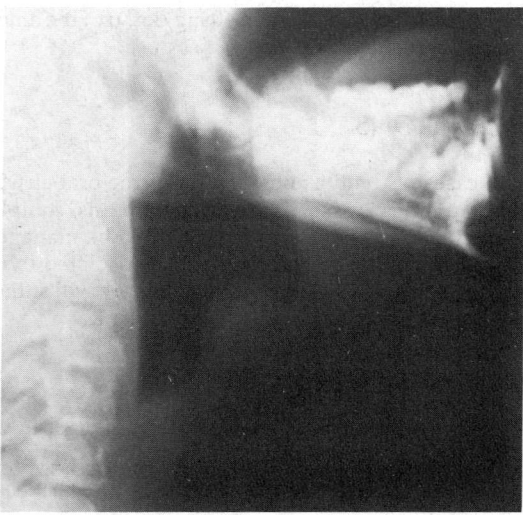

**Figure 36-15.** Lateral neck radiograph showing a positive "thumb" sign and ballooning of the hypopharynx.

## CLINICAL MANIFESTATIONS

The child with typical epiglottitis usually has been completely well or has had a limited prodrome of mild upper respiratory symptoms before the onset of sore throat and dysphagia. High temperature (39 °C to 40 °C) generally is noted almost simultaneously. Within a short time, evidence of toxemia and respiratory distress develops. The youngster appears extremely anxious and prefers to remain sitting up, usually leaning forward with the chin hyperextended. The respiratory effort is slow and labored; drooling as a manifestation of dysphagia begins. Cough, hoarseness, and stridor are belated symptoms if they occur at all. The interval from the onset of clinical symptoms until appearance at the emergency department because of fever and progressive respiratory distress generally is less than 12 hours.

## DIAGNOSIS

If the diagnosis of epiglottitis is unclear but suspected and the degree of respiratory distress is moderate, a lateral neck radiograph can be performed. The characteristic finding in cases of epiglottitis is the so-called thumb sign, reflecting the dimensions of the swollen epiglottis. In addition, there may be ballooning of the hypopharynx as a nonspecific indication of upper airway obstruction (see Fig 36-15).

When a child has classic signs and symptoms of epiglottitis, the diagnosis is straightforward and should be confirmed in the operating room under direct vision when intubation of the airway is accomplished. In these cases, a lateral neck radiograph may delay airway establishment. The tentative diagnosis of epiglottitis constitutes a medical emergency. Every effort is made to keep the child calm and comfortable; manipulations are kept to a minimum. Under no circumstance is the child placed in the supine position. Parents are encouraged to accompany the youngster until definitive treatment is accomplished. After very rapid assembly of a team that includes an otolaryngologist, an anesthetist, and a pediatrician, direct inspection of the upper airway should be undertaken (in a setting in which intubation can be accomplished) to confirm the diagnosis. After the airway has been secured, a blood culture and a surface culture of the epiglottis should be performed. Blood culture results almost always are positive for *H influenzae* type b.

## DIFFERENTIAL DIAGNOSIS

When a child presents with acute onset of fever, dysphagia, and labored respirations, diagnostic considerations include laryngotracheobronchitis with secondary bacterial infection (bacterial tracheitis), uvulitis, diphtheria, and retropharyngeal or peritonsillar abscess. Severe laryngotracheobronchitis occasionally can be caused by parainfluenza or influenza viruses without bacterial superinfection; however, patients with uncomplicated viral croup usually have a more indolent presentation, with lower-grade fever and slower progression of respiratory distress. In croup, barking cough and hoarseness are prominent, the respiratory rate is rapid, and the patient spontaneously assumes the supine position.

If the child is cooperative, inspection of the mouth and throat should be undertaken gingerly, without a tongue blade. This may reveal a peritonsillar abscess, uvulitis, or a diphtheritic pharyngeal membrane. Diphtheria is a rare infection seen only in certain geographic areas of the United States. A history of immunization against diphtheria and the absence of a pharyngeal membrane on physical examination make the diagnosis unlikely.

Retropharyngeal or peritonsillar abscess also may cause fever, dysphagia, and respiratory obstruction. Cough, hoarseness, and stridor usually are absent, although the child characteristically has a muffled or "hot potato" voice. Examination of the throat may reveal the peritonsillar abscess. A lateral neck film will show the presence of a retropharyngeal abscess. In severe cases, endoscopy and airway placement may be necessary.

Another consideration is foreign body aspiration in a child with an upper respiratory infection. This may result in the acute onset of respiratory distress, but fever and dysphagia usually are not prominent. The onset of an upper respiratory infection in a child with a congenital airway problem (such as tracheal stenosis, laryngeal webs, or vascular ring) may cause apparent severe respiratory distress with pronounced hoarseness, cough, and stridor; however, fever is low-grade or absent.

Two rare causes of noninfectious swelling of the supraglottic area are thermal injury (hot food or drink) and allergic edema (insect bite).

## COMPLICATIONS

Complications of supraglottitis can be classified into those that accompany the bacteremic phase of the disease and those that are associated with therapy. Children with supraglottitis almost always are bacteremic. The usual cause is *H influenzae* type b. Occasionally, *S pyogenes* may be recovered from the bloodstream. In either case, other distant foci may become infected. In cases of *H influenzae* type b epiglottitis, pneumonia and cervical lymphadenopathy have been reported as extraepiglottic complications. Rarely, septic arthritis and pericarditis may occur. Of interest, *H influenzae* meningitis has been a very rare complication of epiglottitis in the United States. Meningitis has developed during therapy for epiglottitis in a few children; in each case, the dose of antimicrobial agent being given was well below that which ordinarily is recommended.

The most serious complication of supraglottitis is complete airway obstruction leading to respiratory arrest and hypoxia before arrival at the hospital. Potential therapeutic complications of supraglottitis include aspiration, tube dislodgment, irritation or erosion of the trachea, and extubation. Pneumomediastinum and pneumothorax also may occur. Pulmonary edema may complicate epiglottitis either before or after artificial airway placement. This results from an increase in pulmonary capillary hydrostatic pressure and from increased pulmonary capillary permeability.

# TREATMENT

The most important component of treatment of epiglottitis is se-curing the airway. This can be accomplished by nasotracheal intubation or tracheostomy, depending on the facilities available at the receiving hospital. In general, intubation is accomplished with a tube that is slightly smaller than that which ordinarily would fit the airway. After the child has been intubated suc-cessfully, intravenous antimicrobial agents are initiated. Preferred agents include cefuroxime, 150 mg/kg/d in three divided doses; cefotaxime, 100 mg/kg/d in four divided doses; or ampicillin/ sultamicillin, 200 mg/kg/d in four divided doses. Intravenous hydration and positive-pressure ventilation are provided as re-quired. Extubation generally can be accomplished in 24 to 48 hours. Criteria for extubation include decreased erythema and swelling of the epiglottis on direct inspection, the development of an air leak around the nasotracheal tube, or an empiric 24-hour period of intubation. Prompt defervescence generally occurs after the initiation of appropriate antimicrobial treatment; oral medication can be used to complete a 7- to 10-day course of therapy as soon as extubation has been accomplished and oral intake is assured. The index case should receive rifampin (20 mg/kg/d as a single daily dose for 4 days [maximum 600 mg/ d]) to eradicate colonization with _H influenzae_ type b if there are susceptible children in the household or child-care setting. Inti-mate contacts of the child with epiglottitis also may require ri-fampin prophylaxis if they are susceptible to invasive _H influenzae_ type b disease.

## Selected Readings

Blackstock D, Adderly RJ, Steward DJ. Epiglottitis in young infants. Anesthesiology 1987;67:97.
Gonzalez C, Reilly JS, Kenna MA, Thompson A. Duration of intubation in children with acute epiglottitis. Arch Otolaryngol Head Neck Surg 1986;95:477.
Lacroix J, Ahronheim G, Arcand P, et al. Group A streptococcal supraglottitis. J Pediatr 1986;109:20.
Mauro RD, Poole SR. Lockhart CH differentiation of epiglottitis from laryngotracheitis in the child with stridor. Am J Dis Child 1988;142:679.
Molteni RA. Epiglottitis: Incidence of extraepiglottic infection: Report of 72 cases and review of the literature. Pediatrics 1976;58:526.
Travis KW, Todres ID, Shannon DC. Pulmonary edema associated with croup and epiglottitis. Pediatrics 1977;59:695.

_Principles and Practice of Pediatrics, Second Edition._
edited by Frank A. Oski et al. J. B. Lippincott Company, Philadelphia © 1994.

# 36.11 _Croup_

Ellen R. Wald

The term _croup_ describes a clinical syndrome characterized by a barking cough, hoarseness, and inspiratory stridor. This discussion of infectious non-diphtheritic croup is divided into four sections: (1) acute infectious laryngitis, (2) laryngotracheitis, (3) laryngo-tracheobronchitis (bacterial tracheitis), and (4) spasmodic croup.

## ACUTE INFECTIOUS LARYNGITIS

Acute infectious laryngitis is an illness experienced primarily by older children, adolescents, and adults during the respiratory virus season. The principal symptom of infection is hoarseness, which may be accompanied by variable upper respiratory symptoms (coryza, sore throat, nasal stuffiness) and constitutional symptoms (fever, headache, myalgias, malaise). The presence of associated complaints varies with the infecting virus: adenoviruses and in-fluenza viruses may cause more systemic disease; parainfluenza viruses, rhinoviruses, and respiratory syncytial virus most often cause mild illness.

The diagnosis of acute laryngitis is made on clinical grounds, and laboratory evaluation is unnecessary. In the febrile school-age child with hoarseness who complains of sore throat and has tender anterior cervical adenopathy, a throat culture to detect _Streptococcus pyogenes_ may be appropriate. Hoarseness without any other respiratory symptoms may represent voice abuse.

Acute infectious laryngitis virtually always is self-limited. Treatment consists of symptomatic therapy with fluids and hu-midified inspired air. Voice rest is beneficial. Protracted episodes of hoarseness (no improvement after 7 to 10 days) suggest an underlying anatomic abnormality.

## ACUTE LARYNGOTRACHEITIS

The term _croup_ usually refers to acute laryngotracheitis, a respi-ratory disease that is prevalent in preschool children. Acute lar-yngotracheitis is seen in children of any age, but is most common between the first and third years of life; boys are affected more often than are girls. The causative agents are respiratory viruses exclusively, and the illness frequently occurs in epidemic patterns. The viruses most frequently implicated are parainfluenza 1 and 3, but influenza A and B, respiratory syncytial virus, parainfluenza 2, adenoviruses, and _Mycoplasma pneumoniae_ also may cause croup. In areas of endemic measles, severe croup may dominate the clinical picture. In summertime croup, the enteroviruses (coxsackievirus A and B and echovirus) are the usual cause.

### Pathophysiology

Transmission of the causative virus is by the respiratory route, either direct droplet spread or hand-to-mucosa inoculation. After acquisition, primary viral infection involves the nasopharynx. Viral replication ensues, producing nasal symptoms, and infection spreads locally to involve the larynx and trachea. Endoscopically, the mucosa is erythematous and swollen. Histologic evaluation reveals mucosal edema with cellular infiltration of the lamina propria, submucosa, and adventitia. The cellular constituents include lymphocytes, histiocytes, and polymorphonuclear leukocytes.

### Clinical Manifestations

The usual onset of croup is with the signs and symptoms of a common cold: coryza, nasal congestion, sore throat, and cough, with variable fever. The cough becomes prominent, with a bark-like quality (akin to that of a puppy or seal), and the voice becomes hoarse. Many children with this syndrome do not ever visit a physician. The child may begin to have evidence of respiratory distress, however, with the onset of tachypnea, stridor (when agitated or crying), nasal flaring, and suprasternal and intercostal retractions. The increase in respiratory distress prompts a visit to the physician or emergency department. Usually, the illness peaks in severity over 3 to 5 days and then begins to resolve. Most characteristically, the signs and symptoms worsen in the evening.

In typical cases of acute laryngotracheitis, the diagnosis is made easily on clinical grounds and no radiographs or blood tests are required. If an anteroposterior radiograph is performed, a so-called steeple sign may be seen as a consequence of subglottic swelling. The blood count usually is less than 10,000 cells per cubic millimeter, with a predominance of lymphocytes. Indications for hospitalization, which is undertaken in about 10% of children with laryngotracheitis, include the presence of stridor, anxiety or restlessness, cyanosis, or retractions at rest. Children with a history of croup or previous airway intubation also may benefit from hospitalization. Children for whom close follow-up cannot be arranged or whose families cannot provide the necessary observation and care also should be admitted to the hospital.

As laryngeal inflammation increases and secretions accumulate, respiratory distress increases and complete obstruction may occur. Almost always, this progression is gradual and is signaled by slowly increasing respiratory rate and effort, increased stridor at rest, and pallor or cyanosis. Agitation increases and air entry is poor. In about 5% of hospitalized patients, intubation is required to overcome the respiratory obstruction. Children who have a deteriorating respiratory status should be monitored in an intensive care unit (ICU) by staff who are skilled in the care of pediatric patients.

One of the most important principles of treatment of patients with croup or other upper airway problems is minimal disturbance. Any stimulus that upsets the child will result in crying, which causes hyperventilation and an increase in respiratory distress. The parents should be encouraged to hold and comfort the child whenever possible and invasive procedures should be kept to a minimum.

Treatment strategies for acute infectious laryngotracheitis have included mist, racemic epinephrine, and corticosteroids. Although not subjected to study until recently, mist therapy has been considered standard management. Several small investigations have suggested that mist is of no demonstrable benefit; however, this remedy still is employed routinely. Racemic epinephrine, in use since 1971, is a potentially lifesaving therapy in patients with croup who are in moderate to severe respiratory distress. Racemic epinephrine is an equal mixture of the *d*- and *l*-isomers of epinephrine. The dose is 0.5 mL of a 2.25% solution diluted with 3.5 mL of water (1:8), delivered via a nebulizer with a mouthpiece held in front of the child's face. Administration results in rapid clinical improvement; by its β-adrenergic vasoconstrictive effects on mucosal edema, racemic epinephrine increases the airway diameter. Because the effect may be only temporary, with reappearance of the same degree of respiratory distress that prompted its initial use, a trial of racemic epinephrine mandates hospital admission for at least 24 hours. The dosing interval depends on the severity of the laryngotracheitis; it can be administered every 20 to 30 minutes in the ICU where monitoring is possible, but usually is spaced 3 to 4 hours apart when the patient is in a regular hospital unit.

The use of steroids in acute laryngotracheitis has been controversial for 3 decades. They appear to offer neither great benefit nor excessive risk when used for a short period. There seems to be a subgroup of patients (perhaps those with spasmodic croup) who may benefit from steroid use, although they are not easy to identify before treatment. Accordingly, some investigators recommend that, if the clinical syndrome of croup is severe enough to warrant the use of racemic epinephrine, a single dose of steroids (dexamethasone 0.30 to 0.50 mg/kg per dose) should be employed as a test dose. Although steroids do not have an immediate effect, improvement within 6 hours of their use suggests efficacy, and a repeat dose may be given. If no improvement is noted in 6 hours, subsequent doses are withheld. Antibiotics are not indicated in the routine treatment of children with this croup syndrome.

Most patients who are hospitalized for acute laryngotracheitis are treated with supportive therapies (mist and, occasionally, ox-

ygen and intravenous fluids) and can be discharged in a few days. If intubation is required, the nasotracheal tube frequently must remain in place for 3 to 4 days until an air leak develops around it, reflecting subsidence of the inflammation. Hospitalization for several days after extubation is desirable to ensure respiratory stability and the reintroduction of oral feeding.

## SEVERE LARYNGOTRACHEOBRONCHITIS (BACTERIAL TRACHEITIS)

Bacterial tracheitis is a recently re-described example of upper airway obstruction that was recognized more regularly in the era before antibiotics. Initial reports in 1979 emphasized the clinical presentation and bacterial component of the infectious process. Recent investigations, which have had the benefit of more complete microbiologic evaluation, indicate convincingly that the process represents a secondary bacterial infection of a primarily viral process.

### Etiology

The consensus is that bacterial tracheitis represents a secondary bacterial infection of viral laryngotracheitis. The specific agents that have been implicated include parainfluenza and influenza viruses, and enterovirus. The secondary bacterial invaders most often are coagulase-positive staphylococci. Group A *Streptococcus*, *Streptococcus viridans*, *Haemophilus influenzae*, and gram-negative enteric bacteria also have been implicated however.

### Epidemiology

Bacterial tracheitis occurs principally during the respiratory virus season, overlapping the seasonal occurrence of laryngotracheitis—fall and winter. This pathologic entity affects all age groups from young infants to school-age children, with a predominance in 1- to 2-year-olds. Boys and girls are affected equally.

### Pathophysiology

The site of infectious inflammation is the mucosa of the subglottic area and upper trachea. In some cases, autopsy material reveals a necrotizing inflammatory reaction with mucosal ulceration and microabscess formation. In other cases, a thick pseudomembrane is described. The membrane is attached loosely and is easy to remove without hemorrhage. The membrane may become detached from the mucosa spontaneously, leading to further obstructive symptoms. The purulent exudate that frequently is suctioned from patients with bacterial tracheitis shows abundant polymorphonuclear leukocytes. Gram's stain usually will reveal the involved bacterial species. Bacteremia is absent in these cases, but pneumonia is a frequent accompaniment.

### Clinical Manifestations

The onset of croup is variable. Some children become ill acutely and have severe respiratory distress within hours of onset of the illness. In others, there is a 1- to 5-day prodromal period of mild upper respiratory symptoms and the onset of cough, stridor, and hoarseness that is characteristic of typical croup; then, within just a few hours, higher temperature, a toxic appearance, and a remarkable increase in respiratory distress develops. As distress becomes apparent, it is notable that these patients do not respond to the inhalation of racemic epinephrine. Typically, high temperature, prominent cough, and stridor are noted at the time of clinical presentation. Clinical differentiation of this illness from epiglottitis may be helped by the usual absence of dysphagia and drooling in bacterial tracheitis. When signs of airway obstruction escalate, however, the key issue, as in cases of suspected epiglottitis, is securing the airway.

## Diagnosis

The diagnosis of bacterial tracheitis may be suspected clinically, but it is confirmed endoscopically. At the time of intubation or bronchoscopy, the epiglottis is found to be normal. The pathologic process involves the subglottic area, with extension into the trachea. Abundant purulent exudate and pseudomembranes may be present. If radiographic studies have been performed, the anteroposterior radiograph will show the steeple sign and, occasionally, the detached pseudomembrane may be seen as a soft-tissue shadow or shadows of irregular configuration in the upper trachea. Pneumonia frequently is a complication in cases of bacterial tracheitis. Leukocytosis may be prominent, but blood culture results are negative.

## Treatment

The appropriate treatment of bacterial tracheitis includes securing the airway and instituting antimicrobial therapy. Tracheal intubation is recommended for patients in whom bacterial tracheitis has been diagnosed. This can be accomplished with nasotracheal intubation or tracheostomy. In either case, observation in an ICU is essential. The copious and thick secretions may lead to blockage of the artificial airway, necessitating meticulous respiratory toileting. As the most common bacterial species implicated has been the *Staphylococcus*, nafcillin therapy is indicated in cases in which gram-positive cocci or no organisms at all have been seen on a smear. In patients in whom gram-negative rods or mixed flora are observed, an advanced-generation cephalosporin, such as cefotaxime or ceftriaxone, may be best. Parenteral therapy should be continued for the duration of intubation or for several days after the patient has undergone defervescence. Oral antimicrobial agents may be used to complete a 10-day course of therapy in cases in which the clinical improvement has been prompt. Typically, the clinical course of bacterial tracheitis is longer than that of uncomplicated croup or epiglottitis, and requires a mean of 10 days of hospitalization.

## Complications

Complications of croup occur before and after intubation. The most serious is complete respiratory obstruction leading to respiratory arrest. A number of cases of severe hypoxia and, ultimately, death have occurred in patients with bacterial tracheitis. Pneumomediastinum and pneumothorax also may be seen as complications of intubation. Pneumonia occurs in about 50% of cases.

## SPASMODIC CROUP

Acute spasmodic croup is a clinical entity that is seen in exactly the same age group and during the same season, and is caused by the same viruses, as is acute infectious laryngotracheitis. Typically, children experiencing an episode of acute spasmodic croup go to sleep well or with the mildest of upper respiratory infections. They awaken in the night with a barking cough, hoarseness, inspiratory stridor, and variable degrees of respiratory distress. They always are afebrile. Most patients respond to mist therapy, provided by the bathroom shower or a cool-water vaporizer. Occasionally, the night air inhaled en route to the hospital is sufficient to reduce the dyspnea. Although most episodes are mild to moderate, airway support occasionally is required. Recurrences

may be observed during the same evening or on the subsequent 2 to 3 nights.

This condition may be differentiated from infectious laryngotracheitis endoscopically. Whereas examination of the mucosa in the former reveals an erythematous, inflamed, velvety appearance, the mucosa is pale and boggy in the latter. Although viral cultures yield the same agents as in laryngotracheitis, the mucosal appearance and clinical course suggest an allergic component of the pathophysiologic process. This group of patients usually benefits from racemic epinephrine if the degree of respiratory distress mandates its use. Likewise, these patients may do well with corticosteroid therapy, reflecting either the allergic nature of the process or the natural history of a self-limited disease.

## DIFFERENTIAL DIAGNOSIS

The differential diagnosis in patients who have upper airway obstruction includes both infectious and noninfectious problems. The noninfectious causes are foreign body aspiration and angioneurotic edema. Foreign body aspiration occurs most often in children 2 to 4 years of age. If the aspiration is observed, the diagnosis is straightforward. The ambulatory preschooler, however, often is unobserved when the aspiration occurs. There is an initial choking and gagging episode, usually followed by a "silent" period during which the child is asymptomatic. The recurrence of symptoms may include the acute onset of cough, wheezing, stridor, or dysphagia in variable combinations. The child usually has no upper respiratory symptoms or fever. Auscultation of the lungs may reveal differential aeration and wheezing. Most aspirated foreign bodies are vegetable matter (eg, peanuts, carrots, corn) and, therefore, plain radiographs may not reveal their presence. The sudden onset of upper respiratory tract obstruction in a previously well child always should arouse concern about foreign body aspiration. Endoscopy is diagnostic and therapeutic in this situation.

Angioneurotic edema may cause sudden respiratory obstruction in a previously well child of any age. There may be an allergic history or previous episodes of respiratory tract obstruction. The angioneurotic edema may be based on a hereditary C1 esterase deficiency; in these cases, there may be a positive family history. Alternatively, a sudden allergic reaction to ingested material or inhalants may cause swelling of the tongue, epiglottis, or larynx. In any case, if severe reactions do not respond to injected or inhaled epinephrine, endoscopy and airway intubation may be necessary.

The infectious causes of upper airway obstruction include, in addition to laryngitis, laryngotracheitis, laryngotracheobronchitis, and spasmodic croup, laryngeal diphtheria. Currently, this infection is rare in the United States, occurring in limited geographic regions. Fully immunized individuals should be immune. Partially immunized or non-immunized children will have symptoms of low-grade fever and sore throat. The illness is slowly progressive, but toxicity is out of proportion to the degree of fever. Respiratory difficulty develops over 2 to 3 days, and usually is characterized by hoarseness and barking cough, as in the usual case of croup. Dysphagia commonly is present in diphtheria, however, in contrast to viral croup. Physical examination of the throat reveals a membranous exudative pharyngitis; the membrane is tightly adherent to the underlying tissue and removal is difficult. Smear and culture of the membrane will disclose the infecting *Corynebacterium diphtheriae*.

The remaining causes of acute infectious obstruction in the region of the larynx are contrasted in Table 36-15. Laryngitis is not included, as it rarely presents difficulty in differential diagnosis. Acute epiglottitis is a medical emergency that must be dif-

**TABLE 36-15.  Differential Diagnosis of Acute Infectious Obstruction in the Region of the Larynx**

| Category | Epiglottitis | Acute Laryngotracheitis | Laryngotracheobronchitis | Spasmodic Croup |
|---|---|---|---|---|
| Prodrome | Usually none or mild upper respiratory infection | Usually upper respiratory symptoms | Usually upper respiratory symptoms | None or minimal coryza |
| Age | 1–8 y | 3 mo–3 y | 3 mo–8 y | 3 mo–3 y |
| Onset | Rapid; 4–12 h | Gradual | Variable | Sudden, always at night |
| Fever | High (39.5 °C) | Variable | Usually high | None |
| Hoarseness/barking cough | No | Yes | Yes | Yes |
| Dysphagia | Yes | No | No | No |
| Toxic appearance | Yes | No | Yes | No |
| Microbiology | Blood culture positive for *Haemophilus influenzae* type b | Viral infection | Viral infection with bacterial superinfection | Viral infection with allergic component |

Modified from Cherry JD. Croup. In: Feigin RD, Cherry JD, eds. Textbook of pediatric infectious diseases, ed 2. Philadelphia: WB Saunders, 1987.

ferentiated from the remaining croup syndromes to enable appropriate airway management. Severe laryngotracheobronchitis (bacterial tracheitis) may require immediate airway placement. In both situations, the child is highly febrile, appears to be in a toxic condition, and is in marked respiratory distress. Immediate endoscopy is diagnostic and allows proper airway management.

## Selected Readings

Baugh R, Gilmore BB. Infectious croup: A critical review. Arch Otolaryngol Head Neck Surg 1986;95:40.
Cherry JD. Croup (laryngitis, laryngotracheitis, spasmodic croup, and laryngotracheobronchitis). In: Feigin RD, Cherry JD, eds. Textbook of pediatric infectious diseases, ed 2. Philadelphia: WB Saunders, 1987:237.
Davis HW, Gartner JC, Galvis AG, et al. Acute upper airway obstruction: Croup and epiglottitis. Pediatr Clin North Am 1981;28:859.
Donnelly BW, McMillan JA, Weiner LB. Bacterial tracheitis: Report of eight new cases and review. Rev Infect Dis 1990;12:729.
Kairys SW, Olmstead EM, O'Connor GT. Steroid treatment of laryngotracheitis: A meta-analysis of the evidence from randomized trials. Pediatrics 1989;83:683.
Taussig LM, Castro O, Beaudry PH, et al. Treatment of laryngotracheitis (croup): Use of intermittent positive-pressure breathing and racemic epinephrine. Am J Dis Child 1975;129:790.
Tunnessen WW Jr, Feinstein AR. The steroid-croup controversy: An analytic review of methodologic problems. J Pediatr 1980;96:751.

*Principles and Practice of Pediatrics, Second Edition.*
edited by Frank A. Oski et al. J. B. Lippincott Company, Philadelphia © 1994.

# 36.12 *Cervical Lymphadenitis*

### Carol J. Baker

Cervical adenitis is inflammation of one or more lymph nodes of the neck. In children, the most common causes of cervical lymph node enlargement exceeding 10 mm are reactive hyperplasia in response to an infectious stimulus in the head or neck and infection of the node itself. Self-limited cervical lymph node inflammation occurs in association with upper respiratory tract infection as the lymphatic channels drain proximally affected sites. In 80% of children with acute cervical adenitis, the submaxillary, submandibular, and deep cervical nodes are inflamed, because these are the routes by which much of the lymphatic drainage of the head and neck proceeds. Malignancy is the second most common cause of lymph node enlargement in children, but neoplasia constitutes a minority of neck masses. Children with malignant lesions tend to have systemic complaints and firm, nontender nodes that are located characteristically in the posterior triangle or supraclavicular regions.

## EPIDEMIOLOGY

Although patients at any age may be affected, the majority of children with cervical adenitis are 1 to 4 years of age. This age restriction and peak in incidence reflects the prevalence of infections caused by *Staphylococcus aureus*, group A *Streptococcus*, and atypical mycobacteria. The sexes are affected equally, with two exceptions. Some studies indicate a female predominance for granulomatous lymphadenitis caused by atypical mycobacteria, and young infants with the cellulitis-adenitis syndrome caused by group B *Streptococcus* are predominantly male (75%). Droplet-borne transmission is the route of acquisition for most viral causes of cervical adenitis and for bacterial disease caused by group A *Streptococcus* and *Mycobacterium tuberculosis*. The remaining bacterial agents are normal inhabitants of the mouth, oropharynx, and nose, or are soil bacteria inoculated by trauma to the skin. There is no racial predilection for acute bacterial cervical adenitis (Table 36-16). In contrast, adenitis caused by atypical mycobacteria occurs commonly in whites, whereas that caused by *M tuberculosis* tends to have a greater incidence in blacks and Hispanics. For children living in temperate climates, an increase in incidence occurs during the winter and spring months. A history of dog or cat contact, bite, or scratch may be a helpful clue in suggesting specific causative agents, such as *Pasteurella multocida*, *Toxoplasma gondii*, or the gram-negative pleomorphic rod that causes cat-scratch disease (CSD). Similarly, a history of a minor inoculation wound of the skin proximal to affected cervical lymph nodes should suggest the possibility of soil organisms such as *Nocardia brasiliensis*, atypical mycobacteria, and gram-negative enteric organisms. Finally, the human immunodeficiency virus (HIV) should be added to the list of agents causing cervical adenopathy, and, because most HIV-infected children are infected perinatally, the epidemiology reflects that of the mothers.

**TABLE 36-16.   Differentiation of Bacterial and Mycobacterial Cervical Adenitis**

| Clinical Characteristics | Bacteria | Atypical Mycobacteria | *Mycobacterium tuberculosis* |
|---|---|---|---|
| Onset | Acute (<2 wk) | Subacute to chronic | Subacute to chronic |
| Age (y) | 1–4* | 1–4 | All |
| Race | All | White | Black, Hispanic, or Asian |
| Regional node distribution | Unilateral | Unilateral | Unilateral or bilateral |
| Focal tenderness | Mild to marked | Usually absent | Usually absent |
| Exposure to adult with tuberculosis | Absent | Absent | Present |
| Abnormal chest radiograph appearance | Never | Never | Sometimes |
| Mantoux test (PPD-S) result > 15 mm induration | Never | Rare | Often |

\* Seventy percent to 80% of cases.

Modified from Butler KM, Baker CJ. Cervical lymphadenitis. In: Feigin RD, Cherry JD, eds. Textbook of pediatric infectious diseases, ed 3. Philadephia: WB Saunders, 1992:221.

## PATHOGENESIS AND PATHOLOGY

The pathogenesis of cervical adenitis is elucidated poorly. Apparently, a microorganism first must infect asymptomatically the upper respiratory tract, anterior nares, mouth, or skin of the head or neck before spreading to the cervical lymph nodes. Overt infection of the skin, teeth, or oropharynx may occur in association with cervical adenitis, but clinically evident infection proximal to the affected nodes is not a requisite. For example, asymptomatic colonization of the anterior nares routinely precedes the development of cervical adenitis resulting from *S aureus*. The common occurrence of group A streptococcal adenitis in children younger than 2 years, in contrast to the infrequency with which streptococcal pharyngitis is observed in infants, suggests that adenitis may result when host defense mechanisms are insufficient to limit this organism to mucous-membrane sites in the pharynx. Some investigators consider group A streptococci to be responsible for invasion of the nodes, with *S aureus* playing a secondary role in patients who have both agents isolated from infected cervical lymph nodes. Dental caries or abscesses may predispose to the development of anaerobic cervical adenitis; however, when proper culture techniques are employed, mixed aerobic-anaerobic infections are diagnosed frequently. This suggests that elaboration of extracellular enzymes by mixed flora may have a role in the pathogenesis of these infections. Certain infections are characterized by direct inoculation of skin proximal to regional lymph nodes (eg, group A *Streptococcus, Nocardia,* cat-scratch bacillus). Finally, viral cervical adenitis may reflect either a local response to a virus invading the oropharynx or respiratory tract (eg, adenovirus) or a more generalized reticuloendothelial response to systemic viral infection (eg, Epstein-Barr virus or HIV).

The increased size of lymph nodes in response to infection is the result of an increase in the number of cells in response to infection. While it is filtering pyogenic microorganisms, chemoattraction of neutrophils to the lymph node may result in the formation of microabscesses and small areas of necrosis, or in frank suppuration. Granuloma formation with a delayed cellular immune response that may lead over a period of weeks or months to the formation of a "cold" abscess is characteristic when the infection is caused by acid-fast organisms, fungi, or the gram-negative organism that is implicated in CSD. With both *M tuberculosis* and atypical mycobacteria, biopsy material usually reveals extensive replacement of normal architecture by caseating granulomas surrounded by epithelioid cells and giant cells, and acid-fast organisms are demonstrable in stained sections in about 50% of cases. Epithelioid granulomas that are infiltrated with neutrophils, forming large pus-filled sinuses, are characteristic of the lymph nodes excised from children with CSD.

## CLINICAL MANIFESTATIONS

Cervical adenitis may be classified according to its mode of presentation as acute, in which symptoms are of less than 2 weeks in duration, or subacute to chronic (Table 36-17). The causative agents tend to fall into one of these two categories, although there may be overlap. Overall, about three fourths of all the infections have an acute presentation. The duration of lymph node swelling is less than 2 days in half of all children with acute adenitis, and less than 1 week in the majority of them. Acute bilateral cervical adenitis generally is associated with upper respiratory tract viral infection or with streptococcal pharyngitis. Lymph nodes may be tender, but none of the other signs of inflammation are found. Recognition of exanthem and focal findings such as gingivostomatitis are features that suggest either a respiratory viral or a streptococcal cause.

Children with acute unilateral cervical lymphadenitis generally have a paucity of systemic manifestations. A history of upper respiratory tract symptoms such as sore throat, earache, coryza, or impetigo can be elicited from one fourth to one third of patients. The infected node usually ranges in diameter from 2.5 to 6.0 cm, is tender, and exhibits varying degrees of warmth and erythema. *S aureus* and group A *Streptococcus* are the causative agents in 50% to 90% of infections. Less commonly, other bacteria residing in the oropharynx are implicated (see Table 36-17). Streptococcal adenitis occurs in younger children, is accompanied more often by generalized adenopathy, has a shorter duration of symptoms (4 versus 10 days), and is less likely to suppurate than are nodes infected by *S aureus*. Overall, one fourth to one third of involved nodes suppurate, and 90% of these become fluctuant within 2 weeks after the onset of symptoms. Concomitant lymphadenopathy at other sites is observed in as many as one third of children with acute unilateral cervical adenitis, most commonly in association with a generalized viral process or a group A streptococcal

TABLE 36-17. Infectious Agents or Diseases Associated With Cervical Adenitis

| Agent or Disease | Frequency* | Onset Acute (A) or Subacute to Chronic (S) | Generalized Adenopathy |
|---|---|---|---|
| **Bacterial** | | | |
| *Staphylococcus aureus* | +++ | A | − |
| Group A *Streptococcus* | +++ | A | + |
| Anaerobes | +++ | A/S | − |
| Cat-scratch disease bacillus | +++ | S | − |
| Atypical mycobacteria | +++ | S | − |
| *Mycobacterium tuberculosis* | ++ | S | ± |
| *Nocardia brasiliensis* | ++ | S | − |
| Gram-negative enteric organisms | ++ | A | − |
| Group B *Streptococcus*† | ++ | A | − |
| *Pasteurella multocida* | ++ | A | + |
| *Haemophilus influenzae* | + | A | − |
| *Yersinia pestis* | + | A | + |
| *Actinomyces israelii* | + | A | − |
| Diphtheria | + | A | − |
| Tularemia | + | A | − |
| Syphilis | + | S | + |
| Anthrax | + | A | − |
| **Viral** | | | |
| Epstein-Barr virus | +++ | A/S | + |
| Herpes simplex | +++ | A | − |
| Cytomegalovirus | +++ | A/S | + |
| Adenovirus | +++ | A | − |
| Varicella | ++ | A | + |
| Enterovirus | +++ | A | + |
| Human herpes virus-6 | + | S | + |
| Measles | + | A | + |
| Mumps | + | A | − |
| Rubella | + | A | + |
| Human immunodeficiency virus | + | S | + |
| **Fungal** | | | |
| Histoplasmosis | + | S | + |
| *Cryptococcus* | + | S | − |
| Aspergillosis | + | S | − |
| Candida | + | S | − |
| Coccidioides | + | S | − |
| Sporotrichosis | + | A | − |
| **Parasitic** | | | |
| *Toxoplasma gondii* | + | S | + |

\* Key: +++, common; ++, uncommon; +, rare.
† Neonates and young infants only.
*Modified from Butler KM, Baker CJ. Cervical lymphadenitis. In: Feigin RD, Cherry JD, eds. Textbook of pediatric infectious diseases, ed 3. Philadephia: WB Saunders, 1992:224.*

infection. Hepatomegaly or splenomegaly is rare, however, and, if found, should suggest a generalized process (eg, HIV infection, Epstein-Barr virus, tuberculosis, reticuloendotheliosis, etc.).

In infancy, *S aureus* is the most common isolate from unilaterally infected cervical lymph nodes. The presentation is similar to that in older infants and children, except that irritability and other systemic symptoms may be observed more frequently. Infants 1 to 2 months of age who have facial or submandibular adenitis, particularly male infants with ipsilateral otitis media, may have the cellulitis-adenitis syndrome that is caused by group B streptococci. In contrast to infants with staphylococcal adenitis,

those with group B streptococcal infection have a high likelihood (94%) of concomitant bacteremia.

The most common causes of subacute to chronic cervical adenitis are mycobacteria, cat-scratch bacillus, *Nocardia*, and Epstein-Barr virus. Less frequently, fungal infections, syphilis, and *T gondii* may present as subacute or chronic cervical lymphadenitis (see Table 36-17). The features that aid in differentiating atypical mycobacterial adenitis from that caused by *M tuberculosis* are found in Table 36-16. Nontuberculous adenitis has an age distribution similar to that of acute bacterial adenitis, and almost invariably is unilateral and localized to a single submandibular or tonsillar node. Although marked erythema may develop, these masses are "cold" and there is less tenderness than would be expected given the degree of erythema. There is some geographic variation, but *Mycobacterium avium-intracellulare* is the species most often isolated from affected nodes. The regional findings are similar in atypical and typical mycobacterial adenitis, but the latter is distinguished by bilateral involvement in 10% of patients, by almost invariable (>90%) exposure to a household adult contact with tuberculosis, and by abnormalities on chest radiography in about 30% of cases. Mantoux skin testing is a helpful discriminator, because the diameter of the reaction usually exceeds 15 mm when infection is caused by *M tuberculosis*, whereas reactions of smaller diameter commonly are found in children with infection caused by atypical mycobacteria.

CSD is a lymphocutaneous syndrome in which regional lymph nodes proximal to the subcutaneous inoculation of the cat-scratch bacillus become inflamed. The interval between the cat scratch (or bite) and the development of adenitis ranges from 1 week to 2 months. Sixty percent of patients or parents describe a papular lesion at the inoculation site, but this may have resolved at the time the adenitis is most severe. Lymph nodes of the head or neck were involved in 58% of the 548 patients described in one large series. Fever, persisting for as long as 1 week, occurs in 25% of children, but constitutional symptoms of malaise, anorexia, and headache are mild or absent in the majority of them. In 15% (range, 10% to 30%), the lymph nodes suppurate. Adenitis usually resolves within 2 weeks to 2 months, but it may persist for a more protracted interval in a minority of children (up to 20%).

Another lymphocutaneous syndrome that may present with cervical node involvement is that caused by *N brasiliensis*. Traumatic introduction of *Nocardia* from soil produces a pustule or localized cellulitis on the face or head, followed several days later by lymph node enlargement. These nodes typically are moderately inflamed, and mild systemic symptoms may accompany the early phase of illness. Clues to this causative agent include the presence of the inoculation lesion and failure of the syndrome to respond to the antibiotics usually used to treat cervical adenitis.

Acquired toxoplasmosis may present with generalized adenopathy (see Table 36-17), but more often it appears as regional adenitis, typically restricted to a single node in the posterior cervical chain. Contact with cats or their litter or with undercooked meat usually is elicited in the history. In most children, the disease is asymptomatic, resolution is complete, and specific therapy is not required.

A rare disorder of unknown cause that may present as painless cervical adenopathy is necrotizing lymphadenitis, or Kikulehi's disease. The typical patient is an adolescent female or young woman, and the course is benign, with resolution over 3 to 4 months. Characteristic histopathologic findings confirm this diagnosis.

## DIFFERENTIAL DIAGNOSIS

Noninfectious causes of cervical adenitis include a variety of benign and malignant entities (Table 36-18). Their duration is an aid to diagnosis, because most tumors and miscellaneous conditions that cause cervical adenitis are characterized by chronicity. These lymph nodes usually are painless, are not inflamed, and are firm in consistency. Location also is a helpful distinguishing feature, because about half of all masses located in the posterior triangle are malignant tumors, whereas masses found in the anterior triangle, with the exception of those involving the thyroid, tend to be benign. Masses that extend across the sternocleidomastoid muscle to involve both the anterior and the posterior triangles should be viewed as potentially malignant. Finally, age

**TABLE 36-18.   Noninfectious Causes of Cervical Adenitis**

| Causes | Frequency* | Associated With Generalized Adenopathy |
|---|---|---|
| **Neoplasm** | | |
| Hodgkin's disease | ++ | + |
| Lymphosarcoma, rhabdomyosarcoma | ++ | − |
| Non-Hodgkin's lymphoma | ++ | + |
| Neuroblastoma | ++ | + |
| Leukemia | + | + |
| Metastatic carcinoma | + | − |
| Thyroid tumor | + | − |
| **Collagen Vascular Disease** | | |
| Lupus erythematosus | + | + |
| Juvenile rheumatoid arthritis | + | + |
| **Miscellaneous** | | |
| Kawasaki disease | +++ | + |
| Drug-associated | ++ | + |
| Sarcoidosis | + | + |
| Histiocytosis X | + | + |
| Reticuloendotheliosis | + | + |
| Sinus histiocytosis with massive lymphadenopathy | + | + |

\* Key: +++, common; ++, uncommon; +, rare.

*Modified from Butler KM, Baker CJ. Cervical lymphadenitis. In: Feigin RD, Cherry JD, eds. Textbook of pediatric infectious diseases, ed 3. Philadelphia: WB Saunders, 1992:225, and from Margileth AM. Cervical adenitis. Pediatr Rev 1985;7: 13.*

is a discriminator to some extent, because lymphoreticular malignant tumors occur more frequently among older children, in contrast to the infectious causes that predominate in children 1 to 4 years of age.

Lymphoid neoplasms and neuroblastoma constitute two thirds of all malignant neck masses seen in children (see Table 36-17). Lymphomas, both Hodgkin's and non-Hodgkin's, are more common than is neuroblastoma in older children, whereas neuroblastoma is the most common malignant lesion in young children. With the exception of thyroid tumors and metastatic carcinoma, which may present as isolated cervical masses, the conditions included in the differential diagnosis of cervical adenitis have generalized adenopathy or other systemic features. Kawasaki disease deserves special mention, as it is a common cause of unilateral anterior cervical adenitis for which the causative agent is undefined. This syndrome is diagnosed by clinical criteria that include persistence of fever for longer than 5 days and the presence of other major features (conjunctivitis, truncal exanthem, oral manifestations, and involvement of the hands and feet). An enlarged lymph node (>1.5 cm) in the cervical chain is the major feature of this disease that is noted least often, and this is present in one half to two thirds of patients.

Congenital lesions of the neck may simulate cervical adenitis. The most common of these is the thyroglossal duct cyst, which may be distinguished by its midline location and movement with tongue protrusion. These cysts may become infected secondarily, and even may progress to frank suppuration. The existence of a pit, dimple, or draining sinus along the anterior margin of the sternocleidomastoid muscle serves to differentiate between branchial cleft cyst and cervical adenitis, although the distinction may be difficult if the cyst becomes infected secondarily. Cystic hygromas are soft masses that transilluminate, aiding in their differentiation from inflammatory or malignant neck masses.

## DIAGNOSIS

As stated previously, a detailed history to ascertain the duration of the illness (acute or subacute to chronic), the presence or absence of associated systemic symptoms, animal exposures, preceding trauma, contact with an adult with tuberculosis, the presence of maternal risk factors for HIV infection, drug usage (especially phenytoin [Dilantin]), ingestion of unusual substances (undercooked meat, unpasteurized milk), or recent travel may yield important diagnostic clues regarding the cause of cervical adenitis. The physical examination reveals the location of the adenitis (anterior or posterior triangles), the presence of dental disease, non-cervical lymphadenopathy, oropharyngeal or skin lesions, and evidence of generalized or localized involvement.

In patients with acute infection, needle aspiration of the largest or most fluctuant affected node is the best way to establish a specific cause. In 60% to 88% of patients with acute cervical adenitis caused by aerobic agents or mycobacteria, a causative agent is recovered by this diagnostic maneuver. Only inflamed nodes should be aspirated, however. These need not be fluctuant, and the clinician should make sure that the cervical mass is not a vascular structure. The skin should be cleansed and anesthetized, and an 18- or 20-gauge needle attached to a 10- to 20-mL syringe should be used for aspiration. If no material is aspirated, 1 to 2 mL of sterile, non-bacteriostatic saline should be injected into the node, and it should be aspirated again. Gram's and Kinyoun stains of the aspirated material should be performed. Then, it should be inoculated from the syringe into aerobic and anaerobic media, and onto cleaned glass slides for Gram's and acid-fast stains. If *Nocardia* is suspected, the laboratory should be informed and asked to hold the blood agar plates for up to 7 days. If mycobacterial or fungal infection is suspected, processing of the aspirate by appropriate culture media should be requested. Cultures of infected skin lesions or exudates on tonsils (if present) also should be performed.

If purulent material is not obtained, cultures for aerobic bacteria are negative, and the patient fails to respond to antibiotics that are active against staphylococci and streptococci, the following laboratory evaluation should be considered: throat culture; Mantoux intradermal purified protein derivative (PPD) test; complete blood count; antistreptolysin O test; rapid plasma reagin test for syphilis; and serologic tests for Epstein-Barr virus, cytomegalovirus, toxoplasmosis, human herpesvirus 6, HIV, tularemia, *Brucella*, histoplasmosis, and coccidioidomycosis. Intradermal (Mantoux) testing for *M tuberculosis* with 5 TU of tuberculin always should be done in patients with subacute or chronic adenitis; induration greater than 15 mm is strongly suggestive of infection with *M tuberculosis*, whereas smaller reactions are more consistent with atypical mycobacterial infection. Patients with a PPD reaction exceeding 10 mm should undergo a chest radiograph and be subjected to further questioning about exposure to tuberculosis in the recent past. Intradermal skin testing using atypical mycobacterial antigens and materials from patients infected with CSD agents also has proved useful in the diagnosis of these infections. Unfortunately, neither of the latter tests is available commercially.

The diagnosis of CSD still is based on clinical criteria, although a gram-negative bacillus recently has been established as the causative agent. This agent has been identified in lymph node and inoculation site biopsy materials. The typical child with CSD is not a candidate for a biopsy, but if one is done, the specimen should be stained appropriately and interpreted by someone familiar with the techniques necessary for identifying the CSD bacillus. The clinical diagnosis is made if three of the following four criteria are present:

1. A subacute or chronic adenitis not responding to antimicrobial therapy
2. Cat contact and the presence of a scratch or primary dermal or eye lesion
3. A negative laboratory evaluation for other causes of adenitis
4. Characteristic histopathologic features in a lymph node biopsy sample, if a biopsy is performed.

If the evaluation outlined above does not reveal the cause of the adenopathy and it persists, enlarges, or is hard or fixed to adjacent structures, excisional biopsy should be considered strongly. Ideally, the pathologist should be aware of the patient's clinical history before receiving the surgical specimen. Furthermore, the surgeon should be aware of the need to excise the entire node routinely, if possible, because atypical mycobacterial infection is so common in children and this surgical approach is necessary for therapeutic reasons. Biopsy material should be submitted for the microbiologic studies listed above, as well as for routine histology and Ziehl-Neelsen or auramine O, Giemsa, periodic acid–Schiff, Warthin-Starry (cat-scratch bacillus), and methenamine silver stains. In select cases only, viral cultures can be requested. If histologic examination reveals noncaseating granulomas and the child has a history of cat exposure, the most likely diagnosis is CSD. Sarcoidosis involving the lymph nodes has a similar histologic appearance, but this illness is rare in children.

Older children are more likely to be candidates for excisional lymph node biopsy. These also are the patients more likely to have lymphomas. Thus, it is important that a biopsy of the appropriate node is performed and that it is removed intact for proper fixation, cutting, and staining. The largest node should be chosen and, if several sites of involvement are present, specimens from the lower neck and supraclavicular area should be removed, because these have the highest diagnostic yield. Other areas, including the upper cervical, submandibular, axillary, and parotid nodes, are more likely to have reactive hyperplasia that may or may not be related to the underlying process. Reactive hyperplasia is the final diagnosis in about half of all cases. In these children, particularly when no improvement is noted, a repeat biopsy performed at a later time may offer additional information. For example, the lymphocyte-predominant variety of Hodgkin's lymphoma, which is readily confused histologically with reactive hyperplasia, may become apparent. If lymphoma is suspected, needle biopsies or frozen sections are useless for diagnosis.

## TREATMENT

Many infants and children with cervical lymphadenopathy accompanying viral infections of the respiratory tract never see a physician because of the self-limited nature of these infections. In others, cervical adenitis resolves during the course of antimicrobial therapy given for a primary diagnosis of otitis media, streptococcal pharyngitis, or impetigo of the face or scalp. Another group of patients has acute inflammation of cervical lymph nodes as the primary site of infection; in these, empiric antimicrobial therapy without prior needle aspiration may be given. If no clinical response occurs within 48 hours, however, aspiration should be performed. This empiric therapy should be directed against *S aureus* and group A *Streptococcus*, and it should include such agents as dicloxacillin (25 mg/kg/d) or cloxacillin (50 mg/kg/d), or, for penicillin-allergic patients, clindamycin (30 mg/kg/

d), cephalexin (50 mg/kg/d), or cephradine (50 mg/kg/d). A combination of amoxicillin and clavulanic acid (Augmentin) provides good activity for staphylococci and streptococci, as well as for oral anaerobic bacteria. This expanded activity combined with its palatability make amoxicillin/clavulanic acid a good alternative to penicillinase-resistant penicillins. Cefixime, an oral third-generation cephalosporin, is inactive against staphylococci and has no place in empiric therapy for presumed bacterial adenitis.

In children with acute suppurative cervical adenitis, surgical drainage is key to appropriate resolution. Some patients have progression of local inflammation and persistence of systemic symptoms despite oral antimicrobial therapy. These children require parenteral therapy, and methicillin, nafcillin, or oxacillin (150 mg/kg/d) is recommended. In the penicillin-allergic patient, cefazolin (100 mg/kg/d) or clindamycin (40 mg/kg/d) may be substituted. Ceftriaxone (50 to 100 mg/kg/d) given once daily is an excellent alternative to the parenteral antibiotics, which require more frequent administration. Antimicrobial therapy can be modified once a causative agent is identified (for example, group A streptococcal infection can be treated with penicillin G or V), and may need to be modified if there is an obvious primary infectious focus, such as a dental abscess, in which therapy active against anaerobic organisms is mandatory. In the latter circumstance, penicillin V (50 mg/kg/d), clindamycin, or amoxicillin/clavulanic acid (30 mg/kg/d) may be used.

Adenitis caused by group A *Streptococcus* should be treated for a minimum of 10 days, or about 5 days after signs of local inflammation and systemic symptoms have disappeared. If the child is penicillin-allergic, erythromycin ethylsuccinate (40 mg/kg/d) or cephalexin can be used. Warm, moist dressings over the inflamed area give symptomatic relief, but probably do not aid in the localization process. If abscess formation occurs late in the first or early in the second week of antibiotic therapy, incision and drainage are indicated, and therapy should be continued for another 5 to 7 days.

Clinical improvement in bacterial adenitis is expected within 48 to 72 hours of the initiation of treatment, but the size of the node or nodes usually does not regress at this stage, and low-grade fever may persist. Regression of lymph node enlargement is slow. As a general guideline, however, significant enlargement that persists beyond 4 to 8 weeks demands exclusion of an underlying disorder and consideration of excisional biopsy.

Rational therapy for cervical lymphadenitis when organisms other than staphylococci or streptococci are involved or when lymph node enlargement is the result of noninfectious processes depends on the cause of the condition. Disease caused by *M tuberculosis* requires specific chemotherapy for that infection as well as family contact tracing for the infected adult. Disease caused by atypical mycobacteria requires complete surgical excision without medical therapy, because these organisms are resistant to most antituberculous drugs. *Nocardia* infections are treated with trimethoprim/sulfamethoxazole orally, but therapy for as long as 3 or 4 weeks often is required for resolution. CSD usually is a benign, self-limited process, and no specific therapy is recommended. In certain patients, however, ongoing local discomfort may be an indication for aspiration to hasten resolution and relieve discomfort. Surgical excision is reserved for the occasional patient who has ongoing systemic symptoms, persistence of significant adenopathy, or development of draining sinuses.

## OUTCOME

Cervical adenitis generally resolves without complication when the infection is caused by agents that are susceptible to antimicrobial therapy (staphylococci and streptococci). Delay in diagnosis or initiation of therapy, however, may prolong the clinical course. In this situation, complications or sequelae may occur, including sinus tracts (mycobacteria and CSD), abscess formation, cellulitis and bacteremia (S aureus and group A *Streptococcus*), acute glomerulonephritis (group A *Streptococcus*), and disseminated infection (M tuberculosis). Untreated suppurative cervical adenitis usually drains exteriorly; rarely, this process may extend internally, producing thrombosis of the jugular vein, rupture of the carotid artery, mediastinal abscess, or purulent pericarditis. Compression of the esophagus or larynx also has been described.

These complications, with the exception of abscess formation, are rare. In children with abscess, appropriate drainage and specific antimicrobial therapy result in prompt resolution of signs and symptoms, and relapse is rare. In the unusual patient with repeated adenitis caused by S aureus, chronic granulomatous disease should be excluded.

The availability of effective antibacterial and antituberculous agents has resulted in an excellent prognosis for almost all children with cervical adenitis. Without surgical excision, however, 84% of those with atypical mycobacterial infection have ongoing morbidity. Appropriate surgical intervention as sole therapy produces cure in 92% to 98% of patients.

## PREVENTION

The elimination of predisposing conditions such as dental caries or abscesses, group A streptococcal upper respiratory infection, bacterial otitis media, and impetigo of the scalp or face should reduce the incidence of adenitis. Minimizing the exposure of infants and young children to adults with active tuberculosis is an obvious means of preventing this extrapulmonary manifestation of tuberculosis. Likewise, lack of exposure to dogs and cats has been hypothesized by some as a means by which reduction in infections resulting from zoonoses may be achieved, but data are lacking. Clearly, our poor understanding of the pathogenesis of many of the causative agents of cervical adenitis limits insight concerning prevention.

## Selected Readings

Butler KM, Baker CJ. Cervical lymphadenitis. In: Feigin RD, Cherry JD, eds. Textbook of pediatric infectious diseases, ed 3. Philadelphia: WB Saunders, 1992.

Huebner RE, Schein MF, Cautheu GM, et al. Usefulness of skin testing with mycobacterial antigens in children with cervical lymphadenopathy. Pediatr Infect Dis J 1992;11:450.

Knight PJ, Mulne AF, Vassy LE. When is a lymph node biopsy indicated in children with enlarged peripheral nodes? Pediatrics 1982;69:391.

Lai KK, Stottmeier KD, Sherman JH, McCabe WR. Mycobacterial cervical lymphadenopathy. Relation of etiologic agents to age. JAMA 1984;251:1286.

Marcy SM. Infections of lymph nodes of the head and neck. Pediatr Infect Dis J 1983;2:397.

Margileth AM. Cervical adenitis. Pediatr Rev 1985;7:13.

Margileth AM, Chandra R, Altman RP. Chronic lymphadenopathy due to mycobacterial infection. Clinical features, diagnosis, histopathology, and management. Am J Dis Child 1984;138:917.

Schaad UB, Vottler TP, McCracken GH Jr, et al. Management of atypical mycobacterial lymphadenitis in childhood: A review based on 380 cases. J Pediatr 1979;95:356.

*Principles and Practice of Pediatrics, Second Edition.*
edited by Frank A. Oski et al. J. B. Lippincott Company, Philadelphia © 1994.

# 36.13 *Herpangina*

Sarah S. Long

Herpangina is a specific, common, acute, febrile viral illness that usually occurs in epidemic form in young children in the summer and fall in temperate climates. Although the clinical symptoms and signs were referred to in 1906, Zahorsky introduced the name *herpangina* in 1924 to distinguish the clinical entity. Although coxsackieviruses of group A were the first known, and thought to be the only, causative agents, it is apparent now that infection with coxsackieviruses of group B and many echoviruses can result in herpangina. At least 24 enteroviral agents have been isolated in epidemic or sporadic cases of herpangina.

## ETIOLOGY

At about the time that Enders, Weller, and Robbins discovered that the first known enterovirus, poliovirus, could be propagated in tissue culture in the late 1940s, Dalldorf and Sickles recovered agents after the inoculation of newborn mice with fecal extracts from two children with paralytic disease. Later shown to be viruses, the new group was called coxsackieviruses after the township in New York State where they were isolated. Two main groups, A and B, were distinguished by histopathologic characteristics in mice and then by the inability to propagate most type A viruses in tissue culture. Later, additions were made to the enterovirus group that did not include poliomyelitis, and this group now contains a total of 23 group A coxsackieviruses, 6 group B coxsackieviruses, 31 echoviruses, and 4 numbered enteroviruses (68 to 71). Hepatitis A virus is classified as enterovirus type 72.

Interpretation of the role of these agents in causing herpangina reflects the evolution of clinical viral diagnostic techniques. Group A coxsackieviruses were associated definitively in the early 1950s with summer epidemics of herpangina, when suckling mice were inoculated for virus isolation. With the increasing use during the next decade of tissue culture techniques to replace the use of animals, seven echoviruses and five group B coxsackieviruses were associated with both epidemic and sporadic cases of herpangina. Other viruses, such as herpes simplex virus and polioviruses, are occasional causes of nonepidemic herpangina. Group A coxsackieviruses probably continue to be the most common cause of herpangina.

Cosackieviruses are 30-nm particles composed of a single strand of RNA with a protein coat of icosahedral symmetry. They are indistinguishable morphologically from each other and from other enteroviruses, are stable at a pH of 3, and are resistant to inactivation by ether. Assignment of a virus to group A or group B is based on its chemical properties, ability to grow in tissue cultures, pathogenicity for laboratory animals, and serologic reactivity.

## EPIDEMIOLOGY

Enteroviruses have a worldwide distribution and produce disease in both sporadic and epidemic forms, particularly in summer in temperate climates. Sporadic cases occur throughout the year.

The majority of enteroviral infections cause either no symptoms or mild nonspecific febrile illnesses. Illness is reported most commonly in children aged 1 to 4 years. It is not clear whether infections occur more frequently, disease manifestations are more common, or recognition and reporting of diseases reflect greater concern for illnesses at this age. In epidemic disease, all age groups are represented.

## PATHOPHYSIOLOGY

In experimental infection with coxsackievirus A4 in rhesus monkeys, oropharyngeal lesions typical of herpangina developed 2 to 7 days after inoculation. The data suggest that, regardless of the site of inoculation, oropharyngeal lesions occur and represent the secondary site of infection after viremia rather than the primary site of virus replication.

Transmission in humans of the viruses that cause herpangina is fecal-oral or oral-oral. Airborne transmission probably occurs, but is less common. Virus can be isolated from throat and fecal specimens in the acute phase of illness, and from fecal specimens for weeks after recovery. Infection elicits the production of type-specific humoral and secretory antibody. Infection appears to elicit lifelong immunity from clinical illness caused by the same agent. Local reinfection with brief periods of virus replication occurs. The role of cellular immune responses is not well defined.

## CLINICAL MANIFESTATIONS

The diagnosis of herpangina is suggested by the presence of lesions in the oropharynx. Herpangina usually is manifested by the sudden onset of fever with no prodrome or only a few hours of anorexia or listlessness. Temperature varies from normal to 41°C, and onset can be accompanied by a seizure. Headache, backache, sore throat, and dysphagia are noted by older patients. The oropharyngeal lesions usually are present at the onset of fever or occur in the subsequent 24 hours. The characteristic lesion evolves from a small papule to a 1- to 2-mm vesicle with surrounding erythema and then to an ulcer. Lesions remain discrete and enlarge to only 3 to 4 mm over 3 days. The average number of lesions is 5, with more than 20 being distinctly unusual. The sites of the lesions are characteristic in their involvement of the anterior tonsillar pillars, tonsils, soft palate, uvula, and pharyngeal wall. Occasionally, posterior buccal surfaces and the tip of the tongue are involved. The diagnosis of herpangina should be made only when the enanthem on the posterior oral cavity is obvious. Other diseases associated with enanthems usually can be distinguished by careful attention to the number, size, and nature of the lesions involved. Features differentiating herpangina from other diseases with enanthems are shown in Table 36-19.

The diagnosis of herpangina is made on clinical grounds. Delineation of a specific cause is helpful to define an epidemic or confirm an unusual case. Throat and stool specimens are the best source of viruses. An increase in specific serum antibody can be demonstrated between acute and convalescent serum samples. The lack of a common enteroviral antigen and the large number of serotypes that are etiologic possibilities make serologic confirmation of the pathogen feasible only when a virus is isolated concurrently from the patient.

## TREATMENT AND PREVENTION

No specific antiviral therapy is available for the treatment of herpangina due to enteroviruses. Treatment is focused on maintaining comfort and adequate hydration, and on observing patients

TABLE 36-19. Features Differentiating Herpangina From Other Diseases With Enanthems

| Disease | Etiology | Occurrence | Character of Oral Lesion(s) | Site of Oral Lesion(s) | Number of Lesions | Size of Lesions | Other Features |
|---|---|---|---|---|---|---|---|
| Herpangina | Coxsackieviruses, echoviruses | Acute | Vesicles, ulcers with erythema | Anterior pillars, posterior palate, and pharynx | 1–5 | 1–2 mm | Dysphagia |
| Herpes stomatitis | Herpes simplex 1 | Acute | Vesicles, shallow ulcers | Gingival/buccal mucosa, tongue, lips | Any | >5 mm, coalescent | Drooling, nodes |
| Hand-foot-mouth | Coxsackieviruses, enterovirus 71 | Acute | Vesicles, shallow ulcers | Tonsillar fauces, buccal mucosa, tongue | Any | 1–3 mm, coalescent | Vesicles on hands and feet, maculopapular rash |
| Aphthous stomatitis | Unknown | Acute, recurrent | Ulcers with rim of erythema, gray exudate | Buccal mucosa, lateral tongue | 1–2 | >5 mm | Pain, no fever |
| Behçet's syndrome | Unknown | Chronic, recurrent | Ulcers with rim of erythema, gray exudate | Any | 1–5 | >5 mm | Ulcers of genital mucosa, uveitis |
| Stevens-Johnson syndrome | Many, unknown | Acute | Ulcers, hemorrhagic ulcers, pseudomembranes | All, lips | Confluent | Confluent | Systemic illness, rash, drug history |
| Mucositis (ulcerative gingivitis) | Neutropenia, chemotherapy, bacteria | Chronic | Ulcers, exudate, pseudomembranes | Gingiva, buccal mucosa | Confluent | Confluent | Fetid breath, pain, other gastrointestinal mucosal lesions |
| Kawasaki disease | Unknown | Acute | Erythema, strawberry tongue | Diffuse | — | — | Prolonged fever, rash, conjunctival hyperemia, cracked lips |
| Toxic shock syndrome | Staphylococcus aureus toxin | Acute | Erythema, strawberry tongue | Diffuse | — | — | Erythroderma, conjunctival hyperemia, hypotension |
| Streptococcal pharyngitis | Group A Streptococcus | Acute | Erythema, exudates, strawberry tongue, palatal petechiae | Tonsils, pharynx | — | — | Sore throat, dysphagia |
| Adenoviral pharyngitis | Adenoviruses | Acute | Follicles, erythema, exudate | Tonsils, pillars, pharynx | — | — | Dysphagia, nodes, conjunctivitis |
| Epstein-Barr pharyngitis | Epstein-Barr virus | Acute | Exudate, palatal petechiae | Tonsils | — | — | Nodes, fatigue, splenomegaly |

for the involvement of other organ systems. The prognosis is excellent, except in rare instances when herpangina is associated with hepatitis, encephalitis, or myocarditis, or with disseminated disease in the neonate. Oral secretions and feces are infectious during acute phases of the illness, and virus can be recovered from feces for weeks after symptoms abate. Asymptomatic infected individuals probably are the primary sources for the spread of infection. Care with handling diapers, good hand-washing practices, and attention to personal hygiene limit the spread of these viruses.

## Selected Readings

Cherry JD, Jahn CL. Herpangina: The etiologic spectrum. Pediatrics 1965;36:632.

Enteroviral infections. In: Krugman S, Katz SL, Gershon AA, Wilfert C, eds. Infectious diseases of children, ed 9. St Louis: CV Mosby, 1992:68.

Nakayama T, Urano T, Osano M, et al. Outbreak of herpangina associated with coxsackievirus B3 infection. Pediatr Infect Dis J 1989;8:495.

Parrott RH, Ross S, Burke FG, et al. Herpangina. Clinical studies of a specific infectious disease. N Engl J Med 1951;245:275.

Simkova A, Petrovicova A. Experimental infection of rhesus monkeys with Coxsackie A4 virus. Acta Virol (Praha) 1972;16:250.

Wenner HA, Ray CG. Diseases associated with coxsackieviruses and echoviruses. In: Kelley VC, ed. Practice of pediatrics, vol 4. Chapter 10. Philadelphia: Harper & Row, 1987.

Zahorsky J. Herpetic sore throat. South Med J 1920;13:871.

*Principles and Practice of Pediatrics, Second Edition.*
edited by Frank A. Oski et al. J. B. Lippincott Company, Philadelphia © 1994.

# 36.14 *Pharyngoconjunctival Fever*

Sarah S. Long

Pharyngoconjunctival fever is an acute viral illness defined by the presence of fever, conjunctivitis, and pharyngitis. It occurs in epidemic and sporadic fashion. Several distinct serotypes of adenovirus are causative agents.

## CHARACTERISTICS OF THE VIRUS

Forty antigenically distinct adenoviruses have been described. These viruses have a diameter of 80 nm and contain double-stranded linear DNA. They have an icosahedral structure with 252 capsomeres, and are resistant to ether and acid but are destroyed if exposed to a temperature of 56 °C for 30 minutes. Important antigenic determinants include those associated with hexons, pentons, and fibers of the virion.

These viruses appear to be harmless commensals at times, but cause highly contagious disease associated with significant morbidity in many individuals. Major epidemics of acute febrile adenoviral respiratory illnesses were noted in recruits during World War II. A highly immunogenic enteric-coated adenovirus vaccine incorporating types 4 and 7 has been used routinely by the military since 1970. Studies of civilian populations showed that diseases caused by adenovirus types 4 and 7 were less contagious and less symptomatic, with a less severe clinical course, than in the military population. These adenoviruses have been suggested to play a very minor role in respiratory illnesses in children. It has been estimated that the vaccine used for the armed forces would reduce the number of respiratory illnesses experienced by the average child in the first 10 years of life by only 6% if universal immunization were recommended for children.

The name *adenoviruses* was assigned after these viruses were recovered from cultures prepared from normal human adenoid tissue in 1953. This finding, together with subsequent documentation of periods of latency and reactivation, makes it difficult to assign specific pathogenic roles in many clinical situations. Human adenoviruses are not infective for laboratory animals. Studies of epidemic disease coupled with the use of serologic techniques have documented that adenoviruses are related causally to illnesses that are characterized by fever, conjunctivitis, lymphadenopathy, rash, and respiratory tract symptoms. Adenoviruses also can infect the lungs, heart, liver, central nervous system, and urinary tract, and can result in severe systemic disease that may be fatal. Epidemic conjunctival and respiratory infections have been documented with increasing frequency in staff and children in hospital and day-care settings. Recently, several new species of adenovirus that cannot be recovered after usual tissue culture inoculation techniques have been identified by immune-electron microscopic techniques in fecal specimens of patients with gastroenteritis. These viruses are associated with acute diarrheal illnesses.

Infections with adenoviruses occur early in life. Serologic surveys suggest that the majority of children acquire at least one adenovirus infection during the first 5 years of life. Adenoviruses can be recovered from most samples of adenoidal or tonsillar tissue removed from young children. It is during this period of high acquisition that infections are most likely to cause no symptoms or only minor respiratory illness. Recent studies, however, using special nasal wash collection techniques, antigen detection methods, virus isolation, and virus neutralization of acute and convalescent serum, have suggested a more important role for adenoviruses in diseases of childhood. Multiple acquisitions occur in infants who spend time in day-care centers, and these are associated highly with episodes of acute otitis media. Disseminated adenovirus infection with fatal hepatic necrosis or necrotizing pneumonia has been reported in multiple patients with congenital or acquired immunodeficiency, such as after organ transplantation or infection with human immunodeficiency virus. Commonly found serotypes are causative. Fatal infection can follow new acquisition or prolonged asymptomatic shedding.

## ETIOLOGY

Pharyngoconjunctival fever has been associated most often with adenovirus type 3, followed by adenovirus type 7. Epidemics of pharyngoconjunctival fever have been caused by four other adenovirus types. Sporadic disease has been associated with more than 11 different antigenically distinct adenoviruses.

## EPIDEMIOLOGY

Pharyngoconjunctival fever occurs in large community epidemics (usually associated with public swimming facilities), in local outbreaks (such as in hospitals, schools, and camps), and sporadically. It is primarily a disease of school-age children. The increase in frequency noted in outbreaks that occur in the summer probably reflects the risk of conjunctival inoculation in swimming pools. Water that was chlorinated inadequately was implicated in one epidemic of adenovirus disease.

Secondary cases may be the result of respiratory spread of large droplets to the conjunctiva, or contamination of the hands with eye or respiratory secretions of the infected individual and then autoinoculation of the conjunctiva.

Conjunctival infection usually is the result of direct inoculation. The same serotypes of adenovirus that cause pharyngoconjunctival fever associated with swimming pool outbreaks rarely cause sporadic cases of conjunctivitis. Volunteer studies have documented that pharyngoconjunctival fever occurs after conjunctival but not after nasopharyngeal inoculation. Outbreaks of adenovirus type 8 have been associated with inadequately decontaminated ophthalmologic equipment.

## PATHOPHYSIOLOGY

The route of inoculation of adenoviruses causing pharyngoconjunctival fever determines the pathophysiologic sequence. Biopsies of conjunctivae in infected volunteers reveal, predominantly, infiltration of lymphocytes in the submucosa. Biopsy material from tonsils and involved lymph nodes reveals hypertrophy and hyperplasia of the lymphoid tissue, with congestion and edema of connective tissue. Primary infection, regardless of the clinical syndrome, generally confers protection against clinical illness caused by that strain. Adenoviruses do not destroy the cells they infect in vivo. Virus can persist in the nuclei of cells and replicate intermittently to detectable levels. Recurrent shedding of virus probably is not associated with symptoms.

## CLINICAL MANIFESTATIONS

Patients with pharyngoconjunctival fever have fever, pharyngitis (hoarseness, sore throat, cough, or local signs of pharyngeal inflammation), and conjunctivitis (eye pain, itching, excessive tearing, hyperemic conjunctivae). Fever is abrupt in onset and the temperature is greater than 39.2 °C (102.6 °F) in more than 50% of patients. Throat complaints range from mild irritation to severe pain and dysphagia. Tonsils usually are enlarged, and about one third of patients have follicular exudates. Conjunctival abnormalities are more severe than are symptomatic complaints. Disease usually is bilateral. Itching, aching, and soreness are common; photophobia, exudate, and keratitis occur less frequently. Conjunctivae are erythematous and edematous. The palpebral conjunctiva appears granular, and 1- to 3-mm yellow-gray collections of lymphocytes on hyperemic epithelium sometimes are visible (so-called follicles). During epidemics or school or family outbreaks, not all infected individuals have the triad of signs and symptoms. Common additional symptoms and signs include nasal complaints related to adenoid infection and hypertrophy (coryza, stuffiness, epistaxis), systemic complaints (headache, malaise, achiness, anorexia), tender cervical lymph node enlargement, and flushed appearance of the face.

Compared to other viral respiratory illnesses, adenoviral infections are quite protracted. High fever generally is sustained for 4 to 5 days. Although eye findings improve by the end of the first week of illness, symptoms of burning or irritation and dryness of the throat, as well as general malaise, persist into the second week. The peripheral white blood cell count frequently is elevated, and an increase in polymorphonuclear leukocytes may be noted. Conjunctival swabs, throat swabs, and nasal wash specimens are excellent sources of virus for isolation. Viruses replicate in a variety of commonly employed tissue culture systems. Characteristic cytopathic effect and intranuclear inclusions can be seen in tissue culture cells as well as in infected human tissue. Routine histologic examination of conjunctival scrapings does not provide a sensitive means of diagnosis. Rapid detection methods seeking the presence of adenovirus hexon antigens in clinical specimens frequently are useful and are used routinely to confirm isolates from culture.

## DIFFERENTIAL DIAGNOSIS

The differential diagnosis is not problematic, because the triad that leads to the appellation is unique. Epidemic hemorrhagic conjunctivitis, caused by coxsackievirus A24 and enterovirus 70, is associated with subconjunctival hemorrhages ranging in size from small petechiae to large blotches. Chemosis and hyperemia of the bulbar conjunctivae, serous discharge, and fine corneal erosions also can be observed. In addition, patients usually are febrile and have preauricular lymphadenopathy. Conjunctivitis caused by herpes simplex virus is much more serious, and usually is distinguished by its unilateral involvement, vesicular lid lesions, corneal involvement, and preauricular lymphadenopathy. Eye complaints occur with some viruses that cause fever and pharyngitis, such as Epstein-Barr virus, parainfluenza viruses, and influenza viruses, but abnormal conjunctival findings are minimal and infection of other sites predominates in the clinical appearance of these disorders. The hallmark of bacterial infections of the conjunctivae, such as those caused by *Haemophilus influenzae*, *Streptococcus pneumoniae*, and *Neisseria gonorrhoeae*, is purulent exudate. In these infections, infection at other body sites frequently is present. Infection caused by *Chlamydia trachomatis* causes nonspecific findings and cannot be diagnosed on the basis of conjunctival abnormalities alone. The predilection of *C trachomatis* for certain age groups, the lack of associated fever and systemic illness, and the accessibility of highly sensitive diagnostic tests help to establish a diagnosis of *Chlamydia* infection in most cases. The distinctive systemic manifestations of Kawasaki disease, toxic shock syndrome, tularemia, and leptospirosis aid in differentiating these disorders that may cause conjunctival hyperemia or suffusion from the conjunctivitis that is caused by adenoviruses. The degree of lower respiratory tract involvement noted in patients with psittacosis or infection caused by *Mycoplasma pneumoniae* helps to suggest infection with these agents when they cause conjunctivitis. The history and physical examination should separate patients with pharyngoconjunctival fever from those with cat-scratch disease, Newcastle disease, or allergic conjunctivitis.

## TREATMENT AND PREVENTION

No specific form of therapy shortens the course of pharyngoconjunctival fever. The prophylactic use of antibiotics administered topically has no proven efficacy. Steroid-containing ophthalmic ointments should not be used. If purulent conjunctival discharge appears, culture to exclude a bacterial cause should be performed. The prognosis for complete recovery is excellent. Even when keratitis occurs, permanent scarring is rare.

Swimming pools are the predominant sources of epidemics of pharyngoconjunctival fever. Appropriate chlorination, adequate water filtration systems, and exclusion of infected individuals can eliminate this as a source of infection. Care in handling secretions of infected individuals, scrupulous hand washing, and careful personal hygiene habits should be practiced to reduce transmission in hospitals, within families, and in camps.

### Selected Readings

Cherry JD. Pharyngoconjunctival fever. In: Feigin RD, Cherry JD, eds. Textbook of pediatric infectious diseases, ed 3. Philadelphia: WB Saunders, 1992:232.

D'Angelo LJ, Hierholzer JC, Keenlyside RA, et al. Pharyngoconjunctival fever caused by adenovirus type 4: Report of a swimming-pool-related outbreak with recovery of virus from pool water. J Infect Dis 1979;140:42.

Edwards KM, Thompson J, Paolini J, et al. Adenovirus infections in young children. Pediatrics 1985;76:420.

Gigliotti F, Williams WT, Hayden FG, et al. Etiology of acute conjunctivitis in children. J Pediatr 1981;98:531.

Gold E. Adenoviruses. In: Kelley VC, ed. Practice of pediatrics, vol 4. Chapter 2. Philadelphia: Harper & Row, 1987.

Krilov LR, Rubin LG, Frogel M, et al. Disseminated adenovirus infection with hepatic necrosis in patients with human immunodeficiency virus infection and other immunodeficiency states. Rev Infect Dis 1990;12:303.

Matoba A. Ocular viral infections. Pediatr Infect Dis 1984;3:358.

Pacini DL, Collier AM, Henderson FW. Adenovirus infections and respiratory illnesses in children in group day care. J Infect Dis 1987;156:920.

Ruuskanen O, Meurman O, Sarkkinen H. Adenoviral diseases in children: A study of 105 hospital cases. Pediatrics 1985;76:79.

*Principles and Practice of Pediatrics, Second Edition.*
edited by Frank A. Oski et al. J. B. Lippincott Company, Philadelphia © 1994.

# 36.15 *Parotitis*

### Ellen R. Wald

Inflammation of the parotid gland may result from infectious or noninfectious causes. In children, most single attacks of parotitis result from viral infection of the gland. This section is divided into considerations of viral parotitis, suppurative parotitis, and recurrent parotitis.

## VIRAL PAROTITIS

Before the availability of the Jeryl Lynn vaccine that was licensed in 1967, the most common cause of parotitis in children was infection with mumps virus, a myxovirus categorized in the same group of RNA viruses as influenza and parainfluenza viruses. After vaccine licensure, it became apparent that other viruses could cause parotitis, namely, parainfluenza types 1 and 3, influenza A and B, coxsackieviruses A and B, echoviruses, and lymphocytic choriomeningitis virus. Parotitis also may be seen as one of the protean manifestations of infection with the human immunodeficiency virus.

Transmission of a myxovirus is by the respiratory route. After it is acquired, the virus replicates in the epithelial cells of the nasopharynx; subsequently, a viremia occurs, with ultimate localization of virus in the parotid gland.

In the typical case of viral parotitis, the preschool or school-age child may have a brief prodrome of constitutional symptoms such as fever, headache, anorexia, and malaise. The initial local complaint is ear pain near the lobe of the ear that is accentuated by chewing movements. Initially, when the parotid gland begins to swell, the sulcus between the mastoid and the mandible is obliterated. The gland enlarges symmetrically in front of and behind the ear, obscuring the angle of the mandible and displacing the lobe of the ear upward and outward (Fig 36-16). The entire parotid gland becomes swollen in a uniform fashion. The gland peaks in size in 1 to 3 days, and can be quite tender and painful. The swelling is impressive visually. On occasion, the swelling is boggy to the touch and the parotid gland is difficult to delineate precisely by palpation. In other patients, the gland is firm and indurated, with a well-demarcated posterior edge. The skin overlying the gland is neither erythematous nor warm, remaining nearly normal in appearance. The orifice of Stensen's duct opposite the second molar may be prominent as a consequence of erythema and swelling. Expressed secretions appear clear. Generally, the parotid on one side swells first and then, in several days, the contralateral gland also becomes involved. Unilateral involvement is seen in 25% of cases. Pain, trismus, and dysphagia are commonplace, leading to poor oral intake. The swelling may take a week or 10 days to subside.

The diagnosis of viral parotitis usually is clinical. Culturing the throat for virus may allow delineation of the precise causative agent. Surprisingly, the amylase level is not always elevated in cases of parotitis. Treatment of viral parotitis is symptomatic. Analgesics may be prescribed. A fluid or soft diet is preferable when the parotid swelling is maximal.

## SUPPURATIVE PAROTITIS

Suppurative parotitis is an unusual clinical problem in the pediatric age group. It is most common in neonates, and occurs sporadically in children older than 10 years. The usual predisposing cause is stasis of secretions in the parotid gland. This may be secondary to dehydration or to an abnormality of Stensen's duct—either a congenital or an acquired malformation, including a sialolith (stone). Clinically, the child is highly febrile (temperature = 40.5 °C) and toxic, and the gland becomes swollen, hot, and very tender to the touch. The overlying skin is erythematous. Purulent secretions can be expressed through Stensen's duct by milking the gland.

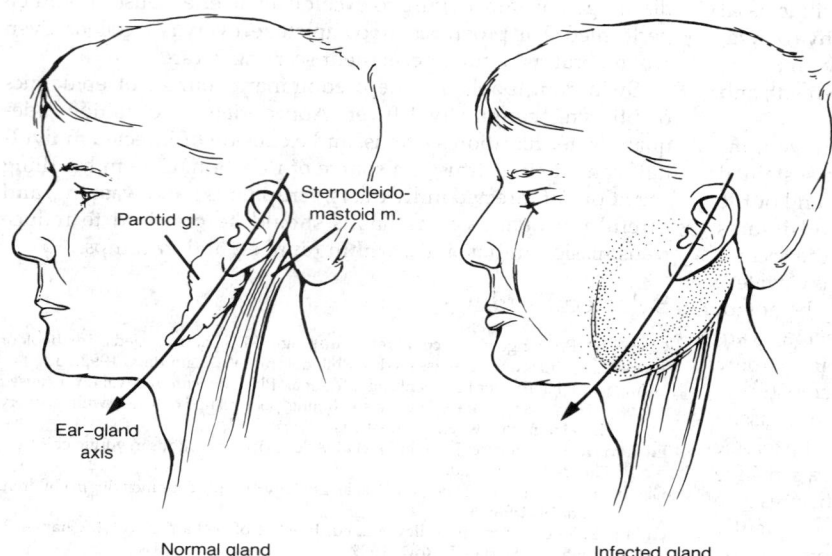

Parotid gl.

Sternocleido-mastoid m.

Ear–gland axis

Normal gland

Infected gland

**Figure 36-16.** Schematic drawing of parotid gland infected with virus (*right*), compared with normal gland (*left*). An imaginary line bisecting the long axis of the ear divides the parotid gland equally. These anatomic relationships are not altered in the enlarged gland.

The most common bacterial isolate in cases of suppurative parotitis is *Staphylococcus aureus.* Other bacterial species that have been implicated include *Streptococcus pneumoniae,* α- and β-hemolytic streptococci, enteric gram-negative bacilli, and *Haemophilus influenzae.* An important role for anaerobic bacterial species (*Bacteroides melaninogenicus* and *Peptostreptococcus* spp.) recently has been emphasized. The path of infection is thought to be the ascending route; the oral flora gain access to Stensen's duct, and stasis of secretions prevents the organisms from being washed out again. Although cases occasionally occur by the hematogenous route, this is much less common.

Treatment of suppurative parotitis consists of providing appropriate parenteral antibiotics and supportive therapies such as fluids and analgesics. Gram's stain of parotid secretions and ultimate culture and sensitivity tests should direct the selection of an antimicrobial agent. If gram-positive cocci in clusters are observed, nafcillin at 150 mg/kg/d in four divided doses is appropriate initial treatment. Alternatively, clindamycin at 30 mg/kg/d in four divided doses provides excellent coverage for staphylococci and respiratory anaerobes. Rarely, incision and drainage of the parotid gland are required if medical management does not result in a clinical cure. Response to therapy should occur in about 48 hours. Treatment of the neonate should be extended for 10 to 14 days. The older child's treatment may be completed with an oral antimicrobial agent for a total course of 7 to 10 days.

## RECURRENT PAROTITIS

Recurrent parotitis of childhood, which is characterized by rapid and repeated swelling of one or both parotid glands, is accompanied by constitutional symptoms of fever and malaise, and by local symptoms of pain and tenderness. The episodes may last for 3 to 7 days. The usual age of onset is between 3 and 6 years. Attacks recur at variable intervals, but every 3 to 4 months is typical. Recurrent juvenile parotitis frequently appears in multiple members of a single family. In most cases, there is spontaneous remission of episodes in late adolescence. The duration of attacks appears to be independent of antibiotic therapy; consequently, this condition is presumed to be noninfectious. First and second episodes often are thought to be examples of suppurative parotitis and, accordingly, are treated with antimicrobial agents.

In cases of recurrent parotitis, it is appropriate to perform sialography. Before this examination is undertaken, a scout film should be performed to scan for the presence of a stone. If a stone is found, sialography is not indicated. Stones in the parotid duct are located most often close to the orifice of the duct; they usually can be removed by milking the gland and duct. Surgical incision made through the ostium of the duct may be required. If no stone is found in the scout film, sialography should be performed. The sialogram will demonstrate diminished acinar components of the gland, partial destruction of the ductal system, and impaired clearance of contrast material. Follow-up studies when attacks remit ultimately may show improvement in the glandular elements and the ductal system. The sialogram appears to exert a therapeutic effect in some patients; fewer recurrences may be seen after the procedure.

When cultures of the parotid saliva are performed in cases of recurrent parotitis, the usual isolate is alpha streptococcus, which is presumed to be normal flora.

## DIFFERENTIAL DIAGNOSIS

When the parotid gland swells initially, the diagnosis of either viral or suppurative disease is made based on the findings of the physical examination. The presence of systemic toxicity and overlying cutaneous changes suggests a suppurative process. Microscopic examination of the drainage emerging from Stensen's duct should clarify the process further: purulent material consisting of polymorphonuclear leukocytes is seen in suppurative parotitis.

Acute suppurative lymphadenitis occasionally may be difficult to distinguish from suppurative parotitis. When the lymph node in the parotid or buccinator area becomes inflamed, the distinction may be impossible. Identifying a site of drainage from the oral cavity, teeth, facial skin, eyes, or external auditory canal may help to clarify the issue. In suppurative submandibular lymphadenitis, the swelling is firm and tender. The overlying skin is erythematous, and the swollen lymph node is easy to delineate. In about half of the patients, there is fever and an obvious focus of infection being drained by the node. The peak age group is 2 to 4 years.

Other causes of persistent salivary gland swelling include amyloidosis, sarcoidosis, disseminated lupus erythematosus, Sjögren's syndrome, and Mikulicz's syndrome. Infectious causes of persistent parotitis include actinomycosis, *Mycobacterium,* toxoplasmosis, melioidosis, and cat-scratch disease. Otherwise, asymptomatic salivary gland swelling may accompany drug therapy with supersaturated potassium iodine or the thiouracils. Symptomatic parotitis may accompany high-dose etoposide and autologous bone marrow transplantation. Toxic parotitis may occur secondary to copper, lead, or mercury poisoning.

## Selected Readings

Brook I, Frazier EH, Thompson DH. Aerobic and anaerobic microbiology of acute suppurative parotitis. Laryngoscope 1991;101:170.
Ericson S, Zetterlund B, Ohman J. Recurrent parotitis and sialectasis in childhood. Ann Otol Rhinol Larygol 1991;100:527.
McNally T. Parotitis: Clinical presentations and management. Postgrad Med 1982; 71:87.

*Principles and Practice of Pediatrics, Second Edition.*
edited by Frank A. Oski et al. J. B. Lippincott Company, Philadelphia © 1994.

# CHAPTER 37
# *Sports Medicine*

## Gregory L. Landry

Pediatricians involved in primary care encounter sports medicine on a daily basis. In most practices, at least one patient each day is involved in athletic pursuits and brings to the physician an agenda related to sports participation. Athletically inclined children and their parents ask difficult questions that are different from those of other patients seeking primary medical care. Recent advances made in the diagnosis and treatment of medical problems in athletes have provided answers to many of those questions.

Sports medicine in the United States traditionally has been a subspecialty of orthopedic surgery. It developed from the evaluation and treatment of injuries occurring to professional and Olympic athletes. Techniques were discovered in the diagnosis and treatment of these athletes that minimized time lost from their sport as a result of injury. These techniques were applied quickly to college athletes, trickled down to high school athletes, and currently have many applications in youth sports. More and more families are demanding the same kind of treatment and care for younger patients that is provided for college and professional athletes. It no longer is acceptable simply to explain the diagnosis of and treatment for a particular injury or illness. Young athletes want to know how soon they can return to participation in their sport and what they can do to speed their recovery. When an illness or injury strikes, "When can I . . .?" becomes the patient's chief concern in the disposition. To maximize safe return to activity, a physical therapist or an athletic trainer may assist with rehabilitation of the injury. In addition, if the child cannot perform a favorite athletic activity, an alternative activity should be suggested to enable the patient to maintain some degree of fitness during rehabilitation.

To care for young athletes, physicians need not be knowledgeable about sports (although it helps), but they must be sensitive to the importance of sports activities in the lives of athletic children. Similar, in a sense, to children with special educational needs, young athletes also have special needs. Athletes may be physically talented, and medical illness or injury may take on more significance than it would in children who are less physically talented. The principles of sports medicine have applications in pediatrics in a broader sense, however. For example, young musicians who are ill or injured and are working toward a musical performance have needs similar to those of injured athletes who are working toward an athletic performance.

Once thought to be a passing fad, sports medicine has become an important area of health care. This chapter addresses some of the most common medical questions that may be encountered by a pediatrician who cares for children who participate in athletic activities.

## THE PRE-PARTICIPATION HEALTH INVENTORY

Children should have a yearly health check-up with a primary care health provider that includes a pre-participation health inventory for those patients who participate in sports activities.

Unfortunately, this is not always possible. Adolescents tend to seek health care infrequently and often only when they are required to do so by an employer or when it is a contingency for athletic participation. Most states require that athletes obtain a physician's statement of approval before they participate in sports activities, and this pre-participation visit provides an opportunity to address many health issues that may not come up at visits made for injuries.

The goals of a pre-participation health inventory vary somewhat from those of a routine health inventory in a non-athlete. In addition to assessing general health and diagnosing treatable conditions, it is important to identify conditions that may interfere with athletic participation or worsen as a result of it, especially any condition that may cause sudden death. Education related to the prevention of athletic injuries also should be included in the inventory process.

## Group Examinations

Some physicians are faced with providing evaluations for a large number of athletes at one time. The most inefficient method practiced traditionally is for one or two physicians to perform a cursory examination of each athlete in a locker room. Instead, when a large number of athletes require examination, the use of revolving stations provides the opportunity for more thorough and highly efficient evaluation. If additional health providers are recruited, the physical examination can be divided by organ systems into stations, and the tasks can be divided among the examiners. A list of possible stations appears in Table 37-1. Parents and coaches may help in administration of the process.

A few drawbacks to the station method deserve consideration. In a large group, the athletes face multiple examiners; with little time available in which to develop rapport, it is difficult to address sensitive topics such as sexual issues or drug use, or to perform examinations of breasts and external genitalia in females. For this reason, one-on-one evaluation by the primary care provider always is preferable.

## Areas of Highest Yield

The history and orthopedic examination portions of the pre-participation inventory yield the most useful information. Most important in the history are questions pertaining to past injuries and to risk factors for sudden death. It is important to question athletes regarding any family history of premature, non-accidental death, and about fainting or dizziness with exercise. Some of the cardiac causes of sudden death in the young athlete can be prevented (Table 37-2). The low prevalence of these problems in the general population makes it difficult to justify the cost of an electrocardiogram and echocardiogram for every athlete. Some

---

**TABLE 37-1.    Stations for the Pre-Participation Evaluation***

1. *History*: parent or coach—must be completed before athlete proceeds to any station
2. *Blood pressure*: trainer or nurse—must have thigh cuffs available for large athletes; should be right arm, sitting
3. *Visual acuity*: trainer or nurse—Snellen chart best; need well-lighted area
4. *Head and neck*: physician or nurse practitioner—disposable specula, extra batteries
5. *Heart and lungs*: physician or nurse practitioner—need quietest area available
6. *Abdomen*: physician or nurse practitioner—gloves for male genitalia and hernia examinations
7. *Orthopedic*: physician or trainer—large examination table
8. *Laboratory*: medical or nursing assistant—gloves and specimen containers
9. *Review and disposition*: physician—best if it is the team physician

* A list of stations, with suggestions about personnel, equipment, and space needs.

---

**TABLE 37-2.    Cardiac Causes of Sudden Death in Young Athletes**

Cardiomyopathy
Hypertrophic cardiomyopathy*
Congenital heart disease
Anomalous left coronary artery
Aortic rupture*
Hypoplastic coronary arteries
Prolonged QT syndrome*
Unknown

* Causes of death that are potentially preventable through detection of a family history of sudden, unexplained death or symptoms during exercise.

common causes of sudden death in athletes are familial, such as hypertrophic cardiomyopathy, prolonged QT syndrome, and aortic rupture associated with Marfan syndrome. Because athletes with Marfan syndrome are at risk for sudden death caused by aortic rupture, examiners should scrutinize tall, thin athletes for findings consistent with the syndrome, such as scoliosis, pectus excavatum, hyperextensible joints, and a click and murmur consistent with mitral valve prolapse. Sudden, unexplained death in the family, fainting with exercise, or findings consistent with Marfan syndrome warrant further evaluation.

A good screening orthopedic examination can be performed in 90 seconds by primary care physicians as part of a general physical examination. The screening orthopedic examination is outlined in Table 37-3. If there is a history of any injury or a positive finding on the screening orthopedic examination, a more thorough evaluation is necessary.

## Disposition

Most athletes fear that something will be discovered during the evaluation that will result in their disqualification from sports participation. Examiners should work toward allowing participation and should not disqualify any youngster who is physically and emotionally fit. In the group setting, it is important to make the disposition very clear. Ideally, the disposition should be written. If further medical evaluation is necessary, it should be made clear to the athlete that this either precludes participation or simply is a recommendation for further care.

## ROLE OF THE TEAM PHYSICIAN

Immediate, and often ongoing, care of injuries in the estimated 20 million young athletes in the United States falls into the hands

### TABLE 37-3. The Orthopedic Screening Examination

| Athletic Activity (Instructions) | Observation |
|---|---|
| Stand facing examiner | Acromioclavicular joints; general habitus |
| Look at ceiling, floor, over both shoulders; touch ears to shoulders | Cervical spine motion |
| Shrug shoulders (examiner resists) | Trapezius strength |
| Abduct shoulders 90° (examiner resists at 90°) | Deltoid strength |
| Rotate arms fully externally | Shoulder motion |
| Flex and extend elbows | Elbow motion |
| Arms at sides, elbows 90° flexed, move wrists into pronation and supination | Elbow and wrist motion |
| Spread fingers; make fist | Hand or finger motion and deformities |
| Tighten (contract) quadriceps; relax quadriceps | Symmetry and knee effusion; ankle effusion |
| "Duck walk" four steps (away from examiner with buttocks on heels) | Hip, knee, and ankle motion |
| Back up to examiner | Shoulder symmetry; scoliosis |
| Knees straight, touch toes | Scoliosis, hip motion, hamstring tightness |
| Raise up on toes, raise heels | Calf symmetry, leg strength |

*Garrick JG. Sports medicine. Pediatric Clin North Am 1977;24:737.*

of coaches. Eighty percent of the sports injuries that occur in this country may be evaluated and treated first by coaches. This statistic points to a need to promote greater involvement by health professionals and to educate coaches regarding sports injuries. Pediatricians may feel unqualified to help with athletic teams because of the number of orthopedic injuries that occur. Actually, pediatricians make excellent team physicians because of their broad knowledge of primary care and their sensitivity to the young athlete psychologically. Most college and professional sports teams involve both a primary care physician and an orthopedic surgeon in team care. Very few of the injuries that occur require extensive musculoskeletal evaluation on the field, but many do require a physician who is knowledgeable about sports injuries.

The basic requirements for a team physician are interest and a willingness to read about problems that are unique to the field of sports medicine. Team physician duties typically are voluntary, and most of us do the job because it is fun!

The specific duties of a team physician must be defined. Some medical–legal problems can be avoided if these responsibilities are delineated clearly in writing. Physicians' responsibilities vary greatly from team to team, and defining them protects a physician to some extent from incurring an excessive time commitment. Most coaches and athletic directors welcome physician involvement because they recognize their expertise in caring for medical problems and injuries. Occasionally, however, an overzealous coach cannot understand why an athlete with a particular injury cannot participate. To minimize this problem, the team physician's authority regarding the ability of the athletes to play in the event of any medical illness or injury should be clarified in writing.

Ideally, the school or team should enlist the services of a certified athletic trainer. The expertise of an experienced certified athletic trainer in assessing an injury and evaluating a player's ability to participate can be invaluable. In addition, a trainer can provide rehabilitation for the injury. If a school or team does not have one, hiring a trainer should be one of the first investments they make toward improving the medical care of their athletes. The trainer will make the job of a team physician much easier.

The equipment that will be available to a physician on the field is limited by cost considerations. The minimum requirements include a first aid kit, a water jug, and an ice chest containing plastic bags. These items are inexpensive, and the importance of having water available for hydration and ice available for injuries cannot be emphasized too strongly to both coaches and athletes.

The supplies included in the medical bag can be extensive, especially if those that usually are available in a trainer's bag are provided. A checklist for the medical bag appears in Table 37-4. Not all these items are required, but the team physician may want to consider them for adequate on-the-field coverage.

## MANAGEMENT OF ATHLETIC INJURIES

### Emergencies

When physicians provide medical coverage for any event, they must be prepared for any eventuality. They should have a plan in the event of a catastrophic injury, such as a spinal cord injury or cessation of pulse and breathing in an athlete. Team physicians also should be prepared to care for spectators in the event of a crisis. The ability to communicate with sources of emergency help can be critical. The location of the nearest telephone always should be known. If it is a pay telephone, loose change must be available to those individuals who are responsible for the care of the spectators and athletes; medical help can be delayed if coins for a pay telephone are not available. Determining in advance those individuals who will call for help if an ambulance is needed and those whom should be called, including the location

**TABLE 37-4.** The Sports Medicine Bag*

| Airway Supplies | Medications | Equipment | Dressings |
|---|---|---|---|
| 1. Oral airways<br>2. Nasal airways<br>3. Ambu bag with face mask and endotracheal tube adapter<br>4. Endotracheal tubes<br>5. Laryngoscope with light source and blades<br>6. Cricothyrotomy kit with tracheostomy tubes | 1. Epinephrine 1:10,000, for resuscitation<br>2. Lidocaine hydrochloride, 100-mg vial for arrhythmias<br>3. Lactated Ringer's solution with IV tubing and IV catheters<br>4. Epinephrine 1:1,000 for endotracheal tube installation or subcutaneous use for anaphylaxis<br>5. Diazepam, 10-mg vial, for seizures<br>6. Dexamethasone, 4 mg, for spinal cord injury<br>7. Ophthalmologic saline for irrigation<br>8. Antibiotic ointment<br>9. β-agonist inhaler | 1. Stethoscope<br>2. Otoscope/ophthalmoscope<br>3. Thermometer<br>4. Penlight<br>5. Swiss Army knife<br>6. Sphygomomanometer<br>7. Tongue blades<br>8. Surgical towel clip | 1. White bandage tape<br>2. Sterile gauze pads<br>3. Cotton swabs<br>4. Elastic bandages<br>5. Sterile suture kits (gloves, suture material, syringes, and lidocaine)<br>6. Ster-I-Strips<br>7. Tincture of benzoin<br>8. Povidone-iodine solution<br>9. Bandage scissors<br>10. Finger splints<br>11. Plaster bandages and cotton-web roll |

\* A checklist of items that the team physician may want to include in the on-the-field medical bag for sports-event coverage.

of the closest ambulance service, saves valuable time. This information probably should be written on the medical bag and the coach's first aid kit.

## Management on the Field

Management of injuries on the field really is applied first aid. When an athlete "goes down" on the playing surface, physicians should remain calm, because other people look to them for direction. Whenever it is possible, using the athlete's name will have a calming effect. Once the athlete's attention is gained, the physician should ask the child to indicate where the pain is located. If the athlete is unresponsive, basic principles of life support (ie, A, B, C [airway, breathing, circulation]) should be followed.

An unconscious athlete who has been injured in a contact sport, such as football, should be treated as if a fracture of the cervical spine has been sustained. If there is any pain in the neck or back, palpation of the cervical spine and back should be performed before the athlete is allowed to move. If there is any suggestion of a significant neck or back injury, the athlete should be transported by an emergency vehicle to the nearest emergency facility for radiography. Injuries to the extremities should be assessed by visual observation and palpation, and by determination of range of motion and stability. Immediate swelling, bony tenderness, deformity, lack of range of motion, or instability indicates that the athlete may need assistance in leaving the field of play.

An examination should be repeated after the athlete has left the playing surface. In the absence of suspicion of fracture, ligamentous instability, or any neurovascular compromise, the question of the child's ability to play arises.

## Determining an Athlete's Ability to Play

Determining an athlete's ability to play can be a challenge, even to a physician who has vast experience in sports injuries. Simple guidelines are helpful in dealing with medical problems that arise in the heat of the action.

Once the injury has been evaluated and determined to be relatively minor, the athlete's ability to play is assessed by functional evaluation. The athlete should be asked to perform a function that is similar to, or related to, actions that are required during the athletic event. If any pain, weakness, or instability is experienced during the functional examination, participation should be disallowed. For example, the athlete with a mildly

sprained ankle can be asked to jump up and down on the toes of the injured foot while avoiding weight bearing on the uninjured foot. If this task can be performed without difficulty, return to play is reasonable. Other functional tests may be added, such as running in a figure-of-eight pattern or in zigzag sprints. Playing when an injury is present can increase the risk of further injury, and a functional examination shows the athlete that some degree of impairment exists. Functional testing takes some of the guesswork out of this sometimes difficult decision.

Stability should be assessed immediately after an injury occurs, because a ligament examination can be obtained best before swelling, hemorrhage, and inflammation have started to cause pain and protective muscle guarding. Any instability or increased joint laxity precludes athletic participation. Whereas the first examination is best for determining stability in regard to the athlete's ability to return to play, the extent of the injury may become clearer 15 to 20 minutes after the injury has occurred, when tissue damage has caused more inflammation. Protective taping or bracing will not, and should not, be used to permit an athlete with a significant injury to participate, but it may be used to protect a mild injury from exacerbation when the athlete returns to play.

## HEAT ILLNESS

Heat illness is relevant to physicians in both cool and warm climates, because sporting events occur indoors as well as outdoors. Our understanding of the pathophysiology of heat illness has improved markedly in recent years, which is important, because life-threatening heat illness (heat stroke) probably is entirely preventable.

The terminology in this area can be confusing and often is misunderstood. Heat cramps, heat syncope, heat exhaustion, and heat stroke are part of a continuum.

## Heat Cramps

Heat cramps are painful and forceful muscle contractions that usually occur in the gastrocnemius or hamstring muscles. They probably are not related to electrolyte balance or inadequate salt intake, but to heat, dehydration, and lack of training. Treatment includes rest and the ingestion of copious amounts of cold water.

## Heat Syncope

Heat syncope is a term often used to describe a phenomenon that is common in runners in which they stop running at the end of a race and experience hypotensive syncope as a result of venous pooling. This is not life-threatening, but is indicative of hypovolemia and the redistribution of blood volume that is caused by sweating and mild hyperthermia. Treatment is rest and the ingestion of generous amounts of cold water.

## Heat Exhaustion

Heat exhaustion is manifested by pale skin color, vasoconstriction, dizziness, visual disturbances, syncope, and a moderately elevated rectal temperature (38 °C to 40 °C, or 101 °F to 105 °F). As with muscle cramps, treatment involves rest and rehydration. Ice packs and a fan may speed recovery. In some cases, intravenous fluid therapy may be required because of nausea and vomiting. Most authorities recommend 0.5% normal saline, which approximates the composition of the sweat that has been lost.

## Heat Stroke

The presence of central nervous system symptoms such as delirium, convulsions, and coma is indicative of heat stroke. A rectal temperature greater than 41 °C (106 °F) characteristically is seen in acute exercise-induced heat stroke. In the absence of exercise, heat stroke is associated with the absence of sweating and the presence of warm, flushed skin. The young, exercising athlete with heat stroke, however, usually still is sweating profusely and has peripheral vasodilation. The central nervous system symptoms are more specific for heat stroke and indicate a medical emergency. Heat stroke can be fatal if it is not treated. The athlete should be packed in ice bags applied to the head, neck, and groin areas. Intravenous fluids (0.5% normal saline) should be administered as soon as possible, and immediate transport to a hospital is imperative. Because heat stroke may cause multi-system failure, the athlete may require admission to the hospital for observation.

## Prevention of Heat Illness

It is important to consider the environmental conditions that cause the greatest heat stress. These include high environmental temperatures, high levels of relative humidity (as measured by a wet-bulb thermometer), and high levels of solar radiation (as occurs during the hottest part of the day). Evaporation is less effective when there is little wind. The greatest risk probably occurs on relatively warm days that follow cooler weather, especially in the early spring when athletes have not had time to adjust to the temperature change.

## Susceptible Individuals

Certain types of individuals are at greater risk for sustaining heat injury, including those who are obese, poorly trained, dehydrated, or not used to heat. Age also is a risk factor, primarily for young children and the elderly. Anyone with a history of heat stroke is at risk for recurrence.

Football players are more susceptible to heat illness than are other athletes because their ability to lose heat through evaporation is abolished almost completely. Football uniforms cover most of the body, and practices start during some of the hottest days of the summer. Because coaches often are the only ones in contact with these athletes, they bear the main responsibility for preventing heat illness. Football players often have two practices a day, and they may not rehydrate their bodies before each prac-

tice. To address this problem, many coaches require that weight measurements be taken before and after each practice. The weights are recorded on a chart in the locker room next to the scales. At the beginning of a practice session, athletes who have lost 3% or more of their body weight are observed carefully and may not be allowed to participate because they are at higher risk of the development of heat illness. Most coaches modify practices on hot days and allow the players to wear shirts and shorts for all or part of the practice session.

In addition to identifying risk factors, unlimited water should be provided to the athletes. Salt tablets should not be used, because they increase the risk of hypernatremia. Sweat is hypotonic, and athletes are depleted primarily of water.

# COMMON MEDICAL ILLNESSES IN ATHLETES

## Common Viral Infections

Exercise causes changes in the immune system, the significance of which is unknown. Exercise causes a transient granulocytosis and lymphocytosis as well as an increase in circulating endogenous pyrogen. Despite these changes, athletes are just as susceptible to the common viral illnesses as are non-athletes. For individuals participating in team sports, the exposure rate probably is as high as it is for other children and adolescents attending school.

Few scientific data exist regarding common viral illnesses in relation to the ability of a child to participate in sports activities. The objective finding of fever is helpful. Excellent studies have shown increased cardiopulmonary effort and reduced exercise capacity in response to fever. Fever also is associated with poor tolerance of orthostatic stress, poor tolerance of submaximal exercise, and abnormal temperature regulation. For these reasons, fever should preclude participation in most instances.

Some physicians are extremely conservative because of the fear of precipitating myocarditis in an athlete who exercises in the presence of viral infections. The only suggestion of this occurred in an animal study, which showed that a coxsackievirus B27 infection in mice produced a significant incidence of myocarditis when exercise was forced. No studies in humans have proven this connection. If exercise is a precipitating factor, it would seem that a much higher incidence of myocarditis would be seen in athletes. Most physicians use the presence of fever and the severity of symptoms to determine an athlete's ability to play.

It is well known that many of the common cold viruses can cause significant impairment of small airways for several weeks after the infection. Viral respiratory infections in any athlete who has known reactive airways are more likely to make the individual symptomatic. Exercise-induced asthma is as common in athletes as it is in non-athletes. Rather than restricting the athlete from competition because of cough, wheezing, and shortness of breath, the bronchospasm should be treated aggressively with a $\beta_2$-sympathomimetic aerosol, such as albuterol. This will control asthmatic symptoms in at least 80% of children who have exercise-induced symptoms.

Exercise-induced chest tightness or cough should alert the physician that reactive airways may be impairing the athlete's performance. Treatment with albuterol can safely provide marked improvement in symptoms. Additional agents such as cromolyn or a corticosteroid may be necessary for adequate treatment of the athlete with symptoms caused by bronchospasm.

## Infectious Mononucleosis

At least once a year, most practicing pediatricians are faced with an athlete who has infectious mononucleosis. In almost all sports, this usually has a significant impact on the individual's ability to participate in sports activities. It is of special concern in collision and contact sports because of the high incidence of splenomegaly and the risk of splenic rupture. A review of the reports regarding splenic rupture demonstrates that most ruptures occur during the first 3 weeks of the illness. Also, in more than 50% of the splenic ruptures reported, the spleen was not palpable during the initial examination.

Palpation on physical examination is a poor method of assessing splenic size. In dealing with an athlete, especially one who is participating in collision sports such as football or hockey, radiologic evaluation should be considered. Plain radiographs of the abdomen are about 70% accurate in assessing splenic size. Ultrasound, if it is available, provides an accurate measurement of splenic volume.

The duration of illness and degree of splenomegaly vary greatly from person to person. Rather than setting an arbitrary interval during which an athlete must not participate in a sport, each individual should be observed on a weekly basis, with the ability to play determined by clinical symptomatology and physical examinations. Most athletes with mononucleosis are too ill to consider resuming competition before 3 to 4 weeks after the onset of the illness. By the 3-week mark, they are past the period of high risk for splenic rupture and should be allowed to play sports if they feel able to do so.

Occasionally, athletes have a mild case of mononucleosis and their symptoms have abated as early as 2 weeks after the onset of the illness. With documentation by radiography or sonography that the spleen is not enlarged, return to competition probably carries little risk. The athlete certainly should avoid physical stress early in the illness when fever and other symptoms are present. Light workouts probably can be resumed when the athlete feels able; however, the effects of exercise on the severity and duration of mononucleosis have not been studied. In a study of infectious hepatitis in army personnel, there was no difference in recovery time (4 weeks) or relapse rate between patients who performed regular exercise and light work and those who were kept at rest.

## SPORTS NUTRITION

Nutrition is an increasingly important aspect of sports medicine. Unfortunately, many athletes do not ask for nutritional information from health professionals, but seek advice from their coaches and teammates. Many experts in the field of sports medicine feel that the most significant advances made in sports medicine in the future will be in the area of nutrition. The pre-game meal, fluid replacement, and weight gain and loss methods are common topics that pediatricians may be asked to address by athletes and coaches.

### The Pre-Game Meal

The meal that is eaten just before an athletic contest is important to athletes who want to be at their best at game time. Most athletes are not comfortable exercising on a full stomach. Ideally, the meal should be consumed 2 to 3 hours before exercise, and it should consist mostly of complex carbohydrates. High-fat meals tend to prolong the full feeling and take longer to digest.

A "quick energy" candy bar or simple sugar snack consumed immediately before an event is more likely to be detrimental than helpful to an athlete. A rebound hypoglycemia may occur during athletic activity as a result of the relative hyperinsulinemia that occurs after the sugar load. This has been demonstrated in studies of patients who underwent aerobic exercise on a treadmill after sugar loading.

### Fluid Replacement

During most athletic events, the best fluid to use for rehydration is cold water. It certainly is the cheapest and most easily obtainable fluid. Although most of the commercial sports drinks are pleasant tasting, they are hypertonic and relatively expensive. The carbohydrate and electrolyte composition of the replacement fluid probably is important only in endurance events that involve 30 minutes or more of continuous exercise. Hypertonic solutions once were thought to impede gastric emptying and intestinal absorption. Recent research has shown that oral solutions containing as much as 6% glucose are absorbed rapidly and provide an important source of carbohydrate for endurance athletes. Cold liquids appear to be absorbed in the stomach faster than are lukewarm liquids. Athletes should be reminded that thirst is not a sensitive indicator of hydration status and that they should replace fluid before they feel thirsty.

### Weight Gain

An athlete who is interested in gaining weight to improve performance in a particular sport, such as football, should be trying to achieve a gain in lean body mass. The athlete may be tempted to buy all kinds of nutritional products that are claimed to promote rapid weight gain. Numerous amino acid supplements are available, but studies have not shown them consistently to have any effect other than being an additional source of calories.

Free amino acid supplements cause both proven and theoretic harm to the athlete. The osmotic load is associated with a significant incidence of diarrhea and abdominal pain. Physiologically, polypeptides are absorbed more efficiently in the gut than are free amino acids. Animal studies on amino acid supplementation show a high incidence of nephropathy, but this never has been shown in humans.

A careful dietary analysis often is helpful in assessing the daily caloric intake of an athlete, and it may reveal a level of caloric intake that is insufficient for adequate weight gain. If the athlete needs to increase the total daily caloric intake, ingesting more carbohydrates should be emphasized because the diets of most Americans already are rich in protein. While attempting to gain weight, the athlete should be involved in a strength training program so that the gain is more likely to be in lean body mass.

### Weight Loss

For some athletes, thinness is vital to their success. Ballet dancers, wrestlers, gymnasts, and distance runners often feel pressured to stay thin or to lose weight. These athletes are just as prone as are non-athletes to use unhealthy rapid weight loss methods, and they may be at risk for the development of eating disorders.

In general, athletes should use the same sensible weight loss methods as non-athletes, decreasing their caloric intake while increasing their caloric expenditure. For most athletes, a reasonable maximum weight loss per week is 0.90 kg (2 lb). Faster weight loss probably will result in ketosis, loss of muscle mass, and dehydration. Use of saunas, rubber suits, or diuretics to lose weight should be discouraged strongly because of the associated risks of electrolyte disturbance and excessive dehydration. Fortunately, many of the unhealthy eating behaviors seen in athletes are transient, practiced only during participation in the particular sport, and do not become integrated permanently into their behavior patterns.

## DERMATOLOGIC CONCERNS IN ATHLETES

Few skin problems disqualify athletes from playing sports, but contagious skin infections do rule out competition in sports that involve close contact, such as wrestling or rugby. Impetigo and herpesvirus infections are seen most commonly, although scabies also is contagious enough to warrant disqualification. Impetigo and herpes infections can spread through a team quickly unless the athletes and coaches are cognizant of the importance of early diagnosis and treatment. With aggressive treatment, the amount of time lost from participation can be minimized.

## Impetigo

The athlete with impetigo usually is infected by the same organism as is the non-athlete, predominantly *Staphylococcus aureus* or *Streptococcus pyogenes*. The diagnosis of impetigo may be more difficult in the wrestler because any bulla or crust may be rubbed off during a match or in the shower. Also, the lesions occur anywhere on the body, and they may not look much more impressive than do fresh abrasions. Early in the course of infection, an athlete with recurrent impetigo may be able to tell the physician when the condition began. Skin cultures do not distinguish pathogens from flora, and probably need not be performed unless recurrences are frequent or treatment response is poor.

Treatment involves good local care, including scrubbing with an antiseptic soap and applying an antibacterial ointment such as mupirocin. Systemic antibiotics should be used more liberally in most athletes, to speed recovery and decrease contagiousness to the other participants.

The ability of an athlete with impetigo to participate in a sport is subjective, but a waiting period of at least 24 hours after the initiation of a systemic antibiotic is necessary. Covering lesions with an occlusive dressing often is impractical because of perspiration and constant trauma to the dressing.

Impetigo can be prevented by frequent washing of the mats that serve as fomites. Athletes with impetigo should be disqualified promptly from competition. It may be reasonable for some athletes who are particularly susceptible to impetigo to take an antibiotic prophylactically during a designated period of time. This may be especially useful toward the end of the season, just before tournaments. The use of a prophylactic antibiotic increases the risk that resistant bacteria will develop, however, and this possibility should be weighed against the benefit of preventing an outbreak.

## Herpes Simplex

Herpetic infections in athletes who are involved in high-contact sports such as wrestling sometimes are called "herpes gladiatorum." Lesions develop anywhere on the trunk or extremities and are more likely to occur in a break in the skin caused by an abrasion. The signs and symptoms are the same as for herpes simplex infections occurring elsewhere on the body, except that the lesions often are more widespread.

Treatment includes disqualification until all vesicles are crusted over. As with impetigo, evaluation of a player's ability to participate is somewhat subjective. Some athletes have outbreaks that last for 5 to 7 days, which is a significant time away from competition. Acyclovir has been extremely helpful in treating herpes simplex, especially in individuals with recurrent outbreaks. Acyclovir ointment can be applied locally every 2 hours at the beginning of an outbreak, and it may speed recovery. A more effective treatment is oral acyclovir, 200 mg given five times a day until the lesions are gone.

As athletes become better educated about acyclovir, they are quicker to seek treatment because it speeds recovery. Some collegiate wrestling teams are using acyclovir prophylactically, especially at tournament time. Although its use in athletes has not been studied specifically, prophylactic acyclovir has been shown to be effective against recurrent herpetic lesions in various areas of the body.

# COMMON INJURIES INVOLVING THE HEAD AND NECK

Head and neck trauma can be quite anxiety provoking for the athlete, the family, and the physician covering an athletic event. Fortunately, in most sports, severe injuries occur infrequently, but mild head and neck traumatic injuries are common occurrences in contact sports such as football and ice hockey. In sports that involve the use of protective helmets, the team physician should be prepared to remove the face mask in case of a head or neck injury requiring access to the airway. Using a screwdriver or knife to remove the fasteners connecting the face mask to the helmet allows quick removal of the face mask and access to the airway without moving the athlete's neck.

## Assessment on the Field

When physicians evaluate the extent of an athlete's injury while he or she still is on the field, they should ask the individual whether any neck pain is present. Even when neck pain is denied, if the athlete has sustained a concussion, the neck should be palpated carefully along the cervical spine for any area of tenderness. It also is important, before the athlete is allowed to sit up or to stand, to ask him or her whether any neurologic symptoms are felt in the extremities, such as numbness, tingling, or weakness. If there is any neck pain, especially any cervical spine tenderness, the athlete must be considered to have sustained a neck fracture and must not be moved. After being immobilized properly, the athlete should be transported by trained personnel to an emergency facility. If the individual is unconscious, he or she must be assumed to have a neck fracture, and should be treated accordingly. If an airway must be established, this potential injury must be assumed.

## Concussions

Concussions occur frequently in contact sports, and determining an athlete's ability to return to play afterward can be difficult. Some physicians unnecessarily disqualify athletes with even the mildest of head trauma. The diagnosis of a concussion should be made in any athlete who sustains a transient loss of cognitive ability as a result of trauma to the head. The mildest form of concussion is commonly referred to as the "ding," and it consists of a few seconds of confusion, loss of balance, and "seeing stars." This can be brief enough to go undetected by teammates and coaches.

Criteria for return to play after concussion are similar to those after other injuries; the athlete must pass a functional examination. Gait analysis and balance should be evaluated on the sideline. The most sensitive examination is a test for memory. In addition to asking simple information about the athlete's address or events that took place earlier in the day, it is helpful to have a teammate discuss the higher cognitive aspects of the game. If the athlete stumbles when being asked questions about the game plan or the assignments, then return to competition is forbidden. These cognitive abilities may return during the event, and the athlete may return to competition at that time if there is no nausea, vomiting, or headache.

The longer the athlete experiences loss of higher cognition, the more severe the concussion is. The athlete should be questioned carefully about events that occurred earlier in the day. The presence of retrograde amnesia signals a more severe concussion, even without a history of loss of consciousness. The athlete with evidence of retrograde amnesia will be unlikely to regain full cognition during the game, will have a headache, and should not be allowed to compete.

Any athlete who loses consciousness during a competition should be disqualified from further participation in that competition. No matter how insistent the athlete may be, the loss of consciousness signals a more severe concussion, and the athlete probably will have a severe headache within an hour after injury. When an athlete is restricted from competition, especially for head injury, the coach should be informed. In sports that require headgear for participation, non-participation almost is guaranteed if the physician retains the athlete's headgear. In the heat of the moment, especially if he or she is not thinking clearly, the athlete may try to resume competition against medical advice. In contrast to other sports injuries, it usually is not a good idea to send to the showers an athlete who has sustained a head injury, because medical personnel may not be available to accompany the individual. The athlete must be observed closely after sustaining a concussion, and the team physician can best keep an eye on the athlete on the sidelines.

The headache that an athlete experiences after sustaining a concussion can last for days or weeks. Because headache indicates some cerebral dysfunction, an athlete should not be allowed to participate in sports in the presence of headache after a concussion. When the headache resolves, the athlete may be allowed to do some light jogging and, eventually, sprinting. If running produces headache, the athlete should not be allowed to proceed to competition. Occasionally, an athlete will have a postconcussional syndrome, with frequent headaches, poor concentration, irritability, and loss of certain cognitive abilities for days to weeks after the injury. An athlete with a persistent headache or a progressively worsening headache warrants a computed tomographic (CT) scan and a neurosurgical evaluation.

Once an athlete has received a concussion, his or her risk of sustaining another concussion is increased. Traditionally, physicians have disqualified athletes from participating in a sport when they have sustained three concussions. The "three concussions and you are out" rule may be appropriate in some cases, but every patient must be approached individually. Both the severity of the concussions and the time between their occurrence should be considered. The possibility of delayed cerebral dysfunction, which has been documented in boxers who have sustained recurrent concussions, should be kept in mind when counseling the athlete and the family.

## Brachial Plexus Injuries

Many spectators of football, ice hockey, or wrestling are familiar with the athlete who comes off the field dangling or shaking an arm. Frequently, this athlete has sustained an injury commonly known as a "burner" or "stinger," which is a stretch of the brachial plexus. The burning pain with associated shoulder and arm weakness usually abates in a few minutes; in a few instances, weakness may persist for a few days to a few months. This injury is thought to be caused by a blow that hyperextends the neck, or causes lateral flexion of the neck away from the side of the injury, with or without a concomitant blow to the shoulder. Traction of the brachial plexus produces paresthesias in the shoulder, radiating down the arm and frequently into the hand. The athlete may complain of pain in the area of the trapezius muscle, but the injury seldom, if ever, should be associated with true neck pain. Bilateral symptomatology is strongly suggestive of cord injury rather than plexus injury. The athlete should be removed from the game and appropriate radiographs should be taken to rule out the possibility of spinal stenosis in an individual with bilateral paresthesias or weakness.

Occasionally, symptoms of a "burner" are caused by pinching of a cervical root resulting from compression from a blow to the head. If cervical spine tenderness is present, this should *not* be considered a "burner," and the athlete should be disqualified from participation until further evaluation of the neck can be performed. Cervical disc herniation also may present as a "burner." Careful questioning of the athlete may reveal pain originating from the cervical spine. Manual axial compression of the head and neck often reproduces the symptoms. Suspicion of cervical disc pathology warrants further evaluation such as a magnetic resonance imaging scan and consultation with a neurosurgeon.

Brachial plexus injuries have been classified as first-, second-, or third-degree, based on clinical and electromyographic study results. Most brachial plexus nerve injuries fall into the category of grade I and last for seconds to minutes. Theoretically, an interruption in function has occurred without anatomic damage. The decision regarding return to play is based on a careful strength assessment of the upper extremities. When the athlete feels completely recovered, his or her head and neck should be put through a range of motion against resistance. The shoulder girdle musculature and forearm muscles also should be tested against resistance. If no pain or weakness is reported by the athlete, return to competition may be allowed. Occasionally, an athlete may have persistent weakness that lasts for several weeks or several months. This indicates that a grade II injury with anatomic axonal damage has been sustained. A grade III brachial plexus nerve injury produces motor and sensory deficits of at least 1 year's duration. Fortunately, this injury appears to be rare.

Any persistent weakness disqualifies an athlete with a brachial plexus injury from further sports activity. The trapezius pain frequently persists beyond the paresthesia and need not disqualify an athlete from competition. The cause of trapezius pain probably is significant stretching of the muscle at the time of the injury. The athlete should be reexamined 24 to 48 hours after injury, because neuronal dysfunction resulting from edema may be delayed. Appropriate cervical spine films, including anteroposterior (AP), lateral, oblique, and flexion and extension lateral views, should be taken the first time any athlete sustains this injury, to ascertain whether congenital anomalies are present.

The athlete who sustains a "burner" in football or hockey should be fitted with a protective collar over the shoulder pads to limit neck movement. Other methods of limiting neck motion (eg, straps) also exist and probably offer some protection against brachial plexus injury. Increasing overall neck strength is an important aspect of preventing these injuries.

## INTRODUCTION TO ORTHOPEDIC INJURIES

In general, musculoskeletal problems are the most common reason for athletes to seek medical attention. Athletes are likely to delay seeking care until significant disability is present because they are taught to deny pain at an early age. In other words, most athletes tend to disregard minimal injuries and to obtain health care only when something is seriously wrong. Although the majority of injuries are exacerbated and recovery is prolonged by continued participation in a sport, there are some injuries that do not preclude participation and with which the athlete may play safely in the presence of pain.

## Definitions

The terms *strain* and *sprain* frequently are used incorrectly; often, the former is meant to suggest a minor injury and the latter to indicate a more significant injury. A sprain is defined accurately as any injury to a ligament or joint capsule. A strain is any injury to a muscle. Acute traumatic orthopedic injuries may warrant a visit to the pediatrician, but many of the visits are prompted by overuse injuries caused by cumulative microtrauma instead of one single impact, or macrotrauma. Strenuous athletic activity frequently produces microscopic tissue breakdown, but the body's capacity to heal usually repairs this breakdown before significant injury occurs. When the tissue trauma exceeds the body's healing capacity, inflammation and edema result in pain, a signal that a clinical injury has occurred. Repetitive microtrauma to a tendon may produce tendinitis. Once thought to be a tenosynovitis, a painful tendon in an athlete usually is a result of tissue damage and inflammation within the substance of the tendon, rather than inflammation of the synovial sheath. With repeated loading of bone, a stress fracture may be produced. In the skeletally immature athlete, especially during a period of rapid growth, muscle-tendon overload at the traction growth plate apophysis may produce a stress reaction. This injury is called an apophysitis. Tibial tubercle apophysitis (Osgood-Schlatter syndrome), calcaneal apophysitis (Sever syndrome), and iliac crest apophysitis are but a few examples of this phenomenon. With most overuse injuries, simple rest will help, but a rehabilitation program will speed recovery and aid in preventing recurrences. Many overuse injuries develop when a change in the training regimen causes an increase in repetitive microtrauma. For example, in a runner with an overuse injury, it is important to inquire about any change in weekly mileage, terrain, or intensity of the workout. Identifying the cause of the overuse injury is important in providing treatment and preventing repetitive injury.

## Grading

Quantifying the severity of a sports injury is somewhat subjective, but grading systems do exist that make classification reasonably objective for most injuries. A sprain is graded as being either first-, second-, or third-degree. A grade I sprain is one in which a few fibers within a ligament are torn. Clinically, there is little pain and swelling, a full range of motion, and no increased joint laxity. In a grade II sprain, a significant number of fibers are torn and there is a detectable increase in joint laxity, but at least a few fibers are intact. Clinically, there is significant pain and swelling, with impairment of range of motion. In a grade III sprain, the entire ligament has been disrupted, and marked laxity is evident when the ligament is stressed.

Strains, or injuries to the muscle, are more difficult to evaluate than are sprains. Grading is based primarily on the clinical findings. In a grade I strain, only a few fibers are torn and, clinically, only a little pain or contraction of the muscle against resistance is present. Strength testing reveals little, if any, loss of strength. In a grade II strain, a significant number of muscle fibers have been injured and, clinically, marked pain is noted on palpation and muscle contraction against resistance, as well as significant loss of strength (resulting more from a protective inhibition of recruitment than from actual muscle injury). A grade III strain involves a complete rupture of the muscle. This rupture actually occurs most commonly at the muscle-tendon junction, and it usually requires surgical repair.

Overuse injuries, such as tendinitis, are graded from I to III based on symptomatology. A grade I injury produces pain only during athletic activity. A grade II injury produces pain for some time after the athletic activity. A grade III injury causes pain throughout the day and may disrupt sleep.

## Treatment Modalities

Cryotherapy often is administered effectively by placing ice cubes in a resealable plastic bag and applying the bag to the site of injury. The application of ice reduces edema and inflammation by causing vasoconstriction. Maximal vasoconstriction is produced in 15 to 20 minutes. Heat should not be applied to any acute injury for at least 72 hours, because the vasodilation it produces may increase bleeding and edema.

Anti-inflammatory medications are used liberally in sports medicine in an effort to reduce inflammation and edema in patients with acute and chronic injuries. Although they have not been studied well for use in soft-tissue injuries in athletes, these agents seem to be especially helpful during the rehabilitation period. Aspirin is the least expensive anti-inflammatory medication, and it works best taken four times a day for a minimum of 10 to 14 days at a time. Ibuprofen is more effective in some athletes. More expensive prescription agents are more effective in selected patients, and most of these offer the advantage of longer half-lives, which improve compliance.

## BACK INJURIES

Low back pain in athletes can be quite disabling, but the pain generally resolves within 2 weeks, often before medical care is sought. Athletes who seek medical care for back pain often have had pain for several weeks or intermittently for months, and have tried to continue their sport until they are unable to compete. The differential diagnosis of back pain in the athletically active child or adolescent is very broad. In addition to mechanical causes, metabolic, neoplastic, and infectious origins should be kept in mind. In young athletes, however, the most common causes of back pain are mechanical.

### Muscle Strain

Probably the most likely cause of low back pain in young athletes is an acute or chronic muscle strain. This tends to occur in children who have a functional hyperlordosis of the lumbar spine in the standing position. The athlete usually has loss of flexibility and benefits from regular back exercises that increase flexibility. Significant hamstring muscle tightness also is a common finding and contributor. A flexibility program should include these muscles.

### Spondylolysis

Spondylolysis is another significant cause of low back pain in the adolescent athlete. Young athletes who participate in sports that involve repetitive hyperextension of the low back, such as gymnastics, may sustain stress fractures of the pars interarticularis of the lower lumbar spine. While bending, these patients frequently can touch their toes or even put their palms on the floor with their knees extended, yet most will have marked hamstring tightness. The spondylolysis may be unilateral or bilateral. When radiographs are ordered, they always should include oblique views, as these may provide the only means of detecting this lesion (Fig 37-1).

Lifters of heavy weights and football linemen who sustain loading of the spine in extension may experience pain from spondylolysis. When the pars defect is bilateral, there may be some slippage of the vertebrae on occasion, which is called spondylolisthesis. Increased slippage is uncommon, but should be evaluated by an orthopedist.

### Epiphyseal Injury

A less common condition in an athlete is Scheuermann's epiphysitis, which typically occurs in the thoracic area. Irregularities of the epiphyses may be evident on radiography. Scheuermann's disease is associated with a kyphotic deformity and wedging of the vertebrae. The athlete must limit athletic activities. Occasionally, a brace is necessary to halt progression of the deformity.

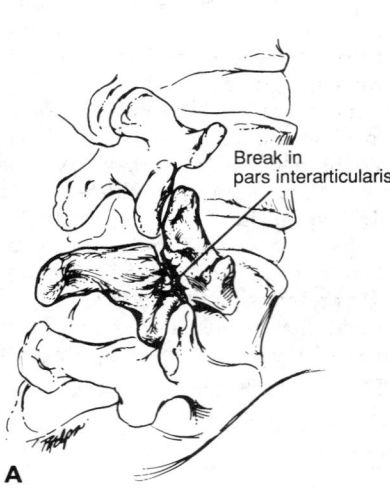

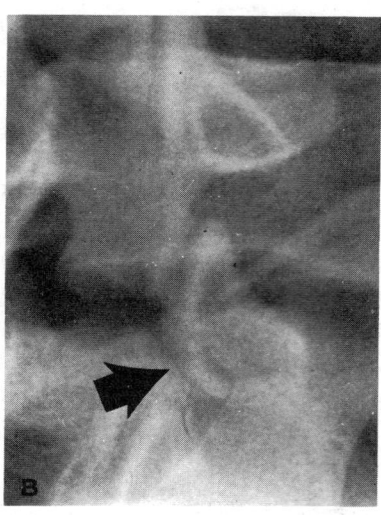

Break in
pars interarticularis

A

B

**Figure 37-1.** (**A**) Anatomy and (**B**) radiographic evidence of spondylolysis. *Spondylolysis* is a break in the continuity of the pars interarticularis, which can be seen as a lucency on one of the oblique radiographs.

## The Herniated Disc

Disc protrusion should be considered in the evaluation of an adolescent with low back pain. Although it occurs less frequently in young athletes than in adults, disc protrusion tends to occur in athletes who are loading the spine repeatedly, predominantly during participation in the sports of football and basketball. The diagnosis can be difficult to make in adolescent athletes because they often do not have sciatica, which is the radiating pain down the sciatic nerve that is associated with disc disease in adults. Avoidance of heavy lifting, use of an anti-inflammatory agent, bed rest, and a regular back exercise program often will allow the individual to resume athletic activities once the symptoms abate.

## Evaluation of Back Pain

In evaluating the athlete who has low back pain, the history may not be as helpful as the physical examination. The athlete may not volunteer neurologic symptoms, and these must be inquired about specifically. In addition, the physician should ask about any changes in bladder or bowel control that the patient may have experienced. Pain that occurs only with athletic activity, especially in hyperextension, is suggestive of spondylolysis. A family history of back pain, especially that caused by disc pathology, may be indicative of a familial predisposition to the problem.

The examination of the athlete with low back pain should begin with careful observation of the individual standing as well as walking. Assessment of range of motion should be performed in the standing position. The presence of pain with flexion, extension, or lateral movement should be noted. The athlete also should be asked to twist in both directions to see whether this produces pain; pain produced with this maneuver is suggestive of spondylolysis or disc protrusion. Pain that occurs when the patient extends the back while standing on one leg ("single leg hyperextension test") also is suggestive of spondylolysis.

The athlete should be asked to lie prone on the examining table for palpation of the entire spine and back. Deep palpation to localize the maximal area of tenderness may be diagnostic (Fig 37-2). The neurologic status of the lower extremities should be examined with the athlete in the supine position. Straight leg raising tests should be performed to determine whether stretching of the sciatic nerve reproduces pain. Care should be taken not to confuse the discomfort produced on stretching of the hamstrings with stretching of the sciatic nerve. This test also will enable an assessment of hamstring tightness to be made. Many athletes with low back pain of various origins have inflexible hamstrings that either contribute to or are a result of the pathology that is present.

Radiographs of the spine should be performed in most cases. In a patient with acute low back pain and no history of trauma, it may be reasonable to wait for 2 weeks after the injury before obtaining radiographs, because the pain often will resolve within that interval. Studies of back pain in children and adolescents, however, have shown that the yield of pathology on plain radiographs is much higher than that in adults with low back pain. If the history and physical examination are suggestive of spondylolysis, oblique views of the lumbosacral spine should be obtained to look for a pars interarticularis defect. A technetium bone scan may be necessary to confirm the clinical suspicion of acute spondylolysis.

## Treatment

In general, even when the cause of low back pain is unclear, a trial of rest, anti-inflammatory medication, and a back exercise

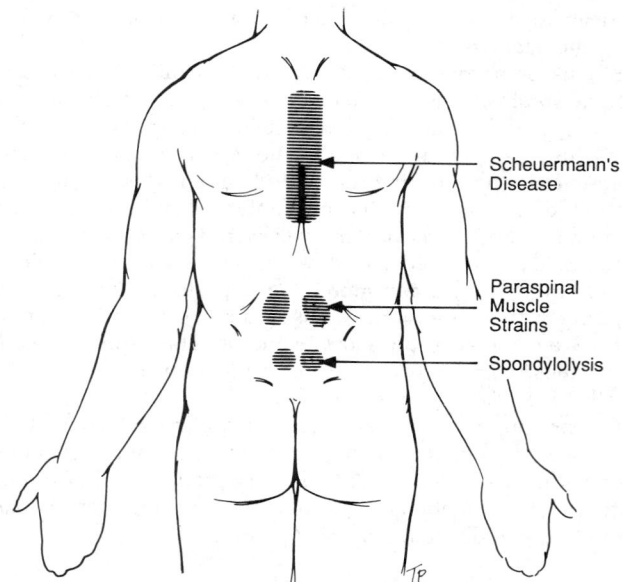

Scheuermann's
Disease

Paraspinal
Muscle
Strains

Spondylolysis

**Figure 37-2.** Palpation of the back and mechanical causes of low back pain. Pictured are the sites of pain and tenderness in the following causes of mechanical low back pain: Scheuermann's epiphysitis, muscle strain, and spondylolysis. (Modified from Keene JS, Drummond DS. Mechanical low back pain in the athlete. Compr Ther 1985;11:7.)

program is helpful. Because of the poor flexibility of many of these athletes, consultation with a physical therapist often is beneficial for instruction in a back exercise program. As with adults, young athletes benefit from sleeping on their side in a fetal position on a very firm mattress. Occasionally, significant muscle spasm is associated with the low back pain. Heat usually relieves the spasm, but muscle relaxants may be warranted in a few cases. In terms of competition, as with many other injuries, athletes can use pain as their guide, avoiding maneuvers that produce pain. It is important to help the athlete understand that back pain usually does not resolve quickly, and that the exercise program probably is the most important part of the treatment.

## INJURIES TO THE UPPER EXTREMITY

### Acromioclavicular Sprains

The most common acute shoulder injury is the acromioclavicular (AC) sprain, also known as a shoulder separation. The mechanism of injury of the AC sprain involves a blow to the superior aspect of the shoulder or a blow laterally to the deltoid. The sprain also may be caused by landing on an outstretched arm. Abduction of the arm produces pain that is so acute that the athlete may not want to move the shoulder at all. The physical examination will demonstrate well-localized swelling and marked point tenderness over the AC joint. There may be a palpable step-off at the joint that can be appreciated best when the injured and normal shoul-ders are compared. It is difficult to assess ligament stability at this particular joint. With a second-degree sprain of the AC lig-ament, the adjacent stabilizing ligaments (the trapezoid and con-oid ligaments) also must be torn (Fig 37-3). If there is tenderness over these ligaments, at least a second-degree sprain of the AC joint has occurred.

Radiographs may show an elevation of the distal clavicle. In the presence of a second-degree or greater injury, the AP views probably should be performed with and without weights. The athlete should not be allowed to grasp the weights because this will make him or her shrug the injured shoulder, and the liga-ments will not be tested.

Treatment of the AC sprain involves immobilization for pain relief. As soon as possible, as pain improves, range of motion and strengthening exercises should be started. The athlete should be warned that there may be some cosmetic defect after an AC sprain, and there may be a noticeable bump with callus formation.

Surgical management of third-degree sprains is controversial, but it usually is performed for cosmetic reasons only. Anti-inflammatory medication for pain relief and intermittent icing are helpful adjuncts to the exercise program. With collision sports such as hockey and football, additional padding such as a foam doughnut pad or a more rigid Orthoplast (a moldable plastic) splint under the shoulder pad helps the athlete feel more secure in competition and helps to prevent repeat injury. To return to competition, the athlete must have full range of motion of the shoulder with no pain, and be able to abduct the arm against resistance with no weakness and minimal or no pain.

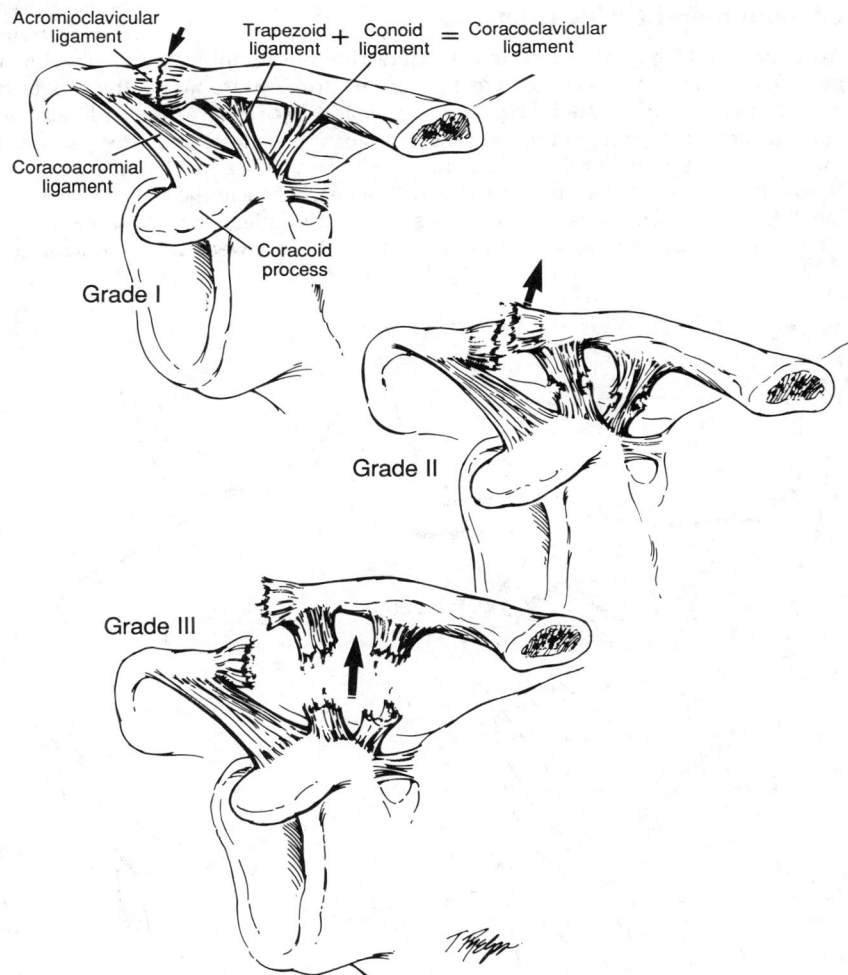

**Figure 37-3.** Acromioclavicular (AC) sprains. A *grade I sprain* implies damage to the AC ligament without dis-placement of the clavicle. A *grade II sprain* means sub-luxation of the AC joint caused by disruption of the AC ligament and damage to the trapezoid and conoid liga-ments. In the *grade III sprain,* all three of these ligaments are disrupted completely.

## Sternoclavicular Sprains

Although it is significantly less common than the AC sprain, the sternoclavicular (SC) sprain can be just as painful and disabling, and in some cases it can be life-threatening. If there is complete disruption of the ligaments, anteriorly or posteriorly, dislocation of the clavicle may occur. If the dislocation is posterior, it can be life-threatening as a result of compression of the trachea and great vessels in the neck. To treat this injury, outward traction on the arm and posterior shoulder traction may reduce the posterior dislocation. If that is unsuccessful, grasping the proximal clavicle with a surgical towel clip and pulling the clavicle anteriorly should reduce the dislocation. For this life-threatening injury, a towel clip should be kept in the medical bag on the field. In the skeletally immature individual, an SC injury usually is not a dislocation but a physis fracture of the proximal clavicle, with anterior or posterior displacement of the fracture.

The physical examination is remarkable for well-localized tenderness and swelling over the SC joint, and any movement of the shoulder, especially adduction, may produce pain. The SC joint and proximal physis of the clavicle are difficult to see on plain radiographs, but generally are seen best on the serendipity view (an AP view of the SC joint, with 30° of cephalad tilt of the x-ray beam). Tomograms or CT scanning may be required for differentiation of fracture and dislocation.

Treatment of a first-degree SC sprain is entirely symptomatic. A sling is used for the first few days, and then the patient is provided with range of motion exercises. A second- or third-degree sprain is treated with a figure-of-eight appliance for about 3 to 6 weeks, as is a reduced fracture.

## Glenohumeral Dislocation

Anterior shoulder dislocations are far more common than are posterior dislocations, and they have a high recurrence rate no matter how they are treated. There still is a great deal of controversy regarding the best method of conservative management of these injuries. Recent studies document that the recurrence rate is no different between patients treated with an early functional rehabilitation program that is begun as soon as the patient can tolerate it and those who are rigidly immobilized for 3 weeks.

Return to competition is not allowed in either case until there is full range of motion and essentially equal strength in comparison with that of the uninjured shoulder.

## Glenohumeral Subluxation

Glenohumeral subluxation probably is more common than is frank dislocation in young athletes. Shoulder subluxation can be more difficult to diagnose, but it can cause just as much pain and disability as can dislocation. Subluxations may occur anteriorly, posteriorly, and, occasionally, interiorly.

Anterior subluxations occur as a result of a forceful abduction and external rotation, such as happens in making an arm tackle. The athlete is aware immediately that the shoulder "slid." There may be actual dislocation with spontaneous reduction. Treatment is the same as for the anterior dislocation and the recurrence rate is similarly high.

Posterior subluxation usually occurs with the arm outstretched, such as when a baseball player slides headfirst. This produces posterior pain, but the athlete may not have noticed any pop or feeling of instability at the time of the injury. It is important to note that subluxation of the shoulder posteriorly probably can be produced in more than 50% of normal individuals on clinical examination. With this in mind, the normal shoulder always should be evaluated as well.

Examination of the shoulder reveals guarding, with marked tenderness over the glenohumeral joint in the area of the subluxation. After an anterior subluxation, the athlete often has apprehension when the shoulder is taken into abduction and external rotation. Pain is produced when there is traction on the humeral head in the direction of the subluxation. This can be demonstrated by performing a shoulder drawer test (Fig 37-4).

Treatment consists of rest and pain relief. As soon as possible, the athlete should begin range of motion exercises and a shoulder girdle strengthening program. The athlete should be advised that recurrences are common, but that they can be prevented most effectively with an aggressive rehabilitation program that focuses on strength training. The athlete should be withheld from competition until he or she is free of pain and strength in the injured shoulder girdle is the same as that in the uninjured shoulder.

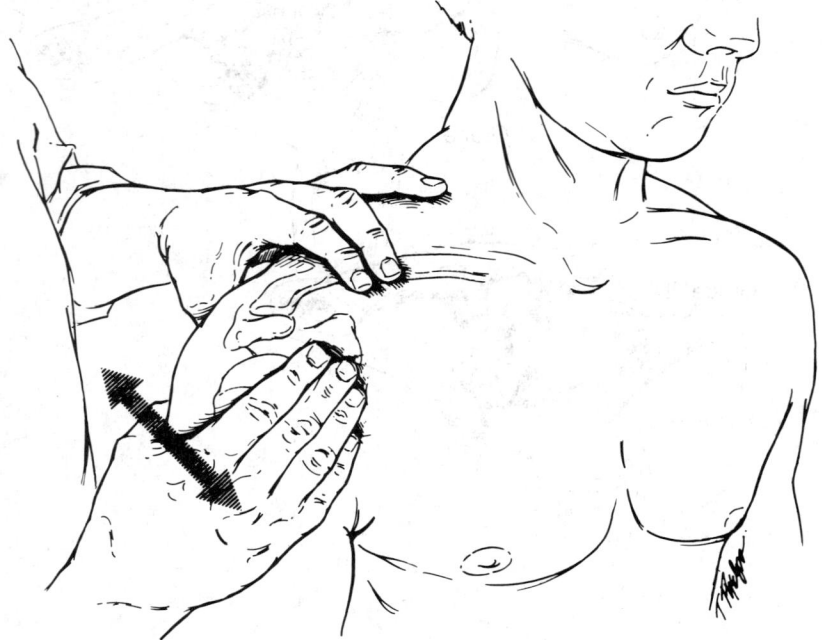

**Figure 37-4.** The shoulder drawer test (also called the glide test). To demonstrate anterior and posterior glenohumeral instability in the right shoulder, the left hand is placed on top of the shoulder so that the clavicle and the scapula are stabilized. The right hand is free to create traction on the humeral head to push or pull it in and out of the glenoid fossa.

## Impingement Syndrome

The most common cause of chronic shoulder pain in the young athlete often is referred to as impingement syndrome, also known as pitcher's shoulder, swimmer's shoulder, and tennis shoulder. The single common denominator is that the pain is present only when the shoulder is abducted to 90°. The athlete seldom experiences any pain with movement if the shoulder is not abducted to 90°. Although many clinicians believe that this injury occurs as a result of compression of the rotator cuff and subacromial bursa by the coracoacromial ligament and the overlying acromion (Fig 37-5), it actually is the result of a supraspinatus tendinitis. When the patient has pain, it is the inflamed supraspinatus tendon that is the major source. Whether the cause was the impingement or accumulated overload seldom is possible to determine. On occasion, it may be that an inflamed bursa is the only problem. A large number of athletes with impingement syndrome also have evidence of chronic anterior glenohumeral instability. Some clinicians believe that the instability plays a significant role in the pathophysiology of impingement syndrome.

Onset usually is insidious, and the pain continues to worsen as the duration and intensity of the workouts increase. The athlete complains of anterior shoulder pain and may have referred pain in the deltoid muscle.

On examination, the athlete usually experiences the greatest tenderness to palpation over the greater tuberosity, just anterior and lateral to the edge of the acromion. Typically, the athlete has pain with tests for impingement. One impingement test requires taking the shoulder up to 180° of forward flexion actively or passively. This may produce pain, especially if the shoulder is adducted across the face. Another impingement test is performed by placing the shoulder at 90° of forward flexion with the arm held in internal rotation. Forced internal rotation may reproduce the pain. Palpation of the bicipital groove may reveal tenderness, because biceps tendinitis also may occur in those with chronic impingement syndrome. An athlete with impingement syndrome may have relatively weak muscles involved in external rotation, with poor flexibility. Pain may be produced with strength testing of these muscles, especially the supraspinatus, which is the most superior muscle in the rotator cuff group. This is tested best by placing the arms in internal rotation, elevated to 90° and abducted 70°. Resistance to further elevation selectively tests the supraspinatus (Fig 37-6). Tests for glenohumeral instability also should be performed.

Treatment of impingement syndrome involves rest, or at least a decrease in activity. Ice applied to the subacromial area for 15 to 20 minutes after activity helps to reduce pain and inflammation. Anti-inflammatory medication also provides some relief. As in many overuse injuries, rehabilitation is the key to treatment of this injury. A strengthening and stretching program for the supraspinatus usually is different from any exercises the athlete previously has been taught. The strengthening program is especially important in the athlete with glenohumeral instability as well as impingement syndrome. As in many overuse injuries, it may take 6 to 8 weeks to resolve this problem entirely. After 3 or 4 weeks of intense rehabilitation, however, the athlete usually will note significant improvement. In the absence of improvement, injection of a soluble corticosteroid into the subacromial bursa should be considered. Because it is almost impossible to differentiate between subacromial bursitis and supraspinatus tendinitis, injection of the bursa is reasonable. In the presence of subacromial bursitis, the injection often provides the athlete with marked relief.

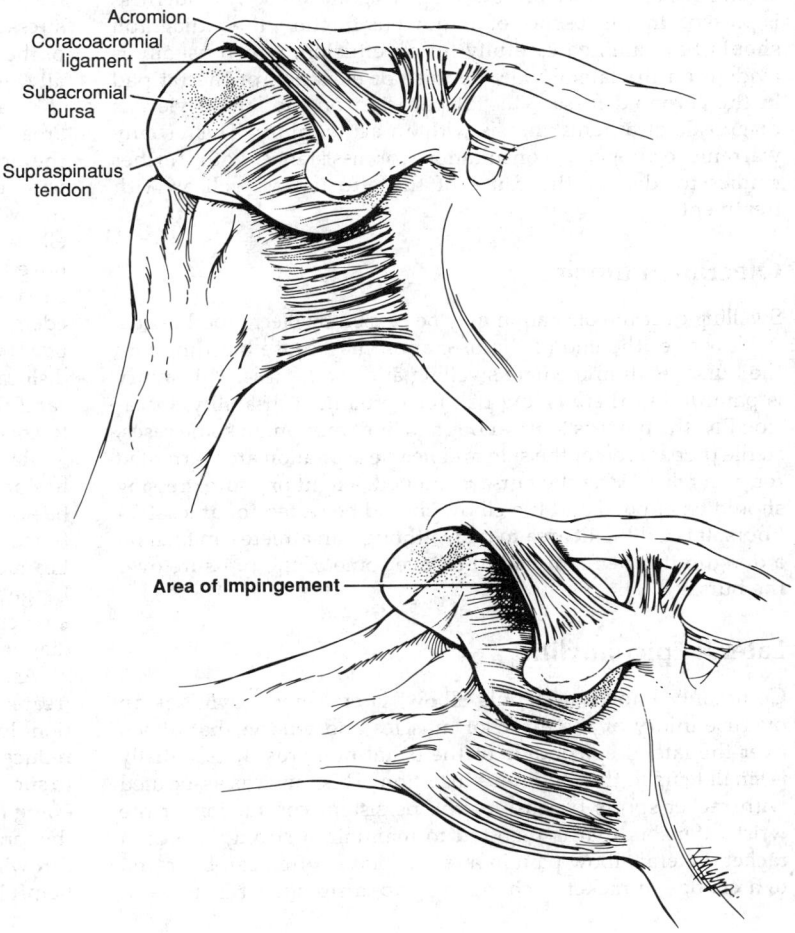

**Figure 37-5.** Anatomic basis for impingement syndrome. *Impingement syndrome* involves the compression and inflammation of the subacromial bursa and the supraspinatus tendon between the humerus and the coracoacromial ligament along the inferior edge of the acromion.

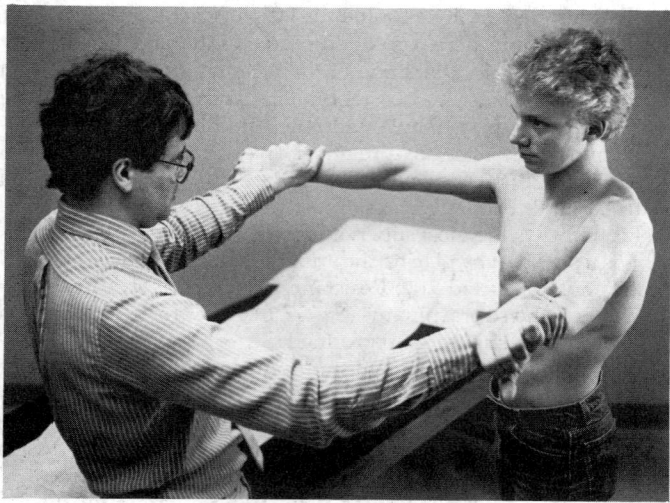

**Figure 37-6.**   Strength assessment of the supraspinatus muscle. With the patient standing and facing the examiner, the arms are elevated to 90°, abducted 70° (20° of adduction to the parasagittal plane), and placed in internal rotation. Resistance to further elevation (forward flexion) selectively tests the supraspinatus muscle.

In a small percentage of patients, conservative management fails and a surgical procedure for decompression is required.

## Acute Elbow Injuries

Acute trauma to the elbow is important because fractures of the elbow tend to involve the physes. Radiographs of the elbow should be performed if any swelling or significant bony tenderness is present. In the absence of an obvious fracture, the radiograph should be examined carefully for an effusion, which usually is evident on the lateral view because of elevation of the fat pad in the coronoid fossa. The fat pad sign on the lateral view is diagnostic of a hemarthrosis with an acute injury. This usually warrants orthopedic consultation for assistance with further studies to identify the cause of the effusion as well as with treatment.

## Olecranon Bursitis

Swelling over the olecranon may be caused by olecranon bursitis. A blow over the end of the olecranon may cause bleeding into the bursa, with immediate swelling and tenderness. This injury is painful, but there is low risk for permanent disability. Occasionally, the bursa is tense enough to limit motion. In some cases, sterile preparation of the skin and needle aspiration are warranted for pain relief. After the bursa is drained, a tight pressure dressing should be applied and the elbow should be rested for at least 24 hours. It is a difficult area to pad, although an athlete can fashion a doughnut-type foam pad to relieve some of the pressure over the bursa.

## Lateral Epicondylitis

Commonly known as tennis elbow, lateral epicondylitis is an overuse injury of the extensor muscles and tendon that attach over the lateral epicondyle of the distal humerus. It essentially is small tears in the tendinous insertion. This injury is associated with racket sports because of the persistent contraction of the wrist extensors that is required to maintain a strong grip on a racket. Lateral elbow pain in a tennis player often can be traced to a change in racket, a change in grip, a significant increase in

playing time, or an attempt to learn to put topspin on the ball. It should be kept in mind, however, that it is unusual for lateral epicondylitis to develop in an adolescent athlete. Subacute or chronic lateral elbow pain needs to be evaluated for Panner's disease (osteochondrosis of the humeral capitellum), especially in a gymnast or pitcher who has lateral elbow pain.

Point tenderness over the lateral epicondyle at the insertion of the extensor mass in the elbow is indicative of lateral epicondylitis. Forced resistance to extension also produces pain. There should be no swelling about the elbow and no loss of range of motion. Radiographs probably are not necessary early in this problem, unless there is a history of an injury.

The key to the treatment of lateral epicondylitis is a diligent rehabilitation program outlined by a physical therapist or trainer. This involves regular stretching and strengthening of the extensor muscle-tendon unit. Ice applied after exercise helps to reduce some of the pain and inflammation. An anti-inflammatory medication helps to make the athlete more comfortable. Rest speeds healing, although it is not always necessary for the athlete to refrain totally from activities. This problem takes at least 6 to 8 weeks to resolve, and the athlete often needs a lot of encouragement along the way. Most experts feel that local injection of corticosteroid or surgery rarely are necessary.

## Flexor-Pronator Tendinitis

Flexor-pronator tendinitis usually is seen in patients who are involved in throwing and racket sports. Athletes complain of pain over the medial aspect of the elbow. This condition is seen often in young pitchers when they are learning to throw breaking pitches. This throwing motion creates valgus stress, loading the medial aspect of the elbow, including the ulnar collateral ligament (UCL) and the pronator teres muscle and tendon. Associated with stress and inflammation of the medial structures is inflammation of the ulnar nerve. Ulnar nerve symptoms in the adolescent usually are indicative of dislocation or subluxation of the ulnar nerve.

Examination of the elbow usually demonstrates the maximal area of tenderness to be the pronator mass and, to a lesser extent, the area at the medial epicondyle. Pain frequently is present, with resistance to pronation and flexion of the wrist. Occasionally, the MCL may be inflamed, and stress of the ligament with the elbow flexed at 30° to 40° may produce pain. Pain may be produced with palpation of the ulnar nerve and the groove. Percussion of the nerve may reproduce paresthesia if there is any edema or inflammation of the nerve in the groove. If tenderness over the ulnar nerve is found, the nerve should be examined for dislocation or subluxation when the elbow is flexed past 90°. A careful neurologic examination of the hand should be performed to check for evidence of ulnar nerve dysfunction.

Radiographs should be performed in any young athlete who has acute medial pain to determine whether the medial physis has been disrupted. Stress of the physis may cause an avulsion fracture, which classically has been associated with excessive Little League pitching and has been called Little League elbow. Little League elbow is a misused term that has been applied to virtually any child with elbow pain, however, and is not a specific diagnosis.

As with lateral epicondylitis, flexor-pronator tendinitis is treated with rest, anti-inflammatory medication, and rehabilitation. Ice applied to the elbow after any kind of activity helps to reduce some of the pain and swelling. Rehabilitation is the key to successful treatment in the long term. Stretching and strengthening of the pronator teres muscle will help the athlete resolve the problem and prevent recurrences. In sports that involve throwing, a change in the athlete's throwing mechanics often is helpful as well.

## Wrist Sprains

The most common injury to the wrist involves the disruption of one or more of the numerous ligaments in the wrist. Many mechanisms of injury may cause ligament damage to the wrist, but there may not be much swelling or pain with this injury. Pain to palpation and pain with stress of the corresponding ligaments is consistent with the diagnosis of a sprain (eg, tenderness dorsally and pain with hyperflexion of the wrist). Radiographs should be performed because it may be very difficult to distinguish a fracture from a sprain based on physical examination alone. Treatment involves immobilization in the form of a wrist splint, application of ice, and use of anti-inflammatory medication. The time required for healing is variable.

## Navicular Fractures

Falling on an outstretched hand may cause a fracture of the carpal navicular (scaphoid) bone. This fracture may not always produce noticeable swelling, but palpation of the anatomic "snuff box" will produce pain. The navicular bone has a marginal blood supply, and this may lead to delayed healing or, on occasion, to avascular necrosis, especially when the diagnosis of fracture is delayed. Radiographs should be performed with navicular views. When tenderness is present, even if the radiograph results are negative, the patient should be cast in a thumb spica cast for 2 weeks. Physical and radiographic examination should be repeated at that time. Orthopedic consultation should be considered if the diagnosis is unclear. Navicular fractures usually require a minimum of 8 weeks of immobilization in a thumb spica cast.

## Hamate Fractures

The hook of the hamate bone may be fractured during a fall or while gripping a bat or club. The fracture produces wrist pain, a poor grip, and tenderness over the hamate bone. Routine radiographs may not reveal the fracture, so a carpal tunnel view should be obtained. Treatment is immobilization in a cast with incorporation of the little finger. An orthopedist should be consulted, because the rate of nonunion is high.

## Finger Injuries

The most common injury involving the hand is the finger sprain. Sometimes called a "jammed" finger, it usually is the result of hyperextension of the proximal or distal interphalangeal joint. The sprain may produce moderate swelling and tenderness, with some limitation of motion. Careful palpation of the finger reveals tenderness about one or both of the collateral ligaments and, frequently, tenderness over the volar plate (palmar ligament). Flexion and extension should be examined carefully at each joint in the finger to rule out a disruption of the flexor or extensor mechanisms, such as mallet finger (disruption of the terminal extensor mechanism) or the boutonniére deformity (rupture of the insertion of the central extensor tendon). Stability of the joint should be assessed, comparing ulnar and radial laxity with stress and anterior-posterior laxity with stress with the contralateral joint in the other hand.

Radiographic evaluation should be considered in all patients with significant finger injuries. The degree of swelling or tenderness does not distinguish sprains from fractures. One should be quick to obtain films of the dominant hand in an athlete, especially of the thumb and index finger, which are so important functionally.

Finger sprains are treated in a position of function, with splints applied for comfort. As soon as it is comfortable, the finger should be taken out of the splint to allow for range of motion exercises. If the finger is left in the splint indefinitely, the fibrosis that occurs after hematoma can cause stiffness and loss of motion. Splints should be used to protect the finger from further injury as long as any tenderness remains over the joint. One of the easiest and most comfortable methods used to splint the sprained finger is by buddy taping (taping the injured finger to the adjacent finger).

The athlete's ability to return to play should be determined on a individual basis, because the severity of the sprain, the athlete's position on the team, and the type of sport being played are important considerations. Sometimes it is easy to protect the injured finger. For example, a football lineman can have the entire hand bandaged in a fist, giving the injured finger a great deal of protection.

One particular sprain in the hand can be quite troublesome. The "skier's thumb" or "gamekeeper's thumb" is a sprain of the ulnar collateral ligament of the metacarpal-proximal phalangeal joint. This sprain is produced when an athlete lands on an outstretched hand and the thumb is deviated excessively radially. If a third-degree sprain occurs and is treated inadequately, the result may be long-term instability of the joint. The third-degree sprain warrants orthopedic consultation, because open repair or casting may be required.

# INJURIES TO THE LOWER EXTREMITY

## Iliac Crest Contusion

In contact sports, a blow to the iliac crest may produce a periosteal hematoma, which often is very painful and disabling. Commonly known as a "hip pointer," this injury can cause the athlete to miss several days or weeks of practice time and games. Usually, the contusion involves the anterior superior iliac crest. Treatment consists of ice and rest. When the athlete can sprint at full speed without a limp, return to competition is allowed. Reinjury is painful but is unlikely to result in any permanent disability. Padding of the area can be achieved with a large foam doughnut pad.

## Iliac Apophysitis

Iliac apophysitis is seen almost exclusively in adolescent cross-country and distance runners. The aching pain over the iliac crest is insidious in onset. There usually is marked tenderness to palpation of the iliac crest, most often at the anterior superior iliac crest. AP and oblique radiographs should be performed in any patient who has an acute onset of symptoms to rule out an avulsion fracture of the anterior superior iliac spine.

Treatment of this entity involves rest, ice application, and anti-inflammatory medication. The athlete should discontinue running until there is no pain to palpation of the involved area. The pain usually will resolve completely after 4 to 6 weeks of complete avoidance of running. Permanent sequelae from this injury have not been reported.

## Quadriceps Contusion

A blow to the thigh may result in a large contusion within the quadriceps muscles. There may be massive bleeding to the point that shock may be induced. This injury can be very painful and debilitating. On physical examination, a large, tender mass can be palpated within the muscle, and pain is produced with flexion of the knee. The severity of the damage cannot be assessed until 24 to 48 hours after the injury has occurred, but it correlates highly with the expected amount of time that will be lost from play and the risk that myositis ossificans will develop. If knee flexion is greater than 90°, the injury is categorized as being grade I. If flexion is 45° to 90°, it is grade II, and if there is less than 45° of knee flexion, the injury is considered to be grade III. The incidence of myositis ossificans in grade III injuries is high, even if they are treated properly. Application of ice to the area and cessation of athletic activity are important to stop the acute bleeding. For at least 72 hours after the injury occurs, rest, ice, compression, and elevation should be used to minimize bleeding and edema. The use of heat may increase bleeding. Crutches should be used if the patient limps. The key to rehabilitation of this injury is the initiation of gentle, painless stretching of the quadriceps muscles as the hematoma resolves. Strengthening of the quadriceps also is important. Return to competition is based on full and painless range of motion, no pain to palpation, a minimum of 85% strength of the quadriceps compared to that in the uninjured leg, and completion of the running program (Table 37-5).

## Femoral Stress Fracture

If a young running athlete has persistent vague thigh pain, a femoral stress fracture should be considered strongly. Usually seen in high-mileage distance runners, the injury can be overlooked for weeks. The aching pain occurring with exercise has an insidious onset, and the physical examination often is non-localizing or the pain appears to be muscular in origin. If the pain has persisted for several weeks, the periosteal reaction may be seen only on oblique radiographs. If the results of plain radiographs are negative, a technetium bone scan is necessary to make the diagnosis.

Vague anterior groin pain may represent a femoral neck stress fracture. Prompt diagnosis with radiographs or a technetium bone scan is important, because delay in diagnosis can lead to a displaced fracture, which is associated with a high risk of poor long-term outcome.

## Medial Collateral Ligament Sprains

In contrast to ankle injury, knowledge of the mechanism of injury can be helpful in determining the diagnosis of the acutely injured knee. The MCL sprain probably is the most common knee ligament injury to occur in contact sports. It occurs with valgus stress, such as happens with a blow to the lateral aspect of the knee. If the injury is mild, it may not produce much immediate disability, and the athlete may be able to continue to play for several more minutes. With significant bleeding and inflammation over the ligament, the athlete usually has a limp and must leave the game or practice.

In patients with an isolated MCL injury, examination of the knee reveals a trace to mild effusion. The presence of a large and tense knee effusion usually is indicative of an intra-articular injury or a patellar dislocation, and is not consistent with an isolated MCL sprain. There is point tenderness over the MCL, often at the middle portion of the ligament. Full extension may be limited because it stretches the MCL, and the ligament is more relaxed at 30° of flexion. Pain is produced with stress of the MCL, which is examined best with the patient lying supine and the knee in 20° to 30° of flexion. With the table supporting most of the weight of the leg, the femur is stabilized with one hand and the ankle is grasped with the other hand. Outward stress is applied gently to the ankle to produce valgus stress to the knee, and the severity of the sprain is graded according to the degree of laxity noted. The knee should be examined for other ligament injury as well.

Radiographs should be performed to rule out a fracture. If the physes are open, stress radiographs must be taken. The MCL sprain is treated in a fashion similar to the ankle sprain. Rest for 2 to 3 days and the use of crutches often will provide pain relief, along with anti-inflammatory medication, ice, compression, and elevation. As with the ankle sprain, rehabilitation is the key to ensuring a quick return to competition. Even with a third-degree sprain, rehabilitation is vital, and MCL injuries no longer are treated surgically unless another injury is involved. The criteria for an athlete's return to play are similar to those for ankle sprain. The athlete must have no pain, full range of motion, strength equal to at least 85% of that of the uninjured leg, and no swelling, and he or she must have completed the running program without pain or limp (see Table 37-5).

## Anterior Cruciate Ligament Sprain

In contrast to the MCL sprain, an anterior cruciate ligament (ACL) sprain produces swelling of the knee in the first several hours after the injury occurs. Bleeding from the ligament usually produces a tense hemarthrosis. The ACL sprain almost always is a third-degree sprain, meaning that the ligament is disrupted completely.

The ACL tear usually is a non-contact injury caused by hyperextension of the knee or sudden deceleration of the leg with the foot flexed. Frequently, the athlete hears a loud pop. The injury is very painful, and the athlete seldom is capable of continuing to play.

If the athlete is evaluated on the field, stability testing for the ACL injury is extremely important. In the absence of bleeding or inflammation, the athlete will have less guarding and the examination will be more accurate. Several hours after the injury, the knee is very tender and swollen, and the athlete may object to any movement of the knee, which makes examination difficult. The large, tense effusion that is seen 24 hours after the injury is grossly bloody on aspiration. More than 85% of all acute tense hemarthroses are caused by ACL disruptions. (Patella dislocations are the second most common cause of acute hemarthroses.)

On physical examination, the most important test to perform is the Lachman test. The traditional anterior drawer test, performed with the knee at a 90° angle, is not very reliable. The Lachman test is an anterior drawer test with the knee held in 20° to 30° of flexion. One hand is placed on the femur to stabilize it, the other hand is used to grasp the proximal tibia, and anterior

---

**TABLE 37-5.  The Running Program***

1. Jog ½ to 1 mile. Stop immediately if you are limping or if there is pain. Wait until tomorrow to start to the program again. If there is no pain or limp during your jog, you may proceed to:
2. Six to eight 80-yard sprints at half speed. If no pain or limp, then do:
3. Six to eight 80-yard sprints at three-quarter speed. If no pain or limp, then do:
4. Six to eight 80-yard sprints at full speed, followed by 4 to 6 full-speed starts. If no pain or limp, then do:
5. Six to eight 80-yard cutting sprints (changing directions) every 10 yards at half speed. Then do:
6. Six to eight 80-yard cutting sprints at full speed.

After every workout, ice should be applied immediately to the injured area. (Do not stand around).

Once you can perform all the above tasks with no pain and minimal swelling, you may return to competition. If you short-cut this program, you are only fooling yourself, and are risking reinjury or possibly a more serious injury and a much longer time out of competition.

* This is a running program that can be given to the athlete so that the criteria for return to competition are clear and the athlete can work toward a goal.

stress is applied (Fig 37-7). Loss of ACL integrity allows excessive anterior motion, compared to motion in the normal knee. Any hamstring spasm will negate the results of this test. Occasionally, the athlete may injure the MCL in addition, and examination for this injury should be performed also.

Radiographs should be performed, especially in an adolescent with open physes who may have a tibial plateau fracture instead of an ACL tear. (This is an avulsion fracture of the ACL, and it requires urgent attention from an orthopedic surgeon.) For an ACL tear, treatment with a knee immobilizer, crutches, and pain relief is reasonable; a surgical consultation should be obtained within the next several days. Arthroscopy or magnetic resonance imaging often is used to examine the menisci, because a meniscus tear also will be demonstrated in 30% to 40% of patients with ACL tears.

Treatment of the acute ACL tear in most, but not all, cases requires surgery. A patient with an ACL-deficient knee is likely to have recurring instability and probably is at risk for early traumatic arthritis. Recent surgical advances have led to excellent results in patients who have chosen surgical stabilization. Careful evaluation and discussion with the athlete about his or her preference is critical. Cast immobilization of an isolated ACL tear is to be condemned; it does not allow for healing and only adds to muscle atrophy and prolongs the rehabilitation process.

## Posterior Cruciate Ligament Sprain

Far less common than the ACL sprain, injury to the posterior cruciate ligament (PCL) also is not as disabling. The injury is caused by a forceful blow to the tibia that drives it posteriorly, usually with the knee flexed. For example, sustaining a fall on the knee with the foot in plantar flexion, striking the tibia, may disrupt the PCL. The athlete usually complains of posterior knee pain, but does not have instability. On physical examination, an effusion is found, but it usually is small. The Lachman test results seldom are positive; a positive finding may indicate a more extensive injury. With the knee flexed to 90°, on palpation of the medial and lateral femoral condyles and the anterior tibial plateau, an 8- to 10-mm plateau step-off is noted in the normal knee. If there is complete loss of the step-off, the tibia is displaced posteriorly and the diagnosis of a complete PCL injury is made readily. It is important to obtain radiographs of patients with

suspected PCL injuries, as bony avulsion of the PCL may occur in the pediatric age group. Patients with bony avulsion of the PCL should be treated surgically, because excellent static results can be achieved.

Treatment for a PCL injury is similar to that for an MCL sprain, including rest, ice, anti-inflammatory medication, and a rehabilitation program. Isolated PCL deficiency rarely is a problem of functional instability once the athlete has completed a rehabilitation program, although some athletes have significant early traumatic arthritis. Surgical treatment of isolated PCL injury is controversial, because the prevalence of traumatic arthritis in athletes with a PCL-deficient knee is unknown. The results of surgical stabilization are not yet satisfactory.

## Patellar Dislocation/Subluxation

Although it is not as common as the ACL tear, patellar dislocation/subluxation is the second leading cause of acute hemarthrosis. The athlete occasionally says that the kneecap "went out of joint." With the knee flexed and some degree of valgus stress applied, the athlete will feel the knee give way and may report an audible pop; he or she may indicate that the knee went back into the joint when it was straightened.

The diagnosis often can be made based on the physical examination alone. With careful palpation, marked tenderness will be demonstrated over the medial aspect of the patella, the medial retinaculum, or the adductor tubercle. For subluxation or dislocation of the patella to result, there must be disruption of the medial retinaculum and the vastus medialis muscle, which is attached to the adductor tubercle and the intermuscular septum. The adductor tubercle is located just superior to the proximal attachment of the MCL (Fig 37-8). The knee also should be examined for any ligament injury. Radiographs should be performed, because subluxation/dislocation can produce an avulsion fracture. If a fracture is present, surgical intervention may be required if it is intra-articular in location.

Treatment of the athlete for pain relief consists of the use of a knee immobilizer and crutches. Anti-inflammatory medication or a narcotic agent may be necessary to achieve adequate pain relief during the first few days after injury. Although the risk of recurrence is high, few surgeons operate for a first episode unless there is a significant fracture. Regaining range of motion and

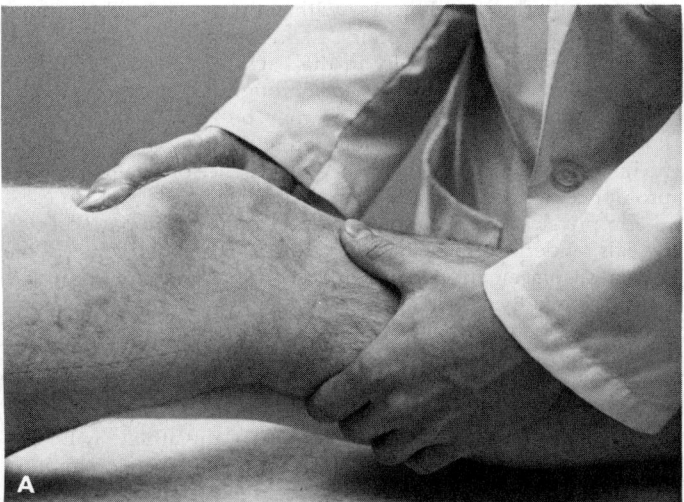
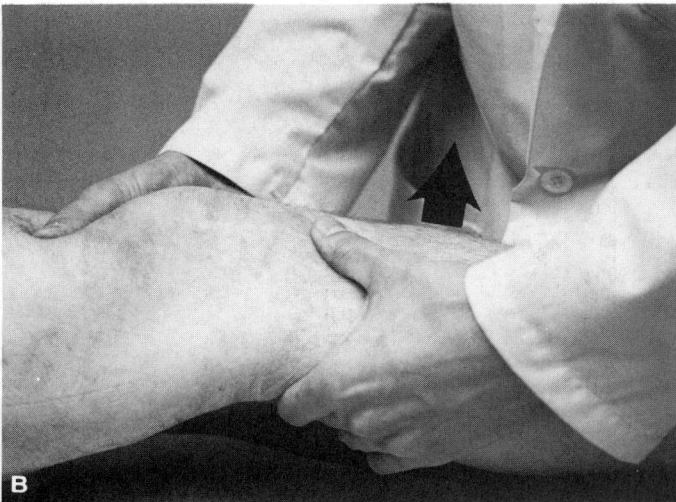

**Figure 37-7.** Lachman test. With the patient supine, the knee is flexed to 20° to 30°. (**A**) While the femur is stabilized with one hand, the tibia is grasped with the other hand. (**B**) When pulled anteriorly in the absence of the anterior cruciate ligament, the tibia moves excessively anteriorly.

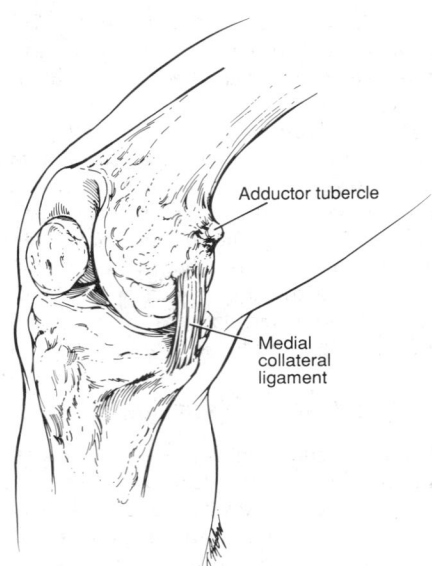

**Figure 37-8.** Adductor tubercle. When the patella is dislocated, the medial retinaculum often is torn at its attachment to the adductor tubercle. The adductor tubercle can be palpated easily just superior to the proximal attachment of the medial collateral ligament.

strengthening the upper leg muscles are imperative for an athlete to be able to resume play. Each patient must be assessed individually, but knee immobilization usually is maintained for only 7 to 10 days. The time required for full rehabilitation is variable. When the knee is rehabilitated completely, a patellar stabilizing device such as a Palumbo or a Richards knee sleeve helps to prevent recurrences (Fig 37-9). These knee sleeves are designed to give the patella lateral pressure to prevent lateral excursion of the patella in the femoral groove.

## Prepatellar Bursitis

A blow to the patella can cause contusion of the prepatellar bursa and bleeding within the bursa. Sometimes the injury is called turf knee or wrestler's knee because it usually results from a fall that strikes the patella on hard turf or a wrestling mat.

Physical examination reveals marked anterior swelling directly

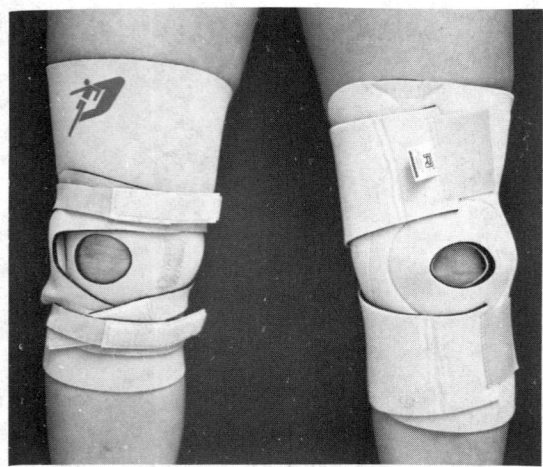

**Figure 37-9.** Patellar stabilizing devices. Shown are the Palumbo (on this athlete's right knee) and Richards (on the left knee) knee sleeves, which are designed to give the patella lateral pressure to prevent subluxation/dislocation.

over the patella. Palpation of the center of the patella reveals ballotable fluid; in contrast, joint effusion demonstrates fluid around the patella but not directly anterior to it. Flexion of the knee is painful. Treatment includes ice, compression, and, rarely, aspiration of the bursa. Aspiration of the bursa invites infection, and the injury usually can be managed conservatively. Padding the area is difficult and recurrences are common. The swelling does not preclude participation if the athlete has full range of motion and symmetric strength, and can pass a functional examination.

## Peripatellar Contusion

A blow to the soft tissues around the patella can cause a large hematoma to develop. A second mechanism of this injury is forced knee flexion while the quadriceps muscles are contracted. A tearing in the distal vastus medialis muscle causes bleeding into the subcutaneous tissue about the knee. The resolving hematoma in either case may develop into a large fluid collection around the patella. When the contusion is severe, the large amount of blood may take weeks to reabsorb, slowing efforts at rehabilitation. If the hematoma is aspirated, hemorrhage frequently recurs unless significant compression is applied, and the patient must refrain from activities involving knee flexion. Management is similar to that for the quadriceps contusion (see above).

## Patellofemoral Stress Syndrome

The most common complaint heard in most sports medicine clinics is that of chronic patellar pain. Sometimes known as chondromalacia, this entity also is called runner's knee, peripatellar pain syndrome, patellalgia, and patellofemoral stress syndrome (PFSS). Chondromalacia is an inappropriate term for most of these chronic pain conditions, because it is a specific pathologic diagnosis. When patients with this problem are examined surgically, no abnormality of the articular surface is found in more than 50% of them. The most appropriate term for the condition is PFSS. This syndrome is a common problem in athletes who run; many chronic injuries to the lower extremity occur in distance runners or in athletes who participate in sports that involve running, such as soccer.

The origin of the pain in patients with PFSS is thought to be subchondral stress or synovial inflammation. Patients typically have a history of dull, achy knee pain that is difficult to localize. Movement of the knee may be associated with a clicking or popping sound. The pain is worse with activity, especially running and going up and down stairs. Exacerbations may occur with prolonged sitting, especially in the back seat of a car with the knees fully flexed. The pain also is brought on or aggravated by any trauma to the patella. There may be "giving way" of the knee, which commonly is associated with pain. There usually is no history of swelling. The history or presence of swelling should prompt consideration of another diagnosis.

On physical examination, firm palpation of the patella often reveals tenderness over the medial facet. This may require some medial displacement of the patella with palpation of its undersurface medially. There also may be tenderness over the lateral facet of the patella or at any point along the patellofemoral joint line. Compression of the patella in the femoral groove produces pain, which sometimes is called a positive compression test result. Patellofemoral pain is associated with hypermobile patella as well as patella alta (high-riding patella). Often, the athlete will have evidence of malalignment, such as femoral anteversion and external tibial torsion. Gait analysis often reveals ankle valgus and excessive pronation of the foot (Fig 37-10). This also may be seen by examining the patient's worn shoes, which show breakdown of the heel counters medially and a worn sole medially.

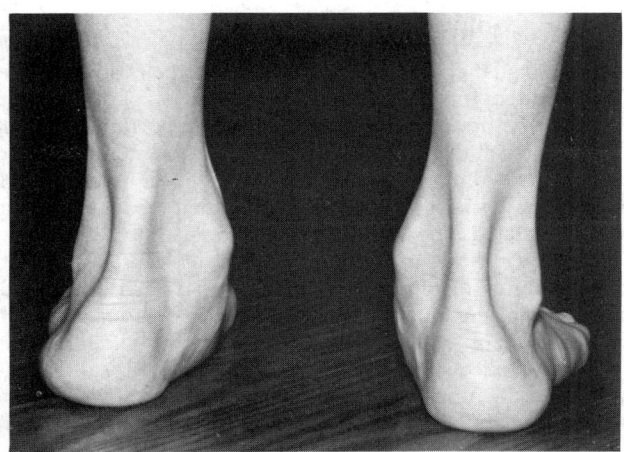

**Figure 37-10.** Ankle valgus and excessive foot pronation. This patient has marked ankle valgus bilaterally and excessive foot pronation standing.

Radiographs should be performed in any athlete with more than 4 to 6 weeks of pain. Any history or evidence of swelling also warrants radiography. AP, lateral, tunnel, and patellar views should be obtained for complete evaluation of the knee. The sunrise view no longer is considered optimal for assessment of the patellofemoral joint. The Laurin, Hughston, or Merchant views are more helpful in diagnosing patellofemoral disorders, especially patellar subluxation. Performed with less knee flexion, each of these views is obtained using a different radiologic technique. The tunnel view is especially important for the growing adolescent, who is at risk for osteochondritis dissecans, usually of the medial femoral condyle.

The treatment of PFSS usually is not surgical. Modification of activities to avoid full flexion of the knee and stress of the patellofemoral joint is imperative. A strengthening program for the quadriceps mechanism and a stretching program, especially for the hamstring muscles, often improve the patient's symptoms. In the athlete with excessive foot pronation, treatment should include the use of flexible orthoses. Judicious use of ice and anti-inflammatory medication usually is helpful. The athlete should be warned that patellar pain tends to be chronic, with exacerbations and remissions. The pain can be a lifelong problem, depending on the patient's activities. The goal is to educate the athlete regarding means of controlling the pain and still being able to enjoy some degree of athletic activity.

## Patellar Tendinitis

Another common cause of chronic anterior knee pain in an athlete is patellar tendinitis. Also known as jumper's knee, it is seen most often in athletes who participate in sports that involve running and jumping, especially basketball and volleyball. The onset of pain is insidious and it rarely is disabling. The injury consists of a microscopic fatigue tear at the insertion of the patellar tendon into the inferior pole of the patella.

The physical examination reveals point tenderness of the patellar tendon at the infrapatellar pole in 80% to 90% of patients. The remaining patients have tenderness of the quadriceps tendon at the superior attachment to the patella. Frequently associated with this problem is poor flexibility of the quadriceps and hamstring muscles.

Treatment includes rest, ice, anti-inflammatory medication, and frequent stretching of the quadriceps muscles. The athlete may continue to engage in the sport, but this may prolong the course of the tendinitis. With complete rest from running or jumping for 6 to 8 weeks, an athlete may be able to recover fully.

Recurrences are common, and the pain can become more resistant to treatment as a result of scarring within the tendon.

## Osgood-Schlatter Disease

In skeletally immature athletes with open tibial physes, swelling and point tenderness at the tibial tubercle are indicative of Osgood-Schlatter disease, which is associated with running and jumping in these individuals. This condition probably represents tiny stress fractures in the apophysis, and it is associated with a rapid growth spurt. Ice, anti-inflammatory medication, and a decrease in activity help the young athlete to manage this problem. The only permanent sequela is a prominence of the tibial tubercle, which rarely represents a cosmetic problem. Immobilization through the use of a knee immobilizer or crutches occasionally is necessary in patients who have severe pain. A few athletes continue to play until they are unable to walk without a limp. Regardless of the severity of the condition, the long-term prognosis is excellent and chronic pain or disability are uncommon.

## Iliotibial Band Friction Syndrome

The most common cause of lateral knee pain in a runner is known as iliotibial band (IT) friction syndrome. The IT band crosses the lateral femoral epicondyle before inserting into the tibia. Friction and pain can be produced when the IT band is taut, such as occurs in the downside leg when the athlete runs on banked roads consistently against traffic. There is no history of swelling or giving way, but the runner describes dull, achy pain associated with the activity.

On occasion, it may be difficult to demonstrate tenderness in this area on physical examination, so it may be helpful to examine the runner after he or she has completed a workout. It should be possible to reproduce the patient's symptoms by applying firm pressure over the IT band at the lateral femoral epicondyle while flexing and extending the knee (Noble test).

Treatment for this problem consists of rest, a course of anti-inflammatory medication, and the use of a flexible orthosis with a ⅛-in medial heel wedge. Probably the most important aspect of treatment is instruction of the patient in IT band stretching, which must be done faithfully. This problem seldom resolves without a minimum of 6 weeks of rest from running. The athlete should be cautioned about running consistently on only one side of the road, with its inherent drainage pitch. Running on alternating sides of the road or on level ground is encouraged. A tight IT band also may produce a friction syndrome over the greater trochanter at the hip (trochanteric bursitis). The pathophysiology of this condition is similar, and stretching of the IT band again is an important part of the treatment regimen. In both areas, the chronic bursitis may persist; if rest and stretching fail to provide relief, a local injection of soluble corticosteroid into the bursa should be considered.

## Shin Splint Syndrome

Lower leg pain is a common reason for a young runner to seek medical attention. The most common cause of this pain is shin splint syndrome, which also is known as medial tibial stress syndrome and posterior tibialis tendinitis. The athlete complains of achy pain that increases gradually in intensity throughout the exercise regimen. The pain improves greatly with rest. Shin splints often are related to overtraining, especially in the school-age athlete who has not been doing much distance running before cross-country or track season begins. On physical examination, there is marked diffuse tenderness over the posteromedial aspect of the tibia at the insertion of the posterior tibialis and soleus muscles (Fig 37-11). The tenderness with shin splint syndrome usually is

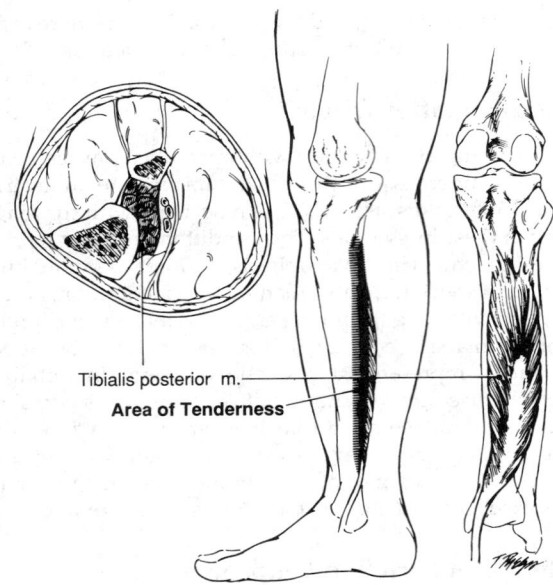

Tibialis posterior m.

**Area of Tenderness**

**Figure 37-11.** Shin splint syndrome. The pain and tenderness may be present throughout the entire posteromedial aspect of the tibia, corresponding to the fascial attachment of the tibialis posterior (and soleus) medially on the tibia.

present over the distal half of the tibia, as opposed to a tibial stress fracture, which tends to produce tenderness somewhere in the proximal half of the tibia. Ankle valgus and excessive pronation of the foot frequently are seen on gait analysis. Mechanically, the excessive pronation stresses the posterior tibialis and soleus muscles at their origin at the posterior medial aspect of the tibia. Treatment of the excessive pronation with better footwear or flexible orthoses usually is key to producing resolution and preventing recurrences. Rest, ice, and anti-inflammatory medication also speed recovery. Frequent calf stretches, which stretch all the ankle plantar flexor muscles, also are helpful. Athletes usually do not have to stop running completely, but must decrease significantly the intensity and duration of their workouts.

## Tibial and Fibular Stress Fractures

If the athlete with shin pain has a well-localized area of tenderness over the tibia or fibula, a stress fracture should be considered. An athlete with this condition often complains of pain at the start of the running activity that lasts for the duration of the workout. On physical examination, diffuse tenderness may be noted along the medial aspect of the tibia or lateral aspect of the fibula, but one area usually is significantly more tender than are the rest. A stress fracture may be difficult to demonstrate radiographically, because the only abnormality seen may be a small area of periosteal reaction at the site of the fracture, without an actual cortical defect. Also, plain radiographs will not reveal evidence of a stress fracture until it has caused pain for at least 2 weeks. When there is serious suspicion of a stress fracture, AP, lateral, and both oblique views should be obtained, because more of the periosteum is visualized tangentially. A technetium bone scan may be required to make the diagnosis. Most tibial stress fractures heal with rest from running and do not require cast immobilization. When point tenderness on palpation or pain with running has abated, the athlete may resume training. The fracture usually takes about 6 to 8 weeks to resolve, but there is some individual variability in the rest period required for healing. To maintain cardiovascular fitness while allowing the fracture to heal, the athlete should bike, swim, or run in water, as long as these activities do not produce pain.

## Chronic Compartment Syndrome

Lower leg pain that is worse *after* running should raise the concern of a chronic compartment syndrome. Instead of pain that occurs during the entire workout, the athlete will report that the first 5 to 10 minutes of the run are essentially pain-free. Once the muscles are warmed up, however, there will be achy, pounding leg pain that may persist for several minutes to hours after the workout is completed. The athlete localizes the pain to a diffuse area of one of the muscle compartments. The pain is caused by elevated pressure within the muscle compartment resulting from a relative inadequacy of the musculofascial compartment size. The athlete may complain of numbness or weakness corresponding to nerve compression in that compartment. For example, the anterior lateral compartment may involve the peroneal nerve, with tingling over the dorsum of the foot and weakness to dorsiflexion of the great toe.

Physical examination may reveal tenderness to palpation of the medial tibia or anterior fibula, but careful palpation will reveal that the maximum area of tenderness really is a diffuse area of one of the muscle compartments. To confirm the diagnosis, the athlete requires compartmental pressure measurements after exercise. If the pressure is elevated, fascial release is necessary to allow the patient eventually to train without pain. Rarely, an athlete may have an acute compartment syndrome and require an emergent fascial release.

## Ankle Sprains

The most common acute injury to the lower extremity is the ankle sprain. The athlete usually reports twisting the ankle, but may not remember the details of the injury. There may be an audible pop at the time of the injury. Unlike in other sports injuries, knowledge of the mechanism of injury of an ankle sprain is not very helpful. A fair amount of swelling often is noted, with disruption of the ankle ligaments as a result of bleeding. About 90% of ankle sprains are of the lateral ligaments, caused by inversion of the ankle or a combination of inversion and plantar flexion of the ankle. A small percentage are medial sprains involving eversion of the ankle.

Physical examination of the ankle involves the application of applied surface anatomy. Careful palpation of the structures reveals the maximal area of tenderness to be over the ligaments. If any bony tenderness is present, a fracture should be suspected and radiographs should be obtained. Stability testing may be difficult to perform if the athlete is seen a day or two after the injury, because of marked pain and muscle spasm. The most common ankle sprain involves one or both of the lateral ligaments, which are the anterior talofibular and the calcaneofibular ligaments. The anterior talofibular ligament is examined with the anterior ankle drawer test. With the tibia stabilized with one hand and the calcaneus grasped with the other hand, traction is placed on the talus anteriorly (Fig 37-12). Increased laxity, as compared to laxity in the uninjured ankle, implies that at least a second-degree sprain has occurred. If there is a poor end point (ie, a marked diminution in resistance to stress of the ligament), a third-degree sprain of that ligament has occurred. Inversion testing with the ankle in slight plantar flexion tests the calcaneofibular ligament. Comparison to the patient's uninjured ankle is imperative, because ligament laxity varies a great deal from athlete to athlete. Eversion testing with the ankle in a neutral position reveals any instability of the deltoid ligament. In some ankle sprains, there may be a great deal of pain but no increased laxity. Careful palpation may reveal tenderness over the deltoid ligament, the lateral ligaments, and anteriorly over the inferior tibiofibular ligament. This type of sprain at first may appear to be minor because there is no appreciable ankle laxity, but the sprain also involves

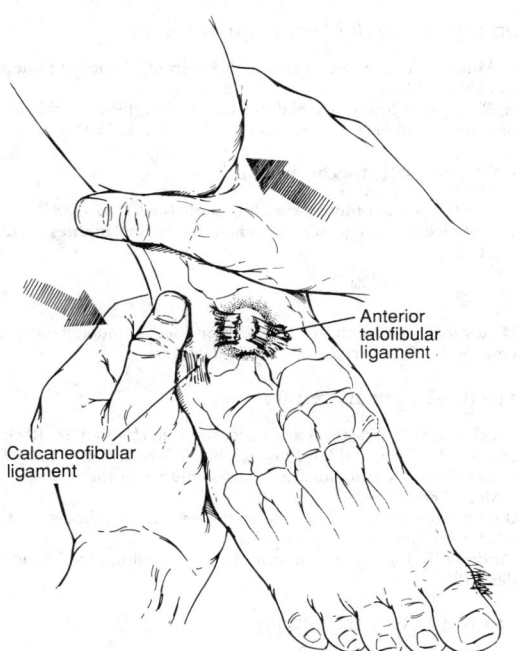

**Figure 37-12.** Anterior ankle drawer sign. To test the integrity of the anterior talofibular ligament, the tibia is stabilized with one hand and the calcaneus and talus are grasped with the other. With the ankle in slight plantar flexion and internal rotation, the talus is given traction anteriorly. Excessive motion with this maneuver with a poor end point is a *positive drawer sign,* and implies a third-degree sprain of the anterior talofibular ligament.

a tear of the interosseous membrane between the tibia and the fibula. Sometimes descriptively called the "ring-around-a-rosy" or "high" sprain, this injury usually takes longer to rehabilitate than do other, mild sprains.

Radiographs should be performed in any ankle injury that produces more than minimal swelling or pain with weight bearing. AP, lateral, and mortise views should be included to enable adequate assessment of the ankle mortise. Careful examination of the talar dome radiographically is important because any small fracture seen on the radiograph is indicative of a larger chondral defect.

Treatment of the ankle sprain initially is designed to minimize the hematoma and swelling. The mnemonic RICE is a helpful way to remember rest, ice, compression, and elevation as the important modalities with which to achieve this goal. Most athletes benefit from 48 to 72 hours of avoidance of weight bearing through the use of crutches. Compression bandages take many different forms, but a snug elastic wrap will suffice. The elastic wrap is even more effective if a U-shaped felt pad is placed over the malleolus to add pressure beneath the wrap. Elevation of the extremity above the level of the heart increases venous return. The worst thing that an athlete with an ankle sprain can do is to continue playing despite the pain. Contrary to popular belief, the common ankle sprain is associated with a significant amount of pain and disability.

The second aspect of treating an ankle sprain concerns resolution of the hematoma. This involves range of motion exercises, along with protective weight bearing. An ankle sprain will resolve much more quickly with the help of a physical therapist or an athletic trainer who can direct an exercise program. It also is helpful for athletes to have an exercise program provided in writing, to outline goals as well as to provide instruction regarding reasonable progression through the program. It must be emphasized that athletes should not ignore pain, but should use it as a

guide regarding their ability to engage in weight-bearing activities. As soon as they can hop up and down on the affected ankle several times without pain, the athletes are ready to begin the running program (see Table 37-5). Athletes may progress through sprinting and changing directions on the ankle, and must not be allowed to return to competition until they are able to change direction at full speed on the ankle without experiencing pain or instability.

Protective taping has been shown to be effective in preventing recurrent ankle sprain. Because tape can be expensive and many young athletes do not have access to a coach or trainer who is skilled in ankle taping, a lace-up ankle brace will help to prevent recurrences. High-top shoes probably are helpful in giving the ankle some stability. Surgical intervention rarely is indicated for third-degree ankle sprains. Surgery should be considered in an elite ballet dancer or gymnast, however, because an athlete engaging in this type of activity is less tolerant of ankle instability.

## Achilles Tendinitis

Chronic aching pain over the Achilles tendon in a runner usually is caused by Achilles tendinitis, which once was thought to be a tenosynovitis. Most cases probably do involve inflammation of the synovial sheath, but, more importantly, they represent tiny tears in the substance of the tendon.

The examination reveals tenderness located a distance corresponding to the width of about 2 to 3 fingers above the calcaneal insertion of the tendon. Minimal swelling and crepitus to dorsal and plantar flexion of the ankle may be noted.

Appropriate treatment includes rest, ice, anti-inflammatory medication, and gentle static stretching of the muscle-tendon unit. Heel lifts placed in the footwear add relief and help to reduce stress to the tendon. The athlete who is not a runner may continue to engage in sport but must lighten workouts, especially if they involve any running activity. An athlete who is a runner usually must rest from running for a minimum of 12 to 14 days. When the area no longer is tender to palpation, gradual return to training may be resumed. On occasion, it may take as long as 6 to 8 weeks before the athlete can resume running.

## Calcaneal Apophysitis

A school-age or adolescent athlete who has heel pain associated with exercise in a running sport usually has apophysitis of the calcaneus, also known as Sever disease. It frequently is bilateral and rarely produces swelling or discoloration. Examination reveals tenderness on medial and lateral heel compression. Radiographs usually are not necessary initially, but should be considered to rule out other diagnoses if the pain does not respond to treatment. Ice, anti-inflammatory medication, rest, and heel lifts usually provide relief. Flexible orthoses with a ⅛-in medial heel wedge should be considered instead of heel lifts for pronated feet. Total rest from weight-bearing activities is not imperative, but will speed relief.

## Plantar Fasciitis

Chronic heel pain in the older adolescent or teenage runner, located over the plantar surface of the heel, often is caused by plantar fasciitis. This may not come to the attention of a physician until it has been going on for several weeks or months. Typically, an athlete will complain that the pain is most problematic on rising in the morning. After warming up, he or she may be able to run with minimal pain. Palpation reveals marked tenderness over the calcaneus at the insertion of the plantar fascia.

Treatment for this condition consists of rest, anti-inflammatory medication, ice, and, most importantly, flexible orthoses with a

⅛-in medial heel wedge to relieve the stress on the plantar fascia at its insertion on the calcaneus. Some runners do well with new running shoes, which provide a better arch support. Plantar fasciitis usually takes a minimum of 6 to 8 weeks to resolve totally, even with complete rest.

## CONCLUSION

Sports medicine has become an important area of concern in ambulatory pediatrics because the young athletic patient expects the same care that is provided to college and professional athletes. It is important to recognize that the ability to return quickly to play and competition frequently are first on the agenda of the athlete who is seeking medical care. The most common injuries confronting the pediatrician often require the help of a physical therapist or trainer to instruct the athlete in a proper rehabilitation program. Rehabilitation frequently shortens the time that it is necessary for the athlete to spend away from competition and maximizes his or her safety on returning to the sport.

## Selected Readings

### General

Committee on Sports Medicine and Fitness, American Academy of Pediatrics. Dyment PG, ed. Sports medicine: Health care for young athletes, 2nd ed. Elk Grove Village, Illinois: American Academy of Pediatrics, 1991.
Garrick JG, Webb DR. Sports injuries: Diagnosis and management. Philadelphia: WB Saunders, 1990.
Grana WA, Kalenek A, eds. Clinical sports medicine. Philadelphia: WB Saunders, 1991.
Kulund DA, ed. The injured athlete, 2nd ed. Philadelphia: JB Lippincott, 1991.
Strauss RB, ed. Sports medicine, 2nd ed. Philadelphia: WB Saunders, 1991.

### The Pre-Participation Health Inventory

Committee on Sports Medicine and Fitness, American Academy of Pediatrics. Sports preparticipation examination. In: Dyment PG, ed. Sports medicine: Health care for young athletes. Elk Grove Village, Illinois: American Academy of Pediatrics, 1991:48.
Hara JH, Puffer JC. The preparticipation physical examination. In: Mellion MB, Walsh WM, Shelton GL, eds. The team physician's handbook. St Louis: Hanley & Belfus, 1990:18.
Maron BJ, Roberts WC, McAllister HA, et al. Sudden death in athletes. Circulation 1980;62:218.

### Role of the Team Physician

Committee on Sports Medicine and Fitness, American Academy of Pediatrics. The team physician. In: Dyment PG, ed. Sports medicine: Health care for young athletes. Elk Grove Village, Illinois: American Academy of Pediatrics, 1991:48.
Lombardo JA. Sports medicine: A team effort. The Physician and Sports Medicine 1985;13:72.

### Management of Athletic Injuries

McKeag DB. On-site care of injured youth. In: Kelley VC, ed. Practice of pediatrics, vol 10. Philadelphia: Harper & Row, 1984:1.

### Heat Illness

Squire DL. Heat illness: Fluid and electrolyte issues for pediatric and adolescent athletes. Pediatr Clin North Am 1990;37:1085.

### Common Medical Illnesses

Eichner ER. Infectious mononucleosis: Recognition and management in athletes. The Physician and Sports Medicine 1987;15:61.
Simon HB. Immune mechanisms and infectious diseases in exercise and sports. In: Strauss RB, ed. Sports medicine, 2nd ed. Philadelphia: WB Saunders, 1991:95.

### Sports Nutrition

Clark N. Sports nutrition guidebook. Champaign, Illinois: Leisure Press, 1990.
Loosli AR, Benson J. Nutritional intake in adolescent athletes. Pediatr Clin North Am 1990;37:1143.

### Dermatologic Concerns

Bergfeld WF, Helm TN. The skin. In: Strauss RB, ed. Sports medicine, 2nd ed. Philadelphia: WB Saunders, 1991:117.

### Common Injuries to the Head and Neck

Cantu RC. Minor head injuries in sports. Adolescent Medicine: State of the Art Reviews 1991;2:141.
Hershman EB. Injuries to the brachial plexus. In: Torg JS, ed. Athletic injuries to the head, neck, and face. St Louis: Mosby-Year Book, 1991:338.

### Introduction to Orthopedic Injuries

Micheli LJ. The traction apophysitises. Clin Sports Med 1987;6:389.
Risser WL. The acute management of minor soft tissue injuries. Pediatric Ann 1992;21:170.

### Back Injuries

Andrish JT. Overuse syndromes of the back and legs in adolescents. Adolescent Medicine: State of the Art Reviews 1991;2:213.

### Injuries to the Upper Extremity

Curtis RJ, Rockwood CA. Fractures and dislocations in children. In: Rockwood CA, Matsen FA, eds. The shoulder. Philadelphia: WB Saunders, 1990:991.
Ireland ML, Andrews JR. Shoulder and elbow injuries in the young athlete. Clin Sports Med 1988;7:473.
Pappas AM. Overuse syndromes of the shoulder and arm. Adolescent Medicine: State of the Art Reviews 1991;2:181.
Zarins B, Andrew JR, Carson WG. Injuries to the throwing arm. Philadelphia: WB Saunders, 1985.

### Injuries to the Lower Extremity

Garrick JG. Knee problems in adolescents. Pediatr Rev 1983;4:235.
Hergenroeder AC. Diagnosis and treatment of ankle sprains: A review. Am J Dis Child 1990;144:809.
Jacobson KE, Flandry FC. Diagnosis of anterior knee pain. Clin Sports Med 1989;8:179.
Jones DC, James SL. Overuse injuries of the lower extremity: Shin splints, iliotibial band friction syndrome, and exertional compartment syndromes. Clin Sports Med 1987;6:273.
Markey KL. Stress fractures. Clin Sports Med 1987;6:405.
Santopietro FJ. Foot and foot-related injuries in the young athlete. Clin Sports Med 1988;7:563.
Waters PM, Millis MB. Hip and pelvic injuries in the young athlete. Clin Sports Med 1988;7:513.

*Principles and Practice of Pediatrics, Second Edition.*
edited by Frank A. Oski et al. J. B. Lippincott Company, Philadelphia © 1994.

## CHAPTER 38
# Bone, Joint, and Muscle Problems

### Paul D. Sponseller

Physicians caring for children require a knowledge of orthopedics to treat injuries, recognize skeletal manifestations of systemic diseases, and provide or suggest therapy for congenital or developmental abnormalities. This chapter is designed to help in the initial understanding of the broad range of orthopedic conditions that are encountered in children; as a result, it is intended to have breadth rather than depth. Conditions that are isolated to one anatomic region are presented first, followed by generalized musculoskeletal conditions. Table 38-1 lists the differential di-

## TABLE 38-1.  Differential Diagnoses of Common Pediatric Symptoms

The following are presented to guide in the use of sections of this chapter and in the selection of references for further reading.

**Differential Diagnosis of Limp**

A. *Pain*
   Septic arthritis/osteomyelitis
   Transient synovitis
   Juvenile rheumatoid arthritis
   Migratory polyarthritis (immunologic)
   Legg-Calvé-Perthes disease
   Slipped capital femoral epiphysis
   Meniscus tear
   Idiopathic chondrolysis of the hip
   Osgood-Schlatter disease
   Impacted fracture
   Spinal disorder
B. *Weakness*
   Congenital dislocation of the hip
   Myopathy
   Polio
   Cerebral palsy/myelomeningocele
   Spinal cord compression
C. *Limitation of Motion*
   Legg-Perthes disease/slipped capital femoral epiphysis (old)
   Posttraumatic muscle contracture
   Posttraumatic joint contracture
D. *Leg-Length Inequality*
   Idiopathic hemihypertrophy
   Posttraumatic malunion or growth plate closure
   Neuromuscular
   a. Cerebral palsy
   b. Polio
   Neurofibromatosis
   Congenital limb deficiency
   Ollier's disease
   Arteriovenous malformation

**Knee Pain**

A. *Musculotendinous*
   Patellofemoral stress syndrome
   Osgood-Schlatter disease
   Patellar/quadriceps tendinitis
   Iliotibial band syndrome
B. *Bony–Cartilaginous*
   Meniscus tear
   Discoid meniscus
   Osteochondritis dissecans
   Tibial spine fracture/physeal injury
C. *Miscellaneous*
   Infection
   Tumor
   Connective tissue disorder
   Hip disorder

**Childhood Back Pain**

A. *Developmental/Acquired*
   Scheuermann's kyphosis
   Spondylolysis/spondylolisthesis
   Herniated nucleus pulposus
   Fracture of vertebral body
   Muscle strain
B. *Infectious*
   Vertebral body osteomyelitis
   Discitis
   Tuberculosis
C. *Neoplastic*
   Osteoid osteoma
   Osteoblastoma/osteosarcoma
   Leukemia/lymphoma
   Eosinophilic granuloma
   Ewing's sarcoma/neuroblastoma
   Spinal cord tumor

**Internal Rotation of the Lower Extremity: Toeing-In**

A. *Femoral*
   Anteversion
   Muscular/capsular
B. *Tibial Torsion*
C. *Metatarsus Adductus*
D. *Clubfoot, Partially Treated*
E. *Neuromuscular Disorder*

**Flatfoot**

A. *Flexible/Idiopathic*
B. *Tarsal Coalition*
C. *Juvenile Rheumatoid Arthritis*
D. *Congenital Vertical Talus*
E. *Marfan Syndrome*
F. *Neuromuscular Disorders*

agnoses of certain presenting signs and symptoms, and is meant to aid in the organization of a diagnostic plan. The selected readings listed at the end of the chapter are provided to guide further study of any particular condition.

Orthopedic terminology often is idiosyncratic; a few definitions are provided to assist the reader. The term *congenital* refers to a condition that is present at birth, regardless of whether it is inherited. *Developmental* refers to findings that occur or increase with time and growth, irrespective of their cause. *Physis* refers to the growth plate; therefore, the *epiphysis* is that portion of a bone that is "on top of" the physis (ie, nearer to the joint), *the metaphysis* is the widened portion of the shaft that is adjacent to and arises from the growth plate, and the *diaphysis* is the narrow portion of a tubular bone that is midway between two physes. The Greek root words *genu*, *coxa*, and *pes* refer to the knee, hip, and foot, respectively. When two bones or two fracture fragments form an angle, they are in *varus* when the apex of the angle points away from the midline and in *valgus* when it points toward the midline. Alternatively, *angulation* may be stated in any of the three standard anatomic planes by the direction of the apex (ie, genu valgus is medial angulation of the lower extremity at the knee). *Dislocation* refers to complete loss of contact of two joint surfaces, and it is specified by the direction of displacement of the most distal part. *Subluxation* is an incomplete dislocation. *Abduction* refers to movement away from the midline; *adduction* denotes movement toward the midline.

## REGIONAL ABNORMALITIES

### Hip/Femur

#### Developmental Dysplasia of the Hip (DDH)

The normal hip develops from a common anlage resulting from reciprocal contact between the femur and acetabulum during growth. Loss of this contact may occur as a result of abnormal in utero positioning; neuromuscular abnormalities such as myelodysplasia, arthrogryposis, or Larsen's syndrome; or intrinsic abnormalities in the cartilaginous anlage of the hip. The earlier this loss of relationship occurs, the more marked are the femoral and acetabular abnormalities that result; the later it is corrected, the less the remodeling potential.

The cause of congenital dislocation of the hip in an otherwise normal child is multifactorial. Mechanical factors play a role, and the frequency is increased greatly in fetuses with breech presentation (a factor in 30% of all cases of DDH), in firstborn children, and in infants with oligohydramnios. The left hip is involved more commonly than the right. These factors are associated with increased forces across the hip or positioning in adduction-hyperflexion, causing the femur to be directed out over the edge of the acetabulum. Hormonal factors may play a role, as there is generalized ligamentous laxity around the time of birth caused by increased circulating estrogens and relaxin. The incidence of DDH is sixfold greater in girls than in boys. Evidence for hereditary control of these and other factors lies in the fact that more than 20% of patients have a positive family history.

There are three degrees of hip dysplasia: subluxatable, dislocatable, and dislocated hips, in order of increasing severity. In the first degree, the femoral head rests in the acetabulum and can be dislocated partially by examination. The second degree involves a hip that can be dislocated fully with manipulation but is located normally when the baby is at rest. In the third degree of hip dysplasia, the hip rests in the dislocated position. The combined incidence of these three conditions is 1:60 births; the incidence of true dislocation is only 1.5:1000 births. A change in terminology from CDH to developmental dysplasia of the hip (DDH) has become widely accepted. Dysplasia better describes the spectrum of severity of this disorder, which ranges from malformation to dislocation of the hip. The term developmental is meant to acknowledge the fact that some cases cannot be detected at birth and may occur later; the anatomic findings are evolving continually. The pathologic anatomy includes capsular laxity, which progresses to capsular malformation with time if the hip remains dislocated. The acetabulum becomes shallow as a result of lack of concentric contact with the femoral head. A false acetabulum may form where the femoral head contacts the lateral wall of the ilium above the normal location. The outer rim of the acetabulum becomes rounded during the period when the femoral head is able to slide in and out of the acetabulum. The movement over this ridge is felt as the "clunk" of Ortolani's and Barlow's tests. The femur remains rotated anteriorly (anteverted) as the head rests against the lateral iliac wall.

Physical examination remains the key to the diagnosis of DDH. The signs in the newborn period usually include instability without significant fixed deformity; in later months, untreated dis-

location becomes more fixed and there is less instability and more limitation of certain motions. Specifically, Barlow's and Ortolani's signs should be sought in the newborn. These signs are considered to be positive when the hip can be dislocated and relocated, respectively. The child should be relaxed when the tests are performed, and only one hip should be examined at a time. The pelvis should be enclosed and stabilized with one hand, while the femur is controlled with the other hand, with fingers placed on the greater and lesser trochanters (Fig 38-1). With adduction and pressure directed posteriorly, the femur can be felt to slide in a posterosuperior direction over the rounded limbus in the abnormal hip (Barlow's sign, see Fig 38-1A) and then back in with abduction, causing a dull clunk to be heard (Ortolani's sign, see Fig 38-1B). Thus, these signs indicating dislocation and relocation are alternate phases of the same process of hip instability.

A common error made in DDH diagnosis is examining both hips at once, which impairs proprioception and may cause insignificant soft-tissue "clicks" to be mistaken for the more important and palpable "clunk." These innocent clicks may result from movement of fascia over the greater trochanter, the meniscus or the patella, or from the stretch of a normal labrum. Routine screening of neonates in the past 3 decades has resulted in a dramatic increase in the early diagnosis of DDH and, thus, more successful treatment of the disorder.

About 60% of all unstable hips seen in newborns normalize spontaneously within the first 2 to 4 weeks after birth as perinatal laxity resolves. A hip that is severely dysplastic may have negative results on examination because of the lack of an acetabular shelf. Not all hips can be reduced at birth, however, presumably because of earlier development of dislocation in utero, with fixed joint contractures. Similarly, some cases of dysplasia are believed to develop after birth. In most large series, it has been shown that not all abnormal hips can be detected by screening, even when it is done by skilled examiners.

If the hip remains dislocated, it can be relocated on examination in less than 15% of patients by the time they are 6 months of age. Findings of asymmetry, such as limitation of abduction and of full extension (see Fig 38-1C), as well as apparent shortening of the femoral segment are more sensitive at this time. This last sign, known as Allis' sign or the Galeazzi sign, is noted best by comparing the lengths of the two flexed thighs when they are held together. Asymmetry of skin folds by itself is an unreliable finding. When the child begins to walk, a positive Trendelenburg sign is noted: when weight is borne on the unstable side, the pelvis inclines to the other side.

Radiographs should not be used commonly before 6 months of age because of a lack of apparent bony changes during this time, except in infants with teratologic conditions; physical examination remains more reliable. Many centers use ultrasonography as an objective tool, but accurate interpretation of these studies requires extensive experience and should be done by a pediatric radiologist or orthopedist. Ultrasonography is indicated if the neonatal examination is abnormal or questionable, as well as to guide initial treatment. After 6 months of age, plain films may show cephalad and lateral migration of the femur with a break in Shenton's line (Fig 38-2), delayed appearance of the femoral ossific nucleus, a shallow and more vertical acetabulum, and later formation of a false acetabulum.

Treatment involves different measures at different ages. The aim of all therapy is to restore contact between the femoral head and the acetabulum. Because of the high percentage of patients who experience spontaneous improvement of lax hip capsules in the early perinatal period, most orthopedists recommend observing a hip that is subject to subluxation and reexamining it 3 to 4 weeks after birth. Dislocated hips should be treated at the time of diagnosis. If the hip remains unstable, an abduction-flexion device such as a Pavlik harness may be used. This al-

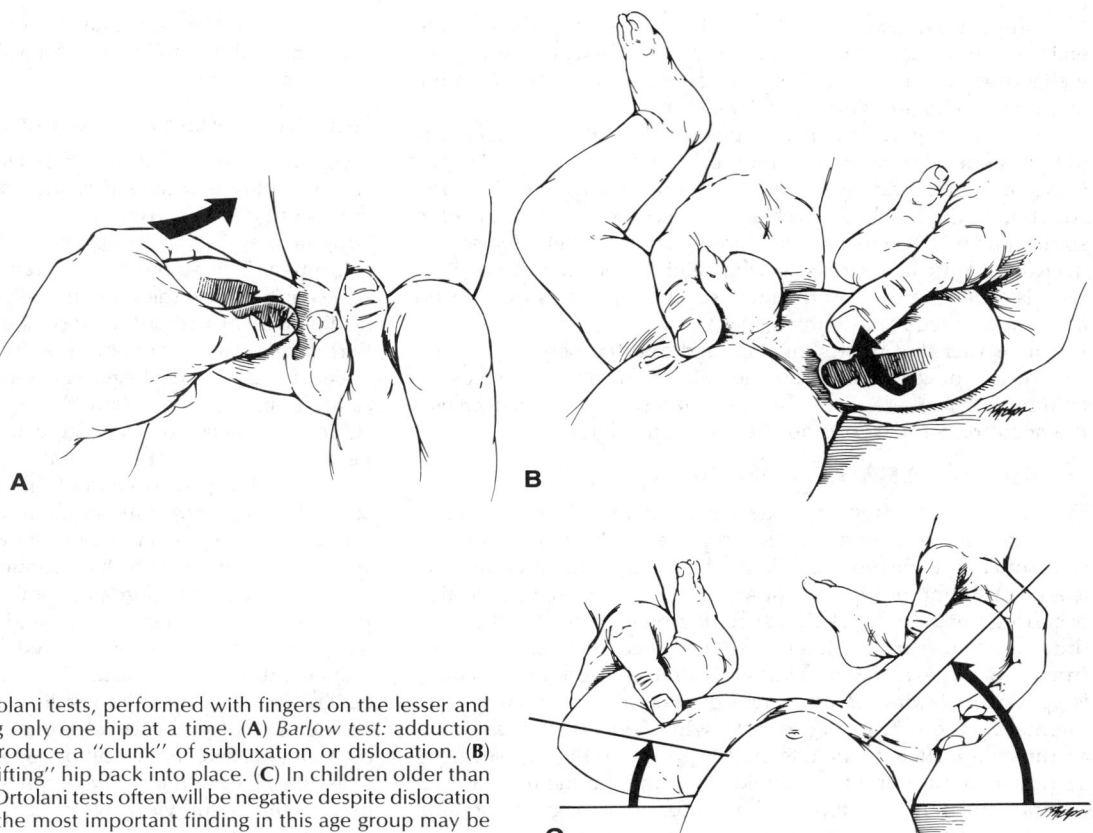

**Figure 38-1.** Barlow and Ortolani tests, performed with fingers on the lesser and greater trochanters, examining only one hip at a time. (**A**) *Barlow test:* adduction and posterior pressure may produce a "clunk" of subluxation or dislocation. (**B**) *Ortolani test:* abducting and "lifting" hip back into place. (**C**) In children older than age 3 to 6 months, Barlow and Ortolani tests often will be negative despite dislocation because of diminished laxity; the most important finding in this age group may be limitation of abduction.

lows some motion while it promotes the appropriate femoral-acetabular contact. The alignment should be checked by radiography in 1 to 2 weeks. The brace is worn until the results of clinical and radiologic examinations are normal, an interval that is equal to about 1 to 2 times the child's age at diagnosis. If treatment is begun after the child has reached 6 months of age, he or she usually is too large and strong to tolerate the brace. At

that point, reduction must be preceded by traction to bring the femoral head down toward the acetabulum, decreasing the muscle forces that could contribute to avascular necrosis. If closed reduction is unsuccessful, open reduction should be carried out. This involves tightening the lax superior capsule and releasing the tight psoas tendon and inferior capsule, allowing the femoral head to be brought down to its appropriate location.

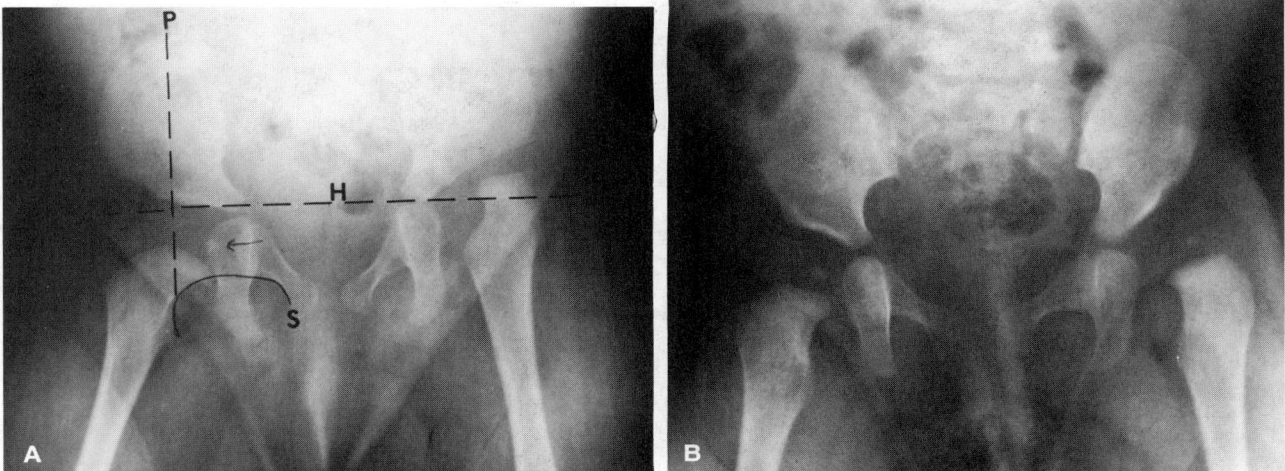

**Figure 38-2.** (**A**) Radiographic examination of congenitally dislocated hip. The femoral head ossific nucleus should be within the lower inner quadrant formed by Perkin's vertical line (P) at the outer edge of the acetabulum and Hilgenreiner's horizontal line (H). The nucleus appears at age 5 months, on the average. *Shenton's line* is the arc of the femoral neck, which should continue smoothly into the superior public ramus. This is a teratologic hip dislocation; note extreme height and rounded false acetabulum. (**B**) A more subtle example of congenital dislocation of the left hip.

If there is extensive distortion of the bones (ie, a shallow acetabulum or a rotated femur), a femoral or pelvic osteotomy as well as open reduction might be indicated. This is more common in patients who are more than 2 years of age.

Possible complications include persistent dysplasia from failure of normal development, recurrent dislocation, and avascular necrosis of the femoral head. The latter condition is caused by obstruction of the epiphyseal vessels by excess pressure or capsular stretch and it is the most serious complication of DDH. Avascular necrosis is more likely to occur when a hip is reduced in a patient who is older than 6 months and requires excessive traction or abduction to reduce the hip.

The earlier that treatment is carried out, the better is the resultant hip development and the safer is each of the steps in treatment. Thus, careful, methodical, early screening can decrease the need for complex orthopedic procedures later on.

### Transient (Toxic) Synovitis of the Hip

Transient (toxic) synovitis of the hip is a diagnosis of exclusion; it is a self-limited condition that represents the most common cause of an irritable hip in children. The usual clinical presentation is a painful limp or hip pain of acute or insidious onset, usually occurring unilaterally. The most common age range for the condition is 2 to 6 years, but it has been described in patients ranging from 1 to 15 years in age. Males are affected more often. There is spasm on testing of hip range of motion, particularly with internal rotation. The temperature, white blood cell count, and erythrocyte sedimentation rate may be normal or slightly elevated. The cause of the condition is unknown; an immune mechanism or viral infection is postulated. The differential diagnosis should include septic arthritis, osteomyelitis, and Legg-Calvé-Perthes disease, which usually is associated with a subchondral crescent of lucency or further changes in the femoral head on radiography. Juvenile monoarthritis, rheumatoid arthritis, and slipped capital femoral epiphysis (SCFE) also should be considered. Admission to the hospital, observation, and possible early aspiration should be undertaken if septic arthritis cannot be ruled out. Treatment consists of bed rest with analgesic agents provided as needed for 2 to 7 days. Therapy sometimes can be accomplished on an outpatient basis with frequent follow-up if the diagnosis is clear.

Persistence of the symptoms beyond 1 week should prompt reevaluation, although bed rest for as long as 1 month occasionally has been required.

### Legg-Calvé-Perthes Disease (Coxa Plava)

Legg-Calvé-Perthes disease first was differentiated from tuberculosis within a decade after the popularization of radiography, but its cause still is unknown. The condition is characterized by ischemic necrosis of the proximal femoral epiphysis with later resorption. The amount of the femur that is rendered ischemic varies and affects the outcome. Ischemia is followed by reossification with or without collapse of the femoral head. Legg-Calvé-Perthes disease usually, but not exclusively, affects children between 4 and 8 years of age. Males are affected four times as often as are females. As a group, these patients have slightly shorter stature and delayed bone age compared to their peers. Fifteen percent of all cases are bilateral.

The clinical presentation of this disorder usually is a limp (ie, an abductor lurch) with minimal pain of either short or long duration. The pain is not as acute or severe as that of transient synovitis or septic arthritis. Motions that are especially limited include internal rotation and abduction. Internal rotation is performed with the patient supine and the hip flexed, and the angle to which the leg may be rotated laterally is measured. These movements may be resisted by mild spasm or guarding. In the earliest stage, radiographic results may be normal or reveal slightly smaller size of the affected femoral epiphysis compared to the contralateral side as a result of its failure to grow after becoming avascular. Later, there may be a narrow crescentic lucency, seen best on the lateral view, which is the result of a tiny fracture of the subchondral bone. This reveals the extent of bone involved (Fig 38-3A). In some cases, revascularization may occur without collapse, but in others, revascularization of the femoral head is accompanied by progressive resorption and deformation, often with lateral and superior migration (see Fig 38-3B). Reossification follows, and the femoral head continues to grow. Whether this further growth occurs spherically depends on the patient's age, the amount of collapse, and the method of treatment.

The differential diagnosis should include transient synovitis, septic arthritis, hematogenous osteomyelitis, various types of he-

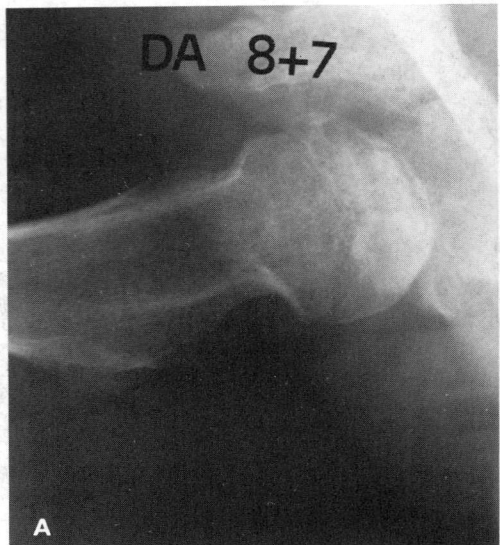
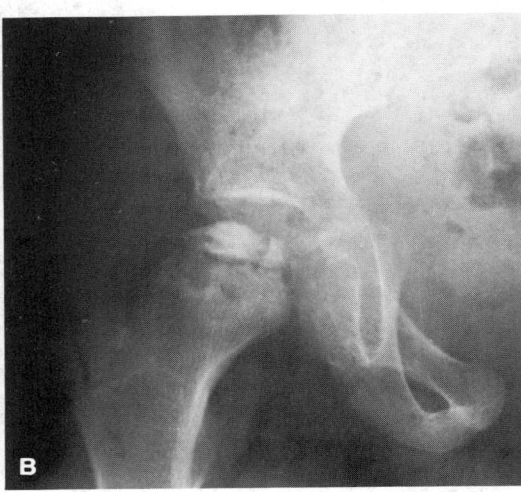

**Figure 38-3.** (**A**) Early Legg-Calvé-Perthes disease, showing subchondral "crescent." (**B**) Later, there is resorption and apparent collapse of the femoral head.

moglobinopathy, Gaucher's disease, hypothyroidism, and the epiphyseal dysplasias. The latter two conditions often are temporally symmetric bilaterally, whereas Legg-Calvé-Perthes disease is not.

Treatment follows two principles: functional containment of the femoral head within the acetabulum and maintenance of range of motion. During the vulnerable phase, the avascular portion of the femoral head is less likely to become severely deformed and is more likely to reconstitute spherically if it is contained within the "mold" of the acetabulum by abduction. Children younger than 6 years of age who have involvement of less than half the femoral head may be observed without active treatment if a full range of motion is preserved, because this signals containment and patients in this age group have a good prognosis. Aggressive treatment is indicated of patients who have involvement of more than half the femoral head or are more than 6 years in age.

Containment may be achieved by the use of an orthosis or by surgery. Orthoses produce abduction with or without internal rotation. The most commonly employed orthosis is the Scottish Rite brace, which does not extend below the knees (Fig 38-4). Containment should be documented radiographically. The child is allowed to perform any activity that is possible in the brace. The orthosis should be worn until early reossification is seen. Surgical treatment is used if an orthosis is not desirable because of the size of the child, the anticipated duration of wear (as long as 18 months in an older child), or lack of acceptance. Either a femoral osteotomy to redirect the involved portion within the acetabulum, or an innominate osteotomy or shelf procedure may be performed. The femoral osteotomy may cause slight shortening

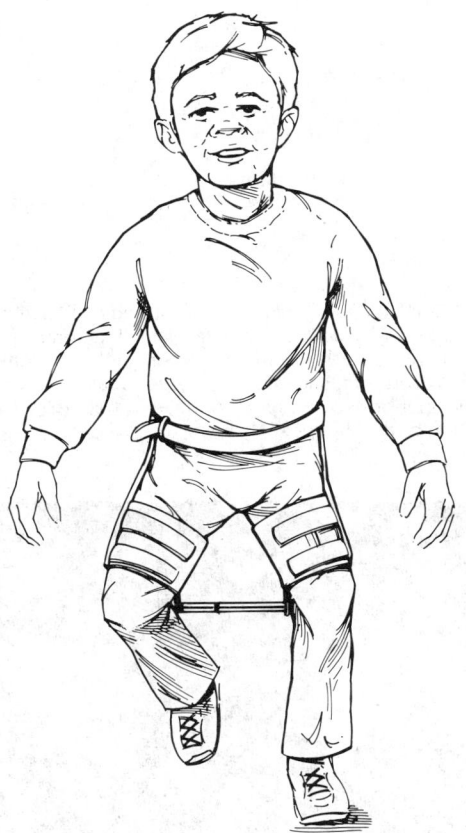

**Figure 38-4.** Scottish Rite brace for Legg-Calvé-Perthes disease produces containment by abduction and allows free knee motion.

and an increased likelihood of a limp, but it can be controlled more precisely. The two procedures produce about equal results.

## Slipped Capital Femoral Epiphysis

SCFE is a disorder of the growth plate that occurs near the age of skeletal maturity; it involves a three-dimensional displacement of the epiphysis posteriorly, medially, and inferiorly. In other words, the femur is rotated externally from under the epiphysis. The cause is unknown, but may involve mechanical as well as biologic factors. SCFE usually occurs without severe sudden force or trauma. Mechanically, there is increased stress as a result of obesity in most affected children and abnormal retroversion (posterior rotation) of the femoral head and neck. The periosteum at this age is thin and less able to resist the shearing forces. Possible biologic causes include delayed growth plate maturation and hormonal factors, which may account for the associated obesity. Increased growth hormone levels have been associated with decreased physeal shear strength, and hypothyroidism has been found in some cases. SCFE usually occurs during the growth spurt, and before menarche in girls. The condition is rare, with a frequency of 1:100,000 to 8:100,000. It is more common in males and in blacks. About one fourth to one third of all affected children have bilateral involvement, but usually not simultaneously.

The clinical presentation varies with the acuity of the process. Most children have a limp and varying degrees of aching or pain. The discomfort may be in the groin, but often is referred to the thigh or knee. Many patients are dismissed for an apparent knee complaint with no obvious cause only to have the true hip pathology discovered later with worsening of the slip. This paradoxic distribution of pain is attributed to referral within the femoral nerve distribution, which involves both the hip and knee joints. Some patients have acute, severe pain and inability to walk or move the hip. Again, abduction, internal rotation, and flexion are the motions that are most limited. A characteristic finding is external rotation of the hip with flexion, which is caused by the preexisting retroversion and the slip itself (Fig 38-5). There may be apparent limb shortening as a result of the proximal displacement of the metaphysis.

The earliest radiographic findings are widening and irregularity of the growth plate and osteopenia of the femur. Later, there is displacement of the epiphysis. This is seen best on the frog-leg lateral view of the pelvis. A line on the anteroposterior (AP) view drawn through the upper margin of the narrowest portion of the neck should intersect at least 20% of the epiphysis (Fig 38-6). This is an important point, because, with remodeling during chronic slipping, there may not be a step-off at the junction of the epiphysis and metaphysis. The severity of the slip is graded as mild (<33%), moderate (33% to 50%), or severe (>50%). Later changes may include avascular necrosis of the epiphysis or chondrolysis (ie, joint space narrowing).

Treatment centers on preventing further slippage, usually by placing the patient immediately at bed rest and obtaining a prompt orthopedic consultation. Surgery is intended to stabilize the upper femur and cause the growth plate to close. Realignment of the slip is not safe in chronic cases, because the forces necessary to accomplish realignment may produce avascular necrosis by disrupting the blood supply to the epiphysis. The gold standard of treatment is pin fixation in situ. Long-term follow-up reveals some remodeling of the slip. The pins should not penetrate the joint. Open epiphysiodesis using bone graft avoids the risk of pin penetration and produces faster growth plate closure, but it is a longer surgical procedure and requires cast stabilization in acute slips. Osteotomy of the proximal or distal neck to correct the deformity has been performed occasionally, but it carries a high risk of avascular necrosis. The contralateral side should be monitored

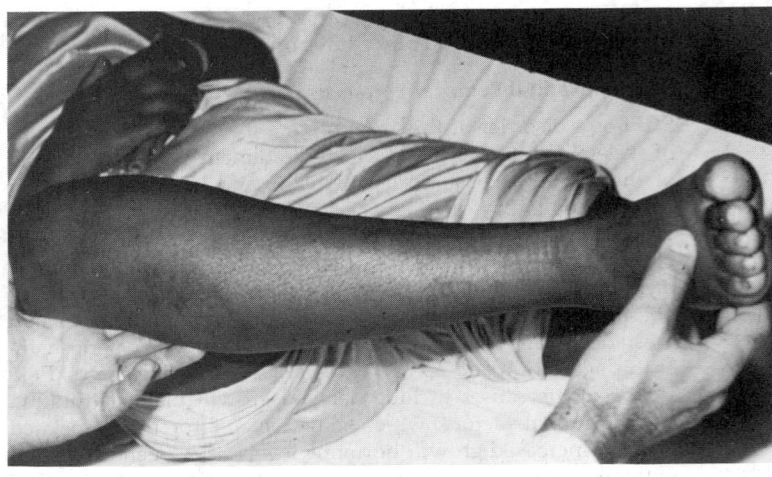

**Figure 38-5.** In slipped capital femoral epiphysis, the hip rotates externally as it is flexed by the examiner.

for SCFE and should be pinned early if symptoms occur. Long-term follow-up reveals no early degenerative change unless chondrolysis or avascular necrosis occur; each has an incidence of 1% to 5%.

### Increased Femoral Anteversion

Increased femoral anteversion is one of a spectrum of torsional deformities that affect the alignment of the knee and foot with the body. The differential diagnosis of toeing-in includes this as well as internal tibial torsion and foot deformities such as metatarsus adductus (see Table 38-1). Increased anteversion of the femur is defined as an increase in the angle between the plane of the femoral neck and the plane of the posterior femoral con-

dyles (Fig 38-7). This normally is about 30° at birth and declines to 15° by 10 years of age. The increasing pressure of the anterior hip capsule, as the child loses the physiologic flexion contracture, causes the change. Increased femoral anteversion persists in some neuromuscular conditions, presumably as a result of lack of these remodeling forces. The type discussed here is isolated idiopathic femoral anteversion.

On physical examination, the patient appears to toe in unless compensatory external tibial torsion is present. The patellae also face medially ("squint"). Internal rotation of the hip is much greater than external rotation in both flexion (supine) and extension (prone). Anteversion usually is not clinically significant unless external rotation at the hip is less than 15°.

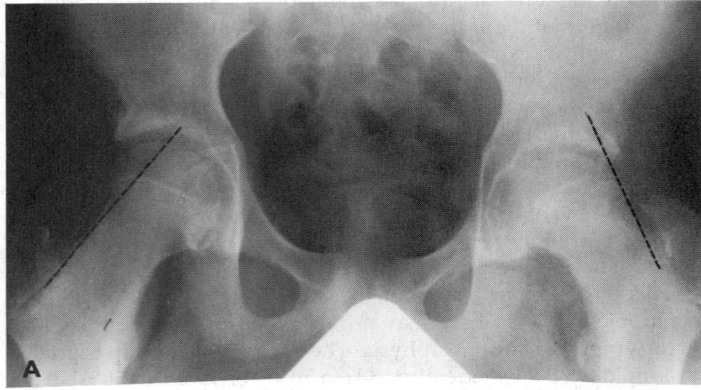

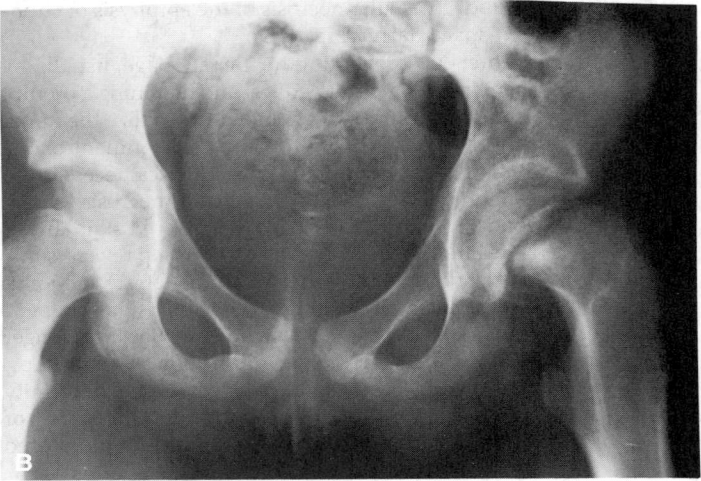

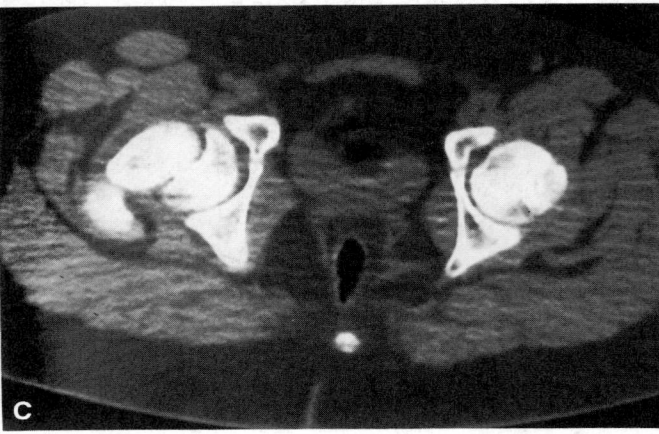

**Figure 38-6.** Radiographic findings in slipped capital femoral epiphysis. (**A**) A line drawn along the superior-lateral femoral neck intersects less than the normal 20% of the epiphysis on the left (affected) side. (**B**) A more severe slip, showing that the femoral neck subluxates laterally and superiorly with respect to the epiphysis. (**C**) CT scan shows the direction of the slip most clearly.

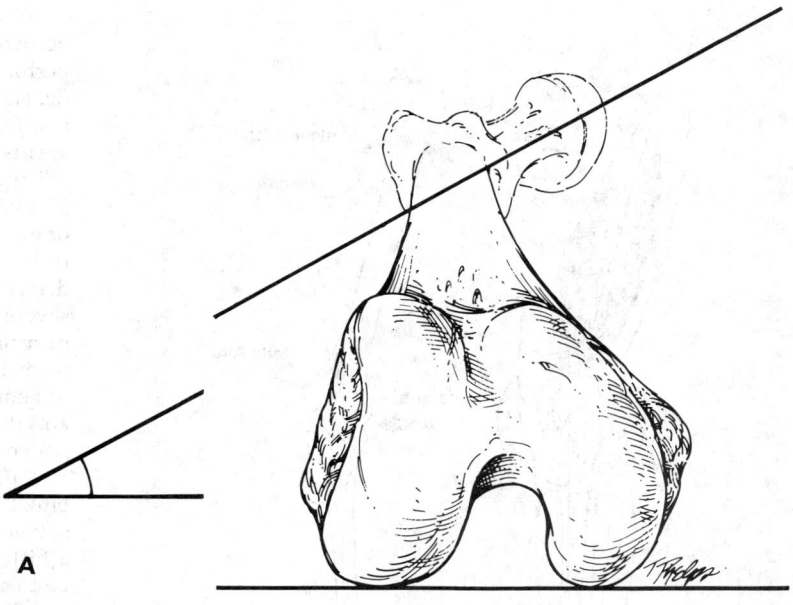

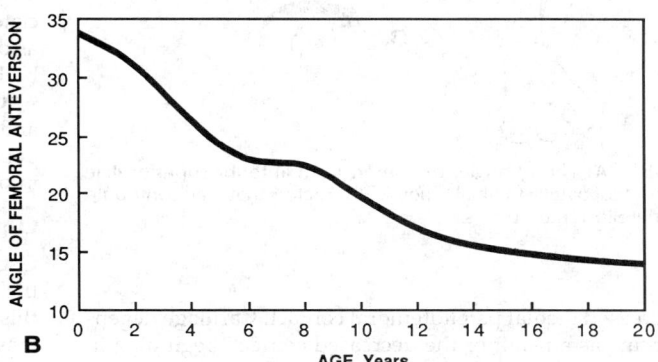

**Figure 38-7.** (**A**) Femoral anteversion is defined as the rotation of the femoral neck forward (in comparison with the distal condyles), as seen in this view down the axis of the femur. (**B**) The curve shows the normal decrease in femoral anteversion with age.

Radiographically, the femoral head and neck appear to be relatively straight on an AP film with the patella forward. This is a one-plane projection of a three-plane deformity. Computed tomography (CT) is best for measuring femoral anteversion directly.

The natural history of femoral anteversion is benign. In a few patients, it may contribute to patellar malalignment. Anteversion later in life has been found to be unrelated to arthritis of the hip or knee. Anteversion does not impair function. Treatment of increased anteversion consists of observation at least until the patient is 8 years of age and restriction from W-sitting, which may impair remodeling. The child instead should sit in the tailor position. Cables and bars are not effective in de-rotating the femur, and no orthotic method of treatment affects anteversion. In fact, most cases need no treatment. Femoral osteotomy, proximally or distally, is the only truly effective therapy. It should be performed rarely, however, and only in children more than 8 years of age who have functional disability as a result of patellar malalignment or, rarely, a persistent concern regarding their appearance.

## Knee

### Extensor Mechanism Disorders (Patellofemoral Problems)

The patellofemoral joint is subject to repeated high loads of laterally and posteriorly directed forces. A number of conditions involving this joint have been described in children and adoles-

cents, and they are treated by attempting to improve the basic forces.

Chondromalacia refers specifically to the appearance of softening and degeneration of the patellar cartilage. Patellar subluxation refers to partial lateral displacement of the patella. The terms patellofemoral stress syndrome, patellar malalignment, and excessive lateral pressure syndrome refer to the abnormal mechanics causing stress concentration and pain.

The patellofemoral force may be as great as 2.5 times body weight and is greatest in flexion. The average tibiofemoral angle is angled about 6° outward, which the patella must follow. The quadriceps–patella mechanism itself is angled away from the midline of the body, as measured by the "Q" (quadriceps) angle from the anterosuperior spine to the patella to the tibial tubercle (Fig 38-8A). These high forces and asymmetric loads cause minor variations to become significant, especially when they are coupled with high numbers of repetitions as a part of daily living. Possible factors contributing to patellar pathology (see Fig 38-8B) include increased outward angulation of the knee, abnormal rotation in the form of increased anteversion of the femur or external torsion of the tibia, a high patella ("alta"), abnormal shape or development of the quadriceps, or flattening of the femoral groove. Laxity of the medial side of the patellar restraints contributes to subluxation or dislocation. Women normally have slightly greater genu valgum than men. The above-mentioned factors usually cause greater stress on the lateral side of the patella and, some-

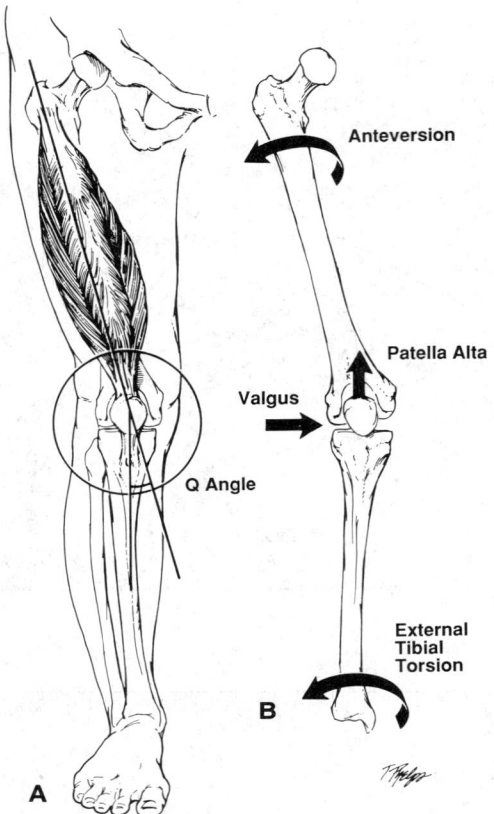

**Figure 38-8.** (**A**) The Q angle, measured from anterior superior iliac spine to center of patella to tibial tubercle. (**B**) Factors that may contribute to excess patello-femoral stress.

times, decreased medial patellofemoral contact. Cartilage degeneration occurs as a result of the decreased contact, beginning in the deep layers centrally and medially and becoming visible later.

Clinically, problems with the patella cause aching that is greatest in the anteromedial knee region, on the medial side or center of the patella. This usually is worse with stair climbing or prolonged sitting, as flexion increases patellofemoral force. Crepitus may be felt, but this may be painless in some patients and is not pathologic in itself. "Catching" or "locking" may be noted and might represent pain-induced inhibition or mechanical phenomena. A feeling of "giving way" may be described by the patient, especially with subluxation of the patella.

On physical examination, the most reliable way to test patellar tenderness is by direct compression of each facet against the femur. Palpation under the patella is not diagnostic. Contraction of the quadriceps and patella against resistance is nonspecific, because it may be painful even in normal persons. Effusion is present only if patellar degenerative changes or extreme overuse have occurred. Reproducing patellar subluxation with laterally directed pressure may cause apprehension. The "Q" angle, femoral anteversion, and tibial torsion should be checked. Radiographic results usually are nonspecific, but lateral displacement or tilt of the patella may be seen occasionally on the sunrise view.

The natural history of patellofemoral stress disorders is that they are common between the ages of 10 and 20 years, but often become less symptomatic later. They usually do not progress to osteoarthritis.

The differential diagnosis includes a synovial fold or "plica" that may snap over the medial femoral condyle, a medical meniscus tear, tendinitis of the quadriceps or patellar tendon, or osteochondritis dissecans of the patella or distal femurs.

Treatment consists of altering the abnormal stresses that are occurring. Modification may include decreasing activities that are performed with the knees flexed, especially those that cause pain (ie, stair climbing, prolonged sitting, and bicycling). Temporary rest from sports and the use of nonsteroidal anti-inflammatory agents may be necessary. Exercises to strengthen the medial (stabilizing) part of the quadriceps include resisted extension from 0° to 30°, most practically by lifting weights within this range or extending the knee on a pillow, flattening it. Hamstrings and rectus femoris muscles should be stretched if they are tight to decrease preload on the extensors. Arch supports may help if severe flexible flatfoot is contributing to tibial torsion. Surgical measures include release of a tight lateral patellar retinaculum, medial soft-tissue tightening, tibial tubercle transfer, or correction of genu valgum, knee anteversion, or patella alta if it is severe, and these all produce satisfactory pain relief in 75% to 90% of patients.

Patellar dislocations may be acute, recurrent, or, rarely, habitual. They almost always are lateral. Acute dislocations are associated with significant swelling and medial knee pain, and with a history of significant outward or rotating force. They should be treated for 4 to 6 weeks in extension with a lateral knee immobilizer, except in skeletally mature patients with bony avulsion. Recurrent subluxation is common, causes less pain and swelling, and often occurs with minimal force. There usually is an associated extensor mechanism abnormality. A realignment operation as described above is the only effective way to stop frequent and bothersome episodes.

Osgood-Schlatter disease, patellar tendinitis (jumper's knee), and quadriceps tendinitis all are manifestations of excessive, repetitive stresses on the extensor mechanism. They are listed here in order of decreasing frequency in children.

### Osgood-Schlatter Disease

Osgood-Schlatter disease is a traction-induced inflammation of the tibial tubercle. It is a reaction of the bone and cartilage of this region to high stress. The tibial tubercle is a downward extension of the proximal tibial epiphysis. It develops an ossification center between 9 and 13 years of age, but does not ossify completely until 15 to 17 years of age. It is within this age range that repetitive stresses gradually can deform the tubercle plastically, causing it to enlarge and become locally inflamed. Tenderness and swelling are localized to this region. Symptoms are worse with running, jumping, or kneeling. Treatment involves decreasing activity to a tolerable level and occasionally using a knee immobilizer, crutches, and ice after activity in severe cases. The patient may be vulnerable to recurrence for up to 2 years until the tubercle matures. If the child and family are informed of this likelihood, individual regulation of activities can be effective. Usually, activities of daily living and even some sports are tolerated, using daily stretching of tight quadriceps and hamstrings, and occasional anti-inflammatory agents. Complete avulsion of the tubercle is extremely rare and seems to be related more to sudden stress than to apophysitis.

### Patellar Tendinitis

Inflammation at the origin of the patellar tendon (which is at the inferior pole of the patella) is known as patellar tendinitis and is related to the same type of overuse as is Osgood-Schlatter apophysitis. It is seen most often in basketball players and also is called jumper's knee. The duration of pain serves as a guide to the severity of involvement. Pain that is present during both rest and activity is more worrisome than pain that occurs only after activity. Treatment is the same as for Osgood-Schlatter disease. Warm packs before and cold packs after activity also may be beneficial. Rarely, pain may occur at the proximal pole of the patella; in this case, the condition is termed quadriceps tendinitis.

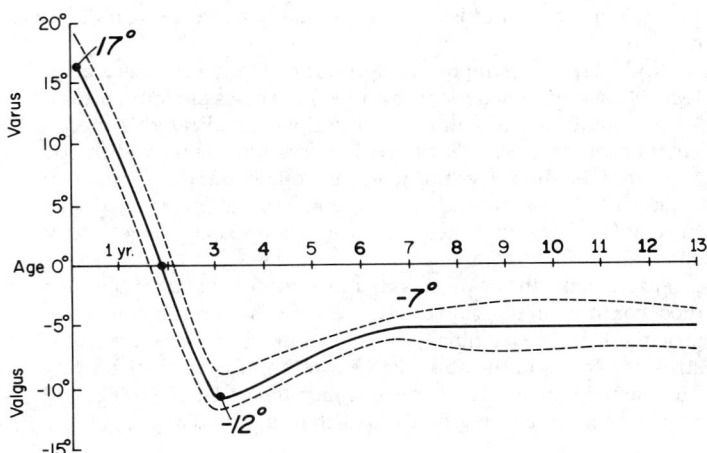

**Figure 38-9.** Normal change in the tibiofemoral angle during growth. (Reproduced with permission from Salenius P. Development of the tibiofemoral angle in children. J Bone Joint Surg 1975;57A:260.)

Treatment is the same as that described above for Osgood-Schlatter apophysitis.

## Tibiofemoral Disorders

### Popliteal Cysts

Popliteal cysts in children are localized behind the knee on the medial side. They occur most commonly in boys less than 9 years of age. Unlike in adults, these cysts in children usually are not associated with any intra-articular pathology and they tend to regress spontaneously with time. The recurrence rate actually is higher after surgical excision. The origin of these cysts is a slit-like communication between the knee joint and the gastrocnemio-semimembranous bursa.

### Discoid Meniscus

An acquired flattening of the lateral meniscus is known as discoid meniscus. In some cases, this flattening occurs as a result of the absence of normal peripheral attachments. Symptoms such as pain, clicking, and locking often develop in the absence of trauma in children from the age of 2 years to adulthood. The meniscus should be trimmed or excised if symptoms become severe. If the attachments are intact, no removal is necessary unless a tear is seen.

### Genu Varum

Genu varum, or "bowed leg" of up to 20° is normal in children until the age of 18 months (Fig 38-9). It normally does not increase significantly after walking begins. After the age of 24 months, genu valgum develops. Radiographs are indicated if genu varum is present after this age or is progressive after the age of 1 year, if it is unilateral, if it appears to be severe, or if it occurs in a high-risk group such as obese black children who walk early. Radiographic findings of benign genu varus include symmetric bowing of the tibia and femur, a normal-appearing physis without narrowing or step-off, and a generalized, rather than focal, outward angle.

Treatment involves observation to verify resolution. Measurement of the angle on physical examination should be performed with the child standing and may also be accomplished by measurement of the distance between the femoral condyles or of the AP tibiofemoral angle. These methods are not as accurate as are radiographs, but they are a practical way of observing change in patients when the presumptive diagnosis is physiologic genu varum.

The differential diagnosis of physiologic genu varum includes Blount disease, rickets, post-traumatic growth plate disturbance, enchondromatosis, achondroplasia, and other skeletal dysplasias.

### Tibia Vara (Blount Disease)

Tibia vara, also known as Blount disease, is an idiopathic, probably mechanical deficiency in the medial tibial growth plate that may be unilateral or bilateral. It may present initially in two different age groups, infants and adolescents.

Untreated infantile tibia vara almost always is progressive and, in addition to outward angulation, includes flexion, internal rotation, and, often, abnormal lateral knee laxity. Radiographs demonstrate progressive depression of the medial metaphysis, the growth plate, and the epiphysis, and, eventually, fusion of the medial metaphysis to the epiphysis in severe cases. A helpful early distinction in tibia vara is the focal nature of the change, with sharp angulation of the proximal tibial metaphysis resulting in a metaphyseal–diaphyseal angle of 11° or more, measured as shown in Figure 38-10. This is a specific sign, because such localized angulation occurs in fewer than 5% of children with

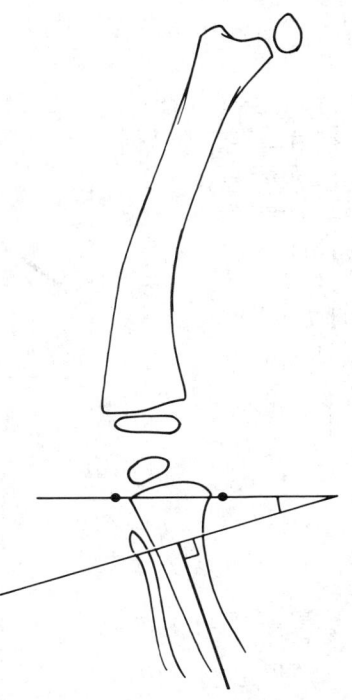

**Figure 38-10.** Metaphyseal–diaphyseal angle. The angle is formed by the line of the tibial shaft and the line between the medial and lateral beaks of the proximal tibial metaphysis. (Redrawn with permission from Levine AM. Physiologic bowing and tibia varum. J Bone Joint Surg 1982;64A:1159.)

physiologic varus, but is seen in essentially all those with Blount disease.

Night brace treatment, though not formally proven to be effective, usually is used for mild but definite cases of Blount disease. Valgus rotational osteotomy of the tibia is indicated if the angulation progresses, or if physeal depression occurs and the patient is older than 3 years. Recurrence is common if treatment begins after 4 years of age, if the epiphysis is fragmented, or if the child is obese. Persistent tibia vara leads to early degenerative change.

Adolescent tibia vara has its onset after 9 years of age. It is most common in obese males. It probably is caused by decreased growth of the medial tibial physis resulting from excessive medial stresses. Radiographs show medial femoral and tibial bowing. Treatment involves osteotomy to realign the limb or lateral growth plate closure to allow growth to "catch up" medially.

### Genu Valgum

Genu valgum of the knee is normal after 2 years of age, reaches a mean of 12° at 3 years of age, and remains constant at a mean of about 7° in boys and 9° in girls after 8 years of age. Night bracing may be helpful in children with angulation exceeding 20°. If it remains greater than 15° at 10 years, early growth plate stapling or later osteotomy of the affected region may be indicated

to prevent patellofemoral problems and degenerative changes. Valga of the proximal tibia often follows medial metaphyseal fractures, but frequently corrects spontaneously.

## Tibia

### Internal Tibial Torsion

Internal tibial torsion is the most common cause of toeing-in in children between 1 and 3 years of age. Tibial torsion is determined by measuring the angle between the foot and the thigh with the ankle and knee positioned at 90°. The foot normally rotates externally with age (Fig 38-11). The differential diagnosis includes metatarsus adductus, femoral anteversion, and neuromuscular disorders. To make these distinctions, the foot as well as the hip should be examined (see Fig 38-11, *A*, *B*, and *C*). Tibial torsion improves naturally with growth, but this often takes years. Because of our improved knowledge of the benign natural history of this condition, bracing with devices such as the Denis-Browne bar is used only rarely now. Studies have shown that external braces cannot apply significant rotational force to the tibia, because it is taken up in the foot, knee, and hip joints. The improvement that previously was attributed to the brace is primarily the result of normal growth patterns. Correction is a slow process and often frustrates parents. Knowledge that braces were used

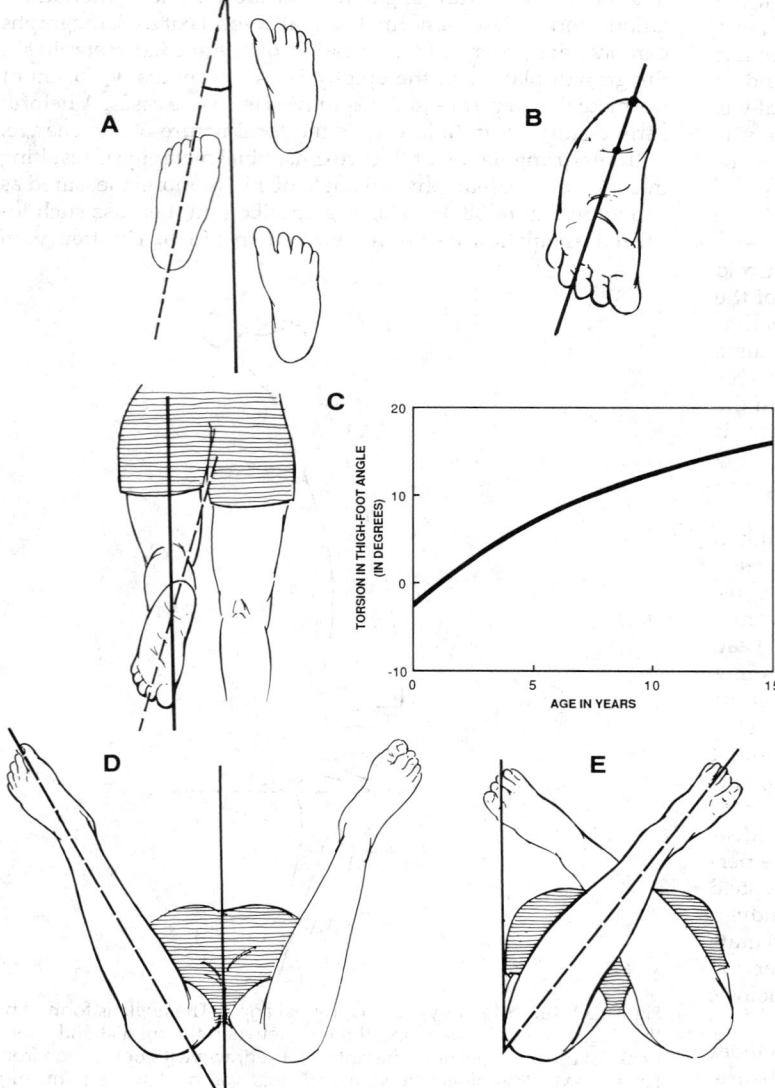

Figure 38-11.   Assessment of torsional deformities. (**A**) Angle of progression: the angle between the foot and the line of gait—summation of femoral, knee, tibial, and foot relationships. (**B**) Assessment of metatarsus adductus. The heel bisector normally falls between second and third toe space. (**C**) Thigh–foot angle, and its variation with age. This is a reflection of tibial torsion. (**D, E**) Measurement of internal (**D**) and external (**E**) rotation of the hip. If external rotation is less than 20°, "in-toeing" may come from femoral anteversion or hip capsular contractures. (Redrawn with permission from Staheli LT, et al. Lower-extremity rotational problems in children. J Bone Joint Surg 1985;67A:41.)

heavily in the past, reinforced by grandparents and friends, often drives anxious parents to visit the doctor to make sure they are not missing a golden opportunity to avoid problems. The physician should be confident in allaying their anxiety and should tell them something similar to the following: "Your child is toeing-in because of inward twisting of the tibia (or leg bone). This is a normal stage in resolution of the position in the womb. Some children have more toeing-in than others. Although your child occasionally may catch his foot when he runs, this will improve. As the bone grows longer, it will grow straighter. It may take a few years to correct. Doctors used to use braces for this, but we found that children were getting better by themselves. You can reassure friends and relatives that he will outgrow it." Use of the graph shown in Figure 38-11C may prove convincing. Although very little evidence exists regarding the efficacy of a brace or of any orthotic method, it is a very widely used treatment. Some feel that its main value lies in preventing turning-in of the leg during sleep in the prone position, facilitating spontaneous correction (Kling, 1983). Minor persistent internal torsion has not been shown to be detrimental.

### External Tibial Torsion

External tibial torsion is less common. Few data exist regarding the course of the condition, but no treatment is indicated and some spontaneous improvement can be expected.

### Mild Anterior and Lateral Bowing

Mild anterior and lateral bowing of the tibia are common in infancy and should be observed to make certain that spontaneous straightening occurs. Focal sclerotic defects in the tibia may be seen with severe anterolateral bowing. Fractures are present or develop in affected tibias (congenital pseudarthrosis), and patients may be found to have neurofibromatosis. If the severe anterolateral bow is present but the tibia is not fractured, it should be braced for protection. If the bone is fractured, attempts to gain union by electrical stimulation, vascularized fibula grafting, and bone grafting have similar success rates that range from 50% to 75%. Anterolateral bowing also may be seen with congenital absence of the fibula.

### Posterior/Medial Bowing

Posterior/medial bowing of the tibia is more benign, usually straightens by the time the child reaches 4 years of age, and is not associated with fracture. Between 2 and 6 cm of shortening commonly are seen by maturity, however. Treatment involves stretching of the tight dorsiflexor muscles and length equalization as indicated.

## Foot

### Isolated Idiopathic Adduction

Isolated idiopathic adduction of the forefoot or metatarsals is designated by terms that carry different meanings for different individuals: metatarsus adductus, metatarsus varus, or "C"-foot. In contrast to clubfoot, the hindfoot is normal or angled outward slightly. The ankle joint itself has normal dorsiflexion and plantar flexion (Fig 38-12). The hypothesized cause of this condition is increased medially directed intrauterine pressure. Children with metatarsus adductus also may have an increased incidence of other molding deformities, such as congenital dislocation of the hip or torticollis. Metatarsus adductus deformity should be differentiated from skewfoot, in which there also is severe outward bending of the hindfoot that is much harder to treat. A rough measure of the degree of adduction can be obtained by determining the position of an imaginary line that would bisect the sole of the hindfoot. Normally, the line falls between the second and third toes; in patients with severe adduction, it is lateral to the fourth toe (see Fig 38-11B).

The natural history of untreated metatarsus adductus is spontaneous correction in 85% of children, with the persistence of mild adduction in 10% and severe adduction in 5%. Unfortunately, those cases that will resolve spontaneously cannot be predicted, even on the basis of severity or rigidity. Manipulative correction is equally successful anytime during the first 8 months of life. Thus, the author's preferred treatment is observation with stretching for the first 4 to 6 months, followed by corrective casts or splints if the condition persists beyond this time. The casts are changed every 1 to 2 weeks until the defect is corrected clinically, then a "holding cast" is applied for 2 weeks. Capsulotomy or osteotomy for very late deformities occurring in children more than 3 years of age rarely is necessary.

### Clubfoot

Talipes equinovarus congenita, or clubfoot, is a more complex disorder involving not only metatarsal adduction, but also abnormalities of the hind part of the foot, including malrotation of the calcaneus under the talus and equinus (plantar flexion) of the ankle. The incidence is 1:1000 and it is more common in males than in females. Clubfoot may be unilateral or bilateral. Its cause is unknown, but appears to be related to a primary defect in or a very early insult to the leg muscles or tarsal bones. Muscle biopsy results are abnormal, which is consistent with the observation that the leg muscles are underdeveloped, even in treated cases.

Physical examination reveals a small foot, and the combination of deformities often results in a 90° rotation of the forefoot in all planes so that the leg and foot truly resemble the shape of a club. There is a deep crease on the medial border of the foot. The deformity may be correctable to neutral initially only in the neonatal period, and the range of motion in all planes is limited. Radiographs show an abnormal parallelism of the talus and calcaneus, but they are not necessary in the typical case. Neuromuscular disorders (especially lipomeningocele, myelomeningocele, or arthrogryposis) may produce similar deformities. Also, the condition of diastrophic dwarfism includes a deformity similar to clubfoot.

Clubfoot ranges from a mild, "postural," and easily correctable condition to one that is severe and resistant to treatment. A trial of cast correction is indicated in all cases, however. This is most successful in the perinatal period when ligamentous laxity is greatest, with the casts being changed every few days. Overall, casting is effective in about one third of all patients. Surgery is indicated in the others and involves complete release of all bony malalignments and tendon contractures; it is performed most commonly between the ages of 6 and 12 months.

### Flatfoot (Pes Planovalgus)

The condition called flatfoot must be divided into flexible and rigid types. The flexible type is very common in children and usually causes no symptoms. Development of the arch of the foot occurs spontaneously during the first 8 years of life in most children. The arch of the foot is restored when weight bearing is relieved. Inward-outward motion is normal. In contrast, rigid flatfoot may be caused by tarsal coalition, a vertical talus, neuromuscular imbalance (which occasionally also may be flexible), or arthritis of the foot. These conditions should be considered in the differential diagnosis.

The cause of the usual type of flexible flatfoot is ligamentous laxity with mild secondary bony changes. No primary muscle abnormality exists. Occasionally, a tight heel cord may contribute by pulling the foot into greater outward angulation. Treatment is not indicated in asymptomatic cases of flexible flatfoot; prospective studies have shown that no orthotic or shoe configuration

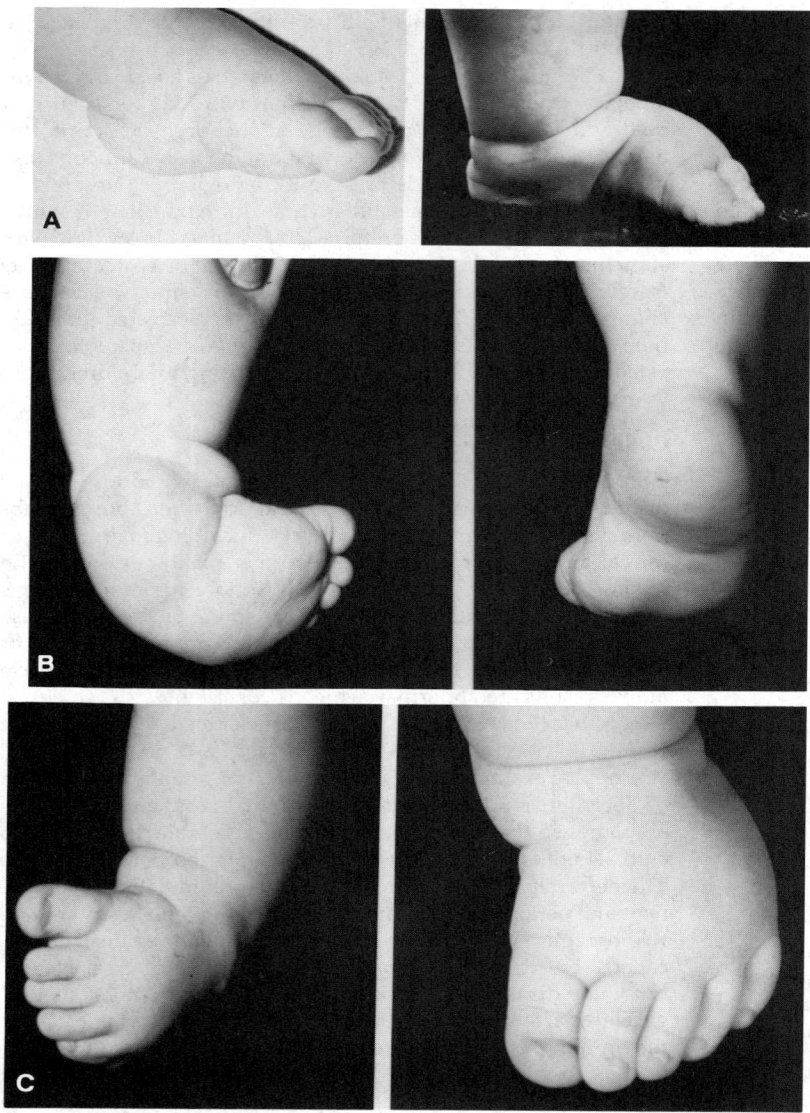

**Figure 38-12.** Comparison of clubfoot (*left*) and metatarsus adductus (*right*). (**A**) Lateral view, showing the equinus present only in clubfoot. (**B**) Posterior view, showing the hindfoot varus in clubfoot but not in metatarsus adductus. (**C**) Anterior view, showing adduction in both feet, with the varus also present in clubfoot.

can produce a lasting change in pediatric flatfoot. Such devices may be indicated for rigid or neuromuscular flatfoot, but not in asymptomatic children who have flexible flatfoot. The heel cord should be stretched if it is tight. Rarely is soft-tissue reconstruction or osteotomy indicated.

General principles that a physician should stress to parents when asked about shoes are summarized in an article by Staheli. In short, shoes are primarily for protection; "corrective shoes" have no effect on flatfoot; and shoes should be flat, flexible, porous, and high-topped to prevent them from slipping off the foot. These characteristics are available in most reasonably priced footwear found in regular shoe stores.

### Tarsal Coalition

Failure of complete separation of hindfoot bones with persistence of a bridge or coalition between two of them that may be fibrous, cartilaginous, or bony is known as tarsal coalition. This anomaly is transmitted in an autosomal dominant fashion and is present in about 5% of the population. Many individuals with tarsal coalition are asymptomatic. The presence of symptoms seems to be related to the degree of outward angulation that is present, which places more shear strain on the abnormal junction.

The diagnosis usually is made during the second decade after an ankle "sprain" with persistent pain or the spontaneous onset

of pain in the ankle. The reason for this presentation probably is that the ossification that occurs at this time, near the point of skeletal maturity, makes the coalition more stiff. The hindfoot shows limitation of the inward-outward motion, but it is tender to palpation. Sometimes there is manifested pain over the peroneal muscles, which contract excessively to stabilize the foot.

An oblique radiograph of the foot can illustrate reliably the most common type of coalition, the calcaneonavicular bar, if it has ossified. If it is fibrous or cartilaginous, there may not be a bony connection, but an irregularity of the cortices might be seen. Negative radiographic results combined with clinical suspicion indicate the need for a coronal CT of the foot to search for a talocalcaneal coalition, which is the next most common type of deformity.

With rest or casting, many cases of tarsal coalition will stabilize and become painless. If pain persists, the coalition can be excised if it is not large and if no degenerative change has occurred. If these conditions are not met, fusion of the hindfoot is indicated.

### Spine

Back problems in children generally fall into two categories: those associated with spinal deformity and those associated with pain in various parts of the back. When these conditions exist in the same child, determining the cause of the pain is more urgent than treating the deformity.

### Childhood Back Pain

Generally, pain in the back in a child is indicative of a problem that requires further attention and evaluation. Whereas low back pain in adults often has no demonstrated cause, about 75% of cases in children have a definite cause. Careful neurologic examination is necessary when evaluating children for back pain, as is an assessment of spinal flexibility and deformity. The differential diagnoses listed in Table 38-1 are the conditions that are encountered most commonly.

*Musculoligamentous Pain.*    All the components of a child's spine (ie, discs, ligaments, muscles, and joint capsules) are flexible and conform easily to the extreme spinal positions that are encountered daily in the schoolyard or on the playing field. After about 12 years of age, the spine generally loses some of its flexibility, and during the teenage years, further "stiffening" may take place. Muscular or ligamentous back pain almost never is seen in children who are less than 10 years of age. This diagnosis should be reserved for an older child, often one who is involved in a new physical activity, who has pain in the lumbar area for which no other specific cause can be elucidated. To warrant this diagnosis, the child should have pain localized to the lumbar area, a normal neurologic examination, normal results on radiography of the lumbar spine, and, in some instances, normal bone scan results.

Once the diagnosis has been made, the treatment of musculoligamentous pain involves rest from any activity that causes the pain. The use of ice in the first 24 hours after onset is helpful, but thereafter, heat usually is more efficacious. Once the pain has resolved, exercises to strengthen the abdominal musculature and the lumbar muscles should be used before sports activity is resumed. A lumbosacral corset often is helpful in the acute stage and for a few months thereafter when the child is participating in sports to protect the low back and its muscles from the extremes of spinal movement. The long-term use of a corset or other brace rarely is needed if the diagnosis of musculoligamentous back pain is correct. Once low back pain has resolved, it is important to stress to affected children that warming up before participating in sports activities is more important for them than for their teammates. The persistence of pain requires further investigation for unusual causes of back pain.

*Spondylolysis and Spondylolisthesis.*    A relatively common cause of childhood back pain, spondylolysis usually is a stress fracture of the pars interarticularis segment of the vertebra. This thin segment of bone between the facet joints is subjected to high forces, especially with marked lordosis of the lumbar spine or with heavy lifting. The overall incidence in the general population is about 6%. Most of these stress fractures likely occur in the early school years, though symptoms occur most frequently when children are in their early teenage years. There is a much higher frequency of spondylolysis in children who participate in gymnastics, wrestling, and weight-lifting activities, at times approaching 20% for participants in these sports.

Symptoms most commonly include pain in the lumbar area after or during a sports activity and a concomitant limitation of lumbar spine motion. If the child has a chronic spondylolysis, the pain often is intermittent; if the spondylolysis is acute, the pain is more severe the first time it is noted. Radiation of pain along the sciatic nerve distribution into the lateral calf or dorsum of the foot occasionally may be present.

The physical examination may not be remarkable. Usually, there is limitation of lateral spine flexion toward the side of the spondylolysis, often associated with limited forward flexion from

back pain, not hamstring tightness as in some other conditions. Back pain may be produced by straight leg raising, but radiation of pain into the legs with this maneuver is rare. The results of the neurologic examination are normal.

The diagnosis usually can be made by lumbar spine radiographs (Fig 38-13). The most common location of spondylolysis is at L5, with L4 being the next most frequent site. Spondylolysis often can be visualized by AP and lateral radiographic views, but oblique views usually are more definitive. In addition, oblique views reveal the unilateral or bilateral nature of the defect. If a lytic defect is observed, the age of the lesion should be determined if possible. The spondylolysis generally is old if the defect has sclerotic edges. A technetium 99m bone scan, with pinhole collimator views, is helpful to determine the age of the stress fracture. If the scan is cold and sclerotic edges are present on radiography, it will not be possible to obtain bone union nonoperatively. If the scan shows increased uptake at the lytic area and the radiographs reveal no sclerotic edges, however, the stress fractures might heal if the child is placed in a body jacket brace or cast.

If the scan shows no increased uptake, the treatment of spondylolysis is similar to that of a musculoligamentous problem. Initially, rest from activity should be instituted. A lumbosacral corset often is helpful for a few weeks until pain resolves. Some teenagers with spondylolysis prefer to wear the corset during sports activities as added protection even after acute back pain resolves. Fusion for spondylolysis without spondylolisthesis generally is not needed. With the exception of occasional episodes of low back pain, teenagers are able to participate in any sport that does not lead repetitively to back pain after playing.

Spondylolisthesis occurs in some children who have spondylolysis. This condition results from forward slipping of a superior vertebra on the inferior vertebra, most commonly slipping of L5 on the sacrum (Fig 38-14). Worsening of this slip coincides with growth of the spine and generally subsides once growth is completed. As the slip of the vertebra progresses forward, the posterior elements (ie, the spinous process and inferior facets) remain behind, attached to the adjacent vertebrae by ligaments.

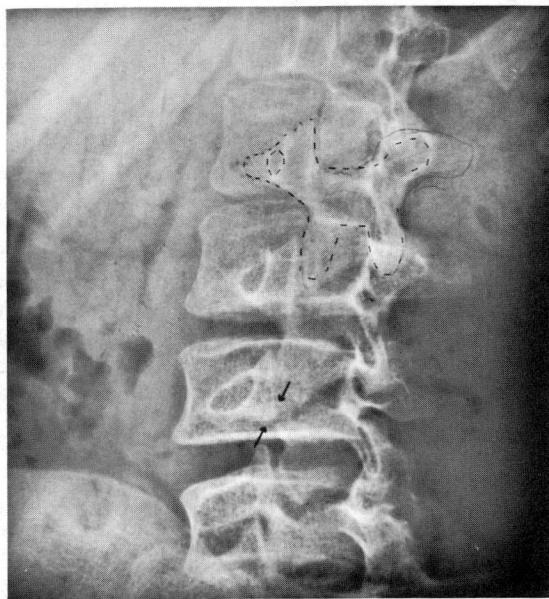

**Figure 38-13.**    Spondylolysis. Oblique film of lumbar spine shows defect in pars interarticularis of L4 (*arrows*). Note that the posterior elements of a vertebra resemble a "Scotty dog" in this view, as outlined. The nose, eyes, ears, neck, and body are the transverse process, pedicle, pedicle superior articular process, pars interarticularis, and lamina, respectively. Spondylolysis appears as a break in the "neck" region.

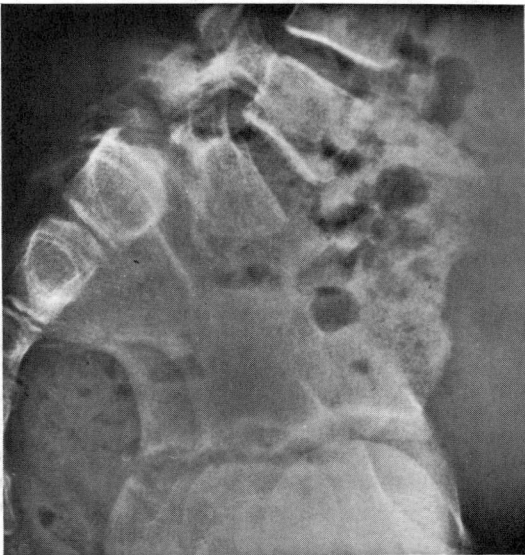

**Figure 38-14.**   Severe slips, as shown here, lead to hamstring spasm and leg pain as well as to back pain. Surgery is needed.

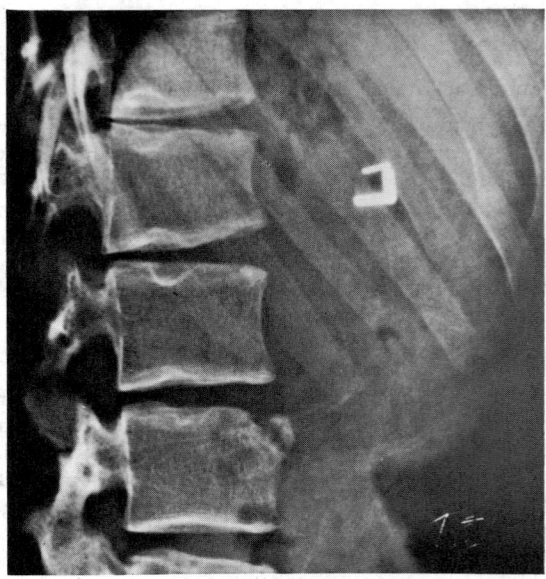

**Figure 38-15.**   A disc rupture in the skeletally immature child will lead to disruption of the apophysis or vertebral growth area, as shown here.

The combination of excessive motion of the posterior elements and forward vertebral slipping may lead to irritation of L5 or S1 nerve roots. As this slipping usually is slow, the nerve root irritation may present only as progressive tightening of the hamstrings. The child may note difficulty in touching his toes or reaching objects on the floor. If one side of the spine is affected more than the other, scoliosis also may be present.

On physical examination, the most striking finding is limitation in straight leg raising because of the hamstring spasm. Radiation of pain into the calf or foot with straight leg raising may indicate more advanced nerve root irritation. At times, the ankle jerk reflex is diminished.

A definite diagnosis can be made based on plain radiographs, most easily on the lateral view. The amount of slip should be estimated between grade 1 and grade 4 (ie, grade 1, up to 25%, grade 2, up to 50%, and so on). If the slip is greater than 50%, posterior lumbosacral fusion is indicated. If the slip is less than 50%, initial management is directed toward relief of back pain and hamstring spasm, using rest and corset therapy as with spondylolysis. If the pain does not respond to conservative treatment, fusion may be needed. If the pain improves with conservative treatment, a corset may be used for sports activities, and follow-up lateral lumbosacral radiographs at 6- to 9-month intervals are recommended until growth is complete or a worsening slip can be identified. If there is progression of the slip, fusion is indicated.

The use of a brace does not prevent further slipping. If a child does not have hamstring tightness and is pain-free, there usually is no need to restrict activities, provided the child and the parents are aware that periodic back pain is likely to occur. There is no evidence that increased physical activity causes an increase in vertebral slip.

*Intervertebral Disc Herniation.*   Herniation of the intervertebral disc is a common cause of back and leg pain in middle-aged adults. In this age group, disc protrusion occurs posteriorly, with the protruded disc compressing the nerve roots or the cauda equina. If similar forces are applied to the spine of a skeletally immature child, the disc will not rupture posteriorly, but a fracture of the ring apophysis of the vertebral body will occur, causing the extrusion of disc material anteriorly (Fig 38-15) or into the vertebral body itself (Schmorl's nodes). Most affected children

have back pain without radiation into the leg or calf. If nerve root pain occurs also, a small avulsion fracture of the ring apophysis posterolaterally might be present in such a position as to cause nerve root compression. The diagnosis of an old disc injury in a child can be confirmed by radiographic findings of a narrowed lumbar disc adjacent to a vertebral end plate that has some irregular pattern of ossification.

If no neurologic defect is present, treatment consists of symptomatic care, usually rest until the pain resolves. If the condition is the result of a vehicular accident, evaluation for the development of an ileus should be performed. If there is leg pain as well as back pain, a magnetic resonance image (MRI) or CT/myelogram should be performed to localize any neural compression, which could be relieved by surgical treatment.

*Discitis.*   Discitis may present in a wide variety of ways. Severe back pain with limitation of back movements is common in older children, whereas younger children simply may refuse to walk or may limp. The cause of this disc inflammation is variable, but bacterial infection is suspected most commonly. The vascular anatomy of the growing disc varies from that of the adult, and the common bacteremias of childhood can infect the disc more readily than the vertebral body itself. About 50% of these children have positive blood culture results at the time of their acute pain, with the most common organism identified being *Staphylococcus aureus.* Despite this, milder forms of discitis often appear to resolve without the need for antibiotics.

The most striking finding on physical examination in patients with discitis is marked stiffness of the spine that is notable with attempts at flexion. Fever often is present. The results of the neurologic examination are normal. In the early stages, radiographs of the spine appear normal. Usually, a few weeks after the onset of pain, narrowing of a single disc may be seen on radiography. The sedimentation rate and white blood cell count often are elevated. A technetium 99m bone scan virtually always reveals increased uptake at the involved level and should be performed whenever discitis is suspected. If the bone scan results are positive and the age and clinical presentation are typical, needle aspiration or open biopsy of the involved disc generally is not necessary.

Treatment decisions in cases of discitis revolve around whether to use antibiotics or a body jacket brace or cast. If a positive blood culture result has been obtained, antibiotics should be used for

3 to 6 weeks. We prefer to use antibiotics in children who have a positive bone scan result, even if no bacteremia has been demonstrated. Bed rest should be instituted at the time of presentation to decrease the spasm. If the spasm persists for more than a few days, a body jacket brace or cast will allow for immobilization and ambulation on a limited basis. It is extremely rare for discitis to develop into vertebral osteomyelitis with local bone destruction.

*Spinal Cord Tumors.* Back pain and limitation of spinal movement also may be seen as the presenting problem in patients with spinal cord tumors, even without a demonstrable neurologic deficit. In one large series of spinal cord tumors, the presenting complaint was back pain or scoliosis in almost one third of the children. The hallmark of the physical examination is severe limitation of forward flexion of the spine. Pain may be worsened by neck flexion. Neurologic changes may be very subtle and difficult to detect.

In patients with back pain and marked limitation of spinal motion, especially if scoliosis also is present, an MRI or CT/myelogram is needed if the bone scan and plain radiographs do not elucidate the cause. The most common tumor is an ependymoma. Treatment is neurosurgical. If the tumor is benign and can be removed, the pain, scoliosis, and back stiffness generally resolve.

## Spinal Deformity

In about 5% of children, some degree of spinal deformity will occur as they grow. Scoliosis, a lateral curvature of the spine, is the most common condition, although increased thoracic kyphosis or round back is not rare. School screening programs for spinal deformity, which are mandated in many states, have served to increase the public's awareness of these conditions. Whereas formal school programs generally are targeted toward children in the sixth or seventh grades, routine evaluation of the back should be a feature of each child's annual examination.

*Scoliosis.* Scoliosis is a lateral curvature of the spine. The two forms of scoliosis are postural and structural. Postural scoliosis results from spinal factors outside the spine, such as leg length discrepancy. In these cases, if the leg lengths are equalized or if the child sits, the spine becomes straight, indicating that no structural change has occurred. Structural scoliosis is of greater concern, because it involves not only a lateral spinal curvature, but also a rotation of the vertebrae involved in the lateral curve.

Although numerous conditions are associated with scoliosis, the most common groups include idiopathic (80%), congenital (5%), neuromuscular (10%), and miscellaneous (5%) disorders. The miscellaneous disorders encompass connective tissue disorders, genetic diseases, and other, less common, conditions.

Congenital scoliosis is present at birth, though the diagnosis often is not made at that time (Fig 38-16). It may be associated with other birth defects or present as an isolated condition. Because the genitourinary system arises embryologically from the same region as does the spine, about 30% of children with a congenital spinal deformity have an associated genitourinary abnormality. The most common anomaly is unilateral renal agenesis, so a sonogram or intravenous pyelogram should be performed on all patients who have congenital scoliosis or kyphosis. Although active treatment of unilateral kidney absence may not be necessary, appropriate cautioning against the child's participation in contact sports that may lead to kidney injury is important. The treatment of congenital scoliosis consists of serial radiographic follow-up to determine whether the deformity is worsening. If no curve progression occurs, further treatment generally is not needed. If worsening of 5° to 10° or more is documented, surgical fusion is necessary, no matter what the child's age. Brace treatment may be useful to prevent worsening of curves above or

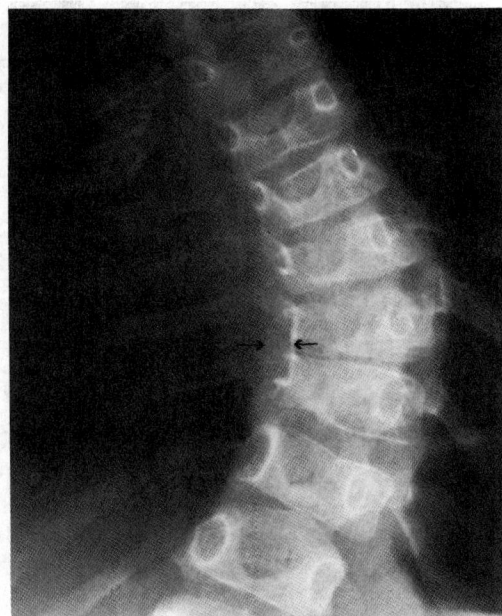

**Figure 38-16.** Congenital scoliosis results from incomplete vertebral segmentation in utero. Genitourinary abnormalities are frequently associated with these bony deformities.

below the congenital scoliosis, but it seldom is successful or indicated for the congenital scoliosis itself.

Neuromuscular scoliosis is the deformity that is associated with a wide variety of neurologic or muscular diseases, such as cerebral palsy (CP), muscular dystrophy, and poliomyelitis. Spinal curvature that is secondary to muscular imbalance classically is C-shaped and extends to include the pelvis (Fig 38-17), which is not usually the case in idiopathic scoliosis. Scoliosis is present more often and tends to worsen most quickly in patients who do not walk because of their neuromuscular disease. With continued progression, sitting balance becomes impaired further and it may be necessary for the child to use one arm or hand to assist in sitting. Treatment centers on preservation of sitting ability and pulmonary function. Although brace wear often is useful, surgical fusion frequently is indicated to preserve function.

Idiopathic scoliosis generally is found in otherwise healthy children. Although idiopathic scoliosis requiring treatment is about eight times more frequent in girls than in boys, the incidence of mild curves is about equal between the sexes.

A family history of curvature of the spine is found in as many as 70% of all children with scoliosis, though the exact mode of inheritance has not been determined definitely. Although the cause of idiopathic scoliosis remains elusive, a combination of growth asymmetry and postural imbalance is believed to be important. Minor abnormalities in the postural control center in the brain stem have been demonstrated in children with mild scoliosis. Once the curve begins to develop in response to this impaired postural feedback, growth asymmetry likely occurs. Growth is slower where increased pressure is exerted on the growth areas. Because there is more pressure on the concave growing areas than on the convex side, the convexity grows more quickly, leading to increasing curve size. This theory accounts for the observation that curves worsen most during the rapid adolescent growth spurt, which is the time when most of these curves are diagnosed. Muscles, discs, and bone appear to be normal in the young patient with idiopathic scoliosis.

The key to early detection of scoliosis is careful assessment of the entire trunk for asymmetry. The child should be examined with the back clearly exposed. The examination should include

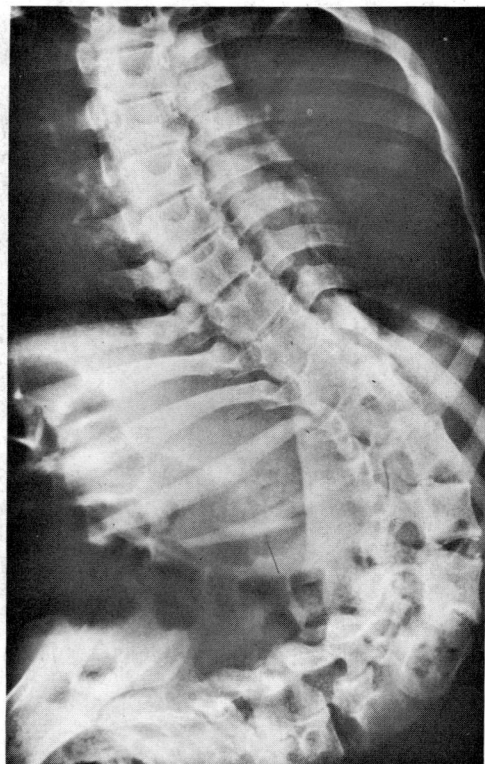

**Figure 38-17.** Sitting anteroposterior radiograph of a child with cerebral palsy and severe scoliosis. Note the C-shaped curve and the pelvic tilt characteristic of neuromuscular scoliosis.

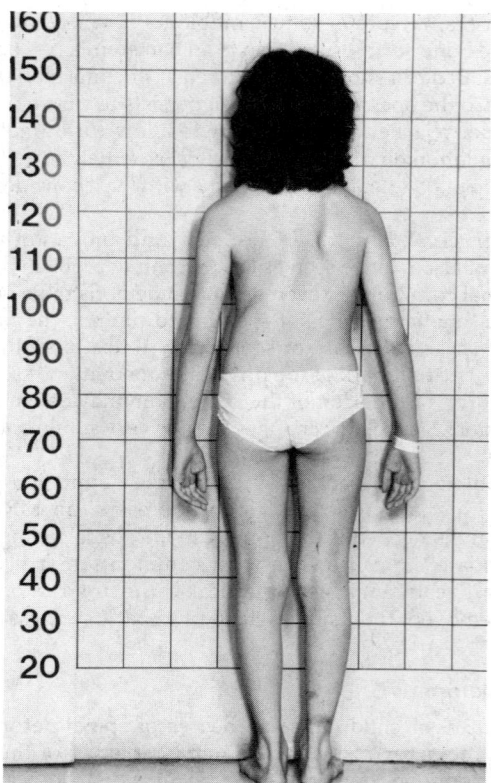

**Figure 38-18.** In examining for scoliosis, asymmetry of the trunk (shoulders, scapular height, waist area, pelvic height) should be noted carefully.

evaluation of shoulder height, scapula position and prominence, waistline symmetry, and levelness of the pelvis (Table 38-2). Asymmetry in any of these areas may indicate a scoliosis (Fig 38-18). In about 50% of children with uneven shoulder height, no spinal deformity is present on radiography. To define further whether a structural scoliosis is present, the child should be examined bending forward (Fig 38-19). Viewed from the caudal aspect, prominence of the thoracic ribs can be detected readily, whereas further bending or viewing from the head down is better for suspected lumbar curves. Both thoracic and lumbar regions should be checked. This "forward-bending" test is very sensitive in demonstrating the vertebral rotation that takes place in a

structural scoliotic curve. It is possible to measure the amount of rib hump by means of an inclinometer placed at the apex of the curve with the child bending forward. If the inclinometer measurement is 5° or less, the scoliosis rarely is significant and radiographs usually are not needed. If the inclinometer reading exceeds 7°, standing posteroanterior and lateral radiographs are indicated for better assessment.

The magnitude of the scoliosis is measured radiographically by the Cobb method (Fig 38-20A). This measurement always

| TABLE 38-2. Spinal Deformity Evaluation |
| --- |
| Examine in swimming suit or similar clothing so back is exposed. |
| Observe asymmetry on trunk examination: shoulder height, scapular height, waistline equality, levelness of pelvis, leg length difference, forward bending, both side and front/back. |
| Measure rib prominence with inclinometer (optional). |
| Assess skeletal maturity (eg, age of menses onset). |
| Obtain standing posteroanterior radiograph of the spine if asymmetry is seen. |
| Measure using Cobb method. |
| Recommend follow-up or treatment. |
| None if the curve is less than 25° and growth is complete. |
| If growth remains and the curve is less than 25° obtain repeat radiographs in 4 to 15 mo (see text). |
| If scoliosis more than 25° is seen and growth remains, consider a brace. |
| If scoliosis more than 40° is seen, consider surgery. |

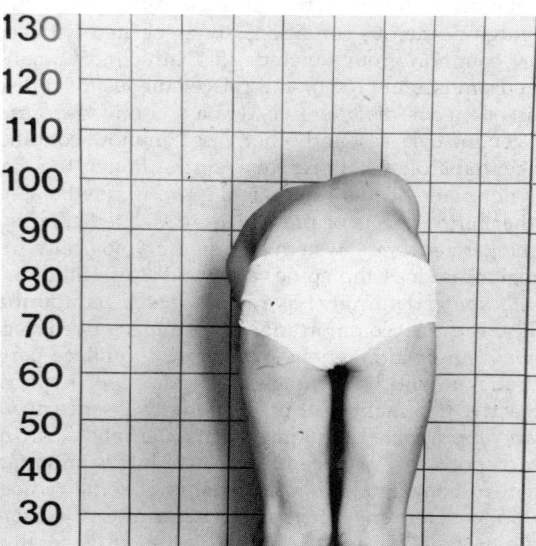

**Figure 38-19.** The forward bending examination will detect even very small curvatures. The prominence is produced by chest-wall asymmetry, caused by vertebral-body rotation in the curved segment of the spine.

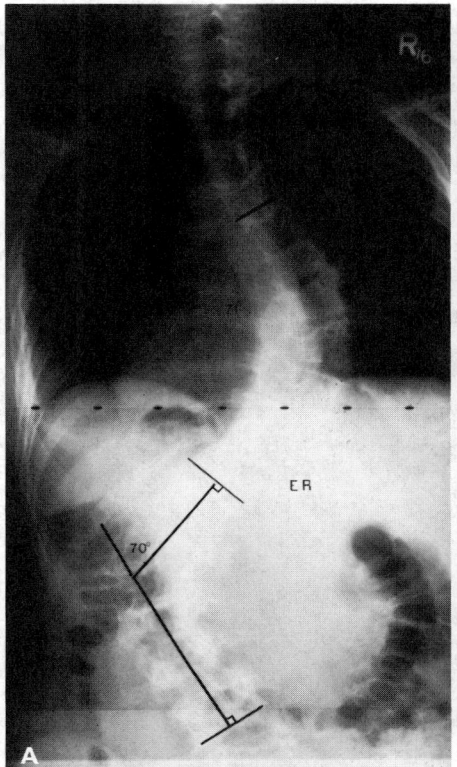
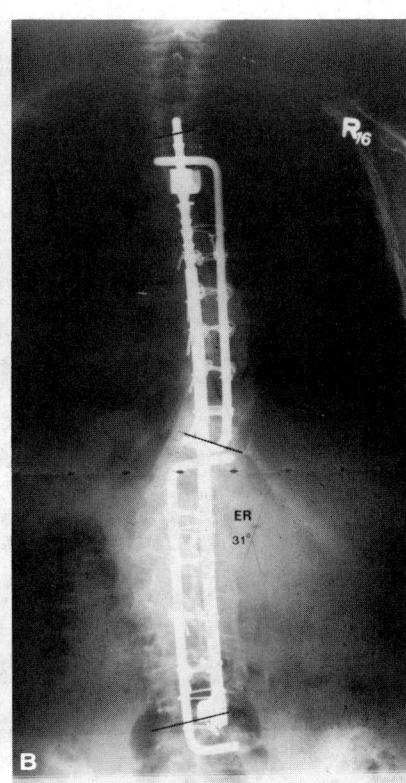

**Figure 38-20.** A standing postero-anterior radiograph of the spine is the correct film to use in quantitating the magnitude of scoliosis. (**A**) The Cobb method of measurement is used routinely, and is obtained as shown on this radiograph. (**B**) This is the postoperative result after spinal correction and fusion in the same patient.

should be performed on an erect posteroanterior spine radiograph. The error of measurement for this method is about ±5°. Because no active treatment is needed until the curve reaches 25°, the time estimate for a follow-up radiograph, once the diagnosis has been made, is 25 minus the present curve magnitude. This provides an estimate of the number of months that may pass until another radiograph is indicated. For example, if a child has a scoliosis of 15°, waiting about 10 months before repeating the posteroanterior radiograph to check for progression is appropriate. This time estimate is based on the premise that, during the adolescent growth spurt, annual curve progression is 5° to 10° or about 1°/mo.

Completion of growth or skeletal maturity can be assessed most accurately with bone age radiographs of the hand and wrist. From the clinical standpoint, girls who have been menstruating for 2 years essentially have completed their spinal growth.

The treatment of scoliosis is based on three fundamental principles:

1. Curves of more than 25° are likely to increase if the child is still growing.
2. Curves of 40° to 50° are likely to increase even after growth is complete.
3. Some degree of clinical pulmonary restriction may begin to be noted in thoracic curves of more than about 75°.

If a child is skeletally mature and has a curvature of less than 25°, no further evaluation or treatment of scoliosis is needed. If the scoliosis is 25° or more and the child is still growing, brace treatment generally is recommended and is successful in about 80% of the patients who actually wear the brace as prescribed. Spinal exercises alone will not be successful in stopping curve progression. Once the brace treatment begins, it is continued until growth is complete. The brace usually is worn 18 to 23 hours daily. Physical activity is not limited by scoliosis and affected children often can participate in sports activities while wearing their brace. Brace wear is considered to be successful if it prevents

further progression rather than providing correction of the curve, as long-term follow-up studies have shown that the final size of the curve is virtually the same as before brace treatment begins. Although children and parents often are dismayed by our inability to straighten the spine nonoperatively, if curves can be kept at less than 35° to 40° by the time growth is completed, most cases of scoliosis will not worsen in adult life. If the thoracic curve is greater than 50° or the lumbar curve is greater than 40° at the time growth is completed, progression usually will continue at a rate of about 1° annually and surgery often will be required.

Surgical treatment is recommended for curves that are greater than 40°, particularly in a child who is not fully grown. The surgical treatment usually employed consists of instrumentation of the curved area of the spine, combined with posterior spinal fusion of the instrumented area (see Fig 38-20, A and B). Correction of the scoliosis generally is about 50%. Failure of fusion occurs in only about 1% of teenagers. Fusion is complete by 6 months after surgery, at which time the teenagers can return to almost all physical activities, except tackle football, wrestling, and gymnastics. They should be encouraged to return to activity, including physical education class in school, to de-emphasize the psychologic potential for disability after this surgery.

If the thoracic scoliosis exceeds 50°, patients commonly have diminished vital capacity and residual lung volumes on pulmonary function testing. Arterial blood gas levels and forced expiratory volume in 1 second are normal except in children with severe curves. Vital capacity is decreased further if a thoracic lordosis is associated with the scoliosis. Even with surgical correction of the scoliosis, pulmonary function postoperatively will change little because of the persistence of chest wall or rib deformities that have occurred as a result of the scoliosis. Therefore, scoliosis should be prevented from progressing to this point if possible.

Pain is rare in adolescents who have idiopathic scoliosis. Although it may result from degenerative changes that are present by the time the patient is middle-aged, pain that occurs during

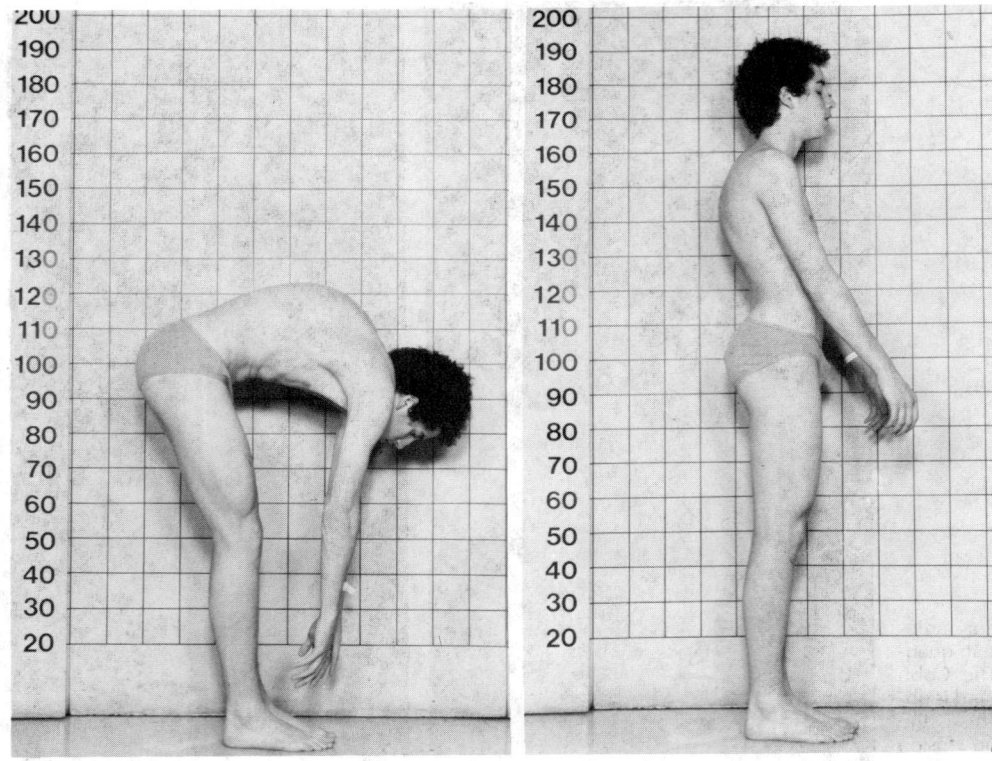

**Figure 38-21.** The examination for kyphosis should also include a forward bending test to help to determine the rigidity and severity of the kyphosis, which may be hidden more easily in the upright position.

adolescence is an indication for further evaluation. If the neurologic examination is normal, a technetium 99m bone scan should be performed to screen for discitis, stress fracture, osteoid osteoma, or other bone tumors. If there is limited spinal flexion and a neurologic deficit is discovered, an MRI or CT/myelogram is necessary to rule out intraspinal pathology. Although all these conditions may cause scoliosis, the curvature will straighten as soon as its underlying cause is treated. Therefore, physicians should evaluate a patient thoroughly for treatable causes of scoliosis before making a diagnosis of idiopathic scoliosis and instituting brace treatment or recommending spinal fusion.

*Kyphosis.* Normal spinal sagittal contours consist of lordosis in the cervical and lumbar spinal segments to balance the kyphosis that is present in the thoracic area. The term *kyphosis* sometimes is used to describe those abnormal conditions in which there is increased rounding of the back in the thoracic or thoracolumbar area. The parents usually complain about the child's posture. Assessment of apparent excessive kyphosis should include a forward bending examination, viewed from the side, to determine if the back is flexible or rigid in the rounded segment (Fig 38-21). The kyphosis may be discovered to be a rib prominence that is associated with a scoliosis. Similarly, mild to moderate scoliosis is seen commonly with moderate and marked kyphosis, so careful examination for both of these conditions is necessary.

The least serious of these conditions is postural round back. This is seen most commonly in the preadolescent years. It occurs more often in children who are taller than their peers and in girls who have had breast development earlier than have their friends. This condition is a flexible, increased kyphosis that can be straightened voluntarily by the child and can be corrected well with hyperextension positioning. This is one group of spinal deformities that can be treated with exercises alone. Active hyperextension of the trunk and sit-ups to decrease lumbar lordosis are useful in improving trunk control. As long as no fixed deformity is established, as the teenager's body image improves, so will the rounding of the upper back.

A more fixed and less flexible thoracic or thoracolumbar kyphosis usually is referred to as Scheuermann's disease. This condition occurs most commonly in teenage boys. Attempts to correct this kyphosis passively are unsuccessful, and there often is a large lumbar lordosis associated with it. A lateral radiograph of the spine will demonstrate irregularity of numerous disc spaces and anterior vertebral body wedging (Fig 38-22). To establish the diagnosis of Scheuermann's kyphosis radiographically, at least 5° of wedging in three adjacent vertebrae should be demonstrated. The Cobb method also is used to measure the amount

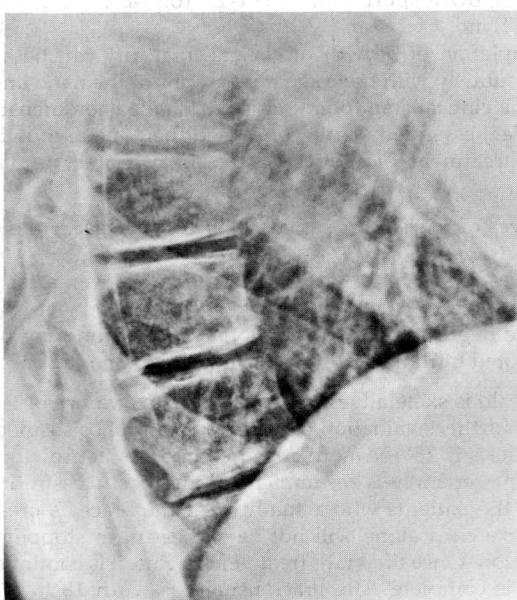

**Figure 38-22.** This lateral spine radiograph demonstrates the disc irregularities and anterior vertebral body wedging seen in Scheuermann's disease.

of kyphosis present. Normally, the amount of kyphosis from T3 to T12 is between 20° and 40°. If the kyphosis is present in the thoracolumbar area, which normally appears straight on a lateral radiograph, measurements greater than 25° are abnormal.

If wedging is present, little correction can be achieved with thoracic spine hyperextension, and if the lateral thoracic kyphosis is 55° to 60°, bracing is indicated if the child is still growing. A Milwaukee brace, which employs a neck ring in addition to trunk pads, should be used. Unlike scoliosis, in which little correction results from bracing, in kyphosis, about 50% improvement can be anticipated after 1 year of full-time brace wear. Once this degree of correction is obtained, nighttime brace wear generally is sufficient until growth is complete.

Increased thoracic kyphosis does not cause abnormalities in pulmonary function. The principal problem seen later in Scheuermann's disease is pain in the low thoracic spine after the patient has been standing for some time. If the kyphosis exceeds 70° by the time the patient has stooped growing, spinal instrumentation and fusion, as with scoliosis, can provide excellent correction with a significant improvement in appearance.

Congenital kyphosis is less common than congenital scoliosis, but almost always requires early spinal fusion surgery. If the congenital kyphosis progresses unchecked, spinal cord compression at the apex of the kyphosis is common. As with congenital scoliosis, evaluation for associated genitourinary abnormalities should be performed.

### The Cervical Spine

Because of its many normal variations in radiographs, the cervical spine often is a confusing area to evaluate. On the lateral cervical spine radiograph, the anterior and superior corner of each vertebral body normally is the last part to ossify, sometimes giving the appearance of a small compression fracture. Full ossification and development of the odontoid process is not complete in the young child and may give the appearance of being maldeveloped. The spine of a child less than 10 years of age is much more flexible than that of a teenager or an older adult. As much as 3 mm of anterior movement of C2 on C3 with flexion is normal in this group, whereas no such movement should be present in adults. In fact, under experimental conditions, the newborn spine can stretch about 5 cm (2 in) before it fails, whereas the adult spinal cord can stretch only 1.25 cm (½ in) before it ruptures. Because of this difference in elasticity, infants who are involved in automobile accidents may sustain spinal cord injury without apparent spinal fracture. The proper use of car seating supports for these very young children decreases the risk of these devastating injuries (see Chapter 24.3).

Children with Down syndrome comprise a special group that commonly has instability of the altantoaxial region. If this instability persists unrecognized, spinal cord compression with myelopathy may result, leading to leg weakness and lessened walking ability. Lateral cervical flexion/extension radiographs should be performed at the age of 3 to 4 years in all children who have Down syndrome. Although about 15% of these children will have some evidence of atlantoaxial instability, the majority do not need emergent fusion surgery, but can have periodic follow-up by neurologic examination. If the first radiograph reveals increased laxity, films should be repeated every 2 years. If no laxity is seen, there is no recommendation for repeat radiographs as long as there are no signs of spasticity or symptoms of neck pain. Atlantoaxial posterior fusion is recommended if a neurologic deficit or excessive instability is present.

Instability of the upper cervical spine also may result from os odontoideum or from odontoid hypoplasia. Os odontoideum occurs most commonly as the result of an early childhood fall that causes a fracture through one of the two synchondroses of the odontoid process. This unrecognized fracture develops into a fibrous nonunion (Fig 38-23), which gradually becomes unstable over the ensuing months and years. The diagnosis usually is made when the patient is being evaluated for neck pain or other head or neck trauma. Neurologic symptoms rarely are present, but atlantoaxial fusion generally is indicated to stabilize this region and to protect the spinal cord from sudden, catastrophic injury that may result in death. After fusion union is accomplished, the child will be able to participate in normal activities, although mild to moderate limitation of head rotation will be present. Odontoid dysplasia occurs periodically, but it is associated most often with genetic disorders, such as Morquio syndrome and spondyloepiphyseal dysplasia congenita. Fusion generally is necessary.

### Torticollis

Torticollis most commonly is present at or near the time of birth and results from a contracture of one of the sternocleidomastoid muscles. The child's head will be tilted toward the side of the contracture, with the chin rotated away from the contracted side, because the origin of the contracted muscle is on the mastoid process. The cause of torticollis is not well defined, but the incidence is higher in children with breech presentation and forceps delivery. Commonly, a fusiform, firm mass is palpable in the body of the contracted muscle. These children often have plagiocephaly, or asymmetry of face and skull development. If the neck range of motion can be returned to normal by the age of 1 year, this facial asymmetry will disappear. If the torticollis is untreated until later in childhood, the eyes and ears never will become level.

Cervical spine radiographs should be evaluated to ensure that the position of the head is not the result of congenital spine abnormalities, such as hemivertebrae. If the bony cervical spine is normal, stretching exercises should be instituted shortly after birth. These exercises are designed to stretch the contracted sternocleidomastoid muscle and should be taught to the parents by a knowledgeable physical therapist. Although one of the parents should be asked to do these stretching exercises at home, initial weekly check-ups by the therapist or the physician can help to ensure compliance. If a significant contracture persists by the time the patient reaches 1 year of age, despite stretching exercises, surgical treatment to lengthen the sternocleidomastoid muscle is appropriate. Even after surgical release, some stretching and, at times, bracing will continue to be needed as the child grows.

Torticollis may present later in childhood after an upper re-

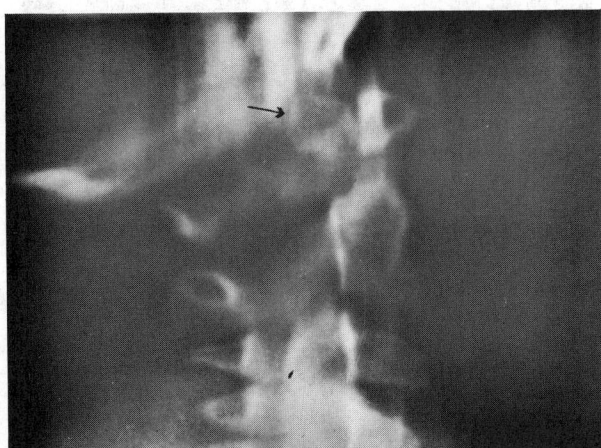

**Figure 38-23.** An unsuspected injury to the synchondrosis of the odontoid in early childhood may lead to high cervical instability due to an os odontoideum. This child required atlantoaxial fusion, and is now asymptomatic.

spiratory infection or trauma. Torticollis that occurs after an upper respiratory infection is thought to result from retropharyngeal edema that leads to malposition at the atlantoaxial level, causing a rotatory deformity. Similarly, after muscular neck trauma, the child may have a persistent torticollis for several days or weeks, secondary to an unsuspected rotatory subluxation at the atlantoaxial level. If torticollis from either of these causes persists, the child should be treated with traction, followed by either bracing or atlantoaxial fusion. The likelihood that surgical fusion will be necessary increases with the duration of symptoms, so prompt treatment is required.

### Klippel-Feil Syndrome

Failure of normal vertebral segmentation in the cervical spine is known as Klippel-Feil syndrome (Fig 38-24). In the milder forms, when only one or two levels are involved, diagnosis may be delayed until the teenage years and, even then, may be made only when the neck is examined radiographically for other reasons. In more severely involved children, however, the neck is very short and webbing appears to be present. Often, Klippel-Feil syndrome is associated with Sprengel's deformity, which is failure of normal descent of the scapulae. Associated genitourinary abnormalities may be present, and a sonogram or an intravenous pyelogram is indicated when the diagnosis of Klippel-Feil syndrome is made. Little specific treatment is available for this syndrome. Because of the congenital fusion of several segments of the cervical spine, instability may occur at the levels that move. If this instability is excessive or if neurologic deficits are present, it is necessary to fuse the unstable segment. Surgical fusion also may be needed in adult life for degenerative changes at the moveable segments.

Particularly in more involved cases, contact sports should be avoided, because any neck injury in a child with Klippel-Feil syndrome is more likely to be serious as a result of the limited flexibility of the cervical area.

## Upper Extremity

Congenital and developmental abnormalities of the upper extremities of children are less common than those of the lower extremities, perhaps partly because of the greater stresses that are imposed on the lower extremity in utero and later during standing.

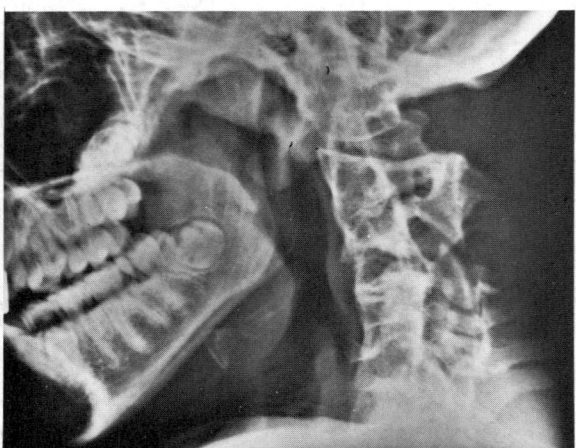

**Figure 38-24.** Klippel-Feil syndrome results from incomplete segmentation of the cervical vertebrae. Sprengel's deformity of the scapulae is often associated with this syndrome.

### Obstetric (Brachial Plexus) Palsy

The brachial plexus is composed of contributions from C5 to T1. Most severe injuries to the area involve lateral flexion of the neck or downward pressure on the shoulder, such as may occur during a difficult delivery. Therefore, the upper portions of the plexus (C5 to C7) are stretched most commonly in a manner similar to that which causes the "burners" that occur during blocking maneuvers made in sports activities. This stretching causes denervation of the shoulder abductors and elbow flexors, which results in gradual joint contractures if it is not treated. These are known as Erb-Duchenne palsies. The lower plexus (C7 to T1) can be affected by excessive abduction–traction and has a poorer prognosis; this is the rarest occurrence and it is called Klumpke's palsy. In these cases, loss of function of the elbow extensors, wrist flexors, and finger muscles, and possibly a Horner's syndrome result. The entire plexus occasionally may be involved.

Factors associated with brachial plexus palsy include shoulder dystocia, breech position, high birth weight, and prolonged labor. The incidence is 1:1000 to 3:1000 births. The incidence and severity of this condition gradually have declined as obstetric care has improved. The site of injury may be at any level from the origin of the nerve roots to the plexus itself, but even root lesions may resolve spontaneously. On physical examination, the early typical Erb's palsy appears as an arm that is rotated internally at the shoulder, extended at the elbow, and flexed at the fingers. Passive range of motion initially should be full.

Skeletal injuries such as clavicle fractures and proximal humerus separations should be ruled out radiographically, although they often can be differentiated by guarding on testing of passive motion and the presence of Moro's response. Because of the trauma, palsy and skeletal injury may coexist.

Treatment involves maintenance of motion and transfers of tendon in those rare, severe cases in which function does not return. With current obstetric practice, 92% of palsies resolve completely by the time the infants reach 3 months of age, and 95% of infants eventually recover fully. Physical therapy should be used initially to maintain range of motion. Splinting in most cases results in contractures, although there may be a role for later functional splinting of the hand. For patients with persistent weakness at 3 months of age, electromyography and, possibly, myelography may help to identify those rare cases in which nerve grafting is required. Cases that are detected later may benefit from osteotomy or contracture release and tendon transfer, especially to restore shoulder external rotation.

### Sprengel's Deformity

Sprengel's deformity, or congenital elevation of the scapula, actually represents embryonic failure of complete descent, rotation, and development of the scapula. This realignment normally occurs predominantly between the 9th and 12th weeks of gestation. The cause is unknown.

On physical examination, the upper pole of the scapula may be visible in the base of the neck. Abduction is limited. The pectoralis major muscle may be underdeveloped. Scapular winging may occur as a result of serratus anterior muscle palsy. The scapula may be connected to the vertebrae by an abnormal omovertebral bone, which is named for the two structures it connects. Associated congenital anomalies such as cervical or thoracic vertebral fusions, anal abnormalities, or cardiac abnormalities may coexist. Treatment is indicated in moderate and severe cases to improve abduction and appearance. The most effective means of treatment involves detaching and lowering the midline origins of the rhomboid and trapezius muscles (Woodward procedure), combined with a clavicular osteotomy.

## Congenital Pseudarthrosis of the Clavicle

Congenital pseudarthrosis of the clavicle is a tapered defect in the continuity of this bone that presumably is caused by pressure from the more cephalad position of the right subclavian artery. It almost always involves the right clavicle unless the patient has dextrocardia or a cervical rib. Bone grafting and pin fixation before 6 years of age usually are indicated.

## Radial Clubhand

Longitudinal failure of formation of many tissues on the radial side of the forearm and hand is known as radial clubhand. The severity of this condition varies. About 50% of cases are bilateral. Associated abnormalities may include VATER syndrome, hydrocephalus, and clubfoot. The upper arm also may be short and the shoulder girdle may be underdeveloped. The radial-sided muscles, radial carpal bones, thumb, and radial artery may be absent. The hand is deviated radially up to 90° because it lacks its normal radial support, and the ulna may be bowed. Treatment involves centralization of the wrist on the ulna, transfer of tendon, and, possibly, straightening of the ulna and creation of a thumb, as long as reasonable elbow flexion is present. Untreated cases are problematic cosmetically, although, surprisingly, they pose less functional difficulty. Congenital absence of the ulna is only one third as common. In most cases, some remnant of the proximal ulna provides elbow stability.

## Radioulnar Synostosis

Often inherited, radioulnar synostosis (fusion) results in a fixed position of forearm rotation, usually in pronation. At times, the synostosis may be only fibrous. Shoulder motion usually can compensate for the lack of rotation, and rotational osteotomy should be done only if clear-cut functional deficit can be demonstrated.

## Congenital Constriction Bands (Streeter's Bands)

Congenital constriction bands most likely are the result of intrauterine encirclement by amniotic bands or the umbilical cord. They may be located anywhere, and also may be associated with the amputation of parts. The bands can be released with Z-plasties after the patient reaches 2 years of age, or urgently if they are associated with neurocirculatory compromise.

## Polydactyly

Polydactyly, or the presence of an extra digit, varies in spectrum from a hypoplastic addition of soft tissue to a fully developed digit with all phalanges and metacarpals. Fifth finger polydactyly is ten times more common in black than in white individuals. Therefore, a white child with this finding should be examined for other abnormalities, especially of the cardiovascular system. The simple, small, non-skeletal duplications can be excised or tied off. If there is significant skeletal stability, all the digits should be reexamined to determine which is the least functional, and this should be excised.

## Congenital Trigger Thumb

Congenital trigger thumb presents as a clenched digit and is not always recognized at birth. It usually is the result of excessive tightness of the annular ligament at the metacarpal head. This causes swelling of the tendon, which later becomes firm. Treatment consists of 6 to 8 weeks of stretching if the condition is diagnosed early, and surgical release if it persists or is diagnosed later.

## Nursemaid's Elbow

Radial head subluxation, known as nursemaid's elbow, consists of elbow pain after longitudinal traction on a pronated, extended elbow in children between the age of 2 and 7 years. A snap may or may not be heard. Radiographs usually show no bony abnormality or displacement. Only one case report describes actual exploration of this pathology (Salter, 1971). This report and laboratory studies suggest that the annular ligament of the radial head slips partially over the radial head, the narrowest portion being prominent when pronated (Fig 38-25). An elbow fracture or septic arthritis should be ruled out. Treatment usually is reduction by stabilizing the elbow with one hand, with a finger placed over the radial head for palpation, followed by gentle firm flexion until a click is felt. The child should begin using the elbow within minutes. Immobilization usually is not carried out and is not necessary in first-time cases. It can be done with 2 to 3 weeks in a cast if the episode recurs. Parent education regarding the mechanism of this condition is most important.

# GENERALIZED ABNORMALITIES

## Bone Dysplasias

### Osteocartilaginous Exostoses (Osteochondromas)

Osteochondromas, which can be single or multiple, are sessile or pedunculated bony masses located on the metaphysis and directed away from the growth plate that appear to move away from it over time (Fig 38-26). These outgrowths have their own growth plates. Osteochondromas are thought to arise from defects in the perichondrial ring that encircles the growth plate, permit-

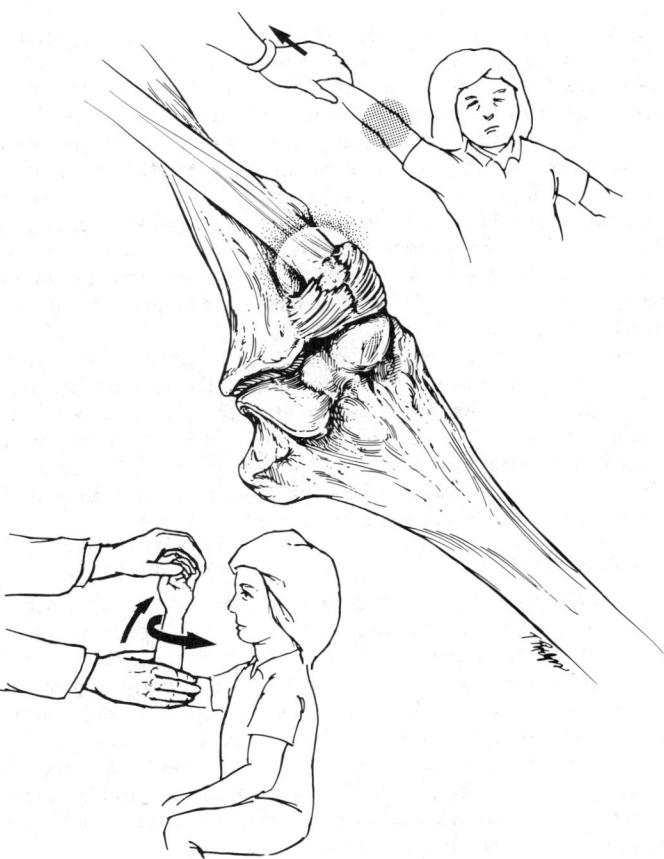

**Figure 38-25.** ''Pulled elbow'' represents subluxation of the radial head through a partially torn annular ligament. The method of injury is shown above, and the method of reduction is shown below.

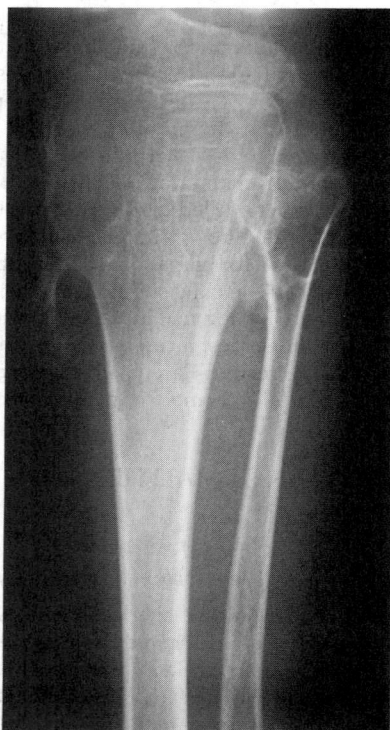

**Figure 38-26.** Osteocartilaginous exostoses are metaphyseal pedunculated or sessile lesions directed away from the growth plate.

ting lateral growth rather than the usual organized distal growth. The condition of multiple exostoses usually is distinct and is transmitted in an autosomal dominant manner, and affected persons frequently are somewhat short in stature.

Any bone with endochondral growth may be affected, but the long bones of the extremities are involved most often. Because of asymmetric growth plate activity, angular growth often ensues, resulting in outward angulation of the knees and ankles, and in ulnar deviation of the forearm and wrist. These conditions should be corrected by partial epiphyseal stapling in young children, or by osteotomy in older patients. Leg length inequality is significant in 50% of patients.

The indication for excision of the lesions themselves is pain or compromise resulting from pressure on the tendons, nerves, or spinal cord. Malignant transformation should be suspected if continued growth occurs after skeletal maturity is reached or if there is new onset of pain. A bone scan may be helpful, because absence of uptake indicates a benign lesion; however, increased uptake does not always mean malignant change.

### Fibrous Dysplasia

Fibrous dysplasia is a disorder in which bone formation in the medulla and cortex is altered, and the marrow contains much fibrous tissue. Radiographically, the bone has a uniform "ground glass" consistency, and the cortex is thin and often deformed. One bone (the monostotic form) or several bones (the polyostotic form) can be affected. Pathologic fractures occur often, but usually heal in a normal period. Proximal femoral ("shepherd's crook") bowing is the most difficult to manage. Deformities and fractures of the lower extremities usually require internal fixation, whereas those in the upper extremities require casting.

Irregular café au lait spots occur in 30% of patients with the polyostotic form of fibrous dysplasia. When polyostotic lesions and café au lait spots are associated with precocious puberty, the condition is called Albright's syndrome. Other types of endocri-

nopathy (thyroid, parathyroid, or adrenal problems) may occur. Malignant transformation to fibrosarcoma or osteosarcoma is rare.

### Osteogenesis Imperfecta

Osteogenesis imperfecta encompasses a spectrum of diseases that are the end result of defects in collagen or proteoglycan synthesis. These result in bones that have thin cortices and multiple fractures. Short stature, blue sclerae, middle ear deafness, abnormal dentition, and thin skin may coexist. Inheritance usually is dominant, occasionally is recessive, but frequently is the result of spontaneous mutation. Tiny fractures occur to cause bowing of long bones and scoliosis. Child abuse should be considered in the differential diagnosis, and the absence of pelvic deformities or wormian cranial bones in children who are subjected to abuse may be helpful.

Aids to mobility and preventive bracing can be very helpful in preventing fractures. Occasionally, intramedullary rods that elongate with growth are needed. Fortunately, the frequency of fractures diminishes with age.

### Tumors

A complete discussion of musculoskeletal tumors is beyond the scope of this section; instead, an attempt is made to describe an appropriate differential diagnosis and evaluation.

Benign or malignant musculoskeletal tumors can be classified according to their tissue of origin (Table 38-3).

The history and physical examination rarely are definitive. Many tumors become evident after trauma, when a new prominence is noted, or when pathologic fracture occurs through weakened bone. For example, osteoid osteoma, a benign condition, frequently produces pain that is relieved by nonsteroidal anti-inflammatory agents. Very early sarcoma may be painless. Unexpected presentations may occur, such as Ewing's sarcoma, various types of histiocytosis, and leukemia, each of which may present with fever and malaise.

Some idea of the benign or malignant nature of a tumor can

**TABLE 38-3. Musculoskeletal Neoplasms**

| Origin | Benign | Malignant |
|---|---|---|
| Cartilage | Chondroblastoma | Chondrosarcoma* |
| | Enchondroma | |
| | Chondromyxoid fibroma | |
| | Osteochondroma | |
| Bone | Osteoid osteoma | Osteosarcoma |
| | Osteoblastoma | |
| Marrow elements | Lipoma | Ewing's sarcoma |
| | | Reticulum cell sarcoma |
| | | Liposarcoma* |
| | | Plasma cell myeloma |
| Fibrous connective tissue | Desmoplastic fibroma | Fibrosarcoma |
| | Fibrous cortical defect | |
| Skeletal muscle | | Rhabdomyosarcoma |
| Neurogenous tissue | Neurilemma | Neuroblastoma |
| | Neurofibroma | |
| Unclear | Giant cell tumor* | Adamantinoma |

\* Rarely occurs in children.

be gained from the following radiographic features. Lesions associated with rapid spread and lack of local containment should heighten the suspicion of malignancy. A vague zone of transition between the lesion and normal bone is worrisome, as is a soft-tissue mass in the presence of a bone tumor. Periosteal lamellar change is a response to spread outside the cortex, and may occur with benign or malignant tumors. Rapid growth is suggested when periosteal lamellation is extensive, and there is no formation of definite new cortex. Thinning of the cortex itself is not pathognomonic of malignancy; this also occurs with fibrous cortical defects and unicameral cysts. Internal stippling suggests calcification of a cartilage matrix; fluffy opacification usually represents new bone formation, as in osteosarcoma. Lesions crossing the epiphyseal plate usually are infections or malignant tumors. Leukemia presents with musculoskeletal complaints 20% of the time, and radiographic findings include osteopenia, sclerotic or lytic lesions, lucent metaphyseal bands, or periosteal new bone.

Certain general radiographic studies can be helpful. Radiographic studies must be tailored to the differential diagnosis. CTs may show internal consistency, soft-tissue spread, and extent of the lesion. Technetium bone scans reveal lesions in the remainder of the skeleton, bony involvement with soft-tissue lesions, and bone turnover or activity of questionable lesions. Angiograms may be helpful to determine whether the tumor involves a vascular bundle. MRI is helpful in assessing soft-tissue involvement.

The location of a lesion is meaningful and a diagram of the location of common bone lesions is presented in Figure 38-27. Laboratory studies generally are not specific; the sedimentation rate and complete blood count are abnormal in several of the

above-mentioned tumors, and the alkaline phosphatase level often is elevated in patients with osteogenic sarcoma.

The treatment of musculoskeletal tumors defies simplification. The most important generalization is that any patient requiring surgery should be cared for by a surgeon who has had experience in this area. Errors related to biopsy placement or specimen adequacy are 3 to 5 times more frequent in centers where the surgeons do not specialize in tumor treatment.

### Unicameral Bone Cyst

Two common, benign bone tumors deserve brief mention. A unicameral bone cyst is a smooth, well-marginated lucency that is located fairly centrally near the growth plate in the metaphysis of a child who is 2 to 15 years of age. The lesion can be observed if it is small and is located in a bone that does not bear weight; otherwise, it can be curetted or injected with steroids. The latter two treatments produce about equal results. The natural history of these defects is spontaneous regression during adolescence.

### Fibrous Cortical Defects

Fibrous cortical defects are well-marginated lucencies located in, and occasionally slightly expanding, the cortex. Usually, one radiographic view can show that these lesions are not central in bone (Fig 38-28). They are present in as many as one third of all young children at some time and disappear with age. In a weight-bearing bone, the risk of fracture is appreciable if the lesion is greater than about 3 cm in length and more than half the width of the bone. Lesions this large should be protected by limiting activities if possible or by performing bone grafting.

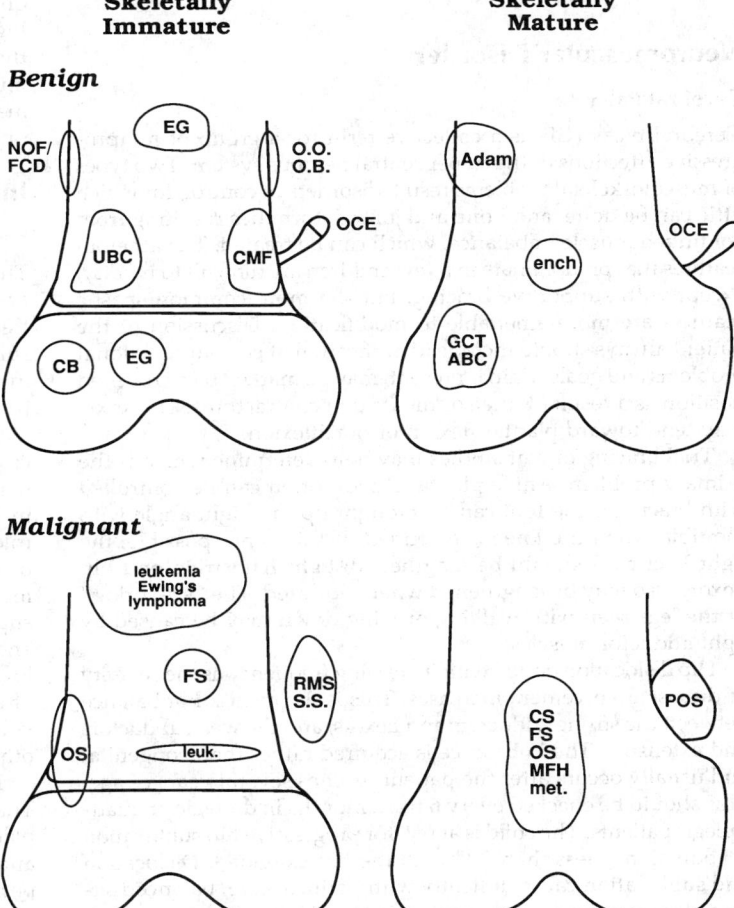

**Figure 38-27.** Location of tumors in immature and mature skeletons. Abbreviations: *Adam,* adamantinoma; *ABC,* aneurysmal bone cyst; *CB,* chondroblastoma; *CMF,* chondromyxoid fibroma; *CS,* chondrosarcoma; *EG,* eosinophilic granuloma; *ENCH,* enchondroma; *FCD,* fibrous cortical defect; *FS,* fibrosarcoma; *GCT,* giant cell tumor; *NOF,* nonossifying fibroma; *MFH,* malignant fibrous histiocytoma; *OB,* osteoblastoma; *OCE,* osteocartilaginous exostosis; *OO,* osteoid osteoma; *OS,* osteogenic sarcoma; *P,* parosteal; *RMS,* rhabdomyosarcoma; *SS,* synovial sarcoma; *UBC,* unicameral bone cyst.

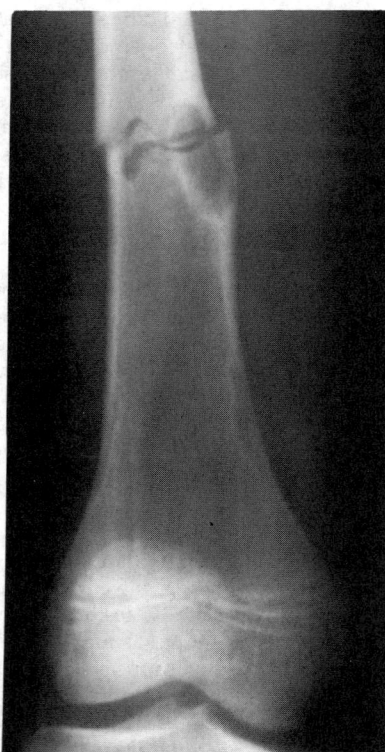

**Figure 38-28.** Fibrous cortical defects with pathologic fracture. Note two lesions on the medial side, *within* one wall of the cortex and expanding it.

## Neuromuscular Disorders

### Cerebral Palsy

Cerebral palsy (CP) is a collective term for a group of nonprogressive affections of the upper central nervous system. Two types of musculoskeletal problems result: disorders of control, for which little can be done; and bone and joint deformities resulting from continued muscle imbalance, which can be treated. The athetoid features that predominate in a few children are difficult to modify, except with supportive bracing, but the more common spastic features are more amenable to modification. Discussion of the patient always should include identification of current functional problems and goals. Gait, if present, may be marked by a crouched position as a result of knee or hip flexion contractures. The ankle may tend toward plantar flexion or dorsiflexion.

Trial bracing or gait studies may help determine which is the primary problem. Ankle plantar flexion often can be controlled with bracing if the foot can be brought up to a right angle with the tibia when the knee is extended. If this is not possible, the tight heel cord should be lengthened; tight hamstring and hip flexors also may be lengthened when indicated. The "scissoring" of the legs seen with walking or lying down may be caused by tight adductor muscles.

Hip dislocation occurs with increasing frequency as the severity of disease involvement increases. This is the result of imbalance between the strong adductors and flexors, and the weak abductors and extensors. The imbalance is acquired rather than congenital and usually occurs after the patient reaches several years of age. This should be checked every 6 to 12 months in diplegic or quadriplegic patients. The child is at risk for progressive hip subluxation if abduction is less than 30° with the hip extended. Dislocation and subluxation cause difficulty with perineal care, balanced sitting, degenerative joint disease, pain, and increased spasm. Consequently, they should be treated aggressively. Even in severely involved patients, they can be prevented by early muscle release or later osteotomy.

Scoliosis also is encountered more frequently with increasing severity of CP. It is present in as many as 69% of severely affected children, perhaps because of persistent primitive reflexes, an inclined pelvis, or asymmetric muscle tone. Bracing should be tried, but it is less effective than in idiopathic scoliosis. Surgery may be necessary.

The upper extremity may be flexed at the elbow, wrist, and fingers. The decision to correct this condition is based on the patient's intelligence, ability to control the hand voluntarily, and degree of sensation. The thumb may be clenched and early bracing may be helpful, with surgery performed later if the digit has potential for use.

The benefits of physical therapy in general are debated. Positioning and hand and heel cord stretching may produce increased range of motion. The severity of involvement probably is more important than therapy in determining the patient's ability to walk, however.

Myelodysplasia or spinal dysraphism involves malformation of the embryonic neural tube with paralysis below a certain thoracic or lumbar level of innervation. The functioning muscles usually allow more control than is possible in patients with CP. The goal of orthopedic treatment is optimizing mobility and socialization, which does not always mean enabling the patient to walk. The quadriceps are the most important muscles for mobility. Severely affected children with poor intelligence and weak quadriceps muscles are more mobile in wheelchairs. In most cases, joint deformities are treated by surgical release and bracing. In contrast to CP, hip dislocations usually are not painful and should not be reduced unless they are unilateral or the child has good quadriceps muscles. Scoliosis also may occur, especially with higher-level spinal defects. One of the most important roles of the pediatrician is to observe the child for loss of lower extremity muscle power as he or she grows. This loss of muscle strength may be caused by tethering of the cord distally as the child grows or by a disturbance of cerebrospinal fluid pressure.

## Infections

### Hematogenous Osteomyelitis

The incidence and presentation of hematogenous osteomyelitis are changing following the introduction of newer imaging and treatment methods, but certain principles remain constant. The summary presented here should be coupled with that provided in the chapter regarding infectious diseases to illustrate the spectrum of treatment philosophies.

Acute hematogenous osteomyelitis by definition includes processes that have been operating for a week or less at the time of diagnosis. After infancy, this condition occurs more frequently in males than in females, presumably because trauma plays a role in increasing susceptibility. The peak ages of occurrence are infancy (less than 1 year) and preadolescence (9 to 11 years). The incidence declines in adulthood because of the change in vascular supply of bone. The most commonly affected sites are the femur and tibia, each of which accounts for one third of all cases, followed by the humerus, calcaneus, and pelvis. Any bone may be affected, however. The metaphysis is the region most often involved, and spread may occur from this point to involve any other portion. Rarely, the process may begin in the epiphysis.

Its pathophysiology explains some features of this disease. The metaphyseal vascular channels form loops near the growth plate. Blood flow is slowed, and the capillary basement membrane and reticuloendothelial system are deficient in these regions. Experimental bacteremias have been shown to produce foci of infection only in these areas. Trauma likely plays more than a circumstantial role, as experimentally traumatized areas are more susceptible to the development of osteomyelitis. Only about one fourth of all cases have a demonstrable source, such as cutaneous, aural, or respiratory seeding. Direct traumatic inoculation is a different disease process.

After a focus of infection is initiated, local inflammation is followed by spread up and down the medullary canal. The growth plate in children has no bridging vessels and acts as a barrier to spread in most cases. The germinal cells are on the epiphyseal side and, therefore, are spared. In the first year of life, however, transphyseal vessels do exist that allow spread to proceed up to the epiphysis and into the joint. These facts have two implications. First, growth plate damage is more likely during the first year of life. Second, in children of this age, septic arthritis may follow osteomyelitis in any metaphyseal location, whereas in older children without transphyseal vessels, it occurs only in locations where the joint capsule extends over the growth plate (ie, the shoulder, elbow and hip). At skeletal maturity with growth plate closure, this barrier again is eliminated, although hematogenous osteomyelitis is rare after this point. As intramedullary pressure increases, pus dissects through the haversian system to elevate the periosteum and produce a subperiosteal, then soft-tissue, abscess. The elevated periosteum may be radiographically apparent within 1 to 2 weeks.

Unlike septic arthritis, the organisms involved in hematogenous osteomyelitis vary slightly with the age of the patient (Fig 38-29). In all age groups, the predominant organism is *Staphylococcus aureus*, although *Streptococcus pneumoniae* and *Haemophilus* must be considered. *Staphylococcus* is associated with a higher recurrence rate than other organisms. *Salmonella* should be considered in patients with sickle cell anemia, although *Staph-*

*ylococcus* still is more common in these patients. Blood culture results during the acute phase are positive about 40% to 50% of the time, and direct cultures of pus or bone are positive only 60% to 80% of the time. This may be the result of prior antibiotic use, errors in sampling or processing, or autoeradication of the organism.

Clinical diagnosis remains key despite the availability of new imaging techniques. The child may appear well or may have systemic involvement ranging from malaise to shock. Often, refusal to bear weight is an early symptom. The very earliest sign is fever and local bone tenderness, followed later by a fluctuant mass if a subperiosteal or soft-tissue abscess has developed. Spread to adjacent joints should be ruled out by palpation and range of motion evaluation. Passive motion of the extremity usually is not resisted significantly unless a soft-tissue abscess or joint involvement is present. Increased suspicion should be aroused with neonates, who more often are afebrile and first may be noted to have a swollen or motionless limb. Vertebral or pelvic osteomyelitis may present as abdominal pain and can resemble the more common septic arthritis of the hip.

The differential diagnosis primarily includes neoplasm, contusion, non-displaced fracture, and sickle cell crisis. Elevated white blood cell counts and sedimentation rates are helpful, but not diagnostic. Serum antibody titers may be helpful, but their sensitivity is a problem. Radiographs at the earliest stage may show soft-tissue swelling. Osteopenia or lysis may appear after 7 to 10 days, followed by new bone formation at the borders of the process. Bone scanning has been used widely in the past 2 decades, but the subtleties of its use have been recognized only recently. The tracer that is used most widely is technetium 99m methylene

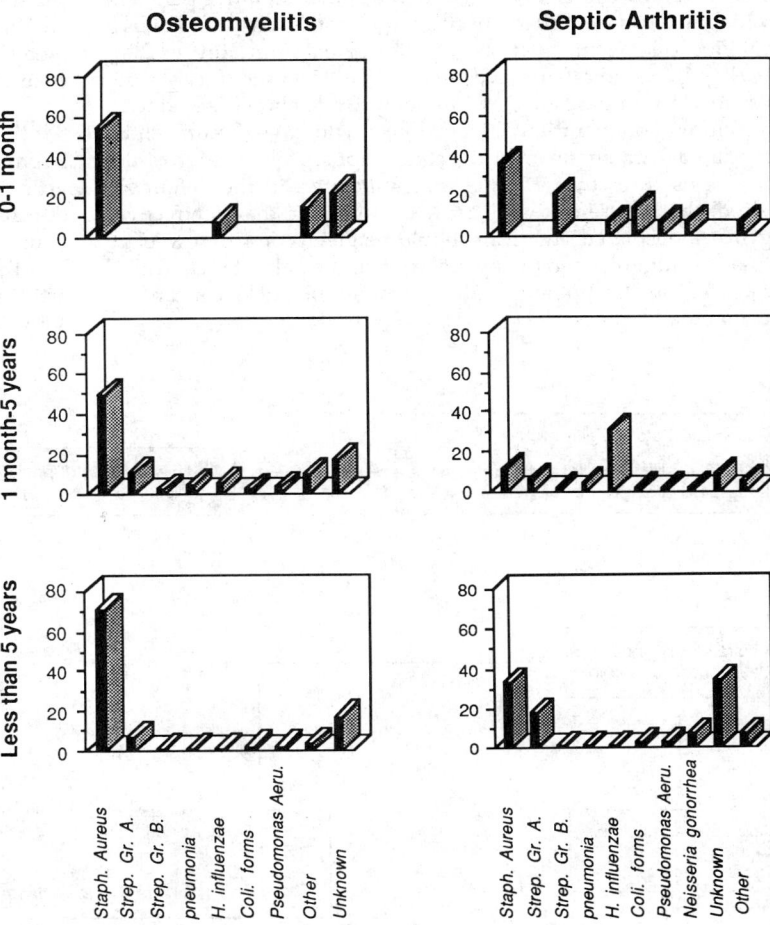

**Figure 38-29.** Frequency of occurrence of organisms involved in acute hematogenous osteomyelitis and septic arthritis in three age groups. (Drawn from table, with permission, from Jackson MA. Management of the bone and joint infections. Pediatr Orthopaed 1982;2:315.)

diphosphonate because of its speed, cost, and sensitivity (Fig 38-30). Immediate scans for flow and blood pool should be obtained, as well as later skeletal images. Results of the scan may be normal in the very early stages. It should be repeated after 48 hours if clinically indicated.

Cold or photopenic areas are important because they may indicate avascular sites, especially when they are accompanied by adjacent areas of increased uptake. Cellulitis may cause confusion, but usually does not show bony localization on delayed images. The overall accuracy of nuclear imaging is about 60% to 90%. It may be much lower in neonates, however, according to some reports. Gallium citrate may be sensitive, but it requires a minimum of 24 hours; indium-labeled white cell studies require similar amounts of time, including preparation of the tracer. Because of the above-mentioned limitations, radionuclide scans should not be relied on in all instances, especially when the clinical diagnosis is clear. These studies have their greatest value when localization for aspiration is difficult. The role of MRI has yet to be defined.

Aspiration is indicated in all cases to identify the pathogen and in some cases to decompress localized purulence. It should be performed with a large-diameter needle. The anesthetic may be local, intravenous, or general, as indicated. In sequence, the extraosseous soft tissues, periosteum, and, if necessary, intramedullary canal should be assessed for purulent localization. Fluoroscopy may be useful in deep lesions if radiographic changes are evident. Experiments in animals have shown that aspiration of bone by itself does not cause a bone scan result to become positive.

Treatment involves the delivery of an appropriate antibiotic to all infected tissue. Therefore, avascular abscesses may require surgical decompression if aspiration cannot accomplish this. Antibiotic therapy can be divided into initial and definitive periods. In the initial phase, broad-spectrum antibiotics, including antistaphylococcic agents such as nafcillin or oxacillin (150 to 200 mg/kg/d) are indicated. Vancomycin should be used if resistance is suspected. In neonates, an aminoglycoside should be added. In children younger than 3 years of age who have osteomyelitis associated with septic arthritis, chloramphenicol or cefuroxime may be used to cover *Haemophilus influenzae*. In the definitive period, the most effective, least toxic antibiotic that is effective against the isolated organism should be given for 4 to 6 weeks. It may be administered by the oral route if the patient is clinically improved and compliant, and if adequate blood levels can be documented.

Surgery is reserved for those cases in which the child is systemically ill or worsening under medical treatment, or in which an abscess has been demonstrated. Abscess or avascular tissue should be removed to allow antibiotic penetration, and the wound usually is closed over a drain. Complications include recurrence (20% overall; 6% at 6 months), minor growth acceleration, growth plate damage, and fracture through weakened bone.

### Subacute Osteomyelitis

Subacute osteomyelitis is a more subtle condition. No systemic signs may be evident and, in Roberts' series, fewer than one fifth of all patients had a fever, an elevated white blood cell count, or a positive blood count result. Abnormal radiographic and bone scan results, however, were more common than in the acute form. Treatment follows the principles discussed above.

### Chronic Recurrent Multifocal Osteomyelitis

Chronic recurrent multifocal osteomyelitis is a rare syndrome involving low-grade systemic manifestations that are ongoing for several years, with reports of up to 12 areas of lytic–sclerotic juxtaepiphyseal involvement. No organism has been isolated, and treatment is supportive.

### Fungal Osteomyelitis

Fungal osteomyelitis may be disseminated (sporotrichosis, candidiasis) or direct (eumycetoma). Aggressive debridement is more important in these conditions than in bacterial infections.

### Puncture Wounds

Puncture wounds to the foot are significant in that they may involve *Pseudomonas* infection. The wound should be inspected and foreign material removed. If the bone or joint is contaminated, full debridement and antibiotic therapy for recovered organisms should be begun. Otherwise, the patient should be seen in 3 to 5 days or at least be instructed to return if symptoms of infection occur.

### Septic Arthritis

Slightly more common than hematogenous osteomyelitis, septic arthritis may have more disastrous long-term consequences if effective treatment is delayed. Most cases occur in infants and younger children, with nearly half of all affected patients being less than 3 years of age. A high index of suspicion for septic arthritis should be maintained in sick neonatal patients, for they show few signs. The hip is the joint most commonly involved in

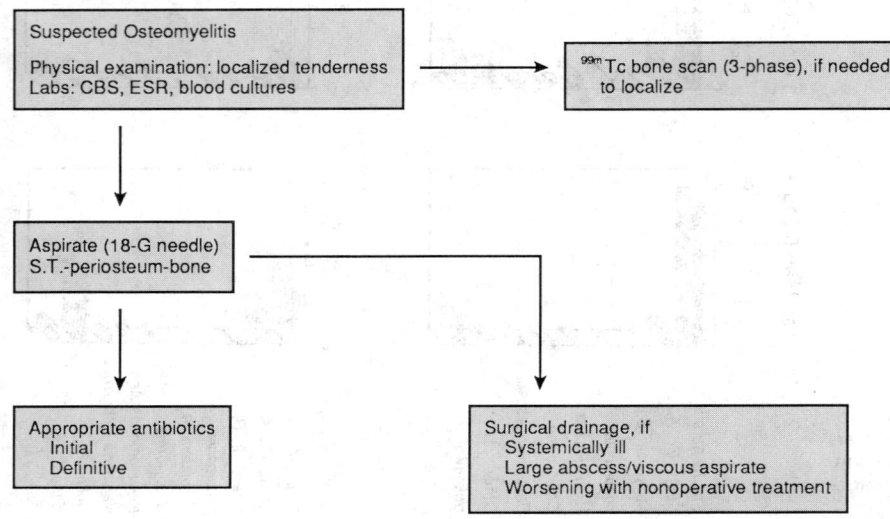

Figure 38-30. Diagnosis and treatment algorithm for hematogenous osteomyelitis.

the infant compared to the knee in the older child. The spread may be from the bloodstream or from an adjacent osteomyelitis, especially in the hip and shoulder where the capsular insertion extends over the growth plate onto the metaphysis. Many theories have been advanced for the pathogenesis of joint destruction, including alteration of joint fluid by toxins from both the neutrophils and the bacteria.

The spectrum of causative organisms in septic arthritis is somewhat broader than that of hematogenous osteomyelitis (see Fig 38-29), which may be related to the greater frequency of this condition. Overall, *S. aureus* still is the most common causative organism. In patients between 1 month and 5 years of age, however, *H influenzae* is more common than *Staphylococcus*. The streptococci, *Escherichia coli*, *Proteus*, and other organisms also should be considered. The yield of organisms from aspiration is about 60% to 80%.

Clinical findings vary with the age of the patient. In the infant, there may be fever, failure to feed, and tachycardia. Subtle changes in position may serve as clues, as well as unilateral swelling of an extremity or a joint, asymmetry of soft-tissue folds, and pain with range of motion. In the older child, the signs are more localized.

Aspiration with a large needle should be performed if any reasonable suspicion of septic arthritis exists, both for diagnosis and, in some cases, for treatment. In deep joints such as the hip, injection of radiopaque dye should be used to confirm the position of the needle, especially if the aspirated fluid is normal. This assures that joint fluid actually was obtained, and it also helps to distinguish joint infection from septic involvement of the bursa underneath the nearby psoas muscle. The white cell count in fluid obtained from patients with septic arthritis ranges from 25,000 to 250,000. Elevated lactate levels may be helpful in cases in which white cell counts are borderline.

The differential diagnosis includes toxic synovitis of the hip, in which pain, fever, leukocytosis, and spasm are more moderate and do not escalate on serial observations. At times, however, the two conditions are indistinguishable and aspiration should be performed. Rheumatoid arthritis, cellulitis, traumatic synovitis, and the migratory multiple arthralgias of rheumatic fever should be considered. A sympathetic effusion also may occur from adjacent osteomyelitis.

The role of arthrotomy versus aspiration in confirmed cases of septic arthritis is controversial. The key feature is removal of deleterious enzymes and restoration of effective synovial perfusion. Because the decision not to operate requires the ability to monitor and aspirate repeatedly as needed, it probably is preferable to use arthrotomy in joints that are deep and difficult to assess such as the hip and shoulder, in young patients who are difficult to examine, and when the fluid obtained is viscous.

The surgical procedure should include irrigation, drainage, and closure. This may be done arthroscopically in the knee, shoulder, and ankle. Direct instillation of antibiotics has no benefit. Some investigators feel that the femoral metaphysis should be drilled whenever the hip is aspirated to decompress any possible femoral osteomyelitis.

Early effective treatment is very important. The chance of achieving good results declines dramatically if treatment is initiated after the symptoms have been present for 4 days. Antibiotics should be continued for 4 to 6 weeks. Controversy exists regarding whether the joint should be immobilized or treated with continuous passive motion; however, the latter is practiced less commonly. Contractures should be prevented, and abduction of the hip decreases the likelihood of dislocation. Complications include permanent destruction of cartilage and, in the hip, avascular necrosis with resorption or overgrowth of the femoral head. Complications are more frequent in young infants.

Gonococcal arthritis also occurs in children. It usually becomes evident after the systemic and febrile phase of the illness and should be distinguished from the more common gonococcal migratory multiple arthralgia or tenosynovitis. An average of 2 to 3 joints are affected, most commonly the wrists and knees. Treatment is aspiration and closed irrigation followed by 3 days of intravenous penicillin and 4 days of ampicillin or amoxicillin. Oral treatment alone with one of these drugs for 7 days is acceptable in compliant patients after a loading dose has been given.

## INJURIES

A comprehensive discussion of musculoskeletal trauma is beyond the scope of this chapter. Some problems are discussed in the chapter regarding sports medicine, and the reader is referred to the works by Rockwood and by Rang for further information. Basic principles of injury evaluation and common injuries and emergencies are discussed here.

Children's bones differ from those of adults both biomechanically and physiologically. Mechanically, immature bone is more porous, and the pores serve to limit crack propagation. Instead of complete fractures, children often have involvement of only part of the cortex, such as in a buckle fracture from compression or a greenstick fracture from tension. The most extreme example is plastic deformation of bone without fracture. This should be corrected if it is 20° or greater.

Another biomechanical feature of the child's skeleton is that the ligaments are stronger than either the bone or the growth plate. Injuries that would produce dislocations or sprains in adults (ie, elbow dislocation or medial collateral ligament tear of the knee, respectively) produce different patterns in children (ie, supracondylar humeral fractures or femoral physeal separations, respectively) (Fig 38-31). Thus, the presence of non-displaced fractures and separations should be sought on physical examination and radiographs in children. In the knee, gentle stress radiographs may show a non-displaced separation, which should be immobilized.

Physiologic differences include union rates, remodeling, overgrowth, and growth plate injuries. Nonunion is nearly unheard of in children, occurring only in open fractures with extensive soft-tissue loss and periosteal stripping. Bone union times range from 2 weeks in infants to 3 months in adolescents. Remodeling of angulation and displacement is an impressive tendency until the early teen years. This occurs through alterations in physeal growth as well as local periosteal resorption on the convex side and deposition on the concave side. This is most effective in the metaphysis, where angulation does not create as much deformity as in the mid-shaft.

Compensation for any residual deformity is much better if it is in the plane of joint motion. For example, posterior angulation of a distal femur fracture can be compensated for by knee flexion, whereas the knee has no ability to compensate for outward angulation at this site. In the upper extremity, overlap of fracture segments is acceptable as long as the angulation is not excessive.

Another physiologic feature of the child's fracture is growth stimulation. This occurs because of hyperemia and continues for about 18 months after the fracture occurs. It is most significant in the femur, where it averages 1 cm, but it occasionally becomes significant in the tibia. In contrast, growth arrest may occur if the growth plate is crushed or crossed by the fracture. The Salter-Harris classification (Fig 38-32) was developed to predict the risk for growth arrest. It also is helpful in communicating with consulting physicians. Because types I and II do not cross the germinal layers, the risk of growth plate damage with these injuries is minimal. In types III and IV, the fracture crosses the plate, but anatomic reduction may diminish the risk of plate closure. In type V, the crushing cannot be reversed. Combinations of types may occur, especially with irregular growth plates. Such injuries

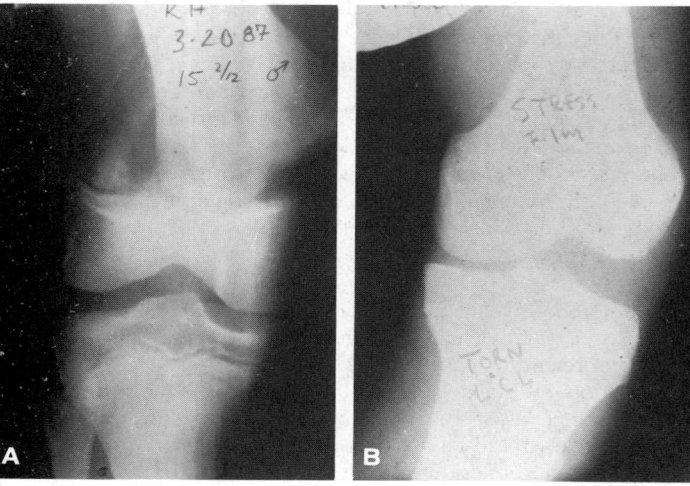

Figure 38-31.   A valgus stress to the knee produces failure at the weakest spot. (**A**) The growth plate in a child. (**B**) The medial collateral ligament in an adult.

should be observed carefully, because, if a limited growth plate bar forms, it can be resected to restore normal growth.

Basic evaluation of specific injuries should include three features: (1) assessment of the entire limb to rule out other fractures or dislocation above or below the joint; (2) assessment of neurovascular status, including sensation and motor function as well as pulses, capillary refill, and temperature (the possibility of compartment syndrome [tissue pressure greater than capillary perfusion pressure] should be considered in the forearm or leg; and (3) assessment of the site of injury. A surprising amount can be learned regarding known structures (ie, growth plates, ligaments, and so on) by palpating carefully in an attempt to identify the injured area. For example, lateral ankle swelling may be caused by fibular growth plate injury, ligament sprain, or peroneal tendon

subluxation, and all these conditions can be differentiated by palpation.

## Hand Injuries

Injuries to the hand are common in children. Fractures of the phalangeal and metacarpal shafts can be splinted if they are minimally angled and stable, but rotational alignment should be checked by observing the fingernails with the fingers flexed and extended. They should be aligned similarly if there is no malrotation. "Buddy taping" helps to minimize malrotation. Growth plate or epiphyseal fractures may be splinted if they are non-displaced, but should be referred if they are displaced. Dorsally dislocated interphalangeal joints may be reduced and radiographed to rule out fracture. If they are stable enough to allow active range of motion, they should be splinted for 3 weeks with an aluminum splint. Immobilization of the metacarpophalangeal joints should be in 50° to 90° of flexion to minimize stiffness, and the interphalangeal joints should be in mild flexion of about 20°.

One problematic injury is an avulsion of the base of the nail bed, which often is associated with open separation of the nearby phalangeal growth plate, which may become infected and stop growing. This should be distinguished from a Kirners' deformity, which is a bilateral, idiopathic irregularity of the distal phalangeal growth plate.

## Scaphoid Fractures

The scaphoid bone ossifies when a child is 6 years of age. Scaphoid fractures may occur in children and develop nonunion if they are not recognized. This occurs less often in children than in adults, however. Laceration of the palm and digits may sever a flexor tendon, and active range of motion of each joint should be checked to assure that this has not occurred.

## Forearm Fractures

Forearm fractures are very common in children. Non-displaced buckle fractures of one or both bones should be treated with a short arm cast for 3 or 4 weeks. Greenstick fractures represent tension or rotational failures with less intrinsic stability, and these should be held in a long arm cast for 6 weeks. Completion of the greenstick fracture is not necessary as long as angulation can be controlled. With any forearm fracture, the wrist and elbow joints should be checked, because dislocation may occur at one of these locations to compensate for fracture malalignment (Fig 38-33A).

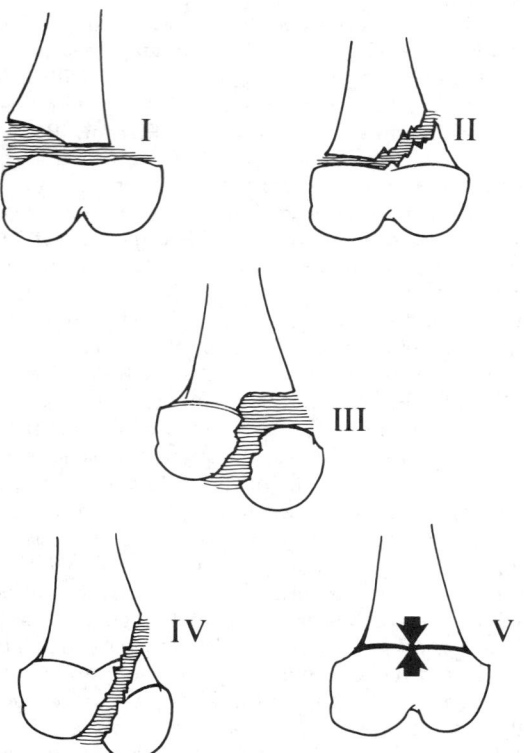

Figure 38-32.   Salter-Harris classification of fractures involving the growth plate.

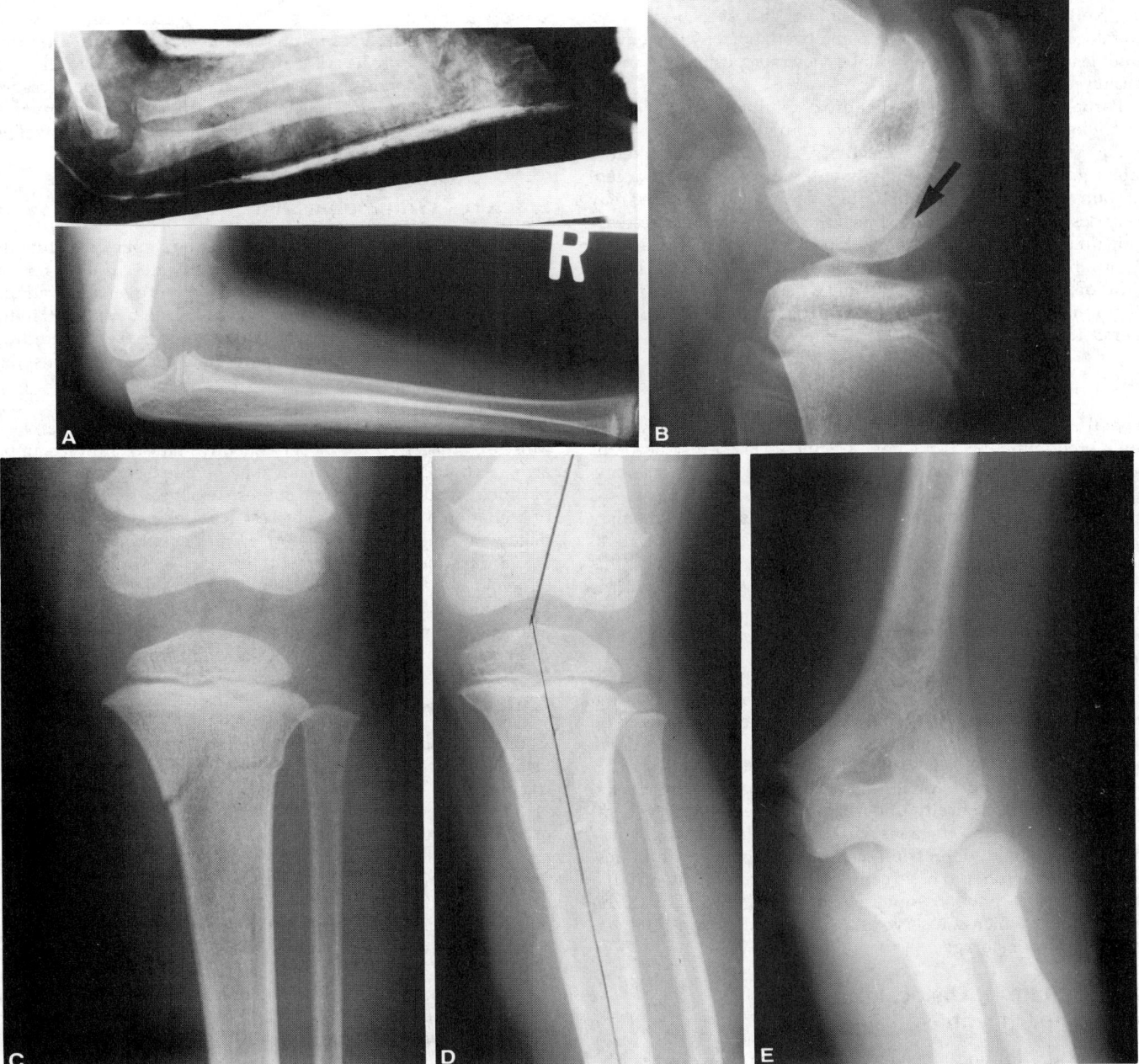

**Figure 38-33.**    Avoiding four common pitfalls in evaluating musculoskeletal trauma. (**A**) Always check the joint above and below a fracture. This Monteggia fracture of the ulna is reduced, but the radial head fracture was missed. The radial head should line up with the capitellum, as it does in the elbow on the right. (**B**) In a child's swollen knee, check the lateral film for a tibial spine avulsion fracture. It may be partially obscured by the overlying femoral condyles. (**C, D**) A proximal tibial fracture may result in valgus deformity even when initially reduced well. (**E**) Obtain comparison views when uncertain. This round ossicle in the medial joint space looks like it belongs there and was missed by an orthopedist, but actually represents the medial epicondyle trapped inside the joint.

## Clavicle Fractures

The clavicle usually fractures at the junction of the middle and distal thirds. Neurovascular damage to the underlying brachial plexus and subclavian vessels is rare, but should be considered. Usually, the periosteal sleeve is intact and remodeling is excellent. Treatment consists of preventing movement with a sling for 4 weeks in children and 6 weeks in teenagers.

## Knee Ligament Injuries

Knee ligament injuries are rare in children. Femoral growth plate separation usually occurs instead of collateral ligament damage. The tibial growth plate is protected because the collateral ligaments insert distal to it. Any trauma resulting in a swollen knee in a growing child (one that is 7 to 13 years old) should be examined to rule out avulsion of the tibial intercondylar eminence because this eminence represents the insertion of the anterior cruciate ligament and is a serious injury. It is seen best on the lateral view, but may be pulled up and overlapped by the femoral condyles (see Fig 38-33B). Oblique views or positioning in extension may help.

Partial fractures of the medial proximal tibial metaphysis are notorious for later developing outward angulation as a result of medial tibial growth plate overactivity. Care should be taken to obtain good initial fracture alignment, and parents will accept this outward angulation better if they are forewarned that it may occur despite adequate care. Some of the angulation may decrease with time, but osteotomy may be performed near maturity if significant deformity persists (see Fig 38-33, C and D). The ossification patterns of the elbow and wrist are complex. If a radiographic text is not available, comparison films of the contralateral side may clarify abnormalities (see Fig 38-33E).

## Ankle Injuries

Several ankle injuries are common, with injuries of the distal fibula predominating. If the bone fragment is non-displaced, diagnosis is made by palpating for tenderness at the growth plate, not by obtaining stress films. Three weeks in a short leg cast is the usual treatment; the intent is more to increase patient mobility than to decrease instability. On the tibial side, the anterolateral quadrant of the distal tibial physis is the last to close, and this area may be avulsed with rotation. It should be reduced if it is displaced.

## Soft-Tissue Injuries

Soft-tissue trauma of the extremities may be encountered in the emergency department, and foreign body penetration should be considered. Occasionally, palpation and radiography at soft-tissue settings may help. Glass is seen only if it has a high lead content. Exploration for deeper foreign bodies may be very frustrating unless it is done surgically under adequate regional or general anesthesia. Contusions to areas with thick subcutaneous fat may produce permanent depression of the area secondary to fat necrosis; the family should be so counseled. Injuries involving large amounts of soft-tissue loss may be able to be covered with the patient's skin, which can serve as a split-thickness graft if it can be saved in cool storage.

## Open Fractures, Dislocations, and Compartment Syndromes

Open fractures, dislocations, and compartment syndromes (the latter in particular), should be treated as quickly as possible for best results. Open fractures allow bacteria to come in contact with damaged tissue, which is an ideal culture medium. They should be irrigated down to bone within 6 hours to decrease the rate of infection and should be left open for several days for drainage and further debridement unless they are small and clean.

Dislocations of almost all major joints constitute emergencies because nerves and vessels are stretched, and further swelling can add to the problem. The ulnar, median, and radial nerves, and the brachial artery are involved at the elbow; the sciatic nerve is involved at the hip; and the popliteal artery is involved at the knee. Fractures that occur near these areas have similar implications.

Compartment syndromes have been recognized increasingly in the past 2 decades. Such syndromes occur when injury increases the tissue pressure within a closed fascial compartment, such as the forearm, leg, and buttock, above the capillary perfusion pressure (usually 30 to 45 mm Hg), resulting in ischemia and swelling. The earliest sign is excessive pain on passive stretch of the involved muscles within the compartment, followed by sensory loss and paresthesias of the involved nerves, and weakness of the muscle. Loss of pulses is a very late sign, and it indicates that pressure has risen above large arteriolar systolic pressure. Confirmation is obtained by measurement of the pressures using a hydrostatic or electronic apparatus. Treatment involves release of the tight fascia, with later skin closure when swelling resolves, if possible, or skin grafting, if not.

## Fractures With Malposition

Fractures with malposition may need to be stabilized so that the child can be transported to a consultant. Materials used for this purpose may be improvised, or plaster splints over soft wadding may be employed. In general, fractures should be splinted in the position in which they present, with the exception of femur fractures, which can be placed in longitudinal traction with a splint.

## Muscle Contusions

Muscle contusions occur most frequently in the quadriceps, upper arm, or shoulder muscles. They may be intensely painful. Compartment syndromes are rare in these regions. Treatment consists of limitation of hemorrhage by rest, ice packing, and elastic bandage wrapping. Active range of motion should be instituted in 1 to 3 days, but passive range of motion (ie, stretching) should be avoided because it may cause further damage. Strength rehabilitation is instituted after motion is regained. Myositis ossificans (ie, intramuscular calcification and ossification) may follow this injury, but usually does not limit function.

## Child Abuse

About 1% of all children in the United States are abused. Most victims are under 3 years of age. In children under 1 year of age, fracture more often than not may be non-accidental. One third of victims are reinjured if the initial diagnosis is missed. Fractures occur in about one third to one half of all abused children. The most common sites include the long bones, skull, and ribs. Most fractures that are specific for abuse are those of the metaphysis near the growth plate, the posterior ribs, the scapula, or the sternum. Unfortunately, there are no completely diagnostic radiographic signs of abuse. It is most helpful to use the radiograph to look for inconsistency, and to guide the investigation into the mechanism of fracture. Although long bone fractures may occur from a spontaneous fall out of bed or from a counter, they are rare. It is useful to get an idea of the "age" of a fracture by radiography. Periosteal new bone forms 6 to 10 days after a fracture in infants. At 10 to 14 days, there is blurring of the fracture lines and soft, mobile (poorly defined) callus. Hard callus occurs at 14 to 21 days. The differential diagnosis includes osteogenesis imperfecta, Caffey's disease, syphilis, scurvy, rickets, leukemia, and congenital insensitivity to pain.

If abuse is suspected, reporting is mandatory and the reporter is protected by law. The initial search for other fractures should be done by skeletal survey (AP and lateral views of the skull and spine, an AP view of the extremities), with bone scanning in selected cases. Admission to the hospital usually is the best means of protecting the child and further evaluating the family. Keeping careful records and being willing to advocate for the child may be the most important steps a physician can take to help.

## Selected Readings

### General

Morrissy RT. Pediatric orthopaedics, ed 3, vol 2. Philadelphia: JB Lippincott, 1990.
Rang M. Children's fractures. Philadelphia: JB Lippincott, 1983.

Renshaw TS. Pediatric orthopaedics. Philadelphia: Saunders, 1986:192. (Written for the primary care physician.)

Rockwood CA, Wilkins KE, King RE. Fractures in children. Philadelphia: JB Lippincott, 1991.

## Congenital Dislocation/Developmental Dysplasia of the Hip

Harcke HT, Kumar SJ. Role of ultrasound in diagnosis and management of congenital dislocation and dysplasia of the hip. Current concepts. J Bone Joint Surg 1991;73A:622.

Ilfeld W, Westin GW, Making M. Missed or developmental dislocation of the hip. Clin Orthop 1986;203:276.

Mubarak S. Pitfalls in use of Pavlik harness for treatment of congenital dysplasia, subluxation and dislocation of the hip. J Bone Joint Surg 1981;63A:1239.

Zionts LE, MacEwen GD. Treatment of congenital dislocation of the hip in children between the ages of one and three years. J Bone Joint Surg 1986;68A:829.

## Transient Synovitis of the Hip

Haueisen DC, Weiner DS, Weiner SD. The characterization of transient synovitis of the hip in children. J Pediatr Orthop 1986;6:11.

## Legg-Calvé-Perthes Disease

Catterall AM. Legg-Calve-Perthes disease. Edinburgh: Churchill-Livingstone, 1982.

Salter RB. Current concepts review: The present status of surgical treatment for Legg-Perthes disease. J Bone Joint Surg 1984;66A:961.

Salter RB, Thompson GH: Legg-Perthes disease. CIBA Clinical Symposia, 1986.

## Slipped Capital Femoral Epiphysis

Weiner DS, Weiner S, Melby A, Hoyt WA. A thirty-year experience with bone graft epiphysiodesis in the treatment of slipped capital femoral epiphysis. J Pediatric Orthop 1984;4:145.

## Popliteal Cysts

Dinham JM. Popliteal cysts in children. J Bone Joint Surg 1975;57B:69.

## Discoid Meniscus

Dickhaut SC, DeLee JC. The discoid lateral meniscus syndrome. J Bone Joint Surg 1982;64A:1068.

## Genu Varum/Tibia Vara/Genu Valgum

Kling TF, Hensinger RN. Angular and torsional deformities of the lower limbs in children. Clin Orthop 1976;176:136.

Levine AM, Drennan JC. Physiological bowing and tibia vara. J Bone Joint Surg 1982;64A:1158.

Salenius P, Vankka E. The development of the tibiofemoral angle in children. J Bone Joint Surg 1975;57A:259.

## Tibial Deformities

Morrissy RT. Congenital pseudarthrosis of the tibia. J Bone Joint Surg 1981;63B:367.

Pappas AM. Congenital posteromedial bowing of the tibia and fibula. J Pediatr Orthop 1984;4:525.

Staheli LT. Torsional deformities. Pediatr Clin North Am 1977;24:799.

Staheli LT, Corbett M, Wyss C, King H. Lower extremity rotational problems in children. J Bone Joint Surg 1985;67A:39.

## Metatarsus Varus

Bleck EE. Metatarsus adductus: Classification and relationship to outcomes of treatment. J Pediatr Orthop 1983;3:2.

Rushforth GF. The natural history of hooked forefoot. J Bone Joint Surg 1978;60B:8.

## Talipes Equinovarus

Simons GW. Complete subtalar release in club feet. J Bone Joint Surg 1985;67A:1044.

## Flatfoot

Staheli LT. Shoes for children. A review. Pediatrics 1991;88:371.

Wenger DR, Mauldin D, Speck G, Morgan D. Corrective shoes as treatment for flexible flatfoot. J Bone Joint Surg 1989;71(A):800.

## Tarsal Coalition

Mosier KM, Asher M. Tarsal coalitions and peroneal spastic flat foot. J Bone Joint Surg 1984;66A:976.

Scranton PE Jr. Treatment of symptomatic talocalcaneal coalition. J Bone Joint Surg 1982;69A:533.

## Spinal Disorders

Bradford DS, Hensinger RN. The pediatric spine. New York: Thieme, 1985.

Moe JH, Winter RB, Bradford DS, Lonstein JE. Scoliosis and other spinal deformities. Philadelphia: WB Saunders, 1987.

Tredwell SJ, et al. Instability of the upper cervical spine in Down syndrome. J Pediatr Orthop 1990;10:602.

## Upper Extremity

Bora WF. Pediatric upper extremity. Philadelphia: WB Saunders, 1986.

Dobyns JH, Wood V, Bayne LG. Congenital hand deformities. In: Green D, ed. Textbook of hand surgery. New York: Churchill- Livingstone, 1982.

## Brachial Plexus Birth Injuries

Hoffer MM, Wickenden R, Roper B. Brachial plexus birth palsies. J Bone Joint Surg 1978;60A:691.

Tada K, Tsuyuguchi Y, Kawai H. Birth palsy: Natural recovery course and combined root avulsion. J Pediatr Orthop 1984;4:279.

## Sprengel's Deformity

Carson WF, Lovell WW, Whitesides TE Jr. Congenital elevation of the scapula. J Bone Joint Surg 1981;63A:1199.

## Radial Clubhand

Bora FW. Radial clubhand deformity. J Bone Joint Surg 1981;63A:741.

## Radioulnar Synostosis

Cleary JE, Omer GE. Congenital radioulnar synostosis. J Bone Joint Surg 1985;67A:539.

## Pulled Elbow

Salter RB, Zaltz C. Anatomic investigations of the mechanism of injury and pathologic anatomy of "pulled elbow" in young children. Clin Orthop 1971;77:134.

## Bone Dysplasia

Lange RH, Lange TA, Rao BK. Correlative radiographic, scintigraphic and histologic evaluation of exostoses. J Bone Joint Surg 1984;66A:1454.

## Fibrous Dysplasia

Harris WH, Dudley R, Barry RJ. The natural history of fibrous dysplasia. J Bone Joint Surg 1962;44A:207.

## Osteogenesis Imperfecta

Albright JA. Management overview of osteogenesis imperfecta. Clin Orthop 1981;159:80.

Bleck EE. Nonoperative treatment of osteogenesis imperfecta. Clin Orthop 1981;159:111.

## Musculoskeletal Tumors

Lange TA. Ultrasound imaging as a screening study for malignant soft-tissue tumors. J Bone Joint Surg 1986;69A:100.

Mankin HJ, Lange TA, Spanier SS. Hazards of biopsy in patients with malignant primary bone and soft tissue tumors. J Bone Joint Surg 1982;64A:1121.

Rogalsky RJ, Black GB, Reed MH. Orthopaedic manifestations of leukemia in children. J Bone Joint Surg 1986;68A:494.

## Neuromuscular Disorders

Bleck EE. Locomotor prognosis in cerebral palsy. Dev Med Child Neurol 1975;17:18.

Bleck EE. Orthopaedic management in cerebral palsy. Philadelphia: JB Lippincott, 1987.

Menelaus MB. Orthopaedic management of spina bifida cystica. Edinburgh:Livingstone, 1980.

## Osteomyelitis

Green NE. Pseudomonas infections of the foot following puncture wounds. In: American Academy of Orthopaedic Surgeons Instructional Course Lectures. 1983:43.

Jackson MA, Nelson JD. Etiology and medical management of acute suppurative bone and joint infections in pediatric patients. J Pediatr Orthop 1982;2:313.

Nade S. Acute hematogenous osteomyelitis in infancy and childhood. J Bone Joint Surg 1983;65B:109.

Scoles PV, Aronoff SC. Current concepts review: Antimicrobial therapy of childhood skeletal infections. J Bone Joint Surg 1984;66A:1487.

Septic Arthritis

Green NE. Disseminated gonococcal infections and gonococcal arthritis. In: American Academy of Orthopaedic Surgeons Instructional Course Lectures. 1983:48.
Nade S. Acute septic arthritis in infancy and childhood. J Bone Joint Surg 1983;65B: 234.

Injuries

Dent JA, Paterson CR. Fractures in early childhood: Osteogenesis imperfecta or child abuse? J Pediatr Orthop 1991;11:184.
Jackson DW, Feagin JA. Quadriceps contusions in young athletes. J Bone Joint Surg 1973;55A:95.
Sanders WE, Heckman JD. Traumatic plastic deformation of the radius and ulna. Clin Orthop 1984;188:58.

*Principles and Practice of Pediatrics, Second Edition.*
edited by Frank A. Oski et al. J. B. Lippincott Company, Philadelphia © 1994.

# CHAPTER 39
# *Failure to Thrive*

## Rebecca T. Kirkland

Failure to thrive (FTT) is a term descriptive of a particular problem rather than a diagnosis. The term is used to describe instances of growth failure or, more specifically, failure to gain weight in childhood, although in more severe cases linear growth and head circumference may be affected. It differs from other causes of poor weight gain or growth failure because of its lack of obvious organic etiology. Failure to thrive describes a child usually younger than 2 years whose weight is below the fifth percentile for age on more than one occasion or whose weight is less than 80% of the ideal weight for that age, using the standard growth charts of the National Center for Health Statistics (NCHS).

## INCIDENCE

Failure to thrive is a problem common in pediatric practice and accounts for 1% to 5% of all referrals to children's hospitals or tertiary centers. In a rural primary-care setting, 10% of children in the first year of life have had failure to thrive. Failure to thrive occurs more frequently among children living in poverty.

## ORGANIC VERSUS NONORGANIC ETIOLOGIES

The distinction between organic causes of FTT and nonorganic or psychosocial etiologies has limited usefulness. In the child with congenital heart disease or other chronic disease, the nonorganic or environmental factors also may contribute to the failure to thrive and should not be overlooked. Likewise, the child within an emotionally disturbed family also may have an organic problem. One third to more than 50% of cases of FTT investigated in tertiary-care settings and almost all the cases in primary-care settings have nonorganic etiologies. About one fourth of all cases have involved a combination of organic and psychosocial factors.

## APPROACH TO THE SIGNS AND SYMPTOMS

A careful, thorough history and physical examination (Table 39-1) of the child whose only sign may be a diminished weight allow a logical, rational approach to ordering of laboratory tests and other investigations. Observation of the infant and of the interaction of the child with the guardian or parent, and an assessment of the social and environmental factors yield valuable information regarding the psychosocial milieu. In the absence of evidence for an organic problem in the initial history and physical examination, subsequent laboratory investigation is unlikely to reveal an organic cause.

### History

The pediatric history of the patient who fails to thrive should include an elicitation of symptoms suggesting organic diseases. A detailed environmental assessment is essential. Adverse psychosocial circumstances are known to have an association with diminished weight gain and growth in infancy.

The history should include a detailed dietary and feeding history, including information related to breast-feeding in the breast-fed infant. Deficient caloric intake due to increased losses of nutrients in the stool (malnutrition or diarrhea), vomiting or regurgitation, or impaired utilization can be clarified. If a psychosocial problem is suspected, caution should be used when interpreting a dietary history, because parental guilt may result in inaccuracies.

The psychosocial history should include an assessment of the family composition (absent parents), employment status, financial

TABLE 39-1.   Clinical Approach and Management for Failure to Thrive

| Approach | Immediate Support | Long-Term Support |
|---|---|---|
| Careful history | Nutritional support (plot daily intake and weights) | Frequent follow-up visits (well-child maintenance, plot heights and weights, developmental assessments) |
| Thorough physical examination (plot height and weight on curves) | Team approach (pediatricians, nurses, social workers, developmental specialists, community service workers, health educators, child-life workers, volunteers) or temporary/permanent foster home | |
| Observation of infant's behavior | | |
| Psychosocial evaluation (family and environmental factors) | | |
| Judicious approach to laboratory testing, radiology, and imaging | Treatment of uncommon underlying organic illness | |

state, degree of social isolation (absence of a telephone or of nearby neighbors), and family stress. Poverty indicators including eligibility for the Supplemental Food Program for Women, Infants and Children (WIC) should be sought. Maternal factors relating to the pregnancy, such as planned or unplanned pregnancy, use of medications for illness, substance abuse, physical or mental illness, postpartum depression, or inadequate breast milk, may be significant. Assessment should be made of levels of knowledge about parenting and about how to provide an adequate diet. Predisposing factors in the infant are intrauterine growth retardation, perinatal stress, prematurity, chronic disease, and frequency of intercurrent illness such as diarrhea, vomiting, or otitis media. In the dynamic interaction between the parent and the child, factors in the child, such as being "difficult" or chronically ill or giving diminished feedback, may contribute to the overall problem. Questions regarding the child's sleep pattern, other behaviors, and the amount of time spent alone may be helpful.

Family members' heights and weights, their history of illness, and any developmental delay in family members that may contribute to slow growth or constitutional short stature should be included in the assessment. Support systems available to the family and frequency of changes of home address should be examined. Initially, parents may avoid mentioning psychosocial problems such as marital discord; discussions of such issues should take place during several visits. These conversations should be conducted in a nonthreatening manner, demonstrating concern and compassion.

## Simple Observation

The infant's behavior can give valuable clues regarding his or her ability to interact appropriately for age. Behavioral features suggestive of psychosocial or environmental deprivation may include avoidance of eye contact, absence of smiling or vocalization, and a lack of interest in the environment. The negative response of the child to cuddling, and an inability to be comforted, may indicate a problem. The child may exhibit repetitive motions such as head-banging or self-stimulatory activity such as anogenital manipulation, or may be relatively immobile, with infantile posturing. The infant may be withdrawn and socially unresponsive, even to the mother, and actually may look away from her. Some infants inappropriately seek affection from strangers. Historically, these behaviors have been described in institutionalized infants who suffer from lack of care and affection.

Observing the mother feeding the child may be helpful. Does she cuddle the infant or merely "prop" the bottle? Does she allow sufficient time for feeding? The parents' level of concern may be inappropriate if they are eager to relinquish the child to the health team quickly. Observing the parents' interactions with each other will indicate whether they are supportive of each other.

## Physical Examination

Accurate assessment of the child's height, weight, and head circumference is essential. In the child younger than 2 years, the recumbent length rather than the standing height should be obtained carefully. This figure, along with weight and head circumference, should be plotted on the NCHS growth charts and related to previous measurements. The NCHS growth charts are gender specific and appropriate for all races and nationalities. Attention to the percentile curves of length, weight, and head circumference may give valuable clues as to the etiology of failure to thrive. When all measurements are below the third percentile, the incidence of organic disease has been noted to be 70%. Gastrointestinal disorders are more common when only the weight is below the third percentile. The single assessment of height and weight may have limited usefulness without an indication of

whether the child's pattern is deviating from the percentile or of how far below the curve the measurement may be. In intrauterine growth retardation, the child initially is small for height and weight; weight gain and growth velocity may be adequate, yet continue to be below the third percentile. Also, 3% of the normal population has had growth patterns at or below the third percentile (constitutional short stature). Therefore, determining the median age for the child's length (height or length age) and the median age for the child's weight (weight age) may be useful.

The complete developmental assessment is important. Careful evaluation should be made for dysmorphic features (clinical or genetic syndromes) and for signs of central nervous system (hypotonia or spasticity), pulmonary, cardiac, or gastrointestinal (swallowing disorders, gastroesophageal reflux) disorders. Isolated defects in the soft or hard palate may indicate a feeding problem.

Signs of neglect may be indicated by a diaper rash, impetigo, flat occiput, poor hygiene, protuberant abdomen, lack of appropriate behavior, and inappropriate infantile postures. Child abuse may result in bruises and fresh lesions or healed, unexplained scars. Notation of drooling and bowel habits is essential.

## MANAGEMENT

Most experience in the evaluation and initial management of FTT has been in the inpatient setting in tertiary centers. Exhaustive investigations for organic causes and prolonged hospitalizations to evaluate family dynamics and poor infant weight gain have resulted in inefficiencies and often the lack of a diagnosis.

### Laboratory Investigation and Evaluation

A careful history and physical examination in the child with FTT may suggest clues to organic disease in the child who has received an organic diagnosis. The search for organic disease should be guided by the signs and symptoms found in the initial examination. Laboratory studies not suggested on the basis of the initial examination rarely are helpful. Simple routine testing, including hematocrit, urinalysis and culture of urine, blood urea nitrogen, calcium, electrolyte levels, HIV ELISA antibody test, and Mantoux tuberculin skin testing, is appropriate. Additional testing, radiographs, and imaging may be indicated specifically by the clinical examination.

Hospitalization may not be helpful or necessary unless the child is seriously ill or is at risk of physical or sexual abuse, or parental concern and anxiety warrant it. Separation of the child from the family by hospitalization may promote anxiety and anorexia in the child, and cause a delay in feeding and supporting the child within his or her environment. Psychosocial factors should also be examined in children with organic problems.

In the past hospitalization was considered essential to demonstrate rapid weight gain in the child with FTT, in order to distinguish between organic and nonorganic etiologies. However, although immediate, rapid weight gain suggests evidence for a nonorganic cause of FTT, failure to gain weight does not rule out the nonorganic etiology. Children in whom the initial history and physical examination suggest an organic basis for FTT can either be admitted to an acute-care hospital or be evaluated as outpatients, if indicated. The child who has no evidence of organic disease or who may have a combination of organic and psychosocial problems can be evaluated and supported in either outpatient or inpatient settings.

Effective evaluation, whether inpatient or outpatient, requires involvement of the parents from the beginning with the support provided by an interdisciplinary program. In addition to the pediatrician, the program may involve social workers, nurses, developmental specialists, nutritionists, child-life workers, psychiatrists, and workers from social and educational services in the community. The low self-esteem that many parents have suggests that the health-care providers should not focus blame, but should work with the strengths of the family to encourage development of a nurturing environment.

The many possible causes of FTT are listed in Table 39-2.

## Nutrition and Growth Recovery

Nutritional requirements for the healthy infant younger than 1 year are an average of 100 kcal/kg of body weight per day. A child who fails to gain weight normally and whose weight is below the third percentile will not experience "catch-up," and therefore a caloric intake that is higher than normal is required. In such cases, intake requirements may be 50% higher than normal, or 150 kcal/kg/day. A higher caloric intake may be needed when the infant's normal energy requirements in the state of good health are considered.

Malnourished infants require extra concern because of the anorexia that may accompany the malnutrition state. The anorexia occurs early in the process and may last for up to a week. Malnutrition can result in transient malabsorption during the refeeding process. Environmental deprivation can result in the physiologic changes of hypopituitarism. The response of these secondary changes to treatment should be observed.

An aggressive approach to nutritional therapy is suggested. Supernormal caloric intake may be required to achieve catch-up, but frequently this increased intake is achieved by the child's own demands after entering the recovery phase. The following points may be a guide:

- Feeding and appropriate nutritional intake should be based on age and weight.

- In the nutritionally deprived child, feeding should be allowed to proceed ad libitum as the child demands.
- After a child goes into the recovery phase, the ad libitum intake frequently will achieve 150% of the daily requirement or greater.
- The child should be the guide as to when to increase the intake. This guideline applies to the child who is nutritionally deprived as a primary problem with no other abnormalities and who can take food by mouth.

Hospital volunteers, when available, may provide valuable role modeling, support, and aid in feeding. Home visitation may be helpful. Eligibility for WIC, food stamps, and Aid to Families with Dependent Children (AFDC) should be considered and facilitated.

During the nutritional recovery, some children may experience the symptoms of a nutritional recovery syndrome, including sweatiness, hepatomegaly (due to increased glycogen deposition in the liver), widening of the sutures (the brain growth is greater than the growth of the skull in infants with open sutures), and fidgetiness or a mild hyperactivity.

## FOLLOW-UP AND PROGNOSIS

Close follow-up and frequent contact with the health-care team are essential for reinforcing nutritional recommendations and psychosocial support. Involvement with the family by community social service workers, visiting nurses, and nutritionists is important. Although the prognosis with respect to weight gain and growth is good, one fourth to one half of infants with FTT remain small. The possibility that caloric deprivation in infancy will pro-

### TABLE 39-2. Causes of Failure to Thrive

| Inadequate Caloric Intake | | | Inadequate Caloric Absorption: No Weight Gain During Refeeding; Increased Losses | Increased Caloric Requirements |
|---|---|---|---|---|
| **Weight Gain During Refeeding** | **No Weight Gain During Refeeding** | **Inadequate Appetite or Inability to Eat Large Amounts** | | |
| Inappropriate feeding technique | Psychosocial problems* | Psychosocial problems (apathy)* | Psychosocial problems (refeeding diarrhea, intercurrent illnesses, rumination, regurgitation)* | Hyperthyroidism |
| Disturbed mother/child relationship* | Maternal/infant dysfunction, economic deprivation | Cardiopulmonary disease | Malabsorption—diarrhea (lactose intolerance, cystic fibrosis, cardiac disease, malrotation, inflammatory bowel disease, milk allergy, parasites, celiac disease) | Cerebral palsy |
| | Mechanical problems | Hypotonia | | Malignancy |
| | Insufficient lactation in mother | Anorexia of chronic infection or immune deficiency diseases (AIDS or AIDS-related complex) | Vomiting or "spitting up" or diarrhea | Chronic systemic disease (juvenile rheumatoid arthritis) |
| | Cleft palate | Endocrine disorders (hypothyroidism, diabetes insipidus) | Intestinal tract obstruction (pyloric stenosis, hernia, malrotation, intussusception, chalasia) | Chronic systemic infection (UTI, tuberculosis, toxoplasmosis) |
| | Nasal obstruction | CNS tumors | CNS problems—increased intracranial pressure (subdural hematoma) | |
| | Sucking or swallowing dysfunction (CNS, neuromuscular, esophageal motility problems) | Genetic syndromes | Chronic metabolic problems (hypercalcemia, storage diseases, and inborn errors of metabolism such as galactosemia, methylmalonic acidemia, renal acidosis, diabetes mellitus, adrenal insufficiency) | |
| | Regurgitation (gastroesophageal reflux) | Metabolic conditions (lead toxicity, iron deficiency, zinc deficiency) | | |
| | Malformation | Anemia | | |
| | Congenital syndromes (alcohol, phenytoin, drugs) | | | |
| | Genetic syndromes (Turner) | | | |

* Environmental causes are the most common source of problems.

duce severe, irreversible developmental deficits is the reason why treatment should begin expeditiously. Cognitive function is below normal in half of the children with FTT, and a high incidence of behavior problems is found on follow-up. Whether these findings are a direct result of the failure to thrive or of the contribution of continued adverse social circumstances is not known. The families need education and community services to help them to cope and to provide a nurturing environment for the children.

## Selected Readings

Berwick DM. Nonorganic failure to thrive. Pediatrics in Review 1980;1:265.

Berwick DM, Levy JC, Kleinerman R. Failure to thrive: diagnostic yield of hospitalization. Arch Dis Child 1982;57:347.

Bithoney WG, Dubowitzh H, Egan H. Failure to thrive: growth deficiency. Pediatrics in Review 1992;13:453.

Goldbloom RB. Growth failure in infancy. Pediatrics in Review 1987;9:57.

Hannaway PJ. Failure to thrive: a study of 100 infants and children. Clin Pediatr 1970;9:96.

Homer C, Ludwig S. Categorization of etiology of failure to thrive. Am J Dis Child 1981;135:848.

Mitchell WG, Gorrell RW, Greenberg RA. Failure to thrive: a study in a primary-care setting. Epidemiology and follow-up. Pediatrics 1980;65:971.

Pollitt E, Eichler A. Behavioral disturbances among failure-to-thrive children. Am J Dis Child 1976;130:24.

Sills RH. Failure to thrive: the role of clinical and laboratory evaluations. Am J Dis Child 1978;132:967.

*Principles and Practice of Pediatrics, Second Edition.*
edited by Frank A. Oski et al. J. B. Lippincott Company, Philadelphia © 1994.

## CHAPTER 40
# Sudden Unexplained Death and Apparent Life-Threatening Events

## 40.1 Sudden Infant Death Syndrome

John L. Carroll and Gerald M. Loughlin

The sudden unexpected death of a baby is a devastating event, both for the family and for the infant's pediatrician. Sudden unexpected death may occur in infants with an occult disorder such as infant botulism, in chronically ill children whose illness was not expected to be fatal (such as infants with bronchopulmonary dysplasia), or in apparently completely healthy infants. When postmortem examination fails to reveal an adequate cause of death in an infant who has unexpectedly died, it is called *sudden infant death syndrome* (SIDS).

SIDS remains the most common cause of postperinatal death in infants during the first year of life. It is not a diagnosis but a syndrome based on not finding a diagnosis. Despite over 2000 published articles on the subject, with nearly 1000 addressing etiology, no cause has been identified. After the rise and fall of countless hypotheses, years of intensive research, and years of experience with pneumograms and home infant monitoring, physicians can neither predict SIDS nor prevent it.

Whatever the cause or causes may be, the pediatrician in practice is faced with frustrating practical management dilemmas. These include trying to understand why one of his or her infant patients has suddenly and unexpectedly died, helping the surviving parents and siblings, and counseling the parents about the risk of SIDS in subsequent siblings. Despite the lack of definitive information about the causes of SIDS, the pediatrician must still cope with the death of a baby (Did I miss something? Could I have prevented this death?), the questions of the parents (What did we do wrong?), the questions of siblings (Why was my little brother taken away?), and the questions of extended families (Was this anyone's fault?).

In addition, with a new definition that *requires* a death scene investigation (see below), parents must cope with police or other authorities (eg, the medical examiner) coming into their home to interrogate them and to investigate the scene where the death occurred. Pediatricians can play a major role in helping parents through this difficult and trying period.

Finally, several new developments in the 1980s and early 1990s have yielded the potential for active prevention of some, if not most, SIDS deaths. Through preventive interventions, such as decreasing maternal smoking, improving prenatal care, and changing child-care practices (eg, infant sleeping position), pediatricians can have a major impact on child health.

## DEFINITION

SIDS is what remains after a thorough postmortem examination fails to reveal a cause of death; in other words, it is a diagnosis of exclusion. Since the early 1970s SIDS has been formally defined as "the sudden death of any infant or young child, which is unexpected by history, and in which a thorough postmortem fails to demonstrate an adequate cause for death." This definition has now been supplanted by one produced by an expert panel convened at the National Institutes of Health: "The sudden death of an infant under 1 year of age which remains unexplained after a thorough investigation, including a performance of complete autopsy, examination of the death scene, and review of the clinical history." The new definition restricts the age to infants less than 1 year of age and requires a thorough investigation; it explicitly states that if no death scene investigation is performed, a diagnosis of SIDS *cannot* be made.

The definition of SIDS is still controversial. Although everyone seems to agree that a worldwide standard definition is desirable and necessary, no definition has been agreed on, even within the United States. This situation is further complicated by the fact that the definition of SIDS actually used by medical examiners in the United States is a matter of local preference, not policy. Thus, the meaning of a SIDS diagnosis varies widely according to locality. Pediatricians should find out what criteria their local medical examiner uses to make this diagnosis.

There is controversy concerning whether SIDS should include infants with serious illness. A baby with bronchopulmonary dysplasia (BPD) may die suddenly. Was the infant *expected* to die from BPD? Difficulty arises when evidence of disease is found on the postmortem exam but it is not clear that the disease could have caused the death. For example, an infant who has suddenly died may have evidence of bronchial inflammation. Was bronchitis the cause of death? In reality pathologists can find very few clues that allow definitive statements about the cause of death in such cases. The best they can offer is to suggest what "adequate'' causes of death might be. In an individual case, however, it is usually impossible to delineate the role of apparently minor disease in the infant's death. When an infant with chronic illness dies suddenly and unexpectedly and no *adequate* cause of death is found on autopsy, some medical examiners will classify the death as SIDS; others will not. The highest risk occurs after discharge from the hospital in infants with BPD, of whom as many as one in 10 may die suddenly without sufficient explanation.

## EPIDEMIOLOGY

Most deaths caused by congenital anomalies occur during the first week of life, leaving SIDS as the most common single cause of death between 7 days and 365 days of age. About 35% of postperinatal deaths in the United States are attributed to SIDS. Each year between 5200 and 5500 infants die of SIDS in the United States, making the overall incidence about 1.4 SIDS deaths/1000 live births. Around the world incidence figures vary, ranging from less than 0.5 SIDS deaths/1000 live births in Sweden to more than five SIDS deaths/1000 live births in other parts of Europe. In most countries, the incidence falls between one and three SIDS deaths/1000 live births. In reality, the SIDS incidence depends heavily on precisely how SIDS is defined and how thorough is the search for a cause of death.

SIDS is uncommon during the first week of life. Most deaths occur between 1 and 5 months, peaking at about 3 months postnatal age. The apparently unimodal age distribution of SIDS, with a single peak at about 12 weeks, does not mean that SIDS is due to a single cause. Males have a higher incidence of SIDS in all racial groups (female:male ratio, 1:1.6). The reason for sex differences in SIDS is unknown.

SIDS is more common during the winter. In Europe and North America, the January SIDS rate is about double the incidence during July, while in the southern hemisphere, the July SIDS incidence is nearly double that during January. Many believe that all SIDS deaths occur during sleep (or at least when the infant was supposed to have been asleep), but deaths are known to have occurred in awake infants. Several studies have reported that most SIDS infants are found between 6 a.m. and noon, suggesting that the baby died during the night while asleep. However, it is possible that an infant may have been seen alive early in the morning and then found dead later. A British study found that when infant deaths were classified according to "time last seen alive," SIDS deaths were less likely during the night and more likely during the day.

Some factors, such as time of death, appear to vary with age at death. A study from Australia found that younger SIDS infants (<6 weeks of age) were just as likely to be discovered day or night. Beyond 6 weeks of age, increasing age at death correlated with the likelihood of the infant being found dead between 10 p.m. and 10 a.m. Several studies have suggested that an excess number of SIDS deaths occurs on weekends and "movable holidays." As anticipated, the interpretation of this finding is controversial. Some argue that excess SIDS on weekends results from decreased accessibility to medical care on weekends, while others point to the importance of environmental factors such as disruption of family routines. The meaning and importance of these findings remain unknown.

## RISK FACTORS

### Environmental Risk Factors

#### Infection

The role of infection as a risk factor remains in dispute. A variety of bacteria and viruses have been identified from SIDS victims, but no consistent association has been found between SIDS and infection with any particular organism. Parents often report that the infant showed "cold symptoms" just before a SIDS death, giving a general impression that infection is associated with SIDS. However, the National Institute of Child Health and Human Development (NICHD) SIDS Cooperative Epidemiological Study analyzed 800 SIDS cases with respect to matched control infants. They found that 29% of SIDS cases had a cold on the day of death, but so did about the same proportion of control infants. SIDS infants were more likely to be droopy and listless or suffer diarrhea or vomiting during the 2 weeks before death compared with control babies. A key finding, however, was that these symptoms were reported in less than 20% of the 800 SIDS cases. Numerous studies have made exhaustive attempts to identify symptoms that could be used to identify SIDS infants before death, but none have been found so far.

#### Nutrition

SIDS infants are smaller than normal at birth and smaller than normal at death, and growth velocity is decreased (even controlling for prematurity) compared with normal infants, suggesting a role for inadequate nutrition. Serum prealbumin levels, which reflect recent poor nutrition, and mineral content of bone, an indicator of chronic poor nutrition, have been reported to be normal in SIDS infants.

#### Family, Home, and Child-Care Practices

Numerous studies have shown an association between SIDS and maternal and socioeconomic factors such as young maternal age, mother unmarried, less than high-school education, low income, inadequate or no prenatal care, crowded living conditions, multigravidity, lack of breast-feeding, parental drug use, and smoking during pregnancy. The United States Collaborative Perinatal Project and the NICHD SIDS study found several prenatal, neonatal, maternal, and postnatal risk factors to be significant (Table 40-1). Similar studies from England have found a strong association between SIDS and such factors as "housing in poor repair," parents unemployed, poor financial circumstances, and the family not owning their house or not having a telephone. Such associations suggest that parental or environmental factors are important.

#### Infant Sleeping Position

Because of fear of suffocation, infants in Hong Kong usually are positioned supine to sleep. Parents in Western countries, afraid of vomiting and aspiration, put their babies to sleep in the prone position. Without any scientific evidence to support the practice, so-called baby experts have been strongly recommending the prone infant sleeping position for years. Recently, a study from Hong Kong reported that the SIDS incidence there was extremely low and noted that SIDS babies were much more likely to have slept in the prone position than control infants. From the Netherlands, another report indicated that infants who usually were placed prone to sleep showed an increased relative risk for SIDS. Several large controlled studies have now confirmed the association between the prone sleeping position and an increased risk of SIDS (odds ratios between 3 and 12).

If it is true that the prone sleeping position increases the risk of SIDS, what is the mechanism? Several investigators believe that it is related to a developmental vulnerability to upper airway obstruction, leading to asphyxia and suffocation. After about 6 months of age, when an infant can spontaneously change head, face, and body position, he or she is likely to be past the vulnerable period. Other possibilities include widespread alveolar collapse with hypoxemia and bronchoconstriction or impaired body heat loss and hyperthermia. However, the mechanism by which prone positioning could lead to SIDS is unknown.

TABLE 40-1.   Reported Risk Factors for Sudden Infant Death Syndrome (SIDS)

**Maternal Risk Factors**

Cigarette smoking during pregnancy*
Drug use during pregnancy
Inadequate prenatal care*
Lack of breast-feeding*
Low education level*
Mother unmarried*
Multiparity*
Young maternal age (<20 years)*
Young maternal age with first pregnancy
(<20 years)*

**Neonatal Risk Factors**

Cyanosis
Fever
Hypothermia
Irritability
Poor feeding
Respiratory distress
Tachycardia
Tachypnea

**Newborn Risk Factor**

Black race, Native Americans*
Low Apgar score (<7)
Low birth weight*
Male sex*
Prematurity*
Small-for-gestational-age*

**Postneonatal Factors**

History of cyanosis or apnea
History of diarrhea or vomiting in 2 weeks before
SIDS death
History of listless/droopy in 2 weeks before SIDS
death

**Prenatal (Pregnancy) Factors**

Anemia*
Low prepregnancy weight
Poor weight gain
Urinary tract infection
Venereal disease

**Socioeconomic Risk Factors**

Crowded living conditions*
Dwelling in poor state of repair
Family problems
Multiple child deaths in one family (no known
medical cause)
Poor family finances

**Miscellaneous Risk Factors**

Previous SIDS death in family
Previous SIDS infant older than 6 months
Multiple births (eg, twins)

* Widely accepted, general agreement among investigators.

There is no scientific evidence, at least with respect to SIDS, that there is any advantage to the prone sleeping position for healthy infants. There is also no scientific evidence, despite "common sense" fears of aspiration, that the supine sleeping position is harmful to a healthy infant. However, since evidence *is* accumulating that the prone sleeping position may increase the risk of SIDS, it seems reasonable to stop recommending the prone sleeping position for newborn infants and to recommend the side-lying or supine position for healthy infants. Recently the American Academy of Pediatrics recommended that healthy infants be positioned on their side or back when being put down for sleep. Of course, in certain medical conditions, such as gastroesophageal reflux, the prone sleeping position might be the more appropriate recommendation.

These recommendations concerning infant sleeping position are meant to apply to newborn and young infants who cannot yet change position on their own. Once an infant has advanced developmentally such that he or she can roll over back to front, parents need not force the infant to sleep in the supine or side-lying position.

## Illicit Drugs

Cocaine exposure may affect neurologic development, possibly leading to postnatal abnormalities of cardiorespiratory control, sleep, and arousal. Several studies to date indicate that the SIDS risk is higher in infants of substance-abusing mothers; the incidence figures range between nine and 150 deaths/1000 live births. Another study, however, found no difference in the SIDS rate between cocaine-exposed and nonexposed infants. Although drug-exposed infants may exhibit disordered sleep, respiratory

control abnormalities, and an increased risk of sudden unexpected death, no study has shown that these factors are causally related to SIDS, and no study has shown that death is related to drug exposure per se.

## Over-the-Counter Medications

In the NICHD SIDS study, 43% of SIDS victims had a history of a cold within 2 weeks before death and 29% reported cold symptoms within 24 hours before death. Sick infants are likely to be treated with over-the-counter medications containing antihistamines, phenothiazines, or other powerful sedatives. One study found that SIDS victims and matched controls had the same incidence of cold symptoms, but infants dying of SIDS were much more likely to have received cold medicine before death. About 25% of SIDS infants had been given phenothiazine-containing cold remedies within 48 hours of death, compared with only 2% of control babies.

## Immunization

Several controlled studies have now shown that DPT immunization does *not* increase the risk of SIDS. An infant should not be denied the protection of standard immunizations because of perceived risk factors for SIDS.

## Infant Risk Factors

### Race

Blacks and Native Americans have the highest rates of SIDS in the United States; babies of Asian origin have the lowest. However, no study has been able to sort out an increased SIDS risk due to race per se as opposed to differences in environmental or child-care practices.

### Birth Weight and Prematurity

Birth weight and prematurity are two of the strongest risk factors for SIDS. The NICHD SIDS study found that infants with birth weights below 2500 g and below 1500 g were about five and 18 times, respectively, more likely than controls to die of SIDS. Similarly, infants with preterm birth at less than 37 weeks and less than 33 weeks were five and 16 times, respectively, more likely to die of SIDS than controls. Increased SIDS risk also was found in that study for small-for-gestational-age full-term infants, and 1- or 5-minute Apgar scores below 7. In another study, even when gestational age was controlled for, infants destined for SIDS appeared to be lighter and shorter than controls. This suggests that SIDS infants are not perfectly healthy before death and that prenatal factors may be important.

## Neonatal Risk Factors

### Apnea

Despite widespread beliefs about infant apnea and SIDS, to date no properly controlled study has shown that apnea of prematurity is a risk factor for SIDS. The NICHD SIDS study found that other neonatal factors such as hypothermia, tachypnea, poor feeding, cyanosis, irritability, fever, and respiratory distress were statistically more likely to have occurred in SIDS infants but were not of predictive value. The medical literature has linked infant apnea strongly with SIDS for decades. However, several studies now have shown that infant apnea does *not* correlate with subsequent SIDS death.

### Maternal Smoking and Fetal Hypoxia

Maternal cigarette smoking is a major risk factor for SIDS. One large study found that 70% of mothers in the SIDS group smoked during pregnancy. A cigarette consumption/SIDS dose-response curve was demonstrated more than 15 years ago. Even after controlling for other risk factors, maternal smoking roughly doubles the risk of SIDS. According to the NICHD SIDS study, if a mother smokes during pregnancy the SIDS risk is 3.4 times higher than for controls. Another recent controlled study showed that maternal smoking of one to nine cigarettes per day doubled the risk, and smoking 10 or more per day tripled the risk of SIDS death. Thus, maternal smoking is a potent risk factor for SIDS and possibly one about which pediatricians can do something.

Maternal anemia greatly enhances the SIDS risk for infants of smoking mothers. An anemic smoking mother appears to be about four times more likely to have an infant die of SIDS than a nonanemic, nonsmoking mother. Such a strong interaction with anemia and smoking during pregnancy suggests that fetal hypoxemia, prenatal nutrition, or other toxicity may play a role in SIDS.

## PATHOLOGY

### Autopsy

For many years, pathologists have searched unsuccessfully for pathologic markers that would positively identify these infants. SIDS remains a pathologic diagnosis of exclusion. Table 40-2 lists several proposed subtle pathologic findings in SIDS, but many of these so-called "subtle" pathologic findings of SIDS are matters of great debate. *No pathologic finding has been found to be diagnostic of SIDS.*

---

**TABLE 40-2.   Reported Pathologic Findings in Sudden Infant Death Syndrome (SIDS)**

**Main Finding**
No pathology that explains death

**Currently Accepted "Subtle" Findings***
Brain stem gliosis
Frothy secretions at nose or mouth†
Hepatic erythropoiesis†
Intrathoracic petechiae
Minor inflammatory changes (respiratory tract)
Periventricular leukomalacia†
Persistence of dendritic spines in "respiratory centers" of brain stem
Pulmonary congestion†
Pulmonary edema†
Retention of periadrenal brown fat
Unclotted blood in left ventricle†

**Unconfirmed to Date**
Abnormal development of vagus nerve
Abnormal pulmonary surfactant
Abnormalities of carotid body
Decreased laryngeal cross-sectional area
*E coli* toxin
Elevated hypoxanthine levels in vitreous humor
Increased immunoglobulin levels in lung washings

**Validity Seriously in Question**
*C difficile* toxin (not different from controls)
Retained hemoglobin F (conflicting results from different studies)

* Agreement between several different investigators
† Some investigators question whether these differ significantly from deaths due to other causes.

---

### Death Scene Investigation

The unexpected death of an infant always raises the question "why?" Such a question cannot be answered fully without all available information concerning the circumstances of death. Clinical history from caretakers is important but insufficient. A variety of environmental factors would not be recognized by untrained observers and are likely to be missed even by a physician taking a thorough history. Despite disagreement about the proportion of SIDS cases that are due to nonaccidental injury or neglect, most investigators would agree that at least some deaths are nonnatural. Especially in these cases, there is no substitute for a thorough professional death scene investigation.

The widely accepted belief that SIDS has nothing to do with environmental factors, child-care practices, accidents, neglect, or intentional injury was not based on scientific data. Recent reports suggest that if a more complete death circumstances inquiry were conducted, many SIDS deaths could be explained. The death scene investigation may be more important than autopsy in some cases. Without a thorough death scene investigation as part of every SIDS investigation, we will never determine the actual proportion of SIDS cases that are related to environmental factors, neglect, or intentional injury. Without all available information, the true proportion of preventable SIDS deaths cannot be known.

## PATHOGENESIS

The cause or causes of SIDS are unknown. The search for the causes of SIDS has been further complicated by the study of so-called infants at risk or high-risk infants, since identification of groups that are at risk is a matter of dispute. Much of the scientific data that have been proposed or assumed to describe infants at risk may or may not actually apply to most SIDS victims.

## Respiratory Control

Many investigators believe that some abnormality of respiratory control underlies SIDS in most cases. As pointed out in 1987 by Hunt and Brouillette, early reports associating SIDS with prolonged apnea encouraged an excessive emphasis on apnea per se. A more broadly formulated "cardiorespiratory control hypothesis" proposes that SIDS could result from developmental abnormalities in cardiorespiratory control, including the brain stem control centers, chemoreceptor responses, autonomic control, autoresuscitative gasping mechanisms, arousal from sleep, and upper airway control. Several large prospective studies have now reported that in general there are subtle findings concerning respiratory and cardiac variability, higher mean heart rates, and sinus tachycardia. These studies may be most significant, however, for what they did *not* find; no study has found characteristic respiratory control abnormalities in babies destined to die of SIDS. One recent study, using sophisticated breathing analysis techniques, was unable to find breathing pattern abnormalities suggestive of respiratory control system instability in babies who later died of SIDS.

## Upper Airway and Small Airways Occlusion

It has been suggested that SIDS may sometimes be caused by nasal/oral occlusion or suffocation of an infant with the face pressed into a pillow or mattress. However, to date no scientific study has confirmed these hypotheses. Several studies have suggested that pulmonary surfactant was abnormal in SIDS victims compared with control infants who died of non-SIDS, nonpulmonary causes. Abnormal surfactant may lead to widespread alveolar collapse, causing hypoxia and death. Much more study is needed in this area before a conclusion is possible.

## Cardiovascular

The long QT syndrome and hypersensitivity to vagal stimulation have both been suggested as causes, but neither has been proved to be associated with SIDS. Tachycardia and decreased heart-rate variability have been found in infants who later die of SIDS, but the meaning of these findings is unknown.

## Defects of Metabolism

Underlying metabolic abnormalities such as medium-chain acyl-CoA dehydrogenase deficiency, ethylmalonic-adipic aciduria, multiple acyl-CoA dehydrogenase deficiency, long-chain acyl-CoA dehydrogenase deficiency, and systemic carnitine deficiency may account for some SIDS deaths. However, the proportion of SIDS cases that may be attributable to metabolic disorders is probably small, and firm conclusions cannot be reached at present. An underlying metabolic disorder should be strongly considered in cases of apparent SIDS in older infants (>6 months) or when multiple cases occur in one family.

## Infection

Acute bacterial and viral infections, intrauterine and perinatally acquired chronic infections, and various toxins elaborated by infectious organisms have all been proposed as possible causes or predisposing factors for SIDS. Although infection may play an indirect role, to date there is no evidence linking SIDS to any specific infectious etiology.

## Delayed Neural Development

An hypothesis involving abnormal neural maturation is attractive because it could at least partially explain developmental vulnerability to SIDS. Abnormalities described so far include delayed central nervous system myelination, astrogliosis, periventricular and subcortical leukomalacia, delayed dendritic pruning, and other suggestions of abnormal nervous system development. However, no neuropathologic finding has been causally linked with SIDS or shown to be specific for SIDS.

## Impaired Arousal Responses

It is well known that children and adults tend to sleep more when sick. This is not simply a matter of feeling bad but involves infection-related increased levels of somnogenic substances that exaggerate the tendency to sleep and may impair arousal. Such somnogenic substances include muramyl peptides, the lipid-A moiety of endotoxin, poly(I C), interleukin-1, and others. It has been suggested that infection leads to increased levels of somnogenic substances, increased sleep, impaired arousal, and an increased vulnerability in the infant to airway obstruction or other causes of asphyxia. This is a promising area in need of further exploration.

## Developmental Vulnerability

After birth the infant does not simply grow larger; rather, many (if not all) systems show continued structural and morphologic maturation. The lungs are not fully developed until about 8 years of age. The central nervous system continues to undergo significant structural modification for years. Just as motor skills and reflexes are primitive in the newborn and develop slowly in the infant, many physiologic responses are incompletely developed at birth. These include major changes in cardiorespiratory control that occur during the first 6 months of life. The infant's ability to "defend" himself or herself against hypoxia or asphyxia changes during the first 6 months of life. In this sense, all infants are vulnerable to a variety of postnatal insults at certain times. Vulnerability could be increased in some infants due to prenatal injury (smoking, substance abuse, poor nutrition, anemia during pregnancy), abnormal development (eg, delayed central nervous system maturation), or postnatal factors (eg, illness or medication with sedative drugs).

The "developmental vulnerability" hypothesis proposes that SIDS may result from a variety of insults (eg, infection, thermal stress, accidental occlusion of oronasal airway) to a vulnerable infant. Any one factor, occurring in isolation, may not lead to death, but particular combinations of stresses or a particular insult at a vulnerable time may be lethal for 1.5/1000 infants. Thus, there would be no single cause of SIDS. SIDS could result from a variety of stresses and multiple causes of vulnerability that vary with age. Such an etiology would be consistent with variable pathologic findings, multiple risk factors, parental and environmental factors that appear to play a variable role, and risk factors that vary depending on the age at death.

## GROUPS PROPOSED TO BE AT INCREASED RISK

Traditional groups said to be at increased risk include premature infants, subsequent siblings of SIDS victims, survivors of apparent life-threatening events (ALTE), and recently infants of substance-abusing mothers. Prematurity is a potent risk factor for SIDS and one of the few that is not in dispute.

## Siblings of SIDS Victims

If a physiologic abnormality is operative in SIDS, it could be hereditary (eg, defects in metabolism). If family factors, child-care practices, or environmental factors play a role, these would probably be similar for subsequent siblings of a SIDS victim. Finally, if intentional injury is a factor in a particular SIDS case, subsequent siblings in the same family are likely to be at increased risk. A family in which multiple SIDS death occur should be investigated for all of these possibilities.

The literature on the risk to a subsequent sibling after one SIDS death is unclear at present. Some studies describe an increased risk of recurrent SIDS, while others say that there is no increased risk. A 1990 article by Guntheroth and colleagues reported a recurrence rate of 13/1000 live births among a group of 385 subsequent siblings, but also found a similar recurrence rate among siblings of non-SIDS infant deaths. They concluded that the overall recurrence risk for SIDS is low but still significant.

## Apparent Life-Threatening Event

ALTE is the new designation for a group of infants that some call "near-miss" for SIDS. This term applies to infants who have been observed to have pallor, cyanosis, apnea, choking, or other indications that they might be in danger of dying. Are infants who experience an ALTE at higher risk of SIDS? A study from Boston found that babies who experienced ALTE episodes requiring cardiopulmonary resuscitation were at increased risk of sudden death. The NICHD SIDS study found that 7% of mothers of SIDS victims recalled a previous episode of "baby turned blue or stopped breathing" compared with 3% of matched controls. Although this was statistically significant, the most important finding was that 93% of mothers of SIDS infants recalled no ALTE. Available data suggest that ALTE infants constitute only a small number of SIDS cases, and that most infants dying of SIDS do *not* experience a prior ALTE.

## PREDICTION

At present, SIDS risk cannot be predicted for an individual infant. No test, including a pneumogram or polysomnography, is useful for determining SIDS risk. No test can predict SIDS risk for a family or a subsequent sibling. No test can determine which infants should use home apnea monitoring or when a home monitor can be appropriately discontinued. However, we *can* predict increased risk for groups such as premature infants, infants of smoking mothers, and so forth, opening the door for a variety of preventive interventions.

## MANAGEMENT

As Mandell and colleagues have described in several articles, the management of SIDS is the management of the surviving parents and the extended family, surviving siblings, and subsequent siblings. The parents and siblings have no warning and are frequently in a state of shock when they come into contact with the medical system. Parents often cannot believe what has happened. They may become hostile and angry, guilty, and self-blaming.

The pediatrician's role varies as the case evolves. Immediately after the death, the pediatrician can help the family cope with the initial shock and arrangements for death scene investigation

and autopsy. The pediatrician should be an advocate for the proper investigation, as discussed above. Parents will ask, "What did we do wrong?" Since in most cases the parents did nothing wrong, appropriate counseling during this time can be of tremendous benefit to confused, self-blaming, self-questioning families. When death scene investigation results and autopsy results are available, the pediatrician should review these in detail with the family. Most often these results will reassure the family that the death was not their fault. If some evidence of accident or injury is found, then disclosure of such information, as painful as it may be, could only be in the best interest of future children.

In addition to self-blaming, parents often have their own beliefs about SIDS, perhaps expressing concerns about environmental factors and risk to their other children. The father's reaction may be quite different from the mother's and may require a different counseling approach. All parents will be concerned about hereditary factors and the risk to subsequent children, and the pediatrician will be called on to counsel parents on these issues.

The pediatrician also experiences grief and anxiety when a patient dies of SIDS. It is natural to wonder what serious medical problem he or she might have missed. Fear of being held responsible may lead to intense self-questioning. One study of pediatricians' reactions to SIDS revealed sadness, shock, frustration, anger, guilt, regret, hurt, and feelings of inadequacy.

The reaction of a surviving sibling to SIDS in the family should not be overlooked. Young children do not understand. Older siblings are suddenly deprived of the role of older brother or older sister, often with devastating results. Surviving siblings may feel responsible, thinking that something they did caused the baby's death. Others deny their feelings. The pediatrician should anticipate these problems, inform parents, and if necessary counsel the children. Professional counseling may be necessary.

The pediatrician's role extends to when the parents decide to have subsequent children. One should anticipate that the birth of a subsequent child will raise many concerns and questions. A danger for the subsequent sibling is overprotection or the "vulnerable child" syndrome. The pediatrician can evaluate any actual risk and advise the parents appropriately. The articles by Mandell and colleagues provide a wealth of useful information concerning SIDS and the family.

## HOME MONITORING

The question of home monitoring is still unsettled. Home cardiorespiratory monitoring, as currently used in the United States, is intended to improve the outcome of any infant perceived to be at increased risk of sudden death. However, after decades, home monitoring has not decreased the incidence of SIDS. In 1986 the Consensus Development Conference on Infantile Apnea and Home Monitoring found that there were no reports of scientifically designed studies of the effectiveness of home monitoring on ALTE, subsequent siblings of SIDS victims, premature infants, or other pathologic conditions, and in 1993 this remains true. Current recommendations are summarized in Tables 40-3 and 40-4, and the reader is referred to the summary statements of the 1986 NIH conference report.

Pediatricians often have questions concerning when to discontinue home monitoring. There are no tests, including pneumograms or polysomnography, that will answer this question. Discontinuing monitoring is a clinical decision based on the overall clinical picture. In general, monitoring can be discontinued when there have been no significant abnormal cardiorespiratory events for 2 or 3 consecutive months. We use memory monitors, which provide a hard-copy printout of all alarm events, on all patients. Although the monthly cost is higher than for conventional car-

## TABLE 40-3. Indications For Home Monitoring

**Monitoring Recommended For:**

Any infant perceived to be at increased risk of unexpected sudden death, including:

Infants with one or more severe apparent life-threatening events (CPR or vigorous stimulation required)

Subsequent siblings in family with SIDS case

Symptomatic premature infants (abnormal apnea or bradycardia at time of discharge)

Infants with central hypoventilation

Infants on supplemental oxygen

**Not Recommended For:**

Normal infants

Asymptomatic premature infants

**Individualize Case-by-Case For:**

Infants who have experienced less severe apparent life-threatening events

Infants who have bronchopulmonary dysplasia

Infants who have tracheostomies

Infants of substance-abusing mothers

---

diorespiratory monitoring, the overall cost is often lower because most alarm events are false (artifact). Much of the guesswork is taken out of monitor decision-making because the physician and parents can review the hard copy, be reassured that serious cardiorespiratory events did not occur, and discontinue the monitor sooner than it would have been using conventional monitoring.

## PREVENTION

Can pediatricians prevent SIDS? Monitoring does not appear to have much impact on the incidence of SIDS. Improved technology

## TABLE 40-4. Discontinuing Home Monitoring

Monitoring may be discontinued when the infant is no longer thought to be at increased risk of sudden death.

**Suggested Criteria for Discontinuation of Monitoring (Assuming Good Compliance With Monitor Usage):**

No significant apparent life-threatening event (no color change, no CPR or vigorous stimulation required) for 2 or 3 consecutive months

Infant has tolerated at least one viral infection without significant alarms or events

**Factors That May Affect Decision:**

Not sure if alarms are "true" or "false"

Infant on medication to treat apnea (eg, theophylline)

Infant on medication related to indication for monitoring (eg, bethanechol for gastroesophageal reflux)

Age of infant

Other indications to continue (eg, infant on supplemental oxygen)

Family's anxiety level

**Testing (Pneumogram, Polysomnography):**

Obtaining a normal pneumogram is unnecessary.

Polysomnography (sleep study) is unnecessary.

Documented monitoring is the best way (currently) to distinguish "true" from "false" alarms.

## TABLE 40-5. Possible Approaches to Prevention of Sudden Infant Death Syndrome (SIDS)

**Risk Reduction**

Abandon recommendation of prone sleeping position for all infants (prone sleeping position still recommended for infants with specific clinical indication)

Recommend side-lying or supine sleeping position for healthy infants

Advocate better and more standardized policy concerning death scene investigation

Better educate public about dangers of over-the-counter remedies to young infants

Decrease parental smoking, before and after birth of child

Decrease parental drug use (eg, crack cocaine smoking), before and after birth of child

Improve access to and use of postnatal medical care

Improve prenatal care (anemia, smoking, nutrition)

Improve recognition of and services for dysfunctional families at risk for intentional injury of infants

Improve services to young mothers living in poor socioeconomic conditions

Improve targeting of very high risk groups (eg, Native Americans with very high maternal smoking rates)

Improve understanding of child-care practices that may increase SIDS risk

**Physiologic Component**

Improve diagnosis of metabolic disorders leading to SIDS

Increase understanding of possible sources of postnatal vulnerability

Increase understanding of the role of infant sleeping position in increasing SIDS risk

**Increase Efficacy of Home Monitoring**

Improve compliance with monitor use

Improve monitoring technology

Improve selection of candidates for monitoring

---

of conventional cardiorespiratory monitoring may be helpful but is probably not the answer. Some investigators are now stressing the importance of hypoxemia and recommending that all high-risk infants be placed on saturation (oximeter) monitors at home. Whether this will be more effective than standard monitoring remains under investigation. Risk profiles are not of predictive value for individual infants. Possible strategies for SIDS prevention are listed in Table 40-5. For the most part, these involve improving the general health and well-being of mothers and infants. Major risk factors such as maternal smoking, prematurity, and possibly infant sleeping position present the pediatric community with a tremendous opportunity for preventive intervention.

## Selected Readings

American Academy of Pediatrics—Task Force on Prolonged Infantile Apnea. Prolonged infantile apnea: 1985. Pediatrics 1985;76:129.

American Academy of Pediatrics—Task Force on Infant Positioning and SIDS: 1992. Pediatrics 1992;90:1120.

Bulterys MG, Greenland S, Krauss JF. Chronic fetal hypoxia and SIDS: interaction between maternal smoking and low hematocrit during pregnancy. Pediatrics 1990;86:535.

Dwyer T, Ponsonby AL, Newman NM, Gibbons LE. Prospective cohort study of prone sleeping position and SIDS. Lancet 1991;337:1244.

Golding J, Limerick S, Macfarlane A. Sudden infant death: patterns, puzzles and problems. Seattle: University of Washington Press, 1985.

Guntheroth WG. Crib death: the sudden infant death syndrome, ed 2. Mount Kisco, NY, Futura Publishing Co., 1989.

Guntheroth WG. Theories of cardiovascular causes in SIDS. J Am Coll Cardiol 1989;14:443.

Guntheroth WG, Lohmann R, Spiers PS. Risk of SIDS in subsequent siblings. J Pediatr 1990;116:520.

Guntheroth WG, Spiers PS. Sleeping prone and the risk of SIDS. JAMA 1992;267:2359.

Harper RM, Hoffman HJ, eds. Sudden infant death syndrome: risk factors and basic mechanisms. New York: PMA Publishing Corp., 1988.

Hoffman HJ, Damus K, Hillman L, Krongrad E. Risk factors for SIDS: results of the National Institute of Child Health and Human Development SIDS cooperative epidemiological study. Ann NY Acad Sci 1988;533:13.

Hunt CE, Brouillette RT. SIDS: 1987 perspective. J Pediatr 1987;110:669.

Kraus JF, Greenland S, Bulterys M. Risk factors for SIDS in the US Collaborative Perinatal Project. Int J Epidemiol 1989;18:113.

Mandell F, Dirks-Smith T, Smith MF. The surviving child in the SIDS family. Pediatrician 1988;15:217.

Mandell F, McClain M. Supporting the SIDS family. Pediatrician 1988;15:179.

Mandell F, McClain M, Reece RM. Sudden and unexpected death: the pediatrician's response. Am J Dis Child 1987;141:748.

Mitchell EA, Scragg R, Stewart AW, et al. Results from the first year of the New Zealand cot death study. N Z Med J 1991;104:71.

Nicholl JP, O'Cathain A. Epidemiology of babies dying at different ages from SIDS. J Epidemiol Community Health 1989;43:13.

NIH Consensus Development Conference of Infantile Apnea and Home Monitoring, 1986. Pediatrics 1987;79:292.

Smialek JE, Lambros Z. Investigation of sudden infant deaths. Pediatrician 1988;15:191.

Taylor EM, Emery JL. Categories of preventable unexpected infant deaths. Arch Dis Child 1990;65:535.

Thach BT, Davies AM, Koenig JS. Pathophysiology of sudden upper airway obstruction in sleeping infants and its relevance for SIDS. Ann NY Acad Sci 1988;533:314.

*Principles and Practice of Pediatrics, Second Edition.*
edited by Frank A. Oski et al. J. B. Lippincott Company, Philadelphia © 1994.

# 40.2 *Apparent Life-Threatening Events*

Gerald M. Loughlin and John L. Carroll

Infants who are unexpectedly discovered with some combination of pallor, hypotonia or hypertonia, cyanosis, apnea, and bradycardia, usually leading to vigorous stimulation or resuscitation by the caretaker, are often perceived by the person who witnesses the event to be at significant risk of dying. In the past, these frightening events were inappropriately called near-miss SIDS or aborted SIDS, based on the unproved assumption that the infant would have died of SIDS if intervention had not occurred. Such episodes are now called *apparent life-threatening events* (ALTE), a term that, like SIDS, describes a clinical syndrome that may result from a multitude of disorders. The absence of respiratory airflow, termed apnea, may be caused by absence of respiratory effort (central), obstruction of the airway (obstructive), or a combination of both mechanisms (mixed). Occasional short apnea, a pause of 15 seconds or less, may be a normal finding at any age. When it is prolonged for 20 or more seconds or is accompanied by cardiac arrhythmias, pallor, hypotonia, or cyanosis, it is termed *pathologic apnea* and warrants further investigation. *Periodic breathing*, recognized as alternating periods of apnea and regular breathing, is defined as three or more breathing pauses of more than 3 seconds' duration, with less than 20 sec-

onds of breathing between pauses. Small amounts of periodic breathing may occur normally during infancy. Brief (<15 seconds) central apnea events are often misinterpreted by anxious parents as being dangerous, adding to the dilemma. Some degree of variability in respiration is common in infants and children.

Whatever the cause, the pediatrician is presented with a frustrating management problem when faced with one of these infants. Despite the absence of definitive information on the etiology and exact nature of the event, evaluation and therapeutic decisions must be made. This chapter will focus on how these children should be evaluated, what tests if any should be ordered, who should be treated and how, and finally who should be monitored at home.

The term ALTE describes a complex of observations and events that are perceived by the child's caretaker to be life-threatening (Table 40-6). Older terms for this problem (aborted SIDS, near-miss SIDS) are a source of confusion and should not be used; the persistence of such terms reflects a failure to understand the epidemiologic implications of the definition of ALTE. Two points will serve to illustrate this. Since an ALTE must by definition be observed, any cause of death that was truly quiet, such as sudden cardiac arrhythmia, would be less likely to appear as an ALTE and more likely to result in quiet unexpected death. Likewise, since observation is required, ALTEs are most likely to occur when the parents or caretakers are awake (9 a.m. to 9 p.m.), which selects events more likely to occur when the infant is awake.

Since it is impossible to ascertain whether an episode was actually life-threatening, the incidence of ALTE is unknown or, at best, crudely estimated. Three percent of 1514 parents of control infants in a SIDS risk factor study reported observing an ALTE or apnea. Oren and colleagues analyzed more than 13,000 referrals and found 1153 with idiopathic sleep apnea, of which only 76 had received CPR for the event. If we assume that the need for CPR actually indicated imminent danger of death, this places the incidence of ALTE, even in a selected population, at about six per 1000.

## ETIOLOGY

ALTE merely describes a manner of presentation for many different disorders (Table 40-7). In most studies of ALTE, a possible cause of the event is discovered in about 50% or more of cases. Previously, an ALTE with no definable etiology was termed apnea

**TABLE 40-6. History of Infants With Unexplained Apparent Life-Threatening Events**

| Symptom | % of Infants |
|---|---|
| Apnea | 82 |
| Pallor | 70 |
| Limpness | 60 |
| Cyanosis | 48 |
| Pallor and limpness | 47 |
| "Lifelessness" | 41 |
| Coldness | 16 |
| Not clear if breathing | 14 |
| Stiffness | 11 |
| Staring/rolling eyes | 10 |
| Shallow breathing | 4 |

*Modified from Dunne KP, Matthews TG. Near-miss sudden infant death syndrome: clinical findings and management. Pediatrics 1987;79:889.*

### TABLE 40-7. Some Causes of Apparent Life-Threatening Events

| | |
|---|---|
| Cardiac disease | CNS neoplasm |
| Respiratory disease | CNS structural abnormalities |
| Upper airway obstruction | Seizures |
| Gastroesophageal reflux | Infection |
| Laryngeal chemoreflex apnea | Metabolic disorders |
| Anemia | Poisoning |
| Hypoventilation syndromes | Prematurity |

of infancy. We find this term confusing and prefer the designation ALTE of unknown etiology.

In both term and preterm infants, about 90% of unexplained ALTEs occur before the infant is 16 weeks old. Apnea with periodic breathing is common in infants born before 37 weeks' gestation (Table 40-8) and is termed apnea of prematurity (AOP) when a treatable cause cannot be found. Since it generally resolves by 37 to 38 weeks after conception, it was formerly a problem almost exclusively encountered in the newborn nursery. However, the move toward earlier discharge of these infants has resulted in increasing numbers of preterm infants who are at home while still vulnerable to this disorder. Consequently, the pediatrician must be aware of this entity, as episodes of AOP may occur after the infant has been discharged and thus considered as an ALTE. It has been estimated that half of premature infants exhibit periodic breathing, and that at least half of those infants will develop AOP.

In the past, AOP was thought to be due to immaturity of central (brain stem) respiratory control and peripheral chemoreceptor function, but this explanation is incomplete. Obstructive or mixed apnea is also common in premature infants, especially during sleep, indicating that the complex mechanisms maintaining upper airway patency and coordinating diaphragm and upper airway, chest, and abdominal muscle function may also be immature in these infants.

AOP should resolve by 37 to 38 weeks of gestational age and usually does not recur, but occasionally AOP may not resolve, even by the time the infant is otherwise ready to be discharged to home. Such *persistent apnea of prematurity* may warrant treatment or continued monitoring at home.

Although apnea may be one component of an ALTE, some apnea is a normal finding at all ages, not all episodes of apnea, even if abnormal, are life-threatening, and not all ALTEs involve apnea. Similarly, although about 18% of SIDS victims are preterm infants, there is no evidence that a history of apnea per se increases the risk for SIDS.

### TABLE 40-8. Specific Causes of Apnea in Preterm Infants

| | |
|---|---|
| Hypoxemia | Temperature sensitivity |
| Respiratory distress | Anemia |
| Sepsis | Patent ductus arteriosus |
| Metabolic disorders | Gastroesophageal reflux |
|   Electrolyte imbalance | Reflex stimulation by catheters |
|   Hypoglycemia | Upper airway obstruction (eg, due to positioning, secretions) |
|   Hyperammonemia | |
|   Acid–base disturbances | Swallowing incoordination during feeding |
|   Amino acid disorders | Hiccups |
| Seizure disorders | |
| CNS malformations | |

## APPROACH TO THE INFANT WITH ALTE

Our lack of understanding of the pathogenesis of SIDS, coupled with our inability to predict who is at risk for a sudden unexplained death, places the physician responsible for these infants in a compromised position. Unfortunately, the limitations of our knowledge have resulted in confusion and controversy surrounding the management of infants who are perceived as being in danger of dying suddenly and unexpectedly. This discussion will focus on a practical approach to the diagnosis and management of infants with ALTE, based on the information currently available. As new information is added and clinical experience expands, these recommendations will undoubtedly change.

The goal of the initial approach to the patient is to rule out treatable causes of life-threatening events, in order to minimize the number of infants left in the idiopathic category. This can be done in about half of the cases.

The pediatrician should remember that in many instances parents have witnessed a normal physiologic variation that appears to be life-threatening to the inexperienced layperson. Normal infants can experience respiratory pauses lasting for up to 15 seconds during sleep. Many of these are unassociated with color change or disruption of oxygenation, and frequently they are preceded by a sigh. However, to a parent waiting for a baby to start breathing again, 10 seconds seems like an eternity. Thus, this infant may be brought to medical attention in an urgent fashion and labeled as abnormal. The physician is confronted by an anxious parent or caretaker who has witnessed an event that is perceived as endangering the child's life. Somehow, the infant at true risk must be identified and the family reassured.

A detailed history of the event must be obtained. Table 40-9 summarizes the important features of this history. A description of the circumstances preceding the event is essential. Was the patient awake or asleep? If the infant was awake, this raises concern about seizures or laryngospasm due to reflux or aspiration. Were these associated with body movements or unusual posturing? This suggests the possibility of a seizure disorder or gastro-

### TABLE 40-9. ALTE Diagnostic Evaluation

**History**

Detailed description of the event from all observers: infant asleep or awake; position infant found in; duration of event; action required to terminate event; association with feeding, choking, formula in nose, body movement; infant's state after event

Perinatal history: labor and delivery, neonatal respiratory problems

Review of systems: infection, feeding, weight gain, vomiting, diarrhea, diet

**Physical Examination**

Vital signs

General appearance, growth parameters

HEENT: fontanelle, eye grounds, nose, mouth and throat

Neck: masses, rigidity

Chest: respiration rate, respiratory noises, signs of upper airway obstruction

Cardiac: rate, rhythm, murmurs

Abdomen

Neurological exam: developmental milestones, tone, reflexes, strength, sensorium, affect

Feeding and sleep patterns

**Screening Labs**

Hgb/Hct

Acid–base status

esophageal reflux. Was the child struggling to breathe (suggestive of airway obstruction), or were respiratory efforts absent?

An accurate description of the intervention required to reestablish normal respirations is very important. Oren and colleagues have demonstrated a strong association between the need for vigorous resuscitation and increased risk of recurrent severe spells and even death. Recovery spontaneously or with minimal intervention (ie, touching the infant) is reassuring and may suggest that what was witnessed was most likely a normal physiologic event. Information about the time required to reverse the event and the infant's mental and physical status after the event is also important.

Establishing a potential relationship between feeding and the apnea event is useful. Dysfunctional swallowing is a common problem in preterm infants, but also can be seen in term infants. Reflex apnea and bradycardia can be triggered not only by aspiration but also by reflux of formula into the nasopharynx. Apnea may be central or obstructive.

Was the infant premature? Was there difficulty with delivery? Was respiration initiated in normal fashion at birth? Has the infant had evidence of prior respiratory difficulties? Have the child's growth and development been appropriate? These questions help establish a predisposition to abnormalities in control of respiration and also help to identify a chronic condition.

Is there a family history of sudden unexplained death in other siblings or relatives, including children and adults? Is there a family history of snoring or obstructive sleep apnea? This information suggests a possible familial predisposition to respiratory control disorders. In the physical examination (see Table 40-9), signs of acute illness such as sepsis and meningitis should be sought. Assessment of growth and development, along with a focus on cardiac, neurologic, and respiratory systems, is necessary to identify subtle signs of chronic conditions that may predispose to life-threatening events.

## Laboratory Studies

Laboratory studies should be reserved for infants whose history and physical examination suggest that this was a significant event. The extent of the initial evaluation has changed dramatically. The minimum evaluation should include a complete blood count with differential, looking for either anemia or polycythemia and signs of acute infection. A hematocrit in the high 30s or 40s in an infant aged 2 to 3 months whose hematocrit should be at physiologic nadir suggests underlying chronic hypoxemia. On the other hand, hematocrit values in the 20s have been associated with apnea and bradycardia in the preterm infant. Measurement of blood glucose (if the infant has not been fed recently) and some measure of acid–base status should also be obtained. A serum bicarbonate level is a particularly useful test. A low value suggests that the event may have been severe enough to result in a metabolic acidosis, or may suggest the presence of an underlying metabolic disorder. On the other hand, elevation of serum bicarbonate is consistent with chronic compensation for respiratory acidosis.

Based on results of these tests, the history and physical examination, or subsequent observations, other studies may be indicated (Table 40-10). However, these tests are not necessary for all infants with life-threatening events, since their yield without specific indications is generally low. For example, evaluation for gastroesophageal reflux should be reserved for infants with spells associated with emesis or the finding of gastric contents in the oropharynx at the time of the event. Similarly, events temporarily related to feedings or associated with choking and obstructive breathing, particularly when the infant is awake, require study of the esophageal function. Apnea with feeding is best evaluated using a dilute barium solution. However, many infants will have

| Study | Possible Diagnosis |
|---|---|
| Chest radiography | Respiratory symptoms, screen for cardiac disease |
| Barium swallow | Dysfunctional swallowing, gastroesophageal reflux, upper airway obstruction |
| EEG | Seizure disorder |
| ECG and echo | Rule out cardiac disease or cor pulmonale |
| pH probe | Suspicion of gastroesophageal reflux |
| Sleep studies (pneumograms or polysomnograms) | Unusual apnea, recurrent alarms, need to assess oxygenation, obstructive apnea |

TABLE 40-10. Other Studies Possibly Indicated in Children with ALTE

brief episodes of reflux on barium swallow, and this finding does not indicate a causal relationship to the ALTE. A pH probe study to document abnormal amounts of reflux or an association between a reflux episode and clinical symptoms may be helpful in defining a potential relationship.

Similar logic must be applied to decision-making regarding other tests, such as the EEG and ECG. If an initial workup is negative and the infant is quite stable, it is appropriate to defer additional testing pending the child's subsequent clinical course.

## Assessment of Cardiorespiratory Patterns

Stimulated by the hypothesis that some aberration of cardiorespiratory control was involved in a significant number of ALTEs, attempts have been made to record heart rate and respiratory rate over extended periods in these infants to identify underlying abnormalities in cardiorespiratory control that may predict recurrences.

### Pneumograms

This technique records cardiac rate and respiratory effort by transthoracic impedance. These two channels of data can be recorded on tape, paper, or more recently on a computer chip. The latter technique is referred to as *documented monitoring*. Advantages of this approach are that it records all the events that triggered alarms, provides invaluable data on parent compliance with use of the monitor, and provides a longer window of recorded monitoring than the standard pneumogram, which typically is performed for 24 to 48 hours. These procedures are minimally invasive, and the study can be performed at home without disrupting the infant's routine or introducing extraneous stimuli.

Unfortunately, there are limitations to these studies. They cannot predict the risk for SIDS or recurrent ALTE. Obstructive apnea cannot be identified. No behavioral information is provided other than a brief parental diary. Sleep/awake state must be either assessed from the diary provided by the parents or inferred from heart and respiratory patterns. The pneumogram can detect prolonged central apnea and bradycardia, but it cannot provide data on the physiologic significance of less dramatic events, such as periodic breathing or brief apneas.

At present, the role of the pneumogram is evolving. Many centers obtain pneumograms before, during, and at the completion of monitoring. However, review of decision-making practices demonstrates that in most instances the decision to initiate monitoring is based on clinical rather than pneumogram data, since a normal pneumogram does not rule out the possibility that another life-threatening event could occur. The recent NIH Consensus Conference reached similar conclusions regarding pneumograms. Thus, pneumograms should not be considered a routine part of the evaluation of an ALTE, and they are not required either to initiate or discontinue home monitoring; both of these decisions can be made on clinical grounds alone.

Documented monitoring may be quite helpful and has been found to be useful in situations in which parents report recurrent alarms. An extended home recording may provide both extremely useful information about the nature of these spells and corroboration of the parents' reports. It also provides information on compliance with use of the monitor.

### Polysomnography

Alternatively, cardiorespiratory patterns can be studied with standard nocturnal polysomnography in a sleep laboratory. The following parameters are monitored: respiration (using abdominal and thoracic strain gauges in conjunction with a monitor of nasal and oral airflow), oxygenation (by pulse oximetry), ECG, EEG, and sleep state; activity during sleep usually is also recorded by videotape. These studies are generally performed overnight, but have also been used effectively in young infants during daytime naps. There is concern, however, that nap studies may miss abnormal events that occur only at night.

Polysomnograms provide extensive physiologic information. Not only can obstructive apnea be identified, but the physiologic consequences of events such as periodic breathing, hypopnea, and short apnea spells can be identified because oxygenation can be monitored. Significant gas-exchange abnormalities can occur in some infants during episodes of periodic breathing or short apneas (<10 seconds). Neither the duration nor the frequency of these respiratory events would distinguish these infants from those who experience no change in oxygenation during these respiratory pauses. Polysomnograms also provide important information on the relationship between breathing patterns and sleep states. Since a technician is present and the study is frequently videotaped, it is possible to correlate behavioral events with physiologic recordings. This is especially useful if seizures are considered as a cause of the apnea.

Limitations of polysomnography include the fact that it is more disruptive to usual routines. Studies are performed in strange surroundings, and many more wires are attached to the infant than in the home setting. These studies are also more expensive. Unfortunately, as with pneumograms, polysomnography has not been shown to be predictive of subsequent risk for SIDS or ALTE. However, only a few studies have used polysomnography in a large number of infants with ALTE. Obstructive and central apneas have been identified in some infants thought to be at risk for SIDS, and these obstructive spells would not have been detected by pneumograms.

In summary, studies of cardiorespiratory patterns cannot be used to predict subsequent risk for death from SIDS. However, if used judiciously, these studies can provide important information useful in the management of infants who have recurrent ALTE or recurrent alarms while on home monitoring.

## MANAGEMENT

For infants who required minimal intervention and who appear quite normal on physical examination, discharge from the emergency room or clinic may be possible without an extensive workup. However, sufficient time must be spent with the family to answer questions, explain the normal variations in respiratory patterns, and reassure them that their baby does not demonstrate evidence of underlying disease. Follow-up should be provided for the family in the event of questions or if the child has another event.

An infant who experiences a severe ALTE should be monitored in a hospital for 48 hours after the event. Hospitalization allows for a period of close observation. All infants should be placed on both cardiac and respiratory monitors and should be easily observable by the medical and nursing staff. This initial monitoring must be done quite carefully, since undocumented false alarms will lead to increased anxiety for the family and may lead to additional and unnecessary studies. Hospitalization also allows the nursing staff to obtain important information on parent/child interactions and on feeding skills of the infant and parents, and to observe the development of clinical symptoms of an underlying disease. Hospitalization allows time for initial laboratory data to be analyzed and if necessary for secondary tests to be ordered.

Finally, many parents are frightened by these events and are quite concerned about the future; a brief hospital stay gives the appropriate medical and other support personnel enough time to talk with the family and to establish relationships that will form the basis for continuity of outpatient support. Furthermore, if a decision is made to initiate cardiorespiratory monitoring, there will be enough time to train the family in the use of the monitor and CPR.

## Conditions Associated With Life-Threatening Events

If a particular condition is identified as the probable cause of the event, therapy should be directed at the underlying disease process, recognizing that the life-threatening event is merely a consequence of this disorder. In that context, the more common conditions associated with life-threatening events or apnea are discussed individually below.

### Acute Infections

In general, infections, including meningitis, sepsis, and pneumonia, should be treated as in routine practice. Bronchiolitis caused by respiratory syncytial virus is frequently associated with apnea early in the course of the illness, often before the usual manifestations of bronchiolitis are apparent. Therapy is supportive. Occasionally, ventilatory support is required. The role of theophylline as a respiratory stimulant is unclear in these conditions. The pathogenesis of the apnea is unknown, but is probably related to effects of the virus on respiratory control.

There are limited data on the indications for home monitoring in this population. Since the condition appears to be self-limited, monitoring is generally unnecessary. However, if there is significant concern about subsequent events, then the recommendations for ALTEs with no definable etiology should be used.

### Gastroesophageal Reflux

If an association between the ALTE and gastroesophageal reflux is established either by laboratory studies or by clinical observation, simple standard medical management should be initiated, including use of the prone position with head elevated, thickened feedings, and avoidance of infant or car seats for 1 to 2 hours after feeding. Persistence of spells after institution of this therapy, or an initial spell that results in a need for vigorous resuscitation, is an indication for use of metoclopramide (0.1 mg/kg/dose four times a day p.o.) or bethanechol (3.0 mg/m$^2$/dose every 8 hours p.o.). Only limited clinical research data support their use, but experience has documented a positive response to these agents in terms of a reduction in episodes in some patients.

If the ALTE was severe or there is concern about the effectiveness of therapy, home apnea/bradycardia monitoring should be instituted in addition to medical management of reflux. Although fundoplication is generally not needed, there are some infants who have persistent spells and documented reflux despite medical management. Surgery may be indicated if it can be established that control of reflux by use of continuous low-volume nasogastric feeding results in cessation of the episodes, and that these spells are severe enough to represent a continued threat to the child's life. Since reflux is in general a self-limited condition, a conservative approach is usually justified. Maturation of gastroesophageal sphincter function generally results in a cessation of ALTE in these children.

### Seizures

Seizures can present as apnea spells, especially awake apnea. Frequently, the diagnosis of seizure is not readily apparent because these infants may not have tonic-clonic movements. Therapy should focus on seizure control. Home monitoring may be indicated for a limited time until seizure control can be ensured.

### Feeding

Events related to feeding are most common in premature infants and represent a maturational delay in the development of the suck-swallow mechanism. Improvement is predicated on the assumption that substantial CNS injury has not occurred. In the most severe cases, avoidance of oral feedings is necessary until maturation occurs. Occasionally, apnea during feeding is associated with marked gastroesophageal reflux. Monitoring is generally not required for apnea associated with feeding, since the events are almost exclusively related to feeding, a time when the infant is being observed.

### Disorders of Respiratory Control

In respiratory control disorders, the episodes generally occur during sleep. Apnea with secondary bradycardia occurs. The events are central in origin and if recurrent can result in marked hypoventilation. Occasionally, obstructive or mixed apnea occurs. Therapy includes a variety of pharmacologic agents (methylxanthine, medroxyprogesterone, doxapram). In more severe cases, mechanical ventilation during sleep may be necessary. These infants require nocturnal cardiorespiratory monitoring. Methylxanthine and caffeine therapy have been tried in this setting, but their effectiveness in infants with structural abnormalities or brain stem injury appears limited.

### ALTE With No Definable Cause

Infants who have ALTE with no definable cause represent the major management dilemma for the practitioner. The data on the risks of subsequent spells and possible death are limited and somewhat biased by interventions. The physician has, at best, three therapeutic options: no intervention, the use of respiratory stimulants, or home monitoring. Because monitoring has not been demonstrated to reduce the incidence of SIDS, some have recommended a nonintervention approach once treatable or diagnosable conditions are eliminated. This choice is not popular with many families, but it is an option, assuming the family can be reassured and the physician is comfortable that the event is not severe. Unfortunately, many families and physicians are extremely uncomfortable with doing nothing.

An alternative approach includes the use of respiratory stimulants such as theophylline or caffeine. They have been used effectively in AOP and have been shown to correct potential abnormalities found on pneumograms (ie, reduction of periodic breathing and short apneas). They also have been used successfully in infants who have recurrent apnea alarms while on home monitoring. However, since the clinical significance of increased periodic breathing and short apneas is unclear, the use of respiratory stimulants may constitute treating a laboratory tracing rather than the patient.

The recommended dosage of theophylline is between 1 and 2 mg/kg every 8 hours. A level of about 10 $\mu$g/dL is generally adequate to control symptoms. Because no readily accessible oral caffeine preparation is available, theophylline is generally the drug of choice. Since metabolism in young children may be unpredictable, it is important that levels be followed. Also, theophylline has been shown to decrease lower esophageal sphincter tone, and thus may make reflux worse. It is also a general CNS stimulant and may lower the seizure threshold. Because both of these conditions can result in ALTE, the physician should be reasonably comfortable that these conditions are not present before using theophylline. If ALTEs increase after theophylline has been started, these conditions should be reconsidered. Considering the potential side effects, theophylline therapy should be reserved for infants with recurrent spells (apnea) documented by monitor alarms. Therapy should be continued until the spells have been absent for several weeks. Weaning from the medication is unnecessary, but home monitoring should continue for at least 6 weeks after the drug is stopped.

## Home Monitoring

Although technically not a treatment, the third option, home cardiorespiratory monitoring, has emerged as the most widely used approach to the problem. The use of monitoring has increased out of a sense of frustration about the unknown and unpredictable nature of these spells, coupled with an effort to alleviate parental fears and stress. Current indications for home monitoring are listed in Table 40-11. This discussion focuses on the first indication, since the others are relatively straightforward.

There are no clear-cut guidelines on which to base the decision to initiate home monitoring. As discussed in the section on pneumograms, there are no tests that clearly define the subgroup of infants with ALTE who are truly at risk of sudden death. About 60% of infants who required vigorous resuscitation have been noted to have a second severe spell; consequently, this group should be monitored. However, for most infants reported to have an ALTE, the circumstances are unclear.

The following basic guidelines can be used to approach the problem. Considering all the unknown variables, an infant who is reported to have had a life-threatening event and in whom an etiology cannot be established should be considered at increased risk of a subsequent event. Unless there is evidence to suggest otherwise, the parents' or caretakers' observations must be considered valid and accurate. In addition, a negative laboratory evaluation does not necessarily indicate that a significant event did not occur or that it will not happen again.

The physician responsible for the child is frequently asked about the chances that an event will recur at a time when no one is watching the child. Since this question cannot be answered with certainty, home monitoring has evolved as a way, albeit an

---

**TABLE 40-11. Current Indications for Home Monitoring**

Infants with severe ALTE requiring vigorous resuscitation and for whom no treatable cause can be identified (monitoring for infants with milder spells and siblings of SIDS victims is somewhat controversial)

Infants with tracheostomy under 1 year

Infants with BPD on supplemental oxygen

Infants with potential treatable causes of ALTE in order to assess response to therapy

Premature infants discharged on methylxanthine therapy for persistent apnea

imperfect one, of providing some security for the family. Thus, if the parents' observations suggest that an event occurred that apparently threatened the child's life and for which a correctable cause cannot be found, home monitoring should be used for the period of presumed increased risk. This decision is based on clinical judgment.

Instituting home monitoring is a medical recommendation with advantages and disadvantages that must be discussed in detail with the family. Home monitoring should be instituted only after a careful assessment of the home environment, including the skills and abilities of those responsible for the infant. The individuals responsible for the infant must be instructed in the use of the monitor and in infant CPR. The family should be prepared to recognize and deal with subsequent spells, including making provisions for contacting emergency services.

Follow-up for the infant and access to support systems are essential to the success of any home monitoring program. Frequently, these infants are referred to centers with resources dedicated to management of infants on home monitoring. These centers, in conjunction with primary-care physicians, can provide the appropriate level of support for these families. Contact with the family should be fairly frequent initially, and then can be tapered as the family settles into the routine.

Home monitoring is not without problems. False alarms are a significant nuisance. Despite attempts on the part of manufacturers to minimize them, they are still an unavoidable problem or necessary evil of monitoring. Monitoring systems must be sensitive to disturbances in normal cardiorespiratory patterns. As a result, shallow breathing episodes, which are a regular occurrence during deep sleep, are frequently interpreted by the monitor as apnea, and alarms are triggered. The monitor cannot distinguish between these events and something pathologic; thus, it must err on the side of caution. In addition, heart-rate norms are not clearly established, and as the infant matures isolated bradycardia alarms may increase in frequency. After the alarm, parents usually find the infant sound asleep and breathing normally. Readjusting the low-heart-rate alarm often alleviates this problem, but these spells must be distinguished from bradycardia associated with obstructive apnea. Any evidence of increased respiratory effort with these alarms is an indication for polysomnography.

The characteristics required for a basic monitor for home use are summarized in Table 40-12. Many monitors in use today have these characteristics, but none of the commercially available home monitors can detect obstructive apnea. Unexplained bradycardia can be presumed to be secondary to obstructive apnea, but polysomnography, or at least recording flow in addition to chest wall movement, is required to detect this event reliably. State-of-the-art monitors should be able to recognize central pauses of varied duration as well as bradycardia and tachycardia.

---

**TABLE 40-12.  Characteristics of an Acceptable Monitor**

Ability to detect both bradycardia and tachycardia

Ability to detect central apnea

Ability to detect monitor dysfunction

Ability to identify what triggered the alarm (monitor dysfunction, bradycardia, loose lead, apnea)

Simplicity of operation

Safety

Portability

Powered by battery and AC

Ability to detect unauthorized changes in settings (generally due to siblings) or loss of power

---

The monitor also should be able to tell when it is not working or when a lead is loose. Since parents are asked to provide information about what triggered alarms, the monitor should indicate what initiated the alarm.

The home monitor should not require an engineering degree to be used safely. It should have a simple operating manual, and the supplier must be able to provide troubleshooting services and personal instruction in use of the monitor. Infants at risk for life-threatening events frequently must be monitored in settings other than the home. Events have been reported in car seats, for example, and therefore the monitor must be portable and operate from a reliable battery source.

Safety is an additional factor. Reports of infants who have been electrocuted because a monitor lead was inadvertently plugged into an AC outlet by a sibling, and of infants who have become entangled in monitor wires, demonstrate the need to minimize these electrical and mechanical hazards. Active and inquisitive siblings pose a particular problem. Monitors can be turned off and alarm settings changed by curious siblings, so the monitor alarm should sound if the power is turned off or the settings are changed inadvertently. Many monitors have been childproofed by requiring that any change must occur in a certain sequence or while a second button is depressed, essentially preventing the average toddler from making unauthorized and unrecognized changes in the monitoring status.

The reliability of the supplier is as important as the equipment. The number of monitoring companies has increased without real controls or standards. The physician prescribing the machine must monitor the supplier to ensure the quality of the equipment delivered and the adequacy of training and of company responsiveness to families' requests and needs.

In general, families are relieved to have something to fall back on, especially if the event occurred during a nap or at night, times when infants usually are unobserved. Occasionally, after a thorough discussion of the risks and benefits, parents may choose not to initiate monitoring. This is not unreasonable, since monitoring has not been clearly shown to prevent death or subsequent severe events. The one instance in which this noninterventionist position is not appropriate is in the case of an infant who required vigorous resuscitation to overcome the first event. These infants appear to be at significant risk for subsequent life-threatening spells and should be monitored.

When a treatable cause of the event has been identified, appropriate therapy initiated, and the problem controlled, home monitoring should not be necessary. Exceptions to this recommendation can be made if the treatment efficacy is questionable or if compliance with drug therapy may be a problem. In these instances, temporary use of the monitor may be helpful. Also, if the cause of a life-threatening spell is not readily amenable to therapy, home monitoring may be useful to protect the child until a therapeutic plan can be developed. Home monitoring should not be necessary for infants who have had spells associated with an acute infection, once treatment or time has resulted in resolution of the acute illness.

An area of particular concern and confusion is that of the risk of siblings of SIDS victims. Previous data suggested that these infants were at increased risk for SIDS, but recent studies have indicated that this risk is not increased over that in the general population. Based on these data, the recommendation of the recent NIH Consensus Conference was that siblings should not be monitored automatically until there have been two deaths in the family. This conference recommendation may be the most controversial and difficult to follow. Considering the uncertainty surrounding SIDS and the effects on a family of the fear of losing a second child to this unknown syndrome, it would seem that despite the limitations of monitoring, this is a situation in which monitoring an infant through the first several months of life may reduce stress in the family. If the second child should have a life-threatening episode, the presence of a system in the home that may detect the problem could be a factor in preventing mortality and reducing morbidity and anxiety in the home. However, this is certainly an unproven therapeutic intervention.

Our recommendation for subsequent siblings of SIDS victims is that home monitoring should be considered, and the pros and cons should be discussed with the family. Monitoring may alleviate stress in the family through a difficult period. If a decision is made to monitor, the monitoring should continue several weeks beyond the age at death of the sibling. However, some families may opt for shorter periods of monitoring, especially if there are no alarms within the early weeks or months of monitoring.

Other situations in which home monitoring has been used are for infants who have experienced AOP and infants with bronchopulmonary dysplasia. Current available data, as well as the recommendation of the NIH Consensus Conference, suggest that a history of AOP does not increase the risk of SIDS beyond that of prematurity itself. Thus, home monitoring is generally not indicated for infants with AOP unless apnea persists at the time of anticipated discharge or the infant continues on theophylline therapy. Monitoring in either the home or the hospital should be continued for several weeks after theophylline or caffeine is discontinued. On the other hand, infants with bronchopulmonary dysplasia who require supplemental oxygen have an increased risk of sudden unexplained death. Whether or not these children should be considered in the SIDS population is irrelevant; this increased risk appears significant, and these children should be monitored until several weeks after oxygen therapy has been stopped.

Home monitoring is not a panacea. Despite its extensive use, its effect on the incidence of SIDS has been minimal. However, monitoring has had some influence on the outcome for infants who were observed to have had a life-threatening event requiring vigorous intervention. Several studies have demonstrated a reduction in subsequent deaths in this high-risk population.

Monitoring is also a mixed blessing for the family. The frequent false alarms are a particular problem because there is no way to know that the alarm is false until the infant is checked. Monitors change the family's lifestyle. The mother often bears the major burden of responsibility for the child. Routine daily procedures like vacuuming and showering must be scheduled around times when someone is available to monitor the infant. Locating babysitters is a problem. This is not totally related to the monitor, since the idea of caring for a child who is at risk for a life-threatening event generally frightens away caretakers. Many babysitters are not CPR-certified. Thus, families often find themselves isolated.

Respite care or help in identifying and training alternate caretakers is an important component of any comprehensive monitoring program. Parent support groups are often helpful in this area. However, the stress imposed by this invasion of technology is less than that created by the lack of a diagnosis and the fear of repeat events that might not be detected until it is too late. In general, monitors provide a sense of security for families and, despite the limitations and nuisance, many families would rather have the monitor.

The decision to discontinue monitoring is influenced by a va-

riety of factors. If monitoring was initiated for an ALTE, it should be continued for at least 2 months beyond the last event or "real" alarm. Bradycardia due to inappropriate alarm-setting or shallow breathing interpreted as apnea by the monitor should not be counted. The infant should be at least 6 months old (the incidence of SIDS decreases rapidly after 6 months) and have had at least one DPT immunization and one upper respiratory infection before discontinuing the monitor; these are considered to be stress tests. (The DPT vaccine has *not* been shown to increase the risk of SIDS, but there is an apparent association between viral upper respiratory tract infections and SIDS.)

Cessation of monitoring for other conditions is based on the natural course of the disease and the response to therapy. If drug therapy (methylxanthine, antireflux or seizure medication) has been used, monitoring usually should be continued for at least 1 month after the drug therapy has been stopped. This is somewhat arbitrary, and decisions must be individualized. Monitoring for a sibling of a SIDS victim generally continues until several weeks beyond the age at which the other child died.

Discontinuing the monitor is difficult for parents. Many families become dependent on it, so the physician and support team frequently must increase their involvement with the family to support them through the weaning process. Families anxious about stopping the monitor should start by not monitoring the infant during naps to facilitate the transition to no monitoring.

## THE FUTURE

Much work remains to be done in improving our understanding of the pathogenesis of life-threatening events. This work must include studies of respiratory control during both sleep and wakefulness, better methods of identifying the population at true risk, and improved monitoring if it remains a cornerstone of management.

## Selected Readings

Ariagno RL, et al. Near-miss for SIDS infants: a clinical problem. Pediatrics 1983;71: 726.

Brazy JE, et al. Central nervous system structural lesions causing apnea at birth. J Pediatr 1987;111:163.

Dunne KP, Matthews TG. Near-miss SIDS: clinical findings and management. Pediatrics 1987;79:889.

Golding J, Limerick S, Macfarlane A. Sudden infant death: patterns, puzzles, and problems. Seattle: University of Washington Press, 1985.

Hunt CE, et al. SIDS: 1987 perspective. J Pediatr 1987;110:669.

NIH Consensus Development Conference Proceedings: Infantile Apnea and Home Monitoring. NIH publication No. 87-2905. US Department of Health and Human Services, NIH, 1986.

Oren J, et al. Identification of a high-risk group for SIDS among infants who were resuscitated for sleep apnea. Pediatrics 1986;77:495.

Petersen DR, et al. Infant mortality among subsequent siblings of infants who died of SIDS. J Pediatr 1986;108:911.

Shannon DC, et al. SIDS and near-SIDS, parts 1 and 2. N Engl J Med 1982;306: 959.

Southall DP. Home monitoring and its role in SIDS. Pediatrics 1983;72:133.

Southall DP, et al. Identification of infants destined to die unexpectedly during infancy: evaluation of predictive importance of prolonged apnea and disorders of cardiac rhythm or conduction. Br Med J 1983;286:1092.

Valdes-Dapena MA. SIDS: a review of the medical literature, 1974–1979. Pediatrics 1980;66:597.

Werthammer J, et al. SIDS in infants with bronchopulmonary dysplasia. Pediatrics 1982;60:301.

Weese-Mayer DB, et al. Assessing validity of infant monitoring alarms with event recording. J Pediatr 1989:115:702.

*Principles and Practice of Pediatrics, Second Edition.*
edited by Frank A. Oski et al. J. B. Lippincott Company, Philadelphia © 1994.

# 40.3 *Obstructive Sleep Apnea Syndrome*

## Carole L. Marcus and John L. Carroll

The obstructive sleep apnea syndrome (OSAS) is an important cause of morbidity in children. If left untreated, it can result in cor pulmonale, neurologic impairment, and even death. Pediatric OSAS was recently rediscovered when it was described in detail by Christian Guilleminault in 1976. However, the earliest descriptions of this syndrome date back to the writings of William Osler, more than a century ago.

Obstructive apnea is defined as the cessation of airflow at the nose and mouth, despite continued respiratory effort, secondary to airway obstruction. This is distinct from central apnea, where cessation of airflow is associated with absent respiratory effort. Many children with OSAS exhibit continuous partial airway obstruction, associated with hypoxemia and hypoventilation, rather than complete airway obstruction; this has been termed *obstructive hypoventilation*.

The prevalence of OSAS in the pediatric age group is unknown. The peak incidence, mirroring the peak incidence of adenotonsillar hypertrophy, is at 3 to 6 years of age, but OSAS can occur at any age, from the neonatal period on. In children, OSAS occurs equally among boys and girls.

## PATHOPHYSIOLOGY

The upper airway (naso-, oro-, and hypopharynx) is usually patent, but it has the potential to collapse in order to facilitate speech and swallowing. In patients with OSAS, the upper airway remains patent during wakefulness, but collapses abnormally during sleep.

OSAS results from a combination of abnormal neuromuscular control and anatomical narrowing of the upper airway. During wakefulness, the patient with a narrow airway can compensate by augmenting upper airway muscle tone. However, during sleep there is a decrease in ventilatory drive and in neuromuscular tone, facilitating upper airway collapse. In children, the anatomical narrowing is usually due to adenotonsillar hypertrophy. Other common causes of structural narrowing include nasal obstruction, micrognathia, fat deposition around the airway, or craniofacial anomalies. Obstruction at or below the level of the epiglottis results in stridor and persistent airway obstruction rather than OSAS. Children with syndromes encompassing developmental delay, hypotonia, obesity, and upper airway narrowing (eg, children with trisomy 21) are at very high risk for OSAS.

## HISTORY

Most children present with a history of snoring and difficulty breathing during sleep. The onset is usually insidious. Children with OSAS have persistent, loud snoring that often can be heard outside the bedroom. During sleep, the child has labored breathing, retractions, and paradoxical inward motion of the chest wall during inspiration. During periods of complete obstruction, the child can be observed to be making respiratory efforts, but no snoring is heard and no airflow is detected. Obstructive episodes are usually terminated by gasping, motion, or arousal. The child

sleeps restlessly and may adopt bizarre sleeping positions, such as sleeping in a seated position or with the neck hyperextended. Enuresis is common. Diaphoresis, pallor, or cyanosis may be present. The appearance of the child during sleep can be so alarming that it is not unusual for parents to maintain bedside vigils, or to continually stimulate or reposition the child throughout the night. Despite this, many parents do not volunteer a history of their child's sleep symptoms unless specifically asked. Most parents can mimic their child's breathing pattern when asked to do so.

During wakefulness, the child breathes normally. Symptoms of tonsilloadenoidal hypertrophy may be present, including mouth breathing, rhinorrhea, and recurrent otitis media. Severely affected patients may have dysarthria or dysphagia. There is often a family history of snoring or OSAS.

## PHYSICAL EXAMINATION

In most children with OSAS, the physical examination during wakefulness is entirely normal. This commonly leads to a delay in diagnosis, as the physician often does not have the opportunity to see the child asleep.

Physical examination should include an assessment of the child's growth. Failure to thrive or, conversely, obesity may be present. Allergic stigmata, mouth breathing, adenoidal facies, midfacial hypoplasia, retro/micrognathia, or other craniofacial abnormalities may be present. The patency of the nares should be assessed. The pharynx should be evaluated for tongue size, palatal integrity, oropharyngeal diameter, redundant palatal mucosa, tonsil size, and uvula size. The lungs are usually clear to auscultation. Cardiac examination may reveal signs of pulmonary hypertension such as an increased pulmonic component of the second heart sound and a right ventricular heave. Neurologic examination should be performed to evaluate muscle tone, developmental status, behavior, and excessive daytime somnolence.

## COMPLICATIONS

Patients with severe OSAS can have failure to thrive. Neurobehavioral complications, which result from sleep fragmentation and nocturnal hypoxemia, include hyperactivity, personality changes, excessive daytime sleepiness, poor school performance, and developmental delay. Seizures, asphyxial brain damage, and coma have been reported. Pulmonary hypertension is a common complication of OSAS and can progress to cor pulmonale and congestive heart failure. This resolves following successful treatment of OSAS. Respiratory arrest and sudden death have been reported.

## DIAGNOSTIC TESTS

The diagnosis of OSAS should be established by polysomnography (sleep study). History alone is inadequate, as it cannot distinguish between OSAS and primary snoring or other causes of sleep-related symptoms. In addition, polysomnography provides objective measures of severity, and provides a baseline for those children whose condition does not resolve postoperatively. During polysomnography, noninvasive monitoring of sleep architecture, chest and abdominal wall motion, airflow, oxygenation, and carbon dioxide tension is performed. Polysomnography should be performed in a laboratory used to studying children, as both techniques and normative values differ widely between children and adults. Home audio/video recording can be a useful screening test. Adenoidal size can be assessed by lateral neck x-ray. An electrocardiogram and echocardiogram should be obtained to evaluate the patient for pulmonary hypertension.

## TREATMENT

Most children are cured by adenotonsillectomy. OSAS results from the relative size and structure of the upper airway components, rather than the absolute size of the tonsils and adenoids. Therefore, both the tonsils and adenoids should be removed, even if one or the other appears to be the primary abnormality. By the same logic, adenotonsillectomy should be the initial treatment of OSAS in children with other predisposing factors (eg, obesity, Down syndrome), although further treatment may be necessary. Although frequently considered to be minor surgery, adenotonsillectomy can be associated with significant complications. Therefore, primary snoring without OSAS is not an indication for surgery. Children with OSAS are at risk for postoperative complications, including upper airway edema, pulmonary edema, and respiratory failure. Perioperative deaths have been reported, so the patient should be monitored closely in the postoperative period. OSAS may not resolve fully until 6 to 8 weeks after surgery.

Occasionally, children present with severe OSAS that requires emergency admission to the hospital. Monitoring in the hospital should include pulse oximetry, as cardiorespiratory monitors alone will not detect obstructive apnea until bradycardia occurs. Sedative drugs should be avoided, as these may aggravate OSAS. Supplemental oxygen should not be given without simultaneous monitoring of $P_{CO_2}$, as it may precipitate respiratory failure. Obstructive episodes can be terminated by awakening the patient, but this is obviously only a very temporary solution. Nasopharyngeal tubes can be placed to bypass the obstruction pending definitive treatment. Vigilant nursing is necessary, as the tubes frequently clog with mucus. If nasopharyngeal tubes are unsuccessful in relieving the obstruction, the patient should be intubated. Alternatively, nasal continuous positive airway pressure may be given. Steroids shrink lymphoid tissue, including adenoidal tissue, and can relieve OSAS within 24 hours. This effect usually lasts only a few days or weeks, but may be useful in patients who cannot undergo immediate surgery.

A minority of patients with OSAS do not respond to adenotonsillectomy. When applicable, specific surgery should be performed at the site of obstruction (eg, lip-tongue adhesion procedures in patients with Pierre Robin syndrome). Some patients benefit from uvulopharyngopalatoplasty. Obese patients should be encouraged to lose weight. Continuous positive airway pressure, delivered by nasal mask, is used widely in the treatment of OSAS in adults. It can be used effectively in children, although compliance and mask size can be problematic with young children. Children with severe OSAS unresponsive to the above treatments, especially children with craniofacial anomalies, may require tracheostomy.

## PROGNOSIS

Most children experience a dramatic resolution of their symptoms following adenotonsillectomy. However, the natural course and the long-term prognosis of pediatric OSAS are unknown. Children with treated OSAS may be at risk for recurrence during adulthood.

## Selected Readings

Brouillette RT, Fernbach SK, Hunt CE. Obstructive sleep apnea in infants and children. J Pediatr 1982;100:31.

Guilleminault C, Eldrige F, Simmons FB, Dement WC. Sleep apnea in eight children. Pediatrics 1976;58:23.
Hudgel DW. Mechanisms of obstructive sleep apnea. Chest 1992;101:541.
Mallory GB Jr, Fiser DH, Jackson R. Sleep-associated breathing disorders in morbidly obese children and adolescents. J Pediatr 1989;115:892.
Marcus CL, Keens TG, Bautista DB, von Pechmann WS, Ward SLD. Obstructive sleep apnea in children with Down syndrome. Pediatrics 1991;88:132.

*Principles and Practice of Pediatrics, Second Edition.*
edited by Frank A. Oski et al. J. B. Lippincott Company, Philadelphia © 1994.

# 40.4 *Central Hypoventilation Syndromes*

Carole L. Marcus

Central alveolar hypoventilation is defined as an increase in arterial carbon dioxide tension (>45 mm Hg) due to a decrease in CNS ventilatory drive. It is usually associated with hypoxemia. Patients with central hypoventilation fail to breathe normally despite having normal lungs, upper airway, and chest wall. Central hypoventilation may be congenital or acquired, and primary or secondary. Causes of central hypoventilation are listed in Table 40-13.

**TABLE 40-13. Causes of Central Hypoventilation**

**Primary**
Congenital central hypoventilation syndrome (CCHS)
Central hypoventilation syndromes associated with endocrine dysfunction

**Secondary**
*Obesity Hypoventilation Syndrome*
*Increased Intracranial Pressure*
Arnold-Chiari malformation
Ventriculoperitoneal shunt malfunction
Achondroplasia
Other causes
*Central Hypoventilation Associated With Brain Stem Lesions*
Hypoxic-ischemic encephalopathy
Trauma
Hemorrhage
Tumor
Congenital anomalies
Moebius syndrome
Meningoencephalitis
Poliomyelitis
*Central Hypoventilation Associated With Other Neurologic Syndromes*
Autonomic neuropathies (familial dysautonomia)
Subacute necrotizing encephalomyelopathy (Leigh's disease)
Mitochondrial defects
Neurodegenerative syndromes
*Miscellaneous*
Drugs
Hyperthermia
Hypothyroidism
Metabolic dysfunction, inborn errors of metabolism

## CLINICAL FEATURES

Patients with congenital central hypoventilation usually present in the neonatal period with cyanosis or apnea. Although they may present at a later age, symptoms usually can be traced to infancy. Patients with acquired central hypoventilation can present at any age. Patients may initially have nonspecific symptoms, such as lethargy, poor sleep, irritability, or morning headaches. These subtle signs are frequently overlooked, and it is not unusual for patients to be diagnosed only following catastrophic events, such as apparent life-threatening events, seizures, or congestive heart failure resulting from cor pulmonale.

Patients with central hypoventilation do not have signs of respiratory distress or increased respiratory effort even when severely hypoxemic or hypercapnic; the term "happy hypoxia" has been applied. This is in marked contrast to patients with respiratory failure secondary to pulmonary mechanical abnormalities or ventilatory muscle weakness, who have subjective distress, tachypnea, and thoracic retractions. Patients with central hypoventilation usually have shallow breathing rather than bradypnea or frank central apnea. The patient may be able to transiently breathe adequately when instructed to do so. The breathing pattern may be abnormal only during sleep, especially in children with the congenital central hypoventilation syndrome (CCHS).

On physical examination, growth failure or signs of pulmonary hypertension may be present. In children with secondary central hypoventilation, the underlying condition or associated neurologic abnormalities are usually evident.

## LABORATORY DIAGNOSIS

The presence of hypoventilation is established by arterial blood gas analysis. Gas exchange can also be assessed noninvasively by polysomnography. It is essential to assess gas exchange during both wakefulness and sleep. Potential diagnostic tests are shown in Table 40-14; the choice of tests must be individualized for each patient. Pulmonary and neuromuscular causes of hypoven-

---

**TABLE 40-14. Diagnostic Evaluation of Suspected Hypoventilation**

**Establishing the Presence of Hypoventilation**
Arterial blood gas
Polysomnography

**Establishing the Etiology**
Chest x-ray
Pulmonary function tests
Ventilatory responses to hypoxia and hypercapnia
Diaphragm fluoroscopy
Ventilatory muscle strength evaluation
Fiberoptic laryngoscopy
MRI of brain stem
Brain stem auditory evoked potentials
Endocrine evaluation
Serum glucose, ammonia, pyruvate, lactate
Serum and urinary amino acids, organic acids

**Assessing the Severity**
Hematocrit/hemoglobin
Serum bicarbonate
ECG, echocardiogram

---

tilation must be excluded. In particular, isolated diaphragmatic paralysis should be excluded. The hypoventilation can be assumed to be central in origin if tests of pulmonary function and ventilatory muscle strength are normal. MRI of the brain stem is recommended for all patients with central hypoventilation of undetermined etiology. The diagnosis of CCHS is made primarily by exclusion, according to the following criteria: persistent hypoventilation during sleep ($P_{CO_2}$ consistently >60 mm Hg), onset of symptoms from birth or early infancy, and absence of primary pulmonary, cardiac, CNS, neuromuscular, or metabolic dysfunction.

## TREATMENT

The aims of treatment are to prevent respiratory failure, cor pulmonale (the usual cause of death in patients with central hypoventilation), and hypoxic neurologic damage. Whenever possible, the primary cause of the hypoventilation should be treated. The mainstay of treatment, for those in whom the primary cause of hypoventilation cannot be successfully treated, is ventilatory support. This can be provided by positive pressure ventilation via tracheostomy or nasal mask, diaphragm pacing, or negative pressure cuirass ventilation. Pharmacologic therapy has not been shown to be efficacious. Supportive care includes prompt treatment of respiratory tract infections, avoidance of sedative medications, and nutritional support. With modern techniques for home ventilation, children with central hypoventilation can lead fulfilling lives.

## SPECIFIC DISEASE CONDITIONS

### Congenital Central Hypoventilation Syndrome

CCHS is a rare condition in which patients have intact voluntary control of ventilation but lack automatic control. Previously, this syndrome was named "Ondine's curse" after a German fable; this is no longer used due to its negative connotations. Classically, children with CCHS were described as having normal breathing during wakefulness, but severe hypoventilation during sleep. It is now recognized that many patients with CCHS cannot breathe adequately even when awake. Patients with CCHS can have normal cognitive function if hypoxemic episodes are prevented. Associated abnormalities that may be present include autonomic dysfunction, Hirschsprung's disease, and neural tumors. Rare instances of familial occurrence have been reported. The etiology of CCHS is unknown, and no specific pathologic lesions have been determined. The older literature described substantial morbidity and mortality in children with CCHS. Death usually resulted from cor pulmonale, aspiration, or sepsis. Recent reports describe prolonged survival, with a good quality of life; our oldest patient is currently 16 years of age. However, children continue to need ventilatory support and do not outgrow their disease.

### Obesity Hypoventilation Syndrome

The obesity hypoventilation syndrome (Pickwickian syndrome) occurs in patients with primary obesity or with obesity secondary to other conditions. These patients have a decreased ventilatory drive, resulting in hypercapnia and hypoxemia during both wakefulness and sleep. Cor pulmonale is a common complication. Additional pulmonary problems that may be present include the obstructive sleep apnea syndrome and restrictive lung disease (secondary to obesity). The pathophysiology of the obesity hypoventilation syndrome is not fully understood. Patients with the syndrome have a decreased ventilatory drive in response to hypoxia and hypercapnia. This normalizes with weight loss. It is hypothesized that obese patients have chronic hypoxemia and hypercapnia due to mechanical limitation of ventilation, and therefore develop secondary blunting of their ventilatory drive.

The treatment for the syndrome is weight loss. If the patient has potentially life-threatening complications, such as respiratory failure or cor pulmonale, hospital admission for supervised weight loss is justifiable.

## Arnold-Chiari Malformation

Children with Arnold-Chiari malformations have central hypoventilation secondary to abnormal central chemoreceptor function. The type I Arnold-Chiari malformation consists of caudal herniation of the cerebellar tonsils through the foramen magnum. The type II malformation consists of caudal displacement of the cerebellar vermis, brain stem, and fourth ventricle, and is associated with brain stem compression or dysplasia. The type II malformation is present in the vast majority of patients with myelodysplasia; it is this population that the pediatrician is most likely to encounter. An estimated 6% to 13% of children with myelodysplasia have either vocal-cord paralysis or clinically apparent ventilatory control abnormalities, but subclinical abnormalities are probably present in most patients. Patients with Arnold-Chiari malformation and severe ventilatory control dysfunction may have normal intellectual function. Clinical manifestations of ventilatory control dysfunction include central apnea, cyanotic spells, breath-holding spells, respiratory failure, and sudden death. In addition, children with myelodysplasia are predisposed to other pulmonary problems, such as restrictive lung disease secondary to ventilatory muscle weakness, scoliosis, and aspiration. Bilateral vocal cord paralysis can occur as a result of traction on the vagus nerve roots. An increase in apnea or stridor indicates an increase in intracranial pressure, and "croup" in children with Arnold-Chiari malformation should always be regarded as a sign of increased intracranial pressure until proven otherwise.

Patients with Arnold-Chiari malformation and hypoventilation or vocal cord paralysis usually improve following ventriculoperitoneal shunting or posterior fossa decompression. However, some patients with chronic or severe abnormalities may have dysplasia or necrosis of the brain stem, and require tracheostomy or prolonged ventilatory support.

## Miscellaneous Causes of Central Hypoventilation

Central hypoventilation can result from any congenital or acquired CNS lesion that results either in severe and diffuse neurologic damage, or selective brain stem damage. In patients with hypoventilation secondary to severe CNS dysfunction, palliative treatment (eg, supplemental oxygen) may be preferable to invasive measures that will prolong life without enhancing the quality of life. However, supplemental oxygen alone should be given with caution, as it may suppress the hypoxic ventilatory drive and therefore worsen hypoventilation.

## Genetic Factors

The CNS ventilatory drive in response to hypoxia and hypercapnia varies widely in the normal population and is largely determined by genetic factors. An individual with a congenitally low ventilatory drive may remain asymptomatic as long as he or she does not encounter a stress to the system. However, if asymptomatic individuals with a congenitally low ventilatory drive develop lung disease or are in an hypoxic environment (eg, high altitude), they may not increase their ventilation in response to the stress. This can result in hypoxemia or hypercarbia that appears disproportionate to the degree of illness.

## Selected Readings

Garay SM, Rapoport D, Sorkin B, Epstein H, Feinberg I, Goldring RM. Regulation of ventilation in the obstructive sleep apnea syndrome. Am Rev Resp Dis 1981;124:451.

Hays RM, Jordan RA, McLaughlin JF, Nickel RE, Fisher LD. Central ventilatory dysfunction in myelodysplasia: an independent determinant of survival. Dev Med Child Neurol 1989;31:366.

Marcus CL, Jansen MT, Poulsen MK, et al. Medical and psychosocial outcome of children with congenital central hypoventilation syndrome. J Pediatr 1991;119:888.

Mellins RB, Balfour HH, Turino GM, Winters RB. Failure of automatic control of ventilation (Ondine's curse). Medicine (Baltimore) 1970;49:487.

Rochester DF, Enson Y. Current concepts in the pathogenesis of the obesity-hypoventilation syndrome. Am J Med 1974;57:402.

Swaminathan S, Paton JY, Davidson Ward SL, Jacobs RA, Sargent CW, Keens TG. Abnormal control of ventilation in adolescents with myelodysplasia. J Pediatr 1989;115:898.

Weese-Mayer DE, Silvestri JM, Menzies LJ, Morrow-Kenny AS, Hunt CE, Hauptman SA. Congenital central hypoventilation syndrome: diagnosis, management, and long-term outcome in 32 children. J Pediatr 1992;120:381.

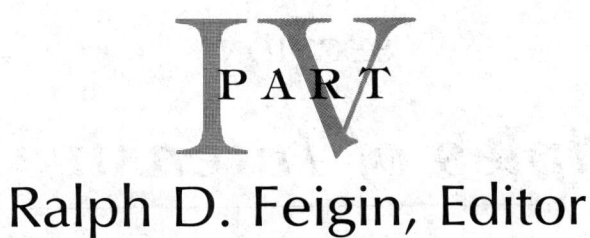

PART

IV

Ralph D. Feigin, Editor

# *The Sick or Hospitalized Patient*

# SECTION I

# Principles of Intensive Care

*Principles and Practice of Pediatrics, Second Edition.*
edited by Frank A. Oski et al. J. B. Lippincott Company, Philadelphia © 1994.

## CHAPTER 41
# Equipment and Techniques

## 41.1 Physical Environment

### Fernando Stein

The pediatric intensive care unit is only as good as the people who work in it. Although excellent equipment is important, the major emphasis should always be the quality of the staff. An area of 120 square feet per child or adolescent patient is a minimum; 144 square feet per patient is ideal. This area is necessary because of recent innovations and additions in equipment, such as ventilators, dialysis machines, suction and infusion pumps, continuous EEG monitoring, and other computerized equipment that can be brought to the bedside.

Each bedside should be equipped with continuous display monitors with at least four channels: heart rate, respiratory rate, and two channels for other aspects of monitoring, such as pressure, $CO_2$, temperature, and respiratory patterns.

The headboard should have sufficient oxygen outlets, compressed air, suction, and three different sets of electrical outlets, as well as 12 or more electrical outlets of standard amperage. At least two 220-amperage outlets and sufficient grounding sockets also should be available.

In areas in which patients are being ventilated with an endotracheal tube, a person who is capable of intubating should be immediately available. Thus, a call room located inside or in immediate proximity to the intensive care unit is strongly suggested.

*Principles and Practice of Pediatrics, Second Edition.*
edited by Frank A. Oski et al. J. B. Lippincott Company, Philadelphia © 1994.

## 41.2 Electrocardiographic and Respiratory Monitors

### Thomas A. Vargo

The monitoring of cardiorespiratory parameters is an integral part of the care of critically ill children. Life-threatening arrhythmias frequently occur as a result of cardiac surgery, electrolyte disturbances, systemic infections, toxic ingestions, cardiomyopathies, antiarrhythmic therapy, cardiac trauma, and various shock states. Seriously ill children should be monitored routinely by continuous oscillographic display of the ECG to detect changes in heart rate, the early development of arrhythmias, and other ECG abnormalities associated with myocardial and metabolic derangements.

## ECG MONITORING

Continuous ECG monitoring of the hospitalized patient most commonly uses a simplified system of three or four electrodes located on the right and left upper chest and the left hip. If a fourth electrode is used, it is placed in the right hip and is usually a grounded lead, but usually the fourth electrode is not needed. The electrodes may have to be moved if an adequate ECG tracing is not obtained. The lead that gives the best visualization of the P, QRS, and T waves should be used. When monitoring specifically for arrhythmias, the lead that shows the P wave best should be used.

Most bedside ECG monitors use a standard oscillometric display at the bedside and a remote display screen at a central location for additional monitoring. Monitors in the ICU should allow permanent graphic recording of the ECG.

A common error in monitoring ECGs is for the clinician to diagnose atrial enlargement from a single lead displayed on an oscilloscopic tracing, not realizing that this tracing usually has a high sensitivity and gives the P waves an exaggerated height. Similarly, abnormal ST segment elevations are sometimes erroneously diagnosed from these ECG recordings. Continuous monitoring of ECG tracings is especially helpful in detecting sinus tachycardia, sinus bradycardia, and widening of the QRS complex. The last two ECG recordings may be due to life-threatening processes such as hypoxemia or hyperkalemia.

## RESPIRATORY MONITORING

Routine monitoring of the respiratory rate and depth of respiration is done by transthoracic bioimpedance. This technique involves placing one electrode on either side of the thorax and a reference electrode over the hip or the apex of the heart. In most pediatric ICUs, the same electrode and oscilloscope used for the ECG also measure respiration. Changes in intrathoracic lung and intravascular blood volumes cause proportional changes in electrical resistance. This information then is used to monitor the respiratory rate and depth of respiration. Alarm systems are incorporated to identify periods of respiratory inactivity. These instruments have been used principally for apnea monitoring, both at home and in the ICU. Respiratory monitors are much less accurate than ECG monitors and are more easily altered by mechanical ventilators, motion of the patient, and so forth.

## PULSE OXIMETRY

Pulse oximetry can be used to monitor the heart rate and to determine indirectly the oxygen saturation of cutaneous blood. A disposable transducer containing a photoelectric diode and light source is attached to an exposed finger or toe. Light emitted by the diode is absorbed in proportion to the level of oxygen-saturated hemoglobin. Erroneous readings occur with anemia, hypotension, polycythemia, and hypothermia. Since pulse oximetry, in essence, measures color, the "redder" the blood is, the higher the oxygen saturation will be because oxyhemoglobin is red. Pulse oximetry is relatively accurate at the 70% to 100% saturation range. It is less accurate at lower ranges, but at the lower ranges it is almost always necessary to check the patient and make changes in his or her therapy to correct any underlying reason for the low saturation.

Since the first edition of this textbook, the use of pulse oximetry has become routine in many situations. It should be used in almost every child where the oxygen saturation may suddenly diminish, such as children receiving general anesthesia, children receiving sedation, intubated patients, mechanically ventilated patients, newborns with cyanotic heart disease, and patients with acute lung disease.

## Selected Reading

Kouffman RE, Banner W Jr, et al. Guidelines for monitoring and management of pediatric patients during and after sedation for diagnostic and therapeutic procedures. Pediatrics 1992;89:1110.

*Principles and Practice of Pediatrics, Second Edition.*
edited by Frank A. Oski et al. J. B. Lippincott Company, Philadelphia © 1994.

# 41.3 *Infusion Devices*

### Fernando Stein

It is a standard of pediatric intensive care to give medications with a short half-life through an infusion device. These devices also are considered for accurate administration of intravenous fluids and to guarantee the constant infusion of volume administered in a given period of time. These devices help to maintain the viability and patency of catheters such as central lines, pulmonary artery catheters, or arterial pressure lines.

In addition to the infusion device, there should be a fluid reservoir that ensures accurate recording of infused fluids. This type of receptacle is available in different sizes according to the patient's age. There are three types of infusion devices: peristaltic infusion by compression of the tubing through a rotatory device, peristaltic infusion through sequential compression of the tubing, and a syringe type of infusion device.

Because many of the pumps are insensitive to obstruction of flow, the site of catheter or needle insertion should be monitored to avoid the complications of extravasation and infiltration.

The standard infusion device can measure up to 999 mL by 1-mL increments. Infusion devices that can deliver fluid in one tenth of National Formulary milliliter increments also are available.

*Principles and Practice of Pediatrics, Second Edition.*
edited by Frank A. Oski et al. J. B. Lippincott Company, Philadelphia © 1994.

# 41.4 *Temperature-Controlling Devices*

### Fernando Stein

Three types of temperature-controlling devices are commonly used in the ICU: the cooling/heating blanket, the radiant warmer, and the incubator. The cooling/heating blanket can be placed between the patient and the bed, thus controlling the temperature while maintaining easy access to the patient. The blanket is particularly useful in children who weigh more than 6 kg, since radiant warming devices are not made to fit children this size. The radiant warming device is an electronic heating apparatus. A heated coil above the patient radiates heat toward him or her; the temperature can be preset or regulated through a servomechanism connected to the child. The standard incubator provides warming by circulating humidified warm air.

All three devices must be checked regularly by the hospital's biomedical instrumentation department for accuracy in the delivered temperature. Patients must be monitored when connected to a warming or cooling device and should have temperature checks every hour. Overheating is the most serious complication of any type of warming device, and it can lead to permanent neurologic damage. Specific recommendations from the manufacturer should always be observed, and personnel should be thoroughly familiar with the details of operation of all warming and cooling devices in use in their units.

Changes in temperature are characteristic of many pathophysiologic processes, so temperature monitoring is crucial in the ICU. There are three basic temperature-sensing devices. The most common is the thermal-expansive thermometer, the standard glass thermometer filled with mercury that is applied to the mouth, axilla, or rectum. It continues to be the most consistently reliable form of monitoring body temperature. When temperature is being monitored hourly, irritation may occur in the area where the thermometer is being applied, particularly the rectum.

Another commonly used device, the thermal-resistive electronic thermometer, produces a reading in about one third to one tenth of the time of the standard mercury thermometer (depending on the patient's temperature), and it has a digital display. This device must be calibrated and checked regularly and must be approved by the biomedical instrumentation department.

The temperature probe is a thermal-sensitive device used to monitor changes in temperature on a minute-by-minute basis. This thermal-resistive thermometer is connected to the rectum or the esophagus; it also can be applied to the axilla.

The main pitfall of monitoring temperature in the ICU is related to accuracy in technique. False elevations may occur when the probe is placed in the axilla or too close to a warming blanket, or when the probe is located near a large blood vessel. An esophageal probe may read the temperature of the cool gases or warm gases that are being circulated in the trachea through the respirator. Meticulous attention to detail is necessary to maintain an appropriate standard in measuring temperature in the ICU setting.

*Principles and Practice of Pediatrics, Second Edition.*
edited by Frank A. Oski et al. J. B. Lippincott Company, Philadelphia © 1994.

# 41.5 *Vascular Catheters*

## Thomas A. Vargo

## PERIPHERAL VENOUS CATHETERS

Venous cannulation is the most common procedure performed in pediatric hospital practice. It is indicated for the administration of drug therapy and intravenous fluids in the child in whom oral therapy is inadequate or contraindicated. In infants, favored sites for intravenous lines include scalp, external jugular, hand, antecubital, foot, and saphenous veins. In older children and adolescents, catheter placement in the lower extremities generally is avoided to promote ambulation.

In infants, 22- and 24-gauge catheters are large enough for most purposes. Larger catheters are used in older children and adolescents. Care should be taken when restricting patient movements during the placement of scalp or external jugular intravenous lines, so as not to compromise the patient's airway.

Site preparation is dictated by the patient's immune status and the purpose of line placement. In general, if the catheter is used for hyperalimentation purposes or if the patient is immunocompromised, site preparation should include a povidone-iodine solution, which is allowed to air dry. For routine administration of fluids and medications or if emergency venous access is required, skin preparation with denatured alcohol is considered

adequate. Covering materials should not obscure easy inspection of the cannula.

In children with right-to-left intracardiac shunts, intravenous lines should be equipped with microfilters inserted distal to all administered fluids to reduce the risk of systemic embolization of air and particulate matter.

Hypertonic medications and solutions should not be given routinely through peripheral catheters. If emergency administration of hypertonic medications becomes necessary and central venous line access is unavailable, peripheral line use is indicated. In such situations, the intravenous line should flush easily and the skin must be observed for any evidence of extravasation or change of skin color over the vein. If practical, catheters used for this purpose should be replaced as soon as possible to avoid the risk of subsequent extravasation.

Risks of peripheral venous catheter placement are related to the patient's underlying clinical illness, to difficulty in catheter insertion, and to the duration of cannulation. A patient with an underlying coagulopathy is at risk for hematoma formation, which can even be life-threatening in rare cases. Sepsis from peripheral venous catheters occurs and is more common in children who are immunocompromised or who have untreated systemic infection before catheter placement. Catheter-related infections can be reduced if the intravenous sites are changed every 2 or 3 days and if catheters are removed after they are no longer medically needed. In many infants and children, it is necessary to use an intravenous cannula longer than this; in these instances the cannula should be inserted sterilely and meticulous attention should be paid to maintaining sterility.

## ARTERIAL CATHETERS

Arterial catheter placement is frequently necessary in the pediatric and neonatal ICU. Continuous systemic pressure monitoring by arterial cannulation is indicated in cases of hypotension that do not respond to initial therapy, and most other cases where the cardiovascular status is unstable. Arterial cannulation also is indicated whenever frequent monitoring of gas exchange is necessary, such as in children receiving mechanical ventilation.

In most cases, the clinician should avoid cannulating the artery in a limb with compromised arterial supply. Examples include arteritis, coarctation of the aorta, previous arterial cutdowns, and any arm that has had a classic Blalock-Taussig shunt.

Preferred sites of arterial cannulation in newborns include the umbilical and radial arteries. In children, the radial and dorsalis pedis arteries are favored cannulation sites because of the collateral circulation supplied by the ulnar and posterior tibial arteries, respectively. Other frequently used sites in children are the femoral and brachial arteries. The brachial artery has limited collateral vessels and if used for arterial cannulation, that limb must especially be observed for any evidence of arterial compromise. Of course, a compromised arterial supply should be observed for in any limb that has an arterial catheter in it.

Catheter insertion is performed using various percutaneous techniques or direct cutdown. The method used is determined by the artery and the technician's expertise. If possible, the smallest catheter that allows easy sampling and gives a good pressure waveform is used. In general, we use a 24-gauge cannula in the extremities of premature infants and a 22-gauge cannula in full-term infants. We usually use a 20-gauge catheter in children weighing more than 10 kg.

## CENTRAL VENOUS CATHETERS

Central venous catheters are indicated when treating hypovolemic or septic shock or myocardial failure, when administering large amounts of fluid or medications, and when transvenous pacing of the heart is necessary. Central venous access is also used in the administration of vasoactive drugs such as dopamine. Hypertonic drugs such as mannitol, 3% saline solution, calcium chloride, and concentrated potassium chloride should be given by central line access. Central venous lines are also useful in children in whom peripheral access is impossible to obtain.

In the newborn, the umbilical vein is the central vein used most frequently. Often the tip of an umbilical vein catheter will be in the left atrium even though on a chest x-ray the catheter may appear to be in the right atrium. This is because the left atrium is essentially behind the right atrium, rather than to the left of it. To help prevent systemic embolization, the umbilical vein catheter tip should be in the right atrium, at or just cephalad to the diaphragm. However, even if the catheter is in the right atrium, paradoxic embolism can still occur.

In older infants and young children, the internal jugular, brachial, median basilic, and femoral veins are the sites used most frequently. The subclavian route also is used in children and adolescents.

In our institution, the femoral vein is the site used most frequently in children. The internal jugular route also is used frequently but requires more technical mastery, and complications arising from accidental puncture of local structures are associated with a higher risk of morbidity and mortality. In a child with coagulation abnormalities, the antecubital region is the preferred insertion site. In older children and adolescents, large-bore central catheters often can be inserted through an antecubital vein.

Before catheter placement, the patient should be placed in a position that favors cannulation. The Trendelenburg position is used for insertion of catheters into the internal jugular or subclavian veins, whereas the reverse Trendelenburg position is often used for brachial and femoral cannulation. Again, rigorous attention should be focused on minimizing the risk of infection, especially if lines are left in place for a long time.

The insertion techniques used most frequently include percutaneous and direct cutdown methods. The percutaneous method is usually preferable, but direct cutdown is sometimes used for catheterization of the superficial saphenous and median basilic veins. Arteries and nerves in the cutdown site should be identified to avoid accidental puncture. After catheter insertion, blood return by aspiration with a syringe is necessary to confirm catheter location inside the vessel. A chest radiograph should be obtained in all cases to confirm an appropriate intrathoracic location.

In infants, including premature infants, very narrow Silastic catheters can be inserted through a small needle, but this technique is difficult. Whenever any intravascular line is inserted through a needle, the catheter should *never* be withdrawn through the needle, as the catheter may shear and embolize.

The insertion site should be dressed using antiseptic gels and should be covered with a sterile dressing. The cannulation site should be inspected daily. If the site develops clinical evidence of infection (ie, erythema, swelling, or induration), the tip of the catheter should be removed and cultured. Intravenous antibiotic therapy often is given empirically until culture results are available.

Complications common to all central venous lines include local and systemic infection, hemorrhage, thrombus formation, arrhythmias, and accidental arterial or nerve puncture. Internal jugular and subclavian vein catheter insertions can cause pneumothorax or cardiac tamponade. Catheter-related infection can be reduced by controlling line manipulation and by performing daily dressing changes. The number of infants and children with central lines who develop endocarditis and thrombi in their lines seems to be increasing recently. However, this apparently increased incidence may be due to an increased use of central lines,

a higher index of suspicion, and the improvement of echocardiography in detecting thrombi.

Catheter life depends on the indications for placement. For instance, a catheter sometimes must remain in place for weeks or months for parenteral hyperalimentation. Changing catheter sites is often impractical in chronically ill infants and smaller children in whom every vein seems to have been already used and is often unnecessary, especially if strict adherence to sterile technique can be maintained.

## INTRAOSSEOUS INFUSIONS

In life-threatening situations where fluid replacement must be given and an intravascular line cannot be obtained, fluids can be given by an intraosseous infusion. In most children, fluids can be given temporarily via a spinal or bone-marrow needle inserted into the tibia or distal femur. As soon as an intravenous line is inserted, the fluids should be given intravascularly rather than intraosseously.

## PULMONARY ARTERIAL CATHETERS

Pulmonary artery (PA) catheters provide a plethora of data defining hemodynamic, respiratory, and metabolic function. Most commonly they are used to monitor hemodynamic indices in children after corrective cardiac procedures or in medical conditions such as septic shock, congestive heart failure, or severe respiratory failure. Information that can be determined with a diagnostic Swan-Ganz catheter includes direct measurement of PA pressure, pulmonary capillary wedge pressure, right atrial pressure, and central venous pressure.

With a thermodilution catheter, cardiac output, vascular resistances, and ventricular function can be estimated. Simultaneous determination of cardiac output and paired mixed venous and arterial blood oxygen contents can be used to calculate intrapulmonary shunt fraction, oxygen consumption, oxygen extraction ratio, and the arterial mixed venous oxygen difference. These data help in bedside interpretation of cardiopulmonary and metabolic interrelationships during serious illness and help gauge the success of cardiotonic agents, afterload reduction, mechanical ventilation, and positive end-expiratory pressure.

While a central venous pressure measurement should be obtained from a port in the right atrium or the superior vena cava, measurement with the tip in the innominate vein or distal in the inferior vena cava will be essentially equal to a "true" central venous pressure.

The PA catheter used most commonly is a balloon-tipped, four- lumina catheter with a thermistor at the tip for measuring cardiac output. This catheter is available in No. 5 or No. 7 French sizes. The four lumina are a distal port for the measurement of PA pressure and pulmonary capillary wedge pressure, a proximal port for measuring right atrial pressure and central venous pressure, a thermistor for determining cardiac output, and a port for inflating the balloon. Two- and three-lumina catheters are also available and are usually easier to manipulate into the PA, but they are more limited in the amount of physiologic information that can be obtained because they do not have a thermistor at the tip for measuring cardiac output. Catheter size is determined by patient size and the insertion site. The No. 5 French catheter typically is used in the child with a body weight of 18 kg or less, while the No. 7 French catheter is used in larger children and adults.

In the pediatric ICU, PA catheters are usually placed through the femoral vein, which I believe is the preferred site for infants and most children. The femoral vein approach occasionally results in knotted catheters, but most of these can be untied under fluoroscopic guidance. Using the femoral vein, the catheter can cross the foramen ovale to enter the left side of the heart, but this is relatively rare. Other insertion sites routinely used are the internal jugular or brachial veins. In adolescents and adults, the subclavian veins frequently are used.

Catheter insertion typically is performed at the bedside. Portable fluoroscopy rarely is needed to guide catheter placement. Catheter insertion is performed by using the flow-directed approach and by monitoring the characteristic pressures and waveforms recorded on the bedside oscilloscope from the distal lumen as the catheter passes through the systemic veins, right atrium, and right ventricle, and finally into the main pulmonary artery. The final resting position for the catheter tip is a point at which near-maximal balloon inflation produces damping of the PA pressure.

Complications of PA catheter placement include puncture of major systemic vessels or cardiac chambers, ventricular arrhythmias, PA rupture, pneumothorax, catheter knotting, and bacteremia. A chest radiograph should be obtained frequently enough to identify catheter location and ensure that catheter migration has not occurred. The duration of catheter placement is dictated by the need for hemodynamic monitoring and the difficulty of

subsequent PA catheter reinsertion. If practical, PA catheters should be changed every 3 to 5 days.

## LEFT ATRIAL CATHETERS

In critically ill patients with myocardial dysfunction or those who are receiving positive pressure ventilation, monitoring of central venous pressure and pulmonary capillary wedge pressure may not accurately reflect the volume status of the left-sided cardiac chambers. In these patients, left atrial filling pressures are more accurate. Left atrial catheters can be inserted only during cardiac surgery.

The major risk of left atrial catheters is direct systemic embolization from gas bubbles or particulate matter. Significant systemic emboli occur with left atrial lines, so they are not routinely used after most cardiac operations. They should be used only by physicians and nurses experienced in their use.

### Suggested Reading

Ponamem ML, White L. Intraosseous infusions. In: Levin DL, Morriss FC, eds. Essentials of pediatric intensive care. St. Louis: Quality Medical Publishing, 1990.
Pope J. Pulmonary artery catheters. In: Blumer JL, ed. A practical guide to pediatric intensive care. St. Louis: Mosby Year Book, 1990.

---

*Principles and Practice of Pediatrics, Second Edition.*
edited by Frank A. Oski et al. J. B. Lippincott Company, Philadelphia © 1994.

# 41.6 *Measurement of Cardiac Output*

### Thomas A. Vargo

Cardiac output is an important physiologic variable commonly measured to assess hemodynamic function. Serial determinations of cardiac output are useful in guiding fluid and vasoactive drug therapy in patients with compromised myocardial function. Numerous methods to measure cardiac output exist, but only a few are applicable in the critically ill child. The most frequently used methods of measuring cardiac output are indicator dilution techniques and the Fick method.

## INDICATOR DILUTION METHODS

### Thermodilution

The thermodilution method, a form of the indicator dilution technique, is the most commonly used method of measuring cardiac output in the ICU setting. The thermodilution method requires placement of a pulmonary artery catheter with a proximal injection port and a thermistor at the catheter tip. Thermodilution is accurate, reproducible, and easily performed. The technique requires minimal subjective interpretation of collected data, and serial measurements can be repeated rapidly.

A 3- to 10-mL volume of normal saline or 5% dextrose solution is injected into the proximal port, which is in the right atrium or one of the vena cava, and the temperature is measured at the thermistor, which is in the pulmonary artery. The injectate is

cooled either to room temperature or to 0 °C by placing it in an ice bath; the thermistor in the pulmonary artery is obviously at body temperature. The cold water injected "upstream" causes a transient mild temperature drop "downstream" when this bolus of cold water passes through the pulmonary artery. The thermistor is connected to a commercial cardiac output computer, and the change in pulmonary arterial blood temperature is recorded. The computer automatically constructs the thermal dilution curve and calculates the cardiac output in liters per minute.

Despite the relative reliability of this method, a 10% to 15% variance is seen frequently between measurements. Therefore, three to five serial measurements should be obtained and averaged.

### Vascular Resistance

Once the cardiac output (CO) is determined by the thermodilution technique, it is easy to measure both the pulmonary (PVR) and systemic (SVR) vascular resistances by the following formulas:

$$PVR = \frac{PA_P - PCWP_P}{CO}$$

$$SVR = \frac{SA_P - RA_P}{CO}$$

$PA_P$, $PCWP_P$, $SA_P$, and $RA_P$ are the mean pressures in the pulmonary artery, pulmonary capillary wedge position, systemic artery, and right atrium, respectively. With a thermodilution catheter, the mean pressures in the wedge position can be determined when the Swan-Ganz balloon is inflated; when the balloon is deflated, the mean pressure in the pulmonary artery can be determined. The right atrial pressure is almost always the pressure recorded from the proximal port of the catheter. The mean systemic arterial pressure is determined from either an arterial line or an automated cuff blood pressure measurement.

### Green Dye

The use of various nontoxic, water-soluble dyes as indicators is reserved primarily for the cardiac catheterization laboratory. Indocyanine green (Cardiogreen) is the most frequently used dye. A centrally placed venous catheter at the injection site and a peripheral arterial catheter are used simultaneously for continuous sampling of blood. A small, precise quantity of dye is injected into the central catheter, and the concentration of dye is determined at the arterial sampling site. Cardiac output then is calculated by the following formula:

$$CO = \frac{I \times 60}{C \times T}$$

$I$ represents the amount of dye injected in milligrams, $C$ represents the mean concentration of dye in the arterial blood sample in milligrams per liter, and $T$ is the time it took for the dye to pass by the arterial sampling site in seconds; 60 is needed to convert seconds to minutes.

Because of the simplicity of performing thermodilution cardiac outputs, green dye dilution curves are rarely used in the pediatric ICU and today are performed relatively infrequently even in the cardiac catheterization laboratory.

## FICK PRINCIPLE

The Fick method is the oldest method for determining cardiac output and is considered the gold standard. While still performed commonly during cardiac catheterization, measuring the cardiac output by the Fick principle has limited applicability in the pediatric ICU. This technique requires indwelling pulmonary and systemic arterial catheters for the simultaneous sampling of mixed venous and arterial blood. Oxygen consumption ($VO_2$) is measured by using commercial instruments that automatically determine oxygen consumption. Arterial ($CaO_2$) and venous ($CvO_2$) oxygen contents are determined either by color spectrophotometry or by calculation of the oxygen content from blood gas samples. Calculation of cardiac output by the Fick principle uses this formula:

$$CO = \frac{VO_2}{(CaO_2 - CvO_2)}$$

The Fick principle can be used to estimate qualitatively the changes in cardiac output. Assuming $VO_2$ remains constant in a given patient, the cardiac output is inversely proportional to the difference between arterial and venous oxygen content. In most cases this also means that whenever a patient's venous saturation decreases, the cardiac output also is decreased.

## NONINVASIVE DETERMINATION OF CARDIAC OUTPUT

Noninvasive methods for determining cardiac output are sometimes used in the management of critically ill children. Echocardiography can be used to estimate cardiac output. The technique consists of measuring the cross-sectional area of the aorta by two-dimensional echocardiography, then determining the velocity of the blood flow in the aorta by Doppler sampling. The volume of blood flow can be calculated readily whenever one knows how fast the blood is flowing across a known area. It is difficult to measure the aortic wall diameter accurately in children; this often results in large errors in calculation of cross-sectional area.

Another echocardiographic method of estimating cardiac output is to determine end-systolic and end-diastolic left ventricular chamber volumes to calculate stroke volume. Again, difficulties in obtaining precise and accurate measurements of cardiac chambers by echocardiography can cause significant errors in measuring ventricular volumes. Because of this, echocardio-

graphic measurements of cardiac output are not routinely used in the pediatric ICU.

Exercise physiology and pulmonary function laboratories can reliably estimate cardiac output in children at rest and during exercise by measuring inhaled tracer gas uptake using several methods or by transthoracic electrical bioimpedance. Recent attempts to apply these methods in critically ill children have given poor results when compared to values obtained by the thermodilution technique.

## Selected Reading

Vargo TA. Cardiac catheterization—hemodynamic measurements. In: Garson A Jr, Bricker JT, McNamara DG, eds. The science and practice of pediatric cardiology. Philadelphia: Lea & Febiger, 1990.

*Principles and Practice of Pediatrics, Second Edition.*
edited by Frank A. Oski et al. J. B. Lippincott Company, Philadelphia © 1994.

# 41.7 *Echocardiography*

## Thomas A. Vargo

The use of ultrasonic imaging techniques to determine cardiac anatomy and myocardial function is one of the most rapidly advancing technologies in pediatric cardiology. The popularity of echocardiography in evaluating the child with suspected heart disease is due to its safety, portability, ease of use, continued improvement in imaging, and the ability to estimate cardiac function. Because of these and other reasons, the use of echocardiography has resulted in a significant reduction in the number of diagnostic cardiac catheterizations performed in children.

In children, essentially every congenital cardiac defect can be diagnosed by echocardiography. However, a "negative" echocardiogram does not necessarily rule out a cardiac defect. For example, in some newborns it may be impossible to determine if the infant has anomalous pulmonary venous return or a coarctation of the aorta. Echocardiographic diagnosis may be impossible in children who are difficult to image (eg, some children with marked chest wall abnormalities). In children who are difficult to image by standard echocardiographic techniques, transesophageal echocardiography (TEE) can be performed. TEE almost always gives excellent cardiac imaging, but the esophageal probes are large and TEE in children usually must be done using general anesthesia.

Cardiac contractility can easily be defined by echocardiography, because ventricular wall motion is seen so well. Almost all ventricular muscle abnormalities, such as depressed contractility, ventricular dilatation, or infarcted areas, can usually be seen well. Because precise, accurate measurements of ventricular volumes are difficult to obtain, we believe the best way to measure contractility is to determine the difference between the left ventricular systolic and diastolic diameters. Normally, the left ventricular systolic diameter is about two thirds of the diastolic diameter (ie, a shortening fraction of 33%). Shortening fractions less than 25% suggest a significant reduction in left ventricular function.

Pericardial effusions are especially well seen by echocardiography. Because pericardial effusions are more common than generally realized, I believe an echocardiogram should be done in any sick child who has unexplained cardiomegaly.

Doppler echocardiography can be used to estimate the pressure in most cardiac chambers by the following formula:

$$PG = 4 \times (m/s)^2$$

PG is the pressure gradient in mm Hg, and m/s is the velocity of the intracardiac jet in the heart in meters per second.

The Doppler technique usually estimates intracardiac pressures accurately. For example, if the velocity across a stenotic pulmonic valve is 5 m/s, then the gradient across the pulmonary valve would be 100 mm Hg. In this case, the right ventricular (RV) systolic pressure would be about 115 mm Hg, because the pulmonary artery systolic pressure is about 15 mm Hg in most children with pulmonic stenosis.

The RV pressure also can be estimated in a patient with a ventricular septal defect (VSD). Let us suppose that the velocity of the flow across the VSD is 4 m/s and the systemic blood pressure is 104/60; in this case, the RV systolic pressure will be 40 mm Hg. This calculation is done by assuming that the left ventricular (LV) systolic pressure is the same as the arterial systolic blood pressure and that the LV systolic pressure is 64 mm Hg greater than the RV systolic pressure.

*Principles and Practice of Pediatrics, Second Edition.* edited by Frank A. Oski et al. J. B. Lippincott Company, Philadelphia © 1994.

# 41.8 *Intracranial Pressure Measurements*

Fernando Stein

Elevation of the intracranial pressure (ICP) is a common complication in patients with head injury, neoplasia, or cerebral vascular accidents, and with infections or metabolic processes. ICP is monitored in the pediatric ICU when one or more of the indications listed in Table 41-1 are present.

Normal ICP in children is 15 mm Hg or less. However, the goal in controlling ICP is not necessarily to preserve this ideal number, but to preserve cerebral perfusion pressure (CPP). CPP is the difference between the mean arterial pressure (MAP) and the ICP: CPP = MAP − ICP. In a normal child, CPP of 40 mm Hg or more is sufficient to maintain normal blood flow and appropriate delivery of nutrients.

There are three basic types of intracranial pressure monitors: hydrodynamic monitors, electronic fiberoptic monitors, and cuff pressure monitors. Hydrodynamic monitors contain a fluid-filled column connected to a transducer that in turn connects to an

oscilloscope or digital display. The fluid-filled column is usually a catheter implanted in the ventricle or a bolt that sits in the subarachnoid space or in the epidural space. The intraventricular cannula allows CSF to be withdrawn in case of an extreme increase in ICP. In an electronic fiberoptic monitor, a sensor sits directly in the brain and measures the pressure by fiberoptic oscillation. Cuff monitors apply the principle of an air- or fluid-filled bag that transmits the pressure by compression of the bag or cuff. These monitors must be implanted through a bur hole and are usually big and cumbersome to insert and remove.

Regardless of the type of ICP monitor used, equipment failure may occur. Close neurologic observation with frequent pupillary checks are mandatory whenever ICP is being monitored.

*Principles and Practice of Pediatrics, Second Edition.* edited by Frank A. Oski et al. J. B. Lippincott Company, Philadelphia © 1994.

# 41.9 *Intubation*

Fernando Stein

Intubation of the trachea is a skill every pediatrician should have, because most cardiac arrests in children are due to respiratory failure. Except for acute upper airway obstruction with arrest, intubation of the trachea should be a carefully planned and preconceived procedure. All the necessary equipment should be checked regularly and should be available; Table 41-2 lists the minimal equipment necessary for intubation.

Ventilatory assistance can be provided for most children with a bag and mask, and during that time the physician should give clear, concise commands as to the orderly performance of procedures and administration of medications.

Semiconscious or alert patients who require endotracheal intubation should receive appropriate sedation and cardiovascular protection, and they should be paralyzed for the procedure (Table 41-3). An intravenous line is recommended with rare exceptions.

Various sedatives are available, and an individualized decision must be made depending on the patient's condition. Opiates are a satisfactory alternative, as they provide both analgesia and narcosis; an antagonist drug (naloxone) is available, if required. Barbiturates are used commonly in anesthesia, and either the short-acting or the intermediate-acting kinds are suitable for intubation of the trachea. Some of the benzodiazepines also are acceptable,

**TABLE 41-1. Indications for ICP Monitoring**

Acute shifting of the midline brain structures indicated by CT scan
Rapid depression in the Glasgow coma score of 4 points or more
Evidence of increased ICP by physical examination in a condition that consistently leads to brain edema
Presence of space-occupying lesions with increased ICP
Hydrocephalus under certain circumstances
Other individual cases in which monitoring of the ICP is necessary for accurate and successful treatment

**TABLE 41-2. Intubation Equipment**

Laryngoscope with several sizes of blades, curved and straight
Endotracheal tubes, several sizes (2.5–8.0)
Ambu bags, several sizes (infant, child, adult)
Masks, several sizes (infant, child, adult)
Malleable metal stylet
Oral airways, six sizes
McGill forceps
Suction tube and suction catheter, all appropriate sizes to fit endotracheal tubes
Bite lock
Adhesive tape
Suction device (wall or portable unit)
Oxygen (tank or central)

## TABLE 41-3.   Drugs for Intubation*

| Drug | Dose |
|---|---|
| **Cardiovascular Protection** | |
| Atropine sulfate | 0.01 mg/kg |
| **Sedation** | |
| Morphine | 0.1–0.3 mg/kg |
| Diazepam | 0.1–0.3 mg/kg |
| Barbiturates | |
| Thiopental (short-acting) | 5–10 mg/kg |
| Pentobarbital (intermediate-acting) | 3–5 mg/kg |
| **Paralyzation** | |
| Succinylcholine (depolarizing; short-acting) | 1 mg/kg |
| Dimethyltubocurarine (nondepolarizing) | 0.2–0.4 mg/kg |
| Pancuronium (nondepolarizing) | 0.1 mg/kg |

\* The physician should be thoroughly familiar with the action, half-life, pharmacologic interactions, and pharmacokinetics of all drugs administered.

but they have been associated with sporadic reports of elevation of the pulmonary artery pressure.

Cardiovascular protection is provided by administering atropine, 0.01 mg/kg per dose. This should be done intravenously and is recommended in patients beyond the neonatal age. Atropine is specifically contraindicated in patients with glaucoma.

Once the patient is sedated appropriately and cardiovascular protection has been provided, the physician should ensure that all the necessary equipment is ready and that the patient is monitored appropriately (electronic cardiac monitoring). Only then can the paralyzing agent be given.

The patient's head is placed over a 1″ to 2″ pillow or folded piece of cloth, and an artificial oral airway is inserted to remove the tongue from the normal anatomical air passages. The bag and mask are then applied. A tight seal should be created between the mask and the face, and the bag should be compressed at a rate no slower than 15 times per minute. Expansion of the chest should be noted and a stethoscope used to determine that breath sounds are satisfactory.

After 2 to 3 minutes of bagging with 100% oxygen (except in neonates), the laryngoscope is inserted in the mouth, trying to lift it to a 45° angle in reference to the horizontal axis. If intubation is performed with a straight blade, the blade should be moistened, inserted through the right side of the mouth, and advanced toward the epiglottis on the right side of the tongue. The epiglottis then is visualized, and the laryngoscope blade tip lifts the epiglottis. This provides visualization of the larynx with a lift forward, as described, at a 45° angle. Visualization should never be forced by angling the laryngoscope blade against the teeth; this is a leading cause of dental trauma.

The endotracheal tube then is inserted with the concavity lateral to the angle of the mouth. It is advanced toward the larynx until it disappears beyond the vocal cords. Sometimes it is necessary to rotate the tube 90° to 150°. After intubation is accomplished, the tube is advanced 3 to 5 cm beyond the vocal cords, depending on the patient's size and age.

The technique with a curved blade is slightly different in that the epiglottis is not elevated. With the curved blade, the tip is positioned in the fold between the base of the tongue and the epiglottis. An upward motion stretches the ligaments and folds the epiglottis up, thereby allowing visualization of the vocal cords.

After intubation has been accomplished, bilateral and equal breath sounds should be noted. The endotracheal tube is secured, a mouth block or oral airway is applied, and a chest radiograph is obtained to check for satisfactory position of the tip of the tube.

## Selected Readings

Applebaum EL, Bruce DL. Techniques of tracheal intubation. In: Applebaum EL, Bruce DL, eds. Tracheal intubation. Philadelphia: WB Saunders, 1976.

Dripps RD, Eckenhoff JE, Vandam LD. Intubation of the trachea. In: Dripps RD, Eckenhoff JE, Vandam LD, eds. Introduction to anesthesia: the principles of safe practice. Philadelphia: WB Saunders, 1977.

*Principles and Practice of Pediatrics, Second Edition.*
edited by Frank A. Oski et al. J. B. Lippincott Company, Philadelphia © 1994.

## 41.10 *Extubation*

### Fernando Stein

When the indications that prompted endotracheal intubation no longer exist, extubation should be carefully executed. There are three major areas of concern when a tube is going to be removed: avoiding laryngospasm, maintaining airway patency, and ensuring adequate ventilatory function.

The tube should be removed when the patient has adequate reflex control. Therefore, paralyzing agents, sedatives, and narcotics must be discontinued before extubation.

Laryngospasm occurs in a state of semi-alert/semi-asleep consciousness when droplets of secretions fall on the vocal cords and they, in turn, approximate and occlude the airway. Although this may be short-lived, it is potentially fatal, so extubation should be conducted as if the patient were to require intubation at the same time.

Laryngospasm is better prevented than treated. The treatment includes administering oxygen under pressure with reservoir bag and mask and perhaps paralyzing the patient completely. Laryngospasm is best prevented by keeping the patient as alert as possible and by careful attention to aspiration of secretions. Before the tube is removed, the lungs should be inflated with 100% oxygen for a few minutes; after removal of the tube, the patient should be given oxygen.

In infants and small children, the administration of racemic epinephrine has been shown to be helpful in the control of postintubation subglottic edema. After the endotracheal tube has been removed, a chest radiograph should be obtained to check for postintubation atelectasis.

*Principles and Practice of Pediatrics, Second Edition.*
edited by Frank A. Oski et al. J. B. Lippincott Company, Philadelphia © 1994.

## 41.11 *Tracheostomy*

### Fernando Stein

The indications for tracheostomy in children are divided into three categories: airway obstruction, pulmonary toilet, and mechanical ventilation. In a 12-year review of indications for tracheostomy at Children's Hospital of Pittsburgh, the indication for 80% of the procedures was assisted ventilation and pulmonary toilet; the rest were performed for upper airway obstruction. With small variations this is true for most children's hospitals in the United States.

Whenever time and conditions allow, the tracheostomy should be performed by the most expert personnel available, and the procedure should be done in the operating room. An endotracheal tube should be present before the tracheostomy procedure begins, except for extreme obstructive emergencies. Local anesthesia usually is inappropriate, and this procedure should be performed under general controlled anesthesia. After the tracheostomy has been performed, it is important to provide warmed, filtered, and humidified air, because the tube bypasses the nasopharynx.

Some of the most important complications following tracheostomy are hemorrhage, air entry, anatomical damage, tracheostomy tube problems, respiratory arrest, and pulmonary edema. Any of these problems can be fatal; most of them can be prevented.

When the patient returns to the ICU after tracheostomy, the equipment required to perform a new tracheostomy should be placed at the bedside and should remain there in a sterile package for 3 to 5 days after the procedure. An appropriate light source for the performance of emergency surgery should be available at the bedside. Physical and pharmacologic restraint of the patient is necessary to avoid accidental intubation or dissection of air between superficial and deep tissue planes. Suction and ventilation with a mask should be performed by personnel who are appropriately trained in the complications of recent tracheostomy.

## Selected Readings

Dammert W, Mast CP. Tracheostomy. In: Levin DL, Morris FC, Moore GC, eds. A practical guide to pediatric intensive care. St. Louis: CV Mosby, 1979.
Stool SE, Eavey R. Tracheostomy. In: Bluestone CD, Stool SE, eds. Pediatric otolaryngology. Philadelphia: WB Saunders, 1983.

*Principles and Practice of Pediatrics, Second Edition.*
edited by Frank A. Oski et al. J. B. Lippincott Company, Philadelphia © 1994.

# 41.12 *Abdominal Paracentesis*

### Penelope Terhune Louis

In abdominal paracentesis, the abdominal cavity is entered to obtain diagnostic information for the differential diagnosis of ascites, peritonitis, and intraperitoneal hemorrhage, or to institute therapeutic measures such as dialysis, abdominal decompression to relieve respiratory compromise secondary to diminished diaphragmatic excursion from large amounts of gas or fluid in the abdomen, decompression of chylous ascites, and internal cooling.

There are no absolute contraindications to paracentesis. However, bleeding disorders, disruption of abdominal wall integrity, and marked distention of the bowel (which predisposes to puncture and leakage of the bowel wall) require prudent evaluation before beginning the procedure.

Abdominal paracentesis in all abdominal quadrants is obsolete and less informative than either peritoneal lavage or abdominal CT scan.

## TECHNIQUE

The technique for peritoneal lavage is as follows:

1. Empty the bladder spontaneously or with catheterization.
2. Place the patient in a supine position with the head slightly elevated.
3. Prepare the area by aseptic technique.
4. Infiltrate the chosen area with lidocaine.
5. Introduce an 18- to 22-gauge needle and catheter set perpendicular to the skin in either flank, in line with the nipples and below or at the level of the umbilicus, or in the midline below the umbilicus. The risk of intestinal perforation may be reduced by avoiding areas where the bowel may be adherent to the abdominal wall, such as near scars from previous abdominal operations.
6. Advance the needle until the peritoneum is entered. The needle then is withdrawn and the catheter advanced. Suction should be applied with a syringe during advancement.
7. Sample contents of the peritoneal cavity, including culture (aerobic, anaerobic, acid- fast, viral, and fungal), Gram stain, cell count with differential analysis, specific gravity, glucose, total protein, amylase, ammonia, and cellular morphology.
8. Peritoneal lavage can be used to diagnose intra-abdominal hemorrhage or other trauma. A standard dialysis catheter is inserted with infusion of 20 mL/kg of fluid of balanced salt solution.
9. Affix the catheter to the skin and apply a sterile dressing.
10. The fluid is withdrawn and sent for analysis.

## FLUID ANALYSIS

### Appearance

The fluid is normally straw-colored. Turbidity is associated with chemical or infectious peritonitis. Milky or yellow-white fluid is associated with chylous ascites. Green-stained fluid may be associated with pancreatitis or gallbladder or common duct perforation. Blood-tinged fluid is associated with visceral disruption or a traumatic tap.

### Cytology

A positive test is the presence of more than 100,000 red blood cells/mL or 500 white blood cells/mL (with greater than 50% polymorphonuclear leukocytes). A lymphocytic predominance may be seen with chylous ascites or tuberculous peritonitis.

### Chemical Analysis

Fluid glucose is low if less than 60 mg/dL or less than two thirds of the serum glucose. The total protein helps to classify the fluid collection as transudate or exudate. A total protein level of less than 2.5 g/dL, a fibrinogen level of 0.3% to 4.0% of the total protein, and a fluid-to-serum protein level of 0.5 or less are consistent with a transudate. The fluid's specific gravity also reflects the protein content. A specific gravity less than 1.015 is consistent with a transudate. An alkaline phosphatase level elevated to twice normal may be seen in a patient with perforated or necrotic viscera. The fluid ammonia level is elevated to twice normal in strangulated bowel or duodenal ulcer perforation. Children with urinary ascites have increased fluid levels of ammonia, creatinine, and potassium. Fluid amylase levels are elevated in excess of serum amylase levels in patients with pancreatitis, pancreatic pseudocyst, intestinal perforation, or strangulation.

## COMPLICATIONS

Complications of paracentesis include perforation of a hollow viscus, perforation of a blood vessel, introduction of contaminants, and extraperitoneal hematoma formation secondary to trauma of the deep epigastric vessels in the lateral aspect of the recti muscles.

## Selected Readings

Damment W. Abdominal paracentesis. In: Levin DL, Morriss FC, eds. Essentials of pediatric intensive care. St. Louis: Quality Medical Publishing, 1990.
Harris BH. Management of multiple trauma. Pediatr Clin N Am 1985;32:175.
Pokorny WJ. Abdominal trauma. In: Raffensperger JG, ed. Swenson's pediatric surgery, ed 5. Chicago: Appleton & Lange, 1990.
Rice TB, Pontus SP. Diagnostic and therapeutic centeses. In: Fuhrman BP, Zimmerman JJ, ed. Pediatric critical care. St. Louis: Mosby Yearbook, 1992.
Yaster M, Haller JA. Multiple trauma in the pediatric patient. In: Rogers MC, ed. Textbook of pediatric intensive care, ed 1. Baltimore: Williams & Wilkins, 1987.

*Principles and Practice of Pediatrics, Second Edition.*
edited by Frank A. Oski et al. J. B. Lippincott Company, Philadelphia © 1994.

# 41.13 *Acute Peritoneal Dialysis*

Penelope Terhune Louis

Peritoneal dialysis first was used to treat children with acute renal failure more than 40 years ago. It is a simple and safe technique that is easily adapted for use in patients of any age or body size. Peritoneal dialysis can be effective in the treatment of infants and children suffering from acute or chronic renal failure, from intoxication with certain dialyzable poisons, from severe hypernatremia due to sodium chloride poisoning, or from any of a small group of congenital metabolic disorders.

The peritoneal cavity functions as a dialysis system when it acts as a semipermeable membrane across which solute and fluids are exchanged between the peritoneal capillary blood and the dialysis solution that bathes the surface of the peritoneal membrane. Peritoneal dialysis is more efficient in infants and children than in adults; the relative area of the peritoneal membrane in young children is two to three times as large as it is in adults.

There are few absolute contraindications to peritoneal dialysis. In some situations, the relative inefficiency of peritoneal solute transfer makes hemodialysis the preferred therapy. Certain intraabdominal lesions are relative contraindications to peritoneal dialysis: intestinal adhesions, recent abdominal surgery, major abdominal trauma, bowel distention, colostomy, organomegaly, or a diaphragmatic defect.

## TECHNIQUE

Before the dialysis catheter is introduced, the bladder should be emptied either spontaneously or by catheterization. The abdomen then is prepared by sterile technique. Soft multihole catheters have been found to be associated with a lower incidence of intraabdominal bleeding and have a low rate of obstruction. If there has been prior abdominal surgery or bowel distention, or if the patient is less than 2 years old, has poor abdominal muscle tone,

or needs long-term peritoneal dialysis, then the catheter should be placed under direct vision by a surgeon in the operating room. If there are no contraindications, the catheter may be placed by a percutaneous method. The chosen puncture site is infiltrated with 1% lidocaine. The optimal puncture sites are in the midline 2 to 3 cm below the umbilicus or lateral to the rectus muscle in the left lower quadrant.

After the needle is withdrawn, the trochar and catheter are advanced together perpendicularly through the abdominal wall, using a twisting motion. The trochar is withdrawn as the catheter is advanced in the direction of the lower quadrants. The skin incision then is closed and the catheter affixed to the skin with suture or tape.

After the catheter is advanced into the peritoneal cavity, a volume of prepared dialysate is instilled. Instillation of this initial volume should be terminated if fluid accumulates in the abdominal wall, if significant abdominal pain is noted, if returned fluid is frankly bloody, or if hypotension, tachypnea, or tachycardia occurs.

If dialysis is anticipated for longer than 3 days, implantation of a more permanent catheter under sterile conditions should be considered. Placement of the peritoneal dialysis catheter for chronic use differs from placement for acute use in that the catheter is tunneled under the skin, reducing the likelihood of infection. In addition, an omentectomy may be performed to decrease the incidence of obstruction of the catheter. If chronic peritoneal dialysis is planned, healing should be allowed to occur for 3 to 5 days before beginning dialysis with full fluid volumes. This allows fibroblastic growth to fix the catheter and to seal the tissues around the catheter, reducing the likelihood of leakage or infection.

## DIALYSATE

If fluid removal is an important objective, the dialysate concentration used should be 2.5% to 4.25% dextrose. A 1.5% dextrose solution is standard if fluid removal is unnecessary. Dialysate containing lactate is favored over acetate solutions because of decreased peritoneal scarring. Most dialysis solutions contain no potassium, but solutions can be made with concentrations of 3 mEq/L if the serum potassium level falls. Heparin, 100 to 500 units/L, is added to the initial dialysate to prevent clots from obstructing the catheter.

All dialysate should be warmed to 38 °C by a peritoneal dialysis cycler. Using this device allows fewer entries into the system and reduces the risk of infection. Administering cold dialysate can cause arrhythmias. Warming the dialysate prevents heat loss, decreases discomfort, and improves urea clearance by increasing peritoneal blood flow.

## MANAGEMENT

During acute peritoneal dialysis, a functioning intravenous cannula is necessary. Resuscitation drugs, equipment for emergency airway management, and anticonvulsants should be readily available. Meticulous accounts of intake and output with daily weights must be maintained to prevent hypovolemia due to excessive fluid removal. Electrolytes, serum calcium, phosphate, blood urea nitrogen, and creatinine are monitored frequently. The ECG should be monitored continuously with analysis for hyperkalemia. If hypertonic glucose dialysate is used for fluid removal, abdominal pain may be severe and additional analgesia may be necessary. Cultures of drained fluid are obtained daily. If positive cultures are obtained in association with increased fluid white cell count, antibiotics may be added to the dialysate.

The incidence of infection associated with catheters placed percutaneously is high, especially if the catheter stays in place longer than 3 days. Precautions taken to reduce the incidence of peritoneal infections include the following:

1. Use aseptic technique during catheter insertion.
2. Maintain all of the catheter holes within the peritoneal cavity.
3. Maintain sterile dressings over the catheter site.
4. Remove peritoneal catheters after 48 hours.
5. Avoid prophylactic use of antibiotics that may predispose to *Candida* peritonitis.
6. Obtain surveillance cultures and Gram stain of dialysate fluid every 24 hours.
7. Use closed dialysate delivery systems when available.
8. Soft, pliable plastic (Silastic) dialysis catheters (Tenckhoff catheters) may be used in children with acute renal failure who are probable candidates for multiple dialysis procedures.

## COMPLICATIONS

In children, the most common complication of peritoneal dialysis is peritoneal infection. The incidence of peritonitis has been reported to be as high as 68% in children less than 2 years old and 30% in older children. In several large studies, the incidence of peritonitis has been found to be directly proportional to time on dialysis. There is a dramatic increase in the incidence of peritonitis when temporary catheters are left in place for more than 72 hours. Most episodes of peritonitis are due to inoculation of the peritoneal dialysis fluid during the exchange procedure, or to local seeding from infections involving the tissue along the catheter tunnel or at the skin exit site. The pathogens isolated most commonly are *Staphylococcus epidermidis* and *Staphylococcus aureus*, although gram-negative organisms and *Candida* may cause as much as 30% of the episodes of peritonitis.

Careful attention to the cardiorespiratory status is necessary when peritoneal dialysis is initiated. Instilling large volumes of dialysate can compromise cardiac output by decreasing venous return. The increase in intra-abdominal volume and pressure may cause an elevation of the diaphragm, with a decline in the functional residual capacity and expiratory reserve volume. This may lead to atelectasis and a decline in the $PaO_2$, with an increased alveolar-arterial oxygen gradient. Decreased chest wall compliance and a decline in diaphragmatic mobility may be due to fatigue or pain associated with the instillation of dialysate.

Potentially serious derangements of fluid and electrolyte balance can result from peritoneal dialysis in children. Most of these can be anticipated and avoided through careful monitoring and appropriate therapy adjustments.

## Selected Readings

Alexander SR. Peritoneal dialysis. In: Levin DL, Morriss FC, eds. Essentials of pediatric intensive care. St. Louis: Quality Medical Publishing, 1990.

Donaldson MD, Spurgeon P, Haycock GB, et al. Peritoneal dialysis in infants. Br Med J 1983;286;759.

Gaudio KM, Siegel NJ. Pathogenesis and treatment of acute renal failure. Pediatr Clin N Am 1987;34:771.

Lattouf OM, Ricketts RR. Peritoneal dialysis in infants and children. Am Surg 1986;52:66.

Maxwell LG, Firush BA, McLean RH. Renal failure. In: Rogers MC, ed. Textbook of pediatric intensive care, ed 1. Baltimore, Williams & Wilkins, 1987.

Reznik VM, Griswold WR, Peterson BM, et al. Peritoneal dialysis for acute renal failure in children. Pediatr Nephrol 1991;5:715.

*Principles and Practice of Pediatrics, Second Edition.*
edited by Frank A. Oski et al. J. B. Lippincott Company, Philadelphia © 1994.

# *41.14 Acute Hemodialysis*

### Penelope Terhune Louis

Hemodialysis is a treatment used to augment or replace renal excretory function. Most water-soluble substances that are not protein- or tissue-bound in the extracellular fluid can be effectively removed by hemodialysis. Hemodialysis may be combined with charcoal hemoperfusion to remove certain drugs and toxins. In general, the management of acute renal failure consists of supportive care until the kidney recovers from the acute renal insult. Acute dialysis or continuous arteriovenous hemofiltration is necessary in the following instances: volume overload with pulmonary edema or hypertension refractory to pharmacologic therapy; hyperkalemia greater than 6.5 mEq/L despite ion exchange therapy; metabolic acidosis with pH below 7.20 or $HCO_3$ less than 10; blood urea nitrogen above 150 (or less if rapidly rising); calcium/phosphorous imbalance; or neurologic symptoms secondary to uremia or electrolyte imbalance.

The principle of hemodialysis is that solutes diffuse across a semipermeable membrane from blood to dialysate or vice versa along their concentration gradients. If the concentration of a substance is the same on both sides of the membrane, the concentration of the substance will not change. Small molecules can be removed from or added to the blood by lowering or raising the concentration in the electrolyte solution. The steeper the concentration gradient, the more efficient is the removal of the substance from the blood. Larger molecules such as protein, protein-bound substances, blood cells, and bacteria cannot cross the membrane.

Urea, creatinine, and potassium travel from the blood to the dialysate, and acetate travels from the dialysate to the blood, helping to correct the metabolic acidosis. The rate at which this diffusion occurs depends on the temperature of the solutions, the membrane surface area, the permeability of the membrane, and the rate of blood and dialysate flow. By instituting positive pressure, water can be forced through the pores of the membrane. Water can be pulled out by creating negative pressure or by increasing the concentration of an osmotically active molecule.

Today, most dialysis machines can provide up to 1 L/min of dialysate with a constant osmolarity at body temperature, effect a wide range of positive and negative pressures within the system for water removal (ultrafiltration), detect air in the column of blood as it passes through the dialyzer, and detect the presence of hemoglobin within the dialysate to predict membrane rupture.

In emergency hemodialysis, intravascular access may be obtained via the femoral or subclavian veins using the Seldinger technique. If longer-term dialysis is planned, the subclavian vein is the preferred site because of better patient mobility. There is a 4% to 12% incidence of infection. The catheter must be flushed with heparinized saline to prevent thrombosis. Surgically created arteriovenous fistulae cannot be used in the acute situation, because 6 weeks are needed for the shunt to mature.

The availability of pediatric dialysis tubing and dialyzers of small volume has made hemodialysis more feasible even in neonates. The volume of the dialyzer and connecting tubes must approximate no more than 10% of the child's blood volume. This prevents the removal of too much volume, which can result in cardiovascular instability. The appropriate rate at which the patient's blood must be pumped through the artificial kidney is determined by the rate that the blood can be returned, by membrane characteristics of each artificial kidney, and by the patient's hemodynamic status. In general, the minimum blood flow of 2 to 3 mL/min/kg provides an adequate clearance rate of urea or creatinine.

Hemofiltration devices are available that depend on ultrafiltration rather than simple diffusion for removal of solutes. Water and solutes are extracted from the blood by the development of a hydrostatic pressure gradient produced by negative pressure applied to the dialysate side of the membrane, or positive pressure in the circuit is generated by clamping the return line. These devices are more efficient in removing larger molecules. Ultrafiltration may be combined with the use of a charcoal cartridge for removing some poisons. Ultrafiltration also may remove large volumes of fluid; therefore, it can be used in the treatment of patients with fluid overload.

Careful monitoring of the patient's cardiovascular status, body weight, hematocrit, activated clotting time, body temperature, dialysate osmolarity, and serum electrolytes must be performed for early detection of any unexpected changes produced by the therapy. Complications that may occur in association with hemodialysis include hemorrhagic hypotension secondary to blood loss during machine malfunction, circulatory shock secondary to rapid changes in intravascular volume, tissue ischemia, air embolism, hemolysis, and wide variation in body temperature.

## Selected Readings

Arant BS. Hemodialysis. In: Levin DL, Morriss FC, eds. Essentials of pediatric intensive care. St Louis: Quality Medical Publishing, 1990.

Gaudio KM, Siegel NJ. Pathogenesis and treatment of acute renal failure. Pediatr Clin N Am 1987;34:771.

Maxwell LG, Fivush BA, McLean RH. Renal failure. In: Rogers MC, ed. Textbook of pediatric intensive care, ed 1. Baltimore, Williams & Wilkins, 1987.

Vanherweghem JL, Drukker W, Schwarz A. Clinical significance of blood-device interaction in hemodialysis: a review. Int J Artif Organs 1987;10:219.

*Principles and Practice of Pediatrics, Second Edition.*
edited by Frank A. Oski et al. J. B. Lippincott Company, Philadelphia © 1994.

# 41.15 *Continuous Arteriovenous Hemofiltration*

## Penelope Terhune Louis

Continuous arteriovenous hemofiltration (CAVH) was introduced in 1977 as a method for emergency fluid removal in overhydrated patients resistant to diuretics. The use of CAVH has been emphasized for treating uremia in acute renal failure. It has proven to be a relatively simple technique that can be used in patients with marked vascular instability.

The technique consists of inserting a hemofilter in an extracorporeal blood circuit between an artery and vein. In this technique, ultrafiltration occurs in the absence of a blood pump, thus taking advantage of the spontaneous pressure gradient that results from arterial and venous cannulations. Ultrafiltration rates of 5 to 20 mL/min are obtained. The gravity draining the ultrafiltrate away from the filter creates negative pressure in blood chambers

of the filter, resulting in further ultrafiltration. The ultrafiltrate is balanced by a continuous infusion of replacement fluid.

This method also has been described as continuous hemofiltration, slow continuous ultrafiltration, and spontaneous arteriovenous hemofiltration.

Patients with mild forms of acute renal failure do not require CAVH and are probably best treated by traditional intermittent dialysis. However, critically ill patients with multiple-organ failure or traumatic injuries are good candidates for CAVH. CAVH can be used when peritoneal dialysis is contraindicated, as in paralytic ileus or respiratory failure, or when abdominal drains are present.

Hypercatabolic patients with acute renal failure may require hyperalimentation, during which large amounts of fluid must be given to provide adequate nutrition. Therefore, CAVH helps to accomplish adequate total parenteral nutrition because it allows the administration of large volumes of fluids. Fluids can be given freely instead of being restricted. Careful records of intake and output must be kept to avoid significant errors in fluid and electrolyte management.

The difficulties and complications encountered with this technique are related to anticoagulation, the establishment of adequate vascular access, and the selection of an appropriate hemofilter for the system.

## Selected Readings

Leone MR, Jenkins RD, Golper TA, et al. Early experience with continuous arteriovenous hemofiltration in critically ill pediatric patients. Crit Care Med 1986;14:1058.

Maxwell LG, Fivush BA, McLean RH. Renal failure. In: Rogers MC, ed. Textbook of pediatric intensive care. Baltimore: Williams & Wilkins, 1987.

Pascual JF, Lopez JD, Molina M. Hemofiltration in children with renal failure. Pediatr Clin North Am 1987;34:803.

Zobel G, Ring E, Trop M, et al. Arteriovenous hemodiafiltration in children. Int J Pediatr Nephrol 1986;7:203.

Zobel G, Trop M, Ring E, et al. Continuous arteriovenous hemofiltration in critically ill children with acute renal failure. Crit Care Med 1987;15:699.

*Principles and Practice of Pediatrics, Second Edition.*
edited by Frank A. Oski et al. J. B. Lippincott Company, Philadelphia © 1994.

# 41.16 *Continuous Drip Feeding*

## Fernando Stein

Continuous drip feeding is used in patients who cannot tolerate boluses of food or in patients in whom the presence of a large quantity of volume in the stomach is deemed inadvisable. Continuous infusion of liquid nutrients or formula can be achieved through a nasogastric, gastrostomy, or duodenal tube.

Because of circadian rhythms, bowel function is not optimal during the late hours of the evening and early hours of the morning (11 p.m. to 5 a.m.). This is why some practitioners give the 24-hour continuous drip requirement over a 16-hour period.

Formula and liquefied foods that remain at room temperature longer than 4 hours may become contaminated with pathogenic organisms, so they should not hang in the bag longer than 4 hours. The bag and the connecting tubes should be changed at least every 8 hours, and residuals should be checked by aspirating the stomach contents every 2 to 4 hours. There is no universal agreement on what constitutes an acceptable residual. I believe that residuals in an amount greater than that of the previous 3 to 4 hours of continuous feeding should be noted carefully, and reasons for these findings should be sought. Aspirates that are the same in quantity as those of the previous 1 or 2 hours are probably insignificant in the child beyond the neonatal period.

The mattress of the bed or crib should be elevated between 15° and 30° with the head up to prevent gastroesophageal reflux in patients receiving continuous feedings.

*Principles and Practice of Pediatrics, Second Edition.*
edited by Frank A. Oski et al. J. B. Lippincott Company, Philadelphia © 1994.

# CHAPTER 42
# *Shock*

## M. Michele Mariscalco

## DEFINITION

Shock is a clinical syndrome that has been characterized in cardiovascular terms. It now is recognized that shock states reflect a disruption in and eventual loss of normal metabolic function at the cellular level. Cellular derangement occurs because of either inadequate delivery or impaired use of oxygen, termed *cellular hypoxia*, and other essential substrates. Cellular hypoxia causes the cell to shift to anaerobic metabolism with accumulation of lactic acid and other metabolic by-products, which can lead to further cell dysfunction. Shock can be recognized clinically by evidence of acute disruption of circulatory or other organ function, particularly the brain, lungs, and kidneys. Hypotension is a late manifestation of shock because the body has a host of mechanisms to maintain adequate perfusion to the central vascular bed. To develop a logical treatment plan, the dynamics of the shock state must be understood.

The cardiovascular system can be likened to a pump that generates pulsatile flow through a series of tubes. The pressure (blood pressure) generated by the pump (the heart) depends on the amount of fluid flowing through the tubes (cardiac output) and the resistance to that flow (systemic vascular resistance). Thus, as in Figure 42-1:

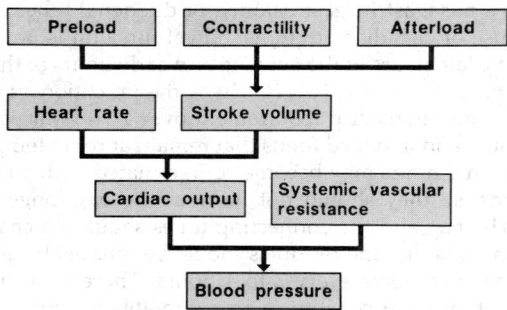

**Figure 42-1.** Regulation of blood pressure.

Blood pressure = cardiac output × systemic vascular resistance *(Equation 1)*

If a decrease in cardiac output occurs (as in cardiogenic shock or hypovolemic shock), there is a compensatory increase in systemic vascular resistance to maintain blood pressure. This increase is mediated by the sympathetic nervous system and endogenous catecholamines. Clinically, the patient's periphery appears cool and mottled. In patients with septic shock, one of the primary defects is loss of systemic vascular resistance; the periphery is warm and appears vasodilated. To maintain blood pressure, cardiac output increases to compensate for loss of vascular tone.

According to the model, the pulsatile flow generated by the pump depends on the rate and volume of each stroke:

Cardiac output = stroke volume × heart rate *(Equation 2)*

Therefore, tachycardia should be present in most forms of shock as a compensatory mechanism to increase cardiac output. Severe bradyarrhythmias or tachyarrhythmias may themselves result in shock if the stroke volume is insufficient to compensate for the reduced cardiac output.

*Stroke volume*, the amount of blood ejected with each heartbeat, is determined by three factors (see Fig 42-1): ventricular preload, the volume of blood in the ventricle at the end of diastolic filling, which reflects venous return to the right heart; ventricular afterload, the impedance to the ejection of blood; and intrinsic myocardial contractility. According to Frank-Starling mechanisms, the stroke volume is directly proportional to the preload. For the myocardium to contract, the contractile proteins of the myocardial fibril, actin and myosin, must overlap. The greater the degree of stretch of the myocardial fibrils at the end of diastolic filling (ie, increased preload), the greater the overlap of the contractile proteins and the greater the increase in stroke volume. Stroke volume will decrease with increased preload if the myofibrils are stretched to a point when the contractile proteins no longer overlap (Fig 42-2).

At a given preload and afterload, the force that a myocardial fibril can generate depends on its intrinsic contractility. Contractility can be increased by release of endogenous catecholamines, increased sympathetic stimulation of the nervous system, and infusion of exogenous inotropic agents, such as epinephrine, dopamine, and dobutamine (see Fig 42-2). Afterload is the composite of factors that oppose ventricular ejection. These factors include resistance to flow by the arterial tree, as reflected by aortic blood pressure, and left ventricular cavity size. Afterload is inversely proportional to stroke volume. An increase in afterload will de-

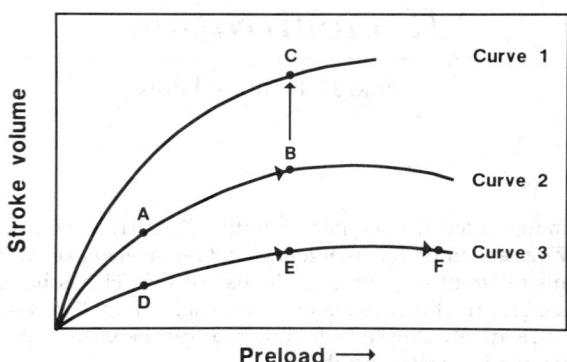

**Figure 42-2.** The Frank-Starling curve. Curve 2, normal heart. Moving from A to B, stroke volume increases with an increase in preload. Curve 3, depressed contractility or increased afterload. Stroke volume can increase if preload is increased from D to E. Further preload increase to F will not increase stroke volume and may lead to increased hydrostatic pressure and pulmonary edema. Curve 1, increased contractility or decreased afterload. Stroke volume can increase from B to C with same preload by increasing contractility or decreasing afterload.

crease stroke volume unless either preload or contractility increases concomitantly. Because blood pressure is a clinical estimate of afterload, increases in blood pressure may decrease cardiac output in certain hemodynamic states. Thus, support of blood pressure does not guarantee adequate delivery of blood and oxygen to the tissues.

Oxygen delivery to the tissues is defined as:

Oxygen delivery = hemoglobin × saturation × cardiac output
(*Equation 3*)

In addition to cardiac output, the hemoglobin content of the blood and the oxygen saturation of the hemoglobin are important in oxygen delivery. If delivery is inadequate for cellular needs, hypoxia will result. Examples of inadequate delivery of oxygen from decreased cardiac output include cardiogenic and hypovolemic shock. In contrast, in septic shock, cellular dysfunction occurs secondary to an intrinsic inability to use oxygen and other substrates, as well as a decrease in oxygen availability from peripheral vasodilation and decreased preload.

With these basic principles, it is possible to understand and therefore treat the initial hemodynamic derangements seen in various shock states. In cardiogenic shock, the underlying hemodynamic dysfunction is in cardiac contractility; in hypovolemic shock, there is a decrease in preload volume; and in septic shock, the initiating event is a decrease in systemic vascular resistance. Hypoxia (absolute oxygen deficit) and ischemia (oxygen and substrate deficit) occur at some time in all types of shock. Either of these insults leads to lactic acidosis, release of vasoactive metabolites and other mediators that are responsible for a host of cellular injuries. Some metabolites and mediators can cause an increase in capillary permeability, leading to a decrease in intravascular volume; others are direct depressants of myocardial contractility, leading to further hemodynamic compromise and multiorgan dysfunction. Thus, the shock cycle perpetuates itself.

Unfortunately, there is little the physician can do to interrupt the mediators of the cellular injury. Support of oxygen delivery and blood pressure, along with any specific measures to treat the underlying injury or infection, is critical to stopping the shock cycle. Success is greatest when recognition of shock occurs and appropriate therapy is begun before the onset of hypotension.

## DIAGNOSIS

The key to making an early diagnosis of shock is a high index of suspicion and a knowledge of which conditions predispose children to shock. A correct diagnosis can be made only after patient history has been obtained. Given the exigencies of the case, the history may be brief initially, but it is crucial in providing optimal stabilization.

Hypotension may be difficult to diagnose in a child without knowing normal values of blood pressure for the child's age. In the adult, a systolic blood pressure less than 90 mm Hg or a fall of 30 to 40 mm Hg is considered hypotension. In addition, one must assess the adequacy of perfusion to the core circulation, because inadequate perfusion precedes hypotension. Oliguria (0.5 to 1.0 mL/kg/hour) accompanies diminished renal perfusion from insufficient cardiac output. Altered mental states such as confusion and agitation occur in early shock. With advanced hypoperfusion, patients classically exhibit obtundation and stupor. Vasoconstriction and diminished flow to the skin manifests as pallor, mottling, and poor capillary refill. In early septic shock, however, a decrease occurs in systemic vascular resistance, the skin is warm, often flushed, and one must rely on other signs, symptoms, and laboratory values to make the diagnosis.

Tachycardia and tachypnea are almost invariably present in patients with shock. As discussed earlier, tachycardia is a compensatory mechanism to increase cardiac output. If cardiac output is diminished, the pulses are rapid, weak, and thready. In early septic shock, cardiac output initially is increased; the pulses are bounding. Severe bradycardia may be the cause of shock if stroke volume cannot increase to maintain cardiac output. In advanced shock, bradycardia is a result of severe hypoxia and acidosis. It usually heralds circulatory arrest unless appropriate and timely interventions are made. Because of limited reserves in stroke volume, the younger child is more dependent on heart rate to increase cardiac output. Extremely rapid heart rates can occur in neonates, infants, and small children before hypotension occurs.

Lactic acidosis, the consequence of tissue hypoxia and ischemia, elicits a compensatory increase in alveolar ventilation, resulting in a fall in $PaCO_2$. The patient exhibits tachypnea (rapid breathing) or hyperpnea (deep breathing). The ensuing respiratory alkalosis will compensate for the metabolic acidosis. However, the rise in minute ventilation increases the proportion of cardiac output that must be supplied to the respiratory muscles. This increase occurs at a time when cardiac output is limited. Relative hypoventilation will occur as the respiratory muscles tire. The acidosis worsens, and the patient will decompensate with increasingly shallow and ineffective respirations, leading to respiratory arrest.

Several laboratory investigations can assist in the further assessment of the severity and cause of shock states. Probably the most common and useful investigation is the blood gas analysis. Adequacy of ventilatory function can be evaluated by monitoring the arterial oxygen and carbon dioxide content. The degree of metabolic acidosis can be a useful indicator of tissue hypoxia or ischemia and of efficacy of therapeutic support. Other laboratory investigations, such as serum electrolytes, blood cell counts, platelet counts, and hematocrit levels, are important in detecting the extent of metabolic disturbances. Calcium should be determined in all shock states because hypocalcemia occurs frequently and can further compromise myocardial, respiratory muscle, and metabolic function. Ionized calcium determinations are preferable to serum calcium levels.

## MONITORING

The most effective and sensitive physiologic monitoring available is the frequent, repeated examination of the child by a competent, careful observer. Minimal monitoring of the child in shock or at risk for shock should include continuous ECG monitoring, frequent blood pressure and temperature measurements, and blood glucose levels in younger infants. Sphygmomanometer readings often can be misleading, and most children require intra-arterial pressure monitoring. Urine production is a sensitive indicator of core perfusion; hourly monitoring of urine output is essential. Central venous and intrapulmonary catheters can also be extremely useful in patients who require close monitoring and manipulation of ventricular filling pressures and cardiac contractility, but they must be used as an adjunct to the physical examination, never as a replacement.

## TREATMENT

For all forms of shock, treatment of the underlying cause and optimization of oxygen and substrate delivery to critical vascular beds (ie, cerebral, renal, and coronary vascular beds) are the cornerstones of therapy. The ultimate goal is to prevent or reverse the defects in cellular metabolism until homeostasis is restored and adequate nutritional support can be instituted to allow healing to begin.

An adequate airway, oxygenation, and ventilation are crucial to maximizing oxygen delivery (see Equation 3). The hemoglobin saturation (% saturation) at a partial pressure of oxygen, $PaO_2$, depends on the oxyhemoglobin dissociation curve (Fig 42-3). Acidosis, hyperthermia, and hypercarbia shift the curve to the right and decrease hemoglobin oxygen affinity or hemoglobin saturation, thus releasing more oxygen to the tissues. Because of the shape of the curve, increases in $PaO_2$ above 65 mm Hg have little effect in increasing oxygen saturation of the hemoglobin. But $PaO_2$ less than 60 mm Hg can cause large decreases in hemoglobin saturation. Therefore, providing supplemental oxygen is part of the initial management of the child in shock.

As discussed above, the respiratory effects of shock can tax an already compromised cardiovascular system severely. Assisted ventilation decreases oxygen transport needs, thereby allowing available oxygen to be delivered to other organs. In addition, positive pressure ventilation helps decrease left ventricular afterload and thus may be useful to the patient with myocardial compromise. However, positive pressure ventilation may also increase intrathoracic pressure enough to decrease venous return to the right side of the heart, decreasing preload and ultimately compromising cardiac output and oxygen delivery. Thus, the effects of mechanical ventilation must be monitored closely.

The most important maneuver in reestablishing circulation is to place an intravascular catheter of an adequate bore for the child's size or an intraosseous catheter. Cardiac output and blood pressure are optimized based on the principles outlined earlier in the section. Preload augmentation often is adequate to restore perfusion and blood pressure in children. Rapid intravascular expansion is guided by clinical examination and urine output. Volume expansion of 20 mL/kg of either normal saline or 5% albuminized normal saline over 10 minutes is generally safe. When volume resuscitation greater than 50 to 70 mL/kg in the first 4 to 6 hours is required, more invasive monitoring should be considered. Modifications of fluid resuscitation must occur to replace ongoing losses due to excessive urine output, stool output, or hemorrhage.

The use of colloid versus crystalloid replacement for shock is an ongoing debate in pediatrics. For simple dehydration, replacement of estimated fluid and electrolyte loss should be sufficient. In sepsis or trauma, difficulties with vascular leak, intravascular oncotic pressure maintenance, and pulmonary edema complicate the picture. To maintain colloid oncotic pressure, a judicious mix of crystalloid, blood products to maintain hemoglobin and clotting factors, and colloid (albumin and hetastarch) should be used. In patients with sepsis, large volumes are often required to maintain adequate preload; volumes of more than 70 to 100 mL/kg are not uncommon.

Preload augmentation is limited in children when there is evidence of an elevated ventricular filling pressure without an in-

crease in cardiac output. Clinically, this condition can be monitored by observing for signs of cardiac congestion: jugular venous distention, enlarging liver associated with a previously undetected cardiac gallop rhythm, and continued evidence of hypoperfusion. Central venous pressure lines may be helpful to prevent further volume overload in these patients. A central venous pressure that is rising or exceeds 7 to 10 mm Hg indicates either myocardial dysfunction, volume overload, or increased right ventricular afterload. In these cases, further management may require more invasive monitoring and the use of inotropic or afterload-reducing agents. Aggressive fluid administration in patients who are on the downward slope of the Starling curve (see Fig 42-2) will result in increased venous pressure and decreased perfusion of several critical beds. Increased venous pressure may worsen vascular leak, leading to increased tissue edema (most notably pulmonary edema) and contributing to the likelihood that the adult respiratory distress syndrome will develop.

When evidence suggests myocardial dysfunction with persistence of shock, interventions must be taken to augment cardiac output. Specific inotropic and afterload-reducing agents are discussed in the section on myocarditis. As mentioned earlier, cardiac dysfunction can occur with any shock state, and the physician must be prepared to intervene at its occurrence. The inotropic agents commonly used have variable effects on heart rate and vascular tone depending on the dose used, the child's age, and the physiologic disturbance. Given this fact, it is misleading to label these agents vasopressors; indeed, one rarely wishes to use a pure vasopressor in most forms of shock.

Managing the multisystem deterioration with shock states is as important as treating the underlying condition. Renal, gastrointestinal, hematologic, and central nervous system derangements should be anticipated, searched for, and treated.

Coagulation abnormalities are common to some extent in all forms of septic shock but are also likely in hypoperfusion states from any cause. Monitoring of prothrombin time, partial thromboplastin time, fibrinogen, fibrin split products, platelet count, and evidence of excessive bleeding is crucial. Use of vitamin K, fresh-frozen plasma, and platelet transfusions will correct most abnormalities.

Gastrointestinal disturbances include paralytic ileus and bleeding from gastritis or ulcer. The ileus may lead to severe fluid and electrolyte disorder, complicating the management of the shock. Gastrointestinal blood loss may be prevented by the use of antacids or $H_2$-receptor blockers such as cimetidine and ranitidine hydrochloride. Liver dysfunction often accompanies shock. Monitoring of liver enzymes will indicate the severity of injury, but usually elevations in the levels occur after the first 24 hours of presentation. Modification of drug therapy should be considered when there is evidence of liver involvement.

Renal support is essential to avoid prolonged periods of anuria or oliguria during hypoperfusion states. Volume augmentation and the use of diuretics such as mannitol, furosemide, and ethacrynic acid have been advocated to maintain renal blood flow and renal tubular function. Low-dose dopamine (3 to 5 $\mu g/kg/$minute) increases renal blood flow and sodium excretion and is used to preserve kidney function. Acute renal failure can lead to oliguria or anuria and may require treatment with peritoneal dialysis, hemodialysis, or ultrafiltration. High-output renal failure can occur without a previous oliguric phase.

Acid–base disturbances are usually severe. A base deficit greater than 10 mEq/L with a pH of less than 7.2 should probably be corrected in acute shock states. Acidosis itself can be an acute, life-threatening event. Hepatic conversion of lactate or acetate to correct acidosis is inadequate. Bicarbonate supplementation can be given by repeated slow-infusion boluses of sodium bicarbonate, 1 to 2 mEq/kg. In infants, 0.5 mEq/mL of solution is used to decrease the risk of intraventricular hemorrhage. Large

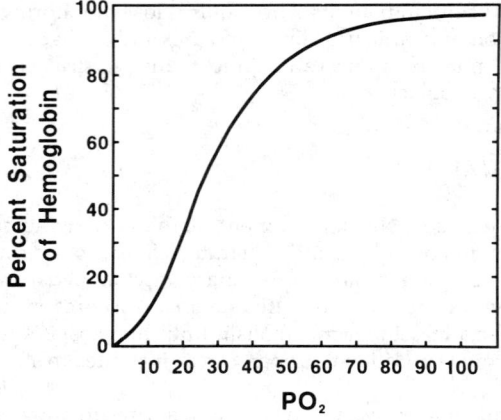

**Figure 42-3.** Oxyhemoglobin dissociation curve.

amounts of bicarbonate may be required. The major limitations to bicarbonate replacement are sodium overload and hyperosmolarity. Overzealous administration of bicarbonate can lead to alkalosis, shifting the oxyhemoglobin curve to the left, increasing oxygen-hemoglobin affinity and thereby worsening oxygen delivery at the tissue level. Close monitoring of serum sodium, pH, and $Paco_2$ is indicated.

A fall in serum ionized calcium is common as the pH returns to normal. Decreased serum ionized calcium can lead to alterations in the level of consciousness, tremors, seizures, hypotension, myocardial depression, and acidosis. Serum ionized calcium bears little relationship to total serum calcium. Either calcium gluconate, 100 mg/kg IV, slow-infusion bolus, or calcium chloride, 20 mg/kg, will rapidly restore serum ionized calcium.

Hyperglycemia or hypoglycemia can accompany severe stress states in children. Hypoglycemia is common in the small or malnourished child. It can be corrected by bolus injection of 25% dextrose, 0.5 to 1 mL/kg, or continuous infusion of glucose, 4 to 8 mg/kg/minute. Hyperglycemia can cause difficulties with osmotic diuresis. Correcting the underlying stress usually will resolve the hyperglycemia without the use of insulin.

## Selected Readings

Edwards JD. Oxygen transport in cardiogenic and septic shock. Crit Care Med 1991;19:658.

Notterman DA. Pharmacology of the cardiovascular system. In: Furhman BP, Zimmerman JJ, eds. Pediatric critical care. St. Louis: Mosby Year Book, 1992.

Perkin RM. Shock states. In: Furhman BP, Zimmerman JJ, eds. Pediatric critical care. St. Louis: Mosby Year Book, 1992.

Shapiro BA, Cane RD. Interpretation of blood gases. In: Shoemaker WC, ed. Textbook of critical care. Philadelphia: WB Saunders, 1989.

Shoemaker WC. Shock states: pathophysiology, monitoring, outcome prediction and therapy. In: Shoemaker WC, ed. Textbook of critical care. Philadelphia: WB Saunders, 1989.

Spivey WH. Interosseous infusion. J Pediatr 1987;111:639.

Zaritsky A. Selected concepts and controversies in pediatric cardiopulmonary resuscitation. Crit Care Clin 1988;4:735.

*Principles and Practice of Pediatrics, Second Edition.*
edited by Frank A. Oski et al. J. B. Lippincott Company, Philadelphia © 1994.

# CHAPTER 43
# *Adult Respiratory Distress Syndrome*

## M. Michele Mariscalco

The adult respiratory distress syndrome (ARDS) is a common form of acute lung failure that occurs in adults, children, and infants. It occurs after a catastrophic event and is characterized by diffuse injury of the capillary-alveolar unit that leads to an increase in extravascular lung water. The syndrome first was described in 1967 by Ashbaugh and Petty, who had observed a series of 12 adult patients suffering from a syndrome similar to hyaline membrane disease in newborns.

Diagnosis of ARDS is based on four criteria: a catastrophic pulmonary or nonpulmonary event in the patient with previously healthy lungs; respiratory distress with hypoxemia, decreased pulmonary compliance, and increased shunt; radiologic evidence of diffuse pulmonary infiltrates; and exclusion of left heart disease and congestive heart failure.

Physicians have recognized for decades the adverse pulmonary effects of both thoracic and extrathoracic trauma, as well as of other kinds of catastrophic events. ARDS has been described by many different names, including Danang lung, hemorrhagic lung syndrome, shock lung, and postperfusion lung. ARDS can occur at any age, even in newborns. Retrospective reports of pediatric ARDS indicate an incidence of 8.5 to 10.4 cases per 1000 pediatric ICU admissions. In the United States, the incidence in adults is estimated at 150,000 cases per year.

Shock, sepsis, and near-drowning are the most common causes of ARDS cited in published pediatric studies. All types of shock have been reported to cause ARDS, as have surface burns, smoke inhalation, infectious and aspiration pneumonias, and disseminated intravascular coagulopathy. Other causes include drug overdose, cardiopulmonary bypass, fat embolism, high altitude, toxic gas inhalation, pancreatitis, and massive transfusion. The mortality rate of patients with ARDS in adult studies ranges from 50% to 80%, with numbers approaching 100% in patients with ARDS who show evidence of failure of two other organ systems. In a study performed by Montgomery in 1985, only 16% of the deaths were attributable to irreversible respiratory failure; the majority were attributed to sepsis syndrome or multiple organ system failure. The mortality rates from two 1991 studies in children with ARDS were 44% and 75%.

Pathologically, within the first 24 to 96 hours after injury, interstitial and then alveolar edema develops. Erythrocytes, neutrophils, and macrophages begin to move into the interstitium and alveolus (Fig 43-1). The thin type I alveolar cells that form the normal epithelial lining of the lung are destroyed, leaving denuded basement membranes. Histologically, the epithelial

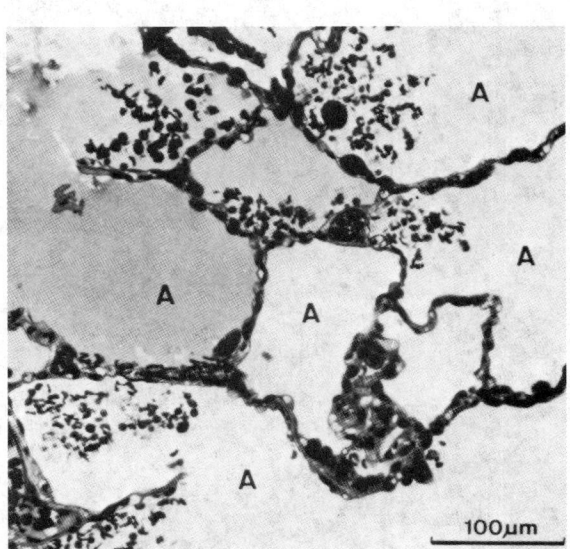

**Figure 43-1.** Light-microscopic view showing pulmonary edema and alveolar spaces (*A*) inhomogeneously filled with proteinaceous fluid. The alveolar walls are edematous and the capillaries are congested. Red blood cells and leukocytes have spilled into the alveolar spaces. (Bachafen M, Weibel ER. Structural alterations of lung parenchyma in the adult respiratory distress syndrome. Clin Chest Med 1982;3:35. Reproduced with permission.)

damage appears to be more severe at this stage than the damage to the capillary endothelium. Within 72 hours of the injury, type II alveolar cells proliferate dramatically (Fig 43-2). These cells are thick, enzymatically active, and responsible for the production of surfactant. Hyaline membranes form over the denuded alveolar surface (Fig 43-3). Over the next 3 to 10 days, the alveolar septum becomes markedly thickened and is infiltrated by proliferating fibroblasts, plasma cells, leukocytes, and histiocytes. The first endothelial changes can be seen as irregularities of the luminal surface. However, significant capillary injury can occur with little morphologic change in the endothelial cells. By the end of 1 week, fibrotic changes may develop in both the alveolar septa and the hyaline membranes. The alveolar structure is no longer recognizable (Fig 43-4). This diffuse alveolar damage is the pathologic hallmark of ARDS.

Noncardiogenic pulmonary edema is a central feature of ARDS. On gross inspection, the lungs with ARDS appear red, heavy, and airless. Ultrastructural evidence supports the notion that disruption of the alveolar capillary membrane is responsible for the pulmonary edema in ARDS. The high protein content of edema fluid in ARDS patients suggests that the restrictive properties of the capillary membrane have been disrupted. Noncardiogenic pulmonary edema floods the lungs more rapidly than hydrostatic pulmonary edema because of the increase in capillary permeability and consequent loss of the protective osmotic gradient between capillary and interstitium.

Patients with ARDS demonstrate reduced lung volumes, large intrapulmonary shunt fractions, and hypoxemia. Alveolar flooding and surfactant abnormalities decrease alveolar volume and lead to widespread atelectasis. Areas of the lung that are perfused either are not ventilated (intrapulmonary shunt) or are ventilated

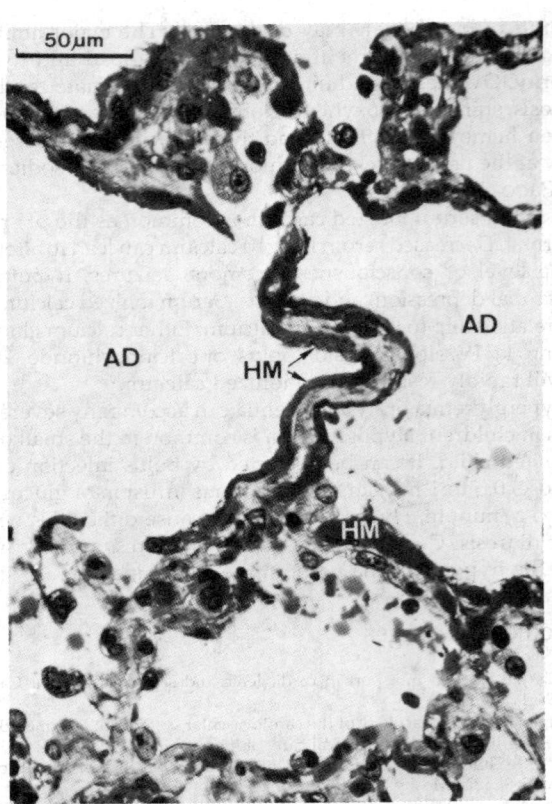

**Figure 43-3.** Light-microscopic view of hyaline membranes (HM) lining alveolar ducts (AD). (Bachafen M, Weibel ER. Structural alterations of lung parenchyma in the adult respiratory distress syndrome. Clin Chest Med 1982;3:35. Reproduced with permission.)

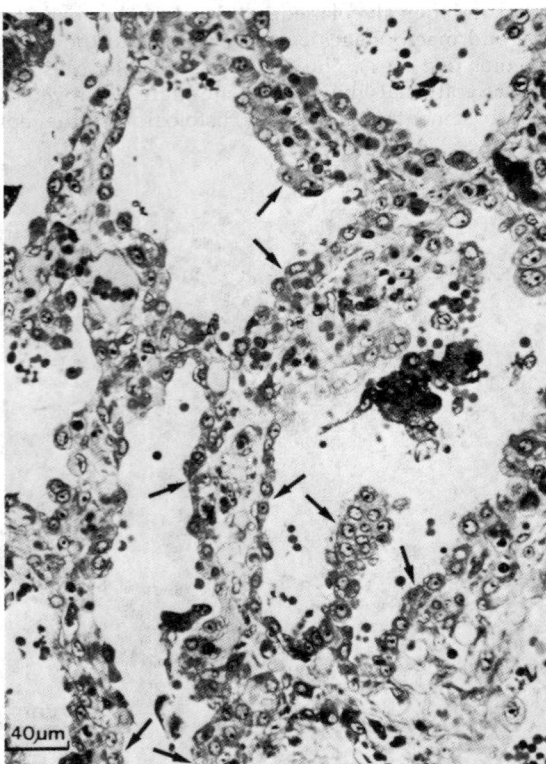

**Figure 43-2.** Light-microscopic view showing proliferation of type II alveolar cells and a markedly thickened septum with cellular proliferation. Arrows show pronounced epithelial transformation. (Bachafen M, Weibel ER. Structural alterations of lung parenchyma in the adult respiratory distress syndrome. Clin Chest Med 1982;3:35. Reproduced with permission.)

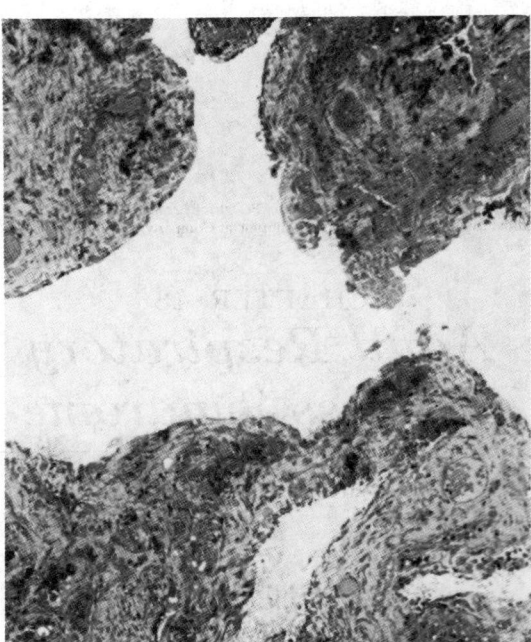

**Figure 43-4.** Light-microscopic view demonstrating markedly distorted pulmonary architecture. The alveolar septae are markedly thickened, and the alveolar spaces are almost obliterated. Hematoxylin and eosin stain, low-power view. (Bachafen M, Weibel ER. Structural alterations of lung parenchyma in the adult respiratory distress syndrome. Clin Chest Med 1982;3:35. Reproduced with permission.)

inadequately (V/Q inequalities), both of which lead to hypoxemia. The decreases in lung volume are reflected by decreases in functional residual capacity and lung compliance. The work of breathing is elevated markedly due to the change in lung compliance. In patients in whom the disease course is protracted, marked pulmonary artery hypertension and lung fibrosis develop.

There is no unifying hypothesis for the pathogenesis of ARDS. Experimental data from various studies have implied that the activation of complement causes activated granulocytes to adhere to and damage pulmonary microvascular endothelial cells via the release of lysozymes and toxic oxygen radicals. Increased permeability of pulmonary capillaries results. Nonetheless, there are inadequate clinical data to confirm this. Other mediators, such as the metabolites of arachidonic acid, prostaglandins, thromboxanes, and leukotrienes, have also been implicated in the increase in vascular permeability and pulmonary artery changes. There is evidence that pulmonary endothelial injury can occur via neutrophil-independent mechanisms, as is the case in oxygen toxicity or endotoxin-induced ARDS models. Clearly, many complex permutations underlie the phenomenon of ARDS, and therapy probably should be directed at more than one of them if morbidity and mortality rates are to improve.

The common complication in ARDS of multiple organ failure has led to the hypothesis that ARDS is part of a spectrum of diseases of diffuse organ injury. In both ARDS and multiple organ failure there is an oxygen demand/supply imbalance at almost all levels of oxygen delivery, thought to be secondary to either altered blood flow distribution or direct endothelial or parenchymal injury. Thus, there is abnormal gas exchange in both the pulmonary and systemic vasculature, leading to oxygen debt.

The history of the patient with ARDS varies, depending on the inciting event. Once direct or indirect injury has occurred, there usually is a latent period during which the patient's respiratory status appears stable. Tachypnea and tachycardia usually develop during the first 12 to 24 hours. As the syndrome progresses, the work of breathing increases dramatically, with nasal flaring and intercostal and accessory respiratory muscle activity. Auscultation of the chest reveals either no abnormality or high-pitched end-expiratory crackles throughout the lung fields. The chest radiograph demonstrates diffuse bilateral alveolar infiltrates. Once respiratory failure occurs, the patient may die from acute respiratory failure (occasionally) or other associated causes (more commonly), or the patient may develop severe fibrotic lung disease requiring prolonged ventilation.

When possible, treatment of the underlying etiology is the first step in the management of ARDS. Currently, no therapeutic modality can halt or reverse either the capillary leak or the pulmonary fibrosis. Neither corticosteroids nor the prostaglandin $PGE_1$ has been shown to be of use in increasing survival in ARDS. Ongoing multicenter trials are evaluating the use of ibuprofen and inhaled surfactant in these patients.

The basis of therapy is supportive at present. The goal of supportive care in ARDS is to deliver sufficient oxygen to satisfy the metabolic demands of tissue. Because these patients are in a state of oxygen debt, oxygen delivery should be maintained in the supranormal range. Oxygen delivery depends on the percentage of saturation of the hemoglobin by oxygen, the hemoglobin content of the blood, and the cardiac output. Therapy is directed at increasing the saturation of oxyhemoglobin without compromising cardiac output. All patients with respiratory failure require supplemental oxygen, which may be supplied by face mask or nasal prongs. However, when an oxygen concentration of up to 50% to 60% is no longer sufficient to prevent hypoxemia, endotracheal intubation usually is required to provide positive end-expiratory pressure (PEEP) without incurring the risks of oxygen toxicity.

PEEP or continuous positive airway pressure (CPAP) increases the compliance of the lung. *Lung compliance* is defined as the transpulmonary pressure ($P_1$) that must be achieved to obtain a certain lung volume ($V_1$). With decreased compliance, as in ARDS, a higher pressure ($P_2$) must be achieved to maintain the same volume ($V_1$). PEEP increases lung compliance by opening and stabilizing atelectatic alveoli and airways, thereby allowing $V_1$ to be achieved at the lower transpulmonary pressure ($P_1$). As compliance increases, lung volume and functional residual capacity increase. Shunt fraction—those lung units with decreased or absent ventilation with normal blood flow—decreases and hypoxemia improves.

PEEP and CPAP do not retard or reverse the development of pulmonary edema. They also can have deleterious effects on cardiac output by decreasing venous return to the right ventricle, decreasing right ventricular compliance, and compromising left ventricular filling and emptying. Thus, PEEP may improve the hemoglobin saturation but decrease cardiac output; ultimately, oxygen delivery may be either not improved or actually worsened.

Several unconventional ventilatory strategies have been advocated for use in patients with ARDS. High-frequency ventilation has been shown to have no advantage over conventional ventilation. Other therapies such as inverse-ratio ventilation, permissive hypercapnia, and airway pressure release have all been advocated as salvage techniques or as routine alternatives, although no controlled trials support their use. A 1979 study using extracorporeal membrane oxygenation (ECMO) showed no improvement in survival; both groups had a survival rate of 10%. Recently an adult ARDS study using extracorporeal $CO_2$ removal ($ECCO_2R$) demonstrated that conventional therapy and $ECCO_2R$ were equal in survival (50%). Although ECMO is used in some centers on children with ARDS, and claims have been made that it improves survival, again no controlled trial supports its use.

Careful fluid and blood-product management remains crucial to the stabilization of patients with ARDS. There is controversy over whether crystalloid or colloid replacement should occur. At present, volume expansion with blood clearly seems to be preferable to crystalloid, as oxygen delivery is improved by increases in both hematocrit and cardiac output. Because of the permeability of the alveolar-capillary membrane, some fluid will leak into the pulmonary interstitium or alveoli, ultimately worsening the intrapulmonary shunt. Cardiac filling pressures should be monitored so that overhydration can be scrupulously avoided. Right atrial pressure catheters or pulmonary artery catheters to measure pulmonary capillary wedge pressure are helpful in fluid management and support of cardiac output. Inotropic agents are also used to maximize cardiac output.

Nutritional repletion is vital in patients with ARDS and should be instituted as early as possible in the clinical course. Often gastrointestinal motility is impaired in ARDS, usually from a variety of factors including CPAP/PEEP, inactivity, and sedatives, requiring parenteral nutrition. Calories are maximized while fluid administration is minimized. Excessive intake of carbohydrates is avoided, as carbohydrates are metabolized into fat in the liver, leading to large amounts of $CO_2$ production. Patients with respiratory failure may not be able to increase minute ventilation sufficiently to excrete this excess $CO_2$ load.

Other supportive measures include diligent surveillance for secondary infections and the use of sedatives and occasionally muscle relaxants to ventilate the patient effectively.

The complications of therapy for ARDS include oxygen toxicity to the lungs and the risk of barotrauma. Inspired oxygen concentration should be kept at the lowest point with adequate tissue oxygenation by the judicious use of CPAP/PEEP. Alveolar rupture from overdistention can lead to pneumothorax, pneumoperitoneum, pneumomediastinum, pneumopericardium, and subcutaneous air. Pneumothorax should be suspected whenever

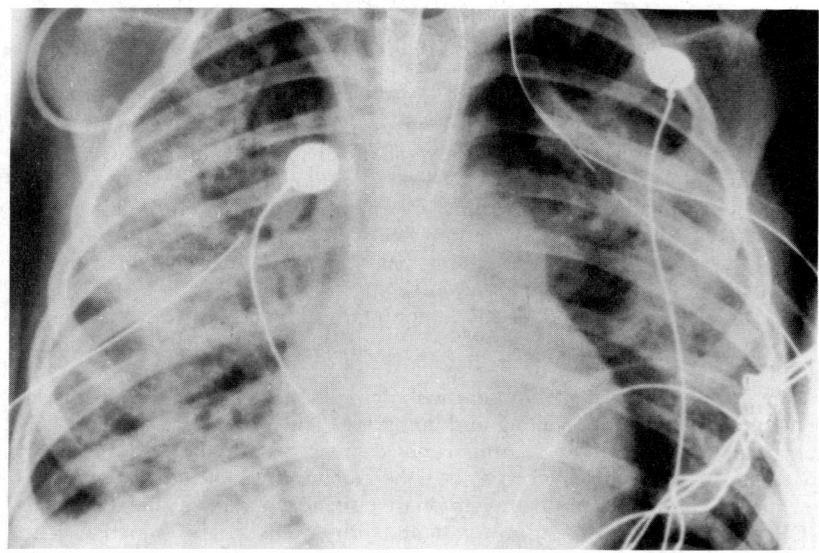

**Figure 43-5.** Severe ARDS and pneumothoraces in a 4-year-old boy who required multiple chest-tube drainage.

the ARDS patient on CPAP/PEEP exhibits an unexplained sudden deterioration in clinical appearance, arterial oxygen tension, or hemodynamic stability (Fig 43-5). Successful management of the pneumothorax almost always requires closed-chest thoracostomy tube evacuation of air to an underwater seal.

Adult long-term survivors of ARDS are likely to have normal chest radiographs and minimal respiratory symptoms. Data suggest that the gas-exchanging surface area of the lung is adequate to meet oxygen requirements of the patient at rest; during exercise, however, efficient oxygenation is impaired, and $PaO_2$ may fall. Although there are few follow-up data on children after severe ARDS, they tend to support the premise that children who have had ARDS are more likely than adults to be left with significant respiratory abnormalities, including resting hypoxemia, cough, and exertional dyspnea. Long-term follow-up is required.

## Selected Readings

Dorinksy PM, Gadek JE. Multiple organ failure. Clin Chest Med 1990;11:581.

Fuhrman BP, Dalton HJ. Progress in pediatric extracorporeal membrane oxygenation. Crit Care Clin 1992;8:191.

Morris AH, Wallace CJ, Clemmer CJ, et al. Final report: computerized protocol controlled clinical trial of new therapy which includes $ECCO_2R$ for ARDS. Am Rev Resp Dis 1992;145:A184.

Petty TL, Bone RC, Gee MH, Hudson LD, Hyers TM. Contemporary clinical trials in ARDS. Chest 1992;101:550.

Royall JA, Matalon S. Pulmonary edema and ARDS. In: Fuhrman BP, Zimmerman JJ, eds. Pediatric critical care. St. Louis: Mosby Year Book, 1992.

Stoller JK, Kackmarek RM. Ventilatory strategies in the management of the ARDS. Clin Chest Med 1990;11:755.

Tamburro RF, Bugnitz MC, Stidham GL. Alveolar-arterial oxygen gradient as a predictor of outcome in patients with neonatal pediatric respiratory failure. J Pediatr 1991;119:935.

Timmons OD, Dean JM, Vernon DD. Mortality rates and prognostic variables in children with ARDS. J Pediatr 1991;119:896.

---

*Principles and Practice of Pediatrics, Second Edition.*
edited by Frank A. Oski et al. J. B. Lippincott Company, Philadelphia © 1994.

# CHAPTER 44
# *Hypertension*

## J. Timothy Bricker

## ARTIFACTS IN BLOOD PRESSURE MEASUREMENT

Physicians who care for children monitored by indwelling arterial lines must understand how to zero, calibrate, and prevent artifacts in the system. An artifact from an underdamped indwelling arterial line is a common source of apparent hypertension in the critically ill child. Inaccurate calibration or inappropriate zeroing of a manometer may result in artifactual hypertension. An overdamped system, a partially occluded arterial line, or an arterial spasm may cause a low measured arterial blood pressure, with

the diagnosis of an acute increase in blood pressure when the arterial line is discontinued and cuff measurements are begun. Periodic cuff pressures should be recorded for the patient being monitored with an indwelling arterial line.

Oscillometric methods of pressure measurement have been shown to correlate well with other methods, including indwelling arterial lines, and have come into general use on many pediatric inpatient units. Patient motion can cause artifactual hypertension when motion artifact is confused with pulse-wave oscillation by the pressure-measurement device. Another common cause of artifactual hypertension is a cuff too small for the patient. The width of the cuff bladder should be about 40% to 50% of the circumference of the child's upper arm at its midpoint. This principle applies to both oscillometric and auscultatory methods of blood pressure determination.

Another type of artifact with auscultatory measurement of the systemic arterial pressure is the missed auscultatory gap. The auscultatory gap is a silent pressure interval between the onset of Korotkoff sounds and their final disappearance or muffling. Failure to inflate the cuff to a high enough pressure (ie, 20 mm Hg above the point at which Korotkoff sounds are heard on the first measurement, confirmed by disappearance of the radial pulse) or failure to listen for Korotkoff sounds all the way down to zero can result in the appearance of a sudden increase or decrease in blood pressure when it is measured accurately.

## EFFECTS OF ELEVATION OF SYSTEMIC ARTERIAL BLOOD PRESSURE

Systemic arterial hypertension can be an acute pediatric emergency because of the impact of a severely elevated pressure on vital organ systems. The most prominent effects of severe, acute hypertension are on the neurologic and the cardiovascular systems.

### Neurologic Complications

Neurologic abnormalities due to hypertension can include lethargy, headache, confusion, stupor, focal motor deficits, visual loss, seizures, and coma. In a retrospective study of hypertension with neurologic complications, convulsions were the initial feature in 42% of the children. Two of the patients had altered consciousness alone, and two had cranial nerve findings. Nausea and vomiting may be present in the early stages. Physical findings often include advanced hypertensive retinopathy with papilledema, retinal hemorrhages, and retinal exudates, as well as abnormalities on neurologic examination.

Evidence of cerebral edema is likely on CT scanning. If features such as a stiff neck and fever mandate a lumbar puncture, both the CSF pressure and the CSF protein content will probably be elevated. Most cases of hypertensive encephalopathy can be managed without a lumbar puncture, and the risk of lumbar puncture in the presence of an elevation in intracranial pressure is increased.

Treatment of the hypertension typically results in very rapid improvement in the neurologic signs and symptoms, although some findings may require several days to resolve.

Pathologic features include brain swelling, hemorrhages (punctate to massive), and microinfarctions. In some cases, there may be enough swelling of the brain for herniation to be apparent.

It is important to pursue the differential diagnosis of hypertensive encephalopathy (Table 44-1) because treatment for hypertensive encephalopathy (ie, abruptly lowering the blood pressure to normal) can be detrimental in some patients with chronic hypertension. For example, the patient with severe renal artery stenosis may have diminished flow distal to the obstruction, which may result in renal ischemia if the arterial pressure is lowered abruptly by a systemic arteriolar dilator.

For patients with hypertension that is chronic and not extremely severe, and for patients in whom there is an alternative explanation of the encephalopathy, the diagnosis of hypertensive encephalopathy should be viewed with some skepticism. It may be necessary to lower the systemic arterial blood pressure in many of the chronically hypertensive patients admitted to the ICU, but it is not safe to do so as abruptly as one would with acutely hypertensive patients who usually are normotensive.

Children who recover from hypertensive encephalopathy can be expected to do well. In a 10-year study of 45 children with neurologic complications of hypertension, no neurologic or cognitive sequelae were noted on long-term follow-up.

Another neurologic problem associated with severe hypertension is the development of intracranial hemorrhage. Massive hemorrhage due to hypertension may occur in a child with a berry aneurysm of the circle of Willis, or in one who has undergone neurologic surgery recently. Systemic hypertension in profoundly premature infants is thought to put them at risk for subependymal bleeding from the germinal matrix.

### Cardiopulmonary Complications

Acute and severe hypertension can be associated with cardiac dilation, elevation of the left ventricular end-diastolic pressure, and symptomatic pulmonary edema. The normal myocardium handles the acute increase in left ventricular afterload relatively well. Children with acute glomerulonephritis do not typically have findings of a low cardiac output state as a result of increased afterload, and typically symptomatic pulmonary edema resolves rapidly without residual cardiac abnormality when the excessive intravascular blood volume associated with acute glomerulonephritis is lowered by diuretic therapy.

Some children have a limited cardiac reserve due to severe prematurity, congenital cardiac disease, or acquired cardiac disease. Under these circumstances, a hypertensive crisis may result in cardiovascular decompensation. Abruptly lowering the systemic arterial pressure is required in this setting. Cardiovascular decompensation with hypertensive crisis is more common in adults than in children because of the prevalence of overt or subclinical coronary artery atherosclerotic disease among adults with hypertension. Most children with hypertension will have a hyperdynamic apex impulse, a dilated heart with an apex impulse displaced laterally, and a diastolic filling sound during a hypertensive crisis. Chronic hypertension may be associated with left ventricular hypertrophy and arterial abnormalities. Acute aortic dissection has occurred in severely hypertensive children who did not have features of Marfan syndrome or other abnormalities of connective tissue. The degree of left ventricular hypertrophy ascertained by ECG and echocardiography can give a clue as to the chronicity of hypertension.

### Complications in Other Organ Systems

Renal abnormalities may develop or progress in the child with extremes of hypertension. Ophthalmic abnormalities may be re-

---

**TABLE 44-1. Conditions That May Be Confused With Hypertensive Encephalopathy***

| | |
|---|---|
| Illicit or therapeutic drugs | Reye's syndrome |
| Uremic encephalopathy | Diabetic ketoacidosis |
| Encephalitis or meningoencephalitis | Seizure disorder |
| Hypoglycemia | Hyperthyroidism or |
| Hypocalcemia | hypothyroidism |
| Trauma | Psychosis |
| Low cerebral blood flow | Cerebritis |
| Hepatic causes | |

* Hypertensive encephalopathy is defined as a hypertensive state with alternative (superimposed) explanation of encephalopathic features.

---

**TABLE 44-2. Hypertensive Emergencies and Urgencies in the Pediatric Intensive Care Patient**

**Hypertensive Emergencies**
Hypertension causing neurologic symptoms
Hypertension causing congestive heart failure
Hypertension associated with aortic dissection

**Hypertensive Urgencies**
Hypertension in the postoperative cardiac patient
Hypertension in the postoperative neurosurgery patient
Hypertension after renal transplantation
Hypertension in the profoundly premature infant
Hypertension in the child who must be taken to the operating room for a surgical emergency
Extreme asymptomatic hypertension
Severe hypertension in the patient with risk of bleeding (eg, following renal biopsy)

lated to severe hypertensive retinopathy. Nonneurologic manifestations of the effects of severe, acute hypertension in children are lower in frequency and severity compared with effects on the brain. Urgent therapy for hypertension might be considered in the child whose hypertension is associated with bleeding after cardiac surgery or whose hypertension might compromise the success of a renal transplant (Table 44-2).

# BLOOD PRESSURE ELEVATION OF DIAGNOSTIC IMPORTANCE IN THE PEDIATRIC ICU

In many pediatric ICU patients, hypertension is neither an emergency nor of urgent significance, but it provides insight into the

## TABLE 44-3.   Differential Diagnosis of Hypertension in Children

### Iatrogenic, Factitious, Accidental

Acute Na overload: $NaHCO_3$, glucose and electrolyte mixtures, Scholl's antibiotics (Na-penicillin or Na-carbenicillin), Kayexalate, phosphate replacements, contrast media (Hypaque = 786 mEq/L), IV fluids

Licorice and related compounds (similar to aldosteronism)

Exogenous steroids

Nonsteroidal anti-inflammatory drugs: mineralocorticoid-like effect, probably mediated by prostaglandins

Antidepressant drugs: MAO inhibitors (with other drugs), tricyclics, lithium

Other sympathomimetics (direct and indirect): phenylephrine eye or nose drops, appetite suppressants, cold medicines, thyroid medications, street drugs

Anesthetics: ketamine, cyclopropane, local anesthetics, pancuronium, narcotics (esp. Narcan)

Ergot alkaloids (for migraines, in obstetrics, from plants)

Antihypertensive drug therapy (beta blockers, saralasin, clonidine, postganglionic blockers, methyldopa) with catecholamine excess or rebound

Poisons: heavy metals, spider bites, drugs, plants

Accidents: burns, orthopedic accidents, trauma

### Cardiovascular Etiology

Coarctation of the aorta: preop, acute postop, residual, recurring.

Causes of "diastolic runoff" (systolic hypertension with a wide pulse pressure): PDA, AV fistula, aortic regurgitation, AP window, ruptured sinus of Valsalva aneurysm, large aorticopulmonary anastomosis

Infective endocarditis (renal mechanism)

Arteritis (radiation, Takayasu's disease, connective-tissue disease)

Peripheral atherosclerosis (systolic only with wide pulse pressure)

### Renovascular Hypertension

*Intrinsic Renal Artery Disease*

Intimal fibrosis (postinjury, idiopathic)

Medial (fibromuscular dysplasia, muscular hyperplasia)

Subadventitial (fibrosis or dysplasia)

Arteritis

Thrombotic

Embolic

Aneurysms, dissecting aneurysms

Fistulae

Neurofibromatosis

Associated with other congenital defects:

   Renal artery stenosis with coarctation

   Uteropelvic junction obstruction

   William's syndrome

   Atherosclerotic lesions

*Extrinsic Compression*

Renal parenchymal tumors

Para-aortic tumors:

   Neurofibroma

   Pheochromocytoma

   Ganglioneuroma

Para-aortic lymphatics:

   Lymphoma

   Chronic granulomatous

Ectopic kidney position

Iatrogenic (ligature involving a normal or aberrant renal artery)

### Renal Parenchymal and Structural Disease

Cystic disease:

   Infantile polycystic kidneys

   Adult polycystic kidneys

   Medullary sponge kidney (juvenile nephronophthisis) with Zellweger's, Jeune's, Goldenhar's, trisomies D and E, and orofacial digital syndromes, short-rib polydactyly, Ehlers-Danlos syndrome, various chromosome translocations

Segmental hypoplasia (Ask-Upmark kidney)

Hydronephrosis

Pyelonephritis

Glomerulonephritis

Renal vein thrombosis (uncommon)

Trauma

   Page kidney (cellophane), resultant parenchymal compression

   Transient hypertension after blunt abdominal trauma

Nephrotic syndrome (lowers, probability of minimal lesion)

Hemolytic-uremic syndrome

Sickle-cell disease

### Endocrine Causes

Congenital adrenal hyperplasia

   11-Hydroxylase deficiency

   17-Hydroxylase deficiency

Cushing's syndrome

   Iatrogenic

Hyperaldosteronism

   Primary (Conn's nodular hyperplasia, dexamethasone suppressible)

   Exogenous

   Secondary

Tumors

   Pheochromocytoma, neuroblastoma, ganglioneuroblastoma, argentaffinoma, Wilms' tumor, JGA tumors

Thyrotoxicosis

Hyperparathyroidism

Turner's syndrome patients taking estrogens

Birth-control pills, SIADH

### CNS Hypertension

Elevated ICP, ischemia

Riley-Day syndrome (familial dysautonomia)

Quadriplegia, polio, Guillain-Barré syndrome

Absent corpus callosum, increased ADH-hypertension syndrome

### Other Causes

Volume excess from polycythemia

Stevens-Johnson syndrome

Cyclic vomiting with dehydration

Intussusception

Femoral nerve traction

*After Inglefinger J. Hypertension in childhood. Philadelphia: WB Saunders, 1982.*

patient's disease process and assists the astute clinician in diagnosis and patient management.

A very common cause of hypertension in the pediatric ICU is pain or agitation. An example is the child who requires neuromuscular-junction blocking agents for adequate mechanical ventilation and who is not well sedated. Hypertension may be noted before the next dose of sedatives is due, and it will respond to an increase in dose or in frequency of administration of sedatives. The child who has a physiologic narcotic dependency due to a prolonged need for sedation in the ICU may manifest withdrawal by hypertension. Hypertension is also commonly associated with an increase in intracerebral pressure. The concomitant findings of sinus bradycardia and irregular breathing may give the clue to the etiology of hypertension in this setting. Hypertension may be present in the early phase of septic shock and may be noted as a response to chronic ventilatory insufficiency.

The differential diagnosis of hypertension in children is given in Table 44-3.

## TREATMENT

The standard agent for lowering blood pressure in patients with hypertensive encephalopathy is diazoxide. The usual dose range is 3 to 5 mg/kg IV; however, a dose of 1 to 2 mg/kg has been found to be adequate in many cases, so an initial dose in the lower range is recommended. A dose of 10 mg/kg may be required in some cases. Diazoxide must be given in a rapid bolus, because slow IV infusions result in binding of the drug by plasma proteins and loss of effect. Diazoxide is unlikely to lower the blood pressure to an excessive degree, but it is wise to monitor the pressure immediately after a bolus dose. Appropriate management of excessive hypotension includes a volume infusion (eg, 10 mL/kg of normal saline). Hyperglycemia is a side effect of diazoxide and is of particular concern when repeated doses are required.

Other agents that may be helpful for treatment of acute hypertension are hydralazine and nitroprusside (Table 44-4). It may be necessary to treat cerebral edema with an osmotic agent such as mannitol or glycerol and with hyperventilation sufficient to maintain the arterial $PCO_2$ in the low 30-mm Hg range in some cases of hypertensive encephalopathy associated with profound brain swelling, but lowering blood pressure alone is sufficient in the vast majority of cases.

Treatment with diazoxide of a hypertensive crisis with cardiovascular manifestations is reasonable. Volume reduction by diuretic therapy alone may ameliorate the findings of pulmonary edema in some of these cases. Diuretic therapy should be included for most patients with a hypertensive crisis that includes pulmonary edema. Patients in renal failure with a hypertensive crisis may not be responsive to diuretics; if they have a severe degree of volume overload, they may need dialysis or plasmapheresis if there is evidence of cardiac dysfunction and cardiogenic pulmonary edema. Pericardial effusion is a common cause of radiographic cardiomegaly in the uremic patient, and cardiac tamponade in the uremic patient can be the cause of symptoms of heart failure. Abrupt volume reduction without treatment of cardiac tamponade is likely to cause hemodynamic deterioration.

Hydralazine is a common choice for the management of a hypertensive crisis after emergency treatment with diazoxide. Hydralazine can be given at a dose of 0.2 to 0.8 mg/kg IV or 1.0 to 5.0 mg/kg/day PO. A lupuslike syndrome occurs in some patients given hydralazine, but this typically is reversible when the drug is discontinued. Hydralazine is used commonly for patients who have hypertension associated with systemic lupus erythematosus, including the emergency treatment of a hypertensive crisis.

Propranolol and other beta blockers may be useful adjuncts in the treatment of chronic hypertension. The use of intravenous beta blockers in children is considered relatively hazardous, and the physician should be prepared to pace the rhythm if excess bradycardia occurs. Intravenous beta blocker therapy rarely is required for pediatric hypertension.

Intravenous verapamil and other calcium channel blockers have been used to treat hypertension. Rarely, they are also required in the emergency treatment of hypertension. As with the beta blockers, the role of calcium channel blockers in hypertension is primarily as an adjunct in chronic therapy.

Nitroprusside is an arteriolar dilator that lowers blood pressure by dropping the systemic vascular resistance. A nitroprusside infusion acts rapidly to lower the pressure and can be titrated to the arterial pressure desired. The usual dose range is from 0.5 to 8.0 $\mu$g/kg/minute. High-dose and prolonged infusions are associated with toxicity from cyanide and thiocyanate. Nitroprusside

## TABLE 44-4. Drugs and Dosages for Use in the Treatment of Hypertensive Emergencies in Children

| Drug | Dose | Comments |
| --- | --- | --- |
| Diazoxide | 1.0–10.0 mg/kg/dose IV | Start at lower range, rapid infusion. Watch for hypotension and hyperglycemia. |
| Hydralazine | 0.2–0.8 mg/kg/dose IV | Concerns about development of lupuslike phenomenon |
| | 1.0–5.0 mg/kg/day PO | |
| Nitroprusside | 0.5–8.0 $\mu$g/kg/min infusion | Cyanide and thiocyanate toxicity with prolonged high-dose therapy |
| Propranolol | 0.1–2.0 mg/kg/dose | IV use with slow infusion and with capability to pace if bradycardia is excessive |
| Verapamil | 0.1–0.2 mg/kg/dose | Not if patient is under age 6 months, is on beta blockers, or has congestive heart failure |
| Hydrochlorothiazide | 0.5–2.0 mg/kg/day PO | More often for chronic therapy |
| Methyldopa | 10.0–40.0 mg/kg/day | More often for chronic therapy |
| Reserpine | — | No longer available |

can be useful during the period between the initial lowering of pressure with diazoxide and the initiation of long-term antihypertensive therapy.

## Selected Readings

David Y. Basic science of blood pressure measurement. In: Garson A Jr, Bricker JT, McNamara DG, eds. The science and practice of pediatric cardiology. Philadelphia: Lea & Febiger, 1990.

Inglefinger J. Hypertension in childhood. Philadelphia: WB Saunders, 1982.

Park MK, Menard SM. Accuracy of blood pressure measurement by the Dinamap monitor in infants and children. Pediatrics 1987;79:907.

Trompeter RS, Smith RL, Hoare RD, et al. Neurologic complications of arterial hypertension. Arch Dis Child 1982;57:913.

*Principles and Practice of Pediatrics, Second Edition.*
edited by Frank A. Oski et al. J. B. Lippincott Company, Philadelphia © 1994.

# CHAPTER 45
# *Acute Hepatic Failure*

## Penelope Terhune Louis

Acute hepatic failure is a clinical syndrome that occurs within 8 weeks of the onset of liver disease in patients in whom liver function is presumed to have been normal before the illness. Acute hepatic failure is a rare but devastating event, with a mortality rate of 80% or higher. However, full recovery to normal hepatic structure and function is possible even after massive injury. In view of this potential for full recovery, all patients with acute hepatic failure should receive intensive support.

Acute hepatic failure implies either acute massive destruction of liver tissue or other processes that cause rapid deterioration in function. The diagnosis of acute hepatic failure in children must be differentiated from that of hepatic failure that occurs as a complication of underlying congenital, anatomical, and metabolic abnormalities. In addition, hepatic encephalopathy with hyperammonemia is necessary for the diagnosis of acute hepatic failure, as is coagulopathy with prolongation of the prothrombin time (PT) and partial thromboplastin time (PTT).

## ETIOLOGY

Acute liver failure in the pediatric ICU is usually associated with viral hepatitis, drugs, or toxins. Although hepatitis A virus usually affects children, hepatitis B virus infection is most likely to cause fulminant hepatic failure, representing as much as 75% in some series. Patients exposed to hepatitis B virus who develop fulminant failure tend to have an enhanced antibody response, with an earlier appearance of antibodies to the hepatitis B surface antigen and hepatitis B e antigen and a more rapid clearance of the surface antigen than in patients who do not develop fulminant failure. Work with the delta agent indicates that delta agent

markers occur more frequently in patients with fulminant hepatitis B viral infection than in patients with uncomplicated hepatitis B disease. Other less common infectious agents include hepatitis C viruses, Epstein-Barr virus, cytomegalovirus, echoviruses, herpes simplex virus, adenoviruses, leptospires, and *Toxoplasma gondii.*

Accidental ingestion of toxic amounts of acetaminophen, iron, and vitamin A can cause acute hepatic failure. Halothane can cause hepatic failure in children. Idiosyncratic hypersensitivity to isoniazid, α-methyl-dopa, and some anticonvulsants and antibiotics also can cause acute fulminant hepatic failure.

## CLINICAL MANIFESTATIONS

Mild to moderate nausea, anorexia, and fatigue are common with acute hepatitis. The presence of protracted vomiting, altered behavior, bruisability, or ascites alerts the clinician that the case may be associated with acute hepatic failure. Other associated symptoms include jaundice, abdominal pain, fever, and rash. Throughout the course of the illness, the degree of neurologic deterioration is one of the most reliable means of assessing and following the severity of the hepatic failure.

Liver function tests monitored include measurements of transaminases, alkaline phosphatase, bilirubin, albumin, and PT. The transaminases become elevated with altered hepatocellular integrity. The absolute height of transaminase elevation does not correlate with the severity of the disease. The pattern of change in transaminase levels with time can be useful in following the activity of the disease, as long as the liver still can produce transaminase. There may be such rapid destruction of hepatocytes that the transaminases can fall precipitously as a premorbid event.

Alkaline phosphatase is produced in the bile canaliculus in response to increased pressure within the canaliculus. Thus, alkaline phosphatase of liver origin rises with any extrahepatic or intrahepatic obstruction to bile flow. An assay of 5'-nucleotidase may be useful to differentiate between bone and liver alkaline phosphatase.

Neither the transaminases nor alkaline phosphatase defines liver function as well as does serum bilirubin, albumin, or PT. The prolonged PT observed is not responsive to parenteral vitamin K in the face of acute hepatic failure. The albumin level is often below 4 g/dL despite the long half-life of this protein. Mixed hyperbilirubinemia is variable, with levels ranging from 15 to 40 mg/dL.

## COMPLICATIONS
### Coagulopathy

An elevated PT is present by definition in acute hepatic failure. This coagulopathy is the result of inadequate synthesis of Factors V, VII, and X. Patients with acute hepatic failure given a trial of phytonadione (AquaMEPHYTON) show little or no change in the PT. Low-grade disseminated intravascular coagulation, prolonged PT, PTT, and thrombin time, lowered fibrinogen and platelet counts, and the presence of fibrin split products all are common in acute hepatic failure.

### Gastrointestinal Bleeding

Up to 70% of patients with acute hepatic failure may experience GI bleeding, and as many as 30% of those die from this complication. Bleeding is the result of stress gastritis and portal hypertension exacerbated by the coagulopathy of liver disease.

## Renal Failure

One complication of acute hepatic failure is an oliguric form of renal failure described as the hepatorenal syndrome. This condition is characterized by a urine sodium concentration of less than 10 mEq/L in a euvolemic patient. The cause of the hepatorenal syndrome is unknown. Functionally, patients with acute hepatic failure behave as if they have depletion in the intravascular volume, rendering them particularly sensitive to any further decrease such as that associated with septic shock, diuresis, or GI hemorrhage. Any of these events can push these patients into progressive renal failure. The kidney in these patients is histologically normal and can function normally when transplanted into another patient.

## Electrolyte Imbalance

Profound alterations in serum sodium and potassium levels are common. Patients with acute hepatic failure may require large doses of intravenous potassium to maintain a normal serum level because of the kaliuresis associated with secondary hyperaldosteronism. Decreased serum sodium is noted because of an antidiuretic-like activity combined with increased total body sodium and fluid retention due to a hyperaldosterone-like activity. In addition, in some patients there is a shift of sodium into intracellular compartments. Profound hypoglycemia is found in as many as 40% of the children with acute hepatic failure. Severe hypoglycemia occurs because of the liver's impaired ability to store glycogen. Respiratory alkalosis is also a common phenomenon, occurring in the presence of central hyperventilation.

## Infection

Sepsis is a common problem in any acutely ill hospitalized patient, and may be the precipitating event when hepatic coma develops in the face of acute hepatic failure. Infection in patients with liver disease consists of bacteremia of gut organisms due to poor hepatic clearing of organisms seeded from the edematous bowel of portal hypertension; urinary tract infections; and aspiration pneumonia. Worsening encephalopathy, sudden development of hepatorenal syndrome, and new onset of fever and leukocytosis should raise suspicion of infection.

## Respiratory Failure

There are many reasons for respiratory failure and the need for respiratory support in fulminant hepatic failure. Neurologic dysfunction in hepatic coma may warrant intubation and mechanical ventilation independent of respiratory failure. Encephalopathic changes produce inappropriate secretion of antidiuretic hormone and potentiate the development of pulmonary edema. Hepatic failure also has been implicated in the production of respiratory failure by intrapulmonary shunting secondary to the effect of vasoactive substances normally metabolized by the liver.

## MANAGEMENT

Initial, specific therapy for treatable conditions that cause hepatic failure must be instituted as rapidly as possible. Otherwise, the aim of therapy in patients with acute hepatic failure is to maintain cerebral, renal, cardiac, and pulmonary function until hepatic regeneration can occur. Basic maintenance includes monitoring, intravenous alimentation, respiratory support, control of cerebral edema, prevention of and intervention for hepatorenal syndrome, prevention of bleeding disorders (including GI bleeding), and aggressive therapy during infectious complications.

Attempting to correct the coagulopathy associated with fulminant hepatic failure is generally nonproductive, except in the presence of active bleeding or in preparation for an invasive procedure.

The high mortality rate for all cases of fulminant hepatic failure despite intensive medical therapy has led to the investigation of several methods and devices to support the patient until hepatic function returns. Exchange transfusion, charcoal hemoperfusion, plasmapheresis, peritoneal dialysis, and hemodialysis have resulted in occasional temporary improvement in the patient's condition. However, many of these procedures place the patient at increased risk for bleeding and have not improved the survival rate.

Liver transplants have been successful in some patients with fulminant hepatic failure, but specific indications for this procedure have not been established. Transplants generally are not advocated in patients with systemic viral infections, or in patients with irreversible neurologic damage.

Artificial hepatic support systems have been developed but have not been tested in clinical trials; their use at present is experimental.

## Selected Readings

Balknap WM. Acute hepatic failure. In: Levin DL, Moriss FC, eds. Essentials of pediatric intensive care. St. Louis: Quality Medical, 1990.

Bismuth H, Samuel D, Gugenheim J, et al. Emergency liver transplantation for fulminant hepatitis. Ann Intern Med 1987;107:337.

Chapman RW, Forman D, Peto R, et al. Liver transplantation for acute hepatic failure? Lancet 1990;335:32.

Kocoshis SA. Disorders and diseases of the gastrointestinal tract and liver. In: Fuhrman BP, Zimmerman JJ, eds. Pediatric critical care. St. Louis: Mosby Year Book, 1992.

O'Brady JG, Alexander GJM, Hayllar KM, et al. Early indicators of prognosis in fulminant hepatic failure. Gastroenterology 1989;97:439.

Partin JC. Acute hepatic failure in children. Pediatr Ann 1985;14:446.

Psachanopolous HT, Mowat AP, Davies M, et al. Fulminant hepatic failure in childhood. Arch Dis Child 1980;55:252.

Riely CA. Acute hepatic failure in children. Yale J Biol Med 1984;57:161.

Rogers EL, Perman JA. Gastrointestinal and hepatic failure. In: Rogers MC, ed. Textbook of pediatric and intensive care. Baltimore: Williams & Wilkins, 1987.

Rogers EL, Rogers MC. Fulminant hepatic failure and hepatic encephalopathy. Pediatr Clin North Am 1980;27:701.

*Principles and Practice of Pediatrics, Second Edition.*
edited by Frank A. Oski et al. J. B. Lippincott Company, Philadelphia © 1994.

CHAPTER 46
# *Acute Renal Failure*

M. Michele Mariscalco

Acute renal failure (ARF) is defined as an abrupt decline in the renal regulation of water, electrolyte, and acid–base balance of sufficient magnitude to result in the retention of nitrogenous waste. Renal failure is potentially fatal but often is reversible if a prompt, accurate diagnosis is made and close attention is paid to the wide variety of predictable and preventable complications. Oliguria is defined as urine output of below 0.5 mL/kg/hr or below 300 mL/m$^2$/day. In the past 15 years, there has been an increasing recognition of the occurrence of nonoliguric renal failure in adults. This is thought to be secondary to increased use of nephrotoxic drugs (aminoglycosides in particular), improved resuscitation and survival of trauma victims, and conversion of oliguric to nonoliguric renal failure with the use of potent diuretics. The pediatric series reflect a very low incidence of nonoliguric renal failure, with most cases occurring in postoperative patients.

The process of ARF can be divided into three phases:

1. The *initiation phase*, in which ischemia or a toxin sets in motion a sequence of events that produces an injury to tubular epithelial cells
2. The *maintenance phase*, during which the glomerular filtration rate (GFR) remains relatively low for several days or weeks, depending on the severity of the initiating insult
3. The *recovery phase*, characterized by gradual and progressive restoration of GFR and tubule function.

Experimental evidence suggests three factors that may account for the development of ARF: renal hemodynamics, nephronal factors, and metabolic/cellular mechanisms.

Under normal circumstances, when the functional capacity of the renal tubule is exceeded and there is excessive excretion of solute and water, a negative feedback cycle initiates an increase in cortical vascular resistance, diminishing renal blood flow and GFR. During an acute renal insult, however, tubular epithelial injury results in altered reabsorption of solute and water in the proximal nephron, the feedback cycle is activated, renal blood flow is decreased further, and tubule injury is perpetuated. Several vasoactive compounds such as the renin-angiotensin system, vasodilatory prostaglandins, and adenosine have been implicated as the mediators in this feedback cycle. Although the specific compounds involved in the renal vasoconstriction have not been identified conclusively, it is clear that these hemodynamic factors play an important role in the initiation of the acute renal insult. Therefore, in the initiation phase of ARF, efforts should be made to maximize renal blood flow and to enhance renal perfusion.

In contrast, renal hemodynamic factors do not play a dominant role during the maintenance phase of ARF. Once the renal insult has been established, attempts to increase the renal blood flow do not result in a sustained increase in GFR, nor do they lessen the degree of cellular damage.

As the nephronal tubular epithelial cells sustain lethal injury, they become detached from the basement membrane, are sloughed into the tubule lumen, and can ultimately obstruct the lumen. Concomitantly, there is a loss of tubular integrity. Solute and fluid that should be retained within the tubule lumen leak back across the damaged membrane into the peritubular fluid and eventually into the plasma. Thus, progressive necrosis of epithelial cells can result in obstruction of some nephrons and the loss of tubular integrity in others, causing the tubular flow rate to diminish and GFR to be reduced. The end result is oliguria and ARF.

The mediators of the renal injury itself are not well delineated. Compounds such as oxygen-free radicals, high intracellular levels of calcium, and adenosine have been implicated in experimental models of ARF.

Oligoanuria may be the result of anatomical obstruction of the kidneys, a pathophysiologic response to impaired renal perfusion, or an established acute renal injury. Oliguria does not result from occlusion of the artery, the vein, or the ureter of a single kidney unless the contralateral kidney is absent or nonfunctioning. Renal artery stenosis and renal vein thrombosis are rare in children, but they do occur in the newborn period. Renal artery stenosis usually occurs as a complication of umbilical artery catheterization and presents with hypertension. Renal vein thrombosis should be suspected in a neonate with hematuria, proteinuria, or an enlarging abdominal mass. An early ultrasound diagnosis is imperative in establishing this diagnosis or other causes of obstruction, such as bilateral ureteral obstruction or bladder outlet obstruction. Obstruction of these anatomical sites must be considered before evaluation for any pathophysiologic causes of oliguria.

A scenario for oligoanuria more commonly encountered in the ICU is a child with decreased intravascular volume or cardiac output that leads to impaired renal perfusion. Renal responses to a decrease in intravascular volume and to a primary decrease in perfusion are similar. Renal tubular function remains intact, but there is a marked increase in the reabsorption of solutes and water throughout the nephron. By the increased release of renin, aldosterone, and antidiuretic hormone, the nephron is under maximal stimulation to conserve both salt and water. Consequently, the urinary sodium and fractional excretion of sodium are low (<10 mEq/L and <1%, respectively) and the urine osmolarity and urine/plasma osmolar ratio are high (>500 mOsm/L and >1.5, respectively). There is also an increased tubular reabsorption of urea. Creatinine is not reabsorbed by the tubule, and therefore an increased blood urea nitrogen (BUN)/creatinine ratio results.

## DIAGNOSIS

The renal failure indices listed in Table 46-1 can be helpful in distinguishing between oliguric patients with decreased per-

---

### TABLE 46-1.    Clinical Evaluation of Acute Renal Failure

| | Volume Depletion/ Decreased Renal Perfusion (Adolescents/Children) | Acute Renal Failure (Adolescents/Children) |
|---|---|---|
| $U_{Na}$ (mEq/L) | <10 | >50 |
| $FE_{Na}$ (%)* | ≤1 | >2 |
| $U_{osm}$ (mOsm/L) | ≥500 | ≤300 |
| $U/P_{osm}$ | ≥1.5 | 0.8–1.2 |
| BUN/Cr | >20 | Progressive increases in both |

* $FE_{Na} \% \neq (U/P)_{Na} \div (U/P)_{(Cr)} \times 100$

fusion to the kidneys and those with intrinsic renal failure. Clinical conditions associated with a decreased effective intravascular volume in children include both dehydration secondary to vomiting, diarrhea, or nasogastric drainage, and the peripheral pooling of fluid. In such a clinical setting, repletion of the intravascular volume through appropriate fluid therapy results in an increased urine output. Children with nephrosis occasionally become oliguric because of a decreased circulating volume secondary to a reduced plasma oncotic pressure. Conversely, children with myocardial failure may have an adequate blood volume but diminished cardiac output, with a consequent decrease in their renal blood flow. Therapy in these children is aimed at improving cardiac function.

Patients with intrinsic renal failure manifest an acute decrease in GFR and paralysis of tubular function. A decrease in GFR is reflected by a progressive increase in both the BUN and the serum creatinine concentrations. The rate of BUN change is not a specific index of the level of the GFR because it can be affected by a variety of factors, including catabolic rate, protein load, and medications. With diminished tubular function, the small volume of urine that is produced has a high level of urine sodium (usually >50 mEq/L) and there is an elevated fractional excretion of sodium (>2%). The urine is isotonic compared to plasma, with a urine osmolality of 280 to 300 mOsm/L and a urine/plasma osmolality of 0.8 to 1.2.

Clinical conditions associated with the development of ARF include hypotension, shock, renal ischemia, nephrotoxicity, drug toxicity, hyperuricemia, asphyxia, and sepsis. In children, more than 50% of ARF cases can be attributed to acute parenchymal disorders such as glomerulonephritis and hemolytic-uremic syndrome. Most ARF in the newborn period is secondary to major perinatal insults. More than 60% of neonatal ARF is reported to be secondary to perinatal asphyxia, hypoxia, and sepsis.

Nonoliguric ARF has been described in association with the nephrotoxic aminoglycoside antibiotics. The presentation is that of a gradual onset of nonoliguric renal failure that frequently is preceded by polyuria and decreased urine osmolality. In patients with nonoliguric renal failure, clinical studies show more normal urinary indices, a lower BUN, and a higher measured GFR, as well as fewer complications and lower mortality rates.

Once the diagnosis of ARF is made, all aspects of patient care must be monitored closely. Survival and return of renal function in 1 to 3 weeks are likely if the patient does not succumb from the underlying disease process or suffer from infectious, metabolic, or hemorrhagic complications of ARF or its treatment. The basis of therapy is careful monitoring of fluid and electrolyte balance, nutritional management directed at preventing a catabolic state, and meticulous care to avoid infections. The physiologic consequences of ARF include edema, pericarditis, electrolyte abnormalities including acidosis, anemia, thrombocytopenia, coagulopathy, gastrointestinal bleeding, poor nutrition, and sepsis.

## TREATMENT

The first step when confronting a patient with oliguria is a careful assessment of volume status. Physical examination may reveal hypovolemia (dry mucous membranes, tachycardia, "tenting" of the skin) or volume overload (peripheral edema, rales, gallop rhythm, hypertension, liver enlargement). A chest radiograph should be taken, looking for pulmonary edema or cardiomegaly, and an ECG performed, looking for changes associated with hyperkalemia. If there is no evidence of hypervolemia, a fluid challenge of 10 to 20 mL/kg of normal saline should be given. Central venous pressure catheters and pulmonary artery catheters are invaluable in monitoring the adequacy

of blood volume when it is in question. Neither diuretics nor vasopressors should be given until the adequacy of circulating volume has been ascertained.

Although it is controversial, some recommend the use of a diuretic early in the course of acute oliguria, as a few studies have shown a conversion from oliguric to nonoliguric renal failure with diuretic use. Diuretics can increase urine flow in human ischemic and nephrotoxic renal failure; however, increased urine flow is not necessarily the equivalent of improved renal function. Diuretics appear to be of limited value in preventing, reversing, or hastening recovery from renal failure. The conversion of oliguric to nonoliguric renal failure helps to simplify fluid management.

The rapid intravenous administration of 0.5 g/kg of mannitol should result in a urine output of more than 0.5 mL/kg within 1 hour. Mannitol may cause hypervolemia and pulmonary edema in patients who cannot excrete it, so it is best to avoid its use if there is any question of incipient volume overload or congestive heart failure. Furosemide also may be given, not only as a provocative test to generate urine production but also to attenuate ARF due to its vasodilating and natriuretic properties. Furosemide should be given to euvolemic patients in a dose of 1 mg/kg intravenously. If there is no response within 30 minutes, incrementally higher doses up to 10 mg/kg have been used, although the risk of ototoxicity increases dramatically. The use of these agents may have deleterious effects on renal blood flow and GFR if intravascular volume is inadequate.

Low-dose dopamine also has been advocated to improve urine output in adults with ARF. Dopamine increases renal blood flow, GFR, and sodium excretion independently of its effects on cardiac output. In adults, a dose of 1.0 to 2.5 μg/kg/min is favored to improve urine output through dopaminergic effects on the renal vascular bed and tubules. Doses higher than 10 μg/kg/min may result in vasoconstriction of the renal vascular bed. In children, doses of 2.5 to 5.0 μg/kg/min appear more effective. Some experimental animal and human data suggest that there is a synergistic response between low-dose dopamine and furosemide in converting oliguric to nonoliguric renal failure. Other inotropic agents, such as epinephrine and norepinephrine, should be avoided because these agents reduce renal blood flow even in the face of increased systemic blood pressure.

Once fixed renal failure occurs, conservative management should be used. This includes normalizing intravascular volume, systemic blood pressure and renal blood flow, sodium and potassium levels, and acid–base balance, and minimizing accumulation of nitrogenous wastes by restricting protein intake moderately while maximizing caloric intake. Prophylaxis for gastrointestinal bleeding should be initiated. Special care must be taken to avoid infectious complications.

Strict attention to physical examination, an accurate record of input and output, and daily weight and serum sodium determinations will maintain correct fluid balance. Fluid administration, both oral and parenteral, should be restricted to the sum of insensible losses (400 mL/m²/day) plus measured urine output and any other losses (eg, gastrointestinal, respiratory, evaporative secondary to burns). Hyponatremia can occur in the patient with volume overload; management entails further fluid restriction. Hyponatremia also can be seen in the patient with increased urinary sodium excretion who is in the diuretic phase of recovering ARF. Sodium replacement then is indicated.

Hyperkalemia is often encountered in ARF patients. Serum potassium does not reflect total body potassium content adequately, as potassium may move into or out of cells in exchange for hydrogen ions. Therefore, serum potassium must be interpreted on the basis of the patient's acid–base status. Hyperkalemia is a life-threatening complication of ARF and must be treated promptly to avoid cardiac toxicity. ECG changes range from the mild (peaked T waves) to the ominous, including widened QRS complex and arrhythmias. Measures to decrease serum potassium levels rapidly include sodium bicarbonate, 1 to 2 mEq/kg over 15 to 30 minutes; glucose, 0.5 to 1.0 g/kg, and insulin, 0.1 to 0.2 units/kg; and 10% calcium gluconate solution (0.5 mL/kg) over 5 to 10 minutes. These measures will drive potassium into the cells and antagonize the effects of hyperkalemia, but they will not remove potassium from the body. Sodium polystyrene sulfonate (Kayexalate) is an ion-exchange resin and reduces the total body burden of potassium by exchanging equal milliequivalent amounts of sodium and potassium. The dose is 1 g/kg in 70% sorbitol PO or in 30% sorbitol PR. Dialysis may be necessary to control hyperkalemia. Continuous ECG monitoring and repeated glucose and potassium determinations should be done as therapy proceeds.

A consequence of impaired renal function is retention of hydrogen ions, sulfate, and phosphate and development of a mild metabolic acidosis with an increased anion gap. Usually respiratory compensation is adequate and no intervention is required. If acidosis is severe or contributing to the development of hyperkalemia, or if the patient's respiratory compensation is impaired, sodium bicarbonate can be given. Sodium bicarbonate is effective as a buffer only if the $CO_2$ produced can be removed by adequate ventilation; also, rapid correction of acidosis in these patients, who often have hypocalcemia, limits the availability of ionized calcium and may induce tetany or seizures.

Hypertension is frequently a complication in children with ARF. Hypertensive encephalopathy may present as headache, irritability, or seizures. Papilledema is not necessarily present in these patients. Volume overload is often an inciting event and must be addressed early in the management. Acutely, a rapid-onset, short-acting agent is used such as diazoxide, nitroprusside, or hydralazine. The agent chosen depends on the clinical circumstances and the monitoring capabilities available. Diazoxide, often chosen for the severely symptomatic patient, is an arteriolar vasodilator with a peak-effect of less than 5 minutes and a duration of action of up to 4 to 12 hours. The initial dose is 3–5 mg/kg, up to 300 mg per dose. The dose can be repeated in 5–15 minutes until a satisfactory blood pressure has been achieved. If this is ineffective and the patient remains symptomatic, sodium nitroprusside may be initiated, carefully titrated with the blood pressure. In asymptomatic children with severe hypertension, treatment can be initiated with parenteral hydralazine, 0.1 to 0.5 mg/kg IM or IV every 4 to 6 hours; the adult dose is 20 to 40 mg. Once the blood pressure has been lowered, a long-term therapeutic regimen can be initiated.

Children with ARF are usually catabolic. High rates of catabolism lead to increased accumulation of potassium, phosphate, and urea, and may necessitate earlier dialysis. If calories are supplied and the breakdown of endogenous proteins is spared, the need for dialysis may be delayed. There has been concern in recent years that the administration of parenteral amino acids to patients with ARF worsens the degree of azotemia, but current data do not support this concern. No study performed to date has shown that hyperalimentation leads to an increase in morbidity or mortality. Because of fluid restriction in these patients, it often is difficult to provide adequate calories without the use of parenteral hypertonic glucose, amino acids, and intralipids. Protein requirements of these patients may range from 0.5 g/kg to 1.5 g/kg in the severely catabolic patient. Hypertonic glucose can be given relatively safely through central venous catheters. Complications such as sepsis, acidosis, and hyperglycemia may occur. Once the patient is no longer oligoanuric or is on an artificial kidney, fluid administration may be liberalized, and nutritional management becomes easier and safer. Enteral alimentation should be initiated as soon as clinically feasible.

There are six indications for dialysis: volume overload with evidence of pulmonary edema or hypertension refractory to pharmacologic therapy; hyperkalemia despite conservative measures; severe metabolic acidosis (pH <7.20); BUN above 150, or lower if rising rapidly; neurologic symptoms secondary to uremia or electrolyte imbalance; and calcium/phosphorus imbalance (hypocalcemia with tetany or seizures in the presence of a very high serum phosphate).

Both peritoneal dialysis and intermittent hemodialysis have been used for many years in children in ARF, but often these modes of therapy have been less than optimally effective in the critically ill child. Hemodialysis is difficult to maintain in the patient with cardiovascular instability, and its intermittent mode of administration makes removal of extravascular fluid difficult without causing further fluctuations in blood pressure. Effective peritoneal dialysis also requires an adequate cardiac output, which may not be present in these children, and peritoneal dialysis can lead to respiratory embarrassment.

Recently there has been an opportunity to use continuous renal prosthetic therapy in both adults and children. Two of these modes, slow continuous ultrafiltration (SCUF) and continuous arteriovenous hemofiltration (CAVH), are gaining widespread use. With these therapies, patients who are oligoanuric can receive the drugs and nutrients they need without fear of causing fluid excess. In addition, both of these modes are characterized by ease of application and hemodynamic stability, so therapy is instituted earlier. Both require the insertion of arterial and venous catheters. The driving pressure supplied by the arterial bed provides the flow through the dialysis membrane. With SCUF, fluid removal or only ultrafiltration is done, but this has been found to be helpful in maintaining fluid volume while decreasing plasma volume. Azotemia is not controlled as effectively with this method. With CAVH, azotemia, fluid, and electrolyte balance can be maintained. CAVH can be seen as the replacement of plasma water with sterile fluid. Modifications may need to be made in the hypercatabolic patient to compensate for the rapidly rising urea nitrogen.

In most series of childhood ARF, mortality is associated with the irreversible nature of the underlying disease rather than the renal failure itself. Treatment modalities are largely supportive, and successful therapy requires meticulous attention to the details of the clinical setting.

## Selected Readings

Badr KF, Ichikawa I. Prerenal failure: a deleterious shift from renal compensation to decompensation. N Eng J Med 1988;319:623.

Gaudio KM, Sigel NJ. Pathogenesis and treatment of ARF. Pediatr Clin North Am 1987;34:771.

Jones DP, Chesney RW. Glomerulotubular dysfunction and ARF. In: Fuhrman BP, Zimmerman JJ, eds. Pediatric critical care. St. Louis: Mosby Year Book, 1992.

Paganini EP. Continuous renal prosthetic therapy in ARF, an overview. Pediatr Clin North Am 1987;34;165.

Zobel G, Trop M, Ekkehard R, Hans-Michael G. Continuous arteriovenous hemofiltration in critically ill children with ARF. Crit Care Med 1987;15:699.

*Principles and Practice of Pediatrics, Second Edition.*
edited by Frank A. Oski et al. J. B. Lippincott Company, Philadelphia © 1994.

# CHAPTER 47
# *Hemolytic-Uremic Syndrome*

Penelope Terhune Louis

The hemolytic-uremic syndrome (HUS), first described in 1955, is characterized by the triad of nephropathy, thrombocytopenia, and microangiopathic hemolytic anemia. HUS is a heterogenous group of disorders that have a common end result. To differentiate the pathogenesis and clinical outcome, the following classification has been proposed:

1. The *classical* form presents in infants or small children following a prodrome of bloody diarrhea that may involve the verotoxin-producing strain of *Escherichia coli.*
2. The *postinfectious* form is associated with an identified infectious agent such as *Shigella* or *Salmonella* or with endotoxemia.
3. *Hereditary* forms have been recognized that have both autosomal dominant and recessive modes of inheritance; these patients probably lack a plasma factor necessary for prostacyclin production or have a prostacyclin inhibitor.
4. An *immunologically mediated* form is characterized by low plasma C3 and activation of the alternative pathway; this form also may be familial.
5. A *secondary* form is related to known predisposing conditions such as lupus, scleroderma, chemotherapy, malignant hypertension, and renal irradiation.
6. A form related to *pregnancy or oral contraceptives* is characterized by arterial microangiopathy.

## PATHOGENESIS

The pathogenesis of HUS can be explained by several mechanisms. The anemia is characterized by negative direct and indirect Coombs tests, a falling haptoglobin, and a reticulocyte response. There is strong evidence that hemolysis is secondary to mechanical destruction of erythrocytes by fibrin strands in small renal vessels. There is also evidence that the redox state of the red cell is altered, leading to increased oxidation of the red-cell membrane.

Thrombocytopenia is present universally and is secondary to peripheral destruction. The mechanisms implicated are increased platelet activation and enhanced platelet aggregation as a result of prostaglandin imbalance. The degree of thrombocytopenia does not predict morbidity or length of illness.

The nephropathy of HUS is characterized by glomerular capillary endothelial injury. The endothelium separates, and the subendothelial space is littered with debris such as fibrin strands and erythrocyte fragments. As a result of the thickening of the endothelial space, the capillary narrows, predisposing to capillary thrombosis. Fibrin is demonstrated with immunofluorescent techniques. There has been no consistent evidence that immune complexes are involved with renal injury, since immunoglobulin deposits usually are not found using immunofluorescent techniques.

The role of prostaglandins in HUS has been studied with increased interest. Prostacyclin ($PGI_2$) is a potent depressor of platelet aggregation. Prostacyclin production may be decreased by damage to endothelial cells, or there may be a circulating inhibitor to prostacyclin. The platelet aggregator thromboxane may be elevated in HUS, with the imbalance of decreased prostacyclin and increased thromboxane leading to enhanced platelet aggregation.

## EPIDEMIOLOGY

HUS is largely a disease of infants and children. The syndrome is endemic in Argentina, southern Africa, and the western United States. There is no predilection for either sex. In southern Africa, it is more common in white children. Age of onset is between 2 months and 8 years in most cases and is usually less than 5 years.

There is no one causative factor, and etiologic agents may be viral (coxsackieviruses, echoviruses, influenza viruses, Epstein-Barr virus), bacterial (*Shigella, Salmonella, Streptococcus pneumoniae, Escherichia coli* 0157:H7), or drugs (oral contraceptives and cyclosporin A) and complement abnormalities. There seems to be a genetic predisposition. Familial illness with the typical prodrome has a low mortality rate. If there is no typical prodrome, the mortality rate is high and the predisposition seems to be autosomally transmitted.

## CLINICAL FEATURES

The syndrome typically has a prodrome of diarrhea or an upper respiratory illness. The diarrhea may be bloody. The prodrome occurs 5 days to 2 weeks before the onset of the classic syndrome.

At initial examination, the child is pale and irritable, with petechiae and edema. Dehydration may be present if there is severe diarrhea. Hypertension also is common.

The mildly affected patient may have only anemia, thrombocytopenia, and azotemia. The severely affected patient has the complications of metabolic derangement, including hyperkalemia, metabolic acidosis, hypocalcemia, and hyponatremia or hypernatremia. Neurologic dysfunction will be manifested by seizures, coma, and stroke. Infection may be either primary or nosocomial. Cardiac failure may result from hypertension, volume overload, or severe anemia. Bleeding also may be present in the severely affected patient.

Laboratory features include hemoglobin concentrations of 2 to 10 g/dL, platelet counts of less than $100,000/mm^3$, and an increased prothrombin time due to consumption of Factors II, VII, IX, and X. A decrease in fibrinogen and an increase in fibrin split products also appears early in the illness.

## TREATMENT

Management of the HUS patient is mainly supportive. The mainstay of therapy is meticulous control of fluid and electrolyte balance, control of hypertension, careful use of red-cell transfusions, and early initiation of dialysis for hyperkalemia, metabolic acidosis, severe uremia, or volume overload. The aim of red-cell transfusions during the period of hemolysis should be to prevent heart failure and not to return the hematocrit to normal. Thrombocytopenia may be severe but only rarely results in significant bleeding; therefore, platelets should not be given unless clearly needed to stop bleeding or in anticipation of invasive procedures. Fluid restriction to $400 \text{ mL/m}^2$/day is standard.

The difficulty in management is distinguishing between mild

disease, which responds to the previously mentioned therapy, and severe disease, which requires more aggressive treatment.

Other therapies used include heparin, streptokinase, aspirin, dipyridamole, vitamin E, intravenous immunoglobulin G (IgG), and plasmapheresis. The use of heparin and streptokinase has declined because of hemorrhagic complications. Aspirin and dipyridamole have been used because of their effects on prostaglandin synthesis. Dipyridamole interferes with phosphodiesterase, which results in the slower metabolism of cyclic AMP. Aspirin inhibits cyclooxygenase, which leads to decreased platelet-aggregating thromboxane. In general, studies report little benefit from the use of heparin, fibrinolytics, and antiplatelet therapy. Vitamin E therapy has been proposed after reports of abnormal lipid peroxidation and low vitamin E activity in patients with HUS, but controlled studies have shown no benefit at present. Intravenous IgG infusions have received attention based on studies performed in adults showing that IgG can inhibit platelet aggregation. This presumably would diminish thrombotic microangiopathy and reduce the period of time of thrombocytopenia. Controlled studies have not been completed, and preliminary data suggest that the period of thrombocytopenia is shortened but morbidity is not altered. Fresh-frozen plasma infusions have been suggested because of findings that serum from HUS patients cannot generate normal amounts of prostaglandin or does not demonstrate normal amounts of antithrombotic and antiplatelet function. There also have been anecdotal reports of experience with plasmapheresis in the treatment of childhood HUS, but because there have been no prospective clinical trials, plasmapheresis remains untested and is not recommended.

## PROGNOSIS

The prognosis for the most common forms of HUS is good. Most studies report 3% to 5% mortality, and another 3% to 5% of patients experience chronic renal disease.

## Selected Readings

Bell WR, Braine HG, Ness PM, et al. Improved survival in thrombocytopenic purpura-HUS. N Engl J Med 1991;325:398.

Drummond KN. HUS—then and now. N Engl J Med 1985;312:116.

Friedman AL. Acute renal disease. In: Fuhrman BP, Zimmerman JJ, eds. Pediatric critical care. St. Louis: Mosby Year Book, 1992.

Havens PL, O'Rourke PP, Hahn J, et al. Laboratory and clinical variables to predict outcome in HUS. Am J Dis Child 1988;142:961.

Kaplan BS, Ceary TG, Obrig TG. Recent advances in understanding the pathogenesis of HUS. Pediatr Nephrol 1990;4:276.

Maxwell LG, Fivush BA, McLean RH. Renal failure. In: Rogers MC, ed. Textbook of pediatric intensive care. Baltimore: Williams & Wilkins, 1987.

Neill MA, Tarr PI, Clausen CR, et al. Escherichia coli 0157:H7 as the predominant pathogen associated with HUS: a prospective study in the Pacific Northwest. Pediatrics 1987;80:37.

Rizzoni G, Clari-Appiani A, Facchin P, et al. Plasma infusion for HUS in children: results of a multicenter controlled trial. J Pediatr 1988;112:284.

Siegler RL. Management of HUS. J Pediatr 1988;112:1014.

*Principles and Practice of Pediatrics, Second Edition.*
edited by Frank A. Oski et al. J. B. Lippincott Company, Philadelphia © 1994.

# CHAPTER 48
# *Epiglottitis*

## Johnny Ray Griggs and Fernando Stein

Epiglottitis (supraglottitis) is a pediatric emergency. What may begin as an apparently mild upper airway infection can progress rapidly to a life-threatening airway obstruction. It usually has an abrupt onset. The temperature may increase rapidly to 38° to 40 °C, and mucus formation usually leads to moderate respiratory distress and then total airway occlusion within hours. In its classic presentation, the patient has an anxious appearance and prefers the sitting position, with the neck in hyperextension. Inability to handle secretions secondary to the pain of swallowing also may be noted. Nasal flaring and suprasternal, intercostal, and subcostal retractions with use of the accessory muscles of respiration may occur. If epiglottitis is not recognized appropriately, the likelihood of a fatal outcome or permanent neurologic damage is high.

Individuals of any age may be affected, but 75% of the cases occur in 1- to 5-year-olds. In general, patients with epiglottitis are older than patients with laryngotracheitis.

The offending organism in most cases is *Haemophilus influenzae* type b; the organism can be cultured from the epiglottis directly as well as from blood.

Pathologically, the epiglottis, arytenoids, arytenoepiglottic area, vocal cords, and subglottic regions are inflamed and edematous. This can be appreciated with direct visualization of the airway via laryngoscopy. However, visualization should be done only in a controlled environment in which both personnel and equipment are readily available to perform immediate endotracheal intubation or tracheostomy. Marginal airway patency can be compromised by a physician with good intentions who inserts an instrument into the oral cavity or airway for examination. Laryngeal spasm may lead to airway occlusion.

In a patient with marked respiratory distress and clinical features of epiglottitis, even roentgenographic studies of the airway should be omitted, and direct examination should be performed in the operating room. Appropriate personnel include an anesthesiologist, an otolaryngologist, or a pediatric surgeon able to perform rigid bronchoscopy or urgent tracheostomy.

When a child presents with mild respiratory distress and a questionable diagnosis of epiglottitis, a lateral neck radiograph may be helpful in differentiating epiglottitis from other forms of airway obstruction. The classic "thumb sign" appearance of the swollen epiglottis on lateral neck films is diagnostic. The patient should be taken to the imaging department only by personnel capable of performing endotracheal intubation. The total and differential white-cell studies show a leukocytosis with a left shift in most patients. Serum chemistries are usually normal and often are not helpful.

Associated infections such as meningitis, septic arthritis, and pericarditis are uncommon.

Treatment of the child with epiglottitis starts when the diagnosis is entertained. A calming, nonthreatening environment that allows the child to stay in the arms of the parent or caretaker is recommended. Parents or a caretaker may be with the child in the operating room until the induction of anesthesia is complete. Once anesthetic induction is achieved and intravenous access is secured, blood cultures, a complete blood-cell count, and clotting studies can be obtained. Endotracheal intubation is performed with direct visualization of the epiglottis. Rigid bronchoscopy and tracheostomy equipment should be available.

We recommend nasotracheal intubation. Intubation is achieved with an endotracheal tube 0.5 to 1.0 mm smaller than the tube diameter usually recommended for the patient's age. This is an ideal time to obtain cultures of the epiglottis.

Ampicillin (200 mg/kg/day) and chloramphenicol (100 mg/kg/day) or cefotaxime (150 mg/kg/day) are recommended for initial therapy. Antibiotic therapy can be modified when culture and sensitivity data on the organism are known. Length of therapy usually is 7 to 10 days. *H influenzae* prophylaxis for household contacts is recommended.

The usual length of time for intubation in acute epiglottitis is 2 to 4 days. Extubation can be performed when the patient is alert and able to handle secretions and when visual inspection of the epiglottis shows a significant improvement in the degree of edema. An agitated child can become extubated easily, so four-point physical restraints should be ordered. Adequate sedation for control of movement and agitation also should be provided (see Chap. 41.9).

Complications associated with epiglottitis usually are those associated with endotracheal intubation.

## Selected Readings

Daum RS, Smith AL. Epiglottitis (supraglottitis). In: Feigin RD, Cherry JD, eds. Textbook of pediatric infectious diseases. Philadelphia: WB Saunders, 1987.

Fried MP. Controversies in the management of supraglottitis and croup. Pediatr Clin North Am 1979;26(11):4.

*Principles and Practice of Pediatrics, Second Edition.*
edited by Frank A. Oski et al. J. B. Lippincott Company, Philadelphia © 1994.

CHAPTER 49

# *Syndrome of Inappropriate Secretion of Antidiuretic Hormone*

Penelope Terhune Louis
and James D. Fortenberry

## PATHOPHYSIOLOGY AND DIAGNOSIS

Fluid management in the acutely ill child may be complicated by alterations in the regulatory mechanisms of sodium and water homeostasis. Antidiuretic hormone (ADH) plays an important role in responding to changes in extracellular volume by altering the renal clearance of free water to maintain appropriate serum tonicity. ADH release from the posterior pituitary gland is influenced primarily by changes in plasma osmolality and effective circulating blood volume. Hypothalamic osmoreceptors maintain osmolality over a narrow range, with 1% to 2% changes altering ADH secretion. The response to volume changes by the carotid body and left atrial stretch receptors is less sensitive, requiring 10% differences to stimulate or suppress ADH release.

Many disease states, medications, and pathophysiologic processes can alter ADH excretion and secretion (Table 49-1). In some of these entities, ADH release may be an appropriate response to the alterations sensed by body receptors, as in the decreased venous return produced by positive pressure ventilation. However, if ADH release is excessive or inappropriate in relation to either normal osmolality or volume status, the typical findings of the syndrome of inappropriate ADH secretion (SIADH) ensue. SIADH is often recognized in children and is established by five classic clinical criteria: hyponatremia with corresponding serum hypo-osmolality; urine osmolality that is greater than appropriate for concomitant serum osmolality (ie, less than maximally dilute); continued urine sodium excretion that is excessive for the degree of hyponatremia, with elevated urine sodium concentrations; normal renal, adrenal, and thyroid function; and absence of volume depletion.

Urine needs only to be submaximally dilute to establish a diagnosis of SIADH. The kidneys normally can dilute urine up to 50 to 150 mOsm/kg. It is possible, with urine hypotonic to plasma, for the tonicity of serum to fall below normal and to be maintained at subnormal levels, producing hyponatremia. Hyponatremia may not be present early in the process and develops only when fluid retention occurs.

The associated increase in urinary sodium excretion is an interesting finding. Aldosterone secretion is typically normal and the filtered sodium load does not increase; therefore, a third factor, possibly atrial natriuretic peptide, has been proposed that may suppress proximal tubular reabsorption of sodium in response to expanded extracellular volume.

SIADH must be differentiated from the many clinical conditions that cause hyponatremia in children. Physical examination and evaluation of simultaneous urine and serum sodium concentrations and osmolalities, urine specific gravity, and serum electrolytes will help exclude disorders such as hyponatremic dehydration, congestive heart failure, and renal insufficiency. Serum cortisol levels are recommended because patients with adrenal insufficiency may demonstrate a component of inappropriate ADH secretion and present a similar picture if well compensated. Thyroid function tests should also be considered. Water-loading procedures are dangerous and unnecessary for diagnosis.

Physical findings in SIADH are related to the associated disease process. Despite mildly increased total body water, edema formation is not typically seen. Symptoms are related to the presence and duration of hyponatremia. Anorexia, nausea, mental status changes, and convulsions are more likely to be seen with serum osmolality below 240 mOsm/kg $H_2O$ and serum sodium concentration below 120 mEq/L of acute onset.

## DISORDERS ASSOCIATED WITH SIADH

SIADH in children occurs most often in association with CNS disorders. Laboratory evidence of SIADH was noted in almost 60% of the children presenting with bacterial meningitis. ADH levels in patients with meningitis were also significantly elevated in comparison with normal and febrile controls. The duration and degree of hyponatremia were shown to correlate significantly with subsequent development of seizures, subdural effusions, and development. A leak of endogenous ADH across inflamed meninges has been suggested to explain these findings, but lab-

**TABLE 49-1.   Disorders and Agents Associated With SIADH**

| | |
|---|---|
| **CNS** | **Intrathoracic** |
| Meningitis | Tuberculosis |
| Encephalitis | Viral/bacterial/fungal pneumonia |
| Head trauma | Mycoplasma pneumonia |
| Tumor | Empyema |
| Hypoxia-ischemia | Asthma |
| Guillain-Barré syndrome | Pneumothorax |
| Subarachnoid hemorrhage | Cystic fibrosis |
| Acute intermittent porphyria | Positive pressure ventilation |
| Cavernous sinus thrombosis | Positive end-expiratory pressure (PEEP) |
| Anatomical abnormalities | Tumor |
| Vasculitis | Patent ductus arteriosus ligation |
| Brain abscess | **Miscellaneous** |
| Hydrocephalus | Pain |
| Acute psychosis | Stress (postoperative) |
| Rocky Mountain spotted fever | Nausea, vomiting |
| Spinal fusion | Bacterial endocarditis |
| Craniopharyngioma (triphasic postoperative response) | Malignancy |
| **Drugs** | Infant water intoxication (postulated) |
| *Enhance ADH Release* | Idiopathic |
| Morphine | |
| Vincristine | |
| β-adrenergic agonists | |
| Cyclophosphamide | |
| Carbemazepine | |
| Barbiturates | |
| Halothane | |
| Clofibrate | |
| Nicotine | |
| Phenothiazines | |
| Adenine arabinoside (ARA-A) | |
| *Potentiate ADH Action* | |
| Chlorpropramide | |
| Indomethacin | |

*Adapted from Kaplan SL, Feigin RD. SIADH in children. Adv Pediatr 1980;27:247.*

oratory markers of inflammation did not show a correlation with arginine vasopressin (AVP) levels. SIADH is seen with other CNS infections, including brain abscesses and encephalitis, and with Rocky Mountain spotted fever, most likely secondary to hypothalamic involvement from rickettsial vasculitis. CNS disturbances such as head trauma, perinatal hypoxia, brain tumors, subarachnoid hemorrhage, anatomical defects, and Guillain-Barré syndrome may produce SIADH.

Intrathoracic disturbances are less common causes in children. Pulmonary tuberculosis is well recognized, but viral, fungal, bacterial, and mycoplasma pneumonias have also been cited. Disorders that lead to decreased left atrial pressure, such as positive pressure ventilation or pneumothoraces, can induce excessive ADH release by diminishing venous return. This is inappropriately perceived by stretch receptors as evidence of decreased circulating blood volume. ADH levels are probably elevated by a similar mechanism in status asthmaticus, leading one to reconsider the vigorous use of intravenous fluids often recommended in initial management.

Many drugs have been implicated in the production of SIADH, acting either by increasing endogenous central ADH release or by enhancing its renal tubular effects (see Table 49-1). Frequently used agents include chemotherapeutic agents, morphine, β-adrenergic agonists, and indomethacin. Carbamazepine-induced

SIADH was reportedly reversed by concomitant use of phenytoin, which inhibits ADH secretion. Phenytoin may minimize SIADH while treating seizures associated with CNS insult.

Many other disorders can induce SIADH. Ectopic production of ADH may be seen in adults with bronchogenic carcinoma, leukemia, and thymoma. Transient increases in ADH secretion are also seen as part of the triphasic ADH response following resection of craniopharyngiomas. ADH secretion may be excessive in the general postoperative setting due to the effects of increased epinephrine release from pain or stress, nausea and vomiting, the use of morphine, or the surgical procedure itself; posterior spinal fusion for scoliosis is a common association. A syndrome of hyponatremia with water intoxication has been described in otherwise normal infants receiving dilute formula at home; inappropriately increased AVP levels were found in some of these infants.

## MANAGEMENT

Appropriate treatment of the underlying disease process is essential to the resolution of SIADH. However, fluid restriction remains the cornerstone of acute therapy and prevention of symptoms in patients at risk. Intake should be limited to insensible losses (800 to 1000 mL/m²/day) with appropriate sodium content to allow the slow excretion of excess fluid, diminishing extracellular volume and thus decreasing urinary sodium excretion.

The fluid management of patients with meningitis has undergone increasing scrutiny. While SIADH may occur in this setting, many patients with meningitis may be volume-depleted and have associated hyponatremic dehydration. In a recent study by Powell and associates, children with meningitis were randomly assigned to receive either fluid restriction (two-thirds maintenance) or maintenance fluid therapy plus estimated deficit replacement during the initial 24 hours of therapy. Plasma AVP concentrations were initially elevated in both groups but returned to normal after 24 hours of therapy in patients who received maintenance and deficit therapy; levels were unchanged in fluid-restricted patients. ADH reduction was presumed to be secondary to correction of hypovolemia and sodium deficits. Fluid restriction in an animal model of bacterial meningitis also produced decreased cerebral flow and increased CSF lactic acidosis. Therefore, it is probably appropriate to give maintenance plus replacement fluids to patients with meningitis who do not initially demonstrate laboratory evidence of SIADH. Close monitoring of electrolytes should continue during the first 24 to 48 hours of therapy, and the presence of hyponatremia should prompt the evaluation of urine osmolality and sodium concentration to rule out SIADH.

Hypertonic (3%) saline infusion should be used only in patients whose hyponatremia has induced seizures or coma. Concomitant use of furosemide can act to increase free water excretion relative to sodium excretion and diminish the volume expansion induced by hypertonic saline. The use of furosemide alone, with replacement of measured urine electrolyte losses, has also been suggested. Corticosteroids have been used in combination to increase sodium retention, but their use remains controversial. Lithium carbonate and demeclocycline inhibit ADH effects on the renal tubule and can correct hyponatremia, but significant complications limit their use in children.

## Selected Readings

Bartter FC, Schwartz WB. SIADH. Am J Med 1967;42:790.

Burrows FA, Shutack JG, Crone RK. Inappropriate secretion of ADH in a postsurgical pediatric population. Crit Care Med 1983;11:527.

David R, Ellis D, Gartner JC. Water intoxication in normal infants: role of ADH in pathogenesis. Pediatrics 1981;68:349.

Feigin RD, Kaplan S. Inappropriate secretion of ADH in children with bacterial meningitis. Am J Clin Nutr 1977;30:1482.

Hartman D, Rossier B, Zohlman R, et al. Rapid correction of hyponatremia in SIADH. Ann Intern Med 1973;78:870.

Kaplan SL, Feigin RD. SIADH in children. Adv Pediatr 1980;247.

Kaplan SL, Feigin RD. SIADH in children with bacterial meningitis. J Pediatr 1978;92;758.

Powell KR, Sugarman LI, Eskenazi AE, et al. Normalization of plasma AVP concentrations when children with meningitis are given maintenance plus replacement fluid therapy. J Pediatr 1990;117:515.

Rascher W, Tulassay T, Lang RE. Atrial natriuretic peptide in plasma of volume-overloaded children with chronic renal failure. Lancet 1985;2:303.

Sordillo P, Sagransky DM, Mercado R, et al. Carbamazepine-induced SIADH. Arch Intern Med 1978;138:299.

Robertson GL, Shelton RL, Athar S. The osmoregulation of vasopressin. Kidney Int 1976;10:25.

Tureen JH, Tauber MG, Sande MA. Effect of hydration status on cerebral blood flow and CSF lactic acidosis in rabbits with experimental meningitis. J Clin Invest 1992;89:947.

*Principles and Practice of Pediatrics, Second Edition.*
edited by Frank A. Oski et al. J. B. Lippincott Company, Philadelphia © 1994.

# CHAPTER 50
# *Multiple Trauma*

## M. Michele Mariscalco

Since therapeutic measures for patients with congenital anomalies and serious infections have become increasingly successful, trauma has become the leading cause of death and disability during childhood and adolescence. In 1989, injuries caused about 16,000 deaths, a relatively stable 23% of all childhood deaths. In adults, 3.7% of deaths are traumatic in origin. For each child who dies, there are four survivors who suffer some form of permanent physical disability. The vast majority of serious trauma occurs in conjunction with motor-vehicle accidents, and vehicular accidents are the most common single cause of pediatric trauma deaths, accounting for 61% of the total.

Blunt trauma accounts for 80% to 90% of pediatric trauma. It differs from other forms of injury in that multiple organ injuries are common, as is occult head injury. Progressive organ damage occurs frequently in blunt trauma because of continuing hemorrhage or edema formation. Acidosis and hypoxia are often more prominent than the dysfunction from the primary injury.

The causes of injury in children differ from those in adults, reflecting the differences in activities, size, and intellectual maturity. The patterns of injury in children also differ from those in adults. Head trauma occurs in 80% or more of severely injured children. Abdominal injuries occur more frequently because poorly developed abdominal muscles offer little protection of the viscera. Both the spleen and the duodenum are more likely to be injured. Elasticity of the chest wall makes rib and sternal fractures rare, but also permits severe crush injuries of the heart and lungs without apparent deformation of the chest wall.

Children's physiologic responses also differ from those of adults. The vascular system can compensate for a greater blood volume loss (20% to 25%) before hypotension occurs, but tachycardia presents earlier than in adults. The maintenance of normal blood pressure masks impaired tissue perfusion and may lead to a delay in treatment. The young child becomes hypothermic easily, which greatly increases the difficulty of resuscitation. Since the child is a growing organism, uncorrected injury may lead to progressive deformity and disability.

## PREHOSPITAL CARE

Treatment of multiple trauma begins at the scene by prehospital attendants. There is a fundamental difference between medical delivery and surgical delivery of prehospital emergent care. In medical prehospital care, in which the vast majority of patients are adults with cardiac dysfunction, the working premise is to take time to stabilize the patient and achieve a stable rhythm, and then slowly transport the patient to the hospital. For trauma patients, the definitive management is available only in the hospital. Once the airway is stabilized, the patient is ventilated adequately, and bony injuries are stabilized, the patient should be transported to the hospital as soon as possible.

In children, the concept of stabilization should be confined to airway control and cervical spine and long bone immobilization. Hemorrhage control can be obtained by primary pressure or by a pediatric pneumatic antishock garment. Peripheral intravenous access is the preferred route, but may be technically difficult in children. Intraosseous infusion is technically easy and safe and is recommended in children younger than 6 years, although it may be used in older children and adults. Once vascular access is established, care must be taken to avoid overtransfusion of crystalloid. Transport must not be delayed while vascular access is established in the pediatric trauma patient.

## THE PRIMARY SURVEY

Successful initial management of a critically injured, multiple-trauma pediatric patient depends on the expertise of a well-coordinated team consisting of physicians, often headed by surgeons familiar with pediatric trauma, and emergency medical personnel. Management begins with a systematic approach to the ABCs (airway, breathing, circulation). Within the first 20 to 30 minutes at the hospital, the patient should receive a primary survey with initial resuscitation, a secondary survey consisting of a complete examination from head to toe, and a plan for definitive care.

The initial focus of the primary survey is the airway. The goals are to relieve anatomical obstruction, prevent the aspiration of gastric contents, and promote adequate gas exchange with protection of the cervical spine. Any child with significant trauma is assumed to have cervical spine injury. These goals may be met by maneuvers as simple as a chin lift or a jaw thrust, with careful attention to avoiding hyperextension of the cervical spine. Use of a rigid collar, sandbags, and tape, or manual immobilization with the head in a neutral position, prevents manipulation of the cervical spine that may result in spinal cord injury with quadriplegia. The mouth may be suctioned for retained secretions, but care must be taken to avoid precipitating vomiting and regurgitation. Nasopharyngeal and oropharyngeal airways are poorly tolerated and often induce gagging. A child who tolerates them usually has compromised protective reflexes and requires definitive airway management with an endotracheal tube.

The second goal of the primary survey is to maintain breathing. The patient should receive 100% inspired oxygen. If ventilation is inadequate or absent, if arterial hypoxemia unresponsive to increased inspired oxygen is present, if there are burns of the face and neck, or if the patient is hemodynamically unstable, the airway should be secured. Oral tracheal intubation is the preferred route. These patients are at high risk for vomiting and aspirating. Also, their airways may be made more inaccessible by traumatic injury to the bones and soft tissue. Intubation is performed by the most experienced personnel and under controlled conditions using rapid sequence and cricoid pressure to prevent passive regurgitation. Manual cervical in-line immobilization is performed to counter the flexion and extension during intubation if cervical injury is suspected.

Once the patient is intubated, ventilation is begun with 100% inspired oxygen at rates of 10 to 20 breaths per minute. If head injury is suspected, the minute ventilation rate should be increased to lower arterial carbon dioxide pressure. If ventilation is impaired, malposition of the endotracheal tube or tube plugging with secretions is suspected. If inadequate ventilation continues, a pneumothorax, hemothorax, or other thoracic injury is suspected, evaluation is completed, and treatment is given. This usually entails the use of needle thoracentesis or tube thoracostomies.

The third goal of the primary survey is to ensure effective circulation. Initially this may be done by artificial support with chest compressions. At the same time, basic steps for hemorrhagic shock are undertaken, including control of active hemorrhage, placement of intravenous lines, and aggressive crystalloid and blood replacement. Control of obvious hemorrhage is most important. In most situations, direct pressure is adequate. Fractures of the pelvis or long bones produce hidden blood loss that can be massive in both adults and children. Pneumatic antishock garments can be used to control hemorrhage following fracture of the long bones of the lower extremities. Antishock garments are available in several pediatric sizes, and they must be used with extreme caution following truncal wounds.

In the patient with hemorrhage and shock, there is no substitute for volume and blood replacement. The debate about the use of crystalloid versus colloid for volume replacement continues. In the few studies in young adult, previously healthy trauma patients, there seem to be no differences in the development of pulmonary edema and pulmonary dysfunction when either crystalloid or colloid are used. Some physicians prefer the use of D5 lactated Ringer's solution or lactated Ringer's solution over the use of normal saline because the chloride concentration more closely approximates that in normal plasma and the lactate serves as a source of buffering base. The volume infused should be 20 to 30 mL/kg initially, with an observation for improvement in circulatory status; if no improvement is noted, another 20 to 30 mL/kg is given. Balanced salt solution is not intended as a substitute for blood. Loss in excess of 30% of total circulating blood volume must be replaced with red blood cells in addition to fluid. Blood volume is 60 to 80 mL/kg of optimal body weight. In the emergent phase of resuscitation, time may not allow for a full type and crossmatch. When using uncrossmatched blood, it is best to obtain at least an ABO-Rh type and a partial crossmatch. This is preferable to the use of type O, Rh-negative uncrossmatched blood, although this may be used if type-specific uncrossmatched blood is unavailable. If large amounts of crystalloid and red blood cells are required, hemostatic defects occur. Fresh-frozen plasma to replete circulating coagulation factors and platelets should be given when 100% to 200% of the circulating blood volume has been replaced.

If a child with blunt trauma is in cardiorespiratory arrest despite an adequate airway and ventilation, immediate insertion of bilateral thoracostomy tubes and a large fluid bolus are critical, followed by pericardiocentesis if there is no improvement. Failure to respond indicates irreversible shock, traumatic myocardial injury with pump failure, or severe CNS failure.

The final phase of the primary survey is monitoring, including vital signs, temperature, urine output, and possibly filling pressures measured by central venous pressure catheter. Because of surface area/mass ratios in children, increased minute ventilation with accompanying heat of vaporization loss, and, usually, resuscitation in a cold environment, the child may become quite hypothermic, complicating resuscitation. Temperature can be supported by warming administered fluid and blood, by using external heating elements, and by wrapping all exposed parts in plastic.

The last step in the primary survey is a rapid neurologic evaluation to establish a Glasgow coma score; more extensive neurologic evaluation is not indicated at this time.

After the primary survey, initial stabilization of the cardiorespiratory system, and aggressive management of shock, a complete physical examination and reassessment, including examination of the child's back, take place; this process is called the secondary survey. A history of the injury is obtained. Roentgenograms of the cervical spine, chest, abdomen, skull, and long bones are taken.

By now, the child should be either hemodynamically stable with a controlled airway or rapidly on the way to the operating room because of continued instability. If the child's condition is stable, appropriate specialized radiographic studies are performed on the way to the ICU. Now, definitive care can be provided for each of the child's injuries.

## THORACIC INJURIES

Thoracic injuries are less common than intra-abdominal injuries in children. In children with multiple trauma, only 4.5% have thoracic injuries; however, associated mortality is 25%. Childhood chest injuries differ from those of adults in two ways. The more compliant chest of the child contributes to a low incidence of rib fracture, although serious intrathoracic injury may be present in the absence of obvious chest wall injury. In addition, the mediastinum of the child is more mobile, which contributes to a low overall incidence of major vessel and airway injury, but cardiovascular and ventilatory compromise can occur rapidly with excessive mediastinal shifting.

There are five immediately life-threatening injuries of the chest wall and parenchyma. They should be diagnosed in the initial primary assessment.

Either penetrating or blunt trauma can produce an *open pneumothorax*. The inability to generate negative intrathoracic pressure causes lung collapse and ventilatory insufficiency. In addition, there is a to-and-fro movement of the mediastinum, with interference of venous return to the right side of the heart. Treatment consists of immediately covering any hole in the chest with an airtight dressing, and inserting a chest tube through a separate incision.

*Flail chest* results from the paradoxical movement of a portion of the chest wall because of multiple rib fractures. As in open pneumothorax, generation of negative intrathoracic pressure is prevented. The chest wall is unstable, moving inward with inspiration and outward with expiration. Definitive treatment is positive pressure ventilation for internal stabilization of the chest wall. Often flail chest is complicated by underlying pulmonary contusion.

*Massive hemothorax* occurs from injuries to the aortic arch, pulmonary hilum, or systemic vessels, such as the internal mammary or intercostal arteries. Most of the bleeding that occurs with thoracic injuries is not from the lung, but from the systemic arteries in the chest. Chest tubes must be placed early in any patient with intrathoracic blood loss. Total blood loss of more than 20% or 30% of total blood volume or more than 2 to 3 mL/kg/hr usually indicates the need for surgery.

A laceration in the pulmonary parenchyma may act to allow ingress of air into the chest cavity with no egress, creating a *tension pneumothorax*. Pleural pressure rises, the lung collapses, the mediastinum shifts into the opposite hemithorax, the opposite lung becomes compressed, and venous return to the heart is compromised. Treatment is immediate tube thoracostomy.

Children with *pericardial tamponade* present with paradoxical pulse, distended neck veins, and muffled heart sounds. Lethal hypotension may result from inadequate filling of the ventricles. Pericardiocentesis is used as temporizing treatment and definitive diagnosis. Treatment ultimately requires surgical exploration.

Several common occult and potentially serious injuries to the chest and its contents are usually diagnosed on the secondary survey. *Pulmonary contusion* with or without *laceration* or *hemorrhage* is the most common serious chest injury. Pulmonary contusion from blunt injury is common and is often associated with both pulmonary edema and atelectasis. Pulmonary contusion presents with respiratory distress, hypoxemia, atelectasis, and roentgenogram changes almost immediately. Small areas of lung involvement require no specific therapy other than pulmonary toilet, but extensive injuries usually mandate mechanical venti-

lation. If a laceration is associated with the contusion, chest tube insertion is required for expansion of the pneumothorax.

*Tracheobronchial rupture* is characterized by respiratory distress, subcutaneous emphysema, and hemoptysis. Depending on the nature of the injury, some patients have airway obstruction, some have a tension pneumothorax, many have a simple pneumothorax, and all have mediastinal air on chest roentgenogram. A chest tube is inserted to evacuate the pneumothorax. Thoracotomy is usually required to control the tear.

*Myocardial contusion* is a bruise or intramural hematoma of the myocardium that occurs after blunt trauma of the anterior chest. The diagnosis is made on the basis of arrhythmias or on routine ECG. Because these children may be at risk of life-threatening arrhythmias, they require cardiac monitoring.

*Rupture of the diaphragm* may be difficult to diagnose unless the physician has a high index of suspicion. It occurs more often on the left side. Treatment is urgent diaphragmatic repair.

*Esophageal injury* may occasionally result from penetrating trauma. Esophageal perforation produces mediastinitis, a potentially lethal, rapidly progressive infection in the mediastinal space. Treatment is primary repair and drainage.

Most patients who suffer from rupture or *injury of the great vessels* die at the scene of the accident. If the patient has a wide mediastinum or obliteration of the aortic knob on roentgenogram, prompt angiographic diagnostic studies are required. As with the more recent adult literature, associated fractures of the first and second ribs do not correlate with injury to the great vessels.

*Traumatic asphyxia* is a dramatic but rare complication of blunt chest trauma. It results from sudden intense compression of the chest wall with the glottis closed. The intrathoracic pressure is suddenly increased, and this increase is reflected in the veins of the upper torso. The child presents with petechial hemorrhages in the sclerae, conjunctiva, and skin of the upper extremities and head. The hemorrhages resolve over several days. Traumatic asphyxia implies severe, blunt forces to the chest wall.

## ABDOMINAL TRAUMA

Intra-abdominal injuries account for a significant percentage of the traumatic deaths in children. The liver and spleen are the two organs most commonly injured. The main purpose of the primary and secondary survey is not to obtain a specific diagnosis of organ injury, but to determine the next course of action. Immediate laparotomy is indicated in patients with frank peritonitis or signs of massive hemorrhage. In the more stable child, CT scanning has become a standard technique of evaluation. It has replaced many of the other time-consuming radiographic procedures and the need for peritoneal lavage in most patients.

With the recognition of problems of postsplenectomy infection, nonoperative management of splenic injuries and splenic preservation have become increasingly common. Nonoperative management of splenic injury includes close observation of the patient in the ICU, with frequent measurements of hematocrit. Observation without operative treatment is not contraindicated by the need to administer a blood transfusion.

Liver injuries are usually the most serious injuries, although many liver injuries are now detected by CT scan that in the past would have gone unrecognized. Major hepatic resections are undesirable, and conservative operations are now recognized as the most appropriate treatment.

Small intestine and pancreatic injury in children occurs secondary to high-speed deceleration, as when the child crashes against the handlebars of a bicycle or after blunt trauma from child abuse. The injuries include duodenal hematoma, traumatic rupture of the jejunum near the ligament of Treitz, and pancreatic contusion or transection. The most common cause of pancreatitis and pseudocyst formation in children is pancreatic trauma. Serum amylases should be monitored for several hours after presentation and for several days after the event. When laparotomy for trauma is performed, exploration of the pancreatic bed is mandatory. Symptoms of duodenal hematoma may develop gradually, with abdominal pain, bilious vomiting, epigastric tenderness, and leukocytosis occurring hours to even days after the initial event. Expectant therapy with bowel rest, nasogastric tube placement, and parenteral nutrition is required for 7 to 10 days. Occasionally, expectant therapy fails and evacuation of the hematoma is indicated. Diagnosis of traumatic jejunal rupture is usually based on clinical signs of peritonitis; abdominal roentgenograms show free air in fewer than half of the cases.

Injury to the urinary tract is seen in about 5% of pediatric trauma patients. A catheter should not be passed in patients with pelvic fracture until a gentle retrograde urethrogram has excluded a urethral tear. Other contraindications for catheter insertion are blood at the urethral meatus, a high-riding prostate, gross hematuria, and labial, scrotal, or perianal ecchymosis or hematoma. Intravenous pyelography is recommended when the urinalysis demonstrates gross hematuria with physical evidence of renal injury, when there is an unstable clinical course with blood loss, or when renal artery injury is suspected. In many centers, the CT scan has replaced intravenous pyelography for evaluation of renal trauma. Most renal injuries do not require operation. Ureteral injuries are rare in children but should be suspected if there is extravasation of contrast material in the presence of good renal function and an intact pelvicalyceal system.

## INJURIES TO THE SPINE AND CRANIUM

Vertebral column and spinal cord trauma must be presumed to have occurred in any child with a head injury who is rendered unconscious. Up to 10% of spinal cord injuries develop cord compression during the initial period of emergency care. Great care must be taken during transport and in-hospital resuscitation not to move the head until fractures and dislocations have been excluded by appropriate films. The initial workup incorporates lateral cervical spine films that include the C7-T1 junction. Often in pediatric trauma, spinal cord injury can exist even if roentgenograms appear normal. Initial evaluation must include careful neurosensory examination. Prognosis for spinal cord injury is poor if the lesion remains complete 24 hours after the initial injury. Recent work supports the use of high-dose methylprednisolone in adults with spinal cord injury.

Management of the child with closed head injury begins, as for any child with trauma, with attention to the ABCs. The evaluation of the child during the primary survey focuses on the Glasgow Coma Scale (Table 50-1). The scale briefly evaluates best eye, motor, and verbal responses, giving a score that is reproducible and of prognostic significance. Severe head injury is found in patients with a Glasgow coma score of 11 or less. A more thorough exam is done in the secondary survey, with documentation of level of consciousness, spontaneous reactions, and response to stimuli. Cranial nerve examination should concentrate on movements of the eyes and face, particularly pupillary size and reactivity. Doll's-eyes maneuvers or caloric responses should not be attempted because of the possibility of an unstable cervical spine or ruptured eardrums.

### TABLE 50-1. Glasgow Coma Scale

| | | |
|---|---|---|
| Eyes opening | 4 | Spontaneously |
| | 3 | To verbal command |
| | 2 | To pain |
| | 1 | No response |
| Best motor response | 6 | Obeys |
| | 5 | Localizes pain |
| | 4 | Flexion withdrawal |
| | 3 | Flexion abnormal (decorticate) |
| | 2 | Decerebrate extension |
| | 1 | No response |
| Best verbal response | 5 | Oriented and converses |
| | 4 | Disoriented and converses |
| | 3 | Inappropriate words |
| | 2 | Incomprehensible sounds |
| | 1 | No response |
| Total score | 3–15 | |

If the child has a significant head injury, initial treatment should be directed at maintaining normal blood pressure and intracranial pressure. Intravenous fluid should be iso-osmolar and nonhypotonic and given at baseline infusion rates, unless the child has associated injuries requiring fluid resuscitation. Mannitol is frequently given in the seriously head-injured child to reduce intracranial pressure. It should be reserved for patients with acute neurologic dysfunction or transtentorial herniation, and used as a lifesaving measure while definitive diagnostic or surgical options are being carried out. The dose of mannitol is 0.25 to 1.0 g/kg, rapid IV.

CT scanning is the most important diagnostic modality in the management of pediatric head injury. The CT scan can make it possible to diagnose a surgically treatable mass lesion (epidural or subdural hematoma), diffuse cerebral swelling, or increased CSF volume. While definitive diagnostic studies are undertaken, hyperventilation to a $P_{CO_2}$ in the 25- to 30-mm Hg range will decrease intracranial pressure by decreasing cerebral blood volume. Control of seizures is essential for the management of acute head injury. Other treatments will best be predicated on the results of diagnostic studies.

## Selected Readings

Better OS, Stein JH. Early management of shock and prophylaxis of acute renal failure in traumatic rhabdomyolysis. N Engl J Med 1990;322:825.
Bracken MB, Shepard MJ, Collins WF, et al. A randomized, controlled trial of methylprednisolone or naloxone in the treatment of acute spinal cord injury: results of the second national acute spinal cord injury study. N Engl J Med 1990;322: 1405.
Jaffee D, Wesson D. Emergency management of blunt trauma in children. N Engl J Med 1991;324:1477.
Pepe PE. Antishock garments: more harm than good? J Crit Illness 1992;7:166.
Peclet MH, Newman KD, Eichelberger MR, Gotschall CS, Garcia VF, Bowman LM. Thoracic trauma in children: an indicator of increased mortality. J Pediatr Surg 1990;25:961.
Young GM, Eichelberger M. Evaluation, stabilization, and initial management after multiple trauma. In: Fuhrman BP, Zimmerman JJ, eds. Pediatric critical care. St. Louis: Mosby Year Book, 1992.
Ziegler MM. Major trauma. In: Fleisher GR, Ludwig S, eds. Textbook of pediatric emergency medicine, ed 2. Baltimore: Williams & Wilkings, 1988.

# SECTION II

# Infectious Diseases

*Principles and Practice of Pediatrics, Second Edition.*
edited by Frank A. Oski et al. J. B. Lippincott Company, Philadelphia © 1994.

## CHAPTER 51
# Assays for the Diagnosis of Infectious Diseases

James A. Wilde and Robert H. Yolken

The accurate diagnosis of an infectious disease is a crucial initial step in the proper management of an infectious process. Rapid laboratory diagnosis of infections is particularly important to pediatric practitioners in that infections in the pediatric age group often present with few specific signs or symptoms. Diagnostic assays frequently are applied to the diagnosis and management of infections in children, and pediatricians are often the first clinicians called on to interpret the results of these assays.

A number of diagnostic assays have been developed recently, such as those incorporating the polymerase chain reaction, that are applicable to the diagnosis and monitoring of infectious diseases in children, and it is likely that more will be developed and applied to this population in the future. The goal of this chapter is not to review specific assays for the diagnosis of specific diseases, but rather to present the general principles involved in the performance and interpretation of assays used to diagnose pediatric infectious diseases.

## GENERAL PRINCIPLES OF DIAGNOSTIC ASSAYS

Assays for the diagnosis of infectious diseases can be divided into two general categories: those that directly identify microbial products in a body fluid site and those that measure immunoglobulins specifically directed at microbial antigens. The general principles of these assays are presented in Table 51-1.

### Direct Assays

The direct assays generally are most useful for the diagnosis of an active infection, because they involve the direct measurement of microbial components. Furthermore, direct assays can be

Work supported by Grant #5 U01 AI30420 from the National Institute of Allergy and Infectious Diseases of the National Institutes of Health

quantitative, so they can also be used to monitor the level of the infecting microorganism and to assess the course of the infection and the response to antimicrobial treatment.

A principal limitation of direct assays is that the level of the infecting microorganism in some disease states may be quite low, in which cases, only assays capable of the detection of very small quantities of microorganisms would be able to make accurate diagnoses in all infected patients. Another limitation is that direct assays require the presence of the organism or its antigens in an accessible body site for a diagnosis to be made. This makes it difficult to diagnose some infections, such as those caused by hepatitis A, *Mycoplasma pneumoniae* and HIV, in which symptoms generally occur after microbial replication has reached its peak.

### Antibody Detection Assays

Some of the problems of direct detection assays are overcome by the use of assays that measure the immune response to microbial infection. In such assays, serum (or, in some cases, urine or other body fluids) is tested for the presence of immunoglobulins directed at specific microbial organisms or at microbial components. The advantage of this procedure is that the organism need not be present in the sampled site when the measurement of an immune response is performed. Furthermore, since even a small quantity of infecting antigen can give rise to a large number of activated B-cells, high degrees of sensitivity generally are not required for the detection of specific antibodies. Finally, since the immune response to an infecting microorganism persists for an extended period, antibody detection assays allow for the diagnosis of an infection after microbial replication has declined. These assays can thus be used for the diagnosis of infections that lead to chronic disease processes, such as infections with hepatitis C virus, Dengue viruses, *Borrelia burgdorferi*, and *Treponema pallidum*.

In the case of lifelong infections such as those caused by HIV, the detection of antibody (in the absence of maternal antibody derived prenatally) is diagnostic for the disease process. In many other cases, however, this persistence of detectable antibody constitutes one of the principal limitations of antibody detection assays, the fact that the antibody can be present long after the infectious process is completed or the patient has undergone successful treatment. For this reason, the detection of antibody often cannot, by itself, be considered diagnostic of a current infection. For example, a child with antibodies to enteroviruses might at the time of testing have acute bacterial meningitis; a patient with antibodies to Epstein-Barr virus might be undergoing an acute streptococcal pharyngitis; and a patient with a high antibody titer to histoplasmin antigen might have tuberculosis. This problem can be partially overcome by the measurement of antibody classes such as IgM and IgA that are associated with an early immune response to infection. Such measurements are particularly useful in the diagnosis of infections that occur during the prenatal period. Because IgM and IgA class antibodies do not

## TABLE 51-1.   Assays Used in Diagnosis of Infectious Diseases

| Assay | Results |
|---|---|
| **Antigen Detection** | |
| Counterimmunoelectrophoresis (CIE) | Line of precipitation produced when test specimen containing antigen migrates in gel toward anode and antigen specific antibody migrates toward cathode |
| Latex Particle Agglutination (LA) | Antigen-specific antibody-coated latex beads agglutinate when test specimen containing specific antigen is added. In some cases, erythrocytes or other particles are used in place of latex beads. |
| Enzyme Immunoassay (EIA, ELISA) | Antigen in specimen binds to antigen specific antibody bonded to plastic plate. Antigen specific antibody labeled with enzyme is added, binds antigen in "sandwich." Substrate for the enzyme is added; rate of reaction as measured by color change reflects quantity of antigen in specimen. |
| Fluorescent Antibody (FA) | Fluoresceinated antigen specific antibody binds antigen from specimen. Fluorescence after unbound antibodies washed away indicates presence of antigen. |
| DNA Probe | Enzyme or radiolabeled segment of target-specific DNA binds to homologous nucleic acid in sample. Signal remaining after unbound probe is washed away reflects quantity of target. |
| Polymerase Chain Reaction (PCR) | Uses thermostable DNA polymerase and specific primers to amplify target nucleic acid from undetectable to detectable levels. Variety of methods to detect products of reaction. |
| **Antibody Detection** | |
| Complement Fixation (Comp Fix) | Sample containing antibody is combined with target antigen and known amount of complement. Ag-Ab complexes cause fixation (consumption) of complement. Sensitized red cells are added, unfixed complement causes lysis. Degree of complement fixation reflects quantity of antibody. |
| Radioimmunoassay (RIA) | Iodine 125 is used to label target immunoglobulins in a sample. Reaction with antigen and unlabeled immunoglobulin (competitively inhibits labeled Ig) as measured by radioactivity level reflects amount of labeled immunoglobulin. |
| Enzyme Immunoassay | Antibody in specimen binds to antigen bound to plastic microtiter plate or a similar surface. Anti-human immunoglobulin labelled with enzyme is added. The bound enzyme is reacted with substrate. The rate of reaction as measured by color change reflects the quantity of antibody in the clinical sample. Immunoglobulin class or subclass can be measured by the use of the specific enzyme-labelled anti-human immunoglobulin (eg, anti-human IgM or anti-human IgG$_1$). |
| Neutralization Reactions | Serial dilutions of sample containing antibody is added to viral culture media along with target virus. Presence of antibody neutralizes virus, preventing growth in tissue culture. |
| Hemagglutination Inhibition | Antibody in sample is reacted with specific antigen. The amount of unreacted antigen is quantitated by binding of the antigen to erythrocytes. In some cases, the antigen contains a hemagglutinin and can bind directly to the erythrocytes (eg, influenza virus). In other cases, binding of the erythrocytes to the unreacted antigen is accomplished by the coating of the erythrocytes with specific antibody. |

cross the normal placenta in appreciable quantities, the detection of these antibodies in the infant can be used to distinguish maternal from fetal infections. This method has been used to detect perinatal infections with cytomegalovirus, rubella virus, toxoplasmosis and, more recently, HIV. It should be noted that in the case of infections that occur later in life, the persistence of these "acute phase" antibodies can be variable, making their detection unreliable as specific indicators of recent infection. This is particularly important to remember when more sensitive assays are used because they can detect small concentrations of IgM antibody long after the initial infection. The possibility of false positive results due to the presence of rheumatoid factors and other autoimmune reactants also limits the specificity of these reactions for the definitive diagnosis of the infectious process.

One approach to improving the specificity of antibody detection assays for the diagnosis of recent infectious diseases takes advantage of the fact that certain components of infecting microorganisms often are selected by the immune system as the initial targets of the immune response. The measurement of antibodies to such "early antigens" is thus a reflection of a recent infection, especially if it occurs in the absence of antibodies to other components of the organism that develop later in the course of infection (late antigens). Such assays are particularly useful for the diagnosis of infections due to cytomegalovirus, Epstein-Barr virus, and other herpesviruses, in which the viral targets of an early and late immune response have been well characterized. The recent characterization of the timing of the immune response to *Borrelia burgdorferi* also indicates that the measurement of antibodies to different microbial components can be used as a more accurate way to characterize the status of patients presumed to have Lyme disease. As the immune response to other microbial organisms becomes better characterized, the measurement of early antigens will play a more important role in the diagnosis of a recent infection in children.

Most antibody assays involve the measurement of immunoglobulins in blood or serum specimens. Recently it has become possible to measure antibodies in mucosal body sites. Studies have indicated that antibodies to infectious antigens can be measured accurately in mucosal sites such as saliva and urine (Harcourt et al, 1990). These antibodies can arise either from transudation from the systemic circulation or in response to antigenic stimulation at the mucosal surface. In either case, the measurement of antibodies at the mucosal site provides an assessment of the immune response to the infecting microorganism.

Being able to measure a range of antibodies in readily accessible body fluids would be of great help in diagnosing infections in young infants and in monitoring immune responses in a clinical practice setting.

## SPECIFIC ASSAYS FOR ANTIBODY DETECTION

A wide variety of assays are available for the detection of antibodies to infectious agents. Although these assays are named for the method that is used for the measurement of the antigen–antibody reaction, all of the assays make use of a similar basic reaction—that is, the binding of the patient's immunoglobulin to a defined microbial antigen. The main reason for the multiplicity of tests that are available is that several methods can be used for measuring this antigen–antibody reaction. Current assay methods vary a great deal in terms of their ability to detect specific antibodies, and hence in their sensitivity and specificity. In general, the solid phase immunoassays (exemplified by solid phase enzyme immunoassays, also known as enzyme linked immunosorbent assays or ELISA) offer the highest degree of sensitivity while allowing for objective quantitation and the inclusion of controls for the maintenance of specificity. The explosion of

knowledge on the antigenicity of microbial proteins and techniques for their cloning and production in recombinant forms should lead to the availability of more sensitive and specific solid phase assays for detecting antibodies to a wide range of infecting microorganisms.

Older assays such as complement fixation and immunofluorescence are still of use in situations in which highly purified components of the infecting microorganism are not widely available, which is generally the case with bacteria and *Mycoplasma*. In infections with these microorganisms, the components against which antibodies are directed have not been well characterized, and hence cannot be used as antigens for the solid phase assays.

Another group of widely used assays are those that rely on agglutination. In most agglutination assays, particles made of latex or similar materials are coated with antigen. When these react with serum that contains antibody, cross-bridging causes the beads to bind to each other in a recognizable pattern of agglutination. Antibody-coated erythrocytes also can be used in place of synthetic particles, in which case a pattern of hemagglutination in reaction with antibody is observed. Although the particle agglutination assays are less sensitive than solid phase immunosorbent assays, they are rapid and simple to perform and can be used outside central laboratory settings. They are ideal for use in situations in which qualitative, rather than quantitative, results are needed. For example, such assays are useful to determine whether an individual is lacking antibody to rubella virus and is thus susceptible to infection with this virus.

One problem inherent in the use of assays for the detection of antibodies is the way in which the results are reported by the laboratory and interpreted by the clinician. Traditionally, results are reported in terms of a "titer," in which the maximum dilution that results in a positive reaction is reported (ie, a titer of 1:8 means that the sample gave a reaction when diluted 8-fold but not when diluted 16-fold.) The disadvantage of this system is that it does not take into account the inherent sensitivity of the assay that is used for the antibody measurement. This is particularly problematic when the more sensitive immunoassays are employed for antibody measurement; a serum that has a titer of 1:8 as measured by an insensitive complement fixation assay may have a titer of more than 1:1000 when measured by means of a solid phase immunosorbent assay. This variation can cause problems in interpreting laboratory tests and can complicate the comparison of assays performed in different laboratories. Another problem with endpoint titers is that, regardless of the assay, they are difficult to attain in a reproducible manner. If a laboratory reports a change in titer in samples obtained over time, it is not always clear whether the change is due to the generation of antibody in the patient, indicating an active infection, or day-to-day variations in the sensitivity of the assay system used for the performance of the measurements.

Fortunately, the solid phase immunosorbent assays are quantitative in nature and lend themselves to the performance of standard curves and accurate reproducibility. In addition, they allow for reporting assay results in standard units, thus allowing for the performance of control reactions and the standardization of results between different test runs and among different laboratories. The use of standard units also allows for higher degrees of accuracy since it does not require the traditional 4-fold increase to achieve clinical significance; cut-off values and levels of significance can be established for each assay system. Although the units may be less familiar to the clinician than titer measurements, assays reported in terms of standard units are generally more reproducible and allow for more reliable comparisons with reference values. The universal reporting of antibody values in standard units, therefore, would represent a major step forward in the clinician's ability to interpret serological data and to use the results in the management of the pediatric patient.

Until standard unitage becomes universally available, clinical laboratories should provide clinicians with data indicating the sensitivity of the assay used for the measurement and the expected assay-to-assay variation in the test results. Also, when using a four-fold rise in titers over time to make a diagnosis, it is essential for acute and convalescent samples to be tested simultaneously to avoid the problems associated with day-to-day variability.

## ADVANTAGES OF DIRECT DETECTION ASSAYS

Although assays that measure the immune response to an infecting organism are useful in many situations, there are several advantages inherent in assay systems that directly assess the presence of microbial organisms in body fluids. Until recently, the direct detection of microbial pathogens was accomplished by immunoassay systems designed to detect antigenic components of the infecting microorganism. These assays are similar in design to the immunoassays for measurement of antibodies described above in that they involve the measurement of the interaction between antigens and antibodies. However, antigen detection assays differ in that they involve the interaction of antigens in a patient's sample with an antibody of known specificity. This generally is accomplished by labeling the antibody with a suitable marker such as a radioactive isotope, an enzyme or a latex particle (see Table 51-1). In general, the enzyme-based assays offer the highest levels of sensitivity and specificity; the particle-based assays, however, can be useful in situations outside clinical laboratories in which rapid results are needed. For example, particle agglutination assays are widely used in clinical settings for rapid detection of antigens from group A streptococci.

Assays for the direct detection of microbial agents offer a number of advantages in the diagnosis of acute infections. Because they do not require the generation of an active immune response, they can be used to ascertain the presence of an infectious process before the patient has had sufficient time to generate detectable antibodies. Furthermore, these assays can be used for the diagnosis of infections in immunocompromised individuals, neonates, and other patients who would not be expected to generate a predictable immune response to infection. The principal drawback of antigen-detection assays is that they are limited by the kinetics of the antigen–antibody reactions used to make the diagnostic measurement. Although this limitation can be partially overcome by the selection of antigens that are present in multiple copies in microbial organisms (such as the capsular polysaccharide of *Haemophilus influenzae),* many important pathogens do not contain antigens that can be used for this purpose. In such cases, the presence of more than 1000 organisms might be required before a detectable signal could be obtained, meaning that the assays would not be useful for the diagnosis of infection early in the course of disease, when the antigen load is low. In addition, the generation of an effective immune response to infection generally leads to the production of antibodies that bind to the microbial antigens that are the targets of the immunoassay reagents. Such antibodies can interfere with the sensitivity of the immunoassay, decreasing the utility of these assays late in the course of a chronic infectious process.

### Nucleic Acid Assays

Recently, a new class of diagnostic assays that has sufficient sensitivity for the early diagnosis of a wide range of infectious diseases has been developed. These assays are based on the measurement of microbial nucleic acids in the body fluids of infected infants and children. Like the antigen assays, assays for the direct detection of nucleic acids measure components of the infecting microorganism. Instead of measuring antigens derived from the organism, however, they rely on the detection of genetic material specific for the pathogenic agent. In the case of viruses, the detection of virions requires the detection of the appropriate genomic nucleic acid. This is DNA in the case of DNA-containing viruses such as herpesviruses, hepatitis B virus, and adenoviruses, and RNA in the case of viruses such as influenza, parainfluenza, measles, rotavirus, hepatitis A and hepatitis C viruses. Retroviruses such as HIV and HTLV require RNA detection for the identification of intact virions, but since retroviruses undergo integration into the cellular genome in the form of a reverse transcribed copy of DNA, such agents also can be detected in infected cells in the form of DNA. Conversely, viruses with a DNA genome, such as the herpesviruses, usually generate messenger RNA when they are undergoing active replication and can thus be detected in their RNA form in infected cells. The ability to detect both DNA and RNA provides a great deal of information, not only in terms of the presence of the microbial agent, but also in terms of the stage of infection.

The detection of nucleic acids offers a number of striking advantages in terms of the rapid diagnosis of infectious diseases in the pediatric age group. First, the fact that nucleic acids from all microorganisms are made up of combinations of the same 4 nucleotides (A, T, G, and C for DNA and A, U, G, and C for RNA) allows for the detection of virtually any infectious pathogen in the same reaction format. It should be possible, for example, to detect viral, bacterial, mycoplasmal, fungal, and chlamydial agents of pneumonia using the same set of reactions, varying only the order of the nucleotides and the size of the probes. Second, since nucleic acids can be extracted free from blocking immunoglobulins and other agents that might interfere with immunoassays, nucleic acid detection methods can be used to detect microorganisms in virtually any body fluid and at any stage in the disease process. Third, as discussed above, the measurement of DNA or RNA can be used to determine whether an agent is undergoing active replication and thus whether it is latent or is actually contributing to the acute disease process. Finally, the repetitive nature of nucleic acids allows for the performance of amplification reactions in which small quantities of nucleic acid are amplified by means of controlled chemical reactions to amounts that are easily detectable. Nucleic acid amplification assays, exemplified by the polymerase chain reaction (PCR), offer extreme degrees of sensitivity, theoretically allowing for the million-fold amplification of nucleic acids and hence the detection of very small numbers of infectious microorganisms. Furthermore, the nucleic acid amplification reactions can be performed with very small amounts of blood or other body fluids, making them well suited for the diagnosis of infections in infants and small children.

The extreme sensitivity of nucleic acid amplification assays also results in a number of problems in assay interpretation. Because very small amounts of genetic material can be amplified to a great extent, contamination of samples by as little as one organism or a single copy of amplified DNA during the collection or processing steps can lead to false positive results. For this reason, great care must be taken to prevent contamination. This is monitored through the processing of multiple negative controls in the extraction and amplification steps. In addition, a number of modifications to the nucleic acid amplification format are being included to minimize the chances of false positive results due to sample contamination. Until such modifications are shown to obviate the problem of contamination, it is imperative that clinicians who use these assays demand from the laboratory that appropriate controls for contamination be included in each assay run and that data be reported only from assay runs certified to be free from contamination.

Additional limitations of currently available nucleic acid amplification assays is that they must be performed in specialized laboratories, require extended periods of time to complete, and cost significantly more than other assay systems. For this reason, the use of nucleic acid amplification assays is not warranted for detection of infectious agents in which sufficient quantities of antigen are present to allow for detection by means of antigenic assays. It is thus unlikely that nucleic acid detection assays will replace antigenic assays for the detection of antigens from group A streptococcus, hepatitis B virus, or rotavirus. However, nucleic acid amplification assays are likely to play an important role in the diagnosis of diseases in which the microbial load is below that which can be detected by immunoassay systems. It is thus likely that such assays will play an important role in the diagnosis of HIV infection in the first year of life, the detection of hepatitis C virus in the blood, and the detection of herpes viruses in the cerebrospinal fluid. In addition, nucleic acid amplification assays will play a crucial role in the identification of new pathogens and in their characterization as agents of disease in the pediatric population.

## INTERPRETATION OF ASSAY RESULTS

The performance characteristics of individual assays are generally expressed in terms of sensitivity, specificity, and positive and negative predictive values. Understanding these concepts is crucial to the proper interpretation of laboratory tests for the diagnosis of infectious diseases. *Sensitivity* is a measure of the assay's ability to identify a true positive accurately—that is, to detect the microorganism or antibody in situations in which it is actually present (Table 51-2). *Specificity* is a measure of the assay's ability to identify a true negative accurately—that is, to yield a negative result in situations in which the microorganism or antibody is absent. In practice, no diagnostic assay achieves 100% sensitivity or specificity, so clinicians often have to determine whether a positive result means that the infection is actually present or a negative result means that an infection is truly absent. This is the question addressed by the predictive value of the test: given a positive result, what is the likelihood of a true positive (positive predictive value), or given a negative result, what is the likelihood of a true negative (negative predictive value)? Predictive values depend directly on the prevalence of the condition in the study population. As prevalence goes down, positive predictive value goes down but negative predictive value goes up. As prevalence goes up, positive predictive value goes up but negative predictive value goes down.

An example will help to illustrate this important point (Table 51-3). Suppose in two populations of 1000 people you wanted to test for disease X. In population A, the prevalence of X is 20%, whereas in population B it is 0.1%. Now suppose you wanted to test for disease X using an assay with 90% sensitivity and 95% specificity. What are the predictive values of positive and negative results in these populations?

As can be seen in Table 51-3, the predictive value of a positive test is highly dependent on the prevalence of the disease in the population. In population A, most of the positive results occur in persons who actually have the disease (220 are positive and 180 have the disease; positive predictive value = 82%). The occurrence of a positive result, therefore, has a reasonable correlation with the presence of the disease state. On the other hand, in low prevalence population B, of 59 persons who test positive, only 9 (15%) will actually have the disease. In this population, there will be many false positive results for each true positive, despite the apparently high specificity of the test. Note that in both cases, the negative predictive value is high; an individual whose test result is negative is unlikely actually to have the disease. It should also be noted however, that the negative predictive value goes down as the prevalence in the population increases. Since no assay can be assumed to be 100% sensitive, the presence of an infectious disease cannot be completely ruled out by a negative assay. Further diagnostic tests and treatment may be indicated if the clinical state of the patient does not match the test results.

What are the implications of these points about positive predictive value and negative predictive value? The most important is that the role of the physician is of paramount importance in deciding which tests to order on a patient. Many infectious diseases occurring in the developed world have very low prevalence rates. If the test for disease X were used indiscriminately on all

### TABLE 51-2. Definition of Assay Sensitivity and Specificity

| | Test Positive (+) | Test Negative (−) | Total |
|---|---|---|---|
| Disease Present | a (true +) | b (false −) | a + b |
| Disease Absent | c (false +) | d (true −) | c + d |
| Total | a + c | b + d | a + b + c + d |

$$\text{Sensitivity} = \frac{a}{a + b} = \frac{\text{true positive}}{\text{total with disease}}$$

$$\text{Specificity} = \frac{d}{c + d} = \frac{\text{true negative}}{\text{total without disease}}$$

$$\text{Positive predictive value (PPV)} = \frac{a}{a + c} = \frac{\text{true positive}}{\text{all test positive}}$$

$$\text{Negative predictive value (NPV)} = \frac{d}{b + d} = \frac{\text{true negative}}{\text{all test negative}}$$

### TABLE 51-3. Predictive Values of An Assay System in a High-Prevalence and Low-Prevalence Population

**High-Prevalence Population (n = 1000)**

Prevalence = .2
Sensitivity = .90
Specificity = .95

| | *Test Result* | | |
|---|---|---|---|
| | + | − | Total |
| Disease Present | 180 | 20 | 200 |
| Disease Absent | 40 | 760 | 800 |
| Total | 220 | 780 | 1000 |

PPV = 180/220 = 82%
NPV = 760/780 = 97%

**Low-Prevalence Population (n = 1000)**

Prevalence = .01
Sensitivity = 90
Specificity = .95

| | *Test Result* | | |
|---|---|---|---|
| | + | − | Total |
| Disease Present | 9 | 1 | 10 |
| Disease Absent | 50 | 940 | 990 |
| Total | 59 | 941 | 1000 |

PPV = 9/59 = 15%
NPV = 940/941 = 99.9%

children in the United States to test for infection, the predictable result would be that most of the people identified as infected would, in fact, be from the false positive category. If, however, the test were used only on people who had signs and symptoms known to be characteristic of infection with disease X, the prevalence rate in this group would be greater and thus the predictive value of a positive reaction would be higher. Thus assays for the detection of antigens from group A streptococcus are of more use when employed on samples from individuals with pharyngitis than when they are used on samples obtained from asymptomatic individuals, and assays for the detection of HIV are more predictive when employed for the analysis of samples from high-risk populations. It is important that assays for infectious diseases not be ordered on a routine basis or in the form of a large battery, but rather only following careful consideration of the likelihood of disease in light of the patient's clinical condition and the epidemiology of the suspected infectious process.

Another issue involved in the interpretation of laboratory results involves the study population in which the assay's original sensitivity and specificity data are collected. The problem is this: data derived from the sampling of one population may not be applicable to the interpretation of assay results in another. For example, assays with high degrees of sensitivity for the detection of chlamydia infections in symptomatic males may not be appropriate for the detection of infection in asymptomatic females. Similarly, assays for the diagnosis of Epstein-Barr virus infection based on the heterophile reaction are quite sensitive when applied to adolescents, but lack sensitivity for the detection of this infection in infants. Similarly, antigenic assays with high degrees of specificity in samples obtained from unselected infants can display false positive results in individuals with autoimmune reactivity.

For each assay, the manufacturer may claim a certain sensitivity and specificity, but these numbers may come from study populations quite different from the one in which you are interested. The appropriateness of the study group should always be considered when interpreting the results of a laboratory test, especially when the patient has underlying immune activation or is from an age group or a geographic area in which the assay system has not been evaluated.

The concepts of sensitivity and specificity imply that there is a gold standard by which new assays can be assessed. In some cases, such as the diagnosis of acute bacteremia and meningitis, currently available culturing techniques, although slower than direct detection assays, possess good levels of sensitivity and specificity and can generally be used to assess the performance characteristics of newer assay systems. However, in the case of infections due to viruses, mycobacteria, and other slower growing microorganisms, current assays do not detect every case of infection and, thus, a gold standard does not yet exist. In such cases, a rapid test can be truly positive in situations where the standard test does not detect the presence of the infecting agent. This is particularly likely to happen with the nucleic acid amplification assays, in light of their high degrees of sensitivity. For example, a physician may have to decide what plan of action to follow in the case of a patient who tests positive for a sexually transmitted disease by a nucleic acid amplification assay but negative by a less sensitive antigen-detection assay. This question can only be addressed if the true sensitivity and specificity of both assays can be determined.

Documentation that a more sensitive assay can detect a microbial pathogen not detected by a less sensitive assay requires experiments using animal models, sequential analysis of infected individuals, and the study of disease transmission in defined outbreaks of infection. Although such studies can be difficult and expensive to design and perform, they are crucial to the development of a data base on the performance characteristics of the newer, more sensitive assay systems. Such studies also are necessary to distinguish microbial carriage from disease, since the more sensitive assays may detect the presence of microorganisms in clinical situations not previously recognized by less sensitive assays. Carefully controlled clinical trials are thus essential for obtaining these data and represent a crucial step in making these assays useful for the pediatrician.

In the next few years, a large number of new diagnostic assays will become available to the pediatric practitioner. These assays will have degrees of sensitivity and specificity substantially greater than those currently available. The development of guidelines for using these assays and interpreting assay results will undoubtedly pose challenges to the pediatric community. The successful application of these assays to the detection of microbial pathogens, however, will provide pediatricians with unique tools for the diagnosis and management of children with suspected infectious diseases.

## Selected Readings

Baseler MW, Stevens RA, Metcalf JA. Immunologic monitoring of patients with human immunodeficiency virus infection. In: Rose NR, deMacario EC, Fahey JL, Friedman H, Penn GM (eds). Manual of clinical laboratory immunology, ed 4. Chapter 59. Washington, DC: American Society for Microbiology, 1992.

Benenson AS, Peddecord KM, Hofherr LK, Ascher MS, Taylor RN, Hearn TL. Reporting the results of human immunodeficiency virus testing. JAMA 1989;262:3435.

Bobo L, Coutlee F, Yolken RH, Quinn T, Viscidi RP. Diagnosis of *Chlamydia trachomatia* cervical infection: an enzyme immunoassay for detection of DNA amplified by the polymerase chain reaction. J Clin Microbiol 1990;28:1968.

Dienstag JL, Feinstone SM, Kapikian AZ, and Purcell RH. Faecal shedding of hepatitis A antigen. Lancet 1975;i:765.

Feldman WE. Diagnostic and prognostic values of bacterial antigen detection. In: Wicher K (ed). Microbial antiginodiagnosis, Vol 2: Practical applications. Boco Raton, FL: CRC Press, Inc, 1987:143.

Fleisher G, Henle W, Henle G, Lennett ET, Bigger RJ. Primary infection with Epstein-Barr virus in infants in the United States: clinical and serologic observations. J Infect Dis 1979;139:553.

Fuccillo DA, Vacante DA, Sever JL. Rapid viral diagnosis. In: Rose NR, deMacario EC, Fahey JL, Friedman H, Penn GM (eds). Manual of clinical laboratory immunology, ed 4. Chapter 81. Washington, DC: American Society for Microbiology, 1992:545.

Harcourt GC, Best JM, Banatvala JE. Rubella-specific serum and nasopharyngeal antibodies in volunteers with naturally acquired and vaccine-induced immunity after intranasal challenge. J Infect Dis 1980;142:145.

Hollinger FB, Dienstag JL. Hepatitis viruses. In: Lennett EH, Balonis A, Hausler WJ Jr, Shadomy HJ (eds). Manual of clinical microbiology, ed 4. Washington, DC: American Society for Microbiology, 1985:813.

Juto P, Settergren B. Specific serum IgA, IgG, and IgM antibody determination by a modified indirect ELISA-technique in primary and recurrent herpes simplex virus infection. J Virol Methods 1988;20:45.

Kenny GE, Kaiser GG, Cooney MK, Foy HM. Diagnosis of *Mycoplasma pneumoniae* pneumonia: sensitivities and specificities of serology with lipid antigen and isolation of the organism on soy peptone medium for identification of infections. J Clin Microbiol 1990;28:2087.

Lieu TA, Fleisher GR, Schwartz JS. Cost-effectiveness of rapid latex agglutination testing and throat culture for streptococcal pharyngitis. pediatrics 1990;85:246.

Nahmias A, Yolken R, Keyserling H. Rapid diagnosis of viral infections: a new challenge for the pediatrician. In: Barness LA (ed). Advances in pediatrics, Vol 32. Chicago: Yearbook Medical Publishers, 1985:507.

Pang J, Modlin J, Yolken R. Use of modified nucleotides and uracil-DNA glycosylase (UNG) for the control of contamination in the PCR-based amplification of RNA. Mol Cell Probes 1992;6:251.

Pepple JM, Moxon ER, Yolken RH. Indirect enzyme-linked immunosorbent assay (ELISA) for the quantitation of the type specificntigen of Haemophilus influenzae B: a preliminary report. J Pediatr 1980;97:233.

Relmer CB, Black CM, Phillips DJ, Logan LC, Hunter EF, Fender BJ, McGrew BE. The specificity of fetal IgM: antibody or anti-antibody? Ann NY Acad Sci 1975;254:77.

Saiki RK, Gelfland DH, Stoffel S, Scharf SJ, Higuchi R, Horn GT, Mullis RB, Ehrlich HA. Primer-directed enzymatic amplification of DNA with a thermostable DNA polymerase. Science 1988;239:487.

Schacter J, Cles L, Ray R, Hines P. Failure of serology in diagnosing chlamydial infections of the female genital tract. J Clin Microbiol 1979;10:647.

Schmid GP. Epidemiology and clinical similarities of human spirochetal diseases. Rev Infect Dis 1989;2:S1460.

Schwartz JS, Dans PE, Kinosian BP. Human immunodeficiency virus test evaluation, performance, and use: proposals to make good tests better. JAMA 1988;259:2574.

Sever JL, Tzan NR, Shekarchi IC, Madden DL. Rapid latex agglutination test for rubella antibody. J Clin Microbial 1983;17:52.

Tobin Jr, Berkowitz ID, Yolken R. The clinical laboratory and pediatric clinical care. Critical Care Report 1991;2:406.

Viscidi RP, Yolken RH. Molecular diagnosis of infectious diseases by nucleic acid hybridization. Mol Cell Probe 1987;1:3.

Watts NB. Medical relevance of laboratory tests: a clinical perspective. Arch Pathol Lab Med 1988;112:379.

Weiner AJ, Kuo G, Bradley DW, et al. Detection of hepatitis C viral sequences in non-A, non-B hepatitis. Lancet 1990;335:1.

Wilde J, Yolken R, Willoughby R, Eiden J. Improved detection of rotavirus shedding by polymerase chain reaction. Lancet 1991;337:323.

Yolken RH. Solid phase immunoassays for the detection of viral diseases. In: van Regenmortel MHV and Neurath AR (eds). Immunochemistry of viruses. The basis of serodiagnosis and vaccines. Amsterdam: Elsevier, 1985.

Yolken RH. Nucleic acids or immunoglobulins: that are the molecular probes of the future. Mol Cell Probes 1988;2:87.

Yolken RH. Laboratory diagnosis of viral infections. In: Galasso GJ, Whitley RJ, Merigan TC (eds). Antiviral agents and viral diseases of man, ed 3. Chapter 5. New York: Raven Press, 1990:141.

Yolken RH. New methods for the quantitation of microbial nucleic acids. Pure & Appl Chem 1991;63:1127.

Yolken RH. Gastroenteritis viruses. In: Lennett EH (ed). Laboratory diagnosis of viral infections, ed 2. New York: Marcel Dekker, 1992:381.

Yolken RH, Coutlee F, Viscidi RP. New prospects for the diagnosis of viral infections. Yale J Biol and Med 1989;62:131.

Yolken RH, Hart W, Perman J. Viral infection and gastrointestinal dysfunction in children with HIV infection. In: Pizzo PA, Wilfert CM (eds). Pediatric AIDS: the challenge of HIV Infection in infants, children, and adolescents. Baltimore: Williams & Wilkins, 1990:277.

Yolken RH, Stopa PJ. Analyses of non-specific reactions in enzyme-linked immunosorbent assay testing for human rotavirus. J Clin Microbiol 1979;10:703.

*Principles and Practice of Pediatrics, Second Edition.*
edited by Frank A. Oski et al. J. B. Lippincott Company, Philadelphia © 1994.

# 51.1 *Pathogenesis of Fever and Its Treatment*

Martin I. Lorin

Fever often is defined simply as an elevation of body temperature above normal, or above an arbitrary upper limit. However, a more exact definition would be an elevation of body temperature as part of a specific biological response mediated and controlled by the central nervous system (CNS). This definition distinguishes fever from other types of elevated body temperature such as heat stress and heat illness.

## PATHOPHYSIOLOGY

Fever is one of a large array of responses elicited by chemical mediators involved in the inflammatory process. The most important substance currently identified as mediating the febrile response is interleukin-1 (IL-1), a polypeptide, or group of peptides, synthesized by blood monocytes, phagocytic cells lining the liver and spleen, and other tissue macrophages. IL-1 also is the major currently identified mediator of the acute phase inflammatory response. Before its widespread metabolic, endocrinologic, and hematologic effects were recognized, IL-1 was called *endogenous pyrogen*. In addition to fever, IL-1 or related mediators increase the synthesis of acute phase proteins by the liver, decrease serum iron and zinc levels, provoke leukocytosis, and accelerate skeletal muscle proteolysis. IL-1 also induces slow-wave sleep, perhaps explaining the somnolence and lethargy frequently associated with a febrile illness. Keratinocytes, renal mesangial cells, gingival epithelial cells, and brain astrocytes also produce IL-1-like substances, but it is believed that these have primarily a local rather than a systemic effect.

Fever is the result of a highly coordinated series of events that begins peripherally with the synthesis and release of IL-1 by phagocytic cells in the blood or tissues. Molecules of IL-1 enter the blood and are carried to the CNS, where they induce an abrupt increase in the synthesis of prostaglandins, especially prostaglandin $E_2$, in the region of the anterior hypothalamus. This increase results in elevation of the set-point (or reference point) of the thermostat mechanism in this area of the brain. The temperature control region of the anterior hypothalamus then reads the current body temperature as too low in comparison to the new set-point and initiates a series of events to elevate body temperature to a height equal to the new set-point. This adaptation involves an augmentation of heat production by increased metabolic rate and increased muscle tone and activity. It also involves decreased heat loss, primarily through diminished perfusion of the skin. Body temperature rises until a new equilibrium is achieved at the elevated set-point.

## FEVER: FRIEND OR FOE?

How important is fever as a defense mechanism? Klastersky and Kass expressed it well when they wrote that despite recognition and study for more than 2000 years, it remains unclear "whether fever is an essential defensive mechanism or is a relatively trivial and unimportant biological response to infection." Generally, it is assumed that such a complex mechanism would represent an integral and functional part of the inflammatory response and not an incidental or accidental biological effect. Whether this response is always beneficial, however, is a more difficult question. Defense mechanisms can go awry. Fluid retention in congestive heart failure and antidiuretic hormone secretion in increased intracranial pressure are examples of situations where, in excess, the defense mechanism may do more harm than good.

The question often posed is, "Is fever a friend or a foe?" A more appropriate question would be, "Under what conditions is fever beneficial and under what conditions is it harmful?" Little doubt exists that, biologically, fever has some role in defending the host against infection and possibly against other diseases as well. However, it may be that fever is a less important protective mechanism in higher animals with well-developed immunologic systems, such as mammals, than in those with more primitive immunologic systems, such as fish and reptiles. Indeed, if one reviews the animal experiments purporting to demonstrate a survival benefit due to fever, most instances are in lower animals such as fish and lizards. Studies in higher animals have been more equivocal; indeed, some mammals have shown better survival in the euthermic than the febrile state. Cold-blooded animals (poikilotherms) develop fever in response to infection. They do so strictly by behavioral mechanisms, by moving to the warmest external environment available. Despite the lack of similarity of their immunologic systems to that of humans, these animals often have been selected as laboratory models for the study of fever because of the convenience with which fever can be prevented in them without confounding the study by the introduction of drugs such as aspirin. In view of our current knowledge of the immunosuppressive effects of aspirin, studies that have used this drug to study the effect of fever reduction on morbidity or mortality, either in animals or humans, must be considered highly suspect.

The growth or survival of a few pathogenic bacteria or viruses is impaired at temperatures in the range of 40 °C (104 °F). Many pathogenic bacteria require iron for their growth, and it has been shown that fever is associated with a decrease in serum iron and increase in serum ferritin, resulting in minimal levels of free iron in the blood. Because these bacteria have an enhanced need for iron at high temperatures, it has been suggested that this response is a coordinated host defense mechanism to deprive bacteria of free iron when they need it most. Studies in lizards and goldfish infected with *Aeromonas hydrophila* have shown a higher mortality when these animals are denied access to a warmer environment, thus preventing the febrile response. In vitro studies have demonstrated enhancement of several human immunologic functions at moderately elevated ambient temperatures. These functions include increased lymphocyte transformation response to mitogen, increased bactericidal activity of polymorphonuclear leukocytes, and increased production of interferon. However, as temperature approached 40 °C (104 °F) in these experiments, most of the functions decreased to below baseline levels.

Kluger and Vaughn studied rabbits infected with *Pasteurella multocida* and found that although survival increased with moderate fever, fevers greater than 2.25 °C above baseline were associated with lower survival rates than was the euthermic state. Banet demonstrated increased mortality associated with fever in rats infected with *Salmonella enteritidis*. Thus, it appears that fever, especially fever of moderate degree, can enhance several aspects of the immunologic response. At high body temperatures, however, these effects may be diminished or even reversed.

Fever may have undesirable effects other than the immunologic changes described earlier. Fever often makes patients uncomfortable. It is associated with an increased metabolic rate, increased oxygen consumption and carbon dioxide production, and increased demands on the cardiovascular and pulmonary systems. For the normal child, these stresses are of little or no consequence. However, for the child with an underlying disorder, especially of the heart or lungs, these increased demands may be significantly detrimental.

Fever clearly can precipitate febrile convulsions in susceptible children between 6 months and 5 years old. Although these seizures generally are benign, they are disturbing to the parent and child and may lead to invasive procedures such as lumbar punctures as well as considerable expense. Experiments in monkeys demonstrated a deleterious effect of fever on injured cerebral tissue. Clasen and colleagues introduced a standardized insult to one cerebral hemisphere in each experimental animal. Half of the animals were maintained in the euthermic state and half were maintained at a core temperature of 40 °C (104 °F) for 2 hours after the injury. All animals were then killed. A 40% increase in edema was found in the traumatized hemisphere of the hyperthermic animals compared with the euthermic animals. Bleeding also was more profuse in the experimental group.

## TREATMENT

Although our current state of knowledge does not permit dogmatic pronouncements regarding the symptomatic treatment of fever, we can make some reasonable recommendations. Clearly, fever need not always be treated and body temperature need not always be restored completely to normal. I advocate treating high fever (40 °C [104 °F] or greater), fever in children at risk for febrile convulsions, fever in children with underlying neurologic or cardiopulmonary disease, and any situation in which there is consideration of a component of heat illness. Until more data are compiled, the treatment of fever when necessary to establish patient comfort should not be condemned.

Once a decision is reached to treat the patient's fever symptomatically, the choice of a specific therapeutic modality should be based on several considerations. Because fever is the result of an elevation of the set-point in the hypothalamic thermoregulatory center, the most rational way to treat fever is to restore this set-point to normal; agents such as aspirin, acetaminophen, ibuprofen, and naproxen work on this basis. Aspirin and acetaminophen have been studied extensively and are equally effective at similar doses. Ibuprofen and naproxen are newer agents that appear to be of about the same effectiveness as aspirin or acetaminophen, but at lower dosages and perhaps with longer duration of action.

The selection of one of these agents should be based on potential toxicities and cost rather than efficacy. In therapeutic dosage, aspirin is the most toxic of these agents. Gastritis, gastrointestinal bleeding, impaired platelet function, diminished urinary excretion of sodium, and blunted immune response occur relatively frequently with aspirin, less often with ibuprofen and naproxen, and not at all with acetaminophen. Indeed, therapeutic doses of acetaminophen are remarkably free of side effects. Considerable evidence has associated aspirin with Reye's syndrome and has led to the virtual abandonment of this drug for antipyretic therapy in infants and children. This association is not shared by acetaminophen; whether it is shared by ibuprofen is not yet clear, although to date no cases of Reye's syndrome in association with ibuprofen have been reported.

Although the mechanisms are different, massive overdose of any of these agents can be lethal. Fatal aspirin overdose has been associated primarily with a mixed metabolic acidosis and respiratory alkalosis; the major cause of death in cases of acetaminophen overdose has been hepatic necrosis. It is difficult to say which of these poisonings is less dangerous. However, the kinetics of acetaminophen excretion favor the use of this drug because there is less risk of overdose with excessive repeated *therapeutic* dosage. Although overdose of ibuprofen appears less severe and more easily managed than overdose of either aspirin or acetaminophen, deaths in children from CNS depression and apnea have been reported. From the point of view of toxicity with ordinary therapeutic dosage, acetaminophen clearly is preferable to aspirin. Acetaminophen probably also is preferable to ibuprofen because of less potential toxicity and a longer history of use and familiarity.

Although acetaminophen often is prescribed on the basis of age, about 60 mg/day/year of age, a weight-based dosage is more accurate. In general, the dose of acetaminophen is 10 to 15 mg/kg every 4 hours. The half-life of acetaminophen is prolonged significantly in the newborn and very young infant; therefore, it should be used with caution and at a reduced dosage in these age groups.

Under certain circumstances it is necessary or advisable to use external cooling, generally by sponging, as a means of reducing

**TABLE 51-4. Use of External Cooling in Treating Elevated Temperature**

| Cooling Method | Indications |
| --- | --- |
| Tepid sponging *instead of* antipyretic drugs | Very young infants |
| | Severe liver disease |
| | History of hypersensitivity to antipyretic drugs |
| Tepid sponging *plus* antipyretic drugs | High fever (>40°C [>104°F]) |
| | History of febrile seizures, neurologic disorders, or brain damage |
| | Infection plus suspicion of overheating or overwrapping |
| | Septic shock* |
| Cold sponging *alone* | Heat illness |

* May require cold sponging.

body temperature, either in addition to or instead of antipyretic drugs (Table 51-4). External cooling is the treatment of choice for heatstroke and other forms of heat illness. However, in cases of fever, external cooling is indicated only in specific situations. External sponging is advisable in any situation in which suspicion exists that the cause of the elevated temperature may be a form of heat illness. Some patients with infection also have a component of heat illness from overwrapping, dehydration, or drugs.

For the previously well child with a non–life-threatening febrile illness, sponging adds little other than patient discomfort. Sponging with tepid water plus acetaminophen is only slightly more rapid in its antipyretic effect than is acetaminophen alone. Sponging with ice water is more rapid, but obviously more uncomfortable, and is indicated only when treating heat illness. Sponging often is useful in patients with neurologic disorders, because many of these children have abnormal temperature control and respond poorly to antipyretic agents. Sponging also would be preferable to antipyretic agents in children with hypersensitivity to these agents and in patients with severe liver disease. As mentioned above, in very young infants, the half-life of acetaminophen is prolonged, and sponging may be preferable to use of this agent.

Sponging should be done with tepid water (generally around 30 °C [85 °F]). Rubbing alcohol should not be used, because its fumes are absorbed across the alveolar membrane and possibly across the skin as well, resulting in CNS toxicity.

## Selected Readings

Banet M. Fever and survival in the rat. The effect of enhancing the cold defense mechanism. Experientia 1981;37:985.

Cashman TM, Starns RJ, Johnson J, Oren J. Comparative effects of naproxen and aspirin on fever in children. J Pediatr 1979;95:626.

Clasen RA, Pandolfi S, Laing I, Casey D. Experimental study of relation of fever to cerebral edema. J Neurosurg 1974;41:576.

Dinarello CA. Interleukin-1 and the pathogenesis of the acute-phase response. N Engl J Med 1984;311:1413.

Klastersky J, Kass EH. Is suppression of fever or hypothermia useful in experimental and clinical infectious diseases? J Infect Dis 1970;121:81.

Kluger MJ, Vaughn LK. Fever and survival in rabbits infected with *Pasteurella multocida*. J Physiol 1978;282:243.

Lorin MI. The febrile child: clinical management of fever and other types of pyrexia. New York: John Wiley & Sons, 1982:27.

Roberts NJ, Steigbigel RJ. Hyperthermia and human leukocyte function. Infect Immun 1977;18:673.

Rumack BH. Aspirin versus acetaminophen: a comparative view. Pediatrics 1978;62(suppl):943.

Steele RW, Tanaka PT, Lara RP, Bass JW. Evaluation of sponging and of oral antipyretic therapy to reduce fever. J Pediatr 1970;77:824.

*Principles and Practice of Pediatrics, Second Edition.* edited by Frank A. Oski et al. J. B. Lippincott Company, Philadelphia © 1994.

# CHAPTER 52
# *Fever Without Localizing Signs*

## Mark W. Kline and Martin I. Lorin

Fever is one of the most common pediatric complaints. In the first few years of life, fever is second only to routine care as the cause of office or clinic visits. Between 5% and 20% of febrile children have no localizing signs to explain the fever. Fever without localizing signs (FWLS), like febrile illness in general, is most common in children less than 5 years old, with a peak prevalence between 6 and 24 months of age. We define FWLS as unexplained fever of relatively brief duration, arbitrarily less than 5 or 7 days. If the unexplained fever persists longer than 7 to 10 days, it is commonly referred to as fever of undetermined origin (FUO). Although overlap exists between FWLS and FUO, the differential diagnosis and the clinical approach are quite different for children with FWLS or FUO.

In many cases, FWLS resolves spontaneously without a specific diagnosis being established. In other cases, a relatively minor infectious process, either focal (eg, otitis media, pharyngitis) or nonfocal (eg, varicella, roseola), becomes apparent as the cause for the fever. Examples of infections with long prodromal periods, during which fever may be the only manifestation, are roseola, cytomegalovirus infection, typhus, and typhoid fever. Not all

cases of FWLS are due to acute infectious diseases; some cases herald the onset of chronic disorders. However, because FWLS is by definition of relatively brief duration, and because so many children with self-limited viral infections present with FWLS, the percentage of children with FWLS who have serious persistent infections or other inflammatory conditions such as juvenile rheumatoid arthritis is much lower than that of children with FUO. Rarely, FWLS in an infant or child represents a drug reaction, an allergic or hypersensitivity disorder, or heat illness. In recent years, a number of young children presenting with FWLS have manifested features of Kawasaki syndrome after a few days. It is not currently known whether Kawasaki disease is an infectious disorder.

## OCCULT BACTEREMIA

Except in the very young infant, most serious infections can be recognized by a careful history and physical examination. However, a small but significant percentage of children with bacteremia cannot be identified by the ordinary clinical examination alone. These children have occult bacteremia, which we define as the presence of a positive blood culture in a child who looks well enough to be treated as an outpatient and in whom the positive result is not anticipated. Specifically, the child does not have any soft-tissue infection or local infection that ordinarily would be associated with bacteremia, (eg, pneumonia or epiglottitis), but he or she may have a minor infection such as otitis media. Although only about 5% of children with FWLS have occult bacteremia, somewhat more than 50% of the children with occult bacteremia come from the pool of children with FWLS (Fig 52-1).

The organism most frequently responsible for occult bacteremia is *Streptococcus pneumoniae*, the second most common organism is *Haemophilus influenzae* type b, and salmonellae and *Neisseria meningitidis* make up most of the remaining small per-

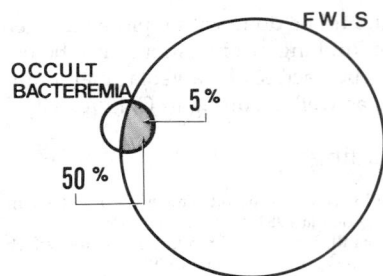

**Figure 52-1.** Numerical interrelation of fever without localizing signs (FWLS) and occult bacteremia. Many more cases occur of FWLS than of occult bacteremia. Only 5% of the cases of FWLS have occult bacteremia (*shaded area*), but more than 50% of the patients with occult bacteremia have FWLS.

centage. The predominance of pneumococcus is related to age. In series that focus on children from 3 to 24 months of age, *S pneumoniae* generally accounts for more than 80% of the cases of occult bacteremia; in series that include febrile children of all ages, *S pneumoniae* is found to account for only 60% to 70% of the cases of occult bacteremia. Because *S pneumoniae* is the predominant cause of occult bacteremia, it is not surprising that many of the characteristics of occult bacteremia associated with *S pneumoniae* are statistically true for occult bacteremia in general—peak prevalence between 6 and 24 months, association with high fever and high leukocyte count, and association with the absence of evident focal soft-tissue infection. These criteria are met much less consistently in cases of occult bacteremia due to *H influenzae*, *N meningitidis*, and salmonellae.

Initially, occult bacteremia was believed to be a disease of the underprivileged, because it first was described in inner-city hospitals serving mostly indigent patients. Subsequent studies have shown that occult bacteremia occurs with essentially the same frequency in the middle- and upper-class populations as it does in the underprivileged. No racial, geographic, or socioeconomic predilection for occult bacteremia is apparent. Although the exact prevalence of occult bacteremia in different series of outpatients varies, figures generally have been in the range of 3% to 6% of significantly febrile young children. The actual prevalence appears to vary more with the selection criteria for study than with the geographic or socioeconomic base of the study population. The highest frequency of occult bacteremia is in children younger than 2 years. Children with FWLS are more likely to be bacteremic than are children with minor outpatient infections. In one series, blood cultures were obtained from all febrile children under the age of 2 years presenting to the emergency department. The prevalence of bacteremia in children with infections such as otitis media and pharyngitis was 1.5%; in those with FWLS, the prevalence was 3.9%. It is unfortunate that the authors chose to include children with evidence of upper respiratory tract infections in the FWLS group, because children with upper respiratory infections have a lesser prevalence of bacteremia. In one series, febrile children with evidence of upper respiratory tract infections had a prevalence of occult bacteremia of 3%, in contrast to those with FWLS, for whom the prevalence was 9%.

Although it is clear that most patients with high fever do not have bacteremia and that some patients with bacteremia are afebrile, a trend exists for higher fever to be associated with a greater risk of bacteremia. This trend is most pronounced for *S pneumoniae*.

About 75% of children with occult bacteremia recover completely. Of the remaining 25%, some 5% develop purulent meningitis and another 5% develop other significant soft-tissue infections such as periorbital cellulitis or osteomyelitis. The remaining 15% are found to have persistent bacteremia at the

time of reexamination; most of these patients do well with treatment. The 5% figure for subsequent bacterial meningitis has been remarkably consistent from series to series. However, since the risk of subsequent meningitis is greater with *H influenzae* bacteremia than with *S pneumoniae* bacteremia, it is possible that the relatively recent introduction of routine *H influenzae* immunization in infancy will decrease the number of cases of occult bacteremia due to *H influenzae* and, therefore, decrease the overall incidence of meningitis following occult bacteremia.

## DIAGNOSIS

Many of the diagnostic studies used to evaluate children with FWLS are directed at excluding the presence of bacteremia. Failure to identify bacteremic children accurately subjects them to the potentially adverse sequelae of undiagnosed and untreated bacteremia. Conversely, the indiscriminate use of diagnostic tests represents unnecessary effort, expense, and discomfort for the patient.

Several investigators have suggested that careful clinical evaluation of children with FWLS may permit the selection of a subgroup of patients who appear well and have a small or negligible risk of bacteremia or other serious bacterial illnesses. These clinical features include the child's appearance (eg, normal hydration, lack of apparent toxicity, and lack of distress) and behavior (eg, alert, playful, eating and drinking well). The studies on which this suggestion is based, however, all involved the full spectrum of febrile children presenting to the emergency department; none focused specifically on children with FWLS. It is likely that a child with bacteremic pneumonia or bacteremic meningitis would look and act more ill than would a child with occult bacteremia. Although these clinical features can be helpful, they are not completely accurate.

Febrile children without localizing signs of infection who are at greatest risk of bacteremia are those between 6 and 24 months of age with temperatures above 39.4 °C (103 °F). These children should be considered for diagnostic laboratory studies. In addition, diagnostic studies to exclude bacteremia or other serious bacterial diseases (eg, meningitis) may be indicated routinely in the febrile neonate and in immunocompromised hosts, where the consequences of unrecognized infection can be devastating.

Two types of laboratory tests are used in the evaluation of a child for bacteremia: indirect tests, such as the white blood cell (WBC) count and erythrocyte sedimentation rate (ESR), which reflect the body's response to infection, and direct tests, such as blood culture and rapid tests for the detection of bacterial antigens, which detect the organism itself. Indirect laboratory tests, such as the WBC count, serve only as screening tests to identify a subgroup of children at high risk of bacteremia. These tests cannot diagnose specific children as bacteremic. In a population with low prevalence of a disease—as is the case with febrile children and bacteremia—even a sensitive and specific screening test will have a low positive predictive value. In other words, the test might identify most bacteremic children accurately, but it would not discriminate between these few patients and the many children with positive test results but without bacteremia. For children with FWLS, a WBC count of 15,000/μL or greater has sensitivity and specificity of about 85% and 75%, respectively, for the detection of bacteremia. The positive predictive value, however, is only about 15%. Nevertheless, the WBC count is the most widely used and probably the most practical screening test currently available. Other screening tests, such as the ESR and WBC morphology, suffer from the same low positive predictive value that affects the WBC count. Whether rapid tests for bacterial antigens eventually will prove useful as screening tests for occult bacteremia remains to be determined.

TABLE 52-1.  Risk of Occult Bacteremia

|  | Low Risk | High Risk |
|---|---|---|
| Age | >3 years | <2 years |
| Temperature | <39.4°C (<103°F) | >40°C (>104°F) |
| WBC (per mm³) | >5,000 *and* <15,000 | <5,000 *or* >15,000 |
| Observational variables | Normal | Abnormal |
| Other |  | History of contact with *Haemophilus influenzae* or *Neisseria meningitidis* |
|  |  | History of bacteremic illness |
|  |  | Immunologic impairment |

Blood culture is an important diagnostic tool in the child with FWLS. It is technically easy to perform and unlike screening tests is a direct and precise means of diagnosing bacteremia. Reserving blood culture for children deemed to be at high risk for bacteremia by clinical criteria and by the finding of a WBC count above 15,000/µL will result in substantial cost savings.

Other laboratory tests may be indicated in certain situations. Young infants in particular may fail to manifest signs of meningeal irritation even in the presence of confirmed bacterial meningitis, so a high index of suspicion for that disease must be maintained and a lumbar puncture performed if any concern for meningitis exists. Urinalysis is indicated in the female infant with unexplained fever to exclude "occult" urinary tract infection. Beyond the neonatal period, boys with unexplained fever appear to be at low risk of urinary tract infection. In infants, pneumonia often does not produce obvious auscultatory findings, although some clue to pulmonary involvement (cough, tachypnea, retractions) almost always is present, and a chest roentgenogram may be necessary to exclude that diagnosis. Chest roentgenogram is not indicated routinely for all infants and children with FWLS but should be considered for young infants and those patients with very high fever, signs of toxicity, or markedly elevated WBC counts.

## ANTIBIOTIC TREATMENT

Expectant antibiotic therapy may be justified for the child with FWLS and high fever, WBC count above 15,000/µL, or risk factors for serious bacterial disease (Table 52-1). Several retrospective studies as well as prospectively collected data from one study of occult bacteremia show that children treated expectantly with antibiotics at the time of the initial visit fare better than do those who do not receive antibiotic therapy. Children who appear seriously ill, and those with underlying diseases predisposing to serious bacterial infection (eg, immunodeficiency states, sickle-cell disease), should receive an initial course of parenterally administered antibiotics in the hospital. In most other cases, expectant therapy may be given on an outpatient basis.

Antibiotic therapy should be directed against the most common bacterial pathogens, *S pneumoniae* and *H influenzae* type b. Amoxicillin (40 to 60 mg/kg/day) is a reasonable choice. In areas with a high prevalence of *H influenzae* type b resistant to ampicillin, reasonable alternative therapy includes erythromycin-sulfisoxazole, trimethoprim-sulfamethoxazole, or amoxicillin-clavulanic acid. A single injection of ceftriaxone in a dose of 50 to 75 mg/kg will theoretically provide coverage against the common pathogens causing occult bacteremia without concern about

compliance or vomiting; studies to evaluate such a regimen currently are underway. Penicillin V does not have useful activity against *H influenzae*.

Regardless of therapy, careful follow-up care is essential, and the child should be reevaluated immediately if the clinical condition deteriorates, if signs or symptoms of serious focal infection develop, or if the blood culture yields a pathogen.

## CLINICAL MANAGEMENT

Decisions regarding diagnostic investigation and expectant antibiotic therapy should be based on careful analysis of all available data and thoughtful weighing of the risks and cost/benefit ratio for each patient. The physician should be cognizant of the costs of diagnostic procedures and expectant therapy. Cost includes not only the dollar amount of the tests and the medication, but also the physical and emotional trauma of blood-drawing, the side effects of antibiotics, and the time and distress involved in clarifying false-positive results, lost specimens, and laboratory errors. On the benefit side are possible decreased morbidity (eg, prevention or early detection of subsequent meningitis and other serious bacterial illness) and mortality (low in all series). Table 52-1 serves as a framework for assessing the risk of bacteremia in the individual patient.

## Selected Readings

Carroll WL, Farrell MK, Singer JI, et al. Treatment of occult bacteremia: a prospective randomized clinical trial. Pediatrics 1983;72:608.

Lorin MI. The febrile child: clinical management of fever and other types of pyrexia. New York: John Wiley & Sons, 1982:69.

McCarthy PL, Grundy GW, Spiesel SZ, Dolan TF. Bacteremia in children: an outpatient clinical review. Pediatrics 1976;57:861.

McCarthy PL, Lembo RM, Baron MA, et al. Predictive value of abnormal physical examination findings in ill-appearing and well-appearing febrile children. Pediatrics 1985;76:167.

Pantel RH, Bergman DA. Epidemiology of fever in infants and young children. In McCarthy PL, ed. Dialogues in pediatric management, vol 1. Norwalk, CT: Appleton-Century-Crofts, 1985.

Roberts KB, Charney E, Sweren RJ, et al. Urinary tract infection in infants with unexplained fever: a collaborative study. J Pediatr 1983;103:864.

Teele DW. Bacteremia and the use of blood cultures in febrile children. In McCarthy PL, ed. Dialogues in pediatric management, vol 1. Norwalk, CT: Appleton-Century-Crofts, 1985.

Teele DW, Pelton SI, Grant MJA, et al. Bacteremia in febrile children under 2 years of age: results of culture of blood of 600 consecutive febrile children in a walk-in clinic. J Pediatr 1975;87:227.

Waskerwitz S, Berkelhammer JE. Outpatient bacteremia: clinical findings in children under 2 years with initial temperatures of 39.5 °C or higher. J Pediatr 1981;99:231.

Wright PF, Thompson J, McKee KT, et al. Patterns of illness in the highly febrile young child: epidemiologic, clinical and laboratory correlates. Pediatrics 1981;67:694.

*Principles and Practice of Pediatrics, Second Edition.*
edited by Frank A. Oski et al. J. B. Lippincott Company, Philadelphia © 1994.

CHAPTER 53

# Fever of Undetermined Origin

## Martin I. Lorin and Ralph D. Feigin

The definition of fever of undetermined origin (FUO) in children has evolved over the past few decades so that a prolonged period of documentation of fever and in-hospital workup no longer are required as criteria for use of this label. These rigid criteria arose primarily from studies in adults and were appropriate in earlier days when our understanding of this entity was primitive and modern diagnostic technology was unavailable. It now is acceptable to use the term FUO to describe the condition of children who are febrile for 8 or more days and in whom careful history, physical examination, and preliminary laboratory evaluation fail to reveal probable cause for the fever. Youngsters who have been febrile without explanation for fewer than 5 days should be considered as having fever without localizing signs, which carries a different set of diagnostic probabilities as well as a different clinical diagnostic approach (see Chap. 52). Youngsters evaluated between the fifth and seventh day of fever constitute an overlap group and must be approached with thought given to both entities.

## GENERAL PRINCIPLES

Most children with FUO do not have rare or exotic diseases. This finding has been true even in series from major pediatric referral centers. For example, in a series of 100 children evaluated at the Children's Hospital Medical Center in Boston, only three had diseases that would be considered rare—undefined vasculitis, Behçet syndrome, and ichthyosis.

Although the relative frequencies are somewhat different, the three most commonly identified causes of FUO in children are the same as in adults—infectious diseases, connective tissue disorders, and malignancies. Although the prognosis in children is somewhat better than in adults, FUO often represents a serious condition even in children. The mortality rate was 9% in Pizzo and colleagues' 1957 series and 17% in Lohr and Hendley's 1977 series. McClung reported in 1972 that 40% of the children in his study had "serious or lethal diseases." Infection, the leading cause of FUO at all ages, is even more common in children than in adults, accounting for more than 50% of the cases in some reports. Connective tissue diseases occur with roughly the same frequency in pediatric and adult series, and neoplasms are a less common cause of FUO in children than in adults.

The percentage of specific etiologies in different reports varies with factors such as criteria for inclusion in the study, availability of diagnostic expertise, and classification of patients with probable but uncertain diagnoses. In many cases of FUO in children, a specific diagnosis is never established and the condition resolves spontaneously.

## INITIAL APPROACH TO CLINICAL EVALUATION

The clinical approach to the child with FUO must be organized and individualized for each patient. A diagnostic evaluation may be initiated in the office or clinic for the child beyond early infancy who has been febrile for 7 to 14 days and who looks well. Conversely, a young infant or child who has been febrile for a more prolonged period, or a youngster who appears significantly ill should be hospitalized for evaluation. Hospitalization is useful not only for the purpose of expediting laboratory tests, but it also provides an important opportunity for continued history-taking, repeated physical examination, and constant observation.

Documentation of prolonged or recurrent fever helps to exclude certain relatively acute infections such as viral influenza and group A streptococcal pharyngitis. The child's age affects both the probability of certain disorders and the urgency with which workup is undertaken. Young infants present a more urgent problem; bacteremia and meningitis cannot be safely excluded without appropriate cultures. Neonates and young infants also are susceptible to certain organisms such as group B streptococci and *Listeria monocytogenes*, which are rare in older patients. On the other hand, *Neisseria gonorrhoeae* as a cause of prolonged fever usually is seen in adolescents. Connective tissue diseases are more common in older children; Pizzo and colleagues reported an incidence of connective tissue disease about four times greater in children over 6 years of age than in those younger than 6 years. The patient's sex also is relevant. Autoimmune disease is more common in girls, and certain immunologic deficiencies, such as Bruton's agammaglobulinemia and classic chronic granulomatous disease, are restricted to boys. Pelvic inflammatory disease, of course, occurs only in girls.

The patient's history should be searched carefully for any possible clues, however trivial or remote. A history of transfusion or the use of blood products would raise the possibility of a variety of transmitted viral and parasitic agents, including HIV. Animal contact always is important. Dogs may harbor brucellosis or leptospirosis, and cats are vectors for cat-scratch fever and toxoplasmosis. Birds are a source of ornithosis and histoplasmosis. Rodents carry tularemia, leptospirosis, *Spirillum minus*, and *Streptobacillus moniliformis*. A history of travel, even in the distant past, is notable. Endemic diseases in Africa, India, and Asia include malaria, amebiasis, and schistosomiasis, which may be manifest months to years after returning from an endemic area. Coccidioidomycosis is endemic in the southwestern portion of the United States.

## IN-HOSPITAL EVALUATION

Inpatient evaluation of the child with FUO can be seen as three processes proceeding simultaneously: follow-up of all diagnostic clues, screening tests, and observation and reexamination.

### Follow-Up of All Potential Clues

The most important aspect of the evaluation of a youngster with FUO is meticulous and complete follow-up of all potential clues, however insignificant they may appear. The results of the history and physical examination and all available laboratory data must be scrutinized closely for any abnormalities or positive features. Pizzo and coworkers noted that failure to use existing laboratory data correctly occurred in one half of the cases in their series and was a major reason for failure to establish the proper diagnosis before hospitalization. A history of an episode of abdominal pain or diarrhea even weeks before the onset of the fever may be a clue to an enteric infection or an intra-abdominal abscess. The slightest tenderness over the sinuses or mastoid area may be indicative of underlying chronic infection. Even a mild peripheral eosinophilia may be a clue to parasitic infection, immunodeficiency, or occult malignancy. Perseverance in following each potential clue is the most efficient and cost-effective method of evaluating a youngster with FUO.

## Screening Tests

When there are no clues to guide the workup, the physician must rely on an initial battery of screening tests. Even when clues are present, it is not unreasonable to proceed with some preliminary screening tests while following up on specific clues. Screening tests include those that detect organ dysfunction as well as those that identify specific diseases. Basic screening tests to evaluate organ function and to look for clues as to which systems may be involved include serum levels of hepatic enzymes and alkaline phosphatase, renal function tests such as blood urea nitrogen and creatinine, urine analysis, chest roentgenogram, and complete blood count. The erythrocyte sedimentation rate is a useful test in assessing the severity of tissue inflammation but generally is of little help in identifying specific diagnoses, although a normal ESR does weigh against diseases characteristically associated with high ESRs, such as inflammatory bowel disease. The EEG and ECG are unlikely to yield useful information in the absence of specific findings pointing toward these systems and therefore are not cost-effective as screening tests. A lumbar puncture should be considered in every child with FUO but need not necessarily be performed in all patients.

Screening tests for certain specific diseases should be done in all children hospitalized for the evaluation of FUO: blood culture, tuberculin skin test, urine culture, febrile agglutinins, serum rheumatoid factor, and antinuclear antibody titers. Because they are invasive, expensive, or infrequently positive, other screening tests should be considered as second-stage tests and generally not ordered at the time of admission unless there are specific indications or unless basic laboratory investigation had been completed before hospitalization. Such tests include bone marrow aspiration, abdominal ultrasound or CT examination, gallium scan, bone scan, radiographic skeletal survey, and roentgenograms of the sinuses and mastoid.

## Observation and Reexamination

Hospitalization should be used as an opportunity to obtain additional historical data from the patient and parents, and even other family members who may visit. It is surprising how often parents will recall a pertinent event, such as travel or animal exposure, or relevant family history only after days in the hospital. The patient must have a relatively complete physical examination at least daily, but obviously it is unnecessary to repeat items such as funduscopic examination, detailed neurologic examination, or rectal examination every day unless specifically indicated. Often, pulmonary rales, cardiac murmurs, skin rashes, areas of tenderness, pain on motion of a joint, and even abdominal masses will appear during the hospitalization. All available data should be reviewed continually for clues that were not initially apparent. The pattern of fever should be observed. A high spiking fever once or twice a day may be a clue to an occult abscess or to the systemic form of juvenile rheumatoid arthritis (JRA). The patient should be examined during an episode of fever; the rash of JRA may be present only at this time.

A youngster who looks well, has no tachycardia, and does not feel warm at the time of alleged fever may have factitious fever. In the age of the electronic thermometer, it has become routine for the nurse to remain at the bedside during the temperature measurement, making it difficult for the patient or parent to factitiously elevate the temperature reading. However, it still is possible to influence the oral reading by ingesting hot liquids before the temperature measurement. The ingenuity of these patients or parents in falsifying temperature readings and feigning illness is extraordinary, and undoubtedly such individuals will find ways to circumvent modern technology.

The response to antipyretic agents should be noted. Lack of response may indicate factitious fever or a CNS basis for the fever. Temperature elevations secondary to neurologic dysfunction often are unresponsive to antipyretic drugs. Children with recurrent periodic fever frequently respond poorly or not at all to antipyretic drugs.

## ETIOLOGY

### Infectious Causes

In the United States, the most common infectious diseases implicated in children with FUO include brucellosis, tularemia, tuberculosis, salmonellosis, diseases due to spirochetes (leptospirosis, rat-bite fever, syphilis), rickettsial infections, cytomegalic inclusion disease, infectious mononucleosis, hepatitis, and HIV infection. The most common causes of localized infection that may present as FUO include sinusitis, otitis media, tonsillitis, urinary tract infection, osteomyelitis, and occult abscesses, including those of the subdiaphragmatic, hepatic, pelvic, or perinephric region.

#### Brucellosis

The presentation of brucellosis as a disease that causes FUO is explained by the nonspecificity of its symptomatology and by the chronicity of the untreated infection. Physicians tend to ignore the possibility of this disease and often neglect to ask for a history of exposure to animals or animal products.

#### Leptospirosis

Leptospirosis is caused by a family of organisms of which multiple serogroups and serotypes exist. Transmission of infection from animals to humans may follow direct contact with the blood, tissue, urine, or organs of infected animals, or indirectly by exposure to an environment contaminated by leptospires. The organism may be acquired from soil or from fresh water after ingestion. Reports suggest that leptospirosis is not rare. Most infections are no longer associated with occupational exposure; rather, urban and suburban cases are now more prevalent than are cases reported from rural areas.

The clinical manifestations of leptospirosis are not specific. A variety of laboratory tests are available, but appropriate handling and collection of specimens is imperative. In many cases, it is impossible to establish a definitive diagnosis because of negative culture results and failure to demonstrate a rise in antibody titer to these organisms. These factors do not exclude the possibility of active infections, because the organism may not be in the specimens that have been cultured. Moreover, the antibody titer may have peaked before the collection of an acute-phase specimen, and antibiotic therapy can suppress the development of positive titers or delay their appearance.

#### Salmonellosis

*Salmonella* spp. have been found as contaminants in most food products in recent years. The nonspecificity of signs and symptoms that may be associated with salmonellosis is one reason why it is associated with FUO in children. Repetitive blood and stool cultures are most helpful in establishing a diagnosis; serologic evidence of infection also should be sought.

#### Tularemia

*Francisella tularensis* may be acquired from contact with a variety of animal species, as well as from mosquitoes, lice, fleas, ticks, flies, and contaminated water. The organism may penetrate mucous membranes and unbroken or broken skin. It also may be inhaled or swallowed. It is crucial to ask patients and their parents not only about the ingestion of rabbit and squirrel meat, but about other animal contact and a history of tick bite.

## Tuberculosis

Tuberculosis is a common cause of FUO in children. Nonpulmonary tuberculosis presents as FUO more frequently than does pulmonary tuberculosis. FUO is most common with disseminated tuberculosis that involves the peritoneum, pericardium, liver, or genitourinary tract. Active disseminated tuberculosis has been documented in children with normal chest radiographs and negative tuberculin test results. Funduscopic examination may reveal choroid tubercles in these individuals. The bone marrow and liver are involved frequently in children with miliary tuberculosis. Liver specimens and bone marrow aspirates should be obtained and processed for morphologic evaluation and appropriate cultures. Gastric aspirates should be cultured in patients suspected of having miliary tuberculosis, even in the presence of a normal chest roentgenogram. Culture material must be prepared by the newer, rapid culture techniques that can provide an answer within 7 to 10 days. The demonstration of acid-fast organisms on smears of gastric secretions does not necessarily indicate *Mycobacterium tuberculosis* infection because nontuberculous *Mycobacterium* spp. may be present in the gastric contents of normal individuals.

## Bacterial Endocarditis

Infective endocarditis is an infrequent cause of FUO in children. Acute bacterial endocarditis tends to be explosive in onset. Subacute bacterial endocarditis is rare in infants, increasing in frequency with advancing age. The absence of a cardiac murmur does not exclude the possibility of endocarditis and is particularly common when infection involves the right side of the heart. Endocarditis also may occur in the absence of positive blood culture results, particularly in association with the following factors: right-sided cardiac lesions; use of antibiotics for an undefined febrile illness; prolonged duration of disease; infection by organisms that are not readily apparent on culture, such as *Brucella* spp. or *Coxiella burnetii*; and inadequate culture methods for the detection of an infection with anaerobic organisms. Associated laboratory findings include anemia, leukocytosis, and elevated ESR. Five or six blood cultures should be obtained both aerobically and anaerobically over a period of several days. Echocardiograms may reveal vegetations, but negative study results do not exclude endocarditis.

## Bone and Joint Infections

Infections of the bones and joints usually can be diagnosed clinically but occasionally may present as FUO. This situation is more common with osteomyelitis than with septic arthritis. Infection of the pelvic bones most often is implicated in this regard. Radioisotopic bone scanning is more sensitive than radiographic examination of the bones.

## Liver Abscess and Other Hepatic Infections

Pyogenic liver abscesses are encountered most frequently in the immunocompromised child, but they also may be seen in the normal child. In some children, fever is the only finding. Blood cultures are usually sterile, and liver function tests are within normal limits. Hepatomegaly and right upper quadrant abdominal tenderness may be present in some patients. Diagnosis can be established by examination of the liver by ultrasound, by CT scan, or by radioisotopic scanning techniques. Bacterial hepatitis as well as cholangitis can occur in the absence of jaundice.

Granulomatous hepatitis is a syndrome characterized by granuloma formation within the liver, rather than a specific disease. In many cases, the specific etiology is never determined. Most cases have been reported in adults, but examples in children have been seen. Diagnosis can be established only by liver biopsy.

## Intra-Abdominal Abscesses

Subphrenic, perinephric, and pelvic abscesses all may present as FUO. A history of intra-abdominal disease, abdominal surgery, or vague abdominal complaints should heighten suspicion that an intra-abdominal collection of pus may be present. The organisms involved most commonly include *Escherichia coli*, anaerobic flora, *Staphylococcus aureus*, and streptococci.

Perinephric abscesses generally develop during the course of bacteremia, and fever may be the only sign. *S aureus* is the organism most often recovered. Urinalysis generally is normal; the intravenous pyelograph may fail to demonstrate a mass. Both pyuria and mass effect on radiographic study of the kidney are late findings. The results of examination by ultrasound or CT scan may be positive earlier in the course of infection.

Deep pelvic abscesses are an important cause of FUO in children. Possible sources of deep pelvic abscesses in children include osteomyelitis of the pelvic bones, previously infected skin lesions with associated lymphadenitis, mesenteric salmonellosis, pelvic thrombophlebitis, and appendiceal infection. Careful pelvic and rectal examinations are important in suspecting or diagnosing pelvic abscesses. Ultrasound examinations and CT scanning may be used to help confirm the diagnosis.

## Viral Infections

Infection by most viruses produces an illness that is self-limited and brief, but hepatitis viruses, cytomegalovirus, Epstein-Barr virus, and certain arboviruses are exceptions to the general rule. In all of these disorders, the symptomatology may be variable and signs and symptoms nonspecific. Thus, these viral infections should be considered in the differential diagnosis of patients with FUO.

## Upper Respiratory Tract Infection

Infections of the upper respiratory tract and related organs frequently present as FUO. Although obvious symptoms and signs might be expected, the complaints are often trivial and thus ignored. Physical findings may be absent even in cases of mastoiditis or sinusitis. Thus, chronic or recurrent pharyngitis, tonsillitis, peritonsillar abscess, and otitis media should be considered in the differential diagnosis of patients with FUO.

## Immunodeficiency

A variety of immunodeficiency states, both congenital and acquired, can present as FUO. HIV infection may present as FUO before specific signs or symptoms of individual organ systems are noted. In other patients, malaise, listlessness, fever, and generalized lymphadenopathy are noted but the precise etiology is not considered. Diagnosis can be established by serologic evaluation for HIV infection.

## Parasitic Infections

Malaria should be considered in children as a cause of FUO. In addition to fever, splenomegaly usually is present. A history of travel to endemic areas should be sought. Several months may pass between infection and the onset of symptoms. If an appropriate mosquito vector is present, infection may be transmitted from an individual who has visited an endemic area to one who has not. Malaria also may be acquired by blood transfusion or by the use of needles and syringes contaminated by the parasite. Demonstration of the organism on appropriately stained thin or thick smears of blood is diagnostic.

Toxoplasmosis, caused by *Toxoplasma gondii*, should be considered in any child with persistent fever. Supraclavicular or cervical lymphadenopathy is present in most cases, but fever is sometimes the only manifestation. The diagnosis is established by demonstrating a rising serologic titer. Antibody to *T gondii* is so common that demonstration of a single high titer alone is not diagnostic of acute infection. Demonstration of *Toxoplasma* spp. in tissue secretions or body fluids is highly suggestive, but the organism may persist in tissue for years. Therefore, isolation of the parasite is not absolutely diagnostic of acute toxoplasmosis.

## Connective Tissue Diseases

Connective tissue disorders and vasculitis are the second leading cause of FUO in children. Within this group of disorders, JRA accounts for most cases in all pediatric series. Although all three clinical forms of this disorder—acute systemic, pauciarticular, and polyarticular—may be associated with fever, the acute systemic form is most likely to present as FUO. The classic fever pattern in this disorder is one or two temperature spikes daily. Most serologic test results for rheumatoid factor are negative in children with the acute systemic form of JRA, so the disease can be difficult to diagnose. The diagnosis often is made clinically by observation over a prolonged period. A therapeutic trial of a nonsteroidal anti-inflammatory drug can be useful both in controlling the symptoms and in confirming the diagnosis.

## Malignancy

Malignancies are the third most frequent cause of FUO in children. The most common is the leukemia-lymphoma group and, less often, neuroblastoma; rarely, other cancers such as hepatoma, rhabdomyosarcoma, and atrial myxoma may present as unexplained fever.

## Factitious Fever

Factitious fever always must be considered in the evaluation of a child with FUO. When the patient is an infant or young child, it is a parent or other caretaker who is fabricating. In bizarre cases, the parent actually may induce fever by injecting the child with infectious or noxious materials. In the case of the older child or adolescent, it is the patient who is falsifying information. In most cases, factitious fever can be excluded by having the nurse or physician stay in the room as the temperature is taken. Occasionally the temperature must be taken rectally to ensure that the youngster has not ingested or rinsed the mouth with hot liquids before the temperature measurement. In rare cases, measuring the temperature of a freshly voided urine specimen may be helpful.

## Periodic Disorders

Familial Mediterranean fever is an exceedingly rare, autosomal recessive disorder seen mostly in Arabs, Armenians, and Sephardic Jews. It is characterized by acute episodes of fever and inflammation of serosal tissue such as the peritoneum, pleura, or joint synovia. Attacks occur at irregular intervals.

Reimann and McCloskey called attention to a group of disorders characterized by recurrent episodes of fever at fairly regular intervals. At first the febrile attacks tend to occur 3 or 4 weeks apart, but as the illness persists the interval between attacks often lengthens to 5 or 6 weeks. Between episodes, the patient is normal and asymptomatic. Some patients in the series had neutropenia at the time of fever, suggesting a relationship to the entity of cyclic neutropenia. Others had arthralgias or evidence of peritoneal inflammation. More recently, Marshall and coworkers described 12 children with periodic fever, pharyngitis, aphthous stomatitis, and no hematologic abnormalities. The nature of most of these periodic disorders remains unknown.

## Other Causes

Other causes of FUO include serum sickness, drug reactions, inflammatory bowel disease, thyrotoxicosis, Behçet syndrome, histiocytosis, sarcoidosis, ectodermal dysplasia, diabetes insipidus, chronic brain syndrome, subdural hematoma, and immunodeficiency.

Mucocutaneous lymph node syndrome (Kawasaki syndrome) should be considered in the differential diagnosis of any young child with FUO, but usually can be diagnosed or ruled out by the presence or absence of clinical features. Occasionally, however, fever and irritability may be the only findings for up to 10 days. The cause of this presumably infectious disease has not been determined.

Infrequently, the apparent FUO is only an exaggerated normal circadian temperature pattern, a misinterpretation of normal temperature readings in infants or young children, which may be as high as 38°C (100.4°F), or an unfortunate (but not remarkable) series of self-limited viral infections.

Finally, in up to one quarter of all the cases of FUO in children, no definite diagnosis is ever established. Most of these cases resolve spontaneously.

## Selected Readings

Brewis EG. Child care in general pediatrics: undiagnosed fever. Br Med J 1965;1: 107.

Feigin RD, Shearer WT. Fever of unknown origin in children. Curr Probl Pediatr 1976;6:2.

Lohr JA, Hendley JO. Prolonged fever of unknown origin: a record of experiences with 54 childhood patients. Clin Pediatr 1977;16:768.

Lorin MI. The febrile child: clinical management of fever and other types of pyrexia. New York: John Wiley & Sons, 1982:94.

Marshall GS, Edwards KM, Butler J, Lawton AR. Syndrome of periodic fever, pharyngitis and aphthous stomatitis. J Pediatr 1987;110:43.

McClung HJ. Prolonged fever of unknown origin in children. Am J Dis Child 1972;124:544.

Pizzo PA, Lovejoy FH, Smith DH. Prolonged fever in children: review of 100 cases. Pediatrics 1957;55:468.

Reimann HA, McCloskey RV. Periodic fever: diagnostic and therapeutic problems. JAMA 1974;228:1662.

Steele RW, Jones SM, Lowe B, Glasier CM. Usefulness of scanning procedures for diagnosis of fever of unknown origin in children. J Pediatr 1991;119:526.

*Principles and Practice of Pediatrics, Second Edition.*
edited by Frank A. Oski et al. J. B. Lippincott Company, Philadelphia © 1994.

# *53.1* **Sepsis and Septic Shock**

Kenneth M. Boyer and William R. Hayden

United States Supreme Court justice Potter Stewart once wrote, "I can't define obscenity; but I know it when I see it." Most pediatricians would feel that statement could equally well be applied to "sepsis", "septic shock", and the related life-threatening systemic infections that occur in children.

In the last decade, intensive study has led to an improved understanding of the basic biochemistry and pathophysiology of serious infection. Fundamental to this new knowledge is the discovery that a great variety of illnesses—including non-infectious conditions such as immune-mediated organ injury, multiple trauma, and malignancy—have in common with infection the endogenous production of certain key inflammatory mediators that result in similar physiologic consequences.

## TERMINOLOGY

A vigorous debate is underway among subspecialists in infectious diseases and critical care medicine regarding the terminology that should be used to classify serious infections. The American College of Chest Physicians and the Society of Critical Care Medicine recently convened a consensus task force to consider appropriate terminology for sepsis. Their classification system is a start in the process of organized thought about these potentially life-threatening events. Their proposed definitions include the following:

- *Systemic inflammatory response syndrome (SIRS).* The systemic inflammatory response to a variety of severe clinical insults. The response is manifested by two or more of the following conditions:
  Temperature >38°C or <36°C
  Heart rate >90 or >2 SD above normal for age
  Respiratory rate >30 or >2 SD above normal for age or $Paco_2$ <32 mm Hg
  WBC >15,000 cells/mm$^3$, <5,000 cells/mm$^3$, or >10% immature (band) forms
- *Infection.* Microbial phenomenon characterized by an inflammatory response to the presence of microorganisms or the invasion of normally sterile host tissue by those organisms.
- *Bacteremia.* The presence of viable bacteria in the blood. Viremia, fungemia and parasitemia are the terms to be used when the corresponding organisms are isolated.
- *Sepsis.* The systemic response to documented infection. (Sepsis = SIRS + infection).
- *Severe sepsis.* Sepsis associated with organ dysfunction, hypoperfusion, or hypotension. Hypoperfusion and perfusion abnormalities may include, but are not limited to, lactic acidosis, oliguria, or an acute alteration in mental status.
- *Septic hypotension.* A blood pressure <2 SD below normal for age, associated with sepsis.
- *Septic shock.* Sepsis with hypotension that persists after adequate fluid resuscitation, along with the presence of perfusion abnormalities that may include, but are not limited to, lactic acidosis, oliguria, or an acute alteration in mental status. Patients who are on inotropic or vasopressor agents may not be hypotensive at the time that perfusion abnormalities are measured.
- *Multiple organ dysfunction syndrome (MODS).* Presence of altered organ function in an acutely ill patient such that physiologic homeostasis cannot be maintained without intervention.

Unlike the situation in adult medicine, SIRS and sepsis as defined above are common "problem statements" in pediatrics. Although the categories apply well to older children and adolescents, there is a need for clearer diagnostic criteria for SIRS in infants and younger children (we have made a few modifications for the purposes of this chapter). Pediatric patients compensate well for shock states with tachycardia and vasoconstriction, so septic shock and MODS by these definitions become relatively uncommon (and ominous) clinical entities. Note that the term "septicemia" is no longer used, in favor of categories with a definable physiologic status. The term "multiple organ system failure" has not been replaced by MODS. The term "sepsis syndrome" has now been replaced by "severe sepsis." This is the category that should serve as an early warning of a life-threatening pediatric infection.

## ETIOLOGY

Sepsis and the various septic syndromes are typically caused by bacterial infections of an advanced nature. Contrary to popular belief, the majority of patients with sepsis do *not* have documented bacteremia. This was a major reason for the recent changes in definitions, although the probability of positive blood cultures increases as one progresses down the classification list

to septic shock and MODS. Even with negative blood cultures, however, bacterial etiology can generally be established by positive Gram stains and cultures of purulent exudates, characteristic alterations in hematologic parameters, tests for the presence of capsular polysaccharide antigens, or clinical responses to empiric antimicrobial therapy.

The common, and some of the unusual, bacterial etiologies of sepsis in the previously normal child are presented in Table 53-1, according to the presence or absence of a focal source and according to the presence of accidental or surgical alterations in integumentary and mucosal barriers. A working knowledge of these organisms and the clinical settings in which they are most likely to present provides a rational basis for organism identification and selection of an empiric antibiotic regimen. The causes of neonatal infections are discussed comprehensively in Chapters 12.15.1 and 12.15.2. A complete description of the causes of community-acquired and nosocomial sepsis in compromised hosts

---

**TABLE 53-1. Bacterial Etiologies of Sepsis in Previously Normal Pediatric Patients, by Apparent Source**

**Occult**

*Streptococcus pneumoniae, Haemophilus influenzae* type b, *Neisseria meningitidis, Staphylococcus aureus*

**Focal Source**

Skin and musculoskeletal: *S aureus, Streptococcus pyogenes, H influenzae* type b
Respiratory tract: *S pneumoniae, H influenzae, S aureus,* oral anaerobes,* *S pyogenes*
Gastrointestinal tract: *Salmonella* spp., *Shigella* spp., *Yersinia enterocolitica*
Peritoneum: Enteric gram negative rods†, enteric anaerobes‡, *Enterococcus faecalis*
Heart or pericardium: *S aureus, H influenzae* type b
Urinary tract: Enteric gram negative rods
Genital tract: *Neisseria gonorrhoeae,* enteric anaerobes
Meninges: *H influenzae* type b, *N meningitidis, S pneumoniae*

**Acquired Barrier Disruption**

Abdominal surgery or penetrating trauma: Enteric gram negative rods, enteric anaerobes, *Enterococcus faecalis*
Cardiac surgery: Staphylococci§, multiply-resistant gram negative rods‖
Orthopedic surgery or compound fracture: Staphylococci
Craniofacial surgery: Staphylococci, *S pneumoniae, H influenzae,* oral anaerobes
Vascular access device-related: Staphylococci, multiply-resistant gram-negative rods, *Acinetobacter* spp., *Candida albicans*
Burn wounds: *S pyogenes, Pseudomonas aeruginosa*

**Bite Wounds**

Human: *Eikenella corrodens,* staphylococci, oral anaerobes
Dog: *Capnocytophaga canimorsus* (DF-2), *Pasteurella multocida,* staphylococci, oral anaerobes
Cat: *P multocida,* oral anaerobes
Rat: *Streptobacillus moniliformis, Spirillum minus*
Flea: *Yersinia pestis*
Tick: *Francisella tularensis*

---

* *Peptostreptococcus, Fusobacterium* spp., *Bacteroides melaninogenicus, Veillonella.*
† *Escherichia coli, Klebsiella* spp., *Enterobacter* spp.
‡ *Bacteroides fragilis, Clostridium perfringens, Clostridium septicum, Fusobacterium* spp.
§ *Staphylococcus aureus,* coagulase-negative staphylococci.
‖ *Enterobacter* spp., *Pseudomonas aeruginosa, Klebsiella* spp., *Xanthomas maltophilia, Serratia marcescens.*

can be found in Chapter 55, and particularly in Tables 55-1 and 55-3. It is important to recall that sepsis of a critical nature, even in a previously normal child, should prompt consideration of an important defect in host defense. For example, meningococcemia should suggest an abnormality in the terminal complement pathway.

The encapsulated organisms—*Streptococcus pneumoniae, Neisseria meningitidis,* and *Haemophilus influenzae,* type b—are the most common causes of sepsis (and bacteremia) of occult origin. These organisms are most frequent in children aged 3 months to 5 years and correspond to the nadir in transplacentally-acquired maternal IgG antibodies. Such infections are commonly preceded by a viral upper respiratory illness that results in a mucosal portal of entry for the organism (eg, meningococcemia preceded by influenza).

A focus of infection should always be sought in patients with occult bacteremia. Often, the identity of a blood stream isolate can be a clue to the origin. *Staphylococcus aureus* bacteremia, for example, should always suggest the possibility of osteomyelitis, endocarditis, or pericarditis.

In sepsis of focal origin, likely bacterial etiologies are suggested by the site of the infection and often are determined by normal flora of a contiguous surface. Urinary tract infections, for example, often are caused by enteric flora. First episodes generally are due to antibiotic susceptible *Escherichia coli*. Recurrent episodes separated by periods of prophylactic antibiotics—to the extent that prophylaxis has altered enteric flora—will be due to *Klebsiella spp., Enterobacter spp.,* or *Pseudomonas aeruginosa* with multiple-drug resistance. Sepsis associated with bacterial enteritis generally is caused by salmonella, shigella, or *Yersinia enterocolitica. Salmonella* enteric fever often is associated with bacteremia. Shigellosis, on the other hand, rarely is bacteremic, but may be associated with sepsis and septic shock, especially if *Shigella dysenteriae* is involved.

Disruption of skin or mucosal barriers may be accidental or surgical. Bite wounds can be associated with unusual oral pathogens, depending on the source. Dog bites, for example, generally are inoculated with staphylococcus and oral anaerobes, but may also be contaminated with *Pasteurella multocida* or *Capnocytophaga* DF-2. The latter two species often are associated with bacteremia and sepsis. Infections affecting surgical sites generally involve normal flora at the site of operation that contaminate surgically-damaged tissue. Sepsis complicating craniofacial surgery, for example, is caused by the normal flora of the skin, scalp, and upper respiratory mucosal surfaces, including staphylococci, *Haemophilus spp., S pneumoniae,* and oral anaerobes.

Sepsis has a broad differential diagnosis, as summarized in Table 53-2. Included are nonbacterial infections, such as viral, rickettsial, and spirochetal infections, as well as responses to bacterial products, such as vaccines. Although it is not a final diagnosis, sepsis is an appropriate problem statement for such conditions. Shock states that may be confused with septic shock include tachyarrhythmia with cardiogenic shock (often triggered by acute febrile illness) and gastroenteritis with hypovolemic shock (also commonly associated with fever). The former is particularly important to recognize, because aggressive fluid resuscitation can lead to deterioration rather than improvement in cardiovascular status.

## PATHOGENESIS

Septic shock has in the past been considered synonymous with "endotoxin shock." Lipopolysaccharides purified from the cell membranes of a variety of gram negative organisms such as *E coli, Salmonella, Pseudomonas,* and *N meningitidis* are capable of eliciting the characteristic picture of sepsis in experimental animals. Accidental infusion of contaminated intravenous fluids

containing large amounts of endotoxin (but without viable organisms) has been found to trigger septic shock in humans. Experimental infusion of low doses of endotoxin in volunteers elicits characteristic physiologic and laboratory changes. Anti-endotoxin antibodies in pooled sera or in the form of specific monoclonal antibodies can block the response and improve outcome in crit-

---

**TABLE 53-2.** Differential Diagnosis of Sepsis

**Infection**
Viral illness (influenza, enteroviruses, dengue hemorrhagic fever, disseminated herpes)
Encephalitis (arbovirus, enterovirus, herpes)
Rickettsial infection (Rocky Mountain spotted fever, *Ehrlichia,* Q fever)
Spirochetal infection (syphilis, relapsing fever; Jarisch-Herxheimer reaction)
Vaccine reaction (pertussis, whole-virus influenza, typhoid)

**Cardiopulmonary**
Pneumonia (bacterial, viral, mycobacterial, fungal, pneumocystis)
Pulmonary emboli
Congestive heart failure
Arrhythmia (with cardiogenic shock)
Pericarditis (with pericardial tamponade)
Myocarditis

**Metabolic-Endocrine**
Adrenal insufficiency (adrenogenital syndrome, Waterhouse-Friderichsen syndrome, steroid withdrawal)
Diabetes insipidus
Diabetes mellitus
Inborn errors of metabolism (organic acidosis, urea cycle, carnitine deficiency)
Hypoglycemia
Reye syndrome

**Gastrointestinal**
Gastroenteritis with hypovolemic shock (viral, bacterial, parasitic)
Malrotation with midgut volvulus
Intussusception
Appendicitis or appendiceal abscess
Peritonitis (spontaneous, perforation, dialysis)
Hepatitis
Hemorrhage

**Hematologic**
Anemia (sickle cell, blood loss, nutritional)
Splenic sequestration crisis
Leukemia, lymphoma

**Neurologic**
Intoxication (drugs, carbon monoxide, intentional or accidental overdose)
Intracranial hemorrhage
Trauma (child abuse, accidents)
Guillain-Barré syndrome
Myasthenia gravis

**Other**
Collagen-vascular disease (systemic lupus erythematosus, juvenile rheumatoid arthritis)
Anaphylaxis (food, drug, insect sting)
Kawasaki syndrome
Erythema multiforme
Hemorrhagic shock–encephalopathy syndrome
Heatstroke
Malignant hyperthermia

ically ill patients. Thus, there is no question that endotoxin is one of the trigger mechanisms of sepsis.

Other organisms can clearly produce septic syndromes either by virtue of their production of exotoxins or by sheer force of numbers. Staphylococcal and group A streptococcal toxic shock syndromes are both potentially lethal conditions whose clinical picture is caused by the circulation of well-characterized exotoxins from the site of an occult infection. Bacteremia infrequently accompanies these conditions. Although the clinical features differ somewhat, toxemias arise in association with *Shigella dysenteriae* dysentery and with the acute hemorrhagic colitis caused by verotoxin-producing *E coli* 0157. Their exotoxins are biochemically similar and lead to the hemolytic uremic syndrome. Like staphylococcal and streptococcal toxic shock, blood cultures are generally negative. Finally, it has been found in experimental animals that high level intravenous infusion of even relatively nonvirulent gram positive bacteria, such as *Staphylococcus epidermidis*, can induce the physiologic changes of sepsis and septic shock. Thus, endotoxins can no longer be considered the common pathway of sepsis and septic shock.

It is now recognized that septic shock results from the sequential release of endogenous mediators. These substances, referred to as cytokines, are products of monocytes, macrophages, T-lymphocytes, endothelial cells, mast cells, polymorphonuclear leukocytes, and an increasingly lengthy list of other cell types. These substances are the signals that comprise the inflammatory cascade. Presumably these substances evolved as part of the mechanisms for controlling relatively localized infections or trauma. When a human host is confronted by a more massive challenge, however, it appears that these substances may be produced excessively—leading to a response so vigorous so as to be potentially fatal. One of the most extensively studied substances in the inflammatory cascade is tumor necrosis factor (TNF), a product of the monocytes and macrophages. Injection of TNF in experimental animals completely mimics the clinical response (fever, hypotension, coagulopathy, multiple organ failure, and death) seen after injection with endotoxin, but with a reduced latency time. Circulating levels of TNF may correlate with prognosis, as has been demonstrated in meningococcal disease.

Other mediators appear to be responsible for other familiar elements in the sequence. The interleukins (particularly IL-1, IL-2, and IL-6) mediate hypotension and fever. Hageman factor (factor XII) and platelet activating factor (PAF) mediate coagulopathy. Interferon-gamma (IFN-γ) activates macrophages. The colony-stimulating factors (G-CSF and GM-CSF) stimulate production of phagocytic cells. The integrins (CD11 and CD18) and the intercellular adhesion molecules (ICAM-1 and ICAM-2) control leukocyte migration. Endothelium-derived relaxing factor (nitric oxide) is a potent vasodilator of the microcirculation. The complement system produces substances (C3a and C5a) that are the major chemotactic stimuli for leukocytes. The list of mediators is ever increasing, with a clear picture of the complete sequence only beginning to emerge.

The consequence of the release of these mediators is the development of sepsis. Progression to septic shock and multiorgan system dysfunction or failure depends on the pathogens involved and the degree to which the host mediators and effector cells are capable of localizing and killing them. The most prominent physiologic features of septic shock are fever and cardiovascular compromise or collapse. The cardiac response to sepsis is characterized by an initial increase in cardiac output followed by a period of poor myocardial performance probably due to one or more myocardial depressant factors. The effect of sepsis on the vascular bed is quite complex but is characterized by direct injury to the endothelium. This results in alterations in vascular tone and capillary leak. The alterations in tone result in decreased systemic vascular resistance, abnormal perfusion patterns to var-

ious organ systems, and may lead to organ dysfunction or complete organ failure. The capillary leak allows the egress of fluid and proteins from the vascular system and results in hypovolemia and the severe edema often encountered in severe cases.

The effects of compromised perfusion and capillary leak are unique to each organ system. The mortality rate is directly proportional to the number of organs that fail. Capillary leak and intrapulmonary right-to-left shunting may lead to the adult respiratory distress syndrome (see Chap. 43). Decreased renal perfusion initially leads to oliguria. In the presence of uncorrected hypotension, acute tubular necrosis may supervene (see Chap. 46). Decreased cerebral circulation leads to confusion, disorientation and obtundation. Compounding these changes is the frequent development of disseminated intravascular coagulation (see Chap. 94), which can further reduce perfusion or, by depletion of clotting factors, lead to major hemorrhage.

## Clinical Manifestations

Recognition of the septic child is difficult. The pediatrician's fundamental dilemma is how to detect the child with a potentially life-threatening infection among the many children with self-limited or readily-treated infections that are not life-threatening. An awareness of the presence of predisposing conditions to infection in an individual child is probably the most helpful guide. Unfortunately, not all seriously ill children have identified defects in their host defenses, particularly in infancy.

Most children with sepsis have obvious and significant elevated temperatures. In the very young and in advanced disease, however, temperatures may actually be in the hypothermic range. Rigors and hyperthermia (temperature >41°C [105.8°F]) imply bacteremia.

Behavioral changes may be helpful indicators of serious illness. Four of the six items on the Yale Observational Scale—quality of cry, reaction to parent stimulation, state variation, and response to social overtures—are behavioral. The child with febrile illness, a weak cry, poor responsiveness, no smile, and lack of facial expression is likely to be septic. These changes in most cases reflect compromised cerebral circulation; occasionally they indicate complicating meningitis.

Although changes in respiratory pattern generally point to pulmonary disease, tachypnea and acrocyanosis also may reflect metabolic acidosis and poor peripheral perfusion—both characteristic of sepsis.

A careful evaluation of circulatory adequacy is important. Measurement of blood pressure is basic, but it should be recognized that children often compensate well for early shock states, so that blood pressure may be in the normal range. Note, however, that difficulty in measuring a child's blood pressure is more likely to be a reflection of marginal circulation than it is of a technical problem with the blood pressure apparatus. Even if measured blood pressure is in the normal range, circulatory inadequacy is usually manifested by cool extremities, acrocyanosis, absent or diminished peripheral pulses, and capillary refill times of >3 seconds. Although it is said that "warm shock" may be seen early in sepsis, this is relatively unusual in children.

Cutaneous manifestations of sepsis may be externally helpful as warning flags. Between 8% and 20% of patients with fever and petechiae have a serious bacterial infection, and 7% to 10% have meningococcemia or meningococcal meningitis. Purpuric lesions or ecchymoses of the distal extremities (purpura fulminans) raise these probabilities even higher. Diffuse erythroderma in the presence of fever and shock should suggest toxic shock syndrome.

## Laboratory Abnormalities

Laboratory manifestations of sepsis include positive blood cultures and positive cultures from other sites such as urine, cerebrospinal fluid, stool, joint or bone aspirates, exudates, abscesses, and cutaneous lesions. Continuing efforts should be made to identify the site of origin of a septic process, using multiple cultures of multiple sites if necessary. Blood cultures that are persistently positive in spite of treatment imply resistant organisms or an endovascular origin of infection.

Hematologic parameters are useful in initial and continuing evaluation. Leukocytosis is the norm; leukopenia is more prognostically ominous. Often leukopenia is the initial response, with remarkable leukocytosis the paradoxic response to successful therapy. Elevated band counts, toxic granulation, and Döhle bodies imply bacterial sepsis. Thrombocytopenia implies the presence of disseminated intravascular coagulation, which should be confirmed with documentation of prothrombin time, partial thromboplastin time, fibrinogen levels, and the presence of fibrin split products. Band counts (decreasing) and platelet counts (increasing) are useful serial studies implying successful treatment.

Metabolic acidosis, manifested by decreased serum bicarbonate, pH, and increased serum lactate, is a frequent biochemical manifestation of diminished end-organ perfusion. Persisting metabolic acidosis during therapy is an ominous indicator of inadequate tissue oxygen delivery. Compensatory respiratory alkalosis is a common early abnormality. Prerenal azotemia or uremia are the usual manifestations of diminished renal perfusion and acute tubular necrosis, respectively. Hypoalbuminemia often develops during management of severe sepsis, the consequence of both a catabolic state and capillary leak of colloid into the interstitium.

## THERAPY

The cornerstones of treatment for sepsis and septic shock are eradication of the infecting organisms and maintenance of adequate oxygen and nutrient delivery to vital organs. After recognition of the situation, an orderly—but rapid—sequence of initial interventions to achieve these goals is mandatory.

Patients with severe sepsis should be monitored for all five vital signs: respiration, heart rate, blood pressure, temperature, and oxygen saturation (by pulse oximetry). An adequate airway and peripheral oxygen saturation are top priorities. If abnormal, they should be immediately supported by oxygen administration and, if necessary, by an endotracheal tube and mechanical ventilation.

Circulation also should be assessed rapidly and, if marginal or inadequate, vascular access must be achieved by peripheral or central venous catheter or by the intraosseous route. Initial blood cultures should be obtained when access is achieved. If cardiogenic shock can reasonably be excluded, then 20 to 40 mL/kg of normal saline should be administered as bolus infusions.

Initial empiric antibiotic therapy is then indicated by the parenteral route. An assessment of probable etiology should be made, with consideration of the likely infecting organisms as presented in Table 53-1. The other key element in antibiotic choice is the likelihood of encountering resistance, the two major determinants of which are whether the infection was acquired in the hospital and whether the patient has received recent antimicrobial therapy.

**TABLE 53-3.  Recommended Dosage Schedule for the Antimicrobial Agents Most Frequently Used in Empiric Treatment of Pediatric Patients With Sepsis**

| Agent | Dosage (mg/kg/d) and Intervals of Administration | Maximum Daily Dosage | Most Common Target Organisms |
|---|---|---|---|
| Amikacin | 30 div q 8 hr | —* | Hospital gram-negative rods |
| Ampicillin | 100–300 div q 4–6 hr | 10–12 g | Community encapsulated organisms |
| Ampicillin/sulbactam† | 150–200 div q 4–6 hr | 10–12 g | Community encapsulated organisms, anaerobes |
| Amphotericin B | 0.5–1.5 once daily | —* | Invasive fungal infection |
| Aztreonam† | 75–150 div q 6 hr | 6–8 g | Hospital gram-negative rods |
| Cefotaxime | 150–200 div q 6 hr | 8–10 g | Community encapsulated organisms |
| Ceftazidime | 100–150 div q 8 hr | 4–6 g | Hospital gram-negative rods |
| Ceftriaxone | 50–100 div q 12–24 hr | 2 g | Community encapsulated organisms |
| Cefuroxime | 100–250 div q 6 h | 4–6 g | Community encapsulated organisms, staphylococci |
| Chloramphenicol | 75–100 div q 6 h | 2–4 g* | Rickettsiae, salmonella |
| Clindamycin | 30–40 div q 8 hr | 2–4 g | Anaerobes, community staphylococci |
| Flucytosine | 100–150 div q 6 hr | —* | Invasive fungal infections (with ampho B) |
| Gentamicin | 5–7.5 div q 8 hr | —* | Community gram-negative rods |
| Imipinem/Cilastatin† | 60–100 div q 8 hr | 2–4 g | Hospital gram-negative rods, anaerobes |
| Metronidazole | 30 div q 6 yr | 2–4 g | Anaerobes |
| Mezlocillin | 200–300 div q 4–6 hr | 18–24 g | Hospital gram-negative rods |
| Nafcillin | 150–250 div q 4–6 hr | 8–12 g | Community staphylococci |
| Tetracycline | 20–30 div q 8–12 hr | 1–2 g | Rickettsiae |
| Ticarcillin | 200–300 div q 4–6 hr | 18–24 g | Community pseudomonas |
| Tobramycin | 5–7.5 div q 8 hr | —* | Hospital gram-negative rods |
| Trimethoprim/Sulfamethoxazole | 8–20 trimethoprim div q 12 hr | 1–2 g* | Salmonella, Shigella, pneumocystis |
| Vancomycin | 40 div q 6–12 hr | 2–4 g* | Hospital staphylococci |

* Serum concentration and/or toxicity monitoring desirable.
† Not licensed by FDA for pediatric use (< age 12). Use should be limited to critical illness with high probability of resistant microorganisms.

In the former instance, knowledge of previous bacterial isolates from a hospitalized child may be very helpful. In the latter, one can suspect an overgrowth phenomenon requiring an alternative drug or combination. The parenteral antibiotics most frequently used in treatment of sepsis, their dosages, and their usual indications are summarized in Table 53-3. Sepsis that is occult and of community origin is appropriately treated with cefuroxime, cefotaxime, or ceftriaxone. Cefuroxime has superior activity against staphylococci, but should not be used if the physician has not excluded the presence of meningitis. Nosocomial sepsis is best treated with multiple agents. Vancomycin, a third generation cephalosporin, and an aminoglycoside are a commonly used combination.

The goals of initial empiric antimicrobial therapy are clearing of the bloodstream, penetration to infected sites, and control of the progress of the infectious process. With more definitive microbiologic data, regimens should be changed to the specific drugs of choice for the organisms isolated—as single agents or synergistic combinations depending on identity. Gram-positive organisms often are treated effectively with single agents; gram-negative rods are best managed with combinations. With the exception of children with bacterial meningitis (see Chap. 54), corticosteroid therapy is not beneficial. Clarification of the source of a problem may mandate surgical drainage or removal of hardware as therapeutic adjuncts. When a source or infecting organism is not defined or results are delayed, modification of regimens may be necessary based on clinical response criteria alone.

The elements of supportive care after intensive care unit admission include continued monitoring of vital signs and oxygen saturation (see Chap. 41). In addition, invasive monitoring of central venous pressure and arterial pressure generally are indicated. Pulmonary artery catheters are used aggressively in adult critical care, but more selectively in pediatric patients. Multiple organ system dysfunction, in which the pressure demands of mechanical ventilation may adversely affect cardiovascular performance, is the usual setting in which PA catheters are considered. They enable rational management of intravascular volume status, ventilator settings, and pressor infusions.

Management of pressor infusions (see Chap. 42), ARDS (see Chap. 43), acute tubular necrosis (see Chap. 46), and disseminated intravascular coagulation (see Chap. 94) are discussed elsewhere in this book. Subspecialist consultation and team management of septic shock are essential. Conflicting priorities are common in managing these complex patients. One common situation is the need for administration of multiple blood products, total parenteral nutrition, and numerous drugs and infusions—in the face of pulmonary edema, marginal myocardial performance, and renal failure. This situation may be handled readily by the use of slow continuous ultrafiltration (SCUF) or continuous arteriovenous hemofiltration (CAVH), which can maintain euvolemia despite massive infusion volumes. Because they are continuous, they are much more physiologic approaches than intermittent hemodialysis.

Another major issue is maintenance of adequate nutrition. Sepsis mediators create a hypermetabolic state that rapidly depletes body stores and exceeds the caloric content of conventional intravenous fluids. Early and aggressive parenteral nutrition is necessary to keep up with these demands and to provide sufficient calories to promote tissue regeneration and healing.

The most exciting recent advances in therapy for sepsis and septic shock involve the use of monoclonal antibodies directed against gram-negative endotoxin or receptor antagonists of the mediators of the sepsis inflammatory cascade. Monoclonal antibodies against lipopolysaccharides have shown some promise in clinical trials, but only in population subgroups who have proven gram-negative infection. Their benefit may be mitigated by the fact that they are administered at a time at which pathogenic pathways are already far advanced. Perhaps more promising is the possibility of using recombinant proteins that closely resemble the naturally occurring antagonists of TNF and IL-1, or monoclonal antibodies directed against these mediators. Such products are in advanced clinical trials in adult patients. Extension of these studies to pediatric patients is in the near future.

## PREVENTION

Dramatic reductions in the incidence of invasive *H. influenzae* type b disease are the welcome result of the widespread use of polysaccharide conjugate vaccines in infancy. Meningococcal and pneumococcal polysaccharide vaccines also have had an impact on the incidence of invasive infection in high-risk children older than age 2. Conjugate vaccines are under development, and may permit immunization of young infants in the future. Prevention of sepsis in compromised hosts is discussed in Chapter 55.

## Selected Readings

Beutler B. Endotoxin, tumor necrosis factor, and related mediators: new approaches to septic shock. New Horizons 1993;1:3.

Bone RC. The pathophysiology of sepsis. Ann Intern Med 1991;115:457.

Bone RC, Balk RA, Cerra FB, et al. Definitions for sepsis and organ failure and guidelines for the use of innovative therapies in sepsis. Crit Care Med 1992;20:864.

Bone RC, Fisher CJ, Clemmer TP, et al. The methylprednisolone severe sepsis study group: a controlled clinical trial of high-dose methyl prednisolone in treatment of severe sepsis and septic shock. N Engl J Med 1987;317:653.

Dinarello CA, Gelfand JA, Wolff SM. Anticytokine strategies in the treatment of the systemic inflammatory response syndrome. JAMA 1993;269:1829.

Jacobs RF, Hsi S, Wilson CB, et al. Apparent meningococcemia: Clinical features of disease due to *Haemophilus influenzae* and *Neisseria meningitidis*. Pediatrics 1983;72:469.

Jacobs RF, Sowell MK, Moss MM, et al. Septic shock in children: bacterial etiologies and temporal relationships. Pediatr Infect Dis J 1990;9:196.

Lowry SF. Anticytokine therapies in sepsis. New Horizons 1993;1:120.

McCarthy PL, Sharpe MR, Spiesel SZ, et al. Observation scales to identify serious illness in febrile children. Pediatrics 1982;70:802.

Nelson JD: 1993–94 Handbook of pediatric antimicrobial therapy. Baltimore: Williams & Wilkins, 1993.

Parillo JE. Pathogenetic mechanisms of septic shock. N Engl J Med 1993;328:1471.

Thomas L. The Lives of a Cell. New York: Viking, 1974:75.

Uauy R, Mize CE. Starvation in the PICU. In: Levin DL, Morriss FC, eds. Essentials of pediatric intensive care. St. Louis: Quality Medical, 1990:586.

Ziegler EJ, Fisher CJ, Sprung CL, et al. Treatment of gram negative bacteremia and septic shock with HA-1A human monoclonal antibody against endotoxin. N Engl J Med 1991;324:429.

*Principles and Practice of Pediatrics, Second Edition.*
edited by Frank A. Oski et al. J. B. Lippincott Company, Philadelphia © 1994.

## CHAPTER 54
# *Bacterial Meningitis Beyond the Newborn Period*

### Ralph D. Feigin

## ETIOLOGY

Any organism can cause meningitis. Etiologic agents responsible for 95% of cases that occur in children over 2 months of age have been *Haemophilus influenzae* type b, *Streptococcus pneumoniae* (most commonly serotypes 1, 3, 6, 7, 14, 17–19, 21, and 23), and *Neisseria meningitidis* (particularly serotypes A, B, C, Y, and W135). Immunization with *H influenzae* conjugate vaccines beginning at 2 months of age already has been associated with a decrease in the frequency of meningitis caused by *H influenzae* type b. Organisms that colonize the skin should be suspected in a child with a dermoid sinus or meningomyelocele, or in patients with hydrocephalus in whom devices for CSF diversion have been placed. The child with cystic fibrosis or the burn victim may develop bacteremia and meningitis secondary to colonization with *Staphylococcus aureus* or *Pseudomonas aeruginosa*. Patients placed in a humidified atmosphere are at special risk to develop infection with *P aeruginosa* or *Serratia marcescens*. *H influenzae* bacteremia and meningitis are seen with increased frequency in children with diabetes mellitus, Cushing syndrome, and coma secondary to drug overdose. The child with sickle-cell disease is particularly susceptible to infection with *H influenzae*, *S pneumoniae*, and *Salmonella*. These same organisms also may be encountered in patients with congenital asplenia or splenosis. In addition to the more common organisms, patients with reticuloendothelial malignancy, as well as those undergoing chemotherapy, may be threatened by other organisms of low virulence rarely encountered in normal children.

## EPIDEMIOLOGY

In 1972 in the United States, 29,000 cases of meningitis were attributed to *H influenzae* type b, 4800 to *S pneumoniae*, and 4600 to *N meningitidis*. However, meningococci were more common than *H influenzae* as a cause of meningitis in Great Britain from 1968 to 1977. The frequency of meningitis continued to increase through 1989, most notably because of an increase in the incidence of disease caused by *H influenzae* and group B streptococci. Recent reports, however, have documented a sharp diminution in the number of cases of *H influenzae* type b meningitis since 1990. At one center, a tenfold increase in the number of cases of meningitis due to *H influenzae* was noted from 1945 to 1971. During the same period, admissions for meningitis of all etiologies increased only twofold. Between 1935 and 1968, deaths due to bacterial meningitis decreased by only 50%.

The highest risk period for bacterial meningitis is between 6 and 12 months of age. Ninety percent of all cases occur between 1 month and 5 years of age. In a prospective study of 235 patients aged 1 month to 15 years, 64% of cases were caused by *H influenzae*, 15% by *S pneumoniae*, and 11% by *N meningitidis*; 10% of cases involved other organisms. The incidence of disease caused by *Haemophilus* spp. in all children in the United States less than 5 years of age has been 32 to 71 per 100,000 population. The risk of invasive disease due to *H influenzae* type b (including meningitis) in household contacts less than 6 years of age was similar to the risk of subsequent meningococcal disease in contacts of patients with meningococcal septicemia and meningitis.

Sepsis and meningitis occur most frequently with pneumococcal serotypes 1, 3, 6, 7, 14, 17, 18, 19, 21, and 23. The black population in the United States is at a five- to 36-fold greater risk of acquiring pneumococcal meningitis than is the general population. An estimated one in 24 children with sickle-cell disease will develop *S pneumoniae* meningitis by 4 years of age. This incidence is 36 times greater than that in black children who do not have sickle-cell disease and 314 times greater than the risk in the white population.

The carriage rate for *N meningitidis* is 1% to 15% in the civilian population in the United States. Carriers are generally over 21 years of age and harbor the organisms for months. Significantly greater carriage rates are noted in military personnel, particularly during epidemic periods. The likelihood that severe meningococcal disease will occur simultaneously with the first (index) case is 1% in family contacts, a rate 1000 times greater than the risk in the community. The risk of meningitis in day-care center contacts is one per 1000 population. The disease appears to be more prevalent in urban than in rural settings. Most cases of meningococcal meningitis in recent years have been caused by serogroups B and C and generally have been acquired by young children or adults who have been exposed in a day-care setting, to an adult carrier in the family, or to individuals with meningococcal disease who are carrying the organism.

## PATHOLOGY AND PATHOPHYSIOLOGY

Bacteremia generally antedates the occurrence of meningitis. Bacterial invasion from a contiguous focus of infection (mastoiditis, osteomyelitis of the skull) also may occur. Meningitis following otitis media usually is not a result of direct invasion from the middle ear; rather, bacteremia from this site is the mode of spread. Anatomical defects secondary to trauma (eg, fracture through the cribriform plate) or congenital defect (eg, a defect in the stapedial footplate) should be suspected, particularly in cases of recurrent meningitis.

The sequence of events leading to meningitis has been elucidated in experimental rat and monkey models. Initially, the upper respiratory tract becomes infected. A bacteremic phase follows with eventual seeding of the meninges. The organisms initially are detected in the lateral and dorsal longitudinal (sagittal) sinuses. Inflammation of the dura disrupts normal flow from the subarachnoid space to the sinuses, permitting spread of infection through this stagnant fluid.

Descriptions of pathologic features of the disease in the preantibiotic and post-antibiotic era do not differ significantly. A meningeal exudate of varying thickness is noted, particularly over the convexity of the brain (most marked in pneumococcal meningitis), in depths of the sulci, in the sylvian fissures, in the basal cisterns, and around the cerebellum. Purulent material accumulates about the veins and venous sinuses. The spinal cord may be encased in pus. Ventriculitis is a common finding in fatal cases and may be found frequently in survivors of neonatal meningitis. Perivascular collections of purulent material may be noted in the ventricular wall. Disruption of the ependymal membrane and subependyma also may be observed. Subdural empyema is described rarely.

Meningeal signs are attributed to inflammation of spinal nerves and roots. Early pressure on peripheral nerves may lead to residual motor or sensory deficit: cranial and spinal nerves coursing through the subarachnoid space often become involved in the inflammatory process. Deafness and vestibular disturbances are observed most commonly, but optic nerve involvement also may occur. Inflammation and swelling of the facial nerve (as it passes through the stylomastoid foramen) and auditory nerve (entering the temporal bone through the internal acoustic meatus) may cause a compromise of their blood supply. Transtentorial herniation may cause extravascular nerve compression.

Communicating hydrocephalus is the result of adhesive thickening of the arachnoid about the basal cisterns. Fibrosis and reactive gliosis obliterating the aqueduct of Sylvius or the foramina of Magendie and Luschka will lead to obstructive hydrocephalus. Hydrocephalus is a rare complication of meningitis beyond the neonatal period.

Thrombosis of small cortical veins results in necrosis of the cerebral cortex. Cerebral necrosis also has been noted in the absence of evidence of small vessel thrombosis. Cerebral necrosis, secondary to obliteration of veins and arteries, and combined with increased intraventricular pressure, may lead to total dissolution of the cerebrum. Vascular changes noted at necropsy of patients with meningitis are characterized by polymorphonuclear infiltrates that extend to subintimal regions of small arteries and veins. Major vascular events, such as occlusion of a major venous sinus or subarachnoid hemorrhage secondary to necrotizing arteritis, have been observed. Pathologic changes in the cerebral cortex (reactive microglia and astrocytes) are noted without evidence of invasion by infectious agents. Toxic or circulatory factors, in concert with fever, systemic hypoxia, and changes in cerebral circulation secondary to increased intracranial pressure (ICP), are of potential importance as causes of this encephalopathy. Damage to the cerebral cortex, as described above, provides an adequate explanation for the neurologic sequelae of the disease, such as impaired consciousness, seizures, retardation, and motor and sensory deficits.

ICP often exceeds 300 mm $H_2O$, but values of 500 to 600 mm $H_2O$ may be encountered. Papilledema is rare because of the brief duration of increased pressure.

Inflammation involving the veins that traverse the subdural space and capillaries found within the dura leads to an increase in vascular permeability and loss of albumin-rich fluid into the subdural space. With resolution of the inflammatory process, this increase in vascular permeability may resolve, but continued transudation from newly formed capillaries in the subdural membrane persists. This mechanism of fluid production provides an adequate explanation for the formation of subdural effusion. In this light, subdural effusion is best considered a condition concomitant to meningeal inflammation rather than a complication of the disease.

The precise contribution of the cellular inflammatory response to brain damage is unclear. Arachidonic acid is a potent inducer of cerebral edema; however, the increase in water content of the brain in experimental meningitis is similar in neutropenic and normal animals. Currently available data suggest that activated neutrophils potentiate cerebral edema produced by microorganisms via products of activation.

Prostaglandin $E_2$, interleukin-1, tumor necrosis factor, and many other soluble mediators undoubtedly contribute to the damage and cerebral dysfunction seen in patients with bacterial meningitis. Prostaglandin $E_2$ has been found in the CSF in increased concentrations in experimental meningitis, and administration of indomethacin (an inhibitor of prostaglandin $E_2$ production) reduced its concentration within CSF and reduced cerebral edema. The inflammatory mediators undoubtedly contribute to the increased vascular permeability, increased ICP, and

reduction in absorption of CSF by the arachnoid villae that have been noted.

Inappropriate secretion of antidiuretic hormone also may occur with meningeal inflammation. Resultant water retention increases the risk of developing increased ICP. Depolarization of neuronal membranes occurs as a result of cellular electrolyte balance and predisposes to seizure activity.

Hypoglycorrhachia results primarily from decreased transport of glucose across the inflamed choroid plexus, coupled with increased glucose use by the host. This condition is found in bacterial disease (meningitis, partially treated meningitis, parameningeal foci of infection, and endocarditis), viral disease (herpes simplex, mumps, and lymphocytic choriomeningitis), fungal meningitis, parasitic disease (*Naegleria* and *Plasmodium* organisms), hemorrhage, and malignancy. Increased oxidation of glucose results in excess production of lactate with depletion of the high-energy compounds, ATP, and phosphocreatine. Resultant tissue acidosis may lead to a loss of autoregulation of cerebral blood flow. Autoregulation may be restored by inducing hypocapnea in some cases.

## CLINICAL MANIFESTATIONS

The patient with bacterial meningitis typically presents with signs of meningeal inflammation, including nausea and vomiting, irritability, confusion, anorexia, headache, back pain, hyperesthesia, photophobia, and nuchal rigidity. These signs are usually secondary to the effects of increased ICP and inflammation of sensory nerves. No satisfactory pathophysiologic explanation for photophobia has been found. Fever is generally present, but its absence is not unusual in the face of bacterial meningitis. Infants display restlessness, irritability, and poor feeding. Nuchal rigidity is not a reliable sign.

In one review of children with bacterial meningitis beyond the neonatal period, 1.5% had no meningeal signs throughout the hospital course, despite the presence of CSF pleocytosis. Common clinical signs associated with meningeal irritation are Kernig's sign (flexion of the leg 90° at the hip with pain on extension of the leg thereafter) and Brudzinski's sign (involuntary flexion of the legs when the neck is placed in flexion). Increased ICP also is a common finding. In infants, this condition is seen as a bulging fontanelle with or without diastasis of sutures. In older children, increased ICP is frequently exhibited as headache. Papilledema is rare; if it is present, a search for other processes (eg, brain abscess, subdural empyema) should be made.

Transient or permanent paralysis of cranial nerves such as deafness, vestibular disturbance, or optic nerve pathology with blindness in rare cases, as well as paralysis of the extraocular or facial nerves, may be seen. Ataxia also is noted as a presenting sign.

In one series, 14.9% of the patients were semicomatose or comatose at admission. This condition was seen more commonly with pneumococcal or meningococcal than with disease caused by *Haemophilus* spp. Sixteen percent of all children with bacterial meningitis presented with focal neurologic signs (34.3% of children with pneumococcal meningitis). Focal signs indicate a poor prognosis correlating with persistence of neurologic deficits and varying degrees of mental retardation.

Seizures occur in 26% of the patients during the first or second hospital day. Seizures occur in 30% of patients with bacterial meningitis when those with seizures noted before diagnosis are included. The occurrence of seizures does not herald the onset of a permanent seizure disorder. Seizures that are difficult to control or persist beyond the fourth hospital day are of greater significance and do not bode well. Focal seizures, in particular, are associated with a greater likelihood of development of sequelae. Seizure frequency is similar for meningitis due to *H influenzae* type b and *S pneumoniae*; seizures occur twice as often in these cases as in children with meningococcal meningitis.

Subdural effusion is noted in up to 50% of the patients during the acute illness. In one prospective study, subdural effusions were observed in 32.9% of the patients with meningitis caused by *Haemophilus* spp., 19% of the patients with pneumococcal meningitis, and 8% of the patients with meningococcal meningitis. With appropriate correction to normalize for age, the incidence of subdural effusion proved to be independent of the causative organism. Subdural effusion also may be associated with a rapidly increasing head circumference, abnormal transillumination, vomiting, seizures, full fontanelle, focal neurologic signs, or persistent fever. However, these findings are noted as frequently in children without documented subdural effusion; thus, the findings cannot be attributed directly to the effusion.

Meningomyelitis and spinal cord infarction may lead to spastic paraparesis with or without extremity sensory loss. Optic nerve arachnoiditis may lead to optic atrophy and eventual blindness. Arthritis occurs most commonly during meningococcal meningitis. Arthralgias and myalgias also may be noted during the course of bacterial meningitis. Petechiae or purpura may occur in any process with accompanying vasculitis. Half the patients with meningococcal disease may have purpura or petechiae during their course. Purpura accompanied by shock and hypothermia indicates a poor prognosis. Pericardial effusions accompanying bacterial meningitis usually resolve with antibiotic therapy. Rarely, however, persistent fever in the face of pericardial effusion may require a pericardiocentesis or an open drainage procedure.

Of children with meningococcal meningitis, 3.8% develop profound hypotension, and 5.5% of the patients with meningitis due to *H influenzae* type b develop shock. Shock occurs most frequently in patients with fulminant meningococcemia, but it may be associated with any form of overwhelming bacteremia. Disseminated intravascular coagulation may accompany shock in these patients.

## PROGNOSIS AND SEQUELAE

Prognosis depends on many factors, including the patient's age at the onset of meningitis; the duration of the disease before appropriate antibiotic therapy was started; the specific microorganism involved; the number of organisms (or quantity of capsular polysaccharide antigen present in CSF and meninges); disorders that may compromise host response to infection; the presence of focal neurologic findings (not postictal) at admission; and the presence of inappropriate secretion of antidiuretic hormone.

The worst prognosis is in younger patients with higher bacterial colony counts. If more than $10^7$ organisms grow from the CSF, more frequent seizures, subdural effusion, bacteremia, and a prolonged period of fever are noted. These patients are also more likely to have hearing loss and speech disturbance.

Although the mortality rate has been reduced to 1% to 5% beyond the neonatal period, up to 50% of the survivors may have some sequelae of the disease.

Relapse following therapy for meningitis has been noted, particularly in cases of bacterial meningitis caused by *H influenzae* type b that were treated with ampicillin. Relapses noted after chloramphenicol therapy were related in most cases to an inappropriate (intramuscular) route of administration. The current relapse rate is stated to be less than 1% when ampicillin, chloramphenicol, or third-generation cephalosporins are used for treatment of bacterial meningitis.

A previous prospective study of 50 infants and children following meningitis due to *H influenzae* type b revealed that 50% of the survivors were neurologically normal, 9% exhibited behavioral problems only, and 28% presented with significant neurologic handicap. The major handicaps noted were hearing loss in 10% to 11%, language disorder or delay in 15%, vision impairment in 2% to 4%, mental retardation in 10% to 11%, motor abnormalities in 3% to 7%, and seizures in 2% to 8%. Twenty-one patients who had completed therapy for meningitis were paired with sibling controls. Their IQs, measured by the Wechsler Intelligence Scale, were 86 on average versus 97 in the control group ($p < .05$).

Prospective studies of bacterial meningitis performed by this author revealed that 32.8% of the survivors had abnormalities detected by neurologic examination at discharge. By 5 years after discharge, however, only 11.1% had a neurologic deficit detectable by neurologic examination. Even major neurologic deficits may resolve unpredictably with time. Therefore, cautious optimism must be maintained in discussing the long-term complications of meningitis with parents.

All children with bacterial meningitis should have hearing evaluations with evoked-response audiometry (or pure-tone audiometry in older, cooperative children) before or soon after discharge from the hospital. It is important to distinguish children with conductive hearing loss from those with eighth cranial nerve deficits. Any child identified as having a hearing deficit should have repeated audiometric evaluation after discharge. Children presenting with ataxia may be identified as those at high risk for later development of hearing loss. In these cases, vestibular and auditory branches of the eighth cranial nerve may be assumed to have been affected simultaneously. A markedly depressed CSF glucose:blood glucose ratio has been associated with patients at increased risk for developing deafness. Evoked-response audiometry has revealed a deficit of auditory nerve function in 6% of the patients with *H influenzae* type b meningitis, 10.5% of the patients with meningococcal meningitis, and 31% of the patients with pneumococcal meningitis. Deafness often is noted early in the course of bacterial meningitis and occurs despite the rapid institution of appropriate therapy. The time interval over which the relative risk of developing severe sensorineural hearing loss increases remains unclear.

Cerebral infarction has been diagnosed by CT scanning within 1 or 2 days of onset of febrile illness. Although some cases of cerebral infarction are related to profound hypotension occurring with endotoxemia, most are attributable to significant changes in cerebrovascular dynamics. Cerebral infarction generally is not related to a delay in the institution of appropriate therapy or a delay in diagnosis. Spinal cord infarction as an acute or delayed event may result in quadriplegia or respiratory arrest. The speed of diagnosis and institution of therapy has not been related to the likelihood of this complication. Other specific sequelae of meningitis include diabetes insipidus (transient or permanent), transverse myelitis without evidence of vascular occlusion, and polyarteritis.

Brain abscess as a complication of bacterial meningitis is extremely unusual; indeed, if an abscess is found, one should consider the probability that it preceded the onset of meningitis. In this case, infection at other locations (such as endocarditis) should be sought. Brain abscess should be anticipated, particularly in cases of bacterial meningitis due to *Citrobacter diversus*. Response of the abscess to antimicrobial therapy can be followed by serial CT scans. Other indications for CT scan include prolonged obtundation, focal seizures, focal neurologic signs, rapidly increasing head circumference, persistently increased CSF protein, persistent CSF granulocytosis, or chronically recurring meningitis.

## DIAGNOSIS

Clinical acumen is the best tool in the diagnosis of bacterial meningitis. No one clinical sign is pathognomonic of meningitis.

The differential diagnoses for bacterial meningitis are as follows: mycobacterial meningitis; fungal meningitis; aseptic (viral) meningitis; protozoal meningitis; brain abscess; spinal, epidural, or intracranial abscess; bacterial endocarditis with embolism; subdural empyema with or without thrombophlebitis; ruptured dermoid cyst; ruptured spinal ependymoma; and brain tumor. Careful examination of the CSF obtained at lumbar puncture will help differentiate between the diagnostic possibilities.

Lumbar puncture is performed when the diagnosis is known or expected. The occluded lumbar puncture needle is passed into the intervertebral space at the L3-L4 interspace or L4-L5 interspace. This area is defined anatomically by a line drawn between the iliac crests (Tuffier's line).

In children who present with known positive blood culture results, a lumbar puncture is performed if the fever persists or signs of meningeal reaction are present. Bacteremia may progress to meningitis within hours. Culture results may be positive with otherwise normal CSF findings. Therefore, cultures should be performed on CSF regardless of the appearance of the fluid or its cell count. In 225 children who had lumbar punctures performed for febrile seizures, 5% had meningitis, but most of these patients presented with physical findings suggestive of meningitis. For all children presenting with their first febrile seizure, a lumbar puncture should be considered unless the physician is confident that the child is alert and well.

Adverse reactions to lumbar puncture include pain at the lumbar puncture site, headache, and bleeding in the area surrounding the lumbar puncture. Herniation may result if there is an intracranial mass with accompanying increased ICP.

There are three reasons to withhold lumbar puncture: cardiopulmonary compromise, signs of increased ICP (such as papilledema), or infection in the area overlying the lumbar puncture location.

Chemical or infectious meningitis may follow spinal anesthesia, myelography, or pneumoencephalography. Several investigators have reported the development of meningitis following lumbar puncture that presumably was performed during the course of bacteremia, particularly in children younger than 1 year. These data suggest that children younger than 1 year with possible bacteremia who have undergone lumbar puncture should be observed closely.

## Laboratory Tests

When a lumbar puncture is done, CSF pressure should be measured whenever possible. When ICP is significantly elevated, the minimum amount of fluid necessary for all desired laboratory determinations should be removed. The color of the CSF should also be recorded. Xanthochromia indicates increased bilirubin from hemorrhage or icterus (eg, in neonates, leptospirosis), or increased CSF protein.

Immediate microscopic examination of the fluid should be done, including a total leukocyte count and a differential count performed on a Wright-stained smear. If the lumbar puncture is traumatic, the cell count is done in a counting chamber, the red blood cells are lysed with acetic acid, and the count is repeated. If the ratio of leukocytes to red blood cells exceeds whole blood ratios, pleocytosis of the CSF should be assumed. If the peripheral red blood count and leukocyte count are normal, one leukocyte per 700 red blood cells in the CSF is subtracted.

In children between 1 and 12 years of age, a normal leukocyte count in the CSF is less than six cells/mL. When examining the differential count, 95% of healthy individuals have no polymorphonuclear cells in the CSF. CSF protein and glucose should be measured. Glucose in the CSF should be compared to the blood glucose obtained just before the lumbar puncture. CSF glucose is normally greater than two thirds of the blood glucose; CSF glucose concentration less than two thirds of the blood glucose concentration is the rule in bacterial meningitis.

Separate smears for Gram stain and Kinyoun carbol-fuchsin stain (for mycobacteria) should be done. The probability of visualizing bacteria in a Gram stain is as follows: up to $10^3$ colony-forming units per milliliter (CFU/mL), 25% of Gram stain results will be positive; between $10^3$ and $10^5$ CFU/mL, 60% will be positive; and more than $10^5$ CFU/mL, 97% will be positive. False-positive Gram stain results may be obtained when contaminated reagents are used or if an unoccluded needle is used to obtain CSF. In the latter case, one may visualize skin organisms. CSF cultures always should be made for bacterial pathogens.

Antibiotic treatment, in dosages smaller then those usually used to treat meningitis, provided orally 4 hours to 3 days before the initial lumbar puncture will not significantly alter the chemical or morphologic findings within the CSF. Pretreatment for the same period generally will not impair the growth of H influenzae type b. Pretreatment may, however, preclude the recovery of pneumococci or meningococci in selected cases. Blood culture results are positive in almost 90% of the patients with H influenzae meningitis and 80% of the patients with S pneumoniae meningitis. Ninety percent of patients with meningococcal meningitis also have positive blood culture results. In the child younger than 1 year of age, efforts should be made to obtain urine for culture before beginning antibiotic therapy, but this is not a reason to delay therapy. Purpuric or petechial lesions on the skin may be scraped and a Gram-stained specimen prepared. These smears may reveal the causative organism.

## Rapid Diagnostic Tests

Countercurrent immunoelectrophoresis (CIE) may be used for the rapid identification of H influenzae type b, S pneumoniae, and N meningitidis types A, C, Y, and W135. A commercially available group B meningococcal antiserum is available but generally is considered unreliable. Concurrent evaluation of the CSF, urine, and serum is recommended to enhance the likelihood of establishing an etiologic diagnosis rapidly. A negative CIE result does not exclude the diagnosis of bacteremia or meningitis caused by these organisms.

Latex particle agglutination (LPA) tests may be used for the rapid diagnosis of H influenzae type b, S pneumoniae, and N meningitidis. LPA testing is more sensitive than CIE because it permits the detection of antigens at lower concentrations; however, this increase in sensitivity is accompanied by loss of specificity. The H influenzae type b polysaccharide vaccine may cause urine to be positive by CIE for up to 10 days after vaccination.

Enzyme-linked immunosorbent assays (ELISA) have been developed to detect bacterial antigen within CSF. To date, the use of ELISA to detect polyribose phosphate (PRP) of H influenzae type b has received the most detailed evaluation. ELISA is comparable in sensitivity to radioimmunoassay for detecting PRP (sensitivity 0.1 ng/mL) and is more sensitive than either CIE or LPA tests. The major disadvantage of the ELISA technique described to date is the time it takes. LPA or CIE can be performed within 30 to 60 minutes, but ELISA techniques require from 3 to 6 hours to complete. The future development of homogeneous assays may permit the use of ELISA for rapid identification of microorganisms, because time-consuming incubation and separation steps are eliminated.

An enzyme radioisotope assay has been developed to measure the activity of $\beta$-lactamase, an enzyme produced by many bacteria. This assay offers the potential for rapid diagnosis of $\beta$-lactamase-producing bacteria.

The CSF lactate level is significantly elevated in patients with bacterial meningitis, secondary to decreased cerebral blood flow, hypoxia, and a change to anaerobic metabolism in the brain. The same degree of elevation of lactate may be seen in selected patients with aseptic (viral) meningitis. Thus, viral and bacterial meningitis cannot be differentiated reliably by this technique.

## Differential Diagnosis

Bacterial meningitis must be differentiated from parameningeal infections and the suppurative diseases of the CNS and meninges. Initial CSF findings in suppurative diseases of the CNS are shown in Table 54-1.

## TREATMENT

Treatment of bacterial meningitis is essential and should be instituted before definitive culture results are available. Previously, therapy with ampicillin and chloramphenicol was preferred for children over 3 months of age. This therapeutic regimen still is used in some centers, and its long-term results are at least as good as those with third-generation cephalosporins. If this regimen is used, ampicillin should be given in six divided doses with a total daily dose of 300 mg/kg body weight. An initial bolus of 100 mg/kg body weight of ampicillin should be given intravenously. No loading dose of chloramphenicol should be given; it is provided in a total daily dose of 100 mg/kg body weight in four divided doses. For children more than 3 months of age, most centers now use cefotaxime or ceftriaxone as single agents (see dosages below). If organisms other than *H influenzae*, *S pneumoniae*, or *N meningitidis* are suspected, alternative initial therapy should be considered.

Chloramphenicol should be avoided in patients with persistent hypotension or shock. Concomitant administration of chloramphenicol with phenobarbital, phenytoin, or rifampin also should be avoided unless prompt serum chloramphenicol levels can be obtained. Serum levels of chloramphenicol from 15 to 30 μg/mL have been determined to be safe and efficacious. Studies using oral chloramphenicol (after a 2- to 5-day initial period of intravenous therapy) have demonstrated its effectiveness in the treatment of bacterial meningitis. A total oral daily dose of 75 to 100 mg/kg body weight in four divided doses is recommended, but the patient should remain hospitalized to ensure compliance. In addition, the increased serum half-life of oral chloramphenicol may lead to drug accumulation. Therefore, routine measurement of chloramphenicol concentrations should be performed whenever possible, regardless of the route of administration.

About 5% to 20% of *S pneumoniae* strains are relatively resistant to penicillin. All pneumococcal strains should be tested for penicillin susceptibility. Chloramphenicol may be used for treatment of patients with penicillin-resistant pneumococci. Resistance of *S pneumoniae* to chloramphenicol has been encountered on rare occasions. Vancomycin is an acceptable alternative for multiply resistant strains of *S pneumoniae*. Cefotaxime or ceftriaxone also is generally effective against penicillin-resistant pneumococci, but caution is urged. Although these strains are susceptible to these newer agents in vitro, this may not always be the case in vivo. In one study performed in 1983, the minimal inhibitory concentration for 90% of penicillin-susceptible strains ($MIC_{90}$) was 0.03 μg/mL and 0.06 μg/mL for cefotaxime and ceftriaxone, respectively. The $MIC_{90}$ for cefotaxime and ceftriaxone were 0.25 and 0.5 μg/mL, respectively, for pneumococcal isolates that were relatively resistant to penicillin. In addition, recent reports from South Africa document that up to 20% of penicillin-resistant pneumococci are resistant to third-generation cephalosporins in that country. At present, vancomycin should be considered the drug of choice for these organisms.

Cefuroxime is a second-generation cephalosporin shown to be effective in vitro against *H influenzae* type b, *S pneumoniae*,

and *N meningitidis*. Cefuroxime readily crosses the blood–brain barrier and enters the CSF when meninges are inflamed. Experience with the use of cefuroxime in the treatment of meningitis to date documents that it is not as effective as ampicillin plus chloramphenicol, cefotaxime, or ceftriaxone. We do not recommend the use of cefuroxime for the treatment of bacterial meningitis in children.

Cefotaxime is a third-generation cephalosporin with a broad spectrum of activity against both gram-positive and gram-negative organisms. It has a high level of resistance to hydrolysis by β-lactamase. It is metabolized to desacetyl cefotaxime, a derivative with four- to eightfold less activity. However, the combination of cefotaxime and desacetyl cefotaxime is synergistic against 75% of the clinical isolates. The antibiotic penetrates the blood–brain barrier well, and the bactericidal activity in the CSF is equivalent to or greater than that of antibiotics used for conventional treatment of meningitis. When this antibiotic is given, a daily dose of 200 mg/kg body weight in four divided doses should be given intravenously.

Ceftriaxone is another third-generation cephalosporin with broad antimicrobial activity against organisms that cause bacterial meningitis. Ceftriaxone readily penetrates the CSF of patients with inflamed meninges. Because of its long serum half-life, the antibiotic may be given every 12 to 24 hours; for meningitis, we prefer administration every 12 hours. This antibiotic should be given in a daily dose of 100 to 150 mg/kg body weight. A higher incidence of mild, self-limited diarrhea was noted in children who received ceftriaxone compared with those who received conventional therapy. Biliary pseudolithiasis also has been reported in patients receiving this agent.

Cefoperazone and cefoxitin do not reach concentrations within the CSF required to kill susceptible strains of *Haemophilus* and pneumococcus; therefore, these antibiotics cannot be recommended for treatment of bacterial meningitis in children.

The duration of antibiotic therapy for meningitis depends on the causative agent and clinical response to therapy. The minimal duration of therapy for meningitis due to *H influenzae* type b and *S pneumoniae* is 10 days. Seven to 10 days generally is required as a minimum treatment course of meningitis due to *N meningitidis*. In addition, the development of certain complications (such as subdural empyema, delayed sterilization of CSF, prolonged fever, persistent meningeal signs, or development of nosocomial infections) may require longer therapy.

Patients who have received prior antibiotic therapy should receive the same initial empiric antibiotic regimen recommended for all patients. If the organism cannot be isolated, therapy may be continued beyond the initial 72-hour period with an antibiotic identical or similar to that given before the diagnosis of meningitis. If clinical improvement is slower than anticipated or is not noted, a repeat examination of CSF may be indicated at any time.

## ADJUNCTIVE THERAPY

Corticosteroids have been suggested as an adjunct to therapy of bacterial meningitis for three reasons: they may decrease ICP by decreasing meningeal inflammation and brain water content; they may modulate the production of lymphokines, which in turn lessens the meningeal inflammatory response; and they may decrease the incidence of sensorineural hearing loss or other neurologic sequelae in patients with meningitis.

When increased ICP is suggested by signs such as progressive lethargy, increased muscle tone, or bulging anterior fontanelle, elevating the head about 30° may be helpful. Increased ICP associated with deterioration in mental status or by signs of cerebral herniation may be treated more vigorously by intravenous mannitol (0.5 g/kg) infused over 30 minutes and repeated as nec-

TABLE 54-1. Initial CSF Findings in Suppurative Diseases of the CNS and Meninges

| Condition | Pressure (mm H₂O) | Leukocytes/mm³ | Protein (mg/dL) | Sugar (mg/dL) | Specific Findings |
|---|---|---|---|---|---|
| Acute bacterial meningitis | Usually elevated; average, 300 | Several hundred to more than 60,000; usually a few thousand; occasionally fewer than 100 (especially meningococcal or early in disease); PMNs* predominate | Usually 100 to 500, occasionally more than 100 | <40 in more than half of cases | Organism usually seen on smear or culture in more than 90% of cases |
| Subdural empyema | Usually elevated; average, 300 | Fewer than 100 to a few thousand; PMNs predominant | Usually 100 to 500 | Normal | No organisms seen on smear or culture unless concurrent meningitis |
| Brain abscess | Usually elevated | Usually 10 to 200; fluid is rarely acellular; lymphocytes predominate | Usually 75 to 400 | Normal | No organisms seen on smear or culture |
| Ventricular empyema (rupture of brain abscess) | Considerably elevated | Several thousand to 100,000; usually more than 90% PMNs | Usually several hundred | Usually <40 | Organism may be seen on smear or culture |
| Cerebral epidural abscess | Slightly to modestly elevated | Few to several hundred or more cells; lymphocytes predominate | Usually 50 to 200 | Normal | No organisms seen on smear or culture |
| Spinal epidural abscess | Usually reduced with spinal block | Usually 10 to 100; lymphocytes predominate | Usually several hundred | Normal | No organisms seen on smear or culture |
| Thrombophlebitis (often associated with subdural empyema) | Often elevated | Few to several hundred; PMNs and lymphocytes | Slightly to moderately elevated | Normal | No organisms seen on smear or culture |
| Bacterial endocarditis (with embolism) | Normal or slightly elevated | Few to fewer than 100; lymphocytes and PMNs | Slightly elevated | Normal | No organisms seen on smear or culture |
| Acute hemorrhagic encephalitis | Usually elevated | Few to more than 1000; PMNs predominate | Moderately elevated | Normal | No organisms seen on smear or culture |
| Tuberculous infection | Usually elevated; may be low with dynamic block in advanced stages | Usually 25 to 100, rarely more than 500; lymphocytes predominate, except in early stages when PMNs may account for 80% of the cells | Nearly always elevated, usually 100 to 200; may be much higher if dynamic block | Usually reduced; <50 to 75% of cases | Acid-fast organisms may be seen on smear of protein coagulum (pellicle) or recovered from inoculated guinea pig or by culture |
| Cryptococcal infection | Usually elevated; average, 225 | Average, 50 (0 to 800); lymphocytes predominate | Average, 100; usually 20 to 500 | Reduced in more than half the cases; average 30; often higher in patients with concomitant diabetes mellitus | Organisms may be seen in India ink preparation and on culture (Sabouraud's medium); will usually grow on blood agar; may produce alcohol in CSF from fermentation of glucose |
| Syphilis (acute) | Usually elevated | Average, 500; usually lymphocytes; rare PMNs | Average, 100; γ globulin often high, with abnormal colloidal gold curve | Normal (rarely reduced) | Positive results of reagin test for syphilis; spirochetes not demonstrable by usual techniques of smear or culture |
| Sarcoidosis | Normal to considerably elevated | 0 to <100 mononuclear cells | Slight to moderate elevation | Normal | No specific findings |

* Polymorphonuclear leukocytes.

Feigin RD, Cherry JD, eds. Textbook of pediatric infectious diseases, vol 1. Philadelphia: WB Saunders, 1987:488. Reprinted with permission.

essary. Steroids may play a role in the management of the child with increased ICP, although no data specifically indicate that corticosteroids decrease cerebral edema caused by bacterial meningitis in children. If steroids are used for this purpose, the recommended steroid is dexamethasone in a total daily dose of 10 to 12 mg/m$_2$ in four divided doses. Generally, steroids should not be used for more than 4 or 5 days. Prolonged administration has been associated with persistently positive CSF cultures in children with pneumococcal meningitis.

Dexamethasone given 1 hour before or simultaneously with *H influenzae* type b lipo-oligosaccharide significantly reduced tumor necrosis factor activity and meningeal inflammation in rabbits. Dexamethasone administration has been associated with decreased concentration in CSF of prostaglandin E$_2$ and decreased leakage of some proteins from serum into CSF in rabbits with experimental pneumococcal meningitis. Interleukin-1 concentration in CSF obtained after 24 hours of therapy in patients with bacterial meningitis also was lower in steroid-treated patients than in controls who received a placebo. This finding correlated inversely with CSF protein, lactate, and glucose concentrations and with the presence of some neurologic sequelae on follow-up examination of these children.

Although our understanding of the pathophysiologic events associated with initiation of the acute inflammatory response has been enhanced by recent data, a meta-analysis of all nine available controlled trials of corticosteroids for adjunctive therapy of bacterial meningitis before the 1991 report by Odio and associates failed to document that corticosteroid administration reduced the risk of death or neurologic abnormality at hospital discharge or follow-up examination. Odio and associates reported that the administration of dexamethasone immediately before the initiation of cefotaxime therapy was associated with a lower incidence of neurologic sequelae (14%) than that noted when cefotaxime alone was given (38%). However, there was no significant difference in the frequency of hearing loss in this study when dexamethasone-treated patients were compared with members of a control group who had been given a placebo. Moreover, the frequency of neurologic sequelae in placebo-treated patients (38%) was considerably higher than that noted in patients in several studies performed in recent years (11% to 14%) in which steroid therapy was not used.

Sensorineural hearing loss is an important sequelae of bacterial meningitis. A recent study examined the use of short-term dexamethasone administration (0.15 mg/kg every 6 hours for 4 days) as a possible method of decreasing the incidence of moderate to severe hearing loss. In a double-blind placebo-controlled trial, 100 infants and children with bacterial meningitis were treated for 10 days with cefuroxime and either a placebo or dexamethasone for 4 days. An additional 100 infants and children with bacterial meningitis were treated with ceftriaxone for 10 days and either a placebo or dexamethasone for 4 days. A significant reduction in moderate to severe hearing loss in children with *H influenzae* type b meningitis (*p* <.001) was reported. There were no significant differences between the two groups in other neurologic sequelae, in the resolution of clinical signs, or in the duration of hospital stay. Two patients receiving dexamethasone developed gastrointestinal bleeding severe enough to require transfusion and two others developed heme-positive stools. One patient in the steroid group had a positive culture for *H influenzae* at the end of 10 days of antibiotic therapy. These investigators concluded that dexamethasone was beneficial in diminishing the incidence of deafness in infants and children with bacterial meningitis.

Dodge and associates reported the results of studies of bacterial meningitis in children in which detailed evoked-response audiometry and careful follow-up evaluations were performed on all patients for 5 years. With this approach, 5.5% of the children

with *H influenzae* meningitis treated with ampicillin and chloramphenicol but not steroids developed a hearing deficit. The incidence of hearing loss noted by Schaad and associates in patients treated with ceftriaxone and not steroids also was only 4%. In a large nationwide study of more than 140 children performed in 1991, preliminary analysis suggests that steroids have neither a beneficial nor a detrimental effect on neurologic sequelae of bacterial meningitis.

The Committee on Infectious Diseases of the American Academy of Pediatrics has recommended individual consideration of dexamethasone for bacterial meningitis in infants and children 2 months and older after the physician has weighed the benefits and possible risks. The committee recognizes that some experts have decided not to use dexamethasone therapy until additional data are available. The effect of dexamethasone administration or lack thereof on neuropsychological function of children with meningitis has not been assessed. Dexamethasone should not be used for suspected or proved aseptic or nonbacterial meningitis. No data are available on which to recommend the use of dexamethasone for the treatment of bacterial meningitis in infants younger than 2 months of age. If dexamethasone is utilized, it should be given immediately prior to antibiotic administration in a dose of 0.15 mg/kg/dose intravenously every 6 hours for no more than 4 days. Whether shorter or longer courses of steroid therapy would yield different results with regard to the occurrence of deafness is unknown; longer courses, however, are likely to increase the rate of complications referable to steroid therapy.

## Supportive Care

The first 3 or 4 days of treatment of bacterial meningitis are the most critical. Vital signs should be taken every 15 to 30 minutes during the initial period until the patient is stable. They then should be repeated hourly for the first 24 to 48 hours. The patient's body weight, urine specific gravity, serum sodium, chloride, carbon dioxide, and potassium should be measured on admission, and a repeat serum sodium determination should be made every 12 to 24 hours for the first 2 days.

A complete neurologic evaluation should be performed on admission, followed by frequent brief neurologic checks for the first 24 hours or more. Complete neurologic evaluation may be performed daily throughout hospitalization. Monitoring of neurologic status is considered to be a minimal requirement for management of the patient with meningitis.

All patients with meningitis should be evaluated and treated, if necessary, for development of inappropriate antidiuretic hormone (ADH) secretion. Inappropriate ADH secretion was noted in 56% of the patients with bacterial meningitis in one prospective trial. Initially, the patient should receive nothing by mouth in order to prevent vomiting and aspiration and also to enable better assessment of fluid intake. A careful record of intake and output is required. The best indicators of inappropriate ADH secretion are increased body weight, decreased serum osmolality, and hyponatremia. The rate of fluid infusion initially should be restricted to 800 to 1000 mL/m$^2$/24 hours. Fluid administration can be liberalized toward normal maintenance requirement (1500 mL/m$^2$/24 hours) as evidence of inappropriate ADH secretion dissipates.

In patients with septic shock accompanying meningitis, sufficient fluid must be provided to maintain adequate circulation and blood pressure. In these patients, brain swelling may ensue. Sufficient fluids should be given to maintain a blood pressure of 80 to 90 mm Hg systolic, a urine output greater than 500 mL/m$^2$/24 hours, and adequate cerebral perfusion as evidenced by improvement in mental status. Monitoring of central venous pressure helps to avoid fluid overload. The use of fluids such as plasma or albuminized saline and agents such as isoproterenol and dopamine may promote improvement in blood pressure while minimizing the total amount of fluid required for resuscitation.

A CT scan or MRI should be obtained in children with focal neurologic signs. CT scans also can be obtained in children with papilledema or on an emergency basis before initial lumbar puncture in patients suspected of having increased ICP. CT scanning also is helpful in detecting large subdural effusions, hydrocephalus, or possible cerebrovascular abnormalities in patients with focal neurologic deficits. Daily measurements of the patient's head circumference and head transillumination also are recommended. Head transillumination is best performed in children younger than 18 months. These simple procedures may permit detection of developing subdural effusion or hydrocephalus.

## PREVENTION

### Passive Prevention

Vaccines are currently available for immunization against *S pneumoniae*, *N meningitidis* (A, C, Y, W135) and *H influenzae* type b. The pneumococcal polysaccharide vaccine (Pneumovax 23) is a 23-valent vaccine: 0.5 mL of vaccine contains 25 µg of each polysaccharide antigen (capsular types 1–5, 8, 9, 12, 14, 17, 19, 20, 22, 23, 34, 43, 68, and 70 [U.S. nomenclature]). These pneumococcal serotypes are responsible for nearly all the cases of bacteremia and meningitis in children and are effective in children older than 17 months. The vaccine is recommended for children at high risk for pneumococcal infection (eg, children with sickle-cell disease, functional or anatomical asplenia, nephrotic syndrome, and children about to undergo cytoreduction therapy for Hodgkin's disease). The pneumococcal vaccine is not recommended for prevention of respiratory tract infection or otitis media in young children.

The meningococcal vaccine is recommended for high-risk groups (as described earlier) and children with defects of the terminal components of the complement cascade (C5–C9). A quadrivalent vaccine consists of 50 µg of capsular polysaccharide A, C, Y, and W135 in each 0.5-mL dose. The vaccine is also available in monovalent A, monovalent C, and bivalent A and C forms. The quadrivalent vaccine is given to all members of the American armed services. Monovalent or quadrivalent vaccine may be recommended for people traveling to hyperendemic areas (eg, Brazil) or in the case of an epidemic of known type.

Two *H influenzae* conjugate vaccines currently are licensed for use beginning at 2 months of age. All infants should be immunized with either HbOC or PRP-OMP beginning at 2 months of age or as soon as possible thereafter. HbOC is given at 2, 4, and 6 months of age, with a booster at 15 months of age. PRP-OMP is given at 2 and 4 months of age, with a booster at 12 months of age. Because there is no current data on whether these vaccines are interchangeable, the vaccine product used for the first dose in children less than 15 months of age should be used for subsequent doses. For the most current information on recommendations for prevention of *H influenzae* type b disease, the reader is referred to the periodic reports of the Committee on Infectious Diseases of the American Academy of Pediatrics.

### Prevention (Antibiotic Prophylaxis)

Prophylactic antibiotic therapy with rifampin or sulfisoxazole should be offered to household, day-care center, and nursery school contacts as soon as possible after a patient with meningococcal disease is identified. A 2-day course of rifampin is recommended, preferably beginning within 24 hours of recognition of the primary case. The dose of rifampin recommended for meningococcal prophylaxis is 10 mg/kg body weight (600 mg maximum) given every 12 hours for 2 days. All patients taking rifampin should be advised that their urine, sweat, and tears may become orange; contact lenses may be stained permanently. Prophylaxis with sulfisoxazole should be given only in cases involving strains of *N meningitidis* proven to be sensitive to sulfa. Sulfasoxazole (500 mg) should be given once daily for 2 days to infants younger than 1 year and every 12 hours to patients 1 to 12 years of age. The dose for children over 12 and for adults is 1 g every 12 hours.

Rifampin prophylaxis for disease caused by *H influenzae* also is recommended. A dose of 20 mg/kg body weight (600 mg maximum) given once daily for 4 days eradicates *H influenzae* type b in 95% of carriers. Rifampin prophylaxis is recommended for all household contacts (including adults) if an unvaccinated child younger than 48 months of age lives in the home. Prophylaxis is also recommended if the child younger than 48 months was given the vaccine at less than 24 months or within the 3 weeks preceding the contact. The Committee on Infectious Diseases of the American Academy of Pediatrics suggests that rifampin prophylaxis be given to day-care center or nursery school contacts if two or more index cases occur in a unit within 60 days of each other. If the decision is made to give prophylaxis in the home or day-care setting, children who have received vaccine for *H influenzae* type b should not be exempted.

Recent prospective studies in Minnesota and Texas have confirmed the low incidence of subsequent disease in the day-care setting. Many authorities have concluded that it is premature to recommend rifampin prophylaxis in contacts of a single day-care center case. They estimate a cost of $750,000 for the prevention of a maximum of two cases of meningitis caused by *H influenzae* if rifampin prophylaxis is to be given to all day-care center contacts.

## Selected Readings

Dodge CR, Davis H, Feigin RD, et al. Prospective evaluation of hearing impairment as a sequela of acute bacterial meningitis. N Engl J Med 1984;311:869.

Feigin RD. Bacterial meningitis beyond the neonatal period. In: Feigin RD, Cherry JD, eds. Textbook of pediatric infectious diseases, ed 3. Philadelphia: WB Saunders, 1992.

Feigin RD, Stechenberg BW, Chang MJ, et al. Prospective evolution of treatment of *Haemophilus influenzae* meningitis. J Pediatr 1976;88:542.

Kaplan SL, Catlin FI, Weaver T, et al. Onset of hearing loss in children with bacterial meningitis. Pediatrics 1984;73:575.

Kaplan SL, Mason EO, Mason SK, et al. Prospective comparative trial of moxalactam versus ampicillin or chloramphenicol for treatment of *Haemophilus influenzae* type b meningitis in children. J Pediatr 1984;104:447.

Klein JO, Feigin RD, McCracken GH Jr. Report of the task force on diagnosis and management of meningitis. Pediatrics 1986;78(suppl):959.

Lebel MH, Freij BJ, Syrogiannopoulos GA. Dexamethasone therapy for bacterial meningitis. Results of two double-blind, placebo-controlled trials. N Engl J Med 1988;319:964.

Odio CM, Faingezicht I, Paris M. The beneficial effects of early dexamethasone administration in infants and children with bacterial meningitis. N Engl J Med 1991;324:1515.

Odio CM, Faingezicht I, Salas JL, et al. Cefotaxime versus conventional therapy for the treatment of bacterial meningitis of infants and children. Pediatr Infect Dis 1986;5:402.

Schaad UB, Suter S, Gianella-Borradori A. A comparison of ceftriaxone and cefuroxime for the treatment of bacterial meningitis in children. N Engl J Med 1990;322:141.

Sell SH. Long-term sequelae of bacterial meningitis in children. Pediatr Infect Dis 1983;2:90.

*Principles and Practice of Pediatrics, Second Edition.*
edited by Frank A. Oski et al. J. B. Lippincott Company, Philadelphia © 1994.

## CHAPTER 55
# *Opportunistic Infections in the Compromised Host*

## Ralph D. Feigin and Britton M. Devillier

Infection by organisms generally considered to be nonpathogenic may occur when host defenses are compromised. Congenital or acquired defects in the physical barriers through which microorganisms may enter or defects in the immune system predispose the host to infections by these organisms. Changes in the environment or indigenous flora increase the likelihood of colonization with resistant organisms, which may cause disease when host defenses are impaired. To choose the proper therapy, the physician must know the identity and antibiotic sensitivity of the organisms most likely to cause disease in a particular patient.

Opportunistic infections resulting from defects or interruption in normal anatomical barriers are listed in Table 55-1. The pathophysiologic basis for the occurrence of opportunistic infections in selected organ systems is discussed in the following section.

## PATHOPHYSIOLOGY

### Heart

Malformations, surgery, trauma, and prior infection of the heart are associated with an increased incidence of acute and subacute endocarditis. Eighty percent of children with endocarditis have congenital heart disease. Of patients with congenital heart disease, 24% have tetralogy of Fallot and 18% have a ventricular septal defect. Most cases of endocarditis in children are caused by viridans streptococci. Other opportunistic organisms responsible for endocarditis include *Staphylococcus aureus, Haemophilus aphrophilus, Streptococcus faecalis, Streptococcus pneumoniae*, other β-hemolytic streptococci, *Corynebacterium* spp., *Neisseria flava, Pseudomonas cepacia, Aerococcus viridans, Staphylococcus epidermidis*, gram-negative aerobic bacilli, and *Aspergillus fumigatus*. Opportunistic infection in patients following cardiac surgery most often is due to *S epidermidis*, diphtheroids, pseudomonads, *Candida albicans*, and *Mimeae* spp., *Acinetobacter*, and *Aspergillus* spp.

Infections of prosthetic heart valves and vascular grafts can be divided into early- and late-onset disease. *S aureus*, enteric gram-negative organisms, pseudomonads, *S epidermidis*, diphtheroids, and *Candida* spp. are common causes of early-onset infection; α-hemolytic streptococci, *S faecalis*, staphylococci, and gram-negative bacilli more often are found in late-onset disease.

Fungal endocarditis most commonly occurs after cardiac surgery or prolonged intravenous antibiotic therapy and is uncommon in children. *Candida* spp. are the most common fungal causes of endocarditis.

Disruption of the endocardium followed by platelet aggregation and fibrin clot formation is the initial event in the devel-

---

**TABLE 55-1.** Opportunisitic Infection in the Host Compromised by Changes in the Skin or Mucous Membrane Barrier to Infection or by Anatomical Defects

| Predisposing Causes: Defects in Anatomical Barriers | Opportunistic Organism Isolated Most Frequently | Suggested Mechanisms |
|---|---|---|
| Dermal sinus tracts | *Staphylococcus epidermidis*, diphtheroids | Bypasses skin as barrier to infection |
| CSF shunts | *S epidermidis, Staphylococcus aureus*, diphtheroids, *Bacillus* spp. | Bypasses skin as barrier to infection; acts as nidus for infection |
| IV catheters | *S epidermidis; Acinetobacter; Bacteroides, Pseudomonas, Candida*, and *Cryptococus* spp. | Bypasses skin as barrier to infection; may serve as nidus for infection |
| Urinary catheters | *S epidermidis; Pseudomonas, Serratia, Acinetobacter*, and *Candida* spp. | Serves as nidus for infection and new portal of entry for microorganisms |
| Inhalation therapy equipment | *Pseudomonas* and *Serratia* spp. | Serves as new portal of entry for microorganisms; equipment and medication frequently contaminated with opportunistic organisms |
| Burns | *Pseudomonas, Serratia, Staphylococcus, Candida*, and *Mucor* spp. | Changes skin flora ecology and physiochemical properties of skin; neutrophil dysfunction, abnormal responses to antigenic stimulation, impairment of delayed hypersensitivity |
| General surgery | *S epidermidis; Alcaligenes fecalis; Pseudomonas* and *Candida* spp. | Prophylactic antibiotics alter normal flora; bypasses skin as barrier to infection |
| Cardiac surgery | *S epidermidis*; diphtheriods; *Mimea; Pseudomonas, Candida*, and *Aspergillus* spp. | Prophylactic antibiotics may alter normal flora; foreign bodies inserted may serve as nidus of infection |
| Congenital cardiac defects | Viridans streptococci; *Corynebacterium; Pseudomonas* and nonpathogenic *Neisseria* spp. | Damaged tissue serves as nidus for infection |
| Retained foreign body | *S aureus*, enterics, *Mycobacterium* spp., *Nocardia, Vibrio* spp. | Serves as nidus for infection; bypasses skin as barrier to infection |

Feigin RD, Matson DO. Opportunistic infections, the compromised host. In: Feigin RD, Cherry JD, eds. Textbook of pediatric infectious diseases, ed 3. Philadelphia: WB Saunders, 1992:961.

opment of endocarditis in patients with congenital or acquired cardiac disease. Transient bacteremia from any cause then leads to adherence of bacteria to the fibrin clot. Proliferation of organisms results in deformation of the involved endocardium or valve. The clinical features of endocarditis are related primarily to embolic events originating from infected endocardium. Prophylactic administration of antibiotics to patients at risk for endocarditis is recommended (Table 55-2) based on evidence that antibiotics can prevent endocarditis and reduce the incidence of bacteremia in patients requiring cardiac surgery.

## Skin

Organisms normally colonize the skin or mucous membranes by attaching to epithelial cells (including hair follicles) or to mucus. The attachment may be specific (bacterial attachment to a host receptor) or nonspecific. The skin provides protection by elaborating fatty acids that impair bacterial growth and by undergoing desquamation. In addition to being a physical barrier, mucous membranes contain cellular and humoral elements of the immune system that help control potentially infectious agents.

Any disruption of the normal integrity of the skin or mucous

---

TABLE 55-2. Conditions and Procedures Related to Endocarditis Prophylaxis

**Cardiac Conditions for Which Endocarditis Prophylaxis is Recommended**

Prosthetic cardiac valves (mechanical and biosynthetic)
Most congenital cardiac malformations
Surgically constructed systemic-pulmonary shunts
Rheumatic and other acquired valvular disease
Idiopathic hypertrophic subaortic stenosis
History of bacterial endocarditis
Mitral valve prolapse with insufficiency
Foreign material in the heart

**Cardiac Conditions for Which Endocarditis Prophylaxis is Not Recommended**

Isolated secundum atrial septal defect
Secundum atrial septal defect repaired without a patch 6 or more months earlier
Patent ductus arteriosus ligated and divided 6 or more months earlier

**Procedures for Which Endocarditis Prophylaxis is Recommended**

All dental procedures likely to induce gingival bleeding
Tonsillectomy or adenoidectomy
Surgical procedures or biopsy involving respiratory mucosa
Bronchoscopy, especially with a rigid scope
Incision and drainage of infected tissue
Selected genitourinary and gastrointestinal procedures (cystoscopy, urethral catheterization, urinary tract surgery, gallbladder or colonic surgery, esophageal or anal dilataion, colonoscopy, upper GI tract endoscopy with biopsy, proctosigmoidoscopic biopsy)
Cardiac surgery

**Procedures for Which Endocarditis Prophylaxis is Not Routinely Recommended**

Orotracheal intubation
Cardiac catheterization
Cesarean section
Therapeutic abortion
Intrauterine device insertion or removal

*Friedman RA, Starke JR. Infective endocarditis. In: Garson A, Bricker JT, McNamara DG, eds. The science and practice of pediatric cardiology. Philadelphia: Lea & Febiger, 1990;1568.*

---

membranes such as cracking, peeling, desquamation (congenital ichthyosis), burning, ulcer formation, or insertion of transcutaneous intravenous catheters impairs host defenses against infection that are normally provided by the skin. Patients with intravenous catheters have a 2% to 5% chance of experiencing bacteremia or fungemia. *S epidermidis, S aureus,* and *Bacteroides, Mimeae, Pseudomonas, Candida,* and *Cryptococcus* spp. are among the organisms seen most often as a cause of catheter-related bacteremia. Central lines also may become infected, and patients receiving total parenteral nutrition (versus standard intravenous fluids) through these central lines are at increased risk of infection with *S epidermidis, S aureus, C albicans,* pseudomonads, *Bacteroides, Serratia, Citrobacter,* and *Torulopsis* spp. *Malassezia furfur,* a lipophilic yeast, has been associated with long-term lipid infusions. The time after insertion, quality of sterile technique, and type of catheter used are factors affecting the incidence of line-associated infections. Stainless-steel needles are preferable to plastic catheters.

Use of contaminated intravenous solutions also may result in opportunistic infection. The organisms reported most commonly include *Enterobacter cloacae, S epidermidis, Pseudomonas maltophilia, Pseudomonas stutzeri, Erwinia* and *Bacillus* spp., and yeast.

Surgical incisions, sutures, burns, traumatized and devitalized tissue, foreign bodies (after penetration), dermal sinus tracts, and dermoids are well-known examples of factors predisposing any individual to opportunistic infection of the skin. Factors that increase the chance of infection in surgical wounds include malnutrition, coexisting disease, wound contamination, foreign bodies, devitalized tissue, or any condition that impairs circulation to the incision site. The chances of infection are related to the degree of contamination of the surgical site at the completion of the procedure.

Most wound infections occur with organisms indigenous to the patient, including staphylococci, *Enterobacteriacae* spp., pseudomonads, and anaerobes. Community-acquired organisms generally are more sensitive to antibiotics than are organisms acquired in the hospital. Postoperative infection also can result from instrumentation with intravenous, intra-arterial, or Foley catheters.

Patients with burns are known to have abnormalities of neutrophil function, including altered chemotaxis, diminished NADH-NADPH activity, decreased lysosomal enzyme content, and decreased oxygen consumption. In addition, the lymphocyte response to antigen stimulation is abnormal, and delayed hypersensitivity is impaired. After a burn, bacteria grow on nonviable surface tissue and ultimately enter the bloodstream. *S aureus* has been replaced by gram-negative organisms such as *Pseudomonas aeruginosa, Serratia* spp., and *Aeromonas hydrophila* as the most common causes of bacteremia in these patients.

## Brain

CNS infection may follow insertion of shunts, or it may be the result of communication between the skin and subarachnoid space through sinus or mucosal defects. Suppurative foci adjacent to the CNS also predispose the patient to CNS infection. Meningitis rarely occurs after lumbar puncture, myelography, or other transient invasive procedures; however, postoperative meningitis and ventriculitis are associated more often with shunts or indwelling monitoring devices. Before isolation and identification of the etiologic agent, treatment should include coverage for gram-positive penicillin-resistant and gram-negative microorganisms, including *Pseudomonas.*

Most infections associated with shunt implantation occur within the first 2 months after shunt placement. In one study, half of the infections occurred within 2 weeks of insertion. Bacteremia is uncommon following placement of ventriculoperitoneal shunts. It is more frequent when a ventriculoatrial shunt has been implanted. Children usually present with fever, irritability, vomiting, and abdominal complaints. Shunt malfunction may occur, and erythema overlying the shunt tubing is highly suggestive of bacterial infection.

Perioperative use of antistaphylococcal antibiotics has proved efficacious in reducing the incidence of shunt infection. Direct aspiration of the shunt bubble is usually helpful in diagnosing the bacterial agent responsible for the infection. Removal of the infected shunt increases the likelihood of cure, and replacement with a new shunt should be delayed until sufficient time has elapsed to sterilize the CSF. The incidence of infection has been related to the number of shunt operations performed by the neurosurgeon; those who frequently perform the operation have lower rates of infection.

Other conditions that may predispose patients to CNS infection include CSF leakage associated with penetration of normal anatomical barriers. Some 10% to 60% of patients with basilar skull fracture and persistent CSF leakage develop meningitis. Most of these infections are caused by S pneumoniae. Children with dermal sinus tracts or dermoids that communicate with the subarachnoid space or neural tissue have developed meningitis due to S epidermidis, Corynebacterium spp., P aeruginosa, Proteus mirabilis, and Alcaligenes faecalis. Other conditions predisposing patients to opportunistic infection of the CNS include foreign bodies, myelomeningocele, encephalocele, treated or untreated local infections of sinuses or the middle ear that spread to contiguous structures (potentially resulting in epidural abscesses, subdural empyema, brain abscesses, venous sinus thrombosis, or meningitis), intravenous drug abuse, infective endocarditis, heart disease, lymphoma, leukemia, immunosuppression, and transplantation.

## Genitourinary System

Factors that predispose patients to infection of the genitourinary system are obstruction at any level of the urinary tract, reflux, incomplete emptying of the bladder, foreign body (catheter), and instrumentation. Intrarenal causes of obstruction include nephrocalcinosis, polycystic kidney disease, sickle-cell disease, and other nephropathies.

Normal fecal flora cause most infections of the genitourinary system. Escherichia coli is the most common cause of infection of the urinary tract, but other organisms are noted frequently, including S epidermidis, pseudomonads, Torulopsis glabrata, and Serratia, Acinetobacter, and Candida spp.

Vulvovaginitis due to Candida spp. is a complication of prolonged antibiotic therapy. Children with uncontrolled diabetes mellitus may have frequent episodes of mycotic vaginitis.

## Pulmonary System

Any impairment of defense mechanisms of the upper or lower respiratory tract may predispose children to infection. Defense against respiratory tract pathogens is provided by filtration, bacterial interference, secretory IgA, mucociliary clearance, cough, secretion of immunoglobulins, complement and pulmonary macrophages, polymorphonuclear leukocytes, and lymphocytes.

Many conditions predispose patients to pulmonary infection, including prolonged hospitalization (allowing oropharyngeal colonization with nosocomial organisms), intubation, smoking, gastroesophageal reflux with aspiration, ciliary defects (Kartagener's syndrome), neurologic impairment, chemotherapy, viral infection, inhalation burns, and inhalation therapy equipment. Viral infections (particularly influenza $A_2$ virus) predispose patients to infection with S pneumoniae, Haemophilus influenzae, and S aureus. Viral infection in patients with previous chronic lung disease is devastating and may lead to bacterial superinfection, especially with respiratory syncytial virus infection in patients with bronchopulmonary dysplasia, cystic fibrosis, pulmonary hemosiderosis, and bronchiolitis obliterans.

The use of respiratory life-support systems, particularly in neonates, has been associated with an increase in opportunistic infections. Serratia marcescens and P aeruginosa are the organisms found most commonly in respiratory tract infections in intubated patients. Microaerosols generated by reservoir nebulizers pose a greater threat than cascade humidifiers. The careful use of all equipment used for ventilation of respirator-dependent patients involves a specific maintenance regimen, including replacing disposable tubing according to a predetermined schedule and cleaning parts that cannot be replaced. Periodic surveillance cultures should be used. The chances for opportunistic infections are related to the general oral hygiene of the patient, the technical care provided by the staff, the patient's specific disease, and the presence of other infections in the intensive care area.

Patients hospitalized for prolonged periods acquire gram-negative bacilli and fungi in the mouth and pharynx. Most nosocomial respiratory infections are due to Klebsiella, Enterobacter, Serratia, E coli, Proteus, and Pseudomonas.

## Gastrointestinal Tract

Normal bowel flora may help protect the host by producing antibodies that cross-react with potential pathogenic microorganisms. Bowel flora also may compete with true pathogens for food (bacterial interference). The indigenous flora in the gastrointestinal tract may be altered by situations predisposing to overgrowth. For example, irradiation of the head, tooth extraction, changes in peristalsis, hospitalization, and antibiotic usage (especially poorly absorbed drugs) allow for overgrowth of organisms that generally are not abundant in the normal host. Pseudomembranous colitis can develop after antibiotic therapy, and overgrowth with Candida, staphylococci, or Clostridium difficile may occur.

## Blood and Blood Products

Opportunistic infection may be acquired following infusion of blood or blood products. Infections with cytomegalovirus (CMV), Epstein-Barr virus (EBV), non-A, non-B hepatitis, and human immunodeficiency virus (HIV) are most common. Screening for HIV antibody has reduced greatly the number of individuals acquiring infection with HIV by this route.

CMV infection may be transmitted via blood that is culture-negative. Screening of blood by DNA hybridization techniques will help minimize transmission of CMV in CMV-culture-negative blood. Neonatal CMV acquisition is more likely to occur in babies with a birth weight below 1250 g. It is also more common in babies born to CMV-seronegative mothers, in infants hospitalized for more than 4 weeks, in those who have received multiple blood transfusions or a single transfusion with a total volume greater than 50 mL, and in babies who receive blood from a seropositive donor.

## CONGENITAL AND ACQUIRED HOST DEFENSE DEFECTS

The immune system is composed of cellular and humoral elements. The cellular arm is defined by the granulocytes (or phagocytes) and B and T lymphocytes. Humoral factors include serum complement, serum and secretory immunoglobulins, and the circulating mediators of the immune response. Table 55-3 summarizes the diseases that result from an impairment of the in-

**TABLE 55-3.   Opportunistic Infection in Inherited and Acquired Disorders That Diminish Host Resistance**

| Predisposing Causes: Inherited and Acquired Disorders of Inflammation or Immunity | Opportunistic Organisms Isolated Most Frequently | Suggested Mechanisms |
|---|---|---|
| Chronic granulomatous disease | Gram-negative enteric organisms; Staphylococci; Serratia and Nocardia spp. | Impaired production of $H_2O_2$ with defective bactericidal function |
| Job syndrome | Staphylococcus aureus, Haemophilus influenza | Unknown |
| Myeloperoxidase deficiency | Candida spp. | Failure to kill Candida spp. |
| Glucose-6-phosphate dehydrogenase deficiency | Catalase-positive organisms; S aureus; Chromobacterium and Serratia spp. | Deficient cellular NADH and NADPH, deficiency HMPS activity, impaired $O_2$ generation, decreased $H_2O_2$ production, defect in bacterial killing |
| MAC-1 deficiency | Gram-negative enteric organisms; pseudomonads; S aureus | Deficient surface glycoproteins |
| Hereditary specific granule deficiency | Pseudomonads; S aureus, Escherichia coli, Candida albicans; Proteus, Klebsiella, Enterobacter, and Acinetobacter spp. | Defective intracellular killing, deficient chemotaxis and adherence |
| Lazy leukocyte syndrome | Staphylococci | Unknown |
| Actin dysfunction | S aureus, C albicans | Exact mechanism unknown |
| Chédiak-Higashi syndrome | S aureus | Defective bactericidal activity, impaired chemotaxis, neutropenia |
| Kartagener's syndrome | Endogenous respiratory flora | Defect in ciliary motility secondary to improper dynein arm structure |
| Periodontitis | Fusobacterium and Capnocytophaga spp. | Impaired chemotaxis |
| Neutropenia (any cause) | Pyogenic bacteria or fungi | Decreased neutrophil numbers |
| Complement deficiencies (C1, C2, C3, C4 and factor B) | Streptococcus pyogenes, Streptococcus pneumoniae. S aureus, H influenzae, Neisseria meningitidis; Klebsiella spp. | Defective chemotaxis, impaired opsonization |
| C5-C8, CI-Cg, properdin deficiencies | N meningitidis, Neisseria gonorrhoeae | Defective membrane attack mechanism |
| Splenic insufficiency | Salmonellae; S pneumoniae | Defective opsonization, defective clearing of organisms |
| Sickle-cell disease and other hemoglobinopathies | Salmonellae; S pneumoniae; Edwardsiella spp. H influenzae type b | Reticuloendothelial blockade, defective opsonization |
| Humoral immunodeficiency syndromes (predominantly B-cell defects) | Bacterial pathogens; pseudomonads | Reduced phagocytic efficiency, failure of lysis and agglutination of bacteria, inadequate neutralization of bacterial toxins |
| Cellular immunodeficiency syndromes (predominantly T-cell defects) | CMV, VZV; Strongyloides stercoralis; Mycobacterium, Listeria, Nocardia, Cryptococcus, Candida, and Pneumocytosis spp. | Absence or impaired delayed hypersenstivity response, absent T-cell cooperation for B-cell synthesis of antibodies to T cell-specific antigens |
| Severe combined immunodeficiency syndrome | Many bacteria, fungi, and viruses; Pneumocystis spp. | Absence of T- and B-cell responses |
| Wiskott-Aldrich syndrome | Gram-negative enteric organisms; CMV, HSV; staphylococci; S pneumoniae, H influenzae, Pneumocystis carinii | Decreased antibody production to carbohydrate antigens |
| Ataxia-telangiectasia | Sinopulmonary infection with saprophytes | T-helper cell deficiency, immunoglobulin deficiency |
| AIDS | HSV types 1 and 2, CMV, VZV, adenovirus, EBC, HBV; Candida albicans, Giardia lamblia, Entamoeba histolytica, Mycobacterium tuberculosis, Mycobacterium avium–intracellulare, Mycobacterium kansasii, Toxoplasma gondii, Cryptococcus neoformans, P carinii; Campylobacter, Legionella, Candida, Isospora, Aspergillus, Nocardia, Strongyloides, and Cryptosporidum spp. | Retrovirus infection transmitted by blood that impairs T-cell response, impaired T-helper cells |
| Cancer* | VZV, HSV; E coli; Pseudomonas, Klebsiella, Listeria, Cryptococcus, Pneumocystis, and Mycobacterium spp. | Granulocytopenia, decreased neutrophil chemotaxis, decreased bacterial activity of neutrophils, lymphopenia, defective cell-mediated immunity, impaired antigenic response to challenge |
| Immunosuppression | HSV, VZV, CMV, EBV, papovavirus, hepatitis virus; pseudonomads, E coli; Klebsiella, Acinetobacter, Serratia, Candida, Apsergillus, Mucor, and Cryptococcus spp. | Depends on agent used |

TABLE 55-3.    *(Continued)*

| Predisposing Causes: Inherited and Acquired Disorders of Inflammation or Immunity | Opportunistic Organisms Isolated Most Frequently | Suggested Mechanisms |
|---|---|---|
| Transplantation | CMV, HSV, VZV, hepatitis virus; staphylococci, pseudomonads; *Klebsiella, Candida, Aspergillus, Nocardia,* and *Pneumocystis* spp. | Probably related to use of immunosuppressive agents or graft-vs.-host disease |
| Malnutrition | Measles, HSV, VZV; *Mycobacterium* spp. | Impaired T-cell function, reduction in complement activity, impaired migration of phagocytes, reduced bactericidal activity |
| Cystic fibrosis | Staphylococci, pseudomonads | Presence of ciliary dyskinesia factor, impaired phagocytosis of *Pseudomonas* spp. |
| Diabetes | Staphylococci, *E coli; Proteus, Clostridium; Actinomyces, Candida, Mucor, Torulopsis* | Impaired phagocytic activity, decreased serum opsonizing capacity, decreased chemotaxis of neutrophils |
| Polyendocrinopathy | *Candida* spp. | Unknown |
| Nephrotic syndrome | Enteric bacteria; *S pneumoniae* | Unknown |
| Uremia | HSV, VZV; staphylococci; *Bacteroides, Serratia, Enterobacter, Candida* and *Mucor* spp. | Defects in early phases of inflammatory response, lymphopenia, impaired T-cell function |
| Peritoneal dialysis | Gram-negative enteric organisms; staphylococci, streptococci; *C albicans, Candida tropicalis* | Presence of foreign body |
| Exudative enteropathy | Enteric bacteria; *S pneumoniae, Giardia lamblia* | Low levels of IgG, depressed T-cell function in intestinal lymphangiectasia |
| Inflammatory bowel disease | HSV, VZV; *Candida* and *Mucor* spp. | Probably not related to basic disease but to use of corticosteroids |
| Colllagen disease | CMV, HSV, VZV; diphtheroids; staphlococci, pseudomonads; *Candida, Mucor, Aspergillus, Pneumocystis, Listeria, Serratia,* and *Nocardia* spp. | Probably related to use of immunosuppressive agents, may relate to involvement of reticuloendothelial system |

\* Incidence of infection with gram-negative organisms increases in presence of neutropenia.
*CMV,* cytomegalovirus; *EBV,* Epstein-Barr virus; *HBV,* hepatitis B virus; *HSV,* herpes simplex virus; *VZV,* varicella-zoster virus.
*Feigin RD, Shearer WT. Opportunistic infection in children. J Pediatr 1975;87:677.*

flammatory or immune response to infection, opportunistic organisms causing infection in these disorders, and the mechanism by which disease is produced.

## Phagocytic Defects

Phagocytes (primarily neutrophils and monocytes) are often the first cells to interact with infectious organisms in any tissue. The cumulative effect of phagocytic action is either intracellular killing or inactivation of bacteria, viruses, or fungi. Any defect in the processes of adherence, aggregation, chemotaxis, migration, motility, ingestion, or intracellular killing may result in an increased frequency of infections.

### Defects of Intracellular Killing

*Chronic Granulomatous Disease.* Ingestion of organisms by granulocytes is not impaired but intracellular killing is defective in children with chronic granulomatous disease; all other neutrophil and monocyte functions are normal. The response of the hexose monophosphate shunt to phagocytosis is reduced, resulting in decreased free oxygen radicals and peroxide. The defect is present in neutrophils, eosinophils, monocytes, macrophages, and lymphocytes. The disease is X-linked recessive in boys with cytochrome b245 deficiency. This enzyme catalyzes the reaction generating superoxide anion.

Other patients with similar clinical syndromes may have defects of other enzymes associated with oxygen metabolism such as glucose 6-phosphate dehydrogenase, NADPH oxidase, or glutathione peroxidase. These patients are at risk for infection with catalase-positive organisms that do not produce hydrogen peroxide.

Patients may present with infections of the skin, pulmonary system, and bones of the hands and feet, as well as with abscesses of the liver, appendix, and subphrenic or retroperitoneal spaces. The most frequently encountered organism responsible for infection is *S aureus*. Patients also are infected commonly with gram-negative, catalase-positive organisms such as *S marcescens, E coli,* and *Enterobacter* and *Klebsiella* spp. Other organisms identified in abscesses include salmonellae, pseudomonads, *Providencia* spp., *A fecalis,* and *Proteus, Acinetobacter,* and *Chromobacterium* spp. Aspergilli are the most common fungal isolates and have been implicated with increasing frequency in patients with chronic granulomatous disease who have pneumonitis.

Therapy of chronic granulomatous disease involves abscess drainage and appropriate intravenous antibiotic therapy. When serious infections are under control, consideration of prophylactic antibiotic therapy may be warranted. However, despite several reports of a decline in frequency of infections, no prospective study of the effect of prophylactic antibiotics has been performed.

*Job Syndrome (Hyper-IgE Syndrome).* Patients with Job syndrome have repeated bouts of abscess formation of the subcutaneous tissue, skin, muscle, or lymph nodes associated with otitis media or externa, chronic nasal discharge, chronic eczematoid rashes, coarse facies, mild eosinophilia, mucocutaneous candidiasis, and serum IgE levels above 2000 mg/dL. The organisms isolated most frequently are *S aureus* and *H influenzae*. Bronchitis and pneumonia occasionally occur; septicemia, osteomyelitis, meningitis, and endocarditis occur infrequently. The etiology of the disease is unknown. The abscesses often have been described as cold because they do not exhibit the warmth, redness, and swelling usually seen with infected abscesses.

*Myeloperoxidase Deficiency.*    Myeloperoxidase is a component of primary granules. Its deficiency in monocytes and neutrophils leads to a disease in which there is defective killing or inactivation of intracellular phagocytized organisms. The respiratory burst is normal, but chemiluminescence is initially low during phagocytosis. Case reports of intermediate myeloperoxidase abnormalities in relatives support the expected autosomal recessive mode of inheritance of the disease. Patients with myeloperoxidase deficiency should be considered at risk for opportunistic infections by bacteria as well as by fungi such as *Candida* spp.

*Severe Glucose 6-Phosphate Dehydrogenase Deficiency.* Patients with this deficiency have ineffective hexose monophosphate shunt activity and reduced generation of peroxide that results in an inability to kill bacteria. Patients may be unable to kill gram-positive or gram-negative organisms.

### Defects of Adherence and Aggregation

*MAC-1, LFA-1, p150,95 Deficiency.*    Patients with this disorder may have severe or moderate levels of deficiency of surface glycoproteins that mediate adhesion between granulocytes, monocytes, and lymphocytes and effector surfaces such as fibroblasts and endothelium. Cell migration and phagocytic ingestion are affected. Patients exhibit recurrent soft-tissue infections and markedly impaired pus formation. A spectrum of disease is seen based on the degree of deficiency, with severely affected patients dying in infancy and moderately affected individuals surviving considerably longer (mean age of death, 20 years). The diagnosis may be entertained when at least one of the following findings is noted: recurrent cutaneous, periodontal, or other soft-tissue infections, or delayed separation of the umbilical cord. Delay or failure in wound healing is a consistent feature. Patients also may have ulcerative stomatitis, gingivitis, or periodontitis. Granulocytosis of 15,000 to 69,000 cells/mm³ when patients are healthy and 100,000 cells/mm³ or greater when patients are infected also has been observed. *S aureus, Pseudomonas,* and other gram-negative enteric bacteria are the organisms most often responsible for infection.

*Hereditary Specific Granule Deficiency.*    Specific granules are neutrophilic granules containing inflammatory mediators. In addition, the granules contain receptor molecules for chemotactic factors and adhesive glycoprotein (MAC-1). Thus, these patients not only have defects in intracellular killing but also in adherence and chemotaxis. Patients with this disorder experience recurrent destructive infections of skin, mucous membranes, and lung. *S aureus, E coli, C albicans,* pseudomonads, and *Proteus, Klebsiella, Enterobacter,* and *Acinetobacter* spp. are the predominant organisms isolated from infected patients. Diagnosis is suggested by a history of recurrent infection and can be documented by appropriate leukocyte function studies. Appropriate antibiotics and supportive medical care are essential.

### Abnormalities of Leukocyte Migration

*Lazy Leukocyte Syndrome.*    Patients with this syndrome have recurrent episodes of otitis media, stomatitis, gingivitis, rhinitis, and profound neutropenia despite normal cellularity and

maturation of the bone marrow neutrophilic pool. Recurrent staphylococcal skin infections are seen most commonly.

*Chédiak-Higashi Syndrome.*    This autosomal recessive disorder is characterized by partial oculocutaneous albinism, photophobia, nystagmus, and the presence of neutrophils with giant cytoplasmic granules. The disease occurs with variable severity. The susceptibility to infection may be related to impaired microtubular function or cyclic nucleotide metabolism. Defective chemotaxis and delayed postphagocytic fusion of phagosomes with lysosomes results in the inability to kill gram-positive and gram-negative organisms. Infections in these patients usually are caused by *S aureus*; group A streptococci, *H influenzae,* and gram-negative enteric organisms are noted in a few patients. Patients in the accelerated phase of the disease (characterized by tissue infiltration by lymphoid and histiocytic cells) are particularly susceptible to neutropenia.

*Kartagener's Syndrome.*    Kartagener's syndrome (immotile cilia syndrome) is an autosomal recessive disorder characterized by chronic or recurrent sinusitis, otitis media, and pneumonia associated with situs inversus. The basis of the clinical features is a defect in ciliary motility attributable to improper structure of the dynein arms. Despite findings of defective chemotaxis in vitro, patients with Kartagener's syndrome are at risk only for infections caused by indigenous respiratory flora that are removed ineffectively from the respiratory tract.

*Periodontitis.*    Periodontitis is one of the clinical manifestations often found in patients with defects of neutrophil function or number. Maintenance of normal periodontal integrity depends in part on the presence of leukocytes within the gingival areas. In the normal host, these infiltrates are mostly neutrophils. Neutrophils from patients with periodontitis exhibit defects in chemotaxis in vitro.

Immunocompromised or diabetic patients as well as those with poor oral hygiene are at increased risk for gingivitis; progression to periodontitis is possible. Anaerobes including *Fusobacterium* are the leading infectious agents isolated from periodontal infections. *Capnocytophaga* has been isolated from patients with chemotactic defects.

*Protein-Calorie Malnutrition.*    Impaired wound healing, decreased bacterial killing, poor inflammatory responses (probably related to decreased complement concentration), and poor mobilization of leukocytes are noted in patients with protein-calorie malnutrition. Infection with viruses (measles, herpes simplex), fungi, parasites, and bacteria are common, and any organ system may be affected. Patients with glycogen storage disease type 1b, Shwachman-Diamond syndrome, congenital ichthyosis, and mannosidosis also exhibit increased susceptibility to infection as a result of defects in leukocyte migration.

*Neutropenia.*    Patients with Shwachman-Diamond syndrome and type 1b glycogen storage disease also may have neutropenia. Neutropenia predisposes a patient to pyogenic or fungal infection of the skin and respiratory tract as well as to sepsis. Disorders or conditions associated with neutropenia are listed in Table 55-4.

## Complement or Lymphokine Deficiency

### Humoral Complement Deficiency and Disorders of Decreased Production of Chemotactic Factors

C3b is the most important opsonic factor in serum, and C5a and C5a des-arg are potent chemotactic factors. Defects of synthesis (absence of gene) of C3 or C5 and the presence of inhibitors of

| TABLE 55-4. Disorders or Conditions Associated With Neutropenia | |
|---|---|
| Vitamin B$_{12}$ or folate deficiency | Infantile lethal agranulocytosis |
| Copper deficiency | Acyclic neutropenia |
| Felty's syndrome | Drug-induced neutropenia |
| Gaucher's disease | Transient neutropenia |
| Sarcoidosis | Familial benign neutropenia |
| Shwachman-Diamond syndrome | Opportunistic infection |
| Type 1b glycogen storage disease | Radiation treatment |
| Overwhelming sepsis | Hypersplenism |
| Chédiak-Higashi syndrome | Malignancy with and without bone marrow failure |
| Aplastic anemia | Chemotherapy treatment |
| Lazy leukocyte syndrome | |

these factors in serum or plasma have been reported. Some patients with systemic lupus erythematosus have been shown to have impaired production of C5a in serum.

Patients with C1, C2, C3, C4, or factor B deficiency are susceptible to infection by *S pneumoniae, S aureus, Streptococcus pyogenes*, aerobic gram-negative bacilli (*Klebsiella aerogenes*), *N meningitidis*, and *H influenzae*. Patients with C5, C6, C7, or C8 deficiency are at increased risk for infection with *N meningitidis* or *Neisseria gonorrhoeae*. Recurrent, localized soft-tissue infections, sepsis, meningitis, pneumonia, and septic arthritis are more common in these patients with complement deficiency.

Patients with malnutrition or nephrotic syndrome and newborn infants have a relative deficiency in the activity of the complement system and are probably at increased risk for opportunistic infection.

### Chronic Mucocutaneous Candidiasis

Defective production of lymphokines by T cells and thus lack of T-cell response to specific antigens has been observed in several patients with chronic infection of mucocutaneous surfaces with *Candida*.

### Splenic Insufficiency

The normal spleen removes bacteria from the bloodstream (especially encapsulated organisms) and produces antibodies (especially IgM), properdin, and tuftsin. In the infant, the spleen probably removes bacteria by phagocytosis and begins forming opsonizing antibody soon after contact with an infectious agent. A defect in these abilities in the newborn could lead to overwhelming infection. Congenital asplenia and splenosis have been associated with recurrent or fulminant infections.

Patients with sickle-cell disease are extremely susceptible to systemic or focal infection (pneumonia, osteomyelitis, meningitis, genitourinary infection) by encapsulated organisms such as *S pneumoniae, H influenzae* type b, salmonellae, *Shigella* spp., and *Edwardsiella tarda*. This susceptibility is related to the progression of splenic dysfunction in sickle-cell patients. By 6 months of age, the spleen is nonfunctional, primarily because of splenic enlargement as a result of phagocytosis of defective red blood cells and impaired phagocytic functions. Reduced flow or stasis due to increased trapping of abnormally shaped red blood cells causes further infarction of the spleen. The greatest susceptibility to infection with encapsulated organisms is from 6 months to 6 years of age; however, the risk is always greater than for normal patients.

A patient with sickle-cell disease and fever should be considered to have a potentially life-threatening bacterial infection. All patients with sickle-cell disease should be placed on penicillin at 6 months of age, and pneumococcal vaccine should be given at 2 years of age.

Splenectomy predisposes patients to infectious agents to which the body has not yet made antibody. Complement-mediated opsonization is defective in patients without antibody to the bacterial cell wall.

## B- and T-Cell Immunodeficiency

Humoral immunodeficiency is confined primarily to B cells (X-linked agammaglobulinemia, selective IgA deficiency), whereas cellular immunodeficiency is primarily a T cell (HIV infection, thymic dysplasia) disorder. Combined immunodeficiency disorders involve both B and T cells and may be noted if a common essential enzyme is defective or if cellular interaction is impaired. The function of the cellular immune system depends on the interaction of many cellular and humoral elements. Insufficient involvement of B or T cells may impair their function and predispose the host to opportunistic infections.

The clinical features attributable to immunodeficiency of either T- or B-cell origin are difficult to segregate completely. Infections with unusual organisms are common to both. T-cell defects usually are suspected when a patient has frequent viral infections or prolonged and unusual infection with viruses such as CMV or varicella-zoster virus. Chronic mucocutaneous candidiasis, oral or esophageal candidiasis, and infections with *Mycobacterium, Listeria, Nocardia, Cryptococcus*, or *Pneumocystis* organisms may be observed.

In X-linked agammaglobulinemia (Bruton's disease) the concentrations of all serum immunoglobulins are decreased markedly. Although normal numbers of pre-B cells exist in the marrow, plasma cells are nonexistent in lymphoid tissues. As one would expect, there is defective opsonization and phagocytosis of cells. Recurrent infections with encapsulated organisms (*S pneumoniae, H influenzae, N meningitidis*) and *P aeruginosa* are common, and disease caused by these organisms may rapidly overwhelm the host. Infections with viral or parasitic agents have been reported, including vaccine-associated polio, enterovirus encephalitis or arthritis, *Giardia* diarrhea, and *Pneumocystis carinii* pneumonia.

Half of patients with selective IgA deficiency have recurrent infections, and about 25% have a collagen-vascular disease. Selective IgA deficiency can be an autosomal recessive or autosomal dominant inherited disorder, and patients usually have a deficiency of both secretory and serum IgA. IgA normally is secreted into the respiratory and gastrointestinal systems. The absence of secretory IgA is associated with recurrent progressive respiratory infections. The most common agents encountered are *H influenzae* and *S pneumoniae*. The occurrence of IgG subclass deficiency in association with partial or complete IgA deficiency has recently been described and may explain why some patients with IgA deficiency experience more sinopulmonary infections than others.

DiGeorge syndrome, or thymic aplasia, predictably results in T-cell defects but no impairment of serum immunoglobulin production or T cell-independent antibody responses. Patients with this syndrome have an increased susceptibility to a wide variety of organisms including *S pneumoniae, H influenzae, Mycobacterium tuberculosis, Listeria monocytogenes* (facultative intracellular organisms), *Nocardia asteroides*, viruses (CMV, measles, varicella-zoster, vaccinia), and fungi (*Cryptococcus neoformans, Histoplasma capsulatum*).

## Combined Immunodeficiencies

Severe combined immunodeficiency disease refers to an X-linked recessive disorder with a severe deficiency in the activity of the T- and B-cell systems. The clinical features characteristically associated with severe deficiency of both T and B cells include failure to thrive, morbilliform rash in the first few days of life, chronic oral thrush, intractable diarrhea, alopecia, and fulminant or prolonged pneumonia (most often due to *P carinii*). Fatal infections with varicella-zoster, herpes simplex, or CMV are common. Other findings include skin and joint laxity, large umbilical hernias, and hematologic abnormalities. Bone marrow transplantation has been successful in restoring T- and B-cell lineages. Both HLA-compatible and HLA-incompatible bone marrow transplants have been attempted.

*Common variable immunodeficiency syndrome* is the term used to describe a group of autosomal recessively inherited disorders with a variable degree of activity of T and B cells. Usual symptoms vary from frequent but mild upper respiratory tract infections to more serious systemic disease.

Orotic aciduria, adenosine deaminase deficiency, and purine nucleotide phosphorylase deficiency are disorders of DNA metabolism carrying a predisposition to opportunistic infections. Patients with purine nucleotide phosphorylase deficiency are predominantly susceptible to fatal viral infections. A drastic T-cell paucity is present despite normal B-cell numbers and immunoglobulin.

Defective vitamin $B_{12}$ intracellular transport results in megaloblastic anemia in infancy of those patients with transcobalamin II deficiency. Progressively impaired B-cell differentiation occurs with resultant agammaglobulinemia.

Cell-mediated immunity is altered in some patients with multiple biotin-dependent carboxylase deficiency.

### Wiskott-Aldrich Syndrome

Patients with Wiskott-Aldrich syndrome, an X-linked recessive disorder, have thrombocytopenia, upper respiratory tract infections (sinusitis, otitis media), and eczema. Antibody production in response to carbohydrate antigens is impaired. Progressive T-cell dysfunction is evident as the disease evolves. Leukemia or Hodgkin's disease frequently complicates the syndrome. Recurrent infection due to bacterial and viral agents is noted and accounts for two thirds of all deaths.

### Ataxia Telangiectasia

Clinical findings in ataxia telangiectasia include cerebellar ataxia, developmental arrest at 10 years of age, drooling, and telangiectasias of the sclera, ear, lateral aspect of the nose, and antecubital and popliteal fossae.

T-cell deficiency (primarily helper cells) with deficiency of one or more of the immunoglobulins or subclasses (repaired in vitro with addition of T-helper cells) and recurrent sinopulmonary infections are noted. The T-cell defect may be related to an immature thymus gland. Patients often have auto-antibodies to immunoglobulin G. Tumors, particularly of the lymphoreticular system, are the most common cause of death.

## Acquired Immunodeficiency Syndrome

Opportunistic infection is common in children with AIDS due to infection with HIV or other retroviruses. AIDS is acquired in children by blood or blood-product transfusion (hemophiliacs), vertical transmission (baby of a mother with HIV infection), sexual contact with an infected partner, transplantation of an infected donor organ, or intravenous drug abuse.

HIV-1 and HIV-2 (formerly HTLV-III or LAV) are known to infect a particular subset of T lymphocytes, the T4 lymphocyte, as a result of the interaction between the virus and a specific receptor on the cell surface. Abnormal but increased production of serum immunoglobulins, inability to make antibody to new antigens, delayed T-cell responses to mitogens or antigens, impaired release of interleukin-2, and difficulties in monocytic ability to process antigen or interact with T cells are noted.

In children with AIDS, the major opportunistic infections noted are pneumonia, meningitis, encephalitis, esophagitis, enterocolitis, and mucocutaneous herpes infection. Table 55-5 lists agents of opportunistic infections in patients with AIDS. Malignant neoplasms such as Burkitt's lymphoma, diffuse undifferentiated non-Hodgkin's lymphoma, or Kaposi's sarcoma may further impair the patient's immune status.

Many patients with AIDS present with symptoms of opportunistic infection. They also may present with failure to thrive, chronic interstitial pneumonitis, hepatosplenomegaly, fever, generalized adenopathy, thrombocytopenia, protracted or recurrent diarrhea, developmental delay, or microcephaly. Immunization of children who have AIDS with live-virus vaccines is not recommended.

## Malignancy

The occurrence of opportunistic infections in these patients is related to the type of malignancy, the stage of disease, and the status of the immune system during and after treatment. For example, a patient undergoing bone marrow transplantation can be expected to pass through a predictable pattern of susceptibility to infectious agents. Initially, granulocytopenia and mucosal damage result in bacterial and fungal infections in the pretransplantation and immediate posttransplantation period. Cellular immune deficiency in the initial postengraftment period results

### TABLE 55-5.    Reported Agents Responsible for Opportunistic Infection in Patients With AIDS

**Viruses**

Herpes simplex (types 1 and 2)
Cytomegalovirus
Varicella
Adenovirus
Epstein-Barr
Hepatitis B
Polyoma

**Fungi**

*Candida albicans*
*Cryptococcus neoformans*
*Histoplasma capsulatum*

**Protozoa**

*Pneumocystis carinii*
*Toxoplasma gondii*
*Isospora* spp. (including *Cryptosporidium*)
*Giardia lamblia*
*Entamoeba histolytica*
*Nocardia* spp.

**Other Microorganisms**

*Mycobacteria*
*M tuberculosis*
*M avium-intracellulare*
*M kansasii*

*Spirochetes*
*Treponema* spp. (including *T pallidum*)

*Bacteria*
*Campylobacter* spp.
*Legionella* spp.
*Neisseria* spp. (including *N gonorrhoeae*)
*Shigella* spp.
*Salmonella* spp.
*Streptococcus pneumoniae*
*Staphylococcus aureus*
Various gram-negative organisms

in infections due to *P carinii* and CMV. Infections with *S pneumoniae* are more common a year or more after the transplant because previous antibody made by prior exposure is depleted and not renewed. Patients with lymphomas treated with radiation have a high risk of developing infections due to varicella-zoster virus during the year following immunosuppression.

Children with leukemia are particularly susceptible to gram-negative organisms. Patients with solid tumors have the lowest risk of infection. Children in relapse from leukemia are susceptible to bacterial and fungal infections, whereas those children in remission are infected with *P carinii* and *Toxoplasma gondii*.

Almost any procedure such as bladder catheterization, transfusion, intubation, broad antibiotic coverage, or surgery in a patient with cancer carries more risk than for the patient who does not have cancer. In all patients, the most important factor is the peripheral granulocyte count. Granulocytopenia (<1000/mm³) has been associated with an increased fatality rate and an increase in culture-positive bacteremia. Despite normal numbers of granulocytes, children with malignancy (Hodgkin's and myelocytic leukemias) may have impaired chemotaxis or digestive capacity of neutrophils. Defects of T-cell function have been observed

(especially in lymphoma) and may be responsible for the increased incidence of viral and fungal infections. Patients with prolonged fever often have fungal infections. Common viral infections (chicken pox, herpes simplex) carry increased morbidity and mortality in patients with malignancy.

## Immunosuppression

In general, the immunosuppressed host is infected with aerobic gram-negative organisms (*E coli, P aeruginosa,* and *Klebsiella, Acinetobacter, Serratia* and *Proteus* spp.) more frequently than with aerobic or anaerobic gram-positive organisms. Viral infections with herpes simplex, varicella-zoster, CMV, EBV, and measles are common. Infections due to saprophytic molds such as *Fusarium solani, Paecilomyces lilacinus, Aspergillus* spp., Zygomycetes (including *Mucor, Rhizomucor, Rhizopus, Absidia, Apophysomyces,* and *Cunninghamella* spp.), *Penicillium, Alternaria, Exophiala, Wangiella,* and *Drechslera* spp. are becoming more common. Infections due to *Acanthameba* spp. also have been reported to be increased in patients treated with corticosteroids, radiotherapy, or chemotherapy. Granulomatous encephalitis is the usual in-

**TABLE 55-6. Opportunistic Infection in Apparently Normal Children**

| Organism | Frequent Type of Infection | Suggested Treatment |
|---|---|---|
| *Actinomyces israelii* | Cellulitis, pneumonia, osteomyelitis | Penicillin; alternate: tetracycline |
| *Aeromonas hydrophila* | Abscesses, cellulitis, diarrhea, peritonitis, pneumonia, septicemia, urinary tract infection | Chloramphenicol, gentamicin, kanamycin |
| *Alcaligenes fecalis* | Abscesses, cellulitis, otitis media, septicemia | Chloramphenicol, gentamicin, kanamycin |
| *Bacteroides* spp. | Abscesses, peritonitis, septicemia | Chloramphenicol; alternate: clindamycin |
| *Fusobacterium gonidiaformans* | Peritonsillitis, subdural empyema | Penicillin; alternates: tetracycline, erythromycin |
| *Bacillus subtilis* | Abscess, cellulitis, conjunctivitis, septicemia | Penicillin; alternate: chloramphenicol |
| *Chromobacterium* spp. | Abscess | Carbenicillin—sensitivity varies and should be checked |
| Diphtheroid | Endocarditis, meningitis | Penicillin; alternate: erythromycin |
| *Aerococcus* | Meningitis | Penicillin |
| *Haemophilus parainfluenzae* | Endocarditis, meningitis, otitis media, septicemia | Ampicillin; alternate: chloramphenicol |
| Hepatitis B group | Brain abscess, cellulitis, meningitis, otitis media, pneumonia | Chloramphenicol, tetracycline; alternate: ampicillin—sensitivity varies |
| *Lactobacillus* spp. | Lung abscess | Check sensitivities |
| *Mimeae; Moraxella, Acinetobacter* spp. | Cellulitis, conjunctivitis, endocarditis, meningitis, pneumonia, septicemia, septic arthritis, stomatitis | Gentamicin; alternate: kanamycin; oxidase-positive strains may be sensitive to penicillin |
| Nonpathogenic *Neisseria* spp. | Meningitis, septicemia, otitis media | Penicillin, ampicillin |
| *Nocardia* spp. | Osteomyelitis, pneumonia, septicemia | Sulfonamides or sulfonamides plus penicillin |
| Nonpathogenic *Pasteurella* spp. | Brain abscess, meningitis | Penicillin, chloramphenicol |
| Pseudomonads | Abscesses, otitis media, pneumonia, septicemia | According to sensitivity studies |
| *Serratia* spp. | Diarrhea, pneumonia, otitis media, osteomyelitis | Gentamicin; alternate: kanamycin or chloramphenicol according to sensitivity studies |
| Nonpathogenic *Spirillum* spp. | Septicemia | Penicillin; alternate: tetracycline or chloramphenicol |
| *Staphylococcus epidermidis* | Meningitis, otitis media, osteomyelitis, septic arthritis, septicemia, urinary tract infection | Penicillin, or semisynthetic penicillin derivative if strain resistant to penicillin |
| Nonhemolytic streptococci | Abscess, cellulitis, endocarditis, gingivitis, pneumonia | Penicillin; alternate: erythromycin, ampicillin, or penicillin plus streptomycin |
| *Vibrio* spp. | Abscess, pneumonia, septic arthritis | Chloramphenicol |
| *Aspergillus* spp. | Abscess, endocarditis, pneumonia, osteomyelitis | Amphotericin B |
| Cryptococcacea | Oropharyngeal candidiasis, pneumonia, meningitis | Amphotericin B |

*Feigin RD, Shearer WT. Opportunistic infection in children. J Pediatr 1975;87:852.*

TABLE 55-7. Selected Prophylactic Treatment Regimens Useful in Children With Disorders in Which the Immune System Is Compromised

| Predisposing Cause | Opportunistic Organisms Isolated Most Frequently | Prophylactic Regimen* | Comments |
|---|---|---|---|
| Chronic granulomatous disease; leukocyte glucose-6-phosphate dehydrogenase deficiency | Gram-negative enteric organisms; staphylococci; *Serratia* and *Nocardia* spp. | Sulfisoxazole, 50 mg/kg/day (1.4 g/m²/day) bid PO | No controlled trials have been performed. |
| Job syndrome | *Staphylococcus aureus* | Dicloxacillin, 25 mg/kg/day q 12 h PO (700 mg/m²/day in 2 daily doses) | No controlled trials have been performed. |
| Chédiak-Higashi syndrome, neutropenia | Pyogenic infection | Dicloxacillin, 25 mg/kg/day q 12 h PO (700 mg/m²/day in 2 daily doses) or penicillin V, 250 mg bid PO | Choice of regimen depends on sensitivities of organisms with which patient has been infected. |
| Complement deficiency syndromes | *Streptococcus pneumoniae, Streptococcus pyogenes, Neisseria meningitidis* | Penicillin V, 250 mg bid PO; pneumococcal vaccine; meningococcal vaccines | |
| Sickle-cell anemia | Influenza virus; *S pneumoniae, Haemophilus influenzae; Salmonella, Shigella,* and *Mycoplasma* spp. | Amoxicillin, or penicillin 20 mg/kg/day (560 mg/m²/day) bid PO; pneumococcal vaccine; annual influenza virus vaccine | |
| Humoral immunodeficiency | Encapsulated microorganisms (*S pneumoniae, S aureus, H influenzae, N meningitidis, Pseudomonas aeruginosa*) | Maintenance γ-globulin, 0.7 mL/kg | Chronic recurrent respiratory disease demands vigorous attention to postural drainage. In selected cases such as recurrent or chronic pulmonary infections or otitis media, prophylactic administration of ampicillin or penicillin is recommended. |
| Cellular and combined immunodeficiency syndromes | Encapsulated microorganisms (*S pneumoniae, H influenzae*); facultative organisms (*Mycobacterium tuberculosis, Listeria monocytogenes*); viruses (CMV, measles, VZV, EBV, influenza virus); fungi (*Cryptococcus neoformans, Histoplasma capsulatum, Candida* spp.); *Pneumocystis carinii, Nocardia asteroides* | 1. Trimethoprim, 2 mg/kg/day (56 mg/m²/day), and sulfamethoxazole, 10 mg/kg/day (280 mg/m²/day) bid PO; *or* nonabsorbable antibiotics: vancomycin, 20–40 mg/kg/day (560–1120 mg/m²/day) q 6 h; *or* gentamicin, 7.5 mg/kg/day (210 mg/m²/day) q 8 h; *or* polymyxin B, 2.5–4.0 mg/kg/day q 6 h PO<br>2. Isoniazid, 10 mg/kg/day (max 300 mg)<br>3. Immune globulin, 0.25 mg/kg up to 15 mL IM within 6 days of exposure to measles<br>4. Varicella-zoster immune globulin, 125 U/10 kg up to 625 U IM within 5 days of exposure<br>5. Amantadine, 1–9 years: 4.4–8.8 mg/kg/day (125–250 mg/m²/day) q 12 h PO (max 150 mg/day); 9–12 years: 100 mg q 12 h PO<br>6. Maintenance γ-globulin, 0.7 mL/kg/month | 1. Trimethoprim-sulfamethoxazole combination is used for prophylaxis against both bacterial and infection with *Pneumocystis*.<br>2. Nonabsorbable antibiotics are most useful in protected environment in preparation for bone marrow transplant in certain intestinal infections.<br>3. Isoniazid is indicated for patients with positive skin test results or with significant exposure; in these syndromes, option for treatment is suggested.<br>4. Gamma globulin is added in combined immunodeficiency syndromes.<br>5. Patients receiving pentamidine by aerosol remain susceptible to disseminated *Pneumocystis* infection. |
| Malignancy, active immunosuppression and transplant recipients | **Bacteria:** Streptococci, *P aeruginosa* and other pseudomonads, *Escherichia coli, S aureus, Staphylococcus epidermidis; Serratia* spp., other gram-negative bacilli, *Bacteriodes* spp. and other anaerobes, *Enterobacter, Klebsiella, Proteus,* and *Listeria* spp.; diphtheroids<br>**Viruses:** VZV, CMV, HSV, HAV, HBV, EBV, adenoviruses, measles, influenza viruses | 1. Trimethoprim, 5 mg/kg/day (56 mg/m²/day), *and* sulfamethoxazole, 30 mg/kg/day (280 mg/m²/day) bid PO; *or* nonabsorbable antibiotics: vancomycin, 20–40 mg/kg/day (560–1120 mg/m²/day) q 6 h; *or* gentamicin, 7.5 mg/kg/day (210 mg/m²/day) q 8 h; *or* polymyxin B, 2.5–4 mg/kg/day (70–112 mg/m²/day) q 6 h PO<br>2. Pneumococcal vaccine | 1. Trimethoprim-sulfamethoxazole given during periods of granulocytopenia; oral prophylaxis effective in combination with regimen of protected environment; several oral regimens have been used.<br>2. Pneumococcal vaccines are given at the time of diagnosis and at least 10 days before chemotherapy for patients with Hodgkin's disease. |

TABLE 55-7.    (Continued)

| Opportunistic Organisms Isolated Predisposing Cause | Most Frequently | Prophylactic Regimen* | Comments |
|---|---|---|---|
| | **Fungi:** *C. neoformans, Candida albicans* and other *Candida* spp., *Aspergillus* spp.<br>**Protozoa:** *P carinii, Toxoplasma gondii* | 3. Isoniazid, 10 mg/kg/day (max 300 mg)<br>4. Varicella-zoster immune globulin, 125 U/10 kg up to 625 U IM within 5 days of exposure<br>5. Acyclovir, 15–45 mg/kg/day (420–1350 mg/m²/day) q 8 h IV for 18 days after induction of immunosuppression<br>6. Immune globulin, 0.25 mg/kg up to 15 mL IM within 6 days of exposure<br>7. Annual vaccination with influenza virus; amantadine, 1–9 years: 4.4–8.8 mg/kg/day (125–250 mg/m²/day) q 12 h PO (max, 150 mg/day); 9–12 years; 100 mg q 12 h PO<br>8. Amphotericin B, 1.0 mg/kg/day (56–225 mg/m²/day q.i.d. PO; *or* ketoconazole, 3.3–6.6 mg/kg/day (90–180 mg/m²/day); PO; *or* miconazole, 20–40 mg/kg/day (560–1120 mg/m²/day) qid PO<br>9. Pentamidine 4 mg/kg IV or by aerosol once monthly | Antipneumococcal prophylaxis for postsplenectomy is given during the period of chemotherapy and at least 3 years thereafter.<br>3. For patients with positive tuberculin skin test results and normal chest radiographs during prolonged periods of corticosteroid or immunosuppressive therapy<br>4. For immunocompromised patients known or likely to be susceptible with close or prolonged exposure to VZV; time after exposure may be extended in special circumstances.<br>5. Acyclovir is given to bone marrow recipients seropositive for antibodies to HSV.<br>6. Influenza vaccine is not indicated routinely; amantadine is reserved for high-risk patients.<br>7. Prophylaxis against fungal disease for this indication is not recommended routinely; it is most likely to be of significant benefit in neutropenic patients.<br>8. Pentamidine usually provided as secondary prophylaxis |
| Cystic fibrosis | Respiratory viruses; pseudomonads; *S aureus*, nontypable *Haemophilus* spp. | Cephalexin, 20 mg/kg/day; amantadine, 6 mg/kg/day (168 mg/m²/day); annual influenza virus vaccine | Cephalexin is of demonstrated benefit on short-term basis in patients not colonized with pseudomonads. Patient-specific prophylactic antimicrobial therapy based on sputum culture is under investigation. |
| Chronic renal disease | Influenza virus, *S pneumoniae* | Penicillin V, 250 mg bid PO; pneumococcal vaccine; annual influenza virus vaccine. | |

* Consult drug product information sheets (package inserts) and other sources for more complete data.
*CMV*, cytomegalovirus; *EBV*, Epstein-Barr virus; *HAV*, hepatitis A virus; *HBV*, hepatitis B virus; *HSV*, herpes simplex virus; *VZV*, varicella-zoster virus.

Feigin RD, Matson DO. Opportunistic infections, the compromised host. In: Feigin RD, Cherry JD, eds. *Textbook of pediatric infectious diseases, ed 3.* Philadelphia: WB Saunders, 1992:978.

fectious presentation of *Acanthameba* organisms in the immunosuppressed host.

Bacterial pneumonia and intrathoracic infections are common problems in patients receiving cyclosporine A after heart transplantation. Infections with CMV, EBV, and herpes simplex virus also occur; fungal and protozoan infections are less common. Posttransplant CMV infections may be acquired from donor organ, donor blood, or nosocomial sources. Patients with primary CMV infection have a more difficult course than those in whom infection has been reactivated. Superinfection with bacteria, fungi, or protozoan organisms may occur in cardiac patients infected with CMV; however, infection due to *Coccidioides immitis* is rare in patients with transplants receiving cyclosporine A, presumably because of its antifungal activity.

Recipients of renal transplants often have urinary tract infections. CMV infection is also common. Respiratory virus infections,

wound and skin infections, and local fungal infections are less common.

Cyclosporine inhibits interleukin-2 production by T-helper cell populations, which in turn impairs B-cell activation and cytolytic T-cell generation and impedes expansion of T-helper/inducer cell populations. In contrast, cyclosporine has no effect on mature granulocytes.

Steroids impair inflammation by blocking the action of migratory inhibiting factor and chemotactic factors. They decrease lymph node size, cause thymic involution, suppress production and activity of interleukin-1 (which stimulates T cells to release interleukin-2), and thereby impair lymphocyte function. Steroids also interfere with the function of polymorphonuclear leukocytes. Patients receiving corticosteroids and other immunosuppressive agents are particularly susceptible to reactivation of tuberculosis and latent viral infections (herpesvirus, papovavirus, CMV, EBV).

TABLE 55-8. Selected Prophylactic Treatment Regimens Useful When Indicated for Surgery or When Disruption of the Skin or Mucous Membrane Barriers to Infection Occurs*

| Predisposing Cause | Prophylactic Regimen | Comments |
|---|---|---|
| **Congenital or Acquired Cardiac Defects** | | |
| Dental and other procedures of upper respiratory tract | 1. Usual regimen: Amoxicillin 50 mg/kg (1400 mg/m²) PO 1 h before procedure, then 25 mg/kg (700 mg/m²) 6 h after initial dose, *or* ampicillin 50 mg/kg (1400 mg/m²) IV or IM 30 min before procedure, then 25 mg/kg (700 mg/m²) IV or IM (or amoxicillin PO) 6 h after initial dose<br>2. With amoxicillin/penicillin allergy: erythromycin ethylsuccinate, 20 mg/kg (560 mg/m²) PO *or* clindamycin 10 mg/kg (280 mg/m²) PO or IV, before procedure, then half the dose 6 h after initial dose.<br>3. With high risk (eg, cardiovascular prosthesis): ampicillin 50 mg/kg (1400 mg/m²) plus gentamicin 2.0–2.5 mg/kg (55–70 mg/m²) IV or IM 30 min before procedure, then amoxicillin 50 mg/kg (1400 mg/m²) alone 6 h or repeat of parenteral combination 8 h after initial dose<br>4. With high risk and ampicillin/amoxicillin/penicillin allergy: vancomycin 20 mg/kg (560 mg/m²) IV over 1 h, beginning 1 h before procedure | IM injections should be avoided in patients receiving anticoagulants. |
| Gastrointestinal or genitourinary tract surgery or instrumentation | 1. Amoxicillin 50 mg/kg (1400 mg/m²) PO 1 h or combination of ampicillin 50 mg/kg (1400 mg/m²) and gentamicin 2.0–2.5 mg/kg (55–70 mg/m²) IV or IM 30 min before procedure, then amoxicillin 50 mg/kg (1400 mg/m²) alone 6 h or repeat of parenteral combination 8 h after initial dose<br>2. With ampicillin/amoxicillin/penicillin allergy: vancomycin 20 mg/kg (560 mg/m²) IV over 1 h plus gentamicin 2.0–2.5 mg/kg (55–70 mg/m²) IV or IM 1 h before procedure and 8 h after initial dose | |
| **General Surgery** | | |
| Head and neck | Ampicillin 20 mg/kg (560 mg/m²) q 4 hr IV, or cefazolin 12.5 mg/kg (350 mg/m²) q 6 h IV, with first dose 30–60 min before procedure, to be given for 2 days | |
| Cardiovascular | Oxacillin 50 mg/kg (1.4 g/m²) q 4–6 h IV, *or* cefazolin 12.5 mg/kg (350 mg/m²) q 6 h IV, *or* vancomycin 20 mg/kg (560 mg/m²) q 6 h IV, with first dose 30–60 min before procedure, to be continued for 2 days | |
| Gastroduoenal with preexisting abnormal gastric motility | Cefazolin 12.5 mg/kg (350 mg/m²) q 6 h IV, with first dose 30–60 min before procedure, to be continued for 2 days | |
| Biliary tract obstructive disease | Cefazolin 12.5 mg/kg q 6 h IV, or gentamicin 2.5 mg/kg q 8 h IV, with first dose 30–60 min before procedure, to be continued for 2 days | Recommended only for patients with acute cholecystitis or ductal obstruction |
| Colon | Oral: Erythromycin 15–50 mg/kg (420–1400 mg/m²) and neomycin 25 mg/kg (700 mg/m²) PO, given at 1 p.m., 2 p.m., and 11 p.m. the day before the procedure<br>Parenteral: Cefazolin 12.5 mg/kg (350 mg/m²) q 6 h IV or cefoxitin 40 mg/kg (1120 mg/m²) q 4–6 h IV, or metronidazole 15–50 mg/kg/day (420–1400 mg/m²/day) q 6 h IV | Oral antibiotics are part of preparative program lasting over several days; parenteral medication given in cases of emergency surgery or when enteral route is prohibited. In cases of "dirty surgery," antibiotic therapy should be continued for full therapeutic period. |
| Elective splenectomy | Pneumococcal vaccine before procedure | |
| Orthopedic | Cefazolin 12.5 mg/kg (350 mg/m²) q 6 h IV or vancomycin 20 mg/kg (560 mg/m²) q 6 h IV, with first dose 30–60 min before procedure, to be continued for 2 days | For internal fixation of fractures or placement of other devices |
| CSF shunts | Methicillin, oxacillin, or nafcillin, 100–200 mg/kg/day (2.8–5.6 g/m²/day) q 4–6 h IV or cefazolin 50 mg/kg/day (1400 mg/m²/day) q 6 h IV, to be given for 2 days; first dose 30–60 min before procedure | |
| Urinary tract obstructive lesions | Trimethoprim 2 mg/kg (56 mg/m²) and sulfamethoxazole, 10 mg/kg (280 mg/m²) qid PO 3 day/wk, or ampicillin 20 mg/kg (560 mg/m²) qid PO, or nitrofurantoin 2 mg/kg/day (56 mg/m²/day) q.d. PO | |

| TABLE 55-8. *(Continued)* | | |
|---|---|---|
| Predisposing Cause | Prophylactic Regimen | Comments |
| Cleft palate | Sulfisoxazole 50 mg/kg/day (1.4 g/m²/day) bid. PO, or ampicillin 20 mg/kg (560 mg/m²) qid. PO, or trimethoprim 2 mg/kg (56 mg/m²) and sulfamethoxazole 10 mg/kg (280 mg/m²) qid. PO | |
| Burns | Penicillin 50,000 U/kg/day (1.4 U/m²/day) q 4 h IV or q 6 h PO, plus 0.5% silver nitrate solution or 10% mafenide acetate cream to area of burn with dressing changes | |

\* See Table 55-7 for organisms isolated most frequently and for suggested mechanisms by which infection may be initiated.

Consult drug product information sheets (package inserts) and other sources for more complete data.

Feigin RD, Matson DO. Opportunistic infections, the compromised host. In: Feigin RD, Cherry JD, eds. Textbook of pediatric infectious diseases, ed 3. Philadelphia: WB Saunders, 1991:980.

Patients treated with ionizing radiation and antilymphocyte globulin also are at increased risk of opportunistic infection.

Chemotherapeutic agents suppress replication of cells. Cell populations undergoing rapid turnover and DNA synthesis, such as those in bone marrow and intestine, are particularly susceptible. The greatest risk factor for infection in patients receiving chemotherapeutic agents is granulocytopenia. In addition, primary and secondary antibody responses may be suppressed, and delayed hypersensitivity may be affected.

## Transplantation

Since the advent of cyclosporine and other immunosuppressive agents, the use of transplantation in the management of end-stage disease has become more common. The use of immunosuppressive agents increases the risk of opportunistic infection in these patients. In addition, the process of transplantation itself predisposes the patient to infection, particularly with viruses.

Bone marrow transplant patients are at risk for infection with all classes of organisms. In general, the period when granulocytopenia is most likely is early (1 to 2 weeks) after transplantation, whereas decreased humoral antibody production and decreased cellular immunity is impaired later (1 to 3 months after transplantation). Infections caused by bacteria and fungi occur early in the pretransplantation and posttransplantation period. CMV and *P carinii* infections occur in the initial postengraftment period. *S pneumoniae* infections are common a year or more after the transplant because prior antibody is depleted and not renewed.

Infections associated with renal and heart transplants have become less common in recent years for four reasons: the use of less toxic immunosuppression regimens, effective screening of blood products for hepatitis B and HIV, closer tissue matching (decreased rejection), and antimicrobial prophylaxis.

CMV infection is common in all transplant recipients and may be the cause of unexplained pneumonia with or without obstructive airway disease. CMV infection also may alter T-cell function and be associated with decreased renal function.

## Protein-Calorie Malnutrition, Vitamin Deficiency, and Specific Metal Deficiencies

Children with protein-calorie malnutrition are susceptible to disseminated infections with measles, herpes simplex, bacteria, and parasites. Diarrhea, pneumonia, urinary tract infection, tuberculosis, and gram-negative infections predominate. The susceptibility to infection is higher in infants born to nutritionally deprived mothers. Continued malnutrition is associated with alterations of the skin or mucosal barriers to infection, or alterations in the immune system that predispose to infection.

Atrophy or deterioration of skin and mucous membranes and immunologic components contained therein may be noted in the following nutritional deficiency syndromes:

Avitaminosis A—hyperkeratosis
Riboflavin and pyridoxine deficiency—dermatitis, cheilitis, and angular stomatitis
Pellagra—mucosal atrophy and dermatitis
Kwashiorkor—atrophy of skin and gastrointestinal mucosa
Scurvy—spongy gums and subcutaneous hemorrhages.

Malnutrition also may be associated with decreased secretory IgA, decreased complement and complement-derived chemotactic factors, decreased cellular immunity coincident with decreased T-cell numbers, decreased intracellular bacterial killing, and decreased chemokinesis of phagocytes.

Viral infections may be more severe in malnourished children than in healthy children. Septicemia is common and usually is caused by gram-negative bacteria.

The role of iron in host resistance to infection depends in large part on the individual's ability to use or sequester it from use by pathogens.

## Cystic Fibrosis

Patients with cystic fibrosis primarily experience respiratory tract infections. *S aureus* and mucoid *P aeruginosa* (and *P cepacia*) are isolated frequently from sputum cultures of these patients. Other organisms isolated commonly include anaerobes, atypical mycobacteria, and *H influenzae*. The humoral and cellular immune systems of these patients are normal. A factor present in the serum of patients with cystic fibrosis may inhibit ciliary motility. The precise mechanism underlying persistent colonization with pseudomonads in the pathology of cystic fibrosis is unknown.

## Diabetes Mellitus

Children and adults with diabetes mellitus have decreased resistance to bacterial and fungal infections. The response of the diabetic patient to infection is impaired. Sluggish polymorphonuclear leukocyte response to infection, ineffective phagocytosis, poor fibroblast proliferation, decreased opsonizing capacity of serum, and decreased chemotactic activity have been observed in juvenile diabetics.

TABLE 55-9. Selected Agents Useful in Treating Severe Bacterial Infections in Immunocompromised Children

| Agent | Dose* | Usual Susceptible Organisms | Comments |
|---|---|---|---|
| Amikacin | 15–40 mg/kg/day (420–1100 mg/m²/day) q 8 h IM or IV (30-minute infusion) | *Pseudomonas aeruginosa, Escherichia coli, Klebsiella pneumoniae; Proteus, Providencia, Serratia, Acinetobacter,* and *Enterobacter* spp., nontuberculous mycobacteria, resistant *M tuberculosis* | Blood levels 1 hour and 8 hours (peak and trough) after administration are necessary to ensure adequate concentration without toxicity.† |
| Ampicillin | 100–300 mg/kg/day (2.8–8.4 g/m²/day) q 4 h IM or IV (5-minute infusion) | Salmonellae, enterococci; *Listeria monocytogenes, E coli, Proteus mirabilis, Haemophilus influenzae; Shigella* spp. | When given in conjunction with an aminoglycoside, synergism frequently occurs. |
| Carbenicillin | 200–500 mg/kg/day (5.6–14.0 g/m²/day) q 4 h IV (5-minute infusion) | *Bacteroides* spp. and other anaerobes; with gentamicin, amikacin, or tobramycin for *P aeruginosa* and other gram-negative bacilli | Should always be used in conjunction with an aminoglycoside antibiotic |
| Cefazolin | 25–50 mg/kg/day (0.7–1.4 g/m²/day) q 6 h IM or IV (5-minute infusion) | Gram-negative bacilli, *Staphylococcus aureus* | When given in conjunction with an aminoglycoside, synergism frequently occurs. |
| Chloramphenicol | 50–100 mg/kg/day (1.4–2.8 g/m²/day) q 6 h PO or IV (30-minute infusion) | Anaerobes, gram-negative bacilli, salmonellae, *H influenzae, Shigella* spp. | |
| Clindamycin | 10–40 mg/kg/day (280–1120 mg/m²/day) q 6 h IM or IV (30-minute infusion) | Anaerobes | |
| Erythromycin | 30–50 mg/kg/day (840–1400 mg/m²/day) q 6 h PO or IV (1-hour infusion) | Streptococci; *S aureus, Mycoplasma pneumoniae; Chlamydia* and *Legionella* spp. | |
| Ethambutol | 25 mg/kg/day (700 mg/m²/day) for 2 months, then 15 mg/kg/day (420 mg/m²/day) PO | *Mycobacterium* spp. | |
| Ethionamide | 15 mg/kg/day (420 mg/m²/day) (max 500 mg/day) bid PO | *Mycobacterium* spp. | |
| Gentamicin | 5.0–7.5 mg/kg/day (140–210 mg/m²/day) q 8 h IM or IV (30-minute infusion) | *E coli, K pneumoniae, P aeruginosa; Proteus, Providencia, Serratia, Acinetobacter,* and *Enterobacter* spp. | Blood levels 1 hour and 8 hours (peak and trough) after administration are necessary to ensure adequate concentration without toxicity.† |
| Isoniazid | 10–20 mg/kg/day (280–560 mg/m²/day) (max 500 mg/day) PO or IM | *Mycobacterium* spp. | Use in conjunction with ethionamide or rifampin; three-drug therapy with ethambutol, streptomycin, or pyrazinamide.† |
| Kanamycin | 15–20 mg/kg/day (420–560 mg/m²/day) q 8 h IM or IV (30-minute infusion) | *E coli, K pneumoniae; Proteus, Providencia, Serratia, Acinetobacter,* and *Enterobacter* spp. | |
| Metronidazole | 15–50 mg/kg/day (420–1400 mg/m²/day) q 6 h IV | Anaerobes | |
| Nafcillin | 100–200 mg/kg/day (2.8–5.6 g/m²/day) q 4–6 h IM or IV (5-minute infusion) | *S. aureus* | |
| Oxacillin | 100–200 mg/kg/day (2.8–5.6 g/m²/day) q 4–6 h IM or IV (5-minute infusion) | *S. aureus* | |
| Penicillin | 50,000–300,000 U/kg/day (1.4–8.4 million U/m²/day) q 4 h IM or IV (5-minute infusion) | *Streptococci*; oropharyngeal anaerobes; *Streptobacillus moniliformis, Pasteurella multocida; Neisseria* and *Clostridium* spp. | |
| Piperacillin | 200–300 mg/kg/day (5.6–8.4 g/m²/day) q 4 h IV or IM (30-minute infusion) | Anaerobes; pseudomonads, streptococci including enterococci; *K pneumoniae, Enterobacter* and some *Providencia* and *Serratia* spp. | Frequently used in combination with an aminoglycoside |
| Pyrazinamide | 20–30 mg/kg/day 560–840 mg/m²/day) or 20 mg/kg (560 mg/m²) twice weekly PO | *Mycobacterium* spp. | Fourth drug in tuberculous meningitis; used in selected patients with isoniazid-resistant *Mycobacterium tuberculosis* |
| Rifampin | 10–20 mg/kg/day (280–560 mg/m²/day) (max 600 mg/day) | *Mycobacterium* spp., other susceptible organisms | For tuberculosis, use in conjunction with isoniazid or ethionamide; three-drug therapy with streptomycin or ethambutol. |

TABLE 55-9. *(Continued)*

| Agent | Dose* | Usual Susceptible Organisms | Comments |
|---|---|---|---|
| Streptomycin | 15–30 mg/kg/day (420–840 mg/m²/day) IM | *Mycobacterium* spp. | Use in three-drug therapy with isoniazid and rifampin; has synergistic role in therapy of bacterial endocarditis. |
| Tetracycline | 20–40 mg/kg/day (560–1120 mg/m²/day) q 6 h PO or IV (2-hour infusion) | *M pneumoniae;* other susceptible organisms | |
| Tobramycin | 3–5 mg/kg/day (84–140 mg/m²/day) q 8 h IM or IV (30-minute infusion) | *P aeruginosa, E coli, K pneumoniae; Proteus, Providencia, Serratia, Acinetobacter,* and *Enterobacter* spp. | Blood levels 1 hour and 8 hours (peak and trough) after administration are necessary to ensure adequate concentration without toxicity.† |
| Trimethoprim-sulfamethoxazole | Trimethoprim, 10–20 mg/kg/day (280–560 mg/m²/day); sulfamethoxazole, 50–100 mg/kg/day (1.4–2.8 mg/m²/day) q 12 h PO or IV | Salmonellae; *Providencia, Serratia,* and *Shigella* spp. | Useful when organism is resistant to aminoglycosides |
| Trisulfapyrimidines | 120 mg/kg/day (3.4 g/m²/day) q 6 h PO for 4 weeks | *Nocardia* spp. | |
| Vancomycin | 20–40 mg/kg/day (560–120 mg/m²/day) q 6 h IV (30-minute infusion) | *S aureus, Streptococcus* spp. | Oral route restricted to intraintestinal infections. Blood levels 1 hour and 6 hours (peak and trough) after administration are necessary to ensure adequate concentration without toxicity. |

\* Consult drug product information sheets (package inserts) and other sources for more complete administration and toxicity data.

† Patients with cystic fibrosis frequently require higher doses of aminoglycosides to achieve therapeutic blood levels.

Feigin RD, Matson DO. Opportunistic infections, the compromised host. In: Feigin RD, Cherry JD, eds. Textbook of pediatric infectious diseases, ed 3. Philadelphia: WB Saunders, 1992:974.

Pyelonephritis and perinephric abscesses due to *S aureus, S epidermidis, E coli,* and *Proteus, Clostridium,* and *Actinomyces* spp. have been reported. *T glabrata* and *Mucor* and *Candida* spp. infect diabetics more often than they infect normal individuals.

## Other Endocrine Disturbances

Hypoparathyroidism with and without associated polyendocrinopathy may be associated with an increased frequency of infection of the skin, nails, and mucous membranes with *Candida* spp.

## Nephrotic Syndrome

Patients with nephrotic syndrome lose many proteins in the urine, including albumin, IgG, transferrin, and others of low molecular weight. Increased susceptibility to infection, particularly with *S pneumoniae,* probably is related to decreased serum IgG concentration and loss of factor B in the urine (resulting in decreased opsonization). Opportunistic infection also may occur as a result of the risks associated with therapeutic intervention in the disease process (corticosteroids, instrumentation, chemotherapy). Patients develop peritonitis, sepsis, or cellulitis with greater frequency than do normal individuals. Peritonitis is caused primarily by *S pneumoniae,* group A streptococci, and *S aureus.* Other agents include *E coli, Bacteroides* spp., and *H influenzae* type b.

## Uremia

Herpes simplex virus, staphylococci, and *Enterobacter, Serratia, Bacteroides, Candida, Mucor,* and *Pneumocystis* spp. are the primary infectious microorganisms in patients with uremia. Decreased T-cell function (delayed skin tests), abnormal proliferative responses to antigens, decreased granulocyte chemotaxis, and decreased acute inflammatory response have been documented in patients with uremia. Patients with end-stage renal disease have dry, excoriated, pruritic skin and ulcerated mucous membranes that provide a portal of entry for organisms that commonly inhabit the skin.

Patients undergoing peritoneal dialysis are at increased risk of peritonitis. Infections with staphylococci, streptococci, pseudomonads, *Enterobacter* and *Acinetobacter* spp., and fungal organisms have been reported in these patients over the past several years. *C albicans* and *C tropicalis* are the primary fungal pathogens, but infection with *C parapsilosis, Rhodotorula rubra, Fusarium, Drechslera spicifera, T glabrata, Aspergillus flavus, A. fumigatus,* and *Mucor, Candida,* and *Trichosporon* spp. have been described.

Removal of the Tenckhoff catheter increases the likelihood of cure of fungal peritonitis regardless of antifungal antibiotic administration. Previous bacterial peritonitis and prior antibiotic therapy provided within 1 month before development of peritonitis are risk factors in patients who develop fungal peritonitis.

## Miscellaneous

Patients with intestinal lymphangiectasia may have decreased serum immunoglobulin concentrations, lymphopenia, and skin anergy. Persistent giardiasis has been noted in these patients.

Cirrhosis with ascites and hepatic failure predisposes patients to infection. Fulminant hepatic failure or hepatitis also predisposes patients to infection by decreasing serum opsonizing activity as a result of complement deficiency.

**TABLE 55-10.  Agents Useful in Treating Viral Infections in Immunocompromised Children**

| Agent | Dose | Usual Susceptible Viruses | Comments |
|---|---|---|---|
| Acyclovir | 15–45 mg/kg/day (420–1350 mg/m²/day) q 8 h IV for 5–10 days (1-h infusion); 5% ointment 6 times/day for 7 days | HSV, VZV | Oral therapy may be beneficial in certain situations. |
| Amantidine | 1–9 years: 4.4–8.8 mg/kg/day (125–250 mg/m²/day) q 12 h PO (max 150 mg/day); 9–12 years: 100 mg q 12 h PO | Influenza A | Most effective when given within hours of first symptoms |
| Ganciclovir | 7.5 mg/kg/day (210 mg/m²/day) q 8 h IV for 14–30 days | CMV | Symptoms likely to recur when therapy is stopped |
| Idoxuridine | 0.1% solution q 1 h; 0.5% ointment q 4 h | HSV (keratitis) | |
| Methisazone | 200 mg/kg/day (560 mg/m²/day) q 6 h PO (initial dose 200 mg/kg) | Vaccinia | |
| Ribavirin | Ribavirin (Virazole) supplied as 6 g of lyophilized drug per vial; to reconstitute the therapeutic concentration (20 mg of ribavirin/mL of sterile water), add by sterile technique 300 mL of sterile USP water for injection or inhalation. Important: This water should not have any antimicrobial agent or other substance added. Pour solution into clear, sterilized 500-mL wide-mouth Erlenmeyer flask (reservoir). Ribavirin is not to be given with any other device or in conjunction with any other drugs using SPAG-2 aerosol generator. Dose of ribavirin given is controlled by concentration of drug actually aerosolized, by amount of drug retained in lungs, and by time of exposure to aerosol, as shown in the following equation:  Dose = (AC) × (MV) × (t) × (Rf)  Where AC = aerosol drug concentration (ug/mL); MV = patient minute volume (L/min); t = time of exposure (minutes); and Rf = pulmonary retention factor. Using recommended drug concentration of 20 mg/mL of ribavirin as starting solution in drug reservoir of SPAG unit, average aerosol concentration for 12-h period would be 190 ug/L (0.19 mg/L) of air. Pulmonary retention factor has been demonstrated to be 0.70, which will provide retained dose of 50–55 mg/hr of exposure. Usual dose based on exposure to aerosol 12–18 hr/day for at least 3 days; aerosol dose will vary by minute volume and weight. See product insert for additional information. | RSV | Has proved useful in therapy of respiratory syncytial viral infection in children and adults. Has shown efficacy in vitro against influenza, parainfluenza, and measle viruses; clinical studies of this agent for treatment of influenza and parainfluenza viruses are in progress. |
| Rimantidine | 6.6 mg/kg/day (185 mg/m²/day) q 12 h PO for 5 days | Influenza A | Experimental for this indication |
| Trifluridine | 1% solution q 2 h (max 9 drops/eye/24 hr) | HSV (keratitis) | |
| Vidarabine | 15–30 mg/kg/day (420–740 mg/m²/day) IV (12-h infusion) for 10–14 days; 3% ointment, 0.5", 5 times/day for 7 days after complete reepithelialization for HSV keratitis | HSV, VZV | |
| Zidovudine | 3 mg/kg/day (85 mg/m²/day) in 6 doses PO for 1 month, then 1.5 mg/kg/day in 6 doses PO thereafter | HIV-1 | Optimal dosage as yet uncertain; other dideoxy analogues under study |

\* Consult drug product information sheets (package inserts) and other sources for more complete administration and toxicity data.

HSV, herpes simplex virus; RSV, respiratory syncytial virus; SPAG, small particle aerosol generator; VZV, varicella-zoster virus; CMV, cytomegalovirus.

Feigin RD, Matson DO. Opportunistic infections, the compromised host. In: Feigin RD, Cherry JD, eds. Textbook of pediatric infectious diseases, ed 3. Philadelphia: WB Saunders, 1992:976.

Patients with inflammatory bowel disease may present with chronic bacterial or parasitic bowel infections; however, opportunistic infection with *Candida, Aspergillus, Mucor,* and *Pneumocystis* organisms may occur more commonly in patients receiving steroids.

## Prolonged Hospitalization and Prolonged Antibiotic Therapy

Patients who are hospitalized may acquire organisms peculiar to the hospital from contact with fomites, invasive indwelling intravenous or intra-arterial lines, surgery, ventilator support equipment, and staff. The most common mode of transmission is hand to hand. In general, hospital-acquired organisms are more resistant to antibiotics than those acquired from the community.

Treatment with antibiotics changes the microflora of the body, and patients often acquire organisms that are resistant to multiple antibiotics. Attention to spread of infection is particularly important when contacts are made with multiple patients.

## The Neonate

Chemotactic activity of neutrophils is decreased significantly in most newborns, as is their ability to generate chemotactic stimuli. Neutrophils also have poor locomotion to f-met-leu-phe and show decreased adherence. Phagocytosis is thought to be well developed by 32 weeks' gestation, but minor defects in attachment and ingestion can be found if appropriate tests are done. Metabolic

responses to phagocytosis are normal or increased; however, the bactericidal activity of neutrophils from infants under stress at any gestational age may be reduced.

After 16 weeks' gestation, maternal IgG in the fetus rises, and low levels are reached by the fourth to sixth month of gestation. Although the duration of intrauterine life has no effect on the onset of IgG production by the infant, premature infants start life with lower maternally acquired IgG levels. The ability of transplacental IgG to protect the infant is related to its ability to opsonize microorganisms. Other opsonins such as complement are not passed transplacentally. Serum concentrations of opsonins correlate with gestational age. Hemolytic complement and factor B activity in the fetus are about half of maternal concentrations. A direct correlation can be made between concentrations of complement and opsonizing activity in newborn infants.

## Opportunistic Infection in the Apparently Normal Host

Saprophytic microorganisms may cause infection in normal, healthy children. The indigenous flora of the host or organisms commonly found in the environment during the neonatal period carry the greatest risk for infection of the normal individual.

Saprophytic microorganisms that have produced infection in normal children, the types of infection encountered most frequently, and the antibiotic therapy most likely to be effective (to be modified on the basis of specific sensitivity testing) are shown in Table 55-6.

TABLE 55-11. Selected Agents Useful in Treating Fungal Infections in Immunocompromised Children

| Agent | Dose* | Usual Susceptible Fungi | Comments |
|---|---|---|---|
| Amphotericin B | 0.8–1.5 mg/kg/day (22–42 mg/m²/day) q.d. or q.o.d. (4- to 6-h infusion) | *Coccidioides immitis, Cryptococcus neoformans, Histoplasma capsulatum; Mucor, Aspergillus, Blastomyces,* and *Candida* spp. | Initial dose should be 0.25 mg/kg; increase dosage daily over 4 days to 1.0 mg/kg. For fungal meningitis, intrathecal administration may be necessary. In severely ill patients, the first four doses can be given 6 to 12 h apart, then dosing may be adjusted to q 24 h or q 48 h. Serum potassium, BUN, creatinine; hepatic enzymes, and urinalysis should be monitored frequently. |
| Clotrimazole | 1% ointment or solution bid to qid | *Candida* spp. | |
| Fluconazole | 3–6 mg/kg/day (85–170 mg/m²/day) PO qd or IV | *Candida, Cryptococcus* | Primary use is in suppressive therapy. |
| Flucytosine | 50–150 mg/kg/day (1.4–4.2 g/m²/day) q 6 h PO | *C neoformans, Candida* spp. | Use in conjunction with amphotericin B. |
| Ketoconazole | 3.3–6.6 mg/kg/day (100–200 mg/m²/day) q.d. PO | *C immitis, C neoformans, H capsulatum; Blastomyces* and *Candida* spp. | CSF penetration inadequate for treatment of fungal meningitis |
| Miconazole | 20–40 mg/kg/day (600–1200 mg/m²/day) q 8 h IV (30- to 60-min infusion) | *C immitis, C neoformans; Candida* spp. | In treatment of fungal meningitis and cystitis, IV infusion alone is inadequate. |
| Nystatin | Cream, ointment, powder, oral suspension, oral tablets, and vaginal tablets, 100,000–1,000,000 U/day qid | *Candida* spp. | |

* Consult drug product information sheets (package inserts) and other sources for more complete administration and toxicity data.

*Feigin RD, Matson DO. Opportunistic infections, the compromised host. In: Feigin RD, Cherry JD, eds. Textbook of pediatric infectious diseases, ed 3. Philadelphia: WB Saunders, 1992:976.*

# PROPHYLAXIS AND TREATMENT OF OPPORTUNISTIC INFECTIONS

## Prophylaxis

Prophylactic regimens are aimed at four targets: enhancing host defense mechanisms, minimizing damage to mucosal barriers, reducing colonization, and suppressing potentially pathogenic organisms currently colonizing the patient. The most important factor in the prevention of colonization is effective hand-washing by staff.

Tables 55-7 and 55-8 detail selected prophylactic regimens useful in patients when their immune systems are compromised, before surgery, or when skin or mucous membrane barriers are disrupted. In some cases, the efficacy of prophylactic antibiotics is controversial, and a program of therapy for an immunocompromised patient requires considerable attention to detail. Goals of therapy may need to be limited to prevention of infection by only a few organisms. Clear efficacy of antifungal prophylaxis has not been demonstrated.

Patients with malignancy may benefit from administration of trimethoprim-sulfamethoxasole. Although 68 cases were predicted on the basis of previous experience, no cases of pneumocystic pneumonia occurred in 1983 at St. Jude Hospital in Memphis, Tennessee, 4 years after routine antibiotic prophylaxis of all patients on cancer chemotherapy with trimethoprim-sulfamethoxasole was instituted.

**TABLE 55-12.** Selected Agents Useful in Treating Parasitic Infections in Immunocompromised Children

| Agent | Dose | Usual Susceptible Parasites | Comments |
|---|---|---|---|
| Amphotericin B | 1 mg/kg/day (28 mg/m² day) IV | Acanthamoeba and Naegleria spp. | Investigational for this indication |
| Chloroquine phosphate | 10 mg base/kg/day (280 mg/m²/day) PO for 2–3 weeks | Entamoeba histolytica | Maximum dose 300 mg/day in combination therapy |
| Dehydroemetine | 1.0–1.5 mg/kg/day (28–42 mg/m²/day) bid IM, for up to 5 days | E histolytica | Maximum dose 90 mg/day; followed by chloroquine or iodoquinol |
| Emetine | 1 mg/kg/day (28 mg/m²/day) bid IM for up to 5 days | E histolytica | Maximum dose 50 mg/day; followed by chloroquine or iodoquinol |
| Iodoquinol | 30–40 mg/kg/day (0.8–1.1 g/m²/day) tid PO for 20 days | E histolytica and others | Maximum dose 2 g/day; dosage and duration should not be exceeded because of possibility of causing optic neuritis. |
| Mebendazole | 100 mg bid PO for 3 days | Ascaris and others | |
| Metronidazole | 15–50 mg/kg/day (420–1400 mg/m²/day) q 8 h PO | E histolytica, Giardia lamblia | For E histolytica use 50 mg/kg/day; for G lamblia use 15 mg/kg/day. |
| Pentamidine | 4 mg/kg/day IV (112 mg/m²/day) for 14 days | Pneumocystis carinii | |
| Praziquantel | 40 mg/kg/day (112 mg/m²/day) bid PO for 14 days | Cysticercosis, schistosomiasis | Single day for schistosomiasis |
| Pyrantel pamoate | 11 mg/kg/day (310 mg/m²/day) PO for 3 days | Ascaris, hookworm | Single dose for Ascaris |
| Pyrimethamine | 2 mg/kg/day (56 mg/m²/day) for 3 days, then 1 mg/kg/day (28 mg/m²/day) PO | Toxoplasma gondii, Isospora belli | Use with trisulfopyrimidines or sulfodiazine. To prevent hematologic toxicity, give leucovorin 10 mg/day PO or IV; give with triple sulfonamides (150 mg/kg/day q 6 h). For ocular toxoplasmosis, give corticosteroids to reduce ocular inflammation. |
| Quinocrine hydrochloride | 6 mg/kg/day (56 mg/m²/day) t.i.d. PO | G lamblia | Maximum dose 300 mg/day |
| Spiramycin | 50–100 mg/kg/day (1.4–2.8 g/m²/day) PO for 3–4 weeks | T gondii | Use with pyrimethamine |
| Thiobendazole | 50 mg/kg/day (1400 mg/m²/day) bid PO for 2–5 days | Creeping eruption, Strongyloides | |
| Trimethoprim-sulfamethoxazole | Trimethoprim, 20 mg/kg/day (560 mg/m²/day); sulfamethoxasole, 100 mg/kg/day (2.8 g/m²/day) q 6 h PO or IV | I belli, P carinii | For Isospora, quadruple dose for 10 days, then double dose for 3 weeks |
| Trisulfapyrimidines | 100–200 mg/kg/day (2.8 to 5.6 g/m²/day) q 6 h PO for 4 weeks | T gondii | Use with pyrimethamine |

\* Consult drug product information sheets (package inserts) and other sources for more complete administration and toxicity data.

Feigin RD, Matson DO. Opportunistic infections, the compromised host. In: Feigin RD, Cherry JD, eds. Textbook of pediatric infectious diseases, ed 3. Philadelphia: WB Saunders, 1992:977.

Nafcillin or oxacillin administration may help prevent staphylococcal infection of prosthetic devices following cardiac surgery.

The efficacy of antimicrobial prophylaxis in the patient with granulocytopenia may be more difficult to prove; however, some benefit may be achieved using trimethoprim-sulfamethoxasole as one component of the regimen.

Inactivated vaccines, immunoglobulin, and hyperimmune globulin appear to offer effective prophylaxis for viral diseases caused by varicella-zoster, measles, and hepatitis B. Serious viral infections may be diminished in frequency by providing a course of acyclovir for infection caused by herpes simplex virus and possibly CMV in patients undergoing allogeneic bone marrow transplantation; amantadine to prevent infection by influenza A viruses; and α-interferon to delay infection with CMV and reduce superinfection in recipients of heart and kidney transplants.

## Treatment

Despite attempts at prevention, some patients succumb to opportunistic infection. Management of these infections and the patient outcome are often more favorable when potential pathogens are known before isolation of the offending organism. Routine baseline throat and stool cultures of the patient should be obtained so that comparisons can be made to identify new flora that emerges subsequently. Blood cultures from intravenous or intra-arterial lines as well as cultures from tracheostomy tubes may be helpful.

The possibility of opportunistic infection can be anticipated in association with certain clinical situations, and the physician may be able to predict the organisms most likely to cause infection. For example, the stage of bone marrow transplantation influences the host's susceptibility. Suspicion of fungal or parasitic infection

increases in the settings of prolonged immunosuppressive therapy, culture-negative febrile episodes in neutropenic patients, poor response to broad-spectrum antibiotics, culture-negative or antimicrobial-resistant diarrhea, prolonged violation of mucosal barriers, or when any of these conditions are noted in patients with a preexisting defect in humoral or cellular immunity.

Definitive antibiotic therapy should be based on culture results when available. However, when cultures are pending, antibiotic therapy can be initiated based on recognition of the clinical syndrome and knowledge of those organisms that more often produce diseases in early situations. Tables 55-9 through 55-12 detail selected agents useful in treating bacterial, viral, fungal, and parasitic infections in immunocompromised children.

## Selected Readings

Anderson DC. Infectious complications resulting from phagocytic cell dysfunction. In: Feigin RD, Cherry JD, eds. Textbook of pediatric infectious diseases, ed 2. Philadelphia: WB Saunders, 1987.

Brooks RG, Hofflin JM, Jamieson SW, et al. Infectious complications in heart-lung transplant recipients. Am J Med 1985;79:412.

Feigin RD, Matson DO. Opportunistic infections, the compromised host. In: Feigin RD, Cherry JD, eds. Textbook of pediatric infectious diseases, ed 3. Philadelphia: WB Saunders, 1992.

Feigin RD, Shearer WT. Opportunistic infection in children. J Pediatr 1975;87:507.

Meyers JD. Infection in bone marrow transplant recipients. Am J Med 1986;81(suppl 1A):27.

Newman KA, Schimpff SC. Hospital hotel services as risk factors for infection among immunocompromised patients. Rev Infect Dis 1987;9:206.

Nusinow SR, Zuraw BL, Curd JG. The hereditary and acquired deficiencies of complement. Med Clin North Am 1985;69:487.

Peter G, Geibank GS, Hall CB, Plotkin SA. Report of the Committee on Infectious Diseases, ed 20. Am Acad Pediatr 1986;420.

Peterson PK. Host defense abnormalities predisposing the patient to infection. Am J Med 1984;76(5A):2.

Scherer LR, West KW, Weber TR, et al. *Staphylococcus epidermidis* sepsis in pediatric patients: clinical and therapeutic considerations. J Pediatr Surg 1984;19:358.

*Principles and Practice of Pediatrics, Second Edition.*
edited by Frank A. Oski et al. J. B. Lippincott Company, Philadelphia © 1994.

# CHAPTER 56
# *Bacterial Infections*

## *56.1* Aeromonas

### Ralph D. Feigin

*Aeromonas* species are causes of opportunistic infections and are increasingly identified as pathogens in healthy persons. *Aeromonas* organisms are found as normal flora in nonfecal sewage and can be isolated from rivers, streams, canals, and tap water. These organisms cannot be recovered from water sources in which the saline content approaches that of sea water. *Aeromonas* can survive readily on work surfaces and can be recovered from moistened paper towels.

*Aeromonas* are asporogenous, gram-negative, motile rods that contain a single polar flagellum. These organisms are oxidase and catalase positive and produce acid or gas during carbohydrate fermentation. *Aeromonas* grow well on blood agar, and most strains produce a large zone of β-hemolysis on this medium. *Aeromonas* also grow on *Salmonella-Shigella*, MacConkey, eosin-methylene blue, and triple sugar-iron media.

*Aeromonas* are confused most often with Enterobacteriaceae. The oxidase tests aid in differentiation: *Aeromonas* generally are oxidase positive, and Enterobacteriaceae are oxidase negative. *Aeromonas* species are susceptible to cefamandole, chloramphenicol, gentamicin, streptomycin, and trimethoprim-sulfamethoxazole. *Aeromonas* are consistently resistant to penicillin, ampicillin, cephalothin, and carbenicillin.

## PATHOGENESIS

*Aeromonas hydrophila* produces α- and β-hemolysins that are significant virulence factors in the pathogenesis of *A hydrophila* infection. α-Hemolysin, released from cells, can produce dermonecrosis and may be cytotoxic to HeLa cells and human embryonic lung fibroblasts. β-Hemolysin also may produce dermonecrosis and is cytotoxic to HeLa cells and to human diploid lung fibroblasts. Antibodies to either hemolysin neutralize both toxins.

*Aeromonas* elaborate a cytotonic enterotoxin that stimulates the cyclic adenosine monophosphate-mediated sequence of events in cells. This enterotoxin may cause diarrhea in humans.

*Aeromonas* also produce endopeptidase, fibrinolysin, leukocidin, proteinase A and B, and staphylolytic enzyme.

Agglutinating, precipitating, and antihemolysin antibodies to *A hydrophila* have been detected in patients with systemic *Aeromonas* infections but not in those with superficial infections. Antihemolysin titers as high as 1:1280 and agglutinin titers up to 1:640 have been found. A specific opsonizing antibody in normal serum and the normal bactericidal activity of neutrophils are required to prevent invasive *A hydrophila* infections.

## CLINICAL MANIFESTATIONS

Septicemia caused by *Aeromonas* has been reported in more than 40 children. Because this infection is not a reportable disease, the total number of affected children is unknown. Although septicemia caused by *Aeromonas* has occurred in normal children, most have had a disorder known to impair the normal host response to infection. Clinical manifestations of septicemia are similar to those of other gram-negative enteric bloodstream infections. High fever and shock are common, and ecthyma gangrenosum, seen more commonly in *Aeromonas* infections, has been described. The reported fatality rate has been 50% despite the introduction of antibiotic therapy. The high fatality rate may be related to the severity of the underlying disorder and does not reflect an unusual virulence of this microorganism.

Meningitis due to *Aeromonas* has been reported in children. In all cases, the course has been fulminant, and the patients have died despite antibiotic therapy.

Gastroenteritis due to *Aeromonas* has been described in a newborn nursery and in older children. Because *Aeromonas* is carried in the stool of normal persons, its isolation from a patient with diarrhea does not necessarily imply an infection due to *Aeromonas* organisms. In a prospective study of 1156 children with diarrhea and an equal number of age- and sex-matched controls, enterotoxigenic *Aeromonas* was isolated from 10.2% of children with diarrhea compared with 0.6% of healthy children. The same study described three clinical syndromes of *Aeromonas* gastroenteritis: vomiting, low-grade fever, and watery diarrhea in 41% of patients; diarrhea with blood and mucus in the stool in 22%; and prolonged diarrhea of more than 2 weeks' duration, in 37%.

*A hydrophila* has been recovered from skin and wound infections in children. Most were normal hosts. Exposure to some water source was documented in 40% of these patients. I have recovered *Aeromonas* from skin lesions resulting from tick bites. In each case, an area of purple discoloration surrounded the bite, and nonpurulent drainage from the center of the lesion yielded the organism.

*Aeromonas* has been described as a cause of osteomyelitis, myositis, urinary tract infections, and ocular infections in normal and immunocompromised children.

*A caviae* and *A sobria* have been isolated from stool specimens of patients with gastroenteritis. *A punctata* has been recovered from the stool of patients with gastroenteritis. Bacteremia caused by *A sobria* and *A punctata* has been described.

## DIAGNOSIS

*Aeromonas* can be considered as a possible cause of infection in children who have any disorder in which the immune system has been compromised. It should always be considered as a possible cause of bacteremia, gastroenteritis, and skin infections in compromised hosts.

## TREATMENT AND PROGNOSIS

In vitro, *Aeromonas* generally are susceptible to trimethoprim-sulfamethoxazole, chloramphenicol, aminoglycosides, and the third-generation cephalosporins. Chloramphenicol and moxalactam have proved efficacious. A drug to which the organism is sensitive should be provided intravenously in most cases. The duration of treatment depends on the site of infection and clinical response to therapy.

## Selected Readings

Feigin RD. *Aeromonas.* In: Feigin RD, Cherry JD, eds. Textbook of pediatric infectious diseases, ed 3. Philadelphia: WB Saunders, 1992, 1035.
Gracey M, Burke V, Robinson J. *Aeromonas*-associated gastroenteritis. Lancet 1982;2:1304.
Gracey M, Burke V, Rockhill RC, et al. *Aeromonas* species as enteric pathogens. Lancet 1982;1:223.
Hazen TE, Fliermans CB, Hirsch RP. Prevalence and distribution of *Aeromonas hydrophila* in the United States. Appl Environ Microbiol 1978;36:731.
Kuijper EJ, Peeters MF, Steigenwalt AG, et al. Clinical and epidemiologic aspects of members of *Aeromonas* DNA hybridization groups isolated from human feces. J Clin Microbiol 1989;27:1531.
McCracken AW, Barkley R. Isolation of *Aeromonas* species from clinical sources. J Clin Pathol 1972;25:970.
Meeks MV. The genus *Aeromonas.* Methods for identification. Am J Med Technol 1963;29:361.
Shackelford PG, Ratzan SA, Shearer WT. Ecthyma gangrenosum produced by *Aeromonas hydrophila.* J Pediatr 1973;83:100.

*Principles and Practice of Pediatrics, Second Edition.*
edited by Frank A. Oski et al. J. B. Lippincott Company, Philadelphia © 1994.

# 56.2 *Actinomycosis*

Jeffrey R. Starke

Actinomycosis is a rare infection in children, marked by chronic granulomatous or suppurative inflammation and formation of external sinus tracts. Another hallmark of this infection is contiguous spread unimpeded by the usual anatomic tissue barriers. Metastatic spread to distant sites also occurs. Infection occurs when these endogenous oral commensal organisms invade tissues of the face and neck, thorax, or intestines.

Actinomycosis occurs worldwide and usually is not an opportunistic infection. The organism can be isolated from the saliva, dental surfaces, gingiva, or tonsillar crypts of 30% to 50% of normal adults, if specimens are cultured properly, and may be part of the normal intestinal flora. Sex, race, season, and occupation are not important epidemiologic factors. The infection is reported less frequently in children than in adults, probably because the major predisposing factor for invasive infection is chronically poor oral hygiene. Children who are predisposed to aspiration may be at higher risk of developing thoracic actinomycosis.

Actinomycosis in humans was first reported in 1857 by Lebert. The organism *Actinomyces bovis* (literally, ray fungus of the cow) was first seen in 1877 in granules from cattle with lumpy jaw syndrome. In 1878, Israel saw similar granules in human autopsy material, and by 1885, he had characterized actinomycosis in humans. For decades, the etiologic agents of actinomycosis in cattle and humans were thought to be the same, but in 1940,

Erikson showed that *A bovis* and *Actinomyces israelii* were distinct species.

Before the 1940s, the term *actinomycosis* designated infection from any actinomycete. In 1943, Waksman and Henrici separated the pathogenic Actinomycetaceae using oxygen requirements and mycelial fragmentation. Microaerophilic and anaerobic actinomycetes were placed in the genus *Actinomyces,* and aerobic pathogens were assigned to the genus *Nocardia.* Current classification places the aerobic actinomycetes in a separate family, Nocardiaceae.

## ETIOLOGIC AGENTS

Actinomycosis may be caused by any of several agents, which have been placed in the genera *Actinomyces* and *Arachnia.* These organisms are gram-positive, facultative or strict anaerobes, with a morphology that varies from diphtheroid to mycelial. Branching is a characteristic feature, but it may be difficult to demonstrate in clinical samples. Members of both genera are oral commensals.

A characteristic of all organisms that cause actinomycosis is the propensity to form sulfur granules (Fig 56-1). These granules are hard, gritty, yellow or white, and average 2 mm in diameter. They are usually round basophilic masses with a fringe of eosinophilic clubs. Granules caused by other organisms, such as fungi, *Nocardia, Streptomyces,* and *Staphylococcus,* usually lack the characteristic clubbed fringe. Granules may be difficult to find, especially in chronic infections and may be in an abscess wall or sinus tract rather than in the pus or drainage. The granule represents a mycelian mass held together by host calcium phosphate and therefore cannot form in vitro.

The most common agent of human actinomycosis is *A israelii.* Grown on artificial media, the early colonies are branched filaments radiating from the center "spider" colony. The mature colonies are usually white, opaque, and rough. In enriched thioglycolate broth, discrete breadcrumb-like colonies form, and after 7 to 10 days of growth on solid media, they have a heaped and lobulated appearance like the surface of a molar tooth.

Several other species of *Actinomyces* have been isolated from human cases of actinomycosis. *Actinomyces naeslundii* has been isolated from blood, thoracic abscess, cervicofacial infection, gallbladder, and pleural empyema. Granules are less common and free mycelia more common than in infection due to *A israelii.*

*A naeslundii* and *A israelii* have similar biochemistries, although *A naeslundii* may be slow or difficult to grow on artificial media.

Other species that have been implicated in human actinomycosis include *Actinomyces viscosus, Actinomyces odontolyticus,* and *Actinomyces meyeri.* The organism *Arachnia propionica* was originally called *Actinomyces propionicus* until it was discovered to be part of a serologically distinct genus. It is similar morphologically and biochemically to *A israelii* and has been implicated in cervicofacial, intracranial, and pleuropulmonary infections, bite wounds, and renal abscess.

The pathologic lesions and sulfur granules of actinomycosis usually contain other bacteria and species of *Actinomyces* or *Arachnia.* Some investigators have found these aerobic and anaerobic associates in all lesions, but others have found them in many but not all. The most common associates are other oral commensals, including *Actinobacillus actinomycetem-comitans, Haemophilus* sp, *Eikenella corrodens,* streptococci, and oral anaerobes. Antibiotic therapy directed at *Actinomyces* usually effects a cure, even if the associates are resistant to the drug used. The pathogenic role of these associates is unknown.

## CLINICAL MANIFESTATIONS

Although actinomycosis may affect almost any organ in the body, there are three major areas of infection, in decreasing frequency, in adults and children: cervicofacial, abdominal, and thoracic.

Cervicofacial actinomycosis is caused by the organisms entering the tissue through trauma to the mucous membranes of the mouth, carious teeth, or the tonsils. Poor dental hygiene usually is a predisposing factor. In children, tooth eruption, especially of a molar, may provide a portal of entry. Two distinct patterns of cervicofacial actinomycosis occur. The first, commonly referred to as lumpy jaw, is a slowly enlarging, painless, fluctuant swelling, usually located at the lower border of the mandible. The second form is painful and widespread and may simulate an acute pyogenic infection of the submandibular area. Both forms spread slowly, without regard to tissue planes, which differentiates cervicofacial actinomycosis from most other head and neck infections. Trismus can occur and one or more sinus tracts may form (Fig 56-2). In the acute, rapidly progressive form, the degree of trismus and tissue edema may be disproportionate to the amount of inflammation. Lymphadenopathy usually does not develop,

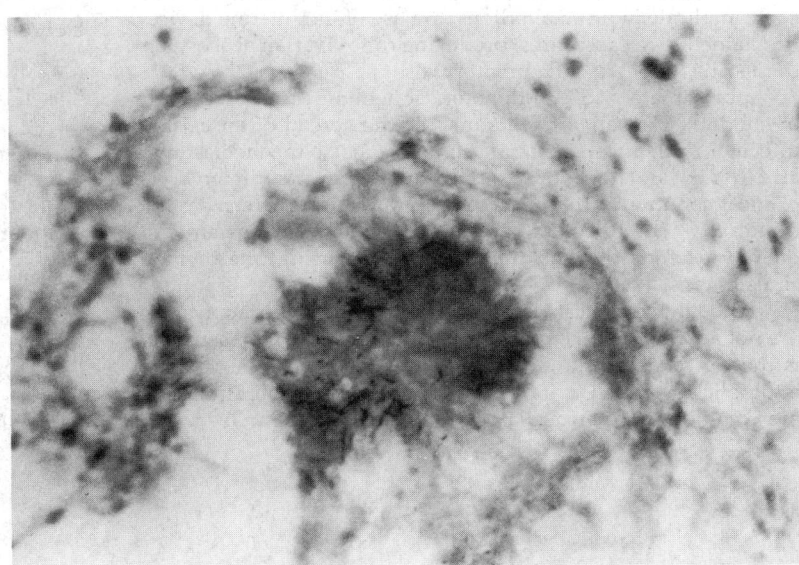

**Figure 56-1.** Sulfur granule found in a lung biopsy taken from a child with thoracic actinomycosis caused by *A naeslundii.* The central core, made up of mycelian mass and calcium phosphate, is surrounded by a fringe of eosinophic clubs. (Courtesy of David Hines, Director of Microbiology Laboratory, Texas Children's Hospital, Houston, TX.)

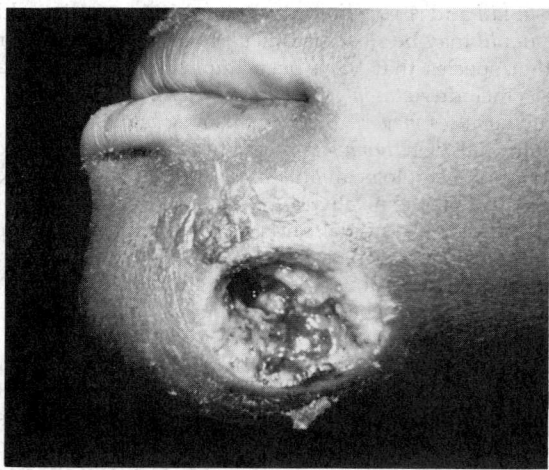

**Figure 56-2.**   Large draining sinus tract caused by cervicofacial *A israelii* infection. (Courtesy of Carol J. Baker, Baylor College of Medicine, Houston, TX.)

but a cold abscess or pseudotumor may form. There is no bone involvement in the early stages of the disease, although as infection progresses, radiographs of involved bone may reveal periosteal reaction, sclerosis, or lytic destruction.

Primary infection can occur in the scalp, palate, lacrimal gland, orbit, tongue, hypopharynx, larynx, trachea, salivary glands, paranasal sinus, or maxilla. Infection may spread through the sinus tracts to the cranial bones, eventually causing meningitis.

Abdominal actinomycosis, which is unusual in children, usually results from previous abdominal surgery, acute perforating gastrointestinal disease, or blunt or penetrating abdominal trauma. A hallmark of abdominal actinomycosis is delayed diagnosis, frequently due to a latent period of many months between the precipitating event and the development of infection. Abdominal actinomycosis occurs most frequently in the ileocecal region and may cause chronic appendicitis. The infection may spread in any direction, involving other areas of the bowel or abdominal organs, the pelvis, the retroperitoneum, or the abdominal muscles. Bone involvement is uncommon. Frequently, the first clue to the diagnosis of this illness is a sinus tract to the rectum, back, or abdominal wall. Primary pelvic actinomycosis can complicate induced abortions, the use of intrauterine devices, or retained surgical sutures, producing tubo-ovarian abscess, endometritis, or pelvic inflammatory disease.

Approximately 25% of the thoracic actinomycosis cases occur in children. Causative factors include the spread of an existing infection, such as cervicofacial actinomycosis, to the mediastinum and thorax; hematogenous seeding; inhalation of a foreign body; or most commonly, inhalation or aspiration of organisms in the oral cavity. The infection spreads across tissue planes and frequently extends through the chest wall, causing one or more sinus tracts.

Although the clinical manifestations and radiologic appearance are not specific for this infection, the most common presentation is that of an indolent, chronic pneumonitis that is resistant to antibiotic therapy. Cavitation of the lung and pleural effusion are common, but pericardial involvement occurs rarely. Symp-

toms include fever, productive cough, weight loss, chest pain, and retrosternal or back pain, which may accompany mediastinal lesions. Thoracic actinomycosis can resemble tuberculosis, lung abscess, and malignancy, but actinomycosis commonly involves the adjacent ribs or vertebral bodies, and bone involvement is rare with other infections. Distant sites of metastatic infection can occur in as many as 40% of thoracic actinomycosis cases. Diagnosis rarely is established before detection of a sinus tract, soft tissue mass, bony lesion, or metastatic site of infection.

Other forms of actinomycosis are rare in children. Actinomycosis of the central nervous system (CNS) may result from direct extension from the paranasal sinuses but usually develops secondary to infections at distant sites. The most common forms are brain abscess (67%), meningitis or meningoencephalitis (13%), actinomycoma (7%), subdural empyema (6%), and epidural abscess (6%). Unfortunately, the prognosis is poor, usually because of delayed diagnosis and treatment. Primary actinomycosis of an extremity usually develops secondary to penetrating trauma from a knife, toothpick, or other object, but most extremity infections are caused by hematogenous spread from another focus.

## TREATMENT

The basic principles for treating actinomycosis have remained unchanged since the early 1960s, when Peabody and Seabury emphasized intense and prolonged antibiotic therapy combined with surgical drainage of abscesses and excision of sinus tracts. Penicillin, in large doses given over weeks or months, is the drug of choice. Cervicofacial infection usually responds to antibiotics alone, as do some cases of thoracic and abdominal disease. The usual dosage schedule for intravenous penicillin G is 200,000 to 300,000 units/kg/day for 4 to 6 weeks, followed by oral penicillin for an additional 6 to 12 months. Specific considerations, such as dissemination, inoperability, or CNS disease, may alter this treatment schedule. Occasionally, penicillin alone is ineffective, usually because of an undrained abscess or the persistence of a resistant bacterial associate. Tetracyclines, erythromycin, clindamycin, sulfadiazine, and chloramphenicol are effective if penicillin cannot be used or is not effective.

Although some cases of extensive abdominal or thoracic actinomycosis have been cured with antibiotics alone, most require extensive surgical resection of affected tissues, excision of sinus tracts, and drainage of suppuration.

## Selected Readings

Bates M, Cruickshank G. Thoracic actinomycosis. Thorax 1957;12:99.

Berardi RS. Abdominal actinomycosis. Surg Gynecol Obstet 1979;149:257.

Bramley P, Orton HS. Cervico-facial actinomycosis. A report of eleven cases. Br Dent J 1960;109:235.

Dobson SRM, Edwards MS. Extensive *Actinomyces naeslundii* infection in a child. J Clin Microbiol 1987;25:1327.

Golden N, Cohen H, Weissbrat J, et al. Thoracic actinomycosis in childhood. Clin Pediatr 1985;24:646.

Smego RA Jr. Actinomycosis of the central nervous system. Rev Infect Dis 1987;9: 855.

Spinola SM, Bell RA, Henderson FW. Actinomycosis. Am J Dis Child 1981;135: 336.

Thompson AJ, Carty H. Pulmonary actinomycosis in children. Pediatr Radiol 1979;8: 7.

Waksman SA, Henrici AT. The nomenclature and classification of the actinomycetes. J Bacteriol 1943;46:337.

Weese WC, Smith IM. A study of 57 cases of actinomycosis over a 36-year period. Arch Intern Med 1975;135:1562.

*Principles and Practice of Pediatrics, Second Edition.*
edited by Frank A. Oski et al. J. B. Lippincott Company, Philadelphia © 1994.

# 56.3 *Nocardiosis*

### Jeffrey R. Starke

Nocardiosis is a localized or disseminated infection caused by an aerobic actinomycete. It was first described in humans in 1890, 2 years after Nocard observed an aerobic actinomycete in bovine farcy, an emaciating disease of cattle that causes pulmonary lesions and cutaneous abscesses. In humans, the soil-borne agent usually causes a pulmonary lesion that may be clinically silent or may provoke chronic bronchopulmonary disease. Hematogenous dissemination from the lungs may infect the central nervous system (CNS), bones, liver, spleen, or other soft tissues. Reports suggest an increasing incidence or recognition of primary lymphocutaneous forms of nocardiosis in children, usually involving the face or an extremity.

Most reported cases of nocardiosis have occurred in immunocompromised hosts, especially in patients with hematologic malignancy or those being treated with immunosuppressive drugs, with chronic granulomatous disease, or with chronic underlying pulmonary disease. Patients with pulmonary alveolar proteinosis have an especially high incidence of positive cultures for *Nocardia asteroides* from lung secretions. Only the lymphocutaneous form of nocardiosis occurs commonly in immunocompetent patients.

## EPIDEMIOLOGY

*Nocardia* are distributed widely in nature. Their natural habitat is soil and decaying vegetable matter. Infection in humans occurs by inhalation or direct skin inoculation of soil or organic particles. Because these organisms rarely are part of the normal flora of humans and are not a common laboratory contaminant, their isolation from a clinical specimen suggests disease. Some studies support the concept that *Nocardia* can be respiratory saprophytes. There is no definite evidence for animal-to-person or person-to-person transmission, although one cluster of cases has suggested

the latter possibility. Tick bites have been proposed as the cause of several cases of cutaneous nocardiosis. Nosocomial cases have been described, including an outbreak of nocardiosis in renal transplant patients that was related to organisms in the dust and air of the hospital unit.

Between 500 and 1000 recognized cases of nocardiosis occur in the United States each year, of which 85% are serious pulmonary or systemic infections. Cases occur in a random geographic distribution, with no seasonal or occupational predilection. Affected males outnumber females by 3 to 1. Although persons of any age can develop nocardiosis, most patients are between 21 and 50 years of age.

## ETIOLOGIC AGENTS

Before 1943, cases of nocardiosis were included under the term *actinomycosis*. Waksman and Henrici separated the pathogenic Actinomycetaceae into two groups: the microaerophilic and anaerobic actinomycetes were placed in the genus *Actinomyces*, and aerobic forms were assigned to *Nocardia*. Current classification places the aerobic actinomycetes in a separate family, Nocardiaceae.

*Nocardia* reproduce by fragmentation into bacillary and coccoid elements but are differentiated by their propensity for filamentous growth with true branching. The organisms grow over a wide range of temperatures on simple laboratory media, such as blood agar. Colonies on agar may be smooth and moist or rough with a velvety surface. Their color varies from cream to brick red. *Nocardia* may grow poorly on antibiotic-containing media used for isolation of fungi. Colonies in pure culture often grow after 48 hours of incubation, but growth can take up to several weeks in mixed cultures from clinical material.

The usual microscopic appearance of *Nocardia* is a delicate, weakly gram-positive, beaded branching filament (Fig 56-3). Most *Nocardia* are acid fast but retain fuchsin less avidly than mycobacteria. Acid and alcohol solutions (ie, Ziehl-Neelsen stain) decolorize *Nocardia*, but more basic solutions do not. A modified Ziehl-Neelsen stain using 1% sulfuric acid is the best solution to demonstrate *Nocardia* in clinical specimens.

*Nocardia asteroides* is the predominant pathogen, involved in as many as 90% of human nocardiosis cases. *Nocardia brasiliensis* is now recognized as a common cause of lymphocutaneous nocardiosis in immunocompetent patients and is the major cause

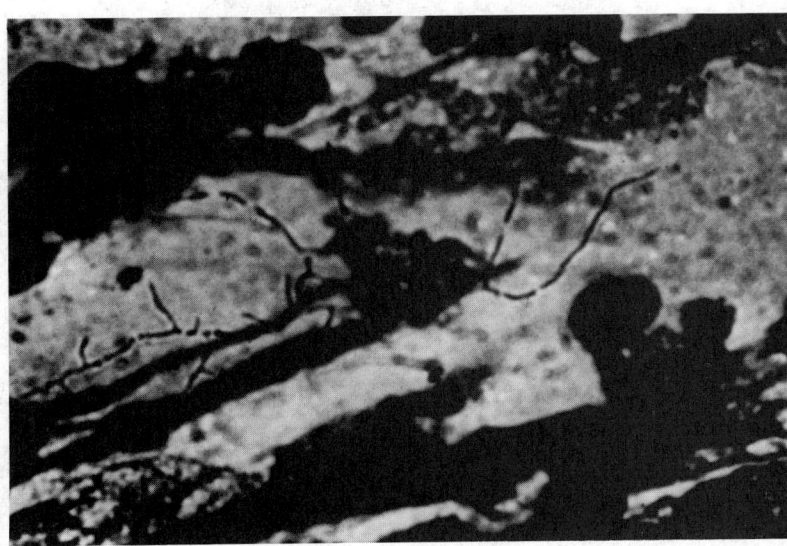

**Figure 56-3.** Microscopic appearance of *Nocardia brasiliensis.* Beaded, branching filaments are visible in pus from a cutaneous abscess.

of mycetoma in Central and South America. In experimental animals, *N brasiliensis* is more virulent than other *Nocardia* species. The association of skin trauma with lymphocutaneous nocardiosis suggests that, once beyond the skin barrier, *N brasiliensis* can cause local disease despite normal host defenses. Other species, including *Nocardia caviae*, *Nocardia nova*, and *Nocardia transvalensis*, are rarely involved in human disease.

## PATHOGENESIS AND PATHOLOGY

*N asteroides* usually infects humans through the respiratory tract, although the intestines—especially the appendix—may be the site of entry. Dissemination from the initial site is common and can involve the liver, spleen, kidneys, CNS, or skin. Primary cutaneous nocardiosis is preceded by trauma and can take the form of mycetoma, cellulitis, pyoderma, or infection of a compound fracture.

Although most nocardiosis cases before 1961 were primary infections, 85% of the current cases are associated with an array of debilitating diseases and conditions, especially lymphoreticular neoplasms, chronic granulomatous disease, long-term steroid usage, organ transplantation with associated immunosuppressive treatment, dysgammaglobulinemias, and alcoholism. Many of the antecedent conditions involve dysfunction of cellular immunity, but immunoglobulin and leukocyte defects also predispose to this infection.

The host reaction to *Nocardia* infection is complex and poorly understood. The major responses in animals include macrophage activation, development of cell-mediated immunity, inhibition of growth by polymorphonuclear leukocytes, and induction of a T-cell population capable of direct lymphocyte-mediated toxicity to *N asteroides*. Which components of the immune system are most important in defense against nocardiosis in humans remains to be determined.

Histologically, nocardiosis causes a suppurative lesion with abscess formation and necrosis. Pulmonary lesions usually consist of multiple abscesses, although a single abscess or nodule may occur. The suppuration resembles that seen with bacterial pyogenic infections. There is little evidence of encapsulation, which may account for the ready dissemination of *Nocardia* from the pulmonary focus.

## CLINICAL MANIFESTATIONS AND DIAGNOSIS

The most common form of nocardiosis in immunocompromised patients is pulmonary infection. Specific presentations include bronchopneumonia, lobar pneumonitis, and necrotizing pneumonia with single or multiple abscesses or empyema. Endobronchial nocardiosis occurs rarely. Pulmonary involvement usually is chronic but can be acute, with rapid dissemination. Clinical symptoms are nonspecific and include fever, anorexia, weight loss, productive cough, pleural pain, dyspnea, and hemoptysis. Chest radiographs show great variability, but the most common findings are alveolar or interstitial infiltrates, segmental bronchopneumonia (with or without thin-walled cavitation), subpleural plaques, and single or multiple nodules; rarely, there are miliary lesions or thick-walled cavities. The radiographic pattern is often confused with tuberculosis, metastatic malignancy, bacterial pneumonia, or pyogenic abscess.

Clinical manifestations frequently occur in sites distant to the lung as a result of direct extension or hematogenous dissemination. Related problems seen most often include tracheitis, peritonsillar abscess, pericarditis, peritonitis, muscle abscess, perirectal abscess, endophthalmitis, sinusitis, mediastinitis with superior vena cava obstruction, septic arthritis, osteomyelitis, and a disseminated miliary form. *Nocardia* infection of virtually every organ has been reported.

The skin, subcutaneous tissues, and lymph nodes are common sites for *Nocardia* infection in children. Lymphocutaneous infection can occur secondary to dissemination from a silent pulmonary lesion or direct inoculation through traumatized skin. *N brasiliensis* is the most common species involving the skin. Subcutaneous abscesses related to disseminated disease can be single or multiple, are usually firm (but may be fluctuant), and usually lack induration, extensive erythema, or warmth. In children, a cervicofacial syndrome usually consists of a pustular facial lesion associated with submandibular or cervical adenitis. This presentation can be confused with tularemia, cat-scratch disease, actinomycosis, or cutaneous diphtheria. *Nocardia* occasionally form multiple subcutaneous nodules on an extremity, mimicking sporotrichosis. Primary cutaneous infection usually involves the inoculation site and the regional lymph nodes (Fig 56-4), although dissemination from the skin to other organs can occur.

The CNS is involved in about one third of the immunocom-

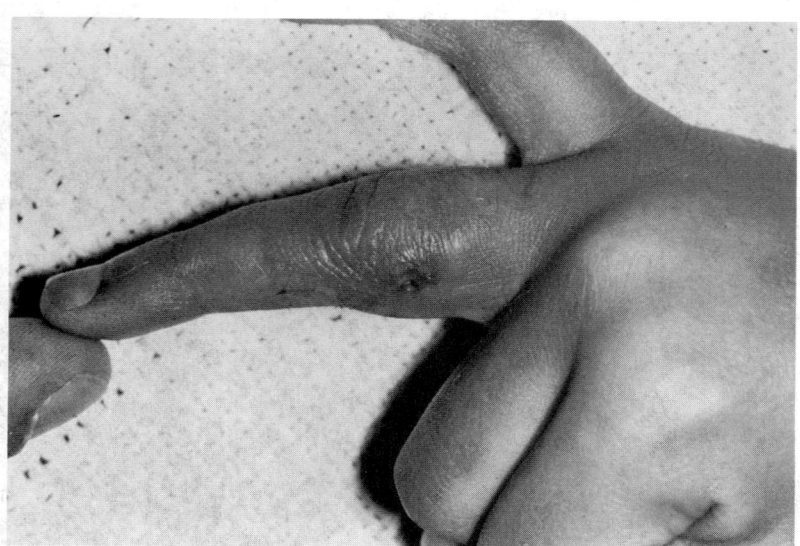

**Figure 56-4.** Cutaneous lesion caused by *Nocardia brasiliensis* in a 4-year-old girl. This lesion was accompanied by markedly tender epitrochlear adenitis. (Courtesy of Moise L. Levy, Department of Dermatology, Baylor College of Medicine, Houston, TX.)

promised patients with disseminated nocardiosis. The fatality rate of CNS nocardiosis is 40% to 70%, with most deaths resulting from delay in diagnosis and institution of specific therapy. Brain involvement may dominate the clinical presentation, although it usually is associated with other manifestations. Multiloculated brain abscesses are most common, although meningitis occurs rarely. Involvement of the CNS can also be secondary to penetrating trauma of the skull or placement of a ventriculoperitoneal shunt.

Diagnosing pulmonary nocardiosis may be difficult, because the organism is seen in the sputum of only one third of affected patients. Bronchoalveolar lavage or open lung biopsy frequently is required to establish the diagnosis and to differentiate nocardiosis from the myriad other infections that have a similar clinical and radiographic appearance in an immunocompromised host. *Nocardia* are usually isolated from lymphocutaneous lesions and can be detected microscopically by using the appropriately modified weak acid-fast stain of pus. *N asteroides* may be recovered from blood cultures in immunosuppressed patients. Tests for humoral antibodies or delayed cutaneous hypersensitivity are not useful clinically.

## TREATMENT

Sulfonamides have been recognized as the drugs of choice in nocardiosis since their release in the 1940s. Previous therapy had been supportive, and spontaneous remissions were rare. Cure of *Nocardia* infection can be expected in most cases if appropriate antibiotics are used in conjunction with surgery for drainage of suppurative foci.

A variety of antibiotics have been used to treat nocardiosis. Ideally, in vitro susceptibility testing can be used to direct therapy. Tube dilution susceptibility testing is best but is usually available only at reference laboratories. Disk diffusion susceptibility testing can be difficult, because as many as one third of *Nocardia* isolates do not grow adequately on agar plates, and test procedures are not well standardized. The relative rarity of *Nocardia* infections makes controlled antibiotic trials almost impossible.

The treatment of choice for *Nocardia* infections is sulfisoxazole at a dose that achieves serum levels of 12 to 15 $\mu g/dL$ (usually 100 to 150 mg/kg/day). The combination of sulfamethoxazole-trimethoprim has proved synergistic against some strains of *Nocardia*. Although this combination is used frequently, it is unclear whether it has any advantage over sulfisoxazole alone. Occasionally, a second antibiotic, such as chloramphenicol, tetracycline, or ampicillin, is necessary to effect a cure. For patients who cannot tolerate sulfa drugs, minocycline, erythromycin, and amikacin may be used. Some of the other $\beta$-lactam antibiotics (eg, cefotaxime, cefuroxime, ceftriaxone) are active in vitro against *Nocardia*, but clinical data are lacking.

The optimal duration of therapy is uncertain. A minimum of 6 weeks is recommended, but sulfonamide therapy usually is continued for as long as 6 months because of the likelihood of relapse or appearance of metastatic abscesses with shorter treatment duration. The appearance of a metastatic abscess during appropriate therapy usually represents the evolution of a previously seeded metastasis, which may progress until adequate surgical drainage is achieved. Most lymphocutaneous sites of *Nocardia* infection require surgical drainage for cure, but pulmonary, brain, and other deep-seated infections often can be cured with antibiotics alone.

## Selected Readings

Beaman BL, Burnside J, Edwards B, et al. Nocardial infections in the United States, 1972–1974. J Infect Dis 1976;134:286.

Bross JE, Gordon G. Nocardial meningitis: case reports and review. Rev Infect Dis 1991;13:160.

Curry WA, Human nocardiosis. Arch Intern Med 1980;140:818.

Idriss ZH, Cunningham RJ, Wilfert CM. Nocardiosis in children: report of three cases and review of the literature. Pediatrics 1975;55:479.

Lampe RM, Baker CJ, Septimus EJ, et al. Cervicofacial nocardiosis in children. J Pediatr 1981;99:593.

Law BJ, Marks MI. Pediatric nocardiosis. Pediatrics 1982;70:560.

Smego RA Jr, Gallis HA. The clinical spectrum of Nocardia brasiliensis in the United States. Rev Infect Dis 1984;6:164.

Smego RA Jr, Moeller MB, Gallis HA. Trimethoprim-sulfamethoxazole therapy for *Nocardia* infections. Arch Intern Med 1983;143:711.

Stites DP, Glezen WP. Pulmonary nocardiosis in childhood. Am J Dis Child 1967;114:101.

Wallace RJ Jr, Septimus EJ, Musher DM, et al. Disk diffusion susceptibility testing of Nocardia species. J Infect Dis 1977;135:568.

*Principles and Practice of Pediatrics, Second Edition.*
edited by Frank A. Oski et al. J. B. Lippincott Company, Philadelphia © 1994.

# 56.4 *Anaerobic Infections*

Lisa M. Dunkle

Diseases caused by anaerobic infection or intoxication have been known since the time of Hippocrates, when tetanus was first described. The existence of anaerobic microbes was recognized centuries later by Pasteur in his observations of bacterial fermentation. In 1896, Welch began the process of identifying specific etiologic agents with the description of what now is recognized as *Clostridium perfringens*. Disease is caused by relatively few representatives of the vast taxonomic spectrum of anaerobic organisms. The genus *Clostridium* includes several of the most prominent pathogens and causes the most characteristic disease patterns of all anaerobic infections, mainly by the production of potent toxins. Nonclostridial anaerobic bacteria cause less typical disease patterns, and their clinical importance has been recognized only within the last half of the 20th century.

Organisms of the genus *Clostridium* are characterized as anaerobic, gram-positive, spore-forming bacilli, although there are a few exceptions to each of these characteristics. Clostridial spores are found worldwide and are ubiquitous in soil, dust, street dirt, and human and animal feces. They have been found as contaminants of heroin solutions. Most species are considered nonpathogenic, although it may be difficult to differentiate pathogens from nonpathogens in a polymicrobial infection. The protein exotoxins produced by some of these organisms are among the most potent poisons known, and the toxin-produced diseases frequently occur without tissue inflammation.

## CLOSTRIDIUM TETANI

### Etiology and Epidemiology

Tetanus is an ancient disease, the clinical course and prognosis of which have changed little over centuries. The disease is caused by the exotoxin tetanospasmin, a 67,000-d protein elaborated by the vegetative form of *Clostridium tetani*. Tetanospasmin is a potent neurotoxin that is lethal to humans at a dose of less than 150 $\mu g$. Because the spores of *C tetani* are ubiquitous and are resistant to heat and disinfection, they can readily contaminate wounds. Most tetanus occurs in patients without a history of apparent wound contamination, although puncture wounds and grossly contaminated, ragged lacerations commonly are characterized as tetanus prone.

The incidence of tetanus varies widely throughout the world; recent figures in the United States reveal 50 to 100 cases reported annually, with an average incidence of 0.03 cases per 100,000 persons. This is one tenth of the incidence in 1947, when reporting began. In the United States, 95% of cases occur outside the pediatric age group, and 70% occur in patients older than 50 years of age. Neonatal tetanus has not been reported in this country in the 1980s. These figures reflect the efficacy of the aggressive immunization program in the United States, especially compared with developing countries, for which the World Health Organization reported more than 600,000 cases of neonatal tetanus in 1980 and 1981. During the source period, there were an estimated 100,000 to 120,000 deaths from tetanus worldwide. Unhygienic childbirth practices in most of the developing world and inadequate immunization of mothers explain most cases of neonatal tetanus. Other health practices, such as frequent nonmedical abortions in Africa and lack of attention to penetrating wounds in much of the world, are often responsible for tetanus in adults. Climate and soil pH in the tropics probably contribute to the prevalence of C tetani and its availability to contaminate wounds. In the absence of vigorous hygiene and immunization programs, tetanus remains a major killer.

## Pathophysiology

After introduction into tissues, spores convert to vegetative forms, multiply, and elaborate tetanospasmin. There is often no associated inflammation or apparent local infection. The conversion to vegetative bacilli with the production of toxin and disease occurs only if the oxidation-reduction potential of the inoculated tissue is sufficiently low to allow anaerobic growth, as in nonviable umbilical cord tissue or in wounds with significant tissue damage or imbedded foreign material.

Because the tetanus toxin is elaborated in distal tissues, the mechanism of transport of the toxin to the central nervous system (CNS) is critically important for establishing the disease. Data support the theory that tetanospasmin enters the peripheral nerve and travels through the nerve to the CNS. The toxin's effect on the nervous system is seen centrally and peripherally. At the presynaptic nerve ending, the toxin binds to gangliosides in the neuronal membrane, prevents release of neurotransmitters, and affects polarization of postsynaptic membranes in complex polysynaptic reflexes. The resultant lack of inhibitory impulses is manifested in the characteristic spasms, seizures, and sympathetic overactivity of tetanus. The toxin has no apparent effect on mental status, and consciousness is not impaired directly by this disease.

The neuronal transport of the toxin is consistent with the observation that the time between injury and disease correlates with the distance between the wound and the CNS. The incubation period is usually between 3 days and 3 weeks; the most severe cases develop after the shortest incubation periods. In some instances, the toxin remains localized to the neurons associated with the wound, producing a localized form of tetanus. More commonly, the toxin affects the entire nervous system, causing generalized tetanus. In rare cases, the toxin affects only cranial nerves, a condition known as cephalic tetanus.

Tetanospasmin binds irreversibly to neurons and cannot be neutralized by antitoxin thereafter. The course and duration of established disease are determined by the location and "dose" of bound toxin. The complete course of tetanus is usually from 2 to 4 weeks but is influenced greatly by patient age and complications. The worldwide mortality rate is in the range of 45% to 55%; the mortality rate is approximately 1% in localized tetanus, but mortality rates of more than 60% are reported for tet-

anus neonatorum. Observations of tetanus in heroin addicts suggest greater susceptibility of these hosts to disease and virtually uniform mortality. Although survivors generally experience no neurologic sequelae, prolonged convalescence with residual muscle rigidity is observed for several months.

## Clinical Manifestations

The clinical presentation of tetanus usually falls into one of three categories: localized, generalized, or cephalic. Neonatal tetanus, a generalized form of the disease, warrants discussion because of its occurrence worldwide.

### Localized Tetanus

An unusual manifestation of tetanus, localized disease is thought to occur when circulating antitoxin is sufficient to prevent general spread of the toxin but insufficient to prevent local uptake at a wound site. The condition results in prolonged, steady, and painful muscle contraction in the region of the wound. The duration of this painful rigidity is several weeks, with eventual complete resolution. The condition has a low mortality rate (<1%). Some investigators have suggested that localized tetanus may go unrecognized or be mistaken for pain-induced muscle spasms. The local form of the disease may be unrecognized before generalized tetanus supersedes.

### Generalized Tetanus

The most common form of clinical tetanus, generalized disease may occur after relatively minor injuries and commonly follows wounds not characterized as tetanus prone. Although the onset may be insidious, the typical initial complaint of trismus due to spasms of the parapharyngeal and masseter muscles is seen in 50% of cases. Common complaints include pain and difficulty with swallowing, unilateral or bilateral neck stiffness, and stiffness of other muscle groups, such as abdominal or thoracic musculature. The finding of trismus is so characteristic of tetanus that this diagnosis must be strongly considered when a patient presents with this complaint. Persistence of trismus is responsible for the risus sardonicus that long has been considered a classic finding of tetanus.

With progression of the disease, additional muscle groups become involved; perhaps the most striking is paraspinal musculature involvement. Tonic spasm of these muscles may result in severe opisthotonos; in young infants, the soles of the feet may touch the head. Vertebral fractures are not uncommon in this situation. Tetanic contractions progress over the course of several days; recruitment of additional muscle groups and significant worsening of symptoms are to be expected after the initial presentation.

In addition to the tonic contractions, tetanospasmin causes painful spasms of contraction that further contort and distort the patient's posture. These affect all voluntary muscles and may involve the larynx, a complication that can be fatal. The force of the spasms may be great enough to produce fractures of vertebrae or other bones and hemorrhage into muscles. Although these spasms are often referred to as seizures, they are not associated with the characteristic electroencephalographic changes of convulsions and are more appropriately called tetanus spasms. They are extraordinarily painful and constitute the major horror of full-blown tetanus. The spasms are stimulus dependent, but the stimuli may be minor; light, drafts, noises or voices, and light touch are all sufficient to cause spasms, which makes management challenging. Because patients remain fully conscious throughout these spasms, anxiety and pain further complicate management and contribute to the severity of the untreated disease.

The effect of tetanospasmin on the autonomic nervous system

results in characteristic cardiovascular instability. Labile hypertension, sometimes of a marked degree, is common, as are episodes of tachycardia or other tachyarrhythmias. Fever can also result from sympathetic overactivity, although its occurrence should prompt a search for superinfections, such as pneumonia. In the modern intensive care setting, where ventilatory support and therapeutic paralysis are routinely available, cardiovascular complications are the primary problem in management. As is the case with spasms, cardiovascular complications are most common during the first week of the illness and resolve slowly during the ensuing 2 to 4 weeks.

### Cephalic Tetanus

A rare manifestation of disease, cephalic tetanus exclusively involves the cranial nerves after entry of C tetani into wounds or chronic infections of the head and neck. Cranial nerve VII is involved most frequently, although any of the cranial nerves may be affected, singly or in combination, causing weakness of the affected nerve(s). Cephalic tetanus may precede generalized disease, and isolated cephalic tetanus can occur and follows a chronology similar to generalized disease. The mortality rate is significant for these patients, but survivors demonstrate no sequelae.

### Neonatal Tetanus

Tetanus in the newborn is a generalized form of the disease that warrants special comment because of its importance worldwide and the potential for its occurrence in the United States. Infants delivered vaginally to mothers who have not been immunized are at significant risk for neonatal tetanus. Birth practices in developing countries, such as applying mud or feces to the umbilical stump, greatly increase risk and can be considered responsible for a large proportion of the many cases seen throughout the world in recent years. The mortality rate in these cases is high, with infants dying of complications such as pneumonia and pulmonary hemorrhage, CNS hemorrhage, and laryngeal spasms.

The risk of neonatal tetanus in the United States should not be dismissed, particularly in unusually contaminated deliveries and if the maternal immunization status is uncertain. Passive immunization should be administered in these circumstances.

## Differential Diagnosis

Tetanus is uncommon in developed nations, where immunization and hygiene practices have largely eliminated the disease. The classic presenting complaint of trismus and of muscle spasms, stiffness, and pain with dysphagia and cranial nerve weakness can be seen in other conditions, although the classic picture is sufficiently characteristic to support the diagnosis of tetanus. Other conditions that can mimic some manifestations of tetanus include parapharyngeal and peritonsillar abscesses, poliomyelitis and other forms of viral encephalomyelitis, Bell's palsy, meningoencephalitis (including rabies), hypocalcemic tetany, and dystonic reactions to phenothiazines. These other conditions are relatively easily differentiated from tetanus by specific laboratory or radiographic evaluations or by the clinical course. The absence of altered consciousness in tetanus is an important point of differentiation from CNS infections, and a parapharyngeal inflammatory process can be suspected from clinical examination or radiographs of the airway. Hypocalcemic tetany usually is confirmed by low serum levels of calcium; idiosyncratic dystonia caused by a phenothiazine resolves promptly after intravenous diphenhydramine.

It is difficult to confirm a specific diagnosis of tetanus by routine laboratory tests. Routine blood counts are normal or slightly elevated; CSF evaluations are normal; and electroencephalogram (EEG) and electromyogram (EMG) are normal and nonspecifically abnormal, respectively. Gram stains and anaerobic cultures of wounds reveal the characteristic gram-positive bacilli with terminal spores in as many as one third of tetanus patients. Although positive wound cultures may support the diagnosis in patients with clinical disease suggestive of tetanus, a positive culture from a contaminated wound in the absence of symptoms does not indicate that tetanus intoxication will develop.

## Management and Prognosis

Without specific confirmatory laboratory tests, the clinician must institute appropriate treatment based on the clinical diagnosis. The goals of therapy are to eradicate and neutralize C tetani and its toxin and to provide appropriate supportive care, which is often a more complex task than the medical treatment.

Specific therapy should include intramuscular administration of tetanus immune globulin (TIG) to neutralize circulating toxin before it binds to neuronal cell membranes. Antitoxin given early in the disease may prevent spread of the toxin within the CNS. The dosage of TIG does not appear to be critical, but a range of 500 to 3000 U is recommended. Although a dosage recommendation based on body weight is not available, it appears reasonable to give a considerably smaller dose to newborn infants with tetanus, probably a single vial of TIG (250 U). The efficacy of additional intrathecal administration of TIG has not been proven, although some have advocated this regimen.

Additional specific therapy should include antimicrobial therapy for C tetani, preferably penicillin G administered as 200,000 U/kg/day in four divided intravenous doses for 10 days. Alternative agents for patients allergic to penicillin include oral tetracycline (40 mg/kg/day; maximum of 2 g) or intravenous vancomycin (30 to 40 mg/kg/day). The cephalosporins are not reliably active against C tetani.

Local wound care, including surgical debridement, is essential. Foreign bodies must be removed and wounds irrigated well and left open. Local antibiotic or TIG instillation is not warranted. Excision of necrotic tissue may be required, but excision of the umbilical stump is no longer recommended in cases of neonatal tetanus.

Supportive care of tetanus patients always involves meticulous nursing care. Ventilatory support and dramatic pharmacologic intervention to stabilize vital signs may be necessary. If possible, patients should be managed in an intensive care setting of a tertiary-care center. Transfer to such a setting should be accomplished early in the disease, before the severity of spasms precludes moving the patient; the clinical condition deteriorates during the first week after the onset of the disease.

Equipment and facilities that should be available include a quiet darkened room, suction equipment and oxygen, cardiac and respiratory monitors, a ventilator, and tracheostomy equipment. In the initial days of the illness, minimizing external stimuli and maintaining intravenous hydration may be sufficient supportive care. Sedation and muscle relaxation should be instituted, usually with diazepam. Diazepam in a dose of 0.1 to 0.2 mg/kg given intravenously every 4 to 6 hours provides smooth, safe muscle relaxation and may be adequate for relatively mild cases. Additional sedation with phenothiazines may be used, although these drugs alone are less effective than diazepam. If spasms are not adequately controlled, therapeutic paralysis is necessary. These patients must be treated by experienced caregivers highly skilled in ventilatory support and maintenance of cardiovascular stability.

Neuromuscular blockade can be accomplished with the curariform drugs. The agents used most often are pancuronium and vecuronium. Vecuronium, an intermediate-acting neuromuscular blocking agent in an initial dose of 0.08 to 0.1 mg/kg intravenously, with maintenance doses of 0.01 to 0.15 mg/kg every 30 to 60 minutes, as needed, appears to have fewer adverse effects on blood pressure and heart rate—a significant benefit in patients for whom hypertension and tachycardia are major complicating factors. Doxacurium, a long-acting agent of the same class with similar safety profile for the cardiovascular system, may offer more prolonged effect with each dose and smoother patient management. The recommended initial dose is 0.03 to 0.05 mg/kg intravenously, followed by 0.01 mg/kg in 60 to 90 minutes, as needed. Subsequent intervals between maintenance doses may be lengthened or shortened by the administration of smaller or larger doses. Patients who undergo therapeutic paralysis must be sedated to avoid the anxiety that occurs in a conscious patient.

Therapy also may be required to manage the hypertension that results from sympathetic overactivity. Beta-blocking agents appear to be the agents of choice, with propranolol used most commonly (usual dose, 0.01 to 0.10 mg/kg every 6 to 8 hours). Propranolol may be useful for the management of tachyarrhythmias. For either indication, the dosage must be titrated to achieve optimal effect. The duration of these pharmacologic manipulations is dictated by the duration of effect of tetanospasmin, but it is in the range of 2 to 3 weeks. Careful monitoring of all vital signs and activities and their correlation with drug effect will indicate when the toxin's effects have resolved.

Maintenance of adequate nutrition and hydration is mandatory. Because of the likely duration of the disease and the undesirability of oral or nasogastric feedings, parenteral nutrition is usually required for children with tetanus. Optimal nutritional support can minimize the tremendous weight loss that traditionally has been considered an expected outcome, and maintenance of adequate electrolyte balance can improve management of arrhythmias. Careful attention must be paid to skin care, especially in the paralyzed patient, and excretory functions must be monitored closely for urinary retention or serious constipation.

In the absence of optimal tertiary-care facilities and personnel for modern management, minimal stimulation, muscle relaxation, sedation short of respiratory depression, and adequate hydration may be the best that can be achieved. Tracheostomy may be required (preferably on an elective rather than emergency basis) to avoid fatal laryngospasm. Laryngospasm greatly increases the mortality rate of the disease.

An important aspect of treatment is initiation of active immunization with tetanus toxoid. Patients must be immunized to prevent further disease, because the amount of toxin required to produce disease is far less than that needed to stimulate immunity.

Although tetanus is still a very serious disease, the prognosis with modern techniques of intensive care is markedly better than that predicted by earlier statistics. The overall mortality rate for 1950 to 1959 was 66% in the United States, but the mortality rate for 1982 to 1986 was between 26% and 31%. Age plays an important part in outcome, with only 5% mortality for patients younger than 50 years of age treated in recent years compared with 42% for those older than 50 years. There were no deaths among five infants with tetanus neonatorum managed in a medical center intensive care nursery in 1979. Survivors are left largely without sequelae of tetanus, although it can be predicted that the sequelae of modern intensive care will be seen in time.

The primary predictors of prognosis remain the rapidity of symptom onset and the rate of progression from trismus to severe spasms. Poor outcome is predicted by an interval between injury and trismus shorter than 7 days or by progression from trismus to spasms in less than 3 days. These statistics come largely from developing countries, where there are sufficient cases to draw such conclusions, but the data appear to have predictive value for disease severity in the United States. With appropriate intensive care, the ultimate mortality of tetanus in the United States has been reduced greatly.

| TABLE 56-1. Tetanus Prophylaxis in Wound Management | | |
|---|---|---|
| Immunization History | Type of Wound | |
| | Clean, Minor | All Others |
| Three or more doses of tetanus toxoid | No TIG; toxoid only if >10 y since last dose | No TIG; toxoid only if >5 y since last dose |
| Fewer than three doses or uncertain history | No TIG; toxoid, 0.5 mL | TIG, 250–500 U; toxoid, 0.5 mL |

*Adapted from the Report of the Committee on Infectious Diseases, ed 20. Evanston, IL: American Academy of Pediatrics, 1986.*

## Prevention

Tetanus is an entirely preventable disease, and the fact that fewer than 5% of cases in the United States in the 1980s were in children attests to the efficacy of vigorous primary immunization. The primary series of tetanus toxoid, administered as DTP vaccine at 2, 4, and 6 months and a booster 12 months later, virtually ensures protection in childhood. Additional boosters of tetanus toxoid should be administered each decade throughout life, with further tetanus prophylaxis after acute wounds, as advocated by the American Academy of Pediatrics Advisory Committee on Immunization Practices (Table 56-1).

Patients who have documentation of full primary immunization and appropriate boosters need no tetanus prophylaxis beyond appropriate local wound care for clean minor wounds but should receive a toxoid booster after a dirty, tetanus-prone injury if the most recent dose was received more than 5 years previously. Patients who are not known to have completed the primary series require a tetanus toxoid booster after any penetrating wound and TIG after a tetanus-prone injury. The prophylactic dose of TIG is 250 to 500 U, given intramuscularly. A human γ-globulin product, TIG does not carry the risk of serum sickness seen with equine antitoxin, and skin testing for hypersensitivity is unnecessary. U.S. statistics reveal that only 13% of patients who subsequently developed tetanus received appropriate tetanus toxoid boosters at the time of injury and that TIG was not given to any of the patients who should have received it. A continuing effort to educate the public about the need for tetanus immunoprophylaxis after childhood is necessary to prevent this disease. Prevention is much less costly than treatment.

## CLOSTRIDIUM BOTULINUM

### Etiology and Epidemiology

Botulism represents acute neurologic disease caused by another potent clostridial toxin, elaborated by *Clostridium botulinum*. Botulinal toxin is the most potent poison known, causing death in mice that receive as little as 10 pg. Disease is caused in humans by less than 100 ng. There are seven antigenically distinct botulinal toxins (ie, types A through G), which are produced by four groups of *C botulinum*, each distinguished by its characteristic biochemical activities. The production of each toxin appears to depend on the presence of a plasmid that encodes the toxin gene. Elimination of the plasmid renders the bacteria nontoxigenic. The molecular weights of the toxins, which now are believed to be cellular proteins that are released during lysis, vary within the range of 130,000 to 150,000 d. The active moiety of the protein may be as small as 10,000 d. The toxin is destroyed by heat and pressure (ie, 100°C for 10 minutes or 80°C for 30 minutes) but is resistant to chemical deactivation. The bacterial spores are highly resistant to heat but may be killed by autoclaving at 120°C for 20 minutes.

Botulinal toxin acts at the neuromuscular junction, where it inhibits the release of acetylcholine, producing a flaccid paralysis. There is no effect on the CNS or on mentation, although the earliest effect is seen on the cranial nerves. Progression of paralysis occurs in a characteristic descending fashion, ultimately affecting the entire peripheral nervous system. Respiratory failure is the major cause of death, as the paralytic effect of the toxin reaches the muscles of respiration.

Botulinum spores are common in soil, dust, lakes, and other environmental matter and can contaminate fruits, vegetables, meats, and fish. Honey has become recognized as a potential source of *C botulinum* spores and one form of botulism.

In view of the widespread occurrence of *C botulinum* spores and their remarkable resistance to destruction, the epidemiology of the disease correlates most closely with circumstances in which contaminated foods are inadequately heated and the preformed toxin is ingested. The contaminated food often correlates with geographic location and the type of botulinal toxin involved. Most cases of botulism in humans are caused by types A, B, and E; more than half of food-borne cases in the United States are type A, and 25% are type B. Type A causes two thirds of cases in the western half of the United States, and type B a exhibits similar prevalence east of the Mississippi. Cases of type E botulism usually involve fish from the Pacific Northwest and Alaska; worldwide, most type E disease occurs in Japan, Scandinavia, and the former Soviet Union, presumably because of dietary habits.

Most outbreaks of botulism in the United States are associated with food products (eg, home-canned vegetables), in which spores generate and form toxins, that are not adequately heated before consumption. Other food products that have been incriminated include smoked meats, raw and fermented fish products, and potato salad and commercial frozen pot pies prepared improperly at home.

Ingestion of *C botulinum* spores may lead to generation of toxin in the intestine of susceptible hosts and to botulism. This mechanism is operative in infantile botulism, which has been linked to the addition of honey (a natural, unpasteurized product) to infant formula. This form of botulism, which represents two thirds of reported cases in the United States, first was recognized and still predominates in the western United States among families favoring "natural" food products, although it is now recognized throughout the country. A similar mechanism of acquisition of botulinal toxin has been implicated in rare cases in older children and adults. Prolonged or recurrent paralysis in some patients with typical food-borne botulism may be due to intestinal infection with *C botulinum* and resultant continued elaboration and absorption of toxin. Contamination of wounds with *C botulinum* rarely results in parenteral absorption of botulinal toxin and in "wound botulism."

## Pathophysiology

Botulism is caused by the binding of botulinal toxin to the neuromuscular junction. Whether from absorption of toxin from the gastrointestinal tract or from locally infected wounds, the toxin enters the lymphatics and bloodstream to circulate and gain access to neuromuscular junctions. The toxin does not cross the blood–brain barrier but is bound to the cytoplasmic membrane of peripheral cholinergic nerve endings, where it inhibits the exocytosis of acetylcholine, resulting in flaccid paralysis. The toxin is bound irreversibly, like tetanus toxin, and recovery occurs only with regeneration of nerve endings. Unbound toxin may be neutralized

with antitoxin early in the disease, indicating the importance of early diagnosis and therapy.

The incubation period, duration, and severity of botulism are related directly to the quantity of toxin absorbed and bound to nerve endings. Speed of recovery depends entirely on the extent of involvement of nerve endings, which must be regenerated to replace those inactivated by botulinal toxin.

## Clinical Manifestations

The clinical manifestations of botulism are related in some measure to age, with considerably less specific symptoms in infants than in older patients. The typical patient with botulism presents 18 to 48 hours after ingestion of tainted food, with cranial nerve dysfunction manifested by diplopia, dysphagia, and difficulty speaking. Patients remain lucid, although anxiety and agitation may develop. Fever typically is absent unless there is superinfection. Additional signs may include pupillary dilatation, vertigo, tinnitus, and dry mouth and mucous membranes. The descending progression of paralysis in botulism occurs at various rates, spreading to involve muscles of respiration and most voluntary musculature. The major manifestation is respiratory embarrassment, which may appear gradually or suddenly. If progression is slow, repeated measurements of tidal volume and other pulmonary function tests may be useful to predict the need for ventilatory support.

Involvement of the gastrointestinal tract varies and is related somewhat to the toxin serotype. Types A and B, the most common causes of botulism in the United States, cause abdominal complaints (eg, abdominal pain, bloating, cramps, diarrhea) in approximately one third of patients. These complaints are quickly replaced by constipation or obstipation. Type E produces more significant gastrointestinal complaints than the other types. Gastrointestinal complaints do not accompany wound botulism. The incubation period is 4 to 14 days and the progression of paralysis is otherwise similar to that in food-borne disease.

Botulism in infants may present suddenly with respiratory failure, and infant botulism has been implicated in some cases of apparent sudden infant death syndrome. More commonly, weakness and flaccidity are insidious, with slow progression from poor feeding and constipation to weakness, hypotonia, and respiratory insufficiency. Most parents describe a weak cry and diminished movement. Ptosis, loss of gag reflex, and poor head control are common findings.

The duration of flaccidity and respiratory embarrassment in all forms of botulism may be quite prolonged. The typical duration of symptoms exceeds 1 month, and full recovery from weakness and fatigability may require as long as 1 year. Recovery usually is complete. Although there are no additional specific complications of botulism intoxication, it is obvious that the potential complications of prolonged paralysis, assisted ventilation, and nutritional support are significant. Patients who progress to significant respiratory compromise should be cared for in tertiary-care centers where experienced ventilatory support teams are available. The susceptibility to hospital-acquired infections of skin, respiratory tree, urinary tract, and indwelling intravascular devices defines the additional clinical signs and symptoms that may be present in these patients.

## Differential Diagnosis

The clinical constellation of acute onset of symmetric descending flaccid paralysis, initially involving cranial nerves but sparing mentation and unassociated with fever, should be considered botulism, regardless of whether a history of tainted food can be obtained. The entities most frequently confused with botulism are Guillain-Barré syndrome, myasthenia gravis, cerebrovascular accidents, other paralytic food poisonings, and some drug toxicities. Infectious encephalomyelitis may be confused with botulism in older children. Infant botulism is easily mistaken for septicemia, hypoglycemia, encephalitis, Werdnig-Hoffmann disease, or congenital myopathies.

Infectious conditions of the CNS can be differentiated from botulism by inflammatory changes in the CSF. Neither CSF pleocytosis nor chemical changes are characteristic of botulism. Similarly, Guillain-Barré syndrome is differentiated by its characteristic elevated CSF protein (ie, albuminocytologic dissociation). The diagnosis of myasthenia gravis rests on a positive response to edrophonium (ie, Tensilon test), and radiographic or nuclear imaging of the CNS usually demonstrates cerebrovascular accidents. Other forms of paralytic food poisonings (eg, ciguatera) may be difficult to differentiate without a positive ingestion history but are probably extraordinarily rare in the United States. Toxicity due to aminoglycosides, phenothiazines, or atropine can be determined by the patient's history.

Electromyography may reveal suggestive changes in the form of diminished amplitude of muscle action potentials or brief, small, abundant motor-unit action potentials. Absence of these changes, however, does not rule out the diagnosis of botulism. Electrophysiologic studies may help in identifying other possible diagnoses, such as primary myopathy. Routine hematologic and biochemical testing does not produce diagnostically useful findings, although changes suggesting acute infection may direct the clinician's attention toward some other condition.

## Management and Prognosis

Management of botulism involves optimal supportive care and specific therapy directed at neutralizing unbound toxin and eradicating any infection with C botulinum. Speed is of the essence in establishing the diagnosis with a reasonable degree of certainty so that circulating toxin can be neutralized before it binds to nerve endings. Because the only available antitoxin is of equine origin and therefore carries a significant risk of serum sickness, every effort should be made to substantiate the diagnosis, including EMG, Gram stain, and culture of any infected wounds and an exhaustive history of food intake in the previous 7 to 10 days. Suspected cases of botulism must be reported to local and state health authorities and to the Centers for Disease Control (phone: 404-329-3753 days; 404-329-2888 nights), from whom trivalent antitoxin for types A, B, and E is available. Blood and stool samples should be obtained and refrigerated for transport to a laboratory (usually state health departments) equipped to determine botulinal toxin. These specimens must be handled with utmost care, because percutaneous or mucous membrane exposure to minute quantities of the toxin may cause fatal disease. Patients with botulism should be treated with appropriate health care precautions, probably including blood and enteric isolation. Stool should be cultured for Clostridium because C botulinum is not normal flora, and its identification in stool confirms the clinical diagnosis.

Treatment with penicillin G has been advocated to eradicate C botulinum from wounds and to treat enteric infection in infant botulism. For wounds, intravenous penicillin G in a dose of 250,000 U/kg/day for 10 days is appropriate. For infants, a similar dose of penicillin administered enterally is suggested, although efficacy has not been demonstrated. There are no data on the safety or efficacy of oral vancomycin for the eradication of enteric C botulinum, despite its demonstrated efficacy in Clostridium difficile enteric infections. Additional systemic antibiotic therapy is warranted only if superinfection occurs. Because aminoglycosides can affect the neuromuscular junction and potentiate the effect of botulinal toxin, they should be avoided.

Supportive care for patients with botulism involves the availability of equipment and experienced personnel for the meticulous and prolonged maximal ventilatory support of a totally paralyzed patient. Because the ultimate extent of paralysis cannot be predicted early in the patient's course, patients should be transferred to tertiary intensive care facilities when the diagnosis is entertained. Monitoring with pulmonary function studies is a sensitive means of assessing the progression of paralysis and determining the need for ventilatory support. These patients also need nutritional support, usually with total parenteral nutrition because of the prevalence of adynamic ileus. Every effort should be made to ensure optimal caloric intake because paralysis may be quite prolonged. Careful attention to skin care and to bowel and bladder function must be maintained to minimize complications.

The prognosis of botulism is related to the dose of toxin acquired and the duration and severity of paralysis. The patient's age is relevant. The overall mortality rate is 30% to 35%, but for patients younger than 20 years of age, the mortality rate is 10%. The mortality rate for infant botulism is less than 5%. There may be a correlation with antigenic type; type B appears to have a lower mortality rate than type A. Most deaths from botulism occur in hospitals and can be attributed to failure to recognize the need for ventilatory support, failure of ventilatory equipment, and nosocomial pulmonary or systemic infections. Early recognition of the disease, provision of adequate supportive care, and meticulous attention to life support systems markedly improve the outcome of botulism. Survivors ordinarily recover without neurologic or neuromuscular sequelae, although full recovery may require many months. Weakness and easy fatigability are prolonged.

## Prevention

Although botulinal toxoid is immunogenic and presumably protective, the rarity of this disease makes active immunization impractical. The best preventive measure is to ensure adequate care of food products and infant feedings. After a case has been recognized, health authorities must be notified so that other potential cases can be identified and treated expectantly.

Because the commercial food industry is attentive to appropriate temperatures and aseptic conditions, few cases of botulism are traced to these sources. In the home preparation of food, all hot foods should be brought to the appropriate temperature before consumption, with particular attention to canning and preserving foods. The use of sterile containers and pressure cookers in which temperatures of 120 °C can be reached and maintained for 30 minutes ensures the elimination of viable C botulinum spores. Boiling home-preserved foods for 10 minutes before consumption inactivates the toxin. Neither microwaves nor the temperatures commonly achieved in microwave ovens are adequate to kill C botulinum spores or inactivate the toxin. Home-preserved foods should be cooked in traditional equipment.

Prevention of infant botulism appears simple: eliminate honey and other uncooked or inadequately preserved foods from the diets of young infants. C botulinum spores have been recovered from corn syrup, although no cases have implicated this source. Breast-feeding apparently diminishes the severity of infant botulism, although cases have occurred in breast-fed infants receiving honey in supplemental feedings. Adhering to standard recommendations for infant feeding practices can eliminate this risk.

## CLOSTRIDIUM PERFRINGENS

C perfringens is a ubiquitous bacterium associated with several exotoxin-mediated clinical diseases. There are 12 recognized toxins (ie, alpha through nu), and the species is divided into types A through E based on the spectrum of toxins produced. Disease syndromes that are caused by *C perfringens* include food poisoning, necrotizing enteritis, and gas gangrene.

## Clostridial Food Poisoning

Acute self-limiting gastroenteritis due to contaminated food products is often associated with *C perfringens* and its toxins. In some years, *C perfringens* has been documented as the third most common etiologic agent in outbreaks of food-borne disease (following *Salmonella* and *Staphylococcus aureus*). This variety of food poisoning occurs as a result of ingestion of vegetative forms of *C perfringens* that have developed in foods (eg, meats and gravies) that have been allowed to reach and stand at a temperature between 30°C and 50°C.

Primary contamination of meat with *C perfringens* spores is common, and temperatures of cooked meat must exceed 120°C to ensure that spores are killed. At lower temperatures, spores may be converted to vegetative forms during cooling of the food, risking *C perfringens* growth in the gastrointestinal tract. The toxins produced by these organisms are responsible for subsequent symptoms.

### Pathophysiology

Although the symptoms of *C perfringens* food poisoning are attributable largely to the action of enterotoxins, these usually are formed in the gut after ingestion of the whole organisms. Ingestion of preformed toxin only results in diarrhea if gastric acidity has been neutralized. The enterotoxin formed in vivo is a 35,000-d peptide that is heat and acid labile and is inactivated by some proteolytic enzymes. In animals, the toxin inhibits glucose absorption and secretion of water, sodium, and chloride, and it strips the epithelium of villous tips. The in vitro cytotoxic effect is similar to that of *Shigella* toxin but differs from that of cholera or *Escherichia coli* enterotoxins. Adenylcyclase appears not to be involved in the mediation of *C perfringens* toxin activity. The resultant gastroenteritis demonstrates components of secretory and inflammatory diarrhea.

### Clinical Manifestations

*C perfringens* food poisoning is an acute, self-limiting diarrheal illness with an onset 8 to 24 hours after ingestion of contaminated food. Crampy abdominal pain commonly accompanies watery diarrhea, which does not contain blood or mucus. Fever, nausea, and vomiting rarely occur. The duration of disease commonly is less than 24 hours, and medical intervention usually is not warranted or sought, except in the case of outbreaks. Occasionally, fluid loss sufficient to require intravenous rehydration may occur, particularly in young infants.

### Differential Diagnosis

Differentiating this acute diarrheal disease from the numerous other viral, bacterial, and toxic causes of diarrhea may be difficult on clinical grounds unless an outbreak has occurred. The absence of fever, nausea, vomiting, or blood or mucus in stools makes *Salmonella*, *Shigella*, *Campylobacter*, *Yersinia*, or rotavirus unlikely. The duration of infection caused by these agents is usually more prolonged than is *C perfringens* food poisoning. Diagnosis can be substantiated reliably only by culture of large quantities of *C perfringens* from the suspect food and the patient's fecal samples. Immunologic testing for enterotoxin may be used to detect contaminated food but is not useful in clinical diagnosis.

### Management and Prognosis

By virtue of the self-limiting nature of this disease, medical intervention rarely is warranted. Oral rehydration with hypotonic fluids generally suffices, although in unusual circumstances, particularly in infants, intravenous hydration may be required. Symptomatic antidiarrheal therapy is used infrequently because of the short duration of symptoms but probably is not contraindicated and may be useful in large outbreaks. Antibiotics serve no useful purpose in this disease and should not be used; no antitoxin is available.

### Prevention

As is the case in most food-borne diseases, the best means of prevention is appropriate handling of cooked foods, especially meats. Meats should reach at least 120°C during cooking and, if not consumed while hot, should be stored at less than 5°C. Meat allowed to stand at room temperature is prime material for contamination with vegetative forms of *C perfringens*. Preformed toxin is destroyed with reheating to serving temperature, although spores are not affected by this temperature. Inhomogeneous heating, as may occur in microwave ovens, can leave some toxin undestroyed and should be avoided.

## Necrotizing Enteritis

Necrotizing enteritis due to *C perfringens* (ie, pig-bel) is a rare, frequently fatal condition seen almost exclusively in highland natives of New Guinea. The disease is caused by *C perfringens* type C; this organism elaborates the potent β-toxin, which is responsible for extensive cytotoxicity and tissue necrosis. The β-toxin is highly susceptible to proteolysis, and the disease is seen in hosts who lack intestinal proteolytic enzymes, presumably because of a largely vegetarian diet. Pig-bel is seen after ritual feasting on roast pig.

Although the equivalent of pig-bel has not been described in the developed world, the pathology and pathophysiology of the disease have led to speculation about the role of *C perfringens* in other forms of necrotizing enteritis. In pig-bel, the β-toxin causes extensive destruction and gangrene of the jejunum and ilium. Intramural gas (ie, pneumatosis cystoides intestinalis) is a common accompaniment, an observation that has long interested pediatricians and neonatologists. The clinical manifestations of pig-bel include anorexia, severe abdominal pain, hematochezia, prostration, shock, and death. Diagnosis is clear-cut and specific in the appropriate epidemiologic setting. Proof that the same pathophysiology is operative in developed societies has not been obtained.

The management of pig-bel is largely supportive; no antitoxin or antibiotics are available or useful. Treatment of necrotizing enteritis of any type in the developed world requires supportive care, management of hypovolemia, and probably antimicrobial therapy directed at potential secondary invading organisms from the gastrointestinal tract. The prognosis is relatively poor; New Guinea natives rarely recover from pig-bel. Protective antibodies for the prevention of pig-bel can be induced by immunization with a β-toxoid. The role of this observation in the larger context of *C perfringens* food-borne diseases is unclear.

## Gas Gangrene

Skin and soft-tissue infections are caused infrequently by clostridial organisms; when this manifestation occurs, it is usually in the context of a polymicrobial infection involving other anaerobes, aerobes, and frequently both. Clostridial myonecrosis (ie, gas gangrene) is a rare but extraordinarily serious condition caused largely by *C perfringens*. More than 90% of cases of gas gangrene are caused by this species, although *Clostridium novyi*, *Clostridium septicum*, *Clostridium histolyticum*, *Clostridium sordellii*, and *Clostridium fallax* have rarely been associated with the disease.

Gas gangrene affects muscle tissue that has been compromised by surgery, trauma, or vascular insufficiency and contaminated with *C perfringens* spores, usually from foreign material such as clothing, dirt, or hardware. The ubiquitous nature of *C perfringens* spores in dirt, soil, clothing, and on skin, especially of the lower trunk, ensures availability of these organisms for inoculation into tissues with appropriate wounds. The metabolic requirements of *C perfringens* for growth are the major factors in the establishment of clostridial myonecrosis. *C perfringens* will not replicate in a redox potential $(E_h) > -80$ mV; the $E_h$ of healthy muscle is $+120$ to $+160$ mV. With vascular embarrassment or tissue death due to trauma, the $E_h$ may fall to $-150$ to $-250$ mV and allow clostridial growth. Prior bacterial infection lowers tissue pH and promotes clostridial growth because the tolerable $E_h$ for *C perfringens* at low pH ($<7.0$) is significantly higher than at physiologic pH. The occurrence of clostridial myonecrosis depends much more on appropriate physiologic conditions for growth than on the likely presence of *C perfringens*. Observations in military and civilian life have determined that the wounds usually producing gas gangrene are those involving missiles, severe compound fractures, and crush injuries. These wounds occur in adults more often than children, although motorcycle injuries in adolescents provide a fertile physiologic field. The threat of uterine myonecrosis is very real after septic abortion and may be encountered in pediatric and adolescent practice.

After infection with *C perfringens* is established in the muscle, the severe, rapidly progressive myonecrosis results from the toxins elaborated by the organism, principally the $\alpha$-toxin. The $\alpha$-toxin is a lecithinase that rapidly lyses cell membranes and causes hemolysis, myofibrillar injury, and vascular permeability. The absence of detectable circulating $\alpha$-toxin suggests that this toxin is not responsible for the overwhelming systemic toxicity, vascular collapse, shock, and mental status changes that characterize gas gangrene. These symptoms appear to be caused by undefined toxins or by products released from the necrotic muscle. Although toxins elaborated by the other infrequent causative agents of gas gangrene are not all lecithinases, the pathophysiology of the disease appears similar.

## Pathophysiology

After inoculation of *C perfringens* into an appropriate wound and generation of replicative organisms from the spores, toxins are produced that rapidly lyse myofibers and increase vascular permeability, and marked edema is an early concomitant of the ongoing tissue destruction. Gas that is produced within the disrupted myofibers is responsible for the more familiar name of the syndrome. Vascular congestion in the area of infection does not occur and no inflammatory exudate is observed, but there is a thin, watery, foul-smelling interstitial fluid. Pathologic examination of affected tissues reveals myofiber destruction, marked edema, gas formation, and extensive invasion with the characteristic large, blunt-ended, gram-positive bacilli of *C perfringens*. No spores are present when the organism grows in tissue.

Massive tissue death occurs at the site of local gas gangrene, but death from the disease is usually caused by resultant systemic symptoms. Tachycardia, hypotension, vascular collapse, and shock occur late in the course of the disease; massive hemolysis may occur, and renal failure may result from shock or hemoglobinuria. The latter symptoms have not been clearly associated with specific clostridial toxins, and only removal of necrotic muscle has been effective in ameliorating the symptoms. Inflammatory mediators (eg, interleukins, cachectin) have yet to be studied in this disease.

## Clinical Manifestations

The clinical picture of gas gangrene is so characteristic that the diagnosis can be made with fair certainty on clinical grounds. The major problem is that the rarity of the disease may lower clinical suspicion and hamper decisive action before massive destruction and systemic disease have occurred. The disease char-

acteristically begins 6 hours to 5 days after an injury. Approximately 70% of cases follow trauma, 20% to 30% follow controlled surgical procedures, and the remainder arise spontaneously in compromised hosts or after intramuscular injections. The initial symptom is pain in the affected area and an accompanying "heaviness" of the limb. The overlying skin appears normal at the onset but quickly becomes cool, pale, and waxy. Pain remains the most prominent symptom as the pallor and edema progress; serous fluid begins to exude from wounds and into spontaneously appearing blisters that are filled with clostridia. Frank necrosis of the skin is preceded by blotches of brown discoloration, both of which spread within hours to involve ever larger areas of skin. Underlying crepitus usually is obscured by the severe edema. Uterine myonecrosis generally presents as an intra-abdominal crisis, the diagnosis of which rests on the history of recent abortion.

The systemic symptoms of tachycardia, widespread myalgia, anxiety, and diaphoresis despite low-grade fever appear early and progress rapidly to hypotension, poor perfusion, and mental status changes. Without definitive therapy, the disease progresses inexorably to high fever (often with rigors), shock, renal failure, coma, and death. Clostridial septicemia may be a terminal event.

Surgical excision of affected tissues is the definitive therapy for gas gangrene and must be done early to minimize the extent of muscle necrosis. At operation, the muscle initially is pale and watery appearing, with greatly diminished contraction after transection. Hours later, the tissue is dull red and lacking in contractility and does not bleed from cut surfaces. Necrosis of overlying skin and soft tissues occurs late and generally is an indication for amputation or, in areas for which amputation is not possible such as the abdominal wall, wide excision.

## Differential Diagnosis

The major conditions from which gas gangrene must be differentiated are other forms of severe, progressive necrotizing cellulitis (eg, progressive synergistic gangrene, necrotizing fasciitis). The laboratory evaluation most likely to differentiate these entities is a Gram stain of tissue fluid revealing the sheets of gram-positive bacilli, without associated leukocytes, characteristic of gas gangrene. Progressive synergistic gangrene is a polymicrobial infection, usually involving gram-positive and gram-negative anaerobes, aerobic streptococci, and staphylococci, all of which are seen on gram-stained smears of tissue aspirates. The exudate recovered from necrotizing fasciitis reveals the etiologic agents of *Staphylococcus aureus* and *Streptococcus pyogenes*. Necrotizing fasciitis results in dissolution of the fascia; the overlying skin is no longer anchored and can be elevated easily. Both of these conditions may be associated with systemic toxicity, shock, and death, but the mental status changes characteristic of gas gangrene are not seen. At operation, the typical picture of myonecrosis is absent. Additional laboratory evaluation is not particularly useful for confirming the diagnosis of gas gangrene or eliminating the alternatives. Endometritis and septic shock due to septic abortion may be clinically indistinguishable, although the characteristic distribution of gas in the myometrium may be apparent radiographically.

## Management and Prognosis

The cornerstone of management is early and complete surgical debridement of the affected muscle. Delay in diagnosis or surgery allows progression and spread of the myonecrosis, leading to extensive tissue loss and worsening systemic toxicity. The extent of debridement depends on the viability of muscle, which is determined at operation. Commonly, several surgical procedures must be performed before all nonviable tissue is removed, because surgeons understandably attempt to save as much tissue as possible, and subsequent operations are needed to remove tissue that proves to be nonviable. Aggressive surgical management must be encouraged early in the disease if a successful outcome is to be achieved.

Specific antimicrobial therapy directed at *Clostridium* should be administered to minimize the growth of the bacterium, recognizing that the anoxic and acidic environment of dead muscle is not conducive to antimicrobial efficacy. The drug of choice is penicillin G in a dose of 200,000 to 400,000 U/kg/day intravenously, divided for administration every 4 hours. Alternatives for penicillin-allergic patients include chloramphenicol, advanced-generation cephalosporins, and vancomycin. Treatment should be continued until bacteremia has cleared and symptoms have resolved.

Supportive care is essential to the management of gas gangrene, and patients should be treated in centers capable of supporting vital signs, cardiovascular output, and renal function. Although no controlled data are available and pediatric studies are lacking, it appears that hyperbaric oxygen is useful in treating gas gangrene in centers capable of managing its complications. The major advantage may be in minimizing tissue loss and diminishing the extent of debridement required. Complications, including oxygen toxicity, mental status changes, and tympanic membrane perforation, are significant, and the prognosis for survival may not be improved over the aggressive surgical approach. The use of specific antitoxin has been advocated, but substantive supportive data are not available. The polyvalent antitoxin is of equine origin, carrying the risk of serum sickness, and has not been shown to improve outcome.

The prognosis for survival from gas gangrene depends on the location and extent of disease and rapidity of appropriate debridement. Mortality rates range from 5% with early diagnosis and aggressive debridement to virtually certain death if surgical treatment is delayed (eg, in a wartime situation). The overall survival rate appears to be 75% to 90% with competent treatment.

### Prevention

The key to preventing clostridial myonecrosis is adequate cleaning and debridement of contaminated wounds. Antimicrobial treatment, best considered therapeutic rather than prophylactic in this setting, should be administered to patients with heavily contaminated wounds, and care should be taken to avoid the anaerobic environments created by closing the wounds. Meticulous attention to the principles of surgical wound management prevents most cases of surgical wound gas gangrene.

## CLOSTRIDIUM DIFFICILE

Antibiotic-associated colitis is a potentially serious diarrheal illness that was initially attributed to the direct toxic effect of some antibiotics but has been shown conclusively to be caused by toxigenic *C difficile*. The etiologic role of this organism and its toxins was confirmed in the hamster model of antibiotic-induced cecitis, which parallels the disease in humans. In hamsters, the disease is always associated with an overgrowth of *C difficile*. *C difficile* toxin is detected in fecal extracts, which can produce the disease in healthy animals. Specific antitoxin neutralizes the toxic effect and prevents the disease.

*C difficile* produces two toxins, A and B, both of which cause disease. A toxin C has been described, but its role in disease production is not yet clear. The prevalence of *C difficile* in the gastrointestinal flora seems to vary widely depending on patient age, underlying disease, and history of hospitalization or antibiotic usage. Carriage rate in asymptomatic neonates and infants may reach 50%, but the organism exists in fewer than 2% of older children and adults without diarrheal disease. Patients with cystic fibrosis demonstrate higher than average rates of asymptomatic

carriage. Positive assays for *C difficile* toxin suggest that factors providing protection against *C difficile* colitis may be operative in infants and patients with cystic fibrosis.

Symptomatic *C difficile* colitis is unusual in pediatric patients, although one investigator suggested that this organism is second only to *Salmonella* as a cause of bacterial diarrheal disease in the United States. Whatever host factors play a role in protecting newborns and infants probably influence the incidence of symptomatic infection throughout childhood.

Virtually all antibiotics with antibacterial properties, except vancomycin, have been associated with the development of *C difficile* colitis. The association of this disease only with clindamycin has been disproved. The drugs most commonly implicated are ampicillin, the cephalosporins, and clindamycin. Dose, route of administration, and duration of treatment are not related to the development of colitis. Antitubercular and antiparasitic drugs without antibacterial effect are not associated with the disease.

### Pathophysiology

*C difficile* colitis is caused by the toxins produced by intestinal infection with *C difficile*. Ingestion of preformed toxin does not seem to play a role in the disease. Symptoms may occur during administration of an antibiotic or as long as 6 weeks after its discontinuation. It is presumed that overgrowth with *C difficile* occurs after suppression of the normal enteric flora with antibiotics and, with the production of toxin, colitis occurs. The predominant effect is on the colon, with erythema and edema visible on sigmoidoscopy. The characteristic lesion (lending the condition one of its names) is that of pseudomembranous plaques that appear as gray-white exudates in a nodular configuration. The characteristic plaques are loosely adherent and composed of fibrin, inflammatory cells, bacteria, mucus, and sloughed epithelial cells. If plaques are not visible to the naked eye, pathologic examination of biopsy material is diagnostic.

### Clinical Manifestations

Some degree of watery diarrhea, infrequently with blood or mucus, develops in virtually all patients. The extent of other abdominal complaints or systemic symptoms varies from mild to severe. The disease may be fatal. Abdominal pain, cramps, and lower quadrant tenderness are common, as are fever and leukocytosis. Severe dehydration and vascular collapse are rare at any age and virtually unheard of in children, but they should be considered. The duration of symptoms in those with mild disease not requiring specific therapy generally ranges from 7 to 10 days after discontinuation of the instigating antibiotic. More prolonged symptoms or significant toxicity may indicate specific antimicrobial intervention. Additional complications may include toxic megacolon, intestinal perforation, and arthritis.

### Differential Diagnosis

*C difficile* pseudomembranous enterocolitis must be differentiated from all the other infectious causes of diarrheal disease, especially hospital-acquired infections. *Salmonella, Shigella, Campylobacter, Yersinia,* and rotavirus can be differentiated by culture or antigen assay of stool. A history of having received antibiotics in the 4 to 6 weeks before onset with the detection of *C difficile* toxin in fecal samples strongly supports the diagnosis of *C difficile* colitis. Sigmoidoscopic examination revealing characteristic pseudomembranous plaques confirms the diagnosis. In extremely ill patients, necrotizing enterocolitis and toxic megacolon should raise the question of Hirschsprung's disease, and the abdominal pain and tenderness of *C difficile* colitis may occasionally mimic peritonitis.

## Management and Prognosis

Overall, the prognosis is excellent, with most patients recovering after discontinuation of the instigating antibiotic, with replacement of fluid and electrolytes as needed. In patients whose symptoms are more severe or prolonged, treatment with oral vancomycin is effective. Infection is eradicated in approximately 80% of patients; relapses may occur in the remainder. Vancomycin, which is not absorbed from the gastrointestinal tract, is administered in doses of 10 to 40 mg/kg/day in four divided doses for 7 to 14 days; the lower dose is adequate in most patients. Bacitracin has demonstrated modest efficacy, but no agent has been superior to vancomycin for this condition.

Supportive care, especially rehydration, is required by many patients; antidiarrheal agents are probably ill advised.

Retreatment with vancomycin is indicated for relapses. Metronidazole has been used with some success in adult patients, although there is not a sufficient pediatric experience on which to base recommendations. Cholestyramine, an ion-exchange resin, has been used in patients with a chronic low-grade disease or multiple relapses to suppress symptoms over several weeks while normal bowel flora are reestablished.

## Prevention

C difficile colitis is an endogenous infection that is induced to produce symptoms by antibiotic therapy. There are few means by which to predict in whom it may occur, and no active or passive immunity has been shown to be protective. Epidemiologic studies of C difficile in hospitals have demonstrated that this organism is spread within health care institutions and that outbreaks can occur with relative ease. Because patients in hospitals may be at significant risk by virtue of prior antibiotic treatment and underlying disease, every effort should be made to prevent spread of C difficile within the hospital setting. Patients who are known to be excreting C difficile should be maintained in enteric isolation.

## NONCLOSTRIDIAL ANAEROBIC INFECTIONS

When sought, anaerobes have been found to cause 5% to 10% of all clinically significant bacteremic episodes in infants and children. Other infections, such as peritonitis, abscesses, and a variety of soft-tissue infections, are also caused by anaerobes. Although anaerobic infections occur less frequently in children than in adults, they should be considered in high-risk situations or cases of unexplained clinical sepsis.

## Epidemiology and Pathophysiology

Infection by nonclostridial anaerobic organisms usually involves endogenous flora. The species most commonly encountered and their most likely locations are listed in Table 56-2. Anaerobic infection usually follows some alteration in the physical barrier to endogenous microbes and further compromise in the viability of infected tissues. Devitalized tissue provides the necessary reduced environment for the growth of anaerobic organisms. The anaerobic environment is enhanced by concomitant inoculation with several microbes, resulting in a symbiotic infection involving organisms generally considered nonpathogenic and recognized pathogens. Other deficiencies in host defense mechanisms caused by malignancy, prematurity, and drug- or disease-induced immunosuppression are associated with serious anaerobic infections. Compromise of tissues in the otherwise normal host by surgery, injury, or vascular embarrassment predisposes the patient to anaerobic infection.

| TABLE 56-2. Anaerobic Species Commonly Encountered in Clinical Infections | | |
|---|---|---|
| Site of Infection | Gram-positive Species | Gram-negative Species |
| Upper half of body | Peptostreptococcus Eubacterium | Bacteroides melaninogenicus Porphyromonas sp. Fusobacterium sp. |
| Lower half of body | Clostridium sp. Peptostreptococcus | Bacteroides fragilis Fusobacterium sp. Veillonella |

Anaerobic bacteria are isolated most frequently from children with peritonitis due to appendicitis or gastrointestinal perforation. The organisms recovered represent fecal flora, with Bacteroides fragilis the most common isolate. In most children with peritonitis, the infection is polymicrobial, and E coli is often isolated concurrently. Virtually all cases of secondary peritonitis and associated wound infections yield anaerobic organisms. Anaerobic bacteremia in children follows dissemination from a focus in the gastrointestinal tract, including the oral cavity. Alternatively, it may occur in patients with chronic disease or compromised host defenses (eg, leukemia). The organisms recovered from patients with septicemia are Bacteroides, Fusobacterium, Clostridium, and Peptostreptococcus. Osteomyelitis and septic arthritis occasionally complicate anaerobic bacteremia. The clinical manifestations do not differ from those of bone and joint infections caused by more common aerobic pathogens. Specimens for anaerobic culture should be obtained if drainage or biopsy procedures are performed, and anaerobic infections should be seriously considered in osteomyelitis of unknown cause.

Brain abscesses almost invariably yield anaerobic organisms in children, as in adults. These uncommon infections usually occur in patients with chronic otitis, mastoiditis, or sinusitis or in children with cyanotic congenital heart disease. Other forms of anaerobic CNS infection are rare and have usually been reported as a complication of surgery or foreign body implantation.

Cutaneous abscesses and wounds in sites proximal to gastrointestinal and genitourinary tracts often yield anaerobic organisms, as do chronic or acute infections of mastoids, paranasal sinuses, and middle ear. Beta-lactamase–producing anaerobes exist in substantial numbers in tonsillar crypt abscesses, deep within chronically inflamed tonsils, and in parapharyngeal abscesses. Whether these organisms interfere with the action of the penicillins on other sensitive anaerobic or aerobic strains remains to be proved, but it seems prudent to consider penicillin-resistant anaerobes as potential etiologic agents in serious parapharyngeal infections.

In addition to the sites associated prominently with anaerobic infection, virtually any local infection may yield anaerobes. Specific cultures for these organisms should be performed in cases of deep-seated infection, particularly in patients with underlying diseases that predispose to opportunistic infection and in sites involving devitalized tissue.

The pathogenesis of anaerobic infections reflects the complex interaction of host defense mechanisms, including tissue blood supply and viability, and the virulence factors peculiar to each organism. The multiple proteolytic exotoxins and enzymes elaborated by many of the anaerobic organisms are probably responsible for the necrotizing nature of many anaerobic infections, such as pneumonia and cellulitis. These toxins may contribute to the pathogenesis of the synergistic infections common to anaerobes, in which several relatively nonpathogenic organisms contribute to each other's virulence.

Some cell wall virulence factors have a direct role in the pathogenesis of clinical manifestations. The extensively studied animal model of peritoneal infection after gastrointestinal perforation has shown that the capsular polysaccharide of *B fragilis* is solely responsible for the promotion of abscess formation. There is a T-cell-mediated immune reaction to the polysaccharide capsule of *B fragilis*, and lymphocytic cellular reaction is crucial in the development of intra-abdominal abscess after fecal contamination of the peritoneum. Cellular immunity to the polysaccharide can be induced, and protection from abscess formation may result.

Interaction with host defenses contributes to pathogenesis but is incompletely understood. Certain strains of *Bacteroides* and *Fusobacterium* can activate complement by classic and alternate pathways, resulting in the generation of chemotactic factors and local accumulation of leukocytes. Most strains of *B fragilis* are resistant to killing by serum mediated by complement.

## Clinical Manifestations

The common clinical syndromes in children that may be caused by nonclostridial anaerobic organisms are listed in Table 56-3. In general, the clinical appearance of these infections is not different from similar infections caused by facultative organisms. Gas formation may be seen with facultative organisms, as with *Clostridium* and other anaerobes. The major clinical distinction is the foul odor associated with anaerobic infection. Anaerobic organisms may cause infection in most of the same sites seen in adults, although pleuropulmonary and pelvic anaerobic infections are unusual in children. Anaerobic osteomyelitis, soft-tissue cellulitis and abscesses, and perinephric and scrotal abscesses occasionally develop in children. Meningitis caused by anaerobic organisms is rarely reported in children.

Because of the toxins produced, significant systemic disease may accompany local anaerobic infections. Endotoxin is elaborated by gram-negative anaerobes, and typical endotoxic shock can occur in serious anaerobic infections. Hemolysis, vascular collapse, jaundice, and severe toxigenic diarrhea may also occur.

---

**TABLE 56-3. Infections Commonly Associated With Anaerobic Bacteria**

**Associated With Organisms Indigenous to Upper Half of Body**

Brain abscess
Sinusitis
Chronic otitis
Parapharyngeal abscess
Dental abscess and periodontitis
Ludwig's angina
Branchial cleft cyst infection
Human bite wound infection
Necrotizing pleuropulmonary infection
Septicemia secondary to any of the above

**Associated With Organisms Indigenous to Lower Half of Body**

Peritonitis and peritoneal abscess
Abdominal surgical wound infection
Ascending cholangitis
Cellulitis, particularly perirectal
Blood infection after gastrointestinal disease or immunocompromise

---

The classic syndromes of gas gangrene, progressive synergistic gangrene, synergistic necrotizing cellulitis, nonclostridial crepitant cellulitis, chronic burrowing ulcer, and necrotizing fasciitis are manifestations of anaerobic or mixed soft-tissue infections that are rare in children. This probably reflects the generally healthy vascular supply to the tissues of children. If the blood supply is compromised, these characteristic infections can occur as they do in adults.

The specific anaerobic strains isolated from anaerobic infections are usually those endogenous flora common to the anatomical site involved. Abdominal infections and associated septicemia commonly are due to *B fragilis*, *Fusobacterium*, and *Clostridium*. Primary anaerobic septicemia in immunocompromised children is caused most frequently by these organisms, probably from invasion by gastrointestinal microbes. Ascending cholangitis in infants who have undergone surgical palliation for biliary atresia is a complication that may involve anaerobic and aerobic gastrointestinal organisms. Certain strains of *B fragilis* may elaborate an enterotoxin that may cause diarrhea.

Deep cellulitis and abscess formation around the oropharynx, including peritonsillar abscess, periodontal disease, dental abscess, and secondary facial cellulitis, most commonly involve *Bacteroides melaninogenicus*, *Fusobacterium*, *Peptostreptococcus*, and *Porphyromonas*; occasionally, *B fragilis* or other *Bacteroides* species are involved. Aerobes are often isolated concomitantly. The syndrome of Ludwig's angina has a characteristic clinical picture of rapidly progressive, submental, spreading cellulitis that elevates the tongue from the floor of the mouth and may encroach on the airway. Systemic toxicity usually is severe. The organisms involved usually are *Fusobacterium* and anaerobic cocci. Spirochetes may be seen in aspirated material. Wounds contaminated with anaerobic organisms may result in polymicrobial soft-tissue infections. Wound infections of human or animal bites typically involve anaerobes among their polymicrobial flora.

The clinical manifestations of brain abscess due to anaerobic organisms are indistinguishable from those involving only aerobes. The predominant anaerobes in these abscesses include *Peptostreptococcus*, *B fragilis*, *Veillonella*, and *Fusobacterium*.

## Diagnosis

The diagnosis of anaerobic infection requires an alert physician and Gram stain and culture of appropriately collected material. Culture of the organisms is the only method of confirming clinical suspicion. In obtaining material to be cultured, care must be taken to aspirate the infected site directly, avoiding contamination by endogenous flora of mucous membranes. Pus obtained after incision of abscesses may yield unreliable results. Similarly, expectorated sputum or drainage from mastoids and sinuses may be contaminated by mucosal flora, rendering culture results unreliable. These materials should be obtained by aspiration that bypasses the oropharyngeal mucosa. Gram-stained smears of all aspirated material should be examined for characteristic forms and used to complement culture results, which may be compromised by the fastidious nature of many anaerobic pathogens. Radiographs demonstrating gas in infected tissues may be helpful but are nonspecific.

Methods of processing cultures for anaerobic organisms are evolving and incorporating new techniques for the identification of organisms. Commercialized kits using DNA probes or monoclonal antibodies to specific sites of certain strains are being developed. The field of anaerobic microbiology is undergoing rapid change, and considerable controversy exists about the best procedures to be employed in the clinical microbiology laboratory. Nonetheless, most hospital laboratories are equipped to identify organisms or groups of organisms from clinical specimens with the degree of certainty and specificity required to assist a clinician in managing patients with anaerobic infection.

## Management and Prognosis

The treatment of anaerobic infection usually involves appropriate debridement and antibiotic therapy. Other therapeutic modalities, including hyperbaric oxygen, have been used in certain instances, but experience in children is limited, and clear-cut recommendations are not available.

Anaerobic abscesses usually require incision and drainage. Deep abscesses in the abdominal cavity should be opened and drained, and the area should be irrigated with physiologic saline, if possible. Generalized peritonitis may also respond best to this therapy. Anaerobic lung abscess and empyema (rare in children) require drainage, but irrigation rarely is indicated. Oropharyngeal abscesses respond to incision and drainage without irrigation, although excision of malformations such as branchial cleft cyst should be performed. Large abscesses in the brain respond best to drainage, although computed tomography has documented the resolution of some large abscesses with medical therapy alone. The occurrence of multiple or loculated abscesses may make surgical drainage impractical. Most authorities agree that abscesses larger than 2 cm in diameter have improved outcome if drainage is performed and that excision is the treatment of choice for well-encapsulated lesions. Smaller lesions and those documented before encapsulation commonly respond to prolonged medical therapy alone.

Management of anaerobic cellulitis frequently requires prompt and extensive debridement and antibiotic therapy to prevent spread and lessen tissue loss. This is particularly true of clostridial gas gangrene but is also necessary in progressive synergistic gangrene, necrotizing fasciitis, and anaerobic myositis. Unlike aerobic soft-tissue infections, severe anaerobic cellulitis frequently does not respond to antibiotics alone, probably because most antibiotics function poorly in the markedly reduced pH and molecular oxygen tension of anaerobic infections.

Because susceptibility testing is time-consuming, costly, and often unreliable, the choice of antibiotics is based on recognizing the organisms likely to be involved in various anatomical sites and on known trends in antimicrobial susceptibilities. Specific antimicrobial susceptibility may be available in specialized laboratories.

Most non-*Bacteroides* species of anaerobes are sensitive to clinically achievable levels of penicillin. Semisynthetic penicillin derivatives, such as ampicillin, methicillin, oxacillin, and nafcillin, are less active than the parent compound, but the very high levels of these drugs achieved with the parenteral administration of large doses may be adequate in some cases. Nonetheless, if infection due to anaerobes thought to be penicillin sensitive is suspected, penicillin G should be used in dosages of 200,000 to 400,000 U/kg/day. Penicillin V is less effective. The comparable dosage of intravenous ampicillin, oxacillin, and methicillin is 200 mg/kg/day and of nafcillin is 100 mg/kg/day. Penicillin-resistant strains present a significant problem with *B fragilis* and a growing proportion of *B melaninogenicus*, other *Bacteroides* species, and some *Clostridium* species.

Alternative antibiotic therapy to penicillin includes several agents that exhibit high degrees of activity against the penicillinase-producing anaerobic strains. These include chloramphenicol, amoxicillin with clavulanic acid, imipenem with cilastatin, metronidazole, and clindamycin. The ticarcillin and clavulanic acid and comparable combinations are active against most strains of anaerobic organisms. Cephalosporins of all varieties exhibit various degrees of activity against anaerobic strains and should not be relied on for empiric therapy. For most pediatric infections thought to involve anaerobic organisms, the ampicillin or ticarcillin and clavulanic acid combinations are probably the drugs of choice. Oral therapy with ampicillin and clavulanic acid in a dose of 40 mg/kg/day may be used for relatively uncomplicated infections, but more serious infections above the diaphragm should be treated with intravenous ampicillin with sulbactam in doses of 200 mg/kg/day. Ticarcillin with clavulanic acid in doses of 200 to 400 mg/kg/day should be chosen for infections below the diaphragm that are presumed to involve anaerobic organisms. The dose of imipenem with cilastatin, when chosen for broad coverage of aerobic and anaerobic organisms, is 50 mg/kg/day divided in four daily intravenous doses.

The third-generation cephalosporins exhibit variable efficacy against anaerobes and should not be relied on without culture results demonstrating susceptibility to these agents. Newer ureidopenicillins demonstrate broader activity than the cephalosporins, but their inhibitory concentrations are significantly higher than those of the first-line drugs. First-generation cephalosporins and aminoglycosides, frequently used for aerobic gram-negative infections, have no activity against *B fragilis*.

If there is CNS involvement, chloramphenicol succinate in a dose of 100 mg/kg/day remains the proven drug of choice, despite the need for monitoring blood levels, modification of doses, and monitoring for potential toxicities. Because of its excellent penetration of the CNS and its bacteriocidal activity, metronidazole is an attractive alternative for these infections. For children, the dose of metronidazole is estimated at 30 mg/kg/day, administered in four divided doses after a single loading dose of 15 mg/kg/day. Accumulation of metronidazole may occur in the face of significant hepatic dysfunction.

The duration of therapy for anaerobic infections is the same as that for comparable infections caused by aerobic organisms, ranging from 10 to 14 days for minor soft-tissue infections, 10 to 21 days for septicemia, 6 weeks or more for bone infections, and 6 to 8 weeks for brain abscesses.

Hyperbaric oxygen has been recommended for the treatment of rapidly progressive anaerobic infections, but the potential toxicity of this therapy is significant and its value in children is uncertain. It should be administered only by experienced physicians in adequate facilities and does not obviate the need for standard therapy with surgery and antibiotics.

The outcome of severe anaerobic infections generally is related to the rapidity with which effective antibiotic or surgical treatment is administered and to the severity of underlying disease. Peritonitis, peritoneal abscess, and abdominal wound infection in otherwise normal hosts carry a good prognosis if their anaerobic cause is recognized, surgical drainage and debridement are carried out, and an antibiotic effective against *B fragilis* is administered. This is also true of secondary septicemia associated with intra-abdominal anaerobic infection. If endotoxic shock, disseminated intravascular coagulopathy, or metastatic foci of infection supervene, the chances of a favorable outcome diminish, reflecting the effectiveness of treatment for these complications. Anaerobic septicemia in patients with malignancy or other immunosuppressive conditions carries a poor prognosis, as does any generalized bacterial infection.

Data on the prognosis of anaerobic bacteremia in infants are conflicting and probably reflect the different circumstances under which cultures are obtained. Transient anaerobic bacteremia in newborns occurs approximately one tenth as often as does aerobic bacteremia and appears to carry little or no morbidity or mortality, but anaerobic bacteremia associated with significant underlying clinical disease such as necrotizing enterocolitis carries a mortality rate as high as 30% to 40%.

Abscesses and cellulitis surrounding the oropharynx have an almost uniformly good prognosis with adequate drainage and antimicrobial therapy. The complications of airway compromise, spontaneous rupture into the pharynx or trachea, carotid artery invasion, jugular venous thrombosis, and dissection into the neck or mediastinum are rare. Cavernous sinus thrombosis is a potentially fatal complication of sinusitis. All of these complications are exceedingly rare because most children with suppurative infections of this nature receive some form of penicillin to which anaerobes are sensitive, even if anaerobic infection is not suspected.

Superficial anaerobic cellulitis and abscesses respond well to debridement and appropriate antibiotics. However, in progressive soft-tissue infections caused by toxin-producing anaerobes such as *Clostridium*, the prognosis for saving the affected limb is poor, and as many as 15% of patients die despite vigorous therapy.

Anaerobic cholangitis in patients who have undergone the Kasai procedure is difficult to eradicate, primarily because of the underlying biliary pathology. The poor prognosis of this disease reflects this problem.

The prognosis in patients with brain abscesses is related almost entirely to the location of the abscess, the ease with which it can be surgically drained, and the degree to which the mass effect of the abscess and surrounding edema compromises intracranial contents. The mortality rate overall approaches 20%; lesions in the cerebral hemispheres carry a significantly better prognosis than those in the cerebellum or brain stem structures. Death commonly follows rupture of the abscess into the ventricular system, brain stem herniation, or iatrogenic intracranial hemorrhage, which occurs in approximately 10% of patients undergoing needle aspiration. Patients with severely altered mental status have a very poor prognosis.

## Prevention

Because most anaerobic infections are caused by endogenous flora, prevention through isolation techniques or immunization usually is not possible. Severe anaerobic infections caused by bowel flora after gastrointestinal compromise or perforation can often be prevented by early, judicious surgery combined with appropriate antibiotic coverage for *B fragilis* and for any aerobic pathogens involved. This therapy constitutes early treatment for infection rather than prophylaxis. Similar management of other potentially contaminated sites may prevent the development of severe infection.

Superficial wounds that are thought to be contaminated by anaerobes should be irrigated copiously and allowed to heal by secondary intention. This is particularly true of the ragged lacerations caused by animal or human bites. Appropriate antibiotics may help to prevent severe infection.

## Selected Readings

Arnon SS, Midura TF, Clay SA, et al. Infant botulism: epidemiological, clinical and laboratory aspects. JAMA 1977;237:1946.
Bartlett JG. *Clostridium difficile*: clinical considerations. Rev Infect Dis 1990;12 Suppl 2:S243.
Brook I. In vitro susceptibility vs in vivo efficacy of various antimicrobial agents against the *Bacteroides fragilis* group. Rev Infect Dis 1990;13:1170.
Busch DF. Anaerobes in infection of the head and neck and ear, nose and throat. Rev Infect Dis 1984;6:S115.
Dunkle LM, Brotherton TJ, Feigin RD. Anaerobic infection in children: a prospective survey. Pediatrics 1976;57:311.
Gorbach SL, Bartlett JG. Anaerobic infections. N Engl J Med 1974;290:1177.
Hofstad T. Current taxonomy of medically important nonsporing anaerobes. Rev Infect Dis 1990;12 Suppl 2:S122.
Hughes JM, Blumenthal JR, Merson MH, et al. Clinical features of types A and B food-borne botulism. Ann Intern Med 1981;95:442.
Mellunby J, Green J. Commentary—how does tetanus toxin act? Neuroscience 1984;6:S242.
Myers LL, Shoop DS, Stackhouse LL, et al. Isolation of enterotoxigenic *Bacteroides fragilis* from humans with diarrhea. J Clin Microbiol 1987;25:2330.
Nord CE, Hedberg M. Resistance to β-lactam antibiotics in anaerobic bacteria. Rev Infect Dis 1990;12(Suppl 2):S231.
Onderdonk AB, Cisneros RL, Finberg R, et al. Animal modes system for studying virulence of and host response to *Bacteroides fragilis*. Rev Infect Dis 1990;12(Suppl 2):S169.
Trujillo MJ, Castillo A, Espuna JV, et al. Tetanus in the adult: intensive care and management experience with 233 cases. Crit Care Med 1980;8:419.

*Principles and Practice of Pediatrics, Second Edition.*
edited by Frank A. Oski et al. J. B. Lippincott Company, Philadelphia © 1994.

# 56.5 *Bartonellosis*

### Barbara W. Stechenberg

Bartonellosis is caused by *Bartonella bacilliformis*, which produces two illnesses that are distinctive clinically and temporally. They are Oroya fever, a disease characterized by severe, febrile, hemolytic anemia, and verruca peruana, an eruption of hemangioma-like organisms. *B bacilliformis* also may cause subclinical asymptomatic infection. Carrión's disease, an eponym that refers to both forms of the disease, is found only in an area of South America that includes parts of Peru, Ecuador, and Colombia.

## ETIOLOGY AND PATHOGENESIS

*B bacilliformis* is a small, gram-negative, motile organism with a brush of 10 or more unipolar flagella. It is an obligate aerobe that grows best at 28 °C in semisolid nutrient agar with 10% rabbit serum and 0.5% rabbit hemoglobin.

The vector of this disease is the sand fly, *Phlebotomus noguchi*. After inoculation, *Bartonella* enter the endothelial cells of the blood vessels, where they proliferate during the incubation period. These organisms, which can be found throughout the reticuloendothelial system and in many specific organs, then reenter the bloodstream and parasitize the erythrocytes. The resulting hemolytic anemia is caused by the destruction of these parasitized cells, which may constitute as many as 90% of the erythrocytes. Patients who survive the acute phase of Oroya fever may or may not develop the cutaneous manifestations of the disease, which appear as nodular hemangiomatous lesions or verrucae ranging in size from a few millimeters to several centimeters.

## CLINICAL MANIFESTATIONS

The incubation period ranges from 2 to 14 weeks. Patients who are totally asymptomatic can be diagnosed only by blood culture. Other patients may develop symptoms such as headache, malaise, and occasional fever without anemia despite recovery of *B bacilliformis* from blood cultures. Patients with severe anemia or Oroya fever are febrile, and *Bartonella* can be seen parasitizing the erythrocytes. The anemia develops rapidly, and patients present with a peculiar discoloration of the skin and sclera caused by the combination of slight icterus and severe anemia. Other symptoms referable to severe anemia are often present. Clouding of the sensorium and delirium are rather common symptoms that are usually mild but may progress to overt psychosis. On physical examination, the signs of severe anemia and icterus may be accompanied by generalized lymphadenopathy.

The anemia is macrocytic and hypochromic, with anisocytosis and poikilocytosis. The erythrocyte count may drop to 500,000 cells/mm$^3$ in the first 2 to 4 weeks of the disease, and the reticulocyte count may increase to 50%. The pathognomonic sign of the disease is the identification of *B bacilliformis* in Giemsa-stained erythrocytes, appearing as red-violet rods. The critical stage of the anemia is the period of transition when the organisms suddenly disappear from the erythrocytes. During this time, the organisms change from the rod shape to more coccoid forms. The anemia may decrease at this time, but in some cases, illness may become more severe, suggesting the development of intercurrent infection (usually with *Salmonella*).

In the preeruptive stage, patients may complain of pain in the joints, muscles, and bones, and cramps or paresthesias may occur. Inflammatory reactions such as phlebitis, parotitis, pleuritis, erythema nodosum, and encephalitis may occur. The anemia and lymphadenopathy of the invasive stage usually disappear. The appearance of verrucae is pathognomonic of the development of the disease in the eruptive stage. These are usually in the skin but may be found in mesenchymal tissue.

## DIAGNOSIS

The diagnosis of bartonellosis is based on the clinical manifestations in conjunction with a blood smear showing typical organisms or blood cultures. In the preanemic stage and for patients without the typical anemia who reside in an endemic area, the diagnosis can be made on the basis of blood cultures alone. In the eruptive phase, the diagnosis may be made by the appearance of the typical verruca.

## TREATMENT

*B bacilliformis* is sensitive to many antibiotics, including penicillin, tetracycline, streptomycin, and chloramphenicol. Treatment usually takes effect rapidly, lowering fever and eradicating the organisms from the blood. The choice of antibiotics should be guided by considerations other than simple eradication of the organism, including the risk of intercurrent infection. Chloramphenicol is considered the drug of choice, because it is also useful in the treatment of salmonellosis. Blood transfusions may be necessary during the period of severe anemia. Treatment for verruca peruana is not necessary unless particularly large lesions interfere with function and therefore require surgery. Oral tetracycline may be used to aid in healing the lesions.

## PREVENTION

In endemic areas, people can protect themselves by avoiding particular areas at night and by using insect repellents. Insecticide use has been effective in controlling the disease by eliminating the vector.

*Principles and Practice of Pediatrics, Second Edition.*
edited by Frank A. Oski et al. J. B. Lippincott Company, Philadelphia © 1994.

# 56.6 *Borrelia*

## 56.6.1 *Relapsing Fever*

Barbara W. Stechenberg

Relapsing fever is a vector-borne, spirochetal infection characterized by recurring febrile episodes of a remitting nature. It is caused by several species of *Borrelia*.

*Borrelia* are loosely coiled spirochetes that easily stain with Wright or Giemsa stain, allowing diagnosis by examination of the blood smear. They also can be grown on artificial media. The organism undergoes spontaneous antigenic variation in vivo and in vitro. Different antigenic variants result in repeated episodes of dense spirochetemia and account for the cyclic nature of the disease. With each remission, antibodies are produced to a specific strain, which is then immobilized and removed from the circulation.

## EPIDEMIOLOGY

Louse-borne epidemic relapsing fever is caused by *Borrelia recurrentis*. Lice become infected by feeding on spirochetemic humans. Transmission to humans takes place when the bite wound is contaminated with the infectious hemolymph of the louse as it is crushed or wounded. This form of relapsing fever is no longer found in the United States, but it occurs in Africa and South America, particularly in areas of crowding, cold weather, and poor hygiene.

Endemic relapsing fever is transmitted by ticks of the genus *Ornithodoros*. After the tick becomes engorged on an infected host, borreliae invade all tissues, and the tick remains capable of transmitting infection for years. These ticks occur in many areas of the world, but in the United States, they are primarily seen in forested mountain areas of the western states, particularly in areas or dwellings with large rodent nests.

## CLINICAL MANIFESTATIONS

After an incubation period of 5 to 11 days, the illness begins abruptly with high fever (39 °C to 41 °C), chills, prostration, headache, myalgia, and arthralgia. Diarrhea, chest pain, and cough may occur. Splenomegaly is common; other physical findings may include conjunctival suffusion, hepatomegaly, and abdominal tenderness. Some patients experience a fleeting, truncal rash, especially at the end of the primary episode. Neurologic involvement is sometimes seen, particularly in louse-borne disease.

The primary febrile episode characteristically lasts from 3 to 6 days and is followed by a period of 7 to 10 days of decreased symptoms (ie, patients are afebrile but weak). Relapses are associated with similar influenza-like symptoms but can be shorter than the primary episode. Louse-borne disease may relapse up to four times and tick-borne disease 10 to 12 times.

## DIAGNOSIS

The most important aspect of diagnosis is clinical suspicion of the disease in patients who have traveled to or live in an endemic area. The diagnosis can be established by demonstrating the organism by Wright or Giemsa stain of a peripheral blood smear. Examination of dehemoglobinized thick smears or buffy coat smears may increase the yield. Intraperitoneal injection of infective blood into young mice, with demonstration of the organism in 1 to 14 days, may be used to confirm the diagnosis.

Serologic testing usually is not clinically helpful, although patients with relapsing fever may have elevated *Proteus* Ox-K agglutinins. Other laboratory findings may include thrombocytopenia, hyperbilirubinemia, and elevated liver function tests.

## TREATMENT

Relapsing fever has been treated successfully with tetracycline, which is usually considered the drug of choice, and with chloramphenicol, erythromycin, or penicillin. In louse-borne disease, single-dose regimens of tetracycline and erythromycin have proved to be effective. A single dose of tetracycline (500 mg or 10 mg/kg for children older than 8 years of age) or of erythromycin (500 mg or 10 mg/kg for children younger than 8 years old) may eradicate the organism.

Antibiotic therapy typically induces a Jarisch-Herxheimer reaction, with severe rigors, fever, and hypotension. It may be prudent when treating tick-borne disease in children in the United States to use a more conservative regimen. A single, initial oral or parenteral dose of penicillin may attenuate this reaction, because penicillin kills the organisms gradually. Because of the Jarisch-Herxheimer reaction, supportive measures are particularly important during the first few hours of treatment. This reaction cannot be prevented by prior administration of hydrocortisone. After defervescence, a 10-day course of erythromycin (40 to 50 mg/kg/day) is given to prevent relapse.

Prevention of relapsing fever requires the avoidance or elimination of the arthropod vector. Cases should be reported immediately, particularly if they can be traced to public recreational settings.

### Selected Readings

Butler T, Jones PK, Wallace CK. *Borrelia recurrentis* infection: single dose antibiotic regimens and management of the Jarisch-Herxheimer reaction. J Infect Dis 1978;137:573.
Le CT. Tick-borne relapsing fever in children. Pediatrics 1980;66:963.

*Principles and Practice of Pediatrics, Second Edition.*
edited by Frank A. Oski et al. J. B. Lippincott Company, Philadelphia © 1994.

## 56.6.2 *Lyme Disease*

Barbara W. Stechenberg

Lyme disease, recognized in 1975, was first brought to medical attention by two women from Lyme, Connecticut, who were concerned about an illness spreading in their community. Their inquiries sparked an intensive investigation of this disorder and its protean manifestations.

Because of epidemiologic characteristics, such as geographic and seasonal case clustering, and reports of resolution of the early rash (ie, erythema migrans [EM]) with empiric treatment, an infectious cause that was probably bacterial and associated with a vector was sought. In 1982, Burgdorfer and colleagues isolated a spirochete from the midgut of the tick *Ixodes dammini*. This organism causes EM-like disease in laboratory animals, and its etiologic role was soon confirmed by isolation of the spirochete from blood, skin, and cerebrospinal fluid of patients with Lyme disease.

The spirochete has irregular coils and is 10 to 30 $\mu$m long and 0.18 to 0.25 $\mu$m in diameter. It grows on artificial media, particularly a modified Kelly medium. It was designated *Borrelia burgdorferi*.

## EPIDEMIOLOGY

The best documented vector is the deer tick, *I dammini*, whose geographic distribution correlates with the endemic foci in the eastern United States. The major areas where this organism is found are the Eastern Seaboard (eg, Massachusetts, Rhode Island, Connecticut, New York, New Jersey, Maryland), the upper Midwest (eg, Wisconsin, Minnesota), and the West (eg, California, Nevada, Utah, Oregon). In the West, the tick associated with this disease is *Ixodes pacificus*. In Europe, cases of EM, with or without neurologic findings, have occurred primarily in the geographic range of the *Ixodes ricinus* tick. The disease is more widespread than previously thought, implicating other potential vectors, such as *Amblyomma americanum* ticks.

The occurrence of Lyme disease peaks during summer and early fall. Cases cluster in sparsely settled and wooded areas. As many as 67% of the patients in many studies do not report a history of tick bite, probably because of the small size (ie, no larger than a pinhead) of the unengorged tick.

## PATHOGENESIS

Lyme disease results from direct infection by *B burgdorferi* and the host's response to infection. The spirochete is probably injected into the bloodstream through the saliva or fecal material of the tick. After an incubation period of 3 to 32 days, the spirochete may invade or migrate to the skin, causing EM, or it may enter the bloodstream and migrate to distant sites. The isolation of the organism from patients with later manifestations and their positive response to antibiotic treatment support the direct effect of viable organisms in these late complications. Humoral and cell-mediated immunologic changes in patients with late disease suggest the involvement of immunologic mechanisms in the pathogenesis of Lyme disease.

## CLINICAL MANIFESTATIONS

The clinical findings in Lyme disease can be seen in isolation or recurrently. The most common clinical finding is the skin rash (EM) (Fig 56-5), which usually begins 4 to 20 days after the tick bite. An erythematous macule or papule forms at the site of the bite and gradually enlarges to form a large, plaquelike erythematous annular lesion with a median diameter of 16 cm. The middle of the lesion is often clear but can be indurated. These lesions can occur anywhere on the body, but the usual sites are the thigh, buttocks, and axillae. Multiple secondary annular lesions are seen on approximately half of the patients. The average duration of the untreated skin lesion is about 3 weeks. Often, EM is associated with systemic symptoms, most commonly malaise, fatigue, headache, stiff neck, and arthralgia. Fever is usually low grade but may be as high as 40 °C. Lymphadenopathy, which is usually regional and associated with EM, and anicteric hepatitis, conjunctivitis, or pharyngitis may also occur. These symptoms

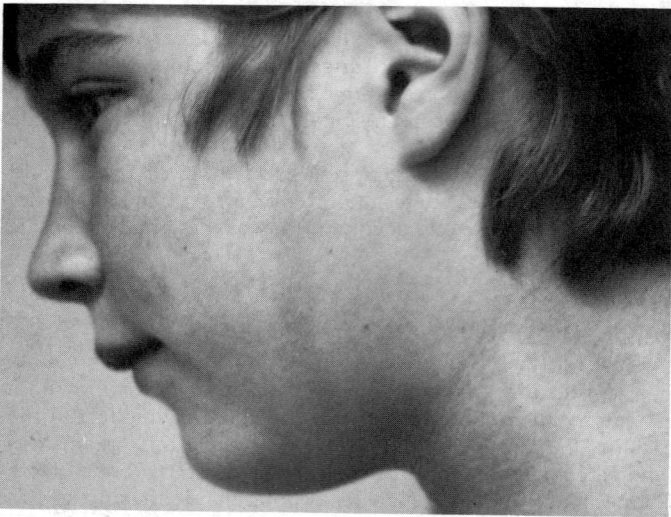

**Figure 56-5.** An enlarging lesion and multiple smaller annular lesions on the face of an 11-year-old boy diagnosed with Lyme disease who had been hiking in Westchester, NY.

usually resolve over several days but may occur intermittently for several weeks.

Neurologic involvement usually occurs within 4 weeks after the tick bite. Meningitis, cranial nerve palsies, and peripheral radiculoneuropathy constitute the triad of neurologic Lyme disease. Aseptic meningitis is characterized by excruciating headache and stiff neck, often associated with nausea and vomiting, emotional lability, and sensory disturbance. The seventh cranial nerve is involved most frequently, in association with meningitis or as the sole neurologic manifestation. Less common neurologic abnormalities include meningoencephalitis, chorea, cerebellar ataxia, Guillain-Barré syndrome, pseudotumor cerebri, and myelitis.

Cardiac abnormalities occur in a small percentage of patients (primarily young men) within several weeks after the bite. These abnormalities range from fluctuating degrees of atrioventricular block to myocarditis and left ventricular dysfunction. The cardiac involvement is usually brief but may be associated with other late findings.

The second most common manifestation of Lyme disease after EM is arthritis, which occurs in approximately half of the patients. Typically, it begins 4 weeks after EM, although the time varies from less than 1 week to many months. Some patients with arthritis do not recall any skin lesions. The arthritis is usually of sudden onset, monoarticular or oligoarticular, and occasionally migratory. Large joints, particularly the knee, are affected most frequently. The first attack usually lasts about 1 week but can persist for several months; recurrent attacks are common. Children experience complete remissions between attacks. Approximately 10% of all the patients with Lyme disease develop a severe, erosive arthritis; this appears to be associated with the B-cell alloantigen HLA-DR4.

Maternal–fetal transmission has been documented. Studies of Lyme disease during pregnancy have not documented a consistent pattern of adverse outcome.

## DIFFERENTIAL DIAGNOSIS

Differential diagnosis depends on the presentation of the illness. When the characteristic EM rash is recognized, the diagnosis should be fairly obvious. If the rash is not identified as EM, it may be confused with streptococcal cellulitis, erythema multi-

forme (if there are multiple lesions), or erythema marginatum. It is important to differentiate Lyme disease from acute rheumatic fever. Fortunately, the specific characteristics of rheumatologic and cardiac involvement differ, and in Lyme disease, there is no evidence of antecedent streptococcal infection.

Forms of arthritis that may be confused with Lyme disease are pauciarticular juvenile rheumatoid arthritis; reactive arthritis associated with *Salmonella, Shigella,* or *Yersinia;* Reiter's syndrome; or postinfectious arthritis associated with several viral illnesses.

The major neurologic manifestation of aseptic meningitis may be confused with enteroviral, leptospiral, or early tuberculous meningitis. If neurologic signs and symptoms are chronic, the physician must consider sarcoidosis, Mollaret's meningitis, Behçet's syndrome, and multiple sclerosis.

## DIAGNOSIS

The diagnosis of Lyme disease is best made on clinical and epidemiologic grounds; early in the illness the, gross appearance of the skin lesions is diagnostic. Routine laboratory tests are usually nonspecific and not useful. The yield from culture or direct visualization techniques is too low to be practical. Specific serologic diagnosis can be used for patients with late complications or with no history of EM. Enzyme-linked immunosorbent assay is more sensitive than indirect fluorescent antibody testing. However, there is no standardization of testing, and marked interlaboratory variability in results has been documented. It is important to consider the clinical picture in the interpretation of serologic results. If a false-positive result is suspected, an immunoblot (ie, Western blot) assay may be helpful. Elevated antibody (ie, IgG) response to *B burgdorferi* persists for years.

## TREATMENT

Even before the causative agent was identified, antibiotic treatment with penicillin or tetracycline was shown to be associated with more rapid resolution of the rash and with prevention of late complications. For children older than 8 years of age who are in the early stages of Lyme disease, the treatment is oral tetracycline in a dosage of 250 mg four times a day or doxycycline 100 mg twice a day for 10 to 30 days. In younger children, amoxicillin administered orally in a dose of 30 to 50 mg/kg/day in three divided doses for 10 to 30 days is recommended, with phenoxymethyl penicillin in a dose of 50 mg/kg/day in four divided doses as an alternative. For penicillin-allergic children, oral erythromycin administered as a dose of 30 to 50 mg/kg/day in four divided doses may be used. The duration is based on clinical response.

For patients with Bell's palsy or early arthritis, a similar regimen can be used for the longer duration. Children with other neurologic manifestations or established arthritis may be treated with ceftriaxone or high-dose parenteral penicillin. The sensitivity of the *Borrelia* to ceftriaxone makes it an attractive choice. Parenteral therapy should be continued for a minimum of 14 days.

## PREVENTION

The prompt recognition of this disease, with its diverse manifestations, should lead to early treatment and resolution. Avoiding contact with the tick vector prevents infection, and awareness of the brushy, wooded locations where the tick is found and prompt removal of the tick after a bite can contribute to prevention. Detachment is particularly important, because at least 24 hours of attachment may be required to allow transmission of the organism. Judicious use of insect repellents such as DEET for skin and permethrins for clothing may be helpful.

## Selected Readings

Burgdorfer W, Barbour AG, Hayes SF, et al. Lyme disease—a tick-borne spirochetosis? Science 1982;216:1317.

Echenfield AH, Athreya BH. Lyme disease: of ticks and titers. J Pediatr 1989;114: 328.

Markowitz LE, Steere AC, Benach JL, et al. Lyme disease during pregnancy. JAMA 1986;255:3394.

Steere AC. Medical progress: Lyme disease. N Engl J Med 1989;321:586.

Steere AC, Bartenhagen NH, Craft JE, et al. The early clinical manifestations of Lyme disease. Ann Intern Med 1983;99:22.

Steere AC, Grodzicki RL, Kernblatt AN, et al. The spirochetal etiology of Lyme disease. N Engl J Med 1983;308:733.

Szer IS, Taylor E, Steere AC. The long-term course of Lyme arthritis in children. N Engl J Med 1991;325:159.

*Principles and Practice of Pediatrics, Second Edition.*
edited by Frank A. Oski et al. J. B. Lippincott Company, Philadelphia © 1994.

# 56.7 Campylobacter *and* Helicobacter

G. M. Ruiz-Palacios, Robert W. Frenck, Jr., and Larry K. Pickering

## CAMPYLOBACTER

Since 1909, *Campylobacter* has been recognized as an animal pathogen associated with abortion in cows and sheep. *Campylobacter* was discovered to cause infections in humans in 1947, when a pregnant woman was found to have bacteremia due to *Campylobacter fetus*. Originally regarded as a rare, opportunistic pathogen, *Campylobacter* has been shown to be one of the leading causes of bacterial enteritis in the world. The incidence of diarrhea due to *Campylobacter jejuni* in the United States parallels that of *Salmonella* and surpasses that of *Shigella*. Type B gastritis has been associated with chronic infection with *Helicobacter pylori*. This spiral-like organism, isolated from the stomachs of patients with peptic disorders, was initially named *Campylobacter pylori*, based on its morphology and similar culture conditions. Profound differences were found in DNA structure, and the organism was moved to the newly proposed family Helicobacteriaceae.

## Etiology

*Campylobacter* are slender, spirally curved, motile, gram-negative bacilli with a flagellum on one or both ends. The organism was originally classified as *Vibrio* because of a similar shape. It was later renamed *Campylobacter* (Gr. *kampylos*, curved; *baktron*, rod), because it cannot ferment sugars like *Vibrio* and the DNA content differs from *Vibrio*.

Fifteen species of the genus *Campylobacter* have been identified, but only five (ie, *C fetus, C jejuni, C coli, C laris, C upsaliensis*) cause human disease (Tables 56-4, 56-5). *C fetus* is an infrequent cause of systemic illness in debilitated hosts. *C jejuni* and *C coli* are almost identical biochemically and in the diarrheal disease

Supported by grant HD13021 from the National Institutes of Health.

### TABLE 56-4. Taxonomy of Campylobacteriaceae

| Organism | Reservoir |
|---|---|
| **Genus *Campylobacter*** | |
| C jejuni subsp *jejuni* | Poultry, cattle, dog, cat, sheep |
| C jejuni subsp *doylei* | Pig |
| C coli | Swine and poultry |
| C laris | Seagull, dog, cat, poultry, monkey, fur seal |
| C upsaliensis | Dog, cat |
| C fetus subsp *fetus* | Cattle, sheep |
| C fetus subsp *veneralis* | Cattle, sheep |
| C hyointestinalis | Pig, cattle, hamster |
| C concisus | Human oral cavity |
| C mucosalis | Pig |
| C sputorum bv *sputorum* | Human oral cavity |
| C sputorum bv *bulbulus* | None known |
| C sputorum bv *faecalis* | Humans |
| C curvus | None known |
| C rectus | None known |
| **Genus *Arcobacter*** | |
| A cryoaerophila | Cattle and swine |
| A nitrofigilis | Roots of plants |
| A butzleri | None known |

they produce, although they can be differentiated by hippurate hydrolysis screening and DNA hybridization. A thermophilic strain, *C laris*, has been differentiated from *C jejuni* by its nalidixic acid resistance and halo tolerance. Otherwise, *C laris* appears to be clinically, epidemiologically, and microbiologically similar to *C jejuni* and can be mistaken for it if nalidixic acid susceptibility or hippurate hydrolysis screening is not performed. The species name *C laris* was proposed because most isolates are from sea gulls. This organism rarely causes diarrhea in humans. *C upsaliensis* is a weak catalase producer and is susceptible to cephalothin. It has been isolated from dogs and cats and has been associated with episodes of diarrhea in humans.

## Epidemiology

Animals serve as the reservoir for *C jejuni* and *C coli*, which have been isolated from the gastrointestinal tracts of cattle, sheep, pigs, and numerous commercially raised fowl. Contamination of meat during slaughter may be the way bacteria enter the human food chain. The main source of *C jejuni* and *C coli* infection in humans

### TABLE 56-5. Species of *Campylobacter* and *Helicobacter* That Infect Humans

| Species | Affected Human Hosts | Common Disease Produced in Humans |
|---|---|---|
| C fetus | Extremes of age; immunocompromised | Bacteremia, meningitis, intravascular infections |
| C jejuni/C coli | All ages; cases tend to cluster | Diarrhea |
| C laris | All ages | Diarrhea |
| C upsaliensis | All ages | Diarrhea, bacteremia |
| H pylori | All ages | Gastritis |

is poultry, although pet dogs, cats, and hamsters are potential sources. Transmission occurs by the fecal-oral route through contaminated food and water or by direct contact with fecal material from infected animals or people. *C fetus* causes abortion in sheep and cattle and has been isolated from bile, blood, intestine, and placenta of these animals. Venereal transmission of *C fetus* has been suggested as a cause of perinatal infections in animals, including humans.

Outbreaks of diarrhea caused by *C jejuni* and *C coli* have been associated with consumption of undercooked poultry or red meat, unpasteurized milk, and contaminated water. Person-to-person transmission of *Campylobacter* has been reported, specifically when the index cases were young children who were incontinent of stool (eg, children in day care, neonates of infected mothers). Intrafamilial spread has occurred but is uncommon.

Of all *Campylobacter* species isolated from persons with diarrhea, 98% have been *C jejuni*. In the United States, *C jejuni* is thought to be the cause of 5% to 8% of all episodes of infectious enteritis, twice the rate of isolation of *Salmonella* and five times greater than that of *Shigella*. The annual incidence of *Campylobacter* diarrhea has been estimated to be 1 in 1000 in the general population, similar to figures found in the United Kingdom. The rate of asymptomatic carriage is low in developed countries, but may be as high as 40% in developing nations. In developing countries, *Campylobacter* is isolated from 20% to 40% of children with diarrhea, with an annual incidence of two infections per child; two thirds of these infections are asymptomatic. *C jejuni* has a bimodal age distribution, with peaks in children younger than 5 years of age and in people 15 to 29 years of age. Males and females have equal rates of infection. In temperate climates, infections occur more frequently during warm months, but in tropical climates, there appears to be greater incidence during the rainy season.

Perinatal infections due to *C fetus* have been related to maternal infections during pregnancy or at the time of delivery. Because of the uncommon occurrence of the disease, the incidence of *C fetus* infection in this setting is unknown.

## Pathogenesis

After ingestion, *C jejuni* are rapidly killed by hydrochloric acid, indicating that gastric acid is an effective barrier against infection. Controlled studies have shown a wide variation in the number of *C jejuni* organisms needed to produce an infection. Although some people have symptoms after ingesting 500 organisms, others ingest more than $10^6$ organisms without effect. If the organisms survive the gastric milieu, they must attach to the intestinal mucosa for the infection to persist. This apparently occurs because of the ability of *C jejuni* to penetrate the mucous layer and to adhere to epithelial cells. In vitro adherence may occur through actions of the flagella, lipopolysaccharides and surface structures of the outer membrane of the bacteria. The attachment and subsequent uptake of *C jejuni* into enterocytes is regulated at least by nonfimbriated bacterial surface proteins that bind to specific fucosylated oligosaccharide cell receptors. The latter mechanisms are similar to those described for *Shigella* and *Escherichia coli*.

After *C jejuni* adhere to the epithelial cells, the organisms are capable of causing illness by three postulated mechanisms. The first involves cell attachment and production of an enterotoxin, similar to cholera toxin, with subsequent secretory diarrhea. Second, like *Shigella*, the bacteria can penetrate and proliferate within the intestinal epithelium, causing cell damage and death, which can be manifested as bloody diarrhea. In the third mechanism referred to as translocation, the bacteria may penetrate the epithelial lining without cellular damage and proliferate in the lamina propria and mesenteric lymph nodes, reaching the bloodstream to cause extraintestinal infection such as mesenteric adenitis, ar-

thritis, meningitis, and cholecystitis. In vitro, *Campylobacter* have been able to survive in monocytes for as long as 7 days, but the clinical significance of this is unknown. *C jejuni* also produces a cytotoxin, but its role in the pathogenesis of disease is unknown. The lack of a simple animal model has hampered further characterization of the pathogenesis of *Campylobacter* infections. The models available are too cumbersome, expensive, or require surgical alteration of the animal to produce disease.

## Clinical Manifestations

Clinical manifestations of infection caused by *Campylobacter* depend on the species involved and characteristics of the host, such as age, immunosuppression, or underlying chronic and debilitating diseases. Acute diarrhea is the most common clinical presentation, and more than 90% of the cases are caused by *C jejuni*. After an incubation period of 1 to 7 days, patients typically experience prodromal symptoms of fever, headache, and myalgia. Diarrhea, accompanied by nausea, vomiting, and abdominal cramps, usually occurs within 24 hours, with stools that vary from loose and watery to grossly bloody. Substantial differences in the clinical presentation of diarrhea occur between children from developed and developing countries. The incidence of bloody diarrhea is greater than 50% in most studies conducted in developed countries, but in developing nations, watery diarrhea is the most frequent presentation; bloody diarrhea occurs in only 20% of cases. However, *C jejuni* is the most commonly isolated pathogen in children with dysentery, followed by *Shigella* and *Entamoeba histolytica*. The frequency of stools varies, but many patients have at least 1 day with more than 10 stools. Acute resolution is the rule, but diarrhea lasts longer than 2 weeks in 20% of cases, and chronic diarrhea accompanied by failure to thrive has occurred.

Abdominal pain affects more than 90% of patients older than 2 years of age, and it can be severe enough to mimic appendicitis. Acute colitis with bloody stools, tenesmus, and low-grade fever has been reported. When this symptom complex occurs in an adolescent, the illness can easily be confused with ulcerative colitis, and it is important to exclude *C jejuni* if a diagnosis of inflammatory bowel disease is suspected. Immunoreactive complications such as Guillain-Barré and Miller-Fisher syndromes, reactive arthritis, Reiter's syndrome, and erythema nodosum have been described.

Bloodstream and extraintestinal infections, which are uncommon events, are mostly caused by *C fetus*, a pathogen that infrequently causes diarrhea. *C fetus* bacteremia can be self-limited and readily responsive to antimicrobial agents, or it can be a secondary bacteremia associated with endocarditis, phlebitis, meningitis or pneumonia. It also can occur as chronic bacteremia affecting mostly immunosuppressed patients and can persist for several months. *C fetus* infections in children occur mainly during the perinatal period. This predilection may be due to the ability of *C fetus* to colonize the genital tract and colon and by tropism for fetal tissue. Perinatal *C fetus* infections can induce abortion, stillbirth, premature labor, or neonatal sepsis and meningitis, with considerable morbidity and a mortality rate that can be as high as 80%. Extraintestinal infections caused by *C jejuni* are rare. Septicemia, meningitis, cholecystitis, urinary tract infection, and septic arthritis have been reported.

## Diagnosis

Clinical diagnosis of *Campylobacter* diarrhea is difficult because of the variation in the clinical presentation, from watery to grossly bloody diarrhea. However, when it occurs as inflammatory diarrhea, with bloody stools, fever, and abdominal pain, *Campylobacter* should always be considered first in the differential diagnosis. A microbiological diagnosis is needed to differentiate this from other causes of colitis, such as *Salmonella, Shigella, Escherichia coli* 157:H7, or *E histolytica*. Direct examination of stool with Wright stain often shows the presence of fecal leukocytes. A Gram stain of stool may show spiral and curved organisms, which may lead to a tentative diagnosis. For detection of *C jejuni* by stained stool smears, 1% aqueous basic fuchsin is superior to Gram stain, to Gram stain counterstained with carbol-fuchsin, and to phase-contrast microscopy. Rectal swabs can be cultured for *C jejuni*, but are less effective than stool samples for growing the organism.

*Campylobacter* are microaerophilic, requiring 5% oxygen, 10% carbon dioxide, and 85% nitrogen for optimal growth. A candle jar can support growth but is not optimal. A gas-generating envelope that reproducibly provides the correct environment is available commercially. Although all *Campylobacter* species grow at 37 °C, the optimal temperature for growth of *C jejuni* is 42 °C. The slow growth of *Campylobacter* requires selective media that allow its isolation from more rapidly growing enteric flora. Several isolation methods have been developed, generally based on two principles. For the optimal isolation of all species, including *C upsaliensis* and *C laris*, clinical laboratories should use one of each of the methods. The first is a filtration method using a cellulose triacetate membrane of 0.45 μm, and the second is the use of selective media (eg, Skirrow, Butzler, Blaser-Wang, Campy BAP, CSM, or CCDA media). Although enrichment media have been developed, the large number of organisms shed in human intestinal infections (ie, $10^6$ to $10^9$ colonies/g of stool) usually makes their use unnecessary. Because *C jejuni* is the species that usually causes intestinal illness, many laboratories place stool specimens on one of the media and incubate stool cultures at the higher temperature to help select for this organism. Agglutination, complement fixation, bactericidal selection, immunofluorescence, enzyme-linked immunosorbent assays, and DNA probes have been used for serologic diagnosis of *C jejuni* infection but are of limited value for clinical purposes.

Isolation of *Campylobacter* from blood and other sterile body sites does not present the same problem as isolation from feces. Growth occurs on standard blood culture media, but slow growth requires that bottles be kept at least 2 weeks. *C fetus* is usually diagnosed by blood culture; these organisms are rarely isolated from stool.

## Treatment

Rehydration and correction of electrolyte abnormalities are the mainstay of treatment for patients with *C jejuni* enteritis. There is debate over the use of antimicrobial agents in uncomplicated infections. When antibiotic therapy is indicated, erythromycin has been the recommended agent because most *Campylobacter* strains are susceptible. Erythromycin shows little propensity to select for plasmid-mediated antibiotic resistance. Erythromycin-resistant strains have been reported in developing countries but are not a problem in the United States. Several placebo-controlled studies have shown erythromycin therapy to be of no clinical benefit if given late in the course of disease, although it does decrease fecal shedding of the organism. Excretion of the organism can persist for 2 weeks to 3 months in immunocompetent hosts not treated with antibiotics. If antibiotic therapy is initiated early in the illness, reduced excretion of the organism and rapid resolution of symptoms occur (Table 56-6).

Symptoms in patients who have been exposed to someone with known *Campylobacter* diarrhea may warrant empiric treatment pending culture results. Treatment of toddlers in day-care centers may be reasonable to prevent secondary spread of the disease. Macrolides such as azithromycin and clarithromycin, which have a longer half-life, may simplify management, with shorter courses and fewer side effects. Enteritis due to *C jejuni* has been treated with furazolidone and, in patients older than 9 years of age, tetracycline. The fluoroquinolone compounds (eg, ciprofloxacin, ofloxacin) may be useful agents in treating *C jejuni* infections of the gastrointestinal tract in adults, although emergence of resistance during treatment has been documented in immunocompromised patients.

Infections with *C fetus* are usually systemic and require antibiotic therapy. Although *C fetus* is often susceptible to erythromycin, the preferred drugs are aminoglycosides, chloramphenicol, or third-generation cephalosporins, depending on the susceptibility pattern (see Table 56-6).

## HELICOBACTER

*H pylori* has been implicated as a cause of type B gastritis and an important contributing factor in the pathogenesis of peptic ulcer disease and gastric carcinoma. Spiral-like bacteria were first seen in human gastric mucosa by Bizzozero in 1893. In 1975, Steer reported the association of spiral structures in gastric mucosa with histologic changes in chronic gastritis, although this work received little attention. In 1982, Warren and Marshall isolated a gram-negative spiral bacterium from a biopsy of gastric mucosa from a patient with gastritis and determined the association of this microorganism with type B gastritis and peptic ulcer.

## Etiology

The newly proposed family of Helicobacteriaceae (Gr. *helicos*, spiral; *baktron*, rod) comprises gram-negative, microaerophilic bacteria with multiple, sheathed flagella that are unipolar or bipolar and lateral with terminal bulbs. The cells have a smooth

| | Antibiotic Therapy | |
|---|---|---|
| Species | *Children* | *Adults* |
| C fetus | Aminoglycoside or chloramphenicol | Aminoglycoside or chloramphenicol or cefotaxime |
| C jejuni/C coli | None or erythromycin, 40 mg/kg/d in 4 divided doses for 5 d | None or erythromycin, 250 mg 4 times each day for 5 d or ciprofloxacin |
| H pylori | Bismuth subsalicylate plus amoxicillin plus metronidazole | Bismuth subsalicylate plus amoxicillin plus metronidazole |

TABLE 56-6. Treatment of *Campylobacter* and *Helicobacter* Infections

surface and rounded ends, unlike *Campylobacter* species, which have ruffled surfaces and tapered and depressed ends with a single, polar flagella.

There are seven recognized species of the family Helicobacteriaceae, including *H pylori*, affecting humans, *Helicobacter mustelae* of ferrets, *Helicobacter nemestrinae* from the pig-tailed macaque, *Helicobacter acimonyx* from cheetahs with gastritis, and a new species isolated from mucosa of rodents. Phylogenetic studies of 16S ribosomal RNA homologies indicate that *Campylobacter fennelliae* and *Campylobacter cinaedi*, which were originally isolated from homosexual men and classified as members of the family Campylobacteriaceae, should be reclassified as *Helicobacter*.

## Epidemiology

*H pylori* has been isolated from patients with gastrointestinal tract symptoms and asymptomatic persons from different parts of the world. It is a ubiquitous pathogen, with prevalence rates that differ among populations and ethnic groups. Seroepidemiologic studies in different countries have shown an age-related increase in the prevalence of antibodies to *H pylori*. Antibodies are uncommonly found among asymptomatic children from industrialized countries, although children from developing regions acquire the infection early in life, as seen by a prevalence of up to 50% among children younger than 10 years of age. Although only 40% of adults from developed countries have antibodies, the prevalence among adults is greater than 80% in developing countries.

Serologic studies of Australian aboriginals, who are known to be free of duodenal ulcer, have demonstrated a prevalence of *H pylori* antibody of less than 1%, but in regions where a high prevalence of duodenal ulcer and gastric cancer exist, such as in Hawaii, central Africa, southern China and Mexico, the antibody prevalence is high.

Transmission of *H pylori* to humans is not well understood. Available information suggests at least three modes of transmission: person-to-person spread, contact with domestic animals, and dissemination through contaminated medical equipment, including fiberoptic endoscopes and nasogastric tubes. The importance of crowding has been suggested by several studies, which have consistently shown that the chance of *H pylori* infection is greater in crowded conditions. Several studies have demonstrated a clustering of *H pylori* infection in families, with a significantly higher proportion of infected household members when a child is found to be colonized with this organism, suggesting that there may be person-to-person spread of the infection. A higher prevalence of *H pylori* antibodies in institutionalized mentally retarded persons also suggests person-to-person spread. In both cases, the existence of a common source of infection, such as contaminated food, cannot be ruled out. Studies in Africa found a greater risk of infection in children when food was premasticated by the mothers to feed their infants. The presence of *H pylori* DNA in saliva suggests the role of saliva in person-to-person transmission.

*H pylori* may be transmitted by animals, as suggested by the higher prevalence of infection among slaughterhouse workers, who have direct contact with freshly cut animal parts; among persons exposed to cattle; or persons who consume internal organs. Transmission by the fecal-oral route and through contaminated water has been postulated by several investigators.

## Pathogenesis

*H pylori* has been associated with type B gastritis and peptic ulcer. There is sufficient evidence to consider this pathogen as a cause of gastritis, although its role in the pathogenesis of peptic ulcer disease is not universally acknowledged. There are enough data to suggest that *H pylori* is a conditioning factor in ulcer production. *H pylori* overlays only gastric epithelium and is always associated with active inflammation of the mucosa. Gastritis associated with *H pylori* affects primarily the mucus-secreting antral-type gastric epithelium and eventually involves the stomach fundus. These lesions are known as type B or nonspecific gastritis. *H pylori* has not been associated with atrophic autoimmune fundal (type A) gastritis, in which parietal cells are destroyed but mucus-secreting cells are not affected. It has not been related to gastritis secondary to medication or to bile reflux. *H pylori* gastritis has been reproduced experimentally in volunteers and several animal models have been developed. The histologic changes of gastritis associated with detection and isolation of *H pylori* revert with specific antimicrobial treatment, and after reinfection occurs, the changes return.

The presence of gastric-like tissue in the duodenum provides a supportive milieu for *H pylori* colonization. The active inflammation results in the development of duodenal ulcer. In patients with recurrent duodenal ulcers, *H pylori* is always found in the margins of the ulcer and in the inflamed antral mucosa. Several putative virulence factors of *H pylori* have been implicated in the pathogenesis of gastritis, including flagella that allow penetration into the mucous layer, production of protease with mucolytic activity, the ability to attach to epithelial cells, production of a potent urease, and production of a cytotoxin.

It has been postulated that *H pylori* is a conditioning factor in gastric cancer, because an association has been found between a high incidence of gastric cancer and a high prevalence of *H pylori* infection in the general population in endemic areas. The organism has been consistently isolated from the margins of healthy tissue surrounding the tumor, and some carcinogenic products (eg, amine derivatives) liberated by *H pylori* have been identified.

## Clinical Manifestations

The spectrum of clinical manifestations in children has not been well defined, because this is a chronic infection and the diagnosis is made after the infection has occurred. Reports on the early stages of infection come from anecdotal cases. One of the most frequent clinical symptoms in children is chronic, recurrent abdominal pain. However, the infection in young infants can present as an acute illness characterized by protracted vomiting that can be confused with upper gastrointestinal tract obstructive disorders. Three clinical entities have been associated with *H pylori* infection: acute active gastritis; chronic gastritis, duodenitis and peptic ulcer, and asymptomatic gastritis.

### Acute Active Gastritis

After infection, symptoms may initiate with epigastric pain, nausea, and vomiting that may last for a few days. Patients may improve rapidly and remain asymptomatic. The pH of gastric juice is usually neutral or alkaline as a result of a decrease in gastric acid output. This hypochloridia may persist for several weeks and may present with halitosis and mild gastrointestinal tract disturbances.

### Chronic Gastritis, Duodenitis, and Duodenal Ulcer

The triad of antral gastritis, duodenitis, and duodenal or gastric ulcer seen by endoscopy is associated with chronic and more severe gastrointestinal tract symptoms. Children may present with severe chronic and recurrent abdominal pain, anorexia, and failure to thrive or with persistent vomiting. Occasionally, hematemesis may be the first symptom.

If *H pylori* infection is associated with chronic gastritis alone, the only symptom may be recurrent abdominal pain or symptoms associated with nonulcerative dyspeptic syndrome (NUD) or, occasionally, chronic diarrhea associated with NUD. Frequent endoscopic findings are nodular antritis and pyloric hyperemia, although it is not unusual to observe normal gastric mucosa with histologic findings of active gastritis.

### Asymptomatic Gastritis

The frequency of asymptomatic gastritis is unknown, but according to seroepidemiologic studies in which a high prevalence of antibodies has been found in the general population, it does not seem to be a rare event, particularly in older children and adults. There are no explanations for the absence of symptoms, although factors related to the pathogen and to the host have been postulated.

## Diagnosis

For isolation of *Helicobacter* species from clinical specimens, at least two homogenized biopsies from the gastric antrum should be placed in a selective and enriched medium at 37 °C under microaerobic conditions for 2 to 5 days. The organism has been isolated almost exclusively from gastric mucosa; only a few isolates have been obtained from stool specimens. It has not been isolated from oral mucosa, including gums, although *H pylori*-specific DNA has been retrieved from saliva and gastric biopsy material using the polymerase chain reaction method. Organisms usually can be visualized easily on histologic sections using Gram, hematoxylin-eosin, silver, Giemsa, or acridine orange staining.

For a presumptive diagnosis, several commercial tests are available for detection of urease production in biopsy specimens, although their sensitivity and specificity are lower than those of silver stains of histologic preparations. Noninvasive, commercially available tests include serology and detection of $^{14}$C-urea in expired air. Detection of antibodies in saliva have had promising results and may simplify the diagnosis. Serology can be used to follow the response to treatment.

## Treatment

Treatment is indicated only in symptomatic children in whom *H pylori* infection has been confirmed by culture or serology. It is not recommended in asymptomatic children or in those with nonspecific gastrointestinal tract symptoms, although close follow-up is recommended. Success in the treatment of *H pylori* infection depends on several factors. It is important to determine susceptibility of the isolate or at least to know the resistance pattern in the specific geographic area where the patient lives. For instance, in the United States, resistance to metronidazole, a rarely used antibiotic, is low, but in Mexico, where this antibiotic is widely used, resistance is greater than 40%.

The required high concentrations of antibiotics in the gastric mucosa can be achieved with metronidazole, the new fluoroquinolones (which are not FDA approved for people < 18 years old), newer macrolides with long half-lives, and bismuth salts (eg, colloidal bismuth subcytrate, bismuth subsalicylate). Antibiotics should be acid resistant, such as those just described and amoxicillin.

Treatment should be given for long periods. The highest eradication rates occur after 4 weeks of treatment, although high rates of side effects are expected and treatment compliance limits long-term regimens. Monotherapy with bismuth salts or amoxicillin is ineffective. The combination of several antimicrobial agents has proved more efficacious than the use of single-drug regimens. Triple therapy for 2 weeks is recommended.

There is little experience in treating *H pylori* infection in children, but the regimens that have proved more efficacious for eradication should be used. These include metronidazole plus bismuth salts, amoxicillin plus bismuth salts, and a combination of the three drugs. The outcome of treatment should be followed using serology. A significant decrease in antibodies should occur by 6 months after therapy was started. Microbiological relapse correlates with a rise in antibody concentrations, and failure of eradication correlates with a lack of significant decrease in the antibody level.

## Selected Readings

Blaser MJ, Perez GP, Smith PF, et al. Extraintestinal *Campylobacter jejuni* and *Campylobacter coli* infections: host factors and strain characteristics. J Infect Dis 1986;153:552.

Blaser MJ, Taylor DN, Feldman RA. Epidemiology of *Campylobacter jejuni*. Epidemiol Rev 1983;5:157.

Blaser MJ. *Helicobacter pylori* and the pathogenesis of gastroduodenal inflammation. J Infect Dis 1990;161:626.

Calva JJ, Ruiz-Palacios GM, Lopez-Vidal AB, et al. Cohort study of intestinal infection with *Campylobacter* in Mexican children. Lancet 1988;1:503.

Fiedorek SC, Malaty HM, Evans DL, et al. Factors influencing the epidemiology of *Helicobacter pylori* infection in children. Pediatrics 1991;88:578.

Hentschel E, Brandstätter G, Dragosics B, et al. Effect of ranitidine and amoxicillin plus metronidazole on the eradication of *Helicobacter pylori* and the recurrence of duodenal ulcer. N Engl J Med 1993;328:308.

Lee A, Fox J, Hazell S. Pathogenicity of *Helicobacter pylori*: a prospective. Infect Immun 1993;61:1601.

Penner JL. The genus *Campylobacter*: a decade of progress. Clin Microbiol Rev 1988;1:157.

Simon AE, Karmali MA, Jadavji T, et al. Abortion and perinatal sepsis associated with *Campylobacter* infection. Rev Infect Dis 1986;8:397.

Walker RI, Caldwell MB, Lee EC, et al. Pathophysiology of *Campylobacter* enteritis. Microbiol Rev 1986;50:81.

*Principles and Practice of Pediatrics, Second Edition.*
edited by Frank A. Oski et al. J. B. Lippincott Company, Philadelphia © 1994.

# 56.8 *Clostridial Infection and Intoxication*

Ralph D. Feigin and Linda D. Parsi

## BOTULISM

Botulism is an acute, descending, flaccid paralysis caused by ingesting food that contains a toxin elaborated by *Clostridium botulinum*. The three forms of botulism are food-borne, wound, and infant botulism. Chapter 56.4 offers a complete description of the clinical manifestations, diagnosis, treatment, and prevention of this disease.

## TETANUS

Tetanus (ie, lockjaw) is often fatal. It is characterized by tonic spasms of voluntary muscles and occasional spasm of the glottis and larynx, associated with slight or no fever. It is induced by a potent neurotoxin elaborated by *Clostridium tetani*. The disease resembles diphtheria in that absorption of exotoxin produces systemic disease.

### Etiology

*C tetani* is a gram-positive, slender, nonencapsulated, motile, endospore-forming strict anaerobe. This bacterium has terminal spherical spores, giving it a "drumstick" appearance. It is nonproteolytic and does not ferment glucose, sucrose, or lactose. *C tetani* usually inhabit the superficial layers of soil, especially in cultivated fields fertilized with manure. The spores are distributed widely in nature. The vegetative, nonsporulating forms are destroyed by heat or disinfectants, but the spores are resistant to boiling, phenol, cresol, or other disinfectants. The spores may be destroyed by heating at 120 °C for 15 to 20 minutes. If not exposed to sunlight, spores can survive for months or years. Spores often are ingested with vegetables, but because they are incapable of germinating in the aerobic environment of the gut, they produce no exotoxin. Tetanus usually results from the contamination of wounds with spores that germinate in the presence of anaerobic conditions to produce exotoxin. There are three nonpathogenic clostridia, *Clostridium tetanomorphum*, *Clostridium tertium*, and *Clostridium tetanoides*, that are morphologically similar to *C tetani*, and they occur in human and animal feces and in soil.

## Epidemiology

Tetanus occurs throughout the world. In developing countries, it is a significant cause of neonatal death. In the United States, fewer than 200 cases of tetanus have been reported annually since 1968. The annual incidence is approximately 1 case per million inhabitants. The annual incidence of neonatal tetanus in the United States is 10 to 14 cases per 10 million live births. Despite a significant reduction in the incidence of tetanus, fatality rates have remained unchanged (50% to 65%) for the last two decades. Approximately 66% of cases in the United States occur between May and November, and the highest incidence is in the southern states.

## Pathogenesis

Under suitable conditions, tetanus bacilli produce two exotoxins: tetanolysin and tetanospasmin. Tetanolysin is a hemolysin and plays no role in the pathogenesis of tetanus. Tetanospasmin, a neurotoxin, is one of the most powerful exotoxins known and causes the typical symptoms of tetanus.

Tetanospasmin acts at four different sites in the nervous system, including the motor end plates in skeletal muscles, medullary centers, anterior horn cells, and the sympathetic nervous system. Neurotoxin is thought to affect the motor end plates in skeletal muscle by inhibiting the release of acetylcholine from the nerve terminals. It has been suggested that the tetanospasmin interferes with contraction coupling or with the mechanisms involved in contraction–relaxation, because tetanospasmin is found in the transverse and terminal sacs of the longitudinal elements of the sarcotubular system of skeletal muscle. This probably explains the pathogenesis of local tetanus.

In the spinal cord, the effect of tetanospasmin resembles that of strychnine. The effects of this neurotoxin on the central nervous system (CNS) resemble those of strychnine. The toxin apparently acts by inhibiting release of acetylcholine, blocking the normal central inhibition of the anterior horn cells and causing exaggerated motor responses to all types of stimuli, muscle spasm, and tonic seizures. The toxin, by virtue of its action on the medullary respiratory center, can cause respiratory depression. Combined with spasm of respiratory muscles, this can result in asphyxia, a common cause of death among patients with tetanus. After the toxin combines with receptor cells, it cannot be neutralized by antitoxin, and its effects persist until it is metabolized by the body. In the brain, tetanospasmin may be responsible for the typical seizures of tetanus, partly explained by the fact that cerebral gangliosides fix the toxin. Tetanospasmin can cause sympathetic nervous system dysfunction, which can be manifested by profuse sweating, peripheral vasoconstriction, labile hyper-

tension, cardiac arrhythmias, tachycardia, increased output of carbon dioxide, elevated urinary concentrations of catecholamines, and hypotension late in the course of the disease.

The mechanism by which toxin is transferred from the site of production to the CNS is unclear. Presumably, toxin is absorbed by muscles and travels in a retrograde manner along the axis of peripheral nerves to the CNS. Hematogenous spread also can play a role in toxin transmission. The incubation period usually is between 7 and 14 days but can be as long as several months, depending on the local wound conditions and the distance between the entrance site and the CNS. In general, the greater the distance between the local area and CNS, the longer is the incubation period. In local wounds, tetanus does not always develop after a simple inoculation of spores, because it depends on the degree of tissue necrosis. The reduction in oxidation-reduction potentials and oxygen tension is greater in necrotic tissue, which creates more favorable anaerobic conditions for the spores to germinate and produce tetanospasmin.

## Clinical Manifestations

Three forms of tetanus are recognized: local, cephalic, and generalized tetanus. Local tetanus is characterized by painful, tonic spasm of the muscles closest to the entrance site of the *C tetani* spores. Local tetanus often results when the dose of antitoxin given after wound infection is inadequate to inactivate all the toxin at the entrance site. Symptoms may persist for several weeks or months and finally resolve without sequelae. Local tetanus may be the only manifestation of the disease, with a fatality rate of about 1%, or it may be followed by a generalized disorder.

Cephalic tetanus results from contamination of a scalp, eye, face, ear, or neck wound; from chronic otitis media; or rarely after tonsillectomy. Insect bites of the face or head also can serve as portals of entry for the organism, especially if the bites are secondarily infected by pyogenic organisms. The incubation period of cephalic tetanus is short, frequently 1 to 2 days. Cranial nerve involvement, the most significant clinical feature of this entity, carries a high mortality rate. Paralysis of cranial nerves III, IV, VII, IX, X, and XII may occur singly or in any combination. However, after recovery, there are no sequelae unless the patient has suffered hypoxic insult. In some instances, generalized tetanus may develop during the course of the cephalic form of the disease.

Generalized tetanus is the most common form of tetanus. Trismus, caused by spasm of the masseters, is the presenting symptom in more than 50% of patients. Trismus may be associated with nuchal rigidity and difficulty swallowing. Restlessness, irritability, and headache are other early symptoms. Within 1 to 2 days after the onset of symptoms, muscle spasm may spread rapidly and involve the trunk and extremities. The characteristic facial expression, created by wrinkling of the forehead and distortion of the eyebrows and corners of the mouth, has been re-

TABLE 56-7. Differential Diagnosis of Tetanus

Strychnine poisoning
Dystonic reaction to dopamine blockage (eg, phenothiazine administration)
Meningitis
Rabies
Other encephalitides
Peritonitis
Alveolar abscess
Tetany
Hysteria

**TABLE 56-8.  Recommended Schedule for Tetanus Immunization**

| Recommended Age or Timing | Vaccine* |
|---|---|
| **Regular Schedule** | |
| 2 mo | DTP |
| 4 mo | DTP |
| 6 mo | DTP |
| 18 mo | DTP§ |
| 4–6 y | DTP§ |
| 14–16 y | Td† |
| **Alternate Schedule‡** | |
| First visit | DTP |
| 2 mo later | DTP |
| 3 mo later | DTP |
| 4 mo later | DTP |
| 10 to 16 mo later | DTP |
| Preschool | DTP |
| Age 14–16 y | Td† |

\* DTP, Diphtheria and tetanus toxoids with pertussis vaccine; Td, adult tetanus toxoid (full dose) and diphtheria toxoid (reduced dose.)
† Repeat every 10 years.
‡ For infants and children not initially immunized at regular time (2 months).
§ DTP with acellular pertussis component may be used.

ferred to as risus sardonicus. The abdominal wall becomes rigid, the extremities are stiff and extended, and the patient assumes an opisthotonoid posture caused by spasm of the neck and back muscles.

In moderate and severe cases of generalized tetanus, the patient experiences generalized, acute, paroxysmal, uncoordinated muscle spasms that can last from a few seconds to several minutes. These spasms may occur spontaneously or be precipitated by stimuli such as a cold draft, minor noises, and light or attempting to drink or move. These spasms or tonic convulsions can cause dysphagia, dyspnea, urinary retention, compression fractures of the spine, hemorrhage into a muscle, or even death due to sudden respiratory failure. During the illness, the patient usually has a normal sensorium. Temperature is usually normal or mildly elevated, although temperatures as high as 104 °F have been reported. Signs and symptoms usually increase during the first week, plateau during the second week, and gradually resolve, with complete resolution within 2 to 6 weeks.

Heroin addicts develop different clinical features of generalized tetanus from patients who do not abuse drugs. Heroin addicts usually have higher levels of fever and no trismus throughout the course of disease, or trismus may also appear well after other manifestations. Marked stiffness of the neck and back and early

onset of coma may develop. In addicts, prophylaxis is less effective, and the fatality rate approaches 100%.

Neonatal tetanus, although rare in developed areas of the world, is a major cause of death in infants in Africa, the Middle East, Asia, India, Southeast Asia, and the Philippines. The high frequency of neonatal tetanus in these areas probably is related to the environmental conditions in which most of the babies are born. For example, dirty instruments are used to sever the umbilical cord, mud and manure are applied directly to the umbilical stump, and rags, contaminated with soil or feces, are used as dressings.

The most common cause of death in neonatal tetanus is pulmonary disease. Bronchopneumonia, hemorrhage in the lungs, or both were the most frequent finding at autopsy. Complications involving the lungs probably are related to aspiration associated with laryngoglottal spasm, characteristic of the disease. Other possible features of neonatal tetanus are hepatitis, omphalitis, cerebral hemorrhage, and thrombosis or rupture of the renal vein.

## Diagnosis

The diagnosis of tetanus is primarily clinical. Most cases occur in persons who are not immunized or in infants born to unimmunized mothers. Tetanus rarely has been reported in patients who were fully immunized. The combination of trismus, muscle spasms, increased deep tendon reflexes, clear sensorium, low-grade or no fever, and a normal sensory examination should suggest the diagnosis. Cerebrospinal fluid studies, electroencephalography, and electromyography are not helpful in making the diagnosis. Disorders that must be differentiated from tetanus are listed in Table 56-7.

## Management

The management of tetanus consists of the removal of the toxin source, inactivation of circulating toxin, and supportive care until the fixed toxin is metabolized.

Aggressive debridement of the infected wound and the removal of any foreign body that might facilitate growth of *C tetani* is imperative. Amputation should be considered for gangrenous lesions. Close monitoring of fluid, electrolytes, and caloric balance is essential because they are frequently abnormal, especially if a patient is unable to eat or drink because of severe trismus, dysphagia, or hydrophobia. Antimicrobial agents are of little value if there is tissue necrosis, because they fail to reach the site of infection in sufficient concentration. Nevertheless, large doses of penicillin G (200,000 U/kg/day) should be given to increase the amount of penicillin reaching the gangrenous tissues. Tetracycline or erythromycin should be used in penicillin-sensitive patients.

Human tetanus immune globulin (TIG) is used to neutralize circulating toxin. A total dose of 500 to 3000 U of TIG is given intramuscularly in three divided doses at three different sites. TIG is available only as an intramuscular preparation, but in-

**TABLE 56-9.  Guide to Tetanus Prophylaxis in Wound Management**

| History | Non–Tetanus-Prone Wounds | | Tetanus-Prone Wounds | |
|---|---|---|---|---|
| Previously received tetanus toxoid | Td (0.5 mL IM) | TIG (250 U IM) | Td (0.5 mL IM) | TIG (250 U IM) |
| Unknown or received <3 doses of tetanus toxoid | DTP (complete primary immunization) | TIG not required | DTP (complete primary immunization) | TIG, as above |
| Received ≥3 doses | DTP not required unless ≥10 years since last dose | TIG not required | DTP not required unless ≥5 years since last dose | TIG not required |

trathecal administration has been tried with some success. TIG does not cross the blood–brain barrier and does not neutralize fixed toxin. If TIG is not available and the patient's tetanus skin test is negative, tetanus antitoxin (50,000 to 100,000 U) may be given in two divided doses. The first half of the dose is given intramuscularly, and if well tolerated, the remainder is given slowly intravenously. Local instillation of antitoxin around the wound may be of value before surgical removal or if excision is not possible.

The patient should be placed in a quiet environment with few or no visual stimuli. Because respiratory complications are the most common cause of death in patients with generalized tetanus, tracheostomy should be seriously considered for all patients. The patient must be monitored for the development of atelectasis, aspiration, pulmonary emboli, cardiac dysrhythmias, and respiratory failure. The patient should be followed for urinary retention and catheterized if necessary. Feeding is accomplished either by a nasogastric tube or intravenously. Parenteral hyperalimentation may be employed.

For treatment of spasms, the ideal drug should control seizures and decrease spasticity without impairing respiration, voluntary movement, or consciousness. Diazepam (Valium) is the muscle relaxant of choice, because it is metabolized rapidly and has sedative properties. Enough should be given to control spasms. If this does not control spasms, neuromuscular blockade and artificial ventilation may be required. The management of tetanus often consists of two of the following agents: a phenothiazine, a barbiturate, mephenesin, meprobamate, morphine, dantrolene sodium, tribromoethanol, or paraldehyde. One agent provides basic sedation, and the second is given intravenously to titrate the level of sedation. Some successful combinations are the tranquilizer chlorpromazine with a barbiturate, mephenesin, meprobamate, or tribromoethanol. A combination of any or all of these drugs may be required.

## Prevention

With adequate immunization and wound care, tetanus can be prevented. Proper immunization entails a series of three doses of adsorbed tetanus toxoid given no less than 1 month apart, followed by a booster every 10 years (Table 56-8). Even fully immunized persons may require a booster of tetanus toxoid after 5 years or more if they are at risk for getting tetanus. For a serious injury with significant tissue destruction, tetanus toxoid should be given even if the last dose was provided more than 1 year previously. If the initial immunization series was given in infancy, a fourth dose should be given 12 months after the third and a fifth on school entrance. The failure rate in fully immunized persons is less than 4 in 100 million. A circulating tetanus antitoxin level of at least 0.01 U/mL is considered protective. Persons with tetanus-prone wounds whose immunization status is suboptimal should receive 250 U of TIG. A guide to tetanus prophylaxis in wound management is presented in Table 56-9. If human immune globulin is not available for prophylaxis, horse serum antitoxin (3000 U) may be substituted for unimmunized persons.

Pseudomembranous colitis, gas gangrene, and other clostridial infections are discussed in Chapter 56.4.

## Selected Readings

Black TP. Pharmacology of tetanus. Clin Neuropharmacol 1986;9:103.
Cornblath DR. Disorders of neuromuscular transmission in infants and children. Muscle Nerve 1986;9:606.
Edlich RF, Silloway KA, Haines DC, et al. Tetanus. Compr Ther 1986;12:12.
Weinstein L. Tetanus. N Engl J Med 1973;289:1283.
Weinstein L. Tetanus. In: Feigin RD, Cherry JD, eds. Textbook of pediatric infectious diseases, ed 2. Philadelphia: WB Saunders, 1987:1126.

*Principles and Practice of Pediatrics, Second Edition.*
edited by Frank A. Oski et al. J. B. Lippincott Company, Philadelphia © 1994.

# 56.9 *Diphtheria*

Ralph D. Feigin

Diphtheria is an acute infectious disease caused by the bacteria *Corynebacterium diphtheriae*. Symptoms follow production and elaboration of a toxin that is an extracellular protein metabolite of toxigenic strains of *C diphtheriae*.

## ETIOLOGY

*C diphtheriae* are gram-positive, nonmotile, nonsporulating, pleomorphic bacilli. Their club-shaped appearance results from attempts to grow the bacillus on media that are nutritionally inadequate (eg, Loeffler media). The organism can be recovered most readily on media containing selective inhibitors that retard the growth of other microorganisms (eg, tellurite agar).

Three colony types of *C diphtheriae* have been identified: mitis, intermedius, and gravis. The exotoxins elaborated by the three strains appear to be identical. Diphtheria toxin is produced by strains of *C diphtheriae* that are lysogenic for β-prophage, or a phage closely related to it, and that carry the gene for toxin production. Phage multiplication is not a prerequisite for toxin production. The most important factor affecting the amount of toxin produced is the concentration of inorganic iron in the culture medium: high concentrations of iron inhibit toxin production. Toxin production can be increased by use of ultraviolet radiation. Diphtheria toxin is lethal to humans in an amount of approximately 130 µg/kg of body weight. Although toxigenic and nontoxigenic strains of *C diphtheriae* can produce disease, only strains that produce toxin cause symptoms of myocarditis and neuritis.

## EPIDEMIOLOGY

Diphtheria is encountered in every country of the world. Since 1976, an average of 56 cases has been reported annually in the United States. More than 80% of *C diphtheriae* infections occur in persons younger than 15 years of age, who usually are unimmunized. In countries where infants and children are immunized routinely, diphtheria occurs relatively more frequently in adults.

Diphtheria is acquired by contact with a person with the disease or by contact with a carrier. The bacteria can be transmitted by droplets during conversation with an infected or colonized person or when an infected person coughs or sneezes. Infection of the skin with *C diphtheriae* may predispose to respiratory tract colonization and infection. Dust and fomites also serve as vehicles of transmission.

## PATHOGENESIS AND PATHOLOGY

*C diphtheriae* can enter the nose or mouth, where they may remain localized on the mucosal surfaces of the upper respiratory tract. The skin, ocular, or genital mucous membranes can serve as sites of localization. After an incubation period of 2 to 4 days, lysogenized strains may elaborate toxin.

Toxin is adsorbed initially to the cell membrane, and it then penetrates the membrane and interferes with protein synthesis. The toxin excreted by the bacteria is in the form of a single polypeptide chain with a molecular weight of 63,000. Protein synthesis ceases because the toxin produces an enzymatic cleavage of nicotinamide adenine dinucleotide, with the subsequent formation of an inactive transferase, adenosine diphosphoribose.

Necrosis of tissue is most notable in the area of colonization. The local inflammatory response, coupled with the necrosis, causes a patchy exudate that can be removed in the early stages of disease. As toxin production increases, the area of infection becomes deeper, and a fibrinous exudate develops. A black or gray adherent membrane is formed that contains inflammatory cells, erythrocytes, and epithelial cells. The membrane sloughs spontaneously during the recovery period. Edema of soft tissues in the area beneath the membrane and in surrounding areas may be extensive. Secondary bacterial infections develop, usually due to group A $\beta$-hemolytic streptococci. The membrane and edematous tissue may impinge on the airway, causing suffocation.

Toxin produced at the site of infection can spread hematogenously or enter the lymphatic system. Toxin reaches the bloodstream readily from the pharynx and tonsils when they are covered by diphtheritic membrane. C diphtheriae may also contaminate wounds, producing a gray ulcer with a membranous base that has sharply defined edges.

Diphtheria toxin can damage any organ, but lesions of the heart, kidneys, and nervous system have been described most frequently. Diphtheria antitoxin is capable of neutralizing circulating toxin or toxin that is adsorbed to cells but is ineffective after cell penetration has occurred. Myocarditis may be observed 10 to 14 days after the onset of illness. Nervous system manifestations of disease generally do not appear until 3 to 7 weeks after the onset of disease.

The most striking pathologic findings are toxic hyaline degeneration of various organs and tissues, with associated necrosis. Cardiac findings include mononuclear cell infiltration and fatty accumulation in muscle fibers in the conducting system and generalized edema and mononuclear cell infiltration. If the patient survives, cardiac muscle regeneration and interstitial fibrosis are seen. Fatty degeneration of myelin sheaths, toxic neuritis, liver necrosis, acute tubular necrosis of the kidney, and adrenal hemorrhage have also been reported.

## CLINICAL MANIFESTATIONS

The symptoms and signs of diphtheria depend on the immunization status of the host, the site of infection, and whether toxin has disseminated by the bloodstream to other organs and tissues.

The incubation period varies from 1 to 6 days. Diphtheria is classified clinically by the anatomical location of the initial infection and of the diphtheritic membrane (eg, pharyngeal, laryngeal, nasal, tonsillar, conjunctival, skin, genital). Several anatomical sites may be involved concomitantly.

Nasal diphtheria initially produces symptoms that mimic those encountered with the common cold. Nasal discharge gradually becomes serosanguineous and then mucopurulent and finally excoriates the upper lip and nares. A foul odor may be apparent, and careful inspection may detect a white membrane on the nasal septum. The slow absorption of toxin, coupled with the lack of systemic symptoms, may delay an accurate diagnosis. This form of disease is most common in infants.

Pharyngeal or tonsillar diphtheria begins as a more insidious but more severe form of the illness. Malaise, anorexia, low-grade fever, and pharyngitis occur initially. Within 1 to 2 days, a membrane may appear, but in those who are partially immune, the membrane may not develop. This white or gray adherent membrane may cover the pharyngeal walls, tonsils, uvula, and soft palate and extend into the larynx and trachea. Attempts to remove the membrane produce bleeding. Cervical lymphadenopathy is a variable finding. In selected cases, lymphadenopathy may be associated with edema of the soft tissue of the neck and is severe enough to give the characteristic appearance of "bull neck." "Erasure" edema of the neck has affected patients with pharyngeal diphtheria. Patients with erasure edema do not have a classic bull neck appearance; instead, the edema is characterized by obliteration of the border of the sternocleidomastoid muscle, the mandible, and the median border of the clavicle. Areas of edema may be brawny, warm to the touch, pitting, and tender to palpation. Erasure edema is observed more commonly in children older than 6 years of age and usually is associated with the gravis or intermedius strains of C diphtheriae.

The course of pharyngeal diphtheria depends on the extent of the membrane and the amount of toxin elaborated. In severe cases, circulatory collapse and respiratory failure may occur. The pulse rate is increased disproportionately to body temperature, which generally is normal or only slightly elevated. Unilateral or bilateral paralysis of the palate is associated with difficulty in swallowing and regurgitation. Stupor, coma, or death may occur within 7 to 10 days. In less severe cases, recovery is often slow and may be complicated by neuritis or myocarditis. In milder cases, the membrane sloughs over a period of 7 to 10 days, and recovery is otherwise uneventful.

Laryngeal diphtheria is the result of a downward extension of the membrane from the pharynx. In the patients with laryngeal involvement only, the toxic effects are less prominent. The clinical findings in primary laryngeal diphtheria are indistinguishable from other forms of infectious croup. Noisy breathing, hoarseness, a dry cough, and progressive stridor may be noticed. Suprasternal, subcostal, or supraclavicular contractions reflect severe laryngeal obstruction and can be fatal unless alleviated. In severe cases of laryngeal diphtheria, the membrane may extend downward and invade the entire tracheobronchial tree. Signs of generalized illness are few in children with primary laryngeal diphtheria.

Conjunctival, aural, cutaneous, and vulvovaginal diphtheria have been reported. The skin lesion is ulcerative and has a sharply defined border and membranous base. Conjunctival lesions usually are limited to the palpebral conjunctiva, which is red, edematous, and membranous. These lesions have been associated with corneal erosions in selected cases. Aural diphtheria is characterized by a persistent, purulent, foul-smelling discharge and the development of otitis externa.

## DIAGNOSIS

The diagnosis of diphtheria is based on clinical findings. Definitive diagnosis depends on the isolation of C diphtheriae on appropriate media. Direct smears of diphtheritic lesions are generally unreliable, and identification by fluorescent antibody technique is reliable only in the hands of experienced personnel.

Cultures should be obtained from material beneath the membrane or from a portion of the membrane itself. Laboratory personnel should be notified about the possibility of diphtheria, because special media are needed. A tellurite plate, a Loeffler slant, and a blood agar plate should be inoculated. Diphtheria bacilli that are recovered should be tested for toxigenicity. Typically, two guinea pigs are inoculated intracutaneously with a broth suspension of the microorganisms. One of the animals is given diphtheria antitoxin before intracutaneous challenge. This animal should show no skin reaction, but a lesion appears within 24 hours at the site of inoculation in the other animal and becomes necrotic in 72 hours.

Leukocyte counts may be normal or elevated. Anemia may occur on rare occasions as a result of rapid hemolysis. Examination of cerebrospinal fluid may reveal a minimal elevation of protein or a mild pleocytosis in patients who have diphtheritic neuritis. Hepatic toxicity resulting from the diphtheria toxin may be reflected by hypoglycemia. An elevated blood urea nitrogen suggests the possibility of acute tubular necrosis. Electrocardiographic studies may reveal ST and T wave changes or dysrhythmias suggestive of myocarditis.

The Schick test, used extensively in previous decades, has now fallen into disuse. It is not helpful in early diagnosis and was used previously to determine the patient's immune status. In this test, a measured amount of diphtheria toxin is injected intracutaneously. The injected toxin causes a local inflammatory response that peaks at about 5 days in persons who have no circulating antitoxin. If sufficient antitoxin is present, no reaction should occur. Because hypersensitivity may develop to the toxin itself, a control injection of tetanus toxoid (0.005 Lf) is administered intradermally in the opposite arm. Patients who are immune but sensitive to the toxin preparation reacts to the toxin and the toxoid. These persons have skin reactions that generally are maximal at 48 to 72 hours and then fade; the skin reaction in the positive Schick test persists for many days. If a person has no circulating antitoxin but is allergic to the toxin, a reaction is observed on both arms, but the reaction at the site of toxin injection peaks on day 5 and persists. The reaction to toxoid subsides by 5 to 7 days. A positive Schick test, defined by documentation of 10 mm of induration, suggests susceptibility to diphtheria.

Pharyngeal diphtheria must be differentiated from streptococcal pharyngitis, infectious mononucleosis, primary herpetic gingival stomatitis, Vincent's angina, thrush, and erosions of the pharynx and tonsils that occur as a result of agranulocytosis or leukemia. It also must be differentiated from oropharyngeal involvement caused by cytomegalovirus, tularemia, salmonellosis, or toxoplasmosis. Appropriate smears, cultures, and serologic tests aid in the diagnosis of these disorders.

Laryngeal diphtheria must be differentiated from spasmodic or nonspasmodic croup, epiglottitis, foreign body aspiration, peripharyngeal and retropharyngeal abscesses, and laryngeal papillomas, hemangiomas, or lymphangiomas.

## TREATMENT

Treatment of diphtheria is based on neutralization of free toxin and eradication of the organism by the use of antibiotics. The only specific antitoxin is of equine origin. Antitoxin should be administered on the basis of the size and site of the membrane, the degree of toxicity, and the duration of illness.

Antitoxin should be given intravenously as quickly as possible and in sufficient doses to neutralize all free toxin. A single dose is usually given to avoid risking sensitization from repeated doses of horse serum.

Tests for sensitivity to horse serum should be performed before administering antitoxin. This may be done by giving 0.1 mL of a 1 : 1000 dilution of antitoxin in saline intracutaneously or by placing it in the conjunctival sac. A positive reaction is heralded by greater than 10 mm of erythema at the injection site within 20 minutes or the development of conjunctivitis and tearing. If the patient is sensitive to horse serum, desensitization should be provided by slowly increasing doses given at 20-minute intervals, as in this commonly employed regimen:

0.05 mL of a 1 : 20 dilution subcutaneously
0.1 mL of a 1 : 20 dilution subcutaneously
0.1 mL of a 1 : 10 dilution subcutaneously
0.1 mL undiluted subcutaneously

0.3 mL undiluted intramuscularly
0.5 mL undiluted intramuscularly
0.1 mL undiluted intravenously

If there is no reaction, the remaining material is given by slow intravenous infusion. Intravenous administration results in a more rapid secretion of antitoxin into saliva. Possible reactions to horse serum administration can be treated with aqueous 1 : 1000 epinephrine given intravenously.

The dosage of antitoxin is empiric. Limited nasal or pharyngeal diphtheria can be treated with 40,000 U of antitoxin; a dose of 80,000 U is used for moderately severe pharyngeal diphtheria; and extensive pharyngeal or laryngeal diphtheria should be treated with 120,000 U. The 120,000-U dose should be given to patients with mixed clinical symptoms and to those who have severe edema of the soft tissues or disease lasting longer than 48 hours' duration.

Penicillin and erythromycin are effective against most strains of *C diphtheriae*. Penicillin is given as aqueous procaine penicillin G (600,000 U) intramuscularly once daily for 7 days. Patients who are allergic to penicillin should be given erythromycin (40 mg/kg/day) in four divided doses for 7 to 10 days. The end point of therapy is three consecutive negative cultures taken at least 24 hours apart. Clindamycin, amoxicillin, and rifampin in appropriate dosages may also be effective. The carrier state has been treated effectively with oral benzathine penicillin G or erythromycin.

Bed rest is important and is recommended for a period of 2 to 3 weeks. An electrocardiogram should be obtained two to three times each week for the first 6 weeks to detect myocarditis as quickly as possible.

A high-calorie liquid or soft diet should be provided and adequate hydration maintained. Secretions must be suctioned. Laryngeal diphtheria that progresses to obstruction may require release by tracheostomy.

Bed rest is particularly important if myocarditis is detected. Sudden death has been precipitated by excessive activity. Patients with diphtheritic myocarditis may be digitalized if congestive heart failure develops. However, digitalization may be contraindicated if the patient has dysrhythmias. In severe cases of diphtheria, prednisone (1 to 1.5 mg/kg/day) for 2 weeks has diminished the incidence of myocarditis.

Immunization always is indicated after recovery of the patient with diphtheria. Almost 50% of the patients with diphtheria fail to develop adequate immunity after recovery from their infection and remain susceptible unless immunized.

## COMPLICATIONS

Penicillin should be used to eradicate *C diphtheriae* and to prevent secondary streptococcal disease. Despite the use of antibiotics, complications remain the greatest cause of morbidity and mortality associated with diphtheria. Respiratory obstruction and death may occur in young children with tracheal or laryngeal involvement as a result of airway occlusion by the diphtheritic membrane. Edema of the peripharyngeal tissue can also compromise the airway.

Myocarditis may follow mild or severe cases of diphtheria. It is most common in patients with extrinsic local lesions in whom administration of antitoxin was delayed. Myocarditis generally occurs in the second week of the disease but can appear at any time between the first and sixth weeks. Muffled heart sounds, dysrhythmias, murmurs, and tachycardia may suggest myocardial involvement; myocarditis may be followed by cardiac failure.

Neurologic complications may occur after a latent period that varies from days to several weeks. The neurologic findings are generally bilateral and more often affect the motor system than the sensory system. Paralysis of the soft palate is most common, appearing in the third week of illness and is characterized by a nasal quality to the voice, nasal regurgitation, and difficulty swallowing.

Ocular paralysis usually is characterized by blurring of vision and difficulty with accommodation. This is most common during the fifth week but may appear as early as the first week of illness.

Diaphragmatic paralysis may result from neuritis of the phrenic nerve and can appear between the first and seventh weeks. Loss of deep tendon reflexes and paralysis of limbs may be associated with elevated cerebrospinal protein, and a diagnosis of Guillain-Barré syndrome may be entertained inappropriately. Hypotension and cardiac failure may occur 2 to 3 weeks after the onset of disease. Selected patients may experience hepatitis, nephritis, or gastritis.

## PROGNOSIS

The mortality rate from diphtheria before the availability of antibiotics and antitoxins was 30% to 50%. Death occurred most often in patients younger than 4 years of age, as a result of suffocation. The mortality rate has diminished to less than 5% and is not associated with patient age.

The prognosis is always guarded until recovery is apparent, because laryngeal obstruction may develop unexpectedly. Myocarditis can be associated with congestive heart failure, which may respond poorly to digoxin. Diphtheritic myocarditis may be followed by permanent cardiac damage. Phrenic nerve paralysis, which may occur late in the course of disease, can produce respiratory paralysis.

The prognosis depends on the virulence of the organism, the immunization status of the host, the location and extent of the diphtheritic membrane, and the rapidity with which treatment is initiated. Diphtheria caused by the gravis strains carries a poor prognosis. The more extensive the diphtheritic membrane, the more severe is the disease. Laryngeal diphtheria is more likely to be fatal in patients whose respiratory status is not monitored closely and in infants. Although there are few laboratory parameters that indicate the severity of diphtheria, the development of megakaryocytic thrombocytopenia and leukocytosis greater than 25,000/mm$^3$ have been associated with a poorer outcome.

If specific treatment is provided on the first day of disease, mortality is less than 1%. Delaying treatment until day 4 is associated with a 20-fold increase in mortality.

## PREVENTION

Prevention is accomplished by active immunization. The immunizing agent for children younger than 6 years is diphtheria toxoid, given in combination with tetanus toxoid and pertussis antigen (DTP). Primary immunization should be carried out by giving DTP vaccine at 2, 4, and 6 months of age, with booster doses at 18 months and again at 4 to 6 years.

Primary immunization of children who are older than 6 years may be carried out using the adult-type adsorbed diphtheria and tetanus toxoids (Td). This preparation contains no more than 2 Lf of diphtheria toxoid per dose, compared with 7 to 25 Lf in the pediatric DTP adsorbed preparations used for younger children. Two doses are given subcutaneously or intramuscularly at least 4 weeks apart, with a booster dose 1 year later. The administration of Td is not followed by the high incidence of reactions associated with pediatric DTP. Td may be given safely without prior skin testing. Booster doses of Td should be given at 10-year intervals.

Primary immunization against diphtheria for infants who have progressive neurologic disease and completion of the primary immunization series in patients who have experienced untoward reactions to an earlier DTP immunization can be safely carried out using diphtheria and toxoid (DT) with adjuvant rather than DTP.

Diphtheria immunization is not always followed by complete protection; persons who are fully immunized may be carriers or may develop mild disease. The most important health consideration in the United States today is inadequate immunization rates in adults resulting from failure to maintain adequate immunity through booster immunizations.

Prevention of diphtheria may depend on managing contacts of known cases of diphtheria and carriers of the organism and on isolating patients to minimize the spread of disease. The patient is no longer infectious when the bacillus can no longer be cultured from the site of infection. Three consecutive negative cultures are required before a patient can be released from isolation.

Intimate contacts of patients with the disease are at risk for infection if they are not immune. Carriers who have been immunized should be given a booster injection of diphtheria toxoid. They can also be treated with aqueous procaine penicillin (600,000 U/day) for 4 days; benzathine penicillin G (600,000 U) given intramuscularly as a single dose; or erythromycin (40 mg/kg/day) for 7 to 10 days.

Asymptomatic carriers who have not been immunized previously should be cultured and given diphtheria toxoid, penicillin, or erythromycin as previously described. If daily surveillance by a physician is not possible, diphtheria antitoxin (10,000 U) may be administered intramuscularly. The risk of allergic reactions to this horse serum preparation limits its usefulness, and skin testing for sensitivity at a site separate from that of the toxoid injection is necessary. The efficacy of chemoprophylaxis for diphtheria has not been established conclusively. A contact who is experiencing symptoms when first seen should be treated as a case of diphtheria.

## Selected Readings

Brooks GF. Recent trends in diphtheria in the United States. J Infect Dis 1969;120: 500.

Centers for Disease Control. Diphtheria, tetanus and pertussis: guidelines for vaccine prophylaxis and other preventive measures. MMWR 1981;30:392.

Collier RJ. Diphtheria toxin: mode of action and structure. Bacteriol Rev 1975;39: 54.

Feigin RD, Stechenberg BW. Diphtheria. In: Feigin RD, Cherry JD, eds. Textbook of pediatric infectious diseases, ed 2. Philadelphia: WB Saunders, 1987:1134.

Miller LW, Older JJ, Drake J, et al. Diphtheria immunization. Effect upon carriers and the control of outbreaks. Am J Dis Child 1972;123:197.

*Principles and Practice of Pediatrics, Second Edition.*
edited by Frank A. Oski et al. J. B. Lippincott Company, Philadelphia © 1994.

# *56.10* Escherichia coli

## John J. Mathewson and Larry K. Pickering

*Escherichia coli* inhabits the human gastrointestinal tract and accounts for the largest proportion of the facultative aerobic, gram-negative bacteria in fecal flora. In this ecologic setting, *E coli* is part of the normal bacterial flora, except for a few strains that

This work was supported by NIH Grant HD-13021.

TABLE 56-10. Characteristics of *Escherichia coli* Associated With Diarrhea

| Type of E coli | Epidemiology | Type of Diarrhea | Diagnosis |
|---|---|---|---|
| Enteropathogenic | Acute and chronic endemic and epidemic diarrhea in infants | Watery | Serotyping, HEp-2 cell adherence, DNA probe |
| Enterotoxigenic | Infantile diarrhea in developing countries and travelers' diarrhea | Watery | Animal models, tissue culture, ELISA, DNA probe |
| Enteroinvasive | Dysentery with fever | Bloody | Biochemical characteristics, animal model, tissue culture, gene probe, PCR |
| Enterohemorrhagic | Hemorrhagic colitis, hemolytic uremic syndrome and thrombotic thrombocytopenic purpura | Bloody | Sorbitol plate, serotyping, cytotoxin production, DNA probe, PCR |
| Enteroadherent | Not fully defined | Watery | HEp-2 cell adherence, gene probes |

*ELISA*, enzyme-linked immunosorbent assay; *PCR*, polymerase chain reaction.

can cause gastrointestinal tract illness. The diarrhea-associated *E coli* strains possess specific virulence properties that can produce disease. Pathogenic stains resemble normal flora when cultured on media routinely used in clinical microbiology laboratories. To identify pathogenic strains, *E coli* must be shown to possess a recognized virulence property, to possess the genes that encode the property, or to belong to a specific serotype.

At least five different classes of diarrhea-associated *E coli* are recognized (Table 56-10). Each class has a distinct group of somatic (O) and flagellar (H) antigens and has specific virulence characteristics that are usually plasmid-mediated. There are 164 O and 56 H groups. Enteropathogenic *E coli* (EPEC) cause disease by adherence to the intestinal mucosa, and enterotoxigenic *E coli* (ETEC) adhere to the small bowel by a different mechanism and elaborate enterotoxins. Enteroinvasive *E coli* (EIEC) invade the mucosa of the colon. Enterohemorrhagic *E coli* (EHEC) cause grossly bloody diarrhea by adhering to the colonic mucosa and producing cytotoxins that are referred to as Shiga-like toxins. Enteroadherent or enteroaggregative *E coli* are a class of diarrhea-associated *E coli* that adhere to HEp-2 tissue culture cells but do not belong to EPEC serotypes.

These five classes of *E coli* are important causes of diarrhea in children around the world and are among the most common causes of endemic diarrheal disease of children in developing countries, where diarrheal illnesses are the leading cause of morbidity and mortality. Except for EHEC, these classes of *E coli* are less frequently associated with sporadic episodes and with outbreaks of diarrheal disease in the United States than in developing countries.

## ENTEROPATHOGENIC *ESCHERICHIA COLI*

The enteropathogenic class contains specific *E coli* serotypes that have been epidemiologically incriminated as causes of infantile diarrhea. These serogroups do not produce traditional *E coli* enterotoxins and are not enteroinvasive. EPEC consists of 12 different serogroups (Table 56-11) that are identified by serotyping.

EPEC were the first recognized diarrhea-associated *E coli*. In the late 1940s and early 1950s, certain serogroups of *E coli* were associated with outbreaks of severe, protracted diarrhea with a

high mortality rate among children in hospital nurseries. After discovery that some *E coli* were enterotoxigenic and others were enteroinvasive, the pathogenicity of EPEC was questioned. Some investigators claimed that during storage these original outbreak strains had lost the plasmids that encoded for invasion or toxin production and that EPEC should not be considered as a separate group. However, EPEC strains that were not invasive and did not produce enterotoxins caused diarrheal illness when fed to adult volunteers. There is no doubt of the enteropathogenicity of EPEC strains.

### Epidemiology

Infection with EPEC usually occurs in children younger than 2 years of age and results in acute or chronic diarrhea. In developing countries, EPEC strains are a common cause of endemic pediatric diarrheal disease, but in industrialized countries EPEC is a less frequent cause of diarrhea. In the United States, outbreaks have occurred in hospitals and day-care centers, but community outbreaks and sporadic cases have been described. Knowledge of the epidemiology of this organism has been limited by the fact that identifying EPEC requires serotyping all *E coli* strains to demonstrate that they belong to specific serogroups. This technique is too costly and labor intensive for large-scale field studies.

TABLE 56-11. Serogroups of *Escherichia coli* Associated With Diarrhea

| Types of E coli | Serogroups |
|---|---|
| Enteropathogenic | O44, O55, O86, O111, O114, O119, O125, O126, O127, O128, O142, O158 |
| Enterotoxigenic | O6, O8, O12, O15, O20, O25, O27, O63, O78, O80, O85, O115, O139, O148, O149, O153, O159, O167 |
| Enteroinvasive | O11, O28, O29, O32, O42, O112, O115, O124, O136, O143, O144, O152, O164, O167 |
| Enterohemorrhagic | O157:H7, O26:H11, others |

## Pathogenesis

EPEC infection produces a characteristic lesion in the intestinal tract, called an attaching and effacing lesion. Attaching and effacing lesions are also produced by EHEC and *E coli* that produce diarrhea in suckling and weaning rabbits, such as the RDEC-1 strain. These organisms adhere to the intestine and form microcolonies, with destruction of microvilli and pedestal formation. Localized adherence to HEp-2 and HeLa tissue culture cell lines has become the in vitro model of EPEC adherence but not of EHEC adherence. Adherence is mediated by plasmid and chromosomal genes and and associated with a 94-kd protein. A DNA probe has been developed to detect adherent EPEC strains and is referred to as EPEC adherence factor.

The microcolony forms because of bundle-forming pili that bind the bacterial cells together. Attaching and effacing histopathology is characterized by close attachment of the bacterium to the enterocyte, effacement of the microvilli, disruption of the cellular cytoskeleton at the site of attachment, and cupping of the enterocyte membrane around the bacterium. Actin polymerization occurs in the host cells to which the EPEC adhere. Invasion of the intestinal epithelium in the HEp-2 cell model suggests that mucosal invasion may be part of the disease process. Non-EPEC *E coli* strains also adhere to HEp-2 cells, but they are a distinct class of diarrhea-associated *E coli* referred to as enteroadherent or enteroaggregative *E coli*. The adherence patterns in HEp-2 cells of the enteroadherent and enteroaggregative *E coli* are not localized.

The EPEC strains do not produce the traditional *E coli* enterotoxins, but concentrated supernatants have toxic effects in some animal models. Some EPEC strains produce low or moderate levels of Shiga-like cytotoxin, and some EHEC strains adhere to HEp-2 cells. The importance of toxin production in the pathogenicity of EPEC is unknown. The relation of EPEC and EHEC strains needs further investigation.

## Clinical Manifestations

Children with EPEC infection often develop chronic, watery diarrhea. Most patients are younger than 2 years of age, and most are younger than 1 year. The diarrhea is often severe (ie, 10 to 20 stools a day) and lasts 10 days to 2 weeks if untreated. The mortality due to this infection can be high. Dehydration is common and is the most important complication. Vomiting and fever occur in about 60% of these children. Fecal leukocytes and gross blood usually are not present in stool, but occult blood is sometimes found.

## Diagnosis

Diagnosis of infection due to EPEC is a problem for clinicians. EPEC infections are diagnosed based on isolation of *E. coli* belonging to a serogroup considered to be an EPEC strain. Because these strains are biochemically the same as strains of *E. coli* that are part of the normal flora, identification is established by serotyping the isolate. This specialized technique is generally available only in reference laboratories. Commercially available *E. coli* typing sera may be used for presumptive identification, but a definitive identification can be made only by a reference laboratory. An HEp-2 cell adherence assay can be used to detect adherent strains. The DNA probe for genes that mediate adherence has proven to be a valuable tool for epidemiologic studies of EPEC diarrhea. Electron microscopy of involved intestinal tissue may demonstrate the characteristic attaching and effacing lesion of EPEC infection.

## Treatment

Therapy involves management of dehydration by oral administration of a fluid and electrolyte solution and eradication of the organism. Many EPEC strains are resistant to multiple antimicrobial agents. Agents effective for treatment of these infections include trimethoprim-sulfamethoxazole (TMP-SMX), to which EPEC may be resistant, systemically administered aminoglycosides, and the fluoroquinolones, which are approved for use only in adults.

## ENTEROTOXIGENIC *ESCHERICHIA COLI*

ETEC cause disease in animals and humans, particularly in travelers and in infants and young children in tropical, developing countries. Strains of ETEC cause disease by adherence to the mucosa of the small intestine, followed by elaboration of one or more enterotoxin. Heat-labile (LT) and heat-stable (ST) enterotoxins are produced, both of which increase net secretion in the small intestine. Strains can produce one or both toxins. Toxin production is plasmid mediated and associated with relatively few *E coli* serotypes (see Table 56-11).

### Epidemiology

ETEC have been associated with several large food-borne and water-borne outbreaks in the United States. In developing countries, these organisms are major causes of endemic pediatric and travelers' diarrhea. ETEC strains are one of the most common causes of diarrhea in children in developing countries. Prolonged exposure to these agents probably produces immunity, because adults in these areas rarely develop illness due to ETEC.

### Pathogenesis

Specific pili that mediate adherence in the small intestine are characteristic of ETEC. These colonization factor antigens (CFA) are species specific; the most commonly recognized antigens from strains that infect humans are CFA types I through IV, but others are likely to be identified. These pili are encoded by plasmids and are detected by specific antisera or by their ability to agglutinate erythrocytes of different animal species in the presence of D-mannose.

After adhering to the small intestine, ETEC elaborate ST, LT, or both toxins. LT is a large molecule (ie, 84 kd) that resembles cholera toxin biologically, structurally, and antigenically. This toxin consists of five A subunits and one B subunit. The B subunit is involved in binding of the enterotoxin to the epithelial cells of the intestine; the A subunits enter the cell, causing accumulation of cyclic adenosine monophosphate, which results in secretion of fluids and electrolytes into the intestinal lumen. ST enterotoxin is a smaller molecule (ie, 6 kd) that, unlike LT, does not elicit a serum antibody response. Although less is known about how ST acts, it causes intracellular accumulation of cyclic guanosine monophosphate in the intestinal epithelial cells, resulting in an outpouring of fluid and electrolytes into the intestinal lumen.

### Clinical Manifestations

ETEC infection is characterized by secretory diarrhea. Stool specimens are watery and do not contain blood or fecal leukocytes. Fever is rare. As with most diarrheal diseases, dehydration is the major complication, especially in infants. The severity of ETEC disease varies widely. Mortality is almost always associated with dehydration, usually in smaller, malnourished infants.

## Diagnosis

The diagnosis of ETEC infection can only be accomplished by isolation of *E coli* from stool and demonstration that the isolate has the ability to produce enterotoxin or contains the genes encoding for enterotoxin production. Enterotoxin production can be detected biologically, immunologically, or genetically. LT causes rounding of Y-1 adrenal cells in culture, which can be neutralized by specific antisera against LT. ST causes fluid accumulation in the intestinal tracts of suckling mice. Enzyme-linked immunosorbent assays (ELISA) have been developed to detect ST and LT. The genes that encode the enterotoxins can be detected by hybridization with DNA probes. This probe technology has proven extremely useful in large field studies and is the most commonly used technique for detecting ETEC strains. Unfortunately, none of these methods is available in the routine diagnostic laboratory. If ETEC infection is suspected, *E coli* should be isolated and sent to a reference laboratory for evaluation.

## Treatment

Treatment of patients with ETEC infection consists of rehydration and eradicating the organism by administration of antimicrobial agents. ETEC-induced dehydration is usually managed with oral rehydration solutions. Studies of adult travelers and children have shown that antimicrobial agents such as TMP-SMX and fluoroquinolones in adults are effective in treating patients with ETEC diarrhea.

## ENTEROINVASIVE *ESCHERICHIA COLI*

EIEC strains are a cause of diarrhea and dysentery in children in developing countries and have been implicated in food-borne outbreaks in industrialized countries. The *Shigella*-like EIEC cause disease indistinguishable from shigellosis. Strains of *E coli* in this group resemble *Shigella* biochemically and have the same genes that encode for colonic invasion. These diarrhea-associated *E coli* strains belong to relatively few serotypes (see Table 56-11).

## Epidemiology

Little is known about the prevalence and epidemiology of EIEC, because the organisms are difficult to identify. They have a worldwide distribution, and the highest isolation rates have been reported from Brazil. EIEC infections have been associated with about 5% of the episodes of diarrhea among travelers to Mexico. Several large U.S. outbreaks of food-borne diseases have been associated with EIEC, but the role of this organism in sporadic cases of diarrhea in the United States remains undetermined.

## Pathogenesis

EIEC cause bacillary dysentery by invasion of colonic epithelium. These organisms spread laterally in the epithelial cells, resulting in ulcer formation, which accounts for the blood and mucus in the stools of patients infected with EIEC. Penetration through the intestine is rare. The invasion is mediated by the same *Shigella* plasmid that encodes the virulence-associated polypeptides necessary for expression of the invasive phenotype.

## Clinical Manifestations

EIEC infection is similar to that seen with *Shigella*. Much of what is known about clinical disease is based on challenge experiments in adult volunteers and from outbreaks. Stool specimens are grossly bloody and contain mucus and fecal leukocytes. Fever is a common finding. All of these signs and symptoms are characteristic of infection due to an invasive bacterial enteropathogen.

## Diagnosis

Definitive diagnosis of EIEC infection can be difficult. It is necessary to isolate *E coli* from stool and demonstrate that the strain has the ability to invade epithelial cells. Biochemically, EIEC are distinct from most other *E coli* strains and tend to resemble *Shigella*. Most EIEC strains are late or nonlactose fermentors, are lysine decarboxylase negative, and are not motile. This biochemical profile can be used for presumptive identification of EIEC. Strains with this biotype should then be tested for their ability to invade or for the genes that encode for the invasive phenotype. The classic test for colonic invasion is the Sereny test, in which an organism is considered invasive if it produces keratoconjunctivitis when inoculated into an eye of a guinea pig. EIEC possess a large plasmid containing the genes that encode for several outer membrane proteins involved in epithelial cell invasion. DNA probes can detect *Shigella* and EIEC strains, and the probes help in understanding the epidemiology of this type of diarrhea-associated *E coli*. Tests using the polymerase chain reaction to detect EIEC have been performed on crude DNA isolated from feces.

## Treatment

Little is known about the treatment of patients with EIEC disease, because the infection is usually not diagnosed. Because antimicrobial agents have shortened the course of illness and reduced the severity of shigellosis, it seems reasonable that similar antimicrobial therapy would be appropriate for diarrhea caused by EIEC.

## ENTEROHEMORRHAGIC *ESCHERICHIA COLI*

In 1982, there were two large outbreaks of diarrhea associated with the consumption of hamburgers. The signs and symptoms of disease were unique and consisted of grossly bloody diarrhea with little or no fever. This clinical syndrome, called hemorrhagic colitis, was later associated with a rare *E coli* serotype, O157:H7. Other serotypes of *E coli*, including O26:H11, have been implicated as a cause of hemorrhagic colitis, but *E coli* serotype O157:H7 is the most prevalent; these strains are collectively referred to as enterohemorrhagic *E coli* (EHEC). EHEC strains also are associated with hemolytic uremic syndrome and thrombotic thrombocytopenic purpura.

## Epidemiology

The prevalence of EHEC infection varies among regions. *E coli* O157:H7 is a common enteric pathogen in Canada and parts of the northern United States, but it appears to have a worldwide distribution. These *E coli* strains have caused food-borne outbreaks in schools, child day-care centers, nursing homes, and communities. Many of these outbreaks have been associated with the consumption of beef that was contaminated with O157:H7. The reservoir of these organisms is thought to be cattle because of outbreaks associated with beef and dairy products and because cattle have been shown to harbor the organism. Spread among siblings within a family has been documented. These organisms cause sporadic cases of diarrhea disease in children and adults in the United States.

## Pathogenesis

Two potential virulence traits have been identified. First, EHEC adheres to intestinal cells by means of specific receptors, with resultant attachment and effacement lesions visible by electron microscopy. Second, EHEC strains produce high concentrations of cytotoxins, referred to as Shiga-like toxins (SLT) or verotoxins, which inhibit protein synthesis and cause cell death. These cytotoxins are structurally and functionally related to Shiga toxin produced by *Shigella dysenteriae* serotype 1. Genes coding for three of these cytotoxins (ie, SLT-I, SLT-II, and SLT-II variant) have been cloned and sequenced. The receptor for SLT-I and SLT-II is the glycolipid, globotriosyl ceramide (Gb$_3$), and the receptor for SLT-II variant is the related Gb$_4$.

## Clinical Manifestations

When first described, the disease caused by EHEC was thought to be a distinct clinical syndrome characterized by grossly bloody diarrhea, with little or no fever. It is now known that there is a spectrum of disease caused by these organisms. The illness usually begins as a watery diarrhea, which may or may not develop into grossly bloody diarrhea. Fever affects 20% to 50% of patients, and severe abdominal pain is typical. Barium studies have shown a characteristic "thumb-print" pattern in the transverse colon of some patients. This is often a relatively severe illness, and many patients require hospitalization. After infection with O157:H7, children may develop hemolytic uremic syndrome. Adults can sometimes develop thrombotic thrombocytopenic purpura as a sequela of EHEC infection.

## Diagnosis

The recovery of *E coli* O157:H7 from stool specimens depends on the timing of collection and antibiotic status of the patient. Recovery of organisms is optimal early in the course of illness in patients who have not received antimicrobial agents. The clinical laboratory can screen for *E coli* O157:H7 by using MacConkey agar base with sorbitol substituted for lactose. Approximately 90% of *E coli* rapidly ferment sorbitol, but *E coli* O157:H7 strains do not. The sorbitol-negative *E coli* strains can be tested to determine if they belong to the O157:H7 serotype. Other detection methods used in research or reference laboratories include testing strains and stool specimens for Shiga-like toxin production, using DNA probes derived from genes that code for toxin production, and using polymerase chain reaction methods to detect SLT. ELISAs for rapid detection of SLT-I employ Gb$_3$ or P1-glycoprotein from hydatid cyst fluid from animals infected with *Echinococcus granulosus* as the capture molecule for the toxin.

## Treatment

Little is known about the effect of antimicrobial therapy on clinical outcome or on the development of hemolytic uremic syndrome. Antimotility agents are thought to amplify morbidity and should not be used.

## ENTEROADHERENT *ESCHERICHIA COLI*

Enteroadherent or enteroaggregative *E coli* are defined by their adherence pattern in tissue culture-based assays. Three distinct patterns of adherence in the HEp-2 cell assay have been described: localized, diffuse, and aggregative. The gene sequences coding for each type of adherence pattern suggest that each pattern is associated with a defined pathogenic mechanism of diarrheal disease in humans. The localized phenotype is characteristic of strains of the EPEC category. Strains exhibiting diffuse and aggregative adherence patterns represent new categories of *E coli* associated with diarrheal disease. They are referred to as diffuse adherence *E coli* and enteroaggregative *E coli*. In Mexico, locally adherent *E coli* were found more frequently among children with acute diarrhea. In the same study, diffusely adherent *E coli* were found in the same proportion of children with and without diarrhea, although diffuse adhering *E coli* were significantly associated with diarrheal disease in another study. Studies of adult volunteers have not supported the pathogenic potential of diffusely adherent *E coli*.

Enteroaggregative *E coli* have been associated with acute and chronic diarrhea in infants in developing countries and in animal models. These organisms cause shortening of intestinal villi, edema, and mononuclear cell infiltration of the submucosa.

Probes can detect diffuse and enteroaggregative *E coli* and should greatly facilitate epidemiologic and clinical studies assessing the role of these types of *E coli* in diarrheal disease.

## Selected Readings

Belongia EA, Osterholm MT, Soler JT et al. Transmission of *Escherichia coli* O157: H7 infection in Minnesota child day-care facilities. JAMA 1993;269:883.

Donnenberg MS, Kaper JB. Enteropathogenic *Escherichia coli*. Infect Immun 1992;60: 3953.

Karmali M. Infection by verocytotoxin-producing *Escherichia coli*. Clin Microbiol Rev 1989;2:15.

Krogfelt KA. Bacterial adhesion: genetics, biogenesis, and role in pathogenesis of fimbrial adhesions of *Escherichia coli*. Rev Infect Dis 1991;13:721.

Levine MM, Kaper JB, Black RE, Clements ML. New knowledge of pathogenesis of bacterial enteric infections as applied to vaccine development. Microbiol Rev 1983;47:510.

Levine MM. *Escherichia coli* that cause diarrhea: enterotoxigenic, enteropathogenic, enteroinvasive, enterohemorrhagic and enteroadherent. J Infect Dis 1987;155: 377.

Mathewson JJ, Carvioto A. HEp-2 cell adherence as an assay for virulence among diarrheagenic *Escherichia coli*. J Infect Dis 1989;159:1057.

*Principles and Practice of Pediatrics, Second Edition.* edited by Frank A. Oski et al. J. B. Lippincott Company, Philadelphia © 1994.

# 56.11 *Haemophilus influenzae*

Sheldon L. Kaplan

*Haemophilus influenzae* is a fastidious, gram-negative, pleomorphic coccobacillus that is responsible for serious systemic and local infections in children.

## MICROBIOLOGY

*H influenzae* is differentiated from other *Haemophilus* species by its requirement of factors X (ie, heat-stable hematin) and V [ie, heat-labile nicotinamide adenine dinucleotide (NAD)] for growth. Encapsulated strains of *H influenzae* are classified by capsular polysaccharides types a through f. The polysaccharides are negatively charged, high-molecular-weight polymers that comprise repeating subunits of a disaccharide. Approximately 95% of invasive diseases are caused by the type b strain, for which the repeating subunit is polyribosyl ribitol phosphate (PRP). Unencapsulated strains (ie, nontypable strains) are primarily etiologic agents in upper respiratory tract infections such as otitis media and sinusitis, but they also cause systemic disease, especially in the neonate or immunocompromised host.

*H influenzae* can be subdivided into seven biotypes based on biochemical characteristics (eg, indole production, urease activity, ornithine decarboxylase activity). Because over 90% of the type b strains belong to biotype I, biotyping is not particularly helpful for epidemiologic studies.

*H influenzae* organisms have several outer membrane proteins (OMP) that can be differentiated by sodium dodecylsulfate–polyacrylamide gel electrophoresis. Based on the OMP pattern, 21 subtypes of *H influenzae* type b can be described, although 5 subtypes account for more than 90% of the systemic isolates. OMP patterns have proven useful for epidemiologic investigations, such as studies indicating that most cases of recurrent invasive *H influenzae* type b disease are caused by the same organism responsible for the first infection. Unlike type b strains, the OMP patterns of nontypable *H influenzae* are highly variable. *H influenzae* type b strains also have been characterized by the electrophoretic mobility of 16 metabolic enzymes (ie, multilocus enzyme electrophoresis). Most invasive disease in the United States is caused by clonal isolates of two related multilocus genotypes.

*H influenzae* contain a lipopolysaccharide (LPS) that differs from LPS of Enterobacteriaceae in that it lacks repeating O side chains and is classified as a lipooligosaccharide (LOS). The lipid A component and core oligosaccharide of *H influenzae* LPS are similar in structure to enteric LPS. LPS is an additional virulence factor for *H influenzae* type b.

*H influenzae* produce an IgA1 protease that can specifically cleave the hinge region of the heavy chain of human IgA1. Similarly, strains of *Neisseria meningitidis* and *Streptococcus pneumoniae*, which are also encapsulated and cause serious systemic infections, produce IgA1 proteases. The contribution of IgA1 proteases to the pathogenesis of nasopharyngeal colonization or actual infection by these organisms is unknown.

Some nasopharyngeal isolates of *H influenzae* type b express pili or fimbriae, filamentous surface appendages that promote the adherence of microorganisms to epithelial surfaces. Enrichment procedures can be used to obtain a piliated subpopulation of *H influenzae* type b from systemic isolates, which are not piliated when recovered from blood or cerebrospinal (CSF) cultures. The role of pili in the pathogenesis of *H influenzae* type b infections is unknown. Nontypable *H influenzae* may also express pili.

## EPIDEMIOLOGY

In the United States, approximately 20,000 cases of systemic *H influenzae* type b infection occurred yearly before the introduction of the *H influenzae* type b protein conjugate vaccines. Most cases were bacterial meningitis. The estimated annual age-specific attack rate of *H influenzae* type b infection was 100 cases per 100,000 children younger than 5 years of age. The highest age-specific attack rate occurred in children between the ages of 6 and 11 months; the next highest rate was among those between the ages of 12 and 17 months (Table 56-12). Overall, approximately 1 in 200 children developed a systemic infection due to *H influenzae* type b by 5 years of age. Worldwide, the incidence of invasive *H influenzae* infection is highly variable.

Certain risk factors for systemic *H influenzae* type b infections have been identified. Black, Hispanic, and Native American children have higher rates of infection than do white, non-Hispanic children. The highest endemic incidence of disease occurs among native Alaskan Eskimos. Children younger than 4 years of age who are household contacts of a patient with *H influenzae* type b disease have a much higher risk for this disease than the general population. Children with underlying immune deficiencies and anatomical or functional asplenia (eg, hemoglobinopathies) are more likely to develop systemic *H influenzae* infections. Other risk factors for invasive *H influenzae* type b infections are socioeconomic in nature, such as day-care attendance, crowded households, frequent infections, and socioeconomic status.

Breast-feeding for infants between 2 and 5 months of age appears to be a relatively protective factor.

## PATHOGENESIS

Unencapsulated *H influenzae* are common inhabitants of the upper respiratory tract under normal conditions in children and adults. *H influenzae* type b can be isolated from as many as 5% to 7% of young children at any time. Higher colonization rates occur among children in day-care centers, and much lower rates are observed in children after immunization with the *H influenzae* protein conjugate vaccines. The factors that promote the nasopharyngeal surface colonization of *H influenzae* type b have not been delineated. Piliated or fimbriated strains adhere more avidly to buccal or pharyngeal epithelial cells in vitro than do nonpiliated strains. In studies employing surgical specimens of nasopharyngeal tissue from children, the piliated and nonpiliated strains of *H influenzae* attach to nonciliated epithelial cells. Other unknown surface structures may act as adhesins.

Invasive disease due to *H influenzae* type b frequently follows a viral upper respiratory infection, which may disrupt mucosal barriers and interrupt the normal activity of respiratory cilia. In infant rats, prior intranasal inoculation with influenza virus promotes bacteremia after the intranasal administration of *H influenzae* type b. In human nasopharyngeal organ cultures infected with *H influenzae* type b, organisms can be identified within the epithelium in an intercellular location by 24 hours. This invasion is preceded by disruption of the tight junctions between nonciliated cells. Presumably, after it is passes the mucosal barrier, the organism can directly invade the bloodstream. In a susceptible host, bacteria multiply readily, and after a critical bacterial density is reached, dissemination occurs.

For local infections caused by unencapsulated strains, a preceding viral upper respiratory infection frequently disrupts the normal physiologic clearance mechanisms and permits invasion of the sinuses or middle ear by normal respiratory flora (eg, *S pneumoniae*, nontypable *H influenzae*, *Moraxella catarrhalis*).

**TABLE 56-12.** Estimated Age-specific Attack Rate for *Haemophilus influenzae* type b Disease in U.S. Children, 1984

| Age (Months) | Meningitis* | Nonmeningitic Infections | Total Attack Rate |
|---|---|---|---|
| 0–5 | 112 | 41 | 153 |
| 6–11 | 192 | 106 | 298 |
| 12–17 | 113 | 49 | 162 |
| 18–23 | 59 | 63 | 122 |
| 24–35 | 33 | 23 | 56 |
| 36–47 | 17 | 30 | 47 |
| 48–59 | 8 | 16 | 24 |
| Total | 60 | 40 | 100 |

* Annual cases per 100,00 children in age group.

*Modified from Cochi ST, et al. Immunization of U.S. children with Haemophilus influenzae type b polysaccharide vaccine: a cost-effectiveness model of strategy assessment. JAMA 1985;253:521.*

# HOST IMMUNITY

Antibody to the capsular polysaccharide is a major component of the host defense against *H influenzae* type b. The inverse relation between PRP antibody concentrations and susceptibility to systemic infection is well known. Children who develop serum anti-PRP antibody concentrations at least 1 $\mu$g/mL 3 weeks after immunization with PRP are protected against invasive disease. Antibody to PRP is an important opsonin, is bactericidal in combination with complement, and promotes neutrophil chemotaxis. Functional differences exist for IgG and IgM and for the IgG subclasses (eg, IgG1, IgG2) antibodies directed against PRP, but the relative contributions of the immunoglobulin classes to host defenses are unclear. Mucosal anti-PRP antibody (IgA) develops after natural diseases and parenteral immunization with PRP, but the clinical significance of IgA anti-PRP is unknown.

Antibodies to other noncapsular polysaccharide antigens such as OMPs and LOS may play some role in immunity against *H influenzae*. These antigens are immunogenic in young infants, and antibodies directed against them in studies using animals are protective, although not uniformly. *H influenzae* type LOS is an important inducer of the inflammatory response, related to the production of cytokines such as tumor necrosis factor or interleukin-1. The macrophages of the reticuloendothelial system are key components for intravascular clearance of *H influenzae* type b.

Immunity to nontypable *H influenzae* has not been as extensively studied as that for type b strains. Human serum contains opsonizing and bactericidal activity for nontypable *H influenzae*, a substantial portion of which is contributed by antibody to surface-exposed OMP.

# INFECTIONS CAUSED BY *HAEMOPHILUS INFLUENZAE* TYPE B

After *H influenzae* type b bacteremia develops, invasion of most sites in the body can occur, but certain sites of infection predominate.

## Meningitis

*H influenzae* type b was the leading cause of bacterial meningitis in children between the ages of 1 month and 4 years in the United States. *H influenzae* type b meningitis cannot be clinically differentiated from that caused by *N meningitidis* or *S pneumoniae*. Among children with *H influenzae* type b meningitis, 5% to 10% develop septic shock.

## Pneumonia

The true incidence of *H influenzae* type b pneumonia in children is unknown, but the infection is more common among children 4 years of age or younger. The mean age of patients is 26 months. The signs and symptoms are similar to those of pneumonia caused by other organisms, except that the course of illness may be more prolonged. Associated infections, such as otitis media, meningitis, and epiglottitis, are common. There is no characteristic pattern on the chest radiograph; segmental infiltrates, single or multiple lobe involvement, lobar consolidation, pleural effusion, and pneumatoceles may be observed.

## Septic or Pyogenic Arthritis

*H influenzae* type b is the organism most often responsible for septic arthritis in children younger than 2 years of age. Large joints, such as the knee, hip, ankle, and elbow, are affected most often. Single joints are infected more frequently than multiple joints. Associated infections are common. An immune complex or noninfectious arthritis associated with systemic *H influenzae* type b infections, predominantly meningitis, may develop several days after appropriate antibiotic therapy has been initiated. *H influenzae* type b is an uncommon cause of osteomyelitis.

## Cellulitis

Cellulitis due to *H influenzae* type b characteristically develops in children younger than 2 years of age. These children often have an upper respiratory infection that is followed by the acute onset of cellulitis. There is usually no history of trauma to the involved area. The cheek or buccal region and the periorbital area are the most common sites of infection. Why *H influenzae* type b is so frequently related to buccal cellulitis is unknown. There is conflicting evidence for the role of lymphatic seeding of the buccal soft tissues from otitis media. The area of cellulitis generally has indistinct margins and is tender and indurated. A violaceous or blue-purple color is common but not diagnostic. Concomitant infections, especially meningitis, may complicate the diagnosis. In young children with a buccal cellulitis thought to be due to *H influenzae* type b, lumbar puncture is indicated if meningitis cannot be excluded clinically. Blood cultures are positive in as many as 80% of the patients, and *H influenzae* type b can often be recovered from an aspirate of the cellulitis.

## Pericarditis

*H influenzae* type b is the cause of bacterial pericarditis in as many as 15% of the children with this infection. These patients usually are between 2 and 4 years of age and often have had an antecedent upper respiratory tract infection. Fever, respiratory distress, and tachycardia are consistent findings. Associated infections are also common. The etiologic diagnosis may be established by blood culture or by culture, Gram stain, or antigen detection of pericardial fluid. Optimal management includes pericardiectomy, which effectively drains purulent material from the pericardial sac and minimizes the chances of pericardial tamponade and constrictive pericarditis.

## Acute Epiglottitis

Acute epiglottitis is a dramatic, rapidly fulminating infection. It occurs predominantly in children 2 to 7 years of age.

## Miscellaneous Infections

Urinary tract infections, epididymo-orchitis, cervical adenitis, acute glossitis, uvulitis, bacterial tracheitis, infected thyroglossal duct cysts, endocarditis, endophthalmitis, primary peritonitis, soft-tissue abscess, periappendiceal abscess, brain abscess, and neonatal infections can be caused by *H influenzae* type b. See Chapter 52 for a detailed discussion of nonspecific bacteremia.

# INFECTIONS CAUSED BY NONTYPABLE *H. INFLUENZAE*

## Upper Respiratory Tract Infections

Unencapsulated *H influenzae* is second only to *S pneumoniae* as a cause of acute otitis media and acute sinusitis in children. In older children and adults, nontypable *H influenzae* is associated with bronchitis. A syndrome of concomitant purulent conjunctivitis and otitis media due to nontypable *H influenzae* occurs in young children. Spread among family members is common.

## Neonatal Infection

Nontypable *H influenzae* is a more common pathogen than type b strains in the neonate. Septicemia, pneumonia, and respiratory distress syndrome with shock, meningitis, and conjunctivitis have been reported.

## Miscellaneous Infections

Bacteremia, meningitis, lung cyst, thyroglossal duct cyst infection, rectal abscess, septic arthritis, and CSF shunt infections may be caused by nontypable *H influenzae*. Systemic infections due to unencapsulated *H influenzae* occur predominantly in immunocompromised hosts. Invasive infections due to non-type b *H influenzae* should prompt an investigation for an underlying anatomical or immune defect.

## DIAGNOSIS

Cultures of blood, CSF, and other body fluids and sites yield *H influenzae* type b in most children with invasive infections. Gram stain of appropriate specimens frequently demonstrates the characteristic pleomorphic coccobacilli of *H influenzae*, although other organisms can have similar morphology. Polysaccharide antigen is detected readily by latex agglutination in a variety of body fluids, especially CSF, urine, and serum. Because antigen may be detected in urine for as long as 1 month after some *H influenzae* type b vaccines, it is not a reliable predictor of systemic infection in this instance.

## TREATMENT

Strains of *H influenzae* type b may be resistant to commonly employed antibiotics, and several different mechanisms may be involved in this resistance. Since 1974, an increasing incidence of ampicillin-resistant strains has been observed in the United States. Approximately one third of *H influenzae* strains isolated from systemic infections are resistant to ampicillin. The predominant mechanism of ampicillin resistance is the production of the β-lactamase enzyme. The gene coding for the production of this enzyme is usually contained within a plasmid that can be transferred. In some strains, this gene is located on a chromosome. A small percentage of ampicillin-resistant strains have a mechanism of resistance related to altered penicillin-binding proteins. These strains are β-lactamase negative but resistant to ampicillin by standard laboratory techniques.

In the United States, fewer than 1% of *H influenzae* type b isolates are resistant to chloramphenicol on the basis of the plasmid-mediated production of the enzyme chloramphenicol acetyltransferase (CAT). CAT production can be rapidly detected in isolates by using commercially available kits. A few CAT-negative, chloramphenicol-resistant unencapsulated isolates have been described and are thought to have a relative barrier to chloramphenicol transport into the cell.

Because β-lactamase and CAT enzymes are plasmid-mediated, strains of *H influenzae* type b can be resistant to ampicillin and chloramphenicol. Although this is not yet common in the United States, it is a major problem in some parts of the world. Approximately 60% of *H influenzae* type b isolates in Spain are resistant to ampicillin and chloramphenicol.

Several other classes of antibiotics have excellent activity against *H influenzae* isolates (Table 56-13). Cefuroxime, cefotax-

| TABLE 56-13. In Vitro Susceptibility for Selected Antibiotics Against *Haemophilus influenzae* type b | |
|---|---|
| Antibiotic | Minimal Bactericidal Concentration (μg/mL) |
| Ampicillin | 0.5–0.2 |
| Ampicillin-sulbactam | <0.03/0.02–4/2 |
| Amoxicillin/clavulanic acid | 0.8–1.6/0.8 |
| Chloramphenicol | 2.0–8.0 |
| Cefaclor | 6.25–12.5 |
| Cefixime | 0.06* |
| Cefuroxime | 0.3–0.6 |
| Cefotaxime | 0.04 |
| Ceftriaxone | <0.03 |
| Ceftazidime | 0.8 |
| Rifampin | 0.125–0.25* |
| TMP/SMX | 0.15/0.008–19/1 |
| Imipenem | 0.5–2 |

*\* Minimum inhibitory concentration (MIC).*

ime, and ceftriaxone are parenteral cephalosporins with proven efficacy in the treatment of systemic *H influenzae* type b infections. Ampicillin- and chloramphenicol-resistant strains remain susceptible to these cephalosporins. Trimethoprim-sulfamethoxazole, cefaclor, cefixime, cefuroxime axetil, erythromycin-sulfisoxazole, and the combination of amoxicillin and clavulanic acid (a β-lactamase inhibitor) are oral agents useful for treating upper respiratory infections due to ampicillin-resistant *H influenzae* type b.

Several treatment options are available for the initial management of the child with suspected infection due to *H influenzae* type b. Traditionally, ampicillin and chloramphenicol have been initiated in children older than 2 months of age with bacterial meningitis until the culture results are available. Single-agent treatment with cefotaxime or ceftriaxone is most commonly recommended treatment (see Chap. 54).

Cefuroxime is a convenient antibiotic for initial therapy of a variety of non-CNS infections (eg, pneumonia, septic arthritis, buccal cellulitis) in normal children. In addition to it activity against *H influenzae* type b, cefuroxime is active against *Staphylococcus aureus* and *S pneumoniae*, the other most commonly encountered pathogens in these infections. Cefotaxime combined with an antistaphylococcal penicillin is also appropriate. After *H influenzae* type b is isolated and the antimicrobial susceptibility is determined, the most appropriate antibiotic can be continued. Ampicillin remains the treatment of choice for infections due to susceptible strains. Chloramphenicol, cefuroxime, cefotaxime, or ceftriaxone should be used if ampicillin-resistant strains are identified. Chloramphenicol should be avoided if the child has underlying liver disease or is in shock; both processes alter the pharmacology of chloramphenicol. The inability to monitor the concentrations of chloramphenicol is another reason to avoid this agent. Cefotaxime or ceftriaxone should be used to treat infections due to strains of *H influenzae* type b resistant to ampicillin and chloramphenicol. Ceftriaxone is particularly convenient for once-daily administration if home parenteral therapy is considered.

In some instances, after the signs and symptoms of the acute non-CNS infection have resolved, therapy can be completed with an oral agent. The duration of therapy is discussed in the sections describing specific infections.

The initial treatment of upper respiratory infections possibly due to *H influenzae* is usually with amoxicillin. If the physician

TABLE 56-14.    *Haemophilus influenzae* type b Protein Conjugate Vaccines

| Source | Abbreviation | Commercial Name | Polysaccharide | Carrier Protein | Spacer Molecule | Recommended Ages for Administration |
|---|---|---|---|---|---|---|
| Connaught | PRP-D | Prohibit | Native | Diphtheria toxoid | Yes | 15 mo |
| Lederle-Praxis Biologicals | HbOc | HibTITER | Oligosaccharide | CRM$_{197}$ mutant | No | 2, 4, 6, 15 mo |
| Merck, Sharp and Dohme | PRP-OMP | PedvaxHib | Native | Outer membrane protein of *N meningitidis* group B | Yes | 2, 4, 12 mo |
| Pasteur Merieux-Connaught | PRP-T | Act Hib | Native | Tetanus toxoid | Yes | 2, 4, 6, 15 mo |

suspects that ampicillin-resistant strains are involved, any one of the oral agents previously mentioned can be administered. The choice of a specific agent is based more on preference, cost, and ease of administration than on efficacy.

## PREVENTION

The development of the *H influenzae* type b protein conjugate vaccines is one of the most important recent advances in preventive pediatrics. Children younger than 2 years of age do not develop protective antibodies after immunization with the purified polysaccharide capsule (PRP) of *H influenzae* type b. However, conjugating PRP to a protein enhances the immunogenicity of PRP in infants, presumably by converting a T-cell-independent antigen to a T-cell-dependent one. The four available *H influenzae* type b protein conjugate vaccines differ in composition (Table 56-14). The HbOc (ie, oligosaccharide conjugate *H influenzae* type b vaccine) and PRP-OMP vaccines prevented systemic *H influenzae* type b infection in large field trials and were licensed for administration to infants in the United States. The American Academy of Pediatrics and the Centers for Disease Control recommend routine immunization with the HbOc or PRP-OMP vaccine beginning at 2 months of age. The vaccine administration schedules are different because of differences in the kinetics of antibody response to HbOc or PRP-OMP. In March 1993, the FDA approved the PRP-T vaccine for administration to infants at 2, 4, 6, and 15 months of age. PRP-D can be used for the booster dose at 15 months of age in the HbOc schedule. The administration of DTP (ie, diphtheria, tetanus, and pertussis vaccine) and a PRP conjugate vaccine in the same syringe appears to be equivalent to separate-site administration with regard to safety and immunogenicity and has been approved for the HbOc vaccine by the FDA. After one PRP conjugate is administered, the series should be completed with the same vaccine, although studies are examining the interchangeability of PRP conjugate vaccines.

In areas where the *H influenzae* type b protein conjugate vaccines are administered routinely to infants, the incidence of systemic *H influenzae* type b disease is declining dramatically. In Finland, where PRP conjugate vaccines have been offered in infancy since 1988, invasive *H influenzae* type b infections have virtually disappeared. Preliminary observations from surveillance studies in Connecticut, Pittsburgh, and United States Army beneficiaries demonstrate that the annual incidence of invasive *H influenzae* type b infections has declined approximately sixfold to eightfold.

To prevent secondary infection, rifampin prophylaxis is indicated for all family contacts of persons with *H influenzae* type

b disease if there is another family member younger than 4 years of age residing in the same household. Rifampin is administered to children at a dose of 20 mg/kg (not to exceed 600 mg) for 4 consecutive days. Parents are given 600 mg/day for 4 days. The index patient should receive rifampin because systemic antibiotics do not reliably eradicate nasopharyngeal colonization of *H influenzae* type b. Parents should be told that there is an increased risk of secondary infection in the household and should seek prompt medical attention for any suspicious signs or symptoms in their child. Parents of children exposed to a single case of systemic *H influenzae* type b infection in a day-care center or nursery school should be similarly warned. Rifampin should be administered to all infants and day-care personnel if two or more cases of invasive disease have occurred among the children or employees within 60 days. Although not perfect, rifampin prophylaxis is effective in preventing secondary infections.

## Selected Readings

Black SB, Shinefield HR, Fireman B, et al. Efficacy in infancy of oligosaccharide conjugate *H influenzae* type b (HbOc) vaccine in a United States population of 61080 children. Pediatr Infect Dis J 1991;10:97.

Bodor FF, Marchant CD, Shurin PA, Barenkamp SJ. Bacterial etiology of conjunctivitis-otitis media syndrome. Pediatrics 1985;76:26.

Campos J, Garcia-Tornel S, Gairia JM, et al. Multiply resistant *Haemophilus influenzae* type b causing meningitis: comparative clinical and laboratory study. J Pediatr 1986;108:897.

Committee on Infectious Diseases, American Academy of Pediatrics. *H influenzae* type b conjugate vaccines: recommendations for immunization of infants and children 2 months of age and older: update. Pediatrics 1991;88:169.

Dajani AS, Asmar BI, Thirumoorthi MC. Systemic *Haemophilus influenzae* disease: an overview. J Pediatr 1979;94:355.

Epidemiology, pathogenesis, and prevention of *H influenzae* Disease. J Infect Dis 1992;165(suppl 1):S1.

Farley MM, Stephens DS, Kaplan SL, Mason EO Jr. Pilus-and non-pilus-mediated interactions of *H influenzae* type b with human erythrocytes and human nasopharyngeal mucosa. J Infect Dis 1990;161:274.

Gilsdorf JR: *H influenzae* non-type b infections in children. Am J Dis Child 1987;141:1063.

Ginsburg CM, Howard JB, Nelson JB. Report of 65 cases of *Haemophilus influenzae* b pneumonia. Pediatrics 1979;64:283.

Jorgensen JH: Update on mechanisms and prevalence of antimicrobial resistance in *Haemophilus influenzae*. Clin Infect Dis 1992;14:1119.

Murphy TF, Apicella MA. Nontypable *Haemophilus influenzae*. A review of clinical aspects, surface antigens, and the human immune response to infection. Rev Infect Dis 1987;9:1.

Rotbart HA, Glode MP. *Haemophilus influenzae* type b septic arthritis in children: report of 23 cases. Pediatrics 1985;75:254.

Santosham M., Wolf M, Reid R, et al. The efficacy in Navajo infants of a conjugate vaccine consisting of *H influenzae* type b polysaccharide and *Neisseria meningitidis* outer-membrane protein complex. N Engl J Med 1991;324:1767.

Todd JK, Bruhn FW. *Haemophilus influenzae* infections. Spectrum of disease. Am J Dis Child 1975;129:607.

Wallace RJ, Baker CJ, Quinones FJ, et al. Nontypable *Haemophilus influenzae* (biotype 4) as a neonate, maternal, and genital pathogen. Rev Infect Dis 1983;5:123.

Ward JI, Fraser DH, Baraff LJ, et al. *Haemophilus influenzae* meningitis: a national study of secondary spread in household contacts. N Engl J Med 1979;301:122.

Weinberg GA, Granoff DM. Polysaccharide-protein conjugate vaccines for the prevention of H influenzae type b disease. J Pediatr 1988;113:621.

Wenger JD, Hightower AW, Facklam RR, Gaventa S, Broome CV, and the Bacterial Meningitis Study Group. Bacterial meningitis in the United States, 1986: report of a multistate surveillance study. J Infect Dis 1990;162:1316.

*Principles and Practice of Pediatrics, Second Edition.*
edited by Frank A. Oski et al. J. B. Lippincott Company, Philadelphia © 1994.

# 56.12 *Legionella*

## Morven S. Edwards

A constellation of illnesses due to *Legionella* has been defined during the past decade. When epidemic pneumonia was diagnosed among delegates attending the 1976 American Legion convention in Philadelphia, Pennsylvania, the descriptive term "legionnaires' disease" was coined. An estimated 182 people developed pneumonia and 29 died. A 3-year-old child was among those with documented seroconversion. Within months, a "new" bacterium was discovered: *Legionella pneumophila*. Serologic testing revealed that the bacillus had existed for decades and accounted for a number of previously unexplained outbreaks of pneumonia.

Many of the members of the genus *Legionella* are recognized agents of human infection (Table 56-15). Legionnaires' disease and Pontiac fever are caused by *L pneumophila*. The former is a long-incubation, lower respiratory tract infection, and the latter is an influenza-like illness without pneumonia, named for an outbreak in Pontiac, Michigan, in 1968. In 1979, the Pittsburgh pneumonia agent, now designated *Legionella micdadei*, was isolated from the lung tissue of two renal transplant patients. Most infections due to *L micdadei* are nosocomial and occur in immunocompromised patients.

## MICROBIOLOGY

*Legionella* are small, pleomorphic, gram-negative bacilli that are approximately 0.5 μm wide and 3 μm long. Their ultrastructural features are typical of gram-negative bacilli and include a cell wall with trilaminar cytoplasmic and outer membranes. *L pneumophila* has a single polar flagellum; other species, except *Legionella oakridgenesis*, have polar or subpolar flagella.

The best medium for isolating *Legionella* species is buffered charcoal-yeast extract agar, supplemented with α-ketoglutarate. Cysteine and amino acids are required for growth. Growth occurs optimally at 35 °C in 5% $CO_2$. Colonies of *L pneumophila* and other species are 1 to 2 mm in diamter, have a ground-glass appearance, are gray to gray-white, and have a sticky consistency when lifted with a loop. The addition of dyes to the agar, use of fluorescence, and modification of L-cysteine requirements may be used in the laboratory to differentiate species.

Of the more than 30 species of *Legionella*, at least 18 have been associated with human disease (see Table 56-15). *L pneumophila* has 14 serogroups, each of which has been associated with human infection. Serogroups 1, 4, and 6 account for most infections.

*Legionella* from clinical specimens are not visible by Gram stain. Special stains, such as the Gimenez stain and Dieterle's silver-impregnation stain, can be used for visualization. When obtained from tissue specimens, *L micdadei* is acid fast by a modified Ziehl-Neelsen stain or Kinyoun carbol-fuchsin technique. Other species are not acid fast.

## EPIDEMIOLOGY AND TRANSMISSION

*Legionella* spreads by the airborne route, and legionnaires' disease is transmitted by inhalation, particularly of water vapor containing aerosolized bacteria. Outbreaks have been linked to the evaporative condensers of air cooling systems, which amplify spread of the bacteria, and to soil-associated sites of excavation, whirlpool spas, showers, respiratory therapy equipment, and the ultrasonic humidifier of a grocery store mist machine.

The incidence of legionnaires' disease peaks in the late summer and early fall and has a male predominance. Person-to-person spread has not been documented. The incidence peaks is in the sixth decade of life, and infection is uncommon in the first two decades. Risk factors for infection in adults include smoking and alcoholism. Major predisposing features for all ages include organ transplantation, immunosuppression, malignancy, and renal disease. Underlying respiratory disease may be a risk factor in childhood.

Seroconversion to *L pneumophila* or a closely related or cross-reacting organism in association with mild or inapparent clinical infection appears to be common among young children. In one longitudinal 5-year study, more than half of the participants who were younger than 4 years of age at enrollment developed a fourfold or greater rise in titer that was not associated with acute illness. In another investigation, the frequency of reciprocal antibody titers of at least 256 was 25% among children 2 to 9 years of age, some of whom were tested during episodes of respiratory tract infection. The infrequency with which *L pneumophila* can be implicated as a cause of acute pneumonia in normal children was illustrated by a study of 110 children ranging in age from 1 week to 17 years who were hospitalized with pneumonia. Only two cases of legionnaires' disease—one confirmed and one possible—were identified.

## PATHOPHYSIOLOGY

Legionnaires' disease is initiated by inhalation of *L pneumophila*. The bacillus gains entry into the cytoplasm of macrophages through phagocytosis and has the capacity to resist monocytic microbicidal mechanisms and to replicate intracellularly. The resultant cellular infiltrate in the alveolar spaces consists of macrophages and neutrophils. Because the organisms are clustered in macrophages rather than in lung tissue, pulmonary tissue is not severely damaged. The predominant sites of involvement are the terminal bronchioles and alveoli. Radiographically, this mode

| TABLE 56-15. Clinical Forms of Infection Due to *Legionella* Species and Their Causative Organisms | |
|---|---|
| Clinical Form of Infection | Causative Organisms |
| Legionnaires' disease | *L pneumophila* |
| Pontiac fever | *L pneumophila* |
| Pittsburgh pneumonia | *L micdadei* |
| Bronchopneumonia | *L pneumophila, L micdadei, L bozemanii, L dumoffi, L longbeachae*, and others |

of invasion causes a patchy lobular consolidation, which may progress to severe multilobular and bilateral consolidation. A nodular infiltrate occurs in about 20% of the patients. Small abscesses may occur, but frank abscess formation that is evident radiographically is rare.

Bacteremic spread is the proposed route for dissemination of infection in immunocompromised patients. The reticuloendothelial system is often involved in fatal infections. Focal involvement of other organs, such as the heart (eg, myocardium, pericardium, endocardium), kidneys, brain, and peritoneum, has been observed. Cellular rather than humoral immunity has a major role in host defense.

## CLINICAL MANIFESTATIONS

The incubation period for legionnaires' disease is 2 to 10 days. Prodromal symptoms include malaise, myalgias, and headache. The illness is characterized by the sudden onset of high fever and shaking chills, with systemic toxicity. Nonbloody, watery diarrhea occurs in one third to one half of the patients and may begin with the onset of fever or at any time during the first week of illness. A dry, nonproductive cough usually is apparent by the second day of illness. The sputum is nonpurulent or minimally purulent. Without intervention, pulmonary signs become more prominent and progress to evidence of consolidation, with or without pleuritis. Dyspnea is a prominent feature at the peak of illness. In the normal host, spontaneous resolution of symptoms begins on day 7 to 10 of the illness.

Most symptomatic pediatric infections have been diagnosed in children with specific risk factors for legionnaires' disease, who are unlikely to recover spontaneously. Symptoms may progress to respiratory failure with fatal outcome, often presaged by renal failure and neurologic manifestations. Among pediatric renal or bone marrow transplant recipients or those with leukemia in relapse, the initial features of legionellosis are similar to those enumerated for normal hosts, but the disease is likely to progress rapidly, resulting in opacification of an entire hemithorax, or to have produce findings of extrapulmonary foci of infection. Five of eight adult heart transplant recipients had consolidation with eventual cavitation. In one report, seven adult patients acquired Legionella prosthetic valve endocarditis in the perioperative period.

The usual laboratory features include leukocytosis (ie, 10,000 to 20,000 leukocytes/mm$^3$) with a neutrophil predominance, hyponatremia due to inappropriate secretion of antidiuretic hormone, hypophosphatemia, and abnormal liver function tests. Arterial blood gases document hypoxemia and hypocarbia. Abnormalities of renal function are unusual. Chest radiographs reveal distal air space disease, usually in a segmental or lobar distribution. Initially, infiltrates are typically unilateral, but bilateral involvement may be a feature of progressive disease, even after the initiation of therapy. Small pleural effusions may be evident, particularly early in the course of infection.

Pontiac fever is a self limited disease and has been diagnosed only in epidemic situations. The onset of influenza-like symptoms occurs so rapidly after exposure (ie, 6 hours to 2 days) that symptoms may represent a toxic or allergic response to the bacillus rather than a response to replication of the bacteria in pulmonary macrophages.

## DIAGNOSIS

Legionellosis can be diagnosed by isolation of the organism, by direct staining techniques, or by demonstration of a rise in specific antibody titer in paired sera. For laboratories with experience in isolating the organism, blood, lower respiratory tract secretions, and lung tissue are the best sources, and after 2 to 6 days, Legionella may be recovered from 50% to 70% of patients. Direct fluorescent antibody (DFA) techniques employ fluorescein-labeled antibodies to L pneumophila to detect the organism in sputum, pleural fluid, and fresh or formalin-fixed lung specimens. For patients able to produce sputum, the technique has a sensitivity ranging from 25% to 75% and specificity exceeding 90%, and it may provide a diagnosis within hours. The test has limitations among pediatric patients, particularly because sputum is often not available early in the course of illness.

Legionellosis is most often diagnosed by indirect fluorescent antibody (IFA) techniques. The polyvalent reagents were developed and standardized by the Centers for Disease Control. A fourfold rise between acute and convalescent sera obtained at least 3 weeks after the onset of illness to a titer of 1 : 128 or more is diagnostic. Among some patients, seroconversion may not occur until the sixth week of illness. For L pneumophila serogroup 1, the sensitivity and specificity of the IFA assay in adult patients are 70% and 95%, respectively. Because of the low prevalence of disease in children, the predictive value of seroconversion probably is lower, but this has not been investigated. A single convalescent titer of 1 : 256 or greater establishes a presumptive diagnosis when clinical findings are compatible.

Newer commercially available diagnostic tests include a DNA hybridization test for L pneumophila ribosomal RNA and tests to detect L pneumophila serogroup 1 antigen in urine. Results of both tests are available within hours. Sensitivity of the DNA probe assay is comparable to DFA methods, but false-positive results have been reported. Commercially available urine latex agglutination assays (Dupont, Wilmington, DE; Binax, South Portland, ME) have high sensitivity (>90%) and high specificity (99%) with the advantage of low cost. Antigen remains detectable in urine for days or weeks, even during the administration of antibiotics.

Community-acquired Legionella may resemble Mycoplasma infection, psittacosis, Q fever, influenza, or other viral lower respiratory tract infections. The differential diagnosis for sporadic infection in hospitalized children also includes the fungal, mycobacterial, and protozoan agents that cause atypical pneumonia in immunosuppressed hosts.

## TREATMENT

Erythromycin is the drug of choice for the treatment of Legionella infections. Initially and for the first week of therapy, it should be administered intravenously at a dosage of 40 mg/kg/day (maximum, 2 to 4 g/day), in divided doses every 6 hours. The 2- to 3-week course of treatment may be completed using the same regimen orally. Rifampin (15 mg/kg/day) may be used with erythromycin as adjunctive therapy for patients with severe infection but should not be given as the sole therapy because resistant strains may emerge. Trimethoprim-sulfamethoxazole, clarithromycin, minocycline, tetracycline, imipenem, and ciprofloxacin are active in vitro or have been used successfully in anecdotal reports. Penicillins, cephalosporins, and aminoglycoside antibiotics are ineffective for Legionella infections.

Appropriate supportive care should be provided for lower respiratory tract infection, respiratory failure, or inappropriate secretion of antidiuretic hormone.

## OUTCOME

Clinical response usually is evident within 2 to 5 days after initiation of therapy. Fever may persist for as long as 1 week. The resolution of pneumonia proceeds slowly and may require 1 month. Among immunocompetent adults, fatality rates are as low as 4% to 7% with appropriate treatment. The overall fatality rate for patients managed appropriately is 15% to 25%, but rates as high as 80% have been reported for immunocompromised patients. Apparent relapses have been encountered with a 2-week treatment course and are an indication for reinitiation of erythromycin therapy.

## Selected Readings

Andersen RD, Lauer BA, Fraser DW, et al. Infections with *Legionella pneumophila* in children. J Infect Dis 1981;143:386.

Carlson NC, Kuskie MR, Dobyns EL, et al. Legionellosis in children: an expanding spectrum. Pediatr Infect Dis J 1990;9:133

Dowling JN, Pasculle AW, Frola FN, et al. Infections caused by *Legionella micdadei* and *Legionella pneumophila* among renal transplant recipients. J Infect Dis 1984;149:703.

Edelstein PH. Legionnaires disease, Pontiac fever, and related illnesses. In: Feigin RD, Cherry JD, eds. Textbook of pediatric infectious diseases, ed 3. Philadelphia: WB Saunders, 1992:1141.

Finegold SM. Legionnaires' disease—still with us. N Engl J Med 1988;318:571.

Fuller J, Levinson MM, Kline JR, et al. Legionnaires' disease after heart transplantation. Ann Thorac Surg 1985;39:308.

Kovatch AL, Jardine DS, Dowling JN, et al. Legionellosis in children with leukemia in relapse. Pediatrics 1984;73:811.

Kugler JW, Armitage JO, Helms CM, et al. Nosocomial Legionnaires' disease. Occurrence in recipients of bone marrow transplants. Am J Med 1983;74:281.

Mahoney FJ, Hoge CW, Farley TA, et al. Community wide outbreak of legionnaires' disease associated with a grocery store mist machine. J Infect Dis 1992;165:736.

Muldoon RL, Jaecker DL, Kiefer HK. Legionnaires' disease in children. Pediatrics 1981;67:329.

Nguyen MH, Stout JE, Yu VL. Legionellosis. Infect Dis Clin North Am 1991;5:561.

Orenstein WA, Overturf GD, Leedom JM, et al. The frequency of *Legionella* infection prospectively determined in children hospitalized with pneumonia. J Pediatr 1981;99:403.

Schwebke JR, Hackman R, Bowden R. Pneumonia due to *Legionella micdadei* in bone marrow transplant recipients. Rev Infect Dis 1990;12:824.

Winn WC Jr. Legionnaires disease: historical perspective. Clin Microbiol Rev 1988;1:60.

*Principles and Practice of Pediatrics, Second Edition.*
edited by Frank A. Oski et al. J. B. Lippincott Company, Philadelphia © 1994.

# 56.13 *Leptospirosis*

Ralph D. Feigin

Leptospirosis is a disease caused by a single family of organisms, of which there are multiple serogroups and serotypes. The disease is characterized by a broad spectrum of clinical findings.

## EPIDEMIOLOGY

Virtually all mammals can be infected by leptospires and can transmit disease caused by this genus of organisms. In various parts of the world, field mice, rats, moles, gerbils, hedgehogs, dogs, skunks, raccoons, opossums, and cattle have been implicated as sources of human infection. A host species may serve as a reservoir for one or more serotypes of leptospires, and a particular serotype may be hosted by many different animal species. Two or more animal hosts for the same serotype may exist in the same geographic area. Virtually any animal that is susceptible to infection by leptospires (ie, tightly coiled spirochete) may become a temporary urinary shedder of the organisms.

Transmission of leptospires to humans follows contact with urine, blood, tissues, or organs of infected animals or exposure to an environment that has been contaminated by leptospires. Humans represent a dead end in the chain of infection, although person-to-person transmission is theoretically possible. Leptospires may enter breaks in the skin or may penetrate the mucous membranes of the conjunctiva, nasopharynx, or vagina.

Leptospires may be transmitted from soil or water to humans. A warm climate (>25°C), moisture, and pH values of soil or surface water between 6.2 and 8 are optimal for survival of leptospires. These conditions are common in many tropical regions throughout the year and in temperate zones during the late spring, summer, and autumn months.

The role of occupation as a major risk factor in leptospirosis was emphasized in the 1960s. During the past several decades, however, an increasing number of cases have been reported among children living in urban areas who have participated in outdoor recreation. In rural areas, leptospires may be acquired from swimming in farm ponds or in contaminated rivers and streams.

In recent years, leptospirosis has become increasingly prevalent among children, students, and housewives. Cases from urban and suburban communities have been reported more frequently than cases from rural areas. The dog has been incriminated increasingly as an important vector and reservoir of this disease.

## PATHOPHYSIOLOGY

Leptospires penetrate the skin or mucous membranes and then invade the bloodstream and spread throughout the body to produce a wide variety of manifestations. The organism appears to bore through connective tissue and invade various tissues, including the anterior chamber of the eye and the subarachnoid space, without eliciting a significant inflammatory response.

Avirulent and virulent strains of leptospires are taken up by fixed phagocytes and reticuloendothelial tissue in vivo. The severity of the lesions produced correlates positively with the number of organisms. Specific resistance is apparently mediated by antibodies. Antibody increases the efficacy of clearance of leptospires from the bloodstream by improving phagocytosis by enhancing opsonization. Polymorphonuclear leukocytes are not an efficient defense factor against pathogenic leptospires in nonimmune hosts. The virulence of leptospires appears to be related to their ability to resist killing by neutrophils and by serum.

Selected clinical and histologic findings in human leptospirosis suggest that pathogenicity may partially result from enzyme, toxin, or other metabolites that are elaborated by or released by lysed leptospires. Endotoxin has been demonstrated in extracts of leptospires, but its precise role in the pathogenesis of leptospirosis remains unknown.

The development of jaundice and hemolytic anemia in patients with leptospirosis suggests the possibility that hemolysis plays a role in the pathogenesis of this disease. Hemolysis may persist during leptospirosis, suggesting that circulating hemolysin is adsorbed by erythrocytes early during the course of leptospirosis and that the erythrocytes subsequently lyse despite the development of serum antibody.

In humans, a profound derangement in hepatic function has been associated with leptospirosis. Necrosis of liver cells is infrequent, however, and the activity of serum glutamic oxaloacetic and pyruvic transaminases generally is elevated only slightly. The most prominent clinical manifestations of hepatic dysfunction include icterus and impaired production of the clotting factors dependent on vitamin K, decreased serum albumin, and increased serum globulins. These abnormalities have occurred in icteric and anicteric patients with leptospirosis.

Renal failure is an important cause of death in patients with leptospirosis. In patients who died during the first week of disease, renal changes included cloudy swelling or isolated tubular epithelial cell necrosis. In those who died during the second week of illness, numerous foci of tubular epithelial necrosis were apparent. When patients die after the 12th day of illness, an inflammatory infiltrate in the kidney is widespread, involving the medulla and the cortex. Impaired renal blood flow appears to constitute a fundamental alteration of the nephropathy associated with leptospirosis. Diminution in renal perfusion is suggested by hypotension, hypovolemia, and circulatory collapse. Reversible oliguria observed during the course of leptospirosis has been attributed to reduced renal blood flow resulting from hypotension, a deficit of extracellular fluid, or both. Rarely, adrenal insufficiency may follow hemorrhagic infarction of the adrenal glands.

Cardiac dysfunction can lead to hypoperfusion in severe leptospirosis. Focal hemorrhagic myocarditis, pericarditis, and cardiac arrhythmias have been documented. Cardiac malfunction may occur secondary to hypotension, electrolyte imbalance, hypovolemia, or uremia. Other pathologic alterations of leptospirosis include acute hemorrhagic lobar pneumonia and massive hemoptysis, meningitis, meningoencephalitis and encephalitis, radiculitis, myelitis, and peripheral neuritis.

The intraocular fluid provides a protective environment for leptospires. Despite the development of high antibody titers in serum, leptospires may remain viable in the anterior chamber of the eyes for many months. This phenomenon appears to be responsible for the recurrent, chronic, or latent uveitis syndromes of patients with leptospirosis.

Myalgia is a common complaint in patients with all forms of leptospirosis. Myalgia appears to be the result of pathologic changes, including vacuolation of the cytoplasm of the myofibrils.

## CLINICAL MANIFESTATIONS

### Common Leptospirosis

Leptospirosis is an acute systemic infection characterized by generalized vasculitis. Diminished awareness of this disorder, coupled with the diversity and nonspecificity of its presentation, accounts for the significant number of cases that go unrecognized.

The incubation period is usually 7 to 12 days, but a range of 2 to 20 days has been reported. The variation in incubation period is not serotype specific and has no prognostic significance.

The first (septicemic) stage of leptospirosis is characterized by the development of an acute systemic infection with an abrupt onset of symptoms. This phase terminates in about 4 to 7 days with symptomatic improvement and defervescence. These changes coincide with the disappearance of leptospires from the blood, cerebrospinal fluid (CSF), and all other tissues except the aqueous humor of the eye and renal parenchyma. Antibody titers to leptospires develop rapidly, heralding the onset of the second (immune) stage of the illness. This stage lasts 4 to 30 days. Leptospiruria is common and continues for 1 week to 1 month. This immune phase of the disease generally is unaffected by antibiotic therapy. Meningitis and hepatic or renal involvement reach peak intensity during this stage of disease.

Clinical leptospirosis can follow an icteric or anicteric course. At least 90% of all the patients with leptospirosis are anicteric. They therefore escape definitive diagnosis, largely because icterus and azotemia are absent. The onset of the septicemic phase of anicteric leptospirosis is heralded by fever, malaise, myalgia, headache, chills, and abdominal pain. Fever abates by lysis, and other symptoms resolve. Death is rare in the first stage of anicteric leptospirosis. The second stage of anicteric disease is characterized by fever, uveitis, rash, headache, and meningitis. The fever is usually of brief duration and has a lower peak than during the septicemic phase.

Physical examination during the septicemic stage may reveal muscle tenderness, conjunctival suffusion, dehydration, generalized lymphadenopathy, hepatosplenomegaly, and skin rashes, which can be macular, maculopapular, urticarial, erythematous, petechial, purpuric, hemorrhagic, or desquamating. The skin lesions are most prominent over the trunk, but any area of the body can be affected. Pharyngitis, rales, arthritis, nonpitting edema, and tachycardia may occur. Hypotension is rare in anicteric disease. Muscle pain and tenderness may be generalized, but the muscles of the calf, lower spine, and abdomen are affected most frequently. Conjunctival suffusion, photophobia, ocular pain, and conjunctival hemorrhage are more helpful diagnostic signs. Suffusion is more marked on the bulbar than on the palpebral conjunctiva. A nonobstructive, toxic dilatation of the gallbladder requiring cholecystomy often occurs in children with leptospirosis. Pain associated with this problem must be differentiated from myositis, subperitoneal or subserosal hemorrhages, pancreatitis, or abdominal wall causalgia, all of which may occur in patients with anicteric or icteric leptospirosis. Other signs and symptoms of the septicemic phase of anicteric leptospirosis include parotitis, orchitis, epididymitis, prostatitis, arthralgia, arthritis, and otitis media.

The immune phase of anicteric disease is reflected by a CSF pleocytosis, with or without meningeal signs or symptoms. As an antibody titer develops, leptospires are cleared rapidly from the CSF. If examination of the CSF is performed during the second week of illness, a meningeal reaction can be demonstrated in more than 80% of the patients with anicteric disease, but only 50% have clinical signs and symptoms of meningitis.

Lumbar punctures may reveal various CSF pressures, with mean values less than 200 mm $H_2O$. Cell counts within the CSF vary from normal to 500 cells/mm$^3$. Polymorphonuclear leukocytes predominate early during the immune phase, but mononuclear cells predominate subsequently. Protein concentrations within the CSF range from normal to 300 mg/dL. Glucose concentrations generally are normal.

Encephalitis, spasticity, paralysis, cranial nerve paralysis, peripheral neuritis, nystagmus, radiculitis, seizures, visual disturbances, myelitis, or Guillain-Barré syndrome may appear during or after the immune stage of anicteric disease. Leptospiruria is the rule during the immune stage of anicteric leptospirosis, and it is not associated with impaired renal function.

### Icteric Leptospirosis

The icteric form of leptospirosis is also known as Weil's syndrome. This form of leptospirosis is a distinctive clinical expression describing severe leptospirosis, but it does not refer to a specific serotype. Weil's syndrome is dominated by symptoms of renal, hepatic, or vascular dysfunction. Icterus and azotemia may be so severe that the biphasic course of illness is not observed.

Icterus remains the hallmark of Weil's syndrome, with bilirubin concentrations as high as 60 to 80 mg/dL, although concentrations are usually less than 20 mg/dL. Direct and indirect reacting bilirubin increase, and modest elevations in serum alkaline phosphatase and depressed activity of plasma prothrombin occur. The hypoprothrombinemia responds to the parenteral administration of vitamin K. Serum albumin generally is depressed.

Hepatomegaly develops in approximately one quarter of these patients, a frequency no greater than that in anicteric cases. Transient intrahepatic biliary obstruction may occur, but acholic stools generally are not observed. Acalculous cholecystitis occurs in about 55% of children with icteric leptospirosis.

Renal dysfunction may be seen in all forms of leptospirosis, regardless of the severity of disease or the serotype causing infection. Proteinuria is the most frequent abnormality, but it is usually mild. Hyaline or granular casts and cellular elements may be found in the urinary sediment. Gross or microscopic hematuria probably reflects a hemorrhagic diathesis rather than glomerular injury. Oliguria or anuria may develop early and may persist. Renal failure is generally reversible, but it is also the principal cause of death in patients with leptospirosis.

Cardiac involvement occurs relatively infrequently. Congestive heart failure and cardiovascular collapse are seen, and cerebrovascular accidents are observed in patients with leptospirosis.

Hyponatremia is a consistent finding in patients with severe icteric leptospirosis. The hyponatremia appears to result from the failure of the sodium pump that causes sodium to move intracellularly in exchange for potassium and from a redistribution of fluid such that the extracellular fluid space is expanded at the expense of the intracellular space. Hyponatremia in these patients may be unresponsive to sodium replacement and fluid restriction. It is best treated by fluid restriction, which can be continued unless hypotension ensues. Clinical improvement generally follows a spontaneous increase in serum sodium, which may be seen before any other evidence of clinical improvement.

## LABORATORY DIAGNOSIS

A confirmed case of leptospirosis, as defined by the Centers for Disease Control, must fulfill the following criteria: clinical specimens that are culture positive for leptospires or clinical symptoms compatible with leptospirosis and either seroconversion or a fourfold or greater rise in the microscopic agglutination titer between acute and convalescent serum specimens obtained 2 or more weeks apart and studied at the same laboratory.

Presumptive leptospirosis is defined as showing clinical symptoms compatible with leptospirosis and a microscopic agglutination titer of at least 1 : 100, a positive macroscopic agglutination slide test reaction on a single serum specimen obtained after the onset of symptoms, or a stable microscopic agglutination titer of at least 1 : 100 in two or more serum specimens obtained after the onset of symptoms.

Leptospires can be recovered from blood or CSF during the septicemic stage of illness and from urine during the immune phase. Media for the inoculation of leptospires usually contain a buffered solution, with or without peptone, and with or without 0.1% or 0.2% agar to which rabbit serum has been added to provide a final concentration in the medium of 5% to 10%. A pH between 7.2 and 7.8 is essential. For routine use, Fletcher semisolid medium or EMJH semisolid medium is recommended. Polysorbate 80–albumin medium is available commercially. This medium appears to be superior for primary isolation of leptospires.

Multiple cultures should be obtained because the concentration of organism at any given time may be very low. Urine is the main source from which leptospires can be isolated during the immune and convalescent phases of leptospirosis. A clean-voided urine specimen can be inoculated directly into an appropriate semisolid medium. It is imperative to dilute urine specimens with sterile buffered saline solution to ensure growth. The best results are obtained by adding 0.1 mL of urine to 0.9 mL of buffered saline before inoculation into 5 mL of semisolid medium.

Leptospires may be observed by dark-field examination, but a concentration of 10,000 to 20,000 leptospires per 1 mL of fluid is needed to observe these organisms. Leptospires can be stained by several silver impregnation techniques.

Fluorescent antibody techniques have been applied successfully to the detection of leptospires in urine or tissues. It is important to run a positive and negative control specimen at the time that the unknown specimen is being tested. Positive results are considered presumptive evidence of infection.

Serologic tests are available for the diagnosis of leptospirosis. The microscopic agglutination test performed with live organisms at the Centers for Disease Control is one of the methods of choice. The enzyme-linked immunosorbent assay (ELISA) has been compared with the microscopic agglutination test for the serologic diagnosis of leptospirosis. The results suggest that this test is a sound alternative to the microscopic agglutination test because of its sensitivity, standardization, and simplicity.

A fourfold increase in titers between acute and convalescent sera is indisputable evidence of active leptospirosis when this result is obtained using any of the specific serologic tests. Other tests that may be used for the serologic diagnosis of leptospirosis include a complement fixation assay, a hemolytic test, an indirect immunofluorescent test, an erythrocyte sensitizing substance test, and countercurrent immunoelectrophoresis.

## TREATMENT

Treatment is most beneficial when administered early. Treatment with penicillin or tetracycline (except in children younger than 8 years of age) should be initiated if the diagnosis of leptospirosis is suspected. Parenteral aqueous penicillin G administered as 6 to 8 million U/m² body surface/day in six divided doses is optimal. For patients sensitive to penicillin, tetracycline administered as 10 to 20 mg/kg/day should be provided intravenously, or 25 to 50 mg/kg/day can be given orally in four divided oral doses for 1 week.

Management of leptospirosis requires attention to supportive care. Fluid and electrolyte balance must be meticulously maintained. Dehydration, acute renal failure, and cardiovascular collapse require prompt and specific treatment.

## PREVENTION

Hygienic conditions should be encouraged in farmyard buildings, swimming pools, and slaughter houses. Immunization of workers at high risk for leptospirosis has been used successfully in other parts of the world. Leptospire bacterins are available commercially and have been evaluated for safety and efficacy in laboratory animals and in domestic livestock. The degree of protection attained in these animals depends largely on the antigenic potential of the immunizing agent.

## Selected Readings

Feigin RD, Anderson DC. Leptospirosis. In: Feigin RD, Cherry JD, eds. Textbook of pediatric infectious diseases, ed 3. Philadelphia: WB Saunders, 1992:1167.

Feigin RD, Lobes LA, Anderson DC, et al. Human leptospirosis from immunized dogs. Ann Intern Med 1973;79:777.

Heath CW Jr, Alexander AD, Galton MM. Leptospirosis in the United States. N Engl J Med 1965;273:857.

Peter G. Leptospirosis: a zoonosis of protean manifestations. Pediatr Infect Dis 1982;1:282.

Sulzer CR, Glosser JW, Rogers F, et al. Evaluation of an indirect hemagglutination test for the diagnosis of human leptospirosis. J Clin Microbiol 1975;2:218.

*Principles and Practice of Pediatrics, Second Edition.*
edited by Frank A. Oski et al. J. B. Lippincott Company, Philadelphia © 1994.

# 56.14 *Listeriosis*

## Morven S. Edwards

*Listeria monocytogenes* was first described in 1911 as a bacillus that produced minute nodular lesions in the liver of a rabbit. It was shown to have infective capacity in laboratory animals in 1926 and was isolated from the blood of a patient with a mononucleosis syndrome in 1929. The first perinatal infection due to *L monocytogenes* was described in 1936. The organism was called *Listerella* at that time; the current designation was adopted in 1939 in honor of Lord Lister.

## MICROBIOLOGY

*L monocytogenes* is a short, non-spore-forming, gram-positive bacillus. In young cultures and in cerebrospinal fluid (CSF), organisms may appear predominantly coccoid and may form short chains, and they may be mistaken for pneumococci or group B streptococci. Older cultures may Gram stain variably and can be confused morphologically with *Haemophilus influenzae*. *L monocytogenes* grows well on most laboratory media. On sheep blood agar, the colonies at 24 to 48 hours are 1 to 2 mm in diameter, gray-white, and translucent, with a narrow zone of $\beta$ hemolysis that may be most evident on lifting a colony from the plate. Almost all strains of *L monocytogenes* are motile, a feature most pronounced at room temperature in semisolid motility medium. The organism is catalase positive and oxidase negative, and it hydrolyzes esculin. Optimal temperatures for growth range from 20°C to 37°C and, although growth is faster at 30°C to 37°C, the organism's capacity to replicate at low temperatures is a helpful differentiating feature. *L monocytogenes* may be confused in the laboratory with corynebacteria, group B streptococci, enterococci, and diphtheroids.

Somatic and flagellar antigens were used to classify *L monocytogenes* into four serotypes, designated numerically. Subsequently, more serotypes were added, and there currently are at least 11. Types 1a, 1b, and 4b account for 90% of the clinical infections.

## EPIDEMIOLOGY AND TRANSMISSION

*Listeria* is almost ubiquitous in nature. The organism is found in dust, soil, water, sewage, and vegetation. It has caused naturally acquired infection in more than 50 species of animals, including mammals, birds, rodents, crustaceans, and fish. It has been isolated from insects, but they are not considered an important vector of infection. The organism's capacity to withstand dry, alkaline conditions may account for its persistence in soil and widespread distribution in nature. Between 1% and 5% of asymptomatic adults may harbor *L monocytogenes* among the normal flora of the gastrointestinal tract.

The incidence of human infection is highest in the spring and summer months, but infection in animals is more prevalent during the winter months. Most cases of infection in humans are sporadic and cannot be traced to animal contacts. Most cases are probably dirt-borne infections. The acquisition of *L monocytogenes* beyond the neonatal period probably results in asymptomatic colonization or infection of the mucous membranes of the throat or gastrointestinal tract, with transient or persistent fecal shedding. Among neonates, infection may be acquired transplacentally or perinatally after delivery through a colonized birth canal. *Listeria* may be transmitted genitally from person to person, but transmission by the respiratory route has not been documented. Epidemic neonatal listeriosis may be transmitted between infants by contact with the hands of hospital personnel. A nosocomial outbreak has been associated with contaminated mineral oil used for infant bathing. Clusters of infections with no evident source have also been described in newborn nurseries and among hospitalized immunocompromised hosts.

In three food-borne outbreaks, listeriosis probably arose from domestic animals. In one outbreak, cabbage used in coleslaw was contaminated, presumably from the manure of a flock of sheep, one of which had died from listeriosis. Pasteurized milk was the source in another outbreak. The milk came from dairy cows that had suffered from *Listeria* encephalitis. Mexican-style cheese contaminated with *L monocytogenes* serotype 4b was implicated in the third outbreak, in which 58 of 86 cases were among mother and infant pairs.

## PATHOPHYSIOLOGY

Fecal carriage rates and serologic assessment indicate that many people are exposed to *L monocytogenes*, although few develop invasive infection. Most infections are observed in neonates and older persons, suggesting a host-associated immune deficiency. Also predisposed are persons with reticuloendothelial dysfunction caused by diabetes, alcoholism, or cirrhosis; those requiring immunosuppressive or corticosteroid therapy; patients with malignancy, particularly lymphoma or Hodgkin's disease; solid organ transplantation patients; pregnant women; and patients with acquired immune deficiency syndrome. The propensity for listeriosis seen in persons with T-cell dysfunction demonstrates the critical role of thymus-derived lymphocytes and mononuclear phagocytes in host response to this intracellular pathogen. Although cell-mediated immunity is of central importance, immune globulins and complement also function in host defense, but only limited protection is conferred by these T-cell-independent mechanisms.

*L monocytogenes* can invade the eye and skin of humans by direct exposure or inoculation, but bloodstream invasion from a gastrointestinal tract source is the most likely route. The organism has tropism for the central nervous system (CNS), particularly the meninges. Among neonates, hematogenous maternal infection is presumed to seed the placenta and cause fetal infection through the umbilical vein, with dissemination to multiple organs. Human listeriosis is characterized by the formation of nodular granulomas that vary in site and number according to the mode of infection, the dose of organisms, and the age and resistance of the host. In neonates, the liver is usually diffusely involved, and granulomas also are observed in the lungs, spleen, adrenal glands, and lymph nodes. The organisms cause necrosis followed by proliferative activity of cells of the reticuloendothelial system. After granulomas form, the central part of the granulomas undergo necrosis. At the periphery of the necrotic focus, chronic inflammatory cells and organisms may be seen.

## CLINICAL MANIFESTATIONS

*Listeria* infections affecting children can be divided into three broad categories: maternal infections, neonatal infections, and infections beyond the neonatal period in children with or without predisposing conditions.

## Maternal Infections

Maternal infection is manifested as an influenza-like illness with chills, fever, vomiting, myalgia, and headache that occurs in the days or weeks before abortion or delivery. These symptoms were present in 60% of 37 women reported in two recent outbreaks of perinatal listeriosis. Other patients had (with decreasing frequency) abdominal or urinary symptoms, cough or upper respiratory tract congestion, or fever alone. Only 5 women (14%) who delivered affected infants had no symptoms. Intrauterine infection can cause amnionitis, premature labor, spontaneous abortion, stillbirth, or early-onset neonatal infection. Green or brown staining of the amniotic fluid is often observed.

## Neonatal Infections

There are three syndromes of listeriosis in neonates: granulomatosis infantisepticum, early-onset sepsis with or without pneumonia, and late-onset meningitis.

Granulomatosis infantisepticum is the designation for classic disseminated listeriosis, with generalized septicemia, extensive pustular or petechial rash, and marked hepatomegaly. This overwhelming form of listeriosis frequently results in death in utero. Liveborn infants with granulomatosis infantisepticum often are depressed at birth and usually die in the first hours of life due to respiratory distress, meningitis with seizures, or shock. In one report (Larsson, 1979), 15 of the 21 infants born alive had fatal outcomes.

Early-onset listeriosis is defined by the onset of symptoms within the first 5 days of life. Most infants are symptomatic at or within hours after delivery. Also referred to as the "septicemic" form of the illness, early-onset listeriosis is associated with obstetric complications and premature onset of labor. Respiratory distress and shock, with cardiac dysfunction, are the predominant symptoms. In one report, 10 of 14 liveborn infants with listeriosis had respiratory symptoms at delivery; 3 infants developed illness at 12 hours, 3 days, and 4 days of age, respectively; and 1 infant was asymptomatic. Meningitis occurred in 4 patients, all of whom were symptomatic at birth. Nonspecific findings of neonatal sepsis, such as hypothermia, fever, cyanosis, poor feeding, and vomiting, may accompany early-onset infection. Type 1a and 1b strains predominate in early-onset disease, although outbreaks due to type 4b also have been described. The mortality rate, even in series reported within the past decade, ranges from 20% to 40%.

Late-onset listeriosis occurs 2 to 4 weeks (mean, 2 weeks) after delivery through a colonized birth canal. Also referred to as the meningitic form of disease, late-onset listeriosis generally occurs in full-term infants whose mothers have had a benign obstetric course. It is almost always manifested as meningitis or meningoencephalitis, with symptoms typical of purulent meningitis, including fever, irritability, and poor feeding. Presenting features include bulging fontanelles, seizures, respiratory distress, and vomiting or diarrhea. Cerebrospinal fluid examination reveals pleocytosis, usually ranging from 100 to several thousand cells per cubic millimeter, an elevated protein, and depressed glucose level. Neutrophils or mononuclear cells may predominate, and the predominant cell type may shift to neutrophils or mononuclear cells during the course of illness. Serotype 4b strains predominate in late-onset disease. With proper treatment, the fatality rate is less than 10%, but some infants sustain neurologic damage after meningitis.

## Infection After the Neonatal Period

Listeriosis in childhood or adolescence is uncommon. Among 87 patients between the ages of 2 months and 20 years for whom sufficient data are available, 54% had no underlying diseases known to predispose to Listeria infections. Approximately one fourth had hematologic malignancies, were organ transplant recipients, or were receiving medications that caused immunosuppression. Miscellaneous predisposing conditions, including juvenile cirrhosis, portal hypertension, diabetes mellitus, tuberculosis, renal disease, systemic lupus erythematosus, and pregnancy, may have enhanced susceptibility in the remainder. Infection may consist of bacteremia with no focus; focal infection such as bacterial endocarditis, osteomyelitis, peritonitis, or ocular infection; or CNS infection. The manifestations of meningitis for this older group of children are similar to those of neonates.

Several CNS manifestations of listeriosis have been described. With its propensity to affect the brain or brain stem, Listeria may cause a diffuse encephalitis or rhombencephalitis, characterized by dizziness, vomiting, and cranial nerve palsies. Primary involvement of the brain stem follows a biphasic pattern in which a nonspecific prodrome of headache, vomiting, and fever is followed by cranial nerve palsies most commonly involving the sixth, seventh, ninth, and tenth nerves. Among 14 cases of L monocytogenes brain abscess, 7 occurred in patients with leukemia or renal allografts and 4 in patients without predisposing features. With the exception of an unusually high frequency of associated bacteremia and meningitis, the features of Listeria brain abscess were not distinctive.

## DIAGNOSIS

The only means by which L monocytogenes infection can be diagnosed reliably is by isolating the organism from clinical specimens. Cultures should be obtained, as indicated, from blood, CSF, purulent collections, and bone marrow. For suspected early-onset neonatal infection, the placenta, amniotic fluid, and maternal vagina and lochia may provide evidence of infection. Neonatal surface cultures from the throat, conjunctivae, or feces are indicative only of colonization, which may or may not be associated with invasive infection. A Gram stain of normally sterile sources such as CSF or purulent collections that reveals short, gram-positive coccobacillary organisms supports the diagnosis. Cultures usually yield the organism in 24 to 48 hours, but a longer interval from inoculation may be required. Rapid diagnostic testing procedures such as countercurrent immunoelectrophoresis have been evaluated but are not in general use. Serologic tests have not been useful for establishing a diagnosis of Listeria infection in individual patients. The presence of peripheral blood monocytosis or a mononuclear cell predominance in CSF should enhance the suspicion of L monocytogenes infection. However, the absence of these findings does not exclude the diagnosis.

Although other in utero infections such as disseminated cytomegalovirus infection should be considered in the differential diagnosis, the features of granuloma infantisepticum usually are so distinctive as to be pathognomonic. The septicemic form of early-onset listeriosis, with or without respiratory distress, cannot be differentiated clinically from septicemia associated with other bacteria that cause early-onset infection, particularly group B streptococci and the Enterobacteriaceae. Similarly, Listeria meningitis cannot be differentiated from other bacterial infections of the meninges. CSF Gram-stained smears may be confused with group B streptococci, Streptococcus pneumoniae, Corynebacterium, and H influenzae. Listeria meningitis, particularly rhombencephalitis, has been misdiagnosed as tuberculous meningitis. Among immunocompromised patients, Listeria meningitis may present in a manner similar to cryptococcal or pneumococcal meningitis. If the T-cell function is abnormal, Nocardia asteroides should be considered in the differential diagnosis of brain abscess.

# TREATMENT

There are reports of successful treatment of *L monocytogenes* infection with ampicillin or penicillin alone. However, because of reported in vitro tolerance or resistance to penicillin alone and studies showing in vitro synergy and increased clinical efficacy, combination therapy with ampicillin and gentamicin is the regimen of choice. In neonates, an ampicillin dose of 150 to 200 mg/kg/day for nonmeningeal infections or 300 to 400 mg/kg/day for *Listeria* meningitis is indicated. The higher dose is appropriate for treating infection in immunocompromised hosts. Treatment should be continued for 10 days for bacteremia without a focus, 14 to 21 days for meningitis or meningoencephalitis, and 4 to 6 weeks for serious focal infections such as brain abscess or endocarditis.

Alternative antibiotics to which *Listeria* is susceptible include tetracycline, chloramphenicol, trimethoprim-sulfamethoxazole, and erythromycin. There are insufficient data on which to base a recommendation for vancomycin as alternative therapy. Cephalosporins are ineffective and have no role in treatment. Trimethoprim-sulfamethoxazole is active against *L monocytogenes*, achieves good penetration of the CNS, and may be an alternative for penicillin-allergic patients. Newer antibiotics that appear to be effective include mezlocillin, imipenem, and ciprofloxacin.

# COMPLICATIONS

Untreated, listeriosis is usually fatal within 4 days. With treatment, the usual duration of illness is 10 days for septicemia, 2 to 3 weeks for meningitis or meningoencephalitis, and 4 to 6 weeks for more severe illness, such as brain abscess or endocarditis.

Among patients with underlying immunosuppression and those with granuloma infantisepticum, the fatality rates are 60% to 70%. Proportionately lower rates are found among neonates and otherwise healthy older children. The bacteremic and meningeal forms of listeriosis can be cured, but complications may develop despite prompt antimicrobial treatment. Sequelae such as hydrocephalus, strabismus, and retardation may occur after CNS infections.

## Selected Readings

Bortolussi R, Seeliger HPR. Listeriosis. In: Remington JS, Klein JO, eds. Infectious diseases of the fetus and newborn infant, ed 3. Philadelphia: WB Saunders, 1990:812.

Boucher M, Yonekura ML. Perinatal listeriosis (early-onset): Correlation of antenatal manifestations and neonatal outcome. Obstet Gynecol 1986;68:593.

Dee RR, Lorber B. Brain abscess due to *Listeria monocytogenes:* case report and literature review. Rev Infect Dis 1986;8:968.

Evans JR, Allen AC, Stinson DA, et al. Perinatal listeriosis: report of an outbreak. Pediatr Infect Dis 1985;4:237.

Larsson S, Cornberg S, Winblad S. Listeriosis during pregnancy and neonatal period in Sweden 1958–1974. Acta Paediatr Scand 1979;68:485.

Lennon D, Lewis B, Mantell C, et al. Epidemic perinatal listeriosis. Pediatr Infect Dis 1984;3:30.

Linnan MJ, Mascola L, Lou XD, et al. Epidemic listeriosis associated with Mexican-style cheese. N Engl J Med 1988;319:823.

Schuchat A, Lizano C, Broome CV, et al. Outbreak of neonatal listeriosis associated with mineral oil. Pediatr Infect Dis J 1991;10:183.

Schuchat A, Swaminathan B, Broome CV. Epidemiology of human listeriosis. Clin Microbiol Rev 1991;4:169.

Tim MW, Jackson MA, Shannon K, et al. Non-neonatal infection due to *Listeria monocytogenes*. Pediatr Infect Dis 1984;3:213.

*Principles and Practice of Pediatrics, Second Edition.*
edited by Frank A. Oski et al. J. B. Lippincott Company, Philadelphia © 1994.

# 56.15 *Neisseria Infections*

## 56.15.1 *Meningococcal Infections*

Carol J. Baker and Morven S. Edwards

Great strides have been made in our understanding of the meningococcus since the initial descriptions of "epidemic cerebrospinal meningitis" by Vieusseux in 1805 and of "petechial or spotted fever" the following year by Elisha North. It has been more than a century since the causative organism, then called diplococcus intracellularis meningitidis, was described by Weichselbaum, who observed that it was found almost exclusively within neutrophils and that it could be differentiated morphologically from the pneumococcus.

The introduction of serum therapy in 1907, the later addition of sulfonamides and penicillin, and the current availability of intensive care support have dramatically improved the outcome of these infections. However, *Neisseria meningitidis* still causes fulminant infections that are fatal within hours after the onset of symptoms, and many problems must be resolved before meningococcal disease can be successfully eradicated.

# MICROBIOLOGY

*Neisseria* is a member of the family Neisseriaceae, which also contains the genera *Branhamella, Acinetobacter, Kingella,* and *Moraxella. N meningitidis* is differentiated from *Neisseria gonorrhoeae* and the less pathogenic *Neisseria* species on the basis of carbohydrate fermentation reactions. *Neisseria gonorrhoeae* ferments only glucose, but most strains of *N meningitidis* ferment glucose and maltose. The few strains that fail to produce acid from either carbohydrate may be particularly difficult to identify in the laboratory.

Meningococci have fastidious cultivation requirements. For optimal growth, they require enriched media such as chocolate, blood, or Mueller-Hinton agar and a 3% to 10% $CO_2$ atmosphere. Colonies are 1 to 5 mm in diameter, translucent, and nonhemolytic. *N meningitidis* is a gram-negative, biscuit-shaped or coffee-bean–shaped diplococcus with rounded outer and flattened inner margins.

Specific capsular polysaccharide antigens allow the classification of meningococci into at least 13 serogroups, of which three—designated A, B, and C—are responsible for 90% of human disease. The other 10 groups are designated D, X, Y, Z, W135, 29-E, H, I, K, and L. The principal noncapsular cell wall antigens include the lipooligosaccharides (LOS), which is analogous to the lipopolysaccharide of enteric gram-negative bacilli, and the outer membrane proteins (OMP). There are at least 12 different LOS serotypes. Groups B and C can be subdivided into at least 15 protein types based on antigenically distinct OMPs. Endemic disease appears to be caused by a broad, heterogeneous group of serotypes. The outer membrane proteins are part of a lipoprotein-lipopolysaccharide complex that is responsible for the endotoxin effect observed in invasive infection. Meningococci also contain pili or fimbriae, which enhance attachment to nasopharyngeal epithelial cells.

## EPIDEMIOLOGY

Meningococcal infection is primarily a disease of childhood. In general, there is an inverse relation between age and attack rate, with the exception of an increased incidence among 15- to 19-year-old adolescents. More than 50% of the patients are younger than 4 years of age, and the highest age-specific attack rate is found among infants younger than 1 year. Infection is unusual within the first 2 months of life. Approximately two thirds of the cases occur during the winter and spring months, and increased disease activity may follow an outbreak of influenza A. Among children, the sexes are affected equally.

Meningococcal disease has a worldwide distribution. The incidence of disease varies from year to year because of the superimposition of 3- to 5-year epidemic cycles of disease on a base of endemic disease activity. Since the classification of *N meningitidis* into serogroups in 1950, epidemic and endemic serogroups have been identified. Historically, group A strains were associated with worldwide epidemics in the preantibiotic era and until 1963, when a serogroup shift occurred and epidemic group B disease was observed. These shifts have continued, to group C in 1967 and to groups A and B in 1976. Clusters of group C disease have been reported in school children after epidemic influenza or a preceding viral-like illness, supporting antecedent upper respiratory tract infection as a feature predisposing to meningococcal disease.

Reasons for shifts in serogroup prevalence are unclear. One group of investigators described the clonal population structure of more than 400 strains of *N meningitidis* group A isolated from 23 outbreaks by starch-gel electrophoresis of seven cytoplasmic enzymes and SDS-gel electrophoresis of two outer membrane proteins. Most epidemics or outbreaks were characterized by a single or predominant clone. A limited number of clones have been responsible for the epidemics since 1915. Similar clonal analysis has been carried out for serogroups B and C. It is hypothesized that epidemic outbreaks may begin only when changes in herd immunity coincide with appropriate seasonal and climatic conditions that promote carriage and transmission of one or more strains.

Endemic or sporadic disease is usually caused by groups B and C meningococci. Until recently, endemic or sporadic disease was likely to be caused by group B strains in the 6- to 24-month age group and by group C strains in older children. Since the mid-1980s, serogroup C strains have predominated in endemic disease. Infection due to less common serogroups such as Y or W-135 is often associated with a complement deficiency.

## PATHOGENESIS AND PATHOLOGY

Humans are the only natural host for meningococcal infection, and the oropharynx is its reservoir. Acquisition of nasopharyngeal infection by inhalation or direct contact results in transient, intermittent, or chronic carriage. The prevalence of asymptomatic carriage during nonepidemic periods ranges from 2% to 38%, and the median duration of carriage is 9.6 months. In most hosts, infection of the upper respiratory tract elicits formation of serum bactericidal antibody 7 to 10 days later. This immune response does not eliminate the nasopharyngeal carrier state, but it does protect the host from symptomatic infection. Susceptibility to invasive disease exists in the interval between acquisition of the

organism in the nasopharynx and development of bactericidal antibody in the serum. Pili mediate the attachment of meningococci, and parasite-directed endocytosis promotes their entry into nonciliated cells of the nasopharyngeal mucosa. Dissemination occurs when the organism penetrates the nasopharyngeal mucosa of the nonimmune host into the bloodstream, where it replicates. From there, it may disseminate to the meninges, joints, myocardium, or elsewhere. Injury to the nasopharyngeal mucosa by preceding respiratory viral infection may promote invasiveness, but this hypothesis is contested.

The prevalence of passively or naturally acquired bactericidal antibody is inversely related to the incidence of invasive infection. Maternally derived antibody provides protection for most infants during the first months of life. Passively acquired antibody levels reach a nadir between the ages of 6 and 24 months, when the incidence of invasive infection is greatest. Nasopharyngeal carriage of meningococci from serogroups with low pathogenicity may elicit cross-reactive antibodies that protect against invasiveness of pathogenic serogroups A, B, and C. Similarly, gastrointestinal colonization with bacteria containing antigens that cross-react with meningococci may contribute to the development of naturally acquired immunity.

Specific antibody and complement are important for immunity to meningococci. Specific bactericidal IgG antibodies bind to meningococci and may activate the classic or alternative complement pathways. Bacterial killing can be mediated by serum bactericidal activity, which requires the membrane attack complex, or by phagocytes. Patients who are deficient in specific antibody must rely more heavily on the integrity of complement-dependent bactericidal activity. Fatal meningococcemia has been associated with congenital deficiencies of properdin or of terminal pathway components C5 through C9. These hosts must kill the organism by phagocytic rather than complement-mediated mechanisms. Partial compensation for this opsonic deficiency can be provided by eliciting specific antibodies through immunization. Some people develop serum IgA antibody (ie, blocking antibody) that renders the bactericidal IgG or IgM antibody ineffective and results in disease susceptibility.

The predominant pathologic feature of fulminant meningococcemia is diffuse vascular damage and disseminated intravascular coagulation. Bleeding into any organ may occur. Histopathologically, the vascular changes consist of endothelial damage, vessel wall inflammation, necrosis, and thrombosis. These changes presumably are mediated by the effects of endotoxin and are quite similar to the pathologic changes that can be observed in animals given endotoxin. A correlation between C3 activation products and the level of endotoxin supports the concept that complement activation may contribute to multiple organ failure in overwhelming disease. Endotoxic shock resulting in circulatory collapse and myocardial dysfunction is the major cause of death.

## CLINICAL MANIFESTATIONS

The clinical expression of meningococcal disease in children was categorized in 1987 by Sullivan and La Scolea: bacteremia without sepsis, meningococcemia without meningitis, meningitis, and other manifestations. The initial replication of meningococci in the bloodstream usually causes the nonspecific symptoms of fever, malaise, myalgias, and headache. Bacteremia without a focus may be considered as a possible diagnosis, and depending on degree of toxicity, these patients may be sent home, with or without oral antimicrobial therapy. Among 13 children with the diagnosis of occult bacteremia, 6 received amoxicillin at the time of initial evaluation. At reexamination, the bloodstream had cleared in 3 patients without antimicrobial therapy; 4 patients had developed meningitis; and the remainder were clinically improved.

Acute meningococcemia without meningitis begins with influenza-like symptoms, but within hours to days, these children are septic. Most have cutaneous manifestations, which initially may take the form of a nonspecific maculopapular, morbilliform, or urticarial rash. Evolution to a petechial or purpuric rash within hours or days is the rule. Purpura, usually most extensive on the buttocks and lower extremities, is a feature of fulminant disease. In fulminant disease, hypotension, oliguria, disseminated intravascular coagulation, myocardial dysfunction, and vascular collapse (often irreversible) lead to death in approximately 20% of the patients. When the course is less fulminant and shock is responsive to therapy, the occasional fatal infection is usually due to the consequences of direct invasion of the myocardium, manifested by congestive failure, poor contractility, and pulmonary edema.

Only one third to one half of the children with meningococcal meningitis have petechiae or purpura at the time of initial evaluation. Among the remainder, the clinical presentation is that of bacterial meningitis, characterized (except in very young infants) by nuchal rigidity, altered level of consciousness, and signs or symptoms of increased intracranial pressure. Most children (95%) with meningococcal meningitis survive. The most common cause of death is cerebral edema with herniation.

Children with meningitis or meningococcemia have quantitatively higher-grade bacteremia than do those with occult bacteremia or other manifestations of infection. However, at the time of hematogenous dissemination, other sites may be seeded. The primary presentation reflects the particular focus in which a nidus for infection was established. Primary meningococcal pneumonia, periorbital cellulitis, pericarditis, peritonitis, cervical adenitis, endocarditis, purulent conjunctivitis, and endophthalmitis are rare but have been reported in children. Occasionally, manifestations of disease usually attributed to *N gonorrhoeae,* such as vulvovaginitis or pelvic inflammatory disease, prove to be caused by *N meningitidis.* The syndrome of chronic meningococcemia, in which persistent meningococcal bacteremia is associated with fever, skin lesions resembling gonococcemia, and arthritis, is also extremely rare in childhood.

## DIAGNOSIS

The diagnosis of infection due to *N meningitidis* is established by growth of the organism from blood, cerebrospinal fluid (CSF), skin lesions, or other sites of infection. The diagnosis can be determined presumptively by the presence of gram-negative diplococci in stained smears of centrifuged CSF or cutaneous lesions. The procedure of pressing a clean glass slide against a lanced petechial or purpuric lesion is simple and yields the organism in as many as 83% of the attempts when performed before or promptly after initiation of antimicrobial therapy. A presumptive diagnosis can also be established by rapid tests for antigen detection. Commercially available reagents are sensitive and specific for the detection of groups A, C, D, and Y meningococcal polysaccharides by latex agglutination or countercurrent immunoelectrophoresis techniques. Concentrated urine and CSF are most likely to contain detectable levels of antigen, although serum and other normally sterile fluids can be submitted for testing. Unfortunately, reagents for detecting group B meningococcal polysaccharide have poor sensitivity and specificity.

Meningococcemia should be considered a possible diagnosis in any child with fever and a petechial rash. In one review of 129 children with the findings of fever and petechiae, 20% had invasive bacterial disease, including 11% with meningococcal infection. Rocky Mountain spotted fever, epidemic typhus, *Ehrlichia canis* infection, atypical measles, staphylococcal sepsis, and viral infections (particularly ECHO and adenoviral infections) are other infectious causes of fever and petechial rash. The noninfectious or unclassified disorders that should be considered in the differential diagnosis are Kawasaki disease, idiopathic thrombocytopenic purpura, Henoch-Schönlein purpura, vasculitis, drug reactions, and leukemia.

Among 42 children who had sepsis with coagulopathy, purpura, or adrenal hemorrhage, with or without shock, Jacobs and associates found that 30 infections were caused by *N meningitidis* and 12 by *Haemophilus influenzae.* Patients with meningococcal disease were older, more often male, more likely to have contracted the disease in winter or spring, and had a more protracted duration of symptoms before admission. Children with infection due to *H influenzae* were younger and significantly more likely to die, emphasizing the importance of initially providing broad-spectrum antimicrobial therapy in young children.

Early in the course of infection, meningococcal skin lesions may be exclusively macular or maculopapular. Meningococcemia should be considered in any child who shows signs of toxicity, even if the rash appears benign. Urticarial rash occurring soon after the initiation of penicillin therapy is likely to be a manifestation of meningococcemia rather than penicillin allergy. In the absence of rash, the features of meningococcal meningitis are not distinctive, and the presenting findings are similar to those of other types of bacterial meningitis.

## TREATMENT

Aqueous penicillin G administered intravenously at a dose of 300,000 U/kg/day remains the treatment of choice for meningococcal infections. Ampicillin (300 mg/kg/day) is also effective, as is cefotaxime (200 mg/kg/day) or ceftriaxone (100–150 mg/kg/day). For the penicillin-allergic child, in whom a cephalosporin may pose some risk for cross-allergenicity, chloramphenicol (100 mg/kg/day) is an alternative antimicrobial. Strains of *N meningitidis* with reduced sensitivity or resistance to penicillin (minimal inhibitory concentration 0.1 $\mu$g/mL to 1.0 $\mu$g/mL) have been recovered with increasing frequency since 1986 in Spain and parts of Africa. Penicillin-resistant strains remain susceptible to chloramphenicol, cefotaxime, and ceftriaxone. These strains have not been reported in the United States.

Meningococcemia constitutes a medical emergency. The initial dose of antimicrobial therapy should be administered before transport of an acutely ill patient with a petechial or purpuric rash. Supportive care should be directed toward managing shock. Many patients develop shock shortly after the initiation of antimicrobial therapy, and this LOS-mediated course should be anticipated. Continuous monitoring of vital signs, including blood pressure by the Doppler method, and of clinical status (eg, urine output, peripheral perfusion) in an intensive care setting is mandatory. Anticipatory therapy with volume resuscitation or pressor agents should be provided as indicated. The advisability of administering hydrocortisone (10 mg/kg initially, followed by a divided dose of 10 mg/kg/day for 2 days) to patients with possible adrenal hemorrhage is debated, but it probably does not favorably affect the outcome in critically ill patients. Treatment should be provided as indicated for control of increased intracranial pressure, seizures, and correction of anemia. Dexamethasone therapy (0.6 mg/kg/day) in four divided doses for 4 days should be considered for children and infants more than 2 months of age with meningitis. The usual duration of treatment for meningococcemia or meningococcal meningitis is 7 days of parenteral drug therapy.

## OUTCOME AND COMPLICATIONS

Approximately 20% of the children with meningococcemia die. The usual cause of death is irreversible shock, and most deaths occur within the first 48 hours after hospital admission. Fatality rates for children with meningococcemia plus meningococcal meningitis are lower (approximately 5%), presumably because these patients constitute a subset who have survived meningococcemia long enough to develop meningeal seeding. Several prognostic signs recognized at the time of hospital admission predict poor survival: meningococcemia without meningitis, shock or coma, extensive purpura, neutropenia, thrombocytopenia, disseminated intravascular coagulopathy, and myocarditis.

The complications of meningococcal infections may be classified as early and late (Table 56-16). Early complications are the direct result of infection and include myocarditis, pericarditis, pneumonia, hemorrhage, and arthritis. Meningococcal meningitis may be complicated acutely by seizures, cranial nerve palsies (particularly of the third, fourth, and sixth cranial nerves), ataxia, or cerebral herniation. Subdural effusion, almost universally sterile, may be seen during convalescence. The most common neurologic residual of meningococcal meningitis is deafness, which is usually bilateral, sensorineural, and permanent. Reported for 5% to 10% of the survivors, hearing loss occurs significantly more often among children with leukocytosis (>20,000 cells/mm$^3$) or leukopenia (<5000 cells/mm$^3$) at the time of admission and in those with CSF leukocytosis (>10,000 cells/mm$^3$) than in

patients with an uncomplicated course. Neurologic sequelae are generally limited to deafness, but residual cranial nerve palsy or retardation occur occasionally.

Late, allergic, hypersensitivity, immune complex-mediated, and reactive are all terms that have been employed to describe the complications of meningococcal disease that occur during recovery from infection. Late complications, manifested as cutaneous vasculitis, arthritis, pericarditis, or rarely as episcleritis, occur in 10% of the survivors. Although these survivors present with inflammatory features, the clue to the noninfectious cause of the complications is the timing of onset—usually 7 to 10 days into therapy. Pericardial or joint fluid may contain leukocytes in excess of 50,000/mm$^3$ with a neutrophil predominance, but the fluid invariably is sterile. Patients with the admission findings of shock, extensive rash, leukocytosis, or leukopenia and those with fever persisting more than 5 days into therapy are at significant risk for these complications. The treatment consists of drainage (only if needed for symptomatic relief) and administration of anti-inflammatory agents such as aspirin (60 mg/kg/day). Occasionally, prednisone (60 mg/m$^2$/day initially) may be required to reduce inflammation in patients with pericarditis. Antimicrobial therapy should not be prolonged beyond the duration required for uncomplicated infection. Arthritis and vasculitis usually resolve fully within 2 to 3 weeks, but recovery from pericarditis may require several months.

## PREVENTION

### Antimicrobial Prophylaxis

Chemoprophylaxis to eradicate the meningococcal carrier state interrupts the spread of meningococcal infections. Among household contacts, the secondary attack rate varies from 3 per 1000 for endemic or sporadic disease to 3 per 100 exposed persons in epidemic situations. Contacts who are at sufficient risk to warrant antimicrobial prophylaxis include household members and the day-care center contacts who are in the "secretion-sharing" preschool age range. Prophylaxis is not required for school contacts of endemic cases. However, a few outbreaks among school classmates have been reported, and prophylaxis is indicated in this setting. Hospital contacts do not require prophylaxis. Because high-dose penicillin suppresses colonization of the nasopharynx only transiently, the index patient should receive treatment for carrier state eradication at the conclusion of parenteral therapy.

Rifampin is the antimicrobial most often used for chemoprophylaxis in children (Table 56-17). Rifampin eradicates the carrier state rapidly, but resistant strains have emerged. It is usually well tolerated, but recipients should be alerted that it stains urine and tears red-orange. Sulfisoxazole has proved efficacy for eradication of colonization and prevention of secondary disease, but widespread sulfa resistance has resulted in the restriction of its use to situations in which the disease-producing strain has documented susceptibility. Ceftriaxone, given as a single intramuscular dose of 125 mg for children younger than 12 years of age and 250 mg for adults, has been shown more efficacious than rifampin for interrupting carriage of group A meningococcal strains. It is not recommended for routine use, because efficacy has not been documented for other serogroups.

Monthly injections of benzathine penicillin G have prevented recurrence of invasive disease in patients with a terminal complement protein deficiency.

### Immunoprophylaxis

Commercially available vaccines that are safe and immunogenic for children older than 2 years of age include monovalent prep-

**TABLE 56-16.    Relative Frequency of Complications of Meningococcal Infection**

| Complication | Frequency* |
|---|---|
| **Early** | |
| Cardiovascular | |
|   Pericarditis | + |
|   Myocarditis | +++ |
| Pulmonary | |
|   Pneumonia | ++ |
|   Pleural effusion or empyema | + |
| Neurologic | |
|   Seizures† | ++++ |
|   Cranial nerve palsy | + |
|   Ataxia | ++ |
|   Cerebral herniation | + |
|   Subdural effusion | +++ |
|   Hearing loss | +++ |
| Miscellaneous | |
|   Arthritis | ++ |
|   Hemorrhage | +++ |
| **Late** | |
| Arthritis | +++ |
| Vasculitis | ++ |
| Pericarditis | ++ |
| Episcleritis | + |

\* +, rare; ++, 1% to 5%; +++, 5% to 10%; ++++, more than 10%.
† At hospital admission.

Ross SC, Rosenthal PJ, Berberich HM, et al. Killing of *Neisseria meningitidis* by human neutrophils: implications for normal and complement-deficient individuals. J Infect Dis 1987;155:1266.

Stephens DS, Farley MM. Pathogenic events during infection of the human nasopharynx with *Neisseria meningitidis* and *Haemophilus influenzae.* Rev Infect Dis 1991;13:22.

Sullivan TD, LaScolea LJ Jr. *Neisseria meningitidis* bacteremia in children: quantitation of bacteremia and spontaneous clinical recovery without antibiotic therapy. Pediatrics 1987;80:63.

Van Esso D, Fontanals D, Uriz S, et al. *Neisseria meningitidis* strains with decreased susceptibility to penicillin. Pediatr Infect Dis J 1987;6:438.

Van Nguyen Q, Nguyen EA, Weiner LB. Incidence of invasive bacterial disease in children with fever and petechiae. Pediatrics 1984;74:77.

Wong VK, Hitchcock W, Mason WH. Meningococcal infections in children: a review of 100 cases. Pediatr Infect Dis J 1989;8:224.

## TABLE 56-17. Antimicrobial Prophylaxis of Contacts

| Age of Contact | Dose and Duration |
|---|---|
| **Rifampin** | |
| <1 mo | 5 mg/kg bid for 2 days |
| 1–12 y | 10 mg/kg bid for 2 days (600 mg/dose maximum) |
| >12 y | 600 mg bid for 2 days* |
| **Sulfisoxazole†** | |
| <1 y | 500 mg/day for 2 days |
| 1–12 y | 500 mg bid for 2 days |
| >12 y | 1 g bid for 2 days |

\* Dose based on weight in kilograms should be employed if an adolescent's weight does not warrant use of the adult dose.
† Isolate must be known to be sulfa susceptible.

*Principles and Practice of Pediatrics, Second Edition.*
edited by Frank A. Oski et al. J. B. Lippincott Company, Philadelphia © 1994.

arations containing polysaccharides of groups A or C, a bivalent A-C vaccine, and a quadrivalent preparation containing polysaccharides of groups A, C, Y, and W135 *N meningitidis.* Because the duration of eradication of pharyngeal colonization may be as short as 6 weeks after chemoprophylaxis and the time required to elicit an immune response after immunization is approximately 10 to 14 days, administration of vaccine should be considered as an adjunct to chemoprophylaxis among household and intimate contacts. Immunization is recommended for persons with anatomical or functional asplenia and deficiencies of terminal components of the complement system. Travelers to areas with hyperendemic or epidemic meningococcal disease should be immunized.

Vaccines have been used successfully to halt the spread of epidemic disease. The usual dose is 50 µg, administered once. The group A polysaccharide vaccine has proved efficacy for infants as young as 3 months of age, but the current group C vaccine has poor immunogenicity for children younger than 2 years. However, group C polysaccharide as contained in a tetravalent A, C, Y, W135 vaccine elicits good responses in infants as young as 6 months of age when a second dose is administered 3 months after primary immunization. Preparations of group B polysaccharide with sufficient immunogenicity for commercial use have not been developed. Preparations in which the polysaccharide is conjugated to an outer membrane protein carrier are under investigation and may resolve the problem of poor immunogenicity in young children.

## Selected Readings

Edwards MS, Baker CJ. Complications and sequelae of meningococcal infections in children. J Pediatr 1981;90:540.

Feigin RD, Baker CJ, Herwaldt LA, et al. Epidemic meningococcal disease in an elementary-school classroom. N Engl J Med 1982;302:1255.

Harrison LH, Armstrong CW, Jenkins SR, et al. A cluster of meningococcal disease on a school bus following epidemic influenza. Arch Intern Med 1991;151:1005.

Jacobs RF, Hsi S, Wilson CB, et al. Apparent meningococcemia: clinical features of disease due to *Haemophilus influenzae* and *Neisseria meningitidis.* Pediatrics 1983;72:469.

Olyhoek T, Crowe BA, Achtman M. Clonal population structure of *Neisseria meningitidis* serogroup A isolated from epidemics and pandemics between 1915 and 1983. Rev Infect Dis 1987;9:665.

Peltola H. Meningococcal disease: still with us. Rev Infect Dis 1983;5:71.

Peltola H, Safary A, Käyhty H, et al. Evaluation of two tetravalent (ACY W135) meningococcal vaccines in infants and small children: a clinical study comparing immunogenicity of O-acetyl-negative and O-acetyl-positive group C polysaccharides. Pediatrics 1985;76:91.

Potter PC, Frasch CE, van der Sande WJM, et al. Prophylaxis against *Neisseria meningitidis* infections and antibody responses in patients with deficiency of the sixth component of complement. J Infect Dis 1990;161:932.

## 56.15.2 Gonococcal Infections

Lori E. R. Patterson

The term *gonorrhea* refers to several clinical conditions caused by *Neisseria gonorrhoeae.* Gonorrhea is the most common reportable infectious disease in the United States, and the increasing prevalence of antibiotic-resistant strains has necessitated substantial changes in therapy.

## MICROBIOLOGY

*N gonorrhoeae* is an aerobic, gram-negative, nonmotile, oxidase-positive bacterium that appears as small diplococci with flattened adjacent surfaces. In clinical specimens, the organism is usually seen within neutrophils. The ultrastructure of the gonococcus is typical of that seen in the gram-negative organisms: the outer membrane contains pili, lipopolysaccharide, and several distinct proteins. The most prevalent of these, the outer membrane protein I (OMP I), acts as an anion channel through the hydrophobic cell membrane. This protein demonstrates antigenic variability and is useful for serotyping. Certain serotypes are more frequently associated with invasive disease. By virtue of its role in adherence, protein II (OMP II) appears to be a virulence factor. Pili also facilitate adherence; strains that lack pili are avirulent and are more susceptible to phagocytic action.

Other characteristics help to differentiate gonococcal strains. Auxotype is a designation that describes the ability of a particular isolate of *N gonorrhoeae* to grow on various nutrient deficient media. Combined auxotype and serotype data have revealed more than 100 distinct strains of *N gonorrhoeae.* The antibiotic resistance pattern can also differentiate strains, although this property may not remain fixed. These patterns may be conferred by plasmid-mediated penicillinase production or by chromosomal alterations that produce intrinsic resistance to penicillin or other antibiotics. Plasmid-mediated resistance to tetracycline also occurs.

## PATHOPHYSIOLOGY

On exposure to mucosal surfaces, the gonococcus adheres to the host cell, aided by cell-surface pili. By endocytosis, the bacteria penetrate through or between epithelial cells, disrupting the mucosal integrity. Lipopolysaccharide exerts a toxic effect on the ciliated epithelial cells. An intense inflammatory response produces the characteristic profuse exudate. As gonococci are released into the subepithelial space, deeper tissue destruction occurs through the action of extracellular enzymes and the cytotoxic and endotoxin-like effects of lipopolysaccharide. Invasion of local blood vessels and lymphatics leads to dissemination. Eventually, scarring and fibrosis develop in the untreated patient.

Although the host defense against gonococcal infection is not fully understood, clinical and laboratory observations give important clues about its nature. Humoral and secretory immunoglobulins against *N gonorrhoeae* are produced at the time of infection, but they are not fully protective. One possible reason for this is that gonococci can readily alter the antigenic structure of pili (ie, phase variation) and OMP II and evade recognition by the host. Pili themselves appear to protect against phagocytosis. All gonococci produce a protease that cleaves IgA1, thwarting the protective action of this mucosal surface antibody.

The production of mucus, pH, hormonal milieu, and normal flora probably influence the infection in its early stages. Prepubertal girls, whose vaginal secretions are alkaline and whose epithelium lacks the effect of estrogen, are more likely to develop vaginitis than are adolescents, in whom cervicitis is more common. Disseminated or complicated gonorrhea is more common during menses and with the use of intrauterine devices and less common during pregnancy or with the use of oral contraceptives.

Complement activation may play a role in protecting against disseminated disease, because complement-deficient patients appear to be at increased risk for the development of gonococcemia. The role of cellular immunity in defense against the gonococcus is undetermined.

Most strains of *N gonorrhoeae* are susceptible to the bactericidal action of normal serum. However, strains that cause invasive disease lack this serum sensitivity, have different growth characteristics and nutritional requirements, and are more likely to be highly sensitive to penicillin than serum-sensitive strains.

## EPIDEMIOLOGY

Despite the remarkably high prevalence of gonorrhea, a significant proportion of cases are not reported. Slightly under 500,000 cases were tallied by the Centers for Disease Control and Prevention in 1992, but because of asymptomatic infection, authorities estimate that about 2 million cases actually occur annually in the United States. Cases are concentrated in young adults, followed closely by older adolescents. The incidence is higher in girls until early adulthood, when the sex ratio reverses. Demographic risk factors for gonococcal disease include young age, unmarried status, non-Caucasian race, urban residence, low socioeconomic status, and male homosexuality. Recent declines have been seen in rates among homosexual men, presumably due to alterations in sexual behavior resulting from the epidemic of acquired immune deficiency syndrome. Asymptomatic men and prostitutes are important reservoirs of infection and are likely to contribute to difficulty in eradicating the disease. Nonetheless, gonorrhea incidence rates have been falling since the 1970s, and the United States' 1990 health objective of fewer than 280 reported cases of gonorrhea per 100,000 population was fulfilled. In the 3 years since new treatment strategies were announced, the reported cases of gonorrhea have fallen an additional 30%.

Transmission of gonorrhea generally occurs through direct physical contact with infected mucosa. In adolescents and young adults, this spread is mainly venereal. Neonates and young children are usually infected intrapartum or by sexual abuse, respectively. Conjunctivitis in older children is usually from autoinoculation. Rectal gonorrhea may be acquired by receptive anal intercourse or by perineal contamination by genitourinary

secretions. Transmission by fomites occasionally occurs and has been implicated during nursery outbreaks. Strain identity of gonococcal isolates may be particularly useful in epidemiologic studies.

Of concern is the rapidly increasing prevalence of antibiotic-resistant strains of the gonococcus. The United States' Gonococcal Isolate Surveillance Project monitors trends in antimicrobial susceptibility patterns, and data are used to formulate treatment strategies. Penicillinase-producing *N gonorrhoeae* represented 2.2% of isolates for the period ending in 1988 and accounted for more than 3% in some regions. One percent of isolates had plasmid-mediated tetracycline resistance. Of all other isolates, 16.8% exhibited chromosomally mediated resistance to various antibiotics (eg, tetracycline, penicillin, cefoxitin). Overall, 21% of isolates were classified as resistant to one of these antibiotics or spectinomycin. This proportion continues to rise: by 1991, over 10% of gonococcal isolates were resistant to penicillin. These patterns prompted recent changes in therapeutic recommendations, because empiric therapy must now address these resistant strains.

## CLINICAL PRESENTATION AND COMPLICATIONS

Although the gonococcus is most familiar as a cause of genital tract infection, the organism may cause disease at many other sites. These infections may be localized to a mucosal surface (often with production of a thick, yellow-white, purulent exudate) or hematogenously disseminated. Most infected adults are asymptomatic, but the proportion of infected children who lack symptoms is unknown.

### Ophthalmia Neonatorum and Other Neonatal Disease

Ophthalmia neonatorum is the most common form of neonatal gonorrhea. It usually occurs after intrapartum contact with the mother's infected genital secretions, but cesarean delivery does not preclude development of the condition. Risk factors include prematurity and prolonged rupture of amniotic membranes. Onset of the conjunctivitis usually occurs at 2 to 5 days of age, but earlier and later cases are not uncommon. The conjunctival discharge is classically bilateral, mucopurulent, and profuse, and marked lid edema and chemosis are present. Unilateral and milder cases are also seen. Without treatment, corneal ulceration and invasion of deeper ocular structures may occur, with subsequent loss of vision.

Other localized forms of disease in the neonate include rhinitis, funisitis, vaginitis, anorectal infection, and scalp abscess after fetal electrode monitoring. Invasive infection (sepsis, meningitis) also occurs, albeit rarely. A form of neonatal septic arthritis usually appears 1 to 4 weeks after delivery and after several days of prodromal symptoms, involves one to four joints, and is not associated with skin lesions.

### Vaginitis and Cervicitis

Uncomplicated gonococcal infection of the female genital tract presents with mild symptoms of vaginal discharge, local pruritus, and dysuria. Urinary symptoms may predominate in the young child. Nonmenstrual bleeding and pelvic pain are common. However, many infections produce no symptoms. Pelvic examination may or may not reveal a purulent endocervical discharge in postpubertal girls. Edema, erythema, and tenderness of the vulva are common in young children. Labial swelling and tenderness may reflect infection of Bartholin's gland. Systemic symptoms and signs are rare.

The most serious complication of genital gonorrhea, seen in 10% to 20% of infected female patients, is pelvic inflammatory disease (PID). Children and adolescents are more likely to develop this syndrome than are adult women. Risk factors include multiple sexual partners, use of an intrauterine device, and vaginal douching. Ascent of the gonococcus from the vagina or cervix leads to endometritis, salpingitis, and occasionally to pelvic or abdominal abscesses. Other genital microbes (particularly *Chlamydia* and anaerobes) are frequently found in the diseased structures, with or without gonococci; the relative role of each of these organisms in the pathogenesis of PID is undefined. The resultant fallopian tube fibrosis leads to obstruction and sterility in 12% of first-time infections. This increases to 50% to 75% after three episodes. Other patients later have an increased incidence of ectopic pregnancy or chronic pelvic pain. PID is suggested clinically by lower abdominal pain, fever, unexplained genital bleeding or discharge, and pain on palpation of the cervix and adnexal structures, which may show a mass-like enlargement. However, symptoms may be minimal or absent. Further upward spread of the gonococcus, with or without other organisms, can lead to a perihepatitis (ie, FitzHugh-Curtis syndrome), with fever and right upper quadrant tenderness.

## Urethritis

Purulent urethral discharge and dysuria are the hallmarks of urethral infection. A significant percentage of infected males are asymptomatic. Epididymitis and prostatitis are unusual complications, but scarring may result in urethral strictures.

## Other Localized Disease

The clinical picture of gonococcal conjunctivitis in older children and adolescents resembles that in neonates. Pharyngeal and anorectal gonorrhea are most often asymptomatic, although the latter may present with tenesmus, rectal bleeding or discharge, and pruritus. Cervical adenitis may result from gonococcal pharyngitis. Mucopurulent exudate may be seen with pharyngitis or proctitis.

## Disseminated Gonococcal Infection

Hematogenous spread of the gonococci to joints and other sites after localized mucosal infection occurs more frequently in children and adolescents than in adults. In males, disseminated gonococcal infection usually occurs after asymptomatic infection. In females, the preceding genital infection is also often unnoticed, but a temporal association between menses and dissemination has been reported. Unlike the pattern of arthritis in neonates, joint symptoms in older children mimic the adult presentation and take one of two forms, which may represent a continuum. The first is a syndrome of tenosynovitis, polyarthralgia, skin lesions, and systemic symptoms. Knees, ankles, and wrists are most commonly involved. The skin lesions are usually sparsely distributed on the dorsal extremities and appear as painful papules or petechiae that rapidly become hemorrhagic, pustular, necrotic, or ulcerated. Blood and skin biopsy cultures are usually positive, but no growth is obtained from synovial fluid. The second syndrome is characterized by a monoarticular purulent arthritis without systemic signs. A joint aspirate is likely to show gonococci on smear or culture, but bacteremia is not demonstrable. This is the most common form of septic arthritis in young adults.

Other forms of disseminated gonorrhea are extremely rare in childhood. Meningitis and endocarditis with valvular involvement have been reported.

## DIAGNOSIS

A prerequisite in diagnosing gonorrhea is a high index of suspicion on the part of the physician. Many health care practitioners have a psychosocial aversion to the thought of sexually transmitted disease in the pediatric population. This reluctance does a disservice to the increasing number of sexually abused and sexually active young patients. The history should include notations about the risk factors (eg, young age, unmarried status, non-Caucasian race, urban residence, low socioeconomic status, male homosexuality) and details of alleged abuse of the child. In adolescents, information must be obtained about sexual activity and symptoms in sex partners. *N gonorrhoeae* in other siblings or adult household members should be recorded.

The patient should be examined gently but thoroughly for urogenital discharge and for signs of trauma, such as perineal bruising or lacerations. Confirming the presence of gonorrhea requires isolation of *N gonorrhoeae* from the infected site. Samples should be collected from the urethra in males, the vagina in prepubertal females, the endocervix in older females, and other sources (eg, rectum, pharynx, joint fluid, blood, skin biopsy) as appropriate. Use of gel lubricants or cotton swabs may interfere with isolation of the gonococcus and should be avoided; warm water and synthetic swabs are suitable alternatives.

Gonococci are somewhat fastidious in their growth requirements, and do not tolerate drying. Success in isolation requires immediate plating of clinical specimens. Specialized transport systems, nutritive or nonnutritive, may be useful if this is not feasible. Modified Thayer-Martin medium (ie, chocolate agar plus vancomycin, colistin, trimethoprim, and nystatin) is generally used for isolation. The added antibiotics suppress growth of accompanying normal flora, but may also impair isolation of certain vancomycin-sensitive strains of *N gonorrhoeae*. If the specimen is taken from a normally sterile site (eg, synovial fluid), chocolate agar alone is sufficient. Optimal growth generally occurs at 35°C to 37°C in an atmosphere enriched with 5% carbon dioxide, which may be obtained with use of an incubator and a candle jar. If disseminated gonococcal infection is suspected clinically but blood cultures are negative, isolation of gonococci from mucosal surfaces (eg pharynx, rectum, urogenital tract) may lend support to the diagnosis.

A Gram stain of purulent secretions that shows gram-negative diplococci is helpful in diagnosing gonococcal urethritis and conjunctivitis but less useful in other clinical conditions because of the presence of similar appearing microbes. It is impossible to differentiate *N gonorrhoeae* from the nonpathogenic *Neisseriae* by appearance alone. After isolation, oxidase-positive, gram-negative diplococci should be speciated in the laboratory by carbohydrate fermentation pattern (ie, the gonococcus metabolizes glucose but not maltose, lactose, or sucrose). Several variations on this method are available commercially. Other methods available for definitive identification include chromogenic enzyme substrate systems, rapid coagglutination techniques using monoclonal antibodies against the gonococcus, and fluorescence-tagged polyclonal antibodies. Enzyme immunoassay or nucleic acid probes may be used to detect the gonococcus directly in clinical specimens, but their utility is limited to populations with a high prevalence of gonorrhea.

Gonococcal ophthalmia neonatorum may be differentiated by time of onset and by Gram stain from infection by *Chlamydia*, herpes simplex, or other bacteria such as staphylococci and from the chemical conjunctivitis caused by silver nitrate. Nongonococcal urethritis, with a discharge that is typically less purulent than that caused by *N gonorrhoeae*, may be caused by chlamydial or trichomonal infection and perhaps by *Ureaplasma*; these agents can also cause vaginitis, as does *Candida albicans*.

The arthritis of disseminated gonococcal infection may be

TABLE 56-18.    Treatment of Gonococcal Infection in Childhood

| Patient Group | Treatment of Choice | Penicillin-Sensitive Isolate |
|---|---|---|
| **Neonates*** | | |
| Ophthalmia neonatorum† | CTX, 50–100 mg/kg/d in divided doses q 8–12 h IV or IM × 7 d *or* CTR 25–50 mg/kg IM once (max, 125 mg) | Pen G, 100,000 U/kg/d in divided doses q 6–12 h IV × 7 d |
| Sepsis, arthritis, abscess | CTR, 25–50 mg/kg IV or IM q 24 h for ≥7 d *or* CTX, 50–100 mg/kg/d in divided doses q 8–12 h IV or IM for ≥7 d | As above |
| Meningitis | CTR, 50 mg/kg IV or IM q 24 h × 10–14 d *or* CTX, 50–100 mg/kg/d in divided doses q 8–12 h IV or IM × 10–14 d | Pen G, 150,000–200,000 U/kg/d in divided doses q 6–12 h IV × 10–14 d |
| **Older Children‡** | | |
| Urethritis, vaginitis, cervicitis, proctitis§, pharyngitis§ | CTR, 125 mg IM once (250 mg if >45 kg) *or* Spectinomycin 40 mg/kg IM once (max, 2 g) *or* Cefixime, 400 mg PO once‖ | Amoxicillin, 50 mg/kg (max, 3 g) PO once + probenecid, 25 mg/kg (max, 1 g) PO once |
| Conjunctivitis† | CTR, 50 mg/kg (max, 1 g) IM once | Pen G, 75,000–100,00 U/kg/d (max, 10⁷ U) in divided doses q 6 h IV for ≥7 d |
| Sepsis, arthritis | CTR, 50 mg/kg (max, 1 g) IM or IV q 24 h × 7 d *or* CTX, 150 mg/kg/d (max, 3 g) in divided doses IV q 8 h × 7 d *or* Spectinomycin, 80 mg/kg/d (max, 4 g) in divided doses IM q 12 h × 7 d | Ampicillin, 150 mg/kg/d (max, 4 g) in divided doses IV q 6 h × 7 d |
| Meningitis | CTR, 100 mg/kg/d (max, 2 g) in divided doses IV q 12 h × 10–14 d | Pen G, 250,000 U/kg/d in divided doses q 6 h IV × 10–14 d |
| Pelvic inflammatory disease | Therapy individualized for polymicrobial infection, but includes cefoxitin and doxycycline or clindamycin with an aminoglycoside | |

*CTX*, cefotaxime; *CTR*, ceftriaxone; *Pen G*, aqueous penicillin G; U, units.
\* Patients should be cultured and treated.
† Accompany with frequent saline eye washes; a formal eye examination for complications should be performed.
‡ Children weighing > 100 lb (45 kg) should receive the adult dose. Coincident treatment (with doxycycline 100 mg bid × 7 d in patients ≥ 8 years old) for presumptive chlamydial infection is recommended. Younger patients beyond the neonatal period should be treated with erythromycin instead.
§ Ceftriaxone is the drug of choice.
‖ For older adolescents. May be effective in younger children, but not evaluated in this group.

confused with other septic arthritides (eg, those caused by *Staphylococcus aureus*, group A or B streptococci, or *H influenzae* type b) or with that found in various collagen-vascular diseases. Associated tenosynovitis or the characteristic rash suggests a gonococcal cause. It may be difficult to differentiate PID from other intra-abdominal conditions such as appendicitis, ectopic pregnancy, ovarian cyst, mesenteric adenitis, and urinary tract infection. Laboratory indicators of inflammation, such as elevated sedimentation rate and leukocytosis, are common, but normal values do not exclude the diagnosis of PID. Ultrasound of pelvic structures, endometrial biopsy, or laparoscopy may be helpful in difficult cases. Failure to identify another cause for arthritis or for abdominal pain in a sexually active or abused female should prompt an investigation for gonorrhea.

## TREATMENT

Historically, penicillin has been the drug of choice for most gonococcal infections. Trends in antibiotic resistance have forced the abandonment of this approach for all but infections proven to be caused by penicillin-susceptible strains. Treatment strategies now focus on using drugs that have an efficacy approaching 100% for all strains after a single dose, are well-tolerated, and are preferably inexpensive. Treatment recommendations are listed in Table 56-18; many other regimens have proven effective. "Test of cure" cultures are generally unnecessary after standard therapy, but it is advisable to perform follow-up cultures several weeks after treatment of a sexually active patient, because reinfection is common.

Regardless of the disease form, it is medically and legally imperative that the source of pediatric gonorrhea be found and treated. The possibility of prior sexual abuse must always be considered, and all household members should be evaluated for gonorrheal infection. Because other sexually transmitted infections (eg, syphilis, *Chlamydia*) frequently coexist with gonorrhea, they should be sought in all patients. Serologic testing for human immunodeficiency virus should also be considered. Because the detection of chlamydial infection is often difficult, concurrent empiric therapy for this condition is recommended.

### Neonates

Infants born to mothers with untreated gonorrhea should receive a single parenteral dose of 50 mg ceftriaxone/kg (maximum, 125 mg) after gastric and rectal cultures are obtained. If signs of infection develop, the appropriate regimen should be instituted (see Table 56-18).

### Older Children

A single dose of any of several different antibiotics listed in Table 56-18 is effective in the treatment of uncomplicated genitourinary infection. Pharyngeal or rectal gonorrhea is also treatable by any of these regimens, although ceftriaxone is the drug of choice.

Disseminated gonococcal infection requires intravenous therapy in the hospital. Bacteremia and arthritis should be treated for 7 days; some experts believe that oral therapy with cefuroxime axetil or amoxicillin with clavulanic acid can be substituted after clinical improvement is seen, usually within 2 to 3 days. Intra-articular antibiotics and surgical drainage of an infected joint (except perhaps the hip) are not necessary, although serial joint space aspirations may be needed in occasional patients.

Because PID usually results from polymicrobial infection, therapy must be individualized. Culture results and clinical response should be considered. Therapy in an inpatient setting is generally recommended for adolescents. Suggested antibiotic regimens include cefoxitin and doxycycline or clindamycin and an aminoglycoside for at least 48 hours after improvement is seen. Doxycycline or clindamycin should be continued at least 10 to 14 days.

## PROGNOSIS

When treated promptly with appropriate antibiotics, most gonococcal infections can be cured. Permanent sequelae (eg, blindness from ophthalmia neonatorum, sterility from PID) are usually the result of delay in seeking medical attention or receiving correct antimicrobial therapy.

## PREVENTION

Preventing the spread of gonorrhea from mother to neonate may best be accomplished by identifying the women who harbor the infection at the time of the first prenatal visit. Every culture-positive woman and her sexual partner(s) must be treated at that time. High-risk persons, such as adolescents and promiscuous young adults, those of low socioeconomic level, and those with previous history of any sexually transmitted disease, should be cultured again in the third trimester and retreated if reinfection has occurred. Extensive experience has proven the efficacy of the Crede procedure (ie, instillation of 1% silver nitrate solution into the conjunctival sac shortly after birth) in preventing gonococcal ophthalmia neonatorum. The use of topical 1% tetracycline ophthalmic ointment or 0.5% erythromycin ophthalmic ointment has been advocated as an alternative to silver nitrate, because these agents do not cause chemical conjunctivitis and appear to be as effective. In communities with chromosomally mediated resistance to tetracycline, use of that antibiotic may be contraindicated. None of these agents can reliably protect against non-ocular infection or chlamydial conjunctivitis in the neonate.

Educating school children and adolescents about sexually transmitted diseases may be another way of interrupting spread. Among sexually active adolescents, the use of condoms and spermicides should be encouraged as a means of preventing spread of gonorrhea and other sexually transmitted diseases. Every effort should be made to identify and treat the sexual contacts of known gonorrhea patients. Unfortunately, persons with asymptomatic infection rarely seek or receive treatment, which promotes spread and increases their own risk of complications.

## Selected Readings

Britigan BE, Cohen MS, Sparling PF. Gonococcal infection: a model of molecular pathogenesis. N Engl J Med 1985;312:1683.

Centers for Disease Control. Pelvic inflammatory disease: guidelines for prevention and management. MMWR 1991;40:RR5.

Centers for Disease Control. Sexually transmitted diseases: treatment guidelines. MMWR 1989;38:S8.

Dallabetta G, Hook EW. Gonococcal infections. Infect Dis Clin North Am 1987;1: 25.

Hammerschlag MR, Cummings C, Roblin PM, Williams TH, Delke I. Efficacy of neonatal ocular prophylaxis for the prevention of chlamydial and gonococcal conjunctivitis. N Engl J Med 1989;320:769.

Handsfield HH, McCormick WM, Hook EW, et al. A comparison of single-dose cefixime with ceftriaxone as treatment for uncomplicated gonorrhea. N Engl J Med 1991;325:1337.

Morello JA, Janda WM, Doern GV. Neisseria and Branhamella. In: Balows A, ed. Manual of clinical microbiology, ed 5. Washington, DC: American Society for Microbiology, 1991:258.

Rawstron SA, Hammerschlag MR, Gullans C, Cummings M, Sierra M. Ceftriaxone treatment of penicillinase-producing Neisseria gonorrhoeae infections in children. Pediatr Infect Dis J 1989;8:445.

Schwarcz SK, Zenilman JM, Schnell D, et al. National surveillance of antimicrobial resistance in Neisseria gonorrhoeae. JAMA 1990;264:1413.

*Principles and Practice of Pediatrics, Second Edition.*
edited by Frank A. Oski et al. J. B. Lippincott Company, Philadelphia © 1994.

# 56.16 *Pasteurella multocida*

## Morven S. Edwards

The organism now designated *Pasteurella multocida* was first isolated by Kitt in 1878 and subsequently by Pasteur, who identified it as the causative agent of fowl cholera. Originally, *Pasteurella* species causing "hemorrhagic septicemia" were classified according to the animal source from which they were isolated. Recognition of interspecies transmission of infection and common biochemical features led to the grouping of isolates from all sources as *P multocida* in 1939. These organisms are common commensals in the respiratory tract of animals, and human infection usually can be linked to contact with animals.

## MICROBIOLOGY

*Pasteurella multocida* is one of several *Pasteurella* species, most of which are more commonly associated with animal than human disease. *P multocida* includes the three subspecies: *multocida, septica* and *gallicida*. *P multocida* is the most virulent species in animals. It is indole- and urease-positive and is characterized by absence of hemolysis when grown on blood agar. *P multocida* grows well on a variety of routine media that do not contain bile, including blood, chocolate, and Mueller-Hinton agar; it will not grow on the bile-containing MacConkey agar. On blood agar, its colonies resemble enterococci. Optimal growth occurs at 37°C under aerobic or facultatively anaerobic conditions.

*P multocida* is a small, nonmotile, gram-negative rod that occurs singly, in pairs, or in short chains and may exhibit bipolar staining. These organisms may be confused microscopically with *Haemophilus influenzae*, *Neisseria* species, and *Acinetobacter*. Serotypes based on heat-stable O antigens, including six that have caused disease in humans, have been identified. Oberhofer (1981) divided 48 isolates of *P multocida* into 10 biotypes based on fermentation reactions. Although no pattern was evident for isolates from dog bites, most cat bite isolates were biotypes A or B.

## EPIDEMIOLOGY AND TRANSMISSION

The incidence of asymptomatic respiratory tract or oral cavity colonization with *P multocida* ranges from 70% to 90% in cats and 50% to 70% in dogs and approximates 50% in pigs and 15% in wild rats. Carriage has been documented in larger felines (eg, lions, tigers, leopards, panthers, lynx) and a variety of other animals, including horses, cattle, sheep, rabbits, and water buffaloes.

Most *P multocida* infections in humans are the result of direct inoculation by animal bites or scratches, and this pathogen has been implicated in 80% of infected cat bites and 50% of infected dog bites. There is no seasonal or sexual predilection for infection. *P multocida* infections for which specific bite exposure cannot be elicited usually are the result of contact with animal secretions. Occasionally, asymptomatic upper respiratory tract colonization may precede dissemination of infection in humans, and *P multocida* has been isolated from asymptomatic persons with frequent animal contacts. Close contact with the family cat during breast feeding has been described as the source for transmission through oropharyngeal colonization to an infant who developed meningitis and bacteremia due to *P multocida*. In rare cases, no animal contact can be established for diagnosed *Pasteurella* infection. Although exquisitely susceptible to direct sunlight, the organism can survive in water or soil for approximately 3 weeks. Human-to-human transmission has not been documented, but an animal-soil-human route could account for some cases that cannot be linked directly to animals.

## PATHOGENESIS AND PATHOLOGY

The pathogenesis of *P multocida* infections may be best understood by examining the several potential routes of inoculation. The most common way in which infection is established is direct implantation of organisms beneath the skin from an animal bite or scratch. Inoculation is likely to be deeper and more likely to penetrate the periosteum or a joint space if the source is a cat bite (ie, puncture wound injury) than if it is a dog bite (ie, laceration wound). The rapidly established and intensely painful local cellulitis that results may be attributed in part to the production by *P multocida* of neuraminidase and endotoxin. The discharge from wounds is gray and serosanguineous. Localized infections are characterized by an infiltration of neutrophils that may manifest as abscess formation, osteomyelitis, septic arthritis, or tenosynovitis.

Nasopharyngeal colonization with *P multocida* may precede respiratory tract infection. Invasive infection occurs almost exclusively in the setting of underlying respiratory tract disease, such as chronic bronchitis or bronchiectasis.

In animals, intraperitoneal or parenteral inoculation promotes rapid replication in extracellular tissues, with subsequent hematogenous dissemination and invasion of reticuloendothelial organs that has a fatal outcome. Bacteremic infection in humans is a particular risk in the setting of hepatic dysfunction. Weber (1984) found focal infection (most commonly intra-abdominal), meningitis, pneumonitis, or wound infection in 88% of 47 cases of bacteremic infection.

## CLINICAL MANIFESTATIONS

The three major clinical manifestations of *P multocida* infections are focal soft-tissue, respiratory tract, and disseminated infections. Cellulitis due to *P multocida* characteristically has a rapid onset, often within a few hours after an animal bite or scratch. The average time of onset is 12 to 24 hours, with a range of 3 hours to 3 days. Erythema, exquisite pain, edema, and discharge described as watery and gray, odorous, or serosanguineous are the predominant local features, and 20% to 30% of patients have regional adenopathy. Depending on the location and extent of the wound, infection may be complicated by abscess formation, tenosynovitis, arthritis, or osteomyelitis. Direct inoculation presumably is required to establish infection in the tendon sheath, joint, or bone. The extremities are usually affected, but osteomyelitis and brain abscess have complicated bite wounds to the heads of children. Joint stiffness with cellulitis of the hand is a sign of tendon sheath involvement, and surgical exploration should be undertaken. Even with appropriate drainage, wound infections due to *P multocida* heal slowly, particularly if poorly vascularized tissues such as the tendon are involved.

Respiratory tract infections occur in the setting of chronic pulmonary disease, such as bronchitis or bronchiectasis, and are rare in children. Organisms colonizing the nasopharynx are of low virulence and have minimal invasive potential unless there is preexisting injury.

Meningitis with or without bacteremia is the most common manifestation of disseminated infection in children. Of 14 reported cases, 12 occurred in infants younger than 1 year of age. A history of nontraumatic animal contact, such as facial licking by household pets, was elicited for 10 children. Presenting symptoms for infants with *Pasteurella* meningitis were those of purulent meningitis and included lethargy, vomiting, irritability, and fever.

*P multocida* has been isolated from the female genital tract, and neonatal sepsis associated with maternal chorioamnionitis has been described. Bacteremia is a rare complication of wound infection. A few patients have had appendicitis due to *P multocida*. The isolates were recovered from peritoneal fluid, appendiceal abscess, or incisional wound abscess. The source and pathogenesis of infection in these patients is uncertain; at the time appendicitis was evident, bacteremia did not coexist in the patients who underwent blood culture.

## DIAGNOSIS

The diagnosis of *P multocida* infection is established by culture of the organism from blood, wound drainage material, focal abscess, or in the case of meningitis, from cerebrospinal fluid. When cultures are obtained from wound infections, laboratory personnel should be alerted to the possibility of *Pasteurella*. The Gram stain may produce confusion with *H influenzae*, which, unlike *Pasteurella*, requires factors X and V for growth; with *Neisseria*, which is differentiated by indole production; and with *Acinetobacter* species, which grow on bile-containing media. Clinically, the features of rapid onset and grayish drainage aid in differentiating cellulitis due to *P multocida* from staphylococcal or streptococcal wound infections. With exposure to cats, tularemia, plague, and cat-scratch disease are differential considerations. Each of these occurs more often after an incubation period longer than that for *Pasteurella* infections.

## TREATMENT

Penicillin is the drug of choice for *P multocida* infections. For uncomplicated wounds managed on an outpatient basis, penicillin V at a dosage of 50,000 U/kg/day administered four times daily is recommended. If wound severity warrants hospitalization, aqueous penicillin G should be employed at a dosage of 200,000 U/kg/day, given every 4 to 6 hours. Parenteral therapy always is indicated if bite wounds are associated with signs of systemic toxicity; if involvement of tendon, bone, or joint is a consideration; if wound cellulitis has progressed despite oral therapy; and in children with impaired immune function, particularly splenic dysfunction. In patients allergic to penicillin, chloramphenicol or tetracycline (which should not be given to children younger than 9 years) may be employed.

*P multocida* strains are almost universally susceptible to penicillin, having a median minimal inhibitory concentration of approximately 0.1 $\mu$g/mL. However, penicillin susceptibility testing should be confirmed in serious infections or in those failing to show the expected response to therapy, because rare isolates may be penicillin-resistant. Other antimicrobials to which isolates of *P multocida* are susceptible include the penicillin derivatives ampicillin, ticarcillin, piperacillin, mezlocillin, and carbenicillin; the second- and third-generation parenteral cephalosporins. Ciprofloxacin has good activity in vitro, but the clinical experience is limited. Antibiotics that are inadequate for treating *P multocida* infections include the antistaphylococcal penicillins, orally administered cephalosporins, erythromycin, clindamycin, vancomycin, and the aminoglycosides. If *P multocida* may be one of several pathogens in an infected animal or human bite wound, ticarcillin with clavulanate, administered parenterally, and amoxicillin with clavulanate, given orally, are ideal antimicrobials for empiric treatment.

The usual duration of parenteral treatment for cellulitis or a localized wound abscess due to *P multocida* is 5 to 10 days. A 10- to 14-day course of treatment with penicillin V often can be completed on an outpatient basis after signs of inflammation have abated. With adequate drainage, 2 to 3 weeks of parenteral treatment usually are required for arthritis or tenosynovitis, and 3 to 4 weeks of therapy are required for osteomyelitis. Recovery among infants and children with meningitis due to *P multocida* has been reported with regimens including ampicillin (200 to 300 mg/kg/day) or penicillin G (300,000 to 600,000 U/kg/day) for a 14-day (mean) course of therapy.

## OUTCOME

Recovery is the rule, but bone and joint infections due to *P multocida* may have residua consisting of decreased joint mobility or ankylosis and chronic osteomyelitis, depending on the extent of the initial injury. Most survivors of meningitis have had a normal outcome, but hemiparesis has been reported.

## Selected Readings

Arons MS, Fernando L, Polayes IM, et al. *Pasteurella multocida.* The major cause of hand infections following domestic animal bites. J Hand Surg 1982;7:47.

Clapp DW, Kleiman MB, Reynolds JK, et al. *Pasteurella multocida* meningitis in infancy. An avoidable infection. Am J Dis Child 1986;140:444.

Kumar A, Devlin HR, Vellend H. *Pasteurella multocida* meningitis in an adult: case report and review. Rev Infect Dis 1990;12:440.

Oberhofer TR. Characteristics and biotypes of *Pasteurella multocida* isolated from humans. J Clin Microbiol 1981;13:566.

Raffi F, David F, Mouzard A, et al. *Pasteurella multocida* appendiceal peritonitis: report of three cases and review of the literature. Pediatr Infect Dis 1986;5:695.

Thompson CM, Pappu L, Levkoff AH, et al. Neonatal septicemia and meningitis due to *Pasteurella multocida.* Pediatr Infect Dis 1984;3:559.

Weber DJ, Wolfson JS, Swartz MN, et al. *Pasteurella multocida* infections. Report of 34 cases and review of the literature. Medicine (Baltimore) 1984;63:133.

*Principles and Practice of Pediatrics, Second Edition.*
edited by Frank A. Oski et al. J. B. Lippincott Company, Philadelphia © 1994.

# 56.17 *Pertussis*

James D. Cherry

Pertussis (ie, whooping cough) is an acute, communicable, respiratory illness that affects susceptible persons of all ages but is particularly serious in infants. The illness can be effectively controlled by immunization.

## ETIOLOGY AND EPIDEMIOLOGY

Pertussis is caused by *Bordetella pertussis*, a gram-negative aerobic coccobacillus that is 0.2 to 0.8 $\mu$m long. Pertussis-like illness can also be caused by several types of adenoviruses, *Bordetella parapertussis*, and *Bordetella bronchiseptica*.

The epidemiology of pertussis is extensively affected by the degree of vaccine use. Pertussis occurs in all parts of the world, and humans are the only known hosts of *B pertussis*. Transmission occurs from person to person by respiratory secretion droplets, and contagion is extremely high in unimmunized populations. Spread occurs from patients with disease to susceptible contacts; asymptomatic carriers are not thought to be important in transmission. Adults with protracted cough illnesses (ie, atypical pertussis) are an important source of *B pertussis* infection among unimmunized or partially immunized children.

In unvaccinated populations, about 10% of the cases occur in children younger than 1 year of age, 40% in children 1 to 4 years of age, 45% in children 5 to 9 years of age, and 5% in children 10 to 14 years of age. Typical pertussis in persons older than 15 years is rare. In highly immunized populations, such as in the United States, about 50% of the reported cases occur in the first year of life, another 25% occur before age 5, and 15% occur in teenagers and adults.

Pertussis is an endemic disease with epidemic cycles occurring at intervals of 2 to 5 years. In the prevaccine era in the United States, the average yearly reported attack rate was 157 per 100,000 members of the population. If an allowance is made for underreporting, the actual rate can be estimated to be about 900 cases per 100,000. During the vaccine era, the reported rate of illness has ranged from 0.5 to 1.5 per 100,000 persons. The major mortality from pertussis occurs among infants. Of reported pertussis cases in the United States, about 0.6% of the patients younger than 1 year of age die. The clinical attack and mortality rates of pertussis are higher for females than males.

## PATHOPHYSIOLOGY

Pertussis is predominantly a disease of the ciliated epithelium of the respiratory tract. The *B pertussis* organism has many unique, biologically active antigens, and studies have suggested roles of these antigens in the pathogenesis of disease. In the pathogenesis of pertussis, four steps are important: attachment, evasion of host defenses, local damage, and systemic disease.

After the airborne transmission of respiratory secretions containing *B pertussis*, the organisms attach to the cilia of the respiratory epithelial cells of the new host. Filamentous hemagglutinin (FHA), lymphocytosis-promoting factor (LPF), pertactin (ie, 69-kd outer membrane protein), and possibly agglutinogens are *B pertussis* antigens that are important in the attachment process. After attachment, the infection proceeds because of the profound adverse effect on host immune effector cell function by organism adenylate cyclase and LPF. Another *B pertussis* toxin, tracheal cytotoxin, disrupts normal clearance mechanisms, allowing infection to persist.

Three *B pertussis* toxins contribute to local tissue damage of the ciliated respiratory epithelium: tracheal cytotoxin, dermonecrotic toxin, and adenylate cyclase. Pertussis is a unique disease in that systemic manifestations are rare. The characteristic lymphocytosis is caused by LPF.

## CLINICAL MANIFESTATIONS

Pertussis is a lengthy illness, commonly lasting 6 to 8 weeks, and characterized by three stages: catarrhal, paroxysmal, and convalescent. The catarrhal stage has its onset after an incubation period of 7 to 10 days; incubation usually does not exceed 14 days. The onset of illness is subtle and resembles a mild upper respiratory tract infection with coryza, mild conjunctival injection, and mild cough. The upper respiratory symptoms continue, and during the next 7 to 10 days, coughing becomes more persistent and frequent. Fever usually is not a feature of this stage.

The paroxysmal stage is manifested by increasingly forceful

coughing in the form of episodic paroxysms, which are particularly frequent at night. In classic pertussis, episodes of repetitive severe coughing are followed by a single sudden massive inspiration. The characteristic "whoop" sound results from the forceful inhalation and a narrowed glottis. Each coughing paroxysm consists of 10 to 30 forceful coughs in a staccato series. The patient's face becomes increasingly cyanotic, the tongue protrudes to the maximum, and mucus, saliva, and tears stream from nose, mouth, and eyes. There may be 20 or more paroxysms each day. The paroxysmal episodes are exhausting, and young children appear apathetic and dazed after attacks. Paroxysms are precipitated by eating, drinking, and physical activity. Between attacks, patients usually show few signs of illness, and fever is not characteristic of uncomplicated cases. In young infants, a whoop is less likely to occur after a paroxysm.

After the paroxysmal stage, which lasts from 1 to 4 weeks or more, the convalescent stage is heralded by a lessening in the severity and frequency of paroxysms. The duration of the convalescent stage varies. Paroxysmal-type coughing often occurs for 6 months or more after pertussis associated with other respiratory infections. Weight loss or failure to gain weight is a conspicuous feature of severe pertussis, especially in infants.

## COMPLICATIONS

Complications in pertussis are common and can be grouped into the three categories of respiratory, central nervous system (CNS), and secondary pressure effects. The rate of complications is inversely related to age. Bronchopneumonia, the most common complication, is caused by secondary infection with common respiratory pathogens (ie, *Haemophilus influenzae*, *Streptococcus pneumoniae*, *Streptococcus pyogenes*, and *Staphylococcus aureus*), or it can be caused by a more extensive *B pertussis* infection. If pneumonia is the result of secondary infection, significant fever and tachypnea are the usual findings. Other respiratory complications include atelectasis, bronchiectasis, interstitial or subcutaneous emphysema, and pneumothorax. Although atelectasis may persist for months after illness, there is little evidence from carefully done follow-up studies that permanent pulmonary sequelae occur. Otitis media is a frequent complication, especially in infants.

CNS complications are relatively common during the paroxysmal stage of pertussis. Data from the Centers for Disease Control indicate that 3% of infants have seizures with pertussis, and about 9 of 1000 are thought to have more serious neurologic illness (eg, encephalopathy). Severe disease is usually manifested by convulsions and then semicoma or coma. Hemiplegia, paraplegia, ataxia, aphasia, blindness, deafness, and decerebrate rigidity may occur. After encephalitis-like illness, permanent sequelae are common. About one third of patients die, one third survive with residua, and one third survive and appear normal. Sequelae include mental retardation, seizure disorders, and changes in personality and behavior.

Secondary pressure effects during the paroxysmal stage of severe pertussis may cause epistaxis, melena, petechiae, subdural hematoma, spinal epidural hematoma, umbilical or inguinal hernias, and rectal prolapse.

## DIAGNOSIS

Typical pertussis can be reliably diagnosed clinically on the basis of characteristic history and physical findings. However, for infants, adults, and cases modified by immunization, the diagnosis may be difficult. Because asymptomatic infection is not thought to be important in transmission, a careful history usually reveals contacts with illnesses characterized by prolonged coughing spasms. These contact cases are likely to be young adults.

The absence of or only minimal fever is strong evidence for the diagnosis of pertussis rather than a similar type of illness caused by a respiratory virus. In classic pertussis, the leukocyte count is elevated, and lymphocytosis occurs. Leukocytosis develops at the end of the catarrhal and during the paroxysmal stage of disease. Absolute lymphocyte counts usually are greater than 10,000 and often reach more than 30,000 cells/dL. Young infants and patients with mild or modified disease may not have the typical lymphocytosis.

The specific diagnosis of pertussis depends on the isolation of the organism or its demonstration by a rapid identification method. B pertussis can be isolated from nasopharyngeal secretions during the catarrhal and early paroxysmal stages of disease. With optimal specimen collection, fresh culture medium, and experienced technicians, 80% of the suspected cases can be confirmed by culture in outbreak situations. Specimens for culture should be obtained from the nasopharynx with the use of Dacron or calcium alginate swabs. These specimens should be directly plated onto selective media (eg, Regan-Lowe charcoal agar, modified Stainer-Scholte agar, or fresh Bordet-Gengou medium). Alternatively, Regan-Lowe transport medium should be inoculated, and the specimen transported to a diagnostic laboratory. Prior antibiotic treatment may markedly reduce the isolation rate.

Direct fluorescent antibody identification of B pertussis in nasopharyngeal specimens is a reasonably accurate procedure when performed with good reagents by experienced personnel. This technique is particularly useful if antimicrobial therapy has been given, decreasing the likelihood of obtaining a positive culture. Studies using the polymerase chain reaction (PCR) suggest that this technique may be available for the diagnosis of pertussis in the next few years.

Pertussis can also be diagnosed serologically, but because all standard tests depend on the demonstration of an increase in antibody titer, these techniques are not useful for early diagnosis. The only routinely available procedure is the agglutination test. The demonstration of a fourfold rise in agglutinin titer is firm evidence that the illness was pertussis. False-positive test results are rare, but the sensitivity of this test is limited. Enzyme-linked immunosorbent assay (ELISA) techniques that use several different pertussis antigens (eg, LPF, FHA, whole cell) and measure antibody in different immunoglobulin fractions (eg, IgA, IgM, IgG) have been used in research and investigational settings. The sensitivity of ELISA techniques is better than agglutination, but no routine test is available.

## TREATMENT

B pertussis is susceptible to erythromycin, and the administration of this antibiotic to a child during the incubation period or the catarrhal stage may prevent or modify clinical disease. Erythromycin therapy can also alter the clinical course of pertussis if treatment is initiated early in the paroxysmal stage. Treatment initiated later in the paroxysmal stage does not lessen the duration or severity of clinical illness, although patients should be treated to reduce the risk of spread to other susceptible contacts. The dosage of erythromycin is 40 to 50 mg/kg/day (adults, 1 g/day), given in four doses for a total of 14 days. This regimen should be used for treatment and prophylaxis. Trimethoprim-sulfamethoxazole is a suggested alternative to erythromycin, but its efficacy has not been documented.

Because pertussis is a highly contagious infectious disease, patients should be placed in respiratory isolation, which should be maintained for 5 days after the initiation of erythromycin

therapy. If erythromycin therapy is not given because of a contraindication, the patient should remain in isolation until 3 weeks after the onset of paroxysms. The younger the child, the more likely is the need for hospitalization. In severe cases, respiratory therapy may be lifesaving. Most infants should receive oxygen, and gentle suction should be used to remove secretions. Supportive care includes avoidance of situations that provoke attacks of coughing and maintenance of hydration and nutrition. Although corticosteroids and salbutamol (albuterol) have been used as adjuncts to therapy and, in uncontrolled studies, have reduced coughing paroxysms, there are no controlled data to indicate the usefulness of either type of medication.

## PREVENTION

Universal immunization with pertussis vaccine in children has been extraordinarily successful in controlling epidemic pertussis in the United States. Until recently, the only available vaccines in the United States and in all areas of the world except Japan were suspensions of inactivated B pertussis cells (ie, whole cell vaccines). Pertussis vaccines are routinely available in the United States only in combination with diphtheria and tetanus toxoids (ie, DTP vaccine); the combination products are adsorbed with aluminum salts. A successful immunization program for children consists of five doses of DTP. The primary immunization series consists of an initial three doses given at approximately 2, 4, and 6 months of age and a fourth dose at 15 to 18 months. The fifth dose (ie, booster) is given at the time of school entry, at 4 to 6 years of age.

In December 1991, the FDA licensed one DTP vaccine with an acellular pertussis component (DTaP) for use as the fourth and fifth doses of the recommended DTP series. This vaccine was efficacious in 2-year-old children in Japan, and the immune response in United States children is similar to or better than that after conventional DTP vaccine. In August 1992 a second DTaP vaccine was also licensed for similar use.

If pertussis is prevalent in a community, the immunization schedule can be adjusted so that the first dose is given during the third week of life and the next two doses at monthly intervals. Vaccine efficacy after three doses of DTP varies from 60% to 95%, depending on study methods. The duration of vaccine-produced immunity is relatively short, although illness is usually less severe in previously vaccinated than unvaccinated persons.

The DTP vaccine is given intramuscularly in a volume of 0.5 mL per dose. In the past, physicians often gave fractional doses in an attempt to reduce vaccine reactions. This dosage plan should not be used, because it is based on the false premise that neurologic disease occurring at the time of the immunization is caused by the vaccine. There is considerable risk that underdosing produces inadequate protection.

Pertussis immunization is not done routinely in persons age 7 years of age or older, because severe pertussis is a disease of young children, and it is thought that reactions to immunization increase with age. In the future, the successful control of pertussis will probably necessitate booster immunization in adolescents and adults, as is recommended for diphtheria and tetanus toxoids.

Reactions associated with DTP immunization are common and occasionally quite alarming. Redness, swelling, and pain at the injection site occur in a third to a half of those vaccinated. Approximately 50% of children have temperatures of 38°C (100.4°F) or higher during the 48-hour period after immunization, and 3 of 1000 have temperatures of 40.5°C (104.9°F) or higher. Fretfulness occurs in about 50% of children; other systemic complaints and their frequencies are drowsiness (32%), anorexia (21%), vomiting (6%), and persistent crying for 3 to 21 hours (1%).

Febrile convulsions are a disquieting event after DTP vaccination, occurring in approximately 1 of every 1750 immunizations. Because convulsions usually occur in children older than 6 months of age, the rate associated with the fourth immunization increases to more than 1 per 1000. Another vaccine-associated complication is the hypotonic-hyporesponsive state (ie, collapse or shock), which complicates approximately 1 of every 1750 immunizations and is most commonly associated with the first three DTP immunizations.

Of most concern to parents and physicians are so-called pertussis vaccine encephalopathy and sudden infant death syndrome (SIDS) after immunization. Instances of alleged pertussis vaccine encephalopathy are actually neurologic diseases of other causes and are only temporally related to immunization. There is no evidence to support the concept of pertussis vaccine encephalopathy. SIDS is a catastrophic event that occurs at a rate of 1.4 to 1.9 per 1000 live births. Because DTP immunization is carried out at the age of peak occurrence of SIDS, it is evident that by chance alone many cases occur after DTP immunization. Carefully conducted, large, controlled epidemiologic studies during the last 10 years have shown no correlation between DTP immunization and SIDS.

Contraindications for immunization have evolved over the past 30 years because of the presumed complications of the pertussis component of DTP vaccine. Although there is no evidence of the validity of these contraindications, it is prudent to observe them to avoid misunderstandings about the cause of temporally associated events. Children who have had an immediate anaphylactic reaction after DTP immunization should not have further immunization with this product. After immunologic evaluation and possible desensitization, further immunization with tetanus toxoid may be carried out. Children with unexplained encephalopathy within 7 days after DTP should not receive additional pertussis vaccine. In children who have a febrile illness at the time of scheduled immunization, the immunization should be deferred until the child is well. The child with an evolving neurologic disease should have immunization deferred until further observation and study have clarified the child's neurologic status. Physicians should seek up-to-date immunization advice from the Report of the Committee on Infectious Diseases of the American Academy of Pediatrics or Reports of the Immunization Practices Advisory Committee (ACIP), because recommendations change frequently.

Immunization programs can be successful only if virtually all infants are immunized. When contraindications are overinterpreted and a large percentage of children remain unimmunized, a significant risk of disease exists for those who most need protection. The benefits of pertussis immunization substantially outweigh any possible risks of immunization.

Certain control measures are necessary in situations of exposure. In day-care centers and in families, those exposed should be given erythromycin (40 to 50 mg/kg/day orally) for 14 days. Booster doses of vaccine should be given in many instances.

## Selected Readings

American Academy of Pediatrics, Committee on Infectious Diseases. Pertussis (whooping cough). In: Report of the Committee on Infectious Diseases, ed 22. Elk Grove Village, IL: American Academy of Pediatrics, 1991:266.

Centers for Disease Control. Pertussis vaccination: acellular pertussis vaccine for reinforcing and booster use—supplementary ACIP statement. MMWR 1992;41:RR1.

Centers for Disease Control. Diphtheria, tetanus and pertussis: guidelines for vaccine prophylaxis and other preventive measures. MMWR 1991;40:RR10.

Cherry JD. The epidemiology of pertussis and pertussis immunization in the United Kingdom and the United States: a comparative study. Curr Probl Pediatr 1984;14:1.

Cherry JD, Karzon DT, Brunell PA, Golden GS. Report of the Task Force on Pertussis and Pertussis Immunization—1988. Pediatrics 1988;81(suppl):939.

Cody CL, Baraff LJ, Cherry JD, Marcy SM, Manclark CR. Nature and rates of adverse reactions associated with DTP and DT immunizations in infants and children. Pediatrics 1981;68:650.

Feigin RD, Cherry JD. Pertussis. In: Feigin RD, Cherry JD, eds. Textbook of pediatric infectious diseases, ed 3. Philadelphia: WB Saunders, 1992:1208.

Mortimer EA. Kimura M, Cherry JD, et al. Protective efficacy of the Takeda acellular pertussis vaccine combined with diphtheria and tetanus toxoids following household exposure of Japanese children. Am J Dis Child 1990;144:899.

*Principles and Practice of Pediatrics, Second Edition.*
edited by Frank A. Oski et al. J. B. Lippincott Company, Philadelphia © 1994.

# 56.18 *Plague*

Ralph D. Feigin

Plague, which is caused by *Yersinia pestis*, has caused the most devastating epidemics in human history. The epidemic spread of this disease through most of Europe in the 1300s became known as the Black Death. One third of the population of Europe died as a result of this epidemic.

The bacillus responsible for plague was first identified in 1894, and at about the same time, the role of fleas and rats in transmitting the disease was recognized. In 1900, plague was introduced in San Francisco, California, by rats aboard ships. The disease rapidly spread to rodents of the American Southwest, and plague is now enzootic throughout the western United States, Central and South America, and other parts of the world.

## MICROBIOLOGY

*Yersinia pestis* is a pleomorphic, nonmotile, gram-negative bacillus of the family Enterobacteriaceae. When the bacillus is stained with Gram, Giemsa, or Wayson stains, it reveals a bipolar morphology.

*Y pestis* grows optimally at 28 °C. Organisms can be isolated from blood, sputum, or aspirates of enlarged nodes. These body fluids can be examined for the typical bacilli. Bacteria that are isolated can be identified by their nonmotile activity at 37 °C and 22 °C. The organism is usually negative for urea hydrolysis but may be positive in freshly isolated specimens. The response is positive for catalase, methyl red, esculin, and β-galactosidase. The indole, oxidase, and Voges-Proskauer reactions are negative. *Y pestis* ferments maltose, xylose, glucose, arabinose, salicin, dextrin, mannitol, and trehalose. It does not produce acid from lactose, sucrose, rhamnose, melibiose, adonitol, cellobiose, sorbose, or dulcitol. It does not use citrate or grow in potassium cyanide. *Y pestis* does not respond to lysine, ornithine decarboxylase, and arginine dihydrolase.

The organism can be identified by lysis of the isolate by known strains of bacteriophage, agglutination with specific *Y pestis* antiserum, animal inoculation, and fluorescent antibody staining.

The strains of *Y pestis* vary in their virulence. Virulence depends on the development of the envelope of fraction I antigen, absorption of hemin from medium, production of V and W antigens, synthesis of purines, and generation of toxins. The presence of a fraction I envelope or V and W antigens renders the strain resistant to phagocytosis and permits the organism to multiply. Toxins have been produced by all strains that are fully virulent. Endotoxin and exotoxin appear to contribute to the morbid effects of plague. A plasmid of 9-kb pairs contains the determinant of secretory protein that kills other bacterial strains. A plasmid of 72-kb pairs, which all pathogenic *Y pestis* strains contain, confers the requirement for environmental calcium ($Ca^{2+}$), which is necessary for the organism to grow at 37 °C. When grown under this condition, *Y pestis* produces the V and W antigens necessary for virulence.

## TRANSMISSION

Historically, plague was typically transmitted by fleas that had fed on infected rats. This form of transmission is rare today, especially in the United States, where plague is transmitted to humans after contact with an enzootic focus. Wild rodents perpetuate the plague bacillus by virtue of their ability to withstand an inoculum of *Y pestis* many times greater than that which causes disease in domestic animals or humans. After inoculation, the wild rodent becomes bacteremic and can infect the fleas that feed on it. The fleas can transmit the plague bacillus to another rodent. Animals that are hibernating are particularly resistant to clinical infection. Animals inoculated before going into hibernation may survive the winter and succumb to the infection only after they emerge from their burrows, carrying the bacillus into a new season.

Cats and dogs are susceptible to natural and experimental plague. Because of their more extensive contact with humans, domestic animals may be responsible for some cases of human plague.

Plague is transmitted to humans by the bite of an infected flea, the inhalation of infected droplets from a patient with pneumonic plague, or the skinning and evisceration of infected animals. Rarely, *Y pestis* can enter through the conjunctiva and the pharynx.

Fleas of domestic animals are more likely than rodent fleas to bite humans. The Oriental rat flea is the most efficient transmitter of the plague bacillus because of the frequency with which it bites humans and its propensity for regurgitating large numbers of *Y pestis* in the process of biting.

Sylvatic plague depends on the rodent flea as a vector. This flea is not as efficient as a rat flea in transmitting *Y pestis* but may itself become a reservoir of the organism by surviving for a year or more after the original host dies. *Y pestis* can survive in soil during interepizootics, which may serve as a mechanism for transmission of plague.

In urban areas, the organism usually is introduced from an enzootic focus into a susceptible rat population. In areas where humans and rats live in proximity, an epizootic in rats may be followed by an epidemic in people. In the United States, children become infected by direct contact with a sylvatic reservoir of this infection. Adult cases are the result of working or hunting in plague-infected areas.

## PATHOGENESIS AND PATHOLOGY

The portal of entry of the *Y pestis* organism determines the form that the disease takes. The most common site of entry is the skin, after the bite of an infected flea. Broken skin provides an easy route for direct inoculation while handling infected animals. After the organism has bypassed the skin barrier to infection, it moves by lymphatics to regional lymph nodes. The infection may be localized at this site, with subsequent antibody formation and ultimate recovery of the patient. This form of the disease has been called pestis minor.

*Y pestis* is frequently disseminated through the bloodstream. Involvement of the liver, spleen, lungs, kidneys, and meninges may occur. Disseminated intravascular coagulation is a common finding in fatal cases. Coagulation defects reported include an elevation of split-fibrin products, thrombocytopenia, and fibrin deposition in the glomeruli.

The major determinant of disease severity appears to be the presence of high levels of circulating endotoxin. Virulent *Y pestis* organisms are phagocytized but are not killed. They replicate unimpeded in macrophages, permitting the accumulation of endotoxin.

If the primary portal of entry is the lung, the resulting disease is usually fulminant. Plague bacilli can replicate freely in the alveolar spaces, resulting in severe, overwhelming pneumonitis, septicemia, and endotoxemia. In fatal cases, lymph nodes in the thoracic region have shown infarction, liquefaction necrosis, and pus formation. The mucosa of the trachea and bronchi may be covered by a frothy, bloody exudate. Submucosal hemorrhages and necrotic areas surround the trachea. Pleural surfaces contain hemorrhagic lesions and fibrinous adhesions. The lung may show signs of acute edema or consolidation. The most prominent histologic feature is an alveolar exudate consisting of polymorphonuclear leukocytes and histiocytes. The kidneys may appear grossly hemorrhagic, and there may be areas of necrosis. Glomeruli with fibrin thrombi are found frequently in patients who have disseminated intravascular coagulation.

## CLINICAL MANIFESTATIONS

The incubation period of *Y pestis* is about 3 or 4 days but can be as short as 1 to 2 hours or as long as 2 weeks. The onset of illness usually is abrupt, beginning with malaise, headache, fever, and weakness. Fever is often accompanied by shaking chills. A visible or palpable mass of nodes, known as a bubo, may be preceded by tenderness or pain at the site.

On physical examination, the patient appears to be apprehensive, toxic, and tachycardiac. The site of inoculation at the skin may or may not be evident. In some cases, the inoculation site is covered by a carbuncle. In bubonic plague, large, fixed, tender, and edematous lymph nodes are evident at one anatomical site. The areas of nodal involvement are the groin, axilla, and neck, in decreasing order of frequency. Any involved lymph node can suppurate, including the intra-abdominal nodes, which may produce the picture of an acute abdominal emergency.

Neurologic manifestations resulting from the effects of toxin on the brain are common. Patients with plague may report insomnia or suffer from weakness, delirium, stupor, gait disturbances, disorders of speech, loss of memory, and vertigo. Meningitis may occur. Intravascular coagulation may herald the onset of renal involvement, which can present clinically as an acute cortical or tubular necrosis. Involvement of the liver is evidenced by mildly elevated liver enzymes.

Pneumonic plague has identical constitutional symptoms, but the course is more fulminant and the pulmonary component more pronounced. Within 20 to 24 hours after the onset of illness, dyspnea, tachypnea, and a bloody mucopurulent productive cough are evident. If effective treatment is not instituted immediately, most patients die.

## DIAGNOSIS

Bubonic plague can be confused with any other disorder of the skin or lymph nodes. The diagnosis of staphylococcal or streptococcal lymphadenitis is established by appropriate culture. A more indolent disorder known as lymphogranuloma venereum usually presents with mild localized or systemic disease and commonly is associated with anogenital ulcers. Adenitis due to *Treponema pallidum* (ie, syphilis) is usually not tender. Adenopathy as a result of *Pasteurella multocida* infections or cat-scratch fever usually is associated with few constitutional symptoms and a history of exposure to animals. The adenopathy associated with *Francisella tularensis* infection (ie, tularemia) is more gradual in onset. The ulcerated skin lesions of anthrax may resemble those of plague in the later stages.

The buboes of plague are quite tender. Bacterial staining of lymph node tissue by Wright, Gram, or Wayson stains should show bipolar plague organisms. Fluorescent antibody staining of direct smears and tissues can provide a rapid presumptive diagnosis of plague.

## TREATMENT

Definitive diagnosis can be made only by culture of *Y pestis* from infected tissue or body fluid. Therapeutic decisions must be carried out before culture results are available.

The Centers for Disease Control recommend treatment of all suspected cases of plague. Patients who do not require hospitalization can be treated with tetracycline or chloramphenicol. Tetracycline can be given to patients 8 years of age and older at a dosage of 30 to 40 mg/kg/day in four or six divided doses, up to a total dose of 2 g in children and 6 g in adults. If outpatient treatment is provided, the patient should be followed for the first 3 days to ensure resolution of disease. For acutely ill patients, streptomycin remains the drug of choice. Streptomycin should be administered intramuscularly at a dosage of 20 to 30 mg/kg/day in two divided doses. If plague meningitis is considered, chloramphenicol, administered as 50 to 100 mg/kg/day intravenously in four divided doses, is the treatment of choice. Other intravenous antibiotics that can be useful, particularly in the presence of hypotension, are kanamycin, administered as 15 mg/kg/day in three divided doses up to a maximum dose of 1.5 g/day, and gentamicin, administered as 7.5 mg/kg/day for children or 3 to 5 mg/kg/day for adults in three divided doses. The duration of therapy must be determined by the severity and length of disease. Treatment should be continued for at least 7 days for patients with uncomplicated disease.

## PROGNOSIS

Mortality rates for untreated cases of plague range between 40% and 70%. Pneumonic plague is almost invariably fatal without treatment. If antimicrobial therapy is provided promptly, the overall mortality rate for plague should be as low as 5%. Complications of plague during convalescence may include lung abscess, suppuration of buboes (which may be delayed), and polyarthritis. Secondary infection with *Pseudomonas* species and *Staphylococcus aureus* may occur, particularly within lymph node tissue.

## PREVENTION

Eradication of rats and their removal from areas inhabited by humans are the best means for limiting urban epidemics of plague. Vector control is achieved by the use of insecticides in fields and housing areas. Rodent control can be carried out by trapping, fumigation of burrows, and poisoning. Education of the public is important. Children should be taught not to handle sick or dead rodents, and care must be exercised in removing fleas from household pets. Trash should not be permitted to accumulate near living areas.

Victims of plague should be isolated until they are bacteriologically sterile. Contacts of patients who have pneumonic plague should receive chemoprophylaxis with tetracycline if they are older than 8 years of age (0.5 g, four times each day for 7 days) or with streptomycin (20 mg/kg/day in two divided doses) if they are younger than 8 years. There is a 6-day quarantine period for contacts of patients with regard to international travel.

Plague vaccines have been available for many years but are not fully effective. The plague vaccine licensed in the United States consists of a formaldehyde-inactivated *Y pestis* that has been preserved in 0.5% phenol. The Centers for Disease Control recommend plague vaccine for workers who reside in areas of enzootic or epidemic plague where avoidance of rodents and fleas is impossible and for laboratory and field personnel who regularly work with *Y pestis* or plague-infected rodents. Primary immunization for adults and children who are 11 years of age and older consists of three doses of vaccine. The first dose of 1.0 mL can be followed by a second dose of 0.2 mL 4 weeks later and a third dose of 0.2 mL 6 months after the first dose. Three booster doses follow at 6-month intervals. Additional doses can be given at 1- to 2-year intervals. Children younger than 1 year of age receive one fifth of the adult dose; those 1 to 4 years of age should receive three fifths of the adult dose. The dosage schedule is the same as that for immunization of adults. Persons who have been vaccinated but who experience a definite exposure to plague should receive chemoprophylaxis because the vaccine is not completely protective, even when high levels of circulating antibody are demonstrable.

## Selected Readings

Cantey JR. Plague in Vietnam. Arch Intern Med 1974;133:280.
Centers for Disease Control. Plague vaccine. MMWR 1982;31:301.
Centers for Disease Control. Plague in the United States, 1982. MMWR 1983;32:SS19.
Finegold MJ. Pathogenesis of plague. Am J Med 1968;45:549.
Goldstein MD. Plague. In: Feigin RD, Cherry JD, eds. Textbook of pediatric infectious diseases, ed 3. Philadelphia: WB Saunders, 1992:1218.
Kaufmann AF, Boyce JM, Martone WJ. Trends in human plague in the United States. J Infect Dis 1980;141:522.
Mann JM, Schaudler L, Cushing A. Pediatric plague. Pediatrics 1982;69:762.

*Principles and Practice of Pediatrics, Second Edition.* edited by Frank A. Oski et al. J. B. Lippincott Company, Philadelphia © 1994.

## 56.19 *Pneumococcal Infections*

### Ralph D. Feigin

Disease caused by *Streptococcus pneumoniae* remains one of the leading causes of morbidity and mortality in children. Almost all children experience some manifestations of pneumococcal infection during childhood. *S pneumoniae* are the leading cause of otitis media and a frequent cause of pneumonia in children.

## MICROBIOLOGY

S pneumoniae are gram-positive, lanced-shaped cocci that usually occur in pairs. Under certain conditions, pneumococci may form chains, the length of which depends on the type of media in which the organism has been grown. S pneumoniae are encapsulated, and capsular size varies considerably. With Gram stain, pneumococci may resemble other organisms, particularly $\alpha$-hemolytic streptococci.

On solid media, encapsulated pneumococci produce round, shiny colonies approximately 1 mm diameter. Serotypes 3, 8, and 37 form larger, mucoid colonies. As the cultures age, the center of the colony regresses, creating a central dimple. When grown on media containing blood, all pneumococci cause $\beta$-hemolysis of the surrounding erythrocytes. Pneumococci are facultative anaerobes and may be grown aerobically or anaerobically. Rarely, strains of S pneumoniae are obligate anaerobes.

Optochin is helpful in identifying pneumococci because these $\alpha$-hemolytic organisms are sensitive to this agent, and $\beta$-hemolytic streptococci are resistant. Discs impregnated with optochin are laid on pneumococci, and the plate is incubated overnight. With the discs that are currently available, inhibition with a zone of greater than 18 mm identifies the colony as a pneumococcus with greater than 90% accuracy.

Pneumococci may also be identified by a bile solubility assay. When bile is added to a broth culture of pneumococci, prompt dissolution of the cocci is seen.

The Quellung reaction permits rapid identification of pneumococci. This reaction is carried out by mixing equal volumes of the suspension of bacteria, antiserum, and methylene blue on a slide and examining the bacteria by light microscopy. Capsular swelling identifies genus, species, and serotype. The use of the quellung reaction permits immediate identification of pneumococci from cultures or body fluids.

A rapid test to identify pneumococci growing in liquid culture employs latex particles coated with antibodies to all 83 currently identified serotypes. This is an extremely useful test, although selected strains of $\alpha$-streptococci may cross-react with pneumococci.

## EPIDEMIOLOGY

Pneumococci are typically found in the pharynx of healthy people. S pneumoniae is spread from person to person in droplets from respiratory secretions. Infection of the upper respiratory tract aids the spread. Colonization and disease due to pneumococci are more common in the winter and spring in temperate climates. Rates of colonization depend on the age of the patient, the population studied, and their rate of exposure to young children. The highest colonization rates occur among young children who are receiving care in an institutional setting. The prevalence of colonization has been as high as 97% in selected studies, but most reports estimate the rate at 25% to 50%. In one study, 63% of otitis media and 76% of pneumococcal bacteremia occurring in children were caused by types 6, 14, 18, 19, and 23. Disease in children is more commonly due to serotypes numbered 6 and above than to serotypes 1 through 5.

Immunity to S pneumoniae depends on the presence of type-specific antibody to the capsular antigen of the organism. Immunity during the first few months of life apparently is derived from maternal antibody that is transferred passively to the fetus. Children younger than 2 years of age respond poorly to pneumococcal antigens in the available vaccines. This may explain the frequency of pneumococcal bacteremia in children between 6 and 24 months of age.

Pneumococcal infection occurs more frequently in blacks than in whites, a finding that is not explained fully by the frequency of sickle cell disease in the black population.

## PATHOGENESIS

Pneumococci may invade from a site of colonization by hematogenous spread or direct extension. Pneumococcal meningitis follows pneumococcal bacteremia in most cases. In some persons, pneumococcal meningitis can result from direct spread to the meninges as a result of a temporal or basilar skull fracture. Pneumococcal otitis media usually results from the spread of pneumococci colonizing the nasopharynx by the eustachian tube into the middle ear. Pneumococcal pneumonia is caused by aspiration of pneumococci that reside in the pharynx. Several studies document that preceding viral infection may compromise pulmonary defense mechanisms and predispose to invasion by pneumococci. Although pneumococci most commonly produce otitis media, pneumonia, bacteremia, and meningitis, any organ system can be affected.

The specific factors responsible for injury to the host remain unknown. Many studies have sought but failed to find toxins capable of producing disease. The capsule of S pneumoniae aids the pneumococci in resisting phagocytosis, but the capsule itself is nontoxic. Specific serotypes associated with large capsules appear to be particularly virulent and cause greater morbidity and mortality than do serotypes characterized by smaller capsules. Rough strains of pneumococci that lack a capsule are avirulent.

Deficiency of the terminal components of complement has been associated with recurrent pyogenic infection, including that caused by S pneumoniae. Deficiency of complement factor C2 also appears to be associated with S pneumoniae infection. Pneumococcal disease is much more prevalent among persons with anatomical or functional asplenia. Pneumococcal disease is particularly prevalent in patients with sickle cell disease and other hemoglobinopathies. These patients appear to be unable to activate C3 by the alternative pathway or to fix opsonin to the pneumococcal cell wall. Ineffective clearance of blood-borne bacteria in the absence of type-specific antibodies and abnormal activation of the alternate pathway for complement metabolism are factors that place the asplenic patient at risk for overwhelming infection. The efficacy of phagocytosis for S pneumoniae is diminished in patients with B-cell and T-cell deficiency syndromes, who lack opsonic anticapsular antibody and fail to produce agglutination and lysis of bacteria. These observations suggest that opsonization of the pneumococcus depends on the classic and alternate complement pathways and that recovery from pneumococcal disease depends on the development of anticapsular antibodies that act as opsonins and enhance phagocytosis and intracellular killing of the pneumococcus.

Low levels of factor B or impairment of the properdin pathway and defective opsonization occur in normal persons during acute pneumococcal disease. These findings suggest that pneumococcal infection may develop in some people because of a transient preexisting depression of factor B or that acute pneumococcal infection may be accompanied by consumption of this component of the complement system. Complement factors C3 through C9 produce chemotaxic, anaphylatoxic, and opsonic properties in serum, and each plays an important role in protection against pneumococcal infection.

Within body tissues, particularly the lung, the spread of infection is enhanced by the antiphagocytic properties of the capsular-specific soluble substance. An edema-promoting factor also plays an important role in the pathogenesis of infection within the lung. After infection is established, the alveoli fill with serous fluid. Subsequently, polymorphonuclear leukocytes accumulate in the infected alveoli, causing consolidation. Ultimately, macrophages replace the leukocytes, and the exudate resolves. This sequence of events evolves over 7 to 10 days but can be modified by the use of appropriate antimicrobial therapy.

## CLINICAL MANIFESTATIONS

The clinical manifestations are related to the site of infection. Otitis media, sinusitis, pharyngitis, abscesses, pericarditis, laryngotracheobronchitis, bacteremia, empyema, peritonitis, mastoiditis, epidural abscess, and meningitis have been reported as a result of infections with S pneumoniae. Bacteremia may be followed by septic arthritis, osteomyelitis, endocarditis, or brain abscess. Epiglottitis due to S pneumoniae has been observed in immunocompromised children.

Pneumococcal bacteremia may occur in children between 6 months and 2 years of age who have unexplained fever and no localizing signs or symptoms. Subcutaneous abscesses have been reported after occult pneumococcal bacteremia, and endocarditis has been documented. Renal glomerular and cortical arterial thromboses have been associated with pneumococcal bacteremia. Gangrenous lesions of the skin on the face or extremities, localized gingival lesions, and disseminated intravascular coagulation also have been reported as manifestations of pneumococcal disease.

## DIAGNOSIS

The isolation of pneumococci from the nasopharynx does not permit a diagnosis of pneumococcal disease because pneumococcal carriage is so prevalent. Blood cultures should be obtained from all children with pneumonia, septic arthritis, osteomyelitis, meningitis, peritonitis, pericarditis, and gangrenous skin lesions. Blood cultures are also necessary in children 6 to 24 months of age who have unexplained high fever and leukocytosis without localized signs of infection. Urinary excretion of S pneumoniae presumably represents seeding of the urine from a remote site of pneumococcal infection. Pneumococci should be sought in cerebrospinal fluid (CSF), pleural fluid, or effusions from the middle ear.

Pneumococci can be identified in selected body fluids as gram-positive, lancet-shaped diplococci by Gram strain. A direct quellung test using pneumococcal omniserum helps to establish a definitive diagnosis rapidly. Countercurrent immunoelectrophoresis of serum, CSF, and urine using pneumococcal omniserum may be helpful in diagnosing pneumococcal bacteremia or meningitis. Pneumococcal antigen may be detected in blood or urine of patients with localized pneumococcal disease, such as pneumonia or otitis media. The use of type-specific antisera enhances the sensitivity of the technique, and its value is not altered significantly by previous antimicrobial therapy. Countercurrent immunoelectrophoresis of sputum has been helpful in differentiating patients with pneumococcal pneumonia from those in whom pneumococcal colonization has occurred, because the test is usually positive in the former circumstance and negative in the latter. Latex particle agglutination tests can also rapidly establish a diagnosis and are more sensitive than countercurrent immunoelectrophoresis in detecting polysaccharide capsular antigen. Early in the course of pneumococcal meningitis, numerous S pneumoniae may be revealed by Gram stain in relatively acellular CSF.

## TREATMENT AND PROGNOSIS

Penicillin is the drug of choice for most patients with pneumococcal disease. The dose and duration of therapy vary with the site of infection. Pneumococci with a decreased susceptibility to penicillin (0.1 to 1 μg/mL) have been isolated repeatedly. S pneumoniae showing this type of resistance and pneumococci that are resistant to penicillin, tetracycline, and chloramphenicol have been isolated from as many as 20% of the patients in several regions of the United States. The existence of these organisms makes it necessary to use high-dose penicillin therapy in all patients with meningitis. All pneumococci isolated from the CSF of patients with meningitis and from blood should be tested by tube dilution techniques as a guide to the most appropriate therapy. If the S pneumoniae is resistant to penicillin but sensitive to chloramphenicol, chloramphenicol is the drug of choice. Strains of pneumococci resistant to many other antibiotics and to sulfonamides have been reported. When a multiply resistant S pneumoniae is encountered, intravenous treatment with vancomycin (60 mg/kg/day in four divided doses) can be used. Many other agents are active against pneumococci, but none is superior to penicillin. Third-generation cephalosporins, such as ceftriaxone or cefotaxime, usually are effective against penicillin-resistent pneumococci isolated in the United States. Reports from South Africa have documented that up 15% of penicillin-resistant pneumococci are resistant to third-generation cephalosporins isolated in that community and 5% of isolates in some regions of the United States are resistant to third-generation cephalosporins.

For most patients, penicillin G or V remains the drug of choice for pneumococcal infection. Sensitive strains of pneumococci are inhibited and killed by a concentration of between 0.001 and 0.1 μg/mL of penicillin. The recommended dosages of penicillin G for pneumococcal infections in childhood are as follows: for infections such as otitis media, 50,000 U/kg/day; for more serious infections other than meningitis (eg, septicemia), 200,000 to 250,000 U/kg/day; and for meningitis, 300,000 U/kg/day. Penicillin V is only available for oral use and should be used only for infections such as otitis media and pneumonia. The recommended dosage of penicillin V is 50 to 100 mg/kg/day. Other penicillins, such as ampicillin, methicillin, and related compounds, show excellent activity against pneumococci, but these agents add nothing but additional cost and toxicity and are not the drugs of choice for pneumococcal disease.

Erythromycin may be used for mild pneumococcal disease in children who are allergic to penicillin. It can be provided in a dosage of 40 mg/kg/day in four divided doses. Chloramphenicol is the drug of choice for patients who are penicillin-sensitive and have meningitis or septicemia requiring hospitalization.

The prognosis of pneumococcal disease depends on the age of the host, integrity of the immune system, virulence of the infecting organism, site of infection, and adequacy of therapy.

## PREVENTION

A 23-valent pneumococcal polysaccharide vaccine is commercially available. Current recommendations are to provide pneumococcal vaccine to children 2 years of age and older with anatomical or functional asplenia, including patients with sickle cell disease and other hemoglobinopathies, and to children with nephrotic syndrome. Most pneumococcal serotypes are poor immunogens in young children, although type 3 antigen produces an excellent response.

Several reports suggest successful prevention of recurrent otitis media by chronic administration of sulfisoxazole or ampicillin. Studies reporting success with use of these regimens do not delineate the mechanisms by which preventive therapy works. Penicillin or ampicillin should be given to children 3 years of age or younger who are anatomically or functionally asplenic. Controlled studies suggest that the use of penicillin G or V, administered as 25,000 to 50,000 U/kg/day in four divided oral doses, may be effective in reducing the incidence of pneumococcal bacteremia in these patients.

## Selected Readings

Applebaum PC, Scragg JN, Bowen AJ, et al. *Streptococcus pneumoniae* resistant to penicillin and chloramphenicol. Lancet 1977;2:995.

Austrian R, Gold J. Pneumococcal bacteremia with especial reference to bacteremic pneumococcal pneumonia. Ann Intern Med 1964;60:759.

Coonrod JD, Rytel M. Detection of type-specific pneumococcal antigens by counterimmunoelectrophoresis. II. Etiologic diagnosis of pneumococcal pneumonia. J Lab Clin Med 1973;81:778.

Fraser DW, Darby CP, Koehler RE, et al. Risk factors in bacterial meningitis: Charleston County, South Carolina. J Infect Dis 1973;127:271.

Teele DW. Pneumococcal infections. In: Feigin RD, Cherry JD, eds. Textbook of pediatric infectious diseases, ed 2. Philadelphia: WB Saunders, 1992:1223.

Teele DW, Pelton SI, Grant MJA, et al. Bacteremia in febrile children under two years of age: result of cultures of blood in 600 consecutive febrile children seen in a "walk-in" clinic. J Pediatr 1975;87:227.

Topley JM, Cupidare L, Vaida S, et al. Pneumococcal and other infections in children with sickle cell-hemoglobin C (SC) disease. J Pediatr 1982;101:176.

Ward J. Antibiotic-resistant *Streptococcus pneumoniae*: clinical and epidemiologic aspects. Rev Infect Dis 1981;3:254.

*Principles and Practice of Pediatrics, Second Edition.*
edited by Frank A. Oski et al. J. B. Lippincott Company, Philadelphia © 1994.

# 56.20 *Pseudomonas Infections*

### Ralph D. Feigin

*Pseudomonas* species are strict aerobes. Aerobic pseudomonads can use any carbon source, and they multiply readily in a moist environment containing minimal concentrations of organic compounds. Most *Pseudomonas aeruginosa* strains possess fine projections called pili and a single, polar flagellum, and most strains are motile. These organisms grow readily on standard laboratory media. When strains are obtained from a clinical specimen, β-hemolysis may be observed on blood agar. A blue-green phenazine pigment and fluorescein are produced by more than 90% of *P aeruginosa*. *Pseudomonas* strains can be differentiated from one another by phage, serologic, and pyocin typing.

## EPIDEMIOLOGY

*Pseudomonas* organisms are ubiquitous and may be found in water or soil and on vegetation. Many normal persons carry *Pseudomonas* in their gastrointestinal tracts. The organism is found frequently in the hospital environment on the skin, clothes, and shoes of patients or hospital personnel. These organisms can be found growing in distilled water, antiseptic solutions, and often in equipment used for inhalation therapy or respiratory care.

## PATHOGENESIS

*Pseudomonas* organisms usually are noninvasive, even after colonization and infection of the skin. *Pseudomonas* produces endotoxin, but it is weak compared with the endotoxins produced by other gram-negative organisms. Endotoxin produced by *Pseudomonas* may produce a diarrheal syndrome. A *Pseudomonas* enterotoxin also has been described, but its role in causing diarrhea in humans is undefined.

*Pseudomonas* produces many extracellular products, including caseinase, collagenase, elastase, exotoxin A, gelatinase, hemolysin, lecithinase, and lipase. Localized necrosis of skin, lung, or cornea may result from the elaboration of proteolytic enzymes. These proteases can degrade complement and coagulation factors. Destruction of lecithin and solubilization of this material (ie, surfactant) may play an important role in the atelectasis seen in pulmonary infections caused by *Pseudomonas*. A leukocidin has been described, and exotoxin S has been identified as still another virulence factor.

The glycocalyx and other surface structures are involved in the attachment of *P aeruginosa* to mucosal surfaces. The organism binds preferentially to normal respiratory mucin compared with other Enterobacteriaceae. Elevated serum concentrations of IgG4 antibodies to opsonic determinants may inhibit normal pulmonary clearance of *P aeruginosa* by pulmonary macrophages in vivo. The pathogenicity of *P aeruginosa* depends on its ability to resist phagocytosis. The persistence of these organisms in the lungs of patients with cystic fibrosis may be related to factors in the sputum that interfere with the bactericidal activity of fresh, normal serum against this organism.

## CLINICAL MANIFESTATIONS

*Pseudomonas* can produce disease in healthy normal children. This occurs after the organism has been introduced into a minor wound, and a localized abscess develops that exudes blue or green pus. The skin lesions, which may be caused by direct inoculation or secondary to septicemia, begin as pink macules, progress to small hemorrhagic nodules, and eventually become necrotic, with associated eschar formation. The central area may be surrounded by an intense red areola (ie, ecthyma gangrenosum). Rarely, *P aeruginosa* causes septicemia, meningitis, endocarditis, pneumonia, corneal infections, or urinary tract infections in normal children. Osteomyelitis caused by *P aeruginosa* or other *Pseudomonas* strains may follow puncture wounds of the foot or other bones.

Outbreaks of urinary tract infections and dermatitis caused by *P aeruginosa* have been reported in healthy children after the use of community swimming pools, family-owned hot tubs, or other recreational whirlpool baths. Skin lesions may develop several hours to 2 days after contact with these contaminated water sources. The skin lesions may be macular, pustular, or erythematous. In selected cases, nodules develop. Illness may vary from extensive truncal involvement in some patients to only a few scattered lesions in others. Occasionally, malaise, vomiting, sore throat, conjunctivitis, rhinitis, fever, and breast swelling may be associated with the skin lesions. Multiple serotypes of *P aeruginosa* have been associated with these outbreaks.

Otitis externa caused by *P aeruginosa* has been reported in healthy persons who swim competitively in a pool contaminated with this organism. *Pseudomonas* has been found in patients with a malignant form of otitis externa that is associated with high fever and necrosis of portions of the external ear. These patients may also have paralysis of the facial nerve and mastoiditis. Most children with malignant forms of otitis externa suffer from leukopenia or disordered leukocyte function with normal numbers of leukocytes, malnutrition, or diabetes mellitus.

*P aeruginosa* produces infection somewhat more often during the neonatal period than later in life. This form of septicemia is associated with high rates of mortality and morbidity.

Disorders reported with other *Pseudomonas* species in healthy children include pneumonia and abscesses due to *Pseudomonas cepacia*, abscesses due to *Pseudomonas fluorescens*, otitis media due to *Pseudomonas putrefaciens* or *Pseudomonas stutzeri*, and cellulitis and septicemia due to *Pseudomonas maltophilia*. Septicemia and endocarditis associated with *P maltophilia* have been primarily seen in intravenous drug abusers. Septicemia and peritonitis caused by *P cepacia* have been associated with contamination of equipment used for peritoneal dialysis.

## Cystic Fibrosis

Death of patients with cystic fibrosis usually results from obstructive, chronic pulmonary disease (see Chap. 72). *P aeruginosa* can be recovered from cultures of the respiratory tract of most children with cystic fibrosis. Recovery of *P aeruginosa* from the sputum of these patients does not imply infection and pneumonitis. Colonization of sputum may reflect the extensive use of mist tents and continuous broad-spectrum antibiotic therapy. However, some observations suggest a more specific correlation between cystic fibrosis and *Pseudomonas*.

*P aeruginosa* organisms isolated from patients with cystic fibrosis are almost all mucoid. These organisms produce excessive amounts of capsular slime. It is almost impossible to eradicate the organism by continuous antibiotic therapy. Recovery of mucoid *P aeruginosa* is unusual in patients without cystic fibrosis (0.5% to 1.7%).

Bacterial infection in cystic fibrosis is limited almost entirely to the lung, and septicemia is rare. The pulmonary infection is chronic, and bronchitis, bronchiectasis, and bronchiolitis are common. Some patients develop necrotizing pneumonitis.

*P cepacia* is an increasingly frequent cause of pneumonia and septicemia in patients with cystic fibrosis. The frequent colonization of the respiratory tract with *P cepacia* in patients with cystic fibrosis has been associated with increased morbidity and mortality rates in some cystic fibrosis centers during the past decade.

## Burns and Wound Infection

The surfaces of burns and wounds are often colonized by *P aeruginosa*. Colonization does not imply infection but is a prerequisite to invasive disease. Septicemia due to this organism is a major problem in burned patients. The administration of antibiotics may diminish the susceptible microbial flora but permits selective strains of *Pseudomonas* to grow and become more numerous. In burned patients, abnormalities of neutrophil function precede the onset of septicemia. Thermal injury is also associated with abnormalities in the killing of *Pseudomonas* by neutrophils, delayed rejection of homografts, abnormal responses to antigens, impaired delayed hypersensitivity responses, and diminished uptake of particles by the reticuloendothelial system.

## Malignancy and Immunosuppression

Neutropenic patients, particularly children with leukemia who are receiving immunosuppressive therapy, are susceptible to *Pseudomonas* septicemia. Infection is usually a result of invasion of the bloodstream by *Pseudomonas*, with which the patient is already colonized (eg, in the gastrointestinal tract). A generalized vasculitis may develop, and hemorrhagic necrotic lesions may be found on the skin as purple nodules or ecchymotic areas that become gangrenous. Gangrenous perirectal cellulitis or abscesses may occur. Anorexia, nausea, vomiting, diarrhea, fever, ileus, and profound hypotension may develop. The single most important factor predisposing children with cancer to infection is granulocytopenia. Heat-stable opsonins specific for *P aeruginosa* may be depleted in children with acute leukemia who are receiving combination chemotherapy; fatal infections with this organism may be related to deficiencies of a specific opsonin.

Infection by *P aeruginosa*, particularly septicemia and pneu-

monia, is more common in children receiving immunosuppressive therapy than in normal healthy children or adults.

## Other Predisposing Conditions

*Pseudomonas* septicemia occurs with increased frequency in children who have indwelling intravenous or urinary catheters. Pneumonia and septicemia due to *Pseudomonas* also are increased in frequency in children receiving respiratory support or inhalation therapy. Children with dermoid sinus tracts or dermoids that extend down to or communicate with the meninges or neural tissue are prone to develop abscesses and meningitis due to *Pseudomonas*. *Pseudomonas* septicemia may occur in children with congenital or acquired neutropenia and in any person with deficient leukocyte function.

## Glanders

Glanders, a zoonotic disease that primarily infects horses and other equine animals, is caused by *Pseudomonas mallei*. Glanders is spread from diseased to healthy animals directly or indirectly. Human infection is seen primarily in persons with direct or indirect contact with diseased animals or their tissues. Infection is particularly prevalent among veterinarians or laboratory workers. Infection in children is unusual but has been reported.

The incubation period is usually 1 to 14 days, but extended incubation periods have been described. The prodrome may consist of fever, anorexia, nausea, vomiting, myalgia, and icterus. An erysipelas-like swelling of the face or limbs and painful nodules may be observed. The nodular eruption spreads rapidly and is followed by a generalized pustular skin eruption. Nasal involvement may include a thick, purulent discharge and erosion of the nasal structures. Lymphadenopathy and pneumonia are common. Severe septicemia with metastatic abscesses, pneumonitis, and death in 2 to 4 weeks may occur with the acute forms of glanders. A chronic form of this disorder with acute exacerbations also has been described.

The most important feature in the history is animal contact. The clinical manifestations are not specific and may resemble typhoid fever, melioidosis, erysipelas, tuberculosis, or syphilis.

Diagnosis is made by direct smear of discharges and exudates and identification by staining or use of fluorescent antibody techniques, bacteriologic isolation from purulent material or biopsy, intraperitoneal inoculation of guinea pigs or hamsters with exudates, or skin testing. Agglutination and complement fixation tests are available. The agglutination test is more sensitive, but complement fixation is more specific.

Before the antibiotic era, human glanders was fatal. Most strains of *P mallei* are sensitive to sulfonamides and tetracyclines. The efficacy of these agents in children with glanders is difficult to establish because of the paucity of cases.

## Melioidosis

Melioidosis is a rare disease found predominantly in Southeast Asia. It increased in frequency in the United States with the return of Americans from Vietnam and is seen rarely in immigrants from Southeast Asia. The causative agent is *Pseudomonas pseudomallei*. Infection with this organism follows direct contamination of abrasions or wounds or inhalation of dust contaminated by this organism. Transmission from animals to humans has not been reported.

Melioidosis may remain latent for months or years before the clinical manifestations appear. The disease may present as a single primary skin lesion (eg, vesicle, bulla, pustule, urticaria) in a patient who has no other underlying disease. Occasionally, septicemia and multiple abscesses develop in every organ of the body. Meningitis and endophthalmitis have been observed in normal and immunocompromised hosts during or after an episode of septicemia. Myocarditis, endocarditis, pericarditis, intestinal abscesses, acute gastroenteritis, cholecystitis, septic arthritis, osteomyelitis, urinary tract infections, and generalized lymphadenopathy may be caused by *P pseudomallei*.

Chronic melioidosis is more common in Caucasians than in Asians. Chronic melioidosis may involve every organ in the body except the brain. Melioidosis may remain dormant, with exacerbations occurring years after primary infection when host defenses are impaired as a result of burns, steroid use, or other processes. Diagnosis is established by culture of blood, skin lesions, or other purulent material. The organism grows in any media commonly employed for isolation of gram-negative bacteria.

Serologic tests are more useful in establishing the diagnosis of melioidosis in latent or asymptomatic forms of the disease. Hemagglutination, indirect hemagglutination, and complement fixation tests are available. Diagnostic titers are 1 : 40 or greater for the hemagglutination test and 1 : 10 or greater for the complement fixation test. Both tests should be performed because the sensitivity of serologic tests varies. Hemagglutination antibodies are usually evident within 7 to 14 days after the onset of illness, but the complement fixation test does not become positive until 4 to 6 weeks into the disease process. Peak titers for both tests are observed at 4 to 6 months. An enzyme-linked immunosorbent assay that detects specific IgG and IgM antibody to *P pseudomallei* is available as a screening test for melioidosis; it is more sensitive than the indirect hemagglutination test melioidosis.

## DIAGNOSIS

The diagnosis of *Pseudomonas* infection depends on recovery of the organism from a localized site of infection or from the blood or cerebrospinal fluid (CSF). Recovery of the organism from the surface of the skin, throat, or bronchial secretions may reflect colonization and is not diagnostic of infection. Although the bluish, nodular skin lesions and ulcers with ecchymotic and gangrenous centers (ie, ecthyma gangrenosum) had been considered pathognomonic of *Pseudomonas* infection, similar lesions may be seen after septicemia due to Enterobacteriaceae, *Aeromonas*, *Serratia*, and other gram-negative organisms. Immunoglobulin antibodies to *P aeruginosa* surface antigens in serum have been detected reliably by enzyme-linked immunosorbent assay. Antibody titer increases are associated with active disease due to *P aeruginosa* in patients with cystic fibrosis. Antibody titers normalize after *Pseudomonas* infections is controlled by effective antimicrobial therapy. This assay is helpful in differentiating early infections from colonization. Antibodies to *P aeruginosa* also may be detected by immunoblotting (eg, Western blot).

## TREATMENT AND PROGNOSIS

*Pseudomonas* infections should be treated promptly with an antibiotic to which the organism is sensitive in vitro. Septicemia usually can be treated with gentamicin in a dosage of 5 to 7.5 mg/kg/day in three divided doses every 8 hours. The higher dose may be used after the first week of life. Gentamicin can be given intramuscularly or intravenously (infused over a period of 1 hour). Therapy with carbenicillin (200 to 400 mg/kg/day in six divided doses) or ticarcillin (200 mg/kg/day in six divided doses) can be provided concomitantly by the intravenous route. Carbenicillin and ticarcillin may be synergistic with gentamicin

in their effect on *Pseudomonas*. It is not advisable to use carbenicillin or ticarcillin alone for treating *Pseudomonas* septicemia, because strains of this organism rapidly become resistant to these agents. Tobramycin (3.5 mg/kg/day) or amikacin (15 to 25 mg/kg/day) in three divided doses given intramuscularly or intravenously over 1 hour may be used instead of gentamicin. Ceftazidime has proved useful in selected patients with this disease and can be provided in a dosage of 150 to 200 mg/kg/day in three or four divided doses. Azlocillin and piperacillin have proved effective against *P aeruginosa* when combined with an aminoglycoside. These antibiotics can be given intramuscularly in dosages of 300 mg/kg/day in three or four divided doses. Abscesses due to *Pseudomonas* should be incised and drained.

Ciprofloxacin has been evaluated for the treatment of acute and chronic *P aeruginosa* infection in adolescents and adults with cystic fibrosis. This antibiotic can be given orally or intravenously. Ciprofloxacin should not be used until after puberty because it may bind to cartilage and arrest growth. If it is used, it may be given in a dose of 4 to 6 mg/kg administered intravenously twice daily. Oral dosage should not exceed 1000 mg/day for patients who weigh less than 40 kg or 1500 mg/day for patients who weigh more than 40 kg.

*Pseudomonas* meningitis can be treated with gentamicin and carbenicillin given intravenously in the doses previously indicated. Concomitant intraventricular or intrathecal treatment with gentamicin may be required to sterilize the CSF. Gentamicin can be placed into the ventricular or lumbar CSF in a total dosage of 1 or 2 mg once daily.

Melioidosis is treated with tetracycline or chloramphenicol given for several months. In patients with systemic melioidosis, chloramphenicol (50 to 75 mg/kg/day) plus an aminoglycoside (eg, kanamycin, 20 to 30 mg/kg/day; amikacin, 15 to 20 mg/kg/day) should be administered for 4 weeks. Alternatively, a third-generation cephalosporin may be used. Ceftazidime has shown greater activity against *P pseudomallei* than other third-generation cephalosporins. Recent data suggests that ceftazidime in a daily dose of 120 mg/kg, administered intravenously in three divided doses, is the drug of choice for treatment of severe melioidosis.

Soft-tissue infections due to *P pseudomallei* should be treated for 4 to 6 months with tetracycline (in children older than 8 years of age) in a dosage of 50 mg/kg/day in four divided doses. In younger children, trimethoprim-sulfamethoxazole (6 mg/kg/day of trimethoprim and 30 mg/kg/day of sulfamethoxazole) in two divided doses can be used. The duration of therapy must be guided by clinical findings. Therapy for many months may be required for patients with *Pseudomonas* osteomyelitis.

Prognosis depends on the nature of the underlying disease process. Septicemia is a leading cause of death in children with leukemia, and *Pseudomonas* is responsible for half of these deaths.

## PREVENTION

The prevention of *Pseudomonas* infection depends on continuous surveillance of the hospital environment and eradication of the source of *Pseudomonas* as quickly as possible. The prevention of follicular dermatitis is possible by maintaining pool water at a pH of 7.2 to 7.8 and free available chlorine concentrations at 70.5 mg/L.

*Pseudomonas* infection in newborn nurseries is usually transmitted by the hands of hospital personnel. Strict attention to hand washing, preferably with a liquid iodophor, before and between contacts with newborn infants can prevent transmission. The growth of *Pseudomonas* on suction catheters can be prevented by rinsing the catheter in an acetic acid solution.

Solutions used for total parenteral alimentation should be prepared meticulously, and similar care should be exercised in the insertion and maintenance of other catheters.

The efficacy of active immunization of burn patients with specific strains of *Pseudomonas* or the administration of hyperimmune globulin to prevent *Pseudomonas* septicemia has been demonstrated. *Pseudomonas* infection in burn patients has been minimized by the use of topical applications of 10% mafenide acetate cream or topical silver nitrate (0.5% solution). *Pseudomonas* vaccine has been suggested as a possible method for preventing septicemia in patients with acute leukemia or cystic fibrosis.

## Selected Readings

Feder HM Jr, Grant-Kels JM, Tilton RC. *Pseudomonas* whirlpool dermatitis. Clin Pediatr 1983;22:638.

Feigin RD. *Pseudomonas* infections. In: Feigin RD, Cherry JD, eds. Textbook of pediatric infectious diseases, ed 3. Philadelphia: WB Saunders, 1992:1229.

Horn KL, Gherini S. Malignant external otitis of childhood. Ann J Otol 1981;2:402.

Neu HC. The role of *Pseudomonas aeruginosa* in infections. J Antimicrob Chemother 1983;11(suppl):B1.

Patamasucon P, Pitchyangkura C, Fischer GW. Melioidosis in childhood. J Pediatr 1975;87:133.

Pennington JE, Reynolds HY, Wood RE, et al. Use of *Pseudomonas aeruginosa* vaccine in patients with acute leukemia and cystic fibrosis. Am J Med 1975;58:629.

Stechenberg BW, Feigin RD. Glanders. In: Feigin RD, Cherry JD, eds. Textbook of pediatric infectious diseases, ed 2. Philadelphia: WB Saunders, 1987:1140.

Vishwanath S, Ramphal R. Adherence of *Pseudomonas aeruginosa* to human tracheobronchial mucin. Infect Immunol 1984;45:197.

White NJ, Chaowagul W, Wuthiekanum V, et al. Solving of mortality of severe melioidosis by ceftazidime. Lancet 1989;2:697.

Zuravleff JJ, Yu VL. Infections caused by *Pseudomonas maltophilia* with emphasis on bacteremia: case reports and review of the literature. Rev Infect Dis 1982;4:1236.

*Principles and Practice of Pediatrics, Second Edition.*
edited by Frank A. Oski et al. J. B. Lippincott Company, Philadelphia © 1994.

# 56.21 *Rat-Bite Fever*

Brenda S. Harvey and Ralph D. Feigin

Rat-bite fever comprises two distinct clinical syndromes, the spirillary form and the streptobacillary form. Spirillary rat-bite fever, also called soduku, usually follows the bite of a rat or other rodent, although cases have been reported in the absence of a bite or scratch. Streptobacillary rat-bite fever may also follow a rat bite but can occur after ingestion of contaminated, unpasteurized milk. Rat-bite fever is seen worldwide, occurs more often in children and laboratory workers than other groups, and is more common in urban areas with large rat populations.

## SPIRILLARY RAT-BITE FEVER

*Spirillum minus*, the organism responsible for the spirillary form of rat-bite fever, is a gram-negative, short spirochete with terminal flagella. It cannot be grown consistently on current media but may be seen by darkfield microscopy in exudate from the inoculation site or regional nodes. Animal inoculation is necessary to isolate the organism.

## Clinical Manifestations

The spirillary form of rat-bite fever has an incubation period of 14 to 18 days. The bite may heal superficially but then becomes erythematous and indurated, with ulceration and eschar formation. Fever, chills, severe myalgias, and a reddish-brown macular rash are common at the onset of the disease. Lymphangitis and lymphadenitis are usually prominent around the area of the bite. If the infection is untreated, symptoms subside in 3 to 4 days. However, after several days without symptoms, the fever may recur, with exacerbation of the rash. This cycle can continue for 3 weeks to several years, although the disease is eventually self-limiting. Fatalities are uncommon, and the only major complication is endocarditis.

## Diagnosis

Diagnosis of the disease in a patient with a history of rat bite depends primarily on differentiation from the streptobacillary form of this disease. *S minus* can be identified by animal inoculation or darkfield microscopy. Mild or moderate anemia and an elevated leukocyte count may occur; 50% of the patients have false-positive serologic tests for syphilis.

## Treatment

*S minus* is extremely sensitive to penicillin. *Streptobacillus moniliformis*, the cause of Haverhill fever, is less sensitive, and larger doses of penicillin usually are recommended because of the difficulty in differentiating the diseases caused by these organisms. Procaine penicillin (600,000 U every 12 hours for 10 days) is effective. Oral tetracycline (2 g/day) or intramuscular streptomycin (15 mg/kg/day in two divided doses) can be administered if the patient is allergic to penicillin.

## STREPTOBACILLARY RAT-BITE FEVER

*S moniliformis*, the organism responsible for the streptobacillary form of rat-bite (ie, Haverhill fever) is a pleomorphic, nonmotile, unencapsulated, gram-negative rod that can be grown on current media supplemented with serum, ascitic fluid, or blood. The organism grows best in a $CO_2$-enriched environment; sodium polyanethol sulfonate, a substance sometimes added to culture media to inhibit the antibacterial activity of human blood, impedes growth. The organism may produce L-forms (ie, variant growth forms that do not produce rigid peptidoglycan cell walls) in the presence of penicillin or suboptimal growth conditions, but these usually revert to the parent bacterial form. A variety of morphologic forms may be seen with Gram or Giemsa stain, depending on the growth conditions used. Transmission occurs through a rat bite or contaminated milk. The organism produces the same clinical syndrome regardless of the source, but the strains can be differentiated by gel-protein electrophoresis.

## Clinical Manifestations

The incubation period of rat-bite fever caused by *S moniliformis* is 2 to 3 days. The original inoculation site has often healed by the time fever, chills, vomiting, and headache begin. A diffuse morbilliform rash that involves the palms and soles appears several days later. Arthritis develops in about half the patients, but lymphangitis and lymphadenitis are uncommon. If the infection is not treated, the symptoms resolve but usually relapse with fever, rash, and arthritis. Complications are uncommon but include endocarditis, pneumonia, brain abscess, amnionitis, and severe persistent arthritis.

## Diagnosis

Diagnosis depends primarily on the clinical history of a rat bite and differentiation from the spirillary form. The streptobacillary form of this disease has a shorter incubation period, the bite heals without secondary ulceration, arthritis is common, and lymphangitis and lymphadenitis are rare. *S moniliformis* grows readily from the patient's blood, joint fluid, and sometimes from the wound itself. Fatty acid profiles may be of value in the rapid identification of *S moniliformis*.

## Treatment

Penicillin is the treatment of choice for the streptobacillary form of rat-bite fever. Procaine penicillin G (600,000 U every 12 hours for 10 days) is effective against most strains of *S moniliformis*. Streptomycin may be used for strains that are resistant to penicillin or for patients who are allergic to penicillin. Tetracycline is effective for patients older than 8 years of age who are allergic to penicillin.

## Selected Readings

Anderson LC, Leary SL, Manning PJ. Rat-bite fever in animal research laboratory personnel. Lab Anim Sci 1983;33:292.

Costas M, Owen RJ. Numerical analysis of electrophoretic protein patterns of *Streptobacillus moniliformis* strains from human, murine and avian infections. J Med Microbiol 1987;23:303.

Dijkmans BA, Thomeer RT, Vielvoye GJ, et al. Brain abscess due to *Streptobacillus moniliformis* and *Actinobacterium meyerii*. Infection 1984;12:262.

Edwards R, Finch RG. Characterisation and antibiotic susceptibilities of *Streptobacillus moniliformis*. J Med Microbiol 1986;21:39.

McHugh TP, Bartlett RL, Raymond JI. Rat bite fever: report of a fatal case. Ann Emerg Med 1985;14:1116.

Mandel DR. Streptobacillary fever: an unusual cause of infectious arthritis. Cleve Clin Q 1985;52:203.

Savage N. *Streptobacillus*. In: Krieg NR, Holt JG, eds. Bergey's manual of systematic bacteriology. Baltimore: William & Wilkins, 1984:598.

Shackelford PG. Rat bite fever. In: Feigin RD, Cherry JD, eds. Textbook of pediatric infectious diseases. Philadelphia: WB Saunders, 1987:1257.

Shanson DC, Midgley J, et al. *Streptobacillus moniliformis* isolated from blood in four cases of Haverhill fever. Lancet 1983;42:92.

Speck WT, Toltzis P. Rat bite fever. In: Behrman RE, Vaughan VC, eds. Nelson's textbook of pediatrics, ed 12. Philadelphia: WB Saunders, 1983:736.

Washburn RG. *Streptobacillus moniliformis* (rat-bite fever). In: Mandell GL, Douglas RG, Bennet JE, eds. Principles and practice of infectious disease. New York: Churchill-Livingstone, 1990:1762.

*Principles and Practice of Pediatrics, Second Edition.*
edited by Frank A. Oski et al. J. B. Lippincott Company, Philadelphia © 1994.

# *56.22 Salmonella Infections*

Larry K. Pickering and Douglas K. Mitchell

*Salmonella* organisms cause disease in humans and other animals. Salmonellosis is a term that refers to infections caused by the genus *Salmonella*, which contains more than 2000 serotypes. Humans are infected by ingesting contaminated food or water. This mode of transmission can result in large outbreaks of disease. Clinical manifestations vary, ranging from a carrier state to gastroenteritis to extension beyond the gastrointestinal tract with severe disease.

This work was supported by grant HD-13021 from the National Institutes of Health.

## ETIOLOGY

*Salmonella* organisms are gram-negative bacilli of the Enterobacteriaceae family. *Salmonella* that cause human disease may be divided into groups A through E on the basis of their O (somatic) and H (flagellar) antigens; serotypes may also be designated by their Vi (capsular) antigens. Most hospital laboratories biochemically differentiate the salmonellae as one of three species: *S choleraesuis*, *S typhi*, and *S enteritidis*. *S choleraesuis* (group C1) and *S typhi* (group D) each consist of a single serotype; the remainder (>2000) are designated as serotypes of *S enteritidis*. The numerous strains of *S enteritidis* are familiarly named as species. For example, *S enteritidis* serotype *paratyphi A* is commonly referred to as *S paratyphi* or *S paratyphi A*.

*S typhimurium* (group B) is the most common cause of human *Salmonella* infections in the United States. Other common serotypes include *S enteritidis* serotype (group D), *S newport* (group C2), *S heidelberg* (group B), *S infantis* (group C1), *S hadar* (group C2), and *S agona* (group B).

## EPIDEMIOLOGY

Animals, including poultry, livestock, and pets, are the major reservoirs for nontyphoidal *Salmonella*. Other sources include contaminated animal products, meat processing plants, contaminated water, and infected humans; rarely, fruits and vegetables are sources. *S typhi* infects only humans; *S paratyphi A*, *S schottmuelleri* (paratyphi B), and *S hirschfeldii* (paratyphi C) have reservoirs primarily in humans. Methods of transmission include ingestion of contaminated food, milk, water, medications, or dyes; contact with an infected animal; fecal-oral transmission resulting in person-to-person spread; and contact with contaminated medical instruments. Volunteer studies using adults have shown that between $10^5$ and $10^6$ viable organisms must be ingested for clinical disease to occur, although data from food-borne outbreaks of salmonellosis indicate that the infective dose for various *Salmonella* serotypes may be much lower.

Infections with nontyphoidal strains of *Salmonella* are common, with approximately 50,000 cases reported to the Centers for Disease Control and Prevention in 1992. *Salmonella* is the most frequently reported cause of food-borne outbreaks of gastroenteritis in the United States. There has been a steady increase in the reported rates during the past 30 years, which is thought to reflect increasing incidence of the disease rather than more efficient reporting. Because these figures are derived from a passive surveillance system, it has been estimated that 800,000 to 3.7 million infections occur annually in the United States.

Age-specific attack rates peak in the first year of life and are higher for children younger than 5 years of age and for persons older than 70 years of age. Most reported cases of *Salmonella* infection are sporadic, but transmission by contaminated food and water frequently results in outbreaks of disease. There have been many outbreaks of *S enteritidis* associated with ingestion of contaminated eggs. The possible transovarian infection of eggs by *S enteritidis* has been inferred from the recovery of the same serotype from the contents of intact shell eggs. Morbidity and mortality after infection are more common in certain groups (Table 56-19).

There were 382 cases of typhoid fever (ie, systemic infection with *S typhi*) reported in the United States in 1992; over half of these were acquired during foreign travel. In 1990, six typhoid fever outbreaks in the United States were reported to the Centers for Disease Control. Two outbreaks were associated with foods prepared in restaurants, two with home-cooked food, one with imported shellfish, and one with an unknown source. The source of domestically acquired typhoid usually is a person who is a

**TABLE 56-19. Conditions That Predispose to Invasive Salmonellosis**

Acquired immune deficiency
Bartonellosis
Collagen vascular disease
Diabetes mellitus
Extremes of age
Hemolytic anemia, including sickle cell disease
Malaria
Malignancy
Recipients of immunosuppressive therapy
Schistosomiasis

chronic carrier of *S typhi*. Groups at risk for typhoid fever include persons in developing countries, visitors from industrialized countries who travel to endemic areas, and technicians in clinical microbiology laboratories. Typhoid fever is uncommon in the United States, but is a frequent problem in developing countries, where typhoid fever affects mainly persons between the ages of 5 and 25 years. The incubation period for *Salmonella* gastroenteritis is 6 to 72 hours (usually less than 24 hours) and that for enteric fever is 3 to 60 days (usually 7 to 14 days).

## PATHOGENESIS

Symptoms associated with *Salmonella* gastroenteritis are caused by mucosal invasion with inflammation, a cholera-like enterotoxin, and a cytotoxin that inhibits protein synthesis. Only *Salmonella* strains that invade the ileal epithelium can cause enteritis or intestinal fluid secretion and subsequent diarrhea. *Salmonella* do not multiply in epithelial cells as do *Shigella*, and ulcer formation in salmonellosis is rare. Within 24 hours of ingestion, *Salmonella* may pass through the epithelium into the lamina propria, where an intense inflammatory cell reaction occurs. Most *Salmonella* serotypes elicit a polymorphonuclear leukocyte response that eliminates the organisms and limits the clinical illness to gastroenteritis, although infection outside the gastrointestinal tract can occur. *S typhi* and *S paratyphi* elicit a mononuclear response, and the clinical syndrome is called enteric fever. The Peyer patches of the distal ileum are the primary site of bacterial penetration, with infection spreading to regional lymph nodes. The more virulent strains enter the thoracic lymph from the intestinal lymph nodes, reach the systemic circulation, and disseminate to the liver, spleen, and other parts of the reticuloendothelial system.

## CLINICAL MANIFESTATIONS

There are several clinical syndromes associated with *Salmonella* infection: the carrier state; acute gastroenteritis; bacteremia and enteric fever, including typhoid and paratyphoid fevers; and dissemination with localized suppuration, which manifests as abscesses, osteomyelitis, arthritis, or meningitis. These clinical syndromes may overlap.

Every serotype can produce any of the clinical patterns, but certain *Salmonella* serotypes are consistently associated with specific clinical syndromes. The transient asymptomatic carrier state may be more common than gastroenteritis. By the third month after infection, more than 90% of infected persons have stopped excreting the organism. Persons who excrete the organism for longer than 1 year are considered to be chronic carriers. Asymptomatic fecal excretion of *S typhi* for longer than 1 year occurs in

approximately 3% of adults after an episode of acute typhoid fever. The severity of the initial infection has no relation to the duration of *Salmonella* carriage. Gallbladder disease predisposes to chronic carriage.

The most common manifestation of disease caused by *Salmonella* is gastroenteritis, which is most frequent in infants during the first year, decreases abruptly in early childhood, and remains relatively constant throughout the adult years. Manifestations include diarrhea, abdominal cramps and tenderness, and fever. The most prominent symptom is usually diarrhea, ranging from a few stools to profuse bloody diarrhea to a cholera-like syndrome. In uncomplicated gastroenteritis, bacteremia occurs in 5% to 10% of cases.

Enteric fever is most often produced by *S typhi* and the paratyphoid bacilli, *S paratyphi A*, *S paratyphi B* (*S schottmuelleri*), and *S paratyphi C* (*S hirschfeldii*), but it may be caused by any serotype. Clinical manifestations are usually more severe when the causative organism is *S typhi*. *Salmonella* bacteremia may occur in any patient with *Salmonella* gastroenteritis, but it is more common in groups at high risk (see Table 56-19). The major significance of nontyphoid or nonparatyphoid *Salmonella* bacteremia is the risk of developing disseminated focal infections. *S choleraesuis* and *S typhimurium* are the nontyphoid serotypes that most often cause *Salmonella* bacteremia. The onset of enteric fever is typically gradual, with systemic symptoms, including fever, headache, malaise, anorexia, rose spots, and lethargy, and abdominal symptoms, including initial constipation and then diarrhea, abdominal pain and tenderness, and hepatosplenomegaly. Typhoid fever has been associated with the late complications of intestinal hemorrhage and perforation. Chronic *Salmonella* bacteremia has been associated with concomitant *Schistosoma mansoni* infection.

Focal infections occur in approximately 10% of patients with *Salmonella* bacteremia. Osteomyelitis, meningitis, and pneumonia are the most common focal infections, followed by pyelonephritis, endocarditis, and arthritis.

## DIAGNOSIS

The diagnosis of *Salmonella* infection is made by obtaining cultures of stool in patients with gastrointestinal tract infections and stool, urine, blood, bone marrow aspirate, and material from any foci of infection in patients with systemic illness. More than 90% of untreated patients with typhoid fever have positive blood or bone marrow cultures during the first week of illness. This slowly diminishes over time, with a concomitant increase in positive stool and urine cultures. Bone marrow culture is the most sensitive procedure for recovery of *S typhi*. Fecal leukocytes in a stool smear stained with methylene blue suggest enterocolitis, but the finding is not diagnostic for a specific organism. Serologic tests for *Salmonella* agglutinins are often part of the febrile agglutinin panel, which includes the Widal test. This procedure, which measures the antibody response to somatic and flagellar antigens of *Salmonella*, is unreliable because of frequent false-positive and false-negative results. Many typhoid carriers may have antibody titers against the Vi capsular polysaccharide of *S typhi*. The test is useful for identification of chronic carriers associated with outbreaks of typhoid fever. DNA probes and monoclonal antibodies against protein antigens of *S typhi* may soon be of value in diagnostic testing for *S typhi* in samples of body fluid from patients suspected of having typhoid fever.

## TREATMENT

Table 56-20 illustrates the antimicrobial therapy for various clinical manifestations of *Salmonella*. The specific syndrome asso-

### TABLE 56-20. Antimicrobial Therapy for *Salmonella* Infections

| Clinical Manifestation | Agent | Dosage |
|---|---|---|
| Carrier state | None | None |
| Acute gastroenteritis* | None | None |
| Bacteremia or fever | Ampicillin | 200 mg/kg/day, IV, divided every 4 h for 2 wk; maximum, 8 g/day |
| | *or* | |
| | Chloramphenicol | 75 mg/kg/day, orally or IV, divided every 6 h for 2 wk; maximum, 3 g/day |
| | *or* | |
| | Trimethoprim-sulfamethoxazole | TMP, 10 mg/kg/day, plus SMX, 50 mg/kg/day, divided every 12 h for 2 wk; maximum, 160 mg TMP plus 800 mg SMX every 12 h |
| | *or* | |
| | Cefotaxime for resistant organism | 200 mg/kg/day, divided every 6 h for 2 wk; maximum, 12 g/day |
| | *or* | |
| | Ceftriaxone for resistant organism | 100 mg/kg/day, given once or twice a day for 2 wk; maximum, 4 g/day |
| Dissemination with localized suppuration (osteomyelitis) | Ampicillin *or* chloramphenicol *or* Trimethoprim-sulfamethoxazole *or* Cefotaxime for resistant organism *or* Ceftriaxone for resistant organism | Same doses as above; administer for 4–6 wk for osteomyelitis and meningitis or other infection showing slow response to treatment |

* Patients with hyperpyrexia and systemic signs or symptoms should be treated for bacteremia.

ciated with *Salmonella* infection influences the selection and duration of antimicrobial therapy. Antibiotics should not be used in persons who are nontyphoid *Salmonella* carriers or in most patients with mild gastroenteritis. The use of antimicrobial agents should be considered in patients with gastroenteritis if the disease appears to be evolving into enterocolitis or into one of the systemic syndromes. Antibiotics should be considered for treating neonates; patients with hemoglobinopathies, malignancies, or human immunodeficiency virus infection; and those receiving immunosuppressive therapy because of the increased incidence of invasive disease occurring in these groups (see Table 56-19). These patients are at high risk of developing bacteremia or metastatic infection.

The selection of antimicrobial agents for therapy is complicated by the emergence of *Salmonella* strains that are resistant to multiple antibiotics. Antibiotics used to treat patients with various *Salmonella* syndromes include chloramphenicol, ampicillin, trimethoprim-sulfamethoxazole (TMP-SMX), cefotaxime, ceftriaxone, and fluoroquinolones. Candidates for antibiotic treatment of *Salmonella* infection include patients with typhoid fever, bacteremia caused by nontyphoid strains, dissemination with localized suppuration, and gastroenteritis. Chloramphenicol, ampicillin, cefotaxime or ceftriaxone are the antibiotics of choice for enteric fever in children. The response to treatment is gradual, with temperatures returning to normal within 3 to 5 days in most patients. Ampicillin, chloramphenicol, TMP-SMX, cefotaxime, or

ceftriaxome can be used in patients with disseminated infections. For intravascular localized infection, such as endocarditis or infection of an aneurysm, ampicillin or cefotaxime are preferred over chloramphenicol because of their bactericidal activity. For *Salmonella* meningitis, cefotaxime or ceftriaxone is recommended. Ciprofloxacin is the drug of choice for chronic adult carriers. In children with normally functioning gallbladders without cholelithiasis, ampicillin or amoxicillin combined with probenecid is the treatment of choice for chronic enteric carriers.

Broad selective pressure appears to affect rates of resistance for *Salmonella* serotypes in various reservoirs. This pressure includes antibiotic use in poultry, which is a reservoir for *S heidelberg*, and in cows, which is a reservoir for *S typhimurium*. Nontyphoidal *Salmonella* species have become progressively more resistant in recent years to chloramphenicol, ampicillin, and TMP-SMX. This is thought to be the result of the chronic use of antibiotics in the feed of many livestock and poultry and the indiscriminate use of antibiotics in humans. This trend includes *S typhimurium*, which is the most common isolate in the United States and Europe. Other serotypes that are commonly implicated in human disease and are frequently multiresistant include *S heidelberg*, *S agona*, *S muenchen*, *S enteritidis*, and *S hadar*. Although most strains in the United States remain susceptible to chloramphenicol and TMP-SMX, several outbreaks of multiresistant infections have occurred.

Chloramphenicol-resistant strains of *S typhi* that are susceptible to ampicillin have occurred worldwide, as have multiresistant strains of *S typhi*. Clinical experience indicates that cefotaxime, ceftriaxome, and the fluoroquinolones (eg, ciprofloxacin, ofloxacin) appear to be useful for treatment of patients with typhoid fever, bacteremia, meningitis, osteomyelitis, and the chronic carrier state. Cefotaxime and ceftriaxone are the third-generation cephalosporins most frequently studied in the treatment of typhoid fever and other systemic salmonelloses. The quinolones are not approved for use in people younger than 18 years old because of their potential for causing arthropathy. Despite in vitro activity, first- and second-generation cephalosporins have been ineffective in the therapy of patients with *Salmonella* infection and should not be used.

Antipyretics can cause precipitous declines in temperature and shock and should be avoided in patients with enteric fever syndromes. Corticosteroids may be administered to patients with severe typhoid fever, for whom prompt therapy for toxemia may be lifesaving. The duration of steroid therapy is 48 hours. Dexamethasone (3 mg/kg), followed by eight doses of 1 mg/kg every 6 hours, is the usual regimen.

## PREVENTION

The most important aspects of prevention of *Salmonella* infection are education and avoidance. Proper food handling and storage techniques should be employed, especially for raw eggs, which should be thoroughly cooked and never eaten raw. Travelers should be advised to follow appropriate practices when eating abroad.

Several vaccines are available for the prevention of typhoid fever, but the degree of protection they provide is limited and can be overcome by ingestion of a large inoculum of *S typhi*. Two vaccines are licensed in the United States. The oral live-attenuated Ty21a vaccine has a protective efficacy of 42% to 96%. The parenteral heat-phenol-inactivated whole-cell typhoid vaccine is 51% to 77% effective in preventing typhoid fever.

The oral vaccine has minimal adverse reactions, but the parenteral vaccine causes frequent adverse reactions, such as fever, headache, pain, and swelling. Either vaccine is recommended for travelers to areas where typhoid fever is endemic, persons with intimate exposure to a documented *S typhi* carrier, and laboratory workers in frequent contact with *S typhi*. The oral vaccine has not been adequately tested in children younger than 6 years of age and therefore cannot be recommended in this age group (Table 56-21). It is contraindicated in immunocompromised persons, including those known to be infected with human immunode-

ficiency virus. The parenteral vaccine should be used for both of these groups when indicated. Booster doses are recommended every 3 years for the parenteral vaccine and every 5 years for the oral vaccine. Vaccine trials with the purified Vi capsular polysaccharide of *S typhi* are underway.

## Selected Readings

Asperilla MO, Smego RA, Scott LK. Quinolone antibiotics in the treatment of *Salmonella* infections. Rev Infect Dis 1990;12:873.

Bhutta ZA, Naqvi SH, Razzaq RA, Farooqui BJ. Multidrug-resistant typhoid in children: presentation and clinical features. Rev Infect Dis 1991;13:832.

Cárdenas L, Clements JD. Oral immunization using live attenuated *Salmonella* spp. as carriers of foreign antigens. Clin Microbiol Rev 1992;5:328.

Centers for Disease Control. Outbreak of *Salmonella enteritidis* infection associated with consumption of raw shell eggs, 1991. MMWR 1992;41:369.

Chalker RB, Blaser MJ. A review of human salmonellosis: III. magnitude of *Salmonella* infection in the United States. Rev Infect Dis 1988;10:111.

Cohen ML, Gangarosa EJ. Nontyphoid salmonellosis. South Med J 1978;71:1540.

Edelman R, Levine MM. Summary of an international workshop on typhoid fever. Rev Infect Dis 1986;8:329.

Hornick RB, Greisman SE, Woodward TE, et al. Typhoid fever: pathogenesis and immunologic control. N Engl J Med 1970;283:686.

MacDonald KL, Cohen ML, Hargrett-Bean NT, et al. Changes in antimicrobial resistance of *Salmonella* isolated from humans in the United States. JAMA 1987;258:1496.

Soe GB, Overturf GD. Treatment of typhoid fever and other systemic salmonellosis with cefotaxime, ceftriaxone, cefoperazone, and other newer cephalosporins. Rev Infect Dis 1987;9:719.

Telzak EE, Budnick LD, Greenberg MSZ, et al. A nosocomial outbreak of *Salmonella enteritidis* infection due to the consumption of raw eggs. N Engl J Med 1990;323:394.

Typhoid immunization recommendations of the Immunization Practices Advisory Committee (ACIP). MMWR 1990;39:1.

Wittler R, Bass J. Non-typhoidal *Salmonella* enteric infections and bacteremia. Pediatr Infect Dis J 1989;8:364.

*Principles and Practice of Pediatrics, Second Edition.*
edited by Frank A. Oski et al. J. B. Lippincott Company, Philadelphia © 1994.

## *56.23* Shigellosis

David Prado and Thomas G. Cleary

Dysentery has been recognized since the time of Hippocrates, and bacillary dysentery has profoundly affected the course of history. Dysentery epidemics during times of war have often played a greater role in the outcome of military campaigns than physical injuries. Because of its frequency, morbidity, and high mortality, dysentery was one of the diseases investigated by the early microbiologists. In 1898, Kiyoshi Shiga described the causative organism of the yearly summer and autumn epidemics of dysentery that plagued Japan, and bacillary dysentery was differentiated from amebic dysentery. Although the same organism had been described 10 years earlier by Chantemese and Widal, the genus eventually was named after Shiga because his description and serologic data strongly linked the organism to the disease.

## MICROBIOLOGY

Shigellosis denotes the enteritis syndromes resulting from infection with any of the four serogroups of *Shigella*. The shigellae are gram-negative, aerobic, nonmotile bacteria that do not use lactose or use it only during prolonged incubation.

### TABLE 56-21. Typhoid Vaccines

| Age (years) | Vaccine and Dose |
|---|---|
| <6 | Parenteral Inactivated Vaccine; 0.25 mL subcutaneously, given on two occasions separated by 4 or more weeks |
| 6–9 | Parenteral Inactivated Vaccine; 0.25 mL subcutaneously, given on two occasions separated by 4 or more weeks |
| | *or* |
| | Oral Ty21a Vaccine; One enteric-coated capsule on alternate days for a total of 4 capsules |
| ≥10 | Parenteral Inactivated Vaccine; 0.5 mL subcutaneously, given on two occasions separated by 4 or more weeks |
| | *or* |
| | Oral Ty21a Vaccine; One enteric-coated capsule on alternate days for a total of 4 capsules |

The *Shigella* genus consists of four species that are biochemically differentiated. Group A contains the 12 serotypes of *Shigella dysenteriae*. Group B includes *Shigella flexneri* serotypes, numbered 1 through 6, and 13 subserotypes called 1a, 1b, 2a, 2b, 3a, 3b, 4a, 4b, 5a, 5b, 6, X variant, and Y variant. Group C incorporates the 18 serotypes of *Shigella boydii*. Group D contains *Shigella sonnei*, which has one serotype. A clinically indistinguishable illness is caused by some *Escherichia coli* (enteroinvasive *E coli*) that carry the *Shigella* virulence genes. Although there are some clinically important differences between *S dysenteriae* serotype 1 (ie, *Shiga* bacillus) and the other shigellae, these organisms are traditionally discussed together because of their microbiologic and clinical similarities.

## EPIDEMIOLOGY

Shigellae are spread by the fecal-oral route. They are hardy organisms that can survive in water for up to 6 months. Unlike most other agents that cause diarrhea, the number of ingested organisms required to cause illness is very low. Some adult volunteers have become ill after ingesting only 10 shigellae. Although shigellae are like other enteric pathogens in that they can be spread through contaminated food or water, they are atypical in that they are passed easily from person to person.

The peak incidence of symptomatic *Shigella* infection occurs during the first 4 years of life. Despite the small inoculum required to produce disease, infants in the first few months of life rarely are infected symptomatically with shigellae. The reason for this is unclear. The exact incidence of symptomatic *Shigella* infection is unknown because many cases are not diagnosed or reported. Only about 5% of cases are reported in the United States, for which an incidence of 270 per million children between 1 and 4 years of age was estimated for 1988. The overall rate for all persons living in the United States was 100 per million for the same year.

In 1987, reported isolation rates of *Shigella* species began to increase dramatically in all regions of the United States after more than a decade of relatively low rates. Some settings, such as custodial care institutions and Indian reservations, had unusually high rates. American Indians have a risk of shigellosis that is about four times greater than that of the rest of the population.

In the developing world, where carriers are common, the frequency of infection is even greater, and infants are routinely exposed to *Shigella* early in life. Studies by Leonardo Mata of 45 Guatemalan infants whose stools were cultured weekly during their first 3 years of life documented 1032 positive cultures for *Shigella*. Although these studies were done 20 years ago, there is good reason to believe that the risk has not decreased.

Day-care centers are an important focus for outbreaks of shigellosis in the United States. The small inoculum required for disease production, the pooling of susceptible children, and the frequent lack of adherence to basic hygienic procedures contribute to this situation.

There are seasonal variations in the frequency of shigellosis in the United States; the peak occurrence is between July and October. In tropical regions, the peak period is during the rainy season.

There are important geographic variations in the prevalent serotypes of *Shigella*. In the United States, most shigellosis is caused by *S sonnei*, with *S flexneri* the second most important cause. In most of the developing world, *S flexneri* is more common than *S sonnei*. Serogroup A and C infections are much less common, although massive outbreaks associated with *S dysenteriae* serotype 1 often occur.

## PATHOGENESIS

Because the shigellae have been studied for almost 90 years, much is known about their virulence and the host responses to infection. The most fundamental virulence property shared by all shigellae and by the enteroinvasive *E coli* is the ability to invade mammalian cells. This trait is coded for by a large plasmid (120 to 140 Md). Shigellae that lack this plasmid are consistently avirulent. The predilection of shigellae to invade is conventionally studied in tissue culture (eg, HeLa cell invasion model), animal intestine, or rabbit or guinea pig eyes (ie, Sereny test). A small number of polypeptides are coded for by the virulence plasmid. The exact function of each of these proteins has not been determined, although there is little doubt that they allow shigellae to enter and kill eukaryotic cells.

There are chromosomally encoded traits that enhance pathogenicity. In studies of *S flexneri*, three specific regions of the chromosome are required for the organism to be fully virulent. The gene product is known for only one of these regions. The region is involved in the synthesis of lipopolysaccharide. Precisely how lipopolysaccharide is involved in the pathogenesis of shigellosis is undefined. The shigellae produce at least two types of cytotoxins that kill cells in tissue culture. The clinical significance of these toxins is debatable, although there is good evidence that the toxin produced in high amounts by *S dysenteriae* serotype 1 is important; this Shiga toxin may account for the severity of infection due to *S dysenteriae* serotype 1 compared with other shigellae. There is strong evidence that this toxin is involved in the pathogenesis of the hemolytic uremic syndrome (HUS), a major complication of *S dysenteriae* serotype 1 infection. A second cytotoxin produced by shigellae has not been characterized fully, although data suggest that it also may be clinically relevant.

Immune responses to shigellae are primarily humoral. Although there is some evidence for the involvement of cell-mediated immunity, most data describe serum or mucosal antibodies. Antibodies to lipopolysaccharides and the virulence plasmid-coded polypeptides are produced during natural infection. Although serotype-specific immunity follows infection, the serum titers to the lipopolysaccharides do not correlate with protection during experimental infection. The role of antibodies to virulence polypeptides and toxins in preventing subsequent infection also remains uncertain.

## PATHOLOGY

The most obvious pathologic changes in shigellosis are those found in the colon. The rectosigmoid and distal colon are typically more involved than proximal areas. Erythema, mucosal edema, friability, focal hemorrhages, and adherent mucopurulent pseudomembranes all may be found. The microscopic findings include edema, capillary congestion, capillary thromboses, focal hemorrhages, crypt hyperplasia, crypt abscesses, goblet cell depletion, mononuclear and polymorphonuclear infiltrates, shedding of epithelial cells, and ulcerations. In animals, fluorescent antibody stains have demonstrated that shigellae penetrate intestinal epithelial cells.

## CLINICAL MANIFESTATIONS

The usual incubation period in outbreaks and volunteer studies is 12 to 48 hours, although illness may be delayed for a week or more. There are several typical clinical presentations of *Shigella* enteric infection. Some children have a biphasic illness, presenting with severe abdominal cramps associated with fever and watery diarrhea, followed in 24 to 48 hours by small-volume, bloody stools whose passage is associated with tenesmus and pain. Other children do not have the early watery diarrhea and present with a colitic picture. In still others, watery diarrhea never progresses to the colitic phase. It is not known why some children have predominantly watery diarrhea and others have dysentery. In adult volunteer studies, the dose of organisms that causes watery diarrhea in some patients causes dysentery in others. *S dysenteriae* serotype 1 typically is more likely to produce severe colitis. Overall, only about 40% of children with *Shigella* infection have blood in their stools. About half have emesis and 90% have fever, which is often quite high.

Physical findings include fever (ie, more than two thirds have rectal temperatures greater than 38.9°C [102°F]), evidence of toxicity, dehydration, and lower quadrant abdominal tenderness. Because the disease involves the most distal segments of colon more than the proximal areas, rectal examination may demonstrate an unusual degree of tenderness. Without therapy, fever and diarrhea may persist for a week or more. Dehydration and electrolyte disturbances are common in children with shigellosis, but severe dehydration is an infrequent event. Despite frequent bowel movements, less than 30 mL/kg/day of fluid is lost during the dysenteric phase.

There are several important complications of shigellosis. Hyponatremia and hypoglycemia are the two major metabolic abnormalities that occur with shigellosis. Hyponatremia is most common with *S dysenteriae* infection. Because stool sodium losses do not appear to account for the degree of hyponatremia, it has been postulated that the abnormality is produced by an inappropriate antidiuretic hormone secretion. The prevalence of hypoglycemia is higher among patients with shigellosis than among patients with non-*Shigella* diarrhea. The appropriately low concentrations of insulin and the appropriately elevated concentrations of glucose counter-regulatory hormones (eg, growth hormone, glucagon, epinephrine, norepinephrine, cortisol) suggest failure of gluconeogenesis as the cause of hypoglycemia. Hyponatremia and hypoglycemia have been associated with the deaths of patients with shigellosis.

In various series, 10% to 35% of the affected children have seizures or other neurologic symptoms. Seizures have been considered the most frequent extraintestinal manifestation of shigellosis. Their frequency is disproportionate to the expected incidence of febrile convulsions, which suggests that shigellae produce a neurotoxin. *Shigella* isolated from patients with seizures did not produce Shiga toxin. Lethargy and seizures often precede development of diarrhea. In patients whose course is complicated by seizures, the outcome is usually good. Although a few patients have died, most children recover and have no neurologic residua, even if the convulsions were prolonged or focal. Encephalopathy is a more ominous complication than convulsion. Patients can present with obtundation or coma or with abnormal neurologic signs, such as decorticate or decerebrate posturing. Cerebral edema, necrosis, and hemorrhage have been described.

The development of hemolysis or hemolysis with uremia (ie, HUS) is particularly associated with *S dysenteriae* serotype 1 and rarely associated with *S flexneri* infection. These complications are probably triggered by vascular damage caused by inhibition of protein synthesis due to Shiga toxin. Some *E coli* (eg, *E coli* O157:H7, *E coli* O26:H11) are like *S dysenteriae* serotype 1 in that they produce massive amounts of Shiga toxin or a closely related cytotoxin. These *E coli* are associated with an afebrile hemorrhagic colitis and HUS. During a retrospective case-control study, it was observed that treatment with certain antimicrobial agents was associated with an increased risk of development of HUS, but this association remains equivocal.

Sepsis (often with disseminated intravascular coagulation) complicates enteritis in more than 10% of dysentery cases. In about half of the bacteremic cases, shigellae are isolated from the bloodstream, with other enteric organisms found in the remainder. Children infected with *S dysenteriae* serotype 1 are at least twice as likely to develop bacteremia as those infected with other serotypes. Overall, bacteremia-associated mortality is almost 50%, although for *S dysenteriae*, the mortality is 85%. Those at highest risk of death include infants in the first year of life and children who are not breast-fed, are malnourished, or are afebrile. Extraintestinal localization of infection during bacteremia is rare. The bacteriology of the bronchopneumonia that is common among bacteremic children has not been well defined. Evidence obtained at autopsy suggests that the pneumonia is often caused by pathogens other than *Shigella*.

There are a few reports of a syndrome affecting children that is characterized by extreme toxicity, seizures, obtundation or coma, extreme hyperpyrexia (sometimes above 41.7°C [107°F]), hypotension, and a rapidly fatal course, without sepsis or severe dehydration. The pathogenesis of this syndrome, called Ekiri syndrome in the Japanese literature, is not well understood, although some data suggest that hypocalcemia may be important. Ekiri was predominantly associated with *S sonnei* infection and was responsible for many deaths in Japan before and immediately after World War II.

Focal nonbacteremic extraintestinal shigellosis occurs rarely. Vaginitis with a bloody discharge with or without associated diarrhea is more commonly associated with *S flexneri* than with other serogroups. In some girls, symptoms last for months if systemic therapy is not given. Keratitis, conjunctivitis, iritis, and iridocyclitis are other rare complications of shigellosis in young children. In a few cases, eye involvement has occurred without diarrhea. Patients positive for HLA-B27 are at risk of developing the Reiter syndrome (ie, arthritis, urethritis, conjunctivitis) after a bout of shigellosis.

The mortality rate of isolated enteric infection is less than 1% in industrialized societies. However, in preindustrial societies, 10% to 30% of the children with shigellosis die. Although complications have been most commonly reported in patients infected with *S dysenteriae* type 1, infection with any species of *Shigella* may be fatal. Complications that can lead to death include intestinal perforation, toxic megacolon, dehydration, sepsis, hyponatremia, hypoglycemia, encephalopathy, HUS, pneumonia and malnutrition.

Shigellosis can aggravate or provoke malnutrition and lead to death. Shigellosis is probably the most frequent enteric infection resulting in the progression of marginal malnutrition to overt protein calorie malnutrition. Protein-losing enteropathy may develop. This is probably the reason that dysentery, rather than diarrhea, is frequently associated with growth stunting in infants. The major impact of shigellosis on global public health is on nutritional status.

## DIAGNOSIS

Often shigellae are not isolated from patients who have shigellosis. Adult volunteer studies have shown that even daily stool cultures fail to yield the organism in about 20% of the ill patients who have ingested shigellae. Optimal recovery of shigellae from stool or rectal swab specimens is achieved by promptly inoculating selective and nonselective media. There are serotype-related differences in yield with common media. *S dysenteriae* serotype 1, unlike other shigellae, is isolated more consistently on MacConkey media than on *Salmonella-Shigella* agar. Complete identification of shigellae depends on biochemical and serologic criteria. Most mannitol nonfermenters are classified as *S dysenteriae*. Although these organisms are grouped together, their lipopolysaccharide antigens are not closely related; there is no shared group antigen for this "serogroup." Polyvalent antisera are useful in confirming that a *Shigella* belongs to serogroup A. The ornithine decarboxylase-positive, slow lactose fermenters are *S sonnei*. There is a single serotype (ie, O antigen defined) that all *S sonnei* share. The shigellae that are mannitol fermenters but do not decarboxylate ornithine or ferment lactose belong to serogroups B and C. Those that have immunologically related lipopolysaccharides have been grouped together as *S flexneri*, and those not immunologically related have been grouped together as *S boydii*. Because all but 2 of the 37 serotypes of *Shigella* have O antigens related to common *E coli* O antigens, serology alone is inadequate to define a *Shigella*.

Ancillary laboratory studies are sometimes helpful in making a presumptive diagnosis before culture results are available. The fecal leukocyte examination is commonly positive in children with bacillary dysentery. Leukocyte counts show leukocytosis often with a left shift; about one third of the children have more than 25% band forms. Leukemoid reactions with leukocyte counts greater than 50,000 occur in as many as 10% of the patients in some series. *S dysenteriae* serotype 1 characteristically is associated with higher leukocyte counts than other serotypes of *Shigella*. Cerebrospinal fluid examinations of children who have seizures are usually normal, although a few have a mild lymphocytic pleocytosis.

The clinical picture of colitis can be caused by shigellae and by enteroinvasive *E coli*, enterohemorrhagic *E coli*(eg, *E coli* O157:H7), salmonellae, *Campylobacter jejuni*, *Yersinia enterocolitica*, *Clostridium difficile*, *Entamoeba histolytica*, and inflammatory bowel disease. Definitive diagnosis of these illnesses on presentation is difficult, although there may be differential points in some cases. Epidemiologic evidence of person-to-person spread suggests shigellosis. Convulsions are common with *Shigella* but uncommon with the other forms of colitis. Bloody diarrhea in the first few months of life is more likely to be caused by salmonellae than *Shigella*. A history of antibiotic use (particularly clindamycin or ampicillin) suggests *C difficile*. A negative fecal leukocyte examination may suggest *E histolytica*, particularly if the patient is afebrile; the fecal leukocyte examination often is positive with the other illnesses included in the differential diagnosis. Negative study results for the routine bacterial pathogens listed and *E histolytica* suggest a hemorrhagic colitis caused by *E coli* O157:H7, particularly if the child is afebrile. Negative studies may suggest an enteroinvasive *E coli*, particularly if only nonmotile, lysine decarboxylase-negative *E coli* are isolated. The differentiation of *Shigella* from other causes of watery diarrhea may not be possible on presentation.

## TREATMENT

Antibiotics have a major role in the management of bacillary dysentery. Shigellosis should be treated routinely with antibiotics. Treatment clears the organism from the feces, diminishing the chances of secondary cases, and gives relief from an illness that typically makes the child feel miserable. Children who are treated recover more rapidly and are able to absorb nutrients more efficiently. It is not known whether treatment prevents complications such as hemolysis or HUS, but it is thought that treatment prevents the Ekiri syndrome. The major disadvantage associated with treatment is the development of resistance to the antibiotic used and to antibiotics to which the patient is not exposed. This peculiar finding is explained by the fact that drug resistance is usually a plasmid-coded trait. Plasmids are transferred easily between enteric bacteria. A single plasmid commonly carries the genes for resistance to multiple antibiotics. The selective pressure of a single antibiotic may allow a strain to emerge that is resistant

to many drugs. The cost associated with drug therapy and occasional side effects have prompted some authorities to not recommend routine treatment of *Shigella*.

The choice of drugs for eradicating shigellosis is problematic. The emergence of resistant shigellae has been a recurring theme during the last 40 years. Until recently, ampicillin was the drug of choice, but in the United States, 30% to 50% of *S sonnei* and a few *S flexneri* are resistant to ampicillin. The usual choice of therapy is trimethoprim-sulfamethoxazole (TMP-SMX), but the incidence of isolates resistant to TMP-SMX has also been increasing worldwide. In the United States, the frequency of resistance to this drug is higher among patients with a history of foreign travel. Most children treated with TMP-SMX improve within 1 or 2 days, although normal stools may not be seen for as long as 9 days. This response appears to be better than that seen in patients treated with ampicillin, who typically remain ill for several days despite therapy. Patients with *S dysenteriae* serotype 1 infection respond more slowly to antibiotic therapy than do others with bacillary dysentery.

Nalidixic acid is commonly used to treat shigellosis due to strains that are resistant to ampicillin and TMP-SMX. The rate of clinical cure associated with the use of nalidixic acid is equivalent to that achieved with ampicillin, although eradication of *Shigella* from the stool may take longer. The newer quinolones have been successfully used in the treatment of shigellosis in adults. Because of their potential toxicity, they are not approved for use in children. A third-generation cephalosporin such as ceftriaxone is occasionally appropriate.

The timing of therapy is important. If there is a strong clinical suspicion of shigellosis, the patient should be started on antibiotics before culture data become available. The patient who has high fever, severe abdominal pain, small and frequent stools with blood and mucus, and a positive fecal leukocyte examination should be treated without delay. If an outbreak of one of the other organisms known to cause these symptoms is in progress, it may be reasonable to withhold treatment directed at shigellae. In areas where *Campylobacter* infection is particularly common, it may be advisable to start therapy directed at shigellae and Campylobacter. If *Shigella* was not suspected initially because of a watery diarrhea syndrome without colitis, therapy should be started after cultures suggest that *Shigella* is the likely cause.

The duration of therapy required for shigellosis is shorter than that for many other common infections. Although in older children single-dose regimens are almost as effective as multiple-dose regimens in relieving symptoms, they are less effective in clearing the feces of the organism. Because one of the goals of therapy is the prevention of intrafamilial spread, multiple doses are typically used. This strategy is debatable in developing nations, where asymptomatic excretion is common and eradication of a single focus of infection may have little impact on secondary cases. Whether the choice of antibiotics is ampicillin, TMP-SMX, or nalidixic acid, a 5-day course of therapy is recommended. The dose is 10 mg/kg/day of the trimethoprim component and 50 mg/kg/day of the sulfa component, given orally in two equally divided doses. The maximum dose is 160 mg of trimethoprim and 800 mg of sulfamethoxazole given twice daily. If administered intravenously, the drug is given in three divided doses, each over a 1-hour period. For a patient who is unable to take TMP-SMX because of glucose-6-phosphate dehydrogenase deficiency, deficient folate reserves, or drug sensitivity and who has an ampicillin-sensitive shigellosis, the usual dose of ampicillin is 100 mg/kg/day given orally or parenterally in four divided doses. The usual maximum is 500 mg four times each day. The dose of nalidixic acid is 55 mg/kg/day in four divided doses.

Some measures occasionally recommended by physicians for the treatment of diarrhea are dangerous in patients with bacillary dysentery. Antimotility agents such as diphenoxylate hydrochloride with atropine (Lomotil) appear to prolong fever and excretion of the organism.

## PREVENTION

Because day-care centers represent a major source of *Shigella* infection in young children in the United States, attention to basic infection control measures should be encouraged. These measures typically include emphasis on hand washing, exclusion of sick children, and exclusion of food preparers from diaper changing duty. Excluding children who are convalescing is controversial because adherence to infection control strategies prevents further spread, even if convalescent children are allowed to return to the center. The parents should be instructed about the importance of hand washing. In developing nations, the best means of preventing infection of the young child appears to be prolonged breast-feeding. Whether breast-feeding decreases shigellosis by preventing the consumption of contaminated food, by secretory IgA, or by nonspecific gut flora-modifying factors remains uncertain.

## Selected Readings

Ashkenazi S, Dinari G, Zevulunov A, et al. Convulsions in childhood shigellosis: clinical and laboratory features in 153 children. Am J Dis Child 1987;141:208.

Bartlett AV, Prado D, Cleary TG, et al. Production of shigatoxin and other cytotoxins by serogroups of *Shigella*. J Infect Dis 1986;154:996.

Bennish ML. Potentially lethal complications of shigellosis. Rev Infect Dis 1991;13(suppl 4):319.

Nelson JD, Kusiemsz H, Shelton S. Oral or intravenous trimethoprim-sulfamethoxazole therapy for shigellosis. Rev Infect Dis 1982;4:546.

Salam MA, Bennish ML. Antimicrobial therapy for shigellosis. Rev Infect Dis 1991;13(suppl 4):332.

Sansonetti PJ, Kopecko DJ, Formal SB. *Shigella sonnei* plasmids: evidence that a large plasmid is necessary for virulence. Infect Immunol 1981;34:75.

Speelman P, Kabir I, Islam M. Distribution and spread of colonic lesions in shigellosis: a colonoscopic study. J Infect 1984;150:899.

Struelens MJ, Patte D, Kabir I, et al. *Shigella* septicemia: prevalence, presentation, risk factors and outcome. J Infect Dis 1985;152:784.

*Principles and Practice of Pediatrics, Second Edition.*
edited by Frank A. Oski et al. J. B. Lippincott Company, Philadelphia © 1994.

# 56.24 *Staphylococcal Infections*

## Christian C. Patrick

Staphylococci are ubiquitous bacteria that colonize humans and animals. *Staphylococcus aureus* is a major etiologic agent causing human disease, and coagulase-negative staphylococci (CoNS) have emerged as pathogens in patient populations with impaired host defense.

## MICROBIOLOGY

Staphylococci are gram positive, nonmotile, aerobic or facultatively anaerobic. They are not fastidious and grow well on ordinary media. All members are catalase positive. Staphylococci are categorized by their ability to produce coagulase; *S aureus* is always coagulase positive. There are 27 recognized species of staphylococci, and 25 are CoNS. *S aureus* and some CoNS produce a capsule, but its clinical importance is unclear. Some CoNS, especially *Staphylococcus epidermidis*, produce a slime layer or glycocalyx, which is a virulence factor and is distinct from the capsule. *S aureus* produce a unique cell wall protein, protein A, which possesses antiphagocytic properties and has a high affinity for the Fc portion of certain immunoglobulin subclasses.

## INFECTIONS DUE TO *STAPHYLOCOCCUS AUREUS*

Infections due to *S aureus* are common in children. The organism causes skin infections (eg, furuncles, carbuncles, impetigo, wound infections), pneumonia, septicemia, osteomyelitis, meningitis, pericarditis, and endocarditis. *S aureus* is also a major cause of toxin-induced food poisoning.

### Epidemiology

Staphylococci are common organisms of the normal human flora. *S aureus* are carried by 20% to 40% of adults; of these patients, approximately 30% are long-term carriers, and 50% are intermittent carriers.

Staphylococci are usually tolerated by the human body, causing disease in patients compromised locally (eg, open wounds, intravenous catheters) or systemically (eg, immunosuppression, diabetes mellitus). Viral respiratory infection may alter the natural host defense and allow the development of staphylococcal pneumonia. Recurrent staphylococcal infections and autoinfection are common because of the asymptomatic carriage rate. *S aureus* often colonizes the infant's umbilicus and groin.

Staphylococcal infections can occur as an epidemic or as a sporadic event. Person-to-person spread appears to be the most common form of transmission, although airborne transmission is possible. The person-to-person spread can be compounded by hospital personnel taking care of immunocompromised patients, such as neonates.

### Pathogenesis

The pathologic effects of *S aureus* can be attributed to tissue invasion or toxin production. Surface components with possible virulence attributes include teichoic acid, protein A, and the capsule. Teichoic acid, which comprises 40% of the cell wall weight, mediates adherence *S aureus* to nasal mucosa cells. Protein A, located in the cell wall, is antiphagocytic. The capsule of *S aureus* may impair phagocytosis by stearic hindrance.

Some enzymes and toxins produced by *S aureus* are known virulence factors, and others have an indeterminant status. Enzymes involved in pathogenesis include coagulase, catalase, hyaluronidase, and $\beta$-lactamase. DNAse and lipase have an unknown role in pathogenesis. Coagulase causes plasma to clot and may cause bacterial clumping aiding phagocytosis. Catalase converts $H_2O_2$ to $H_2O$ and $O_2$, reducing $H_2O_2$ as a host defense mediator in phagocytosis. Hyaluronidase or spreading factor can allow the spread of an infection by digesting the connective tissue ground substance. The $\beta$-lactamase inactivates benzylpenicillin and several cephalosporins.

*S aureus* produces a variety of toxins. Five are membrane-damaging toxins (ie, $\alpha$, $\beta$, $\gamma$, $\delta$, leukocidin). Others are exfoliation toxins, enterotoxins, and toxic shock syndrome toxin. Although four hemolysins (ie, $\alpha$, $\beta$, $\gamma$, $\delta$) are produced, only the $\alpha$-toxin is involved in pathogenesis. The $\alpha$-toxin damages human and rabbit skin and causes platelet aggregation, contraction of smooth and skeletal muscles, tissue necrosis, and lysis of macrophages. Leucocidin has several biologic effects, but its foremost action is the lysis or granulocytosis of macrophages.

Exfoliative toxin exists in at least two forms, and the toxin acts by dividing the epidermidis at the stratum granulosum layer. It primarily affects newborns.

Five serologically distinct enterotoxins (ie, A through E) produced by S aureus cause food-borne disease. The mechanism of action of these enterotoxins is unknown, but intestinal peristalsis is increased.

## Pathology

The formation of an abscess is characteristic of staphylococcal infections in humans, and the skin is the usual portal or entry. Invasion and spread of the organism is promoted by increased connective tissue permeability secondary to local multiplication and production of hyaluronidase. There is exudation of plasma and migration of granulocytes to the area of invasion. After invasion with staphylococci, rapid liquefaction necrosis and destruction of tissue ensues. Thrombosis of the blood vessels with formation of fibrin clots can occur. Fully developed local lesions consists of a central necrotic area that is filled with dead leukocytes and organisms surrounded by a fibroelastic, avascular wall. The lesion may contain viable bacteria and leukocytes. Trauma that breaks the fibroelastic barrier may spread the infection, often initiating bacteremia.

## Clinical Manifestations

The clinical manifestations vary with the portal of entry of the organism and with the immune status and general health of the patient.

S aureus infections of the skin are among the most common bacterial infections. Lesions caused by this organism include furuncles (ie, boils), carbuncles, paronychia, folliculitis, cellulitis, bullous impetigo, scalded skin syndrome (ie, Ritter's disease), and toxic epidermal necrolysis.

Muscle abscesses usually are associated with the subacute onset of moderate muscle pain, followed several days or weeks later by fever. There is an associated increase in serum muscle enzymes, without evidence of septicemia. The abscesses are found deep in the striated muscle and are bound by the overlying fascia. The use of appropriate antibiotics and surgical drainage produces a high rate of cure. These lesions are seen much more often in tropical areas (ie, "tropical pyomyositis") but have been described in the United States.

Sources of staphylococcal bacteremia are varied and often obscure, but the skin, respiratory tract, and genitourinary tract usually are the primary sites of infection. Staphylococcal bacteremia may be slowly progressive, with shaking chills, fever, metastatic abscesses in organs such as lung, bone, kidney, heart, and brain. Disseminated staphylococcal disease is marked by bone and joint pain, fever, and urticarial, petechial, maculopapular, or pustular skin rashes. Hematuria, jaundice, seizures, nuchal rigidity, and cardiac murmurs occur less frequently. Laboratory findings include leukopenia or leukocytosis, proteinuria, and erythrocytes or leukocytes in the urine sediment.

Staphylococcal organisms are the most frequent cause of acute osteomyelitis. In most cases, the bacteria reach the bone by hematogenous spread from a skin lesion. S aureus usually localizes in the metaphyseal ends of the long bones because of increased circulation in this area. The clinical syndrome may be preceded by trauma, pyoderma, or other antecedent infection. It is associated with irritability, fever, anorexia, vomiting, local warmth, and point tenderness.

Renal involvement, with the formation of cortical abscesses, perirenal abscesses, and pyelonephritis, can be associated with bacteremia. Diffuse proliferative glomerulonephritis is a renal manifestation of staphylococcal bacteremia that is not thought to be associated with actual bacterial seeding of the kidney. Urinary tract infections caused by S aureus seldom occur.

The most common source of staphylococcal enterocolitis is contaminated food. When left at room temperature, certain foods (eg, meats, dairy products, bakery products) are fertile soil for the formation of bacterial enterotoxin. The illness has a sudden onset, occurring 1 to 6 hours after ingestion of preformed toxin in contaminated food. It is manifested by profuse diarrhea, abdominal cramps, and nausea. The symptoms improve within 8 to 24 hours, but weakness may last several days. Staphylococcal enterocolitis can be caused by bacterial overgrowth in the bowel after antibiotic therapy. The symptoms are the same as those of food poisoning, with the addition of fever.

Peritonsillar abscesses, otitis media, retropharyngeal abscesses, sinusitis, and parotitis can be caused by S aureus. Staphylococci can cause aseptic cerebral emboli, cerebral venous thromboses, brain abscesses, and meningitis. Meningitis due to S aureus generally results from hematogenous dissemination but may occur as an extension of otitis media, sinusitis, mastoiditis, or osteomyelitis of the skull and vertebrae. Brain abscesses usually are small, without focal neurologic signs.

Staphylococcal endocarditis is manifested by high fever, progressive anemia, and metastatic abscesses to the skin and deeper structures. Staphylococcal bacteremia may lead to acute necrotizing ulcerating lesions of the endocardium. The lesions are found most often on the mitral and aortic valves.

Staphylococcal pneumonia occurs as a primary infection or secondary to a viral infection. The highest incidence is seen among children. The illness begins as an upper respiratory tract infection with fever, nasal discharge, cough, and anorexia. This often leads to increasing cough, tachypnea, dyspnea, and retractions. Radiographic findings associated with staphylococcal pneumonia include pneumatocele, empyema, pneumothorax, abscesses, and consolidation.

## Diagnosis

A presumptive diagnosis of staphylococcal infection can be obtained by identifying gram-positive cocci in clusters on a Gram stain of clinical material (eg, abscess or joint fluid, sputum, blood). A definitive diagnosis depends on isolation of the organism on liquid or solid media from an otherwise sterile site or aspiration from a wound or lesion.

Serologic assays are used to evaluate the host antibody response to multiple staphylococcal antigens, including teichoic acid and $\alpha$-toxin. The sensitivity of each assay depends on the type of disease.

The diagnosis of staphylococcal food poisoning is usually made on a clinical basis. Suspicion of the disease can be substantiated by a Gram stain and culture of the presumed food source and by demonstration of toxin-producing staphylococci. Enterotoxin determination can be done by the Centers for Disease Control.

The diagnosis of staphylococcal pneumonia should be suspected if two or more of the following are observed: acute respiratory distress in a young infant; history of recent pyoderma, omphalitis, or mastitis followed by symptoms of respiratory tract disease; and radiographic evidence of pneumatoceles, empyema, or pyopneumothorax. The presenting symptoms of pneumococcal pneumonia, coliform bacillus pneumonia (due to E coli, Pseudomonas, Klebsiella, or Enterobacter), acute bronchiolitis, or aspiration of a foreign body may mimic those of staphylococcal pneumonia. Staphylococcal osteomyelitis may be confused with rheumatic fever, septic arthritis, cellulitis, poliomyelitis, fractures, and sprains. Other enteric infections, such as shigellosis and salmonellosis, may cause symptoms similar to those of patients with staphylococcal food poisoning. It is often difficult to differentiate clinically between skin lesions due to staphylococci and those due to group A $\beta$-hemolytic streptococci.

## Treatment

The therapy for staphylococcal infections depends on the general health and immune status of the patient, the site of infection, and the results of antimicrobial susceptibility testing. Focal infections with collections of purulent material require adequate drainage. Serious staphylococcal infections require systemic bactericidal antibodies.

Penicillin G (100,000 to 250,000 U/kg/day given intravenously every 4 hours) is active against penicillin-sensitive, non–penicillinase-producing organisms. However, 90% of community and hospital-acquired staphylococci are penicillin-resistant.

For organisms resistant to penicillin, the semisynthetic penicillins, such as methicillin, nafcillin, or oxacillin, should be used. Aminoglycosides, such as gentamicin and amikacin, act synergistically with the penicillinase-resistant penicillins. Methicillin-resistant S aureus is widespread, necessitating the use of vancomycin in some geographic areas. Vancomycin (40 mg/kg/day given intravenously every 6 hours) is the drug of choice for organisms resistant to penicillinase-resistant penicillin and is recommended for treating severe infections empirically before antimicrobial susceptibility tests are known.

Because staphylococcal infections can persist and recur, prolonged antibiotic therapy is required. Staphylococcal pneumonia should be treated with intravenous antibiotics until the patient is afebrile for 72 to 96 hours. The drug(s) should then be switched to an appropriate oral antibiotic for at least 3 weeks. Osteomyelitis due to staphylococcal infections should be treated for a minimum of 3 to 4 weeks, depending on the clinical course. Staphylococcal endocarditis should be treated for 6 weeks, along with surgery in the acute phase if needed.

Oral therapy is acceptable in the treatment of mild soft-tissue or upper respiratory tract infections. Dicloxacillin (12 to 25 mg/kg/day in divided doses given orally every 6 hours) is a reasonable drug because of its penicillinase resistance, reliable gastrointestinal absorption, and adequate serum levels.

Penicillin-allergic patients should be treated with alternate antibiotics. Alternative therapy for skin, soft tissue, bone, and joint infections due to staphylococci includes clindamycin. This drug can be given intravenously or orally at a dose of 20 to 30 mg/kg/day in four divided doses. In treating endocarditis, brain abscesses, or meningitis due to S aureus, vancomycin can be used, but serum antibiotic levels should be monitored.

## Complications

Staphylococcal bacteremia may be complicated by disseminated intravascular coagulation and thrombocytopenia. Staphylococcal osteomyelitis can lead to pyogenic arthritis, sterile arthritis, subperiosteal abscesses, or subcutaneous abscesses. Untreated staphylococcal osteomyelitis may be complicated by the formation of a Brodie abscess. This low-grade infection, which produces a necrotic core surrounded by granulation tissue, can persist for years. Staphylococcal endocarditis can lead to septic pulmonary emboli if the infection is right sided. Infection in the nasolabial areas of the face may be associated with cavernous sinus thrombosis and infection. Staphylococcal pneumonia can be complicated by congestive heart failure, fibrothorax secondary to inadequate drainage of an empyema, bronchopleural fistulas with subsequent pneumothorax, abscess formation, or empyema. Staphylococcal enterocolitis can result in shock and dehydration due to excessive fluid loss.

## Prevention

Preventing staphylococcal infections is difficult because of this organism's ubiquitous nature. However, because most infections are caused by direct contact from staff to patient or patient to patient, hand washing with a detergent containing hexachlorophene or an iodophor is effective in preventing the spread of disease.

Bacterial interference is successful in arresting nursery outbreaks of staphylococcal infections. This procedure of implanting a penicillin-sensitive, nonpathogenic strain of S aureus onto the nasal mucosa and umbilical stump of newborns is done to prevent colonization of these areas with epidemic strains of S aureus and to interrupt the transmission of S aureus from infant to infant. It is important to alert the infection control committee at the hospital when a nosocomial staphylococcal infection has occurred.

Food poisoning can be prevented by excluding persons with staphylococcal infections from the preparation and handling of food. Optimal cooking and refrigeration of meat, dairy products, and bakery goods help to prevent the disease.

## INFECTIONS DUE TO COAGULASE-NEGATIVE STAPHYLOCOCCI

CoNS have been historically regarded as harmless, commensal saprophytes, but this group of organisms are now implicated in a wide range of nosocomial infections prevalent among immunocompromised patients, particularly those with indwelling medical devices.

CoNS, especially S epidermidis, have been implicated in a variety of clinical infections. They are the primary cause of nosocomial bacteremia in some centers and the prominent pathogens causing bacteremia in neonates and immunocompromised patients with cancer or after bone marrow transplantation. CoNS are the major pathogens in patients with central venous catheters, central nervous system shunts, or peritoneal dialysis catheters. Two nonnosocomial infections caused by CoNS are recognized; S epidermidis can cause native valve endocarditis, and S saprophyticus causes urinary tract infections in young, sexually active women.

The coagulase-negative organisms adhere to catheters and secrete a slime substance or glycocalyx that coats the staphylococci and perhaps protects them from host defenses. Several exoproteins are produced by CoNS, but their role in disease is unclear. Opsonophagocytosis is the most important immune defense against CoNS.

Antibiotic therapy against CoNS should be accompanied by susceptibility testing because these organisms are often resistant. There is a degree of cross-resistance between the semisynthetic penicillinase-resistant penicillins and the cephalosporins; as a rule, methicillin resistance can be interpreted as resistance to all $\beta$-lactam antibiotics. Vancomycin is the drug of choice for organisms resistant to penicillinase-resistant penicillin and is also recommended for treating severe infections.

## TOXIC SHOCK SYNDROME

Toxic shock syndrome (TSS) is an uncommon but potentially devastating illness. TSS was first described in a series of 7 children in 1978.

### Etiology

Toxic shock syndrome toxin-1 (TSST-1), produced by S aureus, is a significant mediator of the pathogenicity of TSS. Other mediators include *S aureus* enterotoxins A through E, exotoxins, and endotoxin from gram-negative bacteria. Although TSS is mainly caused by *S aureus*, certain CoNS can produce TSST-1, and group A β-hemolytic streptococci can produce a syndrome similar to TSS.

## Epidemiology

TSS was first described in 1978, but in 1980, it was recognized with increasing frequency in young, menstruating women using a particular brand of tampon. TSS can occur at any age but has been more commonly described in healthy children and young adults. About 1% of the patients hospitalized with a *S aureus* infection are at risk of developing TSS. The high-risk group of nonmenstruating patients with TSS include patients with surgical wound infections, those with focal staphylococcal infections, postpartum women, and patients after nasal surgery.

## Pathology

The most striking finding is a lack of inflammation. Skin biopsies reveal a mild lymphocytic dermal perivasculitis; an epidermal cleavage plane is occasionally seen. There is evidence of a shock state in the kidneys, liver, and lungs.

## Clinical Manifestations

Patients with TSS usually describe a prodrome of nausea and vomiting, sore throat, watery diarrhea, and myalgia. The typical patients present with fever greater than 38.9 °C, hypotension, diffuse sunburn-like macular erythroderma, and multiple organ dysfunction. The rash is more prominent on the trunk and is usually not pruritic or painful; petechiae, vesicles, or bullae are uncommon. The Nikolsky sign is usually negative. Desquamation of the palms, soles, fingers, and toes occurs 2 to 4 weeks after the onset of the illness. Pharyngeal hyperemia with a strawberry tongue and conjunctival hyperemia without purulent exudate are common.

## Diagnosis

The diagnosis of TSS should be considered when a patient meets all of the major criteria and at least three of the minor criteria. Major criteria include fever (temperature ≥38.8 °C), rash (eg, diffuse, macular erythroderma), skin desquamation (particularly palms and soles), and hypotension (ie, below the fifth percentile by age for children under 16 years of age). Minor criteria include muscular, mucous membrane, gastrointestinal, renal, hepatic, hematologic, and central nervous system involvement. The isolation of *S aureus* from a normally sterile site in a nonmenstruating female supports the diagnosis. Serologic assays for TSST-1 in acute and convalescent sera are supported in a retrospective diagnosis. The detection of TSST-1 is feasible, but not all cases of TSS involve TSST-1, making diagnosis by this route confusing.

The differential diagnosis of TSS includes sepsis, septic shock (eg, meningococcemia), leptospirosis, Rocky Mountain spotted fever, scarlatiniform eruptions, staphylococcal infections (including staphylococcal scalded skin syndrome), streptococcal infections, viral infections, urinary tract infections, toxin-induced diarrhea, erythema multiforme major (ie, Stevens-Johnson syndrome), and Kawasaki disease.

## Treatment

Prompt intervention is mandatory for shock and multiorgan involvement. Drainage of the infected sites or removal of a poten-

tially infectious medical device is imperative. Appropriate antibiotics, usually a penicillinase-resistant penicillin such as nafcillin, should be administered intravenously at a dose of 150 mg/kg/day (maximum dose, 10 to 12 g/day) for 7 to 10 days. The administration of intravenous immune globulin should be considered for severely ill patients, because the preparation contains high levels of antibody to TSST-1.

## Selected Readings

Chesney PJ. Clinical aspects and spectrum of illness of toxic shock syndrome: overview. Rev Infect Dis 1989;11:51.
Melish ME. Staphylococcal infection. In: Feigin RD, Cherry JD, eds. Textbook of pediatric infectious diseases, ed 2. Philadelphia: WB Saunders, 1987:1260.
Patrick CC. Coagulase-negative staphylococci: pathogens with increasing clinical significance. J Pediatr 1990;116:497.
Patrick CC. Staphylococci. In: Patrick CC, ed. Infections in immunocompromised infants and children. New York: Churchill-Livingstone, 1992:421.
Resnick SD. Toxic shock syndrome: recent developments in pathogenesis. J Pediatr 1990;116:321.
Waldvogel FA. *Staphylococcus aureus* (including toxic shock syndrome). In: Mandell GL, Douglas RG Jr, Bennett JE, eds. Principles and practice of infectious diseases, ed 3. New York: Churchill-Livingstone, 1990:1489.

*Principles and Practice of Pediatrics, Second Edition.*
edited by Frank A. Oski et al. J. B. Lippincott Company, Philadelphia © 1994.

# 56.25 *Group A Streptococcal Infections*

Ralph D. Feigin

## MICROBIOLOGY

*Streptococcus pyogenes* (group A *Streptococcus*) is a gram-positive coccus that produces clear (beta) hemolysis on blood agar. This bacteriologic feature aids in the recognition and in the differentiation of *S pyogenes* from viridans (alpha) streptococci and from nonhemolytic (gamma) streptococci. Selected strains of group A streptococci hemolyze slowly and produce a greenish hemolysis on the surface of blood agar plates, similar to that produced by viridans streptococci. These strains can be identified by their ability to produce a clear hemolysis under anaerobic conditions.

Group A hemolytic streptococci can be differentiated from other hemolytic streptococci by their sensitivity to bacitracin. Definitive identification of group A streptococci is established by the use of serologic techniques that employ group-specific antisera.

More than 60 types of group A streptococci have been identified on the basis of their serologically distinct surface proteins (ie, M proteins). The M protein plays a role in the pathogenesis of infection due to the group A *Streptococcus* because it renders this organism resistant to phagocytosis.

Protruding from the surface of the group A streptococcal cell and into a hyaluronic capsule layer are hair-like fimbriae that are responsible for adhering group A streptococci to epithelial cells. These fimbriae contain lipoteichoic acid. The M protein also is associated with these fimbriae. Other surface proteins that have been identified are the T and R proteins, which bind nonspecifically to the Fc fragment of γ-globulins, and serum opacity reaction proteins. The specific function and precise location of each of these proteins on the surface of the organism have not been identified. However, evaluation of these characteristics has proven useful in the course of epidemiologic studies of streptococcal infections.

The carbohydrate substance that is responsible for group specificity is found in the cell wall. The group A carbohydrate is a polymer of rhamnose units with side chains of *N*-acetyl-glucosamine, which is responsible for its group specificity. The cell membrane lies within the cell wall and is composed primarily of lipoprotein complexes or lipid and protein. This membrane is the outer surface of the protoplasts or L-forms of streptococci. The groups of streptococci that lack cell walls are resistant to penicillin and other cell wall-inhibiting antibiotics.

The group A streptococci release into surrounding media many biologically active extracellular products. Streptolysin O (ie, oxygen-labile hemolysin) and streptolysin S (ie, oxygen-stable hemolysin) can injure cell membranes. Streptolysin O is antigenic, but streptolysin S is not. Three erythrogenic or pyrogenic toxins may be elaborated. These substances, identified as A, B, or C, are similar to endotoxin in their ability to exhibit primary toxicity or a secondary toxicity that results from the acquisition of host hypersensitivity. The outbreak in the late 1980s of a toxic shock-like syndrome caused by streptococci is thought to be associated with the reappearance of strains making pyrogenic exotoxin A. Small-molecular-weight proteins (ie, bacteriocins) that can kill other gram-positive bacterial species and play a role in establishing infection are elaborated by group A streptococci. Bacteriocins play a role in the establishment of infection or persistence of colonization.

Other extracellular products of group A streptococci include DNAses (ie, A, B, C, D), the streptokinases, a hyaluronidase, an amylase, a proteinase, an NADase, and an esterase. Several of these are antigenic (eg, streptokinase, DNAase B, hyaluronidase, NADase), and measuring antibodies to these antigens has proven useful in documenting clinical infection.

## TRANSMISSION

Studies of patients with streptococcal pharyngitis suggest that airborne routes of spread and environmental contamination play little or no role in the spread of this form of streptococcal infection. Close contact is required for the spread of streptococcal pharyngitis; direct projection of large droplets or physical transfer of respiratory secretions containing the bacteria is necessary. The spread of group A streptococcal pharyngitis within families or in classrooms is common.

The period of greatest contagiousness for streptococcal pharyngitis or scarlet fever occurs during the acute stage of illness. Penicillin therapy rapidly suppresses the growth of group A streptococci and, if continued, usually eradicates the group A *Streptococcus* from the upper respiratory tract. The patient can be considered much less contagious after 36 to 48 hours of antimicrobial therapy. If they are afebrile, children can return to school by that time with little risk of spread of the organism to close contacts.

Prolonged carriage (weeks to months) of group A streptococci may occur in the throat; prolonged carriage in the entering airways is unusual, and its occurrence suggest the possibility of chronic sinusitis.

Anal carriers of group A streptococci have been identified and have been proven to be the source of epidemic spread of the disease in hospitals. Rectal or anal carriage occurs more often than was suspected previously. Contaminated milk or food may result in outbreaks of streptococcal infection of the throat.

The production of streptococcal skin infections (ie, pyoderma, impetigo) appears to require disruption of the cutaneous epithelium by trauma, preexisting skin disease, or insects. Group A streptococci are often found on normal skin but do not produce disease unless there is some means of access.

## EPIDEMIOLOGY

Group A streptococci are pathogenic for humans but are found infrequently in other species. Streptococcal impetigo occurs with the greatest frequency in preschool children, but streptococcal pharyngitis is predominantly a disorder of school-age children. Outbreaks of streptococcal respiratory tract infections have been observed in day-care centers. Streptococcal impetigo seems to be a recurrent disease in preschool and school-age children.

Tonsillitis and pharyngitis caused by streptococci are particularly common in cold and temperate climates. Streptococcal impetigo and pyoderma occur with greater frequency in tropical climates. Streptococcal pharyngitis is more frequent during the winter and spring, and streptococcal impetigo is generally a disease of the summer months in temperate climates and appears with relatively equal frequency throughout the year in tropical countries.

## PATHOGENESIS

The development of pharyngitis appears to depend on the attachment of group A streptococci to epithelial cells, which is accomplished by their fimbriae. The streptococci must compete with the other pharyngeal flora, which have the ability to interfere with colonization of group A streptococci in the throat.

Skin lipids are lethal for group A streptococci in vitro and may provide a barrier against the establishment of streptococcal infection of the skin under normal conditions. Invasion of tissues by the group A streptococci is facilitated by various toxins and enzymes that attack hyaluronic acid and fibrin. The M protein is antiphagocytic and contains a substance that is cytotoxic in the presence of non–type-specific antibody. Type-specific antibody against M protein enhances phagocytosis, but usually this is not detectable until 6 to 8 weeks after the onset of infection. The primary role of type-specific antibody against M protein may be its prevention of reinfection by the same serologic type. Surface phagocytosis by monocytes and, subsequently, by polymorphonuclear leukocytes appears to be the primary mechanism for defense in the early stages of streptococcal infection.

The spread of streptococci to regional lymph nodes is common, particularly when infection occurs in the pharynx or tonsils. Bacteremia is uncommon in older children and adults, but occurs more frequently in infants with streptococcal disease.

The rash of scarlet fever has been attributed to the elaboration of erythrogenic toxin. Streptococcal toxic shock syndrome may result from a direct influence of the pyrogenic exotoxins on lymphokines (eg, tumor necrosis factor).

## CLINICAL MANIFESTATIONS

Streptococcal pharyngitis and tonsillitis are relatively brief illnesses, with incubation periods of several hours to 3 or 4 days. The infection varies in severity, from subclinical (ie, no symptoms) to relatively extreme toxicity characterized by nausea, vomiting, high fever, and hypotension. The onset is acute and may be characterized by pharyngitis, headache, fever, and abdominal pain, particularly in children. The tonsils and pharynx may appear inflamed and are covered by an exudate in 50% to 80% of patients. The exudate usually appears by the second day of the disease, is characteristically whitish to yellow, and may become confluent. Swollen and tender anterior cervical lymphadenopathy affects 30% to 60% of the patients. Clinical manifestations of the disease subside in 3 to 5 days unless complications such as sinusitis or parapharyngeal, peritonsillar, or retropharyngeal abscess develop. Nonsuppurative complications such as acute nephritis may be seen 10 days and rheumatic fever an average of 18 days after the onset of group A streptococcal pharyngitis.

A form of streptococcal infection known as streptococcal fever may occur in infants. This illness is characterized by a chronic low-grade fever, generalized lymphadenopathy, persistent mucoserous nasal discharge, and little evidence of localized pharyngeal inflammation.

Scarlet fever is unusual in infancy, possibly because of the transplacental transfer of maternal antibody to erythrogenic toxins. It appears that hypersensitivity to these exotoxins must occur before a person can develop scarlet fever as a manifestation of streptococcal disease. The frequency of scarlet fever after infancy has increased since the late 1980s. It usually presents with extreme toxicity, high fever, nausea, vomiting, and the appearance of the typical rash. Abdominal pain and vomiting may precede the development of the rash by 12 to 48 hours. This erythematous maculopapular rash usually begins on the trunk and spreads to cover the entire body within hours to days. The rash has the texture of sandpaper. The forehead and cheeks are flushed, and the area around the mouth is pallid (ie, circumoral pallor). The rash generally fades on pressure and ultimately desquamates. Deep red, nonblanching or petechial lesions may be seen in the folds of the joints (ie, Pastia lines) or in other parts of the extremities. Early in the course of illness, the dorsum of the tongue has a white coat, through which edematous and red papillae project (ie, white strawberry tongue). Several days later, the white covering desquamates, and the tongue becomes swollen, red, and mottled (ie, red strawberry tongue).

A scarlatiniform rash may appear in patients with streptococcal wound infections or impetigo. An enanthema is characterized by bright red or hemorrhagic spots that appear on the interior pillars of the tonsil fossae and the soft palate. The cervical nodes are enlarged and tender, but the pharyngeal signs are usually minimal. The rash may desquamate over 7 to 21 days. Eosinophilia is common during the recovery phases from scarlet fever; the number of eosinophils may reach 30% of the differential leukocyte count in this disorder.

Streptococcal impetigo may develop up to several weeks after a strain of group A streptococci is detected on normal skin. The patient is usually afebrile and the lesion is painless. The lesion initially appears as a superficial vesicle with little surrounding erythema and progresses to a pustule that becomes thick and yellow. The pustule may last for days to a week. A secondary staphylococcal infection occurs commonly in the pustular and subsequently crusted forms of this disease. Removal of the crust, which is a part of local therapy, reveals a moist or purulent undersurface early during the course of the disease. On healing, depigmentation may occur, but permanent scarring is uncommon because the infection does not involve the dermis.

Acute poststreptococcal nephritis follows impetigo or other forms of streptococcal skin infection. This disorder is produced by specific nephritogenic strains of streptococci. Rheumatic fever has not been associated with streptococcal skin infections. The latent period for acute nephritis is longer after skin infection (average, 3 weeks) than after throat infection (average, 10 days). The serologic streptococcal types associated with nephritis after skin infection are usually different from those that produce nephritis after throat infection.

Streptococcal pyoderma may be superimposed on eczema, burns, wounds, scabies, or other diseases that provide access through the barrier of the skin. Ecthyma is a deeper and more chronic form of streptococcal pyoderma found predominantly in tropical areas.

Erysipelas is a form of streptococcal infection involving the skin and the adjacent mucous membranes. It is characterized by an elevated, red lesion, often associated with bullae filled with yellowish fluid that may crust over after rupture. There is a well-demarcated advancing border that appears redder and more edematous at the edge than centrally. The central red area may fade and even appear normal as the lesion progresses. Erysipelas usually involves the face; the extremities and the rest of the body are less often affected. The acute onset of erysipelas often is accompanied by systemic toxicity. The lesion may persist for several days to several weeks, and relapses are common; recurrences usually develop at the same body site.

Other infections that may be caused by the group A *Streptococcus* include otitis media, sinusitis, mastoiditis, pneumonia, empyema, septicemia without localized infection, meningitis, and toxic shock syndrome. The number of cases of toxic shock syndrome caused by group A, $\beta$-hemolytic streptococci has increased significantly in recent years. This syndrome is characterized by high fever (>38.9°C), diffuse macular erythroderma, hypotension, and involvement of at least three of the following organ systems: gastrointestinal, muscular, renal, mucous membranes, hepatic, hematologic, and central nervous system. Group A $\beta$-hemolytic streptococci may be found in 50% of the patients with peritonsillar or retropharyngeal abscesses and may act synergistically with anaerobic bacteria to produce the characteristic clinical picture. Although puerperal sepsis is now rare, nursery outbreaks of bacteremia, omphalitis, and meningitis still occur. Disseminated intravascular coagulation, purpura fulminans, gangrene, perianal cellulitis, and vaginitis have been reported in children as a result of group A streptococcal infection. Streptococcal infections of the thumb have preceded the development of subpectoral abscesses and pleural effusion; this presumably is the result of a spread of streptococci along lymphatic channels that drain the area of the thumb. Streptococci also have been implicated in secondary skin or bone infection in patients who are affected with varicella.

## STREPTOCOCCAL RESPIRATORY CARRIER STATE

Many normal persons harbor group A streptococci in the upper respiratory tract for prolonged periods without evidence of disease or an immunologic response. Carriers only rarely spread the organism to close contacts. The risk of a carrier developing rheumatic fever appears to be significantly less than that of a person with active streptococcal pharyngeal infection.

## DIAGNOSIS

For patients with acute pharyngitis or tonsillitis, the physician must rely on the clinical appearance of the patient, culture results, and epidemiologic findings to confirm the probability of streptococcal infection. The physician's problem in identifying group A streptococcal pharyngitis is difficult, because these organisms are found in the throats of normal children (ie, carriers) and those whose clinical findings are due to many other agents, including gonococci, *Corynebacterium diphtheriae*, and Epstein-Barr virus (EBV). Many viruses produce pharyngitis that closely mimics streptococcal pharyngitis and can be excluded only by the absence of a positive culture for group A streptococci.

Most streptococcal infections are short-term illnesses. Antibody responses appear relatively late, and streptococcal antibody titers are useful only retrospectively in the diagnosis of acute streptococcal infection. However, titers play an important role in supporting the diagnosis of nonsuppurative complications of group A streptococcal disease, such as acute nephritis and rheumatic fever. The measurement of antibody titers may be useful if it is difficult to culture the primary site of infection (eg, osteomyelitis) or during the course of infection in patients who already have been treated with antibiotics to which the group A *Streptococcus* is susceptible.

Clinical manifestations that suggest the streptococcal cause of the disease include high fever, exudative pharyngitis, tender anterior cervical nodes, a history of contact with a documented case of streptococcal infection, and a scarlatiniform rash. The concurrent findings of hoarseness, cough, or conjunctivitis make the diagnosis of streptococcal pharyngitis less likely.

The diagnosis of streptococcal pharyngitis can be confirmed by culture, but recovery of group A *Streptococcus* from the pharynx does not in itself differentiate the streptococcal carrier state from that in which streptococci are actually producing disease. A number of rapid techniques (ie, 5 to 60 minutes) for identifying group A streptococci in the upper respiratory tract are available commercially. These techniques involve extraction of the group-specific carbohydrate from the cell wall of the organism and subsequent identification of the organism by agglutination. Currently available data suggest that the specificity for these tests exceeds 90%, and the sensitivity ranges from 85% to 95%. These tests have the advantage of rapid identification of group A streptococci and are particularly appealing because more rapid treatment is clearly associated with an earlier clinical response. Rapid antigen detection tests can be useful in the detection of group A streptococci from streptococcal pyoderma-like lesions.

Clinically, the pharyngeal exudate of infectious mononucleosis tends to be thicker, whiter, and more extensive than that of streptococcal pharyngitis; the clinical impression of EBV infection can be confirmed by the heterophile "spot test" or other antibody determinations. Diphtheritic pharyngitis can be differentiated by the usually more adherent membrane and the extension of the membrane onto the uvula. The diphtheritic membrane is characterized by a sweet to fetid odor. Simultaneous infection with streptococci and *C diphtheriae* produces the clinical picture of bull-neck diphtheria.

In many patients with impetigo, group A $\beta$-hemolytic streptococci and *Staphylococcus aureus* can be isolated concurrently, but the primary invader is the streptococcus. Occasionally, the vesicles of chickenpox resemble those of a bullous impetigo, but the former are usually less transient and tend to involve the trunk more than the extremities. The lesions tend to itch, and the crusts are not as thick as those of streptococcal impetigo. However, the lesions of varicella can be infected secondarily with streptococci.

Humoral immune responses to a number of somatic components of the streptococcal cell have been demonstrated. Antibody to the M protein is particularly important, because it is the basis of immunity to or protection against reinfection from the same serologic type. Type-specific antibody also may be transferred from the mother to the fetus. The development of type-specific antibody can be inhibited by prompt treatment with penicillin.

Humoral antibody determinations are particularly useful in providing a strict method for defining streptococcal infection in certain clinical and epidemiologic situations and in supporting the possibility of a preceding streptococcal infection in patients with rheumatic fever or glomerulonephritis.

The antistreptolysin O (ASO) titer is the streptococcal antibody test employed most frequently. Because streptolysin O is also produced by groups C and G streptococci, the test is not specific for group A infection. The ASO response is weak in patients with streptococcal impetigo and pyoderma, but the anti-DNAase B and antihyaluronidase responses are good after skin and throat infections.

The Streptozyme agglutination test is based on the antibody agglutination of erythrocytes coated with a mixture of streptococcal extracellular antigens. This test has the appeal of speed, simplicity, and reaction with a variety of streptococcal antigens. Antibody responses measurable by this assay have been demonstrated within the first 7 to 10 days after the onset of infection. This contrasts with the development of neutralizing antibody titers to streptolysin O, which appear after 3 to 6 weeks, and to anti-DNAase B, which appear after 6 to 8 weeks. Because there have been problems with standardization of this reagent, producing variable results with different lots, this test should be interpreted with caution.

## TREATMENT

Penicillin remains the drug of choice for the treatment of group A $\beta$-hemolytic streptococcal infections unless the patient is allergic to this antibiotic. Although penicillin tolerance has been described in group A streptococci, its clinical significance has not been defined. Eradication of group A streptococci from the nasopharynx or the upper respiratory tract may be difficult because of $\beta$-lactamase-producing organisms in the nasopharynx, the production of inhibitory substances by other organisms that may influence the persistence of the group A *Streptococcus*, and the presence of group A streptococci that are tolerant to penicillin.

Erythromycin is the drug of choice in patients who are allergic to penicillin. Group A $\beta$-hemolytic streptococci resistant to erythromycin have been reported, but such resistance is rare except in Japan, where it has increased. Sulfonamides suppress but do not eradicate group A streptococci, and many group A streptococci are resistant to tetracycline.

The rationale for the use of penicillin in the treatment of streptococcal pharyngitis is to prevent the development of acute rheumatic fever. This can be accomplished with low-dose therapy maintained over a rather long period. Administration of a single intramuscular injection of benzathine penicillin G (600,000 U for children weighing less than 27 kg or 1.2 million U for children heavier than 27 kg or for adults) is another method of accomplishing this objective. Alternatively, penicillin V (125 to 250 mg) in three or four divided doses over 10 days is the treatment of choice. In patients who are allergic to penicillin, erythromycin in a dosage of 40 mg/kg/day in four divided doses should be used. Lincomycin (40 mg/kg/day) or clindamycin (30 mg/kg/day) can also be used for the treatment of streptococcal pharyngitis in patients who are allergic to penicillin. Other antibiotics that have been used successfully in the therapy of group A beta hemolytic streptococcal pharyngitis or tonsillitis include amoxicillin, amoxicillin with clavulanic acid, and several cephalosporins.

Patients with scarlet fever, streptococcal bacteremia, deep soft-tissue infections, erysipelas, pneumonia, or meningitis should be treated with penicillin parenterally, preferably intravenously. The dosage and duration of therapy must be based on the nature of the disease process, and daily dosages as high as 400,000 U/kg/day may be required in the most severe infections.

In patients with streptococcal impetigo, oral or parenteral penicillin or oral erythromycin in the dosages prescribed for the treatment of streptococcal pharyngitis should be used. The effectiveness of local skin care, such as removal of crusts and use of special bacteriostatic soaps, probably depends on the thoroughness with which such local care is carried out. These measures, coupled with the use of local antibiotic ointments, may be sufficient for the management of patients with a few skin lesions but are not recommended for those with more widespread impetigo. A topical antibiotic ointment (eg, mupirocin, Bactroban) has proved to be effective therapy for some patients with localized impetigo, even when parenteral therapy has not been initiated.

There is no proof that penicillin treatment reduces the frequency of nephritis after treatment of skin infections, and substantial clinical experience suggests that patients with skin infection due to a nephritogenic streptococcal strain may develop this complication despite penicillin therapy. One study suggests that penicillin therapy may lower the risk of this complication in patients with streptococcal pharyngitis caused by a nephritogenic strain.

## PREVENTION

No satisfactory method has yet been developed to prevent streptococcal disease by immunization. The spread of group A β-hemolytic streptococci is decreased by limiting the density of persons living within the home environment, isolating the contagious patient, and especially by antibiotic treatment of patients known to have this infection. For populations with streptococcal infection occurring at an epidemic level over an extended period (eg, selected military populations), it may be necessary to institute mass prophylaxis, usually with injections of benzathine penicillin.

The administration of penicillin prevents most cases of streptococcal disease if the drug is provided before the onset of symptoms. My colleagues and I obtain throat cultures from children who are close family contacts of patients with streptococcal disease. If cultures are positive, these contacts can be treated with oral penicillin G or V (400,000 U/dose) four times each day for 10 days.

## INFECTIONS DUE TO STREPTOCOCCI OTHER THAN GROUPS A AND B

The classification of streptococci can be confusing because of their separation on the basis of hemolysis and their separate identification by Lancefield typing. These two methods of iden-

---

**TABLE 56-22.** Correlation of Streptococci Identified by Lancefield Grouping and Hemolytic Reactions With Sites of Human Colonization and Disease

| Lancefield Group | Species | Usual Reaction on Sheep Blood Agar | Usual Human Habitat | Most Common Human Disease |
|---|---|---|---|---|
| A | S pyogenes | β-hemolysis | Pharynx, skin, rectum | Pharyngitis, erysipelas, impetigo, septicemia, wound infections, rheumatic fever, acute glomerulonephritis, necrotizing fasciitis, cellulitis, otitis media, meningitis, pneumonia, conjunctivitis, acute endocarditis |
| B | S agalactiae | β-hemolysis | Pharynx, vagina | Puerperal sepsis, endocarditis, neonatal sepsis, meningitis, otitis media, osteomyelitis, pneumonia |
| C | S equi equisimilis dysgalactiae zooepidemicus | β-hemolysis | Pharynx, vagina, skin | Wound infection, puerperal sepsis, cellulitis, endocarditis |
| D | S faecalis* faecium* bovis* equinus | γ | Colon contents | Endocarditis, urinary tract infection, biliary tract infection, intestinal infection, peritonitis |
| E | S infrequens | ? | ? | ? |
| F | S minutus anginosus | β-hemolysis | Mouth, pharynx | Sinusitis, meningitis, brain abscess, pneumonia |
| G | S cariis | β-hemolysis | Pharynx, vagina, skin | Puerperal infection, skin or wound infection, endocarditis |
| H | S sanguist† | α-hemolysis | Mouth | Endocarditis, brain abscess |
| K | S salivarius† | α-hemolysis | Mouth | Endocarditis, sinusitis, meningitis, brain abscess |
| L | | β- or α-hemoylsis | Mouth | Endocarditis, abscess, parotitis, neonatal sepsis |
| M | | β- or α-hemoylsis | Mouth, pharynx, vagina | Endocarditis, septicemia |
| N | S lactis-cremoris | α- or γ-hemolysis | Pharynx | ?Meningitis, ?septicemia |
| O | | α- or β-hemolysis | Pharynx, conjunctiva, vagina | Pneumonia, endocarditis, septicemia |
| Nontypable | S viridans | α-hemolysis | Pharynx | Endocarditis |
| Nontypable | S mutans | α-hemolysis | Pharynx | Endocarditis |

\* "Enterococcus."

† These organisms are frequently isolated from the bloodstream as α-hemolytic streptococci. Along with many nongroupable α streptococci, they are often called *S. viridans*, a term that incorrectly implies a specific species. Nevertheless, as a group, they cause most episodes of endocarditis and are usually exquisitely sensitive to penicillin.

*Reproduced with permission, from Keusch GT, Weinstein L: Streptococcal Disease, Kalamazoo, MI: Upjohn Company.*

tification are not mutually exclusive; Table 56-22 shows classification of streptococci by Lancefield type and by the hemolytic reactions on blood agar and their correlation with human colonization and disease.

As early as 1938, hemolytic streptococci belonging to Lancefield group B (see Chapter 20.15.2) were related causally to severe human disease. Group B streptococcal infection is discussed elsewhere.

Human infections with streptococci groups C to H and K to O and with nontypable strains have been reported in normal infants and children. The classification of these organisms and infections with which they have been associated are shown in Table 56-22. With the exception of group D streptococci (ie, enterococci) and several $\alpha$-hemolytic strains, penicillin G provides effective therapy for non–group-A streptococci. Enterococci are susceptible to ampicillin.

Bacterial endocarditis in children may be related to *Streptococcus viridans*. Some *S viridans* organisms require vitamin $B_6$ or thiol compounds for optimal growth, and supplemental media are necessary for their isolation and sensitivity testing. Some of these organisms are tolerant or relatively tolerant to penicillin, and therapy with penicillin and aminoglycosides is recommended until the results of sensitivity studies are available. If endocarditis is caused by enterococci, therapy with ampicillin plus an aminoglycoside is recommended.

## Selected Readings

Feder HM Jr, Olsen N, McLaughlin JC, et al. Bacterial enterocervicitis caused by vitamin $B_6$-dependent viridans group streptococcus. Pediatrics 1980;66:309.

Gerber MA, Randolph NA, DeMeo KK, et al. The effect of antibiotic therapy on the clinical course of streptococcal pharyngitis. J Pediatr 1985;106:870.

Gerber MA, Spodaccini LJ, Wright LL. Latex agglutination tests for the rapid identification of Group A streptococci directly from throat swabs. J Pediatr 1984;105:702.

Kaplan EL. The group A streptococcal upper respiratory tract carrier state: an enigma. J Pediatr 1980;97:337.

Kaplan EL, Wannamaker LW. Group A streptococcal infections. In: Feigin RD, Cherry JD, eds. Textbook of infectious diseases, ed 3. Philadelphia: WB Saunders, 1992:1296.

Kavey RW, Kaplan EL. Resurgence of acute rheumatic fever. Pediatrics 1989;84:585.

Kim KS. Clinical perspectives on penicillin tolerance. J Pediatr 1988;112:509.

Rammelkamp CH Jr. Epidemiology of streptococcal infections. Harvey Lect 1957;51:113.

Schaffner W, Lefkowitz LB Jr, Goodman JS, et al. Hospital outbreak of infections with group A streptococci traced to an asymptomatic anal carrier. N Engl J Med 1969;280:1224.

Siegel AC, Johnson EE, Stollerman GH. Controlled studies of streptococcal pharyngitis in the pediatric population I. Factors related to the attack rate of rheumatic fever. N Engl J Med 1961;265:559.

Stetson CA, Rammelkamp CH Jr, Krause RM, et al. Epidemic acute nephritis: studies on etiology, natural history and prevention. Medicine (Baltimore) 1955;34:431.

Stevens DL, Tanner MH, Winship J, et al. Severe group A streptococcal infections associated with a toxic shock-like syndrome and scarlet fever toxin A. N Engl J Med 1989;321:1.

Wannamaker LW. Differences between streptococcal infections of the throat and of the skin. N Engl J Med 1970;282:23.

*Principles and Practice of Pediatrics, Second Edition.*
edited by Frank A. Oski et al. J. B. Lippincott Company, Philadelphia © 1994.

# 56.26 *Tularemia*

Richard F. Jacobs

Tularemia is an acute, febrile, zoonotic illness caused by the gram-negative bacterium *Francisella tularensis*. It is widely distributed in the Northern Hemisphere, with numerous infections occurring in humans over relatively large areas of the United States, Europe, and Asia. It is a disease of small animals, but humans are highly susceptible hosts.

## MICROBIOLOGY

*Francisella tularensis* is a small, nonmotile, gram-negative coccobacillary organism that requires cysteine for growth. In 1959, the division of *Francisella tularensis* into *Francisella tularensis* subspecies *tularensis* (type A) and *Francisella tularensis* subspecies *palaearctica* (type B) became the official nomenclature.

*F tularensis tularensis* was believed to be confined to North America and is highly virulent, causing severe disease in mammals and mild to severe disease in humans. *F tularensis palaearctica* has been identified in Asia, Europe, and North America. The species is frequently linked to water-borne disease of rodents and appears to be less virulent in mammals. Descriptions of strains of the organism in Central Asia and Japan added further complexity to the subspecies differentiation. It appears that the biochemical characteristics and virulence of *F tularensis* strains do not reflect their genetic character, as judged by molecular techniques using 16S rRNA. Strains isolated from the Central Asian

area of the former Soviet Union and Japan belong to genotype A, despite the fact that the virulence and some of the biochemical characteristics conform to those of the genotype B strains. This means that strains of *F tularensis* subspecies *tularensis* are not restricted to the North American continent, but it does not exclude the possibility that highly virulent strains of the organism are restricted to North America.

The organism can be cultured on media using glucose-cysteine agar, a temperature of 37°C, and a pH of 6.9, but selected media may be necessary for optimal growth. Clinicians should be aware that the organism does grow on routine blood and wound cultures (eg, lymph node aspirate) and that this may present a health hazard in the microbiology laboratory due to aerosolization among laboratory workers. Clinicians should notify the laboratory if tularemia is included in the differential diagnosis. All strains of *F tularensis* seem to be serologically identical. Despite this serologic homogeneity, future epidemiologic studies will use molecular identification using 16S rRNA to divide the isolates into genotype A and genotype B.

## EPIDEMIOLOGY

Tularemia is a ubiquitous organism found in the Northern Hemisphere between 30° and 71° northern latitude. It has been reported throughout the United States, but it occurs most commonly in the western and south central states, with the highest incidence in regions of Oklahoma, Missouri, Arkansas, Louisiana, Tennessee, Texas, Illinois, and Virginia. Although the incidence peaks during the late spring through summer months, the year-round distribution of cases probably reflects the multiple vectors of transmission of this organism (Fig 56-6). The major vector of *F tularensis* is the tick, and the disease is seen primarily in children and young adults during the major tick season of spring, summer, and early fall. It is transmitted to humans by vector bites (eg, ticks, lice, fleas, deer flies, mosquitoes), animal bites, and ingestion

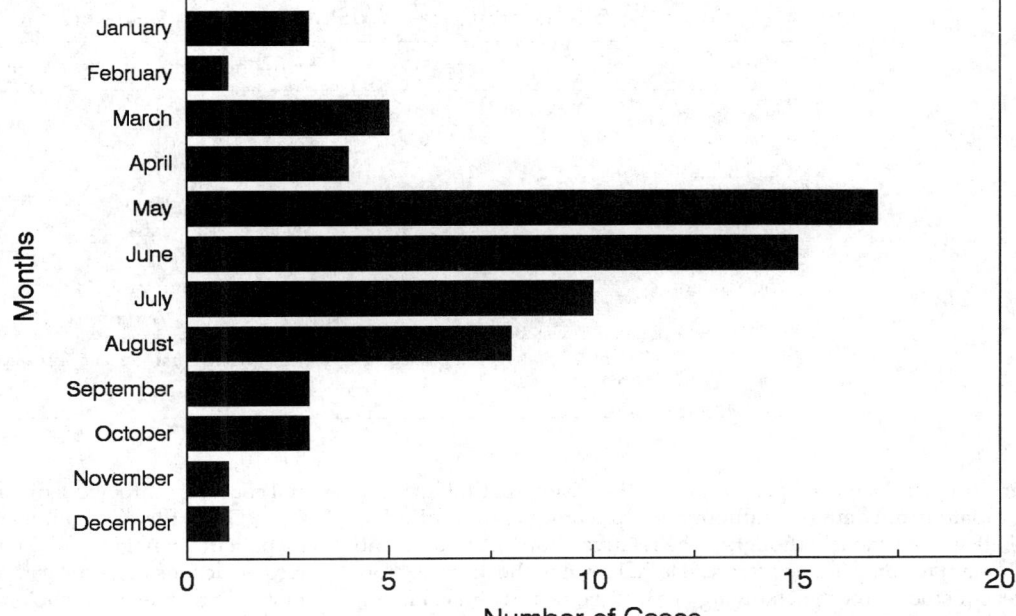

**Figure 56-6.** Distribution of tularemia cases in children. (Adapted from Jacobs RF, Condrey YM, Yamauchi T. Tularemia in adults and children: a changing presentation. Pediatrics 1985;76:818.

of infected, inadequately cooked animal tissues or contaminated water. Inhalation of the organisms, which occurs primarily while skinning animal carcasses and working with the organism in the microbiology laboratory, has been identified as a common cause of tularemia pneumonia. It may be mechanically transferred by claws or teeth of domestic pets that have preyed on infected animals. Rabbits, hares, muskrats, voles, rats, and mice harbor *F tularensis*. Cases of infection in older children and adults in the winter months are typically associated with rabbit or deer hunting or contamination through contact with infected animal tissues.

Contrary to earlier reports of tularemia as "rabbit fever," tick exposure is the vector for 71% of pediatric and adults cases. The reported incidence of rabbit exposure is not different for adults (11%) and children (7%). Tularemia in children has been documented after a cat bite, squirrel bite, and exposure to other domestic animals.

## PATHOGENESIS

*F tularensis* gains access to the human body through the skin, conjunctiva, oropharynx, respiratory tract, or gastrointestinal tract. It spreads by lymphatics or hematogenously, and bacteremia usually develops during the first week of infection. Skin, regional lymph nodes, liver, spleen, and lungs can be involved, and the lesions can occur in the gastrointestinal tract and the central nervous system.

The classic lesion is one of focal necrosis and granuloma formation. After a tick bite, the resultant eschar, ulcer, or papule with regional lymphadenitis is a hallmark presentation for *F tularensis* infection. The organism elicits humoral and cell-mediated immune responses, but seroconversion may take 1 or 2 weeks after infection. Although there have been reports of recurrent disease, the initial attack of *F tularensis* usually confers lasting immunity.

## CLINICAL MANIFESTATIONS

The average incubation period for tularemia is 3 to 4 days (range, 1 to 21 days). The onset of symptoms is usually abrupt, with a temperature usually greater than 39.4°C (103°F), chills, pharyngitis, myalgias, arthralgias, nausea, and vomiting, and patients occasionally have headaches, a cough, and photophobia. The predominant signs of tularemia include lymphadenopathy, an ulcer, eschar, or papule at the site of tick embedment, and hepatosplenomegaly; some patients develop conjunctivitis (Table 56-23). In untreated cases of tularemia, fever may persist for 2 to 3 weeks or longer. There is no characteristic peripheral blood profile for tularemia. A variety of skin rashes have been described, but the predominant feature is that of regional lymphadenopathy or lymphadenitis. Subcutaneous nodules have been reported.

In one study, fever developed in 87% of children, with 48% having temperatures greater than 39.4°C. The mean temperature peak for these patients was 39.2°C (range, 38.3°C to 41.7°C), and the mean duration of fever was 19.4 days (range, 3 to 60 days).

Th classification of six forms of tularemia depends on the portal of entry. The most common forms of tularemia are ulceroglandular and glandular, in which organisms gain access through the skin, usually after a tick bite. Approximately 2 days after the onset of symptoms, the regional lymph nodes become tender and swollen. Within 24 hours, a painful, swollen papule develops distal to the regional nodes. This papule ruptures and progresses to ulceration and eschar. In untreated cases, the ulcer may become indolent, and the lymph nodes may suppurate and drain. In children, regional lymphadenopathy is typically seen in the cervical area, and in adults, it occurs in the inguinal area, probably reflecting the most frequent sites of tick bites. Generalized lymphadenopathy, although uncommon, has been described in cases of tularemia. Glandular tularemia is identical to the ulceroglandular form, except that the portal of entry cannot be identified. The other four forms of tularemia are relatively uncommon compared with the ulceroglandular and glandular types (see Table 56-23). In oculoglandular tularemia, the portal of entry is typically the conjunctival sac. Numerous sharply defined nodules or ulcers are apparent on the palpebral conjunctivae, and regional nodes in the preauricular area are involved, developing as a Parinaud's complex.

After *F tularensis* invades the oropharyngeal route (ie, oropharyngeal tularemia), local involvement consists of pharyngitis, acute tonsillitis, and cervical adenitis. Complaints of sore throat

TABLE 56-23. Clinical Types and Presentation of Tularemia in Children

| Clinical Type | Percentage (%) | Signs and Symptoms* | Percentage (%) |
|---|---|---|---|
| Ulceroglandular | 45 | Lymphadenopathy | 96 |
| Glandular | 25 | Fever (≥38.3 °C) | 87 |
| Oculoglandular | 2 | Pharyngitis | 43 |
| Pneumonic | 14 | Ulcer, eschar, papule | 45 |
| Oropharyngeal | 4 | Myalgias, arthralgias | 39 |
| Typhoidal | 2 | Nausea, vomiting | 35 |
| Unclassified | 6 | Hepatosplenomegaly | 35 |

* Additional signs and symptoms: headache (9%), cough (9%), diarrhea (4%), conjunctivitis (4%).
Adapted from Jacobs RF, Condrey YM, Yamauchi T. Tularemia in adults and children: a changing presentation. Pediatrics 1985;76:818.

are frequently out of proportion to the visible pathology, and exudate is uncommon. Although the pneumonic form of tularemia was previously thought to be relatively rare in children and thought to comprise a severe and lethal form of the disease, more recent studies on the changing epidemiology and clinical manifestations of this disease have shown that pneumonic tularemia is not uncommon. In one study, 14% of children younger than 19 years of age with confirmed tularemia had abnormal chest roentgenograms and were diagnosed with pneumonia. Although most of these children had other clinical forms of tularemia, approximately one third presented with isolated pneumonias unresponsive to traditional antibiotic therapy. The typhoidal form of tularemia is uncommon in children. In typhoidal tularemia, invasion is secondary to ingestion of the causative agent, and there are necrotic lesions throughout the gastrointestinal tract. This form of the disease may present as a fever of unknown origin. The distribution of the clinical manifestations of tularemia in children in one large series was 45% ulceroglandular, 25% glandular, 14% pneumonic, 4% oropharyngeal, and 2% oculoglandular and typhoidal, and 6% of the cases remained unclassified.

## DIAGNOSIS

The diagnosis of tularemia is suggested by the history and aided by the physician's awareness in endemic areas. In nonendemic areas, the diagnosis of tularemia may be difficult. History of contact, although often unavailable, should take into account the season of the year, the clinical manifestations of the disease, the unresponsive nature to antibiotics not effective against tularemia, and the endemic rate of disease in that area.

The diagnosis is confirmed by serologic tests. The commercially available standard agglutination test is preferred and reliable. Unfortunately, it does not provide a diagnosis early in the course of disease. Agglutinating antibody titers often are not detectable until the second week of illness (days 10 to 14). In some cases, seroconversion has not been described until 4 to 6 weeks of illness. In rare cases, patients may never exhibit agglutinating antibodies. A fourfold increase in the specific agglutination titer confirms the diagnosis, but a presumptive diagnosis should be considered with acute titers of greater than or equal to 1 : 160. This titer may indicate current or past infection, but in a clinically compatible case, it should be considered an indication for presumptive therapy. Patients with active disease often develop titers of greater than or equal to 1 : 1280 as the initial manifestation of seroconversion. Other laboratory studies, including a complete blood

cell count, erythrocyte sedimentation rate, urinalysis, and *Proteus* OX2/OX19 titers are not useful in establishing the diagnosis or in patient management. The agglutination test is specific, but cross-reactions do occur with *Brucella* species and have been seen in recent recipients of cholera vaccine. Other serologic tests (eg, enzyme-linked immunosorbent assay, lymphocyte stimulation, antigen detection in urine) have been reliable and confirm the diagnosis early in disease. These tests are not generally available. The Foshay skin test is a relatively accurate and early method of diagnosis, but it is not commercially available.

Gram-stained smears of material from exudates, lymph node aspirates, or sputum do not reveal the organism reliably, but they are useful, because positive smears may rule out other bacterial pathogens. Lymph nodes aspirates from patients with cervical lymphadenitis may be Gram stained safely in the laboratory, and if gram-positive cocci in chains or clusters are identified, the most likely diagnosis of pyogenic cervical lymphadenitis caused by *Staphylococcus aureus* or group A β-hemolytic streptococcus can be confirmed. Cultures of *F tularensis* should not be performed in the usual diagnostic microbiology laboratory because of the danger of aerosolization to laboratory personnel. If confirmation by culture is indicated, appropriate laboratory precautions, with notification of the laboratory of the potential for the specimen to contain *F tularensis*, is the duty of the clinician. Appropriate laboratory precautions can then be maintained, and State Health Department laboratories can perform direct fluorescent antibody testing to confirm the identification of the organisms as *F tularensis*.

The differential diagnosis of tularemia depends on the clinical form of the infection. Ulceroglandular and glandular tularemia must be differentiated from disease due to *Staphylococcus aureus*, *Streptococcus*, *Mycobacterium tuberculosis*, atypical *Mycobacterium*, and the cat-scratch bacillus. In cases of inguinal lymphadenopathy, the diagnosis of lymphogranuloma venereum, granuloma inguinale, and other ulcer adenopathy sexually transmitted diseases should be considered in older patients. Sporotrichosis and infectious mononucleosis are occasionally diagnosed in these patients. Oculoglandular tularemia is more distinctive, but disease due to common pathogens must be excluded. Oropharyngeal tularemia must be differentiated from streptococcal tonsillopharyngitis and corynebacterial disease. Typhoidal tularemia resembles bacteremia and must be differentiated from other more traditional bacterial and enteric diseases and from classic typhoid fever. Tularemia pneumonia may present a significant clinical challenge to the physician. Tularemia pneumonia must be differentiated from other bacterial forms of pneumonia and other forms of lower respiratory tract infection unresponsive to traditional antibiotic therapy. These include *Mycoplasma pneumoniae*,

*Chlamydia pneumoniae, Legionella*, psittacosis, Q fever, fungal infections, viral pneumonia, and rickettsial infections.

## TREATMENT

Streptomycin is classically considered the drug of choice. The recommendation for 30 to 40 mg/kg/day divided into two daily intramuscular injections for a 7-day course is effective. An alternative regimen is streptomycin at a dosage of 30 to 40 mg/kg/day administered intramuscularly for the first 3 days, with subsequent reduction to 15 to 20 mg/kg/day given intramuscularly for the final 4 days. In severe cases or if a child does not establish an afebrile, asymptomatic course within a few days, extension of treatment beyond 7 days is indicated and should be based on clinical assessment. There are reported streptomycin-resistant strains, but they are rare. Defervescence and symptomatic response is prompt, usually within several days. The response may be somewhat delayed if the lymph nodes have progressed to suppuration. Because of the recent shortage of streptomycin within the United States, gentamicin may have to be used. In hospitalized children, intravenous gentamicin at standard dosages of 2.5 mg/kg/dose given every 8 hours for 7 days can be used. If clinical defervescence does occur, outpatient management with intramuscular gentamicin can be pursued. The streptomycin guidelines for length of therapy with time to defervescence and symptom relief should be used in gentamicin therapy.

Although tetracycline and chloramphenicol have activity against *F tularensis*, they are considered to be poor alternatives for children. Although reconsideration of the use of tetracycline in children younger than 8 years of age has been proposed, tetracycline at a dosage of 25 to 50 mg/kg/day, divided four times daily; doxycycline at a dosage of 2 to 4 mg/kg/day, divided twice daily; and chloramphenicol at a dosage of 50 mg/kg/day, divided four times daily, have been used successfully as alternative regimens. Anecdotal reports of an unacceptable rate of relapse of clinical symptoms after discontinuation of tetracycline or chloramphenicol indicate that they should not be used as the standard therapy in children. However, children treated successfully with tetracycline or chloramphenicol with a differential diagnosis that included tick-borne infections (eg, *Rickettsia*) should not be routinely given streptomycin or gentamicin after confirmation of serologic tests for tularemia. The parents should be counseled that relapses have occurred, and if relapse does occur with symptomatic disease, streptomycin or gentamicin should be initiated at that point. Other antibiotics with acceptable in vitro minimal inhibitory concentrations (Table 56-24) have not been proven effective.

The major adverse reaction to streptomycin in children is ototoxicity. Children should be monitored for tinnitus, which indicates the need for a reduction of the daily dose. Hearing screening before initiation of streptomycin or gentamicin therapy should be considered. If there is already hearing loss, the alternative streptomycin regimen or gentamicin therapy with monitoring of serum levels in severe cases can be considered. Audiologic evaluation is indicated after therapy in these cases.

In one study, no deaths occurred in a series of pediatric patients, but suppurative adenitis occurred in 16% of the overall population, with late suppuration after antibiotic therapy occurring in 33% of children with the ulceroglandular or glandular forms. Surgical intervention was required for 19 of these patients, which included repeated needle aspiration in 7, incision and drainage in 8, and excisional biopsy in 4 patients. Cultures of late suppurative nodes did not yield *F tularensis*, and in asymptomatic patients, specimens from the nodes should not be cultured or evaluated.

**TABLE 56-24. Antibiotic Susceptibility to *Francisella tularensis***

| Antibiotic | MIC$_{50}$* ($\mu$g/mL) |
|---|---|
| Penicillin | >8.0 |
| Ampicillin | >8.0 |
| Tetracycline | 2.0 |
| Chloramphenicol | 1.0 |
| Streptomycin | 2.0 |
| Gentamicin | 1.0 |
| Cefotaxime | 2.0 |
| Ceftriaxone | 2.0 |

* MIC$_{50}$ is the concentration ($\mu$g/mL) at which 50% of the isolates are inhibited.

*Adapted from Baker CN, Hollis DG, Thornsberry C. Antimicrobial susceptibility testing of* Francisella tularensis *using a modified Mueller-Hinton broth.* J Clin Microbiol 1985;22:212.

Supportive therapy is indicated for severely ill patients. Although uncommon, patients with typhoidal or pneumonic tularemia with bacteremia have presented with sepsis or the sepsis syndrome. Appropriate monitoring and intensive care therapy are indicated for these patients. The prognosis for appropriately treated patients is excellent. The clinical course of the illness is usually less than 1 month. The mortality rate is less than 1%, except in the subgroups of fulminant pneumonia or typhoidal tularemia.

## PREVENTION

Prevention of human tularemia depends on the prevention of contact with vectors and protection during the handling of contaminated animal tissues. Children should be cautioned against handling sick or dead rabbits or rodents. Rabbit or rodent carcasses should be disposed of by burial or incineration. Rubber gloves should be worn when preparing game animals. Children who live in tick-infested areas should have their skin and hair checked frequently for the presence of ticks, which should be removed carefully and appropriately. Children in an area of tick endemicity should wear clothing with tightly fitting cuffs at the ankles and wrists. Common tick repellents to prevent the attachment and feeding of ticks on children can be used cautiously.

The only tularemia vaccine available in the United States is an attenuated live vaccine that is unlicensed and classified as an investigational product. It is reserved for persons in constant contact with *F tularensis* organisms. Physicians who have patients at risk can obtain information about the vaccine from the Centers for Disease Control and Prevention.

## Suggested Readings

Baker CN, Hollis DG, Thornsberry C. Antimicrobial susceptibility testing of *Francisella tularensis* using a modified Mueller-Hinton broth. J Clin Microbiol 1985;22:212.
Dienst FT Jr. Tularemia: a perusal of 339 cases. J La State Med Soc 1963;115:114.
Jacobs RF, Condrey YM, Yamauchi T. Tularemia in adults and children: a changing presentation. Pediatrics 1985;76:818.
Jacobs RF, Narain JP. Tularemia in children. Pediatr Infect Dis 1983;1:487.
Jacobs RF. Tularemia. In: Nelson JD, ed. Current therapy in pediatric infectious diseases. St. Louis: C. V. Mosby Co. 1986:197.
Mason WL, Figelsbach HT, Little SF, et al. Treatment of tularemia, including pulmonary tularemia with gentamicin. Am Rev Respir Dis 1980;121:39.
Pullen RL, Stuart BM. Tularemia analysis of 225 cases. JAMA 1945;129:495.
Sandstrom G, Sjostedt A, Forsman M, Pavlovich NV, Mishankin BN. Characterization and classification of strains of *Francisella tularensis* isolated in the Central Asian focus of the Soviet Union and in Japan. J Clin Microbiol 1992;30:172.

*Principles and Practice of Pediatrics, Second Edition.*
edited by Frank A. Oski et al. J. B. Lippincott Company, Philadelphia © 1994.

# 56.27 *Syphilis*

M. Melisse Sloas and Christian C. Patrick

Syphilis, a venereal disease of adolescence and adulthood, is of major importance in pediatrics as a congenital infection. Humans are the sole natural host of the etiologic agent of syphilis, *Treponema pallidum.*

Syphilis was recognized as a disease in Europe during the 15th century. Although *T pallidum* was described in 1905, symptoms specific to syphilis were not determined until 1938 because of frequent dual infection with gonorrhea.

## MICROBIOLOGY

*T pallidum* is a member of the order Spirochaetales, which includes five genera; *Treponema, Borrelia,* and *Leptospira* are pathogenic in humans. *T pallidum* is a motile, helical organism that is 0.09 to 0.5 $\mu$m wide and 5 to 20 $\mu$m long. The outer surfaces have polar flagella that wind around the organism. It multiplies by transverse fission.

*T pallidum* is a gram-negative organism but is considered gram indeterminate because its size is below the resolution of the light microscope. Its integument comprises an inner cytoplasmic layer, a cell wall, and an outer envelope. Structural and host-parasite studies are hampered by the inability to grow *T pallidum* in vitro. Although treponeme cultivation in selected tissue cultures has been reported, most studies rely on material from intratesticularly inoculated rabbits.

## EPIDEMIOLOGY

Syphilis is classified as acquired and congenital forms. Acquired syphilis has primary, secondary, and tertiary (ie, late) stages; congenital syphilis is divided into early and late stages. Acquired by adolescents and adults most often by sexual contact, syphilis is rarely transmitted by nonsexual, direct contact with an infectious lesion. Congenital syphilis occurs by transplacental passage of *T pallidum* from an infected mother to her infant or by contact with an infectious lesion in the birth canal.

The incidence of acquired syphilis peaks in persons who are 15 to 30 years of age, coinciding with increased sexual activity. The typical patient profile is that of a sexually promiscuous person with more than five sexual encounters within the incubation period. Syphilis occurs more often in blacks than in whites. Dual infection with gonorrhea occurs in 8% of the cases.

Figure 56-7 shows the number of cases of primary and secondary acquired syphilis per 100,000 women from 1970 to 1990, as reported by the Centers for Disease Control (CDC). The incidence of syphilis reached a nadir around 1977 and was relatively stable until 1987, when there was a sharp increase (ie, 34,834 reported cases compared with 26,818 in 1986). The incidence of syphilis has continued to rise yearly, with over 50,000 cases reported in 1990. The increase is largely the result of the crack cocaine epidemic, in which trading sex for drugs, multiple sexual partners, and poor prenatal care are common.

Figure 56-7 shows the steady increase in the number of cases of congenital syphilis reported to the CDC. This reflects the increase in syphilis among women of child-bearing age and a change in the CDC's case definition of congenital syphilis in 1989.

## PATHOGENESIS

Syphilis is acquired when *T pallidum* penetrates the skin or mucous membrane at a site of exposure. The organism multiplies locally and is spread by the perivascular lymphatic system to the systemic circulation, which disseminates the infection widely even before a primary lesion is evident. Within 3 to 4 weeks, a local inflammatory response is initiated as a result of an invasion by mononuclear leukocytes and plasma cells. This response produces a red, ulcerated lesion with surrounding induration: the chancre. A concomitant cellular proliferation in the regional lymph nodes produces adenopathy.

Secondary lesions of syphilis, a consequence of dissemination, are caused by an inflammatory response in ectodermal tissue of

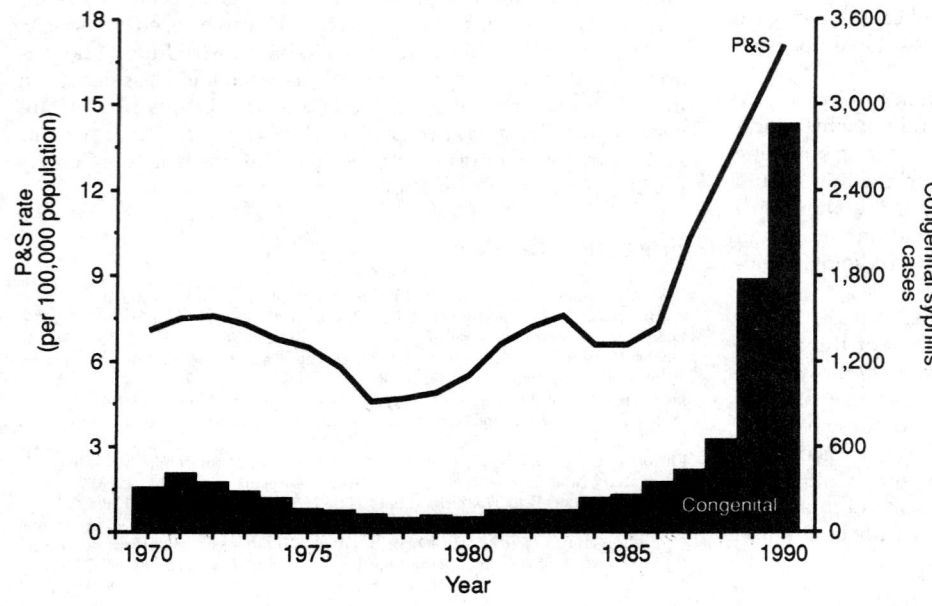

**Figure 56-7.** Incidence of primary and secondary (P&S) syphilis among women per 100,000 population, 1970 through 1990. Bars show the number of cases of congenital syphilis for the same period. (Centers for Disease Control. Graphs and maps for selected notifiable diseases in the United States MMWR 1991;39:42.)

skin, mucous membranes, and the central nervous system (CNS). The host response in these lesions is similar to that in primary lesions.

Tertiary syphilis is caused by the host's hypersensitivity response. This stage is characterized by a diffuse chronic inflammatory response.

Congenital syphilis was previously thought to occur only after 5 months of gestation because of the impediment to transplacental passage of treponemes by Langerhans' cells, which regress after that point. It is now believed that congenital syphilis becomes evident after the fourth month of gestation when immunologic competence begins to develop. The transplacental passage of *T pallidum* occurs during maternal spirochetemia and causes the wide dissemination of the organism in the fetus. The organs most severely affected include bone, brain, liver, lung, and skeletal system. The placenta shows histologic changes, including focal villositis.

## CLINICAL MANIFESTATIONS

The stages of acquired syphilis are based on the different clinical manifestations and underlying pathophysiology. The hallmark of primary syphilis is the chancre, a skin lesion that appears at an inoculation site after a mean incubation period of 21 days (range, 3 to 90 days). The chancre, usually single and nontender, occurs most often on the genitalia and is associated with nontender lymphadenopathy. Regional lymphadenopathy is particularly important in females with a cervical chancre, because the chancre may be the only sign or symptom of syphilis. Primary syphilis heals spontaneously in 3 to 12 weeks.

Symptoms of secondary syphilis appear 6 to 8 weeks after the onset of primary syphilis and are caused by the dissemination of treponemes. The symptoms include low-grade fever, malaise, and diffuse lymphadenopathy. The most notable manifestation is dermatologic, with macular, maculopapular, papular, or pustular lesions that invariably harbor infectious treponemes. The classic rash of this stage is generalized and maculopapular, involving the palms and soles. Secondary syphilis may cause condylomata lata (ie, hypertrophic papular skin lesions found in moist areas, such as the anus or vulva). Neurologic manifestations of meningeal and cranial or spinal nerve involvement appear during secondary syphilis but are reversible with proper therapy. Immune complexes comprising treponemal antigen, fibronectin, antibody, and complement are implicated in the pathogenesis of iritis, anterior uveitis, arthritis, and nephrotic syndrome.

A latent period, defined by positive syphilis serology with no evidence of disease, follows the secondary stage. Patients are immune to reinfection during the latent period.

Tertiary syphilis occurs after a latent period of at least 1 year (usually 3 to 10 years). The classic lesion of tertiary syphilis, called the gumma, comprises a necrotic center surrounded by giant cells with epithelioid cells. The pathogenesis of these lesions is unknown but probably represents a cell-mediated immune response. Involvement of nonvital structures, such as skin, soft tissue, and bone, which is called benign late syphilis, represents 15% of the cases of late syphilis. Cardiovascular syphilis, including syphilitic aortitis with medial necrosis, occurs in 10% of the patients with late syphilis. Neurosyphilis, with multiple presentations that may include tabes dorsalis, paresis, meningitis, or transverse myelitis, develops in 7% of the patients with late syphilis.

Although as many as two thirds of the newborns with congenital syphilis are asymptomatic at birth, early congenital syphilis can affect many organ systems by widespread dissemination of the organisms from maternal spirochetemia. Hepatosplenomegaly occurs in more than 90% of the affected infants, although liver function tests are usually normal. Generalized lymphadenopathy,

including epitrochlear adenopathy, is evident in as many as 50% of the infants and is nonsuppurative. Mucocutaneous lesions produce snuffles (ie, a rhinitis) after the first week of life; the purulent and blood-tinged nasal discharge teems with spirochetes. The nasal cartilage destruction can lead to a saddle nose deformity. The dermatologic lesions consist of pemphigus syphiliticus, condylomata lata, or the classic copper-brown maculopapular rash on the palms and soles. Ocular involvement most commonly presents as chorioretinitis, but congenital glaucoma and uveitis are also seen. CNS disease usually occurs after the neonatal period and ranges from acute syphilitic leptomeningitis to a chronic meningovascular neurosyphilis (Fig 56-8). Pneumonia alba, a fibrotic pneumonia, is seen in congenital syphilis (see Fig 56-8). A slowly resolving, diffuse pulmonic infiltrate may also be documented on the chest radiograph.

The organ system most frequently involved is the skeletal system. Involvement is usually multiple and symmetric and affects the metaphyses and diaphyses of long bones (Fig 56-9). Pain associated with bony involvement can lead to pseudoparalysis (ie, pseudoparalysis of Parrot).

The clinical manifestations of late congenital syphilis may be caused by the changes of progression from early congenital syphilis or by hypersensitivity reactions. Dental anomalies include Hutchinson teeth (ie, notched incisors) and mulberry molars. Eye involvement leads to interstitial keratitis between 4 and 30 years of age, secondary glaucoma, or corneal scarring. Eighth nerve deafness can develop, usually between 8 and 10 years of age. The Hutchinson triad comprises Hutchinson teeth, interstitial keratitis, and eighth nerve deafness. More than 75% of the patients have at least one of these manifestations. The scars that remain after the occurrence of snuffles in early congenital syphilis are called rhagades. Clutton joints are symmetric synovial effusions, usually localized to the knees. Another lesion of bone and joints, saber shins, is secondary to persistent periostitis. A classic sign of late congenital syphilis is perforation of the hard palate. CNS involvement can include meningovascular disease and paresis.

## DIAGNOSIS

Syphilis is diagnosed by clinical findings and direct identification of treponemes in clinical specimens or positive findings on treponemal-specific or nonspecific serology (Table 56-25). The definitive laboratory diagnosis is made by direct visualization of treponemes in exudate by darkfield microscopy. A fluorescent antibody technique is also available. The specimen is usually obtained from a skin lesion in primary, secondary, or congenital syphilis.

The serologic diagnosis of syphilis is accomplished by tests specific for *T pallidum* or its components and by nonspecific, nontreponemal tests that rely on reagins, which are antibodies directed against lipoidal antigens found on treponemal and mammalian cells. The fluorescent treponemal antibody absorption (FTA-ABS) tests and the treponemal-specific microhemagglutination (MHA-TP) tests are positive in more than 85% of the patients with primary syphilis and in 100% of the patients with secondary syphilis. The sensitivity of the treponemal-specific serologic tests results in fewer false positives than do nontreponemal serologic tests. They are also positive earlier in the disease. The disadvantages of using treponemal-specific tests include greater expense and longer assay times, and the FTA-ABS cannot be titered. Investigational tests, such as the Western blot or polymerase chain reaction, may increase the degree of sensitivity and specificity attained.

The nontreponemal tests involve detection of antibodies to cardiolipin, a component of membranes and mammalian tissue.

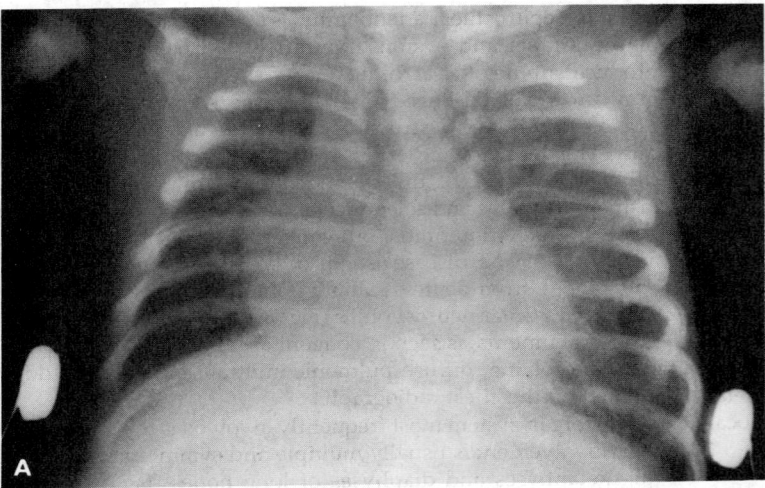

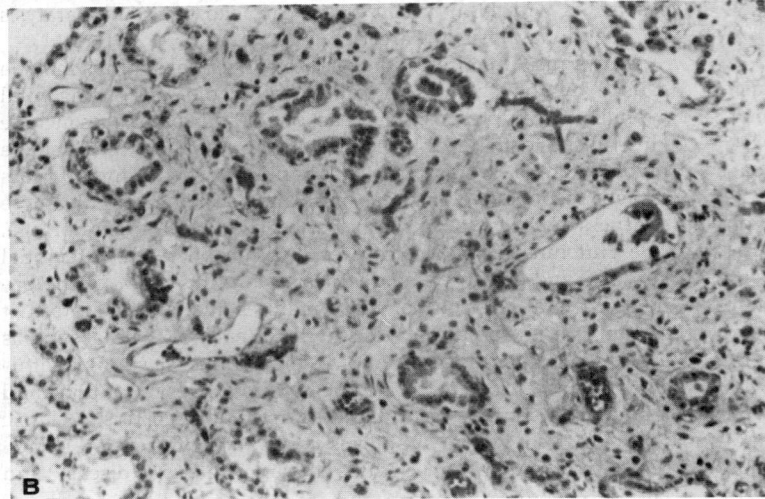

**Figure 56-8.** (**A**) Chest radiograph of an infant with congenital syphilis pneumonia. There are no distinguishing characteristics to differentiate bacterial or certain viral pneumonias of infancy. (Courtesy of Dr. Milton Wagner.) (**B**) Histologic section from a more extensive pneumonia than evident in **A.** Notice extensive fibrosis with loss of normal pulmonary architecture. (Courtesy of Dr. Claire Langston, Baylor College of Medicine, Houston, TX.)

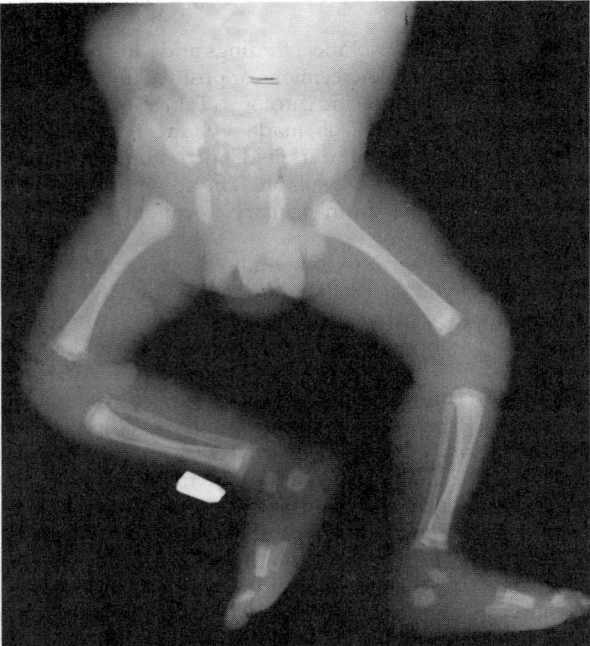

**Figure 56-9.** Skeletal radiograph of legs, showing diffuse metaphysitis in a child with congenital syphilis. (Courtesy of Dr. Milton Wagner, Baylor College of Medicine, Houston, TX.)

The most widely used nontreponemal test, the Venereal Disease Research Laboratory (VDRL), is positive in approximately 75% of the primary syphilis cases and is always positive in secondary syphilis. Titers decrease during latent or tertiary syphilis, which permits monitoring of therapy with the VDRL. In rare cases, a patient's serum demonstrates a serofast state, which is a positive VDRL despite adequate therapy. Autoimmune diseases, certain infections, and pregnancy can produce a false-positive VDRL. False-negative results may occur when a high concentration of antibody inhibits agglutination (ie, prozone phenomenon), and

**TABLE 56-25.  Diagnostic Tests for Syphilis**

**Direct Identification of *T pallidum***
Darkfield examination of exudate
Direct fluorescent antibody to *T pallidum* (exudate)

**Specific Treponemal Serologic Tests**
Fluorescent treponemal antibody absorption test (FTA-ABS)
Microhemagglutination test for *T pallidum* (MHA-TP)

**Nontreponemal Serologic Tests**
Venereal Disease Research Laboratory (VDRL)
Rapid Plasma Reagin (RPR) card test

treponemal-serologic tests are required to confirm the VDRL. The advantages of the nontreponemal tests include reasonable specificity and sensitivity, ease of use, and the ability to follow titers as a guide to therapy.

The diagnosis of congenital syphilis relies on clinical findings and laboratory data and is best achieved through direct identification of *T pallidum* in an exudate smear. Serologic diagnosis is difficult in infants, because transplacentally acquired maternal immunoglobulin G (IgG) may lead to false-positive results. No test for IgM antibody to *T pallidum* is available to diagnose congenital infection. If the infant VDRL is four times the maternal VDRL results, active infection is assumed to be present. The VDRL test becomes negative in 3 months if findings are maternally derived. The FTA-ABS or MHA-TP may be persistently positive but maternally derived for up to 6 months; a positive test at 15 months indicates the probability of an active infection. Figure 56-10 can be used as a guide to help determine the need for therapy. Treatment decisions should largely be guided by the mother's serology and treatment history.

Other laboratory data used to evaluate patients with syphilis include complete blood count, platelet count, liver function tests, and urinalysis. In cases with neurosyphilis, the cerebrospinal fluid (CSF) shows increased leukocytes and increased total protein (including the γ-globulin fraction). It can produce a positive VDRL result, but the CSF VDRL is relatively insensitive and may be negative in as many as one half of the cases of neurosyphilis. A chest radiograph should be obtained if pneumonia is a possibility. Radiographs of the long bones have been reported to be the most sensitive screening assay for congenital syphilis. Figure 56-9 shows the metaphysitis associated with congenital syphilis.

## TREATMENT

Acquired primary, secondary, or early latent syphilis of less than 1 year's duration can be treated with 50,000 U/kg of benzathine penicillin G administered intramuscularly in a single dose (not to exceed 2.4 million U). Tetracycline is the alternate therapy for patients older than 9 years who are allergic to penicillin. The adult dosage of tetracycline is 500 mg, taken orally four times daily for 14 days. If tetracycline cannot be given because of intolerance or the patient's age, erythromycin can be used; the adult dosage is 500 mg, taken orally four times daily for 14 days. Pregnancy mandates treatment with penicillin because insufficient erythromycin may pass through the placenta into the fetus.

Latent or tertiary syphilis existing for longer than 1 year with no evidence of neurosyphilis can be treated with benzathine penicillin G at a dosage of 50,000 U/kg/week, administered intramuscularly for 3 successive weeks (not to exceed 2.4 million U). Erythromycin or tetracycline therapy is an alternative, guided by the caveats described previously. The optimal therapy for neurosyphilis in adults has not been determined, but benzathine penicillin should not be used because of its poor penetration into the CSF.

Treatment programs for congenital syphilis are tailored to the clinical and laboratory data (Figure 56-10). The maternal VDRL should be confirmed by an MHA-TP or FTA-ABS. Because cord blood serology may represent contamination by maternal serum, infant serology should be used to confirm the results. If a baby has a positive MHA-TP result, the treatment strategy is based on the adequacy of maternal therapy, the infant's appearance, and the results of lumbar puncture. If the mother had inadequate or

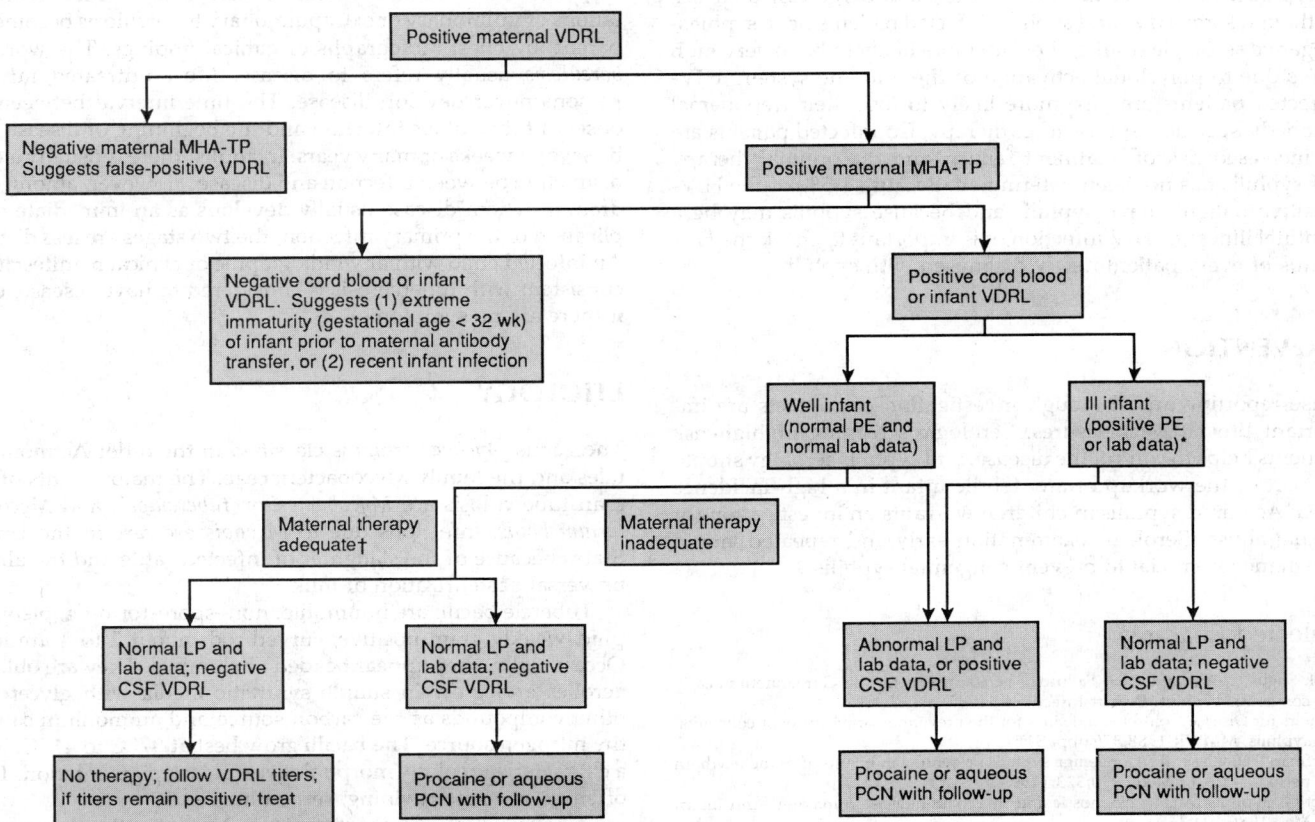

\* See text for positive physical examination (PE) signs and positive lab data.
† Mother with adequate antibiotic therapy and decreasing serologic titers.

**Figure 56-10.** Algorithm for serologic diagnosis of congenital syphilis.

undetermined therapy, received therapy during the last 4 weeks of pregnancy, or was treated with an antibiotic other than penicillin, the infant should be treated. The therapy for congenital neurosyphilis is procaine penicillin administered intramuscularly in a dosage of 50,000 U/kg/day for a minimum of 10 days or aqueous crystalline penicillin G in a dosage of 50,000 U/kg/dose, administered intramuscularly or intravenously two to three times each day for 10 to 14 days. These dosages are also recommended for infants with abnormal CSF data or for those who appear ill and have abnormalities on physical examination or in laboratory data. Some authorities think that a single dose of benzathine penicillin is acceptable treatment if a maternal history of syphilis exists, the mother was treated inadequately or late in pregnancy, the infant's examination and laboratory data are normal, and good follow-up is assured (Zenker, 1991). The use of ceftriaxone to treat syphilis is controversial because the optimal dose and duration remain undetermined.

The Jarisch-Herxheimer reaction of fever, headache, and malaise can occur 2 to 12 hours after therapy for active syphilis. The reaction is thought to be produced by the release of treponemal endotoxin by penicillin.

Follow-up examinations for early congenital syphilis should be at 1, 2, 4, 6, and 12 months after therapy. If titers of repeated VDRLs do not decrease or if signs and symptoms persist, retreatment should be started immediately.

## SYPHILIS AND AIDS

Infection with the human immunodeficiency virus (HIV) can affect the clinical course, diagnosis, and treatment of syphilis. Because HIV infection accelerates disease progression to early neurosyphilis, all co-infected patients should undergo CSF analysis. Although some HIV- and syphilis-infected patients have syphilis-negative serologic results, they are more likely to have very high titers due to polyclonal activation of the immune system. HIV-infected patients are also more likely to lose their treponemal antibody-specific response after therapy. Co-infected patients are at increased risk of treatment failure, and the optimal therapy for syphilis has not been determined. Because 1.5% of the HIV-positive patients have syphilis and because syphilis may be a sentinel illness of HIV infection, it is important to check the HIV status of every patient newly diagnosed with syphilis.

## PREVENTION

Case reporting and thorough investigation of contacts are important preventive measures. Serologic screening of high-risk patients helps to control the disease, and syphilis serology should be part of the workup of any febrile infant in a high-incidence area. Acquired syphilis in children warrants an investigation for sexual abuse. Serologic examination early and repeated late in pregnancy is crucial to prevent congenital syphilis.

### Selected Readings

Beck-Sague C, Alexander ER. Failure of benzathine penicillin G treatment in early congenital syphilis. Pediatr Infect Dis J 1987;6:1061.
Centers for Disease Control. Guidelines for the prevention and control of congenital syphilis. MMWR 1988;37(suppl S1):1.
Dorfman DH, Glaser JH. Congenital syphilis presenting in infants after the newborn period. N Engl J Med 1990;323:1299.
Hart G. Syphilis tests in diagnostic and therapeutic decision making. Ann Intern Med 1986;104:368.
Ikeda MK, Jenson HB. Evaluation and treatment of congenital syphilis. J Pediatr 1990;117:843.
Ingall D, Musher D. Syphilis. In: Remington JS, Klein JO, eds. Infectious diseases of the fetus and newborn infant, ed 2. Philadelphia: WB Saunders, 1983:335.
Musher DM. Syphilis, neurosyphilis, penicillin, and AIDS. J Infect Dis 1991;163:1201.
Wilfert C, Gutman L. Syphilis. In: Feigin RD, Cherry JD, eds. Textbook of pediatric infectious diseases, ed 2. Philadelphia: WB Saunders, 1987:608.
Zenker PN, Berman SM. Congenital syphilis: trends and recommendations for evaluation and management. Pediatr Infect Dis J 1991;10:516.

*Principles and Practice of Pediatrics, Second Edition.*
edited by Frank A. Oski et al. J. B. Lippincott Company, Philadelphia © 1994.

# 56.28 *Tuberculosis*

### Jeffrey R. Starke

Tuberculosis remains the most important chronic infectious disease in the world in terms of morbidity, mortality, and cost. It is estimated that 1 to 2 billion people worldwide are infected with the tubercle bacillus and that there are 1 to 3 million deaths from tuberculosis annually. Children in developing countries account for 1.3 million cases and 450,000 deaths annually from tuberculosis. In the United States, 26,000 people develop tuberculous disease each year, and 2000 die from the disease.

After *Mycobacterium tuberculosis* enters the lung and begins to multiply, the person has tuberculous infection. The hallmark of tuberculous infection is a positive tuberculin skin test, but the chest radiograph is normal, and the child is free of signs and symptoms. Tuberculous disease occurs when clinical manifestations of pulmonary or extrapulmonary tuberculosis become apparent, by chest radiographs or clinical findings. The word *tuberculosis* usually refers to disease. Most untreated infected persons never develop disease. The time interval between the onset of tuberculous infection and the beginning of disease may be several weeks or many years. In adults, there is usually a clear distinction between infection and disease. However, among children, in whom disease usually develops as an immediate complication of the primary infection, the two stages are less distinct. An infected child with any radiographic or clinical manifestations consistent with tuberculosis is considered to have disease, even if there are no symptoms.

## ETIOLOGY

The genus *Mycobacterium* is classified in the order Actinomycetales and the family Mycobacteriaceae. The major agents of human tuberculosis are *Mycobacterium tuberculosis* and *Mycobacterium bovis*. Infections due to *M bovis* are rare in the United States because of the slaughter of infected cattle and the almost universal pasteurization of milk.

Tubercle bacilli are nonmotile, non–spore-forming, pleomorphic, weakly gram-positive, curved rods about 2 to 4 μm long. Occasionally, they appear beaded or clumped. They are obligate aerobes and grow in simple synthetic media with glycerol or other compounds as the carbon source and ammonium salts as the nitrogen source. The bacilli grow best at 37°C to 41°C, have a characteristic colony morphology, and lack pigmentation. They often grow as intertwining, serpentine cords.

A hallmark of mycobacteria is acid fastness (ie, the capacity to form stable mycolate complexes with arylmethane dyes such as carbol-fuchsin, crystal violet, auramine, and rhodamine). The dyes are not readily removed by rinsing with ethanol plus hydrochloric acid. The bacilli appear red when stained with fuchsin (ie, Ziehl-Neelsen or Kinyoun stains) and purple when stained with crystal violet; they exhibit yellow-green fluorescence under ultraviolet light when stained with auramine and rhodamine (ie, Truant stain).

The cell wall of mycobacteria contains 20% to 60% lipids bound to proteins and carbohydrates. This lipid-rich cell wall accounts for hydrophobic properties, acid fastness, and resistance to the bactericidal actions of antibody and complement. True waxes, mycolic acid, and glycolipids are unique to the cell wall of mycobacteria.

Identification of mycobacteria is based on their growth characteristics, staining properties, and biochemical or metabolic characteristics. Speciation depends on temperature of optimal growth; catalase production, which is present in virulent, isoniazid-susceptible *M tuberculosis* but absent in some isoniazid-resistant strains; secretion of niacin, which is characteristic of *M tuberculosis*; sensitivity to sodium chloride; reduction of tellurite; and capacity to produce carotenoid pigments on exposure to light (ie, photochromogen), equally in light and dark (ie, scotochromogen) or not at all (ie, nonphotochromogen).

## EPIDEMIOLOGY

The incidence of tuberculosis in the United States declined 5% to 6% each year for several decades until 1985, when it leveled off. In 1986, the reported number of cases began to increase. The 1991 case total of 26,283 (ie, 10.4 per 100,000 population) was an increase of 2.3% over 1990 and 12% over 1989. From 1985 through 1991, there were more than 40,000 more reported cases of tuberculosis in the United States than would have been expected if the previous decline had continued. Three major factors are often cited to explain the recent increase: the human immunodeficiency virus (HIV) epidemic, because co-infection with HIV infection is the greatest risk factor known for the development of tuberculous disease in an adult infected with the tubercle bacillus; the recent increase in immigrants from countries with a high prevalence of tuberculosis; and the general decline in public health services and access to medical care in parts of the United States, which has hindered rapid diagnosis, treatment, and completion of contact investigations.

In the early 20th century, the risk of exposure to an adult with infectious tuberculosis was higher and more uniform across the entire population. Tuberculosis has retreated into fairly well-defined groups of high-risk persons (Table 56-26). Cities with populations of more than 250,000 account for 18% of the nation's population but more than 42% of its tuberculosis cases. Case

rates also are high in the Appalachian Mountain region and along the southern border of the United States.

Although tuberculosis case rates in the United States have generally increased with patient age, there has been a recent trend toward an increased case rate in young adults, especially among urban minority populations. Case rates are always lowest among children 5 to 14 years of age; most childhood tuberculosis occurs among children younger than 5 years of age.

Certain environments in our society contain sizable numbers of persons at high risk for tuberculosis, which promotes its transmission. Tuberculosis rates in jails, prisons, nursing homes, homeless shelters, and migrant camps are often 10 to 50 times higher than in the general community. Many of these environments house persons at increased risk for HIV infection. While HIV-seronegative adults with untreated tuberculous infection have a 5% to 10% lifetime risk of developing tuberculous disease, HIV-seropositive adults also infected with the bacillus develop tuberculosis at a rate of 5% to 10% per year. Although few cases of children with coexisting HIV infection and tuberculosis have been reported, the increasing rate of childhood tuberculosis can be partially linked to the spread of tuberculous infection from HIV-infected adults with tuberculosis.

Children with tuberculosis represent 5% to 6% of the total annual number of cases. Since 1976, the decline in incidence of childhood tuberculosis had been slower than that for older populations. Between 1987 and 1991, the number of pediatric tuberculosis cases in the United States increased by 39% to 1656 per year. This increase is undoubtedly linked to the increased case rates among young adults. The pediatric tuberculosis case rate reflects the impact of the disease on childhood health and serves as a public health "marker" of ongoing tuberculosis transmission within a community. As long as the disease persists in adults, susceptible children will become infected.

Although the number of cases of childhood tuberculosis has increased recently, the epidemiology in the United States has remained fairly constant. About 60% of childhood cases occur in children younger than 5 years of age. The disease affects the sexes equally. Between 1986 and 1990, the proportion of cases in foreign-born children rose from 13% to 16% among children younger than 5 years of age and from 40% to 49% among adolescents between the ages of 15 and 19. Although most children acquire tuberculosis within their home or neighborhood from relatives or adult family friends, epidemics of childhood tuberculosis—almost always caused by contact with an infectious adult—continue to occur within schools, churches, day-care centers, and nursery schools.

Tuberculosis is transmitted from person to person, usually by droplets of mucus that become airborne when an infected person coughs, sneezes, laughs, or sings. Occasionally, transmission occurs by direct contact with infected discharges (eg, urine or purulent sinus tract drainage) or with a contaminated fomite. The duration of exposure required to transmit tuberculosis depends on the infectiousness of the source case. Adults with cavitary disease harbor the greatest number of tubercle bacilli for the longest time. Most adults are no longer infectious after several days to 2 weeks of therapy, but this period may increase for patients with advanced cavitary disease who continue to cough. Children with primary tuberculosis rarely infect other children. Tubercle bacilli are sparse in the endobronchial secretions of children, who usually do not cough with sufficient force to transmit infection. However, infected children constitute the long-term reservoir of infection for the population.

## PATHOGENESIS

The primary (Ghon) complex of tuberculosis consists of disease at the portal of entry and the regional lymph nodes that drain

**TABLE 56-26. High-risk Groups for Tuberculosis in the United States**

Increased risk of exposure to an infectious adult
  Foreign-born persons from high-prevalence countries
  Residents of correctional institutions
  Residents of nursing homes
  Homeless persons
  Users of intravenous and other street drugs
  Health care workers
  Children living with adults in the categories listed above
Increased likelihood that disease will develop after infection occurs
  Human immunodeficiency virus co-infection
  Medical risk factors (eg, diabetes mellitus)
  Immunosuppressive diseases or therapies
  Malnutrition
  Infancy

the area of the primary focus. The infection may occur anywhere in the body, but the primary site is in the lung in over 95% of cases. Tubercle bacilli on particles larger than 10 μm are usually caught in the mucociliary mechanisms of the bronchi and expelled. Smaller particles are inhaled beyond the clearance mechanisms. In the alveoli or alveolar ducts, bacilli multiply, and there is an inflammatory exudate. Some of the bacilli are carried by macrophages through the lymphatic channels to the regional lymph nodes. While the primary complex is developing, tubercle bacilli spread by the bloodstream and lymphatics to many parts of the body. This dissemination can involve large numbers of bacilli, leading to miliary tuberculosis, or more commonly, small numbers of bacilli that leave tuberculous foci scattered in various tissues. These foci may or may not develop into significant extrapulmonary tuberculosis later in life. After 4 to 8 weeks, cell-mediated immunity usually develops. At this time, the primary complex usually heals to the extent that it is not visible on chest radiographs, and further dissemination is arrested.

The parenchymal portion of the primary complex often heals completely after undergoing caseating necrosis and encapsulation. Further healing occurs by fibrosis or calcification. The nodal component has a decreased tendency to heal completely. Even after calcification, viable tubercle bacilli may persist for many years in the node or in distant sites. Although children usually develop tuberculous disease during the primary infection, most cases in adults are due to endogenous regrowth of persister bacilli resident in the body from the time of the primary infection (ie, adult or postprimary tuberculosis). The most common form of postprimary tuberculosis affects the apical region of the lung. The apex of the lung has the highest oxygen tension, and the many organisms deposited there during hematogenous dissemination are those most likely to reactivate.

Without specific therapy, tuberculosis develops in 5% to 10% of immunologically normal adults with tuberculous infection at some time during their lives. The risk for children is greater; as many as 43% of children younger than 1 year of age with untreated tuberculous infection develop radiographic evidence of disease, compared with 24% of children between the ages of 1 and 5 years and 15% of those between the ages of 11 and 15 years. Although infants and young children are more likely to develop immediate complications of the primary infection, children who are older when infected are more likely to develop postprimary disease as adults.

There is a predictable timetable of primary tuberculous infection and its complications. Massive lymphohematogenous spread leading to miliary or acute meningeal tuberculosis usually occurs around 3 to 6 months after the initial infection. Endobronchial tuberculosis, with segmental pulmonary changes, occurs within 9 months. Clinically important lesions of bones or joints do not appear until at least 1 year after infection, and renal lesions develop 5 to 25 years after primary infection. In general, complications in children occur within the first 5 years (especially the first year) after initial infection. Complications later in life are caused by reactivation of previously dormant persister bacilli at a site of dissemination.

## DIAGNOSIS

The diagnosis of tuberculous disease in adults is mainly bacteriologic, but in children, it is usually epidemiologic and indirect. In the absence of a positive culture, the strongest evidence for tuberculosis in a child is history of exposure to an adult with contagious disease. The importance of an adequate history and exposure tracing cannot be overemphasized. Less direct methods, such as the tuberculin skin test and other laboratory tests, offer supportive information.

## Tuberculin Skin Test

A positive tuberculin skin test is the hallmark of a primary tuberculous infection. Within 8 years of his discovery of the tubercle bacilli, Robert Koch found that subcutaneous injection of a broth culture filtrate of tubercle bacilli, which he called "tuberculin," produced fever, chills, and vomiting in a person with tuberculosis and induration at the injection site. The diagnostic usefulness of this test was described in the early 20th century. In 1934, Florence Seibert developed a purified protein derivative (PPD) from broth cultures, which became the standard known as PPD-S. Commercially produced PPD is still standardized against the original lot of PPD-S.

There are two major techniques for tuberculin skin testing. The first is the multiple-puncture test, which involves the intradermal delivery of tuberculin antigen by metal prongs coated with the antigen. Most commercially available tests use PPD as the antigen (eg, Aplitest, Sclavo Test, Tine Test), but one product uses Old Tuberculin (ie, Mono-Vacc). Because the precise amount of antigen left in the dermis varies among patients, these tests are not standardized well for reaction size. They are qualitative, and results should be read as positive, negative, or questionable. The false-positive rates may be as high as 10% to 20%, and false-negative rates are 1% to 10%. Because of the lack of standardization in dose administration, sometimes low sensitivity and specificity, and their potential to create larger subsequent reactions after repetitive testing (ie, booster phenomenon), the use of multiple puncture skin tests should be eliminated. They should never be used in evaluating patients exposed to tuberculosis or those suspected of having tuberculous disease.

The "gold standard" tuberculin test is the Mantoux, an intradermal injection of 5 tuberculin units (TU) of PPD in 0.1 mL of diluent containing the stabilizing agent polysorbate 80. This test is standardized and quantitative; results are read as the transverse diameter of induration at 48 to 72 hours. The Mantoux test is subject to a variety of influences related to the test procedure (Table 56-27). The testing technique must be precise and consistent. Although experienced health care providers may demonstrate good intraobserver agreement in interpretation, inexperienced observers, especially parents, often report results inaccurately.

### TABLE 56-27. Factors That Can Influence Mantoux Test Results

**Factors Related to the Host**
Presence of other infections (viral, bacterial, fungal)
Recent inoculation with live virus vaccine
Metabolic derangements
Malnutrition
Immunosuppression by disease or drug treatment
Age (very old or young)
Overwhelming tuberculous disease
History of BCG vaccination

**Factors Related to the Environment**
Prevalence of nontuberculous mycobacteria

**Factors Related to the Testing Procedure**
Improper administration or interpretation
Antigen overload with simultaneous tests
Boosting exerted by previous skin tests
Loss of strength of purified protein derivative due to improper storage
Variations in commercial products

A variety of host-related factors, such as age, nutrition, immunosuppression, viral infections or immunization with live viral vaccines, administration of corticosteroids, and the presence of overwhelming tuberculosis, can depress tuberculin reactivity. Approximately 10% of adults and children with culture-documented tuberculosis do not react initially to PPD; delayed hypersensitivity often appears after appropriate treatment is begun. In adults, initial anergy to tuberculin is related to a poor prognosis, but this does not appear to be true for children.

Recent exposure to environmental nontuberculous mycobacteria (NTM) can result in cross-sensitization and a false-positive reaction to PPD. This problem is common in the southeastern United States, where NTM occur in the environment, especially the soil. Cross-sensitization with NTM usually causes a reaction to a 5-TU Mantoux test of less than 10 mm, although reactions up to 15 mm can occur. This cross-sensitization tends to wane over a period of months. Prior immunization with bacille Calmette-Guérin (BCG) also may cause a significant Mantoux reaction, which is usually smaller than 10 to 12 mm and completely wanes within 3 to 5 years. Because the effect of BCG on the skin test is variable and a reaction of 10 mm or more in a previously BCG-vaccinated child usually indicates infection with *M tuberculosis*, the interpretation of the skin test should be the same for a BCG-vaccinated child as it would be for a comparable, nonvaccinated child.

The important issue in interpreting the Mantoux test is the amount of induration that should be considered as truly indicating tuberculous infection. This cut-point varies with the population being tested and depends on epidemiologic factors. For example, in areas of the United States where NTM are common, only 5% of children who have a 5- to 9-mm induration in response to a 5-TU Mantoux test are actually infected with *M tuberculosis*. However, if the child is a contact of a known case of tuberculosis, there is a 50% probability of infection. The critical information is epidemiologic. Has exposure occurred? The only way to answer this question is by vigorous contact tracing in the child's environment.

There is always some overlap in reaction to the Mantoux test between large groups of people with and without tuberculous infection. False positives and false negatives will always occur, no matter what cut-point is selected. Because of the critical contribution of epidemiology to the interpretation of the skin test, the cut-points for a positive reaction should vary for groups according to their risk for tuberculosis. For adults and children at the highest risk—those who are contacts of adults with infectious tuberculosis, who have abnormalities on a chest radiograph, or who have clinical evidence of tuberculosis, or who are HIV-seropositive—induration of 5 mm or more is classified as positive. For other high-risk groups, including all infants, and for children living with adults in high-risk groups, induration of 10 mm or more is a positive result. Although raising the cut-point to 15 mm for children at low risk for tuberculosis may be a scientifically sound practice in some locales, this strategy presents some practical problems. The most important is the difficulty of establishing that a child truly has no risk factors for acquiring tuberculous infection. Many experts continue to recommend that a reaction of 10 mm or more should be considered positive for low-risk children.

Purified protein derivative also is available in 1-TU (first) and 250-TU (second) strengths. The 1-TU strength is used only if the physician suspects that a patient may have a severe reaction to the 5-TU strength. Use of 250 TU of PPD is controversial, because reactions have not been standardized, and appropriate cut-points are not available. A negative 250-TU test after a negative 5-TU test indicates a low probability of tuberculous infection. A positive 250-TU test is less helpful, especially in areas where NTM are common. In such areas, as many as 25% of children not infected with *M tuberculosis* have significant reactions to 250-TU PPD because of cross-sensitization.

## Laboratory Tests

Routine laboratory tests, such as a complete blood count and differential, erythrocyte sedimentation rate, and urinalysis, rarely aid in the diagnosis of tuberculosis. Abnormalities on liver function tests may help diagnose miliary tuberculosis. Analyses of infected body fluids (eg, pleural, joint, cerebrospinal) demonstrating lymphocytes, elevated protein, and decreased glucose suggest tuberculosis. These fluids and sputum should be examined microscopically with acid-fast stain to detect mycobacteria.

The most important laboratory test for the diagnosis and management of tuberculosis is the mycobacteria culture. In adults, isolation of the organism confirms the diagnosis, and susceptibility tests direct therapy. Isolation of *M tuberculosis* is not essential to the diagnosis of tuberculosis in children if epidemiologic, skin test, clinical, and radiographic findings are compatible with the disease. If culture and susceptibility tests are available for the adult source case, cultures from the child add little to management. However, when the source case is unknown, especially in areas of high drug resistance rates, attempts should be made to isolate the organism from the child. Cultures should be obtained in any child with suspected extrapulmonary tuberculosis to confirm the diagnosis.

Sputum produced by an older child or adolescent with pulmonary tuberculosis usually yields *M tuberculosis*. Younger children rarely produce sputum. Gastric aspirates yield the organism in 30% to 40% of patients; the yield is even greater in infants. When obtained correctly, gastric aspirates have a greater yield than bronchial samples. Aspiration should be done early in the morning, as the child awakens, before the overnight accumulation of secretions swallowed from the respiratory tract is emptied from the stomach. The aspirates should be collected using saline-free fluid, and the pH should be neutralized if processing will be delayed for more than several hours.

Traditional culture methods using classic media such as Loewenstein-Jensen or simple synthetic media such as Middlebrook 7H10 require 4 to 6 weeks for isolation of the organism and another 2 to 4 weeks for susceptibility testing. The Bactec radiometric system uses liquid media containing fatty acid substrates labeled with carbon 14. As the mycobacteria metabolize the fatty acids, $^{14}CO_2$ is released and measured as a marker of bacterial growth. A second substrate is used to differentiate NTM from *M tuberculosis*. The Bactec system yields culture and susceptibility results within 7 to 10 days and is more sensitive than traditional media for sputum cultures. Little information is available about the use of Bactec for cultures of gastric aspirates or extrapulmonary sites.

Many laboratories now use DNA probes to identify and speciate mycobacteria after they have been isolated in media. These probes use DNA sequences that are complementary to specific RNA or DNA sequences of *M tuberculosis*. The sensitivity and specificity of these probes when used on isolated organisms approach 100%. Unfortunately, the sensitivity drops precipitously when these probes are used directly on patient samples. The technique of polymerase chain reaction (PCR) markedly increases the sensitivity of DNA testing on patient samples. The target DNA is isolated, replicated thousands of times using DNA polymerase and thermal cycling, and then detected using a nucleic acid probe or specially stained electrophoresis gels. The sensitivity and specificity of PCR for *M tuberculosis* on samples from adults with sputum positive pulmonary tuberculosis have been greater than 95%, and the results are available in less than 48 hours. Adequate studies using PCR for the diagnosis of tuberculosis in children have not yet been reported.

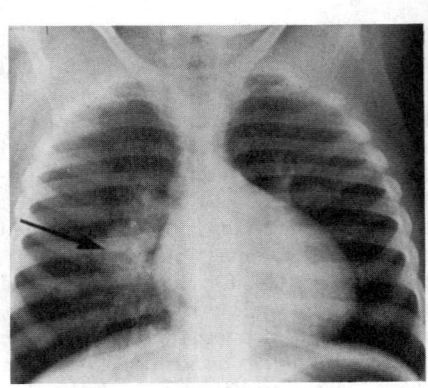
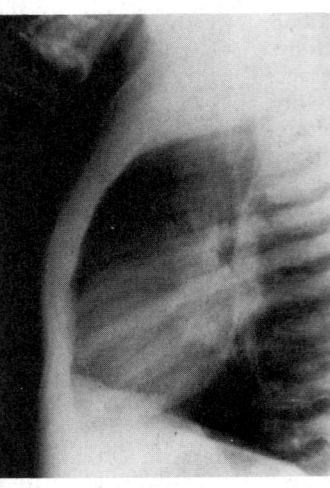

**Figure 56-11.** Chest radiograph of hilar adenopathy (*arrow*) caused by a primary tuberculous infection in an infant. Notice the mass lesion at the hilum, seen best in the lateral view. (Courtesy of Katharine H. K. Hsu.)

## Diagnostic Criteria

The diagnosis of tuberculous disease in children is often based on epidemiologic, clinical, radiographic, and skin test information, rather than mycobacteriological data. The diagnosis of tuberculous disease is confirmed if *M tuberculosis* is isolated from any body site or if the clinical, radiographic, or histologic findings are consistent with tuberculosis and at least two of the following criteria are met: a 5-TU Mantoux test yields more than 5 mm of induration; other disease entities are ruled out and the subsequent clinical course is consistent with tuberculosis; and an adult source case with contagious tuberculosis is discovered.

## CLINICAL FORMS OF TUBERCULOSIS

### Endothoracic Disease

#### Asymptomatic Primary Tuberculosis

Asymptomatic, primary tuberculosis is an infection associated with tuberculin skin reactivity in the absence of clinical or significant radiographic findings. This type of infection is more common in school-age children than in young infants; 80% to 95% of infected older children have silent tuberculous infections, but only 50% to 60% of infected infants are asymptomatic. Children in this category are ideal candidates for preventive chemotherapy. Contact tracing to determine the epidemiology of the infection is important.

#### Primary Pulmonary Tuberculosis

The primary pulmonary complex includes the parenchymal focus and regional lymphadenitis. About 70% of primary foci are subpleural, and localized pleurisy is a common component of the primary complex. The primary infection begins with the deposition of infected droplets into lung alveoli. The initial parenchymal inflammation usually is not visible on chest radiographs, but a localized, nonspecific infiltrate may be seen. All lobar segments of the lung are at equal risk of being seeded. In 25% of cases, there are multiple primary foci in the lungs. The infection spreads early to regional (usually hilar) lymph nodes. If tuberculin hypersensitivity develops within 3 to 10 weeks after infection, the inflammatory reaction in the lung parenchyma and lymph nodes intensifies. The hallmark of primary tuberculosis in the lung is the relatively large size and importance of the hilar adenitis compared with the relatively small size of the initial parenchymal focus. Because of the patterns of lymphatic drainage, a left-sided parenchymal focus often leads to bilateral hilar adenopathy, but a right-sided focus is associated with right-sided adenitis only.

In most cases, the parenchymal infiltrate and adenitis resolve early. In some children, especially infants, the hilar lymph nodes continue to enlarge (Fig 56-11). Bronchial obstruction begins as the nodes compress the associated regional bronchus. Inflammation intensifies, and the nodes may erode through the bronchial wall, leading to formation of thick caseum in the bronchial lumen and eventual occlusion of the bronchus. The common sequence for the development of endobronchial disease is hilar adenopathy, localized emphysema (due to partial obstruction), and then atelectasis. The resulting radiographic shadows have been called collapse-consolidation or segmental tuberculosis (Fig 56-12). The radiographic findings are similar to those seen with foreign body aspiration. Segmental lesions are most common in infants because of the small diameters of their bronchi. These lesions tend to occur within 6 months of the initial infection.

Physical signs and symptoms of hilar adenopathy and segmental lesions are surprisingly uncommon and are usually found in young infants. Occasionally, the initiation of the primary infection is marked by low-grade fever and mild cough. As the

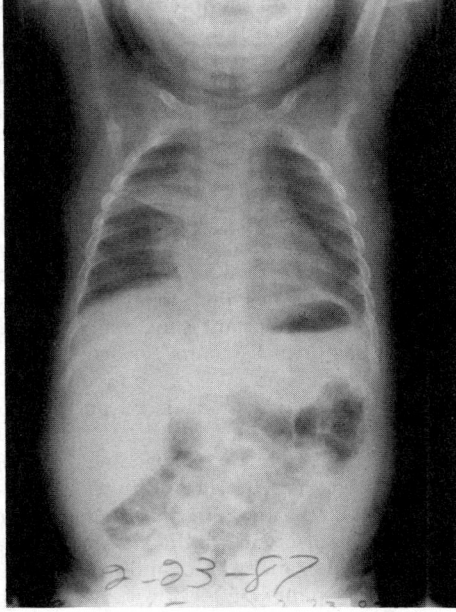

**Figure 56-12.** Chest radiograph shows a segmental lesion during a primary tuberculous infection in an infant. Volume loss on the right is manifested by atelectasis and a displaced horizontal fissure.

primary complex progresses, nonspecific symptoms such as fever, cough, weight loss, and night sweats may occur. Pulmonary signs usually are absent. Some children have localized wheezing or diminished breath sounds, which may be accompanied by tachypnea or rarely by frank respiratory distress. Nonspecific symptoms and pulmonary signs are occasionally alleviated by antibiotics, suggesting that bacterial superinfection may play a role.

Most cases of tuberculous bronchial obstruction in children resolve fully. Occasionally, there is residual calcification of the primary focus or regional lymph nodes. Calcification implies that the lesion has been present for at least 6 months. Rarely, healing of the segment is complicated by scarring or contraction associated with cylindrical bronchiectasis. This occurs primarily in the lower lobes, and is extremely rare in children who have undergone appropriate chemotherapy.

### Progressive Primary Pulmonary Tuberculosis

A rare but serious complication of primary tuberculous infection occurs when the primary focus enlarges steadily and develops a large caseous center. The radiograph shows bronchopneumonia or lobar pneumonia. Liquefaction may result in the formation of a thin-walled primary cavity associated with large numbers of tubercle bacilli. A tension cavity may develop as a result of a valve-like mechanism allowing air to enter but not escape the cavity. The enlarging focus may slough necrotic debris into an adjacent bronchus, leading to further intrapulmonary dissemination. Rupture into the pleural cavity may lead to bronchopleural fistula or pyopneumothorax; rupture into the pericardium or mediastinum can also occur.

Significant signs and symptoms are frequent in locally progressive disease. High fever, severe cough with sputum production, weight loss, and night sweats are common. Physical signs include diminished breath sounds, rales, and dullness and egophony over the cavity. Before the development of tuberculosis chemotherapy, prognosis was poor, with a fatality rate of 30% to 50%. The current prognosis for full recovery is excellent. Superinfection of a simple primary tuberculous focus with a bacterial pneumonia may have a clinical and radiographic presentation similar to progressive primary tuberculosis. Antimicrobial agents effective against *Staphylococcus*, *Klebsiella*, and anaerobes are indicated along with antituberculosis drugs.

### Pleural Effusion

Localized pleural effusion occurs so frequently in primary tuberculosis that it is almost a component of the primary complex. Clinically significant pleurisy with effusion occurs in 5% to 30% of young adults with tuberculosis but is infrequent in children younger than 6 years of age and almost nonexistent in those younger than 2 years of age. Pleurisy occurs within 6 to 12 months of the initial infection and is caused by extension of a subpleural focus. It is virtually never associated with a segmental lesion or miliary tuberculosis. The effusion usually is unilateral and may be small or extensive.

### Chronic Pulmonary Disease

Chronic pulmonary tuberculosis (ie, adult or reactivation tuberculosis) represents endogenous reinfection from a site of tuberculous infection established previously in the body. This form of tuberculosis has always been rare in childhood but may occur in adolescence. Children with a healed tuberculous infection acquired before 2 years of age rarely develop chronic pulmonary disease, which is more common in those who acquire their initial infection after 7 years of age. The most common pulmonary sites are the original parenchymal focus, the regional lymph nodes, or the apical seedings (ie, Simon foci) established during the early bacillemia from the primary focus. This form of disease usually remains localized to the lungs, because the presensitization of the tissues to tuberculin evokes an excellent immune response that prevents further lymphohematogenous spread.

The initial lesion usually is a small area of pneumonia that may progress to caseation, liquefaction, and cavitation (Fig 56-13). The most common clinical features are cough, fever, chest pain, weight loss, and eventually, hemoptysis. This form of tuberculosis is highly contagious if there is significant sputum production and cough. The prognosis is excellent for patients given appropriate antituberculosis therapy.

### Cardiac and Pericardial Tuberculosis

Involvement of the myocardium may occur in miliary disease. Direct extension of tuberculosis to the myocardium from mediastinal nodes or lung parenchyma is exceedingly rare. Tuberculous endocarditis has been described only in several case reports.

The most common form of cardiac tuberculosis is pericarditis, but it is rare, occurring in between 0.4% and 4% of children with tuberculosis. Pericarditis usually arises by direct invasion or lymphatic drainage from subcarinal lymph nodes. Early in the course, the pericardial fluid is serofibrinous or occasionally hemorrhagic. Eventually, fibrosis may obliterate the pericardial sac, with the development of constrictive pericarditis over a period of years. The presenting symptoms are nonspecific and include low-grade fever, malaise, and weight loss; chest pain is unusual. A pericardial friction rub or distant heart sounds with pulsus paradoxus may be present. An acid-fast smear of the pericardial fluid rarely reveals the organism, but cultures are positive in 30% to 70% of cases. Pericardial biopsy may be necessary to confirm the diagnosis. Results of therapy with antituberculosis drugs and corticosteroids are excellent. Partial or complete pericardiectomy may be required when constrictive pericarditis is present.

## Lymphohematogenous Spread

Tubercle bacilli are disseminated to distant sites from the lymphadenitis or primary focus of the primary complex in all cases of

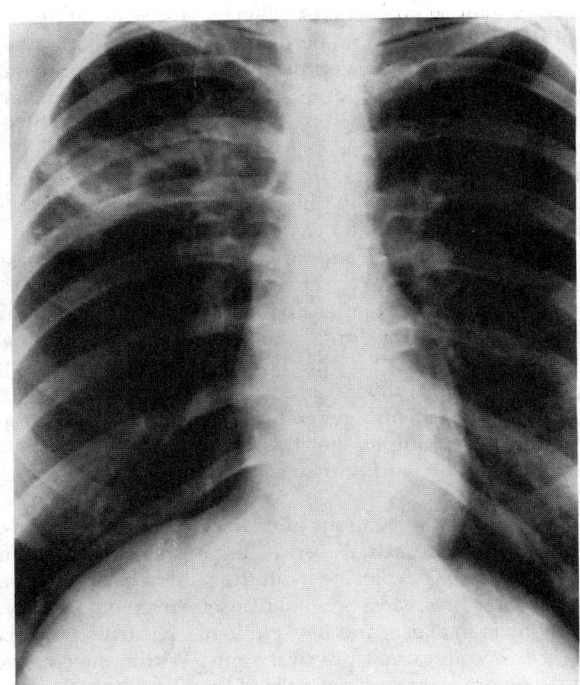

**Figure 56-13.** Chest radiograph shows two tuberculous cavities in an adolescent female.

tuberculous infection. Experimental animals given local injections of bovine tuberculosis develop dissemination within hours. Autopsy studies of people who died within days or weeks after initial infection with *M tuberculosis* have demonstrated organisms in many organs, most commonly the liver, spleen, skin, and apices of the lungs. The clinical picture produced by the lymphohematogenous dissemination depends on the host immune response and the quantity of organisms released. There are three basic clinical forms: occult lymphohematogenous spread, protracted hematogenous tuberculosis, and miliary tuberculosis.

## Occult Lymphohematogenous Spread

Occult lymphohematogenous spread is the most common form, and it occurs in all cases of asymptomatic tuberculous infection. It is this form that leads eventually to the development of extrapulmonary tuberculosis, months or years after the initial infection.

## Protracted Hematogenous Tuberculosis

Protracted hematogenous tuberculosis is now extremely rare. It is probably caused by the intermittent release of tubercle bacilli when a caseous focus erodes through the wall of a blood vessel. The clinical picture may be acute, but more commonly, it is indolent and prolonged. High, spiking fevers accompany the release of organisms into the blood stream. Occasionally, the fever is persistent. Multiple organ involvement is frequent; the most common signs are hepatomegaly, splenomegaly, adenitis of both deep and superficial lymph nodes, and papulonecrotic tuberculids occurring in crops. The skeletal system, joints, and kidneys may become involved. Meningitis occurs late in the course and was often a terminal event before antituberculosis drugs became available. Pulmonary lesions are rare early in the course; diffuse lung disease appears later. The tuberculin skin test usually is markedly positive. Culture confirmation can be difficult and may require bone marrow or liver biopsy. The prognosis is excellent with appropriate therapy.

## Miliary Tuberculosis

Miliary tuberculosis arises when massive numbers of tubercle bacilli are released into the bloodstream, resulting in simultaneous disease in two or more organs. This usually is an early complication of primary infection, occurring within 3 to 6 months after formation of the primary complex. This disease is most common in infants and young children. Adults may develop miliary tuberculosis as a result of the breakdown of a previously healed or calcified lesion that formed years earlier.

The pathologic picture of miliary tuberculosis is caused by tubercle bacilli entering the bloodstream from a caseous focus that erodes through a blood vessel. The organisms lodge in small capillaries in various sites and form tubercles of relatively uniform size, ranging from 2 mm to several centimeters. Different tissues have different susceptibilities to infection. Lesions are larger and more numerous in the lungs, spleen, liver, and bone marrow than in other tissues. This difference may be explained by blood supply and by the numbers of reticuloendothelial cells and tissue phagocytes. The patient's general immune status may play a role, as suggested by findings that this form of tuberculosis is more common in infants and in malnourished or immunosuppressed hosts.

The clinical manifestations of miliary tuberculosis are protean and depend on the actual load of organisms that disseminate. Rarely, the onset is explosive, with the patient becoming gravely ill over several days. Most often, the onset is insidious, with weight loss, anorexia, malaise, and low-grade fever. Early in the course, there are few abnormal physical signs. Within several weeks, hepatosplenomegaly and generalized lymphadenopathy develop in about half the patients. At about this time, there may be a

higher fever, up to 39°C to 40°C. Initially, the chest radiograph may be normal or show evidence only of a primary complex; few respiratory signs or symptoms are observed. Within 3 to 4 weeks after symptom onset, the lung fields usually become filled with tubercles (Fig 56-14). The child may develop respiratory distress and diffuse rales or wheezing. Pneumothorax, pneumomediastinum, and pleural effusion can also complicate miliary tuberculosis. Signs or symptoms of meningitis or peritonitis are found in 20% to 30% of these patients. In a patient with miliary tuberculosis, headache almost always indicates the presence of meningitis, and the presence of abdominal pain or tenderness usually signals tuberculous peritonitis. Cutaneous lesions, including papulonecrotic tuberculids, nodules, or purpuric lesions, may occur in crops. Choroid tubercles appeared several weeks after the onset of disease in 13% to 87% of the patients in various studies.

Diagnosis can be difficult, and a high index of suspicion on the part of the examiner is required. Usually, the patient presents with a fever of unknown origin. As many as 30% of these patients have a negative tuberculin skin test, especially late in the course of disease. The chest radiograph may be characteristic. Early sputum cultures have a low sensitivity; the yield from gastric aspirates or bronchial washings is greater. Biopsy of the liver or bone marrow, with appropriate bacteriologic and histologic examinations, may facilitate a more rapid diagnosis. The most important clue may be history of a recent exposure to an adult with contagious tuberculosis.

Even with proper treatment, the resolution of miliary tuberculosis may be slow. Fever usually declines within 2 to 3 weeks, but the chest radiographic abnormalities may not resolve for several months. Occasionally, corticosteroids hasten symptomatic relief, especially when air block, peritonitis, or meningitis occur. Most patients recover fully with adequate chemotherapy.

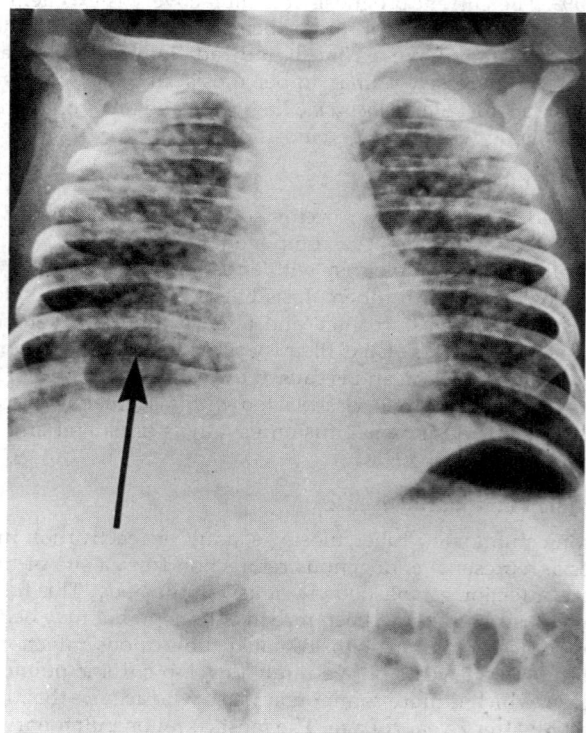

**Figure 56-14.** Chest radiograph of a child with miliary tuberculosis shows typical tubercles and an air-filled cavity (*arrow*). (Courtesy of Katharine H. K. Hsu.)

## Extrathoracic Disease

### Central Nervous System Tuberculosis

Involvement of the central nervous system (CNS) is the most serious complication of tuberculosis in children. Before the development of effective therapy, CNS tuberculosis was uniformly fatal. There are several different forms of CNS tuberculosis, including meningitis, tuberculoma, and brain abscess.

The pathogenesis of CNS tuberculosis results from formation of a metastatic caseous lesion in the cerebral cortex or meninges during the occult lymphohematogenous dissemination of the primary infection. This lesion (ie, Rich focus) may increase in size and discharge tubercle bacilli into the subarachnoid space. A thick, gelatinous exudate may infiltrate the cortical or meningeal blood vessels, producing inflammation, obstruction, or infarction. The brain stem usually is the site of greatest involvement, which accounts for the frequent involvement of cranial nerves III, VI, and VII. The basal cisterns usually become obstructed, leading to hydrocephalus. This is a communicating hydrocephalus because the four ventricles are all open to the flow of cerebrospinal fluid (CSF), but the flow to the spinal column is obstructed.

Tuberculous meningitis complicates 1 of every 300 primary infections. This disease is unheard of in infants younger than 4 months of age because it takes at least that long for the inciting pathologic events to develop. It is most common in children younger than 4 years of age and usually occurs within 3 to 6 months of the primary infection.

The clinical onset of tuberculous meningitis may be abrupt or insidious. The more rapid progression of disease tends to occur in young infants, who may experience symptoms for only several days before the onset of acute hydrocephalus, brain infarction, or seizures. More commonly, the onset is gradual, occurring over several weeks. The usual course can be divided into three stages. The first stage, which may last 1 to 2 weeks, is characterized by nonspecific symptoms such as fever, headache, irritability, drowsiness, and malaise. There are no focal neurologic signs, but infants and young children may experience a loss or stagnation of developmental milestones. The second stage usually begins abruptly, with lethargy, convulsions, nuchal rigidity, positive Kernig or Brudzinski signs, increased deep tendon reflexes, hypertonia, vomiting, and cranial nerve palsies. The appearance of this clinical picture correlates with the development of hydrocephalus and increased intracranial pressure, combined with meningeal irritation. Some patients have relatively few signs of meningeal irritation but show signs of encephalitis, such as disorientation, abnormal movements, and speech abnormalities. The third stage is marked by coma, irregular pulse or respirations, hypertension, hemiplegia or paraplegia, decerebrate posturing, and eventually by death.

The most important aid to the correct diagnosis is a history of recent contact with an adult who has active tuberculosis. The tuberculin skin test is negative in as many as 30% of the patients, especially in infants and young children. The most important test is examination and culture of the lumbar CSF. The CSF leukocyte count ranges from 10 to 500 cells/mm$^3$. Early evaluation may reveal a predominance of polymorphonuclear leukocytes, but in most cases, lymphocytes predominate. The glucose level is typically less than 40 mg/dL but rarely goes below 20 mg/dL, as it does in bacterial meningitis. The protein level is elevated and may be markedly high (>400 mg/dL) because of hydrocephalus and spinal block. The lumbar CSF protein is not indicative of the ventricular CSF protein, which is often normal or only slightly elevated. The success of microscopic examination of stained CSF and mycobacterial culture is directly related to the amount of CSF sampled. If 5 to 10 mL of CSF is obtained, acid-fast stain of spun CSF may be positive in as many as 30% of cases, and culture is positive in 70%. Examination of small (≤1 mL) amounts of CSF is unlikely to yield the organism. Culture of other sites, such as gastric aspirates or urine, may help confirm the diagnosis. Computed tomography may help establish a diagnosis of tuberculous meningitis and aids in evaluating the success of therapy. There may be evidence of brain stem meningitis, hydrocephalus, or focal infarcts. Occasionally, one or several tuberculomas may be present.

### Skeletal Tuberculosis

Skeletal tuberculosis results from lymphohematogenous dissemination of tubercle bacilli early in the course of primary infection. Occasionally, bone infection is initiated by direct extension from a contiguous lymph node or by extension from a neighboring infected bone. Involvement of bone complicates 1% to 2% of untreated primary infections in childhood, usually occurring within 12 to 24 months of formation of the primary complex. The pathologic process begins in the metaphysis because of its rich blood supply. Granulation tissue and caseation develop, destroying bone by direct infection and pressure necrosis. Cold soft-tissue abscesses and extension of the infection through the epiphysis into the joint often accompany the primary bone lesion.

The most commonly affected bones are the vertebrae, causing tuberculosis of the spine (ie, Pott's disease). Although any vertebral body can be infected, there is a predilection for the thoracic vertebrae, especially T12. Involvement of two or more vertebrae is fairly common, and there may be skip areas between lesions. Usually, the body of the vertebra is affected, causing destruction and collapse (Fig 56-15). The progression of tuberculous spondylitis viewed on radiographs is from narrowing of a disc space to collapse and wedging of the vertebral body, with subsequent angulation of the spine (ie, gibbus) or severe kyphosis. Paraspinal abscess, psoas abscess, or retropharyngeal abscess may develop from the bone lesion. The most frequent clinical signs and symptoms of tuberculous spondylitis include low-grade fever, restlessness, pain, and abnormal positioning or gait. Rigidity of the spine is caused by muscle spasm, often initiated by the patient's effort to minimize pain by immobilization. There may be intermittent referred pain caused by associated radiculitis.

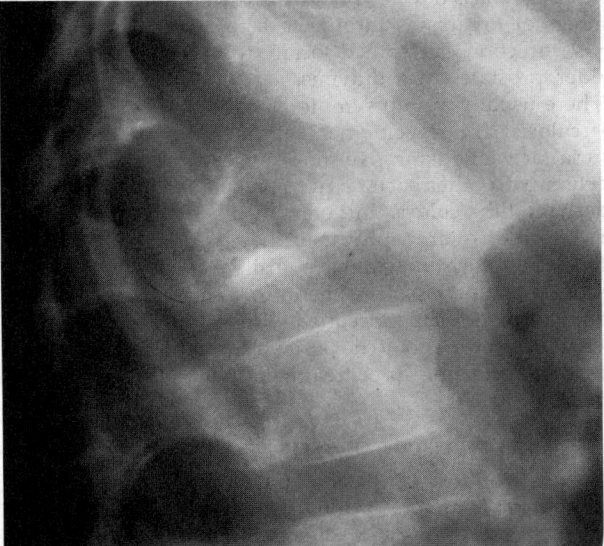

**Figure 56-15.** Radiograph shows destruction and collapse of the twelfth vertebra caused by tuberculous spondylitis. (Courtesy of Gail J. Demmler.)

## Abdominal and Gastrointestinal Tuberculosis

Tuberculosis of the oral cavity and pharynx is quite unusual today; most cases in the past were associated with bovine tuberculosis acquired from infected milk. The usual lesion is a painless ulcer on the mucosa, palate, or tonsil, accompanied by swelling of a regional lymph node. Tuberculosis of the larynx may cause hoarseness. Tuberculosis of the esophagus is exceedingly rare in children.

Tuberculous enteritis is caused by ingestion of infected milk, superinfection of the mucosa caused by swallowed tubercle bacilli discharged from a patient's own lungs, or hematogenous spread. The most commonly affected regions are the jejunum and ileum, especially near the Peyer patches or the appendix. Shallow ulcers are the most common lesions and cause pain, diarrhea or constipation, and weight loss. Mesenteric adenitis accompanying the enteritis may cause intestinal obstruction or may erode through the omentum and cause peritonitis. The clinical presentation of tuberculous enteritis mimics many other conditions; the diagnosis is confirmed by the presence of pulmonary sites of tuberculosis, positive tuberculin skin test, and biopsy and culture of the ulcerative lesions.

Tuberculous peritonitis occurs mainly in young men and is rare in childhood. Generalized peritonitis may occur as a result of hematogenous dissemination. Localized peritonitis is caused by direct extension from a lymph node infection, intestinal focus, or tuberculous salpingitis. The lymph nodes, omentum, and peritoneum are often matted together and are palpated as a "doughy" irregular mass that is relatively nontender. Ascites may occur, usually accompanied by fever. The tuberculin skin test is virtually always positive. Paracentesis may confirm the diagnosis, but the procedure must be done carefully to avoid entering matted, immobilized intestine.

## Renal Tuberculosis

Renal tuberculosis is fairly rare in childhood because it does not develop for several years after the primary infection. Tubercle bacilli reach the kidney during lymphohematogenous dissemination of the primary infection. Organisms can be recovered from the urine in many cases of miliary tuberculosis and in some cases of pulmonary tuberculosis before renal parenchymal disease develops. Small caseous tubercles can develop in the renal parenchyma and discharge tubercle bacilli into the tubules. Occasionally, a large mass develops near the cortex and discharges large numbers of organisms through a fistulous tract into the renal pelvis. Infection can spread locally to involve the ureter, gallbladder, prostate, or epididymis.

There usually are no symptoms early in the course of renal tuberculosis. The development of "sterile pyuria," hematuria, dysuria, or vague flank pain first suggests the infection. Superinfection with other bacteria may cause delay in diagnosing the underlying tuberculosis. Intravenous pyelography may reveal a mass lesion or hydronephrosis if there is ureteral stricture. The urine culture is virtually always positive for M tuberculosis. Microscopic examination of sediment from an adequately large early morning urine specimen frequently reveals acid-fast bacilli. The tuberculin skin test should be positive. Surgical intervention rarely is required for diagnosis or treatment if adequate chemotherapy is given.

## Superficial Lymph Node Tuberculosis

Tuberculosis of the superficial lymph nodes (ie, scrofula) is probably the most common form of extrathoracic disease, occurring in 3% to 6% of primary infections. In most cases, it is an early manifestation of lymphohematogenous dissemination, occurring within 6 to 9 months of the primary infection. Some cases arise years after the initial infection and may herald a reactivation of infection.

Regional lymphadenitis is part of the primary complex of tuberculosis. The nodes most commonly involved are in the tonsillar and submandibular regions because of extension of a primary lesion in the upper lung fields or the abdomen. Enlarged nodes in the inguinal, epitrochlear, or axillary regions result from skin or skeletal infections in the extremities.

In the early stage of infection, the lymph nodes are firm, discrete, and nontender. Multiple nodes in one region often are involved. Scrofula in the neck is usually unilateral, but because of the drainage patterns of lymphatics from the chest, it may be bilateral. Other than low-grade fever, systemic signs and symptoms usually are absent. The lymph nodes may enlarge gradually. Occasionally, there is rapid enlargement, associated with high fever, tenderness, and fluctuance. This picture can be caused by tuberculosis or a bacterial superinfection. The initial presentation is rarely a fluctuant mass with overlying cellulitis or discoloration of the skin.

Many other conditions can be confused with tuberculous adenitis, including infection due to NTM, cat-scratch disease, tularemia, brucellosis, malignant tumor, branchial cleft cyst, cystic hygroma, and pyogenic infection. The most frequent problem in diagnosis is differentiating infection due to M tuberculosis from NTM adenitis in geographic areas where NTM are common. Evidence of thoracic lymph node or pulmonary involvement on chest radiographs is more common in tuberculosis but can occur with NTM disease. The induration caused by a 5-TU PPD Mantoux test usually is greater than 15 mm with M tuberculosis infection and less than 10 mm with NTM disease; reactions of 10 to 15 mm can be caused by either infection. The most important part of an evaluation is determining whether exposure to a tuberculous adult has occurred. In many cases, the correct diagnosis can be established only by biopsy and culture of tissue from the involved lymph node.

If left untreated, tuberculous adenitis causes caseation and necrosis of the lymph node. The capsule may break down, leading to the spread of infection to adjacent lymph nodes. The skin overlying this mass of lymph nodes becomes thin, shiny, and erythematous. Rupture through the skin may result in formation of a sinus tract. Lymphadenitis caused by M tuberculosis responds well to antituberculosis chemotherapy, although the lymph nodes may not return to normal size for months or years. Surgical removal is not adequate therapy, because the lymph node disease is but one part of a systemic infection, and involved nodes frequently extend into the mediastinum, where removal is difficult. However, a surgical biopsy and culture frequently are necessary to differentiate tuberculous adenitis from other entities, especially NTM infection. Excisional biopsy is preferred over incisional biopsy because of an increased risk of subsequent sinus tract formation or severe scarring with the latter procedure.

## Perinatal Tuberculosis

True congenital tuberculosis caused by the spread of infection through the placenta or amniotic fluid has been reported in only 200 infants. Transplacental transmission occurs through the umbilical vein from a mother with primary hematogenous or genital tuberculosis. This hematogenous "inoculation" of the fetus leads to miliary tuberculosis. The major site of disease is the liver, which is enlarged. Pulmonary disease usually has a miliary pattern but may be more localized. Generalized lymphadenopathy and meningitis occur in about 50% of these patients. The exact clinical manifestations depend on the infecting "dose" of bacilli and the time of transmission. Stillbirth has been associated with tuberculosis in the fetus. Although the onset of symptoms may be delayed for several weeks, symptoms most commonly begin around the second week of life and include lethargy, decreased feeding, nasal discharge, jaundice, respiratory distress, and abdominal distention from hepatosplenomegaly.

Several cases of congenital tuberculosis have been caused by aspiration of amniotic fluid infected with *M tuberculosis* from a mother with tuberculous endometritis. Pulmonary symptoms and signs dominate the clinical picture, but hepatomegaly usually is present.

Diagnosis of true congenital tuberculosis is likely to be delayed, especially if the diagnosis of tuberculosis has not been established in the mother. Signs and symptoms in the neonate are similar to those caused by other congenital bacterial or viral infections. The tuberculin skin test is not helpful in diagnosing infants. Demonstration of acid-fast bacilli in a gastric, endotracheal, or bone marrow aspirate or biopsy tissue is required to establish the diagnosis. The mortality rate remains high because of delayed diagnosis and the overwhelming nature of the infection.

Perinatal tuberculosis caused by inhalation of tubercle bacilli expelled by an adult who handles the infant is much more common than true congenital tuberculosis. More than 50% of infants infected with *M tuberculosis* at or near birth can be expected to develop clinically significant disease, usually in the lungs or cervical lymph nodes. The newborn infant should be separated from any adult known or thought to have pulmonary tuberculosis until the disease is no longer contagious. If significant exposure has occurred or is likely to occur at home, the infant should have baseline chest radiography and then be started on isoniazid (10 to 15 mg/kg/day). Isoniazid is continued for 3 months after the last possible exposure, and a Mantoux tuberculin test is then performed. If the test is positive, isoniazid is continued as in standard preventive therapy; if it is negative, the drug is discontinued. Babies who are breast-fed must receive pyridoxine in conjunction with isoniazid. If isoniazid cannot be given or if the adult source case has multiply-resistant tuberculosis, BCG vaccination of the infant should be considered. If the mother or other family members have old cases of treated tuberculosis or untreated inactive infection, there should be no risk to the infant, and treatment is not recommended. However, tuberculin skin tests at 4- to 6-month intervals for the first year of life may be prudent.

## TREATMENT

Approaches to the treatment of tuberculosis have undergone radical changes during the last two decades. Most cases of tuberculosis should be cured, but the limiting factor often is human behavior: poor adherence with treatment, leading to relapse and the emergence of drug resistance.

## Chemotherapeutic Agents

A variety of chemotherapeutic agents are available for treating patients with tuberculosis (Table 56-28). The first-line drugs, which include isoniazid, rifampin, pyrazinamide, ethambutol, and streptomycin, are those most often used for initial treatment. The second-line drugs, including *para*-aminosalicylic acid, ethionamide, capreomycin, kanamycin, and cycloserine, are used when drug resistance or intolerance is encountered.

### Isoniazid

Since its release in 1952, isoniazid has been the mainstay of antituberculosis therapy. At the usual dose of 10 mg/kg, the peak plasma concentration exceeds the minimal inhibitory concentration (MIC) for *M tuberculosis* (0.02 to 0.05 $\mu$g/mL) by a factor of 30 to 80. These high concentrations persist in the plasma and sputum for many hours. Concentrations in the CSF, even in the absence of inflammation, are 50% to 100% of plasma concentrations. Low concentrations are present in breast milk. Tablets frequently are given with food, although there are reports of poor absorption in some children when the drug is given this way. Isoniazid is metabolized in the liver by acetylation. The rate and degree of acetylation are determined genetically, but this

**TABLE 56-28. Antituberculosis Drugs Used in Children**

| Drug | Dose (kg/day) | Route of Administration | Drug Toxicity | Available Preparations |
|---|---|---|---|---|
| Isoniazid | 5–15 mg | Oral, intravenous, intramuscular | Hepatotoxicity; peripheral neuritis; rash | 100-mg and 300-mg scored tablets; 10-mg/mL suspension |
| Rifampin | 10–20 mg | Oral | Hepatotoxicity; staining of contact lenses; flu-like syndrome | 150-mg and 300-mg capsules |
| Pyrazinamide | 20–40 mg | Oral | Hepatotoxicity; arthritis or arthralgias; gout | 500-mg scored tablets |
| Streptomycin | 20 mg up to 1 g total | Intramuscular | Eighth nerve damage (vestibular loss more common than hearing loss) | 1-g vials |
| Ethambutol | 15–25 mg | Oral | Optic neuritis; red-green color blindness | 100-mg and 400-mg scored tablets |
| Ethionamide | 10–20 mg | Oral | Gastric irradiation; teratogenic | 250-mg tablets |
| Capreomycin | 10–15 mg | Intramuscular | Nephrotoxicity; eighth nerve damage (hearing loss more common than vestibular loss) | 1-g vials |
| Kanamycin | 15–30 mg | Intramuscular | Nephrotoxicity; eighth nerve damage (hearing loss more common than vestibular loss) | 100-mg, 500-mg, and 1-g vials |
| Cycloserine | 10–20 mg up to 1 g total | Oral | Neurologic and psychiatric | 250-mg capsules |
| *Para*-aminosalicylic acid | 250–300 mg | Oral | Severe gastric irritation | Available for Centers for Disease Control and Prevention |

usually is of little significance for treatment or drug toxicity in children.

Most children tolerate isoniazid so well that only clinical monitoring is necessary. Transient elevation of hepatic enzymes has been documented in 10% of adult patients, with overt clinical hepatitis occurring in only 1%. Both problems are rare in children, but they are slightly more common in adolescents. Routine serial liver function testing is unnecessary for children taking isoniazid unless they have a history of liver disease or develop clinical signs and symptoms of toxicity. Significant hepatic toxicity is more likely to occur if the dose exceeds 10 mg/kg/day and rifampin also is being given and if the patient has severe disseminated tuberculosis (eg, miliary or meningeal disease).

Peripheral neuritis, caused by the competitive inhibition of pyridoxine metabolism, can occur when isoniazid is given to patients with poor nutrition. Although this problem is fairly common in adults, children's pyridoxine levels are depressed, but clinical manifestations are rare. Children with reasonably balanced diets do not need pyridoxine supplementation. However, breast-fed infants receiving isoniazid should always receive supplementation because of the low pyridoxine concentrations in breast milk.

Infrequent adverse effects of isoniazid include convulsions, psychosis, severe headache, allergic manifestation, and a lupus-like syndrome. Isoniazid can increase phenytoin levels and cause significant toxicity by blocking phenytoin metabolism in the liver.

### Rifampin

A key drug in the modern management of tuberculosis, rifampin is absorbed readily from the gastrointestinal tract. Oral doses of 10 to 15 mg/kg result in peak plasma concentrations of 6 to 32 $\mu$g/mL, far exceeding the MIC for M tuberculosis (0.5 $\mu$g/mL). Rifampin diffuses readily into all body tissues and fluids, achieving CSF concentrations of 60% to 90% of plasma levels. Its metabolism and excretion occur in the liver and kidneys, respectively.

Rifampin usually is well tolerated. However, the preparation is an orange-red dye that stains all body fluids including urine, tears, sweat, and feces. It may permanently stain contact lenses. Hepatic toxicity is rare (<1%) unless rifampin is used in conjunction with isoniazid doses that exceed 10 mg/kg/day. Gastrointestinal irritation, leukopenia, thrombocytopenia, and a peculiar influenza-like syndrome that is immunologically mediated may occur. Rifampin can render oral contraceptives inactive and may interact adversely with several other drugs, including quinidine, solium warfarin, and corticosteroids.

Although the usual dose of rifampin is 10 to 15 mg/kg/day, proprietary formulations include only 150-mg and 300-mg capsules. A suspension can be made by most pharmacies for the desired dose and concentration. Rifampin should not be given with food because its absorption becomes erratic. Rifamate, a capsule with a fixed combination of isoniazid (150 mg) and rifampin (300 mg), may be useful for adults and some children or adolescents.

### Pyrazinamide

First developed in 1949, pyrazinamide has only recently been "rediscovered" as an important antituberculosis. In adults, an oral dose of 30 mg/kg produces plasma levels around 20 $\mu$g/mL. The pharmacokinetics of pyrazinamide are not described adequately for children. Doses of 30 mg/kg are tolerated well by children, and the CSF levels are similar to those obtained in adults—50% to 75% of plasma levels. Pyrazinamide is an unusual drug that is not bactericidal in vitro but does contribute to killing of M tuberculosis in vivo. It is active only at a pH of about 5.5, which is the pH inside macrophages. It is metabolized by the liver, and hepatotoxicity may occur, especially if the dose exceeds 40 mg/kg/day. Pyrazinamide and its metabolites inhibit urinary excretion of uric acid. About 10% of adults develop arthralgias, arthritis, or gout, but these complications are extremely rare in children.

### Streptomycin

Although it is used less frequently than in the past, streptomycin is important for drug-resistant tuberculosis. It must be given intramuscularly. Streptomycin penetrates inflamed meninges well, but CSF levels are low in the absence of inflammation. The principal adverse effect is eighth nerve toxicity. The most common complication is damage to the vestibular branch, resulting in vertigo or ataxia. Hearing loss occurs less frequently, but auditory acuity should be monitored if streptomycin is used for more than a few weeks.

### Ethambutol

At the usual dose of 15 to 20 mg/kg/day, ethambutol reaches a peak plasma concentration of 3 to 5 $\mu$g/mL, a level that is bacteriostatic for M tuberculosis. However, at higher doses, the drug may be bactericidal. It is rapidly absorbed from the gastrointestinal tract and excreted in the urine, mainly as the parent compound. The use of this drug has been limited in children because of its ability to cause optic neuritis or red-green color blindness. At the usual doses, optic toxicity is rare in adults and has not been reported in children. Ethambutol is not used routinely in small children because it is difficult to monitor their visual activity and color perception, but it should be used in cases of drug-resistant tuberculosis.

### Second-Line Drugs

If drug resistance to first-line drugs or toxicity becomes a problem, second-line drugs are used. Para-aminosalicylic acid previously was an important agent for the treatment of tuberculosis. However, it is only bacteriostatic and is associated with severe gastric irritation at usual doses. It is no longer available on a routine basis. Certain aminoglycosides, such as capreomycin, kanamycin, and amikacin, are active against most strains of M tuberculosis, including those resistant to streptomycin. Cycloserine is rarely used in children because of its propensity to cause a variety of neurologic and psychiatric disturbances. Ethionamide is effective and well tolerated by children. It is bacteriostatic but achieves excellent CSF concentrations. It should not be used in pregnant women because of its teratogenic effects in animals.

## Rationale for Multidrug Therapy

The traditional approach to antituberculosis chemotherapy combined use of a potent bactericidal drug—usually isoniazid—with a second drug given to prevent the emergence of resistance to isoniazid. Some drugs, such as pyrazinamide and streptomycin, can kill M tuberculosis but are not as effective in preventing emergence of resistance to other drugs. Rifampin, isoniazid, ethambutol, and para-aminosalicylic acid effectively prevent resistance to other agents. This approach required 12 to 24 months of treatment to produce a bacteriologic cure. Modern methods of combination drug treatment are designed for rapid killing of M tuberculosis to sterilize the lesions as quickly as possible.

## Short-Course Therapy

There are several reasons why it is important to treat patients for the shortest possible period. Expense is markedly decreased compared with longer, traditional therapy—an important consideration in developing countries with limited resources. More time and program resources can be allocated to ensuring adherence with medications and clinic or physician visits, and the patient is exposed to potentially toxic drugs for less time. If a patient quits treatment early, there is a greater likelihood that bacteriologic cure will have been achieved.

There have been numerous short-course therapy trials in adults with drug-susceptible pulmonary tuberculosis. Nine months of treatment with isoniazid and rifampin cures 98% of cases. Both drugs must be given daily for the first 1 to 2 months; thereafter, they can be given daily or twice-weekly, with equivalent results. When given twice weekly, the rifampin dose is the same as the daily dose, but the isoniazid dose is increased to two to three times the daily dose. Twice-weekly therapy is effective because after 2 months the replication of the organisms is slow and the drugs have a long elimination half-life. Twice-weekly medications should be administered under the direct observation of a health care professional because of the adherence problems associated with virtually every tuberculosis control program.

Therapy with isoniazid and rifampin lasting less than 9 months has led to unacceptably high relapse rates (≥10%). Shorter durations can be successful if more than two bactericidal drugs are used initially. Because pyrazinamide and streptomycin have their greatest effect early in therapy, a dualistic approach of intensive three- or four-drug therapy (eg, isoniazid, rifampin, pyrazinamide, streptomycin) for 2 months, followed by isoniazid and rifampin for several months or more, has been suggested. The addition of streptomycin to the initial regimen adds little to efficacy. Unfortunately, regimens shorter than 6 months are not as effective. The current American Thoracic Society recommendation for pulmonary tuberculosis in adults is 9 months of isoniazid and rifampin or a 6-month regimen using isoniazid, rifampin, and pyrazinamide daily for 2 months, followed by 4 months of daily or twice-weekly isoniazid and rifampin.

Intensive, short-course antituberculosis therapy has proven to be highly effective for children with drug-susceptible pulmonary tuberculosis. The best studied regimen consists of isoniazid and rifampin given for 6 months, supplemented with pyrazinamide during the first 2 months. This regimen yields cure rates approaching 100%, relapse rates approaching 0%, and an incidence of mild adverse drug reactions of about 1%. It is desirable to have medications administered daily for the first 1 to 2 months of therapy; thereafter, they can be given daily by the family or twice-weekly under the direct observation of a health care worker. For patients for whom social issues or other constraints prevent reliable daily self-administration of drugs even in the initial phase of treatment, drugs can be given under direct observation two to three times per week from the beginning. If initial isoniazid or rifampin resistance is deemed more likely due to epidemiologic factors, a fourth drug should be added until the drug susceptibility pattern is established.

Most forms of extrapulmonary tuberculosis respond well to the 6-month, three-drug regimen used for pulmonary tuberculosis. One exception may be bone and joint tuberculosis, which often requires 9 to 12 months of treatment to effect a cure, especially if surgical intervention is not undertaken. Although tuberculous meningitis probably can be cured with 6 months of therapy if isoniazid, rifampin, and pyrazinamide are given initially, the lack of data leads many experts to recommend extending therapy to 9 to 12 months. Most experts add a fourth drug initially—usually ethionamide, ethambutol, or an aminoglycoside—to protect against unsuspected drug resistance.

## Drug Resistance

The incidence of drug-resistant tuberculosis is increasing throughout the world, with rates as high as 35% in some locales (eg, Southeast Asia, parts of Central America, South America, Africa). Rates in the United States vary from less than 1% to 15% along the Mexican border and over 30% in New York City. Primary resistance occurs when a person is infected with an organism that is already resistant to a drug. Secondary resistance occurs when drug-resistant organisms emerge as a dominant population during therapy. Poor patient adherence and improper administration of medications by the physician can lead to secondary resistance.

Patterns of drug resistance among children mirror those found in adults in a given population. Certain epidemiologic factors, such as immigration from a country with a high resistance rate or history of prior treatment for tuberculosis, may correlate with drug resistance in adult patients and their contacts. When drug resistance is suspected, initial therapy must include at least three or four drugs. Subsequent therapy must be tailored to the resistance pattern.

For isoniazid resistance, a regimen of rifampin and ethambutol given for 12 to 18 months, supplemented initially with pyrazinamide, is usually effective. For rifampin-resistant tuberculosis, the combination of isoniazid and ethambutol plus initial pyrazinamide is effective. For isoniazid and rifampin resistance, a regimen employing at least two bactericidal drugs must be designed based on the exact susceptibility pattern of the isolate. In this situation, cure rates are usually below 50% even under the best conditions.

## Corticosteroids

Although data on their efficacy are relatively sparse, corticosteroids have found a place in the treatment of some forms of tuberculosis. However, they should never be used unless effective antituberculosis drugs are given simultaneously. Corticosteroids may be of benefit if the host inflammatory reaction is contributing to tissue damage or impairment of function. There is convincing evidence that corticosteroids aid patients with tuberculous meningitis and increased intracranial pressure due to brain stem inflammation and resultant hydrocephalus. Children with endobronchial disease (eg, localized air trapping, collapse-consolidation lesion) frequently benefit from corticosteroids. Other forms of tuberculosis that may benefit from corticosteroids are miliary disease with alveolocapillary block, pericarditis, peritonitis, and pleural effusion. Prednisone is the drug used most commonly, at a dosage of 1 to 2 mg/kg/day for 4 to 6 weeks, with gradual withdrawal over several weeks.

## PREVENTION

Primary prevention, such as BCG vaccination, is designed to prevent the establishment of tuberculous infection. Secondary prevention, such as isoniazid therapy, aims at preventing the development of active disease after infection has occurred.

## BCG Vaccination

Bacille Calmette-Guérin was derived from a strain of *M bovis* that was attenuated through years of serial passage in culture. The many BCG vaccines derived from the original strain vary greatly in antigenicity and efficacy. The BCG vaccine activates host cell-mediated immunity to mycobacterial antigens in an attempt to prevent infection or progression to disease if a subsequent infection with *M tuberculosis* occurs.

Strain variation and lack of experimental standardization have hampered evaluation of many BCG trials. Intradermal injection of BCG is the most precise and effective technique, but multiple-puncture techniques are popular because of the ease of administration. The usual local reaction to an intradermal BCG vaccination is a papule that develops a permanent scar (Fig 56-16). Painless enlargement of the regional lymph nodes frequently occurs but usually resolves within several weeks.

The efficacy of BCG in preventing subsequent tuberculous disease in children has ranged from 0% to 80% in various studies. BCG is given to newborns in some countries, to 1-year-old children in others, and to adolescents in still others. Little is known about the effectiveness of revaccination. The most important and consistent effect of BCG is to limit significantly the development of serious disseminated tuberculosis (eg, miliary disease, meningitis) in young children. Vaccinated children who subsequently develop tuberculosis tend to have localized thoracic disease.

Adverse reactions to BCG are uncommon in immunocompetent children. Localized ulceration, adenitis, and osteomyelitis have been reported. Disseminated infection and death have been reported only in children with severe immunodeficiencies.

The BCG vaccine is used rarely in the United States. A disadvantage is that BCG produces hypersensitivity to tuberculin and a positive Mantoux reaction (usually less than 12 mm) that may persist for as long as 5 years. Because there is no way to differentiate a skin test reaction due to BCG from one caused by infection with *M tuberculosis,* the safest course is to attribute any significant reaction to tuberculous infection, regardless of the BCG status of the patient. In the United States, BCG may be useful in protecting persons likely to have unavoidable exposure to tuberculosis, such as an infant whose mother has active tuberculosis or a child who may become exposed to multidrug-resistant tuberculosis.

## Preventive Therapy

The treatment of asymptomatic, tuberculin-positive patients to prevent development of tuberculous disease is an established practice in the United States. The widespread use of the term *chemoprophylaxis* is unfortunate, because this is actually treatment

of a subclinical infection. Therapy with isoniazid does not alter the tuberculin reaction in most children infected with *M tuberculosis,* but extensive clinical trials have demonstrated that 1 year of daily isoniazid therapy (10 mg/kg/day) prevents the development of active tuberculosis for at least 30 years.

Isoniazid preventive therapy is indicated for children with a positive tuberculin test but no clinical or radiographic evidence of disease; children with a negative tuberculin test who have had known recent exposure to an adult with contagious tuberculosis; and persons of any age who show recent conversion of the tuberculin skin test after exposure to a contagious case. (Children with a negative tuberculin test after known exposure may be an example of primary prophylaxis. Infection may have already occurred, but the skin test has not yet become positive.) Most physicians give isoniazid to any person younger than 35 who has a positive tuberculin skin test but not to older persons unless conversion is recent because of an increased probability of isoniazid-induced hepatotoxicity in the older age group. However, the cutoff at age 35 has been questioned, and some experts would treat tuberculin-positive persons of almost any age. Preventive therapy with rifampin for 6 to 9 months is used for persons known to be infected with isoniazid-resistant strains of *M tuberculosis.* However, data are scarce, and treatment failures have been reported.

A 1-year course of isoniazid preventive therapy is of proven efficacy. A study using data from adults in Eastern Europe with stable, fibrotic tuberculous pulmonary lesions showed that a 6-month regimen was more cost effective than a 12-month regimen. However, no data on the efficacy of 6-month isoniazid preventive therapy for children have been reported. Many physicians and clinics give them preventive therapy for 9 months.

## Selected Readings

American Academy of Pediatrics Committee on Infectious Diseases. Chemotherapy of tuberculosis in infants and children. Pediatrics 1992;89:161.
American Thoracic Society. Diagnostic standards and classification of tuberculosis. Am Rev Respir Dis 1990;142:725.
Bloch AB, Rieder HL, Kelly GD, Cauthen GM, Hayden CH, Snider DE Jr. The epidemiology of tuberculosis in the United States. Clin Chest Med 1989;10:297.
Hsu KHK. Thirty years after isoniazid: its impact on tuberculosis in children and adolescents. JAMA 1984;251:1283.
Lincoln EM, Sewell EM. Tuberculosis in children. New York: McGraw-Hill, 1963.
Miller FJW. Tuberculosis in children. New York: Churchill Livingston, 1981.
Snider DE, Reider HL, Combs D, Bloch AB, Hayden CH, Smith MHD. Tuberculosis in children. Pediatr Infect Dis J 1988;7:271.
Starke JR, Taylor-Watts KT. Tuberculosis in the pediatric population of Houston, Texas. Pediatrics 1989;84:28.
Starke JR, Jacobs RF, Jereb J. Resurgence of tuberculosis in children. J Pediatr 1992;120:839.

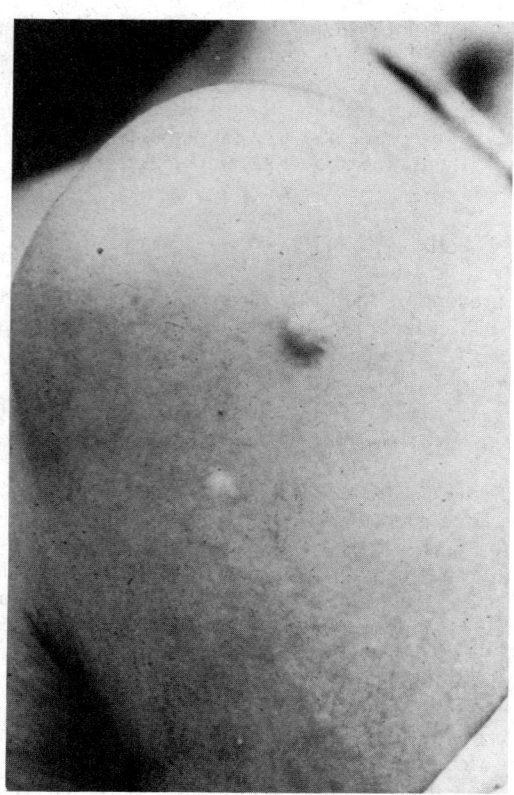

Figure 56-16.   BCG vaccination scar on a young child.

*Principles and Practice of Pediatrics, Second Edition.* edited by Frank A. Oski et al. J. B. Lippincott Company, Philadelphia © 1994.

# 56.29 *Nontuberculous Mycobacteria*

Jeffrey R. Starke

Mycobacteria other than *Mycobacterium tuberculosis* and *Mycobacterium leprae* are known by several names, including nontuberculous, atypical, unclassified, environmental, and opportunistic mycobacteria. Nontuberculous mycobacteria (NTM) is probably the preferred and most accurate nomenclature. These organisms were discovered almost a century ago, but their role in causing pulmonary and lymph node disease was not described until 1948.

## EPIDEMIOLOGY

In the early 1950s, 1% to 2% of the patients in tuberculosis sanatoria in Georgia and Florida had disease that was epidemiologically distinct from tuberculosis. Those with NTM disease were more likely to be older and Caucasian, and they usually had underlying chronic pulmonary disease, such as bronchiectasis or silicosis. Reaction to a tuberculin skin test was less common than among patients with tuberculosis, and close contacts tended to be tuberculin-negative. As more reports of NTM disease were published, it became apparent that there was marked geographic variability in the incidence of NTM disease and in the specific NTM species causing the illness.

Between 1958 and 1970, large numbers of Navy recruits were skin tested with purified protein derivative (PPD) from *M tuberculosis* (PPD-S), *M intracellulare* (PPD-B), and *M scrofulaceum* (PPD-G). The geographic distribution of reactors to PPD-S was very different from that of reactors to PPD-B or PPD-G. Sensitization to NTM antigens was common in recruits from the southeastern United States but less so in recruits from the Northeast, Midwest, or West. None of these sensitized recruits had ever experienced disease, demonstrating that most NTM infections are asymptomatic.

Although it has never been proved, NTM organisms are probably inhaled or introduced into the mouth, nose, or throat. NTM can be found in the environment in soil, water, or vegetation. The organisms may be present in some animals, but animal-to-human or person-to-person transmission has not been demonstrated. Certain mycobacteria that cause cutaneous granulomas may be present in water, including oceans, ponds, swimming pools, aquariums, and hot tubs. Children are more likely to have NTM cutaneous granulomas or superficial lymph node disease, and adults are more prone to pulmonary infections.

A recent change in the epidemiology of NTM infections has occurred because of infections in adults and children with human immunodeficiency virus (HIV) disease. NTM disease is common in HIV-infected patients from all areas of the United States, even those where background infection rates (based on historic skin test results) are low. Their disease tends to be disseminated and is not well controlled with current medications. There is a growing number of reports of instances or clusters of nosocomially acquired NTM infections, most often associated with surgery or an indwelling catheter.

## ETIOLOGY

There are at least 19 *Mycobacterium* species associated with human disease, and several more may be encountered in clinical specimens. In 1959, Runyon proposed a grouping of mycobacteria exclusive of *M tuberculosis*, *M bovis*, and *M leprae* based on pigmentation, growth rate, and colony morphology (Table 56-29). Species are differentiated further by culture characteristics, temperature of optimal growth, enzymatic activity, niacin production, phage typing, and serologic findings. By conventional methods, growth of most of the NTM is slow; exact speciation and susceptibility testing may take as long as 6 to 10 weeks. The Bactec radiometric culture system has reduced the time required for isolation to 2 weeks or less. There is a special Bactec substrate that permits immediate differentiation of NTM from *M tuberculosis*: NTM grow freely in this substrate, but the growth of *M tuberculosis* is inhibited.

| TABLE 56-29. Runyon Classification for Nontuberculous Mycobacteria |
|---|
| **Group I** |
| Photochromogens—grow white in the dark and become bright yellow to orange when exposed to light; colony formation in 2–4 weeks on standard agar. Includes *M marinum*, *M kansasii*, *M simiae*, *M asiaticum*. |
| **Group II** |
| Scotochromogens—produce a yellow-orange pigment in the dark, and become orange to red in the light; colony formation in 1–3 weeks. Includes *M scrofulaceum*, *M szulgai*, *M gordonae*, *M flavescens*, *M xenopi*. |
| **Group III** |
| Nonchromogens—no pigment produced in dark or light; colony formation in 2–4 weeks. Includes *M avium*, *M intracellulare*, *M gastri*, *M malmoense*, *M haemophilum*, *M nonchromogenicum*, *M terrae*, *M triviale*. |
| **Group IV** |
| Rapid growers— no pigment produced in dark or light; colony formation in 2–7 days. Includes *M fortuitum*, *M chelonei*, *M phlei*, *M smegmatis*, *M vaccae*, *M abscessus*. |

## PATHOLOGY

Most people who encounter NTM have asymptomatic infections. Inhaled or ingested mycobacteria may deposit on the mucous membranes of the nose, mouth, and throat. Local manifestations of infection are rare. After disease develops, the histopathologic findings are similar to those caused by *M tuberculosis* infection. Lymph nodes affected by NTM develop necrosis within areas of caseation early in the course. Nonspecific acute and chronic inflammatory changes occur more often than true granulomas. Acid-fast stains of tissue are positive in 30% to 60% of the cases. Even the most experienced pathologist cannot reliably differentiate NTM adenitis from tuberculous adenitis by microscopic or histologic examination.

Pulmonary disease is rare in children, and the clinical picture includes hilar adenopathy, patchy infiltrates of multiple lobes, and lobar pneumonia.

Patients with coexistent NTM and HIV infections tend to have more severe and disseminated disease. NTM infection occurs primarily in the lungs, bone marrow, liver and spleen, gastrointestinal tract, and kidneys. Blood and stool cultures frequently are positive. HIV-infected patients tend not to form granulomas; their inflammatory reaction is a less specific mix of chronic and acute changes. However, infected tissues usually have an enormous number of organisms that are seen readily on acid-fast stain preparations.

## CLINICAL MANIFESTATIONS

### Superficial Lymph Nodes

The most common site of clinically significant NTM infection in children is the superficial lymph nodes of the head and neck. When this clinical picture was first described, *M scrofulaceum* was the most common infecting agent. Most recent cases have been caused by *M avium* and *M intracellulare*, but *M kansasii* and *M fortuitum* occasionally cause this form of disease. Scrofula due to NTM is most common in young children because of their tendency to put objects contaminated with soil, dust, or standing water in their mouths. The younger the child, the more likely it is that scrofula is caused by NTM. Children living in rural or suburban settings are more likely to develop NTM cervical adenitis, but those in cities are more prone to scrofula due to *M tuberculosis.*

Adenitis due to NTM usually involves a group of nodes, most often located in the anterior superior cervical chain or submandibular area. Preauricular, postauricular, and submental lymph nodes also may be infected. In rare cases, infection of an axillary, epitrochlear, or inguinal node occurs secondary to cutaneous inoculation. The disease usually is unilateral. The nodal swelling may be explosive over several days but more often develops insidiously, occasionally after an upper respiratory tract infection. The nodes are usually painless, nontender, and quite firm initially. As the infection progresses, the nodes soften and often develop fluctuance. The skin becomes shiny and thin, with an erythematous or violet hue. Untreated nodes frequently rupture through the skin, causing drainage and eventual formation of a sinus tract that can persist for months or years. Healing is marked by fibrosis and scarring of the skin. Low-grade fever may be present initially, but other systemic signs or symptoms are rare. A high fever or a "toxic" appearance of the child may indicate superinfection with pyogenic bacteria.

The differential diagnosis of NTM adenitis is extensive, including tuberculosis, cat-scratch disease, tularemia, brucellosis, actinomycosis, nocardiosis, toxoplasmosis, mononucleosis, malignancies, cystic hygroma, and rarer conditions. The greatest difficulty is usually the differentiation of NTM adenitis from adenitis due to *M tuberculosis.* The chest radiograph is more often abnormal with tuberculous adenitis, but some children with NTM adenitis have significant mediastinal adenopathy, and rarely, there are segmental pulmonary lesions. Lack of contact with an adult who has tuberculosis, a normal chest radiograph, small reaction to a standard tuberculin skin test, and poor response to antituberculosis therapy suggest the likelihood of an NTM scrofula.

## Pulmonary Infection

Pulmonary disease due to NTM in adults frequently resembles chronic pulmonary tuberculosis, causing upper lobe infiltrates and cavitary lesions. Most of these patients have preexisting chronic lung diseases, such as silicosis, malignancy, cystic fibrosis, or healed tuberculosis. The most frequent etiologic agents are *M kansasii, M avium, M intracellulare,* and *M fortuitum.* Because NTM may be isolated from the sputum of adults with no lung disease, a positive sputum culture is not necessarily sufficient to establish the diagnosis. More invasive procedures, such as bronchial washings or biopsy, may be necessary, especially because more than one pathogenic organism may be present.

Primary childhood pulmonary disease due to NTM is rare. Some affected children have enlarged hilar lymph nodes with endobronchial breakthrough and segmental lesions, similar to those seen in tuberculosis. Others have more diffuse disease, involving all of one or more lobes. Most children do not have underlying chronic pulmonary disease. The onset of illness can be insidious or acute, with fever, cough, and listlessness. Diagnosis is difficult because the clinical, radiographic, and skin test data can mimic tuberculosis, and NTM, especially *M gordonae, M kansasii, M avium,* and *M intracellulare,* can be isolated from the gastric aspirates of healthy children. NTM pulmonary disease should be suspected in a child with the clinical picture of tuberculosis who has no known source case and does not respond well to antituberculosis medications.

## Cutaneous Infection

The most common form of cutaneous NTM infection is the skin granuloma, usually caused by *M marinum* or *M balnei.* The or-

ganisms are introduced by contaminated water that enters a skin abrasion or cut. Direct trauma from contact with shrimp, barnacles, coral, or fishhooks may lead to infection. The granulomatous lesions evolve slowly. They are usually painless and progress from small wart-like nodules to ulcers, with or without drainage, over several weeks. A sporotrichotic form has been described. Regional adenopathy is not routinely part of the primary lesion. The clinical diagnosis is substantiated by biopsy or culture of the ulcer discharge. Usually, no specific therapy is required, but extensive ulcers may require debridement and skin grafting.

The rapidly growing *M fortuitum* and *M chelonei* can cause skin disease resulting from contamination of a wound or needle puncture site. These organisms can be found on the skin, or they may be present in the hospital environment, especially in the operating room. Surgical wound infections, abscess formation after childhood immunizations, and infection complicating puncture wounds to the foot have been described. Seropurulent drainage, poor wound healing, and development of sinus tracts frequently complicate these infections. Diagnosis is established readily by culture of the infected site.

## Disseminated Infection

Disseminated NTM disease was rare before the epidemic of HIV infection. A literature review in 1972 revealed that only 12 cases involving children had been reported. All 12 children had died; 9 had steadily progressive disease, and 3 had periods of remission and reactivation. Lesions of the lungs, long bones, liver, gastrointestinal tract, and bone marrow were common. The histopathology and clinical picture of several children bore a striking resemblance to acute nonlipoid reticuloendotheliosis.

Patients infected with HIV often develop disseminated NTM infection, usually due to *M avium, M intracellulare,* or *M kansasii.* Involvement of the gastrointestinal tract, lungs, bone marrow, liver, kidneys, and rarely of the central nervous system (CNS) with massive numbers of organisms is typical. Blood and stool cultures are usually positive. The most common signs and symptoms are nonspecific, including weight loss, malaise, fever, dyspnea, and diarrhea. Essentially all patients have coexisting infections, and it is difficult to determine which infectious agent is causing a specific problem. It appears that even massive NTM infection rarely is the cause of death in patients with HIV infection, but it contributes to their wasting and the deterioration of immunologic function. Patients with acquired immune deficiency syndrome (AIDS) and disseminated NTM have shorter lifespans than AIDS patients with similar CD4-positive counts who do not have NTM infection. Treatment of the NTM infection leads to clinical improvement in some of these patients.

## Other Sites of Infection

Skeletal NTM infection in the absence of disseminated disease is rare and usually occurs as a complication of surgery or trauma. The rapidly growing mycobacteria are most often the etiologic agents. In children, CNS disease due to NTM is rare, with only 9 cases reported in the pre-HIV era. Meningitis is more common than brain parenchymal disease. Several episodes of infection of indwelling vascular catheters due to *M fortuitum* or *M chelonei* have been described, and porcine heart valves have become infected by these rapid growers. *M chelonei* is a rare cause of postsurgical chronic otitis media.

## DIAGNOSIS

Nonspecific laboratory tests, such as blood counts, urinalysis, and serum chemistry tests, are of no value in diagnosing NTM infection. The most direct diagnostic method is appropriate mycobacterial culture of involved tissue, including lymph nodes, sinus tract drainage, skin granuloma, or bronchial secretions. Unfortunately, culture is positive for only half the cases of probable mycobacterial cervical adenitis. Differentiating NTM isolates from *M tuberculosis* is based on growth characteristics, colony morphology, pigment production, and serum chemistry tests. Drug susceptibility tests should be performed on all mycobacterial isolates. Histopathologic examination of tissues can differentiate mycobacterial infection from other lesions but does not help determine whether the infecting agent is an NTM or *M tuberculosis*.

Skin testing can be a valuable aid in establishing a diagnosis. An immunocompetent person with NTM infection often has a 5 to 12 mm reaction to a 5-TU Mantoux tuberculin (PPD-S) test. Larger reactions are seen but rarely exceed 18 mm. A similar reaction to PPD-S may be caused by infection with *M tuberculosis*, but most patients with tuberculosis have reactions larger than 15 mm. The skin test result is most useful when combined with other information. For example, a 2-year-old child with cervical adenitis who has had no known exposure to tuberculosis but has a normal chest radiograph, has an 11-mm reaction to PPD-S, and lives in the southeastern United States probably has NTM adenitis. Lymph node biopsy may be necessary to confirm the diagnosis. Skin testing with PPD-S is of no value in differentiating the various NTM species. The reaction to PPD-S in persons with NTM infection wanes after resolution of the disease, but patients with tuberculous adenitis retain their delayed hypersensitivity indefinitely. Skin testing is rarely helpful for patients with skin granulomas or infections or in immunosuppressed patients, who usually are anergic.

Skin test antigens more specific for certain NTM species (eg, PPD-B, PPD-G, PPD-Y) are not commercially available. They were used widely until the 1970s, when several studies showed that the available reagents lacked adequate specificity. The Centers for Disease Control conducted a trial with new preparations, and the results for cervical adenitis were encouraging, but the unacceptably high rate of severe skin reactions (eg, blisters) necessitated redevelopment of the antigens.

## TREATMENT

Specific therapy depends on the location and extent of the infected tissue and the species of NTM involved. Surgery usually plays a much more important role in the management of NTM disease than it does for tuberculosis. Most NTM infections are localized in the body and are amenable to surgical removal.

Some cases of NTM adenitis resolve spontaneously, but severe scarring and recurrence are common. Removal of the nodes usually is required for diagnosis and treatment. In the neck, multiple infected nodes located near vital structures, such as the facial nerves and carotid artery, may preclude removal of all involved tissue. Removal of most of the diseased tissue usually leads to resolution, although about 10% to 15% of the infections recur locally, requiring a second surgical procedure. The procedure of choice is excisional biopsy. Incisional biopsy may lead to a chronic sinus tract, poor healing, and increased scarring, although an incision and curettage procedure has been used successfully by some experienced surgeons. The usual agents of NTM adenitis, *M avium*, *M intracellulare*, and *M scrofulaceum*, are resistant to most antimycobacterial drugs. Some cases of NTM adenitis due to *M kansasii* may respond to rifampin and ethambutol.

Most skin granulomas due to NTM heal spontaneously, but some persist and require treatment. Surgical excision has been used frequently, but subsequent skin grafting may be necessary. Lesions caused by *M marinum* or *M kansasii* may respond to rifampin and ethambutol given for 8 to 12 weeks. Minocycline

and trimethoprim-sulfamethoxazole (TMP-SMX) have been effective in a few patients.

Skin and deep tissue infections caused by *M fortuitum* or *M chelonei* require a different approach. Many such lesions heal spontaneously, but systemic therapy may be required. These two species are not susceptible to the typical antimycobacterial drugs. Combinations of drugs, using amikacin, cefoxitin, erythromycin, minocycline, and TMP-SMX, may be effective. Disc susceptibility testing performed in a reference laboratory can help determine the optimal drug regimen. Infected catheters and other implanted devices must be removed to effect a cure.

Treatment of pulmonary or disseminated NTM infections is often difficult. *M avium* and *M intracellulare* usually are resistant to isoniazid, rifampin, streptomycin, and pyrazinamide. Ethambutol, ansamycin, rifabutin, and clofazimine may have some activity against these species. Effective treatment of pulmonary disease usually requires surgery and medical therapy administered for 1 to 3 years. Disseminated infection due to NTM in HIV-infected patients is never eradicated, but many patients improve temporarily after specific therapy is administered.

## Selected Readings

Bass JB Jr, Hawkins EL. Treatment of disease caused by nontuberculous mycobacteria. Arch Intern Med 1983;143:1439.

Bialkin G, Pollak A, Weil AJ. Pulmonary infection with *Mycobacterium kansasii*. Am J Dis Child 1961;101:739.

Contreras MA, Cheung OT, Sanders DE, et al. Pulmonary infection with nontuberculous mycobacteria. Am Rev Respir Dis 1988;137:149.

Horsburgh CR Jr. *Mycobacterium avium* complex infection in patients with acquired immunodeficiency syndrome. N Engl J Med 1991;324:1332.

Lincoln EM, Gilbert LA. Disease in children due to mycobacteria other than *Mycobacterium tuberculosis*. Am Rev Respir Dis 1972;105:683.

Margileth AM, Chandra R, Altman RP. Chronic lymphadenopathy due to mycobacterial infection. Am J Dis Child 1984;138:917.

O'Brien RJ, Geiter LJ, Snider DE Jr. The epidemiology of nontuberculous mycobacterial diseases in the United States. Am Rev Respir Dis 1987;135:1007.

Starke JR. Nontuberculous mycobacterial infections in children. Adv Pediatr Infect Dis 1992;7:123.

Wallace RJ Jr, Swenson JM, Silcox VA, et al. Spectrum of disease due to rapidly growing mycobacteria. Rev Infect Dis 1983;5:657.

Woods GL, Washington JA II. Mycobacteria other than *Mycobacterium tuberculosis*: review of microbiologic and clinical aspects. Rev Infect Dis 1987;9:275.

*Principles and Practice of Pediatrics, Second Edition.*
edited by Frank A. Oski et al. J. B. Lippincott Company, Philadelphia © 1994.

# 56.30 *Yersinia enterocolitica*

## Shai Ashkenazi and Thomas G. Cleary

*Yersinia enterocolitica* first was recognized as a cause of human infection in 1933 by Gilbert and received its current name in 1968. Although initially reported in the cooler regions of Europe and North America, the organism has been recognized worldwide as a cause of human infection. It usually produces acute gastroenteritis in younger children and mesenteric adenitis in older children. It has also been associated with a variety of extraintestinal manifestations.

## ETIOLOGY

The genus *Yersinia,* which belongs to the family Enterobacteriaceae, includes three species that are pathogenic to humans: *Y pestis, Y enterocolitica,* and *Y pseudotuberculosis.* In 1980, three *Yersinia* species, which were previously considered biochemically atypical isolates, were reclassified as *Y fredriksenii, Y kristensenii,* and *Y intermedia.* These strains usually are considered to be non-pathogenic for humans and are usually of animal or environmental origins.

*Y enterocolitica* is an oxidase-negative, non–lactose-fermenting, aerobic, gram-negative coccobacillus. It ferments glucose, galactose, and mannose, reduces nitrates, and does not produce hydrogen peroxide. The organism is motile at 22 °C but not at 37 °C and multiplies more readily at lower temperatures. These properties help to differentiate it from *Y pestis* and other Enterobacteriaceae. *Y enterocolitica* grows well on ordinary media, such as blood, MacConkey medium, heart infusion, and *Salmonella-Shigella* agars, although a selective agar medium has been specifically developed for its isolation. Thirty-four serogroups have been antigenically defined on the basis of the somatic O antigens; most human isolates are serogroups O:3, O:8, and O:9. Twenty flagellar (H) antigens (A through T) have been identified, and serotyping is based on the combined O and H antigens. The pathogenicity of *Y enterocolitica* in laboratory animals and the frequency of immunologic complications in people are related to serotype.

## PATHOLOGY AND PATHOGENESIS

*Y enterocolitica* usually causes diffuse inflammation of the ileum and colon, with infiltrates in the lamina propria and superficial ulcerations in the terminal ileum and colon. Mesenteric lymphadenitis, with reactive germinal centers and sometimes microabscess formation, is often associated. In most cases, the appendix is grossly and histologically normal or shows only mild inflammation.

The pathogenesis of *Y enterocolitica* diarrhea has not been defined fully. Invasiveness, a trait encoded by a 42- to 48-Md plasmid, is a major determinant of the virulence of this organism. The virulence plasmid of *Y enterocolitica* is related to the virulence plasmids of *Y pestis* and *Y pseudotuberculosis.* Plasmid-mediated outer membrane proteins and fimbriae are required for adherence of bacteria to intestinal mucosa and production of infection. The plasmid also endows the organism with other properties, such as calcium dependency, resistance to the bactericidal effect of human serum, and enhanced pathogenicity in laboratory animals. Most clinical isolates of *Y enterocolitica* elaborate an enterotoxin that activates guanylate cyclase and is structurally related to the heat-stable enterotoxin of *Escherichia coli.* Its importance has not been defined because it is produced only when organisms are grown at 30 °C or lower temperatures, and it does not correlate with pathogenicity in animals. Although it has been suggested that toxin preformed in food products may cause diarrhea, the prolonged incubation period makes this mechanism unlikely. The bacteria also produce lipopolysaccharide endotoxin, which has biological properties similar to the endotoxins of other gram-negative bacilli.

Susceptibility to systemic infection is enhanced by visceral iron overload and administration of deferoxamine, an iron-chelating substance. Although *Y enterocolitica* produces no detectable iron-binding compounds (ie, siderophores), it can multiply in the intestine by using siderophores produced by other bacteria. To multiply in tissue, the organism must compete with host iron-binding proteins for the available iron. Extraintestinal infection of *Yersinia* is facilitated by iron overload. Because the organism is capable of using iron bound to deferoxamine, this substance also increases the incidence of systemic infection.

## EPIDEMIOLOGY

The epidemiology of *Y enterocolitica* infections is complex and poorly understood. In Europe and Canada, sporadic cases are quite frequent, outbreaks are rare, and serogroups O:3 and O:9 predominate. In the United States, sporadic cases seem to be less common, and most reported outbreaks are caused by serogroup O:8. Most infections occur in children 5 to 15 years of age, and most series indicate increased incidence during winter months.

The organism has been recovered from a variety of wild and domestic animals, which are probably reservoirs. Water- and food-borne infections have been documented, as has person-to-person transmission in family and community outbreaks. The excretion of the bacteria in stools continues for a few weeks after cessation of the symptoms. In recent years, several food-borne outbreaks of *Y enterocolitica* infection have been reported in the United States, including a large outbreak caused by contaminated pasteurized milk.

## CLINICAL MANIFESTATIONS

Acute gastroenteritis is the most common presentation in young children. Symptoms include diarrhea, usually accompanied by fever, vomiting, and abdominal pain. Stools are usually mucoid, although in 10% to 20% of the patients, there is bloody diarrhea or pus. The severity of diarrhea varies. Fecal leukocytes are commonly present as a reaction to the invasiveness of the organism. The abdominal pain is usually colicky, diffuse, or localized to the right lower abdomen. The disease is self-limiting, usually lasting from 2 to 3 weeks, although prolonged diarrhea has been described. In some children, especially older ones, severe abdominal pain and fever predominate, with minimal diarrhea, suggesting acute appendicitis. The diagnosis of these patients frequently is made only after surgery. Intestinal perforation with peritonitis may be seen in severe cases, especially in adults. Intussusception secondary to *Y enterocolitica* infection has been described in children. The infection may be associated with exudative pharyngitis and headache. In some cases, the infection is entirely asymptomatic, as documented by serologic studies or the recovery of the organism from stool specimens of asymptomatic family contacts.

Extraintestinal manifestations and complications are relatively rare in children. Cutaneous lesions, including erythema nodosum and maculopapular or erythema multiforme-like rashes, appear usually on the trunk and legs several days after the onset of intestinal symptoms and resolve spontaneously. Reactive arthritis appears mainly in adults who have the histocompatibility antigen HLA-B27. Septic arthritis rarely has been reported. Septicemia is unusual but has been described in children with visceral iron overload and patients with underlying diseases, such as diabetes mellitus, malignancy, cirrhosis, or severe anemia, and in a few apparently healthy persons. Rare complications include hepatic or splenic abscesses, osteomyelitis, meningitis, thyroiditis, carditis, and thrombocytopenia. Some of these complications are autoimmune processes, recognized mostly in women.

## DIAGNOSIS

The isolation of the organism from otherwise uncontaminated material, such as blood or lymph nodes, is not difficult, because *Y enterocolitica* grows on ordinary media. Its isolation from stools, the usual source in *Y enterocolitica* infection, is more difficult, because it multiplies more slowly than other enteric bacteria at 37 °C and has no characteristic colony morphology. Recovery can be improved by incubation at a cooler temperature (ie, cold enrichment) and use of selective media, such as cefsulodin-ingasan-novobiocin medium.

Serologic diagnosis has been improved with the use of enzyme-linked immunosorbent assays. Serology can aid diagnosis, especially in outbreaks. Antibodies usually are detected from 8 to 10 days after the onset of clinical symptoms and persist for several months. Serologic response is often absent in infants. *Y enterocolitica* can cross-react with *Y pseudotuberculosis* and with other organisms, such as *Brucella, E coli,* and *Vibrio.*

The differential diagnosis in young children includes the enteric pathogens (eg, *Shigella,* enteroinvasive *E coli, Salmonella, Campylobacter*) that cause a clinically indistinguishable picture. In older children, preoperative differentiation from acute appendicitis may be impossible. *Y pseudotuberculosis* can cause an identical clinical picture. Differentiating these two species can be done only by laboratory identification based on antigenic structure, biochemical activities, and sensitivity to various *Yersinia* phages.

## TREATMENT

The role of antibiotic therapy in the management of children with *Y enterocolitica* enteritis is controversial. Controlled studies have found that antibiotics did not alter the clinical or bacteriologic course of the disease or reduce intrafamilial spread, despite the in vitro susceptibility of the organism. Antibiotic therapy is not indicated in uncomplicated gastroenteritis, which is usually self-limiting; it should be initiated for complicated infections and compromised hosts, especially children with systemic iron overload (eg, those with hemolytic states). The mortality rate for

patients with septicemia is 50% despite antibiotic therapy. *Y enterocolitica* is usually susceptible to trimethoprim-sulfamethoxazole, aminoglycosides, tetracycline, chloramphenicol, and third-generation cephalosporins, and it is resistant to penicillin, ampicillin, carbenicillin, and cephalothin.

Prevention of human infections depends on prevention of food and water contamination, minimizing contact with potentially infected animals, and isolation of infected patients.

## Selected Readings

Black RE, Jackson RJ, Tsai T, et al. Epidemic *Yersinia enterocolitica* infection due to contaminated chocolate milk. N Engl J Med 1978;298:76.

Cornelis G, Laroche Y, Balligand G, et al. *Yersinia enterocolitica,* a primary model for bacterial invasiveness. Rev Infect Dis 1987;9:64.

Foberg U, Fryden A, Kihlström E, et al. *Yersinia enterocolitica* septicemia: clinical and microbiological aspects. Scand J Infect Dis 1986;18:269.

Heesemann J, Keller C, Morawa R, et al. Plasmids of human strains of *Yersinia enterocolitica:* molecular relatedness and possible importance for pathogenesis. J Infect Dis 1983;147:107.

Kohl S. *Yersinia enterocolitica* infections in children. Pediatr Clin North Am 1979;26: 433.

Lee LA, Taylor J, Carter GP, et al. *Yersinia enterocolitica* O:3—an emerging cause of pediatric gastroenteritis. J Infect Dis 1991;163:660.

Marks MI, Pai CH, Lafleur L, et al. *Yersinia enterocolitica* gastroenteritis: a prospective study of clinical, bacteriologic and epidemiologic features. J Pediatr 1980;96: 26.

Pai CH, Gillis F, Tuomanen E, Marks MI. Placebo-controlled double-blind evaluation of trimethoprim/sulfamethoxazole treatment of *Yersinia enterocolitica* gastroenteritis. J Pediatr 1984;104:308.

Robins-Browne RM, Prpic JK. Effects of iron and desferrioxamine on infections with *Y enterocolitica.* Infect Immun 1985;47:774.

Simmonds SD, Noble MA, Freeman HJ. Gastrointestinal features of culture-positive *Yersinia enterocolitica* infection. Gastroenterology 1987;92:112.

Vantrappen G, Geboes K, Ponette E. Yersinia enteritis. Med Clin North Am 1982;66: 639.

*Principles and Practice of Pediatrics, Second Edition.*
edited by Frank A. Oski et al. J. B. Lippincott Company, Philadelphia © 1994.

# 56.31 *Yersinia pseudotuberculosis*

Shai Ashkenazi and Thomas G. Cleary

*Yersinia pseudotuberculosis,* so named because of its ability to cause tuberculosis-like lesions in animals, causes mesenteric lymphadenitis that mimics acute appendicitis. Growing awareness of this entity and improved isolation techniques have increased the number of diagnosed cases.

## ETIOLOGY

*Y pseudotuberculosis* originally was thought to be a transitional form of *Mycobacterium,* because it caused tuberculosis-like lesions when injected into guinea pigs. It now belongs to the genus *Yersinia* and family Enterobacteriaceae with two other human pathogens: *Y enterocolitica* and *Y pestis.* DNA homology studies show that *Y pseudotuberculosis* is closely related to *Y pestis* (90% homology) and more distantly related to *Y enterocolitica.*

*Y pseudotuberculosis* is a non–lactose-fermenting, aerobic, gram-negative coccobacillus. This oxidase-negative, catalase- and

urease-positive organism reduces nitrates and ferments glucose, galactose, maltose, mannose, and xylose. Characteristically, it is motile when grown at 22 °C but nonmotile at 37 °C, and it multiplies better at 22 °C and even at 4 °C in buffered saline than do most other common bacteria. It grows well on ordinary media; colonies are often small after incubation for 24 hours but are apparent after 48 hours. Selective media, such as cefsulodin-ingasan-novobiocin (CIN) medium, are useful, especially for mixed cultures. Growth of this organism may be confused with other organisms, such as *Proteus, Shigella, Salmonella, Brucella,* and other *Yersinia* species, because the organism lacks characteristic colony morphology. Proper identification depends on specific biochemical and serologic reactions.

Six serogroups (I through VI) have been defined antigenically on the basis of somatic O antigens. Four flagellar (H) antigens (A through D) are recognized, and the serotypes are defined by both O and H antigens. Most human infections were previously related to serogroup I, although an outbreak caused by *Y pseudotuberculosis* serogroup III was reported recently. In Canada, isolates from domestic animals were predominantly of serogroup III, and those from wild animals and birds belonged most frequently to serogroup II. Serogroup V has not been involved in human diseases.

## PATHOLOGY AND PATHOGENESIS

Oral infection of guinea pigs with *Y pseudotuberculosis* causes necrotic Peyer's patches in the terminal ileum and cecum, with caseous necrosis in the mesenteric lymph nodes. Parenteral injection of the organism produced granulomatous disease of the liver, spleen, and other organs.

Involvement of the mesenteric lymph nodes, especially those situated at the ileocecal angle, is prominent in humans. The infected lymph nodes are enlarged and inflamed, with hemorrhages on their surface, microabscess formation, and occasional development of a granulomatous reaction with giant cells. The intestinal tract, particularly the terminal ileum, may be involved, with edema, leukocyte infiltration, and superficial ulcerations. The appendix usually is grossly and microscopically normal or is mildly inflamed, but some cases of acute phlegmonous appendicitis associated with this organism have been described.

The pathogenesis of *Y pseudotuberculosis* infection has not been delineated. In vitro studies have shown that the organism can invade mammalian cells and remain viable intracellularly for several days. This invasiveness is the major factor of its virulence and is mediated by a 42- to 48-Md plasmid that codes for outer membrane proteins, fimbriae, and calcium dependency, with decreased cell division in calcium ion-deficient media. The virulence plasmid genes are related closely to those found on the virulence plasmid genes of *Y pestis* and *Y enterocolitica*. A chromosomal gene that encodes a surface bacterial protein may play a role in promoting invasiveness. It appears that after reaching the gastrointestinal tract, the organism penetrates the ileal mucosa, infects the ileocecal lymph nodes, and causes purulent mesenteric lymphadenitis.

Septicemia develops in a few patients, usually those with underlying disorders. Patients with iron overload due to hemochromatosis, hemolytic disease, polycythemia, cirrhosis, and chronic venous congestion are at the greatest risk of septicemia, because this organism, like *Y enterocolitica*, is unable to produce iron-binding compounds. The multiplication of the organism in tissues and the development of septicemia depend on the availability of host iron. The administration of deferoxamine, an iron-chelating substance that is sometimes used in these patients, allows virulent *Y pseudotuberculosis* to thrive, because the organism can use the iron bound to this substance.

## EPIDEMIOLOGY

*Y pseudotuberculosis* is found in animals worldwide. The bacteria have been recovered from a wide range of domestic and wild animals and birds. Rodents and fowl, especially turkeys, pigeons, ducks, and canaries, are frequently infected and represent important reservoirs. The organism is excreted in feces, and animal-to-animal transmission has been documented.

Human infections by these bacteria are infrequent and are reported mainly in northern Europe, generally as sporadic cases for which the source of the infection usually is not found. Direct or indirect contact with infected animals probably represents the major mechanism of infection, as shown epidemiologically in small family outbreaks related to infected domestic animals (eg, chickens, canaries, dogs, cats). The organism has also been recovered from foods, milk, water, soil, and other environmental sources. Most infected patients are children older than 5 years of age or adolescents. Human infections are more frequent during fall and winter months, corresponding to the seasonal peak incidence of the infection in domestic and wild animals.

Epidemics of *Y pseudotuberculosis* are rare, unlike outbreaks of *Y enterocolitica*. One outbreak of undetermined source was caused by serogroup III in Finland. The infected cases were scattered over a large geographic area without clustering in families, leading to the conclusion that the level of infectivity was low, at least for this strain. The disease appeared earlier and in a more severe form in children than in adults.

## CLINICAL MANIFESTATIONS

The most common manifestation of *Y pseudotuberculosis* is mesenteric lymphadenitis, with abdominal pain as the chief complaint. The pain may be diffuse or localized to the right lower quadrant and is usually accompanied by fever. Diarrhea is often absent or mild. Because tenderness in the right lower quadrant is frequent, the clinical picture may be indistinguishable from acute appendicitis. The diagnosis often is considered only after laparotomy reveals the appendix to be normal. The infection is usually self-limiting, with complete recovery beginning around the fifth day of the disease, although symptoms may persist for 1 week to 6 months. In a large, prospective study in England, *Y pseudotuberculosis* was diagnosed by serologic criteria in 11% of patients with nonspecific acute abdominal pain, in 17% with mesenteric adenitis, and in 28% with histologically proven acute appendicitis. It was suggested that this organism plays a greater role in acute abdominal pain than is usually appreciated. Enterocolitis, the usual manifestation of *Y enterocolitica*, is unusual with infection caused by *Y pseudotuberculosis*.

The most lethal complication of the disease is septicemia. It usually occurs in patients with underlying diseases, such as diabetes mellitus, liver cirrhosis, or visceral iron overload (especially with deferoxamine therapy), and in those who are malnourished, receiving immunosuppressive therapy, or undergoing hemodialysis. It is difficult to estimate the frequency of complications, because few large series exist. However, the outbreak of *Y pseudotuberculosis* in Finland was accompanied by a high rate of complications (53%), which included erythema nodosum, arthritis, iritis, and nephritis. Other reported complications are intra-abdominal abscesses, pleural effusion, myocarditis, and hemolytic uremic syndrome. A scarlatiniform rash has been described, and several cases of *Y pseudotuberculosis* fulfilled the diagnostic criteria of the Kawasaki syndrome. Some infected persons identified during investigation of family contacts were completely asymptomatic.

## DIAGNOSIS

*Y pseudotuberculosis* can be recovered from inflamed mesenteric lymph nodes during surgery. The recovery rate of this organism from stools is low because it may be confused with other non–lactose-fermenting organisms that grow faster in culture. Optimal isolation is achieved by incubation at lower temperature (ie, cold enrichment) before culturing on standard media and by use of selective media (eg, CIN). Histologic examination of lymph nodes removed during an operation may aid in the diagnosis.

Serologic examinations, although less definitive than culture, are sometimes helpful. *Y pseudotuberculosis* serogroups II and IV cross-react with *Salmonella* strains and, in some instances, with *Y enterocolitica*, *E coli*, and *Brucella*. Antibody titers during the acute phase may be low, and a second serum antibody titer is needed to demonstrate a fourfold rise. Hemagglutination titers of 1 : 160 or higher are considered significant.

The main differential diagnosis is acute appendicitis; other diseases that may cause enlarged ileocecal lymph nodes or ileitis include tuberculosis, salmonellosis, actinomycosis, *Y enterocolitica*, regional ileitis, and ulcerative colitis.

## TREATMENT

Because mesenteric lymphadenitis is usually self-limiting, with complete spontaneous recovery, antibiotic therapy may not be indicated for all patients. Antibiotics should be used when children with underlying disorders are infected or when septicemia or other complications are suspected. The mortality rate associated with septicemia is high, reaching 70% despite antibiotic therapy. Unlike *Y enterocolitica*, *Y pseudotuberculosis* is usually susceptible in vitro to ampicillin, chloramphenicol, aminoglycosides, cephalosporins, and tetracycline. It is unknown which of these agents represents optimal therapy.

## Selected Readings

Attwood SEA, Mealy K, Cafferkey MT, et al. *Yersinia* infection and acute abdominal pain. Lancet 1987;2:529.
Prober CG, Tune B, Hoder L. *Yersinia pseudotuberculosis* septicemia. Am J Dis Child 1979;133:623.
Saari TN, Triplett DA. *Yersinia pseudotuberculosis* mesenteric adenitis. J Pediatr 1974;85:656.
Sato K, Ouchi K, Taki M. *Yersinia pseudotuberculosis* in children resembling Izumi fever and Kawasaki syndrome. Pediatr Infect Dis 1983;2:123.
Tertti R, Granfors K, Lehtonen O, et al. An outbreak of *Yersinia pseudotuberculosis* infection. J Infect Dis 1984;149:245.
Tertti R, Vuento R, Mikkola P, et al. Clinical manifestations of *Yersinia Pseudotuberculosis* infection in children. Eur J Clin Microbiol Infect Dis 1989;8:587.

*Principles and Practice of Pediatrics, Second Edition.*
edited by Frank A. Oski et al. J. B. Lippincott Company, Philadelphia © 1994.

# 56.32 *Miscellaneous Bacterial Infections*

William C. Gruber

## ACINETOBACTER

*Acinetobacter*, a genus of coccobacillary bacteria in the family Neisseriaceae, is an uncommon human pathogen. The genus includes the clinically relevant species *A. calcoaceticus* var *anitratus* (previously *Herellea vaginicola*) and *A. calcoaceticus* var *lwoffi* (previously *Mima polymorpha*). These aerobic, oxidase-negative, catalase-positive organisms grow on standard agar between 33 °C and 35 °C.

### Epidemiology

*A. calcoaceticus* is distributed widely as a water-dwelling saprophyte and commensal in animals and humans. In hospitals, *Acinetobacter* has been isolated from personnel, mechanical ventilators, room humidifiers, patient mattresses, and water bottles used to warm peritoneal dialysate. These reservoirs are important sources of nosocomial infection.

Most cases of *Acinetobacter* infections occur in patients who require endotracheal intubation or intravenous access. The risk factors include recent surgery, antibiotic therapy, and immunosuppression. Neonates and children with underlying malignancy appear to be particularly vulnerable to infection. A seasonal incidence of infection often is observed, with a peak during the late summer.

### Pathophysiology

Patients with serious underlying illnesses can become colonized rapidly with *Acinetobacter* from a highly contaminated environment. A breach in host defense often allows this relatively avirulent organism to produce disease.

### Clinical Manifestations

*A. calcoaceticus* infection shares several features with other forms of gram-negative infection. Bacteremic patients often present with fever and hypotension; rarely, patients are asymptomatic. The lung is the most common site of primary infection, but infection associated with intravenous catheters occurs frequently. Other microbes are often isolated from blood cultures that yield *Acinetobacter*, a finding that is associated with a poor prognosis. Corneal, dental, meningeal, urinary tract, and wound infections have been described.

### Diagnosis and Treatment

Diagnosis is based on isolation of *Acinetobacter* from clinical material. Because of its coccobacillary shape, this organism may appear similar to *Haemophilus* or *Neisseria* on Gram stain. Its inability to grow anaerobically in any medium readily differentiates *Acinetobacter* from enteric bacteria.

Prompt initiation of appropriate antimicrobial therapy and management of local infection due to *Acinetobacter* usually results in a good outcome. However, selection of an antimicrobial agent may be complicated by the emergence of multiply resistant strains that display high-level resistance to aminoglycosides. Combination antibiotic therapy and third-generation cephalosporins have shown some efficacy in these cases, but the final antibiotic choice should be based on detailed evaluation of the organism's susceptibility.

## CITROBACTER

*Citrobacter*, a genus of enteric, gram-negative rods closely related to *Salmonella*, has been associated increasingly with human disease. This genus includes *C. freundii* (also called *Escherichia freundii*), *C. amalonaticus*, and *C. diversus* (also called *C. koseri*, *Levinea malonatica*). In addition to using citrate, these motile organisms hydrolyze urea and ferment glucose with production of gas.

### Epidemiology

From 1970 to 1979, 4% of neonatal meningitis cases were caused by *Citrobacter*, and *C. diversus* was the species isolated most often. These cases generally occur sporadically, but occasional clusters of *C. diversus* meningeal infection have been reported. The prevalence of neonatal colonization in outbreaks has been as high as 79%.

*Citrobacter* is an unusual cause of infection after the first several months of life and is primarily an opportunistic pathogen in the older child.

### Pathophysiology

The newborn can become colonized in the birth canal of a colonized mother or in the hospital nursery.

Broad use of antimicrobial agents can produce selective pressure leading to increased colonization with *Citrobacter*. Increased bacterial density combined with a blunted immune response may produce invasive disease.

### Clinical Manifestations

Most neonatal *Citrobacter* infections occur within 7 days of birth, but some cases present after 3 weeks of age. The preterm infant is at particular risk. Clinical signs and symptoms are those typical of neonatal sepsis. Fever, lethargy, poor feeding, vomiting, irritability, bulging fontanelles, seizures, and jaundice are common. Umbilical infection and surgical manipulation of colonized umbilical stumps occasionally have preceded bacteremia and meningitis. Neonatal meningitis due to *Citrobacter* is particularly severe and is complicated by multiple brain abscesses in as many as 75% of these patients.

Although *Citrobacter* can be isolated from stools of asymptomatic patients, the organism has been implicated in gastrointestinal disease. Urinary tract, bone, and soft-tissue infections occur but are extremely rare in children.

## Diagnosis and Treatment

*Citrobacter* organisms are isolated readily on standard media as gray, opaque, round colonies that produce a strong fetid odor. Therapy for *Citrobacter* meningitis often includes a systemic aminoglycoside or third-generation cephalosporin. Resistance of *Citrobacter* to aminoglycosides has been common in some institutions, and careful attention should be paid to antibiotic susceptibility when planning therapy. Cranial computed tomography scans are helpful for evaluating complications such as hydrocephalus and multicystic encephalomalacia. Ventriculostomy and craniectomy for open drainage of abscess have been required in some children to effect bacteriologic cure. Therapy for *Citrobacter* infection beyond the neonatal period requires appropriate antibiotic treatment, drainage of abscesses, and debridement of wounds. Outbreaks of neonatal *Citrobacter* infections have been aborted by cohorting patients and caregivers.

## ERWINIA

The genus *Erwinia* has an extended domain as an infectious microbe. The clinically relevant species, *Enterobacter agglomerans*, is a facultatively anaerobic, fermentative, $H_2S$-negative, gramnegative rod that grows well at 37 °C on standard agar.

## Epidemiology

*Erwinia* species are common plant and insect pathogens. *Erwinia herbicola*, also called *Enterobacter agglomerans*, first was isolated in humans from stool specimens of typhoid fever patients in the 1920s. Identification of saprophytic human strains followed, and the first reports of *Erwinia* as a human pathogen appeared in the 1960s. Subsequently, a nationwide outbreak of *E herbicola* was traced to contaminated liners from caps of parenteral solution bottles.

## Pathophysiology

*Erwinia* is commonly associated with other organisms from clinical specimens, but isolation of this organism in pure culture from infected sites leaves little doubt that *Erwinia* can be a human pathogen. Most strains appear to act as saprophytes, but the organism has been isolated from purulent wounds of the extremities acquired by laceration or thorn pricks. Most serious infections have occurred in persons with diminished host defenses (eg, immunosuppressed patients who received contaminated intravenous fluid).

## Clinical Manifestations

*Erwinia* bacteremia often is associated with fever, shaking chills, and systemic toxicity characteristic of gram-negative sepsis. These symptoms have been misinterpreted frequently in hospitalized patients who unknowingly were given contaminated intravenous fluids. Eye and skin infection due to *Erwinia* are particularly prominent, and the organism has been associated with osteomyelitis and neonatal meningitis in rare cases.

## Diagnosis and Therapy

Incorrect identification of *Erwinia* is common, and even when identified in isolates from human sources, *E. herbicola* often is considered a contaminant or saprophyte. The growth of yellow colonies on standard media and the characteristic microscopic spindle-shaped bodies aid identification.

Most localized infections respond to treatment that includes an aminoglycoside. In view of the rarity of bacteremia due to *Erwinia* species, single sporadic cases should be investigated, and clusters of two or more cases should prompt immediate inquiry into a possible common source of infection. Formal surveillance programs have been key to early termination of epidemics.

## ERYSIPELOTHRIX RHUSIOPATHIAE

*Erysipelothrix rhusiopathiae*, also called *E. insidiosa*, was identified definitively by Rosenbach in 1884 as a cause of the cutaneous disease erysipeloid. The organism is a slender, pleomorphic, nonmotile, gram-positive, unencapsulated rod that produces 0.1-mm bluish colonies on blood agar. Some strains produce $\alpha$-hemolysis in 48 to 72 hours. Inoculated gelatin stab culture inconsistently forms a "test tube brush" appearance that is diagnostic for this organism.

## Epidemiology

*Erysipelothrix* is a common commensal of wild and domestic animals and may lead a saprophytic existence in soil. The organism is an important cause of epidemic disease in swine. Not surprisingly, fish handlers, meat processors, poultry workers, veterinarians, abattoir workers, and food handlers are at risk for exposure to *Erysipelothrix*.

## Pathophysiology

Human infection usually results from contamination of skin abrasions while handling colonized material. Males are infected more commonly than females, perhaps because of their increased exposure. The disease is usually self-limiting and most often involves the hands. Biopsy of the skin lesions reveals a marked inflammatory response.

## Clinical Manifestations

Localized cutaneous infection, the erysipeloid of Rosenbach, is the most common manifestation of *Erysipelothrix* disease. After a 1- to 4-day incubation period, an acute, localized, purple-red lesion appears at the side of an abrasion contaminated with *Erysipelothrix*. Absence of suppuration and involution without desquamation help to differentiate this lesion from streptococcal or staphylococcal infections. Fever and other constitutional symptoms are uncommon, occurring in fewer that 10% of cases unless bacteremia supervenes. Untreated infection is usually self-limiting, with an average duration of 3 weeks. Childhood *Erysipelothrix* infection is unusual, but pediatric bacteremia, joint, and pulmonary infections have been reported.

An uncommon but important complication of *Erysipelothrix* infection is endocarditis. Although patients with rheumatic or congenital heart disease are at increased risk for endocarditis, previously normal heart valves can be infected.

## Diagnosis and Therapy

For localized disease, diagnosis depends largely on the clinical appearance of the lesion and an appropriate history of exposure. Attempts to culture the organism from material collected by swab or aspirate from a local lesion are usually unsuccessful. However, biopsies of affected skin cultured in broth usually yield the offending bacteria. *Erysipelothrix* is isolated commonly from the blood of patients with septicemia or endocarditis.

The organism is exquisitely sensitive to penicillin. Localized disease usually can be treated with oral medication, but high parenteral doses are typically necessary for treatment of endocarditis or disseminated disease.

## *FLAVOBACTERIUM*

Members of the genus *Flavobacterium* are not often associated with human infection; most cases follow exposure to a contaminated environmental source. The name *Flavobacterium meningosepticum* was proposed by King in 1959, based on her studies of bacterial isolates primarily associated with neonatal meningitis and septicemia.

These organisms are long, thin, catalase-positive, gram-negative rods with slightly swollen ends. The nonmotile, oxidase-positive, weakly fermentative, proteolytic organisms grow on solid agar as 1-mm, yellow, convex, glistening colonies of buttery consistency. The clinically relevant species include *F. meningosepticum*, *F. balustinum* (FIIB), and *F. odoratum*.

## Epidemiology

Flavobacteria are distributed widely as saprophytes in fresh and salt water. In hospitals, these organisms have been found to be ubiquitous colonizers of the environment, including flower vases, ice machines, vials of intravenous drugs, eyewashes, nebulizers, and sink traps. In some instances, these reservoirs have been implicated in nosocomial outbreaks of disease.

*F. meningosepticum* is an uncommon cause of neonatal infection but can be responsible for nursery epidemics. More than 50% of infected infants weigh less than 2500 g, and more than 50% of the patients manifest illness before 7 days of age.

## Pathophysiology

Most cases of invasive human disease are believed to be caused by heavy environmental contamination with *F. meningosepticum*, which then spreads to compromised newborns or debilitated older patients. Some neonatal infections may be caused by colonization of the infant during passage through the birth canal of a colonized mother. Neonatal flavobacterial infection in underdeveloped countries could be related to the use of contaminated ground water for bathing of newborn infants and poor feminine genital hygiene.

In older persons, the role of *Flavobacterium* is primarily opportunistic. Heavy nosocomial colonization, combined with a blunted immune response, probably accounts for the immunosuppressed patient's poor ability to handle this otherwise noninvasive bacteria.

## Clinical Manifestations

Neonatal sepsis and meningitis caused by *F. meningosepticum* share signs and symptoms with other forms of neonatal bacterial infection. However, the development of meningitis may be insidious, and several days of infection may pass before the symptoms become apparent. The prognosis is extremely poor, with mortality rates exceeding 60%. Half of the survivors develop significant neurologic complications, including hydrocephalus. Childhood flavobacterial infection beyond the newborn period is rare, although this organism has been implicated in meningitis, sepsis, endocarditis, and pneumonia.

## Diagnosis and Therapy

Rapid identification of *Flavobacterium* infection is urgent to ensure proper therapy and to hasten appropriate infection control and forestall epidemic outbreaks. Identification of *F. meningosepticum* is hindered by the characteristically long periods required for oxidation of carbohydrates and weak or delayed indole production. Clinical isolation of an unidentified gram-negative rod that is catalase and oxidase positive and that shows multiple antibiotic resistance should raise the suspicion of *F. meningosepticum* infection.

The treatment of *F. meningosepticum* meningitis represents a true challenge. Flavobacteria are characteristically resistant to ampicillin and aminoglycosides, and a delay in identification of the organism may lead to prolonged periods of suboptimal therapy and consequent persistence of organisms in the cerebrospinal fluid. Drugs that have been used with some success alone or in combination include erythromycin, vancomycin, trimethoprim-sulfamethoxazole, cefotaxime, and rifampin. The complication of hydrocephalus and the possible need for intraventricular therapy make the neurosurgeon an essential part of the management team.

Recovery has been the rule in immunocompetent older patients infected with contaminated materials, often despite treatment with antibiotics to which *Flavobacterium* is insensitive. However, significant mortality and morbidity rates occur among immunosuppressed patients with bacteremia or meningitis. The use of chloramphenicol, vancomycin, erythromycin, or ciprofloxacin has shown some success in these cases, but the final antibiotic choice should be based on detailed susceptibility testing.

## *PROTEUS* AND *PROVIDENCIA*

*Proteus* and *Providencia* (formerly classified as part of the *Proteus* genus) are increasingly associated with pediatric illness. These organisms are motile, gram-negative bacilli that do not ferment lactose and are differentiated from other Enterobacteriaceae by their ability to deaminate phenylalanine and lysine. Rapid and abundant urease production differentiates *Proteus* from *Providencia*.

## Epidemiology

*Proteus* and *Providencia* are found in soil. Although they are normal inhabitants of the colon and perineum, they can be found in greater numbers in patients receiving antibiotic therapy. Approximately 4% of all neonatal meningitis cases are caused by *Proteus mirabilis*. After the first few months of life, *Proteus* infection most commonly involves the urinary tract. Although *Escherichia coli* cause most urinary tract infections in childhood, *Proteus* and *Providencia* species are often implicated in reported series of cystitis and pyelonephritis. *P mirabilis* is particularly common as a cause of male initial urinary tract infections and supplants *E. coli* as the major urinary tract pathogen in children prone to renal stone formation.

## Pathophysiology

Most cases of central nervous system infection due to *Proteus* occur in the neonate. A propensity for brain abscess formation remains unexplained. Several factors may predispose the urinary tract to invasion by *Proteus* and *Providencia*. *Proteus* splits urea, which increases local pH, resulting in toxicity to renal cells and potentiation of urolithiasis. Urinary tract stones provide a refuge for *Proteus* organisms and form a barrier to effective antimicrobial therapy.

## Clinical Manifestations

*P mirabilis* infection of the newborn often presents with typical symptoms of neonatal sepsis; manifestations of sepsis may include encephalitis, septic arthritis, and osteomyelitis. The onset of infection after the first week of life occurs in a few patients, and meningitis may accompany early- or late-onset disease. Brain abscesses rarely may develop for weeks or months before presentation. *Proteus* brain abscesses are associated with a high degree of mortality, frequent complications, and neurologic deficits in the survivors. Hydrocephalus is a frequent complication and should be anticipated. Computerized tomography is especially useful in diagnosing and following the progression of cerebral complications.

Urinary tract infection with these bacteria often is associated with an elevated urinary pH; clinical findings and urine abnormalities in these cases are often less striking than in cases of *E. coli* urinary tract infections. As many as 30% of these patients have recurrent infections more than the 12 months after the initial treatment.

*Proteus* or *Providencia* bacteremia occurs infrequently in the pediatric age group. The genitourinary tract is the most commonly identified source. The mortality rate averages less than 40% and depends on the severity of underlying disease in the host. Osteomyelitis, pneumonia, mastoiditis, and wound infections also occur in these children.

## Diagnosis and Treatment

*P mirabilis* is usually sensitive to ampicillin, and this drug, alone or in combination with an aminoglycoside, is often suitable therapy for neonatal meningitis after identify and susceptibility of the infecting organism are known. A third-generation cephalosporin is often an alternative. Intraventricular antibiotics have not reduced mortality or morbidity significantly but have been used to clear ventricular colonization. Neurosurgical intervention may be required for complications of hydrocephalus or intracranial abscess.

The effective treatment of local infections or septicemia relies on appropriate antibiotic choice, often including an aminoglycoside, combined with surgical debridement and drainage of abscesses. Most *P mirabilis* urinary tract infections respond to ampicillin, but failure to clear bacteria should alert the physician to the possibility of urolithiasis or structural abnormality. Stone removal or surgical correction of anatomical defects often is required for cure.

## Selected Readings

Dooley JR, Nims LJ, Lipp VH, et al. Meningitis of infants caused by *Flavobacterium meningosepticum*. J Trop Pediatr 1980;26:24.

Drelichman V, Band JD. Bacteremias due to *Citrobacter diversus* and *Citrobacter freundii*; incidence, risk factors, and clinical outcome. Arch Intern Med 1985;145:1808.

Du Moulin GC. Airway colonization by *Flavobacterium* in an intensive care unit. J Clin Microbiol 1979;10:155.

Fuchs GJ III, Jaffe N, Pickering LK. *Acinetobacter calcoaceticus* sepsis in children with malignancies. Pediatr Infect Dis 1986;5:545.

Graham DR, Band JD. *Citrobacter diversus* brain abscess and meningitis in neonates. JAMA 1981;245:1923.

Grieco MD, Sheldon C. *Erysipelothrix rhusiopathiae*. Ann N Y Acad Sci 1970;174:523.

Khan AJ, Ubriani RS, Bombach E, et al. Initial urinary tract infection caused by *Proteus mirabilis* in infancy and childhood. J Pediatr 1978;93:791.

Lacroix J, Delage G, Mitchell G. Erysipeloid in an infant. J Pediatr 1981;99:745.

Levy HL, Ingall D. Meningitis in neonates due to *Proteus mirabilis*. Am J Dis Child 1967;114:320.

Von Graevenitz A. *Erwinia* species isolates. Ann N Y Acad Sci 1970;174:436.

*Principles and Practice of Pediatrics, Second Edition.*
edited by Frank A. Oski et al. J. B. Lippincott Company, Philadelphia © 1994.

# CHAPTER 57
# *Viral Infections*

## 57.1 *Arboviruses and Related Zoonotic Viruses*

Theodore F. Tsai

The arboviruses (*arthropod-borne viruses*) are a heterogeneous group of more than 535 viruses that are members of 13 taxonomic families (Table 57-1). Despite their taxonomic diversity, the viruses are studied as a group because of their unique associations with insect or tick vectors. Certain zoonotic infections that spread to humans directly from their vertebrate reservoirs without the agency of a vector often are considered together with the arboviruses because they are related taxonomically or because they share common animal reservoirs.

Although the recognized arboviruses are distributed principally in developing countries, clinicians increasingly encounter exotic infections in travelers, particularly in those returning from remote areas. In the last decade, 269 imported cases of dengue were confirmed in the United States (Table 57-2). Undoubtedly, these cases represent only a small fraction of those that occurred because of inadequacies in obtaining diagnostic specimens and because of difficulties in recognizing the disease. Examples of other arboviral infections occurring in travelers returning to the United States or Canada include cases of Mayaro fever acquired in South America; Toscana and Central European encephalitis acquired in Europe; West Nile viral myelitis acquired in the Middle East; Rift Valley fever viral retinitis, Thogoto viral encephalitis, and Ilesha viral infections acquired in Africa; and Ross River viral arthropathy acquired in Australia. American expatriates and servicemen abroad have acquired Japanese encephalitis, Venezuelan equine encephalitis, hemorrhagic fever with renal syndrome, and many other arboviral infections associated with less distinctive clinical presentations.

The distribution of arboviral diseases is not limited to developing countries. Several arboviral infections indigenous to the United States remain important to the public health. St. Louis encephalitis and western equine encephalitis are the leading causes of epidemic viral encephalitis in the nation and are causes of endemic infections in western states. The incidence of La Crosse

**TABLE 57-1.  Taxonomic and Physical Characteristics of Arboviruses and Certain Zoonotic Viruses**

| Virus (Family) | Arboviruses Causing Human Disease/ Arboviruses Recognized | Genome | Genomic Segments | Size (nm) | Morphology |
|---|---|---|---|---|---|
| Alphaviruses (**Togaviridae**) | 14/29 | Positive, single-stranded RNA | 1 | 60 | Spherical, enveloped |
| Flaviviruses (**Flaviviridae**) | 34/69 | Positive, single-stranded RNA | 1 | 40–50 | Spherical pleomorphic, enveloped |
| Bunyaviruses, phleboviruses, nairoviruses, hantaviruses, uukuviruses (**Bunyaviridae**) | 52/253 | Negative and ambisense single-stranded RNA | 3 | 80–120 | Spherical, pleomorphic, enveloped |
| Orbiviruses, coltiviruses (**Reoviridae**) | 5/77 | Double-stranded RNA | 10/12 | 60–100 | Spherical, nonenveloped |
| Lyssaviruses, Vesiculoviruses, and others (**Rhabdoviridae**) | 6/70 | Negative, single-stranded RNA | 1 | 60–85 × 180 | Bullet-shaped, enveloped |
| Arenaviruses (**Arenaviridae**) | 5/15 | Ambisense, single-stranded RNA | 2 | 50–300 | Spherical, pleomorphic |
| Filoviruses (**Filoviridae**) | 2/2 | Negative, single-stranded RNA | 1 | 80 × 14,000 | Tubular, filamentous |
| (**Orthomyxoviridae**) | 1/2 | Negative, single-stranded RNA | 6–7? | 90–110, up to 1000 | Pleomorphic, enveloped |
| (**Poxviridae**) | 1/3 | Double-stranded DNA | | 200–400 | Pleomorphic, enveloped |
| Others | 3/16 | | | | |

encephalitis in endemic areas of the Midwest equals that of *Haemophilus influenzae* meningitis.

The expansion of residential developments into wooded locations and the increasing popularity of outdoor recreation in remote areas have been associated with the increased occurrence of numerous bacterial, rickettsial, or protozoan vector-borne diseases, such as Lyme disease, ehrlichiosis, and babesiosis. These trends may lead to increased transmission of arboviral infections such as eastern equine encephalitis, which occurs in eastern marshlands, and Colorado tick fever, which is distributed chiefly in the Rocky Mountain states.

## EPIDEMIOLOGY

Most arboviruses are maintained in nature in cycles of alternating infection, from vector insects or ticks to various vertebrates (eg, birds, rodents, marsupials). The viruses may be carried through the winter months by vertical transovarial transmission (TOT) in vector mosquitoes or by transtadial transmission in ticks. In tropical locations, transmission may occur continuously. A common pattern is shown in Figure 57-1. The virus is maintained in an enzootic cycle in a bird-mosquito or rodent-mosquito cycle. The enzootic vector transmits infection to humans or other dead-end

**TABLE 57-2.  Reported Arboviral Infections, United States, 1980–1991**

| Year | Dengue* | California Encephalitis | St. Louis Encephalitis | Western Equine Encephalitis | Eastern Equine Encephalitis |
|---|---|---|---|---|---|
| 1980 | 24 (21) | 49 | 125 | 0 | 8 |
| 1981 | 44 | 91 | 15 | 19 | 0 |
| 1982 | 45 | 130 | 34 | 9 | 12 |
| 1983 | 27 | 64 | 20 | 7 | 14 |
| 1984 | 6 | 89 | 33 | 2 | 5 |
| 1985 | 8 | 68 | 21 | 1 | 0 |
| 1986 | 24 (9) | 64 | 43 | 7 | 1 |
| 1987 | 18 | 87 | 17 | 41 | 3 |
| 1988 | 27 | 42 | 4 | 1 | 2 |
| 1989 | 22 | 57 | 33 | 0 | 9 |
| 1990 | 24 | 61 | 248 | 0 | 6 |
| 1991 | 25 | 57 | 78 | 1 | 10 |
| Total | 294 (30) | 859 | 671 | 88 | 70 |

* Imported cases (indigenous cases).

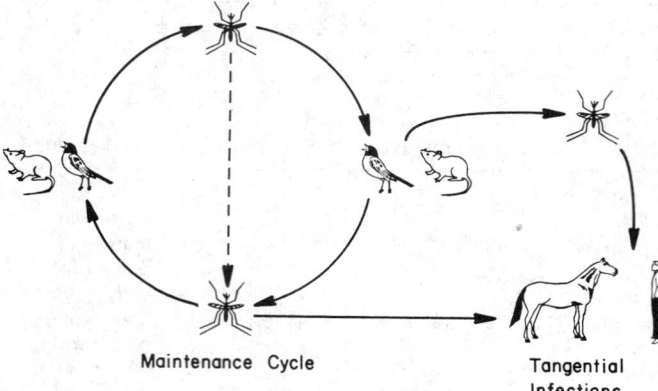

**Figure 57-1.** A typical arbovirus maintenance cycle. The virus is maintained by an enzootic vector among birds (eg, western equine encephalitis [WEE]), rodents (eg, enzootic Venezuelan equine encephalitis virus [VEE]), or monkeys (eg, yellow fever [YF] virus in the jungle cycle). An ancillary vector is needed to bridge the enzootic cycle and humans in eastern equine encephalitis (EEE). Horses and humans are dead-end hosts for western and EEE viruses. Infections occur when humans intrude on the enzootic cycle. Transovarial transmission of the virus in the enzootic vector (*dashed arrow*) may maintain the virus during winter.

hosts, such as horses, when the hosts come in contact with the enzootic cycle. Examples of arboviruses that are transmitted in this way are St. Louis encephalitis and western encephalitis viruses, which are amplified among birds and transmitted to humans by *Culex* mosquitoes; enzootic Venezuelan equine encephalitis viruses, which are maintained in rodent-*Culex* mosquito cycles; and yellow fever virus, which is maintained in its jungle cycle among monkeys and *Hemagogus* mosquitoes in South America and various *Aedes* mosquitoes in Africa. Some enzootic vectors do not bite humans because of their selective feeding preferences, but other vectors with more catholic feeding habits bridge the enzootic cycle and human hosts. Eastern equine encephalitis virus is maintained and transmitted in such a cycle.

Vertebrates that serve as maintenance hosts for arboviruses must sustain viremias of sufficient titers (eg, $\geq 10^4$ pfu/mL) and for sufficient periods (eg, 3 to 5 days) to infect the enzootic vector. Certain arboviruses, notably yellow fever, dengue, chikungunya,

and Oropouche viruses, produce sufficient viremias in humans that interhuman chains of epidemic transmission often follow (Fig 57-2).

In Africa, yellow fever epidemics arise when viremic persons traveling from areas of enzootic virus transmission introduce the virus into urban areas, where an interhuman cycle becomes established, vectored by peridomestic breeding *Aedes aegypti*. If the viruses were to be introduced, a potential would exist for the epidemic spread of dengue and yellow fever in the southeastern United States, where *Ae aegypti* and *Ae albopictus* are established.

Several of the diseases mentioned in this chapter are zoonoses, and human infections arise from direct contact with infectious secretions or excretions of the reservoir host (Fig 57-3). The arenaviruses, which cause Lassa and other hemorrhagic fevers and lymphocytic choriomeningitis, and the hantaviruses, the agents of hemorrhagic fever with renal syndrome, are spread from various persistently infected rodents to humans. Rare cases of human infection from Rio Bravo virus, Duvenhage virus, Mokola virus, and Issyk-kul virus are examples of zoonoses spread from bats. Omsk hemorrhagic fever, Rift Valley fever, and Congo-Crimean hemorrhagic fever may be transmitted from infected muskrats and livestock to trappers and herdsman, respectively, during skinning and slaughter. Person-to-person, often nosocomial transmission of Congo-Crimean hemorrhagic fever and Ebola, Marburg, and Lassa viruses has led to sizable, often fearsome outbreaks.

The transmission cycles of many arboviruses are complex and not fully understood. More detailed characterizations of the individual viruses are given in the selected readings.

## DIAGNOSIS

The key to the diagnosis of arboviral infections is obtaining an accurate epidemiologic history. A detailed list of the dates and places of travel, the kinds of habitats encountered, and the activities in which the patient was engaged provides essential information on the risks of exposure to vectors and of acquiring infection. Other pertinent data include a prior history of military service, travel, or residence in tropical areas (where previous asymptomatic infections may have been acquired) and a history of immunization with yellow fever, Japanese encephalitis, or other arboviral vaccines.

Most arboviral infections produce a nonspecific febrile illness, and specific laboratory tests are needed to confirm the diagnosis. Often, patients are seen after the acute phase of illness, and se-

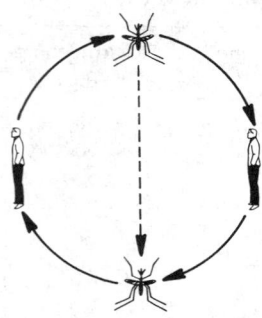

Epidemic Cycle

**Figure 57-2.** Interhuman transmission of certain arboviruses is associated with epidemics (eg, yellow fever, dengue, chikungunya, Oropouche, and Ross River virus). The chief epidemic vector for yellow fever, chikungunya, and dengue is *Aedes aegypti*. In Oropouche virus epidemics, a gnat is the epidemic vector. An interhorse cycle, associated with a variety of vectors, occurs in epizootic Venezuelan equine encephalitis. Transovarial transmission of the virus (*dashed arrow*) in the vector may be needed to maintain the virus between epidemics.

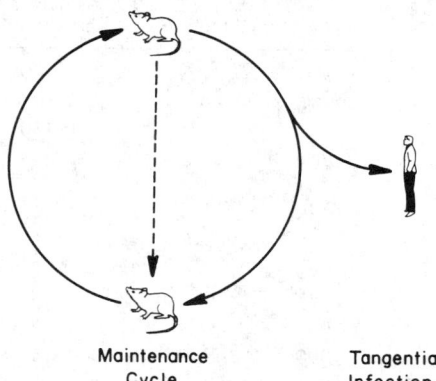

Maintenance Cycle    Tangential Infection

**Figure 57-3.** A typical zoonosis, in which humans are infected after contact with infectious secretions or excretions of persistently infected rodents (eg, arenavirus infections) or bats (eg, Rio Bravo virus, various rhabdoviruses). Infections among the vertebrate reservoir may occur through horizontal or vertical (*dashed arrow*) transmission.

rology is the only means by which the diagnosis can be made. However, clinicians should bear in mind that several arboviruses, including dengue, chikungunya, yellow fever, Venezuelan equine encephalitis, and Colorado tick fever viruses, may circulate in the blood in high titers for several days and that viral isolates can be recovered from the blood in the acute phase of the illness. Suckling mice, primary duck embryo cells, and continuous mosquito cell lines (eg, $C_6 36$) are sensitive systems for recovering most arboviruses, but Vero cells, which are widely available, are an adequate system in most cases. Intrathoracic inoculation of *Toxorhynchites* mosquitoes is a sensitive system for the isolation of dengue and yellow fever viruses.

It may be appropriate to rule out a diagnosis of arboviral infection with viral culture, immunohistochemical studies, or electron microscopy, when a brain biopsy is obtained from a patient with suspected herpes encephalitis.

The serologic diagnosis of an arbovirus infection is confirmed by demonstrating seroconversion (ie, fourfold or greater change in titer) in appropriately timed serum specimens. The diagnosis is presumptive if a high titer is present in a serum pair or in a single serum specimen. Specific IgM in the cerebrospinal fluid (CSF), reflecting an intrathecal antibody response, is diagnostic. Specific IgM in a single serum specimen should be interpreted cautiously because IgM persists beyond a single transmission season after some infections.

Many arboviruses agglutinate goose erythrocytes. The hemagglutination inhibition (HI) test is the most broadly reactive of the serologic assays in common use. Heterologous reactions among the flaviviruses are especially problematic if a patient has had two or more flavivirus infections. Greater specificity is associated with the complement fixation (CF) test, but the CF antibody response is unpredictable, occurring as late as 4 weeks after onset in some cases or not at all in a large proportion of patients. CF antibodies to many arboviruses have a half-life of 2 to 3 years, and their presence is a relatively better indicator of recent infection than HI antibodies, which are long lived in most instances.

The greatest specificity is obtained by measuring neutralizing antibodies. Neutralization tests often are necessary to make a specific diagnosis of a flavivirus infection when previous immunization or infection with a related virus has occurred (ie, flavivirus superinfection). However, in a significant number of superinfections, neutralization tests may fail to differentiate the source of the most recent infection. Competitive binding assays using virus-specific monoclonal antibodies have been used to differentiate tick-borne encephalitis, Japanese encephalitis, and dengue virus infections. Similar problems of specificity are encountered with the diagnosis of some bunyavirus infections, and infections among closely related viruses often cannot be differentiated even in a neutralization test (eg, snowshoe hare and La Crosse virus infections).

Serologic binding assays, such as indirect immunofluorescence (IF) and enzyme-linked immunosorbent assays (ELISA), are available to measure IgM and IgG antibodies. Although IgG assays are sensitive, significant cross-reactions are observed within the alphaviruses, within the flaviviruses, and within serologic complexes of the bunyaviruses. Heterologous IgM reactions may be problematic when IF is used. For example, dengue antibody may cross-react with St. Louis encephalitis viral antigen. IgM capture ELISA is relatively more specific. When IgM is measured, reactions from rheumatoid factors should be controlled.

Direct detection of arboviral antigens in blood or other fluids by antigen-capture ELISA is an important alternative to serologic assays in diagnosing yellow fever and Lassa fever among others. Antigen detection assays offer the advantage of rapid diagnosis in the acute phase of illness, permitting timely decisions to be made about therapy and patient isolation. Antigen detection assays for arboviruses in mosquitoes and ticks have also been described.

Polymerase chain reaction (PCR) amplified assays to detect viral genomic material in blood and other clinical samples have been developed for dengue, yellow fever, St. Louis encephalitis, Lassa fever, hemorrhagic fever with renal syndrome, and several other arboviral or zoonotic diseases. However, clinical experience with this promising technique is limited.

Serologic diagnoses of certain arboviral infections are offered by several private diagnostic laboratories, state health department laboratories, some university laboratories, and by the Division of Vector-Borne Infectious Diseases of the Centers for Disease Control (CDC).

Cases of arboviral encephalitis should be reported to state health departments. The diseases may be epidemic, and control measures can be taken to protect the public health.

## DIFFERENTIAL DIAGNOSIS

Most arboviral infections lead to nonspecific illnesses consisting of fever, headache, musculoskeletal aches, and malaise. These infections cannot be differentiated clinically from a wide variety of viral bacterial and parasitic infections associated with a grippe-like condition. Dengue, West Nile, and certain other arboviral infections are associated with a morbilliform exanthem, although the eruptions may be difficult to detect in dark-skinned persons. Dengue frequently has been misdiagnosed as measles or rubella, because these diseases also may appear in outbreaks. The differential diagnosis of these disorders with maculopapular rash includes infections from enteroviruses, human parvovirus, rhinoviruses, reoviruses, parainfluenza viruses, rotavirus, hepatitis B virus, Epstein-Barr virus (EBV), cytomegalovirus (CMV), various rickettsiae, *Mycoplasma pneumoniae*, roseola, scarlet fever, leptospirosis, relapsing fever, and eruptions associated with medications. Dengue, Colorado tick fever, alphavirus infections, and the hemorrhagic fevers may present with petechial eruptions similar to those seen in tick-borne typhus, epidemic murine typhus, meningococcemia, Brazilian purpuric fever, bacteremia from *H influenzae*, certain enteroviral infections, and Henoch-Schönlein purpura.

Sindbis and other alphaviral infections produce a rash and polyarthritis. Fifth disease, *M pneumoniae* infection, serum sickness, hepatitis B, rubella, rat-bite fever, and enteroarthritis frequently are associated with this combination of signs and should be considered in the differential diagnosis.

Dengue fever frequently produces a mild to moderate hepititis and, in endemic areas, it should be considered in the differential diagnosis of ordinary viral hepatitis.

The central nervous system (CNS) infections produced by arboviruses are not distinctive clinically, although a focal neurologic presentation is atypical. However, focal signs suggestive of herpes encephalitis have been reported in isolated cases of western and snowshoe hare viral encephalitis, and they are a feature in approximately 25% of children with Powassan and La Crosse encephalitis.

In addition to herpes encephalitis, other treatable CNS conditions that should be ruled out are a partially treated bacterial meningitis, *M pneumoniae* infection, Rocky Mountain spotted fever, leptospirosis, tuberculosis, Lyme disease, listeriosis, fungal causes of meningitis, cerebral malaria, toxoplasmosis, cysticercosis, lead encephalopathy, and heat stroke. An important consideration in the differential diagnosis, because a history of exposure to mosquitoes may be given, is encephalopathy from *N,N*-diethyl-*m*-toluamide (DEET), which presents with encephalopathic signs and CSF pleocytosis. Rabies should be retained in the differential diagnosis even if no history of animal bite is given, because the incubation period is variable and may be as long as several months; furthermore, hydrophobia may not be present.

The seasonal distribution of arboviral encephalitis cases in late summer and early autumn may be an important clue to the diagnosis, but this seasonality overlaps the distribution of enteroviral infections, which are probably the leading cause of meningoencephalitis in this season (Fig 57-4). Other viral causes of meningoencephalitis include infections from mumps virus and its vaccine, EBV, CMV, adenoviruses, influenza virus, and postinfectious encephalitis from the viruses associated with childhood exanthems. Polio may be encountered in unvaccinated persons and in immunocompromised persons who are exposed to vaccine strains. Infection with human immunodeficiency virus type 1 (HIV-1) may present with CNS signs before indications of systemic illness are noticed.

Other disorders of the CNS that should be considered in the differential diagnosis of meningoencephalitis include sarcoidosis, reactions to trimethoprim-sulfamethoxazole and other medications, vascular disorders of the CNS, space-occupying lesions, cat-scratch disease, trichinosis, and CNS infections from free-living amoebae and *Baylisascaria procyonis*. Hemorrhagic shock-encephalopathy syndrome, should be considered in the differential diagnosis in infants.

## THERAPY

Research on therapeutic modalities has focused on treatment of the hemorrhagic fevers because of the high fatality rates associated with these infections. In controlled trials, ribavirin reduced mortality and morbidity in Lassa fever and hemorrhagic fever with renal syndrome, and anecdotal experience suggests efficacy in Congo-Crimean hemorrhagic fever. Immune plasma is an effective therapy for Argentine hemorrhagic fever, and immune globulins are available for Congo-Crimean hemorrhagic fever and for tick-borne encephalitis. Passive immunization is used empirically in the therapy or prophylaxis of other hemorrhagic fevers and after laboratory exposure to certain arboviruses. Russian researchers have reported the successful treatment of tick-borne encephalitis with ribonuclease. Specific therapy for other arboviral infections has not been reported.

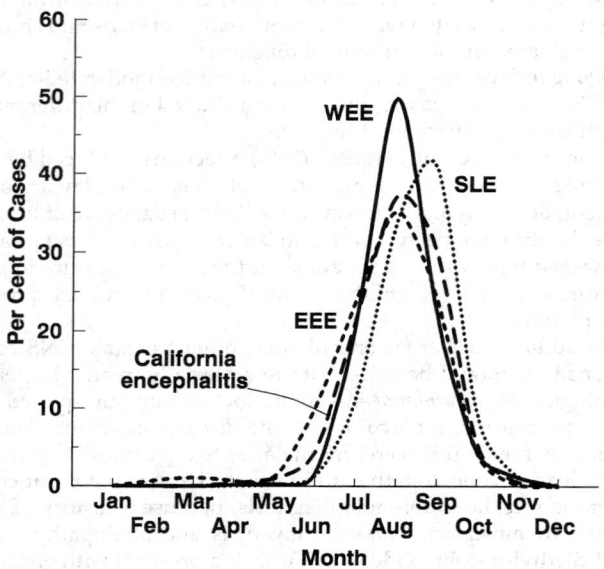

Figure 57-4. Month of onset for reported cases of arboviral encephalitis, United States, 1971–1983.

Supportive therapy for patients with encephalitis necessitates close attention to monitoring intracranial pressure, cardiorespiratory function, and fluid and electrolyte balance. Inappropriate secretion of antidiuretic hormone and hyponatremia is a frequent complication of arboviral encephalitis. Although patients with eastern equine encephalitis, Japanese encephalitis, and other arboviral infections of the CNS frequently exhibit clinical signs of elevated intracranial pressure, in one controlled study of Japanese encephalitis, dexamethasone therapy did not improve outcome.

Convulsions may be the initial presentation in some arboviral CNS infections, and status epilepticus is a complication in some cases. Hypoglycemia and disorders of electrolyte balance should be ruled out or treated before attributing the cause of convulsions to infection. Status epilepticus is a medical emergency, and appropriate cardiorespiratory support and anticonvulsant therapy with lorazepam should be administered promptly.

## PREVENTION

Vaccines are in general use for three arboviral infections: yellow fever, Japanese encephalitis, and Central European encephalitis. In the United States, attenuated yellow fever vaccine and inactivated Japanese encephalitis vaccine (produced in Japan) are licensed and commercially available. Vaccines for Central European encephalitis are produced in Austria, Germany and in Russia, and they are widely available in Europe. However, because risk of acquiring tick-bone encephalitis is low for most travellers, vaccination is not routinely recommended.

**TABLE 57-3.   Preventing Side Effects of Insect Repellents**

Although DEET-containing repellents have been widely used for over 30 years, recently there has been increased attention to their potential for side effects, particularly in children. In high concentrations, DEET can irritate the skin and produce deep ulcerations. More worrisome are rare cases of encephalopathy and seizures, principally in children, that have followed even brief exposures to DEET. To minimize these risks, we recommend the following guidelines for repellent use:

- Apply repellents to clothing and, where ticks are a problem, to shoes and camping gear. Permethrin-containing repellents are best because they kill as well as repel insects and ticks and they are relatively water-fast; treated clothing will remain effective after laundering. Permethrin repellents are not approved for use on skin.
- Use repellents sparingly and apply only to skin not covered by treated clothing. Wear long sleeves, long pants, and a hat when possible.
- Avoid formulations containing >30% DEET.
- Toxicity has occurred after inhalation or ingestion of DEET; use aerosols in an open area. Safeguard containers to prevent accidental ingestion.
- Avoid applying repellent to hands of young children who may rub them into eyes or the mouth.
- Pregnant women and nursing women should minimize use of repellents. Repellents containing ethylhexanediol may be teratogenic and are best avoided by pregnant and nursing women.
- Never use repellents on wounds, irritated skin, or mucous membranes.
- Use repellents sparingly; one application will last 4–6 hours and saturation does not increase efficacy. New formulations of microencapsulated DEET may lengthen effectiveness and reduce potential for absorption and systemic toxicity.
- Wash repellent-treated skin after returning indoors.
- If a suspected reaction to insect repellent occurs, wash treated skin and seek medical attention. Bring the repellent to the attending physician.

**TABLE 57-4.    Examples of Control Strategies to Reduce Transmission of Arboviral and Zoonotic Diseases**

| Disease | Permanent or Long-Term Solutions to Reduce Breeding Sites | Annual or Periodic Maintenance Practices to Reduce Vectors | Emergency Measures to Reduce Vectors | Personal Protective Behaviors |
|---|---|---|---|---|
| Western equine encephalitis | Eliminate natural depressions that hold water<br>Engineer ditches and water impoundments to reduce breeding sites<br>Teach good irrigation water management | Apply larvicides to breeding sites<br>Control irrigation runoff<br>Distribute Gambusia (larvae-eating fish) | Aerial or ground ultra-low-volume (ULV) application of adulticides | Avoid outdoor activity at dusk and dawn<br>Use repellents when outdoors |
| Dengue | Create public awareness to eliminate peridomestic containers | Inspect premises for containers that hold water; destroy, empty, or treat with larvicides | Aerial or ground ULV application of adulticides | Air condition or screen houses<br>Use indoor insecticides |
| Rodent-borne hemorrhagic fevers | Build rodent-proof houses and grain storage facilities<br>Separate human habitation from grain and food stores | Clean up sources of rodent harborage<br>Remove or make garbage and other rodent food sources inaccessible<br>Rodenticides, traps | Rodenticides, traps | Sleep off the ground |

The mainstay for prevention of arboviral infections is the use of repellents and other measures to prevent bites of vector mosquitoes, sandflies, and ticks. Although repellents containing DEET are the most effective formulations, they should be used with caution on children. Six cases of encephalopathy, three of which were fatal, have been reported in children from 17 months to 8 years of age after exposures to formulations containing as little as 10% DEET. Although percutaneous exposure was prolonged in most cases, application of DEET on 2 successive days led to encephalopathy in one child. One child may have had a partial deficiency in ornithyl carbamoyl transferase, suggesting that defects in certain metabolic pathways may predispose to intoxication. Guidelines for the use of repellents are shown in Table 57-3. Dermatitis has been reported after contact exposure to DEET. Ethyl-1,3-hexanediol, an active ingredient in certain repellents, is teratogenic in animals, and these formulations should be avoided by pregnant women.

Permethrin (0.5%, Permanone), sprayed on clothing and bed nets, effectively repels and kills mosquitoes and ticks. Its effectiveness in killing mosquitoes is not reduced even after the impregnated material has been washed several times. Permethrin shampoo (1%, Nix) and permethrin cream (5%, Elimite) are approved for use on children over 2 years of age to treat head lice and scabies, and permethrin has been used topically in powders and soaps to repel or kill body lice and other insects. Presumably, these preparations could be used on skin as protection against mosquitoes and ticks. Citronyl, derived from citronella oil, may be more effective than DEET in repelling certain sandflies. Ordinary insect nets and screens do not have a sufficiently fine mesh to exclude sandflies.

Other simple measures that reduce exposure to vector mosquitoes include covering exposed areas with clothing, avoiding outdoor activities at dusk and dawn when certain vectors are most active, and using mosquito bed nets and insecticidal room sprays. In areas where tick exposures are likely, clothing should be inspected at frequent intervals and adherent ticks removed.

From a public health perspective prevention of arboviral diseases is achieved by combining several approaches: eliminating or reducing sources where vector mosquitoes breed, annual or periodic application of larvicides or adulticides to reduce mosquito populations, and the emergency application of adulticides to lower vector populations in the face of an epidemic. Specific strategies are tailored to the breeding habitat and habits of individual vectors (Table 57-4).

Several arboviruses (eg, St. Louis encephalitis) are transmitted to human populations only after an extensive period of amplification in natural reservoirs (eg, birds). This phenomenon is exploited, and indices of arbovirus activity in nature are surveyed to predict the likelihood of epidemic transmission. Antibody prevalence in birds, the size of vector mosquito populations, and infection rates in vectors are predictive indices that can be followed to trigger emergency vector control measures.

## ARBOVIRAL AND RELATED ZOONOTIC DISEASES

Table 57-5 lists arboviral and related zoonotic diseases that occur after natural exposures. Illnesses have been reported after laboratory exposures to other arboviruses, but these infections may have been associated with unusual routes of infection or with larger viral doses than would be encountered in nature.

Table 57-5 is arranged by geographic distribution, the principal clinical manifestation of infection, vector, and the frequency with which the disease has been recognized. In many instances, only one or two cases of human infection with a given virus have been reported, but often seroprevalence studies suggest the possibility of more widespread infection. Discussions of certain arboviral diseases of public health significance follow.

### Argentine, Bolivian, and Venezuelan Hemorrhagic Fevers

Junin, Machupo, and Guanarito viruses, the etiologic agents, respectively, of Argentine, Bolivian, and Venezuelan hemorrhagic fevers (AHF, BHF, VHF), are the only agents among ten New World arenaviruses that cause human disease in nature. Flexal virus has been reported to cause a simple febrile illness after laboratory exposure. Junin and Machupo viruses are maintained in rodents, *Calomys musculinus* and *Calomys callosus*, respectively. The rodent reservoir of Guanarito virus has not yet been con-
*(Text continues on p. 1275.)*

TABLE 57-5. Arboviral and Zoonotic Viral Infections by Geographic Area

| Virus | Nondescript Febrile Illness | Febrile Illness With Rash | Febrile Illness With Arthritis | Meningo-encephalitis | Hemorrhagic Fever | Other |
|---|---|---|---|---|---|---|
| **North America** | | | | | | |
| *Mosquito-Borne Viruses* | | | | | | |
| Cache Valley | | | | ○ | | |
| California | | | | ○ | | |
| Dengue 1–4 | | ○ | | | | Hepatitis |
| Eastern equine encephalitis | | | | ○ | | |
| Everglades (VEE type II) | | | | ○ | | |
| Jamestown Canyon | | | | ○ | | Respiratory symptoms |
| La Crosse | | | | ● | | |
| St. Louis encephalitis | | | | ● | | |
| Snowshoe hare | | | | ○ | | |
| Tensaw | | | | ○ | | |
| Trivittatus | | | | ○ | | Respiratory symptoms |
| Western equine encephalitis | | | | ● | | |
| *Tick-Borne Viruses* | | | | | | |
| Colorado tick fever | ● | | | ○ | ○ | |
| Powassan | | | | ○ | | |
| *Zoonoses* | | | | | | |
| Lymphocytic choriomeningitis | ○ | | | ○ | ○ | Pneumonia, parotitis, orchitis, arthritis |
| Modoc | | | | ○ | | |
| Rio Bravo | ○ | | | ○ | | Pneumonia, orchitis |
| *Sandfly-Borne Viruses* | | | | | | |
| Vesicular stomatitis (New Jersey and Indiana) | ○ | | | ○ | | Respiratory illness |
| **Central and South America** | | | | | | |
| *Mosquito-Borne Viruses* | | | | | | |
| Bussuquara | ○ | | | | | |
| Catu | ○ | | | | | |
| Cotia | ○ | | | | | |
| Dengue 1–4 | | ● | | ○ | ● | Hepatitis |
| Eastern equine encephalitis | | | | ○ | | |
| Group C viruses (Apeu, Caraparu, Itaqui, Madrid, Marituba, Murutucu, Nepuyo, Oriboca, Ossa, Restan) | ○ | | | | | |
| Guama | ○ | | | | | |
| Guaroa | ○ | | | ? | | Hepatitis? |
| Ilheus | ○ | | | ○ | | |
| Mayaro | | ● | ● | | | |
| Mucambo (VEE type III) | ○ | | | ○ | | |
| Rocio | | | | ● | | |
| St. Louis encephalitis | ○ | | | ○ | | |
| Tonate (VEE subtype III) | | | | ○ | | |
| Tucunduba | | | | ○ | | |
| Tacaiuma | ○ | | | | | Two cases with concurrent malaria fatal |
| Venezuelan equine encephalitis (epizootic subtypes IABC) | ● | | | ● | | |
| Western equine encephalitis | | | | ● | | |
| Wyeomyia | ○ | | | | | |
| Xingu | ○ | | | | | Hepatitis? |
| Yellow fever | ● | | | | ● | Hepatitis |
| *Sandfly-Borne Viruses* | | | | | | |
| Alenquer | ○ | | | | | |
| Candiru | ○ | | | | | |
| Chagres | ○ | | | | | |
| Changuinola | ○ | | | | | |
| Morumbi | ○ | | | | | |

### TABLE 57-5. (Continued)

| Virus | Nondescript Febrile Illness | Febrile Illness With Rash | Febrile Illness With Arthritis | Meningo-encephalitis | Hemorrhagic Fever | Other |
|---|---|---|---|---|---|---|
| Oropouche | ● | ○ | | ○ | | |
| Punta Toro | ○ | | | | | |
| Serra Norte | ○ | | | | | |
| Vesicular Stomatitis (New Jersey and Indiana) | ○ | | | ○ | | |
| Vesicular Stomatitis (Alagoas) | | | | ○ | | |
| *Zoonoses* | | | | | | |
| Guanarito | | | | | ● | |
| Junin | | | | | ● | |
| Machupo | | | | | ● | |
| Rio Bravo | ○ | | | ○ | | Pneumonia, orchitis |
| **Europe** | | | | | | |
| *Mosquito-Borne Viruses* | | | | | | |
| Batai | ○ | | | ○ | | |
| Calovo | ○ | | | | | |
| Inkoo | ○ | | | ○ | | Respiratory illness |
| Sindbis | ● | ● | ● | | | |
| Tahyna | ● | | | ○ | | Respiratory illness |
| West Nile | ○ | ○ | ○ | ○ | | |
| *Sandfly-Borne Viruses* | | | | | | |
| Sandfly fever (Naples) | ● | | | | | |
| Sandfly fever (Sicilian) | ● | | | | | |
| Toscana | ● | | | ● | | |
| *Tick-Borne Viruses* | | | | | | |
| Bhanja | ○ | | | ○ | | |
| Central European encephalitis | ● | | | ● | | |
| Congo–Crimean | | | | | ● | |
| Lipovnik | | | | ○ | | |
| Louping ill | | | | ○ | | |
| Thogoto | ○ | | | ○ | | Hepatitis, optic neuritis |
| *Zoonoses* | | | | | | |
| Encephalomyocarditis | ○ | | | ○ | | |
| Lymphocytic choriomeningitis | ● | | | ● | ○ | Pneumonia, arthritis, orchitis, parotitis |
| Belgrade | ○ | | | | ○ | |
| Puumula | ● | | | ○ | ○ | |
| Seoul | ○ | | | | ○ | |
| **Asia** | | | | | | |
| *Mosquito-Borne Viruses* | | | | | | |
| Chikungunya | | ● | ● | ○ | ○ | |
| Dengue 1–4 | ● | ● | | ○ | ● | Hepatitis common |
| Japanese encephalitis | | | | ● | | |
| Sindbis | ● | ● | ● | | ○ | |
| Snowshoe hare | | | | ○ | | |
| Tahyna | ● | | | ○ | | Respiratory illness |
| West Nile | ● | ● | ● | ○ | | Hepatitis |
| Zika | | ● | | | | |
| *Sandfly-Borne Viruses* | | | | | | |
| Chandipura | ○ | | | ○ | | |
| Sandfly fever (Naples) | ● | | | | | |
| Sandfly fever (Sicilian) | ● | | | | | |
| *Tick-Borne Viruses* | | | | | | |
| Alma-Arasan | ○ | | | | | |
| Banna | | | | ○ | | |
| Congo-Crimean | | | | | ● | |

*(continued)*

## TABLE 57-5. (Continued)

| Virus | Nondescript Febrile Illness | Febrile Illness With Rash | Febrile Illness With Arthritis | Meningo-encephalitis | Hemorrhagic Fever | Other |
|---|---|---|---|---|---|---|
| Ganjam | ○ | | | | | |
| Issyk-kul | ○ | | | | | |
| Karshi | ○ | | | | | |
| Kemerovo | | | | ○ | | |
| Kyasanur Forest | | | | ● | ● | |
| Negishi | | | | ○ | | |
| Omsk hemorrhagic fever | | | | ● | ● | |
| Powasson | | | | ○ | | |
| Russian spring–summer encephalitis | | | | ● | | |
| Syr–Darya valley | | ○ | | | | |
| Tamdy | ○ | | | | | |
| Wanowrie | | | | ○ | ○ | |
| *Zoonoses* | | | | | | |
| Encephalomyocarditis | ○ | | | ○ | | |
| Hantaan | | | | | ● | Pantropic |
| Lymphocytic choriomeningitis | ○ | | | ○ | | Pneumonia, arthritis, orchitis, parotitis |
| Seoul | | | | | ● | Pantropic |
| **Africa** | | | | | | |
| *Mosquito-Borne Viruses* | | | | | | |
| Babanki | ● | ● | ● | | | |
| Bangui | | ○ | | | | |
| Banzi | ○ | | | | | |
| Bhanja | ○ | | | ○ | | |
| Bunyamwera | | ● | | ○ | | |
| Bwamba | ● | | | ○ | | |
| Chikungunya | ● | ● | ● | ○ | ○ | |
| Dengue 1–4 | ● | ● | | ○ | ● | Hepatitis |
| Germiston | | ○ | | ○ | | |
| Ilesha | | ● | | ○ | | |
| Koutango | | ○ | | | | |
| Lebombo | ○ | | | | | |
| Nyando | ○ | | | | | |
| O'nyong-nyong | | ● | ● | | | |
| Orungo | ● | | | | | |
| Pongola | | | ○ | | | |
| Rift Valley fever | ● | | | ● | ● | Hepatitis, retinitis |
| Semliki Forest | | | | ● | | |
| Shokwe | ○ | | | | | |
| Shuni | ○ | | | | | |
| Sindbis | | ● | ● | | ○ | |
| Spondweni | | ○ | | | | |
| Tahyna | ● | | | ○ | | Respiratory illness |
| Tataguine | | ● | | | | |
| Usutu | | ○ | | | | |
| Wesselsbron | ○ | | | | | Hepatitis |
| West Nile | ● | ● | ● | ○ | | Hepatitis |
| Yellow fever | ● | | | | ● | Hepatitis |
| Zika | | ○ | | | | |
| *Sandfly-Borne Viruses* | | | | | | |
| Sandfly fever (Naples) | ● | | | | | |
| Sandfly fever (Sicilian) | ● | | | | | |
| *Tick-Borne Viruses* | | | | | | |
| Bhanja | ○ | | | ○ | | |
| Congo–Crimean | | | | | ● | |
| Dugbe | ○ | | | ○ | | |
| Nairobi sheep disease | ○ | | | | | |

| | TABLE 57-5. (Continued) | | | | | |
|---|---|---|---|---|---|---|
| Virus | Nondescript Febrile Illness | Febrile Illness With Rash | Febrile Illness With Arthritis | Meningo-encephalitis | Hemorrhagic Fever | Other |
| Quaranfil | O | | | | | |
| Thogoto | O | | | O | | |
| *Zoonoses* | | | | | | |
| Dakar bat | O | | | | | |
| Duvenhage | | | | O | | |
| Lassa | | | | | ● | Pantropic |
| Lymphocytic choriomeningitis | O | | | O | O | Pneumonia, arthritis, orchitis, parotitis |
| Mokola | | | | O | | |
| Monkeypox | | O | | | | |
| *Transmission Cycle Unknown* | | | | | | |
| Ebola | | ● | | | ● | Pantropic |
| Kasokero | O | | | | | |
| LeDantec | | | | O | | |
| Marburg | | ● | | | ● | Pantropic |
| **Australia** | | | | | | |
| *Mosquito-Borne Viruses* | | | | | | |
| Barmah Forest | | | ● | | | |
| Dengue 1–4 | ● | ● | | | | Hepatitis |
| Edge Hill | | | O | | | |
| Kokobera | | | O | | | |
| Kunjin | | | O | O | | |
| Murray Valley | | | | ● | | |
| Ross River | | ● | ● | O | | |
| Sepik | O | | | | | |
| Sindbis | O | O | O | | | |

Key: O, rare, sporadic; ●, frequent, epidemic.

firmed, but numerous viral isolates have been recovered from cotton rats (*Sigmodon alstinae*) and rice rats (*Sigmodontomys brevicauda*) in epidemic areas. Humans are infected directly from the rodent reservoir through infected aerosols or by contact with or ingestion of infected excretions.

AHF and BHF occur in relatively localized geographic foci— AHF chiefly in the agricultural pampas of Buenos Aires province and BHF in the tropical savanna of northeastern Bolivia. VHF has been recognized only in the tropical llanos of Portuguesa and adjacent Barinas states in northwestern Venezuela, but the geographic distribution of the infection has not yet been confirmed by systematic study. AHF is almost exclusively an occupational disease of agricultural workers, who become infected during the harvest season in February to May. BHF and VHF are acquired in a peridomestic setting, and cases occur in both sexes and in all age groups. Diseases caused by AHF and BHF were once endemic, with intermittent periods of hyperdemic-epidemic transmission. No BHF outbreaks have been reported since 1975. VHF was first recognized in 1989, and in the following 18 months more than 100 cases including 26 deaths were investigated in residents of the Guanarito municipality of Portuguesa state. The infection evidently is transmitted in an endemic pattern, and several cases are recognized each month without apparent seasonal differences.

The clinical features of the diseases are similar. After an incubation period of 5 to 19 days, fever, malaise, headache, and myalgias develop insidiously. Retroorbital pain, photophobia, and epigastric abdominal pain may occur, but complaints of phar-

yngitis and other respiratory symptoms are uncommon. In the first week, the patients become increasingly toxic and develop a flushed appearance, conjunctival injection, generalized lymphadenopathy, and fine petechial eruptions in the oral pharynx, on the upper trunk, and especially in the axillae. Leukopenia, thrombocytopenia, and proteinuria are characteristic.

Most patients enter into a convalescent phase after the first week of illness, but more than one third develop complications of neurologic abnormalities or hypotension and hemorrhage associated with a capillary leak syndrome. Ten percent to 20% of the patients die. The evolution of an individual infection toward a principally neurologic or hemorrhagic syndrome has been correlated with tropic properties of the infecting virus strain.

Bleeding from the gastrointestinal tract and mucous membranes, increased numbers of petechiae, and a rising hematocrit, indicating hemoconcentration, are manifestations of the hypotensive-hemorrhagic phase. An altered state of consciousness, ataxia, and tremor are common, but even in patients with severe neurologic alterations, the CSF may be normal. Acute renal failure and secondary bacterial infection are additional complications.

In the initial stages of illness, these potentially lethal diseases cannot be differentiated clinically from other acute infections. Illness with hemorrhagic manifestations may be confused with meningococcemia, leptospirosis, yellow fever, dengue hemorrhagic fever, and idiopathic thrombocytopenia. A definitive diagnosis rests on recovery of the virus from blood or demonstration of a specific antibody response by IF, ELISA, or neutralization assays.

Specific therapy for AHF with passively administered immune plasma was proven effective in reducing mortality to less than 1% when 2 U were given within 8 days of the onset of illness. A complication of serotherapy is a neurologic syndrome of fever, ataxia, and tremor that develops in 10% of treated patients 4 to 6 weeks after onset. Full recovery from the late neurologic syndrome is usual. Recognition of and supportive therapy for shock, hemorrhage, and secondary infection are critical in cases with hemorrhagic fever.

Isolation of patients to prevent nosocomial infection is not needed, but patient blood may be infectious, and rare instances of human-to-human transmission are known. An experimental vaccine for AHF (ie, Candid-1) was more than 95% effective in a large-scale human trial. Measures to control rodents reduced BHF outbreaks but are not practical in controlling AHF, which occurs over larger geographic areas.

## Australian or Murray Valley Encephalitis

Intermittent outbreaks of encephalitis have been reported in Australia since 1917, chiefly from the basins drained by the Murray and Darling rivers in southeastern Australia. The principal cause of these cases was shown to be a mosquito-borne flavivirus, subsequently named Murray Valley encephalitis virus, but sporadic human and equine CNS infections also arise from a closely related flavivirus, Kunjin virus.

The viruses are maintained in avian and mosquito cycles and are transmitted to humans by *Culex annulirostris*, the epidemic vector. In northwestern Australia and New Guinea, perennial viral transmission in the enzootic cycle leads to an endemic pattern of human infection; in the southeast, epidemics occur at infrequent intervals in years after heavy spring rainfall in the north. This pattern has been associated with the Southern Oscillation, a climatic phenomenon also related to El Niño. Cases occur in the summer and fall, between January and June.

In endemic areas and especially among Aboriginals, cases are reported principally in children. There is a twofold predominance of cases in males, in whom there is also a slightly higher fatality rate. Overall, the fatality rate is about 30%.

Nonspecific symptoms, including fever, headache, nausea, vomiting, and dizziness, precede the onset of neurologic signs and symptoms. A stiff neck, ataxia, tremor, slurred speech, a confused state, and generalized convulsions are early manifestations of meningoencephalitis. Spasticity and hyperreflexia or, conversely, a flaccid paralysis or hypotonia may develop after infection. Extrapyramidal signs occur in some patients. Bulbar paralysis may lead to respiratory failure. Signs of elevated intracranial pressure are evident in most patients. There is a moderate CSF pleocytosis, with 10 to several hundred leukocytes and with a shift from predominantly polymorphonuclear cells in the first week of illness to a mononuclear pleocytosis.

Permanent brain damage, leading to residual weakness or paralysis, psychomotor retardation, postencephalitic parkinsonism, or lesser disabilities, may occur in one third of the recovered patients.

Destructive changes are prevalent in the cerebellum, particularly in the Purkinje cells, and in the brain stem and spinal cord. Scattered foci of neuronal destruction and inflammation exist in the cortex. Perivascular and meningeal inflammation are pronounced.

It may be difficult to make a specific serologic diagnosis of Murray Valley encephalitis because of heterologous reactions with Kunjin virus and other Australian flaviviruses. Fractionation of CSF or serum to obtain IgM, IgM capture ELISA, CF, or neutralization tests are more specific than HI assays.

Supportive therapy, particularly measures to lower elevated intracranial pressure and respiratory support, may be needed in severe cases.

Public health programs exist to monitor infection rates in vectors and in sentinel animals to anticipate the occurrence of human cases. Long-term forecasting of epidemics based on climatologic data is a goal.

## California Encephalitis

California encephalitis that generally refers to CNS infections occurring in North America from La Crosse, snowshoe hare, Jamestown Canyon, California, or trivittatus viruses. However, infections from related bunyaviruses in Europe (ie, Tahyna and Inkoo viruses), which generally are associated with flulike illnesses, also have produced syndromes of CNS infection.

La Crosse virus is by far the most important disease agent in the group and annually is the cause of more than 100 CNS infections in endemic areas of the upper Midwest (Fig 57-5; see Table 57-2). Most of these cases are in children younger than 15 years of age, and the age-specific incidence of the disease in children in endemic foci approaches the incidence of invasive *H influenzae* disease.

Few CNS infections from Jamestown Canyon (JC) virus have been reported, although high seroprevalence rates in the Midwest suggest that the disease may be underrecognized. (Note: JC virus is also the designation of a human polyomavirus that produces multifocal leuco-encephalopathy.) Aseptic meningitis and self-limited encephalitis syndromes have been described in children and in adults. Snowshoe hare virus infections have been reported almost exclusively from Canada and, in the few reported cases, have been associated with more severe cases of encephalitis or encephalopathy. California virus, distributed in the western United States, and trivittatus virus in the Midwest have been associated with isolated cases of meningoencephalitis. Preliminary reports indicate that meningoencephalitis from snowshoe hare virus and Tahyna virus infections may occur in Asia and in central Russia. Jamestown Canyon and Tahyna viral infections may be associated with respiratory symptoms and pneumonia.

The viruses are maintained vertically in *Aedes* or *Culiseta* mosquitoes and horizontally in a cycle among mammals. *Aedes triseriatus*, the principal vector of La Crosse encephalitis, is a woodland species, breeding in tree holes and discarded manmade containers such as tires and cans. More than two thirds of these infections occur in boys, who are more frequently exposed to the mosquito outdoors.

Most La Crosse virus infections are asymptomatic. The clinical illness ranges from a simple febrile illness with headache to an aseptic meningitis or overt encephalitis. The initial symptoms may be vague, with fever, irritability, headache, anorexia, nausea, and vomiting. Ataxia, confusion, or a seizure may be the first indication of CNS infection. Meningismus, an abnormal sensorium, generalized weakness, abnormal reflexes, and cranial nerve palsies may be present on examination, and focal seizures, weakness, or asymmetric reflexes have been reported in as many as 25% of patients. Patients may have a moderate peripheral leukocytosis with a left-shift. The CSF examination is often unremarkable. A modest pleocytosis (median, 50/mm$^3$) may occur, sometimes with fewer than 10 cells/mm$^3$. The CSF protein concentration is normal in two thirds of patients. The electroencephalogram (EEG) may show evidence of diffuse or focal slowing. A mass effect or signs of localized inflammation may be seen in computed tomographic scans. Convulsions, as a single fit or status epilepticus, occur in 50% of cases. The fatality rate is less than 0.5%. The outcome of recovered patients generally is good, but some adverse effects on psychometric performance can be demonstrated after severe infections. Supportive treatment con-

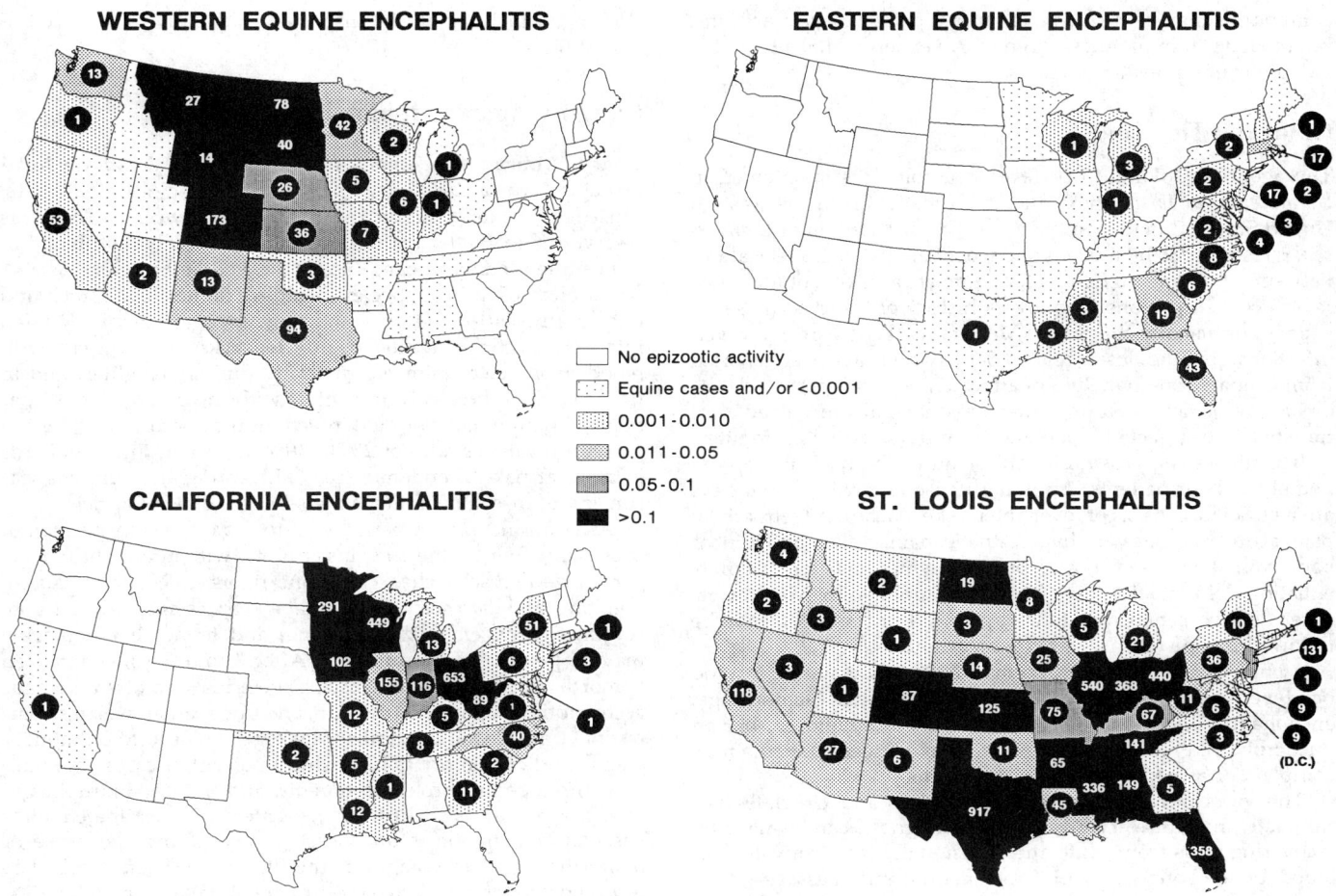

**Figure 57-5.** Reported cases of arboviral encephalitis and incidence per 100,000 by state, United States, 1964–1991.

sists of fluid and electrolyte management and the timely administration of anticonvulsants. In endemic areas, children are advised to use mosquito repellents and to play in open, sunlit areas.

The diagnosis is made serologically with a positive CIE reaction, by identifying specific IgM in CSF or blood by ELISA or IF, or by showing a rise in IF, HI, or neutralizing antibody titers. Heterologous reactions in some serologic systems may prevent the differentiation of La Crosse virus from snowshoe hare virus or other related agents.

## Chikungunya

Chikungunya is an acute viral arthropathy transmitted in an interhuman cycle by *Ae aegypti*. The disease occurs in parts of Asia and Africa in intermittent epidemics and in longer cycles of endemic transmission, followed by disappearance for long periods.

Chikungunya may be confused clinically with dengue and with infections from Sindbis and West Nile viruses, which are present in the same geographic distribution and cause similar syndromes of fever with musculoskeletal pain. Numerous comparative studies of the diseases concur that the presence and severity of arthritis in chikungunya differentiate it from dengue, which is associated with myalgia. The onset of chikungunya may be more sudden, the period of fever somewhat shorter (2 to 4 days versus 3 to 7 days in dengue), and recovery, except for persistent arthritic complaints, more rapid than in dengue.

After the sudden onset of fever, malaise, and generalized

musculoskeletal pain, a symmetric arthritis develops, affecting chiefly the metacarpophalangeal joints, wrists, elbows, shoulders, knees, ankles, and metatarsal joints. Redness and swelling of the pinnae occur in many patients. Infants may remain stiff and motionless, guarding against any movement of their joints. Conjunctivitis, generalized adenopathy, and a maculopapular, often pruritic rash may be detected. The subacute course of articular symptoms is characteristic: joint pain, stiffness, and swelling may persist in a fluctuating course for 6 to 18 months, although resolution without deformity is the rule. Although most patients recover from the acute illness without complication, hemorrhagic fever with severe gastrointestinal, mucosal, and petechial hemorrhages has been described in some cases. Shock was a complication in some patients. In one series, convulsions occurred in a large proportion of affected infants, but these patients had high fevers, and encephalitis could not be differentiated from an encephalopathy arising from another cause. Other cases with extraocular muscle palsy and polyneuropathy suggest the possibility of neurologic involvement. There may be a slight leukocytosis and thrombocytopenia, and the levels of C-reactive protein are elevated.

A specific diagnosis is made by isolating virus from an acute blood sample or by detecting specific IgM or a rise in HI or CF antibody titers. Infants younger than 6 months of age sustain significantly higher levels of viremia than older children or adults, but their clinical course of illness is not more severe.

Treatment is symptomatic. Nonsteroidal anti-inflammatory

compounds may be needed over a long period to treat arthritis, but the long-term prognosis is good. An experimental attenuated vaccine is under evaluation.

## Colorado Tick Fever

The agent of Colorado tick fever is a coltivirus maintained in *Dermacentor andersoni* ticks and small mammals in the western United States, Canada, and Mexico. The distribution of *D andersoni* is restricted to high plains and woodland habitats at elevations between 4000 and 10,000 feet, and most cases of Colorado tick fever occur in persons who give a history of travel to these locations, principally the Rocky Mountains (Fig 57-6). However, infections from the closely related Bannavirus, have been reported from China. More than 90% of affected persons report a tick bite or history of tick exposure. Infections have also occurred after transfusion of infected blood and from ticks carried on fomites.

The illness is a prostrating grippe and is biphasic in approximately 50% of patients. An initial phase occurring 3 to 4 days after a tick bite consists of fever, intense headache, and retroorbital pain, acute myalgias with hyperesthetic, painful skin, and lumbar back pain. The absence of respiratory symptoms aids in differentiating Colorado tick fever from other summertime viral fevers. After defervescence, a 2- to 3-day period of remission may be followed by one or, rarely, more recurrences.

Lymphopenia occurs in two thirds of patients with Colorado tick fever. A moderate thrombocytopenia is usual. Hemorrhage, encephalitis, and death have been reported in children, but an uncomplicated recovery is the rule. Convalescent patients may complain of asthenia for weeks or months.

The virus infects erythrocyte precursors and circulates peripherally in mature erythrocytes. The diagnosis can be made by recovering virus from acute and occasionally from convalescent blood, or serologically by ELISA or neutralization assays.

Colorado tick fever cannot be diagnosed reliably on clinical grounds, but a history of tick exposure in enzootic locations should suggest the diagnosis. Treatment is supportive. Infected persons should not donate blood until viremia is proven to have cleared. Protective measures include impregnating clothing with permethrin and wearing trousers and long-sleeved, light-colored

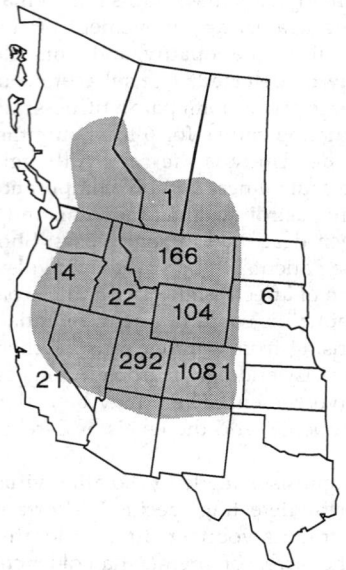

**Figure 57-6.** Distribution of *Dermacentor andersoni* ticks and reported Colorado tick fever cases by state, United States, 1980–1991.

clothing, which should be inspected frequently to remove adherent ticks.

## Congo-Crimean Hemorrhagic Fever

Congo-Crimean hemorrhagic fever (CCHF) is a tick-borne hemorrhagic fever associated with an extremely high fatality rate, caused by a nairovirus in the family Bunyaviridae. The virus reservoir is in *Hyalomma* ticks, which are widely distributed in Africa, the Mediterranean, Russia, the Middle East, and Asia. A wide range of animal species including domestic livestock and dogs are hosts for the ticks and may become viremic. Human infections occur from bites of infected ticks, from contact with blood of infected animals, especially during slaughter, and in nosocomial outbreaks from contact with the blood of index patients. Asymptomatic or mild infections may occur, as evidenced by seroprevalence rates of 2% to 30% in farmers and shepherds in areas at risk. In endemic areas, the spring and summer seasonality of infections follows the seasonal density of ticks.

After an incubation period of 2 to 9 days, a nonspecific but prostrating febrile illness begins abruptly with intense headache, generalized muscle aches, chills, and rigors. Chest pain, nausea, vomiting, and diarrhea may occur at an early stage. Hypotension, conjunctivitis, generalized flushing, and tender hepatomegaly may be present on examination. After 3 to 6 days, generalized hemorrhaging begins with epistaxis, petechial and often dramatic ecchymotic bleeding into the skin, and upper and lower gastrointestinal tract bleeding. Capillary leakage may lead to pulmonary edema and circulatory failure. Thirty percent of cases are fatal.

Lymphopenia, thrombocytopenia, and elevated bilirubin and liver enzyme levels are usually encountered. Disseminated intravascular coagulation is an end-stage event, and the cause of hemorrhage in early stages of the illness has been ascribed to thrombocytopenia, capillary endothelial failure, platelet dysfunction, and other unknown factors.

Pathologic examination discloses disseminated hemorrhages and edema formation in various locations. The liver shows extensive hepatocellular necrosis.

Survival is clearly correlated with an effective antibody response. Passive immunotherapy with immune plasma may be lifesaving if given at an appropriately early stage. For this reason, clinicians should be alert to the possibility of CCHF if ill patients give an appropriate epidemiologic history. Intravenous ribavirin shows therapeutic promise and it may be effective in postexposure prophylaxis. Secondary bacterial infections should be anticipated and treated. Fluid administration and inotropic agents are indicated to treat circulatory failure.

Travelers to endemic areas should take precautions against tick bites and should avoid contact with livestock and freshly slaughtered carcasses. Suspected patients should be isolated, to prevent nosocomial transmission. Secondary cases have occurred frequently in medical staff and tertiary cases in their family members.

The diagnosis is made serologically by demonstrating specific IgM or IgG by IFA, reverse passive hemagglutination inhibition, ELISA, or neutralization assays. Virus and viral antigen may be identified in blood, liver, or other autopsy materials.

## Dengue Fever

Dengue fever ranks as one of the leading infectious causes of morbidity in tropical countries. Epidemic attack rates as high as 50% are not uncommon and, in some outbreaks, 5% of patients may develop hemorrhage and shock, and 1% of these patients may die.

Four dengue virus serotypes (types 1 to 4) circulate in tropical America, Africa, Asia, Australia, and the Pacific. Infections are transmitted from person to person through the agency of *A aegypti* (the principal mosquito vector worldwide), *A albopictus* (an accessory vector in Asia), and various other *Aedes scuttelaris* complex mosquitoes (eg, *Aedes polynesiensis*). Epidemics arise in susceptible populations after the virus is introduced by viremic persons.

In areas where transmission is endemic, dengue is principally a disease of childhood, and infections occur in almost 100% of children before 8 years of age. In the absence of previous immunity, when new virus strains are introduced or among travelers from nonendemic areas, infections occur in all age groups, because exposure to infected vectors is universal. Women may be at higher risk of infection than men, because they are more likely to encounter the vector in peridomestic locations.

The incubation period is 3 to 7 days. Classic dengue is a grippe-like, often biphasic illness that cannot be easily differentiated from influenza, measles, and other acute infections. Fever, muscle and joint pains, chills, headache, and lumbar back pain are the most common early symptoms. However, upper respiratory symptoms, nausea, vomiting, and abdominal pain may occur in one third of patients. In fair-skinned persons, a centrifugally spreading morbilliform rash may be detected. The duration of illness is 3 to 7 days. One clinical study of uncomplicated Dengue found mild or moderate hepatitis in nearly all cases and transaminase levels exceeding 400 U/L in 10% of cases. Thus in endemic areas, Dengue should be included in the differential diagnosis of viral hepatitis. Minor hemorrhagic phenomena may accompany classic dengue, including epistaxis, bleeding from the gums, petechiae, and metrorrhagia.

These self-limited hemorrhagic manifestations should be differentiated from those that constitute the hemorrhagic-shock syndrome. Severe generalized bleeding and edema, pleural and peritoneal effusions, and in advanced cases, hypovolemic shock occur in dengue hemorrhagic fever–dengue shock syndrome (DHF-DSS). A loss of capillary integrity leads to fluid transudation into the extravascular space and microscopic and macroscopic bleeding. The onset of a hypotensive crisis may be precipitous but can be anticipated by serial hematocrit and total serum solids determinations (to find evidence of increasing hemoconcentration), platelet counts, and tourniquet tests. Outpatients should be followed by these simple measures as a means of triaging patients for hospitalization. The pathophysiology of DHF-DSS is not fully understood but may be related to intrinsic virulence properties of viral strains, or it may be associated with enhanced viral replication in persons with preexisting dengue antibody (immune enhancement). DHF-DSS often has been observed in populations sequentially infected with dengue 2 viruses after previous infections with other dengue types. There may be a greater risk of DHF-DSS among Caucasian than among black persons. Neonatal DHF attributed to infection in late pregnancy and transplacental viral passage was reported in three cases.

Classic dengue is self-limited and is treated symptomatically with acetaminophen and bed rest. Hemorrhagic cases must be monitored and treated intensively for hypotension and bleeding. Fluids or blood are needed to maintain cardiorespiratory function. Complications of the syndrome include disseminated intravascular coagulation (DIC), respiratory distress syndrome, and encephalopathy.

Simple dengue cannot be diagnosed accurately on clinical grounds and can be confused with West Nile fever, chikungunya, and commonplace viral illnesses such as influenza and measles. During one epidemic, the positive predictive value of a clinical definition was only 43% (negative predictive value, 95%). Laboratory diagnosis is essential and can be achieved readily by measuring specific IgM in a specimen taken 5 to 90 days after the onset of illness. Acute sera should be processed for viral isolation and by PCR to identify the specific viral type. Alternative serologic tests of paired sera include HI, CF, and indirect measurements of IgG by ELISA or FA. In areas where dengue and other flaviviral infections are endemic, all serologic tests suffer from cross-reactions among dengue serotypes and with other flaviviruses.

Measures to reduce the risk of mosquito bites include the use of mosquito repellents, indoor insecticide fogs, and tightly screened and air-conditioned residences. Reduction of *Ae aegypti* breeding sites in and around houses is the key to community-wide dengue control. Common items, such as flower pots, vases, pet water dishes, bottles, and discarded debris that can hold water, may be exploited by the vector. Public health campaigns aim to reduce the number of discarded containers, and in areas where drinking water is stored, the simple expedient of covering storage containers is effective. Larvicides provide a supplementary control measure. In the event of an epidemic, emergency ultra-low-volume applications of adulticides may be indicated, although the efficacy of this intervention is not proven. Experimental monovalent and multivalent attenuated vaccines have been developed and are being evaluated in human trials.

## Eastern Equine Encephalitis

Eastern equine encephalitis (EEE) is the most fulminant of the arboviral encephalitides, rivaling rabies in the gravity of its outcome. EEE occurs in relatively focal locations on the eastern and Gulf coasts of the United States, in some inland locations, and in the Caribbean (see Fig 57-5). A South American strain of the alphavirus occurs in areas of Central and South America.

EEE virus is maintained in a cycle among birds and *Culiseta melanura*, an ornithophylic mosquito that breeds in specific swampy habitat with mucky peat soils supporting a cedar, red maple, and loblolly bay flora. Other vector species (ie, various *Aedes* species and *Coquillettidia perturbans*) that bite birds and mammals transmit the infection to humans and horses and rarely to other dead-end hosts. In most years, fewer than 10 human infections are reported in the United States (see Table 57-2). The recent isolation of EEE virus from *A albopictus*, an exotic species imported from Asia, signals the potential involvement of a new vector species in EEE viral transmission and the possibility of increased viral transmission to humans.

After an incubation period of 4 to 10 days, the illness begins abruptly with a sudden, intense headache, fever, nausea, vomiting, and myalgias. Infants may present with generalized convulsions after brief intervals of unexplained irritability, anorexia, and fever. Confusion, delirium, and other changes in mentation typically are followed by a further depression in consciousness, eventuating in coma. Patients may develop elevated temperature, meningismus, stupor, and various neurologic abnormalities, including abnormal reflexes, focal weakness or paralysis, and cranial nerve palsies. Patients may exhibit signs of elevated intracranial pressure.

A peripheral leukocytosis with a left-shift differential count and a massive CSF pleocytosis is common. A predominance of neutrophils in the CSF early in the illness may suggest a bacterial meningitis. Later, the composition of the inflammatory cells shifts toward a mononuclear pleocytosis.

Between 30% and 70% of cases are fatal. Serious neurologic sequelae occur most frequently in young children and infants, persisting in more than 50% of surviving children younger than 5 years of age. The consequences of EEE acquired during pregnancy are unknown; one woman who acquired EEE in the third trimester delivered a healthy baby with no evidence of congenital infection. Pathologic findings in the CNS include edema and disseminated foci of neuronal degeneration with neutrophilic or mononuclear inflammatory responses, reflecting the stage of illness when death occurred. An acute pyogenic meningitis may be present. Vasculitis and infarction are seen in some cases.

Because EEE seroprevalence even in endemic areas is well below 1%, the presence of EEE virus antibody demonstrated by HI, CF, ELISA, or neutralization tests in an acute specimen suggests the diagnosis. Brain tissue, obtained by biopsy or at autopsy, should be cultured and examined immunohistologically for evidence of virus or viral antigen.

No specific therapy is available. Intensive supportive care, control of intracranial pressure, and respiratory support are especially important in this fulminant infection.

The risk of acquiring EEE is low, even in endemic areas. In Florida, which has a relatively high EEE incidence, deaths from a lightning strike are reported more frequently than cases of EEE. Nevertheless, the use of mosquito repellents is recommended to reduce the risk of infection.

## Filoviral Hemorrhagic Fevers

The hemorrhagic fevers associated with Marburg and Ebola viruses command attention because of their fulminance and the high fatality rates associated with the illnesses: 26% among the 38 reported cases of Marburg disease and 53% to 88% in outbreaks of Ebola hemorrhagic fever. The similarities in the virions' extraordinary size, tubular morphology, and distinctive physicochemical properties have led to their classification in a new family of RNA viruses, the Filoviridae. Three subtypes of Ebola virus (Reston, Sudan, Zaire), can be differentiated physicochemically and antigenically. The Sudan subtype of Ebola virus is less virulent in animals and is associated with a slightly lower fatality rate in humans than the Zaire subtype. Reston virus was discovered in 1989 as the cause of a highly fatal epizootic hemorrhagic disease of colonized monkeys. Despite explosive, apparently airborne transmission in several colonies, only four humans were infected and none were symptomatic. Reston virus may have limited pathogenicity for humans.

Little is known of the geographic and natural distribution of Marburg or Ebola viruses or of the circumstances leading to human infection in nature. Unlike other hemorrhagic fevers, which are transmitted mainly from natural reservoirs, Ebola and Marburg virus outbreaks, like the initial epidemics of Lassa fever, have arisen exclusively from a relentless, often nosocomial chain of person-to-person transmission through as many as five generations of contacts. Infections have occurred chiefly from contaminated blood or secretions or, in the first Marburg outbreaks, through contact with infected monkey blood, tissues, or cells. Direct contact has been more important than aerosol transmission in epidemic spread, but observations from Reston virus outbreaks in monkeys suggest that the possibility of airborne Ebola viral transmission should not be dismissed.

All cases of human illness have occurred in Africa or, in European outbreaks of Marburg disease, have had their source in that continent through the importation of infected vervet monkeys. The discovery of Reston viral infections in macaque monkeys from Asia suggests a wider, possibly global distribution of Ebola-related viruses. The natural reservoirs of the filoviruses have not been defined, but serosurveys attest to the sporadic occurrence of enzootic and endemic infections among ground-dwelling monkeys and humans in Africa and in free-living Asian monkeys. Bats have been investigated but are unproven as a reservoir for Marburg virus.

Both infections manifest in a similar manner, with an abrupt onset of prostrating fever, headache, and myalgias. Patients may complain of tender adenopathy, pleuritic chest pain, photophobia, and a dry or sore throat, but pharyngitis is not as severe as in Lassa fever.

Patients frequently appear restless and anxious, and they later become disoriented and stuporous and exhibit other encephalopathic signs. After 3 to 8 days, a morbilliform, usually confluent, nonpruritic rash starts on the upper trunk and spreads centrifugally to involve the entire body except the face and neck, which usually are spared. Desquamation occurs in 2 weeks. Profuse vomiting and watery diarrhea commence, accompanied by abdominal pain that may be intense enough to suggest a surgical abdomen. There occur progressively a fall in urine output, hypotension, and severe bleeding, chiefly from the gastrointestinal tract in the form of melena and hematemesis, but also from the vagina and gums. Multisystem failure from pneumonitis, hepatitis, pancreatitis, and tubulointerstitial nephritis combine with generalized bleeding and intractable hypotension, leading to death.

The white blood cell count shows an absolute lymphopenia and a left-shifted differential, and Pelger-Huet anomalies may be seen in some polymorphs. Aspartate and alanine aminotransferase levels are moderately elevated. Proteinuria and chemical evidence of prerenal or renal failure are present.

The pathophysiology of bleeding and events leading to death are not fully understood. Disseminated intravascular coagulation may be a terminal or secondary event, and platelet and endothelial cell dysfunction may be the primary causes of hemorrhage and shock.

The liver shows eosinophilic degeneration with prominent vacuolar changes. Interstitial pneumonia, interstitial nephritis, and follicular necrosis of the spleen are found frequently, but there is pathologic evidence of pantropic infection.

Marburg virus has been recovered from semen, the liver, and the anterior chamber of the eye 2 to 3 months after recovery from the illness, indicating the potential for the virus to persist in some patients.

A rapid confirmation of the diagnosis is important, because isolation of the patient and fluid precautions are critical to prevent nosocomial spread. Viral antigen can be identified readily in autopsy tissues. High titers of the viruses are found in the blood of various organs and occasionally in urine, and virions are often detected directly by electron microscopy. The most widely used serologic test is IFA; CF tests using infected liver antigen produces false-positive reactions.

Attempts at specific therapy with immune plasma and interferon were successful, but experience is limited to a few patients. Anticipation and prophylactic treatment of DIC with heparin was credited with the recoveries of two patients, but there is no consensus regarding the safety and efficacy of this approach.

Prevention of nosocomial transmission through barrier nursing methods and decontamination of clinical specimens is the most critical aspect of prevention.

## Group C Bunyavirus Infections

The group C bunyaviruses are 13 antigenically related viruses occurring chiefly in Central and South America. They are maintained in forested locations in cycles among small mammals and mosquitoes, in a pattern similar to the maintenance cycles for enzootic Venezuelan equine encephalitis viruses. Sporadic infections occur among persons who intrude on the forest, but endemic transmission has been documented among children in exclusively urban locations. Prospective studies of susceptible Dutch soldiers in Surinam disclosed an aggregate annual incidence for group C viral infections of 7%.

Most infections are mild or asymptomatic, but a brief, sometimes prostrating, febrile illness lasting 2 to 7 days has been described. Severe headache, myalgia, photophobia, and leukopenia are the principal clinical findings. Experimental infection of small laboratory animals produces hepatic necrosis. It is unknown if group C viruses are a cause of hepatitis in humans. Heterologous reactions necessitate that the serologic diagnosis be made with a combination of HI, CF, and neutralization tests. Virus can be isolated from the blood of patients in the acute phase illness.

## Hemorrhagic Fever With Renal Syndrome

Hemorrhagic fever with renal syndrome (HFRS) includes a group of diseases caused by rodent-borne hantaviruses in the family Bunyaviridae. The hantaviruses persistently infect small mammals, chiefly rodents (eg, field mice, voles, rats), insectivores (eg, shrews), and carnivores (eg, domestic cats), which remain asymptomatic but shed virus in urine, feces, and respiratory secretions. Humans are infected by direct exposure to infectious aerosols or percutaneously. Infections occur in sylvatic and peridomestic locations with a fall and spring seasonality. Laboratory outbreaks have occurred frequently. Men, particularly agricultural and forestry workers, are at greatest risk for infection in sylvatic locations. Secondary person-to-person transmission does not occur.

Epidemic hemorrhagic fever, the most severe form of HFRS, occurs principally in Asia and eastern Europe and results from infections by Hantaan Seoul or Belgrade viruses. Seoul virus has a worldwide distribution in persistently infected rats, but no cases have been reported in the United States and few cases have been reported in other developed countries. An abrupt, febrile grippe with intense backache, gastrointestinal symptoms, headache, and myalgias marks the initial stage of the illness. With the defervescence of fever, circulatory instability, with periods of abrupt hypotension and hypertension; generalized bleeding from mucous membranes, the gastrointestinal tract, and petechial hemorrhages in the skin; and renal failure from acute interstitial nephritis develop. Recovery follows a diuretic phase. The principal therapeutic challenges are treatment of renal failure and shock, but primary encephalopathy, pneumonia, myocarditis, hepatitis, and pancreatitis may complicate the illness. The fatality rate is less than 5% when good supportive care is available. A residual inability to concentrate the urine may be permanent.

Nephropathia epidemica, a milder form of HFRS caused by Puumula virus, occurs in Scandinavia and western Europe. Most cases are associated with a mild degree of renal insufficiency without significant hemorrhagic phenomena. Epistaxis, macroscopic hematuria, and mild gastrointestinal bleeding may occur in 5% of these patients, but most experience only a febrile grippe with proteinuria. Blurred vision, attributed to edema of the ciliary body, is a variable finding. Meningoencephalitis and death occur rarely. Prospect Hill virus, a vole-associated hantavirus enzootic in the United States and Thailand, and thottapalyam viruses in Asia, have not been associated with human illness.

Pathologic examination in cases of epidemic hemorrhagic fever discloses widespread macroscopic and microscopic hemorrhages, capillary endothelial damage, and associated fluid transudation. Nephritis affecting the medullary interstitium is pronounced.

The diagnosis is made serologically using IFA or an IgM capture ELISA. HI or neutralization tests are needed to differentiate infections among hantaviruses. Virus can be recovered with difficulty from blood and various fluids and tissues. PCR amplification has been used in clinical diagnosis and to differentiate hantaviral strains. Epidemic hemorrhagic fever may be confused with Waterhouse-Friderichsen syndrome, acute glomerulonephritis, pyelonephritis, leptospirosis, or thrombocytopenic purpura. Nephropathia epidemica cannot be differentiated clinically from other viral grippes.

When given early in the illness, ribavirin ameliorates circulatory instability and the course of renal insufficiency and improves survival. Public health measures have focused on the control of rodents and building rodent-proof homes and grain storage facilities.

## Japanese Encephalitis

Japanese encephalitis is the leading cause of arboviral encephalitis worldwide, producing more than 45,000 cases annually in the Far East (ie, China, Korea, Japan, eastern Russia, Taiwan), the Pacific (eg, Philippines and certain western Pacific islands), Southeast Asia, and the Indian subcontinent, (ie, India, Nepal, Bangladesh, and Sri Lanka) (Fig 57-7). Transmission is endemic in the wet season, in tropical locations, and intermittent epidemics occur in temperate locations. Transmission may occur throughout the year in some tropical areas.

The flavivirus, closely related to the agents of St. Louis and Murray Valley encephalitis, is maintained and amplified chiefly in a cycle among domestic pigs and *Culex* mosquitoes, principally *Culex tritaeniorhyncus*. The vector breeds in flooded rice fields, and risk is greatest in rural areas where the vector and domestic pigs coexist.

In endemic areas, high densities of infected vectors lead to exposure at an early age and cases occur principally in young children. Immunologically susceptible visitors of all ages are at risk. The case-to-infection ratio has been estimated to range from 1 : 25 to 1 : 210 in immunologically susceptible persons (eg, military personnel) exposed in endemic settings.

The incubation period ranges from 5 to 14 days. The onset of clinical illness may be gradual, with fever, headache, vomiting, and other nonspecific symptoms appearing over several days. In patients without CNS invasion, the illness resolves over 5 to 7 days. In other patients, the initial symptoms intensify with chills, continued fever and headache, and stiff neck. Occasionally the

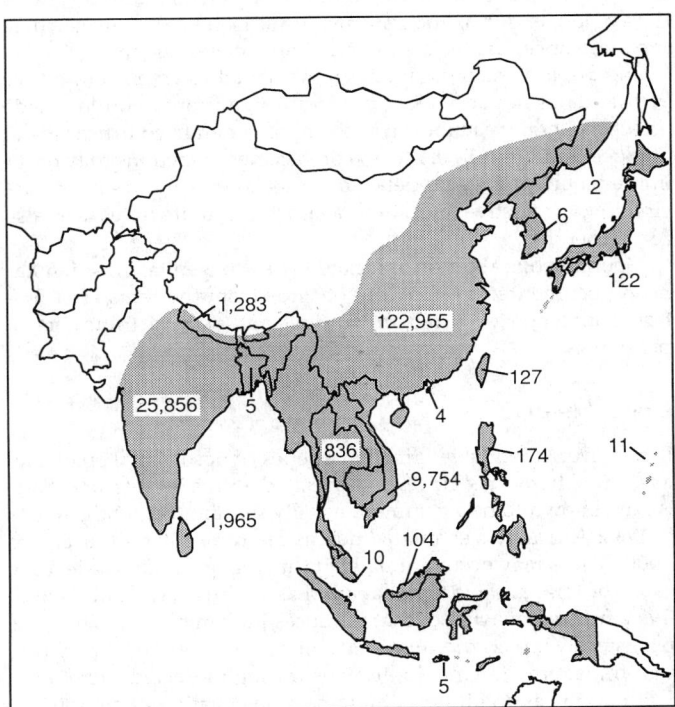

**Figure 57-7.** Reported Japanese encephalitis cases, 1986–1990 and areas of known or suspected viral transmission.

onset is abrupt, leading to hospitalization for delirium, stupor, seizures, or paresis on the initial day of symptoms. Marked changes in the state of consciousness, cranial nerve (especially facial) and oculomotor palsies, generalized or focal spastic or flaccid paresis, tremor, hyperactive or hypoactive deep tendon reflexes, and abnormal plantar reflexes occur with variable frequency. Convulsions occur frequently in children. A peripheral polymorphonuclear leukocytosis may develop early in the illness. The CSF commonly contains up to 500 leukocytes/mm³ and an elevated protein concentration.

The outcome is more grave in children younger than 10 years of age, who have higher fatality rates and a higher rate of sequelae (up to 75%) than older children or adults. The overall fatality rate ranges from 2% to 10% among persons who have ready access to good medical care, but fatality rates remain as high as 25% among children in some endemic areas. Several clinical and laboratory parameters are associated with a fatal outcome: presence of virus and interferon in the CSF, low serum and CSF levels of specific IgG and IgM, and a depressed sensorium on hospital admission. An inverse relation between the proportion of cases that result in death and the proportion of survivors with neurologic sequelae reflects the availability and quality of supportive care. In studies that report high fatality rates (eg, 50%), rates of significant sequelae have been low (eg, 2%). Significant sequelae of psychomotor retardation, paralysis or paresis, convulsions, and extrapyramidal signs are reported in 10% to 30% of recovered patients, and residual EEG abnormalities are common in children.

Neuropathologic examination discloses a panencephalitis with scattered foci of infected neurons in the cerebrum, basal ganglia, brain stem, and cerebellum. Inflammatory cells in the parenchyma chiefly are macrophages, and perivascular lymphocytes are of T-cell and B-cell origin.

Specific therapy is not available. Although clinical signs suggest elevated intracranial pressure in some patients, dexamethasone therapy does not improve outcome.

A purified inactivated vaccine prepared from infected mouse brain (JEVax) is recommended for travelers who plan visits of 30 days or longer during the transmission season to rural areas where Japanese encephalitis is endemic. Three doses, given on days 0, 7, and 30, are recommended. The vaccine has an efficacy above 90% and has not been associated with significant neurologic side effects. Allergic reactions, consisting of generalized urticaria and angioedema occur in 0.1 to 1% of vaccines. Reactions may occur immediately or may be delayed for as long as 9 days after vaccination. Protective measures against mosquito bites are also recommended.

Spontaneous abortion associated with congenital infection has been documented by recovery of virus from the fetus after maternal infection occurred in the first and second trimesters of pregnancy.

## Lassa Fever

Lassa fever, initially described in a series of nosocomial epidemics as a lethal hemorrhagic fever associated with a 50% fatality rate, is now known to be a common, usually self-limited, febrile illness in West Africa. It is estimated that as many as 400,000 cases and 5000 deaths may occur annually in that region, and it is a leading cause of fetal and maternal death. Lassa virus is the only one of five African arenaviruses that produces human disease. The virus persistently infects *Mastomys natalensis*, the rodent host in nature that transmits the virus to humans through infected excretions.

In adults and children, the initial constellation of symptoms, including fever, malaise, headache, and musculoskeletal pain, does not suggest a specific diagnosis. The illness evolves gradually, and painful pharyngitis, cough, chest pain, and abdominal com-

plaints of cramping pain, diarrhea, and vomiting lead progressively to prostration after 4 to 5 days. Patients appear ill, are weak, and may be hypotensive. A purulent pharyngitis, conjunctivitis, edema (particularly of the head and neck), and mucosal bleeding are highly specific signs of Lassa fever. Chest examination may disclose crepitant rales and evidence of pleural or pericardial effusions. Infants younger than 2 years of age evidence few specific signs except for edema, which often is generalized. Frequently, infants are severely ill with diarrhea, abdominal distention, bleeding, or pneumonia, or they have a history of convulsions when they are brought for treatment.

The illness resolves slowly over 8 to 10 days. In severe cases, the illness may be complicated by hypovolemic shock, encephalopathy, and respiratory distress from laryngeal edema, pleural effusion, and pneumonitis. Generalized hemorrhaging from the gums, gastrointestinal tract, and vagina is not a result of DIC but may be related to circulating inhibitors of hemostasis and to platelet or endothelial dysfunction.

An elevated hematocrit may reflect hemoconcentration. Leukopenia and proteinuria may be present. Elevated aspartate aminotransferase levels and high levels of circulating virus ($>10^3$/mL) indicate a poor prognosis. Infants younger than 2 years of age are at higher risk of death (30%) than older patients (15%). Bleeding, temperature above 39 °C, vomiting, and sore throat occur in 90% of fatal cases. Generalized edema in infants is associated with a fatal outcome. Tinnitus and permanent sensorineural hearing loss are late sequelae.

Hepatocellular necrosis, indistinguishable from lesions associated with Marburg, Ebola, and yellow fever viral infections, is the most conspicuous pathologic finding, but splenic and adrenocortical necrosis, interstitial nephritis and pneumonia, and myocarditis often are found. High concentrations of virus are found in the placenta and other organs that do not show distinct pathologic lesions. Circulatory collapse and death result from volume depletion through failed capillary endothelia. Shock cannot be attributed to mucosal bleeding alone in most cases.

Rapid recognition of the disease is essential, because specific therapy in the form of intravenous ribavirin is more effective if administered within 6 days of onset than if it is initiated later. The diagnosis can be made by demonstrating specific IgM antibody by ELISA or IF or by identifying antigen or viral genomic sequences amplified through PCR, in blood. Maintenance of fluid and electrolyte balance and respiratory support are critical elements of supportive therapy. Neutralizing antibodies may not be demonstrable in recovered patients, and the immunologic mechanisms associated with recovery are undefined.

Although nosocomial transmission of Lassa virus has led to numerous deaths, simple barrier nursing techniques may be adequate to protect hospital staff.

## Lymphocytic Choriomeningitis

Lymphocytic choriomeningitis (LCM) is a zoonosis with a worldwide distribution that is associated with the common house mouse, *Mus musculus*, the viral reservoir in nature. LCM virus, an arenavirus, is shed in the urine and other excretions of persistently infected mice and other rodents. Peridomestic infections have occurred among persons living in proximity with wild infected mice, from infected pet rodents, and among scientific workers whose laboratory rodent cell lines were silently infected. Most infections occur during the fall, winter, and spring.

The virus was named after the lymphocytic meningitis that it produces in experimentally infected monkeys and mice, but in humans, 90% or more of patients develop an influenza-like illness without signs of CNS infection. The systemic illness usually is characterized by fever, severe muscle aches, and headache and frequently by nausea, vomiting, pharyngitis, lymphadenopathy, and upper respiratory symptoms. A biphasic fever occurs in one fourth of cases.

A variety of complications may follow the influenza-like prodrome, including arthritis, parotitis, orchitis, pneumonia, myocarditis, mucosal bleeding, aseptic meningitis, and encephalitis. Meningism, an altered mental state, papilledema, cranial nerve palsies, generalized weakness, abnormal reflexes, and focal seizures have been described in patients with CNS infection. Polyneuritis, permanent flaccid paralysis, and a chronic meningoencephalitis have been reported as sequelae. Death has resulted from acute meningoencephalitis and after severe systemic illnesses complicated by pneumonia and generalized hemorrhages.

Patients may have a peripheral leukopenia. Examination of the CSF discloses a pleocytosis with up to 5000 leukocytes/mm³. Lymphocytes predominate, but 25% of the cells may be polymorphs. Hypoglycorrhachia is found in 25% of patients. The diagnosis is made serologically by indirect FA, but LCM virus can be recovered from the CSF, blood, or throat washings in as many as 50% of patients. If mice are used in virus isolation attempts, the colony must be certified to be free of LCM virus.

Infections during the first trimester of pregnancy may produce spontaneous abortion and congenital hydrocephalus or chorioretinitis.

## Monkeypox

Monkeypox is a zoonosis occurring in forested locations of West and Central Africa. The disease produces a generalized vesicular rash indistinguishable from that of smallpox, and illness is associated with a 13% fatality rate. However, unlike smallpox, secondary person-to-person spread occurs in only 3% to 15% of contacts, and all chains of transmission have ended spontaneously. Lymphadenopathy, which is not conspicuous in smallpox, is a characteristic feature of monkeypox.

The natural reservoir is thought to be in forest animals, particularly squirrels, but the mechanisms of viral maintenance and transmission to humans are not defined. Vaccination with modified vaccinia virus (ie, smallpox vaccination) is protective.

## Oropouche Fever

Oropouche fever is a generally mild febrile illness caused by a bunyavirus in the Simbu serogroup. The virus is transmitted in an urban, interhuman cycle by a gnat, *Culicoides paraensis*. The vertebrate hosts and vectors that comprise the sylvatic cycle in which the virus is maintained have not been identified. Major epidemics producing as many as 300,000 cases have occurred in major cities in the central Amazon and in Panama and Peru. The gnat vector exploits decaying banana stalks, discarded cacao hulls, and other peridomestic debris as breeding sites, and infected vectors may be prolific in residential areas.

The incubation period is 4 to 8 days, followed by the abrupt onset of fever, muscle aches, chills, headache, and photophobia. Nausea, vomiting, and diarrhea may occur. An uncomplicated aseptic meningitis has been reported in some cases. The patient may have leukopenia in the acute phase of illness. An uncomplicated recovery after 5 to 7 days is the rule, but in some instances, residual asthenia and a recurrence of symptoms have been reported after stressful activity.

A specific diagnosis is made by recovery of virus from acute-phase blood or serologically by HI, CF, or neutralization tests.

## Phlebotomus or Sandfly Fever

Among the 35 phleboviruses in the family Bunyaviridae, three are important agents of human disease in the Mediterranean littoral and Central Asia. Sandfly fever Sicilian (SFS) and Naples (SFN) viruses caused large epidemics in World War II and remain prevalent agents of endemic infections from June to November in some areas of the Mediterranean, northern Africa, and as far east as India and Pakistan. In some European countries, economic development and large-scale malaria control programs have led to marked declines in SFS and SFN transmission, while Toscana virus infections have become prevalent. Several sandfly-borne viruses of Central and South America produce nonspecific febrile illnesses. Although cases of clinical illness have been reported infrequently, high seroprevalence rates indicate that infections may be widespread.

SFS and SFN viruses are transmitted and maintained vertically chiefly by *Phlebotomus papatasii* sandflies, and Toscana virus is transmitted and maintained by *Phlebotomus perniciosus*, but horizontal transmission among vertebrates may contribute to amplification. The short flight range of the vectors restricts the foci where risk of infection is encountered.

Sandfly fever is a remarkably brief (ie, 2 to 4 days), self-limited illness typified by headache, myalgias, back pain, and photophobia. Nausea and vomiting may occur. Conjunctivitis and leukopenia are hallmarks of the disease. Even milder illnesses and subclinical infections are usual in children. Toscana virus is a frequent cause of meningoencephalitis in Italy and the Mediterranean.

Infections are diagnosed by viral isolation from acute blood or serologically by ELISA or by neutralization tests.

A citronella extract is the most effective repellent, although formulations containing DEET also are effective. Sandflies feed at night, but their small size renders most screens and bed nets ineffective.

## Rift Valley Fever

Before 1977, Rift Valley fever (RVF) was regarded chiefly as a veterinary disease of East and South Africa, where intermittent epizootics, associated with years of heavy rainfall, caused serious losses of domestic livestock from abortions and the death of sheep and cattle. Although sporadic human infections and limited epidemics were recognized, those that occurred in Egypt in 1977 and 1978 were of an unprecedented magnitude, producing 20,000 to 200,000 cases and 600 fatalities; attack rates in some areas reached 27%. A subsequent outbreak in 1987, of hundreds of cases in West Africa, testifies to the changing epidemiology of the disease.

RVF virus is a phlebovirus in the family Bunyaviridae, but it is transmitted by a variety of mosquitoes, and other biting insects may spread the virus mechanically. Mechanical transmission may explain how the virus, which is stable under ambient conditions, can spread so rapidly in an epidemic. Ingestion, direct inoculation, or inhalation of infected aerosols from slaughtered or aborted animals have been the principal modes of transmission in numerous cases among peasants and farmers. Several laboratory outbreaks have been reported.

The usual incubation period is 3 to 6 days, but it may be as brief as 24 hours. In most cases, RVF is a self-limited dengue-like illness with fever, chills, severe muscle aches and backache, and frontal headache that resolve over a 3- to 6-day period. Upper respiratory tract symptoms and conjunctival injection may occur. The major complications of RVF are retinitis, encephalitis, and hemorrhagic fever, which often leads to death. Ocular disease, leading to a decline in visual acuity and scotomas, begins about 1 to 3 weeks after the initial onset of illness. Retinal exudates, usually in a perimacular or macular location, retinal hemorrhages, and edema are the most common ocular findings. These lesions arise from a primary retinitis, and vascular occlusion from vasculitis. A permanent loss or impairment of visual acuity remains in half of these patients.

Meningoencephalitis may develop 3 to 10 days after resolution of the acute grippe. Signs of meningeal irritation, confusion, and other alterations of mentation and extrapyramidal signs may develop. The outcome of meningoencephalitis in children usually is favorable, but fatalities have been reported. The potential for the delayed onset of ocular and CNS findings should be borne in mind by clinicians who attend travelers from endemic areas.

RVF may be associated with a catastrophic illness that is characterized by generalized bleeding, especially from the gastrointestinal tract and into the skin, vomiting, and shock, leading to death in a large proportion of patients. Pathologic examination discloses widespread areas of macroscopic and microscopic hemorrhages. Focal hepatocellular necrosis is a prominent and consistent finding. Fetal death is common in infected livestock but remains an unproven suspicion in human infections.

The diagnosis is made serologically by ELISA or IF. The virus can be isolated from blood, nasopharyngeal washings, and feces.

An experimental inactivated vaccine is not available for general use. No specific therapy is available. Using repellents against mosquitoes and other biting insects and avoiding raw meat and ill animals are recommended as precautions.

## Rocio Encephalitis

The disease was first recognized in a series of outbreaks between 1975 and 1977 in the Ribeira Valley and Santista Lowlands on the southern coast of Brazil, near São Paulo. The outbreaks led to over 1000 cases, principally among men with outdoor exposure to forested areas. Attack rates were high, approximately 35 in 1000 inhabitants, and risk was even higher among poor families. Cases occurred in the fall, late in the wet season, between March and June. The fatality rate was 5% among hospitalized patients. Sporadic cases continue to be reported from the region.

Rocio virus is a flavivirus related antigenically to St. Louis encephalitis virus. The virus maintenance cycle is not defined, but the virus probably is transmitted among birds and mosquitoes, including *Aedes scapularis* or *Psorophora ferox*.

The clinical features of the illness are similar to those of other viral infections of the CNS. After an incubation period of 1 to 2 weeks, there is an initial phase of fever, malaise, nausea, vomiting, and severe headache that lasts several days. These symptoms may resolve, or the illness may lead progressively to a meningoencephalitis with stiffness of the neck, confusion, or a depressed state of consciousness and various neurologic findings, including weakness, pathologic reflexes, ataxia, and cranial nerve (particularly bulbar) palsy.

Neuropathologic lesions are widely distributed in the CNS but are most prominent in the brain nuclei and brain stem. Lesions in the cerebellum and of the anterior horn cells have been described. Major neurologic sequelae were reported in one fourth of survivors.

The diagnosis is made serologically by identifying specific IgM in CSF or the serum of acutely ill patients or by demonstrating seroconversion by HI, CF, or neutralization tests.

Intensive care, particularly of patients with bulbar palsy, may be lifesaving. The use of mosquito repellents and other measures against mosquito bites are recommended. An experimental inactivated vaccine had poor immunogenicity and was not investigated further.

## Ross River Arthropathy

Epidemics of polyarthritis, known in Australia since 1927, were shown in 1963 to be caused by an alphavirus, named Ross River virus. The disease is endemic in Australia, Tasmania, New Guinea, and islands of the western Pacific, principally in rural and sub-

urban locations. Although cases are recognized throughout the year in eastern Australia, transmission occurs principally in the Austral summer and autumn (January to May) after the seasonal densities of *C annulirostris* and *Aedes vigilax*, the principal mosquito vectors, respectively, in inland and coastal locations. The virus is transmitted in nature by these and other species (eg, *Ae camphorhynchus*) in a cycle among mammals and marsupials, but interhuman transmission may contribute to epidemic spread in heavily populated areas in Australia. This type of transmission involving *A polynesiensis* was described in a series of outbreaks in the South Pacific islands. The outbreaks, presumably initiated by viremic travelers, produced attack rates as high as 50%. Introduction of the virus to Hawaii and the continental United States by this means is a possibility.

The clinical illness is mild and principally affects adults. Cases occur more often in females than in males, and children are more likely to have a mild or asymptomatic infection. Increased frequencies of HLA-DR7 and Gma+X+b+ phenotypes have been reported among Ross River polyarthritis patients. Clinical manifestations consist of a maculopapular, usually nonpruritic rash, fever, malaise, myalgia, cervical lymphadenopathy, and polyarthritis. The rash is distributed on the trunk and limbs and may lead to a fine desquamation after 1 week. The affected joints, in decreasing order of frequency, are wrists, knees, ankles, finger joints, elbows, toe and tarsal joints, shoulders, hips, and spine. Pain, limitation of movement, and swelling may remain for more than 6 months (mean, 6 weeks). The period of incapacity tends to be longer in older patients, but permanent deformity does not occur. Congenital infection occurs in almost 100% of fetuses from experimentally infected mice, but observations on transplacental infection in humans are conflicting.

Clinical laboratory examination discloses an elevated sedimentation rate. The joint fluid contains 1500 to 15,000 mononuclear cells. There are no signs of complement activation. Viral antigens can be demonstrated in infected synovial cells. The differential diagnosis includes infections from Barmah forest virus (a related Australian alphavirus); Kunjin and Edge hill viruses (Australian flaviviruses); *M pneumoniae*; rubella and hepatitis B virus; rat-bite fever, Henoch-Schönlein purpura, serum sickness after medication (eg, penicillins), and enteroarthritis. A specific diagnosis can be made serologically by detecting specific IgM in an acute serum or by demonstrating a fourfold rise in HI titer. Symptomatic treatment with nonsteroidal antiinflammatory drugs may be indicated. Use of repellents and other measures to minimize bites of vector mosquitoes are recommended.

## Sindbis Virus Infection

Sindbis virus, an alphavirus, is widely distributed in Africa, Asia, parts of Europe, and Australia. Sporadic human infections result in a self-limited febrile illness with headache, polyarthritis, and a maculopapulovesicular rash. Recent outbreaks in Scandinavia (ie, Ockelbo disease in Sweden, Pogosta disease in Finland), western Russia (ie, Karelian fever), and west and central Africa (ie, Babanki viral infection) have been attributed to variants of the virus.

Sindbis virus is transmitted in an enzootic cycle among birds and principally culicine mosquitoes, among them *Culex univittatus* and *Cx neavei* in Africa, *Cx tritaeniorhyncus* in Asia, and *Cx annulirostis* in Australia. *Culex torrentium* and *Culiseta morsitans* are the principle enzootic vectors in Scandinavia, but certain *Aedes* species that feed on birds and humans may be important as bridging vectors. *Aedes* and *Culiseta* species may be important epidemic vectors in northern Europe. Cases in Scandinavia occur mainly from July to October among persons visiting mosquito infested woodlands to pick berries and mushrooms.

The presenting features of these patients were remarkable because the initial symptoms often were rash or joint pains, and a mild fever was often noted later or not at all. Headache, muscle aches, and lassitude are other early symptoms. The exanthem is not uniform, and discrete macules, papules, and painful or pruritic vesicles appear in crops over several days. The vesicles, filled with clear fluid, appear on an erythematous base and have been described by some observers as varicelliform. The rash appears chiefly over the trunk and lower extremities; the palms, soles, and face also are affected. Enanthems affected some patients. The rash resolves over 5 to 10 days.

The second characteristic feature of the infection is polyarthritis, which appears concurrently or within a few days of the exanthem. Pain in large joints, especially in the ankle and knee, may be disabling. The hips, wrists, shoulders, fingers, and neck also may be affected. Redness, swelling, and a serous effusion may develop. Arthralgias may persist for 3 to 4 years after the onset of illness. A low-grade fever, when present, lasts for a few days. Hemorrhagic manifestations were reported in one case. The diagnosis is made serologically by demonstrating specific IgM in acute serum or a rise in specific HI or CF antibody. Virus has been recovered from vesicular fluid in some patients.

No specific therapy is available. Nonsteroidal anti-inflammatory drugs may be indicated for treating arthritis. Mosquito repellents are recommended as a protective measure against mosquito bites in persons who may visit endemic areas, such as the woodlands in Scandinavia during the summer.

## St. Louis Encephalitis

St. Louis encephalitis is the leading cause of epidemic viral encephalitis in the United States, but epidemic or endemic transmission also occurs in southern Canada, Mexico, and parts of Central and South America (see Fig 57-5, Table 57-2). In the western United States, the flavivirus is transmitted by *Culex tarsalis* in an endemic-enzootic cycle, in common with western encephalitis virus. In the eastern United States and in urban areas of the West, *Culex pipiens*-borne and *Culex quinquefasciatus*-borne epidemics occur intermittently, with the potential for causing thousands of cases. *Cx nigripalpus* is the mosquito vector in Florida. The virus is maintained and amplified by these *Culex* mosquitoes in a cycle among birds.

Fewer than 1% of infections lead to clinical illness. Why neuroinvasive disease develops in such a small percentage of infected persons is unknown, but advanced age is an important risk factor. Morbidity and mortality also are directly associated with age. The spectrum of illness ranges from a simple febrile illness with headache to aseptic meningitis or encephalitis. St. Louis encephalitis generally is a milder illness in children than in adults, but more than 85% of patients younger than 20 years of age develop meningitis or encephalitis. The elderly are at greatest risk of encephalitis and death. The overall fatality rate is 6%, but is less than 1% in children younger than 5 years of age.

The onset often is insidious, with a prodrome of fever, headache, nausea, vomiting, myalgias, mental confusion, and clumsiness. Physical examination may disclose fever, meningism, and an altered state of consciousness. Tremulousness, generalized weakness, hyporeflexia and hyperreflexia, and cranial nerve palsies are the most common neurologic abnormalities. Focal weakness and other localizing signs are reported infrequently.

The CSF may be under pressure. A moderate CSF pleocytosis (ie, 100 to 200 leukocytes/mm$^3$) is typical, but the initial examination may fail to reveal any evidence of inflammation. Pathologic examination of the CNS shows widespread focal neuronal degeneration in the midbrain, thalamus, and brain stem and also in the cerebral cortex, cerebellum, and spinal cord. Inflammatory cells surround foci of infection in the brain parenchyma and in the perivascular cuffs.

Little is known of the risks of St. Louis encephalitis acquired during pregnancy. In a single case acquired during the second trimester, the full-term infant had no viral-specific IgM in cord blood and appeared normal at 1 year of age.

Psychomotor sequelae may result in 25% of recovered infants. In older children and adults, tremulousness, nervousness, headache, and memory impairment are temporary sequelae.

The diagnosis is made serologically by ELISA, HI, or CF, but heterologous reactions with dengue and other flaviviruses may occur. Specific IgM antibody in the CSF is presumptive evidence of infection. Brain tissue from biopsy or autopsy specimens should be examined by IF for evidence of the St. Louis encephalitis viral antigen.

No specific therapy is available. The use of mosquito repellents and air-conditioned and well-screened residences are protective.

## Tick-Borne Encephalitis

Tick-borne encephalitis usually refers to two distinct infections caused by closely related flaviviruses in the tick-borne virus serocomplex. Throughout Europe, including Scandinavia and parts of western Russia, the virus of central European encephalitis (CEE) is transmitted chiefly by *Ixodes ricinus*. Russian spring-summer encephalitis (RSSE) virus is transmitted by *Ixodes persulcatus*, a species distributed in the Far East and Russia. Other viruses of the complex that cause human disease include the agents of louping ill, Omsk and Kyasunur forest hemorrhagic fevers, and Negishi and Powassan viruses.

Tick-borne encephalitis is chiefly an occupational disease of forestry workers and others who have extensive contact with sylvatic habitats of the tick vectors. Most cases of illness are in adults and in males. Infections occur in the spring and summer, with a peak incidence in July. Tick-borne encephalitis may follow the consumption of infected raw cow, sheep, or goat milk products or contact with slaughtered infected animals.

Central European encephalitis typically follows a biphasic course. After an incubation period of 7 to 14 days, a nonspecific febrile illness develops, consisting of fever, head and muscle ache, and upper respiratory symptoms. Defervescence is rapid and complete in 75% to 90% of patients, but in most cases that come to clinical attention, a second phase occurs after 1 week, with the onset of aseptic meningitis or encephalitis. Recrudescent fever, headache, neck stiffness, tremor, somnolence, disturbed mentation, cranial nerve palsies, generalized weakness, and cerebellar signs may occur. In about 3% of patients with CNS involvement, a progressive course of paresis or paralysis affecting the proximal musculature and pharyngeal and respiratory muscles may develop. A fatal outcome, frequently from bulbar paralysis, is reported in fewer than 1% of cases. Minor neuropsychiatric sequelae occur for some patients.

The clinical course of RSSE is more severe. The fatality rate among patients may be as high as 20%, and significant neurologic sequelae follow recovery in half of the survivors. A residual flaccid paralysis of the shoulder girdle is characteristic. The early stages of RSSE do not follow the previously described biphasic pattern. The initial symptoms of fever, intense headache, nausea, vomiting, and photophobia are followed directly by signs of encephalitis, including disturbances in mentation, meningism, weakness in the bulbar musculature and extremities, and convulsions.

Pathologic changes affect chiefly the gray matter of the cerebrum, brain stem, and anterior horn cells of the upper spinal cord. Nodular foci of neuronal necrosis with inflammatory cellular infiltrates, perivascular cuffs, and spongiform rarefaction are the typical pathologic changes.

Treatment of convulsions and ventilatory support in the event of bulbar paralysis may be necessary. No specific therapy is available. Laboratory diagnosis rests on serologic confirmation of infection by ELISA, HI, or CF assays. The differential diagnosis includes borrelial infection and other viral causes of meningoencephalitis. *Ixodes ricinus* is the vector of both Lyme disease and CEE in western Europe. Dual CNS infection was fatal in one case.

Effective inactivated vaccines for CEE are available in Europe and Russia, but vaccination is not indicated for travelers whose exposure to woodlands is limited. Immune globulin for postexposure prophylaxis is available in Austria and Germany; to be effective and to avoid immunopathologic complications, passive immunization must begin within 4 days of exposure.

## Venezuelan Equine Encephalitis

Venezuelan equine encephalitis (VEE) remains an important public health and veterinary problem in Central and South America. VEE outbreaks have led to as many as 30,000 human cases in a single year, with an equal number of fatal cases among horses in contemporaneous epizootics. Epidemics occur at intermittent intervals, principally in rural coastal locations. In 1971, an epizootic spread from Central America into Texas, leading to 110 human and more than 1500 equine cases. No major epizootics have been reported since 1973, but isolated outbreaks among horses periodically are reported from Central America.

During outbreaks, epizootic subtypes of VEE virus (ie, IAB or IC) are spread directly among horses and burros by mosquito vectors. The reservoir of the viruses during interepidemic periods is unknown. Other subtypes of enzootic VEE viruses occur continuously in cycles among forest-dwelling rodents and mosquitoes. Equine and human infections from these subtypes occur sporadically. Subtype II, also known as Everglades virus, is found in Florida and has been responsible for isolated cases of CNS infection.

VEE in humans is manifested chiefly as a prostrating grippe. After an incubation period of 3 to 7 days, the onset of intense headache, fever, and myalgias is so sudden that it can often be documented to an exact hour. Shaking chills, arthralgias, photophobia, ocular pain, nausea, vomiting, and other signs of toxicity force the patient to bed or to the hospital. Recovery follows rapidly; the entire course of the illness lasts less than 1 week. A recrudescence of symptoms and a biphasic fever curve occur in some patients. There are few physical findings; the patient appears flushed and lethargic, has tender muscles, and may have an injected pharynx and conjunctivae.

Neurologic symptoms are rare in adults, but even in children, in whom the risk of CNS infection is greatest, fewer than 5% of of the illnesses lead to meningoencephalitis. Various neurologic abnormalities are reported, including a depressed sensorium, meningism, generalized weakness, focal and generalized seizures, and pathologic reflexes. Twenty percent of the patients with CNS involvement die, and the fatality rate for children younger than 5 years of age is higher.

The clinical laboratory evaluation discloses a panleukopenia with an initial depression of lymphocytes followed by neutropenia. Elevated alanine amino transferase levels have been described in some patients.

The pathologic examination shows lymphoid depletion, follicular necrosis in the spleen and lymph nodes, and an interstitial pneumonia. The brain is congested, and there is evidence of a vasculitis.

A specific diagnosis is made serologically by HI, CF, IF, ELISA, or neutralization tests. However, attempts to isolate virus from pharyngeal secretions or blood during the first 3 days of illness are fruitful in 50% of patients. Identification of the infecting viral subtype with specific monoclonal antibodies provides important epidemiologic information about the likelihood of epidemic spread.

Treatment is supportive. Live attenuated and killed vaccines are available for laboratory workers. Travelers to enzootic areas should take precautions against mosquito bites. Inactivated equine vaccines are administered routinely in some areas; however, inadequate inactivation procedures resulting in residual infectious virus is suspected to have caused livestock deaths and epizootics.

## West Nile Fever

West Nile virus, a flavivirus antigenically related to the viruses of Japanese, St. Louis, and Murray Valley encephalitis, occurs over a broad geographic range that includes Africa, parts of Europe and Russia, the Middle East, and the Indian subcontinent. Significant antigenic differences are demonstrable between Asian and African strains. The virus is maintained in a mosquito and avian cycle chiefly by *Culex* mosquitoes. Although they may be less important in maintaining the virus in its natural cycle, some mammals can be infected, and horses may become ill with encephalitis. High levels of endemic transmission are prevalent in some locations in the virus's geographic range, where the infection is a leading cause of nonspecific summer fevers. In some areas, seroprevalence rates approach 50% to 100% among children 5 years of age. Major epidemics with attack rates as high as 50% have been reported with the introduction of the virus into immunologically susceptible populations.

Most infections, particularly in children, are asymptomatic. The incubation period is 2 to 6 days. Clinical manifestations are generally mild, with fever, malaise, anorexia, headache, and myalgias, and half of the patients develop maculopapular rashes. Nausea, vomiting, conjunctivitis, and pharyngitis may occur. Generalized, mildly tender lymphadenopathy is a characteristic feature, occurring in more than 75% of patients. The skin may be marked by indistinct mottling and macules and a diffuse roseolar eruption, affecting chiefly the trunk and upper extremities. The severity of illness appears to correlate with age. Children usually have asymptomatic or mild infections lasting 5 to 6 days. Meningoencephalitis may complicate the illness in the elderly, but CNS infections, including fatal cases, have been reported in adolescents and children. Hepatitis, pancreatitis, myocarditis, and poliomyelitis with residual flaccid paresis have been reported rarely.

The diagnosis can be made serologically by HI, CF, ELISA, or neutralization tests. However, specimens of acutely ill patients should be submitted for virus isolation, which is successful in almost one third of the attempts.

West Nile fever cannot be differentiated reliably from dengue and Sindbis virus infections, which may occur in the same geographic locations. West Nile infection should also be considered in the differential diagnosis of CNS infections in these areas.

Treatment is supportive. Measures to protect against mosquito bites are recommended.

## Western Equine Encephalitis

Western equine encephalitis (WEE) is an endemic arboviral infection in the western United States, Canada, Mexico, Argentina, and other parts of South America (see Fig 57-5, Table 57-2). The alphavirus is maintained in nature chiefly among birds and *Cx tarsalis*, a mosquito that breeds in rural agricultural locations. Risk of infection is greatest among rural-dwelling persons who spend long hours outdoors and incidence is almost two times higher among males than females.

Infections chiefly are asymptomatic. Clinical manifestations range from a mild illness with headache and fever to meningoencephalitis. The fatality rate is 3%. There usually is a brief prodrome of nonspecific symptoms, including fever, headache, nausea, vomiting, anorexia, and malaise. These symptoms are followed by fluctuations in mental status, signs of meningeal irritation, tremulousness, and weakness. Generalized hyporeflexia or hyperreflexia and focal deficits, localizing to frontotemporal locations, may be present on physical examination. Infants frequently present with convulsions after an abbreviated prodrome of fever and irritability.

A CSF pleocytosis, initially of polymorphonuclear cells and later of mononuclear cells, is elaborated, with a range of 10 to 300 leukocytes/mm$^3$. At autopsy, focal necrosis in various stages of resolution and vasculitis are seen in the white and gray matter, especially of the brain nuclei.

Neurologic sequelae remain in 10% of recovered patients. Postencephalitic parkinsonism has been reported in some instances. Infants have a higher risk of developing psychomotor retardation, paresis, and other sequelae. Third-trimester infection has led to encephalitis in two neonates. Teratogenic effects after infections earlier in pregnancy have not been reported.

The diagnosis usually is made serologically by demonstrating specific IgM in CSF or serum or by showing a rise in HI, CF, or neutralizing antibody in paired serum specimens. The virus has been recovered from blood, CSF, and brain biopsy samples of acutely ill patients.

Treatment is supportive. Avoiding outdoor activities, especially at dusk, and the use of mosquito repellents may offer protection against exposure.

## Yellow Fever

In the late 19th century, yellow fever and cholera were among the most feared causes of epidemic morbidity and mortality in the southern and eastern United States. As recently as 1905, an outbreak in New Orleans produced 5000 cases and 1000 fatalities. Yellow fever is now endemic in tropical western and central Africa between 15°N and 10°S and in parts of Central and South America between 10°N and 40°S (Fig 57-8). Epidemics, often leading to thousands of cases, occur intermittently in Africa; 100,000 cases with 30,000 deaths were reported from Ethiopia in the continent's largest outbreak. *Ae aegypti*, the principal yellow fever virus vector, is prevalent in the southeastern United States and Caribbean, and the introduction of *Ae albopictus*, the Asian tiger mosquito, into the hemisphere potentially increases the risk for epidemic spread if the virus is introduced from its sylvatic source.

Yellow fever is caused by a mosquito-borne flavivirus maintained in nature chiefly in a primate and mosquito cycle. In some locations, the virus may be maintained vertically in mosquito or tick vectors. In South America, the virus is enzootic among monkeys in jungle locations, principally in basins drained by the Amazon, Orinoco, Catatumbo, Atrato, and Magdalena rivers. *Hemagogus* mosquitoes are the primary vectors. Approximately 100 to 200 human infections are reported annually, chiefly among forestry, road, and animal husbandry workers whose occupational activities take them into the jungle. Consequently, most cases occur in persons 15 to 40 years of age and in men. The period of greatest risk is the end of the rainy season.

In West Africa, a similar jungle cycle exists in high forests of the western coast, but inland, in the moist savanna, enzootic and endemic infections occur only in the wet season, when sylvatic *Aedes* mosquitoes emerge to transmit the virus to monkeys and humans. In the dry savanna and in urban areas, yellow fever has the potential of becoming epidemic because water storage practices lead to high densities of peridomestic breeding *Ae ae-*

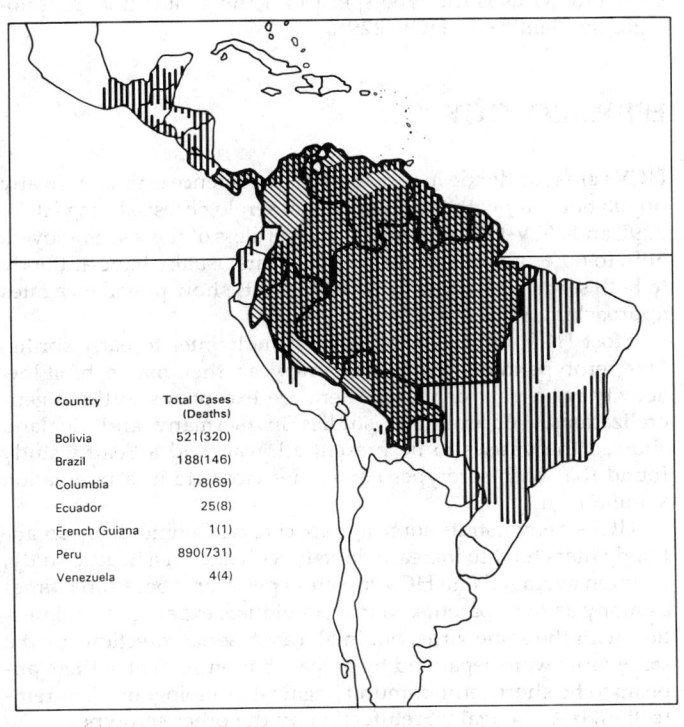

| Country | Total Cases (Deaths) |
|---|---|
| Bolivia | 521(320) |
| Brazil | 188(146) |
| Columbia | 78(69) |
| Ecuador | 25(8) |
| French Guiana | 1(1) |
| Peru | 890(731) |
| Venezuela | 4(4) |

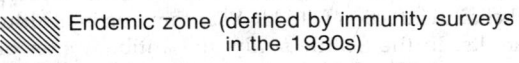 Endemic zone (defined by immunity surveys in the 1930s)

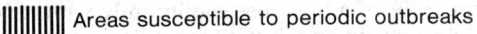 Areas susceptible to periodic outbreaks

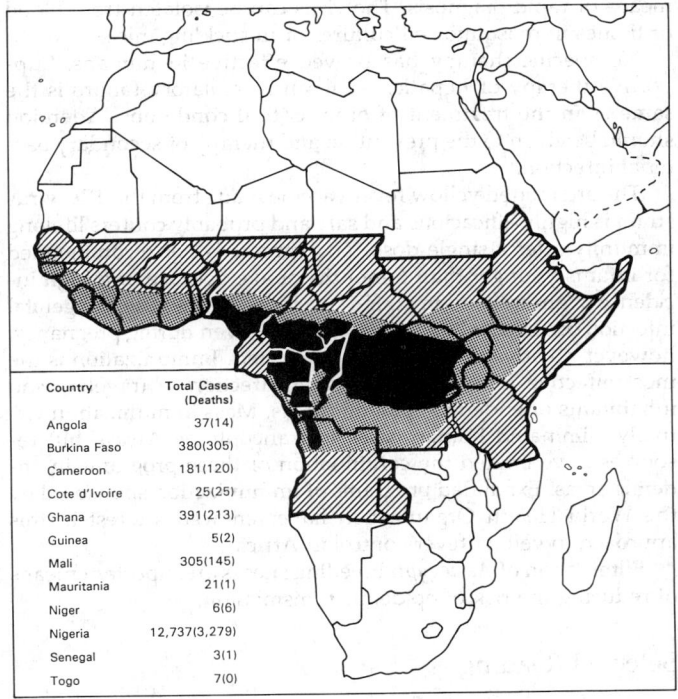

| Country | Total Cases (Deaths) |
|---|---|
| Angola | 37(14) |
| Burkina Faso | 380(305) |
| Cameroon | 181(120) |
| Cote d'Ivoire | 25(25) |
| Ghana | 391(213) |
| Guinea | 5(2) |
| Mali | 305(145) |
| Mauritania | 21(1) |
| Niger | 6(6) |
| Nigeria | 12,737(3,279) |
| Senegal | 3(1) |
| Togo | 7(0) |

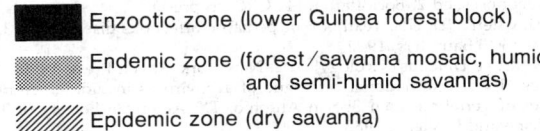 Enzootic zone (lower Guinea forest block)

Endemic zone (forest/savanna mosaic, humid and semi-humid savannas)

Epidemic zone (dry savanna)

**Figure 57-8.** Reported yellow fever cases and deaths, 1980–1990, and risk by geoecologic zone.

*gypti.* Risk of epidemic transmission is associated with the presence of vectors in 5% or more of households. Most infections occur in children younger than 10 years of age.

The disease classically has been divided into three stages: infection, remission, and intoxication. After an incubation period of 3 to 10 days, there is a sudden onset of fever, headache, and musculoskeletal pain. Nausea and weakness occur, but there are few physical signs other than conjunctivitis, flushing of the skin, and Faget's sign, a relative bradycardia. After 2 to 3 days, fever and symptoms remit, and in most cases, the illness resolves. After this brief remission, the illness may resume, with the reappearance of toxicity, fever, vomiting, abdominal pain, jaundice, hematemesis, and other evidence of a hemorrhagic diathesis. Dehydration, hypotension, and a reduction in urine output occur, and proteinuria may develop. Azotemia, encephalopathy, progressive liver damage, and bleeding lead to death in 30% to 50% of patients who develop these signs of severe yellow fever.

The clinical laboratory examination discloses leukopenia, elevated liver enzymes, and abnormalities of coagulation, including prolonged prothrombin, partial thromboplastin, and clotting times and significant reductions of liver-dependent clotting factors. There is evidence of DIC in some patients.

Numerous mucosal, serosal, and subcutaneous hemorrhages are seen at autopsy. The liver may show dramatic parenchymal changes, with widespread necrosis in a midzonal distribution. Councilman bodies, eosinophilic masses representing destroyed cells, are accompanied by a minimal lymphocytic infiltrate. The renal medullae are congested and swollen, and the convoluted tubules are damaged. Evidence of myocarditis may be found.

A clinical diagnosis cannot be made reliably. A specific laboratory diagnosis can be confirmed rapidly by identifying viral antigen or genomic sequences in blood or liver biopsy tissue. Detection of specific IgM by ELISA in serum is an alternative means of rapid diagnosis. The virus can be isolated from blood or tissues in mosquito cell cultures or in suckling mice.

No specific therapy has proved effective in humans. Supportive therapy of hepatic, renal, and circulatory failure is the same as in the treatment of other critical conditions. Attention should be given to the prevention and therapy of secondary bacterial infection.

The attenuated yellow fever vaccine made from the 17D virus strain is highly efficacious and safe and probably confers lifelong immunity after a single dose. The vaccine is not recommended for infants younger than 6 months of age because of a high incidence of encephalitis in young vaccinees. In one case, congenital infection occurred when the vaccine was given during pregnancy; however no adverse effects were reported. Immunization is the most effective means of preventing infection in travelers and inhabitants of endemic-epidemic areas. Mass immunization virtually eliminated human cases in francophone Africa, but resources have limited the continuation of these programs in endemic areas. Expanded programs of immunization sponsored by the World Health Organization have renewed interest in this approach to yellow fever control in Africa.

Elimination of *Ae aegypti* breeding sites is an important means of reducing the risk of epidemic transmission.

## Selected Readings

Beran GW, Tsai TF, Benenson AS, eds. Handbook series in zoonoses. Section B: viral zoonoses, ed 2. Boca Raton, FL: CRC (in press).

Feigin RD, Cherry JD, eds. Textbook of pediatric infectious diseases, ed 3. Philadelphia: WB Saunders, 1992.

Fields BN, Knipe DN, eds. Virology, ed 2. New York: Raven Press, 1990.

Karabatsos N, ed. International catalogue of arboviruses including certain other viruses of vertebrates, ed 3. San Antonio, TX: American Society of Tropical Medicine and Hygiene, 1985.

Monath TP, ed. The arboviruses: epidemiology and ecology. Boca Raton, FL: CRC Press, 1989.

*Principles and Practice of Pediatrics, Second Edition.*
edited by Frank A. Oski et al. J. B. Lippincott Company, Philadelphia © 1994.

# 57.2 *Coronaviruses*

Rebecca L. Byers and Elliot C. Dick

Coronaviruses (CVs) account for 5% to 35% of all upper respiratory tract infections worldwide and are second to the rhinoviruses as a cause of the common cold in children and adults. CVs also have been indicated in lower respiratory tract disease of children and adults, in gastroenteritis, and, possibly, in central nervous system disorders.

## THE AGENT

Human coronaviruses (HCVs) were first isolated in human embryonic trachea organ culture. These agents and other CVs isolated from animals were characterized by electron microscopy as large, pleomorphic, spherical or elliptical, enveloped RNA viruses with a diameter of 80 to 220 nm. The envelope displays distinctive 20-nm-long petal-shaped projections that produce a solar corona appearance. The RNA genome is surrounded by a nucleoprotein, forming a helical nucleocapsid just beneath the envelope. Major antigens are the nucleocapsid and two or three envelope proteins. Based on antigenic relatedness, human isolates are grouped into two serotypes: HCV-229E and HCV-OC43. Avian infectious bronchitis virus is the type species for the genus; it is morphologically identical to HCV-229E.

## EPIDEMIOLOGY

HCVs are worldwide in distribution. Prevalence estimates in any population vary with the sensitivity of serologic tests. Using HCV-229E and HCV-OC43 as antigens, regardless of the test employed, 50% to 60% of adults older than 30 years usually have antibody to both serotypes. The most sensitive tests show prevalence rates approaching 90% to 100%.

Most HCV infections occur from midwinter to early spring. One serotype may predominate one year, then may exhibit low activity for a year or more. There are exceptions to these generalizations. For example, studies in Germany and England showed the viruses to be present all year, and a Seattle study found that both serotypes sometimes circulate in a population simultaneously.

HCVs demonstrate some age specificity. Geometric mean antibody titers tend to increase directly with age. In a Seattle study, children averaged one HCV infection per year–about three times as many as their parents. Many individuals experienced reinfection with the same virus, but in all cases, serial infections by the same virus were separated by at least 8 months. Thus, there appears to be short-term immunity against homologous virus reinfection, but not against reinfection by the other serotype.

Subclinical infection with HCVs is common in healthy children and adults. In the Seattle study, the antibody titer of 40% of children and 36% of adults rose significantly without evidence of illness. Similarly, in an 8.5-year surveillance of healthy older children in Atlanta, only 38% (63/168) of children with HCV-229E seroconversion and 47% (44/93) of those with HCV-OC43 seroconversion reported any illness.

# TRANSMISSION AND PATHOGENESIS

HCVs probably are transmitted only via the respiratory route; however, there is no direct evidence of the natural modes of transmission. Volunteers have been readily infected by intranasal inoculation of virus. A natural transmission experiment in human volunteers using HCV-229E showed aerosol transmission may be most common, but hand-to-face transmission has not been ruled out.

In human volunteers, the incubation period of HCV colds ranges from 1 to 5 days. Viruses replicate in the upper respiratory tract, are shed in nasal washings, and reach detectable levels at symptom onset. Illness generally lasts 6 to 7 days but can persist for 18 days.

Reinfection with HCVs is common. Studies of children in Tecumseh, Michigan, and in Atlanta show a high rate of reinfection in individuals with prior antibodies. In addition, antibody did not appear to modify the severity of clinical illness. As many as 50% of individuals with symptomatic HCV infections do not have diagnostic rises in antibody titer.

Quantity of antibody seems related to protection. A study from England shows that individuals with high concentrations of serum neutralizing antibodies and specific nasal IgA antibodies before challenge had fewer infections, reduced symptoms, and shortened virus shedding. There is also evidence that antigenic variability of HCV-OC43- and HCV-229E-related strains affects level of protection; immunity to a homotypic challenge seems to last at least a year, but immunity to heterotypic strains is slight. Thus, strain-specific antibody, high levels of serum-neutralizing antibodies, and specific secretory IgA antibodies probably all play a protective role, but still may provide only transient immunity.

# CLINICAL MANIFESTATIONS

## Upper Respiratory Disease

HCVs cause typical colds similar to those caused by rhinoviruses but with less cough and more malaise and nasal discharge. Sore throat, cough, malaise, and headache are present in about 50% of adults, 20% of whom have fevers. Cervical adenitis, muscle aches, and rash are less common. Clinical findings in children also are typical of colds; however, manifestations are frequently more severe. In a study of Atlanta children, 40% had fevers above 37.6 °C and one third reported cervical adenitis.

## Lower Respiratory Disease

In children, HCV infections are associated with asthma attacks, pneumonia, and bronchiolitis. A few cases of pneumonia in adults have been reported. The clearest association of HCV infection with lower respiratory tract disease in adults is with chronic obstructive pulmonary disease.

## Gastroenteritis

Coronaviruses are associated with diarrheal diseases in mammals, especially newborns. In 1975, coronavirus-like particles (CVLPs) were found by electron microscopy (EM) in stools from children and adults with nonbacterial gastroenteritis. In subsequent studies, however, CVLPs were found in equal numbers of asymptomatic individuals. It is difficult to propagate CVLPs in vitro, and there is debate whether some EM reports of CVLPs describe true virus particles. There is ongoing controversy on the etiologic role of HCVs as enteric pathogens.

The most convincing association of CVLPs with human enteric disease is with necrotizing enterocolitis in neonates and diarrheal

disease in children. In Arizona, CVLPs were found by EM in 49 of 126 children with diarrhea. Of these patients, 88% were younger than 2 years old, and 71% were younger than 1 year old. Ages ranged from 1 month to 12 years. Peak months for illness were September through January, and median duration of illness was 7 days. Population characteristics, symptoms, and duration of illness were similar to that seen with rotaviruses. Diarrhea occurred in 94%, vomiting in 51%, fever in 63%, and occult blood in stools in 18%, and 18% had at least one other enteric pathogen present. There were no grossly bloody stools. Treatment should center around maintaining fluid and electrolyte balance, just as it is for rotaviruses and other viral-caused gastroenteritis.

## Central Nervous System Disease

Murine coronaviruses JHM and A59 can produce acute encephalomyelitis, subacute demyelinating encephalomyelitis, or chronic asymptomatic demyelinating disease in mice. In humans, viruses are considered possible etiologic agents of multiple sclerosis (MS). In 1976, CV-like particles were identified by EM in tissues from patients with MS. Correlations of MS with upper respiratory infections and HCV-229E infections further stimulate hypotheses of an etiologic role of HCV in this disease; however, the significance of these findings is controversial. A recent study used cDNA probes to detect coronavirus-RNA (CV-RNA) by in situ hybridization. CV-RNA was present in a significantly higher proportion of MS patients than of controls. Thus, the possible causative role of coronaviruses in human central nervous system disease continues to be an intriguing, but unresolved, conjecture.

# LABORATORY DIAGNOSIS

Four approaches are used in the diagnosis of HCV infections. First, the isolation and identification of HCVs in cell and organ culture is difficult and limited to a few research laboratories. Virus often must be detected by EM. Second, serodiagnosis relies on serum neutralization, hemagglutination inhibition, complement fixation, indirect fluorescent antibody, and enzyme-linked immunoassay (ELISA); ELISA tests provide the most sensitive results. Third, viral antigens in clinical specimens are detected using immunofluorescence and ELISA. The ELISA test is sensitive and may require only a single clinical sample. Fourth, the most recent approach is a genetic probe coding for the HCV-229E nucleocapsid protein.

# PREVENTION AND THERAPY

Successful prevention of HCV infection is not imminent. High reinfection rates, limited protective value of circulating antibody, unidentified viral types, and difficulty in propagating the organism in the laboratory make prevention by vaccination unlikely. There has been some success with recombinant alpha interferon nasal sprays. Research toward a recombinant DNA HCV vaccine is underway in several laboratories.

There is no known effective treatment for HCV infections. The role of vitamin C is controversial, and aspirin should be avoided to prevent possible development of Reye's syndrome.

## Selected Readings

Callow KA, Parry HF, Sergeant M, et al. The time course of the immune response to experimental coronavirus infection of man. Epidemiol Infect 1990;105:435.
Dick EC, Inhorn SL. Coronaviruses. In: Feigin RD, Cherry JD, eds. Textbook of pediatric infectious diseases, ed 3. Philadelphia: WB Saunders, 1992:1498.
Kaye HS, Dowdle WR. Seroepidemiologic survey of coronavirus (strain 229E) infections in a population of children. Am J Epidemiol 1975;101:238.

McIntosh K. Coronaviruses. In: Fields BN, Knipe DM, eds. Virology, ed 2. New York: Raven Press, 1990:857.

Mertsola J, Ziegler T, Ruuskanen O, et al. Recurrent wheezy bronchitis and viral respiratory infections. Arch Dis Child 1991;66:124.

Monto AS. Coronaviruses. In: Evans AS, ed. Viral infections of humans, ed 3. New York: Plenum Press, 1989:153.

Mortensen ML, Ray CG, Payne CM, et al. Coronaviruslike particles in human gastrointestinal disease. Am J Dis Child 1985;139:928.

Murray RS, MacMillan B, Cabirac G, et al. Detection of coronavirus RNA in CNS tissue of multiple sclerosis and control patients. In: Cavanagh D, Brown TDK, eds. Coronaviruses and their diseases. New York: Plenum Press, 1990:505.

Schmidt OW, Allan ID, Cooney MK, et al. Rises in titers of antibody to human coronaviruses OC43 and 229E in Seattle families during 1975–1979. Am J Epidemiol 1986;123:862.

Turner RB, Felton A, Kosak K, et al. Prevention of experimental coronavirus colds with intranasal alpha-2b interferon. J Infect Dis 1986;154:443.

*Principles and Practice of Pediatrics, Second Edition.*
edited by Frank A. Oski et al. J. B. Lippincott Company, Philadelphia © 1994.

# 57.3 Rhinoviruses

## Elliot C. Dick and Rebecca L. Byers

Rhinoviruses (RVs) cause about 30% to 50% of all acute respiratory illness. RVs are associated primarily with the common cold, but they also may be involved in bronchitis, sinusitis, pneumonia, and acute exacerbations of asthma.

## THE ORGANISM

The first recognized RV was isolated in 1954; there are now at least 101 serotypes. The genus name was coined in 1963 to reflect the usual prominent nasal involvement. The RVs are one of two genera of human pathogens in the picornavirus family; the other genus includes various enteroviruses (polioviruses, coxsackieviruses, echoviruses, and possibly hepatitis A). Like the other picornaviruses, RVs are small (30 nm), nonenveloped (therefore resistant to lipid solvents), icosahedral (20-sided), and possess a single-stranded RNA genome. At least four RVs have been sequenced completely, and they demonstrate much cross homology among themselves and with the genomes of various other picornaviruses. RVs differ from other picornaviruses in that they become noninfectious at a pH below 5. For all 101 RV serotypes, there are two binding sites where the virus attaches itself to the receptor on the cell; 91 serotypes have one binding site type (the major receptor group), and 10 the other (the minor receptor group). After attaching to a cell, the RV is probably endocytosed within a vesicle, then the RNA is released into the cytoplasm. Viral replication occurs in the cytoplasm, and viruses are released by cell lysis.

RVs have been isolated from natural infections of cattle, chimpanzees, and humans. Human RVs infect only humans and chimpanzees; chimpanzee infections are subclinical.

## EPIDEMIOLOGY

RV infections are found in varying degrees year-round but show the greatest incidence from spring through early fall. This seasonal pattern occurs worldwide. Several RV serotypes usually circulate simultaneously, frequently coincident with other respiratory viruses. All types are not generally equal in prevalence, however, and do not spread to the same degree. In a 1963 to 1965 University of Wisconsin student family study (Eagle Heights village, Madison, Wisconsin), 19 RV types were isolated, but only 3 types (43, 51, and 55) spread beyond the index family, and they spread widely. These dominant RV serotypes occur locally over relatively short time periods but do not extend over large geographic areas or for several years.

Unlike some major respiratory viruses (eg, parainfluenza types 1 and 3 and respiratory syncytial virus [RSV]), individual RV serotypes seldom recur within a population from year to year. At Eagle Heights, 10 RV types were found in 1963 to 1964 and 9 types in 1964 to 1965, but only 1 type, 15, occurred in both years. Also, RV43 and RV55 were predominant in 1963 to 1964, while RV51 prevailed in 1964 to 1965.

The incidence of RV infections is highest in infants and lowest in older individuals. In Seattle, RV infection rates of 0.59 per person-year were found in family members with and without symptoms. Rates ranged from 0.8 to 1.2 for children aged birth to 5 years to 0.2 to 0.3 for adults older than 20 years. Women of childbearing age, however, showed rates 1.2 to 1.5 times higher than men. The true incidence of RV infections is probably higher than reported because RV diagnostic tests often are not very sensitive.

Prevalence studies show RV antibodies begin to appear early, increase throughout childhood and adolescence, peak in early adulthood, then stabilize for years. In Charlottesville, Virginia, fewer than 10% of young children had serum antibodies to any of 56 RV types tested, while adults had antibodies to about 50%.

## TRANSMISSION

Schoolchildren are the most important reservoir of RVs; home and school are locations of the highest rate of transmission. Dissemination within susceptible family members averages about 50%, and within a schoolroom ranges from 0% to 50%. Therefore, long-term association with individuals with RV infections may be required for transmission to occur. Even then, transmission rates only approach 50%. Thus, short contacts such as occur when shopping, attending movies, visiting friends, and visiting a physician's waiting room are reasonably risk-free.

A possible exception to the relative spreading resistance of RV and some other respiratory viruses is among young children in day-care facilities; all respiratory viruses may spread readily in this environment.

Because RVs often seem to disseminate slowly, the route of transmission is important. It may be possible to block transmission in various habitats such as the schoolroom and home. Using an experimental epidemiologic model featuring natural RV16 transmission among human volunteers, it was possible to stop RV16 transmission with virucidal facial tissues, evidently by interrupting aerosol transmission. Aerosol transmission seems predominant over direct contact. It may be possible to interrupt RV transmission with ultrafine, high-volume air filters. Such filters, along with virucidal tissues, are areas of continuing experimentation.

## PATHOGENESIS AND COURSE OF INFECTION

Most infection is presumed to be by the respiratory route, although infection by the conjunctival route has been demonstrated. The incubation period is normally 2 to 3 days. Ciliary dysfunction can predispose to respiratory infection. RVs replicate well in the upper respiratory tract and generally cause rhinorrhea and nasal obstruction. Cough usually is present even in mild RV colds. RVs have been found in the lower bronchi, but there is no compelling evidence of viral replication in the lower respiratory tract.

RVs may be shed in large amounts (1000 to 1,000,000 infectious particles per milliliter of nasal washing) during the first 2 to 3 days of a cold and may continue to be produced for nearly a month. RVs seem to cause only mild pathologic changes in cells of the respiratory tract, even when producing a marked local response. Local secretion of kinins, or products of cell-mediated immunity, such as the interleukins, can cause varied symptoms of inflammation. About 24 hours after infection, there is a sharp increase in nasal IgA secretion. After about 1 week, virus-specific antibody, predominantly IgA, appears in the nasal passages, the tears, and the parotid saliva. Serum antibody, usually IgG, appears at about 1 week and peaks at 1 month; however, specific serum antibody may not form in as many as 50% of cases.

The presence of serum antibody correlates positively with immunity, and resistance to infection is related to amount. Few individuals are infected who have homologous serum antibody levels of about 1:16. The relative importance and specific roles of serum and nasal-secretion antibody, as well as cell-mediated immunity, in protection against RV infection is unsettled. Serum antibody may be simply the indicator of immunity; nasal secretory antibody or cell-mediated immunity may be the active immune component.

Chilling of animals increases the severity and frequency of viral infections; but, experiments with RVs or nasal washings as challenge demonstrate no deleterious effects on human volunteers even after severe chilling.

## CLINICAL MANIFESTATIONS

RV infections in any age group usually cause only mild respiratory tract illnesses (ie, common colds with simple coryza). Complete recovery usually occurs in a week or two. It has been shown since the discovery of the first RV serotypes, however, that these viruses can cause serious lower respiratory illness, especially in young children.

### Asthma

RVs are important precipitants of "wheezy bronchitis" or "infectious asthma." This relationship was first described in 1973 in England. Shortly thereafter, a prospective study of Madison, Wisconsin, children with recurrent episodes of "infectious asthma" showed a clear temporal relation among onset of symptomatic respiratory infection (SRI), asthmatic episode, and presence of viruses—predominantly RVs—in the pharynx. Precipitation of an asthmatic episode occurred more often during severe SRIs than in mild cases, but subclinical infections never precipitated an attack. No specific RV serotypes have been found to be particularly "asthmagenic." It appears that RVs may be the most important cause of asthma attacks in children older than 1 to 2 years, but RSV is most important in the first year of life.

### Other Respiratory Illnesses

RVs are implicated in cases of bronchiolitis, pneumonia, chronic bronchitis, sinusitis, and acute otitis media. There is disagreement on the role of rhinoviruses in severe lower respiratory tract illnesses other than asthma. Nonetheless, in hospitalized infants in Bristol, England, RVs were second in importance to RSV even in patients with bronchiolitis and pneumonia. In Rochester, New York, and Vienna, Austria, RVs were associated with serious lower respiratory disease in hospitalized infants; RV-caused illnesses could not be differentiated clinically from severe lower tract illnesses attributable to RSV.

Acute otitis media (AOM) is primarily a bacterial disease, but is often preceded or accompanied by a viral upper respiratory illness. Clear, comprehensive evidence for viral extension from the nasopharynx to the middle ear is only recent. Antigen detection techniques identified viruses in 44% of 131 Finnish children with AOM. Twenty-four of these children had viruses in the middle ear fluid (MEF), and only 1 of the 24 did not have the same viral antigen in both the MEF and the nasopharyngeal secretions. In 1987–1988, pediatricians in Finland used traditional cell culture methodology to study the role of RVs in children with AOM. Viruses were detected in 42%; RV predominated over RSV—24% over 13%. Subsequent studies found that patients whose AOM is refractory to treatment harbor significantly more viral pathogens than the controls, suggesting that the presence of viruses in the MEFs of children with AOM can delay response to antibacterial therapy.

RVs have also been identified in aspirates obtained by direct puncture of maxillary sinuses, but further information is limited.

## DIAGNOSIS

RV infections cause such a wide spectrum of respiratory illness that it is not possible to diagnose them clinically. RV infections can be isolated year-round, but there is a seasonal pattern of infection recognized internationally; many mild to moderate respiratory infections of the spring-summer-fall months are caused by RVs. RVs have been found in the absence of symptoms, but this is infrequent, at least in industrialized nations. Subclinical shedding from well children in the United States has ranged from 0.8% to 11%, whereas rates up to 50% have been measured in some third world populations. Nasal specimens are superior to throat swabs for RV isolation. The virus can be isolated relatively easily if details of specimen collection and culture procedures are followed; however, there are more than 100 serotypes and none are predictably predominant, so clinical diagnosis by serologic methods is impractical because it is costly. No methods exist for rapid diagnosis of RV infection; research aimed at developing such methods includes use of complementary DNA (cDNA) genetic probes, polymerase chain reaction (PCA), and antigen capture/PCA technique.

## PREVENTION AND THERAPY

Because there are 101 serotypes, a conventional vaccine seems unlikely, but several potential antiviral drugs are in clinical trial. Alpha interferon is a protein produced as part of the host's natural antiviral defense and is now produced by genetic recombinant methods. Alpha interferon is the most effective RV cold preventive described for natural RV colds. It was administered by nasal spray to other members of the family after symptoms appeared in the index case; 80% of secondary RV colds were prevented. A combination of rapid diagnosis and family prophylaxis with alpha interferon would be especially helpful for family members with asthma who are at increased risk for severe complications of RV-caused illness.

Vitamin C and zinc have been proposed as preventives or treatments for colds. Overall, there is no clear indication that treatment or prevention of the common cold is affected by either agent. In 1987, however, three repeated trials showed vitamin C to markedly, consistently, and significantly reduce signs and symptoms of RV16 colds; the verdict is pending.

Environmental controls under study include virucidal tissues and proper air handling and filtration.

## Selected Readings

Arola M, Ziegler T, Ruuskanen O. Respiratory virus infection as a cause of prolonged symptoms in acute otitis media. J Pediatr 1989;116:697.

Dick EC, Inhorn SL. Rhinoviruses. In: Feigin RD, Cherry JD, eds. Textbook of pediatric infectious diseases, ed 3. Philadelphia: WB Saunders, 1992:1507.

Dick EC, Jennings LC, Mink KA, et al. Aerosol transmission of rhinovirus colds. J Infect Dis 1987;156:442.

Fox JP, Cooney MK, Hall CE, et al. Rhinoviruses in Seattle families, 1975–1979. Am J Epidemiol 1985;122:830.

Gwaltney JM Jr. Rhinoviruses. In: Evans AS, ed. Viral infections of humans, ed 3. New York: Plenum Publishing, 1989;598.

Kellner G, Popow-Kraupp T, Kundi M, et al. Clinical manifestations of respiratory tract infections due to respiratory syncytial virus and rhinoviruses in hospitalized children. Acta Paediatr Scand 1989;78:390.

Las Heras J, Swanson VL. Sudden death of an infant with rhinovirus infection complicating bronchial asthma: case report. Pediatr Pathol 1983;1:319.

Pickering LK, Hadler SC. Management and prevention of infectious diseases in day care. In: Feigin RD, Cherry JD, eds. Textbook of pediatric infectious diseases, ed 3. Philadelphia: WB Saunders, 1992:2308.

Schmidt HJ, Fink RJ. Rhinovirus as a lower respiratory tract pathogen in infants. Pediatr Infect Dis J 1991;10:700.

Tyrrell DAJ, Al-Nakib W. Prophylaxis and treatment of rhinovirus infections. In: DeClercq E, ed. Clinical use of antiviral drugs. Boston: Martinus Nijhoff, 1988;241.

*Principles and Practice of Pediatrics, Second Edition.*
edited by Frank A. Oski et al. J. B. Lippincott Company, Philadelphia © 1994.

# 57.4 *Adenoviruses*

James D. Cherry and Lisa M. Frenkel

Adenoviruses cause a diverse array of diseases in children, most commonly respiratory and gastrointestinal illnesses. Certain clinical manifestations of adenovirus infections are distinctive, although most illnesses are difficult to differentiate from those caused by other viral and bacterial pathogens.

## ETIOLOGY

Adenoviruses are DNA viruses; 42 types are known to infect humans. Six subgroups are defined based on the percentage of guanine plus cytosine in their DNA. Adenoviruses can be grown in tissue culture cell preparations of human epithelial origin. Exceptions are enteric adenoviruses types 40 and 41, which were identified by electron microscopy and grow in 293 cells and a few additional cell preparations. Clinical specimens from infected tissues produce a characteristic cytopathic effect in 1 day to 4 weeks. Small eosinophilic intranuclear inclusions can be seen early in infected tissues and cell cultures; later, larger intranuclear basophilic inclusions are seen.

## EPIDEMIOLOGY

Adenoviral infections occur throughout the world. In temperate climates, sporadic disease occurs year-round; epidemic disease commonly occurs in winter, spring, and early summer. Seasonal variation with adenoviral gastroenteritis has not been described.

Transplacental antibody appears to be protective in early infancy. When adenoviral infection occurs in the neonate, however, severe and rarely fatal pulmonary or multiorgan system diseases may occur. Adenoviral infections in children commonly are due to types 1, 2, 3, and 5. Types 6 and 7 occur slightly less frequently. Incidence of adenoviral infection peaks between ages 6 months and 5 years. An increased susceptibility to adenoviruses is reported in neonates and small infants, in immunocompromised patients, and occasionally in males.

Transmission of adenoviruses occurs by small droplets or the oral–fecal route and is facilitated by closed environments. Contaminated swimming pool water has been implicated in the spread of pharyngoconjunctival fever. The incubation period of adenoviruses is between 3 and 7 days. Virus may be shed from the respiratory tract up to 2 days before and 5 days after clinical symptoms develop. Virus may be found in the stool for several months. Adenoviruses are commonly isolated from the throat, conjunctiva, and stool.

## PATHOPHYSIOLOGY

Characteristics of adenoviral infections vary with infecting serotype and immune status of the host. Infection usually involves the upper respiratory tract and the conjunctivae. Spread to the lower respiratory tract may occur by progression or viremia. Rashes and multiorgan infection also may result from viremia. Swallowed virus is thought to cause gastrointestinal infection. Pathologic changes that occur in self-limited respiratory infections are not well studied. Autopsy material from lethal infections have revealed necrotizing bronchitis, bronchiolitis and pneumonia, focal hepatic necrosis, and cerebral edema with perivascular lymphocytic infiltrates. Characteristic small eosinophilic and larger basophilic intranuclear inclusions are seen in all infected tissues.

In humans, adenoviruses can cause lytic and latent infections. Oncogenic cell transformation is reported in animals but not in humans.

## CLINICAL MANIFESTATIONS

### Respiratory Infections

Serologic surveys indicate that 10% of respiratory infections in children are caused by adenoviruses. Rarely, adenoviruses cause common colds. Usually, respiratory infections with adenoviruses are characterized by fever and pharyngitis. Symptoms that occur with acute adenoviral pharyngitis include malaise, headache, sore throat, cough, cervical adenopathy, abdominal pain, and rhinitis, especially in the young. Pharyngeal exudates may be thin and spotty or thick and membranous. Laryngotracheitis, bronchitis, pneumonia, and, rarely, bronchiolitis may occur concomitantly with pharyngeal disease. Illness of 5 to 7 days is common, although symptoms may persist for 2 weeks.

Pulmonary infection with adenoviruses can be severe, especially in infants, toddlers, and immunocompromised patients. High fever, dyspnea, wheezes, and rhonchi are present in these cases, and radiographs may reveal diffuse infiltrates, hyperinflation, lobar atelectasis, and, rarely, pleural effusions. Associated symptoms may include seizures, lethargy, vomiting, diarrhea, and conjunctivitis. Manifestations of extrapulmonary involvement may be present, including meningitis, encephalitis, hepatitis, myocarditis, nephritis, and exanthems. Severe infections result in bronchiectasis, bronchiolitis obliterans, and hyperlucent lung.

Epidemics of adenoviral respiratory disease have been recognized in military populations living in close quarters. The disease, termed acute respiratory disease (ARD), is characterized by an acute, febrile, respiratory infection lasting 1 to 4 weeks with pulmonary involvement in most cases. These epidemics are usually due to adenoviruses types 4 and 7 and occasionally due to types 3, 11, 14, and 21.

## Pertussis-Like Syndrome

Adenoviral infections occasionally are associated with illness characterized by paroxysmal cough with associated post-tussive whoop, vomiting, apnea or hypoxemia, and lymphocytosis. The illness often begins with mild coryza without fever. Convalescence occurs usually in 1 to 3 months. Recent studies suggest that some of these pertussis-like illnesses are *Bordetella pertussis* infections in which the adenovirus is a coinfecting agent.

## Pharyngoconjunctival Fever

The constellation of acute fever, conjunctivitis, coryza, pharyngitis, and cervical adenitis occurring historically in summer epidemics, usually associated with inadequately chlorinated swimming pools, can be ascribed with some certainty to adenoviral infection. Both the bulbar and palpebral conjunctivae are involved. The palpebral conjunctiva may have a granular appearance. Initially, disease may be monocular, although the unaffected eye usually becomes involved. Bacterial superinfection of the conjunctiva is rare and resolution is complete.

## Epidemic Keratoconjunctivitis

A number of adenoviruses have been found to cause epidemics of keratoconjunctivitis, commonly type 8, although more recently type 37 as well. Adenoviral keratoconjunctivitis is nonseasonal, primarily affects adults, and is transmitted by fomites, ophthalmic instruments and solutions, and bodies of fresh water. After 4 days to 2 weeks of incubation, a follicular conjunctivitis develops with symptoms of lacrimation, photophobia, and foreign-body sensation. Hyperemia and edema of the conjunctiva are present and preauricular adenopathy is common. About half of affected persons have rhinitis and pharyngitis. Keratitis with punctate epithelial and sometimes subepithelial lesions develops as the conjunctivitis resolves. Visual disturbances may occur and persist for several years. Similar epidemics of keratoconjunctivitis associated with respiratory and constitutional symptoms have been described in infants and young children.

## Skin

Several types of adenoviruses cause exanthematous disease, usually an erythematous maculopapular rash. Exanthems of confluent morbilliform, petechial, and Stevens-Johnson syndrome have been reported. Other findings of adenoviral respiratory infection are commonly present.

## Genitourinary

Hemorrhagic cystitis due to adenovirus begins acutely with dysuria and frequency; hematuria develops within 24 hours. Occasionally, there is concomitant suprapubic pain, fever, or upper respiratory tract symptoms. Resolution occurs in several days to 2 weeks and appears to be complete. This illness is not seasonal. Boys are affected more frequently than girls.

Nephritis has been reported in cases of disseminated adenoviral infections and in rare instances with respiratory infections.

Adenoviruses reportedly have been isolated from genital lesions that clinically resemble herpes genitalis and from cervicitis occurring with pharyngoconjunctival fever.

## Gastrointestinal

The adenoviral types commonly associated with respiratory illnesses may also cause vomiting and diarrhea. Adenoviruses types 40 and 41 along with rotavirus are thought to cause most gastroenteritis in infants and young children. These enteric adenoviruses are most easily identified by electron microscopy or antibody rapid diagnosis techniques enzyme immunoabsorbent assay (EIA) because they do not grow in commonly used tissue cultures. Watery diarrhea usually lasts 1 to 2 weeks and in the initial days may be associated with vomiting. Mild fever and, uncommonly, respiratory symptoms may occur with enteric adenoviral infection.

Mesenteric lymphadenitis with abdominal pain, fever, and other symptoms suggestive of appendicitis is associated with adenoviral infections. Adenoviruses have been isolated from intraoperative specimens of mesenteric lymph nodes and the appendix. Acute and chronic adenoviral appendicitis occurs. Enlarged mesenteric lymph nodes often are thought to serve as a lead point for intestinal intussusception. Observation of adenoviral intranuclear inclusions and seroconversion has associated a number of adenoviruses with intussusception.

Hepatitis has been reported with adenoviral infection in infants, young children, and immunocompromised patients.

### Neurologic

Central nervous system disease in adenoviral infection is uncommon, but a variety of clinical manifestations has been noted. Both meningitis and encephalitis may be the major manifestations of adenoviral infections. Alternatively, neurologic illness may be associated with marked disease at other body sites.

### Heart

Both myocarditis and periarditis are rare in adenoviral respiratory infections.

## Immunocompromised Host

Comprehensive studies of adenoviral infection in the immunocompromised host are lacking. Reports indicate that severe, disseminated disease occurs, including fulminant disease with multiorgan involvement, notably severe necrotizing pneumonia and hepatitis with disseminated intravascular coagulation. Several different adenoviral types have been recovered from children with immunodeficiency diseases, malignancies, steroid therapy, immunosuppressive therapy, radiation therapy, and transplantation procedures.

## DIAGNOSIS

Differential diagnosis for adenoviral illnesses differs with various clinical manifestations. Pharyngoconjunctival fever and keratoconjunctivitis are often recognized as adenoviral infections based on clinical findings because of their characteristic symptom complex and epidemic nature. Adenoviral pharyngitis must be differentiated from streptococcal, Epstein-Barr, influenza, parainfluenza, and enteroviral infections. Adenoviral pneumonia may be clinically difficult to distinguish from illness caused by other viral and bacterial pathogens. Eye disease must be distinguished from herpes simplex virus keratitis and, in the neonate, from conjunctivitis due to *Neisseria gonorrhoeae* and *Chlamydia* spp. Bacterial and parasitic intestinal infections sometimes produce symptoms like those of adenoviral infections.

Specific diagnosis commonly is achieved by tissue culture methods, specific antigen detection, or seroconversion. Respiratory adenoviruses can be isolated in most clinical laboratories. Specimens for culture should be obtained from the affected conjunctiva or throat by vigorous swabbing with cotton or Dacron; or, respiratory secretions, urine, or tissue may be submitted. Preferably, specimens are placed into viral transport media for transport to the virology laboratory. Rapid diagnostic tests (IFA, EIA,

DNA probes, radioimmunossay) have been developed and will be increasingly available for diagnosis of respiratory and enteric adenoviruses.

The serologic diagnosis of adenoviral infection is achieved by demonstrating a rise in complement-fixing antibody to the adenovirus type-common hexon antigen.

## TREATMENT

No specific treatment exists for adenoviral infections. The patient should be discouraged from strenuous activity and supportive care should be given. Steroid treatment is to be avoided, and immunosuppressive regimens reduced or suspended. Steroid preparations should be administered carefully to patients with pneumonia and wheezing. Steroids may contribute to development of severe disease and may complicate recovery. Experimental treatment of severe adenoviral infections has included administration of immunoglobulins with high titers against the specific adenovirus.

## PREVENTION

Live nonattenuated viruses in enteric-coated capsules are effective and are used to immunize military recruits against adenoviruses types 4 and 7. Subsequent asymptomatic intestinal infection protects against acute respiratory disease. Trials of these vaccines in children show similar efficacy.

## Selected Readings

Brandt CD, Kim HW, Vargosko AJ, et al. Infections in 18,000 infants and children in a controlled study of respiratory tract disease: I. Adenovirus pathogenicity in relation to serologic type and illness syndrome. Am J Epidemiol 1969;90:484.

Cherry JD. Adenoviral infections. In: Feigin RD, Cherry JD, eds. Textbook of pediatric infectious diseases, ed 3. Philadelphia: WB Saunders, 1992:1670.

Ford E, Nelson KE, Warren D. Epidemiology of epidemic keratoconjunctivitis. Epidemiol Rev 1987;9:244.

Krajden M, Brown M, Petrasek A, Middleton P. Clinical features of adenovirus enteritis: a review of 127 cases. Pediatr Infect Dis J 1990;9:646.

Michaels MG, Green M, Wald ER, Starzl TE. Adenovirus infection in pediatric liver transplant recipients. J Infect Dis 1992;165:170.

Pacini DL, Collier AM, Henderson FW. Adenovirus infections and respiratory illnesses in children in group day care. J Infect Dis 1987;156:920.

Ruuskanen O, Sarkkinen H, Meurman O, et al. Rapid diagnosis of adenoviral tonsillitis: a prospective clinical study. J Pediatr 1984;104:725.

Shields AF, Hackman RC, Fife KH, et al. Adenovirus infections in patients undergoing bone-marrow transplantation. N Engl J Med 1985;312:529.

*Principles and Practice of Pediatrics, Second Edition.*
edited by Frank A. Oski et al. J. B. Lippincott Company, Philadelphia © 1994.

# *57.5 Influenza Viruses*

## James D. Cherry

Influenza viruses cause acute respiratory infections that usually occur in outbreaks or epidemics. In contrast to other respiratory viral infections that occur in outbreaks, acute febrile illnesses occur in both adults and children. Influenza viral infections in children are associated with considerable morbidity and mortality, and the spectrum of clinical illness is broad.

Influenza viruses are orthomyxoviruses. There are three major antigenic types—A, B, and C—and multiple antigenic subtypes.

Influenza viruses are irregular, spherical particles 80 to 120 nm in diameter. Their surface is composed of numerous hemagglutinin and neuraminidase "spikes." Inside the virus is a lipid bilayer, a matrix protein, and an RNA nucleocapsid.

There are four important antigenic components. The nuclear protein and matrix protein are antigenically type-specific and stable. The nuclear protein is the antigenic basis for typing strains as A, B, or C. Hemagglutinin and neuraminidase antigens are subtype-specific and variable. There are three separate hemagglutinins, H1, H2, and H3, and two separate neuraminidases, N1 and N2, which have been recognized in influenza A viruses causing infections in humans. Variation in these two antigens (hemagglutinin and neuraminidase) is the basis for antigenic "drift" and "shift" in the prevalent viruses. Drift implies a minor change in an antigen without a change in subtype; shift implies a major change in either hemagglutinin or neuraminidase or both antigens, resulting in a change in subtype. Antigenic drift occurs in influenza A and B viruses, but shift occurs only in influenza A.

In the laboratory, influenza viruses can be cultivated in embryonated chicken eggs, in the MDCK cell line, and in primary monkey kidney tissue cultures.

Nomenclature for the classification of influenza virus strains specifies type, host (for strains of animal origin), geographic source, strain number, and year of isolation. To this, the code designations of hemagglutinin and neuraminidase subtypes are appended. Recently prevalent human influenza viral types are designated A/Texas/36/91 (H1N1), A/Beijing/353/89 (H3N2), and B/Panama/45/90.

## EPIDEMIOLOGY

Pandemics of influenza due to different influenza A subtypes occurred in 1874, 1889, 1900, 1918, 1933, 1946, 1957, 1968, and 1977. The 1918 pandemic resulted in 20 million deaths worldwide. Pandemics of influenza A result from antigenic shift. This shift occurs irregularly, the last being in 1977. After pandemic influenza of a new subtype, epidemics of generally lesser intensity occur approximately every 2 to 3 years in association with antigenic drift. Outbreaks of influenza B are more variable, occur at roughly 4- to 7-year intervals, and are the result of antigenic drift. Infection with influenza C virus is common in children, but the epidemiologic pattern of this virus is not determined.

Populated areas generally experience some influenza viral activity each year. Epidemics and outbreaks usually occur at times of cooler weather; in the tropics, epidemic disease usually occurs during the rainy season. The highest attack rate of influenza usually occurs in children, followed by secondary peaks of illness in adult populations. Case-fatality rates are greatest in infants and the elderly. Influenza is more likely to be fatal in persons with preexisting heart disease, chronic pulmonary disorders, diabetes mellitus, chronic renal disease, neuromuscular disorders, and neoplasms.

Influenza is spread from person to person via the respiratory route. The most common mechanism is inhalation of large airborne particles produced by coughing and sneezing. Spread may also occur by direct or indirect contact with fine-particle aerosols.

## PATHOPHYSIOLOGY

The major site of infection is the ciliated epithelium of the respiratory tract. Extensive necrosis of nasal and tracheal ciliated cells occurs as early as the first day after the onset of symptoms.

This is followed by edema and infiltration with lymphocytes, histiocytes, plasma cells, and polymorphonuclear cells. Repair of affected mucous membranes, indicated by mitoses in the surviving basal cells, begins by the third to fifth day of illness. A pseudometaplastic response of undifferentiated epithelium occurs that reaches a maximum at 9 to 15 days after onset of infection; thereafter, ciliary function and mucus production reappear.

Secondary bacterial infection is common. More extensive inflammatory cell infiltration and destruction of the basal cell layer and basement membrane are seen, and delayed regeneration of the ciliated epithelium results.

Pneumonia may occur as a result of primary influenza viral infection, bacterial superinfection, or combined bacterial–viral infection. Although influenza is predominantly an infection of the respiratory tract, the heart, brain, and lymphoid tissues are sometimes involved in fatal cases. Specifically, focal and diffuse myocarditis, mediastinal lymph node disorganization and necrosis, and diffuse cerebral edema have been observed. In addition, Reye's syndrome (diffuse encephalopathy and fatty degeneration of the liver) is a complication of influenza, particularly that due to type B virus in children.

Influenza viral infection evokes a vigorous and complex immunologic response. Humoral, secretory, and cell-mediated mechanisms are all involved. Hemagglutination-inhibiting antibodies are important for virus neutralization, and antibodies against neuraminidase are associated with diminished illness severity and reduced rates of person-to-person transmission. Local (IgA) antibodies are probably important as a first line of defense, if they are present.

After infection, duration of immunity and degree of protection against challenge by heterologous viral strains vary. In general, natural immunity against influenza A strains lasts about 4 years. As increasing antigenic drift occurs, previously infected persons are likely to have symptomatic reinfections; when antigenic shift occurs, antibody from the previous infection offers no protection.

## CLINICAL MANIFESTATIONS

Clinical manifestations of influenza follow a short, 2- to 3-day incubation period. Although the predominant manifestations of influenza viral infections are respiratory, systemic complaints are an integral part of the illness. In general, the manifestations of influenza in children fall into two categories based on age. In school-aged children and adolescents, the illness is similar to that which occurs in adults (classic influenza). Illness onset is abrupt with fever, facial flush, chills, headache, myalgia, and malaise. Temperature varies between 39 °C and 41 °C and is generally lower in older patients. Systemic complaints, on the other hand, are generally more severe in the older patient. Initially, dry cough and coryza occur, but these symptoms are of lesser concern to the patient than the severe systemic manifestations. About half of patients complain of sore throat, which is associated with a nonexudative pharyngitis. Ocular symptoms are common and include tearing, photophobia, burning, and pain with eye movement. In uncomplicated illness, the fever lasts from 2 to 5 days. Occasionally, the temperature shows a biphasic pattern that may or may not be due to secondary bacterial complications.

The course of illness changes by day 2 to 4 of illness, when the respiratory symptoms become more prominent and the systemic complaints begin to subside. Major coughing—dry and hacking—usually persists for up to a week. Occasionally, coughing persists well after other symptoms have subsided. Influenza A and B infections are generally similar, although B viral infections may have more prominent nasal and eye complaints and fewer systemic findings such as dizziness and prostration than comparable influenza A illnesses. Although influenza C outbreaks are rarely discerned, illness due to this virus is indistinguishable from that due to A and B viral types.

The leukocyte count in uncomplicated influenza usually is normal, but frequently leukopenia (less than 4500 cells/mm$^3$) occurs. About one third of patients have a relative lymphopenia and one third have a relative neutropenia. In general, about 10% of older children have clinical signs and radiographic evidence of pulmonary involvement.

In younger children and infants, the manifestations of influenza viral infections frequently are similar to those of other common respiratory viral infections. Laryngotracheitis, bronchitis, bronchiolitis, and pneumonia all occur. Frequently, primary infection is an undifferentiated febrile upper respiratory illness. Temperature usually exceeds 39.5 °C. Affected children appear mildly toxic and have cough, coryza, and irritability. On examination, pharyngitis is usually noted, and pulmonary involvement is common. Other findings include vomiting, diarrhea, otitis media, and fleeting erythematous or erythematous-maculopapular discrete rashes.

Acute laryngotracheitis due to influenza A virus is occasionally more severe than infection due to parainfluenza viruses. In neonates, influenza infection cannot be distinguished clinically from bacterial sepsis. Lethargy, poor feeding, petechiae, poor peripheral circulation with mottling of skin, and apneic spells all occur.

## COMPLICATIONS

The most common complications of influenza are bacterial infections of the respiratory tract (pneumonia, otitis media, and sinusitis). Acute myositis is a particular complication of influenza B viral infections in children. It is characterized by severe pain and tenderness in the calves of both legs. Onset is sudden, and usually the affected child refuses to walk. Serum creatinine phosphokinase (CPK) and aspartate immunotransferase (SGOT) levels may be increased.

Although the pathogenesis is obscure, Reye's syndrome is a complication of both influenza A and B infections. Outbreaks of Reye's syndrome are related to epidemic activity of influenza.

Other rare complications of influenza viral infections include neurologic manifestations (encephalitis, Guillain-Barré syndrome, and transverse myelitis), pericarditis and myocarditis, and sudden death.

## DIAGNOSIS

During outbreaks and epidemics, the clinical diagnosis of influenza can be made with some reliability. Important in the clinical diagnosis of influenza is the occurrence in the community of similar illness with fever in both adults and children. The definitive diagnosis of influenza depends on either virus isolation from respiratory secretions or a significant rise in serum antibody titer during convalescence. Rapid detection techniques for influenza antigens in nasal pharyngeal epithelial cells recently have been introduced in many laboratories.

The serologic diagnosis of influenza classically employs either complement fixation or hemagglutination-inhibition techniques. Complement fixation detects antibody against soluble nuclear protein antigens common to all strains of influenza A or B. Hemagglutination-inhibiting antibodies, which are subtype-specific, provide more definitive evidence of infection. Recently, the enzyme-linked immunosorbent assay (ELISA) has proved useful for the serologic diagnosis of influenza. With this technique, specific IgM antibodies can be determined so that diagnosis can be made based on a single specimen obtained shortly after the onset of illness.

# TREATMENT

Symptomatic treatment is the cornerstone of management and consists of rest, adequate hydration with oral fluids, control of fever and myalgia with acetaminophen, and maintenance of comfortable breathing by means of humidified air and, occasionally, nasal decongestants. Persistent irritative cough during convalescence often can be relieved with dextromethorphan or codeine.

The physician should be alert to the possibility of secondary bacterial infection. These infections are suggested by a prolonged febrile course or recrudescence of fever during early convalescence. Before antibiotic therapy is begun, the site of infection should be identified and appropriate cultures obtained. Most infections are caused by *Streptococcus pneumoniae*, *Haemophilus influenzae*, *Streptococcus pyogenes*, or, less commonly, *Staphylococcus aureus*.

The antiviral agent amantadine hydrochloride is active in vitro against influenza A viruses and has prophylactic and therapeutic benefits in adults. This drug also has a prophylactic effect in community-acquired influenza A in children, but few studies have considered its therapeutic efficacy in children. Nevertheless, it seems reasonable to administer amantadine therapeutically to severely ill, hospitalized children if the illness is likely to be caused by influenza A virus. Influenza B viruses are not susceptible to amantadine. The prophylactic dose of amantadine for children is as follows: children 1 to 9 years old, 4.4 to 8.8 mg/kg/24 h, administered twice a day; children older than 9 years old, 200 mg/24 h, administered twice a day.

The broad-spectrum antiviral agent ribavirin also is effective in vitro against both influenza A and B viruses. Ribavirin given by aerosol has benefited adult patients with influenza A and B infections. Ribavirin is not approved for treatment of influenza in children.

# PREVENTION

Inactivated influenza viral vaccines are safe and effective in preventing influenza if the antigens in the vaccine correlate with circulating influenza viruses. In general, routine immunization of normal children or adults is not recommended. Vaccine is recommended for children at high risk for complications. Specifically, this includes children with cardiovascular disorders such as rheumatic, congenital, or hypertensive heart disease; chronic bronchopulmonary disease such as tuberculosis, cystic fibrosis, asthma, and bronchiectasis; chronic metabolic diseases such as diabetes; chronic glomerulonephritis; and chronic neurologic disorders in which there is weakness or paralysis of respiratory muscles.

## Selected Readings

Glezen WP. Consideration of the risk of influenza in children and indications for prophylaxis. Rev Infect Dis 1980;2:408.

Glezen WP, Cherry JD. Influenza viruses. In: Feigin RD, Cherry JD, eds. Textbook of pediatric infectious diseases, ed 3. Philadelphia: WB Saunders, 1992:1688.

Glezen WP, Decker M, Joseph SW, Mercready RG Jr. Acute respiratory disease associated with influenza epidemics in Houston, 1981–1983. J Infect Dis 1987;155:1119.

Glezen WP, Six HR, Perrotta DM, et al. Epidemics and their causative viruses: community experience. In: Stuart-Harris CH, Potter CW, eds. The molecular virology and epidemiology of influenza. New York: Academic Press, 1984:17.

Lennon DR, Cherry JD, Morgenstein A, et al. Longitudinal study of influenza B symptomatology and interferon production in children and college students. Pediatr Infect Dis J 1983;2:212.

Troendle JF, Demmler GJ, Glezen WP, Finegold M, Romano MJ. Fatal influenza B virus pneumonia in pediatric patients. Pediatr Infect Dis J, 1992;11:117.

Wright PF, Rose KB, Thompson J, et al. Influenza A infections in young children: primary natural infection and protective efficacy of live-vaccine-induced or naturally-acquired immunity. N Engl J Med 1977;296:829.

*Principles and Practice of Pediatrics, Second Edition.*
edited by Frank A. Oski et al. J. B. Lippincott Company, Philadelphia © 1994.

# 57.6 *Parainfluenza Viruses*

Sarah S. Long

Parainfluenza viruses are second only to respiratory syncytial virus as a cause of significant morbidity and mortality due to respiratory illnesses in infancy. Parainfluenza viruses are responsible for the majority of cases of laryngotracheitis (croup).

## CHARACTERISTICS OF THE VIRUSES

There are four antigenically stable parainfluenza viruses, types 1, 2, 3, and 4. They are ether- and acid-sensitive, RNA viruses of the paramyxovirus family. The glycoproteins of their lipid envelope have hemagglutinating and neuraminidase activity and fusion capacity. These factors are important for attachment to host cells and for cell-to-cell progression of infection. The antigens are used for type-specific identification of the viruses and for detection of immunologic response to infection. The appellation "parainfluenza" was assigned because of characteristics shared with influenza viruses. Unlike influenza viruses, however, parainfluenza viruses have stable antigenic determinants (with some strain variation in type 2), hemolyze certain red blood cells, and can fuse cell membranes.

Primary isolation from respiratory tract specimens is best carried out in monkey kidney tissue culture. The viruses can be identified with immunofluorescent techniques or by their characteristic ability to hemadsorb guinea pig red blood cells with subsequent inhibition by specific antiserum. Antisera suitable for use in rapidly identifying parainfluenza viruses in respiratory tract secretions are becoming more widely available.

## IMMUNE RESPONSE

Primary infection with parainfluenza virus elicits type-specific serum antibody that can be measured as complement-fixing antibody, hemagglutination-inhibiting antibody, or virus-neutralizing antibody. Common antigens are shared among the paramyxoviruses, including mumps virus; thus, heterotypic antibody responses occur after parainfluenza virus infection. Heterotypic antibody responses are more common with increasing age, which suggests that primary infection with a specific agent is required before a boost occurs from exposure to a related agent. Whether heterotypic antibodies contribute to protection against clinical illness is unknown. Development of heterotypic antibodies confounds interpretation of a four-fold rise in antibody titer as evidence of recent infection unless a parainfluenza virus also has been isolated.

Infection with any of the parainfluenza viruses apparently does not confer lifetime immunity because reinfections are common. The decreased severity of reinfection with age suggests that some protection is afforded against clinical disease. The serum concentration of type-specific antibody does not correlate specifically with protection against clinical disease. Demonstration of nasal secretory antibody, on the other hand, strongly correlates with protection against experimentally induced human infection and presumably also against naturally acquired infection.

# EPIDEMIOLOGY

## Seasonal Occurrence

Parainfluenza virus infection occurs year-round. Type 1 parainfluenza viruses produce epidemic disease, recognizable as outbreaks of laryngotracheitis in autumn. Parainfluenza virus type 2 also causes epidemic disease that peaks in the autumn and is milder than that associated with types 1 or 3. A febrile upper respiratory illness is a more common manifestation than laryngotracheitis, and lower respiratory tract infection is unusual. Parainfluenza type 3 predominates in spring and summer and is a major cause of lower respiratory tract disease in infants in the first year of life. Infection due to types 4A and B is less common, more sporadic, and generally mild.

## Age Incidence

Type 3 parainfluenza virus is one of the most common respiratory tract pathogens of infancy. Susceptible soon after birth, most children experience primary infection by age 3 years. Young infants appear to be protected against types 1 and 2 parainfluenza viruses in the first 6 months of life. Primary infection with types 1 and 2 occurs predominantly in children aged 2 to 6 years and is not a universal experience in childhood. Primary infections with parainfluenza viruses and reinfections can occur throughout childhood.

# PATHOPHYSIOLOGY

Any or all respiratory tract sites can be involved in parainfluenza virus infection. Type 1 parainfluenza virus preferentially affects laryngeal and tracheal epithelium, causing the croup syndrome. Parainfluenza types 1 and 3 generally infect more distal sites, causing bronchiolitis or pneumonitis. Parainfluenza type 3 exhibits the least specific tropism with infection occurring from the nose and throat to the alveoli of the lung.

Acquisition and transmission occur by close person-to-person contact, by direct or indirect hand contact with infected respiratory secretions, and by self-inoculation of the recipient's nose. Cells of the nasal and pharyngeal epithelium are infected, and the virus spreads locally to the larynx and trachea. The initial symptoms are nasal stuffiness and throat irritation. Fever is more common than in rhinovirus or other common cold infections. Cilia and respiratory epithelium are destroyed; inflammatory edema and cellular infiltration develop in the lamina propria. Fibrinous exudate, sometimes forming a pseudomembrane, adds to obstruction of the subglottic trachea, which is restricted in its cartilaginous encasement. In some patients, parainfluenza virus infection elicits specific IgE antibody and a bronchiolitis syndrome.

Bacterial complications include infection of the middle ear, paranasal sinuses, trachea, and lower respiratory tract.

# CLINICAL MANIFESTATIONS

Clinical manifestations directly reflect the sites of infection. Type 1 parainfluenza virus causes mild upper respiratory illness but is the virus most commonly associated with croup, accounting for 20% to 40% of cases. The older child or adult experiences laryngitis. Disease due to type 2 parainfluenza virus is generally mild and confined to large airways. Type 3 parainfluenza virus causes disease that varies from symptoms of a common cold to fatal pneumonia. It ranks second to respiratory syncytial virus as a cause of bronchiolitis and bronchopneumonia in infants. Children with immunodeficiency syndromes are prone to severe,

sometimes fatal, pneumonitis. Infection of the pericardium and brain also has been described.

## Laryngotracheitis

### Clinical Manifestations

Acute laryngotracheitis and laryngotracheobronchitis are the most common significant illnesses caused by the parainfluenza viruses. Laryngotracheitis accounts for about 15% of respiratory tract infections below the level of the pharynx in children. Laryngotracheitis occurs in children of all age groups and is noted throughout the year. It occurs more commonly in hosts with predisposing factors such as a structural anomaly of the airway, prior tracheal intubation, or hypotonia. Epidemics reflect community outbreaks of either parainfluenza or influenza virus infection. Laryngotracheitis also may be noted as a manifestation of infection due to adenoviruses and respiratory syncytial virus. The use of the word "croup" as a diagnostic term has led to confusion with respect to specificity of diagnosis and treatment. Initial symptoms are nasal stuffiness and sore throat. Fever ranging from 37.8 °C to 40 °C follows within 24 hours, then the barking cough becomes the predominant symptom. For most patients, the illness progresses no further and symptoms abate over 3 to 5 days. Occasionally within hours, but usually more gradually, upper airway obstruction progresses in some patients and stridor appears. On examination, the child has hoarseness, coryza, and supraclavicular and substernal retractions. Position has no effect on the degree of obstruction. Examination of the pharynx discloses minimal erythema. If infection causes laryngotracheobronchitis or laryngotracheopneumonitis, the respiratory rate is elevated and the child can have a prolonged expiratory phase and wheezing in addition to inspiratory stridor. In severe disease, progressive obstruction leads to hypoxia, restlessness, and cyanosis. Without intervention at this stage, death from asphyxia is likely. In other cases, prolonged incomplete obstruction leads to eventual fatigue and respiratory failure.

Laboratory tests are nonspecifically abnormal. The peripheral white blood cell (WBC) count is frequently greater than 10,000 cells/mm$^3$ with a predominance of polymorphonuclear cells. Cell counts above 20,000/mm$^3$ are infrequent. The lateral neck radiograph shows distention of the hypopharynx and narrowing and haziness of the subglottic trachea. The epiglottis appears normal. Virus can be isolated from nasopharyngeal secretions in tissue culture, usually within 4 to 7 days. Rapid identification of viral antigen in nasopharyngeal secretions is possible by immunofluorescent and enzyme-linked immunosorbent assay (ELISA) methods, but the sensitivity of tests varies.

### Differential Diagnosis

Laryngotracheitis of viral etiology must be differentiated from the more fulminant infectious disease, epiglottitis, from bacterial tracheitis, diphtheria, and retropharyngeal abscess, and from life-threatening obstruction by a foreign body. These distinctions are made on clinical grounds with skillful, unobtrusive examinations and with selective roentgenographic and laboratory tests. The clinical characteristics of infectious causes of upper airway obstruction are listed in Table 57-6.

The patient with epiglottitis generally has a high fever and appears toxic and apprehensive. Characteristically, the child has a clear voice, no cough, and severe dysphagia. He sits forward with the jaw out in a "sniffing position" and refuses to lie down. The child should be disturbed minimally and should be attended at all times by a comforting parent and a person skilled in resuscitation. The swollen red epiglottis can sometimes be seen rising out of the hypopharynx. Roentgenograph of the lateral neck shows distention of the hypopharynx, a swollen thumbprint appearance of the epiglottis, and no abnormality of the subglottic

TABLE 57-6. Clinical Characteristics of Infectious Causes of Upper Airway Obstruction

| | Epiglottitis | Laryngotracheitis | Bacterial Tracheitis | Retropharyngeal Abscess |
|---|---|---|---|---|
| Peak age | 2–7 yr | 7–36 mo | 7–36 mo | 3–24 mo |
| Prodrome | None to nonspecific URI | Coryza, cough | Coryza, cough | Nonspecific URI |
| Onset of fever | Sudden, high | Gradual, variable | Variable, frequently with sudden high rise | Sudden, high |
| Striking feature | Stridor | Stridor/cough | Stridor | Drooling, respiratory distress ± stridor |
| Other major symptoms: | | | | |
|   Hoarseness | – | +++ | ++ | – |
|   Cough | – | +++ | ++ | – |
|   Drooling | +++ | – | – | +++ |
|   Dysphagia | +++ | ± | ± | +++ |
| Major signs | Severe obstruction, toxicity | Obstruction, none to mild toxicity | Obstruction, toxicity | Toxicity, obstruction |
| Associated findings | Visibly swollen epiglottis | Rhinorrhea, mild pharyngitis | Rhinorrhea, mild pharyngitis | Rhinorrhea, bulging posterior pharynx |
| Preferred position | Sitting, sniffing | None | None | Hyperextension of neck |

*URI,* upper respiratory tract infection; ±, sometimes present; ++, frequently present; +++, hallmark of disease.

area. An artificial airway must be rapidly established by an experienced team. Nasotracheal intubation is the preferred method. More than 90% of cases are caused by *Haemophilus influenzae* type b; culture of blood and swab of the epiglottis are positive. As *H influenzae* type b disease diminishes with the widespread use of vaccines, its relative importance in epiglottitis diminishes. Epiglottitis generally can be treated with cefuroxime, 100 mg/kg/d in four doses given intravenously. Antibiotic therapy never supplants the urgent need for securing the airway.

About a decade ago, bacterial tracheitis was rediscovered. Because it is usually a complication of viral respiratory disease, symptoms and signs are rarely confined to the trachea. The tracheal wall is infiltrated with bacteria and inflammatory cells. Ulceration, necrosis, and microabscess formation are common. The patient has symptoms typical of laryngotracheitis but disease suddenly progresses rapidly with heightened fever, toxicity, and severe airway obstruction. The peripheral WBC count is frequently higher than that anticipated in viral infections, with a marked shift to immature neutrophils. A radiograph of the lateral neck demonstrates the subglottic haziness typical of laryngotracheitis, but a tracheal intraluminal mass or pseudomembrane is also seen frequently. Airway obstruction is rapid. This diagnosis is sometimes first considered only during intubation of a patient thought to have viral laryngotracheitis when purulent secretions, pseudomembrane, and epithelial necrosis are seen in the subglottic trachea. Bacterial infection usually is localized to the respiratory tract, but cases of associated toxic shock have been reported. The etiologic agents most commonly recovered from tracheal specimens are *Staphylococcus aureus, Streptococcus pyogenes,* and, occasionally, *H influenzae* or *Streptococcus pneumoniae.* Cefuroxime may be used for initial therapy. Recovery occurs more slowly than in viral tracheobronchitis or epiglottitis. Life-threatening airway obstruction can occur after intubation because of inspissated secretions or accidental extubation. Average length of hospitalization is 9 to 10 days.

Cellulitis, lymphangitis, and abscess can occur in the posterior pharyngeal or retropharyngeal space in infants and probably represent bacterial complications of viral infection of nasal and oropharyngeal tissues. Abrupt onset of fever and upper airway obstruction, refusal to feed, gurgling respiratory sounds, and drooling are the major features. Retropharyngeal abscess is rarely confused with epiglottitis or laryngotracheitis because it generally occurs in children younger than those who develop epiglottitis and without the cough and hoarseness of laryngotracheitis. The neck is held in hyperextension, and bulging of the posterior pharyngeal wall usually is evident on examination. The radiographic appearance of increased paravertebral soft tissue is pathognomonic. Usually caused by Group A streptococcus or *S aureus,* it is a medical and surgical emergency to prevent complete obstruction or rupture, which may cause suffocation.

Spasmodic croup describes an event of poorly understood etiology. It occurs more frequently in young boys of higher socioeconomic status who have a family history of spasmodic croup. Spasmodic croup probably represents an unusual response to minor respiratory viral illnesses. Episodes are recurrent and sudden, usually awakening a child who has gone to bed well. Fever is not a feature of the illness unless the antecedent respiratory infection is significant. Direct laryngoscopy reveals narrowing of the subglottic space due to noninflammatory edema. Whether subtle anatomical factors predispose such children to stridor with minor infections or whether hyperreactivity of the airway is the preeminent factor is unknown. Recurrences with completely normal breathing during intervening periods are hallmarks of the affliction, as are dramatic responses to humidification, comforting, or a trip in the cold night air to seek medical assistance. Episodes cease as the child gets older.

### Treatment

Fewer than 10% of children with acute viral laryngotracheitis require hospitalization, fewer than 10% of these hospitalized children require tracheal intubation, and fewer than 1% of these hospitalized children die. Therapy is primarily supportive. There is controversy among experienced authorities whether other therapies are indicated for most children. Ribavirin, active against parainfluenza virus in vitro, has not undergone adequate clinical trial for use in children with laryngotracheitis.

The following are aspects of management for the more severely affected child:

1. Examinations are performed rapidly with few disturbances. Hospitalization (the main purpose of which is to observe the patient carefully to determine the need for an artificial airway) should not promote worsening of respiratory status.
2. The comforting parent should not be separated from the child.
3. Mist is the cornerstone of therapy. The temperature should be comfortable, not cold. The child's anxiety at being put in a mist tent occasionally overrides the potential benefit of this treatment.
4. Oxygen is administered if hypoxemia is documented.
5. Antibiotics are infrequently indicated. In most cases, epiglottitis, bacterial tracheitis, otitis media, and bacterial pneumonia are easily excluded.
6. Nebulized racemic epinephrine has short-term beneficial effect and is used as an interim measure in hospitalized patients with severe airway obstruction. Assessment of the blinded saline-controlled studies, which minimized enrollment of children with spasmodic croup, suggests that following delivery of racemic epinephrine by nebulization and intermittent positive-pressure breathing, there is likely to be an acute improvement of symptoms of airway obstruction with reversion to pretreatment status within 2 hours. Twenty-four hours after administration, treated and untreated patients are indistinguishable. Outpatients with laryngotracheitis should not be given racemic epinephrine because of the short-lived effect and the potential for a more severe rebound effect.
7. Corticosteroid therapy (a single dose of dexamethasone 0.6 mg/kg given intravenously) seems warranted in hospitalized patients with moderately severe obstruction, and not at all warranted in outpatients. Valid interpretation of studies has been hampered by variabilities in populations, degree of obstruction, etiology of obstruction (eg, spasmodic croup), agents and dosages, and the small size of studies. Recent meta-analysis and a small prospective randomized double-blind study show statistically significant clinical improvement, decreased need for racemic epinephrine, and endotracheal intubation in steroid-treated patients. Rapidly progressive viral pneumonia concurrent with steroid therapy is reported.
8. The decision to perform laryngoscopy, nasotracheal intubation, or tracheostomy should be made by individuals experienced in the care of children with airway problems. Laryngoscopy frequently precipitates a need for an artificial airway and should not be undertaken merely to confirm a diagnosis. On the other hand, emergency intubation of a patient who has suffered respiratory failure or respiratory arrest must be avoided.

## PREVENTION

Parainfluenza virus infection is an unavoidable part of early childhood. Vaccine strategies under investigation include use of live attenuated virus, bovine virus, purified proteins administered intranasally, and vaccinia vector for gene recombination. The major mode of virus transmission is direct hand inoculation of nasal mucosa. Staff of hospitals, schools, day-care centers, and other settings where children congregate, as well as parents and patients, should be careful to wash their hands.

## Selected Readings

Battaglia JD. Severe croup: The child with fever and upper airway obstruction. Pediatr in Rev 1986;7:227.
Denny FW, Murphy TF, Clyde WA, et al. Croup: an 11 year study in a pediatric practice. Pediatrics 1983;71:871.
Gallagher PG, Myer CM III. An approach to the diagnosis and treatment of membranous laryngotracheobronchitis in infants and children. Pediatr Emer Care 1991;7:337.
Glezen WP. Viral infections of the respiratory tract. In: Kelley VC, ed. Practice of pediatrics, Vol 4. Philadelphia: Harper & Row, 1987:1
Heil CA. Respiratory syncytial and parainfluenza viruses. J Infect Dis 1990;161:402.
Kairys SW, Olmstead EM, O'Connor GT. Steroid treatment of laryngotracheitis: A meta-analysis of the evidence from randomized trials. Pediatrics 1989;83:683.
Super DM, Cartelli NA, Brooks LJ, et al. A prospective randomized double-blind study to evaluate the effect of dexamethasone in acute laryngotracheitis. J Pediatr 1989;115:323.

*Principles and Practice of Pediatrics, Second Edition.*
edited by Frank A. Oski et al. J. B. Lippincott Company, Philadelphia © 1994.

# 57.7 *Respiratory Syncytial Virus*

Sarah S. Long

Respiratory syncytial virus (RSV), first isolated in 1956 from a chimpanzee with coryza, takes its name from the characteristic syncytial cell formation of infected tissue culture cells. Of the more than 100 viral agents responsible for acute respiratory tract disease in man, RSV is by far the most important lower respiratory tract pathogen of early life, accounting for the most hospitalizations for acute respiratory disease in children younger than 2 years old and for the most fatal outcomes. Three million children younger than 4 years of age are infected annually; approximately 100,000 require hospitalization, and 2% to 5% of those hospitalized develop respiratory failure. Reinfections continue throughout life. Adults with cold symptoms are important sources of virus for infants. The annual health care costs of disease due to RSV are estimated to be close to $400 million.

## CHARACTERISTICS OF THE VIRUS

RSV is a highly pleomorphic, enveloped, negatively stranded RNA virus of the family of myxoviruses. Its internal structure has helical symmetry, and its outer membrane is studded with glycoprotein spikes. Recent analysis with monoclonal antibodies shows RSV to be of two groups, A and B. Groups differ primarily in the largest surface glycoprotein, the G protein, while the fusion glycoprotein, the F protein, is conserved. The attachment and fusion proteins have special importance in successful infection and cell-to-cell spread of virus by syncytial formation. The virus is labile, surviving poorly in temperatures of 37 °C and higher and after slow freezing and thawing. RSV is rapidly destroyed by acid pH and ether. Unlike influenza viruses, RSV cannot be propagated in embryonated eggs and displays no hemadsorbing or hemagglutinating activity. Humans are the host for RSV, although laboratory animals can be infected. Laboratory tissue cultures of several primary, diploid, and heteroploid human cells as well as heterologous kidney cells have been successfully infected, resulting in formation of multinucleated syncytial areas in the cell layers. Infection elicits thymic-derived lymphocyte memory and antibodies of all classes of immunoglobulins. There is no cross-reactivity with other myxoviruses.

# EPIDEMIOLOGY

## Age Incidence

Infection with RSV is an inescapable feature of infancy. In the Houston Family Study, infection rate was 69 per 100 children in the first year of life and 83 per 100 children in the second year of life. About half the children had a recurrence of RSV infection by age 2 years. Rates of infection, severe disease manifestations, and mortality are highest at age 2 to 6 months in lower socioeconomic groups. Early epidemiologic studies, as well as the adverse clinical experience with the immunogenic killed RSV vaccine, led to the theory that symptoms were immunologically mediated. It was thought that disease was most severe in early infancy because passively acquired maternal antibody persisted. It now seems clear that although maternally derived antibody does not provide complete protection from infection, it does provide some ameliorating effect on symptoms, and certainly does not enhance pathogenic events. Likewise, acquired "immunity" does not provide complete protection from subsequent infection but does lessen the likelihood of repeated febrile or lower respiratory tract disease. A decrease in virus titer in nasopharyngeal secretions and protection from clinical disease correlate best with the presence of virus-specific secretory IgA. The fact that infants and adults can have recurrent RSV infection during the same season attests to the imperfect nature of immunity and the infective power of the virus. The extreme virulence of disease manifestations in infancy is recapitulated in the elderly.

## Seasonal Occurrence

Epidemic disease, easily recognized as outbreaks of bronchiolitis, occurs annually in midwinter to spring peaks (December through April) with virtual absence of RSV activity from August through October. Midwinter epidemics and infection with group A viruses appear to produce more severe disease. During epidemic periods, 80% or more of cases of bronchiolitis are due to RSV; in nonepidemic periods, less than 50% are etiologically related.

## Transmission

Transmission is by infected nasal secretions. Hand transmission of secretions and fomites from infected persons to the nasal or conjunctival mucosa of the recipient is far more important than airborne transmission. The hospital, its patients, and staff are major vectors in the transmission of RSV. Because hospitalized persons are likely to be at increased risk for severe disease, nosocomial transmission carries an inordinate mortality rate. During community epidemics, intensive care nurseries are the site of significant transmission. In infant wards, approximately one half of roommates and one third of staff will be infected from an infant with RSV bronchiolitis. Cohorting of infective patients decreases transmission. Although wearing gowns, gloves, and goggles provides maximal protection, it is likely just as effective to avoid transfer of secretions to clothing, meticulously wash hands, and alter habits conducive to self-inoculation.

# PATHOPHYSIOLOGY

Hallmarks of RSV infection are tropism for ciliated respiratory epithelium, necrosis of respiratory epithelium and destruction of cilia, inflammatory cell invasion of peribronchial tissues, and edema of submucosal and adventitial areas. Obstruction of small airways by edema, necrotic tissue, and inflammatory cells is associated with the classic dichotomous findings of areas of emphysematous overaeration and atelectatic underaeration. Inter-

stitial pneumonitis can be present. In normal children, histologic abnormalities usually are completely reversible.

Knowledge of pathophysiologic mechanisms for wheezing during RSV infection in infancy is evolving. Viral infection confined to the upper respiratory tract of adults and children (atopic and not atopic) results, transiently, in distal small airway dysfunction and in increased constrictive responses to a variety of stimuli. It is possible that virus-induced epithelial damage exposes receptors for environmental irritants that, once bound, elicit release of mediators responsible for the signs and symptoms of reactive airway disease. In support of this theory, infants living in industrialized, urban, or tobacco smoke-contaminated environments who contract RSV disease are more likely to need hospitalization than age-matched infants not living in these environments. A more direct role of damaged tissue is suggested by the finding that epithelial cells infected with virus produce leukotriene $B_4$, a chemotactic factor for neutrophils, which, once recruited, produce leukotrienes $C_4$ and $D_4$, thereby stimulating cyclooxygenase activity and increasing thromboxane production, which is the mediator of hyperreactivity.

Recent attention has been focused on immunopathogenic responses during RSV infection in infancy. Welliver and coworkers (1980) described the appearance of cell-bound IgE antibody to RSV on respiratory tract epithelium during infection and postulated its role in mediating bronchospasm. Circulating RSV-specific IgE and IgG4 antibodies recently have been noted coincident with RSV-associated airway obstruction. There is also evidence that RSV infection, specifically in young infants, has a cell-mediated immune modulating effect that leads to unrestrained production of IgE. This unbalanced response continues for several weeks after the virus disappears.

# CLINICAL MANIFESTATIONS OF INFECTION

Clinical illnesses caused by RSV infection include nonspecific upper respiratory illness, acute otitis media, laryngotracheobronchitis, bronchiolitis, and pneumonitis. Forty percent of infected children younger than 2 years of age have involvement of the lower respiratory tract. Syndromes are related to most significant sites of involvement and to host factors; they are not mutually exclusive. The detection of RSV antigen in middle ear fluid in 15% to 20% of children with acute otitis media in winter months is the first substantial proof of actual causation of otitis media by a virus.

## Bronchiolitis

Bronchiolitis is the most commonly diagnosed illness due to RSV and is almost exclusively confined to children younger than 2 years old. It is a clinical state of acute infection due to RSV (and less commonly to other viruses) in which obstruction of small airways is the predominant feature.

### Clinical Presentation

A time line of bronchiolitis due to RSV is presented in Figure 57-9. The incubation period is 4 to 7 days. Rhinorrhea is the usual initial event, followed by fever in at least 50% of cases, irritability, poor feeding, and cough. Cough progresses over 3 to 5 days, wheezing occurs, and dyspnea ensues. Very young infants and premature infants are less likely to have fever and more likely to have lethargy, apnea, and increased requirements for oxygen if on ventilators. Respiratory distress is the reason for hospitalization of most infants; approximately 20% have cyanosis. Pulse and respiratory rate are elevated, unrelated to the presence or absence of fever. Although retractions and nasal flaring are present during inspiration, the major expenditure of energy is in the

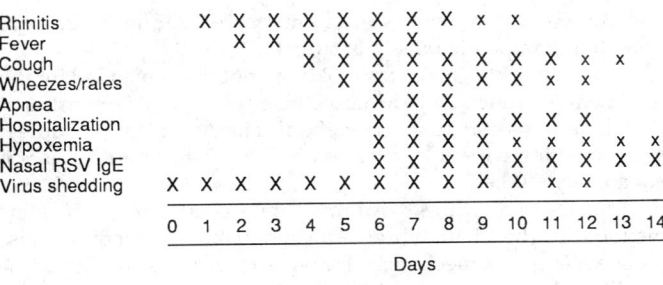

| | 0 | 1 | 2 | 3 | 4 | 5 | 6 | 7 | 8 | 9 | 10 | 11 | 12 | 13 | 14 |
|---|---|---|---|---|---|---|---|---|---|---|---|---|---|---|---|
| Rhinitis | | X | X | X | X | X | X | X | X | x | x | | | | |
| Fever | | X | X | X | X | X | X | | | | | | | | |
| Cough | | | | X | X | X | X | X | X | X | X | x | x | | |
| Wheezes/rales | | | | | X | X | X | X | X | X | X | x | x | | |
| Apnea | | | | | X | X | X | | | | | | | | |
| Hospitalization | | | | | X | X | X | X | X | X | X | | | | |
| Hypoxemia | | | | | X | X | X | X | X | x | x | x | x | x | x |
| Nasal RSV IgE | | | | | X | X | X | X | X | X | X | X | X | X | X |
| Virus shedding | X | X | X | X | X | X | X | X | X | X | X | X | x | x | |

Days

**Figure 57-9.** Average duration of signs, symptoms, and laboratory findings for untreated respiratory syncytial virus bronchiolitis. X, feature; x, diminished feature.

expiratory phase of respiration. The chest is barrel-shaped. Grunting and wheezing are audible. Auscultation reveals bilateral diffuse high-pitched expiratory wheezes and changeable inspiratory rhonchi and rales. Otitis media, pharyngeal hyperemia, and conjunctivitis can be present. Hyperinflation of the lungs pushes the liver and spleen into palpable positions in the abdomen.

### Laboratory Findings

Abnormalities in the peripheral white blood cell (WBC) count are so variable as to be of little use. Although the WBC count is usually less than 10,000 cells/mm$^3$ with a predominance of lymphocytes, higher counts with immature polymorphonuclear cells have been reported. The chest radiograph universally demonstrates overaerated lungs with an increased anteroposterior diameter of the chest, flattened or everted diaphragms, a more horizontal position of the ribs, and, sometimes, a diminished heart size. Peribronchial thickening is common. Overall, hyperaerated lung with areas of atelectatic lung is the radiographic hallmark of the disease. Peripheral interstitial infiltrates are less frequent. Lobar consolidation or pleural effusion is unusual.

Hypoxemia is common and is out of proportion to that expected from the degree of clinical illness. Cyanosis is an insensitive measure of the presence of hypoxemia, whereas the respiratory rate is useful. An increasing resting rate above 60 breaths per minute correlates very well with decreasing PaO$_2$. Fatigue results in retention of CO$_2$ and acidosis.

Apnea appears to occur during RSV bronchiolitis at an increased frequency. Its mechanisms are not understood; neither hypoxemia nor obstruction explains most occurrences. Respiratory pauses of 15 seconds and longer have occurred during hospitalization in nearly 20% of patients in retrospective studies. Apnea is occasionally the reason for hospitalization; almost invariably it disappears within 48 hours of hospitalization. Premature infants, very young infants, and those with a history of episodes of apnea are more prone to this event.

Virus is present in nasal secretions for 24 hours before the onset of symptoms and persists for 4 to 21 days after hospitalization. Laboratory confirmation of specific RSV etiology is useful and is enhanced by the availability of rapid diagnostic tests. Both enzyme-linked immunosorbent assay (ELISA) and a direct fluorescent antibody technique identify about 85% of cases subsequently confirmed by virus isolation. False-positive tests are uncommon. The sensitivity of antigen detection tests and culture is only as good as the specimen. Nasal wash by instillation and aspiration (by aspirator bulb or suction catheter) of 5 mL of isotonic saline is superior to nasal swab. RSV is cell-associated. Epithelial cells must be abundant in the specimen to ensure an adequate examination. Culture media should be inoculated immediately. Virus is identified in tissue culture within 5 to 10 days by appearance of characteristic cytopathic effect, use of antigen detection systems, or both.

### Hospital Course

Course of hospitalization is usually one of defervescence of fever over the first 2 days and diminution of respiratory symptoms between days 2 and 5. The average duration of hospitalization is 7 days.

Mild wheezing is frequently still present at the time of discharge. Oxygenation improves, but minor impairment persists in many children weeks to years after discharge. Virus persists in lower titers in nasal secretions during recovery.

The course of RSV disease is occasionally severe in normal children, but is predictably severe in those with congenital heart disease, especially when pulmonary hypertension exists. Mortality from RSV bronchiolitis in these patients is as high as 30%. Children with bronchopulmonary dysplasia, certain congenital anomalies, neuromuscular disorders, malnutrition, and congenital or acquired abnormalities of immunologic function also have excessive morbidity and mortality.

### Treatment

The administration of oxygen and delivery of general supportive care are the cornerstones of treatment for RSV bronchiolitis. Blood gas values should be determined in hospitalized infants with dyspnea or cyanosis, those with respiratory rates above 60 breaths per minute, and those with protracted courses of moderate severity. Humidified oxygen is given to maintain the PaO$_2$ between 70 and 90 mm Hg, or the O$_2$ saturation greater than 94%. Oxygen should be prescribed and monitored as a drug. Oximetry can be substituted for the arterial blood gas method if measurements are required frequently. Full blood gas determination should be performed at least every 24 hours, however, if the infant continues to require oxygen therapy, lest fatigue or worsening pneumonitis insidiously produce hypercapnia and precipitate respiratory failure.

*Ribavirin Therapy.* With the 1986 licensure of ribavirin for aerosol use in the treatment of RSV bronchiolitis, the first major campaign in the war against respiratory viruses was begun. Ribavirin is a synthetic nucleoside analogue resembling guanosine and inosine. Its exact virostatic mechanism is not known, but it appears to interfere with the capping of messenger RNA, thus inhibiting viral protein synthesis. The spectrum of antiviral activity is broad and includes parainfluenza, influenza, and adenoviruses, as well as RSV. Ribavirin exerts its antiviral effect locally after nebulization to aerosol particle size of 1 to 2 $\mu$m in diameter. Lyophilized ribavirin is reconstituted and diluted in sterile water to a concentration of 20 mg/mL. Aerosol is given by hood, tent, or nasotracheal tube for 12 to 20 hours out of 24 hours. It is not incorporated to a significant degree in host cell RNA or DNA. Teratogenicity was noted when ribavirin was given orally to pregnant rodents for 2 weeks, but this finding has not been duplicated in primates. No toxic effects have been noted in any adult or child treated with aerosolized ribavirin; however, bone marrow toxicity is seen frequently after oral administration of ribavirin. Blood and urine concentrations of ribavirin have been measured in hospital personnel after occupational exposure to treated patients. One study did not detect ribavirin in 18 nurses who worked for 3 days with infants receiving aerosolized ribavirin, whereas ribavirin triphosphate was detected in the erythrocyte fraction of 1 of 30 blood specimens obtained from 10 closely exposed health-care workers in another study.

Clinical studies of aerosolized ribavirin in high-risk and severely ill patients document a decreased duration of respiratory symptoms, decreased duration of hypoxemia, and decreased concentration of virus in nasal secretions soon after therapy was begun. Mortality rates were much lower than in historical controls. In placebo-controlled trials in more standard populations of affected children, ribavirin use had less dramatic effects. Statistically significant improvement in rales and retractions was seen in treated patients, as was statistically significant (but probably clinically insignificant) improvement in arterial oxygenation.

The cost of ribavirin (pharmacy cost of purchase for a course is approximately $1800) and its cumbersome method of administration mandate that ribavirin use be approached on a case-by-case basis. The following guidelines were established in 1987 by the Committee on Infectious Diseases of the American Academy of Pediatrics.

In patients with bronchiolitis proved or highly suspected to be caused by RSV, the following groups should be considered for ribavirin therapy: infants with congenital heart disease, infants with bronchopulmonary dysplasia or other chronic lung disease, certain premature infants (eg, those of postconception age less than 34 weeks and those with a history of apnea), infants with congenital or acquired immune deficiency syndrome as well as older children with disease- or drug-associated immunosuppression, infants with severe illness (eg, $PaO_2$ less than 65 mm Hg, increasing $PaCO_2$, or respiratory rate above 60 breaths/minute), and very young infants (less than 6 weeks old).

Based on these guidelines, approximately 50% of children admitted to an urban primary and tertiary care children's hospital with presumed RSV bronchiolitis qualified for ribavirin therapy. A recent study of high-dose (60 mg/mL) short-duration (2 h three times daily) ribavirin therapy showed 98% reduction of virus titer. Treatment was well tolerated, and it permitted easier accessibility for patient care and less time of environmental exposure of health care workers. Caution and special experience are required to administer ribavirin to patients on ventilators. This drug can precipitate in filters, valves, tubing, and the airway and can interfere with proper delivery of oxygen and pressure. With care, these problems are safely averted.

### Other Therapy

*Humidification.* Humidification should be provided when oxygen is administered. Mist tents and aerosol treatments in themselves are not advantageous and can potentially cause harm due to anxiety, increased fluid volume, or a bronchoconstricting effect on the respiratory epithelium. Hydration should be adequate but not excessive. Pulmonary fluid volume is increased by the disease process. Excessive fluid interferes with gaseous exchange and contributes to obstruction.

*Adrenergic Bronchodilators.* Adrenergic bronchodilators are of questionable benefit in RSV bronchiolitis. Controversy regards use of $\beta$-adrenergic and $\alpha$-adrenergic medications in young wheezing children. Most research has shown that children younger than 2 years do not respond to bronchodilator therapy. Methodologic and technical problems in study design are significant. Two recent double-masked, placebo-controlled trials of 2 doses of 0.10 mg/K nebulized albuterol (Klassen et al; Schuh et al) and a third study of a single dose of 10 mg nebulized metaproterenol (Alario et al) have shown at least short-term clinical effectiveness in relieving respiratory distress of young acutely wheezing children, including those with documented RSV bronchiolitis. Although data are somewhat conflicting, age older than 12 months and early therapies correlate with improvement after $\beta$-agonist therapy. Partial responsiveness to the predominantly $\alpha$-agonist epinephrine (at dose of 0.01 mL/kg of 1 mg/mL solution given for 3 doses subcutaneously) compared to placebo was recently documented in wheezing infants with and without RSV as cause of bronchiolitis. Follow-up study is necessary to confirm whether responders have subsequent evidence of allergic bronchospasm. The heterogeneous population of patients with bronchiolitis represents a continuum of small airways obstruction secondary to an inflammatory process and edema, spasm of the bronchiolar musculature, or both. Multiple studies of the same

and comparative therapies are required before the nuances of potential therapeutic benefit are worked out.

*Corticosteroids.* Corticosteroids are not recommended for the treatment of bronchiolitis. Multiple studies have not demonstrated that their use is particularly beneficial. Their potential usefulness in conjunction with antiviral and bronchodilator therapies is not adequately studied.

*Antihistamine Drugs.* Antihistamine drugs are not recommended for the treatment of bronchiolitis. If IgE-mediated histamine release is a mechanism for wheezing in infants with bronchiolitis, the use of antihistamines is theoretically attractive. Antihistamines are best used before histamine release, however, which is impossible in the wheezing patient. Other infectious and inflammatory mediators of bronchospasm unaffected by antihistamines also contribute to the pathophysiology of bronchiolitis. Furthermore, lower airway obstruction may be worsened by the drying and bronchoconstrictive effects of antihistamines.

*Antibiotic Therapy.* Antibiotic therapy is not warranted for the typical patient with bronchiolitis. Antibiotics do not affect the course of the viral disease. Secondary bacterial infections generally do not occur.

### Outcome

An estimated 1% of patients hospitalized for bronchiolitis die. This relatively high mortality is a reflection of the number of infections in patients with underlying risk factors for severe disease and of the inability to provide antiviral therapy and assisted ventilation. With modern therapy, mortality rates should approach zero in the United States.

The relationship of bronchiolitis in infancy to recurrence of wheezing in infancy and childhood has been appreciated for some time. Excellent long-term studies in patients followed for more than 10 years have documented continued abnormalities of pulmonary function and airway hyperreactivity to chemicals and exercise. Passive and active smoking as well as exposure to other pollutants adversely affect the subsequent health of these patients.

## PREVENTION

The importance of contact with infected nasal or conjunctival secretions in the transmission of RSV and the importance of hand washing to interrupt transmission cannot be overstressed.

If natural disease fails to induce solid protection, vaccine-induced immunity will be difficult to achieve. Attempts to develop a vaccine have been discouraging. When killed RSV vaccine was administered, an antibody response was induced, but subsequently natural infection led to exaggeration of bronchiolitis symptoms, probably related to an imbalance of vaccine-induced lymphocyte and antibody responses. Attenuated live RSV vaccines were not effective in preventing disease. Recently, however, purified RSV glycoprotein attachment (G) and fusion (F) proteins have been shown to be good immunizing agents and to elicit protection against experimental RSV infection in primates. An injectable candidate vaccine is undergoing clinical studies. There is also investigation of recombinant vaccinia virus vaccine for the selective expression of RSV F, G, and N genes. Immunoglobulin preparations with high antibody titers to RSV are being assessed for therapeutic and prophylactic effect.

## Selected Readings

Alario AJ, Lewander WJ, Dennehy P, et al. The efficacy of nebulized metaproterenol in wheezing infants and young children. Am J Dis Child 1992;146:412.

American Academy of Pediatrics, Committee on Infectious Diseases. Ribavirin therapy for respiratory syncytial virus. Pediatrics 1987;79:475.

Bradley JS, Connor J, Compogiannis LS, et al. Exposure of health care workers to ribavirin during therapy for respiratory syncytial virus infections. Antimicrob Agents Chemother 1990;34:668.

Church NR, Anas NG, Hall CB, Brooks JG. Respiratory syncytial virus-related apnea in infants: demographics and outcome. Am J Dis Child 1984;138:247.

Englund JA, Piedra PA, Jefferson LS, et al. High-dose, short-duration ribavirin aerosol therapy in children with suspected respiratory syncytial virus infection. J Pediatr 1990;117:313.

Glezen WP, Taber LH, Frank AL, et al. Risk of primary infection and reinfection with respiratory syncytial virus. Am J Dis Child 1986;140:543.

Hall CB, Douglas RG Jr. Modes of transmission of respiratory syncytial virus. J Pediatr 1981;99:100.

Hall CB, McBride JT, Walsh EE, et al. Aerosolized ribavirin treatment for infants with respiratory syncytial virus infection: a randomized double-blind study. N Engl J Med 1983;308:1443.

Hall CB, Walsh EE, Schnabel KC, et al. Occurrence of groups A and B respiratory syncytial virus over 15 years: associated epidemiologic and clinical characteristics in hospitalized and ambulatory children. J Infect Dis 1990;162:1283.

Klassen TP, Rowe PC, Sutcliffe T, et al. Randomized trial of salbutamol in acute bronchiolitis. J Pediatr 1991;118:807.

Lowell DI, Lister G, VonHoss H, et al. Wheezing in infants: the response to epinephrine. Pediatrics 1987;79:939.

Schuh S, Canny G, Reisman JJ, et al. Nebulized albuterol in acute bronchiolitis. J Pediatr 1990;117:633.

Welliver RC, Kaul TN, Ogra PL. The appearance of cell-bound IgE in respiratory tract epithelium after respiratory-syncytial virus infection. N Engl J Med 1980;303:1198.

*Principles and Practice of Pediatrics, Second Edition.*
edited by Frank A. Oski et al. J. B. Lippincott Company, Philadelphia © 1994.

# 57.8 *Parvoviruses*

James D. Cherry

Parvoviruses infect and cause disease in a great variety of insects and animals. The human parvovirus B19 was serendipitously discovered in 1975 and found to be associated with human disease in the early 1980s. B19 virus is the cause of erythema infectiosum (fifth disease) and transient red blood cell aplasia (aplastic crisis).

Parvovirus B19 belongs to the family Parvoviridae, of which there are three genera: parvovirus, dependovirus, and densovirus. Of these three genera, only parvovirus has been causally related to human disease. In addition to B19 virus, there are currently two other candidate human parvoviruses. These latter viruses include fecal agents, which may be associated with diarrhea, and the RA1 parvovirus, which has been isolated from patients with rheumatoid arthritis.

Parvovirus B19 is a small (22 nm), single-stranded DNA, non-enveloped virus. It has been propagated in suspension cultures of human erythroid bone marrow and in primary fetal liver culture.

## EPIDEMIOLOGY

Most epidemiologic information comes from studies of erythema infectiosum outbreaks. These outbreaks are most prevalent in the winter and spring and last for 3 to 6 months. There is a cyclic pattern to disease, similar to that of rubella. Peak periods of disease occur about every 6 years with increased activity lasting an average of 3 years.

The case-to-case interval of erythema infectiosum is usually between 4 and 14 days, and the attack rate is high. In school-related outbreaks, attack rates of 25% are common. The highest attack rates are in children 5 to 14 years old; secondary cases occur in preschool children, teachers, and parents. In the home, secondary cases are more common in mothers than in fathers.

Limited antibody studies indicate the following prevalence data: in children younger than 5 years old, 2% to 9%; in children and adolescents 5 to 18 years old, 15% to 35%; in adults older than 18 years old, 30% to 60%. The prevalence of antibody suggests that many infections are either asymptomatic or symptomatic but unrecognized as typical B19 viral infections.

The mode of spread is presumed to be by droplet via the respiratory tract. Recent intranasal inoculation studies support this route for the mode of transmission.

## PATHOPHYSIOLOGY

After infection via the respiratory tract, viremia occurs in which $10^{10}$ or $10^{11}$ viral particles per milliliter of blood may be found. Associated with viremia (about 7 to 10 days after infection) a profound reticulocytopenia occurs. In vitro studies indicate that early erythrocyte precursor cells are susceptible to B19 virus infection. Neutropenia, lymphopenia, and a drop in the platelet count occur in conjunction with the reticulocytopenia. During the second week of infection, hemoglobin values drop slightly.

In erythema infectiosum, the exanthem occurs about 17 to 18 days after infection when virus can no longer be detected in throat swabs or blood specimens. At the time of rash, virus-specific IgM antibody is present, suggesting the exanthem may be immune-mediated. The finding of perivascular infiltrations with mononuclear cells in the epidermis of persons with exanthem supports this suggestion.

## CLINICAL MANIFESTATIONS

### Erythema Infectiosum

Although erythema infectiosum is recognized classically by its distinct rash, recent studies in volunteers suggest a biphasic illness. Approximately 1 week after infection, there is a nonspecific febrile illness with headache, chills, malaise, and myalgia. These symptoms last 2 to 3 days, followed by an asymptomatic interlude of about 7 days, then the exanthematous phase of the illness. The exanthem occurs in three stages. The first stage is the appearance of a fiery red rash on the cheeks ("slapped-cheek" appearance) and a relative circumoral pallor. The facial appearance is suggestive of scarlet fever, an allergic reaction, or collagen vascular disease. The facial exanthem may be accentuated when the affected person moves from outdoors to a warm room.

The second stage follows the onset of facial involvement by 1 to 4 days as an erythematous maculopapular rash on the trunk and extremities. Initially, this rash is discrete, but soon it takes on a characteristic lacy or reticular pattern.

The third stage of the exanthem is characterized by changes in the intensity of the rash with periodic evanescence and recrudescence. The duration of the third stage is highly variable; fluctuations are related to environmental factors such as exposure to sunlight and temperature.

The rash is often pruritic, especially in adults, and is generally more prominent on the extensor surfaces. Occasionally, slight desquamation is noted in some patients.

Other symptoms and signs are uncommon in erythema infectiosum. Headache occurs in about one fifth of affected children and one half of affected adults. Enanthem is rare, although children occasionally have pharyngitis. Joint pain and swelling and myalgia are particularly troublesome in adults.

## Arthritis

The most common complication of erythema infectiosum is arthritis. It occurs in 80% or more of affected adults but in less than 10% of children with erythema infectiousum. The illness ranges in severity from mild arthralgia to frank arthritis. Joint involvement is usually transient, lasting only a few days, but in some adults these symptoms may persist for weeks or, rarely, months. Arthritis is more common in women than in men and most often involves the knees, ankles, and proximal interpharyngeal joints; involvement is usually bilateral. The onset of arthritis usually occurs 1 to 6 days after the onset of the rash, but occasionally it has been noted before the exanthem. Many adults have arthritis without skin manifestations of infection.

## Aplastic Crisis

In individuals with hemolytic anemias, the profound reticulocytopenia associated with acute B19 virus infection may result in critical depression of hemoglobin concentrations. This transitory arrest of erythrocyte production is termed aplastic crisis and can occur in any individual whose erythrocytes have a short lifespan. Individuals at risk for aplastic crisis with acute B19 virus infections include those with sickle cell anemia, hereditary spherocytosis, thalassemia, pyruvate kinase deficiency, and acquired hemolytic anemias.

In association with aplastic crisis, most patients have fever, malaise, and gastrointestinal symptoms; some also have respiratory symptoms. Typical erythema infectiosum is rare.

Laboratory studies in afflicted patients reveal reticulocyte counts between 0% and 1% and hemoglobin values 10% to 30% below baseline values. Occasionally, lymphocytosis, eosinophilia, and neutropenia are noted.

## Infection in Immunocompromised Patients

Chronic B19 virus infection occurs in some children with immunodeficiences. Persistent anemia occurs due to a continuous lysis of red blood cell precursors. This has been noted most often in children with acute lymphocytic leukemia.

## Intrauterine Infection

Infection in pregnancy results in fetal hydrops, fetal death, and miscarriage. Recent studies indicate that maternal B19 virus infections results in a transplacental transmission rate of 33% and a fetal death rate of 9%.

## Other Clinical Manifestations

Rarely, erythema infectiosum is complicated by transient hemolytic anemia and encephalitis, with and without residual damage. There are also reports of B19 viral infections associated with thrombocytopenic purpura, Henoch-Schönlein purpura, myocarditis, and pseudo-appendicitis.

# DIAGNOSIS

The exanthem of erythema infectiosum is characteristic, so the diagnosis is easy during epidemics. Sporadic cases can be a problem because rubella, scarlet fever, and enteroviral infections can be confused with erythema infectiosum. Other differential diagnostic considerations are collagen vascular diseases, drug reactions, and allergic responses to environmental substances.

In patients with chronic hemolytic anemia, occurrence of an aplastic crisis generally can be assumed to be due to B19 virus infection. Other causes of moderate degrees of reticulocytopenia and general bone marrow suppression include systemic bacterial infections and marrow-suppressive drugs such as chloramphenicol.

The specific diagnosis of a B19 viral infection can be made by demonstrating B19-specific IgM antibody in the serum of ill or convalescing individuals via enzyme-linked immunosorbent assay, radioimmunoassay, or immunofluorescence. In immunocompromised patients, antigen is detected by DNA hybridization, polymerase chain reaction, or electron microscopy. Past infection and immunity is determined by the demonstration of specific B19 serum IgG antibody.

# TREATMENT AND PREVENTION

There is no specific treatment available for B19 viral infections. Patients with aplastic crisis may require transfusion; otherwise, B19 viral infections rarely require therapy. Arthritis or arthralgia may be painful and can be treated with nonsteroidal anti-inflammatory agents.

In erythema infectiosum outbreaks, pregnant women should, when possible, avoid contact with susceptible school-aged children. If B19 virus infection occurs during pregnancy, the pregnancy should be carefully monitored. At delivery, examination of cord blood or blood from the neonate for virus and IgM antibody will reveal whether in utero infection occurred. Babies infected in utero should be periodically examined for delayed sequelae. Because congenital malformation has not been demonstrated, therapeutic abortion is not indicated for B19 virus infection during pregnancy.

During erythema infectiosum outbreaks, isolation of exanthematous patients is not useful because the patient is no longer contagious by the time the exanthem occurs. On the other hand, patients with aplastic crisis or immunodeficiency may still be excreting virus and should be isolated from other patients when hospitalized.

Intravenous immune globulin treatment should be considered in immunocompromised patients with chronic B19 virus infections.

## Selected Readings

Ager EA, Chin TDY, Poland JD: Epidemic erythema infectiosum. N Engl J Med 1966;275:1326.

Anderson LJ. Human Parvoviruses. J Infect Dis 1990;161:603.

Anderson MJ. Parvoviruses as agents of human disease. Prog Med Virol 1987;34:55.

Anderson MJ, Higgins PG, Davis LR, et al. Experimental parvoviral infection in humans. J Infect Dis 1985;152:257.

Cherry JD. Parvoviruses. In: Feigin RD, Cherry JD, eds. Textbook of pediatric infectious diseases, ed 3. Philadelphia: WB Saunders, 1992:1626.

Chorba T, Coccia P, Holman RC, et al. The role of parvovirus B19 in aplastic crisis and erythema infectiosum (fifth disease). J Infect Dis 1986;154:383.

Public Health Laboratory Service Working Party on Fifth Disease. Prospective study of human parvovirus (B19) infection in pregnancy. BMJ 1990;300:1166.

*Principles and Practice of Pediatrics, Second Edition.*
edited by Frank A. Oski et al. J. B. Lippincott Company, Philadelphia © 1994.

# 57.9 *Polioviruses*

James D. Cherry

Polioviruses are a subgroup of the enteroviruses. When a susceptible person is infected with a poliovirus, one of the following responses may occur: inapparent infection, minor illness (abortive poliomyelitis), nonparalytic poliomyelitis (aseptic meningitis), and paralytic poliomyelitis. Infection with and disease caused by polioviruses can be controlled completely by universal immunization with poliovirus vaccines.

Polioviruses are single-stranded RNA viruses. They are 20 to 30 nm in size and consist of a naked protein capsid and a dense central core of RNA. They grow readily in monkey kidney tissue culture and several different human tissue cultures, and cause illness and pathology in infected monkeys.

The three distinct antigenic types of poliovirus are types 1, 2, and 3. Infection with a poliovirus results in lifelong immunity to the homologous virus type but confers no immunity to the other two viral types.

## EPIDEMIOLOGY

The general epidemiology of polioviruses is similar to that of other enteroviruses and is discussed more fully in Chapter 57.10, Nonpolio Enteroviruses. The spread of polioviruses and the clinical manifestations of infection are markedly affected by the degree of vaccine utilization and the socioeconomic conditions of the population. The epidemiology of poliomyelitis was a mystery until it was discovered that unrecognized infections were the main source of the spread of the virus. Historically, in populations with poor sanitation and hygiene, epidemics of poliomyelitis did not occur, but widespread dissemination of polioviruses occurred continually. In such populations, immunizing infections with all three poliovirus types occurred in infants who were usually protected from significant clinical disease by transplacentally acquired antibodies. In populations with improved standards of hygiene, immunizing infections of infants no longer regularly occur, so pools of susceptible children build up in the population. When poliovirus is introduced into such a population, infection occurs in these older children and poliomyelitis not infrequently occurs. The age spread of cases of poliomyelitis in a population depends on the overall hygienic standards of the population as well as on such things as family size and crowding.

The evolution of poliomyelitis from an endemic to epidemic disease follows a characteristic pattern. Initially, only isolated cases occur. Over the years, the endemic rate gradually increases, followed by periodic, then yearly, severe epidemics with high attack rates. Once a community reaches a socioeconomic situation in which epidemic poliomyelitis occurs regularly, there is a gradual shift in age incidence. Relatively few cases occur in infants, the peak occurs in the 5- to 14-year-old age group, and an increasing proportion of cases occur in young adults.

The universal use of oral polio vaccines during the last three decades has resulted in the virtual elimination of infection with wild polioviruses in the United States. In areas of the world such as developing countries where polio vaccine control measures are not widespread, endemic and epidemic poliomyelitis continue to occur. In the United States, rare cases of poliomyelitis are detected; these are due to imported cases of natural poliomyelitis and cases of vaccine-induced disease.

## PATHOPHYSIOLOGY

The general pathophysiology of enteroviral infections is presented in Chapter 57.10, Nonpolio Enteroviruses.

The virus can be recovered from the blood, throat, and feces of the infected person 3 to 5 days after exposure. At this time, there may be "minor illness," or the infection may be unrecognized. Major illness with central nervous system (CNS) involvement has its onset about 10 days after infection. The blood is most likely the main pathway for viral invasion of the CNS in natural disease. In experimental infections in monkeys, however, it has been demonstrated that the virus can reach the CNS by traveling along axons of peripheral nerves.

The neuropathology of poliomyelitis is usually pathopneumonic. Neuronal damage is directly due to virus multiplication in the cells; there is little evidence of infection in surrounding tissues except for slight histologic evidence of meningitis and perivascular cuffing. Neuronal lesions are most common in the anterior horn cells of the spinal cord.

## CLINICAL FINDINGS

In susceptible persons, 90% to 95% of infections are inapparent, about 4% to 8% are classified as minor illness (abortive poliomyelitis), and rarely does nonparalytic poliomyelitis (aseptic meningitis) or paralytic poliomyelitis develop. In general, older persons are more likely to have severe paralytic disease and higher mortality. Bulbar poliomyelitis may be precipitated by tonsillectomy at the time of inapparent infection; a history of tonsillectomy is also related to a higher rate of bulbar disease.

Abortive poliomyelitis (minor illness) is similar to many other enteroviral infections and frequently is unrecognized as a significant infection. The illness is mild and nonspecific with low-grade fever, malaise, anorexia, and sore throat. On physical examination, no significant abnormalities are noted.

### Nonparalytic Poliomyelitis (Aseptic Meningitis)

Nonparalytic poliomyelitis is similar to aseptic meningitis caused by many other enteroviruses. Initially, illness is characterized by nonspecific fever, malaise, and headache. Other complaints are anorexia, nausea, vomiting, constipation, and diarrhea. Fever is usually moderate (37.8 °C to 39.5 °C) and there is usually aching of muscles. Soon thereafter, the neck, back, and hamstrings become stiff, and sometimes there is hyperesthesia and paresthesia. Occasionally, the illness is biphasic with an initial phase (minor illness) consisting of fever and nonspecific complaints and a second phase (CNS or major illness) with symptoms that indicate CNS involvement.

On physical examination, there are nuchal-spinal signs. For example, when sitting, the patient uses his hands in a tripod supporting position, indicative of spinal rigidity. Nuchal rigidity can be noted by asking the patient to flex the chin to the chest. Kernig's and Brudzinski's signs are usually positive. In nonparalytic poliomyelitis, the reflexes are usually normal. It is important to observe the reflexes over time, however, because changes may indicate impending paralysis. The white blood cell count is usually normal or slightly elevated. Examination of cerebrospinal fluid (CSF) discloses changes similar to those seen in other enteroviral aseptic meningitides. The cell count range usually varies from 20 to 300 cells/mm³. Although the differential cell count usually has a predominance of lymphocytes, greater than 50% polymorphonuclear leukocytes may be seen early in an illness. The CSF glucose level is usually normal, and the protein concentration is normal or slightly elevated. In the usual case, recovery occurs in 3 to 10 days.

## Paralytic Poliomyelitis

The initial findings in paralytic poliomyelitis are similar to those in nonparalytic poliomyelitis, except, occasionally, findings are more pronounced. Fever is likely to be higher and muscle pain is more conspicuous. Before the onset of actual muscle weakness, superficial and deep tendon reflexes diminish or disappear. Patients destined to develop paralytic poliomyelitis often appear acutely ill and are restless, flushed, and have an anxious expression. Biphasic illness with a symptom-free interlude of several days between the initial illness phase and the occurrence of paralysis is common in paralytic poliomyelitis.

The onset of paralysis may be sudden with complete loss of function within a few hours, or it may progress gradually over 3 to 5 days. Asymmetric involvement is typical, particularly in milder cases. About 20% of affected patients have bladder paralysis, which is temporary; paralytic ileus due to bowel atony is common in severe cases. In general, lower limbs are affected more commonly than upper limbs. In severe cases, quadriplegia occurs and there may be functional loss of intercostal, abdominal, and trunk muscles. In affected areas, superficial and deep tendon reflexes are lost, and twitching and diffuse fasciculations of affected muscles may be transiently noted. Sensory abnormalities usually do not occur.

In bulbar disease, the 10th cranial nerve nuclei are most commonly involved, resulting in paralysis of the pharynx, soft palate, and vocal cord. Facial paralysis is less common, and ocular palsies are unusual. There is an encephalitic form of the disease characterized by irritability, disorientation, drowsiness, and coarse tremors. Hypoxia and hypercapnea resulting from respiratory insufficiency due to inadequate ventilation can produce disorientation without true encephalitis.

# COMPLICATIONS

The most important complication of paralytic poliomyelitis is respiratory insufficiency due to inadequate ventilation. Myocardial failure sometimes occurs, either secondary to pulmonary complications or as a direct result of acute myocarditis. Not infrequently, patients who have had paralytic poliomyelitis develop what appear to be new neuromuscular symptoms later in life. The late-onset weakness and muscle atrophy are most likely the results of routine attrition of remaining anterior horn cells associated with aging rather than persistent neural infection with polioviruses.

# DIAGNOSIS

Poliovirus infection should be considered in all unimmunized patients with aseptic meningitis with or without paralysis. If poliovirus infection is suspected, specimens for viral diagnostic studies should be obtained from the throat, stool, and CSF. All diagnostic virologic laboratories have the facilities to isolate polioviruses, and hospitals unequipped for virus isolation should refer specimens to regional laboratories. Poliovirus grows readily in appropriate tissue culture systems, and the presence of an enterovirus is usually noted in 3 to 4 days. Its identification as a poliovirus usually takes another week or so.

Patients infected with polioviruses regularly develop neutralizing antibody to the type-specific virus. Therefore, the cause of the illness can be confirmed by examining acute and convalescent serum antibody titers to the three polioviral types. A fourfold rise in neutralizing antibody titer is indicative of infection. In acute illness, specific IgM neutralizing antibody for a specific poliovirus type is also diagnostic.

The differential diagnosis of nonparalytic poliomyelitis must include other enteroviral infections as well as the numerous other causes of aseptic meningitis. The diagnosis of paralytic poliomyelitis during outbreaks should be no problem. Rarely, however, other enteroviruses (particularly enterovirus 71) cause paralytic syndromes similar to those due to polioviruses. In sporadic instances of paralytic illness, several other diseases must be considered in the differential diagnosis. These illnesses include Guillain-Barré syndrome, peripheral neuritis (postinjection, toxic, herpes zoster), arboviral infections, rabies, tetanus, botulism, and tick paralysis.

Although rare, the consideration that a paralytic illness may be polio vaccine-induced also should be entertained.

# TREATMENT

The treatment of nonparalytic poliomyelitis is nonspecific. In mild cases, analgesics may be given for headache and muscle pain.

All patients with paralytic disease should be hospitalized. Impaired ventilation must be looked for and treated early. Increasing anxiety, restlessness, and fatigue are early indications that intervention is necessary. Mechanical ventilation is often needed. To handle secretions, tracheostomy frequently is indicated in patients with pure bulbar poliomyelitis, spinal respiratory muscle paralysis, and bulbar spinal paralysis. Patients with poliomyelitis are usually fully conscious and aware. All procedures relating to their care should be explained to them to reduce anxiety.

With bladder paralysis, a parasympathetic stimulant such as bethanechol, 5 to 10 mg orally or 2.5 to 5 mg subcutaneously, may induce voiding, but catheterization may be necessary. Bladder paralysis usually lasts only a few days, so catheterization should be temporary. In bed, the patient with poliomyelitis should be in a neutral position with the feet at right angles, knees slightly flexed, and hips and spine straight. This position can be achieved by using boards, sandbags, and, occasionally, light splint shells. Active and passive motions are indicated as soon as muscle pain disappears. Constipation is a common complication and should be treated early to prevent fecal impaction. Consultation with other services (orthopedics and physiotherapy) should be obtained early in an illness so fixed deformities can be prevented.

# PREVENTION

Poliomyelitis is a vaccine-preventable disease. Its control as well as the control of the circulation of wild polioviruses has been achieved in many countries of the world. Recent analysis suggests that with intensified effort and increased international collaboration, global eradication of poliomyelitis is attainable by 1995.

There are two effective poliovirus vaccines, trivalent live oral poliovirus vaccine (OPV) and trivalent formalin-inactivated parenterally administered poliovirus vaccine (IPV). OPV is the usual vaccine of choice for children in the United States. It induces intestinal immunity, is simple to administer, is well accepted by patients, and results in immunization of some contacts of vaccinated persons; its use has eliminated endogenous disease caused by wild polioviruses in the United States. In rare instances—approximately 1 case per 550,000 first doses of vaccine—administration of OPV has been associated with paralysis in healthy recipients or their contacts. IPV is an alternative vaccine to OPV. IPV is not the vaccine of choice in the United States because, from the public health perspective, it is less likely to result in herd immunity in a diffuse and varied population. IPV costs more than OPV, is more difficult to administer, and produces a lesser degree of intestinal immunity; it lacks the ability to immunize contacts of some immunized persons and necessitates booster doses in older children and adults.

OPV is routinely given at ages 2, 4, and 15 to 18 months and at 4 to 6 years of age. Recently, an enhanced-potency IPV became available in the United States. The primary series for enhanced-potency IPV consists of three doses. The interval between the first two doses should be at least 4 weeks, but preferably 8 weeks. The third dose should be given 6 to 12 months after the second dose. A booster dose is given at 4 to 6 years of age before school entry. The need for routinely administered additional booster doses is unknown, but it is likely that adult booster doses will be necessary for continued community protection. Nonenhanced-potency IPV requires a booster dose every 5 years.

Before a child is immunized, the parents should be informed of the availability of OPV and IPV, and the benefits and risks of both polio vaccines for both individuals and the community should be explained. If OPV is refused by the parents, children should be vaccinated with IPV.

Patients with immunodeficiency diseases and adults are at increased risk of OPV-induced paralytic disease. Therefore, patients with immunodeficiency diseases, or household contacts of individuals with immunodeficiency diseases, and adults should receive IPV rather than OPV. Full information regarding polio vaccine immunization practices is in the *Report of the Committee on Infectious Diseases* of the American Academy of Pediatrics (Red Book) and in the recommendations of the Immunization Practices Advisory Committee (ACIP) of the United States Department of Health and Human Services.

Known or suspected cases of poliomyelitis should be reported promptly to county or state health departments so immediate epidemiologic investigation can be undertaken. Specimens should be obtained for viral studies. If a workup suggests wild poliovirus infection, a community immunization plan should be implemented to prevent further cases.

## Selected Readings

American Academy of Pediatrics. Report of the Committee on Infectious Diseases, ed 22. Elk Grove Village, Ill: American Academy of Pediatrics, 1991:381.

Centers for Disease Control. Poliomyelitis prevention: enhanced-potency inactivated poliomyelitis vaccine—supplementary statement of the ACIP. MMWR 1987;36:795.

Cherry JD. Enteroviruses: polioviruses (poliomyelitis), coxsackieviruses, echoviruses, and enteroviruses. In: Feigin RD, Cherry JD, eds. Textbook of pediatric infectious diseases, ed 3. Philadelphia: WB Saunders, 1992:1705.

Hinman AR, Koplan JP, Orenstein WA, et al. Live or inactivated poliovirus vaccine: an analysis of benefits and risks. Am J Public Health 1988;78:291.

Immunization Practices Advisory Committee. Poliomyelitis prevention. MMWR 1982;31:22,31.

Nkowane BM, Wassilak SGF, Orenstein WA, et al. Vaccine-associated paralytic poliomyelitis. United States: 1973 through 1984. JAMA 1987;257:1335.

Strebel PM, Sutter RW, Cochi SL, et al. Epidemiology of poliomyelitis in the United States one decade after the last reported case of indigenous wild virus—associated disease. Clin Infect Dis 1992;14:568.

Wright PF, Klim-Farley RJ, Dis Quadros CA, et al. Strategies for the global eradication of poliomyelitis by the year 2000. N Engl J Med 1991;325:1774.

*Principles and Practice of Pediatrics, Second Edition.*
edited by Frank A. Oski et al. J. B. Lippincott Company, Philadelphia © 1994.

# 57.10 *Nonpolio Enteroviruses*

## James D. Cherry

The nonpolio enteroviruses (coxsackieviruses, echoviruses, and enteroviruses) are responsible for significant and frequent human illness with protean clinical manifestations. These viruses as well as the polioviruses were categorized together and named in 1957 by a committee sponsored by the National Foundation for Infantile Paralysis. They are grouped together because their natural habitat is the alimentary tract and they share common features in their epidemiology, clinical spectrum, and pathogenesis, and have physical and biochemical similarities.

The enteroviruses belong to the Picornaviridae (*pico*, small; *RNA*, ribonucleic acid); they are single-stranded RNA viruses. They are 20 to 30 nm in size and consist of a naked protein capsid and a dense central core of RNA. Most enteroviruses grow in selected primate tissue cultures; some grow only when inoculated into suckling mice less than 24 hours old. A satisfactory system for the primary recovery of enteroviruses from patients includes primary rhesus, cynomolgus, or African green monkey kidney; diploid human embryonic lung fibroblast cell strain; and RD (rhabdomyosarcoma) cell line tissue cultures and the intraperitoneal and intracerebral inoculation of suckling mice less than 24 hours old.

There are 23 coxsackieviruses group A, 6 coxsackieviruses group B, 32 echoviruses, and 5 more recently identified enteroviruses, which are designated enteroviruses 68 to 72 (enterovirus 72 is the hepatitis A virus and is discussed in Chapter 20.14.3).

Although there are some minor serologic cross-reactions between several enterovirus types, there are no common group antigens of diagnostic importance. Individual enteroviral types are identified by neutralization with type-specific antisera.

## EPIDEMIOLOGY

Humans are the only natural host of nonpolio enteroviruses that infect people. Spread is from person to person, by fecal–oral and possibly oral–oral (respiratory spread) routes. Transmission of infection by fomites and the contaminated hands of health-care personnel has been documented in the hospital setting. Contaminated swimming and wading pools may serve as a means of spread of enteroviruses during summer. Children are the main susceptible cohort; therefore, primary spread is from child to child. Secondary spread occurs to susceptible contacts in family groups. The incidence of infection and disease is inversely related to age, and the prevalence of specific antibodies is directly related to age. Epidemics and outbreaks depend on new susceptibles in the population; reinfection with clinical disease with a particular serotype is not thought to occur routinely. In temperate climates, enteroviral infections occur primarily in the summer and fall; in the tropics, infections regularly occur throughout the year.

Although there are 65 nonpolio enteroviral types, excluding hepatitis A virus, usually only a few viral types circulate in a community during any one season. In the last three decades, echovirus type 9 has been the most prevalent of the nonpolio enteroviruses. Other common types in widespread circulation have been echoviruses 4, 6, 11, and 30, all coxsackie B viruses except B6, and coxsackieviruses A9 and A16.

# PATHOPHYSIOLOGY

After exposure, an enterovirus becomes implanted in the pharynx and the lower alimentary tract. The infection quickly spreads to the regional lymph nodes, the virus multiplies, and a minor viremia occurs on about the third day. This viremia results in involvement in many secondary infection sites, and viral multiplication in these sites coincides with the onset of clinical symptoms 4 to 6 days after exposure. As the virus multiplies at the secondary infection sites, a major viremia begins during days 3 to 7 of infection. Central nervous system (CNS) involvement may occur as a result of the initial minor viremia or it may be delayed and be the result of major viremia. Major viremia usually lasts for 3 to 7 days. Cessation of viremia correlates with the appearance of antibody and the beginning of clinical recovery. Infection may continue, however, in the lower intestinal tract for prolonged periods.

Enteroviral illnesses vary from clinically unrecognized to severe fatal illnesses. Pathologic findings are described only in the more severe illnesses. The most striking findings in severe cases are in the heart (myocarditis), the brain and spinal cord (meningitis and encephalitis), the lungs (pneumonitis), the adrenals (cortical necrosis), and the liver (hepatic necrosis).

# CLINICAL FINDINGS

Nonpolio enteroviral infections are exceedingly common in the United States. Virtually all children have one or more infections each summer and fall. There are few specific enteroviral diseases but rather a variety of interrelated syndromes and anatomically associated illnesses. Table 57-7 presents the protean clinical spectrum of disease. Many illnesses and syndromes can be caused by different coxsackieviral, echoviral, and enteroviral types, and most types can produce a variety of clinical syndromes. In a few instances, clinical characteristics indicate one or two specific enteroviral types.

## Asymptomatic Infection

Historically, the finding of enteroviruses in the stool of healthy children led to the assumption that the majority of enteroviral infections were asymptomatic. This reasoning was in error, because enteroviruses may be excreted in stool for months after acute infection, and the finding of an enterovirus on a particular day is no indication of what happened when the infection first occurred. Although most enterovirus infections appear to go unrecognized, it is likely that most affected persons have some symptoms, but usually the illnesses are trivial. The available data suggest that, on average, 50% or fewer of all infections are asymptomatic.

## Nonspecific Febrile Illness

Nonspecific febrile illness is the most common manifestation of nonpolio enteroviral infections. This illness usually has an abrupt onset without prodrome. In young children, frequently only fever and malaise are observed. In older children, headache may be noted. Fever usually lasts days and varies between 38.3 °C and 40 °C. Occasionally, the fever is biphasic. Headache, malaise, and anorexia are generally related to the degree of fever. Additional findings in nonspecific febrile illness include mild nausea, vomiting, diarrhea, and abdominal discomfort. Older patients may complain of sore throat.

In general, the findings on physical examination are benign. The usual duration of illness is 3 to 4 days with extremes of 1 to 6 days.

## Respiratory Manifestations

Respiratory manifestations are common in enteroviral infections. The most common manifestation is pharyngitis; in summer, nonpolio enteroviruses are the most common cause of this illness in children. Enteroviral pharyngitis is usually abrupt in onset. Although physical examination reveals pharyngitis early in infection, the symptoms in younger children often are not particularly referable to the throat. The usual initial complaint is fever, and young children may exhibit malaise and anorexia. Older children may complain of sore throat, headache, and myalgia. Mild vomiting or diarrhea also may occur.

Herpangina is a particular specific enteroviral pharyngitis. In addition to fever, children with herpangina have a characteristic enanthem. Vesicles and ulcers 1 to 2 mm in diameter appear on the anterior tonsillar pillars, soft palate, uvula, tonsils, pharyngeal wall, and occasionally on the posterior buccal surfaces. The lesions are usually discrete and average about five per patient. Some patients have only one or two lesions, others have 14 or more. The lesions are particularly characteristic when they occur on the soft palate. Early virologic studies indicated several coxsackieviruses A as the causative agents. Subsequent study indicated that in addition to coxsackieviruses A, most coxsackieviruses B and many echoviruses also cause herpangina.

The common respiratory viral illnesses of children that involve areas below the pharynx (croup, bronchitis, bronchiolitis, infectious asthma, pneumonia) may in sporadic instances be due to enteroviral infections. Except for pneumonia, these illnesses, when caused by enteroviruses, are generally more mild than their counterparts caused by typical respiratory viral agents.

A specific enteroviral illness of the respiratory tract is pleurodynia (Bornholm disease). Historically, pleurodynia was an epidemic disease with the majority of cases occurring in older children and young adults. Today in the United States, most cases occur sporadically and outbreaks are rare. Most cases in adults are probably diagnosed incorrectly. The onset of illness is characterized by sudden occurrence of pain typically located in the chest or upper abdomen. It is muscular in origin and of variable intensity. Often, the pain is excruciatingly severe and sudden and is associated with profuse sweating. The patient may appear pale, as though in shock. The pain events occur in spasms that last from a few minutes to several hours. During spasms, patients usually have rapid shallow and grunting respirations that suggest pneumonia or pleural inflammation. In older children and adults, the pain is often described as stabbing or knife-like; in adults, the illness can be confused with a heart attack. The symptoms usually last only 1 to 2 days, but frequently the illness is biphasic, so a patient apparently recovers only to have a recurrence several days later.

## Gastrointestinal Manifestations

Gastrointestinal manifestations are almost universal in nonpolio enteroviral infections. Some manifestations such as nausea, vomiting, and diarrhea are very common but usually not severe and are only a part of a more general overall illness. On the other hand, abdominal pain may be a striking specific finding of enteroviral infections in young children.

## Eye Findings

Mild conjunctivitis occurs frequently in many enteroviral illnesses, but in these illnesses it is usually not troublesome. A specific acute hemorrhagic conjunctivitis, however, occurs in major epidemics. This illness is caused mainly by enterovirus 70 but has also been caused by coxsackievirus A24. Most epidemics have occurred in tropical and semitropical countries, but more recently

## TABLE 57-7. Clinical Manifestations of Nonpolio Enteroviruses

| Clinical Categories | Virus Types | | |
| --- | --- | --- | --- |
| | Coxsackieviruses A | Coxsackieviruses B | Echoviruses and Enteroviruses |
| Nonspecific febrile illness | All types | All types | All types |
| Respiratory | | | |
| Common cold | Mainly 21, 24; rarely other types | Mainly 1–5; rarely 6 | Mainly 2, 20; rarely other types |
| Pharyngitis (pharyngitis, tonsillitis, tonsillopharyngitis, and nasopharyngitis) | Probably all types; mainly 9 | Probably all types; mainly 1–5 | Probably all types; mainly 2, 4, 6, 9, 11, 16, 19, 25, 30, 71 |
| Herpangina | 1–10, 16, 22 | 1–5 | 6, 9, 16, 17, 22, 25 |
| Lymphonodular pharyngitis | 10 | | |
| Stomatitis and other lesions in the anterior mouth | 5, 9, 10, 16 | 2, 5 | 9, 11, 20, 71 |
| Parotitis | Coxsackievirus A not typed | 3, 4 | 70 |
| Croup | 9 | 4,5 | 4, 11, 21 |
| Bronchitis | | 1, 4 | 8, 12–14 |
| Bronchiolitis and asthmatic bronchitis | Many types | Many types | Many types |
| Pneumonia | 9, 16 | 1–5 | 6, 7, 9, 11, 12, 19, 20, 30 |
| Pleurodynia | 1, 2, 4, 6, 9, 16 | 1–6 | 1–3, 6–9, 11, 12, 14, 16–19, 23–25, 30 |
| Gastrointestinal | | | |
| Nausea and vomiting | 9, 16 | 2–5 | 2, 4, 6, 9, 11, 16, 18–20, 22, 30 |
| Diarrhea | 1, 9, 16 | 2–5 | 3, 4, 6, 7, 9, 11–14, 16–22, 25, 30 |
| Constipation | 9 | 3–5 | 4, 6, 9, 11 |
| Abdominal pain | 9, 16 | 2–5 | 4, 6, 9, 11, 18, 19, 30 |
| Pseudoappendicitis | | | 1, 8, 14 |
| Peritonitis | | 1 | |
| Mesenteric adenitis | | 5 | 7, 9, 11 |
| Appendicitis | | 2, 5 | |
| Intussusception | | 3 | 7, 9 |
| Hepatitis | 4, 9, 10, 20, 24 | 1–5 | 1, 3, 4, 6, 7, 9, 11, 14, 20, 21, 30, 72 |
| Reye syndrome | 2 | 4 | 14, 22 |
| Pancreatitis | 9 | 3–5 | |
| Diabetes mellitus | | 1–5 | |
| Acute hemorrhagic conjunctivitis | 24 | | 70 |
| Pericarditis and myocarditis | 1, 2, 4, 5, 7–10, 16 | 1–5 | 1, 4, 6–9, 11, 14, 17, 19, 22, 25, 30 |
| Genitourinary | | | |
| Orchitis and epididymitis | | 1–5 | 6, 9, 11 |
| Nephritis | | 4 | 6, 9 |
| Hemolytic-uremic syndrome | 4, 9 | 2–5 | 22 |
| Pyuria, hematuria, or proteinuria | | 5 | 1, 6, 9 |
| Myositis and arthritis | 2, 9 | 4 | 9, 18, 24 |
| Exanthem | 2–5, 7, 9, 10, 16 | 1–5 | 1–7, 9, 11, 13, 14, 16–19, 21, 22, 24, 25, 30, 32, 33, 71 |
| Neurologic manifestations | | | |
| Aseptic meningitis | 1–14, 16–18, 21, 22, 24 | 1–6 | 1–9, 11–27, 29–33, 71 |
| Encephalitis | 2, 4–7, 9, 10, 16 | 1–5 | 1–9, 11–25, 27, 30, 33, 71 |
| Paralysis (lower motor neuron involvement) | 2, 4–7, 9–11, 14, 21 | 1–6 | 1–4, 6–9, 11, 12, 14, 16–19, 25, 27, 30, 31, 70, 71 |
| Guillain-Barré syndrome and transverse myelitis | 2, 4–6, 9, 16 | 1–4 | 6, 7, 19, 22, 70 |
| Cerebellar ataxia | 4, 7, 9 | 3, 4 | 6, 9, 16 |
| Peripheral neuritis | | | 9 |

Modified with permission from Cherry JD. Enteroviruses. In: Nelson's textbook of pediatrics, ed 13. Philadelphia: WB Saunders, 1987:689.

epidemics have occurred in the continental United States. During epidemics, the highest attack rate is in school-aged children. The illness has a sudden onset with severe eye pain, photophobia, blurred vision, lacrimation, erythema and congestion of the eye, and edematous and chemotic lids. Subconjunctival hemorrhages occur, and transient punctate epithelial keratitis, conjunctival follicles, and preauricular lymphadenopathy are noted frequently. Systemic symptoms, including fever, are rare. The illness lasts 7 to 12 days. In a few cases, a paralytic illness that is poliomyelitis-like or Guillain-Barré-like follows enterovirus 70 acute hemorrhagic conjunctivitis.

## Cardiovascular Manifestations

Pericarditis and myocarditis are infrequent but important severe manifestations of nonpolio enteroviruses. The Group B coxsackieviruses have been most frequently implicated. Group B coxsackieviruses are also an etiologic factor in some cases of acute myocardial infarction in young adults.

## Genitourinary Manifestations

Group B coxsackieviruses are second only to mumps as causative agents of orchitis. Orchitis frequently occurs as a second phase in a biphasic illness; the initial phase is usually nonspecific febrile illness, aseptic meningitis, or pleurodynia. Other rare genitourinary findings associated with nonpolio enterovirus infections are listed in Table 57-7.

## Muscle and Joint Manifestations

After intraperitoneal inoculation of suckling mice, Group A coxsackieviruses routinely cause myositis; these viruses, therefore, have been candidates for muscle infection in humans. Although myalgia is a common complaint of illness due to nonpolio enteroviruses, myositis associated with human enteroviral infections has been documented only in persons with immunologic disorders. In particular, dermatomyositis-like syndromes due to echoviral infections have been noted in children with agammaglobulinemia.

Arthritis has occasionally been reported in association with enteroviral infections.

## Skin Manifestations

The nonpolio enteroviruses cause a variety of skin manifestations. Specific exanthematous manifestations by frequency of viral type are listed in Table 57-8. In summer and fall, enteroviruses are the leading cause of exanthem in children.

Echovirus 9 is the agent most commonly associated with exanthem in children. This exanthem is erythematous, maculopapular, and usually discrete. Often it is petechial and is noted in association with aseptic meningitis. The illness mimics meningococcemia. Other enteroviruses cause petechial and purpuric rashes (see Table 57-8), and these can be confused with septicemic illnesses.

The hand, foot, and mouth syndrome, which is most commonly caused by coxsackievirus A16, is a clearly recognizable enteroviral illness. The exanthem is predominantly vesicular and located on the hands, feet, and buttocks. The enanthem usually involves the anterior mouth and consists of large ulcerative lesions.

## Neurologic Manifestations

Neurologic illness is common in nonpolio enteroviral infections; aseptic meningitis is the most common (see Table 57-7). The most

common causes of aseptic meningitis are coxsackieviruses A9, B2, B4, and B5 and echoviruses 4, 6, 9, 30, and 33.

Paralytic illness similar to that caused by polioviruses is also an occasional manifestation of the nonpolio enteroviruses. Paralysis due to the nonpolio enteroviruses is usually less severe and causes less residual damage. Recently, there have been outbreaks of illness due to enterovirus 71.

## Neonatal Infections

Nonpolio enteroviral infections in neonates result in a wide variety of clinical manifestations. Although these neonatal infections may be mild, a significant number are particularly severe, and deaths are not uncommon. In particular, the infections may be generalized with both myocarditis and meningoencephalitis. Outbreaks have occurred in newborn nurseries.

Of particular importance is a sepsis-like illness that can be the manifestation of several different nonpolio enteroviruses. This illness is characterized by fever, poor feeding, abdominal distention, irritability, rash, lethargy, and hypotonia. Patients also may have diarrhea, vomiting, seizures, and apnea. Severe fatal illness is most often due to echovirus 11. In fatal cases, jaundice, hepatitis, disseminated intravascular coagulation, thrombocytopenia, and hypotension occur.

### Chronic Enteroviral Infections in Patients With Agammaglobulinemia

Chronic unusual infections in agammaglobulinemia children due to a variety of enteroviruses have been reported. The most common illness is meningoencephalitis; arthritis and polymyositis also frequently occur. Echovirus 11 has been the most common cause of chronic infection, but 19 other types have also been causative.

## DIAGNOSIS

The clinical differentiation of enteroviral disease is frequently thought to be impossible. When all the circumstances of a particular illness are considered, however, enteroviral diseases can often be suspected on clinical grounds. The most important factors in the clinical diagnosis are the season of the year, geographic location, exposure, incubation period, and clinical symptoms.

Because some enteroviral infections mimic severe but treatable bacterial illnesses (meningitis and septicemia), there are frequent situations in which treatment with antimicrobial therapy should be administered until a bacterial etiology is ruled out.

All hospital viral diagnostic laboratories should have facilities for the recovery of the majority of enteroviruses that cause illness. Laboratories not so equipped should send specimens to a reference laboratory. In general, in suspected enteroviral illness, specimens should be collected from multiple sites. In all cases, material from the throat and a stool specimen should be collected. If possible, the site of the major clinical manifestation should also be cultured (cerebrospinal fluid, pericardial fluid).

Contrary to popular belief, many common enteroviruses grow rapidly in tissue culture, so isolation of an enterovirus as a cause of a specific illness frequently takes less than a week. The identification of an isolated enterovirus is more difficult and can take much longer. Nucleic acid hybridization techniques and polymerase chain reaction hold future promise for rapid detection of enteroviral infections.

Except in special circumstances, the use of serologic techniques in the primary diagnosis of suspected enteroviral infections is impractical; therefore, every effort should be made to culture for virus as early as possible in an illness. Many commercial laboratories offer serologic diagnostic panels for enteroviruses. These

## TABLE 57-8. Clinical Exanthematous Manifestations of Coxsackieviruses and Echoviruses

| Clinical Feature | Virus Subgroup | Associated Viral Agents and Prevalence of Manifestation | | |
|---|---|---|---|---|
| | | Common | Occasional | Rare |
| Macular rash | Coxsackievirus A | | | |
| | B | | 1, 2, 5 | |
| | Echovirus and enterovirus | | 2, 4, 5, 13, 14, 17, 19, 30 | 18, 71 |
| Maculopapular rash | Coxsackievirus A | 9 | 2, 4, 5, 10, 16 | 6, 7 |
| | B | | 1–5 | |
| | Echovirus and enterovirus | 4, 9 | 2, 5–7, 11, 16–19, 25, 30, 71 | 1, 3, 13, 14, 22, 27, 33 |
| Vesicular rash | Coxsackievirus A | 5, 16 | 8–10 | 4, 7 |
| | B | | | 1–3, 5 |
| | Echovirus and enterovirus | | 11 | 6, 9, 17, 71 |
| Petechial or purpuric rash | Coxsackievirus A | 9 | 4 | |
| | B | | 2–5 | |
| | Echovirus | 9 | 4, 7 | 3 |
| Urticarial rash | Coxsackievirus A | 9 | 16 | |
| | B | | 4, 5 | |
| | Echovirus | | 11 | |
| Erythema multiforme or Stevens-Johnson syndrome | Coxsackievirus A | | 9 | 10, 16 |
| | B | | | 4, 5 |
| | Echovirus | | | 6, 11 |
| Exanthem and meningitis | Coxsackievirus A | | 2, 9 | 7 |
| | B | 1, 2, 4, 5 | | |
| | Echovirus and enterovirus | 4, 9 | 6, 11, 17, 18, 25, 30 | 3, 14, 33, 71 |
| Exanthem and pneumonia | Coxsackievirus A | | 9 | 7 |
| | B | | | 1 |
| | Echovirus | | | 9, 11 |
| Hand, foot, and mouth syndrome | Coxsackievirus A | 16 | 5, 10 | 7, 9 |
| | B | | | 1, 3, 5 |
| | Echovirus and enterovirus | | | 71 |
| Hemangioma-like lesions | Coxsackievirus A | | | |
| | B | | | |
| | Echovirus | | | 25, 32 |
| Herpangina and exanthem | Coxsackievirus A | | 4 | 9 |
| | B | | | 2 |
| | Echovirus | | 16, 17 | |
| Roseola-like illness | Coxsackievirus A | | | 6, 9 |
| | B | | 5 | 1, 2, 4 |
| | Echovirus | | 16, 25 | 9, 11, 27, 30 |
| Anaphylactoid purpura | Coxsackievirus A | | | 4 |
| | B | | | |
| | Echovirus | | | 9, 18 |
| Zoster-like rash | Coxsackievirus A | | | |
| | B | | | |
| | Echovirus | | | 5, 6 |
| Pityriasis-like rash | Coxsackievirus A | | | |
| | B | | | |
| | Echovirus | | | 6 |
| Chronic or recurrent rash | Coxsackievirus A | 16 | | |
| | B | | | |
| | Echovirus | | | 11 |

*Cherry JD. Enteroviruses: polioviruses (poliomyelitis), coxsackieviruses, echoviruses. In: Feigin RD, Cherry JD, eds. Textbook of pediatric infectious diseases, ed 3. Philadelphia: WB Saunders, 1992:1720. Used with permission.*

panels are expensive and lack specificity, leading to erroneous diagnoses. In certain circumstances, when specific etiologies are suspected, antibody titer rises or specific IgM enteroviral antibody tests may be useful in confirming a clinical diagnosis.

## THERAPY

There is no specific therapy for any nonpolio enteroviral infection. It has been shown recently that commercially available immune globulins contain antibodies to most enteroviruses. In severe catastrophic enteroviral infections such as those that occur in neonates, it is reasonable to administer intravenous immune globulin to the infant, but there is no evidence that this therapy is beneficial. Immune globulin has a limited beneficial effect in the treatment of subacute and chronic enteroviral infections in patients with immune deficiencies.

## PREVENTION

Because highly effective killed and live viral vaccines for the polioviruses have been extraordinarily effective, it is clear that similar vaccines could be developed for other enteroviruses. If a specifically virulent enteroviral type were to emerge, a new vaccine could be developed.

Passive protection with human immune globulin should be considered in nursery outbreaks of severe enteroviral disease. There is some evidence that immune serum was useful in the management of two nursery enteroviral outbreaks.

### Selected Readings

Centers for Disease Control. Case of paralytic illness associated with enterovirus 71 infection. MMWR 1988;37:107.
Centers for Disease Control. Acute hemorrhagic conjunctivitis caused by coxsackie A24 variant—Puerto Rico. MMWR 1988;37:123.
Cherry JD. Enteroviruses: polioviruses (poliomyelitis), coxsackieviruses, echoviruses and enteroviruses. In: Feigin RD, Cherry JD, eds. Textbook of pediatric infectious diseases, ed 3. Philadelphia: WB Saunders, 1992:1705.
Cherry JD. Enteroviruses. In: Remington JS, Klein JO, eds. Infectious diseases of the fetus and newborn infant, ed 3. Philadelphia: WB Saunders, 1990:325.
Cherry JD. Viral exanthems. Curr Probl Pediatr 1983;13(6):1.
Gilbert GL, Dickson KE, Waters MJ, et al. Outbreak of enterovirus 71 infection in Victoria, Australia, with a high incidence of neurologic involvement. Pediatr Infect Dis J 1988;7:484.
Kinney JS, McCray E, Kaplan JE, et al. Risk factors associated with echovirus 11' infection in a hospital nursery. Pediatr Infect Dis J 1986;5:192.
Rabkin CS, Telzak EE, Ho MS, et al. Outbreak of echovirus 11 infection in hospitalized neonates. Pediatr Infect Dis J 1988;7:186.
Rotbart HA. Nucleic acid detection systems for enteroviruses. Clin Microbiol Rev 1991;4:156.

*Principles and Practice of Pediatrics, Second Edition.*
edited by Frank A. Oski et al. J. B. Lippincott Company, Philadelphia © 1994.

# 57.11 *Infectious Mononucleosis*

### Ciro V. Sumaya

Although there are earlier accounts, the clinical entity of infectious mononucleosis was first clearly identified in the 1920s. A few years later the hematologic abnormalities in lymphocytes that characterize infectious mononucleosis were described in detail. In the 1930s, a heterophil antibody response was detected in patients with infectious mononucleosis, as well as in patients with other illnesses. A differential absorptive step was subsequently developed that distinguished the heterophil antibody response of infectious mononucleosis from that of noninfectious mononucleosis disorders. In 1968, Epstein-Barr virus (EBV), an agent discovered a few years earlier in laboratory cultures of Burkitt lymphoma cells, was first identified as the cause of classic infectious mononucleosis.

## PATHOPHYSIOLOGY

EBV enters the body through salivary exchange and undergoes a replicative cycle in oropharyngeal epithelium. Thereafter, blood invasion occurs by selective infection of B lymphocytes, a cell population that has specific surface receptors for the virus. During acute infectious mononucleosis, 1 in 5000 (.02%) lymphocytes becomes infected with the virus. During convalescence, this number declines to 1 in 10 million or less. Following infectious mononucleosis or other forms of initial (primary) EBV infections, including subclinical infections, a lifelong infection of B lymphocytes is produced regularly by the virus. The latent infection in peripheral blood B lymphocytes and presumably other sites of B cell deposits appears to depend on the continual viral replicative cycle in the oropharyngeal epithelium. EBV also has been detected in cervical epithelium. The role that cervical EBV plays in the replicative or latent phases of EBV infection in the human host is unknown.

An intense host immune response characteristically develops in patients with acute infectious mononucleosis. Specific features of this response include an increase in T8 lymphocytes (suppressor cells), which reduces the T4/T8 (helper/suppressor) lymphocyte ratio (Fig 57-10); the formation of atypical lymphocytes within the T cell population; a transient decrease in IgM- and IgD-bearing B lymphocytes, possibly reflecting interference in the production of these cells or their elimination by activated T lymphocytes; and both viral-specific and heterologous antibody formation. Diminished or absent cutaneous hypersensitivity reactions are noted during the acute episode and for several weeks after the clinical onset of infectious mononucleosis. The onset of symptoms of infectious mononucleosis appears to coincide with the host immune response. Exaggerated immune responses have been theorized to produce serious complications or sequelae from the EBV infection. Excessive T suppressor cell activity is suspected to result in hypogammaglobulinemia or aplasia of various bone marrow elements. Conversely, an abnormally weakened immune response has been considered responsible for the development of disseminated lymphoproliferative lesions or lymphomas.

Several age-related differences exist in the humoral and cellular host immune responses during infectious mononucleosis. Very young children (younger than 4 years old) tend to have less intense T8 responses, smaller numbers of atypical lymphocytes, and less intense EBV-related IgM responses, both EBV-specific and heterophil antibodies. The immune responses that develop in children or adults with subclinical or other forms of EBV infections are not well defined.

EBV is detected in the oropharyngeal salivary secretions in approximately 75% of children with acute infectious mononucleosis. This rate of EBV excretion does not decrease appreciably in the 6 to 12 months after the clinical onset of an infectious mononucleosis episode. The role that this high rate of persistent viral excretion plays in actual transmission of the virus is not known. The prevalence or persistence of oropharyngeal viral excretion associated with other acute clinical or subclinical forms of EBV infections has not been adequately studied. Approximately 6% to 16% of seropositive adults and a smaller percentage of seropositive children in the general population, however, have

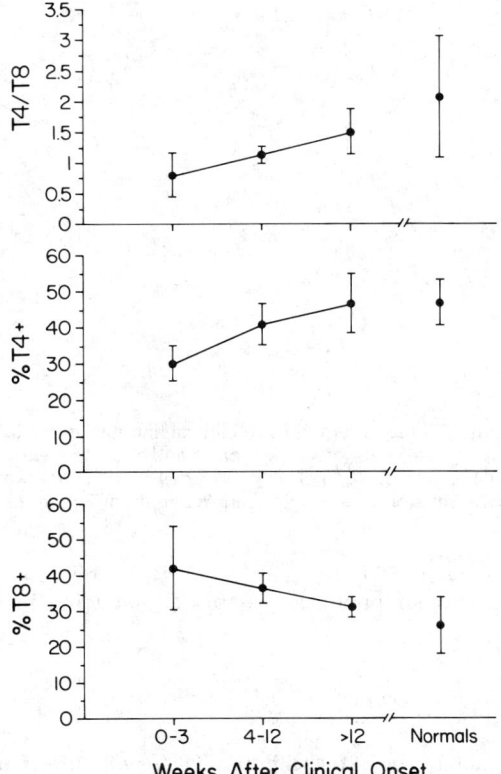

**Figure 57-10.** Changes in lymphocyte subsets in 11 children during the course of infectious mononucleosis. The mean values (±1 SD) for percentage T8+ lymphocytes, percentage T4+ lymphocytes, and ratio of T4/T8 lymphocytes are compared to those for 10 normal children. (Weigle KA, Sumaya CV, Montiel M. J Clin Immunol 1983;3:151. Reproduced by permission of Plenum Publishing Corporation.)

detectable EBV in oropharyngeal secretions. Immunosuppression considerably increases the prevalence of oropharyngeal EBV.

## TRANSMISSION

Factors influencing EBV transmission and the development of symptoms are obscure. For example, EBV infectious mononucleosis occurs uncommonly among intimate contacts of an index patient. In studies in adults, it has been noted that the high proportion of nonimmune persons among these contacts could account for this finding, although it also appears that risk for developing infectious mononucleosis or even an asymptomatic EBV infection is minimal among susceptible family or college student contacts of an adult index patient. In contrast, small outbreaks of EBV infectious mononucleosis in closed populations have been reported. Moreover, EBV must spread efficiently because most of the population is infected during childhood, particularly in developing countries.

One large study notes significant EBV activity in family members with an index case of childhood EBV infectious mononucleosis. This finding suggests that adult family contacts, usually parents, may experience a reactivation of an old EBV infection prior to and, therefore, possibly responsible for the index patient's infectious mononucleosis episode. After the episode of infectious mononucleosis in the index patient, the nonimmune sibling contacts developed EBV infections, as determined by the new development of the viral-specific antibodies, at a slow rate (Fig 57-11). Specifically, 4 (15.4%) of 26 of susceptible sibling contacts developed EBV infection within 2 to 3 months after the index

episode. Overall 9 (34.65%) susceptible children developed infection later after an average observation period of 5.6 contact-months. An unanticipated high rate of infectious mononucleosis was documented with the eventual primary EBV infection of five (55.6%) of these nine nonimmune children. These findings, in addition to the high rate of EBV infectious mononucleosis episodes in sibling contacts (a variable period of time before the enrolled "index" case and at a time before the study was in progress), indicate that the relative risk that a child will develop infectious mononucleosis with a primary EBV infection is substantially increased when a sibling has experienced this disease in the past. The reason is unknown. Why an increased rate of infectious mononucleosis is also manifested in primary EBV infections that do not develop until young adulthood is likewise unknown.

Transmission of EBV via blood products and subsequent development of infectious mononucleosis-like disease occurs, but at a much lower rate than that seen with cytomegalovirus.

The incubation period between viral exposure and development of infectious mononucleosis is usually 5 to 7 weeks. The incubation period is shortened by a few weeks if the exposure to EBV was via a blood transfusion.

Earlier reports on the incidence of infectious mononucleosis usually included cases with positive heterophil antibody responses. Findings from these studies showed the incidence of infectious mononucleosis was highest in young adults between 15 and 22 years of age. Cases in young children, particularly those younger than 4 years of age—a group more likely to lack the heterophil antibody response, may have been excluded from the incidence figures. More recent findings incorporating EBV-specific antibody testing suggest the frequency of infectious mononucleosis in children, including preschoolers, may be more common than previously considered.

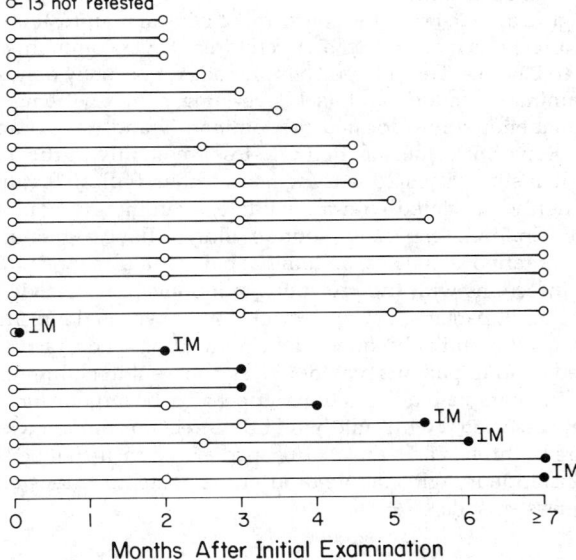

**Figure 57-11.** Surveillance of 39 sibling contacts who lacked antibodies to EBV (ie, seronegative [O]) at the initial examination performed during acute EBV infectious mononucleosis of the index patient. A routine second examination was performed 2 to 3 months after the first. Contacts who remained seronegative may have been examined on later occasions. EBV seroconversion (ie, the development of EBV antibodies) is indicated by ●. Siblings who manifested infectious mononucleosis during the seroconversion event are noted. In one sibling (◑) only, a serum IgM antibody response to EBV capsid antigen was detected at the initial examination, but this child shortly thereafter developed infectious mononucleosis along with other antibody responses typical of a primary EBV infection. (Sumaya CV, Ench Y. J Infect Dis 1986;154:842. Reproduced by permission of The University of Chicago Press.)

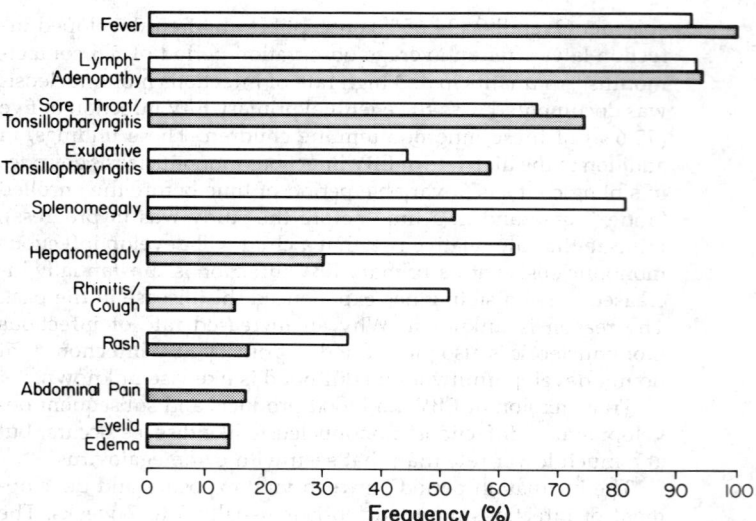

## CLINICAL MANIFESTATIONS

Acute symptomatic primary EBV infection is not synonymous with infectious mononucleosis unless a minimum of typical clinical, hematologic, and serologic findings is present. Clinical manifestations should include fever, malaise, cervical lymphadenitis, tonsillopharyngitis, and spleen or liver enlargement. Minimal hematologic features include a relative lymphocytosis of at least 50% and a relative atypical lymphocytosis of at least 10% of all leukocytes, or at least an absolute concentration of total lymphocytes of greater than or equal to 5000/mm³ or atypical lymphocytes greater than or equal to 1000/mm³. Serologic criterion is a characteristic heterophil antibody response or development of EBV-specific antibodies.

Figure 57-12 shows the spectrum of clinical manifestations of EBV infectious mononucleosis in children. Fever commonly lasts for 1 to 2 weeks. The enlarged lymph nodes are usually nontender or minimally tender and lack overlying skin erythema. The lymphadenopathy is located predominantly and most dramatically along both sides of the neck, less frequently in the axillae or other sites. Tonsillopharyngitis, another typical feature, is commonly associated with an exudate, even in very young patients. Children, especially young children, have a greater rate of "spontaneous" rashes, abdominal pain, and upper respiratory tract infections with the infectious mononucleosis episode than young adult patients. Yet, the correlation between administration of ampicillin and subsequent development of a skin rash as reported in adult patients may not be as apparent in children. Certain uncommon manifestations appear to be unique or more closely associated with childhood EBV infectious mononucleosis: failure to thrive, early-onset otitis media, and recurrent episodes of tonsillopharyngitis before or after the acute infectious mononucleosis episode.

## GENERAL LABORATORY FINDINGS

Although a minimal quantity of atypical lymphocytes (discussed above) is essential for the diagnosis of infectious mononucleosis, the mean relative percentage of these cells in affected children, particularly those younger than 4 years old, tends to be lower than in young adult patients. The concomitant relative neutropenia seen acutely often is quite severe. In one report, a segmented band form count of less than 500/mm³ was detected in 10.6% of children younger than 4 years old and in 6.1% of older children. Serum transaminase levels are moderately elevated, although not

usually above 600 U/dL, in at least 50% of children during an acute infectious mononucleosis episode. Jaundice, however, is rare.

## COMPLICATIONS

Approximately one in five children (20%) with infectious mononucleosis develop one or more significant complications involving mainly the respiratory, neurologic, and hematologic systems (Table 57-9). The thrombocytopenia may be due to increased de-

**TABLE 57-9. Complications Present in Childhood Epstein-Barr Virus Infectious Mononucleosis**

| Complication | No. of Children (%) |
|---|---|
| Respiratory tract | |
| Pneumonia | 6 (5.3) |
| Severe airway obstruction* | 4 (3.5) |
| Neurologic | |
| Seizures | 4 (3.5) |
| Meningitis/encephalitis | 2 (1.8) |
| Peripheral facial nerve paralysis | 1 (0.9) |
| Guillain-Barré syndrome | 1 (0.9) |
| Hematologic | |
| Thrombocytopenia with hemorrhages | 4 (3.5) |
| Hemolytic anemia | 1 (0.9) |
| Infectious | |
| Bacteremia | 1 (0.9) |
| Recurrent tonsillopharyngitis | 3 (2.7) |
| Liver: jaundice | 2 (1.8) |
| Renal: glomerulonephritis | 1 (0.9) |
| Genital: orchitis | 1 (0.9) |
| Total | 31† |

\* Criteria consisted of nasal alar flaring, suprasternal retractions, or stridor.
† Because four children had more than one of these complications, this total is composed of 24 different children, or 21.2% of the study group.

*Sumaya CV, Ench Y. Epstein-Barr virus infectious mononucleosis in children: I. Clinical and general laboratory findings. Pediatrics 1985;75:1003. Reproduced by permission of the American Academy of Pediatrics.*

struction by the enlarged spleen, to antiplatelet antibodies, or to predisposing abnormal platelet function. The airway obstruction is primarily due to the intense inflammation and hypertrophy of lymphoid tissue in Waldemeyer's ring and surrounding areas. It is believed that the virus harbored within B lymphocytes can enter the nervous system to produce the neurologic manifestations. Complications usually develop during or shortly after the peak of clinical illness. They may also develop during early convalescence or, as is not uncommon in the case of petechial rashes and neurologic signs, during the prodrome period. The complications characteristically last only days to a few weeks and rarely produce permanent sequelae. Splenic rupture has been noted in approximately 0.2% of adult patients; the incidence in children is not known.

Despite the frequent occurrence of severe (transitory) neutropenia in children with infectious mononucleosis, significant bacterial superinfections are uncommon. Peritonsillar abscesses have gained increased attention recently as bacterial complications during the infectious mononucleosis episode. Other uncommon complications associated with childhood infectious mononucleosis include hemolytic anemia, renal dysfunction (mainly a glomerulonephritis-like picture), Reye's syndrome, and possibly sudden hearing loss. Earlier (but not later) reports showed an increased rate of Group A *Streptococcus* in throat cultures of children with infectious mononucleosis.

Development of infectious mononucleosis during pregnancy is rarely reported. It appears that development of infectious mononucleosis or an EBV infection during pregnancy in previously susceptible mothers is infrequent. Even if infectious mononucleosis occurred during pregnancy, data indicate that the newborn is at low risk for developing a congenitally symptomatic infection. Few infants have had a documented congenital EBV infection.

## LABORATORY DIAGNOSIS

### Heterophil Antibodies

Heterophil antibodies are serum antibodies of the IgM class that can agglutinate sheep and horse erythrocytes, among others. Horse erythrocytes are the most sensitive agglutination indicators and are used in laboratory tests to detect these antibodies. Heterophil antibodies associated with infectious mononucleosis are differentiated from heterophil antibodies associated with other illnesses by their absorption to beef red blood cells (RBCs) but not guinea pig kidney.

The rapid slide test, a qualitative test, is the most widely used method to detect serum heterophil antibodies of infectious

mononucleosis. Quantitative testing by the traditional Paul-Bunnel-Davidsohn technique rarely is performed except in a research setting. An ox cell hemolysis test that is more specific but less sensitive than the agglutination tests also is rarely performed. Other recently developed techniques using purified forms of heterophil antigen—except, possibly, the immune adherence hemagglutination test—do not offer significant improvement to warrant use in routine diagnostic testing.

In one study, the frequency of serum heterophil antibody responses of children older than 4 years was found to be similar to that of young adult patients (Fig 57-13). Children younger than 4 years have appreciably lower rates of detectable heterophil antibody responses, probably related to the diminished titer of this response generally produced in this young age group. In children younger than 4 years then, the more sensitive quantitative Paul-Bunnel-Davidsohn test and possibly the immune adherence hemagglutination test are more reliable indicators of a heterophil antibody response than the rapid slide test. In the same study, children at least 4 years old had a heterophil antibody response detectable for at least 7 months after the infectious mononucleosis episode in approximately 50% of cases by the quantitative Paul-Bunnell-Davidsohn test and in 30% of cases by the rapid slide test (Fig 57-14). For younger children, the detectable antibody response at 4 months after the infectious mononucleosis episode was 15% by the Paul-Bunnell-Davidsohn test and less than 10% by the rapid slide test.

The absence of a heterophil antibody in patients with an infectious mononucleosis-like illness may pose a diagnostic problem for the clinician. Because EBV can produce an infectious mononucleosis illness without a detectable serum heterophil antibody response, a satisfactory diagnosis may require specific serologic testing for this viral agent. Moreover, some illnesses that exhibit the characteristic clinical and hematologic findings of EBV infectious mononucleosis, although lacking a heterophil antibody response, are not due to EBV.

### EBV-Specific Serologic Testing

Distinct structural or viral-associated antigens—capsid antigen, early antigen, and nuclear antigen, among others—and their corresponding antibodies have been described. The pattern of these antibody responses is an important clue to the temporal onset of EBV infection and allows discrimination of acute, convalescent, or old infection. Antibody responses are determined principally by indirect immunofluorescent techniques.

The acute phase of infectious mononucleosis is characterized by serum IgM and IgG antibody responses to EBV capsid antigen and an IgG response to EBV early antigen (Fig 57-15). The IgM

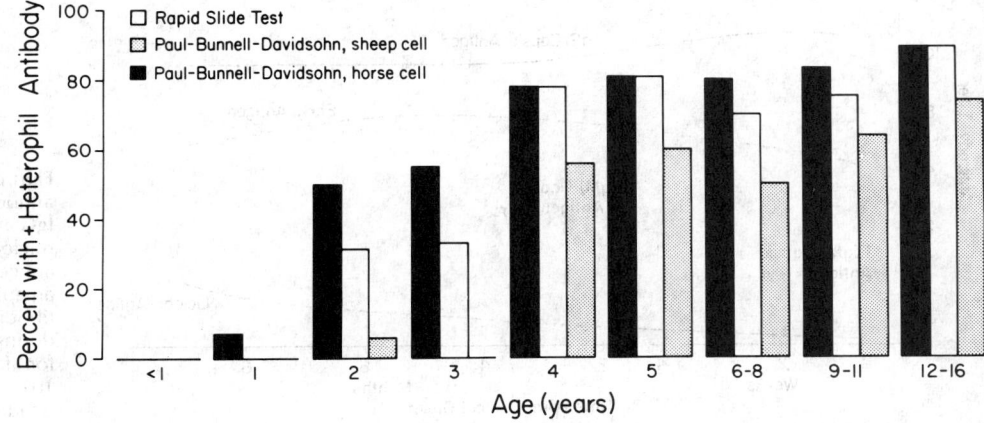

**Figure 57-13.** Frequency of acute heterophil antibody responses detected in children of varying ages with documented EBV infectious mononucleosis. Sera were examined by a qualitative method, the rapid slide test, and by a microtiter modification of a quantitative method, the Paul-Bunnell-Davidsohn differential absorption test using both sheep and horse erythrocytes as agglutination indicator cells. (Sumaya CV, Ench Y. Pediatrics 1985;75:1011. Reproduced by permission of the American Academy of Pediatrics.)

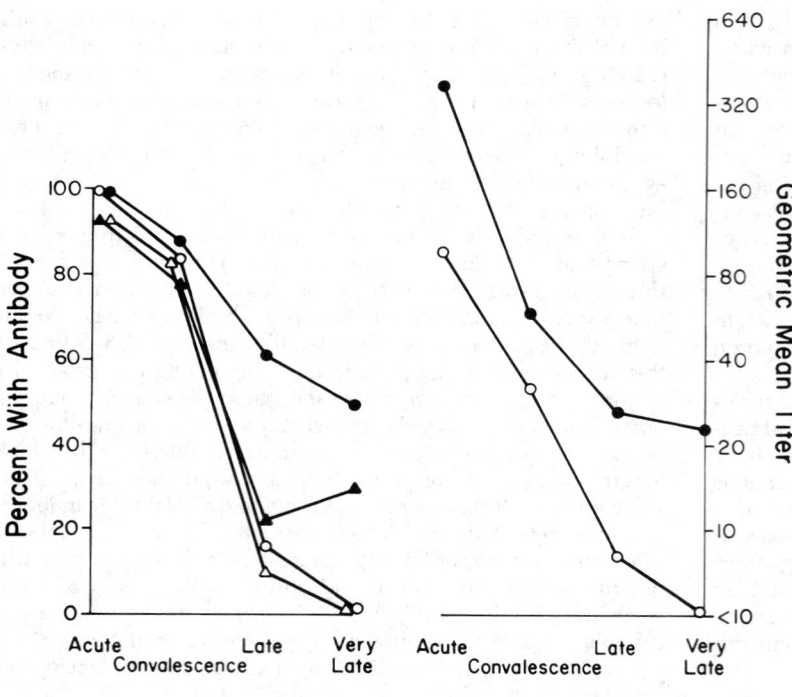

Figure 57-14. Duration of serum heterophil antibodies (left) in 53 children who developed this antibody response during acute EBV infectious mononucleosis. Children are divided into two age groups: those less than 4 years old (open symbols) and those aged 4 years and older (closed symbols). Heterophil antibody responses shown were determined by two techniques—the Paul-Bunnell-Davidsohn (PBD) test, utilizing horse cells (circles), and the rapid slide test (triangles). Results of the PBD test on sheep cells were not included. Detection of serum heterophil antibodies by PBD horse cell test in the acute phase of illness was 100%. Rapid slide test disclosed these antibodies in acute sera of 49 of the 53 children. Geometric mean titers of heterophil antibodies remaining after guinea pig absorption in the PBD horse cell test are shown right. (Sumaya CV, Ench Y. Pediatrics 1985;75:1011. Reproduced by permission of the American Academy of Pediatrics.)

response to EBV capsid antigen is transient, lasting only 1 to 2 months, or even less in very young children, while the IgG response to this antigen probably lasts for life. Of the two components of EBV early antigen, the antibody response in most patients is directed to D component. Responses directed to R component, however, are seen in approximately 20% of very young children. The antibody response to EBV early antigen components may persist for months or years as a normal consequence of the antecedent infectious mononucleosis episode. Antibodies to EBV nuclear antigen are absent usually or present only in low titer during the acute phase of infectious mononucleosis. These "late-onset" antibodies usually begin to develop weeks to months after the clinical onset of the disease and remain for life.

In most cases, a single early serum sample obtained within 3 to 4 weeks, sometimes longer, after the clinical onset of the infectious mononucleosis episode reveals an IgM antibody response and other characteristic antibody responses that can be interpreted reliably to indicate an acute primary EBV infection (Table 57-10). If properly performed, detection of IgM antibody to EBV

capsid antigen alone is probably sufficient to make an accurate diagnosis of an acute infection. It must be ascertained, however, that the serum with the positive IgM reaction to capsid antigen does not contain rheumatoid factor, which can produce false-positive IgM reactions. Commercially available methods are available to detect rheumatoid factor and alert the technician to retest the serum after it has been subjected to an absorption procedure that removes the IgG-rheumatoid factor complex. Because of potential technical problems in performing EBV serologic testing, laboratories should determine at least one more different antibody response to support the IgM antibody results. This other test probably should be determination of antibodies to EBV nuclear antigen (to demonstrate the absence or low-titer presence of this response during an acute primary infection). High titers of IgG antibody to EBV capsid antigen do not necessarily indicate an acute infection.

In the absence of an IgM antibody response, a combination of other antibody responses (or lack thereof) may suggest, although not reliably, a recent infection. Testing a second serum sample 4 to 6 weeks after the first was collected during the acute

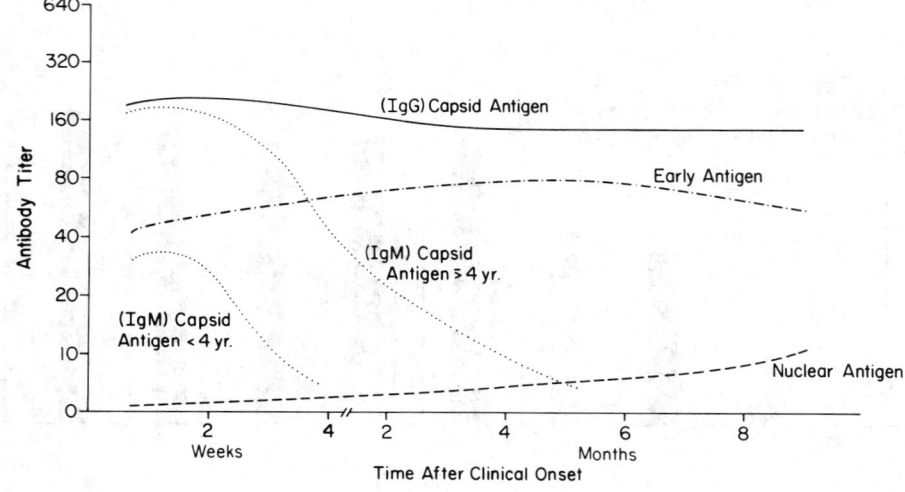

Figure 57-15. Duration of serum IgM and IgG antibody responses to EBV capsid antigen and of IgG antibody responses to EBV early antigen and nuclear antigen. Antibody response to EBV early antigen components may persist for years after an episode of EBV infectious mononucleosis. Antibodies to EBV nuclear antigen may be absent during acute infection but, once present, remain for life. (Sumaya CV, Ench Y. Pediatrics 1985;75:1011. Reproduced by permission of the American Academy of Pediatrics.)

TABLE 57-10. Interpretation of EBV Serum Antibody Patterns

| Interpretation | IgM Capsid Antigen | IgG Capsid Antigen | IgG Early Antigen | | Antinuclear Antigen |
|---|---|---|---|---|---|
| | | | D | R | |
| Susceptible | − | − | − | − | − |
| Acute primary infection (IM presentation) | + | + | + | −* | −† |
| Acute primary infection (non-IM presentation or asymptomatic) | + | + | − | + | −† |
| Old, quiescent infection | − | + | − | −‡ | +§ |
| Reactivated infection | ± | + | + or + | | +‖ |

* A few (<10%) adults and a greater number (10% to 20%) of children with acute IM develop an antibody response directed to R instead of D component.
† A low antibody titer (≤1:5 in our laboratory) may also be detected in acute infection.
‡ Occasionally a weak, probably nonspecific, antibody response to R component is present.
§ Moderate, stable titers of antibody should be present.
‖ Stable levels of antibody, although in low or absent levels in immunosuppressed and immunodeficient patients, are present.

*Sumaya CV. Epstein-Barr virus serologic testing: diagnostic indications and interpretations. Pediatr Infect Dis J 1986;5:337. Reproduced by permission of Williams & Wilkins Co.*

phase of the illness is not of much diagnostic assistance. The titers of IgG antibody to EBV capsid antigen and early antigen usually peak in the early acute serum specimen. Therefore, it is too late to detect significant IgG antibody titer rises, a practice used to retrospectively diagnose recent infections by other viruses.

Enzyme-linked immunosorbent assays (ELISAs) more recently have been developed for the laboratory diagnosis of acute EBV infections. These tests, available as kits, may use the comparative levels of IgM and IgG antibody to a peptide sequence to determine the presence of an acute EBV infection versus an old infection or nonimmune status. The reliability of these commercially available tests is not determined, particularly with sera obtained from children.

## DIFFERENTIAL DIAGNOSIS

The classic presentation of infectious mononucleosis should not produce a diagnostic problem. Diagnostic difficulties may arise early in the clinical course, however, when few typical manifestations are apparent; when a principal typical feature is absent or extremely prominent; or when an organ or system that is uncommonly (or even commonly) affected shows extensive involvement. An example that incorporates some of these difficulties is the child taken to a physician because of the acute onset of hemorrhagic lesions (ie, petechial rash) or facial nerve paralysis. A careful history and physical examination during this visit may reveal other typical signs of infectious mononucleosis; however, some typical manifestations may not be expressed until days later.

Bacterial or viral tonsillopharyngitis is a frequently encountered differential diagnostic possibility. Group A *Streptococcus*, adenoviruses, and *Corynebacterium diphtheriae* may produce a severe tonsillopharyngitis, including an exudate, along with fever and cervical adenopathy—the clinical picture resembling that of EBV infectious mononucleosis. The absence of other typical features and the more transient course of the streptococcal (treated or untreated) or viral (non-EBV) induced tonsillopharyngitis should distinguish these entities from infectious mononucleosis. The symptoms of viral hepatitis may resemble those of early infectious mononucleosis, but the lack of evolution of other characteristic features makes the distinction apparent.

Lymphocytic leukemoid reactions that may occur with pertussis or infectious lymphocytosis, among others, can produce a hematologic picture that resembles that of infectious mononucleosis. On closer examination, the hematologic changes are seen to involve mature rather than atypical lymphocytic forms.

The differential diagnosis sometimes includes lymphoproliferative disorders and acute leukemia. Certain features of these disorders—persistent fever, splenomegaly, and extreme leukocytosis with bleeding from thrombocytopenia—may strongly suggest infectious mononucleosis. Even a positive heterophil antibody reaction has been reported in rare cases.

Drug-induced hypersensitivity reactions from dilantin (phenylhydantoin derivatives) or isoniazid (INH), or serum sickness can produce a clinical picture similar to that of infectious mononucleosis. The lack of significant tonsillopharyngitis and an intense atypical lymphocytosis, or the pronounced migrating arthritis and eosinophilia seen in serum sickness, distinguish these disorders.

Other diseases with manifestations resembling those of infectious mononucleosis include acute brucellosis, secondary syphilis, leptospirosis, and the early stage of an infection with human immunodeficiency virus. Appropriate laboratory testing should differentiate these entities from infectious mononucleosis. About 11% of illnesses that fulfill or nearly fulfill the clinical and hematologic criteria of EBV infectious mononucleosis in children are not caused by EBV. *Toxoplasma gondii* or cytomegalovirus appears to be responsible for some of these infectious mononucleosis-like episodes, but a larger number are due to unidentified agents. From a diagnostic standpoint, the uniform absence of heterophil antibody in these non-EBV illnesses assists in separating them from the usual episode of EBV infectious mononucleosis. On the other hand, a heterophil antibody response may not be detected in some episodes of EBV infectious mononucleosis, particularly in very young children.

The rapid slide test used for detection of heterophil antibodies requires a subjective interpretation of the agglutination reaction. Therefore, the reliability or accuracy of the test depends principally on the experience of the reader. It is estimated that approximately 7% of readings yield false positive results. It is important, therefore, that this test not be performed unless warranted by the clinical and hematologic findings, or unless it is well recognized that this result must be considered in the total context of the clinical and hematologic findings.

## PROGNOSIS

Infectious mononucleosis is almost always a self-limited illness of several weeks' duration. Complications, if they occur, usually are transient and produce no permanent sequelae. Although an accurate figure for the mortality from infectious mononucleosis in either adults or children is not available, fatal cases appear to be rare. When deaths do occur, the causes, in decreasing order, include neurologic complications, splenic rupture, secondary infection, hepatic failure, and myocarditis, as reported in studies of predominantly young adult patients.

In a few selected individuals, often with an underlying immunocompromised state, the infectious mononucleosis episode may be prolonged and lead to serious morbidity and death.

## CHRONIC, SYMPTOMATIC DISEASE

An increasing number of accounts describe EBV infectious mononucleosis episodes that are severe and fatal or that result in significant, long-lasting problems. Patients usually have had an underlying immunologic abnormality. An X-linked lymphoproliferative syndrome characterized by a combined variable immunodeficiency and vulnerability to severe EBV infections has been described in young boys. These patients may develop fatal infectious mononucleosis, or their EBV infection may produce acquired agammaglobulinemia, aplastic anemia, or malignant B cell lymphomas. A deficiency of natural killer cells has been detected that might account for inability to control the EBV infection. Several other patients with a non-X-linked syndrome have experienced a prolonged and severe EBV infection affecting multiple organs. Renal transplant recipients may develop a severe, often fatal, infectious mononucleosis-like illness soon after transplantation or initiation of antirejection therapy, or they may develop solid tumors somewhat later after transplantation. There is increasing evidence that EBV with either its acute primary infection or subsequent activation of a previously latent state may be responsible for these lymphoproliferative lesions or lymphomas. In the more severe form of EBV infection seen with the X-linked lymphoproliferative syndrome, antiviral antibody formation may be poor or absent. Yet, in other types of patients with severe multiorgan EBV infection, the levels of IgG antibody to EBV capsid antigen and early antigen may be extremely high. Regardless of serologic response, EBV, as infectious virus or antigenic markers, may be found in saliva, peripheral blood, lymphoidal deposits, or other body tissues.

Distinct from the chronic, symptomatic disorders discussed above are several reports suggesting that chronic or continually reactivated EBV infections may cause a debilitating syndrome in adults and less commonly in children. The onset of this illness has followed, by a variable period of months or years, a classic episode of EBV infectious mononucleosis or even primary EBV infections not manifested by infectious mononucleosis. The more common clinical manifestations include extreme fatigue, neuropsychological abnormalities, persistent febrile episodes (usually low-grade), recurrent sore throats, and sometimes lymphadenopathy. Less common manifestations include weight loss, arthritis, rashes, significant allergic problems, and hepatosplenomegaly. The EBV serologic findings in these patients consist of significant IgG antibody responses to components of EBV early antigen, often with concurrent elevated titers of IgG antibody to EBV capsid antigen.

The serologic criteria initially considered indicative of this illness may be found in sera from healthy persons long after their infectious mononucleosis episode and even in normal individuals with no history of infectious mononucleosis. Subsequent studies have shown that these patients may have elevated antibody titers

to other viruses as well. Therefore, it appears more likely that the association of EBV and other viruses with this chronic debilitating illness is an epiphenomenon related to some minimal generalized immunologic disturbance.

A consensus group introduced a name for this condition, *chronic fatigue syndrome*, discarding any direct ties to EBV as an etiology. A case definition has been established to identify more clearly individuals with this chronic debilitating illness. Individuals with nonspecific symptoms ascribed to chronic fatigue syndrome should be examined for known diseases that may be serious or treatable, such as collagen vascular disorders, cancer, or psychiatric disturbances.

## TREATMENT

Measures to alleviate symptoms remain the management of choice for children (and adults) with uncomplicated infectious mononucleosis. Reduction of activity and bed rest according to the tolerance of the patient usually are recommended. Contact sports should be avoided while the spleen is palpable (ie, clinically enlarged). Although the rate of Group A *Streptococcus* infections or of tonsillopharyngitis in patients with infectious mononucleosis may be similar to the rate in the general population, and therefore perhaps not intimately involved in the acute inflammatory process, if present, this bacterial infection should probably be treated with oral penicillin or erythromycin. Ampicillin should be avoided because of the potential development of an immunologically mediated rash, although the rash may not be as common a problem in children with infectious mononucleosis as in adults.

Corticosteroids have been administered to alleviate some clinical manifestations such as fever and fatigue, but an adequate, controlled evaluation of their effects has not been performed in children or adults. Corticosteroids also have been administered to patients with severe typical manifestations or with complications such as profound thrombocytopenia and airway obstruction, with reportedly beneficial effects. The therapeutic efficacy of these drugs, however, is unclear because the therapy has been administered in a predominantly uncontrolled fashion.

Life-threatening airway obstruction produced by significant tonsillopharyngeal and upper respiratory tract inflammation commonly is treated by insertion of an artificial airway rather than by emergency tonsillectomy as it was in the past. Nonoperative treatment of splenic rupture also has increased in recent years.

Acyclovir, a new antiviral agent with efficacy against herpesviruses, does not appear to modify the clinical course of uncomplicated infectious mononucleosis, although it does reduce viral excretion. Its use in patients with severe EBV infectious mononucleosis or other severe forms of EBV infections, often due to an underlying immunologic disorder, has yielded variable results. Incidentally, no significant efficacy has been noted in the administration of acyclovir or intravenous formulations of gammaglobulin to children or adults with chronic fatigue syndrome, the condition previously associated with EBV. There have been anecdotal reports of clinical improvement of routine infectious mononucleosis with the administration of cimetidine, metronidazole, and other azole drugs. More critical evaluation of these drugs are needed before they can be indicated for the disease. An experimental EBV vaccine to prevent infection is being tested in animal models.

## Selected Readings

Davidsohn I, Lee CL. The laboratory in the diagnosis of infectious mononucleosis (with additional notes on epidemiology, etiology, and pathogenesis). Med Clin North Am 1962;46:225.

Finch SC. Clinical symptoms and signs of infectious mononucleosis. In: Carter RL,

Penman HG, eds. Infectious mononucleosis. Oxford: Backwell Scientific Publications, 1969:19.

Henle W, Henle G. Epstein-Barr virus: the cause of infectious mononucleosis. In: Biggs IM, de-The G, eds. Oncogenesis and herpesviruses. Lyon: International Agency for Research in Cancer, 1972:269.

Purtilo DT, Linder J. Oncologic consequences of impaired immune surveillance against ubiquitous viruses. J Clin Immunol 1983;3:197.

Sumaya CV. Epstein-Barr virus serologic testing: diagnostic indications and interpretations. Pediatr Infect Dis J 1986;5:337.

Sumaya CV. Serologic and virologic epidemiology of Epstein-Barr virus: relevance to chronic fatigue syndrome. Rev Infect Dis 1991;31:S19.

Sumaya CV, Ench Y. Epstein-Barr virus infectious mononucleosis in children: I. Clinical and general laboratory findings. Pediatrics 1985;75:1003.

Sumaya CV, Ench Y. Epstein-Barr virus infectious mononucleosis in children: II. Heterophil antibody and viral-specific responses. Pediatrics 1985;75:1011.

Sumaya CV, Ench Y. Epstein-Barr virus infection in families: the role of children with infectious mononucleosis. J Infect Dis 1986;154:842.

Van der Horst C, Joncas J, Ahronheim G, et al. Lack of effect of peroral acyclovir for the treatment of acute infectious mononucleosis. J Infect Dis 1991;164:788.

Weigle KA, Sumaya CV, Montiel M. Changes in T lymphocyte subsets in childhood Epstein-Barr virus infectious mononucleosis. J Clin Immunol 1983;3:151.

*Principles and Practice of Pediatrics, Second Edition.*
edited by Frank A. Oski et al. J. B. Lippincott Company, Philadelphia © 1994.

# 57.12 *Postnatal Herpes Simplex Virus*

### Steve Kohl

## THE VIRUS

Herpes simplex virus (HSV) is a moderately large virus consisting of an icosahedral capsid enclosing a core of double-stranded DNA and protein, surrounded by a lipid-containing envelope. There are two serologically distinguishable subtypes—type 1 and type 2—with approximately 50% DNA homology. Although type 1 is regarded as the "oral" type and type 2 as the "genital" type, changing sexual habits and possibly other factors blur this distinction. Thus, the virus type is not a reliable indicator of the anatomic site of isolation.

The large HSV genome (about $100 \times 10^6$ kd) encodes for more than 70 polypeptides. Replication occurs after viral penetration and uncoating by an orderly cascade of gene products. These are encoded by the immediate early genes (alpha, initiation of viral replication), early genes (beta, viral replication peptides), and late genes (gamma, often structural proteins). Several important viral-encoded enzymes (products of beta genes) such as thymidine kinase and DNA polymerase are necessary for viral DNA replication and, as is discussed subsequently, have served as important targets for antiviral compounds. There are several major viral surface structural glycoproteins (gB, gC, gD, gE, gG, gH, gI, gJ, gL), some of which (eg, gG) are type specific. Several are critical for viral-cell interaction (gB, gD, gH), while others form receptors for human complement (gC) or the Fc portion of human immunoglobulin (gE and gI) and may play a role in the pathogenicity of the virus in vivo. Most of these glycoproteins are immunogenic and may be used in type-specific serologic assays (such as gG) or for vaccine candidates (such as gB or gD). The virus is assembled in the nucleus and buds through the nuclear membrane, acquiring its envelope, and is released at the cell surface.

Like all the herpesviruses, HSV assumes a state of persistent latency after primary infection of the host. This occurs in neural tissue (ganglion). It is now clear that a limited number of RNA transcripts occur during latency (latency-associated transcripts—LATs). Their role in maintaining latency and causing recurrence is under intense investigation. Human HSV can be replicated in tissue cultures derived from a variety of species. The ready growth of HSV in the laboratory and the lack of species specificity distinguish this virus from other human herpesviruses. The rapidly progressive and relatively characteristic focal cytopathology induced by HSV in susceptible tissue cultures, coupled with reliable antigen detection techniques, permits simple, inexpensive recovery of this virus and its relatively easy identification.

## EPIDEMIOLOGY

Although highly infectious, HSV is not transmitted casually from person to person. The enveloped virions are relatively unstable at atmospheric conditions, and close interpersonal contact is usually required for transmission. HSV can be transmitted via body fluids such as saliva and certainly can be acquired by direct apposition of infected with uninfected integument or mucous membranes. For example, virus has been transferred directly between wrestlers (herpes gladiatorum), and rugby players (herpes rugbeiorum, or "scrum-pox"). Nurses and respiratory therapists may acquire HSV infections of the paronychial region (herpetic whitlow), presumably from ungloved hand contact with oropharyngeal secretions. Health-care workers may effectively transfer HSV to their patients and actually cause outbreaks of gingivostomatitis. Children may acquire HSV whitlow during gingivostomatitis by nail biting or thumb sucking. Newborns may acquire HSV infection during passage through a virus-infected birth canal. Genital and anal HSV infections are acquired and transmitted through direct contact with infected genitalia or in connection with oral–genital and oral–anal contacts. In all of these cases, transmission may occur even when the infected parties are asymptomatic and unaware of their own HSV infections. The presence of active lesions is associated with high titers of virus, which probably increases the likelihood of transmission. HSV has been isolated from the hands of patients with an oral lesion and has been shown to persist for several hours on inanimate objects or in distilled water. Nevertheless, there are few data to implicate inanimate sources as important reservoirs of virus persistence and spread.

If the uninfected exposed skin or mucous membranes are abraded, damaged, or otherwise altered, the risk of transmission and spread is enhanced. For example, burned skin is more susceptible to HSV infection than is intact skin. Infants may acquire HSV infections in the area of a diaper rash; babies with eczema are at risk for serious disseminated HSV infections (Kaposi varicelliform eruption).

The epidemiology of HSV is dominated by symptomatic and asymptomatic infection with maintenance of a huge pool of latently infected individuals. Symptomatic recurrences and asymptomatic shedding ensure continued spread of HSV. Approximately 1% of individuals shed HSV orally, and 0.2% to 0.5% of women shed HSV genitally at any time. These numbers are higher in high risks or immunocompromised individuals. Seroepidemiologic studies show that HSV infections are found in all populations. There is no definite seasonal pattern to HSV infections.

Most neonatal HSV infections are acquired from maternal genital strains, thus usually are caused by HSV-2. After the neonatal period, HSV-1 infections predominate and, depending on social and economic factors, 40% to 60% of young children of lower socioeconomic status are seropositive by age 5 years. Most of these individuals exhibit HSV-1 antibodies by adulthood.

Recent studies document HSV-1 acquisition in day-care nursery or school settings with clusters of infection and, in some cases, outbreaks of symptomatic illness in as many as 13 children per outbreak. Illness typically occurred in children 1 to 2 years of age with herpetic gingivostomatitis being the major manifestation. Studies of higher socioeconomic populations reveal seroepidemiologic evidence for HSV-1 infection in only 30% of university students. As a reflection of its association with sexual activity, the prevalence of HSV-2 increases at about the time of puberty and early adolescence. The percentage of HSV-2 seropositive adults may range from 20% to 35%.

The incidence of HSV genital infection has increased markedly in the last two decades. About 300,000 new cases a year occur in the United States. In studies of sexually active university students, 4 to 8 per 1000 acquire genital HSV infection annually.

Risk factors for HSV-2 acquisition in North America include gender (female greater than male), race (higher in blacks), lower socioeconomic status, multiple sex partners, and lack of condom use. Transmission of HSV-2 from an infected individual to an HSV-2 seronegative individual in stable heterosexual couples occurs about 10% per year. Higher rates occur from males to females (19%) and from males to HSV-1 and HSV-2 seronegative females (32%).

Reactivation of latent HSV infection is associated with a variety of influences, including exposure to sunlight (ultraviolet), certain febrile illnesses, local trauma, menstruation, and immunosuppression. These influences, therefore, define additional epidemiologic factors pertinent to HSV infections.

## PATHOGENESIS AND PATHOLOGY

HSV tends to infect cells of ectodermal origin, and, in most cases, initial viral replication occurs at the portal of entry, usually in skin or mucous membranes. The infected cells swell with intracellular edema and degenerate. The nuclei of affected cells may undergo amitotic division, leading to formation of multinucleate giant cells. Nuclei of infected cells manifest eosinophilic intranuclear inclusions. Because HSV has a predilection for cells that originate in embryonic ectoderm, these viruses may involve the central nervous system (CNS). Encephalitis may accompany or follow primary HSV infection but can also be connected with reactivation of latent virus.

The incubation period for primary infection varies from 2 to 20 days in most HSV infections. After primary HSV infection, the virus remains latent in sensory neural ganglia innervating portions of the skin or mucous membranes originally involved. Thus, an individual with recurrent HSV almost always experiences reactivation of the HSV lesions in the identical or virtually identical region. The recurrence in immunologically intact individuals is generally less severe than the primary infection. In individuals previously infected with one type of virus (eg, HSV-1, orally), infection with a second type (eg, HSV-2, genitally) is less severe than in a host who has never been infected with either. Similarly, it is possible to acquire a reinfection with the same type (eg, a second infection with a new strain of HSV-2 genitally in a patient with preexisting genital HSV-2 infection). The reinfection is generally mild and often dismissed as an endogenous recurrence. These strains can be differentiated by DNA endonuclease restriction analysis of viral isolates.

After primary HSV infection, most individuals mount a host response consisting of an early nonspecific response followed by a specific immunologic response. The former consists of mobilization of polymorphonuclear and mononuclear leukocytes to the site of infection, release of interferon and other cytokines, and activation of macrophages and natural killer cells. After several days, many types of specific antiviral antibody are produced. In the second to third week of infection, one can detect specific

cellular immunity manifested by lymphocyte blastogenesis, immune lymphokine production (as gamma-interferon, migration inhibitory factor), a positive delayed hypersensitivity skin test, and T cell cytotoxicity. In humans with cellular defects (neonates, severely malnourished infants, patients with Wiskott-Aldrich syndrome and other primary immunodeficiencies, and patients receiving transplants or immunosuppressive chemotherapy), primary HSV infection can be a disseminated, life-threatening syndrome, probably due to a defect in cell-mediated immunity of the nonspecific or specific variety.

The immune response to recurrent infection is less well characterized. It does not appear to be associated with marked alterations in antibody production, although four-fold titer rises and reemergence of IgA and IgM antiviral antibody may occur. Natural killer cell activity and lymphokine production increase, and relative defects in these and lymphocyte blastogenesis may be associated with frequent or severe recurrent infection. In the host with cellular defects, recurrences are common and of long duration and increased severity, although often not causing widespread dissemination.

## CLINICAL MANIFESTATIONS

Most infections do not cause significant or specific symptoms. The largest percentage of seropositive persons (though still harboring latent HSV) are unaware of having ever encountered these viruses. The spectrum of symptomatic HSV infections ranges from minor localized recurrences, usually at mucocutaneous junctions, to severe and even fatal illnesses.

### Gingivostomatitis

Gingivostomatitis is the most common form of HSV-induced primary illness seen in children. Symptomatic illness may occur in 30% or more of seropositive infants. It is usually seen in young children between 6 months and 3 years of age. Before age 6 months, the presence of residual maternal antibody probably modifies or prevents the appearance of recognizable symptoms in association with HSV infection. Primary gingivostomatitis in children is often acquired from a family member with active primary or recurrent oral HSV infection. Though acute gingivostomatitis caused by HSV is relatively infrequent, it is still common enough that most pediatricians become familiar with the condition and learn to distinguish this infection from herpangina.

The incubation period is a few days and the illness is ushered in by fretful behavior and fever. The infant usually refuses to eat and may even refuse fluids. Vesicular lesions appear on and around the lips, along the gingiva, on the anterior tongue, and on the anterior (hard) palate (Fig 57-16). Vesicles break down rapidly and lesions usually appear as 1- to 3-mm shallow gray ulcers on an erythematous base. The gums are generally mildly hypertrophic, ulcerated, and erythematous. They may appear friable and frequently bleed on contact. It is not uncommon for vesicles to extend about the lips and chin or down the neck in the immunologically normal child. There is often a foul smell to the breath (fetor oris). The child experiences extreme discomfort, cannot or will not eat, and if fluids are refused as well, may require hospitalization to maintain adequate hydration. The risk of dehydration is compounded by the fever that usually accompanies this syndrome. The lesions bleed easily and may become covered with a black crust. Cervical and submental nodes are often swollen and tender. The process evolves for 4 to 5 days, and resolution requires at least an additional week.

Autoinoculation may cause lesions on the hands (whitlow) and, less commonly, on the trunk or genital area.

HSV gingivostomatitis is differentiated from herpangina, a

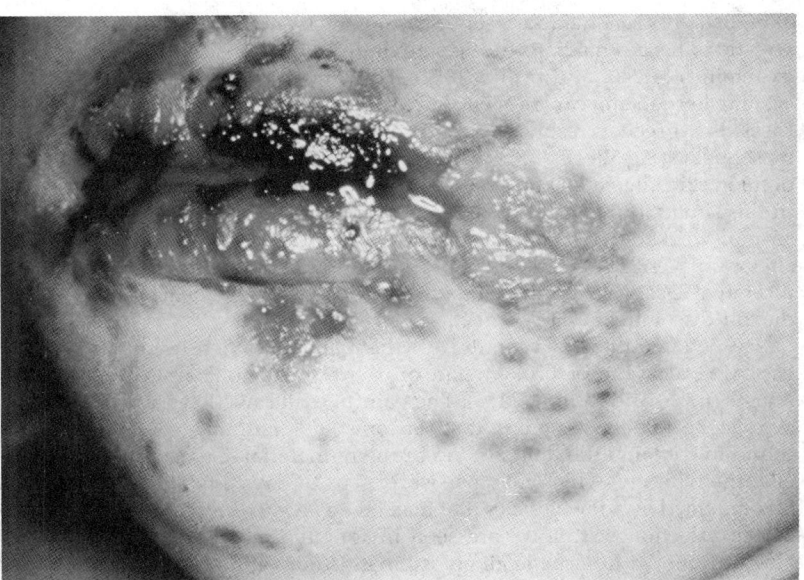

**Figure 57-16.** Primary herpes gingivostomatitis in a normal toddler at the ulcerative vesicular stage. (Kohl S. Postnatal herpes virus simplex infection. In: Feigin RD, Cherry JD, eds. Textbook of pediatric infectious diseases, ed 2. Philadelphia: WB Saunders, 1987:1577. Reproduced by permission.)

manifestation of enteroviral infection, by the predominance of ulcers in the anterior and posterior portion of the oropharynx; herpangina is usually a posterior pharyngeal ulcerative condition. In addition, unlike HSV infection, herpangina often has a more acute onset, shorter duration, and seasonal occurrence. While enteroviral-mediated hand-foot-mouth disease can present with oral ulcers and a vesicular eruption on the distal portion of extremities, the bilaterally symmetric distribution should differentiate it from HSV gingivostomatitis and concurrent HSV autoinoculation of a digit. Severe Stevens-Johnson syndrome (erythema multiforme) may mimic HSV, but the generalized macular rash with "bull's-eye" lesions are characteristic of erythema multiforme. HSV can be associated with erythema multiforme (see Erythema Multiforme and HSV Infection).

In adolescents and especially in college-aged patients, primary HSV infection often manifests as a posterior, occasionally exudative pharyngitis. The characteristic findings are shallow tonsillar ulcers with a gray exudate. In this setting, it must be differentiated from streptococcal, Epstein-Barr virus, adenovirus, and, rarely, diphtheria or tularemia-induced pharyngitis. In one study of college students of high socioeconomic status, HSV was the etiology of acute pharyngitis diagnosed most often (24%). This manifestation is most often due to HSV-1, although with the increasing frequency of oral–genital sexual practices among both heterosexual and homosexual individuals, HSV-2 pharyngitis is becoming more commonly encountered.

In view of the widespread publicity of HSV as a sexually transmitted disease, the physician is advised when making the diagnosis of HSV oral infection to anticipate these anxieties. Unless sexual contact or abuse is suspected, the physician should explain the normal mode of acquisition of oral HSV in young children.

## Vulvovaginitis

Primary herpetic vulvovaginitis may rarely occur in very young infants and children if HSV is introduced inadvertently when handling the genital area with contaminated hands. Moreover, genital herpes may reflect sexual abuse of young children. The occurrence of genital HSV in young children warrants a sensitive and careful appraisal of the family dynamics.

The incidence of genital infection in adolescents and young adults has increased markedly in the past two decades. There is a paucity of data on the incidence in children. Some 35% to 50% of patients with the first episode of genital herpes report a history of genital HSV in their contact. HSV-1 accounts for approximately 25% of primary genital HSV. The incubation period is 2 to 14 days. Primary illness is accompanied by fever, headache, malaise, and myalgias. Other systemic symptoms include an aseptic meningitis syndrome (11% to 35%). Although HSV-2 occasionally may be grown from the cerebrospinal fluid (CSF), aseptic meningitis syndrome differs from HSV-1 encephalitis in that it is generally mild, self-limited, and not associated with neurologic residua. Local genital symptoms include severe pain, itching, dysuria, vaginal or urethral discharge, and tender inguinal adenopathy. In primary illness, lesions begin as vesicles or pustules and progress to wet ulcers and then to healing ulcers with or without crusts. Crusts usually occur only on squamous epithelium. Lesions tend to last for 2 to 3 weeks before complete healing. Virus shedding occurs for a mean of 11½ days.

In addition to aseptic meningitis syndrome, complications of primary HSV genital infection include sacral autonomic nervous dysfunction manifested as poor rectal sphincter tone, constipation, sacral anesthesia, urinary retention, impotence, extragenital lesions, secondary yeast infections in women, and pharyngitis.

Beyond discomfort and embarrassment, the importance of HSV in the female genital tract relates to the potential impact of the virus on offspring, especially when a child is born to a mother with active genital lesions, particularly in connection with a primary maternal infection (see prenatal and neonatal herpesvirus infections in Chapter 20.14.3); genital ulcer lesions, including those due to HSV infection, appear to increase the risk for human immunodeficiency virus (HIV) infection. An additional consideration is the effect of HSV on the self-image of the young, sexually active patient. Although some individuals cope easily with the illness and the likelihood of recurrent disease, a sizable number exhibit profound depression, poor self-esteem, complete abstention from sexual activity, and general withdrawal. Self-help groups of individuals who have genital HSV are useful and are located in many cities of the United States.

## Other Primary HSV Skin Infections

Virtually any part of the skin and mucous membranes may be involved in HSV infections. Altered skin often provides a portal of entry for HSV. Vesicular lesions spread throughout the affected skin, usually crusting and resolving in about 1 week. In normal wrestlers, herpes gladiatorum usually involves the head (73%), extremities (42%), and trunk (28%). The illness accompanying eczema herpeticum can be severe and even fatal, though in most cases, the infection resolves without specific therapy and leaves no sequelae (Fig 57-17). Similar widespread herpetic lesions may occur in skin altered by abrasions or by thermal or chemical burns. In this situation, a secondary fever may occur, usually 1 week to several weeks after the initial insult. Careful inspection of the site or adjacent normal tissue may reveal vesicles or nonspecific ulcerative lesions. Without therapy, several of these patients have died of disseminated HSV infection.

Herpetic whitlow is a painful, erythematous, swollen lesion occurring at a site of broken skin on the terminal phalanx of fingers (69%) and thumb (21%). The painful white swellings appear to be filled with pus but when opened for drainage are found to contain little fluid and no purulent material. Occasionally, the whitlow, which may persist for 7 to 10 days, initially is accompanied by a few vesicles that may give a clue to the etiology of the infection. Whitlows are seen in four typical situations. First, infants with herpetic gingivostomatitis may autoinoculate their fingers (Fig 57-18). Second, whitlows are encountered in infants without obvious oral disease, sometimes due to infected adults kissing their children's fingers. Third, in sexually active patients, the whitlow is more often a manifestation of concurrent genital disease, which should be sought through appropriate history and physical examination. Fourth, dentists, respiratory therapists, nurses, and pediatricians who sometimes examine oral cavities or handle secretion-contaminated material without

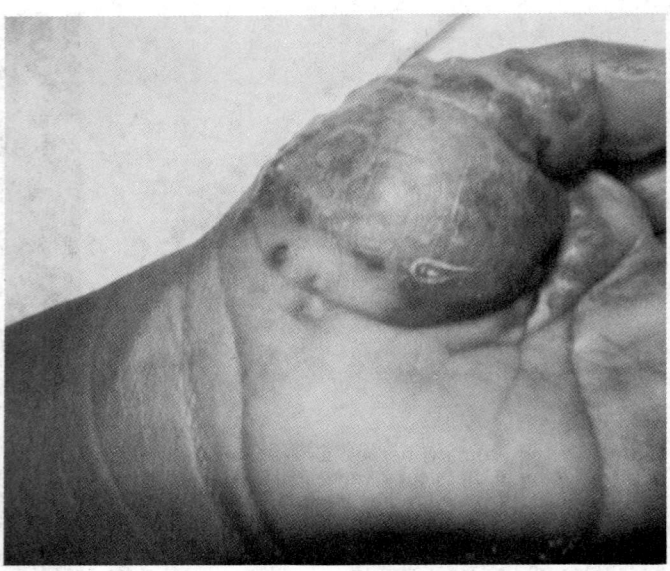

**Figure 57-18.**   Herpetic whitlow in a toddler with oral HSV infection. (Kohl S. Postnatal herpes simplex virus infection. In: Feigin RD, Cherry JD, eds. Textbook of pediatric infectious diseases, ed 2. Philadelphia: WB Saunders, 1987:1566. Reproduced by permission.)

wearing gloves are at risk for herpetic whitlow. Because of the epidemiology of HSV, whitlow in children is usually due to HSV-1. It is important that the herpetic condition be diagnosed because it usually is confused with a bacterial felon or paronychia and is incised and drained. This is not indicated in therapy of HSV whitlow. Only a needle aspiration and culture is necessary for diagnosis of herpetic whitlow. Appropriate infection control measures will lessen the spread of virus due to whitlows.

## HSV of the Eye

Primary HSV infection of the eye may manifest as a blepharitis or a follicular conjunctivitis, often accompanied by preauricular lymphadenopathy. If restricted to the conjunctiva, the infection, which can be accompanied by vesicular herpetic lesions elsewhere on the face or in the nose or mouth, usually resolves without sequelae. Herpetic infection of the eye may, however, progress to involve the cornea with more serious potential consequences. For this reason, an ophthalmologist should always examine and evaluate these cases.

Corneal involvement by HSV may manifest initially with minute vesicles at the corneal margin. The progress of corneal infection (best seen with the use of topical fluorescein dye) is marked by the appearance of branching lesions (a dendritic pattern) or the less diagnostic irregular (ameboid or geographic) ulcer. The affected child complains of severe photophobia, blurred vision, chemosis, and lacrimation. Primary eye infection may include stromal involvement, uveitis, and rarely retinitis. Spontaneous healing, which generally requires 2 to 3 weeks, can be speeded by the use of topical therapy (discussed under Therapy). Corticosteroids are contraindicated. The risk of visual impairment is enhanced with recurrences. With each bout of infection, the dendritic ulcers are more extensive and liable to result in scarring and loss of sight. Rarely in the immunocompromised host, has HSV been associated with retinal necrosis.

## HSV Infections of the CNS

HSV is the most common identifiable cause of sporadic encephalitis and is usually very serious. It accounts for 2% to 5% of all

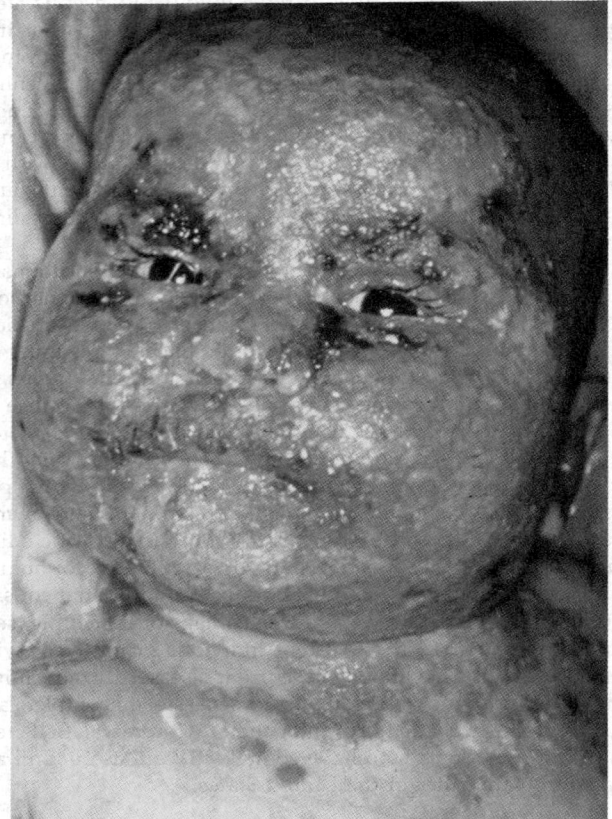

**Figure 57-17.**   Extensive HSV infection in an infant with atopic eczema (Kaposi varicelliform eruption). (Kohl S. Postnatal herpes simplex virus infection. In: Feigin RD, Cherry JD, eds. Textbook of pediatric infectious diseases, ed 2. Philadelphia: WB Saunders, 1987:1577. Reproduced by permission.)

cases of encephalitis in the United States, but for up to 20% of all etiologic diagnoses (60% to 70% of cases of encephalitis remain without a diagnosis). The case-fatality rate associated with untreated HSV encephalitis is approximately 70%, and survivors generally exhibit considerable permanent neurologic disability. The spread of HSV-1 to the CNS seems to proceed via neurogenic pathways. Although HSV encephalitis may involve virtually any area of the brain, it shows a striking tendency to involve the frontal and temporal lobes after the neonatal period.

It is important to differentiate the HSV-induced aseptic meningitis syndrome, usually due to HSV-2 and usually a complication of primary genital infection, from HSV encephalitis. In the former, signs of meningitis, including headache, photophobia, and stiff neck, appear shortly after genital lesions are noted. Seizures and focal CNS findings are usually absent. The CSF examination reveals a lymphocytosis (with 300 to 2600 white blood cells [WBCs] per cubic millimeter) and sometimes a low glucose level. This syndrome may recur with genital recurrences. Usually, there is complete recovery without specific therapy. HSV occasionally may be grown from the CSF.

HSV encephalitis, in contrast to meningitis, is a highly lethal disease. In 96% of cases, it is caused by HSV-1. It may be a result of primary (30%) or recurrent (70%) infection. A larger percentage of HSV encephalitis in younger individuals probably is due to primary infection. One third of cases occur in the pediatric age range. As in most manifestations of HSV infection, but unlike most other common forms of viral encephalitis (enterovirus, arbovirus), there is no seasonality to HSV encephalitis. It is an acute illness with fever, malaise, irritability, and nonspecific symptoms lasting 1 to 7 days, progressing to signs and symptoms of CNS involvement in 3 to 7 days, and finally to coma and death (Table 57-11). Fever and altered behavior in any child should evoke suspicion of encephalitis. Meningeal signs are uncommon. There is no correlation between the isolation of HSV from sites extrinsic to the CNS (such as the oropharynx or genital tract) and the diagnosis of HSV encephalitis. Thus, the presence of oral or genital lesions is of no help in the diagnosis or exclusion of HSV encephalitis. In recent studies, both identical and discordant viruses have been isolated from the brain and oral secretions.

The CSF generally reveals a pleocytosis with up to 2000 WBCs/mm³, usually (80% of cases) greater than 50 WBCs/mm. In 90% of cases, more than 60% of cells are lymphocytes. Early in the infection, neutrophils may predominate. In 75% to 85%

of cases, red blood cells (RBCs), reflecting the hemorrhagic necrosis, are seen in the CSF. Between 5% and 25% of patients have hypoglycorrhachia and 80% have elevated CSF protein levels (median, 80 mg/dL), which rise to striking levels with disease progression. The CSF is normal in 2% to 3% of patients with early HSV encephalitis. HSV almost never is grown from lumbar CSF and rarely from ventricular fluid. Thus, while the CSF examination is helpful, it is not diagnostic of HSV encephalitis unless polymerase chain reaction (PCR) is used to detect HSV DNA.

Neurodiagnostic tests are of limited use. Probably the most useful is electroencephalography (EEG). A "typical" pattern of unilateral or bilateral (poor prognosis) periodic focal spikes against a background of slow (flattened) activity (paroxysmal lateral epileptiform discharges, or PLEDs) is associated with HSV encephalitis. Other findings include large-amplitude irregular slow activity, sharp waves, and variable spikes. In 80% to 90% of patients, the EEG is not only abnormal but also localizing. This is one of the earliest localizing laboratory studies. Less helpful early in the illness is the brain scan or computed tomography (CT). Late in the illness, the CT appearance may be characteristic (ie, low-density contrast-enhanced lesions in the temporal area, mass effect, edema, and hemorrhage [Fig 57-19]), but early in the illness when diagnosis is critical, the CT appearance often is unremarkable. An abnormal CT scan is a poor prognostic factor. Magnetic resonance imaging (MRI) seems to be an early sensitive test for localizing HSV encephalitis (Fig 57-20). It is probably the technique of choice for early diagnosis of HSV encephalitis. The finding of focal abnormality on EEG, MRI, CT, or radionuclide brain scan is significantly more likely to occur in HSV encephalitis than in other illnesses that are confused with it.

The clinical and laboratory data acquired by noninvasive methods are valuable only for increasing the index of suspicion for HSV encephalitis; they do not confirm the diagnosis. The differential diagnosis of this condition is relatively large and includes many treatable conditions (Table 57-12). Therefore, unless reliable HSV DNA detection by PCR is positive, a brain biopsy test is essential in patients with suspected HSV encephalitis, both

### TABLE 57-11. Historical and Clinical Findings in HSV Encephalitis

| Historical Findings | % | Findings at Presentation | % |
|---|---|---|---|
| Alteration of consciousness | 97 | Fever | 92 |
| Fever | 90 | Personality changes | 85 |
| Personality changes | 71 | Dysphasia | 76 |
| Seizures | 67 | Autonomic dysfunction | 60 |
| Vomiting | 46 | Ataxia | 40 |
| Hemiparesis | 33 | Seizures | 38 |
| Memory loss | 24 | Focal | 28 |
| | | Generalized | 10 |
| | | Cranial nerve defects | 32 |
| | | Visual field loss | 14 |
| | | Papilledema | 14 |

*Kohl S. Postnatal herpes simplex infection. In: Feigin RD, Cherry JD, eds. Textbook of pediatric infectious diseases, ed 2. Philadelphia: WB Saunders, 1987: 1577. Reproduced by permission.*

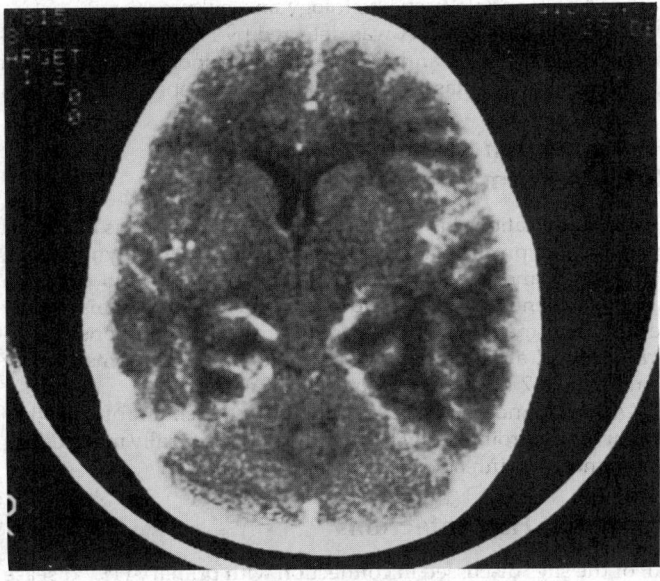

**Figure 57-19.** Computed tomogram obtained 1 week after onset of HSV encephalitis in a 6-year-old child. Note the bilateral temporal low density areas with dye enhancement and the mass effect. (Kohl S. Postnatal herpes simplex virus infection. In: Feigin RD, Cherry JD, eds. Textbook of pediatric infectious diseases, ed 2. Philadelphia: WB Saunders, 1987:1566. Reproduced by permission.)

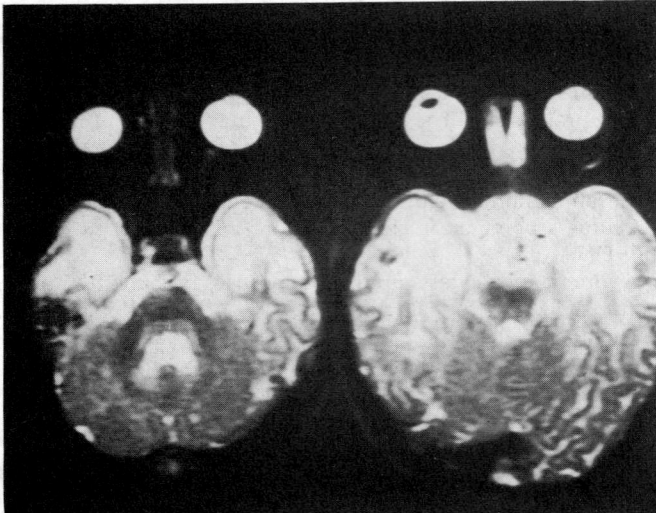

**Figure 57-20.** Magnetic resonance image of patient with early HSV encephalitis. Note the bilateral temporal lobe enhancement. (Kohl S. Herpes simplex encephalitis. In: New topics in pediatric infectious diseases. Pediatr Clin North Am 1988;35(3):465. Reproduced by permission.)

to provide optimal aggressive therapy for that condition and to achieve a diagnosis for the 50% to 60% of patients without HSV infections, roughly one half of whom would benefit from other specific therapies.

The risk of brain biopsy test is low. In a national collaborative study of 182 biopsy tests, there were three complications—hemorrhage in two patients and herniation of brain tissue in a third. Roughly 3% of brain biopsies were false negative, usually due to biopsy of the wrong site.

There are increasingly frequent reports of a postherpetic encephalomyelitis due to a probable autoimmune or demyelinating etiology, and also reports of virus-positive recurrences of HSV encephalitis months after apparently successful therapy. These conditions can be differentiated and documented only by biopsy test and appropriate tissue histology and culture.

Recently, HSV-1 DNA was detected by PCR analysis accompanied by a transient anti-HSV antibody response in the CSF in a patient with the classic syndrome of Mollaret meningitis.

## HSV Infection of the Gastrointestinal Tract in Normal Hosts

Several publications have documented HSV esophagitis in normal patients. The presenting symptoms include severe odynophagia, retrosternal and subxiphoid pain, and the inability to eat. Skin lesions are generally absent. Double contrast esophograms usually reveal abnormalities. Esophagoscopy reveals ulcerations and fibrinous, and at times hemorrhagic exudate. Symptoms usually remit in 5 to 7 days with nonspecific therapy.

Of importance is the delineation of involvement of the other end of the gastrointestinal tract with HSV, especially manifesting as an anorectal infection in homosexual males.

## Recurrent HSV Infections

All of the sites discussed in connection with primary HSV disease may also be involved in recurrent infections. HSV infection may occur without specific lesions. With the aid of co-cultivation techniques, HSV has been recovered from dorsal root ganglia subserving the areas of skin in which individuals have experienced recurrent herpes lesions. HSV-1 has been found in trigem-

**TABLE 57-12.** Differential Diagnosis of HSV Encephalitis

**Infections**
*Fungal*
Especially Cryptococcus
*Bacterial*
Abscess, cerebritis
*Listeria monocytogenes* meningitis
Subdural, epidural empyema
Tuberculosis
Bacterial endocarditis
Lyme disease

Mycoplasma Rickettsial
*Protozoal*
Toxoplasmosis
Amoebic
*Viral*
Mumps virus
Coxsackievirus, echovirus
Arbovirus (especially St. Louis encephalitis)
Postinfluenza encephalitis
Reye's syndrome
Lymphocytic choriomeningitis virus
Rabies virus
Epstein-Barr virus
Rubella virus
Cytomegalovirus
Adenovirus
Tick-borne encephalitis virus
Human immunodeficiency virus-1
Progressive multifocal leukoencephalopathy
Subacute sclerosing panencephalitis

**Noninfectious Disorders**
Tumor
Vascular disease
Arteriovenous malformations
Toxins
Alcoholic encephalopathy
Hematoma
Adrenal leukodystrophy

*Modified with permission from Kohl S. Postnatal herpes simplex virus infection. In: Feigin RD, Cherry JD, eds. Textbook of pediatric infectious diseases, ed 2. Philadelphia: WB Saunders, 1987:1577.*

inal ganglia, and HSV-2 has been recovered from sacral ganglia. By in situ hybridization, HSV DNA also has been detected in ganglia. Concomitant infection of oral and genital sites by HSV is most likely to result in oral recurrences if type 1 and in genital recurrences if type 2 virus.

The most common manifestation of recurrent HSV infection is herpes labialis ("cold sores," "fever blisters"), which is estimated to occur in 25% to 50% of the general population. Most individuals experience a prodrome (pain, burning, tingling, or itching) at the site lasting 6 hours to several days. There is then a progression from papules (lasting 12 to 36 hours) to vesicles (usually gone by 48 hours) to ulcers and crust (lasting 2 to 4 days). Most outbreaks are healed by 5 to 10 days. Most pain occurs during the vesicular stage. Virus is isolated readily from vesicles and less commonly from ulcers and crusts. Maximum virus titer in lesions (to $10^7$ to $10^8$ viruses) are measured in the vesicles.

Recurrences tend to occur at the same location or closely related areas. In general, they occur on the lips, mucocutaneous junction, or other parts of the face. Recurrent lesions inside the mouth are rarely due to HSV and are more likely aphthous lesions. Intraoral HSV recurrences tend to occur on tissue adjacent to bone, such as the gums or palate, and not on the lips or buccal mucosa. A differential diagnosis of the condition also includes pemphigus, lichen planus, ulcers due to cyclic neutropenia, and ulcers associated with celiac disease, ulcerative colitis, Crohn's disease, pernicious anemia, and Behçet's syndrome.

Recurrent genital HSV is probably the second most common manifestation of HSV and one of the most bothersome. Recurrence rates are much more common after primary HSV-2 (90%) than HSV-1 (55%) infection. The mean rate of recurrence is 0.1 episode per month after primary genital HSV-1 and 0.3 episode per month after primary HSV-2 genital infection.

Only 5% to 12% of individuals with recurrent genital HSV have constitutional symptoms. Local symptoms include pain (averaging 4 to 6 days), itching, dysuria, adenopathy, and lesions lasting 4 to 5 days and progressing to crusting and healing by 9 to 11 days. Virus is shed for an average of 3 to 4 days. In dry areas, vesicles are seen, but in wet areas, the vesicles rapidly break down into ulcers. Symptoms are generally milder and of shorter duration than in primary genital disease.

Other cutaneous recurrences may occur at each anatomic site in which primary infection occurs. HSV may recur on the face or trunk in a typical dermatome distribution like that associated with varicella-zoster virus. Frequent repeated attacks of zoster-iform-like lesions on any part of the body in a normal host suggests HSV and not varicella-zoster infection.

## Erythema Multiforme and HSV Infection

Erythema multiforme may be an allergic response to recurrent HSV infection. In several series, approximately 15% of patients with erythema multiforme report recurrent HSV before skin eruption, which may be macular or urticarial. In one series, 5 of 80 patients with recurrent oral HSV experience a rash (presumably erythema multiforme) 8 to 14 days after the onset of a cold sore. Several studies document HSV antigen-antibody immune complexes present in the serum and skin of patients with erythema multiforme after HSV infection.

HSV DNA has been detected in the biopsy samples of skin lesions of patients with erythema multiforme. In a recent study, HSV DNA was detected by PCR analysis of skin biopsy samples from 8 of 10 children with a history of HSV-associated erythema multiforme and from 8 of 10 children with idiopathic erythema multiforme minor (but not in unaffected skin or in biopsy samples from control patients). The skin manifestations may last for 14 to 21 days. Therapy generally is directed toward the allergic and not the viral component of the illness, or toward prevention of herpetic recurrences.

## HSV in the Immunocompromised Host

Table 57-13 lists the states associated with unusually severe HSV infections. HSV infection in the neonatal period is discussed in Chapter 20.14.3. Other than the several cases of HSV encephalitis in patients with agammaglobulinemia (who also had concomitant infections with enterovirus), the common links in these varied groups are either skin abnormalities (eczema, burns) or immunologic defects, primarily in the cell-mediated aspects of the immune system.

The incidence of severe HSV infection in these pediatric groups is poorly defined. In series of adult and pediatric patients with renal, marrow, or cardiac transplants, 70% to 90% of seropositive individuals excreted HSV, usually from the oropharynx and usually at the time of peak immunosuppression, in the first month after transplantation. HSV was isolated from 43% of the pediatric

| TABLE 57-13.   Conditions Contributing to Unusually Severe Herpes Simplex Virus Infection |
|---|
| Newborn period |
| Malnutrition |
| Malignancy |
| Immunosuppressive therapy |
|   Antineoplastic |
|   Transplantation |
|   Corticosteroids or ACTH |
| Primary immunodeficiency disease |
|   Agammaglobulinemia |
|   Common variable hypogammaglobulinemia |
|   Natural killer cell deficiency |
|   Wiskott-Aldrich syndrome |
|   Ataxia telangiectasia |
|   Severe combined immunodeficiency syndrome |
|   Nucleoside phosphroylase deficiency |
| Acquired immune deficiency syndrome (AIDS) |
| Pregnancy |
| Burns |
| Trauma |
| Skin abnormalities |
|   Atopic eczema |
|   Bullous impetigo |
|   Burns |
|   Pemphigus |
| Viral infection |
|   Measles |
| Pertussis |
| Tuberculosis |
| Severe bacterial infection |
|   *Haemophilus* meningitis, pertussis |
| Sarcoidosis |

*Adapted with permission from Kohl S. Postnatal herpes simplex virus infection. In: Feigin RD, Cherry JD, eds. Textbook of pediatric infectious diseases, ed 2. Philadelphia: WB Saunders, 1987:1577.*

renal transplant patients in one series. HSV in cardiac transplant recipients causes symptomatic illness in 45% to 85% of seropositive patients, depending on the intensity of immunosuppression. In bone marrow transplant recipients, HSV (often in the absence of cutaneous or mucous membrane lesions) is one of the causes of interstitial pneumonitis, a disorder that accounts for approximately 5% to 10% of deaths. In children, HSV is both a common cause of acute infection in the leukopenic leukemic patient in relapse as well as accounting for a significant portion of mortality during remission. HSV, typically oral infection, occurs in 5% to 15% of children with AIDS. In developing countries, disseminated HSV infection is not unusual in severely malnourished children.

Several major syndromes are attributable to HSV in immunocompromised patients, with some overlap and occasionally progression from one to another. The first is a local, chronic, often extensive cutaneous or mucocutaneous infection. The second is infection of one organ, usually contiguous to an orifice (eg, esophagitis or pneumonitis). The most serious is widespread dissemination involving distant areas of skin or visceral organs (lungs, liver, adrenals) and the CNS. There is not enough information to be certain, but, except in the most immunosuppressed patients, disseminated disease probably most often represents primary infection, while the local syndromes may represent primary or, more often, recurrent illness.

The typical local syndrome begins in the mouth or about the

lips, often appearing innocuously as an ordinary recurrence of herpes labialis. Over several days, if untreated, the papules and vesicles progress to bullae, often with hemorrhagic fluid. The bullae or vesicles progress to huge, chronic, bloody, coalescing, ulcerated oozing lesions, eroding into the subcutaneous tissue, occasionally destroying underlying structures. The tissue is odorous, and the lesions are painful (Fig 57-21). A similar syndrome may be seen in the perianal or genital area, usually due to HSV-2 infection, and is one of the characteristic syndromes in adolescent and adult patients with AIDS. Untreated lesions may lead to death due to local destruction and hemorrhage or may regress as the immune status of the host improves or as antiviral chemotherapy is used. Poor response to antiviral therapy should prompt viral susceptibility testing to detect acyclovir-resistant virus. This is most typically a problem in patients receiving chronic or frequent courses of therapy.

In patients with burns, eczema, pemphigus, or abrasions, a similar syndrome may occur, often with conversion of second-degree tissue damage to third-degree damage. Possibly as a result of the more severe immunodeficiency occurring with several of these conditions, the local infection may progress to dissemination into visceral organs. The widespread necrotizing lesions are commonly known as Kaposi's varicelliform eruption or eczema herpeticum.

These lesions must be differentiated from bacterial infections due to gram-positive or gram-negative organisms, chronic fungal infections (as seen with *Mucor* species, blastomycosis), other viral infections (vaccinia, varicella), mycobacterial infection, and various noninfectious lesions such as pyoderma gangrenosum or Sweet syndrome.

Esophagitis due to HSV uncommonly has been reported in normal children but is relatively common in immunocompromised patients. Pathologic studies suggest that approximately 25% of cases of autopsy-proven esophagitis are secondary to

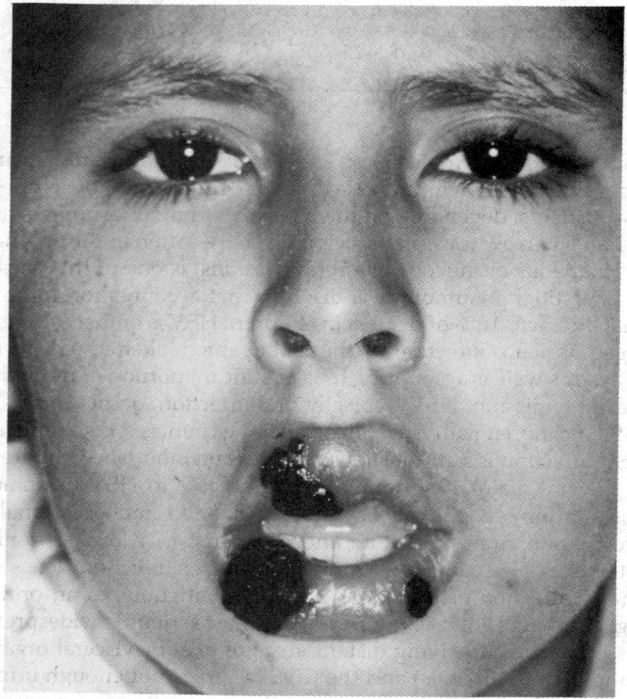

**Figure 57-21.** Chronic hemorrhagic HSV infection in a girl with leukemia and a bone marrow transplant. (Kohl S. Postnatal herpes simplex virus infection. In: Feigin RD, Cherry JD, eds. Textbook of pediatric infectious diseases, ed 2. Philadelphia: WB Saunders, 1987:1577. Reproduced by permission.)

HSV infection. Underlying conditions include burns, aplastic anemia, malignancies, organ transplantation, a variety of other serious medical problems, and nasogastric tube-induced trauma in postoperative patients. Some 20% to 50% of these patients have HSV involvement elsewhere (lungs, trachea, and, less commonly, skin). The esophagitis may be asymptomatic or associated with dysphagia, odynophagia, epigastric discomfort, and retrosternal pain. The characteristic findings in the esophagus are ulcers with raised granular margins. The ulcers are often covered with fibrinous exudate and, in advanced cases, are confluent with progression to complete mucosal loss in large segments of the esophagus. Typically, visceral herpes infection is not suspected premortem. Uncommonly, involvement of adjacent gastric tissue can be documented. Diagnostic evaluation should include barium swallow, which may demonstrate edema, nodules, and ulceration of the esophagus. Esophagoscopy with biopsy and viral culture is diagnostic and helps exclude other common causes of this syndrome, including *Candida*, cytomegalovirus, and possibly other fungal and bacterial infection, or chemotherapy-induced changes.

The second most commonly involved organ in immunocompromised hosts is probably the lungs. HSV pneumonia is a rare premortem diagnosis and occurs almost exclusively in immunosuppressed patients. In one series of 1000 consecutive autopsies, HSV pneumonia was identified in 10 cases. In most cases in adults, the process is a result of endogenous viral mucocutaneous reactivation and involvement of lung tissue by contiguous spread, causing focal pneumonia (60% of cases). Hematogenous spread from an oral or genital site may result in diffuse pneumonitis. Patients had cough, dyspnea, fever, and hypoxia, and 50% had rales. Most had other concomitant pulmonary infections with bacteria, *Candida*, *Aspergillus*, and cytomegalovirus. HSV pneumonia cannot be diagnosed from the association of upper airway cultures with the radiographic picture. The diagnosis must be pursued aggressively using culture and histopathology from involved lung tissue.

Meningoencephalitis due to HSV is not common in immunocompromised patients. It may occur as part of widely disseminated disease or may be a localized condition. In the immunocompromised patient, it may follow a slowly evolving subacute form. The most severe form of HSV infection in the immunocompromised host is widely disseminated disease involving the liver, adrenals, lungs, spleen, kidney, marrow, and, often, the brain. This type of infection occurs in 10% to 25% of children with transplants and HSV infection. The clinical presentation is usually one of initial fever and mucocutaneous involvement, which, instead of healing as expected, disseminates. The cutaneous dissemination may involve a widespread vesicular eruption that looks much like varicella or may involve more local, large, hemorrhagic vesicles and bullae. In approximately 20% of cases of disseminated disease, skin lesions are absent. The major target organs involved give rise to syndromes of hepatitis, pneumonia, shock, bleeding, disseminated intravascular coagulopathy, seizures, coma, renal failure, hypothermia, and death in days to weeks. Laboratory tests may reveal leukopenia, thrombocytopenia, elevated values on liver function tests, hyponatremia, azotemia, pneumonitis, hypoglycemia, CSF pleocytosis, abnormal EEG, and electrocardiographic (ECG) abnormalities. Death is very common in this syndrome, even after the institution of antiviral chemotherapy. Less commonly, isolated organs, particularly the liver, may be involved, resulting in herpetic hepatitis.

## DIAGNOSIS

Since HSV may be shed in response to fever, stress, or immunosuppression, the finding of HSV in certain secretions does not mean that the clinical condition is caused by HSV. In general, the virus must be isolated from the tissue in question to confirm the diagnosis, especially in immunosuppressed hosts.

## Rapid but Nonspecific Methods

Electron microscopy and cytologic examination are rapid and very suggestive diagnostic modalities, but they are not entirely specific. Electron microscopy of vesicular fluid or tissue preparations may reveal the characteristic virus of the herpes family but cannot differentiate HSV from other herpesviruses.

Cytology can reveal the typical multinucleated giant cells and, less commonly, the Cowdry type A intranuclear inclusions characteristic of HSV, but these findings also may be seen with cytomegalovirus and varicella-zoster virus. In most series, 40% to 60% of culture-positive specimens are cytologically positive if examined by an experienced observer. False-positive examinations are unusual but do occur.

## Rapid and Specific Methods

Several rapid, specific tests depend on immunologic reagents for antigen detection. Fluorescent antibody methods, enzyme-linked immunosorbent assays (ELISAs), immunoperoxidase-tagged antibody in ELISA or tissue sections, radiometric tests, and *Staphylococcus* protein A absorption tests are all available or under investigation. These tests generally employ relatively specific hyperimmune serum to HSV or monoclonal antibodies to specific HSV glycoproteins. Most recent studies report a 50% to 90% sensitivity and more than 95% specificity. These tests are of widespread clinical utility but are not yet as sensitive as culture. Reports of successful antigen detection in the CSF of patients with HSV encephalitis have not been confirmed and have been rendered obsolete by PCR technology (see Experimental Methods of Viral Detection).

## Less Rapid but Specific Methods

The reference standard for HSV diagnosis remains tissue culture. HSV grows rapidly (mean, 2 to 3 days) in human and nonhuman cells, producing a typical cytopathic effect. The use of shell vial techniques often allows for definitive diagnosis in 18 to 24 hours. Confusion occasionally is caused by high-titer specimens of varicella-zoster virus or cytomegalovirus. Definitive viral characterization is accomplished by antisera reaction causing neutralization, fluorescent antibody reaction, or several of the antigen detection tests mentioned above. Typing can be accomplished using specific monoclonal antibodies or endonuclease restriction patterns (see Endonuclease Restriction Analysis).

A variety of antibody tests can be used to document primary HSV infection. Classic tests include viral neutralization, complement fixation (CF), indirect hemagglutination (IHA), and fluorescent antibody (IFA) assays. Newer tests are ELISAs to detect antibodies, radiometric assays (RIA), Western blot analysis to detect antibody to specific viral polypeptides, and antibody-mediating cellular cytotoxicity (ADCC) tests.

Several precautions must be observed when analyzing the serologic response. Patients with documented prior HSV infections may have four-fold titer rises with recurrences, and they may have IgM or IgA responses with recurrences. Rarely, severely immunosuppressed patients do not produce antibody. Thus, only when a patient's serum converts from negative to positive can a primary infection be diagnosed with confidence. Patients with prior HSV infection (symptomatic or asymptomatic) generally remain seropositive for life (probably reflecting existing latency) with minor fluctuations. But, in some of the most important conditions—HSV encephalitis or early disseminated HSV in the immunosuppressed host—serology is relatively useless because of

a slow titer rise or late conversion. In addition, a significant percentage of these conditions represents recurrent and not primary disease. Although CSF-to-serum antibody ratios may be diagnostic in HSV encephalitis, they often are not so until several days or weeks into the illness, and thus are of limited clinical use.

## Endonuclease Restriction Analysis

Each HSV DNA has a specific cleavage pattern or "fingerprint" when digested by endonuclease restriction enzymes and electrophoresed in a gel. These cleavage patterns can be used to type the virus and to demonstrate relatedness or differences (strains) between isolates from different persons for epidemiologic purposes ("outbreaks," nosocomial transmission), between isolates obtained from different sites in the same individual during one illness, or between isolates obtained from the same site over time. This has added markedly to the understanding of the epidemiology of HSV, the examination of the possibility of exogenous reinfection versus recurrence, and the recognition of the ability to harbor more than one latent virus at the same site.

## Drug Susceptibility Testing

Although not in uniform use, viral culture and sensitivity testing is increasingly available and important, especially in the care of the immunosuppressed host.

## Experimental Methods of Viral Detection

### Nucleic Acid Hybridization

The development of genetic engineering has permitted production of complementary nucleic acid, enabling genetic probing of tissue. Nucleic acid hybridization may detect virus or incomplete viral DNA or RNA in latent conditions, possibly virus-transformed cells or sites of very low levels of productive infection.

### Polymerase Chain Reaction (PCR)

PCR allows for spectacularly sensitive detection of viral DNA. In most situations, it is not necessary for HSV diagnosis. In unusual settings, such as erythema multiforme, PCR of involved skin lesion biopsy material may establish HSV as the etiology and influence future suppressive therapy. The most useful role for PCR is detection of HSV DNA in spinal fluid of patients with suspected HSV encephalitis. If a reliable laboratory reports positive results, then the need for a brain biopsy test is obviated. The major problem with PCR is false-positive responses, primarily due to poor laboratory technique.

## PROGNOSIS, COMPLICATIONS, AND SEQUELAE

HSV infections occurring after the fetal and neonatal periods are annoying but usually not immediately life-threatening. The outcome of HSV encephalitis can be serious, ranging from extensive and permanent neurologic disability to death. HSV is one of the most common causes of infectious blindness in industrialized countries. In immunocompromised patients, it is a major cause of morbidity and mortality. Genital HSV may not have life-threatening potential but is a significant cause of physical and psychological morbidity.

## THERAPY

The therapy for HSV infection in children is outlined in Table 57-14.

**TABLE 57-14. Therapy of HSV Infection in Children**

**Genital Disease**

*Primary*
Oral acyclovir, 200 mg 5 times a day for 10 days (1 capsule = 200 mg)
Intravenous acyclovir, 15 mg/kg/d in 3 divided doses for 5–7 days

*Recurrent*
Oral acyclovir, 200 mg 5 times a day for 5 days

*Suppressive*
Oral acyclovir, 200 mg 3 to 5 times a day or 400 mg 2 times a day for up to 12 months
Oral dose for children should not exceed 80 mg/kg/d

**Oral Disease (Primary)**

Same as for primary genital infection. Oral dose for children should not exceed 80 mg/kg/d

**Encephalitis**

Intravenous acyclovir, 30 mg/kg/d in 3 divided doses for 10–14 days†

**Neonatal**

Intravenous acyclovir, 30–45 mg/kg/d in 3 divided doses for 10–14 days†
Intravenous vidarabine, 30 mg/kg/d in 1 dose (12-hour infusion) for 10–14 days

**Immunocompromised Patients**

Intravenous acyclovir, 15–30 mg/kg/d in 3 divided doses; duration as warranted clinically
Oral acyclovir, 200 mg 3 to 5 times a day, not to exceed 80 mg/kg/d; duration as warranted clinically*
Intravenous vidarabine, 10 mg/kg/d in 1 dose (12-h infusion)

*Acyclovir Resistant Isolates*
Intravenous foscarnet, 120 mg/kg/d in 3 divided doses*

**Ocular Infection**

Trifluorothymidine (Viroptic), 1% ophthalmic solution; 1 drop every 2 hours to a maximum of 9 drops, then 1 drop every 4 hours (5 drops/d); do not exceed 21 days
Vidarabine (Vira-A), 3% ophthalmic ointment; 5 times a day; change to different agent if no healing in 7–9 days
Iododeoxyuridine (Stoxil), 0.1% ophthalmic solution or 0.5% ophthalmic ointment
*Solution:* one drop each hour during the day and every 2 hours during the night
*Ointment:* 5 times a day every 4 hours and before bedtime; change to different agent if no healing in 7–9 days

* This is an unlicensed use, and controlled trials in children have not been performed.
† The large dose has been found effective and nontoxic in these particular clinical conditions and patients.

*Adapted with permission from Kohl S. Postnatal herpes simplex virus infection. In: Feigin RD, Cherry JD, eds. Textbook of pediatric infectious diseases, ed 2. Philadelphia: WB Saunders, 1987:1577.*

## Oral HSV

There are no controlled, definitive studies regarding the specific antiviral therapy of primary oral HSV infection. This is probably due to its typical occurrence in young children but not in adults. One would expect acyclovir to be as effective in this illness as in primary genital HSV infection (see Genital HSV Infection). Intravenous acyclovir has been used in patients with severe primary gingivostomatitis when hospital admission was required to maintain hydration. In these uncommon cases, the illness responded in several days with defervescence and cessation of new lesions. No data are available to determine whether this therapy would change the risk of recurrences in later life.

Symptomatic therapy includes antipyretics and oral hydration with bland liquids and ice slurries. The use of oral anesthetics is probably not indicated and has resulted in self-injury when children chewed on anesthetized oral mucosa or lips. Topical acyclovir ointment therapy is not indicated in recurrent oral HSV infection except in the immunocompromised patient with mild illness. Oral acyclovir has minimal effects on the course of recurrent oral HSV infection in the normal host and is probably not warranted.

## HSV Keratitis

The pyrimidine nucleoside trifluridine in a 1% ophthalmic solution inhibits HSV DNA synthesis. It is the drug of choice for the local treatment of primary and recurrent HSV such as keratitis, keratoconjunctivitis, and lid lesions, as well as following operations on eyes previously infected with HSV or when using steroid therapy in similar eyes. Keratitis appears to respond more rapidly to trifluridine than to either idoxuridine or vidarabine ointment. Ulcers failing to respond to the latter two agents have responded to trifluridine. None of the local therapies affects the rate of recurrence. Trifluridine is used as one drop per eye every 2 hours while awake (maximum 9 drops daily) until reepithelialization of corneal ulcers occurs, and then one drop every 5 hours while awake (maximum 5 drops daily) for 7 additional days. The maximum duration of therapy is 21 days. Side effects consist of local stinging, burning, and edema (3% to 5% of cases).

The indications for and side effects of vidarabine ophthalmic ointment are similar to those of trifluridine, although the ointment preparation may be more useful in children. Dosage is one-half inch five times per day (at 3-hour intervals). If there is no improvement in 7 days or if there is lack of complete reepithelialization in 21 days, trifluridine is indicated.

It is strongly advised that care of a child with HSV keratitis be undertaken in conjunction with an ophthalmologist familiar with this illness. The use of cycloplegic and anti-inflammatory agents in this illness requires practical experience.

## HSV Encephalitis

Intravenous acyclovir (10 mg/kg/dose three times a day for 10 to 14 days) is the drug of choice in the treatment of HSV encephalitis. As seen in earlier vidarabine studies, the patient's mental status at initiation of therapy markedly influences the outcome of patients with HSV encephalitis treated with acyclovir. Lethargic patients have a 15% mortality rate, while comatose patients have a 40% mortality rate.

In addition to antiviral therapy, meticulous intensive care optimizes the outcome of these patients. Fluid management to prevent overhydration is critical. Often, direct intracranial pressure measurement by ventricular catheter or epidural bolt is necessary to effectively monitor and treat increased intracranial pressure. The use of steroids is common but remains controversial and unstudied. Anticonvulsant therapy to manage the severe and prolonged seizures as well as ventilatory support are usually necessary. The care of a child with HSV encephalitis requires a team of pediatric intensivists, neurologists, neurosurgeons, and infectious disease experts in a tertiary care setting.

## Genital HSV Infection

Acyclovir (Zovirax) is the drug of choice for HSV genital infection. Acyclovir itself is an inactive drug. Inhibition of DNA synthesis requires its phosphorylation. In this regard, HSV thymidine kinase is much more active than its mammalian counterpart. Thus, acyclovir becomes a specific antiviral agent in the presence of thymidine kinase-positive viruses. Thymidine kinase appears to be an important enzyme for viral virulence. While mutant, thymidine kinase-negative acyclovir-resistant isolates of HSV have been recovered from otherwise healthy patients in the course of acyclovir therapy for genital HSV infections. The patients, unlike immunocompromised patients (see HSV Infection in the Immunocompromised Host), generally responded to acyclovir therapy. These viral mutants seem less virulent in animal models, and patients who were culture-positive for such mutants often have thymidine kinase-positive HSV isolates in their next recurrence. Thus, the clinical significance and epidemiologic importance of these mutants in the normal host remain to be established.

Intravenous acyclovir has an impressive effect on primary genital HSV infection. Used in a dose of 5 mg/kg each 8 hours for 5 days, acyclovir decreased duration of viral shedding and shortened local and systemic symptoms by 20% to 50%. Complications such as extragenital lesions and urinary retention were significantly reduced. Although intravenous acyclovir may shorten viral shedding and duration of symptoms in recurrences, it is not recommended for treatment of recurrent genital disease.

Oral acyclovir has therapeutic effects on both primary and recurrent HSV infection in adults. In a dosage of 200 mg five times per day for 5 to 10 days, acyclovir significantly reduced viral shedding, lesion formation, duration of lesions, and duration and severity of symptoms in primary infection. In similar studies of adult patients with recurrent genital HSV infection, acyclovir (200 mg, five times per day for 5 days) decreased the duration of virus shedding, time to healing, and new lesion development, especially when administered early in the recurrence.

In these studies in which patients were cautioned regarding hydration, no significant side effects were noted. Neither oral nor intravenous acyclovir reduces the rate of recurrence when used to treat either primary or recurrent genital infection (see Chemoprophylaxis). Oral acyclovir appears to be the drug of choice for treating genital HSV infection.

Symptomatic therapy of HSV lesions should be directed toward reducing local discomfort, promoting healing, and preventing autoinoculation and superinfection. Nonspecific creams and ointments probably delay healing and increase risk of maceration and infection. Keeping lesions clean and dry is an important local measure. Urination can be made less painful by urinating into a bathtub or sitz bath. Some experts advise Burow's solution sitz baths or short compress treatment. Prolonged soaking delays healing.

## HSV Infection in the Immunocompromised Host

The clinician must make the difficult determination of how serious the manifestation in the immunocompromised host must be before initiating therapy, which may require hospitalization. In addition, no comparative studies are available on the use of vidarabine versus different formulations (topical, intravenous, oral) of acyclovir.

In one study, vidarabine (10 mg/kg/day in a 12-hour intravenous infusion) decreased pain and induced defervescence in immunocompromised patients older than 40 years with mucocutaneous HSV infection. None of the 85 patients developed visceral dissemination of HSV. No controlled studies analyze therapeutic effects of vidarabine in a strictly pediatric population, and the relatively low therapeutic index in the study in adults is not encouraging.

Acyclovir ointment appears to decrease pain, viral shedding, and the time to complete lesion healing in immunocompromised individuals with mild, non–life-threatening mucocutaneous HSV

infection, but essentially has been rendered obsolete by oral acyclovir for mild illness. Patients with more severe illness should be treated with the intravenous preparation in a hospital setting.

Intravenous acyclovir has been analyzed extensively in immunocompromised patients with mucocutaneous HSV infection. When used early, acyclovir arrests progression of infection. It decreases the time to cessation of new lesions, the time to lesion crusting, and the time to healing, and induces more rapid cessation of pain and termination of viral shedding. Intravenous acyclovir is the drug of choice for treating moderate or severe HSV in the immunocompromised host. Dosage is 250 mg/m² or 5 mg/kg/d every 8 hours infused over 1 hour. In very serious disease (eg, dissemination to visceral organs or the CNS), this dosage should be doubled, although there are no controlled studies demonstrating improved efficacy with higher doses of acyclovir in the immunocompromised host. The major toxicity has been renal, with a reversible obstructive nephropathy and transient rises in serum creatinine levels (5% to 10% of patients). Adequate hydration usually prevents this problem. Table 57-15 lists guidelines for dosage in patients with impaired renal function. Less commonly (1%), reversible neurologic symptoms (lethargy, agitation, tremor, disorientation, coma, and transient hemiparesthesia) and laboratory abnormalities (abnormal EEG, increased CSF myelin basic protein) have developed in marrow transplant patients. These patients usually have received interferon and CNS chemoprophylaxis for leukemia. Other less serious problems include phlebitis (14%) and hives (5%).

Oral acyclovir in dosages of 200 mg five times per day effectively promotes lesion healing and inhibits viral shedding. It is useful in treating mild illness in the immunocompromised child. There are few guidelines for treating children with oral acyclovir, and it is not currently licensed for use in children. All studies to date with acyclovir in immunosuppressed patients have noted the marked propensity of these individuals to continue to have recurrences when therapy is withdrawn.

Three HSV mutations give rise to acyclovir resistance. These include altered viral DNA polymerase, altered thymidine kinase, and absent thymidine kinase. The overwhelming majority of significant clinical isolates of acyclovir-resistant viruses is due to absence of thymidine kinase. These isolates have occurred and resulted in acyclovir unresponsive illness in the immunocompromised child who usually is treated with chronic or recurrent courses of acyclovir. This usually manifests as lesions that fail to heal and worsen during the course of adequate acyclovir therapy. While documentation of viral resistance is optimal, in the immunocompromised patient with documented HSV infection who fails to respond after 4 to 7 days of intravenous acyclovir therapy, resistance should be assumed and alternate therapy must be considered. Vidarabine generally has not been efficacious clinically in this setting. A relatively new agent, foscarnet (120 mg/kg/d

**TABLE 57-15. Dosage of Intravenous Acyclovir for Patients With Renal Insufficiency**

| Creatine Clearance (mL/min/1.73 m²) | Dosage (mg/kg) | Dosing Interval (h) |
|---|---|---|
| 50 | 5 | 8 |
| 25–50 | 5 | 12 |
| 10–25 | 5 | 24 |
| 0–10 | 2.5 | 24 |

*Kohl S. Herpes simplex virus infection. In: Kaphan SL, ed. Current therapy in pediatric infectious diseases. Toronto: BC Decker, 1993:209. Reproduced by permission.*

in three divided doses administered intravenously by slow infusion) was efficacious in a controlled trial in a small number of HIV-infected adult patients with acyclovir-resistant HSV infection. It is a relatively toxic drug causing nephrotoxicity, electrolyte imbalance, and bone marrow toxicity and must be used with caution. It is not licensed for use in HSV infection, although approved for therapy of cytomegalovirus retinitis in patients with AIDS. In any event, foscarnet is probably the agent of choice for treating acyclovir-resistant HSV infection in the immunocompromised host.

## PREVENTION

### Environmental Control or Barrier Prevention

Because HSV is sensitive to heat, light, and lipid solvents, the use of antiseptics, soap and hot water, or chlorine decreases the risk of transferring the virus in settings such as the home, spas, pools, and hospitals. Wrestlers with skin lesions should be excluded from participation in practice or competition until herpes infection is ruled out. Medical and dental personnel who handle respiratory or oral secretions and administer oropharyngeal and tracheostomy care should wear gloves and wash carefully before and after working with patients and their secretions. Parents and caretakers of infants with eczema or severe diaper rash should be especially careful to avoid directly or indirectly contacting this altered skin with an active HSV lesion. Burn patients should be protected against exposure to or direct contact with personnel or visitors who have active HSV lesions. Immunosuppressed patients who develop evidence of HSV infection are usually manifesting evidence of reactivation of latent virus. Primary HSV infections in immunosuppressed individuals, as in neonates, may be especially severe, and it is important to protect these susceptible patients against exposure to HSV lesions. Hospital personnel with active cold sores or herpetic whitlow should not care for immunosuppressed patients. Although there are no human data, in vitro experiments have shown that condoms retard the passage of viable HSV. The use of cesarean section to prevent neonatal HSV is discussed in Chapter 20.14.3.

### Immunoprophylaxis

There are no human data on the prevention or successful attenuation of HSV infection by vaccine, but this is an area of active research. Agents such as bacille Calmette-Guèrin (BCG), smallpox vaccine, and many other compounds have been used to attempt to affect herpetic recurrences. They have proved ineffective and, at times, dangerous.

### Chemoprophylaxis

Oral acyclovir administered long-term markedly suppresses recurrences in immunodeficient patients. Oral or intravenous acyclovir used at times of maximum immunosuppression such as in the first weeks after organ transplantation or during periods of neutropenia in individuals receiving antineoplastic chemotherapy nearly completely prevents the predictable rate of HSV recurrence in seropositive individuals. Oral acyclovir (200 mg given two to five times per day) administered long-term decreases recurrence of genital HSV by 50% to 70% in immunocompetent patients with frequent recurrences. Breakthrough recurrences are mild. When oral acyclovir is discontinued, HSV recurrences revert to pretreatment frequency. Thus, oral acyclovir suppresses recurrences without curing the latent infection. Side effects are limited to mild gastrointestinal irritation.

## Selected Readings

Aurelius E, Johansson B, Skoldenberg B, et al. Rapid diagnosis of herpes simplex encephalitis by nested polymerase chain reaction assay of cerebral spinal fluid. Lancet 1991;337:189.
Belongia EA, Goodman JL, Holland EJ, et al. An outbreak of herpes gladiatorum at a high school wrestling camp. N Engl J Med 1991;325:906.
Frenck RW, Kohl S. Herpes simplex virus in the immunocompromised child. In: Patrick CC, ed. Infections in immunocompromised infants and children. New York: Churchill Livingston, in press.
Kohl S. Herpes simplex encephalitis. In: New topics in pediatric infectious diseases. Pediatr Clin North Am 1988;35:465.
Kohl S. Treatment of herpes simplex virus infection. In: Root RR, Sande MA, eds. Contemporary issues in infectious diseases. Viral Infections Vol 10. New York: Churchill Livingston, 1993:31.
Kohl S. Postnatal herpes simplex virus infection. In: Feigin RD, Cherry JD, eds. Textbook of pediatric infectious diseases, ed 3. Philadelphia: WB Saunders, 1992:1558.
Kuzushima K, Kimura H, Kino Y, et al. Clinical manifestations of primary herpes simplex virus type-1 infection in a closed community. Pediatrics 1991;87:152.
Safrin S, Crumpacker C, Chatis P, et al. A controlled trial comparing foscarnet with vidarabine for acyclovir-resistant murocutaneous herpes simplex in the acquired immunodeficiency syndrome. N Engl J Med 1991;325:551.
Weston WL, Brice SL, Jester JD, et al. Herpes simplex virus in childhood erythema multiforme. Pediatrics 1992;89:32.
Whitley RJ, Alford CA, Hirsch MS, et al. Vidarabine versus acyclovir therapy in herpes simplex encephalitis. N Engl J Med 1986;314:144.
Whitley RJ, Cobbs CG, Alford CA, et al. Diseases that mimic herpes simplex encephalitis diagnosis, presentation and outcome. JAMA 1989;262:234.

*Principles and Practice of Pediatrics, Second Edition.*
edited by Frank A. Oski et al. J. B. Lippincott Company, Philadelphia © 1994.

## 57.13 Roseola and Human Herpesvirus Type 6

Julia McMillan and Charles Grose

As early as 1870, the mild illness now referred to as roseola infantum or exanthem subitum was recognized and described as being distinct from other exanthematous diseases of childhood. Roseola affects infants and young children typically between the ages of 6 months and 3 years with 80% of the cases occurring before 18 months of age. Roseola characteristically is manifested by an initial fever that may have an abrupt onset. The fever may reach 40° to 40.5°C (104° to 105°F) and typically persists, either continuously or intermittently, for approximately 3 days. During this febrile period, the affected infant or child typically maintains near normal appetite and behavior, although there may be periods of irritability during times of increased fever.

Physical examination during this preeruptive phase yields few findings to distinguish roseola from other, more worrisome illnesses. Palpebral edema is sometimes described, and careful examination usually reveals suboccipital lymphadenopathy. Mild erythema of the pharynx may be seen in about one third of the patients. A bulging or tense fontanelle is sometimes noted in young infants with roseola. If laboratory studies are undertaken, they will be unrevealing, except that as the febrile illness begins, there may be a brief, slight elevation in the white blood cell (WBC) count with a predominance of neutrophils. During the majority of the febrile period, however, the WBC typically falls to 3000 to 5000 cells/mm$^3$ with a relative lymphocytosis.

The rash of roseola usually coincides with the abrupt termination of the febrile period. Typically, the rash is pale pink (rose) with discrete macules or, less commonly, maculopapules, predominantly on the neck and trunk. Most often the rash persists for 1 to 2 days, but it may last only a few hours. Pruritus and desquamation are not seen.

## COMPLICATIONS

The complication most frequently associated with roseola is febrile seizure. The rapidity of the initial temperature elevation often is cited as the reason for the frequent association between febrile seizures and roseola. Encephalitis and transient hemiparesis have been reported in young infants with a febrile illness, followed by a rash characteristic of roseola. The young age of patients with roseola, combined with their high fever and occasional bulging fontanelle, often indicates the possibility of bacterial infection, including meningitis. Laboratory investigation and hospitalization for treatment with intravenous antibiotics may result.

## EPIDEMIOLOGY

Roseola occurs most frequently in the spring and fall. The nature of the illness suggested its infectious origin, but person-to-person spread resulting in similar clinical illness among household or other contacts is not reported, except for occasional descriptions of outbreaks among institutionalized children. Kempe and associates in 1950 and Hellstrom and Vahlquist in 1951 demonstrated that blood or serum from a child with roseola obtained during the febrile period could produce a similar clinical illness when injected into another child with no history of roseola. These and other investigators had suggested that roseola occurs in infants and young children when a latent virus is shed intermittently by mother and other adults, probably by the respiratory route.

## HUMAN HERPESVIRUS 6

Until 1986, the family of human herpesviruses included five members: herpes simplex viruses type 1 (oral) and type 2 (genital), varicella-zoster virus (VZV), and cytomegalovirus (CMV) and Epstein-Barr virus (EBV). In 1986, two reports described a novel human herpesvirus. The virus was isolated from the white blood cells of six adult patients with various non–AIDS-related lymphomas associated with HIV-1 infection. The virus had several morphologic characteristics in common with other herpesviruses. These included icosahedral symmetry with 162 capsomers covered by a lipid envelope and a diameter of about 200 nm for the mature particle. Like other herpesviruses, the virus had a double-stranded DNA genome. When serologic comparisons were carried out with antisera to the five known human herpesviruses, there was no cross-reactivity. Because this new herpesvirus replicated in human B cells, investigators designated the novel agent as human B-lymphotropic virus (HBLV).

Subsequent reports from other laboratories contained further information about the new virus. One paper from the Centers for Disease Control described the isolation of the novel herpesvirus from white cells of 11 patients who also were seropositive for HIV: 10 with AIDS and 1 with non–AIDS-related lymphoma (Lopez et al, 1988). In contrast to earlier reports, these investigators observed that the virus replicated better in human T cells than in human B cells. The new virus was designated human herpesvirus type 6 (HHV-6) to avoid possibly confusing nomenclature about tropism for either B or T lymphocytes. Because all patients were so ill from their primary illnesses, researchers could not determine whether the novel virus caused specific signs and symptoms in the infected host. A study of a pediatric population finally provided an answer.

In 1988, a group of Japanese researchers isolated HHV-6 from the white blood cells of four otherwise healthy infants with roseola infantum (exanthem subitum) and suggested that HHV-6 is the etiologic agent of the long-suspected viral disease (Yamanishi et al, 1988). Detailed DNA analyses confirmed that HHV-6 is a distinct herpesvirus that is related genetically to CMV. Serologic studies indicated that maternally derived antibody to HHV-6 is present in most infants at the time of birth and that infection with HHV-6 during the first few years of life is common. Frequent isolation of HHV-6 from saliva of healthy, seropositive adults confirmed that intermittent respiratory shedding of the virus occurs after initial infection. The link between HHV-6 and roseola was established by Japanese investigators who isolated HHV-6 from the peripheral blood mononuclear cells of seronegative children during the febrile phase of a clinical illness consistent with roseola. All of the children from whom HHV-6 was isolated had significant antibody response to HHV-6 following the illness.

In addition to roseola, HHV-6 infection now has been associated with a variety of clinical findings in infants and children. Isolation of HHV-6 from peripheral blood mononuclear cells concomitant with a rise in antibody against HHV-6 has been reported for 14% of the children younger than 2 years of age presenting to a pediatric emergency room with fever. Rash following defervescence occurred in the minority of these children, but many of them had otitis media. HHV-6 infection also has been documented during illness associated with rash but no fever. Other findings described in infants and children with what appears to be primary HHV-6 infection include diarrhea, pneumonia, hepatomegaly, hepatocellular dysfunction, seizures, and intussusception. Complete recovery from infection in these patients has been the rule. There is also one report of a fatal hemophagocytic syndrome in an 8-month-old infant infected with HHV-6.

HHV-6 in adults has been found in association with cervical lymphadenopathy and sore throat and with fever, sometimes in association with rash in patients who are immunosuppressed. A relationship between HHV-6 and chronic fatigue syndrome has been sought, but none has been found.

## DIAGNOSIS AND ANTIVIRAL TREATMENT

HHV-6 can be diagnosed by isolating the virus from white blood cells. This technique is cumbersome and performed only in research laboratories. An alternative diagnostic method is polymerase chain reaction amplification of HHV-6 DNA in lymphocytes. The simplest approach, however, is measurement of serum IgM and IgG antibody titers to HHV-6.

Most cases of HHV-6 infection are either unrecognized or only moderately symptomatic (roseola) and, therefore, need no specific antiviral treatment. Antipyretic medication (acetaminophen) may be indicated for amelioration of high fever. In a few instances, such as with severe HHV-6 hepatitis, antiviral treatment is a consideration. Studies in tissue culture have been carried out with three medications already approved for the treatment of other herpesviruses: these agents include acyclovir, ganciclovir, and phosphonoformic acid. Zidovudine also was tested. The results clearly showed that HHV-6 behaved similarly to CMV (ie, HHV-6 replication was readily inhibited by both ganciclovir and phosphonoformic acid, but was not affected by either acyclovir or zidovudine). It should be noted, however, that ganciclovir and phosphonoformic acid are not approved for serious HHV-6 infection in humans (as of May 1993).

## Selected Readings

Berenberg W, Wright S, Janeway CA. Roseola infantum (exanthem subitum). N Engl J Med 1949;241:253.

Hellstrom B, Vahlquist B. Experimental inoculation of roseola infantum. Acta Pediatrica 1951;40:189.

Huang LM, Lee CY, Lin KH, et al. Human herpesvirus-6 associated with fatal haemophagocytic syndrome. Lancet 1990;336:60.

Irving WL, Chang J, Raymond DR, et al. Roseola infantum and other syndromes associated with acute HHV6 infection. Arch Dis Child 1990;65:1297.

Kempe CH, Shaw EB, Jackson JR, et al. Studies on the etiology of exanthema subitum (roseola infantum). J Pediatr 1950;37:561.

Lopez C, Pellett P, Stewart J, et al. Characteristics of human herpesvirus-6. J Infect Dis 1988;157:1271.

Pruksananonda P, Hall CB, Insel RA, et al. Primary human herpesvirus 6 infection in young children. N Engl J Med 1992;326:1445.

Salahuddin SZ, Ablashi DV, Markham PD, et al. Isolation of a new virus, HBLV, in patients with lymphoproliferative disorders. Science 1986;234:596.

Takahashi K, Sonoda S, Kawakami K. Human herpesvirus 6 and exanthem subitum. Lancet 1988,1463.

Veeder BS, Hempelmann TC. Febrile exanthem occurring in childhood, JAMA 1921;77:1787.

Yamanishi K, Shiraki K, Konda T, et al. Identification of human herpesvirus 6 as a causal agent for exanthem subitum. Lancet 1988,1065.

Zahorsky J. Roseola infantalis. Pediatrics 1910;22:60.

*Principles and Practice of Pediatrics, Second Edition.*
edited by Frank A. Oski et al. J. B. Lippincott Company, Philadelphia © 1994.

## 57.13.1 *Human Herpesvirus Type 7*

Charles Grose

In 1990, the discovery of a new herpesvirus was reported. Human herpesvirus type 7 (HHV-7) was isolated from the peripheral blood lymphocytes of a healthy individual. The DNA of HHV-7 has been extensively characterized and found to be distinct from herpes simplex virus types 1 (oral) and 2 (genital), varicella-zoster virus, cytomegalovirus, and Epstein-Barr virus. Even though there is limited DNA sequence homology with human herpesvirus type 6 (HHV-6), the agent that causes roseola in young children, HHV-7 is considered to be sufficiently different to merit classification as a separate virus. The protein antigens of HHV-7 also appear to be immunologically distinguishable from those of HHV-6. In a series of seroepidemiologic studies, seroconversion to HHV-7 was observed in children who were already HHV-6 seropositive. Therefore, prior infection with HHV-6 did not protect against subsequent infection with HHV-7. In an analysis of a large number of children's serum samples, most children older than 2 years were immune to HHV-6, as expected, but a majority of 2-year-old children had no HHV-7 antibody.

The disease caused by HHV-7 infection is not yet apparent, although it is known that HHV-7 seroconversion often occurs in children during their first few years of grade school. Attempts to define transmission of HHV-7 have led to the discovery that HHV-7 can be isolated frequently from saliva of healthy adult individuals in the United States. The virus was shed over periods of at least 4 months, even though the individuals did not complain of any specific illness. The same people were not tested to determine whether their peripheral blood lymphocytes also harbored HHV-7 at the same time. Studies will reveal more about the pathogenesis of this reclusive human herpesvirus. Some of the early studies of HHV-6 may have included patients infected with both HHV-6 and HHV-7 (see Chapter 57.13).

## Selected Readings

Wyatt LS, Frenkel N. Human herpesvirus 7 is a constitutive inhabitant of adult human saliva. J Virol 1992;66:3206.

Wyatt LS, Rodriguez WJ, Balachandran N, Frenkel N. Human herpesvirus 7: antigenic properties and prevalence in children and adults. J Virol 1991;65:6260.

*Principles and Practice of Pediatrics, Second Edition.*
edited by Frank A. Oski et al. J. B. Lippincott Company, Philadelphia © 1994.

## 57.14 *Varicella-Zoster Virus Infections*

Charles Grose

Chickenpox is the common childhood exanthem caused by the human herpesvirus varicella-zoster virus (VZV). Most children acquire chickenpox during early school years, thereby developing lifelong immunity. About 10% of young adults, however, are susceptible to primary VZV infection because they did not contract chickenpox as children. After a person recovers from chickenpox, the virus remains in a latent state in the dorsal root ganglion cells for decades. In late adulthood as immunity wanes, the virus occasionally reactivates and causes the dermatomal exanthem known as shingles or zoster. Zoster also occurs prematurely in children who have had chickenpox, then acquire a disease that must be treated with immunosuppressive chemotherapy and irradiation (eg, leukemia and lymphoma).

## THE VIRUS AND ITS PATHOGENESIS

VZV is one of the seven human herpesviruses. The other six are herpes simplex types 1 (oral) and 2 (genital), cytomegalovirus, Epstein-Barr virus, and the newly discovered human herpesvirus types 6 and 7, which reside within lymphocytes. The herpesviruses are DNA viruses whose genomes are housed in capsids, which, in turn, are covered by lipid envelopes containing biologically important viral glycoprotein antigens. The diameter of the viral particle is approximately 150 nm. The route by which this virus causes disease most likely resembles the schema for pathogenesis described for mousepox (Fig 57-22). The interval between infection and appearance of the vesicular rash (incubation period) is usually 14 to 15 days with a range of 10 to 20 days. The initial site of infection is the conjunctivae or upper respiratory tract. The virus then replicates at a local site in the head or neck for about 4 to 6 days. Thereafter, the virus is transmitted throughout the body during the primary viremia. After a second cycle of replication, the virus is released in larger amounts 1 week later (secondary viremia) and quickly invades the cutaneous tissues. As the virus exits the capillaries and enters the epidermis, characteristic vesicles of chickenpox appear on the skin.

## TRANSMISSION OF CHICKENPOX

Chickenpox is transmitted by virus in water droplets that are carried by air currents from an infected child to a susceptible

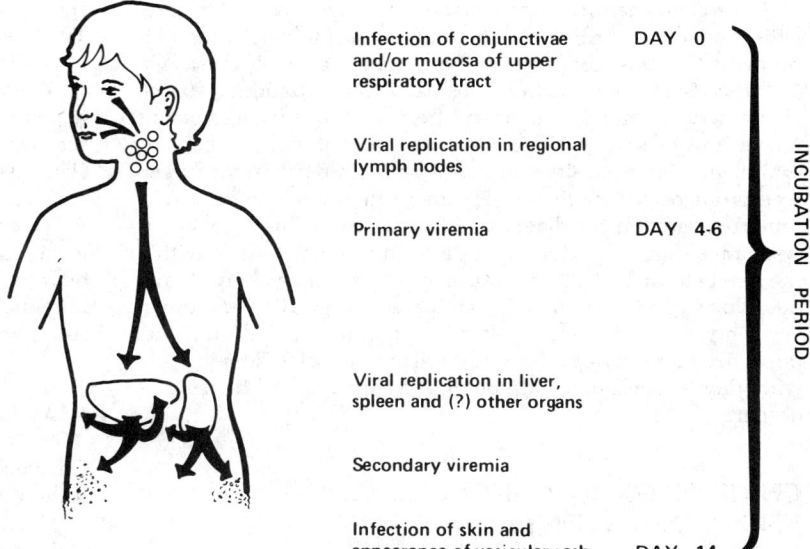

Figure 57-22. The pathogenesis of chickenpox. Primary infection with VZV occurs when virus-laden water droplets contact the respiratory mucosa or conjunctivae of a susceptible host. The pathogenesis most likely includes a biphasic course with a primary and secondary viremia followed by typical vesicular exanthem of chickenpox. Based on this schema, varicella-zoster immune globulin must be given before primary viremia to prevent chickenpox in the exposed host. (Grose C. Varicella-zoster virus infections: chickenpox (varicella), shingles (zoster), and varicella vaccine. In: Glaser R, ed. Human herpesvirus infections. New York: Marcel Dekker, in press.)

individual. Epidemiologic observation studies document that children in the late incubation period may be infectious 1, 2, and possibly 4 days before appearance of the exanthem. They remain infectious through the first few days of the rash, but probably no longer than the sixth day. Therefore, a child can return to school on the sixth day after onset of the rash, or sooner if the child had mild disease with few lesions. Susceptible individuals also can contract chickenpox from patients with zoster, although the period of contagion appears to be much shorter. In this circumstance, the spread of virus again appears to be respiratory and not by direct contact. Finally, VZV in water droplets can be carried by air currents through hospital corridors. Studies within children's wards document the spread of infection from an index case of chickenpox (usually with pneumonitis) in one room to patients housed in separate rooms elsewhere on the ward. The optimal circumstances for this scenario appear to be modern, completely air-conditioned hospitals in which the room of the index case of chickenpox is at positive pressure with regard to the corridor and adjacent rooms.

In most communities in North America and Europe, outbreaks of chickenpox occur annually from January to May. The fewest cases occur in August and September. The periodicity of chickenpox depends on susceptible children being brought together in school every autumn. With an increasing number of young children in year-round day care, this epidemiologic pattern may change. In remote villages where populations are small and isolated, the perpetuation of VZV infection is remarkably different. Outbreaks of chickenpox occur only when one of the elderly develops zoster and subsequently transmits the virus to younger members of the household who develop primary VZV infection.

## CLINICAL FEATURES OF CHICKENPOX

The characteristic feature of chickenpox is the vesicle. In healthy children, the exanthem develops over 3 to 6 days, usually beginning along the hairline on the face. Each lesion begins as a macule that progresses to papule and vesicle, then to a crusted vesicle. The rash subsequently emerges in successive crops over the trunk, then the extremities. Lesions in different stages of development are present throughout the first week. The rash is more confluent wherever the skin is previously abraded, such as the diaper area.

The typical course of chickenpox is documented meticulously in American children. Usually, the prodrome is mild with malaise and low-grade fever. Once the pox appear, the temperature rises, but rarely above 102 °F. The average number of skin lesions ranges between 200 and 300 in the index case within a family. Secondary cases may have a more severe course with up to 500 or more pox, presumably because these patients receive a larger inoculum of virus from the infected sibling. By the end of the first week, the infected child is again afebrile, and the cutaneous lesions continue to form crusts that dry and fall off. Infants younger than 1 year old may have more severe disease; likewise, older teenagers and adults are at greater risk when they develop chickenpox. The mortality rate for chickenpox in otherwise healthy children (ages 1 to 14 years) is about 1:50,000, while that for infants younger than age 1 year is 1:13,000 and that for adults is 1:1400. One subgroup at risk of fatal chickenpox is children on high-dose corticosteroid therapy for diseases such as asthma or rheumatic fever.

The most frequent complication of chickenpox in a healthy child is bacterial infection of a vesicular lesion. The most common infecting organism is Group A *Streptococcus*, although staphylococcal infections also occur. Secondary diseases range from cellulitis and erysipelas to cutaneous abscesses, impetigo, and suppurative lymphadenitis. More serious, but less common, bacterial sequelae include septic arthritis and osteomyelitis, streptococcal necrotizing fasciitis, and staphylococcal pyomyositis. The onset of bacterial disease may be rapid, sometimes within 2 days of the appearance of the exanthem. This complication is usually heralded by a sudden rise in temperature and local signs of inflammation. Diagnosis of fasciitis and myositis, once a difficult procedure, is facilitated by magnetic resonance imaging.

The viral sequelae of chickenpox involve virtually all organ systems. They include pneumonitis, hepatitis, arthritis, pericarditis, glomerulonephritis, orchitis, and involvement of the nervous system. Varicella pneumonitis is one of the most feared complications in an adult with chickenpox; pregnant women are especially prone to develop this complication. Pneumonitis usually develops late in the first week of disease in those patients who have the most florid exanthem. Mild hepatitis is another frequent complication and may account for the nausea often observed during the first few days of illness. Cases of purpuric chickenpox range from mild febrile purpura to the life-threatening condition called purpura fulminans, which is large ecchymoses that appear on the legs and occasionally progress to hemorrhagic gangrene.

Neurologic manifestations include meningoencephalitis, myelitis, and polyneuritis. In particular, the acute cerebellar syndrome is the most common VZV-induced neurologic disease in children. Symptoms include unsteady gait, vomiting, speech changes, nystagmus, vertigo, and tremor. Ataxia usually begins during the second week of the illness, but it can precede the exanthem. Cerebellar signs and symptoms often persist for several weeks but resolve with no permanent neurologic deficits. The preferred method for diagnosis of viral cerebellitis is magnetic resonance imaging, which can detect abnormal signals within the cerebellum better than can computed tomography. Other neurologic conditions include hemiparesis, ascending and transverse myelitis, and facial palsy. Eye findings include unequal pupil size (anisocoria). Chickenpox also is associated temporally with Reye's syndrome, although the etiologic relationship is obscure.

## CHICKENPOX IN CANCER AND AIDS PATIENTS

Although chickenpox is a relatively benign condition in otherwise healthy children, VZV infection is often life-threatening when it occurs in children who are immunocompromised or immunosuppressed. The most relevant data about VZV-related morbidity and mortality were gathered before development of effective antiviral agents. In children with leukemia or lymphoma who were receiving anticancer chemotherapy, chickenpox was a more prolonged disease. New lesion formation lasted an average of 9 days (range 5 to 14 days) rather than 3 to 7 days. Visceral dissemination was apparent in one third of the children, and about 8% of the children died. This severe form of VZV infection often is called progressive chickenpox. Every child who died had varicella pneumonitis (Fig 57-23), which was sometimes associated with hepatitis and encephalitis. The only identifiable risk factor for VZV dissemination was a total lymphocyte count below 500/mm$^3$ on the first day of exanthem. Children in such a risk group

should be treated immediately with acyclovir (see section on Treatment With Acyclovir). Progressive chickenpox was not seen in children in remission who were not receiving chemotherapy.

The variable outcome of chickenpox in HIV-infected children depends on the immunologic status of the patient. In the HIV seropositive child without symptoms of acquired immune deficiency syndrome (AIDS), chickenpox usually follows its typical course. In the child with very low CD4 lymphocyte counts and AIDS, chickenpox may become a progressive disease, as described in children with leukemia. Most HIV seropositive children should be considered in the higher risk category and treated with either immune globulin or acyclovir (see section on Treatment With Acyclovir).

## CONGENITAL VARICELLA INFECTION

Chickenpox in the pregnant woman can lead to intrauterine infection with embryopathy, especially during the first 20 weeks of gestation. The sequelae of VZV infection of the fetus involve mainly ectodermal derivatives and appear to be the consequence of viral destruction within the cervical and lumosacral plexi, as well as the brain. The most common deformities are hypoplasia and paresis of one of the extremities, together with cicatricial scarring over the skin on the involved limb. A more detailed enumeration of the fetal embryopathy is included in Table 57-16. The diagnosis of congenital varicella syndrome is difficult to document because infants usually do not excrete virus and the VZV-specific IgM response is very short-lived postnatally. The risk of fetopathy in the pregnant woman with chickenpox is small, less than 3% by most surveys.

## ZOSTER (SHINGLES)

Zoster is the dermatomal exanthem that occurs when VZV reactivates from its site of latency and travels down a sensory nerve

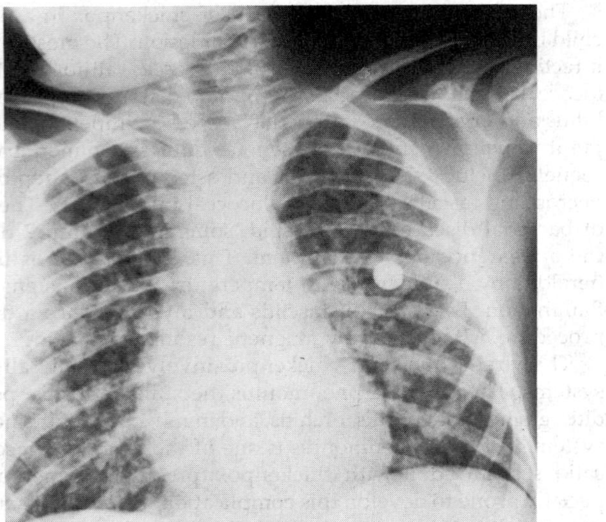

Figure 57-23.   Varicella pneumonitis in a boy with leukemia and chickenpox. Symptoms include cough, dyspnea, tachypnea, and chest pain. Initial roentgenographic findings include peribronchial nodular infiltrates that may extend throughout the lung. Because varicella pneumonitis is a medical emergency, the patient should be admitted for intensive respiratory care as well as administration of antiviral chemotherapy.

| TABLE 57-16.   Neurologic Sequelae of Fetal VZV Infection |
| --- |
| **Damage to Sensory Nerves** |
| Cutaneous manifestations |
|    Zigzag (cicatricial) skin lesions |
|    Hypopigmentation |
| **Damage to Optic Stalk and Lens Vesicle** |
| Microphthalmia |
| Cataracts |
| Chorioretinitis |
| Optic atrophy |
| **Damage to Cervical and Lumbosacral Cord** |
| Hypoplasia of upper/lower extremities |
| Motor/sensory deficits |
| Absent deep tendon reflexes |
| Anisocoria/Horner's syndrome |
| Anal/vesical sphincter dysfunction |
| **Damage to Brain/Encephalitis** |
| Microcephaly |
| Hydrocephaly |
| Calcifications |
| Aplasia of brain |

to the skin. Zoster is unusual in children. Estimated annual rate is about 1 case per 1000 children between ages 1 and 19 years. The younger the child at the time of chickenpox (especially younger than age 2 years), the likelier the same child will develop zoster later in childhood. Localization of zoster is also different in the young child. Rather than the lower thoracic and upper lumbar dermatomes, sites common in adults, zoster in younger children often occurs in dermatomes supplied by the cervical and sacral dermatomes. Thus, the rash frequently is seen on the arms and hands or in the groin and lower extremities.

As discussed, zoster occurs more often in immunocompromised children (Fig 57-24). The incidence in children with leukemia and lymphoma (who have had chickenpox prior to diagnosis of malignancy) is about 20 cases per 1000 per year, which is higher even than the rate in the elderly (6 to 8 cases per 1000 per year). Zoster is rarely a life-threatening illness in these children. The morbidity, however, is appreciable and includes extensive keloid formation, which is both unsightly and deforming when it affects an extremity. Episodes of zoster usually occur between 4 and 24 months after diagnosis of leukemia and are not associated with any particular chemotherapy protocol. Children under treatment for cancer rarely develop zoster more than once, as long as their primary VZV infection antedated their malignancy. Children who contract chickenpox after being placed on chemotherapy for leukemia may have two episodes of zoster. Zoster also occurs with increased frequency in children with AIDS.

## DIAGNOSIS

Because of the characteristic vesicular rash, diagnosis of chickenpox is usually visually apparent. In certain cases, the rash can be confused with herpes simplex virus infection or other skin conditions, particularly when there are few vesicles. Likewise, when zoster occurs in unusual locations, the diagnosis is not always apparent. In these instances, the virus can be identified by obtaining samples of the vesicle fluid for inoculation in cell culture where cytopathic effect usually is observable 3 to 7 days later.

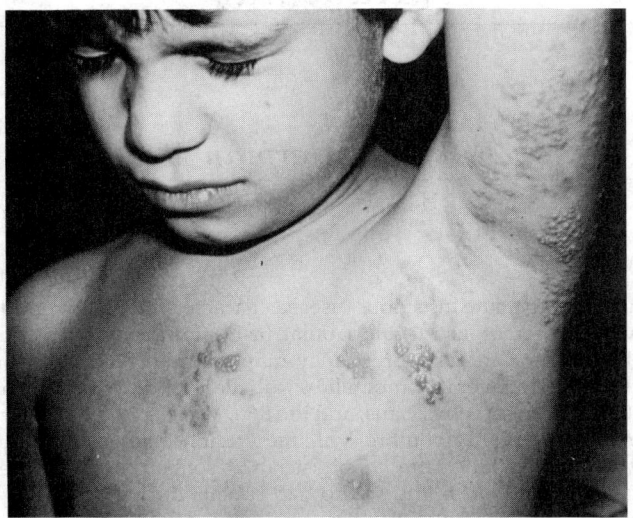

**Figure 57-24.** Zoster (shingles) in a child. The patient was receiving chemotherapy for treatment of leukemia when zoster was observed in the left first/second thoracic dermatome. The child had a history of chickenpox 3 years before the onset of cancer. (Grose C. Varicella-zoster virus infections: chickenpox (varicella), shingles (zoster), and varicella vaccine. In: Glaser R, ed. Human herpesvirus infections. New York: Marcel Dekker, in press.)

The virus infection can be identified more rapidly by antigen detection technique. For this test, cells from the base of a vesicle are dried on a glass slide before probing with a fluorescein-conjugated, VZV-specific monoclonal antibody. Cells containing virus are identified by their brilliant fluorescence.

Recent infection can be documented by obtaining acute and convalescent serum samples and demonstrating a four-fold or greater rise in VZV-specific antibody titer. Likewise, past infection can be demonstrated by persistence of anti-VZV antibody. The most reliable methods for testing VZV humoral immunity are fluorescent antibody to membrane antigen (FAMA) and enzyme-linked immunosorbent assay (ELISA).

## TREATMENT MODALITIES INCLUDING VZIG

Chickenpox in the healthy child is rarely a serious disease. Low-grade fever can be treated with acetaminophen. Aspirin should be avoided in children with chickenpox because of its link with Reye's syndrome. For relief of itching secondary to the vesicular lesions, calamine lotion can be applied liberally to the skin. More severe pruritus, especially at night, may be ameliorated by giving Benadryl Elixir. Most children with chickenpox do not need to be seen by a physician unless they develop symptoms and signs of bacterial skin infection or one of the viral complications previously discussed. Children receiving corticosteroids for diseases such as asthma are in a high risk category and should be seen by a physician.

The approach to the exposed child on corticosteroids or chemotherapy for cancer or AIDS is much more emergent. If the child is known to be susceptible to VZV infection, varicella-zoster immune globulin (VZIG) is the therapy of choice for passive immunization of these children at risk of developing progressive chickenpox. VZIG must be administered by intramuscular injection within 3 to 4 days after exposure to chickenpox (ie, during the early incubation period before the virus has spread throughout the body [see Fig 57-22]). The dose of VZIG is one vial (about 1.25 mL) for each 20 pounds of body weight. Newly available preparations of gamma globulin for intravenous administration may be acceptable substitutes for intramuscular VZIG in the VZV-susceptible adult, but this approach has not been tested extensively.

## TREATMENT WITH ACYCLOVIR

If the VZV-susceptible patient is beyond the fourth day post-exposure, there is no beneficial effect of passive immunization with gamma globulin. Therefore, the physician must wait until chickenpox manifests itself, then treat the patient with acyclovir (Zovirax). Acyclovir is now approved as both an intravenous and an oral formulation for treatment of chickenpox. Acyclovir is administered to high-risk children at a dose of 500 mg/m$^2$ every 8 hours (total daily dose: 1500 mg/m$^2$), usually for 7 days. Within 24 to 48 hours, intravenous acyclovir blocks further viral replication, thus preventing serious complications of progressive chickenpox. Because these complications (eg, pneumonitis) usually appear after the third day, the decision to administer intravenous acyclovir to high-risk children should be made on or before day 3 of the disease. The only serious side effect of acyclovir therapy is renal insufficiency. Therefore, serum creatinine levels should be monitored every 3 days.

In 1992, an oral formulation of acyclovir was approved by the Food and Drug Administration in the United States for treatment of chickenpox in normal children. This recommendation was based on American studies in which acyclovir suspension was administered orally in a dose of 80 mg/kg/d (20 mg/kg four times a day), beginning on the first day of the chickenpox rash. In the largest trial, a total of 367 children received acyclovir, while 357 were in the placebo group. The average age was 5 years (range: 2 to 12 years). The treated group developed 294 vesicles (mean number), while the untreated group developed 347 lesions. The treated group had shorter duration of new lesion formation as well as 1 day less of fever. The median duration of typical chickenpox in the control group, however, was 3 to 4 days, so improvement was not dramatic. Furthermore, acyclovir treatment did not affect the intrafamilial transmission of chickenpox. Because the spread of infection is not altered by acyclovir, treatment of children within a family does not decrease total days of school missed by the children nor does it greatly alter total days of work missed by parents who must care for the children. Thus, there seems to be no strong indication to prescribe oral acyclovir routinely for treating chickenpox in otherwise healthy children. Children with chronic conditions (eg, eczema, asthma, rheumatoid arthritis, diabetes) may benefit more from acyclovir treatment.

No study shows that oral acyclovir shortens the course of chickenpox if begun on day 2 or later of the rash. Thus, the decision to prescribe this antiviral medication should be left to the discretion of physicians. Administration of oral acyclovir may not be adequate for the treatment of chickenpox in immunocompromised children. Zovirax is supplied in 200 mg capsules or as a suspension containing 200 mg per 5 mL.

## VARICELLA VACCINATION

A live attenuated VZV vaccine is undergoing clinical evaluation in the United States. The vaccine was developed in Japan where it already is licensed for administration to children. Results of multiyear assessments of the vaccine experience in Japan are published. In healthy children, nearly all vaccine recipients seroconverted within 1 month after immunization and remained seropositive for years. When these vaccinated children were exposed to chickenpox in other family members or other school children, between 4% and 6% of vaccine recipients developed chickenpox. All had mild disease with fewer than 20 pox lesions. Japanese investigators have followed their vaccine recipient's serologic status for more than 10 years. They observed that humoral immunity was maintained, but speculated that exposure of vaccine recipients to chickenpox cases in the community may provide a booster effect over time. It is well known that VZV antibody titers rise in parents when their children contract chickenpox.

Extensive clinical trials of the VZV vaccine also have been carried out in the United States. Because childhood leukemia patients have a high mortality after chickenpox, this population initially was selected for immunization. Criteria for VZV vaccination was that leukemia be in remission for 9 months and there be no detectable VZV antibody (ie, no evidence of prior chickenpox). Chemotherapy was stopped 1 week before and 1 week after immunization. Most children received two immunizations given 3 months apart to achieve a 95% seroconversion rate. After the first immunization, a mild rash developed within 3 to 6 weeks in 42% of vaccine recipients whose chemotherapy was temporarily suspended. This exanthem, which consists of tiny papules or papulovesicles, is caused by continued multiplication of the vaccine strain (see Fig 57-22). In addition to children with leukemia, varicella vaccine also has been administered to healthy children enrolled in clinical trials in the United States.

At 2 and 3 years postimmunization, at least two thirds of vaccine recipients still had VZV antibody. As in the Japanese trials, community-acquired "breakthrough" chickenpox was observed later in some of the immunized population, but the disease

was always mild. Based on the efficacy data from the clinical trials, the VZV vaccine was estimated to be 80% to 90% effective in children. A few cases of zoster have occurred in the American vaccine recipients; some have been caused by the vaccine strain, while others are associated with nonvaccine VZV strains. Zoster does not occur with increased frequency in immunized children with leukemia. Because of these promising results, the vaccine probably will be licensed in the United States. Critical questions that remain to be answered concern the protective efficacy many years following VZV immunization, especially when the vaccine is given in early childhood, and whether booster immunizations will be required to maintain protective immunity throughout adulthood.

## Selected Readings

Dunkle LM, Arvin AM, Whitley RJ, et al. A controlled trial of acyclovir for chickenpox in normal children. N Engl J Med 1992;325:1539.

Gershon AA, Steinberg SP, Gelb L, et al. Live attenuated varicella vaccine use in immunocompromised children and adults. Pediatrics 1986;78(suppl):757.

Grose C. Varicella-zoster virus infections: chickenpox (varicella), shingles (zoster), and varicella vaccine. In: Glaser R, ed. Human herpesvirus infections. New York: Marcel Dekker, in press.

Grose C, Giller RH. Varicella-zoster virus infection and immunization in the healthy and immunocompromised host. CRC Crit Rev Oncol Hematol 1988;8:27.

Hyman RW. Natural history of varicella-zoster virus. Boca Raton: CRC Press, 1987.

Takahashi M. A live varicella vaccine. In: Lopez C, ed. Immunology and prophylaxis of human herpesvirus infections. New York: Plenum Press, 1990:49.

Zittergruen M, Grose C. Magnetic resonance imaging for early diagnosis of necrotizing fasciitis. Pediatr Emerg Care 1993;9:26.

*Principles and Practice of Pediatrics, Second Edition.*
edited by Frank A. Oski et al. J. B. Lippincott Company, Philadelphia © 1994.

# 57.15 *Rubella (German Measles) and Measles (Rubeola)*

## 57.15.1 *Rubella (German Measles)*

Larry H. Taber and Gail J. Demmler

Rubella is an acute infectious disease characterized by low-grade fever, erythematous maculopapular rash, and adenopathy. Rubella infection in early pregnancy may result in fetal infection with severe congenital anomalies. Rubella was described in the 1700s by German physicians, and in 1866, Veale, a Royal Artillery surgeon, described an outbreak of illness that he named "rubella." In 1941 Gregg, an Australian physician, described congenital defects in infants of mothers who had rubella during pregnancy. Rubella virus was isolated in tissue culture in 1963. Development of the hemagglutination inhibition (HAI) test in 1967 made large-scale surveillance studies and diagnostic testing possible. Attenuated rubella virus vaccine was developed in the late 1960s and was licensed in the United States in 1969. Vaccine use in children and women of childbearing age has reduced the number of cases of postnatally acquired rubella and congenital rubella dramatically.

## ETIOLOGY

Rubella virus is a nonarthropod-borne, RNA-containing, heat labile togavirus, genus *Rubivirus*. It has no antigenic relationship with other togaviruses. Only a single type of rubella virus has been described. Several antigens have been defined, including an envelope antigen, a hemagglutinin, the inhibition of which by rubella-specific antisera is the basis for the HAI test for rubella. Isolation of rubella virus in tissue culture from clinical specimens is achieved by "viral interference." When African green monkey kidney cells are infected with rubella virus, they show no cytopathic effect, and when these same rubella-infected cells then are challenged with an appropriate enterovirus, they resist infection with the enterovirus and again demonstrate no cytopathic effect, or "interference."

## POSTNATALLY ACQUIRED RUBELLA

### Pathogenesis and Epidemiology

Natural infection with rubella virus occurs only in humans, although several different animals have been infected experimentally with the virus. Transmission occurs by oral droplet in acquired rubella and transplacentally in congenital rubella. In human volunteers, infection occurs easily after droplet presentation to the nasopharyngeal mucosa. The sequence of events includes replication of the virus in nasopharyngeal mucosa, involvement of regional lymphatics, and subsequent viremia. The maximum titer of the virus in the nasopharynx is present several days before the rash, and it is during this period that an infected person is most contagious. Periods of maximum communicability include the week before appearance of rash and the week after appearance of rash. Viremia clears quickly after appearance of the rash, but the virus may be shed from the nasopharynx after resolution of the rash. Rubella virus has been isolated from the nasopharynx, blood, skin, synovial fluid, cerebrospinal fluid (CSF), and other specimens. Infected hosts develop both humoral and cell-mediated immunity. After infection, antibodies in both IgM and IgG classes develop rapidly after appearance of the rash. Rubella-specific IgM antibody usually persists approximately 12 weeks and may aid in diagnosis of an acute infection. Antibodies of IgG class persist for life.

In the prevaccine era, major rubella outbreaks occurred at 6- to 9-year intervals, with the highest attack rates in school-aged children (5 to 10 years) and lesser attack rates in preschool-aged children. Rubella occurs worldwide, and outbreaks are seen in winter and spring months in temperate climates. Since widespread immunization with rubella vaccine, incidence rates of reported rubella decreased steadily and reached an all-time low in 1988. Since 1989, however, the number of reported cases has steadily increased each year, marking a moderate resurgence of postnatal rubella. While increases in rubella incidence have been seen in all age groups, rubella has increased most dramatically in persons older than age 15 years. In 1990, 26 rubella outbreaks were reported, and they appeared to fall into two categories. One type of outbreak was associated with settings in which unvaccinated adolescents and adults congregated, such as prisons, colleges, workplaces (especially hospitals), and recreational settings. Another form of outbreak occurred among children and adults in religious communities with low levels of rubella vaccination. Data from both of these types of outbreaks suggest that failure to vac-

cinate, not primary or secondary vaccine failure, is responsible for this increase in rubella.

## Clinical Manifestations

Incubation periods for postnatal rubella range from 14 to 21 days, usually 15 to 18 days. Inapparent infection may occur in 25% or more of infected individuals. Prodromal symptoms, usually appearing 1 to 5 days before the rash, are seen more commonly in older children and adults; they consist of low-grade fever, coryza, conjunctivitis, cough, and lymphadenopathy. An enanthem of rubella, Forschheimer spots, consists of discrete, erythematous, pinpoint or larger lesions found on the soft palate in the prodromal period or on the first day of rash. These lesions are not pathognomonic for rubella.

The lymphadenopathy associated with rubella may appear as early as 7 days before appearance of rash. The suboccipital, posterior auricular, and cervical nodes are most commonly involved, but there may be generalized lymphadenopathy. Maximum swelling of lymph nodes and tenderness usually coincide with the first day of the appearance of the rash.

The exanthem of rubella may be the first indication of this infection in young children. It begins on the face and moves rapidly downward to the trunk and lower extremities. The exanthem lasts approximately 3 days; it may persist for 5 days or disappear within the first day. The rash of rubella is erythematous, discrete, maculopapular, and does not generally coalesce or darken as in rubeola. Fever in rubella is most often low grade (less than 38.8 °C) and does not persist for the length of the exanthem.

Arthritis is seen more commonly in adults and adolescents; females are afflicted more commonly than males. Joint involvement is usually multiple (large and small joints) and appears toward resolution of the rash. It may be accompanied by recurrence of fever. Elevation of the sedimentation rate may occur in rubella arthritis. Symptoms usually abate within 15 days of appearance. Some studies suggest a relationship between rubella arthritis and subsequent development of rheumatoid arthritis.

Encephalitis occurs in approximately 1 in 6000 children, with usual onset after appearance of rash. The encephalitis usually is not fatal, and complete recovery can be expected in most cases. A mononuclear pleocytosis may occur in the CSF along with a normal or slightly elevated protein. Persistent abnormalities in the electroencephalogram have been described. Neuritis may occur during rubella infection with paresthesia being the chief complaint.

Thrombocytopenic purpura has occurred in rubella. In the majority of patients, purpura resolves and platelet count returns to normal within 15 days.

## Differential Diagnosis

There are no pathognomonic findings in rubella, and with the reduced incidence of rubella, the physician must have a high index of suspicion to make the diagnosis. Helpful epidemiologic factors include age of patient, history of contact cases, documented immunization status, season of year, and incubation period.

Included in the differential diagnosis are illnesses associated with enterovirus, mild rubeola, mild scarlet fever, mononucleosis, toxoplasmosis, *Mycoplasma pneumoniae* infection, and human parvovirus B19 infection.

## Diagnosis

Rubella virus may be isolated from nasopharyngeal secretions obtained from individuals with postnatal rubella, and isolation of the virus confirms the diagnosis. Rubella isolation is technically difficult, however, and the virology laboratory must be alerted that rubella virus is suspected so the specimen can be handled appropriately. Because of limitations associated with culture of rubella virus, the diagnosis of postnatal rubella is usually determined by serologic testing of acute and convalescent sera obtained 10 to 14 days apart. The traditional HAI test for rubella has been replaced by commercially available tests that are more sensitive and easier to perform. Serologic tests now performed include enzyme immunoassay (EIA), latex agglutination, and indirect immunofluorescence. One of the most widely used tests is the EIA. Results of this test may be reported as nonimmune or immune, or negative, low-positive, mid-positive, or high-positive. Tests to detect rubella-specific IgM antibody are also commercially available; however, these tests may produce both false-negative and false-positive results.

Test results on paired sera that are reported as nonimmune to immune, a four-fold rise in titer, or the determination of the presence of rubella-specific IgM antibody indicate a recent infection with rubella virus. Tests should be performed on the same sera, simultaneously, in the same laboratory.

## Treatment

Treatment is largely supportive and includes use of acetaminophen for fever. Hospitalization is rarely required but may be necessary when one of the described complications occurs. Rubella arthritis usually responds to aspirin and rest of involved joints.

## CONGENITAL RUBELLA

The initial report of Gregg in 1941 described a triad of congenital cataracts, heart defects, and low birth weight in infants born after maternal rubella during early pregnancy. With the pandemic of rubella in 1964, the complexity of this syndrome was recognized, and the term "expanded rubella syndrome" became standard to describe the more extensive organ involvement observed in infants with congenital rubella.

## Pathogenesis and Epidemiology

The timing of maternal rubella during pregnancy is important as far as the pathogenesis of congenital rubella is concerned. Maternal rubella infection, either apparent or inapparent, in the first month of pregnancy predictably results in maternal viremia with subsequent placental and fetal infection, widespread organ involvement, and persistent infection of the fetus. This risk of fetal infection after maternal rubella is greatest during the first month of pregnancy, and subsequent congenital anomalies are seen in 30% to 60% of offspring. Risk of fetal infection apparently declines thereafter as determined by the reduced incidence of congenital anomalies, although hearing loss, ocular abnormalities, and developmental abnormalities have been described in children in whom maternal rubella occurred in the second trimester of pregnancy. Early fetal infection results in hypoplastic organs with a subnormal number of cells. Rubella virus has been isolated from placental and fetal tissue from aborted fetuses and from nasopharynx, urine, CSF, and almost every organ in infants with congenital rubella, and virus excretion from the nasopharynx and urine may persist until 1 year of age or longer. Infants with congenital rubella develop both humoral and cell-mediated immunity. Differences exist in the immune response in congenital rubella and natally acquired rubella in that the rubella-specific IgM antibody is usually present in sera of infants with congenital rubella until 6 months of age or longer, and HAI antibodies may disappear in later life (after 5 years of age) in infants with congenital rubella.

The number of cases of congenital rubella reported to the Centers for Disease Control declined each year since vaccine licensure in 1969 and reached an all-time low in 1988. Since 1989, however, a major increase in reported cases of congenital rubella syndrome has occurred. This observed increase in congenital rubella parallels the reported increase in postnatal rubella seen since 1989. Because congenital rubella syndrome is the most severe and preventable consequence of rubella infection, congenital rubella cases should be identified and investigated to estimate incidence and identify opportunities to prevent rubella infection in mothers. For example, it is estimated that up to 25% of postpubertal females lack antibody to rubella virus, and continued reports of outbreaks of rubella in populations of childbearing age indicate potential resurgence of congenital rubella.

## Clinical Manifestations

Clinical manifestations include intrauterine growth retardation (the most common manifestation and almost never an isolated finding), hepatosplenomegaly, generalized adenopathy, thrombocytopenia, hemolytic anemia, hepatitis, jaundice, meningoencephalitis (which may persist beyond the first year of life), bone lesions, large anterior fontanelle, pneumonitis, myocarditis, and nephritis.

Eye involvement is manifested by cataracts (usually noted at birth), glaucoma, retinopathy that does not interfere with visual acuity, and micro-ophthalmia, usually associated with cataracts.

Sensorineural deafness is common and may not be apparent until later in childhood. Heart defects are common; patent ductus arteriosus is most common, followed by stenosis of the pulmonary artery. More than one heart defect may coexist.

Numerous delayed manifestations with long-term implications have been described, including deafness, ocular damage, endocrinopathies (diabetes mellitus and thyroid dysfunction), progressive rubella panencephalitis, immunologic defects (particularly low levels of IgG), spastic diplegia, behavioral abnormalities, and learning disabilities.

## Differential Diagnosis

Differential diagnosis includes congenital cytomegalovirus infection, syphilis, toxoplasmosis, neonatal herpes, or enteroviral infection of the newborn. Infants with congenital rubella are much more likely to be symptomatic at birth than infants with the above listed infections.

## Diagnosis

The diagnosis of congenital rubella can be made with isolation in tissue culture of the virus (throat, urine, CSF), demonstration of rubella-specific IgM antibody that may be present until 6 to 12 months of age, or persistence of rubella antibody beyond 6 months of life. When possible, virus isolation from clinical specimens should be performed. It is almost impossible to make a diagnosis of congenital rubella in those infants whose defects are identified in late infancy or childhood. Rubella virus may be isolated from throat, urine, or CSF until 1 year of age and in a small number of children beyond this period. Rubella panencephalitis can be diagnosed by demonstration of rubella IgG antibody in CSF and often of rubella-specific IgM antibody. If tissue from involved organs is available, rubella virus antigen detection can be attempted.

## Treatment

There is no specific antiviral therapy for congenital rubella. Treatment consists of the skillful management of the child and appropriate referrals for identification or correction of defects. Emphasis should be placed on longitudinal assessment of these children for any long-term defects, and in particular, for early recognition of any hearing deficit and referral for training. Children with low levels of IgG might be considered for gamma-globulin replacement therapy.

## Management of the Pregnant Woman

Exposure of the pregnant woman to rubella virus requires immediate assessment of her immune status. If the exposed woman is known to be immune, she can be assured of no risk. If her immune status is unknown and she presents for serologic testing as soon as exposure occurs, the presence of antibody indicates immunity and no risk. If there is no detectable antibody, further testing should be performed in 3 weeks; if antibody is present in the second specimen, infection is documented. If there is no antibody in the second specimen, a third specimen obtained 6 weeks after exposure should be evaluated for the presence of rubella antibody to see whether positive infection occurred. If this third specimen is negative, infection did not occur and no further testing is required. All testing should be performed on all sera simultaneously and in the same laboratory.

Postexposure prophylaxis of the pregnant woman with immune globulin (IG) is not recommended and should be considered only if termination of pregnancy is not an option. The administration of IG 0.55 mL/kg may prevent or modify infection, but congenital rubella has been documented in infants born of mothers who received IG after exposure.

If clinical illness is present (ie, rash), attempted virus isolation and serologic testing should be done. A four-fold rise in titer, the presence of rubella-specific IgM antibody, or isolation of virus indicates a primary infection.

## RUBELLA PREVENTION

### Control Measures

Emphasis should be placed on immunization of children at an appropriate time. Some authorities recommend screening for rubella antibody in all personnel who may have exposure to rubella-susceptible contacts. These include most medical or paramedical personnel. If nonimmune, they should be immunized. Emphasis also should be placed on determination of immunity in women of childbearing age who present for medical service, regardless of anticipated pregnancy.

Patients with natally acquired rubella should be considered contagious for 7 days after appearance of rash and should be isolated when necessary. Infants with congenital rubella should be considered contagious for the first year of life unless virus cultures of nasopharynx and urine prove negative, and they should be isolated (ie, hospitalized) from susceptible contacts (ie, day care, pregnant caretakers) as appropriate. Rubella is a reportable disease, and every effort should be made to diagnose all suspected cases of natally and congenitally acquired rubella and to report them to the appropriate public health agency.

### Vaccine Recommendations

The live rubella virus vaccine distributed in the United States contains the RA 27/3 strain of rubella virus. Serum antibody is induced in more than 98% of recipients of the vaccine and appears to be lifelong. Rubella vaccine is most commonly administered in combination with measles and mumps vaccines (MMR). Recently, there has been a change in the recommended routine

childhood vaccination schedule from a one-dose schedule to a two-dose schedule of MMR vaccine. This change is primarily because of the resurgence of measles, but minor resurgences of mumps and rubella also have occurred. According to the Committee on Infectious Diseases of the American Academy of Pediatrics, the first dose of MMR vaccine should still be administered at 15 months of age, followed by a second dose of MMR vaccine administered at 11 to 12 years of age upon entry to middle or junior high school. Alternatively, the second dose may be administered at 4 to 6 years of age upon entry to kindergarten or first grade, according to the recommendations of the Immunization Practices Advisory Committee from the Centers for Disease Control. While there is flexibility in when the second dose of MMR may be administered, it is important that all children receive a second dose of vaccine. Physicians also should comply with the recommendations of their local public health officials. MMR may be administered at the same time as diphtheria-tetanus-pertussis (DTP) and oral polio vaccine (OPV) with the parenteral preparations given at different sites. Rubella vaccine also may be administered alone when indicated. Adverse reactions to rubella vaccine include rash, fever, and adenopathy in a very small number of children approximately 7 to 10 days after immunization. Postvaccine arthralgias may occur 2 to 3 weeks after vaccine, are transient, and are most likely to occur in postpubertal females. Susceptible children who reside in households with pregnant women may be immunized, as well as children with minor illness.

## Contraindications

Contraindications to rubella vaccine exist in patients with immunodeficiency, those on immunosuppressive therapy including pharmacologic doses of corticosteroids, or any individual considered immunocompromised. The exception is patients infected with the human immunodeficiency virus (symptomatic or asymptomatic), who should be immunized with MMR at the appropriate age. Pregnancy is a contraindication for rubella vaccine, and if a pregnant female is immunized inadvertently or if a female becomes pregnant within 3 months after immunization, she should be advised of theoretical risk to the fetus. Congenital rubella following rubella vaccination in pregnancy has yet to be documented, although it is still a theoretical consideration. Recent administration of immune globulin or blood transfusion (within 3 months) is a contraindication for vaccine administration. Postpubertal women do not need serologic testing before immunization; however, a blood specimen may be stored for future testing if conception occurs within 3 months after immunization.

For detailed recommendations or contraindications for vaccine administration, refer to the 22nd edition of the *Report of the Committee on Infectious Diseases* (Red Book), 1991.

### Selected Readings

American Academy of Pediatrics. Rubella. In: Peter G, Hall CB, Lepow ML, Phillips CF, eds. Report of the Committee on Infectious Diseases, ed 22. Elk Grove Village, Ill: American Academy of Pediatrics, 1991:410.

Best JM, O'Shea S. *Togaviridae:* rubella virus. In: Lennette EH, Halonen P, Murphy FA, eds. Laboratory diagnosis of infectious diseases: principles and practice. Vol 2. Viral, rickettsial and chlamydial diseases. New York: Springer-Verlag, 1988:435.

Centers for Disease Control. Current trends: rubella vaccination during pregnancy—United States, 1971–1985. MMWR 1986;35(17):275.

Centers for Disease Control. Epidemiologic notes and reports: rubella and congenital rubella syndrome—New York City. MMWR 1986;35(50):770.

Centers for Disease Control. Summary of notifiable diseases, United States, 1986. MMWR 1986;35(55):1.

Centers for Disease Control. Current trends: increase in rubella and congenital rubella—United States, 1988–1990. MMWR 1991;40(6):93.

Cherry JD. Rubella. In: Feigin RD, Cherry JD, eds. Textbook of pediatric infectious diseases, ed 3. Vol 2. Philadelphia: WB Saunders, 1992:1792.

*Principles and Practice of Pediatrics, Second Edition.*
edited by Frank A. Oski et al. J. B. Lippincott Company, Philadelphia © 1994.

## 57.15.2 *Measles (Rubeola)*

Larry H. Taber and Gail J. Demmler

Infection with measles virus produces an illness characterized by a prodrome of fever, coryza, cough, conjunctivitis, an enanthem (Koplik's spots), and development of a confluent, erythematous maculopapular rash. The mortality rate associated with measles is approximately 1 in 3000 cases in the United States. A higher mortality and increased morbidity is seen in young infants and in immunocompromised or malnourished children.

Measles epidemics were described in both the Roman Empire and ancient China. By the 17th century, differentiation between measles and smallpox was made, and reports of measles in London and Colonial America were described. In the late 1800s, the pathognomonic enanthem of measles was reported in detail by Koplik.

In 1954, Enders and Peebles isolated measles virus in human and simian tissue culture lines. Cultivation of measles virus in chicken embryo tissue enabled vaccine development to proceed. Vaccine trials occurred in the late 1950s and early 1960s, with vaccine licensure in 1963.

## ETIOLOGY

Measles virus, which has an internal core of RNA and an outer envelope of glycoproteins and lipids, is a member of the family Paramyxoviridae, genus *Morbillivirus.* Two glycoproteins, hemagglutinin (H) and fusion (F), are important in immune protection responses. Immune responses to these two glycoproteins include hemagglutination antibody response in infected individuals (H) and fusion of nucleated cells with formation of multinucleated giant cells (F). Measles virus is monotypic, sensitive to both heat and cold, and inactivated by ultraviolet light.

## EPIDEMIOLOGY

Measles is highly contagious. Transmission of the virus occurs by droplets of respiratory secretions with acquisition of infection by the nasopharyngeal route and possibly the conjunctivae. Person-to-person contact with exchange of infected secretions, particularly in young children, may lead to infection. The highest period of infectivity is the catarrhal period before appearance of the exanthem.

In the prevaccine era, highest attack rates were seen in children 5 to 10 years of age, although in urban populations, a higher incidence was observed in preschool-aged children. In developing countries, the highest attack rate occurs in children 2 years of age or younger. When the widespread use of measles vaccine began in 1965, the incidence of measles fell remarkably and, in 1983, reached an all-time low. Since 1986, however, the incidence of measles has increased. In 1989 and 1990, the incidence of measles increased dramatically in all age groups and reached epidemic proportions in many areas of North America. This increase in measles was most striking among unvaccinated preschool-age children, but outbreaks also occurred in highly vaccinated groups of school-age children, adolescents, and young adults.

In a 1988 outbreak of measles in Los Angeles County, California, the highest attack rate was in children younger than 5 years of age. About half of reported cases of measles were considered preventable. Person-to-person transmission of measles occurred in the home, in medical settings between patients and personnel, and in day-care centers, schools, and colleges.

Measles occurs throughout the world, is essentially a winter/spring disease in temperate climates, and attacks males and females equally, although morbidity is reported to be higher in males.

## PATHOGENESIS AND PATHOLOGY

Measles virus infection of the nasopharynx respiratory epithelium spreads to regional lymphatics, resulting in viremia. This viremia is enhanced by replication of the virus in the reticuloendothelial system. The respiratory tract, skin, and conjunctivae are major sites of infection, but other organs may be involved. Viral replication peaks in all organs and the blood approximately when rash appears, which coincides with development of immune responses and subsequent curtailment of the illness.

Formation of multinucleated giant cells—the result of cell fusion—characterizes the pathologic response to measles virus infection. These cells are found in the skin, respiratory tract, reticuloendothelial system, and other organs. They contain both intracytoplasmic and intranuclear eosinophilic inclusions.

Immune responses to infection with measles include hemagglutination-inhibition (HAI) as well as neutralizing and complement fixing (CF) antibody production. In natural infection, antibody responses appear at approximately 14 days and peak several weeks later with a range of 4 to 6 weeks. CF antibody appears later than HAI and does not usually persist. Antibody in the IgM serum component appears early but rarely persists beyond 90 days.

Infected hosts develop cell-mediated immunity and interferon response in the serum. Delayed hypersensitivity responses are suppressed by infection with natural measles virus as well as by vaccine strains.

Immunocompromised hosts with T-cell lymphocyte dysfunction in particular may have a prolonged course with measles, prolonged excretion of virus, and a high incidence of morbidity and mortality.

## CLINICAL MANIFESTATIONS

Persons with measles virus infection fall into four distinct groups: typical measles in the normal host; modified measles in a host with antibody; atypical measles in the host who received killed vaccine; and measles in immunocompromised persons. The clinical illness may be the same in each group but is usually quite different.

### Typical Measles

The incubation period in typical measles is approximately 10 days, starting with a 3- to 5-day prodrome of malaise, fever, cough, coryza, and conjunctivitis. These symptoms increase over the 3- to 5-day prodrome period. Fever ranges from 39.4° to 40.6 °C, reaching its height at the nadir of the exanthem. About 2 days before the rash, Koplik's spots (white pinpoint lesions on a bright red buccal mucosa) appear opposite the lower molars and quickly spread to involve the entire buccal and lower labial mucosa. Koplik's spots resolve by the third day of the exanthem. The exanthem of measles starts about the 14th day after exposure and appears first behind the ears and the hairline of the forehead. The rash progresses downward to the face, neck, upper extremities and trunk, and reaches the lower extremities by the third day. Initially, the rash is discrete, erythematous, and maculopapular, but it becomes confluent in the same progression as its spread. The rash eventually undergoes a brownish discoloration that does not blanch with pressure and may undergo desquamation. The exanthem lasts 6 to 7 days, and resolution of the rash begins on the third day in the same order as its appearance. In uncomplicated measles, the elevated temperature falls by either crisis or lysis; increased temperature beyond the third to fourth day of the exanthem suggests a complication.

Pharyngitis as well as generalized lymphadenopathy may be seen during the period of the exanthem. Splenomegaly is common. Diarrhea, vomiting, and abdominal pain may be prominent symptoms of measles, especially in young children. Leukopenia is a predictable finding.

## Modified Measles

Modified measles occurs in children who have received immune serum globulin on exposure to measles or in young infants who still have transplacentally acquired maternal measles antibody. In addition, vaccine-modified mild measles, a form of secondary vaccine failure, can occur in individuals who were appropriately vaccinated with the live measles virus vaccine. In mild or modified measles, the prodrome period is shortened, symptoms are not as severe, and Koplik's spots do not usually occur, and, if present, they fade rapidly. The exanthem follows the progression of regular measles but does not become confluent.

## Atypical Measles

Atypical measles usually occurs in persons immunized with killed measles vaccine who are exposed to natural measles. This illness may be observed in adults who received killed measles vaccine from 1963 through 1967 and were not reimmunized with live virus vaccine.

The incubation period for atypical measles is the same as for typical measles. The illness is characterized by sudden onset of fever (39.4° to 40.6 °C). Headache, myalgias, extreme weakness, and abdominal pain may all be present. Almost all patients have a dry, nonproductive cough. The rash of atypical measles appears first on the distal extremities and is pronounced on wrists and ankles. The rash may remain localized or may spread to involve the upper and lower extremities as well as the trunk. The palms and soles are also involved.

The rash of atypical measles may be erythematous and maculopapular (see Color Figure 28); it may be vesicular, petechial, or purpuric in nature. Urticaria has been described. Edema of the hands and feet and severe hyperesthesia have also been described. Koplik's spots are rarely seen.

Pulmonary involvement occurs in almost all cases, with roentgenographic examination revealing pneumonia that frequently appears nodular. Hilar adenopathy and pleural effusion may be seen. Pulmonary involvement is accompanied by respiratory distress with tachypnea, dyspnea, and cough. Pulmonary involvement can occur without the exanthem.

## Measles in the Immunocompromised Host

Giant cell pneumonia is a common complication of measles in the immunocompromised host. It may occur in the absence of an exanthem as has been described in children with symptomatic infection with human immunodeficiency virus (HIV). The pneumonia may have an insidious or fulminant onset. Encephalitis may occur in these patients with a more insidious, protracted course than that seen in the normal host.

## Measles in Pregnancy

Measles occurring in the pregnant female may lead to increased mortality of the pregnant woman and a fetal effect of prematurity, spontaneous abortion early in pregnancy, or increased incidence

of stillbirth. Perinatal measles, which has its onset in the first 10 days of life, is considered to be transplacentally acquired. Perinatal measles has a high incidence of pneumonia with resulting mortality.

## COMPLICATIONS OF MEASLES

Complications of measles include viral pneumonia, laryngitis, laryngotracheobronchitis, and bronchiolitis. It is often difficult to differentiate between the patient who has viral pneumonia associated with measles and the patient who has a superimposed bacterial pneumonia. Therefore, when pneumonia is demonstrated by a chest roentgenogram, antimicrobial therapy should be considered. The bacteria involved include *Streptococcus pneumoniae*, *Staphylococcus aureus*, *Haemophilus influenzae*, and *Streptococcus pyogenes*. Otitis media is a common complication and is caused by the same bacterial pathogens that cause otitis media in children.

Other complications of measles include myocarditis, pericarditis, appendicitis, and corneal ulcerations as well as thrombocytopenic purpura. Hemorrhagic measles, seen frequently in former years, seldom occurs and probably was a result of disseminated intravascular coagulopathy.

Neurologic complications of measles include encephalitis, which occurs in approximately 1 in every 1000 to 2000 cases of measles. A mortality of 15% and morbidity among survivors of 25% has been observed. Encephalitis has its usual onset during the period of the exanthem, but onset may occur in the prodromal period. There is a high incidence of convulsions, cerebral edema, and other neurologic deficits in measles encephalitis. There is usually a mononuclear cell pleocytosis of the cerebrospinal fluid (CSF) and a slightly elevated protein. The electroencephalogram is abnormal in measles encephalitis but may also be abnormal in the absence of clinically diagnosed encephalitis.

Subacute sclerosing panencephalitis (SSPE) is an uncommon degenerative central nervous system (CNS) disease associated with persistent measles virus infection of the CNS. The risk of SSPE is approximately 1 per 100,000 infections with natural measles and 1 per 1,000,000 immunizations in vaccine-associated SSPE. The incubation period is shorter in vaccine-associated SSPE than with natural measles. SSPE has an insidious onset with intellectual deterioration, myoclonic jerks, and progression to dementia and finally decorticate rigidity. The clinical picture, the typical electroencephalogram, and exceptionally high titers of measles HAI antibody in serum and CSF are the basis for the diagnosis.

## DIFFERENTIAL DIAGNOSIS

The differential diagnosis includes infections with those viruses that may cause erythematous maculopapular rashes: the enteroviruses, adenoviruses, rubella, erythema infectiosum, and infectious mononucleosis. Also considered in the diagnosis are infections with *Mycoplasma pneumoniae* and drug eruptions accompanied by fever. It is more likely that these illnesses would be confused with the clinical presentation of modified measles rather than typical measles. In atypical measles, the age of the patient and a history of repeated measles immunizations (killed vaccine may have been administered several times) may help confirm the diagnosis. Atypical measles has been confused with Rocky Mountain spotted fever.

## DIAGNOSIS

Isolation of measles virus conventionally is not used to make a specific diagnosis of measles; however, measles virus may be isolated in tissue culture. Because of the recent resurgence of measles as well as new, commercially available immunofluorescence reagents, many viral diagnostic laboratories are attempting to isolate and identify this virus. The best specimens for isolation of measles are nasopharyngeal washes or swabs and urine sediment. The virus also may be isolated from peripheral blood lymphocytes early in the course of illness and from tissue obtained from biopsy procedures. Specimens must be transported promptly to the virology laboratory for maximum isolation rates.

The HAI test has been widely performed to make a serologic diagnosis of measles. Many laboratories use the enzyme-linked immunosorbent assay (ELISA) technique. Antibodies are usually present in a patient's serum by day 1 to 3 of the exanthem and peak some 2 to 6 weeks later. A patient with suspected measles, either in the prodromal period or with rash, should have a serum obtained immediately and a paired serum in 2 to 3 weeks. Both sera should be evaluated simultaneously in the same laboratory to determine the presence of measles antibody. A four-fold or greater rise in antibody titer in either one of the two tests or the presence of IgM antibody in either serum as determined by ELISA confirms a serologic diagnosis of measles. In atypical measles, a patient's sera may have extremely high titers of HAI antibody. This also occurs in patients with SSPE, in whom HAI antibody is found in the CSF.

Immunofluorescent studies have been performed on exfoliated cells and tissue from different organs to detect measles virus antigen. A paramyxovirus may be seen in lung tissue of patients with giant cell pneumonia.

## TREATMENT

There is no specific approved therapy for measles virus infection. Fever should be controlled by acetaminophen, and room air should be humidified. Careful attention should be given to fluid intake, particularly in young infants. Antibiotics should not be given except when there are bacterial complications. Children with very serious complications of measles (eg, pneumonia, encephalitis, croup) should be hospitalized and treated. Aerosolized or intravenous ribavirin has been used on a compassionate basis to treat measles pneumonia, although its effectiveness has not been rigorously evaluated in clinical trials.

Children with measles are still considered contagious for 5 days after appearance of the rash, and measures should be undertaken to prevent their exposure to susceptible individuals. Immunocompromised persons with measles may be contagious longer.

## MEASLES PREVENTION

### General Considerations

Prevention of measles in the general population is possible by maintaining a high level of immunization among children 15 months of age or older. Many physicians who have recently completed training have not seen a patient with measles and, therefore, must have a high index of suspicion when confronted with a patient with fever and a maculopapular exanthem. A suspected case of measles should be reported immediately to public health authorities, then confirmed serologically. Persons working in medical facilities or matriculating in college should furnish proof of immunization or be screened to determine their immunity to measles. Unless it is contraindicated, nonimmune persons should be considered for immunization.

There remain measles-susceptible persons of all age groups in the United States. Many parents delay immunization of children until they enter school, at which time immunization is re-

quired by law. Therefore, a number of children 15 months to 5 years of age are not immune. Children younger than 15 months of age may have no maternal antibody and, consequently, are susceptible to measles virus infections. Adults born after 1956 may never have been immunized or have had natural measles, and, thus, are susceptible to infection. Persons immunized before 1977 may have been immunized at 12 months of age or younger and may not be immune.

Persons who were immunized with killed measles vaccine (1963 to 1967) may not have been reimmunized with attenuated vaccine. Other reasons for nonimmune persons include vaccine failure (less than 5% of all persons who receive the measles vaccine) and immunization with unknown vaccine between 1963 and 1967. Persons who were immunized with attenuated live virus vaccine (other than Edmonston B) and who received immune globulin (IG) along with the vaccine may not be immune.

Since 1980, a stabilizer has been added to the measles vaccine preparation, making it more resistant to inactivation by heat. Emphasis has been placed on proper handling and storage of the vaccine. Persons immunized before 1980 may have received improperly handled vaccine, which could be ineffective in producing an immune response.

### Vaccine Recommendations

All persons born after 1956 who have no documentation of adequate immunization or natural measles (physician diagnosed) should be immunized unless there is a specific contraindication. Because of the resurgence of measles, there has been a basic change in the recommended routine childhood vaccination schedule from a one-dose schedule to a two-dose schedule, using the combined MMR vaccine. The first dose of MMR vaccine should still be administered at 15 months of age to children in most areas of the country. More than 95% of children who receive the vaccine at 15 months of age will achieve a protective immune response. In areas with recurrent measles transmission, however, the first dose of MMR vaccine should be administered at 12 months of age. During epidemics, a first dose of monovalent measles vaccine should be given at 6 months of age, followed by routine MMR vaccine at 15 months of age, because seroconversion rates are significantly lower among children vaccinated before their first birthday than among older children.

The second dose of MMR vaccine may be administered at 4 to 6 years of age, upon entry to kindergarten or first grade, according to the recommendations of the Immunization Practices Advisory Committee from the Centers for Disease Control. Alternatively, the second dose may be administered at 11 to 12 years of age, upon entry to middle school or junior high school, according to the Committee on Infectious Diseases of the American Academy of Pediatrics. There is flexibility in when the second dose may be administered, but it is important for all children to receive a second dose of vaccine. Because a number of measles cases have occurred in students on college campuses, adolescents and young adults entering institutions for post–high-school education should have received two doses of vaccine or have documentation of physician-diagnosed measles or laboratory evidence of measles immunity before entry into that school. Only constant vigilance controls measles. Physicians caring for children and adolescents should continuously monitor measles epidemiology in their area and comply with the recommendations of local public health officials.

### Vaccine Contraindications

Contraindications to measles vaccine include pregnancy, anaphylaxis to egg or neomycin, compromised immunity (excluding those infected with symptomatic or asymptomatic HIV), or receipt of IG within 3 months. A personal or family history of seizures should be evaluated case by case before vaccine administration. Tuberculosis is not a contraindication for administration of measles vaccine.

## Adverse Vaccine Reactions

As many as 15% of vaccinees may have fever 5 to 12 days after vaccination. Fever usually lasts 1 to 5 days. A small number of vaccinees develop a transient rash. The frequency of CNS complications is 1 per 3,000,000 doses of administered vaccine.

## PREVENTION FOR EXPOSED INDIVIDUALS

If given in the first 72 hours after exposure, live measles virus vaccine may prevent infection. IG may be given to prevent or modify illness in exposed individuals if given within 6 days of exposure. The recommended dose is 0.25 mL/kg (maximum dose, 15 mL). Immunocompromised children should receive 0.5 mL/ kg with a maximum total dose of 15 mL. Children with symptomatic HIV infection should receive IG at time of exposure regardless of vaccination status. IG administration precludes vaccination for 3 months in children in whom there is otherwise no contraindication.

For detailed recommendations or contraindications for vaccine administration, refer to the 22nd edition of the *Report of the Committee on Infectious Diseases* (Red Book), 1991.

## Selected Readings

American Academy of Pediatrics. Rubeola. In: Peter G, Hall CB, Lepow ML, Phillips CF, eds. Report of the Committee on Infectious Diseases, ed 22. Elk Grove Village, Ill: American Academy of Pediatrics, 1991:308.

Cherry JD. Measles. In: Feigin RD, Cherry JD, eds. Textbook of pediatric infectious diseases, ed 3. Vol 2. Philadelphia: WB Saunders, 1992:1591.

Edmonson MB, Addiss DG, McPherson JT, Berg JL, Circo SR, Davis JP. Mild measles and secondary vaccine failure during a sustained outbreak in a highly vaccinated population. JAMA 1990;263:2467.

Fulginiti VA, Eller JJ, Downie AW, Kempe CH. Altered reactivity to measles virus: atypical measles in children previously immunized with inactivated measles virus vaccine. JAMA 1967;202:1075.

Gindler JS, Atkinson WL, Markowitz LE, Hutchins SS. Epidemiology of measles in the United States in 1989 and 1990. Pediatr Infect Dis J 1992;11:841.

Immunization Practices Advisory Committee. Measles prevention. MMWR 1989;38(1):11.

International Symposium on Measles Immunization, Pan American Health Association, Washington, DC, March 16–19, 1982. Rev Infect Dis 1983;5(3):389.

Koplik H. The diagnosis of the invasion of measles from a study of the exanthema as it appears on the buccal mucous membrane. Arch Pediatr 1986;13:918.

Littauer J, Sorensen K. The measles epidemic at Umanak in Greenland in 1962. Dan Med Bull 1965;12:43.

Measles (Rubeola). In: Infectious diseases of children, ed 8. Krugman S, Katz SL, Gershon AA, Wilfert C, eds. St. Louis: CV Mosby, 1985:152.

Measles—Los Angeles County, California, 1988. MMWR 1989;38(4):49.

Minnich LL, Goodenough F, Ray G. Use of immunofluorescence to identify measles virus infections. J Clin Microbiol 1991;29:1148.

Moench TR, Griffin DE, Obriecht CR, et al. Acute measles in patients with and without neurological involvement: distribution of measles virus antigen and RNA. J Infect Dis 1988;158(2):433.

Norrby E. *Paramyxoviridae:* measles virus. In: Lennette EH, Halonen P, Murphy FA, eds. Laboratory diagnosis of infectious diseases: principles and practice. Vol 2. Viral, rickettsial, and chlamydial diseases. New York: Springer-Verlag, 1988:525.

*Principles and Practice of Pediatrics, Second Edition.*
edited by Frank A. Oski et al. J. B. Lippincott Company, Philadelphia © 1994.

# *57.16 Mumps*

Larry H. Taber and Gail J. Demmler

Mumps is a contagious disease characterized by swelling of the salivary glands, particularly the parotid glands. Inapparent infection may occur in 40% of infected individuals. In 1934, experiments by Johnson and Goodpasture demonstrated a mumps-like illness in rhesus monkeys receiving parotid secretions from patients with mumps. Filtered parotid secretions from infected monkeys could be passed to other monkeys with resulting parotitis from a filterable agent, a virus.

Mumps virus subsequently was propagated in eggs, which allowed production of mumps antigen for a complement fixation test. Attenuation of the virus in vitro was accomplished by Enders in the 1940s; this proved useful for vaccine development. A vaccine was prepared and licensed in 1968.

## ETIOLOGY

Mumps is a single-stranded RNA virus and a member of the family Paramyxoviridae, genus *Paramyxovirus*. It has two major surface glycoproteins: the hemagglutinin-neuraminidase and the fusion protein. Mumps virus is sensitive to heat and ultraviolet light.

## EPIDEMIOLOGY

Mumps is transmitted by direct intimate contact or infected droplets from the oropharynx. Communicability is present before parotid swelling (1 to 7 days, but usually 1 to 2 days) and 7 to 9 days after onset of parotid swelling. The incubation period of mumps is approximately 18 days but may be longer. Mumps occurs in winter and spring seasons, and had its highest attack rate in 5- to 9-year-old children in the prevaccine era. Many epidemiologic features of mumps are difficult to ascertain because of the high incidence of inapparent infections.

Not all states have laws requiring mumps immunization; in 1987, the incidence of mumps in 10- to 14-year-old children increased in states with no such law. Overall, there has been a dramatic reduction in cases of mumps since routine use of mumps vaccine was initiated in 1977.

## PATHOGENESIS AND PATHOLOGY

Mumps virus produces a generalized infection. After entry into the oropharynx, viral replication takes place with subsequent viremia and involvement of glands or nervous tissue. The virus may be isolated from saliva, blood, urine, and cerebrospinal fluid (CSF). Affected glands show edema and lymphocyte infiltration.

## CLINICAL MANIFESTATIONS

### Parotitis

The classic illness of mumps is swelling of the parotid gland (ie, parotitis). Systemic symptoms include low-grade fever, headache, malaise, anorexia, and abdominal pain. Acid-containing foods may aggravate discomfort of the parotid gland. Ordinarily, the parotid gland is not palpable, but in mumps cases, it rapidly progresses to maximum swelling over several days. Unilateral swelling usually occurs first, followed by bilateral parotid involvement. Occasionally, simultaneous involvement of both parotid glands occurs. Unilateral parotid disease occurs in fewer than 25% of patients. Fever subsides within 1 week and disappears before swelling of the parotid gland resolves, which may require as long as 10 days. Other salivary glands may be involved, including both submaxillary and sublingual, and orifices of the ducts may be erythematous and edematous.

## Orchitis

About one third of postpubertal males develop unilateral orchitis. It usually follows parotitis but may precede parotitis or occur in the absence of parotitis. It usually appears in the first week of parotitis but can occur in the second or third week. Bilateral orchitis occurs much less frequently and, although gonadal atrophy may follow orchitis, sterility is rare even with bilateral involvement. Prepubertal males may develop orchitis, but it is uncommon in males younger than 10 years of age.

Orchitis is accompanied by high fever, severe pain, and swelling. Nausea, vomiting, and abdominal pain are not uncommon. Fever and gonadal swelling usually resolve in 1 week, but tenderness may persist.

## Meningoencephalitis

Central nervous system (CNS) involvement with mumps is not uncommon and is more often a meningitis than a true encephalitis. It may precede parotitis or appear in the absence of parotitis, but it usually occurs in the first week following parotitis. Headache, fever, nausea, vomiting, and meningismus are common. Marked changes in sensorium and convulsions are not usual.

Pleocytosis of the CSF occurs in a high percentage of persons without clinical evidence of CNS involvement. In clinically diagnosed meningoencephalitis, a CSF mononuclear pleocytosis occurs as does a normal glucose, although hypoglycorrhachia has been reported. Mumps virus may be isolated from CSF early in the illness. Mumps meningoencephalitis has a good prognosis and usually an uneventful recovery.

Other clinical manifestations of mumps include pancreatitis accompanied by severe abdominal pain, chills, fever, and persistent vomiting. Thyroiditis, oophoritis, and mastitis occasionally occur.

## COMPLICATIONS OF MUMPS

Neuritis of the auditory nerve may result in deafness. There is sudden onset of tinnitus, ataxia, and vomiting followed by permanent deafness. Other neurologic complications include facial nerve neuritis and myelitis.

More uncommon complications include arthritis, myocarditis, and hematologic complications.

## DIFFERENTIAL DIAGNOSIS

Parotitis caused by other viruses—coxsackieviruses, influenza viruses, and parainfluenza viruses—cannot be differentiated clinically from mumps parotitis. In suppurative parotitis commonly caused by Staphylococcus aureus or other bacteria, the parotid gland is very tender and the overlying skin is erythematous.

Adenitis, recurrent parotitis, calculus of Stensen's duct, tumors of the parotid gland, and Mikulicz's syndrome may be considered in the differential diagnosis.

Mumps meningoencephalitis is indistinguishable from that caused by many other viruses, unless parotitis is present.

## DIAGNOSIS

The diagnosis of mumps is usually made clinically; however, laboratory confirmation can be helpful, especially in patients with unusual manifestations. The serum amylase level is often elevated when there is salivary gland or pancreatic involvement, and isoenzyme analysis can be performed to distinguish between these two sites of infection. A serologic diagnosis of mumps may be made by testing paired sera for mumps IgG antibody obtained early in illness and 2 to 4 weeks after illness. The diagnosis of mumps also can be made from a single serum specimen if the presence of mumps IgM antibody is detected. Most clinical serology laboratories perform mumps serology using enzyme immunoassay (EIA). In addition, the presence of complement fixing (CF) antibody to the soluble (S) component (composed primarily of the nucleocapsid-associated proteins) of the mumps virus suggests a recent infection within the past 6 months, and this test is available from many reference laboratories. Mumps virus also can be readily grown from saliva or swabs of material expressed directly from Stensen's duct, as well as from urine and CSF. Viral cultures are encouraged because isolation of mumps virus is timely and confirms the diagnosis. Specimens for viral isolation should be collected early in the illness and transported to the virology laboratory on wet ice for maximum isolation rates.

## TREATMENT

Treatment of mumps parotitis and other glandular involvement is largely relief of symptoms. Patients with orchitis may obtain relief with gentle support of the testicle and ice packs. Management of mumps meningitis is similar to that for other forms of viral meningitis. Antibiotics are not recommended. Acetaminophen can be used for fever control, but relief of pain may require a narcotic. Respiratory isolation of the hospitalized patient is advised. Patients are considered no longer contagious 9 days after onset of parotid swelling.

## PREVENTION OF MUMPS

All children should receive measles-mumps-rubella vaccine (MMR) at 15 months of age. More than 95% of persons receiving mumps vaccine develop antibody. Because of recent outbreaks of mumps (as well as measles and rubella virus illnesses) among adolescents and young adults, however, and because of the increased morbidity from mumps in postpubertal individuals, a second dose of MMR vaccine is now recommended by the Committee on Infectious Diseases of the American Academy of Pediatrics at 11 to 12 years of age or upon entry to middle school or junior high school. Alternatively, a second dose of MMR may be administered at 4 to 6 years of age, upon entry into kindergarten or first grade, according to the recommendations of the Immunization Practices Advisory Committee. Flexibility in administration of the second dose allows physicians to comply with recommendations of local public health officials. Contraindications for the administration of mumps vaccine include pregnancy, true egg allergy, altered immunity (excluding persons infected with human immunodeficiency virus), and use of immune globulin (IG) within the past 3 months. Adverse reactions with mumps vaccine administration are uncommon.

For detailed recommendations or contraindications for vaccine administration, refer to the 22nd edition of the *Report of the Committee on Infectious Diseases* (Red Book), 1991.

## Selected Readings

American Academy of Pediatrics. Mumps. In: Peter G, Hall CB, Lepow ML, Phillips CF, eds. Report of the Committee on Infectious Diseases, ed 22. Elk Grove Village, Ill: American Academy of Pediatrics, 1991:328.

Brunell P. Mumps. In: Feigin RD, Cherry JD, eds. Textbook of pediatric infectious diseases, ed 3. Vol 2. Philadelphia: WB Saunders, 1992:1610.

Centers for Disease Control. Epidemiologic notes and reports: mumps—United States, 1985–1988. Morbidity and Mortality Weekly Report 1989; 38(7):101.

Mumps (epidemic parotitis). In: Krugman S, Katz SL, Gershon AA, Wilfert C, eds. Infectious diseases of children, ed 8. St. Louis: CV Mosby, 1985:192.

Orvell C. *Paramyxoviridae*: mumps virus. In: Lennette EH, Halonen P, Murphy FA, eds. Laboratory diagnosis of infectious diseases: principles and practice, Vol 2. Viral, rickettsial, and chlamydial diseases. New York: Springer-Verlag, 1988: 507.

Wharton M, Cochi SL, Hutcheson RH, et al: A large outbreak of mumps in the postvaccine era. J Infect Dis 1988;158:1253.

*Principles and Practice of Pediatrics, Second Edition.*
edited by Frank A. Oski et al. J. B. Lippincott Company, Philadelphia © 1994.

# *57.17 Papovaviruses*

### Gail J. Demmler

The term papovavirus is derived from the names of three viruses originally thought to be similar: *pa*pilloma (wart) virus, *pol*yomavirus, and *va*cuolating agent (SV40) of rhesus monkeys. The Papovaviridae family is considered a heterogeneous family of small DNA viruses that infect a variety of mammals. Human papovaviruses contain two groups: the papillomaviruses, which are responsible for a variety of benign dysplastic and malignant proliferative squamous lesions of the skin and mucosa, and the polyomaviruses, which infect many people subclinically but, in immunosuppressed patients, can produce serious illness. Papillomaviruses are discussed in Chapter 35; this discussion focuses on human polyomaviruses—JC virus (the etiologic agent of progressive multifocal leukoencephalopathy) and BK virus.

## JC VIRUS

Progressive multifocal leukoencephalopathy (PML) is a rare, demyelinating disease of the central nervous system (CNS) seen in immunosuppressed hosts. The causative agent, JC virus, was first isolated in 1971 when the brain homogenate of a patient (initials JC) who died of PML was inoculated into human fetal glial cells.

Although PML is an extremely rare, opportunistic disease, infection with JC virus appears to be common in childhood; 65% of 14-year-old children have antibody to the virus. The JC virus usually causes few or no symptoms, although it has been associated with mild respiratory illness. The virus can reactivate and be detected in the urine of normal pregnant women, renal and bone marrow transplant recipients, and children and adults with malignancies. Evidence for transplacental transmission and congenital infection with this virus, however, is conflicting and requires further study. The JC virus is also oncogenic and neurotropic. It produces medulloblastomas and neuroblastomas when inoculated into animals and may be involved in production of human brain tumors as well.

## Pathology

The histopathologic changes seen in the brains of patients with PML consist of multiple areas of gross demyelination, enlarged hyperchromatic nuclei of the oligodendrocytes, and proliferation of bizarre, neoplastic-appearing astrocytes. Neurons are unaffected. Electron microscopy reveals large numbers of papovavirus particles in the oligodendritic nuclei, and viral antigen can be identified by immunofluorescence. Large quantities of viral DNA can be detected by DNA hybridization assay. There is a striking lack of inflammatory response, however, in the brains of patients with PML.

## Clinical Manifestations

The diagnosis of PML should be considered in any immunocompromised host who develops a progressive, multifocal neurologic illness. Most patients with PML have an immunodeficiency with depressed cell-mediated immunity, resulting from lymphoproliferative diseases, carcinomas, sarcoidosis, tuberculosis, systemic lupus erythematosus, acquired immune deficiency syndrome (AIDS), and renal transplantation. The disease also has been reported in children with severe combined immunodeficiency syndrome. PML begins with personality changes, altered mental status, hemiparesis, ataxia, aphasia, or cortical blindness, and rapidly progresses to coma. Death usually results in 2 to 4 months, although some patients have lived for 1 to 2 years. The cerebrospinal fluid is usually normal. The electroencephalogram shows diffuse and nonspecific slowing. Computed tomography of the brain reveals areas of demyelination.

## Diagnosis

The diagnosis of PML may be suggested clinically in any immunocompromised patient who develops multifocal brain disease. Other neurodegenerative diseases of known or presumed viral etiology include multiple sclerosis, subacute sclerosing panencephalitis, herpesvirus infections of the CNS, and AIDS. A tentative diagnosis of PML can be made if computed tomography or magnetic resonance imaging shows areas of decreased density in the brain. Definitive diagnosis is made by brain biopsy or by examination at autopsy. The unique histopathology usually establishes the diagnosis. Papovavirus particles also may be demonstrated in oligodendrocytes by electron microscopy, the JC virus antigens may be detected in the brain by immunofluorescence, or the viral DNA may be detected by hybridization assays. The virus may also be cultivated from brain tissue or urine when inoculated onto human fetal glial cell tissue culture.

## Treatment

PML is usually fatal within 6 months of diagnosis, although some spontaneous remissions or disease stabilization have been reported. Immunosuppressive regimens should be discontinued, if possible. Nonspecific biologic response modifiers such as levamisole and interferon may provide some benefit. Antiviral chemotherapy with iododeoxyuridine, cytosine arabinoside, and adenine arabinoside has been attempted, but multicenter clinical trials are needed before any definite therapeutic recommendations can be made.

## BK VIRUS

BK virus was first isolated from the urine of a 39-year-old man (initials BK) 4 months after renal transplantation. Infection with BK virus occurs commonly in early childhood and may be asymptomatic or associated with a viral respiratory illness. Ninety percent to 100% of children have antibody to BK virus by age 10 years. BK virus also has been implicated as a cause of viral cystitis in normal children and interstitial nephritis in an immunocompromised child. Up to 40% of renal transplant recipients excrete BK virus in their urine, either as a result of reactivation of their own strain or infection from the allograft if the donor is seropositive for BK virus. Normal pregnant women also may excrete BK virus (and JC virus) in their urine, but there is no conclusive evidence that vertical transmission from mother to infant occurs. The BK virus does not cause PML, although it has been isolated from a brain tumor that occurred in a child with Wiskott-Aldrich disease.

## Clinical Manifestations

The pathologic consequences of BK virus infection have not been fully determined. Certain conditions such as ureteral stenosis, hemorrhagic cystitis, pancreatitis, and pericarditis have been linked to active infection with BK virus.

## Diagnosis

BK virus multiplication in the urine can be suspected by the presence of cytologically atypical cells in the urinary sediment. Virions can be detected by electron microscopy and viral antigen in in-fected cell nuclei can be detected by immunofluorescence. Molecular probes also can detect BK virus DNA sequences in cells or tissue.

BK virus also may be grown in cell cultures. Because BK virus may be shed asymptomatically in the urine, a biopsy of the kidney, ureter, bladder, or other organ suspected to be involved may be necessary to support a pathogenic role.

## Treatment

Recognized BK virus infection is most commonly associated with immunodeficiency or iatrogenic immunosuppression. Therefore, therapeutic efforts should focus on withdrawal of immunosuppression, if feasible. Human leukocyte interferon alpha has been administered to renal transplant recipients with BK virus infection, but no definitive therapeutic recommendation can be made for patients actively infected with BK virus.

## Selected Readings

Norkin LC. Papovaviral persistent infections. Microbiol Rev 1982;46:384.
Padgett BL, Walker D. New human papovaviruses. Prog Med Virol 1976;22:1.
Padgett BL, Walker DL, ZuRhein GM, Eckroade RJ. Cultivation of papova-like virus from human brain with progressive multifocal leucoencephalopathy. Lancet 1971;1:1257.
ZuRhein GM, Padgett B, Walker D, et al. Progressive multifocal leukoencephalopathy in a child with severe combined immunodeficiency. N Engl J Med 1978;299:256.

*Principles and Practice of Pediatrics, Second Edition.*
edited by Frank A. Oski et al. J. B. Lippincott Company, Philadelphia © 1994.

# 57.18 *Reoviruses*

Gail J. Demmler

The term reovirus was coined from *r*espiratory *e*nteric *o*rphan because the first members of this family of viruses inhabited both the respiratory and gastrointestinal tracts of man, but were "orphans" because they were not yet associated with a disease process. The family Reoviridae now contains three genera of viruses that are pathogenic for humans: rotaviruses, a common cause of infantile gastroenteritis; orbiviruses, which include the etiologic agent of Colorado tick fever; and reoviruses (also called ortho-reoviruses), possibly a common cause of mild, self-limited gastroenteritis. Reoviruses are all spherical, viral particles that contain a unique segmented dsRNA genome.

## ROTAVIRUSES

Human rotaviruses were first detected in 1973 by electron microscopy in duodenal biopsy samples of children with acute gastroenteritis. Because the circular outline of the outer capsid of the viruses resembled a double-rimmed wheel, they were named rotavirus from the Latin *rota*, which means wheel. Viral particles are 70 nm in diameter and contain a segmented genome of dsRNA. There are two subgroups (I and II) and six groups (A, B, C, D, E, F) of rotaviruses. Within each group, rotaviruses are classified into serotypes.

## Epidemiology and Transmission

Rotaviruses are ubiquitous and have been isolated from many mammalian and avian species as well as from humans throughout the world. They are a major cause of diarrhea in infants and young children in developed countries and can cause severe morbidity and mortality in children in developing countries. Rotavirus gastroenteritis severe enough to require hospitalization occurs most frequently in infants younger than 1 year of age.

Rotavirus disease has been termed "winter gastroenteritis" because, in temperate climates, it occurs more often in January and February. In tropical climates, it is endemic and may be a cause of traveler's diarrhea. Rotaviruses are also frequent causes of nosocomial infection in hospital nurseries and pediatric wards. Transmission within families and day-care centers often occurs as well.

The virus is shed in large quantities in the feces for 3 to 5 days and probably is spread by contact with virus-infected stool. Water-borne transmission may also occur in community swimming pools because the virus is resistant to chlorination. Many children have a concomitant rhinorrhea, so transmission may also occur by the respiratory route.

## Pathology and Pathogenesis

Rotaviruses multiply in the differentiated columnar epithelium near the apex of the villi of the small intestine. Histopathologic investigation of intestinal biopsy specimens shows blunting and shortening of the villi with infiltration of the lamina propria by mononuclear cells. Disaccharidase deficiency also occurs and may account for the malabsorption commonly seen in rotavirus-induced diarrhea. Although preexisting serum antibody does not protect against infection, local antibody in the intestine, such as IgA antibody from human breast milk, appears to provide protection against disease.

## Clinical Manifestations

Rotavirus infection usually produces clinical illness in children aged 6 months to 2 years. The illness begins with fever, upper respiratory symptoms, and vomiting, followed by a profuse, watery diarrhea that does not characteristically contain blood or fecal leukocytes. The diarrhea can last 3 to 5 days and often causes isotonic dehydration and a metabolic acidosis. Death can occur, especially in malnourished children in developing countries, due to dehydration, electrolyte imbalance, seizures, or aspiration of vomitus. Other clinical manifestations associated either etiologically or incidentally with rotavirus infection include Reye's syndrome, aseptic meningitis, febrile seizures, pneumonia, sudden infant death syndrome, exanthema subitum, Kawasaki disease, hemolytic-uremic syndrome, Crohn's disease, gastrointestinal hemorrhage, and intussusception. Rotavirus has also been detected in the stools of neonates with necrotizing enterocolitis, although many asymptomatic neonates shed rotavirus in their stool as well. Extraintestinal rotavirus infection of the liver and kidney recently has been reported to occur in immunocompromised children. Older children and adults may also asymptomatically shed rotavirus in their stools.

Rotavirus-induced diarrhea is usually associated with a transient disaccharidase deficiency, although chronic or recurrent diarrhea may produce villous atrophy and monosaccharide intolerance. Rotavirus can produce a chronic, symptomatic, even fatal infection in immunosuppressed patients.

## Diagnosis

The diagnosis of rotavirus disease should be considered when a young child presents with vomiting and watery diarrhea, especially if the illness occurs during winter. The presence of rotavirus particles in the stool can be confirmed by direct examination of the stool by electron microscopy or immune electron microscopy. Rotaviruses are shed in large quantities and their appearance is characteristic, making this test both sensitive and specific. A simpler, more available method is detection of rotavirus antigen by enzyme-linked immunosorbent assay (ELISA) or latex agglutination. These antigen detection tests are available commercially, do not require expensive equipment, and can be performed reliably and easily in most clinical laboratories. False-positive ELISA results can occur, especially in stool specimens collected from neonates. Less widely used tests to detect rotaviruses include radioimmunoassay and dot hybridization. Rotavirus is not routinely cultivated in the cell culture systems used in hospital-based diagnostic virology laboratories. A serologic response to rotavirus infection can be measured using ELISA, radioimmunoassay, or complement fixation techniques, but it is used primarily for seroepidemiologic surveys.

## Treatment

The treatment of rotavirus-associated gastroenteritis is restoration of fluid and electrolyte balance. Oral therapy with a glucose-electrolyte solution corrects mild to moderate dehydration and has been lifesaving in developing countries. Intravenous rehydration may be necessary in infants with severe dehydration, shock, or protracted vomiting. Antibiotics and antidiarrheal medications that alter intestinal motility are not indicated. Patients with immunodeficiencies who develop prolonged diarrhea and prolonged fecal excretion of rotavirus have been treated with oral feedings of human milk containing rotavirus antibody. Passive protection has been attempted in low–birth-weight infants by oral administration of human milk or human immune globulin containing rotavirus antibody.

Good hygiene, hand washing, and disinfection are important to prevent spread of rotavirus in families, day-care centers, and hospitals. Improved nutrition and hygiene will help decrease the severe mortality associated with this disease in developing countries.

Immunoprophylaxis using an experimental rotavirus vaccine recently has been shown to induce protective antibody and may be an important step in reducing the worldwide morbidity and mortality associated with this disease.

## ORBIVIRUSES

Because of their large ring- or doughnut-shaped morphology, orbiviruses were named from the Latin *orbis*, meaning ring. In the 1970s, the orbiviruses were removed from the "unclassified arbovirus" group and included in the Reoviridae family of viruses because of their molecular characteristics. Orbiviruses are the only arthropod-borne viruses in the Reoviridae family, and they infect a variety of different animals. Five viruses infect man: the Colorado tick fever virus of the United States, the Kemerova virus of Siberia and Egypt, the Changuinola virus of Panama, and the Orungo and Lebombo viruses of Africa. This discussion is limited to the Colorado tick fever agent, the only orbivirus that causes disease in North America.

## Epidemiology

Colorado tick fever is a zoonotic infection of rodents that occurs in mountainous areas of the western United States, especially Colorado, as well as parts of northwest Canada. The vector is the wood tick, *Dermacentor andersoni*, and human infection occurs when an adult tick harboring the virus bites a human. There is a strong seasonal trend in that cases occur between February and July with most occurring in May and June. The disease also has been reported to be transmitted by blood transfusion.

## Pathology and Pathogenesis

Soon after infection, the Colorado tick fever virus invades the bone marrow and erythrocyte precursors. When the mature red blood cell is produced, it harbors the virus. A prolonged erythrocyte-associated viremia then occurs that peaks during the second and third week of illness and may last many weeks. The infected red blood cells may express viral antigen, as detected by immunofluorescence, for up to 20 weeks. The virus appears to be pantropic and can affect many organ systems, including the testicles, pericardium, lungs and pleura, skin, meninges, brain, and eyes.

## Clinical Manifestations

Colorado tick fever usually occurs in campers or foresters. A history of a tick bite 1 to 2 weeks previously is almost always elicited. The illness begins suddenly with fever, chills, lethargy, headache, severe myalgias, photophobia, and retro-orbital pain. The fever is characteristically biphasic or "saddle-backed;" that is, after the initial 2- to 3-day period of fever, there is a 2- to 3-day remission, followed once again by fever. A maculopapular or petechial rash occurs in 10% of patients. A meningoencephalitis also may occur, especially in children younger than 10 years old. Colorado tick fever is usually a self-limited illness; however, a more severe clinical picture can occur in children with gastrointestinal hemorrhage, disseminated intravascular coagulation, and severe rash. Death is exceedingly rare.

Leukopenia (2000 to 4000 WBCs/mm$^3$) and thrombocytopenia characteristically occur during the acute phase of the illness and may persist for weeks. Also, cerebrospinal fluid findings typical of viral meningitis occur in patients with central nervous system (CNS) involvement.

## Diagnosis

The diagnosis of Colorado tick fever can be established serologically by collecting acute and convalescent sera and demonstrating a seroconversion to the agent by complement fixation, immunofluorescence, or neutralization. A serum IgM test has been recently described and may be available in some laboratories. Some state health department laboratories in endemic areas provide testing. Testing is also performed by the Centers for Disease Control in Atlanta. An immunofluorescence assay can identify Colorado tick fever viral antigen on erythrocyte smears up to 20 weeks after the illness. The agent may also be isolated by inoculating clotted or heparinized red blood cells or cerebrospinal fluid into viral cell culture systems such as Vero cells or into suckling mice.

The differential diagnosis of Colorado tick fever includes Rocky Mountain spotted fever, dengue, acute rheumatic fever, influenza, and North American encephalitides (eg, western equine encephalitis) and other viral agents that can cause encephalitis.

## Treatment

Colorado tick fever is usually a self-limited disease and is probably the most benign febrile illness transmitted by tick bite in the United States. Treatment is aimed at alleviating symptoms of pain, nausea, dehydration, and electrolyte disturbances. There is no specific antiviral therapy available for Colorado tick fever; however, ribavirin has been demonstrated to inhibit the virus in mice. Permanent sequelae are rare but can occur when there is CNS involvement. Preventive measures include avoiding tick-infested areas, use of protective clothing, and prompt removal of any ticks seen on the body or in clothing. To prevent transfusion-transmitted Colorado tick fever, patients recovering from this illness should not donate blood products for at least 1 year after recovery. An experimental inactivated vaccine is under investigation. Because of the relatively benign nature of the disease, however, and the sporadic numbers of cases reported annually, vaccination will probably not be a practical public health measure.

## REOVIRUSES

Reoviruses (*r*espiratory, *e*nteric, *o*rphan), sometimes referred to as orthoreoviruses, were named in 1959 by Sabin because these viruses were typically isolated from the respiratory and enteric tracts, but they were not associated with any known disease (hence, "orphans"). Reoviruses are the third genera of the family Reoviridae, and contain three identifiable serotypes: 1 (Lang), 2 (Jones), and 3 (Dearing).

## Epidemiology

Seroepidemiologic surveys of people from a variety of cultural and geographic settings show the majority of individuals have antibodies against all three reovirus serotypes by 3 years of age. Reoviruses are ubiquitous and are present in water supplies, sewer effluent, and all known species of mammals, as well as humans.

## Pathogenesis

Reoviruses behave primarily as enteric viruses. They naturally enter the host orally and attack and replicate in the gastrointestinal tract. In experimental models in mice, reoviruses can invade the CNS, heart, lungs, hepatobiliary system, and pancreas.

## Clinical Manifestations

Despite the ubiquity of reoviruses, it has been difficult to provide convincing evidence linking these agents to any known human disease. The overwhelming majority of reovirus infections are asymptomatic or, perhaps, produce mild upper respiratory or gastrointestinal symptoms that are so common in infancy and early childhood. Case reports link reoviruses to biliary atresia, other cholestatic liver diseases, exanthemal illnesses, pneumonitis, myocarditis, and meningoencephalitis, but documentation is incomplete in many of these reports. Therefore, the role of reoviruses in serious illness must be considered unproven.

## Diagnosis

Diagnosis of reovirus infections is not routinely sought but can be accomplished by isolation of the virus from stool, throat swabs, nasal washings, cerebrospinal fluid, urine, and tissue. Viral antigens also can be detected by immunofluorescence or immunocytochemistry. Serologic testing, usually neutralization or hemagglutination inhibition (HAI) test, can be used to diagnose acute reovirus infection or to confirm past exposure. HAI antibodies generally appear within 3 weeks of an acute reovirus infection and are lifelong.

## Treatment

Because reoviruses have not been shown to produce any significant human disease, there is no impetus to develop strategies for treatment. Ribavirin has shown antiviral activity in vitro, but no animal model or clinical studies using this antiviral for reovirus infection have been conducted.

## Selected Readings

Bishop RF, Davidson GP, Holmes IH, Ruch BJ. Virus particles in the epithelial cells of duodenal mucosa from children with acute, non-bacterial gastroenteritis. Lancet 1973;2:1281.

Champsaur H, Questiaux E, Prevot J, et al. Rotavirus carriage, asymptomatic infection, and disease in the first two years of life. J Infect Dis 1984;149:667.

Estes MK, Palmer EL, Obijeski JF. Rotaviruses: a review. Curr Top Microbiol Immunol 1983;105:123.

Goodpasture HC, Poland JD, Francy DB, et al. Colorado tick fever: clinical, epidemiologic, and laboratory aspects of 228 cases in Colorado in 1973–1974. Ann Intern Med 1978;88:303.

Kapikian AZ, Wyatt RG, Greenberg HB, et al. Approaches to immunization of infants and young children against gastroenteritis due to rotaviruses. Rev Infect Dis 1980;2:459.

Spruance SL, Bailey A. Colorado tick fever: a review of 115 laboratory confirmed cases. Arch Intern Med 1973;131:288.

Tyler KL, Fields BN. Reoviruses. In: Virology, ed 2. BN Fields, DM Knipe, et al, eds, New York: Raven Press Ltd, 1990;1307.

*Principles and Practice of Pediatrics, Second Edition.*
edited by Frank A. Oski et al. J. B. Lippincott Company, Philadelphia © 1994.

## 57.19 *Retroviruses*

### Mark W. Kline and Ralph D. Feigin

The known human retroviruses include human T-cell lymphotropic virus (HTLV) types I and II and human immunodeficiency virus (HIV) types 1 (formerly HTLV-III) and 2. Retroviruses possess a single-stranded RNA genome. A virus-encoded enzyme known as reverse transcriptase catalyzes the transcription of viral

RNA into proviral DNA, which then integrates into the host cell genome. This characteristic is linked etiologically to several lymphoproliferative, immunosuppressive, and degenerative disorders. Although these disorders have been studied best in adult populations, clinically important pediatric diseases can result from retroviral infection.

## ETIOLOGIC AGENTS AND PATHOGENESIS

All of the human retroviruses belong to a single viral family, the Retroviridae. HTLV-I and HTLV-II belong to a subfamily known as the oncornaviruses, and HIV-1 and HIV-2 belong to the lentivirus subfamily. One other subfamily, the spumaviruses, includes human foamy virus, an agent with no known pathogenicity for humans.

The various retrovirus subfamilies have distinct in vitro and in vivo characteristics. Oncornaviruses transform cells in culture and can produce tumors in animals. Lentiviruses produce syncytia and cytopathic effects in cell culture and cause slowly progressive infections in the host. The spumaviruses induce vacuolization of cells in culture and do not cause apparent adverse effects in the host.

Human retroviruses have a peculiar tropism for lymphocytes. In the case of HIV, this tropism results from the high affinity of the viral envelope protein for the CD4 molecule on the surface of helper/inducer T lymphocytes. A variety of cells in addition to T lymphocytes expresses the CD4 molecule, including monocytes, macrophages, and microglial cells of the central nervous system. The hallmark of HIV infection is progressive loss of CD4$^+$ T lymphocytes with inexorable diminution of immune function. The frequent occurrence of nervous system disease in individuals infected with HIV may be attributable in part to the introduction of virus into the central nervous system via infected monocytes and macrophages.

HTLV-I induces expression of interleukin-2 (IL-2) receptors on CD4$^+$ T lymphocytes. The presence of excessive receptors for IL-2, a recognized T-cell growth factor, may help explain the lymphoproliferation observed in some HTLV-I–infected individuals. HTLV-I and HTLV-II both can cause proliferation in vitro of normal lymphocytes in the absence of exogenous antigens.

This chapter focuses on the epidemiology and clinical features of infection caused by HTLV-I and HTLV-II. For a thorough discussion of pediatric HIV infection and acquired immune deficiency syndrome (AIDS), refer to Chapter 14.

## EPIDEMIOLOGY

Seroepidemiologic studies of HTLV-I and HTLV-II have been hampered by the inability of screening antibody tests to differentiate between infection with the two viruses. HTLV-I infection appears to be most prevalent in southern Japan and the Caribbean basin. Other foci of infection include parts of Africa and Central and South America. The geographic distribution of HTLV-II is unknown. The prevalence of HTLV infection (types I and II) among United States blood donors is about 2.5 per 10,000.

Both HTLV-I and HTLV-II are highly cell-associated, and transmission of either virus is thought to require passage of infected lymphocytes rather than cell-free body fluids. Consequently, the efficiency of transmission of these viruses is thought to be less than that of HIV. The modes of transmission of HTLV-I are identical to those of HIV-1, including sexual activity, transfusion of infected cellular blood products, and breast-feeding. Perinatal transmission has been documented by detection of HTLV-I in cord blood. HTLV-II has been found predominantly among injecting-drug users and their sexual partners; infection also has been documented recently in some non–drug-using native American populations. Preliminary data suggest that mother-to-infant transmission of the virus occurs infrequently.

## CLINICAL MANIFESTATIONS

Individuals infected with HTLV-I have a lifetime risk for development of adult T-cell leukemia/lymphoma (ATLL) or myelopathy/tropical spastic paraparesis (TSP) of about 5% to 10%. It is hypothesized that ATLL results from HTLV-I infection acquired during the first few years of life, with a long period of latency averaging several decades, and the ultimate development of clinically evident disease, usually in middle age. Cases of ATLL attributable to blood transfusion have not been reported.

Clinical features of ATLL result from a malignant proliferation of HTLV-I–infected mature T cells. The disease course may be either indolent or fulminant. The most common findings at presentation include lymphadenopathy, hepatosplenomegaly, and polymorphous skin lesions. Leukocytosis may be present. The diagnosis of ATLL is suggested by the presence in the peripheral blood of abnormal lymphocytes with indented nuclei, but these are not identified in every case. Hypercalcemia and lytic bone lesions are found in most individuals with fulminant disease. Opportunistic infections are common in individuals with ATLL. The spectrum of infectious agents observed is similar to that seen in AIDS caused by HIV-1.

Like ATLL, the clinical onset of HTLV-I–associated myelopathy/TSP typically occurs during middle age. The disease has been reported rarely in children as young as 5 to 10 years of age. The onset of myelopathy after blood transfusion has been reported, with a mean latent period of about 2 years.

The typical presentation of HTLV-I–associated myelopathy/TSP includes slowly progressive spastic weakness of the lower extremities, sometimes associated with numbness or dysesthesia. Physical examination reveals hyperreflexia. Abnormal lymphocytes similar to those seen in ATLL may be found in the peripheral blood or cerebrospinal fluid.

One other condition, the infective dermatitis syndrome, has been linked to HTLV-I infection. Affected individuals typically have been young children with severe exudative eczema, chronic rhinitis, and recurrent infections. Mothers of several of these patients have been found to be HTLV-I–positive, and several of the children have developed ATLL during adolescence.

HTLV-II was isolated initially from a patient with a T-cell variant of hairy cell leukemia, but the association of the virus with this or any other disease is unclear.

## DIAGNOSIS AND TREATMENT

The diagnosis of ATLL or HTLV-I–associated myelopathy/TSP is suggested by compatible clinical findings in a patient from a population with endemic HTLV-I infection. Serologic tests for HTLV-I, including enzyme immunoassay and Western blot assay, also detect cross-reacting anti–HTLV-II antibodies. Therefore, seropositive individuals are referred to as HTLV-positive, and not as HTLV-I–positive. Further discrimination between HTLV-I and HTLV-II infection requires additional testing with newer assays such as polymerase chain reaction or HTLV type-specific peptide serologic assays. Serologic tests for HTLV do not cross-react with those for HIV.

The efficacy of antiretroviral agents for treatment of HTLV-I–associated disease remains to be defined.

### Selected Readings

Blattner WA, Takatsoki K, Gallo RC, et al. Human T-cell leukemia/lymphoma virus and adult T-cell leukemia. JAMA 1983;250:1074.

Bunn PA, Schecter GP, Jaffe E, et al. Clinical course of retrovirus-associated adult T-cell lymphoma in the United States. N Engl J Med 1983;309:257.

Jenson HB. Retrovirus infections and the acquired immunodeficiency syndrome. Adv Pediatr Infect Dis 1990;5:93.

Mofenson LM, Blattner WA. Human retroviruses. In: Feigin RD, Cherry JD, eds. Textbook of pediatric infectious diseases, ed 3. Philadelphia: WB Saunders, 1992.

Salahuddin SZ, Markham PD. Retroviruses: new viral infections in man. Pediatr Infect Dis J 1988;7:S107.

*Principles and Practice of Pediatrics, Second Edition.*
edited by Frank A. Oski et al. J. B. Lippincott Company, Philadelphia © 1994.

# 57.20 *Viral Gastroenteritis*

David O. Matson, Lamia Elerian, and Larry K. Pickering

Acute viral gastroenteritis is a common illness that occurs in both endemic and epidemic forms worldwide. Four categories of viruses are recognized as medically important causes of human gastroenteritis: rotavirus; enteric adenovirus; calicivirus and calicilike virus, including Norwalk virus; and astrovirus. These viruses exhibit important differences in epidemiology and pathogenesis.

## ROTAVIRUS

Human rotavirus was detected by Bishop and associates in 1973 in duodenal biopsies from children with acute diarrhea. Since then, rotaviral gastroenteritis has been reported worldwide, affecting the young of a wide variety of mammalian (including human) and avian species. The virus is 70 nm in diameter; its name is derived from the Latin *rota*, meaning wheel, which it resembles.

Rotavirus is an 11-segmented, double-stranded RNA virus with outer and inner capsids that surround an inner core containing the double-stranded RNA genome segments. The RNA segments can be separated by polyacrylamide gel electrophoresis, which produces an electropherotype pattern used to identify rotavirus strains. The proteins of rotaviruses include a major capsid protein VP6, which forms the inner capsid, two outer capsid proteins, VP4 and VP7, and other proteins that are either nonstructural or associated with the viral core. These proteins allow rotaviruses to be classified into group, subgroup, and serotype categories. The most general category is the group (A, B, C, D, E, F,); the major group antigen is VP6. Subgroups (I, II) are defined by additional antigenic differences in the VP6 protein.

Antibodies directed against VP7 or VP4 neutralize the virus. Changes in VP7 types result in changes in serotype specificity. The VP4 protein, a hemagglutinin, is important for infectivity of rotavirus. Thus, each group A rotavirus strain has both subgroup and serotype designations as well as an electropherotype identified by electrophoresis of its RNA genome segments. Neutralization antigens VP4 and VP7 appear to be more important than other structural antigens in determining host protection from an antigenic type when evaluating immune responses.

Most human rotavirus infections are caused by group A rotavirus, the group detected by commercially available assays. In serologic studies, a high prevalence of antibody to group A ro-

Supported by grants HD-13021 and AI-28544 from the NIH

tavirus occurs by age 3 years, indicating endemic infection. Nongroup A rotaviruses, including groups B and C, also cause human disease, but their distribution is more limited worldwide, and few cases in North America have been recognized.

## Epidemiology

Rotavirus diarrhea occurs in all age groups, with the peak occurrence of severe illness in children 6 to 24 months of age. Rotavirus usually produces sporadic episodes of diarrhea rather than large outbreaks; however, outbreaks are common where young children are housed together, as in day-care settings. The incidence of infection in children has been determined in hospital- and community-based studies. Rotavirus infection accounts for 15% to 50% of cases of acute diarrhea in children presenting to hospitals in tropical countries and for 35% to 60% of cases in temperate areas. The wide range of prevalence reflects differences in age groups studied, methods of detection, geographic locations, and time of year. In community-based studies, rotavirus causes 5% to 10% of diarrheal episodes during the first year of life. Higher prevalence in hospital-based studies reflects the more severe disease caused by rotavirus compared to other agents. In the United States, rotavirus causes about 200,000 hospitalizations each year in children younger than 5 years old. These hospitalizations account for 3% to 10% of all hospital days in this age group. The overall risk for hospitalization by the fifth birthday is about 1 in 50, placing rotavirus as 1 of the top 10 potentially preventable causes of illness among children in the United States.

Rotavirus has a mean incubation period of 2 days (range, 1 to 3 days) in children and in experimentally infected adults. Excretion of rotavirus in stool frequently precedes development of symptoms and continues after symptoms of illness resolve. Asymptomatic rotavirus infection in children beyond the neonatal period has been reported to range from 0% to 50%. In studies of children in day-care centers in the United States, about 50% of infected children excrete rotavirus asymptomatically during outbreaks. The duration of fecal excretion can be up to 10 days. The titer of virus per gram of stool is highest shortly after the onset of illness. The usual duration of illness is 5 to 7 days; chronic infections with rotavirus can occur in immunodeficient children.

Rotavirus diarrhea exhibits a marked seasonality in temperate climates and a lack of seasonality within 10° of the equator. In the United States, the rotavirus season lasts 1 to 4 months. The season begins in October/November in Mexico and the southwest United States, and later a continuous wave of illness spreads across North America from southwest to northeast, ending in May in the Maritime provinces of Canada. The frequency of sequential postneonatal rotavirus infection of individual children by different serotypes is unknown.

Rotaviruses are transmitted by the fecal-oral route, usually from person to person. Transmission within families, day-care centers, and hospital environments has been reported. Increased family size and crowding are significant risk factors for acquiring rotavirus infection. Water-borne outbreaks have been reported, but common source outbreaks of infection are infrequent. The role of asymptomatic excretion of rotaviruses in the transmission of this pathogen is unknown.

## Clinical Manifestations

Symptoms of illness produced by rotavirus vary according to age and range widely within an age group. Newborn infants are usually asymptomatic. When diarrhea does occur, it tends to be mild, although severe illness has been reported among newborns, particularly premature infants. Findings in Australia indicate that neonatal rotavirus infections, even if asymptomatic, may protect children from later, severe rotavirus gastroenteritis. In infants

TABLE 57-17. Characteristics of Viruses That Cause Gastroenteritis

| | Rotavirus | Enteric Adenoviruses | Caliciviruses and Calici-Like Viruses | Astroviruses |
|---|---|---|---|---|
| Age group commonly involved (mo) | 6–24 | 6–24 | All ages | 6–24 |
| Incubation period (d) | 1–3 | 1–3 | 1–2 | 1–3 |
| Duration of illness | 3–7 d | 3–8 d | 12 h–5 d | 1–5 d |
| Method of transmission | Fecal–oral | Fecal–oral | Fecal–oral, foodborne | Fecal–oral, foodborne |
| Method of identification commercially available? | Yes | No | No | Special reference laboratories |
| Immunization available? | Being tested | No | No | No |

and young children, clinical symptoms typically consist of low-grade fever and abrupt onset of explosive, watery diarrhea often associated with vomiting in the early stages. Other common clinical features include isotonic dehydration, compensated metabolic acidosis, and malabsorption, generally of carbohydrate and fat. Dehydration occurs in 40% to 80% of hospitalized patients and usually is less than 5%. Severe dehydration and death have been reported in children and adults, although adults tend to have mild disease. A temperature higher than 38.8 °C occurs in about 30% of pediatric patients and often is associated with dehydration. Rotavirus infection often occurs in adults who are in close contact with young children but also has been reported in adult travelers, hospitalized adults, military personnel, and elderly who are institutionalized.

Watery stools in patients with rotavirus diarrhea usually do not contain blood or fecal leukocytes; mucus is seen occasionally. Stools may be pale and foul-smelling, consistent with fat malabsorption. Concurrent respiratory tract symptoms frequently occur. Whether these reflect coincidental winter infections by other viruses is uncertain. In immunocompromised hosts, rotaviruses may cause a chronic, protein-losing diarrhea, and infection of the liver and kidneys in such individuals has been reported. Rotavirus is associated with, but not proved to be the cause of, several other diseases or conditions, including aseptic meningitis, encephalitis, exanthem subitum, inflammatory bowel disease, intussusception, hemolytic-uremic syndrome, Kawasaki syndrome, neonatal necrotizing enterocolitis, Reye's syndrome, and sudden infant death syndrome. Table 57-17 summarizes several characteristics of viruses, including rotavirus, that cause gastroenteritis.

## Diagnosis

Rotaviruses may be shed in stools in high numbers, up to $10^{11}$ particles/mL of feces. Stools collected early in the course of illness are most likely to contain virus, whereas stools collected 8 or more days after the onset of illness rarely contain virus. Human rotavirus has been isolated in tissue culture, but the technique is cumbersome and is not used as a routine method of detection. Electron microscopy was the original diagnostic technique for identification of rotavirus, but is not suitable for examination of a large number of specimens and requires use of expensive equipment. Electron microscopy enables detection of nongroup A rotaviruses and other viruses.

A number of enzyme immunoassays and latex agglutination tests for detection of rotavirus in clinical specimens are available commercially. They are easy to use, reliable, and more sensitive than electron microscopy. These assay kits have acceptable sensitivities and specificities. In general, the latex assay kits are rapid, do not require complicated or expensive equipment, and are simple to perform, but are not as sensitive as the enzyme immu-

noassays. Table 57-18 lists methods of detection and size of viruses that cause gastroenteritis.

## Treatment and Prevention

Treatment of patients with rotavirus-associated diarrhea is directed toward correction of dehydration and acidosis. Oral fluid replacement with glucose-electrolyte solutions has proved effective in treatment of infants with up to 10% dehydration. Parenteral fluid may be required in severe cases and should be administered when vital signs indicate impending shock. Use of human milk, cow colostrum, and human serum immune globulin, which contains antibodies to rotavirus, may decrease or prevent rotavirus diarrhea in patients with primary immunodeficiencies, healthy infants, and low–birth-weight newborns. Most human colostrum and milk samples tested contain variable concentrations of rotavirus antibody, but the role of human milk antibody in protecting against rotavirus-induced diarrhea remains to be determined. Animal studies suggest that an intact cellular immune system is sufficient to control chronic infections. Rotavirus vaccines that contain several different sources of antigens are being evaluated. Types of vaccines being tested include bovine and rhesus monkey viruses (bovine strain RIT 4237, bovine strain WC3, and rhesus monkey strain MMU 18006) and reassortant rotaviruses, which combine animal and human genes. Rotavirus can be inactivated on surfaces by 70% ethyl alcohol.

## ENTERIC ADENOVIRUSES

Adenoviruses are 70 to 80 nm in diameter, are nonenveloped, and contain a double-stranded DNA viral genome. By measuring antibodies induced by distinct antigenic determinants, 47 serotypes of human adenoviruses have been identified. The enteric

TABLE 57-18. Size of Viruses That Cause Gastroenteritis and Methods of Diagnosis

| Virus | Size (nm) | Methods of Diagnosis |
|---|---|---|
| Rotavirus | 70 | ELISA, LA, EM |
| Enteric adenovirus | 70–80 | EM, ELISA |
| Small round viruses | | |
|    Calicivirus and calici-like | 27–40 | IEM, RIA, ELISA |
|    Astrovirus | 28–30 | IEM, ELISA |

ELISA, enzyme-linked immunoassay; LA, latex agglutination; EM, electron microscopy; IEM, immune electron microscopy; RIA, radioimmunoassay

adenoviruses are members of group F and are designated as serotypes 40 and 41. Unlike other serotypes of adenovirus, enteric adenoviruses do not grow well in conventional cell cultures and require special cell lines for replication. Enteric adenoviruses can be identified by electron microscopy. After rotavirus, enteric adenovirus is the second most common cause of viral gastroenteritis in infants and children.

## Epidemiology and Clinical Features

Failure to cultivate enteric adenoviruses and inability to demonstrate that conventional adenoviruses produce gastroenteritis hampered early studies of these agents. Enteric adenoviruses now can be identified by electron microscopy, by growth in transformed cell lines, and by solid-phase immunoassays. Most episodes of gastroenteritis due to enteric adenoviruses occur in children younger than 2 years of age. Diarrhea is the most prominent symptom, lasting from 4 to 23 days (mean, 7 days). Symptoms are indistinguishable from those associated with rotavirus infection, although generally less severe. Blood and mucus are not present in stools. Dehydration is mild and isotonic, and death is rare. Apparent lactose intolerance occurs in some children with enteric adenovirus infection. In any single region, either type 40 or 41 appears to predominate. The predominant type changes every 1 to 2 years. Seasonality has not been recognized for enteric adenovirus diarrhea.

## Treatment and Prevention

No specific agent for treating children with enteric adenovirus infection is available. Treatment is aimed at replacing fluid and correcting electrolyte abnormalities. Isolation of patients with gastroenteritis in hospitals, day-care centers, and other institutions is the major means of interrupting spread.

Measures that reduce spread of enteric adenovirus are similar to those recommended for all viral gastroenteritis pathogens. These measures include training care providers, routinely cleaning food preparation areas and diaper changing tables, excluding ill care-providers or food handlers, handwashing, and excluding or cohorting ill children.

## CALICIVIRUSES AND CALICI-LIKE VIRUSES

Caliciviruses and calici-like viruses are nonenveloped RNA viruses 27 to 40 nm in diameter. They can be detected in stool specimens from acutely ill individuals with gastroenteritis. The name calicivirus is derived from the characteristic surface cups, or chalice-like indentations, observed by electron microscopy in typical caliciviruses. These viruses include four groups. First, typical caliciviruses include United Kingdom types 1 to 4, Sapporo calicivirus, and a few others lacking assigned names but having typical surface features. Second, Norwalk virus and Snow Mountain agent—the first members of a group of viruses lacking typical calicivirus morphology—are proven to be caliciviruses at the genetic level. Third, other small round viruses, such as Taunton agent, Hawaii agent, and SRSV-9 agent, lack typical calicivirus morphology but share some physical properties that suggest they are caliciviruses; they lack genetic confirmation of their taxonomic status. Fourth, the genomic characterization of hepatitis E virus proves it to be a calicivirus with unique features.

The most extensive information is available for the Norwalk virus, which lacks typical calicivirus morphology, but has been shown to be a calicivirus based on the sequence of its genome. Norwalk virus was identified first in 1972 when immune electron microscopy was applied to samples collected from an outbreak of gastroenteritis in a secondary school in Norwalk, Ohio. It was the first gastroenteritis virus discovered. Caliciviruses with typical morphology, including some fatal cases, were described in human disease in 1976. A large number of caliciviruses cause a wide spectrum of illness in animals, including vesicular exanthem, hemorrhagic pneumonia, a stunting syndrome, aphthous ulcers, myositis, and spontaneous abortion. Initial genetic studies suggest that some human calicivirus strains are related genetically to some of the animal caliciviruses.

## Epidemiology and Clinical Manifestations

Caliciviruses have a worldwide distribution and are a common cause of water-borne and food-borne outbreaks of acute, nonbacterial gastroenteritis. Caliciviruses cause illness more frequently among infants and children, and Norwalk virus causes illness among adults. Typical caliciviruses have been detected in 0.2% to 6.6% of sporadic cases of gastroenteritis requiring hospitalization.

Calicivirus outbreaks tend to occur in closed populations and have a high attack rate. Typical calicivirus infections seem common in day-care centers. Common-source outbreaks occur in association with ingestion of contaminated water and food, particularly shellfish and salads. Secondary transmission presumably is person to person and fecal-oral. Symptoms generally are mild and, especially in adults, of short duration. In children, symptoms are indistinguishable from those of rotavirus gastroenteritis. In adults, symptoms tend to be more sudden in onset and resemble staphylococcal food poisoning. Stools characteristically are not bloody and lack mucus. Leukocytes are not seen in fecal smears. The incubation period is 12 hours to 4 days. Excretion lasts 5 to 7 days after the onset of symptoms in half the infected patients and can extend to 13 days. Virus excretion may continue 4 days after symptoms cease. Persistent excretion may occur in immunocompromised hosts. Asymptomatic, persistent virus excretion has been detected for months after primary calicivirus infections in animals.

Hepatitis E causes epidemics of hepatitis in Asia and Africa. Outbreaks of hepatitis E virus infection have been identified in Mexico, and imported cases have occurred in the United States.

## Diagnosis and Treatment

Electron microscopy is the most widely available diagnostic tool for detection of caliciviruses in stool specimens, but it is fairly insensitive for this virus family. For Norwalk virus and certain other strains, specific diagnostic tests are available in some reference laboratories. Samples submitted for virus detection should be collected early after infection, should be stored at 4 °C, and should not be frozen. Paired serum samples may help establish the diagnosis of infection.

As for the other viral agents, treatment is supportive. Hospitalized patients should be isolated, and infected individuals attending day-care centers or similar institutions should be cohorted. Virus may be inactivated with a 1-minute exposure to 0.1% sodium hypochlorite.

## ASTROVIRUSES

Astroviruses, first described in 1975, are nonenveloped RNA viruses 28 to 30 nm in diameter with a characteristic star-like appearance when visualized by direct electron microscopy. The absence of a central hollow distinguishes astrovirus stars from typical calicivirus stars in direct electron microscopy. Known astroviruses include at least five antigenic types. Human astroviruses are antigenically distinct from animal astroviruses. Initial genetic studies indicate that astroviruses are a unique virus family, distinct from caliciviruses and picornaviruses.

## Epidemiology and Clinical Manifestations

Human astroviruses have been found wherever sought and probably have a worldwide distribution. Outbreaks of gastroenteritis have been detected in all age groups. Multiple antigenic types co-circulate in the same region. Astroviruses have been detected in 3% to 8.6% of sporadic cases of pediatric gastroenteritis requiring hospitalization. Most astrovirus infections have been detected in children younger than 4 years of age. Common-source outbreaks tend to occur in closed populations and have a high attack rate. Astrovirus infections in day-care centers seem common with a high frequency of asymptomatic infection. Transmission presumably is person to person and fecal-oral, although outbreaks associated with contaminated water and shellfish have been documented.

Symptoms generally are mild and indistinguishable from those caused by rotavirus. The incubation period is 1 to 2 days. Excretion lasts 5 days after onset of symptoms in half the infected cases. The duration of asymptomatic excretion after onset of illness is uncertain. Persistent excretion may occur in immunocompromised hosts. Asymptomatic infections also occur.

## Diagnosis and Treatment

Electron microscopy is the most widely available diagnostic tool for detection of astroviruses in stool specimens, but it also is fairly insensitive for this family of viruses. Samples should be handled similarly to methods used for caliciviruses. Enzyme-linked immunosorbent assays (ELISAs) are available in reference and research laboratories. Astroviruses can be cultivated in special cell lines, although this practice is not widely used. Treatment is supportive. Enteric precautions are recommended and control measures are the same as those for rotavirus.

## OTHER VIRAL AGENTS

A number of other enteric viruses are associated with gastroenteritis, including some picornaviruses, coronaviruses, Toroviruses, parvoviruses and parvo-like viruses, pestiviruses, and unclassified small round viruses. Many of these agents are known from single outbreaks of illness and are named for the location of the outbreak, such as Ditchling and Parramatta agents. Information supporting the causative role varies for each agent. For some, lack of diagnostic techniques, inability to cultivate the virus in cell culture, and a paucity of virus-containing samples have limited investigation of their relative importance and features.

## FUTURE TRENDS

Viral gastroenteritis is caused by a number of distinct viruses. Despite intensive investigation, an etiology for most episodes of illness cannot be established. Recent advances in the characterization of individual viral agents have clarified relationships among many of these agents, especially for the caliciviruses. New studies likely will establish the role of and provide diagnostic tools for a number of poorly characterized agents. In general, clinical manifestations are similar for all the agents and the approach to treatment and prevention of infection is the same.

## Selected Readings

Bartlett AV, Reves RR, Pickering LK. Rotavirus in infant–toddler day care centers: epidemiology relevant to disease control strategies. J Pediatr 1988;113:435.

Blacklow NR, Greenberg HB. Viral gastroenteritis. N Engl J Med 1991;325:252.

Conner ME, Matson DO, Estes MK. Rotavirus vaccines and vaccination potential. Microbiol Rev 1992∞ press.

Greenberg HB, Matsui SM. Astroviruses and caliciviruses: emerging enteric pathogens. Infectious Agents and Disease 1992∞ press.

Hermann JE, Taylor DN, Echeverria P, et al. Astroviruses as a cause of gastroenteritis in children. N Engl J Med 1991;324:1757.

LeBaron CW, Furutan NP, Lew JF, et al. Viral agents of gastroenteritis. Morbidity Mortality Weekly Report 1990;39:1.

Matson DO. Calicivirus infections. In: Feigin RD, Cherry JD, eds. Textbook of pediatric infectious diseases, ed 3. Philadelphia: WB Saunders, 1992.

Matson DO, Estes MK. Impact of rotavirus infection at a large pediatric hospital. J Infect Dis 1990;162:598.

O'Ryan M, Matson DO. Viral gastroenteritis pathogens in the day care center setting. Seminars in Pediatric Infectious Diseases 1990;1:252.

Uhnoo I, Wadell G, Svennson L, et al. Importance of enteric adenoviruses 40 and 41 in acute gastroenteritis in infants and young children. J Clin Microbiol 1984;20:365.

Van R, Wun C-C, O'Ryan ML, et al. Outbreaks of human enteric adenovirus types 40 and 41 in Houston day care centers. J Pediatr 1992;120:516.

*Principles and Practice of Pediatrics, Second Edition.*
edited by Frank A. Oski et al. J. B. Lippincott Company, Philadelphia © 1994.

CHAPTER 58

# Mycoplasma *and* Ureaplasma *Infections*

## W. Paul Glezen

Mycoplasmas are classified as bacteria, but are unique because they lack a rigid cell wall. For this reason, their morphology depends on the environment in which they grow, they do not take usual bacterial stains, and they are not susceptible to antibiotics that act on the cell wall, such as the penicillins.

Mycoplasmas are causes of economically important diseases in animals, which may involve the respiratory tract, joints, or central nervous system. The first mycoplasma identified was the bovine pleuropneumonia organism (*Mycoplasma mycoides*), and the species discovered subsequently were called pleuropneumonia-like organisms, or PPLO. These tiniest of free-living organisms were recognized to be similar to bacteria denuded of their cell walls (spheroplasts or L-forms). Only three mycoplasmas have been associated with disease in humans. *Mycoplasma pneumoniae* causes "primary atypical pneumonia" and is the only pathogen of this group that is an important cause of disease in children. *Mycoplasma hominis* and *Ureaplasma urealyticum* are genital mycoplasmas and rarely may cause illness in the neonatal period.

## MYCOPLASMA PNEUMONIAE

### Epidemiology

*M pneumoniae* is the most common cause of pneumonia and tracheobronchitis in school-age children and young adults treated in the outpatient setting. The average annual rate is about 5:1000 school-age children. It is an uncommon cause of lower respiratory tract disease in infants and young children, and usually does not result in hospitalization of children without chronic conditions. College students and military recruits may be confined to bed with M pneumoniae pneumonia.

Epidemics of M pneumoniae disease usually are long and smoldering, and may begin in the summer, with peak activity reached in autumn. Sporadic infections can occur throughout the year. In experimentally inoculated volunteers, the incubation period from the day of infection to the onset of pneumonia was about 14 days, but the average interval between the onset of an index case and the onset of a secondary case in the same household has been closer to 3 weeks and may be as long as 3 months. The longer interval may be explained by the fact that pharyngeal carriage may persist for a similar period, even in patients who have been treated with appropriate antibiotics.

## Pathogenesis

When growing on human respiratory epithelium, the organism is a small, filamentous structure about 0.1 by 2.0 $\mu$m. Infection of a susceptible person probably occurs through contact with M pneumoniae–containing droplet nuclei that are coughed into the environment. Dissemination by aerosol has been demonstrated experimentally and deduced from descriptions of remarkable outbreaks occurring in closed populations. Infection of humans by aerosol may be accomplished by as little as one colony-forming unit (CFU), whereas about 100 CFU are needed to infect volunteers by nose drops. The concentration of organisms in sputum specimens from patients with pneumonia has ranged from $10^2$ to $10^6$ CFU/mL.

The organism attaches to ciliated respiratory epithelial cells by a specialized tip. The attachment protein has been isolated and specific antibodies have been demonstrated in serum and respiratory secretions of immune subjects. It is assumed that these antibodies block attachment and thereby prevent infection. Infection leads to ciliostasis, then loss of cilia, and, eventually, the desquamation of epithelial cells. Mononuclear cells infiltrate the submucosa of affected bronchi and bronchioles. An exudate consisting of debris from the desquamated cells, polymorphonuclear leukocytes, macrophages, and mucus develops as the disease progresses and may lead to a productive cough. Bacterial superinfection may occur; Haemophilus influenzae has been reported in some cases.

## Clinical Features

The main clinical features of M pneumoniae disease are fever, malaise, sore throat, and a dry, hacking cough. The onset usually is gradual over several days. The affected schoolchild may not appear particularly ill, and the examiner may be surprised when chest auscultation reveals rales and rhonchi. The chest roentgenogram may show peribronchial thickening and infiltration of one or both lower lobes, with some subsegmental atelectasis. Pleural effusion is not a prominent finding. The peripheral white blood cell (WBC) count usually is in the normal range. The severity of the illness may be exaggerated in children with sickle-cell disease. These children appear toxic and require hospitalization, with prolonged high fever and peripheral WBC counts greater than 25,000/mm$^3$. The chest roentgenogram may reveal dense infiltrates involving more than one lobe and prominent pleural effusion.

The progress of the infection may be aborted in some children who have fever and pharyngitis. A larger proportion of children have a prominent cough and rhonchi in the larger airways on auscultation; in these children, a diagnosis of tracheobronchitis is warranted.

Some children not known to wheeze previously may have expiratory wheezing on examination. A nondescript rash may accompany the infection. A few children present with acute otitis media or bullous myringitis. The total course of the illness with or without treatment may encompass 2 weeks, with a bothersome night cough persisting even longer.

## Complications

A wide variety of extrapulmonary complications has been attributed to M pneumoniae infection. The complication best documented in children is erythema multiforme bullosum, or Stevens-Johnson syndrome; the organism has been isolated from the skin lesions on occasion. Hemolytic anemia with or without renal failure has been reported in adults. A plethora of neurologic syndromes, including meningoencephalitis, Guillain-Barré syndrome, transverse myelitis, and cerebral infarction, have been attributed to the infection; in most cases, however, the only evidence of infection is either a rise in the level of complement-fixing (CF) antibodies or a single high titer. Some cases have been reported in the absence of evidence of significant respiratory tract infection. The neurologic diseases that occur in the presence of cold agglutinin–positive pneumonia, at least, are more acceptable. Isolation of the agent from respiratory secretions should be required to establish the association between M pneumoniae infection and a neurologic condition.

## Diagnosis

The diagnosis of M pneumoniae infection can be suspected in a child who has the typical clinical picture described above. The clinical impression can be reinforced by the presence of cold agglutinins in the serum at a titer of 1 : 64 or greater. Cold agglutinins are IgM antibodies that may appear early in the course of the infection—probably because the organism has an antigen similar to the I antigen on the red blood cell (RBC) membrane. Cold agglutinins are not specific for M pneumoniae infection and are present in only about 50% of affected persons, but this finding in a child with no chronic underlying condition is helpful, because the likelihood of finding a titer of 1 : 64 or greater increases with the severity of the illness.

A specific diagnosis can be made by isolating the organism. M pneumoniae is relatively easy to grow and identify on enriched PPLO agar containing antibiotics to inhibit normal pharyngeal bacterial flora. About 1 week is required for the growth of colonies on agar when they are incubated in a humidified incubator with 5% $CO_2$. The colonies are small (visible with 10$\times$ magnification), granular, and embedded in the agar without surface growth. When overlaid with a thin layer of sheep blood agar, they produce complete hemolysis in less than 24 hours. This allows presumptive identification, because M pneumoniae is the only respiratory tract mycoplasma that is hemolytic. Another test for presumptive identification is the application of sheep RBCs in suspension that will adsorb to the colonies. In broth culture, M pneumoniae will ferment glucose, so a fall in the pH level is evidence that this bacterium may be present. Specific identification is accomplished by inhibition of growth on agar by a disk soaked with specific antiserum.

Serologic diagnosis usually is accomplished by documenting a fourfold or greater rise in the level of CF antibodies between serum obtained when a patient is in the acute phase of the disease and that obtained when the patient is convalescent. The CF antigen is a lipid that is antigenically similar to that which is found in other organisms and plants; therefore, a rise in the CF antibody titer may not reflect M pneumoniae infection. More specific serologic tests, such as the growth inhibition test, generally are not available.

## Treatment

The treatment of choice for children with *M pneumoniae* infection is erythromycin. Therapy should be started early for optimal response, which may not be dramatic under even the best of circumstances. Controlled clinical trials have shown that either erythromycin or tetracycline will shorten the clinical course and hasten improvement of the chest x-ray findings. The usual dosage of erythromycin is 5–10 mg/kg given every 6 hours for 7 days. Treatment may not eradicate the organism; it often is possible to recover *M pneumoniae* from respiratory secretions after therapy is discontinued. Occasionally, the disease may recrudesce, and it may be necessary to treat the patient again. The prognosis generally is good, and few sequelae of infection have been reported.

*M pneumoniae* has not gained high priority for vaccine development. Although morbidity related to infection is high, the consequences usually are not great. Consideration has been given to incorporating antigens from the attachment protein into an orally administered vector with the goal of stimulating both mucosal and humoral immunity to protect against infection. A safe, effective, and inexpensive vaccine given orally would help to reduce acute respiratory disease in children and young adults.

## GENITAL MYCOPLASMAS

### Mycoplasma hominis

*M hominis* usually is found in the genital tract. This organism grows on routine bacterial media. The colonies are visible on agar without magnification, but often are obscured by bacterial overgrowth. The colonies have the typical "fried egg" appearance, which results from surface growth surrounding the central colony embedded into the agar. *M hominis* has been isolated from the blood of women with postpartum fever and from the cerebrospinal fluid or blood of "septic" infants during the neonatal period. *M hominis* is sensitive to tetracyclines and clindamycin.

### Ureaplasma urealyticum

Organisms of the genus *Ureaplasma* are more fastidious in their growth requirements than are the mycoplasmas. The first strains discovered were called "T" (for tiny) strains. These bacteria have the ability to hydrolyze urea with the production of ammonia; this property is used for presumptive identification by including urea and an indicator in broth cultures. The first suggestion of an association between *Ureaplasma* and human disease came from studies of nongonococcal urethritis; however, subsequent studies have revealed the contemporaneous presence of *Chlamydia*, which clouds the etiologic significance of *Ureaplasma* for this condition. Other investigators have suggested that *Ureaplasma* may be associated with chorioamnionitis and premature labor, but the etiologic significance of these observations remains to be established. This agent has been found along with other genital organisms in the respiratory tract of young infants with pneumonia. It is not certain whether these organisms contribute to the pathology of this disease. Most strains of *Ureaplasma* are inhibited by erythromycin and tetracyclines, which can be given if treatment seems appropriate.

### Selected Readings

Cassell GH, Cole BC. Mycoplasmas as agents of human disease. N Engl J Med 1981;304:80.

Chapman RS, Henderson FW, Clyde WA Jr, et al. The epidemiology of tracheobronchitis in pediatric practice. Am J Epidemiol 1981;114:786.

Collier AM. Attachment by mycoplasmas and its role in disease. Rev Infect Dis 1983;5:S685.

Collier AM, Clyde WA Jr. Appearance of *Mycoplasma pneumoniae* in lungs of experimentally infected hamsters and sputum from patients with natural disease. Am Rev Respir Dis 1974;110:765.

Denny FW, Clyde WA Jr, Glezen WP. *Mycoplasma pneumoniae* disease: Clinical spectrum, pathophysiology, epidemiology, and control. J Infect Dis 1971;123:74.

Hu PC, Fernald GW. Prospects for the development of *Mycoplasma pneumoniae* vaccines. Seminars Pediatr Infect Dis 1991;2:217.

Hu PC, Huang C-H, Collier AM, et al. Demonstration of antibodies to *Mycoplasma pneumoniae* attachment protein in human sera and respiratory secretions. Infect Immun 1983;41:437.

Rudd PT, Waites KB, Duffy LB, et al. *Ureaplasma urealyticum* and its possible role in pneumonia during the neonatal period and infancy. Pediatr Infect Dis 1986;5:S291.

*Principles and Practice of Pediatrics, Second Edition.*
edited by Frank A. Oski et al. J. B. Lippincott Company, Philadelphia © 1994.

## CHAPTER 59
# *Chlamydial Infections*

## Margaret R. Hammerschlag

Chlamydiae are obligate intracellular bacteria that are ubiquitous in nature. Members of the genus possess both DNA and RNA, divide by binary fission, contain their own ribosomes, have a cell wall (but no detectable peptidoglycan or muramic acid), and are susceptible to antimicrobial agents. They lack the ability to generate adenosine triphosphate and, thus, can be considered energy parasites. All members of the genus share a common (group) lipopolysaccharide antigen. They also share a unique developmental cycle involving an infectious, metabolically inactive extracellular form (elementary body [EB]) and a noninfectious metabolically active intracellular form (reticulate body). The EBs, which are 200 to 400 $\mu$m in diameter, attach to the host cell by a process of electrostatic binding and are taken into the cell by endocytosis that is not dependent on the microtubule system. Once within the host cell, the EB remains within a membrane-lined phagosome. Fusion of the phagosome with the host cell lysosome fails to occur. The EBs differentiate into reticulate bodies (RBs), which undergo binary fission. After about 36 hours, the RBs differentiate into EBs. At about 48 hours, release may occur by cytolysis or by a process of exocytosis or extrusion of the whole inclusion, leaving the host cell intact. Thus, there is a biologic basis for prolonged subclinical infection.

Currently, three species are recognized. The first two are *Chlamydia psittaci*, which is primarily a zoonosis and the agent of psittacosis, and *Chlamydia trachomatis*, whose primary reservoir is humans. *C trachomatis* has been subdivided further into two biovars: lymphogranuloma venereum (LGV) and trachoma (the agent of human oculogenital diseases other than LGV). In developed countries, *C trachomatis* probably is the most prevalent cause of sexually transmitted diseases, including urethritis and epididymitis in men, cervicitis and salpingitis in women, and conjunctivitis and pneumonia in neonates. The third species,

*Chlamydia pneumoniae*, strain TWAR, has been identified recently. The name derives from the laboratory designation of the first two isolates. It shares the genus antigen and appears to be a primary human respiratory pathogen. A summary of the characteristics of the three species is shown in Table 59-1.

## INFECTIONS CAUSED BY *CHLAMYDIA PSITTACI*

*C psittaci* is widespread in the animal kingdom, where it is a major cause of both respiratory and genital disease (feline pneumonitis and conjunctivitis; bovine chlamydial abortion; pigeon, turkey, and parrot ornithosis). Humans usually contract the disease from infected birds. The birds may be ill, but inapparent infection also can occur. Psittacosis is a major problem for the poultry industry worldwide. There were several major outbreaks in turkey farms in the United States during the late 1970s. Psittacosis is likely to occur in poultry workers, veterinarians, and bird fanciers. Person-to-person spread is unusual.

The clinical course of psittacosis is variable, with incubation periods of 7 to 15 days or longer. It often starts suddenly with chills and high fever (38 °C to 40.5 °C). Headache, often diffuse and severe, is a common chief complaint, as are malaise and nausea. A persistent dry, hacking cough usually is present. The physical findings may belie the extent of the pulmonary involvement as seen on chest radiographs. Rales may be heard, but changes indicative of consolidation usually are not seen. Chest radiographs reveal soft, patchy infiltrates radiating from the hilum or, less frequently, a reticulonodular pattern.

Once psittacosis is suspected (usually as an atypical pneumonia or epidemiologically because of contact with birds), the best and most available method of diagnosis is serologic. A fourfold rise in the complement-fixing antibody titer between serum obtained when the patient is in the acute phase of the disease and that obtained when he or she is convalescent is diagnostic. A single titer of 1:32 or greater in a patient with a compatible illness is very suggestive of psittacosis. Early treatment may delay antibody response for several weeks. The treatment of choice is tetracycline given for 21 days. Erythromycin may be an alternative. *C psittaci* is resistant to sulfonamides.

## INFECTIONS CAUSED BY *CHLAMYDIA TRACHOMATIS*

### Trachoma

Trachoma probably is the greatest single preventable cause of blindness in the world. It is endemic in the Middle East and Southeast Asia, and there is a small endemic focus among Navajo Indians in the southwestern United States. The disease is spread from eye to eye; flies are a frequent vector. Trachoma starts as a follicular conjunctivitis, usually in early childhood. The follicles heal, leading to conjunctival scarring, which may result in turning of the eyelid so that the lashes abrade the cornea (entropion and trichiasis). Eventually, corneal ulceration secondary to the constant trauma leads to scarring and blindness. Bacterial superinfection also may contribute to the scarring. The end result occurs years after the active disease.

Trachoma can be diagnosed clinically. The World Health Organization suggests that at least two of the following four criteria be met for diagnosis: lymphoid follicles on the upper tarsal conjunctivae, typical conjunctival scarring, vascular pannus, and limbal follicles. The diagnosis is confirmed by culture or staining methods during the active stage of the disease. Serologic tests are not helpful clinically because of the long duration of the disease and high background prevalence of antibody in many populations where trachoma is endemic.

Poverty and lack of sanitation are important factors in the spread of trachoma. As socioeconomic conditions improve, the incidence of the disease decreases substantially.

### Lymphogranuloma Venereum

LGV is a systemic, sexually transmitted disease caused by the LGV biovar. About 20 cases of LGV have been reported in chil-

| TABLE 59-1. Characteristics of the Three Chlamydial Species | | | |
|---|---|---|---|
| Characteristic | C trachomatis | C psittaci | C pneumoniae |
| Number of serovars | 15 | At least 4 avian serovars | 1 |
| Percent DNA homology to C pneumoniae | <5 | <10 | 94–100 |
| Plasmid | Yes | Yes | No |
| Contains glycogen | Yes | No | No |
| Resistant to sulfonamides | Yes | No | No |
| Morphology of elementary body | Round | Round | Round/pear-shaped |
| Natural host | Humans | Birds, mammals | Humans |
| Population | Sexually active adults, infants | Poultry workers, veterinarians, bird fanciers | All ages |
| Mode of transmission | Sexual, mother-to-infant | Aerosol: animal-to-person | Aerosol: person-to-person |
| Diseases | NGU, cervicitis, salpingitis, epididymitis, neonatal conjunctivitis, infantile pneumonia, lymphogranuloma venereum | Pneumonia: "psittacosis" | Pneumonia, bronchitis, pharyngitis |

dren. Fewer than 1000 cases are reported in adults in the United States each year. Unlike the trachoma biovar, LGV strains have a predilection for lymph node involvement.

The clinical course of LGV falls into three stages. The first stage is characterized by the appearance of the primary lesion, a painless, usually transient papule on the genitals. The second stage is characterized by lymphadenitis or lymphadenopathy. Most patients are seen at this time with enlarging, painful buboes, usually in the groin. The nodes may break down and drain. Males are more likely to have this symptom. In females, the lymphatic drainage of the vulva is to the retroperitoneal nodes. Fever, myalgia, and headache also are common. In the tertiary stage, a full-blown genitoanorectal syndrome is seen, with rectovaginal fistulas, rectal strictures, and urethral destruction.

LGV can be diagnosed either through culture of *C trachomatis* from a bubo aspirate or serologically. Most patients with LGV have complement-fixing antibody titers greater than 1:16. The recommended therapy is 2 to 3 weeks of tetracycline or sulfisoxazole. Tetracycline should not be given to children less than 9 years of age.

## Oculogenital Infections in Adults

The trachoma biovar of *C trachomatis* also is responsible for a large spectrum of diseases that occur in sexually active adults. In men, it is the cause of 30% to 50% of all cases of nongonococcal urethritis (NGU). The Centers for Disease Control have estimated that probably 1 to 3 cases of chlamydial urethritis occur for every reported case of gonococcal urethritis. The symptoms are less acute than gonorrhea, and the discharge usually is mucoid rather than purulent. As many as 50% of men with gonorrhea are coinfected with *C trachomatis*, however.

*C trachomatis* also is the major cause of epididymitis in men less than 35 years of age. It also can cause proctitis. Proctocolitis may develop in individuals who have rectal infection with an LGV strain. Asymptomatic urethral infection is frequent in sexually active men. Autoinoculation from the genitals to the eyes can lead to inclusion conjunctivitis in both men and women.

In women, *C trachomatis* infects the endocervix; women may have mucopurulent cervicitis, but frequently are asymptomatic. The prevalence of cervical chlamydial infection among sexually active women has been reported to range from 2% to 35%, depending on the population studied. Some of the highest prevalence rates have been found in adolescent girls. *C trachomatis* also can infect the urethra, leading to the urethral syndrome of dysuria with "sterile" pyuria. Complications of genital chlamydial infections in women include perihepatitis (Fitz-Hugh–Curtis syndrome) and salpingitis. The latter may cause significant morbidity, leading to infertility and ectopic pregnancy. *C trachomatis* appears to be a frequent cause of salpingitis in adolescents.

The definitive diagnosis of genital chlamydial infection in adults is by isolation of the organism in tissue culture, from the urethra in men and the endocervix in women. Care should be taken to obtain cells, not discharge. Alternatively, one of the recently developed non-culture antigen detection methods can be used. The two types currently available are a direct fluorescent antibody (DFA) test, in which chlamydial EBs are identified directly on a specimen smear stained with a conjugated antichlamydial monoclonal antibody, and an enzyme immunoassay (EIA). Both tests perform best for screening in high-prevalence populations (prevalence of infection >7%). A DNA probe also is available and appears to be equivalent in performance to the EIAs and DFA tests.

Tetracycline or doxycycline is the drug of choice for the treatment of uncomplicated genital infection in men and non-pregnant women. Erythromycin or amoxicillin can be used in pregnant women. Uncomplicated genital infection in men and non-preg-

nant women also may be treated with a single 1-g dose of azithromycin, a new azalide antibiotic related to erythromycin. Because *C trachomatis* may be responsible for 25% to 50% of all cases of salpingitis, any therapeutic regimen also should contain tetracycline. Sexual partners should be treated as well.

## Perinatally Transmitted Infections

Cervical chlamydial infection has been reported in 2% to 30% of pregnant women, depending on the population surveyed. An infant may acquire infection during passage through an infected birth canal. The overall risk of transmission is about 50%. The organism can be inoculated into the conjunctivae, nasopharynx, rectum, and vagina. Clinically, the infant may have conjunctivitis or pneumonia.

### Inclusion Conjunctivitis

*C trachomatis* is the most frequent identifiable infectious cause of neonatal conjunctivitis. The risk to an infant born to a mother infected with the organism is about 30% to 50%. The incubation period is 5 to 14 days after delivery. The presentation is extremely variable, ranging from mild conjunctival injection with scant mucoid discharge to severe conjunctivitis with copious purulent discharge, chemosis, and pseudomembrane formation. The conjunctivitis must be differentiated from gonococcal ophthalmia, as there can be overlap in both the incubation period and the clinical presentation of these disorders. At least 50% of infants with chlamydial conjunctivitis also have nasopharyngeal infection. The diagnosis is best made by culture of a conjunctival scraping or by one of the antigen detection methods, both of which perform very well in this setting. Oral erythromycin, 50 mg/kg/d for 10 to 14 days, is the therapy of choice. It permits better and faster resolution of the conjunctivitis and also treats any concurrent nasopharyngeal infection, which will prevent the potential development of pneumonia. Additional topical therapy is not needed.

Although an initial study suggested that neonatal ocular prophylaxis with erythromycin ointment could prevent the development of chlamydial ophthalmia, subsequent studies have not confirmed this. It appears that ocular prophylaxis with silver nitrate, erythromycin, or tetracycline ointments or drops is not effective for the prevention of neonatal chlamydial conjunctivitis or pneumonia. Identification and treatment of pregnant women before delivery appears to be the best method of preventing chlamydial infection in infants.

### Pneumonia

Pneumonia develops in about 10% to 20% of all infants born to women with active chlamydial infection. *C trachomatis* and respiratory syncytial virus probably are the two most common causes of pneumonia in infants less than 6 months old. The clinical presentation of chlamydial pneumonia is distinctive. The onset usually is between 1 and 3 months of age, and is characterized by an insidious course with a persistent cough, tachypnea, and lack of fever. Auscultation reveals rales; wheezing is uncommon. The finding of peripheral eosinophilia (greater than 400 cells per cubic millimeter) is common. The most consistent finding on chest radiography is hyperinflation accompanied by interstitial or alveolar infiltrates. Erythromycin given for 2 to 3 weeks is the treatment of choice and does result in clinical improvement as well as elimination of the organism from the respiratory tract.

### Diagnosis of Chlamydial Conjunctivitis and Pneumonia

Culture of *Chlamydia* from the conjunctiva or nasopharynx is diagnostic. Nasopharyngeal specimens can be obtained with a posterior nasopharyngeal swab or by aspiration. Cotton-tipped swabs with either wire or plastic shafts are preferred. Conjunctivitis also can be diagnosed from examination of Giemsa-stained conjunctival scrapings, but this method had only a 30% sensitivity compared to culture in several studies. DFA and EIA techniques also can be used for conjunctival and nasopharyngeal specimens. These tests appear to perform well at these sites. The diagnosis of chlamydial pneumonia also can be made serologically. An IgM titer greater than 1:32 on the microimmunofluorescence test is very suggestive.

## Infections in Older Children

*C trachomatis* has not been associated with any specific clinical syndrome in older infants and children. Children who have been sexually abused may acquire anogenital infection. These infections usually are asymptomatic. It is not known whether *C trachomatis* causes vaginitis. Evidence is accumulating, however, that perinatally acquired rectal and vaginal infections may persist for at least 3 years; thus, the presence of *C trachomatis* in the vagina or rectum of a prepubertal child cannot be used as absolute evidence of sexual abuse. Cultures should be obtained from these sites only when a prepubertal child is being evaluated. The DFA and EIA tests both have been associated with many false-positive results when used on specimens from these anatomic sites in children and adults, and are not approved by the United States Food and Drug Administration for this indication.

## INFECTIONS CAUSED BY *CHLAMYDIA PNEUMONIAE,* STRAIN TWAR

The first isolates of *C pneumoniae* were obtained serendipitously during studies of trachoma in the 1960s. Subsequent serologic studies demonstrated that the organism was responsible for an outbreak of mild pneumonia among schoolchildren in Finland in 1978. In 1986, Grayston and colleagues at the University of Washington isolated the organism from the respiratory tract of several college students with acute respiratory disease. DNA studies have found less than 5% relatedness between *C pneumoniae* and *C trachomatis* and *C psittaci* (see Table 59-1). Ultrastructural studies demonstrated a unique EB morphology distinct from that of the other two species. *C pneumoniae* shares the *Chlamydia* lipopolysaccharide genus antigen.

*C pneumoniae* appears to be a primary human respiratory pathogen; no zoonotic reservoir has been identified. Transmission is thought to be person-to-person through respiratory droplets. Spread of the infection has been documented among family members in the same household. American studies that have used culture in addition to serology suggest that *C pneumoniae* may be responsible for 10% to 20% of community-acquired "atypical" pneumonia (including acute chest syndrome in children with sickle-cell disease), 10% of bronchitis, and 5% to 10% of pharyngitis. Clinically, infections caused by *C pneumoniae* cannot be differentiated readily from those caused by other agents, especially *Mycoplasma pneumoniae*. Asymptomatic respiratory infection also occurs; however, the frequency is unknown. Serologic surveys have documented a rising prevalence of *C pneumoniae* antibody beginning in school-age children and reaching 30% to 45% by adolescence, suggesting that clinically inapparent infection may be fairly common. Respiratory infection with *C pneumoniae* has been associated recently with reactive airway disease, provoking bronchospasm in patients with no prior history of asthma and possibly causing acute exacerbations of the disease in individuals with asthma.

The specific diagnosis of *C pneumoniae* infection is based on isolation of the organism in tissue culture and serology. The optimum tissue for culture appears to be that of the posterior nasopharynx, and the specimen should be collected with wire-shafted swabs in the same manner as for *C trachomatis*. Few data have been published describing the response of *C pneumoniae* infection to antibiotic therapy. Many of the patients first described by Grayston were treated with erythromycin, 1 g/d for 10 days, with generally poor clinical response. *C pneumoniae* is sensitive in vitro to erythromycin, tetracycline, ofloxacin, and two recently approved macrolide antibiotics, azithromycin and clarithromycin. The latter two drugs are more active in vitro than is erythromycin, with superior pharmacokinetics and tissue penetration, and they may be more effective clinically. Because treatment studies have not been done, however, the optimum dose and duration of therapy are uncertain. Similar to *C psittaci*, *C pneumoniae* is highly resistant to sulfonamides.

## Selected Readings

Alexander ER, Harrison HR. Role of *Chlamydia trachomatis* in perinatal infection. Rev Infect Dis 1983;5:713.

Bell TA, Stamm WE, Wang SP, et al. Chronic *Chlamydia trachomatis* infections in infants. JAMA 1992;267:400.

Centers for Disease Control. Sexually transmitted diseases treatment guidelines. MMWR 1993; in press.

Chernesky MA, Mahony JB, Castriciano S, et al. Detection of *Chlamydia trachomatis* antigens by enzyme immunoassay and immunofluorescence in genital specimens from symptomatic and asymptomatic men and women. J Infect Dis 1986;154:141.

Chirgwin K, Roblin PM, Gelling M, et al. Infection with *Chlamydia pneumoniae* in Brooklyn. J Infect Dis 1991;163:757.

Eagar RM, Beach RK, Davidson AJ, et al. Epidemiologic and clinical factors of *Chlamydia trachomatis* in black, hispanic and white female adolescents. West J Med 1985;143:3.

Grayston JT, Campbell LA, Kuo CC, et al. A new respiratory pathogen: *Chlamydia pneumoniae* strain TWAR. J Infect Dis 1990;161:618.

Hammerschlag MR. Chlamydial infections. J Pediatr 1989;114:727.

Hammerschlag MR, Doraiswamy B, Alexander ER, et al. Are rectogenital chlamydial infections a marker of sexual abuse in children? Pediatr Infect Dis 1984;3:100.

Hammerschlag MR, Roblin PM, Gelling M, et al. Comparison of two enzyme immunoassays to culture for the diagnosis of chlamydia conjunctivitis and respiratory infections in infants. J Clin Microbiol 1990;28:1725.

Miller ST, Hammerschlag MR, Chirgwin K, et al. Role of *Chlamydia pneumoniae* in acute chest syndrome of sickle cell disease. J Pediatr 1991;118:30.

Roblin PM, Hammerschlag MR, Cummings C, et al. Comparison of two rapid microscopic methods and culture for detection of *Chlamydia trachomatis* in ocular and nasopharyngeal specimens from infants. J Clin Microbiol 1989;27:968.

Schachter J, Grossman M, Sweet RL, et al. Prospective study of perinatal transmission of *Chlamydia trachomatis*. JAMA 1986;255:3374.

Yung AP, Grayson ML. Psittacosis—a review of 135 cases. Med J Aust 1988;148:228.

*Principles and Practice of Pediatrics, Second Edition.*
edited by Frank A. Oski et al. J. B. Lippincott Company, Philadelphia © 1994.

## CHAPTER 60
# *Rickettsial Diseases*

Ralph D. Feigin and Marc L. Boom

The rickettsial diseases are caused by microorganisms that have characteristics common to both bacteria and viruses. Rickettsiae depend on the intracellular milieu of animal cells for growth and reproduction, and are considered to occupy a position between bacteria and viruses. They are, however, predominantly bacterial in character, as indicated by the following properties: they contain both DNA and RNA; they multiply by transverse binary fission; they possess enzymes of Krebs' cycle, of protein synthesis, and of electron transport; at least one species contains muramic acid; they are retained by a filter; and their growth can be inhibited by a variety of antibacterial agents. They resemble viruses primarily by virtue of the fact that they grow only within living cells.

Rickettsiae also are agents that are similar in size and shape to one another and can be seen as coccobacillary forms under the light microscope. The characteristic pathologic lesion in all rickettsial diseases is a widespread vasculitis of small blood vessels. The exception is Q fever, in which pneumonitis assumes equal import. The rickettsial agents multiply within cells of susceptible hosts.

All rickettsial diseases are characterized clinically by fever, headache, and rash, with the exception of Q fever, which has no rash, and ehrlichiosis, which frequently has no rash. In the early stages of rickettsial diseases, all infections are susceptible to a number of broad-spectrum antibiotics. All rickettsiae assume a characteristic red color when they are stained by the Gimenez method. All rickettsial infections, with the exception of rickettsialpox, Q fever, and ehrlichiosis, induce agglutinins against strains of the bacillus *Proteus vulgaris*, such as OX19, OX2, or OXK (Weil-Felix reaction). Rickettsial organisms all occur under natural conditions in insects such as lice and fleas or arachnids such as ticks and mites. These arthropods serve as vectors for the transmission of all rickettsial diseases to humans, with the exception of Q fever.

All rickettsial organisms, with the exception of *Ehrlichia* and the heterogeneic strains of scrub typhus and *Ehrlichia*, produce complement-fixing antibodies. The clinical and epidemiologic features of the disease in an individual case supplemented by measurement of complement-fixation titers constitute the principal means for establishing the diagnosis of rickettsial infection.

Immunity produced by any one of the rickettsial infections usually is of long duration against reinfection by the same agent. The single exception to this rule is scrub typhus.

Four major groups of rickettsial disease occur within the tribe Rickettsieae. *Ehrlichia* is a genus within a separate rickettsial tribe, Ehrlichieae. With the exception of *Ehrlichia*, infection by an organism belonging to one of these groups confers partial or complete immunity against infection by any of the other rickettsiae belonging to the same group. In contrast, little or no immunity is conferred by infections that are caused by rickettsiae belonging to different groups. There is, however, a minor degree of serologic cross-reaction between some rickettsiae of the spotted fever groups and typhus. Generally, immunity that follows natural infection is more prolonged than that which follows immunization.

Another general characteristic is that arthropods and mammals serve as natural hosts for rickettsiae. Infection also can occur by an airborne route, however, when infectious microorganisms acquire access to respiratory surfaces or the conjunctivae. The airborne route appears to be the most common method of spread when the infection occurs in laboratories. Humans are an accidental blind-end host for rickettsiae and do not contribute to the survival of the rickettsial species, except for louse-borne typhus.

Rickettsial diseases vary markedly in severity, from benign, self-limited illnesses to severe fulminating diseases. Survival of the patient depends on prompt diagnosis and institution of appropriate therapy.

## THE SPOTTED FEVERS

The spotted fevers are a group of infectious diseases caused predominantly by *Rickettsia rickettsii*. Because most are transmitted by ticks, they are called tick typhuses.

Rocky Mountain spotted fever is the most severe and important disease of the spotted fever group that appears in the temperate zones of North America. An illness almost identical to Rocky Mountain spotted fever occurs in South America, where it is called São Paulo disease. Other, less severe forms of tick typhus occur in Asia, Africa, Australia, and Europe. They can be distinguished by geographic location as well as by differences in the spotted fever rickettsiae that cause them. Important epidemiologic characteristics of the spotted fever group and of other rickettsial diseases are provided in Table 60-1.

## Rocky Mountain Spotted Fever

Rocky Mountain spotted fever is a disease caused by *R rickettsii* that first was recognized in areas of Idaho and Montana. Its occurrence is not limited to the Rocky Mountain area, however; the disease actually is most prevalent in the eastern United States. The incidence of Rocky Mountain spotted fever in the Rocky Mountain region began a steady decline before the introduction of antibiotic therapy in the 1950s and, by 1988, fewer than 20 cases of Rocky Mountain spotted fever were reported in the Rocky Mountain and Pacific coast areas. The majority of cases in the past 10 years have been reported from the southeastern United States. In 1990, 649 cases of Rocky Mountain spotted fever were reported to the Centers for Disease Control and Prevention, representing an incidence of 0.26:100,000 individuals. Forty-five percent of the cases were reported from the South Atlantic region, with the highest incidence rates noted in North Carolina, Oklahoma, Tennessee, and South Carolina. Nearly two thirds of all patients with Rocky Mountain spotted fever are 15 years old or younger.

Despite the use of chloramphenicol or tetracyclines, Rocky Mountain spotted fever has an overall case fatality rate of 3.9%. A considerable number of the deaths can be attributed to failure to consider and establish the diagnosis early enough for appropriate therapy to be beneficial.

### Etiology, Epidemiology, and Transmission

*R rickettsii* is a small coccobacillary microorganism measuring 0.3 to 0.4 $\mu$m in length and 0.3 to 0.5 $\mu$m in diameter. The organisms usually occur singly or in strands. In stained specimens, a diplobacillus with pointed ends and a transparent band between the two bacilli are noted. Rickettsiae must penetrate cells to grow and multiply. They can be grown most readily in the yolk sacs of embryonated eggs. Rickettsiae may remain viable for several days in blood at 4 °C; thus, a specimen of blood from a patient suspected to have rickettsial disease can be held for 1 or more days in a refrigerator before a definitive isolation procedure is performed. Rickettsiae turn red when they are stained with the Gimenez stain. *R rickettsii* organisms have a soluble antigenic moiety shared with all the antigenic variants in the spotted fever group, as well as with rickettsialpox.

Because Rocky Mountain spotted fever rickettsiae primarily are parasites of ticks, human disease generally is associated with the biology of the ticks that transmit it. Disease can be transmitted by the aerosol route in the laboratory, however, or by blood transfusion.

The wood tick (*Dermacentor andersoni*) in the West, the Lone Star tick (*Amblyomma americanum*) in the Southwest, and the dog tick (*Dermacentor variabilis*) in the East all are carriers and vectors of this disease. Rocky Mountain spotted fever rickettsiae do not kill the arthropod host, but can be passed from generation to generation of ticks transovarially. Congenitally acquired rickettsiae in tick eggs can persist through the various larval and nymphal stages into the adult stage of a 2-year cycle of the tick. Infected adult ticks may survive for as long as 4 years.

Important epidemiologic features of Rocky Mountain spotted

## TABLE 60-1. Important Epidemiologic Characteristics of Rickettsial Diseases*

| Disease | Agent | Epidemiologic Features | | |
|---------|-------|------------------------|---|---|
| | | Geographic Occurrence | Usual Mode of Human Transmission | Reservoir |
| **Typhus Group** | | | | |
| Primary louse-borne typhus | R prowazekii | Worldwide | Infected louse feces rubbed into broken skin, or as aerosol to mucous membranes | Humans |
| Brill-Zinsser disease | R prowazekii | Worldwide | Recrudescence months or years after primary attack of louse-borne typhus | |
| Murine typhus | R mooseri* | Scattered pockets, worldwide | Flea bite | Rodents |
| **Spotted Fever Group** | | | | |
| Rocky Mountain spotted fever | R rickettsii | Western hemisphere | Tick bite | Ticks/rodents |
| Tick typhuses (boutonneuse) | R conorii† | Mediterranean, Caspian, and Black Sea littorals; Africa; Southeast Asia | Tick/mite bite | Ticks/rodents |
| Rickettsialpox | R akari | United States, Russia, Korea | Mite bite | Mites/mice |
| Scrub Typhus | R tsutsugamushi | Japan, Southeast Asia, West and Southwest Pacific | Mite bite | Mites/rodents |
| Q fever | Coxiella burnetii | Worldwide | Inhalation of infected particles from environment of infected animals | Ticks/mammals |
| Ehrlichiosis | Ehrlichia canis‡ | United States | Tick bite (presumed) | Unknown |

\* Also *Rickettsia typhi.*
† In addition, in Australia, *Rickettsia australis* (Queensland tick typhus), and in North Asia, *Rickettsia sibirica* (Siberian tick typhus) are both antigenically and geographically distinct entities.
‡ Or a serologically, closely related agent.

*Feigin RD, Snider RL, Edwards MS. Rickettsial diseases. In: Feigin RD, Cherry, eds. Textbook of pediatric infectious diseases, ed 3. Philadelphia: WB Saunders, 1992:1847.*

fever include seasonal characteristics, because most cases occur during the period of greatest tick activity between April and September. Two thirds of the cases in the United States occur in children less than 15 years old. The disease also is focal, that is, relatively small areas within a state may account for a high percentage of that state's recorded cases of Rocky Mountain spotted fever.

## Pathogenesis

The principal pathologic lesion of Rocky Mountain spotted fever is a vasculitis that follows the bite of an infected tick. Rickettsiae multiply within the endothelial cells lining small blood vessels and are disseminated widely by the bloodstream. The rickettsiae can be demonstrated in both the cytoplasm and the nucleus of cells. Numerous mechanisms for cellular injury have been suggested, including injury to cell membranes resulting from penetration by multiple rickettsiae; depletion of adenosine triphosphate by intracellular rickettsiae, causing failure of the sodium pump and an influx of water; damage to the cell by toxic products of the rickettsial metabolism; and competition by R rickettsii for crucial metabolic substrates.

Vascular lesions account for the more prominent clinical features noted, including rash, mental confusion, headache, heart failure, and shock. Pneumonia can be acquired by laboratory inhalation.

The vascular lesions are found everywhere, but are appreciated most readily in the skin, adrenal glands, and gonads. Inflammation accompanies vasculitis of the heart and nervous system. Interstitial myocarditis is demonstrated readily in the location of the rickettsiae by immunofluorescence, which coincides with the

distribution of the myocarditis. In neural tissue, both proliferative glial nodules (which usually are related topographically to inflamed blood vessels) and mononuclear infiltrations are seen. In the kidney, inflammation involves vessels of the interstitium, and acute tubular necrosis may occur in some patients. In the lung, rickettsial involvement of the pulmonary microcirculation results in interstitial pneumonia. Hepatic lesions include portal triaditis, portal vasculitis, and sinusoidal leukocytosis.

Changes in nitrogen balance are extreme. Early in this infection, large amounts of nitrogen may be excreted in the urine. Subsequently, nitrogen imbalances are related to insufficient protein intake. The serum albumin concentration is depressed as the result of protein losses, hepatic dysfunction related to the disease process itself, and protein leakage through the damaged endothelium of blood vessels.

Hyponatremia may be profound. Reported causes of the hyponatremia include a loss of sodium by the urine, a shift in water from the intracellular to the extracellular space, and an exchange of sodium for potassium at the cellular level. The intracellular sodium level increases slightly. The destruction of cells results in an increase in the serum concentration of potassium and in enormous losses of potassium in the urine. Plasma concentrations of antidiuretic hormone and aldosterone have been increased in some individuals with this disease.

## Clinical Manifestations

Fever, headache, and rash are the hallmarks of Rocky Mountain spotted fever as well as of other rickettsial diseases, although the complete triad may be present in only 45% to 62% of all cases. Mental confusion and myalgia are common features of Rocky

Mountain spotted fever. The onset of disease in children usually occurs 2 to 8 days after a bite is sustained from an infected tick. The onset of clinical manifestations may be gradual or abrupt. Body temperature rises rapidly to 40 °C, with a pattern that is characterized by persistence, although many patients do have temperature oscillations over a period of several hours.

The rash associated with Rocky Mountain spotted fever is one of the more pathognomonic features of this disease. It generally appears by the second or third day of illness, although it may be delayed for a week. Initially, the lesions are erythematous macules that can blanch on pressure. The lesions rapidly become petechial and, in untreated patients, even hemorrhagic. Sometimes skin necrosis occurs. The rash appears peripherally on the wrists and ankles, spreading within hours up the extremities and onto the trunk. The rash also appears frequently on the palms and soles. The absence of rash, however, does not exclude a diagnosis of Rocky Mountain spotted fever.

Headache in older children and adults is a characteristic finding. The headache is persistent night and day, and is intractable. Young children, however, may not complain of this symptom. Signs of meningoencephalitis are common and may be appreciated because the patient is irritable, apprehensive, restless, or exhibits signs of mental confusion or delirium. Occasionally, children may become comatose. Meningismus may be present, but is not accompanied always by abnormalities in the cerebrospinal fluid. In fact, the cerebrospinal fluid generally is clear, with minor elevations seen in the lymphocyte count (less than 10 cells/mm$^3$). Seizures (grand mal or focal) have been observed. Central deafness (persistent or transient) and cortical blindness have been described. Other reported neurologic involvement includes sixth nerve paralysis, spastic paralysis, and ataxia. Rocky Mountain spotted fever also seems to exert a consistent effect on intellectual function, and several investigators have suggested that a higher probability of learning disability and difficulty in school performance exists in children who have had this disease.

Cardiac involvement is frequent and requires evaluation of each patient with clinically defined illness by electrocardiography, echocardiography, and other techniques if necessary. Congestive heart failure and arrhythmias are common.

Muscle tenderness is a common feature of Rocky Mountain spotted fever. Characteristically, the patient complains when the calf or thigh muscles are squeezed.

Pulmonary involvement occurs in 10% to 40% of reported cases and may be associated with abnormal chest radiograph results and abnormal arterial blood gas measurements. The chest radiograph may reveal cardiomegaly, focal infiltrates, or pulmonary edema.

Generalized edema of the face and extremities usually occurs and, in occasional cases, nuchal rigidity and conjunctival suffusion are seen. Acute tubular necrosis and glomerulonephritis can occur. Enlargement of the liver and spleen develops, but is infrequent. Other gastrointestinal symptoms and signs, including nausea, vomiting, abdominal pain, and diarrhea, arise frequently during the early course of Rocky Mountain spotted fever. Icterus has been reported, but is relatively rare, except in severe cases.

## Diagnosis

Specific treatment should be initiated promptly because, in most cases, laboratory evaluations do not permit a specific cause to be identified before therapy must be instituted. R rickettsii, however, can be identified by immunofluorescent techniques in skin specimens obtained by biopsy on days 4 through 8 of the illness, and sometimes for a longer period. This is a practical means of confirming the diagnosis during the stages of the disease before positive serologic reactions can be obtained. It must be recognized, however, that an experienced technologist usually is needed to

interpret the immunofluorescent test result and that false-positive and false-negative results do occur. A negative immunofluorescent test result never excludes the diagnosis of Rocky Mountain spotted fever.

Specific serologic results usually are not positive before day 10 or 12 of the illness. At this time, the majority of the 20% of patients who will die if they are not treated already are moribund or dead; therefore, the provision of appropriate therapy can never await a definitive diagnosis.

Selected laboratory clues may be helpful. During the first 4 or 5 days after the onset of disease, the white blood cell count is normal or may reveal a leukopenia. As the disease progresses, secondary bacterial infections may occur, and leukocyte counts may rise to as high as 30,000 cells per cubic millimeter. Thrombocytopenia of varying severity develops in most cases.

Serologic testing is important, primarily to confirm the diagnosis of Rocky Mountain spotted fever. The Weil-Felix test is nonspecific, but is most useful because it is available in almost all medical laboratories and can be performed in 3 to 5 minutes. It also will exhibit positive results as early as or earlier than will any other specific tests in a high proportion of patients with untreated Rocky Mountain spotted fever. This test depends on the fact that rickettsiae possess antigens in common with certain strains of Proteus bacteria. Antibodies to two Proteus strains, OX2 and OX19, regularly have rising titers, singly or together, during the second week of an untreated case of Rocky Mountain spotted fever. It should be noted, however, that Proteus infections of the urinary tract are common and, therefore, low-titer antibodies to Proteus OX strains often are found in normal human serum. Also, the test result can be positive in patients with leptospirosis, brucellosis, Borrelia infections, typhoid fever, and serious liver disease, and occasionally during pregnancy. A rising Proteus OX2 or OX19 titer or a titer of 1:160 or greater of either OX2 or OX19 in a seriously ill patient with signs and symptoms suggestive of Rocky Mountain spotted fever is sufficient reason to initiate therapy immediately.

Other tests that have been used for establishing a specific diagnosis are the complement-fixation test, the indirect hemagglutination reaction, microimmunofluorescence tests, and latex agglutination and microagglutination tests. Each of these tests has limitations with regard to sensitivity or specificity. The complement-fixation and microagglutination tests are highly specific, but lack sensitivity. Indirect hemagglutination and latex agglutination tests are highly sensitive and specific, but are not suitable for seroepidemiologic diagnosis because the immunoglobulins detected by these tests (IgM) are short-lived. The immunofluorescence test is the most specific and sensitive test available, but it is subject to observer bias.

A microtiter enzyme-linked immunosorbent assay (ELISA) has been developed to characterize the IgG and IgM response in Rocky Mountain spotted fever. It is both sensitive and accurate. The value of this test is limited, however, because IgG and IgM seroconversions cannot be demonstrated until 6 days after the onset of illness. This test is useful in seroepidemiologic studies.

More recently, investigators have shown that sera from patients with Rocky Mountain spotted fever have a unique profile when analyzed by frequency-pulsed electron capture-gas liquid chromatography. Typical profiles could be noted as early as 1 day after the onset of disease and before the time that any antibody test result became positive. A polymerase chain reaction assay was developed that enables the detection of specific sequences of DNA at the theoretic limit of one organism. It is a specific and useful screening test and diagnostic tool for the most common rickettsial illnesses in the United States. This test detects as few as 30 organisms per sample, can be completed in 48 hours, and permits therapeutic intervention during the acute illness.

The diagnosis of Rocky Mountain spotted fever can be confirmed by isolation of R rickettsii in embryonated eggs of guinea pigs from blood drawn during the first week of illness, before specific antibodies have developed.

## Differential Diagnosis

Meningococcemia and measles are the disorders most frequently confused with Rocky Mountain spotted fever. A petechial rash involving the palms and soles that spreads in a centripetal manner suggests a diagnosis of Rocky Mountain spotted fever, although the atypical measles syndrome can produce a similar rash. Therefore, a history of previous measles immunization, particularly with killed vaccine, is important. Differentiation from meningococcemia can be difficult because white blood cell counts may be low or normal and signs of meningeal irritation and moderate pleocytosis may be seen in both diseases. The inability to differentiate meningococcemia from Rocky Mountain spotted fever does not justify delaying antimicrobial therapy, because both diseases potentially are fatal. Treatment should be initiated promptly with chloramphenicol and penicillin G if the diagnosis of either disease is entertained and neither can be excluded immediately. When the appropriate diagnosis is certain, the inappropriate drug can be discontinued.

## Therapy

Chloramphenicol and the tetracyclines are highly effective when they are given early in the course of the disease and in an appropriate dosage. In children, we treat seriously ill patients with intravenous chloramphenicol at a dosage of 100 mg/kg/24 h, up to a total dose of 2 g. This dosage must be modified in newborns and in children with serious liver disease as a manifestation of Rocky Mountain spotted fever. It is appropriate to monitor serum chloramphenicol concentrations during the course of this disease. When the patient improves, chloramphenicol can be given orally at 50 mg/kg/24 h in four divided doses. If tetracyclines are provided, 30 to 40 mg/kg/24 h may be given in four divided doses orally or 20 mg/kg/24 h may be given intravenously (maximum dose, 2 g/24 h). Treatment can be terminated 3 to 4 days after the patient's temperature has returned to normal for a full 24-hour period. The duration of therapy usually is 7 to 10 days.

Thrombocytopenia and disseminated intravascular coagulation may develop in the course of Rocky Mountain spotted fever. Adequate antimicrobial therapy is essential to prevent this complication.

Endothelial damage is widespread in Rocky Mountain spotted fever and other rickettsial infections. The need for supportive care cannot be overemphasized. Careful evaluation of serum and urine electrolyte levels, body weight, and renal function is important to guide fluid therapy. Hyponatremia is treated best by providing maintenance fluids (1500 mL/m²/24 h) or, in the case of severe hyponatremia, by instituting modest fluid restriction. The administration of sodium-rich fluids precipitates cardiac decompensation and pulmonary edema in critically ill patients with Rocky Mountain spotted fever without raising the serum sodium concentration substantially. Patients who have concomitant hypotension and hypoalbuminemia may be given albumin (1 g/kg immediately). When the clotting time is prolonged in patients without disseminated intravascular coagulation, the administration of vitamin K (2 mg intramuscularly immediately) has been helpful. Anemia of a severe degree may require blood transfusion. Several investigators have suggested that steroid therapy has been helpful in shortening the febrile period. When steroids are given in sufficient doses to any febrile patient, the febrile period should be diminished, but other specific therapeutic benefits related to this course of action in Rocky Mountain spotted fever have not been proven.

## Prevention

Principal preventive measures that are effective include avoidance of contact with ticks and inoculation with killed vaccines. Individuals who are in a tick-infested area should examine themselves frequently and remove ticks from their bodies and clothing. Frequent removal of ticks is particularly valuable, because infected ticks must be attached and feeding for 4 to 6 hours or more before they can transmit the disease. The application of substances such as dimethyl phthalate to clothes and other exposed parts of the body may provide additional protection against ticks.

Killed vaccines have been valuable in preventing death, but do not reliably protect against the acquisition of disease. The most recently available vaccine is a chicken embryo vaccine that is superior to the more generally available yolk sac vaccine. Recent studies demonstrated that the chicken embryo vaccine is safe and that two doses elicit low levels of antibodies to R rickettsii in 50% of those vaccinated. Although vaccination provides only partial protection against Rocky Mountain spotted fever, it ameliorates the illness when it occurs. An attack of Rocky Mountain spotted fever is followed by solid immunity. No licensed rickettsial vaccine is available.

## Prognosis

The mortality from Rocky Mountain spotted fever was about 25% before appropriate antimicrobial therapy became available. If appropriate antibiotics are provided before the end of the first week of illness, recovery generally is the rule. The overall mortality rate remains 5% to 7%, however, principally because diagnosis and therapy are delayed in many patients until the second week of illness. The case fatality rate in 1990 was 2.4% for persons less than 20 years of age and 6.8% for those greater than 20 years of age. When death occurs, it usually is the result of heart failure, vascular collapse, renal failure, or thrombocytopenia, either alone or in combination. Central nervous system involvement and disseminated intravascular coagulation are common.

Complications are less common in patients who receive appropriate therapy early. Bronchopneumonia may develop in critically ill patients, and the infusion of sodium-rich parenteral fluids may precipitate both cardiac failure and pulmonary edema.

# Mediterranean Spotted Fever

Mediterranean spotted fever first was described in 1910 and is a tick-borne infection caused by Rickettsia conorii. Other names given to this illness include boutonneuse fever, Kenya tick-bite fever, African tick typhus, India tick typhus, and Marseilles fever. There recently has been a resurgence of this disease in Mediterranean countries such as Spain, Italy, and Israel.

## Epidemiology

R conorii is an obligate intracellular parasite of mites, which inoculate the microorganisms directly into the dermis during feeding. In the Mediterranean area, the vector is the brown dog tick, Rhipicephalus sanguineus. Various species of mites may act as vectors in other geographic areas.

The epidemiology of Mediterranean spotted fever is determined by the biology of the tick and results in a consistent seasonal peak that occurs from late June to mid-October. Humans are accidental hosts and become a dead end in the transmission chain. Habitual contact with dogs appears to be the most common factor among people who acquire the infection. Rickettsiae also may be inoculated by scratching and via the conjunctival route. Laboratory infection by accidental inoculation has been described.

The exact prevalence of Mediterranean spotted fever is unknown, although seropositivity rates of antibodies to R conorii have been reported to be as high as 70% in some regions of Spain.

## Clinical Manifestations

The infecting bite passes unnoticed in most cases, and the incubation period varies from 6 to 10 days. Late in the incubation period, a small indurated lesion, called a tache noire (black spot), develops at the site of the tick bite. It is not painful and rarely is pruritic. It becomes necrotic at its center, develops an eschar, and gives rise to enlargement of regional lymph nodes. The tache noire is pathognomonic, but is present in only 30% to 90% of cases. It is localized predominantly on the head of children and on the legs of adults.

The onset of disease usually is abrupt, with severe headache, malaise, and a temperature that reaches 39 °C to 40 °C within the first 2 or 3 days. The fever continues for 6 to 12 days, and antibiotics can shorten the febrile period. Generalized myalgias, especially of the leg muscles, are a prominent feature.

A rash usually appears on the third, fourth, or fifth febrile day. The initial lesions are on the extremities; after 24 to 36 hours, the rash spreads to the trunk, neck, face, buttocks, palms, and soles. The first lesions are macular, pink, and irregularly defined, and they become maculopapular after a few hours. They generally measure 1 to 4 mm in diameter. The rash persists for 10 to 20 days after the remission of clinical symptoms. The cutaneous manifestations result from the involvement of the vascular structures of the dermis by a vasculitis that is similar to the one seen with Rocky Mountain spotted fever.

Bradycardia is the most consistent cardiovascular finding in Mediterranean spotted fever, but other dysrhythmias have been reported. Phlebitis of the lower limbs is the main vascular complication. Venous thrombosis is a recognized complication, particularly in pregnant patients. More seriously ill patients may have pericarditis, heart failure, myocarditis, nephritis with acute renal failure, pneumonitis, pleuritis, the adult respiratory distress syndrome, or involvement of the central nervous system.

The liver is palpable in one third of the patients, and the spleen may enlarge in 20% of children. Tests of hepatic function reveal an increase in levels of serum transaminases in more than half of the cases. Alkaline phosphatase concentrations are elevated in one third of the patients. Needle biopsy of the liver reveals foci of hepatocellular necrosis and a predominantly mononuclear reaction to the necrosis at sites of infection by *R conorii*.

Other systemic symptoms may occur. Photophobia and bilateral conjunctivitis have been reported. Severe unilateral conjunctivitis suggests transmission of the disease via the conjunctival route.

## Diagnosis

If biopsy is performed early in the course of the disease, rickettsial organisms can be detected by immunofluorescence from the tache noire. *R conorii* cannot be isolated from blood cultures by means of routine laboratory procedures. The clinical presentation, geographic location, and epidemiologic considerations are helpful in establishing the diagnosis. Laboratory diagnosis is an important adjunct and involves serologic identification of serum antibody.

The Weil-Felix reaction relies on the antigenic cross-reactivity between certain *Proteus* species (OX19, OX2, and OXK) and rickettsiae. The test is a nonspecific assay for serum antibody response. Single titers of 1:80 strongly support the diagnosis. Antibodies appear on day 7 to 10 and peak during the third week of illness. Results are variable, however, and a high false-negative rate is seen.

Complement fixation, microagglutination, ELISA, and indirect immunofluorescence tests are available. The identification of specific IgM by immunofluorescence helps to differentiate acute infection from a carrier state. A recently developed latex agglutination test for the detection of antibodies to *R conorii* is both sensitive and specific. It is simpler and more rapid than microagglutination.

## Differential Diagnosis

Before the rash appears, differentiation of Mediterranean spotted fever from other acute infections is difficult. Even after the appearance of the rash, the disease can be confused with measles, the rash of meningococcemia, toxicodermatosis, secondary syphilis, and leukocytoclastic angiitis. Other rickettsial diseases should be considered, especially in the absence of a tache noire. Cross-reactions among rickettsiae occur with the Weil-Felix reaction as well as with indirect immunofluorescence testing. Differentiation from typhoid fever is possible when agglutinins against antigens of typhoid or paratyphoid bacilli develop.

## Treatment and Prevention

Mediterranean spotted fever generally runs a benign course, with rare fatalities. Tetracycline is the drug of choice and chloramphenicol is an acceptable alternative. Recommended dosages are 2 g/d for tetracycline hydrochloride and 100 to 200 mg/d for doxycycline. The optimal duration of specific therapy has not been established definitively.

The major effective methods of control are concerned with the avoidance of tick bites. Natural immunity occurs after infection, and specific antibodies have been shown to persist for as long as 4 years after acute illness. Effective vaccines are not available.

# Other Tick Typhus Fevers

Two other antigenically distinct rickettsiae are *Rickettsia sibirica* and *Rickettsia australis*, the causative agents of Siberian tick typhus and Queensland tick typhus, respectively. These agents share the same antigen as *R rickettsii*, but have distinguishing type-specific antigens demonstrated by complement-fixation and neutralization tests. Siberian tick typhus has been diagnosed throughout central Asia, and Queensland tick typhus is found in eastern Australia.

Dogs constitute the principal mammalian reservoir, but ticks also act as reservoirs by virtue of transovarial transmission. Both of these diseases have similar clinical, pathologic, and epidemiologic patterns. They produce a mild disease, similar to that of Mediterranean spotted fever.

Treatment is similar to that of Rocky Mountain spotted fever.

# Rickettsialpox

Rickettsialpox first was recognized in New York City in 1946 as a benign rickettsial infection caused by *Rickettsia akari*. This organism is related antigenically to the spotted fever group. Certain features of the disease that distinguish rickettsialpox from other rickettsial infections include transmission by the body mite, an eschar at the site of the infectious mite bite, a vesiculopapular rather than maculopapular rash, and the absence of Weil-Felix agglutinins.

## Organisms, Epidemiology, and Transmission

The causative agent *R akari* grows in the nucleus as well as the cytoplasm of cells and is a soluble antigen that cross-reacts with Rocky Mountain spotted fever and three other tick typhus rickettsiae. Its clinical, epidemiologic, and serologic features distinguish it from other diseases of the spotted fever group.

Most cases of rickettsialpox in the United States have been reported from New York City, although some have been observed in other cities in the eastern portion of the country. A similar disease has been described in Ukrainian cities in the former Soviet Union. A disease that is clinically consistent with rickettsialpox has been reported in the Republic of South Africa.

House mice are the natural hosts of the mite that transmits rickettsialpox in the United States, but rats have been found to be infected in Russia, and wild rodents are suspected of carrying the disease in South Africa.

## Clinical Manifestations

The incubation period of rickettsialpox is 9 to 14 days, but it is difficult to determine precisely, because most patients have continual exposure to the vector in their homes.

Initially, a red papule develops at the site of the mite bite. The lesion slowly develops into a papulovesicular lesion, which shortly becomes a black scab or eschar at the time the fever begins. The lesion most often is solitary, although two eschars have been described in selected cases. Regional lymphadenopathy related to the primary eschar occurs almost invariably.

The temperature is irregular, fluctuating between 37.8 °C and 39.5 °C, and fever rarely lasts longer than 1 week. The disease characteristically is accompanied by headache, fever, cough, nausea, vomiting, and abdominal pain. The rash develops rapidly from scattered nonpruritic macules that become firm maculopapules in a day or two. In another day, the papules become vesicles. The lesions usually appear on the face, trunk, and extremities, but also may be seen on the palms, soles, and mucous membranes. The number of lesions varies from 5 to more than 100. The characteristic papulovesicular lesions are distributed so haphazardly that this disorder is difficult to distinguish from varicella.

## Diagnosis

The diagnosis can be made with complement-fixation or immunofluorescent tests. Weil-Felix tests are useless because no *Proteus* agglutinins are produced. The major differential diagnostic problem is chickenpox.

## Treatment

Tetracycline is the drug of choice for rickettsialpox, but chloramphenicol is an acceptable alternative. In infants and young children with mild illness, antibiotics can be withheld because the disease is self-limiting.

# TYPHUS GROUP

The typhus group consists of three diseases: louse-borne typhus, Brill-Zinsser disease, and murine flea-borne typhus. These diseases are similar clinically, but distinct epidemiologically.

## Louse-Borne Typhus Fever

Louse-borne or epidemic typhus is an acute infectious disease transmitted by the body louse to humans. Louse-borne typhus has occurred predominantly in Europe, Asia, and Africa, and is seen only intermittently in the United States. It has played a major role in the history of nations over the past 5 centuries: after World War I, more than 30 million people in Eastern Europe were infected with typhus and an estimated 3 million died.

### Etiology, Epidemiology, and Transmission

The etiologic agent of louse-borne typhus fever is *Rickettsia prowazekii*. The morphology, metabolism, growth, toxin production, and staining characteristics of this organism are similar to those of rickettsiae of the spotted fever group.

It has been assumed that the causative agent of epidemic typhus existed only in the human-louse-human cycle, and that individuals who had recovered from typhus constituted the principal reservoir of *R prowazekii* during periods between epidemics.

The findings of sporadic *R prowazekii* infection, particularly in the United States, however, suggest that the agent of epidemic typhus may be perpetuated in an animal reservoir.

The louse becomes infected during a blood meal from a febrile patient. After a 5- to 10-day incubation period in the louse, a large number of rickettsiae can be found in louse feces. Transmission of rickettsiae from an infected louse to a new host can occur in several ways. A louse defecates as it feeds, and infected feces can be rubbed into the louse-bite wound. Dried louse feces can gain access to the mucous membrane of the eye or respiratory tract. The typhus spreads through a community in epidemic fashion, primarily because the louse prefers to feed on people with a normal body temperature. Hence, infected lice leave febrile patients as well as dead patients and prefer to feed on newer hosts who are healthy. Crowding, as occurs during wars or periods of famine, permits ready transfer to new hosts.

## Clinical Manifestations

One to 2 weeks after an infected louse bites a human host, the illness usually begins abruptly. The principal manifestations are fever, headache, and rash. The temperature rises to 40 °C or higher. In an untreated patient, it may remain at this level, fluctuating only minimally until recovery or death ensues.

The rash usually appears on the trunk by days 4 to 7 of the illness, spreading peripherally to the extremities and generally sparing the face, palms, and soles. Initially, the rash is macular and the macules fade on pressure. The rash soon becomes maculopapular and, later, petechial-hemorrhagic. Severe, intractable headache is characteristic of this and other rickettsial diseases.

Typhus fever can present as encephalitis, meningitis, or meningoencephalitis. Severe, untreated cases can progress to prostration, stupor, or delirium with terminal myocardial and renal failure. Uncommon complications include gangrene, parotitis, otitis media, acute pericarditis, myocarditis, pericardial effusion, pleurisy, pleural effusion, and pneumonia.

Case fatality rates in untreated cases correlate with patient age. Mortality is uncommon in young children, but may range from 10% in young adults to as high as 60% to 70% in individuals more than 50 years of age.

## Diagnosis

The rash of louse-borne typhus begins centrally and spreads peripherally, permitting this disorder to be distinguished clinically from Rocky Mountain spotted fever. Whereas the rash of Rocky Mountain spotted fever begins peripherally and spreads to the trunk, the rash of louse-borne typhus behaves in the opposite fashion, beginning centrally and spreading peripherally. Moreover, the rash on the palms and soles, which occurs so frequently in Rocky Mountain spotted fever, occurs rarely in louse-borne typhus.

The Weil-Felix reaction almost always is positive with the *Proteus* OX19 strain and is positive less frequently with the *Proteus* OX2 strain. Complement-fixation and immunofluorescent tests are diagnostic; however, with louse-borne typhus, the *R prowazekii* strains are used as antigens. Antigenic crossing between any members of the typhus and spotted fever groups of organisms occurs frequently.

An ELISA and latex agglutination tests were evaluated and found to be sensitive and reproducible. As a result of the antigenic crossover between the typhus group of rickettsiae, work is under way to isolate the species-specific protein for *R prowazekii* so that it may be used for both immunodiagnosis and immunoprophylaxis. The polymerase chain reaction assay permits confirmation of rickettsial infection within 48 hours, allowing therapeutic intervention during the acute illness.

## Therapy

Treatment with chloramphenicol in young children or tetracycline in older children in the dosages listed for Rocky Mountain spotted fever is recommended.

## Prevention

Vaccination and louse control are the best means of controlling typhus epidemics. Killed vaccines produced from yolk sacs grown in chicken embryos have been highly effective in preventing death, but do not routinely prevent infection.

Dichlorodiphenyltrichloroethane (DDT) and other insecticides such as malathion and lindane have proved effective in reducing louse infestation during typhus epidemics. Insecticides should be dusted onto the clothes of louse-infected populations; when this is done, lice frequently are eliminated from the community.

## Brill-Zinsser Disease

Brill-Zinsser disease is the name given to the relapse or recrudescence of louse-borne typhus that occurs many years after the primary attack. This relapsing form of typhus occurs because the rickettsiae remain dormant somewhere in the body, presumably within cells of the reticuloendothelial system. Many years later, during the course of stress or some other factor, the lice multiply and produce a second acute attack. As a result of partial immunity from the primary typhus attack, recrudescent infection almost always is a shorter, milder, and less debilitating illness. The causative agent is the same as for the primary disease (R prowazekii), and the symptoms and signs are similar in type. Brill-Zinsser disease is rare in the United States, with only one case reported to the Centers for Disease Control and Prevention in the 1980s.

Chloramphenicol or tetracycline is the drug of choice. A single dose of doxycycline may lead to prompt resolution of the clinical symptoms in selected cases. Because recrudescent typhus usually does not occur in young children, tetracycline is the preferred drug for treatment of this disease.

## Murine Typhus

Murine or epidemic typhus is a disease of rats that is passed from rat to rat by the rat flea, and is transmitted only occasionally and accidentally to humans by the bite of an infected rat flea. This disease occurs worldwide and is particularly prevalent along coastal areas and around granaries. It was highly prevalent along the Atlantic seaboard and Gulf coastal areas of the United States during the first half of this century. Murine typhus also is known as urban fever, in reference to the fact that it is the only rickettsial infection that commonly is acquired in cities.

### Etiology, Epidemiology, and Transmission

The causative agent of murine typhus is *Rickettsia mooseri*, which is similar to *R prowazekii* in its metabolism, growth, staining characteristics, and toxin production. It is slightly smaller and more uniform in size than *R prowazekii*.

Murine typhus usually is acquired by humans from the rat flea, *Xenopsylla cheopis*. This flea becomes infected when feeding on an acutely ill rat. The rickettsiae multiply in the flea without causing any ill effects, but the feces of the infected flea are infected for the remainder of the flea's life. Rat fleas prefer to feed on rats, but will feed on people when rats are unavailable. When an infected flea sucks blood, it ejects the rickettsiae into the open wound; alternatively, infected feces may be rubbed into the bite wound or transferred by a dried aerosol to the conjunctivae or respiratory tract. Laboratory-acquired infection also has been documented. In California, sporadic cases have been recorded as a result of the transmission by fleas of *R mooseri* from opossums

to humans. In the early 1940s, about 5000 cases of murine typhus were reported annually in the United States. Currently, only about 60 to 80 cases are reported annually; about 80% of these come from Texas. Most cases occur from April through August.

### Clinical Manifestations

The incubation period ranges from 6 to 14 days. Symptoms and signs include headache, fever, and rash, and the disease appears almost identical to that of louse-borne typhus. The principal difference is that murine typhus is milder and the duration of illness is shorter. The temperature generally does not rise much above 39 °C, and the fever tends to be intermittent. The febrile period terminates after 9 to 13 days. Headache is less severe, and the maculopapular rash is less extensive than in epidemic typhus. Complications are uncommon and the mortality rate is 1% or less.

### Diagnosis

The diagnosis of epidemic typhus can be suggested by a Weil-Felix response with a positive *Proteus* OX19 titer and, less commonly, a positive *Proteus* OX2 titer. Complement-fixation and immunofluorescent tests performed with *R mooseri* antigens are used to diagnose the disease more explicitly. The isolation of *R mooseri* protein antigens has been attempted so that these antigens can be used ultimately to eliminate the problem of an antigenic crossover when complement-fixation reactions are carried out. The use of polymerase chain reaction assays permits confirmation of rickettsial infection within 48 hours and allows therapeutic intervention during the acute illness.

### Treatment

Treatment is similar to that for Rocky Mountain spotted fever or epidemic typhus. Patients with acute illness may be treated with chloramphenicol; those in whom the disease is less acute and those older than 9 years of age can be treated with tetracycline.

### Prevention

Eradication of rats is the principal means of preventing the spread of murine typhus to humans. Rat populations can be reduced by poisoning, trapping, and rat-proofing buildings.

## Tsutsugamushi Fever (Scrub Typhus)

Tsutsugamushi fever is an acute infectious disease transmitted to humans by chiggers. The disease is restricted almost exclusively to a triangular area in Southeast Asia and the southwest Pacific. The points of the triangle are Japan, Pakistan, and the Solomon Islands. Individuals who are seen with scrub typhus infection elsewhere generally have contracted their disease in this area.

### Etiology, Epidemiology, and Transmission

The causative agent, *Rickettsia tsutsugamushi*, is distinguished by antigenic heterogeneity. Antigenic heterogeneity is responsible for the differences seen in the severity of this disease in the same and different locations. This has thwarted all efforts to develop an effective vaccine or a widely specific and applicable serologic test. A modification of the Gimenez method is required to stain scrub typhus rickettsiae bright red.

Trombiculid mites are the reservoirs and vectors of this disease. They transmit rickettsiae to their own progeny by infected ova. They also transmit disease to the small rodents on which they feed.

Because of prolonged persistence of *R tsutsugamushi* in the human host, transplacentally acquired fetal infection is a possibility.

## Pathology

The pathology of scrub typhus is a perivasculitis of small blood vessels similar to that of other rickettsial diseases. An eschar or necrotic inflammatory lesion develops at the site of the mite bite, followed by regional lymphadenopathy similar to that seen with rickettsialpox. Generalized lymphadenopathy is common in scrub typhus, but rare to absent in all other rickettsial diseases.

## Clinical Manifestations

An initial lesion develops into a necrotic eschar in more than 50% of cases. Mites are acquired when people walk through brush; therefore, the initial lesion generally is on the lower limbs. Regional lymphadenopathy accompanies the primary lesion in most cases. The incubation period is 7 to 14 days. At about the time that the initial mite bite, lesion, or eschar is noted, other features of the disease develop, namely, headache, fever, rash, and generalized lymphadenopathy. After regression of the eschar, a scar often remains and may persist for up to 25 years.

A macular rash generally appears on the trunk only for a brief period, between the fifth and eighth days of illness. In selected cases, the rash persists and becomes maculopapular, extending onto the extremities. The generalized lymphadenopathy is prominent. Hepatosplenomegaly and conjunctival injection are seen commonly in patients with this disorder. Deafness and tinnitus may occur and are helpful diagnostic features when they appear. Atypical pneumonia, overwhelming pneumonia resembling the adult respiratory distress syndrome, myocarditis, and disseminated intravascular coagulation have been reported.

## Diagnosis

The Weil-Felix OXK strain agglutination reaction may be the only serologic test result that is positive. It aids in confirming the diagnosis. Only 50% of patients with scrub typhus ever have a positive OXK agglutination titer, however.

Immunofluorescent tests are more diagnostic and reliable. Because of the multiplicity of scrub typhus strains, though, eight or more of the antigenic strains must be included in the immunofluorescent test for scrub typhus. These tests are available in few laboratories.

The antibody to R tsutsugamushi that is measured by immunofluorescence is short-lived; as a result, the true incidence of scrub typhus in endemic areas is likely to be greater than described. An indirect immunoperoxidase test is available and provides specific, sensitive, and reproducible results. There is no cross-reactivity in testing against other diseases; this test is superior to the Weil-Felix reaction and comparable to the immunofluorescent test in the serodiagnosis of scrub typhus.

A dot immunoassay using nitrocellulose sheets that strongly absorb proteins and nucleic acids has been applied to the serodiagnosis of scrub typhus. The results are interpreted easily by untrained personnel because the differences in color intensity between positive and negative reactions can be distinguished readily by the naked eye.

## Therapy

Chloramphenicol and tetracyclines are effective in scrub typhus as described for the other rickettsial diseases. More recently, one study documented that a single 200-mg dose of doxycycline was as effective as a 7-day course of tetracycline in treating patients with this disorder. In that particular study, therapy was not instituted until day 10 of the disease.

Immunity begins to develop only in the second week of illness. Because both chloramphenicol and doxycycline are rickettsiostatic, patients with scrub typhus who are treated during the first week of illness may require intermittent courses of antibiotic therapy to prevent relapse.

## Prevention

Exposed skin surfaces and clothing can be impregnated with dimethyl or dibutyl phthalate.

Short-term control of vectors on camping grounds can be accomplished by cutting, burning, or bulldozing vegetation and spraying insecticides such as lindane or dieldrin.

It also is possible to use chemoprophylaxis for individuals who are in high-risk exposure areas for short periods. Doxycycline given at a dose of 200 mg once a week provides effective chemoprophylaxis for naturally transmitted scrub typhus if treatment is started before exposure to infection and is continued for 6 weeks afterward.

No satisfactory vaccine for this disease has been produced.

# Q Fever

Q fever is a rickettsial disease that occurs worldwide. It is characterized by fever, headache, and pneumonia in more than 50% of cases. It is unique among the human rickettsial infections in that it is primarily a disease of animals that is transmitted to humans by inhalation rather than by an arthropod bite, although it can be transmitted to humans by ticks.

## Etiology, Epidemiology, and Transmission

Rickettsiae that cause Q fever are known as Coxiella burnetii. The organism is highly resistant to heat, a quality that is unique among rickettsial agents, as well as to desiccation and chemicals. It fails to produce cross-reacting Proteus strain agglutinins (Weil-Felix reaction).

Q fever is primarily a zoonosis infecting cattle, goats, sheep, and rodents on a worldwide basis, and marsupials in Australia. Humans acquire the disease when they come in contact with infected animals and materials contaminated by these animals.

Epidemics of Q fever may occur in areas where animals are slaughtered, particularly when infected animals are pregnant, causing contamination of workers and creating aerosols that are carried by air-conditioning systems that may infect personnel far removed from the slaughtering areas. Sheep or cattle used in research increase the possibility of laboratory-acquired infections and, in recent years, outbreaks of Q fever have been reported in many research laboratories. Q fever also occurs commonly in textile plants where wool is processed, and in tanneries or shearing camps. In addition, it is common among children in rural areas who are exposed during the annual spring lambing time. Parturient cuts also have been implicated in outbreaks of Q fever.

The prevalence of Q fever probably is underestimated, because more than 40% of those individuals who have frequent contact with farm animals have been found to be seropositive for antibodies to Coxiella. The disease is being diagnosed in an increasing number of children younger than 3 years of age and should be considered during a workup for fever of unknown origin.

## Pathology

Mortality from Q fever is extremely rare. C burnetii has been documented in lung macrophages at autopsy and in specimens obtained at transbronchoscopic lung biopsy or at the time of lobectomy. C burnetii also may infect the liver, producing hepatosplenomegaly and abnormal liver function test results. Biopsy of the liver in an infected patient demonstrates granulomatous changes, with a dense fibrin ring surrounding a lipid vacuole. Rickettsial organisms are not found in these lesions. Similar granulomas have been noted in bone marrow. Vegetations on heart valves are seen when endocarditis complicates this disease. Rickettsiae have been isolated from the affected valve.

## Clinical Manifestations

After an incubation period of 9 to 20 days, the disease begins with chills, high fever, general malaise, myalgias, chest pain, and an intractable headache, similar to that seen with other rickettsial diseases. This particular rickettsial disorder, however, is not accompanied by a rash.

Physical findings in the chest generally are minimal and a radiograph may be necessary to appreciate the pulmonary pathology. In about 50% of patients, multiple round segmental opacities may be seen on the chest radiograph. Other, less common findings include linear atelectasis, lobar consolidation, or pleural effusion.

Although pneumonitis is a primary characteristic of Q fever, it should be noted that Q fever is a systemic disorder, as are the other rickettsioses. Hepatosplenomegaly occurs frequently, and gastroenteritis and hemolytic anemia have been reported.

The disease usually is mild and self-limited, lasting 1 to 2 weeks, with a mortality rate of 1% or less. Patients in whom Q fever and endocarditis or chronic Q fever develop, however, have a mortality rate between 30% and 60%. Other reported complications include myocarditis, pericarditis, meningoencephalitis, hepatitis, inappropriate secretion of antidiuretic hormone, and glomerulonephritis.

## Diagnosis

Complement-fixation or immunofluorescence tests that measure anti-phase I and anti-phase II antibody are effective in diagnosing Q fever. Specific IgM to *C burnetii* can be measured by ELISA, or by complement-fixation or immunofluorescence tests. Anti-phase II antibody is present early in primary disease. Anti-phase I antibody is present in patients with chronic disease or those who have granulomatous hepatitis or endocarditis.

A polymerase chain reaction test is available now that has the ability to detect as few as 1 to 10 organisms. The assay can distinguish between strains of *C burnetii* that cause acute disease and strains that are associated with endocarditis and chronic Q fever.

An immunoenzymatic test for the detection of anti–*C burnetii* antibodies has proved more sensitive than the indirect fluorescent antibody test for detecting low levels of antibody in individuals who have not developed clinical disease. This test is particularly useful for seroepidemiologic surveys of Q fever.

Attempts to isolate the organism may be successful, but are unrealistic, because they predispose laboratory personnel to infection.

## Therapy

Q fever responds promptly to tetracyclines or chloramphenicol, and relapses are rare. Primary disease should be treated with chloramphenicol in children less than 8 years of age and with tetracycline in those 8 years of age or older. The most appropriate drug and the duration of therapy necessary for patients with endocarditis resulting from Q fever remain unclear. Combination therapy that includes quinolones recently has been shown to be effective. Tetracycline, chloramphenicol, rifampin, lincomycin, co-trimoxazole, and trimethoprim-sulfamethoxazole all have been used, with differing degrees of success.

## Prevention

Experimental Q fever vaccines have been developed and tested in human volunteers, but the development and production of a safe and effective vaccine has not been accomplished.

Controlling infection in domestic animals has proved difficult. Research laboratories that use sheep should be separated physically from other laboratories. Sheep never should be transported through any patient care area, and any transport should be accomplished in a cart that is designed to protect the environment from fomite and aerosol transmission.

## Prognosis

Mortality from uncomplicated Q fever is 1% or less. Most patients recover completely within 30 to 60 days, with or without antimicrobial therapy. Antibiotics shorten the course of infection. When myocarditis, pericarditis, or endocarditis occurs, permanent disability and fatality are reported in 30% to 60% of patients.

# Ehrlichiosis

*Ehrlichia canis* has been recognized as a canine pathogen for many years. Human ehrlichiosis is a febrile illness that is characterized by headache, anorexia, and myalgias, with associated leukopenia or pancytopenia. Most patients have experienced tick attachment or bite within weeks before the onset of illness.

## The Organism

Seven species of the genus *Ehrlichia*, named after Paul Ehrlich, are pathogenic for humans or animals: *E chaffeensis, E canis, Ehrlichia sennetsu, Ehrlichia risticii, Ehrlichia equi, Ehrlichia phagocytophilia,* and *Ehrlichia platys*. Each of these infects the cytoplasm of leukocytes or, in the case of *E platys*, the cytoplasm of platelets. The most extensively studied organism, *E canis*, has been recognized as a cause of acute febrile illness in dogs since 1935.

## Epidemiology and Transmission

Since the initial report of human illness, more than 100 cases of ehrlichiosis in adults and at least 7 cases in children have been described. Seventeen states, primarily in the southeastern and south central areas of the country, have reported infection. Illness occurs in the months when ticks are prevalent, from March to October, and about 80% of the patients diagnosed with infection recall tick contact or bite within the 4 weeks before the onset of symptoms.

The reservoir for human ehrlichiosis has not been clarified. The brown dog tick, *R sanguineus*, is the vector for canine disease, but is unlikely to be the vector for human disease, because this tick rarely feeds on humans. Contact with dogs often is lacking in human infection. Because ticks are the only known vector for *Ehrlichia* species, they are the likely vector for human infection, but documentation requires additional study.

## Pathogenesis and Pathology

*Ehrlichia* enter the cytoplasm of host cells and multiply in phagosomes into elementary bodies. These individual *Ehrlichia* organisms multiply by binary fission into immature inclusions called initial bodies. Mature groups of elementary bodies form morulas that are released by rupture of the cell to reinitiate the infecting process.

Intraleukocytic inclusions have been observed in lymphocytes, monocytes, and neutrophils in some cases of human infection. This has not been a consistent or prominent feature of the disease, however, in part because the majority of infections have been documented by retrospective serologic analysis.

## Clinical Manifestations

The estimated incubation period for human ehrlichiosis is 12 to 14 days. Similar to Rocky Mountain spotted fever, ehrlichiosis is an acute febrile illness that causes fever, headache, anorexia with

TABLE 60-2. Clinical and Laboratory Features of Adult and Pediatric Ehrlichiosis

| Feature* | Percentage of Cases | |
|---|---|---|
| | Adult (N = 46) | Pediatric (N = 6) |
| Fever | 96 | 100 |
| Anorexia | 76 | 83 |
| Headache | 80 | NS† |
| Myalgia | 74 | 75 |
| Rash | 20 | 83 |
| Leukopenia‡ | 61 | 67 |
| Thrombocytopenia§ | 52 | 83 |
| Elevated aspartate aminotransferase levels¶ | 76 | 83 |

\* Some features were not specified for all patients.
† NS, not specified.
‡ White blood cell count less than 4000/mm³.
§ Platelets less than 150,000/mm³.
¶ More than 55 U/L.
Feigin RD, Snider RL, Edwards MS. Rickettsial diseases. In: Feigin RD, Cherry JD, eds. Textbook of pediatric infectious diseases, ed 3. Philadelphia: WB Saunders, 1992:1847.

or without vomiting, and myalgias (Table 60-2). Rash, which may be macular, maculopapular, or petechial, rarely occurs in adults. Among the small number of pediatric infections reported, rash has occurred commonly, with a distribution that often includes both the trunk and the extremities.

Meningitis as a manifestation of ehrlichiosis has been reported in two children, with symptoms ranging from irritability and meningismus to obtundation with response only to painful stimuli. Initial examination of the cerebrospinal fluid revealed pleocytosis ranging from about 50 to 1000 white blood cells, with a predominance of either neutrophils or lymphocytes; between 5 and 40 red blood cells; mildly elevated protein levels (85 to 120 mg/dL); and a normal to slightly low glucose value. Each of the two children recovered fully.

One half to two thirds of affected adults have mild leukopenia and thrombocytopenia. Although the numbers are small, these features also occur with similar frequency in children. One child has had a documented decline in the white blood cell count from 13,000 to 1600 over a period of several hours. Usually, thrombocytopenia is not associated with clinical bleeding; however, disseminated intravascular coagulopathy has been reported. Elevations of aspartate aminotransferase, which usually are modest, peak at about 1 week into the illness, with values ranging from twice normal to several thousand. Other uncommon manifestations of illness include elevation of renal function test results (occasionally of sufficient severity to require dialysis), hyponatremia, and hypoalbuminemia. These manifestations presumably are a consequence of the generalized vasculitis that accompanies the infection.

### Diagnosis and Differential Diagnosis

The diagnosis of human ehrlichiosis is established by documenting a fourfold rise or fall in titer by an indirect fluorescent antibody test that is available through the Centers for Disease Control. The minimum titer required by this method is 80, with a technique in which *E chaffeensis* is used as the source of antigen.

Sera should be collected at the time of diagnosis and then 2 to 4 weeks after the onset of illness for serologic analysis.

Human ehrlichiosis must be distinguished from other tick-borne diseases, especially Rocky Mountain spotted fever. The illnesses are similar in that both have manifestations of diffuse vasculitis. Clinically, ehrlichiosis is less likely to be manifest by rash and more likely to have leukopenia or pancytopenia as a laboratory feature. The similarity of ehrlichiosis and Rocky Mountain spotted fever is emphasized by two retrospective serosurveys in which about 10% of the specimens, taken from patients lacking the serologic criteria for the diagnosis of Rocky Mountain spotted fever, fulfilled the criteria for the diagnosis of ehrlichiosis. Other tick-borne illnesses, such as Lyme disease, babesiosis, Colorado tick fever, relapsing fever, and tularemia, should be included in the differential diagnosis.

Simultaneous infection with *E chaffeensis* and *Borrelia burgdorferi* has been described. Whether this represents dual infection or is an instance of antigenic cross-reactivity is not known. In children, Kawasaki disease may present with features mimicking ehrlichiosis; paired sera from a group of children with Kawasaki disease have failed to react with a panel of *Ehrlichia* antigens.

### Treatment

In adults, the drug of choice for ehrlichiosis is tetracycline. Because this antibiotic is not approved for use in children less than 12 years of age, the optimal therapy for children is unclear. Several children have received treatment with chloramphenicol with apparent improvement, but the experience to date is too limited to advocate chloramphenicol as the treatment of choice for pediatric ehrlichiosis. When tetracycline is employed, the suggested dosage is 25 mg/kg/d in four doses. This should be continued for several days after the temperature returns to normal. Doxycycline, 100 mg twice daily, is an alternative regimen for children more than 12 years of age. The dosage of chloramphenicol that has been used is 75 to 80 mg/kg/d for a 6- to 10-day course of therapy. Mild clinical illness is self-limited, and recovery without specific antimicrobial treatment has been described, although fever may be protracted.

## Selected Readings

Brettman CR, Lewin S, Holymein RS, et al. Rickettsialpox: Report of an outbreak and a contemporary review. Medicine (Baltimore) 1981;60:363.

Brown GW, Saunders JP, Singh S, et al. Single dose doxycycline therapy in scrub typhus. Trans R Soc Trop Med Hyg 1978;72:412.

Centers for Disease Control. Current trends. Outbreak of murine typhus—Texas. MMWR 1983;32:131.

Edwards MS, Jones JE, Leass DL, et al. Childhood infection caused by *Ehrlichia canis* or a closely related organism. Pediatr Infect Dis J 1988;7:651.

Feigin RD, Snider RL, Edwards MS. Rickettsial diseases. In: Feigin RD, Cherry JD, eds. Textbook of pediatric infectious diseases, ed 3. Philadelphia: WB Saunders, 1992:1847.

Hunt JG, Field PR, Murphy AM. Immunoglobulin responses to *Coxiella burnetii* (Q fever): Single serum diagnosis of acute infection using an immunofluorescence technique. Infect Immun 1983;39:977.

Linneman CC. Skin biopsy in diagnosis of Rocky Mountain spotted fever. J Pediatr 1980;96:781.

Liu CT, Hilmas DE, Griffin MJ, et al. Alterations of body fluid compartments and distribution of tissue water and electrolytes in monkeys during Rocky Mountain spotted fever. J Infect Dis 1978;138:42.

Markess JR, Ewing SA, Brumit T, Mettry CR. Ehrlichiosis in children. Pediatrics 1991;87:199.

McDade JE. Ehrlichiosis—a disease of animals and humans. J Infect Dis 1990;161:609.

McDade JE, Shepard CC, Redus MA, et al. Evidence of *Rickettsia prowazekii* infections in the United States. Am J Trop Med Hyg 1980;29:277.

Philip RN, Casper EA, MacCormack JN, et al. A comparison of serologic methods for diagnosis of Rocky Mountain spotted fever. Am J Epidemiol 1976;3:51.

Zinsser H. Rats, lice and history. New York: Blue Ribbon Books, 1943.

*Principles and Practice of Pediatrics, Second Edition.*
edited by Frank A. Oski et al. J. B. Lippincott Company, Philadelphia © 1994.

# CHAPTER 61
# *Fungal Diseases*

## 61.1 *Candidiasis*

### Walter T. Hughes

Candidiasis is the most frequently encountered opportunistic fungal infection of infants and children. The spectrum of the disease extends from benign thrush to life-threatening disseminated (systemic) mycosis.

## ETIOLOGY

Several species of the genus *Candida* may cause infections in humans, but *C albicans* is the usual causative agent. Within recent years, other species have come to prominence as causes of disease, especially in immunocompromised patients. These include *C tropicalis, C pseudotropicalis, C paratropicalis, C krusei, C guilliermondii, C parapsilosis,* and *C stellatoidea.* These yeasts are round to oval vegetative cells that, under conditioned circumstances, produce pseudohyphae. Characteristically, *C albicans* develops chlamydospore formation under stressful, controlled conditions, whereas other species of *Candida* do not exhibit such structures.

## EPIDEMIOLOGY

*Candida* species, which are fairly prevalent in nature, are found predominantly in association with man and other warm-blooded animals. *C albicans* may be isolated from soil, but usually only at sites where human or animal contamination has occurred. One species, *C stellatoidea,* has been isolated only from humans. Within the animal kingdom, *C albicans* has been isolated from a variety of wild and domestic animals.

It is likely that transmission of *Candida* involves direct contact with a colonized site. Oral thrush in neonates results from organisms that are acquired during passage through the birth canal or from colonized nipples of the mother or a nursing bottle. Although *C albicans* has been isolated from the air around patients with cutaneous candidiasis, the extent of airborne transmission has not been established. Colonization with *C albicans* occurs in most infants and children, and is not associated with discernible illness. Receptor sites on epithelial cells of the mucosa permit adherence of the yeast form and the establishment of colonization. Several functions of the immune system actively defend against this organism in the healthy host. Secretory and humoral IgA antibodies are generated, as well as specific anti-*Candida* IgE, IgG, and IgM antibodies. The organism can activate an alternate complement pathway. Neutrophils, monocytes, and eosinophils can ingest and kill the yeast. The organism can induce the formation of suppressor and mitogen-stimulated lymphocytes and produce a lymphokine that will kill it. Lactoferrin has anticandidal activity. Although mucosal surfaces are colonized easily, the normal skin is relatively resistant to colonization and infection with *Candida* species.

Significant disease from *Candida* species is associated almost always with some underlying abnormality in the host. Patients with acquired and congenital immune deficiency disorders, cancer, certain endocrinopathic conditions, diabetes mellitus, burns, trauma, and malnutrition; organ transplant recipients; and individuals receiving immunosuppressive drugs such as corticosteroids are at high risk for infections from *Candida* species. Healthy individuals may be at increased risk for candidiasis of the mucous membranes during infancy, pregnancy, and old age. Disseminated candidiasis has been encountered in 7% of children infected with the human immunodeficiency virus and in 11% of recipients of bone marrow transplants. This invasive form of candidiasis may be found in one third of children with malignant tumors and febrile-neutropenic episodes that are not responsive to antibiotics.

## PATHOLOGY

The initial step in infection is adherence of the yeast form of *Candida* to an epithelial cell surface. The adherent blastospore then develops a filamentous or pseudohyphal form and the organism becomes invasive. In the case of mucous membranes, infection such as thrush develops as an adherent pseudomembrane composed of epithelial cells, leukocytes, keratin, and food debris, as well as both yeast and pseudohyphal forms of *Candida.* Mucosal lesions may progress to well-demarcated ulcers, especially in the intestinal tract, with a base of granulation tissue covered by a fibrinous exudate and granulocytes. Organisms may invade blood vessels, become blood-borne, and disseminate to any organ in the body in immunosuppressed patients. From the mucosal portal of entry, a systemic disease evolves and the kidneys, lungs, liver, brain, and spleen are affected most frequently. In systemic disease, a pyogenic response occurs, with microabscess formation. Granulomatous reactions are infrequent.

## CLINICAL MANIFESTATIONS

The clinical features of candidiasis may be considered in three categories: those associated with mucous membranes, those associated with the skin, and those in which systemic invasion has occurred.

### Mucous Membrane Candidiasis

Oral pharyngeal candidiasis usually is readily recognizable as patches of pearly white pseudomembranes on the mucosal surface that resemble curds of milk. Removal of the pseudomembrane leaves a denuded erythematous lesion. The buccal mucosa, dorsum of the tongue, lateral areas of the tongue, gingiva, and pharynx are involved most frequently. *C albicans* is the species that usually causes thrush.

With esophageal candidiasis, dysphagia and retrosternal pain may be presenting symptoms, but some lesions remain silent, especially in immunocompromised hosts. The inferior third of the esophagus is involved most commonly. Esophagoscopy or esophagography reveals ulcerations of the mucosa producing a cobblestone pattern.

The clinical manifestations of gastrointestinal candidiasis are not well defined. Any portion of the gastrointestinal tract may be affected in severely immunosuppressed patients. Such lesions may provide a portal of entry for systemic disease.

Vaginal candidiasis causes pruritus and a whitish, watery vaginal discharge. Typical thrush lesions may be visualized on the vaginal mucosa. The mucosal surface of the respiratory tract may be colonized with *Candida* at any site. Candidiasis limited to the larynx and bronchi is rare and is associated more often with pulmonary and systemic disease.

## Cutaneous Candidiasis

The most common form of cutaneous candidiasis is dermatitis in the diaper areas of infants. The groin, perineum, and lower abdominal areas usually are involved. The rash often is a confluent papulovesicular reaction with well-demarcated borders. Other sites frequently involved include the intertriginous areas of the axilla and sites around the umbilicus.

Chronic mucocutaneous candidiasis is an uncommon syndrome that reflects an underlying immunodeficiency or, in some cases, an endocrinopathy. Skin, mucous membranes, and skin appendages are involved. Few patients recover from this infection unless the underlying abnormality is corrected.

## Systemic Candidiasis

Systemic or disseminated candidiasis implies hematogenous dissemination to deep organs of the body from a portal of entry at a mucous membrane or skin site. Any organ may be involved, but the lungs, liver, spleen, kidney, and brain are affected most frequently. This form of candidiasis occurs almost exclusively in severely immunosuppressed patients, such as those with cancer, organ transplant recipients, patients with certain congenital and acquired immune deficiency disorders, those receiving immunosuppressive drugs for a variety of reasons, and debilitated, premature infants. Therefore, the clinical manifestations depend on the organs and tissues involved. Suspicion should be aroused in any immunosuppressed patient who has fever of unknown origin. Certain low–birth-weight infants without fever may exhibit nonspecific signs and symptoms such as respiratory abnormalities, hypotensive episodes, endophthalmitis, meningitis, and an erythematous and nodular rash. A chronic disseminated form of candidiasis, with prominent lesions in the liver and spleen, has been reported more frequently in recent years in children with malignant tumors.

## DIAGNOSIS

The lesions of oral thrush are unique and the diagnosis can be made from visual examination in most instances. Infection in mucous membranes and skin, however, can be confirmed by direct examination of materials swabbed or scraped from the surface lesions and by culture of the specimens on the appropriate media. Specimens from surface lesions can be applied to 10% potassium hydroxide or a drop of lactophenol cotton blue solution on a microscope slide with a coverslip and examined for budding yeast forms and pseudohyphae. The diagnosis of systemic candidiasis is difficult and requires at least the isolation of *Candida* species from otherwise sterile body fluids, such as bone marrow, cerebrospinal fluid, or blood, the demonstration of invasive yeasts or pseudohyphae in biopsy specimens, or both. Computed tomography is useful in demonstrating lesions in the liver, spleen, kidneys, and brain. Such lesions often are sufficiently characteristic that a presumptive diagnosis can be made. The usefulness of methods to detect *Candida* antigenemia has been limited, and no generally accepted serologic method has evolved for the diagnosis of invasive disease.

## TREATMENT

The type and location of candidiasis are important in determining the appropriate approach to treatment.

## Mucous Membrane Candidiasis

Oropharyngeal candidiasis is treated with oral nystatin, 200,000 to 500,000 U every 4 to 6 hours, for 1 week or longer. Clotrimazole troches also are effective. Recently, nystatin troches, 200,000 U per tablet, have become available, although comparative studies in children are lacking. Vaginal candidiasis is treated with clotrimazole or nystatin suppositories. Esophageal, gastric, and intestinal candidiasis can be treated in the same manner as oropharyngeal candidiasis, provided the nystatin suspension is swallowed. Fluconazole, given orally or intravenously, has been effective in oral and esophageal candidiasis and should be considered for use in severe cases and in patients who are not responsive to the nonabsorbable drugs.

## Cutaneous Candidiasis

Cutaneous candidiasis can be treated with topical nystatin, amphotericin B, or clotrimazole preparations. Chronic mucocutaneous candidiasis in some cases may be treated effectively with oral ketoconazole.

## Systemic Candidiasis

Candidiasis with deep organ involvement or hematogenous spread is treated with amphotericin B systemically, preferably in combination with flucytosine. The dosage of amphotericin B is 0.5 to 1.0 mg/kg/d as a daily infusion given over 4 to 6 hours. Before this dose is initiated, a test infusion of 0.25 mg/kg/d is given over a period of 6 hours to assess the extent of possible adverse reactions to the preparation. Flucytosine is given orally at a dosage of 150 mg/kg/d in four divided doses. Both compounds should be administered over a period of 4 to 6 weeks, or even longer in some cases. Less well established regimens for treatment include intravenous miconazole or oral ketoconazole. It is especially important to monitor patients who are receiving amphotericin B for adverse effects of the drug, which will be reflected in electrolyte imbalance and nephrotoxicity, and to observe patients who are receiving flucytosine for effects on bone marrow suppression. Liposomal amphotericin B preparations are undergoing clinical trials, but have not been approved by the United States Food and Drug Administration. Fluconazole may be used as an alternative to amphotericin B for systemic cases of candidiasis, other than for patients with *C krusei* infections. The drug may be given orally or intravenously at a dosage of 3 to 6 mg/kg/d with the understanding that studies of its use in children are limited.

## Selected Readings

Baley JE, Kliegman RN, Faranoff AA. Disseminated fungal infection in very low birth weight infants: Clinical manifestations and epidemiology. Pediatrics 1984;73:144.

Meunier F. Fluconazole treatment of fungal infections in the immunocompromised host. Semin Oncol 1990;2:71.

Meyer RD. Current role of therapy with amphotericin B. Clinical Infectious Diseases 1992;14(Suppl 1):S154.

*Principles and Practice of Pediatrics, Second Edition.*
edited by Frank A. Oski et al. J. B. Lippincott Company, Philadelphia © 1994.

# 61.2 *The Dermatophytoses*

## Walter T. Hughes

The dermatophytes are fungi that infect only the epidermis and its keratin-rich appendages—hair and nails. Characteristically, the skin lesions are round with a raised serpiginous border, accounting for the ancient assumption that the cause was worms (the Latin term for which is *tinea*). Modern terminology retains this heritage and designates lesions of the scalp as tinea capitis, lesions of the feet as tinea pedis, lesions of the body as tinea corporis, and lesions of the groin as tinea cruris.

## ETIOLOGY

Terminology for the dermatophytes is not simple. The 39 closely related species are classified into three imperfect genera: *Microsporum*, *Trichophyton*, and *Epidermophyton*. The perfect (sexual) state has been established for 21 of the dermatophytes. The two perfect genera are *Nannizzia* and *Arthroderma*. To a great extent, *Nannizzia* corresponds to the *Microsporum* asexual state and *Arthroderma* to the *Trichophyton* genus.

## EPIDEMIOLOGY

The dermatophytes may be classified on the basis of their predominant habitat. Geophilic fungi (eg, *Microsporum gypseum*) are adapted to an existence in soil, zoophilic fungi (eg, *Microsporum canis*) are found predominantly in domestic animals, and anthropophilic fungi (eg, *Trichophyton rubrum*) reside in humans and may be transmitted from person to person by contact or through fomites.

Age is a determinant for some dermatophyte infections. For example, tinea pedis is common in adults but rare in children. On the other hand, tinea capitis is common in children but rarely occurs after puberty.

Keratin is important to the infection, and fungal invasion is found in tissues that are rich in keratin. The cell walls of the fungi are rich in mucopolysaccharides and stain reddish pink with periodic acid–Schiff stain. These elements are found in the cornified layer of the epidermis, hair, or nails. In skin lesions, lymphohistiocytic infiltrates usually are found loosely disposed about vessels, with or without eosinophils. Acanthosis, hyperkeratosis, epidermal spongiosis, and parakeratosis are found variably in relation to the extent and duration of the infection. In circular lesions of the skin, active fungal invasion and growth occurs at the rim of the lesion; the center of the lesion has relatively few organisms. Generally, the size and duration of lesions are determined by the rate of growth of the fungus and the rate of epidermal turnover.

## CLINICAL MANIFESTATIONS

The clinical features of dermatophytoses depend on the topography of the infection.

## Tinea Capitis

Ringworm of the scalp usually is caused by *Microsporum audouinii*, *M canis*, or *Trichophyton tonsurans*. In *M audouinii* infection, the initial lesion is an erythematous papule at the base of the hair shaft. The fungus spores grow around the hair shaft (ectothrix). The lesions increase peripherally as hairs break just above the level of the scalp, leaving areas of alopecia. Pruritus is common. Patches, sometimes grayish, may appear at separate areas and may become confluent.

Infections with *T tonsurans*, *Trichophyton violaceum*, and certain other dermatophytes are characterized by numerous small, round patches where hair shafts have broken off at the level of the follicle, creating a "black dot" appearance. This is the endothrix type of infection, in which hyphae grow only within the hair shaft.

In some cases of tinea capitis, mild folliculitis or kerion may be seen. A severe inflammatory type of infection may be associated with regional adenopathy.

## Tinea Corporis

The lesions of tinea corporis may be found on the trunk, face, and extremities. The most frequent causes are *Trichophyton mentagrophytes*, *T rubrum*, and *M canis*. The typical ringworm lesion is annular, with an erythematous, elevated, scaly, papular, and sometimes vesicular border spreading in a centrifugal manner and clearing in the control portion. Pruritus is common.

## Tinea Cruris (Jock Itch)

Tinea cruris is similar to tinea corporis. The lesions are localized to the groin and often are associated with tight-fitting underclothing. The condition is found predominantly in adolescent boys. *T rubrum*, *Epidermophyton floccosum*, and *T mentagrophytes* account for most of the cases, but *Candida albicans* also may be a causative agent. The erythematous, slightly indurated patch spreads with tiny vesicles at the peripheral border. The lesions are intensely pruritic. The scrotum usually is involved and the skin often is macerated.

## Tinea Pedis (Athlete's Foot)

Tinea pedis occurs most frequently in adolescent boys and the cause is the same as for tinea cruris. Most commonly, the lesions are chronic, intertriginous, and scaly or macerated. Fissuring is evident. The lateral toe webs are involved initially, then the infection progresses to the sole of the foot. Tinea pedis is acquired in locker rooms, shower rooms, swimming pools, and communal baths.

## Tinea Unguium

Nail infections resulting from the dermatophytes are rare in children, probably because of their fast nail growth.

## Dermatophytid Reaction

Some persons have, in addition to a dermatophytosis, a hypersensitivity-type reaction to the fungal antigens. This reaction may be manifested by dermatophytids, eruptions on the fingers, hands, and arms. These lesions usually are symmetric and may be vesicular, maculopapular, or papulovesicular.

## DIAGNOSIS

The definitive diagnosis of dermatophytosis requires identification of the causative fungus by direct microscopic examination of hair or skin scrapings, or by isolation in culture of these specimens. Processing can be approached in the following manner.

## Skin Lesions

Cells are scraped carefully from the surface of the active margin of the lesion with a scalpel blade, then placed in a drop of 10% potassium hydroxide on a microscope slide and covered with a coverslip. The slide is passed through a flame to heat the preparation gently, which then is examined for hyphae.

Scrapings also can be inoculated into Sabouraud's medium containing chloramphenicol and cycloheximide.

## Hair

Lesions should be examined under ultraviolet light emitted at 365 nm (Wood's light) to locate infected hairs. Hairs infected with *Trichophyton* species do not fluoresce, but those infected with *Microsporum* appear bright blue-green. With precision forceps, infected hairs are plucked out for microscopic examination and culture. A few hair shafts are placed on a microscope slide and covered with 10% potassium hydroxide in 51 Parker's ink and a coverslip.

Arthrospores may be found plastered around the hair shaft as a sheath (ectothrix) or in a mosaic pattern within the hair shaft (endothrix).

The hair can be placed onto Sabouraud's slants and incubated at room temperature.

## TREATMENT

### Tinea Capitis

Tinea capitis is treated with microcrystalline griseofulvin, 15 mg/kg/d given orally for 4 to 8 weeks. Isolation is not necessary after treatment is started.

### Tinea Corporis

Tinea corporis can be treated with any of several topical preparations, such as miconazole, haloprogin, clotrimazole, or econazole for 2 to 4 weeks. Severe cases require griseofulvin orally for several weeks.

### Tinea Cruris

The patient with tinea cruris should wear loose clothing with good aeration. The topical preparations listed for tinea corporis can be used for tinea cruris.

### Tinea Pedis

The patient with tinea pedis should wear clean, absorbent socks and keep the feet as dry as possible. Tolnaftate or undecylenic acid powder is applied twice daily. Severe or unresponsive cases may be treated with griseofulvin. Several topical preparations (miconazole, econazole, clotrimazole) are effective in most infections.

Recent studies show fluconazole given orally in doses of 50 mg/d (adult dose) for 2 to 4 weeks to be highly effective in the treatment of tinea pedis, cruris, and capitis. Also, a single weekly dose of 150 mg of fluconazole has been effective in the treatment of these infections, but further studies are needed to assure proper dosage and efficacy for children.

## Selected Readings

Goslen JB, Kobayashi GS. Superficial dermatophytoses. In: Fitzpatrick TB, ed. Dermatology in general medicine. New York: McGraw-Hill Book Co, 1987.

Hernandez AD. An approach to the diagnosis and treatment of dermatophytosis. Int J Dermatol 1980;19:540.

Montero-Gei, F, Perera A. Therapy with fluconazole for tinea corporis, tinea cruris, and tinea pedis. Clinical Infectious Diseases 1992;14(Suppl 1):S77.

*Principles and Practice of Pediatrics, Second Edition.*
edited by Frank A. Oski et al. J. B. Lippincott Company, Philadelphia © 1994.

# 61.3 *Aspergillosis*

## Walter T. Hughes

Aspergillosis may occur in several diverse disease forms. The clinical features depend on whether the infection results in colonization only, in hypersensitivity to the organism, or in invasive mycotic disease. The latter form is found predominantly in the immunosuppressed host.

## ETIOLOGY

It is likely that any of the some 300 *Aspergillus* species may cause disease in man, but the most common are *A fumigatus* and *A flavus*. Other species involved in human infections include *A niger, A oryzae, A glaucus, A nidulans, A restrictus, A sydowi, A terreus, A versicolor, A candidus, A ustus,* and *A amstelodami.*

## EPIDEMIOLOGY

*Aspergillus* is ubiquitous in the environment in most parts of the world. Aspergilli are found in soil, hay, compost piles, decaying vegetation, water, flour, house dust, bedding, food, chemical solutions, medications, surgical dressings, fireproofing material, and potted plants. Exposure to *Aspergillus* is universal.

Allergic aspergillosis has been reported as a common cause of asthma and pulmonary eosinophilia in the United Kingdom. Such cases also are not uncommon in the United States.

Human-to-human transmission and animal-to-human transmission is not known to occur. Host factors for susceptibility are of prime importance in the acquisition of the infection.

Nosocomial aspergillosis has been associated with airborne organisms in the hospital environment of immunosuppressed patients. The high density of organisms associated with ongoing construction and fireproofing materials has been related to outbreaks of pulmonary aspergillosis in hospitalized patients. Furthermore, primary cutaneous aspergillosis may occur at Hickman catheter sites.

## PATHOLOGY

Aspergillosis in the form of hypersensitivity pneumonitis begins with the inhalation of *Aspergillus* conidia (spores), usually in a patient with asthma. The spores develop into hyphal forms as the bronchi become colonized. A local inflammatory reaction develops. Antigens of the hyphae react with IgG and IgA antibodies as the reaction escalates to bronchial wall damage and eosinophilic infiltration. Histologically, the bronchial wall is infiltrated with mononuclear cells and eosinophils. Inspired mucus and exudate may fill the bronchi, along with segments of the fungus. The lung parenchyma may become involved with granulomatous reactions. Vasculitis is uncommon with this type of pulmonary aspergillosis, and the lack of an acute neutrophil response is compatible with a delayed hypersensitivity response.

The pathogenesis of invasive aspergillosis differs considerably from that of allergic aspergillosis. Although pulmonary aspergillosis is found occasionally in presumably otherwise normal individuals, the usual host for any invasive form of aspergillosis is one whose immune system has been compromised. Normally, inhaled *Aspergillus* conidia that reach the paranasal sinuses and lung are ingested and digested by polymorphonuclear leukocytes or alveolar macrophages. If this arm of the defense mechanism is impaired, as it is in patients with chronic granulomatous disease (who have impaired oxidative intracellular killing) and in those with other phagocytic defects or quantitative deficits, the organism may colonize and develop hyphal and invasive forms. With this type of host-parasite relationship, the outcome often is hemorrhagic infarction and necrosis. The pathologic pattern appears to be related to some extent to the severity of immunocompromise. A fibrosing granulomatous reaction or chronic, nonspecific inflammatory response may be found in an otherwise healthy patient. A severely compromised host exhibits massive hyphal invasion of blood vessels and no granulation tissue. In some patients, the infection may localize, with cavity formation—the aspergilloma. The cavity is occupied partially by a ball of *Aspergillus* hyphae. These lesions tend to be found in the upper lobes. Paranasal sinuses infected with this fungus may exhibit a spectrum of tissue responses similar to the pattern described for the lung, or the site may be colonized only, with hypertrophy of the sinus mucosa.

## CLINICAL MANIFESTATIONS

The clinical features of aspergillosis depend on the host response or, in most instances, on deficits in the host response. The lung and paranasal sinuses are the sites involved most frequently, but disseminated infection may affect several body organs. Another determinant is whether the disease is based on hypersensitivity to the organism or on invasion of tissues by the fungus. The clinical types of aspergillosis are described below.

### Allergic Pulmonary Aspergillosis

An asthmatic patient will have wheezing and dyspnea. Acute attacks may be associated with fever. Cough may produce sputum with plugs of mucus and fungus. Eosinophilia may suggest aspergillosis as a cause of the illness.

### Invasive Pulmonary Aspergillosis

#### Aspergillosis

Aspergillosis is characterized clinically by cough, hemoptysis, obstructive airway signs, and abnormalities associated with the underlying disease, such as neutropenia. Erosion of a major blood vessel may result in fatal hemorrhage.

Pulmonary aspergillosis may progress to a disseminated invasive mycosis involving one or more other deep organs.

#### Sinusitis

Sinusitis may be asymptomatic or associated with chronic symptoms. The maxillary sinus is the site most frequently involved.

#### Otomycosis

The growth of *Aspergillus* in the external otic canal usually is benign, and symptoms should not be attributed to its presence unless other causes are excluded.

### Endophthalmitis

Endophthalmitis may follow trauma or surgery to the eye or it may result from systemic infection. Ocular pain, ciliary injection, and uveitis may occur.

### Cutaneous Lesions

Cutaneous lesions have been described at Hickman catheter sites and under surgical dressings as primary infections. The signs are erythema, induration, and cutaneous or subcutaneous necrosis. Also, cutaneous lesions may follow systemic dissemination of infection from other sites.

## Disseminated Aspergillosis

Hematogenous dissemination is common in severely compromised hosts. It usually is seen in association with invasive pulmonary aspergillosis and neutropenia. The brain, gastrointestinal tract, heart, liver, and kidneys are the sites involved most frequently, but any organ, including bone, can be infected.

The signs and symptoms of aspergillosis are related to impaired function of the organ involved. Although all patients usually have fever, specific signs and symptoms can be absent, despite considerable infection of a deep organ.

## DIAGNOSIS

A definitive diagnosis requires the demonstration of typical septate, branching hyphae in tissues and isolation of the organism in culture. *Aspergillus* species are cultured readily on all standard mycologic media, and growth is apparent within a few days.

Although *Aspergillus* is highly prevalent in the environment and may contaminate laboratory media if care is not taken, it is not found frequently as a part of the normal flora of the respiratory tract. The isolation of *Aspergillus* species from the sputum or nasal swab in an immunocompromised patient with pneumonia suggests the diagnosis of aspergillosis. Even in disseminated disease, the organism rarely is isolated from the blood. Aspirates and biopsies from infected sites should be cultured and studied histologically.

Serologic tests for antibody are helpful in cases of allergic bronchopulmonary aspergillosis and may yield detectable titers in some types of invasive disease. Used alone, however, such tests are not diagnostic.

A radioimmunoassay for *A fumigatus* antigen has been developed and offers promise as an aid to the diagnosis of invasive aspergillosis, but this procedure is not in general use. Also, the detection of the galactomannan of *Aspergillus* in serum and urine may be helpful in the diagnosis of invasive aspergillosis.

## TREATMENT

Treatment of the allergic pulmonary disease is drastically different from treatment of the invasive infection.

In allergic bronchopulmonary aspergillosis, clinical improvement and regression of the infiltrate have followed the administration of corticosteroids. Disease remission has been obtained with prednisone given every other day in a dosage of 0.5 mg/ kg. Larger doses of 60 mg/d (total dose) have been associated with limited tissue invasion by the fungus. The appropriate duration of this therapy is not established, and caution should be practiced in its use. It is currently believed that antifungal drugs are not helpful with this form of aspergillosis.

For invasive infection, amphotericin B is the drug of choice, though it is far from ideal. In vitro susceptibility tests for *Aspergillus* are of no value. A test dose of amphotericin B, 0.25 mg/

kg, should be given intravenously over a 6-hour period while the patient is observed for adverse effects such as hypotension and fever. No premedication to mask reactions should be given with this dose. The next dose should be increased to 0.5 mg/kg/d, and the third dose may be increased to 0.75 mg/kg/d. A final dose then is established at 1.0 mg/kg/d as tolerated until treatment is completed. Limited studies suggest that doses as high as 1.5 mg/kg/d may be warranted in some cases. A course of at least 4 to 6 weeks is needed for all cases, and some may require a longer period. The dose and frequency of administration of amphotericin B usually need modification at times during the course of treatment, based primarily on carefully monitored renal, electrolyte (especially potassium), and hematologic functions. Recent studies indicate that infusion of the daily dose over a period of 2 hours is safe.

Surgical resection of well-localized lesions probably is advisable when possible, but firm guidelines regarding surgical intervention are not available.

The results of treatment of invasive aspergillosis in immunosuppressed patients are poor and depend to a great extent on the reconstitution of immune responses, especially with functional neutrophils in adequate number. The role of recombinant colony-stimulating factors, such as granulocyte colony-stimulating factor, has not been established.

Some experimental evidence suggests that the addition of drugs such as rifampin or flucytosine may be useful, but proof is lacking. A triazole drug, itraconazole, shows promise for efficacy in *Aspergillus* infection, but further studies are needed.

### Selected Readings

Allo MD, Miller J, Townsend T, Tan C. Primary cutaneous aspergillosis associated with Hickman intravenous catheters. N Engl J Med 1987;317:1105.

de Repentigny L. Diagnosis of candidiasis, aspergillosis and cryptococcosis. Clinical Infectious Diseases 1992;14(Suppl):S11.

Graybill JR. Future directions of antifungal chemotherapy. Clinical Infectious Diseases 1992;14(Suppl):S170.

Sheretz RJ, Belani A, Kramer BS, et al. Impact of air filtration of nosocomial *Aspergillus* infections. Am J Med 1987;83:709.

Van Cutsem J, Van Gerven F, Van de Ven M-A, et al. Itraconazole, a new triazole that is orally active in aspergillosis. Antimicrob Agents Chemother 1984;26:527.

Young RL, Bennett JE, Vogel CL, et al. Aspergillosis: The spectrum of the disease in 98 patients. Medicine (Baltimore) 1970;49:147.

*Principles and Practice of Pediatrics, Second Edition.*
edited by Frank A. Oski et al. J. B. Lippincott Company, Philadelphia © 1994.

## 61.4 *Coccidioidomycosis*

### Merrill S. Wise

Coccidioidomycosis is an infection caused by the fungus *Coccidioides immitis*. The disease is endemic in the southwestern United States and in certain areas of Central and South America and northern Mexico. The pulmonary infection caused by *C immitis* usually is self-limited, but disseminated and fatal disease may occur. When amphotericin B became available in 1957, the prognosis associated with disseminated disease improved greatly. Current efforts are directed toward the development of less toxic and more effective therapy, improved diagnostic techniques, and disease prevention.

## ETIOLOGY

As with many pathogenic fungi, the life cycle of *C immitis* demonstrates two distinct phases: a saprophytic or vegetative phase, and a parasitic phase. In nature, the organisms grow as a mycelium with branching, septate hyphae; on most laboratory media, similar morphology is present. After about 1 week, the aerial mycelia develop rectangular spores (arthroconidia) separated by empty cells. The hyphae become very fragile and arthroconidia measuring 2 to 8 $\mu m$ in diameter become airborne. When inhaled, these arthroconidia are capable of reaching the alveolar spaces of the lung. On gaining access to the mammalian host, the arthroconidia begin the parasitic phase through spherule (sporangium) formation. Spherules are round, double-walled structures measuring 20 to 100 $\mu m$ in diameter. Through maturation and reproduction, they form endospores that may reach $10^5$ in number. With rupture of the spherule, endospores are spread into surrounding tissues and may repeat the parasitic phase within the host tissues.

Colonies of *C immitis* grown on laboratory media are white to tan, with a brownish undersurface. Colonial morphology may vary considerably among strains, and a number of nonpathologic fungi have similar colonial and microscopic appearances. Despite variation in colonial morphology, only one species of *C immitis* is recognized; antigenic variation among isolates has been reported, however.

## EPIDEMIOLOGY

The endemic areas of coccidioidomycosis include the San Joaquin Valley of California and scattered regions of southern and northern California, Arizona, New Mexico, west Texas, and certain parts of Central and South America. These areas of increased prevalence generally correspond to the lower Sonoran life zone, which is characterized by flora such as creosote bushes, mesquite, and cacti. The climate is semiarid, with hot summers and brief, wet winters; most fungal growth in the soil occurs during the rainy season. Arthroconidia become airborne through windstorms and with soil disruption during farming or construction work. Local outbreaks have been reported in children who were digging in soil containing the organisms. The organism is very dangerous to laboratory personnel, with epidemics occurring as a result of inadvertent opening of a single culture plate. Primary infection is seen most frequently in summer and fall because of the greater likelihood of arthroconidia dispersal in dry weather.

Susceptibility to primary infection is unaffected by age, sex, or racial background. Because of differences in exposure patterns, incidence rates are much higher in rural areas among older male children. In contrast, susceptibility to disseminated disease is much greater among Filipinos and blacks. Coccidioidomycosis occurs in patients with human immunodeficiency virus (HIV) infection, where it most frequently involves the lungs, but extrapulmonary spread also may occur. Person-to-person spread of coccidioidomycosis rarely takes place, because the arthroconidia are not expelled in sufficient numbers, even when cavitary lesions are present. As a result, patients with coccidioidomycosis do not require isolation, regardless of whether they have draining wounds. In patients with draining wounds, however, dressings should be changed frequently to prevent fungal growth and arthroconidia formation.

## PATHOLOGY

Infection with *C immitis* usually occurs via the respiratory tract, although direct cutaneous inoculation may occur with a contaminated object. An intense inflammatory response develops with growth of the organism and, in most patients, infection remains localized within the lungs and hilar nodes. In a small number of patients, extrapulmonary spread by a lymphatic or hematogenous route may take place.

Acute pulmonary coccidioidomycosis is a bronchopneumonic process that can involve any lobe of the lung. The initial response is predominantly a polymorphonuclear leukocyte reaction. Disseminated coccidioidomycosis involves spread of infection within several weeks or months of initial infection, and resembles progressive tuberculosis of childhood. The tissue reaction in disseminated disease is characterized by granulomatous lesions with giant cells and histiocytes, along with caseous necrosis. Calcification is infrequent, whereas fibrous tissue surrounding areas of inflammation is common.

Disseminated coccidioidomycosis has been reported in infants during the first months of life; almost all these cases occurred after heavy exposure to dust. Disseminated disease may occur during pregnancy, including occasional invasion of the placenta; in most cases, however, infants are born free of infection.

## CLINICAL MANIFESTATIONS

### Primary Coccidioidomycosis

The clinical features of primary infection in children are similar to those observed in adults. Infection is subclinical in 60% of the cases. In the remaining 40%, the severity ranges from a minor flu-like illness of short duration to a severe respiratory illness with lobar pneumonia, pleural effusion, and, occasionally, pericarditis. The incubation period usually is 10 to 16 days, but it may vary from less than a week to almost 4 weeks. Initial symptoms may include fever, nonproductive cough, chest pain, myalgia, headache, and anorexia. Chest pain commonly is pleuritic and occasionally is severe. Hemoptysis occurs in 15% of affected adults, but is rare in children.

Two types of transient rashes are seen in acute disease, with skin manifestations occurring in slightly more than half of all symptomatic children. The early rash seen in primary coccidioidomycosis is a diffuse, erythematous, maculopapular eruption that appears on the first or second day. The rash may vary from an evanescent eruption in the groin to extensive lesions over the lower trunk and thighs that resemble the lesions of measles or scarlet fever. Urticarial lesions also are seen in a small number of cases. The most frequent skin manifestation is erythema nodosum (with or without erythema multiforme), which may appear between the third day and third week of the disease. Erythema nodosum correlates with the development of cell-mediated immunity and is associated with a lower incidence of dissemination. The rash is uncommon in blacks and Filipinos, the populations that are at greatest risk for disseminated disease. Lesions are painful and are distributed maximally over the anterior tibial surfaces. They resolve spontaneously within a few days to several weeks. Acute arthritis or arthralgia can occur as an additional hypersensitivity manifestation.

The radiographic findings in primary infection are not specific and may include bronchopneumonic infiltrates, often with associated hilar node enlargement. Cavities, nodules, or calcifications may develop in a minority of patients, but the lesions generally are asymptomatic and require no specific therapy.

Acute primary infection in neonates may occur, but findings are nonspecific. Radiographs may reveal focal consolidation with diffuse nodular densities, and clinical evidence of mild respiratory tract infection may be evident.

Primary cutaneous coccidioidomycosis has been reported in children, although most cases are found in laboratory workers.

The lesion resembles a chancre and is associated with regional lymphadenitis.

### Disseminated Coccidioidomycosis

In individuals who lack the ability to localize primary coccidioidal infection, dissemination becomes apparent within a few weeks to a few months. Spread of the infection is heralded by persistent fever, toxicity, and the development of lesions outside the chest. Dissemination generally is rare, but it seems to occur more often in very young children, blacks, Filipinos, and patients with HIV infection. Invasion of bone results in chronic osteomyelitis, often with associated fistulas to overlying skin. Bones in the fingers and toes, the ribs, and the vertebrae are affected most often. Cutaneous lesions may occur without bone infection and seem to have a predilection for the face. They begin as papules or pustules and progress to ulceration. The meninges are the most serious extrapulmonary site of infection and, particularly in whites, may be the only site of spread. Coccidioidal meningitis resembles tuberculous meningitis and, before the availability of amphotericin B, this form of disseminated disease was uniformly fatal.

## DIAGNOSIS

Primary pulmonary coccidioidomycosis resembles other lower respiratory tract illnesses, including those caused by viruses, bacteria, mycoplasmas, *Mycobacterium tuberculosis*, and other fungi, such as *Histoplasma*. The diagnosis usually is established without difficulty in endemic areas when appropriate laboratory studies are performed. In other areas, the diagnosis may not be considered unless a travel history is obtained.

The hematologic findings in primary infection are nonspecific, but useful. Elevation of the erythrocyte sedimentation rate, leukocytosis, and eosinophilia are common. A specific diagnosis frequently can be made with the use of skin tests, serologic tests, or examinations of sputum, gastric lavage fluids, or exudates, as well as with culture of *C immitis* from body fluids. Final identification requires conversion of the fungus into the spherule phase by animal inoculation or special culture techniques. If the characteristic double-walled spherules with endospores and no budding are seen on histologic examination, the diagnosis also is certain.

Skin testing with coccidioidin, or the newer antigenic preparation spherulin, can be used to elicit delayed hypersensitivity reactions. A positive skin test result indicates past infection, but is not useful in differentiating recent from distant infection unless a negative test result was obtained just before the onset of symptoms. A negative skin test result does not rule out infection and may be seen frequently in patients with disseminated disease. Occasional cross-reactions may occur in patients with histoplasmosis or blastomycosis. The antigenic preparation is applied intradermally and is interpreted as being positive when 5 mm or more of induration is seen after 48 hours. The standard dose of coccidioidin is 1:100, but patients with erythema nodosum are likely to be hypersensitive and should receive a 1:1000 dilution, whereas patients with disseminated infections are much less sensitive and may require a 1:10 dilution. There is no danger of activating or disseminating infection by using the skin test, although systemic as well as local reactions may occur. Spherulin appears to be a more antigenically active preparation and is given as 0.1 mL of a solution containing 2.8 µg.

The initial antibody response to coccidioidal infection is predominantly in the IgM fraction and is responsible for the positive precipitin test result that accompanies primary infection. Antibodies measured by the complement-fixation test are slower to develop and appear to correlate closely with the severity of infection and the likelihood of dissemination. In most laboratories, titers of 1:16 or greater are highly suggestive of disseminated infection. An antibody response generally is not seen in patients with asymptomatic acute infections. Immunodiffusion and countercurrent immunoelectrophoresis are alternative methods for the detection of antibodies and, when properly standardized, provide another means of monitoring the course of the disease.

Cerebrospinal fluid (CSF) changes during early meningitis may include a polymorphonuclear response, but in chronic meningitis, findings similar to those of tuberculous meningitis are evident. These changes include a predominantly mononuclear cell response, a decreased glucose level, and an elevated protein content. Culture results usually are negative, but the diagnosis often can be made using complement-fixation antibody in the CSF. Patients with vertebral osteomyelitis may have low complement fixation (CF) antibody titers in the CSF without other evidence of meningeal involvement.

Direct examination of infected tissue using hematoxylin-eosin–stained sections may be a useful technique for demonstrating spherules as well as the inflammatory process. Methenamine silver stains highlight the spherule wall, whereas the periodic acid–Schiff stain demonstrates spherule contents.

## THERAPY

The treatment of uncomplicated primary coccidioidomycosis consists of bed rest, analgesics, and, rarely, steroids for severe hypersensitivity reactions. Certain children with primary disease may require treatment with antifungal antibiotics: those with continuous fever for more than 1 month, those with detectable mediastinal adenopathy (in contrast to hilar adenopathy), and those receiving immunosuppressive therapy. Most children of Filipino background and young infants or neonates should be treated. All patients with disease that is disseminated outside the thoracic cavity should receive antifungal therapy. A combination of medical and surgical therapy may be required, especially in patients with progressive pulmonary changes such as recurrent bleeding or advanced cavitation with secondary infection. Treatment should be continued until serologic titers return to normal and radiographic improvement is noted.

Amphotericin B, a polyene antibiotic with strong antifungal activity, has been the mainstay of therapy for disseminated coccidioidomycosis. It should be given mixed only with water and dextrose, at concentrations no greater than 0.1 mg/mL. Bolus injections are contraindicated, but most patients tolerate infusions lasting 1 to 2 hours. The toxicity of amphotericin B is well documented and monitoring for adverse effects must be meticulous during therapy. Nephrotoxic effects occur in most patients and include elevations in serum creatinine and blood urea nitrogen levels, hypokalemia, and diminished ability to concentrate urine. Anemia, thrombocytopenia, and agranulocytosis can occur as a result of diminished bone marrow production. Hepatotoxicity, convulsions, and severe hypersensitivity reactions can occur as well. Thrombophlebitis is common, even with careful intravenous (IV) administration. It is customary to begin therapy with a test dose of 0.1 mg/kg, followed by 0.25 mg/kg. The dose is increased by 0.25 mg/kg until a full daily maintenance dosage of 1 mg/kg has been reached. The total dose of amphotericin B given depends on the patient's age and the severity of the illness. Most patients respond to between 15 and 45 mg/kg, although 7.5 mg/kg may be sufficient in those with mild disease.

Amphotericin B does not cross the blood–brain barrier in quantities sufficient to treat meningitis. Administration into the lumbar area, the cisterna magna, or intraventricular injection through an Ommaya reservoir device is necessary. Intrathecal administration into the cisterna magna is preferable because of the high incidence of arachnoiditis with lumbar injection. The usual starting dose is 0.025 mg, which then is doubled until a maintenance dose of 0.1 to 0.5 mg is reached. After the maintenance dose is achieved, treatment is given every other day, alternating with IV administration. Intrathecal therapy usually exceeds IV therapy and may extend for several years. Therapy commonly is continued until the cellular and chemical characteristics of the lumbar CSF have been normal and the culture results have been negative for at least 1 year. The CSF should be examined at intervals of 1 to 3 months for a period of at least 2 years. With lumbar administration, the patient's head must be tilted down at 30° below the horizontal to minimize the risk of arachnoiditis.

Ketoconazole is an imidazole agent with fungistatic activity that can be administered orally. Studies in adults with disseminated non-meningeal infections suggest that ketoconazole is an effective form of treatment. Patients with chronic pulmonary disease or meningitis have not shown a consistent response after treatment with oral ketoconazole. No clear guidelines have been established with regard to choosing between amphotericin B and ketoconazole in children. Toxicity from ketoconazole appears to be less serious than that of amphotericin B, but hepatotoxicity, abdominal pain, vomiting, and rashes are seen. Decreased adrenal steroidogenesis, blockage of testosterone synthesis, gynecomastia, and reduced spermatogenesis have been reported in patients receiving ketoconazole.

Miconazole, and the newer agents itraconazole and fluconazole, may offer certain advantages to selected patients who fail to respond to or cannot tolerate standard therapy with amphotericin B, but clinical experience with children is limited. The frequency of disseminated fungal disease in patients with HIV infection has led to renewed interest in evaluating antifungal therapy.

## PREVENTION

A killed vaccine prepared from spherules has been efficacious in preventing coccidioidomycosis in experimental animals, but weak and irregular immunity occurred during trials conducted with adult humans. Efforts at prevention through dust control and eradication of the organisms from the soil are impractical, especially in rural areas. Children with negative skin test results should be advised not to engage in field activities or excursions into areas that are highly endemic for coccidioidomycosis.

## Selected Readings

Fish DG, Ampel NM, et al. Coccidioidomycosis during human immunodeficiency virus infection: A review of 77 patients. Medicine (Baltimore) 1990;69:384.

Grant SM, Clissold SP. Itraconazole: A review of its pharmacodynamic and pharmacokinetic properties, and therapeutic use in superficial and systemic mycoses. Drugs 1989;37:310.

Harrison HR, Phil D, et al. Amphotericin B and imidazole therapy for coccidioidal meningitis in children. Pediatr Infect Dis 1983;2:216.

Huntington RW. Coccidioidomycosis. In: Baker RD, ed. Human infection with fungi, actinomycetes, and algae. New York: Springer-Verlag, 1971.

Kafka JA, Catanzaro AT. Disseminated coccidioidomycosis in children. J Pediatr 1981;98:355.

Libke RD, Granoff DM. Coccidioidomycosis. In: Feigin RD, Cherry JD, eds. Textbook of pediatric infectious diseases, ed 2. Philadelphia: WB Saunders, 1987:1949.

Richardson HB, Anderson JA, McKay BM. Acute pulmonary coccidioidomycosis in children. J Pediatr 1967;70:376.

Rippon JW. Medical mycology. Philadelphia: WB Saunders, 1974.

Shaunak S, Cohen J. Clinical management of fungal infection in patients with AIDS. J Antimicrob Chemother 1991;28(Suppl A):67.

Shehab ZM, Britton H, Dunn JH. Imidazole therapy of coccidioidal meningitis in children. Pediatr Infect Dis J 1988;7:40.

Winn WA. The treatment of coccidioidal meningitis: The use of amphotericin B in a group of 25 patients. California Medicine 1964;101:78.

*Principles and Practice of Pediatrics, Second Edition.*
edited by Frank A. Oski et al. J. B. Lippincott Company, Philadelphia © 1994.

# 61.5 *Cryptococcosis*

## M. Melisse Sloas and Christian C. Patrick

Cryptococcosis is a mycosis that occurs in a sporadic fashion. The lung is the portal of entry, and pneumonia is the second most common resulting disease. The most frequent and serious infection caused by cryptococcus is meningitis. Nineteen species of *Cryptococcus* are known; in virtually all human disease, the causative agent is *Cryptococcus neoformans*.

The organism was identified first in 1894, and its relationship to human central nervous system manifestations was described in the early 1900s.

## MICROBIOLOGY

*C neoformans* is a yeast with a spherical shape and a diameter of 5 to 10 μm. Both single and multiple budding may occur (Fig 61-1). The organism is surrounded by a mucopolysaccharide capsule that can be greater than two times the width of the cell; however, the size of the capsule does not correlate with the virulence of the organism.

## EPIDEMIOLOGY

*Cryptococcus* is found worldwide. It resides in soil and is found in high prevalence in avian excreta, especially that of pigeons. Pigeon excreta apparently acts as a reservoir for the organisms, although birds do not appear to acquire the disease.

No evidence supports person-to-person transmission of *Cryptococcus*. *C neoformans* is not considered to be normal flora, but is acquired by inhalation of infected excreta or soil.

In the immunocompetent host, cryptococcosis is primarily a disease of adults more than 30 years of age and it is 2 to 3 times

more prevalent in males. Immunosuppressed individuals with the acquired immunodeficiency syndrome (AIDS), leukemia, lymphoma, sarcoidosis, cirrhosis, or diabetes mellitus; those receiving corticosteroid therapy; or those who have undergone organ transplantation are at increased risk for acquiring the infection. Cryptococcosis develops in as many as 10% of adult patients with AIDS, and this infection often is the AIDS-defining illness. Cryptococcosis is much less common in children with AIDS, however, and was seen in only 4 of the first 307 pediatric cases of AIDS.

## PATHOGENESIS

The major portal of *Cryptococcus* entry appears to be the lung. Lung lesions usually are focal and produce no overt symptomatology in immunocompetent individuals. In immunocompromised patients, dissemination may occur from primary sites in the lungs to other areas of the lungs or to other organ systems. The most frequent site of dissemination is the meninges, where a chronic basilar meningitis occurs. Meningitis develops with a paucity of inflammation. Additionally, small areas of cryptococci can be seeded throughout the brain (cryptococcomas).

The major virulence factor is the mucopolysaccharide capsule. The capsule is inhibitory to phagocytosis and acts as an immunosuppressive factor by means that are unclear.

The major host defense mechanism is cell-mediated immunity. The cell-mediated immunity response involves granuloma formation, with multinucleated giant cells, but with rare necrosis, calcification, or caseation.

The role of humoral immunity is not clear, but most studies provide evidence that antibody does not promote ingestion by phagocytes. A better clinical prognosis is associated with the presence of anticapsular antibody, however. The complement pathway does appear to enhance phagocytosis.

## CLINICAL MANIFESTATIONS

Cryptococcal meningitis causes headache, nausea, vomiting, fever, changes in mental status, and meningeal signs in more than 50% of patients. Cranial nerve involvement with diplopia and

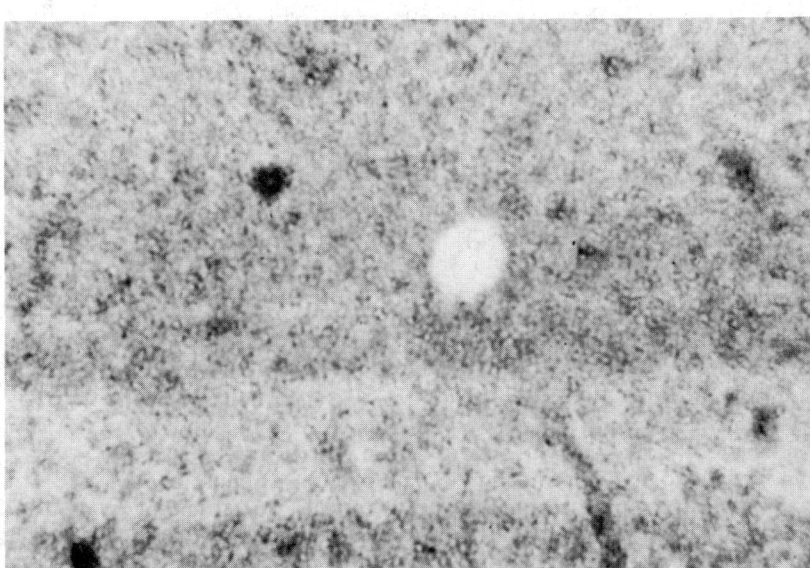

**Figure 61-1.**  India ink preparation of cerebrospinal fluid showing budding yeast with prominent capsule.

blurred vision occur in about one third of all patients with signs of ophthalmoplegia and papilledema. Seizures develop in 15% of patients, and the complete absence of symptoms has been reported in 10% of all affected individuals. Cryptococcal infection in patients with AIDS is even more likely to occur without signs of meningeal irritation; the most common presenting symptoms in this population are fever and headache.

The differential diagnosis of cryptococcal meningitis includes other causes of chronic or basilar meningitis: other fungal agents, brucellosis, syphilis, tuberculosis, and lymphomas or carcinomas (primary or metastatic). Additional noninfectious causes such as sarcoidosis and chronic benign lymphocytic meningitis also must be considered.

Pulmonary cryptococcosis often is asymptomatic in an immunocompetent host and is discovered serendipitously on a chest roentgenogram. Solitary nodules, focal infiltrates, and hilar or mediastinal adenopathy are the most common chest roentgenographic findings in patients with symptomatic pulmonary cryptococcosis. Weight loss, night sweats, chest pain, and a productive cough with or without hemoptysis can occur; in patients with AIDS, fever and cough may be the only symptoms.

Disseminated cryptococcal infection may be seen in immunocompromised patients, especially those coinfected with the human immunodeficiency virus. The central nervous system still is the most frequent site of infection, but the disease is more likely to be accompanied by cryptococcemia, cryptococcal pneumonia, or cryptococcal urinary tract infection. Cryptococcosis may involve almost any organ, including the eyes, heart, gastrointestinal tract, bones, skin, and prostate (which provides a sequestered reservoir for the organism during treatment).

## DIAGNOSIS

The definitive diagnosis of cryptococcal meningitis is made by isolating the organism from the cerebrospinal fluid (CSF). Isolation can be achieved in 75% to 90% of all patients with the disease. Because few organisms may be present, large quantities of CSF should be cultured. India ink preparations to visualize capsule formation surrounding budding yeast yield positive results in 60% of patients (see Fig 61-1). Cryptococci can be isolated from urine and blood in about one third of patients without AIDS and in an even higher percentage of those with AIDS. A number of serologic assays have been used, but latex agglutination (LA) is the method of choice. LA test results in the CSF are positive in more than 90% of the cases and in 50% of the patients. The LA test may reveal extremely high antigen levels in the CSF of patients with AIDS; the titer may fall very slowly or persist in spite of adequate therapy. LA testing also should be done on the serum to detect extraneural disease.

Manometric measurements made during lumbar puncture demonstrate an increased opening pressure in 65% of patients with cryptococcal meningitis. In patients without AIDS, the CSF protein level is increased in 90% and the CSF glucose level is decreased in 75%. The CSF white blood cell count usually is less than 150 cells per cubic millimeter, with a predominance of lymphocytes. In patients with AIDS, CSF findings often are normal or changed only minimally. Any patient with *Cryptococcus* isolated from a site outside the central nervous system should undergo a lumbar puncture, because central nervous system disease may be totally asymptomatic.

The results of as many as 50% of computed tomography scans and magnetic resonance imaging examinations are abnormal in patients with cryptococcal meningitis. Both tests can be helpful in diagnosis or treatment; findings such as hydrocephalus, edema, abscess, and nodular densities, however, are nonspecific.

Pulmonary cryptococcosis is diagnosed by histologic studies, culture of biopsy material, or examination and culture of fluid obtained by bronchial alveolar lavage.

## TREATMENT

Cryptococcal meningitis is invariably fatal if it is not treated. The introduction of amphotericin B in the 1950s increased the cure rate to greater than 50%, with 10% to 25% of patients having relapses after the completion of therapy. The fatality rate in patients with AIDS is nearly 60% in some studies and as much as 65% if these patients experience relapse after treatment. Prognostic factors that have been associated with a poor outcome include high antigen titers, extraneural disease, initial low CSF white count, coexisting infections, and severe underlying disease.

5-Fluorocytosine (5-FC) is an oral fungistatic agent that is inadequate therapy for cryptococcal meningitis when it is used alone because of an associated high frequency of failure and relapse. Used in combination with low-dose amphotericin B, however, the cure efficacy of 5-FC equals that of high-dose amphotericin B without the increased toxicity of the latter agent. 5-FC is given orally at a dosage of 150 mg/kg/day divided every 6 hours, in combination with amphotericin B given intravenously at a dosage of 0.3 mg/kg/d. Serum levels of 5-FC must be monitored. Patients with AIDS often are unable to tolerate 5-FC because of bone marrow suppression, especially with leukopenia, renal toxicity, and gastrointestinal side effects. Amphotericin B used alone may be just as effective in this population. If amphotericin is used alone, a test dose of the drug should be given intravenously at 0.1 mg/kg, with doses increasing to a maximum of 0.5 to 0.6 mg/kg/d. Fluconazole and itraconazole have been used successfully for primary therapy and in patients in whom amphotericin B is not effective.

For the seriously ill, the addition of intraventricular therapy with amphotericin B has been advocated by some authorities.

The duration of therapy for patients with cryptococcal meningitis is a minimum of 4 weeks; patients with neurologic complications, underlying disease, or immunosuppression require at least 6 weeks of treatment. Patients should be examined carefully after treatment, with CSF, blood, and urine cultures performed to document microbiologic cure. Serology also should be used to monitor therapy by decreasing titers. Maintenance therapy is recommended for patients with AIDS because of their high rate of relapse; both amphotericin B and fluconazole can be used for preventive treatment.

Pulmonary *Cryptococcus* infection discovered in an asymptomatic, immunocompetent individual usually is self-limited and requires no therapy. Cryptococcal pneumonia in an immunocompromised host requires amphotericin B, with possible surgical excision of isolated pulmonary lesions. The patient must be receiving amphotericin B before a surgical procedure is undertaken.

## Selected Readings

Bennett JE, Dismukes WE, Duma RJ, et al. A comparison of amphotericin B alone and combined with flucytosine in the treatment of cryptococcal meningitis. N Engl J Med 1979;301:126.

Chuck SL, Sande MA. Infections with *Cryptococcus neoformans* in the acquired immunodeficiency syndrome. N Engl J Med 1989;321:794.

Dismukes WE, Cloud G, Gallis HA, et al. Treatment of cryptococcal meningitis with combination amphotericin B and flucytosine for four as compared with six weeks. N Engl J Med 1987;317:334.

Larsen RA, Leal MAE, Chan LS. Fluconazole compared with amphotericin B plus fluconazole for cryptococcal meningitis in AIDS. A randomized trial. Ann Intern Med 1990;113:183.

Lewis JL, Rabinovich S. The wide spectrum of cryptococcal infections. Am J Med 1972;53:315.

Stockman L, Roberts GD. Specificity of the latex test for cryptococcal antigen: A rapid simple method for eliminating interference factors. J Clin Microbiol 1982;16:965.

Wittner M: Cryptococcosis. In: Feigin RD, Cherry JD, eds. Textbook of pediatric infectious diseases, 2nd ed. Philadelphia: WB Saunders, 1987:1968.

Principles and Practice of Pediatrics, Second Edition.
edited by Frank A. Oski et al. J. B. Lippincott Company, Philadelphia © 1994.

# 61.6 *Histoplasmosis*

## Merrill S. Wise

Histoplasmosis is a common granulomatous infection caused by the dimorphic fungus *Histoplasma capsulatum*. It simulates the varied pathologic picture of tuberculosis. At present, 40 million individuals are estimated to have been infected with this organism at the rate of 500,000 per year. The clinical spectrum of disease ranges from asymptomatic in 50% of the cases to generalized fatal dissemination in less than 1% of the cases. Histoplasmosis occurs worldwide, but is most common in the Ohio, Mississippi, and Missouri River valleys in the United States. The highest density of individuals with positive skin reactions to the fungal antigen is found in Tennessee, Kentucky, Arkansas, and Missouri, with about 90% of the young adults in these states having positive skin test results. Soil contaminated by animal droppings, particularly the excreta of birds and bats, plays a major role in the dissemination of *H capsulatum*. The organism has been isolated from soil near chicken houses, bird roosts, caves infested with bats, and silos inhabited by pigeons. Active disturbance of the environment is necessary for dissemination of the infectious particles or spores. The intensity of inhalation exposure to the airborne particles is one determinant of whether infection will occur, and how serious it will be. Person-to-person transmission of disease is not known to occur.

## ETIOLOGY

The mycelial or saprophytic form of *H capsulatum* has been isolated from soil throughout the world. It grows on Sabouraud's medium at 25 °C with white or tan fluffy colonies. Yeast forms are grown on enriched agar (cysteine glucose) at 37 °C and consist of small, oval, budding yeasts with a diameter of 2 to 4 $\mu$m. The stain of choice for histopathologic sections is Gomori's methenamine silver stain.

## PATHOLOGY

Histoplasmosis usually occurs after the inhalation of microconidia, which reach the alveoli and transform into small budding yeasts. Rarely, the fungus may gain entry through the mucous membranes or the gastrointestinal tract. Within lung parenchyma, the organisms are phagocytosed by macrophages. These prime foci may spread to local lymph nodes and calcify, and they also may disseminate to the spleen, liver, and numerous other organs throughout the body. Within the lung, calcification of a primary focus and adjacent lymph nodes may resemble the Ghon complex of primary pulmonary tuberculosis.

## CLINICAL MANIFESTATIONS

Acute pulmonary histoplasmosis is the most common form of disease. Asymptomatic primary infection occurs in about 50% of adults and children exposed to *H capsulatum* spores, with a positive histoplasmin skin test result being the only manifestation of infection. The incubation period is 7 to 21 days, and the severity of symptoms corresponds to the concentration of inhaled microconidia. Symptomatic disease presents as an influenza-like illness with abrupt onset of fever, malaise, headache, myalgia, and nonproductive cough. Pleural pain and small pleural effusions have been described in a few cases. Results of the physical examination often are normal, although diffuse rales and mild hepatosplenomegaly may be evident. Chest radiographs reveal patchy pneumonic infiltrates and hilar adenopathy. The duration of illness is variable, but most symptoms resolve within 3 to 10 days. In a small number of patients, the illness persists for weeks to months; rarely, the clinical picture of disseminated histoplasmosis may develop. For the great majority of patients, histoplasmosis is a benign, self-limited disease that does not require specific therapy.

In heavily endemic areas, reinfection caused by light or heavy exposure is common. This results in the return of skin test reactivity in patients with asymptomatic infection or a mild influenzal illness in those with symptomatic infection. Chest radiographs frequently reveal uniformly distributed miliary nodules that are indistinguishable from miliary tuberculosis. Symptoms of reinfection usually are less severe and of shorter duration than are those of primary infection.

Epidemic histoplasmosis has been reported after massive exposure to dust or soil that is contaminated heavily with spores of *H capsulatum*. Symptoms appear abruptly within 3 to 20 days and may last for several weeks. The prognosis is excellent, and spontaneous resolution of all signs and symptoms occurs within weeks. On rare occasions, epidemic illness has led to disseminated disease in infants and children.

Two forms of progressive histoplasmosis occur in a small proportion of infected patients. Disseminated histoplasmosis develops in infants, debilitated adults, and patients with defects in cell-mediated immunity. The clinical picture is that of severe systemic infection with widespread involvement of the reticuloendothelial system. The organism may be obtained from cultures of blood, bone marrow, and urine. Dissemination to every organ in the body has been reported, and organisms have been isolated from the central nervous system, gastrointestinal tract, and heart valves. Destruction of the adrenal glands is frequent. The illness begins abruptly with fever, cough, and malaise, but quickly progresses to involve multiple organ systems. Physical examination reveals generalized rales, diffuse lymphadenopathy, and hepatosplenomegaly. The clinical course in untreated patients is progressively downhill, with the frequent occurrence of respiratory failure, disseminated intravascular coagulopathy, and bacterial sepsis. When treatment with amphotericin B is initiated early, the prognosis is good. Most untreated cases are fatal. A significant percentage of patients with this form of disease have facial lesions, usually ulcers of the oropharynx or skin nodules. The finding of facial lesions almost always implies disseminated disease, and treatment should be initiated before the disease progresses further.

Chronic pulmonary histoplasmosis is a disease of middle-aged, white, male smokers with a history of obstructive pulmonary disease; it has not been described in children. Histoplasmoma and mediastinal collagenosis are rare in children and represent an exaggerated immune response to infection. The histoplasmoma is an enlarging, solitary pulmonary nodule with concentrated layers of fibrous tissue and calcium surrounding a healed primary focus. These nodules may reach 3 to 4 cm in diameter and must be differentiated from neoplasms. Mediastinal collagenosis results from fibrocalcification of a mediastinal node with extension through the mediastinum. With time, entrapment and obstruction of mediastinal structures can occur.

Progressive disseminated histoplasmosis is a common opportunistic infection that may represent the acquired immunodeficiency syndrome (AIDS)–defining illness in patients who are infected with the human immunodeficiency virus (HIV). The disease may present as a febrile illness in which the pulmonary component is overshadowed by the severity of the systemic illness, and timely diagnosis requires a high index of suspicion. Treatment that may be effective in immunocompetent individuals seldom is curative in patients with AIDS, and the goals are to suppress rather than to cure the infection in many cases. The growing problem of systemic mycosis in HIV-infected patients has stimulated trials of new antifungal agents such as itraconazole and ketoconazole.

## DIAGNOSIS

The definitive diagnosis of histoplasmosis is made by the isolation and identification of *H capsulatum* in infected secretions or tissues. The most valuable specimen for diagnosing pulmonary histoplasmosis is sputum, usually the first morning collection. Bone marrow, liver, urine, or blood culture results may be positive in infections involving those organs or in disseminated disease. The skin test using histoplasmin is almost useless in diagnosing acute histoplasmosis. Because a high rate of positivity exists in endemic areas, a positive skin test result does not indicate active disease. In addition, the skin test itself can boost antibody titers, making the interpretation of serologic tests difficult. Attempts to see organisms in infected tissue through histologic methods are exceedingly difficult and the results almost always are negative in acute histoplasmosis. Serologic techniques for the diagnosis of histoplasmosis frequently are useful. Seroconversion on the complement-fixation assay or the immunodiffusion test indicates a high likelihood of active disease. An initial titer of 1:16 by complement fixation suggests active disease, but cross-reactivity with the serologic test for blastomycosis is common. An immunoperoxidase technique for the rapid diagnosis of histoplasmosis recently was described. This method allows routinely processed cytologic smears, frozen sections, and paraffin-embedded tissue to be stained to enable *H capsulatum* organisms to be distinguished accurately from other morphologically similar fungi. Radioimmunoassay techniques also have been developed for the rapid detection of *H capsulatum* antigen in urine and serum. The latter two techniques offer obvious advantages in that rapid diagnosis can be made without prolonged delays related to slow growth of the organism in culture.

## TREATMENT

In essentially all cases of histoplasmosis, when the patient does not have overwhelming disease or the inoculum is not large, the disease resolves without therapy. If symptoms persist for more than 3 weeks or if the chest radiograph shows progression of the disease, treatment is indicated. Amphotericin B is the treatment of choice for all life-threatening infections caused by *H capsulatum*. Recent studies, however, demonstrate the effectiveness of ketoconazole in the treatment of immunocompetent hosts with histoplasmosis. The use of ketoconazole in children and adolescents has been clouded somewhat by recent evidence that this drug decreases synthesis of the adrenal and sex hormones. Disseminated disease, particularly in immunocompromised hosts, requires therapy with a total dose of 35 mg/kg of amphotericin B. Shorter courses have been given with good results, especially in infants and young children (less than 2 years of age). Recovery is rapid in most cases; relapses may occur, and repeated cultures should be performed to monitor the success or failure of chemotherapy. In the rare case of cerebral involvement, intrathecal amphotericin B has been recommended.

## Selected Readings

Bennett JE. Chemotherapy of systemic mycoses. N Engl J Med 1974;290:30.
Diamond RD. The growing problem of mycoses in patients infected with the human immunodeficiency virus. Rev Infect Dis 1991;13:480.
Dismukes WE, Stamm AM, Graybill JR, et al. Treatment of systemic mycoses with ketoconazole: Emphasis on toxicity and clinical response in 52 patients. Ann Intern Med 1983;98:13.
Goodwin RA, DesPrez RM. Histoplasmosis. Am Rev Respir Dis 1978;117:929.
Holland FJ, Fishman L, Bailey JD, et al. Ketoconazole in the management of precocious puberty not responsive to LHRH-analogue therapy. N Engl J Med 1985;312:1023.
Klatt EC, Cosgrove M, Meyer PR. Rapid diagnosis of disseminated histoplasmosis in tissues. Arch Pathol Lab Med 1986;110:1173.
Mandell W, Goldberg DM, Neu HC. Histoplasmosis in patients with the acquired immune deficiency syndrome. Am J Med 1981;81:974.
Medoff G, Kobayashi GS. Histoplasmosis. In: Feigin RD, Cherry JD, eds. Textbook of pediatric infectious diseases, ed 2. Philadelphia: WB Saunders, 1987:1974.
Sarosi GA, Johnson PC. Disseminated histoplasmosis in patients infected with human immunodeficiency virus. Clinical Infectious Diseases 1992; 14(Suppl 1):S60.
Weinberg GA, Kleiman MB, Grosfeld JL, et al. Unusual manifestations of histoplasmosis in childhood. Pediatrics 1983;72:99.
Wheat LJ, Kohler RB, Tewari RP. Diagnosis of disseminated histoplasmosis by detection of *Histoplasma capsulatum* antigen in serum and urine specimens. N Engl J Med 1986;314:83.

*Principles and Practice of Pediatrics, Second Edition.*
edited by Frank A. Oski et al. J. B. Lippincott Company, Philadelphia © 1994.

# 61.7 *Sporotrichosis*

Merrill S. Wise and Ralph D. Feigin

Sporotrichosis is a subacute or chronic fungus infection that can involve both superficial and deep tissues. The causative agent is the dimorphic fungus, *Sporothrix schenckii*. Sporotrichosis is worldwide in occurrence, but is found primarily in warm temperate zones. Most cases in the United States have been from the states that border the Mississippi and Missouri Rivers. It is the most common subcutaneous and deep mycosis diagnosed in Mexico as well. With few exceptions, the fungus gains entry into the body through trauma to the skin, causing the lymphocutaneous form of the disease. Most cases of sporotrichosis occur in adults after intradermal inoculation of spores resulting from contact with contaminated thorns, splinters, reeds, or grasses. Floral nursery and tree farm personnel are at highest risk, although epidemic forms have been reported in adults and children. Disseminated sporotrichosis has been reported in patients with human immunodeficiency virus infection, where it usually is associated with diffuse cutaneous lesions and polyarticular arthritis. The pulmonary and extracutaneous forms probably are caused by inhalation of the 2- to 3-$\mu$m spores, causing primary pneumonia. Secondary spread to joints, bone, muscle, and other organs is rare, but may occur in the immunosuppressed host.

## ETIOLOGY

*S schenckii* is a dimorphic fungus that may exist in a mycelial form in culture at 25 °C. The invasive, yeast-like form is grown easily on brain–heart infusion agar at 37 °C and has an oval to cigar-shaped budding appearance. The histologic picture in sporotrichosis is that of an acute inflammatory reaction or microabscesses with necrotic centers. Demonstration of fungi in tissue section is very difficult, and cultures of pus and biopsy material should be performed.

## CLINICAL MANIFESTATIONS

Lymphocutaneous sporotrichosis accounts for more than 75% of all cases reported in the literature. The first sign of infection may appear as soon as 5 days or as late as 6 months after traumatic inoculation; the average incubation time is 3 weeks. The first sign of disease is the appearance of a small, painless, movable subcutaneous nodule. This nodule enlarges to become a fluctuant mass with progression to ulceration. Similar painless subcutaneous nodules appear along the lymphatic channels. The clinical picture of an ulcer on the finger or wrist with an associated chain of nodules along draining lymphatics is pathognomonic of sporotrichosis. These lesions may persist for years if they are not treated. Infection of joints or bone may occur, probably by dissemination via the bloodstream from a cutaneous focus or, less commonly, from a pulmonary source. Bone lesions often are multiple, lytic, and destructive. The tibia is involved most commonly. In sporotrichosis of the joint, thickened synovium with cartilage degeneration is seen. The knee is affected most commonly, with joint swelling, inflammation, and occasional sinus tracts. Extracutaneous sporotrichosis is rare in children, but involvement of the liver, spleen, pancreas, thyroid, myocardium, and central nervous system has been reported.

## DIAGNOSIS

Definitive diagnosis of sporotrichosis requires isolation of *S schenckii* from infected tissue. The sporotrichosis skin test entails the intradermal injection of a diluted culture filtrate of the organism. A 5-mm area of induration constitutes a positive test result and is useful for determining exposure to the fungus, but it is not diagnostic of active disease. The agglutination and immunodiffusion tests are the most specific and reliable aids to diagnosis by serologic tests.

## TREATMENT

Oral potassium iodide is the treatment of choice for cutaneous sporotrichosis. Treatment schedules vary, but all involve the use of rapidly increasing doses until 30 to 40 drops are given three times per day, usually until 4 weeks after symptoms have resolved. Amphotericin B is the most effective drug for pulmonary and disseminated sporotrichosis. With septic arthritis, surgical debridement frequently is necessary. Recent reports suggest that treatment of the lymphocutaneous form with itraconazole or terbinafine may be an acceptable alternative to iodide treatment.

## Selected Readings

Blumer SO, Kaufman L, Kaplan D, et al. Comparative evaluation of the five serologic methods for the diagnosis of sporotrichosis. Appl Microbiol 1973;26:4.

Dahl BA, Silberfarb PM, Sarosi GA, et al. Sporotrichosis in children. JAMA 1971;215:1980.

Heller HM, Fuhrer J. Disseminated sporotrichosis in patients with AIDS: Case report and review of the literature. AIDS 1991;5:1243.

Hull PR, Vismer HF. Treatment of cutaneous sporotrichosis with terbinafine. Br J Dermatol 1992;126(Suppl 39):51.

Lavalle P, Suchil P, DeOrando F, Reynoso S. Itraconazole for deep mycoses: Preliminary experience in Mexico. Infectious Diseases 1987;9:64.

Orr ER, Riley HD. Sporotrichosis in childhood: Report of ten cases. J Pediatr 1971;78:951.

Restrepo A, Robledo J, Gomez I, et al. Itraconazole therapy in lymphangitic and cutaneous sporotrichosis. Arch Dermatol 1986;122:413.

*Principles and Practice of Pediatrics, Second Edition.*
edited by Frank A. Oski et al. J. B. Lippincott Company, Philadelphia © 1994.

# 61.8 *Miscellaneous Fungal Infections*

John Willard Rippon

Over the past 80 or so years, numerous reports have implicated soil-borne and airborne fungi as causative agents for a variety of diseases. Most of the true causative agents are slow-growing and difficult to isolate. The soil and air contaminants are rapid colonizers of culture media as well as human lesions resulting from other causes, so the vast majority of such reports are questionable. Rarely, however, an organism not normally encountered as a pathogen may cause disease in particular circumstances. It also should be remembered that strain variation in fungi is great and mutations occur that may impart pathogenic potential to an otherwise harmless organism. Thus, isolates of soil-inhabiting species of *Aspergillus, Acremonium, Alternaria, Fusarium,* and *Penicillium* that normally do not grow at 37 °C have been recovered from sick patients, and these strains were found to be thermotolerant.

Normally, saprophytic fungi may be involved in disease in at least three situations. The first and most important is the ever-increasing list of opportunistic infections. These occur in the setting of immunologic compromise associated with the use of cytotoxins and steroids to treat neoplasia (particularly hematologic neoplasia), prevent organ transplant rejection, and treat certain collagen, vascular, and arthritic diseases. The degree of immunosuppression often dictates which of the fungal opportunists will be involved. The most common agents are *Candida albicans* and *Candida tropicalis*, which seed in from mucosal reservoirs in the patient. The lungs are the entry portal for the common extrinsic opportunists *Aspergillus,* Zygomycetes, and *Cryptococcus neoformans*. In addition to these commonly encountered opportunistic fungi, infections caused by many other fungi have been documented. *Pseudallescheria boydii* is a strong entry in the list of fungal opportunists; reports of its involvement in infection appear monthly. Fifty reports of *Fusarium* species in human infection have been published. The list is so long that two new disease entities have been defined: phaeohyphomycosis and hyalohyphomycosis. The various types of phaeohyphomycosis are caused by the dematiaceous (having melanin pigment in the cell wall) soil fungi. Some 40 such agents have been documented, 90% of them since 1975 (Table 61-1). The microscopic and histologic appearance of one such agent, *Xylohypha bantianum*, is shown in Figure 61-2; the clinical disease is shown in Figures 61-3 and 61-4. The varieties of hyalohyphomycosis are caused by fungi that lack melanin pigment in their cell walls (Table 61-2). Phaeohyphomycosis tends to be more necrotic and erosive, and the causative agents generally do not respond to treatment with amphotericin B. In contrast, in hyalohyphomycosis, thrombotic phenomena with local invasion are common and most organisms have some sensitivity to amphotericin B.

The second circumstance in which soil organisms may gain entrance to protected organ systems is through a barrier break. This is a much less common predisposing factor than is immu-

**TABLE 61-1. Agents Causing Invasive Systemic and Cerebral Phaeohyphomycosis***

| | |
|---|---|
| *Alternaria* | *Peyronellae (Phoma)* |
| *A alternata* | *glomerata* (a) |
| *A chartarum* | |
| *A dianthicola* | *Phialophora* |
| *A infectoria* | *P bubakii* |
| *A stemphyloides* | *P parasitica* |
| *A tenuissina* | *P repens* |
| | *P richard siae* |
| *Alternaria* species (a) | *P verrucosa* (c) |
| *Anthopsis deltoidea* | *Phialomonium ovovatum* (a) |
| *Arnium leporinum* | *Phoma* |
| *Aureobasidium pullulans* (a) | *P cruris-hominis* |
| | *P eupyrena* |
| *Bipolaris* | *P herbarum* (a) |
| *B hawaiiensis* (c) | *P hibernica* |
| *B australiensis* | *P cava* (a) |
| *B spicifera* (a) | |
| | *Phyllosticta (Phyllostictina)* |
| *Chaetoconidium* species | *citacarpa* |
| *Chaetomium* | *Pseudomicrodochium* |
| *C funicolum* | *suttonii* (a) |
| *C globosum* | *Rhamichloridium schulzeri* |
| *Cladosporium* | *Sarcinomyces* |
| *C cladosporoides* | *phaeomuriformis* |
| *C devriesii* | |
| *C elatum* | *Scolecobasidium* |
| *C oxysporum* | *S humicola* (a) |
| *C sphaerospermum* | *S ishawytschae* (a) |
| *C carrionii* | *Scytalidium lignicola* |
| *Curvularia* | *Trichomaris invadens* (a) |
| *C geniculata* | |
| *C lunata* (c) | *Ulocladium chartarum* |
| *C pallescens* (c) | *Wagiella dermatitidis* (a, c) |
| *Dactylaria (Ochroconis)* | *Xylohypha (Cladosporium)* |
| *gallopava* (a, c) | *bantiana* (a, c) |
| *Exophiala jeanselmeii* (a, c) | |
| *E moniliae* (a) | |
| *E pisciphila* (a) | |
| *E salmonis* (a) | |
| *E spinifera* | |
| *Exserohilum* | |
| *E mcginnisii* | |
| *E rostratum* (a) | |
| *E longirostratum* | |
| *Fonsecaea pedrosoi* (a, c) | |
| *Lecythophora (Phialophora)* | |
| *hoffmannii* and *L mutabilis* | |
| (includes *P mutabilis* and *P* | |
| *luteo-virdis*) | |
| *Moniliella suaveolens* (a) | |
| *Mycocentrospora acerina* | |
| *Oidiodendron cerealis* (a, c) | |

* In this form of the disease, tissue invasion may be localized or may disseminate to other organ systems. Patients usually are immunosuppressed. The primary site of infection is the lungs, sinuses, or a trauma site in the skin. In some cases, the organism enters during surgery, resulting in endocarditis, often with dissemination. In other cases, the organism enters as the result of injection of contaminated material (drugs, etc.). In yet other cases, particularly cerebral disease, no predisposing condition is noted. a, animal infections; c, cerebral involvement.

nosuppression, but such cases do occur. Barrier breaks may be introduced by surgery, indwelling catheters, the use of nonsterile material by drug abusers, intrathecal injections, and ambulatory hemodialysis, among others. There are reports of a mushroom growing on a mitral valve after open heart surgery, of *Scopulariopsis* granulomas in the lung after the injection of crude opium, and of *Aspergillus* meningitis after the intrathecal use of contaminated steroids. Often, the same fungi involved in these diseases are found in the opportunistic categories.

Colonization of injured or debilitated tissue is the third category of infection by opportunistic agents. This commonly is the predisposing situation in reports of *Alternaria* invading the nose after a submucous resection, *Fusarium* colonizing burned skin, Zygomycetes infecting the injured foot of a diabetic, and *Pseudallescheria* infecting the knee after a soccer injury or auto accident. Most patients are not immunosuppressed.

These three categories—opportunism, barrier break, and colonization of debilitated tissue—account for the vast majority of miscellaneous mycoses. Rarely, a case occurs in which no predisposing factor is detected. The patient appears otherwise healthy. Reported cases include *Mycocentrospora acerina* (a plant pathogen) infection of the face (see Fig 61-4), *Aureobasidium* (a soil saprophyte) involvement of the skin, progressive ulceration of the dermis by the water mold *Saksenea vasiformis*, and granuloma of the lung containing the insect pathogen *Beauvaria bassiana*.

Several uncommon fungal infections are described below.

## PSEUDALLESCHERIASIS

*Allescheria boydii* was described by Shear in 1922 as the causative agent of a mycetoma of the foot. The patient lived in western Texas. The fungus was a homothallic (self-fertile) organism that produced sexual spores in a fruiting body. In addition, it produced at least two types of asexual conidia. The asexual phase already had been noted from various types of fungal disease since 1899, and in 1911, it was given the name *Monosporium apiospermum*. In 1944, Emmons realized that the sexual phase and conidia-producing phase were in fact one species. At present, the organism is known as *Pseudallescheria boydii* during the sexual stage and as *Scedosporium apiospermum* in the asexual conidia-producing phase. A second species, *Scedosporium inflatum*, recently was described. Both organisms are soil types. *S. inflatum* has been isolated from a potted spider plant (*Chlorophytum*) and from a dozen bone infections in children. *P boydii* is common in sewage, stagnant water, and barnyard manure.

Since the 1890s, *P boydii* has been isolated from various disease types, particularly ear infections in children. These usually followed a primary bacterial otitis externa and were chronic and difficult to treat. By far the most common form of *P boydii* infection is white grain mycetoma, particularly in the temperate zones of the world. In addition, *P boydii* sometimes produces fungus balls in old pulmonary cavities, just as *Aspergillus* does, and can cause allergic bronchopulmonary pseudallescheriasis, again in imitation of *Aspergillus* (Fig 61-5).

The rarity of *P boydii* infections began to change in the 1960s and 1970s, when the generalized use of high-dose steroids, cytotoxins, and other immunosuppressive agents created a large susceptible patient population. Opportunistic infections of all types became common, and among these were fungus infections. *Candida*, *Aspergillus*, *Cryptococcus*, and Zygomycetes were encountered, in that order. Most affected patients had hematologic neoplasia and, if treatment resulted in neutropenia, fungus infections quickly developed. In the 1980s, an additional population of organ transplant recipients increased the pool of susceptible individuals. The once rare infections caused by *P boydii* have

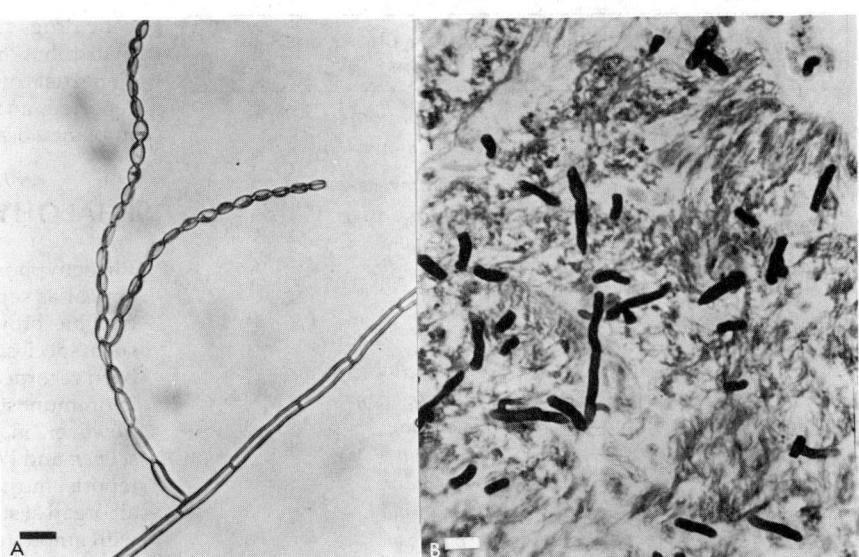

**Figure 61-2.** Phaeohyphomycosis. (**A**) Microscopic section showing conidiation of the agent *Xylohypha bantianum*. (**B**) Typical histologic appearance of dematiaceous septate hyphae in tissue (*Xylohypha bantianum*; original magnification ×450).

increased to the point that this organism now ranks just below the Zygomycetes in number of cases produced.

In the setting of immunosuppression, *P boydii* infections usually begin in the lungs. About 90 such cases have been reported. A variety of changes in the lungs are visible on roentgenogram, ranging from nonspecific infiltrates to cavitating lesions. Dissemination occurs to the brain, thyroid, and other organs. *P boydii* generally is resistant to treatment with amphotericin B and most imidazole drugs. Miconazole has been successful in a few cases. Histologically, the branched, regularly septate mycelia are identical to those of disseminated aspergillosis. The sinuses have been

the portal in several cases. *P boydii* lung infection often leads to brain abscess.

Another form of *P boydii* infection results from the aspiration of contaminated water or sludge, or the introduction of material by injury or accident into immunocompetent patients. In the first form, about a dozen cases have been reported recently in children who aspirated stagnant water, sewer pond sludge, pig manure, or sheep dip, or nearly drowned in swimming pools. An aspiration pneumonia results and the organism disseminates. Often, the course is protracted. Of presently available medications, only miconazole has any efficacy in treatment.

Football injuries, bruises from playing soccer, and motorcycle and automobile accidents have caused lacerations that later were followed by chronic osteomyelitis caused by *P boydii*. Osteomyelitis from this cause is incurable, and amputation is done when necessary.

In 1984, a second member of the genus *Scedosporium* was identified. Initially, all infections with this organism (10 cases) were in children who had suffered trauma. Wound contamination led to a chronic osteomyelitis that was unresponsive to antimy-

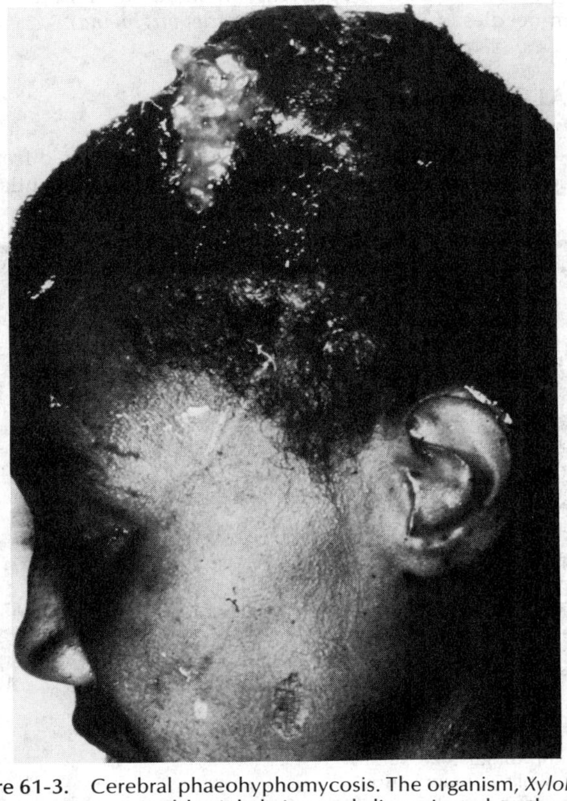

**Figure 61-3.** Cerebral phaeohyphomycosis. The organism, *Xylohypha bantiana,* was acquired by inhalation and disseminated to the brain, producing massive tumor that eroded through the scalp.

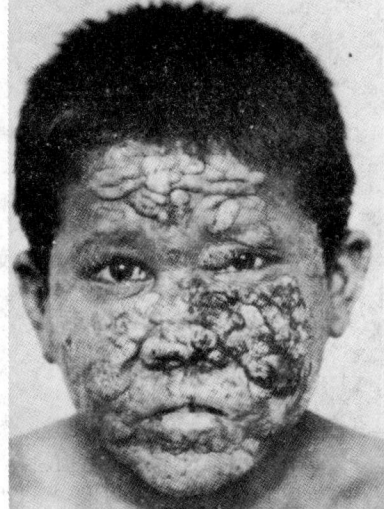

**Figure 61-4.** Phaeohyphomycosis due to *Mycocentrospora acerina,* a pathogen of celery and other plants, in an Indonesian boy. No underlying condition could be detected.

| TABLE 61-2. Agents of Hyalohyphomycosis in Animals and Humans | |
|---|---|
| **Acremonium** | **Myriodontium** |
| A alabamensis | M keratinophylum |
| A kiliense | |
| A potroni | **Paecilomyces** |
| A roseo-griseum | P fumoso-roseus |
| A falciforme | P lilacinum |
| A strictum | P marquandii |
| | P variotii |
| **Anxiopsis** | P javanicus |
| A fulvescens | |
| A sterocaria | **Pencillium** |
| | P chrysogenum |
| **Arthrographis** | P glaucum? |
| A kalrae | P citrinum |
| | P commune |
| **Beauvaria** | P expansum |
| B alba | P spinulosum |
| B bassiana | P marneffei (as a schizo-yeast |
| | and mycelium in tissue) |
| **Chrysosporium** | |
| Chrysosporium species | **Schizophylum** |
| | S commune |
| **Coprinius** | |
| C cinereus | **Scopulariopsis** |
| C delicatulus | S acremonium |
| | S brevicaulis |
| **Cylindrocarpon** | |
| C lichenicola | **Scytalidium** |
| C vaginae | S hyalinum |
| | |
| **Fusarium** | **Trichoderma** |
| F chlamydosporum | T viride |
| F dimerum | |
| F moniliforme | **Tritiachium** |
| F simifectum | T oryzae |
| F oxysporum | |
| F solani | **Volutella** |
| F roseum | V cinerscens |
| | |
| **Microascus** | |
| M cinereus | |

cotic drugs. The organism, *S inflatum*, appears to be worldwide in distribution, having been found in the United States, Australia, Venezuela, and Europe. Infections in horses and a cat have been reported, and in 1987, *S inflatum* was isolated from potting soil in plants located in a hospital corridor.

## PHAEOHYPHOMYCOSIS

Phaeohyphomycosis is a newly described disease entity. The fungi appear as septate branching mycelia in tissue culture with a discernible brown pigment (melanin) in the cell walls. About 40 such species have been described (see Table 61-1). Most have been recorded in only a few cases, almost all of which occurred in immunosuppressed hosts. Two agents are quite common, however, in an entity called pheomycotic cyst. *Exophiala jeanselmeii* and *Wangiella dermatitidis* have been noted in at least 100 reports, mostly in immunocompromised hosts. Dissemination to all organ systems has occurred. A few patients have been treated with amphotericin B. In initial culture, both species occur as black yeasts, only later developing hyphae.

Some agents isolated as opportunists in phaeohyphomycosis also cause other types of infections. The common agents of chromoblastomycosis, *Fonsecaea pedrosoi* and *Phialophora verrucosa*, have come from thousands of cases of that disease. In chromoblastomycosis, they occur as brown, planate-dividing, yeast-like cells in tissue cultures. These same species have been recovered from about a dozen patients with opportunistic phaeohyphomycosis, in whom they appeared as septate, branching, brown hyphae in tissue culture.

A particularly strange form of the disease is cerebral phaeohyphomycosis (see Figs 61-3, 61-4). About 60 cases have been reported, none of which occurred in an immunosuppressed host. Affected patients appear normal, but complain of increasingly severe headache. At autopsy, masses of black–brown hyphae are seen in brain tissue. The agent *X bantiana* has been isolated from fallen needles of juniper trees (*Juniperus virginiana*).

## HYALOHYPHOMYCOSIS

About 20 agents (see Table 61-2) have been recovered from the new clinical entity known as hyalohyphomycosis. Essentially all

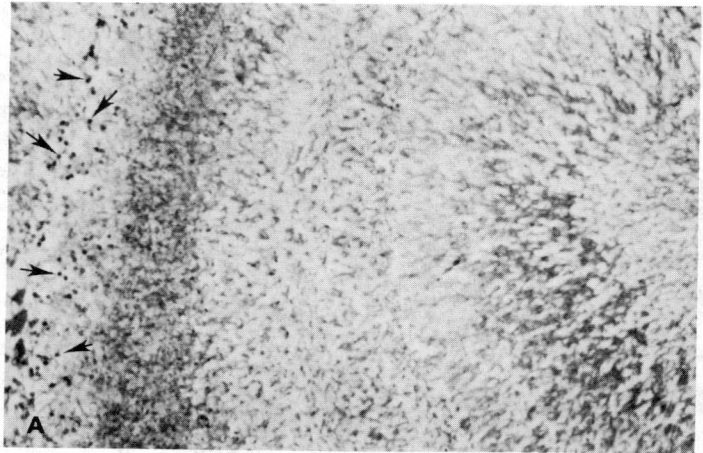
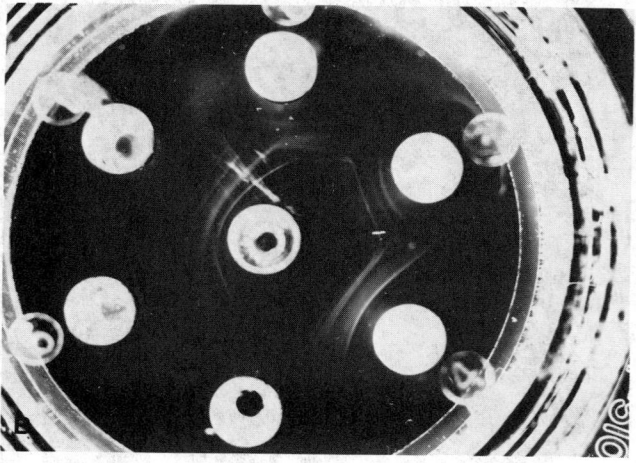

**Figure 61-5.** Pseudallescheriasis. (**A**) Fungus ball in a preformed pulmonary cavity. *Aspergillus* is the most common agent of this disease, but in this section, concentric rings of growth can be seen, topped by single conidia (*arrows*), characteristic of *P boydii*. (**B**) Serology of a patient with fungus ball due to *P boydii*. The patient's serum is in the center well. Five of the six surrounding wells contain various preparations of *P boydii* antigen. Positive reactions have occurred. Well 5 contains antigen to *Aspergillus* and is negative.

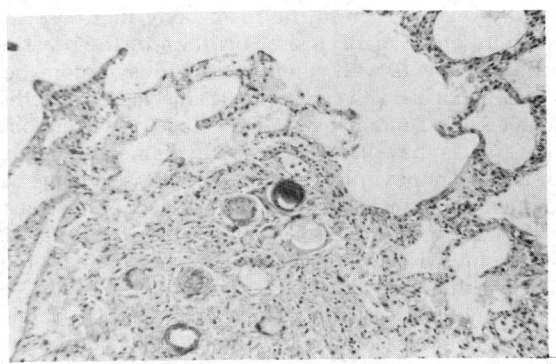

**Figure 61-6.** Adiospiromycosis. Adioconidia (spherule) in lung. The spherules are 150 to 200 μm in diameter in this infection by *Chrysosporium parvum* var *crescens*.

affected patients have been immunosuppressed. The agents gain entrance through the lungs, sinuses, indwelling catheters, dialysis tubing, and gastrointestinal tract (perhaps by the human host eating moldy fruit). In tissue culture, all produce branching, septate, colorless mycelia. The morphology is identical to that seen in invasive aspergillosis. The most common of these agents are *Fusarium* species. About 50 cases have been recorded.

## ADIOSPIROMYCOSIS

Adiospiromycosis denotes the in vivo development without replication of adioconidia (adiospores) from the inhaled conidia of species of the fungal genus *Chrysosporium*. Adioconidia refers to the enlargement without replication of a fungal conidium under the influence of high temperature. Adiospiromycosis is the term used to indicate this development in animal tissue.

The disease first was described in 1942 in desert rodents in Arizona. Examination of museum specimens of rodents and of newly captured animals has revealed that the disease is worldwide in distribution. It has been found in animals captured in the early 1800s.

About a dozen human infections have been described. In general, these infections have been found incidentally at autopsy or in materials, particularly from the lung, in a living host. Cases in children have been noted, particularly in the former Czechoslovakia. One 11-year-old boy had functional impairment of the lung, and a 10-year-old boy required treatment with nystatin and amphotericin B by aerosol.

In tissue, the adioconidia are 10 to 13 μm in diameter when the causative agent is *Chrysosporium parvum* (which is restricted

geographically to the western United States and Canada). Adioconidia as large as 40 μm in diameter can be produced in culture at 37 °C.

The far more widely distributed *C parvum* var *crescens* produces adioconidia as large as 220 μm in diameter in natural infections and as large as 400 μm in culture at 37 °C (Fig 61-6).

## RHINOSPORIDIOSIS

Rhinosporidiosis is an infection of the mucocutaneous tissue caused by the organism *Rhinosporidium seeberi*. The organism has not been grown in culture, but it appears to be a fungus. The disease results in the production of polyps, tumors, papillomas, or wart-like vegetative growths that are hyperplastic, highly vascularized, friable, and sessile or pedunculated (Fig 61-7). The nose and conjunctivae are involved most commonly. Nasal infection is common in damp tropical climates, whereas conjunctivitis is more common in dry, dusty areas. Infection of the anus, penis, vagina, ears, pharynx, and larynx may occur. The disease first was described independently in Tennessee, India, and Argentina. About 4000 cases have been reported from India, where the disease is so common that tabulations are not kept. It also is common in Sri Lanka. Several hundred cases (in horses and humans) have been reported from Argentina and 50 or so have been reported from South Africa and the United States. In both South Africa and the United States, conjunctival disease is more common than nasal infestation. It also is fairly common in dogs (nasal form) in the southeastern United States.

In tissue, the organism grows as a spherule as large as 250 to 350 μm in diameter. The spherules contain endospores that are released at maturity. The endospores then enlarge to produce spherules in a manner similar to that of *Coccidioides immitis*.

Surgical removal is the most common method of treatment, and recurrence is common.

## GEOTRICHOSIS

Geotrichosis is a rare opportunistic infection caused by the yeast-like hyphomycete *Geotrichum candidum*. The organism is ubiquitous in the soil and air, and is part of the normal flora of the skin and gastrointestinal tract. It also has been found in cottage cheese and other dairy products.

Hundreds of reports have linked *G candidum* to a variety of disease types. Unfortunately, in most cases, the pathogenic role of the fungus was not substantiated, and its delineation from *C albicans* often is confusing. There probably are no more than three dozen authentic cases in the literature. A recent report de-

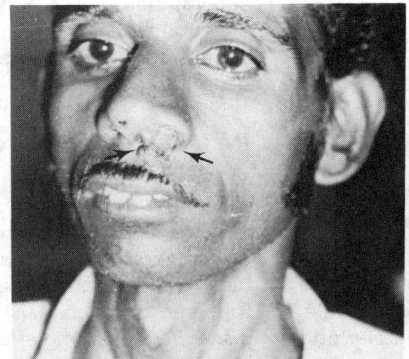
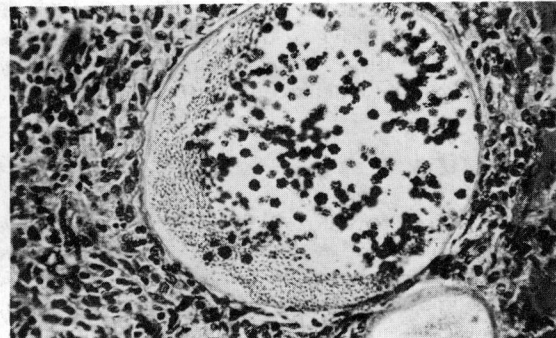

**Figure 61-7.** Rhinosporidiosis. **(A)** Pedunculated lesions have formed on the nasal mucosa (*arrows*). **(B)** Histologic section shows spherule 350 μm in diameter (×450).

scribed a female patient with leukemia in blast crisis after vincristine and prednisone therapy. She developed disseminated fungal disease. Only *G candidum* was isolated from blood, urine, skin biopsy, and autopsy specimens. In tissue, septate hyphae and budding yeasts were seen. *Geotrichum* does not produce yeast-like cells, but it does produce arthroconidia, which resemble yeasts. It is possible that two agents were present—a *Trichosporon* or a *Candida* in addition to *Geotrichum*. This emphasizes the difficulty of assessing fungi in histopathologic sections.

## Selected Readings

Ajello J. Hyalohyphomycosis and phaeohyphomycosis: Two global disease entities of public health importance. Eur J Epidemiol 1986;2:243.

Albassam MA, Bhatnagar R, et al. Adiospiromycosis in striped skunks in Alberta, Canada. J Wildl Dis 1986;22:13.

Kassamali H, Anaissie E, Ro J, et al. Disseminated *Geotrichum candidum* infection. J Clin Microbiol 1987;25:1782.

Milne LJR, McKerrow W, et al. Pseudalleschiasis in northern Britain. J Med Vet Mycol 1987;24:377.

Rippon JW. Medical mycology: The pathogenic and the pathogenic actinomycetes, ed 3. Philadelphia: WB Saunders, 1988.

Woodward BH, Hudson J. Rhinosporidiosis: Ultrastructural study of an infection in South Carolina. South Med J 1984;77:1587.

*Principles and Practice of Pediatrics, Second Edition.*
edited by Frank A. Oski et al. J. B. Lippincott Company, Philadelphia © 1994.

# CHAPTER 62
# *Parasitic Diseases*

## 62.1 *Protozoan Parasites*

### 62.1.1 Entamoeba histolytica

Bradley Howard Kessler and William J. Klish

Amebiasis is defined as infection with *Entamoeba histolytica*, with or without overt clinical symptoms. The disease is worldwide in distribution, affecting as much as 10% of the population. The highest prevalence is seen in underdeveloped areas and tropical regions. It has been estimated that about 1% to 5% of Americans who have never traveled outside the United States have amebiasis; most of these are asymptomatic carriers. Severe disease, such as ulcerative amebic colitis or liver abscess, is relatively rare.

## ETIOLOGY

Two forms of the protozoan parasite *E histolytica*, cysts and trophozoites, are found in stool specimens. Trophozoites are motile, variably shaped organisms that are 7 to 30 μm in diameter and have a single nucleus and a granular, vacuolated cytoplasm. Trophozoites characteristically produce pseudopodia, which are finger-like projections from the main body that participate in both motility and phagocytosis. This form of the parasite may be found in patients with symptomatic or asymptomatic amebiasis. In individuals with symptomatic amebiasis, the pathogenic trophozoites may contain ingested red blood cells in endoplasmic vacuoles and can be as large as 60 μm in diameter. Phagocytosis may be an important virulence factor. Specific isoenzyme patterns or zymodemes obtained from starch gel electrophoresis are indirect markers of virulence. Certain strains of *E histolytica* are associated only with asymptomatic carriage, whereas others are associated with invasive disease.

The nonmotile cyst form is similar in size to the trophozoite, but may contain as many as four nuclei. Infection occurs only with ingestion of cysts. Upon ingestion, after excystation in the small bowel, each single cyst results in eight trophozoites. Unlike the trophozoite, which is destroyed rapidly by external environmental conditions and gastric acid, the cysts are resistant to gastric acid and to the chlorine concentrations commonly used in domestic water purification, as well as to extreme temperature and drying. Cysts may survive outside the host for several weeks in a moist environment.

## EPIDEMIOLOGY

Infection with pathogenic trophozoites is not a major clinical problem in this country, despite prevalence rates ranging from 0.1% to 50% in regional and institutional surveys. Overall, prevalence rates approach 4%. The invasive trophozoites cause diarrhea and dysentery in 2% to 8% of infected patients. Trophozoites that enter the bloodstream may pass to the liver or other organs and cause abscesses. Although amebic hepatic abscess is thought to be less common in children than in adults, it is found as a complication of intestinal disease in all endemic areas. Amebic abscess of the liver has been reported in 1% to 9% of patients with invasive amebiasis. Abscesses are seen more frequently in males, with the highest incidence found in individuals 20 to 50 years of age. Reports from endemic areas also indicate a significant incidence of amebic liver abscess in children less than 3 years of age.

Humans are the natural host and reservoir for *E histolytica*. Fecal–oral transmission occurs frequently through contaminated water or foods such as vegetables. Outbreaks have been associated with pollution of the water supply by sewage. Major outbreaks occur in the United States with person-to-person spread the predominant form of transmission. Infected food handlers play a major role in transmitting the infection. *E histolytica* is a common commensal organism in homosexuals, infecting as much as 30% of this population. Most new infections in the United States are found among foreign travelers and recent immigrants from the developing world. The virulence of the organisms in specific areas, such as South Africa, Mexico, and India, may be explained by the strain of parasite as well as by the nutritional status and bacterial flora in the intestine of the host.

## PATHOGENESIS AND PATHOLOGY

The pathogenesis of invasive amebiasis occurs through a number of steps: colonization in the colonic mucus blanket, penetration or depletion of the mucus layer with disruption of the epithelial barrier, and parasite lysis of responding host inflammatory cells followed by deeper tissue penetration. Cytopathic effects of *E histolytica* on monolayers of mammalian cells in tissue culture have been well described. The factors that determine whether ingestion of *E histolytica* will produce no infection, a commensal state, symptomatic colitis, or hepatic abscess are not well defined. Some factors implicated include the strain of organism, the ability of the organism to produce proteases such as collagenase or phospholipases, the adhesiveness of the organism to epithelial cells through a galactose/$N$-acetyl D-galactosamine lectin binding protein, the ability of the organism to engulf tissue elements through phagocytosis, and the interaction of the organism with the bacterial flora that is indigenous to the gastrointestinal tract. Adherence is necessary for cytolytic activity. The mechanism of tissue invasion is not understood clearly. It is postulated that a toxin or lytic compound from the parasite provokes a generalized inflammatory response that progresses to mucosal destruction. As the process continues, classic flask-shaped ulcers with undermined edges are formed. When amebae move into the bowel wall, some may be picked up in the portal circulation and become disseminated, first to the liver and then throughout the body.

The pathologic lesions described most frequently are ulcers that are scattered throughout the colon, but affect predominantly the cecum and ascending colon. The sigmoid colon and rectum usually are less involved; the terminal ileum rarely is involved. As the disease progresses, the ulcer increases in size and extends into the submucosa and muscular coat. On rare occasions, this can lead to perforation. Histologic examination reveals a diffuse, nonspecific inflammation that is indistinguishable from other forms of idiopathic colitis, such as ulcerative colitis. Amebae frequently can be seen at the leading edge of the ulcer and in the overlying inflammatory exudate.

Amebic liver abscess usually is solitary, but multiple abscesses can occur. The right lobe of the liver is involved most often. The material within an abscess has been described as resembling anchovy paste or chocolate syrup. The parasite rarely is found in aspirated abscess fluid. It is not known whether amebic hepatitis always precedes amebic abscess.

## CLINICAL FEATURES

Most infections are asymptomatic (luminal colonization) and elimination of the parasite from the gut occurs within 12 months. The incubation period for the illness varies, but usually is 2 to 4 weeks. The severity of illness may vary from very mild symptoms to severe fulminating disease with mucosal inflammation, ulceration, and even perforation. Most patients with invasive amebiasis describe a gradual onset of cramping, abdominal pain, malaise, tenesmus (with rectal involvement), and frequent stools. Stools usually are blood-stained and mucoid. Diarrhea may persist for weeks, but can wax and wane with alternating periods of constipation. In some patients, the onset of symptoms may be acute, with fever, profuse bloody mucoid diarrhea, dehydration, and electrolyte abnormalities. This fulminant picture may mimic that seen in toxic megacolon, acute inflammatory bowel disease, and bacillary dysentery. More serious disease is associated with youth, pregnancy, malnutrition, corticosteroid therapy, and underlying systemic disease. Possible complications include intestinal perforation, hemorrhage, stricture, inflammation, peritonitis, and a local inflammatory mass or ameboma. On physical examination, tenderness usually is present throughout the lower abdomen.

Hepatic amebiasis and abscess are characterized by fever, abdominal pain, pleuritic pain, respiratory distress, and hepatomegaly. The pain usually is localized to the right upper quadrant, with radiation to the right shoulder and laterally to the chest. Patients frequently give no history of significant gastrointestinal symptoms. Chest radiographs may show elevation of the right hemidiaphragm. Laboratory evaluation may reveal anemia, with an elevated leukocyte count and a left shift. Amebic abscess develops in less than 1% of patients with intestinal amebiasis. The most common finding on physical examination is a large, tender

liver. Icterus occurs infrequently, and its presence is a ominous sign. Examination of the chest may reveal rales, decreased breath sounds, and a friction rub. Complications involve the pleural cavity or intra-abdominal extension of the abscess.

## DIAGNOSIS

Because medical therapy is highly effective in all forms of amebiasis, the diagnosis should be made as early as possible. It is crucial to distinguish amebiasis from inflammatory bowel disease. The symptoms, findings on colonoscopy, and histologic findings on examination of biopsy material can mimic the findings in ulcerative colitis. Steroids, which frequently are prescribed for ulcerative colitis, may complicate the course of amebiasis and increase the mortality.

Microscopic examination of repeated stool specimens is the definitive diagnostic test. When the test is done correctly, the results of more than 90% of stool examinations are positive in infected patients. Stool samples should be examined immediately after defecation or should be preserved in a fixative such as polyvinyl alcohol or formalin ethyl acetate for later examination. Staining with thimerosal (Merthiolate)-iodine-formalin increases the sensitivity. In addition to direct examination, concentration of the specimen treated with formalin ethyl acetate also increases the sensitivity of the test. An experienced examiner competent in the diagnosis of parasitic infections should be consulted to distinguish the nuclear characteristics of the trophozoites and differentiate *E histolytica* from other amebae that rarely are pathogenic. These include *Entamoeba hartmanni*, *Escherichia coli*, and *Endolimax nana*. It is imperative that the stool be collected before barium studies are done, because barium decreases the yield of positive examination results. Rectal mucosal scrapings collected during proctosigmoidoscopy also can be examined and will increase the positive yield. Trophozoites can be seen on colonic biopsy in about 50% of cases. If stool examination results are negative and a high level of suspicion exists for intestinal amebiasis, serologic testing such as an indirect hemagglutination (IHA) test should be done. IHA test results are strongly positive (titer >1:256) in 85% to 90% of patients with invasive colonic disease or liver abscess. A limitation of the IHA test is that the results can remain positive for more than 20 years and, therefore, may represent earlier illness. The gel diffusion precipitin test has a high predictive value. Other common serologic tests include counterimmunoelectrophoresis, indirect immunofluorescent antibody, complement fixation, and enzyme-linked immunosorbent assay. Colonization with nonpathogenic strains rarely provides a serologic response.

The key to recognizing amebic liver abscess is suspecting the diagnosis in patients with fever and an enlarged, tender liver. It must be remembered that patients with liver abscess usually do not have concurrent diarrhea. Laboratory test results generally are nonspecific. The serum alkaline phosphatase level may be elevated. Bilirubin and liver transaminase levels may be normal or mildly elevated. In addition to serology, liver scanning, including ultrasound, computerized axial tomography scanning, and technetium 99m sulfur colloid, can help detect a liver defect that is consistent with an abscess. Needle aspiration may help to establish a diagnosis, though this is not done commonly for diagnostic purposes.

## TREATMENT

The specific therapy recommended for infection with *E histolytica* depends on the site of involvement (luminal, intramural, or systemic). An asymptomatic carrier should be treated with iodoquinol (formerly diiodohydroxyquin), 30 to 40 mg/kg/d (maximum 2 g/d), in divided doses given every 8 hours for 20 days. Iodoquinol has been reported to cause optic atrophy in rare cases. An alternative regimen is diloxanide furoate (furamide), 7 mg/kg three times a day for 10 days. Invasive amebiasis of the intestine, liver, or other organs requires the additional use of a tissue amebicide such as metronidazole (Flagyl). This is administered at a dosage of 35 to 50 mg/kg/d in divided doses given every 8 hours for 10 days. Because metronidazole is a less effective luminal amebicide, patients should receive iodoquinol as outlined above for 20 days. If iodoquinol or metronidazole cannot be given or the course of illness is severe, dehydroemetine, 1 to 1.5 mg/kg/d (maximum 90 mg/d) in divided doses given every 12 hours by the intramuscular route for 5 days, is an alternative. Dehydroemetine should be used with caution, because it can cause severe side effects. These include cardiotoxicity, which can lead to fatal myocardiopathy, arrhythmias with T wave changes, muscle weakness, and renal complications. Dehydroemetine therapy should be followed by iodoquinol as outlined above for 20 days.

Uncomplicated, deep, unruptured liver abscess may be treated medically. Liver abscess or other forms of extraintestinal disease should be treated with metronidazole followed by iodoquinol as outlined above, or alternatively with dehydroemetine followed by chloroquine, 10 mg/kg/d for 14 to 21 days, plus iodoquinol as outlined above. The patient's clinical condition usually will improve within 72 hours of the initiation of medical therapy. Clinical signs as well as radioisotope scanning or ultrasound of the liver are useful guides to the effectiveness of the therapy. For the refractory case or the patient with impending rupture of the abscess, percutaneous needle aspiration or open drainage may be necessary. Positive contacts should be screened.

Prophylaxis for travelers to endemic areas is not recommended. The best prophylaxis is exercising caution in unsanitary conditions and endemic environments.

Acquired cellular immunity to invasive amebiasis seems to occur. Work is under way using a number of strategies to develop a subunit amebiasis vaccine. Vaccination would be the most cost-effective approach to prevention.

## Selected Readings

Guerrent RL. Amebiasis: Introduction, current status, and research questions. Rev Infect Dis 1986;8:218.

Haffar A, Bolan JFJ, Edwards MS. Amebic liver abscess in children. Pediatr Infect Dis 1982;1:322.

Harrison RH, Crowe CP, Fulginiti UA. Amebic liver abscess in children: Clinical and epidemiologic features. Pediatrics 1979;64:923.

Healy GR. Immunologic tools in the diagnosis of amebiasis: Epidemiology in the United States. Rev Infect Dis 1986;8:239.

Merritt RJ, Coughlin E, Thomas DW, et al. Spectrum of amebiasis in children. Am J Dis Child 1982;136:785.

Pickering LK. Therapy for acute infectious diarrhea in children. J Pediatr 1991;118:S118.

Ravdin JI. Pathogenesis of disease caused by Entamoeba histolytica: Studies of adherence, secreted toxins, and contact-dependent cytolysis. Rev Infect Dis 1986;8:247.

Ravdin JI. Entamoeba histolytica: From adherence to enteropathy. J Infect Dis 1989;159:420.

Ravdin JI. Entamoeba histolytica: Pathogenic mechanisms, human immune response and vaccine development. Clin Res 1990;38:215.

Thompson JE, Forlenza S, Verma Ranesh. Amebic liver abscess: A therapeutic approach. Rev Infect Dis 1985;7:171.

Walsh JA. Problems in recognition and diagnosis of amebiasis: Estimation of the global magnitude of morbidity and mortality. Rev Infect Dis 1986;8:228.

*Principles and Practice of Pediatrics, Second Edition.*
edited by Frank A. Oski et al. J. B. Lippincott Company, Philadelphia © 1994.

## 62.1.2 *Babesiosis*

M. Melisse Sloas and Christian C. Patrick

Babesiosis is a hemolytic disease caused by an intraerythrocytic protozoan known since biblical times. Babesiosis is recognized largely as a disease of livestock, but it occurs occasionally in children in the United States. The first human case of babesiosis was reported in 1957.

## MICROBIOLOGY

The genus *Babesia* belongs to the subphylum Apicomplexa, which includes *Toxoplasma* and the malarial parasite *Plasmodium*. Of the 71 species included in the genus, *Babesia microti* is implicated largely in human disease in the United States, whereas *Babesia divergens* is the major pathogen in Europe.

Microscopically, Babesia appears small and round to pear-shaped. A feature distinguishing *Babesia* from *Plasmodium* is its inability to produce pigment in red blood cells (RBCs) in the later stages of its life cycle.

## EPIDEMIOLOGY

In the United States, the Ixodidae family of hard-bodied ticks is the primary vector of *B microti*, particularly *Ixodes dammini*, the same species of tick that is implicated in Lyme disease; the major reservoir is the white-footed mouse, *Peromyscus leucopus*. The tick's life cycle comprises the larval, nymphal, and adult stages. Only the nymphs are capable of transmitting *B microti* to humans.

Babesiosis occurs most often in this country during late summer and fall, which is the nymphs' major feeding period. Most cases have been confined to the northeast, particularly along the New England coast, although a few have been reported in California and Wisconsin. An acquired form of babesiosis has occurred rarely after blood transfusions.

## PATHOGENESIS

Because of the paucity of human subjects, the pathogenesis of babesiosis has been studied in animals. These studies show that the complement C3b receptor is involved with the parasite's entry into RBCs. Once it is in the cell, the organism reproduces asexually by budding into 2 to 4 merozoites, which are released from the RBCs at varying times. In contrast, the plasmodia that cause malaria are released synchronously from RBCs. Red cell lysis is responsible for most of the clinical manifestations of both babesiosis and malaria. *Babesia*, however, generally produces milder symptoms. Other symptoms of babesiosis, such as hepatomegaly, are secondary to obstruction of vascular access by infected erythrocytes.

The spleen appears to be involved intimately in the disease process. Splenic dysfunction generally causes a more severe case of babesiosis, with removal of the spleen leading to a relapse of the disease in treated patients. The spleen's crucial involvement may be explained by the reticuloendothelial capability to remove deformed (parasitized) RBCs, and by its possible role in the production of anti-*Babesia* antibodies.

## CLINICAL MANIFESTATIONS

In immunocompetent individuals, babesiosis generally is a mild or subclinical infection. Manifestations occur more often and are more severe in immunocompromised patients, including those with the acquired immunodeficiency syndrome, those with asplenia, the elderly, and neonates. After an incubation period of 1 to 4 weeks, the susceptible host experiences a gradual onset of fatigue, malaise, anorexia, and fever, with temperature spikes to 40 °C (104 °F). Other symptoms may include chills, myalgias, arthralgia, nausea, and vomiting. Rash may be present, but is not a constant feature.

Physical examination may reveal mild splenomegaly, hepatomegaly, jaundice (occasionally), and pharyngeal erythema. Laboratory findings include moderately severe hemolytic anemia with an increased reticulocyte count. The erythrocyte sedimentation rate is elevated and the leukocyte count is normal. Elevated liver function test results are found in about half of all patients. The course of the illness can be prolonged, lasting weeks to months. A fulminant course with high fever, hemolytic anemia, hemoglobinuria, jaundice, congestive heart failure, renal failure, and adult respiratory distress syndrome is seen only rarely.

Recent reports have documented simultaneous babesiosis and Lyme disease. Because both are transmitted by the same tick, coinfection should be suspected in severe cases of either disease.

## DIAGNOSIS

Babesiosis is diagnosed from a combination of clinical findings and Giemsa-stained thick and thin blood smears showing intraerythrocytic parasites. Similar to *Plasmodium, Babesia* produces a variety of intraerythrocytic forms. *Plasmodium* can be distinguished by its pigment production and synchronous stages of development, however. In babesiosis, parasitemia can be detected as long as 10 months after the onset of illness.

Serologic assays, which include enzyme-linked immunosorbent assays and complement fixation tests, should not be substituted for pathologic diagnosis. The indirect immunofluorescence tests seem to be the most reliable, but cross-reactions may occur with *Plasmodium* species.

## TREATMENT

No effective therapy for babesiosis is known. Fortunately, the disease largely is self-limited. Chloroquine, which commonly is prescribed when babesiosis is misdiagnosed as malaria, does not eradicate the parasite. A combination of oral quinine and parenteral clindamycin may be efficacious, although one report described a treatment failure.

Exchange transfusions have treated life-threatening cases of babesiosis successfully, but should be reserved for the most severe cases.

### Selected Readings

Benach JL, Habicht GS. Clinical characteristics of human babesiosis. J Infect Dis 1981;144:481.
Centers for Disease Control. Babesiosis—Connecticut. MMWR 1989;38:649.
Grunwaldt E, Barbour AG, Benach JL. Simultaneous occurrence of babesiosis and Lyme disease. N Engl J Med 1983;308:1166.
Jack RM, Ward PA. *Babesia rodhaini* interactions with complement: Relationship to parasitic entry into red cells. J Immunol 1980;124:1566.
Jacoby GA, Hunt JV, Kosinski KS, et al. Treatment of transfusion-transmitted babesiosis by exchange transfusion. N Engl J Med 1980;303:1098.
Krause PJ. Babesiosis. In: Feigin RD, Cherry JD, eds. Textbook of pediatric infectious diseases, 2nd ed. Philadelphia: WB Saunders, 1987:2019.
Krause PJ. Babesiosis. Report on Pediatric Infectious Diseases 1992;2:11.

Rosner F, Zarrabi MH, Benach JL, et al. Babesiosis in splenectomized adults: Review of 22 reported cases. Am J Med 1984;76:696.
Smith RP, Evans AT, Popovsky M, et al. Transfusion-acquired babesiosis and failure of antibiotic treatment. JAMA 1986;256:2726.

*Principles and Practice of Pediatrics, Second Edition.*
edited by Frank A. Oski et al. J. B. Lippincott Company, Philadelphia © 1994.

## 62.1.3 *Cryptosporidiosis*
Walter T. Hughes

Cryptosporidiosis is a common enteric infection caused by the coccidian protozoan *Cryptosporidium*. The first human case was described in 1976. The infection came to prominence in the early 1980s because of its association with the acquired immunodeficiency syndrome (AIDS) and other immunocompromised states. Furthermore, by the mid-1980s, it had become recognized as a frequent cause of diarrhea in otherwise normal children, especially those attending day-care centers.

## ETIOLOGY

*Cryptosporidium* is a small protozoan parasite belonging to the same family as *Toxoplasma gondii, Isospora belli,* and *Sarcocystis*. It completes its life cycle on intestinal and respiratory surface epithelial cells of mammals, birds, and reptiles. The oocyst form of *Cryptosporidium* resides in the feces and is the infective stage. Sporozoites within the oocyst mature, sporulate, and are released into the intestine, where, as trophozoites, they attach to the microvillar surface of epithelial cells. Merogony, gametogony, and sporogony occur. Macrogametes and microgametes develop and, on fertilization, develop into an oocyst with four sporozoites. The oocyst is passed into the feces.

Speciation of *Cryptosporidium* has not been established firmly, but it is likely that several species exist. *Cryptosporidium parvum* is believed to cause the infection in humans.

## EPIDEMIOLOGY

Animal-to-human and human-to-animal transmission of *Cryptosporidium* has been reported. The organism appears to be highly transmissible from human to human, and some outbreaks have been traced to contaminated water supplies. *Cryptosporidium* is a common cause of enteric infection worldwide, and such infections have been reported from 26 countries. Surveys of selected populations reveal prevalence rates ranging from 0.6% to 4.0% in North America and from 4% to 20% in developing countries. About 3% to 4% of patients with AIDS in the United States and 50% of those in Haiti and Africa have the infection. *Cryptosporidium* has been isolated from the stools of 4.1% of hospitalized, immunocompetent patients with diarrhea in Australia, from 1.4% of a similar population in the United Kingdom, from 4.3% of Costa Rican children, and from 8.0% of Liberian children. It has been estimated that diarrhea caused by *Cryptosporidium* occurs in 20 to 30 million children annually in Latin America. Because the oocyst is highly stable in the environment, contaminated supplies of drinking water and swimming pools are sources of outbreaks of infection.

Several outbreaks of diarrhea attributable to *Cryptosporidium* have occurred in day-care centers in the United States, which currently are the setting of highest risk for otherwise normal children. In these outbreaks, other organisms, such as *Giardia lamblia*, also may be found in stool samples. When this occurs, however, *Cryptosporidium* usually is the causative agent of the diarrhea.

Person-to-person transmission has been reported in the hospital environment, suggesting the need for enteric isolation precautions for hospitalized patients with this infection. Animal-to-human transmission may occur, especially from calves.

## PATHOLOGY

The detailed histopathology of cryptosporidiosis in the immunocompetent host is unknown. Limited studies in patients with AIDS have demonstrated the organisms adherent to the surface of enterocytes between the microvilli and often within a parasitophorous vacuole. Although the intestinal mucosa generally is intact, epithelial cell loss, villous atrophy, crypt elongation, and minimal subjacent inflammatory infiltrates of the lamina propria may be seen. The organisms are found only at the surface of epithelial cells. In some cases, *Cryptosporidium* has been found adherent to the epithelium of the gallbladder and biliary duct epithelium. In the few cases studied at autopsy, the jejunum was the most heavily infected area of the gastrointestinal tract. The protozoan has been found in the pharynx, esophagus, stomach, duodenum, ileum, appendix, colon, and rectum, in addition to the jejunum in patients with AIDS.

## CLINICAL MANIFESTATIONS

Infection with *Cryptosporidium* may be asymptomatic or symptomatic. When the infection becomes clinically evident, the extent of the signs and symptoms generally is related to the degree of patient immunocompetence. Normal children and adults have either asymptomatic infection or a self-limited illness.

Patients with AIDS or other severe immunodeficiency states usually have chronic diarrhea, often with cholera-like features. Diarrhea commonly is profuse, watery, and without blood. Fluid losses may be extensive, as much as several liters per day in adults. The pathophysiology of this extensive fluid loss has not been elucidated. These patients also may have abdominal pain, anorexia, nausea, and vomiting, but they rarely are febrile. Symptoms and oocyst shedding persist for months and often until death in patients with AIDS.

In immunocompetent hosts, the illness resembles that of giardiasis, with watery diarrhea, abdominal pain, malaise, myalgias, weight loss, and anorexia. In careful studies of Finnish patients, the incubation period was 1 week and the duration of the illness was about 12 days. Hospitalized children with cryptosporidiosis also have had illnesses of similar duration, and of those with diarrhea, about 50% had fever and about 85% had abdominal pain.

## DIAGNOSIS

The differential diagnosis for cryptosporidiosis includes all causes of diarrhea. Attention should be directed to this protozoan when the patient has AIDS or some other form of immunodeficiency, or when he or she has attended a day-care center. Sporadic cases also may occur in otherwise healthy children, however.

The diagnosis of cryptosporidiosis is established by the demonstration of *Cryptosporidium* oocysts in fecal specimens in the absence of other enteric pathogens. It must be kept in mind that *Cryptosporidium* can be found in asymptomatic individuals. Fecal samples can be examined by several staining methods, including acid-fast stains, fluorescent auramine or rhodamine stains, periodic acid–Schiff stains, and carbolfuchsin-negative stains. Initially, an iodine-stained wet mount and an acid-fast stained (modified Kinyoun or Ziehl-Neelsen) smear should be prepared. If these do not reveal the oocysts, specific concentration techniques should be used. The technique used most frequently is the Sheather sugar flotation method. In this concentrated sugar solution, the oocysts rise to the surface because the specific gravity of the solution is greater than that of the oocyst. A word of caution is in order, however. The original Sheather flotation procedure involved placement of a coverslip on top of the mixture of stool and glucose solution, and removal of the coverslip with adherent organisms for examination. This procedure should not be followed with *Cryptosporidium*, because the organism can be transmitted easily to the laboratory worker and cause infection. Instead, the suspension should be placed in a screw-cap centrifuge tube and, after centrifugation, an aliquot of the supernatant should be transferred by pipette to a slide for examination. With a coverslip applied, the wet preparation can be examined for oocysts, or the dried and fixed specimens can be stained. Two separate specimens studied by acid-fast stain of concentrates are needed to exclude the diagnosis of cryptosporidiosis.

Serologic tests for antibody to *Cryptosporidium* have been developed, but are not in general use at this time.

A fluorescein-labeled antibody test that uses monoclonal antibody to *Cryptosporidium* (Meridian Laboratories, Cincinnati, Ohio) is available and is the most sensitive and specific test for the organism in stool specimens.

## TREATMENT

Because oocyst excretion may persist for as long as 2 weeks after clinical recovery occurs, enteric isolation precautions should be instituted for hospitalized patients, with special efforts made to avoid exposure of immunosuppressed patients.

No specific therapy is available for cryptosporidiosis. Recently, azithromycin has been found to be effective in the prevention and treatment of experimental cryptosporidiosis in rats. In most immunocompetent children, the course is self-limited, but immunosuppressed patients may require intensive and prolonged supportive management.

## Selected Readings

Crawford FG, Vermund SH. Human cryptosporidiosis. Crit Rev Microbiol 1988;16: 113.

Hayes EB, Matte TD, O'Brien TK, et al. Large community outbreak of cryptosporidiosis due to contamination of a filtered public water supply. N Engl J Med 1989;320:1372.

Heijbel H, Slaine K, Seigel B, et al. Outbreak of diarrhea in a day care center with the spread to household members: The role of *Cryptosporidium*. Pediatr Infect Dis J 1987;6:532.

Jokipii L, Kokipii MM. Timing of symptoms and oocyst excretion in human cryptosporidiosis. N Engl J Med 1986;315:1643.

Mata L. *Cryptosporidium* and other protozoa in diarrheal disease in less developed countries. Pediatr Infect Dis 1986;5:S117.

Rehg JE. Activity of azithromycin against cryptosporidiosis in immunosuppressed rats. J Infect Dis 1991;163:1293.

Sorvillo FJ, Fujioka K, Tormey M, et al. Swimming-associated cryptosporidiosis–Los Angeles County. MMWR 1990;39:343.

*Principles and Practice of Pediatrics, Second Edition.*
edited by Frank A. Oski et al. J. B. Lippincott Company, Philadelphia © 1994.

## *62.1.4* Giardia lamblia

William J. Klish

*Giardia lamblia* holds the distinction of being the first protozoan parasite to be recognized. It was described in a letter by van Leeuwenhoek of Delft to the Royal Society of Medicine in 1681 after he observed this parasite in his stool while trying to evaluate his own intermittent chronic diarrhea. He made the important clinical observation that these "animalcules" could be found only in liquid stool, not in normal formed stool.

*G lamblia* is a cosmopolitan parasite of worldwide distribution and an important cause of traveler's diarrhea. Attack rates are particularly high in travelers to Russia, especially St. Petersburg. *Giardia* also is prevalent in the mountainous western United States, where infection can be contracted by drinking water from mountain streams that have been contaminated by feces from humans, dogs, and other species susceptible to *G lamblia*. The beaver acts as a reservoir for the organism during the summer months by becoming infected (presumably from humans) and then defecating directly into the streams. Water can be disinfected by adding 13 mL of a saturated solution of iodine to 1 L of clear water, or 26 mL to 1 L of cloudy water. All organisms are killed after 15 minutes of incubation at 20 °C; at 3 °C, however, this method is not totally effective. Boiling water for 10 minutes kills all organisms.

*Giardia* also can be spread by close person-to-person contact in which fecal contamination may occur, such as in day-care centers and residential institutions. In addition, contaminated food may act as a vector for this parasite.

## THE ORGANISM

Three species of *Giardia* have been described. *G lamblia* is the species that is specific to humans, but it can be cross-transmitted to other animals, such as dogs, cats, rats, gerbils, guinea pigs, beavers, raccoons, bighorn sheep, and pronghorn antelope. *Giardia muris* infects rodents and birds; *Giardia agilis* is specific to amphibians. *G lamblia* is the name used for the species infecting humans in North America. This same organism is called *Giardia intestinalis* in Europe and *Lamblia intestinalis* in Russia and Eastern Europe. It also has been called *Giardia duodenalis* and *Giardia enterica*.

*G lamblia* is a flagellate protozoan belonging to the family Hexamitidae. The trophozoite or motile form is characterized by its symmetry: two oval, dorsally situated nuclei and four pairs of flagella. In addition, it has two median bodies and a ventral adhesive disk by which the parasite adheres to the intestinal mucosa and other surfaces. The organism also exists in a cyst form, which results when the trophozoite rounds up and elaborates a cyst wall. These cysts allow the organism to survive passage out of the host. *Giardia* cysts are resistant to destruction in hypotonic solutions such as water and can survive for more than 2 months in water at 8 °C, but for only 4 days in water at 37 °C. When cysts are ingested, the excystation process is induced by gastric acid and completed in the duodenum with the emergence of trophozoites. Infection is established if the trophozoite can survive, attach to the intestinal mucosa, and multiply. This process may require nutrients within the intestinal fluid.

## CLINICAL FEATURES OF GIARDIASIS

Acute symptoms of giardiasis include watery diarrhea, nausea, bloating, belching (described as "sulfurous"), cramping, abdominal pain, and weight loss; these symptoms usually occur 1 to 2 weeks after the ingestion of cysts. The illness usually is self-limited, lasting 2 to 6 weeks, but may recur intermittently or become chronic. Chronic symptoms can include fatigue, nervousness, weight loss, growth retardation, steatorrhea, lactose intolerance, and, rarely, protein-losing enteropathy. Chronic giardiasis frequently is associated with immune deficiency syndromes such as IgA and IgM deficiencies and the acquired immunodeficiency syndrome. Individuals who are carrying the disease chronically may be asymptomatic.

## DIAGNOSIS

Routine laboratory values such as blood cell counts and electrolyte levels are normal in most patients. Nonspecific radiographic abnormalities that may be seen on barium contrast studies of the upper intestinal tract include thickening of the mucosal folds, hypersecretion with dilution of the barium column, and hypermotility.

Direct examination of feces for the presence of *G lamblia* cysts or trophozoites remains the hallmark for diagnosis. Direct fecal smears in physiologic saline are the easiest way to examine the stool microscopically. Recovery of the organism can be enhanced by a concentrating technique using either formal-ether or zinc sulfate flotation. Permanent slides then can be made using stains such as trichrome. Because *Giardia* cysts and trophozoites are not excreted continuously, however, even the best laboratories report a significant number of stool specimen results as negative in patients with disease. If the diagnosis is suspected strongly, at least three stools should be collected on different days. If both a direct smear and a concentration test are done on each stool, the chance of diagnosis is 75% from one stool, 90% from two stools, and 97% from three stools.

The diagnosis is made readily by examining the upper small intestine directly, either by mucosal biopsy or through the collection of jejunal contents. *Giardia* trophozoites can be seen in histologic sections of the small bowel, particularly if they are stained with trichrome. Their recovery can be enhanced by doing a "touch preparation" of the biopsy material. In this technique, the mucosal surface of the small-intestinal biopsy sample is touched to a glass slide before it is immersed in fixative. The slide then is air-dried, fixed in methanol, stained, and examined microscopically. Jejunal aspirates obtained by intubation or retrieved from a string carried into the intestine within a capsule (Entero-Test, Hedeco, Mountain View, California) also can be examined microscopically for the presence of *Giardia* trophozoites.

Diagnosis of giardiasis using both enzyme-linked immunosorbent assay and counterimmunoelectrophoresis of either stool or serum have become available recently.

## PATHOGENESIS

The pathogenesis of diarrhea and steatorrhea in giardiasis is not understood completely. Initially, it was thought that the organisms damaged the intestinal mucosa, either through direct invasion or through the elaboration of some toxin. Careful histologic studies with light and electron microscopy have shown this to be not true. Mechanical blockage of nutrient absorption resulting from the mass of *Giardia* organisms adhering to the intestinal mucosa also has been postulated. Histologic examination of the intestinal mucosa of diseased individuals, however, usually does not reveal enough organisms to support this hypothesis. *Giardia* appears to have the capability to alter intestinal motility, and this may play a role in the development of symptoms. Finally, careful electron microscopy has revealed that *Giardia* seems to stimulate excessive mucus production by the intestinal mucosa. This causes a thickening of the unstirred layer or glycocalyx adherent to the intestinal brush border and may result in a diffusion barrier for nutrients, ultimately causing diarrhea and malabsorption.

## TREATMENT

Treatment is indicated whenever *Giardia* is found to cause acute diarrhea, chronic intermittent disease, subclinical symptoms, or infection in others. It generally is not recommended that asymptomatic carriers be treated. Children with non-diarrheal giardiasis, however, who exhibit other gastrointestinal symptoms or have evidence of malabsorption should be considered for therapy. Public health considerations also might require that asymptomatic carriers be treated. The treatment of choice in both asymptomatic and symptomatic patients is metronidazole (Flagyl) administered in dosages of 250 mg three times daily for 1 week in adults, or 15 to 20 mg/kg/d, divided into three doses, for children. An alternative drug is quinacrine (Atabrine), 100 mg three times a day for 7 days in adults or 6 mg/kg/d divided into three doses for children (maximum 300 mg/d). Another drug that can be used is furazolidone (Furoxone), 100 mg four times daily for 7 to 10 days in adults or 6 mg/kg/d divided into four doses for children. Tinidazole has been evaluated extensively since the early 1970s and is highly effective in adults when given as a single 2-g dose, but it is not available yet in the United States. It also is effective in children when given by suppository for 1 to 3 days, thereby avoiding upper gastrointestinal side effects.

### Selected Readings

Addiss DG, Juranik DD, Spencer HC. Treatment of children with asymptomatic and non diarrheal Giardia infection. Pediatr Infect Dis J 1991;10:843.

Chandhuri DP, Das P, Bhattacharya SK, Bhattacharya MK, Pal SC. Enzyme immunoassay for detection of immunoglobulin M antibodies to Giardia lamblia. Eur J Clin Microbiol Infect Dis 1991;10:534.

Davidson RA. Issues in clinical parasitology: The treatment of giardiasis. Am J Gastroenterol 1984;79:256.

Forthing MJG, Mata L, Uriutia JJ, Kronmal RA. Natural history of Giardia infection of infants and children in rural Guatemala and its impact on physical growth. Am J Clin Nutr 1986;43:395.

McIntyre P, Boreham PFL, Phillips RE, Shepperd RW. Chemotherapy in giardiasis: Clinical responses and in vitro drug sensitivity of human isolates in axemic culture. J Pediatr 1986;108:1005.

Meyer EA, Jarroll EZ. Giardiasis. J Epidemiol Community Health 1980;111:1.

Solomons NW. Giardiasis: Nutrition implications. Rev Infect Dis 1982;4:859.

Wolfe MS. Giardiasis. Pediatr Clin North Am 1979;26:295.

*Principles and Practice of Pediatrics, Second Edition.*
edited by Frank A. Oski et al. J. B. Lippincott Company, Philadelphia © 1994.

## 62.1.5 *Malaria*

Lori E. R. Patterson

Although rarely seen in the United States, malaria is the most common infectious cause of morbidity in tropical and semitropical regions of the world. An estimated 2 to 3 million deaths annually, mostly of young children, are attributed to the disease. The illness, caused by one of the four species of *Plasmodium* parasite that are specific for humans, is characterized by recurrent paroxysms of high fever, splenomegaly, and anemia.

## THE ORGANISMS

The parasites responsible for malaria are obligate intracellular protozoa. *Plasmodium falciparum, Plasmodium vivax, Plasmodium malariae,* and *Plasmodium ovale* all are similar in their pattern of reproduction. The sexual portion of their life cycle begins when a female *Anopheles* mosquito feeds on an infected human. Malarial gametocytes ingested as part of this blood meal form zygotes in the mid-gut of the insect. These zygotes mature and migrate to the mosquito salivary gland, where they reside as sporozoites until the mosquito's next feeding, at which time they are inoculated into the next human victim.

Leaving the bloodstream almost immediately, the sporozoites invade human hepatocytes. There, nestled in parenchymal tissue, the parasite undergoes multiple asexual divisions to form a cystic structure called a schizont. One to 3 weeks after the initial inoculation, the schizont ruptures, releasing thousands of infective units (merozoites) into the bloodstream. It is at this stage that important species diversity exists: with infection by *P falciparum* or *P malariae,* all the schizonts rupture, effectively ending this exoerythrocytic (ie, intrahepatic) phase. In *P vivax* and *P ovale* infections, however, some of the schizonts remain dormant in the liver, only to rupture months to years later. These dormant forms (hypnozoites) are responsible for the clinical phenomenon of malarial relapse.

On release from the hepatic schizonts, the merozoites initiate the erythrocytic phase by attaching to and invading circulating red blood cells. The age of the erythrocyte influences attachment: *P vivax* and *P ovale* enter only immature erythrocytes, *P malariae* chooses mature cells, and *P falciparum* invades red cells of all ages.

Once inside the erythrocyte, the protozoan, now known as a trophozoite, appears as the characteristic blue "signet ring" against the pink cytoplasm of the blood cell. The organism ingests the host cell cytoplasm and hemoglobin, developing asexually from the ring form to the mature trophozoite. Nuclear division begins, creating schizonts; these ultimately will contain 6 to 24 merozoites, depending on the species. After this process of schizogony occurs (which takes about 72 hours for *P malariae* and 48 hours for the other species), the erythrocyte ruptures. This releases the merozoites, which enter uninfected red cells to start the erythrocytic cycle again. A small percentage of the merozoites diverge from this pattern, differentiating into the sexual gametocytes. These forms circulate in the bloodstream until they are ingested in the next mosquito feeding, thereby completing the life cycle.

## TRANSMISSION AND EPIDEMIOLOGY

Well known even in ancient times, malaria is endemic or hyperendemic in the tropics and subtropics, affecting many of the world's most densely populated regions. At present, malaria is found primarily in Mexico, parts of the Caribbean, Central and South America, sub-Saharan Africa, the Middle East, the Indian subcontinent, southern Asia and Indochina, and certain islands of the South Pacific. Estimates of global prevalence range from 100 to 400 million cases. *P vivax* is the most common species in the temperate and semitropic regions; *P falciparum* malaria predominates in Africa and other tropical areas. Standing water and warm climate (each of which is required for mosquito propagation) favor endemicity. Prerequisites for spread of the disease include the presence of a suitable anopheline vector along with infected and susceptible hosts.

Of particular concern in recent years has been the emergence of plasmodial resistance to chloroquine, the mainstay of pharmacologic therapy since World War II. First detected in the late 1950s, chloroquine-resistant *P falciparum* (CRPF) has spread to most of the areas where malaria is endemic (Table 62-1), sparing only the Middle East, Egypt, Central America west of the Panama Canal, the Dominican Republic, and Haiti. This resistance probably is conferred by the presence of a mutant gene. *P falciparum* resistance to pyrimethamine-sulfadoxine also is seen increasingly in southeast Asia (Thailand, Burma, Cambodia), the Amazon basin in South America, and sub-Saharan Africa. Rare cases of chloroquine resistance also have been reported for *P vivax*, but this phenomenon has not been noted in the other two species.

The United States, Canada, Europe, and Australia are considered to be free of naturally occurring malaria; episodes there usually can be traced to international travelers or immigrants (imported malaria). About 1200 cases are reported to the United States Centers for Disease Control (CDC) annually, although the incidence of *P falciparum* disease, the most serious variety, had been increasing rapidly before recent changes were made in routine chemoprophylaxis recommendations. It is likely that some milder cases go unrecognized by patients and physicians who are unfamiliar with the disease, as symptoms may mimic certain viral illnesses.

In addition to transmission by the mosquito, malaria can be spread through direct exposure to infected blood. Transfusions account for a few cases of malaria in the United States each year, although blood bank screening procedures are designed to prevent this passage. Infected blood also may be exchanged by needle-sharing during intravenous drug abuse. Another form of in-

**TABLE 62-1.  Countries Reporting Malaria***

**Countries With Chloroquine-Resistant Malaria†**

*Africa*

| | | | |
|---|---|---|---|
| Angola | Côte d'Ivoire | Madagascar | Somalia |
| Benin | Djibouti | Malawi | South Africa |
| Botswana?? | Equatorial Guinea? | Mali | Sudan |
| Burkina Faso | Ethiopia | Mauritania? | Swaziland |
| Burundi | Gabon | Mozambique | Tanzania, United Republic of |
| Cameroon | Gambia | Namibia | |
| Central African Republic | Ghana | Niger | Togo |
| | Guinea | Nigeria | Uganda |
| Chad | Guinea-Bissau | Rwanda | Zaire |
| Comoro Islands | Kenya | Senegal | Zambia |
| Congo | Liberia | Sierra Leone | Zimbabwe |

*Americas*

| | | | |
|---|---|---|---|
| Bolivia | Ecuador | Panama | Venezuela |
| Brazil | French Guiana | Peru | |
| Colombia | Guyana | Suriname | |

*Asia*

| | | | |
|---|---|---|---|
| Afghanistan | India | Malaysia | Philippines |
| Bangladesh | Indonesia | Myanmar | Sri Lanka |
| Bhutan | Iran | Nepal | Thailand |
| Cambodia | Lao People's Democratic Republic | Oman | Viet Nam |
| China | | Pakistan | Yemen |

*Oceania*

| | | |
|---|---|---|
| Papua New Guinea | Solomon Islands | Vanuatu |

**Countries Reporting Only Chloroquine-Sensitive Malaria‡**

*Africa*

| | | |
|---|---|---|
| Egypt | Mauritius | Sao Tome and Principe |

*Americas*

| | | |
|---|---|---|
| Argentina | El Salvador | Mexico |
| Belize | Guatemala | Nicaraqua |
| Costa Rica | Honduras | Paraguay |

*Caribbean*

| | |
|---|---|
| Dominican Republic | Haiti |

*Asia*

| | | |
|---|---|---|
| Iraq | Syrian Arab Republic | United Arab Emirates |
| Saudi Arabia | Turkey | |

* Note that only certain areas within a country may be involved; consult references for more specific details.
† Countries for which mefloquine or an alternative drug is recommended.
‡ Countries for which chloroquine prophylaxis is recommended.
?, probable; ??, suspected.
*From Health Information for International Travel. Atlanta, Georgia: Centers for Disease Control, 1991.*

direct spread, congenital malaria, appears in the young infant who was born to a mother who carried the infection during pregnancy. It appears likely that maternal–fetal transfusion, rather than transplacental passage of the parasite, is responsible for transmission, but the mother's immune status also appears to influence whether her fetus becomes infected. In each of these types of induced malaria, merozoites are introduced directly, so the exoerythrocytic phase does not occur.

## PATHOPHYSIOLOGY

Symptoms of malaria in the human host appear only at the time of erythrocyte lysis; the sexual forms and the exoerythrocytic stage seem to be tolerated well. Although fever is the most remarkable of these symptoms, attempts to identify a malarial pyrogen within the red cell debris have not been successful. Evidence also does not suggest that endogenous pyrogen is responsible, but tumor necrosis factor or other cytokines may have a role. Thus, the cause of the fever remains a mystery. Peripheral vasodilation occurs in response to the fever (and perhaps to vasoactive material produced by the parasite). Dilutional hyponatremia results from attempts to correct the diminished effective plasma volume. Decreased glycogen stores and impaired gluconeogenesis appear to contribute to hypoglycemia, as does energy consumption by the parasite.

Splenomegaly is a second key feature of the disease. Plasmodium-infected erythrocytes lose their deformability; this leads to increased trapping in the splenic cords, with subsequent enlargement of the spleen. Marked activation of the reticuloendothelial system also is responsible in part, as splenic macrophages become hyperplastic in their attempts to phagocytize the infected red blood cells and the debris released on hemolysis. Decreased numbers of platelets and neutrophils may be an untoward result. Vascular congestion in this organ greatly increases the risk of splenic rupture.

The anemia seen with malaria primarily is one of consumption as erythrocytes rupture or are phagocytized. The extent of hemolysis depends on the infecting species (eg, it is greatest in *P falciparum* infection, as its parasitemia is the most dense) and on the host's immune status. Nonetheless, the degree of anemia often is more severe than would be explained by the lysis of infected cells alone. Other contributing mechanisms may include autoimmune hemolysis, splenic sequestration of infected and normal erythrocytes, and disordered erythropoiesis. Hyperkalemia and hyperbilirubinemia are seen often; hemoglobinemia and hemoglobinuria occur if hemolysis is massive.

Pathology in the microvasculature accounts for many of the organ-specific aberrations in *P falciparum* malaria. Infected red blood cells become rigid and sticky, impeding passage through the capillaries; adherence to the endothelium of the smallest vessels occurs via "knobs" on the erythrocyte membrane. As cells and debris accumulate, flow becomes sluggish and local tissue hypoxia ensues. Capillary integrity is compromised, and fluid leakage or even hemorrhage into the surrounding tissue may occur. This pathologic chain of events may manifest clinically as cerebral malaria, pulmonary edema, renal cortical disruption and failure, and intestinal malabsorption or sloughing.

Both inherent and acquired factors contribute to host defense against malaria. The inherent factors, which may be particularly important in protecting young children, are those characteristics of the erythrocyte that make it relatively resistant to attachment and growth of the plasmodium. Attachment appears to depend on an interaction between specific organelles on the merozoite and particular erythrocyte surface structures. For instance, erythrocyte glycophorin A seems to be important for the attachment of *P falciparum.* Individuals lacking the Duffy blood group determinant (including most African blacks) are naturally resistant to *P vivax*; this species probably requires the cell-surface protein (or one linked to it) for attachment. The inherent relative resistance of individuals with hemoglobin S to malaria has been well-documented and, in fact, probably selects for that genetic subpopulation in regions where malaria is endemic. Similar selection appears to occur with other types of hemoglobinopathy, certain genetic erythrocyte defects, thalassemia, G6PD deficiency, and pyruvate kinase deficiency. Each of these abnormalities is thought to render the erythrocyte membrane resistant to invasion, or the cytoplasm inhospitable to parasite growth.

Humoral and cellular immunity to malaria are acquired with repeated infection. Although this immunity is not fully protective, it may alter the clinical expression of an infection, leaving an individual asymptomatic for extended periods. Individuals with malaria tend to exhibit a polyclonal hypergammaglobulinemia; the specific antibodies that are produced do provide some opsonic activity against infected erythrocytes, but protection is incomplete and temporary without continued exposure. The tendency of malaria to induce immunosuppression may explain partially the inadequacy of this response. Antigenic heterogeneity among plasmodia probably is a factor also. The monocyte/macrophage is the most important cellular participant in the phagocytosis of infected erythrocytes.

## CLINICAL MANIFESTATIONS

The clinical picture in malaria may vary considerably, depending on the species involved and on the patient's age and immune status. *P falciparum* produces the most severe symptoms; this probably correlates with the degree of parasitemia (up to 500,000 parasites per cubic millimeter of blood in severe cases). The other three species produce milder symptoms and may be considered as a group. In endemic areas, very young infants are relatively protected by virtue of their high concentration of hemoglobin F and their passive acquisition of maternal antibody. Older infants and young children (and their immunologic equivalent, previously unexposed adults) are the most susceptible to severe infection. Individuals who have attained immunity by virtue of repeated exposure to malaria generally have mild symptoms, even in the face of heavy parasitemia.

A quiescent period, corresponding to the exoerythrocytic phase of the parasite, follows the initial inoculation. During the first few cycles of erythrocytic infection, the nonimmune patient exhibits vague influenza-like symptoms of headache, malaise, irritability, anorexia, gastrointestinal complaints, and fever that may be continuous. After a number of infectious cycles, the symptoms often take on the classic "cold-hot-wet" pattern of the periodic fever paroxysm. Coinciding with erythrocytic rupture, the paroxysm consists of a brief episode of chills followed by several hours of sudden high fever, headache, nausea, vomiting, and myalgia, sometimes accompanied by delirium. Abdominal pain is prominent if rapid splenic enlargement has occurred. The patient may be prostrate and, as the ensuing defervescence is accompanied by marked diaphoresis, frequently suffers from dehydration. After a period of hours, the paroxysm ceases rather abruptly; the patient usually is quite fatigued and may rest soundly.

The paroxysm classically returns in 48 to 72 hours (depending on the species of *Plasmodium* involved), producing a fever curve described by the older clinical designations: quartan (*P malariae*), benign tertian (*P vivax* and *P ovale*), and malignant tertian (*P falciparum*). These patterns often are obscured, however, particularly if the patient is infected with more than one species or with more than one brood (leading to asynchronous release of parasites). Children are less likely than adults to show the characteristic fever curve, making the diagnosis less obvious in this age group; their fever more often is continuous or intermittent without pattern.

When it can be observed, the malarial paroxysm is the most characteristic of clinical findings. In its absence, splenomegaly usually is the most striking feature. The spleen may be massively enlarged, and care must be taken in its palpation, as the potential for rupture poses a significant danger. Tender hepatomegaly frequently occurs. Other common physical findings include orthostatic hypotension or other signs of dehydration, herpes labialis, icterus, and the pallor associated with anemia.

Laboratory data in malaria reflect hemolysis, with a normochromic, normocytic anemia, hyperbilirubinemia, and a direct Coombs' test result that frequently is positive. The leukocyte count and differential are unpredictable; an increased proportion of monocytes is common, but eosinophilia usually is not seen. Thrombocytopenia is common. The prothrombin time may be prolonged. Proteinuria often is evident. Hypoglycemia is common in patients with severe *P falciparum* malaria.

The clinical findings in congenital malaria tend to be nonspecific. Onset of the symptoms generally occurs toward the end of the first month of life, although the range is wide. The clinical picture may be indistinguishable from that of sepsis, with fever, irritability, lethargy, anorexia, and diarrhea. Physical examination reveals icterus and hepatosplenomegaly. Hemolytic anemia, reticulocytosis, and thrombocytopenia are common.

The malarial paroxysms finally end after the administration of antimalarial agents or the development of appropriate immunity. With *P vivax* or *P ovale* infection, however, relapse of the disease may occur at irregular intervals. This phenomenon coincides with maturation and rupture of the previously dormant hepatic schizonts, and it may continue for years unless specific therapy is given.

## COMPLICATIONS

Malarial infections from species other than *P falciparum* usually are relatively benign and do not produce significant morbidity or mortality for an otherwise healthy host. The exception to this rule is an infrequently seen immune complex nephritis that occurs in some children with chronic *P malariae* infection. This species also may cause a childhood nephrotic syndrome that is refractory to usual treatment methods and to antimalarial agents. Immune suppression with resultant secondary infection may occur with any species of plasmodia.

In contrast, *P falciparum* malaria is potentially quite severe, and complications occur more frequently. The most serious of these is cerebral malaria, which manifests clinically as headache, persistent mental status changes, diminished level of consciousness, prolonged seizures, coma, or other neurologic aberrations. On lumbar puncture, the opening pressure is elevated, but the cerebrospinal fluid usually is normal. The fatality rate is high, and residual neurologic deficit occurs occasionally, especially in patients who are hypoglycemic when first seen. A good prognosis depends on prompt antimalarial therapy and intensive supportive management.

A second complication of *P falciparum* malaria is "blackwater fever," or hemoglobinuria. The urine appears dark and the patient's condition may progress to acute renal failure. This entity is seen in the face of massive hemolysis. Hypersensitivity to quinine may play a role in some cases. Other conditions seen with severe malaria include adult respiratory distress syndrome, high-output congestive heart failure, dehydration, jaundice, severe anemia, disseminated intravascular coagulopathy, hypoglycemia, and circulatory collapse. "Big spleen disease" (also known as tropical splenomegaly syndrome) generally is seen in children,

and probably represents an abnormal, genetically linked immune response to chronic malaria.

## DIAGNOSIS

In malaria-endemic regions, diagnosis of the disease is not difficult and usually is made on clinical grounds. For individuals outside these areas, however, the key is remembering the disease as part of the differential diagnosis. Travel to endemic areas (even years earlier) and adherence to chemoprophylaxis guidelines are important clues. A history of recurrent high fevers also is helpful, if present. The triad of fever, splenomegaly, and anemia always should suggest the diagnosis. A fever paroxysm is impressive when it is witnessed firsthand by observers who are unfamiliar with the disease.

Examination of Giemsa-stained peripheral blood smears continues to be the primary method of diagnosis for malaria. Because of generally low levels of parasitemia (less than 1% of erythrocytes are infected in cases caused by species other than *P falciparum*), a thick smear is done first for screening. Multiple thick smears performed at 12-hour intervals optimize detection of the parasite. If infected red cells are found, a review of a thin smear by an experienced examiner usually will allow species identification based on the morphology of the intracellular trophozoites. Other diagnostic techniques, such as specific antibody detection and DNA probing, generally are reserved for research and epidemiologic studies.

## DIFFERENTIAL DIAGNOSIS

With its variety of systemic symptoms, malaria may mimic other febrile diseases of childhood, such as meningitis, appendicitis, gastroenteritis, or hepatitis. Milder forms of the disease are mistaken most frequently for influenza or other viral illnesses. A febrile illness in a patient who recently has traveled to an endemic area must be considered to be malaria, however, until proven otherwise.

## TREATMENT

Once the diagnosis of malaria has been made, treatment should be initiated immediately. With severely ill patients for whom the index of suspicion is high, some authorities recommend treating presumptively before laboratory confirmation is available. Delay in treatment may affect prognosis adversely in *P falciparum* infection.

In addition to quinine, currently available antimalarial drugs include the other arylaminoalcohols, synthetic aminoquinolines, and folate antagonists. The exact mechanism of action of quinine and its group and of the related aminoquinolines is unknown. The 4-aminoquinolines (eg, chloroquine) affect the erythrocytic parasites only; the slower-acting 8-aminoquinolines (eg, primaquine) kill both hepatic and erythrocytic parasites. Quinine also attacks both phases. Mefloquine, a 4-quinoline methanol derivative, generally is reserved for prophylaxis (see below) rather than for treatment, because of an increased incidence of side effects at doses required for the latter. A related antimalarial agent, halofantrine, recently has been approved in the United States for the treatment of CRPF, as well as for *P vivax*, but experience with its use in children is limited. Pyrimethamine and the sulfa drugs are representative of the folate antagonists; these generally are used as second-line antimalarial agents. Not currently available in the United States, proguanil is a dihydrofolate reductase inhibitor that often is used for prophylaxis. Doxycycline and clindamycin also are chosen occasionally for prophylaxis or therapy, although their use in malaria is considered to be experimental.

Key issues in deciding on drug(s) of choice for malaria treatment include: species identity (*P falciparum* versus another species); the possibility that the strain is chloroquine-resistant if the infection is with *P falciparum*; and the ability of the patient to take medication orally. Infections with species other than *P falciparum* and those with sensitive strains of *P falciparum* are treated in the same manner in patients with acute infection (ie, with chloroquine [Aralen] orally or quinidine gluconate parenterally). If the history does not clearly suggest the source of a *P falciparum* infection, chloroquine resistance must be assumed and the patient treated accordingly. Oral therapy is standard, but a patient who is comatose, or one who has significant emesis or parasitemia of more than 5% will require parenteral therapy until clinical improvement allows a change to oral medication. Quinine was the parenteral drug of choice for years, but this has been supplanted in the United States by quinidine gluconate, which is more readily available and at least as efficacious. Specific dosage schedules are listed in Table 62-2.

Because they have a persistent exoerythrocytic phase, infections with *P vivax* or *P ovale* require additional treatment with primaquine to prevent relapses ("radical cure"). Primaquine may precipitate hemolysis in G6PD-deficient patients, so the presence of the enzyme should be confirmed before the drug is administered. If deficiency exists, the patient may be given chloroquine prophylaxis continuously over the period of potential relapse, usually 3 to 4 years. Malaria acquired by means other than mos-

quito bite (eg, congenitally) does not require primaquine therapy, as the exoerythrocytic phase is bypassed in these situations.

Supportive care is an important adjunct to antimalarial chemotherapy. Volume depletion should be corrected rapidly, but with care. Analgesics and antipyretics will make the patient more comfortable. If parenteral quinidine is used, an intensive care setting with continuous cardiac monitoring and close attention to fluid status (central hemodynamic monitoring in severe cases) is recommended; frequent determinations of the QT interval (a sensitive indicator of quinidine concentration) and blood glucose level should be made. Some experts advocate the use of exchange transfusion in patients with severe or complicated malaria, as a means of rapidly reducing the level of parasitemia and possibly removing plasmodia-related toxic factors. The total volume of exchange should be based on reaching a parasitemia of less than 1%. The use of corticosteroids in cerebral malaria probably is unwarranted, as they may increase complication rates and the duration of coma.

## PREVENTION

In 1955, the World Health Organization initiated a global strategy for the eradication of malaria. Despite intensive efforts, the program officially was declared a failure 21 years later. Many factors contributed to this lack of success; the development of CRPF, resistance of the anopheline vector to chemical pesticides such as dichlorodiphenyltrichloroethane (DDT), and failure of Third

### TABLE 62-2.   Treatment of Malaria (*Plasmodium* species)

| Species | Oral Therapy | Parenteral Therapy* |
|---|---|---|
| *P vivax, P ovale, P malariae,* or chloroquine-sensitive *P falciparum* | Chloroquine phosphate 10 mg base/kg (maximum 600 mg) immediately, then 5 mg base/kg (maximum 300 mg) 6 h later and once on each of next 2 days† | Quinidine gluconate 10 mg/kg (loading dose) intravenously over 1–2 h, followed by constant infusion at rate of 0.02 mg/kg/min |
| Chloroquine-resistant *P falciparum* | Quinine sulfate 8 mg/kg (maximum 650 mg) 3 times daily × 3 d | Quinidine gluconate as above |
| | PLUS | |
| | Pyrimethamine-sulfadoxine (Fansidar), single dose: 5–10 kg: ½ tablet | |
| | 10–20 kg: 1 tablet | |
| | 20–30 kg: 1½ tablet | |
| | 30–45 kg: 2 tablets | |
| | >45 kg: 3 tablets | |
| | OR PLUS | |
| | Tetracycline‡ 5 mg/kg (maximum 250 mg) four times daily × 7 d | |
| | ALTERNATIVE | |
| | Halofantrine every 6 h × 3 doses§ | |
| | ≤40 kg: 8 mg/kg/dose | |
| | >40 kg: 500 mg/dose | |
| *P vivax* or *P ovale* (for relapse prevention) | Primaquine¶ 0.3 mg base/kg (maximum 15 mg) daily × 14 d | |

\* To be given only if patient is unable to take oral drug or has parasitemia >5%; patient should be monitored in intensive care unit setting (see text). Therapy should be changed to oral form as soon as tolerated by patient.
† Longer therapy may be required for malaria from certain areas (eg, Thailand).
‡ For patients 8 years or older only.
§ Repeat in 1 week for young children and nonimmune travelers; also may be used for *P vivax*.
¶ Determine G6PD status before administration (see text).

World governments to devote the resources necessary for a project of such magnitude often are cited. As a result, the onus for malaria prevention now rests with the individual. The most successful regimens combine personal environmental protection with chemoprophylaxis during exposure in endemic regions. Given the nocturnal feeding behavior of the *Anopheles* mosquito, environmental protection—avoiding mosquito bites—is most important from dusk to dawn. Recommended measures include wearing long clothing, covering exposed areas of the body sparingly with insect repellent (preparations containing N,N diethylmetatoluamide, or DEET, are most effective), remaining in screened-in areas as much as possible, and using fine mesh mosquito netting around beds. Permethrin also may be applied to clothing for extra protection. A flying-insect spray containing pyrethrum also may be useful for living quarters during the evening and nighttime.

The use of drugs to prevent malaria is recommended highly for travelers to regions where the disease is endemic. The risk of exposure generally is higher in rural areas than in cities, and the travel itinerary should be reviewed carefully to ascertain the need for chemoprophylaxis. Unless otherwise noted below, the drug should be taken once weekly, starting 1 to 2 weeks before departure, continuing throughout the trip, and ending 4 weeks after leaving the endemic area. Chloroquine in a dose of 5 mg base per kilogram orally (maximum 300 mg base or 500 mg salt) is the drug of choice for travel to areas that do not have chloroquine resistance. If this drug is not tolerated, one alternative is hydroxychloroquine (Plaquenil), at 5 mg base per kilogram (maximum 310 mg base) weekly.

If exposure to regions with CRPF is planned, prophylaxis with mefloquine (Lariam) should be used, following the same schedule as above. This drug, which is available in a 250-mg tablet, should be taken weekly as follows, based on body weight: 15 to 19 kg, ¼ tablet; 20 to 30 kg, ½ tablet; 31 to 45 kg, ¾ tablet; >45 kg, 1 tablet. Mefloquine is contraindicated in children weighing less than 15 kg, in pregnant women, and in those who have a history of convulsive or psychiatric disorder, or who take beta blockers or other medications that may alter cardiac conductivity. In addition, it should not be taken by those individuals whose daily tasks involve fine coordination or spatial discrimination.

For those travelers to CRPF-endemic areas for whom mefloquine is not appropriate, options for prophylaxis are less satisfactory. One choice is doxycycline taken at 2 mg/kg (maximum 100 mg) daily, but this also is contraindicated in pregnant women and in children less than 8 years of age. If none of the above choices are possible, the traveler should take chloroquine prophylaxis, plus carry a treatment dose of pyrimethamine-sulfadoxine (Fansidar) to be taken immediately in the event of febrile illness. Medical attention should be sought as soon as possible. Fansidar dosing for the treatment of presumptive malaria is based on weight (see Table 62-2).

The above pharmacologic measures will not prevent the establishment of exoerythrocytic infection by *P vivax* or *P ovale*. If there is significant concern about exposure to either of these species, additional prophylaxis with primaquine may be given to eliminate this stage of the parasite. The dose is 0.3 mg base per kilogram (maximum 15 mg base or 26.3 mg salt) orally each day for 14 days, coincident with the last 2 weeks of chloroquine prophylaxis. Prophylaxis with primaquine usually is reserved for individuals with prolonged stays in endemic areas.

Antimalarial agents themselves may produce side effects that should be brought to the attention of the traveler. Chloroquine occasionally causes minor gastrointestinal disturbances, headache, dizziness, blurred vision, and exacerbation of psoriasis; pruritus is one of its most vexing effects. Quinine frequently causes tinnitus, headache, nausea, abdominal pain, and visual changes. Notable effects of parenteral quinidine may include hypotension,

hypoglycemia, and cardiac dysrhythmias. Side effects from mefloquine are minor and transient at prophylactic doses (vertigo, nausea and other gastrointestinal disturbances, headache, and visual disturbances predominate), but more serious neuropsychiatric effects, such as seizures and psychosis, may be seen with higher doses, precluding its routine use for treatment. Coincident or sequential use of quinine or quinidine with mefloquine may potentiate the side effects of the latter drug. Halofantrine generally is well tolerated.

The use of environmental protection and chemoprophylaxis does not absolutely guarantee against the acquisition of malaria. Travelers should be alert to the possibility of infection, and should seek medical attention at the onset of febrile illness both during their trip and after returning. For further questions regarding prophylaxis or treatment of malaria, the physician may contact the Malaria Branch of the CDC at (404) 488-4046; 24-hour information is available on the CDC Malaria Hotline at (404) 332-4555. Current advice on prophylaxis is published yearly in the CDC's *Health Information for International Travel*.

## OUTLOOK

Since the failed attempt at global eradication of malaria, other means of controlling the disease have been sought. Central to this effort has been the attempt to develop an immunization against malaria; several candidate vaccines are in testing at present. In addition, screening programs continue to identify new drugs with promising activity against CRPF. Implementing these new measures will do much to reduce the impact of this serious disease.

## Selected Readings

Bryson HM, Goa KL. Halofantrine: A review of its antimalarial activity, pharmacologic properties and therapeutic potential. Drugs 1992;43:236.

Centers for Disease Control. Health information for international travel, 1991. Atlanta, Georgia: US Department of Health and Human Services, Public Health Service, 1991, DHHS Publication No. (CDC) 91-8280.

Drugs for parasitic infections. Med Lett Drugs Ther 1990;32:23.

Hulbert TV. Congenital malaria in the United States: Report of a case and review. Clin Infect Dis 1992;14:922.

Lynk A, Gold R. Review of 40 children with imported malaria. Pediatr Infect Dis J 1989;8:745.

Miller KD, Greenberg AE, Campbell CC. Treatment of severe malaria in the United States with a continuous infusion of quinidine gluconate and exchange transfusion. N Engl J Med 1989;321:65.

Randall G, Seidel JS. Malaria. Pediatr Clin North Am 1985;32:893.

Wyler DJ. Malaria—resurgence, resistance, and research. N Engl J Med 1983;308:875.

*Principles and Practice of Pediatrics, Second Edition.*
edited by Frank A. Oski et al. J. B. Lippincott Company, Philadelphia © 1994.

### 62.1.6 *Toxoplasmosis*

Christopher B. Wilson

Infection with the coccidian parasite *Toxoplasma gondii* may be asymptomatic or symptomatic. Symptomatic infection produces the disease toxoplasmosis, although in many cases, mild symptomatic infection is not recognized or diagnosed. The disease in humans was recognized first in congenitally infected infants and later in adults. In 1948, Sabin and Feldman described a serologic test, the dye test, that allowed the epidemiology and spectrum of the disease to be determined in humans. In 1969, the organism was found to be a member of the family Coccidia, and its life cycle was defined.

## THE ORGANISM AND ITS TRANSMISSION

*T gondii* exists in three forms: the proliferative form, or tachyzoite; a tissue cyst that contains many bradyzoites; and an oocyst. The cat family is the definitive host of the organism. The tachyzoite and tissue cyst occur in extraintestinal tissues of cats and are the only forms of the parasite in other mammalian and avian hosts. The oocyst forms only during the enteroepithelial stage of infection in members of the cat family.

The tachyzoite form is crescent-shaped or oval, measures about 3 by 7 $\mu$m, and is seen during the acute stage of infection. It invades all mammalian cells except perhaps nonnucleated red blood cells. After penetration, the tachyzoite multiplies by endodyogeny, causing disruption of the cells. It is delicate and cannot withstand freezing and thawing, desiccation, or brief exposure to gastric or duodenal digestive juices.

The cyst form is demonstrable in tissues, particularly muscle, as early as the first week of infection, and varies in size from about 10 to 100 $\mu$m. There usually is no inflammatory reaction around cysts. Because this form may persist in the tissues of infected but clinically normal children and adults for their lifetime, its demonstration in histologic sections does not necessarily signify recent infection. Cysts in the muscle (meat) of domestic animals are one source of human infection. After ingestion of meat containing cysts, peptic or tryptic digestive fluids disrupt the cyst wall. The liberated organisms (which resemble the tachyzoite form morphologically) can survive in these fluids for several hours, which allows time for them to invade local cells. The cyst is destroyed and meat is rendered noninfectious by heating to 66 °C, by freezing to less than −20 °C and then thawing, and by desiccation. The cyst can survive for some months at refrigeration temperatures (4 °C) if it is in tissue.

The oocyst form has been demonstrated only in the feces of members of the cat family, the definitive host for *Toxoplasma*. The oocyst is ovoid and measures about 10 by 12 $\mu$m. Infected cats may shed as many as 10 million oocysts each day, which may be excreted for as long as 3 weeks after primary (acute) infection, but rarely thereafter. Of note, cats that are seropositive for *Toxoplasma* almost never shed oocysts. Thus, the seronegative cat (frequently a kitten) that acquires new infection through ingestion of meat containing viable cysts is the more likely source for transmission of the infection to humans. Excreted oocysts become infectious only after they undergo sporulation (eight sporozoites in each oocyst); this occurs from 1 to 21 days (most commonly 2 to 8 days) after excretion, depending on the temperature and availability of oxygen. The oocyst is far more resistant than the other forms, and can survive for months in water and for a year or more in moist soil. Ingestion of sporulated oocysts transmits the infection.

## EPIDEMIOLOGY

The infection may be transmitted congenitally or acquired after birth.

### Congenital Infection

The congenital infection is considered to occur, with extremely rare exception, only when primary maternal infection with *Toxoplasma* occurs.

The only well-documented cases of transmission from mothers with preexisting *Toxoplasma* infection are three infants born to pregnant women who were immunodeficient as a result of therapy for systemic lupus erythematosus or Hodgkin's disease, or because of the acquired immunodeficiency syndrome (AIDS), respectively. Firm documentation is lacking in other purported cases of transmission from chronically infected mothers. Similarly, data that suggest a causal relationship between chronic infection and spontaneous abortion are insufficient to confirm the significance of such an association. Thus, nearly all perinatal morbidity and mortality related to *Toxoplasma* infection is due to acquisition of primary infection during gestation.

In the United States, about 70% to 85% of women in the childbearing age group lack antibodies and are susceptible to primary infection. The incidence of primary maternal infection during gestation has been estimated to be 6 per 1000 pregnancies in this country. Because about 55% of the women who acquire the infection during pregnancy *and are not treated* give birth to congenitally infected infants, the estimated incidence of congenital infection is 2 to 3 per 1000 live births. This value is similar to the observed incidence of congenital infection (2.2 per 1000 live births) reported in two prospective studies in the United States. Estimated rates of congenital infection in other countries range from 2 to 7 per 1000 live births.

Fetal infection appears not to occur when the onset of maternal infection clearly precedes the time of conception. The high rate of maternal–fetal transmission that is observed when maternal infection is acquired late in pregnancy may be due to transmission of infection during labor. In contrast to the increased risk of fetal infection when maternal infection is acquired late in gestation, the severity of disease in infected offspring is less when maternal infection is acquired late in gestation (see Clinical Syndromes). The greater severity of disease seen in infants whose mothers acquire infection early in gestation may result from the relative immaturity of fetal host defense mechanisms in early compared to late gestation.

### Acquired Infection

Infection with *Toxoplasma* is common in humans. The prevalence of *Toxoplasma* antibodies rises with increasing age, and little or no difference in the prevalence of infection exists between the sexes.

The discovery that feces of infected cats may contain infectious oocysts supports the contention that this household pet may be an important source of transmission. Humans and other mammals are intermediate hosts. If infected tissue (eg, rat) is consumed by a cat, the sexual cycle is induced in the cat intestine; oocysts are excreted and are infectious for mammals and birds, in which the life cycle (tachyzoites and cysts) is perpetuated. Flies, cockroaches, and probably other coprophagic insects can serve as transport hosts for oocysts that may contaminate food consumed by humans. Although inadvertent ingestion of oocysts appears to be the major mode of transmission, this remains to be proved. Meat (particularly pork and lamb) frequently contains *Toxoplasma* cysts and may serve as a source of infection if it is eaten raw or undercooked. It is unlikely that this is the principal mode of spread of infection in most areas of the world, however, because, in the same geographic location, non–meat-eating populations have been found to have the same prevalence of *Toxoplasma* seropositivity as do those who consume meat. The source of infection in seropositive vegetarians is unknown, but felines seem likely. Accidental self-inoculation with a needle contaminated with *Toxoplasma* has resulted in a number of acquired infections in laboratory workers.

Recently, common source outbreaks of acute, acquired *Toxo*-

*plasma* infection have been documented and have been linked to exposure to cats, raw goat's milk, or inadequately cooked meat. Because of the high incidence of common source exposure, the families of patients with symptomatic infection should be evaluated for subclinical infection.

## CLINICAL SYNDROMES

Toxoplasmosis in children may be considered in three categories: congenital, postnatally acquired, and ocular (which may be congenital or acquired). Clinically apparent infection in older children may be recently acquired or due to reactivation of latent congenital or postnatally acquired infection. Both congenital and acquired infections usually are asymptomatic, and the latter rarely result in serious sequelae.

### Congenital Toxoplasmosis

Congenital infection most often is the result of an asymptomatic acute infection in the mother. Spontaneous abortion, prematurity, or stillbirth may result. Congenital toxoplasmosis has a wide spectrum of clinical manifestations and may mimic other diseases of the newborn. In severe cases, fever, hydrocephalus or microcephalus, hepatosplenomegaly, jaundice, convulsions, chorioretinitis, cerebral calcifications, and abnormal cerebrospinal fluid (CSF) findings (xanthochromia and mononuclear pleocytosis) are common. In a series of patients with this syndrome, the mortality rate was 12%; sequelae in survivors included mental retardation (90%), convulsions, spasticity and paresis (about 75%), and severely impaired vision (50%). Other common findings include rash (maculopapular, petechial, or both), myocarditis, pneumonitis and respiratory distress, hearing defect, thrombocytopenia, lymphocytosis, monocytosis, nephrotic syndrome, and a picture similar to that of erythroblastosis.

In a prospective study of mothers who had acquired *Toxoplasma* infection during pregnancy *and who did not receive treatment for their infection during pregnancy*, 9 (6%) pregnancies ended in stillbirth and 85 (55%) resulted in the birth of infected liveborn infants. The risk of infection to the fetus varied significantly with the trimester of gestation during which the mother became infected. For untreated women, it was about 25% in the first trimester, 54% in the second trimester, and 65% in the third trimester. For treated women, the respective percentages of infected offspring were about 8%, 19%, and 44%. The incidence of infection in the offspring of mothers treated during pregnancy was reduced, but the severity of clinical disease was not diminished.

A prospective study of infants born to mothers known to have acquired primary infection during pregnancy revealed significant morbidity in 210 congenitally infected infants (Table 62-3). Overall, 2 cases (0.9%) were fatal, 21 (10.9%) were severe, 71 (33.8%) were mild, and 116 were asymptomatic. About 40% to 45% of the mothers had been treated with spiramycin during pregnancy. Interestingly, clinically overt disease was slightly more common in infected infants born to the treated mothers.

These observations indicate that congenital infection is more likely to be clinically inapparent and rarely fulminant. In infants with clinically inapparent infection, however, intensive examination frequently reveals abnormalities. In one study of 116 infants initially thought to be normal by routine examination, 39 had one or more abnormalities on more careful evaluation; of these 39, 22 (56%) had abnormal CSF, 17 (44%) had chorioretinitis, and 10 (26%) had intracranial calcifications. Furthermore, sequelae develop later in some infected children without overt disease. In three recent studies, chorioretinitis developed sub-

**TABLE 62-3. Prospective Study of Infants Born to Women Who Acquired *Toxoplasma* Infection During Pregnancy: Signs and Symptoms in 210 Infants With Proved Congenital Infection**

| Finding | Number Examined | Number (%) Positive |
|---|---|---|
| Prematurity | | |
| Birth weight <2500 g | 210 | 8 (3.8) |
| Birth weight 2500–3000 g | | 15 (7.1) |
| Dysmaturity (intrauterine growth retardation) | 210 | 13 (6.2) |
| Icterus | 201 | 20 (9.5) |
| Hepatosplenomegaly | 210 | 9 (4.2) |
| Thrombocytopenic purpura | 210 | 3 (1.4) |
| Abnormal blood count (anemia, eosinophilia) | 102 | 9 (4.4) |
| Microcephaly | 210 | 11 (5.2) |
| Hydrocephaly | 210 | 8 (3.8) |
| Hypotonia | 210 | 12 (5.7) |
| Convulsions | 210 | 8 (3.8) |
| Psychomotor retardation | 210 | 11 (5.2) |
| Intracranial calcifications on radiography | 103 | 24 (11.4) |
| Abnormal electroencephalogram results | 191 | 16 (8.3) |
| Abnormal cerebrospinal fluid (pleocytosis or increased protein level) | 163 | 56 (34.2) |
| Microphthalmia | 210 | 6 (2.8) |
| Strabismus | 210 | 11 (5.2) |
| Chorioretinitis | 210 | 46 (21.9) |
| Asymptomatic | 210 | 116 (55.2) |

Adapted from Couvreur J, Desmonts G, Tournier G, et al. Etude d'une serie homogène de 210 cas de toxoplasmose congenital chez des nourrissons ages de 0 a 11 mois et depistes de façon prospective. Ann Pediatr (Paris) 1984;31: 815.

sequently by adolescence in 18% to 75% of such children. Blindness, hydrocephalus and microcephalus, cerebral calcifications, psychomotor or mental retardation, epilepsy, and deafness may develop, but are much less common (<20%). These data indicate that many congenitally infected children, including those with inapparent infection as neonates, suffer untoward sequelae during childhood. At present, it is not possible to predict the outcome in those with inapparent infection as neonates.

Manifestations of clinical toxoplasmosis in the newborn may mimic infection with other organisms and must be differentiated from infections with cytomegalovirus (CMV), herpes simplex virus, rubella virus, *Treponema pallidum* (syphilis), human immunodeficiency virus (HIV) and certain bacteria (eg, *Listeria*), erythroblastosis, and many of the encephalopathies secondary to degenerative disorders.

### Acquired Toxoplasmosis

Acquired *Toxoplasma* infection is most often asymptomatic and goes unrecognized; about 10% of infected individuals have clinical symptoms and signs. In certain recent outbreaks related to infection by oocysts, however, more than half the infected patients were symptomatic. The most common finding is lymphadenopathy and fatigue without fever. The nodes are discrete, may or may not be tender, and do not suppurate. The groups of nodes most commonly involved are the cervical, suboccipital, supraclavicular, axillary, and inguinal nodes. Adenopathy may be localized or it may involve multiple areas. Uncommonly, the lymphadenopathy is accompanied by fever, malaise, fatigue, sore throat, and myalgia, a picture that closely resembles that of infectious mononucleosis, but the heterophil test is negative. The lymphadenopathy also may simulate lymphoma. Chorioretinitis may develop, but is not recognized commonly. In more severe infections, the liver may be involved. In persons with normal immunologic function and without severe underlying disease, the infection usually is self-limited, resolving over 3 to 12 weeks, and rarely requires treatment. In contrast, more severe and frequently fulminant infections are seen in patients receiving immunosuppressive therapy, in those who have disease of the bone marrow or reticuloendothelial system, and in those with congenital immunodeficiencies. Pneumonitis, myocarditis, maculopapular rash, and encephalitis are encountered frequently in acute infection in immunocompromised patients. Although they are uncommon, any of these more serious manifestations may occur in an otherwise normal child.

## Toxoplasma Encephalitis

Toxoplasma encephalitis may occur in the acute phase of a congenital infection or in an infection in an immunocompromised host. It is observed much more commonly now, however, as a recrudescence of latent central nervous system (CNS) infection in patients with AIDS. It is estimated that Toxoplasma encephalitis will develop in as many as 10% of all patients with AIDS in the United States. The predominant neurologic symptoms are headache, disorientation, and drowsiness; the CNS lesion may behave as a mass lesion. In view of the variety of clinical manifestations of CNS involvement, it is important to consider toxoplasmosis whenever there is evidence of CNS damage. Other conditions that produce focal mass lesions in such patients include abscess, tumor, tuberculoma, and Candida, Cryptococcus, or Aspergillus infections. Viral encephalitis may mimic nonfocal infection.

## Toxoplasma Infection in Children With Human Immunodeficiency Virus Infection

To date, nine infants or preschool children with HIV and Toxoplasma infection have been reported. Of these, at least six acquired both infections in utero or perinatally. All but one of these infants had CNS disease in association with hepatosplenomegaly, lymphadenopathy, or chorioretinitis, with manifestations apparent by 4 months of age. Two infants, one of whom was treated for Toxoplasma infection, remained asymptomatic. One other child acquired HIV infection from a blood transfusion at 18 months of age and died with Toxoplasma encephalitis at 5 years of age.

## Ocular Toxoplasmosis

In active congenital toxoplasmosis, retinal lesions commonly are bilateral. In older children, retinochoroiditis may involve only one eye and may be the only manifestation of congenital toxoplasmosis. Even in older children and adults, retinochoroiditis caused by Toxoplasma most frequently is the result of reactivation of a latent congenital infection. In some studies, Toxoplasma has accounted for as much as 5% of severe visual impairments in children.

The patient may present with marked loss of central vision (resulting from a perimacular lesion) or hazy vision (resulting from accumulated exudate from peripheral foci). Neonates or infants with Toxoplasma eye disease may have microphthalmia, small cornea, posterior cortical cataract, anisometropia, strabis-

mus, and nystagmus. Strabismus and nystagmus in any child should raise the possibility of congenital toxoplasmosis. The appearance of lesions in the fundus is not specific, however; the characteristic lesion of ocular toxoplasmosis is a focal necrotizing retinitis. In the acute phase, such lesions appear as indistinct, yellow to white, cotton-like patches in the fundus, usually in association with a vitreous flare; healed lesions are demarcated sharply and are white to gray with accumulations of choroidal pigment. Both acute and healed lesions may be present at birth in infected neonates. Lesions commonly are bilateral and located near the posterior pole. Associated findings may include anterior uveitis, optic atrophy, microphthalmia, nystagmus, strabismus, cataracts, and iritis.

The differential diagnosis of ocular toxoplasmosis in infants includes other congenital infections (CMV, rubella virus, herpes simplex virus, syphilis), birth injury, congenital anomalies, Aicardi's syndrome, congenital vascular malformation, and neoplasms. In older children, Toxocara and Histoplasma infections must be considered.

## LABORATORY DIAGNOSIS

Acute infection is diagnosed by the isolation of T gondii from blood or body fluids, the demonstration of tachyzoites in histologic sections of tissue or cytologic preparations of body fluids, the detection of characteristic lymph node histology or serologic test results, and the demonstration of Toxoplasma cysts in the placenta, fetus, or neonate. The detection of Toxoplasma by amplification of specific portions of its DNA using the polymerase chain reaction is promising, but its value as a diagnostic test remains to be established. Each of these methods is discussed below, with an emphasis on serologic tests, which are the most common techniques of establishing the diagnosis.

### Serologic Methods

#### Tests That Measure IgG Antibody

The most useful tests for the demonstration of IgG antibodies to Toxoplasma include the Sabin-Feldman dye test, the indirect immunofluorescent antibody (IFA) test, modified direct agglutination tests, and the enzyme-linked immunosorbent assay (ELISA). In these tests, IgG antibodies appear within the first week of primary infection and reach peak titers (usually 1:500 or greater) within 1 to 2 months; detectable titers usually persist for life. Although the dye test is the most reliable, it is available only in a few reference laboratories. The IFA and ELISA tests are the most widely available and, when performed properly, they yield results similar to those obtained with the dye test; however, many laboratories use commercially available kits, which are not consistently reliable. False-positive IFA test results occur on some sera that contain antinuclear antibodies. The direct agglutination tests are accurate and simple to perform. Results of ELISAs are reported differently depending on the nature of the reagents or kits used. Thus, it is not possible to describe here which results are meaningful. Consultation with the laboratory providing the test regarding the interpretation and reliability of the results is suggested. Other tests vary in their reliability and are not recommended.

Meaningful interpretation of changes in titer on sequential sera requires that assays on each sample be performed concomitantly by a reliable laboratory.

#### Tests That Measure IgM or IgA Antibody

Because IgG antibodies persist for life, tests that detect antibodies that are induced solely or primarily during acute, primary infection and that persist for shorter periods of time are useful. The detection of IgM antibodies has been used most commonly for this purpose, either by the IgM-IFA, IgM-ISAGA or IgM-ELISA techniques. The IgM-ISAGA and IgM-ELISA techniques are much more sensitive than the IgM-IFA test. These newer tests also are not associated with the false-positive reactions that are observed with the IgM-IFA test when rheumatoid factor or antinuclear antibodies are present. Accordingly, the IgM-ISAGA and IgM-ELISA tests are preferred. Using these more sensitive techniques, IgM antibodies usually are detectable within the first 1 to 2 weeks of primary infection, peak within 1 month, and remain elevated for periods ranging from several months to longer than 1 year.

Recent reports suggest that tests that detect specific IgA antibodies are a useful adjunct to the IgM tests, particularly for the diagnosis of acute, acquired infection in the pregnant woman and for the diagnosis of infection in the fetus and neonate. The detection of specific IgA antibody has been done by ELISA, but these tests are not widely available yet. Consultation with a reference laboratory performing these tests is recommended for assistance in prenatal testing and testing of neonates with suspected congenital *Toxoplasma* infection.

## Diagnosis in Specific Clinical Situations

### Congenital *Toxoplasma* Infection

The demonstration of IgM or IgA antibody in the infant's blood or CSF at any time is diagnostic of congenital infection, with the following caveats: if cord blood is used, maternal contamination is excluded, and if the IgM-IFA test is used, antinuclear antibodies and rheumatoid factor are not present. The IgM-IFA test detects antibodies to *Toxoplasma* in only 25% of congenitally infected children, whereas the IgM-ISAGA and IgM-ELISA tests detect specific antibodies in 75% of these patients. Results with the IgA-ELISA tests are preliminary, but appear to be somewhat better than those with the IgM tests (41 of 46 patients [89%] in one study and 8 of 9 patients [89%] in another). Optimal results in these studies were obtained by the combined use of tests to detect IgM and IgA antibodies to the parasite.

If *Toxoplasma* is not isolated or demonstrated in tissues and IgM or IgA antibodies are not detected, follow-up serologic testing is the only means of establishing the diagnosis. Maternally transmitted IgG antibodies may persist for 6 to 12 months or longer, depending on the original titer. The higher the original titer, the longer maternal antibody will be detectable in the infant. Thus, the presence of IgG antibody at the age of even 8 to 12 months does not necessarily prove that the infant is infected. Synthesis of IgG *Toxoplasma* antibody usually is demonstrable by the third month of life if the infant is not treated; it may be delayed until the sixth or ninth month if the infant is treated. At the time the infant begins to synthesize IgG antibody, infection may be documented by an increasing or stable ratio of specific serum antibody titer to the total serum IgG level in the infant.

### Toxoplasma Infection in the Pregnant Woman

*Toxoplasma* infection acquired during pregnancy is associated with clinical signs (eg, lymphadenopathy) in only about 10% of patients. The fetus is at risk of contracting the infection regardless of whether the mother is symptomatic. To detect acute infection in the pregnant woman in the absence of a routine screening program in which serologic tests are performed each month, the IgM-ELISA or IgM-ISAGA should be performed if other serologic tests for IgG antibody are positive at any titer. If these IgM tests are unavailable and the original serum contains IgG antibodies, the IgG antibody test should be repeated in 3 weeks, in parallel with the original serum, to determine whether the titer is stable or rising. If the IgM test result is negative and the IgG titer is stable and less than 1 : 500, no further evaluation is necessary. Because IgG titers usually stabilize at high levels (eg, ⩾1:500 by

the dye or IFA test) 6 to 8 weeks or longer after acquisition of the infection, if the dye or IFA test titer is less than 1 : 500 and stable (regardless of the IgM antibody titer), the infection was acquired at least 4 weeks and probably more than 8 weeks before the serum was obtained. In the United States, however, it is common for an asymptomatic woman to be evaluated for the first time more than 8 weeks after conception. If her dye or IFA test titer is 1 : 500 or greater, her IgM-ELISA or IgM-ISAGA test result is negative, and no significant rise in titer on any test can be demonstrated, it is almost certain that her infection was acquired before conception. In women with elevated IgM titers or rising dye or IFA test titers, it is possible that infection was acquired during pregnancy. In such cases, the IgA-ELISA test may be helpful. Consultation with a reference serologic laboratory is recommended to settle the question.

Fewer than half of all infants born to mothers who acquire primary *Toxoplasma* infection in the first or second trimesters become infected. Nevertheless, those infants in whom infection develops in association with maternal infection acquired at these times are at greatest risk of severe sequelae. Accordingly, a method by which to determine which fetuses are infected would provide the opportunity to intervene selectively either by termination of pregnancy or by provision of more aggressive therapy in utero. Recent data, derived largely from studies done by one French group, show that prenatal diagnosis is possible with a high degree of precision. These French investigators studied more than 1000 pregnancies with proved primary *Toxoplasma* infection in the first and second trimesters. Of 89 fetuses subsequently proved to be infected after birth or therapeutic abortion, 80 (90%) were diagnosed correctly in utero at 20 to 29 weeks' gestation by isolation of the parasite from fetal blood, amniotic fluid, or both. There were no false-positive results. Importantly, serologic testing of fetal blood was not found to be a useful means of detecting fetal infection: IgM-ISAGA had a sensitivity of less than 25%. Tests to detect IgA antibodies in fetal blood also appear not to be sensitive, and false-positive results have been seen. Thus, a prenatal diagnosis of fetal infection can be established reliably at present only by isolation of the organism. Isolation in tissue culture, although more rapid and widely available, is less sensitive than is inoculation of mice. Preliminary reports using polymerase chain reaction to detect *Toxoplasma* DNA in fetal blood are encouraging, but await confirmation in larger, comparative studies. It also is important to note that the results obtained by the French investigators may not be reproduced easily in other settings, for a variety of reasons: the investigators were able to detect maternal infection soon after it occurred because women were tested monthly during pregnancy; fetal blood and amniotic fluid were sampled on more than one occasion; and optimal laboratory procedures were used by a laboratory with extensive experience. Consultation with a reference laboratory is suggested if fetal diagnosis is contemplated.

In the French studies, ultrasound examination of the fetus in utero, although not sufficiently sensitive to exclude fetal infection, was useful for detecting major CNS lesions. This procedure may be a useful adjunct to the more invasive methods of fetal diagnosis.

Preliminary data from these studies also suggest that aggressive treatment in utero is associated with an improved outcome of disease in infected fetuses. This is discussed in the section on treatment.

### Acute Acquired *Toxoplasma* Infection in the Immunocompetent Child

If antibody is not detectable by the dye or IFA test, the diagnosis of acute *Toxoplasma* infection in an immunocompetent child is virtually excluded. The diagnosis of recently acquired infection is confirmed if there is seroconversion from a negative to a positive titer or if there is a serial two-tube rise in titer to high levels when sera drawn at 3-week intervals are run in parallel. A single high titer in any test is not diagnostic. In an individual with a compatible illness, a dye or IFA test titer of 1:500 or greater in the presence of a high IgM antibody titer probably is diagnostic of recent acute infection. The absence of IgM antibodies in the IgM-ELISA or IgM-ISAGA essentially excludes the diagnosis of acute infection. In contrast, the absence of IgM antibodies in the IgM-IFA test does not necessarily mean the infection is not acute; in one series, 25% of test results in adults with acute infection were negative with the IgM-IFA test.

### Ocular Toxoplasmosis

*Toxoplasma* has been estimated to cause 35% of all cases of chorioretinitis seen in the United States and central and western Europe; most cases represent a recrudescence of latent congenital infection. Although the presence of chorioretinitis should prompt a search for *Toxoplasma* infection, proof that *Toxoplasma* caused the eye disease often is lacking. The titer of antibody in the serum does not necessarily correlate with the presence of active lesions in the fundus, and IgG antibody titers usually are low in patients with active *Toxoplasma* chorioretinitis. IgM antibodies often are absent.

Toxoplasma probably is excluded as a cause of chorioretinitis if the results of serologic tests are negative in undiluted serum. If retinal lesions are characteristic and serologic test results are positive, the diagnosis is likely. If the retinal lesions are atypical and the serologic test results are positive, the diagnosis of *Toxoplasma* chorioretinitis is less certain because of the increasing prevalence of *Toxoplasma* antibodies with age in the normal population. Demonstration of local antibody production obtained by paracentesis of the anterior chamber (the aqueous humor) is useful for establishing the diagnosis of *Toxoplasma* chorioretinitis in equivocal cases.

### Active Infection in the Immunodeficient Child

Serologic tests should be performed to identify individuals at risk of acquiring toxoplasmosis (eg, seronegative organ transplant recipients). The available serologic tests may be inadequate to detect active infection in some immunodeficient patients, because their antibody response may be abnormal. Acute infection may be present in patients with AIDS and in bone marrow transplant recipients without any demonstrable IgM antibody, and in some patients with little or no IgG antibody. These and other immunodeficient patients, as well as, rarely, some apparently normal patients will have progressive, lethal toxoplasmosis. In almost all cases, encephalitis or brain abscesses are the predominant findings; hepatic involvement, pneumonitis, and myocarditis may be present. In these patients, a high index of suspicion is necessary and biopsy of appropriate tissue often is necessary for diagnosis.

## Nonserologic Methods

Nonserologic methods are used less commonly for the diagnosis of *Toxoplasma* infection because they are not widely available or because they require tissue specimens.

### Isolation of the Organism

The isolation of *Toxoplasma* from blood or body fluids (eg, CSF) establishes that the infection is acute. In the case of the neonate, isolation of the parasite from the placenta or the infant's tissues is sufficient to diagnose congenital *Toxoplasma* infection. Isolation from the placenta usually (about 90% of the time) is associated with congenital infection. The isolation of *Toxoplasma* from tissues of older children or adults may reflect only latent infection (cyst form). The organism may be isolated by inoculation into mice or

into tissue cultures. Tissue culture is less sensitive for recovering the organism. Specimens should be processed and inoculated immediately; however, tissue and blood may be stored at 4 °C overnight. Freezing and thawing or formalin treatment kills the organism. Definitive diagnosis by isolation of *Toxoplasma* usually takes 4 to 6 weeks in mice and 1 to 2 weeks in tissue culture.

### Histology

The demonstration of tachyzoites, but not cysts, in tissue sections or smears of body fluids (eg, CSF) establishes a diagnosis of acute infection. The organism may be difficult to see with routine stains. The peroxidase-antiperoxidase technique is exquisitely sensitive and has been used with a high degree of sensitivity and specificity to demonstrate the organism in the CNS of patients with AIDS. In older children and adults, the histopathologic changes in lymphadenitis caused by *Toxoplasma* are sufficiently distinctive to enable pathologists to make a presumptive diagnosis of acute acquired toxoplasmosis. Histologic demonstration of cysts establishes that the patient has *Toxoplasma* infection, but it cannot be concluded that the infection is acute, except as commented on above.

## Demonstration of *Toxoplasma* Antigen or DNA

Because *Toxoplasma* is difficult to isolate and methods of doing so are not widely available, techniques that permit direct demonstration of the organism in blood or body fluids offer the promise of rapid and more widely available means by which to establish the diagnosis of acute infection. Detection of *Toxoplasma* antigen using an ELISA has not proven to be sufficiently sensitive to be of general use. More recently, several groups have demonstrated the potential utility of the polymerase chain reaction for detecting organisms in fetal blood, amniotic fluid, and CSF. The overall value of this technique in clinical practice is unknown, however, and it is not generally available.

## TREATMENT

The need for therapy and the duration of therapy are determined by the nature and severity of the clinical illness and by the host in whom the infection occurs. The optimum dosage and duration of therapy have not been defined. Antibody titers are not useful indicators of therapeutic response, and an increasing antibody titer soon after therapy is discontinued is not an indication of treatment failure.

## Therapeutic Agents

Pyrimethamine (Daraprim) has a half-life in infants of about 3 days. In patients with significant organ involvement, a loading dose of 15 mg/m$^2$ or 1 mg/kg (maximum 25 mg/dose) should be given twice a day for the first 2 days of therapy. Thereafter, a dosage of 15 mg/m$^2$ or 1 mg/kg (maximum 25 mg) usually is given daily for the first week of therapy, but thereafter may be given every other day in less severely infected children. Pyrimethamine is available only in 25-mg tablets. Anticonvulsant agents, particularly phenobarbital, may enhance the clearance of pyrimethamine, necessitating dosage adjustment.

Pyrimethamine is a folic acid antagonist; the most common side effect is dose-related suppression of the bone marrow. In patients receiving pyrimethamine, the peripheral blood cell count and platelet count should be determined twice a week. Less serious side effects of pyrimethamine include gastrointestinal tract distress, headaches, and a bad taste in the mouth. The risk of adverse effects may be decreased by concomitant administration of folinic acid (leucovorin calcium). Unlike folic acid, folinic acid does not inhibit the action of pyrimethamine on tachyzoites. A 5-mg dose may be given at the same time as pyrimethamine.

Because sulfadiazine acts synergistically with pyrimethamine, these drugs usually are given in combination. Sulfapyrazine, sulfamethazine, and sulfamerazine have activity similar to sulfadiazine. All other sulfonamides tested are inferior. Thus, either sulfadiazine or trisulfapyrimidines should be used. The half-life of sulfadiazine is about 10 to 12 hours. A loading dose of 75 mg/ kg (maximum 4 g) is given. Thereafter, 100 mg/kg/d (maximum 6 g/d) is given in two divided doses. Tablets and liquid oral forms are routinely available. A parenteral form is available on special request from Lederle Laboratories in Pearl River, New York.

Other agents, including spiramycin, clindamycin, and trimethoprim-sulfamethoxazole, are less active than is the combination of pyrimethamine and sulfadiazine. Spiramycin, a macrolide antibiotic that is less toxic than are pyrimethamine and sulfadiazine, has been used effectively in the treatment of pregnant women and infants with congenital infection. Although spiramycin is in common use worldwide, it is available in the United States only by special request from the Food and Drug Administration (telephone number 301-443-4310) or through the national collaborative study of the treatment of congenital *Toxoplasma* infection (see below). Clindamycin is concentrated in the ocular choroid and has been used in the treatment of ocular disease; it still must be considered experimental for this purpose. The omission of necessary controls in studies reporting beneficial effects of trimethoprim–sulfamethoxazole in humans leaves it unclear whether the effects observed were caused by spontaneous resolution or by the sulfonamide component alone. It clearly is less active than are pyrimethamine and sulfadiazine in mice. Because sulfamethoxazole is less active than is sulfadiazine, trimethoprim–sulfamethoxazole cannot be recommended at this time. Trimetrexate is an investigational drug that, similar to pyrimethamine and trimethoprim, is a folic acid antagonist. It is highly active against *Toxoplasma* in vitro. It is being tested now in the treatment of *Toxoplasma* encephalitis in patients with AIDS, but sufficient data are not yet available to determine whether it will be useful.

New macrolide-like antibiotics with increased activity against *Toxoplasma* also are undergoing clinical trials, primarily in patients with AIDS and CNS infection.

Importantly, none of the agents described above are active against the cyst form of the parasite. Accordingly, they are effective only in treating active infection and do not result in a radical cure. Recently, agents with activity against the cyst form have been identified and these are being tested in clinical trials. Should they prove to be effective in eliminating cyst forms, they offer the potential to decrease the risk for recurrent infection and would provide an important adjunct to current therapy.

## Therapy in Specific Clinical Settings

### Acquired Toxoplasmosis

Most immunologically normal patients with the form of toxoplasmosis that causes lymphadenopathy do not require specific treatment. Indications for treatment in these cases are the presence of severe and persistent symptoms or damage to vital organs. In such patients, treatment should be given for 2 to 6 weeks until symptoms resolve.

### Ocular Toxoplasmosis

Hypersensitivity appears to play a major role in the pathogenesis in patients with relapse of ocular toxoplasmosis and, in such cases, corticosteroids in addition to specific anti-*Toxoplasma* ther-

apy (at least sulfonamides) have been recommended. Because of the potential untoward effects of corticosteroids, their use should be reserved for cases of retinochoroiditis in which there is involvement of the macula, maculopapillary bundle, or optic nerve. The initial daily dosage of prednisone is 1.5 mg/kg orally (maximum 75 mg) in 24 hours. The equivalent dosage of another corticosteroid may be given. The dosage of corticosteroid may be reduced gradually when the lesion appears to be well demarcated and pigmentation has begun. Systemic or intraocular clindamycin has been used by some to treat patients who do not respond to corticosteroids and pyrimethamine plus sulfadiazine; its efficacy has not been proved in humans.

### The Immunocompromised Host

In patients with *Toxoplasma* encephalitis, which is most common in patients with AIDS, treatment failure at the usual drug dosages, frequent allergic reactions to sulfonamides, and nearly universal relapse of infection when therapy has been stopped have made treatment difficult. In such patients, high dosages (40 to 50 mg/ m²/d of pyrimethamine and 100 to 150 mg/kg/d of sulfadiazine) usually are required; folinic acid in dosages as high as 0.5 mg/ kg/d should be given concomitantly. In those who are intolerant of sulfonamides, high dosages of clindamycin in combination with pyrimethamine and folinic acid have been used, but this approach remains experimental. Initial combination treatment should be given for 4 to 6 weeks after clinical resolution. Thereafter, chronic therapy should be given; the optimal drugs, dosages, and duration of chronic treatment are not known. In patients with AIDS, this regimen probably should be given for their lifetime; in others, it should be prescribed for at least 6 months. Careful follow-up of these patients is imperative, because relapse may occur, requiring prompt reinstitution of therapy.

### The Pregnant Woman

Treatment of the acutely infected woman during pregnancy may prevent transmission of the infection to the fetus. Data from France, where women were treated with spiramycin, and from Germany, where women were treated with pyrimethamine and sulfonamides, indicate that the incidence of congenital infection in the offspring of mothers treated during gestation is about 50% lower than in the offspring of untreated mothers. Neither of these studies was rigidly controlled. Nevertheless, results in the large numbers of women studied by the group from France strongly suggest that treatment does reduce the incidence of congenital infection. It should be emphasized that treatment of pregnant women with recently acquired primary infection should be instituted in the hope of preventing spread of infection to the fetus. Once fetal infection has occurred, it appears that maternal treatment with spiramycin does not alter the development of disease in the fetus.

Although spiramycin appears not to be effective in treating established fetal infection, recent data from Hohlfeld and colleagues suggest that treatment of the mother with pyrimethamine and sulfadiazine may be effective. Of the 80 fetuses that were shown to be infected in utero, 34 were terminated by parental request. These fetuses either had CNS disease detected on ultrasound examination or the onset of maternal infection in the first trimester, and all had detectable brain necrosis at necropsy. An additional 55 infected offspring were carried to term. Of these 55, 43 were diagnosed in utero and were treated aggressively with intermittent pyrimethamine, sulfadiazine, and folinic acid for the remainder of the pregnancy. By comparison to results in infants of mothers treated in previous years with spiramycin alone, treatment with pyrimethamine and sulfadiazine appeared to decrease the rate at which *Toxoplasma* could be isolated at term from placental tissue and also appeared to decrease the incidence

**TABLE 62-4.** Treatment Regimens for *Toxoplasmosis* in the Pregnant Woman and the Congenitally Infected Infant

**Treatment of the Acutely Infected Mother***

Spiramycin, 3 g/d in four doses, or if spiramycin is not available, pyrimethamine, 25 mg every other day† plus sulfadiazine or trisulfapyrimidines, 3 to 4 g/d in two or three doses per day, plus folinic acid, 5 mg daily. During the first 16 weeks of pregnancy, sulfonamides should be used alone if spiramycin is not available. Monitor complete blood counts and platelet counts twice weekly.

**Treatment of the Acutely Infected Mother in Whom Fetal Infection Has Been Proved***

Pyrimethamine 50 mg once daily, sulfadiazine 3 g/d in 2 to 3 doses, and folinic acid 5 mg/d for 3 weeks, alternating with 3 weeks of spiramycin 3 g/d in four doses. Monitor complete blood counts and platelet counts.

**Treatment of the Congenitally Infected Infant* ‡**

*Drugs*
1. **Pyrimethamine plus sulfadiazine:** Pyrimethamine, 15 mg/m² d or 1 mg/kg/d (maximum daily dose is 25 mg) by the oral route.† Although the half-life of the drug is 4 to 5 days, it should be given on a daily basis unless breaking of the tablets is grossly inaccurate during preparation of the smaller doses. In such cases, as for very small infants (eg, when a daily dose of 3 mg is indicated), breaking of a tablet may result in a slightly higher dose, which could be administered every 2 days. Sulfadiazine or trisulfapyrimidines: 100 mg/kg/d by the oral route in two divided doses daily. Monitor complete blood and platelet counts.
2. **Spiramycin§:** 100 mg/kg/d by the oral route in two divided doses.
3. **Corticosteroids** (prednisone or methylprednisolone): 1.5 mg/kg/d by the oral route in two divided doses, daily. The drug is continued until the inflammatory process (eg, high level of cerebrospinal fluid protein, chorioretinitis) has subsided; the dosage then should be tapered progressively and discontinued.
4. **Folinic acid:** 5 mg every 3 days (intramuscularly in young infants) during treatment with pyrimethamine. If bone marrow toxicity occurs at this dose, increase to 10 mg every 3 days. If bone marrow toxicity is severe, discontinue pyrimethamine until the abnormality is corrected and then begin pyrimethamine again using 10 mg of folinic acid every 3 days. In some infants, it may be necessary to administer folinic acid more frequently.

*Indications*
1. **Overt congenital toxoplasmosis:** The course of treatment is for 1 year in all cases. For infants in whom clinical signs of the infection are present, treatment during the first 6 months is with pyrimethamine plus sulfadiazine. During the following 6 months, 1 month of pyrimethamine plus sulfadiazine is alternated with 1 month of spiramycin. Folinic acid should be started as soon as possible. No treatment usually is given after 12 months of age except when there is evidence of evolution of the infection, such as a flare-up of chorioretinitis.
2. **Overt congenital toxoplasmosis with evidence of an inflammatory process** (chorioretinitis, high level of cerebrospinal fluid protein, generalized infection, jaundice): As in number 1 above plus corticosteroids.
3. **Subclinical congenital toxoplasmosis:** Pyrimethamine plus sulfadiazine for 6 weeks; thereafter, alternate with spiramycin. Spiramycin is given for 6 weeks and is alternated with 4 weeks of pyrimethamine plus sulfadiazine to complete a treatment course of 1 year.
4. **Healthy newborn in whom serologic testing has not provided definitive results, but maternal infection was proved to have been acquired during pregnancy:** One course of pyrimethamine plus sulfadiazine for 1 month. Obtain consultation with appropriate authority to determine the necessity for continued therapy and the drug and dosage regimen. This decision must be made on an individual basis and depends on multiple factors, including serologic test titers, immune load, and clinical findings in the infant.
5. **Healthy newborn born to a mother with a high Sabin-Feldman dye test titer—date of maternal infection undefined:** Spiramycin for 1 month. Then as in number 4 above. In certain cases, the indication for treatment is difficult to define because of a lack of information about the pregnancy and lack of isolation attempts from the corresponding placenta.

* The appropriateness of treatment, the treatment regimen, and the duration of treatment must be considered individually (see text).

† Loading dose is recommended in patients with evidence of severe organ involvement.

‡ Modified from the recommendations of Dr. Jacques Couveur, Laboratoire de Serologie Neonatale et de Recherche sur la Toxoplasmose, Institut de Puericulture, Paris.

§ Available in the United States only by request to the U.S. Food and Drug Administration.

*Adapted from Remington JS, Wilson CB. Toxoplasmosis. In: Kass EH, Platt R, eds. Current therapy in infectious disease, 1983–1984. Philadelphia: BC Decker, 1983:149–153, and from Remington JS, Desmonts G. Toxoplasmosis. In: Remington JS, Klein JO, eds. Infectious diseases of the fetus and newborn infant. Philadelphia: WB Saunders, 1990.*

**TABLE 62-5.    Primary Prevention
of *Toxoplasma* Infection**

**Prevention of Acquired Infection**

Cook meat to >66°C (150°F), smoke it, or cure it in brine.

Wash fruits and vegetables before consumption.

Avoid touching mucous membranes of mouth and eyes while handling uncooked meat or unwashed fruits or vegetables.

Wash hands and kitchen surfaces thoroughly after contact with raw meat or unwashed fruits or vegetables.

Prevent access of flies, cockroaches, and other coprophagic insects to fruits and vegetables.

Avoid contact with materials that potentially are contaminated with cat feces, such as cat litter boxes, or wear gloves when handling such materials and when gardening.

Disinfect cat litter box for 5 minutes with nearly boiling water.

**Prevention of Congenital Infection**

Identify women at risk by serologic testing.

Treatment during pregnancy results in about 50% reduction in the incidence of infection in infants.

Therapeutic abortion prevents birth of infected infant; considered only in cases of women who acquired infection in first or second trimester.

*Adapted from Remington JS, Wilson CB. Toxoplasmosis. In: Kass EH, Platt R, eds. Current therapy in infectious disease, 1983–1984. Philadelphia: BC Decker, 1983:149.*

## PREVENTION

Acquired infection may be prevented primarily by the specific hygiene measures listed in Table 62-5. Such measures, if applied to pregnant women, also will prevent congenital infection in their offspring.

## Selected Readings

Couvreur J, Desmonts G, Tournier G, et al. Etude d'une serie homogène de 210 cas de toxoplasmose congenitale chez des nourrissons ages de 0 a 11 mois et depistes de façon prospective. Ann Pediatr (Paris) 1984;31:815.

Daffos F, Forestier F, Capella-Pavlosky M, et al. Prenatal management of 746 pregnancies at risk for congenital toxoplasmosis. N Engl J Med 1988;318:271.

Desmonts G, Couvreur J. Congenital toxoplasmosis: A prospective study of the offspring of 542 women who acquired toxoplasmosis during pregnancy. Pathophysiology of congenital disease. In: Thalhammer O, Baumgarten K, Pollak A, eds. Perinatal medicine, Sixth European Congress, Vienna, 1978. Stuttgart: Georg Thieme, 1979:51.

Eichenwald H. A study of congenital toxoplasmosis. In: Siim JC, ed. Human toxoplasmosis. Copenhagen: Munksgaard, 1960:41.

Hohlfeld P, Daffos F, Thulliez P, et al. Fetal toxoplasmosis: Outcome of pregnancy and infant follow-up after in utero treatment. J Pediatr 1989;115:765.

Remington JS, Desmonts G. Toxoplasmosis. In: Remington JS, Klein JO, eds. Infectious diseases of the fetus and newborn infant, 3rd ed. Philadelphia: WB Saunders, 1990:89.

Wilson CB. Developmental immunology and role of host defenses in neonatal susceptibility. In: Remington JS, Klein JO, eds. Infectious diseases of the fetus and newborn infant, 3rd ed. Philadelphia: WB Saunders, 1990:17.

*Principles and Practice of Pediatrics, Second Edition.*
edited by Frank A. Oski et al. J. B. Lippincott Company, Philadelphia © 1994.

## *62.1.7* **Toxocariasis**

B. Keith English

Human infection with the larval stage of the common dog roundworm, *Toxocara canis*, is the principal cause of two distinct clinical syndromes: visceral larva migrans (VLM) and ocular toxocariasis or ocular larva migrans (OLM). The majority of *Toxocara* infections occur in young children, and though most result in mild or inapparent disease, serious complications may occur. Humans do not act as a definitive host for these nematodes, but the larvae migrate throughout the tissues and provoke an eosinophilic inflammatory response that may result in striking symptoms and laboratory findings.

## EPIDEMIOLOGY AND TRANSMISSION

The epidemiology and pathogenesis of toxocariasis have been reviewed by Glickman and Schantz. *T canis*, a nematode roundworm of the family Ascaridae, is a cosmopolitan parasite, infecting dogs (and other canids) in all tropical and temperate regions of the world. Toxocariasis in domestic dogs is prevalent almost uniformly in North American south of latitude 60 °N and has been reported in all 50 states. The adult worms reside in the proximal small intestine of dogs (the definitive hosts) and live for an average of 4 months. Adult females may produce 200,000 eggs per day; eggs passed in feces are not embryonated and, thus, are not infective. Depending on soil composition, temperature, and humidity, the eggs become infective in 2 to 5 weeks. Dogs may acquire *T canis* infection in five ways:

---

of severe clinical disease in the infants. Because of other known and potential differences in management between the two groups, however, it is not possible to conclude with certainty that the improved outcome resulted solely from the different treatment regimens. Nevertheless, these studies establish the utility of an aggressive approach to prenatal diagnosis, which allowed an accurate, early identification of nearly all infected fetuses. This approach allows for selective intervention in infected fetuses either by therapeutic abortion or by more aggressive antiprotozoal therapy, while avoiding unwarranted intervention in uninfected fetuses.

Suggested treatment regimens are presented in Table 62-4.

### Congenital Infection

Data on the efficacy of postnatal treatment of infants with congenital *Toxoplasma* infection are meager. Uncontrolled studies in humans and controlled studies in experimental animals have been interpreted as indicating beneficial effects of postnatal treatment on the development of sequelae in both symptomatic and asymptomatic infants with congenital *Toxoplasma* infection. Until data from controlled studies in humans are available, postnatal treatment of infected infants for 6 months or more is recommended. Each case should be considered on an individual basis, however.

A controlled national collaborative study, which seeks to determine the optimal therapeutic regimen, is in progress in the United States under the direction of Dr. Rima McLeod at Michael Reese Hospital in Chicago. Physicians may wish to consider enrolling their patients who are less than 2.5 months of age in this study. Until these data are available, we recommend following the treatment regimens used by Couvreur, as outlined in Table 62-4.

Healthy-appearing neonates in whom the diagnosis is suspected, but not confirmed by initial serologic testing should receive 1 month of pyrimethamine plus sulfadiazine, followed by spiramycin or sulfadiazine alone, until the diagnosis is established.

1. By transplacental migration of larvae (the most important method of transmission, resulting in prenatal infection of almost 100% of puppies born to infected mothers)
2. By transmammary passage of larvae to nursing pups in milk
3. By ingestion of infective eggs
4. By ingestion of larvae in tissues of paratenic hosts (see below)
5. By ingestion of late-stage larvae or immature adult worms in vomitus or feces of infected pups.

In adult dogs, embryonated eggs containing second-stage larvae hatch in the stomach and small intestine, penetrate the intestinal mucosa, travel via the portal circulation to the liver, then enter the systemic circulation, reaching the heart and lungs 3 to 5 days after infection. Some larvae penetrate the bronchioles, travel to the trachea and pharynx, are swallowed, and develop into adult worms in the small intestine. Other larvae invade the pulmonary vein, travel back to the heart, and spread via the systemic circulation throughout the body. In puppies, the tracheal route predominates, accounting for their importance in the transmission of disease to other hosts.

In humans and paratenic hosts (including mice, rats, lambs, and pigs), the tracheal route of migration leading to the development of adult worms does not occur. Larvae do travel to the liver via the portal circulation and to the systemic circulation via the lungs, however, lodging in small blood vessels in somatic organs. The larvae then bore through the walls of the blood vessels and migrate through the tissues. As in dogs, most of these larvae become dormant, but may remain viable for many years.

Nearly all human infection occurs by ingestion of infective eggs from soil that is contaminated with excreta from puppies or from contaminated hands or fomites. Ingestion of uncooked organ and muscle meat from paratenic hosts (pigs, lambs, rabbits, snails, and, perhaps, chickens) is a documented, but uncommon, source for human infection. Pica for dirt (geophagia) is the principal risk factor for VLM in children and adults. Because embryonation takes more than 2 weeks, direct transmission from infected dogs presumably is uncommon. Therefore, frequent exposure to dogs (eg, in veterinarians) alone is insufficient to predict an increased likelihood of *T canis* infection. Although puppy ownership is associated with a higher incidence of *T canis* infection, ample exposure may occur in children without a household dog: 10% to 30% of soil samples from public parks, sandboxes, and backyards are contaminated with *T canis* eggs, which may survive for years. Seroprevalence studies using an enzyme-linked immunosorbent assay (ELISA) for antibodies to *T canis* have revealed that 4.6% to 7.3% of kindergarten children from different regions of the United States have been infected. Seroprevalence rates are higher in African-Americans than in whites. For both African-Americans and whites, seroprevalence rates increase with rural residence, crowding, and lower socioeconomic status. In some rural populations in the southeastern United States, seroprevalence rates exceeding 20% have been reported. A positive ELISA for *T canis* also is associated with epilepsy, yet children with epilepsy of undefined origin do not have higher seroprevalence rates than do children with epilepsy of known cause. This suggests that epilepsy is a risk factor for the acquisition of *T canis* (eg, through pica) rather than vice versa.

The epidemiologic features of VLM and ocular toxocariasis are strikingly different. Although both are associated with exposure to puppies, only VLM is associated clearly with pica. Patients with VLM usually are 1 to 4 years old, whereas patients with ocular toxocariasis have a mean age of 7 to 8 years. Most patients with ocular toxocariasis have no history of a syndrome similar to VLM, although ocular involvement may occur concomitantly with VLM, especially in very young children with severe disease, or many years after VLM.

## PATHOGENESIS

The clinical and pathologic features of *T canis* infection in patients with VLM and ocular toxocariasis reflect primarily the brisk inflammatory response of the host, although the migrating larvae may cause direct tissue damage. Dead or dying larvae provoke a particularly intense inflammatory response. As described in the initial report linking *T canis* larvae with VLM, the characteristic pathologic lesions are eosinophilic granulomas that surround larvae in various stages of disintegration; in advanced lesions, no evidence of the larvae remains. The liver is the site of greatest involvement most often in humans, but involvement of the lungs also is frequent. Eye involvement is an important complication of *T canis* infection and occurs in many different forms. Although it is less common, larval infection of the myocardium, brain, pancreas, skin, kidney, intestine, and regional lymph nodes has been documented.

The contrasting epidemiology of VLM and ocular toxocariasis led Glickman to hypothesize that the dose of the organism ingested might determine whether VLM, ocular involvement, both, or neither developed in the patient. In this model, the ingestion of a few larvae would result in initially asymptomatic infection, but could result in ocular disease in some cases. The ingestion of a moderate number of larvae could result in VLM because of a more dramatic inflammatory response; these patients would have a low risk of subsequent ocular involvement if the inflammatory response could prevent migration of larvae to the eye. Finally, ingestion of a very large number of larvae could overwhelm the immune response, resulting in concomitant VLM and ocular disease; these patients would be at higher risk for larval infection of other sites (eg, brain, myocardium) as well. Although there is experimental support for some features of this model, it remains largely speculative. Three human research subjects given a single dose of 100 to 200 larvae had no clinical evidence of disease, but did have moderate eosinophilia.

Experimental infection of paratenic hosts, including mice, rabbits, and the Japanese quail, with embryonated eggs of *T canis* has provided important information regarding the pathogenesis of *Toxocara* infections. These studies have confirmed the importance of the host immune response in the development of tissue injury in this disease. Recent studies in mice (as well as in vitro studies of human T lymphocytes) indicate that the T cell response to *Toxocara* infection is mediated primarily by cells of the T helper 2 (Th2) phenotype. Furthermore, Th2 cell production of the cytokine interleukin-5 appears to be the critical step in the development of eosinophilia during *Toxocara* infection in mice. Future studies in the murine model should lead to an improved understanding of the potential role of antihelminthic and anti-inflammatory agents in the treatment of *Toxocara* infections.

## CLINICAL FEATURES

### Visceral Larva Migrans

The classic manifestations of VLM reflected the fact that only clinical diagnosis of *T canis* infection was possible; fever, hepatomegaly, eosinophilic leukocytosis, and hypergammaglobulinemia defined the syndrome. Many of these patients also had pulmonary involvement (rales or wheezes) and rashes (often pruritic). Seizures were reported in more than 25% of patients in one early series. It is now agreed that the majority of *T canis* infections in children are asymptomatic, and that only a small number of these infections result in the full-blown VLM syndrome. The use of improved serologic tests should define better the clinical characteristics of less severe cases of VLM.

Hepatomegaly remains a common sign in VLM, but the most common symptoms are pulmonary and may mimic those of asthma or pneumonia. Chest radiographs reveal infiltrates in half the patients with pulmonary symptoms, but severe lung disease is uncommon. Fever, adenopathy, rash, and weight loss may occur. Ocular disease is unusual in association with VLM, but may occur in severe cases. Leukocyte counts of 30,000 to 100,000/ mm³ with a pronounced eosinophilia are common. The percentage of eosinophils usually is greater than 20% in acute cases of VLM and may reach 90%; eosinophilia often persists for months or years after symptoms resolve. Hypergammaglobulinemia often is present, with elevations of IgE, IgM, and IgG. Isohemagglutinin titers (anti-A, anti-B) often are elevated because the *T canis* larva expresses surface antigens that cross-react with epitopes of the blood group antigens.

The prognosis in most cases of VLM is excellent, with complete recovery the rule. Severe and even fatal cases have been reported, however. Myocardial involvement is rare, but has been reported in several fatal cases and as an incidental finding at the time of open heart surgery in two patients. *T canis* may cause eosinophilic meningitis; larvae have been found in the brain at autopsy in children with fatal infection and as an incidental finding in children with unrelated causes of death. Although seizures may occur as a complication of VLM, this appears to be a much less frequent complication than early reports suggested. The effects of asymptomatic and mild infection are largely unknown. Both a large cohort study and a large case-control study found small deficits in performance on neuropsychiatric tests in seropositive children as compared with seronegative controls. In the cohort study, confounding variables appeared to explain these differences; in the case-control study, small differences between seropositive and seronegative children remained after careful adjustment for potential confounding factors. Considering the frequency of *T canis* infection in children in the United States, more careful study of the neurologic consequences of *Toxocara* infections is merited.

## Ocular Toxocariasis

An extensive review of ocular toxocariasis has been published. Ocular involvement by nematode larvae first was reported in 1950 and was shown to be caused by *T canis* in 1956. A variety of clinical patterns have emerged, none of which is pathognomonic. Ocular toxocariasis usually occurs in young school-age children (mean age 7 to 8 years), but it may occur in adults and infants. A history of pica frequently is not present and eosinophilia is uncommon. Usually only one eye is involved, but bilateral disease has been reported. Patients commonly complain of decreased visual acuity.

Three clinical patterns are recognized most frequently. The best-known and perhaps most frequent pattern is *Toxocara* endophthalmitis, which is characterized by a yellow-white mass, retinal detachment, and cells in the vitreous; these features are shared by retinoblastoma, and the two disorders often are difficult to differentiate clinically. A feared complication of this condition is the formation of a cyclitic membrane, which may lead to complete visual loss.

The other two syndromes often recognized as consequences of *T canis* ocular disease are posterior retinochoroiditis, which usually occurs in older children or adults, and peripheral retinochoroiditis, which may mimic pars planitis and may cause traction on the retina, resulting in retinal folds, which once were thought to be a congenital malformation. Other clinical patterns include optic papillitis, diffuse unilateral subacute neuroretinitis, the motile chorioretinal nematode syndrome ("true" OLM), keratitis, conjunctivitis, and lens involvement.

## DIFFERENTIAL DIAGNOSIS

The differential diagnosis of VLM caused by *T canis* includes infection by the larval forms of other helminths that have a tissue migratory phase to their life cycle: these include other *Toxocara* species, *Ascaris lumbricoides*, *Strongyloides stercoralis*, *Trichinella*, hookworms, and schistosomes. Eosinophilic leukemia may be considered in some patients with severe eosinophilia. The eosinophilia associated with *T canis* infection may persist for months or years, and it occurs in asymptomatic infected patients. Thus, silent or preceding *T canis* infection should be considered in the differential diagnosis of unexplained persistent eosinophilia.

The differential diagnosis of ocular toxocariasis is broad and depends on the clinical pattern. The most difficult and important problem for the ophthalmologist is the distinction between *T canis* endophthalmitis and retinoblastoma. Although retinoblastoma more frequently is bilateral (30% versus a few case reports) and calcified (commonly versus rarely) than ocular toxocariasis, enough overlap exists to make these features unreliable. *Toxocara* endophthalmitis usually is not associated with much pain or photophobia. *T canis* is one of several causes of pseudo-retinoblastoma; others include Coats disease (retinal telangiectasia with exudation), persistent hyperplastic primary vitreous, retinopathy of prematurity, and ocular toxoplasmosis.

## Laboratory Diagnosis

Although a presumptive diagnosis of VLM can be supported by abnormalities on a variety of laboratory tests (eosinophilia, hypergammaglobulinemia, elevated isohemagglutinin levels), these tests are nonspecific and usually are normal in cases of ocular disease. A variety of immunologic tests have been developed over the years, but have been largely unsuccessful, presumably because they used antigen prepared from adult worms.

Recently, an ELISA test using antigen from larval *T canis* has been developed. The *Toxocara* Excretory–Secretory (TES) ELISA uses an excretory or secretory antigen from the supernatants of *T canis* larvae maintained in vitro. The TES ELISA has proved to be a sensitive and specific test in the diagnosis of VLM, and it appears to be useful in the diagnosis of ocular toxocariasis as well. (A radioallergosorbent IgE test specific for *T canis* also has been developed; preliminary data suggest that it is comparable to the ELISA tests in sensitivity and specificity, but it is not widely available.) Recently, serologic differentiation between *T canis* and *Toxocara cati* infections has been achieved by Ouchterlony's diffusion-in-gel method; this may be helpful in future studies of the epidemiology of *Toxocara* infections.

For the diagnosis of VLM, the TES ELISA is superior to older methods. The reported sensitivity and specificity of the ELISA, with a titer of 1:32 or greater being considered indicative of infection, are 78% and 92%, respectively. This compares with sensitivities of only 18% to 26% for the previously used indirect hemagglutination and bentonite flocculation tests; the former tests also were more than 90% specific. The TES is the serologic test routinely performed by the United States Centers for Disease Control. Evaluation of this test is ongoing and guidelines for interpreting a specific titer should be provided with the results.

The serologic diagnosis of ocular toxocariasis, although promising, is more problematic. In ocular disease, TES ELISA titers usually are lower than are those in VLM. With a titer greater than 1:8 being considered indicative of infection, the ELISA has been reported to be 90% sensitive and 91% specific. Several false-negative results have been reported, however. Elevated titers in the absence of disease or false-positive results (commonly representing asymptomatic *T canis* infection or VLM in association with ocular disease of another etiology) also would be expected to occur, especially in patients from groups with a high seroprevalence. Aspiration of aqueous humor or vitreous humor in affected patients may confirm the diagnosis by allowing the demonstration of antibody to *T canis* in these fluids by ELISA, and positive results have been reported in the face of a negative serum ELISA result. Although the procedure is invasive, aspiration of the aqueous humor may be considered in a patient in whom enucleation of the eye for possible retinoblastoma is planned. Imaging techniques (such as ultrasound and computed tomography) have been used to characterize *T canis* ocular lesions, but do not appear to differentiate these lesions clearly from other diagnoses, including retinoblastoma.

## THERAPY

Discussion of potential therapy of VLM or ocular toxocariasis must begin with consideration of the prognosis of untreated disease. The overall prognosis of VLM is excellent. Even in more severe cases, removal of the patient from the source of exposure usually is adequate to effect satisfactory recovery. Pharmacologic treatment of VLM should be considered only when severe symptoms occur (eg, severe respiratory distress) or involvement of critical organs (myocardium, brain) is noted. In these situations, the use of corticosteroids may be indicated and has been reported to result in dramatic improvement of symptoms. There is no convincing evidence that antihelminthic agents such as thiabendazole or diethylcarbamazine are effective against larval forms in tissues, and these drugs have not been shown to be of clear value in the treatment of any human *Toxocara* infection. Although newer agents, including albendazole and ivermectin, do appear to have activity against larval forms of *Toxocara*, their role in treating human toxocariasis remains uncertain. Indeed, the pathophysiology of these diseases suggests that hastening larval death might be contraindicated. Considering the appreciable toxicity of currently available antihelminthic drugs, these agents should be considered only in patients with severe disease that is unresponsive to corticosteroids.

The prognosis of ocular toxocariasis is more guarded and depends on the clinical pattern. Any child with known or suspected ocular toxocariasis should be referred promptly to an ophthalmologist experienced in the diagnosis and treatment of this condition. Steroids have proved beneficial in severe vision-threatening forms of this disease, and early surgery may prevent some of the complications. Laser photocoagulation may be employed to eradicate meandering larvae if other attempts to remove the larvae fail. Antihelminthic agents have not been demonstrated to be effective and should be used cautiously, if at all, in the treatment of *T canis* ocular infection.

## PREVENTION

Newborn puppies are the principal source of infection in young children. All newborn puppies should be wormed before they reach 2 to 3 weeks of age, and worming should be repeated every 2 weeks until the puppy is 4 months old. Thereafter, fecal examinations should be performed twice yearly, with treatment as indicated. Scoop laws are of some benefit, because eggs that have not undergone embryonation require 2 weeks or more to become infective. Pica should be discouraged and good hygiene practiced. In young children with persistent pica, close supervision is recommended when they play outdoors in parks, backyards, or sandboxes. Once soil is contaminated with *T canis* eggs, it cannot be decontaminated. New agents such as fenbendazole and iver-

mectin appear to be effective against tissue larval forms in pregnant dogs and to interrupt the transplacental infection of puppies. These or other antihelminthic agents may play a future role in the prevention of this common zoonosis.

## Selected Readings

Beaver PC, Synder CH, Carrera GM, Dent JH, Lafferty JW. Chronic eosinophilia due to visceral larva migrans. Pediatrics 1952;9:7.

Del Prete GF, De Carli M, Mastromauro C, et al. Purified protein derivative of mycobacterium tuberculosis and excretory-secretory antigen(s) of *Toxocara canis* expand in vitro human T cells with stable and opposite (type 1 T helper or type 2 T helper) profile of cytokine production. J Clin Invest 1991;88:346.

Glickman LT, Schantz PM. Epidemiology and pathogenesis of zoonotic toxocariasis. Epidemiol Rev 1981;3:230.

Glickman LT, Shofer FS. Zoonotic visceral and ocular larva migrans. Vet Clin North Am Small Anim Pract 1987;17:39.

Marmor M, Glickman L, Shofer F, et al. *Toxocara canis* infection of children: Epidemiologic and neuropsychologic findings. Am J Public Health 1987;77:554.

Schantz PM. *Toxocara* larva migrans now. Am J Trop Med Hyg 1989;41:21.

Schantz PM, Glickman LT Current concepts in parasitology: Toxocaral visceral larva migrans. N Engl J Med 1978;298:436.

Shields JA. Ocular toxocariasis: A review. Surv Ophthalmol 1984;28:361.

Worley G, Green JA, Frothingham TE, et al. *Toxocara canis* infection: Clinical and epidemiological associations with seropositivity in kindergarten children. J Infect Dis 1984;149:591.

Yamaguchi Y, Matsui T, Kasahara T, et al. In vivo changes of hemopoietic progenitors and the expression of the interleukin 5 gene in eosinophilic mice infected with *Toxocara canis*. Exp Hematol 1990;18:1152.

*Principles and Practice of Pediatrics, Second Edition.*
edited by Frank A. Oski et al. J. B. Lippincott Company, Philadelphia © 1994.

# 62.2 *The Nematodes*

## Michael Katz

The phylum Nematoda comprises nonsegmented worms of various sizes, ranging from 1 mm to 1 m. Most species are free-living. A few species are parasitic, and fewer still are parasites of humans.

All nematodes are surrounded by a cuticle that is characteristic of each species. It is a durable, protective structure, complex in composition and involved in active transport of nutrients and water. These worms have a muscular system consisting of cells in an outer ring of tissue just beneath the cuticle, with insertions into the cuticle. There also are muscles in the buccal cavity in the gut tract. The gut is associated with many exocrine glands, which aid in digestion. The excretory function depends on the removal of solid wastes through the gut and the removal of liquid wastes through two tubules connecting a primitive kidney (ventral gland) with an excretory pore. Sexes are separate in most nematodes, and their reproductive organs are highly developed. The egg-laying capacity of the females can be enormous, approaching several hundred thousand per day.

The nematodes have four larval stages. In the parasitic species, some of these stages occur in the host and some occur in the environment. Considerable variation exists in this regard among these parasites. There also is variation in the mode of infection, which can occur by ingestion, penetration of the skin, or through an animal vector.

This chapter considers some of the nematodes parasitic of humans, either because they are quite common or because the diseases they cause are serious.

# INTESTINAL NEMATODES

## *Enterobius vermicularis*

Colloquially known as pinworm, *Enterobius vermicularis* is a nematode with worldwide distribution that probably is the most common of all the helminthic parasites of humans. Most infected individuals are children, and they are of all socioeconomic classes. They become infected by ingesting embryonated eggs that are picked up from the perianal skin by scratching fingers or are inhaled as the eggs float in the air, especially after bedclothes or underwear have been shaken. Swallowed eggs hatch in the duodenum and the liberated larvae undergo additional maturation in the small intestine before reaching the cecum. There, the sexually mature worms copulate and then proceed to the rectum and eventually to the perianal skin, where the gravid females lay eggs. The eggs become infective within 2 to 4 hours after deposition. The entire cycle from ingestion of the egg to the egg-laying phase of the gravid female lasts 4 to 6 weeks. In the rare retrograde mode of infection, eggs hatch on the anal mucosa and the larvae migrate up the bowel and mature there to adult worms.

Communal living, crowded households, and changing of underwear in gymnasiums all promote the acquisition of infection. Adults also can be infected, especially those who are in close contact with infected children.

### Symptoms

*E vermicularis* infection causes no disease in the gut, although the worms can be found in the appendix. They also have been found in the epididymis, associated with inflammation of this structure; in an abscess embedded in an inguinal hernia; and even in the peritoneum. This infection becomes symptomatic only when the adult gravid female lays eggs on the perineal skin. In girls and women, the female worm can crawl into the vagina and cause vulvitis as a reaction to the eggs deposited in that region. The female is 8 to 13 mm in length and usually can be seen with the naked eye as a whitish yellow thread.

Most infected individuals are free of symptoms. Those who have symptoms experience pruritus; its intensity varies from mild itching to acute, intractable pain. In vaginal infections, a discharge and vulval itching can develop. Insomnia, restlessness, irritability, loss of appetite, loss of weight, enuresis, and grinding of teeth all have been attributed anecdotally to pinworm infection, but no evidence of a causal relationship exists.

### Diagnosis

The eggs are identified readily by examination, under a low-power microscope lens, of transparent adhesive tape that previously was applied to the perianal skin and then was affixed to a microscope slide. This specimen is collected best first thing in the morning, when the child awakens.

### Treatment

Equally effective treatments are pyrantel pamoate (11 mg/kg, maximum 1 g) as a single oral dose or mebendazole as a single dose (100 mg, regardless of weight). The dosage of mebendazole for children younger than 2 years of age has not been established; therefore, the drug is not recommended for this age group. None of the complex processes that have been recommended previously, such as intensive laundering of underwear and bedclothes, are necessary, because these drugs are very effective and act rapidly. It is advisable, however, to treat all members of the household, because they all must be presumed to be infected. Repeat treatment in 2 or 3 weeks to destroy any worms that originated from larvae hatched from the eggs swallowed at the time of initial

therapy may be necessary, although there is evidence that mebendazole, in contrast to pyrantel, removes young larvae as well as adult worms. Neither drug destroys the eggs.

Reassuring families that this infection is very common, does not reflect uncleanliness, and frequently recurs (and that its ubiquity virtually precludes its effective eradication) is an important component of therapy.

## *Ascaris lumbricoides*

According to current estimates, more than 1 billion humans worldwide are infected with *Ascaris lumbricoides*. In parts of Africa, the average rate of infection is about 45%. In the rural southern communities of the United States, surveys conducted entirely or predominantly among children have shown prevalence rates of 20% to 67%.

### Symptoms by Life Cycle Phase

Light *Ascaris* infections usually are asymptomatic. Heavy infections tend to be associated with constitutional symptoms during the organism's migratory phase, and with intestinal malabsorption and obstruction after the migration has been completed. The infection begins when embryonated eggs are ingested. They hatch in the upper part of the small intestine, freeing the first stage, or rhabditiform larvae, which penetrate the intestinal wall, reach venules or lymphatics, and pass through the portal circulation to the liver, the right side of the heart, and the lungs. In the lungs, the larvae break out of the capillaries and begin ascending through the respiratory radicles until they reach the glottis; passing over the epiglottis, they enter the esophagus and are carried down to the small intestine, where they mature and become adult worms. The cycle is completed in about 2 months.

Infection is maintained in the community by the deposition of human stools in the soil, which permits embryonated eggs to develop to the infective stage. This takes about 2 weeks. The high prevalence of this infection results not only from deficient sanitary facilities for the disposal of human excreta, but also from the routine use of human feces as fertilizer. *Ascaris* can be found in virtually all human communities, but it is most prevalent in warm climates, in areas where the soil is moist and loose, and in communities where sanitation is deficient. It affects children and adults, but the former are more likely to be exposed, because of their habits, and, therefore, are more likely to be infected.

The eggs in the environment can be destroyed by exposure to direct sunlight for 12 hours and are killed quickly at temperatures in excess of 40 °C. Exposure to cold, on the other hand, does not affect them and, in temperate zones, they can survive ordinary freezing temperatures of the winter months. The eggs also are resistant to chemical disinfectants and are not destroyed readily by sewage treatment.

The migratory phase of the infection is associated with an inflammatory response and eosinophilic infiltration. *Ascaris* antigens released during the molting of larvae evoke an immune response and specific antibodies of the IgG class develop in the host, which are the basis of complement fixation and precipitin tests; however, the primary defense mechanism probably is of the cellular immune type. There appears to be a genetic restriction to the immune repertoire in response to *Ascaris* infection. The major histocompatibility complex limits host response.

During the intestinal stage of the infection, symptoms derive primarily from the physical presence of the worms in the gut, or in other sites to which these worms migrate. There also can be malabsorption, because *Ascaris* secretes antienzymes as a protective mechanism for its own survival, although other mechanisms for the development of malabsorption have been proposed as well.

The majority of infected individuals harbor a small number of worms and rarely are symptomatic. Such individuals become aware of the parasites by passage of the adult worms in the stool or through regurgitation and vomiting up of the adult worms.

During the early phase, if the number of larvae that are migrating simultaneously is small, the patient may be asymptomatic. If the larvae are numerous, the individual is likely to have fever with a temperature in the range of 40 °C, cough, and even dyspnea. Dullness to percussion and rales can be detected on physical examination of the chest. The patient can produce copious blood-tinged sputum containing larvae. Eosinophilia is present. Although fatalities are rare, they have been reported in patients with unusually heavy infections and result from the intensity of symptoms in the migratory phase, or from matting together of the worms, which can form a bolus large enough to cause intestinal obstruction. The incidence of this complication has been estimated at 2 per 1000 infected children per year. When it is recognized early, the obstruction can be treated medically, but surgical intervention is required in many cases.

Intestinal perforation, obstruction of the bile duct, and migration of *Ascaris* to other aberrant sites are rarer manifestations of this infection. These complications also can be fatal. Certain irritants, such as tetrachlorethylene (which was used in the past in the treatment of certain hookworm infections), and increased body temperature have been known to precipitate aberrant migrations.

Although *Ascaris* can induce the malabsorption of fats, proteins, and carbohydrates, there is no clear evidence that this has clinical significance.

### Diagnosis

The diagnosis of *Ascaris* infection is established by the identification of the characteristic ascarid eggs through microscopic examination of the stool. Serologic tests are of no value because of the high frequency of cross-reactions.

### Treatment and Prognosis

For an ordinary *Ascaris* infection, pyrantel pamoate (a single dose of 11 mg/kg, not to exceed 1 g) is extremely effective. Mebendazole (100 mg twice daily for 3 days, regardless of body weight) is equally effective. This agent should not be prescribed for children younger than 2 years of age, however, as mentioned above. The disadvantage of mebendazole is that more than a single dose is required. In cases of intestinal obstruction, piperazine citrate (75 mg/kg, maximum 3.5 g/d, once on each of 2 days) can be used to avert surgery, because the drug paralyzes the myoneural junction of *Ascaris* and leads to relaxation of the worms. It is antagonistic to pyrantel pamoate, and these two drugs should not be given together.

The prognosis is excellent in the great majority of cases of ascariasis. Should obstruction or perforation develop, the prognosis depends entirely on the speed of recognition and therapy.

### Control Measures

Ascariasis could be eliminated entirely through proper disposal of human excreta. Unfortunately, as an isolated means of improving health in the world, this never has been successful. Elimination of *Ascaris* from a community or substantial reduction in the incidence of this infection usually follows a general improvement in the standard of living. Periodic community-wide therapy with pyrantel pamoate or mebendazole has been effective in reducing worm burden.

## Trichuris trichiura

Trichuriasis has a prevalence approximating that of the other major roundworm infections, or some 500 million cases in the world, but the infection usually is asymptomatic because, in the majority of cases, it is light.

Like ascariasis, infection with *Trichuris* is acquired by the ingestion of embryonated eggs, which are picked up from the soil on the hands or through contaminated food. The eggs hatch in the upper part of the small intestine and the emerging larvae penetrate the villi. Unlike the larvae of *Ascaris*, those of *Trichuris* do not migrate, but remain in the intestine for a week or so and then descend into the cecum and the colon, where they mature and become embedded in the mucosa. They derive their nutrients from the colonic contents. About 2 months after the original infection, the infected host begins excreting ova. The persistence of the infection in a community depends on continual contamination of the soil with human feces.

The distribution of *T trichiura* closely parallels that of *Ascaris*. *Trichuris* is most prevalent in the tropics and subtropics. It is found in the United States in the southern states. Eggs incubating in the soil become infective in about 1 month and remain viable for several months. They are killed within 1 hour at temperatures greater than 40 °C, and after several hours at temperatures less than −8 °C. The eggs are relatively resistant to chemical disinfectants.

### Symptoms

No systemic reaction usually is noted, because *Trichuris* does not have a migratory phase through the tissues. In the colon, there is an inflammatory reaction and eosinophilic infiltration as well as evidence of an IgE-mediated mucosal response. Host reaction, however, is insufficient to cause significant expulsion of the parasites. Degeneration of the eosinophils leads to the formation of Charcot-Leyden crystals. *Trichuris* does not cause anemia, contrary to some poorly documented assertions that it does. Neither is there any evidence that it interferes with nutrition.

Clinical disease is limited to heavily infected patients with protracted diarrhea characterized by mucous stools. Many patients experience tenesmus, and rectal prolapse can develop in the younger ones.

### Diagnosis

The diagnosis of trichuriasis is established by identification of the characteristic eggs on microscopic examination of the stool. If a patient with chronic diarrhea has such eggs, it is prudent to consider *Trichuris* as the causative agent. In such a case, a course of therapy for trichuriasis can be prescribed. If the diarrhea abates and the patient is well, no additional studies need be carried out. If the patient continues to be symptomatic, a thorough search for two protozoal pathogens, *Entamoeba histolytica* and *Giardia lamblia*—both of which can elude a casual observer who examines only a single stool specimen—must be made, because children in the endemic areas often are subject to multiple parasitic infections.

### Treatment

Treatment consists of the administration of mebendazole (100 mg twice daily for 3 days). The dose does not need to be adjusted to the weight of the patient because the drug is virtually not absorbable. Although the drug has not been approved officially for use in children younger than 2 years, there is no alternative agent available. Those in this age group who are symptomatic should be treated with mebendazole.

### Control Measures

As with other nematodes, sanitary disposal of human excreta and, even more important, improvement in the standard of living tend to reduce the incidence of infection. Periodic mass treatment with mebendazole reduces the worm burden in a community.

## The Hookworms

Hookworm infection has an estimated prevalence of 700 million cases. The vast majority of infected individuals are free of symptoms. Nevertheless, these parasites are a major cause of anemia in the world. Based on the average blood loss induced by each worm, the average number of worms per infected individual, and the prevalence, these parasites are responsible for an estimated daily loss of more than 1 million L of blood in the world. Besides causing anemia, hookworm infections also result in or contribute to malnutrition, because of the concomitant loss of serum proteins. *Ancylostoma duodenale* and *Necator americanus* are the two hookworm parasites of humans.

Hookworm infection is acquired through the exposure of skin to soil that is infested with the larvae of these worms. This usually happens in shady and moist areas if the soil is loamy or sandy. Thus, infection is most likely to be acquired early in the morning when the ground is moist with dew or after a rainfall. After the larvae penetrate the skin, possibly with aid of a hyaluronidase that they secrete, they are carried by the venous circulation to the right side of the heart and, from there, follow the route described for *Ascaris*.

The larvae mature to adult worms in the small intestine and then become attached by their mouth parts to the intestinal mucosa. They are nourished by consuming the mucosa and by sucking blood, a process that is aided by the secretion of an anticoagulant, which causes continued bleeding from the original site after the worm has moved to a new one. The interval between penetration of the skin to the development of a mature, egg-laying worm in the small intestine is about 6 weeks. Humans are the only reservoir of these organisms, and maintenance of hookworm infection is promoted by continual contamination of the soil by human feces.

The hookworms are most prevalent in the tropics and subtropics; in the temperate climates, they are found occasionally in isolated areas. *A duodenale* predominates in the Mediterranean region, in northern Asia, and on the west coast of South America; *N americanus* is the prevailing species in the western hemisphere, most of Africa, southern Asia, Indonesia, parts of Australia, and certain islands of the Pacific. This differential distribution is not absolute, and small numbers of either species are present where the other predominates.

Left undisturbed, the larvae survive in the soil for 6 weeks. They can be destroyed by drying, freezing, and exposure to ambient temperatures in excess of 45 °C.

During the migratory phase of infection, the larvae evoke an inflammatory response and eosinophilia. In animal models, the host mounts an immune response to the adult worms, and a previously infected host is less susceptible to second infection, probably because of the action of IgA antibody. This is not an efficient defense mechanism; in addition, the worms adsorb host antigens, which mask their true surface composition. In an untreated host, *A duodenale* survives for about 8 years; *N americanus* survives for about 4 years.

### Symptoms

*A duodenale* causes the loss of about 0.2 mL of blood per worm, per day; the respective figure for *N americanus* is 0.02 mL. Rarely, massive bleeding has been reported. The problem of malabsorption in hookworm infection is moot. Although it has been demonstrated in patients infected with these parasites, it appears to be a secondary effect resulting from hypoproteinemia, which can be corrected by the administration of a high-protein diet without deworming the patient.

Penetration by the larvae causes pruritus that is proportional in intensity to the number of infecting larvae. The so-called dew itch, or pruritus of the soles after walking in the morning dew, is an example.

In heavy infections, during the early part of invasion of the intestine, the patient can experience abdominal pain, diarrhea, nausea, and anorexia. Later, anemia develops, particularly in malnourished children, whose hemoglobin levels can be as low as 2 g/dL and in whom edema develops as a result of hypoproteinemia. In patients with light infections, there may be no symptoms and no evidence of anemia or malnutrition.

### Diagnosis

As in the case of ascariasis, the differential diagnosis of pneumonia during the migratory phase suggests a parasitic cause, because of peripheral eosinophilia. Because anemia is the result of blood loss, it must be distinguished from all other causes of intestinal loss of blood. In the developing countries where severe hookworm anemia is common, the probability of the rarer causes of intestinal blood loss (eg, Meckel's diverticulum, polyps) is quite low. The opposite holds true for the regions in which hookworm infections are light or infrequent.

Identification by microscopic examination of the characteristic ova in the stool is the basis of diagnosis of this infection. The species of the hookworm cannot be identified by this method, because the eggs of *Ancylostoma* and *Necator* look alike. It is necessary, therefore, to assume infection by one or the other species on the basis of geographic origin of the patient. Although this decision is not of paramount importance, it does have some therapeutic implications.

### Treatment

Pyrantel pamoate (single dose of 11 mg/kg, maximum 1 g) or mebendazole (100 mg twice daily for 3 days) is equally effective in treating infection with *N americanus*. The former has the advantage of single-dose therapy and, thus, more assured compliance. The latter is more effective in the treatment of *A duodenale* and, therefore, is considered the drug of choice.

### Control Measures

Sanitary control of the disposal of excreta would eliminate the infection entirely, but this is not feasible in most of the world. The popular recommendation for wearing shoes is naive, because large segments of human populations go barefoot for economic and cultural reasons. Moreover, contact with the infested soil through any segment of skin can result in the infection. This is especially a problem for infants, who often are placed on the soil, and for toddlers, who play in it.

## *Strongyloides stercoralis*

*Strongyloides stercoralis* has an estimated prevalence of some 40 million cases in the world. This infection is of major clinical importance even when it is light and the host is well nourished.

Infection is caused by exposure of the skin to infective larvae in the soil. The life cycle of *Strongyloides* resembles those of the hookworms from the moment of penetration of the skin to the arrival of the worms in the intestine. The larvae require the same environmental conditions in the soil for survival as do the hookworm larvae. Differences exist, however, in the behavior of this parasite in the intestine. The adult worms do not attach themselves to the mucosa, but lie embedded in its folds. The eggs embryonate within the intestine, not in the soil, and develop into first-stage larvae there. The larvae are deposited in the soil with human stool and undergo a molt before they become infective. The time from infection to the completion of the cycle is about 28 days.

An alternative pattern permits molting in the human host of the noninfective new larvae into the infective ones, which can penetrate the intestine and set up a new cycle, commonly referred to as an autoinfective cycle. Thus, this nematode, unlike other intestinal nematodes of humans, can increase in numbers without reinfection from the outside world. Moreover, by this mechanism, untreated *Strongyloides* infection can persist for decades. In an immunocompromised host, the autoinfective cycle can become hyperinfective and reach proportions that are lethal for the patient. *Strongyloides* also has a nonparasitic cycle in the soil, which can maintain infestation of the soil indefinitely.

This parasite has a worldwide distribution, but is most prevalent in the tropics and subtropics. It is found also in mental hospitals, prisons, and residential institutions for children, because of the transmission of infection through contamination of the skin by feces. Strongyloidiasis is primarily a human infection, but it also occurs in dogs and anthropoid apes, although the species of the parasite in these animals probably are different.

## Symptoms

During the migratory phase, the larvae evoke an inflammatory response associated with eosinophilic infiltration. Eosinophilia occurs. The adult phase in the intestine, even in moderate infections, can be associated with an inflammatory reaction that is sufficient to cause symptoms. *Strongyloides* induces a malabsorption syndrome that is characterized by steatorrhea. Patients have normal D-xylose absorption; therefore, some researchers have theorized that the abnormality is the result of edema of the lamina propria caused by the release of histamine from mast cells. Malabsorption abates after deworming.

Patients with moderate or heavy infections have intense diarrhea productive of watery, mucous stools that alternates with constipation. In massive infections caused by the hyperinfective cycle, larvae invade all tissues, including the central nervous system (CNS), and can cause sepsis, as they carry with them enteric flora.

## Diagnosis

The differential diagnosis of the diarrhea must include causes of chronic diarrheal disease; associated eosinophilia should suggest strongyloidiasis.

The diagnosis is made by microscopic examination of the stool, which can reveal the characteristic larvae. If the results of the stool examination are negative, the duodenal contents should be examined by means of the string test (Entero-Test). This divulges only the contents of the duodenum, however, and can cause the larvae that are present in the lower small intestine to be overlooked. No specific serologic tests are available. This infection must be ruled out in immunosuppressed individuals, including those treated with corticosteroids for any reason, who have ever been in a geographic locale where *Strongyloides* is found.

## Treatment

Thiabendazole (50 mg/kg/24 h, divided into two equal daily doses on each of two successive days) is the drug of choice, although it still is considered to be an investigational drug for this condition. Its cure rate approaches 100%. Frequent side effects include nausea, vomiting, and vertigo; rare adverse effects are leukopenia, rashes, and even Stevens-Johnson syndrome. Because the drug is detoxified in the liver, its dosage may have to be reduced for patients with liver failure. If the initial course of thiabendazole is only partially effective, the therapy may be repeated. Ivermectin has been tried experimentally in adults and was effective in eliminating *Strongyloides*. It probably will become an alternative drug, or even the drug of choice.

The prognosis is excellent in patients who do not have disseminated infection and who are treated promptly. Unrecognized disseminated infection can be lethal.

## Control Measures

Proper disposal of human excreta will reduce substantially the prevalence of strongyloidiasis in any community. In closed institutions, where control of direct spread is unlikely, the identification and treatment of infected individuals is the only feasible control measure.

# ABERRANT INFECTIONS WITH INTESTINAL NEMATODES

Life cycles of parasites are adjusted precisely through evolutionary selection. In many instances, only one host in which the cycle can be completed is parasitized by the nematode. Infections of an unnatural host in most cases lead to complete failure of development and no disease. In other cases, an infection is established, but the cycle cannot be completed. This often results in aberrant migration of the larvae, which can cause serious disease.

## *Toxocara canis*

Human infection with the dog roundworm, a relative of human *Ascaris*, is an example of aberrant infection with an intestinal nematode. If embryonated eggs of *Toxocara canis*, whose cycle in the dog resembles that of *Ascaris*, are ingested by humans, the larvae will hatch in the small intestine, penetrate the villi, and begin a migration that takes them through every organ and tissue of the body. Because they cannot mature, the larvae tend to migrate for months (hence, the name "visceral larva migrans") until they are overcome by the inflammatory reaction of the host and die. Although larvae of toxocarids such as *Toxocara cati* and *Toxascaris leonina* have been suggested as possible causes of visceral larva migrans, there is no clear evidence that they are involved.

The prevalence of toxocariasis is difficult to assess because many cases probably are overlooked. The disease has been reported from many parts of the world, and is assumed to be present wherever humans and dogs coexist. Several surveys have reported finding eggs of *Toxocara* in as many as 25% of soil samples. Dogs in urban communities are infected frequently; puppies are particularly prone to the infection, which they acquire transplacentally.

Although patients with poliomyelitis have a higher incidence of positive skin test for *Toxocara*, no direct causal relationship between these two conditions has been demonstrated. It is possible that the circumstances that lead to the ingestion of *Toxocara* ova also are conducive to the ingestion of poliomyelitis virus.

### Syndromes and Symptoms

Two distinct syndromes of *Toxocara* infection, visceral and ocular, are recognized. They usually do not coexist and it is possible that different strains of this species exist, with specific tropisms.

As the larvae migrate, they cause protean symptoms. These vary from patient to patient, depending on the intensity of the infection and on which organs or tissues predominantly are infected. The fundamental lesion is a granuloma. The most dangerous manifestation of toxocariasis is retinal granuloma. The lesion mimics retinoblastoma and has been mistaken for this condition. There also can be endophthalmitis or papillitis.

In ocular toxocariasis, the granuloma can be seen readily by ophthalmoscopy. In the visceral variety, the symptoms and signs are those of a multisystem disease associated with fever, hepatosplenomegaly, a high degree of eosinophilia (approaching 80%) and elevated immunoglobulin levels, particularly of the IgM class. The diagnosis must depend on a heightened level of suspicion, and the disease must be distinguished from the migratory phase of the other nematode infections. Because of hepatosplenomegaly and hypereosinophilia, eosinophilic leukemia can be suspected, but it can be ruled out readily by examination of the bone marrow.

### Diagnosis

The diagnosis can be confirmed by demonstration of the larvae in the patient's tissues. Sometimes this can be achieved with liver biopsy, but the yield is low. A magnetic resonance imaging examination of one patient with CNS infection with *Toxocara* revealed lesions in the brain. Often, the diagnosis is made indirectly by recognizing that a multi-system disease associated with elevated IgM levels and hypereosinophilia fits the criteria for toxocariasis. Unusually high levels of blood isoagglutinins, A and B, are found in these patients, if their own blood type does not preclude the presence of these antibodies. Although the currently used serologic test is marred by cross-reactions with *Ascaris* and *Strongyloides*, a new enzyme-linked immunosorbent assay based on an antigen derived from the second-stage larvae has become available. It has a sensitivity of 91% and a specificity of 86%.

### Treatment

Treatment is primarily symptomatic, but thiabendazole (50 mg/kg/24 h in two divided doses for periods of 1 week to 1 month) is claimed to be effective against the migrating larvae. Considering the potential danger of retinal damage, it seems prudent to treat a patient with a suspected case of toxocariasis with this drug until the symptoms subside. The vast majority of patients recover, but those with advanced ocular disease can become blind. Rarely, a fatality will result from the intensity of the acute clinical reaction. Recovery may be slow, lasting as long as 2 years.

### Control Measures

Theoretically, toxocariasis can be prevented by the elimination of dog feces from the human environment, but this has been difficult to implement in practice. Because the infection can be contracted in playground sandboxes, these should be covered when they are not in use.

## Baylisascaris procyonis

*Baylisascaris procyonis*, a parasite of raccoons, also can cause visceral larva migrans syndrome. In the one reported human case, the infection was fatal to an infant. The lesions caused by the larvae are granulomas, which tend to be concentrated in the upper parts of the body and have a particular affinity for the eyes and CNS. The frequency of this infection was not known when the first case was reported. Since then, no series of human infection has been reported. A recent survey of parasites in wild raccoons in Arkansas revealed no evidence of *B procyonis*.

## Other Aberrant Nematode Infections

Other, less severe aberrant infections of importance to humans are those by the larvae of dog hookworms, *Ancylostoma braziliense*, *Ancylostoma caninum*, and *Uncinaria stenocephala*. These infections are acquired in the same fashion as are those by the larvae of human hookworms. Children who expose their whole bodies to the contaminated soil can be infected at any site. Adults are most likely to have infection in the lower extremities, but plumbers in the tropics, who often must crawl beneath houses, acquire infection on the elbows and knees. The larvae migrate within the skin. This is the basis of the terms "cutaneous larva migrans" and "creeping eruption." The interval from exposure to the first symptoms is about 2 weeks. The lesions are serpiginous, erythematous, intracutaneous tunnels leading to papules that are 2 mm in diameter. The involved areas itch intensely.

Cutaneous larva migrans syndrome lasts as long as 2 months. Treatment is symptomatic, with topical ethyl chloride spray, which not only relieves the itching, but also kills some of the larvae. Thiabendazole has been considered effective in the same dosage as for visceral larva migrans, administered for 5 days. Topical therapy with 15% aqueous suspension of thiabendazole also may be effective.

Rarer aberrant infections include those caused by various species of *Angiostrongylus*, *Capillaria*, and *Anisakis*. *Angiostrongylus* species, particularly *Angiostrongylus cantonensis*, whose intermediate hosts are land snails and slugs, are parasites of the rat in which the adult worms are located in the lungs. Ingestion of either the molluscs or of food contaminated by the molluscs can lead to human infection with *Angiostrongylus*. Evidence exists that larvae of this stage can cause infection by penetrating mucous membranes, conjunctivae, or lacerated skin. Infection is limited to the CNS and presents as eosinophilic meningitis. No specific treatment is available, but the disease is self-limited, lasting no more than 2 weeks, although there have been rare deaths. Symptomatic relief has been reported with the use of prednisone.

*Capillaria philippinensis* and *Capillaria hepatica* are common parasites of rodents. Their mode of transmission to humans is unknown, but cases have been reported in which as many as 40,000 adult worms were found embedded in the crypts in the small intestine. No inflammatory reaction occurs, but villous atrophy associated with severe malabsorption has been reported. *C hepatica*, in addition, has been known to disseminate to the lungs, liver, and other viscera. Thiabendazole (50 mg/kg/24 h, in two divided doses, administered for 3 weeks) may be effective in shortening the course of the infection. Mebendazole, in doses comparable to those used in humans, reduced the deposition of eggs by 97% when it was administered to mice that were infected experimentally with *Capillaria*.

*Anisakis* species are parasites of marine fish. Humans ingest the adult worms while eating raw or poorly cooked fish. Thus far, the infection has been reported with any frequency only in adults in Japan, where raw marine fish is eaten commonly, and in Holland, where lightly pickled herring is considered a delicacy. In the United States, only rare, sporadic cases have been reported. The worms become embedded in the gastric and colonic mucosa, and cause an eosinophilic granuloma. One case of acute appendicitis was attributed to intraluminal *Anisakis* worm. The infection can resemble carcinoma of the stomach on clinical grounds and even in the roentgenographic images. This infection has not been reported in children. Diagnosis can be made by radiology and by serology. No specific therapy is available.

## TISSUE NEMATODES

## Trichinella spiralis

*Trichinella spiralis* infects all mammals. Human infections are relatively infrequent compared to those caused by the other parasitic nematodes. Only some 10 million people currently are considered to be infected in the United States. Most countries have reported infections with *Trichinella*, and recent outbreaks have occurred in Southeast Asia and Japan. Puerto Rico and Australia remain the only surveyed areas free of this infection.

This organism is acquired through the ingestion of animal flesh in which the larvae of *Trichinella* are encysted. Depending on the diet of the particular population, the infection usually comes from pork, but it also has been reported from bear meat. The larvae emerge from the cysts in the stomach and are moved by peristalsis to the upper two thirds of the small intestine. After penetrating columnar cells of the epithelium, they develop through four molts, becoming adults in about 30 hours. Five days after the adult worms copulate, the female gives birth to some 1000 live larvae. The newborn larvae penetrate the lamina propria and move via the thoracic duct to the venous circulation, the right side of the heart, the lungs, and—unlike the other migratory nematodes parasitic for humans—through the lungs to the left side of the heart and the systemic circulation. Thus, the larvae can become distributed throughout the body and can enter any cell. Cells penetrated by the larvae die as the result of this invasion. Skeletal myofibrils are an exception, however. They become nurturing cells for these larvae and support their further development until encystment occurs.

## Symptoms

Symptoms caused by *Trichinella* initially are related to the enteritis that is induced during the intestinal phase of the infection, and can include diarrhea. During the subsequent parenteral phase, symptoms are related to the organism's migration through the tissues and indiscriminate penetration of cells. The most problematic symptoms occur from invasion of the heart and the CNS. Myocarditis is mild and transient, because the larvae leave the myocardium soon after penetration. In the CNS, on the other hand, the larvae tend to migrate for a long time and cause granulomas and petechial hemorrhages, with consequent encephalopathy.

Clinical disease is related to the behavior of the larvae. There is fever, general malaise, myalgia, and, in particularly severe cases, myocarditis and encephalopathy. If the extraocular muscles are involved, patients may have diplopia and blurred vision.

## Diagnosis

Diagnosis of *Trichinella* infection depends on clinical suspicion based on the protean nature of the symptoms, an appropriate history of ingestion of suspect meat, and physical findings (muscle tenderness; petechial hemorrhages in the subungual skin, soft palate, and conjunctivae; and edema of the face and eyelids). These findings are supported by the presence of peripheral eosinophilia, which can reach 50% or higher. The absence of eosinophilia or, worse, its gradual disappearance while the disease is acute, indicates overwhelming infection and carries a grave prognosis.

Immunologic tests are helpful, but their results become positive too late to be of immediate clinical usefulness. The best technique is counterimmunoelectrophoresis, which detects antibodies on the 12th day. The bentonite flocculation test result becomes positive after 3 weeks. Both test results remain positive for some 3 months.

Definitive diagnosis is made from biopsy of a skeletal muscle, chosen because of tenderness. The tissue is examined best unfixed and under low microscopic power to detect whole larvae.

## Treatment

The treatment of systemic disease is primarily symptomatic; in severe cases, corticosteroids are recommended. Because there still can be live worms in the intestine generating new larvae at the time when the systemic disease develops, treatment with antihelminthic agents is appropriate. Mebendazole (600 to 1200 mg/24 h in three divided doses for 3 days, followed by 1200 mg/24 h in three divided doses for an additional 10 days) is recommended for adults, although it is considered an experimental drug for this condition. The proper pediatric dosage has not been determined. Thiabendazole (50 mg/kg/24 h in two divided doses for 5 days) has been recommended as well. Experimental infection of mice has been treated with cyclosporin A and with interferon-τ. The former had some beneficial effect; the latter did not.

## Control Measures

Prevention is accomplished best on an individual level by thorough cooking of pork or bear meat until it ceases to be pink. Keeping pork at −15 °C for 2 weeks also is effective, but this method can fail with meat from arctic animals, which contains natural substances that interfere with freezing.

# FILARIAL WORMS

Major filarial parasites are limited in their distribution to the tropics. Some 200 million people are infected by one or more species of these worms. All filarial worms affecting humans are transmitted by vectors, which bite and transfer the infective larvae, or microfilariae, onto the skin of the host. The larvae enter the wound in the skin and make their way to the respective tissue, where they mature into adult worms. The adults invade and occupy the lymphatics, skin, connective tissue, or blood, mate there, and produce live microfilariae, which enter the bloodstream or skin and there undergo further development or remain dormant for weeks or months. They are ingested by blood-sucking insects, in which they undergo metamorphosis through two larval stages until they reach the third, infective stage. The interval from the infective bite to the appearance of microfilariae in the blood of the host can be as long as 6 months. The microfilariae exhibit circadian periodicity, some being diurnal and others nocturnal, depending not only on the species, but also on the different varieties of one species. Some species of the filarial worms cause serious diseases; others do not have any known adverse effects on the host.

Diagnostic tests based on immunodiagnosis are not useful because of cross-reactions to the antigens of other filarial worms and even intestinal helminths. They include intradermal tests, complement fixation tests, and hemagglutination inhibition and fluorescent antibody tests (which still are experimental). Intradermal tests are of value in epidemiologic surveys.

## *Wuchereria bancrofti*

*Wuchereria bancrofti* is prevalent in the tropics. It is spread by various anopheline and culicine mosquitoes in various locales. The microfilariae exhibit nocturnal periodicity everywhere except the South Pacific, where their periodicity is diurnal.

## Symptoms

The microfilariae themselves are fundamentally harmless, although they can cause transient allergic reactions. The adult worms cause the major problem by invoking an inflammatory response, usually associated with a systemic reaction of fever, headache, and general malaise. The infected host has lymphangitis, with the ultimate complications of lymphoid hyperplasia, epithelioid granulomas, and eventual fibrosis, with lymphedema proximal to the obstruction. This leads to the development of classic elephantiasis of the scrotum or labia majora and lower extremities. The obstruction also can lead to chyluria and chylous diarrhea. Clinical manifestations are the result of years of repeated infections. Chronic, recurrent pneumonitis associated with wheezing, cough, chest pain, pulmonary infiltrations, and hypereosinophilia is caused by the migration of microfilariae through the lungs.

## Diagnosis

Diagnosis of this infection depends on finding the microfilariae in the blood, which must be collected at a time when peak microfilaremia is expected. The blood need not be examined immediately, but can be preserved in a large volume of formalin for subsequent concentration and staining. Detection of circulating filarial antigen, as well as its corresponding antibody, is likely to become the basis of a standard immunologic test in the near future.

## Treatment

Diethylcarbamazine (6 mg/kg/24 h in three divided doses for 2 weeks) effectively destroys microfilariae and sterilizes or kills the adult female worms. If microfilariae still appear in the blood after 2 weeks of therapy, treatment for another 2 weeks is advisable. Because the patient can have an allergic reaction to the proteins of the disintegrating worms, and even fever, treatment with antihistamines or corticosteroids is recommended if such reactions develop. Ivermectin, a new drug that is used commonly in veterinary practice, but still is considered experimental in humans, has been introduced recently for the treatment of some filarial worm infections. It has exceptional therapeutic value, few side effects, and the advantage of single-dose administration. It is given at a dose of 0.025 mg/kg once and is repeated semiannually in endemic areas as a prophylactic measure. Without a doubt, it will replace diethylcarbamazine.

The serious manifestations of infection with W bancrofti, such as elephantiasis, do not abate after treatment. Drug treatment prevents complications, but once complications develop, they must be treated surgically if they are disfiguring or interfere with normal life.

## Control Measures

Prevention of filariasis depends on vector control, which has been less than satisfactory. Periodic massive drug treatment of populations at risk has merit, especially because, with the sole exception of Malaysia, there is no known animal reservoir of this infection. The use of salt medicated with diethylcarbamazine substantially reduces, or even eliminates, this infection.

## Brugia malayi

Brugia malayi infection behaves fundamentally as does W bancrofti infection, except that the elephantiasis resulting from Brugia tends to affect mostly the upper rather than the lower extremities.

## Onchocerca volvulus

Infection with Onchocerca volvulus is acquired through the bite of the Simulium fly, which tends to breed along rivers and streams (hence, the common name of the disease, "river blindness"). Onchocerciasis is limited to Africa, Central America, and northern parts of South America. Because many settlements are established alongside rivers, onchocerciasis is highly prevalent wherever there is a high prevalence of Simulium. The development of hydroelectric power with the construction of large dams has increased the breeding sites of Simulium and, as a result, the prevalence of onchocerciasis.

### Symptoms by Life Cycle Phase

Simulium bites and deposits larvae in the subcutaneous tissue, where they develop into adult worms. The adults tend to be coiled, and they become enveloped by fibrous tissues and form nodules, within which they reproduce. The microfilariae invade the skin and remain there for some 30 months, by which time they die. The microfilariae also penetrate the eye and affect every layer from the conjunctiva to the optic nerve. In African onchocerciasis, chorioretinitis and optic atrophy are common; in the Central American disease, iritis is the primary lesion. In Central America, the Onchocerca nodules tend to be located on the upper part of the body; in Africa, they are found predominantly on the lower part.

Migration of the microfilariae through the skin causes a local inflammatory reaction manifested by acute pruritus and chronic changes, such as edema, hypertrophy, and reddish hyperpigmentation (peu d'orange). Eventually, subcutaneous nodules form that contain the adult worms and microfilariae. Microfilariae that have invaded the eyes can be seen readily with an ophthalmoscope. Ocular invasion leads to the development of keratitis, iridocyclitis, chorioretinitis, and eventual blindness.

### Diagnosis

Examination of sectioned and stained tissue obtained by a skin snip will reveal adult worms and microfilariae. An impression smear made from the snip usually shows microfilariae. A complementary DNA fragment coding for an O volvulus antigen (OV-16) has been cloned and expressed in a plasmid vector. This recombinant antigen is capable of detecting antibody to the parasite 1 year before the clinical appearance of onchocerciasis.

### Treatment

The most effective therapy for onchocerciasis is removal by excision of all the visible nodules. This abolishes the source of microfilariae and protects the eyes from further invasion. Diethylcarbamazine has been the standard treatment. The dosage must be started low and built up gradually to the full concentration to protect the eyes from an intense inflammatory reaction to the disintegrating worms. The recommended initial dosage is 1.5 mg/kg/24 h, not to exceed 25 mg/24 h, divided into three doses and administered on each of 3 days. For the following 4 days, the dosage should be increased to 3 mg/kg/24 h; for the 4 days after that, it should be increased to 4.5 mg/kg/24 h. Finally, for the balance of the month's therapy, it should be 8 mg/kg/24 h, not to exceed 150 mg/24 h, administered in three divided doses each day. If the initial reaction is severe, antihistamines or corticosteroids should be used to attenuate it. Because of the complexity of this treatment and its toxicity, diethylcarbamazine will soon be abandoned, and ivermectin soon will become the drug of choice.

### Control Measures

Vector control, periodic treatment of infected individuals, and surgical removal of skin lesions are the only means of prevention, and their success is limited.

## Dirofilaria immitis

Human infections with the filarial heartworm of the dog, Dirofilaria immitis, have been reported, but thus far not in children. The infection is transmitted by culicine mosquitoes. Infected humans can have chest pains, wheezing, and cough, but the majority probably are asymptomatic. Coin lesions are seen on pulmonary roentgenograms. There is no reason to believe that children are spared, and it is possible that lesions in children have been misdiagnosed as representing a Ghon complex. No microfilariae have been demonstrated in peripheral blood in humans. Patients have peripheral eosinophilia, usually not exceeding 10%.

## Suggested Readings

### Intestinal Nematodes

Bundy DA, Cooper ES, Thomson DE, et al. Predisposition to Trichuris trichuria infection in humans Epidemiol Infect 1987;98:65.

Christie JF, Fraser EM, Kennedy MW. Comparison between the MHC-restricted antibody repertoire to Ascaris antigens in adjuvant-assisted immunization or infection. Parasite Immunol 1992;14:59.

Feldmeier H, Fischer H, Blaumeiser G. Kinetics of human response during the acute and the convalescent phase of human trichinosis. Zentralblatt Bakteriologie Mikrobiologie und Hygiene 1987;264:221.

Gam AA, Neva FA, Krotoski WD. Comparative sensitivity and specificity of ELISA and IHA for serodiagnosis of strongyloidiasis with larval antigens. Am J Trop Med Hyg 1987;37:157.

Kolt SD, Wirth PD, Speer AG. Biliary ascariasis—a worm in the duct. Med J Aust 1991;154:629.

Maxwell C, Hussain R, Nutman TB, et al. The clinical and immunological responses of normal human volunteers to low dose hookworm (*Necator americanus*) infection. Am J Trop Med Hyg 1987;37:126.

Newton RC, Limpuangthip P, Greenberg S, et al. Strongyloides stercoralis hyperinfection in a carrier of HTLV-I virus with evidence of selective immunosuppression. Am J Med 1992;92:202.

Pawlowski ZS. Intestinal helminthiases and human health: Recent advances and future needs. Int J Parasitol 1987;17:159.

Pawlowski ZS. Ascariasis. In: Warren KS, Mahmoud AAF, eds. Tropical and geographical medicine, 2nd ed. New York: McGraw-Hill, 1990:369.

Pritchard DI. Antigens of gastrointestinal nematodes. Trans R Soc Trop Med Hyg 1986;80:728.

Schantz PM. Improvements in the serodiagnosis of helminthic zoonoses. Vet Parasitol 1987;25:95.

Shikiya K, Uehara T, Uechi H, et al. Clinical study of ivermectin against Strongyloides stercoralis. Kansenshogaku Zasshi 1991;65:1085.

### Aberrant Infections With Intestinal Nematodes

Glickman LT, Shoifer FS. Zoonotic visceral and ocular larva migrans. Vet Clin North Am 1987;17:39.

Huff DS, Neaffie RC, Binder MJ, et al. The first fatal baylisascaris infection in humans: An infant with eosinophilic meningoencephalitis. Pediatr Pathol 1984;2:1.

Jacquier P, Gottstein B, Stingelin Y, et al. Immunodiagnosis of toxocarosis in humans: Evaluation of a new enzyme-linked immunosorbent assay kit. J Clin Microbiol 1991;29:1831.

Kliks MM, Palumbo NE. Eosinophilic meningitis beyond Pacific Basin: The global dispersal of peridomestic zoonosis caused by Angiostrongylus cantonensis, the nematode lungworm of rats. Soc Sci Med 1992;34:199.

Matsumoto T, Iida M, Kimura Y, et al. Anisakiasis of the colon: Radiologic and endoscopic features in six patients. Radiology 1992;183:97.

Morris PD, Katerndahl DA. Human toxocariasis: Review with report of a probable case. Postgrad Med 1987;81:263.

Richardson DJ, Owen WB, Snyder DE. Helminth parasites of the raccoon (Procyon lotor) from north-central Arkansas. J Parasitol 1992;78:163.

Ruttinger P, Hadidi H. MRI in cerebral toxocaral disease. J Neurol Neurosurg Psychiatry 1991;54:361.

Watson J, Wetzel WJ, Burkhalter J. Human disease caused by dog heartworm. J Miss State Med Assoc 1991;32:399.

### Tissue Nematodes

Cartel JL, Spiegel A, Nguyen L, et al. Double blind study on efficacy and safety of single doses of ivermectin and diethylcarbamazine for treatment of Polynesian Wuchereria bancrofti carriers, results at six months. Trop Med Parasitol 1991;42:38.

Cheirmaraj K, Parkhe KA, Harinath BC. Evaluation of fractionated circulating filarial antigen in diagnosis of bancroftian filariasis. J Trop Med Hyg 1992;95:47.

Liu J, Chen Z, Huang X, et al. Mass treatment of filariasis using DEC-medicated salt. J Trop Med Hyg 1992;95:132.

Lobos E, Weiss N, Karam M, et al. An immunogenic Onchocerca volvulus antigen: A specific and early marker of infection. Science 1991;251:1603.

Partono F. The spectrum of disease in lymphatic filariasis. Ciba Found Symp 1987;127:15.

Pawlowski ZS. Clinical aspects in man. In: Campbell WC, ed. Trichinella and trichinosis. New York: Plenum Press, 1983:367.

Smith HJ. Factors affecting preconditioning of *Trichinella spiralis* native larvae in musculature to low temperatures. Can J Vet Res 1987;51:169.

Subramanyan D. Antifilarials and their mode of action. Ciba Found Symp 1987;127:246.

von Lichtenberg F. Inflammatory responses to filarial connective tissue parasites. Parasitology 1987;94(Suppl):S101.

*Principles and Practice of Pediatrics, Second Edition.*
edited by Frank A. Oski et al. J. B. Lippincott Company, Philadelphia © 1994.

# 62.3 *Schistosomiasis*

## Mark W. Kline

Schistosomiasis is a disease of the circulatory system caused principally by three species of trematodes: *Schistosoma mansoni*, *Schistosoma haematobium*, and *Schistosoma japonicum*. Some 200 to 300 million people worldwide are infected with one of these organisms. Travel to and from endemic areas of Africa, South America, and Asia has spread the disease well beyond its historical geographic boundaries to North America and Europe. In the United States, more than 400,000 people may be infected with one of the human schistosomes. Although transmission of the infection in the United States is not possible because of the absence of snail intermediate hosts, recognition of the clinical features of the disease is key to diagnosis and treatment for the prevention of long-term adverse sequelae.

## LIFE CYCLE

The human is the definitive host for the three principal schistosome species; certain snails serve as intermediate hosts. Deposition of eggs (oviposition) occurs in the venules of the large intestine (S mansoni), small intestine (S japonicum), or urinary bladder (S haematobium) of humans. Female S mansoni organisms release eggs at a rate of several hundred each day. The rate of oviposition for S japonicum may be tenfold higher. Many eggs remain in the tissues or are carried via the bloodstream to the liver or other distant body sites. A minority reach the lumina of the intestine or urinary bladder and are excreted. S mansoni eggs are elliptic, measure roughly 60 by 150 $\mu$m, and possess a lateral spine. S haematobium eggs are of similar shape and size, but possess a terminal spine. The eggs of S japonicum are smaller (about 60 by 90 $\mu$m), more spheroid, and have a vestigial lateral spine.

Free-living miracidia are released when eggs contact warm fresh water. Miracidia swim until they find an appropriate snail intermediate host, then they penetrate its tissues and begin asexual reproduction. In a few weeks, infective larvae, or cercariae, are shed from the snail and may penetrate intact human skin. After penetration, the parasite develops into a worm-like schistosomulum and passes through the skin and to the lungs via lymphatics or the bloodstream. After a total period of 1 to 3 weeks, schistosomula reach the liver, where maturation and sexual reproduction occur. Adult schistosomes descend through the venous system to their preferred sites in the intestine or urinary bladder. Oviposition occurs 4 to 12 weeks after cercarial penetration of the skin.

## EPIDEMIOLOGY

The geographic distribution and prevalence of schistosomiasis change continuously. The transmission of schistosomes depends absolutely on the distribution of susceptible snails. Population shifts and the introduction of irrigation have led to an increased prevalence of infection in many endemic areas. On the other hand, population treatment and snail eradication programs have affected favorably the prevalence of infection in certain areas. Inhabitants of endemic areas usually encounter schistosomes during childhood and may be infected repeatedly throughout their lives. The prevalence of infection may reach adult levels during the first decade of life. The incidence of initial infections, therefore, is low in comparison to the overall prevalence and is restricted largely to children. Most infected humans have a low worm burden and pass only a few eggs in the stool or urine. A relatively small number of individuals are infected heavily, but they contribute disproportionately to environmental contamination and the transmission of infection. Control efforts often have been directed against these heavily infected individuals.

S japonicum is endemic only in the Far East, with foci in China, Japan, the Philippines, Indonesia, Thailand, Laos, and Cambodia. A similar human schistosome of lesser importance, *Schistosoma mekongi*, first was reported from the Mekong River delta and probably is endemic throughout Southeast Asia. S haematobium is endemic throughout Africa and in parts of Southwest Asia and the Middle East. *S mansoni* is widespread in Africa and is the only human schistosome present in the Western hemisphere, with endemic foci in Brazil, Suriname, Venezuela, and the Caribbean. Schistosomiasis in the United States occurs mainly among immigrants from endemic areas.

## PATHOGENESIS AND CLINICAL MANIFESTATIONS

Adult schistosomes mask themselves by adsorption of host antigens onto their surfaces. Consequently, the adult parasites elicit minimal local inflammatory responses. On the other hand, intense local inflammation may accompany cercarial penetration of the skin, and granulomatous inflammation often surrounds schistosome eggs in tissues. The clinical and pathologic features of schistosomiasis are determined in large part by host immune responses to the worms and eggs. Three distinct clinical patterns of disease are noted:

1. Schistosome dermatitis, or swimmers' itch, which is a manifestation of cercarial penetration of the skin
2. An illness similar to serum sickness, which is known as Katayama fever and occurs with the onset of oviposition
3. Fibrosis of the liver (*S mansoni* or *S japonicum*) or of the ureters and bladder (*S haematobium*) and its sequelae.

Cercarial penetration of the skin in a nonsensitized individual usually is an inconspicuous event clinically. Mild erythema and pruritus may develop locally within minutes of skin penetration. This initial reaction is transient. One to 2 weeks later, small (1- to 2-mm) pruritic papules may be noted at the same sites. Individuals previously sensitized to schistosome antigens may have intense reactions on reexposure. Localized urticaria and pruritus occur initially, and pruritic papular lesions are noted within 24 hours. Lesions may persist for 7 to 10 days.

Schistosome dermatitis can be difficult to differentiate from other skin diseases. The diagnosis is suggested by a history of swimming, wading, or bathing in untreated water from areas endemic for schistosomiasis, and by the occurrence of lesions only on water-exposed body surfaces. Biopsy specimens from early skin lesions may demonstrate the organisms.

Individuals heavily infected with *S japonicum* and, to a lesser extent, with *S mansoni*, may experience the abrupt onset of an illness that is similar to serum sickness as oviposition commences. This condition is known as Katayama fever and its clinical manifestations include high spiking fevers, abdominal pain, vomiting, anorexia, myalgias, and headache. Generalized lymphadenopathy and hepatosplenomegaly may be noted, and peripheral blood eosinophilia virtually always is present. Sigmoidoscopy and liver biopsy may be helpful in establishing the diagnosis of Katayama fever. Histopathologically, the liver is infiltrated by eosinophils, and schistosome eggs are seen occasionally. Katayama fever usually is self-limited, but it may persist for weeks to several months.

Much of the long-term morbidity and mortality that is associated with schistosomiasis reflects chronic effects of host immunologic responses to eggs in the tissues. In the wall of the human intestine, eggs of *S mansoni* and *S japonicum* incite granulomatous inflammation, which disrupts tissue architecture and function, and ultimately leads to fibrosis. The clinical manifestations of intestinal schistosomiasis are varied. Many individuals are asymptomatic, whereas others complain of abdominal pain, anorexia, vomiting, diarrhea, or blood in the stool. Children may experience growth failure. Occasionally, symptoms mimic those of cholecystitis or peptic ulcer disease. Colonic polyposis is an uncommon finding seen only in individuals infected with *S mansoni*. Hepatosplenic schistosomiasis occurs when schistosome eggs cause embolization in the liver. A characteristic pattern of scarring,

known as pipestem or Symmers' fibrosis, is found around portal veins, leading eventually to portal hypertension. Hepatomegaly often is the initial clinical manifestation of hepatosplenic schistosomiasis. In advanced cases, congestive splenomegaly and variceal bleeding are noted. Signs and symptoms of hepatocellular disease (eg, icterus, ascites, elevated serum transaminase levels, etc.) usually are absent.

Deposition of *S haematobium* eggs in the bladder and ureters produces granulomatous reactions and scarring, with nodular or ulcerative changes of the bladder and fibrosis of the ureters. Early manifestations of urinary tract schistosomiasis include urinary frequency, dysuria, and terminal hematuria. Intravenous pyelography or ultrasonography may demonstrate hydroureter and hydronephrosis in advanced cases. Carcinoma of the bladder occurs with increased frequency in individuals with *S haematobium* infection.

Schistosome eggs may reach distant body sites via lymphatic or vascular channels. The deposition of eggs in the pulmonary vasculature leads to granuloma formation, obstruction to pulmonary blood flow, and schistosomal cor pulmonale. *S mansoni* and *S haematobium* may produce transverse myelitis by the deposition of eggs in the spinal cord. Mass lesions of the brain caused by *S japonicum* are an important cause of focal seizures in the Far East.

## DIAGNOSIS

Historical and clinical findings suggestive of schistosomiasis already have been described. Definitive diagnosis is based on finding viable eggs in stool, urine, or biopsy specimens. Quantification of eggs in the excreta is desirable, because disease severity correlates with egg counts. Ordinary fecal smears are an insensitive means of diagnosing schistosomiasis. The thick smear method of Kato is simple, accurate, and permits counting of schistosome eggs. Urine samples are collected best around noon to take advantage of the diurnal pattern of *S haematobium* egg excretion. The urinary sediment is examined by routine methods. Eggs, if present, then can be enumerated by the Bell technique. If the results of stool and urine studies are negative, rectal biopsy may assist in establishing a diagnosis, particularly in individuals infected with *S mansoni* or *S japonicum*. Determining the viability of the eggs is important, as nonviable or calcified eggs may persist for long periods after successful therapy or the death of adult schistosomes. Serodiagnostic and antigen detection methods for diagnosing schistosomiasis have not been developed to the level of routine clinical application.

## TREATMENT

Patients with schistosomiasis can be treated safely and effectively with currently available drugs. Praziquantel is the drug of choice for most patients with this infection. A single oral dose of 40 mg/kg is recommended for *S mansoni* and *S haematobium* infections. *S japonicum* and *S mekongi* require a larger total dose: 60 mg/kg, given in two or three divided doses in 1 day. Praziquantel generally is well tolerated. Abdominal pain, nausea, headache, and rashes have been reported, but most adverse reactions are mild.

Oxamniquine is an alternative agent for treating *S mansoni* infections. The usual dose is 15 mg/kg, given once orally. Infections caused by African strains of *S mansoni* require a total dose of 60 mg/kg, given in four divided doses over 2 days. Side effects of therapy include drowsiness, dizziness, and headache. Convulsions may occur in individuals with preexisting seizure disorders. *S haematobium* infections can be treated with metrifonate at a dose of 10 mg/kg, administered on three occasions at 2-week intervals. Reported adverse effects include nausea, vomiting, and bronchospasm. The routine use of other antischistosomal drugs is limited by toxicity.

Treatment of schistosomiasis should not be undertaken unless viable eggs have been demonstrated in excreta or biopsy specimens. Egg counts generally are reduced markedly by therapy, but complete eradication of eggs and schistosomes is not mandatory.

The prognosis of schistosomiasis is excellent when treatment is initiated early. Late effects of chronic schistosomiasis are not entirely reversible with therapy.

## PREVENTION

Contaminated bodies of water in areas endemic for schistosomiasis should be avoided. Waterproof boots offer protection if wading is necessary. Exposed skin should be dried promptly and completely. Personal water supplies can be boiled or stored for several days to eliminate viable cercariae.

### Suggested Readings

DeCock KM. Hepatosplenic schistosomiasis: A clinical review. Gut 1986;27:734.
King CH, Mahmoud AAF. Drugs five years later: Praziquantel. Ann Intern Med 1989;110:290.
Kline MW, Sullivan TJ. Schistosomiasis In: Feigin RD, Cherry JD, eds. Textbook of pediatric infectious diseases, ed 3. Philadelphia: WB Saunders, 1992.
Nash TE. Schistosome infections in humans: Perspectives and recent findings. Ann Intern Med 1982;97:740.
Peters PA, El Alamy M, Warren KS, et al. Quick Kato smear for field quantification of Schistosoma mansoni eggs. Am J Trop Med Hyg 1980;29:217.
Peters PA, Mahmoud AAF, Warren KS, et al. Field studies of a rapid, accurate means of quantifying Schistosoma haematobium eggs in urine samples. Bull World Health Organ 1976;54:159.

*Principles and Practice of Pediatrics, Second Edition.*
edited by Frank A. Oski et al. J. B. Lippincott Company, Philadelphia © 1994.

# 62.4 *Arthropoda*

### Sheldon L. Kaplan

## MYIASIS

Myiasis is the invasion of body tissues or cavities by the larval stage (maggots) of flies. Although myiasis is uncommon in children of developed nations, it may occur in malnourished, neglected children, in travelers to tropical climates, or following accidental exposure. Human myiasis has been linked to warm, humid climates, which provide a favorable environment for the breeding of flies. Epizootics in livestock and inadequate sanitation also are risk factors associated with myiasis.

True flies are arthropods belonging to the order Diptera and have life cycles of four stages: egg, larva, pupa, and adult. Typically, eggs are deposited by a vector such as a mosquito in or around a body site, which ultimately is infested. The eggs, incubated by body heat, hatch, and larvae emerge to burrow into the body tissue or cavity. Some flies require living tissue for the larvae to develop (obligatory myiasis); others successfully adapt to a host–parasite relationship (facultative myiasis), such as occurs

with flesh flies (*Sarcophaga*), which can deposit eggs in wounds or ulcers containing purulent or necrotic material. Facultative myiasis may complicate wounds covered by casts. Accidental myiasis occurs when humans ingest eggs or larvae and the larvae persist and develop in the intestinal tract.

By far the most common form of myiasis in otherwise normal children is cutaneous myiasis, or invasion of the skin by larvae. Pediculosis capitis and pyoderma appear to be predisposing factors for children. The most common fly associated with the cutaneous form is the human botfly or warble fly (*Dermatobia hominis*). After the larvae burrow into the skin, a painful, elevated, pruritic lesion develops. The lesion enlarges and becomes more painful as the larvae increase in size. The lesions are located predominantly on the exposed regions of the body. Serosanguineous material may exude from the lesion, which may be confused with a furuncle. These lesions may have a central, tiny opening at which the larvae may be seen extending and retracting. Scratching resulting from pruritus leads to excoriation of the area; eosinophilia may be noted. Secondary bacterial infection with *Staphylococcus aureus*, *Staphylococcus pyogenes*, or gram-negative bacilli may develop. Early in the infestation, the larvae frequently can be expressed by gentle pressure on the lesion. Cutaneous myiasis should be considered a possible cause of a discrete pruritic lesion that does not resolve with standard therapy.

Intestinal myiasis develops when ingested fly eggs or larvae pass undamaged into the lower gastrointestinal tract. This rarely causes symptoms, however. The child and parent are greatly alarmed when worms or eggs are noted in the stool. Abdominal pain, vomiting, diarrhea, and hematochezia have been reported with intestinal myiasis.

The most serious forms of myiasis involve invasion of the nose and orbit. Nasal myiasis can extend into the sinuses, penetrate the cribriform plate, and reach the meninges and brain. Ophthalmomyiasis may cause massive destruction of orbital tissue, requiring exenteration of the orbital contents. Gonococcal conjunctivitis in children is thought to attract flies and predispose to larval infestation.

The external auditory canal and lower genitourinary tract are other sites of human myiasis.

The treatment of myiasis basically entails the physical removal of larvae from the invaded tissue or cavity. Cutaneous myiasis may require simply gentle pressure to extrude the larvae or more extensive surgical intervention. Occlusive dressings to deprive the larvae of an oxygen supply encourage them to migrate externally. In any case, the maggot should be removed totally and examined under a microscope to ensure that it is intact. Once the larva is removed, the lesion gradually resolves. A more extensive surgical approach may be required for treating nasal or orbital myiasis. Topical or systemic antibiotics are necessary if secondary bacterial infections have developed. No specific treatment of intestinal myiasis is known, although mild cathartics have been recommended.

Human myiasis can be prevented by controlling the source of the larvae, the female fly.

## TICKS AND MITES

Ticks are macroscopic arthropods that may cause local disease after a bite, but, more important, can transmit to man one of several potentially serious infectious diseases (Table 62-6). Mites are microscopic arthropods that also may cause local skin irritation or transmit such diseases as rickettsialpox or scrub typhus.

Dogs and children may be bitten by ticks while playing in wooded areas. Most ticks that feed on humans attach and engorge themselves with blood, then drop off. They may remain attached for several days without causing local discomfort, and are noted

**TABLE 62-6. Infectious Diseases of Humans Transmitted by Ticks**

| Agent | Disease |
|---|---|
| Arbovirus | Encephalitis |
| *Babesia microti* | Babesiosis |
| *Borrelia burgdorferi* | Lyme disease |
| *Borrelia duttonii* | Relapsing fever |
| *Coxiella burnetii* | Q fever |
| *Ehrlichia chaffeensis* | Ehrlichiosis |
| *Francisella tularensis* | Tularemia |
| Orbivirus | Colorado tick fever |
| *Rickettsia conorii* | Fièvre boutonneuse |
| *Rickettsia rickettsii* | Rocky Mountain spotted fever |
| Other rickettsiae | Tick typhus |

only when the child bathes or is undressed. The local reaction due to a tick bite usually occurs within days to weeks of the bite and is thought to be mediated by complement. This reaction may persist and develop into a so-called tick bite granuloma.

The recommended method for removing a tick is to grasp it as close to the skin as possible with curved forceps or protected fingers while exerting a steady pulling force until the tick is withdrawn from the skin. Remaining mouthparts should be removed if practical.

Some pregnant female ticks secrete a neurotoxin that is associated with tick paralysis, a neurologic syndrome that is characterized by an ascending flaccid paralysis. Diminished nerve conduction velocity suggesting peripheral nerve dysfunction has been detected in some children. One to 2 days after the tick attaches, ataxia and areflexia develop in the patient. Subsequently, the syndrome progresses to a gradual ascending flaccid paralysis that ultimately may involve the trunk, upper extremities, pharynx, and tongue. Death may result from respiratory compromise.

Tick paralysis can be diagnosed only by neurologic improvement occurring in a patient with typical features once the tick is removed. Therapy otherwise is supportive, particularly for respiratory function.

In contrast to tick bites, most reactions to mites occur within minutes to hours of the bite. This local reaction is thought to be the result of hypersensitivity to toxins secreted during feeding, which generally takes place at night. Contact with mites in their natural habitat occurs during such activities as hiking and camping. Domestic animals such as dogs and cats as well as wild birds and rodents may harbor mites. Mite bites are treated symptomatically to reduce the pruritus and prevent secondary infections.

## SPIDERS

In the United States, the two spiders that cause severe cutaneous and systemic reactions to envenomation are *Loxosceles reclusa*, the brown recluse spider, and *Lactrodectus mactans*, the black widow spider. The toxin from the venom of the brown recluse spider has been purified and characterized. It has a molecular weight of 31,000 d, is lethal to mice, and induces cutaneous necrosis in rabbits. Envenomation activates complement, which attracts neutrophils into the wound. In addition to this toxin, other proteins and proteolytic enzymes are pooled into the potent venom of *L reclusa*.

## Brown Recluse Spiders

Brown recluse spiders have a characteristic fiddle-shaped marking on the dorsal cephalothorax. This spider lives mainly in the south central United States, especially the Midwest, but can be found in many other areas. It prefers dark, secluded places and often is found in closets, storage boxes, barns, garages, and other little-used areas of the home.

Shortly after sustaining a brown recluse spider bite, the patient may experience itching and tingling; the local area becomes swollen, red, and tender. The lesion may develop central necrosis and blebs. Lymphangitis and regional lymphadenopathy may occur secondarily. Systemic symptoms such as fever, chills, nausea, vomiting, and myalgias may occur 12 to 24 hours after the bite. More severe envenomation may be complicated by thrombocytopenia, disseminated intravascular coagulation, hematuria, hemoglobinuria, renal failure, and shock. In young children especially, a purplish or blanched lesion indicates ischemia, and in these patients, the complete blood cell count, platelet count, and urinalysis should be monitored carefully.

The treatment of uncomplicated cutaneous lesions from a brown recluse spider bite is best approached conservatively. Immobilization of the affected extremity is useful. Frequent cleaning and tetanus prophylaxis, if indicated, are recommended. Administering an antipruritic drug such as diphenhydramine and covering the wound may help prevent further trauma to the area and the development of a secondary infection. Early surgical excision and corticosteroids have not proved beneficial for severe bites. Dapsone, a leukocyte inhibitor, has been shown to reduce surgical complications as well as the time required for the wound to heal. Further studies with this agent are necessary before its general use can be considered in children. Another experimental approach involves a specific antivenin.

## Black Widow Spiders

The black widow spider bite is associated with an immediate sharp pain, followed by burning, swelling, and inflammation of the bite site. Systemic symptoms that may develop shortly include weakness, dizziness, hypotension, tremors, and abdominal muscle cramps. Hemoglobinuria and nephritis have occurred in young children.

Rest and immobilization of the involved extremity are recommended. Pain medication and muscle relaxants are used as necessary. An antivenin (manufactured by Merck, Sharp & Dohme) also can be administered, provided the patient does not have a hypersensitivity reaction to skin testing of this material.

## Selected Readings

Alario A, Price G, Stahl R, et al. Cutaneous necrosis following a spider bite: A case report and review. Pediatrics 1987;79:618.

Chodosh J, Clarridge J. Ophthalmomyiasis: A review with special reference to *Cochliomyia hominivorax*. Clinical Infectious Diseases 1992;14:444.

Elgart ML. Flies and myiasis. Dermatol Clin 1990;8:237.

Gendron BP. *Loxosceles reclusa* envenomation. Am J Emerg Med 1990;8:51.

Honig PJ. Arthropod bites, stings and infestations: Their prevention and treatment. Pediatr Dermatol 1986;3:189.

Kincaid JC. Tick bite paralysis. Semin Neurol 1990;10:32.

Needham GR. Evaluation of five popular methods for tick removal. Pediatrics 1985;75:997.

Rees RS, Altenbern DP, Lynch JB, et al. Brown recluse spider bites: A comparison of early surgical excision versus dapsone and delayed surgical excision. Ann Surg 1985;202:659.

Swift TR, Ignacio OJ. Tick paralysis: Electrophysiologic studies. Neurology 1975;25:1130.

Vallat JM, Hugon J, Lubeau M, Leboutet MJ, Dumas M, Desproges-Gotteron R: Tick-bite meningoradiculoneuritis: Clinical, electrophysiologic, and histologic findings in 10 cases. Neurology 1987;37:749.

Wilson DC, King LE Jr: Spiders and spider bites. Dermatol Clin 1990;8:277.

*Principles and Practice of Pediatrics, Second Edition.*
edited by Frank A. Oski et al. J. B. Lippincott Company, Philadelphia © 1994.

# CHAPTER 63
# *Bacterial Diseases*

## *63.1 Cat-Scratch Disease*

### Kenneth M. Boyer

Cat-scratch disease is a subacute, regional lymphadenitis syndrome that occurs following cutaneous inoculation. Contact with cats, in the form of a scratch by claws or teeth, is associated strongly with the illness, although cases without known cat contact have been reported. Two newly described bacterial organisms, *Rochalimaea henselae* and *Afipia felis*, have been incriminated as causes. Complications of the disease occur, but it generally has an indolent chronic course for 2 to 3 months, followed by spontaneous resolution.

## ETIOLOGY

The two bacteria that are now strongly associated with cat-scratch disease have been isolated over the past decade. The initial breakthrough was the visualization of small, pleomorphic bacilli in biopsy materials obtained from nodes and primary granulomas and stained by the Warthin-Starry silver impregnation technique. In lymph nodes, the bacilli were seen intracellularly in capillaries and in macrophages lining sinuses in or near the germinal centers.

*Rochalimaea henselae* was first identified in 1990 in adult AIDS patients with two unique opportunistic infections, bacillary angiomatosis and bacillary peliosis hepatitis. Lesions in both conditions had been noted to contain argyrophilic bacteria similar to those seen in children with cat-scratch disease. Polymerase chain reaction amplification of ribosomal RNA in such specimens led to identification of bacterial genetic material most closely related to *Rochalimaea quintana*, the rickettsia-like agent known to cause trench fever. After successful cultivation, the new species has been named *R henselae*. Children with cat-scratch disease frequently develop specific antibodies against this organism, which has now been cultured from affected lymph nodes and also from the blood of epidemiologically related cats. In addition, *R henselae*-specific DNA sequences have been amplified from cat-scratch skin test antigen.

*Afipia felis* has also been cultured from the lymph nodes of children with cat-scratch disease—most successfully in tissue culture using human macrophages of HeLa cells. Based on biochemical and DNA-relatedness studies, *Afipia* turns out to be a new genus in the 2-α subgroup of Proteobacteria, along with a number of soil and rickettsia-like organisms. Like *Rochalimaea*, *A felis* appears to be an obligate or facultative intracellular pathogen with phylogenetic relationships to *Bartonella* and *Brucella*. The case for *A felis* as the sole cause of cat-scratch disease is becoming less tenable, since few affected children develop specific antibodies in convalescence. The relative contributions of these two intriguing new organisms to the cause and clinical spectrum of cat-scratch disease will undoubtedly be further elucidated in the near future.

## EPIDEMIOLOGY

Cat-scratch disease is transmitted by cutaneous inoculation. In the great majority of cases, a history of a cat scratch, often by a kitten less than 6 months old, can be elicited. Play may be more frequent with kittens than with older cats, and they are less likely to have been declawed. Interestingly, bacillary angiomatosis in adult patients with AIDS is frequently associated with a history of cat scratch.

Cat-scratch disease is more common in children than in adults, with the peak in case numbers falling between the ages of 5 and 14 years. Clustering of cases within families has been noted frequently, generally in association with the acquisition of new pets. Veterinarians as an occupational group appear to have a greater likelihood of exposure to the disease. An increased prevalence of skin test reactivity among veterinarians and asymptomatic relatives within family case clusters indicates that some infections may be subclinical.

## PATHOLOGY

The pathology of the primary inoculation site and that of the affected lymph nodes are similar. Both show a characteristic central avascular necrotic area surrounded by lymphocytes, with some giant cells and histiocytes. Three evolutionary stages are recognized within affected lymph nodes; all may coexist in the same node. Initially, there is generalized enlargement of the node with thickening of the cortex and hypertrophy of the germinal centers. Lymphocytes are the predominant cell type, and epithelioid granulomas containing Langhans' giant cells may be scattered throughout the node. In the middle stage, granulomas become distributed more densely, fuse, and are infiltrated with polymorphonuclear leukocytes. Central necrosis of the epithelioid granulomas begins at this stage. Progression of the process leads to formation of large, pus-filled sinuses, which are the chief late feature. The capsule of the node may rupture, with drainage of pus into surrounding tissues, resulting in a fibrotic inflammatory reaction and binding of the node to adjacent structures. The early stage of the lesion may resemble lymphoma or sarcoidosis; in later stages, results of histopathologic examination resemble those of tularemia, lymphogranuloma venereum, brucellosis, or infection with mycobacteria.

## CLINICAL MANIFESTATIONS

After an incubation period ranging from 3 to 30 days (usually between 7 and 12 days), one or more red papules measuring 2 to 5 mm in diameter develop at the site of cutaneous inoculation, often within the line of a previous cat scratch. Although they often are overlooked, a careful search uncovered such primary lesions in more than 90% of affected patients in one series. They persist until the development of lymphadenopathy, which generally occurs in 1 to 4 weeks.

Chronic lymphadenitis is the hallmark of cat-scratch disease, most frequently affecting the first or second sets of nodes draining the site of inoculation. Intervening lymphangitis does not occur. The sites affected most frequently, in decreasing order, are the axillary, cervical, submandibular, preauricular, epitrochlear, femoral, and inguinal lymph node groups. Involvement of more than one lymph node group, either within the same regional drainage or at an unrelated site, is present in 10% to 20% of cases. At a given site, about one half of all cases will involve a single node and the other half will involve multiple nodes.

Affected nodes usually are tender, and the overlying skin becomes warm, red, and indurated. Between 10% and 40% of the nodes eventually suppurate, occasionally with formation of a sinus tract to the skin surface. The duration of lymph node enlargement is 4 to 6 weeks, with persistence of up to 12 months in exceptional cases. Nodes that have drained to the skin surface frequently produce some residual scarring. The majority of patients lack constitutional symptoms. Elevated temperatures are documented in about 30% of patients and, when present, are generally in the range of 38 °C to 39 °C. Other nonspecific symptoms may include malaise, anorexia, fatigue, and headache.

A distinctive manifestation of cat-scratch disease is Parinaud's oculoglandular syndrome. The site of primary inoculation is the conjunctiva of one eye or the eyelid. Mild to moderate conjunctivitis accompanies the primary lesion. Preauricular lymph nodes are the corresponding regional site of adenopathy. The involved preauricular nodes may be within the substance of the parotid gland, but exocrine tissue typically is not involved. Although the oculoglandular syndrome may be induced by other agents, notably *Francisella tularensis*, the most common cause appears to be cat-scratch disease.

The most serious complication of cat-scratch disease is involvement of the central nervous system in the form of encephalopathy or encephalitis. High fever and convulsions develop within 6 weeks of the onset of lymphadenopathy, followed by alteration in the level of consciousness, headache, and muscle weakness. The cerebrospinal fluid is normal or shows minimal pleocytosis or elevated protein content. Electroencephalograms reveal diffuse slowing or focal abnormalities in most patients. Recovery has occurred without residua in nearly all the well-documented cases in the literature. A few patients had a prolonged convalescence and required anticonvulsant therapy for persistent seizure foci. The incidence of encephalopathy is low, but it can be the presenting manifestation of cat-scratch disease.

Osteolytic bone lesions have been noted in several well-documented cases. In one affected patient, biopsy of the lesion in the ilium revealed a granulomatous reaction typical of cat-scratch disease. In all the reported cases, the involved bone site was anatomically remote from the site of primary inoculation, suggesting hematogenous spread.

Granulomatous hepatitis is another newly recognized systemic manifestation of cat-scratch disease, and it may present as fever of unknown origin with or without lymphadenopathy. The reported cases have shown characteristic multiple hypodense lesions in the liver on computed tomography scanning.

Other rare complications that have been ascribed to cat-scratch disease include erythema multiforme, thrombocytopenic purpura, mesenteric lymphadenitis, pneumonia, arthralgia, neuroretinitis, iritis, urethritis, lymphedema, thyroiditis, and non-traumatic atlanto-axial dislocation (Grisel syndrome).

## DIAGNOSIS AND DIFFERENTIAL DIAGNOSIS

A number of criteria for the diagnosis of cat-scratch disease have been proposed. In a typical patient with lymphadenopathy that has been present for 3 or more weeks, three of the following four criteria confirm a diagnosis of cat-scratch disease:

1. A history of animal contact about 2 weeks before the onset
2. Negative culture, skin test, and serologic test for other causes of lymphadenopathy

3. A positive skin test with cat-scratch antigen
4. Lymph node or other biopsy material revealing histopathologic features consistent with cat-scratch disease, especially if pleomorphic bacilli are demonstrable by Warthin-Starry silver impregnation staining.

Some difficulties arise with the use of diagnostic (Hanger-Rose) skin tests for cat-scratch disease. Reagents for this purpose are relatively unstandardized and are available only for investigational purposes. Serologic testing for *Rochalimaea henselae* may be helpful and is available from the Viral and Rickettsial Zoonoses Branch, Centers for Disease Control.

The differential diagnosis of cat-scratch disease can include virtually all known causes of lymphadenopathy. As a general rule, the diagnosis is favored by chronicity, unilateral occurrence, tenderness, and characteristic sites of involvement, such as axillary, epitrochlear, and preauricular nodes. Cervical, femoral, inguinal, and generalized lymph node involvement is less specific for cat-scratch disease and necessitates more care in differential diagnosis.

The most common diagnoses in 85 patients with adenopathy and negative cat-scratch skin tests in one series were pyogenic lymphadenitis or abscess (29 patients), benign or malignant neoplasm (12 patients), and cervical adenitis caused by mycobacteria (10 patients). Malignant neoplasm can be ruled out definitively only by biopsy. Other conditions, such as tularemia, toxoplasmosis, plague, and Kawasaki disease, must be considered because of the need for specific therapy.

## TREATMENT AND PROGNOSIS

Controlled studies have not shown any specific antimicrobial agents to affect the course of cat-scratch disease. Uncontrolled experience, however, suggests that rifampin, ciprofloxacin, gentamicin, and trimethoprim-sulfamethoxazole may have some efficacy. The treatment of affected patients is primarily expectant. Suppurative nodes are treated best by needle aspiration, which should be repeated if necessary. Aspirated pus should be cultured, with an emphasis on the recovery of pyogenic organisms and mycobacteria. Surgical excision of affected nodes generally is unnecessary, but is indicated when there is uncertainty about the diagnosis or an atypical or prolonged course. Incision and drainage should not be done, as this leads to prolonged drainage and scar formation. Most patients with cat-scratch disease have a benign course. Systemic symptoms usually last less than 2 weeks. Affected nodes may be painful for several weeks and remain enlarged for a number of months. Patients with such complications as encephalopathy, thrombocytopenic purpura, or bone lesions generally have a more prolonged course, but also have a good long-term prognosis. Reinfection appears to be extremely rare.

## PREVENTION

The only preventive approach to cat-scratch disease might be to avoid cats, particularly aggressive play with young kittens. There seems to be no indication for destroying a family pet to which cases of cat-scratch disease have been attributed, because the capacity for disease transmission appears to be transient. Declawing such a pet might be considered, however.

### Selected Readings

Birkness KA, George VG, White EH, et al. Intracellular growth of *Afipia felis*, a putative agent of cat scratch disease. Infect Immun 1992;60:2281.

Brenner DJ, Hollis DG, Moss CW, et al. Proposal of *Afipia* gen. nov., with *Afipia felis* sp. nov. (formerly the cat scratch bacillus), *Afipia clevelandensis* sp. nov., *Afipia broomeae* sp. nov., and three unnamed genospecies. J Clin Microbiol 1991;29:2450.

Carithers HA. Cat-scratch disease: Notes on its history. Am J Dis Child 1970;119:200.

Carithers HA. Oculoglandular syndrome of Parinaud: A manifestation of cat-scratch disease. Am J Dis Child 1978;132:1195.

Carithers HA, Margileth AM. Cat scratch disease. Acute encephalopathy and other neurologic manifestations. Am J Dis Child 1991;145:98.

Corey B, Corey D. More on pet-associated illness. N Engl J Med 1986;315:461.

Delahoussaye PM, Osborne BM. Cat-scratch disease presenting as abdominal visceral granulomas. J Infect Dis 1990;161:71.

Margileth AM. Cat-scratch disease: Nonbacterial regional lymphadenitis. Pediatrics 1968;42:803.

Margileth AM. Antibiotic therapy for cat-scratch disease: Clinical study of therapeutic outcome in 268 patients and a review of the literature. Pediatr Infect Dis J 1992;11:474.

Relman DA, Loutit JS, Schmidt TM, et al. The agent of bacillary angiomatosis. An approach to the identification of uncultured pathogens. N Engl J Med 1990;323:1573.

Schmidt MJ, Robinson LE, Regnery RL, et al. The role of *Rochalimaea henselae* in cat scratch disease. Ped Research 1993;33:182A.

Schwartzman WA. Infections due to *Rochalimaea*: The expanding clinical spectrum. Clin Infect Dis 1992;15:893.

Wear DJ, Margileth AM, Hadfield TM, et al. Cat-scratch disease: A bacterial infection. Science 1983;221:1403.

*Principles and Practice of Pediatrics, Second Edition.*
edited by Frank A. Oski et al. J. B. Lippincott Company, Philadelphia © 1994.

# 63.2 *Kawasaki Disease*

Ralph D. Feigin, Frank Cecchin, and Guy Randolph

Kawasaki disease is an acute, febrile, multi-system syndrome of unknown etiology that predominantly afflicts children less than 9 years of age. The disease also is referred to as mucocutaneous lymph node syndrome. The diagnosis is based entirely on clinical features because there are no pathognomonic laboratory findings.

The disease first was recognized by Tomisaku Kawasaki in 1961. Subsequently, numerous cases of the disease have been recognized throughout the world in all racial groups. Kawasaki disease is one of the most common causes of acquired heart disease and inflammatory arthritis in North America.

## EPIDEMIOLOGY

Kawasaki disease is seen more often in persons with a Japanese background than in other individuals. The yearly incidence in Japanese in Hawaii is more than 20 cases per 100,000 children.

Cases reported to the Centers for Disease Control (CDC) indicate that the yearly incidence per 100,000 children aged 8 years or younger is three times higher in Asian-American than in African-American children and more than six times higher in Asian-American than in white children. The ratio of affected males to females is 1.5 : 1 in virtually all countries. The mortality rate for Japanese boys with Kawasaki disease is twice that of healthy boys of the same age. There is no significant difference in mortality between girls with Kawasaki disease and healthy girls. The ratio of male-to-female deaths related to Kawasaki disease is much higher in infancy. Japanese data suggest that the combined case-fatality ratio for all children 1 year of age or older may be less than 1%, whereas for infants, it may be as high as 4%.

Kawasaki disease has been seen almost exclusively in children. In several adult cases, the disease reported seems more likely to have been caused by toxic shock syndrome than by Kawasaki disease. The syndrome has not been detected in newborn infants, but the incidence increases steadily to peak at about 13 to 24 months of age and then falls off in almost linear fashion until 12 years of age after which Kawasaki disease is most unusual.

This particular incidence pattern, which has been noted with other infectious diseases, suggests that transplacental antibody may offer some protection in young infants, and that, when maternal IgG levels begin to decline and infants no longer are immune, a cohort of susceptible children is produced. As individuals either have clinical disease or acquire immunity to an as yet unknown agent, the incidence may decline toward zero. The incidence pattern described above, however, cannot be accepted as proof of an infectious cause for Kawasaki disease.

Environmental exposure has been considered and various agents have been sought. Environmental exposure remains a possibility; for example, a similar pattern is seen with lead poisoning, although the peak incidence of this disorder occurs somewhat later in childhood. Lead poisoning is not the cause of Kawasaki disease, however.

Kawasaki disease is seen in all seasons of the year. In the United States and Japan, though, a slight increase in cases occurs in the winter and spring months. There also has been an association noted between Kawasaki disease and residence within 180 m (200 yd) of a body of water.

Clustering of cases of Kawasaki disease has been observed. Often, families of children with the disease have had contact with other children who had it. Outbreaks have been reported in several cities in the United States, Australia, and Japan. One outbreak in Japan started in Tokyo and then spread northward and southward to involve the entire country within 6 months.

In several outbreaks, children with Kawasaki disease had a higher incidence of antecedent illness, primarily of respiratory origin, than did control patients. A report of two cases of Kawasaki disease strongly suggested person-to-person transmission between first cousins, with a latent period of 16 to 18 days. Secondary or co-primary cases are rare, and nosocomial infection has not been reported.

An increased incidence of second cases is seen among siblings of children with Kawasaki disease. During epidemics of the disease in Japan, the rate of second cases among siblings was 10 to 30 times greater than the incidence in the general population.

## ETIOLOGY

The cause of Kawasaki disease is unknown. Most investigators have favored the possibility of an infectious agent or an immune response to an infectious agent or agents. This hypothesis has been supported by the appearance of oropharyngeal inflammation and cervical adenitis, consistent with the acquisition of a replicating agent by droplet transmission; inflammation of the respiratory tract mucosa; the toxic appearance of the child with fever; and involvement of other organ systems. Laboratory features, which may include an elevated white blood cell (WBC) count with a left shift, elevated levels of acute-phase reactants, and pyuria, also suggest an infectious etiology.

Attempts to incriminate specific infectious agents have failed. Several investigators have provided evidence of an agent similar to *Rickettsia*, but others have been unable to substantiate these findings. Kawasaki disease, however, does not respond to treatment with antibiotics known to be effective against rickettsial agents, and most known rickettsial diseases are vector-borne and seasonal. The immunologic and clinical manifestations of Kawasaki disease bear remarkable similarity to diseases that are associated with superantigen production. The classic example is toxic shock syndrome, in which the staphylococcal enterotoxin functions as a superantigen that induces massive expansion of T cells expressing a specific $V_\beta$ region on the T cell receptor. This, in turn, leads to excess cytokine production, causing clinical illness. It has been demonstrated that patients with acute Kawasaki disease have selective expansion of T cells expressing T cell receptor variable regions $V_\beta2$ and $V_\beta8$. Further research to elucidate the source of the superantigen is ongoing.

All attempts to culture bacteria or viruses have been unsuccessful. No culture or serologic evidence of infection with Lancefield group A streptococci or staphylococci exists with respect to the genesis of Kawasaki disease. Although many viruses have been implicated, an abnormal immune response to Epstein-Barr virus (EBV) is postulated. One study of patients with Kawasaki disease in Hawaii, however, showed no association between patients with EBV and control patients. In fact, none of the herpesviruses, including EBV, cytomegalovirus, human herpesvirus 6, varicella-zoster virus, and herpes simplex virus types 1 and 2, display a dominant role in the pathogenesis of Kawasaki disease in Hawaii. Patients studied during two outbreaks in Japan did have increased antibodies to adenovirus type 2, but no supportive data regarding a causative role exist. Some studies have suggested unusual immune responses to leptospires, rubeola, rubella, parainfluenza, and *Mycoplasma*. Single case reports have documented recovery of various bacterial agents, including *Yersinia pseudotuberculosis, Salmonella, Pseudomonas aeruginosa,* and several other organisms.

Several investigators have proposed that a variant strain of *Propionibacterium acnes* may play a causative role in Kawasaki disease, and that house dust mites may play a role as vectors. A causative link has not been established, however, despite multiple investigations.

Investigators have detected RNA-dependent DNA polymerase (reverse transcriptase) activity in cultured peripheral blood mononuclear cells from Kawasaki patients. One study demonstrated that cultures taken between the third and ninth week after the onset of fever are the most likely to be associated with reverse transcriptase activity. The cell can be detected most easily in the early convalescent phase of Kawasaki disease from older patients who mount a marked humoral immune response. All serologic tests for human immunodeficiency virus 1, human T-cell leukemia/lymphoma viruses I and II, however, have been negative. Other studies also rule out any retroviral cause.

Kawasaki disease has not been associated consistently with exposure to environmental pesticides, chemicals, heavy metals, toxins, or pollutants. Poisoning with environmental agents usually does not simulate an acute infectious disease, although similarities between acrodynia (mercury poisoning) and Kawasaki disease have been noted. Children with Kawasaki disease have had normal mercury levels, with the exception of six patients from the Great Lakes area who had increased urinary excretion of mercury.

An outbreak of Kawasaki disease in Denver was felt to be associated with the use of rug shampoo. Eleven of 23 patients with the syndrome had been exposed to rug shampoo in the 30 days before the onset of illness. A total of six case-control studies have been done in an attempt to delineate the association between Kawasaki disease and rug shampooing. Three of the studies demonstrated a significant association, whereas the other three did not.

It also has been suggested that Kawasaki disease may be an allergic phenomenon. Several unpublished studies suggest that there is a higher incidence of allergies in children with Kawasaki disease or in members of their families than there is in control patients. The prevalence of atopic dermatitis is nine times greater in children with Kawasaki disease than in age-matched control children. In addition, a number of children with Kawasaki disease

show a twofold to fourfold elevation in total serum IgE levels during the acute phase of the illness, followed by a decline to the normal range in the ensuing 1 to 2 months. Peak IgE levels do not correlate with the severity of disease or the incidence of arthritis and carditis. The relationship of IgE to the pathogenesis of Kawasaki disease remains unclear.

## Relationship of Kawasaki Disease to Infantile Periarteritis Nodosa

There appears to be a pathologic similarity between infantile periarteritis nodosa and fatal infantile Kawasaki disease. Discussions of the similarities between these disorders have been published by numerous investigators. It cannot be stated that the two diseases are identical, because the cause of both is entirely unknown, and experience with gross and histologic investigation is relatively embryonic. It is impossible pathologically to distinguish infantile periarteritis nodosa with coronary artery involvement from fatal infantile Kawasaki disease. Clinically, most patients with infantile periarteritis nodosa associated with coronary artery involvement have not met the other criteria established by the CDC for Kawasaki disease. When pathologic and clinical criteria are combined, however, the two diseases appear to be indistinguishable, raising a question about the novelty of Kawasaki disease. This is true particularly in the United States, where infantile periarteritis nodosa has been documented since the 1940s, but Kawasaki disease was not recognized as a clinical entity until 1974. A 3 : 1 male : female ratio exists in patients with periarteritis nodosa. Whether any of the cases of periarteritis nodosa with coronary artery aneurysms were examples of Kawasaki disease is speculative, because histories from the past often were scanty and deaths often were attributed, perhaps erroneously, to other disorders, such as scarlet fever.

## PATHOLOGY

Grossly, cardiac hypertrophy is common. Multiple or single beadlike or fusiform aneurysms of the coronary arteries and their branches usually are found in fatal cases. During the various clinical stages, specific pathologic findings are noted, and during days 0 to 9, the coronary arteries have perivasculitis and endarteritis, but medial sparing. Pericarditis, myocarditis, endocarditis, valvulitis, and conduction system inflammation are observed, with polymorphonuclear infiltrates. During days 12 to 25, coronary artery panvasculitis and aneurysm formation occur, with inflammation and necrosis of the media resulting in "true" aneurysms. By the second week, the inflammatory infiltrate has evolved into a lymphocytic and plasma cell dominance. Resolution of the coronary inflammation occurs near day 30, with subsequent granulation formation. Coronary artery scarring, stenosis, and endocardial fibroelastosis are described after day 40. Aneurysms of other arteries, such as the renal, iliac, and brachial arteries, may be found. Phlebitis is common, with vascular inflammation that affects larger musculoelastic arteries in their extraparenchymal portions most often and most severely. Sites of arteritis include the lung, pancreas, spleen, kidney, testis, mesentery, adrenal gland, and gastrointestinal tract.

## CLINICAL MANIFESTATIONS

The clinical manifestations of Kawasaki disease in accordance with the CDC diagnostic criteria are given in Table 63-1.

Kawasaki disease occurs in four discrete phases. In the first phase, the previously healthy child becomes febrile and irritable. Fever is relentless and the temperature frequently exceeds

| TABLE 63-1. Diagnostic Criteria for Kawasaki Disease |
| --- |
| I. Fever of 5 or more days' duration associated with at least four of the five following changes*: <br> 1. Bilateral conjuctival injection <br> 2. One or more changes of the mucous membranes of the upper respiratory tract, including pharyngeal injection, dry fissurred lips, injected lips, and "strawberry" tongue <br> 3. One or more changes of the extremities, including peripheral erythema, peripheral edema, periungual desquamation, and generalized desquamation <br> 4. Rash, primarily truncal <br> 5. Cervical lymphadenopathy <br> II. The disease cannot be explained by some other known disease process. |
| *A diagnosis of Kawasaki disease can be made if fever and any of the changes below are present in conjunction with coronary artery disease documented by two-dimensional echocardiography or coronary angiography. <br> *Modified from previously published diagnostic criteria from the Centers for Disease Control for Kawasaki disease and the American Heart Association Committee on Rheumatic Fever, Endocarditis, and Kawasaki Disease.* |

40.6 °C (105.8 °F) in 40% of the patients at some time. Non-suppurative cervical lymphadenopathy, usually in the anterior triangle and frequently bilateral, may be present, but may disappear rapidly. Within several days, rash and bilateral conjunctival injection appear. It usually is at the end of this phase that the physician first is consulted.

The second phase begins about the fourth day of illness and is characterized by continuing high, spiking fever that is unresponsive to standard antipyretic regimens or to antibiotics. The mean duration of fever is 12 days if the patient is not treated with aspirin or gamma globulin. The child is febrile and irritable, and often appears quite ill. Cervical lymphadenitis usually is present. Bilateral injection of the conjunctivae, primarily bulbar, is impressive, and unilateral subconjunctival hemorrhage may occur. Anterior uveitis may be found in 80% of all patients evaluated by slit-lamp examination. The anterior uveitis is self-limited and the prognosis is good. Other ocular symptoms may include vitreous opacities, punctate keratitis, and papilledema. Chorioretinal and vitreous inflammation have been noted. Purulent conjunctivitis and blepharitis may occur. Photophobia may be apparent.

The lips are bright red, dry, and cracked. A strawberry tongue may be apparent, and the oral mucosa generally is hyperemic.

A rash that is particularly prominent over the trunk consists of maculopapular, ill-defined erythematous plaques of variable size. At times, coalescent areas suggest the possibility of scarlet fever. Vesicles and sterile pustules are seen occasionally. Petechiae, pinpoint rashes, and erythema multiforme have been described in selected cases. The rash also has been noted in the diaper area and on the face.

Hepatomegaly and splenomegaly are detected occasionally, but usually resolve quickly. Diarrhea may occur in the early phases of the illness. Severe abdominal pain, paralytic ileus, and icterus are common. As the second phase progresses, erythema of the palms and soles may develop (Fig 63-1). The hands and feet become edematous, and arthralgia and arthritis of large joints may be noted.

Children with this type of illness usually must be hospitalized. The WBC count is elevated, with a left shift. Counts in excess of 30,000/mm³ are noted in about 15% of patients, and counts in excess of 20,000/mm³ are observed in about 50% of patients. A peripheral smear reveals an increased percentage of toxic neutrophils characterized by cytoplasmic swelling, vacuolation, and toxic granulation, especially with coronary lesions. Toxic granulation and Döhle bodies are seen. The erythrocyte sedimentation rate, C-reactive protein titer, $\alpha_2$-globulin value, and $\alpha_1$-antitrypsin level all are elevated, but normalize by 8 to 12 weeks. An elevated sedimentation rate and C-reactive protein level usually are not present with viral exanthems, hypersensitivity reactions, and measles. Mild anemia may be noted. Severe hemolytic anemia has been described, but is unusual. There often is an acute rise and convalescent fall in the levels of all classes of immunoglobulins. The elevation in the IgG level is predominantly in subclasses IgG1 and IgG3. The serum complement value is normal or high. Transaminase levels may be elevated, but usually are not more than three times the upper limit of normal. Hypoalbuminemia, hyponatremia, and hypophosphatemia have been described. Urinalysis may reveal proteinuria and moderate pyuria, usually reflecting urethritis. In males, meatitis may be visible. Vulvitis has been described.

Meningeal findings are rare, although nuchal rigidity and lethargy have been reported. In patients who have had lumbar punctures performed, 10 to 50 WBCs/mm³, predominantly mononuclear, have been noted, but the cerebrospinal protein and glucose levels have been normal.

Electrocardiograms are abnormal in 77% of patients with Kawasaki disease and in all those who have pancarditis. The most common abnormalities in order of their frequency are flattened T waves initially, followed by peaked T waves in convalescence; first-degree heart block; ST segment elevation or depression; and QT interval prolongation. Auscultation may reveal sinus tachy-

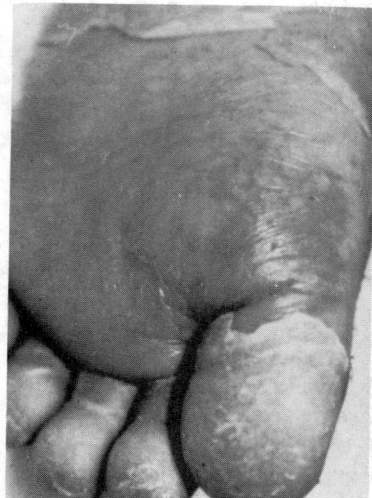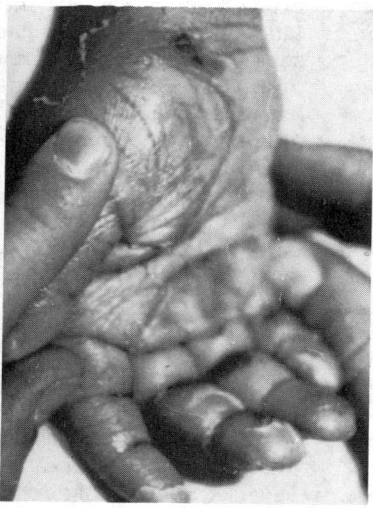

**Figure 63-1.** Erythema and edema of the feet and hands, characteristic of the second phase of Kawasaki disease.

cardia, a gallop rhythm, distant heart sounds, or a frictional rub. Chest radiographs may reveal infiltrates in selected patients and some cardiomegaly. Disappearance of the rash and resolution of the adenopathy herald the end of the second phase of illness.

About day 12 of the illness, the third phase occurs and is dominated by desquamation. Desquamation sometimes can be seen several days before the fever abates, which occurs at a mean of 10 days after the onset of the illness. Desquamation is a constant feature of Kawasaki disease. It usually is noted first in the periungual region, although other parts of the body may be involved. Desquamation may be particularly prominent in the diaper area. During the period of desquamation, arthralgias and arthritis may be noted, even though they were not present earlier. The large weight-bearing joints are involved most often. Thrombocytosis is another constant feature of the third phase of illness, with platelet counts ranging from 500,000 to 3 million/mm$^3$. Thrombocytosis is seen rarely in the first week of illness. It usually appears in the second week, peaks in the third week, and returns gradually to normal about a month after onset in uncomplicated cases.

Bone marrow examination has revealed normal number and morphology of megakaryocytes. Increased fibrinogen levels and prolongation of the partial thromboplastin time have been noted. The third phase of illness is characterized by a gradual return of the patient toward normal. Beau's lines (transverse depressions in the fingernails and toenails) and alopecia may be seen in the weeks and months after recovery.

The fourth phase of illness is recognized in only a minority of cases. This phase is characterized by ongoing inflammation, subacute vasculitis, and an increased incidence of death from cardiac involvement.

## COMPLICATIONS

### Cardiovascular

The most serious complications of Kawasaki disease are cardiovascular and include aneurysms of the coronary arteries and other large arteries, aneurysmal rupture, hemopericardium, myocarditis, coronary thrombosis, pericardial effusions, cardiac tamponade, mitral valve disease, and arrhythmias. Aneurysms of the aorta and the cerebral, vertebral, subclavian, axillary, internal, common and external iliac, hepatic, and renal arteries have been described. In most cases, peripheral aneurysms have been associated with coronary artery aneurysms. (Also see Chapter 87.)

### Other Complications

Acalculous cholecystitis has been noted repeatedly during the second phase of Kawasaki disease. Children with hydrops of the gallbladder usually have abdominal pain, a soft palpable mass in the right upper quadrant, and abdominal distention. The diagnosis can be made by ultrasonography. Most cases resolve spontaneously.

Other complications that have been described include sterile purulent otitis media, mastoiditis, retropharyngeal mass, necrotic pharyngitis, pleural effusion, myositis, renal infarcts, nephritis and nephrosis, gangrene of the fingers and toes, encephalopathy, facial nerve paralysis, hemiparesis, ataxia, and evidence of cerebral aneurysms, cerebral embolus, subarachnoid hemorrhage, and sensorineural hearing loss.

## DIAGNOSIS AND DIFFERENTIAL DIAGNOSIS

The diagnosis of Kawasaki disease is made clinically by exclusion. Children who meet the CDC criteria should be strongly consid-

ered to have Kawasaki disease. Unfortunately, infants are less likely to have a classic presentation than are older children. In fact, children younger than 6 months of age may have coronary involvement, even though they do not fulfill the diagnostic criteria. The most common conditions that mimic Kawasaki disease are measles and group A $\beta$-hemolytic streptococcal infection. Other disorders with which Kawasaki disease can be confused initially include roseola infantum, meningococcemia, Rocky Mountain spotted fever, leptospirosis, rubella, infectious mononucleosis, selected viral infections caused by the enteroviruses, rat-bite fever, toxoplasmosis, acrodynia, collagen vascular diseases (particularly infantile polyarteritis nodosa), Reiter's syndrome, and Behçet's syndrome. Toxic shock syndrome may need to be excluded. Drug reactions also have been confused with Kawasaki disease. Infantile papular acrodermatitis associated with hepatitis B surface antigen (Gianotti syndrome) can be confused with Kawasaki disease during the early stages of the disorder.

## TREATMENT

The goals of therapy for Kawasaki disease are to decrease the inflammatory response and reduce the severity of the cardiovascular complications. The combination of intravenous gamma globulin and aspirin effectively meets these goals.

Corticosteroids appear to be contraindicated. Several investigators have reported a higher incidence of coronary artery aneurysms in patients treated with steroids than in those who received antibiotics or salicylate therapy.

Aspirin appears to be a particularly important therapeutic modality. Although it does not have an immediate antipyretic effect, aspirin can help reduce the height and duration of fever and may serve as an important antithrombotic agent. Experience with patients who receive high-dose aspirin early in the course of disease has demonstrated a lower rate of aneurysm development than in patients who are not given aspirin. The aspirin dosage studied most thoroughly in the United States is 100 mg/kg/d until defervescence of fever, or until the 14th day of illness. Although the optimum dose of aspirin is controversial, Japanese clinicians support an intermediate antipyretic dose of 30 to 50 mg/kg/d in combination with the anti-inflammatory effect of gamma globulin. There appears to be malabsorption of aspirin and enhanced salicylate clearance during the first 3 weeks of illness, and the blood salicylate concentration should be monitored to achieve therapeutic levels in the range of 15 to 25 mg/dL. When fever has abated, absorption of aspirin improves, and the dosage of aspirin can be reduced while therapeutic blood levels are maintained.

Controlled studies of intravenous gamma globulin plus aspirin given within the first 10 days of the onset of fever versus aspirin used alone have shown that high-dose gamma globulin significantly decreases the number of patients in whom aneurysms develop. Recent studies support the use of a single dose of gamma globulin at 2 g/kg given in a 10- to 12-h infusion. Compared to the four-dose schedule of 400 mg/kg/d, the single-dose schedule of 2 g/kg is equally efficacious in reducing the risk of coronary disease and is superior in inducing rapid defervescence of the fever, shortening its duration. Concentrations of phase reactants return to normal more rapidly. Although single-dose therapy is safe, the patient's pulse, heart rate, and blood pressure should be obtained at the beginning of the infusion, then 30 minutes, 1 hour, and every 2 hours thereafter during the infusion. Despite the substantial fluid and protein load that is associated with this dosage, it has not been found to increase the risk of congestive heart failure, even in patients with decreased myocardial function.

The mechanism by which intravenous gamma globulin suppresses coronary artery lesions is controversial. Possible mechanisms include the following: Fc receptor blockade, neutralization of the etiologic agent, an antitoxic effect, alteration of the immune effect via anti-idiotypic antibodies or induction of suppressor T cells, and decreased cytokine production by activated immune cells.

Most children with Kawasaki disease are hospitalized in the initial period after diagnosis because of irritability and fever, and because of the difficulties of administering fluids orally. Intravenous fluids may be required to prevent dehydration. Bed rest generally is suggested until the second or third week after the onset of fever because of the myocarditis that is associated with this disease. Patients may be discharged with restricted activity once they have been afebrile for 3 days and the sedimentation rate and peripheral WBC count are declining. The recrudescence of fever on low-dose salicylate therapy is a poor prognostic sign and usually heralds the onset of cardiovascular complications.

An initial dose of aspirin is given at 30 to 100 mg/kg/24 h, then the dosage is reduced to 30 mg/kg/24 h after the fever has abated and is continued at this level until the end of the fourth week after the onset of illness, or for at least 1 week after fever defervescence has been noted. Subsequently, aspirin therapy can be continued at 3 mg/kg/24 h to maintain an antiplatelet effect.

If there has been any evidence of cardiovascular involvement during the first 4 weeks of illness, we recommend adding dipyridamole at 3 mg/kg/24 h for its ability to induce coronary vasodilation and promote the de-aggregation of platelets.

We generally monitor the peripheral WBC count, sedimentation rate, and platelet count twice each week. The peripheral pulses and capillary circulation should be monitored daily for evidence of vascular insufficiency. During the initial 2 weeks of illness, we recommend performing 1 to 2 echocardiograms, which may reveal early cardiac involvement. Another echocardiogram should be obtained 4 to 6 weeks after the disease onset, but follow-up and monitoring must be individualized for every patient. Angiography is indicated if there is significant coronary dilation or aneurysm formation. If the coronary, renal, and other peripheral arteries appear normal at angiography, it is most unlikely that any signs of vascular insufficiency will appear during the next 10 years. Subtle changes in the coronary endothelium that are not visible on angiography may predispose to the development of coronary atherosclerosis during the second or third decade of life. Long-term evaluation of all patients with Kawasaki disease is recommended to detect the early onset of coronary artery disease or renovascular hypertension.

If coronary or peripheral artery aneurysms are found in the acute or convalescent stages of this illness, we recommend continuing aspirin and dipyridamole, each at 3 mg/kg/24 h, for at least 12 months. At that time, the patient can be studied again by angiography. Regression of aneurysms seen previously occurs in more than 50% of patients; in the others, persistent coronary artery abnormalities, such as thickening of the walls of these vessels or stenosis, may be noted.

The presence of coronary aneurysms predisposes an individual to platelet deposition, embolic phenomena, and progressive intimal fibrosis with luminal obstruction. This may lead to decreased coronary artery blood flow, with resultant angina and myocardial infarction. Fibrinolytic agents, such as streptokinase, urokinase, or tissue plasminogen activator, may be used to treat myocardial infarction. If coronary artery bypass grafting is indicated, internal mammary artery grafts are the best choice, compared to saphenous vein grafts, because of their long-term patency and good growth potential.

Some children have recovered uneventfully from Kawasaki disease, only to have angina and myocardial infarction occur between 1 month and 13 years after the acute illness. Children with persistent coronary artery abnormalities should undergo exercise myocardial perfusion studies with thallium or an exercise stress test on a treadmill or bicycle. Few guidelines are available for the treatment of patients with coronary artery aneurysms. A reasonable approach to the hospitalized child in whom aneurysms form includes a period of 1 to 2 weeks of close observation and cardiac monitoring, with attempts made to assess whether the disease is progressing, has stabilized, or is regressing, as determined by observation of signs and symptoms, performance of serial echocardiograms, and determinations of platelet count, body temperature, WBC count, differential, and erythrocyte sedimentation rate. When the condition has stabilized, the decision may be made to discharge the patient, with plans for regular follow-up and follow-up angiography.

## PROGNOSIS

Kawasaki disease normally is acute and self-limited, although cardiac damage sustained when the disease is active may be progressive. Coronary artery aneurysms are detectable by angiography or two-dimensional echocardiography in 20% of those patients who are not treated with intravenous gamma globulin, as opposed to 3% of those who receive gamma globulin within the first 10 days of illness. These abnormalities occur usually between days 7 and 28 of the illness. For infants less than 1 year of age, however, the risk of coronary abnormalities at 8 weeks still is 15%, even with gamma globulin treatment.

Japanese surveys between 1982 and 1988 of patients with Kawasaki disease suggest an average case-fatality rate of 0.3%. United States surveillance data suggest a 2.8% case-fatality rate in this country, but most investigators believe that this number is inflated artificially as a result of the selective reporting of deaths caused by this disease. It may be assumed, however, that deaths can be expected to occur in about 1% of affected American children. The case-fatality ratio for all infants may exceed 4%; for all patients 1 year of age or older, it probably is less than 1%. Nearly 90% of the infant fatalities occur in males. Most deaths related to Kawasaki disease result from coronary artery thrombosis.

## Selected Readings

Bell DM, Brink EW, Nitzkin J, et al. Kawasaki syndrome: Description of two outbreaks in the United States. N Engl J Med 1981;304:1558.

Chung KJ, Brandt L, Fulton DR, et al. Cardiac and coronary arterial involvement in infants and children from New England with mucocutaneous lymph node syndrome (Kawasaki disease): Angiocardiographic-echocardiographic correlations. Am J Cardiol 1982;50:136.

Fukushigi J, Nihill MR, McNamara DG. Spectrum of cardiovascular lesions in mucocutaneous lymph node syndrome: Analysis of eight cases. Am J Cardiol 1980;45:98.

Furusho K, Nakano H, Shinomiya K, et al. High-dose intravenous gammaglobulin for Kawasaki disease. Lancet 1984;2:1055.

Leung DYM, Kurt-Jones E, Newburger JW, et al. Endothelial cell activation and high interleukin-1 secretion in the pathogenesis of acute Kawasaki disease. Lancet 1989;2:1298.

Melish ME, Hicks RM, Dean AG: Kawasaki syndrome in Hawaii. Pediatr Res 1979;13: 451.

Morens DM, Melish ME. Kawasaki disease. In: Feigin RD, Cherry JD, eds. Textbook of pediatric infectious disease, ed 3. Philadelphia: WB Saunders, 1992.

Morens DM, O'Brien RJ. Kawasaki disease in the United States. J Infect Dis 1978;137: 91.

Yamada K, Fukumoto T, Shinkai A, et al. The platelet functions in acute febrile mucocutaneous lymph node syndrome and a trial of prevention for thrombosis by antiplatelet agent. Acta Hematology Japonica 1978;41:791.

Yanagawa H, Nakamura Y, Yaskiro M, et al. A nationwide incidence survey of Kawasaki disease in 1985–1986 in Japan. J Infect Dis 1988;158:1296.

*Principles and Practice of Pediatrics, Second Edition.*
edited by Frank A. Oski et al. J. B. Lippincott Company, Philadelphia © 1994.

# CHAPTER 64
# *Control of Nosocomial Infections in Children*

## Mark W. Kline and Judith Margolin

The goals and methods of infection control in hospitalized children are no different, in theory, from those in hospitalized adults. In practice, however, the higher percentage of children admitted to hospitals with overt, asymptomatic, or incubating infection; the increased morbidity of certain pathogens in some children; and the close contact required in the care of any young child necessitate modification of traditional methods of hospital infection control. General guidelines by which any hospital or patient care facility may establish a system of infection control are published regularly by the Centers for Disease Control (CDC), the American Hospital Association, and the American Academy of Pediatrics. These guidelines, along with state and local requirements, and those of the Joint Commission on the Accreditation of Hospitals, are the basis for an effective infection control program.

## EPIDEMIOLOGY OF NOSOCOMIAL INFECTIONS IN CHILDREN

Infection acquired by a patient during a hospital stay, which was neither present nor in incubation at the time of hospital admission, is termed nosocomial. In general, nosocomial infection rates are lower for children than for adults hospitalized in comparable facilities. For children, attack rates are highest among infants, lowest among adolescents, and intermediate among toddlers and school-age children. Nosocomial infection rates are highest in large teaching hospitals and lowest in non-teaching hospitals, reflecting, in part, the severity of underlying illnesses and the extent to which invasive diagnostic or therapeutic procedures are performed in the various settings. Children hospitalized in neonatal or pediatric intensive care units are at particularly high risk for acquiring a nosocomial infection.

Virtually any microorganism can act as a nosocomial pathogen under circumstances conducive to its growth and transmission. *Staphylococcus aureus* and coagulase-negative staphylococci lead the list of bacterial isolates found on pediatric and newborn services, followed by *Escherichia coli*, *Pseudomonas aeruginosa*, and miscellaneous enteric gram-negative bacteria. *Candida* is the leading fungal isolate. Viruses are a major cause of nosocomial disease in children. Overall, rotavirus may be second only to *S aureus* as a cause of nosocomial infection in children. Other viral agents, including respiratory syncytial virus, parainfluenza virus, adenovirus, and enteroviruses, contribute substantially to the rate of nosocomial respiratory and gastrointestinal illness. Outbreaks of infections in hospitals occasionally are caused by viruses associated with exanthematous diseases of childhood, including measles, varicella, and rubella.

Direct person-to-person transmission (contact or airborne) is the major mode of spread for most nosocomial pathogens. Prevention of direct transmission is complicated by the social nature of children in hospitals, fecal incontinence and lack of personal hygiene among young children, and mouthing behavior. Intimate contact with visiting parents and siblings provides a portal for entry of infectious agents from the community. Hospital personnel may perform the role of intermediaries in the chain of transmission within the hospital by hand carriage of nosocomial pathogens.

The inanimate environment is implicated less frequently than is person-to-person spread in nosocomial infections. Some respiratory and enteric pathogens in particular, however, may contaminate and survive on surfaces for long periods. Toys may act as vectors for the spread of infection. Building construction has been implicated in the dissemination of fungal spores and disease among immunocompromised patients in hospitals.

## GOALS OF INFECTION CONTROL

Any hospital infection control program should attempt to prevent nosocomial infections and cross-infections (infections spread specifically between patients); provide isolation when required without denying the patient appropriate care; prevent the spread of disease among patients, hospital employees, and visitors; and educate all potential contacts on ways to prevent the spread of infections.

## THE INFECTION CONTROL TEAM

The infection control team is charged most immediately with carrying out the infection control program. Local and state law, and the size and character of an institution (eg, acute versus chronic care patient mix) help determine the size of the infection control team. The team consists of an infection control committee, which sets general policy, receives information, and gives direction to the other members of the team, the hospital epidemiologist, and the infection control practitioner.

An infection control committee generally has representation from all the hospital services that are involved in direct patient care (ie, the various medical and surgical services and nursing), from hospital services that are involved in the hospital environment (eg, housekeeping and laundry), and from other services that are relevant to patient care and health (eg, dietary). Many hospitals either employ a person specially trained in hospital epidemiology or designate a member of the infection control committee to work with both the committee and the infection control practitioner.

The infection control practitioner in most hospitals is a nurse with special training or experience in hospital infection control and epidemiology. This individual has a pivotal role in the daily functioning of the infection control and surveillance programs. The duties and responsibilities of the infection control nurse are quite broad. He or she makes regular rounds through the hospital, seeking out suspected cases of nosocomial infection or cross-infection. The infection control nurse answers questions regarding isolation and other infection control practices during these rounds. He or she works closely with the microbiology laboratory, so that culture results from individual patients and environmental culture results are incorporated in the general infection control plan. The nurse acts as a liaison for any of the hospital services and personnel who have questions regarding infection control issues. The infection control nurse coordinates all activities relating to infection surveillance. Finally, he or she reports on these various activities to the infection control committee. The infection control nurse usually is a full voting and participating member of the infection control committee.

*Strict Isolation*
Visitors—Report to Nurses' Station
Before Entering Room

1. Masks are indicated for all persons entering room.
2. Gowns are indicated for all persons entering room.
3. Gloves are indicated for all persons entering room.
4. HANDS MUST BE WASHED AFTER TOUCHING THE PATIENT OR PO-TENTIALLY CONTAMINATED ARTICLES AND BEFORE TAKING CARE OF ANOTHER PATIENT.
5. Articles contaminated with infective material should be discarded or bagged and labeled before being sent for decontamination and reprocessing.

*Contact Isolation*
Visitors—Report to Nurses' Station
Before Entering Room

1. Masks are indicated for those who come close to patient.
2. Gowns are indicated if soiling is likely.
3. Gloves are indicated for touching infective material.
4. HANDS MUST BE WASHED AFTER TOUCHING THE PATIENT OR PO-TENTIALLY CONTAMINATED ARTICLES AND BEFORE TAKING CARE OF ANOTHER PATIENT.
5. Articles contaminated with infective material should be discarded or bagged and labeled before being sent for decontamination and reprocessing.

*Respiratory Isolation*
Visitors—Report to Nurses' Station
Before Entering Room

1. Masks are indicated for those who come close to patient.
2. Gowns are not indicated.
3. Gloves are not indicated.
4. HANDS MUST BE WASHED AFTER TOUCHING THE PATIENT OR PO-TENTIALLY CONTAMINATED ARTICLES AND BEFORE TAKING CARE OF ANOTHER PATIENT.
5. Articles contaminated with infective material should be discarded or bagged and labeled before being sent for decontamination and reprocessing.

*AFB Isolation*
Visitors—Report to Nurses' Station
Before Entering Room

1. Masks are indicated only when patient is coughing and does not reliably cover mouth.
2. Gowns are indicated only if needed to prevent gross contamination of clothing.
3. Gloves are not indicated.
4. HANDS MUST BE WASHED AFTER TOUCHING THE PATIENT OR PO-TENTIALLY CONTAMINATED ARTICLES AND BEFORE TAKING CARE OF ANOTHER PATIENT.
5. Articles should be discarded, cleaned, or sent for decontamination and reprocessing.

*Enteric Precautions*
Visitors—Report to Nurses' Station
Before Entering Room

1. Masks are not indicated.
2. Gowns are indicated if soiling is likely.
3. Gloves are indicated for touching infective material.
4. HANDS MUST BE WASHED AFTER TOUCHING THE PATIENT OR PO-TENTIALLY CONTAMINATED ARTICLES AND BEFORE TAKING CARE OF ANOTHER PATIENT.
5. Articles contaminated with infective material should be discarded or bagged and labeled before being sent for decontamination and reprocessing.

*Drainage/Secretion Precautions*
Visitors—Report to Nurses' Station
Before Entering Room

1. Masks are not indicated.
2. Gowns are indicated if soiling is likely.
3. Gloves are indicated for touching infective material.
4. HANDS MUST BE WASHED AFTER TOUCHING THE PATIENT OR PO-TENTIALLY CONTAMINATED ARTICLES AND BEFORE TAKING CARE OF ANOTHER PATIENT.
5. Articles contaminated with infective material should be discarded or bagged and labeled before being sent for decontamination and reprocessing.

*Blood/Body Fluid Precautions*
Visitors—Report to Nurses' Station Before Entering Room

1. Masks are not indicated.
2. Gowns are indicated if soiling with blood or body fluids is likely.
3. Gloves are indicated for touching blood or body fluids.
4. HANDS SHOULD BE WASHED IMMEDIATELY IF THEY ARE POTEN-TIALLY CONTAMINATED WITH BLOOD OR BODY FLUIDS AND BEFORE TAKING CARE OF ANOTHER PATIENT.

5. Articles contaminated with blood or body fluids should be discarded or bagged and labeled before being sent for decontamination and reprocessing.
6. Care should be taken to avoid needle-stick injuries. Used needles should be placed in a prominently labeled, puncture-resistant container designed specifically for such disposal.
7. Blood spills should be cleaned up promptly with a solution of 5.25% sodium hypochlorite diluted 1:10 with water.

**Figure 64-1.** Types of isolation and precautions. (Garner J, Simmons B. CDC guidelines for isolation precautions in hospitals. Infect Control 1983;4:245.)

## INFECTION SURVEILLANCE

Knowledge of the rates of infection within a hospital is key to effective infection control. Surveillance data on actual patient infections have proved to be useful in the design of effective infection control programs. Although environmental microbiologic sampling was practiced widely in the past, the data generated often were difficult to interpret and use for infection control planning. Environmental cultures should be obtained only when other factors (eg, *Legionella* outbreaks in patients on ventilators or in certain units) point to a possible common environmental source of infection. Cultures performed to evaluate patient colonization by various microorganisms (especially around invasive appliances and devices) can be helpful not only for patient care, but also to allow the infection control team to monitor the spread of "hospital organisms" before they cause disease. Records are kept on the type of organisms grown in the various cultures, and the antibiotic resistance and susceptibility patterns of these organisms are monitored so that appropriate isolation and antibiotic therapy can be ordered.

In addition to concerns regarding infection that may be present in the hospital at any given time, infection control personnel also should monitor infections that may have been acquired in the hospital, but do not manifest clinically until days or weeks after hospital discharge.

## ISOLATION PRACTICE

Systems of isolation precautions usually are either disease-specific or category-specific. Disease-specific systems apply only to those procedures that are considered necessary to interrupt the spread of specific infectious diseases. The disease-specific systems have the advantage of conserving materials (eg, gowns when they are not absolutely needed) and nursing/physician time in situations in which isolation precautions may not be necessary. The disadvantage of disease-specific systems is that they require a greater level of education for all hospital staff, offer a smaller margin for error, and can be difficult to apply if the patient is not known to have a specific infection on admission.

Category-specific isolation systems are the most common type of isolation systems used in hospitals in the United States. In such systems, all known or suspected types of infections are grouped under several general isolation titles, and a single list of isolation practices for the entire group may be enumerated. The advantages of category-specific systems are that it is easier to

*(Text continues on p. 1446.)*

## TABLE 64-1. Category-Specific Isolation Precautions

| Disease | Category | Infective Material | Apply Precautions How Long? | Comments |
|---|---|---|---|---|
| Abscess, cause unknown | | | | |
|   Draining, major | Contact/isolation | Pus | Duration of illness | Major—no dressing, or dressing does not adequately contain the pus. |
|   Draining, minor or limited | Drainage/secretion precautions | Pus | Duration of illness | Minor or limited—dressing covers and adequately contains the pus, or infected area is very small, such as a stitch abscess. |
|   Not draining | None | | | |
| Acquired immunodeficiency syndrome (AIDS) | Blood/body fluid precautions | Blood and body fluids | Duration of illness | See MMWR 1989;38:1 |
| Actinomycosis, all lesions | None | | | |
| Adenovirus infection, respiratory, in infants and young children | Contact isolation | Respiratory secretions and feces | Duration of hospitalization | During epidemics, patients believed to have adenovirus infection may be placed in the same room (cohorting). |
| Amebiasis | | | | |
|   Dysentery | Enteric precautions | Feces | Duration of illness | |
|   Liver abscess | None | | | |
| Anthrax | | | | |
|   Cutaneous | Drainage/secretion precautions | Pus | Duration of illness | |
|   Inhalation | Drainage/secretion precautions | Respiratory secretions may be | Duration of illness | |
| Arthropod-borne viral encephalitides (eastern equine, western equine, and Venezuelan equine encephalomyelitis, St. Louis and California encephalitis) | None | | | |
| Arthropod-borne viral fevers (dengue, yellow fever, and Colorado tick fever) | Blood/body fluid precautions | Blood | Duration of hospitalization | |
| Ascariasis | None | | | |
| Aspergillosis | None | | | |
| Babesiosis | Blood/body fluid precautions | Blood | Duration of illness | |
| Blastomycosis, North American, cutaneous or pulmonary | None | | | |
| Botulism | | | | |
|   Infant | None | | | |
|   Other | None | | | |
| Bronchiolitis, cause unknown, in infants and young children | Contact isolation | Respiratory secretions | Duration of illness | Various etiologic agents, such as respiratory syncytial virus, parainfluenza viruses, adenoviruses, and influenza viruses, have been associated with this syndrome (Committee on Infectious Diseases, American Academy of Pediatrics. 1991 Red Book); therefore, precautions to prevent their spread generally are indicated. |
| Bronchitis, infective, cause unknown | | | | |
|   Adults | None | Respiratory secretions may be | | |
|   Infants and young children | Contact isolation | Respiratory secretions | Duration of illness | |

*(continued)*

TABLE 64-1. *(Continued)*

| Disease | Category | Infective Material | Apply Precautions How Long? | Comments |
|---|---|---|---|---|
| Brucellosis (undulant fever, Malta fever, Mediterranean fever) | | | | |
|   Draining lesions, limited or minor | Drainage/secretion precautions | Pus | Duration of illness | Limited or minor—dressing covers and adequately contains the pus, or infected area is very small. |
|   Other | None | | | |
| Burn wound | | | | |
| *Campylobacter* gastroenteritis | Enteric precautions | Feces | Duration of illness | |
| Candidiasis, all forms, including mucocutaneous (moniliasis, thrush) | | | | |
| Cat-scratch fever (benign inoculation lymphoreticulosis) | None | | | |
| Cellulitis | | | | |
|   Draining, limited or minor | Drainage/secretion precautions | Pus | Duration of illness | Limited or minor—dressing covers and adequately contains the pus, or infected area is very small. |
|   Intact skin | None | | | |
| Chancroid (soft chancre) | None | | | |
| Chickenpox (varicella) | Strict isolation | Respiratory secretions and lesion secretions | Until all lesions are crusted | Persons who are not susceptible do not need to wear a mask. Susceptible persons should, if possible, stay out of room. Special ventilation for the room, if available, may be advantageous, especially for outbreak control. Neonates born to mothers with active varicella should be placed in strict isolation at birth. Exposed susceptible patients should be placed in strict isolation beginning 10 days after exposure and continuing until 21 days after last exposure. See CDC Guideline for Infection Control in Hospital Personnel for recommendations for exposed susceptible personnel. |
| *Chlamydia trachomatis* infection | | | | |
|   Conjunctivitis | Drainage/secretion precautions | Purulent exudate | Duration of illness | |
|   Genital | Drainage/secretion precautions | Genital discharge | Duration of illness | |
|   Respiratory | Drainage/secretion precautions | Respiratory secretions | Duration of illness | |
| Cholera | Enteric precautions | Feces | Duration of illness | |
| Closed-cavity infection | | | | |
|   Draining, limited or minor | Drainage/secretion precautions | Pus | Duration of illness | Limited or minor—dressing covers and adequately contains the pus, or infected area is very small. |
|   Not draining | None | | | |
| *Clostridium perfringens* | | | | |
|   Food poisoning | None | | | |

## TABLE 64-1.    (Continued)

| Disease | Category | Infective Material | Apply Precautions How Long? | Comments |
|---|---|---|---|---|
| Gas gangrene | Drainage/secretion precautions | Pus | Duration of illness | |
| Other | Drainage/secretion precautions | Pus | Duration of illness | |
| Coccidioidomycosis (valley fever) | | | | |
| Draining lesions | None | Drainage may be if spores form | | |
| Pneumonia | None | | | |
| Coloradio tick fever | Blood/body fluid precautions | Blood | Duration of hospitalization | |
| Common cold | | | | |
| Adults | None | Respiratory secretions may be | | |
| Infants and young children | Contact isolation | Respiratory secretions | Duration of illness | Although rhinoviruses are associated most frequently with the common cold and are mild in adults, severe infections may occur in infants and young children. Other etiologic agents, such as respiratory syncytial virus and parainfluenza viruses, also may cause this syndrome (Committee on Infectious Diseases, American Academy of Pediatrics. 1991 Red Book); therefore, precautions to prevent their spread generally are indicated. |
| Congenital rubella | Contact isolation | Urine and respiratory secretions | During any admission for the first year after birth unless nasopharyngeal and urine cultures after 3 months of age are negative for rubella virus | Susceptible persons should stay out of room, if possible. Pregnant personnel may need special counseling (see CDC Guideline for Infection Control in Hospital Personnel). |
| Conjunctivitis, acute bacterial (sore eye, pinkeye) | Drainage/secretion precautions | Purulent exudate | Duration of illness | |
| Conjunctivitis, *Chlamydia* | Drainage/secretion precautions | Purulent exudate | Duration of illness | |
| Conjunctivitis, gonococcal | | | | |
| Adults | Drainage/secretion precautions | Purulent exudate | For 24 hours after start of effective therapy | |
| Newborns | Contact isolation | Purulent exudate | For 24 hours after start of effective therapy | |
| Conjunctivitis, viral and cause unknown (acute hemorrhagic and swimming pool conjunctivitis) | Drainage/secretion precautions | Purulent exudate | Duration of illness | If patient hygiene is poor, a private room may be indicated |
| Coronavirus infection, respiratory | | | | |
| Adults | None | Respiratory secretions may be | | |
| Infants and young children | Contact isolation | Respiratory secretions | Duration of illness | |
| Coxsackievirus disease | Enteric precautions | Feces and respiratory secretions | For 7 days after onset | |

*(continued)*

## TABLE 64-1.   (Continued)

| Disease | Category | Infective Material | Apply Precautions How Long? | Comments |
|---|---|---|---|---|
| Creutzfeldt-Jakob disease | Blood/body fluid precautions | Blood, brain tissue, and spinal fluid | Duration of hospitalization | Use caution when handling blood, brain tissue, or spinal fluid. (Jarvis WR. Precautions for Creutzfeldt-Jakob disease. Infect Control 1982;3:238.) |
| Croup | Contact isolation | Respiratory secretions | Duration of illness | Because viral agents, such as parainfluenza viruses and influenza A virus, have been associated with this syndrome (Committee on Infectious Diseases, American Academy of Pediatrics. 1991 Red Book), precautions to prevent their spread generally are indicated. |
| Cryptococcosis | None | | | |
| Cysticercosis | None | | | |
| Cytomegalovirus infection, neonatal or immunosuppressed | None | Urine and respiratory secretions may be | | Pregnant personnel may need special counseling (see CDC Guideline for Infection Control in Hospital Personnel). |
| Decubitus ulcer, infected | | | | |
|   Major | Contact isolation | Pus | Duration of illness | Major—draining and not covered by dressing or dressing does not adequately contain the pus. |
|   Minor or limited | Drainage/secretion precautions | Pus | Duration of illness | Minor or limited—dressing covers and adequately contains the pus, or infected area is very small. |
| Dengue | Blood/body fluid precautions | Blood | Duration of hospitalization | |
| Diarrhea, acute—infective cause suspected (see gastroenteritis) | Enteric precautions | Feces | Duration of illness | |
| Diphtheria | | | | |
|   Cutaneous | Contact isolation | Lesion secretions | Until 2 cultures from skin lesions, taken at least 24 hours apart after cessation of antimicrobial therapy, are negative for Corynebacterium diphtheriae | |
|   Pharyngeal | Strict isolation | Respiratory secretions | Until 2 cultures from both nose and throat taken at least 24 hours apart after cessation of antimicrobial therapy are negative for Corynebacterium diphtheriae | |
| Echinococcosis (hydatidosis) | None | | | |
| Echovirus disease | Enteric precautions | Feces and respiratory secretions | For 7 days after onset | |
| Eczema vaccinatum (vaccinia) | Contact isolation | Lesion secretions | Duration of illness | |
| Encephalitis or encephalomyelitis, cause unknown, but infection suspected (see also specific etiologic agents; likely causes include enterovirus and arthropodborne virus infections) | Enteric precautions | Feces | Duration of illness or 7 days after onset, whichever is less | Although specific etiologic agents can include enteroviruses, arthropod-borne viruses, and herpes simplex, precautions for enteroviruses generally are indicated until a definitive diagnosis can be made. |

## TABLE 64-1.  *(Continued)*

| Disease | Category | Infective Material | Apply Precautions How Long? | Comments |
|---|---|---|---|---|
| Endometritis | | | | |
|   Group A *Streptococcus* | Contact isolation | Vaginal discharge | For 24 hours after start of effective therapy | |
|   Other | Drainage/secretion precautions | Vaginal discharge | Duration of illness | |
| Enterobiasis (pinworm disease, oxyuriasis) | None | | | |
| Enterocolitis (see also necrotizing enterocolitis) | | | | |
|   *Clostridium difficile* | Enteric precautions | Feces | Duration of illness | |
|   *Staphylococcus* | Enteric precautions | Feces | Duration of illness | |
| Enteroviral infection | Enteric precautions | Feces | For 7 days after onset | |
| Epiglottis, caused by *Haemophilus influenzae* | Respiratory isolation | Respiratory secretions | For 24 hours after start of effective therapy | |
| Epstein-Barr virus infection, any including infectious mononucleosis | None | Respiratory secretions may be | | |
| Erysipeloid | None | | | |
| Erythema infectiosum | Respiratory isolation | Respiratory secretions | For 7 days after onset | |
| *Escherichia coli* gastroenteritis (enteropathogenic, enterotoxic, or enteroinvasive) | Enteric precautions | Feces | Duration of hospitalization | |
| Fever of unknown origin (FUO) | | | | Patients with FUO usually do not need isolation precautions; however, if a patient has signs and symptoms compatible with (and is likely to have) a disease that requires isolation precautions, use those isolation precautions for that patient. |
| Food poisoning | | | | |
|   Botulism | None | | | |
|   *Clostridium perfringens* or *welchii* (food poisoning) | None | | | |
|   Salmonellosis | Enteric precautions | Feces | Duration of illness | |
|   Staphylococcal food poisoning | None | | | |
| Furunculosis—staphylococcal | | | | |
|   Newborns | Contact isolation | Pus | Duration of illness | During a nursery outbreak, cohorting of ill and colonized infants and use of gowns and gloves is recommended. |
|   Others | Drainage/secretion precautions | Pus | Duration of illness | |
| Gangrene | | | | |
|   Gas gangrene (caused by any bacteria) | Drainage/secretion precautions | Pus | Duration of illness | |
| Gastroenteritis | | | | |
|   *Campylobacter* species | Enteric precautions | Feces | Duration of illness | |
|   *Clostridium difficile* | Enteric precautions | Feces | Duration of illness | |
|   *Cryptosporidium* species | Enteric precautions | Feces | Duration of illness | |
|   *Dientamoeba fragilis* | Enteric precautions | Feces | Duration of illness | |
|   *Escherichia coli* (enteropathogenic, enterotoxic, or enteroinvasive) | Enteric precautions | Feces | Duration of illness | |

*(continued)*

TABLE 64-1. *(Continued)*

| Disease | Category | Infective Material | Apply Precautions How Long? | Comments |
|---|---|---|---|---|
| *Giardia lamblia* | Enteric precautions | Feces | Duration of illness | |
| *Rotavirus* | Enteric precautions | Feces | Duration of illness or 7 days after onset, whichever is less | |
| *Salmonella* species | Enteric precautions | Feces | Duration of illness | |
| *Shigella* species | Enteric precautions | Feces | Until 3 consecutive cultures of feces taken after ending antimicrobial therapy are negative for infecting strain | |
| Unknown cause | Enteric precautions | Feces | Duration of illness | |
| *Vibrio parahaemolyticus* | Enteric precautions | Feces | Duration of illness | |
| Viral | Enteric precautions | Feces | Duration of illness | |
| *Yersinia enterocolitica* | Enteric precautions | Feces | Duration of illness | |
| German measles (rubella) (see also congenital rubella) | Contact isolation | Respiratory secretions | For 7 days after onset of rash | Persons who are not susceptible do not need to wear a mask. Susceptible persons should, if possible, stay out of room. Pregnant personnel may need special counseling (see CDC Guideline for Infection Control in Hospital Personnel). |
| Giardiasis | Enteric precautions | Feces | Duration of illness | |
| Gonococcal ophthalmia neonatorum (gonorrheal ophthalmia, acute conjunctivitis of the newborn) | Contact isolation | Purulent exudate | For 24 hours after start of effective therapy | |
| Gonorrhea | None | Discharge may be | | |
| Granulocytopenia | None | | | Wash hands well *before* taking care of patient. |
| Granuloma inguinale (donovanosis, granuloma venereum) | None | Drainage may be | | |
| Guillain-Barré syndrome | None | | | |
| Hand-foot-and-mouth disease | Enteric precautions | Feces | For 7 days after onset | |
| Hemorrhagic fevers (for example, Lassa fever) | Strict isolation | Blood, body fluids, and respiratory secretions | Duration of illness | Call the state health department and Centers for Disease Control and Prevention for advice about management of a suspected case. |
| Hepatitis, viral | | | | |
|    Type A (infectious) | Enteric precautions | Feces may be | For 7 days after onset of jaundice | Hepatitis A is most contagious before symptoms and jaundice appear; once these appear, small, inapparent amounts of feces, which may contaminate the hands of personnel during patient care, do not appear to be infective. Thus, gowns and gloves are most useful when gross soiling with feces is anticipated or possible. |
|    Type B ("serum hepatitis"), including hepatitis B antigen (HbsAg) carrier | Blood/body fluid precautions | Blood and body fluids | Until patient is HBsAg-negative | See MMWR 1989;38:1. |
|    Non-A, non-B | Blood/body fluid precautions | Blood and body fluids | Duration of illness | Currently, the period of infectivity cannot be determined. |

TABLE 64-1.    *(Continued)*

| Disease | Category | Infective Material | Apply Precautions How Long? | Comments |
|---|---|---|---|---|
| Unspecified type, consistent with viral cause | | | | Maintain precautions indicated for the infections that are most likely. |
| Herpangina | Enteric precautions | Feces | For 7 days after onset | |
| Herpes simplex (herpesvirus hominis) | | | | |
| Encephalitis | None | | | |
| Mucocutaneous, disseminated or primary, severe (skin, oral, and genital) | Contact isolation | Lesion secretions from infected site | Duration of illness | |
| Mucocutaneous, recurrent (skin, oral, and genital) | Drainage/secretion precautions | Lesion secretions from infected site | Until all lesions are crusted | |
| Neonatal (see comments for newborn with perinatal exposure) | Contact isolation | Lesion secretions | Duration of illness | The same isolation precautions are indicated for infants delivered (either vaginally or by cesarean section if membranes have been ruptured for more than 4–6 h) of women with active genital herpes simplex infections. Infants delivered by cesarean section of women with active genital herpes simplex infections before and probably within 4–6 hours after membrane rupture are at minimal risk of developing herpes simplex infection; the same isolation precautions still may be indicated, however. (American Academy of Pediatrics Committee on Fetus and Newborn. Perinatal herpes simplex virus infections. Pediatrics 1980;66:147. Also: Kibrick S. Herpes simplex infection at term. JAMA 1980;243:157.) |
| Herpes zoster (varicella-zoster) | | | | |
| Localized in immunocompromised patient, or disseminated | Strict isolation | Lesion secretions and possibly respiratory secretions | Duration of illness | Localized lesions in immunocompromised patients frequently become disseminated. Because such dissemination is unpredictable, use the same isolation precautions as for disseminated disease. Persons who are not susceptible do not need to wear a mask. Persons susceptible to varicella-zoster (chickenpox) should, if possible, stay out of room. Special ventilation for the room, if available, may be advantageous, especially for outbreak control. Exposed susceptible patients should be placed in strict isolation beginning 10 days after exposure and continuing until 21 days after last exposure. See CDC Guideline for Infection |

*(continued)*

TABLE 64-1. *(Continued)*

| Disease | Category | Infective Material | Apply Precautions How Long? | Comments |
|---|---|---|---|---|
| | | | | Control in Hospital Personnel for recommendations for exposed susceptible personnel. |
| Localized in normal patient | Drainage/secretion precautions | Lesion secretions | Until all lesions are crusted | Persons susceptible to varicella-zoster (chickenpox) should, if possible, stay out of room. Roommates should not be susceptible to chickenpox. If patient hygiene is poor, a private room may be indicated. |
| Histoplasmosis at any site | None | | | |
| Hookworm disease (ancylostomiasis, uncinariasis) | None | | | |
| Immunocompromised status | None | | | Wash hands well *before* taking care of patients. |
| Impetigo | Contact isolation | Lesions | For 24 hours after start of effective therapy | |
| Infectious mononucleosis | None | Respiratory secretions may be | | |
| Influenza | | | | |
| Adults | None | Respiratory secretions may be | | In the absence of an epidemic, influenza may be difficult to diagnose on clinical grounds. Most patients will have recovered fully by the time laboratory diagnosis is established; therefore, placing patients with suspect influenza on isolation precautions, although theoretically desirable, simply is not practical in most hospitals. During epidemics, the accuracy of clinical diagnosis increases, and patients believed to have influenza may be placed in the same room (cohorting). Amantadine prophylaxis may be useful to prevent symptomatic influenza A infections in high-risk patients during epidemics. |
| Infants and young children | Contact isolation | Respiratory secretions | Duration of illness | In the absence of an epidemic, influenza may be difficult to diagnose. During epidemics, patients believed to have influenza may be placed in the same room (cohorting). |
| Jakob-Creutzfeldt disease | Blood/body fluid precautions | Blood, brain tissue, and spinal fluid | Duration of hospitalization | Use caution when handling blood, brain tissue, or spinal fluid. (Jarvis WR. Precautions for Creutzfeldt-Jakob disease. Infect Control 1982;3:238.) |
| Kawasaki syndrome | None | | | |
| Keratoconjuncitivits, infective | Drainage/secretion precautions | Purulent exudate | Duration of illness | If patient hygiene is poor, a private room may be indicated. |
| Lassa fever | Strict isolation | Blood, body fluids, and respiratory secretions | Duration of illness | Call the state health department and Centers for Disease Control and Prevention for advice about management of a suspected case. |

TABLE 64-1. *(Continued)*

| Disease | Category | Infective Material | Apply Precautions How Long? | Comments |
|---|---|---|---|---|
| Legionnaires' disease | None | Respiratory secretions may be | | |
| Leprosy | None | | | |
| Leptospirosis | Blood/body fluid precautions | Blood and urine | Duration of hospitalization | |
| Listeriosis | None | | | |
| Lyme disease | None | | | |
| Lymphocytic choriomeningitis | None | | | |
| Lymphogranuloma venereum | None | Drainage may be | | |
| Malaria | Blood/body fluid precautions | Blood | Duration of illness | |
| Marburg virus disease | Strict isolation | Blood, body fluids, and respiratory secretions | Duration of illness | Call the state health department and Centers for Disease Control and Prevention for advice about management of a suspected case. |
| Measles (rubeola), all presentations | Respiratory isolation | Respiratory secretions | For 4 days after start of rash, except in immunocompromised patients, with whom precautions should be maintained for duration of illness | Persons who are not susceptible do not need to wear a mask. Susceptible persons should, if possible, stay out of room. |
| Melioidosis, all forms | None | Respiratory secretions may be and, if a sinus is draining, drainage may be | | |
| Meningitis | | | | |
|    Aseptic (nonbacterial or viral meningitis) (also see specific etiologies) | Enteric precautions | Feces | For 7 days after onset | Enteroviruses are the most common cause of aseptic meningitis. |
|    Bacterial, gram-negative enteric, in neonates | None | Feces may be | | During a nursery outbreak, cohort ill and colonized infants, and use gowns if soiling is likely and gloves if touching feces. |
|    Fungal | None | | | |
|    *Haemophilus influenzae*, known or suspected | Respiratory isolation | Respiratory secretions | For 24 hours after start of effective therapy | |
|    *Listeria monocytogenes* | None | | | |
|    *Neisseria meningitidis* (meningococcal), known or suspected | Respiratory isolation | Respiratory secretions | For 24 hours after start of effective therapy | See CDC Guideline for Infection Control in Hospital Personnel for recommendations for prophylaxis after exposure. |
|    Pneumococcal | None | | | |
|    Tuberculous | None | | | Patient should be examined for evidence of current (active) pulmonary tuberculosis. If present, precautions are necessary (see tuberculosis) |
|    Other diagnosed bacterial | None | | | |
| Meningococcal pneumonia | Respiratory isolation | Respiratory secretions | For 24 hours after start of effective therapy | See CDC Guideline for Infection Control in Hospital Personnel for recommendations for prophylaxis after exposure. |
| Meningococcemia (meningococcal sepsis) | Respiratory isolation | Respiratory secretions | For 24 hours after start of effective therapy | See CDC Guideline for Infection Control in Hospital Personnel for recommendations for prophylaxis after exposure. |

*(continued)*

TABLE 64-1. *(Continued)*

| Disease | Category | Infective Material | Apply Precautions How Long? | Comments |
|---|---|---|---|---|
| *Molluscum contagiosum* | None | | | |
| Mucormycosis | None | | | |
| Multiply resistant organisms,* infection or colonization† | | | | |
|   Gastrointestinal | Contact isolation | Feces | Until off antimicrobials and culture-negative | In outbreaks, cohorting of infected and colonized patients may be indicated if private rooms are not available. |
|   Respiratory | Contact isolation | Respiratory secretions and possibly feces | Until off antimicrobials and culture-negative | In outbreaks, cohorting of infected and colonized patients may be indicated if private rooms are not available. |
|   Skin, wound, or burn | Contact isolation | Pus and possibly feces | Until off antimicrobials and culture-negative | In outbreaks, cohorting of infected and colonized patients may be indicated if private rooms are not available. |
|   Urinary | Contact isolation | Urine and possibly feces | Until off antimicrobials and culture-negative | Urine and urine-measuring devices are sources of infection, especially if the patient (or any nearby patient) has an indwelling urinary catheter. In outbreaks, cohorting of infected and colonized patients may be indicated if private rooms are not available. |
| Mumps (infectious parotitis) | Respiratory isolation | Respiratory secretions | For 9 days after onset of swelling | Persons who are not susceptible do not need to wear a mask. |
| Mycobacteria, nontuberculous (atypical) | | | | |
|   Pulmonary | None | | | |
|   Wound | Drainage/secretion precautions | Drainage may be | Duration of drainage | |
| *Mycoplasma* pneumonia | None | Respiratory secretions may be | | A private room may be indicated for children. |
| Necrotizing enterocolitis | Enteric precautions | Feces may be | Duration of illness | In nurseries, cohorting of ill infants is recommended. It is not known whether or how this disease is transmitted; nevertheless, gowns are recommended if soiling is likely, and gloves are recommended for touching feces. |
| Neutropenia | None | | | Wash hands well *before* taking care of patient. |
| Nocardiosis | | | | |
|   Draining lesions | None | Drainage may be | | |
|   Other | None | | | |
| Norwalk agent gastroenteritis | Enteric precautions | Feces | Duration of illness | |
| Orf | None | Drainage may be | | |
| Parainfluenza virus infection, respiratory, in infants and young children | Contact isolation | Respiratory secretions | Duration of illness | During epidemics, patients believed to have parainfluenza infection may be placed in the same room (cohorting). |
| Pediculosis | Contact isolation | Infested area | For 24 hours after start of effective therapy | Masks are not needed. |

| | TABLE 64-1. *(Continued)* | | | |
|---|---|---|---|---|
| **Disease** | **Category** | **Infective Material** | **Apply Precautions How Long?** | **Comments** |
| Pertussis ("whooping cough") | Respiratory isolation | Respiratory secretions | For 7 days after start of effective therapy | See CDC Guideline for Infection Control in Hospital Personnel for recommendations for prophylaxis after exposure. |
| Pharyngitis, infective, cause unknown | | | | |
|   Adults | None | Respiratory secretions may be | | |
|   Infants and young children | Contact isolation | Respiratory secretions | Duration of illness | Because adenoviruses, influenza viruses and parainfluenza viruses have been associated with this syndrome (Committee on Infectious Diseases, American Academy of Pediatrics. 1991 Red Book), precautions to prevent their spread generally are indicated. |
| Pinworm infection | None | | | |
| Plague | | | | |
|   Bubonic | Drainage/secretion precautions | Pus | For 3 days after start of effective therapy | |
|   Pneumonic | Strict isolation | Respiratory secretions | For 3 days after start of effective therapy | |
| Pleurodynia | Enteric precautions | Feces | For 7 days after onset | Enteroviruses frequently cause infection. |
| Pneumonia | | | | |
|   Bacterial not listed elsewhere (including gram-negative bacterial) | None | Respiratory secretions may be | | |
|   *Chlamydia* | Drainage/secretion precautions | Respiratory secretions | Duration of illness | |
|   Etiology unknown | | | | Maintain precautions indicated for the cause that is most likely. |
|   Fungal | None | | | |
|   *Haemophilus influenzae* | | | | |
|     Adults | None | Respiratory secretions may be | | |
|     Infants and children (any age) | Respiratory isolation | Respiratory secretions | For 24 hours after start of effective therapy | |
|   *Legionella* | None | Respiratory secretions may be | | |
|   Meningococcal | Respiratory isolation | Respiratory secretions | For 24 hours after start of effective therapy | See CDC Guideline for Infection Control in Hospital Personnel for recommendations for prophylaxis after exposure. |
|   Multiply resistant bacterial | Contact isolation | Respiratory secretions and possibly feces | Until off antimicrobials and culture-negative | In outbreaks, cohorting of infected and colonized patients may be necessary if private rooms are not available. |
|   *Mycoplasma* (primary atypical pneumonia, Eaton agent pneumonia) | None | Respiratory secretions may be | | A private room may be useful for children. |
|   Pneumococcal | None | Respiratory secretions may be for 24 hours after start of effective therapy | | |

## TABLE 64-1.    *(Continued)*

| Disease | Category | Infective Material | Apply Precautions How Long? | Comments |
|---|---|---|---|---|
| *Pneumocystis carinii* | None | | | |
| *Staphylococcus aureus* | Contact isolation | Respiratory secretions | For 48 hours after start of effective therapy | |
| *Streptococcus,* group A | Contact isolation | Respiratory secretions | For 24 hours after start of effective therapy | |
| Viral (see also specific etiologic agents) | | | | |
|   Adults | None | Respiratory secretions may be | | |
|   Infants and young children | Contact isolation | Respiratory secretions | Duration of illness | Viral pneumonia may be caused by various etiologic agents, such as parainfluenza viruses, influenza viruses, and particularly, respiratory syncytial virus, in children less than 5 years old (Committee on Infectious Diseases, American Academy of Pediatrics. 1991 Red Book); therefore, precautions to prevent their spread generally are indicated. |
| Poliomyelitis | Enteric precautions | Feces | For 7 days after onset | |
| Psittacosis (ornithosis) | None | Respiratory secretions may be | | |
| Q fever | None | Respiratory secretions may be | | |
| Rabies | Contact isolation | Respiratory secretions | Duration of illness | See CDC Guideline for Infection Control in Hospital Personnel for recommendations for prophylaxis after exposure. |
| Rat-bite fever (*Streptobacillus moniliformis* disease, *Spirillum minus* disease) | Blood/body fluid precautions | Blood | For 24 hours after start of effective therapy | |
| Relapsing fever | Blood/body fluid precautions | Blood | Duration of illness | |
| Resistant bacterial (see multiply resistant bacteria) | | | | |
| Respiratory infectious disease, acute (if not covered elsewhere) | | | | |
|   Adults | None | Respiratory secretions may be | | |
|   Infants and young children | | | | Maintain precautions for the bacterial or viral infections that are most likely. |
| Respiratory syncytial virus (RSV) infection, in infants and young children | Contact isolation | Respiratory secretions | Duration of illness | During epidemics, patients believed to have RSV infection may be placed in the same room (cohorting). |
| Reye's syndrome | None | | | |
| Rheumatic fever | None | | | |
| Rhinovirus infection, respiratory | | | | |
|   Adults | None | Respiratory secretions may be | | |
|   Infants and young children | Contact isolation | Respiratory secretions | Duration of illness | |

TABLE 64-1.   *(Continued)*

| Disease | Category | Infective Material | Apply Precautions How Long? | Comments |
|---|---|---|---|---|
| Rickettsial fevers, tick-borne (Rocky Mountain spotted fever, tick-borne typhus fever) | None | Blood may be | | |
| Rickettsialpox (vesicular rickettsiosis) | None | | | |
| Ringworm (dermatophytosis, dermatomycosis, tinea) | None | | | |
| Ritter's disease (staphylococcal scalded skin syndrome) | Contact isolation | Lesion drainage | Duration of illness | |
| Rocky Mountain spotted fever | None | Blood may be | | |
| Roseola infantum (exanthemasubitum) | None | | | |
| Rotavirus infection (viral gastroenteritis) | Enteric precautions | Feces | Duration of illness or 7 days after onset, whichever is less | |
| Rubella ("German measles") (see also congenital rubella) | Contact isolation | Respiratory secretions | For 7 days after onset of rash | Persons who are not susceptible do not need to wear a mask. Susceptible persons should, if possible, stay out of room. Pregnant personnel may need special counseling (see CDC Guideline for Infection Control in Hospital Personnel). |
| Salmonellosis | Enteric precautions | Feces | Duration of illness | |
| Scabies | Contact isolation | Infested area | For 24 hours after start of effective therapy | Masks are not needed. |
| Scalded skin syndrome, staphylococcal (Ritter's disease) | Contact isolation | Lesion drainage | Duration of illness | |
| Schistosomiasis (bilharziasis) | None | | | |
| Shigellosis (including bacillary dysentery) | Enteric precautions | Feces | Until 3 consecutive cultures of feces, taken after ending antimicrobial therapy, are negative for infecting strain | |
| Smallpox (variola) | Strict isolation | Respiratory secretions and lesion secretions | Duration of illness | As long as smallpox virus is kept stocked in laboratories, the potential exists for cases to occur. Call the state health department and Centers for Disease Control and Prevention for advice about management of a suspected case. |
| *Spirillum minus* disease (rat-bite fever) | Blood/body fluid precautions | Blood | For 24 hours after start of effective therapy | |
| Sporotrichosis | None | | | |
| Staphylococcal disease (*S aureus*) Skin, wound, or burn infection | | | | |
| Major | Contact isolation | Pus | Duration of illness | Major—draining and not covered by dressing, or dressing does not adequately contain the pus. |
| Minor or limited | Drainage/secretion precautions | Pus | Duration of illness | Minor or limited—dressing covers and adequately contains the pus, or infected area is very small. |

*(continued)*

TABLE 64-1. *(Continued)*

| Disease | Category | Infective Material | Apply Precautions How Long? | Comments |
|---|---|---|---|---|
| Enterocolitis | Enteric precautions | Feces | Duration of illness | |
| Pneumonia or draining lung abscess | Contact isolation | Respiratory secretions | For 48 hours after start of effective therapy | |
| Scalded skin syndrome | Contact isolation | Lesion drainage | Duration of illness | |
| Toxic shock syndrome | Drainage/secretion precautions | Vaginal discharge or pus | Duration of illness | |
| *Streptobacillus moniliformis* disease (rat-bite fever) | Blood/body fluid precautions | Blood | For 24 hours after start of effective therapy | |
| Streptococcal disease (group A *Streptococcus*) | | | | |
|   Skin, wound, or burn infection | | | | |
|     Major | Contact isolation | Pus | For 24 hours after start of effective therapy | Major—draining and not covered by dressing, or dressing does not adequately contain the pus. |
|     Minor or limited | Drainage/secretion precautions | Pus | For 24 hours after start of effective therapy | Minor or limited—dressing covers and adequately contains the pus, or infected area is very small. |
| Endometritis (puerperal sepsis) | Contact isolation | Vaginal discharge | For 24 hours after start of effective therapy | |
| Pharyngitis | Drainage/secretion precautions | Respiratory secretions | For 24 hours after start of effective therapy | |
| Pneumonia | Contact isolation | Respiratory secretions | For 24 hours after start of effective therapy | |
| Scarlet fever | Drainage/secretion precautions | Respiratory secretions | For 24 hours after start of effective therapy | |
| Streptococcal disease (group B *Streptococcus*), neonatal | None | Feces may be | | During a nursery outbreak, cohorting of ill and colonized infants and use of gowns and gloves is recommended. |
| Streptococcal disease (not group A or B) unless covered elsewhere | None | | | |
| Strongyloidiasis | None | Feces may be | | If patient is immunocompromised and has pneumonia or has disseminated disease, respiratory secretions may be infective. |
| Syphilis | | | | |
|   Skin and mucous membrane, including congenital, primary, and secondary | Drainage/secretion precautions, Blood/body fluid precautions | Lesion secretions and blood | For 24 hours after start of effective therapy | Skin lesions of primary and secondary syphilis may be highly infective. |
|   Latent (tertiary) and seropositivity without lesions | None | | | |
| Tapeworm disease | | | | |
|   *Hymenolepis nana* | None | Feces may be | | |
|   *Taenia solium* (pork) | None | Feces may be | | |
|   Other | None | | | |
| Tetanus | None | | | |
| Tinea (fungus infection, dermatophytosis, dermatomycosis, ringworm) | None | | | |
| "TORCH" syndrome. (If congenital forms of the following diseases are being | | | | |

## TABLE 64-1. *(Continued)*

| Disease | Category | Infective Material | Apply Precautions How Long? | Comments |
|---|---|---|---|---|
| considered seriously, see separate listing for these diseases: toxoplasmosis, rubella, cytomegalovirus, herpes, and syphilis.) | | | | |
| Toxic shock syndrome (staphylococcal disease) | Drainage/secretion precautions | Vaginal discharge and pus | Duration of illness | |
| Toxoplasmosis | None | | | |
| Trachoma, acute | Drainage/secretion precautions | Purulent exudate | Duration of illness | |
| Trench mouth (Vincent's angina) | None | | | |
| Trichinosis | None | | | |
| Trichomoniasis | None | | | |
| Trichuriasis (whipworm disease) | None | | | |
| Tuberculosis (TB) | | | | |
|   Extrapulmonary, draining lesion (including scrofula) | Drainage/secretion precautions | Pus | Duration of drainage | A private room is especially important for children. |
|   Extrapulmonary, meningitis | None | | | |
|   Pulmonary, confirmed or suspected (sputum smear result is positive or chest radiograph appearance strongly suggests current [active] TB; for example, a cavitary lesion is found), or laryngeal disease | Tuberculosis isolation (AFB isolation) | Airborne droplet nuclei | In most instances, the duration of isolation precautions can be guided by clinical response and a reduction in numbers of TB organisms on sputum smear. Usually this occurs within 2–3 wk after chemotherapy is begun. When the patient is likely to be infected with isoniazid-resistant organisms, apply precautions until patient is improving and sputum smear result is negative for TB organisms. | Prompt use of effective antituberculous drugs is the most effective means of limiting transmission. Gowns are not important because TB rarely is spread by fomites, although gowns are indicated to prevent gross contamination of clothing. For more detailed guidelines, refer to Guidelines for Prevention of TB Transmission in Hospitals (1982), Tuberculosis Control Division, Center for Prevention Services, Centers for Disease Control, Atlanta, Ga (HHS Publication No [CDC] 82-8371) and CDC Guideline for Infection Control in Hospital Personnel. In general, infants and young children do not require isolation precautions because they rarely cough and their bronchial secretions contain few TB organisms compared to adults with pulmonary TB. |
|   Skin test result positive with no evidence of current pulmonary disease (sputum smear result is negative; radiograph not suggestive of current [active] disease) | None | | | |
| Tularemia | | | | |
|   Draining lesion | Drainage/secretion precautions | Pus may be | Duration of illness | |
|   Pulmonary | None | Respiratory secretions may be | | |
| Typhoid fever | Enteric precautions | Feces | Duration of illness | |
| Typhus, endemic and epidemic | None | Blood may be | | |

*(continued)*

## TABLE 64-1. *(Continued)*

| Disease | Category | Infective Material | Apply Precautions How Long? | Comments |
|---|---|---|---|---|
| Urinary tract infection (including pyelonephritis), with or without urinary catheter | None | | | See multiply resistant bacteria if infection is with these bacteria. Spatially separate infected and uninfected patients who have indwelling catheters (see CDC Guideline for Prevention of Catheter-Associated Urinary Tract Infection). |
| Vaccinia | | | | |
| At vaccination site | Drainage/secretion precautions | Lesion secretions | Duration of illness | |
| Generalized and progressive, eczema vaccinatum | Contact isolation | Lesion secretions | Duration of illness | |
| Varicella (chickenpox) | Strict isolation | Respiratory secretions and lesion secretions | Until all lesions are crusted | Persons who are not susceptible do not need to wear a mask. Susceptible persons should, if possible, stay out of room. Special ventilation for the room, if available, may be advantageous, especially for outbreak control. Neonates born to mothers with active varicella should be placed in strict isolation at birth. Exposed susceptible patients should be placed in strict isolation beginning 10 days after exposure and continuing until 21 days after last exposure. See CDC Guideline for Infection Control in Hospital Personnel for recommendations for exposed susceptible personnel. |
| Variola (smallpox) | Strict isolation | Respiratory secretions and lesion secretions | Duration of illness | Call the state health department and Centers for Disease Control and Prevention for advice about management of a suspected case. |
| *Vibrio parahaemolyticus* gastroenteritis | Enteric precautions | Feces | Duration of illness | |
| Vincent's angina (trench mouth) | None | | | |
| Viral diseases | | | | |
| Pericarditis, myocarditis, or meningitis | Enteric precautions | Feces and possibly respiratory secretions | For 7 days after onset | Enteroviruses frequently cause these infections. |
| Respiratory (if not covered elsewhere) | | | | |
| Adults | None | Respiratory secretions may be | | |
| Infants and young children | Contact isolation | Respiratory secretions | Duration of illness | Various etiologic agents, such as respiratory syncytial virus, parainfluenza viruses, adenoviruses, and influenza viruses, can cause viral respiratory infections (Committee on Infectious Diseases, American Academy |

## TABLE 64-1. (Continued)

| Disease | Category | Infective Material | Apply Precautions How Long? | Comments |
|---|---|---|---|---|
| | | | | of Pediatrics. 1991 Red Book); therefore, precautions to prevent their spread generally are indicated. |
| Whooping cough (pertussis) | Respiratory isolation | Respiratory secretions | For 7 days after start of effective therapy | See CDC Guideline for Infection Control in Hospital Personnel for recommendations for prophylaxis after exposure. |
| Wound infections | | | | |
| Major | Contact isolation | Pus | Duration of illness | Major—draining and not covered by dressing, or dressing does not adequately contain the pus. |
| Minor or limited | Drainage/secretion precautions | Pus | Duration of illness | Minor or limited—dressing covers and adequately contains the pus, or infected area is very small, such as a stitch abscess. |
| *Yersinia enterocolitica* gastroenteritis | Enteric precautions | Feces | Duration of illness | |
| Zoster (varicella-zoster) | | | | |
| Localized in immunocompromised patient, or disseminated | Strict isolation | Lesion secretions | Duration of illness | Localized lesions in immunocompromised patients frequently become disseminated. Because such dissemination is unpredictable, use the same isolation precautions as with disseminated disease. Persons who are not susceptible do not need to wear a mask. Persons susceptible to varicella-zoster (chickenpox) should, if possible, stay out of the room. Special ventilation for the room, if available, may be advantageous, especially for outbreak control. Exposed susceptible patients should be placed in strict isolation beginning 10 days after exposure and continuing until 21 days after last exposure. See CDC Guideline for Infection Control in Hospital Personnel for recommendations for exposed susceptible personnel. |
| Localized in normal patient | Drainage/secretion precautions | Lesion secretions | Until all lesions are crusted | Persons susceptible to varicella-zoster (chickenpox) should, if possible, stay out of room. Roommates should not be susceptible to chickenpox. |
| Zygomycosis (phycomycosis, mucormycosis) | None | | | |

\* The following multiply resistant organisms are included: (1) Gram-negative bacilli resistant to all aminoglycosides that are tested. (In general, such organisms should be resistant to gentamicin, tobramycin, and amikacin for these special precautions to be indicated). (2) *Staphylococcus aureus* resistant to methicillin (or nafcillin or oxacillin if they are used instead of methicillin for testing). (3) *Streptococcus pneumoniae* resistant to penicillin. (4) *Haemophilus influenzae* resistant to ampicillin (β-lactamase–positive) and chloramphenicol. (5) Other resistant bacteria may be included if they are judged by the infection control team to be of special clinical and epidemiologic significance.

† Colonization may involve more than one site.

educate and train hospital staff in the proper practice of a few limited types of isolation, and that these systems are easier to apply in cases of unknown infections. The disadvantages of category-specific systems are that they cost more than do disease-specific systems, and their use tends to result in excessive isolation compared to other systems.

A category-specific system developed by the CDC is shown in Figure 64-1. Seven categories and the isolation precautions for each are listed.

In general terms, strict isolation is designed to prevent the transmission of highly contagious infections spread through both air and contact. Contact, respiratory, and enteric isolation are used to prevent infections transmitted by those routes. Acid-fast bacillus (AFB) isolation is used for patients with contagious respiratory tuberculosis (children with primary pulmonary tuberculosis generally are not contagious and need not be isolated). Drainage/secretion precautions are designed to prevent spread by contact with purulent material or drainage from an infected body site. Because the history and physical examination do not identify reliably all patients with human immunodeficiency virus infection or infection by other blood-borne pathogens, it has been recommended that blood and body fluid precautions be used in the care of all patients (universal precautions). Consistent, meticulous hand washing is essential to prevent the transmission of nosocomial pathogens by any route. Table 64-1, also from the CDC, is a comprehensive list of infectious diseases and conditions, and applicable precautions for each.

## HAND WASHING

Hand washing is the best proven infection control technique. Nevertheless, physicians have been shown to exhibit only 19% to 26% compliance with well-accepted hand washing guidelines; nurses have slightly better compliance rates of 40% to 63%. Hand washing after potential contact with infected material is part of the recommendations for all the isolation categories listed in Table 64-1. The CDC currently recommends hand washing before and after every patient contact. Because these recommendations often are ignored in practice, a system of "washing wisely" (Table 64-2) may be of some benefit. The fact that hand washing compliance can rise above 90% during hand washing campaigns is encouraging; however, compliance usually drops abruptly when the campaign is over.

---

**TABLE 64-2. "Wash Wisely": Summary of Current Strongly Recommended Indications for Hand Washing**

1. Wash before:
   Performing invasive procedures
   Caring for especially susceptible patients
2. Wash before and also after:
   Touching wounds of any type
3. Wash after:
   Situations likely to cause microbial contamination (such as contact with blood or body fluids, secretions, or excretions)
   Touching sources likely to be contaminated with epidemiologically important microorganisms (including urine-measuring devices and secretion-collection apparatus)
   Caring for patients infected or colonized with certain epidemiologically important bacteria (eg, methicillin-resistant *Staphylococcus aureus* or gentamicin-resistant *Klebsiella pneumoniae*)
4. Wash between:
   Contact with different patients in high-risk nursing units

*Bryan C. Editorial. Infect Control 1986;7:446.*

---

## Selected Readings

American Academy of Pediatrics. Infection control for hospitalized children. In: Report of the Committee on Infectious Diseases, ed 21. Elk Grove Village, Ill: American Academy of Pediatrics, 1991:81.

American Hospital Association. Infection control in the hospital, ed 4. Chicago: American Hospital Association, 1979:19.

Cloney DL, Donowitz LG. Overgown use for infection control in nurseries and neonatal intensive care units. Am J Dis Child 1986;140:680.

Donowitz LG. Failure of the overgown to prevent nosocomial infection in a pediatric intensive care unit. Pediatrics 1986;77:35.

Ehrenkranz NJ, Sanders CC, Eckert-Schollenberger D, et al. Lack of evidence of efficacy of cohorting nursing personnel in a neonatal intensive care unit to prevent contact spread of bacteria: An experimental study. Pediatr Infect Dis J 1992;11:105.

Gardner P, Causey W, Beem M. Nosocomial infections. In: Feigin R, Cherry J, eds. Textbook of pediatric infectious diseases, ed 3. Philadelphia: WB Saunders, 1992.

Gardner P, Tipple M, Beem M. Control of infections in the pediatric hospital. In: Feigin R, Cherry J, eds. Textbook of pediatric infectious diseases, ed 3. Philadelphia: WB Saunders, 1992.

Garner J, Simmons B. CDC guidelines for isolation precautions in hospitals. Infect Control 1983;4:245.

Jarvis WR. Epidemiology of nosocomial infections in pediatric patients. Pediatr Infect Dis J 1987;6:344.

Kim M, Mindorff C, Patrick M, et al. Isolation usage in a pediatric hospital. Infect Control 1987;8:195.

*Principles and Practice of Pediatrics, Second Edition.*
edited by Frank A. Oski et al. J. B. Lippincott Company, Philadelphia © 1994.

# CHAPTER 65
# *Use of the Bacteriology Laboratory*

### Edward O. Mason, Jr

A pediatrician's effective use of the bacteriology laboratory is aided by a general understanding of the microbiologic principles involved in the performance of the tests. Good communication with laboratory personnel prevents misunderstanding and promotes good medical care. Pediatric patients may be a minority in many hospitals, and the pediatrician plays an important role in conveying new developments regarding pediatric infections that otherwise might go unnoticed by the microbiology staff.

The laboratory is responsible for the correct and timely implementation and interpretation of culture results. The pediatrician is responsible for seeing that the appropriate specimen for a suspected clinical infection is obtained and delivered quickly to the laboratory in sufficient quantity for optimal study. When possible, the specimen should be obtained before antimicrobial therapy is begun, and it should be accompanied by information indicating the suspected causative agent as well as any special instructions that may help the laboratory to proceed expeditiously. The pediatrician carries the final responsibility of relating the culture results to the clinical condition and treatment of the patient.

# RESPIRATORY CULTURES

## Throat and Nasopharyngeal Cultures

Cultures of material from the throat and nasopharynx are processed for the detection of group A streptococci unless the laboratory is notified differently. Many laboratories use rapid screening procedures to detect group A streptococcal antigen in throat swabs. Positive results obtained with these kits have been shown to correlate with the isolation of *Streptococcus pyogenes* from the nasopharynx. The reliability of a negative result (which depends on the quantity of streptococci present) has not been determined yet. If it is not routine laboratory policy, the physician may be advised to request a standard culture after a negative result is obtained from a screening test. This procedure is being implemented in office settings, with generally good results. Proper performance requires strict adherence to the manufacturer's instructions as well as adequate control procedures. In addition to positive and negative controls supplied with the material, randomly selected specimens should be cultured in parallel with the rapid method on a weekly basis. These tests should be used only to detect group A streptococci in throat specimens. The significance and reliability of results obtained from other sites have not been determined.

If infection with *Bordetella pertussis*, *Corynebacterium diphtheriae*, or *Neisseria gonorrhoeae* is suspected, verbal as well as written requests for these special cultures are necessary. Fluorescent antisera are available to identify both *B pertussis* and *C diphtheriae* directly from culture swabs; however, the results with these reagents should be interpreted with caution. There is a high incidence of false-positive reactions, and these tests should not be used as substitutes for standard culture methods.

## Ear Cultures

The most reliable method for the diagnosis of the causative agent of otitis media is the culture of middle ear fluid obtained directly by tympanocentesis. The next most reliable source of culture material is fluid obtained at myringotomy. Fluid obtained from the middle ear after myringotomy, however, may become contaminated inadvertently with flora from the external ear during collection. Gram stain of this material, followed by prompt processing, is crucial in the subsequent interpretation of culture results.

It is not appropriate to submit nasopharyngeal isolates for culture to determine the cause of middle ear infections. Cultures of nasopharyngeal isolates are poor predictors of the causative agent of otitis media, and the laboratory is not accustomed to processing such specimens for organisms other than group A streptococci.

# STOOL CULTURES

Historically, the microbiology laboratory processed stool specimens exclusively for the detection of *Salmonella* or *Shigella* species. Failure to isolate either of these two species and a subsequent report of "no enteric pathogens isolated" led the physician to search for metabolic causes of gastroenteritis. In the last 10 to 15 years, however, many different bacterial as well as new viral and parasitic causes of diarrhea have been described.

In many cases, the bacteriology laboratory is the primary processor of fecal specimens; therefore, the physician should provide as much clinical information and clinical guidance as possible so that the search for the enteric pathogen can be as complete as possible. Identification of *Salmonella* and *Shigella* as well as *Campylobacter fetus* subspecies *jejuni* should be standard practice in every laboratory.

Other bacterial causes of acute gastroenteritis include the following:

Enterotoxigenic *Escherichia coli*
Enteroinvasive *E coli*
Enteropathogenic *E coli*
Enterocytotoxic *E coli*
*Clostridium difficile*
*Aeromonas hydrophila*
*Bacillus cereus*
*Staphylococcus aureus*
*Vibrio cholerae*
*Vibrio parahaemolyticus*
*Yersinia enterocolitica*

Cost, time, and specialized procedures, some requiring experimental animals, preclude the routine isolation and identification of all causative agents. Thus, if the physician suspects any of the agents listed above to be the cause of gastroenteritis in an individual patient, this should be communicated to the laboratory so that appropriate isolation methods can be employed or the specimen or isolate can be forwarded to a reference laboratory. As an example, *E coli* isolated from appropriately flagged specimens can be retained and referred to a research facility for serotype determination or toxin identification.

# BLOOD CULTURES

Culture of blood can be performed by conventional broth, automated, or lysis filtration/centrifugation methods. The method or combination of methods used in a particular laboratory is a function of the size of the hospital, the type of hospital population, and cost considerations. Each of the different methods requires the dilution of blood to neutralize complement, phagocytes, and lysozyme. In children, the quantity of blood available for culture depends on the size of the child and often is limited to 1 mL in the neonate. This quantity can be diluted in any amount of culture broth as long as the ratio exceeds 1:5 to 1:10. The quantity of blood cultured does influence the ability to detect bacteremia. The level of bacteremia usually is higher in children than in adults, however. Thus, infection of the blood in children is detected reliably even when only small amounts of blood are available for culture. In addition, the timing of obtaining blood for culture in children is not as critical as it is in adults, because, with the exception of abscesses, intermittent bacteremia is uncommon. Because no single standardized blood culture system has been adopted, familiarity with the idiosyncrasies of the several systems in use may be helpful.

## Broth Culture Methods

Conventional blood culture methodology using vented and unvented (anaerobic) blood culture bottles remains a reliable means of detecting septicemia. The broth medium selected must support the growth of a variety of bacterial (and fungal) species. The bottles are inspected daily. Gram-stained smears and subculture of bottles with positive or suspicious results should be performed immediately and preliminary reports telephoned to the physician. All bottles should be subcultured and stained after 6 to 18 hours of incubation, and after 48 hours of incubation if growth has not been detected previously. The bottles generally are not retained longer than 7 days unless the physician indicates the possibility of a fungal or mycobacterial infection.

## Automated Detection

An alternative to conventional broth culture methods is the use of automated systems, which measure periodically metabolites of specific substrates contained in the broth medium. Detection of these metabolites that result from bacterial growth allows more rapid detection of positive culture results coupled with automated sampling. Aerobic and anaerobic media are available, although there is an increasing consensus that, especially in children, routine anaerobic culture of blood may be less preferable to aerobic culture using two different medium formulations or culture techniques. There also are data to support the use of modified systems designed especially for pediatric patients.

## Lysis-Centrifugation

Although the technology of lysis filtration/centrifugation dates back to 1910, this method only now is being developed for use in the clinical laboratory. Red blood cells are lysed by a detergent and the cellular sediment containing any bacteria is collected by centrifugation. The sediment, removed from the possible inhibitory effects of antibiotics, can be measured and plated to several different media. The method is rapid and reliable for detecting anaerobes and is particularly useful in detecting mycobacterial bacteremia in immunocompromised patients.

## Antimicrobial Removal

Synthetic resins in the antibiotic removal device adsorb antibiotics from blood before culture. In theory, this method should lessen the chance that bacterial growth will be suppressed by antibiotics, which often must be given before specimens can be obtained for culture. The system requires several manipulations of the specimen, however, which can introduce contaminating microorganisms. Studies comparing paired samples of blood cultured conventionally and after antibiotic removal have not shown a significant difference between the two systems with all patient populations.

## CEREBROSPINAL FLUID CULTURES

Cerebrospinal fluid (CSF) submitted for any purpose always should be cultured for bacteria, regardless of the clarity of the fluid or the results of the Gram stain or cell count. The specimen should be plated to blood and chocolate agar, and to a broth medium. The preparation of two smears of a centrifuged pellet is advisable. One smear is stained immediately for bacteria, and the other is reserved for staining of mycobacteria if indicated. Any bacteria found in CSF cultures should be identified and reported. CSF (along with serum and urine) also may be submitted for one of the rapid antigen detection methods that are discussed in Chapter 66.

## URINE CULTURES

The proper collection of urine from children is difficult and must be performed with utmost care to ensure meaningful bacteriologic results. Urine collected by any method must be transported to the laboratory and processed within 30 minutes. Refrigeration for as long as 2 hours is permitted if immediate transport is not possible. Quantitative culture results of $10^5$ colony-forming units (CFU)/mL or greater are indicative of infection. Any quantity of bacteria recovered in a bladder aspirate is significant.

Screening devices to exclude bacteriuria rapidly are useful in clinic and office settings. These screening devices are either culture kits or chemical detection devices. Culture kits consist of dipsticks, paddles, or tubes containing a differential agar medium that is inoculated immediately on obtaining the urine sample. The results are semiquantitative and, depending on the individual test, may

indicate the bacterial identity by differential growth or color changes in the agar medium. The specimen can be processed immediately, avoiding refrigeration, and can be transported to a laboratory for identification and susceptibility studies without time and refrigeration constraints. Consistently indeterminate results or a negative test result in the face of persistent symptoms should be investigated by routine quantitative culture procedures.

Chemical screening methods consist of filter paper strips designed to detect either bacterial nitrate, glucose oxidase, or catalase, or leukocyte esterase. Because the first three tests detect products or enzymes of the infecting bacteria, they require a specimen that has been in the bladder at least 4 hours (or overnight). Leukocyte esterase is an enzyme produced by the polymorphonuclear leukocytes that usually are present in response to infection. The leukocyte esterase test is the most reliable of the chemical tests, but it can generate a positive result in the absence of infection. Similarly, it can generate a negative result if no white blood cells are present in the urine, as may occur in patients with asymptomatic bacteriuria.

## ANAEROBIC CULTURES

Proper collection and transportation of specimens for the attempted isolation of anaerobic bacteria is crucial to the successful diagnosis of anaerobic infection. Although some "anaerobic" species can survive prolonged exposure to oxygen, others are killed rapidly by even brief exposure to oxygen. The laboratory should supply adequate sample transportation devices (containers in which all the oxygen has been replaced with nitrogen) to ensure optimal conditions for the recovery of anaerobic organisms. Because many of the procedures that are necessary to obtain material for anaerobic culture are invasive, the laboratory should be advised before the collection procedure to minimize the time between collection and culture. Avoiding normal transportation mechanisms also is advisable, and such samples should be entrusted only to personnel who are aware of their importance. Anaerobic cultures are performed only by request. Because of the difficulty and expense of such cultures, they should be requested only when collection has been optimal and the results will have clinical significance.

## STAINS FOR MICROSCOPIC EXAMINATION

### Gram Stain

Examination of the Gram-stained smear is the most reliable and expedient method of establishing a preliminary diagnosis of bacterial infection. Performed properly, the stain demonstrates the morphology and probable identity of many of the pathogenic bacteria. In addition, the reliability of the specimen can be assessed when that specimen is taken from a nonsterile site (eg, sputum). The results can alert the physician to the presence of polymicrobial infection in specimens from normally sterile sites. Observation of bacteria in stains of specimens from patients who have been given antimicrobial therapy before material is obtained for culture may be the only indication of the infecting bacteria.

Interpretation of the Gram stain by an experienced observer is crucial and should be a joint effort between the physician and the microbiologist. Several clues are helpful in the evaluation of these smears:

1. In sputum and tracheal aspirates, the presence of many polymorphonuclear leukocytes indicates adequacy of the specimen and confirms the source as the lower respiratory tract. The presence of epithelial cells in sputum indicates buccal or salivary contamination, and also indicates that the culture results may be misleading in distinguishing the true pathogen.

2. The staining properties of polymorphonuclear leukocytes can serve as a control of the adequacy of the Gram stain. Leukocytes stain gram-negative; the presence of blue-staining cells indicates inadequate decoloration and should alert the observer to subsequent errors in interpreting the staining reaction of any bacteria.
3. One bacterium per oil immersion field (magnified 1000×) seen on the stained smear of *uncentrifuged* urine corresponds to a colony count of $10^5$ CFU/mL. The staining reaction and morphology also may be a quick guide to the best initial antimicrobial therapy.
4. The predominant location and morphology of bacteria inside the polymorphonuclear leukocyte may be a clue that the bacteria belong to the genus *Neisseria* (gram-negative diplococci) or *Listeria* (gram-positive bacilli).

## Fluorescent Antibody Stains

The use of fluorescein-tagged antibodies directed at specific bacterial antigens can identify specific pathogens rapidly in clinical specimens or confirm the identity of bacteria from cultures. The technique requires a microscope with an ultraviolet light source and conjugated antisera, which may be expensive. The reliability of the results from such examinations is directly dependent on the quality and specificity of the conjugate. Least reliable are tests performed directly on clinical specimens such as throat swabs looking for *C diphtheriae*, *B pertussis*, and *S pyogenes*. The identification of these and other bacterial isolates by this technique is more reliable.

## Wet Mount Preparations

Wet mount preparations for the diagnosis of bacterial infection are performed most often on uncentrifuged urine. The presence of more than 20 bacteria per high-power microscopic field (magnified 400×) corresponds to a colony count of $10^5$ CFU/mL and is a reliable indication of bacterial infection of the urinary tract. The same preparation also can be used to determine the presence of red and white blood cell casts, if they are numerous, but the absence of casts should be confirmed by similar examination of a centrifuged specimen.

## Acridine Orange Stain

The use of the acridine orange stain is helpful because of the extreme sensitivity of this method in detecting bacteria in small quantities and in specimens containing artifacts that can be confused with bacteria using other staining methods. The stain requires ultraviolet microscopy, but is nonspecific and does not require specific conjugated antibody preparations. Bacteria stand out as brightly glowing yellow or red cocci or bacilli, but the stain does not allow determination of the Gram stain reaction.

## AIDS TO THE DETERMINATION OF ANTIBIOTIC THERAPY

### Antibiotic Susceptibility

Antibiotic susceptibility should be determined if the bacterial isolate is obtained from a patient with a serious infectious disease. If the susceptibility of the pathogen is unpredictable, or if the infection has failed to respond to seemingly appropriate antibiotic treatment, then antibiotic susceptibility testing of the isolate is mandatory. In many cases, the antibiotic therapy is selected empirically based on clinical suspicion, Gram-stained smear, and knowledge of antibiotic resistance patterns in an institution. The

manner in which the antibiotic susceptibility is confirmed depends on many factors.

### Qualitative Methods

The disk diffusion susceptibility procedure described by Bauer and Kirby is a standardized, reliable method of assessing the susceptibility of rapidly growing bacteria to a number of antibiotics. Pure cultures of the bacteria are placed on an agar surface, and filter paper disks containing a known and precisely defined amount of antibiotic are applied. Antibiotic diffuses into the agar, and the bacteria grow to an area surrounding the disk to form a "zone of inhibition" correlated to the minimal inhibitory concentration (MIC) of that particular strain. The inhibitory zone is inversely proportional to the MIC. Knowledge of the pharmacokinetics of a particular antibiotic then can be used to define zones corresponding to "susceptible," "intermediately susceptible," and "resistant." In practice, the zone sizes are measured and reported as S (susceptible), I (intermediately susceptible), or R (resistant) in the laboratory report. These assessments of susceptibility are based on the level of antibiotic that can be achieved in the serum. Because antibiotic levels that can be achieved in the meninges, bone, abscesses, and so forth are less than those that can be achieved in serum, caution should be exercised in the use of disk susceptibility data to predict the efficacy of an antibiotic at other body sites.

A 1-$\mu$g oxacillin disk can be used to discern strains of *Streptococcus pneumoniae* that are resistant to penicillin. These strains are not detected readily with penicillin disks, and their presence is confirmed by quantitative methods that reveal the MIC to be greater than 0.1 $\mu$g/mL.

### β-Lactamase Testing

Testing for the presence of penicillin-destroying enzyme (β-lactamase) is useful for rapid determination of resistance to the β-lactam antibiotics. The basis of the test is a colorimetric change in the substrate or indicator on cleavage of the β-lactam ring. With any such test, proper controls consisting of known β-lactamase positive and negative strains should be tested simultaneously. Bacterial species in which this testing is useful include *Haemophilus influenzae*, *N gonorrhoeae*, *S aureus*, and certain anaerobes.

### Quantitative Methods

Bacterial susceptibility can be measured quantitatively by adding a standard inoculum of the bacterial strain to serial twofold dilutions of antibiotic in test tubes. Inhibition is determined by the absence of growth in the broth, and this amount of antibiotic is defined as the MIC. The minimal bactericidal concentration (MBC) is determined by subculture of tubes where inhibition occurred, and is defined as the lowest concentration of antibiotic that was bactericidal for the strain. Knowledge of the antibiotic concentration that can be achieved at different sites of infection and of the MIC and MBC then can be used to guide the choice of antibiotic.

### Automated Methods

Automated antibiotic susceptibility testing is becoming standard practice in large laboratories. The technical specifications and performance of the many systems available are described in detail in reference texts. The two basic methods used are a turbidimetric assay of the bacteria growing in the presence of a carefully selected concentration of antibiotic, compared to bacteria growing without antibiotic; and pre-diluted antibiotics in microtiter trays that are inoculated and read by automation.

Results obtained with these systems have been found to be reproducible and reliable indications of the susceptibility of bacteria encountered in the clinical laboratory. The disadvantage of these systems becomes evident when fastidious strains are tested or the antibiotics requested for testing are not included in standard panels. These disadvantages are compounded when the laboratory has no alternative procedure that can be implemented rapidly and reliably. Examples of the most common problems encountered with automated systems include bacterial strains that require altered growth times, nutritionally fastidious strains, strains with heteroresistant populations, failure to detect the MBC, and failure to detect tolerance. Other difficulties arise when the antibiotics to be tested are selected by the manufacturer and cannot be altered easily, or the susceptibility ranges are predetermined and are not adequate for all bacterial species.

## Antibiotic Combinations

Assessment of the in vitro effect of antibiotic combinations requires specialized testing procedures and best is reserved for reference laboratories. Two or more antibiotics are mixed in multiple concentrations in checkerboard fashion, and the antibiotics alone and in combination are measured for their inhibitory and bactericidal activity. This generates an isobologram, or a fractional inhibitory concentration (FIC) index. Interpretation of the FIC is subject to some disagreement, but synergy generally is represented by an FIC of 0.8 or less and antagonism is represented by an FIC of 1.2 or greater. The antibiotic combination is said to be additive when the calculated FIC falls between 0.8 and 1.2.

## Antibiotic Levels

Measurement of antibiotic levels in serum is indicated routinely when potentially toxic agents such as the aminoglycosides, vancomycin, or chloramphenicol are used in therapy. Knowledge of antibiotic levels also is useful when the patient's altered metabolism (hepatic or renal failure) or disease condition (shock, cystic fibrosis, dialysis) requires modification of standard dosing practices. The procedure can be used to monitor the effects of inadvertent overdoses as well as antibiotic absorption from the gastrointestinal tract and compliance with therapy.

Modern testing methods based on radioimmunoassay, enzyme-multiplied immunoassay, and high-pressure liquid chromatography are highly specific and are not affected by the presence of other drugs or antibiotics. The physician must be cognizant of any reported drug interference, however, and of the procedure used in a particular laboratory.

Regardless of the procedure used to measure the antibiotic level, specimens must be collected and transported correctly if they are to yield accurate information. The timing of the collection is of utmost importance. Trough levels (the lowest level) are determined on specimens collected just before the antibiotic is administered. The time of specimen collection for peak level determination depends on the antibiotic and the route of administration. In general, peak levels of antibiotics administered intravenously are determined on samples collected immediately after completion of the infusion. An exception is chloramphenicol, which must be converted from the inactive succinate to free chloramphenicol by hepatic enzymes; peak levels of this agent, therefore, are reached 1 hour after completion of the infusion. Peak levels for intramuscular antibiotics are reached 1 hour after injection. Peak serum levels for oral antibiotics are determined on samples collected 1.5 to 2 hours after ingestion and can be affected by the timing and content of meals. In any case, deterioration of the antibiotic must be prevented by prompt refrigeration of the blood and delivery to the laboratory. If serum must be held overnight, it should be removed from the clot and frozen.

## Serum Bactericidal Levels

Assessment of the bactericidal level in serum often is useful in evaluating the therapeutic effectiveness of an antibiotic that may be modified by delayed absorption or accelerated excretion. Determination of the serum bactericidal level differs from determination of serum antibiotic concentrations in that it measures the serum dilution that is necessary to inhibit and kill the bacteria that are infecting the patient. Peak and trough levels are obtained at times similar to those described for antibiotic levels. Results are reported as a dilution ratio. A ratio of 1:2 reflects minimal inhibition or killing. Higher ratios, such as 1:64, indicate that the serum may be diluted 64 times and still retain the inhibitory or bactericidal effect. Knowledge of the bactericidal activity is particularly useful in the therapeutic management of endocarditis or osteomyelitis, and in the tailoring of oral antibiotic therapy.

## Selected Readings

Ballows A, Hausler WJ Jr, Hermann KL, Isenberg HD, Shadomy HJ, eds. Manual of clinical microbiology, ed 5. Washington, DC: American Society for Microbiology, 1991.
Lorian V, ed. Significance of medical microbiology in the care of patients, ed 2. Baltimore: Williams & Wilkins, 1982.
Morello JA, Matushek SM, Dunne WM, Hinds DB. Performance of a Bactec non Radiometric medium for pediatric blood cultures. J Clin Microbiol 1991;29:359.
Murray PR, Traynor P, Hopson D. Critical assessment of blood culture techniques: Analysis of recovery of obligate and facultative anaerobes, strict aerobic bacteria, and fungi in aerobic and anaerobic blood culture bottles. J Clin Microbiol 1992;30:1462.
Radetsky M, Solomon JA, Todd JK. Identification of streptococcal pharyngitis in the office laboratory: Reassessment of new technology. Pediatr Infect Dis J 1987;6:556.
Sherris JC, ed. Medical microbiology: An introduction to infectious diseases, ed 2. New York: Elsevier, 1990.
Washington JA III, Ilstrup DM. Blood cultures: Issues and controversies. Rev Infect Dis 1986;8:792.

*Principles and Practice of Pediatrics, Second Edition.*
edited by Frank A. Oski et al. J. B. Lippincott Company, Philadelphia © 1994.

# CHAPTER 66
# *Rapid Diagnostic Techniques in Microbiology*

## Sheldon L. Kaplan

The physician caring for a febrile child with a presumed serious infection frequently must administer antimicrobial agents on an empiric basis until laboratory confirmation of a pathogen is available. Isolation and identification of microorganisms from clinical samples remains the most reliable and accurate means of establishing a causative diagnosis of virtually all infections a child is likely to suffer. Rapid diagnostic techniques for both laboratory and office use are becoming more widely available, however, and are changing the manner in which some infectious diseases initially are approached. For the most part, these techniques have been evaluated carefully for sensitivity (the percentage of positive test results among patients who have the infection), specificity (the percentage of negative test results among patients who do not have the infection), positive predictive value (the percentage of patients who have the infection among all patients with a positive test result), and negative predictive value (the percentage of patients who do not have the infection among all patients with a negative test result). If an infection is relatively common in a given population tested, such as group A streptococcal pharyngitis in school-age children, then the positive predictive value of a test is strengthened. If the infection is not common in the group being tested, such as *Chlamydia* vaginitis in girls less than 5 years of age, the negative predictive value is strengthened.

Several different techniques have been developed to detect microbial antigens rapidly (Table 66-1). All rely basically on an antibody recognizing a specific antigen. For all these tests, false-positive and false-negative results do occur. False-positive results are found most often in urine samples with countercurrent immunoelectrophoresis (CIE) or latex particle agglutination (LA) methods. Cerebrospinal fluid (CSF) appears to be the most reliable source for detecting the polysaccharide antigens of *Haemophilus influenzae*, type b, *Streptococcus pneumoniae*, *Neisseria meningitidis*, and *Cryptococcus neoformans*. These tests are most helpful when the results are positive. A negative result does not exclude a particular pathogen entirely, because a negative result can mean that a pathogen is not present, or that antigen is present, but in concentrations below the detectable limits of the test.

## BACTERIA

Rapid techniques to detect bacterial antigens have been studied extensively for children with bacterial meningitis. The capsular polysaccharides of *H influenzae* type b, *S pneumoniae*, and *N meningitidis* serogroups A, C, and D are detected readily in the CSF of children with bacterial meningitis caused by these pathogens. In general, antigen from *H influenzae* type b is found in 85% to 95% of all children with bacterial meningitis when CIE or LA techniques are used. The value of the LA technique for detecting polysaccharide from *N meningitidis* serogroup B, the most common meningococcal serotype causing meningitis, is not well established. Currently, group B *Streptococcus* and *Escherichia coli* K1 are the only neonatal pathogens included in the routine rapid tests.

In most clinical circumstances, the results of these rapid tests do not alter the antimicrobial treatment of children with suspected bacterial meningitis. That is, despite a positive test result for a specific agent in children more than 3 months of age, empiric antimicrobial therapy with cefotaxime or ceftriaxone should be continued until the isolate is identified and the antibiotic susceptibility pattern is determined. These tests are most helpful when the CSF or blood cultures might be rendered sterile by prior oral antibiotic therapy and LA or CIE is the only way to establish a causative diagnosis. Rapidly determining the causative agent also may help determine the need for isolation procedures or pro-

**TABLE 66-1.    Selected Rapid Microbiologic Tests Useful in Pediatrics**

| Test | Antigen Detected | Comments |
|---|---|---|
| Countercurrent immunoelectrophoresis (CIE) | *Haemophilus influenzae* type b | False-positive reaction most common in urine; cross-reactions occur |
| | *Streptococcus pneumoniae* | |
| | *Neisseria meningitidis*, serogroups A, C, D, Y, W135 | |
| | Group B *Streptococcus* | |
| | *Entamoeba histolytica* | |
| Latex agglutination (LA) | Same as CIE, plus *N meningitidis*, serogroup B | Same as above; more sensitive than CIE for *H influenzae* type b |
| | Group A *Streptococcus* | |
| | *Cryptococcus neoformans* | |
| Enzyme immunoassay (EIA) | Rotavirus | Not practical to run single samples for some; test requires additional time compared to CIE or LA |
| | Respiratory syncytial virus | |
| | Influenza A | |
| | *Neisseria gonorrhoeae* | |
| | *Chlamydia trachomatis* | |
| | Group A *Streptococcus* | |
| Electron microscopy | Rotavirus | Adjunct to standard tests not generally available |
| | Herpesvirus | |
| | Adenovirus | |
| Immunofluorescent assay (IFA) Immunoperoxidase | Respiratory syncytial virus | Requires experienced microscopist |
| | *Bordetella pertussis* | |
| | *C trachomatis* | |
| | *Legionella pneumophila* | |
| | *Pneumocystis carinii* | |
| DNA hybridization | Cytomegalovirus | |
| | Herpes simplex virus | |
| | Epstein-Barr virus | |
| Polymerase chain reaction | Cytomegalovirus | Research applications |
| | Herpes simplex virus | |
| | Parvovirus B19 | |
| | Human immunodeficiency virus | |
| | *Mycobacterium tuberculosis* | |
| | *Toxoplasma gondii* | |

phylactic antibiotics for close contacts of the patient. In experienced hands, the results of Gram stain of CSF are positive in the majority of children with bacterial meningitis. Occasionally, organisms may be seen in CSF by use of an acridine orange stain (a fluorochrome that stains bacterial nucleic acid and requires a fluorescent microscope) when a Gram stain result is negative.

Bacterial capsular polysaccharides are not detected as readily in the serum or urine of patients with infections at sites other than the central nervous system as they are in children with bacterial meningitis. The incidence of positive bacterial culture results from blood or other sources, however, also is less frequent in patients with infections at other sites. Therefore, detecting polysaccharide antigen in the serum, urine, or pleural fluid of a child with pneumonia can be very helpful. Similarly, antigen may be detected in the synovial fluid of children with septic arthritis. Detectable antigenemia or antigenuria is not common in children with bacteremia without a focus of infection. Clinicians need to know that the administration of *H influenzae* type b conjugate vaccines may lead to the excretion of antigen that is detectable in the urine by LA for as long as 1 month.

Group B streptococcal antigenuria in neonates may be the result of true systemic infection or local colonization, or of contamination of urine specimens by group B *Streptococcus* or other cross-reacting streptococci. The interpretation of a positive urine latex agglutination test result for group B *Streptococcus* in a neonate with negative blood or CSF culture results is particularly troublesome and requires that the entire clinical situation be considered. Urine LA for *N meningitidis* serogroup B leads to a very high frequency of false-positive results and should not be performed routinely.

Group A streptococcal pharyngitis is one of the most common infections requiring diagnosis and treatment by the pediatrician. Several kits are available commercially to detect rapidly the presence of group A streptococci in the pharynx of a child with pharyngitis. A positive test result reliably indicates the presence of group A streptococci in the throat. A negative test result, however, does not exclude group A streptococcal pharyngitis. The optimal manner in which to employ this test in an office or outpatient setting is uncertain. One reasonable approach is to treat symptomatic children if the result of the rapid test is positive. If the result of the rapid screen is negative, a throat culture should be done so that the 15% to 40% of these tests that generate false-negative results are detected.

Gram stain of urethral discharge is a time-honored, sensitive, and specific test for *Neisseria gonorrhoeae* infection in males, but not in females. Enzyme immunoassays (EIAs) are available to detect gonococcal antigen in urogenital specimens. Like the Gram stain, the EIA is an excellent technique for males, but is not adequate for females, particularly in populations with a low prevalence of gonorrhea. In adolescents, an EIA for *N gonorrhoeae* infection offers no particular advantage over the Gram stain for males with a urethral discharge. In female adolescents, the prevalence of *N gonorrhoeae* in the population being seen will determine the usefulness of the test. Cervical culture continues to be the most reliable method of diagnosing urogenital infections caused by *N gonorrhoeae*.

## VIRAL INFECTIONS

Commercial reagents for EIAs to detect rotavirus in stool or respiratory syncytial virus (RSV) in respiratory secretions are widely available. Rotavirus antigen is more likely to be detected early in the course of a diarrheal illness. If the initial test result is negative, repeating the test on a second sample will increase the yield of positive results by about 25%. Detecting rotavirus antigen in stool by EIA is not enhanced by testing more than two samples.

A positive test result for rotavirus may eliminate the need for additional diagnostic tests or unnecessary antibiotic administration for a child with diarrhea. Rotazyme, one commercial EIA that is available to detect rotavirus in stools, generated false-positive results when it was tested in asymptomatic neonates and, thus, should not be relied on for screening this population. Positive results in symptomatic neonates appear to be reliable. Electron microscopy can reveal rotavirus particles in stool samples, but is not as sensitive as is EIA. LA procedures for rotavirus are faster to perform, but are not as sensitive as is EIA.

The availability of effective antiviral therapy (ribavirin) for RSV makes the rapid identification of these infections particularly important. Nasopharyngeal aspirates are the most reliable source from which to identify RSV antigen. In comparative studies, the EIA technique usually is more sensitive than is standard isolation by tissue culture for determining RSV infections. Immunofluorescence staining of exfoliated respiratory cells is comparable to EIA for identifying RSV, but requires a highly trained microscopist for valid results.

Monoclonal antibodies to identify herpes simplex directly in clinical specimens by immunofluorescence are available commercially in kit form. These reagents also have been employed for the rapid identification of herpes simplex in viral tissue cultures (ie, shell vial assay). The specificity of these tests is acceptable; however, tissue culture remains the most sensitive, widely available technique with which to document herpes simplex infections. Therefore, the rapid techniques are considered to be only complementary to tissue culture. DNA probes specific for herpes simplex offer great promise for diagnostic testing. Electron microscopy can demonstrate viral particles typical of herpesviruses, but cannot distinguish herpes simplex from other herpesviruses. Perhaps these procedures will be of greatest aid to pediatricians in identifying, just before delivery, pregnant women who are infected with herpes simplex virus. The Tzanck smear of scrapings from the base of a vesicle may demonstrate multinucleated giant cells that are suggestive of infection with herpes simplex or varicella.

Techniques employing DNA probes are valuable for determining rapidly the presence of viruses such as cytomegalovirus and adenovirus in clinical specimens, particularly tissue sections. These techniques are especially important for immunocompromised patients, in whom potentially lethal infections with these viruses may develop. As additional antiviral agents are developed, the rapid identification of viral pathogens will become even more critical for optimal patient care.

Polymerase chain reaction is a highly sensitive technique with which to amplify and detect small quantities of target DNA. This technology is being applied to an ever-increasing number of microorganisms and may be routinely available and reliable for widespread use in the future. The most promising and needed applications for polymerase chain reaction include rapid detection of viral, mycobacterial, and parasitic infection.

## FUNGAL INFECTIONS

Currently, *C neoformans* is the only fungus for which a reliable rapid diagnostic technique is commercially available. The LA test result for *Cryptococcus* polysaccharide in the CSF is positive in more than 90% of patients with meningitis caused by this organism. False-positive results can occur, but these can be minimized by a number of procedures. Measured CSF titers of antigen to *Cryptococcus* provide some prognostic information. The proper interpretation of India ink preparations of CSF requires experience, because lymphocytes can be mistaken for *Cryptococcus* organisms. Both the LA and India ink test results may remain positive after CSF culture results are negative.

A sensitive and specific test for quickly detecting infections with *Candida* species has not been developed. A commercial LA test for *Candida* antigen in sera has been evaluated, but results are conflicting. No studies of *Candida* antigen testing in sera have been performed in children. At present, the clinical significance of a positive *Candida* antigen test result in the sera of children, and especially of neonates, is unknown.

## MISCELLANEOUS PATHOGENS

*Chlamydia trachomatis* is an important cause of conjunctivitis and pneumonitis in infants. The Giemsa stain of conjunctival scrapings may indicate intracytoplasmic inclusions characteristic of *C trachomatis*; however, the technique is not very sensitive. A fluorescein-conjugated monoclonal antibody is both sensitive and specific for detecting *C trachomatis* in conjunctival scrapings of infants with conjunctivitis or in nasopharyngeal secretions of infants with pneumonitis. This commercial test is especially valuable when tissue culture methods are not available. EIAs also can identify *C trachomatis* rapidly in conjunctival and nasopharyngeal specimens collected from infants. The immunofluorescent assay (IFA) and EIA are inferior to tissue cultures for detecting endocervical infections with *C trachomatis* in adolescent girls and should not be used in the evaluation of a child with suspected sexual abuse.

*Legionella* species do not appear to be a common pathogen in normal children with pneumonia. In immunosuppressed children, however, *Legionella* may cause a fatal illness if it is not recognized and treated promptly. Legionellae can be visualized in sputum, tracheal aspirates, and lung tissue by the IFA method. The sensitivity of this test in adults varies between 25% and 80%, but is unknown in children.

As with all immunofluorescent techniques, IFA for *Bordetella pertussis* requires an experienced microscopist. Monoclonal antibodies to *Pneumocystis carinii* enhance the detection of cysts in induced sputum or fluid obtained by bronchoalveolar lavage.

## Selected Readings

Balows A, ed. Manual of clinical microbiology, 5th ed. Washington, DC: American Society for Microbiology, 1991.

Bell TA, Kuo CC, Stamm WE, et al. Direct fluorescent monoclonal antibody stain for rapid detection of infant *Chlamydia trachomatis* infections. Pediatrics 1984;74: 224.

Demetriou E, Sackett R, Welch DF, et al. Evaluation of an enzyme immunoassay for detection of *Neisseria gonorrhoeae* in an adolescent population. JAMA 1984;252:247.

Eisenstein BI. New molecular techniques for microbial epidemiology and the diagnosis of infectious disease. J Infect Dis 1990;161:592.

Gerber MA. Comparison of throat cultures and rapid strep tests for diagnosis of streptococcal pharyngitis. Pediatr Infect Dis J 1989;8:820.

Jones JM. Laboratory diagnosis of invasive candidiasis. Clin Microbiol Rev 1990;3: 32.

Lauer BA, Masters HA, Wren CG, et al. Rapid detection of respiratory syncytial virus in nasopharyngeal secretions by enzyme-linked immunosorbent assay. J Clin Microbiol 1985;22:782.

Radetsky M, Todd JK. Criteria for the evaluation of new diagnostic tests. Pediatr Infect Dis 1984;3:461.

Roblin PM, Hammerschlag MR, Cummings C, et al. Comparison of two rapid microscopic methods and culture for detection of *Chlamydia trachomatis* in ocular and nasopharyngeal specimens from infants. J Clin Microbiol 1989;27:968.

Sanchez PJ, Siegel JD, Cushion NB, et al: Significance of a positive urine group B streptococcal latex agglutination test in neonates. J Pediatr 1990;116:601.

Yolken RH, Leister FJ. Evaluation of enzyme immunoassays for the detection of human rotavirus. J Infect Dis 1981;144:379.

# SECTION
## III
# The Respiratory System

*Principles and Practice of Pediatrics, Second Edition.*
edited by Frank A. Oski et al. J. B. Lippincott Company, Philadelphia © 1994.

## CHAPTER 67
# Lower Respiratory Tract Infections

## 67.1 Acute and Chronic Bronchitis

I. Celine Hanson and William T. Shearer

The term *bronchitis* describes inflammation of the large airways, namely, the trachea and bronchi. Bronchitis can occur throughout the year, but is more likely to be seen in the winter months and in association with viral and bacterial infections. Recurrent episodes of cough that persist almost daily for a minimum of 3 months in 1 year may be noted. Chronic bronchitis is ill-defined in the pediatric literature; commonly, the term is used synonymously with asthmatic bronchitis. Lack of a uniform or standardized definition of chronic bronchitis has led to wide discrepancies in the reported frequency of this disorder. The causative agents associated with chronic bronchitis are similar, but not identical, to those responsible for acute or asthmatic bronchitis. The pathology of acute and chronic bronchitis and results of findings at the time of bronchoscopy are similar to those noted in pediatric asthma, reflecting the inclusion of asthma in the spectrum of the bronchitis complex.

## ACUTE BRONCHITIS

Acute bronchitis is encountered commonly in children. In 1989, the National Health Interview Survey estimated that 1.8 million episodes of acute bronchitis occurred in American preschool children alone. Most clinicians describe acute bronchitis as a febrile illness with cough, rhonchi, and referred breath sounds. Causative agents are many, predominantly adenovirus, influenza viruses, and respiratory syncytial virus. Influenza viruses A and

B have been implicated in epidemics of bronchitis; influenza A is associated with a severe respiratory illness in very young children. Bacterial infections identified include *Bordetella pertussis* and *Haemophilus influenzae* (Table 67-1). Additionally, *Mycoplasma pneumoniae* is a common cause of acute bronchitis in children, especially after 6 years of age.

### Clinical Presentation

By definition, fever and cough are associated with acute bronchitis, almost invariably in connection with upper respiratory congestion (predominantly nasal). The patient's temperature can range from 37 °C to 39 °C (100 °F to 103 °F). Cough usually is dry and harsh without sputum production in young infants. Coughing can be accompanied by gagging and vomiting, leading to poor oral intake and dehydration. Older children with persistent cough occasionally will produce sputum and may complain of chest wall pain. The clinical illness usually is preceded by 24 to 48 hours of lassitude or malaise. Subsequently, fever and cough develop; these findings may persist for as long as 1 week. A relatively slow recovery phase, spanning 1 to 2 weeks, with persistent cough is characteristic. Secondary bacterial infection can complicate the recovery period, causing exacerbation of fever and other clinical findings.

On physical examination, lung auscultation reveals rhonchi and referred upper airway breath sounds. Rhinitis usually is present and may be mucopurulent. Chest radiographs typically are normal unless secondary bacterial infection has occurred. Laboratory data are of limited value, usually suggesting a viral process (ie, the white blood cell count is elevated mildly and only a third of all cases are associated with an increased neutrophil count).

### Differential Diagnosis

Because acute bronchitis rarely is associated with death, little information is available regarding its pathophysiology. The differential diagnosis is somewhat limited, but acute bronchitis should be distinguished from chronic bronchitis, infectious asthma, and asthmatic bronchitis and sinusitis. More serious illnesses associated with recurrent acute upper respiratory tract infections (eg, immunodeficiency states, immotile cilia syndrome, and cystic fibrosis) should be distinguished from acute bronchitis. Acute bronchitis is a self-limited illness, and one bout of clinical disease does not warrant additional investigation.

An epidemiologic history often is helpful in identifying a possible causative agent; pandemics of respiratory viral illnesses occur characteristically during the winter months, and spread of respiratory viruses occurs easily in day-care settings. The age distribution of patients with the illness also can be helpful in sug-

## TABLE 67-1. Infectious Agents Associated With Acute Bronchitis

| Agent | Importance in Causation* |
|---|---|
| **Viruses** | +++ |
| *Adenoviruses types 1–7, 12* | |
| *Enteroviruses* | + |
| Coxsackieviruses B | + |
| Echoviruses 8, 12, 14 | + |
| Polioviruses | + |
| *Herpes simplex* | + |
| *Influenza* | +++ |
| A | ++ |
| B | ++ |
| C | + |
| *Measles* | + |
| *Mumps* | + |
| *Parainfluenza* | +++ |
| 1 | ++ |
| 2 | ++ |
| 3 | +++ |
| 4 | + |
| *Respiratory syncytial* | +++ |
| *Rhinoviruses* | ++ |
| **Bacteria** | |
| *Bordetella pertussis* | + |
| *Bordetella parapertussis* | ± |
| *Haemophilus influenzae* | + |
| *Streptococcus pneumoniae* | ± |
| *Streptococcus pyogenes* | ± |
| **Other** | |
| *Chlamydia psittaci* | + |
| *Mycoplasma pneumoniae* | +++ |

\* +++, very common; ++, common; +, rare; ±, of questionable etiologic significance.

*Modified from Cherry JD. Lower respiratory tract infections: Acute bronchitis. In: Feigin RD, Cherry JD, eds. Textbook of pediatric infectious diseases, ed 2. Philadelphia: WB Saunders, 1987:272.*

gesting the causative agent, as *M pneumoniae* is more common in school-age children. A specific cause can be identified by nasopharyngeal isolation of viruses, bacteria, or *Mycoplasma*.

## Treatment and Complications

Acute bronchitis usually is a benign illness unless secondary infection occurs. Appropriate preventive therapy includes adherence to recommended immunization schedules for children. Accordingly, therapy is palliative (ie, analgesic therapy for febrile episodes, and antitussive, decongestant, and antihistamine agents for cough and rhinitis). The latter approach has not been documented to be helpful in acute bronchitis; in fact, cough-suppressant therapy with codeine or dextromethorphan should be used with great care in these children. When specific respiratory viruses are isolated from nasopharyngeal secretions and the infection is severe enough to warrant hospitalization, then therapy with antiviral agents such as aerosolized ribavirin or amantadine can be considered.

Persistent coughing with gagging and vomiting can precipitate dehydration and serum metabolic changes. Monitoring of these parameters in the severely affected host and reconstitution of deficits by oral or parenteral rehydration are indicated.

When secondary bacterial infection is suggested by exacerbation of fever or by evidence of pneumonia on a chest radiograph, broad-spectrum antibiotic therapy may be indicated. Specific antimicrobial therapy can be provided when *H influenzae* or *Streptococcus pneumoniae* is isolated.

Recurrent acute bronchitis has been associated with reactive airway disease or asthma. Complications of acute bronchitis are few; in the majority of cases, the outcome is excellent, with resolution of disease and return to baseline health.

## CHRONIC BRONCHITIS

Chronic bronchitis, which is described widely in the literature on adults, is ill-defined in children and is described less frequently in this population. The prevalence of childhood bronchitis is variable, ranging from 2% to 40% in selected series.

### Clinical Presentation and Differential Diagnosis

Clinically, chronic bronchitis is characterized by excessive mucus production and by cough that is present on most days for a minimum of 3 months per year. Fever can accompany the cough, and the temperature can range from 37 °C to 39 °C (100 °F to 103 °F). Chronic bronchitis can be a clinical manifestation of a number of disorders, some of which are listed in Table 67-2. Asthma, or reversible obstructive airway disease, can be distinguished by a patient's clinical response to the administration of traditional bronchodilators. Recurrent episodes of acute bronchitis often are interpreted as chronic bronchitis, although the intermittent nature of these episodes and the absence of a persistent cough usually distinguish acute bronchitis clinically. Persistent lower respiratory tract infections, such as pertussis, and *Chlamydia* and *Mycobacterium* infections, can present with a similar complex of symptoms. These entities can be diagnosed by chest radiograph (for example, hilar lymph nodes are more common in *Mycobacterium* infection) and by isolation of the pathogen from nasopharyngeal secretions or sputum. In addition, serologic determinations of antibacterial antibodies assist in the diagnosis. Documentation of a delayed hypersensitivity skin test response to the antigen *Mycobacterium tuberculosis* is helpful in identifying tuberculosis.

Cystic fibrosis, which typically is accompanied by failure to thrive, steatorrhea, and nasal polyps, also is manifested prominently by recurrent lower respiratory tract symptoms. The diagnosis of cystic fibrosis can be established by documentation of abnormally elevated chloride levels (>60 mEq/L), as measured by sweat ionophoresis. Primary ciliary dyskinesia encompasses the immotile cilia disorders and Kartagener's syndrome (rhinosinusitis, bronchitis, or bronchiectasis and situs inversus). These patients have a defect in mucociliary transport, as evidenced by a decrease in ciliary beat frequency. Electron microscopy of bronchial cilia reveals structural defects classically, with absent dynein arms. This diagnosis is made by bronchial or, occasionally, nasal turbinate biopsy.

The immune disorders most frequently associated with recurrent sinopulmonary infection include selective IgA deficiency (serum IgA level 10 mg/dL or less), hypogammaglobulinemia (primary and secondary), IgG subclass deficiencies, and ataxia-telangiectasia. In addition, immunodeficient patients receiving bone marrow reconstitution by transplantation have been described with graft-versus-host disease affecting the lungs and

TABLE 67-2.  Conditions Associated
With Chronic Cough (3 Months or Longer)
or Lower Respiratory Tract Illness

Asthma

Recurrent Episodes of Bronchitis
Infections—*Chlamydia*, Pertussis,
*Mycobacterium*

Cystic Fibrosis

Primary Ciliary Dyskinesia
Kartagener's syndrome
Immotile cilia syndrome

Immunodeficiency
Selective IgA deficiency
Subclass of IgG defiency
Hypogammaglobulinemia (primary and
secondary)
Ataxia-telangiectasia
Graft-versus-host disease after bone marrow
transplant

Anatomic Lesions
Foreign body
Previous esophageal atresia repair
Mediastinal tumors
Congenital heart disease

Irritants
Milk aspiration (gastroesophageal reflux,
tracheoesophageal fistula)
Tobacco smoke
Pollution
Occupational exposure

*Modified from Morgan WT, Taussig LM. The chronic bronchitis complex in childhood. In: The pediatric airway. Pediatr Clin North Am 1984;31:853.*

manifesting itself clinically as a symptom complex suggestive of chronic bronchitis.

Anatomic lesions that lead to obstruction of the respiratory tree can mimic chronic bronchitis. Congenital heart disease should be considered in this patient population, and is evaluated best with clinical examination, chest radiography, electrocardiography, and echocardiography. Mediastinal tumors, although they are uncommon, can produce extrinsic obstruction leading to recurrent cough and wheezing. The infant with chronic cough, poor feeding habits, and failure to thrive should be evaluated for gastroesophageal reflux or a tracheoesophageal fistula, which is identified most easily by barium swallow or pH probe monitoring.

Respiratory tract irritants have been implicated in chronic cough. It is of interest that nonindustrial, rural communities such as the forest zone of Nigeria report virtually no chronic bronchitis, whereas reports from metropolitan New York suggest that an increased risk of respiratory tract infections exists in adults and children who reside in those parts of the city with the highest ambient air levels of sulfur dioxide and particulate air pollution. The correlation between tobacco smoking and reduced ventilatory capacity in adults has been reported by many investigators. Passive smoking also has been implicated as a factor that increases the risk in children of the development of lower respiratory tract infection, and impairment of lung function at the beginning of adult life. The clinician should obtain a history of smoking not only from the patient, but also from other members of the household.

## Pathogenesis and Pathophysiology

Many viral infections have been implicated in the etiology of chronic bronchitis (see Table 67-1). These include rhinoviruses, respiratory syncytial virus, parainfluenza viruses, influenza viruses A and B, adenoviruses, and enteroviruses. Bacterial agents are implicated more commonly in chronic bronchitis. The predominant pathogens isolated from sputum in a group of 40 pediatric patients with chronic bronchitis are shown in Table 67-3. Treatment of exacerbations of chronic bronchitis with antibiotic therapy usually is effective in reducing sputum volume and purulence, but shows no parallel elimination of the cultured microorganisms.

In a review, Smith evaluated 13 children with endoscopically proven chronic bronchitis and noted heterogenous histologic changes, including monocytic and eosinophilic infiltrates in diffuse and, occasionally, localized distributions. Polymorphonuclear cells were noted in endobronchial secretions, and inflammation was localized for the most part to the mucosa. This study was limited by small segmental biopsy sections and may not reflect accurately the histologic changes that occur in this generalized lung disease.

## Treatment

When a specific diagnosis can be identified with chronic cough or wheezing, therapy is directed toward the primary disease entity in addition to the clinical presentation. Hence, bronchodilators (theophylline preparations, $\beta$-adrenergic agents, cromolyn sodium, corticosteroids) are used when deemed appropriate in the treatment of chronic cough associated with asthma. Cough secondary to gastroesophageal reflux can be approached with altered feeding schedules, positioning techniques (prone 30°) and occasional medications (eg, bethanechol). The patient with hypogammaglobulinemia or IgG subclass deficiency may be aided by replacement intravenous immunoglobulin therapy using preparations currently available commercially at appropriate doses and schedules (100 to 400 mg/kg per dose every 2 to 4 weeks).

It is imperative that patients with chronic pulmonary disease as a result of cystic fibrosis or asthma understand the pulmonary irritant effect and possibly additive reduction in pulmonary function caused by tobacco smoking, dust exposure, and air pollution. In addition, parents of these children should be made aware of the effects of passive smoking on the already compromised pul-

TABLE 67-3.  Dominant Pathogens in Washed Sputum
From Patients With Chronic Bronchitis (40 Cases)

| Pathogen | Number of Cases (%) |
|---|---|
| *Haemophilus influenzae* and *Streptococcus pneumoniae* | 21 (52.5) |
| *H influenzae* | 17 (42.5) |
| *Staphylococcus aureus* | 2 (5.0) |
| Superinfection With Gram-Negative Rods | |
| *Pseudomonas aeruginosa* | 4 |
| *Klebsiella pneumoniae* | 2 |
| *Escherichia coli* | 1 |
| *Enterobacter cloacae* | 1 |

*Kubo AS, Funabashi S, Uehara S, et al. Clinical aspects of "asthmatic bronchitis" and chronic bronchitis in infants and children. J Asthma Res 1978;15:99.*

monary function of their children, and should be encouraged to stop smoking.

Antimicrobial therapy in chronic bronchitis is reserved for patients with severe illness in whom the likelihood of secondary bacterial infection is great. In these instances, therapy usually consists of ampicillin (75 mg/kg/d), erythromycin (40 mg/kg/d), or, in adolescents and adults, tetracycline (25 to 50 mg/kg/d). For patients receiving theophylline therapy who also have a bacterial infection, it is important to remember that the use of certain antibiotics (eg, erythromycin) can be associated with elevated serum concentrations of theophylline, making toxicity to the latter more likely. Sequential monitoring of pulmonary function studies is important. The prognosis for the chronic bronchitis complex is varied and depends on the specific diagnosis.

## Selected Readings

American Academy of Pediatrics Committee on Environmental Hazards. Involuntary smoking—a hazard to children. Pediatrics 1986;77:123.

Cherry JD. Lower respiratory tract infections: Acute bronchitis. In: Feigin RD, Cherry JD, eds. Textbook of pediatric infectious diseases, ed 2. Philadelphia: WB Saunders, 1987:278.

Current estimates from the National Health Interview Survey, United States, 1989. Vital Health Stat 1990;176:14.

Glezen WP. Viral respiratory infections. Pediatr Ann 1991;20:407.

Glezen WP, Denny FW. Epidemiology of acute lower respiratory disease in children. N Engl J Med 1979;288:498.

Hallet JS, Jacobs RL. Recurrent acute bronchitis: The association with undiagnosed bronchial asthma. Ann Allergy 1985;55:568.

Irvine D, Brooks A, Walker R. The role of air pollution, smoking and respiratory illnesses in childhood in the development of chronic bronchitis. Chest 1980;77:251.

Kubo AS, Funabashi S, Uehara S, et al. Clinical aspects of "asthmatic bronchitis" and chronic bronchitis in infants and children. J Asthma Res 1978;15:99.

Leibowitz MD, Holberg CJ, Martinez FD. A longitudinal study of risk factors in asthma and chronic bronchitis in childhood. Eur J Epidemiol 1990;6:341.

Love GT, Lan SP, Sky CM, Struba RJ. The incidence and severity of acute respiratory illness in families exposed to different levels of air pollution, New York metropolitan area 1971–1972. Arch Environ Health 1981;36:66.

Morgan WT, Taussig LM. The chronic bronchitis complex in childhood. In: The pediatric airway. Pediatr Clin North Am 1984;31:851.

Peat JK, Woolcock AJ, Leider SR, et al. Asthma and bronchitis in Sydney school children. Am J Epidemiol 1980;111:721.

Pedreira FH, Guandolo VL, Feroli EJ, et al. Involuntary smoking and incidence of respiratory illness during the first year of life. Pediatrics 1985;75:80.

Smith TF, Ireland TA, Zoatari GS, et al. Characteristics of children with endoscopically proved chronic bronchitis. Am J Dis Child 1985;139:1039.

Taussig LM, Smith SM, Blumenfeld R. Chronic bronchitis in childhood: What is it? Pediatrics 1981;67:1.

*Principles and Practice of Pediatrics, Second Edition.*
edited by Frank A. Oski et al. J. B. Lippincott Company, Philadelphia © 1994.

# *67.2 Bronchiolitis*

## I. Celine Hanson and William T. Shearer

Lower respiratory tract infection in children younger than 24 months of age is a common clinical occurrence. The spectrum of pathologic involvement includes large and small airways (tracheobronchitis, bronchitis, bronchiolitis), and alveolar or interstitial lung involvement (pneumonia).

The term *bronchiolitis* was coined in the early 1900s. Criteria for the diagnosis of bronchiolitis include first episode of acute wheezing, age 24 months or younger, accompanying physical findings of viral infection (ie, coryza, cough, fever), and exclusion of pneumonia or atopy as the cause of wheezing.

| TABLE 67-4. Bronchiolitis: Etiologic Agents |
| --- |
| **Viral** |
| Respiratory syncytial virus |
| Adenoviruses (types 3, 7, 21) |
| Parainfluenza virus (type 3) |
| Rhinoviruses |
| Mumps |
| Influenza viruses |
| **Miscellaneous** |
| *Mycoplasma pneumoniae* |

Table 67-4 lists the infectious agents that have been associated with the clinical entity of bronchiolitis. Viruses, particularly respiratory syncytial virus (RSV), account for the majority of pathogens isolated during clinical disease. Epidemics of bronchiolitis almost always are linked to RSV as the causative infectious agent. RSV infection is estimated to be a very common childhood event, affecting almost 60% of infants during the first year of life. Although *Mycoplasma pneumoniae* has been associated with lower respiratory tract disease and episodes of wheezing occasionally in infants and more commonly in older children, no bacterial agents have been implicated as inciting the wheezing.

## CLINICAL PRESENTATION

Bronchiolitis most often affects children between 2 and 12 months of age. The clinical presentation of bronchiolitis is that of a lower respiratory tract viral illness: fever (usually 38.3 °C [101 °F] or less), cough, dyspnea, and rhinitis. Hypoxia with cyanosis and increased work of breathing precipitates most hospitalizations for infants with bronchiolitis, but hypoxia frequently can be documented even without clinical evidence of desaturation (ie, cyanosis or poor peripheral perfusion). On physical examination, tachypnea with chest retractions and wheezing with rhonchi are common findings, and mild conjunctivitis and otitis are not uncommon. Increased respiratory effort, fever, and cough often lead to poor feeding and vomiting. Lethargy and dehydration often are observed.

Radiographic abnormalities usually are nonspecific and may include air trapping, atelectasis, and peribronchial thickening and consolidation. A diffuse interstitial infiltration pattern also has been reported, adding to the spectrum of chest radiographic abnormalities in this disease.

## DIFFERENTIAL DIAGNOSIS

The differential diagnosis of bronchiolitis includes triggering of underlying reactive airway disease or asthma, other infectious lower respiratory tract diseases (eg, pneumonia and chemical irritation, as with reflux or aspiration pneumonia), anatomic abnormalities (vascular ring, lung cysts), and extrapulmonary causes of wheezing (cardiac asthma, acidosis, poisoning). Chest radiographs often are helpful in excluding pneumonia. A barium swallow or pH probe determination can document reflux as a cause of recurrent lower respiratory tract diseases that are accompanied by wheezing. Evidence of cardiac disease may be identified by barium swallow; evidence of extrinsic bronchial constriction may be noted by echocardiography and electrocardiography.

The most difficult diagnostic distinction to make in infants is between intrinsic reactive airway disease and bronchiolitis. Reactive airway disease, or asthma, is a reversible obstructive airway disease; a 20% reduction in pulmonary function (forced expiratory volume in 1 minute, or $FEV_1$) may be noted after cold or methacholine challenge, and is reversible with inhaled bronchodilators. Use of this diagnostic technique is limited to children who are old enough to perform pulmonary function testing (more than 6 years of age), and is not without hazard in that marked bronchospasm can ensue. In small children, the diagnosis of asthma is more difficult; a clinical history or family predisposition, atopy, and recurrent bouts of wheezing that is responsive to bronchodilators assist in making a diagnosis. Recurrent episodes of bronchiolitis have been implicated in the occurrence of reactive airway disease in later childhood. Because the majority of children with bronchiolitis have a viral illness, the diagnosis of bronchiolitis can be made on the basis of clinical and historical findings. Making the difficult distinction between asthma and bronchiolitis may not be crucial, however, because therapy often is similar.

Children with cystic fibrosis can have bouts of bronchiolitis that manifest themselves clinically as prolonged or unusually complicated or severe lower respiratory tract illnesses. The diagnosis of cystic fibrosis can be made by documenting elevated chloride levels (>60 mEq/L) by sweat ionophoresis testing.

IgE-mediated hypersensitivity to foods, airborne allergens, or insect stings can precipitate systemic allergic reactions, including urticaria, wheezing, and hypotension. The history and physical examination can be very helpful in identifying allergies in children. Evidence that the administration of food is followed quickly by diarrhea, vomiting, angioedema, or hives and wheezing clearly suggests food allergy. Radioallergosorbent testing of serum for specific IgE response to food is helpful in confirming this clinical diagnosis. Wheezing with airborne allergen exposure often is accompanied by symptoms of allergic rhinitis, characterized by watery, clear rhinorrhea, nasal and ocular pruritus, and sneezing. Physical examination may reveal the classic stigmata of atopy (eg, an upturned nose with a nasal crease, allergic shiners, follicular conjunctivitis, bluish boggy nasal mucosa, or a cobblestoned appearance of the posterior pharynx). Allergic reactions to insect bites are common, and should be suspected when physical examination reveals either typical lesions, such as vesicular skin lesions after fire ant bites, or an intact stinger still embedded in the skin after bee or wasp stings.

## PATHOGENESIS AND PATHOPHYSIOLOGY

The sites of inflammation in bronchiolitis are the small bronchi and bronchioles; the alveolar spaces are spared. Pathologic changes include necrosis and sloughing of respiratory epithelium with destruction of ciliated cells, lymphocytic infiltration of epithelium and intrabronchiolar plugs of fibrin, and mucus causing either complete or partial obstruction. Usually, 1 to 2 weeks are required before the respiratory epithelium is restored completely.

Airway obstruction from fibrinous debris and mucus plugs combined with the abnormal mechanics of respiration in bronchiolitis increase substantially the work of breathing for these infants, and also lead to mismatching of pulmonary ventilation and perfusion. It is not surprising that arterial hypoxemia can be documented frequently during clinical disease. Carbon dioxide retention is not a common problem, but when it is present, it can result in acute respiratory acidosis and the need for prompt ventilatory assistance. Blood pH level abnormalities can be documented, and may reflect contraction alkalosis related to dehydration associated with poor oral intake and the contraction of extracellular spaces.

Investigation of immunologic responses at the site of injury after viral infection and bronchiolitis has led to speculation re-

garding long-term complications and sequelae of bouts of bronchiolitis, including subsequent reactive airway disease. Inflammatory responses after viral infection traditionally are thought to be cell-mediated, with lymphocytic infiltration and recruitment of macrophages to clear debris. Several investigators have documented immediate hypersensitivity phenomena after viral infection, particularly in patients with RSV infection: an increase in respiratory epithelial cell-bound IgE in patients with RSV infection and wheezing, compared to those without wheezing; detection of RSV-specific IgE in the nasopharyngeal secretions of patients with infection and wheezing, compared to its absence in those without wheezing; and higher nasopharyngeal concentrations of histamine in patients with RSV infection, compared to those without this virus. Similar findings implicating immediate hypersensitivity tissue responses have been documented in patients with parainfluenza virus infections and wheezing. Evidence of histamine release in nasopharyngeal secretions and virus-specific IgE at tissue sites suggests that type I, or IgE-mediated, responses play a role in the pathogenesis of wheezing in patients with these viral infections. Therapeutic intervention aimed at minimizing bronchospasm, therefore, has been suggested in the treatment of bronchiolitis.

## COMPLICATIONS

The vast majority of previously healthy infants infected with RSV and other agents of bronchiolitis have a lower respiratory tract infection of mild to moderate severity that lasts for 3 to 10 days. Most do not seek medical care for their illness. Those who do so, usually are cared for as outpatients. One child in 50 with RSV bronchiolitis requires hospitalization; of these, respiratory failure develops in 3% to 7%, and 1% die. Children with significant cardiopulmonary disease or immunodeficiency, however, are at much greater risk of serious sequelae from bronchiolitis. Mortality from nosocomial RSV infection can reach 20% in ill neonates and infants.

Atelectasis, apnea, and respiratory failure are the most important acute complications of bronchiolitis. Immature ventilatory control and respiratory muscle fatigue lead to apnea and respiratory failure in the youngest patients with bronchiolitis. Once they are intubated and mechanically ventilated, infants with bronchiolitis are at risk for pneumothorax and pneumomediastinum. Intubated patients should be monitored for changes in the amount of tracheal secretions and for secondary fever, which may indicate superinfection and the need for antibiotic therapy.

Infants with bronchopulmonary dysplasia who have been weaned from $O_2$ therapy may require supplemental $O_2$ at the time of discharge from the hospital after a bout of bronchiolitis.

Bronchiolitis obliterans is a complication of bronchiolitis caused by adenovirus types 3, 7, and 21; influenza viruses; M pneumoniae; and Pneumocystis carinii. This disorder is characterized pathologically by diffuse destruction of distal small airways and physiologically by hypoxia and fixed airflow obstruction. Bronchiolitis obliterans has not been described in association with RSV infection.

Recurrent episodes of bronchiolitis in childhood in the absence of underlying pulmonary disease have been implicated as being causative of subsequent pulmonary dysfunction and the development of asthma. Concurrent genetic/environmental factors (including hyperactive airways that are prone to episodic obstruction) and parental smoking have been implicated in the development of recurrent wheezing after bronchiolitis. Significant pulmonary dysfunction noted in these children in adult life may be coupled to subsequent environmental exposures, including adult smoking practices and pollution exposure.

## TREATMENT

The role of bronchodilator therapy in bronchiolitis remains somewhat controversial. Normal infants as young as 4 months of age respond to methacholine with bronchoconstriction and to metaproterenol with bronchodilation. In one series, 30% of the infants with RSV bronchiolitis responded to nebulized albuterol with improvement in their pulmonary function. In a large recent study of RSV bronchiolitis, expiratory flow rates were decreased after the administration of nebulized albuterol, suggesting a deleterious effect from nebulized $\beta_2$-agonists. Prospective trials of theophylline in bronchiolitis have not been performed. Oral or nebulized albuterol given in conjunction with intramuscular dexamethasone appears to reduce the symptoms of bronchiolitis and to protect against progression to respiratory failure. Corticosteroids are not recommended for routine use in patients with bronchiolitis. No complications of corticosteroid use have been described, however, and in patients with severe disease, their addition is not contraindicated. It seems reasonable to use a $\beta_2$-agonist to treat a wheezing infant with bronchiolitis, particularly if one or more doses of a nebulized $\beta$-agonist reduce tachypnea and quiet retractions. Most parents do not have access to a nebulizer, so a $\beta_2$-agonist syrup at traditional doses may be prescribed for outpatient use.

A child with suspected bronchiolitis should be admitted to the hospital if he or she is tachypneic, has marked retractions, seems listless, or has a history of poor fluid intake. Immunocompromised infants and those with underlying cardiopulmonary disease should be hospitalized if bronchiolitis develops.

The inpatient evaluation should include a chest film, arterial blood gas measurements, and $O_2$ saturation ($SaO_2$) monitoring. Nasopharyngeal washings should be obtained for viral cultures and viral immunofluorescent assay. The infant should receive intravenous fluids at maintenance rates, with additional fluids to restore normal hydration. Care to avoid overhydration should be observed. Humidified $O_2$ should be begun at 28% and adjusted to maintain the $PaO_2$ at >60 mm Hg and the $SaO_2$ at >90%. Nebulized $\beta_2$-agonists should be given as needed. If nebulized $\beta_2$-agonist therapy is required more often than every 2 hours (for a falling $SaO_2$ level, marked retractions, or listlessness), the child should be transferred to an intensive care unit.

Intubation and mechanical ventilation are indicated for apnea, for a rising $PaCO_2$ value, and for listlessness and retractions suggesting impending respiratory failure. Corticosteroids, theophylline, and furosemide all have been used in ventilated patients with bronchiolitis. Most patients ventilated for bronchiolitis require 7 to 14 days of mechanical support before they can be weaned from the ventilator.

Ribavirin is an antiviral agent that is effective against RSV and influenza viruses A and B. It is indicated for the early treatment of RSV bronchiolitis in infants with congenital heart disease, bronchopulmonary dysplasia, lung and chest wall anomalies, and immunodeficiency. Infants younger than 6 weeks of age and severely ill patients ($PaO_2$ <65 mm Hg, rising $PaCO_2$) with bronchiolitis also are candidates for ribavirin therapy. This agent is approved for use by nebulization into a hood, mask, or tent. Ribavirin can be used with mechanical ventilators if filters are employed to prevent plugging of the expiratory limb of the ventilator, but only personnel with specific expertise in delivering ribavirin aerosol via a ventilator should use it in this manner. Ribavirin should be delivered by a small-particle aerosol generator for 12 to 18 h/d, and it should be continued for 3 to 7 days until the patient improves.

The role of antibiotic therapy in bronchiolitis is minimal, because no bacterial agent has been described as causative.

Antimicrobial therapy may be administered because of concomitant radiographic evidence of pneumonia. Traditional causative agents should be considered (*Haemophilus influenzae, Streptococcus pneumoniae*) and ampicillin/amoxicillin should be initiated. If secondary bacterial infection is a consideration, nosocomial infectious agents (*Staphylococcus aureus*) should be considered.

## Selected Readings

Committee on Infectious Diseases, American Academy of Pediatrics. Ribavirin therapy of respiratory syncytial virus. Pediatrics 1987;79:475.

Frankel LR, Lewiston NJ, Smith DW, et al. Clinical observations on mechanical ventilation for respiratory failure in bronchiolitis. Pediatr Pulmonol 1986;2:307.

Glezen WP. Reactive airway disorders in children: Role of respiratory virus infections. Clin Chest Med 1984;5:635.

Hall CB, Hall WT, Speers DM. Clinical and physiologic manifestation of bronchiolitis and pneumonia: Outcome of respiratory syncytial virus. Am J Dis Child 1979;133:798.

Hughes DM, LeSouef PN, Landau LI. Effect of salbutamol on respiratory mechanics in bronchiolitis. Pediatr Res 1987;22:83.

Martinez FD, Morgan WJ, Wright AL, et al. Diminished lung function as a predisposing factor for wheezing respiratory illness in infants. N Engl J Med 1988;319:1112.

McConnochie KM. Bronchiolitis: What's in the name? Am J Dis Child 1983;137:11.

Samet JM, Tager, IB, Speizer F. The relationship between respiratory illness in childhood and chronic air-flow obstruction in adulthood. Am Rev Respir Dis 1983;127:508.

Welliver R, Cherry JD. Bronchiolitis and infectious asthma. In: Feigin RD, Cherry JD, eds. Textbook of pediatric infectious diseases, ed 2. Philadelphia: WB Saunders, 1987:278.

Welliver RC, Wong DT, Middleton EJ, et al. Role of parainfluenza virus-specific IgE in pathogenesis of croup and wheezing subsequent to infection. J Pediatr 1982;101:889.

Welliver RC, Wong DT, Sun M, et al. The development of respiratory syncytial virus-specific IgE and the release of histamine in nasopharyngeal secretions after infection. N Engl J Med 1981;305:841.

Wohl ME. Bronchiolitis. Pediatr Ann 1986;15:307.

Wohl MEB. Bronchiolitis. In: Kendig EL, Chernick V, eds. Disorders of the respiratory tract in children, ed 4. Philadelphia: WB Saunders, 1983:283.

*Principles and Practice of Pediatrics, Second Edition.*
edited by Frank A. Oski et al. J. B. Lippincott Company, Philadelphia © 1994.

# 67.3 *Nonbacterial Pneumonia*

### Kenneth M. Boyer

Nonbacterial pneumonias are the most common pulmonary infections encountered in pediatrics. The varied causes of these conditions, excluding bacteria and fungi, cover a broad taxonomic spectrum. With improvement in microbiologic techniques, the number of known causative agents continues to increase. Although most nonbacterial pneumonias have a good prognosis, they occasionally are life-threatening. Defining the cause of these conditions in the past has been the province of the epidemiologist and virologist, but a sufficient body of knowledge has accumulated in recent years to permit the clinician to make informed clinical judgments and rapid specific diagnoses. Moreover, in selected instances, empiric or specific therapies now are available.

## ETIOLOGY

At least 14 different virus groups, three *Mycoplasma* species, one rickettsia, three *Chlamydia* species, and one protozoan parasite have been associated with pneumonia syndromes in children. The overall importance of these agents is not measured simply by their incidence. Some agents, although they are quite common, generally give rise to relatively mild illness; others that are encountered less frequently characteristically cause serious disease. In Table 67-5, the major agents causing disease in various age groups are presented according to their overall frequency, their typical degree of severity, and their usual mode of access to the lung.

Respiratory syncytial virus (RSV) is the most common cause of pediatric pneumonia, particularly if it is associated with bronchiolitis. Although infection with this virus is quite common in all age groups, lower respiratory tract involvement is especially prominent in infancy.

The three parainfluenza viruses (1, 2, and 3) are second only to RSV as causes of lower respiratory tract disease in infants and younger children. Of these agents, parainfluenza virus 3 occurs most frequently in pneumonia; infection by parainfluenza viruses 1 and 2 generally produces laryngotracheitis.

Influenza viruses A and B are not as prevalent overall as are RSV and the parainfluenza viruses, but during periods of epidemic spread, they may become predominant isolates in hospitalized children with lower respiratory tract diseases.

Adenoviruses sometimes are isolated in children with pneumonia and with pertussis syndrome. Although their overall frequency is somewhat less than that of the other common respi-

### TABLE 67-5. Etiologic Agents in Nonbacterial Pneumonia

| Etiologic Agents | Frequency* | | | Usual Degree of Severity† | | | Mode of Access to Lung |
|---|---|---|---|---|---|---|---|
| | 0–3 mo | 4 mo–5 y | 6–16 y | 0–3 mo | 4 mo–5 y | 6–16 y | |
| **Viruses** | | | | | | | |
| Respiratory syncytial virus | +++ | ++++ | + | ++ | ++ | + | Respiratory |
| Parainfluenza viruses | | | | | | | |
| Type 1 | + | ++ | + | ++ | ++ | + | Respiratory |
| Type 2 | + | + | + | ++ | ++ | + | Respiratory |
| Type 3 | ++ | +++ | ++ | ++ | ++ | + | Respiratory |
| Influenza viruses | | | | | | | |
| Type A | ++ | +++ | +++ | ++ | ++ | + | Respiratory |
| Type B | ++ | ++ | + | ++ | ++ | + | Respiratory |
| Adenoviruses‡ | + | ++ | ++ | +++ | ++ | + | Respiratory |
| Rhinoviruses§ | + | + | + | − | ++ | + | Respiratory |
| Enteroviruses¶ | + | + | + | ++ | ++ | + | Respiratory (hematogenous) |
| Coronaviruses | − | + | + | − | ++ | + | Respiratory |
| Measles virus | + | ++ | ++ | +++ | ++ | ++ | Respiratory (hematogenous) |
| Rubella virus | + | − | − | ++ | − | − | Hematogenous |
| Human immunodeficiency virus | + | ++ | + | ++ | ++ | ++ | Hematogenous |
| Varicella-zoster virus | + | + | + | +++ | +++ | +++ | Hematogenous (respiratory) |
| Cytomegalovirus | ++ | + | + | ++ | +++ | +++ | Hematogenous (respiratory) |
| Epstein-Barr virus | − | + | ++ | − | ++ | + | Hematogenous (respiratory) |
| Herpes simplex viruses | ++ | + | + | ++++ | +++ | +++ | Hematogenous (respiratory) |
| **Mycoplasmas** | | | | | | | |
| *Mycoplasma pneumoniae* | − | + | ++++ | − | ++ | + | Respiratory |
| *Mycoplasma hominis* | ? | − | − | ? | − | − | Respiratory |
| *Ureaplasma urealyticum* | ? | − | − | ? | − | − | Respiratory |
| **Chlamydiae** | | | | | | | |
| *Chlamydia pneumoniae* | ? | ? | +++ | ? | ? | + | Respiratory |
| *Chlamydia psittaci* | − | + | + | − | ++ | ++ | Respiratory |
| *Chlamydia trachomatis* | ++++ | − | − | ++ | − | − | Respiratory |
| **Rickettsiae** | | | | | | | |
| *Coxiella burnetii* | − | + | + | − | ++ | ++ | Respiratory (hematogenous) |
| **Protozoa** | | | | | | | |
| *Pneumocystis carinii* | + | + | + | +++ | +++ | +++ | Respiratory |

* ++++, most frequent; +++, frequent; ++, infrequent; +, rare; −, no reported cases; ?, uncertain.
† ++++, often fatal; +++, severe; ++, usually hospitalized; +, home management; −, no reported cases; ?, uncertain.
‡ Types 1, 2, 3, 4, 5, 7, 14, 21, and 35.
§ Ninety or more types known.
¶ Coxsackieviruses A9, A16, B1, B4, and B5; echoviruses 9, 11, 19, 20, and 22.
*Modified from Boyer KM, Cherry JD. Nonbacterial pneumonia. In: Feigin RD, Cherry JD, eds. Textbook of pediatric infectious diseases, ed 3. Philadelphia: WB Saunders, 1992:256.*

ratory viruses, a number of fatal illnesses have been reported. Of the 31 known adenoviruses, types 1, 2, 3, 4, 5, 7, 14, 21, and 35 have been associated clearly with pneumonia. Some degree of lower respiratory tract involvement by rhinoviruses is indicated by their documented role in exacerbations of asthma and bronchitis. Among the enteroviruses, primary virus pneumonia has been documented best with coxsackieviruses A9 and B1, although coxsackieviruses A16, B4, and B5, and echoviruses 9, 11, 19, 20, and 22 also have been reported. Coronaviruses have been implicated as causes of pneumonia in a few seroepidemiologic studies, but recovery of these agents in tissue culture has been rare.

Pneumonia is the most common serious complication of measles. On careful radiographic study, at least half of all patients with a routine case of measles have pulmonary infiltrates early in the illness, suggesting a viral rather than a bacterial cause. Secondary pneumonia in measles results from the common bacterial pathogens, particularly *Streptococcus pneumoniae* and *Haemophilus influenzae*. Progressive, fatal, primary measles pneumonia (Hecht's giant-cell pneumonia) can occur in patients with cell-mediated immunodeficiency, hematologic malignancy, and the acquired immunodeficiency syndrome (AIDS). The characteristic measles rash often is absent.

Viruses that may attack the lungs by hematogenous spread include varicella, Epstein-Barr, rubella, cytomegalovirus (CMV), herpes simplex, and the human immunodeficiency virus (HIV). Rubella, CMV, and herpes simplex viruses may cause interstitial pneumonia in the congenitally or perinatally infected infant. CMV and varicella virus are causes of life-threatening pneumonia in the immunocompromised host. Pneumonia has been noted in adolescents with infectious mononucleosis. Pulmonary infiltration also is a component of the fatal X-linked lymphoproliferative syndrome that is caused by Epstein-Barr virus. Pulmonary lymphoid hyperplasia (lymphoid interstitial pneumonitis) is the most frequent clinical manifestation of pediatric AIDS. Whether this condition is the direct result of pulmonary infection by HIV or is caused by concomitant viral infection (eg, by Epstein-Barr virus) still is unclear.

Of the ten known *Mycoplasma* species that can infect humans, only *Mycoplasma pneumoniae* is a well-established cause of pneumonia. In children younger than 2 years of age, infection is common, but pneumonia is unusual. In children older than 5 years of age, *M pneumoniae* is the most common cause of nonbacterial pneumonia. Genital mycoplasmas, *Ureaplasma urealyticum* and *Mycoplasma hominis* in particular, have been associated with congenital and perinatally acquired pneumonia, although several recent studies have not been confirmatory.

Three *Chlamydia* species have been associated with pneumonia. *Chlamydia psittaci* is the well-recognized cause of psittacosis (ornithosis). *Chlamydia pneumoniae* is a recently described agent that is second only to *M pneumoniae* as a cause of pneumonia in adolescents and young adults. *Chlamydia trachomatis*, the established agent of inclusion blennorrhea in the neonate, causes a characteristic afebrile pneumonitis syndrome in infants aged 3 to 19 weeks. In urban areas in the United States where the condition has been studied extensively—Chicago, Seattle, San Francisco, and Birmingham—it is the most frequent cause of pneumonia in this age group.

Of the rickettsiae, only *Coxiella burnetii* is associated with pneumonia, in the form of Q fever. This infection may be severe, but, because of its restricted ecological niche, it is rare in children.

*Pneumocystis carinii*, a protozoan parasite, is an important cause of pneumonia in children who are receiving chemotherapy and the second major cause of pneumonia in pediatric AIDS. *P carinii* also is known to cause pneumonia in premature and debilitated infants and, with *C trachomatis*, CMV, and genital mycoplasmas, has been associated with the afebrile pneumonitis syndrome of infancy.

## EPIDEMIOLOGY

The major contributors to the overall epidemiology of nonbacterial pneumonia in children are RSV, parainfluenza viruses, *M pneumoniae*, and, to a lesser extent, influenza viruses A and B. Because of their brief incubation periods and high degree of communicability, these agents often spread through communities in well-defined waves. RSV and the influenza viruses occur exclusively in the winter months; parainfluenza viruses 1 and 2 usually are seen in the spring and fall. During intervals between epidemics, *M pneumoniae* and parainfluenza virus 3 tend to persist endemically.

Annual rates of childhood pneumonia show a rough inverse correlation with age, ranging from 40:1000 in children younger than 5 years to 7:1000 in adolescents 12 to 15 years. RSV is the most common causative agent in children less than 5 years of age; *M pneumoniae* is most common in older children.

In children, congenital heart disease and bronchopulmonary dysplasia are associated with viral pneumonia of greater severity, particularly that caused by RSV. Pulmonary deterioration in patients with cystic fibrosis has been shown to be associated with respiratory viral infection. Surprisingly, common respiratory viruses have only moderately greater impact in patients with hematologic malignancy and immunosuppressed states than they have in normal hosts.

Transmission of the more common agents of lower respiratory tract disease most often occurs by means of droplet spread resulting from relatively close contact with a source case. Direct inoculation at the alveolar level probably does not occur in most cases because of the extremely small size of aerosolized particles necessary to accomplish this. Studies of nosocomially transmitted RSV infections have shown the importance of adults with relatively trivial upper respiratory tract infection as intermediates in transmission to susceptible young infants. School-age children often introduce respiratory viral agents into households, resulting in secondary infections in parents and siblings. The increasing use of group day care by working parents has been associated with enhanced transmission of a number of respiratory pathogens, and certainly has extended "school age" to a younger group of children.

## PATHOGENESIS AND PATHOLOGY

After inoculation of the upper respiratory tract, viral agents that cause pneumonia proliferate and spread by contiguity to involve more distal portions of the lower respiratory tract. Infected epithelium loses its ciliary appendages, rounds up, and sloughs into the air passages, resulting in stasis of mucus and accumulation of cellular debris. Relative expiratory obstruction causes hyperinflation and air trapping, with increased dead-space ventilation.

When infection extends to the terminal airways, alveolar lining cells lose their structural integrity, resulting in the loss of surfactant production, hyaline membrane formation, and pulmonary edema. These changes, combined with airway narrowing, lead to atelectasis and increased intrapulmonary shunting. Inflammatory responses at the site of tissue damage and in contiguous submucosal and interstitial structures impair gas exchange further. Four major pathologic expressions have been described in fatal infections, any or all of which may be present in a given case: acute bronchiolitis, necrotizing bronchiolitis, interstitial pneumonia, and alveolar pneumonia.

Two important factors that influence the pathologic expression of nonbacterial pneumonias in children are anatomy and immunity. In the young infant, the small caliber of the terminal airways, their limited cartilage support, and the absence of interconnections between alveolar spaces (pores of Kohn) contribute to wheezing and lobular atelectasis. Immunopathologic mechanisms have been invoked to explain the disparities between clinical expressions of infection by RSV and *M pneumoniae* in infants and in older children. Interaction between RSV-infected epithelial cells and specific IgE, leading to histamine release, has been postulated as an immune mechanism for bronchospasm in RSV disease. Cumulative immunity after repeated natural infections by *M pneumoniae* may account for the more impressive clinical expression of illness that is seen in older children and adults. *Mycoplasma*-specific cell-mediated immunity, which is detectable at low levels in young children but is increased in adults, probably contributes to the pathogenesis.

## CLINICAL PRESENTATION

Acute nonbacterial pneumonia in the infant or young child generally follows 1 or 2 days of coryza, decreased appetite, and low-grade fever. The onset generally is gradual, with increasing fretfulness, respiratory congestion, vomiting, cough, and fever. In the very young infant, fever may be minimal and apneic spells ("near-miss" sudden infant death syndrome or "apparent life-threatening events") the most prominent (and frightening) presenting complaint. The most reliable physical findings of pneumonia are those of respiratory distress: tachypnea, tachycardia, nasal flaring, and retractions, but without the stridor that is characteristic of upper airway obstruction. In the patient with diminished functional residual capacity, grunting may be present. Cyanosis generally accompanies apneic spells or coughing attacks, but it may be present at rest if significant ventilation–perfusion mismatch has developed.

Other physical findings are quite variable and may be normal. Wheezing is present in infants with bronchiolitis. Hyperresonance may be noted if significant air trapping is present. Diminished local percussion or breath sounds may indicate lobar consolidation or atelectasis. In patients with interstitial pneumonia, fine crackling rales may be present diffusely or locally. Also important in the initial assessment is an evaluation of the young child's state of hydration, because increased insensible losses from fever and hyperventilation, coupled with anorexia, can result in significant fluid deficits.

The afebrile pneumonitis syndrome of young infants, in contrast to the usual acute viral pneumonias affecting this age group, is subacute to chronic in its development and is nonseasonal. Characteristic features include the absence of fever, a "staccato" cough pattern, and diffuse rales on auscultation. Radiographic findings usually consist of interstitial infiltrates with subsegmental atelectasis. Hypergammaglobulinemia and mild eosinophilia are common laboratory abnormalities.

Nonbacterial pneumonia in the older child and adolescent occurs clinically more nearly like that in an adult. Premonitory complaints generally include such systemic symptoms as malaise, myalgia, and anorexia in addition to upper respiratory tract symptoms. "Chilliness" may occur, but rigors generally are absent. Cough usually is irritative and nonproductive. A temperature above 39 °C is unusual. Although tachypnea, flaring, and retractions generally are present, they may be less apparent than in the infant or young child. Findings on examination of the chest are more reliable than in infancy, and may include local percussion dullness or diminished breath sounds and local or diffuse fine rales. Because apnea is rare in older patients, cyanosis is an ominous sign of impairment of gas exchange. Although mild dehydration often is present, it generally is not evident on examination.

Radiologic findings in nonbacterial pneumonias vary according to the patient's age and the infecting agent. In the infant and young child, bilateral air trapping and perihilar infiltrates are the most frequent findings. Patchy areas of consolidation may represent lobular atelectasis or alveolar pneumonia. In the older child and the adolescent, lobar involvement can be defined more often, but the affected areas typically are not consolidated completely. Although lobar consolidation may occur in patients with nonbacterial pneumonia, this finding should be distinguished from atelectasis and is more consistent with a bacterial cause of disease. Similarly, although small pleural effusions may be detected in decubitus films in patients with nonbacterial pneumonias, effusions are much more suggestive of bacterial infection.

Peripheral leukocyte counts are variable, but tend to be less than 15,000/mm³ in patients with nonbacterial pneumonia. Gram stains of sputum or tracheal secretions tend to show epithelial cells as the predominant cell type, with a mixed bacterial population representing normal pharyngeal flora. Dominance of polymorphonuclear leukocytes and a uniform bacterial population are more consistent with bacterial infection.

## DIFFERENTIAL DIAGNOSIS

In the differential diagnosis of nonbacterial pneumonias, the following factors must be considered: the status of the host (normal or compromised); the environment (family or school exposure); the age of the patient; and the season of the year. In certain epidemiologic settings, the specific cause of nonbacterial pneumonia may be guessed with relative certainty. Often, however, this category of pulmonary infection is a diagnosis of exclusion. The major conditions to be differentiated include noninfectious pulmonary diseases, bacterial pneumonias that are amenable to conventional antibiotics, and the more unusual bacterial, fungal, or parasitic infections that may require specialized forms of therapy.

Noninfectious conditions that may simulate nonbacterial pneumonia are summarized in Table 67-6. The demarcation between infectious and noninfectious conditions is not always sharp. In a child with sickle cell anemia, for example, pulmonary vascular occlusive crisis presents with fever, leukocytosis, and patchy pulmonary infiltrates. Differentiation from pneumococcal, *Haemophilus*, or *Mycoplasma* pneumonia, to which the child with sickle cell anemia has increased susceptibility, may be difficult or impossible. Early recognition of noninfectious conditions either mimicking or underlying pneumonia may prevent recurrence or improve the prognosis. Recognition of the "snowman in a snowstorm" chest radiograph of total anomalous pulmonary venous return may lead to a curative open heart procedure. Recognition and treatment of cystic fibrosis may prevent early irreversible pulmonary damage.

Pneumonias caused by pyogenic bacteria classically are lobar in distribution and exhibit consolidation on roentgenography. Atelectasis, on the other hand, is common in viral pneumonia and must be distinguished from true consolidation. Pleural effusions, circular infiltrates, consolidations with convex margins, and pneumatoceles all favor a bacterial infection. Because of the association of bacteremic infection with a high fever and significant leukocytosis in the young child, these clinical findings also favor a bacterial cause of pneumonia. The results of a number of other laboratory determinations, such as erythrocyte sedimentation rate, C-reactive protein level, and reduction of nitroblue tetrazolium by leukocytes, frequently are positive in patients with bacterial respiratory infection. These tests add little to a careful initial clinical examination, roentgenographic findings, differential white cell count, and, if accessible, Gram stain of tracheal secretions in excluding a bacterial cause, however. Only positive results of cultures of blood, pleural fluid, or lung aspirates definitely prove the cause of bacterial pneumonia, although the

## TABLE 67-6. Noninfectious Conditions That May Simulate or Underlie Pneumonia in Children

**Technical**
Poor inspiratory chest radiograph
Underpenetrated chest radiograph

**Physiologic**
Prominent thymus
Breast shadows

**Chronic Pulmonary Disease**
Asthma
Cystic fibrosis
Bronchiectasis
Bronchiolitis obliterans
Pulmonary sequestration
Congenital lobar emphysema
Pulmonary hemosiderosis
Desquamative interstitial pneumonitis

**Recurrent Aspiration**
Gastroesophageal reflux
Tracheoesophageal fistula
Craniofacial defect
Neuromuscular disorders
Familial dysautonomia

**Pulmonary Edema**
Congestive heart failure
"Adult" respiratory distress syndrome
Total anomalous pulmonary venous return

**Allergic Alveolitis**
Dusts (farmer's lung)
Molds (allergic Aspergillosis)
Excreta (pigeon-breeder's lung)

**Atelectasis**
Cardiomegaly
Mucus plug
Foreign body

**Damage by Physical Agents**
Bronchopulmonary dysplasia
Lipoid pneumonia
Petroleum distillate ingestion
Near drowning
Smoke inhalation

**Iatrogenic Pulmonary Damage**
Fluid overload
Drugs (nitrofurantoin, bleomycin)
Radiation pneumonitis
Graft-versus-host disease

**Pulmonary Infarction**
Sickle vaso-occlusive crisis
Fat embolism

**Miscellaneous**
Systemic lupus erythematosus
Sarcoidosis
Neoplasms (lymphoma, teratoma, neuroblastoma)
Pleural effusion or reaction
Bronchogenic cyst
Vascular ring
Histiocytosis

*Modified from Boyer KM. Pneumonia. In: Dershewitz RA, ed. Ambulatory pediatric care, ed 2. Philadelphia: JB Lippincott, 1992:621.*

detection of antigenuria (pneumococcal or *H influenzae*, type b) can be helpful.

Among the less common causes of pneumonia, tuberculosis never should be forgotten. Tuberculin testing should be included in the initial evaluation and is especially important in children who live in urban areas, recent immigrants, and Native Americans. Fungal pneumonia, particularly coccidioidomycosis, blastomycosis, and histoplasmosis, should be considered in children who live in or visit endemic areas. Often, a suggestive history may be elicited, such as exposure to excavations (eg, backyard swimming pools, geologic or archaeologic "digs"), clean-up chores in old sheds and barns, and dust storms. Erythema nodosum and eosinophilia are common clinical clues to these entities. Other fungal pneumonias, such as aspergillosis and cryptococcosis, occur in the setting of immunosuppression. These conditions, coupled with the possibilities of infection with *Pneumocystis*, fungi, resistant bacteria, and CMV, may warrant the use of bronchoalveolar lavage or open lung biopsy as definitive approaches to diagnosis in the compromised host.

## SPECIFIC DIAGNOSIS

The methods used for virologic and chlamydial isolation are available in most major medical centers and public health laboratories. With the possible exceptions of herpes simplex viruses and adenoviruses, respiratory viruses rarely are carried asymptomatically. Thus, identification of an agent in upper respiratory tract secretions is strong evidence for its causative role in pneumonia. Conventional virologic techniques provide the most sensitive and specific means of identification. Rapid diagnosis of influenza A virus, parainfluenza viruses, RSV, and *Chlamydia* infections by means of fluorescent antibody techniques, enzyme-linked immunosorbent assays, or DNA probes has proved useful in a number of centers. In an individual case, serologic diagnosis of respiratory viral infection generally is less satisfactory than is virologic diagnosis. The difficulties associated with serology relate to the timing of specimen collection, the choice of antigens to test, and variation in the quality and specificity of available reagents. In contrast, serologic diagnosis of chlamydial pneumonitis can be very helpful. Even at the onset of illness, affected infants have high titers of specific IgG and IgM antibodies. Similarly, a positive antibody test result for HIV infection constitutes strong evidence for either pulmonary lymphoid hyperplasia or opportunistic *Pneumocystis* pneumonia in a child with pulmonary infiltrates and a compatible epidemiologic history for pediatric AIDS.

Laboratory facilities for the isolation of mycoplasmas and rickettsiae are less readily accessible to the clinician. DNA probes have become available for diagnosis of *M pneumoniae*. However, serologic techniques are the most practical means of making a specific diagnosis. Acute-phase reactants (eg, cold agglutinins in *M pneumoniae* infection) are of greatest diagnostic help during acute illness, but are not present invariably. Definitive etiologic identification requires testing of paired sera for specific antibodies. *Pneumocystis* infection usually is diagnosed by visualizing organisms in silver-stained specimens obtained by bronchoscopy or biopsy, although noninvasive serologic diagnosis currently is under investigation.

Because of the epidemiologic behavior of nonbacterial respiratory infections, a reasonable guess as to a specific cause often can be made, based on such factors as patient age, season of the year, and associated clinical features. If the presence of a particular nonbacterial agent in a community can be established by isolation or serologic means, the probability that other patients with similar manifestations have illness caused by that agent is increased greatly. Regional viral surveillance programs, such as those carried out in Rochester, New York, and Houston, Texas, can be particularly helpful to the practicing pediatrician in this regard.

## THERAPY

Therapy for nonbacterial pneumonia is primarily expectant and supportive. The course of uncomplicated viral pneumonia is not influenced by the administration of antibiotics. In the vast majority of cases in which pulmonary involvement is uncovered, however, antibiotic therapy is used because bacterial disease cannot be ruled out with certainty. In all but the most mild cases, this approach is both reasonable and practical. It is important, though, that antibiotic therapy in routine cases be appropriate for the most common bacterial pathogens (*S pneumoniae* and *H influenzae*). In the immunocompromised host or when secondary infection is a possibility, *Staphylococcus aureus* and other hospital-associated and opportunistic pathogens must be considered.

In certain fulminant viral pneumonias, such as varicella in a compromised host, antiviral chemotherapy with acyclovir may be life-saving, but it should be recalled that as many as half of all patients with this condition have complicating bacterial sepsis that is amenable to antibiotic therapy. The treatment of pneumonia caused by CMV in an immunocompromised host now consists of the combination of ganciclovir and intravenous hyperimmune globulin. Inhalational administration of the antiviral compound ribavirin appears to shorten the course of viral pneumonias caused by RSV and influenza. This drug is recommended particularly for the treatment of RSV infection in infants with underlying cardiopulmonary disease. Other infants with proven or suspected RSV disease for whom ribavirin has been recommended include those with severe disease and impending respiratory failure, and those with initially milder disease, but risk factors such as prematurity, young age (<6 wk), and neuromuscular compromise. Crystallization in ventilator valves is a technical difficulty associated with the administration of ribavirin to patients on mechanical ventilation. With protective filtration devices in the circuitry, however, ribavirin has proven to be safe and effective in patients with critical RSV illness.

Specific antimicrobial therapy for mycoplasmal, chlamydial, and rickettsial pneumonias with erythromycin or tetracycline shortens the course of the illness, but generally has a less dramatic therapeutic effect than does specific antibiotic therapy for bacterial infections. The drug of choice for *Pneumocystis* pneumonia is trimethoprim-sulfamethoxazole.

The elements of supportive therapy include adequate hydration, high humidity, maintenance of oxygenation, and mobilization of lower respiratory tract secretions. Because of increased insensible fluid losses as a result of fever, hyperventilation, and anorexia, mild dehydration frequently is observed initially, and continuing losses usually occur during the acute phase of illness. Thus, restoration of deficits and adequate maintenance of fluid intake are desirable. With regard to the latter, it should be remembered that fluid requirements increase by about 12% per °C of fever, and that hyperventilation increases fluid requirements by an additional 15%.

The therapeutic benefits of mist tents are debated because of the negligible amounts of nebulized water that actually reach the bronchiolar level. A high level of humidity is required to prevent the drying effects of supplemental oxygen therapy, however, and, by slowing evaporation, probably also serves to reduce the viscosity of mucus secretions and the magnitude of insensible fluid losses. Mobilization of respiratory secretions by means of vibration and postural drainage is indicated in patients with nonbacterial pneumonia that is complicated by atelectasis, but is not helpful in the absence of excessive secretions or mucus plugging.

Because of ventilation–perfusion abnormalities and alveolocapillary block, most children with nonbacterial pneumonia have some degree of hypoxemia. In a child with respiratory distress, provision of supplemental oxygen reduces anxiety and ventilation rates. Increases in inspired oxygen to about 30% are provided easily in mist tent environments, which are the most convenient means of administering oxygen. More severe respiratory distress or cyanosis requires documentation of the patient's respiratory status by means of arterial blood gas determinations and more exact regulation of inspired oxygen administered by nasal prongs, hood, or face mask. Oximetry, capnography, or transcutaneous monitoring can reduce the need for frequent blood gas sampling and insertion of arterial lines. In patients with respiratory failure, mechanical ventilation is required to maintain oxygenation and control $CO_2$ retention.

Apnea and bradycardia occur commonly in young infants with pneumonia that is caused by RSV, parainfluenza viruses, and influenza viruses, and are particularly frequent complications in those with a history of premature birth. Although the mechanism for these episodes is unclear, continuous monitoring for apnea is prudent in a young infant with viral pneumonia.

Acetaminophen or ibuprofen should be used to control fever.

Expectorants and cough suppressants, although they are prescribed widely for upper respiratory tract infections of children and adults, are not helpful in the initial treatment of nonbacterial pneumonia. Theophylline and aerosolized bronchodilators are used widely in patients with nonbacterial pneumonia that is complicated by apnea or bronchospasm. Controlled trials of their efficacy have been limited to the emergency department setting. During convalescence, a persistent irritative cough that interferes with sleep may be alleviated by judicious use of antihistamines, dextromethorphan, or codeine.

## PROGNOSIS

Children with pneumonia should be reevaluated clinically 2 to 3 weeks after the condition was diagnosed. If the child is asymptomatic, has returned to normal activities, and has benign results on physical examination, a follow-up radiograph is not required. Repeated chest radiographs are indicated in children with complicated clinical courses, underlying cardiopulmonary disease, or prior episodes of pneumonia, or if signs or symptoms of respiratory difficulty persist at the time of follow-up. It should be recognized that about 20% of patients with uncomplicated cases of pneumonia have persistent radiographic abnormalities 3 to 4 weeks after diagnosis, but a selective approach to follow-up films permits the early recognition of atelectasis or chronic disease.

The incidence of long-term complications of nonbacterial pneumonias is unknown. It is likely, however, that these conditions play a role in the development of some cases of bronchiectasis, chronic pulmonary fibrosis, desquamative interstitial pneumonitis, and unilateral hyperlucent lung (Swyer-James syndrome). These complications are well documented sequelae of measles, and of adenovirus and influenza viral pneumonia, but fortunately they are rare now.

## PREVENTION

Nosocomial spread of respiratory viruses occurs readily in pediatric wards and involves intermediate carriage by medical personnel who have acquired mild upper respiratory tract infections. A reasonable approach to interdicting nosocomial transmission is to group patients with pneumonia and exclude personnel with symptomatic respiratory illness from ward duties. With the exceptions of measles and varicella, mask or gown isolation has no effect on transmission. Avoiding close contact, washing hands, and wearing glasses or goggles will minimize respiratory infections of personnel. Regardless of HIV serologic status, blood and secretion precautions ("universal precautions") are recommended for all hospitalized patients.

For the common viral causes of pneumonia, vaccines are available only for influenza viruses and adenoviruses. Annual influenza vaccination using "split-product" vaccines is recommended for children with chronic respiratory disease and other conditions that predispose them to the development of pneumonia. Vaccination of adult health care personnel reduces the number of days they miss work because of illness and can prevent nosocomial transmission. Adenovirus vaccines have been used widely in the military forces, but are not recommended for use in the pediatric population. Attenuated varicella vaccines are immunogenic and have proven protective efficacy, but remain unlicensed in the United States. Attenuated, inactivated, and subunit vaccines against RSV and *M pneumoniae* have received considerable investigative effort, but have not proved yet to be entirely satisfactory.

*P carinii* pneumonia can be prevented in pediatric patients with hematologic malignancy or AIDS by the prophylactic administration of trimethoprim-sulfamethoxazole. This medication has become part of the routine treatment of these conditions and has reduced the incidence of *P carinii* infection dramatically. Note that prophylaxis should be started even in seropositive infants whose HIV infection status is indeterminate. Opportunistic pneumonia caused by CMV, which is a major hazard in seronegative, high-risk, premature infants and in recipients of allogeneic bone marrow transplants, can be prevented effectively by the exclusive use of CMV-seronegative blood products. In marrow transplant recipients who are seropositive and, thus, at risk for reactivated disease, acyclovir, ganciclovir, and intravenous immunoglobulin have been shown to reduce rates of infection and interstitial pneumonia.

## Selected Readings

Beem M, Saxon E. Respiratory-tract colonization and a distinctive pneumonia syndrome in infants infected with *Chlamydia trachomatis*. N Engl J Med 1977;296:306.

Carson JL, Collier AM, Hu SS. Acquired ciliary defects in nasal epithelium of children with acute viral upper respiratory infections. N Engl J Med 1985;312:463.

Dennehy PH, McIntosh K. Viral pneumonia in childhood. In: Weinstein L, Fields BN, eds. Seminars in infectious disease V. Pneumonias. New York: Thieme-Stratton, 1983:173.

Denny FW, Clyde WA Jr. Acute lower respiratory tract infections in nonhospitalized children. J Pediatr 1986;108:635.

Frankel LR, Smith DW, Lewiston NJ. Bronchoalveolar lavage for diagnosis of pneumonia in the immunocompromised child. Pediatrics 1988;81:785.

Hughes WT, Rivera GK, Schell MJ, et al. Successful intermittent chemoprophylaxis for *Pneumocystis carinii* pneumonitis. N Engl J Med 1987;316:1627.

Rubinstein A, Morecki R, Silverman B, et al. Pulmonary disease in children with acquired immune deficiency syndrome and AIDS-related complex. J Pediatr 1986;108:498.

Smith DW, Frankel LR, Mathers LH, et al. A controlled trial of aerosolized ribavirin in infants receiving mechanical ventilation for severe respiratory syncytial virus infection. N Engl J Med 1991;325:24.

Turner RB, Lande AE, Chase P, et al. Pneumonia in pediatric outpatients: Cause and clinical manifestations. J Pediatr 1987;111:194.

*Principles and Practice of Pediatrics, Second Edition.*
edited by Frank A. Oski et al. J. B. Lippincott Company, Philadelphia © 1994.

# 67.4 *Hypersensitivity Pneumonitis*

I. Celine Hanson and William T. Shearer

The term *hypersensitivity pneumonitis* defines a spectrum of pulmonary disorders that includes granulomatous, interstitial, and alveolar filling diseases. These respiratory disorders are associated causally with intense and frequently prolonged exposure to inhaled organic antigens. The range of vegetable and animal antigens implicated is broad. Table 67-7 lists some of the most common offenders. In the United States, bird-breeder's lung, farmer's lung, and ventilator hypersensitivity pneumonitis occur most often. Many of the diseases listed are related to specific adult occupations (eg, pigeon-breeder's lung, farmer's lung disease), but children living in environments rich with these antigens occasionally can be afflicted with these respiratory illnesses also. Medications have been implicated as precipitants of hypersensitivity pneumonitis in adults and children; common offenders include inhaled cromolyn sodium (Spinhalant) and nitrofurantoin.

## CLINICAL PRESENTATION

The clinical presentation of hypersensitivity pneumonitis is variable and traditionally is separated into three somewhat distinct clinical entities: acute, subacute, and chronic. The acute form of hypersensitivity pneumonitis frequently is related to intermittent, intense inhalation of the offending antigen, with symptoms precipitated 4 to 6 h after antigen contact. Typical clinical symptoms include elevated temperature in the range of 38.3 °C to 40.0 °C (101 °F to 104 °F), dry cough, dyspnea, and malaise. Constitutional symptoms can persist for weeks after exposure, but usually resolve within 24 hours. The patient appears ill on physical examination and lung auscultation typically documents bilateral bibasilar rales. Wheezing or evidence of reversible reactive airway disease is uncommon and provides evidence against the diagnosis of hypersensitivity pneumonitis.

Characteristic laboratory findings in patients with an acute episode of hypersensitivity pneumonitis (which can be reproduced by antigen inhalation challenge also) include leukocytosis, with white blood cell counts as high as $25,000/mm^3$; eosinophilia (in about 10% of patients); polyclonal elevation of serum immunoglobulin levels; and nonspecific reactive rheumatoid factor results. Positive evidence of antigen-specific serum precipitins is documented well in both symptomatic and asymptomatic exposed individuals, so using this measure solely to diagnose hypersensitivity pneumonitis is not always valid. The best diagnostic test for this clinical entity is antigen inhalation challenge, although it does have some inherent problems. First, the patient must be able to perform pulmonary function testing adequately, so the procedure is best suited for the evaluation of older children and adults. Second, the patient can exhibit marked decreases in vital capacity and pulmonary function, which are uncomfortable and, if the test is not performed in a controlled setting, can be catastrophic. Third, the delivery of antigen to each individual cannot be measured precisely, so it is difficult to establish the exact dose of antigen that causes a positive response even in asymptomatic exposed individuals. Nevertheless, characteristic pulmonary findings include a restrictive lung pattern, with a fall in the forced expiratory volume and forced vital capacity 4 to 6 hours after inhalation, and a gradual return to baseline capacities over the subsequent 8 to 12 hours.

The subacute presentation of hypersensitivity pneumonitis lacks the characteristic findings of fever, malaise, and dyspnea that are noted in the acute form of the disorder. Clinically, the patient may complain of persistent anorexia or weight loss and malaise. Pulmonary symptoms such as progressive shortness of breath or insidious onset of dyspnea on exertion may be late. The chronic form of hypersensitivity pneumonitis usually is related to long-term, low-dose antigen exposure. Clinical findings include a normal physical examination, with the exception of pulmonary rales detected on auscultation of the chest. Wheezing rarely accompanies chronic hypersensitivity pneumonitis. Lung disease related to the chronic form of the disorder usually is poorly responsive to traditional therapeutic intervention. Initial pulmonary findings include severe restrictive impairment (coupled with a diffusion defect), pulmonary fibrosis (determined radiographically and histologically, with noncaseating granulomas noted), and progressive nonreversible obstructive disease that is characterized by hyperinflation and sometimes is associated histologically with evidence of obliterative bronchiolitis and emphysema.

Chest radiographs of patients with acute hypersensitivity pneumonitis may reveal bibasilar interstitial infiltrates or multibasilar nodular densities. In chronic disease forms, pulmonary fibrosis can be seen, with evidence of contracted lung tissue. When progressive obstructive lung disease complicates hypersensitivity pneumonitis, hyperinflation may be noted radiographically.

## TABLE 67-7.   Causative Agents in Hypersensitivity Pneumonitis

| Antigen | Antigen Source | Name of Disorder |
|---|---|---|
| **Actinomycete and Fungal-Laden Vegetable Products** | | |
| Thermophilic actinomycetes (*Micropolyspora faeni, Thermoactinomyces vulgaris*), *Aspergillus* species | Moldy hay | Farmer's lung disease |
| Thermophilic actinomycetes (*Thermoactinomyces sacchari, T vulgaris*) | Moldy pressed sugarcane (bagasse) | Bagassosis |
| Thermophilic actinomycetes (*M faeni, T vulgaris*) | Moldy compost | Mushroom worker's disease |
| *Penicillium* species | Moldy cork | Suberosis |
| *Aspergillus clavatus* | Contaminated barley | Malt worker's lung |
| *Cryptostroma corticale* | Contaminated maple logs | Sequoiosis |
| *Alternaria* species | Contaminated wood pulp | Wood-pulp worker's disease |
| Thermophilic actinomycetes (*Thermoactinomyces candidus, T vulgaris*), *Penicillium* species, *Cephalosporium* species, amebae | Contaminated humidifiers, dehumidifiers, air conditioners | Humidifier lung |
| *Bacillus subtilis* | Contaminated wood dust in walls | Familial hypersensitivity pneumonitis |
| *Penicillium* species | Cheese casings | Cheese washer's disease |
| *Rhizopus* species, *Mucor* species | Contaminated wood trimmings | Wood trimmer's disease |
| *Saccharomonospora viridis* | Dried grasses and leaves | Thatched roof disease |
| *Streptomyces albus* | Contaminated fertilizer | *Streptomyces*-hypersensitivity pneumonia |
| *Cephalosporium* | Contaminated basement (sewage) pneumonitis | *Cephalosporium* hypersensitivity |
| *Pullularia* species | Sauna water | Sauna taker's disease |
| *B subtilis* enzymes | Detergent | Detergent worker's disease |
| *Mucor stolonifer* | Paprika dust | Paprika splitter's lung |
| **Animal Products** | | |
| Pigeon-serum proteins | Pigeon droppings | Pigeon breeder's disease |
| Duck proteins | Feathers | Duck fever |
| Turkey proteins | Turkey products | Turkey handler's disease |
| Parrot-serum proteins | Parrot droppings | Budgerigar fancier's disease |
| Chicken proteins | Chicken droppings | Feather plucker's disease |
| Bovine and porcine proteins | Pituitary snuff | Pituitary-snuff taker's lung |
| Rat-serum protein | Rat urine and droppings | Rat lung |
| **Insect Products** | | |
| *Ascaris siro* (mite) | Dust | |
| *Sitophilus granarius* (wheat weevil) | Contaminated grain | Miller's lung |
| **Reactive Simple Chemicals** | | |
| Altered proteins (neoantigens) or hapten protein conjugates | Toluene diisocyanate | TDI*-hypersensitivity pneumonitis TMA†-hypersensitivity pneumonitis |
| | Tremetallic anhydride | |
| Hapten protein conjugates | Diphenylmethane diisocyanate | MDI‡-hypersensitivity pneumonitis |
| Hapten protein conjugates | Heated epoxy resin | Epoxy-resin lung |

\* *TDI*, toluene diisocyanate.
† *TMA*, tremetallic anhydride.
‡ *MDI*, diphenylmethane diisocyanate.
*Salvaggio JE. Hypersensitivity pneumonitis. J Allergy Clin Immunol 1987;79:558.*

The differential diagnosis includes all disease states that cause interstitial infiltrates on radiography, such as lymphoid interstitial pneumonitis, which is seen characteristically in human immunodeficiency virus infection and in connective tissue diseases. Infectious causes of granulomatous disease (ie, mycobacteria) should be excluded before a diagnosis of hypersensitivity pneumonitis is made. In the acute form, pyogenic or viral pneumonia often is misdiagnosed because of accompanying fever and leukocytosis. The recurrence of symptoms in characteristic exposure patterns, however, should alert the physician to the possible diagnosis of hypersensitivity pneumonitis. This diagnosis can be made more definitively by obtaining a detailed history of environmental exposure and by observing typical laboratory findings of leukocytosis, a normal serum IgE level, a restrictive pulmonary function pattern, and evidence of offending antigen serum precipitins.

Organic antigens are related causally to hypersensitivity lung disease, so physicians frequently consider clinical patterns of other similar lung diseases to be equivalent. The most common misconception is the equation of acute bronchopulmonary aspergillosis with hypersensitivity pneumonitis. Table 67-8 contrasts the two disease entities and differentiates hypersensitivity pneumonitis by the lack of wheezing noted on auscultation, the negative results of immediate hypersensitivity skin testing for a suspected offending antigen, and the normal serum IgE levels.

## PATHOPHYSIOLOGY

The name *hypersensitivity pneumonitis* and the association of the condition with the inhalation of a foreign antigen suggest that this disease entity is mediated by immunologic phenomena. Gell and Coombs divided immune tissue injury into four types of hypersensitivity reactions. IgE-mediated, or type I, hypersensitivity might seem to be a likely cause of the lung disease that is observed clinically, yet no evidence exists to support this hypothesis. Serum IgE levels are normal in affected individuals; in fact, antigen-specific IgE levels rarely are elevated. Patients affected with hypersensitivity pneumonitis usually are not atopic. After antigen inhalation, rales, not wheezing, are the typical auscultatory finding, and evidence of bronchospasm is exceedingly rare. Pulmonary symptoms of dyspnea and cough rarely respond to the administration of traditional histamine blockers or mast cell stabilizers such as cromolyn sodium. All the information suggests that type I, IgE-mediated hypersensitivity plays little or no role in the pathogenesis of hypersensitivity pneumonitis.

No data conclusively support a role for type II hypersensitivity, or cytotoxic reactions, in hypersensitivity pneumonitis. Much recent data using rabbits as experimental models for hypersensitivity pneumonitis, however, suggest that types III (Arthus reaction or immune-complex) and IV (cell-mediated or delayed) hypersensitivity play a role in the pathogenesis of this disease entity. The role of immune complex–mediated reactions in the pathogenesis of hypersensitivity pneumonitis is supported most significantly by the Arthus-type reactions that are documented histologically after intradermal skin testing with the suspected offending antigen. Circulating serum immune complexes (ie, serum precipitins) suggest that type III hypersensitivity reactions play a significant role in this clinical response to antigen. The absence of immune complexes at sites of inflammation (ie, lung biopsy) suggests that type III responses do not mediate this disease.

Evidence of type IV or cell-mediated hypersensitivity has been derived primarily from work with hypersensitivity pneumonitis induced in guinea pigs and rabbits. In these models, evidence of local T lymphocyte activation has included enhanced local lymphokine production and increased numbers of local activated T cells recovered in bronchoalveolar lavage fluid. Similar findings of activated (DR+) T lymphocytes in bronchoalveolar lavage specimens in affected humans have been documented, and this proliferation is restricted locally (ie, it is not present in peripheral blood analysis). Affected patients have evidence of granuloma formation at lung biopsy (as high as 70% in one review of patients with farmer's lung). Traditional assays for delayed hypersensitivity such as intradermal skin testing typically show anergy in affected patients. One hypothesis regarding granuloma formation is that inhaled organic dusts may have the capacity, much like inert particles, to induce granuloma formation without immunogenic input.

In summary, the majority of immunologic investigation suggests that hypersensitivity pneumonitis probably is mediated by a combination of immunologic events, including immune complex formation and cell-mediated hypersensitivity.

## TREATMENT AND COMPLICATIONS

The therapy of choice for patients with hypersensitivity pneumonitis is avoidance of the offending agent, if it can be identified.

---

TABLE 67-8. Comparison of Hypersensitivity Pneumonitis and Allergic Bronchopulmonary Disease

| Manifestation | Hypersensitivity Pneumonitis | Allergic Bronchopulmonary Disease |
|---|---|---|
| Physical findings | Rales or rhonchi | Wheezing |
| Chest roentgenograms | Interstitial infiltrates | Lobular infiltrates |
| Pulmonary function | Restrictive | Restrictive and obstructive |
| Blood count | Elevated, with increased polymorphonuclear leukocytes | Eosinophilia |
| Sputum findings | Normal | Eosinophils and mycelia |
| Skin test | Delayed | Immediate and delayed |
| IgE | Normal | Elevated |
| Specific antibodies agent | IgG precipitating | IgE skin sensitizing IgG precipitating |

*Slavin RG. When allergic aspergillosis complicates asthma. J Respir Dis 1981;67:57.*

Because causative agents often are related to a person's occupation, however, patients frequently are reluctant to limit their exposure to the offending antigen. For children, this usually is not a difficult problem. For acute and subacute forms of the disease, avoidance alone often is not sufficient to cause clinical improvement. In these instances, corticosteroid therapy has proven useful in controlling pulmonary exacerbations and reversing some restrictive lung components. Antihistamines and bronchodilators are ineffective therapeutic modalities in patients with acute and subacute hypersensitivity pneumonitis.

With chronic lung disease (interstitial fibrosis, obliterative bronchiolitis), steroid therapy usually is not effective in reversing pulmonary function deficits or improving clinical symptoms. Patients with chronic lung disease occasionally have evidence of obstructive lung disease and sometimes benefit from bronchodilator therapy. Given appropriate clinical suspicion and astute and pertinent historical data collection, these affected individuals should be identified before irreversible lung disease ensues.

## Selected Readings

Fink JN. Hypersensitivity pneumonitis. J Allergy Clin Immunol 1984;74:1.

Gell PGH, Coombs RRA. Clinical aspects of immunology, ed 2. Philadelphia: FA Davis, 1968.

Grammer LC, Roberts M, Lerner C, Patterson R. Clinical and serologic follow-up of four children and five adults with bird-fancier's lung. J Allergy Clin Immunol 1990;85:655.

Mornex JF, Cordier G, Pages J, et al. Activated lung lymphocytes in hypersensitivity pneumonitis. J Allergy Clin Immunol 1984;74:719.

Patterson R, Greenberger PA, Castile RG, et al. Diagnostic problems in hypersensitivity lung disease. Allergy Proc 1989;10:141.

Pitcher WD. Hypersensitivity pneumonitis. Am J Med Sci 1990;300:251.

Reyes CN, Wenzel FT, Lawton BR, Emmanuel DA. The pulmonary pathology of farmer's lung. Chest 1982;81:142.

Salvaggio JE. Hypersensitivity pneumonitis. J Allergy Clin Immunol 1987;79:558.

Slavin RG. When allergic aspergillosis complicates asthma. Journal of Respiratory Diseases 1981;67:57.

Wilson BD, Mondloch VM, Katzenstein AL, Moore VL. Hypersensitivity pneumonitis in rabbits. Modulation of pulmonary inflammation by long-term aerosol challenge with antigen. J Allergy Clin Immunol 1984;74:180.

*Principles and Practice of Pediatrics, Second Edition.*
edited by Frank A. Oski et al. J. B. Lippincott Company, Philadelphia © 1994.

# *67.5* Pneumocystis carinii *Pneumonia*

Donald C. Anderson

*Pneumocystis carinii* pneumonia is an opportunistic infection of increasing importance to pediatricians. A marked increase in the prevalence of this disorder in the United States over the past 2 decades has paralleled therapeutic advances in the management of immunologic and neoplastic diseases, resulting in longer survival of children with these underlying disorders. Most important, this infection is occurring now in epidemic proportions in association with the acquired immunodeficiency syndrome (AIDS).

Two schools of thought exist concerning the taxonomic position of *P carinii*. Most investigators consider it a protozoan to be classified with *Toxoplasma*, but some feel it is a fungus that should be classified with the blastomycetes. It behaves as a protozoan in response to antiprotozoal drugs, and as a fungus with respect to its periodic acid–Schiff and silver staining characteristics. Three developmental forms of this organism have been identified by light microscopy: cysts, "sporozoites," and "trophozoites." When they are identified in lung tissue or respiratory secretions, cysts are spherical or crescent-shaped structures about 5 $\mu$m in diameter, containing as many as eight oval bodies or sporozoites that are 1 to 2 $\mu$m in diameter. The successful propagation of *P carinii* in tissue culture in vitro has allowed characterization of the life cycle of this organism.

The natural habitat of *P carinii* and its mode of transmission in humans remain largely unknown. The occurrence of this organism has been recognized in many wild and laboratory animal species over a wide geographic distribution, but an association between animal reservoirs and human infection has not been established. Before and during World War II, epidemics of interstitial plasma-cell pneumonitis secondary to *P carinii* were recognized in debilitated and premature infants throughout European institutions and nursing homes. The interruption of outbreaks by the introduction of strict isolation of affected patients suggested the probable importance of person-to-person spread of disease within that setting. In the United States, *P carinii* pneumonia was not reported until 1956. In contrast to the early European patterns, American cases have been primarily sporadic and have occurred almost exclusively in children with impaired host defenses. Necropsy studies have demonstrated that inapparent (asymptomatic) infection occurs frequently in patients with cancer or other conditions that cause immunocompromise, but the epidemiologic importance of these asymptomatic carriers in the transmission of pneumocystic disease is unknown. *Pneumocystis* organisms are detected frequently in the sputum, pharyngeal secretions, or tracheal aspirates of symptomatic patients, and cysts have been shown to survive for several months in dried lung specimens maintained at room temperature. These observations suggest that infection probably occurs as a result of inhalation of the organism, which justifies respiratory isolation of symptomatic patients who are exposed to other highly susceptible patients.

The dramatic nature of *P carinii* pneumonitis tends to obscure the fact that its severity is the result of the susceptibility of the host rather than the virulence of the parasite. That *P carinii* is an organism of low pathogenicity is emphasized clearly by the rare occurrence of infections in intact hosts. During the past 2 decades, pneumocystic pneumonia has occurred almost exclusively in patients with primary or acquired immunologic disorders or in those receiving immunosuppressive treatment of oncologic disease or organ transplantation. Of 194 cases reported to the Centers for Disease Control from 1967 through 1970, 29 occurred in infants younger than 1 year, 83% of whom had primary immunodeficiency disorders. In contrast, acute lymphocytic leukemia was the most common underlying disease in children older than 1 year. Of 1251 children with malignancies at the St. Jude Research Hospital (1962 to 1971), *P carinii* pneumonia occurred in 51 (4.1%). Within populations of patients with cancer, *P carinii* occurs more commonly in individuals with generalized lymphoproliferative malignancy than in those with solid tumors. The risk of the development of pneumocystic infections rises with the extent of malignant disease and the intensity of chemotherapy or radiotherapy provided. The precise mechanisms accounting for enhanced susceptibility in individual patients are not understood completely. Pneumocystic pneumonia has been reported in association with congenital and acquired hypogammaglobulinemia, severe combined immunodeficiency disease, selective T cell deficiency (DiGeorge syndrome), AIDS, and secondary immunodeficiency states. The development of specific antibodies to *P carinii* in infected patients has been inconsistent. During the course of "epidemic" disease in malnourished infants, IgM values frequently increase markedly, with variable changes in IgG and IgA values. IgG antibody concentrations increase in the serum 4 to 6 weeks after infection, and are thought to provide permanent immunity in those infants. Experimental evidence suggests that specific antibody fixes complement C3 fragments on the surface of *Pneumocystis* organisms, thereby enabling their subsequent phagocytosis by alveolar macrophages. The importance of impaired cellular immunity in the pathogenesis of *P carinii* pneumonia is evidenced by the ability of corticosteroids or cyclosporin A to induce *P carinii* infection in laboratory animals, the remarkable susceptibility of patients with AIDS to *P carinii* pneumonia (it occurs in at least 50% of these individuals), and the occurrence of *P carinii* pneumonia in malnourished hosts with significantly impaired cellular immune responses.

*P carinii* infections are unique in that the pathologic findings, with rare exceptions, are limited to the lungs, even in fatal cases. In the infantile "epidemic" form of the disease, essentially all alveoli contain large numbers of organisms. Extensive interstitial plasma-cell infiltrates distend alveolar walls to 5 to 20 times their normal thickness, and almost no intra-alveolar fibrinous exudate is noted. In the childhood and adult forms of *P carinii* pneumonia, the histogenesis has been described in three stages. An initial stage is characterized by the presence of cysts and trophozoites attached to alveolar walls. No septal inflammatory or cellular responses are evident, and no clinical disease is associated with this stage. A second stage, which may or may not be associated with clinical signs and symptoms, is characterized by the desquamation of alveolar cells and an increase in the number of cysts within alveolar macrophages. A final stage that definitely is associated with clinical manifestations is typified by extensive reactive and desquamative alveolitis, manifested by marked cytoplasmic vacuolation of macrophages, mononuclear and plasma-cell infiltrates within alveolar septa, and clusters of organisms located predominantly within macrophages in the lumina of alveoli.

The natural course of *P carinii* infections in children is highly variable and depends primarily on the status of host defenses in individual patients. Infantile epidemic pneumocystosis is typified in premature, debilitated, or marasmic infants between the ages of 2 and 6 months. These patients often have chronic diarrhea and weight loss before the development of respiratory symptoms. Characteristically, the onset is insidious, with progression of cough, tachypnea, and respiratory distress over a 1- to 4-week interval. Fever is either absent or low-grade in most cases. Symptoms in immunosuppressed children or adults may be more abrupt in onset and more rapidly progressive than in infantile epidemic cases; in these older patients, the severity and duration of disease before diagnosis are highly variable, but the mortality rate is about 100% if treatment is not provided. Unlike in infantile cases, fever generally is present and high-grade, and it often precedes the onset of a nonproductive cough, tachypnea, and severe dyspnea or the appearance of pulmonary infiltrates on radiography. The onset of clinical disease in high-risk patients is unpredictable, but it often has been observed to occur after the discontinuation of corticosteroid therapy or reduction in drug dosage. Observations suggest that the development of clinical disease depends in part on whether inflammatory responses are normal or are impaired somewhat as a result of the patient's underlying disease, therapeutic regimen, or both.

Physical examination at the time of initial presentation may reveal tachypnea, nasal flaring, and intercostal, subcostal, or supracostal retractions. An ashen color or cyanosis may be present or may develop rapidly. Auscultation of the chest frequently is characterized by a conspicuous absence of adventitious sounds despite rapid (80 to 100 per minute), shallow respirations. Scattered rales, rhonchi, or wheezes usually are detected later in the

clinical course as resolution occurs. Aside from variable temperature elevation, few physical abnormalities are noted except those that are referable to pulmonary disease or secondary to the patient's underlying disease or treatment.

Various radiographic abnormalities have been observed in documented cases of isolated *P carinii* pneumonia. These variations in part are a result of observations being made at different stages in the course of the disease. Bilateral diffuse parenchymal infiltrates are seen most commonly, but no pattern is specific enough either to exclude or to confirm a consideration of *P carinii* disease. Although it initially is a reticulogranular interstitial process, *Pneumocystis* pneumonitis progresses to a predominantly alveolar process, with coalescence and air bronchogram formation. Late in the course of the disease, complete opacification of the lung fields may occur. Hilar adenopathy and pleural effusion are not characteristic unless they are a result of an underlying disorder.

Characteristic clinical features are not specific enough to differentiate *P carinii* pneumonia from other opportunistic pulmonary infections in highly susceptible pediatric patients. Furthermore, mixed infections involving viral, bacterial, fungal, or parasitic opportunists along with *P carinii* have been documented. These observations underscore the importance of establishing a definitive diagnosis before the institution of specific therapy. Because clinical features alone are of little value in making a differential diagnosis, a causative diagnosis can be ascertained only by the demonstration of *P carinii* organisms in lung tissue or respiratory secretions.

A variety of techniques have been used to obtain suitable materials for diagnostic purposes. Although specimens obtained by noninvasive methods from sputum or pharyngeal, tracheal, or gastric secretions occasionally reveal *P carinii* in infected patients, these sources are not sufficiently reliable to exclude the diagnosis if organisms are not identified. Bronchoalveolar lavage, endobronchial brush biopsy, and transbronchial lung biopsy have been used successfully to establish a diagnosis of *P carinii* pneumonia in adult patients. Bronchoalveolar lavage has been shown to be safe and effective, especially in patients with AIDS. These techniques have been employed successfully in infants as young as 2 months of age. Their routine use in children is not justified, however, given the limited experience and significant morbidity associated with these procedures in pediatric patients. Invasive techniques, including open lung biopsy, closed needle biopsy, and percutaneous needle aspiration, are the most reliable methods of confirming a diagnosis. Open lung biopsy provides the most reliable specimen for identification of both the organism and the extent of the infection; its chief disadvantage is that it requires general anesthesia. A closed needle biopsy procedure is less reliable for providing adequate tissue and is associated with significantly greater morbidity than is open thoracotomy. Percutaneous needle aspiration has proved to be a reliable and safe procedure in some centers. The methenamine silver nitrate method of Gomori, and the less widely used but more rapid toluidine blue O stain, are most useful for demonstrating cyst forms in tissue section, aspirates, or imprints. For more detailed morphologic study of intracystic sporozoites and trophozoites, polychrome stains, including the Giemsa, Wright, Gram, and methylene blue stains, are more suitable. In tissue sections, the Gomori stain in combination with the hematoxylin-eosin stain enables the study of both the organism and the host tissue.

Serologic methods, including complement fixation, immunofluorescent testing, enzyme-linked immunosorbent assay, and latex agglutination testing, have been developed, but because of a lack of specificity or sensitivity, these techniques generally are not useful for diagnostic purposes. Moreover, the likelihood that impaired immune responses exist in affected patients precludes the interpretation of serologic results in most cases. A method developed for the detection of *P carinii* antigenemia by countercurrent immunoelectrophoresis has proved unreliable as a means by which to confirm or exclude a diagnosis.

Before the availability of specific therapeutic agents, the overall prognosis of patients with *P carinii* pneumonia was poor. Despite supportive care, almost all infected patients with underlying neoplastic or immunodeficiency disorders succumbed, and as many as 50% of affected infants in the European epidemics died as a result of this pulmonary infection. To control the European epidemics, Ivády and Páldy first suggested the use of pentamidine isethionate, a diamidine with previously demonstrated antifungal and antiprotozoal activity. Use of this therapeutic agent in infants during the next several years resulted in a dramatic reduction in the mortality rate, from 50% to 3.5%. Pentamidine became available to investigators in the United States in 1967, through the Centers for Disease Control. Over the next 3 years, of 163 children and adults with documented *P carinii* pneumonia who were treated with pentamidine, 43% recovered. Of 404 patients to whom the drug was administered for suspected or documented *P carinii* infection, however, 189 (47%) experienced significant toxic manifestations. Toxicity ranged from localized reaction at injection sites (18%) to systemic effects, including impaired renal function (24%), liver toxicity (10%), hypotension (10%), and hypocalcemia (1%). Although pentamidine was effective treatment of this disorder, the high incidence of toxicity emphasized the need for an alternative therapeutic agent.

With the advent of the AIDS epidemic, the intravenous administration of pentamidine was initiated. This allowed a marked reduction in the injection site reactions that had been associated with intramuscular administration, but no decrease in the incidence of the other adverse effects.

Early animal studies and limited investigations in human patients suggested that a combination of pyrimethamine and sulfadiazine might be effective in the treatment of *P carinii* pneumonia. When a somewhat similar combination of trimethoprim and sulfamethoxazole (co-trimoxazole) became available, prospective studies demonstrated the efficacy of this agent to be comparable to that of pentamidine in the treatment of *P carinii* pneumonia complicating childhood leukemia. Of great import, no significant toxicity secondary to co-trimoxazole therapy was observed in these investigations. In additional studies in pediatric patients with cancer, co-trimoxazole also was shown to be effective in the prevention of *P carinii* pneumonia. During one 2-year study period representing 30,000 patient days, 17 of 80 placebo-treated patients (21%) contracted pneumocystic pneumonia, whereas no cases were recognized in 80 patients who were given co-trimoxazole prophylaxis. At present, trimethoprim-sulfamethoxazole appears to be the drug of choice for the treatment and prevention of *P carinii* pneumonia. The therapeutic dosage is 20 mg of trimethoprim and 100 mg of sulfamethoxazole per kilogram per day orally in four equal doses. The intravenous dose is 15 mg of trimethoprim and 75 mg of sulfamethoxazole per kilogram per day in four doses.

Patients with AIDS demonstrate a high rate of adverse reactions to co-trimoxazole as well as to pentamidine. Those who cannot tolerate the former should be treated with intravenous pentamidine at a single daily dose of 4.0 mg/kg. Some potential therapies for treating *P carinii* have not been evaluated sufficiently in pediatric patients. Those with evidence of efficacy include trimethylprim-dapsone, pyrimethamine and sulfadoxine, trimetrexate, clindamycin and primaquine, a new hydroxynaphthoquinone (566C80). In addition to antimicrobial agents, the administration of corticosteroids early in the course of moderately severe pneumonitis reduces the occurrence of respiratory failure and improves oxygenation among adult patients with AIDS.

*P carinii* pneumonitis can be prevented effectively by providing chemoprophylaxis with co-trimoxazole given in a daily dosage of 150 mg of trimethoprim and 750 mg of sulfamethoxazole per square meter, or in the same dosage on only 3 days per week. Use of this regimen can prevent this infection in as much as 95% of high-risk patients, including those with cancer and primary immunodeficiency disorders, and recipients of organ transplants. Guidelines for *P carinii* prophylaxis in infants and children with AIDS have been developed recently. Co-trimoxazole given 3 days per week is the preferred drug. For those who are unable to tolerate this agent, aerosolized pentamidine, 300 mg once monthly, is recommended for children 5 years of age and older, and dapsone, 1.0 mg/kg/d, is suggested for those less than 5 years of age. Although no studies have been carried out to evaluate the recommended regimens rigorously, these guidelines provide the most reasonable approach at this time. Although the chemoprophylactic agents may prevent infectious complications, they do not eradicate *P carinii* organisms. Thus, patients at high risk are protected only while they are receiving chemoprophylaxis, and remain susceptible to infection when the drugs are discontinued.

## Selected Readings

Bommer W. Die interstitielle plasmacellulare pneumoniae and *Pneumocystis carinii*. Ergeb Mikrobiol 1964;39:116.

Burke BA, Good RA. *Pneumocystis carinii* infection. Medicine (Baltimore) 1973;52:23.

Centers for Disease Control Working Group on *P carinii* Pneumonitis Prophylaxis. Guidelines for prophylaxis against *Pneumocystis carinii* pneumonia for children infected with HIV. MMWR 1991;40:1.

Doppman IL, Geelhoed GW, DeVita VT. Atypical radiographic features in *Pneumocystis carinii* pneumonia. Radiology 1975;114:39.

Hughes WT. Trimethoprim-sulfamethoxazole therapy for *Pneumocystis carinii* pneumonitis in children. Rev Infect Dis 1982;4:602.

Hughes WT, Feldman S, Chaudhary S, et al. Comparison of pentamidine isethionate and trimethoprim-sulfamethoxazole in the treatment of *Pneumocystis carinii* pneumonitis. J Pediatr 1973;92:285.

Hughes WT, Kuhn S, Chaudhary S, et al. Successful chemoprophylaxis for *Pneumocystis carinii* pneumonitis. N Engl J Med 1977;297:1419.

Hughes WT, Price R, Kim H, et al. *Pneumocystis carinii* pneumonitis in children with malignancies. J Pediatr 1973;82:404.

Perera D, Western KA, Johnson HD, et al. *Pneumocystis carinii* pneumonia in a hospital for children. Epidemiologic aspects. JAMA 1970;214:1074.

Walzer PD, Schultz MG, Western KA, et al. *Pneumocystis carinii* pneumonia and primary immune deficiency diseases of infancy and childhood. J Pediatr 1973;82:416.

*Principles and Practice of Pediatrics, Second Edition.*
edited by Frank A. Oski et al. J. B. Lippincott Company, Philadelphia © 1994.

# *67.6* Toxocara *Pneumonia*

Donald C. Anderson

Pulmonary manifestations may occur in children as a result of visceral invasion by larvae of a variety of nematode species. The dog ascarid, *Toxocara canis*, accounts for the vast majority of these infestations, which generally are referred to as the visceral larva migrans (VLM) syndrome. Rarely, this disorder may be caused by *Toxocara catis*. The life cycle of *T canis* in the dog corresponds to that of *Ascaris lumbricoides* in its natural human host. *Toxocara* ova ingested by dogs develop into mature nematode worms, ultimately resulting in the excretion of potentially infective ova in feces. Ova of *T canis* are ubiquitous in their geographic distribution, and the chances of children being exposed to contaminated soil are great. Serologic studies in the United States indicate that the prevalence and intensity of *Toxocara* infections are greater in children from southeastern states than in those from western, midwestern, or middle Atlantic states; clay soil types and warm and humid climates in the southeastern region that ensure the survival, concentration, and availability of infective *Toxocara* eggs may explain this geographic distribution. Well-documented studies have shown that one fourth to one third of mature male dogs, one third of puppies, and about one tenth of adult female dogs pass *Toxocara* ova indiscriminately in the stool. Furthermore, the ability of infective ova to withstand a variety of environmental conditions for prolonged periods ensures the maintenance of large soil reservoirs.

Seroepidemiologic studies have shown that *T canis* infections occur in canine animals throughout most of the world, and numerous surveys have documented that viable *Toxocara* eggs can be recovered from surface soils collected in parks, playgrounds, and other public places that are frequented by children. Not unexpectedly, human toxocariasis also has been recognized in most countries of the world. Because most individuals with VLM are asymptomatic, the true incidence of infections is unknown. In a seroprevalence survey of *Toxocara* conducted by the National Health and Human Nutrition Examination Survey in the United States, however, 2.8% of the 8500 sera tested were positive for antibody to *Toxocara* excretory–secretory (TES) antigens. The seroprevalence was as high as 4.6% to 7.3% of children aged 1 to 11 years and was associated strongly with black races, rural residence, and low economic status.

The common occurrence of VLM in children 1 to 4 years of age reflects the prevalence of pica and a close association with pet animals in the toddler age group. Most severe cases of VLM are identified among children aged 18 months to 3 years. Children within this age group with geophagic pica (a compulsion to eat dirt) appear to be at high risk in an environment that is contaminated with *Toxocara* eggs. Older children and adults in similar environments generally are not infected or have milder clinical symptoms, presumably because they do not ingest eggs or are exposed less heavily to them.

With infective *Toxocara*, ova are ingested by an unnatural host, such as humans. Larval forms then hatch and migrate through the intestinal wall, gaining access to a variety of tissues, including the liver, lung, and, less frequently, the eye, kidney, heart, or central nervous system. Larvae migrate in host tissues for an indeterminate interval, and eventually are present within granulomatous inflammatory lesions in end organs. Because invasive larvae are unable to complete their life cycle and develop into mature nematodes, *Toxocara* ova and mature nematode forms are not found in the feces of infected children.

The infective worm burden, in addition to variable host responses, determines the extent of infestation. As few as 100 *T canis* ova have been shown to produce prompt eosinophilia, with the subsequent development of pulmonary infiltrates in adult patients. Chronic eosinophilia developed in two pediatric patients (20% to 40% of total white blood cells ranging from 10,000 to 35,000/mm³), but no clinical disease occurred when 200 embryonated ova of *T canis* were administered. In contrast, autopsy studies in some pediatric patients have demonstrated that heavy infestation with extensive multiorgan involvement may occur. Quantitative estimations of granulomatous lesions (with and without larvae) in one reported infant case revealed 60, 5, and 3 to 5 larvae per gram of liver, muscle, and brain, respectively.

Surface protein–polysaccharide complexes of ascarid larvae contain multiple determinants, of which some are antigenic, stimulating host production of precipitating IgM and IgG antibodies, and others are allergenic, being responsible for reaginic IgE production. Clinical features such as urticaria and true asthmatic wheezing correlate with the development of elevated IgE

antibody levels in patients with VLM. Eosinophilic leukocytosis represents a universal, although relatively late, host response in patients with VLM and other forms of visceral parasitism. Elevated circulating eosinophil counts generally are not observed until after peak humoral antibody responses have developed. Antigen–non-IgE antibody complexes are known to activate complement components that are cytotactic for eosinophils, and IgE antigen interactions with mast cells or basophils liberate chemical mediators of eosinophil locomotion. Consideration of these diverse host responses in infested patients suggests that immune mechanisms participate actively in the pathogenesis of VLM. Pulmonary manifestations, it appears, are not only the result of larval migration through lung parenchyma, but also relate to specific immunologic host responses.

VLM generally is characterized by fever, hepatomegaly, irritability, pulmonary symptoms, and anemia, but it may be manifested by localized infection (eg, in the eye) or by eosinophilia without any signs or symptoms. The vast majority of infested patients are clinically asymptomatic. In a large series of symptomatic patients with VLM, cough occurred in 80% and wheezing was documented in 63%. Physical examination in the same group revealed rales, wheezes, or both in only 43%. Cough usually was chronic (of greater than 3 weeks' duration), paroxysmal, more severe at night, and associated with recurrent wheezing. In rare patients in that series, respiratory distress was severe enough to require hospitalization. Radiographic abnormalities, usually characterized as diffuse, bilateral, or migratory infiltrates, often occur in the absence of respiratory symptoms. The occurrence of severe pulmonary symptoms correlates with other generalized features, including eosinophilia, urticaria, and fever.

A specific diagnosis of toxocariasis is difficult to confirm. A positive history of pica in affected children raises the clinician's index of suspicion, but only a presumptive diagnosis can be entertained based on this and other clinical features. Specific diagnostic confirmation depends on the demonstration of larval forms in tissues such as liver or enucleated eye. The most consistent and significant hematologic abnormality is moderate to marked eosinophilia. Total white blood cell counts as high as 100,000 per cubic millimeter may be seen, with the proportion of eosinophils varying between 20% and 90%. Hyperglobulinemia represents another consistent, but nonspecific, feature. Values ranging between 4 and 7 g/dL are common, with the greatest increase occurring in the IgM fraction. A striking increase in isohemagglutinin titers is noted commonly. Patients of blood group O have been found to have anti-A and anti-B titers as high as 1:8 million. Heterophil antibodies absorbed by guinea pig kidney but removed only partially after exposure to beef erythrocytes also have been demonstrated in some patients.

More specific serologic tests to help confirm a diagnosis of toxocariasis include indirect hemagglutination tests, bentonite flocculation tests, radioimmunoassays, and an enzyme-linked immunosorbent assay (ELISA). In the United States, an ELISA that employs TES antigens has proved to be the most useful tool for diagnostic or epidemiologic purposes. Some TES antigens are not species or genus specific, accounting for cross-reactivity in serologic assessments of infected patients. Some sera from patients with ascariasis, filariasis, and strongyloidiasis also show cross-reactivity with TES antigens. Demonstration of a positive ELISA TES titer may reflect only a previous infestation that is not relevant to the patient's clinical illness. The sensitivity of ELISA for the more limited syndrome of ocular larval migrans is significantly less than for VLM.

A variety of anti-inflammatory and antihelminthic agents have been used in the treatment of toxocariasis, but no controlled data are available for adequate evaluation of these regimens. Corticosteroids have been used to attenuate inflammatory responses in patients with severe (life-threatening) pulmonary manifestations, resulting in dramatic resolution of symptoms and radiographic infiltrates. Thiabendazole, an absorbable antihelminthic agent with additional anti-inflammatory, antipyretic, and analgesic properties, has been shown to attenuate the clinical course of VLM in selected patients. Similarly, symptomatic improvement and reduction in eosinophilic leukocytosis have been observed in selected patients after diethylcarbamazine therapy.

The most important consideration in the approach to *Toxocara* infestations in children lies in preventing exposure of the susceptible child to infective ova. Private and public health measures, including control of indiscriminate dog defecation, examination and deworming of pet dogs, and laws to prevent roaming canine populations, are fundamental to the prevention of toxocariasis. In children with active disease, measures must be instituted to prevent the continued ingestion of contaminated soil. Because common-source infections within households have been documented, serologic testing of household members and attempts to identify a source of infective ova also should be considered.

## Selected Readings

Anderson DC, Greenwood R, Fishman M, et al. Acute infantile hemiplegia with cerebrospinal fluid eosinophilic pleocytosis: An unusual case of visceral larva migrans. J Pediatr 1975;66:247.
Dent JH, Nichols RL, Beaver PC, et al. Visceral larva migrans with a case report. Am J Pathol 1956;32:777.
Glickman LT, Schantz PM. Epidemiology and pathogenesis of zoonotic toxocanosis. Epidemiol Rev 1981;3:230.
Herman N, Glickman LT, Schantz PM. Seroprevalence of zoonotic toxocariasis in the United States. Am J Epidemiol 1985;122:890.
Huntley CC, Costas MC, Lyerly AD. Visceral larva migrans syndrome; clinical characteristics and immunologic studies in 51 patients. Pediatrics 1965;36:523.
Huntley CC, Lyerly AD, Patterson MV. Isohemagglutinins in parasitic infections. JAMA 1969;208:1145.
Schantz PM, Glickman LT. Toxocaral visceral larva migrans. N Engl J Med 1978;298:436.
Snyder CH. Visceral larva migrans—ten years' experience. Pediatrics 1961;28:85.
Webb CH. Pets, parasites, and pediatrics. Pediatrics 1965;36:521.
Wodey G, Green JA, Frothingham TE, et al. *Toxocara canis* infection: Clinical and epidemiological associations with seropositivity in kindergarten children. J Infect Dis 1984;149:591.

*Principles and Practice of Pediatrics, Second Edition.*
edited by Frank A. Oski et al. J. B. Lippincott Company, Philadelphia © 1994.

# 67.7 *Bacterial Pneumonia*

## John F. Modlin

In the United States, recognized infection of the lower respiratory tract occurs annually in 15 to 20 per 1000 infants less than 1 year of age and in 30 to 40 per 1000 children 1 to 5 years of age. Although the respiratory viruses and *Mycoplasma pneumoniae* are the most common agents of lower respiratory tract disease in children and young adults, pyogenic bacteria cause a substantial minority of cases of pneumonia; a recent study found that bacteria were responsible for 19% of pneumonia cases among ambulatory children. Bacterial pneumonia is observed most often in the winter and early spring, and occurs almost twice as frequently in males as in females.

Diseases involving the airways, such as bronchopulmonary dysplasia, cystic fibrosis, and bronchiectasis, and anatomic defects, such as cleft palate or tracheoesophageal fistula, predispose to the development of bacterial pneumonia. Pneumonia and lung abscess are common infections in children with severe cognitive neurologic disorders or diminished levels of consciousness. Children with hemoglobinopathies, especially sickle-cell disease, have higher rates of bacterial pneumonia. Children who are immunodeficient on the basis of inherited or acquired disease, or because they are receiving immunosuppressive therapy have an increased risk of pneumonia from a wide spectrum of bacteria in addition to viruses, fungi, protozoa, and parasites. The diagnosis and management of opportunistic pulmonary infections that occur in immunocompromised children are covered in other sections of this book.

In practice, bacterial pneumonia may be difficult to distinguish from other forms of pneumonia. Young children do not produce adequate sputum for Gram stain and culture, and more invasive procedures are not warranted except in a few patients who are severely ill or have underlying immunodeficiency.

## ETIOLOGY

The age of the child and the presence or absence of underlying disease are the two most important patient characteristics determining the cause of bacterial pneumonia. Bacterial pneumonia presenting in the first 2 days of life, which generally is considered to be acquired in utero or intrapartum, is caused by the same organisms that are responsible for generalized neonatal sepsis (ie, group B streptococci, *Listeria monocytogenes*, *Haemophilus influenzae*, and gram-negative enteric bacilli). Most cases of perinatally acquired pneumonia occur among low–birth-weight infants and infants who have peripartum complications. These infants may have an increased risk of nosocomial pneumonia caused by *Pseudomonas aeruginosa*, *Escherichia coli*, or other gram-negative bacilli if they require endotracheal intubation and mechanical ventilation.

After the neonatal period, *Streptococcus pneumoniae*, *H influenzae*, type b, *Staphylococcus aureus*, and group A streptococci are responsible for virtually all cases of bacterial pneumonia in otherwise healthy children. Rare cases may be caused by *Neisseria meningitidis*, anaerobic bacteria, *Salmonella* species, *Bordetella pertussis*, *Legionella* species, *Klebsiella pneumoniae*, and other gram-negative enteric bacilli. In patients older than 4 or 5 years, the spectrum of bacteria causing pneumonia narrows, with *S pneumoniae* and *M pneumoniae* predominating. *Mycoplasma* infections are unusual in young children, but are quite common after the age of 5 years. Recent studies have found that antibodies to the newly identified agent *Chlamydia pneumoniae* begin to be acquired in middle childhood, but disease caused by this agent has not been characterized well in children.

## PATHOGENESIS

The respiratory tract below the vocal cords normally is sterile; microorganisms are excluded from the tracheobronchial tree by nonspecific host defenses, including the blanket of mucus covering the mucosal epithelium, ciliary transport activity, and the cough reflex. Secretory IgA antibody present in mucosal secretions helps to protect against reinfection with specific organisms. Within the lung parenchyma, bacteria are cleared by lymphatic channels that drain particulate matter to regional lymph nodes and by macrophages that line the terminal bronchioles and alveoli. The lung also is protected by systemic humoral and cell-mediated immune mechanisms, including passively acquired maternal antibody, which protects against pneumococcal and *H influenzae*, type b infections in the first few months of life. Alteration of any of these protective mechanisms is likely to predispose the child to the development of bacterial pneumonia.

Most bacterial pathogens that cause pneumonia in children are transmitted person-to-person via close personal contact or airborne spread. Colonization of the upper respiratory tract of young children with pathogenic bacteria is relatively common; the prevalence for carriage of pneumococci, *H influenzae*, type b, and meningococci, is about 40%, 10%, and 2%, respectively. Pneumonia results from the aspiration of pathogenic bacteria into the lower respiratory tract; the process often is aided by concurrent viral infection, particularly with respiratory syncytial virus, measles virus, and the influenza viruses. Careful studies have documented the coexistence of a respiratory virus in 30% to 50% of all children with bacterial pneumonia. Acute viral infection serves to disrupt the normal anatomic and physiologic barriers of the respiratory tract mucosa, and may suppress briefly the activity of phagocytic leukocytes in the airways and lung. Less commonly, bacteria spread to the lung in a hematogenous manner from a distant focus, such as bacterial endocarditis or soft-tissue infection. In these instances, pneumonia may occur in the setting of widespread pyogenic infection of other sites, including the meninges, bones, and joints.

## CLINICAL FEATURES

The signs and symptoms of bacterial pneumonia vary with the age of the child, the infecting organism, and the presence or absence of underlying disease. Older children and adolescents characteristically have fever, chills, headache, dyspnea, productive cough, chest pain, abdominal pain, and nausea or vomiting. Young infants, however, are likely to have the largely nonspecific symptoms of fever, lethargy, poor feeding, vomiting, or diarrhea. Tachypnea may be overlooked by the parents, and cough, if present, often is not a prominent finding in very young infants. Similarly, the findings on physical examination of young infants with pneumonia are less definitive; percussion and auscultation usually do not elicit the characteristic dullness to percussion and decreased breath sounds that are found in older children and adults with pneumonia, and rales may be difficult to distinguish from the sounds produced by a congested upper respiratory tract.

## COMPLICATIONS OF BACTERIAL PNEUMONIA

A parapneumonic effusion, or the presence of fluid in the pleural space, may be caused by congestive heart failure, malignancy, or collagen vascular disease, as well as by infection within the parenchyma of the lung. The composition of a parapneumonic effusion resulting from infection can vary from a thin, serous transudate with few white blood cells (WBCs), a low protein content, and a pH level of more than 7.2, to a thick, purulent exudate (or empyema) in which the WBC count is greater than 15,000/mm$^3$, the protein content is more than 3.0 g/dL, and the pH level is greater than 7.2. A serous exudate and an empyema may represent the extremes in the natural history of pleural space involvement from underlying bacterial infection of the lung, which progresses from an exudative phase, to a fibropurulent phase (empyema) with the accumulation of polymorphonuclear leukocytes and fibrin, then to an organizing, fibrous layer or "peel" that is adherent to the visceral and parietal pleural surfaces and ultimately may restrict expansion of the lung. *S aureus*, *H influenzae*, and *S pneumoniae* represent the major causes of empyema, whereas $\alpha$-hemolytic streptococci, gram-negative enteric bacilli, and anaerobes cause occasional cases. Parapneumonic effusions secondary to viral or mycoplasmal pneumonia are uncommon, and usually are composed of a transudate of low volume when they occur.

Parapneumonic effusions are found more often in young children and in males. The presence of fluid in the pleural space results in continued fever, chest pain, and dyspnea, and in tachycardia, dullness to percussion, and diminished breath sounds on physical examination. A chest radiograph with the patient in the lateral decubitus position demonstrates layering of free pleural fluid. About half the cases are unilateral. Loculation of fluid, which occurs in about 75% of all cases of frank empyema, may inhibit dependent layering of the effusion on the lateral decubitus film. If necessary, computerized tomography of the chest will demonstrate the presence of loculated pleural fluid. Characterization of the pleural fluid is critical in the diagnosis and subsequent treatment of parapneumonic effusions. The character and volume of the aspirated fluid are noted, and samples are sent to the laboratory for WBC and differential count; Gram stain; bacterial culture; assay for pneumococcal and *H influenzae*, type b polysaccharide antigens; pH level measurement; and determination of glucose, protein, and lactic dehydrogenase content. Studies in adults have shown that concentrations of glucose of less than 40 mg/dL, a lactic dehydrogenase level of more than 1000 IU/dL, and a pH level of less than 7.2 are better predictors of a positive bacterial culture and the need for thoracotomy tube drainage than are WBC and protein content.

Management of parapneumonic effusions associated with bacterial pneumonia consists of antibiotic administration and drainage of the pleural fluid. Drainage frequently can be accomplished by needle aspiration during the exudative stage, although more than one aspiration procedure may be required. Empyema requires the insertion of one or more thoracotomy tubes, which sometimes must be repositioned to drain loculated areas of purulent fluid. The tubes generally are withdrawn when drainage ceases, usually after a period of 3 to 5 days. Open thoracotomy and drainage procedures rarely are required in the treatment of empyema in children. The clinical response to the treatment of empyema is characteristically slow; fever, chest pain, and irritability may persist for 1 to 2 weeks, although stabilization of vital signs and improvement of systemic oxygenation occur more rapidly. Clearing of abnormalities on the chest radiograph may take weeks to months. In most children, there is gradual improvement of pulmonary function with little or no long-term restrictive lung abnormality. Surgical decortication of the organized peel no longer is performed in children, except in unusual circumstances. The overall mortality rate for empyema in children is 6% to 12%, but may be higher in young infants and in patients with staphylococcal empyema. Superinfection of the pleural space with other bacteria is an unusual complication of chest tube placement.

Pneumatoceles are thin-walled cavities that develop in the lung during the course of bacterial pneumonia. Pneumatoceles complicate about 40% of all cases of staphylococcal pneumonia and are unusual complications of pneumonia due to *S pneumoniae*; *H influenzae*, type b; group A streptococci; and gram-negative enteric bacilli. Pneumatoceles are asymptomatic except when they rupture into the pleural space, causing a pneumothorax or pyopneumothorax. Most persist for 2 to 3 months and resolve spontaneously.

Lung abscesses arise at the site of a necrotizing pneumonia that follows the aspiration of oropharyngeal secretions containing normal bacterial flora of the upper respiratory tract. Children with severe mental–motor retardation, seizure disorders, poor oral hygiene, and periodontal disease are particularly susceptible to the development of lung abscesses. Dependent segments of the lung are the usual locations of abscess formation, that is, the posterior segment of the right upper lobe and the superior segments of the right lower lobe and the left lower lobe. Anaerobic bacteria play a prominent role in abscess formation. One or more species of oral anaerobes usually are recovered from abscess cavities, with or without aerobic bacteria such as streptococci, staphylococci, or gram-negative enteric bacilli.

Fever, cough, tachypnea, and a fetid breath odor are the major presenting manifestations of lung abscess. Chest radiography reveals a focal infiltrate surrounding a cavity that may contain an air–fluid level; about 10% of all patients have more than one cavity. Fiberoptic bronchoscopy may be employed to obtain a specimen directly from the abscess cavity for diagnostic purposes. Although a 3- to 4-week course of penicillin G is the traditional therapy for lung abscess in children, either metronidazole, clindamycin, or ampicillin combined with a β-lactamase inhibitor (eg, Augmentin, Unasyn) may be preferable, because studies (in adults) indicate that 10% to 20% of lung abscesses now harbor oral anaerobic bacteria that are penicillin-resistant.

## DIAGNOSIS

In practice, the diagnosis of pneumonia is made with the demonstration of infiltrates on anteroposterior and lateral chest radiographs. (Keep in mind that many noninfectious diseases of the lung may mimic the radiographic appearance of pneumonia, including malignancy, collagen vascular disease, congestive heart failure, pulmonary embolus, allergic alveolitis, pulmonary hemorrhage, and hemosiderosis.) A pattern of peribronchial or "patchy" infiltrates (bronchopneumonia) does not distinguish viral or mycoplasmal pneumonia from bacterial pneumonia, but demonstration of hyperinflation is most consistent with viral infection. The presence of lobar consolidation or pleural effusion is suggestive of bacterial infection, whereas pneumatoceles and abscess cavities are diagnostic. Lobar consolidation, which is present in about half of all children with bacterial pneumonia, correlates with the presence of bacteremia. Roentgenograms demonstrate bilateral disease in 20% to 25% of pediatric patients. Spherical infiltrates, which are seen infrequently early in the course of pneumococcal pneumonia, may be confused with a metastatic neoplasm of the lung. Resolution of the pulmonary infiltrates will lag behind clinical improvement of the patient. Routine follow-up radiographs contribute little to the treatment of a child with an uncomplicated course of pneumonia.

A WBC count and differential, and an erythrocyte sedimentation rate test are performed routinely on all pediatric patients with suspected pneumonia. An attempt to determine the cause of the infection should be made in all cases of suspected bacterial pneumonia in hospitalized children. Cultures of blood and pleural fluid, if the latter is present, usually are obtained from children who require hospitalization. Gram stain of expectorated sputum may be of considerable value in the diagnosis of pneumonia in a school-age child or adolescent, especially when a single organism is seen in association with polymorphonuclear leukocytes, and culture of an adequate sputum specimen usually yields the pathogenic organism. Infants and young children are incapable of producing a spontaneous sputum specimen, however, and efforts to induce sputum in younger children generally are unsuccessful. Cultures of the nasopharynx and throat are not useful and should not be attempted because of the risk of producing misleading information. Invasive procedures such as bronchoalveolar lavage or open lung biopsy are justified in cases of pneumonia that are severe or complicated by underlying disease. Transtracheal aspiration is a technique that has proven very useful in adult patients, but most pediatricians have little or no experience with it. Direct transthoracic needle aspiration of the lung has proven to be useful in cases in which recovery of an organism is critical for treatment.

## TREATMENT

The treatment of pneumonia depends on the severity of the illness and the presence or absence of underlying chronic disease. In practice, children with mild to moderate pneumonia often are treated as outpatients. Some physicians choose to withhold antibiotic therapy for cases that, in their judgment, are more likely to have a viral cause. Other physicians prefer to "cover" with an oral antibiotic that is effective against the most likely bacterial pathogens. Oral penicillin V or erythromycin often are used for outpatient treatment of older children and adolescents with pneumonia. Erythromycin often is considered the drug of choice for this age group because of its activity against M pneumoniae, but as many as 5% to 20% of group A streptococci and clinical isolates of S pneumoniae may be resistant. For children less than 5 years of age, amoxicillin-clavulanate (Augmentin) is an excellent choice for oral therapy. Even though ampicillin and amoxicillin are used widely in oral therapy for pneumonia in young children, they are ineffective against 10% to 30% of the strains of H influenzae, type b and β-lactamase–producing strains of S aureus. For hospitalized children with more serious disease, antibiotics and maintenance of adequate oxygenation are the mainstays of treatment of bacterial pneumonia; chest physical therapy and intermittent positive-pressure treatments are of little additional benefit. Antibiotics should be chosen that are effective against the major bacterial pathogens expected, given the child's age. Initial therapy can be guided by the results of a sputum Gram stain and can be modified, if necessary, once the results of cultures of blood, sputum, or pleural fluid are reported. A variety of options are available for parenteral antibiotic treatment of the infant or young child with suspected bacterial pneumonia, including ampicillin-sulbactam (Unasyn), cefuroxime, a third-generation cephalosporin, or the combination of oxacillin and chloramphenicol.

## PNEUMONIA CAUSED BY SPECIFIC BACTERIAL PATHOGENS

S pneumoniae is a common cause of pneumonia in patients of all ages. Serotypes 1, 3, 6, 7, 14, 18, 19, and 23 are the most common of the 84 serotypes found in children, differing slightly from the distribution of serotypes that cause bacteremia pneumonia in adults. Pleural effusion occurs in a minority of cases, but frank empyema is unusual, and pneumatocele formation is quite rare. About 30% of children with pneumococcal pneumonia have positive blood culture results when they are first seen, a finding that is associated with more severe disease. Rapid resolution of fever and dyspnea with appropriate antibiotic therapy is the rule, but prolonged courses occur, especially with extensive lung involvement and with empyema. The mortality rate in children is about 10%, and there is little or no residual impairment of lung function. Rare complications include pericarditis, meningitis, endocarditis, arthritis, and bursitis.

H influenzae, type b pneumonia is indistinguishable clinically and radiographically from pneumococcal pneumonia and is nearly as common in children less than 2 years of age. Seventy-five percent to 90% of children with H influenzae pneumonia have positive blood culture results, however, and 40% to 75% have accompanying pleural effusions. Importantly, 10% to 30% of children with H influenzae pneumonia also have meningitis, epiglottitis, or another serious pyogenic infection. The mortality rate is 5% to 10%.

S aureus pneumonia appears to be less common now than it was in the past, but it remains an important cause of serious pneumonia, especially in infants younger than 6 months. Staphylococcal pneumonia presents initially similar to pneumonia of other causes, but progresses characteristically to pneumatocele formation and empyema, even in the presence of appropriate antibiotic therapy. Although recovery of staphylococci from the blood occurs in only 10% of affected infants, organisms usually are present in large numbers in a gram-stained tracheal aspirate. Mortality resulting from staphylococcal pneumonia is 20% to 30%, and recovery in survivors may take weeks.

## Selected Readings

Ajello GW, Bolan GA, Hayes PS, et al. Commercial latex agglutination tests for detection of *Haemophilus influenzae* type b and bacteremic pneumonia. J Clin Microbiol 1987;25:1388.

Freij BJ, Kusmiesz H, Nelson JD, McCracken GH. Parapneumonic effusions and empyema in hospitalized children: A retrospective review of 227 cases. Pediatr Infect Dis 1984;3:578.

Glezen WP, Loda FA, Clyde WA, et al. Epidemiologic patterns of acute lower respiratory disease of children in a pediatric practice. J Pediatr 1971;78:397.

Hughes JR, Sinha DP, Cooper MR, et al. Lung tap in childhood: Bacteria, viruses, and mycoplasmas in acute lower respiratory tract infections. Pediatrics 1969;44:477.

Jacobs NM, Harris VJ. Acute *Haemophilus* pneumonia in childhood. Am J Dis Child 1979;133:603.

Klein JO. Diagnostic lung puncture in the pneumonias of infants and children. Pediatrics 1969;44:486.

Light RW, Girard WM, Jenkinson SG, George RB. Parapneumonic effusions. Am J Med 1980;69:507.

Mimica I, Donoso E, Howard JE, et al. Lung puncture in the etiologic diagnosis of pneumonia: A study of 543 infants and children. Am J Dis Child 1971;122:278.

Peter G. The child with pneumonia: Diagnostic and therapeutic considerations. Pediatr Infect Dis J 1988;7:453.

Teele D. Pneumonia: Antimicrobial therapy for infants and children. Pediatr Infect Dis 1985;4:330.

Turner RB, Lande AE, Chase P, et al. Pneumonia in pediatric outpatients: Cause and clinical manifestations. J Pediatr 1987;111:194.

*Principles and Practice of Pediatrics, Second Edition.*
edited by Frank A. Oski et al. J. B. Lippincott Company, Philadelphia © 1994.

# CHAPTER 68
# *Foreign Bodies*

## Martin I. Lorin

Foreign bodies in the respiratory tract are a common and important pediatric problem. From the nose to the distal airways, the respiratory tree has been the recipient of a wide range of unnatural, exogenous materials. Aspiration of foreign bodies remains a major cause of morbidity and mortality in children.

## NOSE

Nasal foreign bodies usually are more of an annoyance than a threat to life. The majority are inserted by toddlers or preschoolers, more often mischievously than truly accidentally. Occasionally, a piece of tissue inserted to stop a nosebleed miraculously will avoid dislodgment and stay in place for days to weeks. The classic finding is a persistent, unilateral, purulent nasal discharge that may be blood-tinged. Foul odor is common. Although they generally are not considered to be very dangerous, nasal foreign bodies have dislodged posteriorly and been aspirated, either spontaneously or during an attempt at removal. Although the diagnosis should be readily apparent, the foreign body occasionally is obscured by copious or dried secretions. Alternatively, the foreign object may be misinterpreted as a nasal polyp.

Removal of most nasal foreign bodies is accomplished readily in the office without general anesthesia. Sedation may be required, but even this usually is not necessary.

Soft or irregularly shaped objects that can be grasped easily by forceps are best removed in this way. Removal of a round, hard object, such as a bead, is accomplished best by insertion of an ear curet past the foreign body and then application of gentle forward pressure.

## UPPER AIRWAY (LARYNX AND TRACHEA)

Aspiration of foreign material into the larynx and trachea occurs frequently and, not uncommonly, proves lethal. It has been estimated that aspiration of foreign bodies into the upper airway is the second leading cause of accidental death in the home among children younger than 5 years. In most cases, the diagnosis is immediately evident. Sometimes, however, a child may aspirate while asleep or alone and may be seen either as a sudden, unexpected death or with the sudden onset of severe respiratory distress. Although the aspirated material usually is a piece of food or candy, a variety of other objects have been recovered from the larynx and trachea. The plastic cap of a water pistol, a fragment of balloon, and a piece of bubble gum are examples of objects that have been recovered at autopsy.

Very small foreign objects in the trachea generally are not life-threatening. Although one would imagine that such objects would promptly be coughed out or aspirated more deeply, in reality, this is not always the case; they may remain in the trachea for days or even weeks, often becoming embedded in granulation tissue. Although the predominant clinical feature is inspiratory stridor, associated expiratory wheezing is present in about 25% to 50% of cases. Cases have been misdiagnosed as croup or tumors. Eggshell, plastic toys or parts of toys, and watermelon seeds are examples of objects that have remained in the trachea for extended periods.

Signs and symptoms of an upper airway foreign body may be mimicked by a foreign body in the esophagus that is pressing on the posterior trachea. Remarkably, in some cases, such foreign bodies cause stridor or wheezing without any dysphasia or difficulty in swallowing.

It is not surprising that the treatment of acute, life-threatening upper airway obstruction due to a foreign body is controversial. The great majority of patients with this catastrophic event are treated in the field, usually by someone who is not a physician. By the very nature of the condition, few patients requiring urgent treatment survive to reach the hospital without intervention. Consequently, most "experts" and "authorities" writing about this process have had little direct experience in treating such patients. Obviously, it is not possible to carry out controlled studies in humans. Available data are from anecdotal case reports, studies in anesthetized animals (some of whom had an endotracheal tube in place during the experiment), mechanical models, and theoretic considerations.

Controversy was heightened in 1974, when Dr. Heimlich introduced and popularized the maneuver that bears his name. Before this time, back slaps and blind finger-sweeps of the pharynx were standard emergency treatment of choking children and adults. There is no doubt that some lives were saved by each of these maneuvers.

To perform the abdominal thrust (Heimlich maneuver) with the victim sitting or standing, the rescuer stands behind the patient with his or her arms wrapped around the victim's abdomen and one fist grabbed by the other hand, slightly above the navel and well below the xiphoid process. The rescuer then forces the fist into the abdomen with a quick upward thrust. If the patient is supine, the rescuer places the heel of one hand, with the other hand on top, on the abdomen in the location described above and then exerts a sudden upward pressure in the midline. Back blows are applied with the heel of the hand high between the scapulae. Chest thrusts are similar to external cardiac compression, delivered smartly as four thrusts.

Proponents of the Heimlich maneuver claim that back blows may drive the foreign body further into the airway, whereas proponents of back blows claim that the Heimlich maneuver is dangerous to abdominal viscera, especially the liver in infants. Each group extolls its method as more effective as well as safer.

The current recommendations of the American Academy of Pediatrics are as follows. If the victim can speak, breathe, or cough, all interfering maneuvers are unnecessary and dangerous. The patient should be permitted to try to clear the obstructing object by spontaneous cough while preparations are made for emergency transportation to the nearest medical facility.

If intervention is required for a choking child who is over 1 year of age, the first maneuver should be a series of abdominal thrusts (Heimlich maneuver), as described above. If this fails to relieve the obstruction, examination of the oral cavity and pharynx and removal of the obstructing object under direct visualization are attempted. (Blind finger-sweeps of the hypopharynx are not recommended.) If airway patency and breathing are not achieved by these maneuvers, mouth-to-mouth resuscitation is attempted. If this fails, abdominal thrusts are repeated.

For a youngster who is 1 year of age or less, abdominal thrusts are not recommended. The child is positioned on his or her abdomen, in a head-down position at 60°, and is supported on the rescuer's thigh or forearm. A series of five back blows are delivered rapidly. If this fails to relieve the obstruction, the child is turned over, face up, and five chest thrusts are administered. If this also fails, the pharynx should be visualized, as described above. If the foreign body cannot be seen and removed, mouth-to-mouth resuscitation is attempted. If obstruction persists, the sequence of back blows and chest thrusts is repeated.

## LOWER AIRWAYS (BRONCHI)

The majority of aspirated foreign bodies either are coughed out promptly or lodge beyond the carina, in a major bronchus or more distal airway. The peak incidence of pulmonary aspiration of foreign bodies in children is between the first and second birthdays. More than 90% of foreign body aspiration occurs before the fifth birthday. The variety of foreign bodies that have been aspirated is impressive. The peanut is the most notorious object to be aspirated by young children, accounting for almost 50% of cases in one series of patients. Why the peanut is aspirated so frequently while other objects of similar size such as raisins rarely are aspirated does not appear to have been studied; the relatively hard, smooth, and slippery surface of the nut may be a major contributing factor. Other items commonly aspirated include sunflower seeds, aspirin tablets, pieces of apple (including the stem and pits), teeth, and toys. Unfortunately, most aspirated foreign bodies are radiolucent. Blazer reported that only 4% of pulmonary foreign bodies studied were radiopaque. Some objects, such as eggshell and the aluminum pull tabs from soft-drink containers, are barely radiopaque. These objects can be visualized

on a chest roentgenogram, but often have been missed when the film was not scrutinized closely.

In the classic case (which, of course, is seen only occasionally), a previously well toddler suddenly starts to choke and cough, often while eating, playing with a toy, or crawling on a carpet. The coughing and choking subside, only to be followed by wheezing. Often, however, there is no history to suggest a discrete episode of aspiration, or the episode is recalled only in retrospect when the foreign body has been removed and identified. The onset of symptoms may be gradual. Occasionally, the onset may coincide fortuitously with an upper respiratory tract infection and fever, making diagnosis especially difficult.

If the foreign body is relatively large and, consequently, is impacted in a major or lobar bronchus, symptoms generally are acute, with wheezing and respiratory distress. If the foreign body is relatively small and lodges in a segmental bronchus, symptoms are more likely to be chronic, with persistent cough, wheezing, and signs of pulmonary infection.

Although wheezing is one of the most common signs associated with a pulmonary foreign body, it is far from invariably present. Blazer reported that, in a 1980 study of children with bronchial foreign bodies, wheezing was exhibited in only 60% and stridor in only 13%.

To a large extent, the clinical picture, especially the physical and roentgenographic findings, is dictated by whether the foreign body causes partial or total obstruction of the bronchus in which it resides. Partial obstruction results in wheezing that is predominantly expiratory and may be either unilateral (on the side of the foreign body) or bilateral. In some cases of bilateral wheezing, the expiratory wheeze is clearly louder over the ipsilateral hemithorax. It is not clear whether the contralateral wheezing in these cases represents a generalized reflex bronchoconstriction or merely transmission of the wheezing sound. Partial obstruction results in a check-valve mechanism in the airway, with progressive air trapping in the involved lung, lobe, or segment. On physical examination, breath sounds may be decreased over the involved lung, and the trachea and cardiac impulse are shifted *away* from the involved lung. Tachypnea and retractions are common. Cyanosis generally is seen only in severe cases, usually when the foreign body is obstructing a major bronchus. Radiographically, obstructive emphysema involving a lung, lobe, or segment is the hallmark of a foreign body that is partially occluding an airway. In some cases, the overexpansion of the involved lung is mild and not discernible on an ordinary roentgenogram of the chest. In such situations, fluoroscopy, inspiratory and expiratory roentgenograms, or right and left decubitus films may show an apparent shift of the mediastinum away from the involved lung during expiration. This results from the fact that the uninvolved lung is able to empty and, therefore, gets smaller during expiration, whereas the involved lung is obstructed and remains hyperinflated. Visually, this appears as if the mediastinum were moving away from the involved lung.

When the foreign body occludes the involved airway completely, the result is atelectasis rather than hyperaeration. Clinically, this is evident by decreased breath sounds, with or without rales. Although the trachea and cardiac impulse usually are unchanged, in severe cases, they may be shifted *toward* the involved lung. Chest roentgenography will reveal atelectasis of the affected area.

Fever, rales, purulent sputum, and radiographic evidence of pneumonia can occur with either partial or complete occlusion. Pneumonia may be noted in 15% to 20% of cases.

The mainstay of management of foreign bodies in the lower airways is endoscopic removal. If the presence of a foreign body is unclear, endoscopy can be diagnostic as well as therapeutic. Although, for a time, postural drainage was recommended as a less invasive approach to pulmonary foreign bodies, it quickly was recognized that this form of therapy is fraught with considerable danger. The obstructing foreign body can be dislodged into the opposite main stem bronchus, obstructing that bronchus while the original lung is unable to recover instantly from the insult. Edema of the airway, as well as parenchymal changes in the lung from which the foreign body was just dislodged, may take hours to days to subside. Such instances can be catastrophic.

The gold standard for therapy is endoscopy, usually under general anesthesia with rigid endoscopic equipment. The procedure should be performed in the operating room, and the endoscopist should be familiar with, and comfortable in caring for, the pediatric patient. State-of-the-art endoscopic equipment should be available. Optimal treatment includes assessment by an anesthetist who is skilled in the care of young children and in treating patients during endoscopic procedures. These ideal conditions often are not available and, if the patient's condition is stable, it may be best to transfer the child to a facility where skillful pediatric endoscopic treatment is available. If endoscopy is unsuccessful because the object is too small, or if the object fragments on attempted removal, then a course of postural drainage is reasonably safe and should be undertaken.

With proper treatment, the mortality rate for aspiration of foreign bodies into the lower airways should be exceedingly low.

## Selected Readings

Baker DM. Foreign bodies of the ears and nose in childhood. Pediatr Emerg Care 1987;3:67.

Blazer S, Naveh Y, Friedman A. Foreign body in the airway: A review of 200 cases. Am J Dis Child 1980;134:68.

Cotton E, Yosuda K. Foreign body aspiration. Pediatr Clin North Am 1984;31:937.

Esclamado RM, Richardson MA. Laryngotracheal foreign bodies in children: A comparison with bronchial foreign bodies. Am J Dis Child 1987;141:259.

Greensher J, Mofenson HC. Emergency treatment of the choking child. Pediatrics 1982;70:110.

Halroyd HJ, Aron WR, Greensher J, et al. First aid for the choking child: Committee on Accident and Poison Prevention, American Academy of Pediatrics. Pediatrics 1981;67:744.

Heimlich HJ. First aid for choking children: Back blows and chest thrusts cause complications and death. Pediatrics 1982;70:120.

Kosloske AM. Bronchoscopic extraction of aspirated foreign bodies in children. Am J Dis Child 1982;136:924.

Law D, Kosloske AM. Management of tracheobronchial foreign bodies in children: A reevaluation of postural drainage and bronchoscopy. Pediatrics 1976;58:362.

Pediatric Basic Life Support. JAMA 1986;255:2954.

*Principles and Practice of Pediatrics, Second Edition.*
edited by Frank A. Oski et al. J. B. Lippincott Company, Philadelphia © 1994.

## CHAPTER 69
# *Laryngeal Disorders*

### Nancy M. Bauman and Richard J. H. Smith

The neonatal larynx differs from the adult larynx not only in size, but also in relative dimensions and location. The neonate's larynx is about one third the size of its adult counterpart. The epiglottis is proportionately larger and this relative size difference and the position of the larynx high in the neck are instrumental in allowing the infant to suckle and breathe simultaneously. During swallowing, the epiglottis abuts against the soft palate to create lateral digestive channels that funnel food into the piriform fossae and esophagus while the midline airway remains patent and effectively separated.

Descent of the larynx to a lower position in the neck begins at 2 years of age. During infancy, the inferior border of the cricoid cartilage is located at the fourth cervical vertebra, but by puberty, its location is at the level of the seventh cervical vertebra. This change in position creates a confluence of the digestive and respiratory tracts, and results in a longer vocal tract that is ideal for complex speech and articulation. This lengthening, however, abolishes the ability to suckle and breath simultaneously. Growth of the larynx continues until puberty, by which time full laryngeal development has occurred.

The membranoskeletal framework of the larynx is made up of several cartilages to which are attached muscles and folds of tissue that make respiration, phonation, and deglutition possible. The intricacies and subtleties of these structures are complicated, but their basic anatomy is relatively simple. The major cartilages of the larynx are the cricoid, thyroid, epiglottis, and arytenoids.

Only the cricoid, with a broad arch posteriorly and a narrow arch anteriorly, forms a complete ring. Attached superiorly is the sharply flexed, shield-like thyroid cartilage; its more important features include paired superior and inferior horns, lateral plates or laminae, and the thyroid notch. In lateral profile, the notch forms an anteriorly projecting angle that is known as the laryngeal prominence or Adam's apple. Facets on the inferior horns articulate with the posterior arch of the cricoid, establishing a hinge motion between the two cartilages (Fig 69-1).

The leaf-like epiglottis is tucked within the thyroid cartilage. It is made of fibroelastic cartilage and is attached inferiorly to the thyroid cartilage just above the level of the true vocal cords. From its mid-portion, the epiglottis is attached to the tongue by the median and lateral glossoepiglottic folds. From both lateral borders of the epiglottis, quadrangular membranes arise and arch posteriorly to the arytenoids. So named because of their shape, each quadrangular membrane is as tall as the epiglottis anteriorly and only as high as the ipsilateral arytenoid posteriorly. Both the superior and the inferior borders of each quadrangular membrane are free (Figs 69-2, 69-3).

The arytenoid cartilages are paired paramedian structures. Each has an apex, a concave base that rests on the underlying

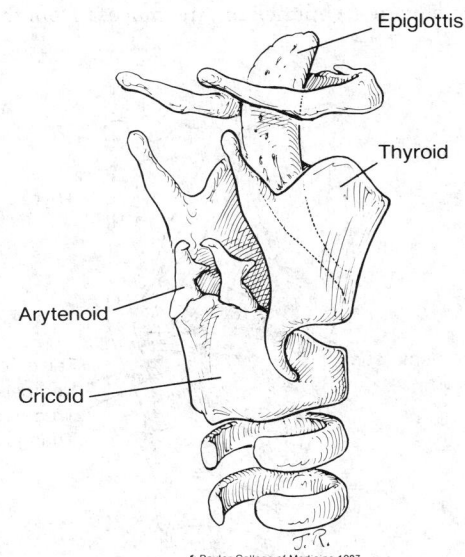

© Baylor College of Medicine 1987

**Figure 69-1.** Posterior oblique view of laryngeal cartilaginous framework.

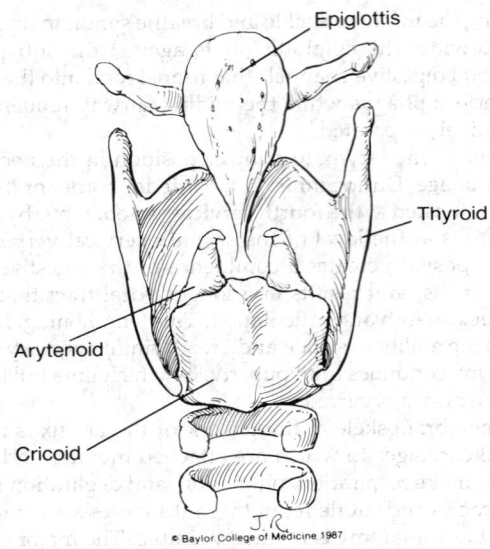

**Figure 69-2.** Posterior view of laryngeal cartilages.

cricoid cartilage, a lateral process to which attach many of the intrinsic muscles of the larynx, and an anteriorly projecting vocal process. A second laryngeal membrane, the triangular membrane or conus elasticus, originates from this anteriorly projecting vocal process and continues anteriorly to the thyroid cartilage. Its superiorly thickened edge forms the vocal ligament. Inferiorly, the triangular membrane attaches to the cricoid cartilage (see Fig 69-3).

Overlying these structures are the laryngeal muscles and mucosa. Although it is somewhat of a simplification, it is helpful to divide the intrinsic muscles of the larynx into two groups. One group, the thyroarytenoid, thyroepiglottic, and aryepiglottic muscles, is associated with the quadrangular membrane. The second group, the posterior cricoarytenoid, lateral cricoarytenoid, and interarytenoid muscles, acts on the arytenoid cartilages. A seventh muscle, the vocal muscle, parallels the vocal fold and is part of the thyroarytenoid muscle (Fig 69-4).

The overlying mucosa forms three important folds: the aryepiglottic folds, the false vocal cords (representing the inferior borders of both quadrangular membranes), and the true vocal folds. With the exception of the true vocal folds, which are covered by stratified squamous epithelium, the mucosa from the trachea

to the aryepiglottic folds is pseudostratified ciliated columnar epithelium (Fig 69-5).

The major functions of the larynx—respiration, phonation, and deglutition—require certain vocal cord positions for optimal operation. On maximal respiration, the vocal cords become flattened. During phonation, they are lightly juxtaposed. During swallowing, maximal closure of the airway occurs by the coordinated apposition of the vocal cords, sphincteric action of the aryepiglottic folds, and elevation of the larynx to the tongue base.

Trauma or pathologic changes involving the larynx may affect vocal cord dynamics; if function then becomes compromised, symptoms such as stridor, hoarseness, and aspiration develop. These are the harbingers of potentially serious laryngeal problems and dictate that an adequate laryngeal evaluation be performed. This may require a simple flexible fiberoptic examination or a more detailed study using rigid laryngoscopes and bronchoscopes under general anesthesia.

## LARYNGEAL TRAUMA

Injuries to the neck resulting in laryngeal trauma are relatively rare in children. The inherent degree of compressibility in the laryngeal cartilaginous framework affords some degree of protection. A blow to the neck from a baseball, injuries sustained by falling against the handlebars of a bicycle, or the garroting that results from riding into a taut line, however, easily can cause life-threatening airway damage. Should disruption of the laryngotracheal complex occur, with or without a fracture or dislocation of the laryngeal cartilage complex, the ensuing edema can result quickly in luminal occlusion and asphyxiation. It is imperative, therefore, to secure an airway in patients in whom a significant laryngeal injury is suspected.

Although the history usually suffices to establish the nature of a cervical injury, the degree of injury must be judged by careful physical examination. The pathognomonic sign of a breach in the airway is the presence of subcutaneous emphysema. A small amount of cervical crepitus usually reflects hypopharyngeal perforation; large amounts imply laryngotracheal injury. Symptoms of laryngeal damage include stridor, dyspnea, and dysphagia, often disproportionate to the degree of anterior cervical contusion and swelling. Concomitant injuries to adjacent structures can occur, and the great vessels, esophagus, and cervical spine must be evaluated. Initial therapeutic steps, however, mandate that the airway be protected.

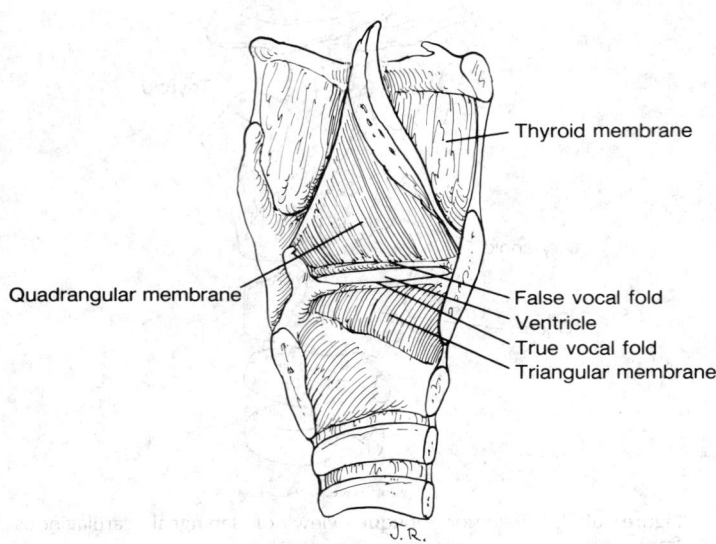

**Figure 69-3.** Quadrangular and triangular membranes as they attach to the laryngeal cartilages.

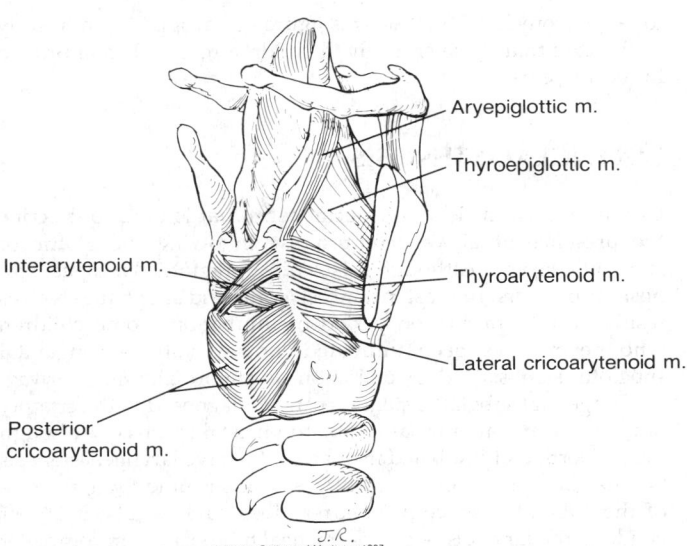

**Figure 69-4.** Laryngeal muscles associated with the laryngeal membranes.

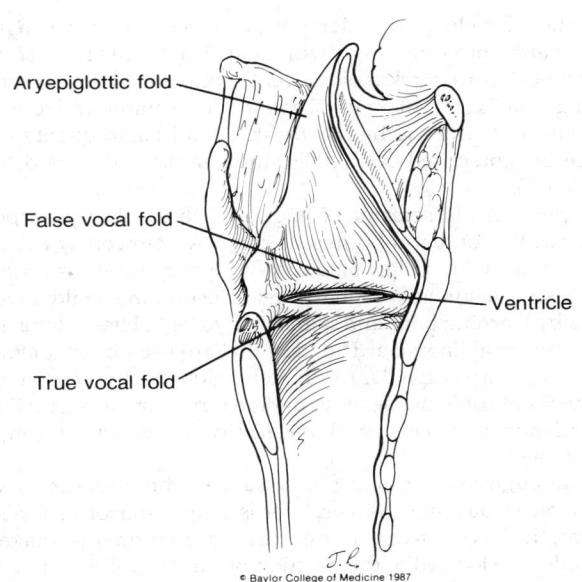

**Figure 69-5.** Overlying mucosa that creates three important folds: the aryepiglottic folds, the false vocal cords, and the true vocal cords.

To avoid long-term morbidity, an accurate assessment of the degree of injury must be made. Standard lateral and anteroposterior neck roentgenograms can confirm the presence of subcutaneous emphysema and permit evaluation of the cervical spine; computed tomography (CT) clearly delineates fractures (Fig 69-6). If possible, indirect or flexible laryngoscopy should be done to assess the extent of supraglottic laryngeal injury and vocal cord mobility. If a vocal cord paralysis is found, the prognosis for ultimate return of function is poor. After the patient has been stabilized, direct laryngoscopy and bronchoscopy should be performed. This is the most important aspect of the evaluation, because the degree of endolaryngeal injury can be determined and treatment decisions can be made.

The treatment objective is to reestablish a mucosa-lined lumen without compromising either arytenoid motion or neuromuscular function. Severe injuries require surgical repair through a laryngofissure. Fractured cartilages are reapproximated and mucosal lacerations are closed to minimize the likelihood of future dysfunction. With minor injuries, after an adequate airway has been

established, the larynx can be reassessed after the edema has resolved. If necessary, an open repair can be performed later.

Occasionally, seemingly trivial cervical trauma can cause laryngeal injury. Symptoms such as vague tenderness, pain, intermittent hoarseness, or intermittent dysphasia may reflect the presence of a small endolaryngeal hematoma. These symptoms resolve in the ensuing weeks and, as fibrosis and healing occur, an asymmetry of the laryngeal cartilages may develop. Years later, hoarseness can recur and the past endolaryngeal injury may be detected as a deformity of the endolarynx at endoscopy.

More common than external cervical trauma is trauma secondary to voice abuse. The anterior two thirds of the vocal cords vibrate synchronously during normal speech, and studies of mucosal dynamics with high-speed videostroboscopy have demonstrated that the vocal cords clearly collide during each cycle of vibration. If vibration is either too forceful or too prolonged, vascular congestion with edema results at the point of maximum trauma. In instances of acute abuse or overuse, only fluid accu-

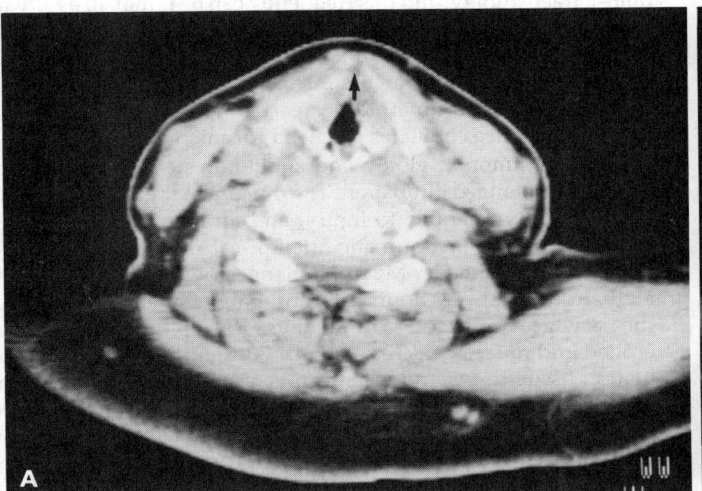

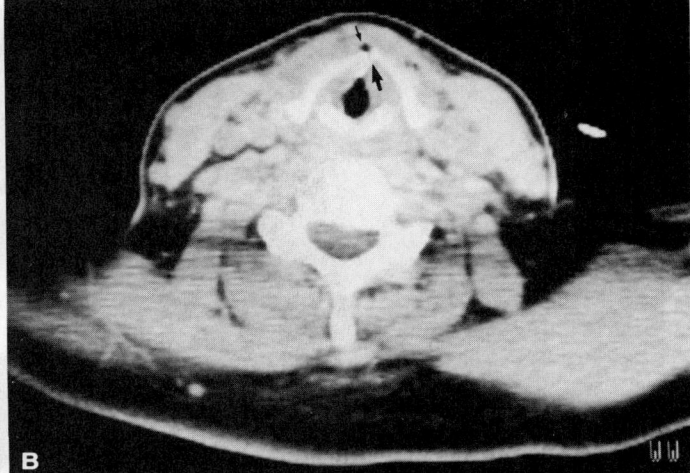

**Figure 69-6.** CT scan showing (**A**) a fracture of the thyroid cartilage (*large arrow*), with (**B**) some air in the adjacent soft tissue (*small arrow*).

mulation develops; with long-term overuse, however, hyalinization and fibrous tissue growth occur. The altered mucosal mass and vocal cord thickness prevent complete glottic closure, a change that is evident on vocalization. Voice timbre and resonance are lowered, and the husky, breathy, and harsh quality of the voice is appreciated easily. Diphthongia often can be detected (Fig 69-7).

Aptly called "screamer's nodules," these changes typically occur in the loud and boisterous child. A noteworthy exception is the child with a cleft palate or velopharyngeal insufficiency. Unable to maintain velopharyngeal closure, this child compensates by learning poor and damaging voice habits—glottal stops and abnormal lingual articulation that are used in an attempt to stop nasal air escape. Unfortunately, glottal stops cause trauma to the vocal cords that leads to nodule formation; incorrect lingual articulation results in speech mechanics that can make language unintelligible.

Although auditory clues may suggest the presence of vocal nodules, visualizing the vocal cords with a mirror or a flexible fiberoptic laryngoscope is essential to confirm the diagnosis. Nodules are located at the junction of the anterior one third and posterior two thirds of the vocal cords, and may vary in size, contour, and color depending on the duration and degree of voice abuse. Papillomas, intracordal cysts, vocal cord polyps, and Reinke's edema may mimic nodules; however, these possibilities are eliminated easily by direct visual examination.

Voice therapy is the cornerstone of treatment and, because nodules are caused by voice overuse, misuse, or abuse, therapy alone may result in a complete cure, especially in acute cases. Surgical removal, however, is an option if nodules remain and the voice continues to be unacceptable despite an adequate period of voice therapy. Precise removal is possible using endoscopic techniques and the carbon dioxide laser to vaporize abnormal tissue. After surgery, a short period of voice rest is necessary and a continued period of speech therapy is essential to prevent the recurrent development of nodules.

The most common form of laryngeal trauma, unfortunately, is iatrogenic. In 1965, McDonald and Stocks suggested long-term intubation as an alternative safer than tracheotomy in the treatment of upper airway problems in neonates. Many neonates sustained airway damage as a sequela; the incidence of chronic subglottic stenosis in the late 1960s and early 1970s was reported to range from 12% to 20%. This figure has dropped significantly as the care that these critically ill children receive has improved in recent years.

## LARYNGEAL STENOSIS

Laryngeal stenosis is a nonspecific term that is used to describe the presence of airway compromise involving the glottic or subglottic larynx. Although it is rare, supraglottic laryngeal stenosis also occurs. In most instances, glottic and subglottic stenosis results from a prolonged period of intubation. Some children who never have been intubated, however, have congenital subglottic stenosis and, by definition, an abnormally small airway.

Congenital subglottic stenosis can be diagnosed with certainty only before any attempt at intubation has taken place. Although the proportion of intubated neonates who have laryngeal stenosis because of a preexisting subglottic stenosis is unknown, the size of the subglottic space in children does vary. In about 1% of children, the larynx is two endotracheal tube sizes (1 mm) smaller than predicted; in 0.06%, the larynx is three tube sizes (1.5 mm) too small. Doubtlessly, some intubated infants have a larynx that is smaller than normal and, therefore, are at higher risk for sustaining damage from an endotracheal tube. Endoscopy is required to assess the larynx properly and determine its size. Using a 3.0 bronchoscope as a gauge, the cross-sectional area of the airway at the level of the cricoid can be estimated. This bronchoscope should pass through the subglottic area if no stenosis is present.

Congenital stenosis at the subglottic level is secondary most often to a cartilaginous abnormality—the cricoid typically is smaller in circumference than normal and somewhat flattened in shape. Another common finding is telescoping of the first tracheal ring within the cricoid cartilage and, as a consequence, narrowing of the airway. Soft-tissue airway compromise occurs when either an increased amount of connective tissue or hyperplastic dilated mucous glands encroach on the subglottic lumen.

Minimal stenosis rarely causes problems except in association with upper respiratory tract infections. In contrast, marked subglottic stenosis produces nearly constant biphasic stridor and sternal retractions. Pulmonary secretions are cleared ineffectively, and a barking cough and recurrent pulmonary infections are common.

Fortunately, most neonates with congenital subglottic stenosis respond to conservative therapy and can be treated with antibiotics and steroids during episodes of upper respiratory tract infection and increased respiratory stridor. Fewer than 50% require a tracheotomy, and this frequently can be removed as airway cross-sectional area increases with growth and development. A weight increase from 2 to 10 kg is associated with an increase in the area of the airway at the cricoid from 20 to 60 mm$^2$. This tripling results in a ninefold decrease in airway resistance, and in many instances obviates the need for major surgery.

More commonly, glottic and subglottic stenosis are the sequelae of prolonged intubation. The mucosa of the larynx is highly reactive and vulnerable to injury, and an inappropriately large tube or repeated or traumatic attempts at intubation cause extensive tissue damage. Mucosal changes occur almost immediately. In the first few hours after intubation, edema develops in the laryngeal mucosa. Within days, the epithelium becomes eroded and mucosal necrosis occurs. At the sites of injury, granulation tissue forms and often can be seen around the endotracheal tube if a direct laryngoscopy is done (Fig 69-8). Attempted extubation at this time often is unsuccessful, as the granulation tissue further narrows an already compromised airway.

If the endotracheal tube is not withdrawn, full-thickness injury to the overlying mucosa may expose the cricoid perichondrium, leading to a perichondritis, and the arytenoid cartilages ultimately

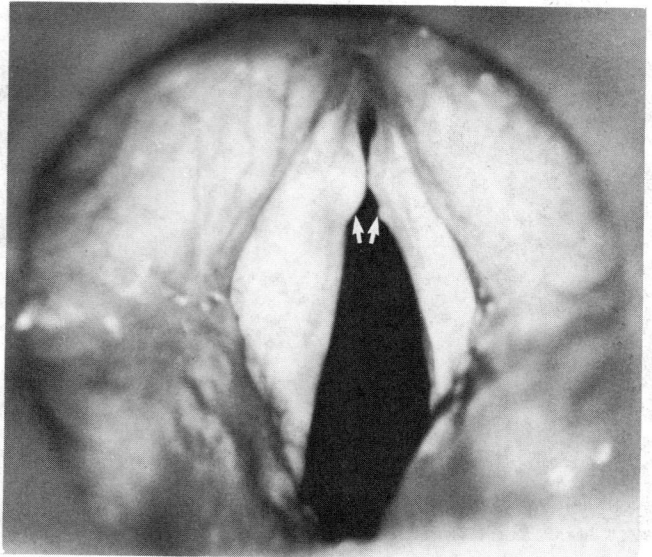

**Figure 69-7.** Vocal nodules (*arrows*).

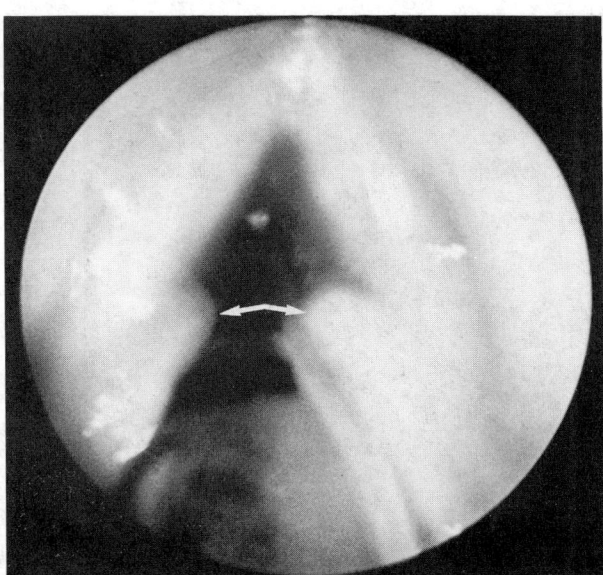

**Figure 69-8.** Intubation granulomas hugging the endotracheal tube, which can be seen inferiorly.

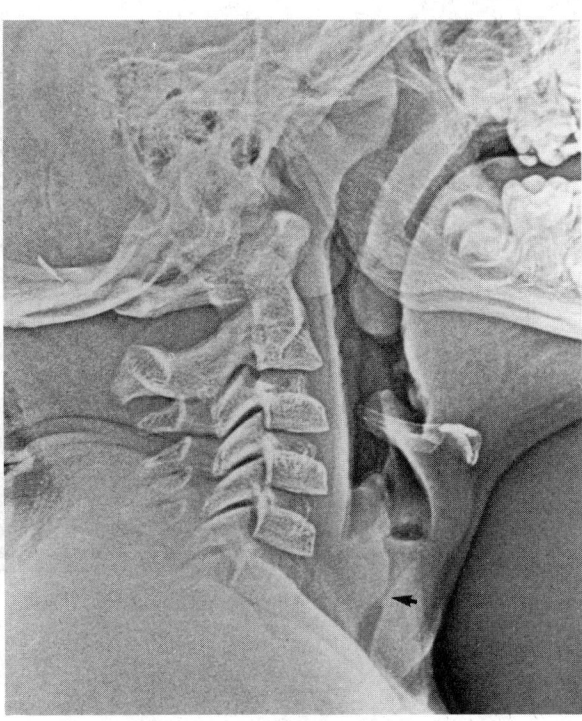

**Figure 69-9.** Xerography of the neck in a child with subglottic stenosis (*arrow*). The tract for the tracheotomy can be seen inferiorly.

may be involved. Progressive damage generally does not continue and, by the end of the first week of intubation, early signs of healing at the margins of the ulcers are present. Re-epithelialization with metaplastic squamous epithelium begins, despite the continued presence of the endotracheal tube; by 4 weeks, fibrous tissue and squamous epithelium mark the site of the old ulcer.

Prolonged intubation, in itself, probably is not followed by subglottic stenosis. Rather, associated risk factors such as the respirator piston action on the endotracheal tube, irritation from chemical constituents of the endotracheal tube, and concomitant bacterial infections lead to increased injury and greater subsequent fibrosis. The reported incidence of subglottic stenosis as a complication of intubation ranges from 0.23% to 8.0%. In many instances, surgery is required before extubation is possible. Treatment possibilities that must be considered in the face of failed attempts to remove the endotracheal tube range from endoscopic laser surgery to cricoid-splitting procedures. If these therapeutic techniques are unsuccessful, a tracheotomy is required.

To assess accurately the location, extent, and severity of the laryngeal stenosis, several steps must be taken. Soft-tissue roentgenograms of the neck and xeroradiography can delineate the length and severity of the stenosis; flexible fiberoptic examination will show endolaryngeal dynamics (Fig 69-9). Vocal cord mobility must be assessed carefully and the presence of interarytenoid fixation considered. An endoscopic examination also should be done. During microsuspension laryngoscopy and bronchoscopy, attention should be focused on the interarytenoid area, and passive cricoarytenoid joint mobility should be evaluated by palpation. The subglottic area should be examined to define the degree and length of stenosis; if the glottic lumen is stenosed completely, the degree of inferior extension must be estimated (Fig 69-10).

In most instances, the stenosis is so severe that conservative treatment will not permit decannulation for several years, if at all. Mortality rates of 11% to 24% have been reported in children less than 3 years of age who are treated conservatively, presumably because the reserve laryngeal airway is not adequate to support respiration if the tracheotomy tube becomes occluded.

Dilatation has been used as treatment, but does not produce an adequate airway if the consistency of the stenosis is firm, mature scar. More aggressive approaches must be taken, including

endoscopic cryosurgery, electrocautery, and laser vaporization of the offending tissue. If these relatively noninvasive techniques are unsuccessful, open techniques must be used. The stenotic segment can be resected and airway continuity restored by end-to-end anastomosis. Alternatively, an extended laryngotracheal fissure procedure can be done. Tissue is interposed in the fissure to increase tracheal circumference and airway size. Sources of tissue include bone harvested from the iliac crest, hyoid, clavicle, and rib; cartilage from the auricle, costal margin, epiglottis, nasal septum, and thyroid ala; and soft-tissue flaps of sternocleidomastoid muscle. Occasionally, the spring of the cricoid ring is too unyielding and the posterior cricoid plate must be divided. A free autogenous graft can be interposed between the halves of the posterior cricoid plate, although this usually is not necessary.

Laryngotracheoplasty with costal cartilage is the preferred treatment method for several reasons: abundant amounts of cartilage can be harvested easily and sculpted to bridge the stenotic defect; the smooth cartilage surface has a minimal effect on airway resistance; and the perichondrium provides a barrier to infection, making resorption less likely. The operation generally is very successful, with the average time from the date of surgery to decannulation being only 7 to 10 days if a one-stage laryngotracheoplasty is performed. If a stent has been placed in the laryngeal lumen, the operation becomes a two-stage procedure, and the average time from the date of surgery to decannulation is 3 months (Fig 69-11).

## SUBGLOTTIC HEMANGIOMA

Hemangiomas are hamartomatous collections of endothelial cells similar to those from which the vascular system is derived. Capillary loops, sinusoidal spaces, or arteriovenous fistulas predominate, and hemangiomas are subclassified accordingly. They are the most common benign tumor of the head and neck in children, with an estimated prevalence of 10% to 12% in whites. This

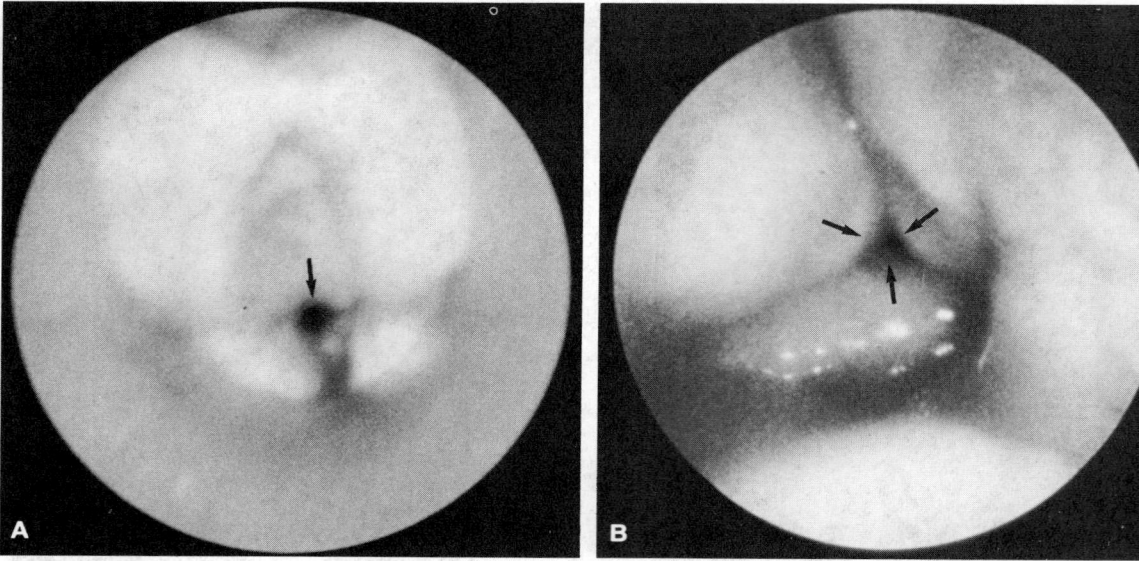

**Figure 69-10.** Two examples of nearly total laryngeal stenosis, one at the glottic level (**A**), and the other in the subglottic area (**B**).

figure increases to 22% in preterm babies weighing less than 1000 g. The female : male preponderance is 3 : 1.

Most commonly, hemangiomas appear in the skin, usually as a single tumor, although multiple cutaneous lesions occur occasionally, often with involvement of other organ systems. If the hemangioma is present in the subglottic area, the lesion potentially can be life-threatening. Subglottic hemangiomas usually are capillary, submucosal, and unencapsulated; in contrast, the rarer supraglottic hemangioma is more likely to be cavernous. Similar to hemangiomas in general, subglottic hemangiomas are more common in females and, in 50% of affected children, are associated with concomitant cutaneous hemangiomas. The site of predilection for these associated hemangiomas is in the head and neck.

Subglottic hemangiomas are present at birth, but typically go unnoticed until several weeks to months have passed. Varying degrees of airway distress develop, bringing these infants to the attention of their pediatrician. The continuum of respiratory problems ranges from mild biphasic stridor that is troublesome

only when it is associated with an upper respiratory tract infection to marked acute stridor that results in dyspnea, failure to thrive, and cyanosis. The natural history is one of progressive enlargement of the hemangioma during the first 12 months of life, followed by autogenous embolization in the ensuing years. Not infrequently, a diagnosis of croup is made initially, and recurrent episodes of croup always should alert the physician to the possibility of an anatomic airway problem such as subglottic hemangioma.

Plain roentgenograms of the neck can reveal an asymmetric subglottic mass, and supplemental studies such as a cine-esophagram can show the extent of invasion of the common tracheoesophageal wall (Fig 69-12). The definitive diagnosis is made under controlled conditions by direct laryngoscopy. A biopsy is not required, as the appearance of the pink to bluish compressible mass in the lateral or posterolateral subglottic space is pathognomonic (Fig 69-13).

Small subglottic hemangiomas do not cause airway compromise and may require no treatment; with larger life-threatening hemangiomas, however, a tracheotomy often is essential. Although this secures the airway, the high mortality rate makes further intervention essential. Local compression is believed to hasten the regression of hemangiomas, and some lesions respond to a 10- to 14-day period of intubation. Systemic steroids may be administered concomitantly, although proof of their efficacy is lacking and their mechanism of action on hemangiomas is not clear. Presumably, steroids enhance the sensitivity of endothelial cells to endogenous circulating vasoconstrictors. Unfortunately, when used alone, they usually are unsuccessful at relieving obstruction and afford only a transient improvement in the airway condition.

Radiation therapy has had some proponents in the past, but its effect on hemangiomas is questionable. Possible treatment complications also are not inconsequential, and the known association of cervical radiation with thyroid malignancies makes this technique unjustifiable. In some countries, gold grains have been inserted in hemangiomas; although regression occurs, the possibly deleterious effects on tracheal and laryngeal cartilages require additional study.

Surgical treatment options include the injection of sclerosants, cryotherapy, laser therapy, and excisional surgery. Of the choices, the precision that is possible and the discrete area of tissue damage

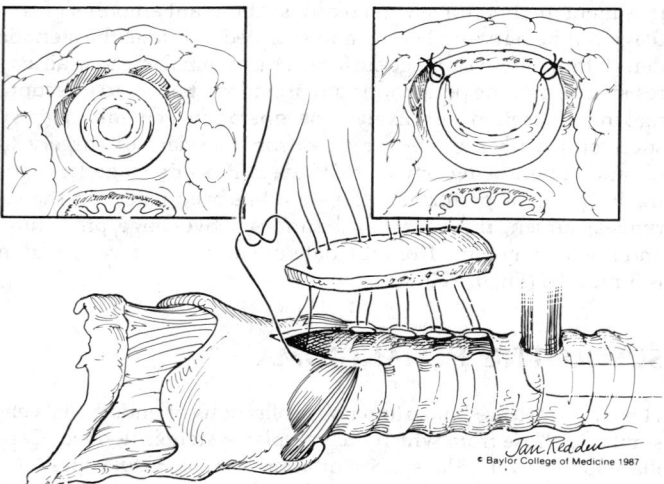

**Figure 69-11.** Illustration of method of repair of laryngotracheal stenosis using costal cartilage.

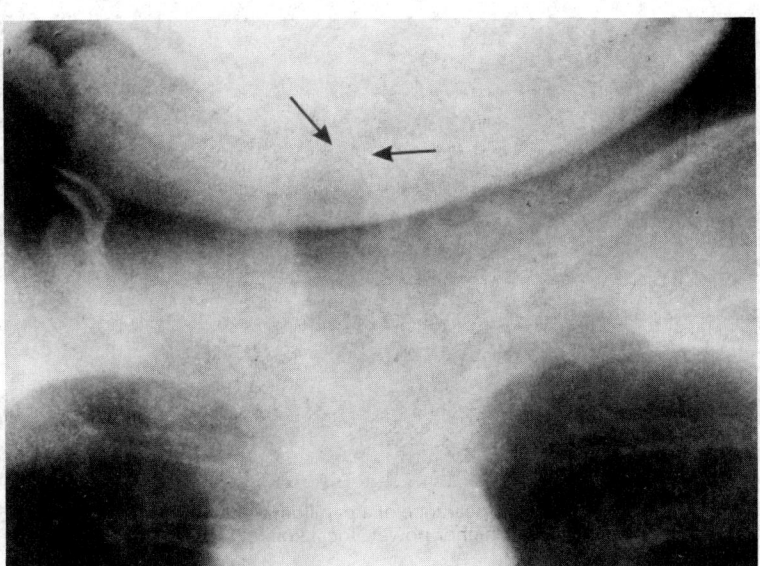

**Figure 69-12.** Soft-tissue roentgenogram of the airway, showing encroachment of the tracheal air column by a right-sided subglottic hemangioma.

that is produced make the $CO_2$ laser especially applicable to endolaryngeal surgery. A beam of coherent light of 10.6 $\mu$m in wavelength is generated. Because this is in the invisible range of the electromagnetic spectrum, a second coaxial helium-neon laser is built into the system; it produces visible light and is used to indicate the site at which the $CO_2$ laser will impact on target tissue. The radiant energy produced by the $CO_2$ laser is absorbed strongly by homogenous water, and the extinction length in soft tissue is only 0.03 mm. Reflection and scattering are negligible. For these reasons, only a small area of tissue destruction results, and the exposed cells absorb energy and are vaporized immediately. Hemangiomas usually must be treated several times before enough scarring and fibrosis form to restore the airway to an adequate size (see Fig 69-13).

Recent studies also have suggested that interferon-$\alpha$2a may be effective in the treatment of hemangiomas. Initially developed as an antiviral agent, interferon-$\alpha$2a has been observed to cause regression of pulmonary hemangiomatosis and life-threatening hemangiomas in infants. Sustained therapy at a dosage of 3 mil-

lion U/m² for 9 to 14 months appears necessary, because early withdrawal is followed by the regrowth of lesions. Regrowth can be halted and reversed by the reintroduction of interferon therapy, however.

## LARYNGEAL PAPILLOMA

The most common benign tumor of the larynx is the papilloma. It accounts for more than 80% of laryngeal growths and, although benign, tends to recur, can be difficult to cure, and can cause fatal airway obstruction. These characteristics are reflected in its common name, recurrent respiratory papillomatosis (RRP). RRP is induced virally, most frequently by human papillomavirus subtypes 6 and 11. The majority of affected individuals are children less than 7 years of age, although papillomas do occur in people of all ages.

Both juvenile and adult forms are described. This distinction is not superfluous, as differences exist in the initial manifestation

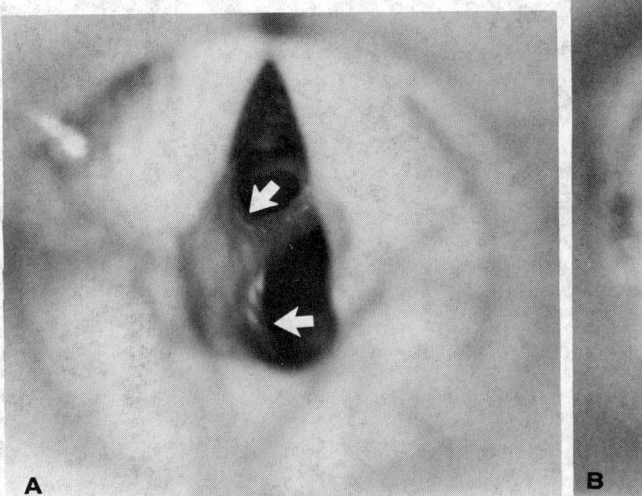
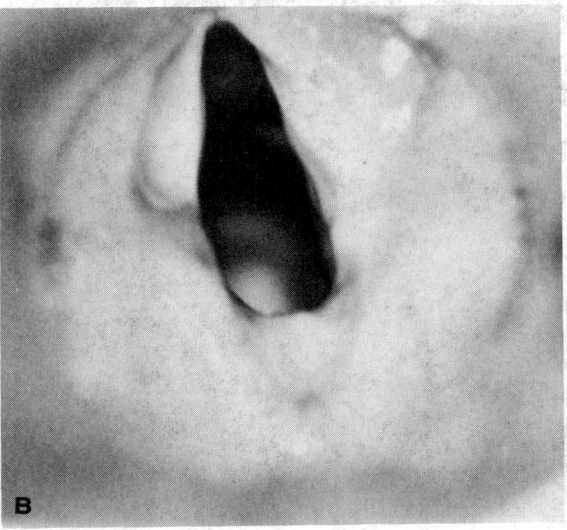

**Figure 69-13.** Endoscopic view of a left posterolateral subglottic hemangioma, before (**A**) and after (**B**) laser therapy.

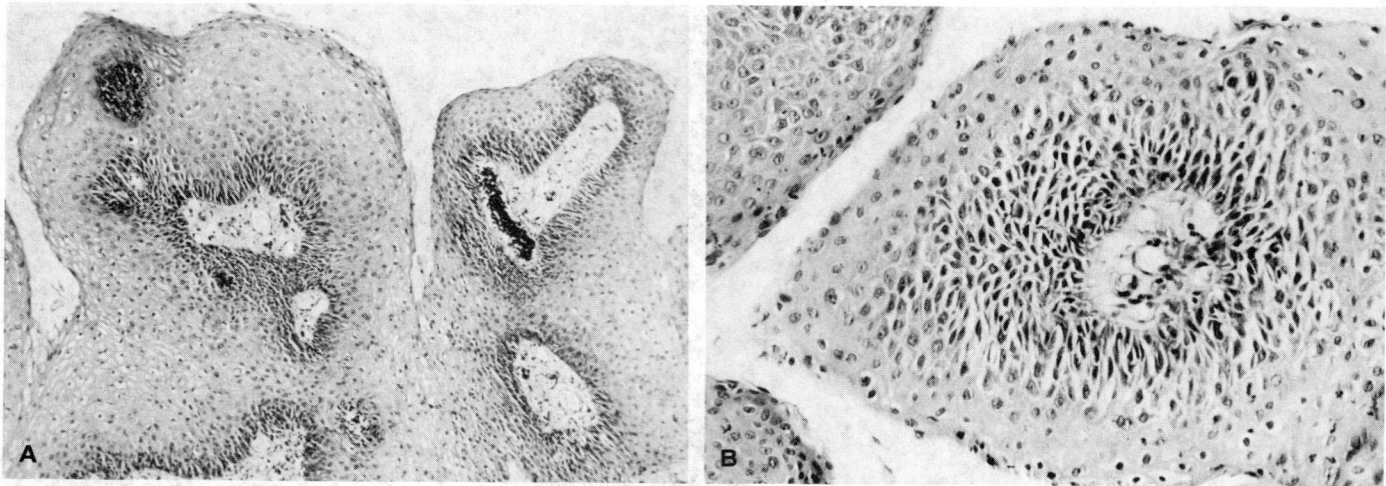

**Figure 69-14.** Histologic appearance of a papilloma, showing (**A**) fibrovascular cores and acanthosis, and (**B**), additionally, under higher power, focal koilocytosis.

and clinical course of the two forms. The adult form has a male predilection, and the papillomas usually are solitary. They generally do not spread and are less likely to recur after surgical removal. A single surgical procedure may be curative.

In contrast, juvenile laryngeal papillomas can be extremely aggressive and resistant to treatment. Most frequently, the anterior portion of the true vocal cords, the false vocal cords, and the laryngeal surface of the epiglottis are involved. Exuberant growth can cover normal anatomy and spread to contiguous areas, which can lead to involvement of the vallecula and hypopharynx, esophagus, trachea, and bronchi. Treatment is extremely frustrating because recurrences are common even after apparently complete removal. Additionally, the clinical course is unpredictable, with spontaneous regression seen occasionally at puberty.

The most common presenting symptoms reflect vocal cord disease and airway compromise. Hoarseness or stridor, a voice change or complete aphonia, a weak cry, and respiratory distress may occur. Occasionally, the degree of papillomatosis is so severe that a tracheotomy is necessary. Tracheotomy increases the like-

lihood of tracheal and bronchial spread, however, and should not be undertaken without serious reflection. Involvement of the lower airways is the harbinger of a particularly bleak prognosis.

The diagnosis of papilloma is made easily by visual examination of the larynx, using either a laryngeal mirror or a flexible fiberoptic laryngoscope. The histologic picture is pathognomonic. Papillary lesions with long, finger-like projections of connective tissue abound. These are covered with acanthotic and hypoplastic ingrowing epithelium. Enlarged stromal vessels lie contiguous to hypoplastic epithelium immediately adjacent to the basement membrane, without apparent intervening stroma (Fig 69-14).

In most cases, surgery is the favored form of treatment. In the past, cryosurgery, ultrasound therapy, and cauterization were popular, but the $CO_2$ laser is preferred now. Laser vaporization of papillomas is performed with the patient under general anesthesia using a direct laryngoscope and a surgical microscope. Papilloma bulk may be so great initially that normal laryngeal landmarks are obscured; with the surgical precision that can be exacted with the laser, however, papillomas can be removed

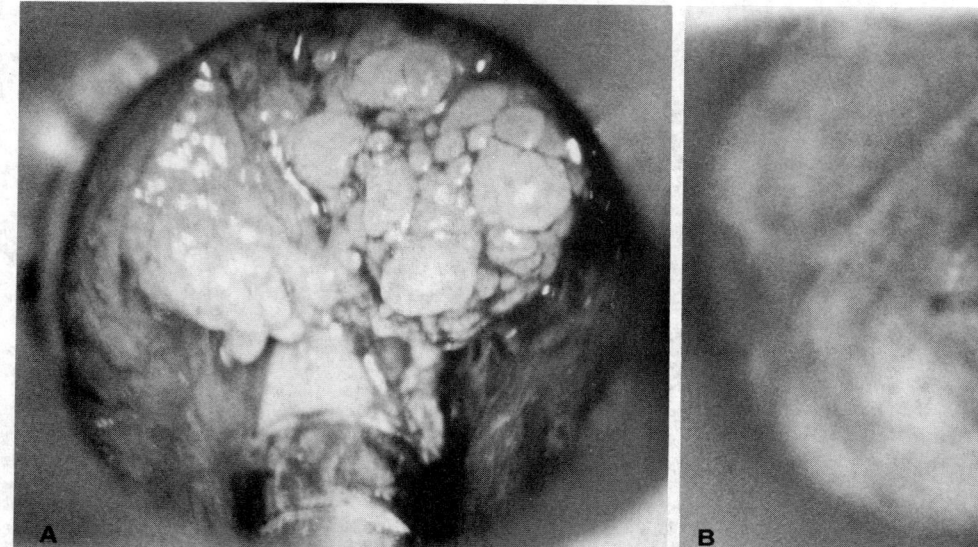
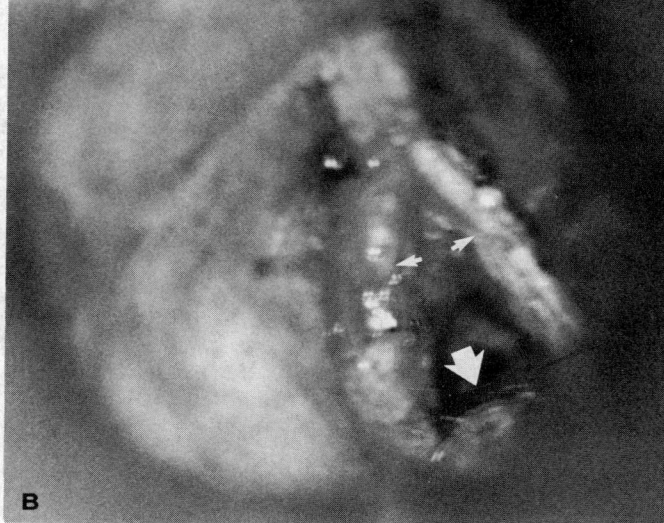

**Figure 69-15.** Marked laryngeal papillomatosis, before (**A**) and after (**B**) laser therapy. *Small arrows,* vocal cords; *large arrow,* endotracheal tube.

length or standardized role of interferon treatment has been formalized, and the long-term role of this form of therapy has not been determined. Side effects include fever, malaise, fatigue, myelosuppression, nausea, vomiting, and elevation of serum glutamic oxaloacetic transaminase levels, but in most instances, the administration of interferon need not be discontinued.

Optimal treatment requires serial laser laryngoscopy with the use of interferon in selected cases. The unpredictable course of papilloma make several procedures the rule, without a guarantee of cure. Recent advances in molecular biology have demonstrated the presence of the viral genome in normal-appearing mucosa in children with laryngeal papilloma. This suggests that the infection is more widespread than is clinically apparent. Advances in medical rather than surgical therapy will be necessary to cure this disorder permanently. Especially promising are the host of antiviral agents that are being developed.

## LARYNGEAL TUMORS

Tumors of the larynx are uncommon in the pediatric population. Nearly all are benign and, of the benign tumors, squamous papilloma is by far the most common. Hemangioma, the second most frequently encountered lesion, is the most common tumor in the subglottic area. A potpourri of other benign tumors has been reported, including neurofibromas, lymphangiomas, chondromas, fibromas, and rhabdomyomas. Malignant tumors are distinctly uncommon; of them, the tumor diagnosed most frequently is rhabdomyosarcoma. Angiosarcoma, fibrosarcoma, chondrosarcoma, neurofibrosarcoma, and squamous cell carcinoma also occur.

Stridor usually is the first symptom of a laryngeal tumor, but this is very nonspecific. In a review by Holinger and Brown of 866 children with stridor, only 2% had a tumor. It is helpful to classify stridor as being either inspiratory, biphasic, or expiratory; the type of stridor that is present can be a clue to the site of the tumor. Inspiratory stridor associated with a muffled cry and poor feeding implies a supraglottic problem; biphasic stridor associated with a normal or slightly hoarse cry and reasonably good feeding implies a subglottic problem; and aphonia or dysphonia accompanied by inspiratory stridor with some expiratory component implies a glottic lesion. In most instances, children with stridor

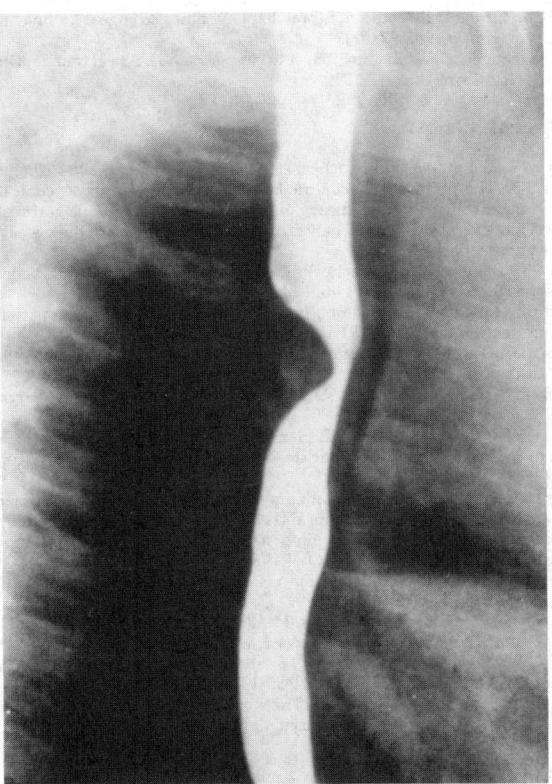

**Figure 69-16.** Barium swallow, showing posterior esophageal compression secondary to a vascular anomaly of the great vessels.

carefully and normal laryngeal anatomy can be preserved. The small underlying vessels also can be cauterized easily (Fig 69-15).

Large trials of interferon therapy have been performed in several centers, and dramatic results have been seen occasionally. Several authors have reported regression or complete disappearance of the papilloma, but with cessation of therapy, exuberant regrowth can occur. There also seems to be a tendency for papillomas to proliferate with dose reduction. No definite

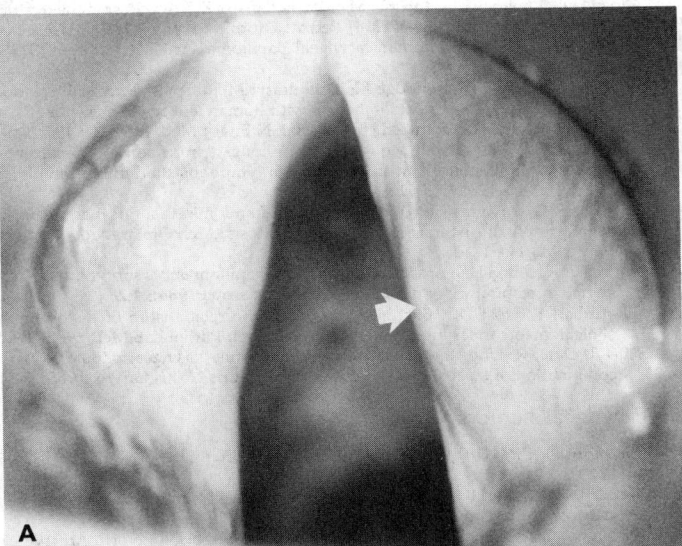 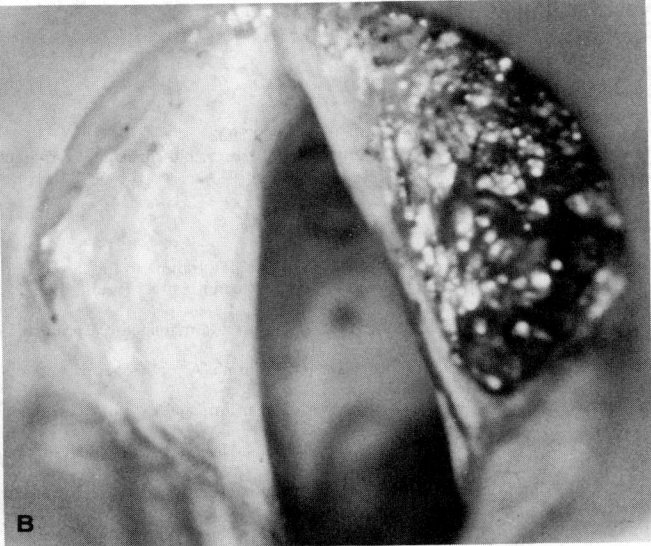

**Figure 69-17.** **(A)** Neurofibroma of the right false vocal fold in a child with neurofibromatosis. **(B)** The laser has been used to remove the bulk of the tumor.

have inflammatory disorders, but a recurrent inflammatory disorder occasionally may mask an underlying neoplasm. For this reason, an anatomic airway problem should be considered if an "infection" occurs far more frequently than expected.

To diagnose the laryngeal pathology, plain roentgenograms of the neck showing the tracheal air column are helpful. A barium swallow should be requested to delineate associated problems such as a vascular ring, and a CT scan can be obtained to demarcate both the extent of disease and the degree of destruction that is present (Fig 69-16). This permits optimal calculation of portals if radiation therapy is required for tumor treatment. Laryngoscopy and bronchoscopy must be done to establish the diagnosis. Squamous papillomas and hemangiomas can be diagnosed with certainty by their visual characteristics. Other tumors may be suspected because of the site of involvement (eg, granular-cell neoplasms have a predilection for the middle to posterior part of the true vocal cords, and chondromas usually occur on the cricoid), but histologic confirmation is necessary to ascertain the diagnosis. Differentiation between chondromas and chondrosarcomas is difficult, and the behavior of chondromas and low-grade chondrosarcomas is so similar that histologic distinction has little practical significance, because neither grows quickly or metastasizes. Most extracardiac rhabdomyomas occur in the head and neck, with a particular affinity for the pharynx and larynx. These tumors can be confused with granular-cell tumors or rhabdomyosarcomas, and must be differentiated from both.

The preferred method of therapy for benign lesions is use of the $CO_2$ laser. This permits tumor ablation and resection with minimal scarring and edema. Removal is precise and relatively atraumatic. More troublesome lesions may require open surgery, and there are occasional reports of the need for supraglottic laryngectomies to treat large cystic hygromas and neurofibromas (Fig 69-17). Small chondromas of the larynx often can be removed by endoscopy, but larger cricoid chondromas require open surgery for adequate treatment. If removal is possible without entering the laryngeal lumen, the likelihood of postoperative subglottic stenosis is minimized.

Malignant tumors often are amenable to chemotherapy and radiation therapy. Occasionally, surgery is employed if a conservative laryngectomy can be curative. Only on rare occasions is a total laryngectomy necessary. Rhabdomyosarcomas are radiosensitive and susceptible to chemotherapy, and results of treatment have shown that most patients are free of disease after therapy.

# Selected Readings

### Infant Larynx

Pracy R. The infant larynx. J Laryngol Otol 1983;97:933.
Too-Chung MA, Green JR. The rate of growth of the cricoid cartilage. J Laryngol Otol 1974;88:65.

### Laryngeal Trauma

Angood PB, Attia EL, Brown RA, et al. Extrinsic civilian trauma to the larynx and cervical trachea—important predictors of long-term morbidity. J Trauma 1986;26:869.
Fuhrman GM. Blunt laryngeal trauma: Classification and management protocol. J Trauma 1990;30:87.
Gusack GS, Jurkovic GJ, Luterman A. Laryngeal trauma: A protocol approach to a rare injury. Laryngoscope 1986;96:660.
Handler SD, Landy M. False vocal cord nodules; an unusual case of hoarseness. Ear Nose Throat J 1984;63:514.
Hanson DG, Mancuso AA, Hanafee WN. Pseudomass lesions due to occult trauma of the larynx. Laryngoscope 1982;92:1249.
Hartman PK, Mintz G, Verne D, Timen S. Diagnosis and primary management of laryngeal trauma. Oral Surg Oral Med Oral Pathol 1985;60:252.
Hirano M, Kurita S, Terasawa R. Difficulty in high-pitched phonation by laryngeal trauma. Arch Otolaryngol 1985;111:59.
Lee SY. Experimental blunt injury to the larynx. Ann Otol Rhinol Laryngol 1992;101:270.

Myer CM, Orobello P, Cotton RT, Bratcher GO. Blunt laryngeal trauma in children. Laryngoscope 1987;97:1043.
Snow JB. Diagnosis and therapy for acute laryngeal and tracheal trauma. Otolaryngol Clin North Am 1984;17:101.

### Laryngeal Stenosis

Cotton RT. Pediatric laryngotracheal stenosis. J Pediatr Surg 1984;19:699.
Cotton RT. The problem of pediatric laryngotracheal stenosis: A clinical and experimental study on the efficacy of autogenous cartilaginous grafts placed between the vertically divided halves of the posterior lamina of the cricoid cartilage. Laryngoscope 1991;101:1.
Donn SM, Blane CE. Endotracheal tube movement in the preterm neonate: Oral vs. nasal intubation. Ann Otol Rhinol Laryngol 1985;94:18.
Gould SJ, Howard S. The histopathology of the larynx in the neonate following endotracheal intubation. J Pathol 1985;146:301.
Koufman JA, Thompson JN, Kohut RI. Endoscopic management of subglottic stenosis with the $CO_2$ surgical laser. Otolaryngol Head Neck Surg 1981;89:215.
Kragina Z, Vecerina S. Chronic stenosis of the larynx in children. J Laryngol Otol 1979;93:81.
Luft JD, Wetmore RF, Tom LWC, Handler SD, Potsic WP. Laryngotracheoplasty in the management of subglottic stenosis. Int J Pediatr Otorhinolaryngol 1989;17:297.
Narcy P, Contencin P, Menier Y, Bobin S, Francois M. Surgical treatment of laryngotracheal stenosis in infants and children. Arch Otolaryngol 1989;246:341.
Papsidero MJ, Pashley NTR. Acquired stenosis of the upper airway in neonates. An increasing problem. Am J Otol 1980;89:512.
Quiney RE, Gould SJ. Subglottic stenosis: A clinicopathological study. Clin Otolaryngol 1985;10:315.
Smith RJH. Laryngotracheal stenosis. Head Neck Surg 1987;10:38.
Smith RJH. Laryngotracheal stenosis: A 5-year review. Head Neck 1991;13:140.
Strong MS, Healy GB, Vaughan CW, et al. Endoscopic management of laryngeal stenosis. Otolaryngol Clin North Am 1979;12:797.
Zalzal GH, Cotton RT, McAdams J. The survival of costal cartilage graft in laryngotracheal reconstruction. Otolaryngol Head Neck Surg 1986;94:204.

### Subglottic Hemangioma

Adzick NS, Strome M, Gang D, et al. Cryotherapy of subglottic hemangioma. J Pediatr Surg 1984;19:353.
Benjamin B, Carter P. Congenital laryngeal hemangioma. Ann Otol Rhinol Laryngol 1983;92:448.
Cleland WJD, Riding K. Subglottic hemangiomas in infants. J Otolaryngol 1986;15:119.
Ezekowitz RAB, Phil D, Muliken JB, Folkman J. Interferon alfa-2a therapy for life-threatening hemangiomas of infancy. N Engl J Med 1992;326:1456.
Healy G, McGill T, Friedman EM. Carbon-dioxide laser in subglottic hemangioma. An update. Ann Otol Rhinol Laryngol 1984;93:370.
Kveton JF, Pillsbury HC. Conservative treatment of infantile subglottic hemangioma with corticosteroids. Arch Otolaryngol 1982;108:117.
Mizono G, Dedo HH. Subglottic hemangiomas in infants: Treatment with $CO_2$ laser. Laryngoscope 1984;94:638.
Narcy P, Contencin P, Bobin S, et al. Treatment of infantile subglottic hemangioma. A report of 49 cases. Int J Pediatr Otorhinolaryngol 1985;9:157.

### Laryngeal Papilloma

Aguado DL, Pinero BP, Betancor L, Mendez A, Banales EC. Acyclovir in the treatment of laryngeal papillomatosis. Int J Pediatr Otorhinolaryngol 1991;21:269.
Ahmed MM. Studies on human laryngeal papilloma. Acta Otolaryngol (Stockh) 1981;92:563.
Healy GB, Gelber RD, Trowbridge AL, Grundfast KM, Ruben RJ, Price KN. Treatment of recurrent respiratory papillomatosis with human leukocyte interferon: Results of a multicenter randomized clinical trial. N Engl J Med 1988;319:401.
Leventhal BG, Kashima HK, Mounts P, et al. Long-term response of recurrent respiratory papillomatosis to treatment with lymphoblastoid interferon alfa-n1. N Engl J Med 1991;325:613.
Leventhal BG, Kashima HK, Weck PW, et al. Randomized surgical adjuvant trial of interferon alfa-n1 in recurrent papillomatosis. Arch Otolaryngol Head Neck Surg 1988;114:1163.
Mounts P, Kashima HK. Association of human papillomavirus subtype and clinical course in respiratory papillomatosis. Laryngoscope 1984;94:28.
Nikolaidis ET, Trost DC, Buchholz CL, et al. The relationship of histologic and clinical factors in laryngeal papillomatosis. Arch Pathol Lab Med 1985;109:24.
Saito R, Date, R, Uno K, et al. Treatment of juvenile laryngeal papilloma with a combination of laser surgery and interferon. Auris Nasus Larynx 1985;12:117.

### Laryngeal Tumors

Abramowsky CR, Witt WJ. Sarcoma of the larynx in a newborn. Cancer 1983;51:1726.
Garud P, Elverland HH, Bostad L, et al. Granular-cell tumor of the larynx in a 5-year-old child. Ann Otol Rhinol Laryngol 1984;93:45.
Healy GB. Neoplasia of the pediatric larynx. Otolaryngol Clin North Am 1984;17:69.
Holinger P, Brown WT. Congenital webs, cysts, laryngoceles, and other anomalies of the larynx. Ann Otol Rhinol Laryngol 1967;76:744.

Keen M, Cho HT, Savetsky L. Pseudotumor of the larynx—an unusual cause of airway obstruction. Otolaryngol Head Neck Surg 1986;94:243.

Moisa II. Neuroendocrine tumors of the larynx. Head Neck 1991;13:498.

Pastore A, Zampano G. Laryngeal chondroma: Case report and surgical technique in a 9-year-old girl. Int J Pediatr Otorhinolaryngol 1984;7:79.

Shipton EA, Van der Linde JC. Paraganglioma of the larynx. A case report and clinical review. S Afr Med J 1984;65:176.

*Principles and Practice of Pediatrics, Second Edition.*
edited by Frank A. Oski et al. J. B. Lippincott Company, Philadelphia © 1994.

# CHAPTER 70
# *Immotile Cilia Syndrome*

Debra A. Cutler and Hal K. Hawkins

The mucus secreted in the respiratory tract is transported to the larynx by the constant synchronized beating of cilia lining the airways. The function of this ciliary apparatus may be disrupted by viral or bacterial agents, gastric acid or other chemicals, smoke, or other irritants that induce squamous metaplasia. Structural abnormalities of respiratory cilia and sperm tails have been described by Afzelius, who studied a group of infertile men with immotile spermatozoa and recurrent respiratory tract infections. Subsequently, several distinct ultrastructural abnormalities were described in the cilia of patients who had deficient mucociliary transport and recurrent respiratory tract infections. Many of these cases were familial, and about half expressed the classic Kartagener's triad of symptoms or signs (chronic sinusitis, bronchiectasis, and visceral situs inversus). Patients also have been described whose cilia are defective but motile, showing abnormal or uncoordinated movements. Thus, a more precise term for the immotile cilia syndrome is primary ciliary dyskinesia. In children, it is appropriate to suspect this condition in any patient who has chronic bronchitis, bronchiectasis, nasal polyposis, or recurrent sinusitis or otitis media. The probability that a given patient has the immotile cilia syndrome is, of course, much higher in children who also have situs inversus or a positive family history.

## STRUCTURE OF CILIA

A normal cilium consists of a tapered cylindric extension of cell surface membrane covering an axoneme that is composed of two central microtubules and nine peripheral pairs of microtubules (Fig 70-1). The outer pairs consist of an "A" microtubule with 13 tubulin monomers arranged in rows, and an incomplete "B" microtubule with 11 monomers. Attached to the "A" microtubule at intervals of 20 nm are inner and outer "arms" of dynein, large polypeptides that function as Ca,Mg-activated adenine triphosphatase. These dynein arms connect adjacent pairs of microtubules under certain conditions. The addition of adenosine triphosphate (ATP) to cilia that have been stripped of their membranes leads to the extrusion of single microtubule pairs. Thus, ATP-dependent sliding of adjacent microtubule pairs,

somehow constrained into a controlled whip-like stroke, appears to be the basis of ciliary motility. The outer microtubule pairs are connected to a central cluster of "sheath" fibers by a series of "radial spokes" that are arranged in a spiral and also show ATPase activity. Links of nexin permanently connect adjacent microtubule pairs.

## STRUCTURAL DEFECTS

In patients with the immotile cilia syndrome, both dynein arms may be completely absent, or either the outer or the inner arms may be absent or incomplete (Fig 70-2). An animal model has been described recently in a strain of rats in which both dynein arms are missing in cilia of the respiratory tract. In addition, several other abnormalities of ciliary structure have been described in familial cases. These include lack of radial spokes with consequent eccentricity of the two central microtubules, and loss of central microtubules with transposition of a peripheral microtubule doublet to the center. Patients with hereditary immotility or dyskinesia of cilia consistently have random orientation of the central microtubule pair, whereas the adjacent cilia of normal individuals usually are oriented in the same general direction. Rare patients have been described whose cilia are immotile, but appear normal by electron microscopy. It is not really surprising that certain essential gene products might not be visible by electron microscopy, because cilia contain numerous distinct polypeptides. Hereditary deficiency in ciliary structure affects all cilia in the same way in all biopsy specimens. It must be noted, however, that abnormal cilia are seen commonly, often together with normal cilia, in patients with respiratory tract infections. These acquired abnormalities must be distinguished carefully from

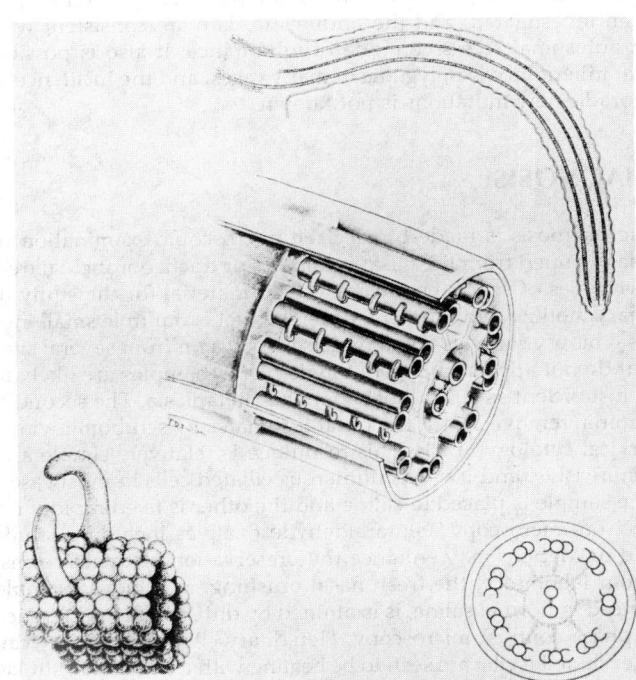

**Figure 70-1.** The fine structure of a cilium is depicted schematically and in longitudinal and transverse section. The nine outer microtubule pairs are built of tubulin subunits, carry inner and outer dynein arms, and are linked to the central structures by radial spokes. (Sturgess JM, Turner JAP. Ultrastructural pathology of cilia in the immotile cilia syndrome. Perspect Pediatr Pathol 1984;8:133. With permission of the authors.)

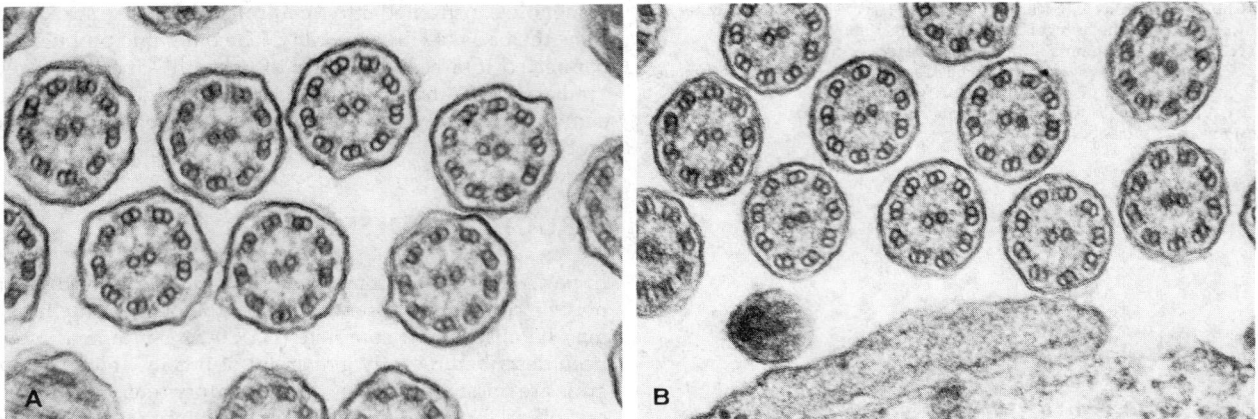

**Figure 70-2.** (**A**) This electron micrograph of a biopsy specimen from human nasal mucosa shows the features that ordinarily are visible in routinely prepared, carefully oriented transverse sections. Note the inner and outer dynein hooks, which are visible in some sections of outer doublets (original magnification ×180,000). (**B**) This micrograph shows cilia from a similar biopsy from a patient who had visceral situs inversus and chronic recurrent sinusitis. The outer dynein arms are abnormal, represented only by a short stub. No other abnormalities were noted (original magnification ×180,000).

genuine hereditary abnormalities of cilia. The secondary abnormalities that have been described include absence of dynein arms, radial spokes, and central microtubules; supernumerary microtubules; an abnormal matrix; "fusion" of adjacent cilia; and abnormal surrounding membranes. These abnormalities are thought to represent stages of ciliary regeneration.

## HEREDITY

Numerous familial cases of the immotile cilia syndrome have been investigated, and the findings to date are consistent with an autosomal recessive mode of inheritance. It also is possible that inheritance is polygenic in many cases, and the incidence of sporadic new mutations is not known.

## DIAGNOSIS

The diagnosis is made by electron microscopic examination of cilia obtained from the nasal turbinates or tracheobronchial tree. Two types of specimen yield excellent material for the study of ciliary motility and ultrastructure. The first is multiple small mucosal biopsy samples taken under direct vision from several sites that do not appear inflamed. Single biopsy samples are likely to be insufficient as a result of squamous metaplasia. The second is material removed from the nasal turbinates by scrubbing with a cervical cytology brush. This technique is relatively simple and noninvasive, and it yields numerous ciliated cells in most cases. One sample is placed in saline and the other is fixed rapidly for electron microscopy. Glutaraldehyde fixatives including tannic acid or $MgSO_4$, may enhance the preservation of dynein arms. In our laboratory, the fresh nasal brushing, or a biopsy sample minced in normal saline, is examined by differential interference or phase contrast microscopy. Hereditary ciliary immotility can be excluded if cilia are seen to be beating with a directional stroke. If cilia are absent, are not beating, or are abnormally motile, electron microscopy is used to evaluate structural abnormalities. It is important to take electron micrographs of numerous groups of cilia with proper orientation (using a goniometer stage) to determine whether any abnormalities are present consistently. Similarly, study of more than one biopsy sample is desirable to establish the diagnosis.

## THERAPY AND PROGNOSIS

Because the respiratory manifestations of the immotile cilia syndrome result from impairment of mucociliary clearance, therapy is directed toward removal of the bronchial secretions and prevention of complications such as infection and atelectasis. Aerosol treatments with normal saline, bronchodilators, and possibly mucolytic agents such as acetylcysteine, followed by chest physical therapy and postural drainage, help to liquefy bronchial secretions, assist in drainage of the airways, and relieve airway obstruction. Oral bronchodilators are used if wheezing associated with reactive airway disease develops. When symptoms of exacerbation of a respiratory tract infection develop, antibiotics are given. In addition, as with all patients with chronic lung disease, yearly vaccination for influenza is recommended.

In general, the prognosis for patients with the immotile cilia syndrome is good. Their lifespan usually is normal, with partial remission of symptoms occurring after adolescence.

### Selected Readings

Afzelius BA. A human syndrome caused by immotile cilia. Science 1976;193:317.

Carlen B, Stenram U. Ultrastructural diagnosis in the immotile cilia syndrome. Ultrastruct Pathol 1987;11:653.

Gonzalez S, von Bassewitz DB, Grundmann E, et al. Atypical cilia in hyperplastic, metaplastic and dysplastic human bronchial mucosa. Ultrastruct Pathol 1985;8:345.

Kartagener M. Zur pathogenese der bronchiektasien i mitteilung: Bronchiektasien bei situs viscerum inversus. Beitrage zur Klinik der Tuberkulose und Spezifischen Tuberkulose-Forschung 1933;83:498.

McDowell EM, Barrett LA, Harris CC, Trump BF. Abnormal cilia in human bronchial epithelium. Arch Pathol Lab Med 1976;100:429.

Rautiainen M, Collan Y, Nuutinen J, Afzelius B. Ciliary orientation in the "immotile cilia" syndrome. Eur Arch Otorhinolaryngol 1990;247:100.

Rossman C, Forrest J, Newhouse M. Motile cilia in "immotile cilia" syndrome. Lancet 1980;1:1360.

Rutland J, Dewar A, Cox T, Cole P. Nasal brushing for the study of ciliary ultrastructure. J Clin Pathol 1981;35:357.

Sturgess JM, Thompson MW, Czegledy-Nagy E, Turner JAP. Genetic aspects of immotile cilia syndrome. Am J Med Genet 1986;25:149.

Sturgess JM, Turner JAP. Ultrastructural pathology of cilia in the immotile cilia syndrome. Perspect Pediatr Pathol 1984;8:133.

Summers KE, Gibbons IR. Adenosine triphosphate-induced sliding of tubules in trypsin-treated flagella of sea-urchin sperm. Proc Natl Acad Sci U S A 1971;68:3092.

Torikata C, Kijimoto C, Koto M. Ultrastructure of respiratory cilia of WIC-Hyd male rats. An animal model for human immotile cilia syndrome. Am J Pathol 1991;138:341.

Van der Baan S, Veerman AJP, Wulffraat N, Bezemer P, Feenstra L. Primary ciliary dyskinesia: Ciliary activity. Acta Otolaryngol (Stockh) 1986;102:274.

*Principles and Practice of Pediatrics, Second Edition.*
edited by Frank A. Oski et al. J. B. Lippincott Company, Philadelphia © 1994.

# CHAPTER 71
# *Respiratory Complications of Burns and Smoke Inhalation (Respiratory Burns)*

## Marianna M. Sockrider and Dan K. Seilheimer

Respiratory complications are a major source of morbidity and mortality from fires. Severe injury to the respiratory tract can occur in the absence of surface burns. Several factors are associated with greater risk of respiratory injury: trapping of victims in confined spaces, unconsciousness of victims, fires involving plastics or steam, and victims who are small children or elderly individuals. The likelihood of asphyxia or respiratory inhalation injury is increased in the presence of cutaneous burn. Unconscious victims are at higher risk of injury due to loss of the protective mechanisms of breath holding and laryngospasm.

Respiratory inhalation injuries account for more than 50% of fire-related deaths. The mortality rate is greater in patients who have both cutaneous burns and inhalation injury. Injuries of the respiratory tract are distributed as follows: 60% upper airway, 30% major lower airway, and 10% parenchymal. Injuries may be seen at several levels simultaneously. Respiratory injuries are classified as thermal, chemical or toxic, and asphyxial. Mechanical interference with breathing may occur, with restricted chest wall movement due to chest burns or airway obstruction due to gastric aspiration. Secondary lung injury may result from sepsis and fluid overload. Hypoxemia may occur as a consequence of carbon monoxide (CO) intoxication, low inspired oxygen tension, or ventilation/perfusion mismatch.

Thermal injury may result from direct flame exposure, inhalation of hot gases, or inhalation of steam. Steam produces the most serious burns because of its higher heat-carrying capacity. Immediate injury to the oropharyngeal area with edema, erythema, and ulceration may lead to life-threatening upper airway obstruction. The normal function of the upper airway as a heat exchanger limits the exposure of the lower airway to thermal injury.

Chemical or toxic injury occurs from exposure to a variety of noxious gases. Chemical injury occurs more frequently than does heat injury. The site of injury depends on the duration of exposure, the size of soot particles, and the solubility of the gases. Damage to the tracheobronchial area results mainly from chemicals that are present in smoke. Toxic gases may be absorbed on small soot particles and carried deep into the lung. The inhaled gases may act as airway irritants or they may be absorbed and become systemic toxins.

Irritant gases, such as hydrogen chloride and oxides of nitrogen and sulfur, combine with water in the lung to form corrosive acids or alkalies. Aldehyde gases lead to the denaturation of surface proteins, resulting in pulmonary edema. Hydrogen cyanide gas causes systemic cyanide poisoning by inhibiting cellular oxidation. Studies of fire victims have revealed toxic cyanide concentrations with increasing frequency.

Carbon monoxide is the gas most commonly produced in fire. CO intoxication and hypoxia may account for as many as 80% of smoke inhalation fatalities, particularly deaths at the fire scene. CO produces its toxic effects by three mechanisms:

1. It has a higher affinity for hemoglobin and displaces oxygen.
2. It alters the ability of hemoglobin to release oxygen to the tissues.
3. It impairs the ability of tissue cells to use oxygen.

Although the oxygen content in the blood is reduced, the arterial pressure of oxygen is normal. The clinical manifestations of CO poisoning vary with the carboxyhemoglobin (COHgb) level. Mild intoxication (level <20%) may lead to headache, dyspnea, decreased visual acuity, and alteration of higher cerebral function. Moderate intoxication (level 20% to 40%) may lead to irritability, nausea, dim vision, impaired judgment, and rapid fatigue. Severe intoxication (level 40% to 60%) may lead to confusion, hallucinations, ataxia, shock, and coma. Concentrations higher than 60% usually are fatal.

The initial clinical assessment of fire victims should include evaluation for upper airway tract obstruction, central nervous system impairment, and cardiac arrhythmias. Respiratory symptoms such as tachypnea, cough, hoarseness, stridor, and chest retractions may be delayed, making them insensitive early indicators of injury. Second- and third-degree burns involving the "respiratory area" between the nose and lips have been associated with both upper airway tract edema and late-onset pulmonary problems, and indicate a need for more aggressive early intervention. Carbonaceous sputum serves only as a marker of exposure, with little diagnostic or prognostic import. The pulmonary examination may reveal diminished breath sounds, wheezes, crackles, and hoarseness. Both physical findings and symptoms may be delayed for as long as 15 hours after the injury.

The laboratory evaluation should include determination of the COHgb level, a complete blood count, and an arterial blood gas analysis. An abnormal $P_{O_2}$ is a strong indication for hospital admission; however, this reading initially may be normal. Soft-tissue radiographs of the neck may demonstrate upper airway tract edema. A chest radiograph should be obtained. Although the initial chest radiograph may be normal or show hyperinflation, subsequent radiographs may demonstrate pneumonitis, atelectasis, or pulmonary edema. Peribronchial infiltrates may persist for weeks. The negative predictive values of normal chest radiographs (38% to 59%) and arterial blood gas measurements (40% to 74%) are low. Normal findings do not exclude inhalation injury. A xenon 133 lung scan or spirometry may demonstrate early obstructive ventilatory defects that imply the presence of airway injury. These defects may have an early onset, antedating radiographic and arterial blood gas abnormalities; however, obtaining these studies may not be practical in young pediatric patients.

Fiberoptic endoscopy allows immediate direct visualization of the airway injury. Early laryngoscopy is recommended to evaluate compromising intraoral edema, especially in patients with facial burns and those who have had significant exposure. Endoscopic findings such as laryngeal or tracheal edema, ulceration or inflammation of airway mucosa, and soot deposits confirm the presence of respiratory tract injury and may antedate radiographic and arterial blood gas abnormalities. The negative predictive value of fiberoptic bronchoscopy is 88% to 100%. It may be particularly helpful in those individuals in whom the results of initial studies are normal or equivocal.

The time course of clinical symptoms depends on the type and severity of injury. CO intoxication, upper airway tract injury, and tracheobronchial obstruction develop in the first 24 hours. During the next 2 to 5 days, noncardiogenic pulmonary edema may develop, particularly in the presence of superimposed sepsis. Nosocomial pneumonia and pulmonary embolism usually occur late, more than 5 days after the event.

The basic tenets of therapy are maintenance of an adequate airway, correction of hypoxia, reversal of ventilation/perfusion abnormalities, clearance of airway debris and secretions, and prompt recognition and treatment of bacterial infection. At the scene, 100% oxygen should be administered and airway patency should be established. Fire victims with any risk of inhalation injury should be observed for the development of respiratory symptoms for at least 24 hours.

Indications for endotracheal intubation include severe burns to the face, laryngeal obstruction, difficulty in handling secretions, and progressive respiratory insufficiency. Swelling increases over the first 8 to 24 hours, and worsening should be anticipated if any degree of laryngeal obstruction is present on early examination. Extubation usually can be accomplished within 2 to 5 days. Tracheostomy commonly is reserved for situations in which there is acute respiratory distress in a child who cannot undergo endotracheal intubation or fails to tolerate extubation. Bronchodilators may be helpful for bronchospasm, and chest physical therapy may enhance the removal of necrotic material and avoid atelectasis. Bronchoscopy may be necessary to clear inspissated secretions. Cautious use of resuscitative fluids is encouraged, because overhydration is associated with a marked increase in pulmonary edema.

Corticosteroids have no established benefit and actually may increase the risk of infection. There is no benefit to the use of prophylactic antibiotics, which may lead to the development of resistant organisms. Daily surveillance of sputum Gram stain may be helpful to detect potential pathogenic organisms should clinical deterioration occur. Pulmonary infection occurs in 15% of patients with respiratory injury alone and in a much greater percentage of patients with surface burns. Treatment should be based on the results of Gram stain and culture of lower respiratory tract secretions.

Treatment of CO intoxication with 100% oxygen leads to reduction of the COHgb level by one half in 40 to 60 minutes. The role of using 2 to 3 atm of oxygen is controversial. Although hyperbaric oxygen does lower COHgb levels more rapidly, it is questionable whether it provides a significant advantage over the administration of an $F_{IO_2}$ of 1.0 and whether it affects the incidence of delayed neurologic complications in patients whose COHgb level already is less than 30 on arrival at the hospital. Although the diagnosis of cyanide poisoning is difficult to establish, it should be suspected in fires in which plastics or chemicals are fuel and in patients who remain comatose after COHgb levels fall to less than 30. Cyanide poisoning is treated with sodium nitrite to induce methemoglobinemia, followed by slow intravenous infusion of sodium thiosulfate.

Most patients who sustain smoke inhalation and survive the initial event regain nearly normal function. Few follow-up studies exist; however, there have been reports of bronchiectasis, bronchiolitis obliterans, tracheal stenosis, and airway granulation tissue formation.

## Selected Readings

Calhoun KH, Deskin RW, Garza C, et al. Long-term airway sequelae in a pediatric burn population. Laryngoscope 1988;98:721.

Charnock EL, Meehan JJ. Postburn respiratory injuries in children. Pediatr Clin North Am 1980;27:661.

Haponik EF, Crapo RO, Herndon DN, Traber DL, Hudson L, Moylan J. Smoke inhalation. Am Rev Respir Dis 1988;138:1060.

Haponik EF, Summer WR. Respiratory complications in burned patients: Pathogenesis and spectrum of inhalation injury. Journal of Critical Care 1987;2:49.

Herndon DN, Barrow RE, Linares HA, et al. Inhalation injury in burned patients: Effects and treatment. Burns 1988;14:349.

Parish RA. Smoke inhalation and carbon monoxide poisoning in children. Pediatr Emerg Care 1986;2:36.

*Principles and Practice of Pediatrics, Second Edition.*
edited by Frank A. Oski et al. J. B. Lippincott Company, Philadelphia © 1994.

# CHAPTER 72
# *Cystic Fibrosis*

## Beryl J. Rosenstein

Cystic fibrosis (CF) is the most common lethal or semilethal genetic disease affecting whites. The triad of chronic obstructive pulmonary disease, pancreatic exocrine deficiency, and abnormally high sweat electrolyte concentration is present in most patients. CF is the major cause of chronic debilitating pulmonary disease and pancreatic exocrine deficiency in the first three decades of life and accounts for a significant number of cases of neonatal intestinal obstruction. The name of the disease is derived from the characteristic histologic changes seen in the pancreas.

## GENETICS

Estimates of the incidence of CF vary according to the population studied, but a reasonable figure for whites is 1 in 2500. The highest incidence is seen in persons of Anglo-Saxon ancestry. The incidence of CF in American blacks is 1 in 17,000. The CF gene is rare in African blacks and Asians. Transmission is autosomal recessive. Based on incidence figures, 4% of whites in the United States are estimated to be carriers (heterozygous) of the CF gene. A heterozygote advantage has been postulated but never documented. Heterozygous persons have no recognizable clinical symptoms. An increased incidence of airway reactivity, however, has been reported in CF carriers, suggesting a subtle abnormality of autonomic function.

### Gene Defect

The gene responsible for CF has been localized to 250,000 base pairs of genomic DNA located on the long arm of chromosome 7. It encodes a protein of 1480 amino acids called the cystic fibrosis transmembrane conductance regulator (CFTR). A 3-base deletion removing a phenylalanine residue at position 508 of CFTR (Δ F508 mutation) is present on about 70% of CF chromosomes. The remaining cases are accounted for by more than 300 mutations, none of which accounts for more than 4% of the cases. The ability to detect CF mutations by direct DNA analysis represents a major improvement in prenatal diagnosis and heterozygote detection, even in families in which DNA is not available from an affected child.

### Ion Transport Abnormality

The CFTR protein contains two nucleotide-binding folds with adenosine triphosphate (ATP) binding sites, a regulatory region with many phosphorylation sites, and two hydrophobic regions that probably interact with cell membranes. The CFTR protein appears to be related to a family of membrane-bound glycoproteins involved in the transport of small molecules across cell membranes; there is evidence that CFTR is a cAMP-activated chloride channel. Functional expression of the CF defect reduces the ability of epithelial cells in the airways and pancreas to secrete chloride in response to cAMP-mediated agonists. Enhanced absorption of sodium across the airway epithelium and failure to secrete chloride (and thereby fluid) toward the airway lumen is thought to lead to dehydration of airway mucus and the abnormal mucociliary clearance and lung disease seen in patients with CF. Complementation of the CF defect has been accomplished in CF airway epithelial cells in vivo in an animal model with an adenovirus vector and in vitro by virus-mediated transduction and plasmid-transfection of a full-length CFTR cDNA.

## PATHOPHYSIOLOGY

Initially, CF was thought to involve primarily the pancreas, but many of the clinical and pathologic findings can be explained by a generalized defect in mucous secretion. When the sweat gland defect was discovered, it became apparent that abnormalities exist in all exocrine glands. Most clinical manifestations can be related to abnormal secretions that result in obstruction of organ passages and to abnormal function of the eccrine sweat glands. Glands are affected in varying distribution and degrees of severity and fall into three types: those obstructed by viscid or solid eosinophilic material in the lumen (pancreas, intestinal glands, intrahepatic bile ducts, gallbladder, submaxillary glands), those that produce an excess of histologically normal secretions (tracheobronchial and Brunner's glands), and those that are histologically normal but secrete excessive electrolytes (sweat, parotid, and small salivary glands). The high concentration of electrolytes in sweat is due to decreased transductal reabsorption of chloride and sodium.

## CLINICAL FEATURES

Table 72-1 is a summary of clinical manifestations of CF.

### Pulmonary

The respiratory tract is invariably involved, and pulmonary complications usually dominate the clinical picture. Manifestations may not appear, however, until weeks, months, or even years after birth. Autopsy studies suggest that the lungs are normal at birth. The initial pulmonary lesion is obstruction of the small airways by abnormally thick mucus secretions. Secondary to obstruction, there is bronchiolitis and mucopurulent plugging of the airways. Bronchial changes are more common than parenchymal changes. Bronchiectasis is present in almost all patients older than age 18 months. It progresses with age and is especially striking in older patients. Emphysema is not common. Figure 72-1 shows a proposed mechanism for pulmonary manifestations seen in patients with CF.

### Infection

Secondary bacterial infection, first due to *Staphylococcus aureus* then to *Pseudomonas aeruginosa*, initiates a cycle of chronic infection, tissue damage, and obstruction. More than 80% of patients with advanced disease consistently harbor strains of *P aeruginosa*, most of which are heavy slime producers known as mucoid variants. These are rarely found in other diseases. The susceptibility of these patients to infection with mucoid *Pseudomonas* strains may be related to a defect in phagocytosis in the lung. Once established, *Pseudomonas* is virtually impossible to eradicate. Systemic defense mechanisms appear to be intact, and infection tends to be localized to the respiratory tract. Septicemia and extrapulmonary infections are rare. In recent years, the incidence of *Pseudomonas cepacia* colonization among adolescent and adult CF patients has increased. Risk factors for colonization include increasing age and severity of underlying disease, ex-

## TABLE 72-1. Summary of Clinical Manifestations

| Upper Respiratory Tract | Nutritional/Metabolic |
|---|---|
| Nasal polyposis | Diabetes |
| Sinusitis | Hypokalemic alkalosis |
| | Hypoprothrombinemia |
| **Pulmonary** | Iron deficiency anemia |
| Allergic bronchopulmonary aspergillosis | Salt depletion syndrome |
| Atelectasis | Protein–calorie malnutrition |
| Bronchiectasis | Vitamin A deficiency |
| Bronchiolitis | Vitamin E deficiency |
| Bronchitis | |
| Cor pulmonale | **Miscellaneous** |
| Hemoptysis | Arthritis/arthropathy |
| Pneumothorax | Absent vas deferens |
| Pneumonia | Aspermia |
| Reactive airway disease | Decreased female fertility |
| Respiratory failure | Delayed puberty |
| | Digital clubbing |
| **Hepatobiliary** | Erythema nodosum |
| Cholecystitis | Failure to thrive |
| Cholelithiasis | Growth retardation |
| Cholestasis | Malnutrition |
| Cirrhosis/portal hypertension | |
| | |
| **Gastrointestinal** | |
| Gastroesophageal reflux | |
| Intussusception | |
| Meconium ileus | |
| Meconium ileus equivalent | |
| Meconium plug syndrome | |
| Pancreatic exocrine deficiency | |
| Pancreatitis | |
| Peptic ulcer disease | |
| Rectal prolapse | |

posure to a sibling colonized with *P cepacia*, and recent hospitalization. Person-to-person transmission has been documented in residential summer camps. Acquisition of this organism, especially by females with moderate or advanced pulmonary disease, may be followed by an unexpectedly rapid decline. The course of disease in some of these patients is characterized by recurrent episodes of fever and bacteremia. If patients do not respond as expected to antimicrobial therapy, then infection with unusual organisms (eg, *Mycobacterium tuberculosis*, atypical mycobacteria) should be considered.

### Inflammatory Lung Damage

Immune-mediated inflammation contributes significantly to lung damage in patients with CF. Recruitment and activation of neutrophils in the airways leads to a high level of elastolytic activity secondary to the release of proteases such as granulocyte elastase and Cathepsin G. This protease burden is associated with breakdown of the lung matrix and with cleavage and inactivation of a variety of opsonins, thereby contributing to the persistence of *Pseudomonas* in the lung. Evidence shows immune complex formation in 20% to 100% of patients with CF, which may also contribute to inflammatory lung damage. The presence of immune complexes correlates with disease severity and prognosis.

### Signs and Symptoms

Half of patients present with pulmonary manifestations, usually consisting of chronic cough and wheezing along with recurrent

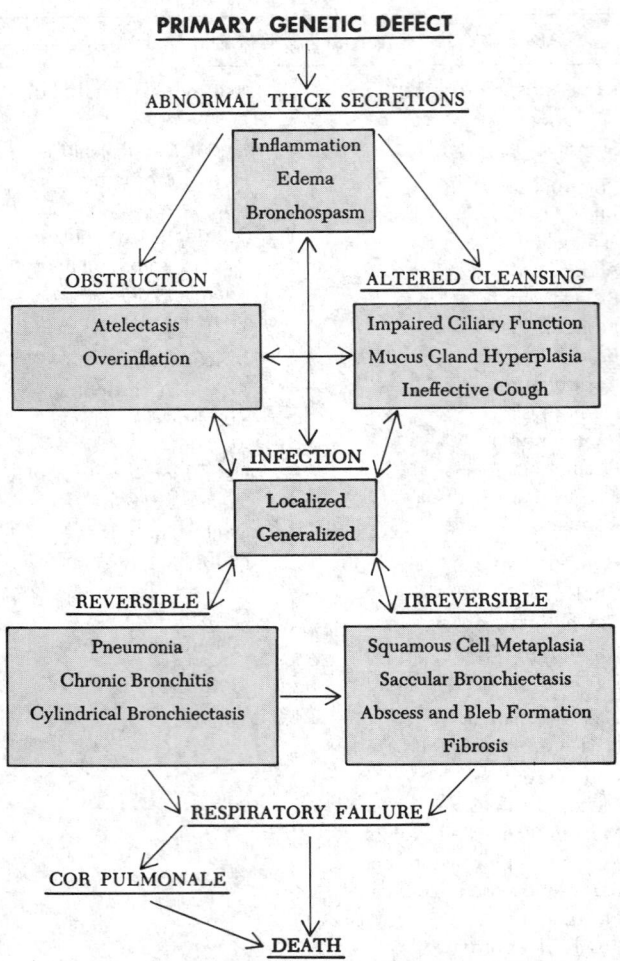

**PRIMARY GENETIC DEFECT**

↓

ABNORMAL THICK SECRETIONS

Inflammation
Edema
Bronchospasm

OBSTRUCTION                    ALTERED CLEANSING

Atelectasis            Impaired Ciliary Function
Overinflation          Mucus Gland Hyperplasia
                       Ineffective Cough

INFECTION

Localized
Generalized

REVERSIBLE                     IRREVERSIBLE

Pneumonia              Squamous Cell Metaplasia
Chronic Bronchitis     Saccular Bronchiectasis
Cylindrical Bronchiectasis   Abscess and Bleb Formation
                       Fibrosis

RESPIRATORY FAILURE

COR PULMONALE

↓

DEATH

**Figure 72-1.** Proposed mechanism for the pulmonary manifestations seen in patients with CF. (With permission from Guide to Diagnosis and Management of Cystic Fibrosis. Bethesda, Md: Cystic Fibrosis Foundation, 1979:8.)

or chronic infections. Young infants can present with atelectasis, often involving the right upper lobe, or a severe bronchiolitic syndrome. The most prominent and constant feature of pulmonary involvement is chronic cough. At first, the cough may be dry, but with progression it becomes paroxysmal and productive. Older patients expectorate mucopurulent sputum, particularly in association with pulmonary exacerbations. Wheezing is often a prominent feature, especially in association with pulmonary exacerbations, but it is unclear if this reflects inflammation and bronchial obstruction or coincidental atopy. A few patients develop allergic bronchopulmonary aspergillosis. Physical findings include a barrel-chest deformity, use of accessory muscles of respiration, growth retardation, digital clubbing, pulmonary hypertrophic osteoarthropathy, and cyanosis.

### Radiographic Changes

Chest x-ray findings can help in the diagnosis of CF. Hyperinflation and bronchial wall thickening are the earliest findings (Fig 72-2). Subsequent changes include areas of infiltrate, atelectasis, and hilar adenopathy. With advanced disease, segmental or lobar atelectasis, bleb formation, bronchiectasis, and pulmonary artery and right ventricular enlargement are seen. Characteristic branching, finger-like opacifications represent mucoid impaction of dilated bronchi.

### Pulmonary Function

Airway obstruction, air trapping, and ventilation–perfusion inequalities are the most important functional changes in CF. Ventilation–perfusion scans usually demonstrate focal areas of inequality. Pulmonary function tests reveal hypoxemia; reduction in forced vital capacity (FVC), in forced expiratory volume in 1 second ($FEV_1$), and in $FEV_1$ to FVC ratio; and an increase in residual volume and in the ratio of residual volume to total lung capacity. Flow–volume loops demonstrate a characteristic "scooped-out" appearance, indicative of small airways disease (Fig 72-3), secondary to flow limitation at lower lung volumes. Airway reactivity, based on broncho-provocative challenges, is present in 50% of patients and may be associated with accelerated progression of pulmonary disease. The response to bronchodilators is unpredictable and varies with time and changes in underlying pulmonary status.

### Pneumothorax

In patients with advanced lung disease, pneumothorax, hemoptysis, and cor pulmonale are frequent complications. Pneumothorax occurs secondary to rupture of apical subpleural blebs. The overall incidence is 2% to 10% and, in adults, may be as high as 16%. Patients typically present with acute onset of chest pain and shortness of breath. After a pneumothorax on one side, there is a 50% incidence on the contralateral side within 6 to 12 months.

### Hemoptysis

Patients often experience blood streaking of their sputum. Bleeding is due to erosion of bronchial arteries into a bronchus, often in association with an exacerbation of the underlying pulmonary infection. Massive hemoptysis is a serious complication associated with significant mortality, a high recurrence rate, and a poor prognosis. The site of bleeding may be localized by bronchoscopy.

### Cor Pulmonale

Cor pulmonale, manifested by hypertrophy of the right ventricle, is seen in 70% of patients dying with CF and occurs in 50% of patients surviving past age 15 years. Chronic alveolar hypoxia

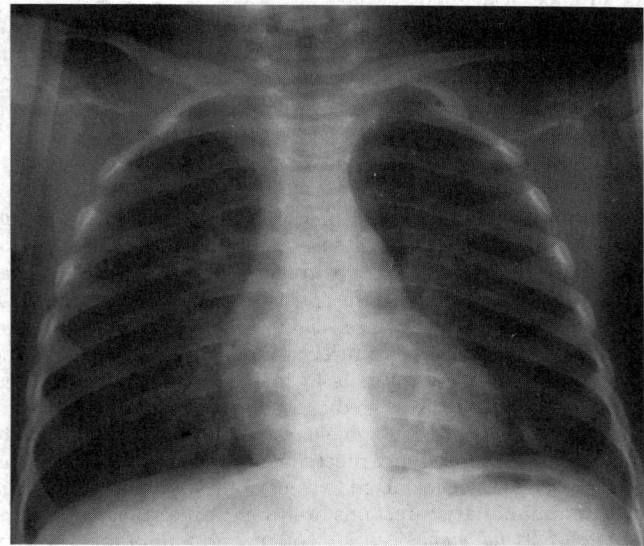

**Figure 72-2.** Chest radiograph from a 6-year-old patient showing increased lung markings and focal areas of peribronchial thickening.

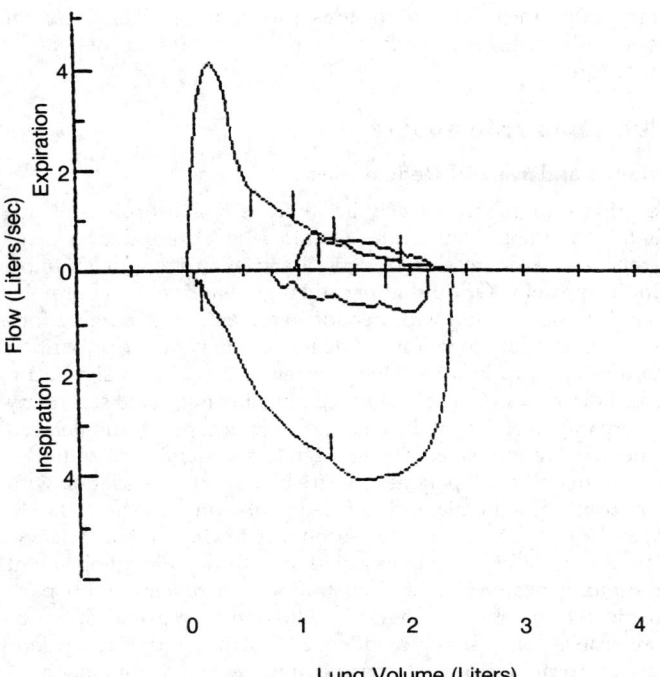

**Figure 72-3.** Flow–volume loop from a 23-year-old patient showing decreased flow at all lung volumes. The "scooped out" appearance is indicative of small airways disease.

and hypoxemia serve as a stimulus to reflex vasoconstriction and medial hypertrophy of the pulmonary arteries. Severe cor pulmonale has been consistently associated with $PaO_2$ values of less than 50 mm Hg. Clinically, cor pulmonale may be difficult to recognize. Peripheral edema is present in only two thirds of cases and is often a late manifestation. Liver tenderness may be an early clue. The electrocardiogram does not correlate consistently with the presence of right ventricular hypertrophy. Echocardiography is probably the most practical and reliable way of documenting cor pulmonale and following its course.

### Course

The pulmonary course is characterized by chronic suppurative bronchitis with recurrent pulmonary exacerbations, often following viral respiratory infections. Infection with respiratory syncytial virus may be an important cause of significant respiratory morbidity in young infants. By age 10 years, 90% of patients have intermittent sputum production; by age 15 years, 90% of patients have daily sputum production. There is progressive shortness of breath and exercise intolerance. Pulmonary involvement advances at a variable rate, usually faster in females than males, but eventually leads to respiratory failure, cardiac failure, or both.

### Upper Respiratory Tract

The upper respiratory tract is usually affected secondary to the hyperactive mucus-secreting glands and the hyperplasia and edema of mucous membranes. Chronic nasal congestion and rhinitis are common. Radiographic evidence of opacification of the paranasal sinuses is present in almost all patients and may be helpful diagnostically in patients with equivocal sweat test results. Clinically significant sinusitis is common and troublesome in some patients. Chronic sinusitis may contribute to infection of the lower respiratory tract. Computed tomography scans of the sinuses help in assessing the extent of sinus involvement and in selecting pa-

tients for a surgical drainage procedure. Slowly progressive unilateral proptosis may occur secondary to formation of an inflammatory mucocele in the underlying maxillary and ethmoid sinuses.

Nasal polyps occur in 6% to 24% of patients. Clinical manifestations include obstruction to nasal airflow, mouth breathing, localized infection, epistaxis, rhinorrhea, and widening of the nasal bridge. Polyps occur at a much younger age in patients with CF as compared with those with underlying atopy, can be differentiated histologically, and tend to recur. The incidence of hearing problems in patients with CF is probably no higher than in the general population.

## Gastrointestinal

### Pancreatic Exocrine Deficiency

The most common gastrointestinal manifestations result from loss of pancreatic enzyme activity and consequent intestinal malabsorption of fats, proteins, and, to a lesser extent, carbohydrates. Complete loss of pancreatic activity is seen in 85% to 90% of patients. Loss of function may be progressive. Clinical manifestations include poor or no weight gain, abdominal distention, deficiency of subcutaneous fat and muscle tissue, rectal prolapse, and frequent passage of pale, bulky, foul-smelling, often oily stools. Steatorrhea and azotorrhea are pronounced. Secondary to pancreatic insufficiency, patients have low serum lipid levels and may be deficient in linoleic acid. Although infants may appear to have a voracious appetite, caloric intake is often deficient. In adolescent patients, there may be absence of a pubertal growth spurt and delayed maturation. In general, growth retardation correlates more closely with the degree of pulmonary involvement. Adolescents and young adults with residual pancreatic function may have recurrent episodes of pancreatitis, sometimes as the presenting manifestation. Patients with residual pancreatic function tend to have lower sweat chloride values, less severe pulmonary involvement, and better survival.

### Evaluation of Pancreatic Function

Tests of fat absorption, including 72-hour fecal fat excretion, provide indirect assessment of pancreatic exocrine function. The most direct measure involves analysis of duodenal fluid before and after intravenous injection of pancreozymin and secretin. In patients with CF, volume and bicarbonate secretion (ductular activity) are grossly reduced, regardless of the presence of steatorrhea. In those patients with steatorrhea, enzyme secretion (acinar activity) is virtually absent. Less invasive means of assessing pancreatic function include: measuring stool trypsin and chymotrypsin, measuring urinary or serum levels of p-aminobenzoic acid after oral administration of synthetic chymotrypsin substrates containing p-aminobenzoic acid, and measuring serum immunoreactive trypsin (IRT) levels. IRT levels progressively decline with destruction of the pancreas.

### Carbohydrate Intolerance

In addition to pancreatic exocrine dysfunction, up to 40% of patients show carbohydrate intolerance that progresses to frank diabetes in 2% to 5% of cases. The incidence of carbohydrate intolerance increases with age, but diabetes has been seen at age 6 months. Diabetes in patients with CF is characterized by insidious onset, mild clinical course, and virtual absence of ketoacidosis. Retinopathy, nephropathy, and vascular changes are infrequent. Evidence shows that CF-associated diabetes does not adversely affect the pulmonary course or shorten survival. The mild diabetic course in these patients may be due to preservation of some endogenous insulin output, decreased glucagon secretion, and compensatory enhancement of peripheral tissue sensitivity to insulin.

## Meconium Ileus

Meconium ileus, in which there is obstruction of the distal ileum by inspissated, tenacious meconium, occurs in 10% to 15% of newborn infants with CF. With rare exception, meconium ileus is always associated with CF. It is probably related to in utero deficiency of proteolytic enzymes along with secretion of abnormal mucoproteins by the goblet cells of the small intestine. Clinically, infants present with evidence of intestinal obstruction. Abdominal films show distended bowel loops with a "bubbly" pattern of inspissated meconium in the terminal ileum. Contrast enema shows a microcolon from disuse secondary to intrauterine obstruction. Associated intestinal complications, including small-bowel atresia, volvulus, and perforation/peritonitis are present in 40% to 50% of cases. Meconium ileus tends to recur in the same family. A delay in the passage of meconium and distal colonic obstruction secondary to the meconium plug syndrome also may be presenting manifestations of CF and are indications for a sweat test.

## Late Intestinal Complications

The intestinal contents tend to be abnormally thick and putty-like as a result of abnormal behavior of intestinal gland secretions, decreased chloride secretion across the colonic epithelium, deficiency of pancreatic enzymes, and prolonged intestinal transit time. This may lead to a variety of late intestinal complications. There may be recurrent episodes of partial or complete obstruction of the small or large bowel, often preceded or accompanied by colicky abdominal pain and a palpable firm mass in the right lower quadrant. This symptom complex is referred to as meconium ileus equivalent or the distal intestinal obstruction syndrome and occurs in as many as 20% of patients. These episodes may be precipitated by decreased fluid intake, change in diet, or cessation of pancreatic enzyme supplements. Precipitated by the abnormal intestinal contents, there may be episodes of small-bowel volvulus or intussusception. The latter complication occurs in 1% of older patients and may be the presenting manifestation. Episodes tend to recur and may be associated with chronic symptoms.

Diagnosis of CF can be suggested by the histology of the appendix; goblet cells are increased in number and distended with mucous, and eosinophilic casts may fill the crypts and extend into the lumen. Mucoid impaction of the appendix may present as a right lower quadrant mass in the absence of other symptoms. Recurrent episodes of rectal prolapse occur in as many as one fourth of patients, who are usually 1 to 2 years of age, most often before the diagnosis is established. Rectal prolapse probably is related to frequent bulky stools, malnutrition, and raised intra-abdominal pressure secondary to paroxysmal cough. The diagnosis of CF should be considered in every patient with rectal prolapse.

## Upper Gastrointestinal Complications

Patients with CF have an increased incidence of gastroesophageal reflux, probably related to chest hyperinflation along with increased abdominal pressure due to coughing. It may be manifested by vomiting and failure to thrive in infants and by abdominal pain, esophageal ulcerations, stricture formation, and blood loss in older patients. Despite increased gastric acid secretion and a low pH in the duodenum (secondary to decreased bicarbonate output), duodenal ulcers have been diagnosed antemortem in only a few patients. A high incidence of peptic ulcer disease, however, has been reported in black adolescents with CF. Radiographically, duodenal abnormalities consisting of thickened mucosal folds, nodular filling defects, and mucosal smudging have been noted in 80% of patients. Because of these abnormalities, peptic ulcer disease may be hard to diagnose radio-graphically. In patients with signs and symptoms suggestive of peptic ulcer disease, endoscopy is the preferred diagnostic procedure.

## Nutritional/Metabolic

### Vitamin and Mineral Deficiencies

Secondary to pancreatic achylia, there is malabsorption of fat-soluble vitamins. Low serum vitamin A levels are due to steatorrhea and a depression of retinol-carrier protein and retinol-binding protein. Xerophthalmia and night blindness occur rarely, usually in association with hepatic involvement. A bulging fontanelle, secondary to vitamin A deficiency, may be the presenting manifestation in infants. Overt rickets is rare, but a significant reduction in vitamin D biologic activity with associated secondary hyperparathyroidism, reduced bone mineral content, and delayed bone maturation is common. Significant demineralization is present in half of all patients. Severe bleeding in association with hypoprothrombinemia and deficiency of clotting factors II, VII, IX, and X may occur in infants secondary to vitamin K deficiency. This is especially likely in association with hepatic involvement or prolonged antibiotic administration. All patients with pancreatic achylia show a marked reduction in plasma alpha-tocopherol levels. Histologic evidence of vitamin E deficiency consists of focal necrosis of striated muscle and ceroid pigment deposition in intestinal smooth muscle. Red blood cells show a moderate decrease in survival although usually not sufficient to produce hemolytic anemia. A progressive spinocerebellar syndrome consisting of ataxia, areflexia, and proprioceptive loss has been seen in patients with prolonged vitamin E deficiency. Clinically, there are no problems associated with deficiency of water-soluble vitamins.

Symptomatic hypomagnesemia has been reported in patients on prolonged aminoglycoside therapy and in those being treated for distal intestinal obstruction syndrome. Decreased plasma levels of zinc and selenium have been reported but do not correlate with clinical evidence of deficiency. Iron deficiency anemia is seen in one third of patients. It is probably related to a variety of factors including inadequate iron intake, impairment of iron absorption, and effects of chronic infection.

### Edema and Hypoproteinemia

The syndrome of edema and hypoproteinemia, secondary to pancreatic enzyme deficiency, may be the presenting manifestation in as many as 8% of patients with CF. It is seen most often in infants 1 to 6 months of age who are breast-fed or receive soy-based formula. Associated findings include hepatomegaly, elevation of liver enzymes, skin rash, and anemia. False-negative sweat test results can be seen in the presence of edema.

### Salt Loss

Clinically, the sweat gland abnormality has important implications. Patients may have a "salty taste" or show salt crystal formation on the skin, findings which are highly suggestive of CF. Patients also may develop dehydration with massive salt depletion, especially in association with gastrointestinal losses or under thermal stress. Profound hypoelectrolytemia, not accounted for by gastrointestinal losses, is particularly suggestive of CF. In arid climates, chronic salt loss can lead to metabolic alkalosis and electrolyte depletion without appreciable dehydration and is a common presenting manifestation of CF.

## Hepatobiliary

### Liver

The liver is extensively involved in CF. Focal biliary cirrhosis—characterized by the inspissation of amorphous, eosinophilic material in the intrahepatic bile ducts, bile duct proliferation, inflammatory reaction, a variable degree of fibrosis, and focal distribution—is pathognomonic of CF. It is associated with and probably due to an excessive accumulation of biliary mucus. This lesion is present in 25% of patients and may appear as early as 3 days of age. It usually produces no clinical manifestations, but secondary to the intrahepatic bile stasis, there may be prolonged neonatal jaundice. Half of such cases occur in association with meconium ileus. In 4% to 6% of patients, the focal biliary cirrhosis progresses to a multilobular biliary cirrhosis that consists of groups of normal-appearing lobules surrounded by dense fibrous septa containing proliferating bile ducts with eosinophilic concretions. This lesion is specific for CF. Hypoalbuminemia in infancy may predispose to later liver complications. Portal hypertension, which is manifested by hepatomegaly, esophageal varices, and hypersplenism, develops in 2% to 3% of all patients and in 5% of adults. Development of thrombocytopenia may be an early clue to the presence of cirrhosis and hypersplenism. Liver failure is rare, and liver function tests may show only mild transaminase elevation until late in the course of disease. Fatty infiltration of the liver secondary to protein–calorie malnutrition may present clinically as massive hepatomegaly. In some patients, liver complications may be the predominant and, at times, presenting features. Liver complications are seen only in those patients with pancreatic insufficiency; there may be a familial pattern to their occurrence.

### Gallbladder

Abnormalities of the gallbladder are common, occurring in 60% of adult patients. The gallbladder is often hypoplastic and filled with thick, colorless mucus (white bile). Calculi are present in about 10% of adult patients, and symptoms referable to gallbladder disease are seen in 3% to 4% of patients.

## Reproductive System

### Male

Aspermia and infertility are seen in 98% of adult males. Histologically, the testes show active but decreased spermatogenesis. There is mechanical obstruction of sperm transport, however, that is secondary to absence or atresia of the vas deferens, along with associated abnormalities of the epididymis and seminal vesicle. The prostate is normal. All postpubescent males should have their semen analyzed for purposes of counseling. Defects of the Wolffian duct structures appear to be specifically related to CF and are a consistent pathologic feature of the disease. An increased incidence of abnormalities associated with testicular descent, (ie, hernia, hydrocele, and undescended testes) has also been reported. A primarily genital form of CF has been described in otherwise healthy men who have congenital bilateral absence of the vas deferens, a high frequency of CF mutations, and normal, borderline, or elevated sweat electrolyte values.

### Female

Although fertility is decreased, many women with CF bear children. Histologically, there is excessive cytoplasmic and extracellular mucus, and there is often plugging of the cervical os by tenacious, dehydrated mucus. This probably acts as a barrier to sperm penetration. The ovaries and endometrium are normal. Among women who become pregnant, there may be deterioration of pulmonary status and there is an increased incidence of spontaneous abortion, prematurity, and stillbirth, possibly related to maternal hypoxemia. Favorable pregnancy outcomes correlate with good nutritional status (more than 85% ideal body weight) and good pulmonary function (FVC more than 80% predicted). In contemplating pregnancy, women with CF need to consider potential health risk to themselves, the genetic risks to their offspring, and child care responsibility associated with impaired health and shortened life expectancy. Oral contraceptives have been shown to be safe in patients with CF.

## Skeletal

### Pulmonary Hypertrophic Osteoarthropathy

Hypertrophic osteoarthropathy, manifested by arthralgias, long bone pain, stiffness, joint swelling, effusion, and radiographic evidence of periostitis is present in as many as 15% of adolescent and adult patients and correlates with severity of the underlying pulmonary disease. The knees, ankles, and wrists are most frequently affected; involvement is usually bilateral and symmetrical. The course is one of chronicity with intermittent exacerbations. Nonsteroidal anti-inflammatory agents provide symptomatic relief.

### Rheumatoid Arthritis

Chronic seropositive arthritis has been reported in patients with CF, probably as a coincidental finding.

### Back Pain and Spinal Deformity

Back pain that is not associated with trauma is present in most patients. It usually affects the mid and lower back, may be exacerbated by coughing, and often interferes with exercise, coughing, daily activities, and physiotherapy. Associated features include decreased range of motion and muscle strength, a "hunched over" posture, and a high incidence of vertebral wedging. Treatment consists of exercise and postural counseling.

### Episodic Arthritis

Unrelated to the severity of the patient's lung disease, recurrent, transient episodes of nondisabling, seronegative, polyarticular arthritis have been described. Associated findings include erythematous and purpuric rashes, erythema nodosum, hypergammaglobulinemia, and elevated levels of circulating immune complexes. Large and small joints are affected; episodes tend to last less than 1 week and may recur at intervals of several weeks to more than a year. Residual joint limitation and joint deformity do not occur. Nonsteroidal anti-inflammatory agents usually provide relief.

## Other Organ Systems

Ocular abnormalities in CF include visual field defects, venous engorgement and tortuosity, hyperemia, and blurring of the nerve head. Acute hemorrhagic retinopathy may occur at high altitudes. Optic atrophy and neuritis have been observed in patients on long-term chloramphenicol therapy. Increased intracranial pressure, manifested by a bulging fontanelle, has been seen in infants with severe respiratory distress, in association with vitamin A deficiency and during recovery from malnutrition. Brain abscesses have been reported in young adults. Posterior column degeneration, in most cases limited to the fasciculus gracilis, is seen in patients dying after 5 years of age. Its occurrence has been related to vitamin E deficiency. In the thyroid gland, there is excessive accumulation of lipofuscin pigment in the follicular epithelial cells. In patients treated with iodide, there is a high incidence of goiter, often in association with clinical or laboratory evidence of hypothyroidism. Puberty is delayed in both boys and girls with CF by an average of 1 to 4 years. Skeletal maturation progresses slowly, but most patients attain near-normal adult height. Maturational delays correlate with the patients' underlying pulmonary and nutritional status. In male adolescents, growth acceleration can be achieved with a brief course of testosterone.

Isolated growth hormone deficiency has been documented in several patients, probably as a coincidental finding. In general, growth hormone levels are normal.

The mucus-secreting salivary glands (ie, submaxillary, sublingual, and submucosal) show morphologic changes similar to those seen in the pancreas, including dilated ducts with inspissated secretions and eventually atrophy of the acini and fibrosis. The serous-secreting parotid gland shows no morphologic changes. Enlarged submaxillary glands are palpable in more than 90% of patients, but there are no important clinical problems related to the salivary glands.

## Psychosocial

### Impact on Family

Cystic fibrosis is accompanied by a series of psychologic crises from the time of diagnosis to the patient's death. The impact on the family is probably related to severity of the disease, rate of progression, stability and mental health of the family before diagnosis, and availability of support systems. Initially, parents may be frustrated and angry by medical delays in making the diagnosis of CF. After the diagnosis is confirmed, there is shock and disbelief, accompanied by the guilt associated with the transmission of a genetic disease. Eventually, there is acceptance of the diagnosis, but denial is used as the overriding defense mechanism. If adaptive, denial enables families to cope; if maladaptive, it can lead to serious problems resulting in denial of the diagnosis by the patient as well as noncompliance with the treatment program. Impact on family functioning is usually significant. Hardest to accept by families is the concept of intensive, long-term care carried out with no guarantee of success. There is often a breakdown in intrafamilial communication and withdrawal from the community. Psychosomatic complaints and depression are common. Siblings often resent the extra care and time required by the patient with CF, but generally function quite well. The occupational goals of the parents may have to be modified and the financial burden can be considerable.

### Impact on Patient

The reaction of the patient to the diagnosis of CF varies with age and parental response. There is often denial of symptoms. There may be maladaptive use of fantasy, repression, and regression. Feelings of anxiety and depression can lead to psychosomatic complaints and problems with discipline and academic work at school. The well-adjusted child is not embarrassed about having CF, discusses it openly with friends, and readily takes medications and treatments in front of others. Adolescence is a critical period for patients, and psychologic problems are prominent. Patients are dissatisfied with their appearance and have to cope with a delay in physical development and maturation. They may be forced to realistically compromise their academic and vocational goals. The extended dependency caused by CF interferes with the normal process of separation from parents. Conflicts during adolescence are often manifested by social withdrawal, noncompliance with medical regimens, and risk-taking behavior.

### The Terminally Ill Patient

In the terminally ill patient, the response to impending death varies with age, developmental level, family support systems, and openness of communication. In younger patients, there may be loneliness and fear of abandonment, while older patients usually experience feelings of anxiety and depression. Open communication decreases feelings of isolation, alienation, and the perception that the dying process is too terrible to talk about. Death is often a lingering process with repeated "final episodes" from which the patient rebounds. The accompanying anger, confusion, and guilt challenge the coping abilities of most families.

## DIAGNOSIS

### Clinical Presentation

The physician should remain vigilant for CF and consider this diagnosis in a wide range of clinical situations. Although two thirds of cases are diagnosed by age 1 year, 10% of cases escape detection until adolescence or adulthood. Overall, 10% to 15% of patients have neonatal intestinal obstruction related to meconium ileus or meconium plug syndrome. In the remaining patients, the diagnosis is suggested because of pulmonary manifestations or steatorrhea, often associated with failure to thrive, a positive family history, or a variety of miscellaneous manifestations related to salt depletion or deficiencies of vitamins, protein, minerals, or calories. The types and severity of CF manifestations somewhat reflect genotypic heterogeneity. Pancreatic sufficiency is seen with increased frequency in those patients with non-Δ-F508 mutations. The spectrum of clinical features is so varied and symptoms may be so minimal that one cannot exclude the possibility of CF even with a normal growth pattern, absence of pulmonary disease, or normal pancreatic exocrine function. A patient should never be deprived of an evaluation because of "looking too well to have CF."

### Sweat Testing

The diagnosis of CF should always be confirmed by documentation of an elevated sweat electrolyte concentration. Indications for a sweat test are outlined in Table 72-2. The standard sweat

| TABLE 72-2. Indications for Sweat Testing | |
|---|---|
| **Pulmonary/Upper Respiratory** | **Metabolic/Other** |
| Atelectasis (especially right upper lobe) | Acrodermatitis enteropathica |
| Bronchiectasis | Aspermia/absent vas deferens |
| Chronic cough | Edema and hypoproteinemia |
| Digital clubbing | Failure to thrive |
| Hemoptysis | Hypoprothrombinemia |
| Mucoid *Pseudomonas* colonization | Metabolic alkalosis |
| Nasal polyps | Positive family history |
| Pansinusitis | Salt depletion syndrome |
| Recurrent/chronic pneumonia | Salty taste/salt crystals |
| Tachypnea/retractions | Vitamin A deficiency (bulging fontanelle) |
| Wheezing and hyperinflation | |
| **Gastrointestinal** | |
| Cirrhosis and portal hypertension | |
| Intestinal atresia | |
| Meconium ileus | |
| Meconium plug syndrome | |
| Mucoid-impacted appendix | |
| Prolonged neonatal jaundice | |
| Recurrent intussusception | |
| Recurrent pancreatitis | |
| Rectal prolapse | |
| Steatorrhea | |

test method is the quantitative pilocarpine iontophoresis sweat test (Gibson-Cooke) in which localized sweating is stimulated by the iontophoresis of pilocarpine into the skin, a sufficient volume of sweat (more than 100 mg) is collected, and the electrolyte concentration is measured. An alternative sweat testing procedure involves collecting sweat with the Macroduct sweat collection system (Wescor; Logan, Utah, 84321) and measuring sweat osmolality or electrolyte concentrations. With this system, samples are not weighed and results are available within minutes. With the Gibson-Cooke test, the chloride concentration is usually measured since it better discriminates between normal individuals and those with CF. A chloride concentration of more than 60 mEq/L is consistent with the diagnosis of CF. The sweat chloride concentration can also be measured by applying a chloride ion electrode directly to the sweating skin. This method is associated with unacceptably high rates of false-positive and false-negative results, however, and should never be the basis of a definitive diagnosis. The sweat electrolyte abnormality is present from birth and persists throughout life. A volume of sweat sufficient for analysis, however, may be difficult to obtain in the neonatal period.

Patients with CF have an abnormality of transepithelial electrolyte transport manifested by increased sodium absorption across epithelium that is relatively impermeable to chloride. Abnormal electrolyte transport has been demonstrated in patients with CF shortly after birth, and measurement of nasal or rectal electrical potential differences may be a diagnostic adjunct to the sweat test in the early diagnosis of CF.

There is no correlation between the magnitude of the sweat gland abnormality and the severity of pulmonary manifestations. Significantly lower, but still abnormal, sweat electrolyte concentrations have been reported in those CF patients with pancreatic sufficiency. Elevated concentrations of sweat electrolytes have been reported in other conditions, including adrenal insufficiency, ectodermal dysplasia, nephrogenic diabetes insipidus, type I glycogen storage disease, anorexia nervosa, hypoparathyroidism, Mauriac syndrome, familial cholestatic syndromes, malnutrition, hypothyroidism, mucopolysaccharidoses, and fucosidosis. Most of these disorders can be differentiated by characteristic clinical features. Transient elevation of sweat electrolyte concentrations has been observed in children with evidence of abuse and neglect. In patients with a "confirmed" diagnosis who do not follow a typical course, it is crucial to repeat the sweat test. Normal sweat electrolyte concentrations have been reported in some patients with CF in the presence of edema and hypoproteinemia. Values become abnormal with resolution of the edema. Most false-positive and false-negative results are due to technical errors, including inadequate sweat collection, sample contamination, and failure to interpret test results correctly. Physiologic variables such as sweating rate, salt intake, and acclimatization may affect the concentration of sweat electrolytes but do not usually interfere with the diagnostic value of the test. Although sweat electrolyte concentrations increase slightly with increasing age, they remain excellent discriminants for CF in adults. The sweat test is not useful in diagnosing CF in heterozygotes.

Intermediate sweat chloride concentrations in the range of 40 to 60 mEq/L have been reported in patients with chronic pulmonary disease and normal pancreatic function (atypical cystic fibrosis). Borderline sweat electrolyte values are otherwise unusual. In such instances, CF mutation analysis may be helpful. Ancillary findings such as radiographic evidence of pansinusitis, aspermia, or the isolation of a mucoid *Pseudomonas* from the respiratory tract also may be helpful. Rarely, CF has been documented in patients with normal sweat electrolyte concentrations. The diagnosis of CF should not be based solely on an elevated sweat electrolyte concentration, but should be made only when

it is associated with pancreatic exocrine deficiency, chronic pulmonary disease, meconium ileus, or a positive family history.

## Newborn Screening

Screening of newborns for CF is now possible. Newborns with CF have elevated blood levels of IRT, presumably due to a secretory obstructive defect in the pancreas in utero. An alternative strategy for newborn screening involves direct mutation analysis on the blood spots of those infants with an elevated IRT value. Screening can be automated by using the dried blood spots routinely collected (in many parts of the world) for metabolic screening. Potential benefits of screening include avoidance of diagnostic delays, decreased early morbidity, improved outcome, timely genetic counseling, and early and complete case detection for clinical and epidemiologic studies. Mass newborn screening programs are not yet recommended for the United States, however, pending results of cost–benefit analysis. The IRT test also may be helpful in evaluating neonates with a positive family history for CF. In such cases, it may yield information 2 to 3 weeks earlier than the age at which an adequate sweat sample can be obtained. In no case should the IRT test be used as a substitute for the sweat test or as the basis of a definitive diagnosis. False-negative IRT results occur in as many as 25% of newborns with intestinal obstruction.

## MANAGEMENT

Because of multisystem involvement, frequency of complications, psychosocial burden, and uncertain prognosis, a comprehensive, intensive therapy program is essential. Patients should be followed at intervals of 2 to 3 months by an experienced, available physician, as well as by nursing, nutrition, physical–respiratory therapy, and counseling personnel. The Cystic Fibrosis Foundation, Bethesda, Md, supports a nationwide network of centers involved in patient care, teaching, and clinical and basic research. Services provided by the centers include sweat testing and confirmation of diagnosis; evaluation and provision of a therapeutic plan; continuity of outpatient and inpatient services; patient and family education; nutrition counseling; instruction in physical and respiratory therapy; psychosocial support, including individual counseling and education/support groups for patients, parents, and siblings; financial counseling; genetic counseling; subspecialty consultative services; and opportunity to participate in clinical research projects. Vocational, educational, financial, and premarital counseling can help the increasing number of adult patients make a smooth transition to independent living. Optimal patient management involves coordination of services between the CF center and the primary care provider who can provide ongoing psychosocial support, offer general medical care, coordinate home, community, and educational services, and interpret the significance of medical developments. Goals of therapy include maintaining adequate nutrition and normal growth, preventing or providing aggressive therapy for pulmonary complications, encouraging appropriate physical activity, and providing psychosocial support.

## Pulmonary

### Antibiotic Therapy

Treatment of pulmonary manifestations of CF is directed at clearing excess mucus from the tracheobronchial tree and providing aggressive antimicrobial therapy. Except in the case of acute respiratory illness, guidelines for the use of antibiotics in these patients are not well established. In some centers, patients are maintained continuously on one or more oral agents, usually directed against *S aureus, Haemophilus influenzae*, or both. In other centers, antimicrobial therapy is used only at times of respiratory exacerbations. Patients who do not respond to outpatient management are usually hospitalized for 10-day to 3-week courses of intensive antibiotic therapy, primarily directed against *P aeruginosa*. Combinations of an aminoglycoside (tobramycin, gentamicin) with an anti-*Pseudomonas* penicillin (carbenicillin, ticarcillin, piperacillin) frequently are used. A third-generation cephalosporin with anti-*Pseudomonas* activity (ceftazidime) as well as Beta lactams (aztreonam, imipenem) may be useful. Patients with CF may require high doses of aminoglycosides to achieve acceptable serum concentrations. Serum concentrations should be monitored and dosage adjusted to achieve a peak level of 8 to 10 $\mu$g/mL and a trough value of less than 2 $\mu$g/mL. Patients also show enhanced renal clearance of penicillins and may require large doses to achieve adequate serum levels. Quinolone derivatives such as ciprofloxacin are absorbed from the gastrointestinal tract and are the first oral agents shown to be effective against *Pseudomonas* pulmonary infections. In controlled trials in CF patients with pulmonary exacerbations, ciprofloxacin was shown to be as effective as intravenous antibiotics; however, it is not approved for use in patients younger than 16 years. Use of ciprofloxacin is limited by rapid development of antibiotic resistance and should be based on results of sensitivity testing.

Improved methods for providing stable venous access have made home intravenous antibiotic therapy an attractive alternative to hospitalization. This type of therapy is cost-effective, is associated with few complications, and does not interfere with normal activity. Long-term daily aerosol administration of anti-*Pseudomonas* agents such as tobramycin and gentamicin may benefit patients with moderate-to-severe lung disease and chronic colonization with *P aeruginosa* who require frequent hospital admission. Aerosol aminoglycoside therapy is well tolerated without significant side effects. There is little systemic drug absorption, and there is no need to monitor serum drug levels. Over time, however, resistance may develop in a significant percentage of patients and should be monitored.

### Physical and Respiratory Therapy

Chest physiotherapy, consisting of postural drainage, manual or mechanical percussion, vibration, and assisted coughing, enhances the removal of bronchial secretions and usually is recommended at the first indication of pulmonary involvement. Other useful methods of secretion removal include autogenic drainage and a variety of forced expiratory techniques. Treatments are carried out several times each day, depending on the degree of pulmonary disease. Although this is a cornerstone of CF therapy, objective assessments of its efficacy have yielded somewhat conflicting, but generally positive results. In adult patients, prolonged coughing in the absence of physiotherapy may yield similar results. Physical activity and exercise programs are useful adjuncts to physiotherapy and should be encouraged.

### Aerosol Therapy

Although a variety of aerosolized agents have been used in CF therapy, evidence to support their use is largely anecdotal. No data document the efficacy of bland aerosols and N-acetylcysteine. In some patients, these agents may lead to reflex bronchoconstriction and worsening of pulmonary function. New approaches to mucolytic therapy include nebulization of amiloride to normalize transepithelial electrolyte transport and increase sputum sodium and water content, and human recombinant deoxyribonuclease (DNase) to enzymatically degrade the high concentration of DNA present in purulent sputum. These agents, however, are not yet approved for clinical use. Bronchodilators, administered either orally or by nebulization, may be useful in

selected patients. The response of CF patients to these agents is highly variable, and they should be used only after observing an obvious clinical response or documenting a beneficial response by pulmonary function testing. Preliminary data indicate $\alpha$-1-antitrypsin administered as an aerosol can neutralize the increased concentration of free proteases that is present in airways of patients with CF.

### Immunotherapy

Evidence supports a role for glucocorticoid therapy in patients with CF. In a double-blind study of alternate-day prednisone given to patients with mild/moderate disease, at the end of 4 years, the treatment group showed significant advantages in height, weight, pulmonary function, sedimentation rate, and serum immunoglobulin G values, and it had fewer hospitalizations for CF-related pulmonary disease. A much larger cohort of patients is being evaluated in an attempt to confirm these results. Until results are available, use of glucocorticoids in the treatment of CF probably should be limited to patients with severe bronchiolitic syndrome, significant airway obstruction that is not responsive to conventional bronchodilators, allergic bronchopulmonary aspergillosis, and evidence of hypersensitivity characterized by recurrent episodes of fever, rash, and joint pain. Patients on long-term glucocorticoid therapy need to be carefully monitored for development of carbohydrate abnormalities, cataracts, and growth retardation.

Infusion of intravenous immune globulin as an adjunct to antibiotic therapy has been shown to enhance short-term improvement in pulmonary function. Intravenous gamma globulin enriched with *P aeruginosa* lipopolysaccharide antibodies has been associated with improvement in pulmonary function in patients infected with antibiotic-resistant phenotypes of *P aeruginosa*. Routine use of these preparations awaits results of further clinical trials.

### Miscellaneous Therapies

Tracheobronchial lavage has been used to remove impacted bronchial secretions, but, in a controlled trial, it was no more effective than conventional therapy. Therapeutic bronchoscopy has been performed in patients with lobar and segmental atelectasis, but results are no better than those obtained with intensified medical therapy. Intermittent positive pressure breathing may worsen chest overinflation and is usually contraindicated. No data support use of oral expectorants, and cough suppressants are contraindicated. Surgical treatment of pulmonary complications is infrequently undertaken because lung involvement usually is generalized, but lobectomy and segmental resection may be useful in some cases of persistent atelectasis and localized bronchiectasis.

### Upper Airway Problems

Patients with symptomatic sinusitis should be treated with a 4- to 6-week course of antibiotics. For patients who do not respond and for those with chronic or recurrent symptoms, a surgical procedure to improve sinus drainage is indicated.

For patients with nasal polyps, intranasal glucocorticoids and oral antihistamines and decongestants may provide transient symptomatic relief but are rarely curative. Antibiotics and immunotherapy are not helpful. Patients with distressing symptoms are best treated by simple polypectomy. Associated sinusitis should be treated as outlined above.

### Pneumothorax

Active intervention is indicated for a pneumothorax greater than 10%. Conventional therapy consists of closed thoracostomy drainage via a chest tube, followed by intrapleural installation of sclerosing agents such as quinacrine and tetracycline. This form of therapy, however, is associated with persistent air leak, prolonged hospitalization, and high rate of recurrence. Because of these complications, an immediate open thoracotomy with pleural abrasion and resection of blebs is recommended as an alternative; it is associated with a less than 5% recurrence rate. Intensive antibiotic therapy usually is used as an adjunct to these measures. Management of pneumothorax is complicated by the availability of heart-lung and bilateral-lung transplantation. Prior sclerotherapy and pleural abrasion significantly increase chest wall bleeding at the time of transplantation, and these procedures are considered as relative contraindications to transplantation. An open thoracotomy with bleb resection and localized sclero-therapy may be an acceptable therapeutic option. This issue should be discussed fully with the patient and family before initiating therapy for a pneumothorax.

### Hemoptysis

Heavy blood streaking of sputum and episodes of hemoptysis usually reflect increased pulmonary infection. The site of bleeding may be localized by bronchoscopy. In patients with heavy blood streaking, intensive antibiotic therapy alone may be sufficient. With massive hemoptysis (more than 300 mL/24 h) or with protracted or recurrent episodes of moderate bleeding, percutaneous catheter embolization of the involved bronchial arteries is the procedure of choice. Bleeding immediately ceases in more than 80% of patients. After the procedure, however, repeat bleeding is common, and one third to one half of patients require repeat embolization.

### Cor Pulmonale

The management of right-sided failure includes therapy of the underlying pulmonary obstruction and infection along with diuretics, salt restriction, and oxygen. Digitalis is not generally useful. Overall, results have not been favorable. In adults with chronic obstructive pulmonary disease, pulmonary hypertension may be reversed by long-term continuous oxygen therapy. This has not been demonstrated in CF cases, however, and the role of oxygen therapy remains poorly defined. It is usually prescribed to relieve symptomatic hypoxemia (ie, headaches and dyspnea) and to improve exercise tolerance.

### Respiratory Failure

In general, assisted ventilation is not indicated for CF patients with progressive respiratory failure; such patients rarely come off of ventilatory support. Its use should be restricted to the occasional patient with good baseline status in whom acute respiratory failure develops, patients awaiting transplantation, or in association with pulmonary surgery. Heart-lung and bilateral-lung transplants have been performed successfully in highly selected patients with chronic cardiorespiratory failure. Results are similar to those seen in non-CF patients with survival rates of 65% to 75% after 1 year and 50% to 60% after 2 years. After successful transplantation, pulmonary function and exercise performance rapidly return toward normal. Airways of the transplanted lungs maintain normal transepithelial ion transport. Early complications include rejection, bleeding, and infection, whereas infection and chronic rejection (bronchiolitis obliterans) are the leading late complications. Daily monitoring of lung function allows early detection of infection and rejection episodes with confirmation of the diagnosis by transbronchial biopsy. Wider application of heart-lung and bilateral-lung transplantation is limited by donor organ availability.

### Immunoprophylaxis of Pulmonary Infections

It is important to follow recommended vaccination schedules, especially for pertussis and measles. The *H influenzae* type B vaccine should be given at the recommended age. Patients should be immunized against influenza starting at age 6 months, followed by a yearly booster. Household contacts should also be immunized. In patients who are exposed to influenza A and have not received vaccine, amantadine prophylaxis can be used until the risk of infection passes. There is no documented increase in susceptibility to or morbidity from pneumococcal infection, and routine use of pneumococcal vaccine is not recommended. *Pseudomonas* vaccines have been used investigationally, but are not available for clinical use.

## Gastrointestinal

### Pancreatic Exocrine Deficiency

Pancreatic enzyme supplements, derived from hog pancreas, constitute the primary therapy of the pancreatic enzyme defect. The most effective preparations consist of capsules containing pancrelipase in pH-sensitive enteric-coated microspheres. The enteric coating prevents gastric acid inactivation of the enzyme. Powdered preparations usually are used in infants. Enzyme supplements are given with all meals and snacks; the dosage is determined by the frequency and character of the stools along with the patient's growth pattern. Development of hard stools while a patient is taking enzymes is usually an indication for more (not less) enzyme. A misguided reduction in enzyme dosage in this situation may precipitate an episode of meconium ileus equivalent. An adverse reaction to increased dose of enzyme is rare.

After enzyme supplementation, fat and nitrogen amounts are reduced in stools, although the values do not return to normal. Persistence of significant steatorrhea after enzyme therapy may be due to enzyme inactivation by gastric acid or to a low duodenal pH. In such cases, addition of bicarbonate or an $H_2$-receptor antagonist may help. Complications of enzyme therapy are rare; skin and mucous membrane irritation may be seen in infants. Hypersensitivity reactions can occur in parents exposed to powdered extracts, but are rare in patients themselves.

### Nutrition

The goal of nutrition therapy is to promote normal growth. Contrary to earlier anecdotal reports of a voracious appetite in patients with CF, most patients have a grossly deficient caloric intake. Because of incomplete correction of steatorrhea and increased metabolic demands, it is recommended that patients receive 50% more calories than usual daily allowances. This usually can be achieved by a well-balanced, high-protein diet with liberal fat. Fat restriction is no longer recommended. Infants can be breast-fed if they are receiving enzyme supplements, but weight gain must be closely monitored. For formula-fed infants, predigested formulas containing medium chain triglycerides (MCT) are advantageous. These preparations are especially useful in infants with liver involvement or persistent steatorrhea, and after intestinal resection.

Older patients should be provided with a high-protein, high-calorie diet consistent with food preferences and lifestyle. Liberal fat should be allowed in the diet. Supplements with MCT oil and polycose can boost caloric intake. In patients who have poor growth and inadequate caloric intake, despite nutritional counseling and attempts at oral supplementation, enteral supplementation may be useful. This is accomplished by nightly infusion of high-calorie elemental formulas via a nasogastric, gastrostomy, or jejunostomy tube. Evidence shows that this type of supplementation, when carried out over an extended period, may stabilize or even improve pulmonary function. Parenteral hyperalimentation has been used but is costly and is associated with complications of prolonged central line infusions. No evidence strongly supports use of artificial elemental diets or supplements with essential fatty acids.

## Vitamin and Mineral Supplementation

Vitamin deficiencies can be prevented by daily administration of a water-miscible vitamin preparation. Patients with achylia should receive a daily supplement of a water-miscible alpha-tocopherol preparation at a dose of 5 to 10 IU/kg up to a maximum daily dose of 400 IU. Routine supplementation with vitamin K is not recommended but may be indicated in patients with extensive liver involvement, at times of surgery, and in patients with demonstrated coagulation problems. Iron deficiency is frequently seen in CF patients. Iron status should be evaluated periodically and appropriate supplementation provided to patients with anemia or low serum ferritin levels. Iron absorption may be impaired in CF patients and response to therapy should be monitored closely. With pancreatic enzyme supplementation, there should be no need for supplementation with other trace metals. Additional dietary salt should be provided at times of thermal stress, including increased activity in hot weather. Supplementation with salt tablets is not usually indicated.

## Carbohydrate Intolerance

Diabetes is managed by modest dietary changes along with low to moderate doses of insulin. Insulin requirements are based on results of daily blood glucose monitoring and periodic glycosolated hemoglobin values. Oral hypoglycemic agents have not been useful. With improved survival, patients should be closely monitored for retinal and renal vascular complications.

## Meconium Ileus

In uncomplicated cases of meconium ileus, the meconium can be removed nonoperatively by hyperosmolar enemas administered under hydrostatic pressure. In patients in whom this procedure is unsuccessful and in those with complications such as volvulus and perforation, it may be necessary to resect the involved segment of bowel. In some cases, mucolytics are used intraoperatively to liquefy the inspissated meconium and may eliminate the need for intestinal resection. Patients who survive the newborn period have a prognosis similar to that for patients without meconium ileus.

## Meconium Ileus Equivalent

In cases of meconium ileus equivalent in which there is no evidence of intestinal obstruction, oral administration of a cleansing electrolyte solution (Golytely) is the treatment of choice. If there is evidence of intestinal obstruction, enemas with hyperosmolar contrast material may be diagnostic as well as therapeutic. Large volume saline and 2% N-acetylcysteine enemas have also been effective. Most episodes can be managed without surgical intervention. For patients with recurrent episodes, helpful measures include increased amounts of pancreatic enzyme, increased fluid intake, and administration of wetting agents, high fiber diet, oral N-acetylcysteine, lactulose, and mineral oil. In patients with intussusception, hydrostatic reduction should be attempted, although surgery may be necessary. Surgery is also indicated for episodes of volvulus.

## Miscellaneous Complications

Gastroesophageal reflux is treated by administration of drugs such as metoclopramide and bethanechol to promote gastric emptying, and, in infants, by positioning and thickened feeds. Antacids and $H_2$-receptor antagonists are indicated in patients with esophagitis. The prokinetic agent cisapride may help reduce symptoms such as crampy abdominal pain, flatulence, and abdominal distention. Episodes of rectal prolapse are usually partial and easily treated by manual reduction. Surgical correction or injection of sclerosing agents is rarely necessary. In patients with recurrent episodes of prolapse, stool wetting agents should be administered and the dosage of pancreatic enzymes increased.

## Hepatobiliary

Although there is no specific therapy for liver complications, administration of the hydrophilic bile acid—ursodeoxycholic acid—has resulted in improvement in liver function and dissolution of cholesterol gallstones in patients with CF. In patients with bleeding secondary to portal hypertension and varices, portal-systemic shunting and splenectomy may be useful. Post-shunt encephalopathy and hepatic failure are not usually a problem. A shunting procedure, however, decreases the patient's suitability for subsequent liver transplantation. The long-term results depend on the degree of underlying pulmonary disease. Endoscopic injection sclerotherapy also can be used to control acute or recurrent episodes of bleeding. In patients with severe liver disease and good pulmonary status, liver transplantation has been carried out; early results indicate excellent 1- and 2-year survival rates. Although gallbladder abnormalities, including cholelithiasis, are common, patients usually are asymptomatic. Cholecystectomy should be reserved for the symptomatic patient who fails a trial of ursodeoxycholic acid.

## Psychosocial

Psychosocial support for the patient and other family members is especially important at the time of diagnosis, with exacerbations, and during the terminal phase of the disease. As with any chronic illness, consistency of medical care providers is essential. Members of the health-care team should allow patients to develop close relationships with them and provide ongoing support throughout life. It is important to know the entire family medically and psychosocially and to be sensitive to individual needs and coping mechanisms. Open communication is essential from the time of diagnosis. Questions should be answered honestly and directly but within a framework of guarded optimism.

Part of every visit should be devoted to a discussion of psychosocial issues. Parents should be encouraged to talk about CF rather than act as if it does not exist. Involvement and support of extended family members should be encouraged. Parents constantly need to be encouraged to treat their child normally and to avoid overprotection. Special treatment and privileges should be discouraged. It is important to work with adolescents to promote independence and to encourage realistic academic and vocational goals. Families can be helped by introduction to a CF family that is coping well, informational/support groups, respite care services, and individual counseling. It is the responsibility of the health-care team to make appropriate referrals to and interface with mental health consultants, interact with the patient's teachers, ensure that the family avails itself of all appropriate community and financial resources, arrange for vocational counseling, and, in the case of adolescents, plan for a smooth transition to adult care. With appropriate support, most patients can make an age-appropriate adjustment at home and school.

## COURSE AND PROGNOSIS

The course of disease varies from patient to patient, possibly related to genetic heterogeneity and environmental factors. Prognosis is largely determined by degree of pulmonary involvement. Some patients retain near-normal lung function over 5 to 7 years but, in general, there is an exponential decline in pulmonary function of about 2% to 3% per year. Early colonization with *Pseudomonas* may be associated with a more severe course.

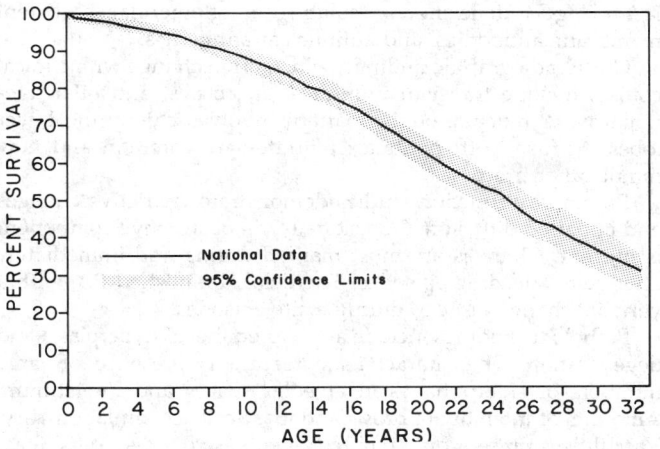

**Figure 72-4.** Survival curve for patients seen in CF centers in the United States in 1990. (Courtesy of Cystic Fibrosis Foundation, Bethesda, MD.)

Passive exposure to cigarette smoke is associated with a more rapid decline in clinical status and should be avoided. Patients with clinically intact pancreatic function have milder pulmonary disease and better survival. Improved prognosis is related to early diagnosis and institution of a comprehensive treatment program before irreversible pulmonary changes are established. Evidence shows that survival may correlate with intensity of the treatment regimen, particularly with antibiotic usage. Clinical scoring systems are available for longitudinal assessment of patients for prognosis counseling and for classifying patients for clinical studies.

There has been steady improvement in prognosis over the past four decades. In 1950, survival past infancy was unusual. By 1990, the median age at time of death was 28 years (Fig 72-4). About one fourth of all patients under care at specialized CF centers are older than 18 years of age. There is a trend toward poorer early survival but better late survival among black patients. For reasons that are not clear, survival of male patients at every age appears better than that of female patients, but in recent years the gap has narrowed.

## Selected Readings

The Cystic Fibrosis Foundation Center Committee and Guidelines Subcommittee. Cystic Fibrosis Foundation guidelines for patient services, evaluation, and monitoring in cystic fibrosis centers. Am J Dis Child 1990;144:1311.

Doring G, Albus A, Hoiby N. Immunologic aspects of cystic fibrosis. Chest 1988;94:109S.

Durie PR, Gaskin KJ, Corey M, Kopelman H, Weizman Z, Forstner GG. Pancreatic function testing in cystic fibrosis. J Pediatr Gastroenterol Nutr 1984;3:S89.

Durie PR, Pencharz PB. A rational approach to the nutritional care of patients with cystic fibrosis. Journal of the Royal Society of Medicine 1989;82:11.

Govan JRW, Doherty C, Glass S. Rational parameters for antibiotic therapy in patients with cystic fibrosis. Infection 1987;15:300.

Hammond KB, Abman SH, Sokol RJ, Accurso FJ. Efficacy of statewide neonatal screening for cystic fibrosis by assay of trypsinogen concentrations. N Engl J Med 1991;325:769.

Kerem E, Corey M, Kerem B, et al. The relation between genotype and phenotype in cystic fibrosis—analysis of the most common mutation (ΔF508). N Engl J Med 1990;323:1517.

Knowles MR, Gatzy J, Boucher R. Increased bioelectric potential difference across respiratory epithelia in cystic fibrosis. N Engl J Med 1981;305:1489.

Knowles MR, Church NL, Waltner WE, et al. A pilot study of aerosolized amiloride for the treatment of lung disease in cystic fibrosis. N Engl J Med 1990;323:1189.

Koletzko S, Stringer DA, Cleghorn GJ, Durie PR. Lavage treatment of distal intestinal obstruction syndrome in children with cystic fibrosis. Pediatrics 1989;83:727.

Lemna WK, Feldman GL, Kerem B, et al. Mutation analysis for heterozygote detection and the prenatal diagnosis of cystic fibrosis. N Engl J Med 1990;322:291.

Michael BC. Antibacterial therapy in cystic fibrosis. Chest 1988;94:129S.

Murphy S. Cystic fibrosis in adults: diagnosis and management. Clin Chest Med 1987;8:695.

Park RW, Grand RJ. Gastrointestinal manifestations of cystic fibrosis: a review. Gastroenterology 1981;81:1143.

Reisman J, Corey M, Canny G, Levison H. Diabetes mellitus in patients with cystic fibrosis: effect on survival. Pediatrics 1990;86:374.

Rosenstein, BJ. Interpreting sweat tests in the diagnosis of CF. Journal of Respiratory Diseases 1990;11:519.

Stern RC. The primary care physician and the patient with cystic fibrosis. J Pediatr 1989;114:31.

Stern RC, Boat TF, Wood RE, Matthews LW, Doershuk CF. Treatment and prognosis of nasal polyps in cystic fibrosis. Am J Dis Child 1982;136;1067.

Stowe SM, Boat TF, Mendelsohn H, et al. Open thoracotomy for pneumothorax in cystic fibrosis. Am Rev Respir Dis 1975;111:611.

Sweezey NB, Fellows KE. Bronchial artery embolization for severe hemoptysis in cystic fibrosis. Chest 1990;97:1322.

Thomassen MJ, Demko CA, Doershuk CF. Cystic fibrosis: a review of pulmonary infections and interventions. Pediatr Pulmonol 1987;3:334.

Tizzano EF, Buchwald M. Cystic fibrosis: beyond the gene to therapy. J Pediatr 1992;120:337.

*Principles and Practice of Pediatrics, Second Edition.* edited by Frank A. Oski et al. J. B. Lippincott Company, Philadelphia © 1994.

## CHAPTER 73
# *Pulmonary Hemosiderosis*

### Marianna M. Sockrider

Pulmonary hemosiderosis is a rare condition characterized by an abnormal accumulation of hemosiderin in the lungs. Hemosiderin deposition results from bleeding into the lungs with diffuse alveolar hemorrhage, rather than from hemorrhage from larger arteries. In chronic pulmonary hemosiderosis, bleeding is usually low-grade, repetitive, or persistent, often with superimposed episodes of brisk hemorrhage. Pulmonary hemosiderosis is classified as primary or secondary, depending on pathogenesis (Table 73-1).

Idiopathic pulmonary hemosiderosis occurs at any age, but usually is seen in childhood. Familial occurrence has been reported. There is no gender difference in incidence. Most cases of pulmonary hemosiderosis in infancy and childhood are primary, and causes are unknown. The idiopathic form is often more episodic, and may be exacerbated by viral illness. Pulmonary hemosiderosis resulting from hypersensitivity to cow's milk is seen mainly in young infants. Other foods have been incriminated in a few cases. There may be associated gastrointestinal or upper respiratory symptoms. Goodpasture's syndrome usually occurs in young adult males, and pulmonary hemosiderosis may precede renal involvement. Acute pulmonary hemorrhage and hemosiderosis are rare features of collagen vascular diseases in children, but may precede other systemic manifestations.

The most helpful clinical features are iron deficiency anemia, recurrent pulmonary symptoms, and characteristic abnormalities on chest radiographs. Any of these features may be the first sign of pulmonary hemosiderosis. Hemoptysis is a helpful clue, al-

**TABLE 73-1.   Classification of Pulmonary Hemosiderosis**

| Primary (Idiopathic) | Secondary |
|---|---|
| Isolated | Cow's milk sensitivity (Heiner's syndrome) |
| With myocarditis | Glomerulonephritis: |
| With celiac disease or pancreatic insufficiency | With antibodies to GBM (glomerular basement membrane) (Goodpasture's syndrome) |
| | Without antibodies to GBM (usually immune-complex) |
| | Collagen vascular: systemic lupus erythematosus, Wegener's granulomatosis, rheumatoid arthritis |
| | Cardiac disease or intrapulmonary vascular abnormalities: pulmonary hypertension, chronic heart failure, pulmonary lymphangioleiomatosis, vascular malformations |
| | Purpuric disease: Schönlein-Henoch purpura, idiopathic thrombocytopenic purpura |
| | Chemicals: D-penicillamine, trimellitic anhydride, toxic hydrocarbon agents |
| | IgA or IgG4 deficiency |

though in young children it may be difficult to discern the source of bleeding. Pulmonary hemosiderosis should be considered when there is unexplained hematemesis. The clinical picture usually is characterized by recurrent episodes of acute pulmonary bleeding. There may be associated fever, tachycardia, tachypnea, and leukocytosis. Sometimes, only long-term observation with awareness of the possibility of pulmonary hemosiderosis leads to the correct diagnosis.

Physical findings vary according to clinical status. There may be pallor or cyanosis. Lung findings include bronchial or suppressed breath sounds, wheezing, crackles, and productive or repetitive cough. Transient hepatosplenomegaly occurs in 20% of cases. Recurrent episodes of pulmonary bleeding may cause signs of chronic respiratory disease, including dyspnea, finger clubbing, and pulmonary hypertension. Poor weight gain and easy fatigability are common in cases with moderate to severe disease.

Microcytic hypochromic anemia is present with a low serum iron despite accumulated iron in the lungs. Reticulocytosis may be seen during active bleeding. Anemia may improve during periods of remission. Eosinophilia can occur, and eosinophil counts fluctuate markedly. Stool hematest is often positive due to swallowed blood. Bleeding studies are usually normal. Transient elevation in serum bilirubin may occur with acute bleeding. Some patients have a positive direct Coombs test and circulating cold agglutinins, suggesting the presence of an unusual immune response. With hypersensitivity to cow's milk, there may be high serum titers of milk precipitins and elevated levels of immunoglobulins, particularly that of IgE or IgA. On the other hand, associated deficiency of IgA, IgG4, or both has been observed.

Iron-laden macrophages (siderophages) provide good presumptive evidence of pulmonary hemosiderosis. Siderophages may be found in gastric fluid, sputum, bronchial washings, or lung biopsy specimens with Prussian-blue staining. Gastric fluid usually contains siderophages from the lungs even when there is no obvious hemoptysis. Other studies are indicated to exclude other primary diseases. Searches should be made for elevated anti-cow's milk protein antibodies of the IgG, IgE, or IgD isotypes,

IgA or IgG4 deficiency, circulating antiglomerular basement membrane antibodies, and antinuclear antibodies.

Chest radiographic findings, which often change with clinical course, include transient infiltrates, atelectasis, and hilar adenopathy. A reticulonodular pattern involves chiefly the lower lobes. Diffuse, soft, perihilar infiltrates are common and may mimic other processes.

Pulmonary function studies demonstrate restrictive changes and impaired diffusion. Occasionally, an obstructive component is present. Changes are most marked during and immediately after acute bleeding episodes. There is a diminished $P_{O_2}$ with a variable change in $P_{CO_2}$ during acute episodes.

Pathologic findings include alveolar epithelial hyperplasia and degeneration. The characteristic feature is presence of large numbers of siderophages in alveolar spaces and interstitium. Amounts of interstitial fibrosis and mast-cell accumulation vary. Vasculitis is present only with collagen vascular disorders. Electron microscopy and immunofluorescent staining may be helpful in cases of Goodpasture's syndrome and connective tissue disorders.

Pulmonary hemosiderosis may mimic other chronic pulmonary conditions of childhood, including asthma, cystic fibrosis, and alveolar filling diseases. Acute bleeding episodes may be confused with bacterial pneumonia. Hemoptysis may be seen in bronchiectasis and tuberculosis.

The clinical course varies and may include periods of remission. Prognosis is difficult to establish because of the disease's rarity and variability. Most deaths are due to acute respiratory failure or shock with massive intrapulmonary bleeding. Repeated exacerbations usually lead to chronic pulmonary disease with interstitial fibrosis, pulmonary hypertension, and right-sided heart failure. Cow's milk hypersensitivity has a good prognosis with dietary restriction. Goodpasture's syndrome has a poor prognosis, with death occurring from renal failure.

When identified, appropriate therapy should be initiated for other primary diseases or factors that might help cause or aggravate pulmonary hemosiderosis. In young patients with idiopathic hemosiderosis, a 2- to 3-month trial of milk-free diet should be considered, even in the absence of high milk precipitins. An attempt can be made to reintroduce milk every 1 to 2 years.

Acute episodes of bleeding should be treated with oxygen. Intermittent positive-pressure ventilation may improve delivery of oxygen. Respiratory failure or persistent bleeding occasionally are reversed with mechanical ventilation using positive end-expiratory pressure (PEEP). Blood transfusions are indicated to correct severe anemia or shock. Superimposed bronchospasm may respond to bronchodilators.

Acute bleeding in pulmonary hemosiderosis may respond to high-dose corticosteroids. ACTH (10 to 25 U/d), methylprednisolone (1 mg/kg every 6 hours), or hydrocortisone (4 to 8 mg/kg/d) intravenously is recommended initially, followed by maintenance oral methylprednisolone at a dosage of 1 to 2 mg/kg/d. Once remission is achieved, steroids should be tapered gradually until discontinued or until symptoms recur. There is little evidence that long-term steroid therapy helps prevent relapse. If maintenance steroids are needed, the minimal dose required to suppress symptoms should be used.

In cases showing an inadequate response to corticosteroids, other immunosuppressant drugs have been used. Azathioprine (Imuran) is used most, and success is reported using 1.2 to 5 mg/kg/d, usually in combination with prednisone. Other drugs that have been reported to have some success include cyclophosphamide, chlorambucil, and chloroquine. An attempt should be made to stop all drugs after 1 year of clinical remission. Intravenous gamma globulin replacement therapy may be considered in subjects with symptomatic immunoglobulin deficiencies. Splenectomy has uncertain value. If other measures fail or with chronic severe disease, iron chelation with deferoxamine may be useful. Close follow-up is important to monitor disease activity.

## Selected Readings

Bush A, Sheppard MN, Warner JO. Chloroquine in idiopathic pulmonary hae-mosiderosis. Arch Dis Child 1992;67:625.
Cutz E. Idiopathic pulmonary hemosiderosis and related disorders in infancy and childhood. Perspect Pediatr Pathol 1987;11:47.
Heiner DC. Pulmonary hemosiderosis. In: Chernick V, Kendig EL Jr, eds. Disorders of the respiratory tract in children, ed 5. Philadelphia: WB Saunders, 1990;498.
Levy J, Wilmott RW. Pulmonary hemosiderosis. Pediatr Pulmonol 1986;2:384.
Soergel KH, Sommers SC. Idiopathic hemosiderosis and related syndromes. Am J Med 1962;32:499.
Turner-Warwick M, Dewar A. Pulmonary haemorrhage and pulmonary haemo-siderosis. Clin Radiol 1982;33:361.

*Principles and Practice of Pediatrics, Second Edition.*
edited by Frank A. Oski et al. J. B. Lippincott Company, Philadelphia © 1994.

## CHAPTER 74
# *Parathyroid Glands*

### John L. Kirkland

Recent advances in understanding calcium homeostasis reveal a rigidly controlled system involving the liver, bone, intestines, kidneys, and parathyroid glands. This system is inherently stable, but diseases of the parathyroid gland or other organs listed above may cause significant clinical and metabolic disorders in children. Transient parathyroid gland dysfunction in the neonate is discussed elsewhere.

## PHYSIOLOGY

Parathyroid hormone (PTH) is secreted from the cell as an 84-amino-acid peptide with a half-life of 5 to 8 minutes. PTH is degraded by the Kupffer's cells of the liver into midregion and carboxy-terminal fragments that have no biological activity but remain in the blood. Previous methods of measuring PTH were complicated by these inactive components. Newer assays using two-site immunoradiometric and immunoaffinity-extraction bioassays facilitate understanding of PTH dynamics in health and diseases. A combination of plasma membrane calcium sensors, as well as calcium selective transmembrane channels, may signal the cell to produce and secrete PTH. PTH exerts its major actions by binding to receptors located in the bone and kidney. PTH indirectly activates the osteoclasts in the bone to increase resorption of mineralized bone, which results in calcium and phosphorus mobilization. PTH activates the proximal and distal tubular cells in the kidney to promote calcium resorption and to inhibit phosphorus resorption. In addition, PTH stimulates production of $1,25(OH)_2$ vitamin D in the kidney. In both the bone and renal cells, PTH acts through two membrane receptor sys-

tems. The first system activates adenylate cyclase with subsequent production of cyclic adenosine monophosphate (cAMP), which acts as a second messenger to mobilize intracellular calcium and increase protein phosphorylation. The second system stimulates breakdown of phosphoinositol to diacylglycerol products. These products then stimulate protein kinase C activation. The two systems promote genomic activation.

PTH closely regulates the concentration of calcium in extracellular fluids. The concentration of calcium throughout the day is stable, but variations exist in the calcium concentration secondary to changes in the concentrations of serum proteins. The usual daily variation of total calcium concentrations is less than 2%. The extracellular concentration of calcium is $10^{-3}$ M, with three major components. The unbound component, or free calcium, composes about 50% of total calcium and is the most important regulator of physiologic processes. The bound components compose the other 50%. Protein binding accounts for about 40%; anion binding for about 10%. Albumin is the most significant protein-binding calcium. Each albumin molecule can bind 12 calcium molecules depending on the extracellular pH. Acidosis decreases binding capacity and increases free extracellular concentration of calcium, whereas alkalosis increases binding capacity and decreases free extracellular concentrations of calcium. These alterations in binding capacity explain variations in clinical signs that occur with disturbances in acid–base regulation. Bicarbonate, citrate, and phosphate complexes make up the anion binding system. The intracellular concentration of calcium is approximately $10^{-6}$ M and is maintained by three intracellular pump-leak transport systems. The rigid control of calcium concentration is due to the role that calcium ions assume in numerous metabolic processes. These processes include permeability of plasma membranes in neural tissue, mineralization of developing bone, and promotion of coagulation, as well as the intracellular role of second messenger for transmembrane hormone signals.

Low levels of serum calcium stimulate release of PTH because of decreased concentrations of intracellular calcium. The calcium selective transmembrane channels may play a role in this process. Low levels of intracellular calcium promote release of PTH, whereas high levels of serum calcium depress release of PTH. Increased levels of PTH stimulate the compensatory mechanisms indicated above.

An understanding of calcium homeostasis includes understanding vitamin D actions. Vitamin D enters the body two ways: by the skin and by dietary supplementation. The skin contains a previtamin D compound, 7-dehydrocholesterol. Ultraviolet waves from the sun or other source convert 7-dehydrocholesterol to a previtamin D compound that is converted by heat sensitive reactions to vitamin D. Vitamin D is transferred by a serum-binding protein to the liver. Dietary supplementation adds vitamin D by irradiated ergosterol, vitamin D2, or vitamin D3. Vitamins D2 and D3 differ slightly in structure but have similar physiologic functions. Vitamin D2 or D3 is hydroxylated in the liver at the 25 position by a 25 hydroxylase enzyme. Diseases of the liver as well as pharmacologic agents, including phenytoin and phenobarbital, have been reported to interfere with this hydroxylation step. Interference in this step may result in vitamin D deficiency. 25(OH) vitamin D is transported to the kidney, where another hydroxylation step occurs in the 1 position. $1,25(OH)_2$ vitamin D is the most active metabolite and is responsible for most actions of vitamin D. Stimulation of 1 hydroxylation is through actions of PTH, estrogen, growth hormone, prolactin, and insulin. Vitamin D exerts its effects through binding to intracellular proteins. Those intracellular proteins exist in most body tissues and must have numerous roles outside the control of calcium metabolism. Once the vitamin D molecule is bound to intracellular vitamin D receptors, the receptor vitamin D complex attaches to a specific part of the DNA, the responsive element, through a DNA-binding domain. This binding to the DNA allows stimulatory regions of the gene to initiate translational events. For example, intestinal cells are stimulated to produce calbindin-D, a calcium-binding protein that facilitates transport of calcium from the intraluminal space of the intestines to the extracellular compartment. Also, osteoclasts are generated from progenitor cells. The osteoclasts enhance release of calcium from bone, thus enabling the body to compensate for acute hypocalcemia. At each level of control, perturbations can occur with predictable consequences to calcium homeostasis.

## HYPOPARATHYROIDISM

Excluding transient hypoparathyroidism in neonates, hypoparathyroidism in children is rare. This disease is recognized clinically by accompanying hypocalcemia. Clinical manifestations of hypocalcemia are secondary to neuromuscular instability. The most common presentation is a seizure, which may be preceded by numbness and tingling sensations in the extremities. Chvostek's sign (stimulation of the upper lip by tapping the facial nerve in front of the ear), Trousseau's sign (carpopedal spasm produced by inflation of the blood pressure cuff greater than the systolic blood pressure for 2 minutes), laryngospasm, bronchospasm, and prolonged QT intervals on the electrocardiogram can occur. Etiologies of hypoparathyroidism are discussed below.

### Autoimmune Hypoparathyroidism

Hypoparathyroidism occurring as part of an autoimmune complex is well described. The basic disease process is known as the polyglandular autoimmune syndrome, type I, or, more recently, as the autoimmune polyendocrinopathy-candidiasis-ectodermal dystrophy (APECED) syndrome. The consistent feature is failure of the parathyroid glands to secrete PTH because of an immunologic destruction of hormone-producing cells.

Affected children usually present with acute signs of hypocalcemia such as tetany, seizures, and neuromuscular irritability. Mucocutaneous candidiasis may precede the hypoparathyroidism. Other endocrinopathies include hypoadrenalism, hypogonadism, hypothyroidism, and diabetes mellitus. Pathologic findings that signal glandular failure include lymphocytic infiltration of the parathyroid glands.

A child with this clinical entity should be examined frequently for other endocrinopathies. Many cases are secondary to an autosomal recessive gene, and genetic counseling should be considered.

## DIGEORGE SYNDROME

DiGeorge syndrome was described originally in infants with congenital absence of the thymus and parathyroid glands and deficient cell-mediated immunity. Later descriptions included cardiovascular malformations. These malformations include truncus arteriosis and aortic arch syndromes. Typical dysmorphic features of the face have been reported. These include low-set ears, short philtrum, micrognathia, and a small "fish-like mouth". Pathologic findings include absent, aplastic, and hypoplastic parathyroid glands.

### Acute Illnesses

In children, acute illnesses (eg, gram-negative sepsis) have been associated with hypocalcemia secondary to a relative hypopar-

athyroidism. The etiology of the relative hypoparathyroidism in critically ill children is unknown, but it may be related to macrophage-generated interleukins that may act as calcium ionophores. The critically ill child admitted to an intensive care unit is a prime candidate. Recognition may be delayed in some severe illnesses due to concern for the primary problem. Correction of hypocalcemia is required for patient improvement, however, because many cardiovascular agents require appropriate concentrations of calcium. Ionized calcium levels, as opposed to total serum calcium levels, reflect the child's true status because disturbances in total calcium determination from hypoalbuminemia, fluctuations in the bicarbonate ion, and radiographic contrast media may complicate total serum calcium measurements.

### Isolated Hypoparathyroidism

Isolated hypoparathyroidism unassociated with other endocrine diseases or as a result of thyroid surgery can occur. The etiology of isolated hypoparathyroidism is unknown, but its clinical and laboratory findings as well as its treatment are identical to other forms of hypoparathyroidism. Familial forms may be due to gene mutations near the PTH gene located on the short arm of chromosome 11.

### Hypomagnesemia

Magnesium deficiency, either congenital or acquired, produces hypocalcemia secondary to diminished production and effectiveness of PTH. Congenital hypomagnesemia is due to urinary or gastrointestinal losses from unknown cellular defects. Infants and children have other metabolic disturbances such as hypokalemia. Acquired hypomagnesemia is usually secondary to another disease. Clinical manifestations usually consist of tetany, carpopedal spasms, or seizures. Laboratory findings consist of serum levels of magnesium less than 1.5 mEq/L. Treatment consists of replacing magnesium intravenously, intramuscularly, or orally. Magnesium levels should be determined frequently to avoid overdosage with parenteral solutions of magnesium. Diarrhea may result from oral administration of magnesium. The replacement amount should be decreased accordingly, then tried at a higher dosage.

## LABORATORY FINDINGS

Characteristic laboratory findings of hypoparathyroidism include hypocalcemia and hyperphosphatemia. The PTH level is low in most situations. Radiographs of bones usually do not show any diagnostic features. The differential diagnosis includes hypocalcemia for other reasons such as phosphate-induced hypocalcemia, renal failure, or hypocalcemic rickets. Clinical history, laboratory assessment, and radiographs can facilitate evaluation. Children with pseudohypoparathyroidism present with hypocalcemia and hyperphosphatemia, but PTH levels are elevated.

## TREATMENT

Acute treatment of hypoparathyroidism in the disorders discussed here can be generalized if modifications are made for each etiology. All untreated patients with hypoparathyroidism have hypocalcemia, which requires immediate medical intervention. Acute treatment of hypocalcemia includes use of intravenous calcium. Numerous preparations have their merits. Pediatricians frequently use 10% calcium gluconate initially as an intravenous solution. One milliliter of this solution supplies 9 mg of elemental calcium. A neonate with seizures and laryngospasm may require an initial dose of 1 to 2 mL/kg, whereas older children may require 5 to 10 mL. Infusion of calcium should be slow with strict attention paid to the heart rate or electrocardiogram monitor. Bradycardia is an indication to discontinue temporarily the infusion of calcium. Subsequent intravenous calcium is administered at a rate of 25 to 100 mg/kg/d of elemental calcium depending on the severity of the hypocalcemia. Intravenous use of calcium may result in skin necrosis if extravasation occurs. This complication may develop despite continuous monitoring of intravenous sites, prompting some physicians to administer intravenous calcium only as an intermittent bolus. A 10% calcium chloride solution also can be used for intravenous treatment but is more irritating to the veins than calcium gluconate. One milliliter of this solution contains 27.3 mg of elemental calcium. Oral treatment with calcium supplementation may be initiated when the patient is stable. Calcium glubionate (NeoCalglucon) contains 23 mg/mL of elemental calcium, while calcium lactate powder is 13% elemental calcium (ie, 100 mg calcium lactate equals 13 mg of elemental calcium). Other commercial preparations contain varying amounts of elemental calcium. The amount of calcium supplementation administered should be regulated closely by serum calcium determinations. The amount of elemental calcium administered to maintain eucalcemia usually ranges from 50 to 150 mg/kg/d. Calcium administration through the gastrointestinal system depends on the presence of 1,25(OH)$_2$ vitamin D or its analogues.

Treatment with various forms of vitamin D is the only method of treating chronic hypocalcemic states such as hypoparathyroidism, because PTH is unavailable in a pharmacologic preparation. Most vitamin D supplementation is undertaken with dihydrotachysterol, 25(OH) vitamin D (Calderol), or 1,25(OH)$_2$D$_3$ (Rocaltrol). Vitamin D itself was used in very large amounts, but its long half-life made corrections in dosage to maintain eucalcemia difficult. Dihydrotachysterol is administered in a dosage of 0.05 to 0.5 mg/d. A solution facilitates small changes in the dosage required to maintain eucalcemia. 25(OH) vitamin D (Calderol) is administered as 20 $\mu$g daily or every other day and is increased slowly. Experience in infants and children is limited. 1,25(OH)$_2$D$_3$ is initiated with a dose of 0.25 $\mu$g/d and increased to several micrograms per day depending on the response of the serum calcium level and the size of the child. Rocaltrol has a more rapid onset of action than dihydrotachysterol, and therapeutic manipulation is easier. The gelatinous material in Rocaltrol can be removed from the capsule to administer smaller amounts to neonates and infants. 1-25(OH)$_2$D$_3$ may be administered intravenously (Calcijex), but its use in children is limited.

The optimal goal of long-term management is to maintain eucalcemia and eucalciuria. Patients with the best control are those who obtain monthly calcium levels and collect 24-hour urine collections twice yearly for calcium content. The optimal serum calcium level is one that is in the low range of normal. The optimal urinary calcium level should be less than 4 mg/kg/d or less than 0.3 mg calcium/mg creatinine. Older children and adolescents may require serum calcium levels lower than the normal range in order to avoid hypercalciuria.

## HYPERPARATHYROIDISM

Hyperparathyroidism is an uncommon disorder for the pediatric patient, but is important because an aggressive approach must be undertaken to prevent chronic renal diseases from nephrocalcinosis. Clinical manifestations of hypercalcemia from any cause are similar. Two systems affected initially are the neuromuscular and gastrointestinal. Muscle weakness, paralysis, or hyporeflexia may be observed in the former, while constipation, anorexia, and vomiting may be observed in the latter. The kidney may be affected adversely with resulting polyuria and polydipsia. Nephrocalcinosis may occur later. The cardiovascular symptoms may reveal bradycardia and a reduced QT interval. The etiologies of hyperparathyroidism are discussed below.

### Neonatal Hyperparathyroidism

A rare form of hypercalcemia in neonates is primary hyperparathyroidism. The etiology is hyperplasia of the parathyroid glands. The PTH levels are increased, and the resorption of bones with demineralization produces hypercalcemia. Phosphate levels are low. Medical treatment is frequently inadequate to manage the hypercalcemia, and total parathyroidectomy may be required. Parathyroid gland autotransplantation to the extremity appears successful in some case reports. The parathyroid tissue can be removed from the extremity as required to maintain eucalcemia. Subtotal parathyroidectomy has a significant risk for the continuation or recurrence of hypercalcemia in neonates.

### Parathyroid Adenoma

Hypercalcemia later in childhood is most likely secondary to hyperparathyroidism from parathyroid adenomas. Presenting clinical signs may include paralytic ileus and personality changes. If the child is asymptomatic, hypercalcemia may be detected when biochemical screening tests are performed for routine physical examinations. The diagnosis can be confirmed biochemically by determining hypercalcemia, hypophosphatemia, and elevated PTH levels. Hypercalcuria may be present. Radiographic findings may consist of osteitis fibrosa cystica. Advances in sonographic techniques allow presurgical localization. Hypocalcemia may occur after surgery, but resolves as the remaining parathyroid glands recover.

### Multiple Endocrine Neoplasia, Type I

Multiple endocrine neoplasia, Type I (MEN-1), or Wermer's syndrome, is an autosomal dominant form of an inherited disease in which hyperparathyroidism, pancreatic tumors, and pituitary adenomas occur. Most affected patients have hyperparathyroidism secondary to enlargement and hyperplasia of all parathyroid tissue. The etiology is unknown, but studies using restriction fragment link polymorphisms have located a potential MEN-1 gene on chromosome 11. Some cases have been reported with an onset in neonates and children. The diagnosis is confirmed by determining hypercalcemia, elevated levels of PTH, and familial incidence. Treatment consists of subtotal parathyroidectomy (3½ glands) with autotransplantation of a small amount of parathyroid tissue to the muscles of one of the extremities.

### Familial Hypercalcemic Hypocalcuria

Familial hypercalcemic hypocalcuria (FHH) is an autosomal dominant form of hypercalcemia known previously as familial benign hypercalcemia. The diagnosis is unsuspected in most children unless other family members are known to have hypercalcemia. The etiology of this disorder is unknown. Numerous investigators have postulated etiologies, but none has explained all biochemical findings.

The cardinal finding is hypercalcemia, occurring from the neonatal period, with relative hypocalcuria for the degree of hypercalcemia. Serum calcium levels usually range from 11 to 12 mg/dL with few levels greater than 14 mg/dL. Urinary calcium expressed in terms of milligrams of calcium per milligram of creatinine is normal or elevated slightly, but is less than would be expected from primary hyperparathyroidism. (Normal levels of urinary calcium are less than 4 mg/kg/d, and calcium-to-creatinine ratio is usually less than 0.3 mg calcium/mg creatinine.) Nephrocalcinosis does not occur. PTH levels are normal, but elevated for the degree of hypercalcemia. Serum magnesium levels are elevated in some children. Other biochemical studies related to calcium and vitamin D metabolism such as $1\text{-}25(OH)_2D_3$, calcitonin, urinary cAMP levels, and radiographic examination of the skeleton do not reveal consistent abnormalities, or they are normal. The diagnosis can be corroborated further by the asymptomatic nature of the disorder, as opposed to the signs and symptoms of hypercalcemia secondary to hyperparathyroidism.

Surgical removal of all parathyroid tissue results in hypoparathyroidism. Removal of only parts of the parathyroid gland does not improve hypercalcemia. No treatment of hypercalcemia is recommended.

## LABORATORY FINDINGS

Hyperparathyroidism from any etiology can be recognized by elevated levels of PTH concomitant with hypercalcemia and hypophosphatemia. Newer assays for the intact (1–84) PTH molecule facilitate measurements that were previously difficult to obtain. Most PTH assays are more helpful, however, when calcium levels are incorporated. The negative feedback system between calcium and PTH allows other causes of hypercalcemia such as hypervitaminosis D to be differentiated. Ultrasound evaluation of parathyroid gland size allows identification of hyperplasia and adenomas. The diagnosis of familial hypercalcemic hypocalcuria usually is based on a normal level of PTH, relative hypocalcuria (frequently the urinary calcium levels are normal), modest hypercalcemia, with the same biochemical findings in other family members.

## TREATMENT

Treatment of hypercalcemia secondary to hyperparathyroidism must include treatment of the underlying disorder. Acute treatment requires hydration. This can be done orally in cooperative children, or by intravenous methods in uncooperative ones. Twice maintenance fluid rates or greater are used. Dehydration secondary to nausea, vomiting, and polyuria can occur with hypercalcemia, and definite amounts to correct dehydration should be added to the total fluid replacement volume. Administration of intravenous saline after rehydration is beneficial because calcium excretion is enhanced by sodium excretion. Furosemide or other loop diuretics increase sodium and calcium excretion. Glucocorticoids such as prednisone in pharmacologic amounts decrease intestinal absorption of calcium, but their effects are minimal in hypercalcemia from hyperparathyroidism. Sunlight, any form of vitamin D, and dairy products should be avoided during hypercalcemia. The above treatments usually suffice in children, but further treatment can be undertaken with calcitonin, phosphorus, mithramycin, peritoneal dialysis, and bisphosphonates. These forms of treatment have been used in adults, and their experience in children is nonexistent or limited.

## Selected Readings

Favus MJ. Primer on the metabolic bone diseases and disorders of mineral metabolism. Richmond: William Byrd Press, 1990.

Harrison HE, Harrison HC. Disorders of calcium and phosphorus metabolism in childhood and adolescence. Philadelphia: WB Saunders, 1979.

*Principles and Practice of Pediatrics, Second Edition.*
edited by Frank A. Oski et al. J. B. Lippincott Company, Philadelphia © 1994.

# CHAPTER 75
# Idiopathic Diffuse Interstitial Lung Disease in Children

Iley Browning and Claire Langston

## IDIOPATHIC DIFFUSE INTERSTITIAL LUNG DISEASE

The term *interstitial pneumonia* describes a variety of pathologic states characterized by a diffuse inflammatory process that involves the interstitium or supporting structures of the lung as opposed to the alveolar spaces. Interstitial pneumonia is a nonspecific reaction to injury that can be a manifestation of infection, drugs, toxic inhalants, collagen vascular diseases, or a variety of genetic, metabolic, or inflammatory disorders. It may present clinically ranging from an acute fulminant to a chronic indolent form. Interstitial pneumonia is generally subdivided, based on histologic pattern, into four groups: usual interstitial pneumonia (UIP), desquamative interstitial pneumonia (DIP), lymphoid interstitial pneumonia (LIP), and giant-cell interstitial pneumonia (GIP). A rapidly progressive form of interstitial pneumonia with a characteristic histologic picture has variously been called acute interstitial pneumonia, rapidly progressive interstitial pneumonia, and Hamman-Rich syndrome. These diseases are unusual in both adults and children, except in individuals with collagen vascular disease or acquired immune deficiency syndrome (AIDS).

The most common pattern of interstitial lung disease seen in children is a cellular interstitial pneumonia without the specific histologic features of the better known interstitial pneumonias, which are more common in adults. Most children with chronic interstitial lung disease have a nonspecific picture of more uniform alveolar epithelial cell hyperplasia and patchy interstitial mononuclear cell infiltration without the features of coexistent hyaline membranes and fibrosis seen in UIP, which suggests both chronicity and activity. This pattern has an unpredictable course. Steroid therapy is the usual treatment. Some patients with this disease pattern do well, while others progress to pulmonary fibrosis.

## USUAL INTERSTITIAL PNEUMONIA

UIP, the most common of these conditions in adults, is a patchy interstitial process with variable microscopic features reflecting progressive infiltration and scarring of the lung parenchyma. These features include the coexistence in the same biopsy specimen of both active lesions with hyaline membranes and cellular infiltration and regions of scarring with collagen deposition. This pathologic picture is described under various names, including fibrosing alveolitis and Hamman-Rich syndrome. The latter term is better reserved for the rapidly progressive variant of interstitial pneumonia, which differs clinically from UIP by its rapid fulminant course and differs histologically by the marked fibroplasia without collagen deposition and the relative paucity of inflammatory cells. The histologic picture of Hamman-Rich syndrome does not show the variability of UIP; its lesions are all of the same age and progression. In UIP, the major signs and symptoms include tachypnea, dyspnea, hypoxia, cough, and failure to thrive. Respiratory and cardiac failure, pulmonary hypertension, and spontaneous pneumothorax are the most common reported major complications. Clinical signs in infancy and childhood are similar to those in adults, but the clinical course is often more rapid in childhood, and fatal if untreated. UIP has been seen in children with rheumatoid arthritis, chronic active hepatitis, ulcerative colitis, thyroid disease, and systemic lupus erythematosus. There are a few familial cases, both children and adults, which suggests an autosomal dominant mode of inheritance. Current treatment is high-dose steroid therapy with a starting dosage of about 2 mg/kg/d, continued for a minimum of 4 to 8 weeks and sometimes for as long as 1 to 2 years. Immunosuppressant therapy has been tried on a limited number of children with mixed results. Those patients with onset of disease before 1 year of age have a shorter mean survival than older patients who may survive for 5 to 10 years. The mortality rate, even with good treatment, may be as high as 50%.

## DESQUAMATIVE INTERSTITIAL PNEUMONIA

DIP is a pathologically distinct type of interstitial pneumonia. It is much less common than UIP and is estimated to account for 10% to 25% of all clinically diagnosed chronic interstitial pneumonias. One review (Stiwell, 1980) found only 28 reported cases in children diagnosed by lung biopsy. DIP is characterized histologically by hyperplasia of type 2 alveolar lining cells and the filling of distal air spaces with numerous macrophages. In contrast to UIP, there is only mild alveolar septal thickening and a sparse interstitial infiltrate. Major signs and symptoms are similar to those of UIP and include dyspnea, tachypnea, failure to thrive, cough, and hypoxemia. Right ventricular hypertrophy and pulmonary hypertension are common findings. DIP has been seen with other disease states, including acute lymphoblastic leukemia, glomerulonephritis with nephrotic syndrome, and trisomy 21. A few familial cases have been reported in children. The primary treatment is steroids, and patients generally respond to therapy. Cytotoxic drugs and chloroquine have been used with limited response in a few children with cases refractory to steroid therapy. The age of onset of disease is divided evenly between children younger than 1 year and older children. There is no difference in mortality rate between the two groups; the overall mortality rate is 35%.

## LYMPHOID INTERSTITIAL PNEUMONIA

LIP was a rare disease in children. With the increase in the number of children with human immunodeficiency virus (HIV) infection, LIP is more prevalent. The incidence of LIP in pediatric AIDS patients is estimated at about 25%. Although LIP was initially grouped with the interstitial pneumonias, it is a manifestation of lymphoproliferative disease involving the lung. LIP is characterized histologically by a prominent interstitial infiltrate of mature lymphocytes with a variable admixture of plasma cells and other lymphoreticular elements; it may be either diffuse or patchy.

Many presenting signs and symptoms are similar to those seen in UIP and DIP. LIP is associated with a variety of immunologic disorders including hypergammaglobulinemia or hypogammaglobulinemia, rheumatoid diseases, Sjögren's syndrome, and, more recently, AIDS in the pediatric age group, for which it is an indicator disease. Familial LIP has been reported. The usual treatment is steroids. Cytotoxic drugs are used when response to steroids is poor.

## GIANT-CELL INTERSTITIAL PNEUMONIA

GIP is a rare condition in adults and is virtually pathognomonic of a hard-metal pneumoconiosis. It is rare in children. GIP is characterized by the presence of many large multinucleate cells in the alveolar spaces. These cells are described as "cannibalistic," (ie, they engulf other cells). In addition, discrete macrophages fill the alveolar spaces and there is hyperplasia of type 2 alveolar epithelial cells and an interstitial infiltrate of lymphohistiocytic cells. The clinical presentation is similar to that of DIP. GIP is associated with immunologic dysfunction. The treatment is steroids, with variable response.

## END-STAGE

End-stage or honeycomb lung represents the final evolution of a variety of inflammatory and proliferative processes, resulting in a cystic and fibrotic lung. While all forms of interstitial pneumonia can progress to this end-stage, other forms of chronic pulmonary disease may also terminate in this picture. It may not be possible at this end-stage to discern which pathologic process led to this entity. The pathologic hallmark of end-stage pulmonary fibrosis is marked remodeling of distal air spaces and obliteration of small airways, leading to the formation of macroscopic cysts separated by areas of dense fibrosis. Steroid treatment is often attempted, but has little or no effect unless there is active inflammation. At this stage of disease, cardiopulmonary dysfunction becomes severe, resulting in high mortality.

### Selected Readings

Carrington CB, Gaensler EA, Coutu RE, et al. Natural history and treated course of usual and desquamative interstitial pneumonia. N Engl J Med 1978;298:801.

Fan LL, Langston C. Chronic interstitial lung disease in children. Pediatric Pulmonology. In press.

Hewitt CJ, Hull D, Keeling JW. Fibrosing alveolitis in infancy and childhood. Am J Dis Child 1977;523:22.

Katkin JP, Hansen TN, Langston C, Hiatt PW. Pulmonary manifestations of AIDS in children. Seminars in Pediatric Infectious Diseases 1990;1:40.

Katzenstein ALA, Askin FB. Surgical pathology of non-neoplastic lung disease. Philadelphia: WB Saunders, 1990:9.

Liebow AA. Definition and classification of interstitial pneumonias in human pathology. In Basset F, Georger R, (eds). Progress in respiration research, alveolar interstium of the lung. Basel, Switzerland: Karger, 1975.

Mak H, Moser RL, Hallett JS, Robotham JL. Usual interstitial pneumonitis in infancy. Chest 1982;82:124.

Nadorra RL, Landing BH. Pulmonary lesions in childhood onset systemic lupus erythematosus: analysis of 26 cases and summary of literature. Pediatr Pathol 1987;7:1.

O'Brodovich HM, Moser MM, Lu L. Familial lymphoid interstitial pneumonia: a long term follow-up. Pediatrics 1980;65:523.

Ohori NP, Sciurba FC, Owens GR, Hodgson MJ, Yousem SA. Giant-cell interstitial pneumonia and hard-metal pneumoconiosis. A clinicopathologic study of four cases and review of the literature. Am J Surg Pathol 1989;13:581.

Stiwell PC, Norris DG, O'Connell EJ, Rosenow EC, et al. Desquamative interstitial pneumonitis in children. Chest 1980;77:165.

*Principles and Practice of Pediatrics, Second Edition.*
edited by Frank A. Oski et al. J. B. Lippincott Company, Philadelphia © 1994.

## CHAPTER 76
# *Pulmonary Alveolar Microlithiasis*

### Carol L. Rosen

Pulmonary alveolar microlithiasis is a rare disorder of unknown etiology characterized by intra-alveolar calcific concretions throughout the lung. Onset can occur in childhood, although most cases occur in adults. About one half of cases are familial, mainly in asymptomatic siblings who are diagnosed incidentally. There is no consistent epidemiologic pattern or exposure history to environmental toxins or infectious agents. Metabolic studies, including those of calcium and vitamin D, have been normal.

Frequently, the illness is discovered in asymptomatic patients when a chest roentgenogram is taken for an unrelated illness. When symptoms develop, cough is often the chief complaint. Patients can remain asymptomatic for years, but most die in middle adulthood from progressive interstitial fibrosis with hypoxemia, respiratory failure, and cor pulmonale. The characteristic chest roentgenogram shows fine sandlike micronodulation diffusely involving both lungs. In children, the differential diagnosis of this miliary pattern includes disseminated tuberculosis, fungal infection (especially healed disseminated histoplasmosis), sarcoidosis, neoplasia, hemosiderosis, and metastatic pulmonary calcification associated with chronic renal failure. The unusual feature of this disease is the striking x-ray changes in contrast to the paucity of physical findings. Computed tomography and technetium $^{99}$m scans have been used to verify diffuse calcification, but neither study provides more diagnostic information than the plain film of the chest. Pulmonary function tests may show restrictive lung disease, the severity of which correlates with the degree of interstitial lung disease. If the clinical history and characteristic roentgenographic findings are present, then lung biopsy and bronchoalveolar lavage are not required. Histologically, numerous laminated calcospherites (0.02 to 3.0 mm diameter) are found within alveolar spaces. While the microliths are intra-alveolar, one ultrastructural study suggests their formation is initiated in the pulmonary interstitium by deposition carboxyapatite crystals produced by membrane-bound extracellular matrix vesicles.

Treatment is supportive. Because there is increased familial incidence, family members should be screened for the disease. Corticosteroids, chelating agents, and bronchoalveolar lavage have no influence on the disease. Because patients are healthy except for this cardiopulmonary problem, heart–lung transplantation may be a future therapeutic consideration.

## Selected Readings

Barnard NJ, Crocker PR, Blainey AD, Davies RJ, Ell SR, Levison DA. Pulmonary alveolar microlithiasis. A new analytical approach. Histopathology 1987;11:639.

Caffrey PR, Altman RS. Pulmonary alveolar microlithiasis occurring in premature twins. J Pediatr 1965;66:758.

Kendig EL Jr. Idiopathic pulmonary alveolar microlithiasis. In: Kendig EL Jr, Chernick V, eds. Disorders of the respiratory tract in children, ed 4. Philadelphia: WB Saunders, 1983:428.

Kino T, Kohara Y, Tsuji S. Pulmonary alveolar microlithiasis: a report in two young sisters. Am Rev Respir Dis 1972;105:105.

Prakash UBS, Barham SS, Rosenow EC III, et al. Pulmonary alveolar microlithiasis: a review including ultrastructural and pulmonary function studies. Mayo Clin Proc 1983;58:290.

*Principles and Practice of Pediatrics, Second Edition.*
edited by Frank A. Oski et al. J. B. Lippincott Company, Philadelphia © 1994.

## CHAPTER 77
# *Emphysema*

### Bruce G. Nickerson

Emphysema is an uncommon but serious problem in pediatrics. It is underrecognized and may masquerade as asthma or some other condition that responds poorly to therapy, or it may be a component of other lung diseases. Emphysema usually is recognized by clinical suspicion in a patient with a hyperinflated chest, prolonged expiratory phase, and wheezing that responds poorly to bronchodilators. It is usually diagnosed by chest roentgenogram with the finding of hyperinflation, dark lung fields, and diaphragms below the 10th or 11th posterior ribs. Diagnosis can be confirmed by measuring lung volumes, flow rates, and compliance in the pulmonary function laboratory. A lung biopsy shows less elastic tissue and simplification of alveolar septation.

## DEFINITIONS

The pathologist defines emphysema as the abnormal, permanent enlargement of air spaces distal to the terminal bronchioles, accompanied by destruction of alveolar walls. The physiologist defines emphysema as the permanent loss of elastic recoil of the lungs. The clinician defines emphysema as overexpansion of a region of the lungs that is not reversible with maximal bronchodilator therapy.

Enlargement of air spaces without destruction of their walls is termed overinflation. The term emphysema is seldom used in pediatrics. Although many children have lungs that fit these descriptions, few come to lung biopsy or autopsy for definitive diagnosis. Furthermore, the rapid increase in the number of alveoli until 8 years of age allows for a dramatic improvement in the clinical status of children with even severe emphysematous changes in the first year of life. A number of clinical syndromes and common pediatric respiratory diseases have significant components of emphysema.

## NORMAL DEVELOPMENT OF THE LUNGS

All airways down to the terminal bronchioles are present by 16 weeks of postconceptual age. Thus, the full complement of airways is developed in the most premature infants who are viable. An acinus is the unit distal to the terminal bronchiole that includes the alveolar ducts and alveoli ventilated by a single terminal bronchiole. Adjacent acini are separated by fibrous septa. Alveoli develop by budding from alveolar ducts. Alveoli increase in number until about 8 years of age. After that, the alveoli continue to expand until the lungs reach adult size, at about 17 years in girls and 20 years in boys. From then on, the alveoli gradually simplify, and the alveolar surface area decreases by about 4% per decade through adult life.

## PHYSIOLOGY OF EMPHYSEMA

At the end of expiration, all respiratory muscles usually are relaxed, and the volume of the lungs is determined by the balance between elastic recoil of lung tissue and compliance of the thoracic cavity. Normally, there is a network of elastic fibers running throughout the lungs in the interstitial spaces that provides the elastic recoil of the lungs. Disruption or destruction of this elastic network occurs in emphysema. Recoil decreases, diminishing the normal tendency for the lungs to shrink, and the functional residual capacity (ie, the lung volume at the end of passive expiration) increases. This causes a number of secondary changes. Diaphragms do not ascend to their normal position at the end of expiration, so they are at a mechanical disadvantage for developing negative pressure in the chest for inspiration. Phrenic muscle fibers are shorter, so they develop less tension. Consequently, diaphragms pull less air into the lungs. Also, because of decreased driving pressure, expiratory flows decrease, particularly at lower lung volumes. This causes a decrease in forced expiratory volume in 1 second ($FEV_1$) and a consequent decrease in maximum minute ventilation, which decreases exercise capacity. With severe emphysema, loss of alveolar surface area decreases the surface area available for gas exchange. This can be measured either as a low diffusion capacity for carbon monoxide or as a fall in oxygen saturation during exercise.

Elastic recoil of the lung can be determined by measuring pulmonary compliance. Almost all pediatric patients with emphysema have regional defects, however, and other regions of the lungs may have restrictive processes. Therefore, the measured compliance reflects the conflicting effects of two different abnormalities. Because of this and because measurement of pulmonary compliance requires swallowing an esophageal balloon, this test is seldom performed in pediatrics.

In clinical practice, useful tests for a patient with emphysema include a forced expiratory flow volume loop that typically shows a mild increase in normal forced vital capacity, a moderate decrease in $FEV_1$, and a more severe decrease in flows at low lung volumes or forced expiratory flow between 25% and 75% of vital capacity. A component of bronchoconstriction may coexist, but the emphysema patient has residual abnormalities even after administration of potent bronchodilators.

Measurements of lung volumes show an increase in functional residual capacity and residual volume. With severe emphysema, there is also an increase in total lung capacity. A test of the diffusion capacity for carbon monoxide can help quantitate the diffusion defect. A progressive exercise stress test with measurement of oxygen saturation often demonstrates a significant fall in oxygen saturation with moderate exercise.

## PATHOLOGIC CLASSIFICATION

Based on the pattern of involvement of alveoli relative to terminal bronchioles, four distinct types of emphysema are recognized by pathologists. These are panacinar, centriacinar, paraseptal, and irregular emphysema (Table 77-1).

In panacinar emphysema, all alveoli, from those close to the bronchioles to those in the lobar septum, are involved with overextension and destruction of their walls. This type of emphysema typically is seen in adults with $\alpha_1$-antitrypsin deficiency. About 1 in 3500 individuals in the North American population has homozygous deficiency in $\alpha_1$-antitrypsin with levels less than 20% of normal. This enzyme protects elastic fibers of the lungs from digestion by proteolytic enzymes released by polymorphonuclear leukocytes and alveolar macrophages.

This type of emphysema takes many years to develop. Most children with this deficiency have no respiratory symptoms and normal pulmonary function. They are more likely to have prolonged neonatal jaundice and symptoms due to liver involvement. Thus, measurement of $\alpha_1$-antitrypsin levels seldom is indicated in the workup of the pediatric pulmonary patient unless there is a positive family history or the child has unexplained liver disease or irreversible overinflation of the lungs.

Individuals with $\alpha_1$-antitrypsin deficiency should be counseled to avoid cigarette smoking, because nearly all smokers with this defect develop emphysema in young adulthood, whereas more than half of nonsmokers escape this complication.

Centriacinar emphysema is characterized by overdistention and destruction of the alveoli near the terminal bronchiole with relatively normal alveoli at the periphery of the acinus. It is seen commonly in adults with a long history of cigarette smoking, but is seldom seen in pediatric patients. This disease, which accounts for disability and premature mortality in adults, is preventable. Because most cigarette smokers start the habit while still in the pediatric age range (as adolescents), pediatricians can influence the course of this disease by helping their patients to avoid starting the smoking habit.

Paraseptal emphysema involves the alveoli most distant from the terminal bronchioles, near the septa between adjacent acini. It is seen most often in tall adolescents and young adults who develop spontaneous pneumothoraces. Generally, these individuals do well with decompression of the pneumothorax by tube thoracostomy. Occasionally, an individual with recurrent pneumothoraces requires sclerosis of the pleural surfaces to prevent

### TABLE 77-1. Pathology of Emphysema

| Pathologic Type | Involvement | Clinical Setting |
| --- | --- | --- |
| Panacinar emphysema | All alveoli involved | $\alpha_1$-antitrypsin deficiency |
| Centriacinar emphysema | Overdistention of the alveoli near the terminal bronchi | Long-time cigarette smokers |
| Paraseptal emphysema | Most distal alveoli | Tall, thin young adults with spontaneous pneumothoraces |
| Irregular emphysema | Alveoli near areas of scar tissue | Bronchopulmonary dysplasia, or following necrotic pneumonia |

recurrence. This can be done with instillation of agents such as tetracycline and its derivatives or hypertonic glucose through the chest tube. Occasionally, surgical abrasion of the pleural surfaces is required. This can be done endoscopically without a thoracotomy.

Irregular emphysema–the overdistention of alveoli seen near scar tissue–can be seen in many patients with pulmonary scarring or a chronic atelectasis. It seems to be caused by overdistention of the alveoli due to local traction from the scarred area. Areas of irregular emphysema may be seen in many pediatric patients with processes that cause scarring, including bronchopulmonary dysplasia, necrotizing pneumonias, cystic fibrosis, and the residuals after mechanical ventilation for adult respiratory distress syndrome.

## CLINICAL SYNDROMES

Clinicians encounter emphysema in a number of clinical syndromes that occur in patients of different age groups. Medical treatment of emphysema is outlined in Table 77-2.

Congenital lobar emphysema actually represents lobar hyperinflation and may present in the first few hours or days of life with increasing tachypnea, respiratory distress, and cyanosis. The chest radiograph shows dramatic overinflation of one or two lobes. The disease usually involves the left upper lobe, but may involve any lobe. If the respiratory distress is significant and of rapid onset and if the overdistended lobe becomes larger and compresses adjacent structures, it is a surgical emergency. The infant should be referred to an experienced pediatric chest surgeon for prompt bronchoscopy to rule out a ball valve obstruction in the bronchus of the affected lobe, and possibly for thoracotomy for removal of the lobe. In a child with a rapidly deteriorating condition, diagnostic tests such as computed tomography, magnetic resonance imaging, or ventilation perfusion scans are superfluous. They should be omitted if they do not add to the surgical decision and involve unnecessary delay, which may cause further respiratory compromise. In the more stable patient, these tests occasionally are helpful in therapeutic decisions. Congenital lobar emphysema may be confused with congenital cysticadenomatoid malformation of the lung, polyalveolar lobe, and sometimes a large pneumothorax.

Occasionally, infants develop giant blebs, which may be congenital or may occur after necrotizing pneumonia or after mechanical ventilation with high inspiratory pressures. Most of these infants do well with conservative therapy, but at times they may be helped by intubating the opposite main stem bronchus to decrease distending pressure on the area affected. One group describes successful surgical obliteration of such blebs at open

thoracotomy. The availability of small thoracoscopes may make this possible without an open thoracotomy. Occasionally, infants with severe overextension of a bleb that compresses more normal lung tissue can benefit from a lobectomy. This surgery results in permanent loss of lung tissue, however, and should be performed only if all options are exhausted.

Infants with bronchopulmonary dysplasia commonly have emphysematous changes that combine focal hyperinflation and destructive remodeling of lung tissue. Older infants who have had episodes of severe respiratory failure due to pneumonia, aspiration, shock lung, or other causes of severe respiratory failure may have a similar picture. There may be a combination of scarring, bronchiolar obstruction, atelectasis, and pleural thickening that reduces lung volumes and increases elastic recoil. At the same time, other areas show loss of elastic recoil, alveolar destruction, and may be significantly overinflated. The incidence of severe hyperinflation seems related to use of high inspiratory pressures. It is tempting to postulate that the elastic fiber network can be damaged by overstretching from high ventilator pressures.

Infants with bronchopulmonary dysplasia who have severe hyperinflation often have a more prolonged recovery than do other infants with this disease. During recovery, they are prone to recurrent exacerbations with viral infections. If gas exchange is marginal, the infants may develop cor pulmonale. Meticulous management of pulmonary status with treatment of reversible airway obstruction with bronchodilators, treatment of interstitial edema with diuretics, and close attention to good oxygenation are essential. These infants frequently require increased caloric intake to make up for the metabolic needs of the chronic inflammation in their lungs. Because resolution of symptoms depends on development of new alveolar growth and repair of damaged airways, excellent nutrition is essential.

Premature infants with respiratory distress syndrome may develop interstitial emphysema, which is the dissection of air into the interstitial spaces of the lungs. Premature infants who develop this lesion have a high incidence of progression to bronchopulmonary dysplasia. Treatment involves lowering the inspiratory pressure for good oxygenation. There have been encouraging results in some, but not all, studies using high frequency ventilation to lower the maximal inspiratory pressures and still obtain adequate gas exchange.

Occasionally, an older child is found to have unilateral emphysematous changes, frequently after a severe viral infection. This syndrome is called the MacLoud or Swyer-James syndrome. It generally occurs in children younger than 8 years during the period of rapid increase in alveolar number. Biopsy studies have shown that these children suffer from a decrease in alveolar number, but there is no true destruction of alveolar walls, so this entity does not fit the pathologic definition of emphysema. Generally, these children do well as they grow older, although, occasionally, they have recurrent infections in the involved area.

Recently, Edell and associates reported an 8 year-old girl with emphysema following Stevens-Johnson syndrome. I am also aware of several other girls who developed severe emphysema following Stevens-Johnson syndrome. Biopsy tests showed severe loss of alveolar septa, and pulmonary function tests showed severe obstructive changes. Long-term follow-up shows these changes are irreversible, and the patients may become permanent pulmonary cripples without a lung transplant.

Occasionally, a child with chronic undertreated asthma is found to have significant deformity of the chest wall and irreversible pulmonary function changes, including severe air trapping. These individuals appear to have a form of emphysema, although lung biopsy seldom has been performed in them. Aggressive treatment of chronic asthma to prevent overinflation might prevent this illness.

---

### TABLE 77-2. Treatment of Emphysema

1. Provide adequate oxygenation at rest and during exercise.
2. Provide adequate nutrition for growth, particularly in the first 8 years when alveolar formation is occurring.
3. Use bronchodilators to treat reversible airway obstruction.
4. Use diuretics to treat interstitial pulmonary edema.
5. Consider anticholinergics for bronchodilating some patients.
6. Use steroids if there is ongoing inflammation.
7. Consider $\alpha_1$-antitrypsin replacement if there is deficiency of this enzyme.
8. Prevent viral infections with flu vaccine, avoidance of day-care centers or exposure to others with respiratory infections.
9. Use agents to thin mucus if it is sticky and a nidus for infection.

## Selected Readings

American Thoracic Society. Chronic bronchitis, asthma, and pulmonary emphysema. Statement by the Committee on Diagnostic Standards for Nontuberculous Respiratory Disease. Am Rev Respir Dis 1962;85:762.

Edell DS, Davidson JJ, Muelenaer AA, Majure MM. Pediatrics 1992;89:429.

Kraemer R, Meister B, Schaad UB. Reversibility of lung function abnormalities in asthma. J Pediatr 1983;102:347

Nickerson BG. An overview of bronchopulmonary dysplasia: pathogenesis and current therapy. In: Lund CH. Bronchopulmonary dysplasia: strategies for total patient care. Petaluma, CA: Neonatal Network, 1990.

*Principles and Practice of Pediatrics, Second Edition.*
edited by Frank A. Oski et al. J. B. Lippincott Company, Philadelphia © 1994.

# CHAPTER 78
# *Diseases of the Pleura*

## James S. Kemp and Dan K. Seilheimer

## STRUCTURE AND PHYSIOLOGY OF THE NORMAL AND INFLAMED PLEURA

The embryonic coelomic cavity is lined by mesothelial cells and fibroelastic tissue. This embryonic mesothelial lining gives rise to the pleura and peritoneum. The parietal and visceral pleural mesothelium are each a single cell layer thick. The visceral pleura is also made up of collagen and elastin connective elements, through which travel its vascular supply, making it thicker than the parietal pleura. Once formed, the visceral pleura adheres tightly to the lung parenchyma and interlobar fissures. The parietal pleura is also firmly anchored—to the ribs, intercostal muscles, and central diaphragm—and is tightly adherent as it reflects over the descending aorta, the esophagus, and the pericardium. Because of the structures that the pleura invests, pressures within the pleural space are important determinants for the transmural pressure of the heart, esophagus, and the lungs.

A fluid layer 10 to 30 $\mu$ thick separates the parietal and visceral pleurae. The total volume of this layer of fluid is small, at most 2 mL in each pleural space of the healthy adult, but the fluid lining allows for direct mechanical coupling between the lungs and the diaphragm, intercostal muscles, and other muscles of the chest wall. This mechanical coupling via the pleural space transmits to the lungs the forces generated by the diaphragm and the lesser muscles of inspiration. Any widening of the pleural space impedes the efficiency of ventilation. There is normally no communication between the left and right pleural cavities, but fluid may enter the pleural space from the peritoneal cavity through pores in the diaphragm.

In healthy children, fluid enters the pleural space from the capillaries, lymphatics, and interstitial spaces of both pleurae. The amount of fluid crossing into the pleural space is approximately 0.01 mL/kg/hr. Recent research on animals with pleurae similar in thickness to that of humans suggests that the visceral pleura, because of its relative thickness, plays a limited role in fluid resorption in both health and disease. The bulk of fluid is resorbed by lymphatics in the parietal pleura, with a maximal rate of resorption of 0.20 mL/kg/hr, which tends to minimize the amount of fluid in the pleural space. The Starling forces equilibrium for the pleural space is defined by permeability of pleural mesothelial cells, hydrostatic pressure differences between the parietal and visceral capillaries and lymphatics, and oncotic pressure of blood compared to pleural fluid.

In addition to allowing coupling to the inspiratory-force generators, fluid in the pleural space permits the pleurae to slide over one another during the respiratory cycle. Glycoproteins, within the matrix formed by mesothelial cell microvilli, also reduce friction during breathing.

The normal cell population within the pleural space is small and includes mesothelial cells, monocytes, macrophages, and lymphocytes. During inflammation, neutrophils also enter the pleural space. Early in inflammation, all pleural space cells aggregate around openings of parietal pleural lymphatics to form "pleural tonsils." There are three clinically recognizable stages during pleural inflammation. First, dry or plastic pleurisy reflect ingress of inflammatory cells with minimal fluid accumulation. Second, pleurisy with effusion indicates that the inflammatory process has increased the permeability of the mesothelial cells, and fluid enters the pleural space at rates exceeding its removal. Third, organizing pleural disease is reached only with bacterial or fungal parapneumonic effusions. The effusion becomes fibrinous, and the accumulating pleural fluid no longer flows freely in the pleural spaces. Instead, pockets of fluid are loculated between gelatinous adhesions. If there is frank pus in the pleural space, the effusion correctly can be called an empyema. Because there is widespread confusion about the proper meaning of the term "empyema," it should be used only after a clear statement of the intended meaning.

## CLINICAL FINDINGS IN DISEASES OF THE PLEURA

### Findings Due to Excess Fluid and Inflammation

Regardless of cause, excess fluid accumulates in the pleural space when production of pleural fluid exceeds resorption. Systemic diseases increasing visceral hydrostatic pressures or decreasing plasma oncotic pressure cause thin transudative effusions. Thicker, exudative effusions (protein concentration more than 50% of serum) result from diseases, usually inflammatory, involving the pleural surfaces themselves. Inflammation increases mesothelial cell permeability and may decrease parietal lymph flow.

Underlying cardiac, hepatic, or renal disease usually causes transudative effusions. Ventilatory function may be impaired by underlying disease, but a large pleural effusion also compresses the lung and deforms the diaphragm and chest wall. Consequently, worsening tachypnea, cyanosis, and retractions with diminished breath sounds and dullness to percussion usually accompany large transudative effusions (see Hydrothorax).

Classic findings of early pleuritis are pain in the chest or shoulder (central diaphragm involved), guarding of the affected side, upper quadrant abdominal pain (costal diaphragm involved), a pleural friction rub, and grunting, shallow respirations. Pain fibers are present in the parietal but not the visceral pleura. Therefore, pleuritic pain reflects an extension of inflammation to the chest wall and indicates that the effusion is exudative. A significant pleural effusion eliminates these signs quickly, except for short, shallow respirations. Later, the child has fever, cough, and dyspnea. Intercostal spaces may bulge outward and the mediastinum may be pushed toward the contralateral side if the effusion is massive. There are "e" to "a" changes on auscultation, and breath sounds are diminished and often tubular. The child with a purulent effusion is febrile and appears ill, often with tachypnea and cyanosis. If the infection is caused by anaerobic bacteria, however, symptoms of a purulent effusion may be less dramatic.

Children with immunodeficiencies and those on steroids may have significant pleural infections with few clinical findings. In these children, thoracentesis should be performed when the radiograph shows an effusion wider than 10 mm on lateral decubitus views. Important conditions in the differential diagnosis of apparent pleuritic chest pain in immunocompetent children include costochondritis, chest pain associated with asthma or gastroesophageal reflux, herpes zoster, and occult trauma.

## Air in the Pleural Space

If the air leak is small and the child has little antecedent lung disease, the only symptom of a pneumothorax may be chest pain. If the pneumothorax is large or the child has severe underlying lung disease, there may be pain, cough, dyspnea, and cyanosis. Breath sounds usually are reduced on the side of the air accumulation. If very large, the trachea and cardiac apical impulse is displaced contralaterally. In a small infant, a large pneumothorax causes subcostal fullness.

## Imaging of the Pleurae and Pleural Space

Pleural effusions usually are detected first on the chest radiograph. Careful use of the chest radiograph, with occasional help from thoracic ultrasound and computed tomography (CT) scan allows identification of pleural disease, characterization of an effusion as free or loculated, and distinction between intrapleural processes and peripheral parenchymal lung disease.

The usual chest radiographic projections used to evaluate pleural disease are the posteroanterior (or anteroposterior), lateral, and lateral decubitus. Several points should be kept in mind when interpreting radiographs:

1. The periphery of pleural masses and pleural loculations generally make an obtuse angle with the chest wall. Pleural lesions can be distinguished from peripheral lung lesions because the latter usually meet the chest wall at an acute angle.
2. Free pleural fluid causes diffuse hazy opacity of the supine anteroposterior radiograph, while on upright films, it causes a meniscus that alters the costophrenic angle.
3. If an effusion is probable, both left and right lateral decubitus radiographs may be ordered to detect fluid moving freely within the pleural space.
4. Pleural fluid may be seen as densities in lung fissures.
5. Pulmonary consolidation usually follows a lobar pattern, thus is distinguished from free pleural fluid, which does not respect lobar boundaries.
6. Lucencies within a pleural effusion before thoracentesis suggest a bronchopleural fistula, or, less often, an anaerobic infection.

Ultrasound is helpful in localizing pleural fluid and in evaluating parenchymal densities abutting the pleura. If a pleural effusion is likely but decubitus views suggest that it is not free in the pleural space, thoracic ultrasound may identify a loculation that can be aspirated under direct ultrasound guidance. Ultrasound often reveals that a pleural process is inhomogeneous with areas of pleural thickening, relatively thin fluid, fibrinous adhesions, and pus within the same pleural space. Because it is portable

and does not require a controlled breathing pattern, ultrasound is relatively easy to use in children.

Although CT scan images portray and define the extent of pleural disease, they can be misleading because they may promote consideration of unnecessary invasive remedies. For example, CT images of parapneumonic inflammation can be worrisome but should not alone alter the traditional clinical approach to these processes. Nonetheless, the CT scan helps in distinguishing between lung abscesses touching the visceral pleura and loculated pus in the pleural space. Lung abscesses rarely require more than lengthy antibiotic therapy, and not tube thoracostomy. Pus in the pleural space, which requires drainage, makes an obtuse angle with the chest wall, and an abscess makes an acute angle. CT scans help detail parenchymal and hilar lymphadenopathy and calcifications accompanying pleural inflammation, and may, therefore, help clarify the etiology of the effusion.

## PNEUMOTHORAX

Free air in the pleural space is detected on a chest radiograph when bronchovascular markings end at the visceral pleural line and do not extend to the chest wall. Air can enter the pleural space by a primary tear in the pleura or by dissection along the bronchovascular sheath after alveolar rupture, with formation and rupture of subpleural blebs. Clinical findings are described above.

A pneumothorax is always a serious complication in children with underlying severe lung disease, but its importance in an otherwise normal child depends on its size. The percentage of the volume of the hemithorax occupied by free air is expressed by the following equation:

$$100\% \times \frac{(\text{diam. of lung})^3}{(\text{diam. of hemithorax})^3} = \% \text{ pneumothorax}$$

Regardless of cause, the recurrence risk after one pneumothorax is 50%, after two, 62%, and after three, 83%. Primary pneumothorax occurs spontaneously in children without previous known lung disease. Secondary pneumothorax occurs as a complication of either chronic or severe acute lung disease. Iatrogenic pneumothorax is the most common type of pneumothorax, particularly during mechanical ventilation or after thoracentesis (Table 78-1).

Children with small primary pneumothoraces should be observed carefully. If they develop respiratory distress, the pneumothorax should be evacuated. A 15% or larger primary pneumothorax can be managed with needle aspiration. Patients with secondary pneumothorax and those on mechanical ventilation usually are treated with tube thoracostomy. Breathing 100% oxygen hastens resorption of free air, but hyperoxia should not be maintained for more than a few hours and must be avoided completely in the premature infant.

Recurrent pneumothorax provokes anxiety and pain, and can be life-threatening. Pleurodesis should be considered in any patient with recurrent pneumothorax and in patients whose underlying lung disease is unremitting. Effective chemical pleurodesis requires lasting adherence of the parietal to the visceral pleura. Tetracycline at doses of 10 to 20 mg/kg should be instilled intrapleurally, with a maximal dose of 1 g. Tetracycline causes intense pain and should be mixed with Lidocaine. Intravenous analgesia also should be considered. Atabrine, if available, can accomplish chemical pleurodesis. Surgical pleurodesis or local pleurectomy with oversewing of subpleural blebs is necessary if chemical pleurodesis fails. Previous pleurodesis, either chemical or surgical, is a relative contraindication for lung transplantation. Because of the risks for life-threatening pleural bleeding after removal of the diseased and adherent lung, pleurodesis should

| TABLE 78-1.   Common Causes of Pneumothorax |
| --- |
| **Primary** |
| Congenital subpleural blebs |
| Familial spontaneous pneumothorax |
| Catamenial |
| Idiopathic |
| **Secondary** |
| Cystic fibrosis |
| Asthma |
| Hyaline membrane disease |
| Trauma—pleural tear, esophageal rupture, or bronchial rupture |
| Bacterial pneumonia with pneumatocele or abscess |
| Tuberculosis |
| Interstitial pneumonia |
| Histiocytosis X and eosinophilic granuloma |
| Marfan's syndrome |
| **Iatrogenic** |
| Mechanical ventilation |
| Thoracentesis with or without pleural biopsy |
| Bronchoscopy |
| Cardiopulmonary resuscitation |
| Radiotherapy |

not be performed if the child is a serious candidate for lung transplantation.

Primary pneumothoraces are not uncommon among adolescents, particularly in a referral practice. A CT scan with intravenous contrast should be obtained in all previously healthy children and adolescents with a pneumothorax. A substantial percentage have five or more subpleural blebs, usually in the apex, despite having normal chest radiographs. Because of a 50% or greater risk for recurrence, surgical pleurodesis with oversewing of blebs should be considered early in this group of patients. Thoracoscopy and thoracoscopic surgery are new techniques for evaluating and treating pneumothorax, and they likely will reduce the morbidity from managing this group of patients, as well as others with recurrent pneumothoraces.

Serious blunt chest trauma can cause tracheobronchial tears with a pneumothorax that persists despite closed-chest tube drainage. These tears should be suspected strongly in a victim of thoracic crush injury. After bronchoscopic identification, tears must be repaired surgically.

A tension pneumothorax results when a large accumulation of intrapleural air leads to hypoxemia and shock. In an emergency, needle aspiration with a large-bore needle, with or without a three-way stopcock, should be done before tube thoracostomy. The needle should be inserted over the second or third rib anteriorally, and the air should be aspirated with a syringe.

If a symptomatic pneumothorax is present for longer than 3 days, particularly in patients with primary pneumothorax, there is a small risk for reexpansion pulmonary edema. This ipsilateral pulmonary edema can be significant and can be prevented by draining the chest tube to water seal only.

## PNEUMOMEDIASTINUM

Air may enter the mediastinum after trauma to the trachea or esophagus, from the neck after facial or dental surgery, from the retroperitoneum after intestinal perforation, and from the lung parenchyma in association with pulmonary interstitial emphy-

sema. The symptoms of pneumomediastinum include stabbing chest pain, cough, dysphagia, sore throat, facial and neck swelling, and a muffled voice. Physical findings include chest-wall and cervical crepitus, distant heart sounds, a crunching sound with cardiac systole (Hamman's sign) and, rarely, low cardiac output. Chest films show streaks of air in the neck and upper mediastinum. There also is a lucency along the left heart border. Lateral chest films show "highlighting" of the mediastinal vessels and much retrosternal air. The most common causes of pneumomediastinum are listed in Table 78-2.

Pneumomediastinum alone usually requires no treatment. In the very sick neonate, however, it is occasionally necessary to evacuate a large pneumomediastinum. Surgical exploration is indicated if tracheal or esophageal rupture is suspected in association with a pneumomediastinum.

## HYDROTHORAX

The term hydrothorax refers to a large transudative pleural effusion. Congestive heart failure, nephrotic syndrome, glomerulonephritis, and hepatic cirrhosis are the most common causes of hydrothorax. Transudative effusions are usually bilateral with heart failure, unilateral or bilateral with nephrosis, or right-sided with cirrhosis. Effusions clearly associated with cardiac, renal, or hepatic disease need not be sampled by thoracentesis unless the child is febrile or respiration is compromised by a large effusion.

The febrile child with hepatic, cardiac, or renal disease and with a pleural effusion usually has an intercurrent infection not involving the pleural space. If another source of fever is not apparent after a period of observation, however, the effusion should be sampled. Most children with low serum osmolarity secondary to cirrhosis do not develop a pleural effusion based on low osmolarity alone. Rather, in a small percentage of cirrhotic children, ascitic fluid leaks across the diaphragm through small defects.

If thoracentesis is done after the transudative pleural effusion is present for several days, the protein content may be equal to that of serum as a result of osmotic equilibration. To treat or prevent circulatory collapse, removal of large quantities of thin pleural fluid should be done with a large-bore intravenous infusion in place. Reexpansion pulmonary edema can complicate removal of large quantities of fluid that have compressed the lung. Closed-chest tube drainage may be indicated if the effusion recurs rapidly. Tetracycline pleurodesis has been used to prevent recurrent symptomatic transudative pleural effusions in adults, but chemical pleurodesis rarely is required in children with transudative effusions.

## FIBROTHORAX

Fibrothorax is a disease of the visceral pleura. Although a dreaded complication of pneumonia in the preantibiotic era, it is now seen rarely after a parapneumonic effusion. Fibrothorax, or "trapped lung," also can occur after hemothorax. The histologic

| TABLE  78-2.   Common Causes of Pneumomediastinum |
| --- |
| Obstructive lung diseases—asthma, cystic fibrosis, bronchiolitis, foreign-body aspiration |
| Trauma, including tracheal and esophageal rupture |
| Screaming |
| Violent emesis |
| Valsalva maneuver while smoking marijuana |

picture in fibrothorax shows fibroblasts in a dense fibrous stroma that covers the lung and replaces the visceral pleura. On the chest radiograph in the presence of a fibrothorax, only a thin density is seen. When present, fibrothorax leads to a large reduction in ipsilateral lung volume and an even more marked reduction in ipsilateral perfusion. Such a thick fibrous "peel," however, should be removed surgically only if all the following criteria are met: the entrapment is unchanged or progressive for 6 months, the patient has exertional dyspnea, and the underlying lung is free of bronchiectasis.

Fusion, or symphysis, of the parietal and visceral pleurae without constriction of the lung is a much more common and predictable result of a parapneumonic effusion. Pleural symphysis does not limit pulmonary function. This may be surprising, because in health, the lung expands and recoils while the pleural surfaces slide over one another. Unlike fibrothorax, pleural symphysis is associated with little reduction in vital capacity or PaO₂.

Because fibrothorax is uncommon after a parapneumonic effusion in children, management is different from that used for adults. Some authors state categorically that decortication, usually meaning the removal of gelatinous adhesions and purulent debris, is never indicated in children. Other writers define decortication as the stripping away of large areas of the visceral pleura with much risk of hemorrhage. The intended meaning of decortication should be defined carefully when surgical intervention is discussed. Recent retrospective studies suggest that limited thoracotomy with debridement of the pleural space, without pleural stripping, hastens defervescence and hospital discharge in children with prolonged illness caused by parapneumonic effusion. Such limited surgical therapy is not mandated to preserve lung function in these cases because lung function usually returns to near normal without surgically opening the thorax. There is striking clinical improvement in most children within 48 hours after pleural debridement through a limited thoracotomy, however, and this intervention should be considered strongly for children who are febrile or bedridden for 2 weeks or longer.

## HEMOTHORAX

Bleeding into the pleural space is unusual in childhood and is most common after thoracic trauma or insertion of a central venous catheter. In adults, hemothorax without trauma raises the possibility of malignancy metastatic to the pleurae or of a pulmonary embolus. Other causes of hemothorax in children include coagulopathies, rupture of a ductus arteriosus, a coarctation, or a pulmonary arteriovenous malformation, and bleeding from a sequestered lobe of the lung. Pleural endometriosis is a cause of nontraumatic hemothorax in young females. Hemothorax often is associated with a pneumothorax, and clinical findings are those of both fluid and air in the pleural space. The diagnosis of hemothorax is supported by chest radiograph and confirmed by thoracentesis. Aspirated fluid is red and has a hematocrit that is either at least 50% of the peripheral blood or is increasing on serial thoracenteses. Pink-tinged pleural fluid is common without pleural bleeding and is of no diagnostic significance. Because red pleural fluid may have a hematocrit less than or equal to 5%, a hematocrit assay should be used to confirm the diagnosis.

Hemothorax after trauma usually is associated with pneumothorax. Blood may not appear for 24 hours, so repeat chest films should be taken 1 day after serious chest trauma causing a pneumothorax. Blood in the pleural space may come from the diaphragm, chest wall, lung, and blood vessels of the thorax. Hemothorax should be treated with a chest tube to drain the pleural space and to allow tamponade of the vessels leaking into the pleura. If the bleeding is greater than 10 mL/kg/h, the thorax should be explored surgically.

Four important complications of hemothorax are retained blood clots, empyema, pleural effusion after chest-tube removal, and fibrothorax. Retained blood clots are important only if they occupy more than 30% of the hemithorax and compress the lung. Empyema is more likely to occur if the pleural space is contaminated at the time of trauma and if the chest tube is left in for many days. Pleural effusion after chest-tube removal usually is benign, although a thoracentesis should be done to rule out pus or recurrent hemothorax. Fibrothorax occurs in less than 1% of hemothoraces and is more likely if there is associated empyema.

## CHYLOTHORAX

Table 78-3 lists the most common causes of chylothorax. Chylothorax may occur on the right or left. Neonatal chylothorax is often bilateral and associated with multiple chyle fistulae entering both hemithoraces.

Nontraumatic chylothorax appears slowly and is associated with dyspnea and "heaviness" of the chest. Traumatic or surgical chylothorax may appear rapidly with severe respiratory embarrassment and shock. Usually, though, surgical chylothorax appears over days, even weeks, because the post-operative patient usually is not fed and is at bed rest, so has minimal chyle flow. When chyle does begin to flow, it then may accumulate first in the posterior mediastinum as a chyloma. Only when this chyloma ruptures into the pleural space is pleural effusion apparent. The appearance of a chylous effusion is usually painless, and there is rarely fever. Chyle is not irritative to the pleura and is bacteriostatic.

Chyle in the pleural space is milky or yellow if the patient has been fed. Thoracic duct fluid is clear in the newborn before the first feeding. In the older child, a chylous effusion is confirmed if the triglyceride level is more than 110 mg/dL of pleural fluid. If the triglyceride level of pleural fluid is less than 50 mg/dL, the fluid is probably nonchylous. If the triglyceride level is between 50 and 110 mg/dL, a lipoprotein electrophoresis should be performed to show a full spectrum of lipoproteins if the fluid is chylous. If a nonchylous effusion is present for several weeks, it may appear milky and have a triglyceride level of more than 110 mg/dL. This is termed a pseudochylothorax and occurs in patients with no obvious risk factors for chylothorax. Lipoprotein electrophoresis distinguishes pseudochylothorax from a chylous effusion.

Chyle contains electrolytes (similar to serum concentrations), 3 g/dL of protein, 0.4 to 0.6 g of fat, and fat-soluble vitamins. If chyle is drained from the pleural space in appreciable quantities, these nutrients should be replaced. Other therapy includes tube thoracostomy and, usually, a diet containing medium-chain triglycerides. If these steps fail, an attempt should be made to stop chyle flow, thus aiding healing of the thoracic duct by starting total parenteral nutrition (TPN). Ligation of the thoracic duct often is not necessary. It should be considered if the daily chyle loss is greater than 100 mL per year of age for 5 days, if chyle flow does not decrease after 14 days of TPN, or if nutrition is poor.

| TABLE 78-3.   Common Causes of Chylothorax |
|---|
| Neonatal "idiopathic" chylothorax |
| Cardiac or great-vessel surgery |
| Penetrating chest trauma |
| Surgery of esophagus, mediastinum, neck, vertebrae |
| Lymphoma |

Sustained lymphopenia due to loss of lymphocytes into the pleural space is a relative indication for TPN or surgical intervention. Tetracycline pleurodesis may be considered if the effusion recurs after ligation of the thoracic duct, or in patients who are not candidates for repeat thoracic surgery.

Recent experience with surgically placed shunts from the pleural space to the peritoneum is encouraging. They have been used in early management of chylothorax and may allow reinstitution of enteral feeding without ventilatory compromise.

## PLEURAL COMPLICATIONS OF THE ACQUIRED IMMUNE DEFICIENCY SYNDROME

Bacterial parapneumonic effusions due to the standard pathogens are the most likely causes of pleural effusions in patients with acquired immune deficiency syndrome. Despite the prevalence of chronic lung disease, however, pleural effusions in general are uncommon in children with AIDS. This may be because *Pneumocystis carinii* infections rarely cause effusions, and although

tuberculosis is common in AIDS patients, effusions are infrequent. Two additional infections causing effusions must be considered in the child with AIDS: disseminated cryptococcosis and severe pneumonia due to atypical mycobacteria. Adults with Kaposi's sarcoma often have effusions, but this malignancy is rare in children.

## Selected Readings

Agostoni E. Mechanics of the pleural space. In: Macklem PT, Mead J, eds. Handbook of physiology. Vol 3. Mechanics of breathing. The respiratory system. Bethesda, MD: American Physiological Society, 1986:531.

Hoff SJ, Neblett WW, Edwards KM, et al. Parapneumonic empyema in children: decortication hastens recovery in patients with severe pleural infections. Pediatr Infect Dis 1991;10:194.

Lesur O, Delorme N, Fromaget JM, Bernadac P, Polu JM. Computed tomography in the etiologic assessment of idiopathic spontaneous pneumothorax. Chest 1990;98:341.

Light RW. Pleural diseases, ed 2. Philadelphia: Lea and Febiger, 1990.

Parrish DA, Seilheimer DK. Chylothorax. In: Garson A, Bricker JT, McNamara DG, eds. The science and practice of pediatric cardiology. Philadelphia: Lea and Febiger, 1990:2512.

Snyder RW, Mishel HS. Mediastinal emphysema after a sex orgy. Letter. N Engl J Med 1990;323:758.

*Principles and Practice of Pediatrics, Second Edition.*
edited by Frank A. Oski et al. J. B. Lippincott Company, Philadelphia © 1994.

# CHAPTER 79
# *Recurrent or Persistent Lower Respiratory Tract Symptoms*

## Peter W. Hiatt

Recurrent cough and wheeze are common symptoms in children. They raise parental and physician concern that an underlying chronic lung disease is present. When confronted with this situation, the physician needs to distinguish between multiple acute unrelated respiratory infections and a significant chronic pulmonary disease. The history and physical examination are extremely important in making this distinction and cannot be overemphasized.

## DETERMINING DISEASE SEVERITY

Although chronic cough and wheeze commonly are found in children with serious pulmonary problems, they are also manifestations of acute self-limited illness. Therefore, the presence of other signs and symptoms is useful in identifying children with an underlying chronic disorder.

Table 79-1 lists signs and symptoms that suggest chronic pulmonary disease. In general, the closer to birth that symptoms first appear, the greater the chance they are a manifestation of inherited disease or are secondary to a congenital malformation.

Malformations such as tracheoesophageal fistula, laryngeal webs, and vascular rings may present shortly after birth, whereas inherited disease such as cystic fibrosis may present a few months after delivery. Table 79-2 presents inherited lung diseases.

Specific points of importance involve the presence of fever, noisy breathing, snoring, grunting, sputum production, and environmental exposure. If acute infection is present, it usually is accompanied by fever, purulent secretions, and an overall toxic appearance of the child. Fever accompanied by grunting often represents a pneumonic process with frequent pleural involvement. Noisy breathing or snoring during sleep is often associated with enlarged adenoids, nasal polyposis, choanal narrowing, nasal

---

**TABLE 79-1. History and Physical Findings Suggesting Chronic Lung Disease**

**History**
Chronic cough
Recurrent wheeze
Decreased activity
Malabsorption symptoms
Fever for longer than 3 weeks
Weight loss
Recurrent pneumonia
Chronic sputum production
Multiple serious bacterial infections

**Physical**
Poor growth and nutritional status
Trachypnea
Cyanosis
Deviated trachea
Increased anteroposterior diameter of chest
Wheezing, crackles
Clubbing
Neurological delay

TABLE 79-2. Hereditary Diseases of the Lungs

| | |
|---|---|
| Agammaglobulinemia (Bruton's disease) | Sex-linked recessive |
| | Autosomal recessive |
| Ataxia-telangiectasia syndrome | Autosomal recessive |
| Chronic granulomatous disease | Sex-linked recessive |
| | Autosomal recessive |
| Cystic fibrosis | Autosomal recessive |
| Familial dysautonomia | Autosomal recessive |
| Homozygous deficiency of alpha₁-antitryspin | Autosomal recessive |
| Familial interstitial fibrosis | Autosomal dominant |
| Familial pulmonary alevolar microlithiasis | Autosomal recessive |
| Familial spontaneous pneumothorax | Autosomal dominant |
| Hunter syndrome | Sex-linked recessive |
| Hurler's syndrome | Autosomal recessive |
| Kartagener's syndrome | Autosomal recessive |
| Lung in Marfan syndrome | Autosomal dominant |
| Tuberous sclerosis | Autosomal dominant |

Waring WW. [*The history and physical examination*]. In Kendig EL Jr, Chernick V, eds. *Disorders of the respiratory tract in children, ed 4*. Philadelphia: WB Saunders, 1983:59.

foreign body, or Pierre Robin syndrome. Sputum production varies in children. Generally, children younger than 5 years of age are unable to expectorate their sputum but rather swallow their secretions after mobilization from the lung. School-aged children begin to expectorate, and the physician should ask about volume, color, viscosity, and odor of the sputum. Clear secretions often are observed in children with asthma, whereas yellow–green sputum is more consistent with a bacterial process. Malodorous sputum can be observed with bronchiectasis and lung abscess or be confused with postnasal drainage from sinusitis. Environmental exposure, with a special emphasis on passive smoke inhalation, should be investigated in all children with chronic or recurrent pulmonary symptoms. Passive smoke exposure may contribute to chronic airway irritation and increase airway reactivity. Other environmental irritants to consider are woodburning stoves, unvented gas stoves or heaters, pesticides, and airborne allergens (animal dander, molds, pollens).

The physical examination can help confirm the presence of underlying lung disease, but normal findings in the examination do not exclude the possibility of significant abnormalities. The physical examination should begin by evaluating the overall nutritional status of the child. This assessment, together with analysis of the growth curve, gives a good indication of the child's recent health. The physical examination should determine the pattern of respiration, adequacy of gas exchange, and location of disease. First, the rate of respiration should be determined. Respiratory rate decreases with age and is best measured in infants and young children by observation with the child in the mother's arms and clothing removed. Rapid rates are observed with anxiety, fever, exercise, anemia, and metabolic and respiratory disease. Slow rates can be seen with metabolic alkalosis and respiratory acidosis (central nervous system depression). An elevated resting respiratory rate should prompt the physician to look for a significant illness, because tachypnea in a child is a sensitive indicator of lung disease. The ease of respiration can be determined by observation. Dyspnea usually represents obstructive lung disease and is readily observed in a child resting in the mother's lap. Head-bobbing can be seen in a sleeping infant and is a sign of dyspnea. The phenomenon probably is explained by use of accessory muscles during respiration. Flaring of the alae nasi, use

of accessory muscles of respiration, wheezing, grunting, and retractions are all signs of dyspnea and indicators of respiratory disease in a child.

Adequacy of gas exchange is more difficult to assess. An observer's ability to detect hypoxia varies and is difficult to determine, even for experienced physicians. Most observers cannot detect hypoxia until oxygen saturation is 80% or less in a child at sea level. Hypercapnia is often associated with hypoxemia and also is difficult to determine by examination alone; it generally requires arterial blood gas to measure the level of carbon dioxide. To aid the health-care worker in assessing gas exchange, pulse oximeters allow easy noninvasive determination of oxygen saturation in infants and young children. Although this instrument works well for measuring oxygenation, a comparable device is not readily available to easily measure carbon dioxide or acid base balance in a noninvasive outpatient setting.

To establish the location of disease, the head, neck, chest, and extremities should be closely inspected. Allergic shiners under the eyes, nasal mucosal swelling, or a crease across the bridge of the nose are commonly observed in children with allergic disease. Enlarged palatine tonsils are observed in some children with obstructive sleep apnea. By palpating the neck, the position of the trachea is determined. Normally midline, the trachea may be shifted to the right or left if there is volume loss in one lung, severe unilateral gas trapping, or a space-occupying lesion. An increase in the anteroposterior diameter of the chest is consistent with severe obstructive lung disease. Auscultation of the chest can reveal crackles, wheezes, or suppression of breath sounds. Clubbing of the extremities is an uncommon finding in children and rarely occurs in asthmatic individuals. If present, an extensive evaluation should be undertaken to rule out chronic liver, heart, and gastrointestinal disease. Clubbing can be familial. If a pulmonary disorder is suspected, however, diseases such as bronchiectasis, cystic fibrosis, immotile cilia syndrome, and disorders causing interstitial fibrosis should be sought.

If a serious respiratory disorder is suspected after the history and physical examination, evaluation should proceed based on an age-dependent differential diagnosis.

## CHRONIC OR RECURRENT COUGH

A chronic cough is defined as a persistent cough lasting for 3 weeks or longer. Cough clears secretions and foreign materials from the lungs. One coughs when the mucociliary and alveolar macrophage systems are overwhelmed with secretions or foreign material, or are compromised after infection. The cough is a powerful way to clear the airway. Cough is a symptom of both upper and lower airway illness and should direct the physician toward identifying the disease responsible for its presence. Table 79-3 lists characteristics of cough and their potential association with disease.

The cough reflex is composed of three parts: the afferent limb, the central cough center, and the efferent limb. The afferent portion of the cough reflex is made up of sensory fibers located in the ciliated epithelium from the pharynx to the small bronchioles. Concentration of these fibers is greatest in the larynx, at the carina, and at the bifurcations of the airways. When sensory fibers in these areas are stimulated, cough is initiated and trapped foreign material may be expelled. Sensory receptors are responsive to both mechanical and chemical stimuli. Impulses generated from these receptors are transmitted to the brain via the vagus nerve.

An impulse from the lungs is received in the central cough center, then is processed and coordinated into a complex set of muscular contractions that result in a cough. The cough center, located in the upper brainstem and pons, is probably the site of action for pharmacologic cough suppressants. Efferent impulses

## TABLE 79-3. General Characteristics of Chronic Cough and Their Potential Significance

| Characteristic | Significance |
| --- | --- |
| Sputum production | |
| Nonproductive | Asthma, foreign-body aspiration, vascular ring, environmental irritants |
| Productive | |
| Purulent | Bronchietasis, cystic fibrosis |
| Clear or white | Asthma |
| Blood-tinged | Tuberculosis, bronchiectasis, cystic fibrosis, hemosiderosis, nasopharyngeal irritation |
| Paroxysms | Foreign body, pertussis |
| Timing of cough | |
| Nocturnal | Bronchospasm, postnasal discharge |
| Upon awakening | Bronchospasm, cystic fibrosis |
| Absent with sleep | Psychogenic cough |
| Seasonal | Allergies, asthma |
| Associated activity | |
| Feeding | Aspiration |
| Exercise | Bronchospasm, bronchiectasis |

## TABLE 79-4. Differential Diagnosis for Chronic Cough in Children

Infant
Aspiration
  Congenital malformations
  Tracheoesophageal fistula
  Vascular ring
  Neuromuscular weakness or pharyngeal incoordination
  Gastroesophageal reflux
Infections
  Congenital
    Cytomegalovirus
    Rubella
  Acquired
    Respiratory syncytial virus
    Adenoviruses
    Influenza and parainfluenza virus
  Other
    *Bordetella pertussis*
    *Chlamydia trachomatis*
    *Mycobacterium tuberculosis*
Cystic fibrosis
Asthma
Congenital heart disease with congestive failure
Acquired immune deficiency syndrome (AIDS)
Environmental irritants

**Preschool-Aged Child**
Aspiration
  Neuromuscular weakness or pharyngeal incoordination
Infection
  Viral
    Adenoviruses
    Influenza and parainfluenza virus
  Other
    *M tuberculosis*
Cystic fibrosis
Foreign-body aspiration
Chronic sinusitis
Asthma
Congenital heart disease with congestive failure
AIDS
Environmental irritants

**School-Aged Adolescent**
Infections
  Other
    *M tuberculosis*
    Histoplasmosis
    Mycotic infections
    *Mycoplasma pneuomiae*
Cystic fibrosis
Chronic sinusitis
Smoking
Psychogenic cough
Hypersensitivity pneumonitis
Kartagener's syndrome
Sarcoidosis

are initiated and are carried by the phrenic, vagus, and spinal motor nerves to the muscles of the larynx, chest, abdominal wall, diaphragm, and pelvic floor. The cough is started by a brief inspiration of air followed by closure of the glottis. Abdominal, pleural, and alveolar pressures are increased, generating extremely high rates of air flow during expiration when the glottis is opened. Foreign particles are loosened and moved into large airways, which aids their clearance from the respiratory tract during the expiratory phase of the cough.

## DIFFERENTIAL DIAGNOSTIC FEATURES OF COUGH BY AGE

The age of a child is important in developing a differential diagnosis of chronic cough. Table 79-4 lists potential etiologies of cough by age group.

### Infancy

A congenital malformation in an infant should be suspected if symptoms of recurrent cough begin at birth. Tracheoesophageal fistula and laryngeal cleft are congenital anomalies first noted in the neonatal period that lead to aspiration of milk during feedings. Symptoms of chronic aspiration, cough, and pneumonia are seen repeatedly in these children, which brings them quickly to the attention of the physician. Similarly, disorders that affect coordination of swallowing are associated with chronic cough and wheeze because of recurrent aspiration. Swallowing dysfunction found during the neonatal period probably represents early symptoms of neuromuscular disease, severe developmental delay, or an esophageal motility problem. If a neurologic disorder exists, associated findings such as muscle tone alteration, abnormal deep-tendon reflexes, weakness, or delayed social adaptive skills can be found.

    Vascular anomalies, another group of congenital malformations, cause chronic cough and feeding disorders. Vascular rings are an assortment of large blood-vessel abnormalities that partially obstruct the trachea and esophagus. Airway or esophageal obstruction results in respiratory distress, cough, and swallowing dysfunction. Vascular anomalies can become symptomatic shortly after birth or during the first year of life.

For all aforementioned congenital anomalies, a careful barium esophagram with special attention to swallowing can reveal the diagnosis by illustrating esophageal compression, aspiration, or tracheoesophageal fistula.

An interstitial pneumonia and cough in a baby in the first 4 to 6 weeks of life generally represent congenital viral infection or *Chlamydia* pneumonia. Rubella and cytomegalovirus (CMV) both can cause an interstitial pneumonia but differ in their effects on other organ systems. CMV infection acquired postnatally produces pneumonitis and hepatosplenomegaly, but is a self-limited disease in most infants. Lung infection from *Chlamydia trachomatis* is acquired from an infected genitourinary tract in the mother at the time of birth. Three to 4 weeks after delivery, the infant can develop conjunctivitis, interstitial pneumonia, and cough. The cough has a characteristic staccato, harsh sound and is accompanied by tachypnea and rales that appear on examination. The chest roentgenogram shows hyperinflation with diffuse interstitial or patchy infiltrates. Both CMV and *Chlamydia* infections are diagnosed most effectively by culture.

A paroxysmal cough in an infant younger than age 12 months suggests infection with *Bordetella pertussis*. Pneumonia, feeding difficulties, and choking spells from thick, tenacious mucus in the upper airway are present during pertussis infection. If secretions are not cleared well by the infant, airway obstruction and hypoxia occur repeatedly. These coughing episodes are potentially life-threatening to the infant, who may require hospitalization for supportive care. The post-tussive whoop can be absent or appear later during the course of illness. A pertussis-like syndrome also has been reported after adenovirus and influenza virus infection.

In infants, cystic fibrosis usually presents with recurrent respiratory symptoms or failure to thrive. In the lungs, abnormally thick mucus predisposes to infection presenting as cough, wheezing, or fever. In a child with respiratory symptoms, particularly when associated with an abnormal chest radiograph and poor growth, the diagnosis of cystic fibrosis should be considered. Infants also may present with only failure to thrive as a result of malabsorption due to pancreatic insufficiency. With either presentation, a pilocarpine iontophoresis quantitative sweat test should be performed to diagnose cystic fibrosis.

Reactive airway disease, or asthma, in infants is characterized by chronic cough, which is typically dry and hacking. The cough worsens with excitement and when the infant is asleep at night. The cough represents the first symptom of airway reactivity and may become prominent after viral respiratory infections. A single diagnostic test is not available to establish a diagnosis of asthma for infants. An atopic family history often is associated with the disorder but is not conclusive. When reactive airway disease is suspected, a trial of symptomatic bronchodilator therapy is reasonable. If the child responds to treatment, a presumptive diagnosis of asthma can be made. If an inadequate response occurs, additional clinical features should be reviewed to exclude other diagnoses.

As with asthma, infants with bronchiolitis usually present with cough or wheeze. Bronchiolitis is caused most commonly by respiratory syncytial virus (RSV) occurring in yearly epidemics in the late fall and winter months. Prodromal symptoms of fever and rhinorrhea are followed by increasing lower airway symptoms of cough, wheezing, or respiratory distress. Using nasal secretions, an enzyme-linked immunosorbent assay (ELISA) confirms a diagnosis of RSV bronchiolitis. It is usually difficult to distinguish clinically between reactive airway disease and bronchiolitis, particularly during an infant's first episode of cough.

A careful history and laboratory investigation are important in establishing the correct diagnosis.

## Preschool-Aged Children

Asthma is the most common disease found in preschool-aged children with chronic cough. It is the most frequently occurring respiratory disorder in childhood, estimated to occur in 5% of the general population. The cough in asthma occurs from both airway irritation and excessive mucus production. In asthma, cough may be triggered by a variety of environmental stimuli, but in young children, most asthma episodes are precipitated by respiratory infections.

Foreign-body aspiration is a common cause of chronic cough in toddlers and preschool-aged children, and should be considered even if a history of choking is not obtained. Peanuts and small plastic objects are common materials seen in foreign-body aspiration. The cough that follows the aspiration event is sudden, violent, and sometimes followed by cyanosis. Conversely, if the object is small and does not obstruct the airway, minimal cough occurs. The cough following aspiration may resolve after 1 or 2 days, only to recur after the buildup of secretions, movement of the foreign body, or development of atelectasis. This period between the foreign-body aspiration and recurrence of cough may be days, weeks, or months. A chest radiograph helps in the diagnosis if a radiopaque object is found or hyperinflation is noted. A normal chest radiograph, however, does not rule out foreign-body aspiration. Fluoroscopy of the chest is a more sensitive, noninvasive method of assessing the dynamics of breathing in a child suspected of foreign-body aspiration; it should be used routinely. Subtle air trapping in a particular lobe of the lung and mediastinal shift are appreciated during this procedure. If foreign-body aspiration is suspected, a rigid bronchoscopy under general anesthesia is indicated for evaluation and removal.

No widely accepted definition of chronic bronchitis in childhood is available. In adults, chronic bronchitis is defined as a daily cough present for 3 months in a year for 2 consecutive years. In pediatrics there is such a strong overlap between airway reactivity with excessive mucus production and bronchitis that the two are difficult to separate. When there is an apparent history of chronic bronchitis, other etiologies for this symptom complex should be entertained. Asthma, cystic fibrosis, bronchiectasis, foreign-body aspiration, infection, and immunodeficiency all should be considered as possible underlying etiologies.

Chronic sinusitis is reported to cause a long-standing cough. Nasal discharge and postnasal drip precipitate cough throughout the day and shortly after lying down at night. In the allergic child, one may see only clear secretions, yet frank mucopus may be observed in other children. Drainage of secretions from the nose to the posterior pharynx results in a sensation of dryness or burning at the back of the nose and an unpleasant taste in the mouth. Morning headaches can be seen in older children, and upset stomachs and vomiting are observed in the younger age group.

## School-Aged Children

Airway reactivity due to asthma is the principal cause of chronic cough in the school-aged child. As the child experiences fewer viral infections with increasing age, other environmental triggers become more important causes of asthma episodes.

An insidious cough that worsens over 2 weeks and is accompanied by headache, malaise, fever, and sore throat generally is observed with infection caused by *Mycoplasma pneumoniae*. The peak incidence for this illness is between 10 and 15 years of age. During epidemics, however, older age groups commonly are infected. There are no specific clinical or laboratory tests that establish a definitive diagnosis of *M pneumoniae* infection early in the course of illness. Clinically, the occurrence of pneumonia in an adolescent and findings of cold hemagglutinins in a titer of 1:64 or greater support the diagnosis. Isolation of the organism by culture or demonstration of specific antibodies help confirm the diagnosis.

A "honking" or "seal-like" cough in an adolescent may represent a psychogenic or habit cough. This usually occurs after a respiratory illness and persists when other clinical symptoms of disease resolve. The cough worsens when the child is under stress or is the focus of attention, yet is absent at night after the child is asleep. Usually, sputum production is absent and there is a paucity of clinical findings on examination. These children are difficult to treat; the intervention of a psychologist or psychiatrist may help with management of the child's cough. Although rare, a similar barking cough can be seen in children with Gilles de la Tourette's syndrome, but verbal or motor tics often accompany the cough. Treatment with haloperidol reportedly decreases the severity and frequency of cough in Tourette's syndrome.

## DIFFERENTIAL DIAGNOSTIC FEATURES OF WHEEZING BY AGE

A wheeze is a high-pitched musical sound produced by rapid vibration of a large bronchial wall. It indicates airflow obstruction from isolated or multiple sites of airway narrowing. High rates of air movement produce bronchial wall vibration, which is achieved only in large airways. Wheeze occurs when expiratory effort exceeds the pressure necessary to achieve maximal flow. Pulmonary disorders that obstruct the airway, whether due to

inflammation, mucosal edema, or bronchospasm, reduce the pleural pressure required to reach maximum flow limitation. Any greater expiratory effort produces a wheeze and fails to improve flow in the obstructed airway. Table 79-5 lists potential etiologies of wheezing by different age groups.

### Infancy

Asthma is the most common disease associated with wheezing in infants and other age groups. Asthma is defined by the American Thoracic Society as increased responsiveness of the trachea and bronchi to various stimuli, resulting in widespread narrowing of the airways that changes in severity either spontaneously or as a result of therapy. Wheezing can be associated with environmental, allergic, and respiratory virus stimuli. In infants, respiratory viral infection is the major trigger of airway reactivity. Environmental irritants such as passive smoking may precipitate wheezing and should be controlled when possible. The role of allergen-induced asthma is unclear in this age group and is difficult both to diagnose and to control.

Bronchiolitis is a common cause of wheezing in infants younger than 12 months of age. It is caused most commonly by respiratory syncytial virus (RSV), but has been reported after infection with adenovirus, influenza, and parainfluenza virus. After 3 days of cold-like symptoms, infants with RSV develop increasing respiratory distress and wheezing. Pathologic specimens from infants who have died from RSV infection demonstrate significant small airway obstruction from submucosal edema, mucus plugging, and peribronchial inflammation. Both partial and complete airway obstruction in these infants lead to air trapping, decreased pulmonary compliance, and increased work of breathing. Airway obstruction allows ventilation and perfusion mismatch to occur,

| TABLE 79-5. Differential Diagnosis for Wheezing in Children | | |
|---|---|---|
| **Infant** | **Toddler/Preschool-Aged Child** | **School-Aged Adolescent** |
| Congenital malformation | Aspiration (less common) | Infection |
|   Tracheobronchial anomalies | Infection |   Viral |
|   Lung cyst |   Viral |     Adenoviruses |
|   Vascular ring |     Adenoviruses |     Influenza |
|   Mediastinal lesions |     Parainfluenza, influenza viruses |   Other |
| Aspiration |   Other |     Tuberculosis |
|   Pharyngeal incoordination |     Tuberculosis |     Histoplasmosis |
|   Gastroesophageal reflux |     Histoplasmosis |     Mycotic infections |
|   Tracheoesophageal fistula |     Mycotic infections | Tumor |
|   Laryngotracheoesophageal cleft |   Parasitic |   Leukemia |
| Infections |     Visceral larva migrans |   Lymphoma |
|   Viral | Tumor |   Lymphosarcoma |
|     Respiratory syncytial virus |   Leukemia | Asthma |
|     Adenoviruses |   Lymphoma | Cystic fibrosis |
|     Parainfluenza, influenza viruses | Foreign-body aspiration | Kartagener's syndrome |
|   Other | Asthma | Hypersensitivity pneumonitis |
|     Tuberculosis | Congenital heart disease with left-to-right shunt | |
|     Histoplasmosis | Cystic fibrosis | |
|     Mycotic infections | Pulmonary hemosiderosis | |
| Asthma | AIDS | |
| Congenital heart disease with large left-to-right shunt | | |
| Bronchopulmonary dysplasia | | |
| Cystic fibrosis | | |
| AIDS | | |

with subsequent hypoxia. Bronchiolitis generally resolves with supportive therapy over 4 to 5 days, but a high incidence of future airway reactivity is reported in children who require hospitalization.

In infants, recurrent aspiration of food (primarily milk) due to poor swallowing coordination can result in wheezing. Choking or cough is reported during feedings, and chest radiographs demonstrate streaky infiltrates, most often in the right upper lobe or right lower lobe. Gastroesophageal reflux with aspiration has a similar radiographic appearance, but the history generally is one of frequent vomiting during or shortly after feedings. Aspiration of formula due to tracheoesophageal fistula is associated with wheezing in infancy, but these episodes characteristically are accompanied by sudden cough and cyanosis. A barium esophagram often reveals the mechanical or structural abnormality leading to aspiration events.

Infants with recurrent wheezing who do not respond well to initial bronchodilator medication should be considered for sweat testing because these symptoms may be the early manifestations of cystic fibrosis.

Vascular anomalies typically cause wheezing during the first weeks of life. Both inspiratory and expiratory wheezing can be heard on auscultation, depending on the severity of airway compression. A pulmonary sling results when the anomalous left pulmonary artery compresses the right main stem bronchus, causing obstruction and hyperinflation of the right lung. A double aortic arch can cause wheezing and swallowing difficulties by compressing the trachea bilaterally and the esophagus posteriorly. A barium swallow demonstrates both bilateral and posterior indentation of the esophagus. A right aortic arch and a ligamentum ductus produces clinical symptoms similar to those of a double arch; on plain chest radiograph, however, the trachea tends to be deviated to the right and an esophagram demonstrates greater indentation on the right side of the esophagus than on the left. Other radiographic findings are similar to those observed with the double aortic arch.

Other infants who have wheezing in the first month of life are those with congenital heart disease and bronchopulmonary dysplasia. Airway compression due to an enlarged heart and pulmonary congestion due to large left-to-right shunts are responsible for the wheeze observed in infants with cardiac defects. Bronchospasm and fibrosis lead to wheezing in babies with bronchopulmonary dysplasia.

## Preschool-Aged Children

Children with cystic fibrosis, bronchopulmonary dysplasia, and congenital heart disease wheeze, but generally become symptomatic in the first 12 months of life. Wheeze associated with aspiration, whether from swallowing dysfunction or gastroesophageal reflux, is less common in preschool-aged children unless a degenerative or neuromuscular disorder is present. A child presenting with an acute onset of wheezing should be suspected of having a foreign-body aspiration.

Disease processes that cause enlargement of the hilar and me-

diastinal lymph nodes can present symptomatically with wheezing by compression of a major bronchus. Enlarged lymph nodes on a chest radiograph should suggest an infectious disease or tumor. Tuberculosis, histoplasmosis, and other mycotic diseases are common infectious agents responsible for lymph node enlargement. Generally, hilar adenopathy from tuberculosis occurs with progressive disease and is associated with symptoms of fever, anorexia, and poor weight gain. A tuberculin skin test, with appropriate controls, aids in the diagnosis of an active tuberculosis infection. Histoplasmosis usually is either a mild self-limited illness or an asymptomatic infection. A more severe illness can occur with malaise, weight loss, hepatosplenomegaly, and hilar adenopathy. Because of the high incidence of positive skin-test reactions in endemic areas, complement-fixation titers and geldiffusion studies are more helpful in making the diagnosis of histoplasmosis disease.

Hilar and mediastinal lymph node enlargement can represent primary or secondary tumor in a child. Leukemia, lymphoma, and lymphosarcoma all can cause hilar nodal enlargement. Any child with hilar lymphadenopathy should receive a careful examination for other signs of malignancy, such as anemia, splenomegaly, bone pain, and fever. A diagnosis may be established in children with mediastinal tumor by the examination of peripheral blood smears, lymph node biopsy, or bone marrow examination. Visceral larva migrans is a clinical syndrome seen in young children with a history of pica, dirt eating, and exposure to dogs. The disease is produced by *Toxocara canis* and occurs following ingestion of ova from contaminated soil. The larvae make their way from the intestine to the lung, where they induce eosinophilic granulomas. Clinically, children have wheezing, bronchitis, hepatomegaly, and eosinophilia on peripheral blood smear. A diagnosis is made from the history, physical findings, and an elevated titer to *Toxocara* antigen (by means of ELISA).

## School-Aged Children

Most school-aged children who wheeze have asthma. Congenital malformations almost always have their first onset of symptoms early in life. Children with neuromuscular disease become weaker with age, losing their ability to protect their airway from secretions. Weakness then predisposes them to aspiration and pneumonia. Immotile cilia syndrome, cystic fibrosis, and congenital heart disease generally are diagnosed at an earlier age.

## Selected Readings

American Thoracic Society, Committee on Diagnostic Standards for Tuberculous Respiratory Diseases. Definitions and classification of chronic bronchitis, asthma, and pulmonary emphysema. Am Rev Respir Dis 1962;85:762.

Eigen H. The clinical evaluation of chronic cough. Pediatr Clin North Am 1982;29:67.

Kamei RK. Chronic cough in children. Pediatr Clin North Am 1991;38(3):593.

Kendig EL Jr, Chernick V, eds. Disorders of the respiratory tract in children, ed 4. Philadelphia: WB Saunders, 1983:275, 283, 835.

Levison H, Tabachnik E, Newth CJL. Wheezing in infancy, croup and epiglottitis. Curr Probl Pediatr 1982;12(3):7.

Parks DP, Ahrens, RC, Hymphries CT, Weinberger MM. Chronic cough in childhood: approach to diagnosis and treatment. J Pediatr 1989;15:856.

# The Cardiovascular System

*Principles and Practice of Pediatrics, Second Edition.*
edited by Frank A. Oski et al. J. B. Lippincott Company, Philadelphia © 1994.

## CHAPTER 80
## Cardiovascular Embryology

### Edward V. Colvin

## STEPS LEADING TO THE FORMATION OF THE HEART TUBE

The cardiogenic area can be seen first on day 15 within the mesoderm, anterior to the buccopharyngeal membrane (prochordal plate). Cells from this area, if moved to a different portion of the embryo, continue to develop to have myofibrils and rhythmic contractions.

The embryo undergoes two major conformational changes. The rapid growth of the brain-vesicle area of the neural tube results in an anterior folding of the cardiogenic area (Fig 80-1). Simultaneously, there is rapid growth of the somite areas, which causes ventral folding of the lateral portions of the embryo. In the process of this folding, the endodermal plate, which has been a flattened structure, is folded to become a tube, giving rise to the embryonic foregut and hindgut. As a part of this process, portions of mesoderm from opposite sides of the embryo are brought together in the midline.

At the beginning of the third week, blood islands form in the visceral mesoderm on the wall of the yolk sac. These clusters of cells exhibit a breakdown of cell-to-cell contact, forming cystic areas. The cells within the cystic areas become rounded, forming blood-forming elements, and the cells on the periphery become flattened, giving rise to the endothelium of the blood islands. These islands approach each other by sprouting endothelial cells, and they fuse to form blood vessels.

In the cardiogenic area, cords and clusters of angioblastic cells in the visceral mesoderm form two strands, one lying on each side of the foregut. When these clefted areas become confluent, forming a lumen, they are called endocardial tubes. These become continuous cephalically with the first arterial arches and caudally with the veins entering the heart. These paired structures have two cellular layers—an inner layer, the endocardium, and an outer layer, the epimyocardium—separated by a layer of hypo-

cellular material, the "cardiac jelly." The paired endocardial tubes fuse to form a single primitive heart tube.

Figure 80-2 shows the primitive heart tube. At the caudal end of the heart tube, the paired sinus venosus, which are embedded in the mesenchyme of the septum transversum, are separated from the common atrium by the sinoatrial groove. The common atrium is separated from the succeeding segment by the atrioventricular canal. The next segment is called the primitive ventricle or, more descriptively, inlet segment. It gives rise to the apical portion of the left ventricle and probably to the inlet portions of both ventricles. The succeeding segment is called the bulbus cordis, the conus, and, more descriptively, the outlet segment. This segment gives rise to the outlet portion of both ventricles and to the apical portion of the right ventricle.

The junction between the inlet segment and the outlet segment has been called the bulboventricular foramen, the primary interventricular foramen, and, most recently, the primary foramen. The external groove corresponding to the site of this junction has been referred to as the bulboventricular groove, the interventricular groove, and, now, the primary groove.

The final segment, the truncus arteriosus, initially is imbedded

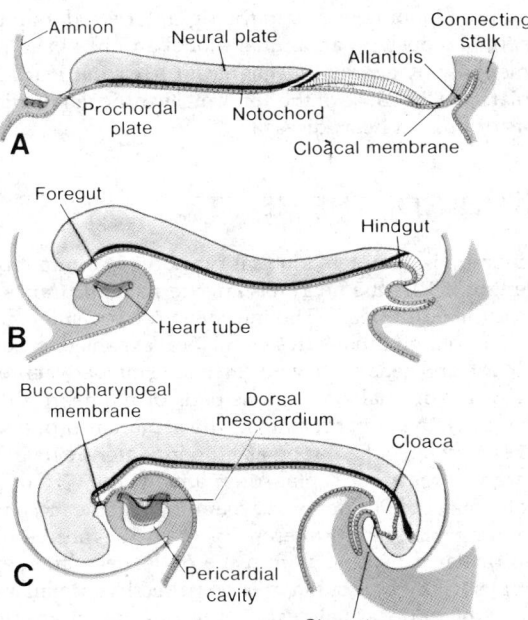

**Figure 80-1.** Cranial caudal midline sections showing anterior rotation of the cardiogenic plate resulting from rapid growth of brain vesicles. (**A**) 18 days, (**B**) 21 days, (**C**) 22 days. (Langman J. Medical embryology, ed 4. Baltimore: Williams & Wilkins, 1981.)

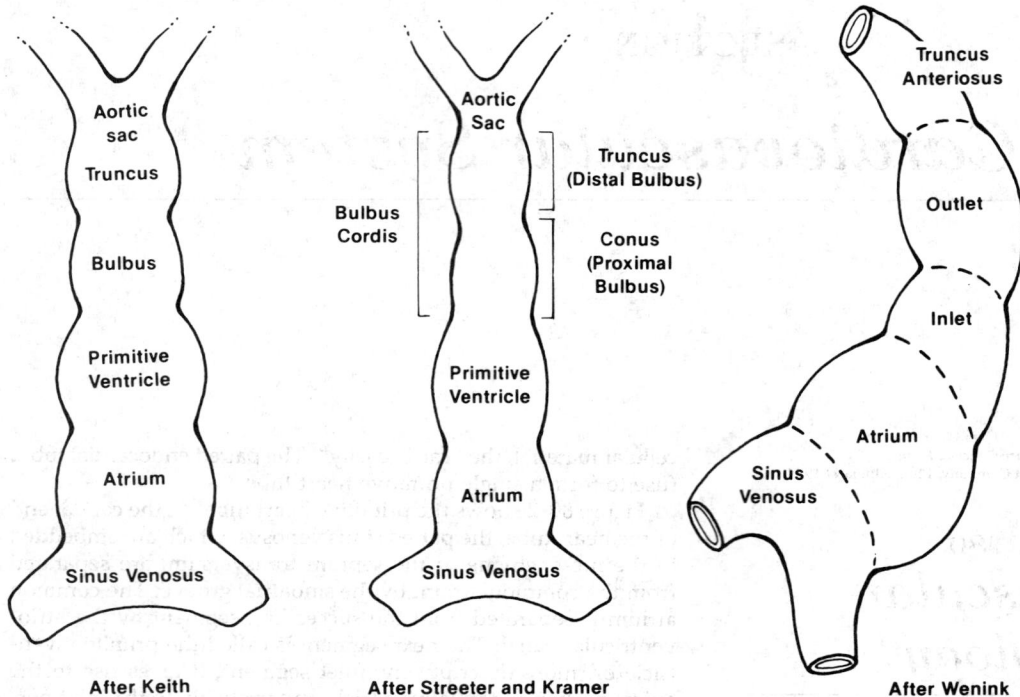

After Keith

After Streeter and Kramer

After Wenink

Figure 80-2. Diagram of the straight primary heart tube as perceived by several different authors. (Anderson RH, Wilkinson JL, Becker AE. The bulbus cordis—a misunderstood region of the developing human heart; its significance to the classifications of congenital cardiac malformations. In: Birth defects. Original articles series 1978;XIV(7): 1; and Wenink ACG. Embryology of the heart. In: Anderson RH, McCartney FJ, Shinebourne EA, Tynan M, eds. Paediatric cardiology. Edinburgh: Churchill Livingstone, 1987.)

in the branchial mesenchyme anterior to the foregut. After looping, this segment elongates and becomes an intrapericardial structure. It becomes angular with respect to the outlet segment. The arterial valves later develop at the site of angulation.

## CARDIAC LOOPING

The primitive heart tube, which is initially quite short and straight, undergoes remarkable growth. The dorsal mesocardium ruptures, freeing the midportion of the primitive heart tube. The tube bends, first ventrally, then with the convexity of a curve to the right. While normal looping occurs to the right, leftward looping does occur spontaneously in an animal model and has been induced experimentally by external mechanical forces. Leftward looping is postulated as the cause of the abnormal ventricular relationships in forms of human heart disease.

## SEPTATION OF THE HEART

When looping is completed in embryos of 5 to 6 mm crown-to-rump length (CRL), the heart has an external appearance similar to that of the adult heart. The internal structure still consists of a single convoluted tube with several local expansions. Septation of the heart proceeds by several mechanisms between days 26 and 37. At the arterial and venous ends of the heart, the extra-cardiac mesenchyme participate in the septation process. These structures may be looked upon as growing into the heart to fuse with purely intracardiac septa. Alternatively, the venous and arterial poles may be considered as expanding into the mesenchyme, incorporating part of the mesenchyme in the process. At the atrioventricular canal and within the outlet segment, septation is accomplished by apposition of large paired hypocellular masses of tissue—the endocardial cushions or ridges that arise only in these areas. Septation also can proceed passively by apposition of the walls of two rapidly expanding chambers. This mechanism appears to account for development of a portion of the interventricular septum—the primary septum—which arises beneath the

primary groove. Finally, the portion of the ventricular septum that arises within the inlet segment appears to arise by coalescence of trabeculae. Although different mechanisms are involved in the septation of the different portions of the heart, the resulting system of septae can be thought of as a continuous system of ridges extending from sinus venosus to truncus arteriosus (Fig 80-3).

## Sinus Venosus and Atria

When the paired heart tubes fuse to form a single endothelial tube, the sinus venosus remain paired. The venous system is symmetrical at this point, and each sinus receives medially a

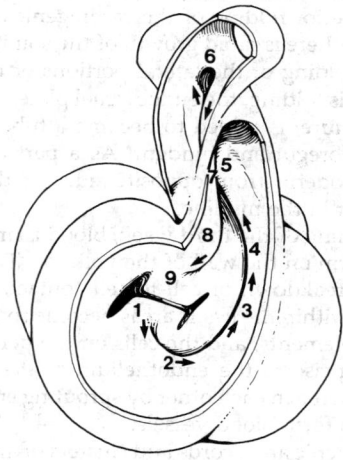

Figure 80-3. Continuity of various components leading to septation. Developmental stages are included; atrial septa are not. 1, Posterior AV cushion; 2, inlet septum; 3, primary septum; 4, left proximal outlet septum; 5, left distal outlet septum; 6, aorticopulmonary septum; 7, right distal outlet septum; 8, right proximal outlet septum; 9, anterior AV cushion. (Steding G, Seidl W. Contribution to the development of the heart. Part I: normal development. Thorac Cardiovasc Surg 1980;28: 386.)

vitelline vein and laterally a common cardinal and an umbilical vein. The paired sinuses eventually fuse to form a transverse sinus with right and left sinus horns. As patterns of venous return change, most venous flow comes to enter the right sinus horn, causing it to become more prominent (Fig 80-4). The entrance of the sinus is shifted to enter the right portion of the atrial mass. This entrance becomes slitlike, with the orifice guarded by invaginations of sinus tissue, which are the right and left venous valves. These valves are initially large relative to the size of the atrium and probably do function as valves. The right sinus venosus is progressively incorporated into the right atrium, and the venous valves become less prominent. The superior portion of the right valve disappears, while the inferior portion persists as the valve of the inferior vena cava (eustachian valve) and the valve of the coronary sinus (thebesian valve). The smooth posterior part of the mature right atrium represents sinus venosus, which is incorporated into the atrium. On the left side, the common pulmonary vein grows out and joins with the pulmonary venous plexus. The common pulmonary vein is later incorporated into the left atrium, giving origin to its smooth posterior portion.

The presence of the distal heart tube creates an external indentation in the roof of the atrium. This corresponds to the internal structure called the septum primum. The inferior border of the septum primum forms an arc concave toward the atrioventricular orifice. The limbs of this arc become continuous with the developing endocardial cushions of the atrioventricular canal. The endocardial cushions fuse and divide the atrioventricular canal into right and left portions, and the septum primum is closed. Just before this closure, a second orifice, the ostium secundum, begins to appear in the posterior portion of the septum primum. This second orifice allows continued flow into the left atrium. As this ostium secundum forms, a second septum also begins to form along the roof of the atrium lying to the right of the septum primum (Fig 80-5). The inferior rim of this septum is an arc, with dorsal and ventral limbs extending more toward the orifice of the inferior cava than toward the atrioventricular orifice. The arc never closes, but forms an oval rim, the limbus of the foramen ovale.

## Atrioventricular Canal

Septation of the atrioventricular canal begins with the appearance of superior and inferior masses of hypocellular tissue. These endocardial cushions enlarge and become impressive structures, which probably do function as valves. Smaller lateral masses—the right and left lateral atrioventricular cushions—appear. In embryos of 10 to 11 mm CRL, the superior and inferior cushions have fused, dividing the atrioventricular canal into right and left orifices.

## Primary and Inlet Septa

In the embryo of about 20 somites, outpocketings of the endocardium appear proximal and distal to the primary foramen in the inlet and outlet segments. These segments undergo progressive enlargement by centrifugal growth. Growth of the inlet and outlet segments takes place much faster than enlargement of the primary foramen. Thus the anteromedial walls of the two segments appose and fuse, giving rise to a portion of the forming interventricular septum—the primary septum. This is the only portion of the septal formation that is intersegmental. Most accounts describe this structure as extending posteriorly to meet with the inferior endocardial cushion. If this was so, the atrioventricular canal would have to shift far to the right of its original position so the right portion of the canal actually enters the outlet segment.

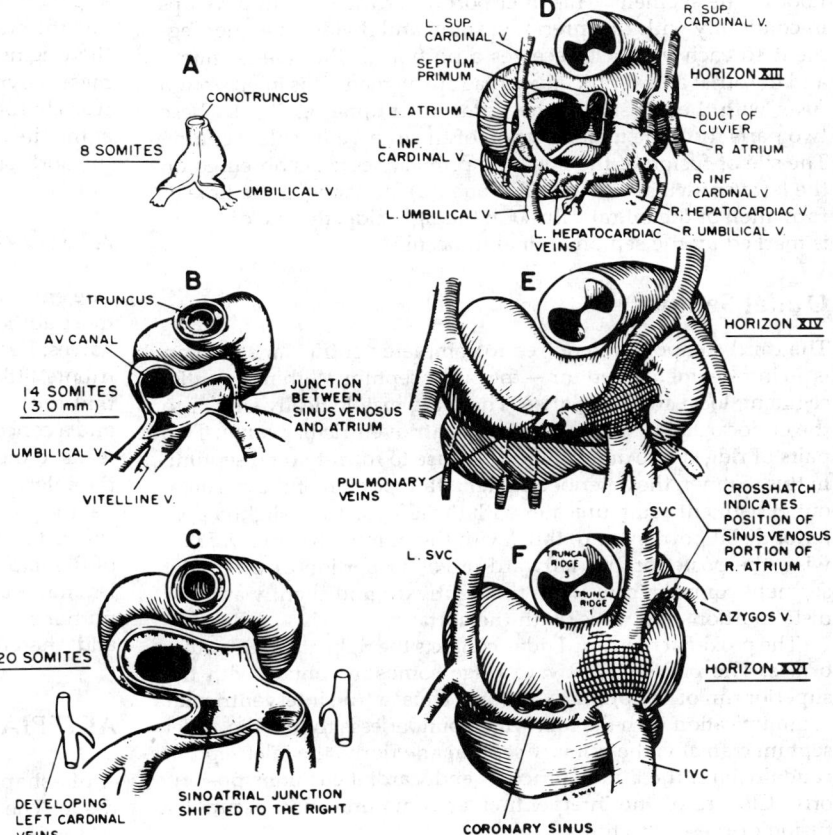

**Figure 80-4.** Dorsal view of changes in the sinus venosus and venous tributaries. (Goor DA, Lillehei CW. Congenital malformations of the heart. New York: Grune & Stratton, 1975.)

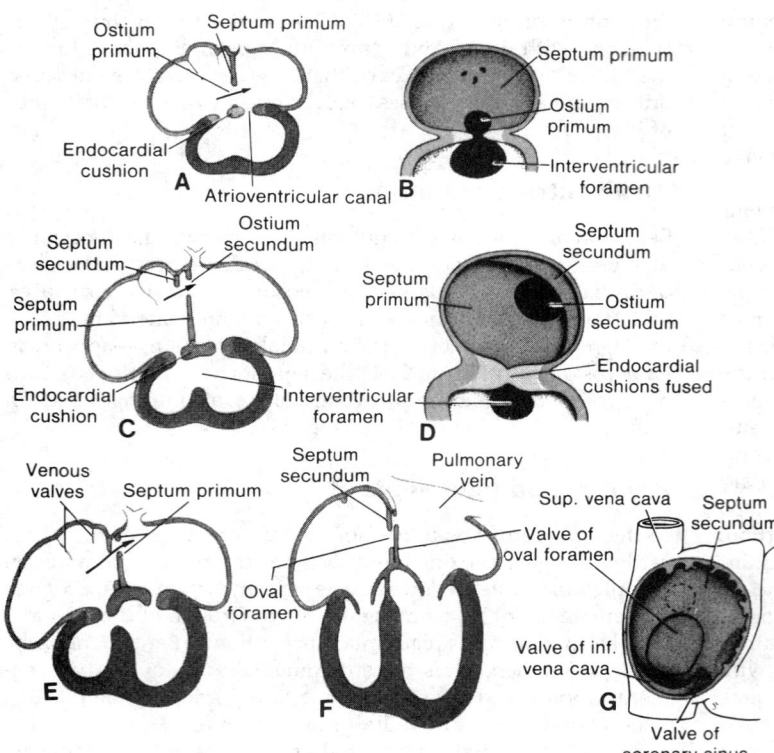

**Figure 80-5.**   Atrial septa at various stages of development. (**A**) At 6 mm (approximately 30 days), (**B**) 6 mm seen from right, (**C**) 9 mm (approximately 33 days), (**D**) 9 mm seen from right, (**E**) 14 mm (approximately 37 days), (**F**) newborn, (**G**) atrial septum seen from right at newborn stage. (Langman J. Medical embryology. Baltimore: Williams & Wilkins, 1981.)

In the description of Wenink, the primary septum is confined to the anterior and apical portion of the two segments and does not extend posteriorly to the inferior endocardial cushion. Instead, a second portion of the forming interventricular septum appears within the inlet segment by a coalescence of trabeculae on the floor of the segment. This inlet portion of the septum develops in continuity with the inferior cushion and divides the inlet segment so each ventricle receives a portion of the inlet segment and the atrial and ventricular septae are aligned. This inlet septum fuses with the left side of the primary septum (Fig 80-6). These two parts form the major portion of the interventricular septum. The site of fusion of the inlet and primary septae is obscured on the left ventricular side by subsequent remodeling at the time of formation of the mitral valve. On the right side, the site of fusion is marked by the septomarginal trabecula.

## Outlet Septum

The third component required to complete ventricular septation is an intrasegmental septum—the outlet septum. Within the outlet segment, local swellings arise. These are histologically similar to the endocardial cushions seen in the atrioventricular canal. Two pairs of ridges, proximal and distal, fuse to form a spiral septum. In this manner, the anterior and rightward portion of the proximal outlet segment communicates with the leftward and slightly posterior distal portion, and, thus, with the pulmonary artery. Likewise, the posterior and leftward proximal portion of the outlet segment communicates with the rightward and slightly anterior distal portion, and, thus, with the aorta.

The proximal rightward ridge contacts the right atrioventricular orifice. The proximal leftward ridge comes in contact with the superior rim of the primary septum. Thus, a true interventricular communication with the following boundaries is found: the outlet septum cranially, the primary septum anteriorly, the inlet septum caudally, and the atrioventricular endocardial cushions posteriorly. Closure of the interventricular communication occurs by fusion of these structures.

## Aortopulmonary Septum

There is disagreement about where the truncus arteriosus begins and ends. It seems practical to define the site of the arterial valves as the distal end of the outlet and to consider the truncus arteriosus as part of the arterial system. The truncus expands asymmetrically into the branchial mesenchyme, with less expansion seen between the origins of the fourth and sixth bronchial arch arteries. The mesenchyme between these arches seems to, and may, grow inward to form the aortopulmonary septum. The outlet ridges fuse at the site of arterial valve formation before complete fusion with the aortopulmonary septum takes place.

## ATRIOVENTRICULAR VALVES

The endocardial cushions have an early valvelike function, and most authors have described the cushions as precursors of the valves. Recently, the endocardial cushions have been felt to contribute little to the mature valve leaflets. Observations confirm that the valves are formed by an invagination of sulcus tissue and a concomitant undermining of ventricular myocardium. This leads to the formation of a three-layered flap hanging down into the inlet. The outer layers of the flap consist of atrial and inlet ventricular myocardium. The middle layer is formed by ingrowing sulcus tissue. Endocardial cushion tissue is confined to the apex of the flap and the atrial aspect. The inlet myocardium becomes less trabeculated as the undermining process proceeds. The apical portions of the two ventricles are not involved in this process, and, therefore, retain their characteristic trabecular patterns.

## ARTERIAL VALVES

An H-shaped outflow channel is formed by mounds of cushion tissue. The two large mounds of tissue correspond to the upper ends of the outlet ridges. The two smaller mounds are called the

**Figure 80-6.** Development of ventricular septal components—right lateral views. (**A**) Before septation. Arrows indicate left and right bloodstreams, which have to pass both the atrioventricular (av) and the primary (*open arrows*) junction; pf, primary foramen. (**B**) Growth of inlet and outlet segments leads to expansion of the intervening primary fold, resulting in the primary septum (ps). At the same time, inlet trabeculations coalesce to form a muscular ridge (r) on the posterior wall of the inlet. (**C**) Posterior ridge grows out to form the inlet septum (is), which fuses with the primary septum. The posterior rim of the latter remains visible as trabecula septomarginalis (ts). (**D**) Endocardial ridges in the distal part of the outlet fuse to form the outlet septum (os). A small interventricular communication (*arrow*) is still present. The left part of the primary fold (stippled line) is in the left ventricle, hidden by the outlet septum. (**E**) As in (**D**), with addition of fused atrioventricular endocardial cushions (ec), which are present in previous stages (although not depicted). Boundaries of interventricular communication are outlet septum (os), primary septum (ps), inlet septum (is), and atrioventricular endocardial cushion (ec). This communication has nothing to do with the primary foramen. Arrows indicate bloodstreams from the right atrium (ra) to the pulmonary trunk (pt) (through right part of primary foramen) and from the left atrium (la) to the aorta (ao) (through left part of primary foramen). (Wenink ACG. Embryology of the heart. In: Anderson RH, McCartney FJ, Shinebourne EA, Tynan M, eds. Paediatric cardiology. Edinburgh: Churchill Livingstone, 1987.)

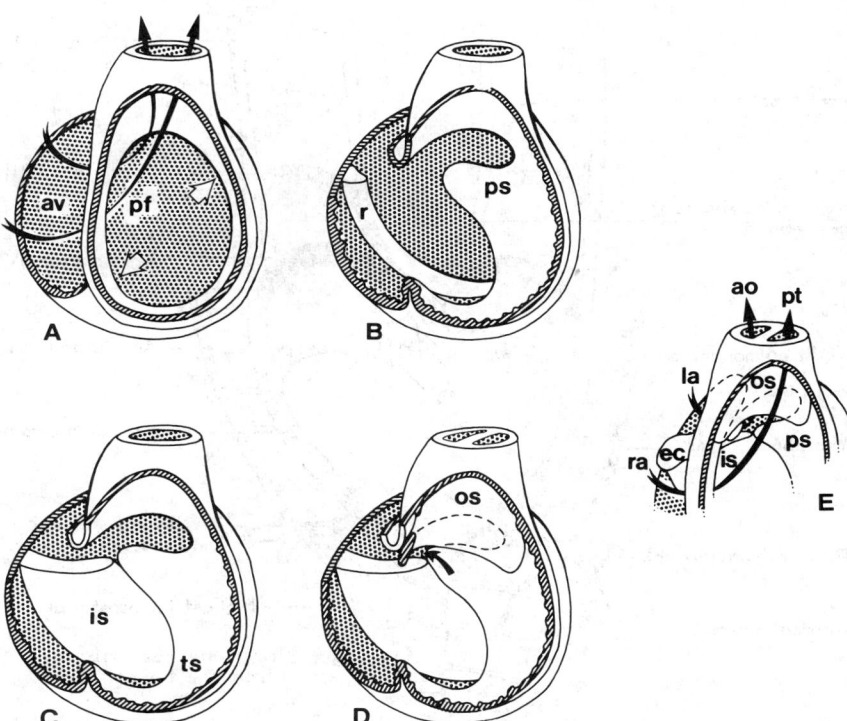

intercalated valve swellings. Growth of the larger ridges divides the aortic and pulmonary outflow tracts. The downstream ends of the intimal mounds acquire a valvelike appearance. Each of the larger cushions divides to give rise to two cusps of each valve; the intercalated valve swelling gives rise to the third (Fig 80-7).

## AORTIC ARCH SYSTEM

The characteristic embryonic segments of the branchial arterial system are the aortic sac, the arterial arches, and the paired dorsal

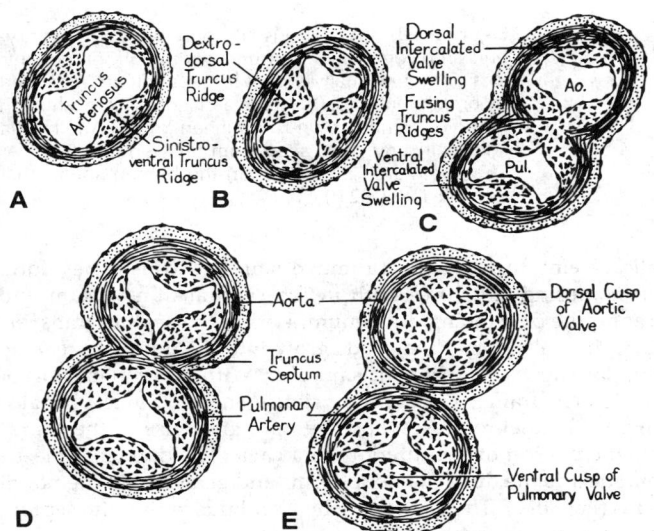

**Figure 80-7.** Origin of semilunar valve primordia. (Kramer TC. The partitioning of the truncus and conus and the formation of the membranous portion of the interventricular septum in the human heart. Am J Anat 1942;71:343.)

aortas. When the heart becomes a tube, the distal end bifurcates into two mesothelial channels—the right and left first arterial arches. These pass on either side of the foregut to become continuous with a pair of dorsal aortas. The aortic sac is the segment that is just upstream from the arterial arches and just downstream from the truncus. The arterial arches are embedded in the branchial arches.

The stream of blood is gradually shifted caudalward in the developing system of arches. The first and second arch arteries, which initially carry the full flow from the heart, regress. Remnants of the first pair of arteries participate in the formation of the maxillary artery from the mandibular artery, and possibly contribute to the external carotid. The second arch arteries participate in formation of stapedial and hyoid arteries. The third pair of arch arteries participate in formation of the common carotids and the proximal portions of the internal carotid arteries. The distal portions of the common carotids are derived from the cranial portions of the paired dorsal aortas.

The right and left fourth arterial arches develop differently. The caudal portion of the right dorsal aorta disappears, but the fourth arch artery persists in continuity with the seventh intersegmental artery to form the distal portion of the right subclavian artery. On the left, the fourth arch gives rise to the portion of the definitive aortic arch between the takeoff of the left common carotid and the entrance of the ductus arteriosus. The fifth arterial arch is not a precursor of normal adult structures in humans.

The sixth or pulmonary arches appear in the middle of the fourth week. They are represented by dorsal and ventral portions, which join each other at an angle. The postbranchial pulmonary arteries join the arches at the angle between the dorsal and ventral portions. The ventral portions of these arches gradually merge, and along with the aortic sac give rise to the main pulmonary artery. The right ventral portion persists as the proximal portion of the right pulmonary artery, while the right dorsal sixth arch is interrupted. The left ventral portion is felt to be largely resorbed, contributing little, if at all, to the left definitive pulmonary artery. The left dorsal portion gives rise to the definitive ductus arteriosus (Fig 80-8).

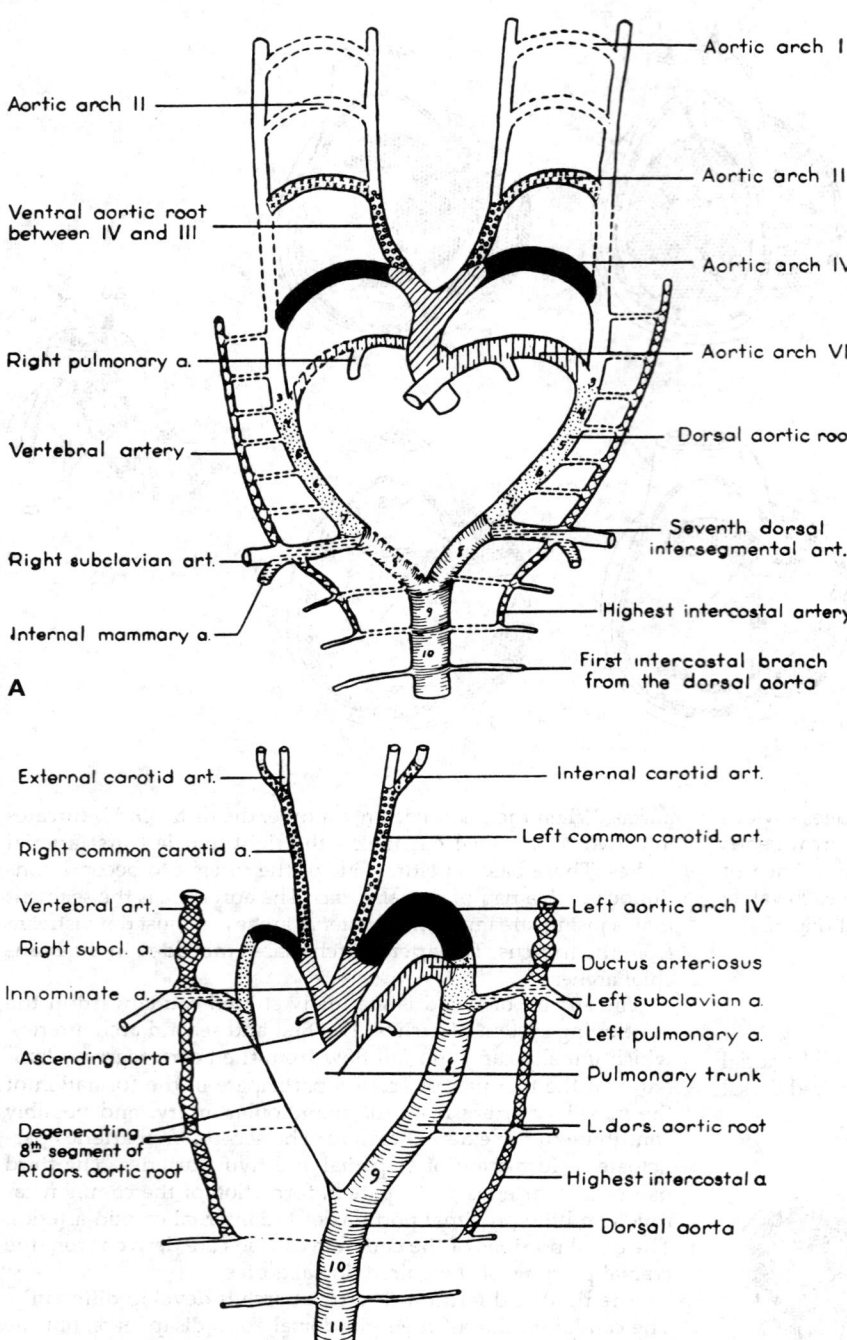

**Figure 80-8.** (A) Various components of the embryonic arch complex in the human embryo. Components that do not normally persist in the adult are indicated by broken outlines. (B) Aortic arch complex in a human embryo 15 mm crown-rump in length. (C) Adult aorta and main branches, seen from left ventral. (Barry A. The aortic arch derivatives in the human adult. Anat Rec 1951;111:221.)

## SYSTEMIC VEINS

Complex changes in the embryonic venous drainage occur with the appearance of whole new systems of veins and the disappearance of parts of previous systems in response to changing needs of the developing embryo. The variability in these processes accounts for the great variability seen in mature venous structures. Two primarily extraembryonic systems, vitelline and umbilical, contribute to the mature venous system. The intraembryonic cardinal veins form the main venous drainage system of the embryo.

## Vitelline Veins

The vitelline veins arise in the yolk-sac wall and pass to the septum transversum where they join with the developing um-

bilical veins to form the primitive sinus venosus. They form anastomosing structures both in the septum transversum and around the developing duodenum. Within the septum transversum, the developing liver buds grow into this plexus, breaking it up into developing hepatic sinusoids. With subsequent shift of the venous drainage to the right sinus venosus, the left hepatocardiac channel regresses, and the right gives rise to the suprahepatic portion of the inferior vena cava. The duodenal plexus remodels as the duodenal loop forms and gives rise to the portal veins (Fig 80-9). The growth of the liver buds within the septum transversum spreads laterally.

## Umbilical Veins

The umbilical veins are broken up into sinusoids, developing communication with the vitelline sinusoids. The right umbilical

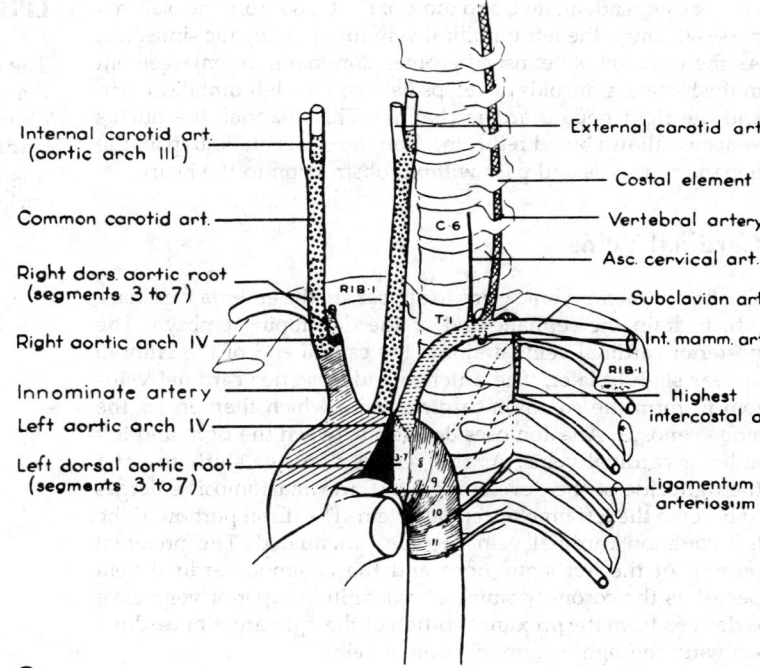

Internal carotid art.
(aortic arch III)

External carotid art.

Common carotid art.

Costal element

Vertebral artery

Right dors. aortic root
(segments 3 to 7)

Asc. cervical art.

Subclavian art.

Right aortic arch IV

Int. mamm. art.

Innominate artery

Highest
intercostal a.

Left aortic arch IV

Left dorsal aortic root
(segments 3 to 7)

Ligamentum
arteriosum

Figure 80-8.   *(Continued)*   **C**

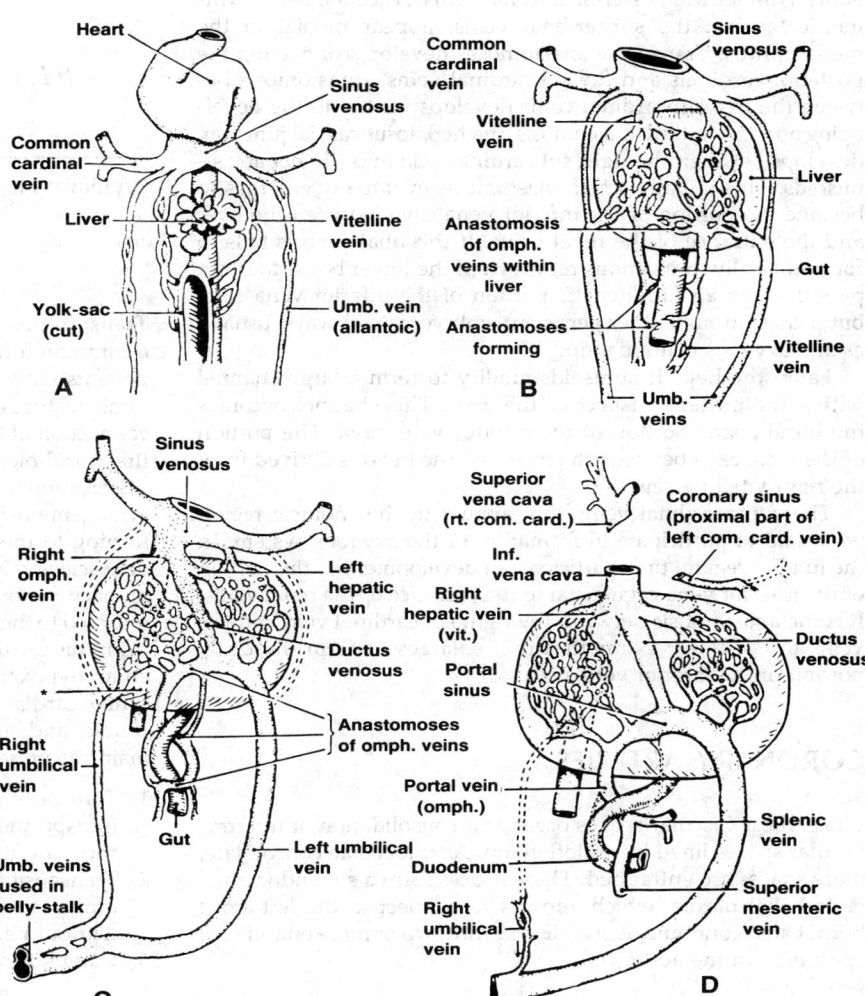

Heart

Sinus
venosus

Common
cardinal
vein

Liver

Yolk-sac
(cut)

Vitelline
vein

Umb. vein
(allantoic)

**A**

Common
cardinal
vein

Sinus
venosus

Vitelline
vein

Liver

Anastomosis
of omph.
veins within
liver

Gut

Anastomoses
forming

Vitelline
vein

Umb.
veins

**B**

Sinus
venosus

Right
omph.
vein

Left
hepatic
vein

Ductus
venosus

*

Anastomoses
of omph. veins

Right
umbilical
vein

Gut

Umb. veins
fused in
belly-stalk

Left umbilical
vein

**C**

Superior
vena cava
(rt. com. card.)

Coronary sinus
(proximal part of
left com. card. vein)

Inf.
vena cava

Right
hepatic vein
(vit.)

Ductus
venosus

Portal
sinus

Portal vein
(omph.)

Splenic
vein

Duodenum

Superior
mesenteric
vein

Right
umbilical
vein

**D**

**Figure 80-9.**   Changes in the vitelline and umbilical venous systems that lead to the development of the hepatic portal circulation. (**A**) Embryos of 3 to 4 mm (fourth week), (**B**) embryos of about 6 mm (fifth week), (**C**) embryos of 8 to 9 mm (sixth week), (**D**) embryos of 20 mm and older. The asterisk in C indicates the hepatic part of the inferior. (Corliss CE. Patton's human embryology. New York: McGraw-Hill, 1976.)

vein becomes attenuated, and most of the blood from the placenta passes through the left umbilical vein into the hepatic sinusoids. As the right sinus venosus becomes dominant, an enlargement in the hepatic sinusoids develops between the left umbilical vein and the right hepatocardiac channel. This channel, the ductus venosus, allows blood returning from the placenta to bypass the hepatic sinusoids and pass without obstruction to the heart.

## Cardinal Veins

The first intraembryonic veins to appear are the anterior cardinals, which drain the cephalic end of the developing embryo. The posterior cardinal veins draining the caudal end of the embryo appear slightly later. The anterior and posterior cardinal veins join to form the common cardinal vein, which then enters the sinus venosus. Anastomoses develop between the right and left anterior cardinal veins. As the venous drainage shifts to enter the right side of the developing heart, the anastomosis enlarges to become the left brachiocephalic vein. The distal portion of the left common cardinal vein becomes attenuated. The proximal portion of the left sinus horn and the common cardinal vein persist as the coronary sinus. The definitive superior vena cava is derived from the proximal portion of the right anterior cardinal vein and the right common cardinal vein.

Development of the venous drainage of the caudal part of the embryo is much more complex. Several sets of veins appear, then partially regress as the definitive venous drainage is formed. Initially, the caudal portion of the embryo is drained by the bilaterally symmetrical posterior cardinal veins. A second set of symmetrical veins, the subcardinal veins, appear medial to the mesonephros. Transverse anastomoses develop, connecting the posterior cardinals and the subcardinal veins. Anastomosis between the two subcardinal veins develops ventral to the developing aorta. A critical anastomosis, the hepatosubcardinal junction, develops between the right subcardinal vein and the hepatic sinusoids. This initially small anastomosis eventually enlarges to become the portion of the inferior vena cava between the liver and the entrance of the renal veins. If this anastomosis fails to form normally, the venous return from the lower body does not pass through an intrahepatic portion of the inferior vena cava but passes through other persistent embryonic pathways, usually as an "azygous continuation."

Later, the hepatic sinusoids modify to form a large channel within the posterior aspect of the liver. This channel becomes the intrahepatic portion of the inferior vena cava. The portion of the vena cava between the liver and the heart is derived from the right vitelline vein.

The supracardinal veins that appear in the thoracic region were said to participate in formation of the azygous system. In the lumbar region, they participate in development of the portion of the inferior vena cava distal to the entrance of the renal veins. It is the anastomosis between the right subcardinal vein and the veins to the lower extremities that enlarges to form the distal portion of the inferior vena cava.

## CORONARY ARTERIES

The earliest vascular spaces occur as a consolidation of intertrabecular spaces lined by endothelium. As trabeculae consolidate, more spaces are entrapped. These spaces form a subendocardial endothelial plexus, which appears to connect to the left sinus horn. Later, continuity is established with two or more endothelial sprouts from the aortic wall.

## EPICARDIUM

The epicardium was initially thought to arise from the same cells that give rise to the myocardium—hence the name epimyocardium. Scanning electron microscopic studies show that the epicardium derives from the mesothelium of the sinus venosus and migrates onto the dorsal and then the lateral and the ventral surfaces of the heart.

*Principles and Practice of Pediatrics, Second Edition.*
edited by Frank A. Oski et al. J. B. Lippincott Company, Philadelphia © 1994.

# CHAPTER 81
# *Cyanotic Congenital Heart Disease*

## *81.1 Transposition of the Great Arteries*

William H. Neches, Sang C. Park, and Jose A. Ettedgui

Transposition of the great arteries, or complete transposition, is a common form of cardiac abnormality found in about 5% of all patients with congenital heart disease. The distinguishing anatomic feature of transposition is the discordant ventriculoarterial connection of the great arteries whereby the aorta originates from the morphologic right ventricle and the pulmonary artery from the morphologic left ventricle. The consequence of this anatomic arrangement is that unoxygenated systemic venous blood returning to the heart passes through the right atrium and right ventricle and is ejected into the aorta. Similarly, oxygenated pulmonary venous blood reaches the left side of the heart and is returned to the pulmonary artery. The clinical situation that results from this cardiac anomaly is characterized by severe, life-threatening hypoxemia early in life. The presence or absence of associated cardiac abnormalities dictates the presentation, clinical course, and surgical approach to the management of the three main categories of patients with transposition:

1. Transposition with an intact interventricular septum (complete transposition). These patients may or may not have left ventricular outflow tract obstruction (subpulmonary stenosis).
2. Transposition with ventricular septal defect, which is complete transposition and an interventricular communication, but without narrowing in the left ventricular outflow tract.
3. Complex transposition, which is complete transposition, ven-

tricular septal defect, and varying degrees of left ventricular outflow tract obstruction. These patients usually have significant subpulmonic stenosis and equal right and left ventricular pressures. This category includes patients with pulmonary atresia.

Other major associated cardiac lesions include patent ductus arteriosus and coarctation of the aorta.

Before the modern era of cardiac catheterization and cardiac surgery, more than 90% of patients with transposition died in infancy. This lesion was one of the most common causes of death from congenital heart disease in the first year of life. In recent years, advancements in cardiac catheterization and cardiac surgery have transformed the devastating natural history of this anomaly so that today, over 90% of patients with this lesion are expected to survive into adulthood.

## PHYSIOLOGY AND HEMODYNAMICS

In the normal heart, the circulation is connected in series. Systemic venous return passes into the pulmonary artery, while pulmonary venous return passes into systemic arterial circulation. In the heart with transposition of the great arteries, the result of the abnormal arterial connection is that there are two parallel circulations (Fig 81-1). Systemic venous return passes through the right heart and is ejected into the aorta, while pulmonary venous return passes through the left heart and is again ejected into the pulmonary artery. This physiologic arrangement is incompatible with life unless blood can be mixed between the two circulations. In the neonate with transposition of the great arteries and an intact interventricular septum, a foramen ovale or atrial septal defect usually is present and facilitates exchange of blood at atrial level. A patent ductus arteriosus enhances this exchange. The ductus

arteriosus is usually a transient neonatal structure, however, and tends to close physiologically within a few days after birth. Closure of the duct precipitates a dramatic change in clinical appearance of an apparently healthy newborn to one with intense cyanosis.

The patient with transposition of the great arteries and a significantly sized ventricular septal defect presents an entirely different clinical picture. These patients often have adequate exchange of blood with a combination of mixing at atrial and ventricular levels. As a result, only mild cyanosis is present in the early neonatal period, and, therefore, a significant cardiovascular anomaly often is not suspected until a few weeks later. As a result of this large ventricular septal defect, patients present with congestive heart failure toward the end of the first month of life and are at risk for subsequent development of pulmonary vascular disease.

The physiology in patients with complex transposition (transposition with ventricular septal defect and pulmonary stenosis) differs from either of the other two clinical forms. In patients with complex transposition, there is a large ventricular septal defect and the balance between pulmonary and systemic blood flow depends on the degree of pulmonary stenosis. When there is severe pulmonary stenosis or pulmonary atresia, patients present with cyanosis and reduced pulmonary blood flow early in life. If pulmonary stenosis is less severe, then clinical presentation is due to the presence of cyanosis or detection of a heart murmur, and may occur even later in infancy.

## DIAGNOSIS

Cyanosis, with or without associated heart murmur, is the most common presenting manifestation of transposition of the great arteries. As previously stated, associated lesions temporarily may provide adequate blood mixing, so the infant may be only mildly cyanotic or have significant cyanosis only during exercise (feeding or crying). In patients with transposition and an intact interventricular septum, there is often no murmur; other than cyanosis, the only abnormalities on physical examination may be a loud, single second heart sound and a prominent right ventricular impulse. In other patients, a murmur may be related to a ventricular septal defect or patent ductus arteriosus, or may be due to pulmonary stenosis.

The electrocardiogram shows right axis deviation and right ventricular hypertrophy, which is a normal pattern in a newborn. Although the classic "egg-on-a-string" radiographic pattern may be seen in about one third of patients, usually the chest roentgenogram is normal in the first few days of life.

Cross-sectional echocardiography has had a dramatic impact on the noninvasive diagnosis of transposition of the great arteries. With this technique, it is possible to demonstrate reliably the atrioventricular and ventriculoarterial connections, thus enabling the diagnosis of transposition of the great arteries. All of the echocardiographic modalities—cross-sectional, M-mode, and Doppler—are important in demonstrating the associated lesions and physiologic derangements that occur in these patients.

Before the 1980s, cardiac catheterization was the only means to make an accurate diagnosis of transposition of the great arteries. This was often performed as an emergency procedure on an extremely ill, hypoxic newborn infant. In many cases, only minimum information was obtained, and a balloon septostomy performed. Since the early 1980s, the use of prostaglandin $E_1$ to maintain patency of the ductus arteriosus has provided the physician with the tool to decrease systemic hypoxemia and acidosis, thereby stabilizing the sick neonate before any procedure. Today,

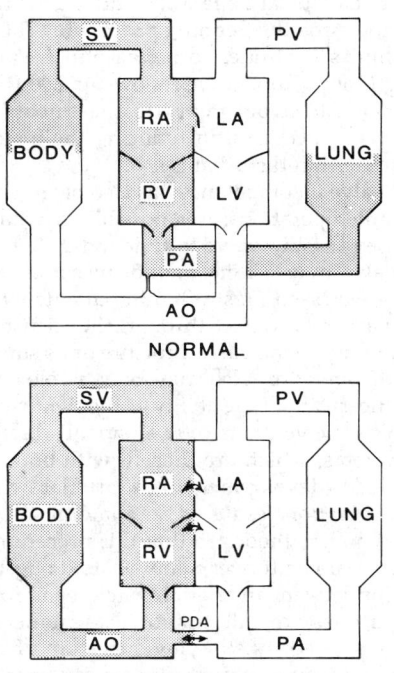

**Figure 81-1.** Circulatory pathways in transposition of the great arteries. *Ao,* aorta; *LA,* left atrium; *LV,* left ventricle; *PA,* pulmonary artery; *PDA,* patent ductus arteriosus; *PV,* pulmonary veins; *RA,* right atrium; *RV,* right ventricle; *SV,* systemic veins.

the anatomic diagnosis usually is established by cross-sectional echocardiography, and cardiac catheterization is required to evaluate the coronary artery anatomy if there is any question about the presence or significance of associated anomalies, or to perform balloon atrial septostomy.

## MANAGEMENT

Introduction of balloon atrial septostomy was the single most important factor influencing survival of the infant with transposition of the great arteries. Other milestones in the two decades before the description of physiologically corrective procedures included development of systemic-to-pulmonary artery anastomoses in the 1940s and the Blalock-Hanlon atrial septectomy and pulmonary artery banding in the 1950s. Although Senning's operation was described in 1959, it was generally unsuccessful in the early years and was abandoned. In the mid-1960s, development of nonoperative palliation by balloon atrial septostomy and physiologic repair by the Mustard operation dramatically altered the survival and prognosis of patients with transposition, especially those with an intact interventricular septum.

Balloon atrial septostomy was the first interventional procedure used in the cardiac catheterization laboratory. It was extremely effective in providing immediate palliation for the patient with transposition of the great arteries. By the early 1970s, successful initial palliation was achieved in more than 85% of patients with transposition. Effective long-term palliation for as long as 2 to 3 years was possible for 65% to 75% of patients who underwent balloon atrial septostomy during infancy. Until development of blade atrial septostomy by Park in 1975, no other nonsurgical option was available for the approximately 25% of patients in whom balloon atrial septostomy was not effective either initially or subsequently during infancy. In an extensive collaborative study reported in 1982, about 80% of these patients who required additional palliation by blade septostomy during infancy and childhood had an adequate result.

Many types of partial and complete atrial redirection operations, including the Senning operation, were suggested but had little success before the description of the atrial baffle repair by Mustard in 1964. Subsequently, this technique was the only procedure used by most centers to repair transposition until the early 1980s when it became popular to use the Senning operation. The goal of both the Mustard and Senning atrial baffle procedures is to redirect the venous inflow to the heart so systemic venous drainage is channeled to the mitral valve, then into the pulmonary circulation, while the pulmonary venous drainage is channeled to the tricuspid valve and, eventually, out into the aorta. In the years before the use of profound hypothermia and circulatory arrest, the Mustard procedure generally performed between 1 and 3 years of age with more than 80% survival in most centers. In the early 1970s when infant surgery became possible, success with atrial baffle procedures progressed even further and many of the preoperative problems associated with hypoxemia and polycythemia were reduced by early repair. In the early 1980s, most centers reported a survival rate of more than 95% for atrial baffle repair of transposition during infancy, usually by the Senning operation.

Concerns about long-term systemic ventricular function, along with problems of atrial baffle obstruction and electrophysiologic abnormalities that are present with both types of atrial baffle repair, led surgeons to consider arterial switch repair. Technically, it is relatively easy to divide the transposed great arteries and re-anastomose the vessels to provide a concordant ventriculoarterial connection. The problem is that the coronary arteries arise from the sinuses of the semilunar valve that is connected to the right ventricle. Because this becomes the pulmonary valve after an arterial switch repair, the coronary arteries would be perfused with low pressure, unoxygenated systemic venous blood, which invariably is fatal. A variety of procedures for connecting one or both coronary arteries to the reconnected aorta has been suggested or attempted. All procedures were unsuccessful until the report by Jatene and associates of survival following an arterial switch repair that included transplantation of both coronary arteries into the reconnected aorta. Although this procedure was associated with high mortality during its initial use, the recent mortality is at more acceptable levels and this anatomic repair is now a worldwide standard.

## LATE RESULTS

Although most patients have good functional results, a number of long-term problems have been identified in patients who have undergone atrial baffle procedures. About 10% to 20% of patients who underwent a Mustard operation developed systemic venous obstruction postoperatively. While some were severe enough to require reoperation, most did not warrant additional surgery. Pulmonary venous obstruction was found less frequently, in about 5% to 10% of survivors, often occurring as a late complication. These were commonly more severe degrees of obstruction that required reoperation. In the 1980s, the Senning operation was popular, and because this operation used the patient's native atrial tissue rather than nonviable material for the atrial baffle, it was hoped that this technique would eliminate most postoperative problems found after the Mustard operation. Systemic venous obstruction generally was uncommon in patients who underwent a Senning operation. Pulmonary venous obstruction occurred with a similar frequency, however, as was found after the Mustard operation.

Atrial arrhythmias (atrial flutter, supraventricular tachycardia, and sick-sinus syndrome) are important problems in patients who underwent a Mustard operation and increasingly in patients who have undergone the Senning procedure. The percentage of atrial arrhythmias continues to increase in frequency with increasing length of postoperative follow-up. Modifications of operative technique to avoid injury to the sinoatrial node or its artery have been successful in reducing the incidence of early postoperative rhythm disturbances.

Tricuspid valve incompetence has also been reported to occur after atrial baffle operations. It is possible that this is caused by inability of the tricuspid valve to function as the systemic atrioventricular valve over a long period. In some series, tricuspid incompetence was seen most often in patients who had closure of a ventricular septal defect through the tricuspid valve. This suggests that injury to the valve structure or its support apparatus at the time of operation also may play a role. Another major problem is concern about the ability of the right ventricle to function as the systemic ventricle over a patient's lifetime.

These problems, which are present with both types of atrial baffle repair, led to development of the arterial switch procedure. Because this operation results in an anatomic as well as physiologic correction, it is theorized that this procedure will provide a better functional result over many years. Long-term results of patients who underwent an arterial switch repair for transposition of the great arteries are still unknown. A number of questions may yet be answered by studying survivors of arterial switch procedure. Maintenance of normal coronary artery blood flow is of major importance, and long-term effects related to growth are unknown. Another concern is the site of anastomosis for reconnection of the great arteries. Stenosis at the site of anastomosis of the great arteries (particularly the pulmonary artery) is fairly common, and some patients have required reoperation to correct this problem. Despite the lack of long-term follow-up to decide questions such as the growth of anastomotic sites and the fate of transplanted coronary arteries, the arterial switch repair is the preferred procedure for surgical management of the patient with transposition of the great arteries.

## Selected Readings

Jatene AD, Fontes VF, Paulista PP, et al. Anatomic correction of transposition of the great vessels. J Thorac Cardiovasc Surg 1976;72:364.
Mustard WT. Successful two-stage correction of transposition of the great vessels. Surgery 1964;55:469.
Park SC, Neches WH, Mathews RA, et al. Hemodynamic function after the mustard operation for transposition of the great arteries. Am J Cardiol 1983;51:1514.
Park SC, Neches WH, Mullins CE, et al. Blade atrial septostomy: collaborative study. Circulation 1982;66:258.
Quaegebeur JM, Rohmer J, Brom AG, et al. Revival of the Senning operation in the treatment of transposition of the great arteries. Thorax 1977;32:517.
Rashkind WJ, Miller WW. Creation of an atrial septal defect without thoracotomy: a palliative approach to complete transposition of the great arteries. JAMA 1966;196:991.
Rastelli GC, Wallace RB, Ongley PA. Complete repair of transposition of the great arteries with pulmonary stenosis: a review and report of a case corrected by using a new surgical technique. Circulation 1969;39:83.
Senning A. Surgical correction of transposition of the great vessels. Surgery 1959;45:966.
Shaher R. Complete transposition of the great arteries. New York: Academic Press, 1973.

*Principles and Practice of Pediatrics, Second Edition.*
edited by Frank A. Oski et al. J. B. Lippincott Company, Philadelphia © 1994.

# *81.2 Truncus Arteriosus*

## Robert Lee Williams

Persistent truncus arteriosus may be defined as a single great artery arising from the base of the heart and giving origin to the coronary, pulmonary, and systemic arteries. The incidence of truncus arteriosus is low; it occurs in approximately 2% of patients with congenital heart defects. There is no apparent gender predilection. Without treatment, truncus arteriosus is usually fatal—the mean age of death is 2.5 months, and 80% of affected children die by 1 year of age.

## EMBRYOLOGY AND ANATOMY

In 1949, Collett and Edwards proposed a classification based on embryologic theory and on their observations of 116 cases of persistent truncus arteriosus. In 1965, a new classification was proposed by Van Praagh; it is more complete and accurate than the earlier one (Fig 81-2). The vast majority of truncal cases have ventricular septal defect and belong to Van Praagh's Group A. Group B indicates the existence of persistent truncus without a ventricular septal defect. Most authors, including Edwards, agree that the type IV Collett and Edwards classification does not represent a persistent truncus arteriosus, but rather an extreme form of tetralogy with main pulmonary artery atresia, commonly described today as pseudotruncus. Another term, hemitruncus, which is similar in nomenclature only, is a distinct anomaly in which a main pulmonary artery gives rise only to one pulmonary artery, the opposite lung being supplied by a branch pulmonary artery arising from the ascending aorta.

Persistence of truncus arteriosus usually occurs in the presence of a ventricular septal defect. The truncal root straddles the ventricular septal defect equally in approximately 60% of cases, with 20% of the remaining cases having either a dominant right or a dominant left ventricular override.

The truncal valve leaflets are usually abnormal and frequently appear to be thick, fleshy, soft, and polypoid. The number of leaflets varies. About 65% have tricuspid valves, 23% have quadricuspid valves, and 9% have bicuspid valves. In 2% of cases, there may be five or more valves. The truncal valve usually has fibrous continuity with the mitral valve, and about 4% to 10% of cases may have a fibrous continuity with the tricuspid valve. Truncal valve regurgitation is present in about 50% of patients and is moderate to severe in half of these. Truncal valve stenosis may be seen in about one third of the patients. The arch is right-sided in about one third of the cases; in Van Praagh type A3, the agenesis of the pulmonary artery is ipsilateral to the site of the arch in 75% of cases. In about 12% of interrupted aortic arch anomalies, there is an associated truncus arteriosus. Noncardiac anomalies are present in about 20% of the cases, with DiGeorge syndrome being one of the more common associated anomalies. Conversely, in patients who have DiGeorge syndrome, which may be an autosomal-dominant inheritance, about 9% have truncus arteriosus; in those who have DiGeorge syndrome with interrupted arch, 33% have truncus arteriosus.

## CLINICAL FEATURES

Patients with truncus arteriosus usually present with severe congestive heart failure during the first few months of life. Cyanosis usually is not visible clinically because increased pulmonary blood flow produces a greater mixing of saturated than of desaturated blood volume, which obfuscates clinical cyanosis. Increased pulmonary flow is due to the perfusion of lungs at systemic pressure from the truncus. This increased blood flow is augmented because pulmonary resistance tends to decrease in early infancy. The severity of congestive heart failure not only depends on pulmonary blood flow volume, but also may be aggravated by truncal valve regurgitation.

Frequently, a systolic murmur that is usually holosystolic is heard at the left sternal border. This is accompanied by an ejection click, followed by a single second heart sound. Occasionally, an early diastolic murmur is present due to truncal valve regurgitation, or a continuous murmur is present if there is a pressure gradient from the truncal root to the branching of the pulmonary arteries or artery. Palpable peripheral pulses may become quickened and sharp in contour secondary to the pulmonary artery run-off. Tachypnea, decreased feeding, and irritability may be the first clinical symptoms. Although symptoms usually occur within the first few days of life, they may be delayed for several weeks, secondary to the delay in the decrease in pulmonary vascular resistance. Clinically, an infant with truncus arteriosus presents similarly to a patient with ventricular septal defect and ductus arteriosus or to one with an aortopulmonary artery window and ventricular septal defect.

The electrocardiogram usually shows biventricular hypertrophy. Isolated right or left ventricular hypertrophy is less common.

The chest roentgenogram shows cardiomegaly after the first day or two of life. Heart size continues to increase as pulmonary overcirculation occurs with regression of fetal pulmonary vascular resistance. The left atrium enlarges to accommodate the increased pulmonary venous return. As congestive heart failure progresses, large pulmonary vessels become indistinct and obscured by pulmonary edema. The position of the aortic arch always should be identified. The finding of a right aortic arch with increased pulmonary vascularity gives an extremely high probability of truncus

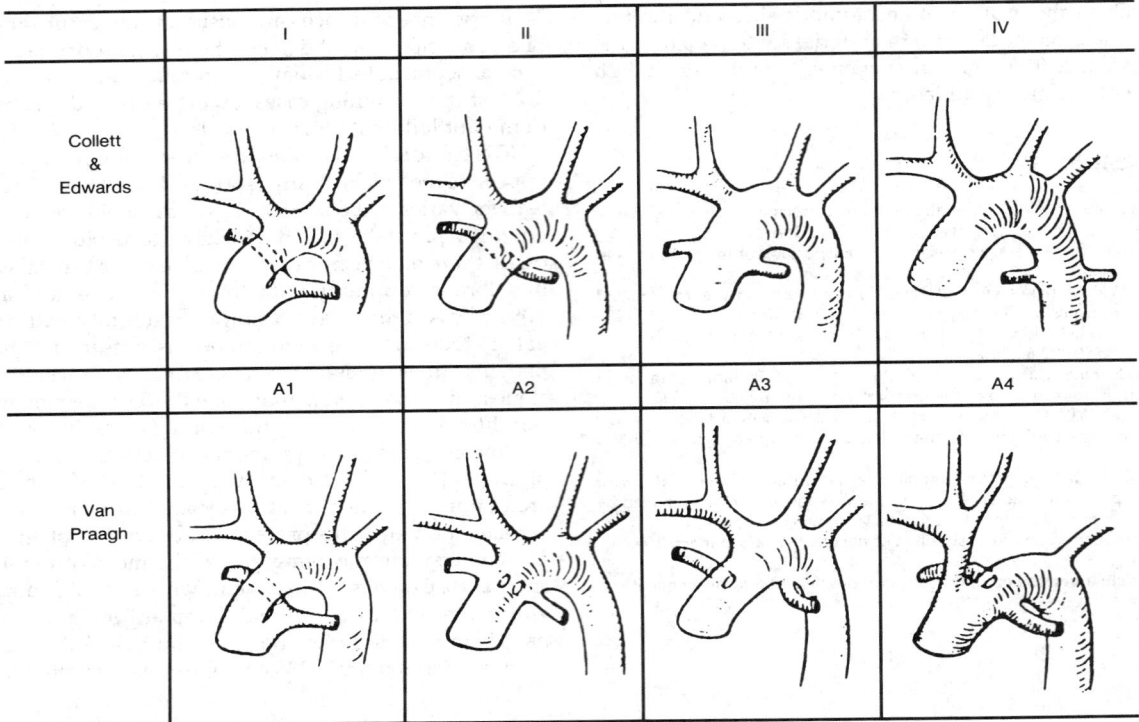

**Figure 81-2.** The classic Collett and Edwards classification of truncus arteriosus is compared with the van Praagh classification. Type I is the same as A1. Types II and III are grouped as a single type, A2. Type A3 denotes unilateral pulmonary artery atresia with collateral supply to the affected lung. Type A4 is truncus associated with and interrupted aortic arch. Type IV is commonly known as pseudotruncus.

arteriosus. If there is atresia of one of the pulmonary arteries (ie, type A3), then there is asymmetry of the pulmonary vascularity associated with hypoplasia of the ipsilateral lung and hemithorax.

## ECHOCARDIOGRAPHIC AND DOPPLER FEATURES

Echocardiogram evaluation usually is the first noninvasive test that can corroborate clinical suspicion of truncus arteriosus. The sine qua non of persistent truncus arteriosus is the demonstration of the pulmonary arteries originating from a common trunk and semilunar valve. Doppler evaluation can accurately indicate the competency of the truncal valve, and color Doppler evaluation can demonstrate better the flow pattern across the truncal valve and the competency of the valve. With parasternal, subcostal, and suprasternal views, differentiation of truncus arteriosus and ventricular septal defect can be made with a high degree of accuracy, but problems may arise in differentiating between truncus arteriosus and pulmonary atresia with ventricular septal defect.

## CARDIAC CATHETERIZATION AND ANGIOGRAPHIC FEATURES

Cardiac catheterization and angiography have long been the definitive way to evaluate the anatomic detail and physiologic variables in truncus arteriosus. Pressures in both ventricles are systemic, and pressure in the left atrium frequently is elevated by increased pulmonary venous return. There may be a drop in pressure in the more distal pulmonary arteries compared to that in the aortic arch. In the past, evaluation of pulmonary arterial resistance was extremely important when patients were older

than 2 years before surgical repair. Surgery was considered not feasible if the pulmonary arteriolar resistance was greater than 8 units · m². The present policy of doing corrective surgery by 6 months of age, however, should prevent the steady increase of pulmonary arteriolar resistance from becoming persistent pulmonary vascular disease.

Truncal angiography is imperative, and an assessment of the valve can be made from the selective truncal angiograms. If the aorta is significantly smaller than the pulmonary artery portion of the truncus, then an interrupted aortic arch is expected. The aortic arch frequently is right-sided, and there may be a persistence of the ductus arteriosus. Anomalous subclavian artery is not unusual. Peripheral pulmonary artery stenosis and origin of one of the pulmonary arteries from a ductus arteriosus with discontinuity of the pulmonary arteries also are not rare.

The ventriculograms, preferably done from both ventricles, can delineate the anatomy and physiology of the truncus arteriosus. The long-axis view delineates the ventricular septal defect directly beneath the truncal valve area where the infundibular septum should be located. The left ventricular outflow tract is formed by the anterior leaflet posteriorly and by the trabecular septum anteriorly. The right ventricular connection to the truncus arteriosus is bound posteriorly by the septal structure and anteriorly by the ventriculoinfundibular fold. The elongated right anterior oblique view may demonstrate the right ventricular outflow to the truncus and may delineate the aortopulmonary septum of the truncus.

Other imaging methods to detect truncus arteriosus may be used more widely in the future. Magnetic resonance imaging can delineate the vessels and chambers in truncus arteriosus accurately without the use of contrast material or exposure of the patient to ionizing radiation, and ultrafast computed tomography eventually may be a useful imaging technique in truncus arteriosus. Neither is used routinely in the workup of truncus arteriosus.

## TREATMENT

The ultimate treatment for truncus arteriosus is surgical. The initial treatment, however, is medical, and should be aimed at cardiac decongestive therapy. In the neonate, diagnosis of classic truncus arteriosus is sufficient to instigate cardiac decongestive therapy, even without signs or symptoms of congestive heart failure. As pulmonary vascular resistance decreases, congestive heart failure occurs. Treatment for congestive heart failure consists of digitalization and aggressive diuretic therapy.

Before 1968, the only surgical palliation available for truncus arteriosus was pulmonary artery banding. Evolution of radical corrective surgery for truncus arteriosus began when it was demonstrated that the right ventricular outflow tract in tetralogy of Fallot could be enlarged with a patch. Rastelli and colleagues (1965) used an artificial, valveless pulmonary artery conduit made of pericardium. In 1967, they used an experimental aortic homograft with a valve conduit for right ventricular pulmonary flow. McGoon and colleagues (1968) used this method for the first successful correction of truncus arteriosus. Homografts were found to calcify and become stenotic, and Malm (1973) used an artificial pulmonary trunk of Dacron containing a valve xenograft. Ebert and colleagues (1976) championed the use of pulmonary artery conduits in infants younger than 6 months of age, with modification of the conduit when the child was older, with a resultant mortality rate of 11%. Some refinements in technique have been suggested, for example, complete division of the truncal root with primary closure using absorbable suture and isolation of the pulmonary orifice as a button to which the valved conduit is attached. Some suggest the use in neonates of valveless conduits as a primary repair. In most patients who have returned for conduit change, repairs were made without the use of a valve conduit.

The alternative to early repair is palliative banding of the pulmonary artery with complete repair as a second stage. Banding of the pulmonary artery in truncus arteriosus frequently requires bilateral banding and is extremely difficult, with a mortality rate approaching 50%. The overall mortality rate for banding with repair later is 75%.

After diagnosis of truncus arteriosus, the challenge to the cardiologist is to determine the optimum time for surgical intervention. Stabilization of the hemodynamics and maturation and growth of the infant need to be balanced with the potential for rapid cardiac deterioration or potential for pulmonary hypertension. With surgical correction in infants at 6 months of age or younger, persistent pulmonary hypertension can be prevented. The exception to this may be in infants with a single pulmonary artery, but the only chance for these infants to avoid persistent pulmonary hypertension is surgery before 6 months of age. Not only is the cardiologist challenged by timing the initial corrective surgery, but close follow-up and deliberation are needed to determine optimal timing for conduit replacement.

Continued advances in surgical therapy for truncus arteriosus in the last two decades allow a lesion previously considered inoperable to be corrected surgically, and the diagnosis and treatment continue to be refined.

## Selected Readings

Bowman TO, Hancock WD, Malm JR. A valve-containing Dacron prosthesis: its use in restoring pulmonary artery-right ventricle continuity. Arch Surg 107: 724.

Ceballos R, Soto B, Kirklin JW, Bargeron LM. Truncus arteriosus: an anatomical-angiographic study. Br Heart J 1983;49:589.

Collett RW, Edwards JE. Persistent truncus arteriosus: a classification according to anatomic types. Surg Clin North Am 1949;29:1245.

Ebert PA, et al. Surgical treatment of truncus arteriosus in the first 6 months of life. Ann Surg 1984;200:451.

Fisher MR, Lipton MJ, Higgins CB. Magnetic resonance imaging and computed tomography in congenital heart disease. Semin Roentgenol 1985;20:272.

Mair DD, et al. Truncus arteriosus with unilateral absence of a pulmonary artery. Criteria for operability and surgical results. Circulation 1977;55:641.

McGoon DC, Rastelli GC, Ongley PA. An operation for the correction of truncus arteriosus. JAMA 1968;205:59.

Moes CAF, Freedom RM. Aortic arch interruption with truncus arteriosus or aorticopulmonary septal defect. AJR 1980;135:1011.

Rastelli GC, Ongley PA, Davis CP, Hinklin JW. Surgical repair of pulmonary valve atresia with coronary pulmonary artery fistulae: report of a case. Mayo Clin Proc. 1965;40:521.

Rice MJ, et al. Definitive diagnosis of truncus arteriosus by two-dimensional echocardiography. Mayo Clin Proc 1982;57:476.

Rohn RD, et al. Familial third-fourth pharyngeal pouch syndrome with apparent autosomal dominant transmission. J Pediatr 1984;105:47.

Van Praagh R, Van Praagh S. The anatomy of common aorticopulmonary trunk (truncus arteriosus communis) and its embryologic implications. Am J Cardiol 1965;16:406.

*Principles and Practice of Pediatrics, Second Edition.*
edited by Frank A. Oski et al. J. B. Lippincott Company, Philadelphia © 1994.

# 81.3 *Tricuspid Atresia*

### David J. Driscoll

Tricuspid atresia, the third most common form of cyanotic congenital heart disease, consists of complete agenesis of the tricuspid valve and absence of direct communication between the right atrium and the right ventricle. The prevalence of tricuspid atresia in clinical series of patients with congenital heart disease ranges from 0.3% to 3.7%. The prevalence rate in autopsy series is 2.9%. Tricuspid atresia occurs in 1 : 17,857 to 1 : 10,000 live births.

## PATHOLOGY

Tricuspid atresia is divided into three types based on the great artery relationship: I, normally related great arteries; II, D-transposed great arteries; and III, L-transposed great arteries (Table 81-1). The three types are subclassified according to the presence or absence and size of the ventricular septal defect and the presence or absence of pulmonary atresia or stenosis. About 70% of cases are type I; 23%, type II; 7%, type III.

An opening in the atrial septum allows egress of blood from the right atrium. The interatrial communication can be or can become restrictive. Additional cardiovascular abnormalities occur in 18% of patients with normally related great arteries and in 63% of patients with transposed great arteries. These include coarctation of the aorta, patent ductus arteriosus, and right aortic arch. Extracardiac anomalies occur in 20% of cases.

In tricuspid atresia, the left bundle of the cardiac conduction system originates early from the bundle of His and is unusually posterior and short. Presumably, this anatomic malformation of the conduction system accounts for the abnormal frontal-plane axis of the electrocardiogram in patients with tricuspid atresia.

## HEMODYNAMICS

In tricuspid atresia, hemodynamics depend on presence or absence of pulmonary atresia, degree of pulmonary stenosis, pres-

TABLE 81-1. Classifications of Tricuspid Atresia

| Type | Description | Relative Frequency (%) | |
|------|-------------|:------:|:------:|
| | | Clinical | Autopsy |
| I | Normally related great arteries | 70 | 69 |
| I-A | No VSD; pulmonary atresia | | 9 |
| I-B | Restrictive VSD; pulmonary stenosis | | 51 |
| I-C | Large VSD; no pulmonary stenosis | | 9 |
| II | D-transposition of great arteries | 23 | 28 |
| II-A | VSD; pulmonary atresia | | 2 |
| II-B | VSD; pulmonary stenosis | | 8 |
| II-C | VSD; no pulmonary stenosis | | 18 |
| III | L-transposition of great arteries | 7 | 3 |

VSD, ventricular septal defect.

*Adapted from Rosenthal A, Dick M. Tricuspid atresia. In: Adams FH, Emmanouilides GC, eds. Moss's heart disease in infants, children, and adolescents, ed 3. Baltimore: Williams & Wilkins, 1983:271.*

ence of normally related or transposed great arteries, and presence or absence of subpulmonary or subaortic stenosis. Because all systemic venous return (blood oxygen saturation low) and pulmonary venous return (blood oxygen saturation high) mix in the left atrium, the level of blood oxygen saturation reaching the left ventricle, and subsequently the aorta, depends on the relative volumes of pulmonary venous return and systemic venous return. Patients with tricuspid atresia and increased pulmonary blood flow (ie, no pulmonary or subpulmonary stenosis) have a relatively larger volume of pulmonary venous return than systemic venous return and have relatively high systemic arterial blood oxygen saturation. In contrast, patients with relatively low pulmonary blood flow (due to pulmonary or subpulmonary stenosis or pulmonary atresia) may have marked systemic arterial hypoxemia. The volume of pulmonary blood flow and the clinical characteristics may change. Patients with pulmonary stenosis may depend on patency of the ductus arteriosus for pulmonary blood flow, and, as the ductus closes, pulmonary blood flow may decrease significantly.

In general, pulmonary or subpulmonary (at the level of the ventricular septal defect) obstruction is present or occurs during the first year of life in most patients with tricuspid atresia and normally related great arteries. In contrast, most patients with tricuspid atresia and D-transposed great arteries (type II-C) have unobstructed pulmonary blood flow. Because of this, patients in the former groups usually have more marked hypoxemia than those with D-transposed great arteries; but, those with D-transposed great arteries are more likely to have pulmonary edema and congestive heart failure and to develop pulmonary vascular obstructive disease. The ventricular septal defect associated with tricuspid atresia tends to become smaller. A restrictive ventricular septal defect associated with normally related great arteries produces progressive subpulmonary stenosis and increasing hypoxemia. A restrictive ventricular septal defect associated with transposed great arteries produces subaortic obstruction. When combined with pulmonary stenosis or the presence of a pulmonary artery band, significant left ventricular hypertension and hypertrophy occur.

## CLINICAL FINDINGS

### History

Because of the presence of cyanosis, congestive heart failure, or growth failure, tricuspid atresia usually is detected in infancy. Cyanosis is the prominent feature in patients whose pulmonary blood flow is limited by pulmonary atresia or pulmonary stenosis. Symptoms of pulmonary edema and congestive heart failure predominate in patients with unobstructed pulmonary blood flow; cyanosis also can be apparent. If pulmonary blood flow depends on the patency of the ductus arteriosus, the degree of cyanosis and arterial hypoxemia may increase dramatically if the ductus arteriosus closes. If pulmonary atresia is present, closure of the ductus arteriosus can produce profound hypoxemia, acidosis, and death. For patients with unobstructed pulmonary blood flow, as pulmonary vascular resistance decreases and pulmonary blood flow increases, signs and symptoms of congestive heart failure and pulmonary edema can increase.

Without surgical intervention, significant pulmonary vascular obstructive disease occurs in patients with unrestricted pulmonary blood flow (types I-C and II-C). Pulmonary vascular obstructive disease is much less common in patients with tricuspid atresia and normally related great arteries than it is in patients with transposed great arteries. This is because most patients with normally related great arteries have or will have (at about 1 year of age) pulmonary or subpulmonary stenosis.

Bacterial endocarditis and brain abscess are relatively common complications of tricuspid atresia. Neurologic complications also can result from cerebrovascular accidents secondary to polycythemia or to intravascular thrombosis or embolic phenomena.

### Physical Examination

Cyanosis is the most common clinical feature of tricuspid atresia. Infants with tricuspid atresia and normally related great arteries may have excessive pulmonary blood flow and little cyanosis but the degree of cyanosis may increase as the ventricular septal defect becomes progressively restrictive, causing subpulmonary stenosis and decreasing blood flow.

The intensity of the second heart sound usually is normal if the great arteries are normally related (ie, pulmonary artery anterior) and the pulmonary artery pressure is normal. Because the aorta is nearer to the anterior chest wall when great arteries are transposed (ie, the aorta is anterior to the pulmonary artery), the second heart sound may be more intense despite normal pulmonary artery pressure.

Cardiac murmurs are present in 80% of patients with tricuspid atresia. A low-frequency holosystolic or, at times, a crescendo-decrescendo murmur is produced by the flow of blood through the ventricular septal defect. A systolic midfrequency crescendo-decrescendo murmur is present in patients with pulmonary stenosis. Patients with pulmonary atresia and a systemic-to-pulmonary collateral blood supply, as well as patients who have had a surgical systemic arterial-to-pulmonary arterial anastomosis, have a continuous murmur. A diastolic mitral murmur may be audible in patients who have excessive pulmonary blood flow.

### Electrocardiogram

First-degree atrioventricular block occurs in 15% of cases and presumably is due to prolonged atrial conduction, because atrioventricular node function usually is normal. Because of early origin of the left bundle from the common bundle, the frontal plane QRS axis usually is leftward or superior and the frontal plane electrocardiographic loop is counterclockwise. Rarely, the frontal plane QRS axis is normal, which suggests the presence of transposed great arteries. The right ventricular electrocardiographic forces are diminished, and there is evidence of left ventricular hypertrophy and, frequently, of discordant QRS and T waves.

## Chest Radiograph

The heart usually is enlarged. The right heart border may be prominent, reflecting enlargement of the right atrium. The pulmonary vascular markings are increased when the pulmonary blood flow is excessive. In 80% of patients with tricuspid atresia, however, the pulmonary blood flow is diminished and the pulmonary vascular markings are decreased.

## Echocardiogram

Basic anatomy, size of the atrial septal defect, size of ventricular septal defect, ventricular function, great artery relationships, and valvular function can be ascertained by using M-mode, two-dimensional, and color flow imaging echocardiography.

## Cardiac Catheterization

In infants, the major use of cardiac catheterization is to determine sources and reliability of pulmonary blood flow. Administration of prostaglandin $E_1$ to maintain ductal patency has improved the safety of cardiac catheterization for babies with decreased or ductal-dependent pulmonary blood flow. Cardiac catheterization may be necessary in infants (2 to 6 months of age) to measure pulmonary artery pressure and resistance as a guide to the need for pulmonary artery banding to prevent development of pulmonary vascular obstructive disease.

In adolescents and adults, cardiac catheterization and angiography define anatomic and hemodynamic details important in surgical management.

## CLINICAL MANAGEMENT

### Infants

Three major considerations should guide the management of infants with tricuspid atresia:

1. The need for manipulating the amount of pulmonary blood flow, either to decrease hypoxemia and polycythemia by increasing pulmonary blood flow or to decrease symptoms of congestive heart failure by decreasing pulmonary blood flow
2. The need to preserve myocardial function, pulmonary vascular integrity, and the pulmonary vascular bed to optimize conditions for future Fontan operation
3. The need to reduce risks of associated cardiovascular complications such as bacterial endocarditis and thromboembolism.

Babies with severe hypoxemia and acidosis should be treated promptly with an infusion of prostaglandin $E_1$ to maintain patency of the ductus arteriosus, thus improving pulmonary perfusion. Cardiac catheterization and angiography establish sources of pulmonary blood flow and help plan for type of surgical systemic-to-pulmonary artery anastomosis.

Infants with transposed great arteries and unrestricted pulmonary blood flow have signs and symptoms of pulmonary edema and congestive heart failure. They benefit from treatment with digitalis and diuretics. Classically, these patients have had a pulmonary artery band surgically placed to decrease pulmonary blood flow. Some investigators suggest, however, that pulmonary artery banding might accelerate ventricular septal defect closure. In tricuspid atresia with transposed great arteries, this would create subaortic obstruction and lead to marked ventricular hyper-

TABLE 81-2. Criteria of Choussat and Fontan for Low-Risk Operation

Age at operation 4 to 15 years
Sinus rhythm
Normal systemic venous return
Normal right atrial volume
Mean pulmonary artery pressure ≤15 mm Hg
Pulmonary arteriolar resistance <4 units·m²
Pulmonary artery/aorta diameter ratio >0.75
Left ventricular ejection fraction ≥0.60
Competent mitral valve
Absence of pulmonary artery distortion

*Adapted from Choussat A, Fontan F, Bosse P, et al. Selection criteria for Fontan's procedure. In: Adams RH, Shinebourne EA, eds. Paediatric cardiology 1977. Edinburgh: Churchill Livingstone, 1978:559.*

trophy. Because marked ventricular hypertrophy is an adverse risk for subsequent successful Fontan operation, surgical procedures to reduce pulmonary blood flow and to bypass potential areas of subaortic obstruction have been recommended. Advantages of these more complicated and riskier palliative procedures have not been established.

### Children and Adolescents

Before 1971, palliative procedures to control pulmonary blood flow (pulmonary artery banding, systemic to pulmonary artery anastomoses, or superior vena cava to pulmonary artery anastomoses) were the mainstay of surgical treatment for patients with tricuspid atresia. In 1971, Fontan and associates described a unique procedure to separate the systemic and pulmonary venous return to eliminate the right-to-left intracardiac shunt and reduce the volume of ventricular overload. They constructed a Glenn anastomosis to direct superior vena caval systemic venous return to the right lung, directed inferior vena caval systemic venous return to the pulmonary artery with a valve-containing conduit connecting the right atrium and the pulmonary artery, inserted a valve into the inferior vena cava, closed the interatrial communication, and obliterated the connection between the pulmonary artery and the ventricle. Since its original description, the procedure has been modified considerably, but the concept of directing systemic venous return directly to the pulmonary artery retains the eponym "modified Fontan procedure."

Ten guidelines for relatively low-risk operation are listed in Table 81-2. Additional criteria include the absence of ventricular hypertrophy, more recent calendar year of operation, absence of subaortic obstruction, shorter operative ischemic time, and absence of incorporation of prosthetic valves into the repair. Although most of these criteria are relative, it is clear that as more of these are violated, operative mortality increases and the chances of excellent long-term results decrease.

In a follow-up study of 125 patients who had a modified Fontan operation between 1973 and 1985, the 30-day, 6-month, 1-, 5-, and 10-year survivorship was 90%, 84%, 84%, 80%, and 70% respectively. Quality of life and exercise tolerance improved after the operation. Preliminary data suggest that the operation prolongs life.

### Selected Readings

Choussat A, Fontan F, Bosse P, et al. Selection criteria for Fontan's procedure. In: Anderson RH, Shinebourne EA, eds. Paediatric cardiology 1977. Edinburgh: Churchill Livingstone, 1978:559.

Dick M, Fyler DC, Nadas AS. Tricuspid atresia: clinical course in 101 patients. Am J Cardiol 1975;36:327.

Driscoll DJ, Danielson GK, Puga FJ, et al. Exercise tolerance and cardiorespiratory response to exercise after the Fontan operation for tricuspid atresia or functional single ventricle. J Am Coll Cardiol 1986;7:1087.

Driscoll D, Offord K, Feldt R, Schaff H, Puga F, Danielson G. Five-to fifteen-year follow-up after the Fontan operation. Circulation 1992;85:469.

Fontan F, Mounicot F, Baudet E, Simonneau J, Gordo J, Gouffrant J. "Correction" de l'atresie tricuspidienne; rapport de deux cas "corrig'es" par 1 'utilisation d 'une technique chirurgicale nouvelle. Ann Chir Thorsc Cardio-Vasc 1971;10(1): 39.

Rao PS. Tricuspid atresia. Mount Kisco, NY: Futura, 1982:13.

Rosenthal A, Dick M. Tricuspid atresia. In: Adams FH, Emmanouilides GC, eds. Moss's heart disease in infants, children, and adolescents, ed 3. Baltimore: Williams & Wilkins, 1983:271.

Tandon R, Edwards JE. Tricuspid atresia: a reevaluation and classification. J Thorac Cardiovasc Surg 1974;67:530.

Vlad P. Tricuspid atresia. In: Keith JD, Rowe RD, Vlad P, eds. Heart disease in infancy and childhood, ed 3. New York: Macmillan, 1978:518.

*Principles and Practice of Pediatrics, Second Edition.*
edited by Frank A. Oski et al. J. B. Lippincott Company, Philadelphia © 1994.

# 81.4 *Tetralogy of Fallot*

### William H. Neches and Jose A. Ettedgui

*Tetralogy of Fallot* refers to a spectrum of anatomic abnormalities that have in common a large, unrestrictive ventricular septal defect and right ventricular outflow tract obstruction—two features of the tetralogy. Clinical presentation varies from the asymptomatic acyanotic child with a heart murmur to the severely hypoxic newborn infant. Severity of presentation largely depends on the nature and degree of the outflow obstruction. The anatomic hallmark of tetralogy of Fallot is the anterocephalad deviation of the outlet portion of the interventricular septum. Apart from producing infundibular pulmonary stenosis, this also accounts for the ventricular septal defect and the third feature of the tetralogy—aortic override (Fig 81-3). The fourth feature of the tetralogy, hypertrophy of the right ventricle, is the result of the underlying anatomic and hemodynamic abnormalities. The severity of the infundibular stenosis ranges from mild to severe pulmonary stenosis and to pulmonary atresia. Further obstruction to pulmonary blood flow often occurs at other levels. Pulmonary valve

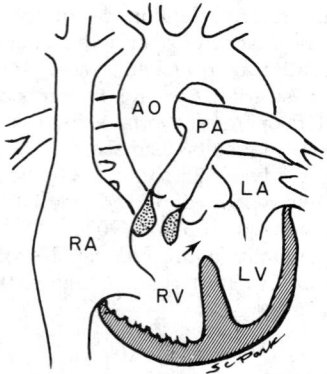

**Figure 81-3.** Anatomic abnormalities in tetralogy of Fallot. *Ao,* aorta; *LA,* left atrium; *LV,* left ventricle; *PA,* pulmonary artery; *RA,* right atrium; *RV,* right ventricle. Note the ventricular septal defect (*arrow*), the infundibular pulmonary stenosis (*stippled area*), and the overriding aorta.

stenosis is common, and stenoses are also often found in the supravalvar region at the bifurcation of the pulmonary artery branches or in the distal pulmonary arteries.

The typical ventricular septal defect in tetralogy of Fallot is large and unrestrictive and is due to malalignment of the outlet portion with the rest of the interventricular septum. Muscular ventricular septal defects, an inlet defect, or a complete atrioventricular septal defect also may be present.

Other possible associated abnormalities include an atrial septal defect (so-called pentalogy of Fallot) or coronary artery abnormalities. About 25% of patients with tetralogy of Fallot have a right-sided aortic arch, an important consideration if a patient undergoes systemic to pulmonary artery anastomosis.

Tetralogy of Fallot occurs in about 6% of infants born with congenital heart disease. The etiology is obscure. Although tetralogy of Fallot and most other forms of congenital heart disease generally occur as isolated abnormalities, children with tetralogy of Fallot are afflicted with additional major extracardiac malformations significantly more often (15.7%) than are patients with other congenital heart defects (6.8%). In addition, the extracardiac malformations may be more serious in patients with tetralogy of Fallot and include cleft lip and palate, hypospadias, and skeletal malformations. Although tetralogy of Fallot is not commonly part of specific hereditary malformation syndromes or chromosomal abnormalities, it is often found in a number of malformation associations, including cardiofacial, VACTERL, and CHARGE associations as well as DeLange, Goldenhar, and Klippel-Feil syndromes.

## PHYSIOLOGY AND HEMODYNAMICS

Equalization of right and left ventricular pressure along with normal or reduced pulmonary artery pressure are the hemodynamic features produced by anatomic abnormalities in patients with tetralogy of Fallot. Because the ventricular septal defect is large and unrestrictive and the right and left ventricles contract simultaneously, the end result is, in effect, a common ventricular chamber ejecting into systemic and pulmonary circulations. Pulmonary and systemic blood flows, therefore, depend on the relation between the pulmonary and systemic resistances. Normally, pulmonary resistance is about 10% of systemic resistance, and these resistances are determined by their respective distal arteriolar beds. In tetralogy of Fallot, however, pulmonary vascular (arteriolar) resistance usually is normal or less than normal, and resistance to right ventricular ejection into the pulmonary vascular bed is related instead to pulmonary stenosis.

The presenting symptoms and severity of clinical manifestations in patients with tetralogy of Fallot depend on the relation between the resistances to systemic and pulmonary outflow. If the total right ventricular outflow obstruction is such that pulmonary outflow resistance is less than systemic resistance, there is a net left-to-right shunt, and clinical manifestations are similar to those of patients with a small to moderate size ventricular septal defect. If pulmonary and systemic resistances are similar, there is a balanced shunt with nearly equal pulmonary and systemic blood flows at rest. Lastly, when resistance to pulmonary outflow exceeds systemic resistance, there is a net right-to-left shunt, and systemic flow is greater than pulmonary flow.

Cyanosis may be mild or undetectable at rest in patients with tetralogy of Fallot but usually becomes apparent or increases with physical activity. With exercise, increased cardiac output and decreased systemic arteriolar resistance result in a considerable increase in the degree of right-to-left shunting. While effective cardiac output is maintained, right-to-left shunting produces a rapid decrease in systemic arterial oxygen saturation and results in exertional dyspnea and decreased exercise tolerance. In contrast to episodes of paroxysmal hypoxemia (tetralogy spells), the systemic desaturation is limited by the duration of exercise and improves as soon as activity ceases.

Squatting is a common posture in patients with tetralogy of Fallot, particularly in young children who easily assume the more comfortable knee–chest position. Squatting is often seen in children after exercise. They also are frequently seen to assume this position while playing quiet games with their peers who are sitting. It is likely that squatting results in an increase in systemic arterial resistance due to kinking and compression of the major arterial circulation to the lower extremities. This increase in peripheral resistance, in the presence of relatively fixed pulmonary outflow resistance, decreases the degree of right-to-left shunting and increases pulmonary blood flow. The result is an immediate increase in systemic arterial oxygen saturation.

Episodes of paroxysmal hypoxemia, also called hypercyanotic or tetralogy spells, often are seen in infants and children with tetralogy of Fallot and other cardiac malformations with similar physiology. These spells are usually self-limited and last less than 15 to 30 minutes, although they may be longer. The spells are seen more often in the morning but may occur during the day and may be precipitated by activity, a sudden fright, or injury or may occur spontaneously without any apparent cause. The spell is characterized by increasing cyanosis and an increased rate and depth of respiration. The physiologic change that produces a hypoxemic spell is an increase in right-to-left shunting and concomitant decrease in pulmonary blood flow. The exact mechanism by which this occurs is unknown.

## DIAGNOSIS

The presentation of patients with tetralogy of Fallot ranges from the small infant with severe hypoxemia to the asymptomatic child with "pink tetralogy." The severity of symptoms is related to the degree of pulmonary stenosis. Cyanosis usually is present in the neonate with severe tetralogy of Fallot or with associated pulmonary atresia. Another relatively common presentation is the asymptomatic infant with a heart murmur. These patients may seem to have only a ventricular septal defect because the murmur of the right ventricular outflow obstruction in the infant with tetralogy of Fallot may be indistinguishable from that of an isolated ventricular septal defect. The presence of significant right ventricular hypertrophy on the electrocardiogram may be a clue to the nature of the underlying abnormality.

Cyanosis and clubbing may be present on physical examination of the child with tetralogy of Fallot. There may be an increased left parasternal impulse, indicating right ventricular hypertrophy. The first heart sound is usually normal, whereas the second sound is single because the pulmonary closure sound is very soft. An ejection systolic murmur is heard at the mid-upper left sternal border and may radiate toward the back. Loudness of the murmur depends on the volume of blood crossing the right ventricular outflow tract. As infundibular stenosis becomes more severe, less blood flows through the right ventricular outflow, and the murmur becomes softer and shorter. In the child having a hypoxemic spell, there is much less antegrade flow into the pulmonary arteries and the murmur disappears.

The chest radiograph in older children with tetralogy of Fallot exhibits the classically described "boot-shaped" heart. This is caused by mild enlargement of the right ventricle and concavity of the upper left heart border caused by absence of the main pulmonary artery segment. In infants, the chest radiograph may be normal or may only show decreased pulmonary vascular markings.

The anatomic features of tetralogy of Fallot are identified by echocardiography. The large ventricular septal defect is easily visualized, and the aorta overriding the ventricular septal defect is apparent. The infundibular narrowing of the right ventricular outflow tract or a thickened and abnormal pulmonary valve usually can be demonstrated. Doppler echocardiography demonstrates an increased velocity of blood flow in the main pulmonary artery and is useful in estimating the gradient across the right ventricular outflow tract.

Cardiac catheterization and angiocardiography are important in the evaluation of the patient with tetralogy of Fallot. In the preoperative patient, it is important to define the levels and severity of stenosis in the right ventricular outflow tract and pulmonary artery and to predict whether the repair is likely to be successful. Associated abnormalities such as multiple ventricular septal defects or coronary artery abnormalities that might adversely affect the success of surgical repair also can be demonstrated. In the postoperative patient with residual defects, cardiac catheterization provides an assessment of the hemodynamic result, ventricular function, severity of residual anatomic abnormalities, and electrophysiologic status.

## MEDICAL MANAGEMENT

Although many patients with tetralogy of Fallot are acyanotic in early infancy, the subpulmonary stenosis tends to be progressive and usually results in the appearance of cyanosis during infancy or early childhood. Before the development of systemic to pulmonary artery anastomoses in the mid-1940s, about 50% of patients with tetralogy of Fallot died in the first year of life, and it was unusual for a patient to survive past the third decade. Mortality was usually a consequence of hypoxia, secondary hematologic changes, or problems such as infective endocarditis or brain abscess. With palliative surgical procedures and complete repair, which is possible even during infancy and early childhood, 90% or more of patients with tetralogy of Fallot are expected to survive to adulthood.

Treatment of significant resting hypoxia or hypercyanotic spells is surgical. Medical management in patients with tetralogy of Fallot, therefore, is directed toward treating associated noncardiac abnormalities, avoiding problems associated with anemia or polycythemia, preventing infectious complications such as bacterial endocarditis or brain abscess, and acutely managing paroxysmal hypoxemic spells. Hypoxemic spells usually are self-limited and last less than 15 to 30 minutes, but can be prolonged. In addition to comforting the patient during one of these episodes, the patient should assume the knee–chest position. Squatting, or assuming the knee–chest position, may cause increased peripheral resistance in the lower extremities, which, in turn, promotes increased pulmonary blood flow. In a hospital situation, oxygen is administered by face mask during a hypoxemic spell. When combined with the above physical maneuvers, this is often sufficient management for a short spell. If this is not successful and the patient's hypoxemic episode does not appear to resolve, morphine sulfate can be administered either intramuscularly, subcutaneously, or intravenously in a dose of 0.1 mg/kg of body weight. The effectiveness of morphine sulfate in treating hypoxemic spells has been known for many years, but its exact mechanism of action is unclear. Because this drug can be administered intramuscularly, it is valuable to use morphine for initial management of a hypoxemic spell when an intravenous route is unavailable. Once an intravenous line is placed, the dose of morphine sulfate can be repeated. Because metabolic acidosis appears quickly after the onset of a hypoxemic spell, sodium bicarbonate in a dose of 1.0 mEq/kg can be given empirically as soon as intravenous access is available. If these measures are unsuccessful, a beta adrenergic blocking agent such as propranolol is valuable in managing a hypoxemic spell. This drug is given intravenously to a maximum total dose of 0.1 mg/kg of body weight. The total calculated dose should be diluted with 10 mL of fluid in a syringe, and no more than half of the calculated dose should be given initially as an intravenous bolus. The remainder can be given slowly over the next 5 to 10 minutes if necessary. Propranolol also has been used in the long-term nonoperative management of paroxysmal hypoxemic spells. It is administered orally in a dose of 1 to 4 mg/kg of body weight per day in four divided doses.

## SURGICAL MANAGEMENT

Surgical management of patients with tetralogy of Fallot consists of either palliative systemic to pulmonary artery anastomoses (shunts) or complete repair. Palliative procedures do not require cardiopulmonary bypass, thus, can be performed in very small infants or in patients with anatomy that is unfavorable for complete repair. In most centers, primary repair is performed electively during infancy or early childhood if the anatomy is suitable.

Surgical palliation became possible in the 1940s with the development of the Blalock-Taussig shunt, an end-to-side anastomosis between the subclavian artery and the pulmonary artery. Other forms of systemic to pulmonary artery anastomoses such as the Potts procedure (between the descending aorta and the left pulmonary artery) and the Waterston shunt (between the ascending aorta and the right pulmonary artery) have either been abandoned or are seldomly performed. Currently, a modified Blalock-Taussig or "H type" shunt is popular. This consists of interposition of a synthetic tube between the subclavian artery and the pulmonary artery, thus preserving blood flow to the arm.

Total correction is preferred, if possible, and consists of patch closure of the ventricular septal defect and relief of the right ventricular outflow tract obstruction. Occasionally, infundibular resection alone relieves the subpulmonary stenosis, but placement of a patch of synthetic material to further widen the right ventricular outflow tract is generally necessary. In patients with severe pulmonary stenosis, it may be necessary to extend this patch across the pulmonary valve annulus onto the main pulmonary artery and even out onto the branches when pulmonary artery hypoplasia is present. In some of these patients, homograft conduits are used instead of synthetic material. When reconstruction of the right ventricular outflow tract is not possible, such as when there is an anomalous coronary artery crossing this area, a palliative procedure may be performed initially, thus delaying definitive repair until the patient is older and surgery is technically easier.

## LATE RESULTS

In most centers, more than 90% of patients who undergo complete repair of tetralogy of Fallot will survive to adulthood and have a good functional long-term result. Postoperative hemodynamic abnormalities such as residual ventricular septal defects, or some degree of right ventricular outflow tract obstruction, are often present, but these usually are not severe enough to require reoperation. Some pulmonary regurgitation is often present, especially in patients who have required a transannular right ventricular outflow tract patch. Even significant pulmonary regurgitation, however, is usually well tolerated. Most patients are free of symptoms, rarely requiring further management, and seem able to tolerate pulmonary regurgitation for many years.

Arrhythmias, particularly ventricular ectopy, are of concern in patients who have undergone repair of tetralogy of Fallot. Sudden unexpected death occurs in a small percentage of postoperative patients and may be caused by a ventricular arrhythmia.

The combination of ventricular ectopy and hemodynamic abnormalities, especially residual pulmonary stenosis with high right ventricular pressure and right or left ventricular dysfunction, is especially worrisome and is treated in most centers.

After complete repair, patients with tetralogy of Fallot are still at risk of subacute bacterial endocarditis and should receive appropriate antibiotic prophylaxis. Preservation of good right and left ventricular function and the possible effects of coronary artery disease in a heart with a repaired congenital defect are potential long-term problems.

## Selected Readings

Anderson RA, Allwork SP, Ho SY, et al. Surgical anatomy of tetralogy of Fallot. J Thorac Cardiovasc Surg 1981;81:887.
Bonchek LI, Starr A, Sunderland CO, et al. Natural history of tetralogy of Fallot in infancy: clinical classification and therapeutic implications. Circulation 1973;48:392.
Castaneda AR, Freed MD, Williams RG, et al. Repair of tetralogy of Fallot in infancy. J Thorac Cardiovasc Surg 1977;74:372.
Daily PO, Stinson EB, Griepp RB, et al. Tetralogy of Fallot: choice of surgical procedure. J Thorac Cardiovasc Surg 1978;75:338.
Fuster V, McGoon DC, Kennedy MA, et al. Long-term evaluation (12 to 22 years) of open heart surgery for tetralogy of Fallot. Amer J Cardiol 1980;46:635.
Garson A Jr, Randall DC, Gillette PC, et al. Prevention of sudden death after repair of tetralogy of Fallot: treatment of ventricular arrhythmias. J Am Coll Cardiol 1985;6:221.
Kramer H, Majewski F, Trampisch HJ, et al. Malformation patterns in children with congenital heart disease. Am J Dis Child 1987;141:789.
Moulton AL, Brenner JI, Ringel R, et al. Classic versus modified Blalock-Taussig shunts in neonates and infants. Circulation 1985;72(suppl):II-35.
Poirier RA, McGoon DC, Danielson GK, et al. Late results after repair of tetralogy of Fallot. J Thorac Cardiovasc Surg 1977;75:900.
Shinebourne EA, Anderson RA, Bowyer JJ. Variations in clinical presentation of Fallot's tetralogy in infancy. Br Heart J 1975;37:946.

*Principles and Practice of Pediatrics, Second Edition.*
edited by Frank A. Oski et al. J. B. Lippincott Company, Philadelphia © 1994.

# 81.5 *Double-Outlet Right Ventricle*

## Michael J. Silka

Double-outlet right ventricle (DORV) refers to a diverse group of congenital heart defects identified by the common origin of both the aorta and the pulmonary artery above the morphologic right ventricle. DORV specifies the anatomic relationship of the great arteries to the ventricles; it does not specify circulatory physiology, which is determined largely by the combination of associated congenital heart defects. Historically, a number of terms have been applied to this malformation and subtypes, including Taussig-Bing complex, origin of both great vessels from the right ventricle, and partial transposition.

DORV is rare, representing 1.5% of congenital heart defects, with a predicted incidence of 1 case per 15,000 live births. Although significant association with trisomy-18 and maternal diabetes is recognized, most cases of DORV occur in infants with no other congenital anomalies. The embryologic basis of DORV involves failure of rotation and shift of the truncus arteriosus from above the primitive right ventricle (bulbus cordis) to a more leftward position, which aligns the anlage of the future aorta above the morphologic left ventricle. Varying degrees of this arrest of conoventricular rotation and leftward shift result in the spectrum of congenital heart defects grouped as DORV.

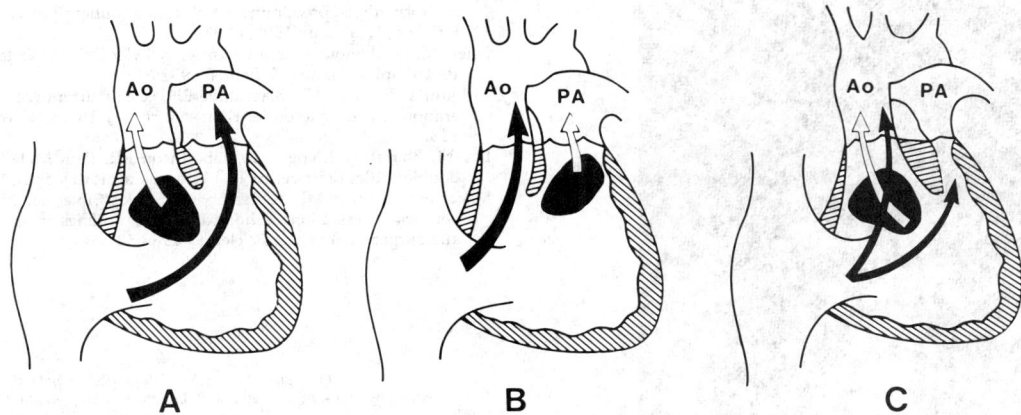

**A**           **B**           **C**

**Figure 81-4.** The three major forms of double-outlet right ventricle, illustrated with the anterior free wall of the right ventricle removed. (**A**) The ventricular septal defect (VSD) is subaortic, and oxygenated blood (*open arrow*) from the left ventricle (LV) is directed preferentially to the aorta (Ao), while the deoxygenated systemic venous return (*solid arrow*) is directed to the pulmonary artery (PA). (**B**) The VSD is subpulmonic, and results in preferential flow of the oxygenated blood from the LV to the PA, while deoxygenated systemic venous return is directed to the aorta, resulting in cyanosis. (**C**) Sub-pulmonic stenosis results in restricted pulmonary blood flow with mixing of both oxygenated and deoxygenated blood in the aorta. The subaortic VSD directs the limited pulmonary venous return to the Ao, resulting in variable degrees of cyanosis.

## ANATOMY AND PHYSIOLOGY

DORV is a specific malformation representing one of the types of malposition of the great arteries. A ventricular septal defect (VSD), which provides the only outlet for the left ventricle, is located beneath either the pulmonary artery or the aorta or, rarely, remote from both great arteries (Fig 81-4). Associated subpulmonic stenosis, which restricts pulmonary blood flow, is present in more than 50% of DORV cases.

The relationship of the VSD to the great arteries and the presence or absence of pulmonic stenosis are primary determinants of the circulatory physiology in DORV. When the VSD is related closely to the aorta (see Fig 81-4A), the resultant physiology is similar to that of a large VSD with a left-to-right shunt and pulmonary hypertension. In this setting, symptoms of congestive heart failure dominate after the anticipated normalization of pulmonary vascular resistance with little or no cyanosis. Conversely, when the pulmonary artery overrides the VSD, without associated pulmonic stenosis (see Fig 81-4B), the hemodynamics simulate those of transposition of the great arteries with a large VSD. Frequently referred to as the Taussig-Bing complex, the clinical features of both cyanosis and congestive heart failure are present. Coarctation of the aorta frequently occurs in association with this form of DORV. In either of these subsets of DORV, natural history is determined by pulmonary vascular resistance and evolution of obstructive pulmonary vascular disease. Severe subpulmonic or pulmonary valvar stenosis occurs most frequently when the VSD is subaortic (see Fig 81-4C). The resultant physiology and clinical manifestations are indistinguishable from tetralogy of Fallot, which is manifested as cyanosis with pulmonary oligemia.

## DIAGNOSTIC CONSIDERATIONS

Clinical features of the types of DORV reflect variations of circulatory physiology and, on physical examination, cannot be differentiated from an isolated large VSD, transposition of the great arteries with a VSD, or tetralogy of Fallot with similar hemodynamics. The chest roentgenogram and electrocardiogram may contain subtle features suggestive of DORV but cannot be considered diagnostic. Accurate diagnosis in each type of DORV is established with two-dimensional echocardiography. The com-

bination of parasternal and apical imaging demonstrates the origin of both great arteries above the right ventricle, the relationship of the VSD to the great arteries, and the presence or absence of pulmonic stenosis and other associated cardiac anomalies (Fig 81-5).

Cardiac catheterization with selective angiography is essential in establishing morphologic details of anatomy before intracardiac repair of DORV. Precise spatial delineation of the relationship of the VSD to the aorta is required, along with determination of the pulmonary vascular resistance and coronary artery anatomy (Fig 81-6).

## SURGICAL PALLIATION AND REPAIR

In the newborn with severe cyanosis due to stenosis of the pulmonary outflow tract in association with DORV, placement of a

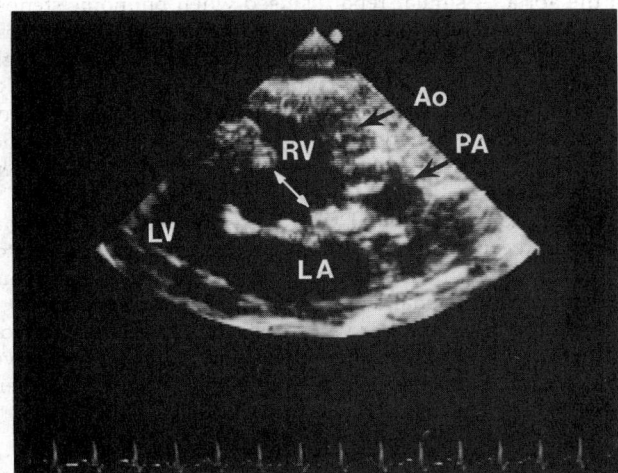

**Figure 81-5.** Echocardiographic features of double-outlet right ventricle. Parasternal long-axis view demonstrating origin of both great arteries above the right ventricle (RV) with the ventricular septal defect (*white arrow*) as the only outlet for the left ventricle (LV). The aorta (Ao) is anterior and remote from the VSD when compared with the pulmonary artery (PA). LA, left atrium.

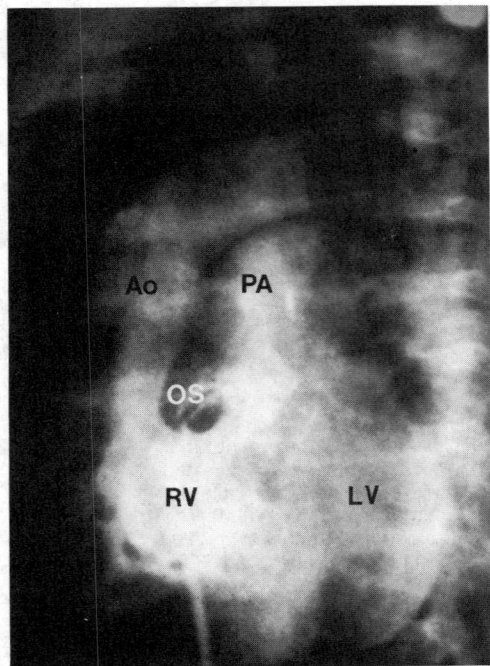

**Figure 81-6.** The angiographic features of double-outlet right ventricle. Lateral view right ventriculogram demonstrating the origin of both great arteries above the right ventricle (RV) with an outlet septum (OS) bifurcating the two outflow tracts. The aorta (Ao) is anterior to the pulmonary artery (PA). The left ventricle (LV) is remote from either great artery.

systemic-pulmonary anastomosis is effective palliation until elective intracardiac repair can be performed at an older age. Similarly, palliative pulmonary artery banding has been used during infancy in types of DORV with unrestricted pulmonary blood flow, in the presence of severe congestive heart failure, and to avoid progression of pulmonary vascular disease. Primary intracardiac repair, however, is increasingly advocated in these subsets of DORV.

Corrective surgical procedures are increasingly successful for most variants of DORV. When the VSD is subaortic, an intraventricular baffle establishes continuity between the left ventricle and the aorta. A similar repair is used when pulmonic stenosis is present, with additional resection of the infundibular stenosis or placement of the homograft conduit to establish right ventricular-pulmonary artery continuity. These forms of DORV are currently managed in accordance with institutional protocols used in patients with a large VSD or tetralogy of Fallot. Experience suggests long-term survival rates exceeding 95% with an excellent functional result.

The surgical approach to DORV with a subpulmonic VSD has evolved in recent years with the development of arterial switch techniques. Ninety percent to 95% operative survival rate and excellent late functional status are reported when the VSD is baffled to the left semilunar valve, followed by arterial and coronary artery translocation. This is significant improvement over repairs based on atrial switch in conjunction with an intraventricular baffle.

## Selected Readings

Bostrom MPG, Hutchins GM. Arrested rotation of the outflow tract may explain double-outlet right ventricle. Circulation 1988;77:1258.

DiDonato RM, Wernovsky G, Walsh EP, et al. Results of the arterial switch operation for transposition of the great arteries with ventricular septal defect. Circulation 1989;80:1689.

Ferenz C, Rubin JD, McCarter RJ, Clark EB. Maternal diabetes and cardiovascular

malformations: predominance of double-outlet right ventricle and truncus arteriosus. Teratology 1990;41:319.

Fyler DC. Double-outlet right ventricle. In: Fyler DC, ed. Nadas' pediatric cardiology. Philadelphia: Hanley & Belfus, 1992:643.

Kirklin JW, Pacifico AD, Blackstone EH, et al. Current risks and protocols for operations for double-outlet right ventricle. J Thorac Cardiovasc Surg 1986;92:913.

Lev M, Bharati S, Meng CCL, Liberthson RR, Paul MH, Idriss F. A concept of double-outlet right ventricle. J Thorac Cardiovasc Surg 1972;64:272.

Macartney FJ, Rigby ML, Anderson RH, Stark J, Silverman NH. Double outlet right ventricle cross sectional echocardiographic findings: their anatomical explanation, and surgical relevance. Br Heart J 1984;52:164.

*Principles and Practice of Pediatrics, Second Edition.*
edited by Frank A. Oski et al. J. B. Lippincott Company, Philadelphia © 1994.

# 81.6 *Eisenmenger's Syndrome*

### Stephen M. Paridon

Eisenmenger's syndrome is a group of cardiac defects that share a common pathophysiology: pulmonary vascular obstructive disease resulting in a right-to-left cardiac level shunting of blood. Although the syndrome has been described since the 19th century, its currently accepted definition generally is credited to Wood (late 1950s). With development of new diagnostic approaches to and surgical therapies for congenital heart defects in the last 30 years, the incidence of Eisenmenger's syndrome has decreased greatly. There is, however, a population with this syndrome that is too old to have benefited from newer medical techniques or is the unfortunate failure of current medical understanding.

## ETIOLOGY AND PATHOPHYSIOLOGY

Eisenmenger's syndrome is not a discrete cardiac defect; rather, it is a group of cardiac defects with the common components of a large cardiac defect that allows the intracardiac shunting of blood with superimposed obstructive pulmonary vascular disease.

Lesions most likely to lead to Eisenmenger's syndrome are those that allow high pulmonary-to-systemic flow ratios in the presence of high pulmonary pressures, such as large defects of the ventricular septum, atrioventricular canal lesions, and patent ductus arteriosus. The presence of hypoxemia, such as occurs in D-transposition of the great arteries with a ventricular septal defect or truncus arteriosus, hastens development of pulmonary vascular disease. Generally, defects with low pulmonary pressures such as atrial septal defects are much less likely to lead to Eisenmenger's syndrome. These lesions, despite their high rate of pulmonary blood flow, usually are tolerated well for decades, whereas high-pressure defects may result in changes in the pulmonary vascular bed in several years or, occasionally, months.

As obstructive pulmonary vascular disease develops, resistance increases in the pulmonary vascular bed. Systemic venous blood, following the course of least resistance, is shunted away from the pulmonary arteries and through the cardiac defect into the systemic circulation. The result is systemic hypoxemia, the degree of which depends on the relative pulmonary-to-systemic vascular resistance. The more severe the pulmonary resistance or the lower the systemic resistance is, the greater is the right-to-left shunting.

At the time of diagnosis of heart disease, the clinical presentation generally is that of congestive heart failure, which results from a high rate of pulmonary blood flow due to large cardiac defects with low pulmonary vascular resistance. In lesions that result in hypoxemia and a high pulmonary blood flow rate, such as D-transposition of the great arteries with ventricular septal defect, cyanosis is superimposed on congestive failure.

As pulmonary vascular resistance increases, signs and symptoms of congestive heart failure decrease. The duration of this change varies from months to decades depending on the presenting cardiac defect and the rate at which vascular changes occur. When pulmonary resistance exceeds systemic resistance, hypoxemia ensues, then progresses as pulmonary vascular resistance rises.

## PHYSICAL FINDINGS

Findings on physical examination of patients with Eisenmenger's syndrome vary depending on the severity of pulmonary obstructive disease. In advanced stages, cyanosis is pronounced. Clubbing of the extremities usually is present. In early cases, cyanosis may be mild or absent, or may become noticeable only when systemic resistance drops, such as with exercise.

Findings of the cardiovascular examination are typical of patients with pulmonary hypertension. The precordium is hyperdynamic, and there may be a right ventricular lift in patients whose defects include a normal right ventricle. The second heart sound is very loud and frequently is palpable at the left upper sternal border due to the pulmonary ($P_2$) component of the second sound. Splitting of the second sound generally is absent or very narrow as a result of the decreased ejection time of the right ventricle in the face of high pulmonary resistance.

Murmurs usually are soft because the intracardiac defects are large, with little pressure gradient between the chambers, and most of the right-to-left shunting of blood in these defects occurs during diastole, which is a period of relatively low pressure. The findings typical of left ventricular failure, such as rales due to pulmonary edema, are absent. In severe cases, evidence of right ventricular failure may be present. Hepatomegaly and peripheral edema may occur in end-stage disease.

## LABORATORY FINDINGS

The chest radiograph in Eisenmenger's syndrome varies with the clinical course. Early in life, before the onset of increased pulmonary vascular resistance, the heart size usually is larger with increased pulmonary vascular markings. There is evidence of flooded pulmonary vasculature and pulmonary edema (Fig 81-7A). The classic chest radiograph for Eisenmenger's syndrome develops after the onset of elevated pulmonary vascular resistance. The cardiac silhouette is small to normal. Proximal pulmonary arteries are dilated and tortuous. There generally is diminished distal pulmonary vasculature giving the lung fields a black appearance in the periphery (Fig 81-7B). Late in the clinical course, cardiomegaly also can be seen where right-sided cardiac decompensation has occurred. Pulmonary vasculature, however, remains sparse and tortuous (Fig 81-7C).

Findings on electrocardiogram are nonspecific and generally reflect the underlying lesion rather than being specific for pulmonary vascular disease. Ventricular enlargement, usually of both chambers if they are present, is common. Enlargement of the atria, especially the right atrium, may occur with the onset of significant atrioventricular valve regurgitation.

Two dimensional echocardiography is useful in delineating the anatomy of the underlying cardiac defects. Doppler echocardiography generally allows accurate prediction of the pulmonary artery pressures. Pulmonary vascular resistance cannot be measured accurately by noninvasive means. In select cases,

however, the evidence of right-to-left shunting through such structures as the ductus arteriosus may be highly suggestive of elevated pulmonary vascular resistance.

In early mild cases, cardiac catheterization frequently is required to enable diagnosis of obstructive pulmonary vascular disease. This is crucial, because there are few cardiac lesions that cannot be corrected or palliated surgically in the absence of advanced pulmonary vascular disease. Pulmonary vascular resistance and reactivity of the pulmonary bed to conditions that result in vasodilatation or constriction must be assessed carefully.

Polycythemia generally is found after the onset of significant right-to-left shunt, and increases as hypoxemia worsens. As a result, the hematocrit frequently increases to the 60% to 70% range. Because of increased red blood-cell production and high iron demands, red-cell indices frequently show indications of a relative iron deficiency anemia despite an overall polycythemia.

## CLINICAL COURSE

The onset of significant vascular changes varies from as early as several months to as late as many years after birth. Large atrial septal defects, for example, seldom result in pulmonary obstructive disease until well into the adult years, while a child with Down syndrome and an atrioventricular canal defect may have significant disease at as early as 2 or 3 months of age.

In patients who initially have large left-to-right shunt lesions, there is a period of hemodynamic stability that follows the onset of obstructive pulmonary vascular disease. During this time, the amount of left-to-right shunting decreases and symptoms of congestive failure improve. Heart size usually decreases and exercise tolerance may improve, as does general well-being. Initially, the predominance of cardiac shunting remains left to right, with evidence of occasional bidirectional flow.

As pulmonary vascular changes progress, the left-to-right shunting decreases and the right-to-left shunting begins to predominate. With the onset of clinically evident hypoxemia, the patient's hemodynamic status usually deteriorates at an accelerated pace. Complications of systemic hypoxemia begin to arise. The effects of polycythemia and hypoxemia on pulmonary vascular resistance further compromise pulmonary blood flow.

Studies examining polycythemia and blood viscosity generally have found that viscosity increases exponentially with hematocrit. The crucial value appears to be the 70% to 75% range. At this hematocrit level, blood viscosity increases dramatically. In addition, studies indicate that both systemic and especially pulmonary vascular resistance increase exponentially with hematocrit as a result of the increase in viscosity. Coronary artery blood flow also decreases significantly as hematocrit increases, although the degree of decrease in oxygen delivery to the myocardium appears to be less than that to systemic tissues.

Generally, the presence of a mild degree of polycythemia resulting in a modest increase in hematocrit to the 55% to 65% range results in increased systemic oxygen delivery. When hematocrit rises above about the 70% range, blood viscosity rises dramatically. This results in decreased oxygen delivery because of decreased cardiac output, despite an increase in the oxygen-carrying capacity of the blood due to the increased hematocrit.

Clinically, the manifestations of polycythemia vary. Some patients may complain only of headaches or general malaise. Anorexia, dyspnea, and visual disturbances have been seen frequently. More severe problems such as thrombi or embolic events are less common but occur often enough to be a significant source of concern to the clinician. This is particularly true of central nervous system events, which may present initially with manifestations seen more commonly in polycythemia than as a frank focal deficit.

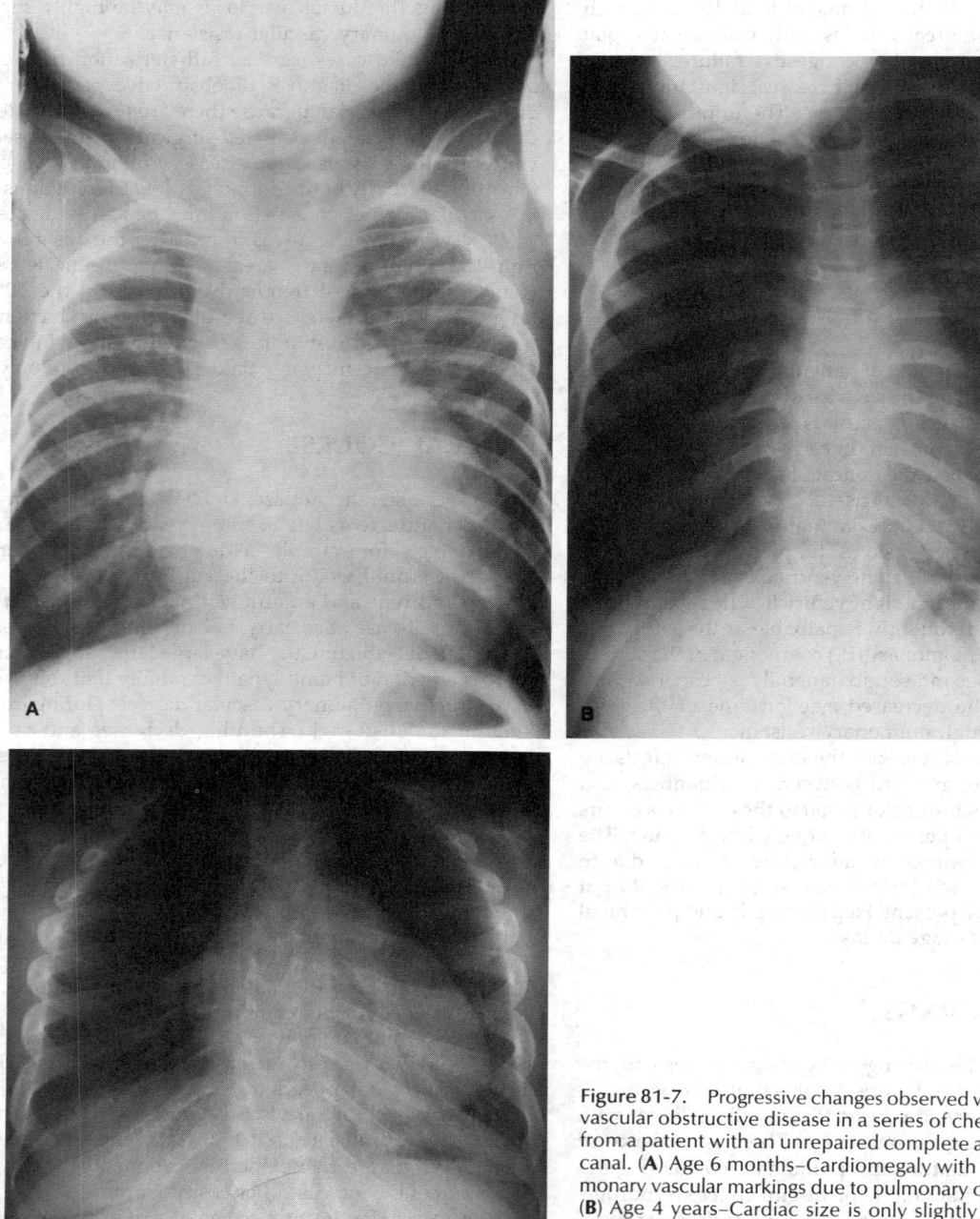

**Figure 81-7.** Progressive changes observed with pulmonary vascular obstructive disease in a series of chest radiographs from a patient with an unrepaired complete atrioventricular canal. (**A**) Age 6 months–Cardiomegaly with increased pulmonary vascular markings due to pulmonary overcirculation. (**B**) Age 4 years–Cardiac size is only slightly enlarged with prominent main pulmonary arteries but diminished peripheral lung field vasculature. (**C**) Age 15 years–Cardiomegaly due to dilated, poorly functioning ventricles. Main pulmonary arteries are prominent but peripheral vasculature remains sparse.

Causes of these findings are not known, although hyperviscosity and red blood-cell aggregation seem to play a major role. In addition, abnormalities of platelet function are noted in these patients. Platelet half-life often appears to be reduced, and an absolute thrombocytopenia is not uncommon. Because of these abnormalities, the incidence of hemorrhage, especially postoperatively, is high in patients with polycythemia and hypoxemia.

Long-term survival rates in these patients vary because of both the age of onset for pulmonary changes and complicating factors, such as Down syndrome, that may affect survival adversely. Usually, death occurs in the second and third decades of life. Variation is great, and survival into the fifth decade has been reported.

Causes of death vary, but often the terminal events result from a combination of hypoxia and the resulting arrhythmia. The occurrence of acute hypoxemic episodes during medical procedures (eg, phlebotomy) that terminate in intractable ventricular arrhythmias lends credence to the notion that sudden death in these patients is probably the result of this mechanism; this is particularly likely if exercise-related sudden death occurs.

Complications of endocarditis, brain abscess, and cerebrovascular accidents are also causes of death related to the patient's hypoxemia and polycythemia. Changes in the pulmonary vascular bed result in increased incidence of hemoptysis and pulmonary hemorrhage. Large pulmonary hemorrhage resulting in increasing hypoxemia as well as systemic hypotension can be fatal in these patients.

## THERAPEUTIC CONSIDERATIONS

Over the last decade, the increasingly successful use of combined heart–lung and isolated lung transplants has offered new hope for a cure to this previously incurable cardiopulmonary problem. A combined heart–lung transplant is used in patients when the nature of the cardiovascular defect is too complex to allow easy surgical repair or if the myocardial function is significantly impaired. In the last 5 years, the use of a single-lung–heart transplant has become increasingly popular, both because of scarcity of donors and of donor recipient size-matching difficulties. The use of either a bilateral or single-lung transplant and repair of the cardiac defect has been undertaken in those patients with relatively simple defects that are readily amenable to surgical repair, such as an isolated ventricular septal defect or patent ductus arteriosus.

Although heart–lung transplantation is a promising area of therapeutic investigation, morbidity and mortality remain considerable and the long-term outcome uncertain. It should generally be reserved for those patients with severe symptomatology. In patients who do not warrant immediate consideration for transplantation or when transplantation is not a therapeutic option, care should consist of monitoring and treating the sequelae that occur as a consequence of chronic hypoxemia as well as the pulmonary vascular changes.

Hemoglobin status of patients should be monitored closely. An increased blood hemoglobin content is required to maintain systemic oxygen delivery in the normal range as hypoxemia increases. This is beneficial as long as the hematocrit does not rise above the 60% to 65% range. Above this level, blood viscosity increases dramatically, and phlebotomy should be performed to lower the hematocrit to a safe range.

Of equal importance, anemia should not be tolerated because it seriously compromises oxygen delivery. Anemia in these patients is relative and occurs with hematocrits in the normal to high–normal range due to the need for increased hemoglobin to expand oxygen-carrying capacity. Regular monitoring of red blood-cell indices alerts the clinician to any evidence of iron deficiency; if present, it should be treated with iron supplements.

An intracardiac right-to-left shunt predisposes patients with Eisenmenger's syndrome to paradoxical embolization and endocarditis. Septic embolization secondary to endocarditis also may occur. Any significant infection should be evaluated for the possibility of endocarditis. The clinician also should be alert to any central nervous system changes that might appear to be due to polycythemia but could be a manifestation of a cerebral embolus or abscess.

Vasodilators of many types have been tried in patients with obstructive pulmonary vascular disease. They have shown limited results, partly because of the lack of responsiveness of the pulmonary bed, which has a relatively fixed obstruction, and partly because these vasodilators have the same or more vasodilating effect on the systemic vascular bed. Currently, calcium channel blockers are the vasodilators used most widely; they have significant effect in less than 15% to 20% of the patient population.

Antiplatelet drugs frequently are used in an attempt to slow progression of pulmonary vascular changes. Histologically, these changes appear similar to the atherosclerotic lesions of coronary artery disease, and the rationale for treatment with antiplatelet drugs is based on the favorable response of coronary artery lesions

to these drugs. Aspirin and dipyridamole are the drugs used most often. Dosage generally is similar to that for adults with coronary artery disease, but remains controversial. Long-term benefits of this therapy remain to be proven.

Last, the physician should be careful when performing any medical procedure on patients with Eisenmenger's syndrome. This can be a time of high risk for cardiac decompensation. Procedures such as phlebotomy and cardiac catheterization, which decrease circulating volume and systemic vascular resistance, can result in increased hypoxemia and tissue hypoxia if circulating volume is not maintained carefully. Surgical procedures and use of general anesthetic agents can result in vascular volume shifts as well as an increased incidence of ventricular arrhythmias. Hypoventilation and resultant acidosis should be avoided during medical procedures. Embolic events, especially air emboli from intravenous lines, should be avoided because of the presence of right-to-left shunt in these patients. Careful monitoring as outlined here can maximize the chances of an uneventful medical procedure in these very labile patients.

## Selected Readings

Beekman RH, Turi DT. Acute hemodynamic effects of increasing hemoglobin concentration in children with a right-to-left ventricular shunt and relative anemia. J Am Coll Cardiol 1985;5:357.

Boerboom LE, et al. Aspirin or dipyridamole individually prevent lipid accumulation in primate vein bypass grafts. Am J Cardiol 1985;55:556.

Kawaguchi A, Gandjbakhch I, Pavie A, et al. Heart and unilateral lung transplantation in patients with end-stage cardiopulmonary disease and previous thoracic surgery. J Thorac Cardiovasc Surg 1989;98:343.

McLeod AA, Jewitt DE. Drug treatment of primary pulmonary hypertension. Drugs 1986;31:177.

Nihill MR. The pathogenesis of pulmonary arteriosclerosis: prophylaxis with drugs that affect platelet aggregation. Cardiovascular Diseases, Bulletin of the Texas Heart Institute 1974;1:137.

Nihill MR. Pulmonary hypertension and pulmonary vascular disease. Chest 1980;77:581.

Packer M. Vasodilator therapy for primary pulmonary hypertension: limitations and hazards. Ann Intern Med 1985;103:258.

Rosenthal A, et al. Acute hemodynamic effects of red-cell volume reduction in polycythemia of cyanotic congenital heart disease. Circulation 1970;42:297.

Sherry S. Aspirin and antiplatelet drugs: the clinical approach. Cardiovascular Reviews and Reports 1984;5:1208.

Steele P, Ellis JH, Weily HS, Genton E. Platelet survival time in patients with hypoxemia and pulmonary hypertension. Circulation 1977;55:660.

Wood P. The Eisenmenger syndrome, or pulmonary hypertension with reversed central shunt. BMJ 1958;2:701.

*Principles and Practice of Pediatrics, Second Edition.*
edited by Frank A. Oski et al. J. B. Lippincott Company, Philadelphia © 1994.

## 81.7 *Single Ventricle*

### Edward V. Colvin

A univentricular atrioventricular (AV) connection is created when both atria are connected to a single chamber within the ventricular mass. Even though most of these hearts have two chambers within the ventricular mass, "single ventricle" is the name most often used.

## NOMENCLATURE

Segmental approach to nomenclature is necessary to describe these hearts (Fig 81-8). Atrial situs may be solitus, inversus, or

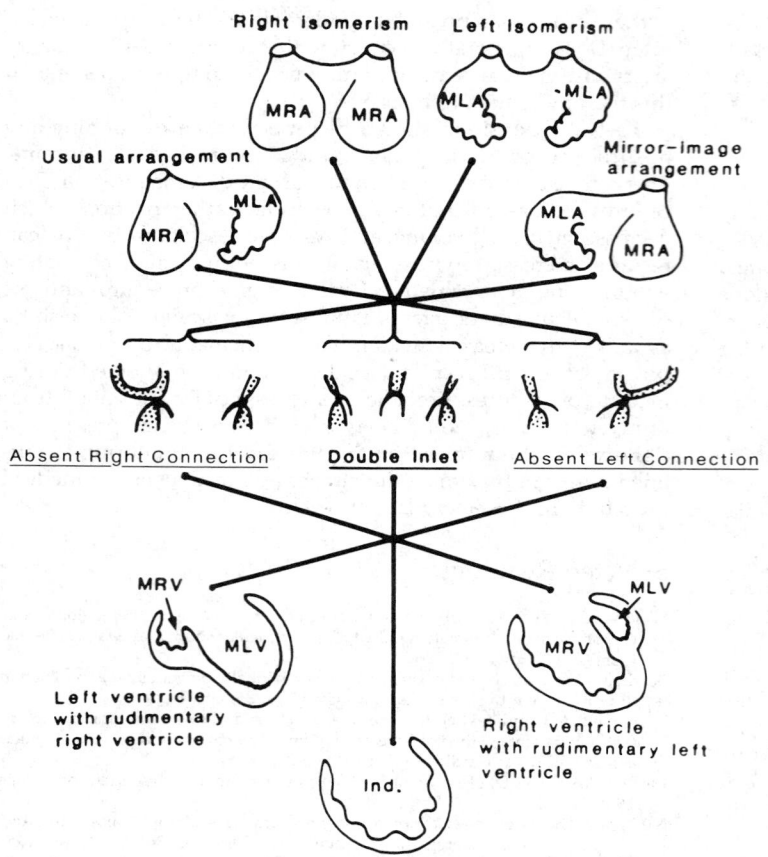

**Figure 81-8.**    Diagram of atrial situs, modes of atrioventricular connection, and types of ventricular morphology. (Becker AE, Anderson RH, Penkoske PA, Zuberbuhler JR. Morphology of double inlet ventricle. In: Anderson RH, Crupi G, Parenzan L, eds. Double inlet ventricle. Tunbridge Wells, Kent: Castle House Publications, 1987:36.)

ambiguous with bilateral right or left morphology. The type of AV connection is, by definition, univentricular. The mode of connection may be double inlet, absent left, or absent right AV connection. In double-inlet connection, the two atria may be connected to the ventricle by two separate AV valves or via a common valve. The two AV valves usually do not have typical characteristics of mitral and tricuspid valves and are, therefore, referred to as *right* and *left* based on the anatomic location of the atrium to which they are connected.

In descriptive morphologic terms, a *complete ventricle* may have inlet, apical trabecular, and outlet components. The apical trabecular portion usually can be used to classify a chamber as being of right or left morphology. In the morphologically right ventricle, the apical component has characteristic coarse trabeculations. In contrast, the apical component of the morphologically left ventricle has much finer crisscrossing trabeculations and a smooth septal surface.

When two chambers are found within the ventricular mass, one has a right and the other a left ventricular apical trabecular component. The ventricle receiving the AV valve or valves usually is larger and termed the *dominant* ventricle. The other ventricle is described as *nondominant*, or rudimentary. The nondominant ventricle usually is small, but size varies. *Outlet chamber* and *trabecular pouch* describe a nondominant ventricle with and without an outlet component, respectively.

The spatial relation of the two ventricles is an important variable and must be specified. This has been designated by various authors as D or L loop, right- or left-hand ventricular architecture, and noninverted or inverted ventricles. When two ventricles are present, the communication between them is properly termed a *ventricular septal defect* (VSD). The terms *outlet foramen* and *bulboventricular foramen* also have been used to describe the VSD.

If two great vessels are present, the ventriculoarterial connection may be concordant, discordant, or double outlet. Single outlet may be present with a common arterial trunk or with aortic or pulmonary atresia.

## ANATOMY

Hearts with univentricular AV connection are subdivided according to ventricular morphology into three basic types: hearts with dominant left, dominant right, or indeterminate ventricular morphology. Dominant left or dominant right ventricular morphology can occur with D loop or L loop (Fig 81-9).

The most common type is called *double-inlet left ventricle*, or single LV. The nondominant ventricle usually is located anteriorly and to the left. It usually gives rise to one or both of the great vessels.

Hearts in which the dominant chamber possesses an apical trabecular portion of right ventricular type are called *double-inlet right ventricle*, or single RV. The nondominant ventricle is located posteriorly. Usually, this chamber has neither inlet nor outlet components.

Hearts in which only one abnormally trabeculated ventricle is found are termed hearts with *univentricular AV connection and indeterminate ventricular morphology*, or single ventricle with morphologically undetermined myocardium.

Hearts have been described in which the ventricular mass contains a trabecular pattern typical of a right ventricle on one side and of a left ventricle on the other with only a tiny rim of apical ventricular septum. These hearts have *biventricular AV connection with a large VSD*.

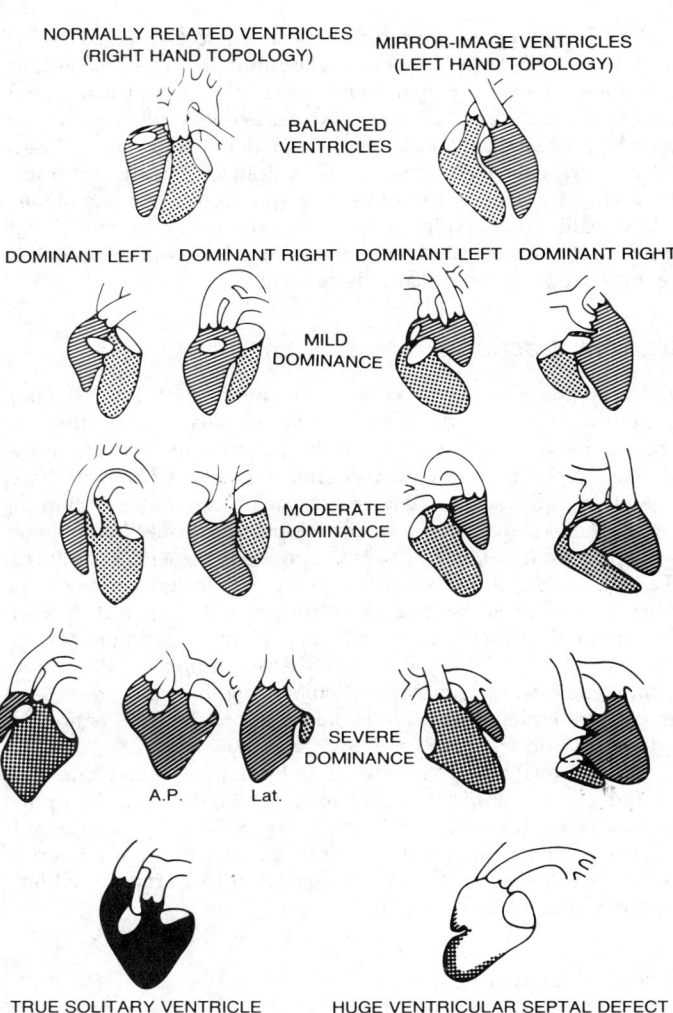

**Figure 81-9.** Spectrum of hearts with one large and one small ventricle. Hearts are traced from angiograms. (Bargeron LM. Angiography of double inlet ventricle. In: Anderson RH, Crupi G, Parenzan L, eds. Double inlet ventricle. Tunbridge Wells, Kent: Castle House Publications, 1987:146.)

## INCIDENCE

Single ventricle is found in about 1% of children with congenital heart defects. While most patients have no chromosomal abnormality, case reports document occasional association. Occurrence in siblings has been reported. Of 237 hearts in one series, 140 had dominant LV, 34 dominant RV, and 41 indeterminant morphology. Associated cardiovascular anomalies are common.

## CLINICAL FINDINGS

Most patients present early in life with cyanosis or congestive heart failure. A few children who are palliated optimally early in life present later in childhood with asymptomatic murmur and mild clinical cyanosis. A few neonates with left outflow obstruction have onset of poor perfusion when the ductus closes in the first few days of life.

Pulmonary stenosis is present in about 67% and atresia in 5% of cases. In earlier series, patients with atresia died without coming to surgery. More recently, the widespread availability of prostaglandin E₁ allows more of these patients to survive to operation. With stenosis, there is a harsh ejection-quality murmur at the base of the heart. With atresia, there is a continuous murmur from ductal patency.

Patients without pulmonary stenosis may present with a murmur or gallop in the first few days of life, but clinical symptoms usually do not become apparent until 3 to 6 weeks of age when the fall in pulmonary vascular resistance allows excessive pulmonary blood flow. The findings at that time are those of congestive heart failure with tachypnea, subcostal retraction, poor feeding, hepatomegaly, and splenomegaly.

In patients with left AV valve atresia or severe stenosis and nearly intact interatrial septum, symptoms of pulmonary venous hypertension may develop as arteriolar resistance falls and pulmonary blood flow increases.

Subaortic obstruction may present early. If present, the fetal circulation pattern usually is quite abnormal, and often there is a reduction in the size of the ascending aorta and severe coarctation or interruption of the aortic arch. If there is associated coarctation and the ductus has closed, femoral pulses decrease. If the ductus is patent, there may be palpable lower-extremity pulses in the presence of severe coarctation or interruption.

### Chest Radiograph and Electrocardiogram

Findings on the chest radiograph depend on the degree of pulmonary outflow obstruction. With moderately restricted pulmonary blood flow, there generally is near-normal heart size and pulmonary vascular markings are normal. When pulmonary blood flow is obstructed severely, the pulmonary vascular markings are decreased. When there is little or no pulmonary stenosis, there is cardiomegaly with increased pulmonary vascular markings. If pulmonary venous return is obstructed severely, the lung fields assume a reticular pattern.

Electrocardiographic findings vary. Usually, there is sinus rhythm and the PR interval is normal, although first-degree heart block is present in about 30% of patients. None of the patients with first-degree heart block have progressed to complete heart block during follow-up. Congenital complete heart block is present in a few patients. Efforts to relate findings on scalar electrocardiogram or the vectorcardiogram with the morphologic type of ventricular mass have been disappointing.

### Two-Dimensional and Doppler Echocardiography

Two-dimensional echocardiography reduces greatly the time required to make the diagnosis. Pulsed range-gated Doppler sampling enables detection of any flow in the ductus and differentiation of venous from arterial structures in complicated cases. Insufficiency of AV valves can be detected and semiquantitated. Color flow mapping provides similar information quickly. Continuous wave Doppler enables quantitation of gradients.

Usually, structure and physiology are demonstrated well by these techniques and catheterization can be directed to obtaining information not available by echocardiography. In many cases, catheterization can be postponed safely until the child is larger and less fragile.

### Catheterization and Angiography

Timing of the catheterization may be dictated by the need in the newborn period for balloon atrial septostomy, shunting, or banding. Catheterization may demonstrate streaming of arterial and venous blood within the heart, so pulmonary and aortic oxygen saturations may differ significantly. The primary determinant of the systemic oxygen saturation is the amount of pulmonary arterial blood flow relative to the systemic blood flow (Qp/Qs).

Angiography has played a major role in the understanding of hearts with univentricular AV connection. Axial angiography enables clearer demonstration of anatomy. In the fragile newborn, interest often is in the anatomy crucial to planning a shunt procedure, and some injections may be deferred until later infancy.

## NATURAL HISTORY

Case reports document survival into adulthood, and female patients have experienced successful pregnancy. Most patients exhibit exercise intolerance and cyanosis. Causes of death include dysrhythmia or sudden, unexplained death, congestive heart failure, thrombotic occlusion of the pulmonary valve, brain abscess, pancreatitis, cerebral infarction, cerebral embolus and hemorrhage, and pulmonary embolus.

## SURGERY

The dismal natural history for this group of patients has motivated development of a number of palliative procedures and two more radical "curative" procedures. Palliative procedures include systemic-to-pulmonary artery shunts, pulmonary-artery banding, atrial septectomy, atrial switch procedures, superior vena caval-to-right pulmonary artery anastomosis, and a number of procedures to relieve subaortic obstruction. The goal is to relieve symptoms and to allow survival to an age when a more "curative" procedure can be performed. It is important to decide early in the life of the patient which "curative" operations are possible to establish the goals of early palliative surgery.

Subaortic stenosis is an ominous finding in this group of patients. When subaortic stenosis is present with or without previous banding, a number of operations have been attempted to achieve palliation, including enlargement of the ventricular defect, placement of a left ventricular-to-descending aorta conduit, and anastomosis of the pulmonary artery to the ascending aorta with placement of a shunt.

### Fontan Procedure Versus Septation

The Fontan-Kreutzer operation used the single ventricle in tricuspid atresia to generate systemic blood flow while allowing pulmonary flow to occur directly from the right atrium to the pulmonary artery. This concept was extended to treatment of other forms of univentricular atrioventricular connection. The risk of operation is 5% to 10%. Presence of a significant subaortic gradient is associated with a high operative mortality rate. For the Fontan procedure in general, death after hospital dismissal is uncommon. Late problems include ventricular dysfunction, atrioventricular valve insufficiency, atrial arrhythmia, and protein-losing enteropathy. Exercise testing in survivors is mildly subnormal.

When two AV valves are present, the single ventricle may be septated by a large patch. Overall operative mortality rates were high during the early experience. Postoperative complete heart block is common. There have been late postoperative sudden deaths. A better outcome has been described for an ideal set of patients. Recently, a two-stage approach has been reported. In infants, a patch is placed at the apex and a second patch between the AV valves. Widely spaced sutures are used. A pulmonary artery band is placed. A second stage is undertaken 6 to 18 months later when the VSD is closed and the band is removed.

The Fontan operation recently has been performed as a two-step procedure, with an initial cavopulmonary anastomosis and subsequent secondary operation to divert the inferior vena caval flow to the pulmonary artery. It also has been modified to include an initial fenestration in the atrial septal defect that can be closed later by catheter techniques, thus avoiding a second operation as a part of a staged procedure. Application of these techniques allows palliation of patients who otherwise would be considered poor candidates for the Fontan operation. Early operative risk is reduced by both these methods as well.

### Current Practice

There is still controversy concerning the best approach to the patient with two good AV valves. For an ideal patient, the operative risks of septation and of the Fontan-type operation are similar. Improved operative risk after the Fontan-Kreutzer–type operation and the good late results make this the operation of choice for patients for whom either operation could be applied.

If pulmonary atresia or severe stenosis is present, a modified Blalock-Taussig shunt is placed. As the patient grows, cyanosis usually progresses and a second shunt may be required. A total cavopulmonary anastomosis may be performed as an initial step toward a Fontan operation. If ventricular function, AV valve competency, and pulmonary vascular structures are acceptable, an elective Fontan operation is planned for when the patient is between 2 and 5 years of age.

If early evaluation reveals no pulmonary stenosis and the anatomy seems unlikely to lead to subaortic stenosis, then pulmonary artery banding may be undertaken. Septation is reserved as an option for older patients with optimal internal anatomy and moderate elevation in pulmonary artery resistance for whom Fontan repair is not advisable.

## Selected Readings

Anderson RH, et al. The univentricular atrioventricular connection: getting to the root of a thorny problem. Am J Cardiol 1984;54:882.

Becker AE, Anderson RH, Penkoske PA, Zuberbuhler JR. Morphology of double inlet ventricle. In: Anderson RH, Crupi G, Parenzan L, eds. Double inlet ventricle. Tunbridge Wells, Kent: Castle House Publications, 1987:36.

Colvin EV. Single ventricle. In: Garson A Jr, Bricker JT, McNamara DG, eds. The science and practice of pediatric cardiology. Philadelphia: Lea and Febiger, 1988.

Crupi G, et al. Palliative surgery. In: Anderson RH, Crupi G, Parenzan L, eds. Double inlet ventricle. Tunbridge Wells, Kent: Castle House Publications, 1987:165.

Danielson GK. Surgical management of double inlet ventricle. In: Anderson RH, Crupi G, Parenzan L, eds. Double inlet ventricle. Tunbridge Wells, Kent: Castle House Publications, 1987:174.

Ebert PA. Staged partitioning of single ventricle. J Thorac Cardiovasc Surg 1984;88:908.

Freedom RM. The dinosaur and banding of the main pulmonary trunk in the heart with functionally one ventricle and transposition of the great arteries: a saga of evolution and caution. J Am Coll Cardiol 1987;10:427.

Huhta JC, et al. Two-dimensional echocardiographic spectrum of univentricular atrioventricular connection. J Am Coll Cardiol 1985;5:149.

Kopf, GS, et al. Fenestrated Fontan operation with delayed transcatheter closure of atrial septal defect. J Thorac Cardiovasc Surg 1992;103(6):139.

Pacifico AD, Stefanelli G, Kirklin JW, Kirklin JK. Septation operation. In: Anderson RH, Crupi G, Parenzan L, eds. Double inlet ventricle. Tunbridge Wells, Kent: Castle House Publications, 1987:183.

Van Praagh R, Ongley PA, Swan HJC. Anatomic types of single or common ventricle in man. Morphologic and geometric aspects of 60 necropsied cases. Am J Cardiol 1964;13:367.

*Principles and Practice of Pediatrics, Second Edition.*
edited by Frank A. Oski et al. J. B. Lippincott Company, Philadelphia © 1994.

# 81.8 *Hypoplastic Left Heart Syndrome*

## Gerald Barber

The term *hypoplastic left heart syndrome* describes a spectrum of congenital cardiac anomalies in which there is an underdeveloped left ventricle and ascending aorta. Severe mitral stenosis, mitral hypoplasia, or mitral atresia is seen in 84% of cases; common atrioventricular canal with the atrioventricular valve malaligned to the right with respect to the muscular ventricular septum accounts for the remaining 16%.

## EPIDEMIOLOGY

The frequency of hypoplastic left heart syndrome is about 0.36 per 1000 live births, and, before surgical palliation was possible, it was responsible for 23% of neonatal deaths due to congenital heart disease. As with other left-sided obstructive lesions, there is a male predominance, with about 60% of cases occurring in males. When hypoplastic left heart syndrome occurs in females, Turner's syndrome should be considered.

## PHYSIOLOGY

Patients with hypoplastic left heart syndrome have complex preoperative physiology. Because of the hypoplasia of the left ventricle and ascending aorta, the right ventricle must maintain both systemic and pulmonary output. This requires both left-to-right shunting of pulmonary venous return and right-to-left shunting of right ventricular output. If the pulmonary veins return normally to the left atrium, as is the usual case, the left-to-right shunt must occur through either a stretched foramen ovale or a true atrial septal defect. The right-to-left shunt must occur through the ductus arteriosus. The carotid, subclavian, and coronary arteries are perfused retrograde via the ductus arteriosus. With the aorta and pulmonary arteries connected in parallel, the percentage of right ventricular stroke volume that goes to the systemic and pulmonary circuits depends on the relative resistances of each of these circuits. Because fetal circulation involves a patent ductus arteriosus with low systemic resistance, high pulmonary resistance, and oxygenation in the placenta, the infant with hypoplastic left heart syndrome develops normally in utero. After birth, lungs are the source of oxygenation. Patency of the ductus arteriosus is required for adequate systemic blood flow. Usually, systemic and pulmonary perfusion remain adequate in the presence of a nonrestrictive ductus. Occasionally, excessive pulmonary blood flow develops when the pulmonary to systemic resistance ratio falls rapidly. In these cases, arterial oxygen saturation increases secondary to the high pulmonary blood flow, but metabolic acidosis ensues because of marginal systemic perfusion. In less than 5% of cases, inadequate pulmonary blood flow and severe cyanosis result from a congenitally small foramen ovale. Metabolic acidosis ensues in these patients because of inadequate oxygen delivery.

## CLINICAL FEATURES

### History

Because systemic perfusion and oxygenation are normal in utero, the infant frequently appears normal at birth and has normal Apgar scores. When hypoplastic left heart syndrome presents with marked cyanosis on the first day of life, severe obstruction to blood flow at the interatrial level (congenitally small or absent foramen ovale) usually is present. More typically, on day 2 or 3 of life, the patient with hypoplastic left heart syndrome develops cyanosis, tachypnea, and respiratory distress. As the ductus arteriosus closes, systemic perfusion is compromised and acidosis develops. If the ductus arteriosus remains patent, however, the onset of cyanosis and respiratory distress could be delayed for weeks.

### Physical Examination

On physical examination, the child with hypoplastic left heart syndrome usually is mildly cyanotic, tachypneic, and tachycardiac. Peripheral pulses are normal to absent depending on the degree of ductal closure at the time of evaluation. Although rales occasionally may be heard, breath sounds are usually normal. The right ventricular impulse is dominant with a diminished left ventricular (apical) impulse. Auscultation usually reveals a normal S1 and a single S2 that is increased in intensity. A nonspecific soft grade 1-3/6 systolic murmur, reflecting relative pulmonic stenosis, is commonly heard at the left sternal border. In rare cases with a dysplastic pulmonary valve, an early systolic ejection click may be heard.

### Electrocardiogram

The underlying pathology is reflected in the electrocardiogram. About 30% to 40% of patients have right atrial enlargement and about 80% to 90% have right ventricular hypertrophy with a qR, rSR', or pure R wave pattern in lead $V_1$. Q waves usually are absent in the lateral precordial leads and 30% to 40% percent of patients have diminished left ventricular forces. A leftward superior axis usually is present in patients with malaligned common atrioventricular canal.

### Chest Radiograph

Cardiomegaly and increased pulmonary vascular markings typically are seen in the chest x-ray of patients with hypoplastic left heart syndrome. A reticular pattern similar to that seen in obstructed total anomalous pulmonary venous connection may be seen in patients with a severely restrictive atrial septal defect.

### Two-Dimensional and Doppler Echocardiography

The diagnosis of hypoplastic left heart syndrome is made by two-dimensional echocardiography (Fig 81-10). Multiple subcostal and suprasternal sweeps should be performed to identify all the features of the lesion. Information obtained from a subcostal window include the relative sizes of the left and right atrium, the pulmonary venous connection, the atrial septal morphology, the right ventricle, the pulmonary artery, the ductus arteriosus and its connection with the descending aorta, the hypoplastic mitral valve, the left ventricle, and the proximal ascending aorta. Both the tricuspid and pulmonic valves should be assessed for evidence of structural anomalies. In cases of malaligned common atrioventricular canal, an ostium primum atrial septal defect and the alignment of the common atrioventricular

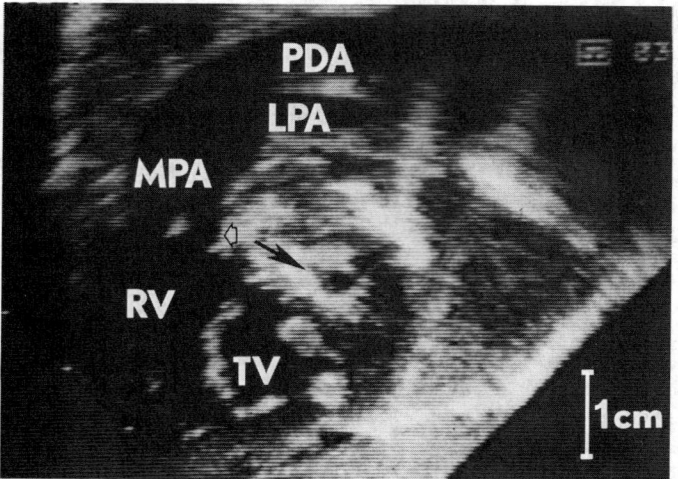

**Figure 81-10.** Echocardiogram demonstrating a subcostal short axis cut in a child with hypoplastic left heart syndrome. *PDA,* patent ductus arteriosus; *LPA,* left pulmonary artery; *MPA,* main pulmonary artery; *RV,* right ventricle; *TV,* tricuspid valve orifice. The solid black arrow points to the hypoplastic left ventricle and the hollow black arrow points to the pulmonary valve.

valve vis-à-vis the muscular ventricular septum should be visualized. From the suprasternal window, the anatomy of the pulmonary veins, ascending aorta, aortic arch, and upper descending aorta should be assessed as well as the continuity and size of the left and right pulmonary arteries. After the anatomic details are determined, physiology is assessed using color flow imaging, pulsed Doppler, and continuous wave Doppler. Detection and quantification of tricuspid (or common atrioventricular valve regurgitation) and pulmonic stenosis are essential. If apparent, the flow pattern across the mitral valve and ascending aorta should be analyzed. Finally, the flow pattern in the ductus arteriosus should be evaluated. Typically, there is systolic right-to-left and diastolic left-to-right flow in the ductus arteriosus. Absence of this diastolic reversal suggests markedly elevated pulmonary resistance, usually secondary to a congenitally small or absent foramen ovale.

## Cardiac Catheterization and Angiography

Because the diagnosis of hypoplastic left heart syndrome is established by echocardiography, cardiac catheterization is not routinely necessary. If cardiac catheterization is performed, a step-up in oxygen saturation is detected in the right atrium consistent with a left-to-right atrial level shunt. Superior vena cava saturations of 23% to 56% with right atrial saturations of 30% to 75% and equivalent right ventricular and aortic saturations of 62% to 80% have been reported (Sinha, 1968). There is usually some obstruction to this left-to-right shunt with elevated left atrial pressure (25 mm Hg) compared to right atrial pressure (12 mm Hg). Right ventricular and pulmonary artery pressures are at systemic levels. An enlarged right atrium, right ventricle, and pulmonary artery are seen on right-sided angiography. The descending aorta fills via the ductus arteriosus. The diminutive stringlike ascending aorta is seen by injecting in the descending aorta.

Although a pressure gradient usually exists between left and right atria, this is usually beneficial for the patient because it limits pulmonary overcirculation and encourages systemic output. Consequently, balloon atrial septotomy during the cardiac catheterization, while it relieves the intra-atrial obstruction, usually results in hemodynamic deterioration.

## NATURAL HISTORY

Patients with hypoplastic left heart syndrome have a poor natural history. If untreated, 90% of affected infants die within the first month of life. Rarely, if the ductus arteriosus remains patent and if pulmonary and systemic resistances are balanced, survival for 4 to 6 years is possible. These latter patients die of pulmonary vascular disease.

## THERAPY

Because patients with hypoplastic left heart syndrome are ductal dependent, therapy consists of preoperative stabilization followed by surgical treatment.

### Preoperative Stabilization

Once the diagnosis of hypoplastic left heart syndrome is made, the infant should be started on prostaglandin $E_1$ or $E_2$ to maintain the ductus arteriosus. Oxygen saturation and acid-base status should be monitored by arterial line, preferably via the umbilical artery to preserve the peripheral arteries for future use. Adequate systemic perfusion needs to be maintained. Because systemic and pulmonary circuits are connected in parallel, systemic perfusion depends on a delicate balance between pulmonary and systemic vascular resistances. Because pulmonary resistance is usually less than systemic resistance, care must be taken not to further decrease it. $PCO_2$ appears to be the chief metabolic factor to influence pulmonary resistance in this group of patients. These patients should, therefore, not be hyperventilated. Because of the effects of oxygen on systemic and pulmonary resistances, hyperoxic ventilation can be harmful. Similarly, unless there is another underlying problem such as sepsis, inotropic agents are usually unnecessary; they can adversely affect the ratio of systemic to pulmonary resistance and may be harmful. Once an adverse pulmonary to systemic perfusion ratio is established, it is often difficult to stabilize the patient. There are successful methods of reversing an abnormal pulmonary to systemic perfusion ratio: by increasing pulmonary vascular resistance either by paralysis and deliberate hypoventilation to a $PCO_2$ of 45 to 50 mm Hg or adding carbon dioxide to the inspired air or by reducing systemic vascular resistance with sodium nitroprusside (Norwood, 1991). In the rare patient with a congenitally small or absent foramen ovale, there may be so much obstruction to pulmonary venous drainage that pulmonary blood flow is inadequate. These patients present early with cyanosis and acidosis. Echocardiography reveals a thick atrial septum with no diastolic reversal by Doppler in their ductus arteriosus. It is usually impossible to either stabilize these patients medically or create an adequate intra-atrial communication by blade/balloon septotomy in the cardiac catheterization laboratory. They require emergency surgery.

Neonatal problems should be recognized and treated. Except for the child with a congenitally small or absent foramen ovale, there is no need to rush a hemodynamically unstable infant to the operating room. Prostaglandin $E_1$ or $E_2$ should be used to maintain ductal patency while the cause of the hemodynamic instability is found and treated. Sepsis must always be considered in the hemodynamically unstable infant. If there is any suspicion of sepsis, antibiotics should be started pending cultures. The sensitivities of organisms associated with neonatal sepsis in each institution should govern the antibiotic choice. Surgery should be delayed until any infection is resolved. Renal failure, hepatic failure, and necrotizing enterocolitis may occur secondary to poor systemic perfusion. They should be recognized and treated before surgical palliation. Because chromosomal abnormalities are seen in 11% of patients with hypoplastic left heart syndrome, a karyotype should be obtained. The infant's neurologic status also should be carefully evaluated in the preoperative period. Major or minor central nervous system malformations, including agenesis of the corpus callosum and holoprosencephaly, have been reported in 29% of autopsy specimens from patients with hypoplastic left heart syndrome.

## Operative Management

Two major surgical approaches exist for this lesion. In one operation, the patient's own cardiovascular tissues are reconstructed to provide for hemodynamics compatible with life until a Fontan procedure can be performed (Norwood, 1983); in the second operation, a cardiac transplantation replaces the hypoplastic heart (Bailey, 1986). The patient's own tissues are used in the reconstructive approach, which eliminates the need for immunosuppression; whereas, a two-ventricular repair is achieved in the transplantation approach. The reconstructive approach typically involves three stages. In the first stage, the main pulmonary artery is transected and the proximal portion anastomosed to the hypoplastic ascending aorta. This allows the right ventricle to continue functioning as the systemic ventricle. The remainder of the aortic arch is then augmented with pulmonary homograph. The ductus arteriosus is ligated and a 4-mm polytetrafluoroethylene shunt is placed between the systemic and pulmonary arterial circuits. This shunt provides for pulmonary blood flow. Potential complications of the first stage reconstruction include development of a restrictive atrial septal defect, neoaortic arch obstruction, pulmonary artery hypoplasia or distortion, and ventricular dysfunction. Long-term survival for the first stage of the reconstructive approach is 70%. At 6 to 12 months of age, the patient undergoes a bidirectional cavopulmonary shunt or "hemi-Fontan." In this operation, the superior vena cava is directly anastomosed to the pulmonary artery and excluded from the right atrium. The shunt is removed and the pulmonary arteries augmented. This prevents the rapid diminution in end-diastolic volume that can occur with removal of the systemic to pulmonary artery shunt during the Fontan operation. About 6 months after the "hemi-Fontan," the Fontan procedure is completed by channeling the inferior vena cava to the pulmonary arteries. There is a 6% mortality from the "hemi-Fontan" and a 7% mortality from the completion of the Fontan procedure. Some patients, because of deterioration in the function of the right ventricle, are not good candidates for a Fontan operation. These patients can be managed successfully by cardiac transplantation. Cardiac transplantation has been adopted by several centers as the treatment of choice for children with hypoplastic left heart syndrome. Children with hypoplastic left heart syndrome account for 38% of heart transplantations for congenital heart disease. Because the hypoplastic heart is replaced in the transplantation approach, the surgical technique is the same as that for any other cardiac transplantation. Complications of transplantation in this age group include rejection (about 1.5 rejection episodes per patient), infection (about 1 episode per patient), and seizures (about 4% of patients). There is a 13% early and an 8% late mortality for neonatal cardiac transplantation. True long-term results from either the reconstructive approach or cardiac transplantation approach remain to be seen, but, with the 60% to 80% intermediate survival, hypoplastic left heart syndrome should no longer be considered a hopeless condition.

## Selected Readings

Bailey L, Conception W, Shattuck H, Huang L. Method of heart transplantation for treatment of hypoplastic left heart syndrome. J Thorac Cardiovasc Surg 1986;92:1.

Barber G, Chin AJ, Murphy JD, Pigott JD, Norwood WI. Hypoplastic left heart syndrome: lack of correlation between preoperative demographic and laboratory findings and survival following palliative surgery. Pediatr Cardiol 1989;10:129.

Bove EL. Transplantation after first-stage reconstruction for hypoplastic left heart syndrome. Ann Thorac Surg 1991;52:701.

Brownell LG, Shokeir MH. Inheritance of hypoplastic left heart syndrome. Clin Genet 1976;9:245.

Glauser TA, Rorke LB, Weinberg PM, Clancy RR. Congenital brain anomalies associated with the hypoplastic left heart syndrome. Pediatrics 1990;85:984.

Jonas RA. Intermediate procedures after first-stage Norwood operation facilitate subsequent repair. Ann Thorac Surg 1991;52:696.

Kawauchi M, Gundry SR, Bailey LL. Infant and pediatric heart transplantation: Loma Linda experience. Japanese Journal of Thoracic Surgery 1991;44:748.

Morris CD, Outcalt J, Menashe VD. Hypoplastic left heart syndrome: natural history in a geographically defined population. Pediatrics 1990;85:977.

Natowicz M, Chatten J, Clancy R, et al. Genetic disorders and major extracardiac anomalies associated with the hypoplastic left heart syndrome. Pediatrics 1988;82:698.

Norwood WI, Lang P, Hansen D. Physiologic repair of aortic atresia—hypoplastic left heart syndrome. N Engl J Med 1983;308:23.

Norwood WI. Hypoplastic left heart syndrome. Ann Thorac Surg 1991;52:688.

Pennington DG, Noedel N, McBride LR, Naunheim KS, Ring WS. Heart transplantation in children: an international survey. Ann Thorac Surg 1991;52:710.

Samanek M, Slavik Z, Zborilova B, Hrobonova V, Voriskova M, Skovranek J. Prevalence, treatment, and outcome of heart disease in live-born children: a prospective analysis of 91,823 live-born children. Pediatr Cardiol 1989;10:205.

Sinha SN, Rusnak SL, Sommers HM, et al. Hypoplastic left ventricle syndrome: analysis of thirty autopsy cases in infants with surgical consideration. Am J Cardiol 1968;21:166.

Watson DG, Rowe RD. Aortic-valve atresia report of 43 cases. JAMA 1962;179:14.

*Principles and Practice of Pediatrics, Second Edition.*
edited by Frank A. Oski et al. J. B. Lippincott Company, Philadelphia © 1994.

# 81.9 *Cardiac Malposition and Heterotaxy*

Howard P. Gutgesell

## CARDIAC MALPOSITION

The term *cardiac malposition* implies location of the heart anywhere other than in its usual position in the left hemithorax, or location of the heart in the left hemithorax when other organs are in abnormal positions, as in situs inversus. Dextrocardia, levocardia, and mesocardia are general terms that indicate the cardiac position only, and do not describe intracardiac anatomy. Dextrocardia denotes a right-sided heart, levocardia a left-sided heart, and mesocardia a midline heart. Situs solitus is the normal or usual arrangement of organs (ie, heart on left, liver on right, stomach on left). Situs inversus is the mirror image of normal (ie, heart on right, liver on left, stomach on right). The term *heterotaxy* designates abnormal arrangements of body organs that are different from the orderly arrangements of situs solitus or situs inversus. Typically, there is duplication or absence of normally unilateral structures (especially the spleen). The terms *situs ambiguous* and *indeterminate situs* are synonymous with heterotaxy. Isomerism indicates presence of paired, mirror-image sets of normally unilateral structures such as the lungs and atria. Left isomerism refers to the presence of two anatomic left lungs and two left atria, while right isomerism implies bilateral right lungs and atria.

## Dextrocardia

The incidence of situs inversus is 1:8000 to 1:7000 living persons. Dextrocardia with situs solitus (isolated dextrocardia) is less common. Incidence estimates are as low as 1:29,000.

Dextroversion, dextrorotation, and pivotal dextrocardia describe dextrocardia with situs solitus. The heart often appears as if the apex has been swung from the left side of the chest to the right side. Isolated dextrocardia similarly connotes that the other organs are in their normal locations and dextrocardia is an isolated finding. Mirror-image dextrocardia generally is applied to more or less normal hearts in subjects with situs inversus. Dextrocardia due to displacement of the heart into the right hemithorax by external causes (pneumothorax, diaphragmatic hernia, or hypoplasia of the right lung) is referred to as secondary dextrocardia or dextroposition.

Although dextrocardia can be diagnosed by physical examination, it usually is detected by chest roentgenography. The clinical presentation may be that of a newborn with cyanosis, respiratory distress, or heart murmur. In cases of secondary dextrocardia, the chest roentgenogram may be the only diagnostic test necessary (for example, in pneumothorax). In the absence of such an obvious cause, the initial step in evaluation of dextrocardia is to determine the situs of the other viscera. The chest roentgenogram frequently is useful in showing the location of the liver and stomach. The situs of the lungs may be inferred from chest films. On the electrocardiogram, a P vector directed leftward and inferiorly suggests situs solitus of the atria, whereas a rightward P axis suggests situs inversus. The details of visceral situs and intracardiac anatomy can be determined by echocardiography, frequently supplemented by cardiac catheterization and angiocardiography.

Dextrocardia in the presence of situs solitus frequently is associated with major intracardiac abnormalities (Fig 81-11). The most common findings are summarized in Table 81-3. Atrioventricular discordance (L-loop ventricles), single ventricle, transposition, and pulmonary stenosis or atresia are often present.

The scimitar syndrome is an uncommon but well-described constellation of cardiopulmonary anomalies consisting of dextrocardia, situs solitus of the atria and viscera, hypoplasia of the right lung, anomalous systemic arterial blood supply to the right lung, and anomalous pulmonary venous connection of the right lung to the inferior vena cava. The anomalous pulmonary vein

**TABLE 81-3.** Incidence of Intracardiac Abnormalities in Patients With Dextrocardia

| | |
|---|---|
| **Dextrocardia With Situs Solitus** | |
| Normal heart | 5% |
| Congenital heart disease | 95% |
| Common lesions: | |
| AV discordance | |
| Single ventricle or VSD | |
| "Corrected" TGA | |
| PS/PA | |
| **Dextrocardia With Situs Inversus** | |
| Normal heart | >95% |
| Congenital heart disease | <5% |
| Common lesions: | |
| VSD, DORV | |
| PS/PA | |
| "Complete" TGA | |
| Right aortic arch | |

Abbreviations: *AV*, atrioventricular; *DORV*, double-outlet right ventricle; *PS/PA*, pulmonary stenosis or atresia; *TGA*, transposition of the great arteries; *VSD*, ventricular septal defect.

is often visible on the chest roentgenogram as a curvilinear shadow in the right lung and resembles a Turkish sword or scimitar (Fig 81-12).

The incidence of congenital heart disease in subjects with dextrocardia and situs inversus is much lower than in those with dextrocardia and situs solitus. Although precise determination is not available, the incidence of congenital heart disease may not differ from that in the general population (about 8:1000). Cardiac abnormalities found in dextrocardia with situs inversus are summarized in Table 81-3. Atrioventricular discordance and transposition complexes are common but occur less frequently than in dextrocardia with situs solitus. Double-outlet right ventricle, pulmonary stenosis or atresia, and ventricular septal defect are

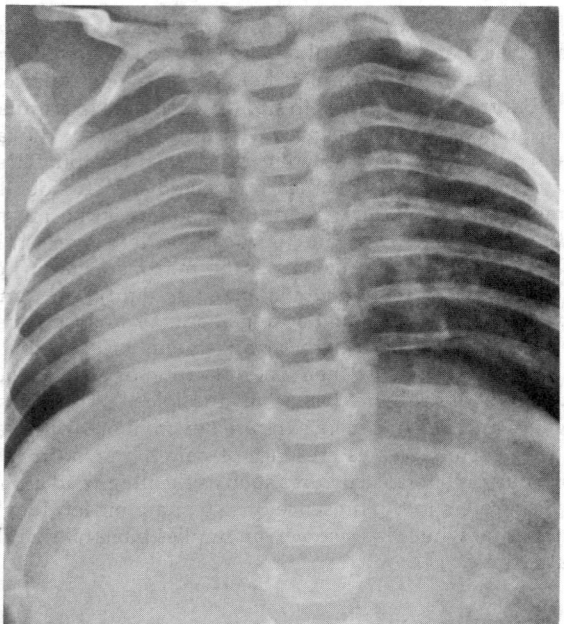

**Figure 81-11.** Chest roentgenogram in a neonate with dextrocardia. Echocardiography revealed situs solitus and normal intracardiac anatomy. The heart has shifted to the right, a process probably related to hypoplasia of the right lung.

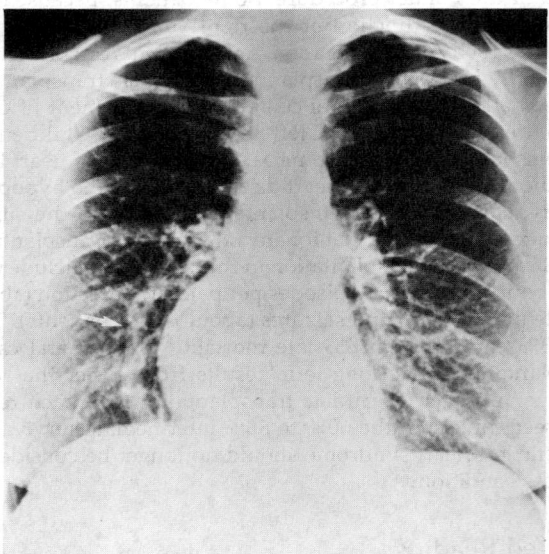

**Figure 81-12.** Scimitar syndrome in young adult with mild dextrocardia (actually mesocardia). Note the vertical shadow in the right lung (*arrow*) made by the anomalous right pulmonary vein's descent toward the diaphragm to join the inferior vena cava.

present in one third to two thirds of reported cases. The aortic arch is usually right-sided.

As many as 15% to 25% of patients with situs inversus have chronic respiratory disease. The most notable is Kartagener's syndrome. In 1933, Kartagener described four patients with situs inversus, chronic sinusitis, nasal polyposis, and bronchiectasis. The ultrastructural basis for the respiratory disease and the male infertility found in this syndrome subsequently was shown to be an abnormality on the dynein arms on the microtubules of the cilia and spermatozoa, with resultant immotility of the spermatozoa and decreased mucociliary transport.

## Levocardia

Levocardia occurring in the presence of situs inversus or heterotaxy almost invariably is associated with major intracardiac anomalies. The most common lesions include atrioventricular canal, transposition complexes, and pulmonary stenosis or atresia. The likelihood of asplenia or polysplenia is high (80%).

## Mesocardia

Mesocardia, or midline heart, is found in less than 1% of autopsied cases of congenital heart disease, but clinicians viewing large numbers of roentgenograms have a somewhat different perspective. Many tall, slender adolescents and adults have an almost vertical heart that might be termed mesocardia. Thus, the setting in which mesocardia occurs is important; a cyanotic newborn with a murmur and a midline heart is likely to have serious heart disease, whereas a midline heart is probably of no concern in an asymptomatic child with no murmur.

## Summary

Four generalizations apply to hearts in abnormal locations within the thorax. First, dextrocardia with situs solitus (isolated dextrocardia) is almost always associated with major intracardiac defects. Scimitar syndrome should be considered even in the absence of obvious intracardiac abnormalities. Second, in dextrocardia with situs inversus, the incidence of congenital heart disease is probably the same as that in the general population. The Kartagener's syndrome is present in 15% to 25% of patients with situs inversus. Third, isolated levocardia almost invariably is associated with major intracardiac abnormalities. Fourth, about one third of patients with dextrocardia and at least two thirds of those with isolated levocardia have either asplenia or polysplenia.

## HETEROTAXY

### Asplenia Syndrome

The usual presentation in asplenia syndrome is that of a cyanotic newborn, often with respiratory distress. The first and second heart sounds are single. There may be an ejection systolic murmur, a continuous murmur, or no murmur. A midline liver often is identifiable by palpation. Clues to the presence of asplenia syndrome are often found on chest roentgenogram (Fig 81-13), and this condition should be considered when the cardiac position is discordant with that of the stomach and liver, especially if pulmonary vascular markings are very diminished (due to pulmonary atresia) or if there is pulmonary edema (obstructed pulmonary veins).

The electrocardiogram generally is abnormal, but the findings are not specific for asplenia. The P-wave axis may be either leftward and inferior (normal) or rightward and inferior because of the frequency of bilateral sinus nodes. Congenital complete heart

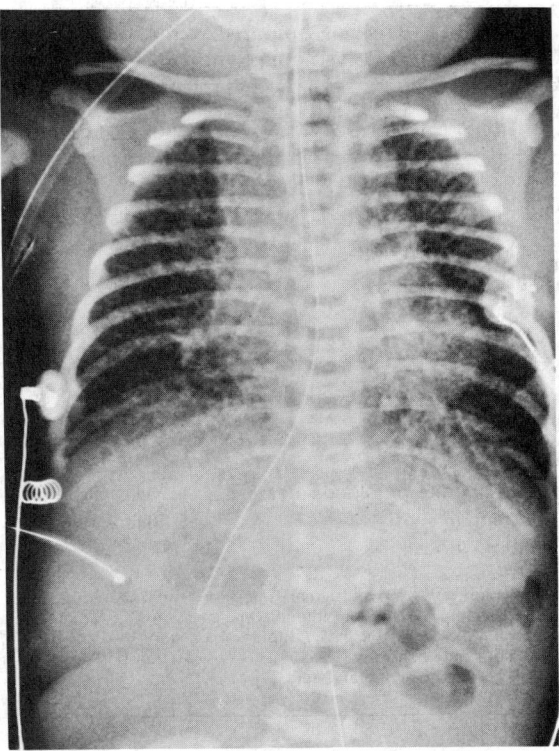

Figure 81-13. Chest roentgenogram in a neonate with asplenia syndrome. Although the heart is on the left, the stomach is on the right. Prominent pulmonary venous markings are the result of the obstructed form of the total anomalous pulmonary venous connection. Intracardial anomalies included complete atrioventricular canal, transposition of the great arteries, and pulmonary atresia.

block is present occasionally. The QRS axis and morphology reflect the cardiac position and intracardiac anatomy; the QRS axis tends to be superior in the presence of two ventricles and inferior when there is a single ventricle.

Details of intracardiac anatomy and systemic and pulmonary venous connections can be established by two-dimensional echocardiography. Additional anatomic and physiologic information can be obtained from cardiac catheterization and angiocardiography. The presence of Howell-Jolly bodies in the red blood cells in a peripheral blood smear suggests asplenia, although they are occasionally present in normal infants in the first week of life. Absence of the spleen can be documented by ultrasonography, computed tomography, or radionuclide scans.

Major intracardiac abnormalities are present in nearly all subjects with congenital asplenia (Table 81-4). Atrioventricular canal, transposition of the great arteries, and pulmonary stenosis or atresia are present almost invariably, and about 75% of cases have total anomalous pulmonary venous connection. Patients with asplenia syndrome typically have two "right" lungs (ie, three-lobed) and two anatomic "right" atria, giving the impression of bilateral right-sidedness, or right isomerism.

Patients with asplenia are at increased risk for overwhelming bacterial infection, and it is recommended that they receive prophylactic antibiotics. In the first 6 months of life, coverage against gram-negative and gram-positive organisms is advised; ampicillin is used most. Penicillin is generally sufficient for older infants and children. Administration of pneumococcal and *Haemophilus influenzae* vaccines likewise is recommended. Serologic testing confirms an adequate response.

Cardiac anomalies typical of the asplenia syndrome occasionally are amenable to intracardiac repair using modifications of

TABLE 81-4. Comparison of Asplenia and Polysplenia Syndromes

| | Asplenia (Right Isomerism) | Polysplenia (Left Isomerism) |
|---|---|---|
| **Incidence of CHD** | >95% | 90%–95% |
| **Common Cardiac Lesions** | AV canal | AV canal |
| | TGA | VSD |
| | PS/PA | DORV |
| | TAPVC | PAPVC |
| | | Absent IVC |
| | Dextrocardia in 40% | Dextrocardia in 40% |
| **Other** | Howell-Jolly bodies on blood smear | Malrotation of bowel |
| | Predisposition to sepsis | Biliary atresia |
| | Malrotation of bowel | |

Abbreviations: *AV*, atrioventricular; *CHD*, congenital heart disease; *DORV*, double-outlet right ventricle; *IVC*, inferior vena cava; *PAPVC*, partial anomalous pulmonary venous connection; *PS/PA*, pulmonary stenosis or atresia; *TAPVC*, total anomalous pulmonary venous connection; *TGA*, transposition of the great arteries; *VSD*, ventricular septal defect.

the Fontan technique or intricate intracardiac and extracardiac baffles, although the operative mortality rate is high. Given the complexity of the intracardiac lesions and the decreased immune function, the prognosis for infants with the asplenia syndrome is poor. The mortality rate is about 80% in the first year of life.

## Polysplenia Syndrome

There is greater variability in the presentation of patients with polysplenia than in those with asplenia. Because pulmonary stenosis and transposition occur relatively infrequently, cyanosis usually is not severe, and symptoms of congestive heart failure from large left-to-right shunts may predominate. Other patients may be asymptomatic, and some have no cardiac disease at all.

Findings on physical examination are not specific for polysplenia and reflect the associated cardiac abnormalities. Chest roentgenogram may provide clues to the presence of polysplenia syndrome. Absence of the hepatic portion of the inferior vena cava with azygous continuation, a common feature in polysplenia, can be predicted from the presence of mediastinal "knuckle," where the azygous vein joins the superior vena cava, especially when coupled with absence of the normal inferior vena cava shadow on the lateral view.

The frontal plane P vector of the electrocardiogram typically is oriented leftward and superiorly. The course of the conduction system is abnormal, and congenital complete heart block is present occasionally. The QRS axis and precordial leads reflect the position of the heart in the thorax and the nature of the intracardiac lesion. A superiorly oriented frontal plane QRS axis reflecting atrioventricular canal defect is common.

The intracardiac and vascular abnormalities occurring in the polysplenia syndrome are summarized in Table 81-4. Although there is considerable overlap, certain features occur with much higher frequency in either asplenia or polysplenia, fostering the notion that these conditions represent syndromes. Atrioventricular canal defect is common to both conditions. In polysplenia, the absence of the hepatic portion of the inferior vena cava is common, as is partial anomalous pulmonary venous connection. Pulmonary stenosis or atresia is uncommon in polysplenia, and normally related great arteries are more common than transposition.

Many of the cardiac abnormalities associated with polysplenia are amenable to surgical correction, with a low mortality rate. Unlike in asplenia, overwhelming bacterial infection is not a risk factor.

## ECTOPIA CORDIS

Ectopia cordis is the rarest and most dramatic of the cardiac malpositions. The heart is either partially or totally outside the thorax. The four types of ectopia cordis are cervical, thoracic, thoraco-abdominal, and abdominal. True cervical ectopia cordis is rare, having occurred only in a few severely deformed fetuses. Sternal cleft, in which the heart may be seen pulsating under the skin due to failure of fusion of the upper sternum, probably should not be considered an example of ectopia cordis because the heart is within the thorax. True abdominal ectopia cordis is likewise rare. The thoracic type is the classical form of ectopia cordis. The entire heart lies outside of the thorax, uncovered by pericardium. Attempts to place the heart into the thorax generally have been unsuccessful because of cardiorespiratory insufficiency due to compression of the heart and lungs within the small thoracic cavity.

The thoraco-abdominal form of ectopia cordis usually occurs as part of a constellation of associated anomalies, including midline supraumbilical abdominal defect, defect in the distal sternum, deficiency of the diaphragmatic pericardium, deficiency of the anterior diaphragm, and intracardiac defect.

Intracardiac abnormalities are common but not invariable in patients with ectopia cordis. The most common lesions are atrial and ventricular septal defect, tetralogy of Fallot, and tricuspid atresia. Additionally, a diverticulum protruding from the apex of the left ventricle is present in 20% of the patients with a thoraco-abdominal defect.

## Selected Readings

Anderson C, Devine WA, Anderson RH, Debich DE, Zuberbuhler JR. Abnormalities of the spleen in relation to congenital malformations of the heart: a survey of necropsy findings in children. Br Heart J 1990;63:122.

Gikonyo DK, Tandon R, Lucas RF Jr, Edwards JE. Scimitar syndrome in neonates: report of four cases and review of the literature. Pediatr Cardiol 1986;6:193.

Ivemark BI. Implications of agenesis of the spleen in the pathogenesis of conotruncus anomalies in childhood: an analysis of the heart malformations in the splenic agenesis syndrome, with fourteen new cases. Acta Paediatr 1955;44(suppl 104):1.

Peoples WM, Moller JH, Edwards JE. Polysplenia: a review of 146 cases. Pediatr Cardiol 1983;4:129.

Rose V, Izukawa T, Moes CAF. Syndromes of asplenia and polysplenia: a review of cardiac and noncardiac malformation in 60 cases with special reference to diagnosis and prognosis. Br Heart J 1975;37:840.

Stanger P, Rudolph AM, Edwards JE. Cardiac malpositions: an overview based on study of sixty-five necropsy specimens. Circulation 1977;56:159.

Toyama WM. Combined congenital defects of the anterior abdominal wall, sternum, diaphragm, pericardium, and heart: a case report and review of the syndrome. Pediatrics 1972;50:778.

Van Mierop LHS. Asplenia and polysplenia syndrome. Original article series. Birth Defects 1972;8:74.

Van Praagh R, Weinberg PM, Matsuoka R, Van Praagh S. Malpositions of the heart. In: Adams FH, Emmanouilides GC, eds. Moss's heart disease in infants, children, and adolescents, ed 3. Baltimore: Williams & Wilkins, 1982:422.

Waldman JD, et al. Sepsis and congenital asplenia. J Pediatr 1977;90:555.

*Principles and Practice of Pediatrics, Second Edition.*
edited by Frank A. Oski et al. J. B. Lippincott Company, Philadelphia © 1994.

CHAPTER 82
# *Acyanotic Congenital Heart Disease or Heart Disease With Infrequent Cyanosis*

## *82.1 Defects of the Atrial Septum Including the Atrioventricular Canal*

G. Wesley Vick III and Jack L. Titus

Congenital defects of the atrial septum are common. They may be located in different anatomic portions of the atrial septum, and the location of the defect generally reflects the abnormality of embryogenesis that led to the anomaly (Fig 82-1). An atrial septal defect (ASD) may be isolated or may be associated with other congenital cardiac abnormalities. Sizes of ASDs vary greatly. Functional consequences of defects of the atrial septum, then, are related to the anatomic location of the defect, size of the defect, and presence or absence of other cardiac anomalies.

Developmental defects resulting from abnormalities in partitioning of the embryologic atrioventricular (AV) canal and in the endocardial cushions often lead to a communication between the right and left atria. Most AV canal (endocardial cushion) malformations have major anomalies of the AV valves in addition to an intra-atrial communication. Defects of the ventricular septum often are present.

## DEFINITIONS AND CLASSIFICATIONS

Interatrial communications are considered in two groups. The first group results from abnormal development of the septa that normally partition the atrial portion of the developing heart into right and left atria. The second group includes interatrial communications that result primarily from maldevelopment of the partitioning of the AV canal and endocardial cushions. The first group may be viewed as isolated ASDs and the second group as AV canal defects.

Isolated ASDs include patent foramen ovale, ASD at the fossa ovalis (secundum ASD), defect superior to fossa ovalis (sinus venosus type ASD, superior vena caval defect), and coronary sinus defects. AV canal defects include complete forms, incomplete forms, and common atrium.

## ISOLATED ATRIAL SEPTAL DEFECTS

### Pathologic Features

#### Patent Foramen Ovale

About 30% to 40% of normal adult hearts have a patent, valve competent foramen ovale, which usually is not considered an ASD. The smallest ASDs are due to incompetence of the valve of the foramen ovale. They may be congenital or may be acquired by stretching of the right or left atria in conditions in which those chambers are enlarged.

#### Defects at the Fossa Ovalis (Secundum Defects)

The typical defect in the fossa ovalis is contained within the area bordered by the limbus of the fossa ovalis. Size of these defects varies greatly. In addition, the floor of the fossa ovalis (valve of foramen ovale) in this region may be fenestrated, so multiple defects are possible. Secundum defects may be associated with or confluent with other defects of the atrial septum such as a sinus venosus defect or ostium primum defect.

#### Sinus Venosus Defect

Sinus venosus defects are located in the part of the atrial septum immediately below the superior vena caval orifice. The right upper and middle lobe pulmonary veins often connect to the superior vena caval and right atrial junction, resulting in partial anomalous pulmonary venous return connection.

#### Coronary Sinus Defect

Coronary sinus ASDs are characterized by absence of part or all of the common wall between the coronary sinus and the left

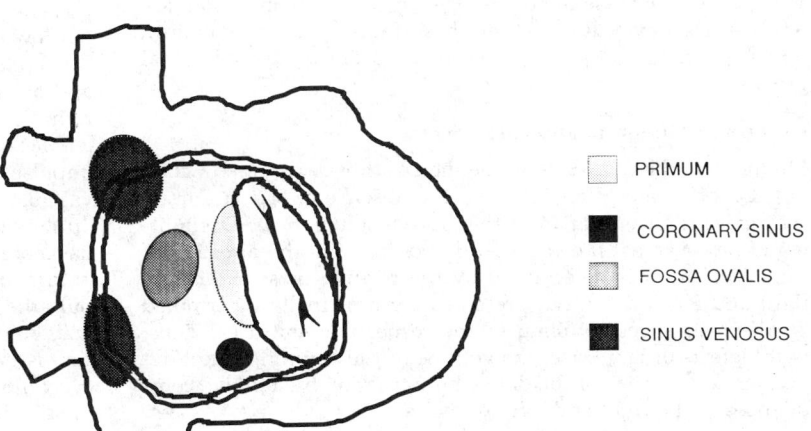

PRIMUM

CORONARY SINUS

FOSSA OVALIS

SINUS VENOSUS

**Figure 82-1.** Atrial septal defects. Only defects within the fossa ovalis region are true defects of the interatrial septum, although all of the defects permit interatrial shunting.

atrium. A persistent left superior vena cava also is present in many cases.

### Associated Cardiovascular Defects

ASDs often occur in conjunction with other congenital cardiac anomalies. In many of these anomalies, the associated defects are lesions of primary importance; however, the ASD may play a major role in the physiologic features of the condition. For example, in complete transposition of the great arteries, an ASD permits mixing between the pulmonary and systemic circulations necessary to sustain life. Another example is in tricuspid atresia in which the entire cardiac output must pass across the ASD.

## Physiology

### Intrauterine and Postnatal

Because pulmonary blood flow is relatively minimal before birth, nearly all blood reaching the left atrium does so by passing across the foramen ovale. When the lungs expand after birth, pulmonary venous return to the left atrium increases substantially concomitant with the fall in pulmonary vascular resistance and increased systemic vascular resistance. As a result, in the normal infant, left atrial pressure rises above the right atrial pressure, and functional closure of the foramen ovale occurs. When an ASD is present, the intrauterine physiology generally is unchanged. The hemodynamic changes occurring after birth, however, do not close the atrial septum, and left-to-right shunting occurs. In some patients, right-to-left shunting via the ASD also may occur and be associated with mild cyanosis in the neonatal period.

### Patent Foramen Ovale

If the flap valve remnant of septum primum of the foramen ovale is competent, shunting at atrial level cannot occur as long as left atrial pressure remains higher than right atrial pressure. Even in normal individuals, however, the right atrial pressure may rise transiently above the left atrial pressure. In this circumstance, right-to-left interatrial shunting may occur if the valve of the foramen ovale is not anatomically sealed or is insufficient to close the foramen ovale. Similarly, blood clots and other emboli may cross the atrial septum from right to left in such circumstances (paradoxical embolism). In patients with pulmonary vascular disease or pulmonary stenosis, enough right-to-left shunting across a patent foramen ovale may occur to cause systemic arterial desaturation.

### Defects of Small Size

Small ASDs are defined as those with a pulmonary-to-systemic flow ratio (Qp : Qs) of less than 2-to-1 in the absence of significant associated cardiovascular anomalies. Presence of a small atrial septal does not cause major changes in cardiac hemodynamics. Small ASDs may be the anatomic basis for paradoxical embolism whenever the right atrial pressure rises above the left atrial pressure.

### Defects of Moderate and Large Size

Moderate and large ASDs are defined as those associated with a Qp : Qs of greater than 2-to-1 in the absence of significant associated cardiovascular anomalies. As a result of the ASD, shunting of blood across the atrial septum occurs, but the direction of the atrial shunt is determined by the relative pressures in the right and left atria. Atrial pressures are principally determined by the resistances to filling of the respective ventricles. Thus, with defects of large size, the volume of the shunting is not dependent on the size of the defect but rather on the relative compliances of the right and left ventricles.

## Natural History

Isolated secundum ASDs do not cause major symptoms in most cases during infancy and childhood. In the absence of unrelated problems, more than 99% of the patients with isolated secundum defects live beyond the first year of life. As noted, mild to moderate cyanosis is sometimes evident during the neonatal period. Children and infants with these defects tend to be smaller than normal, but failure to thrive based on the ASD alone is rare. Exercise intolerance may develop in some patients as early as the second decade of life. Others may remain asymptomatic for several more decades.

Left-to-right shunting tends to increase with age in many patients. Thus, the frequency of congestive heart failure with attendant fluid retention, hepatomegaly, and elevated jugular venous pressure increases with the age of the patient. The large shunts present in many older patients cause stretching of the atria, which presumably predisposes them to atrial arrhythmias, such as atrial flutter, fibrillation, and tachycardia. These arrhythmias are a major cause of morbidity and mortality in older patients with ASDs. Pulmonary vascular disease does develop occasionally in older patients with isolated ASD, but this complication is rare in childhood and adolescence and is unusual in older adults with large defects.

## Atrial Septal Defect and Pregnancy

Pregnancy places additional demands on the cardiovascular system and may cause patients with previously occult ASDs to become symptomatic. In particular, exercise intolerance and congestive heart failure may become apparent during pregnancy. Venous thrombosis, common during pregnancy due to stasis, may lead to paradoxical embolism when an ASD is present. When pulmonary vascular disease is present, pregnancy carries a substantial health risk for the mother and often results in miscarriage.

## Diagnostic Examination: Physical Examination

### Inspection and Palpation

The height and weight of patients with ASDs is often below normal, although usually not substantially so. A precordial bulge may be present in those with a large left to right shunt, and Harrison grooves (transverse depressions along the sixth and seventh costal cartilages at the site of attachment of the anterior part of the diaphragm) may be apparent in some patients. The presence of a hypoplastic thumb, radius, or phocomelia should cause suspicion that the patient has the Holt-Oram syndrome, an autosomal dominant disorder in which an upper limb deformity is found with congenital heart disease, most often an ASD in association with prolonged AV conduction. Cyanosis may be present in infants, particularly in those with right ventricular outflow obstruction of any form.

In patients with a thin body habitus, an uncomplicated ASD, and a large volume of left-to-right shunting, a hyperdynamic right ventricular impulse may be observed. Palpation along the left sternal border and in the subxiphoid area demonstrates this impulse, often termed a *right ventricular heave*. When pulmonary vascular disease exists or when obstruction to right ventricular outflow exists, the right ventricular impulse is less dynamic and has more of a tapping or thrusting quality, suggesting the presence of primarily pressure and not volume overload. An enlarged and pulsatile pulmonary trunk at the second left intercostal space may be palpated in many patients. When pulmonary hypertension is present, the impulse created by the pulmonary artery is even more prominent and a palpable pulmonic component of the second heart sound may be present in such patients.

## Arterial Pulse

The arterial pulse is normal at rest in patients with uncomplicated ASDs. It is possible, however, to demonstrate abnormalities when Valsalva's maneuver is employed. During the straining phase of Valsalva's maneuver, normal persons show a decrease in cardiac output secondary to a decrease in systemic venous return. In contrast, in patients with ASDs and relatively large left-to-right shunts, the large volume of blood pooled in the lungs permits left ventricular output to be maintained.

## Jugular Venous Pulse

Patients with isolated and nonrestrictive ASDs have a jugular venous pulse of normal amplitude. Because the two atria are connected by a nonrestrictive channel, however, the A and V waves of the venous pulse have equal height. When pulmonary vascular disease supervenes, the right atrium contracts more forcefully, causing large A waves to be formed.

## Auscultation

In patients with ASDs, the first heart sound, best heard at the apex and lower left sternal edge, often is split and the second component is increased in intensity. This increased intensity may result from the large volume of diastolic blood flow pressing tricuspid leaflets toward the right ventricular walls so the forceful right ventricular contraction causes an abrupt cephalad excursion of the tricuspid leaflets.

ASDs with moderate to large left-to-right shunts are associated with a pulmonary systolic murmur that begins shortly after the first heart sound, peaks in early systole to midsystole, and ends before the second heart sound. This murmur usually is not associated with a thrill. When a thrill is present, either a very large shunt or pulmonic stenosis usually is present. Rapid flow through the peripheral pulmonary arteries may cause systolic crescendo-decrescendo murmurs that are most prominent at locations in the chest other than the second intercostal space.

The characteristic auscultatory finding in ASD is the wide, fixed splitting of the second sound. This finding is present in patients with large left-to-right shunts and normal pulmonary artery pressure.

The fixed splitting of the second sound results from a combination of factors. In normal individuals, inspiratory splitting of the second sound results primarily from increased pulmonary capacitance during inspiration. The increase causes an inspiratory increase in the "hangout" interval (the time between the descending portions of the right ventricular and pulmonary arterial pressure pulses) and a consequent delay in the pulmonic component of the second sound. With expiration in normal persons, pulmonary capacitance decreases, the "hangout" interval decreases, and splitting of the second sound decreases.

In contrast, in patients with ASD, the capacitance of the pulmonary bed is increased and its impedance is decreased. The increased capacitance causes an increase in the "hangout" interval with a consequent wide splitting between the first and second components of the second heart sound. Because there is little respiratory variation in the pulmonary capacitance, little variation in the "hangout" interval and splitting of the second sound occur in patients with an ASD.

Duration of electromechanical systole is the same in the right and left ventricles of patients with ASDs, because, even though the right ventricle ejects a relatively larger volume than the left ventricle, it ejects it in an accelerated manner. If the pulmonary arterial pressure rises, the "hangout" interval decreases, but the split remains constant regardless of the phase of the respiratory cycle. When the left-to-right shunt is small or negligible, as it is in most neonates with ASDs, fixed splitting of the second sound does not occur. Because relatively wide (but not truly fixed) split-

ting of the second sound is common in the supine position, it is better to evaluate the second sound when the patient is sitting or standing.

The intensities of the pulmonic and aortic components of the second sound are equal in most patients with uncomplicated ASDs. Patients with pulmonary hypertension generally have an accentuated pulmonic component of the second sound. Occasionally, a patient with normal pulmonary pressures has an increased intensity of the pulmonic component of the second sound because of the proximity of the dilated pulmonary artery to the chest wall.

The diastolic murmur most often associated with ASD is a mid-diastolic murmur resulting from the high flow across the tricuspid valve. This murmur becomes apparent when the left-to-right shunt is greater than 2-to-1. The murmur is of low to medium frequency and does not increase with inspiration. Another diastolic murmur sometimes associated with ASD is a low-pitched murmur of pulmonic regurgitation, probably a consequence of dilatation of the pulmonary artery.

Because the pressure gradient across the atrial septum seldom is large, audible murmurs from flow across the ASD itself are rare, though intracardiac phonocardiography can demonstrate them.

In the occasional patient with ASD and right-to-left shunting due to pulmonary hypertension, auscultatory findings differ greatly from those usually found in ASDs. A right ventricular fourth heart sound may be present. The midsystolic pulmonic murmur is softer and shorter because only a normal stroke volume is ejected. The tricuspid flow murmur is not present. The pulmonic component of the second sound is increased in intensity, but the fixed splitting characteristic of ASD is not present. If a murmur of pulmonic insufficiency is present, it is high-pitched. An holosystolic murmur of tricuspid insufficiency also may be present, resulting from right ventricular and atrial enlargement.

## Electrocardiogram

Sinus rhythm is customary in young patients with uncomplicated secundum ASDs. Prolongation of the PR interval is common and sometimes has a familial association. Beyond the third decade of life, patients with ASD have a high frequency of atrial arrhythmias, particularly atrial fibrillation but also including atrial flutter and supraventricular tachycardia.

Patients with secundum ASDs usually have normal P waves. Sinus venosus ASDs often are associated with a leftward frontal plane P wave axis, that is, negative in leads III and aVF and positive in lead aVL. This leftward shift is caused by an ectopic pacemaker, which is the focus of atrial excitation in these patients in whom the ASD is located in the area usually occupied by the sinus node.

The QRS complex in patients with secundum ASDs often has a slightly prolonged duration and a characteristic rSr' or rsR' pattern. The reason for this orientation of the QRS is thought to be disproportionate thickening of the right ventricular outflow tract, which is the last portion of the ventricle to depolarize. The phrase "incomplete right bundle branch block" often is used to describe this QRS pattern but is a misnomer because it is a consequence of hypertrophy and not a conduction disturbance.

With increasing degrees of pulmonary hypertension, patients with secundum ASDs tend to lose the rSr' pattern in V1 and develop a tall, monophasic R wave with a deeply inverted T wave.

A frontal plane QRS axis ranging from +95° to +135° with a clockwise loop is often present. Left axis deviation of the QRS axis with a counterclockwise frontal plane loop suggests the presence of an AV canal defect but can occur with uncomplicated secundum ASD.

## Chest Radiograph

The chest radiograph in patients with secundum ASD and sizable left-to-right shunts generally shows cardiac enlargement and increased pulmonary vascularity (Fig 82-2). Increased pulmonary vascularity typically extends to the periphery of the lung fields, with a dilated pulmonary trunk and central branches. Although the ascending and transverse aorta have normal diameters in these patients, enlargement of the pulmonary arteries causes the aorta not to form the border of the cardiac shape. The consequence is a characteristic triangular cardiac shape. Right atrial and right ventricular enlargement usually are seen, but left atrial and left ventricular sizes usually are normal.

## Echocardiogram

*M-Mode.* The M-mode echocardiogram in patients with isolated secundum ASDs of moderate and large size usually shows right ventricular enlargement. Paradoxical motion of the interventricular septum often is present. Diastolic movement of the anterior mitral valve leaflet stops short of the level of the ventricular septum. In contrast, in patients with AV canal defects, the M-mode echocardiogram shows apparent diastolic motion of the mitral valve through the plane of the ventricular septum.

*Two-Dimensional Echocardiogram.* Two-dimensional echocardiography enables direct, noninvasive visualization of all types of ASDs (Fig 82-3). Reliability of the two-dimensional echocardiogram in demonstrating characteristic dropout in the atrial septum is best when the axis of the echo beam is perpendicular to the atrial septum. For most defects, a subcostal view provides such a perpendicular angle. Depending on the location of the defect, other possible echocardiographic approaches are suprasternal or parasternal views that yield appropriate image planes. ASDs often can be seen in the apical four-chamber view, but as a consequence of the parallel angle of the echo beam to the atrial septum and the thinness of the fossa ovalis, false echo dropout often occurs.

In addition to direct visualization of the ASD, two-dimensional echocardiography also may demonstrate enlargement of the right atrium, right ventricle, and pulmonary arteries, and often shows paradoxical motion of the ventricular septum in a two-dimensional format. In many cases, the pulmonary and systemic venous connections also can be demonstrated.

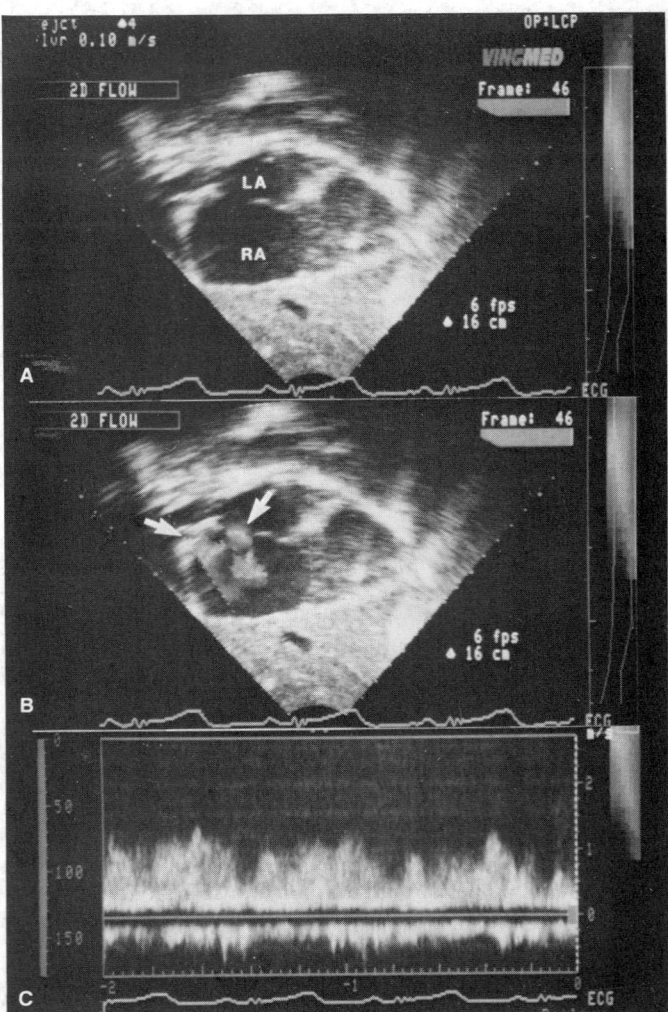

**Figure 82-3.** Two-dimensional echocardiogram demonstrating a fossa ovalis atrial septal defect. (**A**) Note the opening in the fossa ovalis region of the septum between the left atrium (LA) and the right atrium (RA). (**B**) Color Doppler study demonstrating flow across the atrial septum from left to right through the secundum atrial septal defect. (**C**) Pulsed Doppler study demonstrating low-velocity flow from left to right across the defect.

*Doppler Echocardiography.* Abnormal flow across the atrial septum can be detected reliably by pulsed Doppler echocardiography. The accuracy of Doppler identification of flow across the atrial septum can be improved greatly by the use of two-dimensional echocardiographic direction of Doppler sampling. Characteristically, a shunt across the ASD shows turbulent flow in the direction of the shunt and minimal flow in the opposite direction.

Continuous wave Doppler echocardiography can be of assistance in the evaluation of patients with ASD. It is particularly useful in evaluating the gradient across the atrial septum in patients with left atrial hypertension and restrictive ASDs and in evaluating patients for obstruction to pulmonary venous return.

Color Doppler provides useful diagnostic information in patients with ASDs. It allows for direct visualization of the flow across the atrial defect and is particularly helpful in distinguishing normal right superior vena caval flow from left-to-right shunting across the atrial septum.

For additional confirmation of diagnosis, contrast echocardiography using agitated saline or indocyanine green effectively demonstrates the presence of an ASD. A right-to-left shunt can

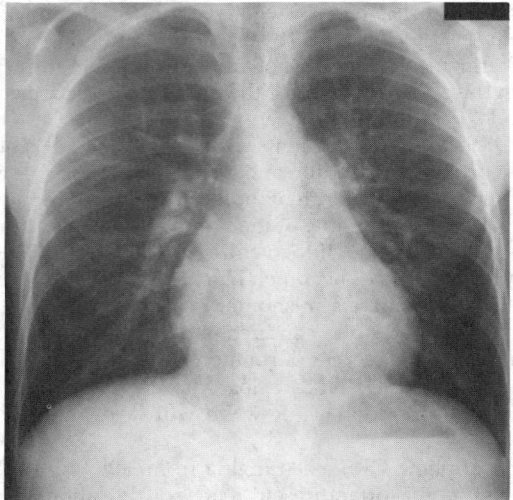

**Figure 82-2.** Chest x-ray of a patient with a secundum atrial septal defect. Note the cardiomegaly and increased pulmonary vascular markings. The main pulmonary artery is enlarged and the aortic knob is small.

be detected by direct visualization of microcavitation bubbles in the left atrium and left ventricle. A left-to-right shunt can be detected as a negative contrast washout effect in the right atrium, if good opacification of the atrium is achieved.

*Transesophageal Echocardiography.* Transthoracic echocardiography is limited by the ability of ultrasound to penetrate to regions of interest. Particularly in older patients and in patients with chest wall deformities and lung disease, transthoracic echocardiographic windows may be so poor that the atrial septum cannot be clearly visualized in its entirety. In such instances, transesophageal echocardiography often is helpful. Two-dimensional anatomic visualization of the atrial septum from the transesophageal approach generally is excellent. Additionally, two-dimensionally directed pulsed, color, and even continuous wave Doppler studies of blood flow can be performed from the transesophageal approach with appropriate equipment. In addition to its diagnostic role in selected cases, transesophageal echocardiography is especially useful for guiding catheter placement of occlusion devices to close ASDs.

### Nuclear Magnetic Resonance Imaging

Isolated ASDs can be identified clearly by noninvasive nuclear magnetic resonance imaging methods. Nuclear magnetic resonance imaging is complementary to other diagnostic methods and is most advantageous for defining extracardiac structures, such as anomalous pulmonary and systemic veins, that may be poorly demonstrated by echocardiography because of surrounding lung tissue. Of particular interest are the recently developed cine methods that facilitate visualization of intracardiac and extracardiac blood flows.

### Cardiac Catheterization

Secundum ASD sometimes can be differentiated from sinus venosus and AV canal defects because characteristic high and low catheter courses across the atrial septum are seen with the latter two defects, respectively. In secundum ASD, the catheter passes across the middle portion of the atrial septum.

Left-to-right shunting across the atrial septum causes an increase (step-up) in oxygen saturation in the right atrium. An increase of 10% over superior vena caval blood in one oxygen saturation series or an increase of 5% in two series generally indicates the presence of a left-to-right shunt at the atrial level.

### Cineangiography

The presence of an ASD with left-to-right shunting can be demonstrated in the AP and lateral projections by injection of contrast medium into the main pulmonary artery. Contrast material passes into the right atrium and ventricle and may reflux into the hepatic veins in patients with ASDs. Pulmonary artery injection also is a good method for evaluating the pulmonary venous return and usually demonstrates any abnormal pulmonary venous connections. Although this technique reveals the presence of an ASD, it does not provide good visualization of the size and location of the ASD. For optimal direct visualization, an injection just outside the orifice of the right upper pulmonary vein in the cranially angulated left anterior oblique projection (often termed the four-chamber view) is the most appropriate approach. With the four-chamber view, secundum ASDs are demonstrated in the middle of the atrial septum, sinus venous defects are demonstrated at the top of the atrial septum, and AV canal defects are shown at the inferior aspect of the atrial septum.

## Treatment

Isolated secundum ASDs associated with a large left-to-right shunt and either symptoms or significant cardiomegaly should be electively closed in childhood. When the findings from a comprehensive noninvasive evaluation demonstrate a classic isolated secundum ASD, many physicians believe that cardiac catheterization for diagnosis is not essential. The noninvasive studies should be of good technical quality, however, so that pulmonary hypertension can be excluded and so that associated anatomic defects such as anomalous pulmonary and systemic venous connections can be excluded.

When pulmonary hypertension is present or the atrial shunt is small, recommendations regarding closure are more controversial. When advanced pulmonary vascular disease is present, operative mortality and morbidity are high and closure of the ASD may worsen the prognosis. Small ASDs cause only a minimal increase in cardiopulmonary stress. Therefore, the hemodynamic gain from closing them may not be worth the hazard of the procedure; however, the risk of paradoxical embolism through a small atrial defect or valve-competent patent foramen ovale is uncertain. This risk may justify closure in selected patients, such as those with a history of cryptogenic stroke. Further clinical studies are required to assess the benefits of intervention in such cases.

Recently, successful catheter closure of secundum ASDs with occlusion devices has been performed (Fig 82-4). Although catheter occlusion of ASDs is investigational, its role in the management of defects of moderate and small size in the fossa ovalis region may be expected to increase. Large secundum defects of greater than about 20 mm in diameter cannot be reliably closed with current catheter devices. Catheter closure has the advantage of avoiding cardiopulmonary bypass, thoracotomy, and atriotomy with their attendant potential problems. Initial results with catheter ASD occlusion are promising, but long-term follow-up studies subsequent to catheter ASD closure are not yet available.

Surgical closure usually is performed with the aid of cardiopulmonary bypass. Patch closure with either pericardium or Dacron is preferred for all but small defects, because closure of large defects by direct suture can distort the atrium.

## Prognosis

Surgical results in uncomplicated secundum ASD are good. Mortality is less than 2% in many large series. Mortality and morbidity are increased with advanced age or congestive heart failure. After the operation, the left-to-right shunt and its consequent cardiac volume overload are eliminated in nearly all patients. Without closure, patients with moderate and large secundum ASDs generally do well until the third decade of life, after which they tend to become progressively more symptomatic with a substantially higher mortality than that for the general population.

## PERSISTENT COMMON ATRIOVENTRICULAR CANAL DEFECTS

AV canal defects include a range of malformations, a central feature of which is usually an ASD of the primum type, and which also involve the ventricular septum and one or both AV valves. A number of terms have been applied to these malformations, including endocardial cushion defect, AV septal defects, and persistent common AV canal.

## CLASSIFICATION

In view of the variety of types of AV canal defects, different classifications exist. In this discussion, the term *complete AV canal* indicates the presence of both atrial and ventricular septal defects

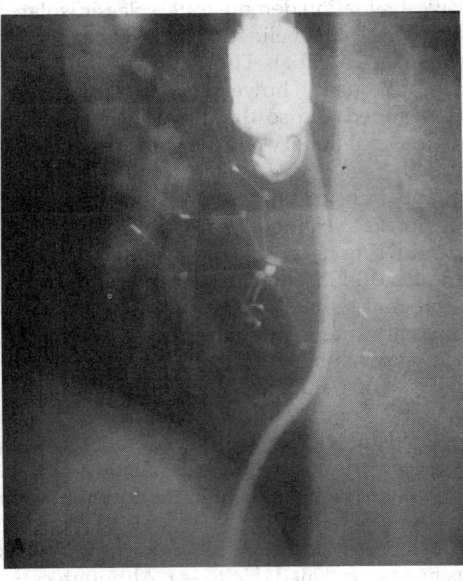
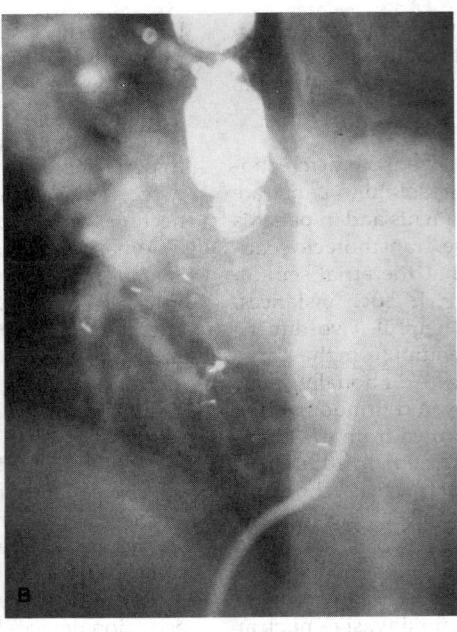

**Figure 82-4.** (**A**) Atrial septal defect occlusion device in place. Note tranesophageal echocardiographic probe positioned immediately superior to device. (**B**) Left atrium opacified by pulmonary artery angiogram. No contrast is seen in right atrium, demonstrating closure of atrial septal defect by device. (Courtesy of Charles E. Mullins, MD)

and a common AV orifice with a common AV valve (Fig 82-5); all other forms that are parts of the spectrum are termed *partial* or *incomplete* forms.

## Pathologic Aspects

### Atrial Septum

Most AV canal defects include an interatrial communication usually labeled ostium primum ASD. They lie at the lowest part of the atrial septum and are variable in size, but usually large in relation to cardiac size. Characteristically, the superior margin of the primum ASD has a concave shape.

### Ventricular Septum

The basal portion of the ventricular septum is deficient in most hearts with persistent common AV canal. In those hearts without interventricular communication, the AV valve tissue attaches to

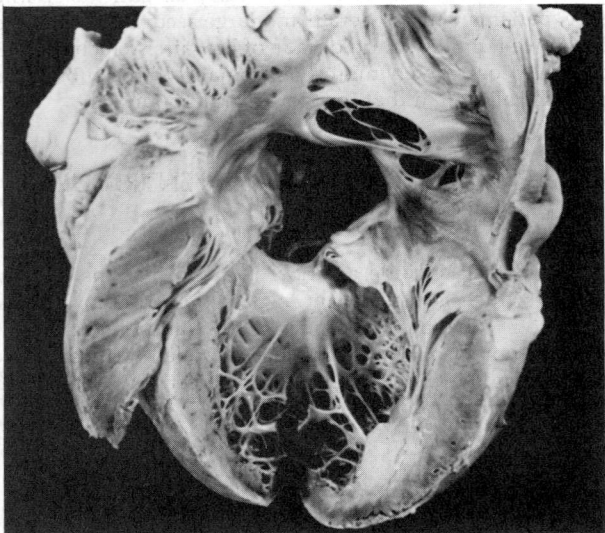

**Figure 82-5.** Complete atrioventricular canal defect. View is from the opened left atrium and left ventricle. Note the large cleft in the anterior mitral leaflet. (Courtesy of Debra Kearney, MD.)

the crest of the deficient ventricular septum in such a way that interventricular communication is precluded. In hearts with interventricular communication, valvular tissue does not attach to the crest of the deficient septum, and interventricular communication exists between the valve tissues superiorly and the crest of the deficient septum inferiorly.

### Atrioventricular Valves

Hallmarks of persistent AV canal defects are abnormal AV valves. Abnormalities involve both the overall configuration and orientation of the valve apparatus and the local structure of the AV valves. Partial forms of AV canal defects usually have two separate AV valve annuli. In this situation, the left and right AV valve leaflets usually are named according to the normal mitral and tricuspid valve components to which they correspond most closely. The anterior (septal) leaflet of the mitral valve is composed of two components, which usually are of approximately equal size, separated by a gap (cleft.)

In complete AV canal defects, a common AV valve exists. Both an ostium primum ASD and a ventricular septal defect of the AV canal type are present and are confluent. The common AV valve has anterior and posterior common leaflets that bridge across the ventricular septum and relate to both ventricles (also called anterior and posterior bridging leaflets).

### Common Atrium

An uncommon form of ASD is that in which almost the entire atrial septum is absent. Often, a band of muscular tissue crosses the atrium, suggesting a vestigial atrial septum. These defects usually are associated with a cleft anterior leaflet of the mitral valve and a deficient summit of the ventricular septum.

## Physiology

### Incomplete (Partial) Atrioventricular Canal

In the absence of pulmonary stenosis or pulmonary vascular disease, there is predominant left-to-right shunting in patients with AV canal defects. When only the ASD is present without substantial left AV (mitral) valvular insufficiency, the physiology is identical to that of an ASD; shunting is primarily determined by the pulmonary vascular resistance. When major left AV valvular insufficiency is present, additional left-to-right shunting occurs directly from the left ventricle to right atrium via the cleft mitral valve as a shunt from a high-pressure chamber to a low-pressure chamber. This additional left-to-right shunt causes volume overload of both the left and right ventricles and is associated with heart failure in early life.

### Complete Defects

When a large interventricular communication is present, additional left-to-right shunting occurs at ventricular level. Such shunts usually are associated with systemic pulmonary artery pressures in the absence of pulmonary stenosis. Left AV valve incompetence compounds the ventricular volume overload in these patients who often have symptoms caused by pulmonary congestion. When pulmonary vascular disease develops, as is likely, patients may improve symptomatically. When advanced vascular disease ensues in later life, the physiology is the same as in patients with Eisenmenger's syndrome, with the additional volume overload imposed by left AV valve insufficiency.

## Natural History

The natural history of AV canal defect primarily depends on the pathologic anatomy of the malformation. In those patients with only an ostium primum ASD and minimal insufficiency of the left AV valve, the clinical course is similar to that of patients with a large secundum ASD. Generally, these patients do well without treatment during infancy, childhood, and adolescence. During adulthood, they have an increasing tendency to develop congestive heart failure, particularly as atrial arrhythmias develop and with the increasing mitral regurgitation that occurs with time.

Those patients with ostium primum ASDs and moderate-to-severe left AV valve insufficiency develop congestive heart failure in early life with a consequent high morbidity and mortality that relates primarily to the severity of the AV valve insufficiency.

Patients with complete AV canal defects generally develop severe symptoms of congestive heart failure in early infancy. They have frequent respiratory infections and poor weight gain. If they survive infancy untreated, they generally develop pulmonary vascular disease with fixed pulmonary hypertension as an additional major deleterious factor.

## Diagnostic Examination: Physical Examination

### Appearance

Patients with partial AV canal defects and minimal mitral insufficiency usually appear normal in infancy and childhood. Patients with partial AV canal and substantial mitral insufficiency may manifest growth failure and other signs of chronic congestive heart failure. Patients with complete common AV canal usually are symptomatic in early infancy with manifestations such as poor physical development, hyperinflated thorax, bulging precordium, Harrison's grooves, and mild or intermittent cyanosis. If there are no signs of chronic congestive heart failure in a patient with known complete common AV canal defect, pulmonary stenosis or pulmonary vascular obstructive disease should be suspected.

The patient with Down's syndrome, which frequently is associated with endocardial cushion defects, has a characteristic physical appearance. Infants with this syndrome have flat facial profiles, oblique palpebral fissures, and a large protuberant tongue. The hands generally are short and broad, with a palmar simian crease, a short, curved fourth finger, and a distal axial triradius. The skin is dry and distinctively pale. There are two distinctive ocular features. The most frequent is an inner epicanthic skin fold that inserts on the lower lid. Brushfield spots (speckled iris) are the second distinctive ocular feature. When Down's syndrome is seen in conjunction with physical signs of chronic congestive heart failure, the coexistence of complete common AV canal should be suspected. Other types of congenital heart disease also occur in Down's syndrome.

### Arterial and Jugular Venous Pulse

In partial endocardial cushion defect, mitral regurgitation sometimes is associated with a water-hammer pulse that is caused by rapid ejection of a large left ventricular stroke volume. Patients with congestive heart failure, however, may have a small pulse volume. When mitral regurgitation is present, the jugular venous pulse may have a dominant V wave because the right atrium receives left ventricular systolic flow.

### Precordial Movement and Palpation

When mitral regurgitation is present in patients with partial endocardial cushion defect, a systolic thrill often is present. This thrill radiates toward the sternum. When a large left-to-right shunt is present, a palpable impulse in the second and third left intercostal spaces often is found, reflecting the presence of a dilated, pulsatile, pulmonary artery trunk. Sometimes, the pulmonic component of the second heart sound is palpable. The right ventricular volume and pressure overload associated with complete AV canal defects causes a prominent systolic impulse or heave at the left sternal border and in the subxiphoid area.

### Auscultation

Complete AV canal defects may be associated with a variety of auscultatory manifestations, depending on the nature of the underlying pathologic physiology. Because one common AV valve is present, the first heart sound is usually single. When the AV conduction time is prolonged, as is often the case, the first heart sound tends to be relatively soft. There is usually constant or fixed splitting of the second sound, although when severe pulmonary hypertension is present, the splitting is narrow. Pulmonary hypertension also may be associated with a loud pulmonic component of the second sound. A murmur of AV valve incompetence frequently is present. This murmur usually is maximal at the left ventricular apex and often radiates toward the sternum rather than toward the left axilla, reflecting the predominance of left ventricular-to-right atrial shunting over left ventricular-to-left atrial shunting. When the ventricular septal defect is restrictive and there is a substantial pressure gradient between the left and right ventricles, a separate murmur of ventricular septal defect may be present, most prominently heard at the lower left sternal border.

Auscultatory findings in ostium primum ASD are similar to those found in fossa ovalis defects with the addition of an apical holosystolic murmur, secondary to AV valve insufficiency, that radiates toward the sternum. A pulmonic flow murmur often is present in the second left intercostal space, and wide, fixed, splitting of the second heart sound occurs.

### Electrocardiogram

The most characteristic electrocardiogram abnormality of AV canal defect is a superiorly oriented QRS frontal plane axis with a counterclockwise depolarization pattern. The mechanism of alteration of the frontal plane QRS axis in these patients is not due to ventricular hypertrophy, but rather is caused by abnormally positioned conduction tissue, which causes abnormal sequences of cardiac activation. Often, AV conduction delay, as evidenced by a prolonged PR interval, exists. Electrocardiographic manifestations of right ventricular hypertrophy also are present often. Electrocardiographic suggestions of biventricular or left ventricular hypertrophy also may occur, particularly if mitral or AV valve insufficiency is severe.

## Chest Radiograph

Cardiac enlargement usually is present in the chest radiograph in patients with ostium primum or complete AV canal defects. In particular, right atrial and right ventricular enlargement often are present. The enlarged right heart may displace the left ventricle making evaluation of left ventricular size difficult.

The main pulmonary artery usually is prominent, and, if a large left-to-right shunt is present, increased pulmonary vascular markings usually exist. With severe pulmonary vascular disease, distal pulmonary vessels may have a lucent, pruned appearance. Severe enlargement of the pulmonary trunk and left atrium may compress the left main stem bronchus and cause atelectasis of parts of the left lung.

## Echocardiogram

*M-Mode Echocardiogram.* In most cases, the M-mode echocardiogram in patients with AV canal defects characteristically demonstrates apparent diastolic movement of the mitral valve through the plane of the ventricular septum. M-Mode echocardiography also shows an enlarged right ventricle and paradoxical motion of the interventricular septum in many patients.

*Two-Dimensional Echocardiogram.* The two-dimensional echocardiogram is highly reliable in identifying AV canal defects. The hallmark of the diagnosis is the demonstration of an absent AV septum. In ostium primum ASDs, the AV valve leaflets appear to originate from the crest of the ventricular septum. In complete AV canal defects, the bridging leaflets of the common AV valve cross the ventricular septum.

*Doppler Echocardiography.* Doppler echocardiography can contribute substantially to the evaluation of AV canal defects. Pulsed Doppler is especially useful in detecting left and right ventricular outflow obstruction and the presence of a ductus arteriosus. Pulsed Doppler examination also helps identify AV valve regurgitation and has been employed to quantitate the degree of AV valve regurgitation. Continuous wave Doppler is useful in quantitating pressure gradients in these patients. When a ventricular defect is present, the instantaneous pressure difference between the right and left ventricles can be determined using the modified Bernoulli formula. Similarly, pressure gradients across the left and right ventricular outflow tracts can be quantitated. Color Doppler studies also may be helpful, particularly for determining the location and for roughly quantitating the degree of AV valve insufficiency.

*Transesophageal Echocardiography.* Excellent images of the AV septum and of the AV valves and their attachments can be obtained with transesophageal echocardiography. Doppler color flow mapping of AV valve flow from the transesophageal approach is also generally excellent. The most extensive use of transesophageal imaging in patients with AV canal is intraoperatively to evaluate postoperative AV valve regurgitation.

## Magnetic Resonance Imaging

Magnetic resonance imaging can demonstrate defects in the AV septum, but the ability of this modality to characterize AV valves is limited by relatively low temporal resolution. Magnetic resonance imaging is helpful as an adjunct to echocardiography to demonstrate extracardiac anatomy and organ situs in patients who have complex anomalies such as heterotaxy syndrome in association with AV canal defects.

## Cardiac Catheterization

AV canal defects can be suspected at cardiac catheterization when the catheter course across the atrial septum is low in the septum.

Oxygen saturation and hemodynamic findings generally are similar to those found in a secundum ASD.

## Cineangiography

Selective left ventricular angiography in the anteroposterior projection demonstrates an elongated left ventricular outflow tract with an abnormally low insertion of the anterior leaflet of the left AV valve, deficiency in the diaphragmatic wall of the left ventricle, and a disproportionately short inlet septum compared to the outlet septum. This combination of characteristics is diagnostic of an AV canal defect and is termed the "gooseneck" deformity (Fig 82-6).

## Treatment

### Medical

When heart failure and associated pulmonary congestion are present, anticongestive measures such as diuretics and digoxin are indicated. Long periods of fluid restriction generally are counterproductive because the patients in distress are usually small infants and such restriction deprives them of calories needed for growth. Hydralazine reduces the magnitude of left-to-right shunting acutely in these patients, but no long-term experience with the drug in complete AV canal defects has been reported. Most cardiologists do not favor prolonged medical therapy in these patients if their symptoms are refractory, but rather refer them for surgical treatment.

### Surgical

Recommendations for surgical treatment depend on the anatomic characteristics of the defect and associated anomalies. Patients with an osium primum ASD, separate AV valves, no ventricular defect, and minimal AV valve insufficiency generally are asymptomatic during infancy and childhood. Because repair of ostium primum ASD is associated with a substantially greater morbidity and mortality than repair of a secundum ASD, many cardiologists do not recommend surgery at any age if cardiomegaly is absent, which usually is the case when AV valve insufficiency is mild and pulmonary-to-systemic flow ratio is less than 2-to-1. Infants with partial AV canal defects that are symptomatic almost invariably have severe AV valve regurgitation. Pulmonary artery banding generally does not help these patients. Therefore, cor-

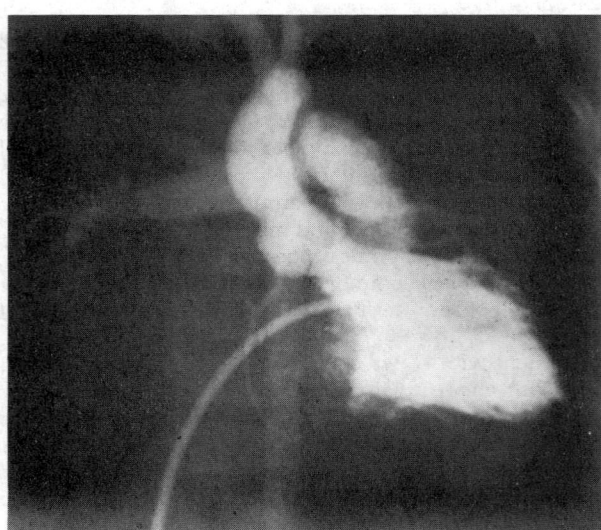

**Figure 82-6.** Frontal view of left ventriculogram in patient with complete atrioventricular canal defect. The "gooseneck" deformity of the left ventricular outflow tract is clearly demonstrated.

rective surgery with mitral valvuloplasty and ASD closure usually is recommended. Asymptomatic patients with ostium primum ASDs that do exhibit substantial cardiomegaly usually are referred for elective surgical repair when they are near school age.

For patients with uncomplicated complete AV canal defects, most centers advocate corrective surgery in early infancy. Palliative procedures such as pulmonary artery banding, however, may be more appropriate in patients who have AV canal defects in association with other anomalies such as hypoplasia of the left ventricle. When pulmonary pressures are near systemic, as they generally are in patients with complete AV canal defects who do not have associated right ventricular outflow obstruction, pulmonary vascular disease usually develops after the first year of life. Therefore, either corrective surgery or a palliative procedure to protect the pulmonary circulation during infancy is recommended in these patients.

## Prognosis

Long-term results of surgical therapy depend greatly on the degree of preoperative pulmonary vascular disease and on the extent of residual left AV valve regurgitation. In many cases, the left AV valve regurgitation is reduced substantially and the left-to-right shunt abolished or reduced to minimal levels by corrective surgery. When pulmonary vascular disease is present preoperatively, however, hospital morbidity and mortality are high, and little

improvement is seen in the late follow-up period for those patients who survive the operation. Postoperative arrhythmias can occur, including complete heart block, and may increase in frequency as patients grow older. With advancing age, patients may require mitral valve replacement.

## Selected Readings

Craig RJ, Selzer A. Natural history and prognosis of atrial septal defect. Circulation 1968;37:805.

Edwards JE. Congenital malformations of the heart and great vessels. A. Malformations of the atrial septal complex. In: Gould SE, ed. Pathology of the heart, ed 2. Springfield, Ill: Charles C. Thomas, 1960:260.

Feldt RH, Edwards WD, Puga FJ, et al. Atrial septal defects and atrioventricular canal. In: Moss AJ, Adams FH, Emmanouilides GC, eds. Heart disease in infants, children, and adolescents, ed 5, Baltimore: Williams & Wilkins, 1989:170.

Moss AJ, Siassi B. The small atrial septal defect—operate or procrastinate? J Pediatr 1971;79:854.

Mullins CE. Pediatric and congenital therapeutic cardiac catheterization. Circulation 1989;79:1153.

Nadas AS, Fyler DC. Pediatric cardiology. Philadelphia: WB Saunders, 1972:317.

Perloff JK. The clinical recognition of congenital heart disease. Philadelphia: WB Saunders, 1987:272.

Rudolph AM. Congenital diseases of the heart. Chicago: Year Book Medical Publishers, 1974:239.

Silverman N, Levitsky S, Fisher E, et. al. Efficacy of pulmonary artery banding in infants with complete atrioventricular canal. Circulation 1983;68(suppl 2):148.

Studer M, Blackstone EH, Kirklin JW, et al. Determinants of early and late results of repair of atrioventricular septal (canal) defects. J Thorac Cardiovascular Surg 1982;84:523.

Titus JL, Rastelli GC. Anatomic features of persistent common atrioventricular canal. In: Feldt RH, ed. Atrioventricular canal defects. Philadelphia: WB Saunders, 1976.

*Principles and Practice of Pediatrics, Second Edition.*
edited by Frank A. Oski et al. J. B. Lippincott Company, Philadelphia © 1994.

# 82.2 *Ventricular Septal Defect*

## Carl H. Gumbiner

Ventricular septal defect (VSD) is the most common cardiac malformation in children. The incidence is estimated at 1.5 to 2.5 per 1000 live births, although this figure varies depending on the method used to identify the defect. VSD accounts for about 20% of patients followed by pediatric cardiologists in the United States.

## ANATOMY

The ventricular septum is a curvilinear, spiraling structure that separates the left ventricle from the right ventricle and, to a small extent, from the right atrium. The ventricular septum consists of a membranous and a muscular portion, and is subdivided into inflow, trabecular, and outflow regions. Defects in the septum may occur in each region. They range in size from "pinhole" defects of 1 mm or less to virtual absence of the septum.

The location of a defect within the ventricular septum is not of great hemodynamic consequence, but is a critical surgical consideration and an important determinant of natural history. The majority of defects are bounded by both a portion of the membranous septum and a portion of muscular septum. The margin of a perimembranous defect, then, is partially membrane and partially muscle. Less common are true muscular defects, which are bounded entirely by muscle. These tend to be multiple and are more difficult to repair. They also have a greater frequency

of spontaneous closure. Defects in a separate category, the doubly committed subarterial defects (formerly designated supracristal or Type I defects), lie in the outflow portion of the muscular septum beneath the pulmonary and aortic valves. They are associated with development of aortic regurgitation and, while infrequently identified in whites, constitute up to 30% of VSDs in Asian children. Malalignment defects in which the crest of the septum lies in a different plane from the anterior portion of the aortic root are found in many complex lesions, but may constitute an isolated VSD as well. Progressive left ventricular outflow tract obstruction is common with such defects.

## PHYSIOLOGY

VSD allows a communication between the systemic and pulmonary circulations. Hemodynamic consequences of this communication depend on the size of the left-to-right shunt, which, in turn, is a function of the anatomic size of the defect and the relative pulmonary and systemic vascular resistances. Left-to-right shunting at the ventricular level results in increased pulmonary blood flow and volume overload of the left ventricle. In accordance with the Frank-Starling principle, increased left ventricular volume work entails increased end-diastolic filling pressure. Consequently, left atrial and pulmonary venous pressures are increased. The combination of increased pulmonary blood flow with elevated pulmonary venous pressure produces increased oncotic pressure within the pulmonary capillary bed and consequent accumulation of pulmonary interstitial fluid. Decreased pulmonary compliance with increased work of breathing accounts for early manifestations of congestive heart failure. More profound failure, causing alveolar fluid collection, can interfere with pulmonary gas exchange as well.

Pulmonary vascular resistance is elevated in the fetus and newborn. Normally, resistance falls during the first several days of life, but may remain high for several months in the presence of a large ventricular communication. Hence, the hemodynamic manifestations of a left-to-right shunt are not evident at birth and may not appear until later in infancy. Elevation in pulmonary artery pressure that invariably is present with large or "unrestrictive" VSD produces characteristic progressive changes in the pulmonary arteriolar bed. Pulmonary vascular obstructive disease (PVOD), with marked, irreversible elevated resistance, may develop as early as 2 years of age. It usually follows a period of low resistance (hence, high pulmonary blood flow with congestive heart failure), but may develop progressively in children whose pulmonary vascular resistance never declines postnatally. The later stage of progressive PVOD in these patients—cyanosis due to reversed shunting through a large interventricular communication—is termed Eisenmenger's syndrome. This well-known late chapter in the natural history of VSD with pulmonary hypertension has made customary the surgical repair of large defects before 1 year of age.

## CLINICAL MANIFESTATIONS

Small VSDs seldom cause significant symptoms and usually come to the attention of a physician because of the associated heart murmur. While the murmur is not present in the immediate newborn period, it may be audible as early as the second day of life and usually is heard at the routine 2-week checkup. It is characteristically a high-pitched, harsh, holosystolic murmur, well localized along the left sternal border. A small VSD may produce a murmur of lower pitch, but a high-pitched murmur strongly suggests that the defect is not large. The precordium is quiet, but a localized thrill may be palpable. The first and second heart sounds are normal, and there is seldom a diastolic murmur. Except finding mild tachypnea in small infants, other physical findings are normal. Small defects, sometimes called maladie de Roger, do not interfere with normal growth. A significant number, estimated from 30% to 70%, undergo spontaneous closure, usually in the first 2 years of life. Small defects that do not close rarely require treatment. Their chief importance lies in their distinction from other anomalies (in young infants, this includes distinction from larger defects) and the risk for developing bacterial endocarditis. Certain types of defects, regardless of size, may predispose to development of secondary conditions, especially secondary aortic regurgitation and left ventricular outflow tract obstruction. For this reason, children older than 2 years of age with physical findings of a small VSD should have an echocardiographic examination to confirm the diagnosis and localize the defect.

Large defects may come to the attention of a physician later than small defects because elevated pulmonary vascular resistance may delay the appearance of a murmur. When present, symptoms are those of congestive heart failure. They include irritability, increased respiratory effort, poor feeding, and poor weight gain. Recurrent respiratory infections are common, and pneumonia is often the preliminary diagnosis.

Signs of congestive heart failure include tachycardia, tachypnea, increased work of breathing, pallor, diaphoresis, and failure to thrive. Pulmonary rales are a late finding. The precordium is hyperactive, and a thrill is often palpable. The second heart sound is single or narrowly split. When audible, it is usually accentuated, but often it is obscured by a loud, low-pitched, harsh, holosystolic murmur. The murmur is loudest along the left sternal border, but is much less well localized than is the murmur of a small VSD. It may radiate to the right of the sternum, but radiates poorly to the back. A diastolic murmur or rumble heard at the lower left sternal border is related to increased mitral flow. Its presence implies a pulmonary-to-systemic flow ratio exceeding

2-to-1. Pulses may be diminished with severe congestive heart failure, but are symmetrical in the absence of aortic coarctation. The liver and sometimes the spleen are enlarged.

Moderately sized defects may produce physical findings suggestive of small defects, although rarely a murmur of high pitch. There is usually some degree of tachypnea and increased respiratory effort. Because of increased volume load of the left ventricle, the precordial impulse is hyperactive and there is often a thrill. When associated with low pulmonary vascular resistance and high pulmonary blood flow, a moderate-sized defect may produce findings similar to a large defect, including those of congestive heart failure.

Large defects with high resistance, and, thus, little increase in pulmonary blood flow, may cause no symptoms or growth failure in the small child. Although the precordial impulse is hyperactive and the pulmonic closure sound is accentuated, an absent or subtle murmur may allow this effect to pass undetected. Older children with more advanced PVOD have resting cyanosis, exercise intolerance, and nail-bed clubbing. A murmur of VSD flow usually is not heard, but a systolic murmur of tricuspid regurgitation or a diastolic murmur of pulmonic regurgitation may be present.

## NONINVASIVE AND INVASIVE STUDIES

Radiographic findings generally reflect the size of the left-to-right shunt. Small defects may produce mild cardiac enlargement on a plain chest roentgenogram, but usually the chest radiograph is normal. Moderately sized defects are associated with cardiomegaly, usually of a predominant left ventricular type. The left atrium may be enlarged on the lateral projection. Pulmonary blood flow is increased. Large defects produce a more diffuse cardiomegaly, increased pulmonary vascular markings, and often signs of pulmonary edema. In patients with large VSD and PVOD, only mild cardiomegaly is shown on the chest roentgenogram. The main pulmonary artery segment usually is prominent and central vascular markings are normal or diminished.

Electrocardiographic changes with small VSD are minimal. Moderately sized defects usually produce some degree of left ventricular hypertrophy. Large defects commonly produce combined ventricular hypertrophy on electrocardiogram. Large defects with PVOD may show more right ventricular hypertrophy than left.

Echocardiography and Doppler echocardiography are the primary modality for anatomic and physiologic assessment of VSD. Real-time two-dimensional echocardiographic imaging in the standard views discloses the presence, location, and size of nearly all defects (Fig 82-7) as well as the presence of associated lesions. Color flow Doppler investigation increases the sensitivity of standard imaging, particularly for small or multiple defects. Pulsed and continuous wave Doppler studies facilitate assessment of right ventricular pressure and pressure gradients between ventricles. Systemic and pulmonary blood flows can be estimated indirectly by measuring semilunar valve diameter and recording flow velocity.

Cardiac catheterization and angiography play a role in evaluation of patients with VSD (Fig 82-8), but are reserved for those patients with unusual or complex anatomy and for those patients who require precise investigation of pulmonary blood flow or vascular resistance beyond Doppler capability. Such evaluation also may entail assessment of response to intervention such as administration of oxygen or vasodilators. The catheterization laboratory is a site for VSD treatment in the form of transcatheter VSD closure devices for selected patients.

Magnetic resonance imaging (MRI) and cine-MRI offer other modes for the anatomic assessment of these defects and are par-

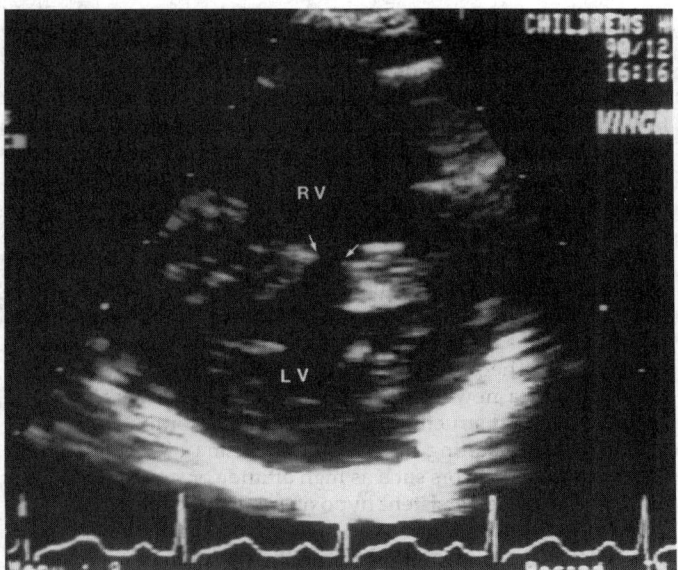

**Figure 82-7.** Short-axis two-dimensional echocardiographic view of a large muscular VSD. Arrows point to margins of the defect. *RV,* right ventricle; *LV,* left ventricle.

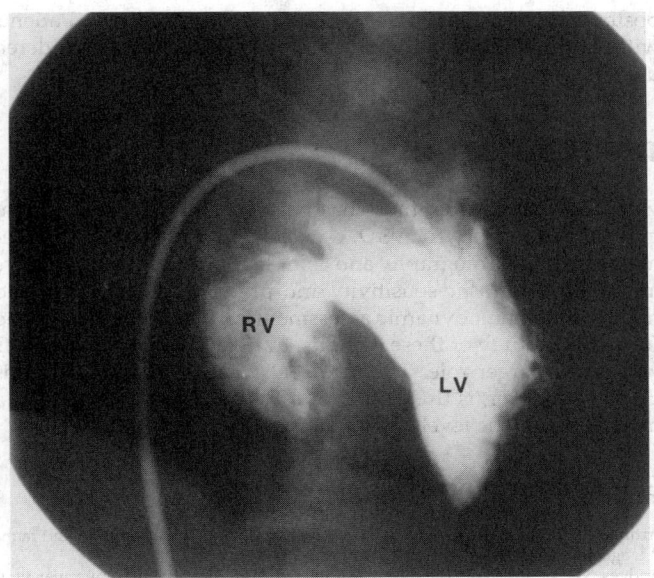

**Figure 82-8.** Left ventriculogram in left anterior oblique cranial projection demonstrating flow of contrast across a moderately sized perimembranous VSD. *RV,* right ventricle; *LV,* left ventricle.

ticularly useful for evaluation of associated extracardiac vascular malformations such as coarctation of the aorta.

## MANAGEMENT

Infants and children with small VSD seldom require treatment. Young infants should be evaluated periodically in the first 6 months of life, when pulmonary vascular resistance is expected to decline. Physical examination and noninvasive studies should be used to ascertain the expected minimal increase in pulmonary blood flow and absence of pulmonary hypertension. Many small defects close spontaneously. Older children with persistent defects should be evaluated periodically, both to screen for acquired lesions (aortic regurgitation, subaortic membrane, right ventricular muscle bundle) and to reemphasize the need for endocarditis prophylaxis.

Infants with moderate-sized and large defects generally have symptoms caused by increased pulmonary blood flow. Most infants with congestive heart failure due to isolated VSD can be treated successfully with conservative therapy. This usually begins with diuretic therapy, usually furosemide 1 to 2 mg/kg twice or thrice daily or chlorothiazide 10 to 20 mg/kg twice daily. Spironolactone 2 to 3 mg/kg/d is often added as a potassium-sparing agent. Digoxin is a conventional component of therapy for these children. Digoxin is used in most centers even though its effects on both the immature myocardium and the pure volume overload state have been questioned. After loading with 0.03 to 0.06 mg/kg over 24 hours, maintenance therapy continues with a dosage of 0.01 mg/kg/d.

Afterload-reduction therapy—hydralazine 0.25 to 1.0 mg/kg three times daily, captopril 0.1 to 0.5 mg/kg three times daily, or enalapril 0.08 mg/kg twice daily—may help patients whose response to diuretic therapy and digoxin is limited. A decrease in systemic vascular resistance can favorably affect relative systemic-to-pulmonary blood flow ratio, especially in patients with low pulmonary vascular resistance.

Even with aggressive medical treatment, infants with excessive pulmonary blood flow may gain weight poorly. Caloric requirements often in excess of 140 kcal/kg/d, concerns about fluid intake, and poor feeding patterns combine to make nutrition a

challenging aspect of care. Standard formulas may be supplemented with carbohydrates and medium-chain triglyceride oil. Nasogastric feeding at home has been employed successfully by many centers.

Goals of medical therapy are relief of symptoms and adequate growth. When these cannot be achieved, early surgical repair should be considered. Palliative surgery in the form of pulmonary artery banding is reserved for rare patients with complicating factors or severe associated lesions. For isolated VSD, intracardiac repair performed under hypothermic circulatory arrest or conventional cardiopulmonary bypass is the operative procedure of choice, even for small infants. Patients in whom medical therapy is successful but pulmonary artery pressure remains elevated should undergo repair before 1 year of age. Children with normal pulmonary artery pressure and persistent significant left-to-right shunt (pulmonary-to-systemic flow ratio greater than 2-to-1) may undergo elective repair in late infancy or in childhood. Surgery generally is not advocated if pulmonary-to-systemic flow ratio is less than 2-to-1.

Markedly elevated pulmonary vascular resistance in the older child makes risk of surgical repair untenable. While there is no treatment for PVOD, antiplatelet agents commonly are used to retard its progression. For cyanotic patients with polycythemia, symptoms often improve with periodic red cell volume reduction by partial exchange transfusion.

## ENDOCARDITIS, PREGNANCY, AND INSURABILITY

Regardless of VSD size, all patients are at risk for developing bacterial endocarditis. Standard recommendations for antibiotic prophylaxis should be used, unless spontaneous closure occurs. Surgical repair reduces the risk but does not eliminate it entirely, especially if there is a residual defect.

Small VSD does not entail risk for pregnancy. Large defects, postoperative defects with compromised clinical status, and pulmonary hypertension all present significant risk for exacerbation of cardiac symptoms during pregnancy.

Life-insurance risk for patients with small VSD or postoperative VSD without residual are standard. Moderate VSD and postoperative residual defect present substandard risk. Patients with large VSD or pulmonary hypertension are considered uninsurable.

## THE FUTURE

Over the past decade, there has been continuing improvement in results of surgery for VSD, especially in small babies. Refinements in echocardiography and color Doppler investigation have improved diagnostic sensitivity and precision. While improved noninvasive hemodynamic assessment further reduces the need for catheter study of these patients, transcatheter closure of VSD will play a larger role. The next real frontier in managing this disease however, is the definition of its etiologies, perhaps on a molecular genetic level, and ultimately its prevention.

## Selected Readings

Artman M, Graham TP. Congestive heart failure in infancy: recognition and management. Am Heart J 1982;103:1040.

Bridges ND, et al. Preoperative transcatheter closure of congenital muscular ventricular septal defects. New Engl J Med 1991;324:1312.

Dickinson DF, Arnold R, Wilkinson JL. Ventricular septal defect in children born in Liverpool 1960 to 1969. Br Heart J 1981;46:47.

Fyler DC, et al. Report of the New England Regional Infant Cardiac Program. Pediatrics 1980;65:377.

Gumbiner CH, Takao A. Ventricular septal defect. In: Garson A, Bricker JT, McNamara DG, eds. The science and practice of pediatric cardiology. Philadelphia: Lea and Febiger, 1990:1002.

Hagler DJ, Edwards WD, Seward JB, Tajik AJ. Standardized nomenclature of the ventricular septum and ventricular septal defects, with applications for two-dimensional echocardiography. Mayo Clin Proc 1985;60:741.

Heath D, Edwards JE. The pathology of hypertensive vascular disease. Circulation 1958;18:533.

Helmcke F, et al. Two-dimensional and color Doppler assessment of ventricular septal defect of congenital origin. Am J Cardiol 1989;63:1112.

Talner NS, et al. Guidelines for insurability of patients with congenital heart disease. Circulation 1980;62:1419A.

Weintraub RG, Menahem S. Early surgical closure of a large ventricular septal defect: influence on long term growth. J Am Coll Cardiol 1991;18:552.

*Principles and Practice of Pediatrics, Second Edition.*
edited by Frank A. Oski et al. J. B. Lippincott Company, Philadelphia © 1994.

# 82.3 *Patent Ductus Arteriosus*

## Charles E. Mullins

The patent ductus arteriosus is a normally occurring essential structure in the fetus and becomes abnormal only when it persists after birth. In the term infant, the persistent ductus probably represents a structural abnormality in the ductus tissues present at birth. The persistent patency of the ductus in the premature infant is a more common problem and usually is a result of immaturity of ductal tissues. The ductus in the premature infant is discussed in Chapter 19.2 and is not discussed here. Persistent patent ductus arteriosus is the second most common congenital heart defect, accounting for about 10% of all congenital heart defects in full-term infants.

The walls of the ductus arteriosus are composed of thick, spiraling elastic fibers and smooth muscles, which, when they con-

tract, cause constriction of the lumen of the ducts. In the fetal circulation, the ductus allows right ventricular blood to bypass the nonexpanded and nonventilated lungs. Both the low $PO_2$ of the blood and a high level of circulating prostaglandins in the fetus inhibit constriction of the ductus. In the normal newborn, lung expansion occurs immediately on delivery. As a result, most of the right heart blood and, in turn, pulmonary artery blood is immediately diverted to the now lower resistant pulmonary vascular bed. This obligatory flow through the lungs allows circulating prostaglandins in the fetus to be cleared by the most effective clearing system, the lungs, and immediately allows oxygenation of the blood, thereby increasing the circulating $PO_2$. Both the decreased prostaglandins and the increased blood $PO_2$ contribute to the normal constriction of the ductus. Normally, the ductus of a newborn functionally is closed by, at most, 72 hours of age and structurally is sealed by 3 months.

All factors resulting in persistent patency of the ductus are not understood. Factors such as high altitude or severe pulmonary disease that cause persistent hypoxia predispose to persistent patency of the ductus. Continued high prostaglandin levels, in the presence of a compromised or inefficient pulmonary clearing function (found in premature infants or in marked decrease pulmonary flow occurring in some pulmonary atresia patients), contribute to the persistent patency of the ductus. Rubella (and possibly other viral infections) during the first trimester of pregnancy frequently results in patency of the ductus. Some evidence shows that a lower socioeconomic status, probably resulting in inadequate perinatal nutrition, may predispose to persistent patency of the ductus.

When the ductus remains open and, with normal lungs, pulmonary resistance drops further, blood flows from the aorta through the ductus into the pulmonary arteries. Eventual flow to the lungs from the ductus depends on size and shape of the ductus and on how close to normal levels the pulmonary vascular resistance drops. With normal pulmonary resistance, the flow through the ductus begins during midsystole to late systole and continues through diastole. This flow pattern corresponds to the timing of the maximal pressure gradient between the aorta and the pulmonary artery during the various phases of the cardiac cycle.

In the usual patient with a left aortic arch, the ductus arteriosus connects the junction of the main and left pulmonary artery to the descending thoracic aorta at a point just distal to the origin of the left subclavian artery. The persistent ductus varies in shape from very short and broad-based at both ends to long and tortuous. The diameter of the clinically detectable ductus ranges from less than 1 mm to more than 1 cm at the narrowest diameter and is independent of the shape of the ductus. Clinical finding depends on the final net flow through the lungs into the left atrium, left ventricle, aorta, and back through the ductus.

The uncomplicated patent ductus places a pure volume workload on the left heart with little or no effect on the right heart. The blood from the aorta flows through the ductus into the pulmonary arteries, through the pulmonary vascular bed into the left atrium, into the left ventricle, and back into the aorta. The total additional workload on the left ventricle depends directly on the size of the persistent ductus arteriosus and the resultant flow through the ductus. The additional blood from the ductus mixes with the blood ejected from the right ventricle into the pulmonary artery; however, in the absence of increased pulmonary resistance, the extra blood does not add significantly to the work of the right ventricle. As a result, in the absence of increased pulmonary resistance, there is little or no additional volume or pressure work placed on the right ventricle and no physical or clinical laboratory signs suggesting right-sided involvement.

## CLINICAL FINDINGS AND DIAGNOSIS

Clinical histories of patients with persistent patent ductus range from florid heart failure in the young infant to incidental murmur in an otherwise perfectly healthy child or, occasionally, adult. The patient with a patent ductus may present as early as the newborn period and anytime thereafter, including late adulthood. The most common presentation of the patient with a persistent patent ductus is a heart murmur discovered incidentally in an asymptomatic young child being examined for some other reason. The infant or child with a moderate-to-large patent ductus may be prone to, or more susceptible to, secondary involvement in the lower respiratory tract or even infections after initial upper respiratory infection. This probably is due to the decreased compliance of the lungs associated with significantly increased pulmonary blood flow.

The murmur and associated clinical finding of a patent ductus usually are characteristic and often pathognomonic of the defect. The typical murmur of a patent ductus is continuous (sounding like machinery) and is maximum in the first and second left intercostal spaces in the left midclavicular line. The murmur begins with the first heart sound, then crescendos throughout systole until the second heart sound. The murmur peaks in intensity at the second sound before trailing off during diastole. Depending on the shape and size of the ductus, the intensity of the murmur varies from grade 1 to grade 6, and the quality ranges from high pitched and blowing to low frequency and rough.

The pulmonary component of the second sound is increased in intensity and delayed in occurrence, which widens the splitting and increases the overall intensity of the second sound, giving it a "slapping sail" quality. The second sound is maximum in the second and third left intercostal spaces. In the larger ductus with a significant increase in pulmonary flow, there is an associated left ventricular lift and an apical diastolic flow rumble from the increased volume flow across an otherwise normal mitral valve.

Peripheral pulses are bounding in quality as a result of both the increased left ventricular stroke volume and the diastolic runoff into the lungs. This combination generates a wide pulse pressure. In the patient with a large persistent ductus, pulses are often visible in the suprasternal, carotid, axillary, and femoral areas.

There are several situations with an isolated ductus in which physical findings of the ductus may be atypical. In the patient with higher pulmonary resistance, the diastolic runoff into the lungs is decreased or stopped, so clinical findings resulting from this runoff are not present. The diastolic component of the murmur, in particular, decreases or disappears, the bounding pulses no longer are present, and there is no mitral flow murmur. These atypical findings may occur in the presence of significant bronchospastic disease or a superimposed severe lower respiratory tract infection.

At the other extreme, in the young infant with very large ductus and low pulmonary resistance, much of the flow through the ductus into the pulmonary arteries occurs during systole, or the ejection phase of the blood, with little continued flow during diastole. In these patients, the murmur is localized further down the left sternal border, and the diastolic component is markedly decreased or absent. The tip-off to the presence of a patent ductus in these patients is the persistence of the split and "slapping" second sound, the bounding pulses, and wide pulse pressure. The atypical persistent patent ductus requires an accurate echocardiogram or, often, a detailed cardiac catheterization for diagnosis confirmation.

The electrocardiogram in the uncomplicated ductus is normal or, in the larger ductus, shows left ventricular hypertrophy and left atrial enlargement. The chest radiograph shows cardiomegaly proportionate to the flow through the ductus with a prominent main pulmonary artery segment, large ascending aorta and arch, increased pulmonary vascular markings, and a "left ventricular" contour to the heart shadow, with possible left atrial enlargement.

The diagnosis can be supported further by the echocardiogram. The ductus usually can be seen on two-dimensional echocardiogram. Turbulent flow by Doppler interrogation in the main pulmonary artery support the echocardiogram. Intracardiac lesions other than persistent ductus can be ruled out, as can lesions that can be confused with the ductus. Continuous wave Doppler detects very small streams of abnormal flow in the pulmonary artery. Even the very tiny ductus that is too small to be audible or visualized by echocardiogram can be detected by continuous wave Doppler, or the flow can be seen using color Doppler.

When all clinical findings of the ductus are assimilated and are absolutely characteristic, the diagnosis is established without further study. If there is even one atypical feature in any part of the clinical assessment, then the diagnosis should be established by cardiac catheterization.

In the catheterization of an isolated patent ductus, the hemodynamic study shows an increase in the oxygen saturation of the mixed venous blood maximized in the main pulmonary artery. Usually, this step-up in saturation is higher in the main pulmonary artery than in the distal pulmonary arteries. This results from the direct stream of blood flowing through the ductus directly toward the main pulmonary artery and pulmonary valve. During catheterization, the cardiac catheter often passes preferentially from the pulmonary artery through the ductus into the descending aorta. Although this adds support to the diagnosis, the catheter passage alone cannot be used to confirm the diagnosis. Similar, if not identical, hemodynamics and course of the catheter can be observed when the catheter passes from the right ventricle through a ventricular septal defect into the ascending aorta and then around the arch to the descending aorta, or when the catheter passes from the pulmonary artery through an aortopulmonary window into the ascending aorta and then around the arch. The presence of a ductus arteriosus should be confirmed by an angiocardiogram recorded in the lateral view with injection of the contrast in the descending aorta immediately adjacent to the usual entrance site of the ductus. This same angiocardiogram provides details about the size and exact shape of the ductus. When a catheterization is performed, it definitively rules out defects that may be confused with a ductus or establishes the presence of other defects that incidentally may be associated with the ductus.

## DIFFERENTIAL DIAGNOSIS

The venous hum is the murmur most often confused with the patent ductus arteriosus; it is the most benign and easiest to clinically differentiate. When carefully examined, the venous hum is a continuous sounding murmur; however, it usually is of a softer "more distant" quality. Most important, it crescendos or peaks in diastole. The venous hum usually is maximum in the first and second right intercostal spaces. It varies in intensity, or it can be eliminated by changes in body position, respirations, or neck rotation. The venous hum can be stopped by placing the patient in the supine position and simultaneously applying compression over the right jugular vein in the right supraclavicular area. With the auscultatory characteristics of the venous hum and the maneuvers to eliminate it, no further diagnostic studies should be necessary.

The lesion that is potentially most difficult to differentiate from the persistent ductus is the aortopulmonary window, which is rare. The aortopulmonary window is a window-like communication between the proximal ascending aorta and the main pulmonary artery that allows systemic blood to flow directly from the ascending aorta into the pulmonary artery. The hemodynamics are virtually identical to those of the ductus, and the site of the abnormal communication is anatomically close to that of the ductus; thus, many clinical findings are similar, if not identical, to the patent ductus.

The aortopulmonary window is usually a large communication resulting in a very large systemic-to-pulmonary shunt. Consequently, these patients usually present early in infancy with significant respiratory distress and signs of congestive failure. Because of the large size of the defect and the proximal location on the aorta, most of the runoff into the pulmonary artery from the aorta occurs during systole. As a result, the murmur may be only systolic and usually is located more over the left sternal border rather than in the infraclavicular area. Because of the more proximal location of the communication, there is a blood "steal" from the more peripheral circulation and vessels; thus, with the large window, all of the palpable pulses may be decreased rather than bounding. The rarer, small aortopulmonary window, on the other hand, has findings indistinguishable from a small persistent ductus. Confirmation of the diagnosis must be by echocardiogram and usually by high quality angiography as well.

A more common lesion that can be confused with a patent ductus if the physical examination is not precise is the combination of ventricular septal defect with associated aortic valve insufficiency. The murmur in these patients is "to and fro" rather than continuous. There is a plateau pansystolic murmur from the ventricular septal defect ending at the second heart sound. This is followed by a higher pitched decrescendo diastolic murmur from the aortic regurgitation. Other physical findings, electrocardiogram, and radiographs may be similar to those of a patent ductus, but the lesions should be distinguishable by astute auscultation, and, if not by the physical examination, then by echocardiogram and cardiac catheterization.

A sinus of Valsalva fistula can create a murmur and clinical findings similar to a patent ductus. On close auscultation, however, the murmur, like the murmur of the ventricular septal defect with aortic insufficiency, is more "to and fro" with separate systolic and diastolic components. Also, the murmur of a sinus of Valsalva fistula usually is localized over the lower left or right sternal border.

Any intrathoracic systemic-to-pulmonary artery or systemic-to-venous fistula can generate a continuous murmur that casually could be confused with a persistent patent ductus. In virtually all of those lesions, the continuous murmur has a markedly different location, depending on the site of the fistulous communication. Over the location of maximum intensity, the murmur of a fistula often has an almost superficial or "close" sounding quality, which is particularly common with a coronary artery camera fistula. This fistula is the most likely fistulous lesion to be localized close to the location of the ductus and, in turn, the most likely to mimic the ductus murmur.

All other lesions with continuous murmurs (eg, truncus arteriosus, pulmonary atresia/ventricular septal defect with systemic collaterals, and stenosed anomalous pulmonary veins) have cyanosis and markedly different associated physical findings, electrocardiograms, and roentgenograms.

## COMPLICATED DUCTUS

When a ductus is present with other congenital heart lesions, it may be difficult to detect. The characteristic murmur and radiographic findings of the ductus may be overshadowed by physical signs, radiographic appearance, and electrocardiogram of the associated lesion. In the absence of the classical continuous murmur of the persistent ductus, the one finding on physical examination

that should make the examiner suspect a patent ductus is the presence of full or bounding pulses that would not be expected with the intracardiac shunts. Associated defects and persistent ductus should be visualized by a carefully performed echocardiogram. When such combination lesions are suspected, however, they should be confirmed by cardiac catheterization. Catheterization determines the relative hemodynamic importance of each lesion as well as documents the presence of the ductus in these cases.

There are two categories of congenital heart lesions in which the associated patent ductus is essential to the survival of the patient—the ductus-dependent lesions. The first category includes those patients with severe coarctation of the aorta or interruption of the aortic arch. In these patients, the blood flow to the lower body may be dependent on the ductus. With the coarctation, the dilated aortic end of the open ductus allows blood flow around or adjacent to the obstruction in the aorta. With complete interruption of the aorta, the blood flow is from the pulmonary artery through the ductus into the descending aorta with the lower body blood flow solely from this route. The second category of ductus-dependent patients includes cyanotic patients with a severely restricted or even totally obstructed pulmonary valve. In those patients, the total or greater amount of pulmonary blood flow comes from the patent ductus. These ductus-dependent lesions must be recognized early and efforts made to keep the ductus open until the appropriate surgical procedure can be performed.

Another complicated ductus arteriosus is the ductus with pulmonary hypertension and associated pulmonary vascular disease. In these patients, none of the characteristic findings of the ductus is present. Because of the high pulmonary resistance, there is little or no flow from the aorta into the pulmonary artery. Thus, physical findings of this flow are absent. There usually is a right ventricular lift, and the second heart sound is single, very loud, and often palpable. There frequently is no murmur or only a short nonspecific systolic murmur. With very high resistance, there is flow of the desaturated pulmonary artery blood into the descending aorta. This latter phenomenon produces the pathognomonic clinical finding of cyanotic lower trunk and lower extremities and, at the same time, normal coloration of the upper trunk, head, and upper extremities. These patients have right ventricular hypertrophy on electrocardiogram. Radiographs reveal a normal to slightly enlarged heart size with prominent main pulmonary artery segment and proximal right and left pulmonary arteries, yet normal or decreased peripheral pulmonary vascular markings. The pulmonary hypertensive ductus should be studied by cardiac catheterization to unequivocally exclude the possibility of any other cause of increased total pulmonary resistance.

Bacterial endocarditis is a potential complication of the patent ductus patient. Since the advent of early surgical correction of the ductus and the use of prophylactic antibiotics in patients with congenital heart lesions, the incidence of this complication has decreased markedly. Its occurrence in patients with patent ductus is now the least of all of the isolated congenital heart defects. The prevention of this complication now is the major indication for correction of most of the small ductus.

## THERAPY

Therapy for patent ductus can be supportive or definitive. Supportive therapy is treatment of symptoms resulting from the patent ductus. Patients with a large persistent ductus have signs and symptoms of pulmonary overcirculation with shortness of breath, dyspnea, even overt pulmonary edema. Symptoms can be treated with digoxin and vigorous diuretic therapy. Occasionally, the young infant with a large patent ductus needs intubation and ventilation with end-expiratory positive pressure to control pulmonary overcirculation. These medical measures help control symptoms but do not treat the underlying anatomic defect.

Definitive therapy for the ductus is complete interruption of blood flow through the ductus. Heretofore, the established definitive therapy for the persistent ductus was surgical ligation and division of the ductus. Definitive therapy is indicated when supportive therapy does not allow normal growth, development, and activity of the infant or child. When no supportive therapy is necessary or when supportive therapy is required and satisfactorily maintains the patient, then elective surgical repair is considered for the patient anytime after 2 to 3 years of age, but usually before the child enters school. The only urgency for repair of the asymptomatic ductus is the anxiety of the child's physician, which often is relayed to the parents.

Surgical repair of the ductus requires a thoracotomy; however, it does not require cardiopulmonary bypass and is a "minor" cardiac surgical procedure. Nevertheless, it is a surgical procedure with the inherent discomfort and morbidity of a surgical procedure. The thoracic surgical patient requires general anesthesia, intubation, and a thoracotomy. There is a 1- to 2-day stay in the recovery ward with a period of continued intubation and with a chest tube in place, followed by 5 to 7 days of hospitalized recovery. The patient has a further 4- to 8-week convalescence before returning to full normal physical activity. In addition to the acute risks of surgery and recovery, there are rare but possible permanent complications. These include vocal cord or diaphragmatic paralysis from intrathoracic nerve injury or even ligation of the wrong vessel or structure within the chest. In addition to the morbidity of the surgery, there is a small, finite mortality associated with surgical repair of the patent ductus.

One year after the ligation and division surgery, the ductus is considered cured. By then, complete healing is ensured, and risk of endocarditis is considered eliminated. After surgical ligation only, there have been cases of "recanalization" of the ductus in as many as 10% of cases. Data accumulated from other ductus occlusion techniques and from high-resolution Doppler studies show that the "recanalization" of the ductus after surgical ligation actually may have been a residual tiny ductus following the initial attempted ligation.

There are alternative, nonsurgical definitive approaches to elective correction of the patent ductus. The first, devised by Werner Portsmann in 1967, is a transcatheter foam plug technique to close the ductus arteriosus. This procedure is complex and requires use of very large catheters in both the artery and vein of the patient. The Portsmann technique is still in use in a few centers outside of the United States, but, because of its limitations, the procedure never was applicable for small children and never achieved wide acceptance.

William Rashkind reported closure of a patent ductus using a tiny single-hooked umbrella in a 3.5-kg infant in 1979. The device was effective in that patient, but because of the attachment hooks, the device is unsatisfactory for general use. As a result, a safer, more usable version was developed. The present Rashkind device is a tiny spring-loaded double umbrella that may be delivered through a relatively small catheter and by either an arterial or venous approach. This device was introduced into a collaborative clinical trial that began in 1981. Both the device and the delivery technique were modified further during the first 2 years of the trials. Initial results of this trial were reported in 1986 when additional centers were added to the study. The study closed in 1988. The experience and data on the use of the Rashkind ductus occluder device were reviewed by the Cardiac Device Panel of the Food and Drug Administration in February 1989, and the device was approved for clinical use at that time. While awaiting final administrative approval, an extension of the trial was initiated and continued until 1991. The device also has been ap-

proved and is in continued routine clinical use in many countries outside of the United States, including the United Kingdom, Canada, Germany, France, and the Netherlands. In this extensive experience of more than 7000 patients and relatively long 12-year follow-up, the device has proved effective and safe. There has been no mortality, little morbidity, and 88% total occlusion with the device. The major remaining problem with the device is the presence of tiny nonaudible residual leaks in about 10% of cases. These tiny leaks have no known clinical consequence, but, theoretically, could be a site for endocarditis. Prototype changes in the device should correct this problem, once the device is clinically available in the United States and official modifications are applied for. Continued changes in the device and improvements in the delivery technique will enhance the ease and success of the ductus device. The device still has not been approved by the Food and Drug Administration and is not available for clinical use in the United States.

In its present configuration, the ductus occluding device is not only an acceptable technique, but also should be the preferred procedure for elective correction of patent ductus arteriosus. If an attempted occlusion with the Rashkind occlusion device is unsatisfactory, then the patient may have to undergo surgical repair of the ductus. While the sick newborn and small infant require surgical closure of the patent ductus, elective correction beyond infancy soon should be relegated to the annals of congenital heart disease history.

## Selected Readings

Alzamora V, Rotta A, Gattilana G, et al. On the possible influence of great altitudes on the determination of certain cardiovascular anomalies. Pediatrics 1953;12:259.
Gittenberger-De Groot AC, Van Ertbruggen I, Moulaert AJMG, et al. The ductus arteriosus in the preterm infant: histologic and clinical observations. J Pediatr 1980;96:88.
Heymann MA, Rudolph AM. Control of the ductus arteriosus. Physiol Rev 1975;55:62.
Portsmann W, Wierny L, Warnke H. Der Verschluss des D.a.p. Ohne Thorakotomie (1 Mitteilung). Thoraxchirurgie 1967;15:199.
Rashkind WJ, Cuaso CC. Transcatheter closure of patent ductus arteriosus: successful use in a 3.5 kilogram infant. Pediatr Cardiol 1979;1:3.
Rashkind WJ, Mullins CE, Hellenbrand WE, et al. Nonsurgical closure of patent ductus arteriosus: clinical application of the Rashkind PDA Occluder system. Circulation 1987;75(3):583.
Rudolph AM, Drorbaugh JE, Auld PA, et al. Studies on the circulation in the neonatal period: the circulation in the respiratory distress syndrome. Pediatrics 1961;27:551.
Swan C, Tostevin AL, Black GHB. Final observations on congenital defects in infants following infectious diseases during pregnancy with special reference to rubella. Med J Aust 1946;2:889.
Thibeault DW, Emmanouilides GC, Nelson RJ, et al. Patent ductus arteriosus complicating the respiratory distress syndrome in preterm infants. J Pediatr 1975;86:120.

*Principles and Practice of Pediatrics, Second Edition.*
edited by Frank A. Oski et al. J. B. Lippincott Company, Philadelphia © 1994.

# 82.4 *Pulmonary Stenosis*

### John P. Cheatham

Obstruction of pulmonary blood flow may occur within the right ventricle, at the valve, or anywhere in the pulmonary arterial system. In general terms, pulmonary stenosis occurs in about 20% to 30% of all patients with congenital heart disease. In about half of these cases, the ventricular septum is intact.

# PULMONARY VALVE STENOSIS

Pulmonary valve stenosis constitutes about 7% to 12% of all congenital heart disease and up to 80% to 90% of all lesions causing obstruction of right ventricular output. The defect originally was described in 1761 by Morgagni. The exact pathogenetic mechanism for its development is not clear. Several authors suggest that an abnormality of the distal bulbus cordis leads to valvar obstruction, with sparing of the proximal bulbus, which participates in closure of the ventricular septum. Fetal endocarditis also is implicated in the etiology of this defect. Genetic factors may play an equally important role, because pulmonary valve stenosis is found often in various syndromes.

The gross and microscopic features of pulmonary valve stenosis are classified in six categories: domed, 42%; tricuspid, 6%; bicuspid, 10%; unicommissural, 16%; hypoplastic annulus, 6%; dysplastic, 19%. The pathology affecting the remaining portion of the right-sided cardiac structures involves changes secondary to the valve obstruction (ie, right ventricular hypertrophy, fibrosis, and tricuspid valve abnormalities).

Clinically, pulmonary valve stenosis with intact ventricular septum is described best as either mild, moderate, or severe. Mild stenosis is defined here as a systolic transvalvular gradient of less than 40 mm Hg or right ventricular pressure of less than half of left ventricular pressure. Moderate obstruction is considered present when the systolic gradient across the pulmonary valve is greater than 40 mm Hg or right ventricular pressure of greater than half of, but less than, the left ventricular pressure. Severe stenosis is classified as a systolic gradient of more than 80 mm Hg or the presence of suprasystemic right ventricular pressure.

Patients with mild stenosis are asymptomatic with normal growth and development and no cyanosis. The jugular venous pulse is normal, and there is no sign of congestive heart failure. Children with moderate stenosis and intact ventricular septum may develop mild dyspnea with exertion, but are frequently asymptomatic. Cyanosis with exertion may be noted occasionally if an atrial septal defect is present. Individuals with severe valvular stenosis usually demonstrate symptoms, although as many as 25% of these patients are asymptomatic. Frequently, dyspnea and fatigue with only a moderate amount of exertion are present. Central cyanosis is one of the most important signs in patients with an atrial communication; it may be present at rest or with minimal exercise. Some evidence shows the degree of cyanosis increases with age. When "squatting" is seen in a cyanotic child suspected of having pulmonary valve stenosis, the diagnosis of tetralogy of Fallot must be considered. Growth and development in infants with severe stenosis are usually normal, without evidence of wasting. "Moon facies" with a chubby phenotype has been described as characteristic of children with pulmonary valve stenosis, but is not pathognomonic and is present in less than 50% of infants with severe obstruction.

The cardiovascular examination helps in the diagnosis of pulmonary valve stenosis. The precordial activity is quiet with mild obstruction, but may be increased with a palpable right ventricular tap in patients with moderate or severe stenosis. A systolic thrill over the pulmonary valve area may be present as the severity increases. The striking auscultatory feature of pulmonary valve stenosis is a prominent systolic ejection murmur. The murmur may vary in length and intensity, but usually ends before the aortic valve closure. The maximum intensity of the murmur is at the upper left sternal border radiating to the back, but it is also heard along the precordium and the neck. As the severity increases, the systolic ejection murmur lengthens, with a later peak in intensity. The murmur of pulmonary valve stenosis increases in duration and intensity after amyl nitrate inhalation, whereas the opposite is true in children with tetralogy of Fallot.

A high-pitched ejection sound or systolic click usually is au-dible along the left upper sternal border. The click probably originates from the sudden opening and doming of the thickened pulmonary valve leaflets. As the severity of obstruction increases, the systolic ejection click occurs earlier, until, in severe stenosis, it may be indistinguishable from the first heart sound. The second heart sound usually is split and of normal intensity in mild stenosis. The degree of splitting is directly proportional to the severity of obstruction. There also appears to be an inverse relationship between the severity of stenosis and the intensity of the pulmonary component of the second heart sound. In severe stenosis, therefore, there is wide splitting of the second heart sound, with a very soft pulmonary component that is often heard as a single second sound.

The electrocardiogram frequently is normal in mild stenosis, whereas it is normal in only 10% of children with moderate obstruction, and it is uniformly abnormal with severe stenosis. Right axis deviation frequently is seen, with right ventricular hypertrophy noted in the anterior precordial leads. In moderate stenosis, the magnitude of the R wave in $V_1$ usually is less than 20 mm, while an upright T wave in $V_1$ is present about 50% of the time. A qR or a pure R wave of more than 20 mm is present in patients with severe stenosis. In some children, there may be ST or T waves suggestive of ischemia.

The most consistent and distinctive radiographic feature is prominence in the main pulmonary artery segment secondary to poststenotic dilatation of the pulmonary trunk and the proximal left pulmonary artery (Fig 82-9). This finding is present in as many as 90% of patients, but does not correlate with the severity of obstruction. In severe stenosis, the cardiac apex may be tilted upward with generalized cardiomegaly and right atrial prominence, especially if right-sided failure is present. The aortic arch is usually left-sided. Presence of a right arch should lead the physician to consider the diagnosis of tetralogy of Fallot.

The noninvasive evaluation of abnormalities of the pulmonary valve by M-mode and two-dimensional echocardiography has been less than satisfactory. With recent advances of Doppler echocardiography and color flow mapping techniques, however, both the sensitivity and specificity of diagnosis of pulmonary valve stenosis have improved. Two-dimensional echocardiog-

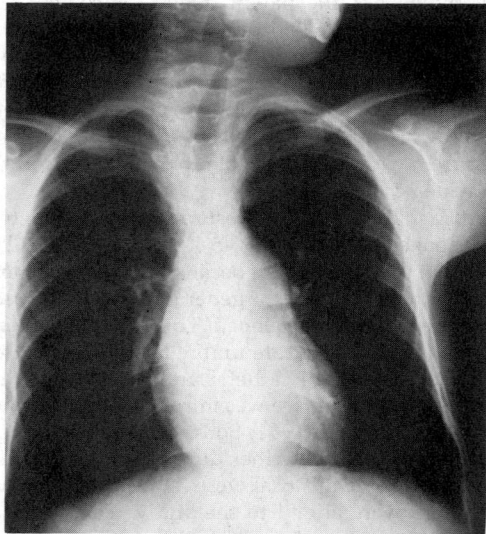

**Figure 82-9.** Chest roentgenogram from an 8-year-old boy with mild stenosis of the pulmonary valve. Heart size is usually normal. Pulmonary vascular markings are unremarkable. The most distinctive radiographic feature of this disease is poststenotic dilatation of the pulmonary trunk, as depicted in this chest film. The degree of dilatation is unrelated to the severity of stenosis.

raphy enables visualization of the thickened and domed pulmonary valve leaflets, pulmonary annulus, dilated pulmonary trunk, hypertrophic right ventricle, and other associated congenital heart defects. Pulsed and continuous wave Doppler echocardiography enable accurate estimation of the location and severity of pulmonary stenosis without invasive procedures. The recorded peak flow velocity on spectral display is converted to estimated transvalvular pressure gradient using the modified Bernoulli equation $PG = 4V^2$, where PG equals instantaneous pressure gradient (mm Hg) and V equals peak Doppler velocity (m/sec). Color-coded Doppler echo may provide additional hemodynamic information about these patients.

The role of cardiac catheterization and angiography in the diagnosis and treatment of pulmonary valve stenosis has changed dramatically over the last 10 years. In the past, information obtained in the catheterization laboratory was a prerequisite for selecting patients for surgical valvotomy. Since the initial use of percutaneous, transluminal balloon pulmonary valvuloplasty in 1982, the catheterization laboratory has become the location for the "treatment" of moderate and severe pulmonary valve stenosis. The most important hemodynamic information obtained during cardiac catheterization is the measurement of right ventricular pressure with simultaneous left ventricular or aortic pressure and the systolic gradient across the pulmonary valve. It is also important to define any associated cardiac defects at this time. The use of biplane cineangiocardiography with high-resolution video discs, recorders, and monitors has helped greatly in the therapeutic techniques during interventional pediatric cardiac catheterization. Angiographic features of pulmonary valve stenosis include thickening and doming of valve leaflets with poststenotic dilatation of the pulmonary trunk (Fig 82-10).

Recent studies demonstrate hemodynamic abnormalities during exercise in children and adults with pulmonary valve stenosis. Both children and adults with severe stenosis had altered myocardial performance during exercise (ie, decreased stroke and cardiac index and increased right ventricular end-diastolic pressure). Adults, however, had a disproportionately lower cardiac index and heart rate at rest and during exercise than did children with obstruction of the same magnitude. There is evidence of myocardial fibrosis in uncorrected moderate to severe pulmonary valve stenosis in adults, which suggests the need for aggressive treatment of this condition during childhood.

The differential diagnosis of pulmonary valve stenosis with intact ventricular septum includes atrial septal defect, pulmonary artery stenosis, ventricular septal defect, idiopathic dilatation of the main pulmonary artery, straight back syndrome, mitral valve prolapse, aortic valve stenosis, and innocent pulmonary flow murmurs. When cyanosis is present, tetralogy of Fallot and pulmonary valve atresia with intact ventricular septum should be considered. The correct diagnosis usually can be made by physical examination, but echocardiography may help distinguish between various congenital heart defects. Pulmonary valve stenosis may be associated with various systemic diseases and syndromes (eg, glycogen storage disease, neurofibromatosis, gout, neoplasm, carcinoid bowel disease, and Noonan's, Williams, Watson, and Leopard syndromes).

The natural history of mild pulmonary valve stenosis is benign. There is little improvement in severe obstruction, however, and often the transvalvular gradient increases with age. There is a definite risk of right-sided congestive heart failure, myocardial fibrosis, and sudden death in these patients. The clinical course of and prognosis for moderate pulmonary valve stenosis is under debate, but recent exercise studies demonstrating right ventricular dysfunction in adults are alarming. The risk of infective endocarditis in patients with pulmonary valve stenosis is low, but all individuals, regardless of the severity of stenosis or whether intervention has taken place, should receive selected antibiotics for infective endocarditis prophylaxis during dental or surgical procedures.

Medical treatment of children with pulmonary valve stenosis usually is confined to neonates with critical obstruction. They present with cyanosis, right-sided congestive failure, and cardiomegaly. Because adequate pulmonary blood flow in these neonates depends on patency of the ductus arteriosus, prostaglandin $E_1$ intravenous infusion (0.05 to 0.10 µg/kg/min) is life-saving. Anticongestive medications (eg, digoxin, furosemide, dopamine) also may be necessary. The treatment of choice in these neonates, as well as in children with moderate to severe stenosis, however, is balloon pulmonary valvuloplasty performed in the cardiac catheterization laboratory.

Since its initial description in 1982, balloon-dilation valvuloplasty for pulmonary valve stenosis has evolved into a fairly standard treatment performed by the pediatric cardiologist with special training. After hemodynamics and angiograms are obtained, a proper-sized balloon is chosen (1.3 times the size of the angio-measured annulus or equal to the echo-measured annulus).

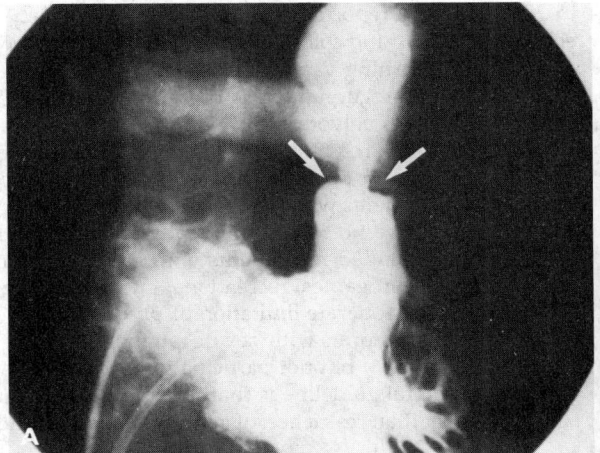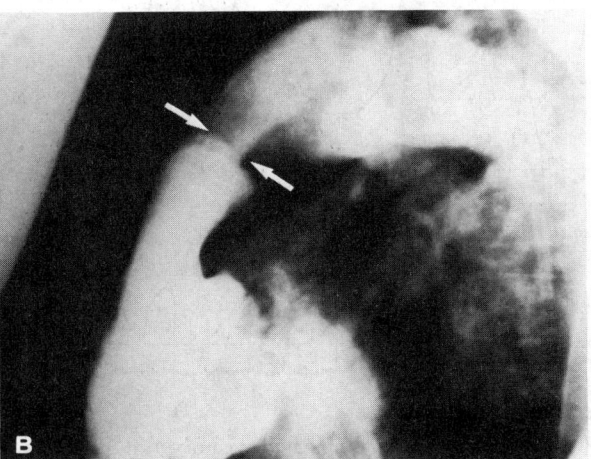

**Figure 82-10.**   Right ventriculogram in a patient with typical features of moderate pulmonary valve stenosis. (**A**) Anteroposterior view demonstrating systolic doming of the stenotic leaflets with a "jet" of contrast material noted (*arrows*). The infundibulum is widely patent and the main pulmonary artery is dilated. (**B**) Lateral projection shows the systolic "jet" that passes through the thickened leaflets (*arrows*).

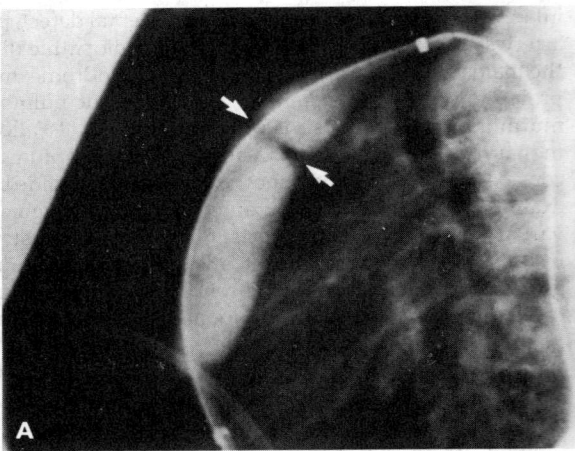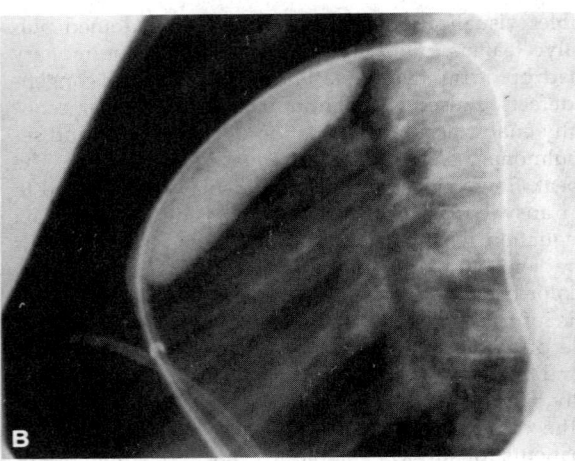

**Figure 82-11.** Proper positioning of the balloon catheter for pulmonary valvuloplasty using the lateral view under fluoroscopy. (**A**) A guidewire passes through the catheter from the right ventricular outflow tract into the left pulmonary artery. The balloon is inflated with diluted contrast (20%) until a "waist" is seen that corresponds to the stenotic valve leaflets (*arrows*). Attempts to maintain the waist at the midportion of the balloon should be made while the catheter is positioned. In this case, the waist is toward the distal third of the balloon. (**B**) The balloon is repositioned more distally and is completely inflated, using a hand-held manometer. Note that the hourglass waist has disappeared.

After positioning the balloon catheter over a guidewire through the stenotic pulmonary valve, the balloon is inflated to 4 to 6 atmospheres of pressure using a hand-held gauge (Fig 82-11). Occasionally, two balloon catheters are required in large children and adults with a pulmonary valve annulus larger than 20 mm in diameter. Immediate relief of the transvalvular gradient is seen frequently (Fig 82-12). Balloon valvuloplasty produces relief of obstruction by commissural splitting of the valve. According to the Valvuloplasty and Angioplasty of Congenital Anomalies (VACA) Registry, the risk of a major complication is 0.6%, including death (0.2%), cardiac perforation with tamponade (0.1%), and severe tricuspid insufficiency (0.2%). Minor complications occur in 1.3% of patients, while 2.6% experience an incident defined as arrhythmia, hypoxemia, or venous bleeding. The incidence of complications and incidents is inversely related to age. It is substantially higher in infants, particularly in neonates.

The response of dysplastic pulmonary valves to balloon dilation varies, but, in general, is less than that of nondysplastic valves. This type of valvar stenosis is present in about 50% of children with Noonan's syndrome. Valve leaflets are unfused, excessively thickened, and demonstrate little motion during the cardiac cycle. Both balloon valvuloplasty and surgical valvotomy usually are inadequate procedures to relieve the obstruction completely. Partial or total surgical valvectomy may be required to relieve the valvar gradient in these children.

Although surgical pulmonary valvotomy is a relatively low-risk procedure (3% to 4% mortality rate), it is seldom necessary because balloon-dilation valvuloplasty is available. When surgery is required, inflow occlusion with transarterial valvotomy or "open" valvotomy using cardiopulmonary bypass is the method usually employed. The incidence of pulmonary insufficiency after surgery varies from 57% to 90%, whereas an incidence of 13% to 20% has been reported after balloon valvuloplasty. Doppler echocardiography and color flow mapping, however, are sensitive methods for detecting valvular insufficiency and suggest that a small amount of regurgitation is present in most patients after surgical or balloon valvotomy.

A special task force committee composed of members of the AHA specializing in cardiovascular diseases of the young recommends that patients with treated or untreated mild pulmonary valve stenosis have no restriction of physical activity. Light exercise is recommended for patients with moderate stenosis (eg, nonstrenuous team games, recreational swimming, jogging, cycling, and golf). Moderate limitation of physical activities is recommended for children with severe pulmonary valve stenosis (eg, attending school but not participating in physical education classes). A general guideline is that treatment of the underlying stenosis, rather than restriction of activity, should be undertaken.

## INTRACAVITARY OBSTRUCTION OF THE RIGHT VENTRICLE

Two types of obstruction are classified as primary infundibular stenosis and double-chambered right ventricle secondary to an

**Figure 82-12.** Pressure recordings obtained at cardiac catheterization before and after balloon valvuloplasty for moderate pulmonary valve stenosis. (**A**) The right ventricular (RV) systolic pressure is somewhat greater than 70 mm Hg before balloon valvuloplasty. Note the triangular appearance of the RV pressure curve indicative of significant stenosis. (**B**) The RV systolic pressure decreases to 30 mm Hg with a completely normal pressure curve. Aortic (Ao) pressure remained unchanged during the procedure.

anomalous muscle bundle. Primary infundibular stenosis is uncommon and is usually secondary to a fibrous band at the junction of the infundibulum and the main body of the right ventricle. Because it closely resembles double-chambered right ventricle, only the latter is discussed here.

The anomalous muscle bundles dividing the right ventricle into double chambers are probably secondary to an arrest of the incorporation of the primitive bulbus cordis into the body of the right ventricle. This would explain the common occurrence of an associated ventricular septal defect, which is present in as many as 93% of cases. Subaortic valve membrane also is seen in association with these defects. The proximal inlet chamber has high pressure, whereas the distal outflow chamber has low pressure that is equal to the pulmonary arterial pressure. Physical examination reveals a systolic ejection murmur lower along the left sternal border than is usually heard with pulmonary valve stenosis. There is no systolic ejection click, and the murmur often is confused with a ventricular septal defect. The electrocardiogram demonstrates right ventricular hypertrophy, depending on the severity. The chest radiograph is unremarkable, but echocardiography may define the intracavitary obstruction. Cardiac catheterization and angiography frequently are used to obtain precise hemodynamic and anatomic information. A selective right ventriculogram is necessary in these children.

Natural history studies indicate the severity of intracavitary obstruction is progressive. Treatment for significant obstruction by an anomalous right ventricular muscle bundle is surgical resection of the bundle, taking care to avoid injury to the tricuspid valve apparatus. Associated ventricular septal defect and subaortic valve membrane may require closure and resection, respectively. Balloon dilation of the intracavitary obstruction is not recommended. Infective endocarditis prophylaxis is recommended for all patients, regardless of treatment.

## PULMONARY ARTERY STENOSIS

Obstruction of pulmonary blood flow along the pulmonary arterial tree may occur at many sites. The overall incidence of pulmonary arterial stenosis is 2% to 3% of cases of congenital heart disease. Isolated pulmonary artery stenosis occurs in one third of the cases, but there are associated cardiac defects in two thirds of the patients. The most common associated defects are pulmonary valve stenosis and ventricular septal defect (ie, tetralogy of Fallot). Multiple peripheral pulmonary artery stenoses commonly are present in rubella and in the Williams syndrome. Several other syndromes also have this associated defect, including Noonan's, Alagille, Ehlers-Danlos, cutis laxa, and Silver-Russell syndromes.

Clinical features of pulmonary artery stenosis may be easily masked by associated defects. Close inspection and auscultation, however, reveal a systolic ejection murmur that is heard over the pulmonary area but is particularly loud in the back and lateral lung fields. A systolic ejection click is absent. A continuous murmur may be present in as many as 10% of patients, indicating a significant diastolic as well as systolic gradient. The degree of right ventricular hypertrophy visible on the electrocardiogram depends on the severity of obstruction. The chest roentgenogram usually is normal. While the echocardiogram may be helpful in defining associated intracardiac defects, it is not reliable in imaging the sites of pulmonary artery stenosis. Therefore, cardiac catheterization and angiography are imperative in these children. Selective right ventriculography and pulmonary arteriography are necessary to define the areas of stenosis precisely.

In isolated cases, the natural history may be benign, but progressive increase in severity with subsequent death in early infancy and childhood has been reported. Because of the poor surgical results in the treatment of isolated and complicated pulmonary artery stenosis, the use of balloon angioplasty began in 1980. A balloon diameter three to four times the stenotic segment of vessel usually is required for successful angioplasty. Studies show significant intimal and medial tears in all successful cases, at times extending into the adventitia. The VACA registry reports a 3% risk of death during this procedure. In addition, complications such as vessel perforation, hemorrhage, and arrhythmias occur in 10% of patients. Balloon angioplasty for pulmonary artery stenosis can provide significant hemodynamic relief for a small group of children in whom conventional operative intervention is unlikely to be successful, but the results of balloon dilation for this lesion are far less spectacular than for pulmonary valve stenosis and there is a significant mortality and morbidity risk. A new method of treating children with failed balloon dilation of pulmonary artery stenosis is the use of endovascular stents to support the vessel wall and eliminate recurrent obstruction. Early results are encouraging with few complications reported. A larger patient experience and a longer period of follow-up are required, however, before this method of treatment can be recommended as the definitive treatment for pulmonary artery stenosis. Regardless of therapy, infective endocarditis prophylaxis is recommended for all patients with this congenital heart defect.

## Selected Readings

Emmanouilides GC, Baylen BG. Pulmonary stenosis. In: Adams FH, Emmanouilides GC, eds. Heart disease in infants, children, and adolescents, ed 3. Baltimore: Williams & Wilkins, 1983:234.

Gallucci V, et al. Double-chambered right ventricle: surgical experience and anatomical considerations. J Thorac Cardiovasc Surg 1980;28:13.

Gikonyo BM, Lucas RV, Edwards JE. Anatomic features of congenital pulmonary valvar stenosis. Pediatr Cardiol 1987;8:109.

Gutgesell HP, et al. Accuracy of two-dimensional echocardiography in the diagnosis of congenital heart disease. Am J Cardiol 1985;55:514.

Gutgesell HP, et al. Recreational and occupational recommendations for young patients with heart disease. Circulation 1986;74:1195A.

Kan JS, et al. Balloon angioplasty-branch pulmonary artery stenosis: results from the Valvuloplasty and Angioplasty of Congenital Anomalies registry. Am J Cardiol 1990;65:798.

Krabill KA, Wang Y, Einzig S, Moller JH. Rest and exercise hemodynamics in pulmonary stenosis: comparison of children and adults. Am J Cardiol 1985;56:360.

Kveselis DA, et al. Results of balloon valvuloplasty in the treatment of congenital valvar pulmonary stenosis in children. Am J Cardiol 1985;56:527.

Lock JE, et al. Balloon dilatation angioplasty of hypoplastic and stenotic pulmonary arteries. Circulation 1983;67:962.

Nugent EW, et al. Clinical course in pulmonic stenosis. Circulation 1977;56:15.

Perry SB, et al. Endovascular stents in congenital heart disease. Progress in Pediatric Cardiology 1992;1(2):35.

Rowe RD. Pulmonary stenosis with normal aortic root; pulmonary arterial stenosis. In: Rowe RD, ed. Heart disease in infancy and childhood, ed 3. New York: Macmillan, 1978:760, 789.

Stanger P, et al. Balloon pulmonary valvuloplasty: results of the Valvuloplasty and Angioplasty of Congenital Anomalies registry. Am J Cardiol 1990;65:775.

*Principles and Practice of Pediatrics, Second Edition.*
edited by Frank A. Oski et al. J. B. Lippincott Company, Philadelphia © 1994.

# 82.5 *Pulmonary Valve Atresia With Intact Ventricular Septum*

## Donald A. Riopel

Pulmonary valve atresia with intact ventricular septum (PA:IVS) results in varying degrees of hypoplasia of the right ventricle and tricuspid valve. The clinical course of severe hypoplasia of the right ventricle can be almost as devastating as that of severe hypoplasia of the left side of the heart. Infants with moderate or mild hypoplasia, however, have a more favorable clinical course.

## INCIDENCE

The defect is estimated to occur in 0.1 to 0.4 per 10,000 births. There is no distinct gender preference.

## ETIOLOGY

At stage 15 of embryologic development, four mounds of endocardial cushion tissue, which eventually form the thin aortic and pulmonary valve cusps, are present in the outflow channel of the developing heart tube. Abnormalities of one valve without abnormalities of the other suggests that the etiology occurs after the valve cusps are formed. The association of pulmonary artery obstruction with rubella infections is an example of indications that a fetal inflammation may be causative.

## PATHOLOGY

The pulmonary valve obstruction is complete. The valve tissue is a membrane, usually with fused commissures depicted by raphes and with three formed cusps. The right ventricular cavity size ranges from tiny to larger than normal, although in most cases, it is smaller than normal.

Frequently seen are communications between the right ventricle and the coronary artery system via myocardial sinusoids. These are unique to this lesion and carry an unfavorable prognosis.

The tricuspid valve, by definition, is patent in all cases, and the size of the tricuspid orifice appears to be proportional to the size of the right ventricular cavity. The deformity of the tricuspid valve results in varying degrees of severity of stenosis or insufficiency.

The size of the right atrium depends on the degree of tricuspid insufficiency and on the presence and size of the communication between the atria.

## PHYSIOLOGY

### Fetal

With no outlet of the right ventricle, the fetus with PA:IVS directs all systemic venous blood to the left side of the heart through a communication in the atrial septum. Therefore, the blood flow through the entire left heart is greater than that in the normal fetus.

### Postnatal

Systemic venous blood enters the right atrium from the vena cavae. With no exit possible through the pulmonary valve, the blood must cross the atrial septum through the foramen ovale or an atrial septal defect. Systemic saturation depends on the amount of pulmonary blood flow, which, in turn, depends on the size and patency of the ductus arteriosus. As the ductus undergoes a natural tendency to close, oxygen tension decreases and symptoms of hypoxia occur.

The presence of communications between the coronary artery system and the right ventricle via right ventricular sinusoids affects coronary blood flow and causes ischemia and subendocardial fibrosis of both ventricles.

## CLINICAL PRESENTATION

### Symptoms

Most of these infants are born at term, have not had growth retardation in utero, and are vigorous. Symptoms of cyanosis occur within a few hours to several days after birth and are dependent on ductal flow. Cyanosis may be intermittent and associated only with the stress of feedings or may be sudden and severe due to sudden closure of the ductus arteriosus. Infants with severe cyanosis also have accompanying acidosis and deep compensatory respirations in an attempt to correct the metabolic acidosis. Hypoxia, acidosis, or hypoglycemia, singly or in combination, can lead to seizure activity.

### Signs

In the symptomatic infant, there is severe cyanosis of the mucous membranes and nail beds, with paleness of the skin secondary to a low cardiac output and peripheral vasoconstriction. Hyperpnea is present, and no rales are heard on auscultation of the lungs. Cardiac auscultation may reveal only the single second heart sound of aortic closure, with no murmur. If there is tricuspid insufficiency, then a long systolic murmur is heard along the lower left sternal border. Rarely is a continuous murmur heard. The liver may be engorged and pulsatile due to passive congestion such as is seen with tricuspid atresia. Pulses are weak and thready. There is cyanosis of the nail beds and clubbing in infants more than 4 months old.

## LABORATORY FINDINGS

Arterial blood gases in infants not on prostaglandins have a low pH, a very low $Po_2$—often in the teens, and a somewhat low $Pco_2$ with a negative base deficit. In infants receiving prostaglandins, arterial blood gas values may approach normal.

Electrocardiographic findings in PA:IVS depend on the anatomy of the defect. The rhythm is sinus with normal time intervals, and the P wave often is tall and peaked. The QRS frontal plane vector tends to be in the lower left quadrant in cases of small right ventricle, whereas it is usually rightward (greater than +120°) in cases with a normal or a large right ventricle. With a severely hypoplastic right ventricle, the R-to-S ratio in the horizontal plane favors the posterior forces, suggesting absent or diminished right ventricular forces (Fig 82-13). The T wave usually is normal, except when there is ischemia of ventricles,

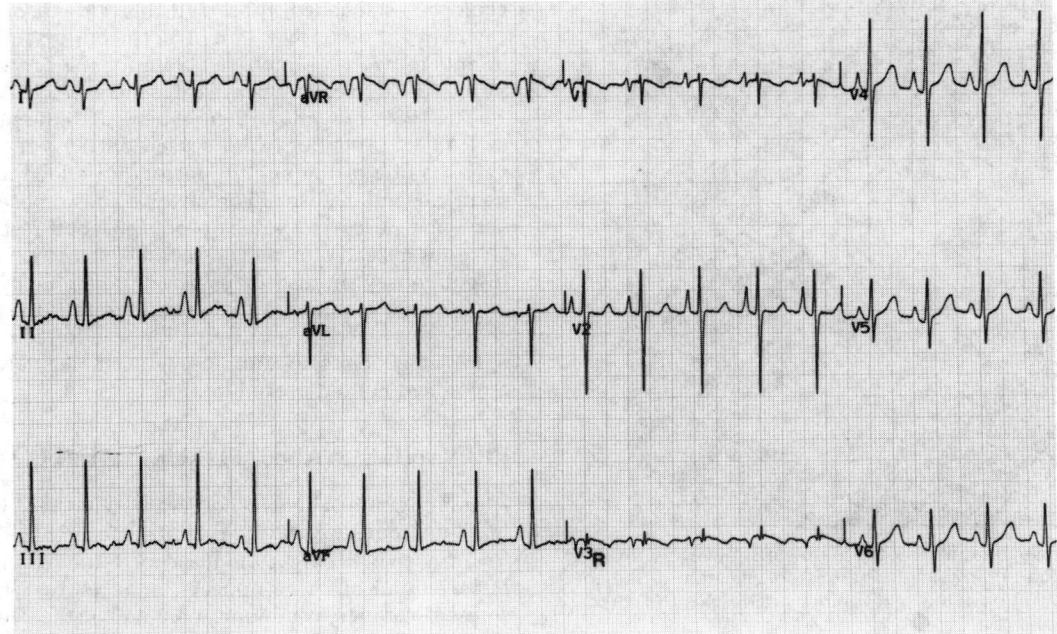

**Figure 82-13.**    Twelve-lead electrocardiogram of a neonate with pulmonary atresia and intact ventricular septum. The tall P waves in lead II indicate right atrial enlargement, and the relative lack of R waves in lead V1 represents the absence of right ventricular forces.

whereupon discordant T vectors are seen and ST changes of strain are present.

Chest roentgenograms in PA:IVS vary with anatomic type. In cases involving a tiny right ventricle and little or no tricuspid insufficiency, the heart is normal in size. The vascularity is reduced but may appear to be normal, depending on the patency of the ductus arteriosus. With tricuspid insufficiency, there is a large right atrium, giving considerable convexity to the right heart border.

Two-dimensional echocardiography, especially in four-chambered views, shows the relative sizes of the ventricles and the atria. The patency and size of the tricuspid valve is seen clearly, and function of the ventricles can be evaluated. In short-axis views, the pulmonary valve membrane and the size of the valve ring can be seen, and the distance of the proximal main pulmonary artery from the distal right ventricular outflow tract is measurable. Color flow Doppler shows the presence and degree of tricuspid insufficiency, the right-to-left shunt across the atrial septum, and the flow into the main pulmonary artery through the ductus.

## Cardiac Catheterization

The use of prostaglandin $E_1$ to dilate the ductus arteriosus and maintain pulmonary blood flow in these infants has enhanced the safety of catheterization greatly. The infant changes from being blue, pale, and acidotic to being pink and well-perfused within minutes of starting an infusion of prostaglandin $E_1$ at the rate of 0.05 to 0.1 µg/kg/min. The infusion is effective given through any vessel. The improved state is maintained as long as the prostaglandins are infused. Administration of prostaglandins allows cardiac catheterization to proceed at a more opportune time and less hurriedly, and allows time for the infant to recover from the catheterization before surgery.

Usually, only a venous catheter is necessary for catheterization because most infants have an umbilical artery monitoring catheter. The left atrium is entered through a patent foramen ovale or septal defect. Manipulation into the left ventricle is possible

from the left atrium. Right atrial pressures are elevated, with tall 'a' waves of 15 to 20 mm Hg. Right ventricular systolic pressures often attain suprasystemic values with a peaked configuration of the pressure curve and may achieve levels of 200 mm Hg. Left ventricular pressures have normal newborn values, unless there is severe hypoxia, acidosis, and hypoglycemia, all of which decrease contractility. Oxygen saturations are invariably very low in infants not on prostaglandins. Due to the large intracardiac right-to-left shunt, administration of oxygen increases systemic saturations very little, if at all.

Balloon septostomy should be performed to ensure a good communication between the atria.

Angiography in the right ventricle establishes the diagnosis, shows the size of the right ventricle, and allows classification of the defect. Communications with the coronary artery system via myocardial sinusoids may be demonstrated (Fig 82-14), as well as the degree of tricuspid hypoplasia and insufficiency.

A left ventricular injection shows the size and function of the left ventricle and eliminates the possibility of a ventricular septal defect. Good opacification of the aorta occurs, and the pulmonary arteries opacify via the ductus arteriosus or other collateral circulation.

## DIFFERENTIAL DIAGNOSIS

Other lesions to be considered in newborns with severe cyanosis include tetralogy of Fallot with pulmonary atresia, severe pulmonary stenosis with intact ventricular septum, tricuspid atresia, and total anomalous pulmonary venous return with obstruction of pulmonary veins.

## TREATMENT

### Medical

Treatment of PA:IVS begins in the neonatal period with the onset of symptoms. As soon as the diagnosis of heart disease with

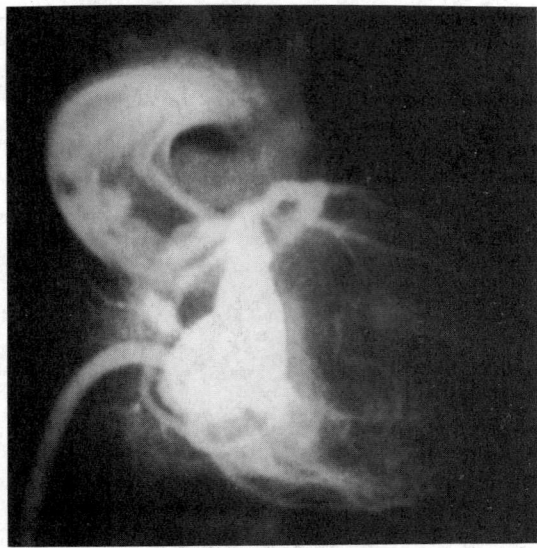

**Figure 82-14.** Angiogram in the right ventricle showing a very small ventricle and a blind outflow tract. There is opacification of the aorta from retrograde flow through the right ventricular sinusoids and coronary arteries.

decreased pulmonary blood flow is made, access to the vascular system should be established and an infusion of prostaglandin started to reestablish pulmonary blood flow. This restores a normal acid–base balance. An arterial line then should be established, most readily in the umbilical artery, because the infant will need frequent determinations of arterial blood gas levels, especially during and after surgery. Abnormalities in glucose or calcium levels should be corrected.

During cardiac catheterization, a balloon atrial septostomy is performed.

## Surgical

Analysis of the anatomy delineated by the catheterization dictates the mode of surgical intervention. Once a balloon septostomy is done, the general goals of surgery are to establish adequate pulmonary blood flow by a systemic-to-pulmonary shunt, to create a communication between the right ventricle and pulmonary artery, or both. The order and timing of these interventions have varied over the years.

Historically, the concept of systemic-to-pulmonary shunting of blood advanced by Blalock and Taussig in 1945 remains an integral part of the treatment of PA:IVS.

Publications of the decade after 1945 generally were more encouraging. Systemic-to-pulmonary shunts combined with a surgical atrial balloon septostomy resulted in improved survival rates. Greater success was achieved by staging surgery. This was accomplished by carrying out atrial septostomy at the time of catheterization, followed by construction of a systemic-to-pulmonary shunt, then relief of pulmonary obstruction several weeks or months later. If blood flow through the right ventricle

could be established, it seemed that growth of the ventricular cavity might occur over time. The use of prostaglandins allowed infants to be in an improved state for the procedures, and late in the 1970s overall survival rates increased.

The 1980s brought further refinement of the surgical treatment of PA:IVS. Attention was focused on the size of the tricuspid valve as one of the limiting factors for allowing growth of the ventricle, and the use of Fontan-type anastomoses in hearts with very small tricuspid valves produced good results. The use of Gore-tex instead of native vessels in construction of the systemic-to-pulmonary shunts is considered preferable by some.

A recent summary article suggests that the tricuspid valve should approach 70% of normal in size for complete correction to have a good result, and those with smaller valves should have a modified Fontan procedure.

## PROGNOSIS AND FUTURE DEVELOPMENTS

Although some patients with PA:IVS have lived into early adulthood without surgery, the prognosis for patients who have this lesion, even with surgery, is guarded. Results continue to improve, but eventual outcome appears to depend on the presence of sinusoid-coronary communications and on the size of the tricuspid valve. The use of newer imaging techniques should improve noninvasive anatomic classification and measurements.

The use of autogenous skeletal muscle to enlarge a hypoplastic ventricle is an experimental concept that has appeal, because the muscle has potential for growth and would not be subject to rejection problems of transplanted tissue. Macoviak and colleagues successfully have used latissimus dorsi muscle, isolated with its neurovascular bundle and stimulated electrically as a neoventricle to provide pulmonary blood flow where the right ventricle was bypassed. The treatment of PA:IVS should continue to improve as techniques to replace or augment the right ventricle are developed.

### Selected Readings

Alboliras ET, Julsrud PR, Danielson GK, et al. Definitive operation for pulmonary atresia with intact ventricular septum. Results in twenty patients. J Thorac Cardiovasc Surg 1987;93:454.

Blalock A, Taussig HB. The surgical treatment of malformations of the heart in which there is pulmonary stenosis or pulmonary atresia. JAMA 1945;128:189.

Bull C, de Leval MR, Mercanti C, et al. Pulmonary atresia and intact ventricular septum: a revised classification. Circulation 1982;66:266.

De Leval MR, Bull C, Stark J, et al. Pulmonary atresia and intact ventricular septum: surgical management based on a revised classification. Circulation 1982;66:272.

Freedom RM, Dische MR, Rowe RD. The tricuspid valve in pulmonary atresia and intact ventricular septum: a morphological study of 60 cases. Arch Pathol Lab Med 1978;102:28.

Freedom RM, Wilson G, Trusler GA, et al. Pulmonary atresia and intact ventricular septum. Scand J Thorac Cardiovasc Surg 1983;17:1.

Fyfe DA, Edwards WD, Driscoll DJ. Myocardial ischemia in patients with pulmonary atresia and intact ventricular septum. J Am Coll Cardiol 1986;8:402.

Kutsche LM, van Mierop LHS. Pulmonary atresia with and without ventricular septal defect: a different etiology and pathogenesis for the atresia in the 2 types? Am J Cardiol 1983;51:932.

Macoviak JA, Stinson EB, Starkey TD, et al. Myoventriculoplasty and neoventricle myograft cardiac augmentation to establish pulmonary blood flow: preliminary observations and feasibility studies. J Thorac Cardiovasc Surg 1987;93:212.

O'Conner WN, Ctorill CM, Johnson GL, et al. Pulmonary atresia with intact ventricular septum and ventriculocoronary communications: surgical significance. Circulation 1982;65:805.

*Principles and Practice of Pediatrics, Second Edition.*
edited by Frank A. Oski et al. J. B. Lippincott Company, Philadelphia © 1994.

# *82.6 Coarctation of the Aorta*

## Mary J. H. Morriss and Dan G. McNamara

Coarctation of the aorta is a congenital malformation characterized by a constriction of a segment of the aorta. Usually, an abrupt narrowing of the lumen of the vessel occurs in the thoracic descending aorta, producing obstruction to blood flow (Fig 82-15). A localized shelflike thickening of the media protrudes into the lumen just beyond the origin of the left subclavian artery, leaving an eccentric orifice displaced toward the usual site of insertion of the vestigial ligamentum arteriosus. To be clinically significant, the narrowing must be marked and must effectively reduce the diameter of the aorta by at least 50%. To maintain flow and adequate perfusion pressure to the kidneys and lower body, blood pressure proximal to the obstruction becomes elevated.

## OCCURRENCE

Coarctation of the aorta is a common congenital defect occurring in frequency just after ventricular septal defect and patent ductus arteriosus in most series. It has a striking male-to-female preponderance in excess of 2-to-1. Patients with the full XO Turner's syndrome with ovarian agenesis and short stature have a high incidence of coarctation in 20% of cases. A more extreme anomaly with complete interruption of the aortic arch in a slightly different location just proximal to the origin of the left subclavian artery has a high association with DiGeorge syndrome and is functionally analogous to severe coarctation with a reverse ductus arteriosus.

## CLASSIFICATION

It is possible to make a clear anatomic distinction between an isolated, discrete coarctation (referred to by some as adult or postductal coarctation) and a more diffuse, long-segment narrowing, usually part of a coarctation syndrome with other more complicated heart defects, resulting in a systemic right ventricle and right-to-left shunting through a persistently patent ductus arteriosus (preductal or infantile coarctation). Rarely, there may be multiple sites of coarctation or an atypical location, such as abdominal coarctation, thought by many to be an acquired disease in association with nonspecific arteritis.

## EMBRYOLOGY

The Skodaic theory of causation is based on an observation that smooth muscle from the ductus arteriosus extends into the aorta and when ductal constriction occurs after birth, traction on the aorta can narrow the lumen and cause coarctation of the aorta. There is general agreement that ductal closure can "unmask" a coarctation lesion, but the theory does not explain the location of the shelflike protrusion of the aorta arising from the wall opposite ductal insertion. It is conceptually easier to accept that alterations in intrauterine flow patterns promote diffuse narrowing in the isthmic region between the origin of the left subclavian artery and the ductus arteriosus, which postnatally is recognized as coarctation. Coexistence of a large ventricular septal defect, or even bicuspid aortic valve with mild obstruction, may divert flow from the aorta into the pulmonary artery with resultant reduction in the amount of flow crossing the isthmus, the point at which natural separation occurs between flow to the upper body and flow to the lower body in utero.

## PHYSIOLOGY

The major physiologic burden imposed by coarctation of the aorta is an increase in afterload of the left ventricle. By the time there is moderate constriction of the aortic lumen, there is an increase in systolic pressure above the obstruction and a lesser degree of elevation in diastolic pressure, with widening of the pulse pressure. Below the coarctation there is a narrowed pulse pressure, with decreased systolic and diastolic pressure (Fig 82-16). These alterations in wave form are reflected by a tactile sensation of delay between radial and femoral pulses. Hypertension is not directly related to the severity of obstruction and may not be extreme. Left ventricular hypertrophy develops and there is stimulation for development of collateral vessels to bypass the obstruction.

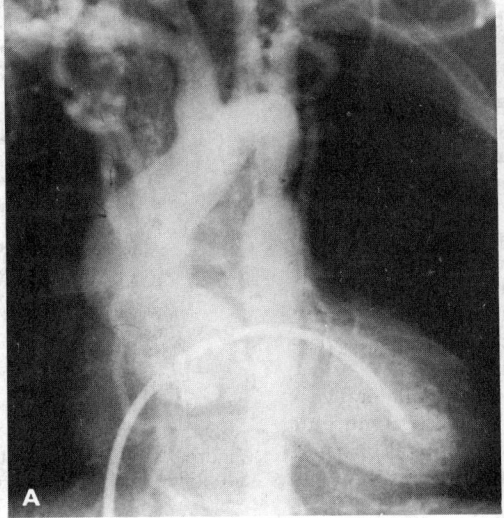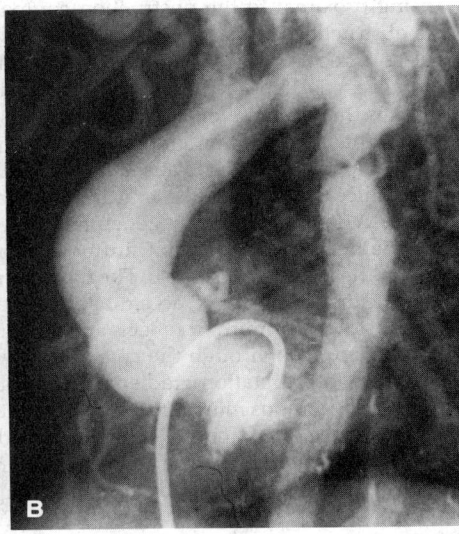

**Figure 82-15.** (**A**) AP and (**B**) lateral frames from left ventricular angiogram. Discrete coarctation is seen in the descending thoracic aorta. Well developed collateral vessels are evident.

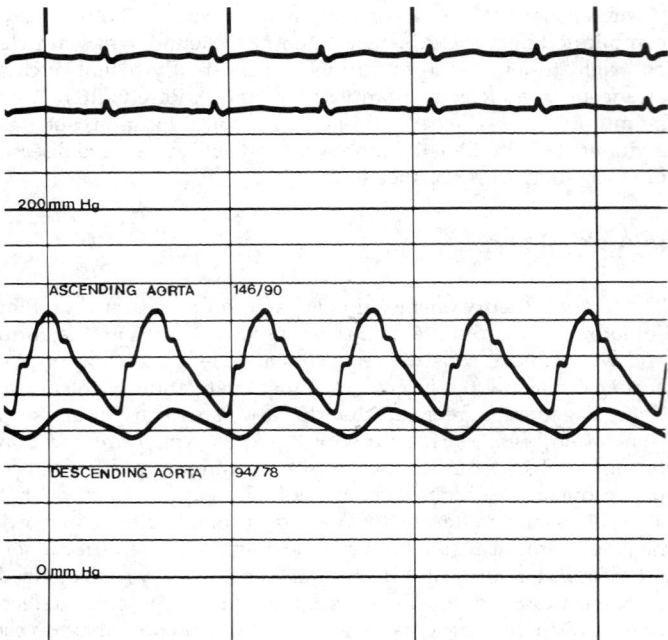

**Figure 82-16.** Pressure recordings simultaneously obtained at catheterization from ascending aorta above coarctation and from descending aorta below coarctation in a 5-year-old child.

## CLINICAL FEATURES

### Coarctation Beyond Infancy

Coarctation of the aorta beyond infancy is recognized clinically when blood pressure recordings are obtained from all four extremities; its hallmark is hypertension in the upper extremities and decreased blood pressure in the lower extremities. It is the discrepancy in blood pressure rather than an absolute level of proximal blood pressure elevation that is most striking; however, evaluation of any patient with hypertension should exclude coarctation as a cause. Most individuals with isolated coarctation have no cardiac symptoms, although minor complaints of cold feet, leg cramps, and nose bleeds are volunteered often. Unilateral headaches, particularly of unusual severity, rarely point to an associated cerebral aneurysm, but may be worrisome enough to prompt a full neurologic evaluation. On physical examination, there is striking inequality in the strength of pulses from vessels arising proximal to the obstruction compared to those distal to the obstruction. Simultaneous palpation of brachial and femoral pulses is recommended; in the presence of well-developed collateral vessels, femoral pulses can be felt easily despite coarctation, and it is the discrepancy in timing and pulse volume that should be sought. Auscultation should be performed systematically in an attempt to explain the auscultatory findings rather than with a prejudice that a particular murmur is always found with coarctation. A systolic murmur generated from the coarctation site may be heard best in the left infraclavicular area, in the axilla, or over the left posterior chest. The murmur may seem to originate after the first heart sound, accentuates in later systole, and extends into diastole. The murmur reflects an apparent lag between cardiac systole and flow through the coarctation site as well as the persistence of a coarctation gradient in early diastole.

True continuous murmurs may be generated by collateral vessels. Presence of an aortic ejection click and an ejection murmur in the aortic area may raise suspicion of an additional bicuspid aortic valve, which is found with high frequency in as many as

85% of patients with aortic coarctation. A thrill at the right upper sternal border or suprasternal notch may accompany significant aortic stenosis, but can also be found with coarctation alone due to rapid ejection into the dilated proximal aorta.

Despite significant aortic coarctation, the electrocardiogram may be normal in older children. When changes occur, they are manifested chiefly by voltage criteria for left ventricular hypertrophy. The rare patient with severe coarctation and left ventricular dysfunction additionally may have ST-T wave changes indicative of ischemia.

The typical radiologic examination of an older child reveals normal heart size, with less common findings of mild enlargement and left ventricular contour. Pulmonary vascular markings are normal in the absence of associated intracardiac defects. There may be dilatation of the ascending aorta. In some patients, radiographic evidence of the prestenotic and poststenotic dilatation resulting from coarctation appears along the left paramediastinal shadow and is referred to as the 3 sign. Reversed 3 sign, or E sign, refers to the mirror-image prestenotic and poststenotic dilatation impinging on a barium-filled esophagus. Rib notching, if present, is pathognomonic of coarctation of the aorta but is related to age, because erosion of the inferior portion of the ribs caused by dilated intercostal collateral vessels is a slow process, rarely seen before a patient reaches school age (Fig 82-17). Unilateral rib notching suggests that one subclavian artery arises below the coarctation in the low-pressure zone, with poor development of collaterals and rib notching on that side. An echocardiogram, particularly when suprasternal notch and high left parasternal views are used, may enable recognition of coarctation, but difficulties in examining the entire aorta throughout its course are well described. Because the diagnosis of coarctation is easier to establish clinically, the justification for the effort and time required to obtain confirmation by echocardiogram may be questioned. The principal values of echocardiography are that associated defects can be assessed, left ventricular function and hypertrophy can be quantitated, and, if visualization of the coarctation site is possible, a more confident recommendation can be made to the surgeon that a typical coarctation is present. Pulsed Doppler echocardiography does reveal patterns of flow thought to be additionally confirmatory of coarctation of the aorta.

Magnetic resonance imaging has a newer application in pro-

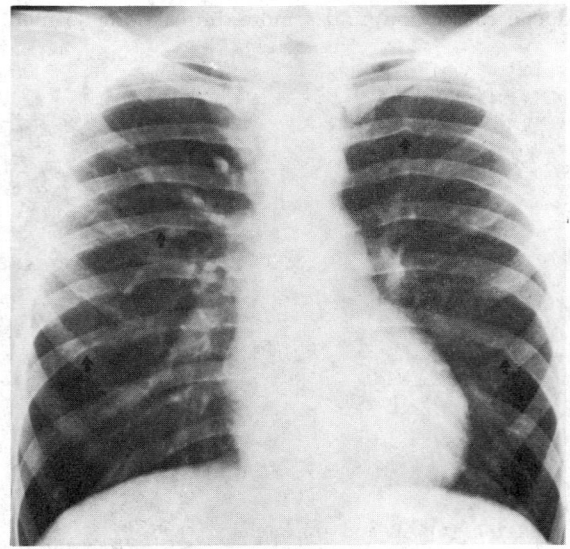

**Figure 82-17.** Posteroanterior chest film with rib notching and "3 sign" identified in a 7-year-old child.

spective identification and follow-up of patients with coarctation of the aorta, and testing of this method's contribution is ongoing.

Catheterization and angiography can confirm the diagnosis, with detailed visualization of the anatomy of the coarctation area directing surgical technique.

## Coarctation in Infancy

Coarctation syndrome in infancy is characterized by a high association with other defects that results in systemic right ventricle, reversed flow from right to left through the ductus arteriosus, and more severe hypoplasia of a greater portion of the aortic arch, although discrete coarctation may be present. Infants with coarctation can appear to be well at birth, but cardiac failure, respiratory distress, and cardiogenic shock may appear rapidly as the ductus constricts. Because of the severe impairment of cardiac output, a murmur may not be detected until the infant is stabilized and treated. The pulse discrepancy may not be apparent in the infant because the widely patent ductus serves as a route for flow to the descending aorta, so coarctation is not excluded even if normal pulses are felt on a routine newborn examination. There is potential for differential cyanosis, with shunting of the blood with a lower saturation to the lower body from the pulmonary artery via the ductus; however, the high frequency of associated defects, particularly left-to-right shunts, may allow pulmonary saturations to be only slightly lower than aortic saturations, masking this difference clinically. Marked benefit can be obtained by dilating the ductus arteriosus with prostaglandin infusion, thus enabling improved renal perfusion and reversal of acidosis and cardiogenic shock.

The electrocardiogram in infants with coarctation of the aorta is normal less frequently because it reflects coexistent anatomic defects. Isolated coarctation of the aorta in infancy is accompanied by electrocardiographic evidence of right ventricular hypertrophy, but left ventricular hypertrophy or left ventricular strain is seen rarely.

The chest film in the ill infant generally correlates with the clinical state, showing dilatation of the heart with congestive heart failure and an increase in pulmonary vascular markings due to either an associated left-to-right shunt or passive venous congestion.

The echocardiogram helps outline additional defects of the heart, enables assessment of left ventricular function, and possibly shows the area of coarctation, which may be difficult in the presence of a widely patent ductus arteriosus.

Response to prostaglandin therapy also has been evaluated with echocardiography to assess ductal patency. Catheterization is undertaken at increased risk in a moribund infant with coarctation, so noninvasive recognition is pursued more urgently.

## TREATMENT

### Surgical

Coarctation of the aorta has been considered a congenital defect amenable to surgical repair since the mid-1940s. The expected result is complete relief of the obstruction so flow to the distal aorta remains unobstructed. Best results are obtained by elective resection and end-to-end anastomosis in a school-aged child, with the single operation providing immediate and long-term relief of hypertension without the need for reoperation. Surgery is performed from a posterolateral thoracotomy incision, spreading the ribs to allow access to the thorax. Mobility of the aorta is improved by ligation and division of a ductus arteriosus or a ligamentum

arteriosum. In the presence of well-developed collaterals, the aorta is safely cross-clamped just above and below the coarctation site, and cardiopulmonary bypass usually is not used. No one method of repair is ideal for all patients (Fig 82-18). Because of the high rate of restenosis when resection and end-to-end procedures were used in infants, with a reoperation rate of up to 60%, a repair using a flap of the subclavian artery was popularized. This vascular flap enables bridging of a long-segment hypoplasia, with the presumption that growth will be permitted. Patch angioplasty and interposition grafts are techniques that can be used when more complex anatomy dictates the need. Complications of surgery include injury to the recurrent laryngeal nerve with resulting hoarseness, diaphragmatic injury from phrenic nerve trauma, bleeding from high-pressure suture lines, chylothorax, and, rarely, spinal cord injury, which is less likely when a well-developed collateral circulation is present.

A special postoperative syndrome of mesenteric arteritis is thought to be related to the duration of preoperative hypertension, the presence of postoperative rebound hypertension, and the introduction of feeding too early postoperatively. Typically, this postcoarctectomy syndrome is recognized by hypertension, abdominal pain and tenderness, vomiting, and, in severe cases, a progression to bowel necrosis. The exact mechanism is unknown, but it appears to be related to vasoconstriction of mesenteric vessels reintroduced to pulsatile flow after successful repair of coarctation. It is because of this described problem that postoperative hypertension is treated vigorously and NPO status is continued for 72 hours, with slow introduction of feeding in these patients.

Infants requiring early repair of coarctation also may require pulmonary artery banding because of associated defects, although enthusiasm for cardiopulmonary bypass even at a young age has enabled complete, definitive repair in some institutions.

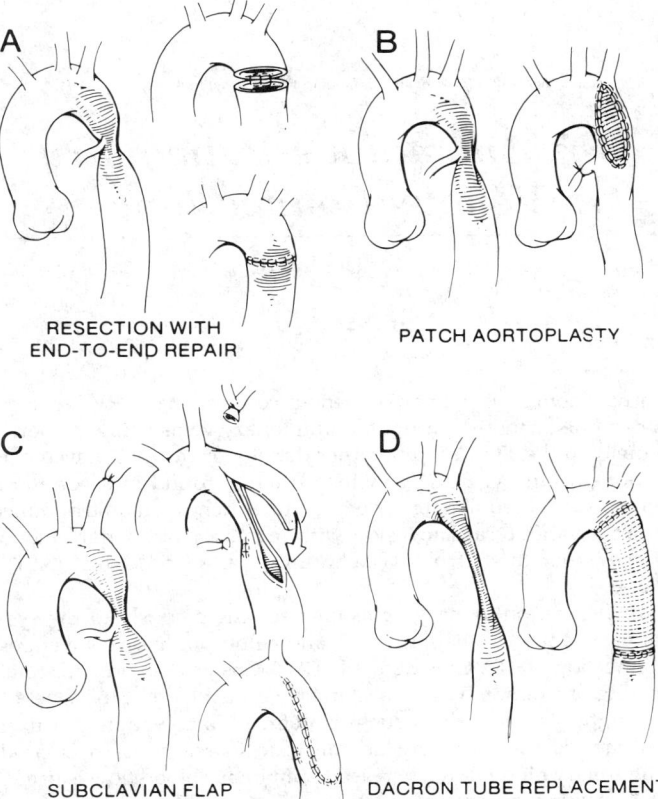

A  RESECTION WITH END-TO-END REPAIR

B  PATCH AORTOPLASTY

C  SUBCLAVIAN FLAP

D  DACRON TUBE REPLACEMENT

**Figure 82-18.** Techniques of repair commonly used for coarctation.

## Therapeutic Catheterization

Therapeutic catheterization using balloon angioplasty techniques has been offered enthusiastically for patients who have restenosis of coarctation sites previously operated on. A dilatation balloon is introduced retrograde from the femoral artery, positioned to straddle the obstruction, and inflated. Application with excellent relief of obstruction also has been available for virgin coarctations. Recent concerns about a higher than acceptable rate of aneurysm formation after successful dilatation may limit use of the technique for native coarctation when surgery offers a safe alternative. These dilatation techniques also have been offered, perhaps more safely, by the umbilical arterial route as a palliative measure for selected critically ill newborns.

## NATURAL HISTORY AND FOLLOW-UP

The former natural history of coarctation of the aorta with an estimated 75% rate of mortality by midadult years has been altered by surgical treatment. Endocarditis with the potential for mycotic aneurysm formation is a lifelong threat, and endocarditis prophylaxis should be observed by all patients both preoperatively and postoperatively. The reversibility of hypertension is thought to be favored by repair in early childhood, avoiding longstanding preoperative hypertension as well as permitting complete relief of obstruction. Considerations based on normal growth of the aorta and concern about reversibility of preoperative hypertension have led pediatric cardiologists to recommend elec-

tive repair of aortic coarctation between the ages of 3 years and 9 years.

A high incidence of congenital berry aneurysms is described, estimated at up to 10% of patients with coarctation. The likelihood of intracranial hemorrhage is thought to be reduced by successful coarctation repair. Follow-up of patients with coarctation for restenosis, recurrent or residual hypertension, endocarditis, and surveillance of aneurysm formation at sites of repaired coarctation continue to be appropriate.

## Selected Readings

Becker AE, Becker MJ, Edwards JE. Anomalies associated with coarctation of the aorta. Particular reference to infancy. Circulation 1970;41:1067.

Campbell M. Natural history of coarctation of the aorta. Br Heart J 1970;32:633.

Gupta T, Wiggers CJ. Basic hemodynamic changes produced by aortic coarctation of different degrees. Circulation 1951;3:17.

Ho ECK, Moss AJ. The syndrome of "mesenteric arteritis" following surgical repair of aortic coarctation. Pediatrics 1972;49:40.

McNamara DG, Rosenberg HS. Coarctation of the aorta. In: Watson H, ed. Paediatric cardiology. London: Lloyd-Luke (Medical Books Ltd), 1968:175.

Messmer BJ, Minale C, Muhler E, Bernuth GV. Surgical correction of coarctation of aorta in early infancy: does surgical technique influence the result? Ann Thorac Surg 1991;52:594.

Morriss MJH, McNamara DG. Coarctation of the aorta and interrupted aortic arch. In: Garson AJ, Bricker JT, McNamara DG, eds. The science and practice of pediatric cardiology. Philadelphia: Lea and Febiger, 1990.

Moss AJ, Adams FH, O'Loughlin BJ, et al. The growth of the normal aorta and of the anastomotic site in infants following surgical resection of coarctation of the aorta. Circulation 1959;19:338.

Rao PS, Chopra PS. Role of balloon angioplasty in the treatment of aortic coarctation. Ann Thorac Surg 1991;52:621.

Rudolph AM, Heymann MA, Spitznas U. Hemodynamic considerations in the development of narrowing of the aorta. Am J Cardiol 1972;30:514.

Van Mierop LH, Kutsche LM. Interruption of the aortic arch and coarctation of the aorta: pathogenetic relations. Am J Cardiol 1984;54:829.

*Principles and Practice of Pediatrics, Second Edition.*
edited by Frank A. Oski et al. J. B. Lippincott Company, Philadelphia © 1994.

# 82.7 *Anomalous Pulmonary Venous Connections*

Kent E. Ward

Partial anomalous pulmonary venous connection (PAPVC) occurs when one or more, but not all, pulmonary veins connect anomalously to the right atrium, either directly or through a systemic venous tributary. PAPVC, which often is found in association with an atrial septal defect, demonstrates hemodynamic findings of an acyanotic cardiac lesion with increased pulmonary blood flow similar to that observed in an atrial septal defect (ASD) alone.

When all pulmonary veins connect anomalously to the systemic venous circulation, total anomalous pulmonary venous connection (TAPVC) is defined. TAPVC is associated with total mixing of pulmonary and systemic venous blood at the level of the right atrium and, as such, is defined as a cyanotic form of cardiac disease that may demonstrate increased or decreased pulmonary blood flow. Increased pulmonary blood flow is usual. Decreased pulmonary blood flow may occur when there is severe obstruction in the anomalous pulmonary venous channel. In ad-

dition, TAPVC always is associated with an interatrial communication, usually a patent foramen ovale.

## EMBRYOLOGY

A review of the embryologic development of the systemic and pulmonary venous systems is necessary to fully understand the abnormalities observed in this spectrum of cardiac defects. In the developing embryo, the primitive foregut gives rise to the lungs, larynx, and tracheobronchial tree. The primordial lung buds share a common vascular plexus (splanchnic plexus) with other derivatives of the foregut and, early on, drain through the paired common cardinal and umbilicovitelline veins. As development proceeds, this splanchnic plexus differentiates into the primitive pulmonary vascular bed, thus becoming committed to draining pulmonary venous blood. This pulmonary vascular bed, however, remains in communication with the cardinal and umbilicovitelline system of veins until later in development. At 27 to 29 days of gestation, a small endothelial outgrowth arises from the posterior superior wall of the primordial left atrium. This outgrowth, called the common pulmonary vein, merges with the splanchnic plexus and begins to drain blood from this region. If development proceeds normally, the pulmonary portion of the splanchnic plexus loses connections with the cardinal and umbilicovitelline venous systems. Tributaries to the common pulmonary vein coalesce to form two pulmonary veins that drain each lung. If the right or left portion of the common pulmonary vein becomes atretic or loses connection with the pulmonary plexus, persistence of the

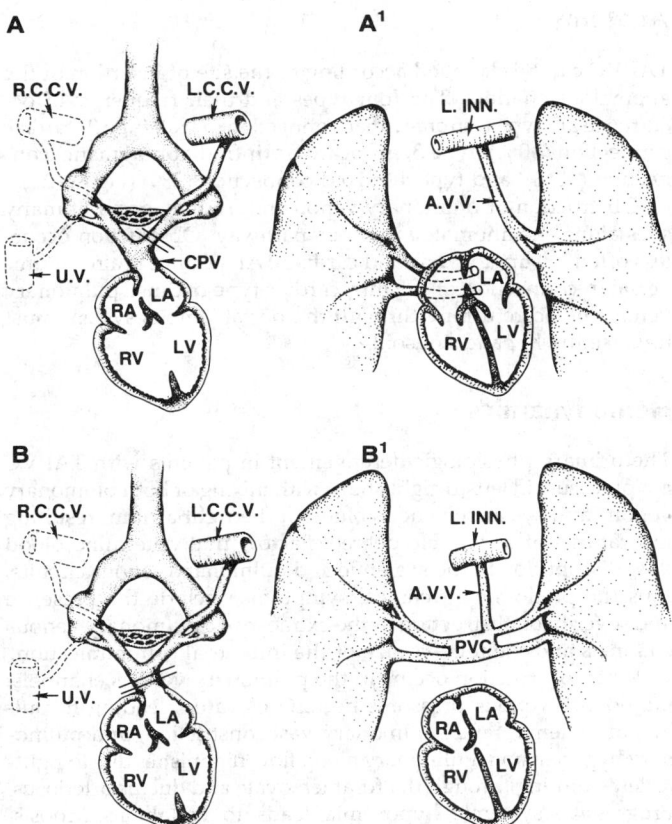

**Figure 82-19.** Embryology of anomalous pulmonary venous connections. (**A**) The primitive left atrium (LA) is connected to the pulmonary venous plexus via the common pulmonary vein (CPV). Partial interruption of this connection early in gestation leads to persistence of ipsilateral systemic venous channels, resulting in partial anomalous pulmonary venous connection (**A¹**). (**B**) Complete interruption of the common pulmonary vein results in total anomalous pulmonary venous connection (**B¹**). A.V.V., anomalous vertical vein; LV, left ventricle; L. INN., left innominate vein; L.C.C.V., left common cardial vein; PVC, pulmonary venous confluence; RA, right atrium; R.C.C.V., right common cardinal vein; RV, right ventricle; U.V., umbilicovitelline vein. (Adapted from Lucas RV. Anomalous venous connections, pulmonary and systemic. In: Adams FH, Emmanouilides GC, eds. Heart disease in infants, children, and adolescents, ed 3. Baltimore: Williams & Wilkins, 1983:458.)

primitive pulmonary venous–systemic venous connection on that side leads to PAPVC. If the common pulmonary vein–left atrium connection is disrupted totally, TAPVC occurs (Fig 82-19).

# PARTIAL ANOMALOUS PULMONARY VENOUS CONNECTION

PAPVC is relatively common and is found in 0.6% of all autopsy studies. The relatively high incidence of this defect observed in autopsy specimens supports the contention that many cases of PAPVC do not produce symptoms and, thus, are not diagnosed during life. In order of decreasing frequency, the most common types of PAPVC encountered are right pulmonary veins to right superior vena cava, right pulmonary veins to right atrium, right pulmonary veins to inferior vena cava, and left pulmonary veins to the left innominate vein. Connection from the right lung anomalously occurs about twice as often as that from the left lung.

Clinically apparent PAPVC usually is found in association with other cardiac defects, most commonly an ASD of the secundum or sinus venosus type. PAPVC from the right lung to the inferior vena cava occurs in the scimitar syndrome, a complex of anomalies that includes pulmonary hypoplasia or sequestration, diaphragmatic abnormalities, and anomalous systemic arterial supply to the right lung.

## Hemodynamics and Clinical Features

The basic hemodynamic alteration that occurs in PAPVC is that of a pretricuspid left-to-right shunt in which fully oxygenated blood is recirculated through the lungs via the right atrium, right ventricle, and pulmonary artery. The increased pulmonary blood flow leads to enlargement of the right atrium, enlargement and hypertrophy of the right ventricle, and dilatation of the pulmonary artery. The left heart chambers are not affected and systemic cardiac output is normal. Most patients with PAPVC, with or without an interatrial communication, do not exhibit symptoms in early life. These patients often are referred with a cardiac murmur or an abnormal chest roentgenogram. When symptoms are elicited at this age, the most common complaint is mild exercise intolerance. Progressive symptoms, if they appear, usually begin when the patient's age is in the mid-30s or early 40s. These consist of dyspnea, recurrent bronchitis, hemoptysis, chest pain, and palpitations associated with supraventricular arrhythmias. Physical examination in patients with isolated PAPVC may be normal if only a single lobe connects anomalously. When multiple lobes are involved or when there is an associated ASD, the findings are typical of an uncomplicated ASD. Occasionally, a low-frequency continuous murmur may be heard over the base, representing flow through an anomalous venous channel. The electrocardiogram usually demonstrates right ventricular hypertrophy, although it may be normal in patients without associated cardiac defects. Atrial arrhythmias are rare in the infant and child but may occur in the third and fourth decade and usually are associated with an ASD or mitral stenosis.

In the presence of an ASD, the chest roentgenogram often shows evidence of right atrial and right ventricular enlargement in addition to increased pulmonary vascularity. Specific radiographic findings related to the insertion or drainage of the anomalous pulmonary vein or veins are described well, the "scimitar sign" being a classic example (Fig 82-20).

PAPVC with or without an ASD has M-mode echocardiographic findings similar to those reported for ASDs, including mild to moderate dilatation of the right ventricle and, usually, paradoxical interventricular septal motion. The anomalous venous connection may be seen by two-dimensional echocardiography. Cardiac catheterization with selective angiography is the definitive diagnostic procedure for most patients with suspected PAPVC with or without associated cardiac defects. Intracardiac pressures are usually normal in patients with PAPVC when less than 50% of the pulmonary veins connect anomalously. Exceptions to this include patients older than 40 years with an associated ASD and those with concomitant mitral stenosis, and patients with scimitar syndrome. In these circumstances, elevation of right atrial, right ventricular, and pulmonary artery pressures may be observed.

## Treatment

Surgical treatment of PAPVC should be considered in the following circumstances:

In the presence of a hemodynamically significant left-to-right shunt (Qp : Qs greater than 2 : 1, cardiomegaly on chest radiograph)—this includes most patients with isolated PAPVC

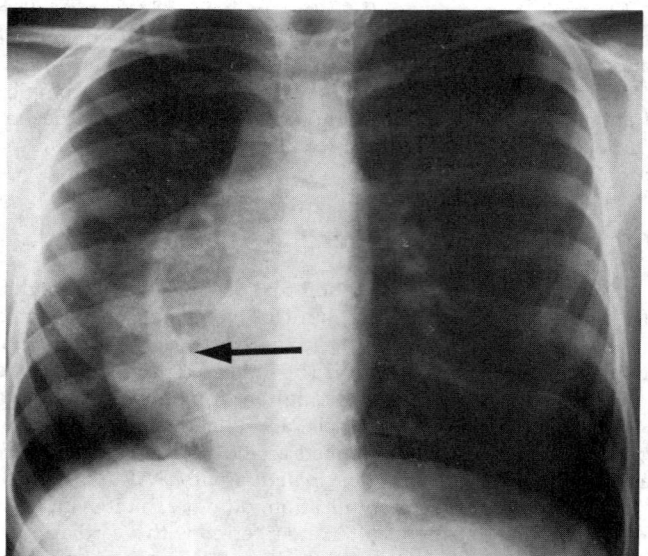

**Figure 82-20.** Scimitar syndrome. Chest radiograph in a patient with dextrocardia and partial anomalous pulmonary venous connection from the right lung to the inferior vena cava. Arrow points to the anomalous "scimitar" vein. (Courtesy of Teresa Stacy, MD.)

in which 50% or more of pulmonary veins connect anomalously.

In patients with recurrent pulmonary infections in association with scimitar syndrome

In conjunction with surgical repair of other major cardiac lesions (ASD, mitral stenosis)

When the anomalous connection affects surrounding structures by compression or obstruction.

Surgical technique involves routing the anomalous pulmonary venous blood to the left atrium, either by transection and direct anastomosis of the anomalous channel or by use of an intracardiac baffle through the right atrium.

Operative results in asymptomatic patients are good, and the prognosis is similar to that observed after closure of an ASD. Late complications following surgery are rare; they include atrial arrhythmias and obstruction of systemic or pulmonary venous return.

## TOTAL ANOMALOUS PULMONARY VENOUS CONNECTION

Total anomalous pulmonary venous connection (TAPVC) affects 2% to 5% of all patients with congenital heart disease. In all cases, systemic blood flow is maintained by way of right-to-left shunting through an interatrial communication, usually a patent foramen ovale. The male-to-female ratio is equal in most types of TAPVC, except there is a strong male predominance (3-to-1) in infants with TAPVC of the infradiaphragmatic type. In the group of patients with this abnormality, about one third have other significant major cardiac malformations, including single ventricle, atrioventricular canal defect, hypoplastic left heart, patent ductus arteriosus, and transposition of the great vessels. Many patients in this group have been found to have abnormalities of atrial and visceral situs associated with the heterotaxy syndromes (asplenia and polysplenia). Most cases of TAPVC are sporadic and are not associated with syndromes or chromosomal abnormalities.

## Anatomy

TAPVC can be classified according to the site of insertion of the anomalous channel. The four types and their frequency of occurrence are type I, supracardiac connection (55%); type 2, cardiac connection (30%); type 3, infracardiac (infradiaphragmatic) connection (13%); and type 4, mixed connection (2%) (Fig 82-21).

Obstruction of pulmonary venous return may occur at many sites along the anomalous venous pathway. Obstruction occurs less often in supracardiac and cardiac TAPVC, but is almost universal in connection of the infracardiac type because pulmonary venous blood returning through the portal venous system must traverse the hepatic sinusoids.

## Hemodynamics

The primary physiologic derangement in patients with TAPVC is a pretricuspid left-to-right shunt with mixing of both pulmonary venous and systemic venous blood in the right atrium, resulting in cyanosis of a variable degree. Factors that determine blood flow distribution in the systemic and pulmonary venous circuits, thus the predominant clinical symptoms, include the presence and severity of obstruction in the extracardiac pulmonary venous channels and the relative size of the interatrial communication.

When obstruction occurs in the pulmonary venous channels, pulmonary venous pressures become elevated, leading to pulmonary edema, reflex pulmonary vasoconstriction, and pulmonary hypertension. Pulmonary blood flow diminishes due to right-to-left shunting through the foramen ovale and ductus arteriosus. Progressive systemic hypoxemia leads to metabolic acidosis, multisystem organ failure, and death within a few days if the obstruction is not relieved.

In infants without significant extracardiac obstruction, the size of the interatrial communication plays a critical role in the development of symptoms after the neonatal period. A patent foramen ovale is found in most infants with uncomplicated TAPVC and results in impedance of left ventricular filling and decreased cardiac output in the first few months of life. The result is massive pulmonary overcirculation, pulmonary hypertension, and congestive heart failure. Surgical or transvenous atrial septostomy relieves both pulmonary hypertension and congestive heart failure in most patients. In the absence of septostomy or total surgical correction, most patients die before 1 year of age.

## Clinical Features

### TAPVC With Obstruction

Infants born with obstruction in the anomalous pulmonary venous channels develop symptoms shortly after birth and demonstrate severe cyanosis and respiratory distress. Physical examination reveals a prominent right ventricular impulse, accentuation of the second heart sound, and, at times, a gallop rhythm over the left lower sternal border. Murmurs are infrequent. Hepatomegaly usually is present and often is dramatic in anomalous pulmonary venous connection to the portal venous system. The electrocardiogram may demonstrate right ventricular hypertrophy and a paucity of left ventricular forces.

The chest radiograph at times is diagnostic in TAPVC with obstruction. The cardiac size usually is normal. Pulmonary vascular markings are striking, characterized by a diffuse, linear reticular pattern radiating from the hilar regions (Fig 82-22). Overt pulmonary edema with Kerley B lines may be present. Hyperinflation of the lungs may be seen, which should differentiate this cardiac anomaly from early hyaline membrane disease. Increased pulmonary vascularity helps distinguish this entity from persistent fetal circulation syndrome.

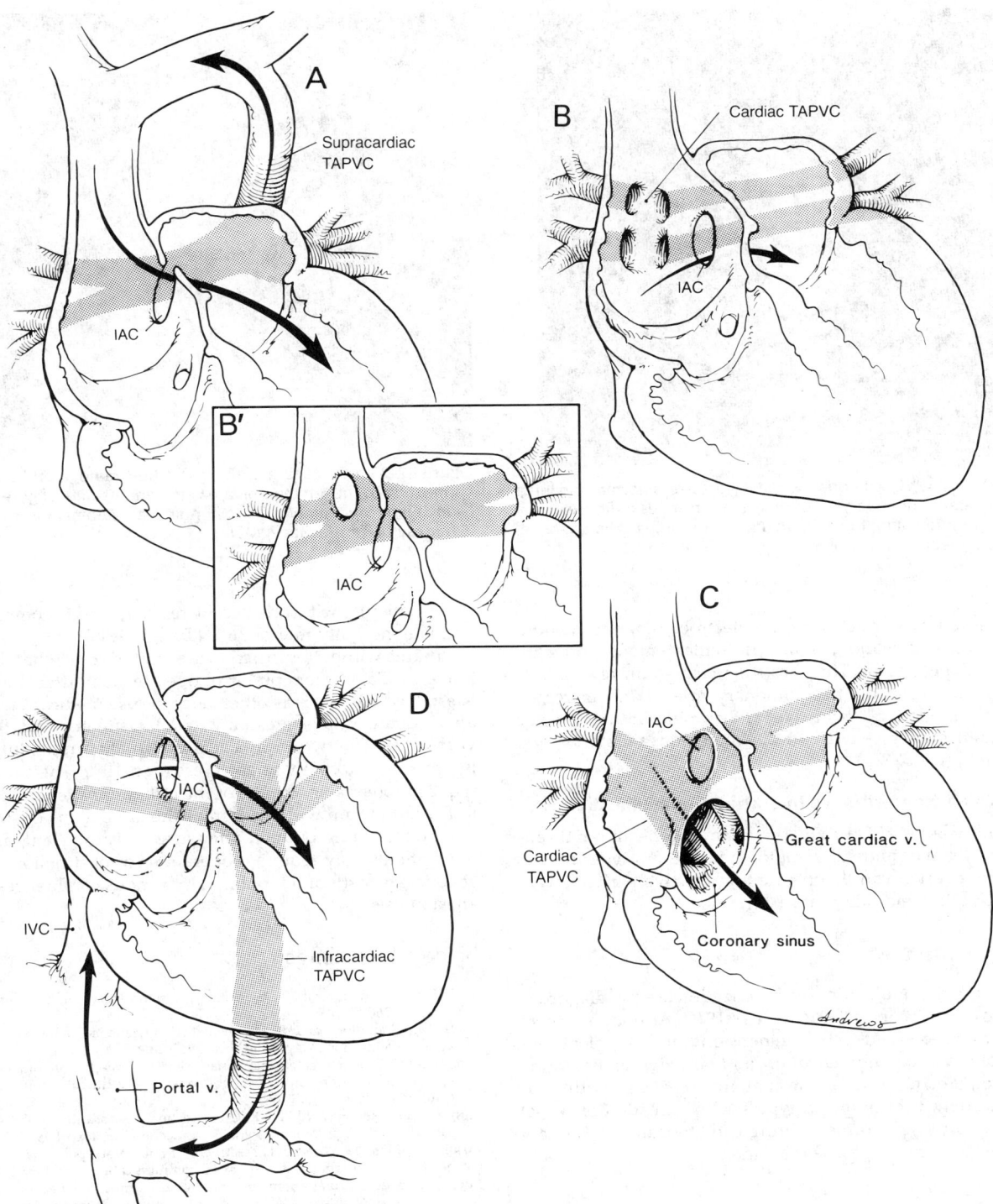

**Figure 82-21.** Types of total anomalous pulmonary venous connection. (**A**) Supracardiac connection to left innominate vein. (**B**) Cardiac connection via four separate veins. (**B'**) Cardiac connection via single common orifice. (**C**) Cardiac connection to coronary sinus. (**D**) Infracardiac (subdiaphragmatic) connection to portal system. *IAC,* interatrial communication. (Adapted with permission from Reardon, et al. Total anomalous pulmonary venous return: report of 201 patients treated surgically. Texas Heart Institute, 1985.)

## TAPVC With a Restrictive Interatrial Communication

Infants born with a restrictive interatrial communication are usually asymptomatic at birth and during the first few weeks of life; then, they develop respiratory distress, feeding difficulties, and poor weight gain. Physical examination reveals tachypnea with perioral duskiness, a hyperdynamic precordium, and hepatomegaly. Auscultation demonstrates a pulmonary systolic murmur, fixed splitting of the second heart sound, and, often, a diastolic murmur over the left lower sternal border. Occasionally, a continuous venous hum may be detected in an area overlying the

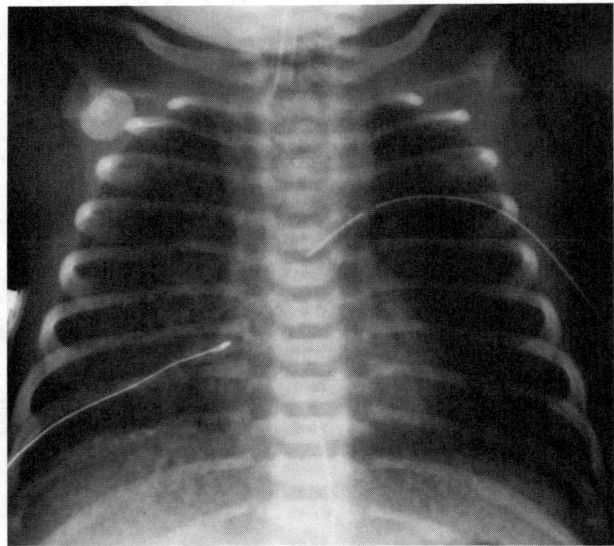

**Figure 82-22.**    TAPVC with obstruction. Heart size is normal and lungs are hyperinflated. Pulmonary vascularity demonstrates a diffuse, linear reticular pattern radiating from the hilum, representing pulmonary venous engorgement.

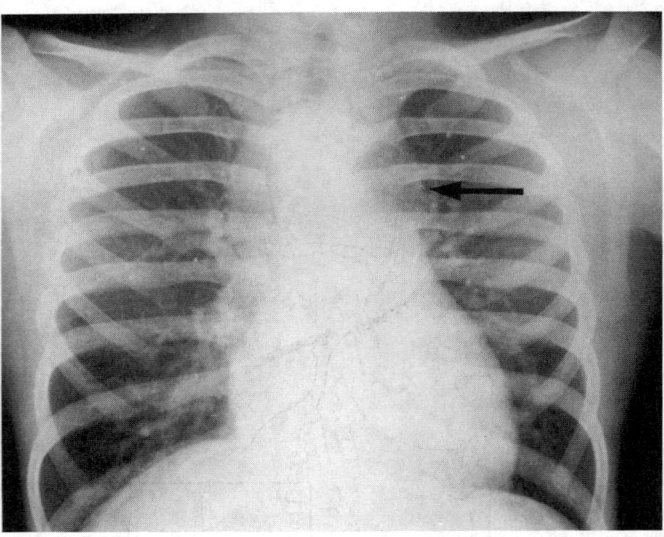

**Figure 82-23.**    Supracardiac TAPVC. Chest radiograph in a child with connection to the left innominate vein demonstrating figure-of-eight or "snowman" appearance. Arrow points to anomalous vertical vein. (Courtesy of Teresa Stacy, MD.)

anomalous venous connection. The electrocardiogram demonstrates right axis deviation, right atrial enlargement, and right ventricular hypertrophy. The chest roentgenogram reveals cardiomegaly, dilatation of the pulmonary artery, and increased pulmonary vascularity. Distinctive radiographic features may be observed, reflecting the course of the anomalous pulmonary venous channel (Fig 82-23).

### TAPVC With a Nonrestrictive Interatrial Communication

Infants with a large ASD or who have undergone an atrial septostomy may have minimal symptoms in the first year of life. These patients often can be operated on electively after 1 year of age, with a low mortality rate.

## Diagnostic Studies

Echocardiography and cardiac catheterization are the diagnostic procedures of choice in patients with TAPVC. Although surgery may be performed based on two-dimensional and Doppler echocardiography alone, catheterization and selective angiography are often required to delineate the anatomy in patients with complex cardiac defects or in mixed-type TAPVC. In addition, atrial septostomy can be performed during catheterization if surgery is to be delayed until the patient is older.

## Treatment

In infants with TAPVC who present with marked cyanosis, respiratory distress, and cardiovascular collapse in the first few days of life, severe obstruction in the extracardiac pulmonary venous channels must be assumed. Surgery must be undertaken immediately after diagnostic studies are performed. Prostaglandin $E_1$ has been used before surgery to dilate the ductus venosus to enhance pulmonary venous return to the portal venous system in patients with TAPVC. Operative mortality rates are high in

these patients, with one recent report citing a combined early and late mortality rate of 36% (Turley, 1980).

Infants without obstruction are treated somewhat differently. Some cardiac centers prefer to operate soon after the diagnosis is established, whereas others elect to use medical therapy after an adequate atrial septostomy to delay surgery until the second year of life. The two approaches are equally successful, resulting in operative mortality rates of less than 10%. The surgical technique involves anastomosis of the pulmonary venous confluence to the left atrium with ligation of the anomalous channel.

The long-term outlook after surgery is excellent, although a few patients may require reoperation for obstruction due to inadequate growth of the pulmonary venous confluence–left atrial anastomosis.

## Selected Readings

Burroughs JT, Edwards JE. Total anomalous pulmonary venous connection. Am Heart J 1960;59:913.

Edwards JE. Pathologic and developmental considerations in anomalous pulmonary venous connection. Mayo Clin Proc 1953;28:441.

Hammon JW. Total anomalous pulmonary venous connection in infancy. Ten years' experience including studies of post-operative ventricular function. J Thorac Cardiovasc Surg 1980;80:544.

Huhta J, Gutgesell HP, Nihill MR. Cross-sectional echocardiographic diagnosis of total anomalous pulmonary venous connection. Br Heart J 1985;53:525.

Kirklin JW, Ellis FH, Wood EH. Treatment of anomalous pulmonary venous connection in association with interatrial communications. Surgery 1956;39:389.

Lucas RV Jr, et al. Total anomalous pulmonary venous connection to the portal venous system. A cause of pulmonary venous obstruction. American Journal Roentgenology Radium Ther Nucl Med 1961;86:561.

Mathey J, et al. Anomalous pulmonary venous return into inferior vena cava and associated bronchovascular anomalies (the scimitar syndrome). Report of three cases and review of the literature. Thorax 1968;23:398.

Turley K, Tucker WY, Ullyot DJ, Ebert PA. Total anomalous pulmonary venous connection in infancy: influence of age and type of lesion. Am J Cardiol 1980;45:92.

Ward KE, et al. Restrictive interatrial communication in total anomalous pulmonary venous connection. Am J Cardiol 1986;57:1131.

Ward KE, Mullins CE. Anomalous pulmonary venous connections. In: Garson A Jr, Bricker JT, McNamara DG, eds. The science and practice of pediatric cardiology. Philadelphia: Lea and Febiger, 1990.

*Principles and Practice of Pediatrics, Second Edition.*
edited by Frank A. Oski et al. J. B. Lippincott Company, Philadelphia © 1994.

# 82.8 *Congenital Mitral Valve Disease*

## Janette F. Strasburger

The left atrioventricular valve (mitral valve) includes the anterior and posterior mitral valve leaflets separated by their commissures, the chordae tendineae, and the anteromedial and posterolateral left ventricular papillary muscles. The annulus, or skeletal support of the mitral valve, is fibromuscular and contracts with the heart. The mitral valve permits egress of blood during diastole and atrial systole from the left atrium to the left ventricle and prevents reflux of blood into the left atrium during ventricular systole. Thus, closure of the mitral valve is the earliest component of the first heart sound. Abnormalities in the development of the mitral valve apparatus can result in hemodynamic and physiologic alterations in blood flow, which can present with either congestive heart failure or pulmonary edema during fetal, neonatal, or later development.

Most abnormalities of the mitral valve, even in the pediatric age group, are acquired as the result of rheumatic carditis, myocardial ischemia or infarction, hypertension, Marfan's syndrome, mitral valve prolapse syndrome, bacterial endocarditis, myocarditis, or cardiomyopathy. Congenital mitral valve abnormalities are much rarer. Because of the severity of obstruction of flow across the valve, valvular regurgitation, or associated cardiac defects, patients with congenital mitral abnormalities often present during infancy. Congenital lesions of the mitral valve are listed in Table 82-1.

Other abnormalities of the pulmonary veins or left atrium also can cause obstruction of left ventricular filling or pulmonary venous egress. These include cor triatriatum, a perforated fibromuscular membrane that subdivides the left atrium; supravalvar stenosing mitral ring, which is a fibrous, shelf-like ridge just above the mitral valve that encroaches on its orifice; left atrial tumor; and unilateral or common pulmonary venous stenosis or atresia. All these lesions can result in pulmonary edema and right-sided cardiac failure secondary to obstructed left-sided flow and pulmonary hypertension.

The physiology of left-sided obstructive and regurgitant lesions is discussed here using mitral valvular insufficiency and mitral valvular stenosis as prototypes, although any of the aforementioned defects can result in similar pathophysiology. Differences between the lesions are described briefly.

## CONGENITAL MITRAL STENOSIS

Mitral valve stenosis presents clinically with right-sided cardiac failure and pulmonary hypertension. The age at presentation depends on the degree of obstruction of left atrial emptying. Because exercise demands greater cardiac output, initial symptoms often are related to exercise. In infants, feeding requires increased cardiac output, and babies often present with dyspnea or cyanosis during feeding and with failure to grow. Because of pulmonary edema, infants and children are at risk for recurring respiratory infections. Tachypnea, hemoptysis, respiratory distress, low cardiac output, and atrial fibrillation can be associated findings of mitral stenosis. Atrial fibrillation and left atrial thrombi are relatively uncommon in children.

The physical examination in mitral stenosis is characterized by a right ventricular lift and by an increased pulmonary component of the second heart sound due to pulmonary hypertension. A fourth heart sound sometimes is audible secondary to enhanced atrial systolic contraction. A long pandiastolic murmur often is audible at the cardiac apex. The chest radiograph usually shows left atrial enlargement with widening of the angle between the left and right main bronchi. In older children, a redistribution of blood flow can be seen, with increased flow to the upper lobes. Kerley B lines and pulmonary edema are also present. The electrocardiogram generally shows left atrial or biatrial enlargement in sinus rhythm, and, rarely, atrial fibrillation is present. Right ventricular hypertrophy with right-axis deviation generally is seen. Two-dimensional and Doppler echocardiography often helps determine the presence of mitral stenosis and detect structural abnormalities of the mitral valve or supporting apparatus. The left atrial size often is enlarged, but the left ventricular volume is usually 70% to 100% of normal. Transesophageal echocardiography, which allows excellent imaging of the left atrium and mitral valve when the patient is under sedation or general anesthesia, frequently is employed during catheterization and surgical valvuloplasty procedures. Cardiac catheterization demonstrates elevation in pulmonary arterial pressure and right ventricular systolic pressure. There is a gradient between the left atrial A wave and the left ventricular end-diastolic pressure. Often, it is necessary to estimate the left atrial pressure using a pulmonary capillary wedge pressure or to enter the left atrium via a transseptal puncture. Injections in the pulmonary artery or left atrium usually demonstrate abnormalities of the mitral valve or adjacent structures.

Mild to moderate mitral stenosis can be managed by diuretic therapy, supplemental nutrition, and aggressive management of respiratory infections. Usually, digoxin is not helpful for right ventricular failure, although it sometimes is used for arrhythmias. Anticoagulation should be considered in patients with longstanding atrial arrhythmias before cardioversion or in whom sinus rhythm cannot be maintained. Rarely, the addition of quinidine, procainamide, or amiodarone to digoxin therapy is necessary to maintain sinus rhythm.

Balloon mitral valvuloplasty to enlarge the mitral valve orifice during cardiac catheterization has been successful in pediatric patients with both congenital and post-rheumatic mitral stenosis. The procedure is technically possible in most patients and is relatively safe. Improvement in exercise tolerance is seen in about 80% of patients initially. Greatest experience with this technique has been gained in the adolescent patient. Five-year follow-up after balloon mitral valvuloplasty has shown that restenosis rates

---

**TABLE 82-1.  Congenital Abnormalities of the Mitral Valve Apparatus**

**Congenital Mitral Stenosis**
Parachute mitral valve
Double-orifice mitral valve
Mitral valve stenosis or hypoplasia

**Congenital Mitral Insufficiency**
Cleft mitral valve
Congenital mitral valve regurgitation
Double-orifice mitral valve
Ruptured chordae tendineae or papillary muscle

vary from 2% to 30% depending on the technique used. Complications have included thromboembolism, endocarditis, atrial septal injury, and mitral regurgitation.

Surgery is indicated for children with low cardiac output, severe symptoms with exercise, and severe pulmonary hypertension who are refractory to or ineligible for balloon mitral valvuloplasty. The preferred treatment is surgical commissurotomy, which is open heart surgery consisting of incision along the mitral commissure. The operation must be considered palliative, because, often, there is either annular hypoplasia or abnormalities in the supports of the mitral valve. When obstruction is due to a fibromuscular ridge or cor triatriatum, these structures must be removed. Whenever possible, mitral valve replacement should be avoided in young children, because anticoagulation is necessary for metallic prosthetic valves in the mitral position. Replacement of the valve often is required in later childhood or adulthood. Unlike isolated mitral stenosis, parachute mitral valve, double orifice mitral valve, and mitral hypoplasia usually occur with other cardiac defects, not as isolated defects. These defects can cause mitral stenosis, mitral regurgitation, or both. Because of the complexity of associated defects, they are less amenable to surgical repair. Shone's complex consists of parachute mitral valve, subaortic stenosis, and coarctation of the aorta with or without a ventricular septal defect.

# CONGENITAL MITRAL REGURGITATION

During mitral regurgitation, the left ventricle decompresses into the left atrium, and half of the regurgitant volume during ventricular systole occurs before the opening of the aortic valve. When the regurgitant volume exceeds the stroke volume of a single systole, cardiac output decreases. This results functionally in an increase in left atrial and left ventricular volume and cardiomegaly. Pulmonary edema develops because of pulmonary venous congestion.

Clinical symptoms of mitral regurgitation are related to the severity of the regurgitation, associated cardiac defects, left ventricular function, pulmonary artery pressure, and rate of development of the regurgitation. Acute mitral regurgitation of moderate or severe degree is tolerated poorly and leads rapidly to acute pulmonary edema and low cardiac output. Chronic mitral regurgitation of mild or moderate degree may be asymptomatic. With increasing severity, symptoms in infants and children include diaphoresis, recurrent respiratory infections, tachypnea, exercise intolerance, and failure to grow because of high caloric requirements.

Children with mitral regurgitation generally have a diffuse left ventricular lift and a palpably enlarged heart. $S_1$ is normal or decreased, and the pulmonary component of the second heart sound is either normal or increased. Mitral regurgitation causes a high-pitched, blowing, apical pansystolic murmur; it must be differentiated from the murmur of a ventricular septal defect, which usually is audible near the left sternal border rather than at the apex. During diastole, the increased flow across the mitral valve results in a low-pitched diastolic flow rumble and sometimes a third heart sound at the apex.

The radiographic appearance of mitral regurgitation consists of cardiomegaly of moderate degree, with increased pulmonary vascular markings. There is enlargement of the left atrial and left ventricular contours of the heart. The electrocardiogram generally shows left atrial enlargement and left ventricular hypertrophy.

Atrial fibrillation is uncommon. Two-dimensional echocardiography helps detect abnormalities of valve appearance, motion, and attachments. The left ventricular systolic function is normal or increased because of Starling's forces. Decreased left ventricular contractility, especially in the presence of cardiomegaly, suggests cardiomyopathy secondary to mitral regurgitation. Color flow mapping is useful in qualitative assessment of the amount of regurgitation. Severe regurgitation occurs over a broad area of the annulus and refluxes far into the left atrium; whereas, in mild mitral regurgitation, only a small jet is noted near the valve.

Mild or moderate mitral insufficiency generally can be managed by diuretic and digoxin therapy. Afterload reduction with nitroprusside has been life-saving in acute mitral regurgitation. Oral afterload-reducing agents, such as captopril and enalapril are used as adjuvant therapy in patients with cardiomyopathy associated with mitral regurgitation.

Surgical intervention is necessary for congestive heart failure and pulmonary edema secondary to mitral regurgitation, which is poorly controlled by medical management, or for progressive left ventricular dysfunction and cardiomegaly. The surgical treatment of choice is mitral valvuloplasty (repair of the mitral valve) or annuloplasty (plication of the mitral annulus). Often, however, it is necessary to replace a damaged valve, so mitral valve surgery should be delayed whenever possible. Because calcification develops on bioprosthetic valves, generally it is necessary to implant a low-profile tilting disk valve in the mitral position. This requires long-term anticoagulation therapy. The smallest valve available is a 16-mm valve that can be implanted in a child at a minimum age of 1 to 2 years. Surgical correction of other lesions such as double orifice mitral valve and parachute mitral valve also is difficult and depends on associated cardiac defects.

Pulmonary hypertension secondary to either mitral regurgitation or mitral stenosis generally is relieved by surgery, because it is uncommon for venous congestion to result in irreversible pulmonary vascular disease. The mortality rate for surgery is 2% to 4% for patients in stable condition, but may exceed 20% when a child has low cardiac output, multiple cardiac defects, or severe pulmonary edema, or requires more than one valve replacement.

## Selected Readings

Babic UU, Grugicic S, Popovic Z, Djurisic Z, Pejcic P, Vucinic M. Percutaneous transarterial balloon dilatation of the mitral valve: 5 year experience. Br Heart J 1992;67(2):185.

Bradley LM, Midgley RM, Watson DC, et al. Anticoagulation therapy in children with mechanical prosthetic cardiac valves. Am J Cardiol 1985;56:533.

Galloway AC, Colvin SB, Baumann FG, et al. A comparison of mitral valve reconstruction with mitral valve replacement: intermediate-term results. Ann Thorac Surg 1989;47(5):655.

Grenadier E, Sahn DJ, Valdez-Cruz LM, et al. Two-dimensional echo Doppler study of congenital disorders of the mitral valve. Am Heart J 1984;107:319.

Grifka RG, O'Laughlin MP, Nihill MR, Mullins CE. Double transseptal, double balloon valvuloplasty for congenital mitral stenosis. Circulation 1992;85(1):123.

Kalke BR, Desai JM, Magotra R. Mitral valve surgery in children. J Thorac Cardiovasc Surg 1989;98(5) Pt 2:994.

Ritter SB. Transesophageal real-time echocardiography in infants and children with congenital heart disease. J Am Coll Cardiol 1991;18:569.

Roberts WC, Perloff JK. Mitral valvular disease: a clinicopathologic survey of the conditions causing the mitral valve to function abnormally. Ann Intern Med 1972;77:939.

Scott WC, Miller DC, Haverich A, et al. Operative risks of mitral valve replacement: discriminant analysis of 1,329 procedures. Circulation 1985;72(suppl II):108.

Solymar L, Rao PS, Mardini MK, Fawzy ME, Guinn G. Prosthetic valves in children and adolescents. Am Heart J 1991;121(2) Pt 1:557.

Spevak PJ, Bass JL, Ben-Shachar G, Hesslein P, Keane JF, Perry S, Pyles L, Lock JE. Balloon angioplasty for congenital mitral stenosis. Am J Cardiol 1990;66(4):472.

*Principles and Practice of Pediatrics, Second Edition.*
edited by Frank A. Oski et al. J. B. Lippincott Company, Philadelphia © 1994.

# 82.9 *Mitral Valve Prolapse*

Victoria E. Judd

Mitral valve prolapse is the most common cardiac diagnosis of childhood, with prevalence estimates of 0.5% to 35%. The overall prevalence in the general population is 4% to 8%. Since Barlow's first report on midsystolic clicks with late systolic murmur in 1963, several reports have documented the syndrome in children.

## DIAGNOSIS

The diagnosis of mitral valve prolapse may be made by auscultatory, echocardiographic, angiocardiographic, and pathologic criteria. Criteria vary according to the examiner and method used. Mitral valve prolapse is divided into normal mitral valve prolapse and pathologic mitral valve prolapse. Normal mitral valve prolapse may have superior systolic motion into the left atrium, which may produce a click. Pathologic mitral valve prolapse has an abnormal valve function and failure of leaflet edge apposition, causing mitral regurgitation.

Perloff and associates propose specific clinical criteria for the diagnosis of mitral valve prolapse. The midsystolic click and the late systolic murmur are diagnostic auscultatory criteria of pathologic mitral valve prolapse. Two-dimensional echocardiogram showing marked superior systolic displacement of the mitral leaflets with failure of leaflet edge apposition, or mild to moderate superior systolic displacement of the mitral leaflets with chordal rupture, Doppler mitral regurgitation, and annular dilatation are echocardiographic diagnostic criteria. The diagnosis may not be made based on symptoms, physical appearance, electrocardiographic abnormalities, chest radiograph abnormalities, or nonspecific echocardiographic abnormalities.

## EPIDEMIOLOGY AND INCIDENCE

Published reports of estimated incidence of mitral valve prolapse reflect different investigative techniques and diagnostic criteria; true incidence is unknown. Based on auscultatory evidence only, the overall incidence of mitral valve prolapse in children is 5%. Evaluation of the presence of mitral valve prolapse solely by echocardiography estimates the prevalence at 13% in children ages 5 days to 18 years with up to 35% prevalence in the 10- to 18-year range. With more stringent echocardiographic criteria, prevalence drops from 13% to 0.5%. True incidence of mitral valve prolapse is probably in the range of 4% with a 2-to-1 female-to-male ratio present at all ages. Why mitral valve prolapse is more common in females is not clear, although smaller left ventricular size and lower body weight may be important. The primary cause of mitral valve prolapse is uncertain. Evidence suggests that most, if not all, cases of mitral valve prolapse are inherited. The likely mode of inheritance is autosomal dominant with variable expressivity.

## ASSOCIATED CONDITIONS

Mitral valve prolapse occurs in patients with a variety of associated conditions or disease. These conditions affect the mitral valve apparatus at the annulus, leaflets, chordae, papillary muscles, or left ventricular wall or cavity. In mitral valve prolapse, underlying associated conditions and mechanisms have one associated factor: the suspension apparatus for the mitral valve is too big, either absolutely or relatively, for the left ventricular cavity to contain. During systole, left ventricular volume progressively decreases. The mitral valve would prolapse in the left atrium if it was not stopped by the support apparatus. If there is too much valve apparatus (eg, as seen in familial mitral valve prolapse, Marfan's syndrome, rheumatic fever, coronary artery disease, and after injury) or left ventricular size is too small (eg, as seen in idiopathic hypertrophic subaortic stenosis, atrial septal defect, straight back syndrome, pectus excavatum, perhaps the normal female heart, and the athlete's heart), then systolic prolapse of the mitral valve may occur.

Mitral valve prolapse may be seen in as many as 40% of patients with an isolated secundum atrial septal defect. This high incidence does not persist after surgical repair of the secundum atrial septal defect. This association probably is based on left ventricular size and geometry, which is changed with correction of the atrial septal defect. Mitral valve prolapse may be a primary condition or secondary to several disorders. Most cases are a primary abnormality of the mitral valve. Secondary abnormalities may be seen in patients with secundum atrial septal defects, anorexia nervosa, and other abnormalities.

## PATHOLOGY

Interchordal hooding is the most consistent gross sign of mitral valve prolapse. The basic microscopic feature of the floppy mitral valve is significant thickening of the spongiosa. The spongiosa encroaches and invades the fibrosa causing focal interruption of the fibrosa. The grading system for quantitating the severity of mitral valve prolapse on a pathologic basis does not necessarily correlate with what is seen on a clinical basis.

## CLINICAL

Most children with mitral valve prolapse are asymptomatic and initially are referred for cardiac evaluation because of a click or a murmur detected during a routine examination. A number of studies report a high incidence of symptoms with mitral valve prolapse, but these are due to selection bias. Small subgroups of patients may be highly symptomatic.

Symptoms may include chest pain, easy fatigability, weakness, palpitations, dyspnea, dizziness, syncope, anxiety, and orthostatic hypotension.

Abnormalities on physical examination include thoracic and skeletal abnormalities such as a tall slender habitus, pectus excavatum, pectus carinatum, scoliosis, or kyphosis. A high arched palate, increased joint laxity, or abnormal dermatoglyphics patterns may be present.

Mitral valve prolapse is characterized by a midsystolic click or a late systolic murmur. The click and murmur vary depending on the patient's position and may vary in auscultatory findings at different times in different patients. The change in the click and murmur is due to alterations in left ventricular geometry. Maneuvers such as moving from a sitting to a supine position, from a standing to a squatting position, passive leg raising, and maximal isometric exercise increase left ventricle volume and decrease the degree of mitral valve prolapse and mitral regurgitation. The click and murmur move toward the second heart sound, and the murmur is shorter.

Administration of amyl nitrate, Valsalva's maneuver, sudden change from a supine to a sitting position, from a sitting to a standing position, from a squatting to a standing position and inspiration, decrease left ventricular size and left ventricular volume. Mitral valve prolapse and mitral valve regurgitation increase, thus the click and murmur move toward the first heart sound, and the murmur becomes longer. Because of the changing intensity or timing with different body positions, auscultation should be carried out with the patient in many positions.

The high-pitched, low-intensity, non-ejection midsystolic click is heard best at the apex of the heart. It may occur from just after the first heart sound to just before the second heart sound. Multiple clicks may be present in certain patients. The crescendo, late systolic murmur of mitral valve prolapse, is usually preceded by a click and is best heard at the apex. Occasionally, the murmur is described as having a honking or whooping quality and may be heard without a stethoscope.

The murmur of mitral valve prolapse may be confused with the murmur of hypertrophic cardiomyopathy. During the strain of the Valsalva's maneuver, the murmur of hypertrophic cardiomyopathy increases in intensity; whereas, the murmur of mitral valve prolapse becomes longer but not louder.

The chest radiograph is usually normal, unless associated cardiac defects are present. If routine chest roentgenogram shows thoracic spine and chest wall abnormalities, then a deliberate search for mitral valve prolapse is indicated.

The electrocardiogram is usually normal. Three types of abnormalities are reported: T wave inversion in leads II, III, and aVF, prolongation of the QT interval, and arrhythmias. The ST segments are usually normal at rest, but ST changes may be induced during standing or exercise.

The exercise test is usually normal. Arrhythmias and ST segment depression have been reported.

Echocardiography is useful in detecting and characterizing mitral valve prolapse. M-mode echocardiography alone should not be used to diagnose mitral valve prolapse; two-dimensional echocardiography should be used as well. M-mode echocardiography may overdiagnose or underdiagnose mitral valve prolapse. The apical four-chamber view in two-dimensional echocardiography is sensitive but not specific for the diagnosis of mitral valve prolapse. Many patients who have a normal auscultatory examination may have mitral valve prolapse as documented by the apical four-chamber view. The mitral valve annulus is not flat but has a saddle shape. The four-chamber view may show superior displacement of the mitral valve leaflets but this may not be true mitral valve prolapse. The long axis view seems to be the most specific view to determine presence or absence of mitral valve prolapse.

Echocardiographic evaluation of patients with possible mitral valve prolapse should include evaluation for mitral annulus dilatation, dysplasia of the mitral valve, mitral valve regurgitation, presence or absence of ruptured chordae and vegetations, and coexistent cardiovascular abnormalities. Prolapse of the tricuspid valve and aortic valve occurs more often in patients with mitral valve prolapse.

Stress radionuclide scintigraphy aids in the differential diagnosis between mitral valve prolapse associated with atypical chest pain and electrocardiogram abnormalities and primary coronary artery disease associated with mitral valve prolapse. A negative test may confirm the diagnosis of primary mitral valve prolapse with unassociated coronary artery disease. A false-positive test, however, may occur in patients with mitral valve prolapse without associated coronary artery disease.

Diagnostic cardiac catheterization with angiography rarely is needed in patients with isolated mitral valve prolapse. If needed, it is used to assess the severity of associated cardiac abnormalities.

# COMPLICATIONS

The prognosis of mitral valve prolapse in children is excellent. Complications such as endocarditis, significant arrhythmias, sudden death, progressive mitral regurgitation, and cerebral ischemia occur infrequently.

## Chest Pain

If patients with mitral valve prolapse have symptoms, the most common presenting symptom is disabling chest pain. The exact mechanism of chest pain is unknown. In some patients with mitral valve prolapse, esophageal motility disorders account for chest pain.

## Infective Endocarditis

Patients with mitral valve prolapse and mitral regurgitation have an increased incidence of infective endocarditis. The Committee on Rheumatic Fever and Bacterial Endocarditis of the Council of Cardiovascular Disease in the Young and the American Heart Association recommend that endocarditis prophylaxis be given to all patients with mitral valve prolapse who have evidence of mitral valve insufficiency. Because patients with mitral valve prolapse may have a murmur on one occasion and not on another, some recommend endocarditis prophylaxis in all patients with mitral valve prolapse whether or not mitral insufficiency is present.

## THROMBOEMBOLISM

Acute hemiplegia, transient ischemic attacks, cerebellar infarcts, amaurosis fugax, and retinal arteriolar occlusion appear to be more frequent in patients with mitral valve prolapse syndrome. They may result from thrombosis formation on the valve or abnormalities in the platelet coagulant activities, shortened platelet survival time, and plasma hyperactivity.

## Arrhythmias

All types of arrhythmias are reported. Premature ventricular contractions are reported to be present in as many as 50% of children with mitral valve prolapse, and complex ventricular arrhythmias are reported in as many as 18.5%. Twenty-four-hour Holter monitoring is more sensitive for detecting arrhythmias. Complex ventricular arrhythmias may be treated with a beta-blocker such as propranolol.

## Sudden Death

Sudden death is a rare complication postulated to be secondary to a lethal arrhythmia. Patients who may be at increased risk of sudden death have complex ventricular arrhythmias, severe mitral regurgitation, left ventricular dysfunction, prolonged QT interval, dysplastic mitral valve, a history of syncope, presyncope, or palpitations, or a family history of sudden death.

## Mitral Regurgitation

Progressive mitral regurgitation is a rare complication. It occurs in about 15% of patients over a 10- to 15-year period. In many patients, it is related to rupture of the chordae tendineae or infective endocarditis. Severe mitral valve regurgitation occurs more frequently in men older than age 50 years with mitral valve prolapse.

# MANAGEMENT

Evaluation of a patient for presence of mitral valve prolapse is first done by a thorough physical examination that includes maneuvers to elicit the click and murmur, a two-dimensional echocardiogram, and a Doppler study.

A resting electrocardiogram is recommended in all patients to look for evidence of ST-T wave changes, a long QT interval, or an arrhythmia. If coexisting cardiac defects are not present, a chest roentgenogram is not needed in patients with isolated mitral valve prolapse. A 24-hour Holter monitor or exercise treadmill is indicated in patients with palpations, light-headedness, dizziness, syncope, arrhythmias on resting electrocardiogram, family history of sudden death, complaints of chest pain, and a long QT interval on resting electrocardiogram. Angiography may be indicated if other cardiac defects coexist.

An asymptomatic patient with an isolated midsystolic click, no evidence of mitral regurgitation, or dysplastic mitral valve should be reassured of the benign nature of mitral valve prolapse and followed up every few years.

Indications for mitral valve replacement are severe mitral regurgitation, severe life-threatening arrhythmias, and uncontrollable chest pain, all unresponsive to medical management.

Prophylactic treatment of patients for cerebral ischemia is not indicated. Patients with mitral valve prolapse who have transient ischemic attacks should receive prophylaxis with antithrombotic and antiplatelet therapy.

Patients with mitral valve prolapse should not participate in competitive athletics if there is a history of syncope or near syncope, a history of disabling chest pain, complex ventricular arrhythmias, significant mitral regurgitation or left ventricular enlargement or dysfunction, prolongation of the QT interval, Marfan's syndrome, or a family history of sudden death. Patients who are asymptomatic and found to have isolated uniform premature ventricular contractions (PVCs) may participate in competitive athletics if there is no history of exercise-induced syncope or increase in ectopic beats with exercise.

## Selected Readings

Bisset GS III, Scwartz DC, Meyer Ra, James FW, Kaplan S. Clinical spectrum and long-term follow-up of isolated mitral valve prolapse in 119 children. Circulation 1980;2:62.

Boudoulas H, Kolibash AJ, Baker P, King BD, Wooley CF. Mitral valve prolapse and the mitral valve prolapse syndrome: a diagnostic classification and pathogenesis of symptoms. Am Heart J 1989;118(4):796.

Cheng TO. Mitral valve prolapse. Annu Rev Med 1989;40:201.

Devereux RB, Kramer-Fox R, Kligfield P. Mitral valve prolapse: causes, clinical manifestations, and management. Ann Intern Med 1989;4:111.

Devereux RB, Kramer-Fox R, Shear K, Kligfield P, Pini R, Savage DD. Diagnosis and classification of severity of mitral valve prolapse: methodologic, biologic, and prognostic considerations. Am Heart J 1987:5.

Krivokapich J, Child JS, Dadourian BJ, Perloff JK. Reassessment of echocardiographic criteria for diagnosis of mitral valve prolapse. Am J Cardiol 1988;61:131.

Perloff JK, Child JS, Edwards JE. New guidelines for the clinical diagnosis of mitral valve prolapse. Am J Cardiol 1986:57.

Savage DD, Garrison FJ, Devereux RB, et al. Mitral valve prolapse in the general population. I. Epidemiologic features: The Framingham Study. Am Heart J 1983: 9.

Warth DC, King ME, Cohen JM, Tesoriero VL, Marcus E, Weyman AE. Prevalence of mitral valve prolapse in normal children. J Am Coll Cardiol 1985;5:5.

Webb Kavey RA, Blackman MS, Sondheimer HM, Byrum CJ. Ventricular arrhythmias and mitral valve prolapse in childhood. J Pediatr 1984:12.

*Principles and Practice of Pediatrics, Second Edition.*
edited by Frank A. Oski et al. J. B. Lippincott Company, Philadelphia © 1994.

# 82.10 *Aortic Arch and Pulmonary Artery Abnormalities*

W. Robert Morrow

Anomalies of the aortic arch and pulmonary arteries constitute a diverse group of malformations. The range of possible deviations from normal morphology of the aortic arch and pulmonary artery is broad. Vascular rings are formed when one or more aortic arch anomalies, with or without a patent ductus arteriosus or ligamentum, produce a ring that completely encircles the trachea and esophagus, leading to symptoms of tracheal or esophageal constriction. A vascular sling, produced by an abnormal origin and course of the left pulmonary artery or abnormal origin and course of a left ductus arteriosus, does not encircle the trachea and esophagus completely, but usually produces severe symptoms of tracheal and bronchial compression.

## EMBRYOLOGY AND EMBRYOPATHOGENESIS

It is possible to describe most anomalies of the aortic arch by postulating regression of a segment of the arch that normally persists or, conversely, persistence of a segment of the arch that normally regresses. In this concept, the normal left aortic arch develops by regression of the eighth segment of the embryonic right dorsal aorta. The remaining elements of the right aortic arch contribute to development of the right innominate artery and the primitive right subclavian artery. The right ductus arteriosus normally regresses, eliminating continuity of the right sixth aortic arch with the aorta. Double aortic arch is postulated to result from persistence of both paired dorsal aortic arches.

A right aortic arch may form by one of two mechanisms, giving rise to right aortic arch with mirror-image branching or without mirror-image branching. The former occurs with abnormal regression of the left eighth dorsal aortic arch segment. When regression of the left arch occurs between the left carotid artery and the left subclavian artery (left fourth primitive aortic arch), the latter arises from the descending aorta and courses posterior to the esophagus. In this situation, the ductus arteriosus arises from the descending aorta at the base of the left subclavian artery or from a retroesophageal diverticulum and produces a vascular ring completely encircling the esophagus and trachea. Regression may occur between the right carotid artery and the right subclavian artery, giving rise to anomalous origin of the right subclavian artery from the descending aorta. Cervical aortic arch probably results from persistence of the third primitive aortic arch, with regression of the contralateral arch between the carotid artery and the subclavian artery (fourth primitive arch).

Anomalous origin of the left pulmonary artery, unilateral absence of one pulmonary artery, and unilateral origin of one pulmonary artery from the ascending aorta result from abnormal regression of the left proximal sixth arch. Alternatively, unilateral origin of one pulmonary artery from the ascending aorta may result from malalignment of the conotruncal ridges. With septation of the conotruncus, one pulmonary artery maintains connection with the ascending aorta and the other is connected to the main pulmonary artery.

## AORTIC ARCH ANOMALIES

### Left Aortic Arch With Anomalous Right Subclavian Artery

Left aortic arch with anomalous origin of the right subclavian artery is the most common aortic arch malformation noted on postmortem examination. The incidence of this abnormality in the general population is about 0.5%. The left arch has a normal course to the left and anterior to the trachea, but the right subclavian artery arises as the last branch of the arch and courses posterior to the esophagus. Most patients with anomalous right subclavian artery are asymptomatic, and the abnormality is discovered incidentally at esophagography or at catheterization. An anomalous right subclavian artery often is seen in patients with tetralogy of Fallot and left aortic arch, and, therefore, have a significant bearing on which systemic-to-pulmonary artery shunt is chosen for palliation of cyanosis. In addition, anomalous right subclavian artery may be present in patients with coarctation of the aorta and often arises distal to the site of coarctation. In these patients, blood pressure in the right arm and legs do not reflect the coarctation gradient. It is necessary, then, to determine blood pressure in both arms as well as the legs when examining patients with suspected coarctation.

Although most patients with an anomalous right subclavian artery are asymptomatic, some older children and adults may experience dysphagia. Routine chest radiography does not demonstrate this anomaly, but barium esophagography is diagnostic. The oblique course of the anomalous vessel posterior to the esophagus in the anteroposterior projection and the posterior indentation of the esophagus in the lateral or left anterior oblique projection are usually diagnostic (Fig 82-24). The diagnosis of anomalous right subclavian artery may be made with two-dimensional echocardiography when the first branch of the aorta is to the right, but the normal bifurcation into a right carotid

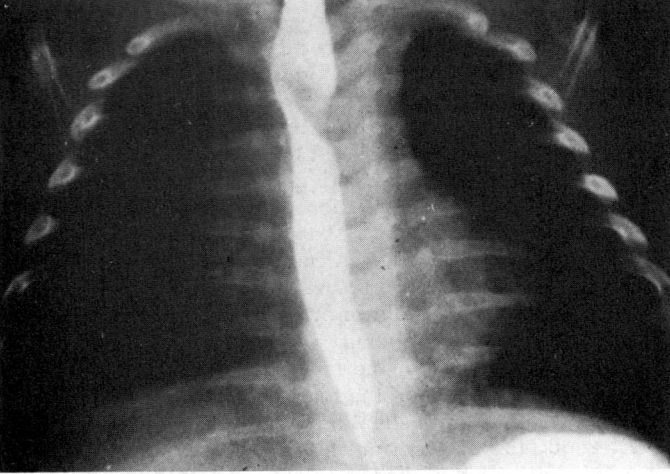

**Figure 82-24.** AP projection of a barium esophagram performed on a patient with tetralogy of Fallot, left aortic arch, and anomalous right subclavian artery. The retroesophageal course of the anomalous right subclavian artery produces an oblique indentation of the esophagus. (Courtesy of Michael Nihill, MD, Baylor College of Medicine, Houston, TX.)

artery and right subclavian artery cannot be demonstrated. An anomalous right subclavian artery may be noted incidentally when aortography is performed in patients with congenital heart disease.

If symptoms of a vascular ring (eg, stridor, wheezing, cough) are present in a patient with an anomalous right subclavian artery, an alternative diagnosis, such as laryngomalacia or tracheomalacia, should be considered. Rarely, an anomalous right subclavian artery in association with a left aortic arch, retroesophageal descending aorta, and right ductus arteriosus or ligamentum produces a symptomatic vascular ring. The retroesophageal descending aorta in these patients results in a large, rounded, posterior indentation on barium esophagram, which usually is distinguished readily from the more shallow indentation produced by an anomalous right subclavian artery without a retroesophageal descending aorta. The diagnosis may be confirmed by magnetic resonance imaging or angiography.

### Double Aortic Arch

Double aortic arch is the most common clinically recognized form of vascular ring. The ascending aorta divides anterior to the trachea into left and right arches, which then pass on either side of the trachea. Usually, the right arch is larger than the left and passes posterior to the esophagus to join the descending aorta to the left of the midline. Uncommonly, the left arch is atretic. A complete vascular ring is formed by the arches on each side of the trachea and esophagus, with the ascending aorta anterior and the retroesophageal arch or descending aorta posterior. The ductus arteriosus is usually left-sided and is not an essential component of the vascular ring, but the length of the ductus arteriosus or ligamentum may affect significantly the severity of symptoms. Associated congenital heart disease may occur in as many as 22% of patients. Cyanotic congenital heart disease predominates, including tetralogy of Fallot and transposition of the great arteries.

Patients with double aortic arch are usually severely symptomatic in infancy, with stridor, dyspnea, cough, and recurrent respiratory infections. Infants feed poorly due to severe respiratory distress and may prefer to assume an opisthotonic posture. Life-threatening episodes of apnea with cyanosis may occur. The diagnosis of double aortic arch often is suggested on routine chest radiography. Both arches may be seen on either side of the trachea in the anteroposterior projection, but usually a right aortic arch with left descending aorta is seen. There also may be evidence of hyperinflation of either or both lungs due to obstruction of the lower trachea and main stem bronchi.

Barium esophagography demonstrates bilateral indentations of the esophagus in the anteroposterior projection (Fig 82-25). Usually, the right arch produces the larger and more superior indentation. In the lateral or left anterior oblique projection, a large posterior indentation is seen and represents the retroesophageal component of the arch. There is also anterior and more inferior indentation of the arch produced by posterior deviation of the trachea. Characteristic findings of bilateral echolucencies of the double arch are demonstrated by suprasternal notch echocardiography in the coronal plane. In double aortic arch, angiography of the ascending aorta demonstrates both arches, establishes the dominant aortic arch, and often differentiates between right aortic arch with anomalous left subclavian artery and double aortic arch with segmental atresia of the left arch. Magnetic resonance imaging also provides sufficient anatomic detail to plan surgical division of the minor arch (Fig 82-26).

Stridor and respiratory distress are usually severe, and affected infants often die without early surgical intervention. The rate of mortality from surgery is low, and eventual long-term relief of symptoms usually is achieved. However, short-term postoperative

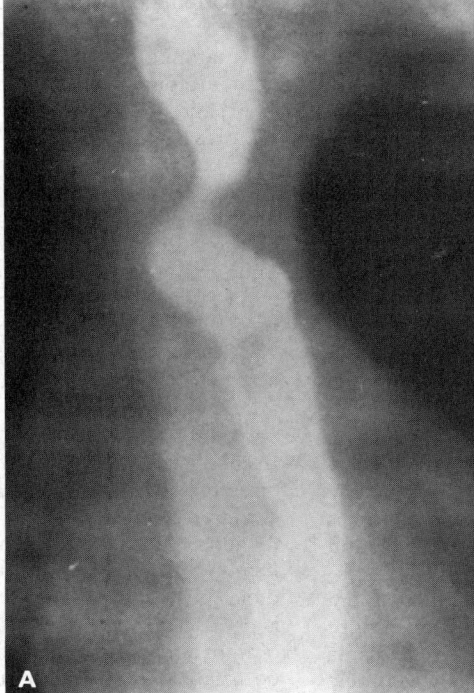
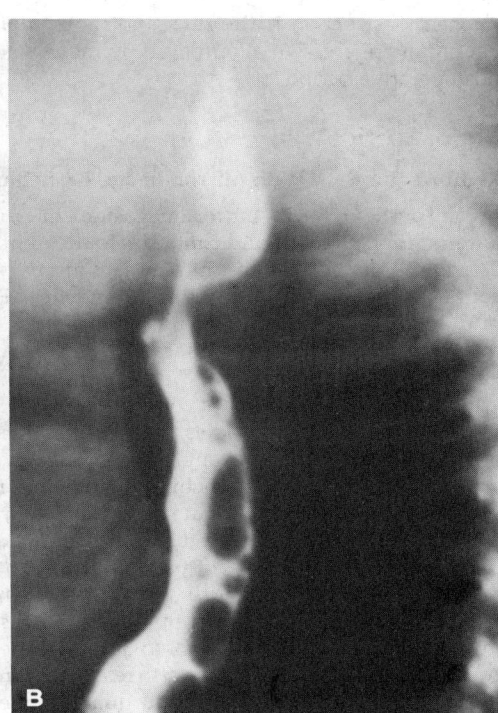

**Figure 82-25.** In double aortic arch, (**A**) bilateral indentation of the esophagus is characteristic in the AP projection with (**B**) a deep posterior indentation on the lateral projection produced by the retroesophageal portion of the arch. The larger and more superior indentation in the AP projection, in this case on the right of the esophagus, usually is produced by the dominant arch. (Courtesy of Michael Nihill, MD, Baylor College of Medicine, Houston, TX.)

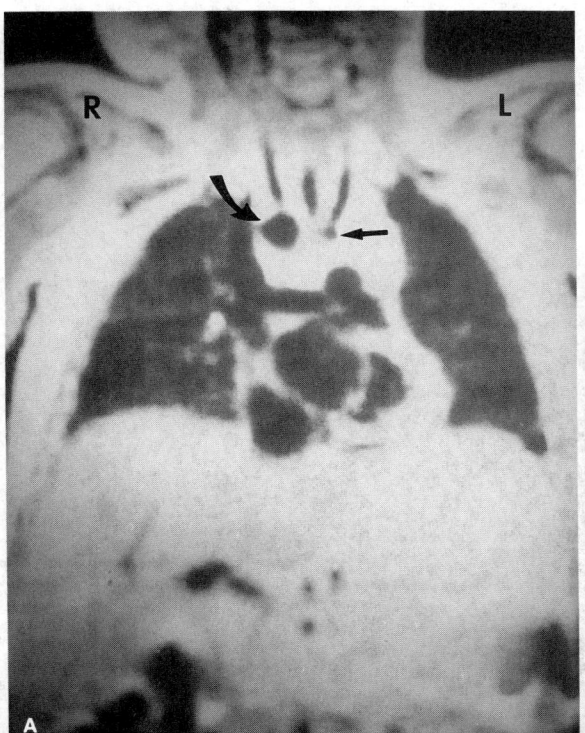
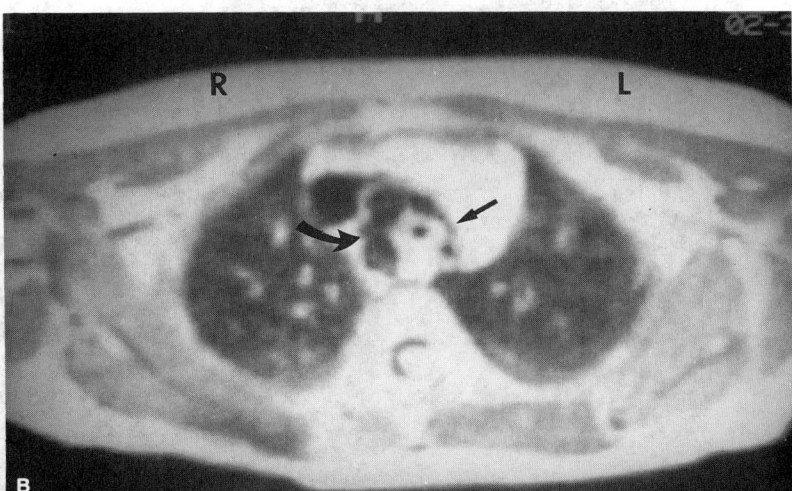

**Figure 82-26.** T1 weighted gated magnetic resonance imaging in a patient with double aortic arch. Coronal images (**A**) demonstrate both the major arch on the right (*curved arrow*) and the minor arch on the left (*straight arrow*). In the axial plane (**B**), the vascular ring is partially demonstrated, and the major arch on the right (*curved arrow*) and the minor arch on the left (*straight arrow*) are clearly seen. The position of the trachea in the center of this ring is seen as the small, dark, circular area of signal loss. (Courtesy of Gary Hedlund, MD, The Children's Hospital, Birmingham, Ala.)

tracheal obstruction is the rule, and most infants require intubation and aggressive attention to pulmonary toilet in the early postoperative period.

## Right Aortic Arch

### Right Aortic Arch With Mirror-Image Branching

In right aortic arch with mirror-image branching, the aorta ascends anterior to the trachea and continues to the right and posteriorly. The first branch is the left innominate artery, which pursues a course to the left and anterior to the trachea. The continuation of the arch to the right of the trachea produces deviation of the trachea to the left. The second and third branches of the arch are the right common carotid artery and the right subclavian artery. The descending aorta continues initially to the right and anterior to the vertebral bodies, then courses obliquely to the left, exiting from the thorax through the aortic hiatus. In right aortic arch with mirror-image branching, the ductus arteriosus usually arises from the left innominate artery at the origin or near the bifurcation. Congenital heart disease, predominantly cyanotic, is present in as many as 98% of patients with right aortic arch and mirror-image branching. With anomalous origin of the left subclavian artery, associated congenital heart disease is uncommon. In tetralogy of Fallot, from 13% to 34% of patients have a right aortic arch. A right aortic arch is also relatively common in patients with truncus arteriosus (36%) and double-outlet right ventricle (20%), but is uncommon in patients with transposition of the great arteries (3%).

### Right Aortic Arch With Anomalous Left Subclavian Artery

Right aortic arch with mirror-image branching does not produce a vascular ring and is usually asymptomatic. Right aortic arch

with anomalous left subclavian artery and left ductus arteriosus is the most common type of aortic arch anomaly that produces an anatomic vascular ring. This group of abnormalities usually is asymptomatic, and, therefore, ranks as the second most common cause of symptomatic vascular ring. The essential pathologic features include course of the arch to the right of the trachea, with the first branch being the left carotid artery. The left subclavian artery arises from the descending aorta, and the ductus arteriosus, which originates from a retroesophageal diverticulum of the descending aorta, courses to the left to connect to the pulmonary artery. Unlike in double aortic arch, the presence of a left ductus arteriosus or ligamentum is an essential component of the vascular ring.

Although patients with right aortic arch, anomalous left subclavian artery, and left ductus arteriosus are usually asymptomatic, symptoms of tracheal or esophageal obstruction, when they occur, are similar to those encountered with double aortic arch. In these patients, however, symptoms are generally milder and often lead to presentation later in life. Nonetheless, affected patients present with stridor, cough, and recurrent respiratory infections. Older patients may complain of dysphagia and may have a history of stridor or wheezing. Anteroposterior chest radiographs demonstrate deviation of the trachea to the left, which is produced by the density of the right aortic arch. The diagnosis of right aortic arch with an anomalous left subclavian artery may be established by echocardiography. Barium esophagography demonstrates an oblique indentation from right to left (Fig 82-27) in the anteroposterior projection and a posterior indentation of the esophagus in lateral views. In symptomatic patients, magnetic resonance imaging confirms the presence of a retroesophageal diverticulum and left subclavian artery (Fig 82-28). Surgery is indicated for patients with symptomatic tracheal or esophageal

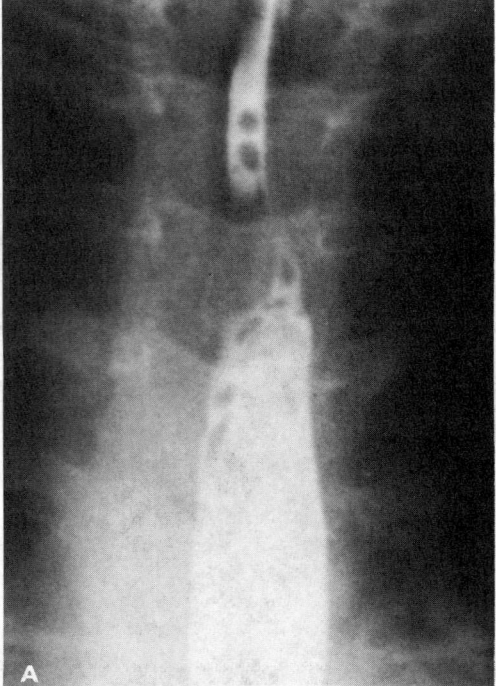
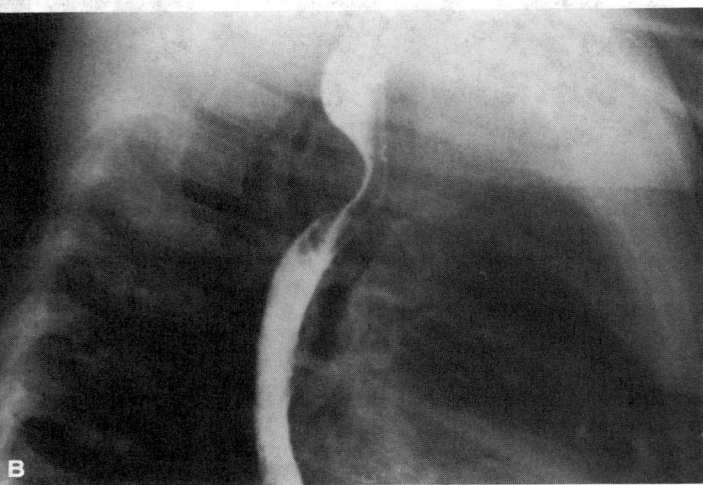

**Figure 82-27.** In right aortic arch with anomalous origin of the left subclavian artery, (**A**) the retroesophageal course of the left subclavian artery produces an oblique impression from right inferior to left superior on the AP barium esophagram. On the lateral esophagram (**B**), a posterior impression is produced by the left subclavian artery or diverticulum of the descending aorta. The large posterior defect in this patient implies the presence of a retroesophageal diverticulum or a retroesophageal course of the descending aorta. (Courtesy of Albert Schlesinger, MD, Wilford Hall Air Force Medical Center, San Antonio, TX.)

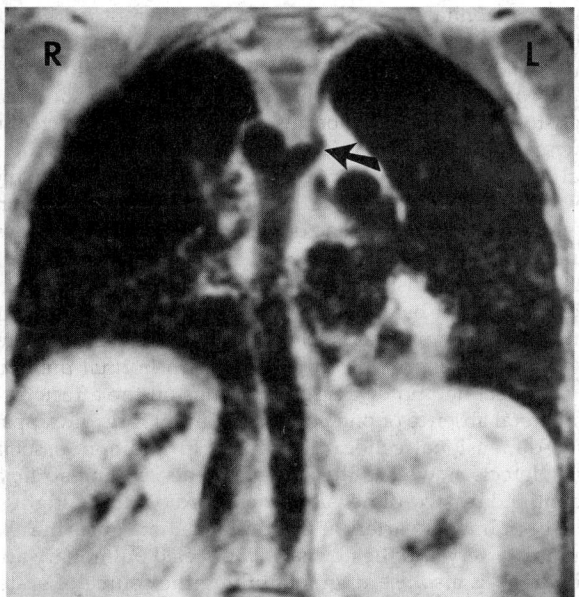

**Figure 82-28.** Gated magnetic resonance imaging study in a patient with right aortic arch and an anomalous left subclavian artery. A T1 weighted coronal image is shown demonstrating the descending aorta with origin of a large Kommerell's diverticulum and left subclavian artery (*arrow*). The point of constriction between the Komerell's diverticulum and left subclavian artery indicates the point of origin of the ligamentum arteriosus. (Courtesy of Gary Hedlund, MD, The Children's Hospital, Birmingham, Ala.)

compression. As for double aortic arch, the surgical mortality rate is low and long-term relief of symptoms is the rule.

## Cervical Aortic Arch

Cervical aortic arch is a rare anomaly characterized by cervical position of the aorta, separate origin of the carotid artery contralateral to the arch, and anomalous origin of the subclavian artery on the side contralateral to the arch. In addition, there usually is separate origin of the internal carotid, external carotid, and subclavian arteries on the side of the arch. There may be a ductus arteriosus or ligamentum originating from the descending aorta on the side contralateral to the arch, producing a vascular ring. Associated congenital heart disease is uncommon.

Most patients with cervical aortic arch are asymptomatic. Symptoms, when present, range from mild dysphagia to significant respiratory distress. The latter occurs when there is a coexisting vascular ring. A pulsatile mass is always noted in the neck. Compression of the mass produces a palpable reduction in leg pulses as well as the arm pulse on the side opposite the arch. This physical finding is pathognomonic for cervical aortic arch. In addition, a thrill and a murmur are present over the mass.

Routine chest radiography demonstrates loss of the normal aortic knob on the left, widening of the upper mediastinum, and an aortic density in the apex of the hemithorax on the side of the arch. There is a large posterior indentation of the esophagus in the lateral projection on esophagography. Although cervical aortic arch is recognized using two-dimensional echocardiography, variations in arterial branching patterns make angiography a prerequisite to surgical repair. In a typical case, aortography reveals an elongated ascending aorta and the apex of the aortic arch above the clavicle. Surgery is reserved for patients with symptoms of tracheal or esophageal compression and for patients with aneurysm formation or coarctation.

## Anomalous Innominate Artery

Patients with stridor and respiratory distress associated with anterior compression of the trachea have been described in infants, with symptoms and compression of the trachea being attributed to an anomalous origin and course of the innominate artery. The role of innominate artery compression in producing symptoms, however, is disputed. The high incidence of coexisting tracheomalacia in affected infants and the frequent finding of anterior tracheal indentation in asymptomatic children undergoing bronchoscopy cast doubt on the primary role of vascular compression in producing symptoms. In addition, Swischuk (1971) emphasized the role of anterior mediastinal crowding, commonly seen on lateral chest radiographs in infancy, in producing apparent anterior tracheal compression. This finding is seen in both asymptomatic and symptomatic infants, and apparently resolves with age.

Symptoms ascribed to innominate artery compression are basically the same as those caused by tracheomalacia. Affected infants have cough, stridor, and dyspnea and may have episodes of apnea and cyanosis. Infants who experience apnea and cyanosis have a relatively poor prognosis. In addition to the findings on chest radiograph and bronchoscopy, echocardiography shows a normal left aortic arch with the first branch being the innominate artery to the right. Barium esophagography is normal, excluding vascular rings and vascular slings. Careful bronchoscopic examination usually demonstrates either local or diffuse tracheomalacia in addition to varying degrees of anterior indentation produced by the innominate artery.

Most affected infants improve without surgical intervention. The surgical procedure performed for symptomatic tracheomalacia is essentially the same as the procedure advocated for symptomatic anomalous innominate artery. The indication for surgery in both conditions is the severity of symptoms. The innominate artery, the aorta, or the anterior mediastinal fascia are sutured to the posterior sternal periosteum to relieve compression. It is likely that the primary diagnosis in most patients is tracheomalacia and that the effect of surgery is to reduce the extrinsic compression produced by "anterior mediastinal crowding."

## PULMONARY ARTERY ANOMALIES

### Anomalous Left Pulmonary Artery-Pulmonary Artery Sling

Anomalous origin of the left pulmonary artery is a rare congenital anomaly that produces severe tracheobronchial obstruction in most affected patients. A normal left pulmonary artery is absent, and the left lung is supplied by an anomalous left pulmonary artery arising from the distal right pulmonary artery. Tracheal and bronchial compression are produced as this artery courses posterior and caudal to the right main stem bronchus and then to the left, posterior to the trachea and anterior to the esophagus. The course of the vessel to the right of the trachea produces deviation of the lower trachea to the left. The resulting compression of the right main stem bronchus and lower trachea leads to airway obstruction, primarily affecting the right lung. Obstruction of the lower trachea and left main stem bronchus may occur, however, resulting in bilateral obstruction.

Associated congenital anomalies are common and are present in from 58% to 83% of patients. Anomalies of the trachea, bronchi, and lung parenchyma are common and include complete cartilaginous rings, tracheomalacia, abnormal pulmonary lobulation, and bronchus suis. Congenital heart defects are present in about 40% to 50% of patients and include persistent left superior vena cava, atrial septal defect, patent ductus arteriosus, and ventricular septal defects, among others.

Symptoms due to anomalous left pulmonary artery occur early in most patients. Two thirds of affected infants are symptomatic by 1 month of age. Symptoms include severe respiratory distress with stridor, wheezing, cyanosis, and recurrent pneumonitis. Obstructive apnea may occur and can be fatal. Unlike aortic vascular rings, dysphagia is rare, because the anomalous left pulmonary artery passes anterior to the esophagus without significant esophageal compression. Although the majority of patients are severely symptomatic, asymptomatic and mildly affected patients have been observed.

On anteroposterior chest radiographs, hyperinflation of the right or left lung is observed often, due to tracheal and bronchial compression. Obstruction of the left bronchus may also produce varying degrees of volume loss (atelectasis) of the left lung (Fig 82-29). Barium esophagography usually demonstrates a characteristic anterior indentation of the esophagus on the lateral projection. The diagnosis of anomalous left pulmonary artery as well as associated cardiac defects is made readily with two-dimensional echocardiography. Pulmonary artery sling may also be recognized by magnetic resonance imaging (Fig 82-30).

Although the presence of a vascular sling can be established noninvasively, pulmonary artery angiography is necessary to delineate the anatomic detail necessary for surgical correction. Catheterization also is indicated to assess the severity of associated cardiac defects. Survival of symptomatic infants is unlikely without early surgical intervention, and surgery should be performed early in infants suffering from severe respiratory obstruction. Although many reports describe successful treatment of this anomaly by surgery, the rate of mortality of surgical procedures is high, at 40% to 50%. Coexisting tracheal or bronchial stenosis is disproportionately prevalent and severe in nonsurvivors, and is undoubtedly a major contributing factor in postoperative death.

## Unilateral Absence of One Pulmonary Artery

Unilateral absence of one pulmonary artery is an uncommon congenital defect. Forty percent of cases occur without associated cardiac defects, whereas the remaining patients usually have tetralogy of Fallot, patent ductus arteriosus, or ventricular septal defect. The absent pulmonary artery usually is opposite the side of the aortic arch. Patients with isolated unilateral absence of one pulmonary artery often are asymptomatic but may experience recurrent pneumonitis, bronchiectasis, or hemoptysis. When as-

sociated congenital heart disease is present, symptoms generally are those of the associated defect. Patients with left-to-right shunts, however, may experience more severe symptoms of pulmonary congestion, because both the normal cardiac output and the left-to-right shunt must perfuse the normally connected lung. Likewise, there are no specific physical findings indicating unilateral absence of a pulmonary artery, although most patients have a nonspecific systolic murmur at the left sternal border. Those with coexisting cardiac defects have compatible physical findings.

Differential perfusion of the lungs with reduced vascular markings may not be apparent in infants on chest radiographs. In older children and adults, chest radiographs demonstrate increased vascular markings on the side with normal pulmonary artery connection and decreased markings on the affected side.

Unilateral absence of one pulmonary artery is readily apparent by two-dimensional echocardiography. In addition, associated cardiac defects as well as the side of the descending aortic arch are identified by two-dimensional echocardiography. Right ventricular or pulmonary artery angiography demonstrates the absent pulmonary artery and the normally connected pulmonary artery. Aortography is also useful in identifying the source of systemic arterial supply to the affected lung. In addition, cardiac catheterization enables assessment of pulmonary artery pressure and resistance in the normally connected lung. About 20% of patients without associated left-to-right shunts demonstrate evidence of pulmonary hypertension, whereas 90% of those with left-to-right shunts have pulmonary hypertension.

Although patients without associated heart defects may escape early recognition, those with coexisting left-to-right shunts usually are recognized in infancy and should undergo early surgical repair to prevent development of irreversible pulmonary hypertension. Older patients with pneumonitis should be treated medically. If severe recurrent lung infections or hemoptysis occurs, however, then pneumonectomy of the affected lung should be considered.

## Unilateral Origin of One Pulmonary Artery From the Ascending Aorta

Unilateral origin of one pulmonary artery from the ascending aorta is rare, occurring in 0.05% of patients with congenital heart disease. In most patients, the right pulmonary artery arises from the ascending aorta and usually is the same size as or larger than

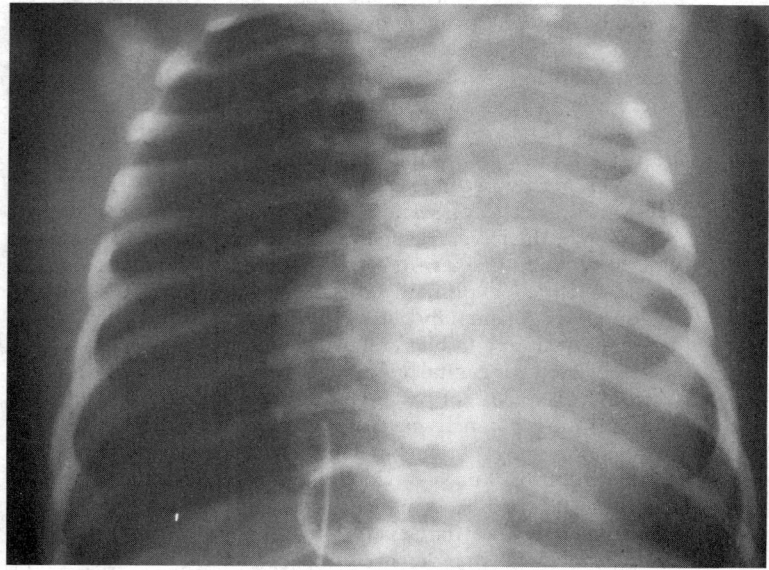

**Figure 82-29.** Posteroanterior radiograph demonstrating loss of volume (atelectasis) with opacity of the left lung field in a patient with a pulmonary artery sling. The course of the left pulmonary artery posterior to the trachea and left bronchus often produce compression with resulting atelectasis of the left lung or hyperinflation of the right. (Courtesy of Gary Hedlund, MD, The Children's Hospital, Birmingham, Ala.)

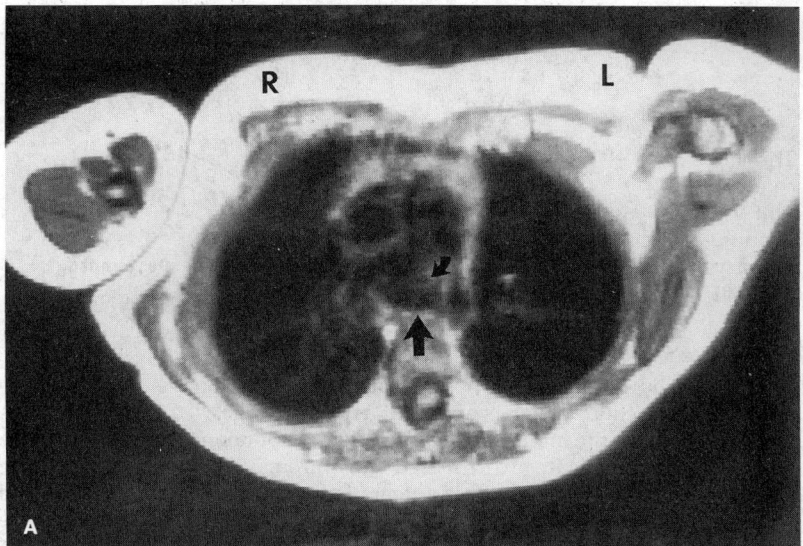

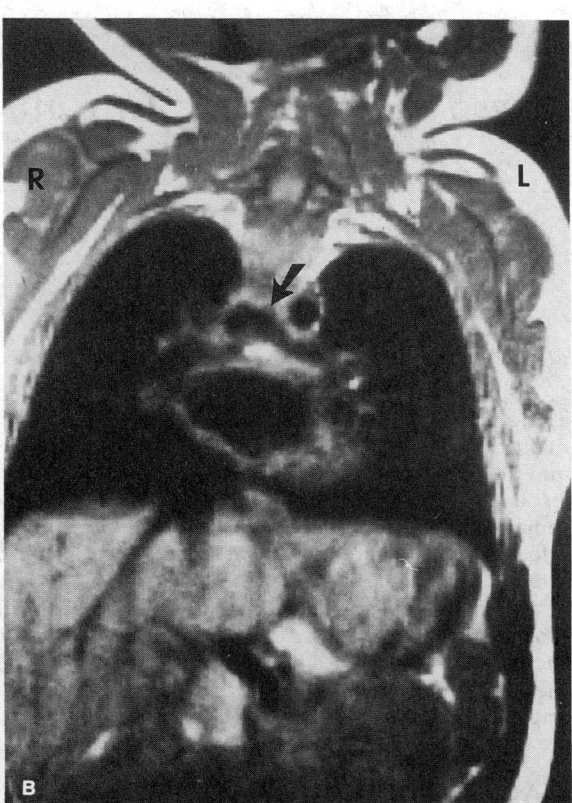

**Figure 82-30.** Coronal and axial T1-weighted magnetic resonance imaging study demonstrating a pulmonary artery sling. The axial image (**A**) demonstrates origin of the left pulmonary artery from the posterior aspect of the right pulmonary artery. The left pulmonary artery (*straight arrow*) courses posterior to the trachea, which is demonstrated by signal loss (*curved arrow*). In the coronal imaging plane (**B**), the origin of the left pulmonary artery (*arrow*) originates from the right pulmonary artery to the right of the trachea.

the left pulmonary artery. The vessel connects to the aorta just above the aortic valve and on the right of or posterior to it, and courses directly to the right hilum. Most patients with origin of one pulmonary artery from the ascending aorta have an associated patent ductus arteriosus to the unaffected pulmonary artery. Cardiac defects associated with origin of the right pulmonary artery from the ascending aorta include ventricular septal defect, coarctation of the aorta, interrupted aortic arch, atrial septal defects, and contralateral pulmonary vein stenosis. Tetralogy of Fallot is often present when the left pulmonary artery arises from the ascending aorta and usually is accompanied by a left aortic arch.

Patients with origin of one pulmonary artery from the ascending aorta but without tetralogy of Fallot characteristically present in early infancy with severe congestive heart failure and cyanosis. Cyanosis results from a right-to-left shunt at the ductal level due to pulmonary hypertension. The heart often is enlarged massively on chest radiographs, and the pulmonary vascular markings are either increased symmetrically or greater on the affected side. The diagnosis may be made by two-dimensional echocardiography. In addition to demonstrating origin of the affected pulmonary artery from the aorta, echocardiographic examination demonstrates two arterial valves, thus excluding truncus arteriosus.

Without surgical intervention, most patients either die or develop significant pulmonary vascular obstructive disease by 6 months of age. Therefore, early surgical repair is indicated when the diagnosis of origin of one pulmonary artery from the ascending aorta is established.

## Selected Readings

Barry A. The aortic derivatives in the human adult. Anat Rec 1951;111:221.

Congdon ED. Transformation of the aortic arch system during the development of the human embryo. Contributions to Embryology 1922;1:47.

Huhta JC. Pediatric imaging; Doppler ultrasound of the chest: extracardiac diagnosis. Philadelphia: Lea and Febiger, 1986.

Kirklin JW, Barratt-Boyes BG. Cardiac surgery. New York: John Wiley & Sons, 1986.

Knight L, Edwards JE. Right aortic arch. Types and associated cardiac anomalies. Circulation 1974;50:1047.

Moes CAF. Vascular rings and anomalies of the aortic arch. In: Keith JD, Rowe RD, Vlad P, eds. Heart disease in infancy and childhood, ed 3. New York: Macmillan, 1978.

Morrow WR, Huhta JC, Mullins CE. Anomalies of the aortic arch and pulmonary arteries. In: Garson A Jr, Bricker JT, McNamara DG, eds. The science and practice of pediatric cardiology. Philadelphia: Lea and Febiger.

Shuford WH, Sybers RG. The aortic arch and its malformations, with emphasis on the angiographic features. Springfield, Ill: Charles C Thomas, 1974.

Stewart JR, Kincaid OW, Edwards JE. An atlas of vascular rings and related malformations of the aortic arch system. Springfield, Ill: Charles C Thomas, 1964.

Swischuk LE. Anterior tracheal indentation in infancy and early childhood: normal or abnormal? Am J Roentgenol Rad Ther Nucl Med 1971;112:12.

*Principles and Practice of Pediatrics, Second Edition.*
edited by Frank A. Oski et al. J. B. Lippincott Company, Philadelphia © 1994.

# 82.11 *Congenital Coronary Artery Abnormalities*

### David J. Driscoll

## NORMAL CORONARY ANATOMY

There are two major coronary arteries—left and right. The left main coronary artery divides into the left anterior descending and the circumflex coronary arteries (Fig 82-31). Branches of the left anterior descending coronary artery include the left conus, septal, and diagonal arteries. Branches of the circumflex coronary artery may include the sinus node artery, Kugel's artery, marginal arteries, and the left atrial circumflex artery.

Branches of the right coronary artery include the right conal branch, the sinus node artery, an atrial branch, the right ventricular muscle branches (including the acute marginal branch), the posterior descending coronary artery, the atrioventricular node artery, and septal branches (Fig 82-32).

## MAJOR CORONARY ANOMALIES

### Anomalous Origin of the Left Coronary Artery From the Pulmonary Artery

Anomalous origin of the left coronary artery (ALCA) from the pulmonary artery may be the most common important coronary anomaly with which pediatricians and pediatric cardiologists must deal. Usually, the anomalous coronary artery arises from the left sinus of the pulmonary artery.

#### Clinical Manifestation

A patient with ALCA may present with signs and symptoms of myocardial infarction and congestive heart failure in infancy, or the condition may be unassociated with myocardial infarction or symptoms of heart disease until detected serendipitously in adulthood or at autopsy. The age at presentation depends on the degree of collateral circulation between the right and left coronary artery systems. Subjects with well-developed collateral connections may not develop myocardial infarction and may do well,

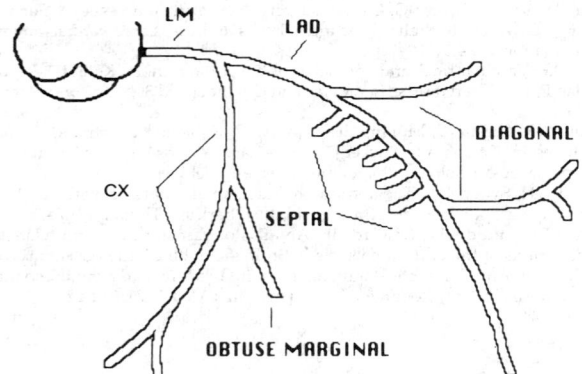

**Figure 82-31.**    Normal left coronary artery system. *CX,* circumflex; *LM,* left main; *LAD,* left anterior descending coronary arteries.

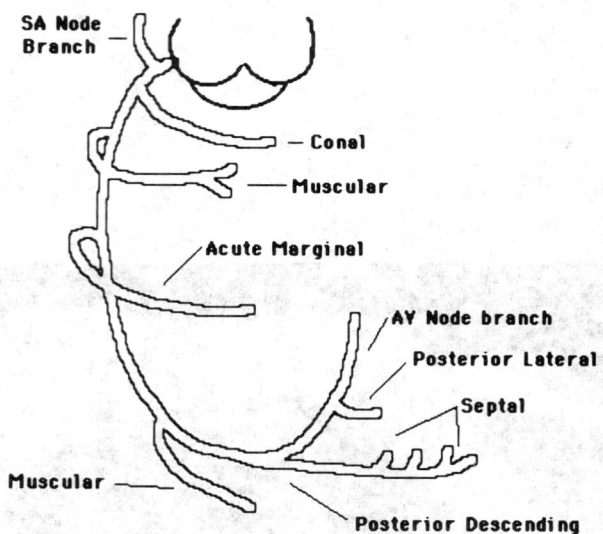

**Figure 82-32.**    Normal right coronary artery system.

but subjects with poor collateral circulation have myocardial infarction, which is apparent at an early age.

In the immediate newborn period, pulmonary artery resistance and pressure are increased, flow through the anomalously arising left coronary artery is antegrade from the pulmonary artery, and myocardial perfusion is adequate. As pulmonary artery resistance and pulmonary pressure decrease, antegrade flow of blood from the pulmonary artery through the left coronary artery decreases. If there is inadequate collateral circulation between the right and left coronary arteries, myocardial infarction probably occurs at this time. If collateral circulation exists, myocardial infarction may occur, depending on the degree of retrograde flow from the right coronary system through the collateral circulation (bypassing the distribution of the left coronary artery) and into the pulmonary artery (ie, coronary steal phenomenon) and on the degree of antegrade flow along the distribution of the left coronary artery (ie, myocardial perfusion).

Clinical features of ALCA in infancy are similar to those of myocarditis and cardiomyopathy, and the diagnosis of ALCA must be considered in the differential diagnosis of unexplained congestive heart failure in infancy. In teenagers and adults, the presence of ALCA may be suspected if there is unexplained cardiomegaly, mitral insufficiency, or continuous cardiac murmur. Angina may occur secondary to a coronary steal phenomenon.

The ideal treatment of ALCA is to detect the presence of the anomaly before myocardial infarction occurs and to establish a coronary system that prevents myocardial infarction. All cases in infancy, however, come to medical attention only after myocardial ischemia and infarction have occurred. Infants with ALCA and poor left ventricular function (ejection fraction less than 20%) do poorly regardless of surgical or medical management at a young age. Infants with ALCA and good left ventricular function do well whether there was an early operation (age less than 1 year) or an operation done after age 1 year. Infants who do poorly occasionally have spontaneous improvement.

Attempts to establish a two-coronary-artery system for patients with ALCA seem warranted. It is unclear which procedure is superior, and the surgeon probably should use the technique with which he or she is most comfortable. For children older than 1 year, adolescents, and adults, it is reasonable to perform an operation to establish a two-coronary-artery system when ALCA is discovered. In infants (age less than 1 year) with ALCA and good left ventricular function (ejection fraction more than 20%) and who are doing well, there are equally persuasive arguments to proceed with an operation or to defer an operation until 12 to 24 months of age. The better option is unclear. For infants with poor left ventricular function (ejection fraction less than 20%), it seems reasonable to intervene surgically because the natural history of the disorder in these children (ie, with poor ventricular function) is poor. As surgical techniques improve and improvement in survival rates of infants who are doing poorly (age less than 1 year; ejection fraction less than 20%) is demonstrated, operating on all infants with ALCA, even on those doing well, may be best.

Patients with ALCA and evidence of congestive heart failure benefit from treatment with digitalis and diuretics. Infants with evidence of acute myocardial infarction should be treated with oxygen, sedation, rest, digitalis, and diuretics.

## Anomalous Origin of the Left Coronary Artery From the Right Sinus of Valsalva

Anomalous origin of the left coronary artery from the right sinus of Valsalva or from the proximal right coronary artery is a rare but important malformation because it is associated with sudden death (Fig 82-33). Patients in whom the aberrantly arising left coronary artery passes between the aorta and the pulmonary artery appear to be at the greatest risk for sudden death. Sudden death presumably is due to myocardial ischemia as a result of compression of the left coronary artery between the aorta and the pulmonary artery and compromise of the lumen of the left coronary artery due to acute angulation near its origin. Patients usually are asymptomatic until sudden death occurs, although some patients may have symptoms of angina or coronary insufficiency. Symptoms may include syncope or light-headedness associated with exercise. This diagnosis must be considered in children and adolescents with angina-like chest pain, syncope, or presyncope. If this condition is suspected, exercise testing may reveal electrocardiographic evidence of ischemia, but a normal result of an exercise study does not exclude the diagnosis. Coronary angiography usually is necessary to establish or exclude the diagnosis. When the left coronary artery passes between the aorta and the pulmonary artery, operative repair is indicated to prevent sudden death.

## Congenital Coronary Ostial Web

A rare but important cause of coronary insufficiency is the presence of a membrane covering the orifice of a coronary artery. Usually, it involves the left coronary ostia and is associated with a dysplastic aortic valve. This diagnosis must be considered in the differential diagnosis of angina pectoris.

## Anomalous Origin of the Right Coronary Artery From the Left Sinus of Valsalva

Anomalous origin of the right coronary artery from the left sinus of Valsalva is detected less often than anomalous origin of the left coronary artery from the right sinus of Valsalva. Except for anecdotal cases, this anomaly is not associated with symptoms of myocardial ischemia or sudden death. Operative repair of this anomaly is indicated if signs and symptoms of myocardial ischemia are present and there are no other apparent causes of the myocardial ischemia.

## Single Coronary Artery

Single coronary artery occurs in approximately 2 of every 1000 patients. It is associated with transposition of the great arteries, coronary artery fistula, and bicuspid aortic valve.

The clinical significance of a single coronary artery is unclear. Patients in whom the single coronary artery arises from the right coronary sinus, with a connecting branch that travels between the aorta and the pulmonary artery, then distributes in the location of a normal left coronary artery, may be at risk for sudden death due to acute angulation of the connecting branch. This is similar to the situation in which the left coronary artery originates from the right sinus of Valsalva.

## CORONARY ARTERY FISTULA

Coronary artery fistula constitutes 0.2% to 0.4% of congenital cardiac defects. Fistulae originate equally from the right and left coronary artery systems. Usually, the fistula connects to the right ventricular cavity. The right atrium is the second most common terminus, and two thirds of fistulae draining into the right atrium originate from the right coronary artery. A fistula also can terminate in the pulmonary artery, left atrium, left ventricle, superior vena cava, coronary sinus, or a persistent left superior vena cava. The involved coronary artery usually is dilated, and the chamber in which the fistula terminates may be enlarged. In childhood and adolescence, the fistula usually does not produce symptoms, but signs and symptoms of congestive heart failure can occur secondary to a large left-to-right shunt. The presence of a fistula usually is detected by the finding of a continuous precordial murmur. There may be a precordial thrill, decreased diastolic blood pressure, and widened pulse pressure. Physical findings may be confused with those of patent ductus arteriosus, but usually the murmur of a patent ductus arteriosus is heard best in the left infraclavicular area and that of a coronary artery fistula at the

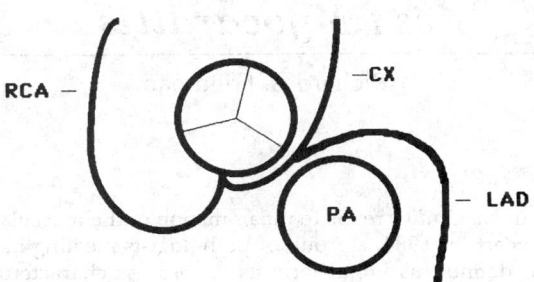

**Figure 82-33.** Origin of left coronary artery from the right aortic sinus of Valsalva. When the left coronary artery passes between the aorta and the pulmonary artery, there is risk of sudden death. *PA,* pulmonary artery; *CX,* circumflex coronary artery; *LAD,* left anterior descending coronary artery; *RCA,* right coronary artery.

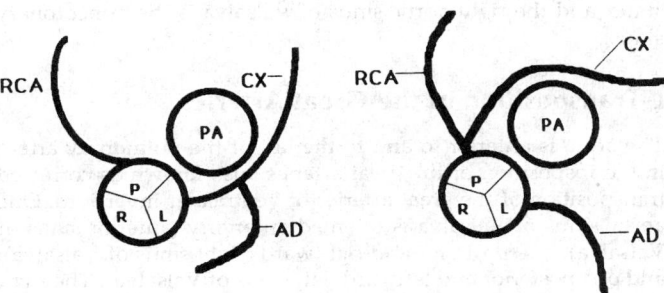

**Figure 82-34.** Coronary artery patterns in D-transposition of great arteries. (**A**) Pattern often found when the great arteries are obliquely related. (**B**) Pattern on right is more common when the great arteries are side by side. *AD,* anterior coronary artery; *P, R, L,* posterior, right, and left aortic cusps; *CX,* circumflex coronary artery; *RCA,* right coronary artery; *PA,* pulmonary artery.

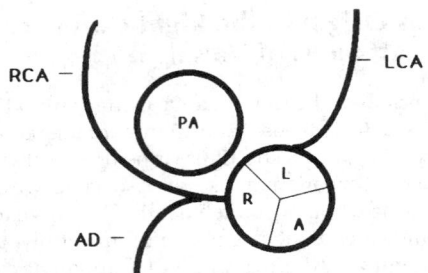

**Figure 82-35.** Coronary artery pattern of L-transposition of the great arteries (or ventricular inversion or corrected transposition). *A,* anterior aortic cusp; *R* and *L,* right and left aortic cusps; *LCA,* left coronary artery; *RCA,* right coronary artery; *AD,* anterior coronary artery; *PA,* pulmonary artery.

midleft sternal border. The presence of a coronary artery fistula is the indication for surgical obliteration of the fistula.

## CORONARY ARTERY PATTERNS ASSOCIATED WITH CONGENITAL HEART DEFECTS

### Tetralogy of Fallot

Although only 4% to 5% of patients with tetralogy of Fallot have associated coronary artery anomalies, these abnormalities should be recognized so damage to essential coronary arteries is avoided during operative repair of tetralogy of Fallot. Origin of the left anterior descending coronary artery from the right coronary artery occurs in 4% of patients with tetralogy of Fallot. Single coronary artery is the second most common coronary anomaly associated with tetralogy of Fallot. Forty percent of cases of tetralogy of Fallot have a long and large right conus artery that distributes to a significant mass of myocardium.

### Transposition of the Great Arteries

There are two major coronary artery patterns in D-transposition of the great arteries (also known as complete or simple transposition of the great arteries). Usually, the right coronary artery arises from the posterior aortic sinus, and the left coronary artery arises from the left coronary sinus and divides into a circumflex and an anterior descending coronary artery (Fig 82-34). The right aortic sinus of Valsalva is the noncoronary cusp. In the second coronary artery pattern, the right coronary artery arises from the posterior aortic sinus and gives rise to the circumflex coronary artery, which passes posterior to the pulmonary artery. The anterior descending coronary artery arises from the left coronary sinus, and the right aortic sinus of Valsalva is the noncoronary sinus.

### L-Transposition of the Great Arteries

The aorta is anterior to and to the left of the pulmonary artery in L-transposition of the great arteries (also known as corrected transposition of the great arteries or ventricular inversion). One aortic sinus of Valsalva is oriented anteriorly (anterior sinus of Valsalva), one posterior and rightward (right sinus of Valsalva), and one posterior and leftward (left sinus of Valsalva). The right coronary artery originates from the right aortic sinus of Valsalva and divides into an anterior descending branch that follows the course of the interventricular sulcus (Fig 82-35). The right coronary artery continues to follow a course in the right atrioventricular sulcus. The left coronary artery originates in the left aortic sinus of Valsalva and follows the course of the circumflex cor-

onary artery in the left atrioventricular sulcus. The left (circumflex) coronary artery produces a marginal branch and continues as the posterior descending coronary artery.

## Selected Readings

Baltaxe H, Amplatz K, Levin D. Coronary angiography. Springfield, Ill: Charles C Thomas, 1975.

Baltaxe H, Wixson D. The incidence of congenital anomalies of the coronary arteries in the adult population. Radiology 1977;122:47.

Bunton R, Jonas R, Lang P, Rein A, Castaneda A. Anomalous origin of left coronary artery from pulmonary artery. Ligation versus establishment of a two coronary artery system. J Thorac Cardiovasc Surg 1987;93:103.

Cheitlin M, DeCastro C, McAllister H. Sudden death as a complication of anomalous left coronary origin from the anterior sinus of Valsalva, a not-so-minor congenital anomaly. Circulation 1974;50:780.

Driscoll D, Nihill M, Mullins C, et al. Management of symptomatic infants with anomalous origin of the left coronary artery from the pulmonary artery. Am J Cardiol 1981;47:642.

Elliott L, Amplatz K, Edwards J. Coronary arterial patterns in transposition complexes. Am J Cardiol 1966;17:362.

Fellows K, Freed M, Keane J, et al. Results of routine preoperative coronary angiography in tetralogy of Fallot. Circulation 1975;51:561.

Hurwitz R, Caldwell R, Girod D, Brown J, King H. Clinical and hemodynamic course of infants and children with anomalous left coronary artery. Am Heart J 1989;118:1176.

Neufeld H, Schneeweiss A. Coronary artery disease in infants and children. Philadelphia: Lea and Febiger, 1983.

Roberts W. Major anomalies of coronary arterial origin seen in adulthood. Am J Cardiol 1986;111:941.

Vlodaver Z, Neufeld H, Edwards J. Coronary arterial variations in the normal heart and in congenital heart disease. New York: Academic Press, 1975.

Vouhe P, Ballot-Vernant F, Tringuet F, et al. Anomalous left coronary artery from the pulmonary artery in infants. J Thorac Cardiovasc Surg 1987;94:192.

*Principles and Practice of Pediatrics, Second Edition.*
edited by Frank A. Oski et al. J. B. Lippincott Company, Philadelphia © 1994.

## CHAPTER 83
# *Diseases of the Myocardium*

## *83.1 Myocarditis*

### Richard A. Friedman

The term *myocarditis* refers to inflammation of the muscular walls of the heart. In 1984, a group of pathologists meeting in Dallas tried to define this broad term as "a process characterized by inflammatory infiltrate of the myocardium with necrosis and/or degeneration of adjacent myocytes not typical of the ischemic damage associated with coronary artery disease." This section deals with proven and presumed infectious causes of myocarditis and describes the clinical presentation and etiology when known.

In general, this disease may go unrecognized in many patients whose illness resolves spontaneously, or it may lead to fulminant disease with a rapid downhill course or to a chronic state, possibly resulting in dilated congestive cardiomyopathy.

Myocarditis may be secondary to many of the common infectious illnesses that affect children and infants (Table 83-1), or may occur as a manifestation of hypersensitivity or as a toxic reaction to drug administration.

Myocarditis is a relatively uncommon finding in children. It was found in only 0.3% of 14,322 patients seen in the cardiology service at Texas Children's Hospital between 1954 and 1977, findings similar to those for a group at the Toronto Children's Hospital between 1951 and 1964. Not all cases of myocarditis are recognized by the clinician, however, and a much higher incidence is noted in autopsy series. During the same two decades at Texas Children's Hospital, an autopsy incidence of 1.15% was found. This is in contrast to the report by Saphir and colleagues who noted an incidence of 6.83% among 1420 autopsies on children. In that series, nearly one third of the cases were felt to have had rheumatic carditis.

One study of 138 cases attempted to estimate the evidence of myocarditis in children who died suddenly and children who died unexpectedly (violently). The control group consisted of 48 children who died a violent death with no history suggestive of myocarditis; the other 90 children died suddenly. The study found that 17 cases (12.3%) revealed evidence of active or healing myocarditis, and that 15 of these cases occurred in children who died suddenly. In contrast, only 4.2% of children dying a violent death had histologic evidence suggestive of myocarditis. Because this was a retrospective study, viral cultures and serologic studies were not routinely obtained at the time of autopsy. Another series found evidence of interstitial myocarditis in 29 of 50 infants and young children who had undergone routine postmortem examination. Several recent investigations found that a significant number of patients undergoing endomyocardial biopsy for unexplained myocardial dysfunction had histologic findings suggestive of myocarditis. Likewise, patients being investigated for occult ventricular arrhythmias for which no etiology could be proved were also found to have evidence of interstitial lymphocytic infiltrates suggestive of myocarditis. A potential for overdiagnosis of myocarditis exists, and one investigator notes that about 5% of "normal" hearts may be found to have minor foci of inflammatory cells. The investigator determined that a normal finding was 25 to 30 interstitial lymphocytes per square millimeter. In that study, the number of lymphocytes per square millimeter in endomyocardial biopsy specimens was lower than that found in autopsy specimens (3.5 versus 7.2 cells/mm$^2$).

In a significant number of cases of myocarditis, manifestations may be subclinical and recognized either through other findings (eg, electrocardiogram changes) or, perhaps, not at all. Myocarditis also may be only one component of a generalized disease and, if the cardiac dysfunction is mild, may be completely overlooked. This could explain the discrepancy between the clinical and the autopsy series.

## EPIDEMIOLOGY

Myocarditis generally is a sporadic disease, although epidemics have been reported. Coxsackievirus B is the most frequently reported cause of epidemics in children. This organism was found to be associated with myocarditis during a nursery epidemic in southern Rhodesia. Reports from Rhodesia, Holland, the United States, Singapore, and South Africa have followed. Infections secondary to coxsackieviruses are common throughout the general population. Target organs include the upper respiratory tract, gastrointestinal tract, liver (hepatitis), lung (pneumonia), central nervous system (meningoencephalitis), lymph nodes (infectious mononucleosis-like syndrome), kidney (hemolytic uremic syndrome), and heart (carditis). Significant titers of type-specific protective antibodies are present in most adults in the United States. After birth, spread occurs by the fecal–oral or airborne route. The coxsackievirus B organisms use receptors that are not shared with other enteroviruses to attach to their target cells. These receptors are felt to be an element essential for viral replication and may help determine tissue tropism. Infections due

TABLE 83-1. Etiologic Agents of Myocarditis

| Viral | Bacterial | Fungi and Yeasts | Hypersensitivity/Autoimmune |
|---|---|---|---|
| Coxsackievirus A | Meningococcus | Actinomycosis | Rheumatoid arthritis |
| Coxsackievirus B | *Klebsiella* | Coccidiomycosis | Rheumatic fever |
| Echoviruses | *Leptospira* | Histoplasmosis | Ulcerative colitis |
| Rubella virus | Diphtheria | *Candida* | Systemic lupus erythematosus |
| Measles virus | Salmonella | **Toxic** | **Other** |
| Adenoviruses | Clostridia | Scorpion (diphtheria) | Sarcoidosis |
| Polio viruses | Tuberculosis | **Drugs** | Scleroderma |
| Vaccinia virus | Brucella | Sulfonamides | Idiopathic |
| Mumps virus | *Legionella pneumophilia* | Phenylbutazone | Cornstarch |
| Herpes simplex virus | Streptococcus | Cyclophosphamide | |
| Epstein-Barr virus | **Protozoal** | Neomercazole | |
| Cytomegalovirus | *Trypanosoma cruzi* | Acetazolamide | |
| Rhinoviruses | Toxoplasmosis | Amphotericin B | |
| Hepatitis viruses | Amebiasis | Indomethacin | |
| Arboviruses | **Other parasites** | Tetracycline | |
| Influenza viruses | *Toxocara canis* | Isoniazid | |
| Varicella virus | Shistosomiasis | Methyldopa | |
| **Rickettsial** | Heterophyiasis | Phenytoin | |
| *Rickettsia rickesii* | Cysticercosis | Penicillin | |
| *Rickettsia tsutsugamushi* | *Echinococcus* | | |
| | Visceral larva migrans | | |

to coxsackievirus B or enteroviruses are subclinical in 50% of cases. During an outbreak of coxsackievirus B in Europe in 1965, cardiac manifestations were noted in 5% of patients. A much higher percentage (12%) of patients in similar outbreaks of the disease that same year in Scotland, Finland, and Austria developed some evidence of myocardial dysfunction. While myocarditis is associated with coxsackievirus B serotypes 1 to 6, the most serious disease is attributed to types 3 and 4. Coxsackievirus B antigens have been demonstrated with the use of an immunofluorescent technique in 41% of 29 infants and children who were found at routine autopsy to have had interstitial myocarditis. Another study found 1299 cases of unexpected death in an autopsy series of 2427 patients; 20 cases of viral myocarditis were identified. Of the 20, nearly half had positive serologic evidence for coxsackievirus B infection. One investigator found a 9% incidence of myocarditis in 67 verified cases of influenza infection during a 1978 epidemic in Sweden. Although much less common, coxsackievirus A and echoviruses are also suspected etiologies.

Rubella virus, a teratogen during the first trimester of pregnancy, is also implicated in myocarditis. Persistence of the virus in the fetus has been shown to produce severe cases of myocarditis. One study found 10 of 47 infants with congenital rubella to have evidence of myocarditis. Seven of these infants had active disease, and four died with severe myocardial failure. Morbidity secondary to chronic cardiac dysfunction was felt to be severe in the survivors. A significant reduction in the number of cases of congenital rubella has occurred because of aggressive immunization programs, and only 28 cases were recorded in 1975.

Herpes simplex virus results in infections of newborns at a rate of 1 in 7500 deliveries. Type 2 virus is the most common and is usually acquired from the genital tract. Herpes virus has been found in the myocardium of autopsy specimens, documenting its association with myocarditis.

During a 1-year period, investigators found a 5.8% incidence of myocarditis in 312 cases of varicella. In that study, patients who complained of skeletal myalgia seemed to have a significantly higher risk of developing cardiac involvement.

Improved diagnostic testing may change the epidemiologic picture of myocarditis over the next decade and may specify the agent responsible for the infection. The most promising technique is that of gene amplification using the polymerase chain reaction (PCR) in tissue that has been obtained via endomyocardial biopsy (see Diagnosis). Not only will this allow determination of the etiologic agent, but also will enable development of specific antiviral therapies.

## PATHOLOGY

### Immunology

Microscopic and immunologic changes seen in humans with viral myocarditis have been described well. To examine the immunopathogenesis of this disease, however, it has been necessary to use animal models, of which, the most thoroughly studied is the murine. Studies using coxsackievirus B and encephalomyocarditis viruses have been used extensively.

After infection with coxsackievirus B, a viremia exists for between 24 and 72 hours, with maximum growth in the tissues at between 72 and 96 hours. Shortly thereafter, virus titers decline, and essentially no organism can be found as early as 7 to 10 days after inoculation. As virus titers decline, antibody concentrations increase, implying an active role by antibodies in viral clearance. Macrophages appear at between 5 and 10 days after infection in the coxsackievirus B model of myocarditis.

Factors that affect severity of myocarditis in the murine model include age, strain of mouse, viral variant, and gender. Several

mechanisms are active in the production of myocarditis in this model. Viruses are associated directly with myofiber destruction. The greatest damage, however, is probably due to an interaction between the myofiber and T cells. Virally induced changes of the myocardial cell produce a neoantigen that is recognized by cytotoxic T lymphocytes that preferentially destroy the myocardial cell. In addition, coxsackievirus may induce cytotoxic T lymphocytes that are autoreactive against antigens on infected myocytes. Mice that are pretreated with antithymocyte serum, thus lacking a normal immunologic response, develop a less extensive myocardial necrosis compared to animals similarly infected and treated with normal rabbit serum. Animals deficient in T cells clear their viremia normally but develop significantly less myocardial injury. The implication is that T cells are not required in elimination of virus, but play a delayed role in the major inflammatory response. Mice that are pretreated with neutralizing antibody fail to develop myocarditis; thus, it appears that a combination of macrophages and antibody suppresses viral infection.

Another type of cell known as the natural killer (NK) cell is important in the pathogenesis of this disease. Animals depleted of NK cells before infection with coxsackievirus develop a more severe myocarditis. Murine skin fibroblasts demonstrate the antiviral activity of activated NK cells. NK cells are activated by interferon, which is an indirect modulator of myocardial injury. When murine skin fibroblasts served as target cells for coxsackievirus B-sensitized cytotoxic T cells, the NK cells limited the nonenveloped virus infection specifically by killing the virally infected cells. This has important implications in host immunity and may help explain why female mice develop a less severe myocarditis than do their male counterparts. Male mice are less efficient in activating NK cells. Presumably, the more efficient viral clearance is, the less opportunity exists for virally induced neoantigen production and recognition by cytotoxic T lymphocytes.

Different ways that T cells effect injury include accumulation of activated macrophages, production of antibody and antibody-dependent cell-mediated cytotoxicity, direct lysis by antibody and complement, and direct action of cytotoxic T cells. The primary importance of cytotoxic T cells in direct myocardial-cell injury was demonstrated in BALB/c mice infected with coxsackievirus B3. Both virus-infected and noninfected myocytes are destroyed in T-cell-deficient animals. Infected host cells stimulate the production of a subset of cytotoxic T cells responsible for injury. These cells then recognize virus-specific and major histocompatibility antigens (modified H2 antigens) present on the cell surface and directly interact, resulting in myocytolysis.

This ongoing injury is considered an autoimmune-type process. To support this concept, investigators studied the CD1 mouse infected with coxsackievirus B3 and demonstrated a KC1-extractable antigen in the hearts of mice previously infected with this virus that was specifically immunoreactive with immune mouse peritoneal-exudate cells (ie, stimulated production of a migration-inhibitory factor). Investigators were unable to demonstrate viral activity in animals that had this extractable antigen. In addition, antigen responsible for cytotoxic T-cell activity cannot be detected by using antiserum-containing antibodies directed at the structural components of the viral capsid. The ineffectiveness of antiviral serum in preventing myocarditis also has been demonstrated.

Susceptibility variation of the BALB/c mouse to coxsackievirus B3 also has been studied. The age of greatest susceptibility was found to be between 16 and 18 weeks, with males having a maximal rate of myocarditis greater than that seen in females. Enhanced myocardial inflammation was seen in older females and was eliminated when they were treated with estradiol. This implies that sex hormones play a key role in host susceptibility. Studies both in vitro and in vivo have shown that testosterone seems to increase the cytolytic activity in males more than in females. Either a preferential stimulation of T-helper cells or an inadequate stimulation of T-cytolytic/suppressor cells could explain why antibody responses to various antigens frequently are enhanced and cellular immune responses depressed in females. Host genetic composition not only affects the severity of disease, but also plays a role in the pathogenic mechanisms involved. With use of coxsackievirus B3 to induce myocarditis in the BALB/c mouse and the DBA/2 mouse, important differences have been found. The BALB/c mouse develops myocarditis in response to cytolytic T cells. Two distinct cytolytic T-cell populations are formed: one recognizing virus-infected cells and producing direct myocytolysis and one that destroys uninfected myocytes and probably is an autoreactive lymphocyte. Complement depletion increases the amount of inflammation in this species, and no reactive immunoglobulin-G antibody is found in the myocytes. In the DBA/2 mouse, however, T-helper cells mediate the course of disease indirectly, and complement depletion reduces inflammation. Cytolytic T cells are produced but apparently are not pathogenic, and immunoglobulin-G antibody is found in the myocytes.

Several other viral agents have been used to produce experimental myocarditis. Induction of myocarditis using influenza A virus (H2N2) in mice has been studied. In one study, mice that were pretreated with radiation or depleted of T lymphocytes did not develop disease. Encephalomyocarditis virus has been used to develop models of acute and chronic myocarditis in mice. This virus is a picornavirus that is similar to the coxsackievirus group. Studies demonstrate a progression from acute myocarditis to dilated cardiomyopathy similar to that seen in humans.

Several studies have been done also in humans. Antibody-mediated cytolysis has been demonstrated in 30% of 144 patients with suspected myocarditis, as well as in 18 of 19 patients with proven viral infections due to coxsackievirus B, influenza A, or mumps. A muscle-specific antimyolemmal antibody (AMLA) was found in these patients and correlated with the degree of in vitro induced cytolysis of rat cardiocytes. Another study used complementary DNA (to coxsackievirus B2 RNA) cloning techniques to develop a coxsackievirus B-specific cDNA "hybridization probe" that detected virus nucleic acid sequences in patients diagnosed as having active or healed myocarditis or dilated cardiomyopathy. Patients with unrelated disorders served as the control group, and no virus-specific sequences were found in those patients. This suggests that, in patients with congestive cardiomyopathy or healing myocarditis, viral particles persist although viral cultures are almost always negative. Thus, a continual viral replication in cells may conceal the antigenicity by an immunologic process that prevents correct post-translational processing of capsid proteins. Adult patients with myocarditis have been found to have been exposed to a greater number of coxsackievirus B1 to B6 organisms, as demonstrated by the number of positive and negative responses to neutralizing antibodies of those viruses. Some authors suggest that immunization against several types of coxsackie B virus is essential in the development of myocarditis. Although they have postulated this "cross-immunization" theory, a few cases of myocarditis in their patients involved exposure to only one type of coxsackievirus B, thus casting some doubt on the validity of this theory.

In summary, the pathogenesis of this disease can be viewed as follows: infection of the mouse with coxsackievirus B3 induces a viremia and replication within the myocardial cells of this virus. Direct viral myocytolysis ensues, with production in other cells of neoantigen in response to viral infection. Cytotoxic T cells directed at both infected and noninfected (autoimmune) cells produce further injury. NK cells attack the virally infected cells only and are responsible for viral clearance. Antibody binding and complement-mediated cell destruction also occur in the de-layed immunologic response. Host factors including age, sex, and immunocompetence play key roles in modulating these processes (Fig 83-1).

## Gross and Microscopic Findings

The pathologic findings are usually nonspecific, with similar gross and microscopic changes noted regardless of the causative agent. Grossly, the weight of the heart is increased. The muscle appears flabby and pale with petechial hemorrhages often seen on the epicardial surfaces. A bloody pericardial effusion, related to the often combined finding of pericarditis, also may be seen. The ventricular wall is frequently thin, although hypertrophy may be found as well. The valves and endocardium usually are spared, although in cases of chronic myocarditis, they may appear glistening white. This suggests to some investigators that the disease process known as endocardial fibroelastosis, which may present with similar clinical findings, could represent an end result of viral myocarditis, possibly induced in utero.

Coxsackievirus B3 has been found in the myocardium of 13 of 28 infants with endocardial fibroelastosis, and echovirus 9 has been found in a 5-month-old infant with myocarditis and severe congestive heart failure who also had histologic findings consistent with endocardial fibroelastosis. Virus was isolated not only in the heart and lungs but also in the liver and lymph nodes.

Mural thrombi have been described in the left ventricles of some patients with myocarditis. Small emboli have been seen in the coronary and cerebral vessels. Coronary emboli, although rare, may produce areas of ischemia or injury, with resultant production of the cardiac arrhythmias that sometimes occur during the acute disease.

The typical microscopic picture of acute myocarditis is that of a focal or diffuse interstitial collection of mononuclear cells, including lymphocytes, plasma cells, and eosinophils. Polymorphonuclear types are noted rarely, except in cases of bacterial myocarditis.

Extensive necrosis of the myocardium, with loss of cross-striation in the muscle fibers and edema, is seen in severe infections. Perivascular accumulation of lymphocytes and plasma cells is described with coxsackievirus B myocarditis, but is usually a minor finding. In disease due to *Rickettsia*, varicella, trypanosomes, or other parasites and in reactions to sulfonamides, this is a much more prominent finding.

Myocarditis secondary to diphtheria infection frequently is complicated with arrhythmias, especially complete atrioventricular block. Diphtheria exotoxin has a particular affinity for the specialized conduction tissue in the heart. The toxin interferes with protein synthesis by inhibition of a translocating enzyme in the delivery of amino acids. Triglyceride accumulation occurs as a result of induction of abnormal carnitine metabolism, and fatty changes in the myofibers occur.

Myocarditis due to bacterial agents usually presents with a different picture than that seen in disease due to viral agents. Microabscesses and patchy focal suppurative changes may be seen.

*Trichinella* sp usually causes a focal infiltrate with lymphocytes and eosinophils. Larvae usually are not identified.

A severe myocarditis may develop in response to *Trypanosoma cruzi* with the development of Chagas' disease. This disease, most commonly found in South America, is uncommon in North America and can affect as much as 50% of the population in an endemic region. Protracted heart failure and death may ensue after acute infection. Microscopic examination may demonstrate the presence of the organism as well as neutrophils, lymphocytes, macrophages, and eosinophils.

Sudden infant death syndrome occurs in as many as 1 in 500 children and could be due to cardiac arrhythmias that may result

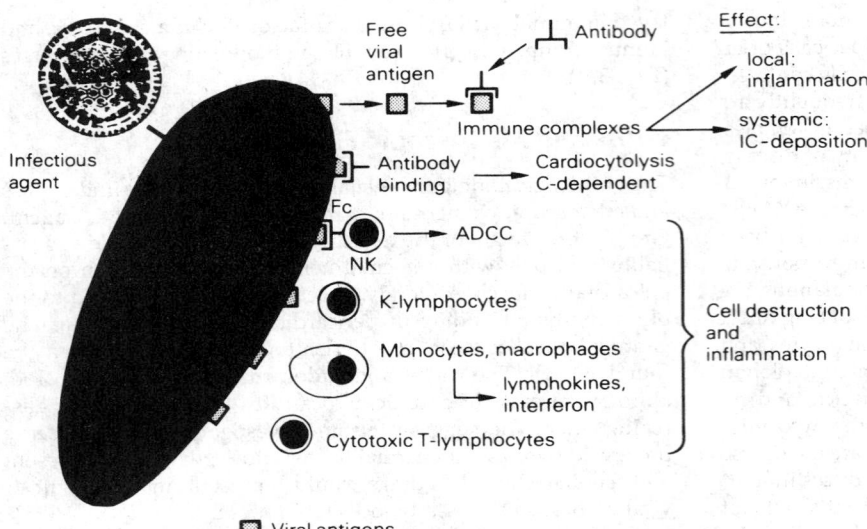

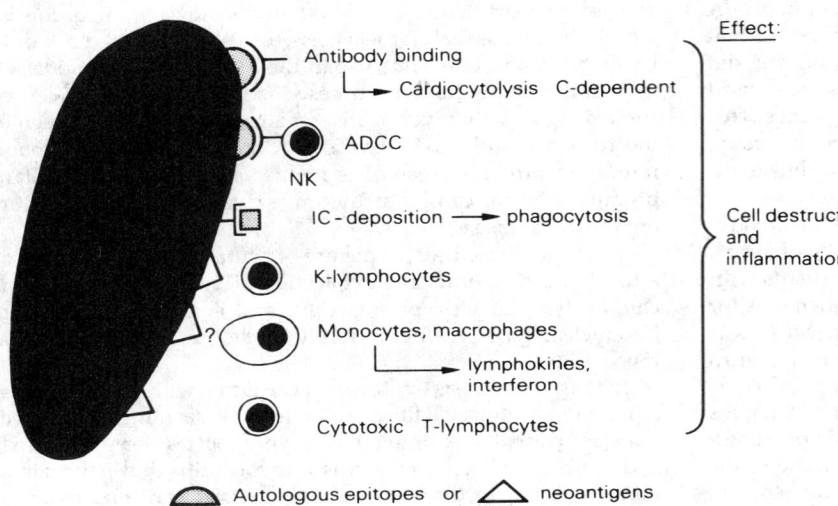

**Figure 83-1.** (*Top*) Early immunopathogenesis. The cell cycle is altered by viral infection. Viral proteins are then expressed on the surface of the cell and become targets of various immunologic effectors. These include the monocytes and macrophages, which release mediators; cytotoxic T lymphocytes and K cells, which lyse the myocardial cell; and NK cells, which together with antibodies also effect cell lysis. Complement-activated antibody-mediated cell destruction also occurs with the production of antiviral antibodies. Formation of immune complexes may occur when circulating viral antigen is coupled with viral antibodies, resulting in local or systemic reactions. (*Bottom*) Delayed immunopathogenesis. In addition to the mechanisms described in early immunopathogenesis, modulation of the inflammatory response by T cells (helper and suppressor types) against autologous heart cells occurs. Complement-activated, antibody-mediated cell destruction is more important than antibody-dependent cellular cytotoxicity (ADCC) in this phase of the injury process. The presence of viral antigens during this phase is negligible compared to that in the early phase of injury. (Maisch B, et al. Immunological cellular regulator and effector mechanisms in myocarditis. Herz 1985;10:11.)

from myocardial inflammation. One study of cases of infants who died in northern Ireland described a resorptive, degenerative process in the His bundle and at the left margin of the atrioventricular node with the absence of inflammatory cells. The investigator postulated that lethal arrhythmias or conduction disturbances could be due to developmental histologic changes in these critical regions of the heart. Lymphocytic infiltrates were demonstrated in the region of the His bundle and left fascicle in a 3-month-old child who died suddenly. No degenerative changes were seen in this heart; thus, the significance of these findings is speculative.

Giant-cell myocarditis is diagnosed when giant cells are found, with or without granulomas. Patients with tuberculosis, syphilis, rheumatoid arthritis, rheumatic heart disease, sarcoidosis, and certain fungal or parasitic infections may all have granulomas found within the myocardium. Giant cells also have been described in idiopathic or Feidler's myocarditis. There are many cases, however, in which giant cells are found but no specific etiology is discovered. There appear to be two types of giant cells, one of which is myogenic in origin and thought to represent transitional forms of myocardial cells. Granulomas usually are not found with this type. The more characteristic type of giant cell probably is derived from interstitial histocytes and usually is found in patients with myocarditis not due to viral agents. Similar cells have been noted in patients who received neomercazole therapy, and there is a report of granulomatous myocarditis associated with ingestion of phenylbutazone.

## Pathophysiology

Myocardial function usually is reduced in the presence of extensive interstitial inflammation or injury. This results in cardiac enlargement and an increase in the end-diastolic volume. Normally, this increase in volume results in an increase in force of contraction, ejection fraction, and cardiac output, as described in the Starling mechanism. In the disease state, however, reduced cardiac output results from the inability of the heart muscle to respond to these stimuli. Congestive heart failure usually ensues with progression of the disease or with intercurrent infections resulting in fever or anemia that further stress the myocardial reserve. Progressive increase in end-diastolic volume and pressure results in increasing left atrial pressure that is transmitted into the pulmonary venous system. The resulting hydrostatic forces overcome the colloid osmotic pressure, which normally prevents transudation of fluid across the capillary membranes. Congestive heart failure with pulmonary edema and systemic venous engorgement is common in more acute forms of myocarditis. Echocardiographic examination may demonstrate severe left ventricular dilatation, and a decreased ejection fraction usually is found. Evaluation of ventricular function using M-mode echocardiography helps establish a baseline at the time of presentation as well as monitor function during therapeutic interventions.

During the healing stages of myocarditis, normal myofibers are replaced with fibroblasts, with resultant scar tissue formation. Reduced elasticity and ventricular performance can result in continuing congestive heart failure. Ischemia may be exacerbated by attempts to preserve cardiac output, with sinus tachycardia further worsening the supply–demand ratio for oxygen in the heart muscle.

## CLINICAL PRESENTATION

The clinical presentation of myocarditis varies in response to host factors, including age and immunocompetence. While the majority of cases probably are unnoticed with no apparent clinical illness, a rapidly fatal illness may occur. Newborn infants are susceptible to infection with coxsackievirus B, which may result in the severe form of myocarditis. Infections with rubella, herpes simplex, and toxoplasmosis also may result in a severe form of illness in infants.

Myocarditis may be merely one component of a more severe generalized illness, with coexisting hepatitis or encephalitis. Myocardial involvement may be only a mild clinical disturbance in these cases. One study found a nursery epidemic of coxsackievirus B5 infection in preterm infants during a virologic survey in one institution. The disease was unnoticed clinically and discovered by chance during this survey. No instance of severe myocarditis was seen, and all infants recovered fully from infection. The major symptoms were lethargy, failure to gain weight, and aseptic meningitis. In a review of 25 infants with myocarditis due to coxsackievirus B, other symptoms of lethargy and anorexia heralded the onset of severe disease. Fever was recorded in more than 50% of the cases, although hypothermia was also noted. Cyanosis, respiratory distress or tachycardia, cardiomegaly, or electrocardiogram changes were present in 19 of 23 infants; vomiting was noted in 4. Initial symptoms in infants include irritability and periodic episodes of pallor, which may precede sudden onset of cardiorespiratory symptoms.

Clinical manifestations of myocarditis generally are less severe in older infants and children than in newborns. Rapidly fatal illness has been reported in association with myocarditis of unknown etiology, enteroviruses, adenoviruses, mumps, varicella, cytomegalovirus, and diphtheria. The usual clinical picture is either an acute or a subacute illness, often beginning with a mild respiratory infection and low-grade fever.

Physical examination usually shows the child to be anxious and apprehensive, although some children appear apathetic and listless. Pallor and mild cyanosis may be present, with the skin cool to the touch and mottled in appearance. Respirations usually are rapid and sometimes labored; grunting may be prominent. The pulse is thready, although blood pressure may be normal or slightly reduced unless the patient is in shock. Palpation of the chest demonstrates a quiet precordium. Tachycardia usually is present. Heart sounds may be muffled, especially in the presence of pericarditis, and a gallop rhythm is heard frequently. With severe ventricular dysfunction, mitral regurgitation with a pansystolic murmur at the apex may be heard. Auscultation of the lungs reveals scattered rhonchi and fine crepitations in the lung

bases. Peripheral edema is rare, but hepatomegaly is found almost uniformly. Some infants may have only mild congestive heart failure without evidence of peripheral circulatory compromise, while others have such a mild illness that the only abnormal finding may be a conduction disturbance visible on surface electrocardiogram.

## Diagnosis

The diagnosis of myocarditis often is difficult to establish but should be suspected in any infant or child who presents with unexplained congestive heart failure. Fever is a common occurrence in children, and the frequency of viral illness may be so high as to invalidate the causal relationship in the history of recent illness in the child who presents with congestive heart failure. If this relationship is found, however, it should be documented for epidemiologic purposes.

A sinus tachycardia out of proportion to the level of fever and in association with a quiet precordium and a gallop rhythm should strongly suggest the diagnosis. A third heart sound, which is a common finding in healthy children, usually is associated with a relatively hyperdynamic precordium with heart sounds that are increased or crisp. When a prominent third heart sound exists without these findings, a significant disturbance in ventricular compliance usually is present and deserves further investigation by chest radiograph, electrocardiogram, and echocardiogram. Children with myocarditis and congestive heart failure usually show cardiomegaly and pulmonary edema on chest radiograph.

In newborn infants whose first sign of illness is acute circulatory collapse, the cardiac size may be normal. This may be true also in children who present with an arrhythmia secondary to myocarditis. Stokes-Adams attacks secondary to complete atrioventricular block also may be a presenting sign in myocarditis in children.

When an arrhythmia occurs after a febrile illness, the clinician should suspect the diagnosis and look for other signs of disease. One study found significant arrhythmias in five infants with isolated myocarditis. Four of the five infants died, and three of them had paroxysmal atrial tachycardia. Paroxysmal atrial tachycardia also has been reported in patients with viral myocarditis. Atrial ectopic-focus tachycardia may mimic sinus tachycardia and should be suspected in a child with persistent sinus tachycardia and congestive heart failure. Careful inspection of the P-wave axis and morphology in a 15-lead electrocardiogram and a 24-hour Holter monitor to observe the variance in rate are essential in establishing the diagnosis. Complete atrioventricular block secondary to idiopathic myocarditis, rubella, coxsackievirus, and respiratory syncytial virus has been described. Some of these patients developed permanent atrioventricular block and required permanent pacing, while the finding was transitory in others.

The electrocardiographic pattern classically described in myocarditis is that of low-voltage QRS complexes (less than 5 mm of total amplitude in all limb leads), with low-amplitude or slightly inverted T waves and a small or absent Q wave in leads $V_5$ and $V_6$. The low voltage also may be present in the precordial leads.

Electrocardiograms of 87 conscripts, 28 of whom had myocarditis, were examined in one study. The most common finding was that of T-wave changes consisting of reduced amplitude or inversion in the left chest leads. Sinus tachycardia was the most common arrhythmia, followed by uniform premature ventricular contractions. Another study described four patterns of electrocardiogram in patients with proven viral myocarditis: normalization even in the presence of severe myocardial damage during the acute stage, "pseudoinfarction" patterns with pathologic-appearing q waves and poor R-wave progression in the precordial leads, conduction disturbances possibly requiring pacemaker support, and chronic arrhythmias consisting of ventricular tachycardia and supraventricular tachycardia.

Animal studies have been performed to investigate the electrophysiologic effects of myocarditis. In one study, coxsackievirus B3 myocarditis was produced in hamsters. ST- or T-wave changes on the surface electrocardiogram were seen in 80% of the animals. Peak changes were seen between days 2 and 4 when mortality was highest. Histologic examination demonstrated that the inner third of the endocardium was primarily involved, suggesting that the subendocardial injury corresponded to the ST- and T-wave changes found on the surface electrocardiogram. In another study, myocarditis was induced in DBA/2 mice with encephalomyocarditis virus. Advanced atrioventricular block, premature atrial contractions, and premature ventricular contractions all were seen acutely. The chronic stage was characterized by sinus tachycardia and low voltage of the QRS complex. In the late chronic stages, QRS voltages returned toward normal, possibly reflective of diminished myocardial edema or compensatory ventricular hypertrophy.

ST-segment and T-wave changes are sensitive indices of myocardial ischemia, but they also appear to be nonspecific findings. This is true prolonged PR segment, which is a common occurrence during fever. One study found a 1.49% prevalence of ST- and T-wave changes and prolonged PR segments in a group of 737 infants and children with respiratory tract infections. PR-segment prolongation and T-wave changes also were demonstrated in infants and children with pneumonia and no signs of myocarditis in another study. Another nonspecific finding, prolonged QT interval, has been noted in acute myocarditis as well as in measles and poliomyelitis without myocardial involvement.

The echocardiogram is essential in establishing the diagnosis. Pericardial effusion, as a cause of cardiomegaly, can be determined using either single-crystal or two-dimensional techniques. Depressed ventricular function with dilatation of one or more chambers in the absence of any structural abnormality helps establish the diagnosis.

Nuclear imaging has been used recently as a screening test to help establish the diagnosis of myocarditis. Screening of patients with dilated cardiomyopathy using gallium 67 may help in selecting a subgroup of patients who could benefit from endomyocardial biopsy. The biopsy sample would be used to confirm the presence of active inflammation and might aid in guiding therapy. In 1 study, 68 patients with a diagnosis of dilated cardiomyopathy underwent 71 parallel studies with gallium 67 scanning and endomyocardial biopsy. A dense gallium uptake was found in 5 of 6 patients whose biopsy samples showed active inflammation. Only 9 of 65 negative biopsy tests had equivocally positive scans. There was a 36% incidence of myocarditis on biopsy tests with positive scans, whereas there was only a 1.8% incidence of myocarditis on the biopsy tests with negative scans. This technique has not been used in children, but may prove to be a relatively safe and effective method of helping select children for biopsy testing.

Acutely ill patients with myocarditis should be stabilized before undergoing cardiac catheterization. Infants may require study to exclude anomalous origin of the left coronary artery, although recent advances in two-dimensional echocardiography have helped to determine origins of the coronary arteries.

Over the past decade, endomyocardial biopsy has become a relatively safe and effective means of sampling heart muscle. The widest application for endomyocardial biopsy is in patients who have undergone cardiac transplantation and who require repeated samples to assess the degree of allograph rejection.

Endomyocardial biopsy helps to establish the diagnosis of myocarditis and possibly to classify the phase of disease (acute,

healed, chronic). Histologic classification is difficult and, at times, controversial. Sampling of small areas precludes accurate diagnosis, especially if the inflammation is focal. In most patients, multiple samples (at least three) should be obtained from the right ventricular septum or apex. Sampling from other areas of the heart (ie, the left ventricle) is felt by some to be more sensitive, but this technique is not applied widely. Sampling error during endomyocardial biopsy has confounded accurate diagnosis of this disease. One study used autopsy specimens from patients who died from myocarditis. These hearts were then subjected to biopsy test using the same bioptome that would have been used in the patient during an actual biopsy procedure. The investigators found only a 63% incidence in these autopsy-proven myocarditis hearts (ie, one third of the cases would have been improperly diagnosed as normal). They concluded that when myocarditis is diagnosed using only the biopsy technique, then only positive findings should be considered diagnostic. A recent study reported the findings of normal myocardium examined with hematoxylin-eosin stain and compared this process to staining with monoclonal antibodies. The findings supported those of previous studies, that fewer than five lymphocytes per high-power field (400X) was normal. No correlation was found between the peripheral lymphocyte count and the lymphocyte count in the myocardium. Specifically, B cells and killer T cells were uncommon, whereas the helper-type T cell (OKT4) predominated over the suppressor/cytotoxic type of T cell (OKT8) in a ratio similar to that found in the peripheral circulation (ie, 1:44).

Immunocytochemical techniques using monoclonal antibodies may be more specific in investigating biopsy samples. A variety of lymphocytes are found within the myocardium. They include the OKT4 (helper/inducer), OKT8 (suppressor/cytotoxic), OKT11 (pan-T cell), $\beta_1$ lymphocyte, NK cell, T200 (pan-leukocyte), and macrophage monocyte cells. Examined in one study were endomyocardial biopsy samples of 80 adult and pediatric patients, 57% of whom had a prebiopsy diagnosis of dilated cardiomyopathy and 29% of whom had a prebiopsy diagnosis of myocarditis. Histologic examination showed that 45% were normal, 3% had active myocarditis, 4% had borderline myocarditis, 6% had dilated cardiomyopathy, and the rest had nonspecific or nondiagnostic findings. Immunocytochemical studies were then performed using the pan-leukocyte marker. Findings in these studies correlated with findings from the hematoxylin-eosin stain and with the sum of the OKT11, $\beta_1$, NK, and macrophage monocyte cells. In 16 patients thought not to have myocarditis (based on findings from examination of tissue stained with hematoxylin and eosin), the immunoperoxidase-positive cells were T lymphocytes of the OKT11 type and monocyte macrophages. In patients with active myocarditis, however, the largest population of cells was that of the OKT8 type, and patients also had an abnormal OKT4/OKT8 ratio. These newer techniques may be used more often to help determine specifically the type of lymphocytic infiltrate present in any case.

As mentioned, a new technique of gene amplification using PCR may aid in the diagnosis of myocarditis, especially in "borderline" cases in which there are significant inflammatory cells but no concomitant myocyte destruction. PCR uses an enzyme known as Taq DNA polymerase that is added to the following: a solution of "target" DNA to be amplified; primers, which are two single-stranded oligonucleotides that are produced to complement known sequences in the target DNA; and excess deoxyribonucleoside bases. This mixture is heated and cooled many times to cycle the following reaction: (1) heating—the target DNA separates into single strands, each of which acts as a template for production of a new double-stranded DNA that (2) when cooled incorporates the primer that is complimentary to the heat denatured strands of target DNA; finally, with (3) further cooling, the Taq polymerase catalyzes the synthesis of the rest of the strand in the presence of excess base. When performed 30 to 50 times, a geometric amplification of the original target DNA occurs. Identification of the target DNA with a specific viral agent can then proceed (Figs 83-2 and 83-3). Several reports link the presence of viral RNA in patients with dilated cardiomyopathy, thus implicating viral myocarditis as a precursor illness.

Recent studies have used endomyocardial biopsy to investigate patients who present with occult ventricular arrhythmias and a clinical picture of dilated cardiomyopathy. Establishment of a diagnosis helped tailor therapy, with improvement of the arrhythmias in some patients.

In one study, endomyocardial biopsy was used to establish the diagnosis of myocarditis in 34 patients who presented with dilated cardiomyopathy. The disease of these patients was classified on the basis of clinical and histologic findings in an attempt to stratify patients who might benefit from immunosuppressive therapy. Three groups—acute, rapidly progressive, and chronic—were formed. Immunosuppressive therapy was beneficial only in the patients with chronic disease. More recently, 27 patients referred for endomyocardial biopsy with the diagnosis of dilated cardiomyopathy were studied. Although two thirds of the patients had a biopsy consistent with myocarditis, there seemed to be no correlation between histologic classification and outcome. More important, there was no difference in outcome between the group receiving immunosuppressive therapy and those who did not receive the drugs. The biopsy was negative in 30% of patients who had clinical criteria of myocarditis and was positive in two of five patients without any clinical evidence of myocarditis.

One investigator reviewed 1200 biopsy specimens from patients with a clinical diagnosis of dilated cardiomyopathy and

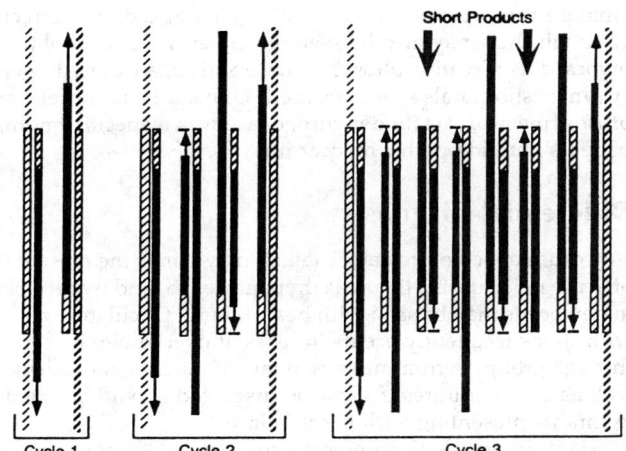

Figure 83-3. Products at the end of the initial polymerase chain reaction cycles. A key element of the polymerase chain reaction is the repetitive thermocycling of the steps shown in Figure 83-2. At each cycle, dark bars denote accumulated DNA that has been synthesized; currently synthesized DNA is indicated by arrows that project in the direction of active DNA polymerization. Because the synthesized products of all previous cycles act as templates for all ensuing cycles, the number of short products increases geometrically at the completion of each cycle. After about 30 cycles, the ratio of short products to other DNA entities is so large that they appear to be the only detectable DNA in the reaction mixture. (Eisenstein BI. The polymerase chain reaction: a new method of using molecular genetics for medical diagnosis. N Engl J Med 1990;322(3):179.)

found that about 25% had a diagnosis of myocarditis based on the critical evaluation of tissue specimens. There are no large series in pediatric patients with myocarditis to help clarify this issue.

## Laboratory Tests

Although rarely successful, an attempt should be made to identify the offending organism for each child with the suspected diagnosis of myocarditis. Early in the course of illness, it is possible to isolate the virus from the stool, throat washings, or, rarely, blood. Active infection is diagnosed when a four-fold increase is found in antibody titer to the isolated virus.

Criteria to help establish a diagnosis of coxsackievirus myocarditis have been suggested. Two high-order associations are identified: isolation of the virus from the myocardium or pericardial fluid and localization of type-specific virus in the myocardium, endocardium, or pericardium at sites of pathologic change. Moderate-order associations are present if the virus is isolated from the pharynx or stool and a four-fold increase in type-specific neutralizing, hemagglutination-inhibiting, or complement-fixing antibodies is demonstrated, or if viruses are isolated from the pharynx or stool with a concurrent serum titer of 1:32 or greater of type-specific IgM-neutralizing or hemagglutination-inhibiting antibodies. IgM specific antibody titers to coxsackieviruses B1, B3, B4, B5, and B6 may be identified and help establish the diagnosis.

Even when a diagnosis of myocarditis is likely, blood cultures should be obtained in any infant with fever and signs of compromised cardiovascular function. A complete blood count should be ordered; a leukemoid reaction may be noted. The erythrocyte sedimentation rate usually is elevated during acute myocarditis, although a normal value does not exclude the diagnosis. Elevated levels of serum glutamic-oxaloacetic and glutamic-pyruvic trans-

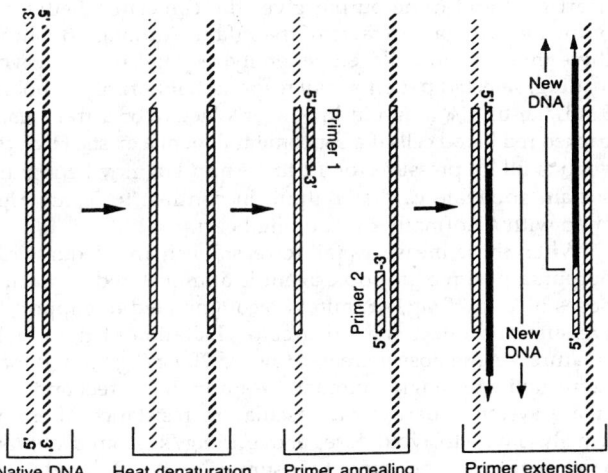

Figure 83-2. First round of the polymerase chain reaction. The basic polymerase chain reaction cycle consists of three steps performed in the same closed container but at different temperatures. The elevated temperature in the first step melts the double-stranded DNA into single strands. As the temperature is lowered for the second step, the two oppositely directed oligonucleotide primers anneal to complementary sequences on the target DNA, which acts as a template. During the third step, also performed at a lower temperature, the Taq polymerase enzymatically extends the primers covalently in the presence of excess deoxyribonucleoside triphosphates, the building blocks of new DNA synthesis. The native DNA target sequences, which will be massively amplified as "short products" in the ensuing cycles, are boxed. The vector of action of the DNA polymerase is denoted by the arrows projecting from the newly synthesized DNA (*dark bars*). (Eisenstein BI. The polymerase chain reaction: a new method of using molecular genetics for medical diagnosis. N Engl J Med 1990;3:179.)

aminase can occur as the result of a generalized viral infection, although they may also be seen during episodes of diphtheritic myocarditis. Creatine phosphokinase and lactate dehydrogenase enzymes should also be measured. One study found elevation of isozyme 1 of lactate dehydrogenase was a specific finding in patients with idiopathic myocarditis.

## Differential Diagnosis

Any cause of acute circulatory failure may mimic the presentation of acute myocarditis. Hypoxia, hypoglycemia, and hypocalcemia in newborns may be seen with heart failure. Circulatory collapse with shock frequently occurs in cases of overwhelming sepsis in this age group. Serum measurements of glucose and calcium as well as blood cultures if sepsis is suspected should be obtained in infants presenting with heart failure.

Many infants with significant structural defects of the heart (eg, hypoplastic left heart syndrome, critical aortic valve stenosis) have no audible murmur when severely ill because of extremely low cardiac output. When cardiac function is improved, however, murmurs may be apparent, as may be hyperactive precordium and clear, not muffled, heart sounds. Echocardiographic diagnosis is essential in the evaluation of these patients to rule out structural abnormalities.

Beyond the immediate neonatal period, many other etiologies are possible. Anomalous left coronary artery arising from the pulmonary artery should be investigated by echocardiography and angiography. Endocardial fibroelastosis, type II glycogen storage disease (Pompe's disease), medial necrosis of the coronary arteries, and left atrial myxoma are among the many diseases that can present a clinical picture similar to that of myocarditis. Murmurs may be audible with anomalous left coronary artery or endocardial fibroelastosis. They are usually apical in location, rarely more than grade 3/6, and usually secondary to mitral insufficiency. Endocardial fibroelastosis is impossible to differentiate from myocarditis by clinical presentation. Endomyocardial biopsy and angiographic changes of the left ventricle help make this diagnosis. The electrocardiogram in anomalous left coronary artery may show a pattern of myocardial infarction, with abnormal q waves in the anterolateral precordial leads. A qR pattern with inverted T waves in limb leads I and aVL may also be noted.

Pericarditis, which may be secondary to viral illness, usually occurs in children rather than infants. The clinical history may be similar to that in patients with myocarditis. Cardiovascular function, however, is usually less severely compromised for the degree of apparent cardiomegaly because of the amount of pericardial effusion. Cardiac tamponade may occur in severe cases and present with circulatory collapse. When pericarditis and myocarditis coexist, "perimyocarditis" results, and a clinical picture consistent with both diseases may be found. An echocardiogram establishes pericardial effusion and left ventricular size and function. Perimyocarditis may be seen with rheumatic fever, collagen vascular disease, other autoimmune diseases, and coxsackievirus B disease. Myocarditis also has been described with rheumatoid arthritis, systemic lupus erythematosus, and ulcerative colitis.

## TREATMENT

The level of care for the patient presenting with a clinical picture and history strongly suggestive of myocarditis depends on the severity of myocardial involvement. Many patients present with a relatively mild disease (ie, minimal or no respiratory compromise and mild signs of congestive heart failure). These patients require close monitoring to assess whether the disease will progress to worsening heart failure and the need for intensive medical care.

Experimental studies in animals suggest that bed rest may prevent an increase in intramyocardial viral replication during the acute stage; therefore, it is prudent to place patients under this restriction at the time of diagnosis.

Although no specific therapy aimed at reversing myocardial injury is recommended widely, maintenance of cardiac output at levels that supply adequate tissue perfusion and prevent metabolic disturbance is essential. In cases of congestive heart failure, digitalis may be used and has effected dramatic improvement in some instances. During periods of acute inflammation, the myocardium may be overly sensitive to digitalis; thus, rapid administration to achieve therapeutic levels should be avoided. Generally, the oral route is preferred, and a dose of 0.03 mg/kg rather than 0.04 mg/kg should be used as a total "digitalizing dose." Half of this should be given initially and the remaining half given in two divided doses at 8-hour intervals. Maintenance therapy should be tailored to achieving adequate serum therapeutic levels.

Diuretics frequently are administered in conjunction with digitalis. Although no direct beneficial effect on the myocardium is achieved, removal of excess extracellular fluid volume may help improve cardiac function. These agents should be administered cautiously; shock may result if extracellular volume is removed too rapidly. Excessive loss of $K^+$ ion secondary to induced diuresis may exacerbate digitalis toxicity and should be avoided. Furosemide should be administered in a dosage of 1 mg/kg/dose. Frequency of administration depends on the clinical state of the patient and may require the addition of spironolactone, a potassium-sparing diuretic agent if t.i.d. dosing is required (total daily dose more than 2 mg/kg/d).

Newborn infants may present initially in shock. Blood pressure usually is maintained at or near normal levels until late in the course and is not a sensitive indicator of the severity of illness. Rather, close attention to the adequacy of peripheral perfusion, heart rate, and urine output gives the clinician a better picture of the hemodynamic status of the infant. Although the hearts of these infants and children generally respond poorly to volume loading, selected patients may respond temporarily to boluses of 5 mL/kg of 5% albumin in Ringer's lactate or a transfusion of packed red blood cells if a concomitant anemia exists. High central venous filling pressures of 12 to 18 mm Hg may be required to sustain adequate cardiac output, in contrast to 5 mm Hg in a child with a normally functioning heart.

When these measures fail to reestablish an adequate cardiac output, a positive inotropic agent is administered. Dopamine in doses of 2 to 10 μg/kg/min is recommended to support blood pressure and effect some degree of dilatation of the renal vasculature. As the dose increases toward 20 μg/kg/min, dopamine exerts an increasingly dominant α-adrenergic effect and may increase systemic peripheral vasculature resistance; therefore, it usually is wise to avoid doses above 15 μg/kg/min. Dobutamine, a sympathomimetic amine that stimulates $\beta_1$-, $\beta_2$-, and α-adrenergic receptors, is used frequently in combination with dopamine. This agent exerts significant positive inotropy while reducing left ventricular filling pressure. It does not effect as positive a chronotropic response as dopamine and seems to result in less ventricular ectopy during administration. When used in combination with dopamine at low doses (more than 10 μg/kg/min), dobutamine, in doses of 10 μg/kg/min, or more, may result in a significant increase in ventricular contractility while avoiding a sinus tachycardia that may compromise cardiac output. For this reason, isoproterenol is best avoided in these patients, as the resultant sinus tachycardia, which in other patients may improve cardiac output, may be affected adversely in this circumstance.

Due to its afterload-reducing effects, sodium nitroprusside recently has been used extensively in children. Cardiac output is improved by reduction of systemic arterial resistance and, thus, ventricular filling pressure. In patients with myocarditis, this agent may be used in conjunction with dopamine or dobutamine if hypotension does not coexist. In addition, bedside assessment of cardiac output using thermodilution techniques after placement of a Swan-Ganz catheter can aid in the pharmacotherapy of the altered hemodynamic profiles. When chronic oral therapy is possible, an afterload-reducing drug such as captopril, an angiotensin-converting enzyme inhibitor, may be used with digitalis and diuretics.

Arrhythmias should be treated vigorously. Supraventricular tachyarrhythmias often are suppressed with digitalis, which usually has been administered previously for the treatment of congestive heart failure. Ventricular arrhythmias usually are responsive to lidocaine, given in a loading dose of 1 mg/kg (up to 50 mg total bolus dose), followed by a continuous infusion adequate to maintain a therapeutic serum concentration (1 to 5 mg/mL). If complete atrioventricular block occurs, a temporary transvenous pacemaker should be inserted. The patient must be observed over 10 to 14 days (in an intensive care unit) for the return of normal atrioventricular conduction. A permanent pacing device should be implanted if complete atrioventricular block persists beyond that time. Implantation can be done as an elective procedure when the patient's condition is stable.

Antibiotic agents should not be given unless a bacterial infection is suspected and cultures are obtained before initiating therapy.

The use of immunosuppressive agents in suspected or proven viral myocarditis is controversial. No controlled studies have been done in humans to prove their efficacy. Some animal studies suggest an exacerbation of virus-induced cytotoxicity in the presence of immunosuppressive drugs, possibly due to interference with interferon production.

Using endomyocardial biopsy to diagnose myocarditis, some investigators followed the inflammatory response to immunosuppressive therapy with follow-up biopsy tests in a series of 10 patients. Eight patients received both prednisone and azothioprine, while two received only prednisone. Clinical and histologic improvement was seen in four patients. Two patients who had their medications discontinued suffered relapses, which were reversed by reinstituting therapy. One patient worsened while on therapy and died. Although this was an uncontrolled study, the authors noted that the reversal of congestive heart failure in the two patients who resumed therapy was highly suggestive of the beneficial effect of immunosuppressive therapy. Another study found definite hemodynamic and histologic improvement in seven of nine patients treated with a combination of prednisone and azothioprine. After discontinuance of therapy for 4 months, however, only four of seven patients still showed improvement. One patient improved with reinstitution of therapy, while two patients deteriorated.

One recent study illustrates the problem of biopsy-directed treatment in myocarditis. Nine patients were treated with single or combined immunosuppressive therapy after a biopsy sample showed evidence of inflammation. Improvement was seen in 4 of 9 patients; however, 6 of 18 patients who did not receive therapy also improved, nullifying any statistically significant difference between the two groups.

One recent study attempted to employ a clinicopathologic description to categorize myocarditis into types that might respond to immunosuppressive treatment. The categories mimicked those of postviral hepatitis syndromes (ie, fulminant, acute, chronic active, and chronic persistent). The only group that seemed to respond to immunosuppressive agents were the patients with acute myocarditis, although some of them went on to develop congestive cardiomyopathy despite the absence of inflammatory cells on their follow-up biopsy samples. Other studies have shown that patients with "borderline" myocarditis respond better (improved left ventricular contractile function) than do patients with unequivocally positive biopsy samples.

A tabulation of results from most studies showing the effects of immunosuppressive therapy revealed that 60% of 82 biopsy-proven cases of myocarditis improved with therapy. Patients who had lower grade changes apparently did better than those with greater involvement. Complications of immunosuppressive therapy, including opportunistic infections and a cushingoid state, should be considered before administration of these drugs. Controlled studies are underway in the adult population to address the usefulness of immunosuppressive therapy, including use of cyclosporine; a similar study in children should be undertaken before firm recommendations can be given to clinicians.

The prognosis for acute myocarditis in newborns is poor. A 75% mortality rate was found in 25 infants with suspected coxsackievirus B myocarditis. The highest rate of mortality occurred in the first week of illness. For the six infants who survived, there were no apparent sequelae, although long-term follow-up was not reported. Older infants and children have a better prognosis, with a mortality rate between 10% and 25% in clinically recognizable cases. Adult patients who recover may be asymptomatic at rest or with light exertion, but may demonstrate a reduced working capacity with exercise stress testing.

The etiology of the disease may affect prognosis. Patients who develop conduction abnormalities or arrhythmias with diphtheritic myocarditis have a poor prognosis. Some investigators report a 100% rate of mortality in the patients with conduction disturbances or supraventricular tachycardia.

## Selected Readings

Daly K, et al. Acute myocarditis: role of histological and virological examination in the diagnosis and assessment of immunosuppressive treatment. Br Heart J 1984;51:30.

Dery P, Marks MI, Shapera R. Clinical manifestations of coxsackievirus infections in children. Am J Dis Child 1974;128:464.

Edwards WD, Holmes DR, Reader GS. Diagnosis of active lymphocytic myocarditis by endomyocardial biopsy: quantitative criteria for light microscopy. Mayo Clin Proc 1982;57:419.

Fenoglio JJ, et al. Diagnosis and classification of myocarditis by endomyocardial biopsy. N Engl J Med 1983;308:12.

Hauck AJ, et al. Evaluation of postmortem endomyocardial biopsy specimens from 38 patients with lymphocytic myocarditis: implication for rule of sampling error. Mayo Clin Proc 1989;64:1235.

Lerner AM, Wilson MF. Virus myocardiopathy. Prog Med Virol 1973;15:63.

Lyden D, Olazewski J, Huber S. Variation in susceptibility of BALB/c mice to coxsackievirus group B type 3-induced myocarditis with age. Cell Immunol 1987;105:332.

Maisch B, et al. Diagnostic relevance of humoral and cell-mediated immune reactions in patients with acute viral myocarditis. Clin Exp Immunol 1982;48:533.

McManus BM, Kandolf R. Evolving concepts of cause, consequence, and control in myocarditis. Current Opinion in Cardiology 1991;6:418.

Saphir O, Simon WA, Reingold MI. Myocarditis in children. Am J Dis Child 1944;67:294.

Woodruff JF. Viral myocarditis: a review. Am J Pathol 1980;101:427.

Zee-Cheng CS, et al. High incidence of myocarditis by endomyocardial biopsy in patients with idiopathic congestive cardiomyopathy. J Am Coll Cardiol 1984;3:63.

*Principles and Practice of Pediatrics, Second Edition.*
edited by Frank A. Oski et al. J. B. Lippincott Company, Philadelphia © 1994.

# 83.2 *Cardiomyopathy*

Marc Paquet and Brian D. Hanna

The term *cardiomyopathy* refers to any structural or functional abnormality of the ventricular myocardium that is not associated with disease of the coronary arteries, high blood pressure, valvular or congenital heart disease, or pulmonary vascular disease. It can be divided into two categories: primary or "heart muscle disease of known cause associated with disorders of other systems" and secondary (Table 83-2). This discussion is limited to primary cardiomyopathies, grouped into four types: dilated, hypertrophic, restrictive, and arrhythmogenic. The most common causes of secondary cardiomyopathy in childhood are listed in Table 83-3.

## DILATED CARDIOMYOPATHY

Dilated cardiomyopathy is characterized by dilatation of the left ventricle (or both ventricles), with resultant cardiomegaly. Dilatation is accompanied by some hypertrophy. Functionally, it impairs systolic function, and the clinical picture is one of congestive heart failure.

### Idiopathic Dilated Cardiomyopathy

Idiopathic dilated cardiomyopathy (IDC) is a disease of infancy. More than 50% of patients present before 2 years of age. Incidence

**TABLE 83-2. Classification of Cardiomyopathy in Children**

Primary
Dilated
  Idiopathic dilated
  Cardiomyopathy
  Endocardial fibroelastosis
Hypertrophic:
  Obstructive
  Nonobstructive
Restrictive:
  Endomyocardial fibrosis
  Löffler eosinophilic endomyocardial disease
  Hemochromatosis
  Fabry's disease
  Pseudoxanthoma elasticum
Arrhythmogenic:
  Arrhythmogenic right ventricular dysplasia
  Oncocytic cardiomyopathy

**Secondary**
Infection
Metabolic
General system disease
Heredofamilial
Sensitivity and toxic reactions

is equal in both sexes. Etiology is unknown. Familial incidence is 600 to 700 times that of the general population, and, in some cases, a hereditary basis has been documented. Histologic examination of endomyocardial biopsy obtained from adult patients with IDC has shown a high incidence of myocardial inflammation, but these findings have not been duplicated in children. Recent clinical and experimental reports suggest that an immunologic abnormality may be implicated in the pathogenesis of the disease. Over the past 5 years, numerous reports have described various cardiovascular abnormalities, including dilated cardiomyopathy, in children infected with the human immunodeficiency virus (HIV). The pathologic process usually involves the myocardium of both ventricles in a uniform fashion, producing generalized cardiac dilatation. The myocardium is pale, and the endocardium is thin and translucent. Microscopic examination shows interstitial fibrosis, myofiber hypertrophy, degeneration, and necrosis.

### Clinical Findings

In one third to one half of reported cases, the initial presentation is preceded by a respiratory or gastrointestinal illness. Symptoms of congestive heart failure—tachypnea, fatigue during feedings, excessive perspiration, and, occasionally, failure to thrive—are usually dominant at the initial presentation. Some patients initially present with ventricular or supraventricular arrhythmias.

Physical examination usually reveals an ill-looking child in moderate to severe respiratory distress. Cyanosis is unusual, but pallor of the skin is common. Peripheral pulses are often weak, blood pressure is low with a narrowed pulse pressure, and *pulsus alternans* is a common finding. Thoracic overdistention and, rarely, prominence of the left hemithorax are apparent on examination of the chest. Auscultation of the lungs often reveals decreased air entry at the base, but inspiratory rales are rare. On palpation of the precordium, the heart usually is quiet, and the apex may be difficult to localize. On auscultation, heart sounds are muffled, but careful auscultation usually reveals the presence of a gallop rhythm. Murmurs often are absent at the time of initial presentation, but the soft apical pansystolic murmur of mitral regurgitation often appears after a few days, once the cardiac function improves. The liver edge is usually palpable well below the right costal margin, and it is rounded as a result of passive congestion. Neck vein distention and peripheral edema are rarely found in infants but are not unusual in older children and young adults.

### Laboratory Findings

The chest radiograph shows cardiomegaly secondary to dilatation of the left atrium and left ventricle, as well as evidence of pulmonary venous congestion that can progress to frank pulmonary edema (Fig 83-4). The electrocardiogram shows sinus tachycardia with ST-T wave abnormalities and left ventricular hypertrophy in most patients (Fig 83-5). The echocardiographic features include dilatation of the left atrium, dilatation of the left ventricle with reduction of the shortening fraction (% Δ LVd), decrease in mean circumferential fiber shortening, and an increase in the distance between the septal surface and the mitral E point (mitral E point–septal separation) (Fig 83-6). Two-dimensional echocardiography usually shows global left ventricular dysfunction and is essential in the early detection of intracavitary thrombi. Doppler examination often demonstrates the presence of mitral regurgitation before it can be clinically detected. Radionuclide angiographic studies confirm dilatation of both ventricles and permit noninvasive measurement of the ejection fraction, which is always decreased.

### Treatment

During the acute phase of illness, treatment is directed at controlling congestive heart failure and includes bed rest, fluid re-

## TABLE 83-3. Secondary Cardiomyopathies

**Infections**

*Viral*
Coxsackie B
Echovirus
Mumps
Rubella
Rubeola
HIV

*Bacterial*
Diphtheria
Meningococcal
Pneumococcal
Gonococcal

*Fungal*
Candidiasis
Aspergillosis

*Protozoal*
American trypanosomiasis (Chagas'
disease) toxoplasmosis

*Rickettsial*
Rocky Mountain spotted fever

*Spirochetal*
Lyme disease

**Metabolic Conditions**

*Endocrine*
Thyrotoxicosis
Hypothyroidism
Diabetes mellitus:
Infant of diabetic mother
Diabetic cardiomyopathy
Hypoglycemia
Pheochromocytoma/neuroblastoma:
Catecholamine
Cardiomyopathy

*Familial Storage Disease*
Glycogen storage disease
   Pompe's disease (type II)
   Cori's disease (type III)
   Andersen's disease (type IV)
   McArdle's disease (type V)
   Hers' disease (type VI)
Mucopolysaccharidoses
   Hurler's syndrome
   Hunter's syndrome
   Morquio's syndrome
   Scheie's syndrome
   Maroteaux-Lamy syndrome
Sphingolipidoses
   Niemann-Pick disease
   Farber's disease
   Fabry's disease
   Gaucher's disease
   Tay-Sachs disease
   Sandhoff's disease
   GM, gangliosidosis
   Refsum's disease

**Nutritional Deficiency**

Protein: kwashiorkor
Thiamine: beriberi
Vitamin E and selenium (Keshan's disease)
Phosphate

*Others*
Carnitine deficiency
   Primary
   Secondary: diphtheritic cardiomyopathy
B-ketothiolase deficiency
Hypertaurinuria

**General System Diseases**

*Connective Tissue Disorders*
Systemic lupus erythematosus
Juvenile rheumatoid arthritis
Polyarteritis nodosa
Kawasaki disease
Pseudoxanthoma elasticum

*Infiltrations and Granulomas*
Leukemia
Sarcoidosis (not in children)
Amyloidosis (not in children)

*Others*
Hemolytic–uremic syndrome
Mitochondrial cytopathy
Reye's syndrome
Peripartum cardiomyopathy
Osteogenesis imperfecta
Noonan's syndrome

**Heredofamilial Conditions**

*Muscular Dystrophies and Myopathies*
Juvenile progressive (Duchenne's disease)
Myotonic dystrophy (Steinert's disease)
Limp-girdle (Erb's disease)
Juvenile progressive spinal muscular
atrophy (Kugelberg-Welander disease)
Chronic progressive external
ophthalmoplegia (Kearns)
Nemaline myopathy
Myotubular myopathy

*Neuromuscular Disorders*
Friedreich's ataxia
Multiple lentiginosis

**Sensitivity and Toxic Reactions**

Sulphonamides
Penicillin
Anthracyclines
Iron (hemochromatosis)
Chloramphenicol
Dexamethasone

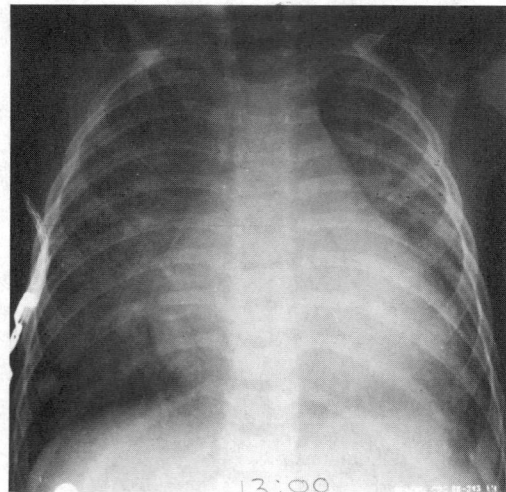

**Figure 83-4.** This chest radiograph of a 12-month-old boy with idiopathic dilated cardiomyopathy shows cardiomegaly and pulmonary venous congestion.

electrolytes and renal function tests should be obtained before institution of diuretic therapy. If potassium depletion occurs, a potassium retaining agent such as spironolactone (1.5 to 3.0 mg/kg/d) may be added to the regimen. Intravenous digitalization (20 to 30 μg/kg over 16 to 24 hours) should be initiated soon after the diagnosis is made. Twelve hours after digitalization is completed, oral maintenance therapy using 7.5 to 10 μg/kg/d in two divided doses should be started. This medication should be continued for many months after the clinical and laboratory evidence of myocardial impairment regresses.

For patients who present with severe congestive heart failure and pulmonary edema, nasotracheal intubation and mechanical ventilation may be lifesaving. Sedation with morphine sulphate often improves the overall condition of these patients. In these acutely ill infants, sympathomimetic amines such as dopamine and dobutamine that have a faster onset of action and a shorter half-life than digitalis, or type III phosphodiestherase inhibitors such as amrinone should be used to improve contractility.

The role of afterload reducing agents in the treatment of patients with IDC is well established. During the acute phase of illness, intravenous sodium nitroprusside or hydralazine is the best agent; for long-term therapy, hydralazine (0.25 to 1.0 mg/kg q.i.d.), prazosin (50 to 100 μg/kg q.i.d.), and captopril (1 to 2 mg/kg t.i.d.) are used orally. At least one clinical study suggests that the addition of the calcium antagonist diltiazem to conventional therapy (digitalis, diuretics, and vasodilators) significantly reduces mortality and improves myocardial function and clinical status in a group of adult patients with IDC; this drug may prove to benefit infants and children as well. While significant atrial or ventricular arrhythmias should be treated according to accepted principles, the question of such arrhythmias representing an independent prognostic factor remains unanswered.

The role of corticosteroids and other immunosuppressive agents such as azathioprine is unclear and controversial in the treatment of children with IDC. Because of the high risk of serious

striction, and use of agents that decrease the cardiac load or improve myocardial contractility.

Infants with severe congestive heart failure should be kept NPO and given intravenous hydration up to 75% to 80% of their calculated maintenance. Infants and children with less severe congestive failure can be fed orally on demand without restriction. Because it renders food unpalatable, sodium restriction usually results in reduced caloric intake in infants and children; low-sodium diets should thus be avoided. Instead, diuretic agents should be used to handle the extra sodium load. Furosemide or ethacrynic acid, 1.0 to 2.0 mg/kg/d, are usually effective. Serum

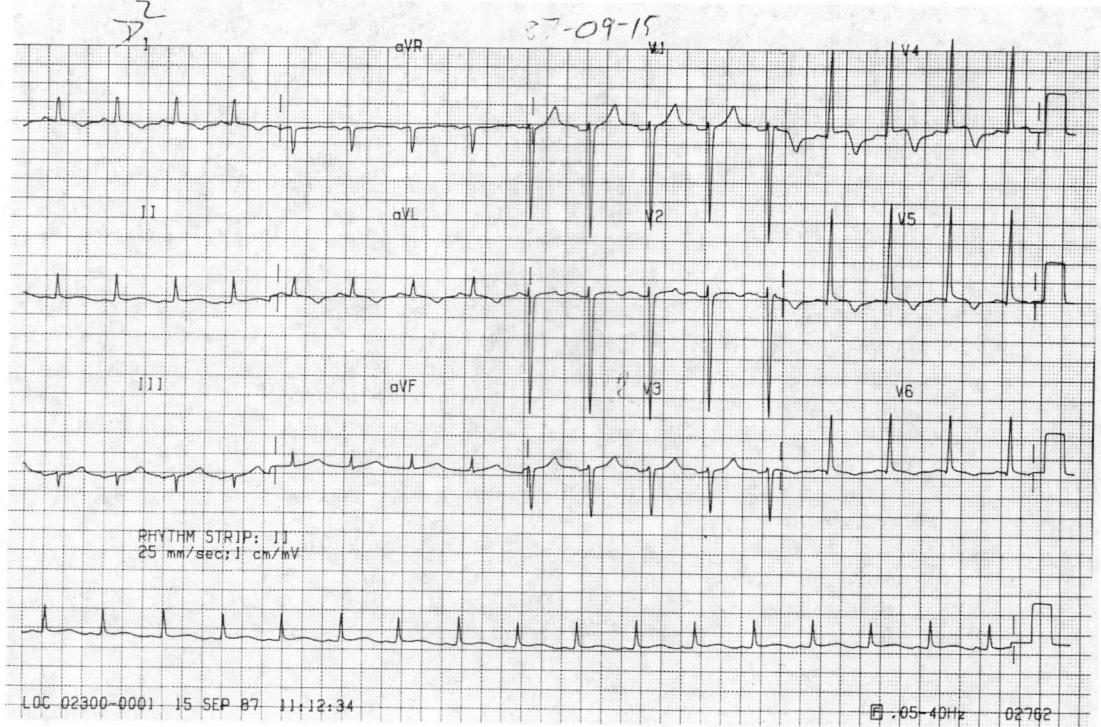

**Figure 83-5.** This 12-lead ECG from a 12-month-old boy with idiopathic dilated cardiomyopathy shows LVH and diffuse ST-T wave abnormalities.

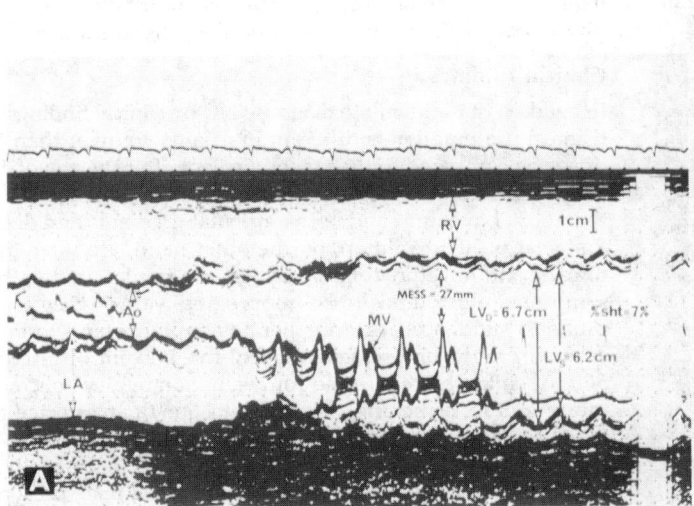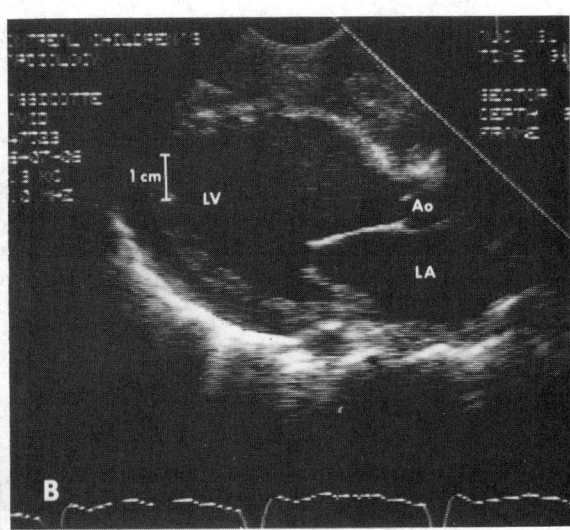

**Figure 83-6.** (**A**) M-mode echocardiogram from a patient IDC. Note dilatation of the left atrium and left ventricle, markedly decreased LV shortening fraction, and increased mitral E point-septal separation. (**B**) Two-dimensional echocardiogram (parasternal long axis) from a 12-month-old boy with IDC shows marked dilatation of left ventricle and left atrium. *LA,* left atrium; *LV,* left ventricle; *MV,* mitral valve; *RV,* right ventricle; *LVd,* left ventricular diastolic dimension; *LVs,* left ventricular systolic dimension; *% sht,* left ventricular shortening fraction; *MESS,* mitral E point-septal separation.

side effects such as growth retardation, bone narrow suppression, and infection, use of corticosteroids and immunosuppressive agents should be restricted to those patients in whom myocardial inflammation is documented by endomyocardial biopsy.

Patients with atrial fibrillation, intracavitary thrombus demonstrated by two-dimensional echocardiogram, or suspected or confirmed arterial embolization should be anticoagulated. Anticoagulation is achieved with heparin 100 U/kg intravenously followed by constant infusion of 10 to 20 U/kg per hour adjusted to maintain the PTT at 1½ times that of the control. After 1 or 2 weeks of this regimen, oral warfarin (0.05 mg/kg/d) should be started, and the heparin should be discontinued over the next 48 to 72 hours. Oral warfarin should be continued for as long as the predisposing factors to thromboembolic episodes (atrial fibrillation or left ventricular dilatation with shortening fraction of less than 20%) are present.

Patients who fail to respond to medical therapy and whose condition deteriorates rapidly are candidates for cardiac transplantation. Indications for cardiac transplantation are New York Heart Association class IV symptomatology and a life expectancy of less than 6 months. It is suggested that patients who present after age 2 years and those who present before 2 years but have persistent cardiomegaly or develop significant atrial or ventricular arrhythmias during follow-up are candidates for transplantation.

### Prognosis

The prognosis for infants with IDC is poor, with mortality rates ranging from 35% to 63%, although in one recent retrospective study, the 5-year survival rate was close to 80%. Most deaths occur during the first year after diagnosis. Few parameters, if any, are useful in predicting the survival of a patient; but, a recent report strongly suggests that patients who present before age 2 years have a better chance of survival than those who present after 2 years of age. Other factors suggestive of poor outcome include persistent congestive heart failure or cardiomegaly and development of significant arrhythmias (ie, atrial fibrillation or flutter, or complex ventricular ectopy) during follow-up. The most common cause of death is intractable congestive heart failure, followed by sudden death secondary to an arrhythmia. About half of the survivors recover completely, while the other half continues to present clinical or echocardiographic evidence of myocardial dysfunction.

## Endocardial Fibroelastosis

Endocardial fibroelastosis (EFE) can be primary (congenital) or secondary to obstruction of the left ventricular outflow tract or to coarctation of the aorta. It is characterized by focal thickening of the endocardium of the left atrium and the left ventricle, giving the appearance of an "iced cake." Histologically, it is characterized by proliferation of collagenous and elastic tissue within the endocardium. There are two varieties of primary EFE of the left ventricle: in the more common dilated type, the left ventricle is enlarged and the walls are hypertrophied; in the less common contracted type, the left ventricular cavity is small. EFE is found in less than 1% of the total number of infants and children with congenital heart disease. Females are affected 1.5 times more often than males. The etiology is unknown. One recent editorial resurrected a concept that questions the existence of primary EFE, but views all EFE as a reactive process set off in the endocardium by various mechanisms producing myocardial stress during fetal life or early infancy. The disease is 700 times as common among siblings of affected patients as in the general population, underlying the importance heredity in its pathogenesis. Risk for a sibling of an affected child is estimated at 4%.

### Clinical Picture, Laboratory Findings, Diagnosis

EFE is a disease of infancy, with more than 75% of cases presenting in the first year of life. Initial presentation is with symptoms of congestive heart failure, which are often preceded by an upper respiratory tract infection. Findings on physical examination, as well as the radiological, electrocardiographic, and echocardiographic features, are similar to those of patients with IDC. A macroscopic or microscopic examination of the left ventricular endocardium is necessary for a definitive diagnosis. Clinically, the differential diagnosis includes myocarditis, Pompe's disease, anomalous origin of the left coronary artery from the pulmonary artery, and medial necrosis of the coronary arteries.

These entities usually can be excluded from the electrocardiogram or echocardiogram.

## Treatment and Prognosis

There is no specific therapy for EFE. Treatment is directed at controlling the effects of myocardial dysfunction as outlined for IDC. The prognosis is poor, although patients who present during the first year of life usually can expect a more favorable prognosis. Familial cases carry a poor prognosis. Most deaths occur during the first year after presentation from congestive heart failure or arrhythmias.

# HYPERTROPHIC CARDIOMYOPATHY

Hypertrophic cardiomyopathy (HC) is characterized by a disproportionate increase in the myocardial mass in the absence of cavity dilatation. The left ventricular cavity may be either normal in size or small. The two types of HC—obstructive and nonobstructive—can be distinguished by the presence or absence of obstruction to left ventricular ejection. HC is rare in children, accounting for 20% to 30% of pediatric primary myocardial disease.

## Pathology

External examination of the heart demonstrates gross hypertrophy of the left ventricle with enlargement of the left atrium in advanced cases. Intracavitary examination reveals hypertrophy of the intraventricular septum with a variable degree of hypertrophy of the left ventricular free wall. On microscopic examination, the myocytes are hypertrophied, varying greatly in size and shape. Myofibers have abnormal branching and are often found in whorls. Myofilaments originate and terminate in the Z bands of different myofibrils.

## Etiology

Most authors believe that the hypertrophy manifests itself in response to altered intramyocardial wall stress, which, in turn, is the result of the primary lesion: myofibril disarray. There is no definite explanation for the myocardial disarray. It has been suggested that it is the result of an arrest in the maturation of the normal myocardial architecture. Although ample evidence supports the possibility of an autosomal inheritance pattern with variable penetrance, the disease manifests itself differently in relatives of patients. Molecular genetic analysis of members of a large kindred has determined that the gene responsible for familial HC is located on chromosome 14 (band ql). About 45% of patients are considered "sporadic cases."

## Physiopathology

HC is associated with significant alterations in systolic function. The left ventricular ejection fraction and the rate of ejection are both increased. These changes are accomplished without an increase in contractility, because the afterload is decreased in proportion to the increase in wall thickness. The existence and significance of left ventricular outflow tract obstruction is debated. When there is a gradient, it is caused by contact between the left side of the interventricular septum and the anterior mitral leaflet, which moves anteriorly as the blood is forced through the narrow left ventricular outflow tract. This systolic anterior motion further narrows the left ventricular outflow tract and is often associated with mitral regurgitation. Left ventricular diastolic dysfunction is evident in all patients whether or not there is left ventricular outflow tract obstruction. The left ventricular end-diastolic pressure usually is elevated secondary to decrease in compliance, and the isovolumic relaxation time is prolonged. Significant abnor-

malities in the small coronary arteries contribute to the pathophysiology of both the systolic and diastolic dysfunctions.

## Clinical Findings

In children, it is difficult to diagnose HC by clinical findings alone. Clinical presentation is different in infants younger than 1 year of age as compared to those who present after the age of 1 year. In general, infants present with congestive heart failure. More than 60% have right and left ventricular gradients and die in the first year of life. Children, on the other hand, are often asymptomatic and have predominantly left ventricular gradients; their symptomatology tends to be nonprogressive, but they are more prone to sudden death. In general, symptoms tend to be more severe in the young patients. Thirty-five percent of infants and 50% of children are referred for evaluation of a systolic ejection murmur or for screening after the detection of an affected family member. In infants, the most common symptoms are tachypnea, tachycardia, and poor feeding; whereas, children usually complain of dyspnea and fatigue on exertion, chest pain, presyncope, syncope, and palpitations.

On physical examination the peripheral pulses present an initial brisk upstroke, followed by a reduction in amplitude in midsystole as the ventricular ejection is impeded. On palpation of the precordium, the apex may be displaced inferiorly and toward the left, and its impulse may be sustained. In some cases, a systolic thrill is felt at the lower left sternal border. On auscultation, S1 is normal and S2 normally is split in most patients, but with significant left ventricular outflow tract obstruction, there is paradoxical splitting. Early (S3) and late (S4) diastolic filling sounds are heard in 37% and 50% of patients, respectively. Systolic ejection murmurs of grade 3/6 or higher are common. The murmur usually begins well after S1 and is loudest between the midretrosternal region and the apex; it radiates widely but not to the carotids. At the apex and into the left axilla, it is often holosystolic, marking the presence of mitral regurgitation. Quality of the systolic murmur varies with the physiologic state of the patient. Maneuvers and agents that increase contractility and/or decrease preload or afterload (ie, exercise, standing, the straining phase of Valsalva's maneuver, digitalis, isoproterenol, amyl nitrate, and nitroglycerin) can be used to augment the gradient and the murmur. On the other hand, the gradient and the murmur are decreased by the following interventions: Mueller maneuver, the overshoot phase of Valsalva's maneuver, squatting, handgrip, alpha-adrenergic stimulation, beta-adrenergic blockade, or general anesthesia.

## Laboratory Findings

Almost all infants and most children demonstrate cardiomegaly on the chest radiograph. Pulmonary vascular markings are usually normal. The electrocardiogram (Fig 83-7) usually shows left ventricular hypertrophy with ST segments of T wave abnormalities as well as abnormal Q waves. In some patients, there is evidence of right ventricular hypertrophy.

The diagnosis often is made based on echocardiography. The M-mode examination reveals asymmetric septal hypertrophy with systolic anterior motion (SAM) of the anterior leaflet of the mitral valve and midsystolic closure of the aortic valve. Two-dimensional echocardiography (Fig 83-8) shows the extent of hypertrophy and the presence or absence of obstruction, and it permits assessment of left ventricular systolic and diastolic function. In general, the presence of SAM of the anterior mitral leaflet, combined with prolonged contact with interventricular septum, is predictive of an left ventricular outflow tract gradient of more than 30 mm Hg. The disease must be differentiated from other causes of myocardial hypertrophy. In infants younger than 1 year of age, the most common cause of myocardial hypertrophy

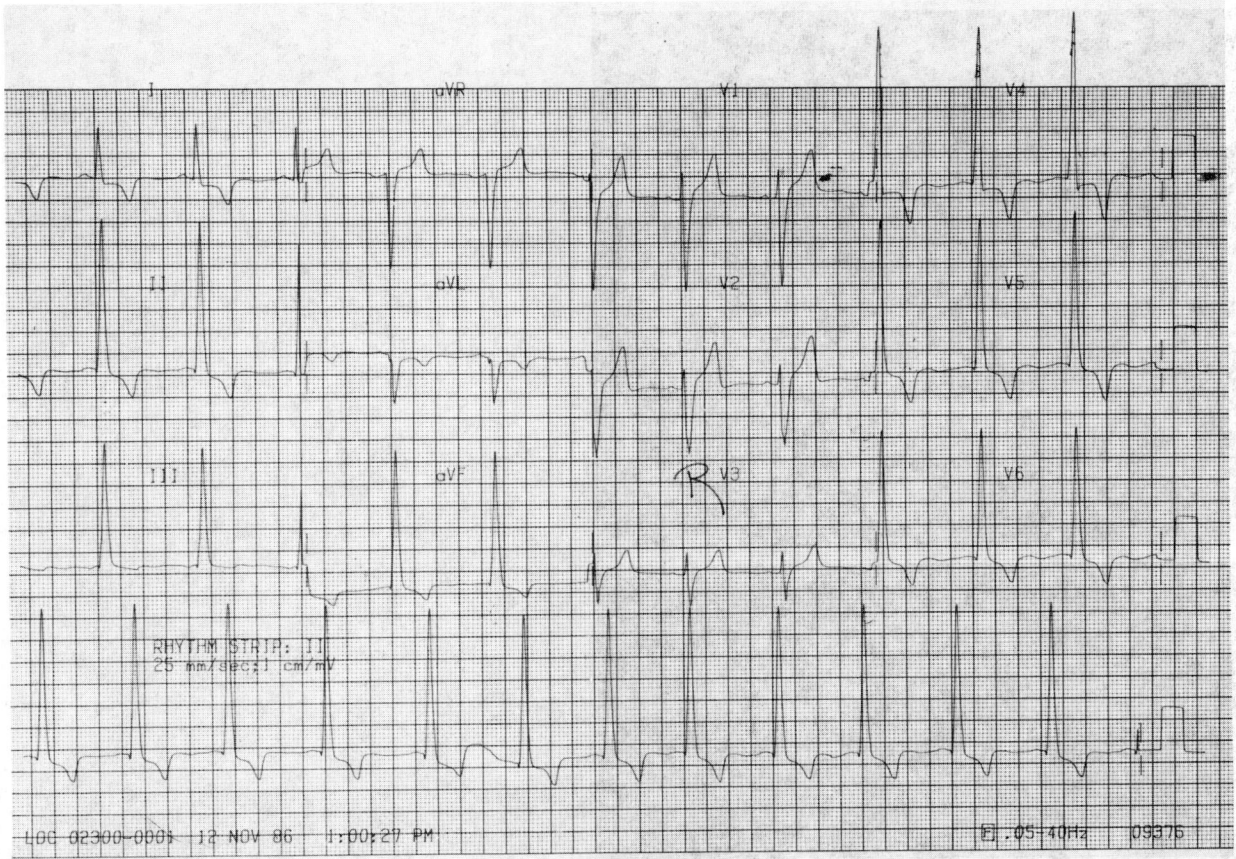

**Figure 83-7.** ECG from a 12-year-old with HC. There are voltage criteria for left ventricular hypertrophy and inverted T waves in the left precordial derivations, as well as in leads I, II, aVL, and aVF.

is maternal diabetes; in older children, causes include Pompe's disease, Friedreich's ataxia, and lentiginosis.

### Treatment

The first-line drug in the treatment of symptomatic children is propranolol, which reduces heart rate, left ventricular contractility, and wall stress. About one third of symptomatic patients obtain complete relief of symptoms with standard doses or oral propranolol. This drug has no effect, however, on the extent of hypertrophy, does not reduce the incidence of ventricular arrhythmia, and, more importantly, does not eliminate the risk of sudden death. Calcium channel blockers such as verapamil and nifedipine are effective in the treatment of HC, even in patients who do not respond to propranolol. Verapamil decreases systolic gradient, improves diastolic filling, and may be effective in decreasing the amount of hypertrophy. The role of amiodarone in the treatment of infants and children with HC is unclear, and its use should be reserved for patients with refractory and potentially lethal arrhythmias. Positive inotropic agents such a digoxin must be used with caution. By increasing contractility, they may produce an increase in systolic gradient and a concomitant deterioration in clinical status. Likewise, by decreasing preload, diuretic agents may worsen the outflow obstruction. Nonspecific therapy includes prophylaxis against bacterial endocarditis at the time of "at risk" procedures. General anesthesia and pregnancy carry increased risk. Active sports participation is not recommended, because most sudden deaths in adolescents with HC occur during or after exercise.

Surgical intervention is indicated when medical therapy fails to alleviate symptoms. Studies show that, in selective patients,

myectomy-myotomy provides symptomatic relief, reduces the gradient, and prolongs life. Mitral valve replacement is recommended only in patients whose septum is too thin to allow adequate resection, in those in whom previous resections have not reduced the obstruction, or when mitral regurgitation is severe.

### Natural History

The prognosis of infants who present at younger than 1 year of age is dismal, especially in those who initially present with congestive heart failure or cyanosis. If the initial presentation is that of an asymptomatic murmur, chances of survival to 1 year are greater than 50%. Of those alive at 1 year, 40% to 50% improve, 30% to 40% die, and 10% to 20% have residual disease. If there is a strong family history of sudden death, children are at increased risk for such an event. Mortality is twice as high in children as in adults. There is no predictive variable to help identify patients at risk for sudden death. One study demonstrated that nonsustained ventricular tachycardia (more than 3 beats) increases the risk for sudden death from 8% to 10% per year, while, in another, the absence of ventricular arrhythmia during ambulatory electrocardiogram monitoring did not correlate with a low risk of sudden death.

## RESTRICTIVE CARDIOMYOPATHY

Restrictive cardiomyopathy (RC) is characterized by impairment of diastolic filling secondary to scarring of the endocardium. The left ventricular end-diastolic volume is usually normal or reduced,

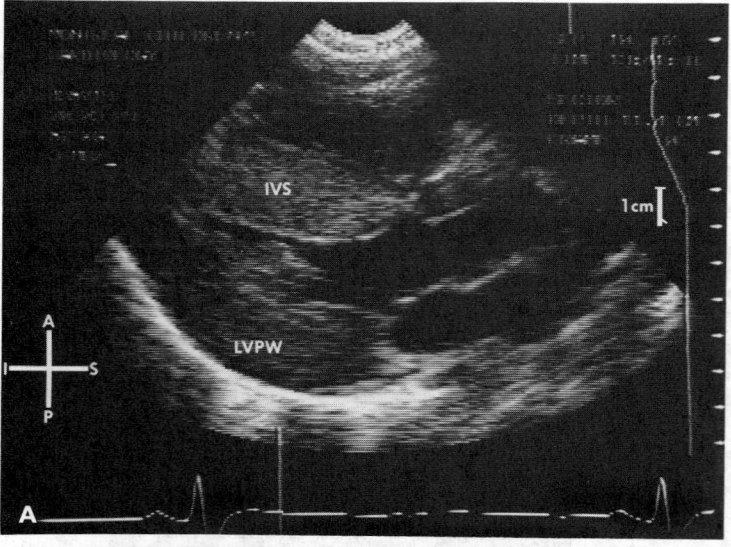

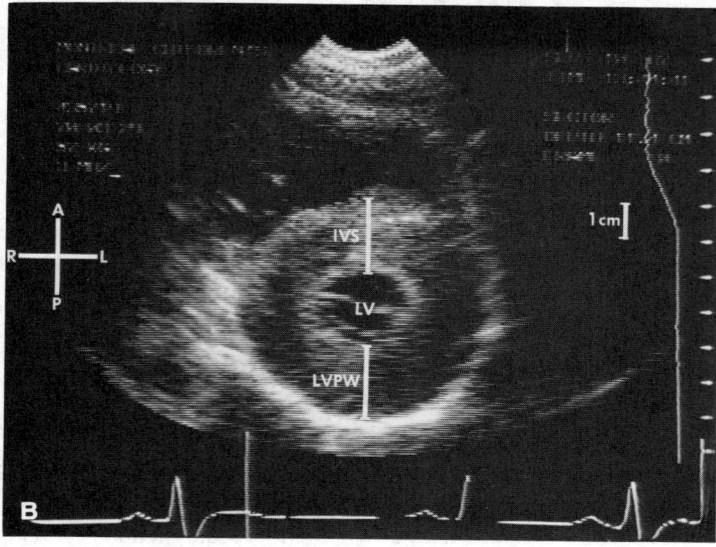

**Figure 83-8.** Two-dimensional echocardiogram of a 17-year-old boy with nonobstructive HC. Systolic frames in parasternal long axis (**A**) and parasternal short axis (**B**) views show concentric hypertrophy of LV wall and near complete cavity obliteration. *IVS,* interventricular septum; *LVPW,* left ventricular posterior wall; *LV,* left ventricle.

and the ejection fraction is only slightly decreased. The primary physiologic anomaly is decreased ventricular compliance.

## Endomyocardial Fibrosis (EMF), Löffler Disease

Endomyocardial fibrosis (EMF) and Löffler disease are the same disease at different stages of evolution. The term "hypereosinophilic syndrome" describes the disease, and the presence of cardiac involvement is described as "endomyocardial disease, with or without eosinophilia." EMF affects adolescents and young adults of both sexes more often, whereas Löffler disease presents at any age and affects males three times more often than females. Although the exact etiology is not identified, the consensus of opinion is that it results from an immunologic reaction involving the eosinophil itself.

The disease is characterized by layers of fibrosis of variable thickness over the endocardium, occurring predominantly in three areas: the left ventricular apex, the mitral valve apparatus, and the right ventricular apex. The histologic picture is characterized by the absence of elastic fibers in the areas of fibrosis. The process can be restricted to either the left or the right ventricle, or both ventricles may be involved simultaneously. In Löffler disease,

intracavitary thrombus and acute myocarditis are more common, and there is often eosinophilic infiltration of extracardiac organs.

### Clinical and Laboratory Findings

The clinical picture depends on whether one or both ventricles are involved. Involvement of the left ventricle results in mitral regurgitation; whereas, disease restricted to the right ventricle produces tricuspid regurgitation. The most common presenting symptom is dyspnea followed by chest pain. Physical findings include nonspecific systolic ejection murmur, holosystolic murmur at the apex, third and fourth heart sounds, jugular venous distention, and peripheral edema.

The chest radiograph often shows cardiomegaly secondary to dilatation of the atria, hypertrophy of the ventricular walls, and pericardial effusion. Electrocardiographic features include nonspecific ST-T wave changes, small QRS voltage, first degree AV block, and variable degree of atrial dilatation and ventricular hypertrophy. Characteristic echocardiographic features include apical obliteration, preserved contractile function of the ventricle, involvement of the papillary muscle and posterior leaflet of the mitral or tricuspid valve, and normal or small ventricles with dilated atria. Intracavitary thrombi are frequently identified on two-dimensional echocardiography. The major diagnostic challenge is to distinguish RC from constrictive pericarditis. The two conditions present similar clinical and hemodynamic features, and, in a significant number of patients, the definitive diagnosis requires endomyocardial biopsy or exploratory thoracotomy.

### Natural History, Prognosis, and Treatment

Because of the low incidence of RC in infants and children, it is difficult to determine the natural history in this age group, but because most cases reported in children were from necropsy studies, the overall prognosis seems poor. There is no specific treatment. Medical treatment with diuretics, venous vasodilators, digitalis glycosides, or arteriolar vasodilators is either ineffective or may be detrimental. In some cases, surgical resection of the subendocardial fibrosis or AV valve replacement has resulted in hemodynamic and symptomatic improvement.

## ARRHYTHMOGENIC CARDIOMYOPATHY

### Arrhythmogenic Right Ventricular Dysplasia

Since first described in 1978, fewer than 20 cases of arrhythmogenic right ventricular dysplasia (ARVD), a rare myocardial disease, have been reported in infants and children. The clinical presentation is one of abrupt onset of syncopal episodes, palpitations, or ventricular tachycardia. The cardiovascular examination is usually normal. Symptoms are secondary to episodes of ventricular tachycardia of left bundle branch block morphology (Fig 83-9). Patients also exhibit a spectrum of right ventricular impairment, ranging from normal function in some to severe dysfunction in others. Arrhythmias originate in areas of localized dysplasia, limited to the right ventricular free wall. On histology, these areas show variable reduction in myofibril number and interstitial infiltration by lipoid cells, histiocytes, and lymphocytes.

Males are affected four times more often than females. The etiology is unknown, but familial occurrence is widely recognized. The electrocardiogram usually shows frequent ventricular premature depolarizations of left bundle branch block morphology, with inversion of the T waves in leads $V_1$ to $V_4$; "epsilon waves" are found in the ST segments in the right precordial leads in 30% of patients. Evidence of right ventricular dysfunction often can be identified on two-dimensional echocardiography and radionuclide angiography.

Combinations of antiarrhythmic drugs frequently are required to control episodes of ventricular tachycardia. Surgical treatment ranging from simple ventriculotomy to total disconnection and resuturing of the right ventricular free wall has been successful in some cases. The usual course is one of slow deterioration in right ventricular function and a reduction in efficacy of antiarrhythmic treatment.

### Oncocytic Cardiomyopathy

Fewer than 25 cases of oncocytic cardiomyopathy have been reported. Females are affected eight times more frequently than males, and the onset is always before the end of the second year of life. In most cases, the initial presentation is with an episode of supraventricular tachycardia. The clinical course is relatively short and is marked by a recurrence of the arrhythmia that gradually becomes refractory to treatment, eventually degenerating into ventricular fibrillation or cardiac arrest unresponsive to therapy. On postmorten examination of the heart, the striking findings are groups of tiny yellowish nodules that merge on the epicardial surface and on the valve leaflets and chordae, as well as areas of yellowish white discoloration of the myocardium. On microscopic examination, the nodules are composed of large (20 to 40 $\mu$) rounded or polyhedral cells containing an abundant, eosinophilic, finely granular cytoplasm with numerous small vacuoles. Ultrastructural examination shows that most of the cytoplasm is

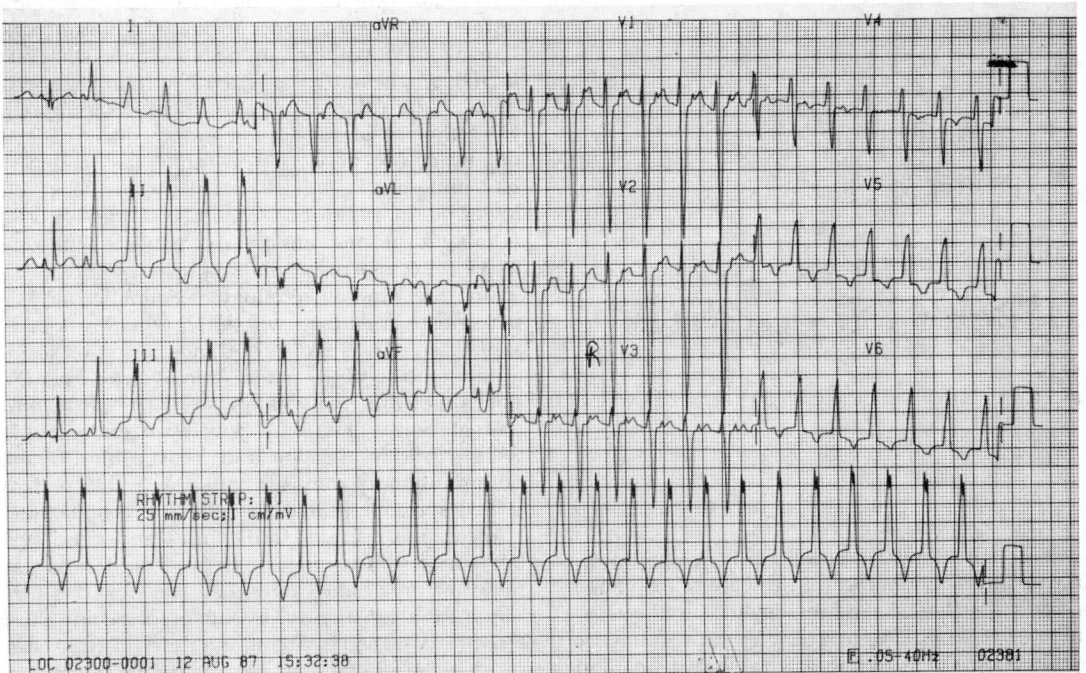

**Figure 83-9.** Twelve-lead electrocardiogram showing ventricular tachycardia with left bundle branch block morphology at a rate of 155/min. The first and second complexes in leads I, II, and III represent a sinus beat and a fusion beat, respectively.

occupied by swollen and distorted mitochondria. Similar changes have been described in the epithelial cells of the anterior pituitary, thyroid, and salivary glands. The etiology is unknown. Because of the early age at presentation, it has been suggested that a viral infection occurring during the first 4 weeks of gestation not only causes the oncocytic changes in the myocytes and in the glandular epithelium, but also is responsible for the eye lesions observed in some patients.

## Selected Readings

Cardiomyopathies: Report of a WHO expert committee. Geneva: WHO Tech Rep Ser 697, 1984.

Benotti JR, Grossman W. Restrictive cardiomyopathy. Annu Rev Med 1984;35:113.

Dungan WJ, Garson, A, Gillette PC. Arrhythmogenic right ventricular dysplasia: a cause of ventricular tachycardia in children with apparently normal hearts. Am Heart J 1981;102:745.

Goodwin JF. The frontiers of cardiomyopathy. Br Heart J 1982;48:1.

Greenwood RD, Nadas AS, Fyler DC. The clinical course of primary myocardial disease in infants and children. Am Heart J 1976;92:549.

Laurie PR. Endocardial fibroelastosis is not a disease. Am J Cardiol 1988;62:468.

Lipshultz SE, et al. Cardiovascular manifestations of human immunodeficiency virus infection in infants and children. Am J Cardiol 1989;63:1489.

Marcus FI, et al. Right ventricular dysplasia: a report of 24 adult cases. Circulation 1982;65:384.

Maron BJ, et al. Hypertrohic cardiomyopathy in infants: clinical features and natural history. Circulation 1982;65:7.

Maron BJ, et al. Hypertrophic cardiomyopathy. Part 1. N Engl J Med 1987;316:780A.

Maron BJ, et al. Hypertrophic cardiomyopathy. Part 2. N Engl J Med 1987;316:844B.

Maron BJ, Roberts WC. Cardiomyopathies in the first two decades of life. Cardiovasc Clin 1981;11:35.

Maron BJ, Spiroto P, Wesley Y, Arce J. Development and progression of left ventricular hypertrophy in children with hypertrophic cardiomyopathy. N Engl J Med 1986;315:610.

Silver MM, Burns JE, Sethi RK, Rowe RD. Oncologic cardiomyopathy in an infant with oncocytosis in exocrine and endocrine glands. Hum Pathol 1980;11:598.

Taliercio CP, et al. Idiopathic dilated cardiomyopathy in the young: clinical profile and natural history. J Am Coll Cardiol 1985;6:1126.

Tripp M. Congestive cardiomyopathy of childhood. In: Advances in pediatrics. London: Year Book Medical Publishers, 1984:179.

Westwood M, Harris R, Burn JL, Barson AJ. Heredity in primary endocardial fibroelastosis. Br Heart J 1975;37:1077.

*Principles and Practice of Pediatrics, Second Edition.*
edited by Frank A. Oski et al. J. B. Lippincott Company, Philadelphia © 1994.

## CHAPTER 84
# Infective Endocarditis

## Richard A. Friedman and Jeffrey R. Starke

Infective endocarditis (IE) refers to a condition in which an organism or organisms infect the endocardium, valves, or related structures. These structures have been previously injured by surgery, trauma, or prior disease. The infecting organism may be bacterial, fungal, chlamydial, rickettsial, or viral. In the first half of the 20th century, many patients with IE had had prior rheumatic heart disease. In the latter part of the century, most children with IE have complex congenital heart defects.

Previous classifications divided cases between acute bacterial endocarditis (ie, rapid, fulminant course with death occurring within 6 weeks) and subacute bacterial endocarditis (ie, slow, indolent course, usually taking several months). The acute form usually was caused by *Staphylococcus aureus*, *Streptococcus pyogenes*, or *Streptococcus pneumoniae*, and the subacute form most commonly involved the viridans streptococci. The newer classification is based on microbiologic cause rather than a description of the course of disease, and the general term infective endocarditis is the name more widely accepted.

## EPIDEMIOLOGY

Widely divergent figures are reported for the incidence of infective endocarditis in children. Most large series are retrospective and do not report the total number of admissions to a given institution during the study period. From 1952 to 1962, 1 of 4500 pediatric admissions to the Hospital for Sick Children in Toronto was for endocarditis. At Boston Children's Hospital, 1 of 1800 admissions from 1963 to 1972 was for endocarditis, but between 1933 and 1963, the incidence was only 1 in 4500. Between 1972 and 1982, 1 of 1280 pediatric admissions to Case Western Reserve–Rainbow Babies Hospital was a child with endocarditis.

The mean age of children with endocarditis is rising, probably because of increases in longevity after corrective or palliative surgery. Between 1930 and 1950, the average age at the time of hospital admission was approximately 5 years, but between 1960 and 1980, this increased from 8.5 to 13 years of age. However, a large retrospective study comparing operated and unoperated children with congenital heart disease (CHD) who developed IE demonstrated no difference in the mean ages of these groups of patients.

The increased incidence of IE among neonates without congenital heart defects seems to be associated with advances in life support in this population and the frequent use of indwelling catheters for nutritional or pharmacologic support.

Virtually any congenital defect may predispose to the development of infective endocarditis. The lifetime risk of developing IE in a patient with an unrepaired, simple ventricular septal defect (VSD) is between 3.2% and 13%. In a large, cooperative study of the natural history of aortic stenosis, pulmonic stenosis, and VSD, the risk of developing endocarditis by 30 years of age was determined to be 9.7% for unoperated patients; if the patient had undergone surgical repair, the incidence of IE was much lower. For aortic stenosis, the risk (1.4%) was slightly increased after surgical intervention, and patients with pulmonic stenosis had a 0.9% risk of developing IE.

In other studies, tetralogy of Fallot accounted for the largest percentage of patients with CHD who developed IE. Ventricular septal defect was the second most common lesion, followed by atrial stenosis (8%), patent ductus arteriosus (7%), and transposition of the great vessels (4%). The most common lesions in patients with CHD who developed endocarditis after surgery were tetralogy of Fallot and transposition of the great vessels with pulmonary stenosis; both occurred in patients who had received systemic-pulmonary shunts. Several other patients had had complex cyanotic CHD with shunts, and 70% of this group developed IE 1 to more than 5 years after surgery. Of patients requiring prosthetic valves, 79% developed infections more than 3 months after surgery. Events predisposing the patient to bacteremia identified in about one third of these cases. Details concerning the unoperated patients with underlying heart disease were not described well, but it appears that most had congenital valve deformities or valve disease secondary to rheumatic fever.

A smaller series from the Yale–New Haven Hospitals showed

a higher incidence of IE in CHD patients who had not undergone surgery than in those who had. Acyanotic lesions were more common in the unoperated group, and cyanotic lesions predominated in the postoperative group. Dacron patches and Gore-Tex grafts were more common sites of infection than prosthetic valves.

It appears that patients with complete correction of tetralogy of Fallot have a low incidence of endocarditis compared with patients who remain palliated. In a large series of patients followed for a mean of 23.7 years, only one patient (1%) developed IE. Tricuspid atresia with diminished pulmonary artery flow commonly is palliated with a shunt procedure; these patients may have an incidence of IE approaching 25%.

A retrospective study looked at the differences in the underlying defects between pediatric patients diagnosed with endocarditis between 1970 to 1990 and earlier studies. As expected, almost half of the patients had undergone surgery for their defect, and many of them had artificial valves inserted at the time of operation. Mitral valve prolapse seems to have become a major risk factor, occurring in 29% of patients with IE.

IE associated with prosthetic materials, especially valves and valved conduits, is likely to increase in the future. Prosthetic valve endocarditis (PVE) has been categorized as early onset (ie, within 3 months of implant) or late onset. The incidence of infection ranges from less than 1% to 10% after implantation. Neither the type of valve nor the site of implant significantly affects the incidence of PVE. *Staphylococcus* species predominate in early-onset PVE, and *Streptococcus* species are the most common cause of infection in late-onset disease. This is probably a reflection of intraoperative contamination. The overall incidence of early-onset PVE has been reduced greatly since the standard administration of perioperative antibiotics was instituted.

## PATHOPHYSIOLOGY

Animal studies and clinical and autopsy investigations have shown that a series of events creates an environment suitable for the establishment of IE. Hemodynamic factors that predispose to turbulence of blood flow and subsequent endothelial damage have been shown to be primary in the development of a nidus of infection in the heart and great vessels. Studies have shown that a Venturi effect is responsible for the fact that the highest yield of bacteria can be found on the low-pressure sink side of a high-pressure jet (ie, left atrial surface of mitral valve in mitral regurgitation, right ventricular side of ventricular septal defect). As a consequence of turbulent blood flow, endothelial damage occurs and initiates the formation of platelet and fibrin deposition. This series of events is similar to that seen in the course of primary plug formation with vascular injury. Exposure to cold, high-cardiac-output states, hormonal manipulations, high altitude, and passage of a sterile catheter across a heart valve in animals also have caused initiation of this lesion.

Growth in fibrin and platelet deposition results in the formation of a nonbacterial thrombotic vegetation (NBTV) that is essential in the pathogenesis of endocarditis. Transient bacteremias that occur as a normal part of daily life may cause colonization of the NBTV. As the NBTV grows in size and bacteria adhere, an infected vegetation develops. The virulence of different bacteria may be directly related to their ability to adhere to the NBTV. A factor that may be important in increased virulence is the ability of certain streptococci found in the oral cavity to produce dextran; the amount of dextran produced by the bacterial strain also may correlate with virulence. Another substance that may be a receptor for certain organisms is fibronectin, a substance found on the surface of NBTV in polyethylene catheter-induced

IE. Organisms such as *S aureus, Candida albicans, Streptococcus sanguis,* and *Streptococcus faecalis* adhere to fibronectin, but nonadherence is the rule for organisms rarely found to cause IE.

After the NBTV is colonized, the size of the vegetation grows by increasing numbers of bacteria and by additional platelet and fibrin deposition. The colonized NBTV produces a constant bacteremia, and reseeding of the vegetation occurs by adherence of circulating organisms to the already enlarging vegetation. Three zones in the vegetation have been described: necrotic endocardium; a broad zone of bacteria, pyknotic nuclear debris, and fibrin; and a thin surface coat of fibrin and leukocytes. Proliferation of bacteria in the protected middle zone is relatively unchecked, because the normal host defense mechanisms are unable to penetrate into the vegetation and penetration of any circulating antimicrobial agent is diminished. Because the internal environment of the middle zone of the NBTV depresses bacterial metabolism, the action of any antimicrobial agent that does penetrate is attenuated.

Pathologic changes observed in the heart are produced by local extension of the infection. Vegetations may be single or multiple, ranging from less than 1 mm to several centimeters. Large lesions may resemble tumors and cause hemodynamically significant stenosis. Certain organisms, such as *Candida* sp, *Haemophilus* sp, and *S aureus*, may produce friable lesions that can embolize. Ulceration of tissue, especially heart valves, may result in perforation and produce the onset of sudden congestive heart failure (CHF). Other complications include rupture of chordae tendineae, abscesses of the valve ring, fistula formation with the development of pericardial empyema and tamponade, aneurysms of the sinus of Valsalva or ventricle, and myocardial infarction secondary to emboli.

Distant organ involvement secondary to emboli may occur. One necropsy review of endocarditis in children found the most common site of distant organ involvement to be the lungs; the kidney was the organ most frequently involved on the systemic side of the circulation. In other studies, cerebral emboli have been found in 30% of adults and children who had IE, with subsequent infarction, abscess, mycotic aneurysm, subarachnoid hemorrhage, and acute hemiplegia of childhood. Microemboli in the cerebral circulation may cause a confused mental state. Strokes usually are secondary to emboli in the middle cerebral artery. Aortic valve infection probably has the highest incidence of embolic complications.

Immunologic mechanisms during subacute IE play an important role in the pathogenesis and sequelae. Cell-mediated and humoral immunity are active in this disease process. A hypergammaglobulinemic state usually exists, caused by polyclonal and antigen-specific B-cell activation. Part of the hypergammaglobulinemia is caused by circulating rheumatoid factors. Levels of rheumatoid factor may decrease with successful therapy and increase with relapse of disease. Antibody responses directed at the infecting organism and nonspecific responses have been demonstrated. It is possible that C3b in conjunction with circulating immune complexes may bind to the surface of B cells and initiate production of antibodies not primarily directed at the infecting organism. Circulating immune complexes are found with increased frequency in patients with long-standing illness, right-sided disease, hypocomplementemic states, and extravalvular manifestations. One study of 29 patients with culture-proven IE found that almost all had levels of circulating immune complexes of higher than 12 μg/mL. A mixed-type cryoglobulinemia occurs in 90% of patients with IE. Renal involvement with focal and diffuse glomerulonephritis has been described, and immune complex deposition is found in both. Other autoantibodies, including antiendocardial, antisarcolemmal, antimyolemmal, and antinuclear, are detected during the course of IE.

# CLINICAL MANIFESTATIONS

The clinical manifestations of IE depend on the underlying pathophysiologic processes of the disease. The extent of local involvement of the myocardium or valves, embolization from vegetations, and activation of immunologic mechanisms play essential roles in clinical expression. Patients with acute IE may present in shock and with a clinical picture consistent with overwhelming sepsis. In some cases, confirmation of endocarditis may be found only at autopsy. The subacute form of the disease may follow an indolent course, and a diagnosis may not be established for weeks or months. Because endocarditis frequently occurs in children with underlying heart disease, subtle changes in their physical examination may be missed unless the examiner is discerning and alert. Table 84-1 lists the major clinical manifestations of IE and their relative frequency of occurrence in children.

The most common finding in IE is fever, although approximately 10% of patients have no fever. It usually is low grade and shows no specific pattern, especially in the subacute form. Other nonspecific complaints include malaise, anorexia, weight loss, fatigue, and sleep disturbances. Involvement of the large joints, with arthralgias or arthritis, occurs in 24% of patients. Nausea, vomiting, and nonspecific abdominal pains are found in 16% of patients. Chest pains, which usually are related to myalgias but are sometimes secondary to pulmonary embolism, especially with tricuspid valve involvement, occur in as many as 10% of older children.

Heart murmurs in patients with infective endocarditis have been accepted as a classic finding. They occur in as many as 90% of affected children, but most of these patients have underlying congenital defects and initially presented with murmurs specific for their lesions. A new or changing murmur occurs in approximately 25% of children. CHF may affect as many as 30% of children with IE and it is especially common in patients who develop a new murmur of valvular insufficiency. Exacerbation of CHF in children with rheumatic or congenital lesions should alert the clinician to consider the diagnosis of IE for patients who previously had been controlled well on medical therapy for their chronic condition.

Signs and symptoms of neurologic involvement are seen in about 20% of children with IE. The sudden development of a clinical picture consistent with cerebral infarction in a child with an underlying heart defect should suggest the diagnosis. Acute hemiplegia, seizures, ataxia, aphasia, focal neurologic defects, sensory loss, and changing mental status may occur as presenting features or even years after the disease process has been treated.

Splenomegaly occurs in about 55% of children with IE, usually in those with subacute disease and activated immune systems. On palpation, the spleen is not tender. Hepatomegaly also is observed in many patients. Infarction of the spleen or abscess formation should be suspected in patients with left upper quadrant pain and tenderness that radiates to the shoulder area. A pleural friction rub or pleural effusion may be observed.

Specific skin lesions associated with IE are more common in adults than in children. Petechiae are seen in about a third of the children, especially in those with a more chronic course. Common sites of involvement are the mucous membranes of the mouth, the conjunctivae, and the extremities. Petechiae are the most common skin manifestation in IE, occurring in as many as 40% of patients; purpura is rare. Osler's nodes, which also have been described in systemic lupus erythematosus and in extremities distal to the sites of prolonged arterial catheterization, are exquisitely tender lesions. They are found most commonly on the pads of the fingers and toes, the thenar and hypothenar eminences, the sides of the fingers, and the skin on the lower part of the arm. There still exists much controversy about whether they represent an immunologic response to infection manifesting as a vasculitis or they are septic emboli. Janeway's lesions are nontender, hemorrhagic plaques that occur frequently on the palms and the soles and represent septic emboli with bacteria, neutrophils, and subsequent necrosis with subcutaneous hemorrhage. Roth's spots are small, pale retinal lesions with areas of hemorrhage that are usually located near the optic disc. Osler's nodes, Janeway's lesions, splinter hemorrhages, and Roth's spots occur in only 5% to 7% of children with endocarditis.

Infants and neonates may present with a clinical picture less specific than that seen in older children. The onset is more acute and clinically mimics overwhelming sepsis. The diagnosis rarely is suspected before death. The use of indwelling vascular catheters has increased the incidence of endocarditis in neonates. Persistent bacteremia associated with a deterioration in pulmonary function, coagulopathies, thrombocytopenia, and the appearance of murmurs should arouse suspicion of possible endocarditis in a neonate.

There are several distinctive features of the clinical presentation of IE in intravenous drug abusers. Previous underlying heart disease is found in one third of these patients. The tricuspid valve is the site most commonly affected, and these patients often have pulmonary complications, including infarction, abscess formation, and signs and symptoms of pleural effusion. Extracardiac sites of infection are found in about two thirds of these patients. Tricuspid insufficiency with findings of a murmur of tricuspid regurgitation, a pulsatile liver, and a gallop rhythm are found in 33% of patients.

# DIAGNOSIS

## Laboratory Investigation

Table 84-2 summarizes the most common laboratory findings in children with IE. Blood cultures are the single most important diagnostic tool for establishing the diagnosis of IE. Because bacteremia usually is continuous and low grade, the timing and site of collection do not affect the yield. In approximately 66% of all cases of IE, the blood cultures grow the infecting organism, and in 90%, the results of the first two blood cultures are positive. If a patient has received antibiotics before the culture is tried, the chance of obtaining a positive culture may be reduced from between 95% and 100% to 64%. If pretreatment has occurred, placing the blood sample in hypertonic media may enhance the

| TABLE 84-1. Symptoms and Physical Findings in Infective Endocarditis | |
|---|---|
| Symptom/Finding | Incidence (%) |
| Fever | 56–100 |
| Anorexia/weight loss | 8–83 |
| Malaise | 40–79 |
| Arthralgias | 16–38 |
| Gastrointestinal problems | 9–36 |
| Chest pain | 5–20 |
| Heart failure | 9–47 |
| Splenomegaly | 36–67 |
| Petechiae | 10–50 |
| Embolic events | 14–50 |
| New/changing murmur | 9–44 |
| Clubbing | 2–42 |
| Osler's nodes | 7–8 |
| Roth's spots | 0–6 |
| Janeway's lesions | 0–10 |
| Splinter hemorrhages | 0–10 |

## TABLE 84-2. Laboratory Findings

| Finding | Incidence (%) |
|---|---|
| Elevated erythrocyte sedimentation rate | 71–94 |
| Positive rheumatoid fever | 25–55 |
| Anemia | 19–79 |
| Positive blood culture | 68–98 |
| Hematuria | 28–47 |

chance of isolating the organism. Patients with fungal endocarditis may have only intermittently positive blood cultures, and the organism may take a week or longer to grow in culture.

Ideally, three to five sets of blood cultures should be obtained within the first 24 hours. These specimens should be taken from different sites and contain 3 to 5 mL of blood. Thioglycolate broth should be used, and the bottles should be kept for 3 weeks to detect slow-growing organisms. Nutritionally variant streptococci should be suspected if a gram-positive coccus is isolated in broth but fails to grow in subculture. The organism should then be subcultured onto media enriched with pyridoxal phosphate or L-cysteine.

Blood cultures may be negative in 10% to 15% of cases of suspected endocarditis. This may occur because of prior administration of antibiotics; endocarditis due to rickettsiae, chlamydiae, or viruses; slow-growing organisms (eg, *Candida* sp, *Haemophilus* sp, *Brucella* sp) or nutritionally variant streptococci; infections due to anaerobic organisms; nonbacterial thrombotic vegetation endocarditis; mural endocarditis; right-sided endocarditis; fungal endocarditis (especially *Aspergillus* sp); or an incorrect diagnosis. Additional sites, including urine, sputum, cerebrospinal fluid, synovial fluid, bone marrow, and lymph nodes, may be infected concomitantly, and cultures of these additional sites should be included if blood cultures fail to demonstrate an infecting agent.

Adjunctive laboratory tests needed include measurement of the erythrocyte sedimentation rate (ESR), which is elevated in as many as 90% of patients and correlates with the hypergammaglobulinemia found in this disease. An artifactually low ESR may be found with renal disease, severe CHF, or polycythemia. The ESR should decrease toward normal if therapy has been successful, and serial measurements may be helpful in monitoring therapy. A positive rheumatoid factor has been found in one fourth to one half of pediatric patients with IE and may be supportive evidence for the diagnosis in cases of culture-negative endocarditis. Immune complex-mediated glomerulonephritis may result in hypocomplementemia. Anemia, usually caused by a chronic disease state, is found in 40% of patients. Because children with cyanotic congenital heart disease frequently develop IE, the finding of a normal or slightly high hemoglobin level should suggest the possibility of anemia. Although leukocytosis is not uncommon, leukopenia may occur in acute cases with overwhelming sepsis. Microemboli and consequent microinfarcts in the kidney produce hematuria with or without proteinuria, casts, and bacteremia in 25% to 50% of patients.

Circulating immune complexes as measured by the Raji cell radioimmune assay or the $^{123}$I-C1q-binding assay are present in most adults with IE, although they may be conspicuously absent in acute disease. Immune complexes may be found in septicemic patients and in as many as 10% of normal adult controls. Although there have been few studies of circulating immune complex levels in children with IE, elevated levels have been found in some patients.

Serologic testing for specific organisms may be helpful in culture-negative endocarditis. Antibodies against teichoic acids, which are major components of the cell wall in *S aureus*, may be present in 85% of adults with IE, although the false-positive rate may be as high as 10%. A teichoic acid antibody titer of >1 : 1 in a bacteremic adult patient correlates with deep-seated infections, including but not restricted to endocarditis. However, teichoic acid antibody levels do not differentiate the type of deep-seated infection. As with circulating immune complexes, serial measurements of teichoic acid antibody levels may correlate with successful therapy. Unfortunately, no data exist concerning teichoatic acid antibody levels in children with IE.

## Echocardiography

The role of echocardiography in helping to establish the diagnosis of IE has grown considerably, because the technology has improved vastly since single-crystal M-mode techniques were first introduced. The M-mode echocardiogram uses a single, narrow ultrasound beam, and the reflected ultrasound echoes are recorded on moving paper. The two-dimensional (2D) echocardiogram uses multiple echo beams and provides a cross-sectional moving image of the heart, which can be recorded from several angles. The 2D technique usually is superior to the M-mode technique in investigating vegetative lesions. Some areas of the heart, such as the pulmonary valve, are visualized better using 2D imaging, and the increased sensitivity of this technique in detecting pulmonary valve endocarditis has been documented. The value of 2D echo in prosthetic valve endocarditis also is superior to that of M-mode echo. An echo-free space found in more than one tomographic plane has aided the diagnosis of perivalvular abscess, which may complicate 30% of the native valve endocarditis cases and even more cases of prosthetic valve endocarditis. Adjunctive use of the Doppler technique to diagnose prosthetic valve regurgitation before it becomes apparent clinically may aid in earlier diagnosis. The sensitivity of echocardiography in detecting vegetative lesions in suspected endocarditis in adults ranges from 13% to 83%, with a greater sensitivity exhibited in the more recently published series using the 2D technique. Several studies have concluded that patients with a "positive echo" were twice as likely to develop serious complications (usually emboli, more commonly cerebral than peripheral) and that patients were at higher risk for death or severe CHF if the vegetation was larger than 1 cm². However, the risk of embolization does not appear to correlate with vegetation size.

The use of transesophageal echocardiography (TEE) to evaluate the patient for vegetations has become important. TEE takes advantage of the proximity of the heart, especially the left atrium to the esophagus. This technique also eliminates the inability to image transthoracically in some patients who do not have good "echo windows" from that approach. The quality of the image is better, making diagnosis more certain. Although this technique can be accomplished using light sedation, our experience has been that heavy sedation, administered by an anesthesiologist is preferable.

One study in adults with endocarditis using the transesophageal approach yielded the following conclusions: when combined with a high clinical suspicion of endocarditis, TEE offers a high sensitivity for properly diagnosing IE, and TEE is significantly better than TTE in imaging vegetations in these patients. Our clinical experience has confirmed these conclusions, and we now routinely use TEE if TTE is equivocal or negative for a patient who we suspect has the disease.

In a study of 15 children with IE using M-mode and 2D techniques, vegetations were detected in 10 (66%) of 15 of patients. Of the 10, 3 had systemic emboli and 2 died, but none of the patients without an echo-proven vegetation had an embolic complication. This suggested that echocardiography may help to identify a high-risk population that could benefit from surgical intervention. Some studies have suggested that the size and mobility of a vegetation may be useful in differentiating bacterial from fungal endocarditis. In our experience, however, this claim is probably not valid, because large vegetations are seen frequently in bacterial or fungal endocarditis.

A negative echocardiographic study does not rule out the presence of vegetations. The limit of resolution on most equipment limits the detection of vegetations to those larger than 2 to 3 mm. Poor technique also may hinder evaluation. Rheumatic heart disease with preexisting valve disease, mitral valve prolapse with thickened leaflets, marantic vegetations, Löffler's endocarditis, Chiari's networks in the right atrium, and valve ring abscesses pose interpretive problems to the echocardiographer.

After a vegetation is detected, it may show no significant change during therapy, and a recurrence of disease cannot be diagnosed unless there is a noticeable increase in size or a new vegetation appears. Attempts to estimate serially the size of a vegetation are fraught with technical and interpretive error and are probably of little value. However, continued growth of a vegetation coexistent with persistent bacteremia or evidence of further endocardial infiltration may indicate a treatment failure or the need for surgical intervention. One study attempted to define risk factors involved with an echocardiographically demonstrable vegetation in adult patients with IE. Significant complications included peripheral and central nervous system (CNS) embolization, failure to respond to therapy, CHF, need for surgery, and death. Using univariate analysis in patients with native left-sided valve endocarditis, the investigators found that vegetation size, extent, mobility, and consistency were all significant predictors of complications. Multivariate analysis demonstrated that size, extent, and mobility could be used to "score" a patient

into a high-risk group. An echocardiogram examination at the time of hospital discharge of a patient after an apparently successful course of antibiotic therapy can be used as a baseline for further evaluation.

## Electrocardiography

Numerous electrocardiographic abnormalities may be found throughout the course of IE. Ventricular ectopy in patients with hemodynamic compromise may be life threatening. Atrial fibrillation in adults and children may be secondary to atrioventricular valve regurgitation. Extension of abscess formation or an inflammatory response may cause direct injury to the conduction system. Complete right bundle branch block, left anterior or posterior fascicular block, and complete atrioventricular block have been reported. Abscess formation in the perivalvular aortic region may cause direct injury to the atrioventricular node because of its proximity to that structure. This may result in sudden death unless temporary and eventually permanent pacing is instituted.

## PROPHYLAXIS

The use of antibiotics before and during any procedure that induces a transient bacteremia has become standard medical practice for the prevention of IE. There are numerous reports of failures, with subsequent development of endocarditis. Although failure often is related to inappropriate drug regimens, infection occasionally develops despite adherence to published guidelines.

TABLE 84-3. Recommended Antibiotic Regimens for Endocarditis Prophylaxis in Children

| For Dental/Respiratory Tract Procedures | | | For Gastrointestinal/Genitourinary Procedures | | |
|---|---|---|---|---|---|
| Regimen | Condition | Dosage | Regimen | Condition | Dosage |
| Standard | For dental procedures that cause gingival bleeding and oral/respiratory tract surgery | Penicillin V (1.0–2.0 g orally 1 h before the procedure, then 0.5–1.0 g 6 h later); for patients unable to take oral medications, aqueous penicillin G (1–2 million U IV or IM 30–60 min before, and 0.5–1.0 million units 6 h later) | Standard | For genitourinary/ gastrointestinal tract procedures indicated | Ampicillin (50 mg/kg IM or IV) plus gentamicin (2.0 mg/kg IM or IV) given 30 min to 1 h before procedure; one follow-up dose may be given 8 h later |
| Special | Parenteral regimen for use when maximal protection is desired (eg, for patients with prosthetic valves) | Ampicillin (50 mg/kg IM or IV) plus gentamicin (2.0 mg/kg IM or IV) 0.5 h before the procedure, followed by oral penicillin V (0.5–1.0 g) 6 h later; alternatively, parenteral regimen may be repeated once 8 h later | Special | Oral regimen for minor or repetitive procedures in low-risk patients | Amoxicillin (50 mg/kg orally 1 h before procedure and 50 mg/kg 6 h later) |
| | Oral regimen for penicillin-allergic patients and those on rheumatic fever prophylaxis | Erythromycin (20 mg/kg orally 1 h before, then 10 mg/kg 6 h later) | | Penicillin-allergic patients | Vancomycin (15–20 mg/kg IV) plus gentamicin (2 mg/kg IM or IV) 1 h before procedure; may be repeated once 8 h later |
| | Parenteral regimen for penicillin-allergic patients and those on rheumatic fever prophylaxis | Vancomycin (15–20 mg/kg IV 1 h before; no repeated dose necessary) | | | |

From Shulman ST, et al. Prevention of bacterial endocarditis. A statement for health professionals by the Committee on Rheumatic Fever and Bacterial Endocarditis of the Council on Cardiovascular Diseases in the Young of the American Heart Association. Am J Dis Child 1985;139:232.

In an attempt to consolidate the current opinion on appropriate antibiotic regimens for endocarditis prophylaxis, the Committee on Rheumatic Fever and Bacterial Endocarditis of the Council on Cardiovascular Diseases in the Young of the American Heart Association published recommendations in 1985 (Table 84-3).

There are numerous theories to explain how antibiotics given prophylactically prevent endocarditis. Two possibilities are that the magnitude of a bacteremia associated with a procedure is reduced by the antibiotic or that bacterial adherence mechanisms are altered such that a nidus of infection would be unlikely to develop. The latter hypothesis is supported by study in which the effects of single-dose amoxicillin and erythromycin after the development of sterile aortic vegetations was evaluated in rats. In this model, periodontally diseased teeth were extracted to produce a bacteremia similar to the conditions that might occur in humans during dental manipulation. Endocarditis developed in 89% of the control group (ie, vegetations but no prophylaxis). The organisms cultivated from the rat's dental plaque were identical to those found in blood culture, confirming the relation between extraction and seeding of the vegetation. The incidence of bacteremia was almost the same for the control and the treated group, but almost none of the treated group developed endocarditis.

Special circumstances can affect the use of antibiotic prophylaxis. Tables 84-4 and 84-5 list various conditions and procedures and the infecting organisms responsible for the development of IE in children and adults. In patients requiring multiple dental procedures who recently have received antibiotic prophylaxis, oral streptococci with reduced susceptibility may flourish, possibly resulting in ineffective prophylaxis. Although 3 g of amoxicillin given once per week does not result in a high incidence of resistant streptococci, erythromycin given at the same frequency may result in a significant number of resistant organisms. If prophylaxis is required twice in 1 month, amoxicillin can be given as recommended. In penicillin-allergic patients who require erythromycin, the interval between dental procedures should be increased if possible. If a dental abscess is found in a patient undergoing treatment for IE, it should be drained surgically.

Patients who develop a condition that must be treated surgically and who are being treated for IE should receive additional prophylaxis specific for the area of surgical interest and in accord with the published recommendations. Patients receiving penicillin prophylaxis for rheumatic fever should receive additional prophylaxis as previously described. Elective surgery, for whatever reason, should be postponed until the treatment of active infective endocarditis is completed. Prophylaxis should be instituted for patients with permanent transvenous pacing leads, cerebral ventriculoatrial shunts, and arteriovenous shunts.

The use of antibiotic prophylaxis in patients with mitral valve prolapse (MVP) is controversial. This condition exists in approximately 5% of the population in the United States. A case-control study comparing persons with MVP to normal controls found that the odds for the association of IE with MVP was 8.2; it increased to 15.2 when a murmur of mitral regurgitation was present. Another study attempted to define the absolute risk (ie, chances of developing IE over a time period) rather than the relative risk. The group with mitral valve prolapse and no mitral regurgitation had an absolute risk for the development of IE of 0.0046% (1 person in 21,950/year), compared with 0.520% (1 person in 1920/year) for the group with MVP and mitral regurgitation. During a 50-year period, 26 of 1000 patients with MVP and mitral regurgitation will develop IE; only 2 of 1000 patients with MVP but without mitral regurgitation will develop IE, which is not significantly greater than the risk to the general population. This analysis suggests that routine prophylaxis should be used only in patients with MVP and mitral regurgitation. This study also showed that male gender and an age greater than 45 years were independent risk factors for the development of IE in patients with MVP, suggesting that they would receive added benefit from routine antibiotic prophylaxis.

Unfortunately, there are not many reports on the natural history of MVP in children that address the risk of developing IE.

---

**TABLE 84-4.    Conditions and Procedures Related to Endocarditis Prophylaxis**

| Cardiac Conditions for Which Endocarditis Prophylaxis Is Recommended | Procedures for Which Endocarditis Prophylaxis Is Recommended |
|---|---|
| Prosthetic cardiac valves (mechanical and biosynthetic) | All dental procedures likely to induce gingival bleeding |
| Most congenital cardiac malformations | Tonsillectomy and adenoidectomy |
| Surgically constructed systemic-pulmonary shunts | Surgical procedures or biopsy involving respiratory mucosa |
| Rheumatic and other acquired valvular disease | Bronchoscopy, especially with a rigid scope |
| Idiopathic hypertrophic subaortic stenosis | Incision and drainage of infected tissue |
| History of bacterial endocarditis | Selected genitourinary and gastrointestinal procedures (eg, cystoscopy, urethral catheterization, urinary tract surgery, gallbladder or colonic surgery, esophageal or anal dilatation, colonoscopy, upper GI tract endoscopy with biopsy, proctosigmoidoscopic biopsy) |
| Mitral valve prolapse with insufficiency | |
| Foreign material in the heart | |
| | Cardiac surgery |
| **Conditions for Which Prophylaxis Is NOT Recommended** | **Procedures for Which Prophylaxis Is NOT Recommended Routinely** |
| Isolated secundum atrial septal defect | Orotracheal intubation |
| Secundum atrial septal defect repaired without a patch 6 or more months earlier | Cardiac catheterization |
| Patent ductus arteriosus ligated and divided 6 or more months earlier | Cesarean section |
| | Therapeutic abortion |
| | Intrauterine device insertion or removal |

From Shulman ST, et al. Prevention of bacterial endocarditis. A statement for health professionals by the Committee on Rheumatic Fever and Bacterial Endocarditis of the Council on Cardiovascular Diseases in the Young of the American Heart Association. Am J Dis Child 1985;139:232.

TABLE 84-5.    Procedures Associated With Bacteremia in Children and Adults

| Procedure | Associated Organism | Positive Blood Cultures (%) |
|---|---|---|
| Dental extraction | Streptococcus, diphtheroids | 30–65 |
| Chewing gum, candy | Streptococcus, Staphylococcus epidermidis | 0–51 |
| Brushing teeth | Streptococcus | 0–26 |
| Tonsillectomy | Streptococcus, Haemophilus, diphtheroids | 28–38 |
| Bronchoscopy (rigid scope) | Streptococcus, S epidermidis | 15 |
| Bronchoscopy (flexible scope) | | 0 |
| Nasotracheal intubation/suctioning | Streptococcus, aerobic gram-negative rods | 16 |
| Orotracheal intubation | | 0 |
| Sigmoidoscopy/colonoscopy | Enterococci, aerobic gram-negative rods | 0–9.5 |
| Upper GI endoscopy | Streptococcus, Neisseria, S epidermidis, diphtheroids, other | 8–12 |
| Percutaneous liver | Pneumococci, aerobic gram-negative rods, S aureus, other | 3–14 |
| Urethral catheterization | Not stated | 8 |
| Manipulation of Staphylococcus aureus suppurative foci | | 54 |

From Everett ED, Hirschmann JU. Transient bacteremia and endocarditis prophylaxis. A review. Medicine (Baltimore) 1977;56:61.

None of the 30 children with MVP followed in one study for an average of 4 to 5 years developed IE, indicating no additional risk for this lesion. However, the relatively short duration of follow-up should preclude such a firm conclusion. A prospective analysis of 300 patients with MVP with a mean follow-up period of 6.1 years found a 6% incidence of IE, which accounted for 15% of all serious complications in these patients.

The intermittent nature of the auscultatory click associated with some cases of mitral valve prolapse implies that the regurgitation associated with this lesion may be intermittent as well. Until additional data for the exact incidence of mitral regurgitation associated with MVP in children are available, we think that the safest course would be to prescribe routine subacute bacterial endocarditis (SBE) prophylaxis for all children who have documented MVP.

TEE may pose a risk similar to orotracheal intubation (ie, no prophylaxis required). There has been one reported case of endocarditis after an apparently uncomplicated procedure. However, a large study looking at the incidence of transient bacteremia after performing TEE did not demonstrate a significant increase in the rate of transient bacteremia and recommended not requiring the administration of prophylaxis for this type of echocardiogram.

## MICROBIOLOGY

Many different organisms have been associated with infective endocarditis in humans. Table 84-6 lists the most common causative agents responsible for the development of infective endocarditis. Gram-positive cocci are the etiologic agents of 90% of cases in which an organism is isolated. Streptococci, especially of the viridans group, remain the bacteria isolated most frequently. Because of the increasing role of surgery and prosthetic material in the correction and palliation of congenital heart disease, the percentage of cases caused by staphylococci, gram-negative bacilli, and fungi have increased. Identification of the

causative agent is the single most important procedure involved in confirming the diagnosis, directing therapy, and predicting outcome and possible complications.

### Streptococci

Streptococci are a heterogenous group of organisms. There are different systems of classification that depend on several features, including patterns of hemolysis observed on blood agar plates, biochemical reactions, growth characteristics, antigenic reaction, and serologic relatedness. The least discriminating system is based on the type of hemolysis produced by a strain of streptococcus when grown on a blood agar plate. In beta hemolysis, there is a clear zone surrounding each colony caused by complete blood cell lysis; in gamma hemolysis, there is no detectable hemolysis;

TABLE 84-6.    Causative Agents in Pediatric Infective Endocarditis

| Organism | Incidence (%) |
|---|---|
| Streptococci | |
|   Viridans | 17–72 |
|   Enterococci | 0–12 |
|   Pneumococci | 0–21 |
|   β-Hemolytic | 0–8 |
| Staphylococci | |
|   S aureus | 5–40 |
|   S epidermidis | 0–15 |
| Gram-negative aerobic bacilli | 0–15 |
| Fungi | 0–12 |
| Miscellaneous | 0–10 |
| Culture negative | 2–32 |

and in *alpha hemolysis*, an inner layer of unhemolyzed cells and an outer layer of hemolyzed cells produce a greenish discoloration in the medium. The term *viridans streptococci* refers to most strains that are α-hemolytic, although other strains such as the pneumococcus also may be α-hemolytic. The group of viridans streptococci is made of many different species that vary considerably in biochemical properties and biological behaviors. For instance, the viridans streptococcus *S milleri* is especially virulent and causes a high incidence of suppurative intracardiac and extracardiac complications in patients with endocarditis. When a viridans streptococcus is isolated in a patient with endocarditis, it may be valuable for species determination to be performed by the laboratory. The most common viridans streptococci isolated from adults with infective endocarditis are *S sanguis*, *S bovis*, *S mutans*, and *S mitior*.

The Lancefield typing system was devised to differentiate β-hemolytic streptococci into serogroups by means of antigenic differences in cell-wall carbohydrates. Certain α- and γ-hemolytic strains also contain group-specific antigen, such as enterococci, which contain group D cell wall carbohydrates. Viridans streptococci may be Lancefield typable or nontypable.

The viridans streptococci are the most common etiologic agents in childhood infective endocarditis, accounting for about 40% of cases. These organisms are part of the indigenous flora of the mouth and gastrointestinal tract. Any procedure, such as dental surgery or extraction, that disrupts the mucosal integrity in these areas predisposes to bacteremia with viridans streptococci. They commonly cause endocarditis in patients with underlying heart disease, but they are less common causes of postoperative infection. Although viridans streptococci usually are associated with a more indolent, subacute clinical presentation, they can cause acute, rapidly progressive disease. Most strains of viridans streptococci are exquisitely susceptible to penicillin, although prior antibiotic administration may promote infection with resistant strains. Recurrences and treatment failures are rare.

Nutritionally variant viridans streptococci are being recognized increasingly as the etiologic agent of IE in children. The organisms grow in broth, but do not grow in subculture unless L-cysteine or pyridoxine is added to the media. These organisms must be looked for in every case of culture-negative endocarditis.

The enterococcus is an unusual strain of streptococci because it is much less susceptible to penicillin; successful treatment requires use of an additional antibiotic, usually gentamicin in children. Enterococcal endocarditis is less common in children than in adults, accounting for only 4% of pediatric cases. This strain of organisms inhabits the gastrointestinal and genitourinary tracts and may enter the blood stream after instrumentation to these areas. Although 40% of adult patients with enterococcal endocarditis have no underlying heart disease, affected children rarely have previously normal hearts. Endocarditis should be considered in all infants and children with unexplained enterococcal bacteremia.

The pneumococcus is an α-hemolytic streptococcus, but the clinical presentation of pneumococcal endocarditis is usually very different from that of endocarditis carried by viridans streptococci. In the preantibiotic era, the pneumococcus accounted for 10% to 15% of cases of endocarditis, but it now causes fewer than 2% of cases. Approximately half of these infections occur in persons without underlying heart disease. The clinical course usually is acute and fulminant, with valvular dysfunction and cardiac decompensation occurring frequently. Early surgical intervention usually is required, because the mortality rate with medical management alone is 75%.

Endocarditis caused by β-hemolytic streptococci also was more common in the preantibiotic era than it is today. Most cases are caused by Lancefield groups B and G strains; groups C and A strains rarely cause endocarditis.

## Staphylococci

Staphylococci are associated with 20% to 30% of the pediatric cases of infective endocarditis, and the incidence is rising. Most are caused by coagulase-positive *S aureus*, but coagulase-negative staphylococci are causing an increased number of infections after cardiac surgery. *S aureus* may attack previously normal heart valves and normal cardiac structures. It is the most likely cause of acute endocarditis in a previously normal child. The course is often fulminant, with frequent suppurative complications in the heart (eg, myocardial abscess, pericarditis, valve ring abscess) and in other organs. *S aureus* causes more than 50% of cases of endocarditis among intravenous drug abusers, but their disease tends to be less severe. The origin of the infecting strain is thought to be the addict's own nose or skin, not the injection paraphernalia. Endocarditis associated with indwelling vascular catheters or prosthetic heart valves frequently is caused by *S aureus* bacteremia, even if a peripheral focus of infection exists. Treatment of *S aureus* endocarditis has been complicated by the emergence of methicillin-resistant strains, which may require synergistic antibiotic combinations such as vancomycin and rifampin for cure.

The incidence of endocarditis caused by coagulase-negative staphylococci, usually *S epidermidis*, is rising rapidly. These organisms rarely cause infective endocarditis in persons without underlying heart disease, but they are common etiologic agents of endocarditis after cardiac surgery. Coagulase-negative staphylococci are the major agents in prosthetic valve endocarditis, causing 25% to 67% of early cases and 25% to 33% of late cases. These organisms can be locally invasive. The mortality rate for adults with *S epidermidis* prosthetic valve endocarditis with no valve replacement may approach 75%.

## Gram-Negative Organisms

Gram-negative bacteria are the etiologic agents in 4% to 5% of pediatric cases of endocarditis. However, the percentage of children with gram-negative bacteremia who develop endocarditis is very low. Burn patients, immunosuppressed hosts, recipients of prosthetic heart valves, and narcotics addicts are at increased risk for gram-negative enteric bacteremia. Many species of gram-negative enteric organisms have caused infective endocarditis in children, but no clear pattern has emerged, because data are limited to case reports and general medicine reviews. Morbidity and mortality rates are high, with frequent development of large vegetations, embolic complications, and cardiac decompensation. Endocarditis should be suspected in patients with gram-negative infection if bacteremia persists despite appropriate antibiotic therapy, especially if an unexplained heart murmur and anemia develop. In the early postoperative period after cardiac surgery, sustained gram-negative bacteremia commonly is secondary to other foci of infection (eg, urinary tract) and does not imply the presence of endocarditis.

*Pseudomonas* sp endocarditis is especially difficult to treat and has a high mortality rate. Most of these patients abuse intravenous drugs. Major embolic complications and CHF are common.

Other gram-negative organisms associated with infective endocarditis are the HACEK coccobacilli—*Haemophilus* sp, *Actinobacillus* sp, *Cardiobacterium* sp, *Eikenella* sp, and *Kingella* sp. Endocarditis due to *Haemophilus influenzae* has been reported in several children, but cases due to *Haemophilus aphrophilus* and *Haemophilus parainfluenzae* are more common. A similar organism, *Streptobacillus moniliformis*, has been linked to endocarditis. All HACEK organisms are fastidious and may require 2 to 3 weeks for primary isolation, needing subculture onto chocolate agar in 5% to 10% $CO_2$ for optimal growth. These organisms should be considered in all presentations of culture-negative endocarditis.

In the preantibiotic era, *Neisseria gonorrhoeae* was responsible for 10% of IE cases. Since 1942, fewer than 40 cases have been reported. The onset usually is acute. It tends to attack previously normal valves, and the need for valve replacement is frequent. Nonpathogenic *Neisseria* species are isolated more frequently in endocarditis than are gonococci, but they usually attack abnormal or prosthetic valves.

## Gram-Positive Bacilli

*Corynebacterium* organisms are unusual agents of infective endocarditis, but they may be found on normal and abnormal heart valves. Both toxigenic and nontoxigenic strains of *C diphtheriae* cause endocarditis in children. *Listeria monocytogenes* endocarditis is rare in children and has a high rate of mortality. Unlike other forms of listeriosis, it is not seen frequently in immunocompromised hosts, and it has not been associated with listeriosis in neonates. Fewer than 30 cases of *Lactobacillus* sp endocarditis have been described. This infection usually follows dental manipulation in a person with underlying heart disease. Embolic phenomena are common, but treatment usually is successful if appropriate antibiotics are used.

## Fungi

The most common predisposing conditions for fungal endocarditis in children are cardiovascular surgery, prolonged antibiotic usage, and an indwelling intravenous catheter. Most infections are caused by *C albicans*, but other *Candida* species, including *C tropicalis*, *C stellatoides*, *C krusei*, *C parapsilosis*, and *C guilliermondi*, have been implicated. Endocarditis caused by intravenous drug abuse is more frequently caused by species other than *C albicans*. The clinical course usually is subacute. Embolic phenomena are extremely common and may be the first clinical indication of infection. Large, friable vegetations occur frequently. Ocular and cutaneous manifestations may aid in the diagnosis. The prognosis for *Candida* endocarditis is poor because of the propensity for septic emboli to major organs, the tendency for invasion into the myocardium, and the poor penetration of antifungal agents into the vegetations. Diagnosis may be delayed by the tendency for blood cultures to be negative or positive only intermittently. Successful therapy usually requires surgical intervention.

*Aspergillus* organisms are the second most common cause of fungal endocarditis in children. Most patients have had underlying heart disease and recent cardiac surgery, although normal valves can be affected. The manifestations seen most frequently are fever and emboli, especially to the central nervous system. Only four cases in children have been diagnosed antemortem, three by culture of peripheral emboli. Blood cultures usually are negative. Surgical removal of all infected material is recommended, although only one child has been treated successfully.

Other fungi that rarely cause infective endocarditis include *Histoplasma capsulatum*, *Coccidioides immitis*, *Cryptococcus neoformans*, *Torulopsis glabrata*, *Hormodendrum* sp, *Mucor* sp, *Paecilomyces* sp, *Phialophora* sp, and *Chrysosporium* sp.

## Other Organisms

Anaerobic bacilli cause 1% of IE in adults, but reports of anaerobic endocarditis in children are exceedingly rare.

Infective endocarditis caused by *Coxiella burnetii* (ie, Q fever) has been documented in more than 100 patients, including several children. Clinical manifestations, including anemia, hepatosplenomegaly, fever, and intracardiac vegetations, are similar in children and adults. The diagnosis is confirmed by serologic and immunohistologic investigation. Although Q fever has been documented in the United States, it is much more common in England, Australia, and France.

## TREATMENT

Several general principles provide the basis for treatment of IE. The preferable route of antibiotic administration is intravenous. Oral antibiotics may be absorbed poorly or erratically, especially in infants, which may result in treatment failure. A course of at least 4 and up to 6 weeks or longer is required to sterilize vegetations and prevent relapse. Bacteriostatic agents are contraindicated, and may lead to failure or relapse if employed. Synergism between certain agents may produce a rapid bactericidal effect and allow smaller doses of each drug to be administered, thereby reducing possible toxic side effects. Certain drug combinations, however, such as penicillin and chloramphenicol, may be antagonistic.

After initiation of therapy, daily blood cultures should be obtained. Although negative blood cultures may not necessarily correlate with a therapeutic success, continued positive blood cultures usually indicate a need for investigation of the serum concentration of the drug in the patient, for the addition of another agent, or for a change in therapy. If the patient has not responded clinically to initial antibiotic therapy within several days, more blood cultures should be obtained. In addition, attention to the patient's clinical course is essential. Patients usually begin to improve within a few days of the initiation of appropriate therapy, although persistent fever may occur occasionally in patients who eventually have a good outcome. Electrocardiographic monitoring should be performed in the early stages to assess for the presence of arrhythmias or the development of conduction disturbances that may require immediate attention. If second-degree atrioventricular block develops during an episode of endocarditis, temporary transvenous pacing should be considered. Pacing always should be instituted for third-degree atrioventricular block. Physical examination to assess for development of regurgitant murmurs or embolic events also is mandatory.

Current recommendations for optimal therapy in pediatric infective endocarditis are based largely on studies from adult patients. These regimens usually are more successful and less toxic in children than in adults (Table 84-7).

The timing of therapy generally depends on the clinical condition of the patient. In a case of suspected IE in a seriously ill child, empirical therapy should begin immediately after obtaining the appropriate blood cultures. In patients in whom *S aureus* is probable (eg, acute presentation, IV drug abusers), a penicillinase-resistant penicillin should be added to the usual regimen of penicillin G and an aminoglycoside. The latter two agents would be employed in a patient with a subacute presentation and would be appropriate for viridans streptococci, enterococci, and most gram-negative organisms. Patients who have recently undergone cardiac surgery would receive vancomycin in addition to an aminoglycoside because of the high incidence of hospital-acquired *S epidermidis*, which may be resistant to methicillin or nafcillin. Once the blood cultures are examined for sensitivity to various antibiotic agents, therapy may be tailored appropriately for the patient.

Several tests are available to determine how sensitive an organism is to treatment with antimicrobials. The *minimal inhibitory concentration (MIC)* is defined as the lowest concentration of the agent that prevents visible growth, usually in broth, after incubation for 18 to 24 hours. The *minimal bactericidal concentration (MBC)* is defined as the lowest concentration resulting in either sterilization or a decline in bacterial count of 99.9%. Monitoring the inhibitory and bactericidal activity of the patient's serum is

TABLE 84-7. Recommended Antimicrobial Therapy for Infective Endocarditis in Children

| Alternate Agent in Infecting Organism | Length of Antibiotic Agent* | Alternate Agent in Allergic Patients* | Length of Therapy (weeks) |
|---|---|---|---|
| Streptococci | | | |
| Susceptible viridans (MIC <0.2 μg/mL penicillin G) | Aqueous penicillin G + streptomycin or gentamicin | Vancomycin ± streptomycin or gentamicin | 2–4 |
| Resistant viridans (MIC <2.0 μg/mL penicillin G) and enterococci | Aqueous penicillin G plus gentamicin | Vancomycin + gentamicin | 4–6 |
| Staphylococci | | | |
| S aureus (methicillin susceptible) | Nafcillin or methicillin ± gentamicin | Cephalothin or vancomycin | 6–8 |
| S aureus (methicillin resistant) | Vancomycin | Same | 6–8 |
| S epidermidis | Vancomycin ± rifampin | Same | 6–8 |
| Gram-negative organisms | | | |
| Enteric bacilli | Ampicillin + gentamicin (based on in vitro susceptibilities) | | 6–8 |
| Pseudomonas aeruginosa | Ticarcillin + gentamicin | | 6–8 |
| Haemophilus | Ampicillin ± gentamicin | | 4–6 |
| Culture negative | | | |
| Postoperative | Vancomycin + gentamicin | | 6–8 |
| Nonoperative | Nafcillin or methicillin + gentamicin ± aqueous penicillin G | | 6–8 |

\* All daily doses for children with normal renal function are as follows:

Aqueous penicillin G: 200,000–250,000 U/kg, in divided doses q 4–6 h.
Streptomycin: 20–40 mg/kg, in divided doses q 12 h.
Gentamicin: 60–90 mg/m², in divided doses q 8 h.
Vancomycin: 40–60 mg/kg, in divided doses q 6 h.
Nafcillin: 100–200 mg/kg, in divided doses q 4–6 h.

Methicillin: 100–200 mg/kg, in divided doses q 4–6 h.
Cephalothin: 100 mg/kg, in divided doses q 6–8 h.
Rifampin: 15–30 mg/kg, in divided doses q 12 h.
Ampicillin: 200–300 mg/kg, in divided doses q 6 h.
Ticarcillin: 200–400 mg/kg, in divided doses q 6 h.

controversial. The *Schlicter test* is an in vitro determination of the maximal serum inhibitory and serum bactericidal levels specific for an infecting organism. However, standardization of this test is poor among different laboratories, which creates problems for interpretation. Studies in rabbits who have experimentally induced endocarditis show that bactericidal titers or 1:8 or greater usually correlate with therapeutic success. In humans with IE, no similar correlation was seen at titers of 1 : 8. Although no formal recommendation exists, prospective studies suggest that therapy should be tailored to achieve peak titers of 1 : 64 or greater and trough titers equal to or greater than 1 : 32. The Kirby-Bauer disc sensitivity test is neither reliable nor quantitative and should not be used to guide therapy. Most viridans streptococci, S pyogenes, S pneumoniae, and nonenterococcal group D streptococci have an MIC for penicillin of less than 0.2 μg/mL in broth. Resistance, as defined by organisms with an MIC of more than or equal to 0.2 μg/mL, occurs in about 15% to 20% of viridans streptococci. Tolerance occurs when growth of the organism is inhibited to an MIC to penicillin of less than 0.1 μg/mL along with an MBC greater than eight times the MIC. Treatment failure may result because of organisms that become tolerant to therapy when penicillin is used as the sole agent. Streptomycin and gentamicin each act synergistically with penicillin or vancomycin in vitro and have been effective in eradicating vegetations in experimentally induced endocarditis in rabbits.

In adults with IE due to penicillin-sensitive viridans streptococci, an unacceptable relapse rate is obtained if penicillin is used alone for 2 weeks. However, if intramuscular procaine penicillin and streptomycin are given together for 2 weeks, 99% of patients are cured, a rate identical to that for a 4-week course of penicillin agents alone or penicillin for 4 weeks with streptomycin administered concomitantly during the first 2 weeks. The most cost-effective and preferred therapy for uncomplicated penicillin-sensitive streptococcal endocarditis in young adults is the 2-week penicillin plus streptomycin regimen. Patients in renal failure or at risk for streptomycin-induced ototoxicity should receive 4 weeks of penicillin. In adults with a complicated course, prosthetic valve endocarditis, infections due to relatively penicillin-resistant organisms, or symptoms lasting longer than 3 months, penicillin with the addition of streptomycin during the first 2 weeks is recommended. Gentamicin is preferred in pediatric patients because its ototoxicity is lower than that of streptomycin. None of these regimens has been evaluated specifically in the pediatric population.

Most strains of enterococci have an MIC to penicillin greater than or equal to 0.4 μg/mL and an MBC greater than or equal to 6.25 μg/mL. Penicillin alone is ineffective and requires the addition of an aminoglycoside to act synergistically to effect a cure. Penicillin plus gentamicin is the preferred initial treatment because of a 20% to 50% resistance (MIC >2000 μg/mL) rate for streptomycin among enterococcal strains. Streptomycin-resistant strains have responded to the synergistic effect of penicillin and gentamicin in vitro. After the susceptibility to streptomycin is determined, therapy should be adjusted accordingly and administered for 4 to 6 weeks.

For patients with IE due to S aureus, a semisynthetic penicillinase-resistant penicillin is given for 6 weeks. A penicillin-susceptible strain (MIC <0.1 μg/mL) is encountered occasionally, and penicillin G can be used. Although in vitro and animal studies have demonstrated enhanced killing of these organisms when gentamicin is added to nafcillin, no real value has been found for most patients, and this combination usually is reserved for seriously ill patients. Vancomycin is used in penicillin-allergic patients or for methicillin resistance. However, a prospective study of adults with methicillin-resistant *S aureus* endocarditis demonstrated a delayed response compared with patients with a methicillin-sensitive strain. The addition of rifampin did not appear to improve the response time or to be more effective than vancomycin alone. Vancomycin is used in patients with hospital-acquired infection due to *S epidermidis* because of the high rate of methicillin-resistant organisms found in this infection. Its bactericidal activity may be increased by the addition of gentamicin or rifampin, and it is recommended in prosthetic valve endocarditis caused by *S epidermidis*.

Infectious endocarditis caused by gram-negative organisms requires individualized therapy determined by the findings of in vitro susceptibility testing. If *Klebsiella* or *Pseudomonas* is involved, a total of 6 to 8 weeks of therapy with two or more agents may be necessary, and surgical therapy frequently is necessary. Infections due to *Haemophilus* organisms usually respond to ampicillin administered for 4 weeks, although the addition of an aminoglycoside may improve the outcome. Most anaerobes are sensitive to penicillin alone, but if resistant *B fragilis* organisms are found, treatment with metronidazole is recommended.

Fungal endocarditis presents the clinician with several difficult problems. The overall survival rate is only 20%, and only rarely is medical therapy reported to be successful in eradicating the disease. A delay in making the diagnosis is encountered frequently because of slow growth in blood culture media. Embolic events often are the first serious sign of fungal endocarditis that may necessitate immediate surgical intervention. The primary antifungal agent used is amphotericin B, alone or in combination with 5-fluorocytosine. Amphotericin B is given at a dose of 0.5 to 1.0 mg/kg/day. Although usually less severe in children than in adults, toxic reactions may necessitate altering the usual regimen. Fevers, chills, phlebitis, anemia, nephrotoxicity, renal tubular acidosis, hypocalcemia, and thrombocytopenia are the toxic effects most commonly reported. Although the optimal dose of amphotericin B is unknown, total dosages of 20 to 50 mg/kg usually are employed. Adults should not receive more than 50 mg/day. Therapy usually continues for at least 8 weeks, and evidence of recurrence must be looked for over a long period because relapses have been observed as long as 2 years after a presumed cure. Amphotericin B penetrates vegetations poorly and may not prevent continued growth of the fungal organism. Reseeding of the vegetation from distant metastatic sites may occur, further complicating attempts at cure. Most physicians agree that the combination of antifungal agents and surgery is the treatment of choice in fungal endocarditis.

In patients with culture-negative endocarditis, empiric therapy with two or more agents is employed for 6 weeks, during which time continuing efforts to identify an organism are pursued. In a study of culture-negative endocarditis in 52 adult patients, survival was correlated with the clinical response to the initial choice of antibiotics, and most deaths were attributable to CHF or systemic embolic events.

Surgery has been a valuable adjunct to medical therapy for IE in certain circumstances. Many studies of the role of surgery recruited mostly adult patients and included a few pediatric patients. In one review of 139 patients who underwent surgical therapy for the treatment of IE, the most common reason for referral was CHF, alone or combined with other conditions (eg, embolization, persistent infection). Aortic valve involvement predominated over mitral valve disease. The early mortality rate was 25%, and the late mortality rate (>30 days) was 8.6%. Only 1.6% of the patients had residual infection, despite the fact that 10% had had a positive valve culture at the time of surgery. One review found that the most common indication for surgical intervention was severe CHF, alone (84%) or combined with other factors (12%). The early and late mortality rates were 30% and 7%, respectively. The most significant factor affecting survival

was severe cardiac failure. In the cases of fungal endocarditis included in the study, recurrent emboli and persistent infection were more common than severe CHF as the indication for surgery.

When aortic valve disease alone is considered, unstable hemodynamics may be the primary reason to perform surgery. Placement of a prosthetic valve during active infection seems to contradict classic surgical techniques. However, there is a surprisingly low incidence of recurrent infection when valve replacement is performed in patients other than intravenous drug abusers. There seems to be no difference in the reinfection rates of bioprosthetic valves and prosthetic valves. Human allograft valves have also been used with success, even in high-risk patients. Double valve replacement (ie, aortic and mitral) has been performed with success when the infection has involved both structures. Extravalvular aortic root infection can be managed successfully with aortic valve replacement, alone or with a Teflon patch attached.

A study of surgical treatment of IE that included 11 patients with congenital heart disease (ie, 7 with ventricular septal defect, 2 with patent ductus arteriosus, 1 with transposition of the great vessels, 1 patient with secundum atrial septal defect) found that the primary indications for intervention were heart failure secondary to valve destruction, removal of a newly leaking prosthetic valve, persistent or recurrent infection, and large left-sided mobile vegetations, regardless of the occurrence of embolism. Overall, the patients with congenital heart disease had the lowest mortality, which the researchers attributed to the primary involvement of the right side of the heart and the low incidence of embolic events. The mortality rate was dramatically lower for surgical therapy for prosthetic valve endocarditis than for native valve endocarditis (10% versus 32%). The investigators concluded that surgery should be considered earlier when medical treatment is failing, when large, mobile vegetations are observed on echocardiographic study, and when fungal endocarditis is encountered. Operative intervention can be performed even during active infection, with good results.

A large series of patients from South Africa was studied prospectively to establish the safety and efficacy of early surgical intervention in native left-sided endocarditis. These patients were referred for surgery if they had CHF from valve dysfunction and vegetations seen on an echocardiographic examination. Despite heart failure and abscess formation, there was only a 4% hospital mortality rate and a 10% late mortality rate. These exceptionally low mortality figures in this high-risk group make a strong case for early intervention after CHF develops rather than following a more conventional, medical approach. Unfortunately, there are no similar studies of the pediatric group with congenital heart disorders.

Patients with infected or contaminated (eg, skin breakdown over the pacemaker site with no evidence of inflammation) endocardial pacemaker or pacemaker leads must have these leads removed and temporary pacing instituted. Permanent pacing leads can be placed safely after successful therapy. Patients who have been treated successfully for endocarditis and who have prosthetic material in the heart should not receive chronic oral "suppressive therapy" in an attempt to prevent a relapse.

## PROGNOSIS

The course and prognosis of patients depends on many underlying factors, including the severity of the primary cardiac lesion, the presence of prosthetic material, the infecting organism, the duration of illness before diagnosis and initiation of appropriate therapy, and the clinical condition at the time of diagnosis (eg, degree of respiratory, neurologic, and cardiovascular or renal compromise). Infective endocarditis was almost 100% fatal in the preantibiotic era. The rate of mortality is now between 20% and 30% because of improved methods of diagnosis and treatment with appropriate antibiotics. Mortality rates are somewhat higher in patients with acute staphylococcal infection, fungal infection, and prosthetic valve endocarditis. Sudden cardiac decompensation due to CHF remains the single most important factor affecting mortality. Several studies of the adult population have directly correlated mortality and uncontrolled CHF. Death may be the result of sudden perforation of the aortic valve with severe aortic insufficiency, chordal rupture with resultant mitral regurgitation, and myocardial necrosis with resultant intracardiac shunting through a ventricular or atrial septal defect or through a atrioventricular communication. Intramyocardial abscess formation with the development of myocarditis may be an important factor determining the ultimate prognosis.

Patients who survive will always be at risk for future development of IE. After an apparently successful course of therapy, the disease may recur early (within 3 months of completion of therapy) or late (3–6 months after completion of therapy), and it should be suspected if fever or other symptoms recur shortly after antibiotics are discontinued. The organism found at relapse may be identical to or different from the organism identified initially.

## Selected Readings

Awadallah SM, et al. The changing pattern of infective endocarditis in childhood. Am J Cardiol 1991;68:90.

Blieden LC, et al. Bacterial endocarditis in the neonate. Am J Dis Child 1972;124: 747.

Clemens JD, Horwitz RI, Jaffe CC, Feinstein AR. A controlled evaluation of the risk of bacterial endocarditis in persons with mitral valve prolapse. N Engl J Med 1982;307:776.

Ivert TS, et al. Prosthetic valve endocarditis. Circulation 1984;69:223.

Johnson DH, Rosenthal A, Nadas A. A forty-year review of bacterial endocarditis in infancy and childhood. Circulation 1975;51:581.

Kaplan EL, et al. A collaborative study of infective endocarditis in the 1970s. Emphasis on infections in patients who have undergone cardiovascular surgery. Circulation 1979;59:327.

Karl T, Wensley D, Stark J, DeLeval M. Infective endocarditis in children with congenital heart disease: comparison of selected features in patients with surgical correction or palliation and those without. Br Heart J 1987;58:57.

Rubinstein E, et al. Fungal endocarditis: analysis of 24 cases and review of the literature. Medicine (Baltimore) 1975;54:331.

Sande MA, Scheld WM. Combination antibiotic therapy of bacterial endocarditis. Ann Intern Med 1980;92:390.

Shulman ST, et al. Prevention of bacterial endocarditis. A statement for health professionals by the Committee on Rheumatic Fever and Bacterial Endocarditis of the Council on Cardiovascular Diseases in the Young of the American Heart Association. Am J Dis Child 1985;139:232.

Van Hare GF, et al. Infective endocarditis in infants and children during the past 10 years: a decade of change. Am Heart J 1984;107:1235.

Weinstein L, Schlesinger JJ. Pathoanatomic, pathophysiologic, and clinical correlations in endocarditis. N Engl J Med 1974;291:832, 1122.

*Principles and Practice of Pediatrics, Second Edition.*
edited by Frank A. Oski et al. J. B. Lippincott Company, Philadelphia © 1994.

# CHAPTER 85
# *Rheumatic Fever*

## Galal M. El-Said

Rheumatic fever (RF) is a delayed, nonsuppurative sequela to upper respiratory infection with group A β-hemolytic streptococci. It is a diffuse inflammatory disease of the connective tissue that involves principally the heart, blood vessels, joints, central nervous system, and subcutaneous tissues.

The term acute rheumatic fever is a misnomer, because it may not be acute, rheumatic, or febrile. Although the term emphasizes involvement of the joints, the disease owes its importance to involvement of the heart. As early as 1884, Lasegue described this feature: "Rheumatic fever is a disease that licks the joints but bites the heart."

## EPIDEMIOLOGY

Numerous investigators have documented the declining incidence of RF, even before the introduction of penicillin. In Rochester, MN, the age-adjusted annual incidence per 100,000 persons was 20 from 1939 to 1949, 12 from 1950 to 1964, and 3 from 1965 to 1978. Several recent outbreaks in military and civilian populations in the United States correlated with the reappearance of virulent M-protein strains belonging to the M serotype associated with previous RF epidemics.

Several factors predispose to RF: age, family history, season, recurrent streptococcal infections, and host factors affecting susceptibility. The first attack usually occurs in patients between 5 and 15 years of age. RF is rare in children younger than 4 years of age. There is no sex preference unless chorea is included, in which case the incidence is slightly greater among girls.

RF may affect more than one member in the same family. It

is possible that the same housing conditions predispose several persons to recurrent streptococcal infections. Constitutional susceptibility may be a factor, but there is no evidence for genetic markers in rheumatic patients, and HLA genotypes do not correlate with the development of RF.

Rheumatic fever occurs more commonly in the winter and spring, a seasonal variation similar to that of streptococcal pharyngitis.

Recurrent streptococcal infections are the most important predisposing factor in the occurrence and recurrence of RF. About 1% to 5% of streptococcal throat infections are followed by RF. The most important factors that may be related to the attack rate of RF after streptococcal pharyngitis are the magnitude of the immune response to the antecedent infections and the duration of convalescent carriage of the organisms. Skin infections are unlikely to produce the disease.

Because RF develops after streptococcal pharyngitis in a relatively small percentage of patients, host predisposition is probably a factor. After RF is acquired, its reactivation after subsequent streptococcal infections is much more likely. The recurrence rate per infection is about 50% during the first year after the initial attack; it decreases sharply after that. The rate levels off after several years to about 10%. This persistently high attack rate after RF suggests acquired hyperreactivity.

## ETIOLOGY

### Streptococci

Streptococci are a large group of gram-positive microorganisms that are distributed widely in nature. When cultured, they are arranged in chains. Their ability to hemolyze erythrocytes to various degrees is an important basis for their classification. The α-hemolytic streptococci form colonies surrounded by an ill-defined, greenish halo in which hemolysis is incomplete. The β-hemolytic streptococci produce a clear zone of hemolysis on blood agar; γ-streptococci do not have any effect on blood-containing media.

The streptococcus (Fig 85-1) is composed of a core of cytoplasm surrounded by three layers: a cytoplasmic membrane, a cell wall, and a capsule that constitutes the external surface of the organism. The capsule is composed of hyaluronate, which is nonantigenic. The cell wall is composed of three layers: the outermost protein, the middle carbohydrate, and the innermost mucopeptide pro-

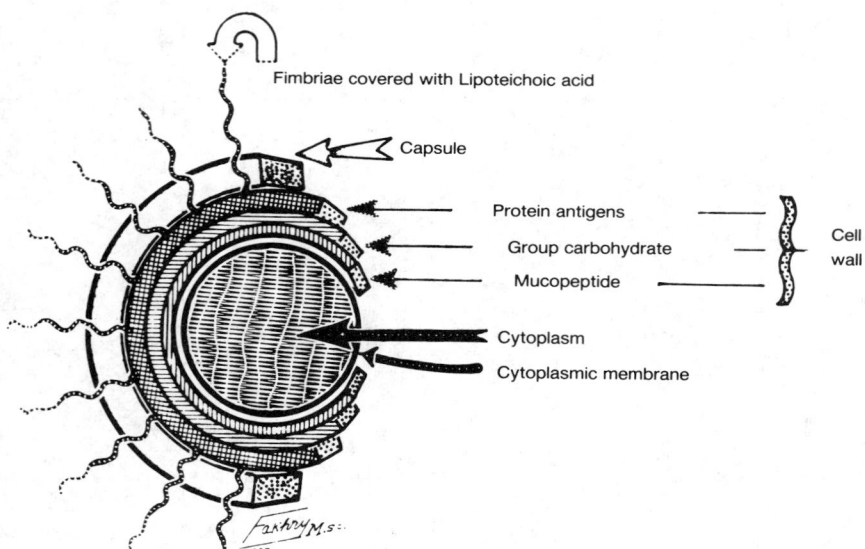

Figure 85-1.   With one end embedded in the protein layer of the streptococcal cell wall, fimbriae covered with lipoteichoic acid help the organism adhere to the throat epithelium (ie, adherence factor). These fimbriae contain M protein (ie, virulence factor). Each of the layers of the cell wall and the cytoplasmic membrane cross-react with several antigens.

toplast. The middle layer of the cell wall, the carbohydrate layer, provides the group specification, given as the alphabetical classification (eg, A through H) of Lancefield. The outer protein layer and its fimbriae, which are attached to the surface of the organism, contain the proteins designated M, T, and R. The M protein is the most important because it determines the virulence of the organism, stimulates formation of opsonizing and precipitating antibodies, and may impede phagocytosis. Lancefield and associates further classified group A streptococci into serologic types on the basis of the M protein. RF can result from infection by many of the serotypes of group A β-hemolytic streptococci, but glomerulonephritis is associated with only a limited number of these serotypes. The cytoplasmic membrane is an antigenic lipoprotein that cross-reacts with several mammalian tissue antigens, including the glomerular basement membrane and sarcolemmal antigen.

The streptococcus produces several extracellular products, some of which are involved in the diseases produced by the microorganism. Erythrogenic toxin is responsible for the rash of scarlet fever. Streptolysin O, which is active only in the reduced state, is cardiotoxic and leukotoxic, is responsible for hemolysis of erythrocytes, and elicits an antibody response, antistreptolysin O (ASO), which is the basis for a useful assay of streptococcal infections. The antigenicity of streptolysin O is inhibited by lipid extracts (probably cholesterol) of skin, and this property may be responsible for the lack of association between streptococcal skin infections and RF. Streptolysin S, an oxygen-stable product, produces the hemolysis characteristic of β-hemolytic streptococci when cultured on sheep blood agar. Streptokinase converts plasminogen to plasmin, an active proteolytic enzyme that digests fibrin. Diphosphopyridine nucleotidase, which determines the ability of the organism to kill leukocytes, elicits an antibody response (ie, antidiphosphopyridine nucleotidase). There are four deoxyribonucleases (ie, A, B, C, D), all of which are antigenic. Deoxyribonuclease B, known as streptodornase, is produced in the largest quantities in response to group A streptococcal infections and is the most consistent of the deoxyribonucleases.

## Mechanism Producing Rheumatic Fever

RF is thought to be an autoimmune disease. The requirements for its development include group A β-hemolytic streptococcal infection in the throat with antibody response indicative of recent infection and persistence of the organism in the pharynx for a period sufficient to produce an immunologic response. The magnitude of the antibody response is a major factor determining the attack rate of RF after streptococcal infection. The predisposing organism has antigens immunologically similar to proteins in the human heart, and the antibodies produced against the streptococci react with the heart (ie, cross-reactive immunity). A plethora of streptococcal cellular components cross-reacting with various mammalian tissues has been described. The hyaluronate capsule is identical to human hyaluronate. Antibodies to the cell wall polysaccharide cross-react with glycoproteins of heart valves. Membrane antigens cross-react with the sarcolemma and smooth muscles of endocardial and myocardial arteries. Antibody to the streptococcal group A polysaccharide persists in the serum of patients with rheumatic valvular disease in contrast to its more rapid decline in patients with RF without cardiac involvement. As with other possible autoimmune diseases, the difficulties of differentiating cause from effect of injury has rendered this hypothesis unprovable.

## PATHOLOGY

### General Pathology

Nonspecific lesions result from fibrinoid degeneration of the connective tissue, inflammatory edema, and inflammatory cell infiltration.

Specific lesions result from a proliferative reaction that forms Aschoff nodules (Fig 85-2). The Aschoff nodules are paravascular nodules consisting of a center of fibrinoid degeneration surrounded by Aschoff cells, lymphocytes, and fibroblasts.

### Cardiac Pathology

RF affects the three layers of the heart, causing endocarditis, myocarditis, and pericarditis (ie, pancarditis). Endocarditis affects the mitral and aortic valves and rarely affects the tricuspid or pulmonary valves. In the active phase, the valves become edematous, and the endocardium is damaged along the contact margins 2 or 3 mm from the free edges. At this site, tiny vegetations consisting of platelet thrombi are formed (Fig 85-3). After inflammation subsides, fibrosis and contracture follow. Similar changes cause shortening of the chordae tendineae. The site of the lesions, at the contact points of the cusps, suggests that trauma determines the position of the damage. The degree of trauma determines the frequency with which the valves are involved.

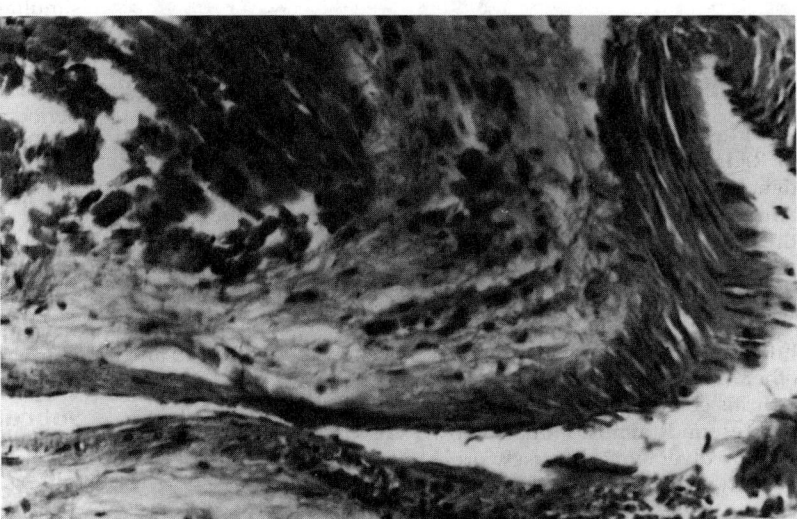

**Figure 85-2.** A paravascular Aschoff nodule (*center*) consists of a central area of fibrinoid change and an Aschoff giant cell surrounded by edematous intermyocardial connective tissue. (Courtesy of Soheir Mahfouz, M.D., Pathology Department, Cairo University).

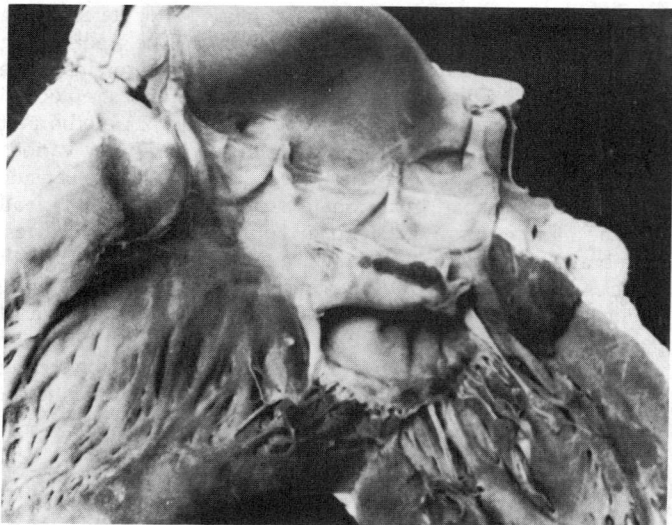

**Figure 85-3.** An opened left ventricle displays the mitral and aortic valves of a patient with acute rheumatic fever. The mitral valve shows small (1 to 2 mm) linear vegetations on the atrial surface of the anterior and posterior mitral leaflet margins. The aortic valve appears to be unaffected. (Courtesy of Soheir Mahfouz, M.D., Pathology Department, Cairo University.)

The mitral valve, closing at the highest pressure ($\approx$120 mm Hg), is subjected to the greatest stress and is the valve most frequently affected. The aortic valve, which closes by systemic diastolic pressure of 80 mm Hg, is the valve next most often involved, followed by the tricuspid valve and the pulmonary valve. If the inflammation is severe, the cusps are damaged, and insufficiency develops. Mild inflammation thickens tissue, and adhesions occur between the cusps. The adhesions gradually increase, producing stenosis of the valve orifice.

## Extracardiac Pathology

Extracardiac pathology includes inflammation of synovial membranes, subcutaneous collections of Aschoff nodules, pleurisy and pneumonitis, meningoencephalitis, and vasculitis. Sydenham's chorea, atrioventricular conduction blocks, and erythema marginatum seem to be related to functional rather than visible lesions.

## CLINICAL MANIFESTATIONS

### Antecedent Streptococcal Infection

The interval between the onset of pharyngitis and the symptoms of RF is 1 to 5 weeks (average, 3 weeks). However, clinical evidence for a preceding streptococcal infection may be lacking. About one third of patients have had no apparent illness during the preceding month.

### Polyarthritis

Inflammation affects the large joints and moves from one to another. The affected joint is hot, red, tender, and swollen. The arthritis characteristically leaves the joints without any sequelae and responds almost immediately to salicylates. The severity of joint involvement is inversely proportional to the severity of cardiac involvement.

## Carditis

In contrast to the seriousness of its prognosis, rheumatic carditis, unless it causes heart failure or pericarditis, produces no symptoms of its own and is usually diagnosed during examination of a patient with arthritis or chorea.

The development of an apical systolic murmur that is propagated to the axilla and is accompanied by a muffled first sound and a third sound indicates the development of mitral insufficiency. A systolic murmur over the apex without these characteristics may be caused by fever and not by mitral valvulitis.

The occurrence of a mid-diastolic murmur over the apex is a definite sign of mitral valvulitis. The diastolic apical murmur is caused by narrowing of the mitral orifice by the thickened, edematous cusps. The murmur may persist, indicating permanent damage, but it frequently disappears for a variable period, followed later by the appearance of the diastolic murmur of stenosis caused by the development of adhesions between the valve cusps.

The occurrence of a high-pitched, early-diastolic murmur over the base indicates aortic valvulitis. As in mitral valvulitis, the occurrence of a systolic murmur over the base may be caused by fever or by aortic valvulitis.

The murmurs of mitral and aortic valvulitis may disappear or may be followed by the establishment of valve regurgitation, stenosis, or both, according to the pathological process occurring in the valve. Regurgitation, the result of damage, takes a short time to develop, but stenosis, the result of union between mobile cusps, takes years to decades to occur.

Myocarditis usually is accompanied by valvulitis and leads to tachycardia (especially if it persists during sleep) that is disproportionate to the patient's fever and can lead to gallop rhythm, rapid cardiac enlargement, and heart failure. Pericarditis accompanies valvulitis in approximately 5% to 10% of patients. The degree of effusion in pericarditis varies from none to moderate.

Electrocardiographic changes characteristically include prolongation of the PR and QT intervals. Second-degree or a complete AV block may occur in response to inflammation of the conduction system. There may be ST wave and T wave changes of pericarditis or myocarditis. Echocardiographic changes can detect valvular and myocardial involvement or pericardial effusion.

## Chorea

Rheumatic or Sydenham's chorea, which is a late manifestation of RF, is more common among female than male patients. Chorea may last from 1 week to more than 2 years. Chorea is never seen simultaneously with arthritis, but it may coexist with carditis. If there is no carditis, the sedimentation rate is not elevated. In such cases, the ASO and other streptococcal antibody titers may not be increased, probably because chorea appears only after a latent period as long as 6 months after the streptococcal infection, and by that time, the acute-phase reactants and the streptococcal antibody titer may have returned to normal.

There are involuntary, incoordinate, jerky movements accompanied by hypotonia and emotional disturbances, with abrupt alterations between laughter and tears. Flexion at the wrist and dorsiflexion of the fingers occur in the outstretched hands. Objects often fall from the hands. The patient, after protruding the tongue for inspection, may withdraw it rapidly, snapping the jaws over it.

## Subcutaneous Nodules

Rarely seen in recent years, subcutaneous nodules usually indicate severe carditis. The nodules are attached to the tendon sheaths

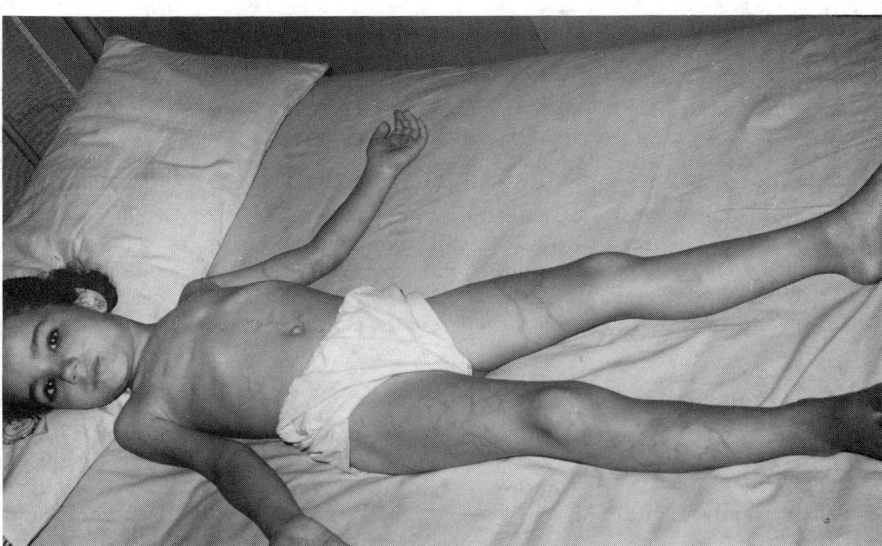

**Figure 85-4.** A 6-year-old girl with erythema marginatum has acute rheumatic fever with severe carditis. (Courtesy of Samir Kassem, M.D., Alexandria Medical School).

and occur on the extensor surfaces and bony prominences of the arms and legs and on the scapula and the mastoid processes. Histologically, they consist of collections of Aschoff bodies.

## Erythema Marginatum

The rash of erythema marginatum generally appears as an area of erythema. The margins progress as the center clears. The rash occurs chiefly over the trunk and the proximal parts of the limbs (Fig 85-4).

## Signs of Inflammation

Pallor, epistaxis, elevated temperature, tachycardia, anorexia, and loss of weight are signs of inflammation. They indicate rheumatic activity in a patient already diagnosed as having rheumatic fever. Pleurisy, pneumonia, and abdominal pain (simulating appendicitis) due to vasculitis have the same significance.

## DIAGNOSIS

Laboratory tests typically show a high erythrocyte sedimentation rate, anemia, leukocytosis, and C-reactive protein. The ASO antibody is elevated abnormally in 70% to 85% of patients with RF. A single value of 500 units indicates recent streptococcal infection, and a value of 333 units is of borderline significance. If the ASO titer is 333 units or less, additional antistreptococcal

antibody assays should be obtained. ASO and anti-DNase are most often used for diagnosis, and antihyaluronidase is a third choice.

The diagnosis of RF is important because serious cardiac disease can be prevented or minimized by long-term antistreptococcal therapy. There is no single diagnostic test for RF. The laboratory tests indicate recent streptococcal infection, but diagnosis of RF rests on the ability to satisfy the Duckett Jones criteria (Table 85-1). It is mandatory to demonstrate recent streptococcal infection (usually by elevation of ASO titer) and to find one major and two minor criteria or to identify two major criteria. The minor manifestations are less specific for the illness.

RF should be differentiated from juvenile rheumatoid arthritis, innocent murmur with a febrile illness, bacterial arthritis, systemic lupus erythematosus, Schönlein-Henoch purpura, acute leukemia, sickle cell anemia, and mucocutaneous lymph node syndrome.

## COURSE AND PROGNOSIS

RF usually follows a characteristic clinical course. The latent period is short for disease complicated with arthritis and erythema marginatum, longest for RF with chorea, and midlength for RF with carditis and subcutaneous nodules. The duration of active disease is usually less than 3 months. Fewer than 5% of patients with RF have disease that remains active for more than 6 months, a condition known as chronic active carditis. The prognosis is

| TABLE 85-1. Duckett Jones Criteria for the Diagnosis of Rheumatic Fever | | |
|---|---|---|
| **Requirements for Diagnosis** | **Major Criteria** | **Minor Criteria** |
| Two major criteria, | Carditis | Previous rheumatic fever |
| *or* | Arthritis | Arthralgia |
| One major plus two minor, | Chorea | Fever |
| *plus* | Erythema marginatum | Raised erythrocyte |
| Evidence of previous streptococcal | Subcutaneous nodules | sedimentation rate |
| infection: (eg, elevated ASO titer) | | Elevated leukocyte count |
| | | Prolonged PR interval |
| | | C reactive protein |

excellent for the patient who does not develop carditis during the initial attack. The prognosis becomes poorer with increasing severity of initial carditis.

Over the years, there have been changes in the epidemiology of RF and in its severity, presentation, and clinical manifestations. RF is less common in developed countries, and when it occurs, it tends to be mild. In tropical and subtropical countries, RF and rheumatic heart disease are common and assume more malignant forms (Fig 85-5). In areas where RF is still common, the course of the disease is subacute or chronic. Joint involvement is less conspicuous. Rheumatic nodules and erythema marginatum are seen less frequently, but chorea is often part of the clinical picture.

## TREATMENT

### Prophylactic Therapy

Prevention of RF is achieved by improving socioeconomic circumstances and sanitation.

The aim of primary prophylaxis is to prevent initial attacks of RF by prompt and accurate recognition and treatment of streptococcal pharyngitis or by antibiotic prophylaxis using benzathine penicillin intramuscularly for members of a susceptible population. Modern outbreaks in the United States were blamed in part on diminished adherence to conventional recommendations for penicillin, which is highly effective in preventing RF due to pharyngeal infections.

Secondary prophylaxis is the prevention of recurrences of RF by continuous chemoprophylaxis. The most effective method is a single monthly intramuscular injection of 600,000 to 1,200,000 U of benzathine penicillin. The incidence of allergic reactions is about 3%, but anaphylaxis occurs after only 1 of 10,000 injections. Oral penicillin prophylaxis can be provided by 500 to 1000 mg of penicillin G administered twice daily. If the patient is allergic to penicillin, prophylaxis can be achieved by 250 mg of erythromycin given twice daily. The injectable form of prophylaxis is more effective than the oral forms, because patient compliance is superior and the medication is not affected by variations in

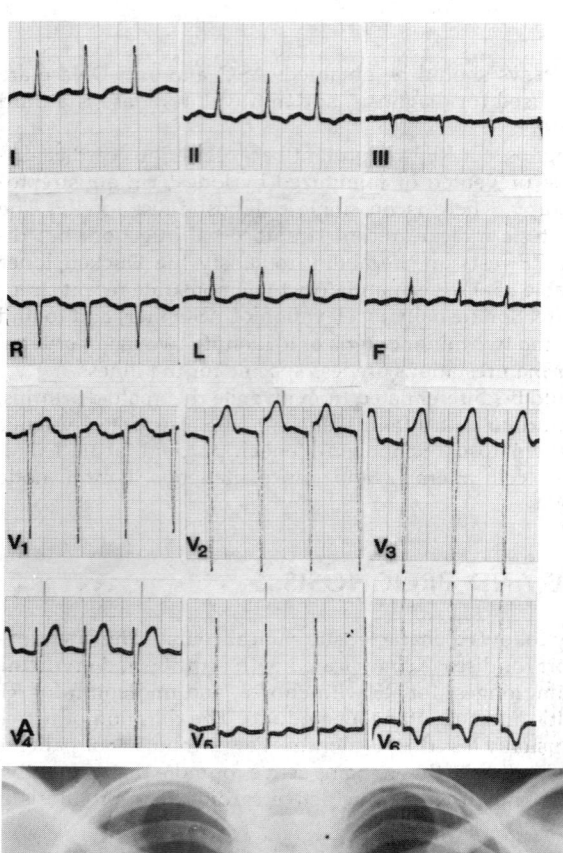

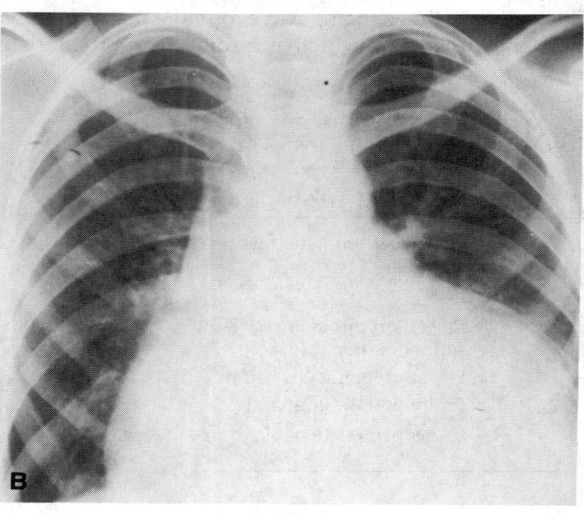

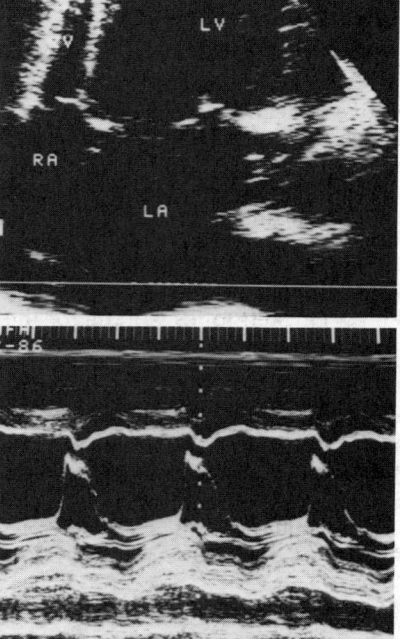

**Figure 85-5.** The electrocardiogram (ECG), roentgenogram, and echocardiogram are from an underdeveloped 11-year-old patient with recurrent rheumatic fever with mitral and aortic rheumatic valve disease. (**A**) The ECG shows sinus tachycardia, a prolonged PR interval, and left ventricular hypertrophy and strain. (**B**) the roentgenogram shows gross cardiomegaly. The apical four-chamber echo view shows a dilated left ventricle and left atrium and a thickened mitral valve. (**C**) The M-mode echocardiogram shows a thickened mitral valve and small pericardial effusion. *LA*, left atrium; *LV*, left ventricle; *RA*, right ventricle.

intestinal absorption. The duration of secondary prophylaxis depends on the variables that influence the recurrence rate and the degree to which the heart has been affected. The risk of recurrence declines with age and with an increased free RF interval from the last rheumatic attack after 10 years.

No vaccine is available, but purification and immunologic study of streptococcal M proteins hold the promise of a streptococcal vaccine in the near future.

## Curative Therapy

Bed rest is required until the signs and symptoms of acute inflammation disappear. Salt is restricted if signs of heart failure are observed.

A course of antibiotics should be initiated after a throat culture has been obtained. Antibiotics should be administered even in the absence of positive throat cultures. One intramuscular injection of benzathine penicillin (600,000 to 1,200,000 U) or a 10-day course of oral penicillin G (500 to 1000 mg, four times daily) is recommended. Patients who are allergic to penicillin should receive erythromycin (250 to 500 mg, four times daily) for 10 days.

The selection of an antirheumatic drug is not critical to the outcome of RF. Salicylates and corticosteroids are valuable symptomatic drugs, but they are not curative and may actually prolong the course of the disease.

Acetylsalicylic acid (aspirin) is analgesic and antipyretic and reduces malaise. It causes such dramatic improvement of the arthritis that it can be given as a therapeutic test, but it has no effect on carditis. Aspirin is given to patients with or without mild carditis, if there are side effects or contraindications to corticosteroids, and during and after withdrawal from corticosteroids. Side effects include tinnitus, gastric irritation, bleeding due to inhibition of platelet function, metabolic acidosis, hyperventilation that may lead to respiratory alkalosis, and hypoglycemia. The dosage is 60 to 120 mg/kg/day, given in six divided doses and administered until a satisfactory clinical response is obtained. The dosage is then reduced by one third and continued until all laboratory findings return to normal, which usually requires 6 to 9 weeks. The dosage is decreased gradually to avoid the rebound that occurs if the drug is stopped abruptly.

Corticosteroids do not markedly shorten the course of illness or diminish the likelihood of cardiac damage. Steroids do produce prompt control of the subcutaneous nodules, erythema marginatum, fever, and arthritis. Corticosteroids are indicated for patients with severe carditis. The dosage of prednisone or prednisolone is 2 mg/kg/day (not to exceed 60 mg/day) for 3 to 4 weeks. Shortly before or at the time steroid therapy is discontinued, aspirin (90 to 120 mg/kg/day) should be given, and it should be continued for 1.5 to 6 months, probably until active inflammation subsides.

## Chorea

The patient with chorea should be maintained in a quiet atmosphere, protected from self-injury, and given a tranquilizer such as phenobarbitone or chlorpromazine. Haloperidol (butyrophenone), a centrally acting drug, is the most effective in controlling chorea, but severe, adverse extrapyramidal reactions have been reported. Patients with concomitant rheumatic activity should be given salicylates.

## Heart Failure

Heart failure may be an indication for the use of steroids or diuretic agents. Operative repair or replacement of a severely compromised cardiac valve may be necessary during acute RF if signs and symptoms of severe congestive heart failure are unresponsive to medical therapy.

## Selected Readings

Annegers JF, Pillman NL, Weidman WH, et al. Rheumatic fever in Rochester, Minnesota, 1935–1978. Mayo Clin Proc 1982;57:753.
Committee Report of the American Heart Association. Jones criteria (revised) for guidance in the diagnosis of rheumatic fever. Circulation 1965;32:664.
Committee Report of the American Heart Association. Prevention of rheumatic fever. Circulation 1977;55:1.
Driscoll DJ. Rheumatic fever In: Brandenburg RO, Foster V, Giulliani ER, McGoon DC, eds. Cardiology fundamentals and practice. Chicago: Year Book Medical Publishers, 1987:1380.
Kaplan MH. Rheumatic fever, rheumatic hear disease, and the streptococcal connection: the role of streptococcal antigens cross-reactive with heart tissue. Rev Infect Dis 1979;1:988.
Stollerman GH. Rheumatogenic group A streptococci and return of rheumatic fever. Adv Intern Med 1990;35:1.
Stollerman GH. Rheumatic fever and other rheumatic diseases of the heart. In: Braunwald E, ed. Heart disease: a textbook of cardiovascular medicine. Philadelphia: WB Saunders, 1992:1721.
United Kingdom and United States joint report. The treatment of acute rheumatic fever in children: a cooperative clinical trial ACTH, cortisone, and aspirin, Circulation 1955;11:343.
Zabriskie JB. Rheumatic fever: a streptococcal-induced autoimmune disease? Pediatr Ann 1982;1:383.

*Principles and Practice of Pediatrics, Second Edition.*
edited by Frank A. Oski et al. J. B. Lippincott Company, Philadelphia © 1994.

# CHAPTER 86
# *Rheumatic Heart Disease*

## Galal M. El-Said

Rheumatic heart disease (RHD), like rheumatic fever, is more common in areas where the standard of living is low. RHD remains one of the leading causes of heart disease in the less developed countries, where rheumatic fever is common. It assumes malignant and chronic forms that can lead to significant valvular heart disease in childhood, often accompanied by significant pulmonary hypertension and may require surgery at an early age (Figs 86-1, 86-2). In children and adolescents, the mitral valve is involved in 85% of RHD cases, the aortic valve in 55%, and the tricuspid and pulmonary valves in fewer than 5%.

## RHEUMATIC MITRAL INSUFFICIENCY

Mitral insufficiency is the most common cardiac defect in children and adolescents with RHD. As the left ventricle (LV) contracts, part of its stroke volume regurgitates into the left atrium (LA) through the incompetent mitral valve. Because of the pressure difference between LV and LA, regurgitation starts during the isometric contraction phase.

Compensation begins with dilatation of the LV to accommodate the increased blood volume. In chronic mitral insuffi-

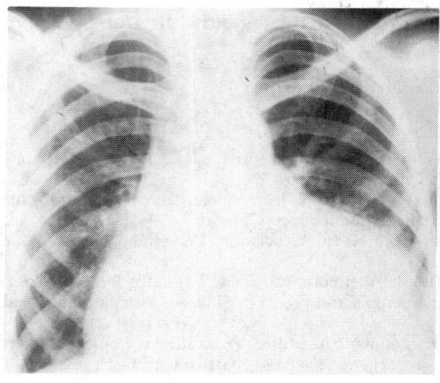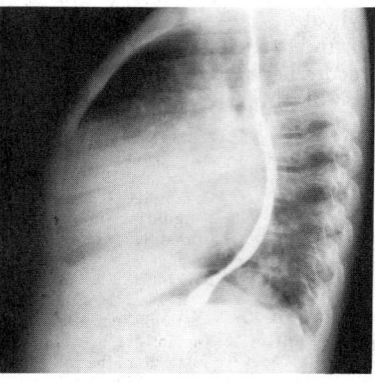

**Figure 86-1.** Posteroanterior and lateral chest radiographs show gross cardiac enlargement.

ciency, the increase in LV end-diastolic volume usually is not accompanied by increased end-diastolic pressure because of increased LV compliance. The increase in LV end-diastolic volume (ie, increased preload) brings the Frank-Starling mechanism into play, which permits a large stroke output. Because the regurgitant mitral orifice is in parallel with the aortic orifice, the resistance to LV emptying is reduced (ie, decreased afterload) (Fig 86-3).

The compensatory mechanisms of increased compliance, increased preload, decreased afterload, and increased wall thickness are not sufficient to overcome persistent mitral insufficiency. Myocardial contractility becomes impaired because of the chronic volume overload. Symptoms of low cardiac output are followed by symptoms of lung congestion due to left ventricular failure (see Fig 86-3).

## Clinical Manifestations

Because symptoms usually do not develop until the LV is compromised, the interval between acquiring rheumatic fever and the development of symptoms of mitral insufficiency tends to be longer than for mitral stenosis, often exceeding two decades. Unlike mitral stenosis, symptoms of low cardiac output (eg, weakness, fatigue) are more prominent and appear before symptoms of lung congestion (eg, exertional, nocturnal, or resting dyspnea, recurrent chest infections, hemoptysis).

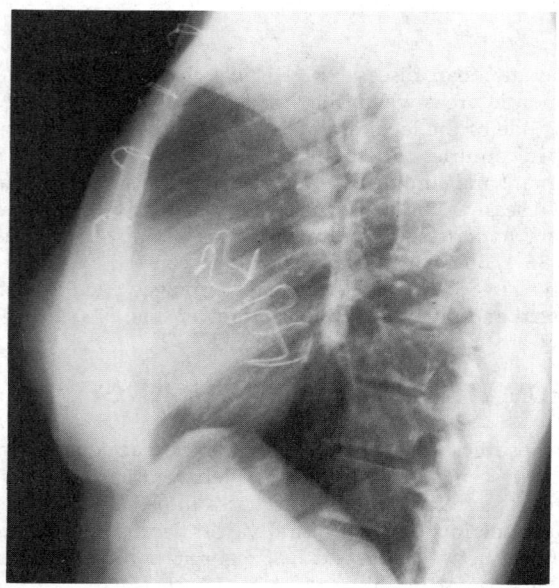

**Figure 86-2.** A lateral chest radiograph shows the mitral and aortic valve stents that were placed at a young age.

The cardiac impulse is diffuse, forceful, and displaced downward and laterally. The first heart sound usually is diminished. A loud apical third heart sound usually is audible; this is caused by the increased transmitral volume flow during the rapid filling phase. The characteristic murmur of mitral insufficiency is a high-pitched holosystolic murmur, beginning with the soft first sound and continuing to the second sound. The second heart sound sometimes is obscured by the murmur. The murmur is loudest at the apex, with radiation to the axilla and left infrascapular area.

## Laboratory Findings

In chronic mitral insufficiency, the electrocardiogram exhibits evidence of LV and LA enlargement. Radiologically, the cardiac shadow is normal early the course of the disease; later, LA and LV enlargement becomes evident.

Echocardiography is useful for identifying the cause and degree of mitral insufficiency and for evaluating LV function. M-mode echo study can show an increase in the LV diastolic dimension and a significant decrease in LV diameter during the pre-ejection phase. The two-dimensional (2D) echo criteria for the diagnosis of rheumatic mitral insufficiency include thickened mitral valve leaflets, incomplete closure of the mitral valve, a relatively immobile posterior mitral leaflet, a dilated LA with systolic expansion, and a dilated LV with hyperdynamic septal and posterior wall motion. The degree of mitral insufficiency can be assessed using echo Doppler, determining the extension and intensity of the Doppler signal of the regurgitant jet in the LA. Color flow Doppler and pulsed techniques correlate well with angiographic methods of estimating the severity of mitral insufficiency.

Gated blood pool imaging may reveal increased end-diastolic volume. The regurgitant fraction can be estimated from the difference between the LV and right ventricular (RV) stroke volumes.

Cardiac catheterization demonstrates elevated LA pressure (particularly the v wave). The diagnosis can be established by left ventriculography. Mitral insufficiency is indicated by the appearance of contrast material in the LA after LV infection through a retrograde aortic catheter and no premature beats.

## RHEUMATIC MITRAL STENOSIS

Stenosis of the mitral valve usually is secondary to rheumatic carditis. Other causes include congenital mitral stenosis, atrial myxoma, infective endocarditis with bulky vegetations, and mucopolysaccharidosis of the Hunter-Hurley phenotype. The combination of mitral stenosis and secundum atrial septal defect frequently is referred to as Lutembacher's syndrome, but the mitral stenosis is almost always rheumatic and the association is fortuitous.

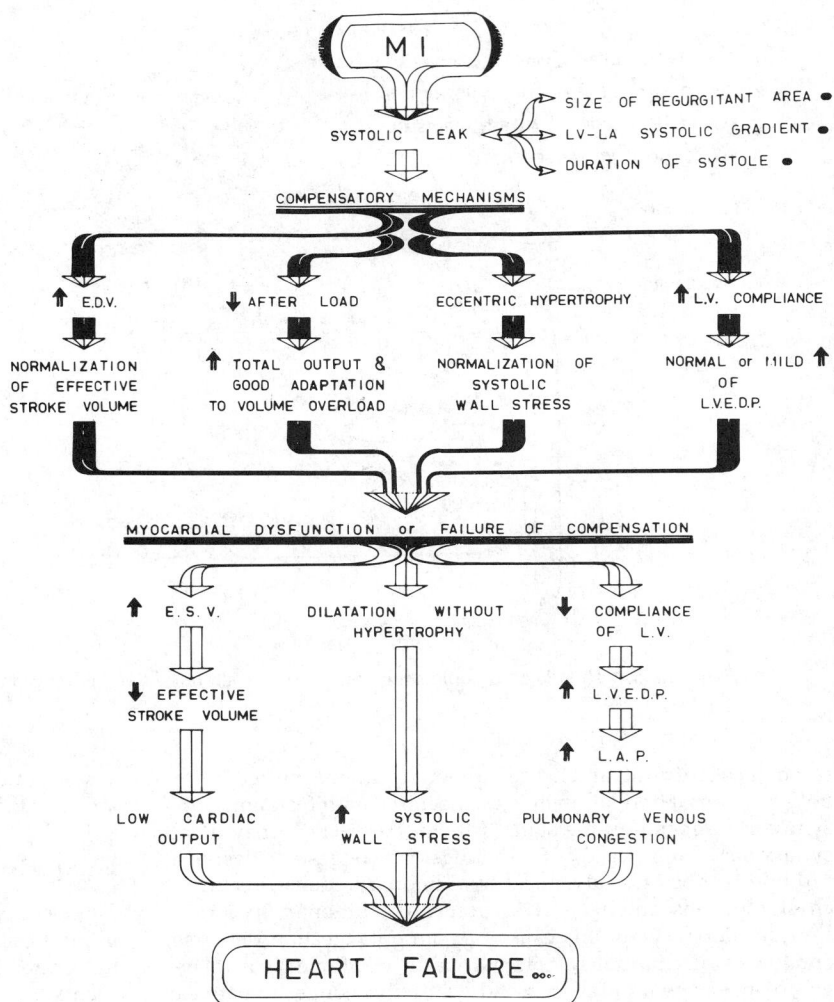

**Figure 86-3.** The diagram depicts factors that determine the degree of regurgitation, compensation, and decompensation in mitral insufficiency. *EDV*, end diastolic volume; *EDP*, end diastolic pressure; *ESV*, end systolic pressure.

Rheumatic fever causes mitral stenosis through fusion of the commissures, cusps, or chordae tendineae of the mitral valve apparatus (Fig 86-4). Obstruction of flow across the narrowed mitral valve produces a diastolic gradient between the LA and LV. Serious circulatory disturbances, with consequent clinical symptoms, occur when the area of the mitral opening is less than 1 cm². As narrowing proceeds, the LA pressure increases, as does the pressure in the pulmonary veins and capillaries, leading to lung congestion. Pulmonary arteriolar vasoconstriction occurs to

"protect" the lungs against congestion, but the protection is at the expense of developing pulmonary hypertension. This produces RV hypertrophy and possible RV failure (Fig 86-5).

## Clinical Manifestations

The symptoms of mitral stenosis may appear insidiously within 3 to 4 years after the attack of acute rheumatic fever, or they may be delayed for as long as 50 years. The onset of symptoms

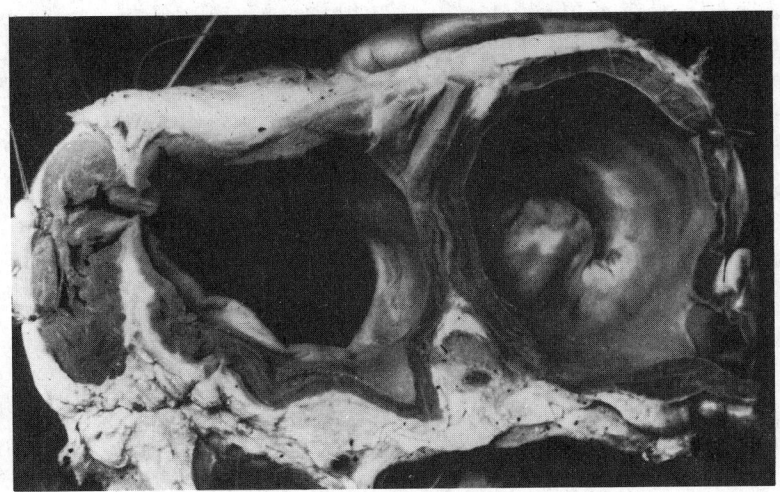

**Figure 86-4.** The cross section shows a stenosed mitral valve (*right*), giving a buttonhole appearance. The tricuspid valve on the left is grossly insufficient. Insufficiency occurs in the later stages of mitral stenosis after long-standing, severe secondary pulmonary hypertension. (Courtesy of Soheir Mahfouz, M.D., Pathology Department, Cairo University.)

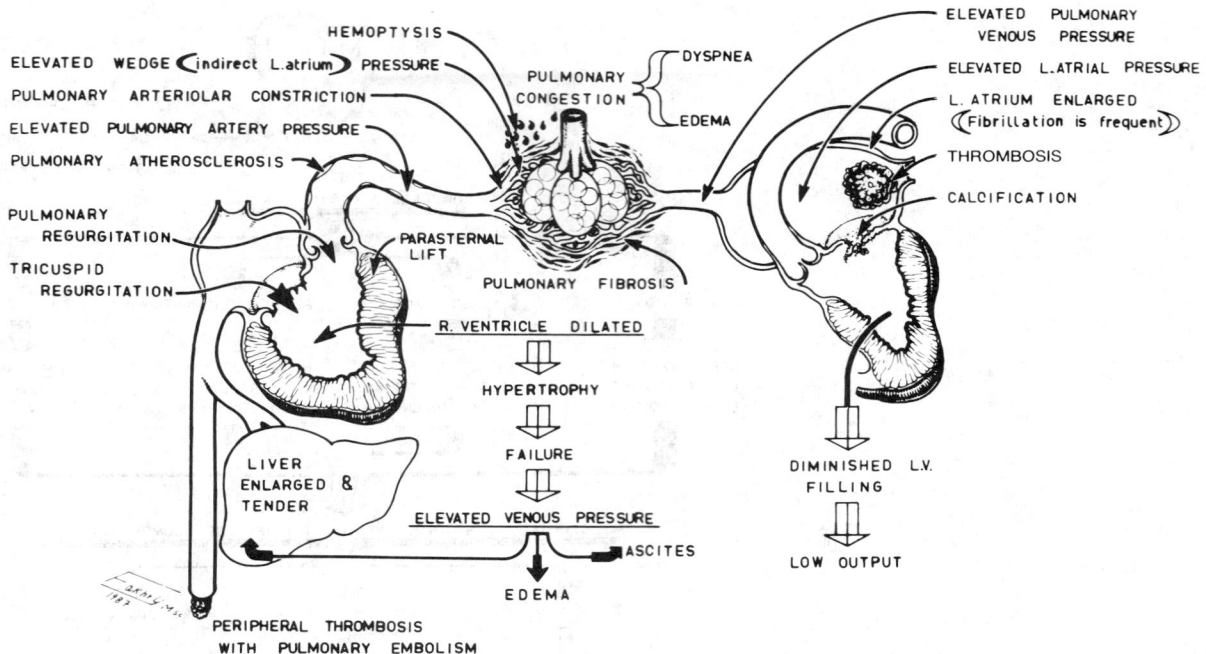

**Figure 86-5.**    The diagram depicts the hemodynamic alterations and complications that occur because of mitral stenosis.

sometimes is abrupt, and acute pulmonary edema, systemic embolism, or atrial fibrillation may be the initial manifestations. The symptoms depend on the state of the disease. There may be no symptoms in mild cases. If the lungs are congested, dyspnea, orthopnea, nocturnal dyspnea or pulmonary edema, recurrent chest infections, and hemoptysis occur. As pulmonary hypertension develops, symptoms caused by lung congestion decrease, and low cardiac output symptoms (mainly exertional fatigue) begin to appear. Symptoms caused by systemic congestion appear if the RV fails.

In a patient with mitral stenosis, the pulse usually is normal unless atrial fibrillation supervenes. The apical impulse is felt at the normal location as a ''hurried, slapping'' impulse. A characteristic diastolic or presystolic thrill ending in a palpable accentuated first sound can be detected over the apex. The first ''mitral'' sound is loud, short, and snappy. The accentuation of the first sound is caused by the open position of the cups in the LV at the end of diastole as a result of the high LA pressure and the incomplete emptying of the LA. There is an opening snap, which is a sharp, clicky sound separated from the second sound by the isovolumic relaxation phase. It is caused by the sudden opening of the rigid mitral valve by the high LA pressure. The murmur characteristic of mitral stenosis is a mid-diastolic or pre-systolic murmur. Developing pulmonary hypertension produces an accentuated pulmonary second sound.

## Laboratory Findings

The electrocardiographic and the cardiac silhouette are normal in mild cases. In patients with moderate or severe obstruction, the principal feature is LA enlargement (Fig 86-6). Right ventricular hypertrophy is seen when pulmonary hypertension develops.

The M-mode echo criteria for the diagnosis of mitral stenosis include a reduced EF slope of the anterior mitral leaflet (reflecting elevated left atrial pressure) and diastolic anterior movement of the posterior mitral leaflet. The latter results from commissural fusion and is considered to be the main diagnostic hallmark of mitral stenosis in M-mode echo studies (Fig 86-7). The feature diagnostic of mitral stenosis in a 2D echo study is doming of the anterior leaflet in diastole (ie, the body of the leaflet separates more widely than do the edges). The posterior leaflet frequently is immobile or severely restricted in diastolic movement (Fig 86-8). The 2D echo-derived mitral valve area often compares favorably with that measured directly at surgery. A Doppler echo study provides information about the flow of blood across the

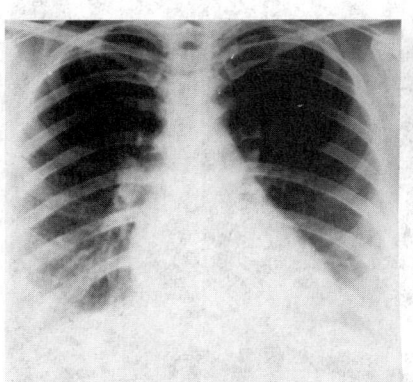
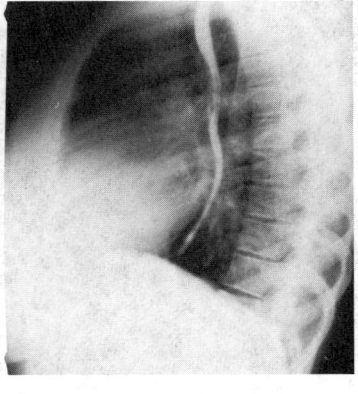

**Figure 86-6.**    Posteroanterior and lateral views from a patient with mitral stenosis show mitralization of the heart, an enlarged left atrium, and lung congestion.

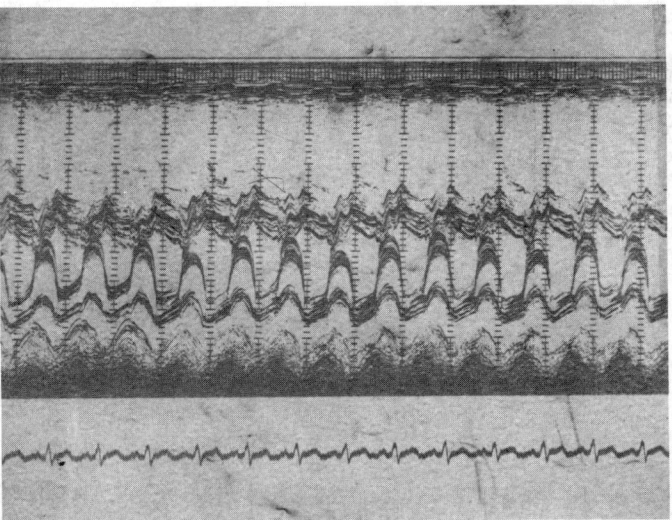

**Figure 86-7.** An M-mode echocardiogram from a patient with mitral stenosis shows a diminished EF slope, thickened mitral leaflets, and concordant movement of the anterior and posterior leaflets. The right ventricle is enlarged, indicating pulmonary hypertension.

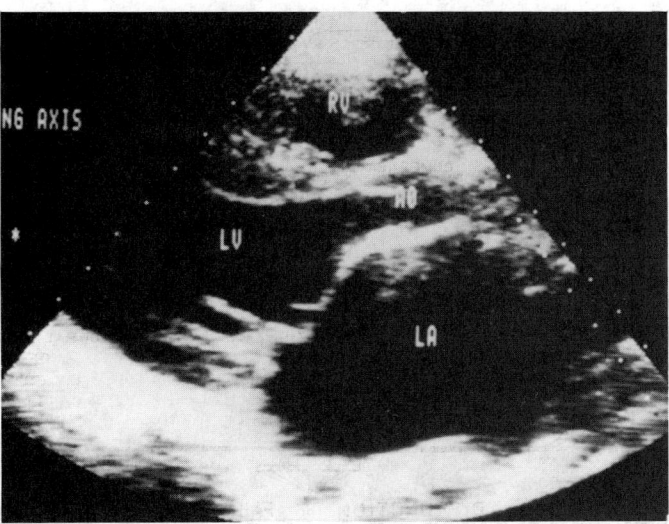

**Figure 86-8.** The two-dimensional echocardiogram from a patient with mitral stenosis shows an incomplete opening of the mitral valve. The anterior leaflet is domed and the posterior leaflet is restricted. The left atrium is markedly enlarged.

mitral valve and can estimate the gradient and the mitral valve area reasonably well.

Cardiac catheterization and angiography usually are unnecessary for evaluating isolated mitral stenosis, but they may be performed for atypical cases. Pressure measurements show elevated LA and pulmonary wedge pressures. In patients with severe stenosis and those in whom the pulmonary vascular resistance is increased, the pulmonary arterial pressure is elevated.

## Differential Diagnosis

Conditions that may mimic mitral stenosis include LA myxoma, cor triatriatum, and pulmonary veno-occlusive disease. The auscultatory findings of the Austin Flint murmur and the Carey Coombs murmur may mimic true mitral stenosis.

## RHEUMATIC AORTIC VALVE DISEASE

Aortic valvulitis, which may develop during rheumatic carditis, may cause aortic insufficiency or stenosis. Aortic insufficiency, which results from damage of the the aortic leaflets, may occur relatively early in the course of the disease and may be exaggerated over time by fibrosis, thickening, and contracture of the aortic leaflets. Aortic stenosis, which results from fusion of the commissures, takes a long time to develop. As a result, aortic valve disease caused by rheumatic conditions in children and adolescents presents usually as isolated or dominant aortic insufficiency with mild or no stenosis. Dominant stenosis at a young age, with or without insufficiency, usually is congenital.

The inability of the scarred and shortened aortic leaflets to coapt and close the aortic orifice completely during ventricular diastole causes diastolic regurgitation of blood from the aorta to the LV, because the normal aortic diastolic pressure approximates 80 mm Hg and the normal LV diastolic pressure is 0 to 12 mm Hg.

With chronic aortic insufficiency, the LV dilates with an increasing volume of blood for many years. The increased LV diastolic volume is not accompanied by an increase in end-diastolic pressure, probably because of an increase in the LV diastolic compliance. The increased LV end-diastolic volume, according to the Frank-Starling principle, results in increased stroke volume

(ie, preload reserve). The stroke volume is also maintained by reduced aortic impedance, which occurs with peripheral vasodilation (ie, decreasing afterload) (Fig 86-9).

The increased LV stroke volume, with consequent elevation in the systolic blood pressure accompanied by a decrease in the diastolic blood pressure (caused partly by regurgitation of a part of the stroke volume and partly by peripheral arteriolar vasodilation), increases the pulse pressure. The classic peripheral arterial pulses of aortic insufficiency have a rapid rise to a high peak, with a collapsing descending limb and a low diastolic pressure.

Because the major portion of coronary flow occurs during diastole, when arterial pressure is lower than normal, coronary perfusion may be reduced. The increased oxygen demand due to hypertrophy in the presence of reduced coronary flow may lead to myocardial ischemia, especially with exercise.

Exhaustion of the compensatory mechanisms (ie, preload reserve, increased contractility, diminished afterload) and myocardial ischemia may result in LV failure (Fig 86-9). In chronic aortic insufficiency, these compensatory changes occur before the onset of symptoms. Symptoms usually start only after the high LV end-diastolic pressure is reflected in the LA and pulmonary capillary pressures.

Associated aortic stenosis causes significant deleterious alterations in the pathophysiology. The increased stroke volume produced by aortic insufficiency causes a corresponding increase in the pressure gradient across the stenotic valve. At the same time, the decreased compliance of the LV secondary to hypertrophy produced by the aortic stenosis prevents the LV from accommodating the regurgitant blood of aortic insufficiency.

## Clinical Manifestations

Early symptoms are unusual, except with gross aortic insufficiency. Patients may complain that they are aware of their hearts' beating, especially with exercise, because of the large stroke volume and forceful contractions. Chest pain may be a prominent symptom during exertion. Disturbing anginal pains may occur at night, accompanied by tachycardia, sweating, and paroxysmal hypertension. The major symptoms, especially breathlessness, are caused by LV disease. Symptoms are exaggerated and occur earlier if aortic insufficiency is associated with aortic stenosis.

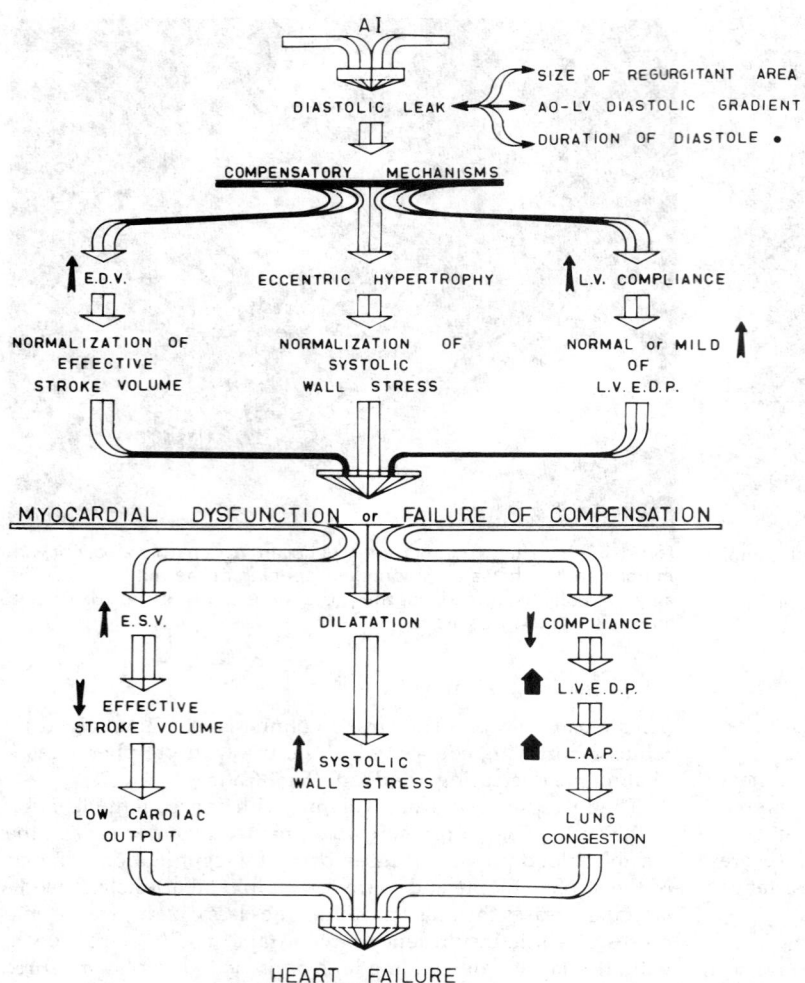

Figure 86-9. The diagram depicts factors that determine the amount of regurgitation, compensation, and decompensation in aortic insufficiency. *EDP,* end diastolic pressure; *ESV,* end systolic volume; *EDV,* end diastolic volume; *LAP,* left atrial pressure.

The characteristic peripheral signs of aortic insufficiency are produced by the combined large pulse volume and peripheral vasodilation. The sharp rise of the pulse gives it a characteristic "water hammer" quality. The visible, jerky arterial pulsations in the neck are known as Corrigan's sign. The blood pressure is normal in patients with very mild aortic insufficiency. With increasing severity of aortic insufficiency, the systolic pressure rises, and the diastole pressure falls. The apical impulse in aortic valve disease is diffuse and hyperdynamic, and it may be displaced laterally and inferiorly.

The typical murmur of aortic insufficiency is an early diastolic, high-pitched, blowing, decrescendo murmur over the base, which begins with the second sound. It is heard best with the diaphragm of the stethoscope in full expiration while the patient is sitting and leaning forward. The duration, rather than the quality or the loudness, of the aortic diastolic murmur correlates with the severity of the aortic insufficiency. An ejection systolic murmur at the base is heard in almost all cases of aortic insufficiency of more than mild degree, due to increased blood flow across the aortic valve in systole. The diagnosis of associated aortic stenosis cannot be based merely on the presence of this systolic murmur. A mid-diastolic or presystolic rumble over the mitral area, the Austin Flint murmur, usually is heard in patients with moderate or severe aortic insufficiency without associated organic mitral stenosis. The Austin Flint murmur may be caused by relative mitral stenosis secondary to improper opening of the anterior leaflet of the mitral valve by the regurgitant bloodstream or by the high LV diastolic pressure. Echocardiography is the most sensitive way to differentiate an Austin Flint from an organic apical diastolic murmur.

## Laboratory Findings

The electrocardiogram is normal in mild cases of aortic insufficiency. Left ventricular hypertrophy develops in severe cases (Fig 86-10). As the severity of aortic insufficiency increases, there is more dilatation and enlargement of the LV radiologically. Typically, the LV enlarges in an inferior and leftward direction and can be seen below the diaphragmatic level.

The most common and characteristic M-mode echocardiographic finding in chronic aortic insufficiency is fine diastolic fluttering of the mitral valve, more frequently the anterior leaflet. The echo study has an important role in the clinical assessment and evaluation of changes in LV function in patients suffering from aortic insufficiency. Serial echo studies can reveal early changes in LV functions. Deterioration is indicated if there is a progressive increase in end-systolic and end-diastolic dimensions accompanied by gradual reduction in LV shortening. Doppler is the most sensitive noninvasive method for detecting aortic insufficiency. Color Doppler flow mapping of the regurgitant jet offers a more precise approach to quantitation of the severity of the aortic insufficiency. Aortography enables diagnosis of aortic insufficiency and grading of its severity, but it is rarely needed.

## Differential Diagnosis

The diagnosis of aortic insufficiency usually is not difficult if the characteristic murmur is detected. After the murmur is heard, its cause must be differentiated from other causes of left parasternal diastolic murmurs, such as the Graham Steell murmur. The Gra-

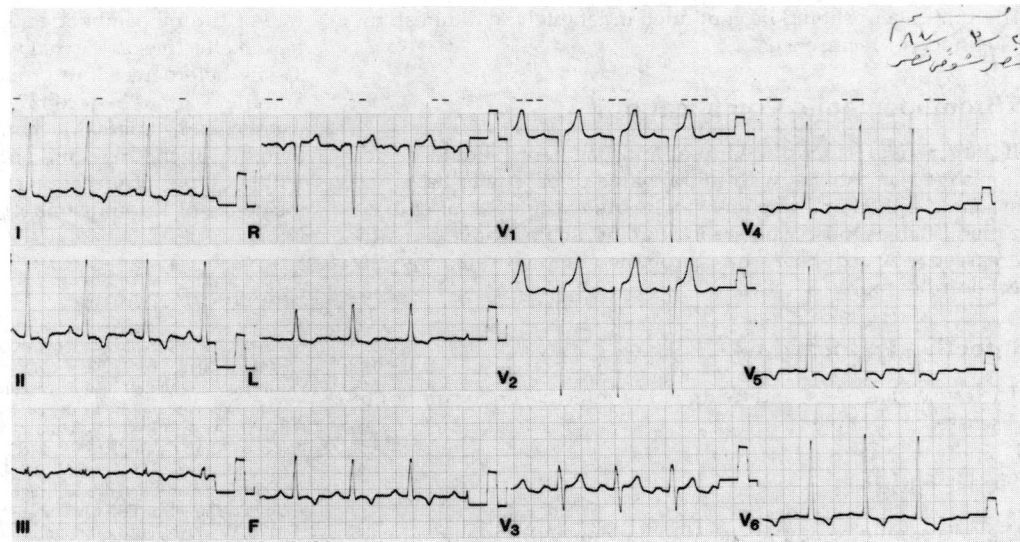

**Figure 86-10.** The electrocardiogram shows severe left ventricular hypertrophy and strain in a patient with gross aortic insufficiency.

ham Steell murmur is a soft, early diastolic, left parasternal murmur caused by functional pulmonary incompetence secondary to dilatation of the pulmonary artery as a result of severe pulmonary hypertension. Aortic insufficiency should be differentiated from other causes of aortic run-off, including patent ductus arteriosus, ruptured sinus of Valsalva, systemic arteriovenous fistula (eg, coronary), and aortic LV tunnel.

After the diagnosis of aortic valve disease is established, a search for the cause is necessary. A history of rheumatic fever or evidence of organic mitral valve disease favors a rheumatic origin. If there is evidence of associated significant aortic stenosis—supravalvular, valvular, or discrete subvalvular—the cause of aortic insufficiency usually is congenital. Isolated congenital aortic insufficiency is rare, but it can occur with aneurysms of the sinus of Valsalva. Aortic insufficiency at a young age can also occur with coarctation of the aorta, ventricular septal defect, or the Marfan syndrome. An important element in the differential diagnosis is infective endocarditis on a congenitally deformed aortic valve.

## RHEUMATIC TRICUSPID VALVE DISEASE

Rheumatic tricuspid valve disease develops in 5% to 10% of patients with rheumatic heart disease and is associated almost invariably with mitral or mitral and aortic valve disease. Organic tricuspid insufficiency can occur alone or with organic tricuspid stenosis as a result of rigidity of the valve edges, shrinkage of leaflet tissue, annular dilatation, or a combination of these abnormalities. Functional tricuspid incompetence is the result of annular dilation and malalignment of papillary muscles secondary to RV failure complicating pulmonary hypertension.

Tricuspid insufficiency permits blood to regurgitate into the right atrium (RA), diminishing the forward flow by the same amount. The larger volume of blood in the RA increases the RA pressure. When the RV relaxes, it is subjected to a higher filling pressure and dilates more to accommodate this extra blood. Right ventricular dilatation intensifies the leak and magnifies the heart failure.

The cardinal feature in tricuspid stenosis is a diastolic pressure gradient across the tricuspid valve with elevation in RA pressure.

### Clinical Manifestations

Symptoms of tricuspid valve disease are dominated by the associated, more severe left-sided lesions. Systemic venous pressure is elevated because of tricuspid valve obstruction or incompetence. The murmur of tricuspid insufficiency is audible at the lower left sternal border, is pansystolic, usually is followed by a third sound, and may radiate laterally. The diastolic murmur of tricuspid stenosis mimics that of mitral stenosis, but it usually is heard best at the lower left sternal border and has a higher pitch. Tricuspid murmurs tend to increase with inspiration, but this usually is difficult to elicit because of gross heart failure and because lung expansion during inspiration interferes with auscultation.

## TREATMENT OF RHEUMATIC HEART DISEASE

Effective prevention of RHD includes prophylaxis against rheumatic fever and its recurrence and against the occurrence of infective endocarditis.

For asymptomatic patients with mild or moderate valvular disease and with normal heart size or insignificant cardiomegaly, normal school activity should be encouraged. Restriction of activity is unnecessary. For symptomatic patients, activities should be limited to those that do not produce symptoms of fatigue, dyspnea, or excessive palpitation. Weight lifting and other isometric exercises should be discouraged. Competitive sports are not encouraged, because the patient tends to ignore symptoms in the excitement of a contest.

### Anemia and Infections

Patients with chronic RHD have diminished cardiac reserves. Cardiac decompensation can be precipitated by anemia or minor infections, which should be treated promptly and aggressively. Because chest infections may be precipitated by pulmonary congestion, a diuretic usually is needed.

### Arrhythmias

In rheumatic mitral valve disease, frequent atrial premature contractions often presage atrial fibrillation, and the administration of antiarrhythmic drugs may be effective in preventing this complication. Atrial fibrillation, flutter, and tachycardia can complicate these cases. The immediate treatment for atrial fibrillation should be directed toward reducing the ventricular rate and, if possible, reestablishing sinus rhythm by pharmacologic treatment and cardioversion, singly or in combination. After reversion to the sinus rhythm, administration of quinidine or a similar antiarrhythmic agent should be continued indefinitely to diminish the likelihood of recurrence.

## Thromboembolic Complications

If surgery is not performed, oral anticoagulants should be administered to patients with mitral valve disease who have had systemic emboli and to patients who are at high risk of embolization, such as those who are in atrial fibrillation, have a greatly enlarged LA, or have LA thrombus demonstrated by 2D echocardiography.

## Infective Endocarditis

The cause, diagnosis, and treatment of infective endocarditis are discussed in Chapter 84.

## Heart Failure

Digitalis should be administered to patients with significant valvular lesions who begin to develop effort fatigue or dyspnea, with or without frank evidence of left-sided or right-sided heart failure. However, if a patient with isolated mitral stenosis does not have right-sided heart failure or atrial fibrillation or flutter, little hemodynamic benefit can be expected from the use of digitalis. Fluid retention in such conditions responds well to treatment with diuretics. A low-sodium diet is advisable, especially if the diuretics are not completely effective. The measures designed to reduce pulmonary venous pressure, including sedation, assumption of upright posture, and aggressive diuresis, are used to treat the hemoptysis of lung congestion. Patients with overt cardiac failure are treated in the usual way. Uncontrollable heart failure in children suggests the possibility of severe valvular afflictions, rheumatic activity, infective endocarditis, or electrolyte imbalance.

For patients with isolated mitral stenosis, $\beta$-blocking agents may increase exercise tolerance by reducing the heart rate.

The response to vasodilator therapy, which diminishes the afterload, is impressive in patients with mitral and aortic insufficiency. By reducing the impedance to ejection in the aorta, the volume of regurgitating blood is reduced. Hemodynamic studies have shown beneficial effects of intravenous sodium nitroprusside in acute mitral insufficiency and oral angiotensin-converting enzyme inhibitors and prazosin in chronic cases. This therapy may be helpful in stabilizing patients who are waiting for surgery. Agents such as sublingual nitroglycerin may be effective in relieving dyspnea brought on by exercise and may permit the same exercise to be undertaken with the pulmonary artery pressure lowered because of venous dilatation, arteriolar dilatation, or both.

## Catheter Balloon Valvuloplasty

Dilatation of a stenosed mitral valve by a balloon valvuloplasty catheter can relieve mitral obstruction. This procedure is used in patients who have pliable, noncalcified mitral leaflets. Left atrial thrombi must be excluded. The best way to determine this is by transesophageal echo studies, especially in patients with atrial fibrillation. The balloon technique is an ideal way for children (who usually have pliable, noncalcified leaflets) to avoid thoracotomy.

## Surgery

Although the only direct therapy for cardiac valve disease is surgical (ie, valvotomy for severe mitral stenosis, replacement for severe mitral insufficiency and aortic insufficiency), the management of children with rheumatic valve disease should conserve the natural valve if possible. There is no prosthesis that is totally free of thromboembolic and anticoagulation problems and that has an effective orifice that will not be outgrown by a small child. Tissue heterografts are prone to calcification and early failure, and they cannot be recommended for children except under unusual circumstances. Mechanical aortic and mitral valves should be used for children, and anticoagulant therapy should be used with all types of mechanical valve prostheses, even though the incidence of thromboemboli in children is much lower than in adults.

## Selected Readings

Bonow RO. Aortic regurgitation: medical assessment and surgical intervention. Adv Intern Med 1983;28:93.

Braunwald E. Valvular hear disease. In: Braunwald E, ed. Heart disease: a textbook of cardiovascular medicine, ed 4. Philadelphia: WB Saunders, 1992:1007.

Dalen JE, Alpert JS, eds. Valvular heart disease, ed 2. Boston: Little, Brown, 1987.

Fuster V, Shub C, Giuliani ER, McGoon DC. Acquired valvular heart disease. In: Brandenburg RO, Fuster V, Giuliani ER, McGoon DC, eds. Cardiology fundamentals and practice. Chicago: Year Book Medical Publishers, 1987:1271.

Shaff HV, Danielson GK. Current status of valve replacement in children. In: Frankl WS, West AN, eds. Valvular hear disease—comprehensive approach and management. Philadelphia: FA Davis, 1986:427.

Wood P. An appreciation of mitral stenosis. Br Med J 1954;1:1051.

*Principles and Practice of Pediatrics, Second Edition.*
edited by Frank A. Oski et al. J. B. Lippincott Company, Philadelphia © 1994.

CHAPTER 87
# Cardiovascular Aspects of Kawasaki Disease

Junichiro Fukushige

Kawasaki disease, or infantile acute febrile mucocutaneous lymph node syndrome (MCLS), is the clinical entity of an acute febrile syndrome of unknown cause that is observed predominantly in children younger than 4 years of age.

## EPIDEMIOLOGY

Kawasaki disease was first described in Japan in 1967. According to national epidemiologic surveys, the number of the patients reached 105,627 (61,211 boys, 44,416 girls) in Japan by the end of 1990, and 383 deaths were reported. In the United States from 1976 through 1985, the Centers for Disease Control reported 2126 confirmed cases, an average of 220 cases per year, with the peak incidence in the winter and spring.

## CLINICAL MANIFESTATIONS

The clinical manifestations include prolonged fever, conjunctivitis, reddening of the lips and oral mucosa, reddening and indurative edema of the palms and soles in the initial stage followed by membranous desquamation from the fingertips in the convalescent stage, polymorphous exanthema, and cervical nonpurulent lymphadenopathy.

The pathologic basis of this syndrome is an acute nonspecific and systemic vasculitis. Cardiovascular lesions of this syndrome are classified into four stages according to the duration of illness. Stage I (days 0 to 12) is characterized by acute vasculitis of the microvessels and small arteries and by acute perivasculitis and endarteritis of the major arteries, especially of the coronary system. Stage II (days 12 to 25) is characterized by panvasculitis and aneurysm formation of the coronary arteries, resulting in embolus formation and local obstruction. In stage III (days 26 to 40), granulation of the medium-sized arteries and the disappearance of inflammation in the microvessels and smaller arteries are evident. In stage IV (day 40 and beyond), scarring, thickening of the intima, calcification, embolus formation, and recanalization are seen. Arteritis is particularly severe and frequently affects the coronary and iliac arteries, but major arterial branches of the aorta, such as mesenteric, renal, celiac, subclavian, carotid, and hepatic arteries, are also sites of involvement. Interstitial myocarditis, pericarditis, inflammation of the sinoatrial and atrioventricular conduction system, endocarditis, and valvulitis also occur.

The similarities of the clinical features and pathological findings in MCLS to those in infantile polyarteritis nodosa have been confirmed by investigators.

The most serious complications of Kawasaki disease are cardiovascular, and they usually occur in the second week of illness. Auscultation of the heart reveals a gallop rhythm and distant heart sound in 80% of the patients, usually in the second week of illness. Rarely, a murmur of mitral regurgitation is heard. Cardiomegaly is revealed on chest roentgenography for more than 30% of the patients. Electrocardiographic (ECG) changes are common and include low-voltage and ST depression in the first week of illness and PR prolongation, $QT_c$ prolongation, and ST elevation during the second and third weeks. Arrhythmias are rare and temporary. Development of paroxysmal supraventricular tachycardia, atrial fibrillation, ventricular tachycardia, or complete atrioventricular block is associated with serious coronary arterial lesions. ECG changes are common in patients with cardiomegaly, congestive heart failure, and heart murmur.

Dilatations or aneurysms of the coronary arteries due to vasculitis are recognized in about 50% of the patients who have not received intravenous γ-globulin therapy beginning on days 7 or 8 of the illness. The left coronary artery is involved in more patients than the right, and the proximal parts of the left or right coronary arteries are involved frequently. More distal parts of the coronary arteries are involved occasionally. The dilatations or aneurysms remain even after the acute phase in 10% to 20%

of these patients. According to Kato and colleagues (1982), of 128 patients who had documented coronary aneurysms during the acute phase, angiographic findings become normal in 73 (57%) within 1 to 2 years, suggesting regression of the aneurysms in 1 to 2 years after the acute illness. A giant coronary aneurysm with a diameter of 8 mm or more and saccular, sausage-shaped, or multiple aneurysms are considered to be important risk factors in the progression to stenosis or occlusion. Ischemic heart disease may develop in fewer than 3% of the patients. Peripheral aneurysms are found in 1% to 3% of the patients, usually with severe clinical symptoms of the acute phase and associated with coronary lesions. Ischemic necrosis of the distal extremities is a rare but potentially severe complication of Kawasaki disease.

## DIAGNOSIS

The diagnosis of Kawasaki disease primarily depends on the clinical manifestations. Diagnosis of coronary artery lesions in Kawasaki disease by two-dimensional echocardiography (2D echo) is well established, and its diagnostic sensitivity is reported to be 80% to 90% (Fig 87-1). Stenotic lesions may be detectable by 2D echo studies, but they are not demonstrable in most cases.

According to Asai and Kusakawa (1983), patients with the following clinical symptoms and signs are more likely to develop coronary artery involvement:

Male sex and age younger than 1 year
A prolonged fever for more than 16 days or recrudescent fever
Peripheral leukocyte count greater than 30,000/mm³
Erythrocyte sedimentation rate (ESR) greater than 101 mm/hour
Elevated ESR or C-reactive protein titer for more than 30 days of illness
Recrudescence of the ESR or C-reactive protein titer
ECG abnormality (eg, abnormal Q wave in leads II, III, aVF)
Symptoms of myocardial infarction.

For the early prediction of coronary involvement in the acute phase, elevated plasma β-thromboglobulin and hypoalbuminemia have been reported to be sensitive indicators for differentiating patients with coronary aneurysms from those with normal coronary arteries. There are no absolute criteria that predict accurately which patient will develop coronary arterial lesions.

The role of selective coronary angiography in evaluating and managing patients with Kawasaki disease is controversial. Although uncommon, aneurysm or dilatation can develop in the more distal part of the coronary arteries, and the normal echocardiographic appearance of the proximal right or left coronary arteries may not exclude coronary lesions completely. Most patients with coronary artery lesions have normal ECGs, chest roentgenograms, and auscultatory findings.

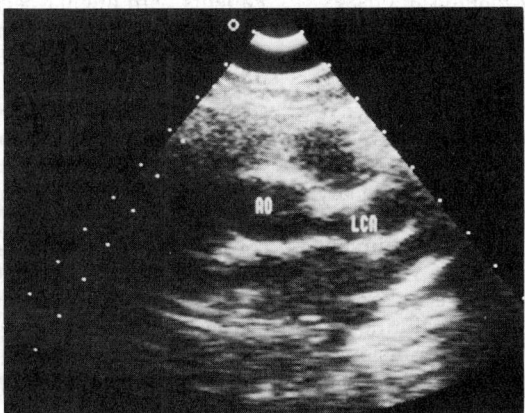 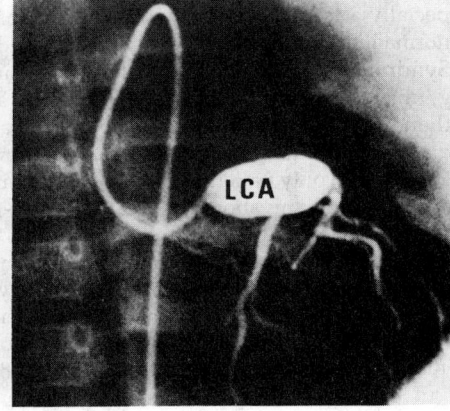

**Figure 87-1.** Two-dimensional echocardiography (*left*) and coronary angiogram (*right*) of a girl at 2 years and 7 months of age, who had Kawasaki disease at 1 year and 5 months. *AO,* aorta; *LCA,* left coronary artery aneurysm.

Pericarditis, usually with a small amount of pericardial effusion, occurs in about 30% of the patients in the first to second week of illness. It progresses to cardiac tamponade rarely, and usually special treatment is not needed. Mitral regurgitation due to valvulitis or ischemia of the papillary muscle is observed in about 1% of the patients in the acute phase. It usually is mild and improves, but in rare cases, congestive heart failure develops and requires digitalis, diuretics, and vasodilators. Aortic and pulmonary regurgitation due to valvulitis occur infrequently.

Myocardial Infarction due to thromboembolic occlusion of aneurysms or progression of the stenotic lesions accounts for most deaths due to Kawasaki disease. Of 104 deaths in Japan, 60 patients (57%) died of acute myocardial infarction, and 7 patients (9%) died of congestive heart failure and myocardial infarction. Infarction developed within 1 year of the onset of the disease in 73% of the cases complicated by myocardial infarction and within 3 months in 40% of those. Asymptomatic myocardial infarction also is common.

## TREATMENT

Japanese investigators have compared the effectiveness of aspirin, flurbiprofen, and prednisolone plus dipyridamole in a total of 306 hospitalized patients with Kawasaki disease. Coronary lesions were recognized in 22% of the patients treated with aspirin, in 39% of those treated with flurbiprofen, and in 27% of those treated with prednisolone and dipyridamole after 1 month of illness. At 1 year after the acute illness began, coronary artery abnormalities were observed in only 1% of the patients treated with aspirin but in 12% of those treated with flurbiprofen and 9% of those treated with prednisolone and dipyridamole. Most Japanese physicians have been using 30 to 50 mg/kg/day of aspirin administered in three divided doses. In the United States, an initial dose of 80 to 100 mg/kg/day has been used for 2 weeks or until the fever defervesces. A controlled, prospective study is needed to decide whether the use of high-dose aspirin is necessary.

High-dose intravenous γ-globulin therapy has been provided with increasing frequency in Japan and the United States. The nationwide survey conducted in Japan revealed that γ-globulin was administered to 39% of the patients in 1986, to 69.3% of the patients in 1990, and to only 3% of the patients in 1982. According to Furusho and colleagues (1984), coronary artery lesions were detected by 2D echo studies within 29 days of the onset of illness in 6 (15%) of 40 patients treated with aspirin plus intravenous γ-globulin and in 19 (42%) of 45 patients treated with aspirin alone. The multicenter study by Newburger and colleagues also concluded that high-dose intravenous γ-globulin, given at a dosage of 400 mg/kg/day for 4 consecutive days, was a safe and effective therapy that was associated with rapid resolution of the fever and other inflammatory manifestations, especially a lower frequency and severity of coronary artery abnormalities. An additional study by the U.S. Multicenter Kawasaki Syndrome Study Group indicated that a single-dose regimen (2 g/kg) of intravenous γ-globulin is as safe as and more effective than the conventional 4-day regimen for patients with Kawasaki disease. To reduce the cost of treatment and the need for hospitalization, only patients who are at risk for developing coronary arterial aneurysms should be treated with γ-globulin. Establishing a method to identify these patients is an important and urgent task. The mechanism by which high-dose intravenous γ-globulin reduces the development of coronary artery lesions is unknown.

Hospitalization and bed rest are the general rule during the acute phase of Kawasaki disease. The use of a single infusion of intravenous γ-globulin (2 g/kg given over 8 to 12 hours) permits hospital discharge much earlier than previously was possible. Patients with coronary artery involvement are at the highest risk for coronary embolism, myocardial infarction, and death during the second and third weeks of illness. For symptoms of myocardial infarction, oxygen, vasodilators (eg, nitroprusside, nitroglycerin), and catecholamines (eg, dopamine, dobutamine) should be administered under close observation, and the patient should be monitored carefully. Anticoagulation with heparin and urokinase, if possible by direct infusion into the coronary arteries, is advised. Defibrillation, cardiac pacing, or the administration of an antiarrhythmic drug such as Xylocaine may be indicated.

A complete blood count, platelet count, C-reactive protein titer, ESR, serum transaminases, serum protein and protein electrophoresis, urinalysis, blood urea nitrogen level, creatinine, ECG, chest roentgenogram, and 2D echo study should be obtained at least once a week, preferably at at twice-weekly intervals. If coronary or peripheral artery abnormalities are detected, dipyridamole (3 to 5 mg/kg/day) may be added to usual dose of aspirin. Patients with coronary artery abnormalities may be discharged unless there is a considerable risk of embolism or infarction.

In patients without coronary lesions (as confirmed by 2D echo or angiography), aspirin should be discontinued after 60 days. No restriction of activities is necessary. Although it is extremely unlikely that these patients will develop any signs or symptoms of cardiovascular abnormalities, yearly follow-up is recommended. Any patient who experienced Kawasaki disease in infancy may be predisposed to the development of atherosclerosis of the coronary arteries early in adult life.

Patients with coronary lesions are provided with a daily dose of aspirin (3 to 5 mg/kg/day in single dose). A dose of 2 mg/kg/day of flurbiprofen may be provided in place of aspirin. Dipyridamole (5 mg/kg/day in three divided doses) often is used in addition, because a single antithrombotic agent may be insufficient. Evaluations by ECG, chest roentgenogram, 2D echo study, and an exercise test on a treadmill or bicycle once every 2 to 3 months should be planned. Symptoms such as chest pain or severe arrhythmias are signs that suggest the need for immediate angiographic evaluation. Coronary angiography may be scheduled every 6 to 12 months after the onset of disease for patients with cardiovascular sequelae but without any symptoms. Regression of the coronary lesions is expected, especially in patients with fusiform dilatation of a mild degree with a diameter less than 8 mm. In patients with coronary abnormalities but without obstructive lesions, no general restriction of daily activities is necessary, but strenuous exercises such as short dashes, marathon runs, and competitive sports should be discouraged or advice should he provided on an individual basis.

Patients with obstructive lesions may be asymptomatic or may suffer from angina pectoris, myocardial infarction, or even sudden death. Antithrombotic therapy is indicated, but dipyridamole may not be recommended in cases with severe obstructive lesions. Patients with angina pectoris may be treated with calcium antagonists, β-blocking agents, and nitrites, or they may require coronary bypass surgery. Patients should be followed closely with ECG, 2D echo studies, an exercise stress test, thallium myocardial scintigraphy, and coronary angiography. The follow-up interval depends on the condition of the individual patient. Some require weekly evaluation, but others need only monthly or quarterly visits. Activities of the patient with obstructive lesions should be determined in light of the clinical symptoms and the results. According to the guidelines established by the Research Committee on Kawasaki disease (1987), coronary artery bypass surgery is considered in patients with severe occlusion of the main trunk of the left coronary artery or of more than one vessel, severe occlusion in the proximal portion of the left anterior descending artery, or jeopardized collaterals.

The great saphenous vein and the internal thoracic artery have been used as autologous graft materials. In view of the long-term patency of the grafts, the internal thoracic artery has been used with increasing frequency. Bilateral use of the internal thoracic artery is recommended whenever indicated, because it does not adversely affect the development of the chest wall in children. The gastroepiploic artery in combination with the internal thoracic artery has been used with favorable early results.

For patients who have a history of Kawasaki disease but who have not been examined by a physician, we recommend a careful history and physical examination, chest roentgenography, an exercise ECG, and 2D echo study. Some of these patients may require selective coronary angiography, but this technique may soon be replaced by digital subtraction angiography, magnetic resonance imaging, and x-ray computed tomography.

## PROGNOSIS

The average mortality rate for Kawasaki disease in Japan is 0.4%. The short-term prognosis is excellent for 99% of the patients. The possible long-term effects of vasculitis and aneurysm formation in the coronary arteries have not been assessed. Although regression of the coronary artery lesions of Kawasaki disease is well known, it is doubtful that the coronary arteries return completely to normal. All patients with a history of Kawasaki disease, including those who have no apparent cardiovascular abnormalities, should be examined at regular intervals. The persistently abnormal lipids in Kawasaki disease may increase the risk of premature coronary disease in young adults.

## Selected Readings

Asai T. Evaluation method for the degree of seriousness in Kawasaki disease. Acta Paediatr Jpn 1983;25:170.

Ettedgui JA, Neches WH, Pahl E. The role of cross-sectional echocardiography in Kawasaki disease. Cardiol Young 1991;1:221.

Fujiwara H, Hamashima Y. Pathology of the heart in Kawasaki disease. Pediatrics 1978;61:100.

Fukushige J, Nihill MR, McNamara DG. Spectrum of cardiovascular lesions in mucocutaneous lymph node syndrome: analysis of eight cases. Am J Cardiol 1980;45:98.

Furusho K, Kamiya T, Nakano H, et al. High-dose intravenous gamma globulin for Kawasaki disease. Lancet 1984;2:1055.

Kato H, Ichinose E, Yoshioka F, et al. Fate of coronary aneurysms in Kawasaki disease: serial coronary angiography and long-term follow-up study. Am J Cardiol 1982;49:1758.

Kawasaki T, Kosai F, Okawa S, et al. A new infantile acute febrile mucocutaneous lymph node syndrome (MLNS) prevailing in Japan. Pediatrics 1977;59:651.

Kawasaki T. Kawasaki disease. Cardiol Young 1991;1:184.

Landing BH, Larson EJ. Are infantile periarteritis nodosa with coronary artery involvement and fatal mucocutaneous lymph node syndrome the same? Comparison of 20 patients from North America with patients from Hawaii and Japan. Pediatrics 1977;59:651.

Mason WH, Schneider T, Takahashi M. The epidemiology and etiology of Kawasaki disease. Cardiol Young 1991;1:196.

Newburger JW, Takahashi M, Burns JC, et al. The treatment of Kawasaki syndrome with intravenous gamma globulin. N Engl J Med 1986;315:341.

Newburger JW, Takahashi M, Beiser AS, et al. Single intravenous infusion of gamma globulin as compared with four infusions in the treatment of acute Kawasaki syndrome. N Engl J Med 1991;324:1664.

Research Committee on Kawasaki Disease. Guidelines for treatment and management of cardiovascular sequelae in Kawasaki disease. Heart & Vessels 1987;3:50.

*Principles and Practice of Pediatrics, Second Edition.*
edited by Frank A. Oski et al. J. B. Lippincott Company, Philadelphia © 1994.

CHAPTER 88

# Abnormalities of Cardiac Rate and Rhythm

## Arthur Garson, Jr.

## THE RANGE OF NORMAL

The normal values for heart rate, PR interval, and QRS duration are shown for different ages in Table 88-1. On any routine electrocardiogram or any rhythm strip taken in the office or emergency room, it is important to examine the tracing for indications of two abnormalities: Wolff-Parkinson-White syndrome and long QT interval. In Wolff-Parkinson-White syndrome, the PR interval is short for the age of the patient; there is slurred upstroke to the QRS complex (ie, delta wave); and there are usually changes in the ST or T waves. These findings may not be found in all leads, and the middle chest leads ($V_2$ to $V_4$) may be the most sensitive

(Fig 88-1). A prolonged QT interval is diagnosed when the corrected QT interval (ie, QT interval in seconds/square root of the RR interval in seconds) is longer than 0.44 (Fig 88-2). Because both of these problems can cause syncope or seizures in a previously well child, an electrocardiogram should be part of the workup of a patient who presents with his or her first nonfebrile seizure or who presents with atypical syncope. Atypical syncope occurs during exercise or without the typical circumstances associated with vasodepressor syncope, such as heat or a crowded room. Atypical syncope frequently occurs without any warning and therefore may result in injury; it may last longer than the 60 seconds associated with the usual faint.

### TABLE 88-1. Heart Rates in Normal Infants and Children*

| Age of Child (Years) | Awake | | Asleep |
|---|---|---|---|
| | Low | High | Low |
| 1 | 90 | 200 | 70 |
| 1–9 | 60 | 180 | 45 |
| 10 | 50 | 180 | 35 |

* Approximate rates; may vary with clinical situation (eg, fever may elevate heart rate).

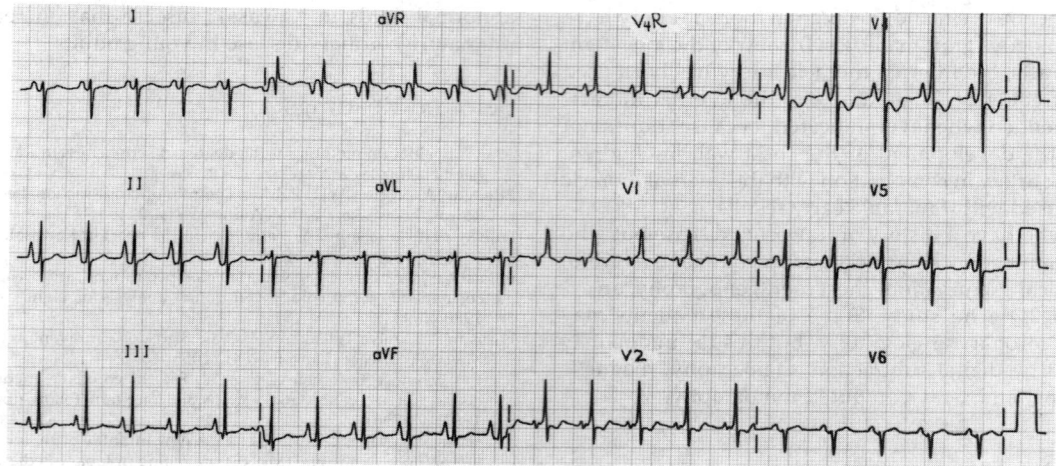

**Figure 88-1.** Electrocardiographic evidence of Wolff-Parkinson-White syndrome in a baby is seen on this strip. In the limb leads, no delta wave is apparent. In lead $V_4$, and the short PR interval (0.075 seconds), the delta wave, and the bizarre QRS morphology are seen most easily. The P waves are tall and broad, indicating atrial enlargement. This patient had just undergone conversion from supraventricular tachycardia to sinus rhythm. Frequently, the P waves show atrial enlargement immediately after conversion.

## VAGAL ARRHYTHMIAS

The arrhythmias that appear with increasing amounts of "vagal tone" are sinus arrhythmia, wandering pacemaker, and junctional rhythm.

In sinus arrhythmia, the P wave axis remains normal (ie, isoelectric or positive in leads I and aVF), but the interval between P waves rate increases with inspiration and decreases with expiration. This variation in rate rarely exceeds 100% (eg, from a rate of 50 to a rate of 100/minute); if it does, it may signify pathology. In sinus arrhythmia, a QRS complex follows every P wave.

In wandering pacemaker, the P wave axis and morphology may change in such a manner that the P wave varies from positive to negative in lead aVF. It is rare for the wandering pacemaker to "wander" to the left atrium, making the P wave negative in lead I. A QRS complex follows every P wave.

In junctional rhythm (ie, nodal premature beats) the P wave occurs within or after the QRS complex. In adults, it is thought that the junctional rhythm may occur with a P wave preceding the QRS. This does not appear to be the case in children; the rhythms seem to originate from the low right atrium.

In most patients, these arrhythmias are entirely normal. If there is excessive variation in the rate, constant sinus bradycardia below the normal limits for age, or constant junctional rhythm, there may be an underlying abnormality. The most common disorder is the "athletic heart," a condition of bradycardia in adolescents. This requires no further workup if the patient is asymp-

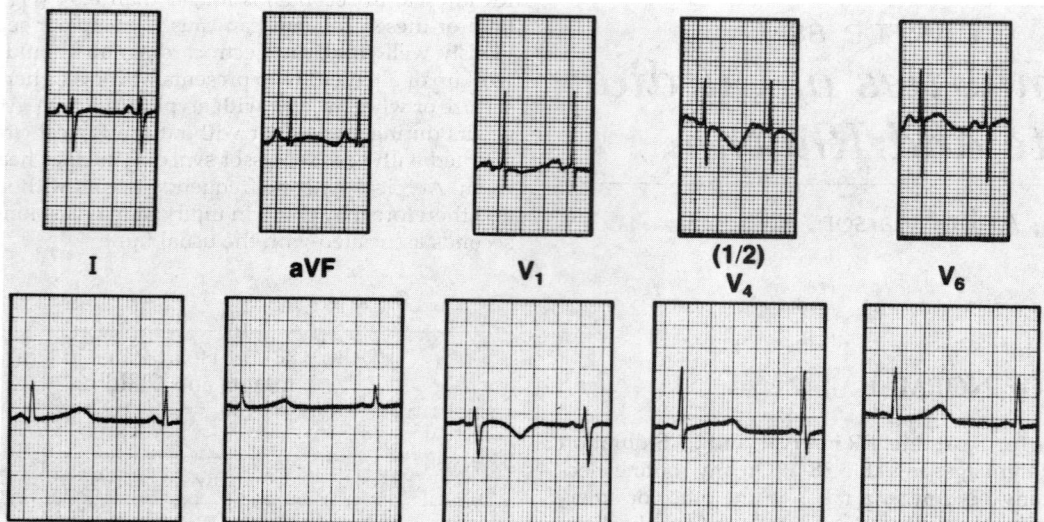

**Figure 88-2.** Congenital prolongation of the QT interval. The top tracings are from a 9-day-old infant with a history of ventricular tachycardia and ventricular fibrillation at the age of 4 days. All the T waves are abnormal; the T waves in lead $V_4$ are especially bizarre. The QT interval is 0.43 seconds, and the RR interval is 0.58 seconds; the corrected QT interval (QT/square root of RR) is 0.56 seconds. The bottom tracings are from a 12-year-old child who had his first episode of syncope at 10 years of age. He was being treated for a "familial seizure disorder," although the actual cause of the "seizures" was ventricular tachycardia. The terminal portion of the T wave in lead $V_4$ is greater in amplitude than the initial portion. The corrected QT interval is 0.55 seconds.

tomatic. Other reasons for excessive vagal arrhythmias are increased intracranial pressure, pharyngeal stimulation, gastric distention, upper airway obstruction, asthma, and drugs that potentiate bradycardia, such as digoxin, propranolol, verapamil, and morphine.

## COMPLETE ATRIOVENTRICULAR BLOCK

In complete atrioventricular (AV) block, the P waves are entirely dissociated from the QRS complexes (Fig 88-3). The QRS complexes usually are extremely regular; there may be a variation in the PP interval (ie, superimposed sinus arrhythmia). In awake newborns with congenital complete AV block, the ventricular rate usually is between 60 and 80 beats per minute. Commonly associated with congenital complete AV block are congenital heart disease (most often "corrected" transposition of the great arteries), long QT syndrome (long QT is also found in second-degree AV block; measure the QT in all patients with AV block), and maternal collagen vascular disease.

The mothers with collagen vascular disease frequently are asymptomatic, although some may have systemic lupus erythematosus or a similar disease. In women with clinical or subclinical disease, there is a high titer of anti-Ro antibodies that seem to cross the placenta and attack the AV node. The infants usually do not have other signs of collagen vascular disease. Despite a low antibody titer, the complete AV block does not reverse in these infants. Some infants born with second-degree AV block may develop complete AV blocks in the first year or two of life, which implies that "congenital" complete AV block may be an evolving process.

Children with complete AV block do not require immediate pacemaker therapy. As long as the ventricular rate is consistently greater than 55 beats per minute and there are no symptoms of congestive heart failure, these infants and children fare quite well. If there is coexistent congenital heart disease, especially with a physiological abnormality such as a ventricular septal defect (frequently associated with corrected transposition), pacing may be instituted earlier. As these children grow, they may exhibit subtle symptoms, such as frequent naps, mild growth failure, night terrors, and lack of full participation in sports. If these subtle symptoms occur, pacemakers usually are implanted. Modern pacemakers that sense the atrium and pace the ventricle can correct the situation physiologically, returning normal variation to the ventricular rate. The development of syncope, presyncope, or even sudden death appears to be more common in patients with extremely low ventricular rates (ie, consistently in the 40s). Consideration should be given to earlier pacing in these patients.

## SUPRAVENTRICULAR ARRHYTHMIAS

### Premature Atrial Contractions

A premature atrial contraction (PAC) is defined as a premature P wave. In most instances, the premature P wave has a different morphology and axis from those of the sinus P waves. If a P wave has a similar morphology and axis to the sinus P wave, there is a regular underlying sinus rhythm and a P wave that occurs obviously early. This may be classified as a PAC. Most PACs are conducted to the ventricles with a normal QRS. As the premature P wave occurs earlier and earlier, there may be conduction to the ventricles with a different QRS (ie, aberrant PAC) from that of the sinus beat; this simulates a premature ventricular contraction (PVC). For any early QRS that has a different morphology from that of the sinus, the preceding T wave should be examined carefully for a hidden P wave. In children, the presence or absence of a compensatory pause is not helpful in differentiating an abberant PAC from a PVC. Occasionally, a premature P wave may occur so early that it does not conduct to the ventricles at all, and it may simulate sinus bradycardia because the premature P wave may conduct into the sinus node, dealying the next expected sinus impulse. In many cases of paroxysmal bradycardia, especially those in which there are conducted PACs on the same tracing, the T wave should be searched carefully for the presence of hidden P waves. This is especially common in newborn infants. Many tracings similar to the one in Figure 88-4 are interpreted as multiform PVCs with PACs and sinus bradycardia, but most of these infants have only PACs, some conducted aberrantly and some not conducted at all.

In the newborn with frequent PACs, it may be useful to obtain a 24-hour electrocardiogram to determine if there are frequent nonsustained episodes of supraventricular tachycardia. If they are observed, the infant should be treated for supraventricular tachycardia. In older children, PACs apparently do not predispose to supraventricular tachycardia, and treatment is unnecessary.

### Supraventricular Tachycardia

Supraventricular tachycardia is defined as an abnormally rapid rhythm that originates proximal to the bifurcation of the bundle of His, is caused by an abnormal mechanism (specifically ex-

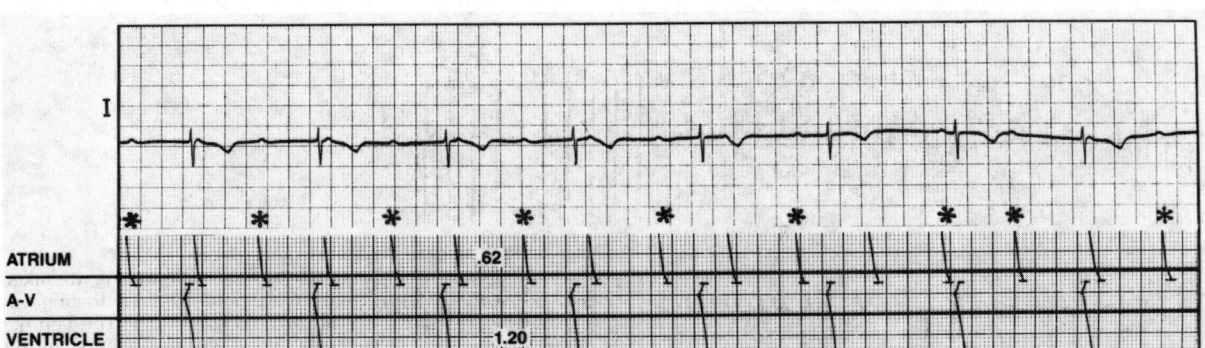

**Figure 88-3.** A complete atrioventricular (AV) block in a 1-month-old child is demonstrated on this strip. The atrial rate is 97/minute (cycle length of 0.62 seconds), and the ventricles are controlled by a junctional, narrow QRS rhythm at a rate of 50/minute (cycle length 1.20 seconds). The P waves with asterisks should conduct to the ventricles; they occur beyond the end of the preceding T wave, and they do not change the ventricular rate. There is complete AV dissociation, with no relation of the P waves to the QRS complexes.

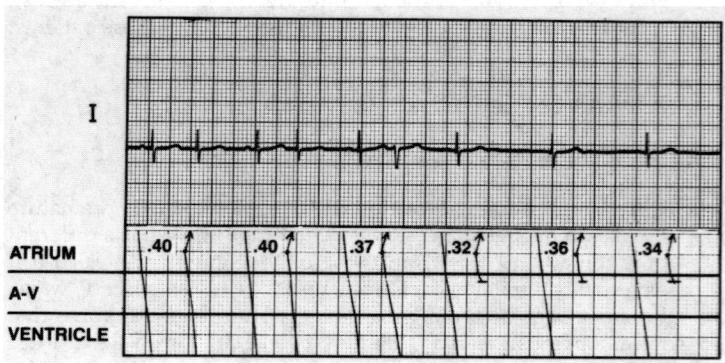

**Figure 88-4.** Blocked premature atrial contractions are demonstrated on this tracing taken from a 1-day-old infant. The first beat is of sinus origin, and it is followed by a premature atrial contraction. The baseline is completely flat immediately after the sinus T wave, after which there is a slight change in the baseline, indicating a premature P wave (ie, premature atrial contraction). This conducts to the ventricles normally. The premature atrial contraction occurs 0.40 seconds after the preceding P wave. This sequence is repeated in the next two beats. The premature P wave that occurs 0.37 seconds after the preceding sinus P wave conducts with a different QRS, indicating QRS aberration. In the last three beats, the sinus T wave has a different shape than do the other sinus T waves, which indicates that a P wave is buried in the T wave. The premature P wave occurs 0.32 seconds after the preceding sinus P wave. Because this is too early for conduction to the ventricles to occur, the premature P wave is not followed by a QRS complex. This "blocked premature atrial contraction" simulates sinus bradycardia.

cluding sinus tachycardia), and does not have flutter waves on the surface electrocardiogram. In most cases of supraventricular tachycardia, the onset is paroxysmal, and the rate is faster than 230 beats per minute; in infants, the most common rate is 300 beats per minute. In approximately half of the patients, P waves may be found, but they are not as obvious as they are in sinus tachycardia.

In 98% of the children with supraventricular tachycardia, the QRS complex during tachycardia (after the first 5 to 10 beats) is identical to the QRS complex during sinus rhythm (Fig 88-5); supraventricular tachycardia with aberration rarely occurs in children. Tachycardias that do not have a broad QRS complex in children are often assumed to be supraventricular tachycardias. This misconception may lead to the underdiagnosis of children who actually have ventricular tachycardia. The major problem in the differential diagnosis of supraventricular tachycardia in children is with sinus tachycardia, because both rhythms usually have a normal QRS complex. If the rate is faster than 230 beats per minute, it is virtually always supraventricular tachycardia; if the rate is slower, the disorder could be supraventricular tachycardia or sinus tachycardia. If the P waves are clearly visible and positive in leads I and aVF, it is likely to be sinus tachycardia. The condition of the patient may be helpful. Most infants or children with very rapid sinus tachycardia have fever, sepsis, hypovolemia, aminophylline intoxication, or another reason for this finding. Most of the children with supraventricular tachycardia are otherwise well.

There are three major predisposing causes in supraventricular tachycardia: Wolff-Parkinson-White syndrome (see Fig 88-1), congenital heart disease, and sympathomimetic drugs (eg, decongestants). It is rare for a child to develop a tachyarrhythmia

associated with the ingestion of caffeine-containing compounds. Because children vary in their responses to the conditions triggering supraventricular tachycardia, we try not to restrict them from any drug or situation unless it is known to lead to the arrhythmia in that particular patient.

The initial treatment of paroxysmal supraventricular tachycardia involves assessing whether the patient has a compromised cardiac output (ie, decreased peripheral pulse volume, decreased capillary refill, diaphoresis, irritability). Many infants with less severe circulatory embarrassment present with mild tachypnea and hepatomegaly. If the infant is judged to be compromised, the following steps should be undertaken to stop the supraventricular tachycardia. Initiate the diving reflex by placing a wet washcloth in crushed ice or filling a rubber glove with crushed ice and placing it on the infant's face for as long as 30 seconds. This always should be done with electrocardiographic monitoring, and the team should be prepared for cardiopulmonary resuscitation because of asystole or ventricular fibrillation, both of which have been reported, although rarely. Other vagal maneuvers, such as Valsalva and carotid sinus massage, are not effective for patients younger than 4 years of age. We do not recommend eyeball pressure, because ruptured retinas have been reported. Injection of adenosine for overdrive pacing, beginning with a dose of 37.5 $\mu$g/kg given by intravenous bolus, can be attempted next. If the drug and vagal maneuvers fail, we then use DC cardioversion, which must be synchronized to the QRS; the dose is 0.5 to 1.5 watt-second/kg.

If the patient is not compromised hemodynamically and if the diving reflex, vagal maneuvers, and adenosine are ineffective, intravenous digitalis may be given. The first dose is 12 $\mu$g/kg. In infants and children older than 6 months of age, the initial in-

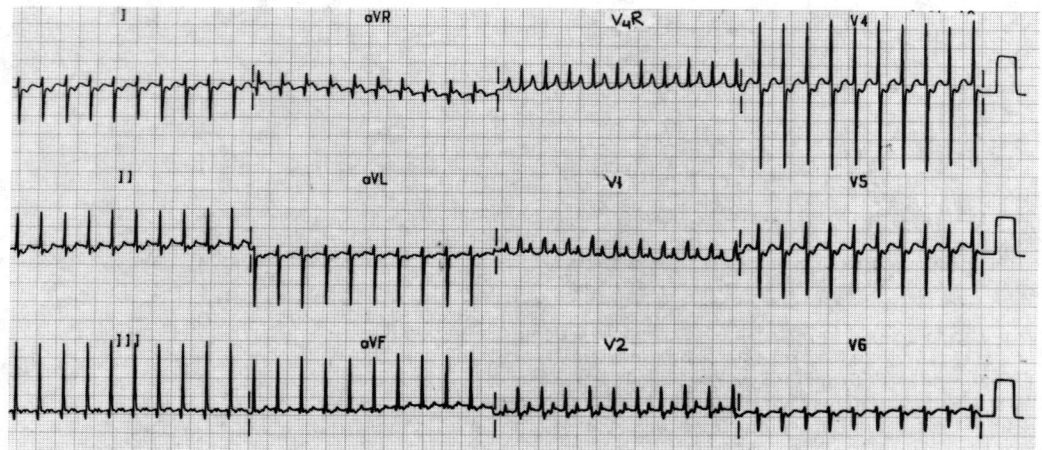

**Figure 88-5.** This tracing was taken from the patient whose tracing was shown in Figure 88-1. The ventricular rate is 250 per minute. In this patient who has Wolff-Parkinson-White syndrome demonstrated during sinus rhythm, the QRS complex during supraventricular tachycardia is normal. There are P waves after the QRS complex, seen best in lead V$_2$.

**Figure 88-6.** This strip demonstrates ventricular tachycardia in an infant. The ventricular rate is 500 per minute, and the QRS duration is only 0.045 seconds. This may be mistaken for supraventricular tachycardia. However, the notched morphology of the QRS complexes, and the discordance between the QRS complexes and the T waves (ie, QRS pointing upward and T waves pointing downward) suggests ventricular tachycardia, even though the QRS duration is normal. In sinus rhythm, this infant had a QRS duration of 0.025 milliseconds with a completely different QRS morphology.

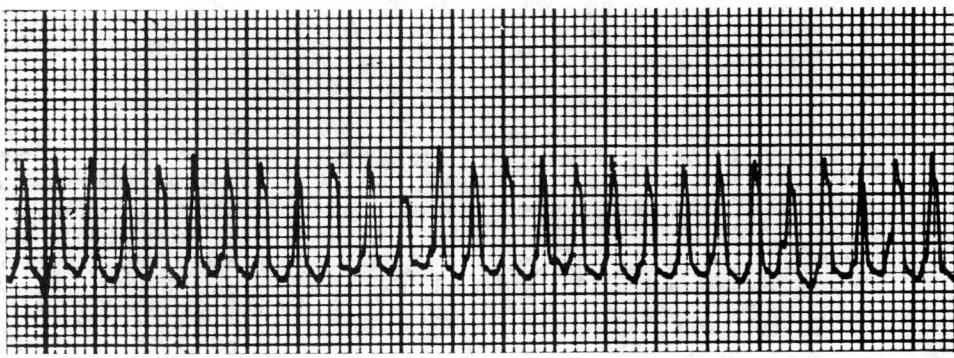

travenous dose is 20 μg/kg. The maximal first intravenous dose for an adult is 0.4 mg. If the hemodynamics are stable, the patient is older than 1 year of age, there is no sign of congestive heart failure, and the patient has not been receiving β-blocking agents, intravenous verapamil (0.05 mg/kg, given in three doses 10 minutes apart) can be administered.

## VENTRICULAR ARRHYTHMIAS

### Premature Ventricular Contractions

A premature ventricular contraction (PVC) is recognized as a premature QRS complex that does not have the same morphology as the sinus complex and is not preceded by a premature P wave. Especially in infants, PVCs may not have a broad QRS complex but may have a different morphology from the sinus QRS. If PVCs have the same shape, they are referred to as uniform, and if they have more than one morphology, they are called multiform. A couplet is two PVCs in a row, and bigeminy is an alternating rhythm in which every other beat is a PVC.

Most children with PVCs have normal hearts. Occasionally, PVCs are associated with long QT syndrome, mitral valve prolapse, hypertrophic cardiomyopathy, congestive cardiomyopathy, and congenital heart disease before or after surgery. If the heart is completely normal, the prognosis for the child with uniform PVCs (even those frequent enough to present as bigeminy) is good, and the condition is entirely benign. For the child with a normal heart and multiform PVCs or couplets, fewer data are available. Because the prognosis may be serious (including sudden death in some children with PVCs and abnormal hearts), it is important to assess whether the heart is normal. This usually involves additional diagnostic testing, such as echocardiography.

### Ventricular Tachycardia

Ventricular tachycardia is defined as three or more PVCs in a row at a rate faster than 120 per minute, and slower rates are referred to as accelerated ventricular rhythms. The QRS complex in ventricular tachycardia is different from the sinus QRS complex, although it may not be broad. In our series of 22 infants younger than 2 years of age with ventricular tachycardia, the QRS duration ranged from 0.06 to 0.11 seconds. The rate may be as rapid as 400 or 500 beats per minute (Fig 88-6). Although ventricular tachycardia is an unusual diagnosis for an infant or a child, it must be suspected in any case in which the QRS complex does

not appear to be similar to the sinus QRS complex. We have found that ventricular tachycardia in young infants usually is associated with a small ventricular tumor or with the long QT syndrome. In older children, ventricular tachycardia is associated with mitral valve prolapse, various forms of cardiomyopathy, and congenital heart disease before and after surgery. In most series, it is rare for a child with ventricular tachycardia to have an entirely normal heart; even if there is no known history of heart disease, many of these children have early cardiomyopathy.

The initial management of ventricular tachycardia consists of intravenous lidocaine (1 mg/kg every 5 minutes for three doses). If the lidocaine is not effective and the patient is hemodynamically unstable, synchronized DC electrical cardioversion should be used (0.5 to 1.5 watt-second/kg). Because most infants and children with ventricular tachycardia have abnormal hearts, additional diagnostic studies should be performed.

## CONCLUSION

Most arrhythmias in children with entirely normal hearts are benign, but for children with abnormal hearts, these arrhythmias may be lethal. In the case of a tachyarrhythmia, it is important to evaluate the patient for hemodynamic stability. If the patient is hemodynamically stable, take time to analyze the electrocardiogram, not mistaking supraventricular tachycardia for sinus tachycardia or ventricular tachycardia for supraventricular tachycardia. If the patient is unstable, synchronized DC electrical cardioversion should be performed and the rhythm then analyzed.

### Selected Readings

Bricker T, Garson A, Gillette PC. A history of seizures in the family associated with sudden cardiac death. Am J Dis Child 1984;138:866.

Esscher E. Congenital complete heart block in adolescence and adult life. A follow-up study. Eur Heart J 1981;2:281.

Garson A Jr. The electrocardiogram in infants and children: a systematic approach. Philadelphia: Lea & Febiger, 1983.

Garson A Jr, Gillette PC, McNamara DG. Supraventricular tachycardia in children: clinical features, response to treatment, and long-term follow-up in 217 patients. J Pediatr 1981;98:875.

Garson A Jr, Gillette PC, Titus JL et al. Surgical treatment of ventricular tachycardia in infants. N Engl J Med 1984;310:1443.

Jacobsen J, Garson A Jr. Irregular heartbeat. In: Garson A Jr, Bricker T, McNamara DG, eds. The science and practice of pediatric cardiology. Philadelphia: Lea & Febiger, 1990.

Scott JS, Maddison PJ, Skinner RP. Connective tissue disease, antibodies to ribonucleoprotein, and congenital heart block. N Engl J Med 1983;309:209.

*Principles and Practice of Pediatrics, Second Edition.*
edited by Frank A. Oski et al. J. B. Lippincott Company, Philadelphia © 1994.

# CHAPTER 89
# *Evaluation of Patients With Heart or Circulatory System Disease*

## *89.1 Echocardiography*

### James C. Huhta

During the past 15 years, echocardiography (ie, ultrasonic imaging) of the heart and cardiovascular system has provided a major advance in pediatric cardiology, allowing imaging of anatomy and appraisal of ventricular function. This noninvasive modality has dramatically altered the assessment of fetal and neonatal congenital heart disease. The technique has slowly changed the practice of pediatric cardiology by replacing cardiac catheterization for the diagnosis of congenital malformations, and combined with the use of prostaglandin for maintaining the patency of the ductus arteriosus, echocardiography has dramatically reduced the need for emergency cardiac catheterization in neonates. Most patients with congenital heart disease detected in the neonatal period can have palliative surgery without cardiac catheterization, and some definitive surgical repairs can be performed successfully without the risks of invasive studies.

## DIAGNOSIS OF CONGENITAL HEART DISEASE

Echocardiography will continue to be the mainstay of the diagnosis of congenital heart disease in neonates, infants, and children and will probably become more important as additional experience is accumulated. Pioneered by Van Praagh (1972) for describing congenital cardiac defects at the autopsy table, the segmental approach has since been applied to cardiovascular diagnosis using various methods, including echocardiography. A logical analysis of cardiovascular anatomy requires a step-by-step segmental approach. This segmental approach is used assessing for complex congenital malformations in which some portions of the heart may be absent or malpositioned and for the angiographic delineation of cardiac anatomy. Data are obtained by combining the findings from several echocardiographic windows. A complete, step-by-step approach to cardiac diagnosis includes atrial situs diagnosis, identification of the chambers and their interconnections, and a systematic assessment of valves, septa, coronaries, systemic and pulmonary veins, and aortic anatomy.

The teams led by Sanders and Silverman pointed out the need for a complete segmental examination inside and outside the heart. The diagnostic accuracy of two-dimensional echocardiographic imaging in children has been proven in several prospective studies, including that of Gutgesell and colleagues (1985).

In 250 consecutive children with congenital heart disease treated at Texas Children's Hospital, there was one surgically significant error in diagnosis.

The segmental approach is based on the condition that all aspects of abnormal cardiovascular morphology can be broken down into discrete, mutually exclusive descriptors, allowing any complex congenital malformation to be described unambiguously. The schema must include information on the presence, position, and connection of each cardiac segment. Classically, three segments have been recognized: the atria, the ventricles, and the great arteries. In complex malformations, it is necessary to have a detailed approach to segmental diagnosis that can be used for noninvasive examination in any setting. By describing the anatomical segments and indicating the normality or abnormality of each, a complete description of the cardiac anatomy is possible.

Echocardiography is a tomographic anatomical tool, but it also provides dynamic information about cardiac function and structure. Doppler echocardiography can provide functional information that is not available from any other method. For example, atrioventricular valve regurgitation can be diagnosed. However, the grading of regurgitation is difficult and depends on many technical and physiologic factors. In addition to seeing a ventricular septal defect (color figure 29), the jet of a left-to-right shunt can be detected by pulsed Doppler, the pressure gradient quantitated by continuous wave Doppler, and the defect spatially oriented by color Doppler. The functional description should be integrated into this approach using the anatomical segment as the finding and the functional aspect as the modifier. For example, a left ventricular shortening fraction is added to the anatomical finding of left ventricular dilation; severe pulmonary valvular stenosis with a peak Doppler velocity of 4 m/second indicates a gradient from the right ventricle to the pulmonary artery of at least 64 mm Hg.

Most early two-dimensional echocardiographic reports were oriented toward a "view approach" to congenital cardiac lesions. The investigators described the appearance of a given cardiac lesion in a standard parasternal, apical, or subcostal scan. However, this approach can lead to diagnostic errors. For example, a scan of an aortopulmonary window from the right ventricular outflow tract can simulate the origin of the aorta from the right ventricle (ie, transposition of the great arteries). The various views must be integrated, scanning from one to another echocardiographic windows to perform a complete anatomical examination. Although the echocardiographic examiner with experience learns to identify the normal appearances of the heart without congenital defects from various echo windows, a structure-oriented or anatomical approach is always superior to one based on standardized views.

### Situs

The diagnosis of cardiac position and atrial-visceral situs using echocardiographic signs is a standard part of the assessment of congenital heart disease. Atrial situs and atrial morphology are diagnosed together, and there are four possibilities: solitus (normal), inversus, and heterotaxy that may be right atrial isomerism or left atrial isomerism. For example, for situs solitus, the morphologic right atrium is on the right, and the morphologic left atrium is on the left. Abnormal atrial situs and cardiac malposition, such as dextrocardia, are frequently associated. Both can be diagnosed by obtaining a short-axis scan of the abdomen, identifying the spine and the left and right chest cavities. The location of the cardiac apex is important for later scanning from the apex. Subcostal scanning above the diaphragm immediately shows the position of the cardiac apex. From this scan below the diaphragm, the position of the inferior vena cava and aorta can usually be identified.

The descending aorta and the inferior vena cava are symmetrically oriented with respect to one another, with the inferior vena cava to the right in situs solitus and to the left in situs inversus. In right atrial isomerism, the aorta and the inferior cava run together on either side of the spine with the cava anterior. A venous structure that courses behind the aorta and does not enter the heart suggests azygos continuation of the inferior vena cava, which is associated with left atrial isomerism. These patients usually have separate, anomalous hepatic venous connections to the heart. Occasionally, atrial appendage morphology can be identified and the diagnosis of atrial situs confirmed directly. A broad-based atrial appendage is usually a morphologic right one, and a narrow-based appendage is morphologic left. Symmetric appendages suggests atrial isomerism. A prospective study of the accuracy of indirect methods showed a sensitivity of 100% and a specificity of 99% for detection of abnormal situs by echocardiography.

## Atrioventricular Connection

The diagnosis of a connection of the atria and ventricles (ie, atrioventricular connection) requires knowledge of the atrial and ventricular morphology. The morphologic left ventricle can be identified by its usual ellipsoidal appearance, two papillary muscles, mitral-semilunar continuity, and the typical mitral valve "fishmouth" appearance. The most reliable criterion for identification of the morphologic right ventricle is tricuspid valve chordal attachments to the septum.

Determination of the atrioventricular and ventriculoarterial connections requires a knowledge of ventricular morphology, and this determination should be one of the first steps in noninvasive diagnosis. The echocardiographic criteria for a morphologic left ventricle include insertion of the mitral valve at the crux of the heart farther from the cardiac apex than the tricuspid valve, two normally placed left ventricular papillary muscles, mitral semilunar continuity, a typical elliptical, smooth wall septum, and a fishmouth appearance of the mitral valve with two commissures. In the absence of the typical offsetting of the atrioventricular valves and with cardiac malposition, the trabecular pattern of the ventricles can sometimes be recognized: the smooth wall pattern of the left ventricle and coarser, more heavily trabeculated pattern of the right ventricle. The appearance of the ventricular outflow tracts may aid in ventricular morphologic diagnosis and should be observed as part of the segmental approach. There normally is continuity between the mitral valve of the left ventricle and the aortic valve, but there is muscle separating the tricuspid and the pulmonary valve in the right ventricular outflow tract.

There are four possibilities for atrioventricular connection: concordant (ie, normal); discordant; univentricular through a single inlet (ie, tricuspid or mitral atresia), double inlet, or common inlet; and ambiguous (ie, two ventricles with atrial isomerism). When the morphologic right atrium connects normally to the morphologic right ventricle and the left atrium connects to the left ventricle, there is atrioventricular concordance. When this connection is reversed and the morphologic right atrium connects to the morphologic left ventricle, there is an atrioventricular discordance that is sometimes referred to as ventricular inversion. Patients with these abnormalities may present with complete heart block and have a high incidence of associated congenital cardiac malformations, such as ventricular septal defect and pulmonary stenosis; they usually also have ventriculoarterial discordance. Rarely, atrioventricular discordance may occur while the ventriculoarterial connection is normal. If most of the atrioventricular connection is to one ventricle, the connection is univentricular through one valve (ie, single inlet with atresia of the other valve), a double inlet (ie, two atrioventricular valves), or a common inlet (ie, common atrioventricular valve). A common

inlet ventricle is part of the spectrum of atrioventricular septal defect (ie, AV canal) in which there is hypoplasia of one of the ventricular chambers and the atrioventricular connection is predominantly to the other.

The accuracy of echocardiographic imaging in the diagnosis of atrioventricular connection is unsurpassed by other modalities. Occasionally, an inexperienced observer may confuse a common inlet with a common (four leaflet) valve with a single inlet. After experience with imaging the variations of atrioventricular septal defect, this should not present problems. Identification of the lower atrial septum unequivocally identifies the crux of the heart and points to a single inlet with atresia of the other valve. There is general agreement that echocardiography in experienced hands is the best method for assessing atrioventricular connection.

## Ventriculoarterial Connection

Ventriculoarterial connection is the manner in which the great arteries and semilunar valves connect to the ventricular outflow tracts. There are four possibilities: concordant (ie, normal); discordant (ie, right ventricle to the aorta and left ventricle to the pulmonary trunk); double outlet (usually the right ventricle); and single outlet (ie, aortic or pulmonary atresia or truncus arteriosus). Normally, the morphologic right ventricle connects to the pulmonary valve, and the morphologic left ventricle connects to the aortic valve.

The most common type of abnormality of ventriculoarterial connection is transposition of the great arteries, in which the morphologic right ventricle gives rise to the aorta and the morphologic left ventricle gives rise to the pulmonary trunk (ie, ventriculoarterial discordance). To diagnose this abnormality, it is necessary to identify the great vessels. The pulmonary artery is identified by its branching pattern into left and right pulmonary arteries and ductus arteriosus, and the aorta is identified by the carotid and subclavian arteries. Both great vessels may originate from either ventricle (usually the morphologic right ventricle), creating a double-outlet right ventricle. If the aortic or pulmonary valve is atretic, a single outlet ventricle is the result. Another example of single outlet is truncus arteriosus, in which there is a single truncal valve originating from the ventricular mass but overrides the ventricular septum. The ventriculoarterial connection is designated as a single outlet with an overriding truncal valve. In complex malformations, including right atrial isomerism with the asplenia syndrome, the atrioventricular septal defect is often associated with a double-outlet right ventricle. In cases of tetralogy of Fallot, there is often overriding of the aortic valve so that almost half of the valve annulus appears to arise from the right ventricle. There is mitral aortic continuity, and except for the rare circumstance in which there is more than 50% overriding of the aortic valve, the ventriculoarterial connection in tetralogy of Fallot is concordant.

Reports of neonates with abnormalities of ventriculoarterial connection and children with transposition of the great arteries show that echocardiography can detect accurately these abnormalities. A newborn with cyanosis due to transposition can be diagnosed without catheterization, and many neonates have had surgery without catheterization.

## Ventricular and Atrial Septa

### Atrial Septum

Before birth, the atrial septum usually bows toward the morphologic left atrium because of the significant blood flow to the left heart through the fossa ovalis. This aneurysmal bowing of the atrial septum after birth may be a clue to right-to-left or left-to-right intra-atrial shunting if it is bowing toward the right atrium. Color Doppler studies have confirmed that left-to-right shunting through a patent foramen ovale is a normal finding soon after birth, particularly if the ductus arteriosus has not closed. After 6 weeks of age, persistent shunting at the atrial level is be considered abnormal.

The results of echocardiographic imaging of atrial septal defects are good. In the prospective study of Gutgesell (1985), there was one false-positive and one false-negative result for diagnosing sinus venosus defects. One practical application of echocardiography is the evaluation of creating an atrial defect by balloon atrial septostomy or blade and balloon techniques.

A thin strand of tissue in what appears to be a common atrium suggests right atrial isomerism. The upper atrial septum where a sinus venosus defect may occur can be difficult to evaluate in an older child, but color flow mapping has improved the results of evaluating all forms of atrial septal defect.

### Ventricular Septum

Defects of the ventricular septum can be analyzed using multiple tomographic imaging approaches, and defects can be separated into those that are perimembranous, muscular, or subarterial. An inlet perimembranous defect (ie, AV canal-type defect) can be differentiated from AV canal by the presence of the central fibrous body at the internal crux of the heart. Small muscular ventricular septal defects and even a significant defect in the perimembranous region may be missed by imaging alone, but color Doppler has substantially improved the ability to detect muscular defects. With multiple ventricular septal defects, color may be crucial for detection. The sensitivity in older children with smaller muscular ventricular septal defects and another large ventricular septal defect was only 72% in one study. The details of complicated interventricular communications in the trabecular septum require angiographic definition. Echocardiography with color Doppler appears adequate to evaluate these patients.

## Valves

### Atrioventricular Valves

A wide variety of malformations may involve the left or right atrioventricular valves. The mitral or tricuspid valve may be abnormally positioned, stenotic, regurgitant, or hypoplastic, or the valve may have a cleft or exhibit prolapse, straddling, or Ebstein's malformation. The pattern of opening on real-time imaging is augmented by the Doppler or M-mode functional assessment. Virtually all forms of congenital abnormalities of the mitral valve can be recognized immediately by imaging alone, with the possible exception of supravalvar mitral ring, in which the ring may adhere to the valve tissue. The normal papillary muscles in this disorder differentiates it from most other congenital forms of mitral stenosis. Color flow mapping and continuous wave Doppler can effectively evaluate the hemodynamics of atrioventricular valve stenosis better than invasive techniques. Regurgitation of atrioventricular valves can be detected with excellent sensitivity, and progress is being made with color Doppler in grading the severity of regurgitation of the atrioventricular and semilunar valves.

### Semilunar Valves

Semilunar valve assessment tries to detect obstruction of or regurgitation at the aortic or pulmonary valve. Because the size of a valve annulus reflects the flow through it, hypoplasia of the valve annulus usually is associated with severe stenosis, and echocardiographic imaging may detect this condition, the doming of a stenotic valve, or the muscular hypertrophy of infundibular stenosis. The abnormal coaptation of the semilunar valve cusps also indicates regurgitation. In assessing congenital heart disease, echocardiography alone detected pulmonary stenosis with a sen-

sitivity of 77% and a specificity of 97%. Sensitivity and specificity approach 100% with the application of color, pulsed, and continuous wave techniques. Because of the variability of cardiac output through a stenotic valve, the flow-independent method may be more useful for looking at the ratio of the mean velocity at the valve to below the valve for assessing stenosis.

## Systemic Veins

### Systemic Venous Connections

A segmental diagnosis of systemic venous connection is possible after birth. Systemic venous return may be typical of the atrial situs (eg, azygos continuation with left atrial isomerism). Systemic venous return that is abnormal in situs solitus may be normal if the situs is not solitus. Normal inferior and superior vena cavae connecting to the right atrium indicate a normal systemic venous connection to the morphologic right atrium. It is important to identify the inferior vena cava connecting to the heart and extending into the abdomen so that hepatic veins connecting separately are not mistaken for it. Each of the systemic venous segments, including the right superior vena cava, the left superior vena cava, the inferior vena cava, coronary sinus, and hepatic veins, should be examined individually. A prospective assessment of this approach showed a sensitivity of more than 95% for assessing each segment, with the exception of the smaller, bridging innominate veins.

### Systemic Venous Anomalies

A persistent left superior vena cava can be detected by echocardiography and confirmed by contrast studies. It is the most common defect in patients with or without congenital cardiac defects. Rarely does this minor defect require attention, except to document its presence in case surgical management is needed for other forms of congenital heart disease. If it appears that the persistent left superior vena cava may connect to the left atrium or drain to this site because of unroofing of the coronary sinus, angiographic confirmation is essential.

## Pulmonary Veins

Each pulmonary vein connecting to the morphologic left atrium must be imaged in a sequential fashion. A four-chamber view often reveals at least two pulmonary veins connecting to the left-sided morphologic left atrium. The suprasternal scan may demonstrate all four pulmonary veins connecting to the left atrium. Total anomalous pulmonary venous connection can be detected with 85% to 97% sensitivity depending on the experience of the examiner. Although accurate diagnosis of an isolated total anomalous pulmonary venous connection can be made in neonates and infants, the ability of any noninvasive tool to exclude an isolated partial anomalous connection of one vein has not been tested. Color Doppler can confirm pulmonary venous flow in the location where the vein is thought to be connecting. Detection of pulmonary venous obstruction and variations depends on Doppler imaging. Direct visualization of all four pulmonary veins is mandatory before corrective surgery for any defect, especially for atrial septal defect or anomalous pulmonary venous connection. Any deviation from the usual anatomy should prompt a complete angiographic study. Patients with atrial isomerism usually have abnormalities of pulmonary venous connection and often require angiography before palliative surgery.

## Coronary Arteries

If intracardiac repair is contemplated, the origin of the coronary vessels must be visualized using a segmental approach. With the exception of aneurysm detection in Kawasaki's disease or the origin of the common left or right coronary artery, ultrasonography is limited in the definition of the abnormalities of the coronary circulation. In the case of fistula, the enlargement of one of the coronaries can usually be detected, and pulmonary atresia with a significant fistula can be diagnosed. Anomalous origin of one or both coronaries from the pulmonary trunk can be detected with high specificity, especially if ultrasonography is combined with Doppler, but the sensitivity is not adequate for these neonates. The use of 7.5- and 10-MHz transducers can improve these results. Any electrocardiographic evidence of coronary insufficiency should prompt immediate coronary angiography if surgical intervention is contemplated. Imaging studies of the coronary artery anatomy in tetralogy of Fallot and transposition may be successful with experience. All patients with tetralogy should have assessment of the coronaries to define the origin of the left anterior descending branch before a right ventriculotomy. In our experience, an isolated coronary fistula can be repaired without bypass, and the entry site can be defined with color Doppler.

## Aorta

Segmental analysis of the aorta and congenital abnormalities that affect it include assessment of the ascending aorta, aortic arch branching, the aortic isthmus, and the descending aorta. Echocardiography is highly accurate (ie, sensitivity of 95%; specificity of 99%) for diagnosing abnormalities of the aorta in neonates, infants, and children. Each segment of the aorta is in a slightly different tomographic plane, requiring a sequential, segmental approach. Normal branching of the right innominate artery indicates a left aortic arch with normal branching. Branching to the left indicates a right aortic arch with mirror-image branching. A patent ductus arteriosus is the most common abnormality of the aorta, and its morphology may help the diagnosis. For example, in pulmonary atresia, the ductus is horizontal, unlike the normal pattern or the ductus of pulmonary atresia with ventricular septal defect. The sensitivity of two-dimensional imaging alone is only 83%. Color and continuous wave Doppler echocardiography and aortic angiography usually agree when ductal shunting is present.

Coarctation of the aorta, which has a typical appearance in the neonatal period that includes hypoplasia of the transverse aortic arch and right ventricular enlargement, can be diagnosed by echocardiography. The typical Doppler pattern confirms the diagnosis. In patients with a large ventricular septal defect, the status of the aorta should always be investigated to exclude coarctation. In adults, the segmental analysis of the aorta is less reliable, but Doppler techniques have significantly improved the detection of aortic obstruction in cases for which imaging was poor.

## Systemic Arteriovenous Fistulas

Systemic arteriovenous fistulas cause enlargement of the artery feeding the fistula and generalized enlargement of the aorta. Sequestration and hepatic and cerebral fistulas are the most common. Sequestration of the lung and other fistulas causing an obligatory shunt can be detected by careful technique. The defect may simulate coarctation of aorta because of the aortic isthmus morphology. Angiography is required for definition of the small vessel anatomy preoperatively.

## Pulmonary Arteries

The most common abnormality of the pulmonary arteries that indicates congenital heart disease is hypoplasia. The pulmonary arteries normally are confluent in the midline, and this detail of anatomy has importance in planning a palliative approach to cyanotic congenital heart disease. Abnormalities of the origin or size of the pulmonary arteries may occur. In severe right ventricular outflow tract obstruction in neonates, pulmonary artery hypoplasia is associated with a reciprocal increase in the size of the aorta, and the ratio of size of the pulmonary arteries to the aorta may be useful in the diagnosis of this abnormality. Assessment of the details of the distal arteries requires angiography. A pulmonary arteriovenous fistula presents with cyanosis and enlargement of the pulmonary arteries and veins on echocardiography and should be confirmed by angiography and pulmonary venous oxygen saturation measurements.

Pulmonary atresia with ventricular septal defect with major aortopulmonary artery collaterals may be difficult to evaluate. The neonate with pulmonary atresia and ventricular septal defect with collaterals can be differentiated from one with ductal-dependent pulmonary supply by the oxygen saturation off prostaglandin and by imaging the ductus and well-developed confluent pulmonary arteries. All patients with collateral arteries and multifocal pulmonary supply must have complete angiographic evaluation before surgery.

## VENTRICULAR FUNCTION ASSESSMENT

The temporal resolution of two-dimensional echocardiography is limited by the scanning rate limits of the equipment. M-mode techniques interrogate the heart at a much higher rate (800 to 1500 times per second) and allow tracking of the ventricular wall and valves at rapid rates of movement. Factors such as the rapidity of the pulse repetition frequency and the depth of the scan alter the maximal rate of ultrasonic sampling. Although M-mode echocardiography has been used for the diagnosis of congenital heart defects in the past, it has been supplanted by two-dimensional imaging. The most useful application of M-mode echocardiography is the measurement of absolute cardiac chamber dimensions and wall thicknesses and their dynamic changes. Normal values for the systolic and diastolic dimensions of the left atrium and ventricle increase with increasing age and body size. M-mode parameters from the left ventricle can be used to estimate the wall stress of the left ventricle and its dynamic changes. Systolic function can be estimated using the concept of shortening fraction. In the case of normovolemia, the dimensional shortening of the left ventricular endocardial cavity correlates well with the stroke volume.

The first attempts at noninvasive measurement of pulmonary artery pressure were made possible by M-mode echocardiography. The systolic intervals of the pulmonary valve (ie, preejection time divided by the ejection time) correlate with the peak systolic pulmonary artery pressure. In transposition of the great arteries, the pulmonary artery pressure can be estimated by the systolic intervals of the left ventricle.

Changes in the pattern of the opening of the pulmonary valve assess by M-mode studies were used to detect pulmonary stenosis, but these methods have been supplanted by Doppler techniques. Quantitation of the peak velocity of tricuspid regurgitation has an excellent correlation with the degree of elevation of right ventricular pressure.

## CONTRAST ECHOCARDIOGRAPHY

An ultrasonic contrast agent is a substance that stabilizes microbubbles in solution, which are large enough to reflect ultrasound but small enough that they disappear rapidly and are physiologically safe. The agent may be as simple as an injection of saline into the circulation during two-dimensional echocardiographic imaging or as complex as precision-engineered microbubbles of polysaccharide that dissolve in the circulation after injection. Contrast can be useful in defining the identity of a structure that is imaged but may be unusual. For example, a structure under the aortic arch may be confusing but can be confirmed to be the innominate vein by an echocardiographic contrast injection in a left arm vein. In congenital heart disease, the major application of contrast echocardiography is for the postoperative patient with residual shunts or in excluding congenital heart disease. Systemic venous injection of contrast fills the right heart sequentially, and the site of residual right-to-left shunting can be defined. A catheter can be advanced retrograde into the left ventricle after closure of a ventricular septal defect, and a contrast injection can diagnose the presence and severity of residual left-to-right shunts. New agents which will cause opacification of the left heart circulation after injection are being studied. In the neonatal intensive care unit, contrast injections using agitated saline can detect right-to-left interatrial shunting in cases of persistent pulmonary hypertension.

## SAFETY OF ULTRASOUND

Significant adverse effects from the use of ultrasound for imaging or M-mode evaluation have not been reported. The potentially negative bioeffects of ultrasound can be classified as those caused by cavitation and those caused by heating. Cavitation refers to the development of tiny, gas-filled bubbles that resonate at the ultrasonic frequency and induce neighboring particles of liquid to vibrate, potentially damaging the ultrasound-transmitting medium. Practically, the intensities for imaging and M-mode (typically 10 $W/cm^2$) are almost an order of magnitude less than those known to produce cavitation. Thermal effects may result from heat generated in the tissue. To reach the thermal threshold for damage using modern ultrasonic intensities for imaging and M-mode, an average intensity of 1000 $W/cm^2$ must be applied for many hours.

Diagnostic ultrasound used at the current pulse intensity levels does not constitute a risk or hazard to the patient. Higher intensities with pulsed Doppler have the potential to cause cavitation, and concerns about the use of Doppler for fetal assessment are being investigated.

## COSTS AND BENEFITS

One of the major reasons that ultrasound is proliferating so rapidly in pediatrics is that it is noninvasive and painless in most examinations. Ultrasound equipment is less expensive than x-ray equipment, and the indications for cardiac catheterization are being reassessed. The development of echocardiography as an extension of the clinician's other assessment skills has decreased the use of catheterization, especially in neonatal patients. If catheterization can be completely avoided, echocardiography has the potential to decrease the cost of medical care for these patients.

For the most effective cardiovascular application of ultrasound, the physician should be involved in the study and its interpretation. A more physician-intensive diagnostic process may benefit the patient but may become more expensive than comparable tests that can be done by technicians.

## TRENDS

Technology has been changing so rapidly that it is difficult to predict which technique will be optimal for a given lesion in 5 years. The rapid development of nuclear magnetic resonance for imaging and spectroscopy is having a major impact on the field.

The emerging areas in echocardiography include the development of contrast agents, some of which will allow myocardial blood flow assessment by ultrasonography; tissue characterization techniques; color Doppler blood flow measurement; invasive imaging probes for intracardiac imaging; transesophageal imaging in neonates for intraoperative functional assessment; and three-dimensional reconstruction of cardiac images from ultrasound data. One thing is certain: continued reevaluation of the roles of the various diagnostic modalities used in assessing congenital heart disease will be needed.

## Selected Readings

Anderson RH, Becker AE, Lucchese FE, Meier MA, Rigby ML, Soto B. Morphology of congenital heart disease. London, Great Britain: Castle House Publications, 1983.

Bansal AC, Tajik AJ, Seward JB, Offord KP. Feasibility of detained two-dimensional echocardiographic examination in adults. Prospective study of 200 patients. Mayo Clin Proc 1980;55:291.

Bierman FZ, Williams RG. Subxiphoid two-dimensional imaging of the interatrial septum in infants and neonates with congenital heart disease. Circulation 1979;60:80.

Daskalopoulos DA, et al. Correlation of two-dimensional echocardiographic and autopsy findings in complete transposition of the great arteries. J Am Coll Cardiol 1983;2:1151.

Freedom RM. Axial angiography in the critically ill infant. In: Friedman WF, Higgins CB, eds. Pediatric cardiac imaging. Philadelphia: WB Saunders, 1984.

Gutgesell HP. Echocardiographic estimation of pulmonary artery pressure in transposition of the great arteries. Circulation 1978;57:1151.

Gutgesell HP, Huhta JC, Latson LA, Huffines D. Accuracy of 2-dimensional echocardiography in the diagnosis of congenital heart disease. Am J Cardiol 1985;55:514.

Gutgesell HP, Huhta JC, Cohen MH, Latson LA. Two-dimensional echocardiographic assessment of pulmonary artery and aortic arch anatomy in cyanotic infants. J Am Coll Cardiol 1984;4:1241.

Gutgesell HP, Paquet M. In: Atlas of pediatric echocardiography. Hagerstown, MD: Harper & Row, 1978.

Gutgesell HP, Paquet M, Duff DF, McNamara DG. Evaluation of left ventricular size and function by echocardiography. Results in normal children. Circulation 1977;56:457.

Hagler DJ, et al. Atrioventricular and ventriculoarterial discordance (corrected transposition of the great arteries). Wide-angle two-dimensional echocardiographic assessment of ventricular morphology. Mayo Clin Proc 1981;56:591.

Hagler DJ, et al. Real-time wide-angle section echocardiography: Atrioventricular canal defects. Circulation 1979;59:140.

Heger JJ, Weyman AE. A review of M-mode and cross-sectional echocardiographic findings of the pulmonary valve (review). J Clin Ultrasound 1979;7:98.

Hirschfeld S, Meyer R, Schwartz DC. The echocardiographic assessment of pulmonary artery pressure and pulmonary vascular resistance. Circulation 1975;52:642.

Huhta JC, Smallhorn JF, MaCartney FJ, Anderson RH. Cross-sectional echocardiographic diagnosis of systemic venous return. Br Heart J 1982;48:388.

Huhta JC, Gutgeseu HP, Murphy DJ, Ludomirsky A, Judd VE. Segmental analysis of congenital heart disease. Dynamic Cardiovasc Imaging 1987;1:117.

Huhta JC, Glasow P, Murphy D, Gutgesell HP, Ott DA. Surgery without catheterization for congenital heart defects: management of 100 patients. J Am Coll Cardiol 1987;9:823.

Huhta JC, Hagler DJ, Seward JB, Tajik AB, Julsrud PR. Two-dimensional echocardiographic assessment of dextrocardia: a segmental approach. Am J Cardiol 1982;50:1351.

Huhta JC, Seward JB, Tajik AJ, Hagler DJ, Edwards WD. Two-dimensional echocardiographic spectrum of univentricular atrioventricular connection. J Am Coll Cardiol 1985;5:149.

Huhta JC, Gutgesell HP, Latson LA, Huffines FD. Two-dimensional echocardiographic assessment of the aorta in infants and children with congenital heart disease. Circulation 1984;70:417.

Huhta JC, Gutgesell HP, Nihill MR. Two-dimensional echocardiographic diagnosis of total anomalous pulmonary venous connexion. Br Heart J 1985;53:525.

Huhta JC, Smallhorn JF, Macartney FJ. Two dimensional echocardiographic diagnosis of situs. Br Heart J 1982;48:97.

Hunter S. Contrast echocardiography. In: Pediatric echocardiography-cross sectional, M mode and Doppler. Amsterdam: Elsevier/North Holland Biomedical Press, 1980.

King DH, Danford DA, Huhta JC, Gutgesell HP. Noninvasive detection of anomalous origin of the left main coronary artery from the pulmonary trunk by pulsed Doppler echocardiography (brief report). Am J Cardiol 1985;55:608.

Kosturakis D, et al. Noninvasive quantification of stenotic semilunar valve areas by Doppler echocardiography. J Am Coll Cardiol 1984;3:1256.

Ludomirsky A, Huhta JC, Vick W, Murphy DJ, Danford DA. Color Doppler detection of multiple ventricular septal defects. Circulation 1986;74:1317.

Meyer RA. Echocardiography. In: Moss AJ, Adams FH, Emmanouilides GC, eds. Heart disease in infants, children and adolescents, ed 2. Baltimore: Williams & Wilkins, 1977.

Miyatake K, Izumi S, Okamoto M, Kinoshita N. Semiquantitative grading of severity of mitral regurgitation by real-time two-dimensional Doppler flow imaging technique. J Am Coll Cardiol 1986;7:82.

Rigby ML, Anderson RH, Gibson D, Jones Owen DH. Two-dimensional echocardiographic categorization of the univentricular heart. Ventricular morphology, type, and mode of atrioventricular connection. Br Heart J 1981;46:603.

Sahn DJ, et al. The utility of contrast echocardiographic techniques in the care of critically ill infants with cardiac and pulmonary disease. Circulation 1977;56:959.

Sanders SP. Echocardiography and related techniques in the diagnosis of congenital heart defects. Part III: Conotruncus and great arteries. Echocardiography 1984;1:443.

Sanders SP, Bierman FZ, Williams RG. Conotruncal malformations: diagnosis in infancy using subxiphoid 2-dimensional echocardiography. Am J Cardiol 1982;50:1361.

Seward JB, Tajik AJ, Hagler DJ, Ritter DG. Peripheral venous contrast echocardiography. Am J Cardiol 1977;39:202.

Silverman MH. An ultrasonic approach to the diagnosis of cardiac situs, connections, and malpositions. In: Friedman WF, Higgins CB, eds. Pediatric cardiac imaging. Philadelphia: WB Saunders, 1984.

Smallhorn JF, Huhta JC, Adams PS, Anderson RH. Assessment of atrioventricular septal defects by two-dimensional echocardiography. Br Heart J 1982;47:109.

Smallhorn JF, et al. Cross-sectional echocardiographic assessment of coarctation in the sick neonate and infant. Br Heart J 1983;50:349.

Smallhorn JF, Tommasini G, Macartney FJ. Two-dimensional echocardiographic assessment of common atrioventricular valves in univentricular hearts. Br Heart J 1981;46:30.

Stark J, Smallhorn J, Huhta JC, de Leval M, McCartney FJ, Rees PG, Taylor JFN. Surgery for congenital heart defects diagnosed with cross-sectional echocardiography. Circulation 1983;68:II-129.

Sutherland GR, et al. Atrioventricular discordance. Cross-sectional echocardiographic-morphological correlative study. Br Heart J 1983;50:8.

Sutherland GR, et al. Ventricular septal defect: two-dimensional echocardiographic morphologic correlations. Br Heart J 1982;47:316.

Suzuki Y, Kambara H, Kadota K, Tamaki S, Yamazato A. Detection of intracardiac shunt flow in atrial septal defect using a real-time two-dimensional color-coded Doppler flow imaging system and comparison with contrast two-dimensional echocardiography. Am J Cardiol 1985;56:347.

Tajik AJ, et al. Two-dimensional real-time ultrasonic imaging of the heart and great vessels: technique, image orientations, structures identification and validation. Mayo Clin Proc 1973;53:271.

Tonkin IL, Tonkin AD. Visceroatrial situs abnormalities: sonographic and computed tomographic appearance. AJR 1982;138:509.

Van Praagh R. The segmental approach to diagnosis in congenital heart disease. In: Bergsma D, ed. Birth defects. Baltimore: Williams & Wilkins, 1972.

Vick GW, et al. Pulmonary venous and systemic ventricular inflow obstruction in patients with congenital heart disease: detection by combined two-dimensional and Doppler echocardiography. J Am Coll Cardiol 1987;9:580.

*Principles and Practice of Pediatrics, Second Edition.*
edited by Frank A. Oski et al. J. B. Lippincott Company, Philadelphia © 1994.

# 89.2 *Therapeutic Cardiac Catheterization*

## Charles E. Mullins

For over four decades, cardiac catheterization has been the definitive diagnostic tool for all cardiac disease. Catheterization has been particularly important for the diagnosis and management of complex congenital heart defects. Cardiac catheterization allows the hemodynamic quantification of normal and abnormal physiology of the heart. With the addition of biplane intracardiac angiography to diagnostic catheterization, the precise anatomical definition of the defects became possible. As techniques for surgical correction of the congenital heart defects appeared, a detailed catheterization with accurate angiography became a prerequisite to the surgery. In the last decade, there has been a proliferation of noninvasive diagnostic techniques that enabled some patients to be sent to surgery without catheterization. During this period,

even more definitive and safer catheterization procedures were developed. Despite the many noninvasive diagnostic technologies, cardiac catheterization still remains the "gold standard" for definitive diagnoses.

Catheter techniques have been used for treating many defects during the last decade. From the first introduction of a diagnostic cardiac catheter, the concept of correcting defects with a cardiac catheter was envisioned. Therapeutic procedures in the pediatric cardiac catheterization laboratory first became a reality with the innovative and courageous development of the balloon atrial septostomy catheter and procedure by Dr. William Rashkind in 1966. This procedure was lifesaving for critically ill infants and demonstrated the feasibility of therapeutic procedures for congenital heart disease in the catheterization laboratory. The balloon atrial septostomy procedure paved the way for all subsequent catheterization procedures aimed at therapy. This particular procedure has served the test of time and still is an essential procedure in the care of infants with complex congenital heart disease. Portsmann (1967) reported on the closure of the patent ductus using a rather large and complex system with a combined venous and arterial approach. The Portsmann procedure still is in use, but because of the size of the delivery catheter and complexity of the procedure, its use is limited, and it is employed only in large patients.

Additional therapeutic catheterization procedures of major importance for congenital heart lesions, particularly for pediatric patients, were slow in coming. However, new procedures proliferated over the last decade to become the most exciting development in the management of congenital heart disease since the introduction of surgery for these patients.

The numerous therapeutic catheterization procedures available for the pediatric cardiac patients can be divided into five main categories: septostomies, catheter removal of intravascular foreign bodies, valve dilations, vessel dilations, and occlusion procedures. Each of these categories contains well-established procedures and those that remain purely investigational. All of the therapeutic catheterization procedures require special equipment and special skills. There is no question that the success and safety of the procedures correlate with the skill and experience of the operators and centers performing the procedures. For these reasons, not every pediatric cardiologist nor every pediatric cardiac center should attempt every therapeutic catheterization procedure.

## ATRIAL SEPTOSTOMIES

The oldest and most established therapeutic catheterization procedure, balloon atrial septostomy, is most effective in infants younger than 1 month of age. It is the one procedure that must be available in all centers caring for infants with congenital heart disease. In newborn infants with transposition of the great arteries in whom no other intracardiac communication exists, balloon septostomy is lifesaving. It provides some immediate mixing of the totally separated systemic and pulmonary venous blood. This is urgently required to correct hypoxemia and acidosis and to stabilize these infants even if an arterial switch procedure is anticipated within hours or days. Balloon atrial septostomy is indicated in many other infants with a variety of other cyanotic lesions in whom an adequate preexisting interatrial septal communication is not present but the continuity of the circulation depends on such a lesion. For example, a septostomy should be performed for infants with mitral atresia to allow the pulmonary venous blood to return from the blind left atrium to the functional circulation. In infants with hypoplastic right heart syndromes, such as pulmonary or tricuspid atresia, all of the systemic venous blood must pass from the right atrium through the atrial septum to return to the effective circulation. In patients with total anomalous pulmonary venous return, the only access of the systemic and pulmonary venous return to the systemic circulation is through the atrial septal defect. If the atrial septal defect is at all restrictive in any of these lesions, a septostomy is indicated.

Although there have been improvements in the balloon catheters available for the balloon septostomy, the procedure is essentially the same as originally described by Rashkind and Miller (1966). A catheter with an inflatable spherical balloon attached at the distal end is used to tear an opening in the interatrial septum. The balloon is inflated carefully in the left atrium and then rapidly and forcefully pulled (ie, jerked) through the atrial septum into the right atrium, which tears an opening in the interatrial septum. The hole created allows free mixing or passage of blood across the atrial septum.

Some patients with these same cyanotic defects or even more complex lesions live for months or years before requiring enlargement of an atrial septal defect or further surgery. When one of these patients who is older than 1 year of age eventually does require an atrial opening, the balloon septostomy procedure alone has no effect or merely stretches the atrial septum and does not create a permanent opening because of the thickened, tougher septa. Dr. Sang Park extended the use of the septostomy procedure for these older patients with the introduction of the blade septostomy catheter in 1975.

The blade septostomy procedure is accomplished using a catheter with a small retractable blade at its distal end. The blade catheter with the blade retracted is advanced through a sheath into the left atrium. The blade is opened carefully in the left atrium. With the blade opened, the blade catheter is withdrawn slowly and forcefully as it is carefully controlled through the atrial septum, incising an opening in the septum. This procedure is repeated, each time changing the side-to-side angle of the blade. After the multiple blade incisions have been completed, a balloon septostomy is performed to further increase the septal opening. In much older patients with septa extremely resistant to further tearing by the septostomy balloon, a dilation balloon may be used after the blading to open the atrial septum. A deflated balloon dilation catheter is advanced over a wire until the balloon is centered in the atrial septum. The dilation balloon is inflated, further extending the previous blade cuts. As with other dilation procedures, two smaller dilation balloons used simultaneously are as effective or more effective than one but cause less trauma to the venous system.

The balloon or blade and balloon septostomies are palliative procedures, but they may be the only procedures available or required for many extremely complex lesions. Although the patients are often extremely ill, the catheter septostomies are effective and safe procedures when performed cautiously and with meticulous attention to the technical details of the procedures.

## CATHETER REMOVAL OF INTRAVASCULAR FOREIGN BODIES

Since they were first introduced purposefully into the vascular system, pieces of indwelling catheters, cardiac catheters, or implantable intravascular devices occasionally have broken off, come loose, or otherwise gone astray in the circulation. The most common of these are the pieces of indwelling tubing from hyperalimentation or chronic chemotherapy lines, which shear off during attempted removal. Most of these loose pieces and devices are on the systemic venous side of the circulation and end up migrating to the right heart or more often to the pulmonary arteries. These foreign bodies originally required surgical removal, often an open heart procedure.

Early in the development of cardiac catheterization, devices were modified from other specialties (eg, urology) or fabricated

by the cardiologists to retrieve the errant objects. The commercially manufactured catheter devices designed specifically for the removal of foreign bodies include simple wire loop snares, wire collapsible baskets, and small grasping forceps, all of which are miniaturized to pass through small catheters or sheaths. With these tools and the use of biplane fluoroscopy to localize the errant object, virtually any item can be grasped within the heart or pulmonary artery and withdrawn from the circulation through a sheath without a cut down over the exit vessel. Foreign body removal in the catheterization laboratory is the standard approach for this problem.

## VALVULOPLASTY

The development, manufacture, and use of tiny, cylindrical, fixed-diameter balloons for dilating renal and coronary arteries began a revolution in the treatment of coronary artery disease. These balloons become hard or rigid and stay at a predetermined diameter when inflated to a specified pressure. The extension of this technology to similar but larger balloons in the early 1980s opened the way to the dilation of stenotic valves and larger vessels in patients with congenital heart disease. Techniques were described with the large balloons for the dilation of pulmonary valves, coarctations of the aorta, pulmonary branch stenoses, and aortic valves. The balloon dilation techniques are still relatively new, with the long-term results still to be determined. However, in a large collaborative study, the methods were immediately effective, safe for the patient, and produced much less morbidity than control procedures. The balloon dilation procedures have achieved acceptance and extensive use in a relatively short period.

A double balloon technique is recommended for virtually all valve dilations and some vessel dilations. The advantages of the double balloon technique are multiple. The greatest advantage is that two smaller balloons with a lower profile of each deflated balloon are easier and safer to introduce into the peripheral vessels than a single, larger deflated balloon that would be required for the same annulus size. Because a "lumen" always persists between the two inflated balloons, blood flow through the lesion being dilated is not totally obstructed as it is with a single balloon, and systemic output is not as drastically reduced while the balloons are being inflated. The two balloons make the larger valve dilations possible if adequate-sized balloons are not available or are too massive.

The pulmonary valve was the first valve to be dilated successfully and is the valve with which the most extensive and valid experience has been accumulated. Shortly after the introduction of the technique in 1982, a voluntary collaborative registry from 27 pediatric cardiology centers was established. By the end of 1986, data on the experience with over 800 patients who had pulmonary valve dilation established the procedure as safe and effective. With such a relatively new procedure, long-term data is just now becoming available. The 10-year follow-up data show the dilation of valvular pulmonary stenosis to be successful. The stenosis does not seem to recur after an initial successful dilation.

Before performing a pulmonary valve dilation, the hemodynamics and exact anatomy are established by cardiac catheterization and selective cineangiocardiography. From previous echocardiograms or the angiocardiograms, an accurate measurement of the diameter of the valve annulus is made. Two long exchange guidewires are passed through two separate catheters previously introduced and maneuvered from the right and left femoral veins into the distal left pulmonary artery. The catheters are removed, leaving the two wires in place. The appropriate balloons are passed over the separate wires, positioned side by side in the valve, with the balloon centers located exactly within the stenotic orifice. They are inflated simultaneously and rapidly to the maximal recommended pressure of the balloons until the circumferential indentation in the balloons created by the stenotic valve disappears; then they are rapidly deflated. To ensure that the balloons were in the optimal position, the positioning of the balloons is changed slightly and the inflation and deflation process is repeated several times. After dilation, the hemodynamics and angiocardiograms are repeated. Pulmonary valve dilation using these techniques has proven to be safe, effective, and probably curative. It has become the accepted therapy for pulmonary valve stenosis.

Valvular aortic stenosis was the next congenital valvular lesion to be treated with dilation. After the first report of this procedure, enthusiasm for aortic valve dilation was limited because of the expected difficulties and dangers of extensive manipulations in the arteries and the systemic circulation. There was fear that significant aortic regurgitation would be created. Eventually, several major centers began dilating valvular aortic stenosis on carefully controlled protocols. With success and complication rates reported from the investigating centers that were comparable to surgical results, the procedure gained a wider acceptance. In many centers, it has become the procedure of choice. Like the surgery for valvular aortic stenosis, dilation is a palliative procedure.

Aortic valve dilation is indicated for patients with pure aortic valvular stenosis that is severe enough to indicate surgery. The goal in aortic valve dilation is to reduce the obstruction from a critical level to a mild degree without producing significant aortic regurgitation. After hemodynamic parameters have been recorded and accurate measurements of the aortic annulus diameter obtained, end-hole catheters are introduced from both femoral arteries, and each is passed retrograde across the stenotic aortic valve. Exchange-length guidewires are passed through the catheters and positioned securely in the left ventricle. The catheters are removed, leaving the wires in place. Two separate balloon dilation catheters are advanced over the wires until the balloons are centered in the stenotic valve orifice. The balloons simultaneously and rapidly are inflated and deflated, which splits the stenotic valve. If a single balloon is used for aortic valve dilation, a long balloon should be used, but its diameter should be no larger than the valve annulus.

The double balloon technique, the use of much longer dilation balloons, and the accurate measurement of the annulus with strict attention to the precise balloon—annulus ratio have made aortic valve dilation safer and more successful. Even these improvements and precautions have not eliminated all the risks nor secured the predictability of the procedure. Although aortic valve dilation is used widely and is no longer considered an investigational procedure, it should be limited to centers with adequate equipment and expertise and centers where long-term data on the technique and results of the procedure can be accumulated.

Because of the better control of rheumatic fever, rheumatic mitral valve stenosis is a rare problem in children and adults in the developed nations of the West. In the Middle East, Far East, and in less developed Western countries, rheumatic fever with resultant mitral stenosis is still rampant. In those areas of the world, there has been extensive, successful experience with the dilation of rheumatic mitral valve stenosis. Congenital mitral stenosis usually results in a grossly deformed mitral valve and valve apparatus. These valves were considered poor candidates for anything except valve replacement, and there was little enthusiasm for and even less experience in valve dilation. The techniques for dilation of the stenotic rheumatic mitral valves eventually were applied to some of the more severe congenital mitral stenoses with satisfactory results. These patients otherwise would have required surgical valve replacement.

The technique for children involves making two separate transseptal punctures through the atrial septum and from there advancing two catheters from the left atrium across the mitral valve and into the left ventricle. Two exchange guidewires are advanced through the catheters and carefully positioned in the left ventricle. The combined diameter of the two dilation balloons is chosen to equal or slightly exceed the annulus diameter or chosen according to the normal estimated valve area for the patient's weight. The balloon dilation catheters are advanced across the atrial septum and into the left atrium. The balloons are advanced across the mitral valve and simultaneously inflated to the maximal recommended pressures and diameters; they are then deflated as rapidly as possible. The inflation and deflation procedure is repeated until the operator is satisfied that there are no residual indentations in the balloons or until the gradient across the valve is abolished.

The dilation procedure for the mitral valve has evolved into a reliable and safe procedure if performed meticulously. The early- and medium-term results of rheumatic mitral valve dilations and the early experience with congenital mitral stenosis dilation have been good. Because of the limited experience and technical difficulties with dilating congenital mitral valves, the dilation of this lesion remains investigational and should be performed only by institutions that are technically experienced and that are collecting data on each case.

Tricuspid valve stenosis of any type is an extremely rare lesion, but it can be dilated successfully and easily using the double balloon technique. Two exchange guidewires are passed from the femoral veins into the apex of the right ventricle or into the distal pulmonary arteries. The dilating balloons are advanced over these wires, centered on the stenosed tricuspid valve and inflated to their maximal pressure or until the balloon's "waist" disappears. Meaningful data on the effectiveness of this technique are lacking, but considering the surgical alternative and the relative ease of this dilation procedure, dilations of stenotic tricuspid valves should be attempted as investigational procedures.

## ANGIOPLASTY

Many congenital and surgically acquired vascular stenoses are amenable to balloon dilation by a catheter technique. The first nonvalvular congenital lesion to be dilated successfully was a recoarctation of the aorta that developed after previous surgical repair. This lesion seems ideally suited for a dilation procedure, because recoarctations are usually discrete, the area of the recoarctation is surrounded by dense (ie, supportive) scar tissue from the original surgery, and the lesion is difficult to remodel surgically. These considerations coupled with the first successful cases reported promoted enthusiasm for the dilation procedure. Many cases were rapidly accumulated in the collaborative Valvuloplasty and Angioplasty of Congenital Anomalies Registry.

The procedure was usually effective in immediately reducing the obstruction to a minimal residual gradient, and during the medium-term follow-up, the obstruction did not seem to recur. There were early complications, mostly involving arterial damage, and there were two deaths related to the procedure. These seemed to be exaggerated vagal-like reactions. Despite the potential problems and with the development of improved equipment and techniques, this procedure has become the preferred procedure for postoperative residual or recoarctation.

The procedure for recoarctation dilation is relatively straightforward. The site and size of the coarctation and adjacent proximal and distal aorta diameter in the area of the coarctation are visualized and accurately measured on an aortogram. A balloon of a diameter equal to the narrowest adjacent "normal" aortic diameter is chosen. A guidewire is passed retrograde through the coarctation, and the balloon dilation catheter is passed over the guidewire to the site of coarctation. The deflated balloon is centered at the narrowing of the coarctation and inflated to its maximal diameter at the recommended pressure for the particular balloon. The waist in the balloon usually disappears with the first inflation and is not apparent on subsequent inflations. Follow-up pressures and angiocardiograms are recorded.

After the success of dilating recoarctation, the same procedure was extended to the dilation of native coarctation. The immediate results of these dilations were even better than for recoarctations, and few immediate complications were encountered. However, infrequent cases of aneurysms developing at the site of the dilated coarctation were reported during follow-up. Although there have been neither acute nor long-term problems from these aneurysms, their presence in a few cases have caused some reservations and prompted a cautious approach to using the procedure. For the few cases of aneurysm, an attempt is being made to determine the cause and the natural history of the aneurysm. With the significantly decreased morbidity and with results apparently equal to those of surgical repair, the dilation of native coarctation is continuing but only as a carefully controlled investigational procedure with long-term monitoring of each patient until the complete information on the long-term results are available.

Success in the dilation of postoperative systemic venous stenosis is second only to the success with coarctation dilation. In the venous switch type of repair for transposition of the great arteries (ie, Mustard or Senning procedures), venous obstruction is sometimes created within the baffle. These severe obstructions previously required a surgical take-down of the baffle, with the inherent risks and morbidity of repeat open heart surgery. Successful dilation of these stenoses has been possible in most cases. Available data indicate that most of these areas will remain open if they initially can be dilated wider than the adjacent normal vessels. The lesions are particularly suited to a double balloon technique because of the small patients and the need for a large dilation diameter. Similar to the double balloon technique in other lesions, two separate guidewires are passed across the stenosis from separate entry veins, and the two balloons are simultaneously inflated in the area of the stenosis. The inflations are repeated until the waists in the balloons disappear. Although usually acutely successful, there have been scattered reports of restenosis of these lesions. The long-term patency of these areas must be determined, but dilation is recommended for all such baffle stenoses, particularly with the use of intravascular stents to ensure patency.

Pulmonary artery branch stenoses, congenital and postsurgically acquired, usually are not amenable to surgery because of the nature of the vessels involved and their location within the lungs. Surgery offers no benefit or worsens the situation. At first, these lesions seemed ideal for a balloon dilation technique. Most can be dilated up to normal or greater than normal vessel size. However, 50% or more of the dilated pulmonary arteries are only temporarily or partially stretched. They often reassume their predilation stenotic configuration and hemodynamics. Complications include pulmonary artery rupture, with a few deaths, and entry vein obstruction secondary to the large, rough dilation catheters. Dilation of pulmonary artery branch stenosis has fallen into disfavor and is reserved for patients with severe obstruction and deteriorating hemodynamics or cardiac function.

A promising approach to vascular stenoses is available. Catheter-delivered, balloon-expandable, intravascular stents are used to support the dilated lesions. The larger stents have been used extensively and successfully in treating atherosclerotic peripheral vascular disease in humans. Experimentally, they were used in the pulmonary arteries, systemic veins, and peripheral arteries of animals with excellent short-term results. The animals were followed for as long as 2 years with neither complications nor adverse effects reported for the stented vessels or the animals. After these favorable studies, a clinical trial of the stents in the

pulmonary arteries and systemic veins of congenital heart disease patients was begun in two centers. The investigation has been underway for 2.5 years, with extremely favorable results reported for the protocol patients. The vascular stents are mounted on a dilation balloon of the desired diameter of the vessel to be stented. The balloon and stent combination is delivered over an exchange wire and through a long, 11-French (3.6-mm) sheath to the area of stenosis. The sheath is withdrawn from the stent and balloon combination. The balloon is inflated, expanding the stent within the stenosed vessel. The balloon is then deflated, leaving the expanded stent in place supporting the vessel in its full open dimension.

The stents have been used successfully in 75 patients and in more than 100 vessels in the protocol study. There have been minimal complications, particularly considering the usually severe disease underlying the lesions being treated. There were two deaths, both of which were more related to the underlying disease than to the stent implant. There has been no evidence for recurrence of the stenosis or significant endothelial proliferation within the stents after implantation within the pulmonary arteries. The stents appear ideal for the pulmonary branch stenoses and the other vascular lesions that develop congenitally or as a result of postoperative restenosis. The stents are approved for human use in adult atherosclerotic vessels and are available for congenital cases on investigational protocols.

Opening of a stenosed cardiac valve or vessel for most patients with congenital heart disease can now be accomplished in the cardiac catheterization laboratory rather than in the operating room.

## OCCLUSION PROCEDURES

Cardiologists have been attempting to close existing abnormal openings or vessels by catheter techniques for as long as the therapeutic catheter procedures have existed for opening structures. However, the development and miniaturization of such devices and the technical problems of implanting these devices have been difficult to overcome. The first clinically successful occlusion technique was developed by Dr. Werner Portsmann in 1967. He developed a device and technique for the closure of patent ductus. His technique is complex, requiring large delivery catheters and a combined arterial and venous approach. Although the technique is still in use in a few centers, it is only useful for larger patients and has never gained widespread popularity. King and Mills developed and used a unique double umbrella device and delivery technique for the closure of atrial defects in 1974. It was successful in several patients, but the technique required a large delivery system, and it never achieved popularity or continued use.

Dr. Rashkind, while still perfecting the balloon septostomy technique, was working on several umbrella-type devices for closing intracardiac defects. The first reported clinical use of these devices was in 1979, with the successful closure of a patent ductus in a 3.5-kg infant. The procedure demonstrated that adequate miniaturization of a catheter-delivered intracardiac device was possible. Although the original device had some significant inherent problems, it led to modifications resulting in the current Rashkind Patent Ductus Occluding Device. The device has been tested in controlled clinical trials in the United States for more than 11 years, and it has proven safe and satisfactory for the closure of ductus in older infants, children, and adults. It was approved by the Food and Drug Administration Medical Device Panel in February 1989, but it has not been released for clinical use in the United States. The device has been approved and has had extensive and successful use in more than 1500 patients in countries outside of the United States, including Canada, the United Kingdom, Germany, France, the Netherlands, Spain, Italy, Greece, Turkey, Mexico, Jordan, and Saudi Arabia.

The Rashkind ductus-occluding device is a miniature double umbrella with a stainless steel frame and polyurethane foam disks. The two umbrella components of the device fold away from each other so that when positioned in the ductus, one umbrella is positioned on the aortic end of the ductus and the opposing umbrella is on the pulmonary side. The central spring mechanism holds the two umbrellas together in the open position and in place in the ductus. The ductus umbrellas are available in two sizes: the standard 12-mm-diameter umbrella and a larger 17-mm-diameter umbrella. In their folded configuration, the umbrellas can be delivered from the venous or the arterial route through an 8-French (2.6-mm) sheath for the smaller device and an 11-French (3.6-mm) sheath for the larger device. The use of a long transseptal sheath as an extension of the metal pod of the delivery catheter makes the delivery of the device to the ductus through the venous route dependable. The venous route has the advantages of not compromising the artery and requiring minimal manipulation on the systemic side of the circulation.

During the diagnostic catheterization, quality angiocardiograms are performed in the anteroposterior and lateral projections with injection into the descending aorta adjacent to the ductus. The angiocardiogram provides an accurate assessment of the exact size and shape of the ductus and demonstrates the exact relation to the surrounding visible mediastinal structures, such as vertebrae and the tracheal air shadow, which can be used as reference structures during implantation of the device. With this information, the size of the ductus-occluding device to be used is chosen, and some idea of the ease or difficulty of delivery can be determined. The long transseptal sheath is advanced from the femoral vein, through the right heart and pulmonary artery, through the ductus, and into the descending aorta. The delivery catheter containing the device is introduced into the sheath and advanced to approximately the area of the tricuspid valve. The occlusion device is advanced out of the delivery catheter and into the sheath until it reaches the tip of the sheath. The sheath is withdrawn to the aortic end of the ductus, and the device is advanced slightly until the legs of the distal umbrella are seen to open fully (ie, 90° to the catheter long axis) in the aorta. The sheath and umbrella are withdrawn together into the ductus until the open legs are seen to bend or flex slightly as the distal umbrella enters the aortic end of the ductus. With the delivery catheter and wire fixed in this position, the sheath alone is withdrawn several centimeters. This allows the proximal legs to open on the pulmonary side of the ductus. After the physician is assured that the device is fixed in this position, the release mechanism is activated leaving the umbrella device fixed in the ductus and occluding it.

In the Texas Children's Hospital series of more than 200 patients treated from January 1984 (when the device and delivery technique were last modified) until 1993, there have been successful total closures in 89% of the patients. There are 13 centers in the United States participating in clinical trials of the improved device, with more than 600 implants performed in these centers. The only complications in all of this experience are hemolysis reported in three patients and endocarditis in two patients. All five patients with complications had significant residual leaks. Two patients with hemolysis had the device surgically removed and the ductus closed at the same surgery; the third patient had the device replaced in the catheterization laboratory; all three had the hemolysis corrected. The two cases of endocarditis were in patients not covered properly for endocarditis with prophylactic antibiotics; these patients were medically cured of their endocarditis.

Large, audible leaks have occurred in approximately 5% of the implants, and these have been corrected with a second device. The one persistent problem with the modified device is the occurrence of tiny, nonaudible, Doppler-detected, persistent leaks in approximately 10% of the patients after otherwise successful implantations. With the introduction of new centers, there have been cases of embolization of the device at the time of implantation. Most of these errant devices were removed by catheter retrieval, and the ductus were closed with a second device. Rarely, these patients require surgery for removal of the embolized device and the closure of the ductus.

The Rashkind occlusion device should be available soon for more routine clinical use in the United States. Once approved, design changes for the device and delivery system will be implemented to further miniaturize and simplify the delivery system and improve the closure rate. With the difficulty of the procedure and the special equipment necessary, the procedure will continue to be limited to centers with special training and expertise.

The ductal occlusion device has been used to occlude other abnormal or unusual persistent communications in patients with congenital heart disease. Some postoperative patients with lesions such as persistent caval communications or small atrial septal defects after the Fontan procedure or persistent systemic-to-pulmonary shunt lesions after other complex intracardiac repairs have been spared further surgery with the use of these devices alone or in combination with other devices. With the increasing numbers of complex, multistage surgical procedures being performed, these atypical uses of the ductal occluding device will probably increase.

Other catheter techniques and devices and combinations of devices are used to occlude abnormal or persistent vascular communications. The abnormal communications include persistent systemic-to-pulmonary collateral vessels to the lungs, arterial-to-venous shunts, pulmonary arteriovenous fistulas, and some surgically created systemic-to-pulmonary shunts. The long, tubular lesions are more suited for one of several embolization devices or materials that, when implanted, stimulate thrombus formation. For communications that end in a capillary bed, Gelfoam bits or the patient's own preclotted blood is used. For slightly larger vessels or communications that do not end in a capillary bed, small detachable balloons or short segments of coiled spring guidewire are used.

The most frequently used device of this type is the Gianturco coil. This is a small coil of spring guidewire with fine fabric embedded within the coils of the wire. The coil is delivered through a catheter as a short, straight segment of wire that, as it is extruded out of the delivery catheter, coils in the vessel at the site of the vessel to be occluded. As thrombus forms within the coil, the abnormal vessel is occluded. These catheter-delivered embolization devices are the standard accepted treatment for most aortopulmonary or arteriovenous lesions. For large communications, the ductal-occluding devices alone or in combination with coils are used. A device consisting of a long "coil" contained within a "bag" is being developed for these larger communications.

The atrial septal occlusion device introduced by King and Mills never was accepted for general clinical use, but it did stimulate further interest in this type of procedure. Rashkind developed a catheter-delivered umbrella device for occlusion of atrial sepal defects. The device was a single umbrella, attached to the septum by tiny hooks at the distal ends of the umbrella arms. The device was used in a few patients under an investigational protocol starting in 1981. Although the delivery catheter was significantly smaller than the King-Mills device, the attachment hooks created problems by attaching to unwanted structures. The device was not accepted for general use, but it helped to stimulate the development of more effective and safer devices for closure of atrial septal defects.

The larger patent ductus arteriosus (PDA) device was used for the closure of small atrial septal defects and led to the development of an even larger PDA device for the larger septal defects. This was only partially effective, primarily because of poor approximation of the legs of the device against the septum. The partially successful experience with the smaller double umbrella rapidly led to the development by Dr. Lock and the engineers of USCI of a effective modification of the double umbrella concept for closure of atrial septal defects. This device, the USCI "Clamshell" ASD Occluder, went into production and clinical trials in five centers in 1989. Within 2 years, the device had been used in 545 patients. Even in these early clinical trials establishing the limitations of the procedure, the results were satisfactory, with minimal complications related to the device. Unfortunately, some clinically nonsignificant structural defects in the devices themselves have appeared, and the trials of this particular device have been stopped while it is being redesigned and reapproved for clinical trials. The device demonstrated definitively the feasibility of closure of small to moderate-sized atrial septal defects, and eventually it will be the standard therapy for these lesions.

As with the PDA device, additional uses became apparent for the ASD clamshell device that were superior to any surgical or other occlusion techniques for those defects. The clamshell device can be used for the closure of muscular interventricular septal defects, the closure of patent foramen ovales (PFO) in patients who have had cerebral vascular accidents from emboli through the PFO, and the closure of fenestrations purposefully left in the baffle during caval pulmonary (ie, Fontan) repairs of complex congenital heart defects. All of these uses have been effective and far safer than the alternative surgical approach, and they will become routine procedures after the device is available again.

# CONCLUSION

Therapeutic procedures that can be accomplished by a catheterization technique rather than by a surgical procedure in an operating room have numerous advantages for the patient and society. The most immediate advantage is the elimination of the physical pain and discomfort of the surgical procedure. The recovery from the catheterization procedure and return to full activity is usually 1 to 2 days, compared with a 1- to 2-week hospitalization plus 6 or more weeks of convalescence to recover from a thoracic surgical procedure. The actual risk of the therapeutic catheterization procedure is far less than the risk of the surgical procedure with the associated general anesthesia, intubation, respirator support, chest tube(s), blood transfusion, and greater risk of wound or systemic infections. Although the catheterization devices and techniques are relatively expensive, there are significant financial savings compared with a surgical operation with its required anesthesia, recovery room, and longer hospitalization expenses.

## Selected Readings

Abele JE. Balloon catheters and transluminal dilatation: technical considerations. AJR 1980;135:901.

Allen HD, Mullins CE. Results of the Valvuloplasty and Angioplasty of Congenital Anomalies Registry. Am J Cardiol 1990;65:772.

Babic UU, Pejcic P, Djurisic Z, et al. Percutaneous transarterial balloon valvuloplasty for mitral valve stenosis. Am J Cardiol 1986;57:1101.

Chuang VP, Wallace S, Gianturco C. A new improved coil for tapered tip catheter for arterial occlusion. Radiology 1980;135:507.

Grifka RG, O'Laughlin MP, Nihill MR, et al. Double transseptal, double balloon valvuloplasty for congenital mitral stenosis. Circulation 1992;85:123.

Gruntzig A. Die perkutane Rekanalisation chronischen arterieller Verschlusse (Dotter-Prinzip) mit einem neuen doppellumigen Dilations kateter. Fortschr Rontgenstr 1976;124:80.

Hellenbrand WE, Allen HD, Golinko RJ, et al. Balloon angioplasty for aortic recoarctation: results of the Valvuloplasty and Angioplasty of Congenital Anomalies Registry. Am J Cardiol 1990;65:793.

Kan JS, White RI Jr, Mitchell SE, et al. Percutaneous balloon valvuloplasty: a new method for treating congenital pulmonary valve stenosis. N Engl J Med 1982;307:540.

Kan JS, White RI Jr, Mitchell SE, et al. Treatment of restenosis of coarctation by percutaneous transluminal angioplasty. Circulation 1983;68:1087.

Khan MA, Mullins CE, Nihill MR. Percutaneous catheter closure of the ductus arteriosus in children and young adults. Am J Cardiol 1989;64:218.

King TD, Mills NL. Nonoperative closure of atrial septal defects. Surgery 1974;75:383.

Labadidi Z, Wu RJ, Walls TJ. Percutaneous balloon aortic valvuloplasty: results in 23 patients. Am J Cardiol 1984;53:194.

Lock JE, Bass JL, Amplatz K. Balloon dilatation angioplasty of aortic coarctation in infants and children. Circulation 1983;68:109.

Lock JE, Bass JL, Castaneda-Zuniga W, et al. Dilation angioplasty of congenital or operative narrowings of venous channels. Circulation 1984;709:457.

Lock JE, Castaneda-Zuniga WR, Fuhrman BP. Balloon dilation angioplasty of hypoplastic and stenotic pulmonary arteries. Circulation 1983;67:962.

Lock JE, Cockerham J, Keane J, et al. Transcatheter umbrella closure of congenital heart defects. Circulation 1987;75:593.

Lock JE, Khalilullah M, Shrivastava S, et al. Percutaneous catheter commissurotomy in rheumatic mitral stenosis. N Engl J Med 1985;313:1515.

Lock JE, Rome JJ, Davis R. Transcatheter closure of atrial septal defects: experimental studies. Circulation 1989;79:1091.

Marvin WJ, Mahoney LT, Rose EF. Pathologic sequelae of balloon dilation angioplasty for unoperated coarctation of the aorta in infants and children. J Am Coll Cardiol 1986;7:117A.

Mullins CE, Latson LA, Neches WH. Balloon dilation of miscellaneous lesions: results of the Valvuloplasty and Angioplasty of Congenital Anomalies Registry. Am J Cardiol 1990;65:802.

Mullins CE, Nihill MR, Vick GW III, et al. Double balloon technique for dilation of valvular or vessel stenosis in congenital and acquired heart disease. J Am Coll Cardiol 1987;10:107.

Mullins CE, O'Laughlin MP, Vick III GW, et al. Implantation of balloon expandable intravascular grafts by catheterization in pulmonary arteries and systemic veins. Circulation 1988;77:188.

O'Laughlin MP, Perry SB, Lock JE, et al. Use of endovascular stents in congenital heart disease. Circulation 1991;83:1923.

Palmaz JC, Sibbitt RR, Reuter SR, et al. Expandable intraluminal graft: a preliminary study. Work in progress. Radiology 1985;156:73.

Palmaz JC, Windeler SA, Garcia F, et al. Atherosclerotic rabbit aortas: expandable intraluminal grafting. Radiology 1986;160:723.

Park SC, Neches WH, Mullins CE, et al. Blade atrial septostomy: collaborative study. Circulation 1982;66:258.

Park SC, Zuberbuhler JR, Neches WH, et al. A new atrial septostomy technique. Cathet Cardiovasc Diagn 1975;1:195.

Portsmann W, Wierny L, Warnke H. Der Verschluss des D.a.p. ohne Thorakotomie (1 Mitteilung). Thoraxchirurgie 1967;15:199.

Rashkind WJ, Cuaso CC. Transcatheter closure of atrial septal defects in children. Proc Assoc Eur Pediatr Cardiol 1977;13:49.

Rashkind WJ, Cuaso CC. Transcatheter closure of patent ductus arteriosus: successful use in a 3.5 kilogram infant. Pediatr Cardiol 1979;1:3.

Rashkind WJ, Miller WW. Creation of an atrial septal defect without thoracotomy: a palliative approach thoracotomy: palliative approach to complete transposition of the great arteries. JAMA 1966;196:991.

Rashkind WJ, Mullins CE, Hellenbrand WE, et al. Nonsurgical closure of patent ductus arteriosus: clinical application of the Rashkind PDA Occluder system. Circulation 1987;75:583.

Ring JC, Bass JL, Marvin W, et al. Management of congenital branch pulmonary artery stenosis with balloon dilation angioplasty: report of 52 procedures. J Thorac Cardiovasc Surg 1985;90:35.

Rocchini AP, Beekman RH, Shachar GB, Benson L, Schwartz D, Kan JS. Balloon aortic valvuloplasty: results of the Valvuloplasty and Angioplasty of Congenital Anomalies Registry. Am J Cardiol 1990;65:784.

Stanger P, Cassidy SC, Girod DA. Balloon pulmonary valvuloplasty: results of the Valvuloplasty and Angioplasty of Congenital Anomalies Registry. Am J Cardiol 1990;65:775.

Tynan M, Finley JP, Fontes V, Hess J, Kan JS. Balloon angioplasty for the treatment of native coarctation: results of the Valvuloplasty and Angioplasty of Congenital Anomalies Registry. Am J Cardiol 1990;65:790.

Waldman JD, Waldman J, Jones MH, et al. Failure of balloon dilation in mid-cavity obstruction of the systemic venous atrium after Mustard operation. Pediatr Cardiol 1983;4:151.

White RI Jr, Kaufman SL, Barth KH, et al. Therapeutic embolization with detachable silicone balloons: early clinical experience. JAMA 1979;241:1257.

Zaibag AM, Kasab AS, Ribeiro AP, et al. Percutaneous double-balloon mitral valvotomy for rheumatic mitral valve stenosis. Lancet 1986:756.

# SECTION V

# Diseases of the Blood

*Principles and Practice of Pediatrics, Second Edition.*
edited by Frank A. Oski et al. J. B. Lippincott Company, Philadelphia © 1994.

## CHAPTER 90
# The Anemias

### Paul L. Martin and Howard A. Pearson

## APPROACH TO THE INFANT OR CHILD WITH ANEMIA

Anemia is among the most frequent laboratory abnormalities seen by a practicing pediatrician. Approximately 20% of all children in the United States and 80% of children in developing countries will be anemic at some time before their 18th birthday. Iron deficiency remains the leading cause of anemia in the United States, despite the success of the Women, Infant and Child program in reducing iron deficiency in urban areas by providing iron-fortified formulas. Screening for anemia, along with administering routine vaccinations, remains an important aspect of preventive medicine for physicians treating infants and children.

In screening for anemia, care must always be taken to compare a patient's hemoglobin or hematocrit with age-adjusted normal values, because all hematologic values vary greatly with age. The causes of anemia also vary with age of the patient. Iron deficiency is rare in the first months of life, but it increases in frequency during the growth spurts of early childhood and adolescence. Similarly, patients with hemoglobinopathies may not manifest anemia until 3 to 6 months of age. Anemia due to glucose-6-phosphate dehydrogenase deficiency usually requires exposure to oxidizing chemicals or medicines before becoming evident.

Documentation of clinically significant anemia is usually simple because of the relative ease of obtaining a hemoglobin or hematocrit measurement in the office setting. On the other hand, determination of etiology is often difficult. If no clues are obtained from the medical history, family history, physical examination, and initial laboratory tests, the clinician should perform erythrocyte indices, reticulocyte count, and an estimation of iron stores. Consultation with a pediatric hematologist may be necessary to determine the cause or to rule out conditions that require intervention. The common causes of anemia in infancy and childhood are outlined in the following sections of this chapter.

*Principles and Practice of Pediatrics, Second Edition.*
edited by Frank A. Oski et al. J. B. Lippincott Company, Philadelphia © 1994.

## 90.1 The Nutritional Anemias

### Paul L. Martin and Howard A. Pearson

The important nutritional anemias result from dietary deficiencies of iron, folic acid, or vitamin $B_{12}$. Deficiencies of other nutrients such as vitamins $B_6$ and E may be associated with anemia, but they are unusual in pediatric practice.

## IRON DEFICIENCY ANEMIA

Anemia due to iron deficiency is the most common hematologic disease of infancy and childhood. The body of the newborn infant contains 0.3 to 0.5 g of iron; the adult's iron content is estimated at 5 g. To make up the 4.5-g difference, an average of 0.8 mg of iron must be absorbed each day during the first 15 years of life. In addition to this requirement for growth, a small amount of iron is necessary to balance normal losses, estimated at 0.5 to 1 mg/day. To maintain a positive iron balance during childhood, 0.8 to 1.5 mg of iron must be absorbed each day from the diet. Because less than 10% of dietary iron is absorbed from the average mixed diet, 8 to 15 mg of iron daily is necessary for optimal nutrition. During the first years of life, when relatively small quantities of iron-rich foods are ingested, it is difficult to attain these amounts. The infant's diet should include iron-fortified foods, such as cereals or iron-supplemented formulas, by no later than 6 months of age.

### Pathophysiology

Most of the iron of the newborn is contained in the circulating hemoglobin. Low birth weight and perinatal hemorrhage are associated with decreases in neonatal hemoglobin mass. As the high hemoglobin concentration of the newborn falls during the first 2 to 3 months of life, iron is reclaimed and stored. These stores are usually sufficient for the first 6 to 9 months of life, but in low-birth-weight infants or those with perinatal blood loss, the transplacental iron endowment may be depleted earlier.

Anemia due solely to inadequate dietary iron is unusual during the first 4 to 6 months of life, but it becomes common from 9 to 24 months of age. The usual dietary pattern of infants with iron deficiency anemia is the consumption of large amounts of milk and carbohydrates not supplemented with iron. Blood loss must also be considered in the genesis of iron deficiency anemia. Chronic iron deficiency anemia from occult bleeding may be caused by a peptic ulcer, Meckel's diverticulum, polyp, or hemangioma. As many as one third of the infants with severe iron deficiency in the United States have chronic intestinal blood loss induced by ingestion of a heat-labile protein in whole cow's milk. This can be prevented by reducing the quantity of whole cow's milk or by using a milk substitute. This gastrointestinal reaction is not related to lactase deficiency or to milk allergy.

## Clinical Presentation

Pallor is the most frequent sign of iron deficiency anemia. In mild to moderate deficiency (ie, hemoglobin level of 7 to 10 g/dL), few symptoms of anemia are seen, but irritability and anorexia may be prominent. As the anemia progresses, tachycardia, cardiac dilation, and systolic murmurs occur.

The spleen is palpable in 10% to 15% of patients, and some chronic cases of anemia are associated with widening of the marrow cavity of the skull. The child with iron deficiency anemia may be obese or underweight with other evidence of undernutrition.

Some children have pica. This and the characteristic irritability may reflect a deficiency in tissue iron-containing enzymes. With iron therapy, striking symptomatic improvement occurs before significant hematologic improvement. In the past, the intracellular enzyme iron compartment was believed to be maintained even in the face of severe deficiency, but this view is no longer supported. Iron deficiency anemia and even iron deficiency without significant anemia may adversely affect the attention span, behavior, and performance of the affected infants.

## Laboratory Findings

A sequence of biochemical and hematologic changes of iron deficiency have been described. First, the iron stores (ie, liver and bone marrow hemosiderin) disappear. The level of serum ferritin provides a biochemical estimate of body iron stores. Serum ferritin levels less than 10 ng/mL indicate iron deficiency. As the serum iron levels decrease to less than 30 g/dL, the iron-binding capacity of the serum increases, resulting in serum transferrin saturation values of less than 15%. As deficiency progresses, the erythrocytes become smaller than normal with decreased hemoglobin content. The reticulocyte count is normal or minimally elevated, and leukocyte counts are normal. Elevated platelet counts (>600,000/mm$^3$) are often seen. The bone marrow is hypercellular, with erythroid hyperplasia. The normoblasts have scanty cytoplasm, with poor hemoglobinization.

Iron deficiency must be differentiated from other hypochromic, microcytic anemias. In lead poisoning, the erythrocytes are morphologically similar, but coarse basophilic stippling of the erythrocytes is prominent. Tests reveal elevations of blood lead and marked elevation of free erythrocyte protoporphyrins. Many cases of lead poisoning have concomitant iron deficiency. $\beta$-Thalassemia trait resembles iron deficiency, but there are characteristic elevations in the level of hemoglobin A$_2$. $\alpha$-Thalassemia trait occurs in about 3% of blacks and in many Southeast Asian peoples, but it is difficult to prove after the neonatal period. Thalassemia

major with its organomegaly, erythroblastosis, and hemolytic component is usually obvious. The erythrocyte morphology of chronic inflammatory or infectious conditions may be microcytic. In these conditions, the serum iron and iron-binding capacity are reduced, and serum ferritin levels are normal or elevated.

## Treatment

The response of iron deficiency anemia to adequate amounts of iron is an important diagnostic and therapeutic feature. Oral administration of simple ferrous salts is satisfactory therapy. Four to 6 mg/kg of elemental iron in three divided doses is optimal; larger doses do not result in a more rapid hematologic response. Medicinal iron should be administered between meals to ensure good absorption. Parenteral iron therapy is almost never indicated unless compliance is poor.

Within 4 days after administration of iron, peripheral reticulocytosis is seen, with the magnitude of the reticulocytic response proportional to the severity of the anemia. The hemoglobin level rises to normal. Iron medication should be continued for 4 to 6 weeks. Iron therapy fails if the child does not receive the prescribed medication or if there is unrecognized continuing blood loss. An incorrect diagnosis of iron deficiency anemia may also be revealed by therapeutic failure.

Because rapid hematologic response can be confidently predicted in typical iron deficiency, blood transfusion is indicated only when the anemia is severe or if concomitant infection may interfere with response. Packed or sedimented erythrocytes should be administered to raise the hemoglobin above 7 g/dL rather than attempting complete correction of anemia. For frank congestive heart failure, an exchange transfusion with packed erythrocytes or the use of diuretics is indicated.

## RARE HYPOCHROMIC MICROCYTIC ANEMIAS

Isolated cases of hypochromic microcytic anemia with other abnormalities of iron metabolism have been described. Some patients have had defects in iron mobilization or reutilization. Congenital absence of the iron-binding protein (ie, atransferrinemia) is associated with severe hypochromic anemia requiring lifelong transfusions. Iron is absorbed normally but is deposited in the visceral organs rather than in bone marrow.

Several patients have had refractory hypochromic anemia associated with lymphatic tumors or lymphoid hyperplasia. Correction of the anemia followed removal of the abnormal lymphatic tissue in these cases.

## MEGALOBLASTIC ANEMIAS

The megaloblastic anemias are uncommon disorders characterized by abnormal erythrocyte morphology and maturation. The erythrocytes are larger than normal. The nucleated erythrocytes have an open, finely dispersed arrangement of chromatin and asynchronous maturation of nucleus and cytoplasm. Megaloblastic anemias are a consequence of disordered syntheses of DNA, and megaloblastic cells have increased amounts of RNA relative to DNA.

Most instances of megaloblastic anemia result from deficiencies of folic acid or vitamin B$_{12}$. Dietary folic acid is converted to tetrahydrofolate; this is a cofactor in several biochemical reactions involving transfer of one-carbon units. Vitamin B$_{12}$ is a component of cobalamin coenzymes that participate in several biochemical reactions, including important interactions with folic acid metabolism.

The currently rare megaloblastic anemia of infancy is caused by a deficient intake or malabsorption of folic acid often aggravated by infection. Goat's milk and powdered cow's milk are poor sources of folic acid, and vitamin C deficiency impairs folate acid absorption. Megaloblastic anemia has a peak incidence at 4 to 7 months of age. In addition to showing pallor, affected infants are irritable, fail to gain weight, and often have chronic diarrhea.

## Laboratory Findings

Megaloblastic anemia is macrocytic (ie, mean corpuscular volume >95 fL). The reticulocyte count is low, but nucleated erythrocytes demonstrating megaloblastic morphology may be seen in the blood. Advanced cases have thrombocytopenia and neutropenia, and many of the neutrophils are hypersegmented (ie, two lobes or more). Serum folate levels are usually reduced, but low levels of erythrocyte folate are a better indication of chronic deficiency. Serum lactate dehydrogenase (LDH) activity is markedly elevated. The bone marrow is hypercellular because of erythroid hyperplasia and shows prominent megaloblastic changes. Large, abnormal neutrophilic forms (ie, giant metamyelocytes) with cytoplasmic vacuolization are also seen.

## Therapy

Initially, folic acid should be administered parenterally in a dosage of 2 to 5 mg every 24 hours and treatment should be continued for 3 to 4 weeks. Antibiotic therapy should be used for superimposed bacterial infection.

Therapy with folic acid should not be started in a patient with megaloblastic anemia until a diagnosis of folate deficiency has been established. Folic acid therapy is contraindicated in Vitamin $B_{12}$ deficiency.

## Folic Acid Deficiency

Because folic acid is absorbed throughout the small intestine, diffuse inflammatory or degenerative disease of the intestine may impair its absorption. Celiac disease, chronic infectious enteritis, and enteroenteric fistulas may lead to folic acid deficiency. Folic acid supplements are indicated in these states.

Many patients have low serum levels of folic acid during therapy with anticonvulsant drugs. Malabsorption of folic acid appears to be induced by these drugs. These patients usually have no anemia or symptoms. However, if anemia develops, it is responsive to folic acid therapy even if administration of the drug is continued. Megaloblastic anemia has been seen in users of oral contraceptives. Drugs such as methotrexate prevent the utilization of folic acid by inhibiting reduction to its active coenzymatic forms.

## Vitamin $B_{12}$ Deficiency

To be absorbed, dietary vitamin $B_{12}$ must combine with a glycoprotein (ie, intrinsic factor) secreted by the parietal cells of the gastric fundus. The $B_{12}$–intrinsic factor complex passes to the terminal ileum, where specific absorptive receptors exist. Vitamin $B_{12}$ deficiency can result from inadequate dietary intake, lack of secretion of intrinsic factor, disruption of the $B_{12}$–intrinsic factor complex, or abnormalities or absence of the receptor sites in the terminal ileum.

Vitamin $B_{12}$ is present in many foods, and pure dietary deficiency is rare. Deficiency may be seen in patients (ie, vegans) subsisting on extreme diets that contain no milk, eggs, or animal products. It has also been reported in breast-fed infants whose mothers were $B_{12}$-deficient because of diet or pernicious anemia.

Because the vitamin occurs in so many foods, most cases of $B_{12}$ deficiency are a consequence of failure to absorb the vitamin.

## Juvenile Pernicious Anemia

Juvenile pernicious anemia (JPA) is a rare disease caused by a genetically determined inability to secrete intrinsic factor. Unlike adult cases of anemia, JPA patients have normal stomach acidity and histology. Consanguinity is often found in parents of affected children, suggesting a recessive inheritance pattern.

Symptoms develop at 1 to 5 years of age, a time consistent with exhaustion of the vitamin $B_{12}$ stores acquired transplacentally from the mother. Progressive irritability, anorexia, and listlessness occur. The tongue is smooth and red. Neurologic manifestations include ataxia, hyporeflexia, and Babinski responses.

The anemia is macrocytic (mean corpuscular volume >95 fL), with prominent macro-ovalocytosis. The neutrophils are hypersegmented, and neutropenia and thrombocytopenia may develop. Serum vitamin $B_{12}$ levels are reduced. Serum LDH activity is markedly increased. Large amounts of methylmalonic acid are excreted in the urine. Unlike pernicious anemia in adults, serum antibodies against parietal cells or intrinsic factor cannot be detected in children. The gastric mucosa is histologically normal, but intrinsic factor is absent in the gastric secretions. Vitamin $B_{12}$ malabsorption is indicated by an abnormal Schilling test and is corrected by exogenous intrinsic factor.

A prompt hematologic response follows parenteral administration of vitamin $B_{12}$. If there is evidence of neurologic involvement, 1 mg should be given intramuscularly daily for several weeks. Maintenance therapy consists of monthly intramuscular administration of 1 mg of vitamin $B_{12}$. Oral therapy is contraindicated.

## Vitamin $B_{12}$ Deficiency in Older Children

Malabsorption of vitamin $B_{12}$ occurs in a syndrome of cutaneous candidiasis, hypoparathyroidism, and other endocrine deficiencies. The serum of these patients contains antibodies against intrinsic factor and gastric parietal cells. Parenteral vitamin $B_{12}$ should be administered regularly to treat and prevent megaloblastic anemia.

## Vitamin $B_{12}$ Malabsorption Due to Intestinal Causes

Familial occurrence (Imerslund syndrome) of a specific intestinal defect in the absorption of vitamin $B_{12}$, in some instances associated with proteinuria, has been described.

Surgical resection of the terminal ileum or an inflammatory disease such as regional enteritis or tuberculosis may also impair absorption of vitamin $B_{12}$. After resection of the terminal ileum, a Schilling test should be done. If this indicates vitamin $B_{12}$ malabsorption, parenteral therapy is indicated. Overgrowth of intestinal bacteria within diverticula or duplications of the small intestine may cause vitamin $B_{12}$ deficiency. In these cases, hematologic response may follow broad-spectrum antibiotic therapy. When the fish tapeworm, *Diphyllobothrium latum*, infests the upper small intestine, deficiency of vitamin $B_{12}$ may occur.

## Selected Readings

Bothwell TH, Charlton RW, Cook JD, Finch CA. Iron metabolism in man. Boston: Blackwell Scientific Publications, 1979.

Chanarin J. The megaloblastic anemias. Oxford: Blackwell Scientific Publications, 1969.

Lukens, JN. Iron metabolism and iron deficiency. In: Miller DR, Baehner RL, eds. Blood diseases in infancy and childhood. St. Louis: CV Mosby, 1990.

*Principles and Practice of Pediatrics, Second Edition.*
edited by Frank A. Oski et al. J. B. Lippincott Company, Philadelphia © 1994.

# 90.2 *The Hemoglobinopathies and Thalassemias*

## Paul L. Martin and Howard A. Pearson

The genetic, molecular, and biochemical characteristics of human hemoglobin are well known. The genes for the polypeptide chains of hemoglobin are located on chromosomes 11 and 16, and their DNA sequences have been determined. Each of the $\alpha$ and $\beta$ chains of adult hemoglobin consist of about 150 amino acids. It is possible to identify and locate the single amino acid substitution in these chains that causes each abnormal hemoglobin syndrome. Although more than 400 types of abnormal human hemoglobin have been characterized, only a few of them are prevalent.

Hemoglobin variants are identified by hemoglobin electrophoresis, a technique that usually permits a specific genotypic diagnosis. The thalassemias are associated with decreased production of the normal polypeptide chains of hemoglobin. The thalassemias are quantitative rather than qualitative abnormalities of hemoglobin.

## SICKLE CELL DISEASE AND TRAIT

The gene for sickle cell hemoglobin (Hb S) is not exclusively African, although there is a broad periequatorial sickle cell belt in Africa. From Africa, the sickle gene was introduced into the Western hemisphere by the 16th through 18th century slave trade. In the United States, sickling disorders are particularly prevalent in the South and in the urban North, reflecting the demography of African-Americans. In Latin America, relatively high frequencies are seen in the Caribbean, Panama, Guyana, and Brazil, but not in Mexico and most of South America. A high incidence of sickle genes, apparently resulting from independent mutational events, is found in Italy, Greece, the Middle East, and India.

### Pathophysiology

In Hb S, a valine residue is substituted for the usual glutamic acid in the $\beta$ chains of the hemoglobin molecule. When Hb S becomes deoxygenated, polymerization occurs with the formation of long, crystalline tactoids. These ultimately form elongated, sickled erythrocytes. Sickled erythrocytes have markedly shortened survival, and they can obstruct small blood vessels and cause distal tissue ischemia and necrosis.

Heterozygosity for a sickle gene has a benign clinical course. About 8% of African-Americans have the trait. The sickle gene is thought to confer a degree of resistance in areas endemic for falciparum malaria in infancy. The erythrocytes in sickle trait contain only 30% to 40% Hb S, and sickling does not occur under physiologic conditions. Rarely, hypoxia resulting from shock or from flying at high altitudes in unpressurized aircraft may produce vaso-occlusive phenomena. Unexpected death has also been observed in military recruits during the extreme exertion of basic training. Spontaneous hematuria, usually from the left kidney, and mild hyposthenuria also occur. Anemia or hemolysis should not be attributed to the sickle trait.

In persons homozygous for the sickle gene, sickle cell anemia is a severe, chronic hemolytic anemia. The clinical course is marked by episodes of pain caused by occlusion of small blood vessels by the spontaneously sickled erythrocytes. These events have traditionally been called crises.

## Clinical Manifestations

Manifestations of sickle cell disease do not usually appear until the second 6 months of life, coincident with the postnatal decrease in fetal hemoglobin (Hb F) and increase in Hb S. The hemolytic process is evident by 6 months of age.

The painful or vaso-occlusive crises are the most frequent clinical symptoms. Symmetric, painful swelling of the hands and feet (ie, hand–foot syndrome) caused by infarction of the small bones of the hands and feet may be the initial manifestation of sickle cell anemia in infancy. Older patients may have painful involvement of the larger bones and joints and severe abdominal pain resembling acute surgical conditions. Strokes may leave permanent paralysis. Extensive pulmonary consolidation occurs, and it is difficult to differentiate infarction from pneumonia. Vaso-occlusive crises are not usually associated with changes in the usual hematologic picture.

A second type of crisis, seen only in young infants and children, is called the sequestration crisis. Large amounts of blood become pooled in the abdominal organs. The spleen becomes massively enlarged, and signs of circulatory collapse develop rapidly. If volume replacement is given, much of the sequestered blood is remobilized. The sequestration crisis is an important cause of death in infants with sickle cell disease.

The third well-characterized type of crisis is the aplastic crisis (see Chap. 90.4).

In addition to these acute crises, a variety of clinical signs and symptoms result from chronic severe hemolytic anemia and vaso-occlusive disease. Impairment of liver function contributes to the jaundice of these patients. Gallstones can occur in children as young as 3 years of age. Renal function is progressively impaired by diffuse glomerular and tubular fibrosis, resulting in hyposthenuria and polyuria.

As many as 30% of children with sickle cell anemia develop pneumococcal sepsis during the first 5 years of life. The increased risk is a result of functional hyposplenia and low levels of specific serum antibodies. Increased susceptibility to *Salmonella* osteomyelitis is also a feature of sickle cell disease.

By mid-childhood, most patients are underweight, and puberty is delayed, particularly in boys. Chronic leg ulcers are common in adolescence and early adult life.

## Laboratory Findings

Hemoglobin levels range from 5 to 9 g/dL. Peripheral blood smears show irreversibly sickled cells, a finding almost diagnostic of homozygous sickle cell disease. The reticulocyte count ranges from 5% to 15%, and nucleated erythrocytes and Howell-Jolly bodies are usually observed. The total leukocyte count is elevated (12,000 to 20,000/mm$^3$), with a predominance of neutrophils. The platelet count is increased, and the sedimentation rate is slow. Other changes include abnormal liver function test results, hyperbilirubinemia, and diffuse hypergammaglobulinemia. The bone marrow shows erythroid hyperplasia.

Diagnostic studies to demonstrate Hb S include the sickle cell preparation and hemoglobin solubility studies. However, hemoglobin electrophoresis is more conclusive and is necessary for a precise diagnosis. After infancy, the erythrocytes of patients with sickle cell anemia contain approximately 90% Hb S, 2% to 10% Hb F, and a normal amount of Hb A$_2$; they do not contain Hb A.

# Treatment

No antisickling pharmacologic agent has proved safe or of consistent value. For mild or moderately painful crises, analgesics are indicated. Parenteral narcotics are often necessary for severe pain. Dehydration and acidosis should be corrected. Bacterial infections require appropriate antibiotic therapy. The risk of sepsis from encapsulated organisms is high enough to justify the use of prophylactic penicillin in all sickle cell patients from 6 months to at least 6 years of age. The value of prophylaxis after 6 years of age is being studied. Blood transfusions are unnecessary for the usual painful crises but are indicated for prolonged or extreme pain, for extensive involvement of lungs or central nervous system, and as preparation for general anesthesia. When the homozygous patient's circulating Hb SS erythrocytes can be diluted to less than 40% by transfusions of normal blood, vaso-occlusive symptoms usually abate. Partial exchange transfusion can be done to rapidly lower the percentage of Hb SS erythrocytes.

Investigational treatments for sickle cell anemia includes the use of hydroxyurea to cause "stress" erythropoiesis, which can increase the percentage of fetal hemoglobin. Bone marrow transplantation from HLA-identical siblings has been performed in at least 21 children with sickle cell disease. The risk of death from toxicity of the transplant and the risk of chronic graft-versus-host disease appears to be 5% to 10%. It is difficult for parents and physicians to weigh the risk of early death from transplant with the risk of death from long-term complications of sickle cell disease until the toxicity of bone marrow transplant can be reduced.

Newborn screening for sickle hemoglobinopathies is mandated in 38 states. Medical counseling of affected families and initiation of prophylactic penicillin for affected infants has been effective in decreasing early mortality from sickle cell disease.

# OTHER HEMOGLOBINOPATHIES

## Hemoglobin C

Hemoglobin C occurs in about 2% of African-Americans. In the heterozygous state (ie, Hb AC trait), there is no anemia, but target cells are seen on the blood smear.

Homozygous Hb CC disease is associated with a moderate hemolytic anemia. The hemoglobin level is 8 to 11 g/dL, and the incidence of reticulocytosis is 5% to 10%. The patients have splenomegaly. The peripheral blood contains striking numbers of target cells and a few spherocytes.

## Hemoglobin SC

When the genes for Hb S and Hb C occur in the same person, a moderately severe anemia with splenomegaly results. Vaso-occlusive episodes are usually less frequent and milder than in sickle cell disease. Aseptic necrosis of the femoral head is an occasional complication, and severe retinal damage also occurs.

Hb SC disease does not usually affect growth and is compatible with extended survival. The hemoglobin concentration averages 9 to 10 g/dL. Target cells are seen in large numbers on blood smears. Hemoglobin electrophoresis reveals an almost equal mixture of Hb S and Hb C, with a slight elevation of Hb F.

## Hemoglobin D

The D hemoglobin syndromes include several varieties of abnormal hemoglobin with electrophoretic mobilities at an alkaline pH similar to that of Hb S, but they do not have the biochemical and physical properties of Hb S. Sickling does not occur in Hb

D syndromes. The homozygous state (ie, Hb DD) is characterized by a mild hemolytic anemia with splenomegaly. Hemoglobin D occurs in Caucasian populations and has a relatively high prevalence in northwest India.

## Hemoglobin E

Hemoglobin E, an electrophoretically slow variant, is prevalent in persons from Southeast Asia, particularly Thailand and Cambodia. The Hb E heterozygote (ie, Hb AE) has increased numbers of target cells on blood smears. Homozygous Hb EE disease is characterized by a mild or moderate hemolytic anemia and by prominent target cells, microcytosis, and splenomegaly.

## Unstable Hemoglobin Syndromes

About 50 varieties of abnormal hemoglobins are characterized by molecular instability and are associated with the precipitation of hemoglobin (ie, Heinz bodies) within the erythrocytes, causing chronic hemolysis. These anemias are inherited as autosomal dominant traits.

Hemolysis is manifested during the first 6 months of life. The patients usually have jaundice and splenomegaly. The abnormal hemoglobin accounts for 30% to 40% of the total, but it may not be detected by electrophoresis. Heating of the hemolysate at 50 °C for 1 hour usually results in a heavy precipitate of the abnormal hemoglobin.

Splenectomy sometimes improves mild or moderately severe hemolytic disease, but severe hemolysis may not be improved by surgery.

## Hemoglobinopathies Causing Cyanosis

A group of abnormal hemoglobins, designated Hb M, are associated with dominantly transmitted familial cyanosis. Because the characteristic amino acid substitutions are strategically located near the heme groups, internal oxidation of heme iron to the trivalent (ie, ferric) form occurs. The Hb M diseases are characterized by cyanosis and mild polycythemia and have sometimes been mistaken for cyanotic congenital heart disease. Hb M can be differentiated from other forms of methemoglobinemia by characteristic changes in the spectral absorption patterns of hemoglobin solutions and by normal levels of erythrocyte methemoglobin reductase (ie, diaphorase). No therapy is indicated.

## Hemoglobinopathies With Altered Oxygen Affinity

More than 20 abnormal hemoglobins are associated with an increase in oxygen affinity. This is indicated by a shift to the left of the oxygen dissociation curve and a low partial pressure of oxygen at which hemoglobin is half saturated ($P_{50}$). Because of the increased affinity for hemoglobin, the decreased release of oxygen to the tissues leads to tissue hypoxia. This accelerates production of erythropoietin and secondary polycythemia.

Six hemoglobin variants with markedly reduced affinity for oxygen have been reported. These are associated with familial chronic cyanosis or pseudoanemia. The oxygen dissociation curve is shifted to the right, with $P_{50}$ values greater than 30 mm Hg.

## THALASSEMIAS

The thalassemias are a group of hereditary hypochromic anemias associated with defective synthesis of one of the polypeptide chains of hemoglobin. In the United States, they chiefly affect persons of Mediterranean and Southeast Asian backgrounds. In the heterozygous state, thalassemia genes produce mild anemia. In the homozygous form, they are associated with severe hematologic disease.

## Pathophysiology

More than 40 separate genetic variants of thalassemia have been identified. These result in quantitative deficiencies of the mRNA of the $\alpha$ or $\beta$ polypeptide chains of hemoglobin. Unbalanced polypeptide chain synthesis results in formation of unstable hemoglobin complexes within the erythrocyte that lead to erythrocyte death, much of which occurs in the bone marrow. The pathophysiology of thalassemia reflects ineffective erythropoiesis with severe hemolysis and compensatory hypertrophy of erythroid tissue in medullary and extramedullary sites.

## Clinical Presentations

Heterozygous thalassemia of the $\beta$-chain variety (ie, thalassemia minor) is a mild familial hypochronic microcytic anemia. Hemoglobin levels are 2 to 3 g/dL below age-appropriate normal values. The mean corpuscular volume averages 68 fL (range, 58 to 75 fL). The erythrocytes are hypochromic and microcytic, with target cells, ovalocytes, and basophilic stippling. Elevation of Hb $A_2$ levels (>3.5%) establishes the diagnosis. No therapy is effective or necessary.

Homozygous $\beta$-thalassemia (ie, thalassemia major, Cooley's anemia) usually becomes symptomatic in the first year of life. The anemia is so profound that regular blood transfusions are necessary to sustain life; untreated, the life expectancy is only a few years. However, about 10% of homozygous patients are able to maintain hemoglobin levels of 6 to 8 g/dL without regular transfusions (ie, thalassemia intermedia). In the untransfused or poorly transfused patient, massive splenomegaly and progressive bone changes become evident during the first few years of life.

## Laboratory Findings

The erythrocyte changes of thalassemia major are extreme. In addition to severe hypochromia and microcytosis, there are many poikilocytes and target cells. Large numbers of nucleated erythrocytes circulate, especially after splenectomy. Typically, the hemoglobin level falls progressively to less than 5 g/dL unless transfusions are given. The unconjugated serum bilirubin level is elevated. The serum iron level is high, with increasing saturation of iron-binding capacity. Lactate dehydrogenase activities are very high, reflecting ineffective erythropoiesis. Large amounts of fetal hemoglobin are contained in the erythrocytes. The level of Hb F exceeds 70% during the early years of life but tends to decline with increasing age.

## Treatment

Transfusions of packed erythrocytes are given to maintain the hemoglobin level above 10 g/dL. This hypertransfusion has striking clinical benefit: it permits normal activity with comfort and prevents progressive marrow expansion and its attendant cosmetic problems and osteoporosis. Transfusions are necessary every 4 to 5 weeks.

Hemosiderosis is an inevitable and fatal consequence of prolonged transfusion therapy, because each 200 mL of erythrocytes contains about 200 mg of iron that cannot be physiologically excreted. The iron burden can be reduced with iron-chelating agents, especially desferoxamine. This must be given parenterally, administered subcutaneously at night over 8 to 12 hours using a battery-driven pump. In many patients, negative iron balance

is possible. A chronic chelation program can reverse the poor prognosis of this disease if patient compliance with the demanding regimen can be obtained. Iron-chelating drugs, especially those which can be taken orally, are undergoing clinical testing. If efficacious and safe, these new drugs will improve compliance with chelation therapy and significantly reduce the incidence of hemosiderosis in chronically transfused patients.

Splenectomy is often necessary because of the size of the organ or because of secondary hypersplenism, but it has no effect on the basic hematologic disease. Immunization with pneumococcal polysaccharide vaccine is indicated, and prophylactic penicillin therapy is advocated by some authorities.

Bone marrow transplantation from HLA-identical and partly mismatched siblings has been performed in over 400 children with thalassemia. Early death from toxicity and graft-versus-host disease is low (<10%) in young patients without hepatic dysfunction. The risk of death is considerably higher for older patients, especially if liver function is already compromised by hemosiderosis. If an HLA-matched, healthy sibling is available, bone marrow transplantation should be considered, especially in a patient without symptoms of hemosiderosis. Introduction of a normal $\beta$-globin gene using gene therapy remains an area of active research.

## Other Thalassemias

### Thalassemia Intermedia

Thalassemia intermedia is a term assigned to patients with thalassemia syndromes intermediate in severity between major and minor. They have jaundice and moderate splenomegaly. The hemoglobin level is maintained at 7 to 8 g/dL. Regular transfusions are unnecessary, but transfusion therapy may be indicated to prevent severe osseous abnormalities. Even without regular blood transfusions, these patients absorb large amounts of iron, and hemosiderosis ultimately occurs.

### Hemoglobin S Thalassemia Disease

The combination of a $\beta$-thalassemia and Hb S gene results in a clinical disease more severe than with either trait alone. Hb S–thalassemia disease is a moderately severe, microcytic, hemolytic anemia with vaso-occlusive symptoms. The proportion of Hb S ranges from 60% to 90%; the remainder is Hb A and variable amounts of Hb F and Hb S–$\beta^+$-thalassemia. Sometimes no Hb A can be detected (Hb S–$\beta^0$- thalassemia). Family studies reveal one parent to have thalassemia trait and the other to have a sickle cell syndrome.

### Alpha Thalassemias

A group of diseases especially prevalent in Southeast Asians results from genetic deletions of $\alpha$-chain genes. There are normally four $\alpha$-chain genes. Five percent of African-Americans have $\alpha$-thalassemia trait associated with deletion of two $\alpha$-chain genes. Clinically, it is characterized by microcytic anemia that is unresponsive to iron. Three and four $\alpha$-chain deletions are rare among African-Americans. The diagnosis is made by excluding other causes of anemia. Hemoglobin electrophoresis is not helpful after the immediate postnatal period. In the newborn period, hemoglobin electrophoresis shows 3% to 6% Hb Barts. Patients are asymptomatic, but should be counseled so that they may prevent well-meaning health providers from prescribing iron for presumed iron deficiency or from performing a workup for anemia.

In Asians, the four distinct $\alpha$-thalassemia syndromes are the silent carrier state, $\alpha$-thalassemia trait, Hb H disease, and fetal hydrops syndrome. These result from increasing numbers of $\alpha$-thalassemia gene deletions, from one to four. Deletion of four $\alpha$-thalassemia genes produces the clinical picture of hydrops fetalis in utero. The predominant hemoglobin is Barts ($\gamma_4$). This variant has abnormal oxygen dissociation properties that make oxygen unavailable to the tissues, causing fetal death.

Deletion of three $\alpha$-thalassemia genes causes the less severe Hb H disease. This is a moderately severe anemia that resembles thalassemia major or intermedia. It is characterized by 5% to 10% of unstable Hb H ($\beta_4$).

## Hereditary Persistence of High Fetal Hemoglobin

Hereditary persistence of high fetal hemoglobin (HPFH) is associated with high levels of normal fetal hemoglobin but few hematologic abnormalities. It occurs predominantly in black and Mediterranean people. The erythrocytes contain 15% to 30% Hb F. There is an even distribution of Hb F in the erythrocyte population, in contrast to the thalassemias, in which Hb F content varies from cell to cell. The HPFH homozygote has 100% Hb F but no significant anemia. If HPFH and a sickle gene affect the same person, only Hb S and Hb F are found. However, the even distribution of Hb F in the erythrocyte population prevents sickling, and hematologic and clinical symptoms are minimal.

## Selected Readings

Bunn HF, Forget BG, Ranney HM. Human hemoglobins. Philadelphia: WB Saunders, 1977.
Charache S, Lubin B, Reid CD. Management and therapy of sickle cell disease. Bethesda: NIH Publication No. 85–2115, September 1985.
Kirkpatrick DV, Barrios NJ, Humbert JH. Bone marrow transplantation in sickle cell anemia. Semin Hematol 1991;28:240.
Lucarelli G, Galimberti M, Polchi P, et al. Bone marrow transplantation in thalassemia. The experience of Pesaro. N Engl J Med 1990;322:417.
Pearson HA. Sickle cell diseases. Diagnosis and management in infancy and childhood. Pediatr Rev 1987;9:121.
Serjeant GR. Sickle cell disease, Oxford: Oxford University Press, 1985.
Weatherall DJ. Bone marrow transplantation for thalassemia and other inherited disorders of hemoglobin. Blood 1992;80:1379.
Weatherall DJ, Cligg JB. The thalassemia syndromes, ed 3. Oxford: Blackwell Scientific Publications, 1981.

*Principles and Practice of Pediatrics, Second Edition.*
edited by Frank A. Oski et al. J. B. Lippincott Company, Philadelphia © 1994.

# 90.3 *The Hemolytic Anemias*

## Paul L. Martin and Howard A. Pearson

After release from the bone marrow, mature, nonnucleated erythrocytes survive for 100 to 120 days in the circulation. In the steady state, about 1% of the senescent erythrocytes are destroyed daily and are replaced by an equal number of new erythrocytes released from the bone marrow. The basic pathophysiology of the hemolytic anemias is a reduced erythrocyte lifespan, ranging from nearly normal to remarkably shortened. In compensation, the bone marrow increases its output of erythrocytes, a response mediated by increased production of erythropoietin. In adults with hereditary spherocytosis, the bone marrow can increase output of erythrocytes sixfold to eightfold. With this maximal response, erythrocyte survival can be reduced to only 20 to 30 days without the onset of anemia (ie, compensated hemolysis). The limits of erythrocyte production in other hemolytic states have not been determined, particularly in infants and children, but they are probably lower in infants than adults.

A hemolytic process can be directly measured by erythrocyte survival rates or indirectly by the presence of increased levels of the metabolic products of hemolysis. Alternatively, a hemolytic process may be inferred by documentation of the increase in erythrocyte production that usually accompanies hemolytic states.

In response to a shortened survival of erythrocytes, the activity of bone marrow increases, and the reticulocyte count exceeds 2% (absolute reticulocyte count >100,000/mm³). Sustained reticulocytosis is presumptive evidence of hemolysis. Hyperplasia of the erythropoietic marrow elements occurs, with reversal of the myeloid erythroid ratio from the normal 3:1. In the severe, chronic hemolytic processes of childhood, hypertrophy of the marrow may expand the medullary spaces, producing bony changes, particularly in the skull and hands.

Elevations of unconjugated bilirubin often occur in children with hemolytic anemias. However, overt jaundice may be absent, and bilirubin levels in excess of 5 mg/dL are unusual if hepatic function is normal. Chronic hemolysis is associated with increased excretion of bilirubin pigments leading to pigmented gallstones that may develop in early childhood.

In any hemolytic state, hemoglobin is released into the plasma, where it combines irreversibly with serum haptoglobin. The large complex is rapidly cleared from the circulation. When haptoglobin use exceeds synthesis, serum levels are decreased (<20 mg/dL) or absent.

Besides these indirect indicators of hemolysis, isotopic techniques can measure erythrocyte survival directly. Sodium chromate ($Na_2{}^{51}CrO_4$) is most often used as a erythrocyte tag. A shortened erythrocyte survival is likely when the $^{51}Cr$ half-life is reduced below 20 days. However, it is rarely necessary to employ such survival studies in clinical practice.

The hemolytic disorders may be conveniently and fairly accurately classified according to whether the shortened erythrocyte survival is a result of an intrinsic abnormality of the erythrocyte or an extrinsic abnormality acting on a normal erythrocyte. Intrinsic hemolytic anemias generally result from inherited abnormalities of the erythrocyte membrane, intracellular enzymes, or hemoglobin. Extrinsic disorders are usually acquired and result from forces or agents that immunologically, chemically, or physically damage the erythrocyte. These two categories are not mutually exclusive, and some hemolytic disorders are caused by a combination of intrinsic and extrinsic mechanisms.

## INTRINSIC HEMOLYTIC ANEMIAS

### Hereditary Spherocytosis

Hereditary spherocytosis (HS; congenital hemolytic anemia, congenital acholuric jaundice) occurs predominantly in persons of North European ancestry, although it has been found in patients of many ethnic groups. The typical features are a familial hemolytic anemia of various degrees of severity, splenomegaly, and spherical erythrocytes found on the blood smear.

In about three quarters of patients, pedigree analysis indicates an autosomal dominant transmission. Sporadic dominant mutations have been invoked and autosomal recessive transmission is suggested in some cases. The gene for HS is located on chromosome 8.

#### Pathophysiology

A deficiency or abnormality of the erythrocyte membrane structural protein spectrin appears to affect most patients with HS. This deficiency is associated with an accelerated loss of the erythrocyte membrane, which reduces the erythrocyte surface area. Because there is no concomitant loss of cellular volume, the erythrocytes assume a spherical shape. Increased membrane cation flux can be demonstrated.

The spleen is intrinsically involved in the hemolytic process. The splenic circulation imposes a metabolic stress on spherocytic cells. The spherocyte is relatively rigid and passes with difficulty through the splenic cords and sinuses. This results in their sequestration and destruction. The hemolytic process regresses after splenectomy, although biochemical and morphologic abnormalities persist.

### Clinical Presentation

The disease may present in the neonatal period with anemia and hyperbilirubinemia that may require phototherapy or exchange transfusion. The anemia varies considerably in severity but tends to be similar within the same family. The patient usually has slight jaundice. Expansion of the marrow cavities occurs to a lesser extent than in thalassemia. The spleen is almost always palpably enlarged after 2 or 3 years of age. Pigmentary gallstones have occurred as early as 4 years of age. Aplastic crises associated with parvovirus infections are the most serious complications during childhood (see Chap. 90.4).

### Laboratory Findings

Indicators of hemolysis include reticulocytosis, anemia, and hyperbilirubinemia. The hemoglobin level ranges from 6 to 10 g/dL and the reticulocyte count from 5% to 20% (average, 10%). The spherocytic erythrocytes are smaller than normal erythrocytes and lack the central pallor of the biconcave disk, but only a relatively small proportion of the cells are spherocytic. There is erythroid hyperplasia in the marrow, but erythrocyte precursors are not spherocytic.

Abnormality of the erythrocyte can be demonstrated by osmotic fragility studies. When erythrocytes are placed in hypotonic saline solutions, water enters the cells, causing them to swell. The normal biconcave erythrocyte can increase its volume, but the spherical cell already has maximal volume for its surface area and hemolyzes at a higher saline concentration (ie, increased osmotic fragility) than normal. In 10% to 20% of HS cases, the osmotic abnormality can be demonstrated only if the blood is incubated at 37 °C for 24 hours.

HS must be differentiated from other congenital hemolytic states. Family history, blood smear, and osmotic fragility studies offer the most diagnostic value. Acquired spherocytosis of the erythrocytes is seen in autoimmune hemolytic anemias, in which the spherocytosis is often more pronounced than in HS, and the direct Coombs' test result is positive. It may be difficult to differentiate HS from hemolytic disease because of ABO incompatibility in the newborn infant. A period of observation may be necessary to clarify the diagnosis.

### Therapy

Splenectomy almost invariably produces a clinical cure, although in a few instances of severe HS with recessive transmission, the operation was not curative. Splenectomy should be deferred if possible until the patient is at least 5 or 6 years of age. If anemia is severe enough to impair growth or normal activity, the operation can be considered earlier after a period of observation. Splenectomy prevents gallstones and eliminates the threat of aplastic crises.

After splenectomy, jaundice and reticulocytosis disappear. The hemoglobin level becomes normal, although the spherocytosis and osmotic fragility abnormalities become more pronounced. Overwhelming sepsis after splenectomy occurs infrequently if the surgery is delayed until the child is 5 or 6 years of age, but the febrile child must be carefully evaluated for sepsis. Polyvalent pneumococcal vaccine should be given before splenectomy. Prophylactic penicillin therapy after splenectomy is advocated by some authorities and is definitely indicated if the operation is done before the child is 6 years of age.

## Hereditary Elliptocytosis

Some oval or elliptical erythrocytes may be seen in a number of conditions, especially thalassemia and iron deficiency; however, they occur in much larger numbers as a dominantly inherited trait in hereditary elliptocytosis (HE; hereditary ovalocytosis). Fifteen percent to 50% of the circulating erythrocytes of these persons are elongated. In most patients, there is no associated hemolysis, and the hematologic values, including reticulocyte counts, are normal. However, in about 10% of patients with elliptical cells, there is evidence of hemolysis, with hemoglobin levels averaging 8 to 10 g/dL and reticulocytes comprising 5% to 15% of the cells.

### Pathophysiology

A structural abnormality of spectrin has been described in erythrocytes from some HE patients with or without hemolysis. The bases for hemolytic HE and HE without hemolysis are unclear. In most family studies of hemolytic HE, one parent has elliptical erythrocytes without hemolysis, and the other parent is hematologically normal.

### Clinical Presentation

HE with hemolysis may be associated with neonatal jaundice, but characteristic elliptocytosis may not be evident at birth. The blood smear instead shows bizarre poikilocytes and pyknocytes. The usual features of chronic hemolytic process, including anemia, jaundice, splenomegaly, and osseous changes, may be seen later. Cholelithiasis occurs in later childhood, and aplastic crises have been reported.

### Laboratory Findings

The morphology of the erythrocytes is the most important diagnostic feature. Elliptical cells characterized by a length more than 1.5 times the diameter account for 15% to 70% of the erythrocytes. The reticulocyte count is increased. Erythroid hyperplasia is evident in the bone marrow, but the erythrocyte precursors are not elliptical. Increased erythrocyte osmotic fragility and increased thermal instability occur in hemolytic HE. This has sometimes led to designating cases of hemolytic HE as pyropoikilocytosis.

### Therapy

If there is significant hemolysis, splenectomy is usually beneficial. Erythrocyte morphology is not changed after the operation, and it may become even more abnormal.

## Paroxysmal Nocturnal Hemoglobinuria

Paroxysmal nocturnal hemoglobinuria is a rare chronic anemia with prominent intravascular hemolysis that may have its onset in late childhood. Hemolysis is characteristically worse during sleep, and morning hemoglobinuria is usual.

The disease is not congenital. It results from an ill-defined acquired defect of the erythrocyte membrane that renders it susceptible to hemolysis by serum complement. In addition to chronic hemolysis, thrombocytopenia and leukopenia may develop. Some cases have been preceded by aplastic anemia.

The diagnosis is established by a positive result in the acidified serum (Ham's) or thrombin or sucrose lysis tests. Therapy is supportive and symptomatic. Bone marrow transplantation has been successful in some cases.

## Hereditary Stomatocytosis

Hereditary stomatocytosis is a rare hemolytic anemia condition associated with erythrocytes that are swollen and cup shaped.

On stained smears, they have a mouth-like slit (ie, stoma) in place of the usual circular central pallor. Hemolytic anemia is associated with extreme permeability of the erythrocyte membrane to cations. Splenectomy may be indicated.

## HEMOLYTIC ANEMIAS RESULTING FROM ABNORMALITIES OF ERYTHROCYTE GLYCOLYTIC ENZYMES

This group of congenital hemolytic anemias was originally classified as nonspherocytic, because spherocytic erythrocytes were not found, and results of the osmotic fragility test were normal.

Most of these anemias are inherited as autosomal recessive disorders. A diagnosis is established by demonstrating reduced levels of the specific glycolytic enzyme. In addition, increased levels of glycolytic metabolites proximal to the deficient enzyme are found. Deficiencies of glycolytic enzyme compromise adenosine triphosphate (ATP) generation. The metabolic energy requirements of the erythrocytes cannot be met, and the erythrocyte lifespan is shortened.

### Pyruvate Kinase Deficiency

An inherited deficiency of pyruvate kinase (PK) is the most frequent of the erythrocyte glycolytic enzyme deficiencies. PK activity, measured in the erythrocytes, is markedly reduced, but the enzyme activity in other blood cells and tissues is normal.

#### Pathophysiology

The disease is caused by homozygosity for an autosomal recessive gene, which results in markedly decreased production of a mutant PK isoenzyme. The PK-deficient erythrocytes are ATP depleted, and their survival is compromised. Levels of glycolytic intermediates, especially 2,3-diphosphoglycerate (2,3-DPG), are greatly increased. The increase in 2,3-DPG causes a right shift of the oxygen dissociation curve that may reduce symptoms of anemia. Heterozygotes for PK deficiency have intermediate enzyme levels.

#### Clinical Presentation

In PK-deficient homozygotes, there is a broad spectrum of clinical and hematologic findings, ranging from a mild, completely compensated hemolytic state to severe anemia. Anemia and hyperbilirubinemia may occur in the neonatal period. In the older patient, pallor, scleral icterus, and splenomegaly are usual findings.

#### Laboratory Findings

The blood smear shows polychromatophilic erythrocytes, indicating an elevated reticulocyte count. A few small spiculated erythrocytes are seen, but no spherocytes are found. Osmotic fragility is normal.

#### Treatment

Hyperbilirubinemia in the neonatal period may require exchange transfusion. Severe disease may require repeated transfusions for anemia during infancy. Splenectomy, although not curative, often improves the anemia and should be considered in patients with severe disease. Marked reticulocytosis occurs after splenectomy.

### Other Inherited Abnormalities of Erythrocyte Glycolytic Enzymes

Deficiencies of several glycolytic erythrocyte enzymes have been described in patients with congenital nonspherocytic hemolytic anemias. These include deficiencies of hexokinase, glucose-6-phosphate isomerase, phosphofructokinase aldolase, triosephosphate isomerase, glyceraldehyde-3-phosphate isomerase, and phosphoglycerate kinase. Most of these diseases are transmitted as autosomal recessive traits, and they are rare.

Chronic hemolysis, often manifested in infancy, is a common feature. Specific erythrocyte morphologic abnormalities are not seen. Diagnosis depends on demonstration of reductions of the specific erythrocyte enzyme. There is no specific therapy, but splenectomy may reduce the rate of hemolysis.

### Deficiencies of Enzymes of the Pentose Phosphate Pathway

The most important function of the pentose pathway is to provide the NADPH necessary for maintaining glutathione (GSH) in the reduced state. This is essential for the physiologic inactivation of oxidant compounds. Without adequate levels of GSH, when oxidant drugs are ingested, hemoglobin becomes denatured and precipitates into erythrocyte inclusions called Heinz bodies. These damage the erythrocyte membrane and cause acute hemolysis.

### Glucose-6-Phosphate Dehydrogenase Deficiency Syndromes

Glucose-6-phosphate dehydrogenase (G6PD) deficiency results in two kinds of hematologic problems: a common, acute condition manifested by hemolytic episodes induced by infection or certain drugs and a rare, chronic, nonspherocytic hemolytic anemia.

The G6PD gene is on the X chromosome. In the hemizygous affected male, the condition results from inheritance of one abnormal G6PD gene. In the affected homozygous female, two abnormal genes are inherited. The normal G6PD enzyme found in most Caucasian populations is designated, G6PD B$^+$. A normal isozyme designated G6PD A$^+$ is common in blacks. More than 100 distinct enzyme variants of G6PD have been documented.

*Pathophysiology.* Thirteen percent of African-American males and 2% of African-American females have a mutant enzyme called G6PD A$^-$ that is unstable and associated with reduced erythrocyte enzyme activity (5% to 15% of normal). Affected persons of Mediterranean, Arabic, and Asian ethnic groups have relatively high frequencies of G6PD deficiency because of a variant designated G6PD B$^-$. The enzyme activity of the homozygous female or the hemizygous male is less than 5% of normal.

G6PD, the rate-limiting enzyme of the pentose phosphate pathway, is crucial for protection of the erythrocytes from oxidant stress. In G6PD deficiency, oxidant metabolites of a number of drugs produce denaturation and precipitation of hemoglobin, causing erythrocyte injury and rapid hemolysis. Hemolysis occurs only if the patient is exposed to oxidant drugs, such as antipyretics, sulfonamides, antimalarials, and naphthaquinolones, or to the fava bean. The degree of hemolysis varies with the drug, the amount ingested, and the severity of the enzyme deficiency in the patient.

*Laboratory Findings.* Hemoglobinemia and hemoglobinuria occur 24 to 48 hours after the ingestion of an oxidant substance. The hemoglobin level may fall as low as 2 to 5 g/dL. Heinz bodies are not visible on stained blood smears. They can be initially demonstrated on supravital preparations, but they disappear after 3 or 4 days. Spontaneous recovery is usual and is heralded by reticulocytosis and an increase in hemoglobin concentration, starting 4 or 5 days after the acute hemolytic episode.

Diagnosis depends on direct or indirect demonstration of reduced G6PD activity in erythrocytes. By direct measurement, enzyme activity in affected persons is less than 15% of normal. The reduction of enzyme activity is more extreme in Caucasians and Asians than in G6PD-deficient blacks. Immediately after a hemolytic event, G6PD activity may be normal. A repeat examination several weeks later may be necessary to prove the diagnosis.

*Therapy.* Prevention of hemolysis by avoiding oxidant drugs is important. Males belonging to ethnic groups in which there is a significant incidence of G6PD deficiency should be tested for the defect before drugs that are known to be potent oxidants are given. After hemolysis has occurred, supportive therapy is indicated, including blood transfusions if the anemia is severe and the patient symptomatic.

### Chronic Nonspherocytic Hemolytic Anemia Associated With Glucose-6-Phosphate Dehydrogenase Deficiency

Instances of chronic hemolytic anemias not associated with oxidant drug ingestion have been associated with profound deficiencies of G6PD due to several enzyme variants. These have occurred predominantly in persons of North European ancestry. For this X-linked disease, splenectomy has been of minimal value.

## EXTRINSIC HEMOLYTIC ANEMIAS

Agents that damage erythrocytes may lead to their premature destruction. The most clearly defined of these agents are the antibodies associated with immune hemolysis. Antibodies directed against specific intrinsic membrane antigens damage the erythrocytes and produce hemolysis. The most important feature of these diseases is the positive Coombs' test, which detects immunoglobulins or components of complement on the erythrocyte surface.

## Autoimmune Hemolytic Anemias

In the autoimmune hemolytic anemias (AIHAs), the patient's antibodies are directed against the erythrocytes. The factors evoking such an autoimmune response are unknown, but they include viral infections and occasionally specific drugs.

### Pathophysiology

AIHAs associated with an underlying disease process such as lymphoma, lupus erythematosus, or immunodeficiency are said to be secondary. In idiopathic AIHA, there is no such underlying disease. Drugs such as penicillin cephalosporins and α-methyldopa evoke the formation of antibodies in some patients.

### Clinical Manifestations

AIHAs occur in two clinical patterns. The first type, a fulminant variety that occurs in infants and young children, is frequently preceded by a respiratory infection. The onset is acute, with pallor, jaundice, and hemoglobinuria. The spleen is enlarged. A consistent response to corticosteroid therapy, low mortality rate, and complete recovery are characteristic. No underlying disease is found. A second type of AIHA has a prolonged course and a significant mortality rate. Underlying diseases are frequently found.

### Laboratory Findings

The anemia may be severe, with hemoglobin levels less than 6 g/dL. Spherocytosis and polychromasia are prominent. Reticulocytosis and nucleated erythrocytes are found, and leukocytosis is common. The platelet count is usually normal; occasionally, there is concomitant immune thrombocytopenic purpura (ie, Evans syndrome).

The direct and indirect Coombs' test results are positive, indicating the presence of antibodies attached to the erythrocytes or free in the serum. These antibodies belong to the IgG class. They are often nonspecific panagglutinins, but they may have specificity for common antigens of the Rh system (eg, LW). Because of spontaneous erythrocyte agglutination, the patient may be mistakenly typed as blood group AB, Rh positive. In acute transient cases, only complement is found on the erythrocytes, chiefly the C3 and C4 components. In chronic AIHA, a pure IgG Coombs' test result is often found.

### Treatment

Transfusion may be required, but it offers only transient benefit. It is difficult to find compatible blood, and it is often necessary to give blood that is "incompatible" as judged by the crossmatch. Prednisone should be administered in a dosage of 2 to 4 mg/kg every 24 hours. Treatment should be continued until hemolysis decreases. The dose can then be gradually reduced. The acute form of disease usually remits spontaneously within a few weeks or months, but the Coombs' test may remain positive for an extended period. Splenectomy may be beneficial in severe refractory cases. Immunosuppressive agents have been used in patients refractory to conventional therapy. In AIHA secondary to lymphoma or lupus erythematosus, the disease tends to be chronic, and the course of the underlying disease determines ultimate prognosis.

## Hemolytic Anemias Associated With Cold Antibodies

Low levels of cold antibodies may exist normally, but after some viral or mycoplasmal infections, they may increase to very high levels. These high titers of cold antibodies induce intravascular hemolysis with hemoglobinemia. The antibodies often have specificity for the I antigen and react poorly with human cord blood cells possessing the i antigen. The antibodies are of the IgM class and require complement for activity. Spontaneous agglutination and rouleaux formation are seen on the blood smear. Patients with infectious mononucleosis may develop acute hemolytic anemia. The antibodies in these cases have anti-I specificity.

## Paroxysmal Cold Hemoglobinuria

Paroxysmal cold hemoglobinuria is a rare condition that is associated with a specific type of cold antibody, the Donath-Landsteiner hemolysin, which has anti-P specificity. Intravascular hemolysis is precipitated by low environmental temperature. About one third of cases are associated with congenital or acquired syphilis.

## Selected Readings

Agre P, Onenger EP. Deficient red cell spectrin in severe recessively inherited hereditary spherocytosis. N Engl J Med 1985;306:1155.

Austin RF, Deforges JI. Hereditary elliptocytosis: an unusual presentation of hemolysis in the newborn period associated with transient morphological abnormalities. Pediatrics 1969;44:196.

Beutler E. Abnormalities of the hexose monophosphate shunt. Semin Hematol 1971;8:311.

Buchanan GR, Boxer LA. The acute and transient nature of idiopathic immune hemolytic anemia in childhood. J Pediatr 1976;88:780.

Geerdnink RA, Hellerman PW, Verloop MC. Hereditary elliptocytosis and hyperhaemolysis: a comparative study of 6 families with 145 patients. Acta Med Sci 1966;179:715.

Habibi B, Homberg JC. Autoimmune hemolytic anemia in children. A review of 80 cases. Am J Med 1974;56:61.

Kruger HC, Burgert EO. Hereditary spherocytes in 100 children. Mayo Clin Proc 1966;41:921.

Lux SE, Becker PS. Disorders of the membrane skeleton: hereditary spherocytosis and hereditary elliptocytosis. In: Scriver CR, Baudet AD, Sly WS, Valle P, eds. The metabolic basis of inherited disease, ed 6. New York: McGraw-Hill, 1989.

Trucco JI, Brown AK. Neonatal manifestations of hereditary spherocytosis. Am J Dis Child 1967;113:263.

Valentine WN, Paglia DE. Erythrocytic enzymopathies, hemolytic anemia and multisystem disease. Blood 1984;64:583.

Young LE. Hereditary spherocytosis. Am J Med 1955;18:480.

*Principles and Practice of Pediatrics, Second Edition.*
edited by Frank A. Oski et al. J. B. Lippincott Company, Philadelphia © 1994.

# 90.4 *The Hypoplastic and Aplastic Anemias*

Paul L. Martin and Howard A. Pearson

## HYPOPLASTIC ANEMIAS

The hypoplastic anemias (ie, pure erythrocyte anemias, aregenerative anemias) constitute an uncommon group of congenital or acquired blood disorders characterized by anemia, reticulocytopenia, and a paucity of erythroid precursors in otherwise normally cellular bone marrow. Unlike the aplastic anemias (ie, pancytopenias), the other formed elements of the blood are usually present in normal or increased numbers.

## Pathophysiology

An understanding of the pathophysiology of the hypoplastic anemias requires a brief review of cellular aspects of erythropoiesis. Insight into the understanding of the nature and interactions of erythropoietic primordial cells has been possible because of the development of techniques for in vitro culture of bone marrow in media such as plasma clots, methylcellulose, and agar. Early committed erythroid progenitor cells can be inferred by their ability to form colonies of erythroid cells using these techniques. Two classes of progenitor cells have been identified: so-called colony-forming units, erythroid (CFU-E), which give rise to compact colonies containing 10 to 100 hemoglobinized erythroid cells after 48 hours of culture, and more primitive erythroid progenitor cells, designated as burst-forming units, erythroid (BFU-E), recognized by their capacity to form large colonies containing as many as 30,000 erythroid cells after 7 to 9 days of culture. Colony formation by CFU-E requires the presence of erythropoietin (EPO), the glycoprotein hormone that regulates erythrocyte formation in the intact animal. BFU-E development does not require the presence of EPO. BFU-E and CFU-E are present in small numbers in the normal bone marrow and morphologically resemble mature lymphocytes.

The next phases of erythrocyte development are represented by cells that can be morphologically identified as belonging to the erythroid series. These include the pronormoblast and the basophilic, polychromatophilic, and acidophilic normoblasts. In the latter stages of maturation of the erythrocyte, nuclear condensation and extrusion occur, resulting in the reticulocyte and finally the mature erythrocyte.

The hypoplastic anemias are a heterogenous group; both congenital and acquired varieties are recognized (Table 90-1).

### TABLE 90-1.    The Hypoplastic Anemias

**Congenital**
Congenital hypoplastic anemia (Diamond-Blackfan syndrome)

**Acquired**
Transient erythroblastopenia of childhood
Parvovirus-induced aplastic crises of hemolytic anemias

## Congenital Hypoplastic Anemia

At the 1938 meeting of the American Pediatric Society, Diamond and Blackfan described four children with severe aregenerative anemia that developed during the first year of life and required regular transfusions for survival. Only about 300 cases of congenital hypoplastic anemia (CHA) have been described in the literature, but many more cases have been recognized.

A familial recurrence in some families suggests that genetic factors may occasionally be operative, but in most cases, no inherited pattern is evident. About 25% of the patients have physical abnormalities of various kinds, including short stature and facial, cardiac, and renal abnormalities. A subset of patients have thumbs with three rather than the usual two phalanges (ie, Wranne syndrome).

### Clinical Presentation

Anemia at or shortly after birth is the presenting manifestation of CHA. About a quarter of the patients are pale at birth. Sixty-five percent are anemic by 6 months of age, and almost all are anemic by 1 year of age. CHA described in older infants, particularly those reported before 1970, must be viewed with some skepticism, because the cases may have represented transient erythroblastopenia of childhood.

### Laboratory Findings

At the time of diagnosis, the hemoglobin levels may be as low as 2.5 g/dL. The erythrocytes are macrocytic and have biochemical properties of fetal erythrocyte (ie, increased levels of Hb F for the patient's age, presence of the i erythrocyte antigen, and increased levels of age-dependent erythrocyte enzymes such as glucose-6-phosphate dehydrogenase). These findings may be of limited diagnostic value in early infancy when fetal cells are still present.

The reticulocyte count is characteristically very low, even in the presence of severe anemia. The remainder of the peripheral blood count is usually normal, although elevated platelet counts and modest neutropenia have occasionally been found.

Serum bilirubin levels are normal. Serum iron levels are usually elevated with increased transferrin saturation. Plasma and urinary levels of EPO are elevated.

In most patients with CHA, erythrocyte adenine deaminase (ADA) levels are two to three times elevated over normal values. However, elevations have also been seen in some cases of acute leukemia, and the enzyme elevation may be an indicator of disordered erythropoiesis rather than a specific marker for CHA.

The most important diagnostic features are found in the bone marrow. The marrow in patients with CHA is normally cellular with normal numbers of megakaryocytes, lymphocytes, and myeloid precursors. However, erythrocyte precursors at every level of development are absent or markedly reduced. The proportion of myeloid to erythroid precursors in the bone marrow (M : E ratio), normally 3 : 1, is markedly increased (10 : 1 to 200 : 1). In some patients, a few primitive pronormoblasts can be recognized, but no more mature erythroid precursors are seen. Bone marrow erythroid cultures consistently have few BFU-E and CFU-E.

### Therapy

The degree of anemia is often so profound at presentation that erythrocyte transfusions are necessary. About 10% to 20% of patients are refractory to therapy and continue to require regular transfusions. Transfusions with packed, leukocyte-poor erythrocytes are given to maintain a hemoglobin level compatible with normal activity and comfort, usually above 8.0 g/dL.

When chronic transfusion therapy is necessary, transfusional hemosiderosis inevitably occurs. Serum ferritin levels should be monitored periodically, and chelation therapy should be begun when there is evidence of tissue iron overload (see Chap. 90.2).

The use of adrenocorticotropic hormone (ACTH) and corticosteroids in CHA was suggested as early as 1949, but it was not until 1961 that a relatively large number of steroid-treated patients were reported. Between 60% and 70% of patients respond to corticosteroid therapy. The mechanism of steroid action may involve an enhancement of the effect of EPO on CFU-E proliferation and maturation. Corticosteroids, such as prednisone, are administered at an initial dose of 2 mg/kg. Response is heralded by the appearance of erythropoietic precursors in the bone marrow within 1 to 2 weeks, followed by reticulocytosis and an increase in the hemoglobin level. The full dose of prednisone is continued until the hemoglobin attains a normal level. The dose can then be gradually decreased until a minimal effective dose is attained. This is often as little as 0.5 to 1 mg/day. In many instances, it is possible to administer corticosteroids on alternate-day schedules that further decrease steroid side effects. Some patients do not respond to the usual dose of steroids and should be given a trial with larger doses (4 to 6 mg/kg). About 20% to 30% of these children are nonresponsive to steroids and require regular blood transfusions.

Children refractory to steroids have usually not responded to other forms of therapy including androgenic and immunosuppressive agents. Bone marrow transplantation has been effective for a few patients.

## Transient Erythroblastic Anemia of Childhood

Transient erythroblastic anemia of childhood (TEC) is a striking syndrome of temporary failure of erythropoiesis, which is increasingly encountered in clinical practice. It is characterized by moderate to severe aregenerative anemia in an otherwise healthy child. The condition is self-limited and usually does not recur.

### Pathophysiology

The disease seems to have an autoimmune basis. A circulating immunoglobulin that inhibits growth of CFU-E or BFU-E in tissue culture has been found in most of these patients. The stimulus that evokes this antibody has not been defined, and the inhibitor disappears from the serum as recovery occurs. TEC has not been associated with parvovirus infection.

### Clinical Presentation

The condition occurs in children older than 1 year of age, but it has been seen as early as 4 months of age. Pallor and symptoms of anemia are the usual presenting manifestations. Because the anemia reflects a complete cessation of erythropoiesis without increased hemolysis, the anemia develops very slowly.

If a patient has a hemoglobin level of 5 g/dL on presentation, it can be assumed that erythrocyte production has been minimal for at least 2 months. Because the anemia develops insidiously, pallor or symptoms may not be noticed by the parents. Except for the features of anemia, the remainder of the physical examination is normal.

### Laboratory Findings

The degree of anemia may be severe, as low as 2.5 g/dL, with a low reticulocyte count. The leukocyte count is normal. The platelet count is usually normal but may be elevated. Other laboratory findings include a high serum iron level reflecting decreased use. The bone marrow shows a paucity of erythrocyte precursors with a high M : E ratio. The other marrow elements are normal.

Recovery occurs spontaneously within a few weeks and is accompanied by a brisk reticulocytosis and rapid increase in hemoglobin level.

The major differential diagnosis of TEC is CHA, particularly in the infant younger than 1 year of age. In contrast to CHA, in TEC the erythrocyte population at presentation has age-appropriate characteristics; a mean corpuscular volume of 70 to 80 fL; Hb F less than 2% to 5%; normal levels of erythrocyte age-dependent enzymes (G6PD); and the usual adult I erythrocyte antigen. Erythrocyte ADA levels are not elevated.

A patient first seen in the recovery state of TEC may be erroneously considered to have a hemolytic process because of the concomitant low hemoglobin and high reticulocyte count. Observation can clarify the diagnosis.

### Therapy

No specific therapy is necessary. Corticosteroid therapy is not indicated. If the anemia is severe, a small erythrocyte transfusion may be considered to sustain the child until recovery occurs. Most children have no recurrence of this disease.

## Aplastic Crisis of Hemolytic Anemias Associated With Parvovirus Infection

Episodes of exaggerated anemia and reticulocytopenia in patients with various kinds of hemolytic anemias have been recognized for many years. Such episodes usually occur in the wake of viral infections and often affect several family members.

A correlation between aplastic crises patients in sickle cell disease and infection by the parvovirus was established in 1981 by the demonstration of virus particles in the blood of these patients. It is likely that most severe aplastic crises in patients with hemolytic anemias are caused by the parvovirus, an organism that also has been established as the cause of erythema infectiosum (ie, fifth disease). Intrauterine parvovirus infection has been invoked as a possible cause of severe anemia and nonimmunologic hydrops fetalis.

### Pathophysiology

The parvovirus directly infects CFU-E, damaging the cells and inhibiting their ability to proliferate. This causes a virtual cessation of erythrocyte production. The inhibition lasts for only 1 to 2 weeks until the virus is cleared. In a normal person whose erythrocyte survival is 100 days, 10 days of erythrocyte aplasia results in an insignificant decrease of the hemoglobin level. However, in patients with hemolytic anemia, whose erythrocyte lifespan is reduced to 10 to 30 days, even 1 week of aplasia results in profound anemia.

During other viral infections, patients with hemolytic anemias may have decreased numbers of reticulocytes, suggesting some degree of marrow suppression. The resultant decrease in hemoglobin is not as severe as that caused by the parvovirus.

### Clinical Presentation

During aplastic crises, the degree of anemia worsens and jaundice decreases. There is profound reticulocytopenia and no erythrocyte precursors in the bone marrow. Early in the aplastic crisis, parvovirus particles can be found in the serum by electron microscopic examination. Later evidence of infection can be documented by changes in antibody titers in acute and convalescent sera.

### Treatment

Supportive blood transfusions are indicated if the degree of anemia is severe or if the patient is symptomatic. Because parvovirus infections evoke protective levels of circulating antibodies, aplastic crises do not recur in the same patient.

## APLASTIC ANEMIAS

The aplastic anemias have diverse causes whose common features are varying degrees of peripheral pancytopenia accompanied by marked hypocellularity of the bone marrow.

### Acquired Aplastic Anemia

#### Pathophysiology

In many instances, aplastic anemia is believed to be a result of destruction or dysfunction of the pluripotential stem cell (CFU-S) that is the progenitor of erythrocytes, platelets, monocytes, and granulocytes. An environmental toxin or agent is believed to cause the stem cell damage, but in as many as a third of patients, aplastic anemia appears to be an autoimmune disorder mediated through an inhibitory process involving T lymphocytes. Other mechanisms, such as an abnormal microenvironment for bone marrow proliferation, have been postulated.

Many drugs, infections, and environmental factors have been associated with the development of aplastic anemia. Some of these agents are directly toxic to the bone marrow and regularly produce marrow hypoplasia in a dose-dependent manner. Such obligate marrow suppressors include ionizing radiation, a variety of chemicals, and many antineoplastic agents.

Another group of drugs produces marrow hypoplasia in only a small proportion of patients who receive them, so that the disease is considered to represent an idiosyncratic reaction. These include a variety of antibiotics, anti-inflammatory agents, and anticonvulsants. Chloramphenicol has been the drug most frequently associated with aplastic anemia. It has been estimated that only about 1 of 20,000 to 50,000 persons taking chloramphenicol develops aplastic anemia, but in as many as 50% of the cases of drug-related aplastic anemia, chloramphenicol has been implicated. A particularly serious form of aplastic anemia occurs in the wake of viral hepatitis. In about half of these patients, no causative factor can be implicated, and their disease is designated idiopathic, although an environmental factor cannot be excluded.

#### Clinical Presentation

The signs and symptoms of aplastic anemia reflect the degree of pancytopenia at presentation. The most common initial manifestations are petechiae and bruising as a consequence of thrombocytopenia. Pallor and bacterial infections develop as anemia and neutropenia ensue. The spleen, liver, and lymph nodes are not enlarged.

#### Laboratory Findings

A variable degree of pancytopenia is found at diagnosis. Platelet counts are moderately to severely reduced (5000 to 50,000/mm$^3$). A moderate to severe, usually macrocytic anemia (Hb of 3 to 10 g/dL; mean corpuscular volume >90 fL) with low reticulocyte counts (<0.1%) and neutropenia (absolute neutrophil count <1500/mm$^3$) are observed at the time of diagnosis or develop within a few months.

Diagnosis is established by examination of the bone marrow by aspiration and biopsy. The marrow is hypocellular due to a loss of hematopoietic elements. Megakaryocytes are reduced, and fat is increased. Bone marrow cultures reveal a marked reduction of progenitor cells of erythroid, granulocytic, and megakaryocytic lines.

The disease is classified as severe if two of the following three peripheral blood value abnormalities occur in combination with severe hypocellularity of the marrow biopsy: neutrophil count of less than 950/mm$^3$, platelet count of less than 20,000/mm$^3$, and a corrected reticulocyte count of less than 1%.

#### Therapy

Anemia and thrombocytopenia may require transfusions of erythrocytes and platelets. These should be used sparingly to prevent isoimmunization that could compromise future bone marrow transplantation. If an HLA-compatible sibling is available, bone marrow transplantation is the preferred treatment. The survival rate after bone marrow transplantation for young, untransfused patients with aplastic anemia is between 85% and 95%. Because the patient is already aplastic, reduction in the conditioning before bone marrow transplantation has allowed most patients to avoid serious long-term side effects, including infertility. Clinical trials with various hematopoietic colony-stimulating factors have been unsuccessful. The use of HLA-incompatible marrow transplantation has been attempted with success in a few patients.

In patients who do not have an HLA-compatible sibling as a donor, various forms of immunosuppressive therapy have been employed, including injections of horse or sheep anti-thymocyte or anti-lymphocyte globulin, high-dose methylprednisone, and cyclophosphamide. Response rates as high as 50% to 60% have been reported. Androgens have been ineffective in severe aplastic anemia but may produce a degree of hematologic improvement in patients with moderate disease.

### Congenital Aplastic Anemia

Congenital aplastic anemia (CAA; Fanconi syndrome, constitutional aplastic anemia) was first described by Professor Fanconi in Switzerland in 1927. More than 600 cases have been reported in many ethnic groups. Although CAA is genetically determined and transmitted as an autosomal recessive disorder, it is not usually hematologically evident during infancy and early childhood. Clinical CAA is characterized by severe pancytopenia, hypoplasia of the bone marrow, and a constellation of physical abnormalities. Some patients do not have obvious physical anomalies.

#### Pathophysiology

CAA is believed to be caused by an ill-defined defect in DNA that renders the patient's cells susceptible to damage by environmental agents. This sensitivity may predispose the patient to bone marrow failure.

The cells of these patients demonstrate abnormal mitotic divisions in tissue culture. This is evident in phytohemagglutinin-stimulated lymphocyte cultures. Structural abnormalities include chromatid breaks, exchanges, and gaps and endoreduplication. These occur in more than 10% of metaphases. Other cell culture lines from these patients, including skin fibroblasts, show similar changes, and this has made prenatal diagnosis possible.

#### Clinical Presentation

Short stature and generalized hyperpigmentation affect most patients. About half of the patients with CAA have congenital skeletal anomalies. The most striking of these include bilateral absence or hypoplasia of the thumb, sometimes accompanied with abnormalities of the radii. About one third of patients have renal abnormalities, including unilateral aplasia and horseshoe kidney. About 50% of patients have no gross anatomic abnormalities.

The onset of progressive bone marrow failure is initially manifested by petechiae and ecchymosis secondary to thrombocytopenia between 2 and 22 years of age (mean age, 7). Anemia and neutropenia develop somewhat later than thrombocytopenia.

## Laboratory Findings

Disordered erythropoiesis is manifested by macrocytosis (mean corpuscular volume >90 fL) and elevated levels of Hb F before the onset of marrow failure. Ultimately, severe pancytopenia develops. Serial bone marrow examinations show progressive hypocellularity and ultimately frank aplasia. The peripheral blood lymphocytes, when cultured in the presence of diepoxybutane, an alkylating agent, consistently show chromosomal abnormalities. This is a useful test when the physical stigmata of Fanconi anemia are absent.

## Treatment

Supportive therapy, including transfusions of erythrocytes and platelets, offers only temporary benefit. In the past, about three quarters of these patients died within 2 years of the onset of marrow failure.

Therapy with pharmacologic doses of androgenic hormones produces a hematologic improvement in more than two thirds of patients. The response to these agents may be sustained for several years, but maintenance therapy is usually necessary. Complications of androgen therapy, including masculinization and liver dysfunction, are common. Ultimately, most patients become refractory to androgens and again require transfusions. Bone marrow transplantation using HLA-compatible siblings who do not themselves have CAA has been successful in many patients.

Long-term complications of the disease and its therapy include androgen-associated hepatic disease and tumors and an increased risk of acute myeloid leukemia and other malignancies.

## Selected Readings

### Congenital Hypoplastic Anemias

Alter BP. Childhood red cell aplasia. Am J Pediatr Hematol Oncol 1980;2:121.
Glader BE, Backer K. Elevated erythrocyte adenosine deaminase activity in congenital hypoplastic anemia. N Engl J Med 1986;309:1486.
Nathan DG, Clark BJ. Erythroid precursors in congenital hypoplastic (Diamond-Blackfan) anemia. J Clin Invest 1978;61:489.

### Transient Erythroblastic Anemia of Childhood

Wang NC, Mentzer NC. Differentiation of transient erythroblastopenia of childhood from a congenital hypoplastic anemia. J Pediatr 1976;88:784.
Wranne L. Transient erythroblastopenia in infancy and childhood. Scand J Haematol 1970;7:76.

### Parvovirus: Induced Aplastic Crisis Complicating Hemolytic Anemias

Brow T, Anan H. Intrauterine parvovirus infections associated with hydrops fetalis. Lancet 1984;2:1033.
Serjeant GR, Topley JM. Outbreak of aplastic crises in sickle cell anemia associated with parvovirus-like agent. Lancet 1981;2:595.

### Aplastic Anemia

Camita BM, Stork R, Thomas ED. Acquired aplastic anemia. N Engl J Med 1982;306:645.

### Congenital Aplastic Anemia

Alter AP. The bone marrow failure syndromes. In: Nathan DG, Oski FA, eds. The hematology of infancy and childhood. Philadelphia: WB Saunders, 1987:159.
Auerback AD, Adler B, Chaganti RSK. Prenatal and postnatal diagnosis and carrier detection of Fanconi anemia by a cytogenetic method. Pediatrics 1981;67:128.
Halperin DS, Grisaru D, Freedman MH, Saunders EF. Severe acquired aplastic anemia in children: 11-year experience with bone marrow transplantation and immunosuppressive therapy. Am J Pediatr Hematol Oncol 1989;11:304.
Sanders JE, Whitehead J, Storb R, et al. Bone marrow transplantation experience for children with aplastic anemia. Pediatrics 1986;77:179.

*Principles and Practice of Pediatrics, Second Edition.*
edited by Frank A. Oski et al. J. B. Lippincott Company, Philadelphia © 1994.

# CHAPTER 91
# *Polycythemia*

## C. Philip Steuber

Polycythemia is an excess of erythrocytes in relation to blood volume (ie, erythrocytosis). Absolute definitions of polycythemia in pediatrics vary with age, as do blood volumes and hemoglobin levels. Hemoglobin and hematocrit values greater than two standard deviations above normal should be considered polycythemia. At any age, if the hematocrit exceeds 60%, the person should be evaluated for polycythemia and its complications.

Traditionally, polycythemic patients are grouped into those with an absolute increase in erythrocytes (ie, primary or secondary polycythemia) and those whose hemoglobin or hematocrit values are elevated but who have a normal erythrocyte mass and decreased plasma volume (ie, relative or spurious polycythemia).

## POLYCYTHEMIA VERA

Primary polycythemia (ie, polycythemia vera) is a hematologic stem cell disorder of clonal origin. It is rare in the pediatric population, and fewer than 20 true cases have been described in the literature. A malignant myeloproliferative disorder, it is characterized by a primary increase in erythrocyte mass. Common presenting complaints include itching, headache, weakness, and dizziness. Patients appear plethoric and often have elevated blood pressures. Enlargement of the spleen and liver is common. Patients are at risk for thrombosis and hemorrhage. In addition to increased hemoglobin and hematocrit values, peripheral blood findings include moderate thrombocytosis and leukocytosis. Bone marrow specimens are usually hypercellular with increased megakaryocytes. Erythropoietin levels are normal or low and do not rise in response to phlebotomy. A normal hemoglobin dissociation curve is often important for the diagnosis in children. A variety of nonrandom cytogenetic abnormalities have been detected in a few patients at diagnosis.

Therapy is directed toward reduction of the erythrocyte mass through phlebotomy, the administration of radioactive phosphorus, or the use of alkylating agents. Phlebotomy to reduce the hematocrit to 45% is probably the initial approach for pediatric patients, unless there are complicating factors contributing to hyperviscosity and vaso-occlusive events. With chronic phlebotomy, attention should be directed at maintaining adequate iron stores. Acute myeloid leukemia may develop during the patient's course, and its incidence may be increased by therapy with alkylating agents.

## SECONDARY POLYCYTHEMIA

In secondary polycythemia, the increase in erythrocyte mass is in response to increased erythropoietin production. Leukocytosis and thrombocytosis do not occur. The increased erythropoietin production may be physiologically appropriate or inappropriate. Table 91-1 lists conditions associated with secondary polycythemia.

Appropriate or compensatory increases in erythrocyte mass are seen in conditions that cause tissue hypoxia and are most often associated with cardiac or pulmonary abnormalities. Diminished delivery or release of oxygen to the tissues by defective erythrocytes may also account for cases of secondary polycythemia. Inappropriate secretion of erythropoietin is not associated with tissue hypoxia and has been related to a variety of benign and malignant tumors, renal abnormalities, and endocrine imbalances due to exogenous or endogenous excesses of various hormones. The remaining category of familial polycythemias is becoming better defined with the recognition of high-oxygen-affinity hemoglobins and erythrocyte enzyme deficiencies.

The physical examination of patients with secondary polycythemia reveals a ruddy complexion, some conjunctival suffusion, and sporadic optic vein engorgement. Enlargement of the liver and spleen is not a common feature, except in some patients with congestive heart failure or tumor.

After the elimination of easily recognizable causes, the evaluation of the child with polycythemia should include measurement of the erythrocyte mass, arterial oxygen pressure ($PO_2$), determination of the oxygen pressure at which the hemoglobin is 50% saturated ($P_{50}$), serum and urine erythropoietin levels, and a radiologic assessment of the genitourinary tract. If the erythrocyte mass is elevated for the patient's age, a reduced $PO_2$ reading should prompt a search for causes of hypoxemia. If the $P_{50}$ is decreased, the patient has a high oxygen affinity hemoglobinopathy. By definition, patients with secondary polycythemia have elevated erythropoietin levels.

Because renal abnormalities are a common cause of increased erythropoietin production, anatomical investigation is warranted early in the evaluation using intravenous pyelography or computed tomography.

Treatment of secondary polycythemia is directed at elimination or correction of the primary or underlying cause. When this is not possible, prevention of vaso-occlusive episodes may be accomplished by periodic phlebotomy designed to keep the hematocrit below 60%. Iron deficiency is a complication of chronic phlebotomy and should be prevented or treated.

## RELATIVE POLYCYTHEMIA

Relative polycythemia is a term applied to conditions with elevated hemoglobin and hematocrit values but a normal erythrocyte mass. The apparent or spurious polycythemia is a result of diminished plasma volume. In pediatrics, this loss of fluid (ie, hemoconcentration) could be associated with decreased fluid intake or increased fluid loss, such as in dehydration secondary to diarrhea or extensive burns. Appropriate fluid and colloid replacement return the erythrocyte values to normal.

*Principles and Practice of Pediatrics, Second Edition.* edited by Frank A. Oski et al. J. B. Lippincott Company, Philadelphia © 1994.

## CHAPTER 92
# *Quantitative Granulocyte Disorders*

### Donald H. Mahoney, Jr.

## NEUTROPENIAS

Neutropenia is defined as an absolute decrease in the number of circulatory neutrophils in the blood. The age and race of the child are important factors for the stratification of normal values. In the normal newborn, the neutrophil comprises approximately 60% of the differential count. However, by 2 weeks of age, lymphocytes assume predominance and retain this until approximately 4 years of age. For normal Caucasian infants between 2 weeks and 1 year of age, the lower limit of normal for the absolute neutrophil count (ANC) including neutrophils and bands is 1000 cells/mm³. After infancy, an ANC of 1500 cells/mm³ is the lower limit. For black children, the lower limits of normal are 100 to 200 cells/mm³ less than those for Caucasian children. Technical factors such as excessive leukocyte clumping or lengthy delays in performance of leukocyte counts may cause false low values.

### Classification

The classification of the neutropenias on a pathophysiologic basis has been problematic. Kinetic, biochemical, and functional studies are difficult to perform because of an insufficiency of circulating neutrophils. Most neutropenia states are transient, and some discretion in the choice of investigations is indicated. Chronic neutropenic syndromes are rare and are largely characterized on the basis of their clinical features.

As a first step, individual cases may be characterized by the severity of neutropenia. Mild neutropenia may be defined as an ANC of 1000 to 1500 cells/mm³, moderate neutropenia as an

---

**TABLE 91-1.   Causes of Secondary Polycythemia**

A. Appropriate erythropoietin response
1. Pulmonary disease
2. Congenital heart disease with right-to-left shunt
3. Hemoglobins with increased oxygen affinity
4. Reduced erythrocyte 2,3-DPG levels
5. Pickwickian syndrome
6. High altitude residence
B. Inappropriate erythropoietin production
1. Tumors
   a. Kidney
   b. Liver
   c. Adrenal gland
   d. Cerebellum
   e. Uterus
   f. Ovary
2. Other renal problems
   a. Cysts
   b. Obstructive uropathy
   c. Bartter's syndrome
   d. After renal transplantation
3. Primary or secondary endocrine imbalance
   a. Excess adrenocorticoids
   b. Excess androgens
   c. Growth hormone therapy
C. Familial polycythemias

ANC of 500 to 1000 cells/mm³, and severe neutropenia as an ANC value of less than 500 cells/mm³. This is a functional classification based on a recognized susceptibility for life-threatening infections, especially in children with persistent, severe neutropenia. For the neutropenic child, infection with *Staphylococcus* or with a gram-negative enteric organism is the greatest danger. However, any organism may become a pathogen. Stomatitis, gingivitis, perirectal inflammation, recurrent otitis media, cellulitis, pneumonia, and septicemia are potential clinical complications. On the other hand, these patients do not have an increased susceptibility to viral or parasitic infections.

As a second step, patients should be initially evaluated for evidence of other hematologic disturbances. The presence of anemia or thrombocytopenia at the outset of the patient's illness should motivate the clinician to consider a broader differential diagnosis. For example, the symptomatic, febrile child, especially with evidence of anemia, hepatosplenomegaly, leukopenia, or abnormal leukocyte forms, may require an immediate bone marrow examination to exclude an infiltrative lymphoproliferative process before a more exhaustive systematic investigation for a cause of neutropenia is pursued.

Using a functional classification scheme, neutropenia of childhood may be categorized as disorders of proliferation of committed stem cells; disorders of proliferation of committed myeloid stem cells; disorders associated with immune dysfunctions, metabolic disturbance, and phenotypic abnormalities; or disorders of neutrophil survival.

## Disorders of Proliferation of Committed Stem Cells

*Reticular dysgenesis* appears to be a defect of the committed stem cell compartment and is characterized by thymic agenesis, severe neutropenia and lymphopenia, and agammaglobulinemia. Infants early in life are vulnerable to fatal bacterial and viral infections.

*Cyclic neutropenia* is a rare disorder characterized by regular, periodic oscillations in the numbers of circulatory neutrophils and is associated with cyclic clinical manifestations. A defect in regulatory mechanisms at the stem cell has been suggested by studies of the gray collie dog, which provides a model for this disease. Transfer of bone marrow from normal dogs to affected animals abolishes the blood count fluctuations.

Cyclic oscillations in the rate of bone marrow production results in neutropenia nadirs at intervals of 19 to 21 days. The specific periodicity is regular and constant for each patient and may be as short as 14 days or as long as 28 to 36 days. A 21-day cycle has been observed in more than 70% of the patients. The neutropenia may persist for 3 to 10 days and then be followed by rising neutrophil counts and normal physical findings. Oscillations of monocytes, platelets, and reticulocytes may also occur, although these elements fluctuate between normal and elevated levels. During the neutropenic phase, patients may suffer with fever, malaise, oral ulcers, stomatitis, pharyngitis, and lymphadenopathy. More serious infections such as mastoiditis, pneumonia, and sepsis have occurred, and an estimated 10% of the patients have died of the complications of infectious diseases.

The diagnosis is established by serial neutrophil counts obtained over a 6- to 8-week period to establish the periodicity. Bone marrow examinations during periods of neutropenia may show granulocytic hypoplasia or an apparent arrest of maturation. Treatment is symptomatic. Androgens, corticosteroids, and lithium have not been consistently successful. Recombinant human granulocyte colony-stimulating factor (G-CSF) produces marked benefits for patients by reducing the duration of neutropenia and substantially decreasing the risk for infection.

## Disorders of Committed Myeloid Stem Cells

*Severe congenital neutropenia* (ie, infantile genetic agranulocytosis of Kostmann) is a rare autosomal recessive disorder, characterized

by a failure of terminal differentiation of the myeloid precursor. The ANC is usually less than 300 cells/mm³. Monocytosis is prominent, and serum immunoglobulins are normal or elevated. The bone marrow morphology reveals a developmental arrest at the promyelocyte or myelocyte stage. Studies of bone marrow in vitro colony-forming units (CFU) reveal a capacity to produce neutrophilic colonies, but with aberrant cells exhibiting bizarre nuclei, excessive cytoplasm, and decreased granules. Monocyte and eosinophilic colonies appear normal.

The clinical presentation is usually one of an acute, life-threatening infection occurring within the first few months of life. Fever, cellulitis, omphalitis, pneumonia, perianal and urinary tract infections, and sepsis have been associated with this disease. Common pathogens include *S aureus, Escherichia coli,* and *Pseudomonas.* Recombinant human G-CSF is effective treatment, leading to increased numbers of neutrophils and decreased infectious complications. Bone marrow transplantation has resulted in partial or complete correction of this disorder. Leukemic transformation has been reported, although the relative risk for this complication is unknown.

*Familial benign chronic neutropenia* is an autosomal dominant disorder characterized by mild to moderate degrees of neutropenia and minimal symptoms. This disorder has been observed in successive generations of Yemenite Jews and in families from Germany, France, the United States, and South Africa. Abnormalities of committed stem cell precursors and reduced marrow neutrophilic reserves have been observed. The illness is benign, and treatment is usually not indicated. A severe form of this disease has been described and has been associated with more severe infections, a more pronounced neutropenia, and bone marrow evidence of depletion of mature granulocyte forms.

*Chronic neutropenia of childhood* is a nonfamilial disorder of variable clinical and laboratory presentation. The total leukocyte count is usually normal. However, the neutrophil numbers fluctuate between fewer than 500 cells/mm³ and 1000 cells/mm³. The risk of infection is proportional to the degree of neutropenia. Bone marrow morphology usually reveals an adequate number of myeloid precursors associated with an apparent arrest at the metamyelocyte or band stage. Studies of bone marrow in vitro CFU have yielded results of normal, decreased, and increased numbers of colonies containing neutrophils. Evidence suggests that the proliferative capacity of the marrow is limited and that rates of maturation may be disordered. These regulatory abnormalities vary among patients.

In the mild form of disease, a neutrophilic response is usually observed in the peripheral blood during the course of infection or in response to an endotoxin challenge. This bone marrow response can be mimicked by the steroid mobilization test. Children with the mild form generally do not experience serious complications with infection. Spontaneous remissions have been reported to occur in children 2 to 4 years after presentation.

Several clinical syndromes have evidence of ineffective granulopoiesis as a common pathophysiologic characteristic. Nutritional deficiencies of vitamin B$_{12}$ or folic acid, in addition to causing megaloblastic anemia, may be associated with neutropenia. Advanced states of malnutrition, such as anorexia nervosa, marasmus in infants, and copper deficiency may be complicated by neutropenia. Ineffective myelopoiesis is an important element in the Chédiak-Higashi syndrome and in a rare condition described as myelokathexis. Increased intramedullary destruction of neutrophils with elevated serum lysozyme levels are part of the clinical spectrum.

Many acquired conditions may be associated with periods of neutropenia (Table 92-1). Infectious diseases are the most common cause of neutropenia in children. The mechanisms responsible for neutropenia include direct marrow suppression, exhaustion of marrow reserves, redistribution of neutrophils from

## TABLE 92-1. Frequently Recognized Causes of Acquired Neutropenia

I. Infection
   A. Viral: Hepatitis A & B, varicella, influenza A, measles, rubella, HSV, RSV, CMV, IM, HIV, and parvovirus
   B. Bacterial: overwhelming sepsis, especially group B streptococci, typhoid, paratyphoid, tularemia, brucellosis, tuberculosis
   C. Rickettsial: rickettsialpox, epidemic typhus, scrub typhus, Rocky Mountain spotted fever
   D. Protozoan: malaria, toxoplasmosis
II. Drugs
   A. Antibiotics: penicillins, aminoglycosides, sulfa, trimethoprim-sulfamethoxazole, cephalosporins, amphotericin, dapsone, griseofulvin, streptomycin, nitrofurantoins, chloroquine
   B. Anticonvulsants: trimethadione, phenytoin, barbiturates, valproic acid, clonazepam, carbamazepine, ethosuximide
   C. Antiinflammatory agents: gold, indomethacin, phenylbutazone, ibuprofen, naproxen, aspirin, penicillamine
   D. Miscellaneous: imipramine, thiazides, acetazolamide, quinidine, procaine amide, propranolol, antithyroid agents, phenothiazines
III. Chemical or environmental toxins
   Benzol, benzene, arsenic, thiocyanate, carbon tetrachloride, insecticides (eg, DDT, chlordane)
   Inadvertent radiation exposure
IV. Anticancer chemotherapy
V. Bone marrow infiltration
   Leukemia, lymphoma, neuroblastoma, rhabdomyosarcoma, retinoblastoma, PNET, myelofibrosis, storage disease

*HSV*, herpes simplex virus; *RSV*, respiratory syncytial virus; *CMV*, cytomegalovirus; *IM*, infectious mononucleosis; *HIV*, human immunodeficiency virus; *PNET*, primitive neuroectodermal tumor.

circulating to marginating pools, and neutrophil aggregation and sequestration after complement activation. Increased destruction of neutrophils may occur as a direct result of interactions with pathogens or indirectly as the result of the formation of antineutrophil antibodies. Overwhelming bacterial sepsis, especially in the neonate, may directly affect the marrow pool. Depletion of precursor and neutrophil pools and degenerative changes in myelopoiesis may occur. Several investigators have suggested that granulocyte transfusions in the face of overwhelming bacterial sepsis and profound neutropenia may be lifesaving.

Drug-induced neutropenias are probably the second most common cause of acquired neutropenia in childhood. Mechanisms of action include direct toxic effects of drugs or metabolites on the bone marrow or the committed stem cells. Induction of an immune response directed at neutrophils has also been implicated.

To list all medications with a potential for producing neutropenia would be an exhaustive exercise. The physician should refer to the product information supplied by the pharmaceutical company when evaluating a neutropenic patient receiving a medication. Idiosyncratic reactions are uncommon but can produce severe neutropenia (ANC <500 cells/mm³). More commonly, neutropenia may follow extended dosing periods and may be aggravated by underlying genetic or metabolic factors. Certain drugs are conspicuous for their frequency of use and are more commonly associated with episodes of neutropenia. These include antimicrobials, particularly the penicillins, trimethoprim-sulfamethoxazole, and certain classes of cephalosporins; anticonvulsants, such as barbiturates, phenytoin, valproic acid, carbamazepine, clonazepam, and ethosuximide; antipyretics such as aspirin; and antirheumatic agents. Certain drugs may act in combination to produce myelosuppression. The onset of drug-induced

neutropenia is unpredictable, but after neutropenia occurs, the most important therapeutic action is to withdraw all drugs that are not essential, especially those with a significant risk for myelosuppression.

### Disorders Associated With Immune Dysfunctions, Metabolic Disturbances, and Phenotypic Abnormalities

*Cartilage–hair hypoplasia* is an autosomal recessive condition associated with short-limbed dwarfism, fine hair, and moderate neutropenia. This condition has been identified frequently in Asian populations. Increased infections and impaired immunologic functions are common complications.

*Dyskeratosis congenita* is an X-linked recessive disease characterized by hyperpigmentation, leukoplakia, nail dystrophy, and in approximately 35% of the cases, mild neutropenia.

Disorders of immunoglobulin production have been associated with neutropenia syndromes. Patients with X-linked agammaglobulinemia may experience neutropenia during the course of their illness. Dysgammaglobulinemia type I (ie, no IgA and IgG, normal to elevated IgM) may be associated with periodic or persistent neutropenia. Bacterial infections, failure to thrive, and hepatosplenomegaly may complicate this condition. A syndrome of neutropenia, eczema, polyarthralgias, eosinophilia, and increased IgA levels has been reported. Depressed cellular immunity and an increased risk for infection, including devastating varicella, has been observed with this disease.

Neutropenia may complicate a number of metabolic disorders. Children with hyperglycinemia, isovaleric acidemia, and methylmalonic acidemia may have significant neutropenia. High concentrations of these metabolites have been proposed as the causative mechanism for impaired myeloid proliferation. Myelofibrosis may be associated with Gaucher's disease. Glycogenesis Ib is an inherited disorder of glycogen metabolism associated with variable neutropenia, abnormal neutrophil motility, and recurrent life-threatening infections. Supportive medical care is the only available therapy for these patients.

### Disorders Associated With Decreased Neutrophil Survival

Infections, particularly viral infections, are the most common cause of transient neutropenia in childhood. Enterovirus infections, respiratory syncytial virus, influenza A, measles, rubella, varicella, hepatitis A and B, and the Epstein-Barr virus are a few of the more common causes of transient neutropenia. The accelerated destruction of neutrophils may cause neutropenia. This may be mediated through the generation of antineutrophil antibodies.

The two classic descriptions for immune neutropenia in childhood are the isoimmune and the autoimmune neutropenias. *Isoimmune neutropenia* is observed in the neonate and is analogous to Rh sensitization. During gestation, fetal neutrophil antigens, most frequently NA1 and NB1, immunize the mother, resulting in an IgG antibody, which crosses the placenta and destroys the infant's neutrophils. At birth, severe neutropenia, monocytosis, and occasionally eosinophilia are observed. Although usually asymptomatic, infants may suffer from cutaneous infections or more serious complications such as sepsis. By 6 to 7 weeks, the neutrophil counts have usually returned to normal. Treatment varies according to symptoms. There have been some responses to high doses of intravenous γ-globulin.

*Autoimmune neutropenia* is a disorder more frequently observed in the 6- to 24-month-old child and may frequently be confused with idiopathic chronic neutropenia. Antibodies of IgG, IgM, or IgA class directed against specific neutrophil antigens (eg, NA1, NA2, NB1), can be detected by direct or indirect immunofluorescent assays in most patients and are proposed as causes of immunomediated destruction of circulatory neutrophils. Patients may generate these autoantibodies for no apparent reason or in response to certain infections (eg, mononucleosis), drugs (eg, penicillins), or in association with certain inflammatory diseases (eg, rheumatoid arthritis, systemic lupus erythematosus, chronic active hepatitis). Treatment is primarily supportive care. Corticosteroids and high-dose intravenous $\gamma$-globulin have been of value in selected cases. Most children with autoimmune neutropenia require no intervention and recover without specific therapy.

## Evaluation

A complete history and physical examination is an essential first step in the evaluation of a child presenting with neutropenia. The history should include a summary of the recent infections, medications, and possible toxic exposures for the child; race and ethnic background, including phenotypic abnormalities; and family medical history for any member with recurrent infections or unexplained deaths in infants younger than 1 year of age. The physical examination should include an assessment of nutritional status and a search for signs of skin or mucous membrane infections, lymphadenopathy, and hepatosplenomegaly. Evaluation for skeletal or cutaneous phenotypic abnormalities is important. The initial laboratory examination should include a complete blood count, with platelets and reticulocytes, to exclude other stem line defects.

In the acutely ill child with fever and severe neutropenia (ANC <500 cells/mm$^3$), a bone marrow aspirate and biopsy may aid in the diagnosis by establishing the extent of marrow neutrophil reserves and by excluding the possibility of a malignant infiltrative process. In the asymptomatic patient, a bone marrow examination may be pursued at a later date and should include electron microscopic, cytogenetic, and in vitro clonogenic analysis.

Patients with a suspected chronic neutropenia should have a leukocyte count obtained at twice-weekly intervals for 6 weeks to determine the periodicity. Further evaluation beyond this point should be dictated by the clinical impression. In infants, quantitative immunoglobulins, T- and B-cell functions, cortisone stimulation tests, and specific antineutrophil antibody assays may help in differentiating the more common causes of chronic neutropenia. In the older child, evaluations for collagen-vascular disorders and folate, vitamin B$_{12}$, copper, and metabolic deficiency states are appropriate.

## Treatment

The management of children with neutropenia must be linked to the presumed diagnosis. Children with fever (with or without specific presenting signs of infection) and with acute-onset (ie, primary) neutropenia of unknown cause or associated with the diagnosis or treatment of a malignant condition require immediate medical attention. In these circumstances, there is a substantial risk of acute, overwhelming, bacterial sepsis. Hospitalization, cultures of blood, urine, and respiratory secretions, and prompt initiation of broad-spectrum intravenous antibiotics are indicated. If cultures fail to yield a pathogen and clinical investigations fail to document evidence of bacterial infection, antibiotics may be discontinued 3 days after the patient has become afebrile.

For the child with mild chronic neutropenia, management recommendations are less clear. The asymptomatic patient requires no specific medical intervention. Good oral hygiene and skin care are important preventive measures. For a child with sustained fever greater than 101 °F or chills or both, it is our usual practice to examine the child for signs of infection, repeat the leukocyte count, and if the ANC value is less than 500 cells/mm$^3$, hospitalize the child and treat with broad-spectrum intravenous antibiotics pending analysis of appropriate cultures. For

the patient with an ANC of 500 to 1000 cells/mm$^3$, clinical discretion must be exercised.

Symptomatic patients with severe chronic neutropenia may benefit from a trial of recombinant human G-CSF. Prophylactic trimethoprim-sulfamethoxazole schedules may be of some value in patients with severe congenital neutropenia or in patients undergoing cancer chemotherapy.

## NEUTROPHILIA

Neutrophilia may result from an increased mobilization of neutrophils from marrow storage compartments or marginating pools, from impaired egress of neutrophils into tissue, or from accelerated proliferation of myeloid progenitor cells.

Increased mobilization of neutrophils from marrow compartments may follow acute stress events, such as acute infection, anesthesia, electrical shock, abrupt temperature changes, hypoxia, or endotoxin exposure. Endogenous release of epinephrine and glucocorticoids under stress conditions mediates the release of neutrophils from storage sites. The administration of pharmacologic doses of glucocorticoids mimic this state.

Increased granulopoiesis and neutrophilia are most frequently the result of acute infections, especially by pyogenic organisms. Profound neutrophilia with a "shift to the left" involving immature myeloid cells (ie, a leukemoid reaction) may occur with infections and with other conditions (Table 92-2).

## EOSINOPHILIA

Eosinophilia is usually defined as an absolute eosinophil count in excess of 500 cells/mm$^3$. Allergy is the most common cause of eosinophilia in children in the United States. Children with bronchial asthma, recurrent urticaria, infantile eczema, serum sickness, and angioneurotic edema often have evidence of eosinophilia. However, symptoms do not directly correlate with the

---

**TABLE 92-2. Disorders Associated With Leukemoid Reactions**

| Infections | Drugs |
|---|---|
| Pyogenic bacteria | Lithium |
| Tuberculosis | Glucocorticoids |
| Brucellosis | |
| Toxoplasmosis | **Others** |
| Leptospirosis | Acute glomerulonephritis |
| Viral (acute phase): herpes simplex, varicella, rabies, poliomyelitis, mononucleosis | Acute liver failure |
| | Functional asplenia |
| | Diabetic acidosis |
| Kawasaki disease | Disorders of neutrophil motility (LFA-1 deficiency) |
| **Chronic Inflammatory Conditions** | Transient myeloprofilerative syndrome in neonatal Down syndrome |
| Rheumatoid arthritis | |
| Polyserositis | |
| **Tumor Invasion** | |
| Lymphoma | |
| Rhabdomyosarcoma | |
| Neuroblastoma | |
| Retinoblastoma | |

degree of eosinophilia. Children with allergic rhinitis have eosinophils in their nasal secretions.

Eosinophilia may be associated with chronic inflammatory diseases of the bowel, including Crohn's disease; tumors such as Hodgkin's disease; and immune deficiency syndromes, especially Wiskott-Aldrich syndrome.

Parasitic infections are the most common cause of eosinophilia outside of the United States. Careful examination of freshly collected feces for evidence of ova or larval forms confirms the diagnosis in most cases. Visceral larva migrans, secondary to *Toxocara canis* or *T cati*, is probably the most common cause for hypereosinophilic syndromes in children. Patients are usually asymptomatic, but some may have fever, occasional wheezing, hepatomegaly, anemia, and hyperglobulinemia. Retinal lesions may be indistinguishable from retinoblastoma lesions. A leukemoid reaction with counts of 100,000 cells/mm$^3$ and 80% to 90% mature eosinophils may occur. The diagnosis cannot be established from stool analysis. Increased isohemagglutinins directed against group A and B substances on erythrocytes and specific serologic tests are necessary to confirm the diagnosis. Specific treatment is usually not needed.

Numerous conditions that may also produce transient eosinophilia are outlined in Table 92-3.

## MONOCYTOSIS AND BASOPHILIA

Monocytosis is an unusual finding in children. Absolute monocyte numbers in normal persons range from 300 to 800 cells/mm$^3$. Infection with intracellular microorganisms or parasites is the most common cause of monocytosis. Infections include malaria, trypanosomiasis, leishmaniasis, rickettsial disease, and *Listeria monocytogenes.* Persistent monocytosis with abnormal forms may precede a variety of lymphoproliferative and histiocytic disorders, such as Hodgkin's disease and acute myelomonocytic leukemia. Monocytosis is frequently associated with granulocytopenic states.

Basophils constitute 0.5% to 1% of the circulatory leukocyte pool. Basophilia is common in myeloproliferative disorders, particularly in chronic myelogenous leukemia. Mild basophilia may also be associated with certain chronic inflammatory diseases, such as ulcerative colitis and rheumatoid arthritis, and with tuberculosis, influenza, and varicella infections.

## Selected Readings

Box LA, Hutchinson R, Emerson S. Recombinant human granulocyte colony-stimulating factor in the treatment of patients with neutropenia. Clin Immunol Immunother 1992;62:539.

Cartron J, Tchernia G, Celton JL, et al. Alloimmune neonatal neutropenia. Am J Pediatr Hematol Oncol 1991;13:21.

Conway LT, Clay ME, Kline WE, et al. Natural history of primary autoimmune neutropenia in infancy. Pediatrics 1987;79:728.

deAlarcon PA, Goldberg J, Nelson DA, et al. Chronic neutropenia: diagnostic approach and prognosis. Am J Pediatr Hematol Oncol 1983;5:3.

Weetman RM, Boxer LA. Childhood neutropenia. Pediatr Clin North Am 1980;27:361.

*Principles and Practice of Pediatrics, Second Edition.*
edited by Frank A. Oski et al. J. B. Lippincott Company, Philadelphia © 1994.

## CHAPTER 93
# *The Spleen and Lymph Nodes*

Richard H. Sills

The spleen and lymph nodes are the major components of the mononuclear-phagocyte system (MPS), which serves as a filter, delivers antigens to the immune system, and removes damaged cells and particulate matter. Originally called the reticuloendothelial system, the MPS consists of fixed phagocytic cells in different organs: macrophages in lymph nodes and the spleen, Kupffer cells in the liver, and histiocytes in connective tissue. These cells all share a common derivation from circulating blood monocytes. Functionally, these phagocytes interact locally with lymphocytes and play an essential role in the recognition and interaction of immunocompetent cells with antigens. The MPS constitutes a crucial component of our immunologic defense mechanisms.

The minimal criteria for inclusion of cells in the MPS are derivation from bone marrow precursors, morphologic characteristics that are common to circulating monocytes and macrophages, and a high level of phagocytic activity mediated by immunoglobulin and complement. Polymorphonuclear neutrophils are excluded from the MPS, although they share many common characteristics, because they do not persist in tissues as do macrophages.

Although components of the MPS occur in most tissues, they are particularly dense in the spleen and lymph nodes. The specialized filtering capabilities of these organs provide ideal locations for contact between antigens and the immune system. Macrophages perching on endothelial cells and reticulum fibers assume the role of immunologic sentries, which are vital in instituting host response.

---

### TABLE 92-3.   Causes of Eosinophilia in Children

**Allergic Disorders**
Asthma, atopic eczema, urticaria, hay fever, drug reactions

**Infections**
Parasitic infections: *Ascaris,* trichinosis, *Echinococcus,* hookworm, *Strongyloides,* filariasis, *Toxocara, Pneumocystis carinii,* malaria, amebiasis
Nonparasitic infections: scarlet fever, tuberculosis, histoplasmosis

**Skin Disorders**
Pemphigus, toxic epidermal neurolysis

**Tumors**
Hodgkin's disease, myeloproliferative syndromes

**Hereditary**
Idiopathic hyper-eosinophilic syndrome

**Miscellaneous Disorders Characterized by Chronic Inflammation**
Chronic hepatitis, regional enteritis, rheumatoid arthritis, periarteritis nodosa, peritoneal dialysis

# SPLEEN

## Anatomy

The spleen is the largest lymph node in the body and contains a rich supply of mononuclear-phagocyte tissue. The supporting structure of the spleen is an external smooth muscle capsule with internal trabeculae that support the major splenic blood vessels. The splenic tissue consists of red and white pulp lying within this support structure. The white pulp contains grossly visible cylindrical or punctate collections of lymphocytes, plasma cells, and macrophages, which are surrounded by red pulp. The red pulp includes splenic sinuses filled with circulating blood which are separated by cylindrical partitions called splenic cords (Fig 93-1).

The splenic artery enters the spleen at the hilum and branches along the trabeculae. Within the white pulp, the arterioles acquire a dense sheath of predominately helper T lymphocytes. Adjacent to these periarteriolar sheaths is a follicular zone of predominately B lymphocytes containing germinal centers made up of B cells and macrophages. The central arterioles supplying these areas tend to branch off at right angles; this anatomical arrangement results in the skimming off of plasma into the white pulp, where antigen processing occurs. The main terminal splenic arteries, which contain hemoconcentrated blood, continue directly forward into the contiguous red pulp.

The red pulp, which constitutes the largest portion of the organ, consists of splenic cords that interdigitate between splenic venous sinusoids. At least 90% of the hemoconcentrated blood

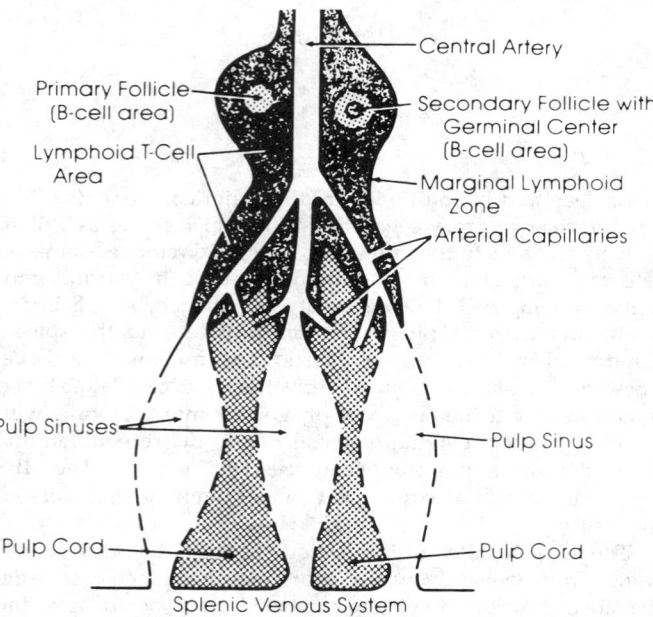

**Figure 93-1.** The spleen is composed of multiple units of red and white pulp around small branches of the splenic artery called central arteries. The white pulp areas of the spleen are lymphoid. Within the white pulp, B cells primarily occupy the follicular zones, and T cells predominate around the follicles and the arterial capillaries. Antigenic stimulation causes primary follicles to become secondary follicles with germinal centers. Most of the circulation to the red pulp enters the pulp cords and reaches the pulp sinuses through the basement membrane fenestrations. (Modified from Hayes B. Enlargement of lymph nodes and spleen. In: Braunwald E, Isselbacher KJ, Petersdorf RG, et al, eds. Harrison's principles of internal medicine. New York: McGraw-Hill, 1987: 276.)

reaching the red pulp enters these splenic cords, which contain a fibrous network of mononuclear-phagocyte tissue. The circulation in the cords is designated as "open" because there is no well-defined endothelial lining. The cords lie between and share a basement membrane with the adjacent splenic venous sinuses. To exit the cords, blood must pass through 1- to 5-$\mu$m slits in this fenestrated basement membrane to reach the sinuses. The circulation through the cords is slow and congested because the blood reaching the red pulp is hemoconcentrated enough to increase its viscosity and because erythrocytes require additional time to pass through the small and limited number of slits that must be traversed to reach the sinuses. This delay provides prolonged exposure of blood cells, bacteria, and particulate matter to the dense mononuclear-phagocyte elements within the red pulp.

After blood reaches the sinuses, it passes into the splenic venous system. Only 10% of the circulation of the red pulp goes directly into the sinuses through a "closed" endothelial-lined channel, bypassing the cords. Blood from the sinuses enters trabecular veins and eventually the hepatic portal vein; there are no valves in this system, which remains at the same pressure as the hepatic portal vein.

## Physiology

The spleen is a large mass of phagocytic and lymphocytic tissue in unique contact with circulating blood. Although none of its individual cells are unique, this distinctive anatomical arrangement provides it with characteristic functional capabilities.

### Resistance to Infection

The spleen provides two important functions of host defense: generation of humoral or cellular responses to intravenous foreign antigens and clearance of circulating microorganisms and other intravenous antigens.

Although the spleen plays a minor role in the formation of antibody to antigens delivered by the subcutaneous or intramuscular routes, it has a major role in the processing of small doses of particulate antigens delivered intravenously. Splenic macrophages efficiently ingest these intravenous antigens and deliver them to the immunocompetent cells of the spleen for antibody production.

The MPS is crucial to the clearance of circulating bacteria. The liver is efficient at removing any bacteria coated with antibody. In the absence of antibody, nonencapsulated bacteria can be effectively removed in MPS tissues other than the spleen. However, the amorphous polysaccharide coat of encapsulated organisms (eg, *Streptococcus pneumoniae* or *Haemophilus influenzae*) greatly impairs bacterial clearance in the absence of antibody. The only effective defense mechanism for the nonimmune host infected with circulating encapsulated bacteria is the spleen, whose highly efficient phagocytic cords are capable of phagocytizing encapsulated bacteria in the absence of antibody. The splenic white pulp processes these intravenous antigens to produce antibody that during subsequent exposures allows for efficient clearance by the remainder of the MPS.

### Filtering of Formed Elements of Blood

Erythrocytes passing through the spleen must endure a slow passage through the hypoxic and acidotic environment of the cords and then squeeze through narrow slits into the sinusoids. Although healthy erythrocytes readily accomplish this, aged and abnormal erythrocytes cannot. They remain behind to be ingested by the macrophages lining the cords. Most aging erythrocytes normally are cleared by the spleen, but in its absence, MPS tissue in the marrow and liver readily accomplish this role. Abnormal cells, such as spherocytes, antibody-coated erythrocytes, or antibody-coated platelets (especially those with light coatings of IgG), are mainly cleared by the spleen. The splenic cords are uniquely capable of removing erythrocytic inclusions, such as nuclear remnants (ie, Howell-Jolly bodies) or precipitated globin (ie, Heinz bodies), without destroying the cell.

The spleen has an ill-defined role in remodeling the membranes of reticulocytes soon after they are released from the marrow. This appears to play a role in decreasing their stickiness and volume.

### Other Functions of the Spleen

The spleen is a site of hematopoiesis until the sixth month of fetal life. Thereafter, splenic hematopoiesis is limited to pathologic extramedullary hematopoiesis associated with disorders such as thalassemia major or Rh incompatibility in the neonate. The spleen also serves as a reservoir for platelets and plasma proteins such as factor VIII. However, its function as a reservoir for erythrocytes is insignificant except in pathologic states such as hypersplenism.

## Physical Examination of the Spleen

The spleen is best palpated by standing on the right side of the child and examining the left side of the abdomen with your right hand. The child should be examined in the supine and the right lateral decubitus position with the knees up. Only light pressure should be used in small children, because the spleen can easily be pushed out of the way without feeling its edge.

The spleen has to enlarge to two or three times its normal size before it can be regularly palpated below the left costal margin. However, in normal children, a palpable spleen is not unusual. A 1- to 2-cm spleen tip is palpable below the left costal margin in 30% of full-term neonates and in 15% of infants younger than 6 months of age. A spleen tip of less than 1 cm is still palpable in at least 1% of older children and adolescents. The normal, palpable spleen is soft and nontender. It can be differentiated from other left upper quadrant masses by the absence of overlying bowel and its movement with respiration.

## Impairment of Splenic Function

Hyposplenism, which is diminished splenic function, is associated with a variety of disorders. Hyposplenism may be anatomical (eg, absence of splenic tissue), functional (eg, impaired function despite an intact spleen), or a combination of both. The most common causes of hyposplenism in children are surgical splenectomy, sickle cell disorders, and congenital absence of the spleen. The functional hyposplenism of sickle cell anemia is readily understood in physiologic terms. The hypoxic and acidotic conditions in the splenic cords are ideal for inducing sickling. Once sickled, the erythrocytes cannot pass adequately from the cords to the sinuses. Splenic circulation becomes so obstructed that splenic function is lost in most patients before 2 years of age.

Congenital asplenia comprises an anatomical lack of splenic tissue as part of a clinical complex of "bilateral rightsidedness." Less common causes of hyposplenism in children include regional enteritis, celiac disease, immune complex glomerulonephritis, and systemic lupus erythematosus.

Normal neonates demonstrate evidence of a physiologic impairment of splenic function that is presumed to represent a developmental phenomenon. This hyposplenism, which resolves in the first few weeks of life, is more severe is premature infants. Its possible role in predisposing neonates to bacterial septicemia has not been determined.

### Diagnosis

Hyposplenism is usually suspected because of the occurrence of a disorder known to cause it. Less commonly, it is detected because of the incidental recognition of erythrocyte inclusions that accumulate when the spleen fails to clear them normally. These findings, which include Howell-Jolly bodies, nucleated erythrocytes, and Heinz bodies, are not pathognomonic of hyposplenism. More specific studies used to confirm hyposplenism are radionuclide scanning using technetium 99m sulfur colloid, which readily labels the liver and spleen and observing increased numbers of erythrocytic vesicles using a specific optical system called interference contrast microscopy. The clearance of these vesicles is impaired in the absence of splenic function, but they appear to provide a more specific marker of hyposplenism than other erythrocytic inclusions.

### Consequences and Treatment

The primary consequence of impaired splenic function is a risk of overwhelming bacterial septicemia. In the absence of specific antibacterial antibody, intravenous encapsulated bacteria are able to elude the remainder of the MPS. Only the spleen, with the tremendous phagocytic capacity of its cords, can clear these organisms. In the absence of splenic clearance, intravenous bacteria reproduce so rapidly in peripheral blood that overwhelming septicemia results. The causative encapsulated bacteria are most often *Streptococcus pneumoniae*, followed in frequency by *Haemophilus influenzae* and *Neisseria meningitidis*.

The risk of septicemia in asplenic patients is approximately 2%, but it varies from less than 1% to 30% or more. In normal children with functioning spleens, the risk is less than 0.1%, and disease is rarely abrupt or severe. Very young children are at the greatest risk for hyposplenia-related septicemia, because they have had less prior exposure to these bacteria and are less likely to produce protective antibody when exposed to the polysaccharide capsular antigens of encapsulated bacteria. The risk of septicemia is twice as great for children younger than 4 years of age, and in the first year of life, it is 30% or higher. The risk is increased when the hyposplenism is concurrent with other immunologic or mononuclear-phagocyte system deficits, as in patients with sickle cell anemia or those undergoing splenectomy with Hodgkin's disease or thalassemia major. The risk of septicemia in these groups is 7% or more, compared with a risk of 2% or less for those undergoing splenectomy for trauma.

These children initially develop high fever without an obvious source of infection. Their ill appearance worsens dramatically with the onset of confusion and irritability. Meningitis is a common complication. Hypotension can rapidly develop as a manifestation of septic shock, and death may occur within 4 to 6 hours from the onset of symptoms. Thirty percent to 50% of these children die. Initially, it is almost impossible to differentiate overwhelming septicemia from the routine febrile viral illness of childhood.

The most important aspect of treatment is prevention, which consists of immunization with vaccines against *S pneumoniae*, given at 2 years of age because it is poorly immunogenic earlier (when the risk of infection is unfortunately highest), and *H influenzae*, which is routinely given to all children starting at 2 months of age. Prophylactic antibiotics (eg, penicillin) are used, and significant febrile episodes (temperature >39.0 °C) are treated aggressively and emergently with high-dose intravenous antibiotics. The antibiotic should effectively cover *S pneumoniae* and *H influenzae* and cross the blood–brain barrier to eradicate organisms that may have seeded the meninges. If treatment of febrile episodes is withheld until the patient looks very ill, the chance of death is high. Careful education of the patient and family should be stressed to encourage them to comply with antibiotic prophylaxis and to seek immediate medical attention in case of fever.

## Excessive Splenic Function

### Splenomegaly

Splenomegaly is the most frequent and important clinical problem involving the spleen. The most important causes of splenic enlargement are listed in Table 93-1.

The usual cause of splenomegaly in children is hyperplasia of the MPS, which can be categorized as excessive antigenic

---

**TABLE 93-1. Causes of Spenomegaly in Children**

**Hyperplasia of the Monocyte-Phagocyte System**
Excessive antigenic stimulation
  Viral infections
    Infectious mononucleosis
    Cytomegalovirus
    Acquired immune deficiency syndrome
  Bacterial infections
    Septicemia
    Endocarditis
    *Salmonella*
  Protozoal infections
    Toxoplasmosis
    Malaria
  Fungal infections
    Histoplasmosis
Disorders of immunoregulation
  Juvenile rheumatoid arthritis
  Systemic lupus erythematosus
  Serum sickness
Excessive destruction of blood cells
  Hereditary spherocytosis
  Sickle cell anemia
  Neonatal Rh or ABO incompatibility

**Neoplastic Infiltration**
Acute leukemias
Hodgkin's disease
Non-Hodgkin's lymphoma
Neuroblastoma
Histiocytosis X

**Disordered Splenic Blood Flow**
Cavernous transformation of the portal vein
Hepatic cirrhosis
Congestive heart failure

**Infiltration With Abnormal Material**
Gaucher's disease
Niemann-Pick disease

**Space-Occupying Lesions**
Hematomas
Pseudocysts
Congenital cysts

**Extramedullary Hematopoiesis**
Thalassemia major
Osteopetrosis

---

stimulation, disorders of immunoregulation, or excessive destruction of abnormal blood cells.

Excessive antigenic stimulation is usually the result of infection, which causes most splenomegaly in children. Viral infections are the most common. Although Epstein-Barr virus and cytomegalovirus are the best known viral agents, many of the more routine viral illness of childhood are probably more frequent causes of splenomegaly. An increasingly important cause of splenic enlargement is acquired immune deficiency syndrome (AIDS). Other common infectious causes include bacterial diseases (eg, septicemia, endocarditis, *Salmonella* infections), protozoal infections (eg, toxoplasmosis), and fungal infections (eg, histoplasmosis). In many areas of the world, malaria and schistosomiasis are routine causes of splenomegaly. Concomitant generalized lymphadenopathy is common in many of these infectious causes of splenomegaly.

Disorders of immunoregulation are much less frequent causes of splenomegaly. Examples include juvenile rheumatoid arthritis (especially in its systemic form), systemic lupus erythematosus, and serum sickness. Excessive destruction of blood cells as a cause of splenomegaly most commonly is the product of hemolytic disorders, including hereditary spherocytosis, sickle cell anemia, and in the neonate, hemolytic anemia caused by Rh or ABO incompatibility.

Splenomegaly is found in approximately one half of children with acute lymphoblastic leukemia, the most common childhood malignancy. It is also a frequent finding in Hodgkin's disease and non-Hodgkin's lymphoma. Although often associated with lymphadenopathy, splenomegaly in both of these disorders may be the sole presenting manifestation. Although acute myeloblastic leukemia is a less common malignancy, splenomegaly is a frequent and prominent finding in this disease. Metastatic involvement of the spleen, which is uncommon in children, is usually produced by neuroblastoma. The spleen can be infiltrated by histiocytes, a condition in children that usually is caused by histiocytosis X.

Many disorders can impair venous blood flow in the splenic or portal venous system and cause splenomegaly. The most common causes include cavernous transformation of the portal vein, hepatic cirrhosis, and congestive heart failure. Children with extrahepatic portal venous obstruction, such as cavernous transformation, often present with splenomegaly as the primary manifestation of their disease. These disorders are discussed later in the section on hypersplenism.

Infiltration of the spleen with abnormal material can cause splenomegaly. Storage diseases such as Gaucher's or Niemann-Pick disease are associated with splenomegaly because of the accumulation of abnormal lipids in splenic macrophages. Splenomegaly may be the first clinical manifestation of these disorders.

After trauma, palpable subcapsular hematomas may develop in the spleen. These hematomas may eventually develop into clinically palpable pseudocysts. Congenital splenic cysts often present with asymptomatic splenomegaly.

Although normally only found during early fetal development, extramedullary hematopoiesis may occur in diseases associated with intense demand on the bone marrow for cell production. Thalassemia major and osteopetrosis are examples of this rare cause of splenomegaly.

### Hypersplenism

Hypersplenism is a clinical syndrome in which normal splenic function becomes excessive as the spleen and its MPS tissues enlarge. The more formal definition includes the following criteria: splenomegaly, a deficiency of at least one or more of the peripheral blood cell lines, normal or increased levels of bone marrow precursors, and an expectation that splenectomy will resolve the cytopenias.

As the spleen enlarges, its minimal erythrocyte reservoir can greatly expand to sequester up to 45% of the total erythrocyte mass. The sequestered cells are not destroyed; they exchange slowly with circulating blood. As plasma volume expands to preserve circulating blood volume, the dilutional effect decreases the hemoglobin concentration in peripheral blood. However, erythrocyte mass remains normal or increases. The anemia is in large part dilutional. There may be excessive erythrocyte destruction by splenic macrophages, but it is limited. Erythrocyte survival is only slightly decreased, and overt hemolysis is rare. The sequestration of leukocytes and platelets may be more severe than that of erythrocytes.

The most common cause of hypersplenism is venous obstruction. Because of the absence of valves in the portal venous system, an increase in portal pressure is reflected immediately in the splenic venous sinuses. This impairs blood flow out of the cords and results in splenic sequestration and hypersplenism.

Hypersplenism in children often is caused by portal hypertension due to extrahepatic venous obstruction, often secondary to thrombosis of the portal vein due to umbilical venous catheterization, septic omphalitis, or thrombosis due to dehydration or shock. Less common causes of extrahepatic obstruction include congenital stenosis, atresia, or aneurysms of the splenic or hepatic portal venous system. Intrahepatic obstructions include cirrhosis due most commonly to hepatitis, cystic fibrosis of the pancreas, galactosemia, Wilson's disease, and alpha$_1$-antitrypsin deficiency. Schistosomiasis and malaria are important causes in endemic areas.

Children with hypersplenism can present with simple fatigue, pallor, and irritability or with unexplained splenomegaly. When the vascular obstruction is beyond the splenic vein, portal hypertension causes increased flow through minor collateral vessels between the portal and systemic circulation. Increased flow through the superficial abdominal and hemorrhoidal veins can cause clinically recognizable dilatation of the superficial veins on the abdominal wall and hemorrhoids, respectively. Dilatation of the short gastric and esophageal veins can result in esophageal varices, which may present with sudden and catastrophic gastrointestinal hemorrhage. Laboratory studies reveal neutropenia, thrombocytopenia, and anemia, singly or in combination, with evidence of active hematopoiesis in the bone marrow. Hepatocellular disease may be evident. Esophagoscopy is the most accurate means for confirming esophageal varices. Angiography, measurements of portal venous pressure, and scans using radioactively labeled blood cells can be used to evaluate the vascular obstruction.

Therapy depends on the site and nature of the vascular obstruction. Splenectomy cures the pancytopenia, but it is usually not indicated. The leukopenia and thrombocytopenia are rarely severe enough to cause sufficient infection or bleeding to justify any therapy. Splenectomy carries significant risks and may limit the potential for subsequent shunting procedures by removing the splenic vein. To prevent esophageal variceal hemorrhage, surgical procedures that relieve the pressure may be helpful by shunting blood from the obstructed hepatic portal system directly to the systemic circulation. In the young child, direct anastomosis between the portal vein the inferior vena cavae (ie, portacaval shunt) is preferred to shunts between the splenic and renal veins.

Hypersplenism occurs less frequently as a result of splenomegaly in the absence of venous obstruction. Specific causes include infections such as malaria and storage diseases such as Gaucher's disease.

The splenic sequestration crisis is a distinct form of acute hypersplenism in young children with sickle cell anemia, and it is an important cause of death. Even after functional hyposplenism develops, young children with sickle cell disease may develop sudden and massive splenic enlargement with sequestration of large portions of blood volume. These children manifest sudden weakness, dyspnea, left-sided abdominal pain, and increasing splenomegaly. So much blood can be trapped within the spleen that death due to hypovolemia can rapidly result. Treatment consists of restoration of blood volume and transfusion. To prevent recurrences, splenectomy is performed after one or two episodes of sequestration.

## Structural Abnormalities of the Spleen

### Congenital Malformations

*Accessory Spleens.*  One or more accessory spleens constitute a normal variant found in approximately 15% of the population. Averaging only 1 to 2 cm in diameter, accessory spleens are usually found in the splenic hilum or adjacent to the tail of the pancreas. Their identification and localization are easily accomplished with radionuclide scanning using $^{99m}$Tc sulfur colloid. Accessory spleens are inconsequential except when they are not removed during splenectomy for disorders such as autoimmune blood diseases or hereditary spherocytosis. The accessory spleen may hypertrophy and cause a recurrence of the clinical manifestations that the splenectomy had initially reversed.

*Congenital Asplenia.*  The spleen is the only organ arising on the left side of the body. Congenital asplenia is usually part of a clinical complex that results from a pathological tendency toward symmetric development of normally asymmetric organs. In this instance, the abnormality is bilateral rightsidedness; the spleen is absent, the lungs are trilobed, and the liver is symmetric and centrally located. Dextrocardia is usually evident, and there is a high risk of other severe congenital cardiac anomalies. Overwhelming septicemia is a common complication because of the absence of the spleen during infancy.

*Polysplenia.*  Polysplenia represents bilateral leftsidedness. Multiple small spleens are found along the greater curvature of the stomach in association with bilateral bilobed lungs and a high incidence of intrahepatic biliary atresia. Congenital heart disease occurs less often and is less severe than in congenital asplenia. The polysplenia itself is rarely of clinical consequence.

*Splenic Cysts.*  Splenic cysts are relatively uncommon. Congenital cysts are true epidermoid cysts lined with stratified columnar epithelium. They are usually recognized as smooth, nontender, left upper quadrant masses. The diagnosis can be established using ultrasonography or computerized tomography. Clinical consequences include a tendency to rupture with associated hemorrhage or to become infected. Larger cysts are usually removed surgically to avoid these complications, but normal surrounding splenic tissue is left intact if possible.

### Acquired Disorders

*Tumors.*  Most neoplastic disorders of the spleen are malignant. Benign tumors of the spleen are rare. Most are hemangiomatous and may be associated with similar tumors of other organs.

*Splenic Trauma and Rupture.*  Splenic injury can result from direct trauma to the left side of the abdomen or the left flank, as commonly occurs in motor vehicle accidents or contact sports. Splenic rupture may occur with relatively minor injury when the spleen is enlarged and friable because of disorders such as infectious mononucleosis. Neonates are particularly susceptible to splenic trauma after difficult (especially breech) deliveries or during cardiopulmonary resuscitation. Trauma often ruptures the splenic capsule and produces intraperitoneal bleeding. If the capsule remains intact, subcapsular hematomas may occur.

When the capsular tear is small, symptoms may be limited to moderate left upper quadrant or generalized abdominal pain; left shoulder pain, which may be elicited only by abdominal pressure during the examination; signs of peritoneal irritation due to intraperitoneal hemorrhage; or fever and emesis. Shifting dullness is rarely elicited. With larger capsular tears, the abdominal pain is severe, and hypovolemic shock rapidly develops. When subcapsular hematomas develop, the symptoms may be mild and overlooked; however, even minor injury may result in sudden rupture of the hematoma days to months later, with a rapid onset of hemorrhagic shock. In the neonate, evidence of shock and abdominal rigidity may be the only clinical signs of splenic rupture. Nonspecific laboratory findings include anemia and leukocytosis. The diagnosis is probably best established with computerized tomography, although radionuclide scanning is helpful.

Before the recognition of the risk of postsplenectomy septicemia, splenic trauma was routinely managed with splenectomy, because the spleen was considered to be a nonessential organ. Splenectomy is now avoided whenever possible. This is especially crucial for children younger than 5 or 6 years of age who are at greater risk for septicemia.

Surgical intervention is often unnecessary, because many hemorrhages from a lacerated spleen stop spontaneously in children. If the child's vital signs are stable and transfusion requirements are moderate (<25 mL/kg), careful observation is reasonable as long as a surgical team is readily available. Serial computerized tomography, ultrasound studies, or radionuclide scans may be helpful in verifying the stability of the lesion. Observation of the hospitalized patient is necessary for 10 to 14 days, with subsequent restriction of physical activity for several months. A pseudocyst may develop as a consequence of the healing of a subcapsular splenic hematoma.

If the hemorrhage is severe enough to result in deterioration in blood pressure, surgical intervention is indicated. Until recently, a simple total splenectomy was performed. Repair of the splenic laceration now is preferred to maintain splenic function and avoid the risk of septicemia. Splenectomy is performed only if safe repair is judged to be hazardous or technically impossible.

*Splenosis.* During the course of splenic rupture or subsequent surgical intervention, splenic tissue may autotransplant onto the peritoneal surface. This process, which is called splenosis, occurs more commonly in children than adults. When the spleen has been surgically removed, these implants enlarge. Splenosis has no serious consequences, but it may present a bizarre surgical picture at subsequent laparotomy. These implants may demonstrate enough splenic function to reverse laboratory evidence of asplenia; Howell-Jolly bodies and erythrocyte vesicles may disappear, and the implants may be visible by radionuclide sulfur colloid scanning. It is not yet known whether splenosis confers protection against overwhelming septicemia; some protection seems to be provided, but patients with splenosis have died of septicemia.

## Indications for Splenectomy

### Surgical Indications

Splenic trauma has been the most common indication for splenectomy. Splenic cysts, tumors, and vascular lesions may require surgical removal. In many instances, adequate normal splenic tissue may be preserved, but total splenectomy is occasionally necessary. Splenectomy may be necessary in disorders such as Gaucher's disease and thalassemia major when splenomegaly is so massive that relief from the mechanical stress is necessary.

Splenectomy may be necessary as part of other surgical procedures. Occasionally, splenectomy is required for adequate surgical exposure of the left side of the abdomen. Shunting procedures for portal hypertension, such as splenorenal shunts, require removal of the spleen. Surgical staging of Hodgkin's disease has routinely included splenectomy. However, the especially high risk of septicemia in this group of patients prompted reassessment of whether this procedure should be done as frequently as in the past.

### Medical Indications

Splenectomy is employed for several medical conditions. It is most effective in hereditary spherocytosis, because the less deformable spherocytes are trapped and destroyed in the splenic red pulp. Splenectomy normalizes erythrocyte survival and results in cure if cholelithiasis has not developed before surgery.

Splenectomy is beneficial in patients with hemolysis due to severe hereditary elliptocytosis and in many patients with severe pyruvate kinase deficiency. Splenectomy may be beneficial in autoimmune hemolytic anemia. Most patients with a warm IgG antibody who are refractory to medical therapy respond to this operation, because IgG-coated erythrocytes tend to be removed by the spleen, and those coated with IgM tend to be removed by the liver. Patients with IgM-mediated autoimmune hemolytic anemia generally do not benefit from splenectomy. Many children with chronic immune thrombocytopenic purpura who are refractory to medical therapy or corticosteroid dependent benefit from this operation, because most childhood immune thrombocytopenia is mediated by IgG. Splenectomy may be helpful in some patients with hypersplenism who develop clinically significant anemia or thrombocytopenia. Splenectomy may ameliorate increasing transfusion requirements caused by hypersplenism in patients with thalassemia major. The risk of splenectomy in these patients is substantially increased because of the excessive demands placed on the MPS by the hemoglobinopathy. Surgical removal of the spleen may be indicated in children with sickle cell anemia who have had an acute splenic sequestration crisis.

## LYMPH NODES

### Anatomy and Physiology

The MPS tissue in the spleen, liver, and bone marrow serves as an immunologic filter for circulating blood and for these organs themselves. However, most foreign antigens enter the body through the skin, gastrointestinal tract, and respiratory tract and then enter the lymphoid circulation rather than blood. Lymph nodes with their widespread peripheral locations provide the common initial site of contact between antigens and the MPS.

Lymph nodes are individual encapsulated anatomical units of the MPS distributed along lymph vessels throughout the body. They are ovoid and vary from a few millimeters to several centimeters long. Each node is surrounded by a connective tissue capsule perforated in several locations by afferent lymphatics. These lymphatics deliver lymphocytes, macrophages, and antigens to the node from the tissues they drain. They empty into peripheral sinuses within the node that are adjacent to the capsule. Branches of these sinuses extend deeper into the node and then terminate at the hilus, where the efferent lymphatics emerge. This allows circulating lymph to be effectively filtered throughout the node. The efferent lymph contains sensitized T and B cells and antibody-secreting plasma cells, which eventually reach the peripheral circulation through the thoracic duct and the right lymphatic duct.

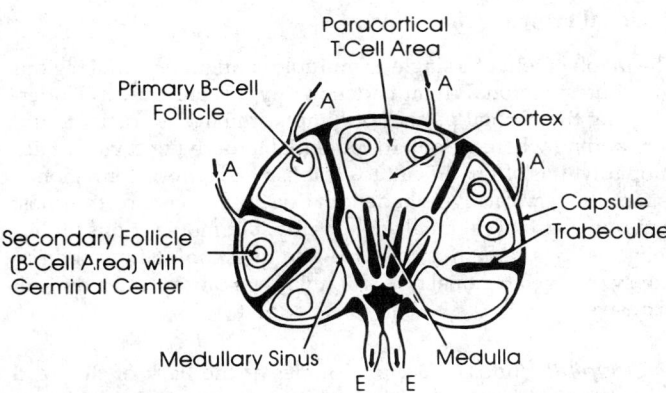

Figure 93-2. Lymph flows into the nodes through afferent lymphatics (A) and enters the cortex. Flow continues through the medulla, and lymph exits the node through the efferent lymphatics (E). B-cell activities are concentrated in the primary and secondary follicles in the cortex, and T cells are concentrated in the paracortical areas. (Modified from Hayes B. Enlargement of lymph nodes and spleen. In: Braunwald E, Isselbacher KJ, Petersdorf RG, et al, eds. Harrison's principles of internal medicine. New York: McGraw-Hill, 1987:276.)

The outer portion of the node is the cortex that contains spherical aggregates of lymphoid tissue called follicles (Fig 93-2). These follicles are centers of B-cell activity. Antigenic stimulation causes the primary follicles to become secondary follicles by enlarging and developing pale-staining germinal centers containing B lymphocytes in various stages of activation, helper T cells, macrophages, and reticulum cells. Surrounding these germinal centers are mantles of small unstimulated B cells. The surrounding paracortical areas between the primary and secondary follicles and the inner medullary region are centers of T-cell activity containing approximately 80% helper T and 20% suppressor T cells. Lymph flows through areas rich in T and B cells in proximity to macrophages. This highly specialized nodal structure provides ideal conditions for delivery of antigens to the immune system, optimizing antigen recognition and the subsequent activation of the cellular and humoral components of the immune response. The ability of lymph nodes to proliferate under immunologic stimulation can be impressive; the nodes can reach 15 times their normal size within 5 to 10 days of antigenic exposure.

Lymph nodes undergo important developmental changes that are essential to understanding the pathophysiology of these organs in children. At birth, there is considerable lymphoid activity throughout the body, but individual lymph nodes usually are not palpable. After birth, continuing exposure to environmental antigens results in a steady increase in the mass of lymphoid tissue, with a peak reached at 8 to 12 years of age. During puberty, lymphoid tissue begins to undergo a progressive atrophy, which continues throughout life. Children respond to new antigens with much more rapid and exaggerated hyperplastic lymphoid responses than do adults. Palpable lymph nodes are therefore much more common in children, especially in the cervical, axillary, and inguinal regions. The supraclavicular, popliteal, and mediastinal nodes rarely enlarge, even in children.

## Lymphadenopathy

By adult standards, almost all children have lymphadenopathy. Absence of palpable cervical or inguinal nodes in children is unusual and even may provide a clinical clue to an underlying immune deficiency. Common viral or bacterial illnesses of childhood often result in additional lymph node enlargement that can be dramatic. These factors explain the difficulty in determining whether enlarged lymph nodes in children represent a normal finding, transient hyperplasia in response to a simple viral illness, or more serious underlying pathology. This decision is based on clinical experience and judgment, but general guidelines are useful. Normal nodes usually do not exceed 2.5 cm in diameter and demonstrate neither warmth, tenderness, fluctuance, overlying erythema, nor any tendency to mat together into less well defined masses. The groups of nodes involved are important. Palpable cervical, axillary, and inguinal nodes are expected; however, supraclavicular nodes, if noticed at all, should be no greater than 1 to 2 mm.

Lymphadenopathy can be caused by an increase in the number of normal lymphocytes and macrophages during a response to an antigen (eg, viral illness such as mononucleosis), nodal infiltration by inflammatory cells in response to an infection localized to the nodes themselves (eg, lymphadenitis), proliferation of neoplastic lymphocytes or macrophages (eg, lymphoma), or infiltration of nodes by metabolite-laden macrophages in storage diseases (eg, Gaucher's disease).

The following sections provide an overview of lymphadenopathy, the most common clinical problem related to lymph nodes and one of the more frequent diagnostic problems in pediatrics. The differential diagnosis of lymphadenopathy has much in common with that of splenomegaly, which is not surprising in view of the common MPS functions of the two organs. Most children with lymphadenopathy have benign disorders, but in a few children, serious and even life-threatening problems will be identified.

### Generalized Lymphadenopathy

Lymphadenopathy is considered to be generalized when it involves enlargement of two or more noncontiguous lymph node regions. Disorders causing generalized lymphadenopathy are usually associated with other findings in the history, physical examination, and laboratory data that usually make it relatively easy to establish a diagnosis. Hepatosplenomegaly often is an associated finding. A careful search for any significant clinical or laboratory abnormalities is essential (Table 93-2).

*Infection.* Viral infections are the most common cause of generalized lymphadenopathy. The nodal enlargement is most often the result of transient responses to common viral upper respiratory infections. Other specific viral infections associated with adenopathy include infectious mononucleosis and cytomegalovirus. Rubella, varicella, and measles are causes readily recognized on the basis of their exanthems. AIDS is becoming an increasingly important cause of lymphadenopathy. Viral infections are usually associated with soft and minimally tender nodes. Bacterial infections are associated with more tender, warm, and sometimes fluctuant nodes with overlying erythema. In some cases, the bacterial infection is acute and associated with toxic symptoms, as with septicemia and typhoid fever. In other instances, such as tuberculosis, systemic symptoms are much less severe. Other infectious causes include *Chlamydia*, protozoa (eg, toxoplasmosis) and fungi (eg, coccidioidomycosis).

*Autoimmune Disorders and Hypersensitivity States.* Many immunologic disorders are associated with lymphadenopathy. Enlarged nodes are a common findings during the acute phases of juvenile rheumatoid arthritis, although other manifestations usually dominate the clinical picture. Children with systemic lupus erythematosus frequently demonstrate generalized lymphadenopathy. Other causes include serum sickness and reactions to specific drugs, such as phenytoin, allopurinol, and isoniazid.

*Abnormal Proliferation of Cells in Lymph Nodes.* Although malignancies are not a frequent cause of lymphadenopathy in

## TABLE 93-2. Causes of Generalized Lymphadenopathy in Children

**Infections**
Viral
  Common upper respiratory infections
  Infectious mononucleosis
  Cytomegalovirus
  Acquired immune deficiency syndrome
  Rubella
  Varicella
  Measles
Bacterial
  Septicemia
  Typhoid fever
  Tuberculosis
Protozoal
  Toxoplasmosis
Fungal
  Coccidioidomycosis

**Autoimmune Disorders and Hypersensitivity States**
Juvenile rheumatoid arthritis
Systemic lupus erythematosus
Serum sickness
Drug reactions (eg, phenytoin, allopurinol, isoniazid)

**Abnormal Proliferation of Cells**
Acute leukemias
Non-Hodgkin's lymphoma
Hodgkin's lymphoma
Neuroblastoma
Histiocytosis X

**Storage Diseases**
Gaucher's disease
Niemann-Pick disease

children, they always must be considered because of the importance of rapidly establishing a diagnosis and instituting therapy. Lymph nodes enlarged because of malignant disease are usually nontender and are not associated with overlying erythema; the nodes may have a rubbery texture, and groups of nodes may become matted together losing their individual character. Acute lymphoblastic leukemia, the most common childhood malignancy, is associated with lymphadenopathy in as many as 70% of these patients, but this is usually an incidental finding and not the presenting complaint. Lymphadenopathy is a frequent finding at presentation of the acute nonlymphoblastic leukemias. Non-Hodgkin's lymphoma is often associated with bilateral adenopathy, and Hodgkin's disease more often presents with unilateral involvement. Occasionally, lymphadenopathy is the presenting sign of neuroblastoma.

Histiocytic infiltration of nodes occurs in a number of disorders, of which histiocytosis X is the most common. In its systemic form, it is frequently associated with lymphadenopathy and hepatosplenomegaly, although these are not usually the presenting manifestations.

*Storage Diseases.* Storage diseases are rare causes of lymphadenopathy. The primary manifestations of these diseases are hepatosplenomegaly or neurologic deterioration. Associated lymphadenopathy is frequently observed in Gaucher's disease and Niemann-Pick disease.

## Regional Lymphadenopathy

The involvement of a single or multiple contiguous nodal regions constitutes regional lymphadenopathy (Table 93-3). Understanding the normal pattern of lymph drainage is crucial to understanding where to look for potential underlying causes of adenopathy. It is often difficult to establish a diagnosis for regional, especially cervical, lymphadenopathy. Infections are the most common cause of regional adenopathy, but more serious underlying diseases remain a concern. The question of how soon to biopsy enlarged regional nodes of unknown cause is often difficult to answer.

*Occipital Nodes.* Occipital nodes at the back of the head drain the posterior scalp. Nodes in this region are palpable in approximately 5% of normal children. Although often enlarged as part of generalized lymphadenopathy, the cause of regional enlargement is almost always infectious and often related to pediculosis capitis, tinea capitis, or seborrheic dermatitis. Roseola infantum and rubella cause enlargement in this region.

*Preauricular Nodes.* Preauricular nodes drain the lateral portions of the eyelid, conjunctiva, and the skin of the temporal

## TABLE 93-3. Causes of Regional Lymphadenopathy in Children

| | |
|---|---|
| **Occipital Nodes** | **Supraclavicular Nodes** |
| Pediculosis capitus | Tuberculosis |
| Tinea capitis | Histoplasmosis |
| Secondary infection of seborrheic dermatitis | Coccidiomycosis |
| | Hodgkin's disease |
| Roseola infantum | Coccidiomycosis |
| Rubella | Hodgkin's disease |
| | Non-Hodgkin's lymphoma |
| **Preauricular Nodes** | |
| Local skin infections | **Axillary Nodes** |
| Chronic ophthalmic infections | Local bacterial infections |
| Cat-scratch fever | Reactions to immunizations |
| | Juvenile rheumatoid arthritis |
| **Tonsillar Nodes** | Non-Hodgkin's lymphoma |
| Viral upper respiratory infection | |
| Streptococcal pharyngitis | **Mediastinal Nodes** |
| Tonsillar abscess | Tuberculosis |
| | Histoplasmosis |
| **Cervical Nodes** | Coccidioidomycosis |
| Viral upper respiratory infection | Acute lymphoblastic leukemia |
| Infectious mononucleosis | Hodgkin's disease |
| Rubella | Non-Hodgkin's lymphoma |
| Streptococcal pharyngitis | Cystic fibrosis |
| Toxoplasmosis | Sarcoidosis |
| Acute lymphadenitis | |
| Acute leukemias | **Abdominal Nodes** |
| Neuroblastoma | Acute mesenteric adenitis |
| Non-Hodgkin's lymphoma | Hodgkin's disease |
| Hodgkin's disease | Non-Hodgkin's lymphoma |
| Rhabdomyosarcoma | |
| Mucocutaneous lymph node syndrome (Kawasaki disease) | **Inguinal and Iliac Nodes** |
| | Local infections |
| **Submaxillary and Submental Nodes** | |
| Local infections of teeth and mouth | |
| Acute lymphadenitis | |

region and cheek. They are not normally palpable. Their enlargement is most often caused by local skin infections, chronic ophthalmic infections (eg, *Chlamydia*, adenovirus), and cat-scratch fever.

*Tonsillar Nodes.* The tonsils undergo the same physiologic hypertrophy as other lymph nodes, reaching a maximal size at approximately age 7. Isolated tonsillar hypertrophy, which has often resulted in unnecessary tonsillectomy, represents an important clinical example of the physiologic lymphoid hyperplasia of childhood. Superimposed viral or bacterial infections (especially simple upper respiratory infections or streptococcal pharyngitis) frequently cause additional, but usually transient, tonsillar enlargement. Bacterial infections can localize to the tonsil and produce a peritonsillar abscess.

*Cervical Nodes.* Areas drained by the cervical nodes include the tongue, external ear, parotid gland, and deeper structures of the neck, including the larynx, trachea, and thyroid. Cervical lymph nodes are normally palpable in all children beyond early infancy. They represent the most common site of abnormal lymph node enlargement. Common viral infections of the upper respiratory tract are the most frequent cause of such enlargement. Other specific viral causes include infectious mononucleosis, cytomegalovirus, varicella, rubella, and measles. Posterior cervical involvement is especially common in infectious mononucleosis and rubella. During viral illness, nodes tend to be soft, are minimally tender, and are usually enlarged bilaterally. β-Hemolytic streptococcal pharyngitis often is associated with bilateral cervical lymphadenopathy, in which the nodes are usually more tender. Toxoplasmosis is a protozoal disease that commonly presents with asymptomatic cervical lymphadenopathy.

Acute lymphadenitis is a common disorder resulting from a regional infection draining into a node or group of nodes and localizes there. The cause is usually bacterial, although viral infections can cause similar, milder symptoms. Frequent primary sites of infection include bacterial infections of the upper respiratory tract, teeth, and gums and severe acne and impetigo. Cervical nodes are most commonly involved, although any region can be affected. Involvement is usually unilateral. The localizing inflammatory response causes involved nodes to become enlarged, warm, and tender. If there is an adequate neutrophilic infiltrate, abscess, acute periadenitis, and inflammation of the overlying skin often develop. Fever, malaise, and leukocytosis are common. Antibiotic therapy is indicated and is directed at the two usual etiologic agents, *Staphylococcus* and β-hemolytic streptococci. Effective oral drugs include cloxacillin, dicloxacillin, or a cephalosporin. If suppuration occurs, surgical drainage may be necessary. Chronic cervical lymphadenitis is much less common. Frequent etiologic agents include cat-scratch disease, *Mycobacterium tuberculosis*, and atypical mycobacteria.

Mucocutaneous lymph node syndrome (Kawasaki disease) is a poorly understood multisystem disorder that is recognized with increasing frequency by pediatricians. Nonsuppurative cervical adenopathy, which can be marked and is often unilateral, occurs in 75% of these patients. The adenopathy represents one of the six diagnostic criteria of this disorder.

Approximately one quarter of childhood malignancies present in the head and neck, and the cervical nodes are the most common site of involvement. During the first 6 years of life, acute leukemias, neuroblastoma, non-Hodgkin's lymphoma, and rhabdomyosarcoma are the most common malignancies. In children older than 6 years of age, Hodgkin's disease and non-Hodgkin's lymphoma predominate. Cervical adenopathy is the presenting manifestation of 80% to 90% of children with Hodgkin's disease; the enlargement is usually unilateral, and the nodes are firm and painless. Approximately 40% of patients with non-Hodgkin's

lymphoma present with cervical adenopathy, which is usually bilateral.

Many nonlymphoid cervical masses may be easily mistaken for lymph nodes. They include cervical ribs, thyroglossal and branchial cleft cysts, branchial sinuses, cystic hygroma, sternocleidomastoid tumors, goiters, thyroid carcinoma, cervical neurofibromas, dermoid cysts, teratomas, and hemangiomas.

*Submaxillary and Submental Nodes.* The areas drained by the submaxillary and submental nodes include the teeth, gums, tongue, and buccal mucosa. Adenopathy is usually caused by localized infections of these structures, including dental abscess, pharyngitis, and herpetic gingivostomatitis. Acute lymphadenitis is a common complication of bacterial infection in this region.

*Supraclavicular Nodes.* The supraclavicular nodes drain the entire head and neck, arms, superficial thorax, lungs, mediastinum, and abdomen. The right supraclavicular nodes drain the mediastinum and lungs. Mediastinal adenopathy, which is usually not otherwise identifiable on physical examination, may be strongly suspected if the patient has right supraclavicular lymphadenopathy. The left supraclavicular nodes are closely related to the thoracic duct. Intra-abdominal processes associated with abdominal adenopathy often spread to the thoracic duct and cause enlargement of the left supraclavicular nodes. Although splenomegaly may be observed, left supraclavicular adenopathy is often the only clinical manifestation of this type of abdominal process.

Right supraclavicular adenopathy can be a manifestation of many pulmonary diseases, including tuberculosis, histoplasmosis, and coccidiomycosis. However, Hodgkin's disease and non-Hodgkin's lymphoma are common causes of enlargement of these nodes, and early biopsy is indicated in the absence of a easily documented pulmonary infection. Left supraclavicular adenopathy is often a manifestation of intra-abdominal Hodgkin's disease or non-Hodgkin's lymphoma, which often skip the mediastinum. Chest radiographs must be obtained for all patients with supraclavicular adenopathy. Thoracic or abdominal computerized tomographic scans may be indicated.

*Axillary Nodes.* Axillary nodes drain the hand, arm, lateral chest wall, lateral abdominal wall, and the lateral portion of the breast. They are normally palpable in 90% of children. Their enlargement is usually a result of infection in these areas. Recent immunizations in the arm, especially with bacillus Calmette-Guérin vaccine, commonly result in axillary adenopathy. Juvenile rheumatoid arthritis can cause adenopathy in this region. Of the malignancies, non-Hodgkin's lymphoma most commonly presents here.

*Mediastinal Nodes.* The thoracic viscera, including the lungs, heart, thymus, and thoracic esophagus, drain through the mediastinal lymph nodes. Because mediastinal nodes are not directly demonstrable on physical examination, they must be examined radiologically. The most common indirect clinical evidence of mediastinal adenopathy is supraclavicular adenopathy; less commonly recognized are direct effects of mediastinal node enlargement, including cough, wheezing, dysphagia, and obstruction of the great vessels, manifested by superior vena cava syndrome.

Malignancies are a common cause of mediastinal lymphadenopathy. Acute lymphoblastic leukemia, Hodgkin's disease, and non-Hodgkin's lymphoma are the most frequent causes. Bilateral hilar adenopathy is also associated with cystic fibrosis of the pancreas, histoplasmosis, coccidioidomycosis, and sarcoidosis. Unilateral hilar adenopathy is most commonly caused by tuberculosis. Common viral or bacterial infections of the lungs are rarely associated with lymphadenopathy. Nonlymphoid structures that may be mistaken for mediastinal adenopathy include the thymus (which can be quite large during early childhood), dermoid or bronchogenic cysts, teratomas, substernal thyroid gland, abnormalities of the great vessels, and neuroblastoma.

*Abdominal Nodes.* Abdominal nodes drain the lower extremities and all pelvic and abdominal organs. Enlargement of abdominal nodes can cause abdominal pain, backache, constipation, increased urinary frequency, and intestinal obstruction due to intussusception. Any disorder causing local abdominal or generalized adenopathy may produce these symptoms. Local disorders include typhoid fever, ulcerative colitis, and acute mesenteric adenitis of childhood. Mesenteric adenitis is thought to be caused by a virus and is characterized by right lower quadrant abdominal pain due to enlarged mesenteric nodes in the region of the ileocecal valve. This may be difficult to differentiate from appendicitis, in which obstruction of the cecal opening is often precipitated by hyperplastic lymphoid tissue. Significant abdominal adenopathy is also a manifestation of Hodgkin's disease and non-Hodgkin's lymphoma.

*Inguinal and Iliac Nodes.* The lower extremities, genitalia, perineum, buttocks, and lower abdominal wall are drained by the inguinal and iliac nodes. They are normally palpable in children. Infection is by far the most common cause of adenopathy. Readily overlooked causes of infection include diaper dermatitis and insect bites. Several nonlymphoid masses that may be mistaken for nodes include hernias, ectopic testes, lipomas, and aneurysms.

*Other Lymph Node Regions.* The popliteal nodes drain the knee and skin of the lateral leg and foot. The epitrochlear nodes, which are 3 cm proximal to the medial humeral epicondyle, drain portions of the forearm and fingers. In both instances, local infection is the only significant cause of lymphadenopathy.

### Lymph Node Biopsy

The evaluation of regional or generalized lymphadenopathy always raises the question of when to consider biopsy. The answer depends on the group of nodes involved, the clinical circumstances, and the appraised relative risk of malignancy or other serious disease. Signs of acute infection, such as tenderness, warmth, erythema, and a site of primary infection support delaying biopsy and treating with antibiotics. If biopsy is indicated, it is important to choose a large node that has been recently enlarging; to avoid a biopsy of the inguinal nodes, because their architecture is frequently distorted by chronic infection; and to avoid choosing a node primarily because of its surgical accessibility. Following these precautions can decrease the risk of obtaining an unrepresentative or reactive node and missing the actual underlying diagnosis. This is particularly a problem in Hodgkin's disease, in which nodes peripheral to the area of primary involvement frequently demonstrate only reactive hyperplasia.

## Lymph Vessels

The lymphatic vessels collect lymph from almost all tissues except the central nervous system, striated muscle, and nonvascular structures, such as cartilage and the cornea. The lymph is essentially colorless extracellular fluid containing large numbers of lymphocytes and material too large to be absorbed into blood capillaries. This fluid and its contents are delivered into blind lymph capillaries and then carried by thin-walled transparent lymph vessels to regional nodes. The lymph enters the nodes by afferent lymphatics, and within the node, the fluid is filtered, and immunologic material is phagocytized and undergoes immunologic processing. The nodes act as protective barriers to prevent the spread of local infections and to facilitate immunologic responses that are effective locally and systemically. Large numbers of lymphocytes are added to the lymph, which exits the nodes through efferent lymphatics and eventually reaches the thoracic duct and the right lymphatic duct. At this point in the base of the neck, the lymph enters the great venous system.

### Acute Lymphangitis

During a local bacterial infection, the lymphatics act as a protective drain that delivers bacteria to regional nodes for clearance and immunologic response. When the infection is not contained locally, it may involve the lymphatic vessels in an acute lymphangitis. Erythematous streaks that are a few millimeters to several centimeters wide may be seen extending from the primary site of infection to regional nodes. Painful swelling of regional nodes usually occurs soon thereafter. Peripheral edema may occur as a result of lymphatic obstruction. Bacteremia may follow as soon as 24 to 48 hours from the onset of the initial lesion. Acute lymphangitis is generally caused by group A streptococci. Rapid institution of penicillin is indicated for local control and to prevent complicating bacteremia.

### Lymphedema

Lymphedema is a diffuse, pitting edema that results from obstruction of the lymphatic flow. It most commonly involves the lower extremities and may be complicated by verrucous hypertrophy of the skin and recurrent infections. Congenital lymphedema occurs in Milroy disease, in which there are multiple congenital obstructions within the lymphatic system, and as part of the syndrome of gonadal dysgenesis. Acquired lymphedema can be the result of inflammatory processes or of surgical or radiologic obliteration of lymphatic channels; it may have no identifiable cause. Treatment is ineffective.

### Tumors of Lymphatic Channels

Benign tumors can arise from lymphatic channels in children, but the lesions are rare. They may be congenital or acquired and usually consist of numerous deep vesicles filled with clear or hemorrhagic fluid.

## Selected Readings

Bedros AA, Mann JP. Lymphadenopathy in children. Adv Pediatr 1981;28:341.
Crosby WH. Hypersplenism. In: Williams WJ, Beutler E, Eslev AJ, Lichtman MA, eds. Hematology. New York: McGraw Hill, 1983:660.
Lewis WM. The spleen. Clin Hematology 1983;12:341.
Margileth AM. Cervical adenitis. Pediatr Rev 1985;7:13.
Shackford RS, Molin M. Management of splenic injuries. Surg Clin North Am 1990;70:595.
Sills RH. Splenic function: physiology and splenic hypofunction. Crit Rev Oncol Hematol 1987;7:1.
Stockman JA. Splenomegaly. In: Stockman JA, ed. Difficult diagnoses in pediatrics. Philadelphia: WB Saunders, 1990:301.

*Principles and Practice of Pediatrics, Second Edition,*
edited by Frank A. Oski et al. J. B. Lippincott Company, Philadelphia © 1994.

# CHAPTER 94
# *Disorders of Coagulation*

## James F. Casella

Abnormalities of the hemostatic system are commonly encountered in hospitalized children, because primary diseases of hemostasis often require hospitalization and systemic diseases severe enough to require hospitalization often produce abnormalities of hemostasis. In addition, pediatricians are frequently called on to evaluate coagulation abnormalities before or after surgery.

Coagulation disorders can be divided into conditions with abnormal bleeding (ie, hypocoagulable states) and those associated with the development of thromboses (ie, hypercoagulable states). Current knowledge of factors necessary for normal clotting to occur and for maintaining blood in a fluid state is sufficiently complex that a full understanding of all the mechanisms involved is a challenge even for an experienced hematologist. New information is being acquired rapidly, especially in the area of hypercoagulability. Despite this surge of new information, most abnormalities of hemostasis can still be approached in an orderly fashion, beginning with a detailed history and physical examination, the evaluation of readily available laboratory tests, and a general overview of hemostatic mechanisms.

## GENERAL APPROACH TO COAGULOPATHIES

Coagulopathies may be secondary to abnormalities of the blood vessels, platelets, or plasma clotting factors, and some hemostatic defects involve more than one of these systems. The result of the history, including the family pedigree, physical examination, and screening laboratory testing, should provide information about which system is responsible for the bleeding abnormality. The following paragraphs summarize the basic functions of each component of the hemostatic mechanism, providing a background for understanding the mechanisms underlying clinical abnormalities. The relative contributions of the history, physical exam, and laboratory testing are then discussed.

### Coagulation Mechanisms

The primary response to bleeding includes a vascular response, platelet activation, and coagulation cascade. Within seconds of injury, damaged blood vessels demonstrate a vasoconstrictive response. During this phase of vasoconstriction, platelets begin to adhere to the damaged endothelium, where collagen, a potent activator of platelet adhesion, is exposed. Adherence and aggregation of platelets appear to be mediated through the action of specific platelet membrane receptors, including glycoprotein Ib (the major von Willebrand's factor receptor) and glycoprotein IIb/IIIa (the fibrinogen receptor). Adherent platelets then release platelet-stimulatory agents, such as thromboxane and adenosine diphosphate, and mediators of platelet interaction, such as fibrinogen and von Willebrand's factor, promoting adherence and activation of more platelets, with the resulting formation of an *unstable hemostatic plug*. Serotonin released from platelet granules

further constricts the large vessels. Platelet factor 4, a substance released from platelet granules, neutralizes heparin. Receptors for activated factor VIII and V are also expressed on the membranes of activated platelets.

Coincident with these events, tissue thromboplastins are released, and activation of the contact-activating factors initiates the coagulation cascade, as illustrated in simplified form in Figure 94-1. The clotting cascade can be activated at two separate levels. Activation of the intrinsic system begins with the surface activation of factor XII, a process that is accelerated by the presence of prekallikrein and high-molecular-weight kininogen. Activated factor XII then activates factors XI and IX in sequence, after which activated factor IX forms a complex with factor VIII, calcium, and phospholipid to activate factor X. Activated factor X then activates factor V, which, in the presence of calcium and phospholipid, cleaves prothrombin to thrombin. Thrombin cleaves fibrinogen to form fibrin monomer, which polymerizes into fibrin. Alternatively, in the extrinsic system, factor VII complexes with tissue factor (factor III), a constituent of the surface of cells in the damaged vessel wall and surrounding tissues and of activated monocytes. Tissue factor–factor VII complex or tissue factor–activated factor VII complex causes the formation of activated factor X, after which the rest of the clotting cascade proceeds as described earlier. This method of activation of clotting obviates the need for factors XII, XI, IX, and VIII. Evidence suggests that tissue factor–factor VII complex or tissue factor–activated factor VII complex can also activate factor IX, providing a redundancy in the activation mechanism of the extrinsic system. This route provides a role for factor VIII and IX in coagulation initiated by tissue factor.

In overview, the coagulation cascade can be thought of as the mechanism by which the soluble protein fibrinogen is converted to an insoluble matrix, fibrin. This fibrin matrix reinforces the primary platelet plug. Fibrin is covalently cross-linked by factor XIII, a transglutaminase that requires the presence of calcium, resulting in stabilization of fibrin. The platelet membrane appears to provide a critical surface for steps in the coagulation cascade that require interaction with phospholipids.

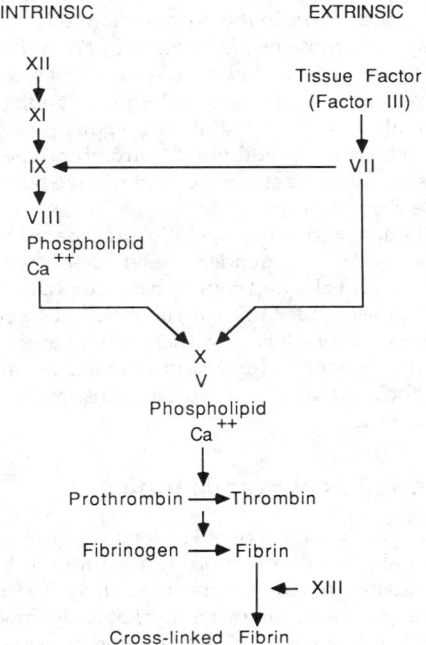

**Figure 94-1.** The coagulation cascade.

## Anticoagulation Mechanisms

The presence of such an elegant system for the formation of blood clots implies that an equally sophisticated system must be in place to prevent the inadvertent formation of blood clots and to provide for their removal and remodeling once formed. Protein C, a recently described anticoagulant protein, plays a primary role in inhibiting the clotting cascade and inducing the dissolution of clots. Like some of the procoagulant factors (eg, II, VII, IX, X), protein C is a vitamin K-dependent factor synthesized in the liver. Unlike the procoagulant factors, activated protein C possesses anticoagulant activity, which is achieved through cleavage and inactivation of activated factors V and VIII. Activated protein C also stimulates fibrinolysis.

Paradoxically, the activation of protein C depends on cleavage of protein C zymogen by thrombin, one of the final products of the clotting cascade. The activation of protein C by thrombin is catalyzed by an endothelial-bound receptor, thrombomodulin, a reaction that requires an essential cofactor, protein S, which is also a vitamin K-dependent factor. Once activated, protein C stimulates fibrinolysis. Protein C and protein S deficiencies are inherited disorders associated with predispositions to thromboses. Thrombin appears to play a pivotal role in both coagulation and anticoagulation, serving as a procoagulant by cleaving fibrinogen and activating platelets and as an anticoagulant by activating protein C in the presence of thrombomodulin. The activity of thrombin is in turn modulated by antithrombin III, in the presence and absence of thrombomodulin. Deficiencies of antithrombin have been reported to result in a tendency toward hypercoagulability. The affinity of antithrombin III for thrombin is enhanced in the presence of heparin, accounting at least in part for the anticoagulant activity of heparin.

Fibrinolysis can be induced by the enzyme plasmin, which is a cleavage product of plasminogen. Plasmin formation is catalyzed by several factors, including urokinase and tissue plasminogen activator. Cleavage of fibrin or fibrinogen by plasmin results in the formation of soluble fibrin degradation products, also referred to as fibrin-split products. Protein C appears to stimulate fibrinolysis by reducing the activity of tissue plasminogen activator inhibitor. Specific antiplasmins also have been demonstrated.

Regulation of the coagulation system can be achieved by other means. Most of the factors in the procoagulant scheme and some of the anticoagulant proteins (eg, protein C) are serine proteases and can therefore be inhibited by a wide variety of serine protease inhibitors in plasma (eg, $\alpha_2$-macroglobulin, $\alpha_1$-antitrypsin). Antithrombin III, also a protease inhibitor, regulates several of the procoagulant molecules in addition to thrombin. Specific inhibitors of the tissue factor–factor VII complex have been described that inactivate the extrinsic system.

The coagulation and anticoagulation mechanisms are delicately balanced and interdependent systems, possessing numerous redundancies, checks, and counterbalances that maintain the blood in fluid phase under normal circumstances yet allow for the rapid formation of clots and their ultimate dissolution in pathological circumstances. Important interactions among these procoagulant and anticoagulant factors are illustrated in schematic form in Figure 94-2.

## History and Physical Examination

Although the search for a possible bleeding disorder is often initiated by an abnormal laboratory test result, the history and physical examination remain the most useful approaches for defining the presence and type of hemorrhagic diathesis. For example, purpura and mucosal bleeding are common presentations of platelet disorders. Abnormalities of the plasma clotting factors

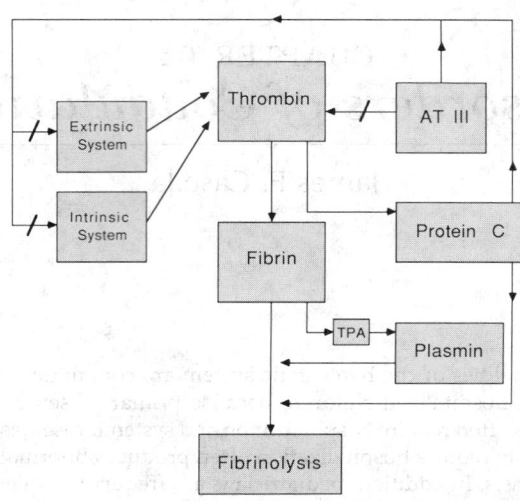

PROCOAGULANT          ANTICOAGULANT

**Figure 94-2.** Interactions among the major factors in the procoagulant and anticoagulant scheme. Prothrombin conversion to thrombin is driven by the intrinsic and extrinsic coagulation cascades. Thrombin causes fibrinogen to be converted to fibrin, the major constituent of clots. Thrombin, once bound by thrombomodulin in the presence of protein S, also activates protein C, which neutralizes the intrinsic and extrinsic systems and induces fibrinolysis. Antithrombin III antagonizes activated factors XII, XI, IX, X, and thrombin, inhibiting the intrinsic and extrinsic pathways. Tissue plasminogen activator (*TPA*), an enzyme that requires the presence of fibrin for activity, cleaves plasminogen to plasmin, which is responsible for clot lysis.

are much more likely to present with deep soft-tissue bleeding or hemarthrosis. The history may indicate that the coagulation abnormality is a secondary phenomenon and lead to the recognition of an underlying systemic illness.

In obtaining a history of abnormal bleeding, the clinician should ask specific rather than general questions. The question, ''Do you or your child bruise easily?'' is answered affirmatively by so many parents that a positive answer is often of little value. The examiner should use specific questions, using recognizable childhood events as a trigger for the parent's memory. Was separation of the cord or circumcision associated with abnormal bleeding? Approximately one half of hemophiliacs have a history of bleeding in the neonatal period, a fact that is often overlooked or unsolicited in the history. Patients with factor XIII deficiency may experience delayed bleeding after cord separation. Did the child bleed at the sites of immunization? Did the child bleed during eruption of teeth or after minor trauma to the mouth (eg, from falling into furniture)? Prolonged bleeding from a torn frenulum suggests factor VIII deficiency. Does the child bleed after minor trauma, such as falling from playground equipment? How frequent are epistaxis, and how long do they last? These questions are useful in gaining positive and negative information. For example, the complaint of frequent nosebleeds often raises concern about a possible coagulation disorder, but nosebleeds that predictably stop within minutes are rarely encountered in patients with significant bleeding disorders. How long does the child bleed from minor cuts? Did the wound heal normally? It is useful to find a scar, which often jogs the parent's memory about a forgotten laceration.

Previous surgical procedures are an extremely important source of information about potential coagulation abnormalities. The child who has had a tonsillectomy or dental extractions without unusual bleeding is less likely to have a serious coagulopathy. In questioning parents about dental procedures, it should be remembered that bleeding for 24 to 48 hours after dental extractions may occur even in normal persons and should not cause undue alarm.

A detailed history of drug administration is essential. Many substances (eg, aspirin, antihistamines) are available in over-the-counter prescriptions and are not reported by parents unless specifically mentioned by the examiner. A history of prolonged antibiotic administration or use of drugs that antagonize or interfere with the absorption of vitamin K (eg, anticonvulsants, antibiotics) may prompt a diagnosis of vitamin K deficiency. Ingestions of rodent poisons containing coumarins may cause coagulopathy.

A careful family history often provides important information. The finding of a sex-linked pattern of transmission of a bleeding tendency may be the first clue to deficiencies of factor VIII (ie, classic hemophilia A) or factor IX (ie, classic hemophilia B). The discovery of an autosomal dominant mode of transmission is characteristic of von Willebrand's disease. Idiopathic thrombocytopenic purpura is commonly encountered in families in which other immunoregulatory abnormalities, such as lupus and thyroid disease, are prevalent.

The physical examination can provide important diagnostic clues. Petechiae, easily overlooked, are an important indication of reduced platelet number or function. Bruises with firm nodular or indurated centers are commonly seen in hemophilia and may be the first sign of a congenital factor deficiency. Poorly healed scars may be seen in patients with factor XIII deficiency. The finding of an enlarged liver may be an indication of a systemic illness or that a coagulation disturbance is secondary to a primary hepatic disorder. An enlarged spleen may reflect significant portal hypertension with consequent hypersplenism and thrombocytopenia. The finding of characteristic angiomatous skin and mucous membrane lesions in a child with gastrointestinal bleeding may lead to a diagnosis of hereditary hemorrhagic telangiectasia. Patients with the stigmata of Ehlers-Danlos syndrome may also manifest purpura.

## Laboratory Evaluation

Excellent screening procedures and tests for specific abnormalities are available for evaluating the patient with a possible coagulation disorder. The physician should first consider whether any laboratory testing is required. The approach advocated by Rapaport is worthy of review. To paraphrase, after the history and physical examination, the physician should be able to reach one of the following conclusions:

The history and physical examination contain sufficient information to conclude that hemostatic function is normal.
The history and physical examination do not contain sufficient information to conclude that hemostatic function is normal.
The history and physical examination suggest the possibility or likelihood of a hemostatic defect.

Appropriate laboratory testing (or no laboratory testing) can then be obtained. A tabulation of all of the available tests of coagulation is beyond the scope of this chapter, but some of the commonly used screening procedures can be discussed. Coulter counter technology is readily available. Numeration and sizing of platelets by this method is routine and inexpensive. A stained blood smear prepared directly from peripheral blood by finger puncture should be examined to confirm the platelet count and size and to search for platelet dysmorphology. This allows an independent cross-check of platelet number, using the rule that an average of one platelet per high-power field on a thin smear viewed with a $10\times$ ocular and a $100\times$ microscope objective indicates the presence of 10 to 15 platelets/mm$^3$. The activated partial thromboplastin time (aPTT) measures functional activity of all of the soluble factors in the classic intrinsic cascade plus those involved in the extrinsic cascade, with the exception of factor VII (Table 94-1). Prolongation of the aPTT can therefore be secondary to an abnormality of one of the contact-activating factors, factors XII, XI, X, IX, VIII, V, II, or fibrinogen. An abnormality of the prothrombin time (PT) occurs with abnormalities of factors X, VII, V, II, or fibrinogen. Abnormalities of the PT or aPTT can also be caused by ingested or endogenous circulating anticoagulants (eg, warfarin, antiphospholipid antibodies) or liver disease.

Bleeding times may be abnormal in diseases of platelet function or number or in diseases affecting vascular integrity. Although the bleeding time is often recommended as a general screening procedure, several points should be recognized when considering its use. The bleeding time is extremely sensitive to platelet number; its use should be restricted to instances in which the platelet count has previously been determined. A history of recently ingested drugs, particularly aspirin, should be obtained before performing the bleeding time. Bleeding times, especially in inexperienced hands, often show considerable test-to-test variability, even when performed with calibrated templates. Citing these and other factors, several authoritative reviews have called into question the usefulness of the bleeding time as a preoperative screen.

Table 94-2 gives the normal values for all of the screening tests discussed.

## DISORDERS OF PLATELETS

Abnormalities of platelets may be quantitative (ie, due to reduced platelet number) or qualitative (ie, due to an intrinsic defect that diminishes function).

## Quantitative Congenital Abnormalities of the Platelets

### Thrombocytopenia–Absent Radius Syndrome

The thrombocytopenia–absent radius (TAR) syndrome is perhaps the most striking and most easily recognized of the congenital thrombocytopenias. Clinical recognition of the disorder occurs soon after birth in the infant with purpura and characteristic limb deformities. Although absence of the radius is the most consistent finding in this condition, cardiac, renal, other skeletal malformations (eg, complete or partial agenesis of other bones or joints, bony synostoses) may also occur. Leukoerythroblastic responses, often associated with severe diarrhea, are often observed in the neonatal period and infancy. The inheritance pattern appears to

**TABLE 94-1. Factors Tested for in the Prothrombin and Activated Partial Thromboplastin Times**

| Prothrombin Time | Activated Partial Thromboplastin Time |
|---|---|
| Factor X | High-molecular-weight kininogen |
| Factor VII | Prekallikrein |
| Factor V | Factor XII |
| Factor II (Prothrombin) | Factor XI |
| Fibrinogen | Factor X |
| | Factor IX |
| | Factor VIII |
| | Factor V |
| | Factor II (Prothrombin) |
| | Fibrinogen |

**TABLE 94-2.** Normal Values for Screening Coagulation Tests

| Assay | Normal Adult | Term | 32–36 Weeks of Gestation | <31 Weeks of Gestation | Age at Which Adult Values Are Reached |
|---|---|---|---|---|---|
| Platelet count ($10^3$/mm$^3$) | 300 ± 50* | 310 ± 68 | 290 ± 70 | 275 ± 60 | |
| aPTT (sec) | 44 | 55 ± 10 | 70 | 108† | 2–9 mo |
| PT (sec) | 13 (12–14) | 16 (13–20) | 17 (12–21) | 23 | 1 wk |
| Bleeding time | 4 ± 1.5 | 4 ± 1.5 | 4 ± 1.5 | NA | |

\* Means ± 1 S.D. or range when available are given.
† Indicates upper limit of normal for cord blood.

be autosomal recessive. Bone marrow specimens exhibit reduced numbers of megakaryocytes, which often appear dysplastic. Transfused platelets survive normally, and with the use of HLA-matched platelets, many patients can be maintained on weekly platelet transfusions for long periods. The thrombocytopenia tends to remit spontaneously in the second and third year of life.

### Amegakaryocytic Thrombocytopenia

Patients with amegakaryocytic thrombocytopenia may present without radial or other congenital abnormalities. Associations with neurologic defects and generalized bone marrow dysfunction developing later in life have been documented. Other syndromes associated with marrow failure or aplastic anemia that may present with thrombocytopenia in the neonatal period include Fanconi's aplastic anemia and the Shwachman syndrome. Although both are associated with major congenital abnormalities, the Shwachman syndrome is differentiated by exocrine pancreatic insufficiency, bony dysostoses, and neutropenia in most cases. In Fanconi's syndrome, a variety of congenital abnormalities may exist in addition to pancytopenia. Many have absent radii, mimicking the TAR syndrome, but in all reported cases of Fanconi's syndrome, absence of the radius is associated with absence of the thumb. In the TAR syndrome, the thumb is invariably present despite the absence of the radius. The phenotype of patients with Fanconi's syndrome often varies within the same family. Some patients exhibit no detectable congenital abnormalities, but the syndrome can be detected on the basis of characteristic chromosomal abnormalities.

### Other Causes of Inherited Thrombocytopenia

Thrombocytopenias transmitted as autosomal dominant traits with and without normal platelet survival have been described. Autosomal recessive inheritance of thrombocytopenia has also been reported. These syndromes may easily be confused with idiopathic thrombocytopenic purpura. Thrombocytopenia also occurs in the Tn-polyagglutination syndrome, a rare clonal disorder caused by an abnormality in glycosylation of the MN blood group antigen. Platelet number may be reduced in the Bernard Soulier, Wiskott-Aldrich, Ebstein, and Hermansky-Pudlak syndromes and the May-Hegglin anomaly.

## Qualitative Congenital Abnormalities of the Platelets

Platelet disorders may arise because of a defect in platelet function despite adequate numbers of platelets. These syndromes are characterized by purpura, abnormal platelet aggregation, and prolonged bleeding times. In some cases, platelet morphology is abnormal.

### Glanzmann's Thrombasthenia

Glanzmann's thrombasthenia is a prototype of the qualitative platelet disorders. This abnormality is inherited as an autosomal recessive trait. Although the number and morphology of the platelets are normal, life-threatening hemorrhagic complications may be encountered. Platelets from patients with Glanzmann's disease do not aggregate in vitro in response to adenosine diphosphate, collagen, epinephrine, and thrombin, but they do agglutinate in the presence of ristocetin and von Willebrand's factor. Clot retraction may be abnormal. These abnormalities are most likely caused by the partial or complete absence of a cytoadhesive protein, glycoprotein IIb/IIIa (the platelet fibrinogen receptor), from platelet membrane. The ability of these platelets to agglutinate in the presence of ristocetin and von Willebrand's factor can be attributed to the presence of normal amounts of another cytoadhesive membrane protein, glycoprotein Ib, the major von Willebrand's factor receptor. Transfusion of platelets is the only effective therapy, but may result in the development of antibodies directed against the glycoprotein IIb/IIIa complex and resistance to further platelet transfusions.

### Bernard-Soulier Syndrome

In Bernard-Soulier syndrome, another autosomal recessive disease resulting in severe hemorrhagic complications, platelets aggregate in vitro in the presence of adenosine diphosphate, collagen, epinephrine, and thrombin. However, agglutination does not occur in the presence of ristocetin, even with von Willebrand's factor. Platelets are often described as large and bizarre. Platelet number is often reduced, sometimes out of proportion to the number observed on peripheral blood smear. Underestimation of platelet counts by electronic techniques can be caused by their abnormal size and density. The primary defect in Bernard-Soulier syndrome appears to be an absence of glycoproteins Ib, V, and IX from the platelet surface. The deficiency of glycoprotein Ib results in the inability to bind von Willebrand's factor or ristocetin. As in Glanzmann's thrombasthenia, platelet transfusion is the only means of therapy. Refractoriness to platelet infusions may occur, caused by the development of antibodies against the glycoprotein Ib in the transfused platelets.

### Gray Platelet Syndrome

Abnormalities of the platelet granules have been described. In the gray platelet syndrome, "washed-out" or gray-appearing platelets are seen on Wright-stained peripheral blood smears, and there is a bleeding diathesis that is usually apparent at birth. A specific deficiency of alpha granules has been implicated as the cause of this disorder. There is a reduction in platelet levels of alpha granule constituents, such as fibrinogen, von Willebrand's factor, factor V, high-molecular-weight kininogen, fibronectin, thrombospondin, $\beta$-thromboglobulin, platelet factor 4, and platelet-derived growth factor.

### Storage Pool Disorders

Deficiencies of the adenine nucleotide-containing dense granules or their contents have been reported in a heterogeneous group of patients. These abnormalities are often referred to collectively as the *storage pool disorders*. Bleeding symptoms are usually not severe. The defect can be demonstrated in vitro by a diminished response of platelets to agonists such as collagen, which depend on the release of endogenous platelet nucleotides (ie, second phase of platelet aggregation) for completion of the aggregatory response or by electron microscopy. Dense body deficiencies have been described as part of the Hermansky-Pudlak syndrome (ie, large, bizarre platelets associated with oculocutaneous albinism and the accumulation of ceroid in bone marrow macrophages), the TAR syndrome, the Chédiak-Higashi syndrome, the Ehlers Danlos syndrome, the Wiskott-Aldrich syndrome, and osteogenesis imperfecta.

### Abnormalities of the Platelet Release Reaction

In addition to the storage pool disorders several abnormalities associated with the defective release of platelet granular contents have been reported. Abnormalities of arachidonic acid metabolism affect some patients, and defects of calcium metabolism have been postulated for others.

### Congenital Disorders Associated With Platelet Dysfunction

Abnormalities of platelet function occur in other congenital disorders, such as type I glycogen storage disease, cyanotic congenital heart disease, pseudoxanthoma elasticum, the May-Hegglin anomaly, and Epstein's syndrome (ie, macrothrombocytopathy associated with deafness and nephritis).

## Quantitative Acquired Abnormalities of Platelets

The acquired disorders of platelets encompass a diverse spectrum of illnesses, including those occurring as primary disorders of the platelets and a larger group secondary to systemic illnesses. An important diagnostic question is whether a thrombocytopenia is occurring as an isolated cytopenia or is accompanying a more generalized marrow failure disorder or systemic illness. One should consider whether the thrombocytopenia is caused by increased destruction or decreased production or is the result of sequestration of platelets. The acquired thrombocytopenic disorders then can be subdivided into immunologic and nonimmunologic events.

### Immunologic Causes of Thrombocytopenia

*Idiopathic (Immune) Thrombocytopenic Purpura.* Idiopathic thrombocytopenic purpura, sometimes referred to as immune or autoimmune thrombocytopenic purpura (ITP or ATP), is perhaps the most commonly encountered acquired platelet disorder of childhood.

*Etiology and Pathogenesis.* Although mounting evidence indicates an immunologic basis for this disease, in most cases the cause of the immunologic aberration is not clear, and the term *idiopathic* is preferred. Clinically, the disease is recognized in acute and chronic forms, and a multitude of pathogenetic mechanisms are probably involved. The immunologic basis of the disease has been suggested by classic experiments demonstrating that homologous and autologously transfused platelets are rapidly removed from the circulation; that the illness in adults can be passively transmitted from one person to another by administration of serum from an affected patient; that platelets from patients with ITP typically show increased amounts of IgG associated with the platelet membrane in several in vitro tests; that in some cases, specific antiplatelet antibodies can be demonstrated by Western-blotting techniques and other assays; and that the disease can be produced in infants by passive transplacental transfer of antiplatelet antibodies from the mother to the fetus. The reticuloendothelial system of the spleen is the major site of destruction

of platelets in ITP, with a less important contribution from the reticuloendothelial system of the liver, bone marrow, and lungs.

Although the concept that there is an immunologic basis for ITP is well accepted, the inciting cause for antibody production often remains obscure. Acute ITP in childhood is often preceded by a viral illness, and it has been postulated that viral antigens may trigger the production of antibodies that cross-react with the platelet membrane. The most convincing evidence for this hypothesis is the finding that postinfectious sera from some patients with varicella contain an antibody that cross-reacts with specific platelet membrane glycoproteins. Specific antiglycoprotein IIb/IIIa antibodies have been demonstrated in the chronic forms of ITP, which often occurs in the setting of other known autoimmune illnesses. However, the exact significance of the autoantibodies demonstrated in ITP remains the subject of debate. Recent studies suggest that much of the platelet-associated IgG (PAIgG) in ITP is not directed against specific platelet antigens. Other serum proteins are associated with platelet membranes in increased amounts, possibly as a nonspecific response to platelet injury. Studies have shown decreased production of platelets in otherwise classic cases of ITP, suggesting that the thrombocytopenia may be the consequence of decreased production and increased destruction in some cases.

*Clinical and Laboratory Features.* Acute and chronic ITP tend to vary considerably in their initial presentations. In acute ITP, the onset of purpuric symptoms is typically abrupt, so much so that parents can often recount the exact hour that they became aware of the problem. In chronic ITP, the onset of purpura is often much more insidious. Acute ITP most often presents in previously healthy children, whereas chronic ITP is more common in patients with other underlying immunoregulatory abnormalities, such as systemic lupus erythematosus, IgA deficiency, autoimmune endocrinopathy, common variable immunodeficiency, or autoimmune hemolytic anemia (ie, Evans's syndrome). Acute ITP tends to occur equally in both sexes, whereas chronic ITP is more common in females. Acute ITP is predominately a disease of early childhood. Chronic ITP is much more common in children older than 10 years of age.

In acute and chronic ITP, purpura and mucosal bleeding are the most prominent symptoms. The fact that the children generally appear well except for the purpuric lesions is helpful in excluding other illnesses associated with severe thrombocytopenia. Gastrointestinal and renal hemorrhage sometimes occur. Central nervous system bleeding is the most feared complication of ITP, but it occurs in fewer than 1% of these patients, usually early in the course of the illness. Such hemorrhages are often fatal. Platelet counts vary from normal (in a compensated phase) to undetectable, but they tend to be lower in acute ITP than in chronic ITP. Bone marrow aspirates should exhibit normal to increased numbers of megakaryocytes. PAIgG on the platelet surface (ie, the direct test) is usually positive if sufficient platelets can be obtained for study, but the patient's serum may or may not increase the amount of IgG on the surface of control platelets (ie, the indirect test). The PT and aPTT should be normal.

The resolution of symptoms and the thrombocytopenia occur in a variety of patterns, from abrupt to slow with frequent relapses. ITP is generally not considered chronic unless symptoms persist for more than 6 months. Relapses are common in chronic ITP. Acute ITP tends not to recur, but relapses have been reported. Improvement of symptoms often precedes a detectable rise in the platelet count.

*Treatment.* Because the spontaneous remission rate for acute ITP is extremely high, a waiting period is usually warranted before attempting therapy if the disease is mild (ie, platelet count >20,000/mm³, no bleeding other than purpura). Platelet counts less than 20,000/mm³ and extensive mucosal hemorrhage indicate a higher risk for internal hemorrhage, and treatment should be considered. If serious complications are present or suspected or if a protective environment cannot be guaranteed, treatment should be initiated. Historically, steroid administration has been the most commonly used therapy. The effectiveness of steroids in this disease is still debated, but the following statements are generally considered to be true:

Steroids may at least transiently increase the platelet count in some patients.

Even if the platelet count is not increased, a lessening of bleeding symptoms may occur, a finding supported by the finding that thrombocytopenic rats show evidence of resistance to basement membrane defects in small vessels after steroid administration.

Steroids do not change the natural history of the disease; they do not induce a true remission or shorten the duration of the disease.

Prednisone is usually administered at an initial dosage of 2 mg/kg orally per day, but higher or intravenous dosages up to 30 mg/kg/day of prednisolone for very short periods may be more effective.

Intravenous γ-globulin is a relatively new but useful modality in the treatment of ITP. The mechanism of action of this agent is not clear, but the best evidence to date suggests that it may act by causing a reticuloendothelial blockade, as evidenced by the reduced splenic clearance of sensitized erythrocytes after administration. Anti-idiotypic or anti-Fc receptor antibodies may be involved. Modulation of T- or B-cell function has been postulated, and it has been speculated that the clearance of infection or antigenemia may play a role. Treatment regimens vary from 1 g/kg/day for 1 to 3 days to 0.4 g/kg/day for 1 to 5 days. The most commonly used dose is 1 g/kg in a single administration. Responses are usually rapid and transitory and should not be expected in all patients. Although side effects appear to be minimal, this therapy is extremely expensive.

Platelet transfusions are generally eschewed in ITP because of the shortened survival of transfused platelets. However, platelet transfusions may be effective in immediately reducing serious bleeding. Splenectomy is effective in resolving the thrombocytopenia in approximately two thirds of patients, but is generally used only in emergencies or in extremely resistant cases. Other therapeutic approaches, such as vinca-loaded platelets or vincristine infusions, other immunosuppressive agents, or danazol, have been used in chronic ITP. In general these therapies should be used after more conventional modes of therapy have failed.

*Drug-Induced Immune Thrombocytopenia.* Acute thrombocytopenia caused by the development of specific antibodies has been attributed to a variety of drugs. These antibodies may be directed against a specific platelet antigen–drug (ie, hapten) complex or may result from absorption of antigen-antibody complexes onto the platelet surface (ie, "innocent bystander" phenomenon). In rare instances, they may represent true autoantibodies that recognize platelet antigens in the absence of the drug. Clinically, the onset of thrombocytopenia tends to be abrupt, within hours after the ingestion or administration of the drug, and ceases with clearance of the drug. The thrombocytopenia is frequently severe enough to be life threatening and tends to recur with repeated administration of the drug. Rechallenge with the offending drug should not be undertaken unless the drug in question is indispensable. In vitro testing to determine whether a drug is responsible for an immune-mediated thrombocytopenia is available. If postrecovery serum from the patient increases PAIgG on the patient's or the control's platelets in vitro only in the presence of the drug, it can be assumed that the drug tested is the causative agent. Drugs that have been convincingly demonstrated to be causes of drug-induced thrombocytopenia include the penicillins, trimethoprim-sulfamethoxazole, digoxin, quinine, quinidine, cimetidine, benzodiazepine, heparin, stibophen, novobiocin, and allylisopropylacetylurea (Sedormid). Many other agents have the potential for causing immune-mediated thrombocytopenia. Withdrawal of the potential offending drug and in vitro testing should be considered in equivocal cases.

*Neonatal Immune Thrombocytopenia.* Severe thrombocytopenia in the neonatal period may occur because of transplacental transfer of antibody from a mother who has ITP (ie, passive autoimmune thrombocytopenia). In these cases, PAIgG can usually be detected on the mother's platelets (ie, direct PAIgG test) and often in the mother's serum (ie, indirect test). The mother's platelet count is not an absolute predictor of thrombocytopenia in the infant. Mothers with normal platelet counts, especially those who have undergone splenectomy for ITP, may deliver severely thrombocytopenic infants. However, thrombocytopenic mothers with ITP often deliver infants with normal platelet counts. In some cases, the platelet count may fall over the first few days of life. The thrombocytopenia may persist for days to months, paralleling the disappearance of maternal antibody from the infant's circulation.

Neonatal thrombocytopenia may occur in mothers who have been sensitized to antigens on the infant's platelets that are absent from her platelets (ie, isoimmune thrombocytopenia). The most common platelet antigen incompatibility involves the PlA1 system. Three phenotypes are possible: PlA(1,1) (ie, homozygous PlA1 positivity), PlA(1,2) (ie, heterozygous PlA1 positivity), and PlA(2,2) (ie, homozygous PlA1 negativity). Approximately 98% of the population is PlA(1,1) or PlA(1,2). If the mother is PlA(2,2), the father is likely to be PlA(1,1) or PlA(1,2), and the infant will be a candidate for isoimmune disease. A number of platelet antigens (eg, Bak, Pen [Yuk], Ko, Plt, Br) less commonly implicated as a cause of isoimmune thrombocytopenia have been described. The mother's platelet count is normal in these disorders. In vitro testing should demonstrate that the direct test for PAIgG on the mother is negative. However, her serum should increase the amount of PAIgG on the father's or the infant's platelets and control antigen-positive platelets (ie, indirect test). Isoimmune thrombocytopenia most often resolves within a few weeks but can persist for longer. As with erythrocyte sensitization, there is a high risk of recurrence with future pregnancies.

Cesarean section should be considered for any delivery in which the child is at risk for passive autoimmune thrombocytopenia, because the risk of intracranial hemorrhage at the time of delivery is high. Platelets should be available in the delivery room. Neonatal immune thrombocytopenia has been treated successfully with transfusion of platelets and exchange transfusion. Steroids may be useful if administered to the mother before delivery or to the infant after delivery. In some infants, intracranial hemorrhages may occur in utero. Several therapies have been proposed to prevent them. Most often used is a corticosteroid preparation that is not inactivated by the placenta, such as dexamethasone. Alternatively, the administration of intravenous γ-globulin to mothers prenatally may be of value. Postnatally, intravenous γ-globulin for autoimmune thrombocytopenia appears to be equally effective as in other forms of ITP, although the experience is much less extensive. In isoimmune thrombocytopenia, transfusion of mother's platelets represents optimal therapy postnatally, because they do not possess the sensitizing antigen and therefore have normal survival. In utero transfusions of maternal platelets have been used to prevent intracranial hemorrhage in isoimmune disease in selected cases.

*Posttransfusion Purpura.* A small percentage of patients, usually adults, respond to erythrocyte transfusions by developing severe thrombocytopenia. The lowering of the platelet count typically occurs abruptly about 1 week after the erythrocyte transfusion. Affected patients are typically $Pl^A(2,2)$ women with a history of one or more pregnancies, who have been transfused with blood from a $Pl^A(1,1)$ or $Pl^A(1,2)$ donor. Recent studies suggest that the thrombocytopenia is secondary to passive absorption of soluble $Pl^{A1}$ antigen from the donor's plasma onto the recipient's platelets.

### Nonimmune Causes of Thrombocytopenia

*Infectious Thrombocytopenia.* Thrombocytopenia may be associated with a variety of infections, viral infections being the most common offenders. The thrombocytopenia may occur during the active infection or as a postinfectious manifestation of the illness. In congenital rubella, for example, the thrombocytopenia can persist for months and often follows a course similar to that of ITP. Other viral infections associated with thrombocytopenia include varicella, Epstein-Barr virus, cytomegalovirus, herpes, and measles. In some cases, thrombocytopenia may be caused by generalized marrow suppression that sometimes occurs after Epstein-Barr viral infections and hepatitis. The mechanism of the thrombocytopenia is not always clear, but in the case of rubella and cytomegalovirus, the virus can be cultured from the marrow. Thrombocytopenia may accompany a number of other systemic infections, including toxoplasmosis, malaria, syphilis, tuberculosis, and overwhelming bacterial or rickettsial sepsis.

Infection with the human immunodeficiency virus (HIV) is an increasingly common cause of thrombocytopenia. Features of immune and nonimmune causes of thrombocytopenia are encountered. Thrombocytopenia can be seen early in the course of HIV infection as the only hematologic abnormality in patients who are otherwise asymptomatic or later in the disease as part of a more generalized bone marrow suppressive process associated with overt acquired immune deficiency syndrome (AIDS). The opportunistic infections suffered by these patients or the administration of antiviral therapy can cause thrombocytopenia. HIV infection has been postulated to cause thrombocytopenia by a variety of mechanisms, including immune destruction of platelets, direct viral invasion of megakaryocytes, and inhibition of stem cells. Increased levels of PAIgG often occur with normal numbers of megakaryocytes, producing a clinical syndrome compatible with ITP. Syndromes mimicking hemolytic uremic syndrome (HUS) or thrombotic thrombocytopenic purpura (TTP) have been reported.

Administration of intravenous γ-globulin is often effective in reversing thrombocytopenia in HIV infection. In many cases, steroids and splenectomy are effective in elevating the platelet count but are less preferred therapies. Antiviral therapy may improve the platelet count. This result may be mediated by direct antiviral effects or an effect on the underlying aberrant immune response. Attention should be directed toward treatment of possible associated opportunistic infections. Therapies specific to the particular disorder should be considered if the symptoms suggest HUS or TTP.

*Microangiopathic Causes of Thrombocytopenia.* Thrombocytopenia is a hallmark feature of hemolytic uremic syndrome and TTP. HUS typically presents with bloody diarrhea, followed by the onset of renal failure, thrombocytopenia, and anemia. Central nervous system involvement, often manifested by seizures, is common. Other extrarenal manifestations include myocarditis, pancreatitis, hepatitis, intussusception, and colitis, which may be followed by colonic strictures. Bacterial and viral infections, toxins, drugs, and prostaglandin abnormalities have been

implicated in the pathogenesis of HUS. A verotoxin-producing *Escherichia coli* (*E coli* O157:H7) identified in several outbreaks of HUS is an important etiologic agent in the epidemic form of the syndrome. Fibrin degradation products are often elevated, but disseminated intravascular coagulation (DIC) is generally not seen. Platelet survival is shortened, presumably secondary to a local microangiopathic process involving fibrin deposition.

The syndrome of TTP overlaps significantly with HUS, to the point that the two syndromes may be different parts of the same spectrum. TTP tends to occur in adults and is more commonly associated with fever than HUS. Neurologic symptoms are prominent, but renal dysfunction is less common and less severe than in HUS. The vascular lesions in the HUS show a predominance of fibrin, but platelet aggregates predominate in the vessels of patients with TTP. However, controversy persists about whether the pathologic lesions are truly distinct in the two syndromes. TTP is usually fatal if treated with supportive care alone, but encouraging results have been produced using plasma exchange as a primary therapy.

Hemangiomas may result in thrombocytopenia (ie, Kasabach-Merritt syndrome). The pathogenesis of this phenomenon involves platelet sequestration and destruction in the hemangiomatous lesion. There is often evidence of fibrin consumption. A variety of treatments have been proposed, including steroid administration, platelet and cryoprecipitate transfusions, epsilon aminocaproic acid, radiation therapy, aspirin, dipyridamole, and surgery. Promising results have been reported with the use of interferon alfa-2a. The ultimate usefulness of each therapy is not clear. Conservative treatment is indicated, because the lesions tend to regress spontaneously.

Thrombocytopenia may be a manifestation of DIC, which is discussed later in this chapter.

*Drug-Induced Thrombocytopenia.* Several drugs cause thrombocytopenia in the absence of an identifiable immune mechanism. In the pediatric population, valproic acid is a common offender. Heparin administration is frequently accompanied by thrombocytopenia, which may be paradoxically associated with arterial thrombosis. Chloramphenicol may produce thrombocytopenia as an isolated finding or as part of a more generalized marrow aplasia. Other agents suppressing megakaryopoiesis and thrombopoiesis include the thiazide diuretics, alcohol, chemotherapeutic drugs, and ionizing radiation.

*Miscellaneous Thrombocytopenias.* Many other clinical conditions may be associated with significant thrombocytopenia. Hypersplenism of any cause, including congestive (eg, Banti's syndrome), infiltrative (eg, Gaucher's disease), sequestrative (eg, sickle cell disease), or rheumatologic (eg, Felty's syndrome), can cause thrombocytopenia. Thrombocytopenia is commonly seen in cyanotic congenital heart disease with polycythemia. Severe liver disease of almost any cause may be associated with a low platelet count. Severe hypothermia or anoxia may induce thrombocytopenia. Thrombocytopenia may be a manifestation of severe iron deficiency or deficiencies of folate or vitamin $B_{12}$. Placement of large vessel catheters, cardiopulmonary bypass, cardiac prostheses, rejection phenomenon, and severe allergic reactions can lower the platelet count. Myeloproliferative and myelodysplastic disorders, including aplastic anemia, are commonly associated with thrombocytopenia.

### Thrombocytosis

Thrombocytosis occurs commonly in children. In most instances, the elevation of the platelet count is attributable to an underlying disorder associated with thrombocytosis. Common causes of thrombocytosis include acute and chronic bleeding, inflammatory or infectious processes, iron or vitamin E deficiency, hemolytic anemia, and asplenia. Thrombocytosis may occur as a result of neoplastic processes, drug administration (eg, vinca alkaloids, epinephrine), nephrotic syndrome, graft-versus-host disease, or during treatment of megaloblastic anemias. Kawasaki disease is frequently associated with extremely high platelet counts. Rarely, thrombocytosis is the result of a primary hematologic disease, essential thrombocythemia. In this condition, platelet production occurs autonomously, with the loss of the normal control mechanisms for thrombopoiesis. Ironically, primary thrombocythemia is associated with bleeding rather than thrombosis. Thrombocytosis may be seen as part of polycythemia vera and chronic myelogenous or megakaryocytic leukemia.

Although an underlying disease causing an elevation of the platelet count frequently requires attention, treatment for the thrombocytosis itself is rarely required. Symptomatic thromboses in children due to elevated platelet counts appear to be extremely rare. Although aspirin and dipyridamole are sometimes prescribed for extreme thrombocytosis, their efficacy in preventing thrombotic complications in children has not been demonstrated. The natural history of thrombocythemia is poorly understood, and the value of treatment of this disorder with chemotherapeutic agents has not been documented.

## Qualitative Acquired Abnormalities of Platelets

Acquired abnormalities of platelet function occur most commonly after the ingestion of drugs that inhibit platelet function. Although a large number of drugs inhibit platelet function in vitro, exposure to aspirin-containing compounds or other cyclooxygenase inhibitors is by far the most common cause of drug-induced platelet dysfunction. Some semisynthetic penicillins, carbenicillin in particular, and valproic acid cause a prolongation of the bleeding time, which may be attributable to impaired platelet function. Acquired abnormalities of platelet function have been demonstrated in uremia and severe liver disease. The exact mechanism of the abnormality in platelet function in these patients is not well characterized but presumably relates to the accumulation of toxins. Interference with platelet function may occur in DIC because of the accumulation of fibrin degradation products. Platelet function may be abnormal in several myeloproliferative disorders. In rare instances, platelet dysfunction may be secondary to the development of antibodies against specific platelet-surface glycoproteins (eg, acquired or pseudo-Bernard-Soulier disease due to antiglycoprotein Ib antibodies). Antibody-induced platelet dysfunction may be present in some cases of ITP.

## DISORDERS OF COAGULATION FACTORS

## Congenital Abnormalities of Coagulation Factors

### Abnormalities of the Factor VIII Complex

Classically, two major congenital disorders have been attributed to abnormalities of the factor VIII molecule: hemophilia A, also referred to as factor VIII deficiency, and von Willebrand's disease. Hemophilia A represents a defect in factor VIII procoagulant activity in which platelet function is normal, whereas von Willebrand's disease involves a defect in platelet function associated with a variable abnormality of factor VIII procoagulant activity. The abnormality of platelet function in von Willebrand's disease is caused by decreased or defective von Willebrand's factor, a substance necessary for platelet adhesion to blood vessel walls and maintenance of a normal bleeding time.

In the past, the relation of factor VIII procoagulant activity to the von Willebrand's factor was poorly understood. Advances in the molecular biology and protein biochemistry of factor VIII

have demonstrated that circulating factor VIII is a complex of two different proteins: the factor VIII procoagulant protein (ie, factor VIII:C) and the von Willebrand's factor (ie, factor VIIIR: vWF or vWF). These proteins are products of separate genes, and each has unique antigenic sites. The von Willebrand's factor is a macromolecular structure (ie, multimer) composed of multiple smaller subunits and appears to act as a carrier protein for the factor VIII procoagulant molecule. Whereas factor VIII procoagulant activity is likely to be reduced when the von Willebrand's factor is not present in sufficient quantities. The designation factor vWF:Ag refers to the major antigen on vWF that is recognized by heterologous antisera against the factor VIII complex; the designation factor VIIIR:C.F. (ie, ristocetin cofactor) indicates the activity of the von Willebrand's factor in vitro, which is the ability of the molecule to support ristocetin-induced agglutination of platelets. An appreciation of these relationships is essential to understanding the clinical disease states.

### Factor VIII Deficiency

*Etiology and Pathogenesis.* Factor VIII deficiency (ie, hemophilia A) is a sex-linked disorder, occurring in about 1 of 10,000 Caucasian male births. The disease results from a deficient or abnormal factor VIII procoagulant molecule. More than 200 discrete mutations or deletions in the factor VIII gene that result in hemophilia A have been described. Spontaneous mutations appear to be common and occur at "hot spots" in the factor VIII gene that structurally favor mutations. Factor VIII levels in affected persons vary from less than 1% to approximately 25% of normal activity. Levels of von Willebrand's factor are normal. Female carriers of the disease are usually asymptomatic and generally have factor VIII levels between 25% and 75% of normal, with normal von Willebrand's factor assays. However, a carrier may have factor VIII:C activity levels higher than 100% of normal (normal range, 50% to 200%); thus, it is not possible to identify the carrier state in all women by use of functional assays of factor VIII:C alone. However, measurements of factor VIII:C and von Willebrand's factor with determinations of DNA polymorphisms among family members can detect more than 95% of the carriers of the abnormal X chromosome. Clinical severity of the disease varies with the degree of deficiency of factor VIII activity and tends to breed true among affected males in a given kindred.

*Clinical and Laboratory Features.* Factor VIII deficiency is characterized by a lifelong tendency toward serious and often life-threatening hemorrhage. Whereas surface bleeding and purpura can occur, deep soft-tissue bleeding and hemarthrosis are the hallmarks of the disease. Hemophiliacs can be divided into three groups based on clinical severity and the level of factor VIII activity: severe (<1% factor VIII activity), moderate (1% to 5% factor VIII activity), and mild ( 5% to 25% factor VIII activity). Severe hemophiliacs are subject to spontaneous bleeding into joints or soft-tissue sites. Moderate hemophiliacs classically develop severe bleeding only after trauma, but mild hemophiliacs may be symptomatic only after surgery or major trauma. Life-threatening bleeding can occur in all groups. Severe hemophiliacs may not bleed excessively immediately after small lacerations or venipunctures due to lack of impairment of platelet function. However, delayed bleeding at such sites is common, particularly if sutures have been placed.

The symptoms tend to vary with age. Approximately 50% of hemophiliacs escape detection in the neonatal period, even if circumcisions are performed. Mucous membrane bleeds in the mouth and bruises, particularly palpable subcutaneous hematomas, are much more common in infancy than later life. The frequency of hemarthrosis tends to increase as the child becomes ambulatory.

Although bleeding may occur at virtually any anatomical site, the most common bleeds encountered in hemophiliacs are hemarthroses, with knees, elbows, and ankles representing the most commonly affected joints; shoulders, wrists, and hips are less frequently involved. The onset of hemarthrosis is often marked by development of pain without other objective findings, followed by acute swelling, warmth, and tenderness of the joint, sometimes accompanied by erythema or discoloration. Bleeding into soft tissues and bursae around the joint may occur. Repeated bleeding into the same joint results in synovial damage and hypertrophy, producing secondary cartilaginous and bony abnormalities. The development of muscular atrophy and contraction of ligamentous structures around such "target" joints is common. The combination of soft-tissue, bony, and cartilaginous abnormalities results in an anatomically abnormal joint that is more susceptible to successive bleeds. Disruption of the epiphyseal structures may result in growth abnormalities. The development of bony cysts represents a late complication of hemarthrosis. Rarely, erosive "pseudotumors" of bone may be seen.

Central nervous system bleeding is one of the most feared complications of hemophilia. It is usually the result of trauma. Symptoms may be minimal immediately after the traumatic event, and the seriousness of the bleeding may not become evident until several days after the initial incident. Even minor episodes of head trauma may be followed by intracranial bleeding, and spontaneous intracranial hemorrhage may occur.

Hemorrhage with dental procedures can be severe. Lip or tongue lacerations occur frequently in toddlers and younger children and can be quite troublesome, possibly because of the high level of fibrinolytic activity of saliva. Excessive bleeding from a torn frenulum can indicate hemophilia, as does the development of a large fleshy clot. Other gastrointestinal bleeding can occur and is usually associated with some type of structural abnormality. Bleeding into retroperitoneal spaces occurs with some frequency and can sometimes be mistaken for an intra-abdominal process. Hematuria is relatively common and can be persistent. Bleeding into muscles or soft tissue can occur at any site. The seriousness of these bleeds is usually dictated by their anatomical location. Entrapment of nerves or blood vessels can be particularly problematic. Bleeding in the area of the airway should be managed as a life-threatening event. Severe hemorrhage may be experienced after surgery if adequate replacement therapy is not administered.

The diagnosis of hemophilia A requires the demonstration of low factor VIII:C activity in the presence of a normal von Willebrand's factor assay. The PTT usually is prolonged, and the PT is normal. However, in some mild forms of factor VIII deficiency, the PTT may be normal. Tests of platelet function are usually normal, although abnormal template bleeding times have been observed in some hemophiliacs. A family history may reveal a sex-linked pattern of inheritance. However, the family history may be negative because of a predominance of females in successive generations or the high rate of spontaneous mutations.

*Treatment.*

PREVENTION AND GENERAL CARE. Prevention of bleeding should be a major goal of treatment, with care taken to avoid an environment of overprotection. Infants should be provided with padded cribs and playpens. Contact sports should be prohibited, but nontraumatic sports such as swimming should be encouraged. Platelet-inhibitory substances such as aspirin should be avoided. Immunizations should be administered after replacement with factor VIII or be given intradermally rather than intramuscularly to avoid hemorrhagic complications. Immunization against hepatitis B should be given as early as possible. Prophylactic dental treatment should be encouraged. Invasive procedures such as lumbar puncture should be performed only under coverage with factor VIII.

Replacement therapy with factor VIII remains the most important part of the care of the hemophiliac. Home therapy has gained widespread acceptance and offers the opportunity for earlier treatment of bleeding episodes and increased autonomy for the hemophiliac. Such programs require close physician supervision.

Blood-borne infections such as hepatitis and AIDS have been major complications of therapy in hemophiliacs. Most hemophiliacs exposed to factor VIII replacement before screening for HIV in blood products was initiated in 1985 are seropositive for HIV. The rate of occurrence of seropositivity in previously uninfected patients has decreased dramatically since the introduction of screening procedures and the introduction of factor VIII concentrates prepared using improved methods of viral inactivation.

DOSAGE AND SCHEDULE OF FACTOR VIII REPLACEMENT. The level and duration of replacement with factor VIII depends on the severity of the bleeding. Replacement doses can be calculated using the rule that 1 U of factor VIII per kilogram of body weight increases circulating factor VIII levels by 2%. For minor soft tissue bleeds, replacement to 20% of normal levels is often sufficient. For hemarthroses or more serious soft-tissue bleeds, at least 40% replacement should be achieved and may be required for several days. Levels of 70% or greater may be required for extensive dental work. Replacement of 80% to 100% is essential in the event of central nervous system bleeding or for surgical procedures. Treatment for 10 to 14 days may be required for surgical procedures or head injury.

With the first dose in a given series, factor VIII tends to disappear with a half-life of approximately 8 hours. Thereafter, the biologic half-life approximates 12 hours, and doses should be given at that interval to maintain a trough level one half of the initial increment. A steady state can also be achieved by continuous infusion of factor VIII when adequate hemostasis at all times is essential (eg, after major surgery or head injury). In these instances, a loading dose of factor VIII sufficient to raise the factor VIII level to between 50% and 100% should be given. A dosage of 3 or 4 U/kg/hour thereafter should maintain a level of approximately 50%. Considerable variation in the biologic half-life of factor VIII may be seen from patient to patient. In the event of serious hemorrhage or prolonged or continuous therapy, levels of factor VIII after transfusion should be measured to determine the adequacy of replacement.

PREPARATIONS OF FACTOR VIII. Several preparations are available for providing factor VIII replacement. Fresh frozen plasma contains approximately 1 U/mL of factor VIII, but volume considerations limit its usefulness. Cryoprecipitate prepared in most blood banks contains approximately 80 to 120 U of factor VIII per bag, which can be resuspended in 10 to 20 mL of plasma or saline. Replacement to 100% of normal for even large persons is possible using cryoprecipitate. Coombs' test positivity with hemolysis due to residual A and B blood group antibodies in cryoprecipitate may occur. The use of cryoprecipitated factor VIII has the advantage of limiting the recipient's exposure to a small number of donors per transfusion. Currently available methods for virus inactivation are not applicable to cryoprecipitate, and cryoprecipitate is much less convenient for home administration. For practical purposes, its use has been supplanted by factor VIII concentrates for the treatment of hemophilia.

Several commercial preparations of concentrated factor VIII are available. These preparations offer the advantages of long shelf-life and ease of administration and are particularly useful for home therapy. Each administration results in exposure of the recipient to tens of thousands of donors, increasing the risk of transmission of blood-borne infections. The risk of transmission of these infections has been minimized by newer techniques of preparation of factor VIII concentrates, such as detergent and wet-heat treatment. Purification and concentration of factor VIII through the use of monoclonal antibodies has resulted in the production of high-purity factor VIII concentrates with low infectious risks. The use of factor VIII concentrates prepared by recombinant DNA techniques may offer the most promising long-term prospects for treating hemophilia effectively with the lowest risk, but such preparations are still in clinical trials. Concern about the high incidence of inhibitors to factor VIII in early trials of recombinant factor VIII need to be allayed before these products replace conventional preparations of factor VIII.

ADJUNCTIVE MEASURES FOR SPECIFIC BLEEDING PROBLEMS. *Joint Bleeds.* Aspiration of joints is generally not necessary, unless extreme distention of the joint capsule is encountered. If aspiration is required, coverage with factor VIII should be instituted before the procedure. Cold compresses may be applied, and brief immobilization of affected joints may provide comfort. Prolonged splinting should be avoided to prevent the development of disuse atrophy and contractures. Physiotherapy should be instituted as soon as possible.

*Hematuria.* Although hematuria may be dramatic in hemophilia, a discrete anatomical source for the bleeding is usually not found. Administration of factor VIII is usually not effective in treating hematuria, and the administration of epsilon aminocaproic acid (EACA) is probably contraindicated because of the risk of clot formation in the ureters. The hematuria usually resolves without specific treatment. The administration of prednisone may be effective in reducing the duration and degree of spontaneous hematuria.

*Dental procedures and mouth bleeds.* Although coverage with factor VIII remains the mainstay of therapy, EACA or tranexamic acid therapy may inhibit clot lysis in the mouth. EACA is usually given as an oral dosage of 75 to 100 mg/kg every 4 to 6 hours, to a daily maximum of 24 g. Tranexamic acid is given orally at 25 mg/kg on the same schedule.

ALTERNATIVE TREATMENTS FOR MILD AND MODERATE HEMOPHILIA. Desmopressin acetate, administered intravenously, increases factor VIII levels twofold to threefold in patients with detectable baseline factor VIII levels. This type of increment may be sufficient to treat minor bleeding episodes in patients with significant levels of factor VIII but is not useful in patients with severe hemophilia A. The usual dosage is 0.3 μg/kg given intravenously every 12 to 24 hours. Tachyphylaxis may occur with repeated administrations. In some patients, danazol therapy has the same effect, but its use has been limited by a high frequency of side effects and unpredictable responses.

*Inhibitors.* The development of circulating inhibitors against factor VIII is a major therapeutic problem, affecting 10% to 15% of hemophiliacs. Failure to reach the expected level of factor VIII activity after infusion of factor VIII or a shortening of the biologic half-life of transfused factor VIII may be the first sign that an inhibitor is present. These inhibitors are IgG antibodies and often show species specificity. Their frequency does not appear to be directly related to the number of transfusions of factor VIII. Affected patients may be low responders, who do not increase their inhibitor level significantly with each administration of exogenous factor VIII, or high responders, who experience a true anamnestic response to factor VIII infusion. Low responders usually can be treated with higher doses of factor VIII. High responders may be treated at least transiently with porcine factor VIII if their antibodies do not cross-react significantly with porcine factor VIII in vitro. Massive transfusions of human factor VIII concentrates can often overwhelm the inhibitor initially if the titer is low. Plasmapheresis may transiently lower the titer of inhibitor. The use of human and porcine factor VIII in high responders is generally restricted to instances of life-threatening emergencies or essential surgery; administration of either preparation may produce within days high titers of inhibitors that persist for long periods.

Prothrombin concentrates and activated products such as FEIBA (Factor VIII Inhibitor Bypassing Activity) and Autoplex

have had some therapeutic effect in controlled, double-blind studies and do not increase inhibitor levels. These products may be helpful in the treatment of non–life-threatening bleeds, but the best results with these products do not approach the effectiveness of factor VIII in patients without inhibitors.

Considerable progress has been reported in the use of "immune-tolerance" regimens in children with high titers of inhibitors. In many cases, tolerance to factor VIII infusions can be achieved without the use of cytotoxic therapy. Continued administration of factor VIII to these patients several times each week appears to be required to prevent the reappearance of the inhibitor. Considerable effort and even greater expense is involved. Whether these patients actually achieve immune tolerance instead of temporary suppression or absorption of their inhibitor is not clear. At this time, this therapy cannot be recommended for all patients with inhibitors but should be considered for recurrent life-threatening hemorrhage or for excessive morbidity caused by an inhibitor.

*Von Willebrand's Disease.* The term von Willebrand's disease encompasses a heterogeneous group of disorders involving primary defects or deficiencies in the vWF portion of the factor VIII complex, with variable deficiencies of factor VIII:C, the procoagulant component of the factor VIII molecule. The abnormalities of vWF result in decreased platelet adhesiveness, impairment of agglutination of platelets in the presence of ristocetin, and prolongation of the bleeding time. Abnormalities of factor VIII procoagulant activity contribute to the coagulation disturbance. Unlike hemophilia A, von Willebrand's disease is usually transmitted as an autosomal dominant trait. Compound heterozygotes have been described. In rare instances, transmission may be autosomal recessive. Studies suggest that 0.8% to 1.6% of the general population show biochemical abnormalities consistent with von Willebrand's disease, making von Willebrand's disease the most common of the inherited coagulation disorders.

Several classifications of von Willebrand's disease have been suggested. All of these schemes recognize that there are two major forms: those due to quantitative abnormalities of vWF and those due to qualitative abnormalities. Mild quantitative deficiencies of vWF and factor VIII:C are referred to as type I or classic von Willebrand's disease. Qualitative abnormalities are classified as type II, and severe quantitative deficiencies as type III. Type II abnormalities can be subcategorized on the basis of abnormalities of vWF subunit and multimer structure, as demonstrated by immunoelectrophoretic techniques and decreased or increased responsiveness to ristocetin in platelet aggregation studies. Quantitative deficiencies of vWF and factor VIII:C may or may not be found in type II disorders. In types I and III, the level of factor VIII:C activity correlates with the amount of vWF. Type III patients are thought to be homozygotes or compound heterozygotes.

Most patients with von Willebrand's disease have a mild to moderate bleeding tendency, usually involving mucocutaneous surfaces. Epistaxis, increased bruisability, and hemorrhage after dental extraction are common manifestations. Melena and menorrhagia may occur. Excessive bleeding after trauma or surgery can develop. Hemarthroses are unusual, except in type III disease, or after significant trauma. Many persons with biochemical abnormalities consistent with von Willebrand's disease report no bleeding symptoms.

The diagnosis of von Willebrand's disease is complicated by the fact that results of laboratory testing sometimes vary, not only within families, but for the same person on repeated determinations. Bleeding times are abnormal at some time for most persons. The PTT may be abnormal, depending on the level of VIII:C activity. Types I and II can usually be differentiated by measuring antigenic vWF (vWF:Ag) and factor VIII:C in conjunction with crossed-immunoelectrophoresis or multimer analysis. Both vWF:Ag and factor VIII:C should be reduced in type I disease, with normal crossed-immunoelectrophoresis or size distribution on multimer analysis. In type II disease, vWF:Ag and or VIII:C may or may not be reduced, but crossed-immunoelectrophoresis or multimer analysis should show abnormal variants or lack of high-molecular-weight multimers of vWF. Assessment of platelet aggregation in response to ristocetin in vitro should define the persons with qualitative abnormalities who show hyper-responsiveness to low doses of ristocetin and are therefore at risk for in vivo platelet aggregation and thrombocytopenia. In type III von Willebrand's disease, vWF:Ag and factor VIII:C are markedly reduced.

Cryoprecipitate contains intact vWF of all molecular weights and appears to be effective in treating most subtypes. The bleeding time is corrected for only a few hours after administration of cryoprecipitate, despite the prolonged increase in factor VIII:C. Factor VIII concentrates may lack the high-molecular-weight forms of vWF and are not consistently effective in correcting the bleeding time in von Willebrand's disease. The treatment of choice for mild to moderate bleeding episodes in type I von Willebrand's disease is 1-desamino-8-D-arginine vasopressin (DDAVP) because of the infectious risks of cryoprecipitate. This therapy is often sufficient for surgical procedures, but adjunctive therapy with plasma products may be required for extensive surgery or serious hemorrhagic episodes. DDAVP should not be given to patients who show increased responsiveness to ristocetin in platelet aggregation studies, because they may be at risk for thrombocytopenia. It may lack effectiveness in some type II patients. The effect of DDAVP on the bleeding time is transient, approximately 3 to 4 hours, and tachyphylaxis may occur. Patients should be tested for efficacy before it is used as a therapeutic agent. In very mild cases of von Willebrand's disease, specific treatment is often not required.

*Platelet-type or Pseudo-von Willebrand's Disease.* A disorder closely related to von Willebrand's disease is platelet-type or pseudo-von Willebrand's disease, in which the primary defect appears to reside in the platelet receptor (ie, glycoprotein Ib) for vWF. Increased amounts of vWF are bound to the platelet membrane because of an abnormally high affinity of the receptor for vWF. This results in depletion of the highest-molecular-weight multimers from plasma. As in type IIB von Willebrand's disease, in which the high-molecular-weight multimers show an increased affinity for the platelet surface, increased responsiveness to ristocetin and thrombocytopenia may be seen. This syndrome is easily confused clinically and biochemically with type IIB von Willebrand's disease. The two syndromes can be differentiated by the fact that cryoprecipitate causes increased aggregation of platelets in pseudo-von Willebrand disease but not in type IIB von Willebrand's disease or by studying the differential binding of the patient's vWF to formalin-fixed platelets.

## Other Inherited Coagulation Abnormalities

*Factor IX Deficiency.* Like factor VIII deficiency, factor IX deficiency (ie, hemophilia B, Christmas disease) is inherited as a sex-linked trait of variable severity. Clinically, it is virtually indistinguishable from factor VIII deficiency. The diagnosis is made in the same way as factor VIII deficiency, except that a factor IX assay is used to confirm the diagnosis. Very low levels of factor IX are occasionally seen in female carriers of factor IX deficiency, in some cases due to abnormality of the chromosomal homolog, such as a deletion in the region of the factor IX gene. Inhibitors occur much less frequently than in factor VIII deficiency.

Treatment with plasma is effective, but larger doses are required than in hemophilia A to achieve the same level of replacement. Commercial concentrates containing factor IX are used more commonly than plasma. Earlier intermediate purity concentrates contained all of the other vitamin K-dependent factors at variable levels. Higher purity products containing only factor

IX have become available and are now the mainstay of therapy. A dose of 1 U of factor IX per kilogram of body weight increases factor IX levels by 1 to 1.5%. This is compensated for by a longer biologic half-life. After an initial loading dose, a subsequent dose is usually given in 4 to 12 hours to account for the shorter initial half-life, and every 24 hours thereafter.

*Factor XI Deficiency.* Factor XI deficiency (ie, hemophilia C) is characterized by an autosomal recessive inheritance pattern and mild bleeding tendency. Heterozygotes also manifest reduced levels of factor XI. The disease occurs most often in persons of Ashkenazi Jewish descent. Symptoms include increased bruisability, epistaxis, menorrhagia, and postoperative bleeding. Hemarthroses and deep soft-tissue bleeds are unusual. Hemorrhagic symptoms in severely deficient patients can usually be controlled with small doses of plasma.

*Other Uncommon Specific Factor Abnormalities.* Selective abnormalities of fibrinogen, factors II, V, VII, X, XII, XIII, prekallikrein, and high-molecular-weight kininogen have been described.

Congenital afibrinogenemia may present with hemorrhagic complications in the neonatal period and is associated with a lifelong bleeding abnormality. The spectrum of symptoms seen in this disorder is similar to that of hemophilia A, but the disease is usually much less severe. Patients with a variety of dysfibrinogenemias have been described. Most of these patients are asymptomatic, but increased bruisability, menorrhagia, wound dehiscence, post-traumatic and surgical bleeding and thrombosis have been reported. Congenital afibrinogenemia appears to be an autosomal recessive disorder, whereas dysfibrinogenemia is an autosomal dominant event in most cases. Therapy with plasma, cryoprecipitate, and fibrinogen concentrates is effective in both disorders.

Congenital prothrombin (factor II) deficiency and dysprothrombinemia result in mild bleeding disorders that usually do not require therapy and are inherited in an autosomal recessive fashion. If necessary, the defect can be corrected with fresh frozen plasma or prothrombin complex concentrates.

Factor V deficiency is also associated with a mild, autosomal recessively inherited bleeding disorder. Replacement with fresh plasma is preferred due to the extreme instability of factor V with storage. It is sometimes associated with renal, cardiovascular, and skeletal abnormalities and the development of inhibitors.

Factor VII deficiency is potentially symptomatic in the heterozygous and homozygous forms. The symptoms include mucosal bleeding, gastrointestinal hemorrhage, menorrhagia, and intracranial hemorrhage. Factor VII deficiency should be suspected in patients in whom the aPTT is normal and the PT is significantly prolonged. Fresh frozen plasma or prothrombin complex concentrates have been effective replacement therapies. However, this situation is now complicated by the depletion of factor VII in many newer prothrombin complex concentrates. This difficulty should be alleviated soon by the commercial availability of purified factor VII concentrates.

Factor X deficiency is similar to factor VII deficiency in its inheritance pattern and symptoms. The aPTT is abnormal, as is the PT. Fresh frozen plasma or prothrombin complexes are used for treatment.

Factor XII (ie, Hageman factor), prekallikrein (ie, Fletcher factor), and high-molecular-weight kininogen (ie, Fitzgerald factor) deficiencies are associated with prolongation of the aPTT, but they do not cause a significant bleeding abnormality. It is important to recognize these abnormalities only to differentiate them from other causes of a prolonged aPTT that are associated with bleeding symptoms. The Passavoy defect causes a prolonged aPTT, and it is associated with variable degrees of bleeding.

Hemorrhage after surgery has been described in patients with the Passavoy defect. In these four disorders, the diagnosis is made by showing that the patient's plasma does not correct the defect in plasma from a patient known to have the disorder. Physicians should understand that routine screening of patients with aPTT will uncover patients with these disorders, many of which have no clinical significance.

Factor XIII deficiency is a heterogeneous disorder that is associated with instability of fibrin clots. Delayed bleeding from the umbilical stump or after trauma is a classic presentation of the disease. Purpura and poor wound healing may be seen. Patients appear to be at higher risk for intracranial hemorrhage and spontaneous abortion. Routine coagulation studies are normal. The diagnosis is established by the relative instability of the patient's clots in urea. Treatment with plasma is effective.

Alpha$_2$-antiplasmin deficiency has been reported as a cause of bleeding diathesis in several families. The results of routine coagulation tests are normal. Bleeding occurs as a result of excessive fibrinolytic activity. Homozygotes have suffered hematomas, hemarthroses, and muscular and central nervous system bleeding. Some heterozygotes may show increased bruisability and postsurgical or dental bleeding.

*Inherited Coagulation Factor Abnormalities Due to Deficiencies of More Than One Factor.*   Several patients have been described who have a deficiency of multiple vitamin K-dependent factors. Deficiencies of factors II, VII, IX, X, and protein C have been demonstrated simultaneously in at least one patient. These patients appear to have a defect in γ-carboxylation of the vitamin K-dependent clotting factors. The hemorrhagic symptoms are consistent with vitamin K deficiency.

Several kindreds have been described in which multiple persons have deficiencies of two or more clotting factors. These reports consist mainly of case histories, the deficiencies are frequently mild and variable, and the underlying defects are poorly understood.

*Inherited Coagulation Abnormalities Resulting in Hypercoagulability.*   Protein C is a vitamin K-dependent factor, which is converted to its activated form by thrombin in the presence of protein S. This reaction is catalyzed by a surface receptor, thrombomodulin, which binds thrombin and increases its affinity for protein C. Protein C is the most potent anticoagulant protein known. Inherited protein C deficiency has been described in heterozygous and homozygous states. Homozygotes usually have no protein C activity and are detected shortly after birth. Purpura fulminans is usually the first recognized symptom. Venous thromboses in the central nervous system and kidneys are common. Thrombosis of the retinal vessels tends to occur early in the illness, followed by secondary vitreous bleeds, resulting in fibrosis and blindness. The disease is fatal if untreated. Patients with apparently homozygous protein C deficiency presenting later in life have been described, but they have detectable levels of protein C activity. Transmission of the disease appears to be autosomal recessive in most kindreds with homozygous protein C deficiency.

Treatment with heparin is not effective, but sufficient protein C can be administered with fresh frozen plasma to reverse the clinical symptoms. Long-term management can be achieved with Coumadin administration, by at least partially restoring the balance between procoagulant and anticoagulant forces. Infusions of purified protein C concentrates have been used to treat this disorder. Successful correction of homozygous protein C deficiency by hepatic transplantation has been accomplished in one patient.

Heterozygous protein C deficiency can be associated with thrombotic disease. Heterozygotes typically manifest levels of

activity between 35% and 65% of normal. Patients with levels of antigenic protein C higher than their activity levels have been described, indicating a qualitative defect of protein C. Most heterozygotes in the best studied kindreds do not become symptomatic until the third decade of life, but children with symptomatic disease in the first and second decade are being recognized with increasing frequency.

Deep venous thrombosis and central nervous system thromboses are among the most common symptoms. Patients with heterozygous protein C deficiency may manifest purpura fulminans shortly after Coumadin administration. This unusual reaction to Coumadin is attributed to the short half-life of protein C relative to some of the vitamin K-dependent procoagulant proteins. Because all of the vitamin K-dependent proteins are reduced after Coumadin therapy, very low levels of protein C may develop quickly in patients with lower than normal levels of protein C at the initiation of therapy, resulting in a procoagulant-anticoagulant imbalance favoring thrombosis.

The transmission of symptomatic heterozygous protein C deficiency appears to be autosomal dominant, but asymptomatic heterozygotes are commonly detected in the families of homozygous patients. Asymptomatic heterozygotes have been detected by random screening of blood bank donors. These observations suggest that protein C deficiency may be caused by a variety of molecular defects. Numerous differing mutations in the protein C gene have been associated with protein C deficiency, but the clinically "dominant" and "recessive" forms of the disease cannot be segregated on the basis of these mutations. The possibility exists of a closely linked second abnormality responsible for expression of the disease in some heterozygotes. Symptomatic heterozygote patients can be treated with Coumadin, but it should be administered simultaneously with heparin until adequate anticoagulation with Coumadin is achieved.

Heterozygous protein S deficiency results in recurrent thromboses with a pattern similar to heterozygous protein C deficiency.

Antithrombin III deficiency is inherited as an autosomal dominant trait. Thromboses occur, beginning in the second decade of life. Heparin resistance can be a feature of antithrombin III deficiency, because antithrombin III is a cofactor for heparin. Anticoagulation can be achieved with Coumadin.

Thrombosis has been associated with qualitative and quantitative abnormalities of plasminogen, impaired plasminogen activator release, dysfibrinogenemias, and reduced levels of heparin cofactor II. The inheritance pattern in these cases is less clear.

## Acquired Abnormalities of Coagulation Factors

### Vitamin K Deficiency

Vitamin K is an essential substrate for the synthesis of procoagulant and anticoagulant proteins, including factors II, VII, IX, X, protein C, and protein S. Identical clinical states can be produced by absence of vitamin K or interference with its action by pharmacologic means. Dietary vitamin K consists mainly of vitamin K$_1$, a fat-soluble naphthaquinone found in leafy vegetables. Intestinal bacteria also synthesize vitamin K compounds. Therapeutically and physiologically, the fat-soluble forms of vitamin K appear to be most useful, and toxicity has resulted from the administration of water-soluble analogues. True dietary deficiency of vitamin K appears to be unusual, except in early infancy or in the setting of prolonged intravenous feedings without supplemental administration of vitamin K. Most cases of apparent dietary insufficiency in older children are caused by malabsorptive syndromes, such as pancreatic insufficiency, biliary obstruction, prolonged diarrhea affecting absorption of vitamin K in the upper small intestine, or the administration of drugs. Drugs that antagonize or interfere with the metabolism of vitamin K include phenobarbital, diphenylhydantoin, some cephalosporins, rifampin, isoniazid, and coumarin. Vitamin K deficiency due to antibiotic suppression of intestinal flora appears to be unusual without a dietary deficiency of vitamin K.

Uncomplicated vitamin K deficiency is characterized by bleeding symptoms (eg, bruising, oozing from puncture sites of the skin, visceral hemorrhage) with an acquired prolongation of the PT and aPTT and a normal fibrinogen. Other clotting factors that are produced in the liver but are not vitamin K dependent (eg, factors V, XI, XII, VIII) are normal. However, the clinical and laboratory picture is often affected by a primary disorder that produces liver disease and malabsorption or decreased utilization of vitamin K, such as biliary atresia, cystic fibrosis, hemolytic anemia with obstructive jaundice, hepatitis, $\alpha_1$-antitrypsin deficiency, or a betalipoproteinemia. In the absence of severe hepatic disease or antagonists, the response to vitamin K is rapid, usually occurring within 6 hours. Anaphylactoid reactions may occur with parenteral administration of vitamin K, but they are unusual. Infusion of plasma is effective in emergent situations.

Hemorrhagic disease of the newborn appears to represent a special case of vitamin K deficiency. As classified by Hathaway, hemorrhagic disease of the newborn can occur in early, classic, and late forms. Early hemorrhagic disease of the newborn often occurs in the setting of maternal ingestion of vitamin K antagonists (eg, anticonvulsants, antituberculous drugs) but may be unassociated with known risk factors. Early disease presents in the first 24 hours of life, often with catastrophic bleeding. Classic hemorrhagic disease of the newborn occurs after the first day of life, usually within the first week. Purpura, oozing from the umbilical cord or circumcision site, hematemesis, hematuria, and gastrointestinal and vaginal bleeding are common symptoms, but intracranial hemorrhage is rare. Premature infants are at increased risk for developing hemorrhagic symptoms. Late-onset disease occurs 1 to 3 months after birth and is associated with a high incidence of central nervous system hemorrhage and mortality. Exclusive breast-feeding without vitamin K supplementation and failure to administer parenteral vitamin K at birth appear to be at least contributing and probably causative factors in classic and late disease. Some cases of early disease may not respond to parenteral vitamin K at birth, and there is some question about whether all cases of late disease can be prevented by a single early dose of parenteral vitamin K alone. The trends toward decreased use of parenteral vitamin K as prophylactic treatment for hemorrhagic disease of the newborn do not appear to be justified, and routine prophylactic treatment of all infants is still recommended.

## Liver Disease

The liver is the major site of production of most coagulation factors and is important for the clearance of activated factors and fibrin degradation products. In pathological states, reduced synthesis of clotting factors is common and often affects the vitamin K-dependent factors most severely. In addition consumption of clotting factors and platelets occurs frequently in liver disease. Essentially all of the laboratory abnormalities seen in DIC may occur in severe liver disease, including prolonged PT and aPTT, increased fibrin degradation products, and thrombocytopenia. Factor VIII appears to be relatively spared in liver disease because of significant extrahepatic synthesis; simultaneous measurements of factor VIII and one or more factors made primarily in the liver (eg, factor VII and IX) can help to differentiate hepatic disease from DIC, in which factor VIII levels are usually depressed. Recent studies have shown that protein C is reduced in many forms of liver disease, which may explain some of the thrombotic complications observed in hepatic diseases.

Treatment of the coagulopathy associated with liver disease usually involves treatment with vitamin K to protect against deficiency or impaired utilization of vitamin K due to hepatocellular disease, fresh frozen plasma to replace factors synthesized in the liver, and platelets as necessary. If volume considerations become important, fibrinogen levels can be raised by administration of cryoprecipitate. Rarely, replacement with vitamin K-dependent factor concentrates may be indicated in patients with life-threatening disease, but administration of these factors to patients with liver disease carries a high risk of thrombotic complications.

## Disseminated Intravascular Coagulation

DIC describes a constellation of clinical and laboratory abnormalities indicative of a combination of accelerated fibrinogenesis and fibrinolysis. Rather than being considered a disease in and of itself, DIC should be thought of as a secondary phenomenon that occurs in response to a variety of stimuli. DIC may be triggered by local or systemic factors. Examples of local problems that can result in systemic DIC include hemangiomas (ie, Kasabach-Merritt syndrome), in which a localized vascular lesion results in consumption of fibrinogen and platelets and in which elevations of fibrin degradation products can be massive, and brain injury, in which release of thromboplastic substances may initiate systemic clotting. Abruptio placenta and massive pulmonary emboli may also produce systemic signs of DIC. Systemic causes of DIC include sepsis, shock of any cause, transfusion of incompatible blood, and injection of snake venom. DIC is encountered in toxemia of pregnancy, respiratory distress syndrome, malignancies, burns, hypothermia, heat stroke, postoperative states, and any situation in which massive tissue damage is encountered. The severity of DIC varies widely, from transient and insignificant to overwhelming. Patients with DIC manifest purpura, and oozing from incisions or venipuncture sites is common. Circulatory collapse may occur.

Purpura fulminans represents a special systemic form of DIC. This rare disorder is characterized at its onset by purpura and DIC, usually in association with viral (eg, varicella), bacterial (eg, meningococcal, streptococcal) or rickettsial infections or severe hypernatremia. Pathologically, this disease is characterized by widespread microthrombi in the vascular bed of a variety of organs. Renal failure is common. The purpuric lesions are often symmetric and show sharply demarcated borders with a surrounding inflammatory reaction. Scarring of the skin and loss of extremities is common, and the fatality rate is high. Rarely purpura fulminans may be seen as a manifestation of protein C deficiency, which was discussed previously.

Laboratory findings in DIC include thrombocytopenia, prolongation of the PT and aPTT, and a reduction of clotting factors, particularly fibrinogen and factors II, V, and VIII. Protein C levels are reduced. Microangiopathic changes in the erythrocytes may be seen in the peripheral blood smear. Plasma levels of fibrin degradation products are usually elevated and may play a pathogenetic role by inhibiting clotting and platelet function. Measurement of fibrinopeptide A, a cleavage product of fibrinogen, and fibrinogen turnover studies increase the diagnostic sensitivity, but these assays are not routinely available.

Treatment of DIC should be aimed primarily at correcting the inciting cause. Concern has been raised about the possibility of "feeding the fire" by administering clotting factors and platelet concentrates. However, the risks of allowing severe thrombocytopenia or hypofibrinogenemia to develop are not warranted on the basis of what are mostly theoretical concerns, and replacement therapy should be given if the consumption has been severe. Heparin may be helpful in some cases if the underlying defect cannot be corrected, but its usefulness is still a matter of debate. Some authors think that heparin is particularly effective in purpura fulminans if initiated early in the illness. EACA may be helpful in cases of DIC with low levels of $\alpha_2$-antiplasmin due to hypergranular promyelocytic leukemia, but it is not considered useful in other forms of DIC.

## Circulating Anticoagulants

Circulating anticoagulants occur most often in children with preexisting specific factor deficiencies; anti-factor VIII antibodies are the most common agents. Anticoagulants are sometimes seen in patients without previous coagulation abnormalities. Many of these patients have underlying immunoregulatory abnormalities or malignancies. Patients infected with HIV frequently develop circulating anticoagulants due to antiphospholipid antibodies. Inhibitors of coagulation occur in otherwise healthy patients after the administration of antibiotics or following viral infections. The true incidence of circulating anticoagulants is difficult to assess, because most patients do not have symptoms. However, in a study of more than 1600 patients in which aPTTs were used as a preoperative screen, 11 patients (0.7%) had circulating anticoagulants.

Acquired anticoagulants are usually IgG molecules and may be directed toward specific coagulation factors. Inhibitors directed against specific factors appear to be more common in adults, and the bleeding disorder can mimic the deficiency state for that factor. Inhibitors occurring in children without underlying disease are often not directed against any one factor and not associated with symptoms. Inhibitors of coagulation are seen in patients with systemic lupus erythematosus. The lupus anticoagulant appears to inhibit intermediate complexes in the coagulation cascade and usually does not inhibit a single specific factor. The lupus anticoagulant and other antiphospholipid antibodies usually are not associated with bleeding symptoms but may be associated with an increased frequency of thrombosis.

Circulating anticoagulants should be looked for in any patient with an unexplained prolongation of the PT or aPTT.

## Miscellaneous Acquired Coagulation Abnormalities

Low levels of clotting factors and elevated fibrin-split products have been reported in children with cyanotic congenital heart disease and polycythemia. Many of these abnormalities are probably explained by concomitant hepatic dysfunction. A variety of coagulation disturbances may be seen after cardiac surgery, including reduced clotting factors and elevations of fibrin-split products, sometimes as a manifestation of DIC. These defects occur most commonly as a result of cardiopulmonary bypass or deep hypothermia, but their exact nature is poorly understood. Depressions of factors VIII and IX have been described in hypothyroidism. The depressions disappear after reinstitution of the euthyroid state. Amyloidosis has been associated with deficiencies of factors V, VII, IX, and X. L-Asparaginase therapy depresses many coagulation factors, including antithrombin III and protein C. These abnormalities may explain the thromboses that occur in children after the use of L-asparaginase therapy. Variable depressions and elevations of specific clotting factors have been described in the nephrotic syndrome, including antithrombin III deficiency. Hypofibrinogenemia has been reported after administration of valproate, and dysfibrinogenemias have been associated with tumors, liver disease, and pseudotumor cerebri.

## Hypercoagulability

Numerous clinical states have been associated with a predisposition to thrombosis. Stasis due to immobilization, hyperviscosity, polycythemia, congestive heart failure, vascular damage or occlusion secondary to sickle cell disease or other causes is a major etiologic factor of thrombosis. Similarly, abnormal intravascular surfaces due to indwelling catheters, artificial heart valves, arteritides (eg, Kawasaki disease, polyarteritis), or homocysteinemia may result in thromboses. A thrombotic tendency may be seen in the setting of malignancies, liver disease, renal disease, infection, inflammatory disease (eg, ulcerative colitis, regional enteritis), diabetes mellitus, paroxysmal nocturnal he-

moglobinuria, contraceptive use, or pregnancy. Hypercoagulability may be seen in patients with the lupus anticoagulant or other antiphospholipid antibodies, nephrotic syndrome, or after the administration of coagulation factors or drugs such as L-asparaginase, warfarin, EACA, or heparin.

Even in patients with hereditary defects predisposing to thromboses, additional factors are often the trigger to clinically evident thromboses. Numerous insights into the possible mechanisms by which other clinical states may result in thromboses are available. Protein C levels, for example, are low in liver disease, DIC, after L-asparaginase therapy and have been shown to decrease after surgery at about the time that deep venous thromboses are found. Antithrombin III levels are depressed in nephrotic syndrome, pregnancy, DIC, liver disease, oral contraceptive use, and after administration of heparin or L-asparaginase. Although it is tempting to assume causality in these instances, it is important to remember that other coagulation factors are dramatically affected in these situations and that the expression of hemorrhage or thrombosis is the result of a complicated interplay among multiple factors.

# VASCULAR ABNORMALITIES

Diseases that affect the integrity of blood vessels may present with hemorrhagic symptoms. The results of coagulation testing usually are normal for these patients, despite the clinical signs of hemorrhage.

## Henoch-Schönlein Purpura

Henoch-Schönlein (anaphylactoid) purpura is an idiopathic vasculitis that results in a distinctive clinical syndrome involving serosanguineous effusions into a variety of tissues. Purpuric lesions involving the buttocks and lower extremities, subserosal hemorrhage of the gastrointestinal tract, periarticular effusions with arthralgias, and glomerulitis with hematuria, proteinuria, and renal dysfunction are its most distinctive features. The skin lesions are often urticarial at their onset and then develop into flat, purpuric lesions. Despite the purpuric nature of the lesions, platelet counts are normal. Painful edema of the scalp, scrotum, or other areas of the body may occur, most frequently in younger children. Gastrointestinal lesions often are accompanied by episodic severe abdominal pain, and intussusception may develop. The joint involvement tends to be periarticular, and true arthritis is usually not found. The renal lesion is of greatest concern and often results in long-standing renal disease. Hypertension is common. A small proportion of patients may display neurologic symptoms, including seizures. A variety of etiologic factors have been postulated, such as streptococcal infections and a number of food allergies, but none has been conclusively demonstrated.

Although the renal lesion does not respond to steroids, symptoms may be controlled, and steroids are generally thought to be indicated if intussusception is suspected. The duration of the illness is quite variable from weeks to months, often with multiple exacerbations.

## Hereditary Hemorrhagic Telangiectasia

Hereditary hemorrhagic telangiectasia is an autosomal dominant condition characterized by localized dilatation and tortuosity of small veins and capillaries of the skin and mucous membranes. The number of telangiectatic lesions tends to increase with age, and they are most commonly seen on the lips, oral mucosa, ears, and palmar and plantar surfaces of the fingers and toes. Telangiectatic lesions may occur in the visceral organs. Symptoms are caused by bleeding from abnormally friable telangiectatic vessels.

Gastrointestinal hemorrhage and epistaxis are common. Pulmonary and urinary bleeding may occur. If bleeding has been excessive, iron deficiency anemia may ensue.

## Miscellaneous Causes of Vascular Abnormalities and Hemorrhages

A wide variety of other insults or underlying diseases can damage blood vessels, with consequent hemorrhagic symptoms. Many viral, bacterial, and rickettsial illnesses can cause vascular purpura with or without thrombocytopenia. Purpuric lesions are a common manifestation of bacterial endocarditis, meningococcemia, and Rocky Mountain spotted fever, and they are sometimes seen in varicella, measles, and enteroviral infections.

Many other infectious processes less commonly produce purpura. Vasculitides (eg, collagen-vascular disorders) may produce purpura and serious bleeding into the lungs, kidneys, and other organs. Cushing's syndrome may be associated with purpuric lesions, as are Ehlers-Danlos syndrome, pseudoxanthoma elasticum, osteogenesis imperfecta, and scurvy. Purpura may be produced by direct mechanical trauma to the skin and its blood vessels. In some patients, self-inflicted trauma is used to cause bleeding to obtain medical attention.

## Selected Readings

Bell WR. Disseminated intravascular coagulopathy. In: Hartmann PM, ed. Guide to hematologic disorders. New York: Grune & Stratton, 1980:159.

Bloom AL. Progress in the clinical management of hemophilia. Thromb Haemostasis 1991;66:166.

Buchanan GR. Overview of ITP treatment modalities in children. Blut 1989;59:96.

Burk CD, Miller L, Handler SD, Cohen AR. Preoperative history and coagulation screening in children undergoing tonsillectomy. Pediatrics 1992;89:691.

Bussel J, Kaplan C. Recommendations for the evaluation and treatment of neonatal autoimmune and alloimmune thrombocytopenia. Thromb Haemostasis 1991;65:631.

Clouse LH, Comp PC. The regulation of hemostasis: the protein C system. N Engl J Med 1986;314:1298.

Furie B, Furie BC. Molecular and cellular biology of blood coagulation. N Engl J Med 1992;326:800.

Hathaway WE. New insights on vitamin K. Hematol Oncol Clin North Am 1987;1:367.

Rapaport SI. Preoperative hemostatic evaluation: which tests, if any? Blood 1983;61:229.

White GC, Montgomery RR. Clinical aspects and therapy for von Willebrand disease. In: Hoffman R, Benz EJ, Shattil SJ, Furie B, Cohen HJ, eds. Hematology: basic principles and practice, ed 1. New York: Churchill Livingstone, 1991:1362.

# SECTION VI

# Neoplastic Diseases

*Principles and Practice of Pediatrics, Second Edition.*
edited by Frank A. Oski et al. J. B. Lippincott Company, Philadelphia © 1994.

## CHAPTER 95
## General Considerations

Donald J. Fernbach

By any measure, cancer in children is a rare disease, accounting for approximately 6000 cases annually among children younger than 15 years of age. There are more than 900,000 cases of cancer annually among adults. This disparity is in no way counterbalanced by the size of the populations of adults and children but reflects the significant role of chronic exposure to environmental toxins, particularly tobacco, in adult cancer. More than 85% of adult malignant neoplasms are carcinomas, but carcinomas are rare in children. Many of the pediatric neoplasms are associated with developmental defects, anomalies, or cytogenetic or chromosomal aberrations. Environmental factors do play a role in pediatric neoplastic disease, but the associations are different for pediatric patients than for adults. Environmental factors may play a role by triggering neoplastic transformation of preexisting defects. The most common cancers in children involve the hematopoietic tissue, the central nervous system, and connective tissues (ie, sarcomas).

Many of the tumors in children can be anticipated on the basis of preexisting immunologic deficiency states, genetic and chromosomal disorders, and congenital anomalies (Tables 95-1 through 95-4). These patients require careful observation and regular evaluation.

Family history of a high incidence of cancer is an important consideration. Some of the syndromes described may not appear until the child is older and need not be considered in the very young infant. Except for these conditions, the detection of cancer in children requires the pediatrician to be alert to the possibility. The seven warning signals of cancer in adults are of limited help in evaluating the pediatric patient. Warning signs in children can include fever, pain, a mass, purpura, pallor, and changes in gait, balance, personality, and the eyes (eg, squint, retinal reflections). Some of these are nonspecific pediatric complaints, but the alert primary physician can quickly sort out the unusual from the usual problems.

Fever is a universal pediatric complaint that brings children to the physician. Unrelenting fever may reflect an occult lymphoma or may be secondary to necrosis within a solid tumor, such as neuroblastoma or Wilms' tumor. In Langerhans' histio-cytosis, persisting fever may be the only presenting complaint. Recurrent or Pel-Ebstein fever, seen in adults with Hodgkin disease, is rarely seen in children. Peripheral blood counts can be helpful in explaining the problem underlying the fever. Neutropenia predisposes patients with leukemia to infection; on the surface, the infection may appear to be routine, except for the failure to respond to appropriate therapy. Peripheral blood counts are a good starting point in evaluating these patients, and leukemic cells often may be seen on the peripheral blood smear. A bone marrow examination can immediately confirm or rule out a disorder of the bone marrow.

Pain is another reason parents seek medical advice. Trauma frequently precedes the bone pain of bone tumors. Localized pain may occur with tumors in any location, but many childhood tumors can grow quite large without complaints of pain. Morning headaches, especially associated with morning vomiting, may indicate increased intracranial pressure. However, in infants, open sutures may permit a natural decompression and mask symptoms of intracranial disease. Unusual irritability may be a symptom in the very young child. Persistent pain in any joint or bone is a common complaint of children with leukemia.

A mass always deserves prompt attention. Regardless of the child's age, all masses in the abdomen should be considered to be malignant until proven otherwise. Computed tomography (CT) or real-time sonography are effective diagnostic clinical aids that may identify the problem quickly. Persistent lymphadenopathy is another common pediatric complaint. If a node increases in size after 2 weeks or fails to regress after 4 to 6 weeks, a biopsy is recommended. Nontender, firm lymph nodes should raise the suspicion of disease, as should any swollen lymph node in an unusual location such as in the supraclavicular area, and should lead to early biopsy.

Purpura and pallor usually reflect bone marrow failure with resultant thrombocytopenia and anemia. A bone marrow examination may be diagnostic.

---

**TABLE 95-1. Immune Deficiency Diseases Predisposing to Neoplastic Disease**

X-linked lymphoproliferative disease
Bruton's agammaglobulinemia
Severe combined immunodeficiency
Wiskott-Aldrich syndrome
IgA deficiency
Common variable immunodeficiency
DiGeorge syndrome
Ataxia telangiectasia
Chédiak-Higashi syndrome

**TABLE 95-2. Genetic Instability and DNA Repair Disorders Associated With Childhood Cancer**

| Disorders | Cancers |
| --- | --- |
| Xeroderma pigmentosum | Basal, squamous cell carcinoma, melanoma |
| Bloom syndrome | Leukemia, lymphoma, gastrointestinal cancers |
| Fanconi's anemia | Leukemia, hepatoma, squamous cell carcinoma |
| Ataxia telangiectasia | Lymphoma, leukemia, Hodgkin's disease, brain, gastric, ovarian, other epithelial cancers |

**TABLE 95-4. Congenital Malformations Associated With Tumors**

| Malformations | Tumor |
| --- | --- |
| Aniridia | Wilms' tumor |
| Hemihypertrophy | Wilms' tumor |
| Cryptorchidism | Testicular tumors |
| Gonadal dysgenesis | Gonadoblastoma |
| Enchondromatosis (Ollier's disease) | Chondrosarcoma |

Changes in gait or balance or other neurologic abnormalities such as head tilt are common complaints in children with posterior fossa tumors. There are a variety of neurologic problems that can result from brain tumors, and some of them may be subtle, such as personality changes in children with supratentorial tumors. Some of these subtle problems may be recognized only by the mother at first. More than a few parents have complained about difficulty in convincing physicians that something was wrong with their child. Fortunately, CT scans of the head are of tremendous diagnostic value and have enhanced the ability of physicians to make an early diagnosis of intracranial lesions. Magnetic resonance imaging has taken this a step further. These techniques have proven invaluable in following these patients.

Changes of vision may be accompanied at first by squinting and later by an obvious yellow-white reflex leukokoria (ie, cat's eye reflex) resulting from retinoblastoma. Complaints about the eye usually warrant an ophthalmologic examination, even if there is no obvious physical abnormality. This often requires sedation or anesthesia in the young child.

After a malignant neoplasm is suspected, the application of many modern imaging techniques can be most helpful in specifying the location and extent of the problem. The approach to the diagnosis should be based on the type of tumor suspected. Many of the lymphomas, and solid tumors such as neuroblastoma and rhabdomyosarcoma, metastasize early. Metastatic disease of the bone marrow may lead to a quick diagnosis and, coupled with the use of electron microscopy, may provide a specific tissue diagnosis in lieu of a major surgical procedure. If the marrow examination is not diagnostic, then the appropriate surgical procedure can be performed.

Knowledge of the precise histologic diagnosis and extent of the disease (ie, staging) is essential before planning any type of therapy. Ideal management usually involves a team approach,

**TABLE 95-3. Constitutional Chromosome Disorders Associated With Childhood Cancers**

| Disorders | Cancers |
| --- | --- |
| Down syndrome | Leukemia, testicular, retinoblastoma |
| Turner's syndrome | Neurogenic, gonadal, endometrial |
| Klinefelter's dynrome | Leukemia, germ cell tumors |
| Other sex aneuploidy | Retinoblastoma |
| SY gonadal dysgenesis | Gonadoblastoma, dysgerminoma |
| Trisomy 13 | Teratoma, leukemia, neurogenic |
| Trisomy 18 | Neurogenic, Wilms' tumor |
| XYY, XYY mosaic | Osteosarcoma, medulloblastoma |

which may include surgeons, pediatric hematologists–oncologists, radiologists, pathologists, radiotherapists, and other specialists, depending on the diagnosis and the complications at the time. The management should consider the effect of the diagnosis on all family members, so that provisions can be made for social service and psychologic counseling as needed.

Pediatric tumors are much more responsive to therapy than adult cancers. Progress during the last 25 years has resulted in a dramatic improvement of the overall survival rate, which is approximately 60% for all children with cancer. Because of the dramatic success with treatment and subsequent reduction of the mortality rate, it is important that each child suspected of or found to have cancer be given a chance to receive the most current available therapy. There are few tumors for which therapy has become standardized, although for specific diseases such as Wilms' tumor, therapy is close to being standardized (survival rate exceeds 90%). Nevertheless, cancer remains the leading cause of death from disease in children between 1 and 18 years of age. Optimal therapy for any of the childhood cancers is most likely to be found in pediatric cancer centers.

*Principles and Practice of Pediatrics, Second Edition.* edited by Frank A. Oski et al. J. B. Lippincott Company, Philadelphia © 1994.

# CHAPTER 96
# *Leukemias*

## 96.1 *Acute Lymphoblastic Leukemia in Childhood*

### Donald H. Mahoney, Jr.

In the past 25 years, there has been dramatic improvement in the treatment of children with acute lymphoblastic leukemia (ALL). ALL once was considered an incurable disease, but approximately 65% of the children newly diagnosed with ALL now survive in complete continuous remission for more than 5 years and remain free of disease.

An expanded understanding of the biologic, immunologic, and genetic heterogeneity of this disease has enabled development of more effective therapeutic strategies. An increased appreciation of the pharmacologic basis for antileukemic therapy has resulted in more successful chemotherapy programs and central nervous system (CNS) therapy. Advance life-support capabilities have permitted the delivery of such therapy. Ongoing comprehensive clinical investigations directed by pediatric cancer centers in cooperation with referring practicing physicians and collaborating basic science laboratories are the principal reasons for this success.

## ETIOLOGY

Acute leukemia is the most common malignancy diagnosed in children. An estimated 2000 cases of leukemia in children younger than 15 years of age occur in the United States each year. Based on mortality statistics, the overall incidence is estimated at 40 per one million children younger than 15 years of age. Approximately three fourths of the cases are ALL and most of the remaining cases of leukemia are acute nonlymphocytic leukemia. In the United States, childhood ALL has a peak incidence between 2 and 6 years of age in white populations but not in blacks. The reason for this difference is unexplained. Childhood ALL occurs more frequently in boys than in girls, and the difference increases with age. Geographic variation in incidence, rates, and subtype of leukemia (ie, leukemic clusters) has been reported in the United States and worldwide. For example, in Turkey, acute myelomonocytic leukemia accounts for approximately 35% of the cases, and in Shanghai, China, almost one half of the children with a diagnosis of leukemia have acute nonlymphocytic leukemia.

The molecular basis for leukemic transformation in humans is unknown. In normal bone marrow, undifferentiated pluripotent "progenitor" cells with a capacity for self-renewal give rise to committed progenitor cells. These are morphologically recognizable cells that give rise to the erythroid, myeloid, megakaryocytic, eosinophilic, and monocytic-macrophage series. In the clonal expansion theory, leukemia arises from a damaged progenitor cell that has the propensity of unlimited self-renewal or has lost the ability to differentiate along the lines of normal committed progenitor cells. The biologic events leading up to the development of this damaged precursor have not been determined.

A variety of environmental, genetic, viral, and immunologic factors may contribute to the development of disease (Table 96-1). Of the possible environmental factors, ionizing radiation has been the most extensively studied. The increased incidence of leukemia in survivors within 1000 m of the atomic bomb explosions during World War II has been well documented. ALL developed most frequently in those younger than 15 years of age at the time of exposure. A more contemporary concern is the relative leukemogenic risk of low-level radiation exposure. Early studies suggested an increased cancer mortality among children of mothers who received diagnostic radiographs during pregnancy. However, questions remain as to what levels of exposure are significant and how estimates of leukemia should be obtained. The relative risk of contracting leukemia or other forms of cancer in persons exposed to electromagnetic fields has been investigated in several studies but no definitive cause and effect association has been established.

Several chemical agents are known to induce or promote leukemia in animals. However, except for benzene exposure, little is known about the importance of such agents in humans. With the exception of second malignancies in children previously treated with chemotherapy, usually including alkylating agents with or without radiation therapy, no clear association for chemical carcinogenesis has been established in children.

A viral cause for leukemia has been sought for several years.

### TABLE 96-1.   Risk Estimates for Developing Childhood Leukemia

| Population at Risk | Estimate Risk | Time Interval (Years) |
|---|---|---|
| U.S. Caucasian children | 1:2800 | 10 |
| Siblings of child with leukemia | 1:700 | 10 |
| Identical twin of a child with leukemia | 1:5 | Weeks to months |
| Children with | | |
| Down syndrome | 1:75 | 10 |
| Fanconi's syndrome | 1:12 | 21 |
| Bloom's syndrome | 1:8 | 26 |
| Ataxia telangiectasia | 1:8 | 25 |
| Exposures | | |
| Atom bomb within 1000 m | 1:60 | 12 |
| Ionizing radiation | ? | 10–25 |
| Benzene | 1:960 | 12 |
| Alkylating agents | 1:2000? | 10–20 |

A small number of RNA viruses, classified as retroviruses, have direct oncogenic potential. These viruses, such as the Rous sarcoma virus and the feline leukemia virus, have caused oncogenic transformations in a variety of animal species but have not been associated with cross-species transmission and cancer in humans. These retroviruses owe their transforming function to a class of nonessential genes called v-onc genes. A number of cellular oncogenes (c-onc) or proto-oncogenes, which are the stable nontransforming counterpart of the viral oncogenes, have been identified in human tissue. The normal functions of many of these genes have not been identified, but in the cancer cell, increased expression or rearrangement of these genes has been observed and appears to be important in malignant transformation. The human T-cell lymphotrophic virus (HTLV-I) is a retrovirus that has been isolated from a subset of patients with adult T-cell leukemia. Whether the HTLV-I agent is a direct cause for leukemia remains to be established.

An unusual susceptibility to leukemia has been associated with certain heritable diseases, chromosomal disorders, and constitutional syndromes. Children with trisomy 21 (ie, Down syndrome) have at least a 10-fold to 15-fold increased risk for developing leukemia compared with normal children. The greatest risk period for leukemia in Down syndrome is before 5 years of age. Before 3 years of age, acute nonlymphoblastic leukemia predominates. Increased chromosomal fragility may predispose these patients to leukemic transformation. Cases of childhood leukemia have been associated with several heritable syndromes, including Klinefelter's syndrome, Rubinstein-Taybi syndrome, Poland's syndrome, Shwachman syndrome, neurofibromatosis, and Kostmann's congenital agranulocytosis. The relation between these syndromes and leukemia and other childhood cancers requires further definition.

Several immunodeficiency states have an associated increased risk for lymphoma and leukemia. These conditions include the syndromes of Wiskott-Aldrich, X-linked agammaglobulinemia, severe combined immune deficiency, and ataxia telangiectasia. The loss of cellular immune surveillance capability for tumor antigens and the inability to self-regulate lymphoproliferative processes may contribute to malignant transformation in these patients. When a child with an identical twin develops leukemia, the risk for leukemia in the other twin is approximately 20%, but the risk diminishes with age. Fraternal twins and siblings of children with leukemia have an estimated fourfold greater risk for leukemia than children in the general population. However, an annual risk that increases from 4 per 100,000 to 16 per 100,000 is not of major clinical significance and should not be a cause for alarm for parents. Epidemiologic studies do not indicate an increased frequency of leukemia in children of leukemic parents, in children breast-fed by mothers who subsequently develop leukemia, in recipients of blood products from donors who develop leukemia, or in households with pets with leukemia.

## CLASSIFICATION AND CYTOGENETIC ASPECTS

Childhood leukemia is a heterogenous disease. Morphologic, immunologic, biochemical, and cytogenetic features are used to characterize the disease, estimate prognosis, and develop successful therapeutic strategies. Under normal conditions, less than 5% of the nucleated marrow is composed of blast forms. *Blasts* are primitive, undifferentiated-appearing precursor cells not normally seen in the peripheral circulation, except in unusual circumstances. With the Wright-Giemsa stain, blasts can be recognized by their large size and high nuclear-cytoplasmic ratio. The nuclear membrane is round or clefted, and the nuclear chromatin appears fine and homogeneous with an occasional small nucleolus. The leukemic lymphoblast frequently reacts with the periodic acid-Schiff stain and with terminal deoxynucleotidyl transferase. The acid phosphatase stain may also be strongly positive in lymphoblasts of T-cell immunophenotype. The lymphoblast is further characterized by the absence of a reaction with myeloperoxidase, Sudan black, and esterase stains.

In 1976, a French-American-British (FAB) cooperative group developed a system for morphologic classification of acute leukemias. The acute lymphoblastic leukemias were divided into three classes:

L1: lymphoblasts are small, have scant cytoplasm and indistinct nucleoli.
L2: lymphoblasts are larger and and more heterogeneous in size, have more abundant cytoplasm, prominent nucleoli, and reniform nuclear membranes.

L3: lymphoblasts are large, with a deep cytoplasmic basophilia, prominent vacuolation, and one or more nucleoli.

Approximately 85% of the children with ALL have lymphoblasts of L1 morphology. Fewer than 15% of the patients have lymphoblasts of L2 morphology. Lymphoblasts with L3 morphology are identical to Burkitt lymphoma cells, ordinarily possess surface immunoglobulin, and are associated with a distinct karyotypic abnormality—a reciprocal translocation between long arms of chromosomes 8 and 14. Specific immunologic phenotypes have not otherwise been associated with L1 or L2 morphology. The FAB classification may have some prognostic value. Childhood ALL with L1 morphology has a high remission induction rate and more prolonged survival, and patients with L3 disease have the worst prognosis.

Immunologic marker analysis has allowed lineage assignment and maturational staging of the lymphoid leukemias and has offered some insight into the pathology of these diseases. Using standard techniques, major subsets of lymphoblastic leukemia have been defined (Table 96-2), revealing several features.

Approximately 65% of the children with ALL have non-T, non-B lymphoblasts. Using monoclonal antibodies directed at specific antigen sites defined as clusters of differentiation (CD), these lymphoblasts were found to express CD10 and CD19 and the HLA-DR antigen (Ia). These lymphoblasts lack surface (sIg) and cytoplasmic (cIg) immunoglobulins, do not react with monoclonal antibodies directed at T-cell antigens, and are usually assigned to an early pre-B lineage.

Pre-B-cell ALL represents approximately 18% to 20% of the new cases of ALL. Morphologic and immunologic features are similar to the early pre-B-cell ALL, except for the presence of heavy chain (cIg) immunoglobulin within the cytoplasm.

B-cell ALL (B-ALL) is rare in children, representing 1% of all cases. The lymphoblasts are characterized by their Burkitt-like appearance and express sIg.

T-cell phenotypes represent 13% to 15% of childhood ALL. Monoclonal antibodies corresponding to different stages of intrathymic differentiation are used to identify these patients, be-

---

**TABLE 96-2. Immunologic Classification of Childhood Acute Lymphoblastic Leukemia Immunophenotypes**

| Characteristic | Early Pre-B Cell | Pre-B Cell | T Cell | B Cell |
|---|---|---|---|---|
| Percent of patients | 63%–65% | 18%–20% | 13%–15% | 1% |
| FAB | L1, L2 | L1, L2 | L1, L2 | L3 |
| E rosette positive | − | − | ++ | − |
| TdT | + | + | + | − |
| Monoclonal antibodies (CD) | | | | |
|   CD2, 5, 7 | − | − | ++++ | − |
|   CD 10 | 90 | 90 | 15–30 | +++ |
|   CD 19 | +++ | +++ | − | +++ |
|   CD20 | ++ | ++ | | ++ |
|   CD 22/24 | ++ | ++ | | ++ |
| Immunoglobulin | − | cIg$^+$ | − | sIg$^+$ |
| Ia | 97%–98% | 97%–98% | 12%–17% | 94% |
| Heavy chain gene rearrangement | ++ | ++ | − | ++ |
| Light chain gene rearrangement | +/− | +/− | − | + |
| Glucocorticoid receptors | ++++ | ++ | + | + |
| Cytogenetics | No specific pattern | T (1; 19) | T (11; 14) | T (8; 22) |

FAB, French-American-British classification; CD, cluster of differentiation, Third International Workshop, Human Leukocyte Differentiation Antigen; Ia, HLA-DR antigen; TdT, terminal deoxynucleotidyl transferase; +, observed; −, absent; ++, observed frequently; ++++, observed in most patients; +/−, observed infrequently.

cause one third to one half of T-ALL cases react with antigens of the early thymocyte state (ie, CD2, CD5, CD7).

Approximately 1% to 3% of patients fail to react with any antigen test system and are classified as undifferentiated, "null," or stem-cell leukemias.

The immunologic subtypes may be important for predicting response to conventional therapy. Patients with early pre-B-cell ALL experience an increased remission induction rate and prolonged remission and survival. Patients with pre-B-cell ALL and the t(1;19)(q23;p13) translocation may not enjoy the same degree of long-term disease control as patients with early pre-B-cell ALL. Patients with T-cell disease are frequently older (average age, 8 to 12 years) and are male (male–female ratio, 4 : 1). They frequently present with a leukocyte count over 100,000/mm³, a mediastinal mass, normal hemoglobin concentration, hepatosplenomegaly, and adenopathy. This disease is more difficult to treat and cure than other forms. Children with B-ALL have an aggressive leukemia (cell doubling time, 24 hours) and require very intensive therapies to achieve a cure. Infants (<1 year of age) frequently fail to express reactivity to any lymphoid antigens, are CD10 negative, and have a poor prognosis. Many of the cases of CD10-negative ALL have been classified in the B-cell lineage, based on immunoglobulin heavy chain gene rearrangements.

Approximately two thirds of the patients with ALL have karyotypic abnormalities involving the leukemic cell. These alterations are broadly defined as changes in chromosome number (ie, ploidy) or chromosome structure (ie, translocations, deletions, inversions). Ploidy can be determined by classic enumeration of chromosome number from metaphase preparations or by analysis of DNA content by flow cytometry. Prognostic significance has been suggested for certain cytogenetic subgroups. Patients with hyperdiploidy (>53 chromosomes/cell) without structural abnormalities have a more favorable prognosis with conventional therapy than other groups. Studies of children with ALL and a blast DNA index greater than 1.16 (approximately 20% to 30% of newly diagnosed ALL cases) report a 90% 4-year event-free survival (EFS) with modern therapy. Most newly diagnosed ALL patients have a diploid or near-diploid chromosome complement. Patients with pseudodiploid or hypodiploid chromosome numbers have a poor prognosis. Multiple leukemic stem lines occur in approximately 9% to 15% of patients. The significance of these complex chromosome combinations is not understood.

Several specific chromosome translocations have been recognized in childhood ALL and are believed to have significance for disease ontogeny and clinical outcome. The t(8;14), t(2;8), and t(8;22) are immunophenotype-specific translocations observed in B-ALL. These translocations produce a rearrangement of the MYC proto-oncogene located on chromosome 8 with the immunoglobulin heavy chain genes located on chromosome 14 or the immunoglobulin light chain genes located on chromosomes 2 and 22. The aberrant expression of these translocated genes is postulated as a critical mechanism in the malignant transformation of B-ALL. The t(9;22)(q34;q11) abnormality (ie, Philadelphia chromosome) is most commonly associated with the adult form of chronic myelogenous leukemia (CML). However, about 6% of the children with ALL present with this abnormality. A rearrangement of the ABL proto-oncogene, distinct from the ABL/BCR rearrangement described in the adult form of CML, has been described. These patients tend to present with higher leukocyte counts and have a poor prognosis.

The t(4;11)(q21;q23) translocation occurs in approximately 5% of childhood ALL and is associated with high leukocyte counts (>150,000/mm³) and often with a CD10-negative phenotype. Cytochemical studies of these leukemic cells frequently reveal monocytic features, suggesting a mixed-lineage or pluripotent leukemic stem cell as the cause of this disease. Infants presenting with ALL frequently demonstrate this translocation and other translocations involving the 11q23 region. The translocation t(11;14)(p13;q11) has been identified in as many as 25% of children with T-ALL that is E-rosette positive. A translocation of the α-chain gene for the T-cell receptor is thought to offer a proliferative advantage for the leukemic transformation. The t(1;19) abnormality has been observed in approximately 30% of the children with pre-B ALL. Loss of chromosome material at 9p21–22 has been associated with a poor prognostic group of children with ALL and lymphomatous features. Other random translocations have been reported in approximately 7% to 10% of pediatric ALL cases.

## DIAGNOSIS AND PROGNOSIS

### Clinical Presentation and Initial Laboratory Findings

In ALL, an uncontrolled proliferation of immature lymphoid cells produces bone marrow failure and may be associated with extramedullary infiltration. The presenting signs and symptoms are a reflection of these events (Table 96-3). The most common presenting symptoms are fever, pallor, purpura, and pain. The onset may be abrupt or insidious. The evolution of symptoms may proceed over a few days, weeks, or months. At first, symptoms may be nonspecific and may mimic other nonmalignant conditions. Fever, although a nonspecific complaint, is a significant symptom in the child with ALL. Fever, particularly if coupled with other nonspecific complaints, may mimic more common pediatric illnesses. Of the first 400 children with ALL treated at Texas Children's Hospital, 6% presented with fever of unknown origin and no other clinical or laboratory evidence for leukemia. The diagnosis was established by bone marrow examination. Because many of these children have absolute neutropenia (neutrophil count <500/mm³) secondary to bone marrow failure, they are at extreme risk for bacterial sepsis.

Anemia occurs in 76% of patients. It is gradual in onset, normocytic, and rarely associated with significant symptoms. In some patients, tachycardia, air hunger, apprehension, and restlessness may signal acute blood loss with impending hypovolemic shock.

Petechiae and bruising are frequently noticed on physical examination and are related to the high incidence (71%) of thrombocytopenia. Epistaxis is not uncommon, especially when thrombocytopenia is severe (platelets <20,000/mm³). Under such conditions, the child may swallow blood, experience gastrointestinal irritation, nausea, and vomiting with hematemesis, followed by melena or bloody diarrhea. All of these symptoms have a profound psychologic effect on the child, parents, and unsuspecting physician.

Symptoms of anorexia and vague abdominal pains are common. Children may present with bone, hip, or joint pain. Ar-

**TABLE 96-3. Frequency of Presenting Complaints in Childhood ALL**

| Symptoms | Frequency (%) |
|---|---|
| Fever | 43–61 |
| Pallor | 39–55 |
| Bleeding | 24–55 |
| Bone/joint pain | 31–38 |
| Abdominal pain | 9–19 |
| Anorexia | 17–33 |
| Fatigue | 30 |

thralgias and refusal to walk may reflect leukemic infiltrations of the bony cortex or the joint compartment. Lymphadenopathy is common, and some degree of hepatosplenomegaly occurs in more than half of the patients. Massive infiltrations can occur but are uncommon.

Clinical laboratory data often reveal a broad spectrum of abnormal findings. In addition to anemia and thrombocytopenia, the leukocyte counts and morphology may be abnormal. Approximately 20% of children present with leukocyte counts greater than 50,000/mm³ (range, 100 to 1,000,000/mm³). About 44% of children have leukocyte counts less than 10,000/mm³. Occasionally, hypereosinophilia has been observed and is thought to be a reactive phenomena. Leukemic blasts may or may not be seen on peripheral smears.

The diagnosis of leukemia cannot be established from peripheral blood examination alone. Osteopetrosis, myelofibrosis, granulomatous infections, sarcoid, Epstein-Barr virus (EBV) infection in the very young, other acute viral infections, and metastatic tumor are conditions that can result in the release of immature-appearing blasts into the circulation.

The diagnosis of ALL is established by bone marrow examination. In children, the bone marrow specimen is usually obtained from the posterior iliac crest rather than by sternal or pretibial puncture. Diagnostic aspirations may be technically difficult to perform because of the density of blast forms or the presence of marrow fibrosis or necrosis. A Jamshidi needle biopsy may be required for diagnosis. For patients for whom the diagnosis of ALL is strongly suspected, my colleagues and I recommend that the diagnostic bone marrow biopsy be performed by an experienced pediatric hematologist to minimize patient discomfort, avoid the necessity for repeat procedures, and maximize the bone marrow sample yield necessary for smears, electron microscopy, cytogenetic studies, and immunophenotype investigations. These studies and special experimental projects that use marrow leukemic blasts are usually required by pediatric leukemic therapeutic protocols.

The normal bone marrow contains less than 5% blasts. A minimum of 25% lymphoblasts on differential examination of the bone marrow aspirate is necessary for the diagnosis of ALL. Most children with ALL have hypercellular marrow with 60% to 100% of the cells as blasts. The presenting characteristics of childhood ALL are outlined in Table 96-4.

## Differential Diagnosis

Because children with ALL present with a variety of nonspecific symptoms, several pediatric nonmalignant conditions may be confused with leukemia. Idiopathic thrombocytopenic purpura is a common cause of bruising and petechiae in children. Anemia, leukocyte disturbances, and significant hepatosplenomegaly are not typical findings. Bone marrow examinations reveal normal or increased numbers of megakaryocytes and no increase in blast forms in children with thrombocytopenic purpura. Children with infectious mononucleosis (ie, EBV) or other acute viral illnesses may present with fever, malaise, adenopathy, splenomegaly, rash, and lymphocytosis. In the young child with EBV, lymphocytosis may be extreme (80 to 100,000/mm³), and thrombocytopenia and immunohemolytic anemia may further confuse the diagnosis. The atypical lymphocytes characteristic of these diseases are larger and pleomorphic, have more abundant pale blue cytoplasm, and may resemble the leukemic lymphoblast. Specific viral serologies can establish the diagnosis, but a bone marrow examination sometimes is necessary.

Leukemoid reactions may be observed in bacterial sepsis, acute hemolysis, granulomatous diseases, vasculitis, and metastatic tumor to the bone marrow. In these circumstances, underlying clinical events may offer some clues to the differential diagnosis.

| TABLE 96-4. Presenting Characteristics of Children With ALL | |
|---|---|
| Characteristic | Frequency (%)* |
| Age (yr) <1.5 | 6–8 |
| >1.5–10 | 72–80 |
| >10 | 15–22 |
| Sex (male) | 54–57 |
| Race (white) | 80–89 |
| Leukocyte count <10,000/mm³ | 44 |
| 10,000–50,000/mm³ | 34 |
| >50,000/mm³ | 22 |
| Platelets <20,000/mm³ | 20 |
| 20,000–100,000/mm³ | 51 |
| >100,000/mm³ | 29 |
| Hemoglobin <7.5 g/dL | 46 |
| 7.5–10 g/dL | 30 |
| >10 g/dL | 24 |
| Hepatomegaly (below umbilicus) | 8–13 |
| Splenomegaly (below umbilicus) | 11–14 |
| Lymphadenopathy | |
| None/minimal | 73 |
| Moderate/marked | 28 |
| Mediastinal mass | 8 |
| CNS symptoms | 4 |
| Immunoglobulin abnormalities (1 or more) | 9 |
| FAB L1 | 82 |
| L2 | 17 |
| L3 | 1 |
| Karyotype abnormality | 45 |

* Percentages are estimates based on accumulated data from large numbers of patients treated by the Pediatric Oncology Group and the Children's Cancer Study Group.

A bone marrow aspirate usually reveals myeloid hyperplasia. The leukemoid reaction resolves as the underlying disease is successfully managed. Isolated neutropenia may also be observed in asymptomatic infants after the use of certain medications for overwhelming bacterial sepsis. In this case, the bone marrow examination may reveal a maturational arrest of the granulocytic precursors, but increased blast forms are not usually seen.

Children with ALL presenting with fever, arthralgias, arthritis, or a limp may frequently be confused with juvenile rheumatoid arthritis (JRA). Anemia, leukocytosis, and mild splenomegaly, all of which may be observed in JRA, can be misleading. Of the first 400 children with ALL treated at Texas Children's Hospital, 4.5% presented with a diagnosis of osteomyelitis or JRA. Several of these patients were receiving anti-inflammatory agents for several weeks before the diagnosis of ALL. Until a reliable positive test for JRA becomes available, a bone marrow examination to exclude ALL should be strongly considered as part of the diagnostic evaluation of patients with atypical presentations of JRA.

Pancytopenia and fever are presenting symptoms for aplastic anemia and ALL in children, but lymphadenopathy and hepatosplenomegaly are unusual findings in aplastic anemia. The bone marrow aspirate and biopsy usually clarify the diagnosis. Patients with aplastic anemia have a hypocellular marrow with cellularity usually less than 10%, no normal marrow precursors, and only small lymphocytes seen on smears. Occasionally, the bone marrow in children with ALL is initially hypocellular, and multiple aspirates and biopsies from additional sites are necessary to establish the diagnosis. Myeloproliferative syndromes and preleukemic conditions are rare in childhood but must be considered in the differential diagnosis whenever a disturbed or dysmyelopoietic bone marrow examination is observed.

Leukemia is a small blue cell malignancy. Other small blue cell malignancies can present in childhood and may produce bone marrow invasion, with the resulting signs and symptoms of fever, pain, petechiae, bruising, and pancytopenia. Neuroblastoma is the most common pediatric solid tumor that is associated with a high frequency (70%) of bone marrow invasion in children older than 2 years of age at diagnosis. The pattern of bone marrow infiltration, including discrete clumps or rosettes, the usual presence of a retroperitoneal mass, and elevated urinary catecholamines help to differentiate this disease from ALL. Other small blue cell tumors that may produce bone marrow infiltration include rhabdomyosarcoma, non-Hodgkin's lymphoma, retinoblastoma, medulloblastoma, and Ewing's sarcoma. Other significant clinical abnormalities characteristic for these diseases help to establish the correct diagnosis.

## Prognostic Factors

The single most important prognostic factor in childhood ALL is effective therapy. Before 1970, the likelihood for long-term survival was less than 10%, but by 1990, the estimated 5-year EFS rate was in excess of 60%. During the 1970s, a poor outcome was documented for a certain subset of patients (ie, patients with high leukocyte counts, older patients, patients with T- or B-ALL) compared with other patients managed on a common chemotherapy protocol. These observations led to the development of clinical prognostic risk categories. These good-risk and poor-risk groups were an attempt to recognize biologically different forms of ALL and have resulted in the development of more aggressive forms of chemotherapy tailored for the different patient populations. As time progressed, many of the unfavorable factors were found to overlap (ie, mediastinal disease and T-ALL) or lost some of their independent significance as therapeutic regimens improved. By administering the most intensive therapy that is biologically tolerable for the patient, some therapeutic programs (eg, West German BFM [Berlin-Frankfurt-Munster] studies) have at-

tempted to cancel the prognostic factors as significant variables for survival.

For childhood ALL, the patient's age at diagnosis and the initial leukocyte count have been the two most reliable indicators for response to therapy. The very young or older child does less well with current therapy. Infants younger than 1 year of age at diagnosis have a particularly poor prognosis. Patients with high leukocyte counts ($>50,000/mm^3$) are thought to have a greater leukemic burden, an increased risk for emergence of resistant clones, and a greater risk for relapse with standard therapy. The Pediatric Oncology Group reported that ploidy of blasts is the strongest predictor for outcome in B-progenitor ALL. Selected leukemic karyotypic abnormalities have been associated with poor prognosis. Patients with the t(9;22) translocation continue to have a poor prognosis with conventional therapy, and some cancer centers now recommend bone marrow transplantation during the first remission for these patients. Other translocations, such as t(4;11) in infant ALL, t(8;14) in B-ALL, and t(1;19), are associated with high-risk diseases and require more aggressive therapy for possible cure. The commonly recognized prognostic factors for childhood ALL are listed in Table 96-5. Prognostic factors will continue to be defined and redefined as therapeutic interventions improve.

## TREATMENT

The treatment of childhood ALL has become progressively complex. Curative therapy for ALL has not been established, and investigational therapy is the treatment of choice. These therapeutic programs recognize that ALL is a heterogeneous disease, that certain risk factors may have importance for response to therapy, that optimal scheduling and delivery of effective chemotherapeutic agents have not been defined, that factors leading to relapse are unknown, and that answers to these and other questions can be obtained only through carefully conducted and critically evaluated cooperative clinical trials. Consequently, the best therapy for the child newly diagnosed with ALL is offered by pediatric cancer centers participating in ongoing clinical therapeutic trials.

Combination chemotherapy is the principal therapeutic modality for childhood ALL. The therapy can be divided into four phases:

Remission induction and consolidation (ie, intensification)
Presymptomatic central nervous system therapy (ie, prophylaxis)
Maintenance
Elective discontinuation of therapy and long-term, late-effects follow-up

## Induction and Consolidation Therapy

The objectives of remission induction are to eliminate as many leukemic cells as biologically tolerable and to reestablish a normal clinical and hematologic state for the patient. Most pediatric cancer centers use at least three drugs to achieve remission: vincristine, prednisone, L-asparaginase with or without doxorubicin or daunorubicin. Rapid cytoreduction is associated with a decreased likelihood of emergence of resistant leukemic clones and increased relapse-free survival. The estimated remission induction rates with this therapy is 95%. Patients who fail to achieve a remission at the end of 4 weeks of induction therapy have a shorter survival even if remission is eventually obtained. Combinations including doxorubicin or daunorubicin have increased remission induction rates and prolonged disease-free survival in childhood ALL in studies reported from the Dana Farber Cancer Institute and else-

TABLE 96-5.   Prognostic Factors
for Childhood ALL at Diagnosis

| Factor | Favorable | Unfavorable |
|---|---|---|
| Cell type | Lymphoid | Nonlymphoid |
| Leukocyte count | $<10,000/mm^3$ | $>50,000/mm^3$ |
| Age | 3–5 yr | <2 or >10 yr |
| Ploidy | >1.16 | <1.16 |
| Karyotype | Hyperdiploid (>53 chromosomes) | Pseudodiploid |
| | | Hypodiploid |
| | | Translocation |
| Cell lineage | CD10 positive | CD10 negative |
| | Early Pre-B cell | B > T > Pre-B cell |
| Race | Caucasian | Black |
| Sex | Female | Male |
| Central nervous system involvement | − | + |
| Organomegaly | − | + |
| Mediastinal mass | − | + |

Symbols: +, present; −, absent.

where. However, the more intensive induction schedules are associated with increased morbidity and mortality, and care must be exercised in the assignment of patients to these schedules.

The assessment of prognostic factors at diagnosis becomes useful at this point. Patients with high-risk leukemia (ie, patients with high leukocyte counts, unfavorable immunophenotypes such as T-ALL, or unfavorable cytogenetic characteristics such as the Philadelphia translocation) are assigned to more intensive treatment regimens at diagnosis. The morbidity of therapy is counterbalanced by the need for more intensive cytoreductive therapies for biologically more aggressive leukemias. At St. Jude Children's Research Hospital, a seven-drug induction schedule including high-dose methotrexate, VM-26, and cytarabine (ie, Total Therapy Study XI) was associated with an overall 4-year EFS rate of 73%, a significant improvement over previous clinical trials.

The concept of intensification of therapy was extended to the period immediately after achievement of hematologic remission. This consolidation phase of treatment was designed to deliver multiple chemotherapeutic agents in a relatively short period. The objective of treatment was to further reduce residual leukemia and minimize the development of cross-resistance. The BFM West German study group employed an intensive eight-drug induction and consolidation program (ie, BFM 76/79) followed by a late reinforcement schedule and achieved an overall disease-free survival rate of 68% at 5.5 years. The Memorial Sloan-Kettering group developed two aggressive chemotherapy regimens (ie, L-2, L-10) for childhood ALL. The overall survival for all patients on the L-2 protocol was 57% at greater than 7 years' median follow-up. The Children's Cancer Study Group (CCSG) is investigating modifications of the BFM and L-10 protocols for children with high-risk ALL. The estimated EFS for both studies is greater than 60%. However, toxic effects, particularly life-threatening infectious complications, have been a major concern in the early developmental phases of these protocols. The Dana Farber Cancer Institute has reported an overall 72% EFS at 7 years for childhood ALL using a schedule of intensive asparaginase during consolidation. Pediatric Oncology Group (POG) studies using intensive courses of intravenous methotrexate and 6-mercaptopurine in children with lower-risk ALL (ie, POG 8399) report a 4-year EFS rate of greater than 90%. Overall, patients with low-risk prognostic features at diagnosis are experiencing a superior response to these forms of intensive therapy and have a better chance for long-term survival.

## Central Nervous System Therapy

Presymptomatic CNS prophylaxis therapy is an integral component of ALL therapy. Effective CNS treatment programs have decreased the incidence of CNS leukemia as a primary site of relapse from 50% to between 6% and 10%. Several regimens have been investigated and include intrathecal methotrexate and cranial irradiation (2400 cGy); intrathecal triple therapy with methotrexate, hydrocortisone, and ara-C; and intrathecal methotrexate coupled with high-dose intravenous methotrexate.

In early studies from St. Jude Children's Research Hospital, cranial irradiation and intrathecal methotrexate were established as effective of preventing CNS leukemia. Subsequent investigations by the CCSG suggested that lower radiation doses (1800 cGy) coupled with intrathecal therapy were as effective and potentially less toxic. Three consecutive studies reported by the POG demonstrated equivalent disease control with triple intrathecal therapy without cranial irradiation in patients with B-progenitor ALL. Potential delayed effects after cranial irradiation, including growth delay and intellectual impairment, prompted further investigations of alternative treatment schedules that exclude irradiation.

## Maintenance Therapy

The rationale for extended treatment during remission is based on historic evidence that patients discontinuing therapy 6 months or less after achieving remission relapsed rapidly. The common element in all maintenance or continuation schedules has been the use of weekly methotrexate and daily 6-mercaptopurine. Pharmacologic investigations suggest marked variability in the bioavailability of orally administered methotrexate and 6-mercaptopurine. Several current protocols seek evidence about whether "pulse" high-dose chemotherapy schedules or regular systemic administration of these agents is more effective therapy.

Additional chemotherapeutic agents have been administered in pulses during maintenance in an effort to prevent relapse. Vincristine and prednisone, VM-26 and ara-C, and methotrexate and ara-C are a few examples of such combinations. Late intensification therapy has also been investigated by St. Jude researchers and other groups. The efficacy of these pulse combinations has not as yet been established.

## Cessation of Therapy

The minimal duration for effective chemotherapy has not been established, partially because of an inability to recognize minimal residual disease. The standard duration of therapy is 2 to 3 years. Improved disease-free survival has not been clearly established for therapy schedules extending beyond 3 years in remission. Historically, 20% to 25% of the children with ALL discontinuing therapy after 3 years relapsed. The risk of relapse was greatest within the first year off therapy, with virtually no relapses occurring 4 years after cessation. Unfortunately, isolated cases of relapsed leukemia have been reported as late as 10 to 15 years after cessation of therapy.

For children who remain in continuous complete remission for 2 to 3 years on therapy, it has been the practice to discontinue therapy and to observe closely during the first 1 to 2 years off therapy for evidence of relapse. Because of the risk for late recurrence, these children require periodic monitoring indefinitely. Whether children will continue to experience this rate of relapse after discontinuation of current protocols remains to be determined.

## Complications of Therapy and Supportive Care

At diagnosis, the critical issues of management relate directly to complications of the leukemic burden. Patients with high leukocyte counts at diagnosis, massive organomegaly, or immunophenotypes such as T- or B-ALL are at greatest risk for these complications (Table 96-6).

Hyperleukocytosis in leukemia is associated with early morbidity and mortality due to complex metabolic complications and leukostasis in the vertebral and pulmonary vasculature. Early introduction of cytoreductive chemotherapy is essential. Exchange transfusion and leukapheresis may also be useful. Life-threatening metabolic complications may result from spontaneous or chemotherapy-induced leukemic cell lysis. Hyperuricemia, hyperkalemia, and hyperphosphatemia with secondary hypocalcemia may develop within hours of the diagnosis and treatment. Careful hydration, alkalinization of the urine, and allopurinol are useful for managing hyperuricemia. A progressive rise in BUN and creatinine, phosphorous, or potassium levels require early intervention with hemodialysis. Drugs such as cyclophosphamide and vincristine may induce a syndrome of inappropriate antidiuretic hormone secretion.

Hemorrhage in children with ALL usually is caused by thrombocytopenia. The skin and mucous membranes are the usual sites

**TABLE 96-6. Potential Complications of Childhood ALL and Its Therapy**

Metabolic complications
  Hyperuricemia
  Hyperkalemia
  Hyperphosphatemia
  SIADH
  Hyponatremia
Hemorrhage (platelets <20,000/mm³)
  Skin: mucous membranes; occasional GI, CNS
Hyperleukocytosis (WBC >100,000/mm³)
  Infarction: pulmonary, CNS hemorrhage
Infection
  Agranulocytic: bacterial (staph, enteric organisms)
  Lymphopenic: *Pneumocystis*, fungal, viral (HSV, CMV, varicella)

Extravasation burns: vincristine, doxorubicin, daunorubucin
Anaphylaxis: L-asparaginase, VP-16, VM-26
Myelosuppression: doxorubicin, daunorubicin, cyclophosphamide, cytosine arabinoside, 6-mercaptopurine, methotrexate, etoposide, nitrogen mustard, procarbazine, dactinomycin
Emetic: High-dose methotrexate, cytosine arabinoside, cyclophosphamide, doxorubicin, daunorubicin, VP-16, VM-26
Dysuria: cyclophosphamide
Mucositis: High-dose methotrexate, cytosine arabinoside, doxorubicin
Hypertension: prednisone
Hepatic dysfunction: methotrexate 6-mercaptopurine, cytosine arabinoside.
Pancreatic dysfunction: L-asparaginase, cytosine arabinoside

of involvement. Significant visceral bleeding is unusual. Intracranial hemorrhages are rare but life-threatening events. Hemorrhagic complications are more commonly associated with acute nonlymphocytic leukemia, especially acute promyelocytic leukemia. Patients with platelet counts less than 20,000/mm³ are at the greatest risk for hemorrhage. The condition of the patient, evidence of active bleeding, and anticipated course of therapy should be used as guidelines for platelet transfusion. The recommended dose of platelet concentrates is 6 U/m². "Prophylactic" platelet transfusion support in the absence of overt bleeding has not been established as necessary care for all patients. Frequent transfusions of platelets may induce alloimmunization to HLA antigens and may reduce the effectiveness of this therapy. Bleeding secondary to a vitamin K-dependent coagulopathy may also occur in patients requiring prolonged broad-spectrum antibiotic support.

Transfusions of packed red blood cells (PRBC) are used frequently in the management of children with ALL, although the indications are not clear. The child who presents with signs or symptoms of acute blood loss clearly requires PRBC and platelet transfusion support. However, guidelines for transfusion of children with anemia without overt bleeding are not established. Patients without overt bleeding have been successfully managed through the remission induction schedule without PRBC support, even with gradual hemoglobin concentration declines to less than 3 g/dL. The final decision for transfusion should be based on the condition of the patient, anticipated problems associated with the induction program, degree of anemia and reticulocytopenia, and presence or absence of bleeding.

Infection associated with granulocytopenia is a potentially life-threatening complication for the child with ALL. Any break in the skin, insect bite, blister, sore, gingival or mucous membrane irritation, or perianal fissure may serve as a portal for bacterial penetration, agranulocytic cellulitis, and sepsis. Overwhelming bacterial sepsis is the greatest threat to the child with ALL receiving intensive antileukemic therapy. Any child who presents with fever of 101 °F or higher and an absolute granulocyte count of less than 500/mm³ must be assumed to have sepsis. This is a medical emergency. These children should be hospitalized immediately; cultures of blood, urine, and respiratory secretions obtained; and broad-spectrum intravenous antibiotics initiated without delay. The principal pathogens include *Pseudomonas*, *Escherichia coli*, and *Staphylococcus*. With increased use of central venous catheters, cutaneous types of organisms (ie, skin contaminants) may be the pathogens.

In addition to bacterial infections, a variety of nonbacterial,

opportunistic infections can cause devastating illness in these patients. Varicella zoster, herpes zoster, and herpes simplex may cause serious systemic complications, including pneumonitis, hepatitis, and cerebritis. Treatment with vidarabine or acyclovir has been successful in controlling these infections. *Pneumocystis carinii* pneumonia is a protozoan infection that occurs in the severely immunosuppressed patient. This illness may present as unexplained fever. The patients are usually lymphopenic but not granulocytopenic. The infection may rapidly progress to cause life-threatening interstitial pneumonia. A program of prophylaxis involving trimethoprim-sulfamethoxazole administered twice daily for 3 days/week is effective in prevention of this disease. Invasive fungal infections continue to be observed in patients receiving intensive immunosuppressive therapy, with prolonged neutropenia and concomitant use of broad-spectrum antibiotics. The major pathogens are *Candida* and *Aspergillus*. Amphotericin B remains the treatment of choice for invasive infections.

Miscellaneous complications related to the choice of chemotherapy agents and routes of administration may be observed. Vincristine, doxorubicin, and daunorubicin are vesicants; care must be taken to avoid extravasation, or serious chemical burns may result. High doses of cyclophosphamide may induce cystitis, with symptoms of dysuria and hematuria. L-Asparaginase and the epipodophyllotoxins (ie, VP-16, VM-26) have associated risks for allergic reactions; appropriate medications should be available within the physician's office to deal with an allergic crisis. High doses of methotrexate, 6-mercaptopurine, and cytosine arabinoside, alone or in combination with other agents, are emetogenic. Hepatic dysfunction may also be associated with these agents. Severe mucositis may be associated with methotrexate and with the anthracyclines.

## Bone Marrow and Extramedullary Relapse and Transplantation

The most serious complication of ALL treatment is bone marrow relapse. Although reinduction of remission is possible, most patients will relapse again and eventually succumb to their disease. Patients who relapse while receiving continuation therapy have the worst prognosis. This event usually signals the emergence of resistant leukemic clones. Remission duration after successful reinduction is usually less than 1 year. In this group of patients, ablative chemotherapy and allogeneic bone marrow transplantation may offer the only hope for long-term survival. The reported experience for the Seattle Transplant Service in this group of patients is a 40% disease-free survival rate with a plateau from 2.5 to 10 years in follow-up.

Transplantation remains a form of investigational therapy. Treatment schedules, bone marrow processing, and post-transplant support measures are undergoing continual refinement. The procedure is risky, with an estimated 15% to 25% mortality rate from all causes during the first 100 days after transplantation. Acute and chronic graft-versus-host disease, interstitial pneumonitis, and relapse of leukemia are some of the many significant complications that may follow the transplantation procedure.

Patients who relapse more than 6 to 12 months after cessation of therapy may have a somewhat better prognosis. Reinduction of remission is usually successful, and long durations of remission have been achieved, with some patients actually discontinuing therapy for a second time.

The CNS and the testes are the most common sites of extramedullary relapse. However, these isolated events should be considered as localized manifestations of recurrent systemic disease; aggressive systemic chemotherapy is an essential part of the management.

Although fewer than 10% of the children with ALL have CNS leukemia at diagnosis, it remains the most common site of extramedullary relapse. Patients with T-ALL or high leukocyte counts at diagnosis have the greatest risk for this event. The clinical signs and symptoms of CNS leukemia may include headache, nausea, and vomiting secondary to increased intracranial pressure; diplopia or blurred vision; nuchal rigidity or hemiparesis with cord involvement; or even hyperphagia and pathologic weight gain. The diagnosis is established by lumbar puncture and analysis of cerebrospinal fluid cytopreparations for leukemic blasts. Symptoms of increased intracranial pressure are not a contraindication for a lumbar puncture.

Treatment for overt CNS leukemia has included intrathecal methotrexate, intrathecal triple therapy, cranial irradiation, craniospinal radiation, intraventricular methotrexate by way of an Ommaya reservoir, high-dose methotrexate, or a combination of these therapies. Significant chronic neurotoxicity is associated with schedules using more than two modalities. Children who develop overt CNS leukemia after adequate presymptomatic CNS therapies have a poor prognosis for survival. The combination of intrathecal methotrexate and cranial or craniospinal irradiation appears to offer the best hope for control of disease.

The increased occurrence of isolated testicular leukemia in children with ALL has paralleled the overall improved survival with this disease. However, testicular leukemia is a manifestation of systemic leukemic relapse and requires aggressive therapy. Patients usually present with a painless swelling. Testicular infiltration may be occult. As many as 15% of asymptomatic boys undergoing testicular biopsies before cessation of therapy have evidence of disease. The diagnosis is established by bilateral testicular wedge biopsies. Patients diagnosed with testicular leukemia should receive radiation therapy to a dose of 2400 cGy to both testes, followed by systemic chemotherapy. The prognosis for these patients remains good. Current chemotherapy regimens incorporating methotrexate at doses of 500 to 1000 mg/m² have reduced the incidence of this complication to less than 4%.

Other sites of extramedullary infiltration with ALL have been observed in children. Renal infiltrates are found in 40% of the children at diagnosis and may contribute to metabolic complications and hypertension during induction therapy. Isolated ovarian involvement has been reported occasionally and may extend to the fallopian tubes, uterus, and pelvic nodes. Radiographic changes in the skeleton, with or without associated symptoms, may be seen in as many as 30% of the patients at diagnosis. Leukemic infiltrates have been observed in the lower gastrointestinal tract, oral and gingival regions, retina and iris, heart, lungs, and skin.

## LONG-TERM SURVIVAL, LATE EFFECTS, AND THERAPEUTIC DIRECTIONS

As with all children with cancer, the management of the child with ALL requires a team approach. Pediatric nurse specialists, psychologists, play therapists, dietitians, and other hospital and clinic personnel play an important role in the total care of these patients. The stresses that frequently are faced by families with a child with ALL include concerns about the discomfort or disfigurement (especially alopecia) associated with chemotherapy, the financial pressures of medical care or disruption of family employment schedules, school performance and peer relationships, particularly for the older child, communication about fears and apprehensions among parents, patient, and siblings, and anxiety preceding the elective cessation of therapy.

With prolonged survival, monitoring for late effects of antileukemic therapy assumes increasing importance. The areas of interest include monitoring for specific organ dysfunction, impaired genetic or immunologic mechanisms, and second malignancies. Several long-term problems have been associated with CNS prophylaxis. These may include a 50% incidence of cranial CT scan abnormalities for children treated with cranial irradiation and intrathecal methotrexate, seizures, neuropsychologic deficits that result in school problems, and endocrine disturbances (eg, growth hormone deficiency). These problems are remediable and are insufficient reasons for altering a successful treatment program. Current leukemia protocols are seeking to obviate some of these complications by the use of high-dose systemic chemotherapy and intrathecal therapy without irradiation. The success of these programs remains to be established.

Delayed sexual maturation may be observed in children receiving irradiation to gonadal tissue, such as boys with testicular leukemia. Male adolescents may be at risk for spermatogenic dysfunction after cyclophosphamide therapy. Successful parenthood in long-term survivors has been reported, but the progeny of survivors of childhood leukemia are few. The data from cooperative late effects studies do not indicate an excess of congenital abnormalities or cancer in the offspring.

Clinical and laboratory-based research for childhood ALL probably will proceed along two principal lines. First, an increased understanding of the molecular and genetic events that regulate normal cellular proliferation and differentiation is essential. By recognizing normal regulatory events in bone marrow and lymphoreticular tissues, it should be possible to identify abnormal regulatory mechanisms and devise strategies for treatment. An increased understanding of the genetic mechanisms that offer the leukemic cell specific and nonspecific resistance advantages against antileukemic therapy will be necessary before we can solve the problem of leukemic relapse. Second, refinements in antileukemic therapy should proceed along more pharmacologically oriented schedules. Early antileukemic therapy was principally based on empiric data. Advances in the technologies of drug pharmacology, immunology, and cell kinetics will contribute to more effective treatment combinations that target specific mechanisms of leukemic proliferation or differentiation and increase the patient's chance for long-term survival.

## Selected Readings

Camitta B, Leventhal B, Lauer S, et al. Intermediate-dose intervenous methotrexate and mercaptopurine therapy for non-T, non-B acute lymphocytic leukemia of childhood: a Pediatric Oncology Group study. J Clin Oncol 1989;7:1539.

Crist WM, Pullen DJ, Rivera GK. Acute lymphoid leukemia. In: Fernbach DJ, Vietti TJ, eds. Clinical pediatric oncology, ed 4. St. Louis: CV Mosby, 1991;305.

Niemeyer CM, Gelber RD, Tarbell NJ, et al. Low-dose versus high-dose methotrexate during remission induction in childhood acute lymphoblastic leukemia (protocol 81-01 update). Blood 1991;78:2514.

Pui CH, Crist WM, Look AT. Biology and clinical significance of cytogenetic abnormalities in childhood acute lymphoblastic leukemia. Blood 1990;76:1449.

Trueworthy R, Shuster J, Look T, et al. Ploidy of lymphoblasts is the strongest predictor of treatment outcome in B-progenitor cell acute lymphoblastic leukemia of childhood: a Pediatric Oncology Group study. J Clin Oncol 1992;10:606.

*Principles and Practice of Pediatrics, Second Edition.*
edited by Frank A. Oski et al. J. B. Lippincott Company, Philadelphia © 1994.

# 96.2 *Acute Myeloid Leukemia*

## C. Philip Steuber

## EPIDEMIOLOGY

Between 350 and 500 new cases of acute myeloid leukemia (AML) are diagnosed in children annually in the United States. The incidence is one fifth to one sixth that of acute lymphocytic leukemia (ALL) in the same age group. The therapy for childhood AML has not reached the degree of success achieved for childhood ALL. Until recently, reports of childhood AML were concerned with limited numbers of patients on various treatment regimens, and they contributed little to understanding the disease process. Current investigations and trials are often lengthy because of the limited numbers of patients available for study. Much of the approach to childhood AML therapy has been the result of studies of adult patients, among whom the disease has a much higher incidence.

## PATHOPHYSIOLOGY

AML is the result of a clonal proliferation of a primitive marrow cell line. The myeloid leukemic subtype is designated by the cell of origin, whether granulocytic, monocytic, erythrocytic, or megakaryocytic. Combined-lineage leukemias of the myeloid-monocytic cell lines occur frequently. As with ALL, morphologic classification is commonly determined in accord with the French-American-British (FAB) guidelines (Table 96-7).

Technologic improvements have enabled recognition of chromosomal aberrations in most children with AML. Many of these abnormal genotypes appear to be disease-subtype specific. Whether these genetic changes precede or are a consequence of the leukemic event is uncertain. The recognized nonrandom disease and genotype associations are listed in Table 96-8. Children with AML-related abnormal cytogenetic studies lose those chromosomal changes when they are in complete remission and regain them on relapse. The cytogenetic abnormality may reappear before overt or clinical relapse is documented. There is growing interest in using cytogenetic criteria rather than morphologic data to define the remission state.

The numbers of malignant cells demonstrating abnormal chromosomes at diagnosis may indicate the ultimate curability of the disease; the greater the percentage of cells demonstrating the abnormality, the poorer is the long-term response.

Much effort is being devoted to studying the role of oncogenes in the leukemic conditions and to correlating molecular and cytogenetic observations with other biologic and chemical measures of disease. However, the data are preliminary and describe only small numbers of patients. There does appear to be a high frequency of *NRAS* and possibly *MYC* activation in adults with AML, but application of this information to children with AML is tentative.

Individuals with specific hereditary or congenital syndromes demonstrate an increased occurrence of AML. These predisposing conditions are listed in Table 96-9 and are themselves rare entities. The reasons for leukemogenesis in these patients awaits the results of molecular studies. As a rule, persons with these conditions who do develop AML respond poorly to chemotherapy and early detection does not seem to impart a therapeutic benefit.

## MORPHOLOGIC CLASSIFICATION

Seven categories (ie, M1 through M7) of AML are determined by morphologic and histochemical criteria. The guidelines of the pathology consortium are most commonly used, and these criteria for the seven AML subtypes are represented in Table 96-7. The combined M1 and M2 morphologies account for about 45% of childhood AML cases, and the M4 and M5 subsets account for another 45%. The remaining subgroups—M3, M6, and M7—comprise 10% to 15%.

When compared with lymphoid leukemia cells, AML cells have a relatively greater amount of cytoplasm, a more reticular nuclear

| | | | |
|---|---|---|---|
| **TABLE 96-7. The FAB Classification System** | | | |
| FAB Type | Morphologic Designation | Myeloperoxidase or Sudan Black | NSE/NaF Inhibition† |
| M1 | Myeloblastic leukemia without differentiation | + | −/− |
| M2 | Myeloblastic leukemia with differentiation | + | −/− |
| M3 | Promyelocytic leukemia | + | −/− |
| M4 | Myelomonocytic leukemia (minor component ≥20%) | + | +/+ |
| M5 | Monocytic | − | +/+ |
| M6 | Erythrocytic | − | +/− |
| M7 | Megakaryocytic* | − | +/− |

\* Recognized by ultrastructural presence of platelet peroxidase activity or immunohistochemical evidence of platelet glycoprotein.

† NSE, nonspecific esterase; NaF, sodium fluoride; +, shows activity; −, lacks activity; +/−, NSE stain positive; NaF inhibition negative.

**TABLE 96-8. Associations of Nonrandom Karyotypic Abnormalities and Leukemic Subtype**

| Abnormality | Leukemic Subtype (FAB Classification) |
|---|---|
| −7 | Acute myelogenous (M1 or M2) |
| t8;21 t6;9 | Acute myelogenous (M2) |
| +8 | AML in general |
| t15;17 | Acute promyelocytic (M3) |
| t4;11 | Acute myelocytic (M1) |
| t1;11 t9;11 | Acute monocytic (M5) |
| t1;11 t9;11 | Acute monomyelogenous (M4) |
| inv or del (16) | |
| t6;9 | |

chromatin pattern, and larger, more numerous nucleoli that are more discrete. Auer rods can be seen in a small percentage of the M1, M2, M3, and M4 cells.

Alternatives or supplements to morphologic classifications and diagnoses have been investigated. Flow cytometry reveals high RNA content in myeloid blast cells and can be helpful in differentiating AML from ALL. Immune phenotyping uses a panel of monoclonal antibodies directed against the surface antigens of monocytes and myelocytes. Most surface antigens are expressed for finite periods during the maturation of normal marrow cells, and the antigens detected on AML cells may indicate the stage at which cell differentiation was arrested in leukemogenesis. Although these data, particularly information about the presence of CD33, CD13, and CD15 antigens, may refine diagnostic capabilities, the prognostic and therapeutic implications of normal myeloid antigen expression on leukemic cells are not clear. The patterns of myeloid antigen expression are often inconsistent with defined stages of maturation and further attest to the heterogeneity of this family of leukemias. It has been suggested that myeloid leukemia cells that express more mature differentiation antigens have a better response to therapy than less differentiated forms.

The erythroleukemias (M6) and the acute megakaryocytic leukemias (M7) require special comment. Acute erythrocytic leukemia is readily definable morphologically by the presence of bizarre erythroblast forms. The cells often have periodic acid-Schiff positivity, and erythrocytic glycoprotein is found in the cell membrane. This entity frequently evolves into one of the other myeloid leukemias, usually M1 or M2. Megakaryoblasts

**TABLE 96-9. Conditions Associated With an Increased Incidence of Childhood AML**

Blackfan-Diamond syndrome
Bloom's syndrome
Chemotherapy for previous malignancy
Down syndrome
Familial myeloproliferative syndromes
Fanconi's anemia
Klinefelter's syndrome
Kostmann's syndrome
Neurofibromatosis
Radiation exposure
Wiskott-Aldrich syndrome

are immature cells of myeloid lineage which do not react to the standard histochemical profile. The diagnosis of acute megakaryocytic leukemia is confirmed by the presence of a distinct enzyme marker, platelet peroxidase, by the immunohistochemical evidence of platelet glycoprotein, or by demonstration of factor VIII antigen in the cells. There is often marked fibrosis in the marrows of these patients. Both of these forms of AML respond poorly to therapy.

## PRESENTING FEATURES AND DIAGNOSIS

As with ALL, children with AML manifest symptoms of bone marrow infiltration and failure. Pallor, bone pain, fever, and bleeding are the most common complaints at diagnosis. There is no sex predominance, and the age-adjusted incidence is constant. Enlargement of the liver and spleen affects approximately half of the children, particularly younger children with M4 or M5 subtypes. Lymphadenopathy is not usually a prominent feature. Testicular involvement at any stage of disease is infrequent. Chloromas or granulocytic sarcomas, particularly of the orbit and skin, may occur in a small percentage of patients. Gingival hyperplasia develops most commonly in children whose disease has a monocytic component (ie, M4, M5).

Cerebrospinal fluid (CSF) studies demonstrate leukemic involvement in 10% of patients at diagnosis. This is higher than for children with ALL. These CSF findings are usually unaccompanied by symptoms. Some reports indicate that the M4 and M5 subtypes have a greater tendency to develop central nervous system (CNS) disease, but this is not a universally reported finding. If detected at diagnosis, CNS leukemia in childhood AML is responsive to specific therapy and does not adversely affect treatment outcome, although as systemic therapy improves, this observation may change. An exception is the infant (<2 years of age) with monocytic leukemia and CNS disease at diagnosis. These patients do not respond well to therapy. In childhood AML, the initial leukocyte count is usually less than 50,000/mm³, but extreme leukocytosis (≥100,000/mm³) is recorded in one of five AML patients and is considered an adverse prognostic factor.

Coagulation studies may indicate a consumptive coagulopathy, particularly in patients with acute promyelocytic leukemia (APL). In contrast to adult APL patients, heparinization may not be necessary to prevent bleeding complications in children with APL. Most respond to transfusion support and early aggressive chemotherapy.

There has not been universal agreement about the prognostic factors in childhood AML because of the generally poor outcome of all subgroups. It has been suggested that extreme leukocytosis, particularly in children younger than 2 years of age at diagnosis and the M5 subgroup are adverse indicators. However, there are considerable data that fail to confirm the importance of these factors in various studies, and the impact of therapy rather than disease as the prognostic factor determinant should not be underestimated.

Studies of leukemic bone marrow growth patterns in various culture systems have been performed in an effort to define the disease and prognosis on the basis of colony and cluster patterns and ratios. The results of these studies were contradictory, and the utility of these observations is questionable. There are ongoing efforts to relate drug sensitivities in culture systems with the results observed in clinical trials.

## THERAPY

The therapeutic concepts of induction, consolidation, maintenance, and CNS prophylaxis or sanctuary therapy that are used in treating ALL cannot be directly applied to the therapy of childhood AML. The initial management concepts for the two major leukemic groups are similar: to deliver a drug or combination of drugs that will achieve in 3 to 4 weeks a reduction in the blast forms to below the detectable level and to reestablish normal marrow function.

For AML patients, successful induction of remission requires regimens more toxic than those used in ALL. It is necessary to create transient marrow aplasia to achieve a complete remission in AML. The therapeutic index for such regimens is narrow, and early death rates are 5% to 15%, although in the past they have been as high as 30%. Complete remissions in childhood AML are being obtained in 70% to 85% of newly diagnosed patients using a combination of an anthracycline (eg, daunorubicin) and cytosine arabinoside, with and without additional drugs. This combination is the standard against which newer induction therapies are measured.

Postremission therapy in patients remains a controversial issue. Multiple therapeutic strategies are being evaluated: repeated courses of alternative, intensive induction therapy regimens; repeated use of the initially successful induction regimen at the same dosage levels; and continuing therapy over a prolonged period using drugs and dosages less toxic than those of the induction regimen (ie, maintenance therapy).

The patients who receive intensive early therapy are not likely to benefit further from prolonged maintenance programs, but the patients who achieve remission on less intense induction therapies are likely to benefit from maintenance therapy. The curability or event-free survival rate for children with AML optimally treated with chemotherapy is approximately 35% to 40%. Approximately 50% of the responders are expected to remain in remission. The median disease-free survival for all patients in most pediatric AML series is 12 to 18 months. An interesting subgroup is patients with Down syndrome and AML. The increased incidence of AML associated with trisomy 21 is well established. The response of these patients to therapy appears to be exceptionally good.

New drugs and drug combinations are being evaluated for use in induction and postinduction therapy with the purpose of improving disease-free survival. They include the epipodophyllotoxins (ie, VM-26, VP-16), amsacrine, azacytidine, and two new anthracycline analogues, mitoxanthrone and idarubicin. Their final value remains undefined.

Alternative postremission therapies using allogeneic bone marrow transplantation or autografting with purged and nonpurged marrows are being compared with chemotherapy regimens (see Chap. 96.4). Although current information supports the use of allogeneic grafts for therapy during the first remission, continuing improvements in chemotherapy regimens may change that recommendation. It may be that one of the many features of the disease can be used to tailor therapy for some patients.

Most chemotherapists agree that there is an indication for CNS prophylaxis or therapy of occult CNS disease in the treatment of childhood AML. The cumulative data show a high incidence of early CNS disease. Effective CNS therapy has been accomplished using radiation therapy or intrathecal therapy with single or multiple agents. Some authorities advocate high doses of systemically administered drugs such as cytosine arabinoside. The impact of CNS therapy on ultimate disease-free survival is unknown because marrow remissions are of short duration in most patients. Refinements of CNS therapy await improvements in systemic therapy.

Improved therapy for childhood AML depends on several factors: a better understanding of the molecular basis of disease, an appreciation of the interactions of malignant cell growth characteristics with the effects of chemotherapeutic agents, and the development of effective new agents or approaches.

## Selected Readings

Bloomfield CD, de la Chapelle A. Chromosome abnormalities in acute nonlymphocytic leukemia: clinical and biologic significance. Semin Oncol 1987;14:372.

Steuber CP, Mahoney DH, Ogden AK. Acute myeloid leukemias and myeloproliferative disorders. In: Fernbach DJ, Vietti TJ, eds. Clinical pediatric oncology, ed 4. St. Louis: CV Mosby, 1991:377.

*Principles and Practice of Pediatrics, Second Edition.*
edited by Frank A. Oski et al. J. B. Lippincott Company, Philadelphia © 1994.

# 96.3 *Chronic Myeloproliferative Disorders Seen in Childhood*

## C. Philip Steuber

The chronic myeloproliferative disorders in children are rare conditions comprising 1% to 2% of all childhood malignancies and 3% to 5% of all childhood leukemias. As with the acute myeloid leukemias, they are the result of uncontrolled clonal proliferation of one or more marrow cell lineages. Each entity listed in Table 96-10 is designated according to the predominant type of cells involved. The term *chronic* is somewhat deceptive in that the prognosis for these disorders is generally worse than that for the acute leukemias.

## JUVENILE CHRONIC MONOMYELOGENOUS LEUKEMIA

Juvenile chronic monomyelogenous leukemia (JCML) is a panmyelopathy most often presenting in children younger than 2 years of age. Boys predominate (>2 : 1). The children present with lymphadenopathy that is often suppurative and with symptoms of thrombocytopenia and fever. They frequently exhibit a chronic eczematoid facial rash and moderate organomegaly. Hematologic abnormalities include a mild anemia, symptomatic thrombocytopenia, and moderate leukocytosis (usually <100,000 cells/mm$^3$). The leukocytosis is caused by immature monocytes and myelocytes, which are identifiable histochemically and in cell culture. Circulating nucleated erythrocytes can also be seen. Fetal hemoglobin levels are markedly elevated. Bone marrow specimens are hypercellular, with elevated numbers of myeloid and monocytoid forms. Dyserythropoietic changes are observed, and megakaryocytes are diminished. Although erythroid, myeloid, and megakaryocytic cell lines are involved, abnormal monocyte forms usually predominate. Marrow cultures demonstrate predominantly monocytic differentiation. Polyclonal elevations of immunoglobulins have been described, and an association with chronic Epstein-Barr virus infection has been reported. Specific cytogenetic patterns have not been associated with JCML, and most patients studied have normal karyotypes.

Children with JCML have responded poorly to therapy. Transient responses have been reported with various antimetabolites. Radiation therapy and splenectomy are not usually helpful. It has been suggested that aggressive therapy similar to that effective in acute forms of myeloid and monocytic leukemia should be employed and that bone marrow transplantation should be considered as the primary therapeutic option. The use of retinoic

| TABLE 96-10.    Chronic Myeloproliferative Disorders Seen in Childhood |
| --- |
| Juvenile chronic monomyelogenous leukemia |
| Chronic myelogenous leukemia |
| Preleukemia (myelodysplasia) |
| Polycythemia vera |
| Thrombocythemia |
| Myelofibrosis |

acid has been proposed to induce maturation of the monocytes and myelocytes. Most children with JCML die within 1 to 2 years of diagnosis, regardless of therapy.

## ADULT CHRONIC MYELOGENOUS LEUKEMIA

The incidence of adult chronic myelogenous leukemia (ACML) in the pediatric age group is approximately twice that of JCML. It is uncommon before 3 years of age and usually is diagnosed between the ages of 10 and 14. As with JCML, males predominate. Common chief complaints include fever, weakness, pain, weight loss, and increasing abdominal girth. Respiratory system complaints are common. Marked splenomegaly is evident.

Peripheral blood counts demonstrate extreme leukocytosis ($\geq$100,000 cells/mm$^3$) usually with thrombocytosis and mild anemia. The circulating leukocyte differential reveals cells at all levels of myeloid differentiation, including eosinophils and basophils. The concentration of leukocyte alkaline phosphatase is reduced or absent. Bone marrow specimens show marked myeloid hyperplasia, increased numbers of megakaryocytes, eosinophilia, and basophilia. Blast counts do not exceed 25%.

Most patients demonstrate the Philadelphia chromosome (Ph[1]) in the malignant cells. This usually results from a reciprocal translocation between the long arms of chromosomes 9 and 22, t(9;22)(q34:q11). In this translocation, the *ABL1* oncogene from chromosome 9 is fused to the breakpoint cluster region (*BCR*) of chromosome 22 and the resultant fusion gene (*BCR/ABL1*) may play an integral part in the development of leukemia. In a few cases, the Ph[1] abnormality involves chromosomes other than 9. About 10% of ACML patients do not have evidence of the Ph[1] chromosome, and they respond less well to therapy. Multiple reports attest to the clonal nature of the proliferative disorder in ACML.

The natural history of ACML is separated into two phases. The initial or chronic phase persists for a limited period (median, 2.5 years) and is followed by an accelerated phase. The accelerated phase is characterized by deteriorating blood counts, progressive neutrophil dysfunction, increasing splenomegaly, and the development of additional chromosomal abnormalities. This phase usually evolves over several months and terminates in acute blastic leukemia. In children, approximately one fourth of the cases of acute leukemia have lymphoid characteristics and patterns of drug response. Occasionally, the transformation phase takes place abruptly and is referred to as a blastic crisis. After transformation occurs, subsequent response to therapy is poor, and most patients die within a few months, regardless of morphologic subgroup.

Management of the chronic phase has consisted of administration of single agents (ie, hydroxyurea or busulfan) to control leukocytosis. The disease was considered to be incurable and acute leukemic transformation inevitable. Efforts at more aggressive therapies in an attempt to eliminate the malignant clone were largely failures. Allogeneic bone marrow transplantation,

if donors were available, has been considered the only truly curative therapy, but the optimal application of such grafts has not been determined. The best results have been observed when the graft is done early in the course of the disease.

Alternative therapies for ACML have included the use of autologous marrow cryopreservation. Marrow is harvested early during the chronic phase, and after the disease accelerates, the patient receives myeloablative therapy followed by reinfusion of the stored marrow. Restoration of the chronic phase in this fashion has had only limited success.

The prolonged use of interferon alpha or gamma has been described as another therapeutic choice. Interferon is capable of suppressing the Ph[1]-positive clone at least temporarily in adults and children with CML. These trials suggest that interferon therapy may prolong the chronic phase but not prevent ultimate blastic transformation. Later trials have combined the biologic response modifiers with other agents.

## MYELODYSPLASTIC SYNDROMES

The myelodysplastic syndromes are a group of loosely defined clinical and laboratory syndromes that often precede the diagnosis of acute leukemia. They have been called preleukemia, myelodysplasia, refractory anemia with excess blasts, and refractory anemia with or without ringed sideroblasts. These entities are characterized by progressive cytopenia and marrow abnormalities. Patients usually present with problems related to marrow failure. The findings at physical examination, with the exception of pallor and bleeding, are usually unremarkable. Circulating bizarre erythrocyte and platelet forms usually are detected. There may be a mild elevation in fetal hemoglobin, probably reflecting ineffective erythropoiesis. Several defects in granulocytic function have been reported.

Cytogenetic abnormalities, particularly involving chromosomes 5, 7, and 8, have been reported for many of these patients. The hematologic abnormalities may persist for months. A significant portion of these patients eventually develop acute leukemia.

Management primarily involves transfusion support and treatment of opportunistic infections. The developing malignancy is usually acute myeloid leukemia, and response to therapy is poor. Marrow growth factors and other biologic response modifiers are undergoing trials. Bone marrow transplantation has been successful in selected patients.

## POLYCYTHEMIA VERA AND PRIMARY THROMBOCYTHEMIA

Polycythemia vera and primary or essential thrombocythemia rarely have been reported in children. They are clonal disorders of the affected progenitors. Children with polycythemia vera have complications related to hyperviscosity (see Chap. 91), and those with thrombocythemia also have problems with vascular occlusion secondary to massive platelet numbers. Splenomegaly is a prominent feature in both entities. Because of the rarity of these disorders in pediatric patients, the causes of secondary polycythemia and thrombocytosis must be carefully investigated. The management guidelines are the same as those used for adult patients.

## PRIMARY MYELOFIBROSIS

Myelofibrosis is characterized by a fibrotic proliferation within marrow spaces. Splenomegaly is common. Hematologic manifestations include bizarre circulating erythrocytes and platelets and immature myeloid cells. Multiple immunologic defects have been observed. Bone marrow aspiration is not diagnostic, and a biopsy is necessary to confirm the diagnosis. Possible causes of secondary marrow fibrosis, malignant and nonmalignant, must be considered. Many cases previously diagnosed as primary or acute myelofibrosis in children are probably instances of acute megakaryocytic leukemia.

Management is primarily by transfusion and infection control. Occasionally, splenectomy is indicated to control symptoms secondary to mechanical dysfunction (eg, hypersplenism, portal hypertension). Steroids have been effective rarely, and the use of aggressive chemotherapy is not established.

## Selected Readings

Schwartz CL, Cohen HJ. In: Pizzo PA, Poplack DG, eds. Principles and practice of pediatric oncology. Philadelphia: JB Lippincott, 1989:397.
Steuber CP, Mahoney DH, Ogden AK. Acute myeloid leukemias and myeloprolif- erative disorders. In: Fernbach DJ, Vietti TJ, eds. Clinical pediatric oncology, ed 4. St. Louis: CV Mosby, 1991:377.

*Principles and Practice of Pediatrics, Second Edition.*
edited by Frank A. Oski et al. J. B. Lippincott Company, Philadelphia © 1994.

# 96.4 *Bone Marrow Transplantation for Childhood Leukemia*

C. Philip Steuber

Bone marrow transplantation is the process of replacing a patient's diseased, defective, or damaged marrow elements with healthy donor marrow cells. In malignancies, marrow grafts offer an opportunity to circumvent the therapeutic dosage limitations imposed by myelosuppressive toxicities and to further intensify therapy.

With improvements in histocompatibility testing, immunosuppressive therapies, and supportive care during the last two decades, bone marrow transplantation is increasingly the therapy chosen for a variety of otherwise fatal conditions. Most marrow transplantations have been performed for patients with leukemia.

The first marrow transplants for leukemia were syngeneic or allogeneic and were given to patients with advanced refractory disease to rescue them from myeloablative therapies. The few successes (5% to 10%) observed at that time outnumbered those seen with other therapies and led investigators to explore the indications for and optimal applications of the transplant procedure.

Current guidelines for considering the use of bone marrow transplantation for childhood leukemia include the following diagnoses:

Acute myelogenous leukemia (AML) in first remission
Selected high-risk acute lymphocytic leukemia (ALL) in first remission (eg, Ph$^1$-positive ALL)
Adult and juvenile forms of chronic myelogenous leukemia during the chronic phase
Recurrent or refractory leukemia of any type

Although conceptually simple, the marrow transplant process and sequelae are complex. Properly matched donor and recipient pairs are needed, appropriate preparative programs are required, and the lengthy period of marrow aplasia, immunosuppression, and graft-versus-host disease (GVHD) after transplantation requires extensive support capabilities.

Most marrow transplantations done for leukemia through 1987 have used HLA/MLC-compatible donor–recipient pairs. These pairs are identical at the A , B, and D loci. The restricted availability of matched, related allogeneic donors reduces the number of patients eligible for transplant by 67%. In an attempt to increase the donor pool for patients without matched siblings, efforts have been directed toward the use of partially matched family members, such as parents (ie, haploidentical). Bone marrow donor registries have been established to catalog unrelated histocompatible persons. Preliminary data suggest that the use of HLA-matched nonrelated donors may result in less GVHD than is seen using partially matched related donors.

To reduce the anticipated increase in the incidence and severity of GVHD under such disparate conditions, methods are used to purge the donor marrow of immunocompetent T cells. Most T-cell depletion procedures involve monoclonal antibodies directed at T cells. These purging methods are effective in reducing the GVHD-related problems, but the incidence of graft rejection and of recurrent leukemia increases. These observations underscore the contribution of immunocompetent donor T cells to engraftment and to disease control.

A multiplicity of bone marrow transplant preparative or conditioning regimens are being investigated. The purpose of these intensive therapies is to eradicate the basic disease and to prevent graft rejection. For malignancies, these goals are usually accomplished by a combination of marrow-ablative chemotherapy and total-body irradiation (TBI). Most preparative regimens use lethal dosages of chemotherapy drugs—usually including an alkylating agent such as cyclophosphamide—and multifraction TBI for a total dosage of 750 to 1500 cGy. For boys with ALL, additional irradiation is given to the testes, which can be a sanctuary site for disease. The patient or recipient is rescued from the results of these myelotoxic therapies by the infusion of healthy donor marrow. The best results are seen in younger patients who are transplanted early in the course of their disease.

There are several obstacles to the ultimate success of bone marrow transplantation: acute and chronic GVHD, recurrent disease, fatal infection (particularly in patients with GVHD), lethal toxicity from the conditioning regimen, and failure to engraft, although engraftment rarely fails with the current preparative regimens.

GVHD is a process in which donor T lymphocytes produce injury in host tissue, particularly the skin, liver, and gastrointestinal tract. The severity of GVHD correlates to some extent with measures of histocompatibility, but it occurs even in complete A-, B-, and D-loci matches, reflecting the limitations of current histocompatibility assessment. Acute GVHD usually occurs within 3 months of grafting. It develops in approximately half of patients receiving allografts. All bone marrow transplant patients receive some form of immunosuppressive therapy in an effort to abrogate or ameliorate the appearance of GVHD. Methotrexate, prednisone, and cyclosporine are the agents most often used in various combinations for GVHD prophylaxis. Attempts can be made to deplete donor marrows of T cells before infusion to reduce the incidence and severity of GVHD, but this process introduces other undesirable complications. Successful, aggressive GVHD prophylaxis may contribute to a greater incidence of relapse.

Chronic GVHD occurs in 15% to 40% of bone marrow transplant patients and is difficult to control. It usually occurs in patients who have experienced acute GVHD but may develop independently, usually more than 3 months after the graft. Chronic

GVHD targets the skin, intestinal tract, liver, and lungs, and may be fatal. Prolonged corticosteroids and azathioprine are the primary treatments. If they are ineffective, there are no established alternative therapies. Thalidomide and antibody immunotoxin conjugates are being explored as alternative therapies for chronic GVHD.

Many transplant investigators recognize a beneficial antileukemic effect from the reaction of the recipient's tissue to the donor T cells, known as the graft-versus-disease (GVD) effect. They cite the improved disease-free survival of allogeneic grafts over that of syngeneic grafts or T-cell-depleted grafts as verification. Data show that patients experiencing some degree of GVHD ultimately fare better with respect to relapse than those who experience none.

In addition to extensive transfusion requirements and parenteral nutrition support, most patients receive frequent infusions of intravenous immunoglobulin (IVIG). Evidence suggests that IVIG reduces the incidence of CMV infection and some types of bacterial infections, and it may reduce the problems related to GVHD. Infection is an almost universal complication of the transplant process, and various strategies to prevent infection, such as isolation procedures and prophylactic antibiotic regimens, are commonly employed.

Hematopoietic growth factors (eg, granulocyte-macrophage colony-stimulating factor) are given to hasten marrow recovery and shorten the period of risk for infection.

Despite these complicating factors and unsettled issues, the successes of bone marrow transplant are substantial. For children with AML in first remission, the disease-free survival rate is approximately 60% to 65% after allogeneic transplants. These figures are markedly reduced if the grafting takes place in second or subsequent remission or at the time of overt relapse. In patients transplanted for AML, most failures are caused by transplant-related causes, and the relapse rate appears to be less than 15%. However, recent advances in drug treatment for childhood AML may require a reevaluation of the timing of bone marrow transplantation for those patients.

The responses of children with ALL to transplant have been somewhat less gratifying. Because more than half of the newly diagnosed patients with ALL respond to chemotherapy regimens, bone marrow transplantation usually is reserved for ALL patients who fail initial therapy and are in second remission. Under such circumstances, long-term, disease-free survivals have been of the magnitude of 30% to 35%, with relapse accounting for the largest number of failures (30% to 50%). Selected patients with ALL in first remission who are considered to be at high risk for chemotherapy failure are considered for transplantation. A widely accepted high-risk feature is the presence of the Philadelphia chromosome (Ph$^1$). Relapse after transplantation reflects the inadequacy of the conditioning regimen. Improved preparative programs use agents more specific for lymphoproliferative disorders and appear to have increased the projected disease-free survival rates to 50%, but the data are preliminary. Bone marrow transplants are not recommended for patients with ALL in frank relapse; previous attempts have not been successful. However, after a relapsed patient is in second remission, every consideration should be given to the possibility of expeditious bone marrow transplant.

In recent years, bone marrow transplants have become the treatment of choice for patients with chronic myelogenous leukemia (CML) while still in their chronic phase. Optimally, marrow grafting for CML patients should be done before acceleration of their disease becomes evident. Although most data reported are the results of treating adult patients, there is sufficient pediatric information to suggest that most affected children can be cured by transplant if a suitable donor is available. The information is even more sparse for children with JCML, but sporadic case reports demonstrate that bone marrow transplantation can also be successful and have been the only instances of probable cure. Long-term follow-up information for patients transplanted for chronic leukemia is forthcoming.

The use of autologous marrow for leukemia patients in remission who do not have matched donors provides another approach to leukemia therapy. Autografting allows for higher-dose chemoradiotherapy without the limitations imposed by marrow-suppressive toxicity, and it enables hematopoietic recovery without the risk of GVHD seen in allografts. There are disadvantages of autografting. If the remission marrow being reinfused remains contaminated with leukemic cells, the disease may recur as a result of the reinfused malignant cells. The therapy regimens used to treat the patient are similar to those used in allogeneic transplants but autografts do not have the added benefit of the GVD effect. There is no accurate method of determining if relapse under these circumstances reflects reinfusion of disease or inadequate systemic conditioning therapy.

The problem of malignant cell marrow contamination is being addressed by a variety of investigative purging techniques using pharmacologic and immunologic tumor cell properties with the goal of isolating and removing the cells with leukemic characteristics.

Marrow autografting is being used to treat increasing numbers of patients with refractory solid tumors. Children with lymphomas, neuroblastoma, sarcomas, and even brain tumors have responded to aggressive myeloablative therapies followed by "rescue" with their own previously cryopreserved marrows. For solid tumors with a proclivity for marrow involvement, the questions of marrow contamination with malignant cells and of the indications and methods for purging remain unsettled.

## Selected Readings

Johnson FL. Bone marrow transplantation. In: Fernbach DJ, Vietti TJ, eds. Clinical pediatric oncology, ed 4. St. Louis: CV Mosby, 1991;213.

*Principles and Practice of Pediatrics, Second Edition.*
edited by Frank A. Oski et al. J. B. Lippincott Company, Philadelphia © 1994.

# CHAPTER 97
# *Lymphomas*

# *97.1 Hodgkin's Disease*

Kenneth L. McClain

Lymphomas comprise the third largest group of childhood malignancies, accounting for about 14% in whites and 11.3% in blacks. The actual incidence is 6.2 cases of Hodgkin's disease (HD) per million Caucasian children per year and 6.9 cases of non-Hodgkin's lymphoma. White children have about half again as many cases of lymphomas as blacks, with an incidence of 16.2 per million whites and 10.2 per million blacks. The differences are most striking in the non-Hodgkin's lymphomas (NHL); the incidence is twice as high for white children as for black children.

## BIOLOGY AND EPIDEMIOLOGY

Hodgkin's disease is a malignancy of the interdigitating, antigen-processing cells, which are found in the paracortical regions of the lymph nodes or spleen. The neoplastic counterpart, known as the Reed-Sternberg cell, can also be found in bone, bone marrow, liver, lung, and in skin and brain in the late stages of disease. The histologic types of HD include nodular sclerosis (46% of patients), mixed cellularity (31%), lymphocyte predominance (16%), and lymphocyte depletion (7%). These histologic patterns suggest an evolution of the disease from early infiltration of lymphocytes to a mixture of monocytes and lymphocytes, with sclerosis and eventual lymphoid depletion. This teleologic order results from a better survival of patients if more lymphocytes are present in the lesion. Because of the important role of the interdigitating cells in antigen processing, it is not surprising that immunodeficiency coincident with HD has been documented. Defective T cells and lymphopenia may also cause the anergy, impaired lymphocyte response to mitogens in vitro, defective T-lymphocyte binding of sheep red blood cells, increased splenic IgG synthesis in vitro, frequent infectious complications, and elevated anti-Epstein-Barr virus (EBV) titers.

HD occurs rarely in children younger than 7 years of age and is diagnosed equally in boys and girls. The incidence increases until the age 25 and then decreases until the mid-thirties.

There has been significant controversy about the possible association of tonsillectomy and incidence of HD. The relative incidence varied from 0.7 to 3.6 in 12 studies seeking to answer the question of an association. The incidence varied with sibship size, and there are probably several confounding variables involved. For example, compared with the general population, more HD patients are single children, although this group is only 12.5% of patients.

Because more patients are from better socioeconomic conditions, it is proposed that delayed exposure to a common infectious agent, such as EBV, may be relevant. Perhaps this is why more Caucasian children in the United States develop these malignancies than other groups. Patients with Hodgkin's disease have a higher titer against the viral capsid antigen than most children do years after infectious mononucleosis. However, this may be secondary to abnormalities of the immune system in HD. Data supporting the contagion theory of HD are controversial. Reported clusters of HD have been discounted on the basis of flawed statistical analysis. However, molecular studies have identified EBV DNA and viral proteins in Reed-Sternberg cells. Of the nodular sclerosis cases studied, 32% are EBV positive. For mixed cellularity cases, 96% were positive.

## CLINICAL FEATURES AND DIAGNOSIS

### Presenting Signs and Symptoms

Most children present with painless lymphadenopathy, usually of the cervical, supraclavicular, axillary, or inguinal nodes. Splenic or hepatic enlargement are infrequently found in early stages of HD. Fewer than 20% of patients have the classic fever and night sweats that adults with HD demonstrate. These initial signs could be caused by a variety of diseases.

A mediastinal mass is seen on chest x-ray films in 17% to 40% of patients and is found more often in children over 12

years of age. It is almost always found when low cervical or supraclavicular nodes are enlarged. Most of the older children have masses less than one third the diameter of the chest, but 30% have mediastinal masses greater than one third of the diameter, which may cause dysphagia, dyspnea, cough, or the superior vena cava syndrome.

There are differences in the histologic type and the stage of disease in children younger than and older than 7 years of age. Almost 75% of the older group have the nodular sclerosing type of HD, compared with 50% of the younger group. The younger group has more cases of lymphocyte predominance and mixed-cellularity histology. Almost 60% of the younger and 33% of older children have limited-stage disease (ie, stage I or IIA). Conversely, 38% of the older group and 12% of the younger group has stage IIIB or IV disease.

### Staging

A complete evaluation of patients with suspected lymphoma is mandatory before beginning treatment. The evaluation and treatment of these diseases should be undertaken at a center where a team of pediatric oncologists, pathologists, surgeons, radiotherapists, nurses, and social workers are experienced in the diagnosis and care of children with cancer. The prompt and efficient care of the child in this setting is the only way to guarantee optimal treatment and the best outcome.

The routine evaluation of a patient with suspected HD should include a complete history with emphasis on constitutional symptoms such as fever and weight loss, previous infections, family exposures to toxins and parental occupational hazards, and evidence for underlying immune deficiencies and familial cancer. A complete physical examination means assessment of general health, height and weight, size and location of lymphadenopathy, liver and spleen size, skin infiltrations, pulmonary findings, and neurologic signs. Laboratory evaluation should include a complete blood count, bilateral bone marrow biopsies and aspirates, erythrocyte sedimentation rate, renal and liver function tests (including lactate dehydrogenase levels), urinalysis, anteroposterior and lateral chest x-ray films, and computerized tomography (CT) scans of the abdomen and chest with oral and intravenous contrast.

Because of increased resolution of CT scans and new treatment regimens, the use and value of bipedal lymphangiography is being questioned. There have been reports of more false-positive and false-negative lymphangiogram results in children than in adults, although investigators at Stanford find lymphangiograms helpful. Gallium scans can also be helpful in defining the disease activity of mediastinal HD. Eighty percent of patients have uptake of gallium 67 ($^{67}$Ga) in their mediastinal masses at the time of diagnosis. After therapy, a residual mediastinal mass that continues to absorb $^{67}$Ga is likely to have active HD.

There are two aspects to staging: clinical and pathologic. Clinical staging refers to an assessment of the disease extent based on history, physical examination, and radiologic tests. Pathologic staging is accomplished by histologic examination of tissues removed at a staging laparotomy and by the bone marrow biopsy. Table 97-1 outlines the Ann Arbor staging system for Hodgkin's disease in children or adults.

The standard evaluation of HD patients with a staging laparotomy for patients without bone marrow involvement includes a staging laparotomy for several reasons: it is the only way to establish involvement of the spleen and enlarged abdominal lymph nodes; it is a better way to assess liver involvement with biopsy of suspicious area; and it is possible to move ovaries out of the potential radiation therapy field.

As many as 30% of patients may have more extensive disease determined by staging laparotomy and histologic examination of

### TABLE 97-1. Ann Arbor System for Staging of Hodgkin's Disease

| Stage I | Involvement of a single lymph node region (I) or a single extralymphatic organ or site ($I_E$) |
|---|---|
| Stage II | Involvement of two or more lymph node regions on the same side of the diaphragm II, or extension to an extralymphatic site and one or more lymph node regions on the same side of the diaphragm ($II_E$) |
| Stage III | Involvement of lymph node regions on both sides of the diaphragm (III), localized involvement by extension to an extralymphatic organ or site ($III_E$), or involvement of the spleen |
| Stage IV | Diffuse or disseminated involvement of one or more extralymphatic organs or tissues with or without associated lymph node enlargement |

All stages are further classified as A or B to indicate the absence or presence, respectively, of systemic symptoms: (1) unexplained fever, (2) night sweats, or (3) weight loss greater than 10% of normal body weight. If laparotomy and histologic review show that disease is limited to spleen, splenic, celiac, or portal nodes, the classification is substage IIIA1. Involvement of the lower abdominal nodes, such as para-aortic, iliac, and inguinal nodes, designates substage IIIA2.

From Carbone PP, Kaplan HS. Report of the committee on Hodgkin's disease staging classification. Cancer Res 1971;31:1860.

the tissues (ie, increased to stage III or IV). This information allows oncologists and radiotherapists to deliver more specific irradiation or aggressive chemotherapy. When patients are confirmed by pathologic staging to have stage I or II HD, limited treatment can achieve a long-term survival rate of more than 90%. Because the toxic effects of extensive therapy are significant, excess treatment is ill advised for patients with stage IA and IIA HD. Patients with clinical stages IIIA2, IIIB, or IV do not require a staging laparotomy because they receive combined therapy regardless of the detailed findings. However, for some patients with equivocal findings by CT scan (eg, abdominal nodes >1 but <3 cm), it may be prudent to confirm the node status by histologic examination. As many patients with a staging laparotomy eventually relapse as those without one, and the ultimate survival rates are equal.

For children, the danger of splenectomy is real. Between 3% and 10% of these patients have sepsis after splenectomy. New combined therapy plans (ie, irradiation plus chemotherapy) have demonstrated convincingly that graded amounts of therapy can "sterilize" areas of hidden disease and probably not increase the risk of complications.

## TREATMENT

Patients with pathologically staged I through IIA disease have until recently been treated primarily with irradiation to involved areas plus an extended field to contiguous regions that are frequently sites of relapse. For a child with a cervical node involvement, this means the neck, supraclavicular, and axillary ("minimantle") regions must be treated. If there is a mediastinal mass, it may require a special boost of radiation if the mass is greater than one third of the chest diameter. Historically, this approach has provided disease-free survival rates of more than 80% for stage I and II HD. Some centers have routinely added extended-field irradiation to para-aortic nodes and to splenic or hepatic regions, even for limited supradiaphragmatic disease. This helped improve survival when B symptoms or extensive mediastinal disease suggested a worse prognosis, but the price paid for this extra therapy was toxicity in the form of musculoskeletal growth problems.

Many centers in the United States and Europe are using graded amounts of radiation therapy (based on age) and chemotherapy for early- and late-stage disease. A report from Stanford showed 100% survival for stage I and II patients and 78% survival for stage III and IV patients. Chemotherapy treatments include 4 to 6 courses of alternating MOPP (ie, nitrogen mustard, vincristine [Oncovin], prednisone, without or without procarbazine) and ABVD (ie, doxorubicin [Adriamycin], bleomycin, vinblastine, and DTIC). (Note: As of 1992, DTIC was no longer available.) The Pediatric Oncology Group is studying the efficacy and long-term effects of treating patients with six courses of MOPP and ABVD compared with the effects of four courses and 2550 cGy of irradiation to involved fields.

Treatment of stage III and IV disease has customarily included chemotherapy (ie, MOPP and ABVD) with radiation therapy. As originally conceived, the chemotherapy consisted of 12 cycles alternating the two groups of drugs. By reducing this to eight cycles and using low-dose radiation (eg, 2100 cGy to lymphoid areas), survival rates are more than 85%. Between 3 and 7% of patients treated with MOPP and ABVD develop second malignancies such as acute myelogenous leukemia or non-Hodgkin's lymphoma. New therapy plans are being investigated to reduce the incidence of second malignancies.

Promising results have been achieved using cytosine arabinoside, cisplatin, etoposide alternating with vincristine, procarbazine, prednisone, and doxorubicin. By combining radiation therapy and these agents, it is hoped that reduced toxicity but equivalent or improved cure rates for HD can be achieved.

## LATE EFFECTS

The toxic side effects of therapy for Hodgkin's disease are many. All patients have alopecia, weight loss, transient pancytopenia, and extreme susceptibility to infections while on therapy. When high-dose radiation therapy is applied to the spinal area, growth is stunted. Twenty to 30 months after receiving radiation to the thyroid, almost 80% of children develop evidence of thyroid dysfunction. This event is dose dependent and usually causes compensated hypothyroidism, with as many as one third needing thyroid replacement therapy.

Patients who receive extensive radiation therapy are at risk for radiation pneumonitis, pericarditis, and enteritis. Radiation pneumonitis and pericarditis have occurred in patients with large mediastinal masses for whom the radiation target size was not decreased as the mass resolved.

Sterility in male patients is a frequent complication, especially after three cycles of MOPP. For female patients, delay and alteration of menstrual cycles have been reported, especially after pelvic irradiation. However, if the ovaries are moved out of the radiation field (ie, oophoropexy) at the time of the staging laparotomy, all patients should have normal menses. If the chemotherapy plans use only MOPP or ABVD, more than 80% of girls have normal menses.

Infections have been one of the main concerns for HD patients because of their underlying immune deficiency, splenectomy, and the toxicity of therapy. Vaccination with pneumococcal, *Haemophilus influenzae*, and *Neisseria meningitidis* antigens should be done routinely in preparation for splenectomy. Prophylactic penicillin is also recommended. Herpes zoster infections occur in as many as 75% of HD patients who receive combined-modality therapy. Thirty percent of those treated with irradiation or chemotherapy alone develop this complication. The use of intravenous acyclovir (9-[(2-hydroxyethoxy)methyl]guanine) has greatly reduced the morbidity of varicella-zoster infections. *Pneumocystis carinii* infection is a constant threat to HD patients, but it can be treated with high-dose trimethoprim-sulfamethoxazole.

*Principles and Practice of Pediatrics, Second Edition.*
edited by Frank A. Oski et al. J. B. Lippincott Company, Philadelphia © 1994.

# 97.2 *Non-Hodgkin's Lymphoma*

Kenneth L. McClain

Non-Hodgkin's lymphomas (NHLs) represent 10% of all tumors in the pediatric age group. The peak incidence occurs among children 7 to 11 years of age, and there is a male predominance. There are three major histologic varieties: lymphoblastic, Burkitt's, and large cell or histiocytic lymphomas.

## TYPES OF NON-HODGKIN'S LYMPHOMA

### Lymphoblastic Lymphoma

The small lymphoblast of the lymphoblastic lymphomas is morphologically similar to the lymphoblast of acute lymphoblastic leukemia. For a child with lymphomatous features of massive lymphadenopathy and hepatosplenomegaly, an arbitrary distinction is made by evaluating the bone marrow aspirate for lymphoblasts. If there are fewer than 25% blasts, the diagnosis is lymphoma if the cells are found in the lymph node biopsy. The cell of origin usually is a T lymphoblast, although non-T, non-B lymphoblasts may rarely be the predominant cell type. The lymphoblastic lymphomas comprise 28% of childhood NHL.

Most children present with cervical lymphadenopathy, a mediastinal mass, and moderate hepatosplenomegaly. The anterior mediastinal mass with or without a pleural effusion may cause respiratory compromise requiring prompt evaluation and therapy. There is a high incidence of central nervous system (CNS) involvement and leukemic transformation in patients with lymphoblastic lymphoma.

### Burkitt's Lymphoma

Burkitt's lymphoma is the most common (39%) type of NHL in childhood. The children usually present with an abdominal mass that may originate in the bowel, kidneys, or gonads and be accompanied by massive ascites. Striking enlargement of the tonsils or thyroid gland and CNS disease may be evident. Bone marrow involvement may show the L3 variety of lymphoblast containing vacuoles staining with oil red O.

Burkitt's lymphoma is a particularly dangerous form of childhood cancer because it frequently masquerades as an apparently "benign" tonsillitis or intussusception from a leading enlargement of cecal, ileal, or mesenteric nodes. Surface marker studies show a mature B cell with surface immunoglobulin. The B lymphoblast is the fastest growing human tumor cell, with doubling times of less than 24 hours. The disease can change from a barely palpable node to massive tumor in a matter of days.

Although the cell of origin and clinical behavior is similar to the African variety originally named after Dr. Denis Burkitt, the association with Epstein-Barr virus is lacking and the source of chronic antigenic stimulation (eg, malaria, parasites) less obvious in western countries. There is a histologic variation of this tumor that causes some confusion; pathologists may report "non-Burkitt's, Burkitt's lymphoma." This designation reflects the heterogeneity of cell size and has little clinical relevance.

Molecular analysis has shown correlations with the frequent chromosome translocations: t(8,14), t(8,22), and t(2,8). The movement of DNA in these translocations bring the *MYC* on-cogene on chromosome 8 into juxtaposition with active immunoglobulin gene-regulating elements on the other chromosomes. These molecular rearrangements may be important in causing the malignant phenotype.

### Large Cell Lymphoma

The third type of childhood NHL is the large cell lymphomas, previously called histiocytic lymphomas. This disease often presents in lymphoid tissue of the tonsils, adenoids, or Peyer's patches. Rarely, it starts as a solitary cervical lymph node enlargement. The cells of origin are usually B cells and rarely T lymphocytes or true histiocytes.

## PATIENT EVALUATION AND DIAGNOSIS

Initial evaluation of NHL patients should include a thorough history and physical examination. Laboratory investigations should include a complete blood count, urinalysis, chest x-ray film, spinal tap, and bone marrow biopsy and aspirate, with samples sent for chromosome and cell marker analysis. Requisite blood chemistry evaluation includes serum electrolytes, including calcium and phosphate; liver function tests and blood urea nitrogen; and creatinine, uric acid, and serum lactate dehydrogenase (LDH) levels. The renal tests are especially important because of frequent kidney involvement in lymphoblastic and Burkitt's lymphomas.

Because of the rapid turnover of these cells and tumor lysis from chemotherapy, the physician must know if cell breakdown has resulted in dangerous levels of uric acid, calcium, or phosphate, which may precipitate in the kidney. This complication is usually preventable by vigorous hydration, alkalinization, and use of allopurinol before the treatment is begun.

The serum LDH is an important marker for following the progress of disease and has prognostic importance. If the LDH level is over 1000, there is a high probability of massive disease and a poor outcome. Chest x-ray and abdominal CT examinations are necessary for determining the extent of intracavitary disease. Lymphangiograms are not helpful.

Removal of abdominal or tonsilar masses or biopsy of mediastinal nodes is required to make the diagnosis. Tissue samples should be sent for cell surface marker studies, chromosome analysis, and special molecular studies for further understanding the tumor biology. A staging laparotomy as is done for Hodgkin's disease is unnecessary for NHL. The clinical staging categories are listed in Table 97-2.

## TREATMENT

### Lymphoblastic Lymphomas

Localized diffuse NHL (ie, stages I and II) responds well to a short induction and consolidation with vincristine, doxorubicin, prednisone, cyclophosphamide, and intrathecal medications. A 33-week maintenance program with mercaptopurine, methotrexate, and intrathecal injections results in a long-term survival rate of more than 95% for stage I patients and 86% for stage II patients.

Stage III and IV NHL present more challenging problems, because the type of therapy depends on the immunologic identification of cell type. For lymphoblastic lymphomas a 12-drug regimen (LSA$_2$L$_2$) lasting 2 to 3 years resulted in 76% disease-free survival rate. Current therapy with eight drugs (ie, ara-C, cyclophosphamide, vincristine, doxorubicin, prednisone, mercaptopurine, VM-26, L-asparaginase) and intrathecal therapy lasts

TABLE 97-2. Staging of Childhood
Non-Hodgkin's Lymphoma

| Stage I | Single tumor in a node or extralymphatic site, excluding the mediastinum or abdomen |
|---|---|
| Stage II | Single extranodal tumor with one regional node positive |
| | Two or more nodal areas on the same side of the diaphragm; two extranodal tumors on the same side of the diaphragm regardless of nodal involvement; or primary gastrointestinal tract tumor plus or minus associated mesenteric nodes, grossly completely excised |
| Stage III | Two single extranodal tumors on opposite sides of the diaphragm; two or more nodal areas above and below the diaphragm; all tumors originating in mediastinum, pleura, or thymus; or all extensive primary intra-abdominal disease (usually many implants, not totally resectable), often with ascites |
| Stage IV | Any of the above with initial central nervous or bone marrow involvement |

*From Murphy SB. Childhood non-Hodgkin's lymphoma. N Engl J Med 1978;299:1446.*

approximately 2 years. The granulocyte colony-stimulating factor (G-CSF) is used to prevent extreme neutropenia and sepsis. This new treatment gives a slightly improved chance of long-term survival.

## Burkitt's Lymphoma

Stage I and II Burkitt's lymphoma patients have been treated with vincristine, doxorubicin, cyclophosphamide, prednisone, and intrathecal medications as induction and consolidation therapy. Some patients continue with maintenance for 33 weeks of mercaptopurine and methotrexate like acute lymphoblastic leukemia patients. A 94% complete remission rate has been reported. Stage III or IV patients had only a 10% chance of survival until the advent of very aggressive chemotherapy treatments. It is now possible to cure 80% of stage III and 50% of stage IV patients. These patients represent an especially challenging group because the high metabolic turnover of their tumor puts them at risk for renal and electrolyte complications (ie, tumor lysis syndrome) before and during induction therapy. Generous prehydration, alkalinization, and allopurinol treatment are necessary. Induction with cyclophosphamide, intrathecal ara-C and methotrexate, doxorubicin, and vincristine is followed by high-dose intravenous methotrexate with leucovorin and high-dose ara-C when the absolute phagocyte count is more than $500/\mu L$. Many patients had life-threatening infections during the initial stages of treatment until their granulocyte production was stimulated with G-CSF. Intensification treatment with VP-16, ifosamide, and intrathecal medications are given to some patients in the current randomized study. Consolidation therapy repeats most of the chemotherapy used in the induction phase. The total time of treatment ranges from 3 to 5 months.

## Large Cell Lymphomas

The standard therapy for large cell lymphomas includes induction treatment with doxorubicin (Adriamycin), prednisone, and vincristine (Oncovin) followed by maintenance therapy with vincristine, mercaptopurine, doxorubicin (to a maximum dose of 300 $mg/m^2$), and prednisone. Intrathecal methotrexate is given as prophylaxis for CNS disease. Radiation therapy is used only if the lymphoma is resistant to initial chemotherapy or for CNS

disease. The disease-free survival rate for patients treated with these therapies is grater than 80%.

For relapsed patients who can be brought back into remission, some centers are now performing bone marrow transplants for hematopoietic rescue after lethal irradiation and chemotherapy for tumor ablation. Some encouraging results have been reported for patients who would otherwise have had a dismal prognosis.

## Selected Readings

### Hodgkin's Disease and Non-Hodgkin's Lymphomas

Donaldson SS, Whitaker SJ, Plowman PN, Link MP, Malpas JS. Stage I-II pediatric Hodgkin's disease: long-term follow-up demonstrates equivalent survival rates following different management schemes. J Clin Onc 1990;8:1128.

Murphy SB. The lymphomas and lymphadenopathy. In: Nathan DG, Oski FA (eds). Hematology of infancy and childhood, 3rd ed. Philadelphia: WB Saunders, 1987:1086.

Pallesen G, Sandvej K, Hamilton-Dutoit SJ, Rowe M, Young LS. Activation of Epstein-Barr virus replication in Hodgkin and Reed-Sternberg cells. Blood 1991;78:1162.

*Principles and Practice of Pediatrics, Second Edition.*
edited by Frank A. Oski et al. J. B. Lippincott Company, Philadelphia © 1994.

CHAPTER 98
# *Malignant Brain Tumors in Children*

## Donald H. Mahoney, Jr.

Primary brain tumors are the second most common type of cancer reported in children and adolescents. In the United States, the annual incidence of primary brain tumors in children younger than 15 years of age is 24 per million persons in the general population or approximately 1200 new cases each year. Unfortunately, progress in the field of pediatric neuro-oncology has been slow compared with that in other childhood malignancies.

Surgery and radiation therapy traditionally constituted the standard therapeutic approach. The tendency has been to manage these children within the general medical community, contrary to the now common practice of referral to a pediatric cancer center for definitive diagnosis and treatment. Pessimism has followed the failure to excise the tumor completely, and chemotherapy has been viewed as noxious, with little justification. However, progress in the comprehensive care of children with malignant brain tumors under the direction of experienced pediatric neuro-oncology teams has provided a rational basis for a departure from a previously gloomy scenario. Tumor heterogeneity, the relatively small numbers of patients with a specific tumor type available for investigation, the limitations of drug delivery across the blood–brain barrier, and the relative biologic resistance to therapy in certain tumors, such as gliomas, are unique technical and theoretical challenges that can be resolved only by continued collaborative clinical and laboratory research.

## SYMPTOMS ON PRESENTATION

Early symptoms of central nervous system (CNS) tumors are frequently nonspecific. In infants with open sutures, these may consist of increased head circumference, irritability, head tilt, and loss of developmental milestones. Older children may present with headache. This symptom usually increases in frequency, becomes more severe in the morning, and is typically followed by vomiting. Approximately 85% of the children with malignant brain tumors have abnormal findings on neurologic or ocular examinations within 2 to 4 months of the onset of headaches.

Children who report an unchanging pattern of headaches without focal neurologic findings for more than 12 months have a low probability for CNS tumors. Specific neurologic symptoms, such as ataxia, somnolence, hemiparesis, seizures, head tilt, cranial nerve palsies, diencephalic syndrome, and diabetes insipidus, may occur later in the illness and may suggest localization of the CNS tumor.

The differential diagnosis for CNS tumors in children is extensive and includes brain abscesses, hemorrhage, nonneoplastic hydrocephalus of any cause, arteriovenous malformations or aneurysm, and indolent virus infections.

## CLASSIFICATION

Traditionally, CNS tumors of childhood have been classified on the basis of location (eg, infratentorial versus supratentorial) and histology. In children between the ages of 4 and 11 years, infratentorial (posterior fossa) tumors predominate. These include cerebellar tumors and brain stem tumors. Supratentorial tumors occur more frequently during the first years of life and during late adolescence and young adulthood. Approximately 45% of the childhood brain tumors arise in the cerebellum. Cerebellar astrocytomas and medulloblastomas are the tumors diagnosed most frequently in this region. Ependymomas that arise in and around the fourth ventricle represent between 3% and 14% of all childhood tumors and have been included as cerebellar tumors by some authorities.

The cerebrum is the next most common site of involvement in children, accounting for 20% to 27% of all brain tumors. The most frequent tumors include astrocytomas, glioblastomas, and ependymomas. Brain stem neoplasms account for 9% to 15% of all intracranial neoplasms. Approximately 75% of all brain stem tumors occur in children younger than 10 years of age. Midline tumors, which include a mix of germ cell tumors, craniopharyngiomas, pinealomas, optic gliomas, and pituitary adenomas, account for another 10%.

The traditional practice of classifying CNS tumors on the basis of location is being reevaluated. An international panel of neuropathologists has proposed a revision of the World Health Organization (WHO) classification system to classify tumors on the basis of histopathologic features alone. For example, medulloblastoma, a highly malignant, poorly differentiated, "small blue cell" tumor was said to arise only within the cerebellum. The revised classification system recognizes this tumor as a primitive neuroectodermal tumor (PNET), with or without elements of astrocytic, neuronal, or ependymal differentiation. Tumors of this identical histologic type arising anywhere within the brain are classified as PNET. The pinealoblastoma arising in the pineal region or the ependymoblastoma or classic PNET arising within the supratentorial regions are all identified by the new classification schema as a PNET.

This proposed classification system recognizes the heterogeneity of tumors arising within a single site and may be useful for future prognostic staging and for the design of new therapeutic strategies. Initially, the revised nomenclature may cause confusion for the clinician who is attempting to establish a specific diagnosis, define a treatment plan, and offer a prognosis.

## DIAGNOSTIC EVALUATIONS

Computed tomography (CT) scanning, with and without contrast enhancement, has been the standard noninvasive diagnostic tool for more than a decade. The unenhanced CT scan can suggest whether a lesion is cystic or solid and whether there are calcifications, hemorrhage, edema, and hydrocephalus. After intravenous contrast, enhancement of the tumor occurs because of a disruption of the blood–brain barrier. This improves detection of small tumors, definition of isodense or hypodense regions within the tumor, and differentiation of areas of edema surrounding the tumor mass. Subarachnoid and leptomeningeal seeding of tumor may also be detected with enhanced scans. Cranial CT scans have a sensitivity of greater than 94% for primary brain tumors, but certain limitations of resolution must be recognized. Small lesions within the posterior fossa, especially within the brain stem, and small midline cystic structures near the base of the skull occasionally escape detection.

Magnetic resonance imaging (MRI) with gadolinium enhancement is a sensitive neuroimaging technology for the diagnosis of CNS tumors and is becoming more widely available. MRI scans are potentially superior to CT scans in the detection and definition of low-grade glial tumors and of lesions at the vertex, within the posterior fossa (especially within the brain stem), near the wall of the middle fossa, and at the base of the skull (Fig 98-1). MRI myelography with gadolinium enhancement is the best method for detecting spinal cord tumors or delineating leptomeningeal tumor invasion. MRI scans use no ionizing radiation and have no calvarium artifact. Limitations include increased cost, longer scan times, an inability to detect calcifications, and limited access to the patient during the actual scan time.

The child with a positive scan may benefit from additional diagnostic procedures. Angiography gives information about blood supply and may assist the neurosurgeon in planning the operative approach. Myelography is important for accurate staging of tumors that tend to disseminate throughout the neuraxis, including all PNETs (eg, medulloblastoma, ependymomas, germinomas) and high-grade astrocytomas. Noninvasive MRI myelography is replacing conventional myelography in pediatric CNS tumor staging. Cerebrospinal fluid examination is of great importance in patients presenting with PNETs, germinomas, and high-grade glial tumors, but it must be performed with great care in patients with increased intracranial pressure. Standard radionuclide scans are no longer of significant value. However, newer methodologies, such as the positron emission tomography scan coupled with 2-deoxyglucose infusions, may help differentiate viable from necrotic tumor after therapy.

The electroencephalogram, visual-evoked potential, and brain stem auditory evoked potential may be useful at diagnosis and in the management of complications of the disease (eg, seizures) or of certain therapeutic strategies (eg, cisplatin-associated ototoxicity). Tumor markers are also important in selected malignant conditions. Alpha-fetoprotein and β-chorionic gonadotropin are useful markers of malignant germ cell tumors that may arise in the pineal or suprasellar regions. Investigations of tumor cytogenetics, monoclonal antibody characterization of specific tumor antigens, and oncogene expression are becoming important aspects of the ongoing studies of the biology of CNS tumors in children, and their use highlights the importance of neurosurgical care at established pediatric cancer centers. Fresh tumor tissue, obtained at the time of surgery, is essential for these biologic studies. Because neuropsychologic testing and endocrine surveillance comprise a critical aspect of the management of long-term survivors, baseline examinations are important.

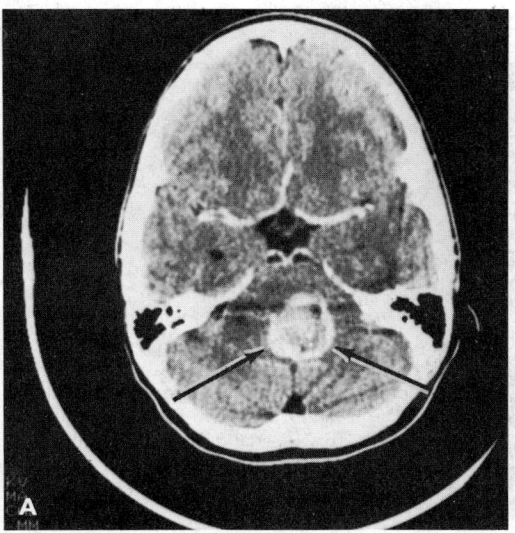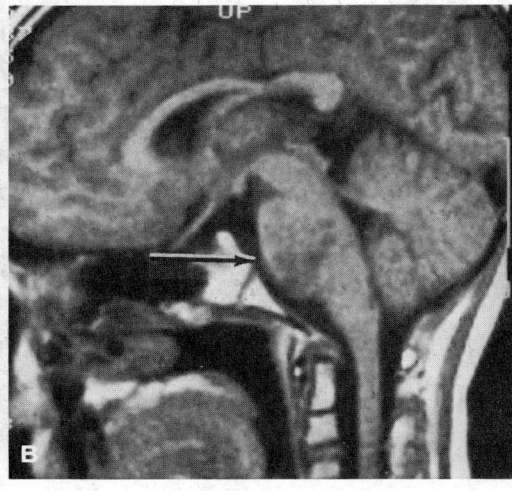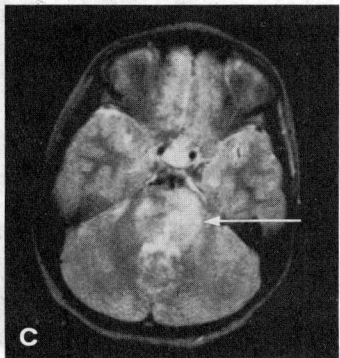

**Figure 98-1.**    CT scan and MRI study of a brain-stem glioma. (**A**) CT scan demonstrating a ring-like enhancing mass (*arrows*) involving the mid pons. (**B**) Six months after the diagnosis and radiotherapy, the MRI sagittal view (T1 weighted) reveals an enlarging mass in the mid pons (*arrows*). (**C**) The axial T2-weighted scan reveals abnormal signal intensity (*arrow*) extending into the left brachium pontis.

## TREATMENT

Published treatment results for various childhood malignant brain tumors vary widely and should be interpreted with caution. The number of patients with specific tumor histologies available for clinical investigations is small, and studies may report results from trials with limited patient entries. Despite this caveat, progress has been made in the treatment of several pediatric CNS tumors. Continued efforts must be made to enroll these patients in prospective, multimodal, cooperative treatment studies and accelerate the development of more effective therapeutic strategies.

### Cerebellar Astrocytomas

Cerebellar astrocytomas account for approximately 20% of all brain tumors in children. Boys and girls are affected equally, and the mean age at diagnosis is 6 years. There are two histologic variants. The juvenile pilocytic astrocytoma accounts for 80% to 85% of the cases. With complete surgical excision, 10-year survival rates of 80% to 95% have been reported. Recurrence may follow a partially excised tumor, but retreatment is usually possible. Diffuse astrocytomas comprise approximately 15% of the cases. The role of radiation therapy in treating incompletely resected tumors is the subject of an ongoing Pediatric Oncology Group and Children's Cancer Study Group (CCSG) survey.

### Medulloblastomas

Medulloblastomas are highly malignant primitive neuroectodermal tumors, usually arising in the roof of the fourth ventricle and cerebellar vermis. They occur more frequently in boys, primarily affect children between 4 and 8 years of age, and account for 20% of all brain tumors in children. Diagnostic studies of these patients should include cranial CT or MRI scans with and without enhancement, cerebrospinal fluid cytology, MRI myelography, and bone marrow examination. Metastatic disease or diffuse subarachnoid involvement may be apparent at diagnosis.

Optimal therapy is multimodal and includes investigational components that seek to improve long-term survival. Therapy includes surgery, irradiation, and chemotherapy in selected cases. The goals of neurosurgery are to establish a tissue diagnosis,

relieve intracranial pressure, and debulk or totally excise gross tumor as clinical conditions permit. Complete tumor excision is achievable in 50% of the patients and may offer a survival advantage. A preoperative staging system developed by Chang and associates, based on a grading scale of T0–4 for extent of local tumor and M0–4 for metastatic disease, has had prognostic value in several studies. Cellular differentiation may have a negative impact on survival.

Medulloblastoma is a radiosensitive and chemosensitive tumor. The conventional radiation therapy schedule has been to administer fractionated doses of more than 5000 cGy to the posterior fossa over 5 to 6 weeks with whole brain and spinal axis irradiation of approximately 4000 cGy and 3600 cGy, respectively. Reports of 5-year disease-free survival rates with radiation therapy alone range from 45% to 60%. Late failures beyond 5 years may continue to occur. Recent data from the Connecticut Surveillance, Epidemiology, and End Result (SEER) registries and from Children's Hospital of Philadelphia indicate that pediatric patients treated at university hospitals have a significantly better prognosis for survival than those treated at community hospitals.

In an effort to improve overall survival, several institutional adjuvant chemotherapy trials have been conducted by pediatric cancer cooperative groups. Three randomized clinical trials have demonstrated that adjuvant chemotherapy after surgery and irradiation increases the survival of children with medulloblastoma. The survival advantages were small (~10%), with patients with locally extensive disease (T3 or T4) or evidence of metastases (M1–3), clearly benefiting from chemotherapy. Additional clinical trials have sought to identify more effective combinations of chemotherapeutic agents. A preirradiation and postirradiation chemotherapy program using eight drugs administered over an 18-hour period (eg, the eight-in-one therapy) has produced a 56% response rate in a CCSG phase II study and is undergoing further clinical trials. Investigators at St. Jude Children's Research Hospital demonstrated excellent responses with preirradiation cisplatin and VP-16. The Children's Hospital of Philadelphia reported a 5-year disease-free survival rate of 88% for children treated with CCNU, vincristine, and cisplatin.

The results of these studies suggest that adjuvant chemotherapy has a role in the treatment of medulloblastoma. Clinical trials conducted by the Pediatric Oncology Group are testing whether preirradiation chemotherapy with cisplatin and VP-16

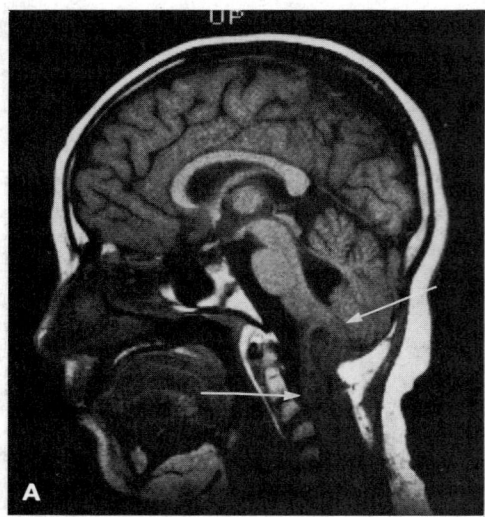
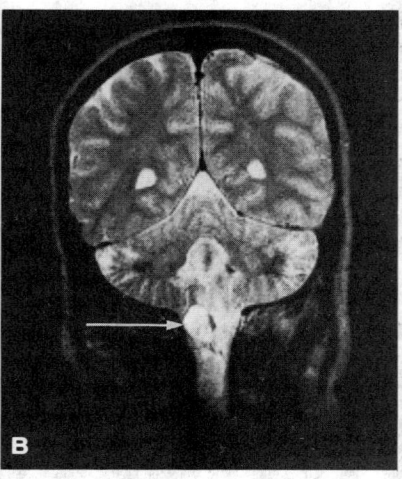

**Figure 98-2.** MRI study of a brain stem and cervical tumor. (**A**) Sagittal view (T1-weighted) reveals enlargement of the caudal brain stem, extending below the foramen magnum to the level of C5-C6 (*arrows*). (**B**) Coronal view (T2-weighted) reveals an increased signal intensity highlighting the cystic component of this lesion as it extends into the cervical cord (*arrow*).

in patients with more extensive disease at diagnosis can enhance the effects of radiation therapy and increase survival. For patients with "standard-risk" medulloblastoma (ie, Chang stage T0–2M0), adjuvant chemotherapy has not been clearly established as beneficial. A clinical trial randomizing patients to surgery and radiation therapy with or without adjuvant chemotherapy may answer this question. Other areas of potential investigation include studies of hyperfractionated irradiation.

## Brain Stem Tumors

Brain stem gliomas have the worst prognosis of all pediatric CNS tumors, with an estimated median survival after local irradiation of less than 12 months and a 5-year disease-free survival rate of 15% to 18%.

Progressive cranial nerve dysfunctions and gait disturbances, coupled with an intrinsic mass in the brain stem as demonstrated by CT or MRI scan are the hallmarks of this disease (Fig 98-2). The staging and surgical management of this disease is controversial. The surgical approach to brain stem lesions is hazardous. Patients with "inoperable" lesions involving the pons or medulla with hypodense regions defined by CT scan or malignant histology have a poor prognosis. Patients with "operable" exophytic components, lower-grade histology, or with lesions arising in higher brain stem regions may experience longer survival.

Conventional therapy has included high-dose steroids and local posterior fossa irradiation to 5500 cGy over 6 weeks. More than 50% of the patients respond, but the tumor invariably recurs. Adjuvant chemotherapy trials have failed to demonstrate any survival advantage for patients. Hyperfractionation radiation techniques for this disease are undergoing trials. Studies from the Brain Tumor Study Group have suggested a significantly improved time to progression for patients receiving hyperfractionated therapy to 7200 cGy. The Pediatric Oncology Group reported a modest survival advantage for patients treated at 7020 cGy. Further studies of hyperfractionated radiation, including potential radiosensitizing agents, are being pursued.

## High-Grade Astrocytomas

High-grade astrocytomas (ie, anaplastic astrocytoma or glioblastoma) represent approximately 25% of childhood tumors. These tumors develop in the cerebral hemisphere (51%), brain stem (37%), and cerebellum (Fig 98-3).

The conventional management of high-grade astrocytomas includes aggressive surgical excision, whenever possible, and ra-

diation therapy to 5500 cGy or greater. The 5-year disease-free survival rate is less than 25%. Adjuvant chemotherapy has been of marginal benefit. In a randomized trial, the CCSG reported a survival advantage for patients treated with CCNU, vincristine, and prednisone after surgery and radiation therapy compared with patients treated without chemotherapy (45% versus 13% 5-year disease-free survival rates). The extent of surgical excision had an important influence on outcome. Favorable pilot experience with the eight-in-one protocol resulted in the incorporation of this treatment regimen into the CCSG control studies for high-grade astrocytoma. The Pediatric Oncology Group is investigating intensive preirradiation chemotherapy schedules with cisplatin and BCNU and with cyclophosphamide and VP-16 followed by hyperfractionated radiation therapy for this group of patients.

## Ependymomas

Ependymomas represent only 9% of all brain tumors in children. These tumors are locally invasive, may be cystic, and demonstrate a spectrum of histologic appearances. Ependymomas occur

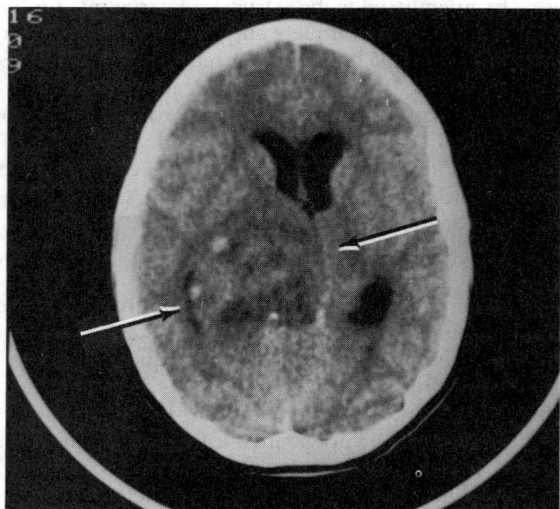

**Figure 98-3.** An unenhanced CT scan demonstrates a large, inhomogeneous mass (*arrows*) involving the right parietal lobe, with a midline shift. Partial excision revealed an anaplastic astrocytoma. Dye sensitivity prevented a contrast study, a problem not encountered with MRI techniques.

equally among boys and girls. Intracranial lesions typically occur in children between the ages of 2 and 6 years, but spinal tumors occur more often during the teenage years. In children, most ependymomas arise in the posterior fossa, about the fourth ventricle. Large supratentorial tumors in paraventricular regions may also occur (Fig 98-4). The incidence of spinal cord seeding at diagnosis has been reported as 10% to 11%, although the actual incidence varies with the location and histology of the primary tumor. Conventional treatment includes aggressive surgery with the goal of gross total excision followed by radiation therapy. The choice of radiation fields (eg, cranial versus craniospinal) is the subject of investigation. Improved disease-free survival has been reported in patients with high-grade ependymomas after craniospinal irradiation. Overall, the estimated 5-year disease-free survival rate with surgery and radiation therapy is 45% to 65%, with an advantage for patients having complete surgical excision. Chemotherapy trials have been limited and inconclusive. Pediatric Oncology Group studies are investigating hyperfractionated radiation therapy for these patients.

## Preirradiation Chemotherapy in Young Children

Effective preirradiation chemotherapy combinations are being investigated for children younger than 3 years of age with malignant brain tumors. Thirteen percent of all brain tumors occur in children younger than 2 years of age, and the standard therapy of surgery and irradiation has produced a dismal 5-year disease-free survival rate of only 18%. Moreover, the quality of life in the few survivors has been poor. Neurotoxicity among survivors has been profound, leaving almost half of the patients retarded or handicapped.

Preliminary experience with postoperative chemotherapy and delayed irradiation for infants has been encouraging. The M.D. Anderson Cancer Center has reported successful management of children younger than 36 months of age with medulloblastoma, treating them with MOPP chemotherapy alone for 2 years. The projected 5-year survival rate was 77%. Neuropsychologic assessment of survivors not receiving radiation therapy indicated average or above-average performance scores. The Pediatric Oncology Group completed a multi-institution study of infants younger than 3 years of age. After surgery, the children with malignant brain tumors were treated with high-dose cyclophosphamide, vincristine, cisplatin, and VP-16, and radiation therapy was deferred. Overall, the 2-year progression-free survival rate was 37%. Many patients received no radiation therapy. Ongoing

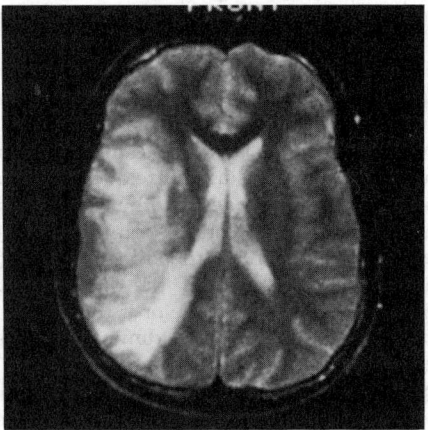

**Figure 98-4.** A T2-weighted MRI scan in the axial projection reveals a large, right frontal-parietal mass, with the central component representing neoplasm (ependymoma) and the peripheral component, probably edema.

clinical trials within the Pediatric Oncology Group and in other institutions will continue to explore optimal chemotherapy schedules for children younger than 3 years of age at diagnosis with poor-prognosis brain tumors.

## Selected Readings

Friedman HS, Oakes WJ. New therapeutic options in the management of childhood brain tumors. Oncology 1992;6:27.

Friedman HS, Oakes WJ. The chemotherapy of posterior fossa tumors in childhood. J Neurooncol 1987;5:217.

Heideman RL, Packer RJ, Albright LA, et al. Tumors of the central nervous system. In: Pizzo PA, Poplack DG, eds. Principles and practice of pediatric oncology. Philadelphia: JB Lippincott, 1989:505.

Van Eys J. Malignant tumors of the central nervous system. In: Fernbach DJ, Vietti TJ, eds. Clinical pediatric oncology, ed. 4. St. Louis: CV Mosby, 1991:409.

*Principles and Practice of Pediatrics, Second Edition.*
edited by Frank A. Oski et al. J. B. Lippincott Company, Philadelphia © 1994.

CHAPTER 99
# *Neoplasms of the Kidney or Suprarenal Area*

## 99.1 *Wilms' Tumor*

C. Philip Steuber and Donald J. Fernbach

Wilms' tumor is a malignant embryonal neoplasm of the kidney of mixed cellular histology. The incidence remains remarkably constant, with 7.8 cases per million children younger than 15 years of age reported annually. It is diagnosed only slightly less often than neuroblastoma, and like neuroblastoma, it is a tumor of young children: 77% occur in children younger than 5 years of age, and 90% occur in children younger than 7 years of age. The incidence peaks in children between the ages 1 and 3 years (median, 3.5 years). The tumors associated with cytogenic aberrations occur at a slightly earlier age. Girls are more frequently affected than boys (2 : 1), and they may present at a slightly older age.

## Etiology

Wilms' tumor is thought to develop from a proliferation of metanephric blastema. Renal blastema develops between 8 and 34 weeks of gestation, and no renal blastema is formed thereafter. The potential for Wilms' tumor to develop from primitive blastema should be determined during that time. This tumor occurs in hereditary and nonhereditary forms. The hereditary form is autosomal dominant, may be multifocal in presentation, and may be associated with other congenital anomalies. Tumors in multiple family members have been reported but are extremely rare.

Cytogenetic analysis of cases associated with aniridia have demonstrated a consistent interstitial deletion of the short arm of chromosome 11. Several congenital anomalies have been associated with Wilms' tumor. Aniridia was found in 1.1% of 547 children evaluated in the National Wilms' Tumor Study (NWTS); 2.9% had hemihypertrophy, and 4.4% had genitourinary anomalies. The most common genitourinary anomalies were hypoplasia, fusion and ectopia of the kidney, duplications in the collecting systems, hypospadias, and cryptorchism. In addition to the aniridia gene, a gene related to normal genitourinary tract development has been localized to chromosome 11p. Patients with aniridia and with genitourinary tract anomalies but not hemihypertrophy are significantly younger at diagnosis.

Closely related to hemihypertrophy and Wilms' tumor is the Beckwith-Wiedemann syndrome, which includes gigantism and macroglossia. It has also been linked to chromosome 11.

## PATHOLOGY

Bilateral tumors occur in about 5% of patients. The first case report of this tumor by Rance in 1814 was of a bilateral tumor. The typical tumor is a solitary, multilobulated lesion that can occur in any part of either kidney. Rarely does it occur outside of the kidney.

Histologically, the tumor is composed of mixed mesenchymal elements in different stages of maturity. Renal blastema denotes epithelial elements that form abortive or embryonic glomerulotubular structures. These structures appear in an undifferentiated stroma, which may also contain differentiated mesenchymal structures such as striated muscles, cartilage, adipose tissue, and bone. The tumors have been referred to as *triphasic* to denote the involvement of blastemal, epithelial, and stromal elements. Individual tumors may have a monomorphic pattern that can be mistaken for a hamartoma.

The use of the terms *favorable* and *unfavorable histology* was derived from the NWTS. Initially, three types of unfavorable histology were identified, which accounted for 10% to 14% of all Wilms' tumors and for more than 60% of the mortality. These are focal or diffuse anaplastic; clear cell sarcoma, often called the bone-metastasizing tumor; and the rhabdoid tumor, often metastasizing to the brain. The rhabdoid histologic type is a highly malignant tumor similar in structure to sarcomatous tumors that occur outside of the kidney. This tumor is no longer considered to be a Wilms' tumor variant by NWTS. It accounts for a small proportion of all tumors that have been registered as Wilms' tumors but a disproportionately high percentage of the fatalities.

The classic, congenital mesoblastic nephroma is a benign tumor that sometimes resembles a clear cell sarcomatous form of Wilms' tumor. Most cases are discovered at birth and in the neonatal period, but some tumors are detected in infants 16 days to 3 months of age. Because of occasional invasiveness, recurrence, and rare distal metastases of tumors with similar histology in older patients, an upper age limit of 3 months has been placed on the diagnosis of this benign tumor.

## CLINICAL AND DIAGNOSTIC FEATURES

The classic Wilms' tumor appears as a silent mass in the abdomen in almost two thirds of the patients. The tumor is often detected accidentally by the parents or incidentally during the course of a physical examination performed for other medical reasons. Abdominal pain occurs in approximately one third of the patients. The mass is usually hard, smooth, and confined to the flank or one side of the abdomen. Occasionally, a patient with Wilms' tumor experiences a sudden hemorrhage into the tumor and pre-

sents with rapid abdominal enlargement and anemia. Hematuria has been observed in 12% to 25% of the patients, and hypertension has been reported for as many as 63%. Nonspecific symptoms such as fever, malaise, constipation, and anorexia may be reported, but weight loss is an uncommon association.

The diagnosis of Wilms' tumor must be suspected in any child who has an abdominal mass. The evaluation includes complete blood counts, liver and kidney function studies, a skeletal survey, a chest radiograph, ultrasonography, and a computed tomography (CT) scan of the abdomen. If the abdominal CT scan fails to substantiate as renal lesion, a bone marrow examination is indicated (see Chap. 99.2) before surgical intervention. CT scans are now used instead of intravenous pyelography to evaluate abdominal masses in children. Areas of hemorrhage and calcification are less common than in neuroblastoma, but intratumoral necrosis does occur and is probably responsible for many of the spillages during surgery. A CT scan of the lungs may identify metastasis not seen on routine chest films and is recommended if the tumor appears to arise in the kidney. A few patients have normal chest radiographs but demonstrate pulmonary nodules by CT scan. The true nature of these nodules is uncertain, and biopsy is encouraged before considering them to be metastatic disease. Imaging studies (usually CT scans) to evaluate the possibility of hepatic parenchymal involvement enable the surgeons to judge how aggressive to be in their attempts to completely excise the disease in all locations.

The differential diagnosis includes neuroblastoma, rhabdomyosarcoma, leiomyosarcoma, renal cell sarcoma, fibrosarcoma, hypernephroma, polycystic kidneys, adrenal hemorrhage, renal vein thrombosis, dysplastic kidney, and renal carbuncle—almost anything that can cause a mass in the upper abdomen.

The final diagnosis depends on a biopsy or a complete excision of the tumor and subsequent histologic examination.

Rarely, syndromes of polycythemia, acquired von Willebrand's disease, and hypercalcemia have been associated with Wilms' tumor. Wilms' tumor occurs rarely in adults, who have a much poorer prognosis than the pediatric patients.

## STAGING

Surgical exploration should be made through a transabdominal approach and should include samples of hilar, periaortic, and other lymph nodes, regardless of their gross appearance. Liver biopsies are performed if there are any unusual hepatic lesions. Exploration of the opposite kidney after opening Gerota's fascia is essential to rule out synchronous bilateral disease.

The staging system developed by the NWTS has been adopted worldwide with minor variations (Table 99-1). The criteria are determined by the anatomical extent of the disease discovered at surgery and by the results of histopathologic examination. The system incorporates the key prognostic variables, which have changed from time to time according to the results of improved therapy. The major factors in staging are distal metastatic disease, involvement of the lymph nodes or other residual disease, and histologic type of tumor (ie, favorable or unfavorable). Other less important factors involved in prognosis have changed somewhat since the initial NWTS. In general, the outlook is better if the child is younger than 2 years of age or if the tumor weighs less than 250 g, but these factors have diminished in significance because of multiple combinations of chemotherapy. Favorable histology and early stage are the crucial good prognostic factors.

Because of a significant number of misdiagnoses after preoperative treatment with radiation therapy or chemotherapy in the European trials (SIOP), clinical investigators in the United States have preferred to establish a tissue diagnosis first. However, for tumors considered to be inoperable based on size or invasion,

## TABLE 99-1. Staging System Developed by the Third National Wilms' Tumor Study

**Stage I**
Tumor limited to kidney and is completely excised. Capsular surface intact; no tumor rupture; no residual tumor apparent beyond margins of excision

**Stage II**
Tumor extends beyond kidney but is completely excised. Regional extension of tumor; vessel infiltration; tumor biopsied or local spillage of tumor confined to the flank. No residual tumor apparent at or beyond margins of excision

**Stage III**
Residual nonhematogenous tumor confined to the abdomen. Lymph node involvement of hilus, periaortic chains or beyond; diffuse peritoneal contamination by tumor spillage; peritoneal implants of tumor; tumor extends beyond surgical margins microscopically or macroscopically; tumor not completely removable because of local infiltration into vital structures

**Stage IV**
Deposits beyond stage III (eg, lung, liver, bone, brain)

**Stage V**
Bilateral renal involvement at diagnosis

## TABLE 99-2. Two-Year Survival Rates for Children With Wilms' Tumor

| Patient Group | Two-Year Survival (%)* |
|---|---|
| Favorable histology | |
| Stage I | 98 |
| Stage II | 95 |
| Stage III | 89 |
| Stage IV | 89 |
| Unfavorable histology | |
| Stages I–III | 79 |
| Stage IV | 55 |
| All patients | 92 |

\* Results of the Third National Wilms' Tumor Study (NWTS-III).

pretreatment with chemotherapy can produce a significant number of successful results. Continued refinements in therapy in the United States and in Europe have brought the results of the two groups closer together.

## TREATMENT

Wilms' tumor is sensitive to chemotherapy and radiation therapy. Nevertheless, the first line of therapy is complete surgical excision of the tumor whenever possible. The NWTS confirmed the value of combined vincristine and dactinomycin therapy and subsequently showed the significant benefit contributed by adding doxorubicin to vincristine and dactinomycin for advanced-stage disease.

The series of NWTS protocols have also shown that postoperative radiation therapy is no longer required for stage I and II disease, eliminating a major cause of some of the most significant late effects of therapy. The NWTS group established that 6 months of therapy is adequate for stage I and II disease, which reduces the morbidity of longer chemotherapeutic schedules. For stage I patients, 10 weeks of two-drug therapy may be adequate.

Stage III patients—those with residual disease in the abdomen—still receive postoperative radiation therapy in addition to the three-drug regimen, but lower dosages of radiation (1000 cGy) with local boosts are adequate. Stage IV patients receive postoperative radiation that can be applied selectively on the basis of substaging of the primary lesions. Stage IV patients receive three or four drugs (including cyclophosphamide) for up to 15 months of therapy. In addition, radiation therapy to both lung fields has been used effectively for treatment of pulmonary metastases. The outlook for children with Wilms' tumor treated along the guidelines of the third NWTS is shown in Table 99-2.

Bilateral tumors can be synchronous or metachronous. The NWTS experience identified 4.2% of patients with synchronous disease and 1.6% with metachronous disease. By use of combined chemoradiotherapy and surgical or multiple surgical procedures, the survival rate of children with bilateral Wilms' tumor has risen impressively. Only in rare instances has it been necessary to perform bilateral nephrectomies, subsequent dialysis, and eventual renal transplantation.

An aggressive approach to metastatic disease has resulted in the salvage of many patients. Pulmonary irradiation plus chemotherapy with multiple agents has achieved survival rates of 40% to 50%. Many institutions excise liver or lung metastases if the lesions are surgically accessible and then administer chemotherapy or combined chemoradiotherapy. The prognosis is poorer for metastatic lesions that develop during the initial therapy, but it is reasonably good for patients off chemotherapy who develop metastatic disease.

The late effects of therapy are being reviewed continuously by the NWTS. The most prominent effects are bone and muscle changes secondary to radiation therapy. Significant among these are degrees of muscle atrophy and impairment of vertebral bone growth, which result in a high incidence of scoliosis. The younger the patient, the more profound is the subsequent damage, and many of these children have required corrective surgery, backbraces, and long-term physiotherapy. Irradiation to the chest can damage mammary tissue in young patients. The incidence of second malignancies is low, but second tumors, benign and malignant, have been described in a few patients. These include exostoses, osteochondromas, mesotheliomas, and leukemia.

## Selected Readings

Beckwith JB, Palmer NF. Histopathology and prognosis of Wilms' tumor. Results from the First National Wilms' Tumor Study. Cancer 1978;41:1937.

Bellasco JB, Chatten J, D'Angio GJ. Wilms' tumor. In: Sutow WW, Fernbach DJ, Vietti TJ, eds. Clinical pediatric oncology, ed 3. St. Louis: CV Mosby, 1984.

D'Angio GJ, Breslow N, Beckwith JB, et al. Treatment of Wilms' tumor—results of the Third National Wilms' Tumor Study. Cancer 1989;64:349.

Ganick DJ. Wilms' tumor. In: Hematology oncology clinics of North America. Philadelphia: WB Saunders, 1987.

*Principles and Practice of Pediatrics, Second Edition.*
edited by Frank A. Oski et al. J. B. Lippincott Company, Philadelphia © 1994.

# 99.2 *Neuroblastoma*

## ZoAnn E. Dreyer and Donald J. Fernbach

Neuroblastoma, ganglioneuroblastoma, and ganglioneuroma are tumors that develop from neural crest tissue and may arise from a number of widely separated anatomical sites along the craniospinal axis. After brain tumors, neuroblastoma is the most common solid tumor in childhood, with an incidence of approximately 10 per million white children per year and 7 per million black children per year. It is slightly more common in boys than in girls. Over half of the tumors occur in children younger than 2 years of age, and 75% are diagnosed during the first 4 years of life.

The actual incidence is probably much greater if based on random sections at autopsy of the adrenal glands of infants younger than 3 months of age, in which the incidence of neuroblastoma in situ has been reported to be as high as 1 in 39. These findings and the propensity for this tumor to regress spontaneously during the first year of life have important implications. Infants appear to possess an innate mechanism to cause regression of active tumor, eliminating a large percentage of the in situ tumors, or there is a biologic difference of the tumors of infants.

Investigations of the chromosome structure, associations with *MYCN* oncogene amplification, and DNA index (ploidy) are ongoing. The early results suggest significant differences in tumor behavior based on these biologic markers. We are just beginning to understand the precise biologic differences between tumors occurring in different age groups. Whatever the explanation is for the remarkable phenomenon of spontaneous regression, it appears to diminish at about 1 year of age.

## ETIOLOGY

The cause of neuroblastoma is unknown. No seasonal variation has been confirmed, but almost all services and surveys report significant variations in the annual incidence of this tumor. It is rare to find more than one case in a family, but there are reports of tumors occurring in siblings or successive generations. The concomitant occurrence of neuroblastoma with congenital anomalies of other organ systems has been described, but no specific defect exceeds the normal expectation of incidence. The findings of increased catecholamine excretion in the siblings of children with neuroblastoma supports the contention that all members of the family should be examined.

## PATHOLOGY

The tumors derive from cells that form the sympathetic ganglia and adrenal medulla. The sympathogonia differentiate along two lines: the pheochromocytoma line and the sympathicoblastic line. The three tumor types that arise from the sympathicoblastic line are the neuroblastoma, ganglioneuroblastoma, and ganglioneuroma.

Neuroblastoma usually consists of closely packed spheroid cells. Cell differentiation is variable, and there may be evidence of differentiation, such as the appearance of rosette-like structures. The centers of these rosettes contain fine neurofibrils that grow from the cells and make up the walls of the pseudorosette. Ultrastructure microscopy aids in the identification of the neurosecretory granules containing catecholamines, by which the diagnosis of neuroblastoma can be confirmed. Often, this can be done with tumor tissue obtained from an aspirated bone marrow specimen. Histologic grade based on calcification and mitotic rate in concert with *MYCN* amplification and ploidy has been proven to have a significant prognostic role in children with neuroblastoma. It is essential to obtain adequate tumor specimens to permit these important tissue examinations. Occasionally, this is possible by bone marrow examination alone, avoiding or postponing extensive surgery.

Ganglioneuroblastoma is a tumor containing recognizable differentiated elements, including ganglion cells. The prognosis is unaltered as long as malignant neuroblastoma cells are present. It is particularly important to examine multiple areas of these tumors to avoid mislabeling a tumor with malignant elements as a benign ganglioneuroma. Ganglioneuroma is composed of mature ganglion cells in a collagen-rich background containing bundles of neurofibrils. This is the benign tumor of this group. After therapy or spontaneous regression, the malignant elements may disappear, and all that remains is the ganglioneuroma tissue. This often is presumed to represent maturation of the malignant neuroblastoma. Ganglioneuroma may be seen in sites of metastatic neuroblastoma and in the area of the primary tumor.

## CLINICAL FEATURES

In almost 70% of the children with neuroblastoma, metastasis has occurred before the diagnosis is made, and the first clinical manifestations may be the result of metastatic disease. Commonly, however, the tumor appears as a large, "silent," intra-abdominal mass, and the signs and symptoms are attributable to compression of other tissues by the primary tumor or by the metastatic deposits. In about 55% of the primary tumors are found in the abdomen, and about 33% arise from the adrenal gland. The abdominal mass is usually firm, irregular, nontender, and crosses the midline. Extrinsic pressure by the tumor on the genitourinary structures may result in increased urinary frequency or a partial obstruction to the flow of urine. The primary abdominal tumor may cause intracranial hypertension and other bizarre neurologic abnormalities.

A primary tumor of the olfactory bulb (ie, esthesioneuroblastoma) can produce a mass in the nasal cavity. The tumor can extend into the intravertebral foramina and compress the spinal cord which, depending on the level, may result in the Horner syndrome or in paraplegia.

Thoracic tumors may displace the chest organs and can compromise the airway or cause superior vena caval obstruction. Unexplained fever is a common presenting complaint. Bone pain may occur in the absence of visible skeletal lesions but may be absent in the presence of widespread, destructive lesions. Unfortunately, this tumor has a predilection for involvement of the skull and facial bones, which may result in bilateral proptosis. This can cause severe deformity later. In association with proptosis, ecchymoses of the upper eyelids are a clue that this symptom is more likely to be caused by infiltrative disease than by trauma.

Skin nodules, which are seen commonly in infants, have a bluish cast and have been given the sobriquet "blueberry muffin." Signs and symptoms occasionally result from the catecholamine production of the tumor and may include flushing, increased perspiration, hypertension, headaches, and tachycardia. Diarrhea unresponsive to medical therapy is rare, as is failure to thrive, but both have been described in association with this type of metabolic activity. Another rare complaint is acute cerebellar ataxia associated with oculogyric crisis (ie, opsomyoclonus). These signs and symptoms, including paraplegia, are all potentially reversible after removal or destruction of the tumor.

## DIAGNOSTIC FEATURES

Peripheral hematologic studies often reveal anemia and reticulocytopenia, which are usually a reflection of metastatic disease involving the bone marrow. A bone marrow examination should be performed in every case of suspected neuroblastoma. Over half of all the children with neuroblastoma have tumor cells in the bone marrow. The tumor cells are seen easily on the bone marrow smears but are difficult to differentiate from other small round cell tumors of childhood such as lymphoma, leukemia, rhabdomyosarcoma, or Ewing's sarcoma. Electron microscopic examination may reveal the neurosecretory granules, which are diagnostic of neuroblastoma.

With the establishment of the relation between neuroblastoma and elevated urinary catecholamine excretion, neuroblastoma became one of a number of malignant neoplasms that have a fairly specific tumor marker. Increased amounts of vanillylmandelic acid or homovanillic acid are detected in the urine in more than 75% of these patients. These tests now can be done on a few milliliters of urine and with much greater accuracy than with the outdated 24-hour urine collection. The newer techniques measure all of the metabolic byproducts of dopamine, norepinephrine, and epinephrine. Urinary metabolites now can be found in the urine of more than 90% of the children with neuroblastoma, with the exception of those with tumors arising from the spinal routes and ganglia, which are nonsecretors of catecholamines. Each laboratory must establish its own range of normal values. The level of catecholamine excretion has little prognostic significance, but the appearance or reappearance of elevated levels in children known to have had neuroblastoma indicates recurrent disease and a poor prognosis.

Japanese investigators first evaluated the use of urinary catecholamine excretion as a screening tool for identifying preclinical neuroblastoma at 6 months of age. Preliminary results are encouraging, but population-based estimates of survival are not available. The Quebec Neuroblastoma Screening Project was initiated to establish a population-based estimate of incidence, stage, and age distribution, and preliminary results are available.

Carcinoembryonic antigen (CEA) reactivity has been found in many children with neuroblastoma, but this is not specific for neuroblastoma and may appear in a number of tumors, including rhabdomyosarcoma.

The complete evaluation of a child suspected of having neuroblastoma should include a total skeletal survey, including the skull. In the skull, osteolytic radiographic lesions and separation of the sutures are practically pathognomonic of neuroblastoma. Lytic lesions of the long bones and pelvis are common, but metastases from neuroblastoma are not easily distinguishable from Ewing's sarcoma, leukemia, or osteomyelitis. Chest radiographs may expose mediastinal or cervical tumors by delineating a mass and displacement of the mediastinal structures. The lateral chest x-ray film may help to reveal tumors in the left chest, where the heart may obscure lesions on routine anteroposterior films. Abdominal tumors may be seen on flat films of the abdomen and may show calcium deposits in many cases. An intravenous pyelogram may help differentiate an extrarenal from an intrarenal tumor.

The computed tomography scan and magnetic resonance imaging (MRI) are particularly useful for examining the abdomen. MRI has replaced standard myelography for the detection of intraspinal tumors and is useful in determining bone disease. Ultrasound examination is a useful tool for diagnosing intra-

abdominal tumors and can also demonstrate calcifications. As a noninvasive imaging tool, sonography is particularly useful in serial follow-up evaluations. Arteriography, myelography, and lymphangiography have almost been replaced by the newer techniques but still may have a role in selected cases. Liver scans may show defects in the liver as an indication of metastatic disease. Regardless of all other findings, the diagnosis must always be confirmed by histologic examination.

## DIFFERENTIAL DIAGNOSIS

Because of the metabolically active products and the propensity for this tumor to metastasize early, the symptoms may be quite variable. Lesions of the skull may resemble those of Langerhans' histiocytosis. Abdominal masses may suggest other diagnoses, including Wilms' tumor, lymphoma, mesenteric cysts, hydronephrosis, and splenomegaly. Occasionally, a mediastinal neuroblastoma may be confused with thymoma. Bone pain may resemble rheumatoid arthritis, osteomyelitis, and leukemia. All things considered, unless the tumor is very undifferentiated, it is usually not a difficult diagnosis to make after a proper biopsy specimen is obtained.

## STAGING

In the past, treatment has been based on the patient's age and the extent and location of the tumor. The evaluation of biologic characteristics of the tumor, such as *MYCN* amplification and DNA content, have added considerably to therapeutic decision making. Unlike other tumors, the degree and extent of metastatic disease is unrelated to the size of the primary tumor. In some cases, it may be difficult to determine the primary tumor site. Two staging systems currently in widespread use are shown in Table 99-3. Surgical exploration for the purpose of excision of the tumor should include sampling of the regional nodes, regardless of their gross appearance, and a liver biopsy if the tumor is in the abdomen. The degree of resectability is included in the revised staging system used by the Pediatric Oncology Group (POG), as shown in Table 99-3. The historic distribution of cases according to the stage at diagnosis is shown in Table 99-4.

## TUMOR BIOLOGY

Age and stage traditionally have had the principal roles in determining therapeutic guidelines for children with neuroblastoma. Despite these factors, therapeutic intensity may have been excessive in certain groups of children, while others continue to fail conventional therapy. To enhance outcome, it has become increasingly important to discriminate potential good responders from poor responders and institute appropriate, tailored therapy for both groups.

Tumor cell DNA content or ploidy first was reported in 1984 as a predictor of response to therapy in infants with unresectable neuroblastoma. All of the patients with hyperdiploid tumors had a favorable response to therapy, and none of those with diploid tumors responded.

*NMYC* proto-oncogene amplification in haploid neuroblastoma cells has clinical relevance. Amplification seems to be strongly associated with aggressive tumor behavior and poor prognosis regardless of stage.

The POG studied 298 children with neuroblastoma, assessing ploidy and *MYCN* gene copy number as combined predictors of outcome. In infants younger than 1 year of age, hyperdiploidy was found in 87% of stage A, B, C, and DS patients, showing

**TABLE 99-3.   Neuroblastoma Staging System**

| Evans | Pediatric Oncology Group |
|---|---|
| **Stage I**<br>Tumor confined to organ or structure of origin | **Stage A**<br>Complete gross resection of primary tumor with or without microscopic residual: intracavitary lymph nodes not adherent to and removed with primary*; histologically free of tumor. If primary in abdomen or pelvis, liver histologically free of tumor |
| **Stage II**<br>Tumor extending in continuity beyond organ or structure of origin but not crossing the midline; regional nodes on homolateral side may be involved | **Stage B**<br>Grossly unresected primary tumor; nodes and liver same as stage A |
| **Stage III**<br>Tumor extending in continuity beyond the midline; regional nodes may be involved bilaterally; bilateral extension of midline disease | **Stage C**<br>Complete or incomplete resection of primary; intracavitary nodes not adherent to primary histologically positive for tumor; liver as in stage A |
| **Stage IV**<br>Remote disease involving skeleton, organs, soft tissue, and distant nodes | **Stage D**<br>Any dissemination of disease beyond intracavitary nodes; for example, to extracavitary nodes, liver, skin, bone marrow, or bone |
| **Stage IVS**<br>Patients who would otherwise be stage I or II (ie, with small or resectable primary tumor), but who have remote disease confined only to one or more of the following sites: liver, skin, or bone marrow (not bone) | **Stage DS**<br>Infants <1 year of age with stage IVS disease |

\* Nodes adherent to or within tumor resection may be positive for tumor without reclassifying patient as stage C.

an excellent correlation with outcome. In stage D patients, ploidy demonstrated remarkable discrimination between those failing early and those with prolonged disease-free survival. The relation of ploidy and outcome with increasing disease stage also was seen in patients 12 to 24 months of age. In stage D, all patients with diploid tumors failed, and 50% of those with hyperdiploidy became long-term survivors. Favorable ploidy was not a predictor of prolonged disease-free survival of children older than 24 months of age at diagnosis.

*MYCN* amplification was seen most often in diploid tumors ($p = 0.001$) and had an overall association with treatment failure ($p <0.001$). Although ploidy becomes much less predictive in patients older than 24 months of age, *MYCN* amplification remains predictive in patients with lower-stage disease. Stage C patients older than 24 months of age with amplification had a high risk of relapse despite favorable tumor ploidy. The combination of age, stage, ploidy, and *MYCN* amplification offer substantial predictive power, and the intensity of the therapy recommended by POG is based on these characteristics.

**TABLE 99-4.   Distribution of Neuroblastoma by Stages***

| Evans Stage | No. of Cases | Percent |
|---|---|---|
| I | 143 | 15 |
| II | 127 | 14 |
| III | 94 | 10 |
| IV | 487 | 51 |
| IVS | 95 | 10 |
|  | 946 | 100 |

\* Composite of three series.

Studies are ongoing to identify other predictors of tumor behavior, such as loss of heterozygosity of certain chromosomes and the occurrence of the multidrug resistance phenotype associated with P-glycoprotein.

## TREATMENT

Almost all treatment programs offer experimental therapy. The prognosis is related to the age of the patient, stage of the disease, and in many cases, the biologic characteristics such as ploidy and *MYCN* amplification at the time of diagnosis. Patients younger than 1 year of age with stage I (stage A) disease have an excellent prognosis, and almost 100% of these children survive. If the tumor is localized (stage I or stage A) at any age, complete surgical excision is the treatment of choice. For metastatic disease, value of surgical excision of the presumed primary lesion is unclear, but second-look surgery is being used more frequently, particularly after initial intensive chemotherapy. The second-look procedure is useful in planning future therapy by identifying residual disease.

Radiation therapy plays an important role in the management of high-risk stage C disease in patients older than 1 year of age. The POG showed that radiation therapy improved initial and long-term disease control in this population compared with standard chemotherapy alone. Radiation therapy is useful in the local control of resistant disease, palliation of pain, and relief of pressure symptoms, such as spinal cord compression.

Chemotherapeutic options include vincristine, cyclophosphamide (Cytoxan), and doxorubicin (Adriamycin) for lower-risk disease, and the epipodophyllotoxins and platinum agents appear essential in treating more aggressive disease.

Allogeneic and autologous forms of bone marrow transplantation have been explored as therapeutic options. Transplantation allows dose intensification for highly resistant and relapsed disease. Allogeneic transplantation appears to offer no advantage over autologous transplantation. The use of autologous transplantation avoids the risk of graft-versus-host disease associated with allogeneic transplantation. The results of autologous bone marrow transplantation for patients with neuroblastoma vary widely. Progression-free survival rates at 2 years are in the range of 20% to 50%. Controversy continues about the utility of marrow purging, the need for total-body irradiation, and the appropriate preparative technique. A large, randomized trial may be necessary to answer the questions raised by transplantation. All investigators agree that intensified therapy is essential in the management of patients with high-risk neuroblastoma. Unfortunately, it is not clear which therapy offers the best opportunity to maximize outcome.

Novel therapeutic techniques include the use of desferrioxamine as an iron-chelating agent, *cis*-retinoic acid as a differentiating agent, and adoptive immunotherapy using tumor-infiltrating lymphocytes. It is hoped that unique agents such as these may offer the therapeutic edge needed to control this disease.

## PROGNOSIS

Age and stage remain important prognostic variables, and biologic markers are becoming increasingly indispensable as additional predictors of outcome. After 1 year of age, the outcome becomes markedly worse, especially for children with stage II, III, or IV disease. Children who develop neuroblastoma after the age of 8 seem to have an improved survival (almost 50%). Patients younger than 1 year of age who have stage III or IV disease have a much more favorable response than those between the ages of 1 and 8. Infants with Evans stage IVS disease probably do as well without chemotherapy but may benefit from chemotherapy if the tumor is rapidly progressive, has unfavorable biologic characteristics, or appears to be acutely threatening the life of the patient. Spontaneous remissions are high in this group of children.

## Selected Readings

Anderson JR. Coccia PF. Is more better? Dose intensity in neuroblastoma (editorial). J Clin Oncol 1991;9:902.

Bernstein ML, Leclerc JM, Bunin G, et al. A population-based study of neuroblastoma incidence, survival, and mortality in North America. J Clin Oncol 1992;10:323.

Brodeur GM, Seeger RC, Schwab M, et al. Amplification of N-myc in untreated human neuroblastomas correlates with advanced disease stage. Science 1984;224:1121.

Castleberry RP, Kun LE, Shuster JJ, et al. Radiotherapy improves the outlook for patients older than 1 year with Pediatric Oncology Group stage C neuroblastoma. J Clin Oncol 1991;9:789.

Joshi V, et al. Correlations between morphologic and other prognostic markers of neuroblastoma: a study of histologic grade (HG), DNA index (DI), N-MYC (NM) gene copy number and lactic dehydrogenase (LDH) in cases from the Pediatric Oncology Group (POG) (abstract). Proc Am Soc Clin Oncol 1992;11:361.

Look AT, Hayes FA, Nitschke R, et al. Cellular DNA content as predictor of response to chemotherapy in infants with unresectable neuroblastoma. N Engl J Med 1984;311:231.

Look AT, Hayes FA, Shuster JJ, et al. Clinical relevance of tumor cell ploidy and N-myc gene amplification in childhood neuroblastoma: a Pediatric Oncology Group study. J Clin Oncol 1991;9:581.

Naito H, Sasaki M, Yamashiro K, et al. Improvement in prognosis of neuroblastoma through mass population screening. J Pediatr Surg 1990;25:245.

Philip T, Zucker JM, Bernard JL, et al. Improved survival at 2 and 5 years in the LMCE1 unselected group of 72 children with stage IV neuroblastoma older than 1 year of age at diagnosis: is cure possible in a small subgroup? J Clin Oncol 1991;9:1037.

Seeger RC, Brodeur GM, Sather H, et al. Association of multiple copies of the N-myc oncogene with rapid progression of neuroblastomas. N Engl J Med 1985;313:1111.

Triche TJ, Askin FB, Kissane JM. Neuroblastoma, Ewing's sarcoma, and the differential diagnosis of small-, round-, blue-cell tumors. In: Finegold M, Bennington JL, eds. Pathology of neoplasm in children and adolescents, vol 19. Philadelphia: WB Saunders, 1986.

Voute PA. Neuroblastoma. In: Sutow WW, Fernbach DJ, Vietti TJ, eds. Clinical pediatric oncology, ed 3. St. Louis: CV Mosby, 1984;559.

*Principles and Practice of Pediatrics, Second Edition.*
edited by Frank A. Oski et al. J. B. Lippincott Company, Philadelphia © 1994.

# CHAPTER 100
# *Soft Tissue Sarcomas*

## Richard L. Hurwitz

The soft tissue sarcomas form a diverse group of malignant neoplasms that arise from embryonal mesenchyma. As a group, these tumors are rare in children, and most of the information known about these diseases is derived from treating adults. The exception is rhabdomyosarcoma, a tumor of embryonal mesenchyma that gives rise to striated skeletal muscle. This malignancy is the most common soft tissue sarcoma of children and accounts for 5% to 15% of all malignant solid tumors in patients younger than 15 years of age. During the past 15 years, successful treatment regimens have been developed, especially for localized disease, using a combination of surgery, irradiation, and chemotherapy.

## RHABDOMYOSARCOMA

The first recorded description of rhabdomyosarcoma was by Weber in 1854, and the histology of these muscle tumors was described by Rakov in 1937. Series of patients, mostly adults, were presented by Stout in 1946 and by Pack and Eberhart in 1952. The histology of these tumors was pleomorphic, a type we now know is rare in children. In 1950, Stobbe and Dargeon described the embryonal form of rhabdomyosarcoma, the most common histologic variety in pediatric patients. In 1958, Horn and Enterline described the four currently recognized histologic subtypes of this malignancy: pleomorphic, embryonal, alveolar, and botryoid.

Surgical removal of the primary tumor was the original therapy, which resulted in some long-term survival, but it was found that the malignancy recurred frequently and early in the course of the disease. Survival varied by the site of the primary disease: head and neck excluding orbit had survival rates of 7% to 14%; orbit, 21% to 48%; trunk or extremity, 22%; bladder, 73%; and vagina, 40%. In retrospect, it was evident that in most cases the metastases had occurred before the diagnosis could be made.

In 1950, Stobbe and Dargeon reported that at least some rhabdomyosarcomas were radiosensitive. D'Angio and coworkers in 1959 observed a synergistic effect using radiation and dactinomycin. Edland in 1965 and Sagerman in 1972 showed that a fractionated total dose of 6000 cGy could locally control this tumor.

During the same time, reports were surfacing that chemotherapeutic agents used singly were successful in producing complete or partial responses in some patients, but the duration of improvement was short. Combined treatment regimens were increasingly more successful. Pinkel and Pickren suggested a coordinated approach to the treatment of rhabdomyosarcoma using surgery, irradiation, and chemotherapy. The utility of this approach has been confirmed repeatedly.

Because rhabdomyosarcoma is such a rare disease, the three pediatric groups studying cancer in children pooled their patients and resources to form the Intergroup Rhabdomyosarcoma Study (IRS). The results from the first three studies have greatly advanced our knowledge and success in dealing with this disease. A fourth study is open to patient registration.

Investigators demonstrated that defects in the short arm of chromosome 11 are associated with the development of rhabdomyosarcoma. Moreover, the loss of the maternal gene with exclusive expression of the paternal gene (ie, genome imprinting) has been found in all embryonal rhabdomyosarcomas that could be conclusively examined. This observation may lead to an understanding of the molecular mechanism underlying this disease.

## Incidence and Epidemiology

Rhabdomyosarcoma is the most common of the soft tissue sarcomas in children, accounting for 4% to 8% of all malignant diseases in children younger than 15 years of age. It is the seventh most common malignant tumor in children. The annual incidence is estimated to be 4.4 per million white children and 1.3 per million black children. The ratio of males to females is 1.4 : 1. Low socioeconomic status has been associated with this disease, implying an environmental role in its pathogenesis.

Relatives of children with rhabdomyosarcoma have a high frequency of carcinoma of the breast and of brain tumors. Rhabdomyosarcoma is a recognized complication of neurofibromatosis and has been associated with other congenital abnormalities as well. Bone sarcoma has been reported as a second malignancy in patients with rhabdomyosarcoma.

## Clinical Manifestations

Rhabdomyosarcoma can occur anywhere in the body. The percentage of cases presenting at each anatomical location is depicted in Table 100-1. The head and neck (including the orbit) are the most common sites of primary occurrence, with 38% of the cases presenting in this region. The orbit accounts for 10% of the total presentations. The genitourinary tract is next in order of frequency, followed by the trunk, extremities, retroperitoneum, and other sites.

Approximately 70% of the tumors occur in children younger than 10 years of age, with a peak incidence between the ages of 2 and 5. The signs and symptoms relate to the primary site of the tumor or the metastases. Usually a painless, enlarging mass is noticed.

Tumors in the orbit can produce proptosis, chemosis, and ocular paralysis. These tumors can begin as a mass in the conjunctiva or eyelid. Tumors in the nasopharynx can cause a nasal voice, dysphagia, airway obstruction, epistaxis, or pain. Tumors in the paranasal sinuses cause swelling, pain, discharge, sinusitis, obstruction, or epistaxis. Laryngeal tumors cause hoarseness. Tumors in the middle ear are associated with a polypoid tumor in the external auditory canal that can cause pain, chronic otitis media, and a facial nerve palsy. Rhabdomyosarcoma may present as a painless facial or parotid mass. Neck masses may present with hoarseness or dysphagia. Parameningeal tumors may extend into the central nervous system, resulting in meningeal symptoms, cranial nerve palsies, or respiratory paralysis.

Tumors arising from the trunk, extremities, or paratesticular region usually occur as painless masses that are noticed by the child or parents. Tumors in the retroperitoneum usually are asymptomatic or are found as large masses that may cause gastrointestinal or urinary tract symptoms. Bladder and prostate tumors usually produce urinary tract symptoms. Tumors from the perineum may involve the bowel or bladder. Botryoid tumors appear as grape-like clusters of clear tissue protruding from the uterus or cervix.

The tumor characteristically grows with indistinct margins along fascial planes and infiltrates into surrounding tissues. Metastases spread hematogenously and by lymphatics to the lung, bone, bone marrow, lymph nodes, central nervous system, heart, and breast.

## Differential Diagnosis

The differential diagnosis of rhabdomyosarcoma reflects the presenting complaint. With orbital tumors, it includes infection (ie, orbital cellulitis), proptosis secondary to hyperthyroidism, hemangioma, metastatic neuroblastoma, optic nerve glioma, retinoblastoma, granuloma, lymphoma, granulocytic sarcoma, fibrous dysplasia of bone, and Langerhans' histiocytosis.

Other tumors that can arise in the nasopharynx and paranasal sinus include inflammatory granulomas, lymphoma, other soft tissue sarcomas, carcinomas, and juvenile nasopharyngeal angiofibroma. Tumors in the neck must be differentiated from inflammatory lesions, branchial cleft cyst, lymphoma, carcinoma, sinus histiocytosis, and Langerhans' histiocytosis.

An intra-abdominal mass must be differentiated from a mesenteric cyst, intestinal duplication, Wilms' tumor, neuroblastoma, hepatoma, hemangioma, lymphoma, teratoma, carcinoma, and other soft tissue sarcomas. A paratesticular mass could be a benign tumor, including a varicocele or hydrocele, a seminoma, teratoma, embryonal carcinoma, lymphoma, or a rare tumor of the spermatic cord. In the bladder, neurofibroma, hemangioma, and transitional cell carcinoma or leiomyosarcoma should be considered. In the vagina, rhabdomyoma, a benign lesion, must be excluded.

Other soft tissue sarcomas can occur on the trunk. Bone tumors and neurogenic sarcoma should be considered in the differential diagnosis of tumors of an extremity.

## Diagnostic Evaluation

Open biopsy of the tumor is the definitive diagnostic procedure for an unexplained mass. Certain tests are performed before the surgical procedure to assess the extent of the disease for staging and therapeutic purposes.

Preoperative assessment should include a complete blood count, urinalysis, measurement of electrolytes (including calcium and phosphorus), liver and renal function tests, and a uric acid determination. Computed tomography (CT) or magnetic resonance imaging (MRI) of the primary tumor should be performed to delineate the involvement of adjacent structures and to aid in the surgical management of the patient. A CT scan of the chest, bone marrow examination, bone scan or skeletal survey, and liver scan should be performed to look for metastases. Patients with cranial parameningeal tumors should also have a CT or MRI scan of the head and an examination of the cerebrospinal fluid (CSF) to look for evidence of meningeal seeding with CSF pleocytosis, elevation in protein, and reduction of glucose. A CT scan may be employed to assess retroperitoneal lymph node involve-

| TABLE 100-1. Primary Sites of Rhabdomyosarcoma | |
|---|---|
| Site | Frequency (%) |
| Orbit | 10 |
| Head and neck | 28 |
| Trunk | 7 |
| Extremities | 18 |
| Genitourinary tract | 21 |
| Intrathoracic tissues | 3 |
| Gastrointestinal and hepatic systems | 3 |
| Perineum and anus | 2 |
| Retroperineum | 7 |
| Other sites | 1 |

ment in patients with lower extremity and genitourinary tumors. Figure 100-1 demonstrates a solid tumor in the pelvis that was shown to be rhabdomyosarcoma after surgical biopsy.

## Histology

Histologically proven rhabdomyosarcoma does not differ from other malignant soft tissue tumors, and with the exception of the grape-like clusters of sarcoma botryoides, the tumors do not differ from each other. The tumors are firm, nodular, and grossly well circumscribed but not encapsulated, and they aggressively invade adjacent tissues.

Four histologic variations have been described. The most common form is the embryonal type, which consists of spindle-shaped myoblasts and small round cells. This type accounts for 57% of rhabdomyosarcomas and 75% of the tumors arising from the head and neck and genitourinary tract. Patients with this histologic variant have a relatively favorable prognosis.

The alveolar type is the second most common type of tumor, accounting for approximately 19% of the cases. It is seen more commonly in children older than 6 years of age and occurs most often in the trunk, extremities, and perianal region. These tumor cells grow in cords that often have cleft-like spaces resembling alveoli. Patients with this tumor have a poorer prognosis than those with the embryonal type.

The botryoid type is most often seen in the genitourinary tract. This tumor accounts for approximately 6% of cases and is seen more commonly in children younger than 6 years of age. A deep, compact zone of spindle-shaped cells resembling myoblasts is found under a layer of myxoid stroma with a layer of small round cells at the periphery. This tumor is associated with a prognosis similar to the embryonal type.

The pleomorphic cell type is found more commonly in adults and is associated with only 1% of all the cases of rhabdomyosarcoma in children. When found, the disease is associated more often with primary tumors of the trunk and extremity. As the name suggests, the cells are large and pleomorphic, and they often contain multiple giant nuclei with cytoplasmic tails.

Two other histologic varieties of mesenchymal tumors have been identified and often are included as rhabdomyosarcoma variants. These tumors arise in the soft tissue adjacent to, but not involving, the bone and have been called soft tissue or extraosseous Ewing's sarcoma because of the morphologic similarities to this bone sarcoma. Type I disease is associated with small round or oval anaplastic cells similar to the small round cells of Ewing's sarcoma of bone. Type II disease has larger, slightly more irregularly shaped cells, similar to the large cell variety of Ewing's sarcoma. Together, these tumors account for approximately 7% of all the patients with rhabdomyosarcoma, and patients with this disease have an overall prognosis similar to that with the embryonal type tumor of the same clinical stage. This malignancy is more frequently found in children older than 6 years of age.

The histologic type frequently is difficult to determine, and mixtures of the various types may occur in the same tumor. Cross striations are not always found under light microscopy and are not necessary to make the diagnosis. Electron microscopy may be of value in certain cases that are difficult to diagnose. Thin myosin filaments and primitive Z bands may be seen and are helpful in making the diagnosis, but the lack of these findings in the presence of other characteristic observations does not preclude the diagnosis of rhabdomyosarcoma.

## Clinical Staging

The IRS Clinical Grouping Classification used in the IRS I, II, and III studies is shown in Table 100-2. This staging system relies on surgical judgment and has had historic utility. Two problems are associated with this system. First, no surgically defined therapeutic questions can be asked, because the extent of surgery defines the clinical stage. One surgeon may perform a biopsy of a tumor, classifying the patient as having stage III disease, and a second surgeon may perform aggressive resection, making a similar patient stage I or II. The biologic role of the particular tumor or the aggressive surgical management of the similar tumor had in patient outcome cannot be assessed. The second shortcoming of this staging system was discovered after analysis of the patient survival curves from IRS I and II. A clear difference in survival is found for patients with metastatic disease (<20% long-term survival) compared with those without metastatic disease (approximately 70% long-term survival). The difference between the other stages is less significant and less useful in defining treatment-related questions.

Several attempts have been made to correct the two inadequacies of the IRS system. By analyzing the same patient survival data from the previous IRS studies, four criteria were found to have statistically significant prognostic implications: primary site

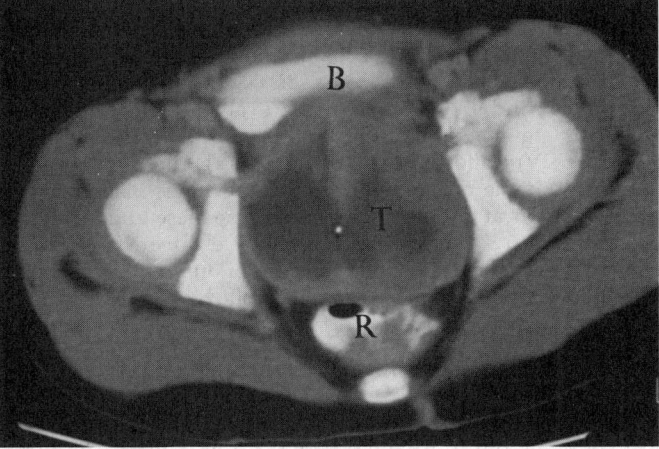

**Figure 100-1.** In the CT scan of a patient with a pelvic mass that was shown to be rhabdomyosarcoma after a surgical biopsy, the large pelvic tumor (*T*) is possibly associated with the prostate, displacing the rectum (*R*) posteriorly, the bladder (*B*) anteriorly, and extending to the side walls bilaterally. Notice the Foley catheter in the center of the tumor and the central area of necrosis depicted by the darker region of the mass.

| TABLE 100-2. | IRS Clinical Classification System |
|---|---|
| Group I | Localized disease, can be completely removed; regional nodes not involved<br>1. Confined to muscle or organ of origin<br>2. Contiguous involvement with infiltration outside the muscle or organ of origin |
| Group II | 1. Grossly removed tumor with microscopic residual disease, no evidence of gross residual tumor, no evidence of regional node involvement<br><br>2. Regional disease, completely removed (regional nodes involved or extension of tumor into an adjacent organ, no microscopic residual disease)<br><br>3. Regional disease with involved nodes, grossly removed but with evidence of microscopic residual disease |
| Group III | Incomplete removal or biopsy with gross residual disease |
| Group IV | Distant metastatic disease present at initial diagnosis |

of tumor, size of tumor at diagnosis, evidence for tumor invasiveness at the time of diagnosis, and the presence or absence of metastases. A staging system incorporating these criteria is shown in Table 100-3. Patients with tumors arising from favorable sites (eg, orbit, head and neck, genitourinary tract excluding bladder and prostate) without evidence of metastases are grouped together as stage I. Stage II contains small tumors from unfavorable primary sites; stage III contains large tumors from unfavorable sites; and stage IV contains all metastatic tumors regardless of the primary site. A further subdivision of stage III includes patients found to have lymph node involvement associated with unfavorable primary disease. A second staging proposal substitutes the degree of tumor invasiveness for the tumor size in patients having primary malignancies in unfavorable sites (ie, stage II and stage III disease).

Either staging proposal enables assessment of the extent of disease independently from the surgical procedure employed, allowing surgical treatment questions to be addressed. The patient survival data from IRS II has been reassessed using this staging criteria in a retrospective approach and was found to have statistically significant differences between each stage. The two objections to the current system have been addressed, and a modification of the staging system presented in Table 3 is being used in the ongoing IRS IV study.

## Treatment

The therapy for rhabdomyosarcoma consists of a coordinated approach using surgery, radiation therapy, and chemotherapy. The surgeon provides tissue for diagnosis and attempts a total resection of the primary tumor, if possible without radical extirpative procedures. A reduction in tumor burden is achieved if total resection is not possible. Current surgical management includes second-look surgery to assess treatment response and the control of complications due to tumor regrowth and metastases. Aggressive excision surgery is not indicated in treating these children.

Radiation therapy is used to lessen the chance of recurrence of the primary tumor and to aid in the control of some metastases. Relatively high doses are recommended (4000 to 5500 cGy). Vital structures such as the lung, liver, and kidney need appropriate shielding to prevent excessive radiation to these organs. Irradiation should be administered using appropriate high-energy equipment by radiotherapists skilled in treating children.

All children with rhabdomyosarcoma receive multiagent, intensive chemotherapy in an attempt to eradicate microscopic residual disease and to reduce macroscopic bulk disease. This approach has improved survival for patients with this malignancy.

## Prognosis

The 5-year survival rates for IRS II are shown in Table 100-4. The differences in survival between patients in group I and group

**TABLE 100-4. Five-Year Survival Rates for Rhabdomyosarcoma\***

| Clinical Group | Five-Year Survival (%) |
|---|---|
| All | 62 |
| I | 82 |
| II | 78 |
| III | 64 |
| IV | 27 |

\* Based on data accumulated in IRS II.

II are not statistically significant and have led to discussion about changing the staging system. Preliminary analysis of patients treated on the IRS III study suggests that disease-free survival in the group III children may be significantly improved from that reported in IRS II. These patients received more intensive therapy. It is clear from this table that the discovery of metastatic disease is an ominous finding. Tumors arising from the orbit, head and neck, and the genitourinary tract have been found to have a significantly better prognosis than do tumors arising from other sites (94% versus 65% 3-year survival rate). Local or distal recurrence carries a grave prognosis. Occasionally, a prolonged remission can be attained, especially if the tumor recurs after the completion of chemotherapy in a site amenable to surgery. Relapses, when they do occur, usually are seen within 2 years of institution of therapy, although a relatively small risk of late recurrences has been reported.

## OTHER SOFT TISSUE SARCOMAS

The other soft tissue sarcomas comprise a histologically heterogeneous group of tumors that arise from undifferentiated mesenchymal cells. These tumors occur in fibrous, connective, lymphatic, or vascular tissue and tend to recur locally. With a combined therapeutic approach, control of local disease is attainable, and prevention of the development of metastases may be possible. Current treatment regimens are testing whether chemotherapy has a role in the treatment of these diseases in children. Preliminary trials suggest that chemotherapy and radiation therapy probably do not have a role in the management of grossly resected, nonrhabdomyosarcoma soft tissue sarcomas in children (ie, groups I and II). Clinical trials are evaluating the role of these treatment regimens in nonresectable (ie, group III) and metastatic (ie, group IV) tumors. Biopsy of the mass is the means to a diagnosis, and the differential diagnosis includes malignant and benign tumors at the site of origin. Because these tumors are rare in children, the diagnosis of a soft tissue sarcoma other than rhabdomyosarcoma is not high on a list of differential diagnoses. A brief description of these sarcomas follows.

### Tendosynovial Sarcoma

Tendosynovial sarcoma is a tumor resembling synovial tissue histologically, but it usually occurs far from a joint. The tumor presents as a painless mass, usually in the extremities. It is the most common malignancy of the hands and feet. The tumor tends to metastasize to the lung and to regional lymph nodes and bone. Treatment consists of surgical removal, irradiation, and chemotherapy. The 5-year survival rate is 40% to 60%, but late recurrences are possible.

**TABLE 100-3. Proposed Staging Criteria for Rhabdomyosarcoma**

| Stage I | Primary tumors found at sites considered to be of favorable prognosis without distant metastases |
|---|---|
| Stage II | All other primary tumors less than 5 cm in diameter without metastases |
| Stage III | 1. All other tumors greater than 5 cm in diameter<br>2. All other tumors with adjacent nodal involvement |
| Stage IV | All tumors with distant metastases at diagnosis |

## Alveolar Soft-Part Sarcoma

Alveolar soft-part sarcoma occurs as a slow-growing asymptomatic mass usually involving the extremities. It seems to occur in a younger age group. Therapy has included local surgery and irradiation; response to chemotherapy has been poor. The tumor commonly recurs locally, and about 50% of the patients develop metastatic disease. Although 60% of the patients in one study were surviving at 5 years, all the patients had died within 20 years after diagnosis.

## Fibrosarcoma

Fibrosarcoma is a tumor of fibrous tissue that has a tendency toward local recurrence but infrequently develops widespread metastases. This tumor has been reported to occur congenitally. Fibrosarcoma tends to occur in the muscles of the extremities. It has been reported in patients with retinoblastoma and glioma in the field of radiation and in patients after prolonged implantation of a plastic prosthesis. Treatment includes surgery of the primary tumor. Irradiation and chemotherapy have been used with some success.

## Dermatofibrosarcoma Protuberans

Dermatofibrosarcoma protuberans is a slow-growing fibrous tumor of the skin characterized by a high recurrence rate locally but with a low incidence of metastases. The condition usually begins as one or more small firm nodules in the skin. They often have a bluish or reddish color and blanch with pressure. The tumors develop slowly but may suddenly grow rapidly. The tumors are found most often on the trunk, arms, or thighs. Surgery is the primary treatment. Chemotherapy has been used with some success in patients with disseminated disease. Because metastases are rare, this disease has a good prognosis.

## Malignant Fibrous Histiocytoma

Malignant fibrous histiocytoma are tumors that occur principally in skeletal muscle or in the abdominal cavity involving deep fascia. Primary tumors of bone have been described. In pediatric cases, girls predominate. Surgery is the primary therapeutic modality. Radiation therapy and chemotherapy have been used to control metastases. The 2-year survival rate is 60%, and the local recurrence rate and metastatic rate are each about 40%.

## Liposarcoma

Liposarcoma is a malignant tumor of adipose tissue. The tumor is rare in children but must be differentiated from the histologically similar lipoblastomatosis, which is a benign disorder occurring in infants and children and which seldom recurs after local excision. Liposarcomas in children have a male preponderance. The liposarcomas occur wherever adipose tissue exists, but the thigh is the most common site. Local recurrence after surgery and metastases have been reported. Surgery and radiation therapy are used most often in the therapy of this tumor; the role of chemotherapy is unclear. The prognosis for children is significantly better than that for adults.

## Angiosarcoma

Angiosarcoma is a rare tumor of the vascular endothelial cells. Vinyl chloride exposure and radiation therapy to hemangiomas have been implicated in its pathogenesis. The duration of symptoms before diagnosis can be weeks or years. The tumor most commonly arises in an extremity but has occurred in the liver, scalp, heart, bone, breasts, and spleen. Angiosarcomas tend to be progressive, multifocal, and rapidly fatal with widespread metastases. Treatment includes surgery, radiation therapy, and chemotherapy.

## Hemangiopericytoma

Hemangiopericytoma is a vascular tumor of the cells that surround capillaries. The most common site of origin is the lower extremity, but the tumor may arise wherever there are capillaries. Local recurrence after surgery and metastases are not uncommon. Surgery, radiation therapy, and chemotherapy are all recommended in the treatment of this disease. Late recurrences of the disease are not unusual.

## Juvenile Nasopharyngeal Angiofibroma

Juvenile nasopharyngeal angiofibroma is a malignant vascular tumor of adolescent boys. Nasal obstruction and epistaxis are the most common presenting symptoms and may be life threatening. These tumors spread locally, and metastases are not seen. Deaths are uncommon but result from intracranial spread or hemorrhage. Surgery with complete excision is the recommended therapy. Radiation therapy has been used in patients with intracranial or orbital invasion and may prevent recurrent epistaxes by reducing the blood supply to the tumors.

## Leiomyosarcoma

Leiomyosarcoma is a rare tumor of the smooth muscle in children. Presenting symptoms depend on the site of the primary tumor. Gastrointestinal tumors may present with abdominal pain, hemorrhage, and associated anemia, but they may be asymptomatic. Intestinal obstruction may occur, especially in the neonatal period. Respiratory tract tumors may cause chest pain, cough, or hemoptysis, although patients may be asymptomatic at presentation. Dysuria and urinary retention may be the presenting symptoms of genitourinary lesions. Pain or swelling can be the symptoms of a patient with leiomyosarcoma of the blood vessels in the extremities. Surgery and chemotherapy have been successful in the treatment of this disease. Local recurrences and metastases are common.

## Epithelioid Sarcoma

Epithelioid sarcoma appears predominantly on the extremities. The median age of patients with this tumor at presentation is 21 years. The tumors occur as firm, slow-growing nodules. Twenty-five percent of the cases are associated with pain and may be accompanied by local numbness and muscle atrophy. There are frequent ulcerations on the overlying skin. Erosion into bone has been reported. Aggressive surgical excision is the treatment of choice, but this therapy frequently is followed by local recurrence; 30% of cases recur with distant metastases. Radiation therapy has been useful in managing pulmonary metastases.

## Malignant Mesenchymoma

Malignant mesenchymoma is a malignant tumor of mesenchymal origin composed of cells that are differentiated into two or more unrelated forms other than fibrosarcoma. These tumors grow rapidly, tend to recur, and occasionally metastasize. They commonly occur in the extremities and retroperitoneum but may occur anywhere. Congenital tumors have been observed, and in children younger than 1 year of age, a 3 : 1 male preponderance has been reported. Surgery has been the primary therapeutic modality, but irradiation and chemotherapy probably will have larger roles in the future. The prognosis depends on the primary cell component of the tumor. Children younger than 5 years of age at diagnosis have the best survival rate.

## Selected Readings

Altman AJ. Management of malignant solid tumors. In: Nathan DG, Oski FA, eds. Hematology of infancy and childhood, ed. 3. Philadelphia: WB Saunders, 1987: 1152

Ensinger PM, Weiss SW, eds. Soft tissue tumors. St Louis: CV Mosby, 1983.

Maurer HM, Ragab AH, Rhabdomyosarcoma. In: Sutow WW, Fernbach DJ, Vietti TJ, eds. Clinical pediatric oncology, ed 3. St Louis: CV Mosby, 1984:622.

Ragab AH, Maurer HM, et al. Malignant tumors of soft tissues. In: Sutow WW, Fernbach DJ, Vietti TJ, eds. Clinical pediatric oncology, ed 3. St Louis: CV Mosby, 1984:652.

*Principles and Practice of Pediatrics, Second Edition.*
edited by Frank A. Oski et al. J. B. Lippincott Company, Philadelphia © 1994.

## CHAPTER 101
# *Retinoblastoma*

### Donald H. Mahoney, Jr.

## INCIDENCE, LATERALITY, AND MORTALITY

Retinoblastoma is a rare, highly malignant tumor of the retina of young children. It is the seventh most common pediatric malignancy in the United States. The worldwide incidence of retinoblastoma is relatively stable at one case per 18,000 to 30,000 live births. There is no significant difference in incidence between sexes or among races. The average age at presentation ranges between 13 and 18 months; more than 90% of the cases are diagnosed before age 5 years. Retinoblastoma is a relatively slow-growing tumor that usually remains confined to the eye for months or even years. With early diagnosis, the overall 5-year survival rate exceeds 90%. However, when disease extends beyond the eye, mortality approaches 100%.

Retinoblastoma occurs unilaterally in 20% to 35% of cases. In more than 70% of cases, the tumor originates from a single focus and, when clinically detected, involves more than half the retina, with extension into the vitreous chamber. Multifocal involvement may be observed with unilateral retinoblastoma but is more common with bilateral disease. Although multiple tumor foci usually present simultaneously, in as many as 25% of cases new foci may develop within weeks to months after the original diagnosis. The potential for metachronous occurrence of retinoblastoma warrants careful follow-up examination, even of the previously unaffected retina. Bilateral disease is detected at an earlier age (median, 13 months) than unilateral disease (median, 24 months). The outlook for bilateral disease is significantly worse than for unilateral disease because of an increased incidence of second, nonocular malignant tumors in bilaterally affected cases.

## GENETICS

Retinoblastoma occurs in both hereditary and nonhereditary forms. Knudson has postulated a "two-hit" mutational event as necessary for the development of disease. The retinoblastoma gene locus resides on human chromosome 13 at band q14. This retinoblastoma gene has been further characterized, mapped, and cloned and is the prototype for a class of recessive human cancer genes (tumor suppressor genes) in which a loss of activity of both normal alleles is thought to be associated with tumor genesis. Retinoblastoma gene mutations also have been found in some osteosarcomas, soft-tissue sarcomas, breast carcinomas, small-cell carcinomas of the lung, and prostatic carcinomas.

More than 90% of the patients have no family history of retinoblastoma and represent the first mutational event within the family. All patients with bilateral retinoblastoma and about 15% of the patients with unilateral retinoblastoma harbor a germinal mutation and have a hereditary form of the disease. According to Knudson's hypothesis, a somatic mutation following the germinal mutation is necessary to form the disease. About 85% of sporadic unilateral cases are nonhereditary; according to Knudson's hypothesis, two somatic mutations are required to produce the disease in these patients. When patients with either bilateral or unilateral retinoblastoma have the germinal mutation, 50% of their offspring will be affected by the disease, and one out of 100 will harbor a gene but not express the disease. Using DNA sequence polymorphism for recognizing the retinoblastoma locus, it is now possible to predict familial predisposition to retinoblastoma in families with two or more affected members. Diagnosis of the hereditary form may now be possible using direct DNA sequence analysis.

Perhaps 5% of retinoblastoma patients present with additional abnormalities, including mental retardation, abnormal dermatoglyphics, imperforate anus, and failure to thrive. Constitutional deletions of the long arm of chromosome 13 have been found in these patients.

## SIGNS AND SYMPTOMS

In the United States, the most common presenting sign is a white pupillary reflex called leukokoria (Fig 101-1). This abnormal reflex, present in 60% of the patients, is the result of a centrally located tumor at the posterior pole. Replacement of the vitreous with tumor or retinal detachment may also be noted.

The second most common sign is strabismus, present in 20% of the patients. In children under age 4, strabismus is usually the result of esotropia. With retinoblastoma, both esotropia and exotropia may occur and usually indicate tumor involvement of the macular area. Other signs include a red, painful eye with glaucoma (7%), poor vision (5%), unilateral dilated pupil, heterochromia (different-colored irises), or nystagmus. Children with advanced stages of disease may present with signs of lethargy, anorexia, failure to thrive, neurologic defects, orbital mass, proptosis, or blindness.

## DIAGNOSIS AND DIFFERENTIAL DIAGNOSIS

The diagnosis of retinoblastoma is made by visual examination alone. The examination is best done by an experienced ophthalmologist using an indirect ophthalmoscope. The patient should be sedated or under general anesthesia, and the pupils should be dilated. Any child presenting with the above signs and symptoms requires prompt attention, with these examinations at a minimum.

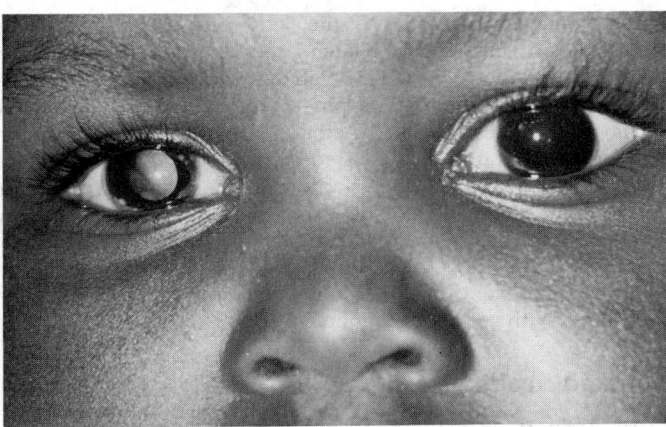

**Figure 101-1.** Abnormal white reflex, leukokoria, in a 7-month-old child with unilateral retinoblastoma.

The most common clinical classification schema for intraocular extent of disease is the Reese-Ellsworth system. At an early stage, the retinoblastoma appears as a hemispheric, localized retinal lesion that is usually pink but may appear gray or white. Larger lesions become pinker with increased vascularization. Tumors originating in the outer nuclear layer may cause retinal detachment. Alternatively, tumors arising from the inner nuclear layers may present as a localized mass or masses. These tumors are friable and may produce vitreous seeding. Intraocular calcifications may be noted with larger tumors. The presence of massive tumor, extensive retinal detachment, or vitreous seeds (group V in the Reese-Ellsworth system) is associated with a poor prognosis for salvage of the affected eye.

Metastatic extension occurs via the systemic circulation, through choroidal blood vessels into the orbit, or directly through the optic nerve tract into the CNS. Sites of metastases include the orbit, CNS, bone, bone marrow, and occasionally the lung. Ancillary noninvasive examinations, including CT scanning and ultrasonography, may help the clinician to make a diagnosis and may be useful in defining extraocular extension of disease (Fig 101-2).

The differential diagnosis for retinoblastoma depends on whether the tumor presents as a solitary mass or underlies an area of retinal detachment. When the tumor presents as a mass, there are two principal considerations: astrocytic hamartomas and granulomas of *Toxocara canis*. If the eye contains a retinal detachment, there are three diagnoses to consider: Coats' disease, retrolental fibroplasia, and persistent hyperplastic primary vit-

reous. The patient's age, past medical history (ie, oxygen exposure for retrolental fibroplasia, tuberous sclerosis for astrocytic hamartomas), and presentation will help the experienced ophthalmologist to distinguish between these disorders.

## TREATMENT

The priorities in treatment for retinoblastoma are to preserve life, to retain the eye, to retain vision, and to ensure favorable cosmetic results. Modalities in current use are enucleation, radiation (external beam and localized radioactive plaques), photocoagulation, cryotherapy, and systemic chemotherapy.

The following indications have been proposed for enucleation: unilateral group V eyes, most bilateral group V eyes, any blind eye with active tumor, any eye with glaucoma from invasive tumor, any eye that has failed all other forms of treatment, and patients who may not be available for future follow-up. At surgery, care must be taken to avoid rupture at tumor insertions, and attempts must be made to remove a long stump of optic nerve.

External beam radiation has been the mainstay of treatment for retinoblastoma. Lateral portal radiation therapy, using a high energy of 6 meV or more for a total dose of 3500 to 4500 cGy, produces tumor regression in virtually all tumors. Radioactive applicators, surgically attached to the sclera and left in place for 2 to 6 days, have produced successful tumor regression in small solitary tumors in 90% of the cases, and with more advanced retinoblastoma have salvaged more than half the eyes.

Photocoagulation, using a xenon laser applied through the pupil under anesthesia, is a highly effective means for treating new tumors that appear after radiation or for treating tumors unresponsive to irradiation. Cryotherapy may also be used to treat isolated lesions. The limiting factor for success for both of these measures is size and location: tumors larger than 3 to 4 DD respond poorly to these treatments.

Retinoblastoma is sensitive to chemotherapy, and nitrogen mustard, vincristine, cyclophosphamide, doxorubicin, cisplatin, and the epipodophyllotoxins have produced objective responses in patients with retinoblastoma. Clinical trials of adjuvant chemotherapy are ongoing. In the only controlled study of adjuvant chemotherapy, no difference in disease-free survival was noted

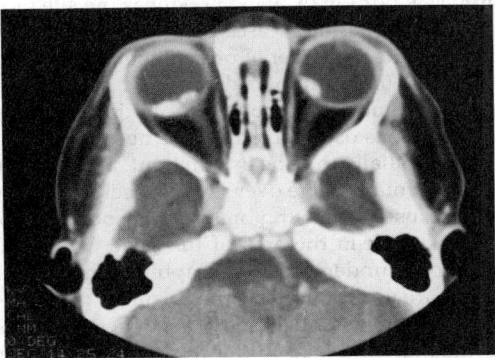

**Figure 101-2.** CT scan of the orbits revealing bilateral, calcified orbital masses, arising from the posterior aspect of the retina and confined to the globe.

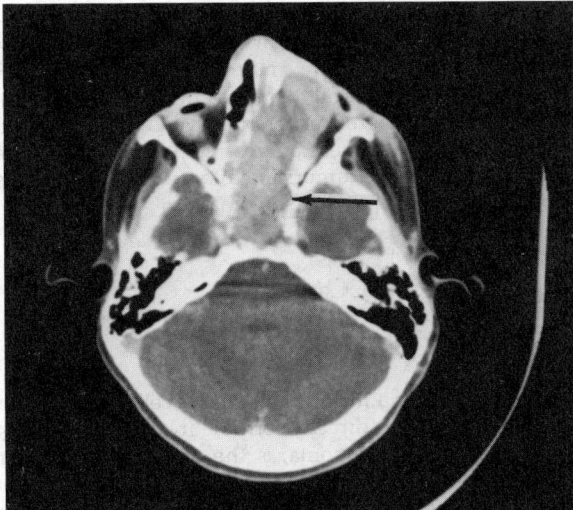

**Figure 101-3.** CT scan of face, sinuses, and orbits of a 14-year-old with bilateral retinoblastoma, treated 12 years prior. Note the large destructive osteosarcoma involving the left ethmoid and sphenoid area.

between patients with group V disease treated with enucleation alone versus patients treated with enucleation plus chemotherapy. However, this study and other investigations have identified risk factors at diagnosis that may contribute to an increased risk for extraorbital relapse, including invasion of the optic nerve beyond the lamina cribrosa, choroidal extension, and extension into the retinal pigment epithelium. Investigators at Cornell report 80% disease-free survival in patients with extraocular retinoblastoma treated with aggressive chemotherapy including cyclophosphamide, vincristine, doxorubicin, cisplatin, and VP-16, together with intrathecal therapy and radiation. Future designs of systemic chemotherapy approaches should take into consideration pathologic staging of this disease.

## SECOND TUMORS

Patients who have the germinal mutation for retinoblastoma and who survive the ocular tumor have a high risk for developing other malignancies. Tumors appear both within and outside the field of radiation. Tumors within the field include osteogenic sarcoma, fibrosarcoma, soft-tissue sarcoma, neuroblastoma, and meningioma. Osteosarcoma of the skull occurs 2000 times more frequently in survivors of bilateral retinoblastoma than in the general population (Fig 101-3). Patients with primitive neuroectodermal tumors involving the pineal region have been described as having "trilateral" retinoblastoma. The most common tumor outside the radiation field is osteosarcoma.

More than 90% of the patients with the germinal mutation who survive retinoblastoma develop a second malignancy within 32 years after treatment. The reason for this extraordinarily high incidence is linked to the retinoblastoma gene, which has been identified in several of these nonocular tumors. The mortality associated with second malignancies is high.

## Selected Readings

Grabowski EF, Abramson DH. Retinoblastoma. In: Fernbach DJ, Vietti TJ, eds. Clinical pediatric oncology, ed 4. St. Louis: CV Mosby, 1991:427.
Knudson AG. Hereditary cancer, oncogenes, and antioncogenes. Cancer Res 1985;45:1437.
White L. Chemotherapy in retinoblastoma: current status and future directions. Am J Pediatr Hematol Oncol 1991;13:189.
Yandell DW, Campbell TA, Dayton SH, et al. Oncogenic point mutations in the human retinoblastoma gene: their application to genetic counseling. N Engl J Med 1989;321:1689.

*Principles and Practice of Pediatrics, Second Edition.*
edited by Frank A. Oski et al. J. B. Lippincott Company, Philadelphia © 1994.

# CHAPTER 102
# *Malignant Bone Tumors in Children*

## Donald H. Mahoney, Jr.

The optimum management for malignant bone tumors arising in children involves a multidisciplinary approach with surgery, radiation therapy, chemotherapy, and rehabilitative therapy. Early diagnosis and prompt referral to an experienced pediatric cancer center will result in a significantly improved clinical outcome in patients presenting with these aggressive tumors. The two most common malignant bone tumors in children and adolescents are osteogenic sarcoma and Ewing sarcoma.

## OSTEOGENIC SARCOMA

### Incidence and Epidemiology

Osteogenic sarcoma is a malignant spindle-cell sarcoma of bone in which the tumor cells directly form neoplastic osteoid. Osteogenic sarcoma, or osteosarcoma, is the most common primary malignancy of bone in children. The estimated incidence in adolescence is 11 cases per 1 million population. The male/female ratio is about 1.5 : 1. The peak incidence occurs within the second decade, during periods of rapid growth spurts, and gradually declines thereafter.

The etiology of osteosarcoma is unknown, but several associations with underlying medical conditions have been reported. Patients who have the germinal mutation for retinoblastoma and who survive the ocular tumor have a 2000-fold increased risk for osteosarcoma in irradiated craniofacial bones. These patients have a 500-fold increased risk for osteosarcoma at any site regardless of prior radiation exposure. This risk appears to be linked to the expression of the retinoblastoma gene, located on chromosome 13, band q14. Radiation-induced osteosarcoma is also being diagnosed with increased frequency in long-term survivors of childhood cancer. Pediatric cancer groups studying late effects estimate a 40-fold risk for bone cancer in survivors who have received more than 6000 rad to the bone. The median time to onset is 10 years. There is also an increased risk associated with alkylating agents, proportional to cumulative doses. In older patients with Paget disease, there is an increased risk for osteosarcoma involving the affected bone. Occasional cases also have been reported in association with chondroma, osteochondromatosis, and nonossifying fibroma.

### Signs, Symptoms, and Diagnostic Studies

The metaphyseal portion of the long bone is the site of predilection. Almost half of all new cases present with involvement in the region of the knee. In order of presentation, the most common sites are the distal femur, proximal tibia, and proximal humerus. However, any membranous bone may be involved, and even cases of extraosseous osteosarcoma have been reported.

Pain, which initially may be intermittent, and swelling of the extremity, which may evolve over several weeks, are the cardinal symptoms. Because these symptoms are nonspecific, adolescents presenting with pain in the area of the knee without a history for trauma should undergo a radiographic examination. Pathologic fractures are uncommon. However, minor trauma with disproportional symptoms of pain may cause these patients to present for evaluation and lead to the recognition of a preexisting pathologic lesion.

The diagnosis of osteosarcoma may be suspected from good-quality radiographs; tumors may appear as lytic, sclerotic, or

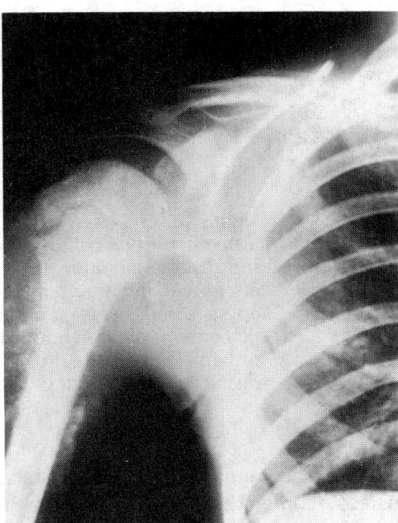

**Figure 102-1.** A large permeative lesion of the proximal right humerus, representing osteosarcoma beginning at the metaphyseal plate, with soft-tissue extension and calcifications due to osteosarcoma.

mixed lesions. Irregular periosteal new bone formation in the metaphyseal region may be an initial observation. In more advanced cases, cortical destruction, sclerosis, a sunburst pattern of periosteal new bone formation, and contiguous, calcified soft-tissue extensions may be noted (Fig 102-1). Submicroscopic extension along the diaphysis can produce "skip" metastases some distance from the primary lesion.

The diagnosis is best made by incisional biopsy and permanent section. A carefully performed needle biopsy also may provide material sufficient for diagnosis. Extreme care must be taken in the biopsy of these lesions, because an incorrectly directed biopsy may produce an inadequate or misleading diagnosis or may leave a tract that will complicate possible consideration for limb salvage therapy. Ultimately, the biopsy tract must be excised en bloc with the tumor at the time of definitive surgery. In view of the rarity of these tumors and because of recent developments in the multimodal management of these patients, referral to a pediatric cancer center for definitive biopsy and diagnosis is in the patient's best interest.

Staging of the disease should include a chest radiograph and a CT scan of the chest. Osteosarcoma may spread by hematogenous routes; metastases involving the lungs or bone are detected at the time of diagnosis in 10% to 20% of the cases (Fig 102-2). Radionuclide scans are more sensitive for detecting foci of osseous disease distant from the primary site. About 2% to 3% of all childhood or adolescent cases of osteosarcoma are multifocal. This rare type, called multifocal sclerosing osteogenic sarcoma, presents with simultaneous or synchronous metastases at multiple metaphyseal regions and has a rapidly lethal outcome.

Patients considered for limb preservation require CT or MRI examinations of the tumor-bearing bone and occasionally angiography. MRI scans are very accurate in the assessment of intraosseous extension of tumor and are the preferred examination for patients undergoing limb salvage procedures.

About 60% of adolescent cases have elevated alkaline phosphatase, but this does not appear to have prognostic significance.

Histologic examination permits a division of osteosarcoma into two broad categories. Low-grade osteosarcomas, including juxtacortical or periosteal and low-grade central osteogenic sarcoma, have a survival of about 70% with amputation or wide local excision alone. High-grade osteosarcomas include fibrosarcomatous, osteoblastic, telangiectatic, and small-cell osteosarcoma.

Patients presenting with these lesions require more aggressive treatment.

## Treatment

Before the 1970s, the prognosis for children with osteosarcoma of the extremity was dismal. Despite control of the primary tumor with amputation, distant metastases developed in most patients, and survival was about 20% at 5 years from diagnosis. Current multimodal treatment strategies for osteosarcoma have reversed this trend, and about 60% to 65% of patients with nonmetastatic disease of the extremities are surviving their disease. Both surgery and high-dose chemotherapy play a significant part in achieving this result.

Surgery has an established role in the treatment of osteosarcoma. Ablative procedures usually involve amputation through the bone above the affected bone. It is generally accepted that the amputation should be 7 cm beyond the most proximal limits of the lesion to minimize the risk for local recurrence. Large lesions involving the proximal femur or humerus occasionally require a disarticulation procedure.

With the availability of more effective chemotherapy programs, limb salvage surgery, after en bloc tumor excision and endoprosthetic replacement, has become a viable alternative for many patients (Fig 102-3). Candidates considered eligible for the limb salvage procedure are generally selected on the basis of the following criteria:

- Attainment of complete or nearly complete physical growth for patients with lesions of the lower extremities
- Anatomical site of the lesion such that no sacrifice of major arteries or nerves is involved
- Absence of metastases at diagnosis, or isolated metastasis that responded to preoperative treatment
- Full understanding by the patient and parents of the nature of the procedure, reasonable expectations for functional outcome, and estimated risks for complications, local recurrence, and possible failure of procedure.

Limb salvage may be performed by immediate en bloc resection or may follow a brief course of chemotherapy. The potential advantages of preoperative chemotherapy are that it allows for planning and acquisition of a custom prosthesis, it may allow some definition of the antitumor efficacy of the chemotherapy regimen to be used as postoperative adjuvant therapy, and the antitumor effects may enhance the safety of the surgical procedure. Several pediatric cancer centers have extended the process of preoperative treatment to all osteosarcoma patients, but the value of this approach remains to be established.

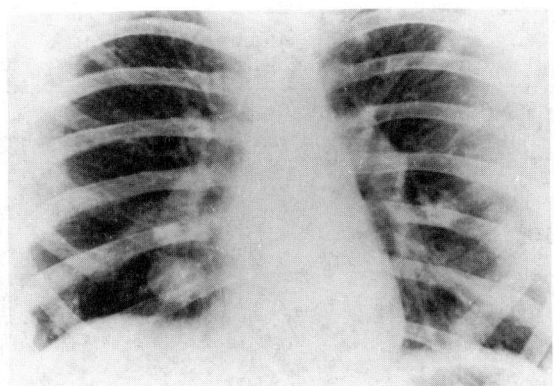

**Figure 102-2.** Chest radiograph demonstrating multiple, bilateral pulmonary nodules of metastatic osteosarcoma.

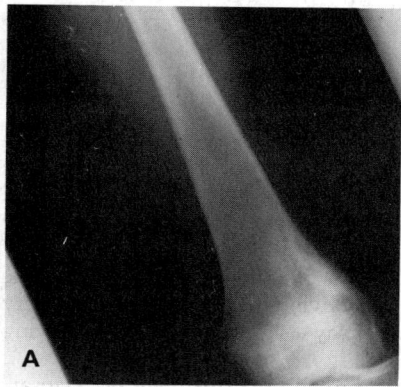
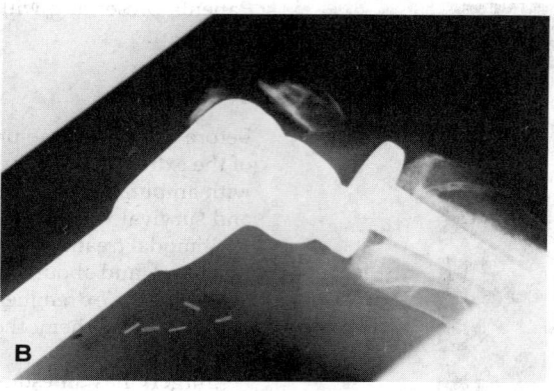

**Figure 102-3.** (**A**) A 14-year-old girl with a small sclerotic osteosarcoma involving the distal left femur. (**B**) Three months after receiving preoperative chemotherapy, she underwent en bloc resection and placement of an endoprosthesis, with proximal insertion into the femur and distal insertion into the tibia.

Over the past 20 years, nonrandomized multicenter chemotherapy trials have established unequivocally the value of high-dose adjuvant chemotherapy for increased relapse-free survival for patients with nonmetastatic osteosarcoma of the extremities. The first successful demonstration of adjuvant chemotherapy was a study by the Pediatric Division of the Southwest Oncology Group in 1970. The COMPADRI-I program, with over 15 years of follow-up, produced an overall 49% disease-free survival (DFS). Studies conducted at the Dana Farber Cancer Center in the 1970s and early 1980s with high-dose methotrexate and doxorubicin produced an overall DFS of more than 55%.

In the early 1980s, randomized studies by the Pediatric Oncology Group (POG 8107) and the University of California–Los Angeles clearly established that postoperative adjuvant chemotherapy improves the DFS of patients with nonmetastatic osteosarcoma of the extremities when compared with surgery alone (64% versus 19%). Since that study, several chemotherapeutic programs have produced long-term DFS in excess of 60% (Table 102-1). Common features of these programs include the use of high doses of methotrexate, doxorubicin, ifosfamide, or cisplatin. New innovations include the use of intra-arterial infusions of cisplatin directed at tumor-bearing sites. Investigations of tumor histology after preoperative chemotherapy suggest that patients who experience tumor necrosis of more than 90% are more likely to remain free of disease.

These chemotherapy programs are potentially very toxic and require considerable expertise in management. Cisplatin may produce difficulties with renal function and hearing. High-dose doxorubicin may be associated with cardiotoxicity. All patients require extensive rehabilitation support to resume normal activities.

Pulmonary metastases remain the major obstacle for cure for patients with osteosarcoma. The number and time of presentation of metastases may have clinical significance: early-appearing, multiple lesions may be associated with drug-resistant disease and poor prognosis. Aggressive surgical treatment, including multiple and occasionally bilateral thoracotomies, coupled with intensive chemotherapy, may salvage 25% to 50% of these patients. Complete removal of all metastatic tumor at the time of the initial thoracotomy may have the greatest importance for long-term survival. Refinement of limb salvage techniques in the future will increase the number of children who might enjoy a more functionally and cosmetically satisfying result from the primary surgical treatment.

## EWING SARCOMA

### Incidence and Epidemiology

Ewing sarcoma is an uncommon primary sarcoma of nonosseous origin that usually arises in children or adolescents. James Ewing is credited with the first description of this tumor in 1921. Ewing sarcoma represents about 1% of all cancers reported in children but about 30% of all bone tumors in this age group. The estimated incidence is two per 1 million population in the United States for Caucasians under age 20; it is rare in the nonwhite population. The male/female ratio is 1.54 : 1.

The etiology for Ewing sarcoma is unknown. Unlike osteosarcoma, ionizing radiation exposure does not represent a significant risk factor.

### Pathology

Ewing sarcoma is a small, round-cell tumor. Because of a poorly differentiated or undifferentiated histology, it may be confused with other undifferentiated round-cell tumors of childhood. The Ewing tumor typically is composed of a uniform population of small polygonal cells with scant cytoplasm and hyperchromatic nuclei. The cytoplasmic borders may be indistinct. Glycogen granules may be present but are not pathognomonic for the disease. The diversity of light microscopic patterns in Ewing sarcoma makes the diagnosis a challenge for even the most experienced pathologist. Recent investigations have demonstrated a cytogenetic abnormality, t(11;22) (q24C2), within tumor cells that may assist in the confirmation of the diagnosis and may be valuable in future research into this disease.

Other round-cell tumors to be considered in the differential diagnosis include non-Hodgkin's lymphoma, rhabdomyosarcoma, neuroblastoma, small-cell osteosarcoma, neuroepithelioma, metastatic medulloblastoma, and the acute leukemias of all types.

| Protocol | DFS ≥ 3 yr (%) | Cancer Programs |
|---|---|---|
| COSS-80, 82 | 68 | German Pediatric Oncology Group |
| HDMTX, IA DDP, ADR | 80 | Instituto Rizzoli Osteosarcoma Study 2 |
| IFOS, ADR, HDMTX | 82 | Mayo |
| ADR, IA DDP | 76 | M. D. Anderson Hospital |
| T-10 | 76 | Memorial Sloan-Kettering |

TABLE 102-1. Summary of Recent Chemotherapy Trials in Osteosarcoma

*ADR*, Adriamycin; *DFS*, disease-free survival; *HDMTX*, high-dose methotrexate; *IA DDP*, intra-arterial cisplatin; *IFOS*, ifosfamide.

## Clinical Presentation and Diagnostic Evaluation

Pain is the most common first symptom in Ewing sarcoma, occurring in more than half of the patients. Swelling associated with a soft-tissue mass may become evident weeks to months thereafter. Fever and an elevated erythrocyte sedimentation rate may develop in time and may confound the diagnosis. Pathologic fractures are uncommon.

The femur is the bone most commonly involved, but any bone of the body may be involved (Figs 102-4, 102-5). The classic radiographic feature is a diffuse, mottled, lytic lesion affecting the medullary cavity and cortical bone. There may be regions of increased density associated with new bone formation. Tumor that penetrates the cortex and extends into the periosteum may produce elevations characterized by multiple layers of reactive new bone formation, creating an "onion-skin" appearance on radiographic examination. The tumor may expand the affected bone and resemble a cystic malformation. A soft-tissue mass, rarely including calcifications, may be associated with the primary bone tumor. Although these radiographic features have been clearly described with Ewing tumors, several conditions can produce similar features, including acute and chronic osteomyelitis, eosinophilic granuloma, osteosarcoma, metastatic sarcomas, and lymphoma. An MRI scan of the affected bone gives the best assessment of intramedullary tumor extension.

An open biopsy is the procedure of choice to establish the diagnosis of Ewing sarcoma. In general, needle biopsies do not provide sufficient material for interpretation and have on occasion produced confusing information. The two conditions most often mistaken for Ewing sarcoma are eosinophilic granuloma and osteomyelitis. The presence of necrosis or inflammatory cells within the tumor can be misleading if the biopsy material is inadequate. Biopsy of cortical lesions should be as small and round as possible, avoiding the tension side of the bone if possible, and should include touch preparations and material for electron microscopy. If a malignant bone tumor is suspected in a child or adolescent, referral to a pediatric cancer center for the definitive diagnosis will ensure the most experienced surgical assessment and optimum biopsy for these patients.

Once the diagnosis of Ewing sarcoma is established, clinical staging is essential, including chest radiographs, a CT scan of the chest, an MRI scan of the bone, a radionuclide bone scan, and

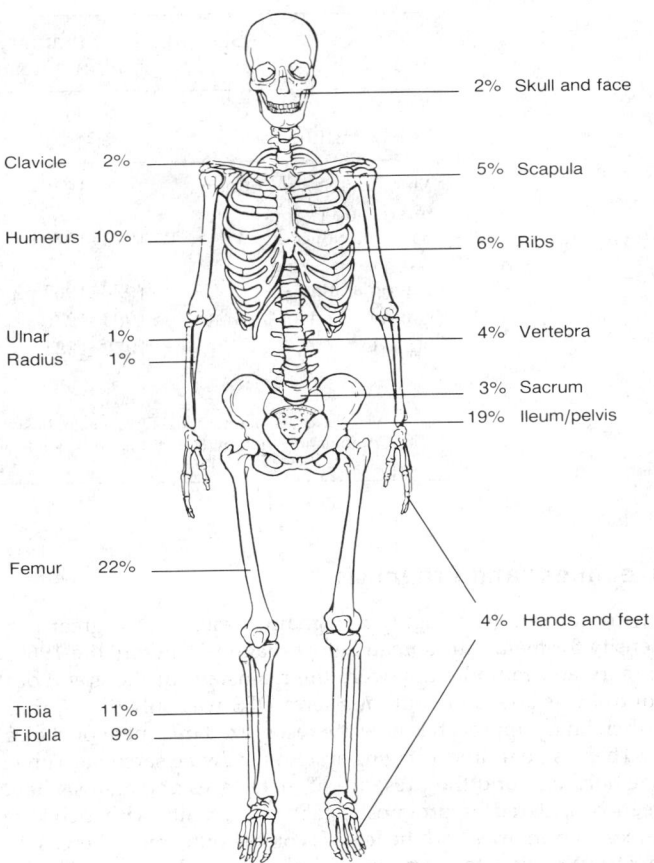

**Figure 102-5.**   Anatomical distribution of Ewing sarcoma, based on 836 cases. (After Sutow WW, Fernbach DJ, Vietti TJ, eds. Clinical pediatric oncology, chap 29. St. Louis: CV Mosby, 1984)

bone marrow aspiration and biopsy. These investigations are pursued because the lungs and bones are the most common sites of metastases (90% of the cases). Other baseline studies are also recommended, including serum lactate dehydrogenase, alkaline phosphatase, and erythrocyte sedimentation rate. These tests may reflect the extent of tumor activity. Urinary catecholamines may be helpful to rule out neuroblastoma in the younger patient.

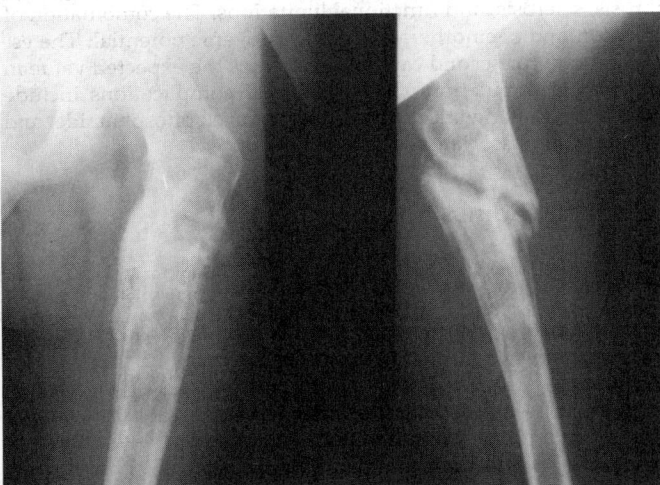

**Figure 102-4.**   Two radiographic views of the left femur demonstrating a diffuse, destructive process due to Ewing sarcoma, involving the intertrochanteric region and extending to the mid-shaft. There is a pathologic fracture.

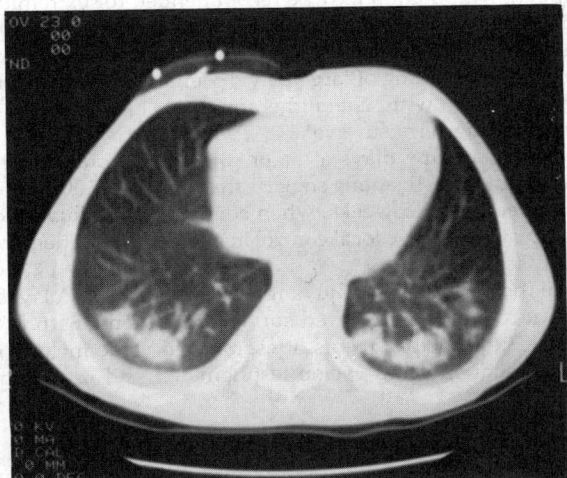

**Figure 102-6.**   CT scan of the chest revealing bilateral pulmonary metastasis, in a child initially treated for a Ewing sarcoma of the femur.

**TABLE 102-2.   Summary of Selected Therapeutic Trials in Nonmetastatic Ewing Sarcoma**

| Institution | Study Period | Local Radiation to Primary | Chemotherapy | DFS > 2 yr (%) |
|---|---|---|---|---|
| Memorial Sloan-Kettering | 1970–1979 | + | T-2/T-6/T-9* | 79 |
| Intergroup Ewing Sarcoma Study-II | 1973–1978 | + | V, A, C, + ADR | 74 |
| Intergroup Ewing Sarcoma Study-I | 1978–1983 | + | V, A, C + ADR | >70 |
| National Cancer Institute | 1983–1986 | + | V, C + ADR | 70 |
| St. Jude | 1978–1981 | + (delayed) | V, A, C | >70 |

V, vincristine; A, actinomycin D; C, cyclophosphamide; ADR, Adriamycin.
* Combination therapy with 4, 6, and 9 agents, including V, A, C + ADR.

## Treatment and Prognosis

Ewing sarcoma is a highly malignant tumor with a great propensity for metastatic spread before diagnosis. Before the 1960s, surgery and radiotherapy were the mainstays of therapy. Local control was adequate, but long-term DFS was only 9%. A multidisciplinary approach is now the recognized treatment of choice.

There is no uniform staging system for Ewing sarcoma. Tumor size, location, and the presence of metastases at diagnosis have been considered as prognostic factors. Patients with pelvic or proximal primaries had the least favorable outcome, whereas the most favorable sites were distal lesions, usually in expendable bones. Patients with large soft-tissue extensions did less well with therapy because of an increased risk for distant, usually pulmonary, metastases (Fig 102-6). Modifications in current therapy may alter the significance of these risk factors.

There is a renewed interest in surgical management of the primary tumor, due to the improved survival in patients with complete removal, the increased risk of orthopedic complications after chemoradiotherapy, the difficulty in confirming that the primary site has been sterilized, and the concern that residual microscopic disease might produce distant metastases. The exact role for surgery in the treatment of Ewing sarcoma is yet to be determined. Possible applications include aggressive surgery for lesions in expendable bones, in which resulting disability is acceptable (ie, lesions in the foot, fibula, rib, forearm bone, clavicle, or scapula). Amputation may be recommended for extremity lesions in which there are huge destructive components, pathologic fractures, or involvement of distal femoral epiphysis in children under age 6. Debulking of large pelvic primaries following initial tumor reduction with chemotherapy may also increase the chances for long-term survival.

Radiation therapy plays a major role in the control of local disease. Most investigations suggest that doses of 5000 to 5500 cGy, divided over 5.5 weeks, when coupled with adjuvant chemotherapy will achieve local control in over 90% of patients with extremity lesions.

Since the early 1970s, adjuvant chemotherapy has played an important role in the improved survival of patients with Ewing sarcoma. The principal agents of established value include vincristine, dactinomycin, cyclophosphamide, and doxorubicin (VACA). Patients with nonmetastatic disease with primary lesions in an extremity have a projected 3-year survival rate of more than 60% and a local recurrence rate of less than 10% with modern therapy (Table 102-2). Ifosfamide and VP-16 are new agents with activity against this tumor. Current clinical trials are investigating the impact of these new agents when given with high-dose vincristine, cyclophosphamide, and doxorubicin. The relapse-free survival for patients with nonmetastatic Ewing sarcoma of the pelvis and sacral bones is 55% following similar therapy.

The presence of metastatic disease at diagnosis has been reported in 14% to 35% of patients and is associated with a poor prognosis. Historically, the median DFS for patients with metastatic disease at diagnosis has been 75 weeks. Patients developing distant metastases while receiving therapy have resistant disease and an expected median survival of 37 weeks.

For survivors of Ewing sarcoma, several late consequences of treatment may have a significant impact. Pathologic fractures may occur at primary tumor sites involving lower extremities at periods of 6 months to 3 years from diagnosis. This complication may be related to impaired bone remodeling following radiation and chemotherapy. Demineralization and radiation-associated delayed healing may aggravate this situation by causing nonunion of the fracture site. Other potential complications of radiation therapy include retarded bone growth, limb-length discrepancy, fibrosis, sclerosis, and functional limitations. The combination of radiation and chemotherapy has carcinogenic potential. The estimated rate for second cancers is 72 times the expected value in the normal population. Other potential complications include sterility associated with prolonged use of cyclophosphamide, and cardiotoxicity associated with doxorubicin.

## Selected Readings

Burgert EO, Nesbit ME, Garnsey LA, et al. Multimodal therapy for the management of nonpelvic localized Ewing's sarcoma of bone: Intergroup Study IESS-II. J Clin Oncol 1990;8:1514.
Eilber FR, Rosen G. Adjuvant chemotherapy for osteosarcoma. Semin Oncol 1989;16:312.
Link MP, Grier HE, Donaldson SS. Sarcomas of bone. In: Fernbach DJ, Vietti TJ, eds. Clinical pediatric oncology, ed 4. St. Louis: CV Mosby, 1991:545.
Meyers PA, Heller G, Healey J, et al. Chemotherapy for nonmetastatic osteogenic sarcoma: the Memorial Sloan-Kettering experience. J Clin Oncol 1989;10:5.

*Principles and Practice of Pediatrics, Second Edition.*
edited by Frank A. Oski et al. J. B. Lippincott Company, Philadelphia © 1994.

## CHAPTER 103
# *Malignant Tumors of the Gastrointestinal Tract, Liver, and Endocrine System*

## C. Philip Steuber

Although many pediatric tumors commonly metastasize to various parts of the alimentary system, primary malignancies of that system are exceedingly rare in children. With the possible exception of hepatic neoplasms, pediatric therapies for these entities are adapted from experience with adult patients, in whom they occur with much greater frequency.

## HEPATOMAS

The most common primary GI tract neoplasms in children are hepatic in origin. Hepatoblastoma and hepatocellular carcinoma, the two main subgroups of primary liver tumors, are clinically indistinguishable at presentation. Symptoms usually are related to the mass and include loss of appetite and weight, and abdominal pain. Physical findings are those of an upper abdominal mass. Jaundice is usually not present, especially with hepatoblastoma. Increased levels of alpha-fetoprotein are associated with both tumor types. When elevated, this tumor marker is a sensitive index of disease presence or activity. Sonography, CT scans, MRI, and rarely angiography can be used to determine operability and to differentiate intrahepatic tumors from other upper abdominal tumors.

Without surgery these tumors are invariably fatal. In fact, unless the tumor can be completely excised at some early point, long-term survival is rare, and most patients die within 12 months of diagnosis. Most liver tumors in children are not amenable to total excision at diagnosis. Liver tumors commonly metastasize to the lungs, brain, and regional lymphatics.

Hepatoblastomas occur almost entirely in very young children (<3 years) and infants. Currently four histologic subtypes are recognized: fetal, embryonal, macrotrabecular, and anaplastic. Those with fetal histology tend to do well if complete excision is accomplished and adjuvant chemotherapy given. The remaining histologic subtypes of hepatoblastoma are most often associated with unfavorable outcome regardless of stage. Hepatocellular carcinomas occur more commonly in very young children but also are diagnosed in early adolescence. Changes in the serum ferritin level may correlate with tumor response.

Liver tumors do not respond well to radiation therapy and only transiently to chemotherapy regimens using cisplatin, 5-FU, doxorubicin, vincristine, etoposide, and cyclophosphamide, either singly or in combination. At present, the greatest value of chemotherapy for primary liver tumors appears to be in converting an inoperable condition to one in which excisional surgery is possible.

Malignant mesenchymoma, cholangiocarcinoma, and hemangiosarcoma are even less common hepatic tumors in children. Management guidelines are much the same as for hepatoblastoma and hepatocellular carcinoma. Aggressive surgery is necessary, but often excision is impossible; even when excision is accomplished, recurrence rates are high.

## OTHER TUMORS OF THE GI TRACT

### Oropharyngeal Tumors

Carcinoma of the oropharynx has been observed in older children. These tumors are primarily mucoepidermoid carcinomas involving the salivary glands. Rare cases of squamous cell carcinoma of the lip or tongue in childhood have also been reported. Esophageal carcinoma has been found in patients as young as age 15.

### Gastric Tumors

Malignant gastric tumors in children are usually lymphomas or sarcomas, but gastric adenocarcinomas have been documented. Most primary tumors found in the stomach are benign, and surgery is the only indicated therapy. For gastric malignancies, surgery is the initial therapy, with postoperative radiotherapy or chemotherapy as indicated.

### Gallbladder Tumors

Primary gallbladder tumors are rare at all ages. When present, they are highly malignant and unresponsive to all forms of therapy. Usually metastatic disease to the liver and lymph nodes is present at diagnosis. The most common childhood cancer to involve the gallbladder is rhabdomyosarcoma.

### Small Intestine

It is unusual to find primary small bowel tumors at any age, but particularly in children. When they do occur they usually present with some manifestations of intestinal obstruction, partial or complete. Occasionally small bowel tumors cause ulceration and intestinal bleeding, rarely even perforation. The most frequently diagnosed small bowel tumor is lymphoma. Therapy after surgery is dictated by the histologic classification and staging, as outlined in Chapter 103.

### Appendix

Carcinoid tumors are the appendiceal tumor recognized most often in children. They usually are detected early before they spread, since they present with signs and symptoms of appendicitis. Appendectomy is the only therapy indicated.

### Pancreas

Pediatric pancreatic tumors fall into three categories: exocrine and ductal tumors, endocrine tumors, and mesenchymal tumors. Most pancreatic tumors in children are benign and are treated by excision. The exception is pancreatic carcinoma, which is highly malignant. Pancreatic carcinoma requires radical surgery, but has often spread to the liver and lung by the time of diagnosis and is thus inoperable. Presenting features include an abdominal mass and pain, GI disturbances, and rarely obstructive jaundice. Chemotherapy and radiotherapy are ineffective.

### Large Intestine

Most cases of colon tumors in children are benign polyps, which can cause rectal bleeding. Adenocarcinomas of the colon and rectum are almost unheard of in the very young child. They are more likely to occur in adolescents and are highly invasive, tending to metastasize early. Several conditions predispose to the development of colon carcinoma in young people, including ulcerative colitis, familial polyposis, ureterocolonic anastomosis, Gardner's syndrome, and Turcot syndrome. Early detection is important. The value of carcinoembryonic antigen determination in childhood colon cancer is not established. Therapy emphasizes aggressive surgery. Effective chemotherapy, with the possible exception of the combination of 5-FU and levamisole, has not been established for colon cancer. Radiation therapy may be helpful for rectosigmoid lesions. Long-term survival rates are dismal.

## ENDOCRINE TUMORS

### Thyroid Carcinoma

Cancer of the thyroid gland is uncommon in children. However, thyroid nodules may be found in 20% to 30% of children who have received external radiation for any reason. Long-term follow-up observation of any patient who has had radiotherapy to the neck region should include examination and evaluation of the thyroid gland. Of children who exhibit nodules, with or without a history of radiation exposure, about 35% to 50% will develop malignancies. The minimum latent period for the development of thyroid cancer is 5 years in males and 10 years in females. Carcinoma of the thyroid in children has a more benign course than in adults, and anaplastic carcinomas are almost nonexistent in children.

Therapy for thyroid carcinoma consists of surgical extirpation or the administration of iodine-131 if there are distal metastases. External radiation and chemotherapy are not indicated in the management of thyroid cancer in children.

Although the overall survival figures appear favorable, there is a notable incidence of late relapses, and patients must be followed for a prolonged time.

### Cancer of the Adrenal Cortex

Cancer of the adrenal cortex has an extremely low incidence. It is often difficult to distinguish between carcinoma and benign adenoma. Such tumors may be hormonally active or inactive. Virilism is the most common complaint in boys or girls. Cushing's syndrome is less common, and feminizing tumors or aldosterone-secreting tumors are extremely rare. Malignant adrenal tumors may metastasize to the liver, lung, and brain. The treatment is surgical, but this should be carefully coordinated with an endocrinologist. Experience in managing disseminated tumor with systemic agents is limited.

### Selected Readings

Ortega JA, Malogolowkin MH. Epithelial and neuroectodermal tumors of the gastrointestinal, genitourinary, and gynecological tracts. In: Fernbach DJ, Vietti TJ, eds. Clinical pediatric oncology, ed 4. St. Louis: CV Mosby, 1991:611.
Pratt CB, Douglass EC. Management of the less common cancers of childhood. In: Pizzo PA, Poplack DG, eds. Principles and practice of pediatric oncology. Philadelphia: JB Lippincott, 1989:759.

*Principles and Practice of Pediatrics, Second Edition.*
edited by Frank A. Oski et al. J. B. Lippincott Company, Philadelphia © 1994.

## CHAPTER 104
# Gonadal and Germ Cell Neoplasms

### ZoAnn E. Dreyer and Angela Ogden

Germ cell tumors are a unique conglomerate of abnormal growths that share a common origin. The germ cells are the precursors of the sperm and egg cells of the gonads and are thus responsible for the production of the entire organism. Because of this, they have the potential to form a multiplicity of neoplasms that vary widely in histology and anatomical distribution. They may be gonadal (occurring in the testis or ovary) or extragonadal (found in the anterior mediastinum, neck, brain, retroperitoneum, or sacrococcygeal regions).

## EMBRYOLOGY

Several hypotheses have been proposed to explain the occurrence of germ cell tumors in extragonadal sites. It has been suggested that during the migration of the germ cells from the yolk sac wall to the hindgut and to the gonadal ridge, some cells are left behind or stray and come to rest at various midline sites of the embryo. If these cell rests remain viable, they may then give rise to tumors in that location. Most investigators currently support this theory of aberrant migration as the likely embryologic explanation for the diversity in germ cell tumor sites.

It is necessary to understand germ cell differentiation to appreciate the relationships of the various germ cell tumors. These cells may differentiate into unipotential primitive germ cells from which germinomas develop; these are called seminomas in males and dysgerminomas in females. Multipotential undifferentiated germ cells may form embryonal carcinomas and these cells may then undergo embryonal differentiation, resulting in teratomas. However, if these multipotent cells follow a path of extra-embryonal differentiation, tumors may arise from structures similar to the yolk sac or placenta, known as yolk sac tumors (endodermal sinus tumors) or choriocarcinoma, respectively (Fig 104-1).

## BACKGROUND

Germ cell tumors of childhood appear to have peak incidences in early childhood, during which sacrococcygeal, head and neck, and retroperitoneal tumors are most common, and in puberty, during which ovarian and testicular tumors are most common. In infancy, germ cell tumors are almost exclusively teratomatous.

Sensitive tumor markers have proven extremely useful in following certain neoplasms for therapeutic response or recurrence. Alpha-fetoprotein (AFP) is a glycoprotein normally synthesized

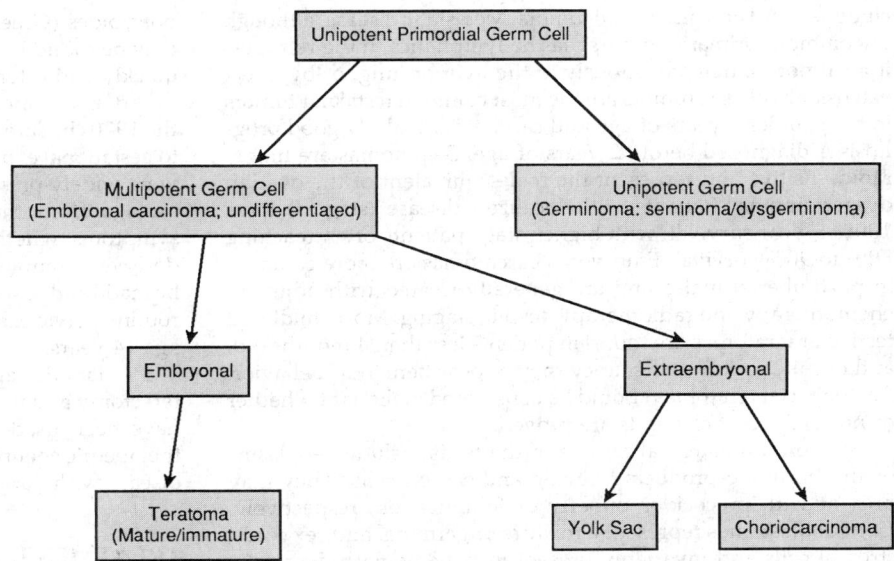

Figure 104-1. Differentiation of germ cell tumors.

in the fetal liver, yolk sac, and GI tract. Its production ceases at birth but normal adult levels of less than 20 ng/mL are not reached until 6 months of age. Hepatomas and tumors with yolk sac elements may secrete AFP, resulting in elevated blood levels. Human chorionic gonadotropin (HCG) is a glycoprotein produced in the trophoblasts of the placenta. The beta-HCG (B-HCG) subunit can be measured, and an elevated level (normal <1 ng/mL) may be seen in trophoblastic tumors (choriocarcinoma) and nontrophoblastic tumors, including embryonal carcinoma, pancreatic carcinoma, breast and GI cancer, as well as malignant melanomas and multiple myeloma.

Obtaining serial AFP and B-HCG determinations in patients with abnormal levels at the time of diagnosis provides a valuable aid in determining the presence of residual or recurrent disease as well as an indication of response to therapy.

## PATHOLOGY

Germ cell tumors can occur as a single histologic type or as a mixed germ cell tumor of two or more cell types. Generally, the tumor's malignant potential is determined by the histology of the most malignant element of the mass. Therefore, meticulous histologic examination must be done to determine what therapy is indicated.

Embryonal carcinomas are highly malignant, with significant anaplasia and frequent mitoses. Cells stain positively for B-HCG. Teratomas are derived from at least two of the three germ cell layers (endoderm, mesoderm, and ectoderm). The tissues may be fully differentiated in the mature teratoma and contain teeth, bone, hair, and skin. The immature teratoma contains tissues more reminiscent of fetal or embryonal structures. The malignant potential of these tumors is determined by the amount of immature neuroepithelium as well as by the presence of other germ cell tumor types. Extra-embryonal yolk sac tumors are the most common malignant germ cell tumors. Microscopically, the tumor resembles normal placenta but with characteristic Schiller-Duval bodies resembling glomeruli. The cells stain for the presence of AFP and rarely B-HCG.

Morphologically, choriocarcinoma resembles the chorion layer of the placenta, with multinucleated syncytiotrophoblasts and cytotrophoblasts, and secretes B-HCG. It can arise from the pluripotent germ cell (nongestational) or from the placenta in a pregnant woman (gestational).

## EXTRAGONADAL SITES

The sacrococcygeal region is by far the most common site of teratomas in childhood (40% to 70% of all cases). Most of these tumors present in the neonatal period. Tumors arising in the sacrococcygeal region are benign in over 95% of those presenting before 1 month of age and in over 60% in all others. The primary therapy is excision of the mass, including the coccyx to avoid recurrence.

The mediastinum is the primary site in 7% of the children with germ cell tumors. Most present with dyspnea and cough due to tracheal compression, and the mass is detected on chest x-ray. Germ cell tumors arising from the heart or pericardium are very rare and are usually detected in the neonatal period due to the mass effect at the lesion.

Less than 5% of the teratomas in childhood originate in the head and neck region. These lesions present with symptoms related to airway compromise from mass compression. Older children are rarely affected. The CNS may be involved due to direct extension or by primary tumor involvement of the pineal gland.

The retroperitoneum is an unusual primary site for germ cell tumors. They may present in early childhood with pain as the most common complaint, followed by vomiting. The mass is often palpated in the upper abdominal quadrants.

## GONADAL SITES

### Genitourinary Tumors in the Male

Testicular tumors represent less than 2% of all pediatric solid tumors, with peak incidences before age 5 years and in the postpubertal population. About 10% occur in cryptorchid testes, with an especially high risk if the undescended testis is in the abdomen. Painless testicular swelling is perhaps the most frequent presenting complaint, and 25% of patients may have an associated hydrocele with positive transillumination often masking the presence of the tumor. Inguinal hernias may be found in 21% of patients.

The normal testis is composed primarily of germ cells (spermatozoa) and the hormone-producing sex cord (Sertoli) and stromal interstitial (Leydig) cells. Thus, two major categories of testicular tumors exist—germinal and nongerminal. Germinal tumors include several varieties of germ cell tumors and represent 70% of all childhood testicular tumors. Nongerminal tumors include sex cord and all stromal tumors. Metastatic disease, although uncommon, primarily occurs via the lymphatics to the retroperitoneal nodes, hematogenously to the liver or lung, or by direct extension. Yolk sac tumors are the most common testicular tumors in boys under 4 years of age and carry a particularly good prognosis if diagnosed before 2 years of age. Seminomas are highly radiosensitive and represent the male equivalent of the ovarian dysgerminoma. Patients with localized disease (stage I) have 100% 5-year survival, with higher-stage patients often reaching 80% to 90% survival. Embryonal carcinomas are more common in postpubertal males and are generally treated with adjuvant chemotherapy and radiotherapy despite staging. Most childhood testicular teratomas are found in patients less than 4 months old, and despite foci of malignancy they appear benign in behavior. Postpubertal teratomas should be considered malignant whether or not malignant elements are proven.

Sex cord and stromal tumors of the testis include neoplasms of the hormone-producing Leydig and Sertoli cells. They may present with precocious puberty or feminization, respectively. Gonadoblastomas represent a mixture of germinal and sex cord/stromal cells and invariably present in patients with dysplastic gonads. Intrascrotal masses arising from the epididymis, spermatic cord, or its coverings are invariably rhabdomyosarcomas, while childhood tumors of the penis usually are hemangiomas or lymphomas.

## Gynecologic Tumors in the Female

Ovarian tumors of childhood represent 80% of the pediatric genital tumors in females, and about one third are malignant. While they may occur at any age, they are seen with increasing frequency in the pubescent population. The risk of malignancy increases with decreasing age. The diagnosis should be considered in any young female presenting with an abdominal mass, vaginal bleeding, and signs of inappropriate hormonal influences. The disease may spread via the lymphatics, hematogenously, by direct extension, or intraperitoneally. Extensive surgical exploration, including multiple biopsies, is required for adequate definition of the disease extent. The prognosis has improved with the addition of adjuvant chemotherapy and, on occasion, radiotherapy. This has allowed the surgical approach to become less aggressive, in most cases preserving fertility.

Yolk sac tumors are rapidly growing ovarian tumors that often present with extensive intra-abdominal and intrapelvic disease with frequent spread to the peritoneal surfaces. Because of this aggressive behavior, combination chemotherapy is mandatory in all stages in addition to surgical resection.

Dysgerminomas are a common ovarian malignancy. They are analogous to testicular seminomas with very high cure rates, particularly with unilateral disease. The least differentiated of the germ cell tumors are embryonal carcinomas, which can be distinguished from yolk sac tumors by the presence of staining for B-HCG. A large percentage of ovarian masses are teratomatous. Of these, 80% are cystic and have a very low malignancy rate, while the remaining 20% are solid and have a much higher risk of malignancy. The prognosis depends on the degree of immaturity and the types of immature cells identified.

Sex cord and stromal cell tumors are much less common and less malignant than germ cell tumors of the ovary. They may exist in pure forms as granulosa (sex cord) or theca (strand) cell tumors, or they may be found as a mixture of these cell types.

Gonadoblastomas (dysgenetic gonadomas) are rare tumors that represent an intimate mixture of germ cell and sex cord/stromal cells, characteristically in patients with dysgenetic gonads.

Lower genital tract tumors include vaginal, cervical, and uterine tumors. Rhabdomyosarcoma is the only lower genital tract malignancy seen with any frequency in young girls. Sarcoma

botryoides (Greek for "cluster of grapes") is such a tumor and may be found in the uterus, vagina, bladder, or cervix. It spreads quickly and often metastasizes early to the lungs.

Adenocarcinoma of the vagina and cervix were rare before the 1970s but are now becoming more common, with most related to gestational exposure to diethylstilbestrol (DES). DES-type drugs were widely prescribed in the 1940s and 1950s to improve fetal salvage from threatened abortion. Young girls with vaginal symptoms, whether or not there is a history of exposure to DES, deserve a complete pelvic examination. Cytologic smears should be made and suspicious lesions biopsied. In DES-exposed patients, routine pelvic examinations should commence at menarche or at age 14 years.

Primary therapy for clear cell carcinoma is radiotherapy. Hysterectomy and vaginectomy, followed by vaginal reconstruction, have been used successfully in several cases. Various chemotherapeutic agents have been used for the treatment of metastatic disease with varied success.

## TREATMENT AND PROGNOSIS

The treatment of germ cell tumors in childhood must be individualized for each patient, depending on tumor histology and the patient's age. The extent of the disease should be evaluated by CT scanning of the chest and abdomen. In males, the testicles should be examined. If there is no apparent mass, a testicular ultrasound should be done. The primary form of therapy is surgery, usually with total excision of the mass, but this is not essential. AFP and B-HCG indicative of malignant elements in the mass should be checked preoperatively and followed serially thereafter. Reappearance or appearance of increased levels of AFP and B-HCG indicates disease activity. Chemotherapy with combinations of vincristine, vinblastine, cisplatin, bleomycin, actinomycin, cyclophosphamide, VP-16, and doxorubicin have been effective in treating advanced-stage disease and tumors with malignant components. Many germ cell tumors are radiosensitive, but radiotherapy must be used cautiously. It is reserved for older patients in most cases due to the deleterious effects of radiotherapy on growth in young children. Prognosis varies widely depending on age, stage, and histologic type at diagnosis.

## TUMORS OF THE BREAST

Less than 0.1% of all breast cancer occurs in patients under 20 years old. Although malignant tumors have been seen in girls as young as 3 years of age, the overwhelming majority of breast tumors in children are benign. Fibroadenoma, the most common of these, may be bilateral and can become massive. Differentiation from virginal hypertrophy can be difficult. Infiltration of the breast can occur in acute leukemia, especially in the postpubertal child, and primary rhabdomyosarcoma of the breast has been reported.

The treatment of juvenile carcinoma of the breast is simple surgical excision. Metastases are unlikely, but since there are some reports of dissemination, it has been suggested that children should be managed the same as adults. Due to these factors, individualized therapy is perhaps the best approach for carcinoma of the breast in a child. The dividing line for the adult type of management may be at puberty, but there are no data to support this. Local recurrences have also been reported, but the final result is good.

## Selected Readings

Altman AJ, Schwartz AD eds. Tumors of germ cell origin: germinomas, embryonal carcinoma, extraembryonal tumors and teratomas. In: Malignant diseases of infancy, childhood and adolescence, ed 2. Philadelphia: WB Saunders, 1983.

Castleberry RP, Kelly DR, Joseph DB, Cain WS. Gonadal and extragonadal germ cell tumors. In: Fernbach DJ, Vietti TJ, eds. In: Clinical pediatric oncology, ed 4. St. Louis: CV Mosby, 1991.

Nichols CR, Fox EP. Extragonadal and pediatric germ cell tumors. Hematol Oncol Clin North Am 1991;5:1189.

*Principles and Practice of Pediatrics, Second Edition.*
edited by Frank A. Oski et al. J. B. Lippincott Company, Philadelphia © 1994.

# CHAPTER 105
# *Histiocytic Proliferative Diseases*

### Kenneth L. McClain

## LANGERHANS CELL HISTIOCYTOSIS

The terminology for histiocytic proliferative disorders is in the process of changing. Experts in the field have suggested that the original terminology for the various syndromes in the "histiocytosis-X" category (Letterer-Siwe disease, Hand-Schüller-Christian syndrome, and eosinophilic granuloma) should be replaced by the term *Langerhans cell histiocytosis* (LCH) because the proliferative cell that causes these entities is known. The cell is the dendritic histiocyte, also called the Langerhans cell, which contains characteristic pentalaminar Birbeck granules seen by electron microscopy (Fig 105-1). These cells also stain with monoclonal antibodies to the T6 antigen of lymphocytes and a neuroprotein stain, S-100. To establish the diagnosis of Lang-

erhans histiocytosis, positive electron microscope identification of Birbeck granules is necessary, and additional data are helpful.

The Langerhans cell diseases are not malignancies, but manifestations of complex immune dysregulation. The proliferation of these "normal" cells causes destruction or impairment of other organ systems. The Langerhans cell is a distinct member of the antigen-processing cells such as monocytes or histiocytes in the bone marrow. Like other antigen-processing cells, it produces a stimulating factor for T lymphocytes (a lymphokine, interleukin-1) that is necessary for the activation and response of T cells. They in turn make interleukin-2, which stimulates other T cells. Feedback stimulation on Langerhans cells (or other histiocytes) results from production of gamma-interferon and prostaglandin $E_2$ by the T cells. Somewhere in the interactive cycle, a regulatory element is lost such that the histiocytes proliferate locally or diffusely.

There is abundant evidence of immunologic abnormalities in LCH patients. Elevation of at least one type of immunoglobulin is found in 75% of patients, with most having high IgM. Although the mitogenic response is normal in most patients' lymphocytes, the number of suppressor T cells is often low. Circulating lymphocytes that were spontaneously cytotoxic to cultured human fibroblasts have been reported.

## Clinical Syndromes

Clinical syndromes of LCH should now be identified according to the degree or number of organ systems involved, such as Langerhans cell histiocytosis, solitary skull lesion, instead of eosinophilic granuloma.

### Solitary Lesions

This is the most benign form of LCH and frequently presents as one or more well-circumscribed lesions in the skull. The patient presents with pain or swelling in the region. Often the defects are easy to palpate. Any bone in the body can be involved, but the other most common sites are the femur, pelvis, vertebra, and mandible. Orbital lesions causing proptosis have been reported. Most children present between 1 and 9 years of age.

Treatments used include curettage or low-dose radiotherapy for resolution of pain, deformity, or danger of pathologic fractures. Some centers treat patients with prednisone or vinblastine sulfate instead of radiotherapy until there is some resolution of the ra-

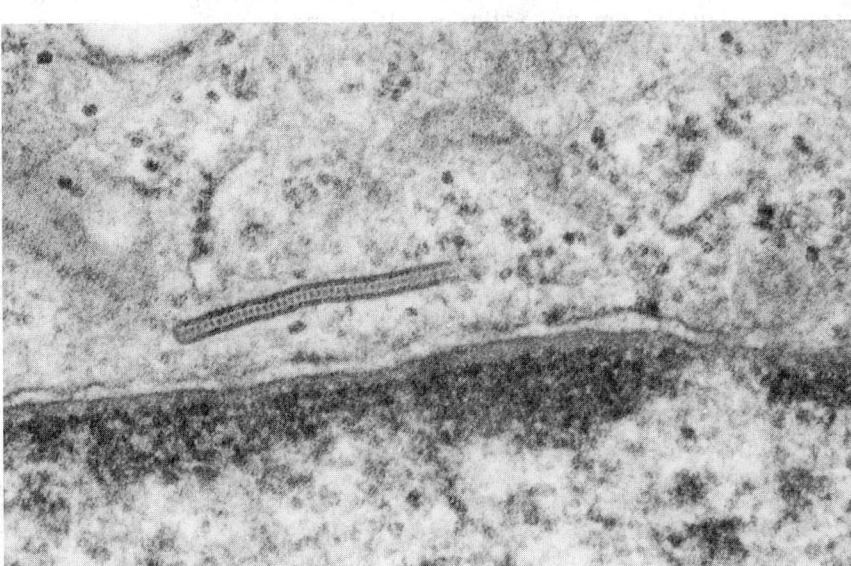

**Figure 105-1.** Electron micrograph of a Langerhans histiocytosis cell showing the striated, multilaminar granule (Birbeck granule) diagnostic of the Langerhans histiocytoses (magnification ×141,831). (Courtesy of Dr. H.K. Hawkins, Department of Pathology, Texas Children's Hospital, Houston.)

diographic findings. Most patients show sclerosis of the margins or more than 75% filling of the defect by 5 months after beginning therapy. Complete healing may take years.

### Multiple Lesions

Multiorgan involvement is more prevalent in children under 5 years of age. Prognosis depends on the age of presentation and whether any organ system function is impaired. A good-risk patient is one older than 2 years with no organ dysfunction; this implies a chance of survival of more than 80%. Those younger than 2 years at diagnosis are by age alone in an intermediate group and have only a 60% to 70% chance of survival. The poorest-risk group includes very young children with multisystem disease, but can include any age with organ dysfunction; this group has an overall survival of less than a 50%.

In these contexts organ dysfunction includes evidence of hepatic failure by total protein less than 5.5 g/dL, albumin less than 2.5 g/dL, total bilirubin over 1.5 mg/dL, edema, and ascites. Hematologic dysfunction includes hemoglobin less than 10 g/dL, leukocyte count less than 4000/mm$^3$, neutrophils less than 1500/mm$^3$, and platelets 100,000/mm$^3$. Pulmonary dysfunction includes tachypnea, dyspnea, cyanosis, cough, pneumothorax, and pleural effusion.

Many of these children will present with a seborrheic rash of the scalp and periauricular regions that mimics "cradle cap" or eczema. The chronic draining ears at first appear to be a chronic otitis externa. Hepatosplenomegaly, anemia, thrombocytopenia, and pulmonary disease make the diagnosis more obvious clinically, but the diagnostic cell type must be confirmed by the methods previously mentioned. Other clinical findings that accompany the various forms of LCH include diabetes insipidus, growth retardation, hyperprolactinemia, hypogonadism, panhypopituitarism, and hyperosmolar syndrome secondary to pituitary involvement. Infiltration of the thyroid and pancreas with resultant organ deficiencies has been reported. Occasionally skull x-rays show evidence of "floating" teeth when the mandible is involved. Gingivitis is also seen.

Of the children presenting with generalized LCH, involvement of various organ systems are found in bone (100%), skin (88%), liver (71%), lung (54%), lymph nodes (42%), spleen (25%), pituitary (25%), bone marrow (18%), and CNS (16%).

The evaluation should include a complete history and physical examination with complete blood count, bone marrow aspirate and biopsy when an abnormal blood count is found, radiographic survey of the complete skeleton and chest, bone scan, lumbar puncture when CNS symptoms are present, careful monitoring of intake and output, serum and urine osmolality, and biopsy of an affected site for confirmatory histologic diagnosis. The biopsy material should be sent for electron microscopy to look for Birbeck granules. The S-100 and T6 stains should be performed as additional confirmatory data.

### Treatment

Standard therapy for disseminated LCH has included prednisone 40 to 60 mg/m$^2$/day orally and vinblastine sulfate 6 mg/m$^2$ (0.1 mg/kg) intravenously weekly. The duration of therapy and need for escalation depend on the patient's response.

Other treatments under study include the use of VP-16 (etoposide), cyclosporine, and a thymic extract. Etoposide is considered a second line of therapy because of recent data linking its use with secondary malignancy in patients with T-cell leukemia. Although this concern may or may not be relevant to LCH patients, it would be prudent to use VP-16 only in patients who do not respond to other modalities. Because cyclosporine blocks the secretion of several lymphokines that affect histiocyte growth, it is often a very good treatment for patients with disseminated

disease. A thymic extract has been reported to result in long-term remissions in nearly as many patients as conventional chemotherapy. The use of alpha-interferon to modulate immune dysregulation in LCH patients has also been reported.

### Long-Term Outlook

LCH is a chronic disease with a waxing and waning nature that tries the patience of all involved. When the disease is active for more than 5 years, many patients will have diabetes insipidus, growth failure, intellectual impairment, neurologic deficit, emotional or orthopedic problems, chronic lung disease, or hearing deficits.

## NON-LANGERHANS HISTIOCYTOSES

This group of diseases results from the aggressive proliferation of normal macrophages and histiocytes in various tissues. These cells do not have the cellular atypia assigned to malignant histiocytes, but represent an uncontrolled growth that causes local problems. One of the major difficulties in understanding the etiology, natural history, and optimal therapy for these diseases is the fact that there is great overlap in the clinical characteristics of each.

### Infection-Associated Histiocytic Proliferations

#### Diagnosis

Evidence for viral infections may be difficult to obtain because some of the children present in the first month of life, are multiply transfused before titers are drawn, and may not respond to infections because of low numbers of T and B lymphocytes. Thus, besides the customary serologic and culture attempts to identify viruses, it is helpful to probe leukocyte DNA for the presence of viral genomes by DNA hybridization studies. Bacteria and other organisms also may cause these diseases.

#### Therapy

Therapy for these children has been frustratingly ineffective. Up to 75% of the patients die from their coagulopathy or secondary infections despite optimal management. One current mainstay of therapy is the chemotherapeutic agent VP-16, which is active against histiocytic proliferative diseases in general. There have been reports of cures using this agent alone. The addition of prednisone, antiviral agents (such as acyclovir), other chemotherapeutic agents, and exchange transfusions has provided little if any additional benefit. Individual patients have benefited from treatment with cyclosporine.

A new approach takes advantage of one possible overreaction of the immune system, in which prostaglandin E$_2$ has been found at high levels. The new therapy may work by shutting off the synthesis of prostaglandins with indomethacin and decreasing lipolysis (which is a factor with liver involvement) by infusing generous amounts of intravenous glucose. Brown and colleagues have reported some excellent therapeutic results when coupling these modalities with VP-16 treatment.

### "Familial" Syndromes

The hereditary forms of nonmalignant histiocytic proliferative syndromes include familial hemophagocytic lymphohistiocytosis, familial erythrophagocytic lymphohistiocytosis, and familial erythrophagocytic reticulosis. These are historical labels attached to clinical syndromes that are hardly distinguishable from the virus-associated hemophagocytic syndrome (VAHS). The familial syndromes are distinct because of the high rate of parental consanguinity, occurrence in identical twins, segregation analysis, presence of CNS disease, and hypertriglyceridemia. However, the same laboratory findings are found in a majority of the VAHS patients. It is my opinion that there is little if any difference between the familial and nonfamilial forms of these diseases, and that much more attention should be paid to finding an underlying etiology and common immune defect. Unfortunately, few of these patients have survived in the past, but bone marrow transplantation has cured over 20 children. Some have temporary remissions with the same therapies as mentioned above for VAHS.

## Sinus Histiocytosis with Massive Lymphadenopathy

These patients present with a marked enlargement of cervical lymph nodes with fever, elevated erythrocyte sedimentation rate, neutrophilia, and eosinophilia. Other sites affected include the orbit, nose, pharynx, and skin. A majority of the fatal cases have underlying immune deficiency such as Wiskott-Aldrich syndrome or autoimmune phenomena. About 7% of all these patients die of secondary infections, bleeding, or malignancy.

## OTHER SYNDROMES

Other rare syndromes of malignant monocytic or histiocytic disorders include monocytic leukemia, chronic myelomonocytic leukemia and "histiocytic lymphoma," and malignant histiocytosis (histiocytic medullary reticulosis).

## Selected Readings

Brown RE, Bowman WP, D'Cruz CA, et al. Endoperoxidation, hyperprostaglandinemia and hyperlipidemia in a case of erythrophagocytic lymphohistiocytosis: reversal with VP-16 and indomethacin. Cancer 1987;60:2388.
McClain K, Gehrz R, Grierson H, et al. Virus-associated histiocytic proliferations in children: frequent association with Epstein-Barr virus and congenital or acquired immunodeficiencies. Am J Pediatr Hematol Oncol 1988;10:196.
Sullivan JL, Woda BA. Lymphohistiocytic disorders. In: Nathan DG, Oski FA, eds. Hematology of infancy and childhood, ed 4. Philadelphia: WB Saunders, 1993: 1354.

*Principles and Practice of Pediatrics, Second Edition.*
edited by Frank A. Oski et al. J. B. Lippincott Company, Philadelphia © 1994.

## CHAPTER 106
# *Hemangioma*

### William J. Pokorny

The term *hemangioma* has been used to describe a continuum that includes obvious malformations, hamartomas, and neoplasms. These vascular tumors are the most common tumors of humans and occur in all parts of the body. The most common cutaneous tumor seen in a pediatric practice is the congenital vascular hamartoma.

Edgerton classifies congenital vascular hamartomas based on the primary involvement of the afferent versus efferent side of the fetal vascular tie. Growth potential, including spontaneous involution and treatment for these vascular hamartomas, can be based on this classification (Table 106-1).

## AFFERENT HEMANGIOMAS

Hemangiomas of infancy affect primarily the afferent capillary bed. Typically not present at birth, they appear several weeks after birth. They are usually bright red and raised. These lesions may show dramatic growth for several months, then the growth slows to parallel the growth of the child. Growth may continue for 2 or 3 years, after which spontaneous involution begins. Involution may continue for several years but usually is complete by age 5 or 6. Complete or partial involution occurs in 85% of the common elevated hemangiomas and appears to be due to progressive thrombosis and sclerosis of vessels. The regression usually begins as a central gray spot, which gradually coalesces to reduce the hemangioma (Fig 106-1).

Hemangiomas of infancy also are classified by their microscopic pattern as capillary, cavernous, and hemangioendothelioma. Capillary hemangiomas are more commonly seen on the skin as "strawberry" birthmarks. They are circumscribed but not encapsulated masses composed of small channels lined by endothelium with scanty intervening stroma. Cavernous hemangiomas are lesions composed of large dilated vessels. When subjected to trauma they may bleed profusely. When completely beneath the level of the skin and consisting predominantly of large vascular channels, there is less tendency for spontaneous regression. Nevertheless, when they involve the face, they should be observed for several years. In other areas of the body they may be removed electively. Hemangioendotheliomas are solid lesions that are microscopically more cellular than capillary or cavernous hemangiomas. They may present as a hard subcutaneous mass. Secondary changes of hemorrhage, thrombosis, ischemic necrosis, and fibrosis are common in all three patterns and account for the frequency of spontaneous involution.

Complications of hemangioma of infancy include superficial ulceration with local infection and bleeding (Fig 106-2). Infection can usually be treated locally with topical antibiotics and a pro-

**TABLE 106-1. Classification of Congenital Vascular Hamartomas**

I. Growing (afferent) with potential for involution
  Hemangiomas of infancy
II. Stationary or slowly enlarging (efferent)
  A. Venous
    1. Port-wine stain
    2. Verruca linearis
    3. Cirsoid (racemose)
  B. Lymphatic
    1. Lymphangioma
    2. Hygroma
  C. Mixed
    1. With regional giantism
    2. Without regional giantism
III. Progressively growing (afferent–efferent)
  A. Congenital arteriovenous fistula
  B. Arterial hemangioma
  C. Angiosarcoma

*After Edgerton MT, Morgan RF. Hemangiomas: congenital hamartomas. In: Welch KJ, Randolph JG, Ravitch MM, et al, eds. Pediatric surgery, Chicago: Year Book Medical Publishers, 1986:1511.*

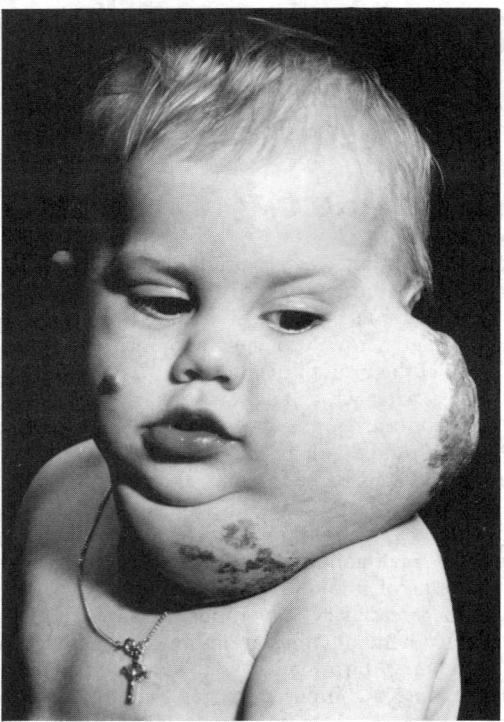

**Figure 106-1.** This 20-month-old girl was first noted to have a 1-cm raised hemangioma at 1 month of age. The mass continued to expand until her third birthday, then the growth leveled off to that of the child for 2 years. At age 5, the mass underwent rapid involution to 10% of its maximum size over a 6-month period.

tective dressing. If cellulitis of the surrounding tissue occurs, systemic antibiotics should be used. Bleeding can usually be controlled with pressure. If the lesion is small or pedunculated, it may be excised. Lesions on the perineum may require excision because of recurrent trauma, bleeding, and infection. Hemangiomas about the eye may interfere with vision and cause amblyopia. When this occurs they should be actively treated and if necessary excised.

Platelet trapping (Kasabach-Merritt syndrome) is occasionally seen and typically occurs during the phase of active growth of the hemangioma. Platelet trapping usually occurs in large cavernous hemangiomas and is attributed to the sequestration of platelets in lacunae and the formation of thrombi in the tumor. Disseminated intravascular coagulation syndrome also may occur. Treatment consists of correction of the coagulation defect followed by surgical excision. Excision returns platelets and other coagulation factors to normal.

Treatment of the majority of uncomplicated hemangiomas consists of observation to allow spontaneous involution to occur. Nevertheless, early consultation should be obtained from a surgeon familiar with the natural history of the various types of hemangiomas. This will allow early excision of those lesions likely to become disfiguring and those unlikely to involute. Although regression may be hastened by injecting sclerosing solutions, freezing, or administering small doses of x-rays, these treatment modalities leave unnecessary scars and should not be used. Pressure therapy with a custom-made elastic dressing has been found to decrease platelet trapping, but it is difficult to keep a growing child correctly fitted for an elastic dressing. Systemic steroids have been used with reported improvement in 30% to 90% of the children with capillary or cavernous hemangiomas. Argon laser therapy has been used to treat superficial port-wine hemangiomas and superficial hemangiomas that have not involuted completely.

## EFFERENT HEMANGIOMAS

Vascular hamartomas that tend to progressively enlarge or remain the same and not to regress include port-wine stains, cirsoid venous angiomas, and lymphangiomas. These lesions commonly are distributed along cutaneous sensory nerves. The port-wine stain (nevus flammeus) usually is located in the distribution of the fifth cranial nerve. Port-wine stain is also associated with Sturge-Weber syndrome and glaucoma. Lesions made up of both venous and lymphatic elements may be associated with regional giantism, Maffucci syndrome, plexiform neurofibroma, and neurofibromatosis.

## AFFERENT–EFFERENT HEMANGIOMAS

Congenital arteriovenous fistulas are hemangiomas in which there are communications between arteries and veins proximal to the normal capillary bed. They may occur anywhere in the body but most often involve the extremities, brain, and liver. Usually, multiple shunts lead into the hemangioma. If the dominant arterial inflow vessel is ligated, others will open and dilate, making surgical intervention difficult and impractical.

During early infancy superficial hemangiomas appear in the extremities. These then grow into extensive hemangiomas. As the blood flow to the extremity increases, bone and soft-tissue growth accelerates and growth discrepancy of the extremities is seen. The lesion is warm to palpation and a bruit can often be felt. Heart failure may develop at any time, even in the newborn. The shunt results in high output failure with an increased cardiac output, increased blood volume, increased heart rate, and left heart failure. If pressure is applied to the lesion, occluding the shunt, the pulse rate will slow (Nicoladoni-Branham sign).

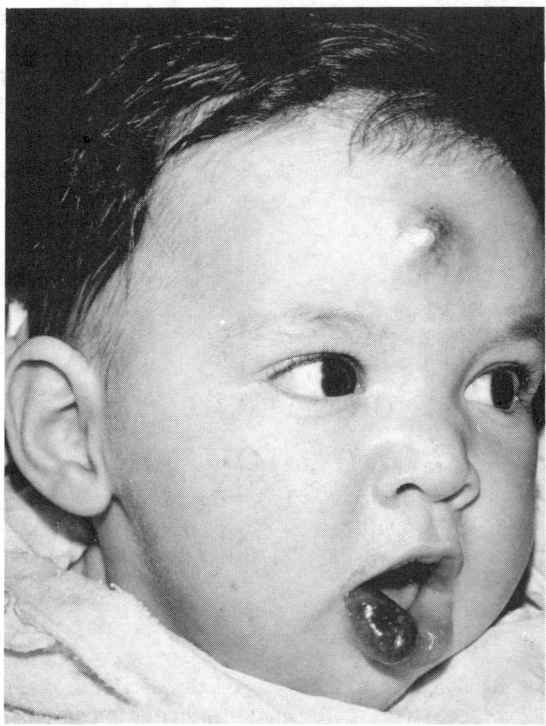

**Figure 106-2.** This infant has hemangiomas of the forehead and lip. The lesion on the forehead was observed and underwent involution. The lesion on the lip required excision because of recurrent trauma and bleeding.

Complications include rupture with severe hemorrhage, cutaneous necrosis, and ischemic pain due to shunting of blood from the skin of the distal extremity, and growth retardation from chronic high output cardiac failure. When the fistula is in the head or neck, the patient may experience persistent tinnitus.

Treatment goals are limb salvage, prevention of hemorrhage, prevention of excessive growth, and cosmetic improvement. If possible, compression should be applied with an elastic custom-made stocking. Ligation may only temporarily control cardiac failure. Embolization has proven helpful in the management of CNS and systemic arteriovenous malformations. Embolization immediately before the resection of large tumors has proven effective in decreasing blood loss.

## HEPATIC HEMANGIOMAS

Hepatic hemangiomas usually are detected during infancy as a mass, as hepatomegaly, or with high output cardiac failure. The latter may be referred to the cardiology service with the diagnosis of congenital heart disease. Treatment depends on the presence or absence of symptoms, resectability of the tumor, and realization that spontaneous resolution does occur. In the unusual situation that an infant in congestive heart failure has a well-localized lesion as defined by CT scanning and ultrasonography, resection should be done. More commonly the lesion is extensive, in which case the patient's congestive failure should be managed medically until involution occurs. If heart failure or thrombocytopenia is not controlled by medical measures, embolization or ligation of the hepatic artery should be undertaken. Steroids and irradiation have been used with varied results. Steroids usually are included in the medical management of symptomatic lesions.

### Selected Readings

Cohen RC, Myers NA. Diagnosis and management of massive hepatic hemangiomas in childhood. J Pediatr Surg 1986;21:6.

Edgerton MT. Vascular hamartomas and hemangiomas: classification and treatment. South Med J 1982;75:1541.

Edgerton MT, Morgan RF. Hemangiomas: congenital hamartomas. In: Welch KJ, Randolph JG, Ravitch MM, et al., eds. Pediatric surgery. Chicago: Year Book Medical Publishers, 1986:1511.

Lofland GK, Filston HC. Giant cutaneous hemangioma associated with axillary arteriovenous fistula causing congestive heart failure in the newborn infant. J Pediatr Surg 1987;22:458.

Pereyra R, Andrassy RJ, Mahour GH. Management of massive hepatic hemangiomas in infants and children: a review of 13 cases. Pediatr 1982;70:254.

*Principles and Practice of Pediatrics, Second Edition.*
edited by Frank A. Oski et al. J. B. Lippincott Company, Philadelphia © 1994.

## CHAPTER 107
# *Congenital Malformations of the Lymphatic System*

### William J. Pokorny

Lymphangioma, cystic hygroma, and congenital lymphedema result from obstruction of the developing lymphatic vessels. Embryologic studies show that the lymphatic system arises from five primitive lymphatic sacs: the paired sacs in the neck, a single sac at the root of the mesentery, and paired posterior sacs near the sciatic veins. The peripheral lymphatic system forms as an outbudding from these five sacs. Lymphangiomas have been classified into three macroscopic forms: lymphangioma simplex, or capillary lymphangioma; cavernous lymphangioma, which consists of dilated lymphatic channels; and cystic lymphangiomas or cystic hygromas. Lesions frequently are mixed.

Cystic hygromas typically occur in or about the neck as the result of sequestration or obstruction of one of the sacs in the neck. Mesenteric or omental cysts result from obstruction of the lymphatics developing from the sac at the root of the mesentery. Congenital lymphedema and intestinal lymphangiectasia may represent variations of these malformations caused by congenital lymphatic obstruction.

Most *lymphangiomas* are present at birth, and nearly all are apparent during the first and second year of life. Although growth of the lesions is unpredictable, rapid growth may occur inter-mittently. Spontaneous regression occurs but is uncommon. The vast majority (95%) occur in the neck or axilla, and 2% to 3% extend into the chest. The rest are found on the extremities or trunk.

*Cystic hygromas* are thin-walled, multiloculated cysts that may or may not communicate and contain clear lymph fluid. The cysts invade the tissue planes and appear to infiltrate normal tissue,

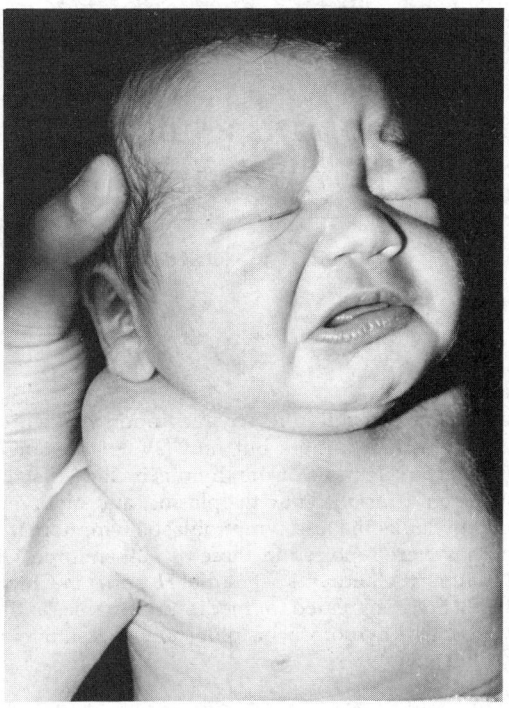

**Figure 107-1.**    This 2-week-old infant presented with a soft, cystic hygroma of the neck at birth. The mass was asymptomatic and transilluminated. Complete excision was done without recurrence.

but they are benign. They vary in size from a few millimeters to huge lesions distorting the face and neck (Fig 107-1). Most cystic hygromas are asymptomatic and present as soft fluid-filled masses in the subcutaneous tissue of the posterior triangle of the neck and axilla. However, depending on their location within the developing fetus and infant, they may be symptomatic and life-threatening. Involvement of the tongue, pharynx, or larynx may result in airway obstruction. Pressure on the periodontal tissue may result in loss of teeth and deformity of the mandible. Mediastinal cystic hygromas also may result in respiratory distress, chylothorax, and chylopericardium. Dysphagia may rarely occur as the result of compression of the superior thoracic outlet. Infection of the cystic hygroma commonly occurs following upper respiratory tract infections. Incision and drainage may result in a long course of lymphatic fluid drainage from the site of the incision. Infection may at times precede spontaneous involution of the lesion.

Treatment is surgical excision when the diagnosis is made. Delay is unwarranted because of the hazards of infection, progressive growth with extension into previously uninvolved areas, and dysphagia or airway obstruction. However, these are not malignant lesions, and although total excision is ideal, one should not damage or sacrifice normal structures or disfigure the child. If all macroscopic tumor is removed, recurrence is rare. On the other hand, if small amounts of cystic tumor are left, the recurrence rate is 10% to 15%. Sclerosing agents such as a solution of iodine, tetracycline, or concentrated glucose have been used to destroy the lining of remaining cysts at the time of operation.

*Omental and mesenteric cysts* result from lymphatic obstruction and are filled with a clear serous or milky fluid. They may be huge, presenting as a distended nontender abdomen, and may be confused with ascites. Ultrasound is diagnostic and treatment is surgical excision.

*Intestinal lymphangiectasia* is also the result of congenital lymphatic obstruction but at the peripheral lymphatics. The bowel wall, including the lamina propria, submucosa, and serosa, is involved by dilated lymphatics. There is malabsorption and loss of protein into the gut; if untreated, malnutrition, growth retardation, anemia, hypoproteinemia, and lymphocytopenia will develop. The diagnosis is suggested by the roentgen findings of thickening of the jejunal folds, flocculation of barium within the lumen of the gut, and dilatation of the small bowel. The diagnosis may be confirmed by duodenal or jejunal biopsy. Treatment consists of high-protein, medium-chain triglyceride diet. Surgical intervention may be of help in confirming the diagnosis and resection of a localized collection of cysts.

*Lymphedema* occurs in three forms: congenital; praecox, which appears in adolescence; and tarda, which occurs in middle age. Congenital lymphedema is usually present at birth and most often involves the lower extremity, but occasionally other areas of the body are affected. The dorsum of the foot is involved most commonly. The extent of swelling due to the lymphedema, compared with body growth, gradually lessens during the first 2 years of life. Therapy during this time should be directed at protecting the extremity from injury and infection. Operative intervention should be reserved for patients with severe congenital lymphedema that persists beyond 3 years of life.

## Selected Readings

Fonkalsrud E. Disorders of the lymphatic system. In: Welch KJ, Randolph JG, Ravitch MM, et al., eds. Pediatric surgery. Chicago: Year Book Medical Publishers, 1986: 1506.

Mollitt DL, Ballantine TVN, Grosfeld J. Mesenteric cysts in infancy and childhood. Surg Gynecol Obstet 1978;147:102.

Phillips HE, McGahan JP: Intrauterine fetal cystic hygromas: sonographic detection. AJR 1981;136:799.

---

*Principles and Practice of Pediatrics, Second Edition.*
edited by Frank A. Oski et al. J. B. Lippincott Company, Philadelphia © 1994.

# CHAPTER 108
# *Thymomas*

## William J. Pokorny

Thymomas are rare in children. Thymic tumors make up 18% of the adult mediastinal tumors but only 3% of the mediastinal tumors in children. Tumors of the thymus include cysts, hamartomas, specific intrinsic thymic neoplasms, and involvement of the thymus by leukemia and lymphoblastic lymphoma.

Thymomas were reported in three of 109 children with mediastinal tumors at Children's Memorial Hospital in Chicago and in two of 188 children treated for mediastinal masses at the Mayo Clinic. Malignant thymomas histologically are similar to lymphoblastic lymphoma and unfortunately have the same clinical course and prognosis. The differentiation depends on the anatomical relationship of the tumor to the thymus. Surgical therapy consists of total excision (although rarely possible), biopsies, and debulking procedures for massive tumors. Surgery may be necessary for the relief of tracheal compression, but relief usually can be achieved with chemotherapy and radiotherapy. Primary therapy is with intensive chemotherapy.

Although 8% to 15% of the adult patients with myasthenia gravis are found to have a thymoma, only one patient under age 19 with myasthenia gravis has been described with a thymoma.

Thymic cysts are usually asymptomatic. They are usually unilocular and may be found in the neck or anterior mediastinum along the embryonic route of descent of the thymus from its pharyngeal origin. They can usually be resected without difficulty.

## Selected Readings

King RM, Telander RL, Smithson WA, et al. Primary mediastinal tumors in children. J Pediatr Surg 1982;5:512.

Pokorny WJ, Sherman JO. Mediastinal masses in infants and children. J Thorac Cardiovasc Surg 1974:5:869.

Pokorny WJ, Sherman JO. Mediastinal tumors. In: Holder TM, Ashcraft KW, eds. Pediatric surgery. Philadelphia: WB Saunders, 1980:241.

*Principles and Practice of Pediatrics, Second Edition.*
edited by Frank A. Oski et al. J. B. Lippincott Company, Philadelphia © 1994.

# CHAPTER 109
# *Splenic Cysts*

## William J. Pokorny

Although splenic cyst is an uncommon condition, it is an important consideration in the differential diagnosis of a left upper quadrant abdominal mass. Splenic cysts increase in frequency in older children, but most nonparasitic cysts occur in patients under age 20. Worldwide nearly two thirds of splenic cysts are echinococcal, but in the United States most splenic cysts are nonparasitic. Most are secondary or pseudocysts without a true lining and usually result from trauma. Primary cysts consist of dermoids, lymphangiomas, cavernous hemangiomas, congenital cysts, and epidermoid cysts. A cyst of malignant or infectious origin is very rare.

Most patients with splenic cysts are in excellent health and are asymptomatic. Many present with a progressively enlarging mass or asymmetric abdominal distention. Nearly 30% report intermittent left upper quadrant pain or fullness. Acute and severe symptoms may result from complications of the cyst, including infection, hemorrhage, and rupture.

Radiographic findings typically demonstrate displacement of the stomach to the right, inferior displacement of the splenic flexure of the colon, inferior displacement of the left kidney, and elevation of the left hemidiaphragm.

Calcification is seen in about 10% of the cases; when present, it suggests primary echinococcal or secondary post-traumatic cysts. Ultrasound effectively demonstrates the intrasplenic location of the cyst and its relationship to other viscera. Splenic cysts are usually relatively free of internal echoes, whereas abscesses and hematomas typically contain internal echoes.

Treatment is surgical. Recent attention has been given to splenic salvage by removing only that portion of the spleen involved with the cyst. Splenic salvage depends on the size, anatomical location within the spleen, and etiology of the cyst. An angiogram may be helpful in planning the operative approach if splenic salvage is to be attempted.

## Selected Readings

Kaufman RA, Silver TM, Wesley JR. Preoperative diagnosis of splenic cysts in children by Gray scale ultrasonography. J Pediatr Surg 1979;4:450.
Touloukian RJ, Seashore JH. Partial splenic decapsulation: a simplified operation for splenic pseudocyst. J Pediatr Surg 1987;2:135.

# SECTION VII

# The Genitourinary System

*Principles and Practice of Pediatrics, Second Edition.*
edited by Frank A. Oski et al. J. B. Lippincott Company, Philadelphia © 1994.

## CHAPTER 110
# *Morphologic Development of the Kidney*

### Edith P. Hawkins

The mature human kidney and ureters are the third set of renal organs derived from the urogenital ridge. The first paired organs, the pronephroi, appear early in the fourth week of gestation. They consist of nests of cells that form primitive tubules. These attach to a ductal system emptying into the cloaca. The pronephroi begin to degenerate as soon as they are formed and are replaced late in the fourth week of gestation by mesonephroi. The mesonephroi develop primitive glomeruli and tubules that connect to the excretory ducts of the pronephroi. These ducts, renamed mesonephric ducts, drain into the cloaca. The mesonephroi are known to function in some lower animals and probably do so in humans as well. They slowly degenerate as the third set of paired organs, the metanephroi, develop.

The development of the metanephroi, the mature kidneys, begins during the fifth week of gestation when a lateral diverticulum appears at the caudal end of each mesonephric duct. These diverticuli, called ureteric buds, grow cephalad. The caudal portions form the ureters, which elongate by cell division, while cephalad portions undergo repeated dichotomous division. The first three to five generations form the major calyces by a similar process of dilatation and coalescence. Generations 10 to 20 form the minor calyces, which due to space limitations are folded inward around their papillae. About 10 to 20 collecting ducts drain into each calyx through pores in the papillary tips.

The generational divisions after the formation of the minor calyces are devoted to induction of nephrogenesis. The leading end of the ureteric bud, now called the ampulla, comes in contact with the metanephric blastema and induces it to form nephrons. The metanephric blastema is composed of nests of primitive cells derived from the mesenchyme of the urogenital ridge. These nests

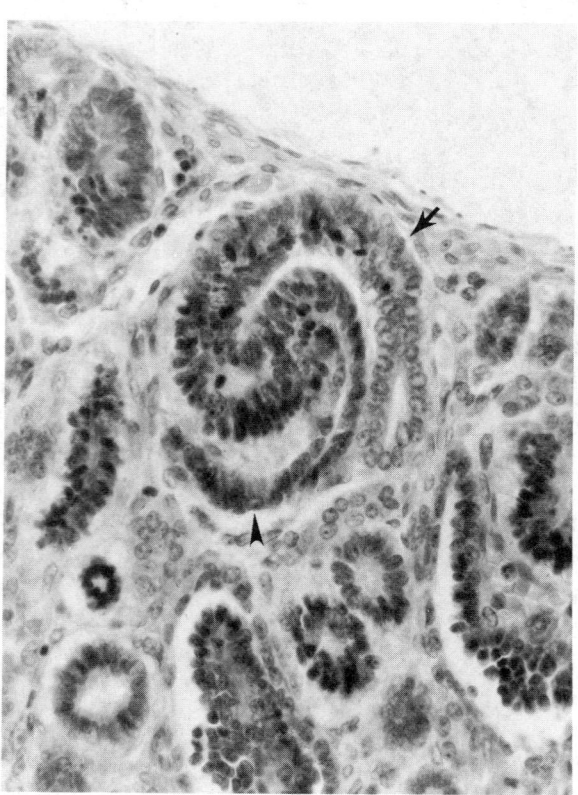

**Figure 110-1.** A small segment of the subcapsular nephrogenic zone. The proximal portion of the S-shaped structure in the center has made connection (*arrow*) with the ureteric bud. The epithelial portions of the glomerulus will form from the distal end (*arrowhead*) (hematoxylin and eosin, magnification ×400).

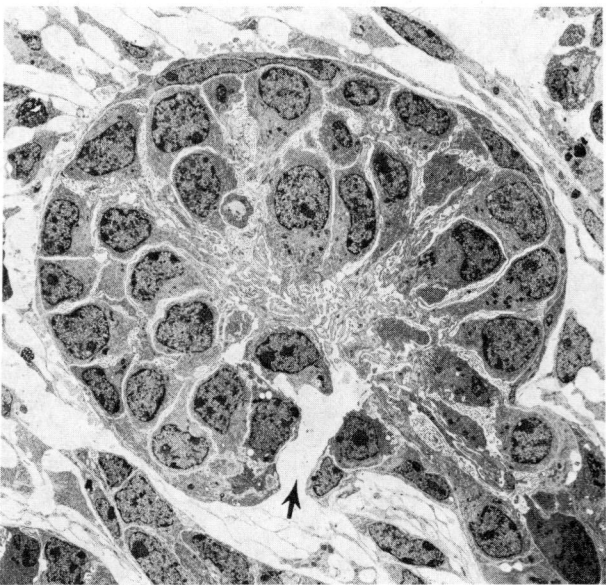

**Figure 110-2.** The epithelial components of a glomerulus are present in this electron photomicrograph of a metanephric culture of mouse blastema. There is a space at the hilum (*arrow*) that appears to be available for vascular penetration. No blood vessels or mesangial cells are seen (magnification ×3000). (Bernstein J, Cheng F, Roszka J. Glomerular differentiation in metanephric culture. Lab Invest 1981;45:183.)

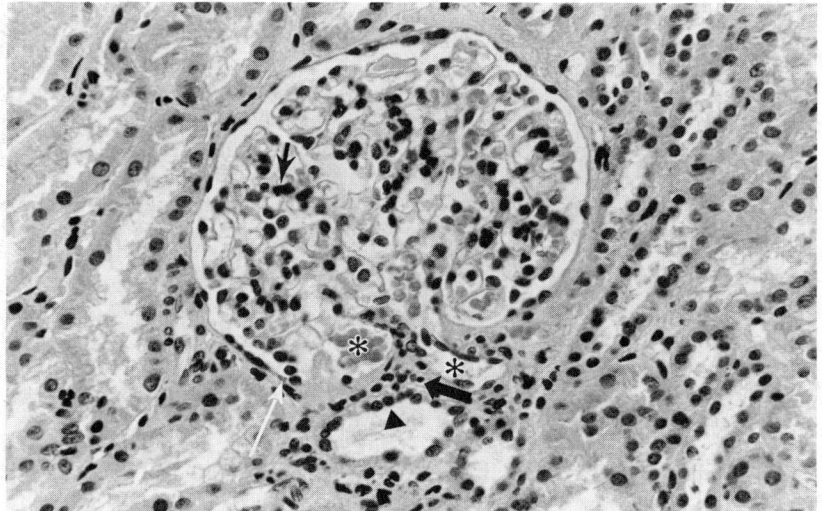

**Figure 110-3.** The glomerulus in this section has wide open capillary loops covered by visceral epithelial cells that are in continuity with the parietal epithelial cells lining Bowman's capsule (*white arrow*). The loops are separated by mesangial cells and mesangial matrix (*small arrow*). Both afferent and efferent arterioles (*asterisks*) are seen at the hilum. The modified epithelial cells (macula densa) of the thick ascending limb of Henle (*arrowhead*) are seen adjacent to the afferent arteriole. The renin-producing cells (the third component of the juxtaglomerular apparatus) are present in the interstitium (*large arrow*) (hematoxylin and eosin, magnification ×315).

in the developing kidney form a continuous subcapsular zone known as the nephrogenic zone.

On induction, the blastemal cells form into a ball, which rapidly elongates and folds to form an S-shaped structure (Fig 110-1). The proximal end of the S-shaped tube attaches to the ampulla of the ureteric bud to connect the collecting tubule (derived from the ampulla) to the distal convoluted tubule (derived from the S-shaped metanephric blastema). The mid-portions of the S-shaped structure elongate and convolute to form the proximal and distal convoluted tubules and the loop of Henle. The distal portion of the S-shaped structure becomes concave to form Bowman's capsule and the epithelial portions of the glomerular tuft. Blood vessels grow between the epithelial cells, and circulating monocytes move into the mesangial region to complete glomerular development. Culture of mouse metanephric cells has shown that the epithelial architecture of the glomerular tufts develops in the absence of vascular stimuli (Fig 110-2). No mesangial cells are found in these cultures, supporting the concept that mesangial cells are derived from circulating hematopoietic elements.

The metanephric kidney becomes functional between 11 and 13 weeks of gestation and begins to contribute significant amounts to the amniotic fluid after the 16th to 18th weeks. Nephrogenesis is completed and the nephrogenic zone disappears between the 35th and 36th weeks of gestation.

The mature kidneys are paired, bean-shaped structures composed of an outer cortex and inner medulla. The cortex contains about 150 million functioning nephrons, except for the portions of the loops of Henle that dip into the medulla. It also contains the outer segments of the collecting ducts. The medulla consists of eight to 18 cone-shaped structures called renal pyramids. The pyramids contain segments of the loops of Henle and the inner portions of the collecting ducts. These ducts drain into the minor calyces through several pores at the tips of the pyramids. The minor calyces empty into the major calyces, which then empty into the renal pelvis.

Microscopically, the mature glomerulus consists of a capillary network derived from the afferent arteriole (Fig 110-3). The capillaries are covered by epithelium and separated by mesangial cells embedded in a basement membrane-like matrix. They rejoin to form the efferent arteriole, which supplies the rest of the nephron and associated collecting duct. The visceral epithelium is continuous with the parietal epithelium lining Bowman's capsule. This epithelium is in turn continuous with the epithelium of the proximal convoluted tubule.

The juxtaglomerular apparatus is a specialized region at the glomerular hilum composed of arteriolar smooth muscle cells, modified tubular epithelial cells of the most distal segment of the thick limb of the loop of Henle (the macula densa), and cells in the interstitium. These latter cells produce renin. This interstitial region, in which lacis cells (macrophages) can also be identified, appears to be an extraglomerular continuum of the intraglomerular mesangium.

## Selected Readings

Barajas L, Salido E. Juxtaglomerular apparatus and the reninangiotensin system. Lab Invest 1986;54:361.

Bernstein J, Cheng F, Roszka J. Glomerular differentiation in metanephric culture. Lab Invest 1981;45:183.

Moore KL. The urogenital system. In: The developing human, ed 3. Philadelphia: WB Saunders, 1982:255.

Risdon RA. Development, developmental defects, and cystic diseases of the kidney. In: Heptinstall RH, ed. Pathology of the kidney, ed 4. Boston: Little, Brown, 1992:93.

*Principles and Practice of Pediatrics, Second Edition.*
edited by Frank A. Oski et al. J. B. Lippincott Company, Philadelphia © 1994.

# 110.1 *Disorders of Renal Development and Anomalies of the Collecting System, Bladder, Penis, and Scrotum*

David R. Roth and Edmond T. Gonzales, Jr.

## DISORDERS OF RENAL DEVELOPMENT

### Anomalies of Position

#### Simple Ectopia

Simple renal ectopia is a condition in which a kidney is located in an abnormal position but remains on its own side of the midline. Often there is associated incomplete rotation of the renal unit. The most common position is in the true pelvis; less common locations are the thorax or iliac fossa. Ectopia occurs in one in 500 to 1200 live births and is more common on the left.

An ectopic kidney is associated with other anomalies in many patients. The most common are other urologic abnormalities and musculoskeletal, cardiovascular, GI, and otolaryngologic anomalies. Treatment, if any, should address pathologic factors (primarily ureteral obstruction) rather than the position of the renal unit.

## Simple Malrotation

During embryogenesis, the kidneys rotate from a position in which the ureters face anterior to their usual postnatal position with the ureter facing medially. Disorders of renal ascent are often associated with persistence of the original orientation. A better term would be *incomplete* rotation rather than malrotation. Unless there are problems such as ureteropelvic obstruction associated with this abnormality of rotation, no treatment is needed.

## Fusion Anomalies

In patients with fusion anomalies, the two renal units are connected either by a large mass of parenchyma (cake kidney) in the midline of the bony pelvis, by a thin isthmus below the inferior mesenteric artery connecting the lower poles (horseshoe kidney), or by crossed fused ectopia in which one renal unit crosses the midline and fuses to the normally positioned contralateral kidney. With crossed fused ectopia, the ureters arise from the appropriate sides of the bladder, but one crosses the midline to enter the lower portions of the fused renal units. The anomaly is slightly more common in boys than girls, and the kidneys reside on the right twice as often as on the left. No treatment is needed, although an increased incidence of ureteral obstruction is associated with this entity.

Horseshoe kidneys are the most common fusion anomalies, accounting for about 90% of these abnormalities. They often are discovered incidentally during evaluation of associated anomalies or urinary infection or at autopsy. The kidneys are positioned lower than normal, with their lower poles joined by an isthmus of tissue. They are incompletely rotated and their axes are more vertical than normal, a consistent and characteristic sign on intravenous urography. The isthmus usually crosses the midline anterior to the great vessels below the inferior mesenteric artery, which blocked further ascent of the kidneys during fetal development. The ureters may be somewhat dilated above the location where they cross in front of the isthmus; however, the need for surgical repair is unusual. Associated anomalies are common but usually are less serious than those related to crossed renal ectopia. Urologic evaluation should include a voiding cystourethrogram because reflux is a common finding. Treatment decisions are based on the same criteria as for a normal kidney (Fig 110-4).

## Anomalies of Renal Parenchyma

### Agenesis

Unilateral renal agenesis is present in one in 450 to 1800 live births. Its etiology is related to maldevelopment of the metanephric duct (primitive ureter) and renal blastema. Often the ipsilateral ureter and vas deferens are absent because their embryologic origins are intertwined. Compensatory hypertrophy of the solitary kidney is common but not pathognomonic for this lesion. Diagnosis often is made during investigation of other anomalies (cardiovascular, GI, musculoskeletal). No treatment is needed, but the child and parents should be cautioned that only a single kidney is present so that they may avoid activities that might put the kidney at undue risk of injury (eg, organized football, riding motorcycles).

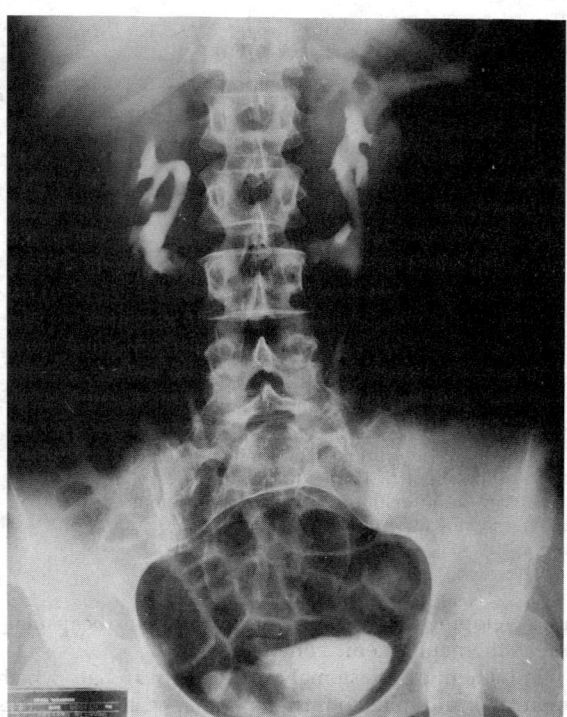

**Figure 110-4.** IVP of a horseshoe kidney. Note the axis deviation and incomplete rotation of the kidneys.

Bilateral renal agenesis is a rare entity that is incompatible with life. There is a high incidence of associated anomalies and, often, developmental abnormalities of the bladder, urethra, and ureters. Pulmonary hypoplasia is common and often the immediate cause of demise. The infants have typical features, described by Potter, that include increased distance between the eyes, flattening or broadening of the nose, a prominent inner canthal fold, spade-like hands, and amnion nodosum. These findings characteristic of Potter's syndrome are the result of severe oligohydramnios, which is caused by the absence of intrauterine urine production. This syndrome is not specific for bilateral renal agenesis, since any condition in which there is markedly decreased amniotic fluid would produce similar findings.

### Renal Hypoplasia

Renal hypoplasia is an unusual condition in which the number of renal lobules is reduced, thereby producing a kidney that is small but with normal nephron differentiation. The number of calyces is decreased, and the renal weight is diminished. If the condition is bilateral, the total nephron mass is deficient, and the result is progressive renal insufficiency with its typical complications of growth arrest and developmental delay. Renal dialysis or transplantation may become necessary at any time from shortly after birth until early adulthood. Unilateral hypoplasia, on the other hand, will not cause any problems or require intervention.

Other, more common causes of small kidneys must be considered before hypoplasia is diagnosed. These include atrophy secondary to reflux nephropathy, atrophic pyelonephritis, vascular ischemia, renal vein thrombosis, and dysplasia.

### Renal Dysplasia

Renal dysplasia is abnormal metanephric differentiation and is a histologic rather than a clinical diagnosis. Dysplastic kidneys may involve both cystic and hypoplastic changes, although both elements are not always present. Histologically, primitive glomerular and tubular elements, cartilage, smooth muscle, and cysts are seen in the parenchyma. The dysplasia may be segmental or involve the entire renal unit. Affected parts of the kidney generally do not function. The kidney may be reniform in shape, or the dysplasia may be so severe that the unit has little resemblance to a normal kidney. Urinary tract obstruction often but not always is associated with dysplasia and may contribute to its formation.

The most common and well-known dysplastic disorder is the multicystic kidney, which consists of numerous fluid-filled cysts that do not communicate. This is one of the two most common renal masses in the newborn and its diagnosis is usually suggested by ultrasound, either prenatally or afterward for evaluation of an abdominal mass. The presence of a multicystic kidney is generally confirmed by the absence of any function on a renal scan. Ureteral atresia is common. Very rarely, long-term complications occur, including urinary tract infection (UTI), rupture of renal cysts, and hypertension. The question of malignant degeneration has been raised but not answered. There is controversy as to whether these lesions require nephrectomy. Some urologists follow these children with ultrasound because, with time, many multicystic kidneys will involute. Others remove these kidneys to avoid the long-term limited risk of complications and the necessity of following the children for an extended time with repeated studies (Fig 110-5).

### Polycystic Kidney

Polycystic kidney disease is an inherited disorder, either autosomal recessive (infantile polycystic disease) or autosomal dominant (adult polycystic disease). The two entities are distinct and should not be confused. The recessive form is found in homozygotes, the dominant form in heterozygotes. Other organs are involved, especially the liver; in the dominant form, cerebral aneurysms are common.

In the recessive form, the kidneys retain their reniform configuration but are enlarged. The parenchyma is filled with dilated renal collecting tubules that appear as small radial cysts. The collecting system (renal pelvis and ureter) is normal, as is the renal pedicle. All children with recessive polycystic kidney disease have involvement of the liver consisting of bile duct dilation and proliferation with varying amounts of periportal fibrosis. Areas of uninvolved parenchyma are interspersed among these involved segments. The degree of renal and hepatic involvement appears to be inversely related, with younger children having more renal but less hepatic involvement. Children who are older when they present usually have more severe hepatic impairment with marked periportal fibrosis. Prognosis is related to age at diagnosis, those children discovered at birth having the worst outcome. Those in whom the disease is found late in childhood do better, but most die before reaching adulthood, often of hepatic complications.

The disease in infants usually is discovered as part of an evaluation for palpable renal masses noted on routine examination. An ultrasound will show enlarged kidneys with increased, diffuse echogenicity. Intravenous urography will show typical radial streaking of the dilated collecting tubules. Although the kidneys function, they do so poorly; without delayed films, visualization of dye in the renal pelvis, ureter, or bladder is unusual (Fig 110-6).

The dominant form is usually noted in adults and is a completely different disease. It too is slowly progressive and ultimately results in renal insufficiency in most cases. The cysts are of various sizes and may be quite large. The kidneys may be huge and fill almost the entire abdomen. Treatment is usually limited to controlling hypertension and any infections that occur and intervention with dialysis or transplantation when necessary. A complete and thorough family history for the past several generations is imperative to identify other affected family members and to assist in the diagnosis. Appropriate genetic counseling should be done.

## ANOMALIES OF THE COLLECTING SYSTEM

### Ureteropelvic Junction Obstruction

Obstruction at the ureteropelvic junction (UPJ) is the most common cause of hydronephrosis in childhood and one of the two most common etiologies for a renal mass in neonates (the other is a multicystic kidney). The obstruction is often caused by an

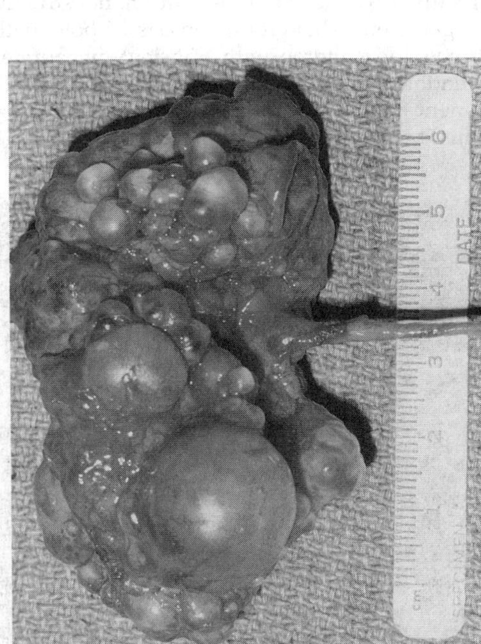

**Figure 110-5.** A gross photograph of a multicystic kidney. (Gonzales ET Jr. Genitourinary disorders in the neonate. In: Whitaker RH, Woodard JR, eds. Paediatric urology. London: Butterworth's, 1985.)

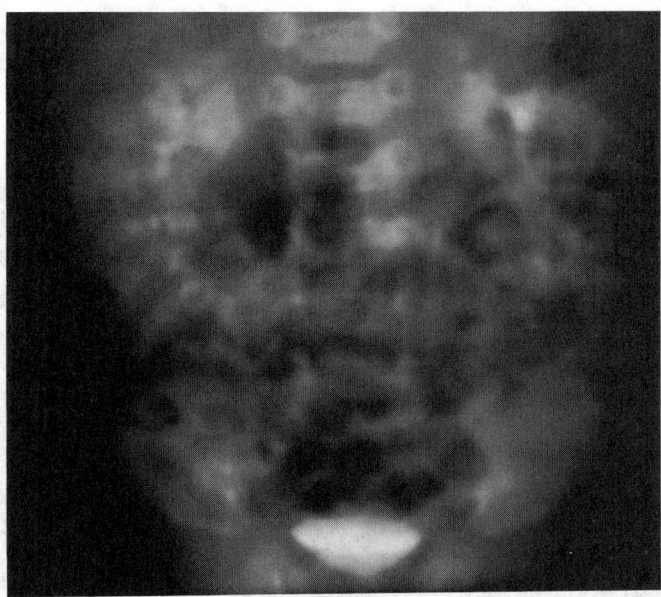

**Figure 110-6.** In this IVP of a child with recessive polycystic kidney disease, note the massive enlargement of the kidneys, good excretion and linear streaking of the contrast material. (Gonzales ET Jr. Genitourinary disorders in the neonate. In: Whitaker RH, Woodard JR, eds. Paediatric urology. London: Butterworth's, 1985.)

intrinsic fibrosis at the junction of the renal pelvis and ureter that disrupts the peristaltic wave across that region. Less common etiologies include a crossing renal vessel, kinking of the ureter, stenosis of the junction, and adhesions or extrinsic fibrosis at the UPJ. The obstruction leads to increased intrapelvic pressure, which causes dilation of the pelvis and calyces. This obstruction predisposes to urinary stasis, infection, hematuria, pain, and gradual destruction of renal parenchyma.

The diagnosis is often suggested by prenatal ultrasound and confirmed by postnatal studies. Other signs and symptoms include UTI, pyelonephritis, abdominal or flank pain, sepsis, palpable masses, nausea, failure to thrive, or an incidental finding during the evaluation of associated congenital anomalies. Investigations should include a renal ultrasound, intravenous pyelogram (IVP), or renal scan. These studies should demonstrate pyelocaliectasis and late emptying of the renal pelvis. Because the IVP often shows poor excretion, delayed films out to 24 hours may be necessary. The renal scan can help estimate the relative contribution of the obstructed kidney to overall renal function, and the addition of diuresis (with furosemide) may show a prolonged washout period that suggests obstruction. A voiding cystourethrogram is necessary because high-grade vesicoureteral reflux can mimic a UPJ obstruction or cause a secondary UPJ obstruction as a result of the large volume of refluxed urine. In both of these cases, control of the reflux will resolve the upper tract difficulties (Fig 110-7).

A pyeloplasty is the surgical repair of a UPJ obstruction. Its goal is to provide a funneled and dependent pelvis leading to the ureter. Reduction of pelvic size may be necessary to facilitate renal emptying. Significant improvement in radiographic appearance and renal function is usual after relief of obstruction, especially in infants. Therefore, efforts should be made to repair even those kidneys with poor function. Currently there is a trend toward earlier exploration and repair of kidneys; some advocate surgery within the first several weeks of life. Neonates tolerate the surgery quite well, and with the use of optical magnification the procedure is technically feasible in even the youngest children. Long-term follow-up is necessary both for confirmation of an adequate postoperative anatomical result and for final assessment of renal function.

## Megaureter

Ureters that are wide and dilated are called megaureters. They are divided into primary and secondary megaureters.

The primary megaureter is dilated, usually more distally than proximally, to the level of the ureterovesical junction, where a stenotic region, or distal inert (aperistaltic) segment, is encountered. Histologic evaluation has shown a deficiency of muscle fibers in this area that disrupts the peristaltic wave and causes functional obstruction. The usual signs and symptoms include hydronephrosis, discovered on prenatal ultrasound or incidentally at the time of evaluation for other congenital anomalies, UTI, flank pain, or hematuria. Diagnosis is generally suggested by pyelography or ultrasound. Confirmation of true obstruction usually requires a diuretic renogram or percutaneous nephrostomy with pressure flow measurements. Ureteroneocystostomy is required to relieve the obstruction. Ureteral narrowing by tapering or tailoring may be required for an adequate repair. Prognosis is generally good but depends on the degree of renal damage present at the time of surgery.

Secondary megaureters are divided into refluxing and non-refluxing units. Those that reflux are either developmentally dysplastic or have become dilated by the volume of urine propelled retrograde by the bladder contraction. In either case, the ureterovesical junction is incompetent and allows the reflux to occur. In most cases, surgical control of the reflux will resolve the problem; however, the fact that the surgical complication rate for refluxing megaureters exceeds that for obstructed megaureters implies an intrinsic ureteral abnormality in some cases that contributes to the ureterectasis.

The nonrefluxing secondary megaureter is dilated secondary to urinary obstruction at a level distal to the ureterovesical junction. The most common causes are posterior urethral valves, urethral strictures, neuropathic bladders, and dysfunctional voiding. Diagnosis may be difficult, and because the surgical approaches are completely different, care must be taken not to confuse the primary obstructed megaureter with the secondary form. The most reliable methods of distinguishing one from the other are diuretic renograms with a catheter in the bladder and pressure flow studies involving a percutaneous nephrostomy. In nonrefluxing secondary megaureters, control of the distal obstructive process will usually solve the problem, and attention should be directed there rather than to the ureterovesical junction.

A final group of patients are those with nonobstructive, nonrefluxing megaureters. This group consists of boys with prune belly syndrome and children with transient megaureters associated with endotoxins from an acute UTI. Neither condition requires treatment for the megaureter itself, and thus an accurate diagnosis must be made to avoid unnecessary surgery.

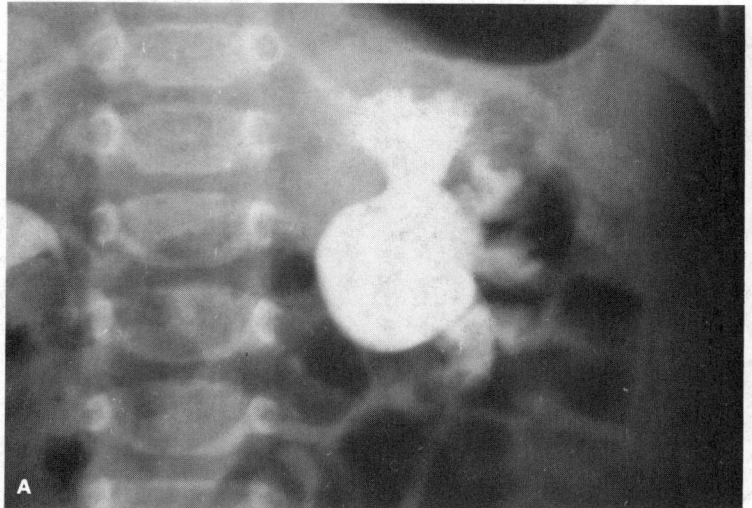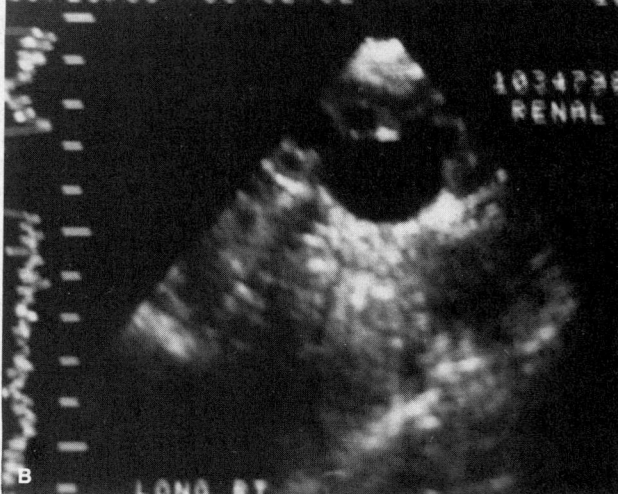

**Figure 110-7.** Ureteropelvic junction obstruction demonstrated by (**A**) IVP and (**B**) renal ultrasound.

## Simple Ureterocele

A ureterocele is a cystic dilation of the intravesical segment of the ureter. A simple ureterocele subtends a single (nonduplicated) renal unit. These anomalies are thought to develop if there is incomplete dissolution of Chwalla's membrane. Many simple ureteroceles are small and asymptomatic, but they can be large and obstruct the ureter or bladder neck. They usually are found when a renal ultrasound or an IVP is done to evaluate a UTI. The radiographic findings are pathognomonic, showing a "cobra-head" deformity within the bladder (Fig 110-8). If obstruction is not present, no treatment is necessary; however, on occasion either a transurethral incision of the ureterocele or ureteroneocystostomy may be required to relieve ureteral obstruction or prevent recurrent infections.

## Retrocaval Ureter

The retrocaval ureter is a rare congenital anomaly in which the right ureter passes medial and posterior to the vena cava. Its etiology is related to persistence of the subcardinal vein ventral to the developing ureter. The ureter then hooks around the future vena cava. The condition is rarely seen in childhood and is significant only if hydronephrosis occurs. Treatment consists of dividing the ureter and reanastomosing it anterior to the great vessels. Prognosis is generally excellent with relief of the obstruction and resolution of the symptoms.

## Ureteral Duplication and Ectopia

### Complete Duplication

Ureteral duplication is the most common congenital urologic anomaly; it affects about one in 150 individuals. Etiologically it can be traced to two ureteral buds arising from a single Wolffian duct. Both buds reach the developing metanephros and stimulate renal differentiation. The ureter to the lower segment is absorbed into the developing bladder earlier and, therefore, travels further along the trigone, finally resting lateral and cephalad to the upper pole ureter, which lies medial and caudal. This relationship is known as the Weigert-Meyer law. The lower pole ureter is prone to reflux, whereas the upper pole ureter (medial and inferior) is more often associated with obstruction from either ectopia or an ectopic ureterocele.

A full spectrum of renal involvement has been observed, ranging from the child with severe bilateral lower pole reflux and bilateral obstructing ureteroceles to the asymptomatic adult in whom duplication anomalies are discovered serendipitously. In the severe case, the diagnosis may be made on the basis of prenatal ultrasound, but more often the diagnosis is made during the workup of a UTI. An IVP may show a nonfunctioning upper pole moiety depressing the functioning lower pole collecting system and pushing it laterally (the so-called "drooping lily" deformity) (Fig 110-9). A renal ultrasound will show similar findings: a hydronephrotic upper pole "cap" of tissue depressing a normal lower pole segment. The bladder may demonstrate a negative filling defect caused by nonopacification of a large ureterocele. A renal scan can estimate the functional capacity of each segment, and a voiding cystourethrogram is required for assessment of possible lower pole reflux.

Treatment is as varied as the presentation. Often when the upper pole has no function, an upper pole partial nephroureterectomy is done. If, on the other hand, there is good function in that segment, a ureteropyelostomy connecting the upper pole ureter to the lower pole renal pelvis is done in conjunction with

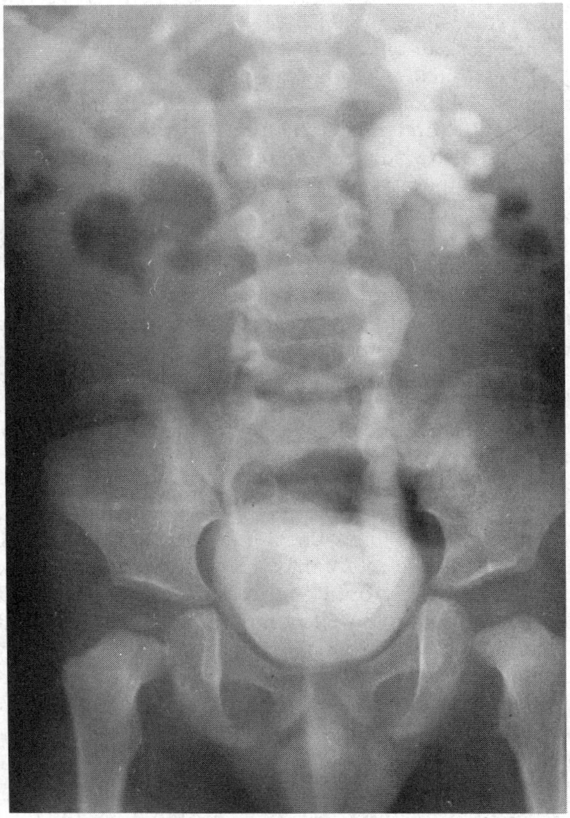

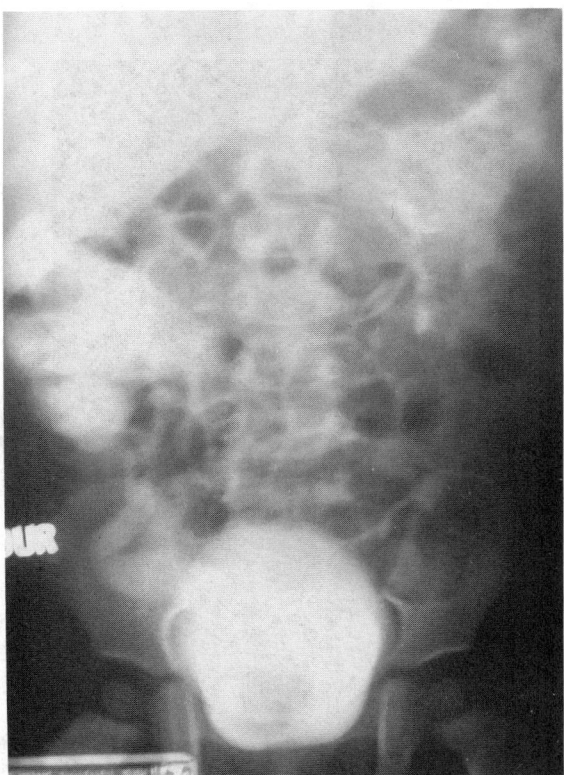

**Figure 110-9.** IVP of a neonate with a right duplication anomaly. There is nonvisualization of the right upper pole with the "drooping lily" deformity of the lower pole moiety. (Gonzales ET Jr. Genitourinary disorders in the neonate. In: Whitaker RH, Woodard JR, eds. Paediatric urology. London: Butterworth's, 1985.)

**Figure 110-8.** A simple ureterocele is shown in this IVP. Note the ureteral dilation and swelling of the distal ureter.

partial resection of the distal upper pole ureter. If lower pole reflux is present with an upper pole ureterocele, some surgeons reimplant the ureters at the same sitting. Other surgeons delay any bladder surgery for several months or years in the hope that the reflux may resolve once the ureterocele, which has been distorting the bladder, has been decompressed. When reflux to the lower pole is present without upper pole obstruction, a common sheath ureteroneocystostomy may be all that is required.

The prognosis depends on the degree of renal damage present at the time of intervention. However, renal function is generally adequate, and further problems are unusual.

### Incomplete Duplication

Incomplete ureteral duplication is caused by division of the ureteral bud after it originates from the Wolffian duct. Two ureteral buds thus promote adjacent renal differentiation but arise from a single ureteral orifice. This condition is generally asymptomatic and does not need attention (Fig 110-10).

### Ureteral Ectopia

Ureteral ectopia occurs when the ureteral orifice lies medial and inferior to its normal location. Its developmental etiology is related to the anomalous development of the terminal segment of the Wolffian duct. The origin of the ureteral bud is more cephalad than normal on the mesonephric system, and this precludes the usual incorporation into the trigone. In the male, the ureter can terminate along the vas deferens, seminal vesicle, prostatic urethra, or distal trigone. Because all these locations are proximal to the external sphincter, continence is preserved. In the female, the analogous structures of the Wolffian duct and urogenital sinus are the bladder neck, urethra, vestibule, and Gartner's duct, some of which are distal to the urinary sphincter. Ureters draining

ectopically at these locations are generally associated with constant urinary leakage (Fig 110-11), a typical presenting symptom.

The clinical features of this disorder depend on the location of the ureteral orifice and the degree of developmental renal damage. The symptoms are usually those of infection or incontinence. In a girl, a history of lifelong constant wetness despite a normal voiding pattern suggests ureteral ectopia. In a male, the diagnosis of ureteral ectopia should be considered whenever a mass is found in the seminal vesicle or epididymitis or prostatitis is encountered in a preadolescent child. Radiographic studies may show either a nonfunctioning renal unit or ureteral dilation, depending on the degree of developmental abnormality. Cystoscopy can be helpful, especially if bilateral ectopia or if a hemitrigone is found.

Treatment generally consists of a nephroureterectomy of the involved renal unit, since renal function is usually poor. However, if kidney function is good or in the case of bilateral ureteral ectopia, reimplantation is appropriate.

## VESICOURETERAL REFLUX

Vesicoureteral reflux is the retrograde regurgitation of urine from the bladder toward the kidney. Reflux is either primary or acquired; in children, primary reflux is more prevalent. Its etiology is embryologically related to a malpositioning of the ureteral bud on the Wolffian duct. This location causes the ureteral orifice to be lateral and cephalad on the trigone, thus foreshortening the submucosal tunnel. The tunnel provides the valvelike mechanism against urinary reflux, and if it is deficient reflux can occur. The degree of reflux may range from very mild (when urine enters the ureter but does not reach the kidney) to very severe (when the ureters are widely dilated and tortuous with gross pyelocaliectasis). An objective system using well-described criteria for grading reflux is used throughout the world and is based on the voiding cystourethrogram.

The diagnosis of reflux is best made with a voiding cystogram (Fig 110-12). Initially, a radiologic study is done because it provides reproducible quantification of the reflux, defines anatomical anomalies at the ureteral insertion area (paraureteral diverticula, ectopia), and also visualizes the urethra, which is imperative in boys to rule out the presence of urethral obstruction causing reflux. In subsequent follow-up studies, a nuclear cystogram may be substituted for the voiding cystourethrogram. The main advantage of the nuclear cystogram is that radiation exposure is lower compared with standard contrast cystography.

Quantification of the reflux is important for prognosis because the lower grades of reflux tend to resolve spontaneously. Higher grades of reflux resolve less often and are more likely to lead to renal injury and scarring.

The basis of treatment for reflux is the premise that sterile reflux is not harmful to the kidney. Therefore, children who have reflux can be treated with a daily low-dose prophylactic antibiotic, generally nitrofurantoin or trimethoprim-sulfamethoxazole, to prevent infection and allow the kidney to grow normally. As the bladder matures, the reflux may spontaneously resolve. While the child is receiving prophylactic treatment, urinalysis and cultures should be done every 3 to 4 months and whenever clinically indicated to monitor for possible infection. Cystography should be repeated at regular intervals so that if resolution of the reflux occurs, the medications can be stopped and the child observed. Normal renal growth and development should follow.

The other treatment option is ureteral reimplantation (ureteroneocystostomy). In uncomplicated cases, the success rate exceeds 98%. After surgery, antibiotics can be discontinued and the child watched. The decision for either medical or surgical treatment is usually made by parents with information and guidance from

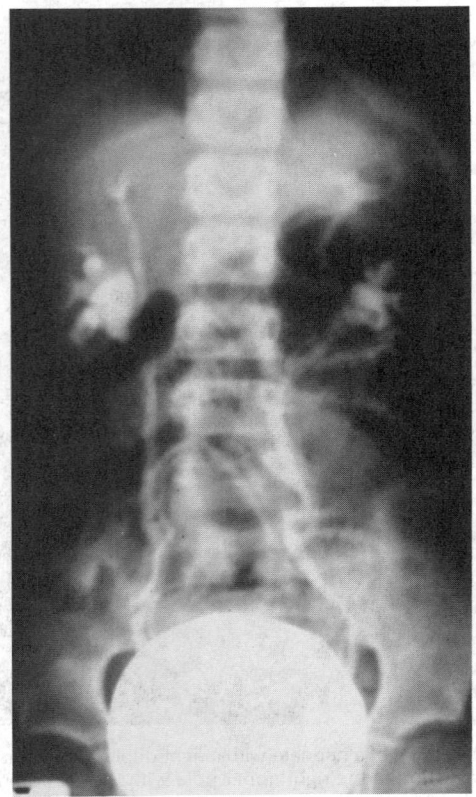

**Figure 110-10.** This voiding cystourethrogram shows bilateral partial duplication anomalies without hydronephrosis or obstruction.

**LOCATIONS OF ECTOPIC URETERS**

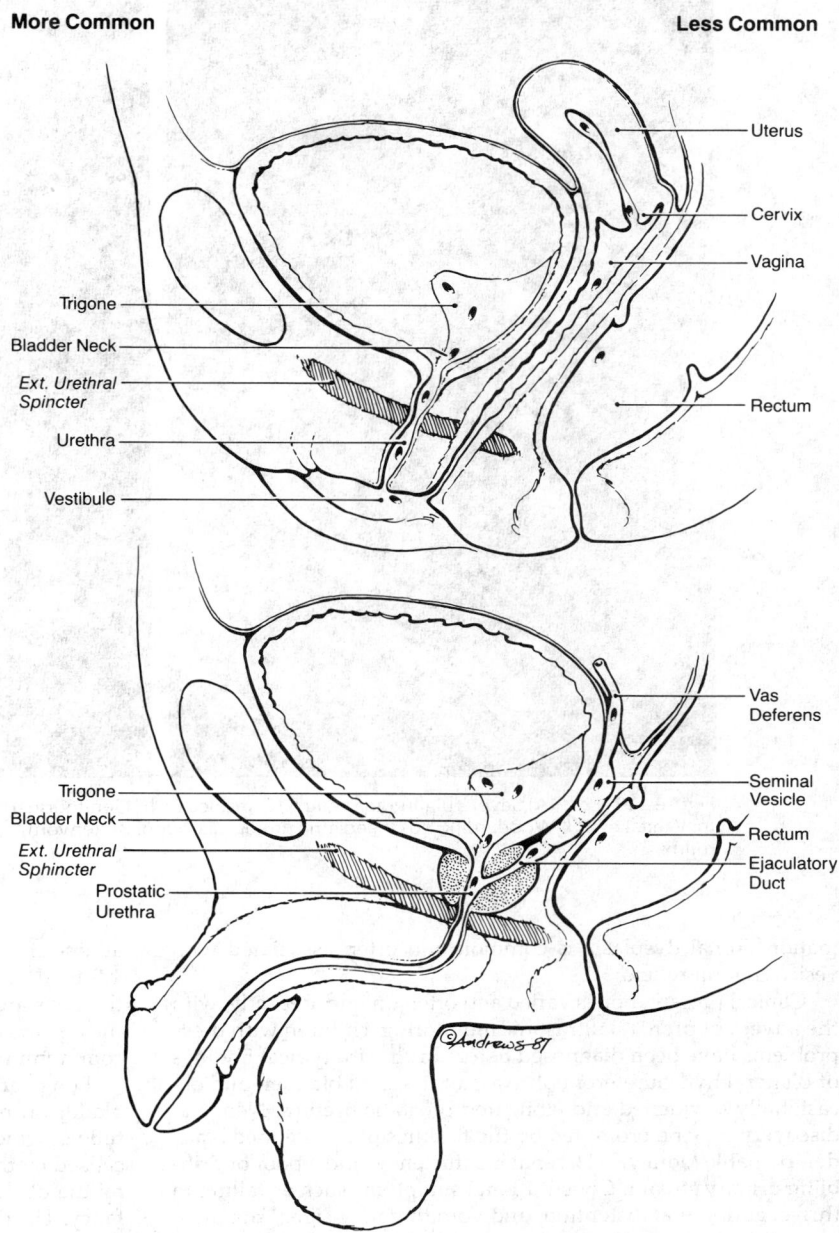

**Figure 110-11.** Possible locations of an ectopic ureter. In the female those locations distal to the urethral sphincter allow constant wetness. In the male, however, all locations are proximal to the sphincter, so incontinence will not occur.

their physicians. The only absolute indication for surgery is a breakthrough infection, a UTI while the child is receiving appropriate chemoprophylactics.

Several other factors, including age, sex, family situation, and presence of renal scarring, may play a role in determining treatment. Location of the ureteral orifices as determined by cystoscopy may predict the likelihood of spontaneous resolution of reflux and can be taken into account when treatment decisions are made. Because of an increased incidence (30%) of reflux in siblings of a refluxer, they also should be investigated. The most accurate screening test is cystography, but in the older asymptomatic child with no history of urinary infection, a renal ultrasound may be adequate. If significant reflux is present, the renal ultrasound will uncover upper tract dilation or scarring. If low-grade reflux is present and missed by ultrasound, the older child is thought to be beyond the age when most renal damage secondary to reflux occurs, and treatment may not be needed. If identified, such a

child should receive the same treatment as anyone else with documented reflux.

## BLADDER AND URETHRAL ANOMALIES

### Posterior Urethral Valves

Posterior urethral valves are rare congenital obstructing leaflets in the region of the verumontanum in the prostatic urethra. There is no analogous structure or pathology in the female. Their etiology is unclear, but they are thought to be related to anomalous development of the urethrovaginal folds. Their pathophysiology stems from their narrowing of the bladder outlet, proximal to the external urethral sphincter. The obstruction they cause increases voiding pressure with dilation of the prostatic urethra, hypertrophy of the bladder neck, bladder trabeculation, and saccule for-

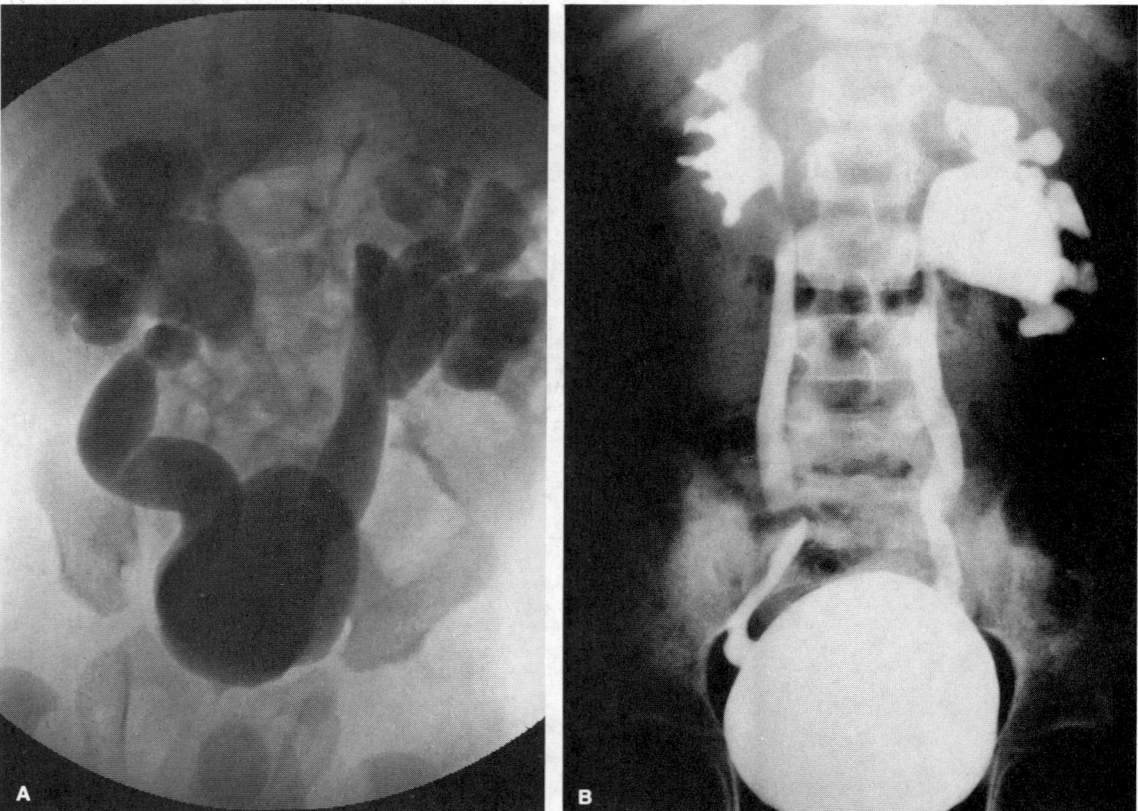

**Figure 110-12.**    (**A**) Severe high-grade reflux. (Gonzales ET Jr. Genitourinary disorders in the neonate. In: Whitaker RH, Woodard JR, eds. Paediatric urology. London: Butterworth's, 1985.) (**B**) More moderate reflux.

mation. Renal dysplasia is common and often associated with vesicoureteral reflux.

Clinical presentation is varied and often unique. Recently, with the advent of prenatal ultrasonic monitoring, children with these problems have been diagnosed before birth with typical findings of bilateral hydroureteronephrosis, a thickened bladder, and occasionally a widened and elongated prostatic urethra. Neonatal discovery may be prompted by the findings of a distended bladder, palpable kidney, UTI, renal insufficiency, and a poor or dribbling urinary stream. Constitutional symptoms such as failure to thrive, abdominal distention, and vomiting may signal the presence of posterior urethral valves. In older boys, voiding problems may predominate and may be obvious. They vary from the expected (poor stream, urinary retention, and bladder distention) to quite subtle (hematuria, enuresis, and hesitancy). The diagnosis is best made on a voiding cystourethrogram (Fig 110-13).

Treatment is directed toward relief of the obstruction. Initial therapy, especially in the neonate, is placement of a transurethral catheter, hemodynamic stabilization, normalization of electrolytes, and treatment of any existing infection. If the renal function is normal or near normal, transurethral ablation of the valves is done within a few days. In neonates with rising creatinine, uncontrollable infection, or a urethra too small to accept an infant cystoscope, a temporary vesicostomy or supravesical diversion is appropriate. The older boy can almost always undergo transurethral surgery because size is not a problem and severe renal insufficiency is rare.

Traditionally, the younger the child is at diagnosis, the poorer the prognosis. This, however, has been modified by prenatal ultrasound, since even mild cases may be discovered before birth. Currently, the best predictor of prognosis is the nadir serum cre-

atinine after treatment. Those in whom the creatinine drops below 1.0 tend to do quite well, but if the creatinine stays above 1.0, the boys are more apt to have difficulties with renal function as they grow. Renal failure with resultant dialysis and transplant is common in the latter group of patients.

Long-range difficulties are associated with both renal and bladder function. The bladder problems include vesicoureteral reflux, which may require surgery, and voiding dysfunction caused by the effects of the high intravesical pressures produced by the obstructing valves during prenatal development and infancy. The difficulties with renal function have been noted above.

## Epispadias–Exstrophy Complex

Classical exstrophy is a rare anomaly (one in 30,000 to 40,000 individuals) of the lower abdominal wall in which a persistent cloacal membrane prevents the medial ingrowth of mesenchyme. The deeper layers of ectoderm and endoderm do not fuse. When rupture of the membrane occurs, there is separation of the midline structures, including the lower abdominal wall, rectus abdominis muscle and fascia, bladder, pubis, urethra, and genitalia.

The degree of exstrophy depends on the size of the cloacal membrane and the time of its rupture. In the most common form, the bladder is open and exposed on the lower abdominal wall. The rectus muscles and fascia diverge to rest on laterally displaced pubic bones. The external genitalia are splayed; in the female, the clitoris is bifid, the labia lateral, and the vagina anterior. In the male, the penis is short and wide with a dorsal urethral strip. There is significant dorsal chordee. The anus is anteriorly displaced and the umbilicus lies at the cephalad portion of the exposed bladder. The pubic bones are divergent in the midline,

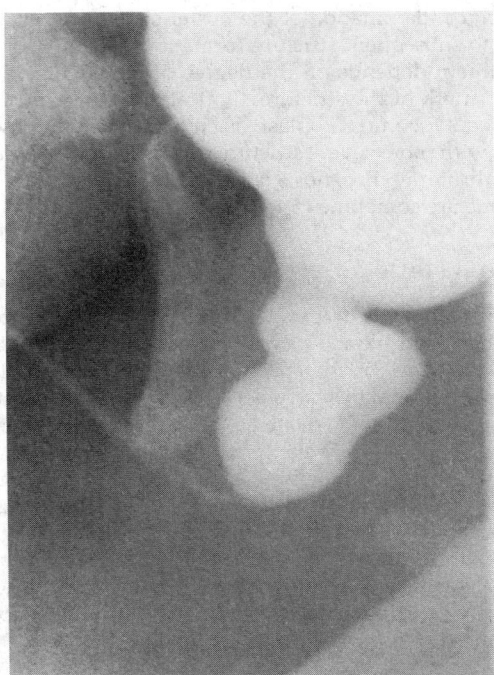

**Figure 110-13.** A newborn boy with typical x-ray findings of posterior urethral valves. (Gonzales ET Jr. Genitourinary disorders in the neonate. In: Whitaker RH, Woodard JR, eds. Paediatric urology. London: Butterworth's, 1985.)

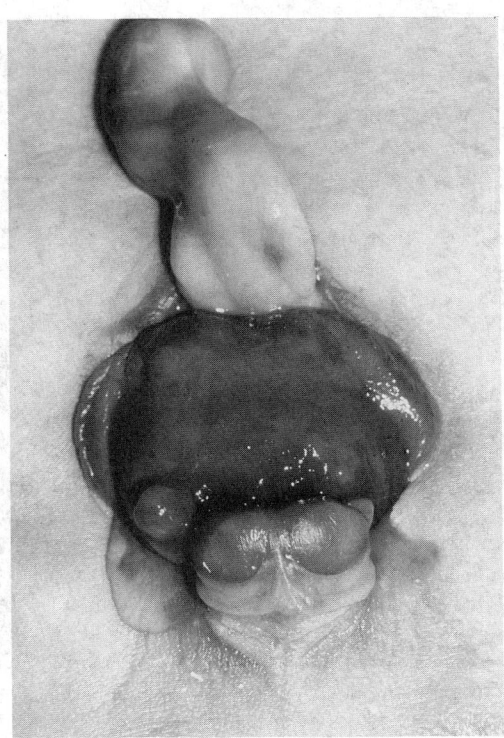

**Figure 110-14.** A typical example of classical bladder exstrophy. (Gonzales ET Jr. Genitourinary disorders in the neonate. In: Whitaker RH, Woodard JR, eds. Paediatric urology. In: London: Butterworth's, 1985.)

leaving the pelvic ring open. The femoral heads are externally rotated and cause a waddling gait if not corrected. Both inguinal and umbilical hernias are common and may require surgery (Fig 110-14).

Diagnosis of the defect is obvious at birth, and prompt attention should be sought from those familiar with such problems. Immediate care is supportive, and there is no recognized pattern of involvement in other organ systems. Uroradiologic evaluation will usually show normally developed kidneys and collecting systems. With time, there may be hypertrophy of the bladder mucosa and prolapse of the ureters, which can lead to hydronephrosis. Initial management of the bladder requires covering of the area with a substance such as cellophane as a protective measure. The cover should remain in place until a more definitive procedure can be undertaken.

Today, the goal of treatment is to provide a functioning bladder capable of social continence, and functional genitalia. Although ambitious, these goals can be reached in most patients over a period of several years. The initial surgical procedure often is closure of the bladder and abdominal wall, leaving an open incontinent epispadiac bladder neck. If possible, this procedure should be attempted within the first 48 to 72 hours of life. If not, consideration should be given to performing iliac osteotomies just before bladder closure. That orthopedic procedure allows the bladder to drop into the abdominal cavity and facilitates closure of the anterior abdominal wall. Several years after bladder closure, most urologists proceed with the second stage of the repair, bladder neck reconstruction and ureteral reimplantation, in an attempt to provide continence and eliminate reflux. Successful results are reported in up to 80% of these children. Subsequently, in the male, epispadias repair is undertaken; a combination of penile lengthening, release of dorsal chordee, and an urethroplasty is used. Individuals who have failed bladder neck reconstruction and remain incontinent must be considered for either a repeat procedure, placement of an artificial urinary sphincter, or urinary diversion.

In some children with exstrophy, the exposed bladder is small and fibrotic. Occasionally, primary closure of the bladder is impossible and urinary diversion to the skin (ileal conduit, nonrefluxing colon conduit, end-cutaneous ureterostomy) or bowel (ureterosigmoidostomy) must be contemplated. Current techniques of continent diversion using nonrefluxing ureterointestinal anastomosis seem much safer than the old ureteroileal cutaneous anastomosis (ileal loop), although long-term studies are not yet available.

Cloacal exstrophy is a more complex and less common anomaly in which the cloacal membrane ruptures before complete descent of the urorectal septum. The resultant defect is much more severe than that of classical exstrophy. The bladder plate on the abdominal wall is split by a strip of open gut. The proximal end leads to the ileum, and the distal opening leads to a blind-ending hindgut. The phallus is widely separated, and regardless of genetic sex the child should be assigned the female gender, as construction of a functional penis is usually impossible. Since associated anomalies are common, a thorough evaluation of other organ systems is mandatory.

In the past, children with cloacal exstrophy rarely survived the neonatal period; however, recent advances in surgical techniques and parenteral alimentation have provided more hope for these babies. Initial management is directed toward stabilizing electrolyte losses from the short gut and meeting nutritional requirements. Diversion of the fecal and urinary streams may be required. Currently, there is enthusiasm for using the rudimentary hindgut to construct a vagina, to extend the bowel (to decrease the effects of the short bowel syndrome), or to serve as a urinary reservoir in a continent diversion.

Epispadias without exstrophy is less common than exstrophy and is classified as balanitic, penile, or penopubic. In boys with this anomaly, the urethral meatus is dorsal, and chordee, if present, is also dorsal (Fig 110-15). Repair of epispadias involves

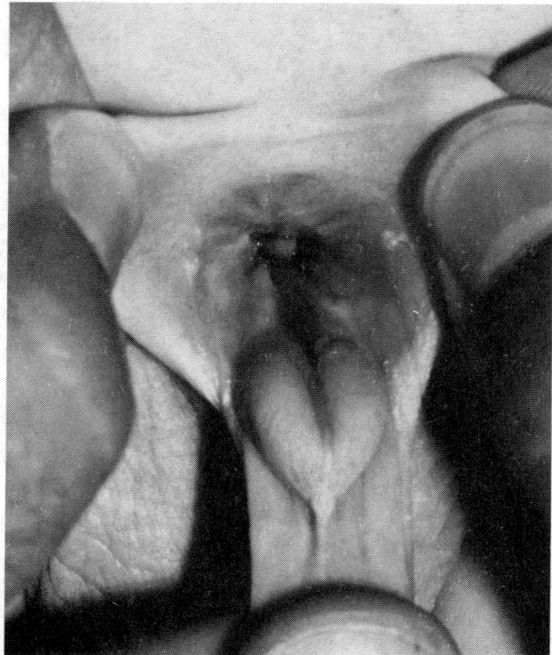

**Figure 110-15.**   Penopubic epispadias with severe dorsal chordee.

correcting the chordee and constructing a neourethra. Female epispadias is more unusual and often goes undetected until a careful genital examination is performed on an older incontinent girl, in whom a bifid clitoris associated with a short and patulous urethra is discovered. If the epispadias extends through the bladder neck, surgery is required to provide continence and will consist of either a bladder neck reconstruction or insertion of an artificial urinary sphincter.

## Anterior Urethral Pathology

### Anterior Urethral Valves

Anterior urethral valves are a rare congenital obstruction of the penile urethra that cause dilation of the urethra proximal to the lesion. Because voiding symptoms are common, this entity should be considered in boys complaining of urgency, frequency, or a poor stream. The diagnosis is made by a voiding cystourethrogram, which shows a urethral diverticulum at the site of stenosis. Treatment consists of transurethral destruction of the lesion or an open excision with reconstruction of the urethral diverticulum. These anomalies can cause severe obstruction and result in severe hydronephrosis with renal failure, similar to changes seen with posterior urethral valves.

### Anterior Urethral Strictures

Strictures of the penile urethra have several etiologies, the most common of which are traumatic, iatrogenic, and inflammatory. Currently, iatrogenic lesions account for more than half of the reported cases. They develop after urologic treatment for congenital anomalies or prolonged catheterization. Traumatic strictures occur after direct injury to the perineum or a straddle injury. Inflammatory strictures are uncommon in childhood, as they usually result from gonococcal urethritis. Whatever the cause, strictures may take years to develop.

Symptoms of a stricture are the same as those associated with other forms of bladder outflow obstruction: strangury, hesitancy, small thin stream with little pressure, and dribbling. Terminal hematuria may occur in conjunction with a stricture or with a

nonspecific inflammation of the posterior urethra that may predispose to subsequent stricture formation.

Treatment depends on the degree of narrowing, symptoms, and the length of the stricture. Optical urethrotomy currently is often used. Open urethroplasty is an option usually reserved for patients with more severe strictures or those unresponsive to optical urethrotomy. Prognosis is generally excellent, but repeated operations are sometimes required.

## Megalourethra

An abnormally wide urethra with deficiency of the corpus spongiosum has been termed *megalourethra*. More severe cases may also have absence of the corpora cavernosa. Fewer than 50 of these rare abnormalities have been reported in the literature. The etiology is thought to be related to a developmental arrest during embryogenesis of the penis. Urethral obstruction is rare. Other associated urologic anomalies are common, and upper tract evaluation by renal ultrasound or IVP is appropriate. Associated anomalies often are more significant and life-threatening. Elective reduction urethroplasty may be required to reduce urinary stasis and improve urethral emptying and cosmetic appearance. In the most severe cases, consideration of a change in the sex of rearing is appropriate.

## Urethral Prolapse

Urethral prolapse occurs in girls and is the protrusion of the urethral mucosa and engorged corpus spongiosum through the external urethral meatus. The most prominent presenting symptom is bleeding, and examination usually suggests the diagnosis (Fig 110-16). This condition is found primarily in preadolescent black females and may be secondary to a transient increase in intra-abdominal pressure. Various treatments have been proposed. Most recent reviews suggest early primary excision as the modality with the fewest complications, lowest recurrence, and shortest hospital stay; however, an initial course of topical estrogens may provide significant improvement and avoid surgical excision.

## Urachal Anomalies

The urachus arises from the bladder dome and extends cephalad to the umbilicus. Embryologically, its origin is either the anterior portion of the cloaca or the allantois. Normally the urachus is a

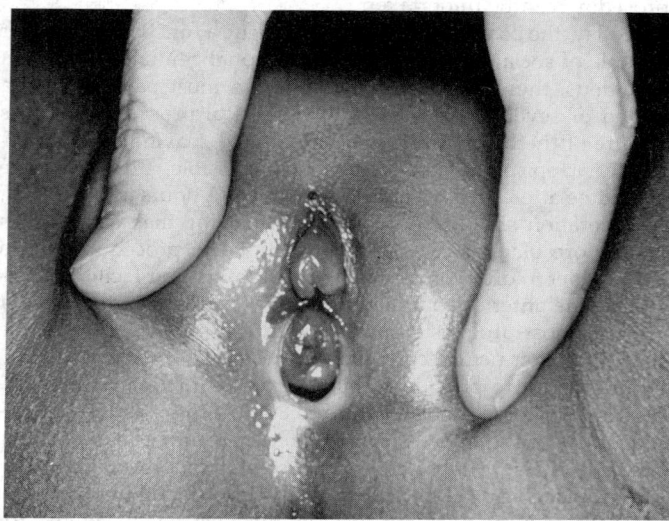

**Figure 110-16.**   Urethral prolapse in a young girl.

fibrous cord with an obliterated lumen; abnormalities of the urachus occur when this obliteration is incomplete. There is a continuum of involvement, from a fully patent urachus to one in which there has been extensive closure of the canal. There is communication between the bladder and umbilicus in a patent urachus. Presentation is usually that of a wet or draining umbilicus. Its presence should alert the clinician to possible bladder outlet obstruction, especially an atretic urethra. Confirmation of the diagnosis can be made by a voiding cystourethrogram, a fistulogram through the draining umbilical site, cystoscopy, or instillation of methylene blue into the bladder and visualization of blue drainage from the umbilicus.

Another urachal abnormality is the urachal cyst, which is usually located in the proximal third of the urachus, closest to the bladder. Intermittent infections most often occur in late childhood. Symptoms are suprapubic pain, tenderness, swelling, a palpable mass, and drainage from the umbilicus. If an infected cyst drains to the umbilicus and a tract is formed, a urachal sinus develops. There often is persistent umbilical drainage and formation of granulation tissue at the umbilicus.

Treatment for these conditions requires antibiotics for any acute infection and subsequent suprapubic exploration and excision of the infected urachal remnant. If not excised, recurrent infections, possibly with abscess formation, are typical.

## ANOMALIES OF THE PENIS

### Hypospadias

Hypospadias is a congenital penile deformity resulting from incomplete development of the distal or anterior urethra. The urethral meatus may be located at any point along the ventral shaft of the penis, midline of the scrotum, or perineum. The more proximal the urethral meatus, the more likely the penis is to be curved because of inelasticity of the dysplastic urethral plate and a foreshortening of the ventral aspect of the paired corpora cavernosa. This curvature is termed *chordee* and may preclude intercourse if severe. The prepuce in these patients is incompletely formed. The ventral foreskin is absent, but there is usually abundant dorsal skin that drapes over the glans as a dorsal "hood."

Hypospadias is the most common congenital anomaly of the penis, affecting about 3.5 boys out of 1000 births. Etiology is thought to be secondary to an in utero disorder of virilization, possibly a temporary deficiency or insensitivity to testosterone. Associated anomalies consist mainly of inguinal pathology, either hernias or undescended testes. Upper tract abnormalities are uncommon unless other organ systems are involved, in which case upper tract screening, by either IVP or renal ultrasound, is appropriate. For boys with bilateral cryptorchidism associated with hypospadias, consideration must be given to an intersex abnormality and appropriate testing should be done. Furthermore, patients with severe hypospadias may have a large utriculus masculinas or vaginal remnant, which can sequester urine and lead to a UTI. In such instances, cystoscopy and cystography may be warranted.

There is a definite familial tendency toward hypospadias. If a boy has hypospadias, his brother has a 14% chance of having hypospadias; if two brothers have hypospadias, the chances of a third brother having the same defect increase to 21%. If a boy has hypospadias, there is an 8% chance that his father is similarly affected. It seems that a multifactorial inheritance pattern is the most consistent explanation for the incidence of hypospadias.

In the initial evaluation of a boy with hypospadias, the position of the urethral meatus (glandular, coronal, distal shaft, mid-shaft, proximal shaft, penoscrotal, scrotal, perineal) should be noted so that the degree of required surgical repair can be estimated. Because almost every hypospadias repair uses preputial skin, documentation of its position and amount is important, and neonatal circumcision is contraindicated. Slight perineal pressure on the corpora cavernosa will mimic an erection by obstructing venous outflow. This erection should help the clinician to assess the degree (mild, moderate, severe) and location (glandular, distal shaft, mid-shaft, or proximal shaft) of chordee. In cases of severe hypospadias, there may be an element of penoscrotal transposition; the scrotal folds envelop or wrap around the proximal penile shaft. This abnormality can be addressed at the same time as the hypospadias and chordee to improve the patient's appearance (Fig 110-17).

The objectives of surgical repair in patients with hypospadias are threefold. The first is to provide a straight penis that is adequate for intercourse. The second is to extend the urethral meatus to the tip of the glans penis, and the third is to make the appearance of the penis that of a normal circumcised phallus. Most pediatric urologists currently suggest that surgery be performed at age 6 to 18 months. Sexual identification is not complete at this age, and the surgical procedure will not be remembered. Today a single surgical procedure is used to correct all but the most severe problems. In instances of penoscrotal or perineal defects, a two-stage procedure remains a reasonable option.

Generally, cosmetic results after hypospadias surgery are excellent, but there is still a significant (15% to 40%) complication rate for patients with proximal defects. These problems consist mainly of fistulas, urethral strictures, and recurrent chordee. Any of these could require a second procedure for revision of the hypospadias repair. Unfortunately, despite our best efforts, some patients will undergo multiple procedures before an acceptable result is achieved.

### Micropenis

Micropenis is a rare condition in which a small but normally developed phallus is present. A micropenis is present if the stretched penile length from the pubic symphysis to the tip of the glans penis is less than 2.5 cm (less than two standard deviations from the mean). Measurement of penile girth (diameter or circumference) is also important, since corporal dimensions will become important when sexual function is considered.

The etiology is thought to be related either to a deficiency of gonadotropin secretion in the last two trimesters of gestation (resulting in deficient testosterone secretion) or—if present with hypospadias—to a local insensitivity to testosterone. Early treatment by local or systemic testosterone may prove helpful to those patients who in utero suffered a deficiency of testosterone or to identify boys with a degree of androgen insensitivity. For those with end-organ failure, consideration of sex reassignment is appropriate, with surgery performed as early as 2 months of age.

### Penile Agenesis

Penile agenesis is a rare defect related to developmental failure of the genital tubercle. The urethral meatus is often situated near the anus. Anorectal deformities and renal malformations are common. Children with these anomalies are best managed by sex reassignment to the female gender in early infancy.

### Difficulties with the Prepuce

#### Phimosis

Phimosis is a condition in which scarring or narrowing of the preputial opening precludes its retraction over the glans penis. In the newborn, the preputial space is not completely developed

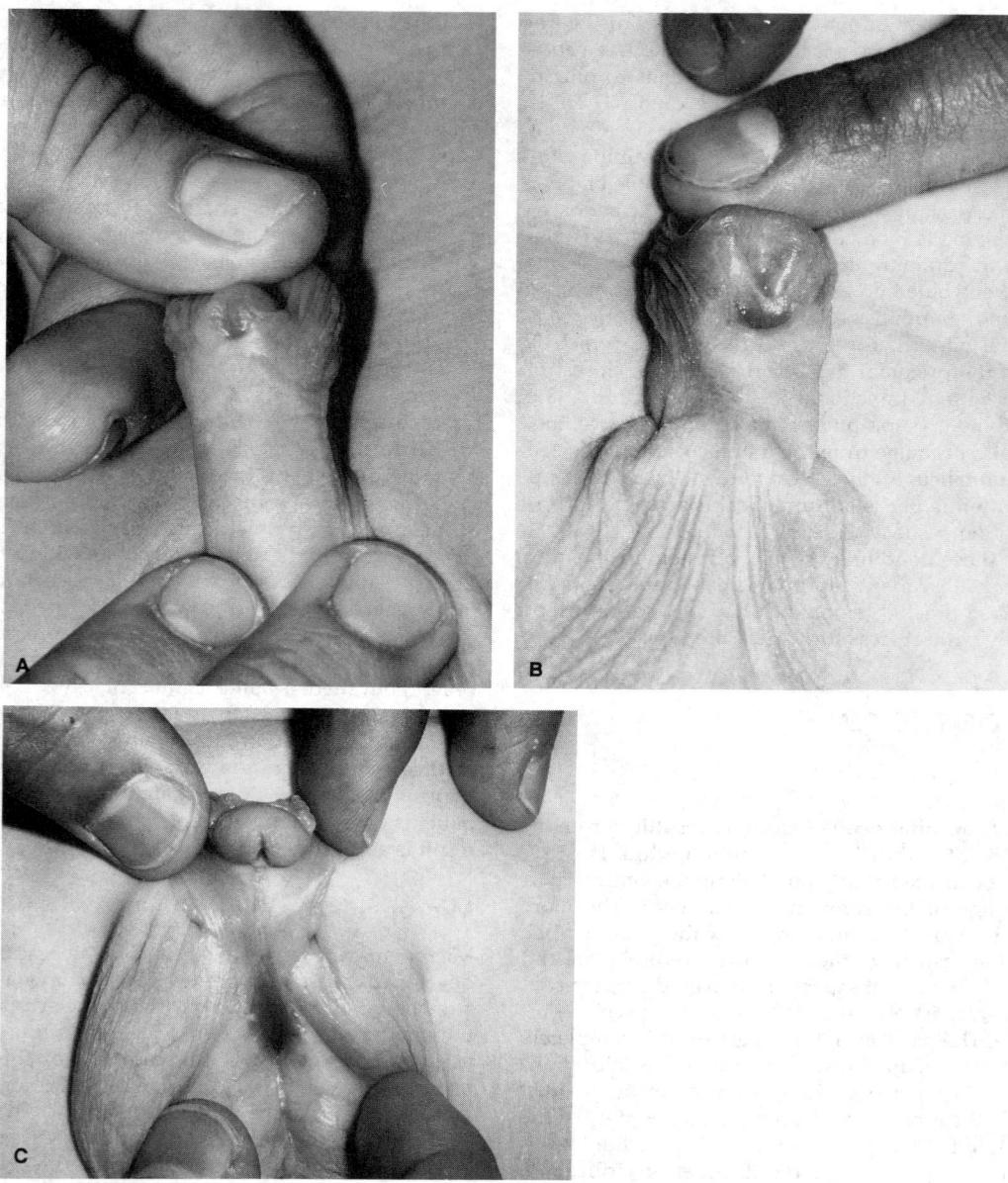

**Figure 110-17.**    Three cases of hypospadias with varying degrees of involvement. (**A**) A distal meatus without evidence of concomitant chordee. (**B**) A more severe case in which there is severe chordee and deficiency of the ventral penile skin. (**C**) A perineal hypospadias with severe chordee.

and there are normal adhesions between the inner aspect of the prepuce and the glans penis. Therefore, in neonates, the foreskin normally is difficult to retract. With normal erections and development, these adhesions will separate to allow retraction of the prepuce. By age 3, the preputial opening should be large enough to allow easy retraction of the prepuce. Boys older than 3 years who have a persistent narrowing of the preputial opening, either congenital or from scarring, are candidates for circumcision. Attempts at blunt retraction and stretching of this opening may lead to tearing, bleeding, and edema, and should be discouraged.

## Paraphimosis

Occurrence of paraphimosis, as distinguished from phimosis, is an emergency that can require surgical reduction. Paraphimosis is a condition in which the prepuce is incarcerated behind the glans penis, producing edema and swelling of the prepuce. Local discomfort is universal and prompt reduction is mandatory. Usually, pressure around the prepuce to reduce edema, followed by

direct pressure to the glans in conjunction with counteraction on the prepuce, will resolve the situation. If not, incision of the restricting band or circumcision is required.

## Infection

Balanitis is a fairly common infection of the prepuce (incidence 6%). It usually responds to oral and topical antibiotics and warm baths. If simple measures are unsuccessful, parenteral antibiotics or circumcision may be required. Most often, mixed flora or organisms are cultured from the exudate. There have been reports of both Group A beta-hemolytic streptococcus and Group B streptococcus causing balanitis. In sexually active teenagers, trichomonal balanitis and candidal infections are possibilities, and if present should prompt investigation of sexual partners.

The first episode of balanitis may not be the last. Repeated episodes of balanitis can lead to preputial scarring and phimosis. Therefore, once an episode of balanitis has occurred, circumcision should be considered as an option for further management.

Several recent studies report greater frequency of UTIs in infant boys who have not undergone circumcision (1.8%) than in circumcised boys (0.2%). Generally, the infections were not severe, but they did require hospitalization and parenteral antibiotics when they occurred in neonates.

## Complications of Circumcision

Neonatal circumcision is safe when done by an experienced practitioner within the first several weeks of life. Reported complications include hemorrhage (1%), infection (0.4%), dehiscence (0.16%), denudation of shaft (0.05%), glandular injury (0.02%), and urinary retention (0.02%). The Gomco clamp, Plastiball, and Mogen clamp are widely used, and there is no significant advantage of one over the other, other than operator preference. Still, there is no medical indication for the procedure. Most pediatric urologists currently suggest circumcision only for boys who have had difficulties with their foreskin (phimosis, paraphimosis, balanitis) or whose parents desire the surgery for personal reasons.

### Meatal Stenosis

Urethral meatal stenosis occurs secondary to glandular irritation or inflammation after circumcision when the glans is allowed to come in contact with the diaper and produce dermatitis. This meatitis is best treated by frequent diaper changes, exposure to the air, and warm baths. As the child grows, meatal stenosis may contribute to dysuria and terminal hematuria. The urinary stream is fine and dorsally deflected, at times making standing to void difficult or embarrassing. The diagnosis should be made on the basis of observed micturition, as the appearance of the glans may be misleading. A narrow, slit-like meatus may stretch significantly during voiding to yield a quite satisfactory opening. If meatal stenosis is present, a meatotomy is usually indicated. This procedure can easily be done in the office with local anesthesia. Because meatal stenosis is a local effect from a limited dermatitis, further urologic investigations are not indicated.

### Unsightly Result

Significant complications from circumcision are uncommon, but parental dissatisfaction with the cosmetic result is much more frequent. Most often the disappointment results from the appearance of excess skin left at the time of the neonatal circumcision. The parents may wish a revision of the circumcision, which must be done under anesthesia when the child is between 6 and 18 months old.

### Circumcision and Hypospadias

Absolute contraindications for circumcision are the presence of hypospadias, epispadias, chordee, or anomalies of the penile skin. Therefore, before circumcision, a careful inspection of the phallus is mandatory. In any anomaly of the penis, the presence of a redundant prepuce may be important to reconstructive efforts, and its absence may turn a rather simple hypospadias repair into a major reconstruction requiring skin grafts from distant sites.

## Priapism

Priapism is rare in healthy children, but it is not uncommon in boys with leukemia or sickle-cell disease. In the first or second incident, resolution is often spontaneous, but with subsequent episodes surgical decompression may be necessary. In cases of sickle-cell priapism, prompt efforts should be directed toward hydration and exchange transfusion with packed normal red blood cells. In boys with leukemia, chemotherapy and radiotherapy are the best initial courses of action. Persistent priapism is often handled by a shunt between the engorged corpora cavernosa and flaccid corpus spongiosum. Impotence is not uncommon following priapism, whether or not surgical decompression is required.

## TESTICULAR AND SCROTAL ANOMALIES

## Cryptorchidism

Testicular descent occurs late in fetal life and is regulated by many factors, including intra-abdominal pressure, hormonal influence, and gubernacular presence. The absence of any one of these elements may contribute to testicular maldescent. The incidence of maldescent depends on fetal age, with up to 30% of premature boys having either one or both testes undescended. In boys born normally at term, the incidence is between 3% and 4%. During the first several months of life, a transient increase in serum gonadotropin and testosterone is responsible for a spontaneous descent in more than half of boys with cryptorchidism at birth. After 1 year of life, testicles have descended in all but about 1% of boys. After that age, descent is rare; the incidence of cryptorchidism in untreated adults is about 1%.

True cryptorchidism must be distinguished from retractile testes, which are believed to be normal testes temporarily drawn into the inguinal canal by a hyperactive cremasteric muscle. With manipulation these can be brought into the deep scrotum. No treatment is needed for these, because given time, the testes will spontaneously descend, remain in the scrotum, and function normally. Therefore, one must accurately differentiate the retractile from the truly undescended testis.

The examination should take place in a relaxed, warm, and nonthreatening environment. The examiner should ensure that his or her hands are warm and should try to make the patient feel at ease. Repeated examinations with the patient in multiple positions (supine, sitting cross-legged, and squatting) may be beneficial. The history is also important, as a parent may remark that the testes are down during baths or diaper changes. The examination should be performed with two hands. One hand should start from the lateral area of the anterior superior iliac spine and sweep caudally along the inguinal canal, thereby "trapping" a testis so that it does not ascend into the abdomen. The second hand should palpate the lower groin and scrotum to identify the gonad.

There is currently some enthusiasm for the "ascending testis," a gonad that at birth appears well descended in the scrotum, but subsequently is found in the inguinal region, often in the superficial inguinal pouch. It is unclear whether these testes were truly descended or were inguinal testes that could be manipulated into the scrotum during infancy.

The position of the testis should be documented as either palpable (80%) or nonpalpable (20%). Palpable testes should be further described as inguinal, low inguinal, high scrotal, or ectopic. Even if the testes are not felt, it is often possible to identify testicular membranes on the spermatic cord; these should be documented for help in planning further therapy.

Treatment is suggested for several reasons. It has been established that progressive injury to the testis occurs as long as the testis remains in an extrascrotal position. Ultrastructural changes have been documented as early as 2 years of age, and it has been reported that after age 6 sperm production is impaired. After puberty, hormonal production has been impaired in a cryptorchid testis, and orchiectomy is often more appropriate than orchiopexy. Fifty percent of adults with a history of unilateral cryptorchidism have oligospermia, but paternity rates approach normal. On the other hand, bilateral cryptorchidism is associated with both oligospermia (80%) and infertility. It is difficult to show, however, that treatment at any age improves ultimate testicular function and fertility.

A second reason for relocating the testes in the scrotum is the increased incidence of malignant degeneration in testes with a history of maldescent. Testicular cancer, which is rare before puberty, affects about three of 100,000 men. In males with a history of cryptorchidism, the incidence is from four to 40 times higher. Yet there is no evidence that an orchiopexy will provide protection against future malignancy. Ideally, a neoplasm in an orthotopic testis will be discovered and treated earlier than one in an inguinal or abdominal position and thus increase the chance of survival, since early, small-volume testicular cancer has a cure rate of better than 95% today.

The last reason for medical intervention is to improve the patient's self-image so that he, like his friends, will have two intrascrotal testes.

Currently, most pediatric urologists suggest treatment of cryptorchidism before the child is 2 years old, preferably when he is between 6 and 18 months. The modalities available are surgical or hormonal. Surgery usually is done on an outpatient basis, and the results generally are excellent. An absent gonad is noted in about 20% of nonpalpable testes and can be confirmed by finding a blind-ending vas deferens and testicular vessels, either at exploration or in some cases by laparoscopy. Laparoscopy has been suggested for evaluation of nonpalpable testes, both to document anorchia and to help plan the surgical approach.

Usually an orchiopexy can relocate the cryptorchid testis into the scrotum without problem; however, when the testis is intra-abdominal or in a high inguinal position, division of the testicular artery and vein may be required so that the testis can reach the scrotum. In such an instance, the blood supply depends on the vasal artery and its supporting mesentery. The success rate in such a procedure drops from 98% to 70% or 80%. Its main complications are that of any orchiopexy—atrophy and retraction. Autotransplantation of the testis (anastomosing the spermatic vessels to the inferior epigastric vessels) can be accomplished by current microsurgical techniques, but it is unclear whether this significantly improves ultimate results over transection of the spermatic vessels alone. A patent processus vaginalis (pediatric hernia) occurs in association with 90% of cryptorchid testes and should be repaired at the same time.

The other treatment modality is hormonal manipulation, based on the observation that increased testosterone may encourage testicular descent. In the United States, intramuscular human chorionic gonadotropin (HCG) is given in a series of injections at varying doses. Success rates with HCG are lower than those with an orchiopexy and at best reach 30%. In Europe, there is a growing trend toward the use of intranasal gonadotropin-releasing hormone (GnRH), given twice daily for a month. Success has been claimed in 80% of the patients, although these data recently have been questioned, with studies in the United States showing only 20% success. No long-term side effects have been observed in association with this short-term hormonal therapy. However, for some patients, orchiopexy is often preferable to repeated injections and hormonal treatment.

When neither testicle is palpable, the question arises as to whether any testicular tissue is present and whether surgical intervention is necessary. Certain observations based on genital appearance and endocrinologic findings can assist in this decision. The presence of adequate levels of fetal testosterone during the first trimester is necessary for normal penile formation. During the last two trimesters, fetal testosterone promotes phallic growth. If the boy has a normal-sized penis, one can deduce that he had functioning testicular tissue until late in gestation; however, the presence of hypospadias or micropenis raises further questions regarding testicular function and development.

Endocrine evaluation of bilateral anorchia consists of measuring serum luteinizing hormone (LH), follicle-stimulating hor-

mone (FSH), and testosterone before gonadotropin stimulation and serum testosterone after HCG administration. To ensure adequate stimulation, HCG should be given over a 2-week period (usually 1000 to 1500 IU every other day for six injections). In the absence of testicular tissue (the penis must be normally developed), one will find an increased FSH but normal LH in young boys and increased FSH and LH in older boys. Serum testosterone levels will be prepubertal before and after HCG administration. When these rigid criteria are adhered to, it is safe to make the diagnosis of bilateral anorchia in this limited subgroup of patients without significant exploration.

## Torsion

### Spermatic Cord and Testes

Torsion of the testicle is one of the few true emergencies in pediatric urology. It is the most common intrascrotal disorder in boys and requires prompt surgical intervention to avoid testicular necrosis. Testicular torsion must be differentiated from epididymitis and torsion of a testicular appendage, since neither of these requires surgery.

Testicular torsion occurs within the tunica albuginea (intravaginal) or includes the tunica albuginea (extravaginal). Intravaginal torsion is more common and occurs most frequently in early adolescence. It is thought to result from the absence of posterior attachments between the tunica vaginalis and testis that normally stabilize the gonad within the scrotum. Signs of testicular torsion consist of the acute onset of severe hemiscrotal pain, nausea, and vomiting. The attacks may be intermittent. Examination reveals an enlarged tender testis and frequently some degree of scrotal edema. The testis may be noted to have an unusual lateral lie. As time goes on, the intrascrotal elements become confluent, and torsion may be difficult to differentiate from acute or chronic epididymitis. Additional investigations that may be beneficial include a nuclear technetium scan of the testes or Doppler examination of the scrotum to assess testicular blood flow.

Prompt surgical exploration and detorsion is mandatory, as irreversible changes in the testis may occur within 4 hours. If treatment is not prompt, orchiectomy may be required. Because the abnormality (absence of posterior testicular attachment) is often bilateral, a contralateral scrotal orchiopexy should be done whenever an intravaginal torsion is diagnosed.

Extravaginal torsion (torsion of the entire spermatic cord and testis, outside the tunica vaginalis) occurs almost exclusively in neonates and often occurs antenatally. Its etiology may be the lack of adhesions between the scrotum and the testicular membranes. It usually presents as a small, hard, nontender mass replacing the testis in a discolored hemiscrotum. Treatment is controversial, since even prompt surgical exploration will reveal a necrotic testis, and an orchiectomy is universal. Although evidence is lacking to show that the defect is bilateral, most surgeons fix the contralateral testis because the result of a subsequent torsion could be devastating (Fig 110-18).

### Torsion of a Testicular Appendage

Torsion of a testicular appendage must be distinguished from testicular torsion. Unless the diagnosis can be made with confidence, one must pursue a more thorough evaluation or surgically explore the acute scrotum. Often the symptoms of a torsed appendage are less severe than those of a testicular torsion. At times the appendage is palpable in the upper aspect of the scrotum, and if infarcted a pathognomonic blue dot may be visible. Appropriate treatment consists of bed rest; the natural course is slow, steady improvement.

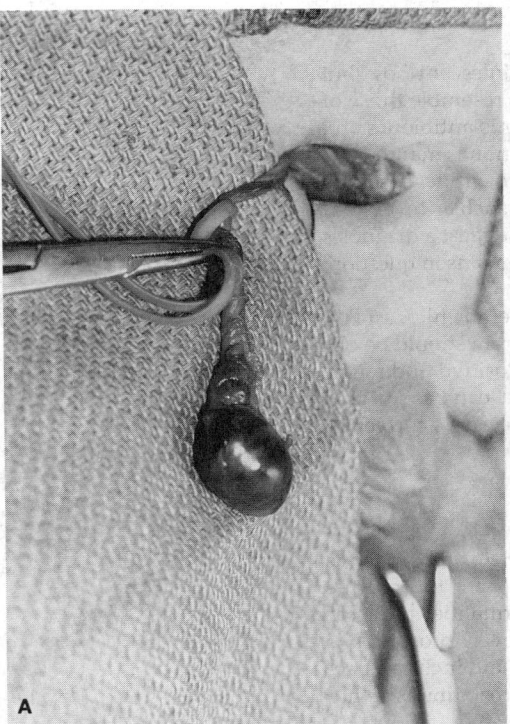 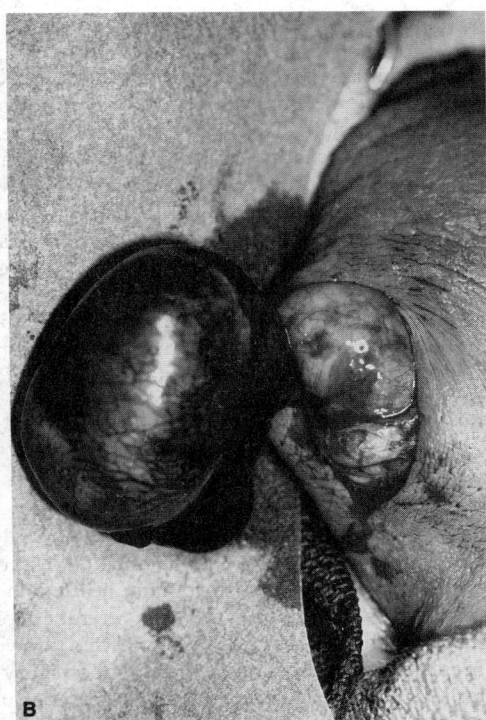

**Figure 110-18.** Testicular torsion. (**A**) Neonatal torsion. Note that the cord twists proximal to the insertion of the tunica vaginalis (extravaginal torsion). (Gonzales ET Jr. Genitourinary disorders in the neonate. In: Whitaker RH, Woodard JR, eds. Paediatric urology. London: Butterworth's, 1985.) (**B**) Intravaginal torsion. The cord twists distal to the vaginal attachments.

## Hydrocele and Hernia

In children, a hernia represents the persistent patency of the processus vaginalis, which normally obliterates before birth. This allows communication of fluid between the scrotum and peritoneum, accounting for both variation in scrotal size and the characteristic inguinal swelling (Fig 110-19). A noncommunicating hydrocele, which is rare in children, represents partial obliteration of the processus vaginalis, leaving a sac of fluid about the testicle but no communication with the peritoneum. A communicating hydrocele is equivalent to a hernia and should be repaired promptly so that incarceration of bowel does not occur. Simple hydroceles, on the other hand, do not need emergency attention; as they tend to resolve spontaneously before age 1, intervention is usually delayed until that time. Reactive hydroceles secondary to infection, trauma, and torsion of an appendage resolve spontaneously and do not need separate attention. In general, the surgical approach to scrotal pathology is through the groin unless an obvious diagnosis of a torsion of the testis or an appendage is made.

## Varicoceles

Varicoceles are the pathologic dilation of the testicular vein and pampiniform plexus, most often on the left side. Their etiology is thought to be an absence of internal spermatic vein valves, which allows a continuous column of blood from the level of the renal vessels to the scrotum. The incidence has been reported to be as high as 15% in adolescent boys, but they are much less common in childhood.

Indications for repair by ligation of the internal spermatic vein are pain, ipsilateral testicular atrophy, or a very large varicocele. Some boys with varicoceles have normal-sized testicles but are found to have abnormalities in testicular hormone function on GnRH stimulation testing. This is considered by some surgeons to be another indication for elective repair. Ipsilateral testicular growth has been reported to increase in adolescents after repair of a varicocele, with subsequent testicular size matching or exceeding that of the contralateral side. In adults, varicoceles are a common cause of infertility, although not all men with varicoceles are so afflicted. It remains unclear whether varicoceles that present in adolescence are more harmful to testicular function and future fertility than varicoceles developing in the adult.

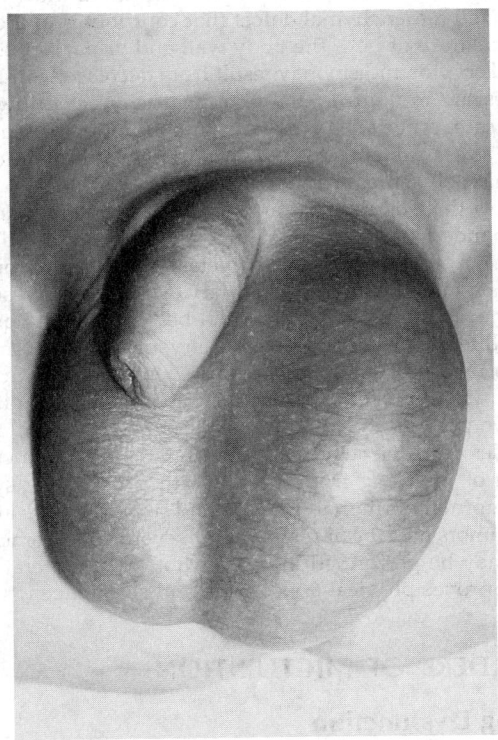

**Figure 110-19.** A large, tense hydrocele.

## Epididymitis

Epididymitis is an unusual finding in a preadolescent boy, but its recognition is important because symptoms resemble those of testicular torsion. The treatment for the former is antibiotics and bed rest; for the latter, prompt surgical exploration is mandatory. The physical findings may be similar for the two entities—scrotal erythema, swelling, and pain. Laboratory data such as fever, leukocytosis, pyuria, and a positive urine culture suggest a diagnosis of epididymitis. Often, because the diagnosis remains in question, a scrotal exploration is done.

Once epididymitis is confirmed in a prepubertal child, an IVP or renal ultrasound and voiding cystourethrogram should be obtained to identify any congenital anomalies. Positive findings—ureteral and vasal abnormalities predominate—can be expected in more than one third of the children. In these cases, correction of the problem often requires surgery.

## Prostatitis

Prostatitis, like epididymitis, is unusual in the sexually inactive male, and investigation for anatomical etiology for the process is appropriate. Again, vasal and ureteral abnormalities predominate. In the sexually active adolescent, however, prostatitis is more common. Prostatitis is a general category and includes bacterial and nonbacterial prostatitis; bacterial prostatitis is either acute or chronic.

The diagnosis of prostatitis is usually made on clinical findings such as perineal pain, dysuria, urinary urgency, or urinary frequency. Fever, back pain, and chills are common in acute bacterial prostatitis but absent in the other forms. Rectal examination may reveal a tender, boggy prostate, and the expressed prostatic secretion often shows leukocytes and macrophages. It may be difficult to differentiate between chronic bacterial and nonbacterial prostatitis, as the findings and symptoms are very similar.

Antimicrobials are the mainstay of treatment for bacterial and nonbacterial prostatitis. Trimethoprim-sulfamethoxazole twice daily or a quinolone in the older child is the preferred therapy for bacterial prostatitis. Prolonged therapy (>30 days) is generally the rule to prevent acute prostatitis from progressing to chronic prostatitis. Treatment of chronic prostatitis may require a course of the same agent for several months. Nonbacterial prostatitis is often more responsive to a course of doxycycline (100 mg twice a day) or minocycline (100 mg twice a day) for several weeks, possibly because chlamydia has been suggested as a causative agent. Warm baths may provide symptomatic relief. Zinc and megavitamins, which have been used in the past, have not shown clinical efficacy.

## PRUNE BELLY SYNDROME

Prune belly syndrome is a rare (one in 30,000 to 40,000) congenital absence of the abdominal musculature associated with severe nonobstructive urinary tract dilation and bilateral intra-abdominal testes. Examination of the newborn usually reveals findings typical of the syndrome that make the diagnosis obvious (Fig 110-20). There is a wide spectrum of involvement, ranging from very minimal changes identifiable only radiographically to a full-blown case manifested as urethral atresia, pulmonary insufficiency, and renal dysplasia. Typical radiographic features include elongated and dilated ureters that cannot produce adequate peristalsis, a large-capacity bladder, and a urachal remnant that in the presence of urethral atresia remains open, forming a patent urachus. The posterior urethra is dilated and the prostate is either absent or hypoplastic. There is often a prominent posterior urethral lip, which is suggestive of posterior urethral valves but is not ob-

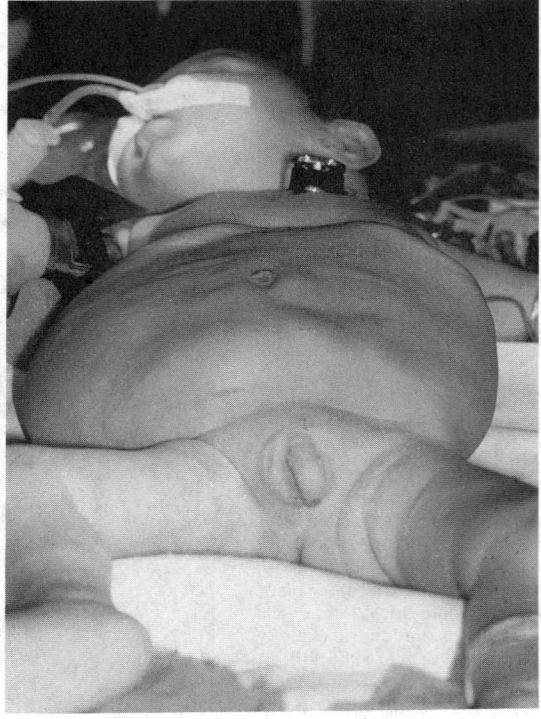

**Figure 110-20.** Typical appearance of a child with prune belly syndrome. (Gonzales ET Jr. Genitourinary disorders in the neonate. In: Whitaker RH, Woodard Jr, eds. Paediatric urology. London: Butterworth's, 1985.)

structive. The penis can be dysplastic, with deficient corpus spongiosum and resultant megalourethra. The kidneys may be dysmorphic, and renal function is often impaired.

The etiology of the prune belly syndrome is thought to be a generalized mesenchymal defect that contributes to the absence of musculature of both the body wall and urinary tract. The associated cryptorchidism may result from decreased intra-abdominal pressure in utero. Initial treatment is directed toward supportive care, especially in patients with pulmonary insufficiency. Despite gross ureteral dilation, true obstruction is uncommon, and renal pelvic pressures are low.

Unless there is urethral atresia, surgical intervention is not recommended in the infant. If infection occurs and is difficult to eradicate, a temporary urinary diversion may be appropriate. In the rare child with anatomical urinary obstruction, a vesicostomy or cutaneous ureterostomies should be considered. Some older boys will require reconstructive surgery, usually performed in an effort to reduce urinary stasis and prevent recurrent urinary infections. These procedures may include ureteral reimplantation, reduction cystoplasty, and urethroplasty. As children grow, orchiopexies are often suggested, although there is no documented incident of offspring from a male with prune belly syndrome despite normal hormonal function and pubertal virilization; testicular tumors have been reported, however. An abdominoplasty, which may be performed in conjunction with ureteral surgery, often improves physical appearance and self-image.

## DISORDERS OF MICTURITION

### Voiding Dysfunction

Abnormal micturition in childhood is not unusual and may take the form of urgency, retention, frequency, dysuria, incontinence, or perineal discomfort. UTI must be ruled out as a cause of these disturbances. Urologic investigation is appropriate in these settings and should include a thorough history, especially a voiding history; physical examination, with emphasis on a possible neurologic etiology for the problem; and urinalysis with culture and sensitivity. If there are no positive findings in a child less than 5 years old, the problem is assumed to be a maturational lag in bladder control, and further investigations are not needed. If the child is older or there are positive findings, appropriate workup and evaluation are necessary. In the older child, a voiding cystourethrogram and some investigation of the upper tracts may be suggested. Some urologists will include urodynamic testing by a cystometrogram and flow rate. If these are negative, maturational delay is suspected, and the treatment, if any, is directed toward symptomatic relief. Medications, usually anticholinergics (oxybutynin, hyoscyamine), have proved to offer significant help to some of these youngsters. Furthermore, because there often is gradual improvement in these symptoms as the children get older, observation alone is a possible approach.

For older children with severe dysfunctional voiding associated with abnormalities revealed by radiographic and urodynamic testing, more involved therapy is indicated both to relieve symptoms and to avoid renal damage. These youngsters may have an abnormal learned response in which the external sphincter contracts in conjunction with a detrusor contraction (bladder-sphincter dyssynergy). This has been termed a "nonneurogenic neurogenic bladder." These children have normal innervation of the bladder and sphincter. The pattern may be difficult to eradicate and requires bladder retraining, usually by biofeedback. The prognosis may be very good, but some children have severe hydroureteronephrosis and renal injury resulting from this disorder. Psychological evaluation and treatment may provide significant help.

## Enuresis

Enuresis is the involuntary loss of urine. Generally, however, it has come to mean the loss of urine during sleep—more appropriately termed "nocturnal enuresis." Enuresis may be either primary or secondary. Primary enuretics have never had a prolonged dry period, whereas secondary enuretics have had a period of at least several months during which they remained dry.

Enuresis was documented in ancient times, and several unusual folk remedies can be found in early medical writings. Its incidence has been estimated to be 15% in 5-year-olds, with a natural resolution rate of about 15% per year. Therefore, by age 10, the incidence has fallen to 5% to 6%, and by age 15 to 1%. The 1% figure remains constant through adulthood. Boys seem to be affected more frequently than girls, and there is a correlation with a family history of enuresis and the child's developmental level at ages 1 and 3. However, factors such as the child's birth order, family's socioeconomic level, maternal and gestational age, changes in parents or residence, and family events have no significant influence on mean age of attaining nocturnal bladder control.

Various theories have been proposed to explain nocturnal enuresis. The most widely accepted is that of delayed maturational control; however, more recent data suggest that some of these patients have an inadequate level of ADH secretion during sleep. Explanations such as sleep disorder, psychological disturbances, transient negative reinforcement, and organic factors are generally discounted, although they may play a role in a specific case.

Appropriate evaluation requires a thorough history, which should include such topics as pattern of wetting, prior UTIs or unexplained high fevers, toilet training (bowel and bladder) history, emotional history, social interactions, and developmental milestones. Especially for males, the physical examination should

include an assessment of the child's urinary stream, either by observation or by a flow rate. The abdominal examination should include a check for the presence of palpable bladder or kidneys. The back examination should include a search for signs of neurologic involvement, such as scoliosis, a sacral dimple, or hairy nevus, that suggest occult spinal dysraphism. A neurologic examination is important; deep tendon reflexes and perineal sensation should be evaluated. During the rectal examination, sphincter tone, bulbocavernosus reflex, and the presence of a sacrum should be evaluated.

The purpose of initial laboratory tests is usually restricted to eliminating infection as a cause of the voiding problem. Therefore, a urinalysis and culture often are the only tests required. For those children with refractory enuresis, a uroradiologic or urodynamic study may be necessary. Additionally, it has been suggested that more involved tests be done for children over 10 years of age.

Many varied and unusual treatments have been proposed, but the first remedy with scientific basis was introduced in the late 19th century. Currently, there are several accepted courses of management. The most successful of these are the use of intranasal desmopressin acetate, behavior modification, and the use of tricyclic antidepressants. Each has advantages and disadvantages. Treatment with imipramine (25 to 50 mg at bedtime) has a success rate of 40% to 60%, but there is a fair degree of recidivism. The physician must be alert for possible side effects: personality changes, GI complaints, nervousness, and sleep disorders. Children appear to be more sensitive than adults to an overdose of this drug, especially cardiac toxicity; therefore, appropriate precautions must be taken to ensure that a younger sibling or patient does not have free access to the medication. If drug therapy is chosen, an adequate trial of several months should be given, but most will respond within the first several days.

The enuresis alarm is the most popular method of behavior modification and gives the best overall success (70% to 90%). It requires more parental support and involvement than medical treatment; often the parent must sleep in the same room for the first week or two of use to ensure that the child is awakened by the alarm. The device consists of two components, the sensor and the sounder. The sensor must be small enough to be positioned near the urethral meatus so that when the child begins micturition, the alarm will sound. Over a period of time (several weeks to months), a conditioned response should occur so that the patient wakes as the bladder gets full before the onset of micturition. A several-month course of treatment is often necessary. As with medical treatment, there is a relapse rate, but it appears to be lower.

Desmopressin acetate, an analogue of vasopressin, has recently been approved by the FDA for use in the treatment of primary nocturnal enuresis. Its efficacy is based on data that show that some enuretics do not experience the normal nocturnal elevation of ADH. Accordingly, the child's nighttime urine remains more dilute and of greater volume than in nonenuretics. The increased volume simply overwhelms the capacity of the bladder, and wetting occurs. By taking an evening intranasal dose of desmopressin acetate (20 to 40 $\mu$g), 70% of enuretics can remain dry overnight. The half-life of the drug is 2 hours and it is gone by morning. Complications are uncommon, but fluids should be restricted after administering the medication to decrease the possibility of water intoxication. A prolonged treatment period of several months is required before attempting to taper the medication. If wetting recurs, desmopressin acetate can be restarted.

Other forms of therapy such as psychotherapy, motivational therapy, and bladder retention training are used, but treatment with either the enuresis alarm, desmopressin acetate, or tricyclic antidepressants holds the greatest promise for those with nocturnal enuresis.

## Selected Readings

Gillenwater JY, Grayhack JT, Howards SS, Duckett JW, eds. Adult and pediatric urology, ed 2. St. Louis: Mosby Year Book, 1991.

Gonzales ET Jr, Roth DR, eds. Common problems in pediatric urology. St. Louis: Mosby Year Book, 1991.

Kelalis PP, King LR, Belman AB, eds. Clinical pediatric urology, ed 2. Philadelphia: WB Saunders, 1985.

Retik AB, Cukier J, eds. Pediatric urology. Baltimore: Williams & Wilkins, 1987.

Stephens FD, ed. Congenital malformations of the urinary tract. New York: Praeger, 1983.

Walsh PC, Gittes RF, Perlmutter AD, Stamey TA, eds. Campbell's urology, ed 5, vol 2. Philadelphia: WB Saunders, 1986.

Whitaker RH, Woodard JR, eds. Paediatric urology. London: Butterworth's, 1985.

Williams DI, et al., eds. Urology in childhood. New York: Springer-Verlag, 1974.

*Principles and Practice of Pediatrics, Second Edition.*
edited by Frank A. Oski et al. J. B. Lippincott Company, Philadelphia © 1994.

# 110.2 Urinary Tract Infection

## David R. Roth and Edmond T. Gonzales, Jr.

The urinary tract ranks second only to the upper respiratory tract as a source of morbidity from bacterial infection in childhood. The neonatal period is the only time that the incidence of male urinary tract infection (UTI) exceeds that of the female. A boy has about a 1% chance of developing an infection during childhood. In male neonates, the incidence of asymptomatic bacilluria is 1.5%, but it decreases to 0.2% by the time boys are of school age. In newborns, the incidence of UTI in uncircumcised boys is about 10 times that of boys who have been circumcised. Still, this is not thought to be an indication for routine circumcision in the newborn, since complications from circumcision potentially negate the benefit of reduced infections. The presence of a foreskin is not currently thought to increase the risk of UTI in older boys. A girl's chance of developing an infection during childhood is close to 3%. Random screening of preschool and school-age girls has shown an incidence of asymptomatic bacilluria in 1%. The incidence peaks between age 2 and 3 years, a time that coincides with toilet training, and then returns to a baseline value of between 1% and 2%.

The signs and symptoms of UTI in an older child are those seen in adults: voiding dysfunction, dysuria, hematuria, incontinence, suprapubic or flank tenderness, lethargy, and fever. In the neonate, however, the symptoms are much more subtle. Weight loss is most often the prominent symptom, followed by irritability, fever, cyanosis, and CNS disorders. Thus, nonspecific complaints or problems should raise the suspicion of a UTI in a newborn but should not lead to hasty conclusions. Fewer than 20% of infants with nonspecific complaints and only 18% of children with specific voiding complaints actually have a UTI.

Documentation of UTI requires that a specimen be properly obtained and cultured. Urinalysis may suggest the presence of an infection, but the final determination should rest on bacterial growth on a culture. Of the several ways to collect an aliquot of urine from a child, the easiest, if a child is toilet-trained, is the midstream clean-catch specimen. If a child is not toilet-trained, that option is unavailable. Three methods remain, each with its advantages and disadvantages. The simplest but least reliable is the U-bag. A negative culture from a U-bag is meaningful, but if the culture grows, the bacteria may be a contaminant from the rectum, skin, or prepuce. Therefore, whenever this method produces a positive culture, the culture should be repeated using a more accurate method. Two other procedures are available; both are somewhat more involved, but each should provide an uncontaminated aliquot of bladder urine. The first is a percutaneous bladder tap. In the neonate and infant, the bladder's intra-abdominal position makes the procedure easier than in older patients. Still, the bladder should be full and preferably palpable. The second method is urethral catheterization. In the small girl, visualizing the urethra may be difficult, but with practice the procedure can be mastered easily. A small feeding tube (5F or 8F) is most appropriate for catheterization. There should be little risk of urethral trauma or introduction of bacteria into the bladder if routine care and antisepsis are used.

Any treatment program should be based on an accurate culture and sensitivity. Consequently, the culture must be obtained before antibiotics are started, because a single dose of medication can give a false-negative result.

UTIs are often divided into categories based on the presumed location of the inflammation. Cystitis is a UTI confined to the bladder, whereas pyelonephritis involves the kidney. Accurate delineation between the two is difficult; clinical signs and symptoms offer the most meaningful clues. High fever, nausea, vomiting, flank pain, and lethargy are usually associated with acute pyelonephritis, whereas dysuria, frequency, urgency, enuresis, suprapubic pain, and a low-grade fever are more common with cystitis, although crossover is common. DMSA renal scanning offers an objective alternative to the subjectivity of clinical acumen, but final determination of the scan's sensitivity is still pending.

Currently, it is recommended that all children with a documented UTI undergo adequate studies to evaluate the anatomy of the urinary tract. Generally, studies should be done to evaluate both the lower tract (urethra and bladder) via voiding cystourethrogram and the upper tracts via renal ultrasound, intravenous pyelogram, or nuclear medicine renal scan. This recommendation is based on the clinical observation that children most likely to sustain renal parenchymal damage from infection are those who have an anatomical defect of the urinary tract. For the older girl with symptoms of simple cystitis, it can be argued that performing only an upper tract study is sufficient because it will reveal any significant pathology. The yield for these evaluations is age- and sex-dependent and ranges up to 50% in young girls with pyelonephritis (primarily from discovery of vesicoureteral reflux). If an anatomical anomaly such as obstruction or reflux is discovered, it must be addressed.

Most UTIs can be treated adequately on an outpatient basis with a 7- to 10-day course of antibiotics. If shorter courses are used, there is a higher recurrence rate. Initial treatment should be begun only after a urine specimen for culture and sensitivity has been obtained. A broad-spectrum generic agent such as amoxicillin (20 to 30 mg/kg/day in three divided doses) or trimethoprim-sulfamethoxazole (1 tsp/10 kg twice a day) is then begun empirically; therapy is adjusted if necessary after the culture and sensitivity results are available. A repeat culture to confirm eradication of the infection should be obtained about 1 week after the completion of treatment. Occasionally a child with severe symptoms accompanying pyelonephritis will require hospitalization for parenteral antibiotics and control of nausea. For the child with frequently recurring infections (at least four per year), a long-term, low-dose daily prophylactic antibiotic is appropriate, usually nitrofurantoin or trimethoprim-sulfamethoxazole at one-quarter to one-half the therapeutic dose. Usually the medications are given for 9 to 12 months. Subsequent follow-up should include regular urinalyses and cultures when indicated.

## CYSTITIS

Most UTIs are limited to involvement of the bladder only. Symptoms are generally local, although they can be socially disabling in older children. Fever can occur, but is usually low-grade and is not associated with systemic toxicity.

The severity of symptoms varies widely, from debilitating frequency and dysuria in some to an apparent lack of symptoms in others. Some authors differentiate between infection (tissue invasion) and infestation (where the organisms are limited to urine), although clear clinical evidence for such a distinction is lacking. Recurrences are common, and in some children they can develop within days of discontinuing antibiotics.

The cause of recurring lower tract infections remains unknown. The belief that urethral obstruction in girls (the so-called "Lyons ring") was a primary anatomical defect and a cause for UTI is no longer accepted, and routine urethral dilation is no longer practiced. Possible factors are an abnormal perineal flora or an abnormality in the glycosaminoglycan layer in the bladder, but neither factor has been shown to be consistently abnormal in controlled studies.

Many children with multiple, rapid recurrences also have symptoms of dysfunctional voiding even when they are not infected, including urgency, frequency, precipitant voiding, and incontinence. When children with dysfunctional voiding are evaluated urodynamically, they have commonly been shown to generate abnormally high voiding pressures. How these parameters might interrelate to cause UTI is unclear, but dysfunctional voiding is currently thought to be a primary cause for the development of bacilluria. The presence of large volumes of residual urine increases the chance that bacteria might establish an infection. Significant postvoiding residual urine might be present in children with large bladder diverticula, neurogenic bladder dysfunction, vesicoureteral reflux, and perhaps dysfunctional voiding.

From a urologic perspective, recurring lower UTI is often viewed as a nuisance, a problem that interferes intermittently with day-to-day activities but rarely if ever results in long-term impairment to urinary tract function. Once it is established that the anatomy is normal, normal renal growth can be anticipated despite numerous symptomatic episodes of cystitis. In most instances, oral antibiotics will resolve the symptoms promptly and sterilize the urine. Occasionally a resistant organism might require parenteral therapy. The decision whether to institute prophylactic antibiotic therapy depends on many factors, but there are no data showing that long-term treatment reduces the long-term risk of recurrences. There is a spontaneous resolution rate throughout childhood, with cessation of most episodes of recurrent infection by puberty.

If the symptoms with each recurrence remain consistent with cystitis, there is no need for repeated invasive evaluations. However, for the child with a persisting problem, it seems prudent to repeat a renal ultrasound every 2 to 3 years to document normal renal growth.

## UPPER TRACT INFECTION

Spread of bacteria into the upper tract is a much more serious problem. First, children with pyelonephritis tend to be very ill and appear toxic. They often require hospitalization for initial control of the fever, nausea, and vomiting. Second, the ultimate outcome may be a focal scar in the renal parenchyma, with subsequent tissue atrophy and loss of segmental renal function.

The potential for bacteria to ascend into the upper urinary tract is a combination of decreased patient resistance and bacterial virulence. While some bacteria can infect the kidney because of their intrinsic virulence, especially those that are P-fimbriated, all bacteria are more likely to cause pyelonephritis rather than cystitis when anatomical abnormalities are present. When children with UTI present with significant fever, 60% are found to

have structural abnormalities, most often vesicoureteral reflux. In addition, children with structural abnormalities are more likely to have pyelonephritis when they have a recurrence than are children who present with symptoms of pyelonephritis but whose initial workup was normal. However, the natural history and ultimate outcome of any episode of pyelonephritis does not seem to differ between children with normal anatomy and those with vesicoureteral reflux.

Acute lobar nephronia is a radiologic diagnosis on the spectrum of renal parenchymal infections ranging from pyelonephritis to renal abscess and ultimately end-stage pyonephrosis. Lobar nephronia is a localized nonliquefactive infection that generally follows the lobular and lobar architecture of the kidney. Its histology is similar to that of pyelonephritis, with acute leukocytic infiltrate, hyperemia, and interstitial edema. Clinical suspicion should arise when a typical pyelonephritis fever curve is prolonged or when the presence of a mass is suggested by upper tract studies. The intravenous pyelogram may suggest a mass by subtle distortion of the renal outline or renal collecting system. The ultrasound may demonstrate a focal or poorly defined region that disrupts the corticomedullary junction. The best diagnostic tool is the CT scan, which shows a wedge-shaped, nonhomogeneous area with poor contrast enhancement.

Treatment for lobar nephronia is prolonged antibiotic therapy, often initiated with parenteral agents and then followed by oral medication, with the drug of choice based on culture results.

Inadequately treated lobar nephronia may progress to renal carbuncle, abscess, or pyonephrosis. These entities are rare and require more extensive therapy. Historically the most common organism has been the staphylococcus, but at present the gramnegative rods predominate. Distinguishing between a carbuncle and an abscess is a matter of degree, with an abscess involving more parenchyma. As with lobar nephronia, the diagnosis requires a high degree of suspicion. Renal ultrasound and CT scanning are the modalities best suited to confirm the diagnosis in a child who has spiking fevers associated with infected urine despite apparently adequate antibiotic treatment. Once the entity is discovered, continuation of antibiotics, combined with drainage of the lesion either percutaneously or surgically, is necessary. Rarely, nephrectomy is required, but in the severely ill child, unresponsive to antibiotics, with a poorly functioning kidney, that procedure should be considered. Once the process has been controlled, the child should be evaluated for both reflux and obstruction as an etiology for the infection.

Not all children who develop pyelonephritis develop renal scars. Among children with vesicoureteral reflux, about 40% have renal scarring. However, most of these scars are noted on their initial evaluation; if additional infections occur, subsequent scarring is often minimal or does not seem to result despite symptoms compatible with renal infection. These observations have led to a theory that the risk of renal scarring depends on the anatomy of the renal papilla. Some papilla ("compound papilla") are more likely to develop severe inflammatory atrophy, and some kidneys have a greater proportion of compound papilla than others. However, the likelihood of developing a renal scar has been shown to correlate with the number of episodes of pyelonephritis.

## CONCLUSION

The recognition of UTI in children requires sufficient workup to place children in categories of "at risk" or "minimal risk." The former are those with structural anomalies, because these children are most likely to develop severe recurrences and renal atrophy. The latter may have multiple recurrences, but with little or no risk of upper tract infection or damage. Their treatment is symptomatic and is driven by social as well as medical factors.

## Selected Readings

Huland H, Busch R. Pyelonephritis scarring in 213 patients with upper and lower urinary tract infections: long-term follow-up. J Urol 1984;132:936.

Jodal U. The natural history of bacteriuria in childhood. Infect Dis Clin North Am 1987;1:713.

Madrigal G, Odio CM, Moks E, et al. Single-dose antibiotic therapy is not as effective as conventional regimens for management of acute urinary tract infections in children. Pediatr Infec Dis J 1988;7:316.

Majd M, Rushton HG, Jantausch B, Wiedermann BL. Relationship among vesicoureteral reflux, P-fimbriated *Escherichia coli*, and acute pyelonephritis in children with febrile urinary tract infection. J Pediatr 1991;119:578.

Parsons CL, Schrom SH, Hanno P, et al. Bladder surface mucin: examination of possible mechanism for its antibacterial effect. Invest Urol 1978;16:196.

Ransley PG. Vesicoureteric reflux: continuing surgical dilemma. Urology 1978;12:246.

Rushton HG, Majd M, Jantausch B, Wiedermann B, Belman AB. Renal scarring following reflux and non-reflux pyelonephritis in children: evaluation with 99m-technetium-dimercaptosuccinic acid scintigraphy. J Urol 1992;147:1327.

Smellie JM, Ransley PG, Normand ICS, et al. Development of new renal scars: a collaborative study. Br Med J 1985;290:1957.

*Principles and Practice of Pediatrics, Second Edition.*
edited by Frank A. Oski et al. J. B. Lippincott Company, Philadelphia © 1994.

CHAPTER 111
# Chronic Renal Failure

Edward C. Kohaut

Two decades ago it was questioned whether any child was a candidate for any form of renal replacement therapy, because the rigors of therapy were not thought to justify the potential benefit. Since that time, dialysis followed by renal transplantation has become routine therapy for the treatment of children with end-stage renal disease (ESRD). The decision is rarely whether to initiate renal replacement therapy, but rather when to do so. Early intervention has become advantageous, placing even more responsibility on the pediatrician to recognize and participate in the treatment of children with renal insufficiency and failure.

The incidence of chronic renal disease in children is unknown, but current data suggest that 1.5 to three children per million population per year develop ESRD. This incidence may increase as more infants with chronic renal failure are recognized and treated.

## SIGNS OF PROGRESSIVE LOSS OF RENAL FUNCTION

The child with chronic renal disease presents in a different manner from a similarly affected adult (Table 111-1). The adult patient with reduced renal function may develop hypertension, edema, and nocturia, but the uremic syndrome is the hallmark of renal failure in most adults. The uremic syndrome includes such nonspecific symptoms as lethargy, drowsiness, itching, nausea, vomiting, and paresthesias. Although at times the pediatrician sees these late symptoms, it is advantageous for the child with renal insufficiency to be diagnosed and to have therapy initiated earlier, when more subtle symptoms occur.

The most common finding that should alert the pediatrician to the possibility of chronic renal disease is growth impairment. Short stature, particularly if associated with other symptoms such as polyuria, frequent bouts of dehydration, salt craving, bone deformities, abnormal tooth development, or anemia, should suggest that the affected patient may have chronic renal disease. A previous history of urinary tract infections or glomerulonephritis adds further support to this suspected diagnosis.

## DEFINITIONS

The nomenclature describing stages of chronic renal disease is confusing. The currently accepted definitions are listed in Table 111-2. The term "impaired renal function" usually refers to an individual who is asymptomatic and has a residual renal function of 40% to 80% of normal. The term "chronic renal insufficiency" (CRI) is associated with a residual function of 25% to 50% of normal. At this level of renal function, distinct biochemical abnormalities may be present only when the patient is stressed. For example, the patient may normally maintain acid–base balance but with stress will develop acidosis. Although serum calcium and phosphorous levels are normal, they remain so at the expense of an elevated serum parathyroid hormone. The child with CRI may develop dehydration early in the course of diarrhea because of reduced renal ability to retain sodium. With this degree of renal impairment, growth is slowed, and although dialysis is not needed, aggressive therapy is indicated.

### TABLE 111-1. Symptoms of Renal Failure

**Symptoms Seen in Adults and Children With CRF**
Hypertension
Edema
Nocturia, polyuria
Lethargy
Itching
Nausea, vomiting
Peripheral neuropathy
Encephalopathy

**Symptoms Unique to Children With CRF**
Growth failure
Bone deformities
Abnormal tooth development
Unexplained dehydration
Salt craving

### TABLE 111-2. Stages of Chronic Renal Disease

| Stage | Residual Renal Function | Symptoms or Metabolic Abnormality |
|---|---|---|
| Impaired renal function | 40% to 80% | None |
| Chronic renal insufficiency (CRI) | 25% to 50% | Asymptomatic; short stature, increased PTH |
| Chronic renal failure (CRF) | <30% | Acidosis, anemia, hypertension, lethargy |
| End-stage renal disease (ESRD) | Usually <10% | Dialysis needed to maintain quality of life |

The term "chronic renal failure" (CRF) is used to describe a patient who has residual renal function of less than 30%. The patient with CRF exhibits biochemical abnormalities even when not stressed. This patient usually has renal osteodystrophy, acidosis, and anemia; hypertension may be present. Vigorous therapeutic regimens may or may not successfully control these biochemical abnormalities.

"End-stage renal disease" is a term reserved for that stage of disease when renal replacement therapy, whether it be dialysis or transplantation, is required. The degree of renal function at which dialysis or transplantation is required varies and depends on many factors, including the cause of renal failure, age of the patient, and the patient's compliance with conservative therapy. Uremia is a symptom complex that includes anorexia, nausea, itching, neuropathy, and malaise. This is not associated with any specific concentration of urea in the blood but usually is considered to be the last stage of renal failure.

## ETIOLOGY

The etiologies of chronic renal failure in children are listed in Table 111-3. Most authors agree that different forms of obstructive uropathy are collectively the most common cause of renal failure in children. Other relatively common causes of ESRD in children that are rare in adults include renal hypoplasia/dysplasia, hereditary nephritis, infantile polycystic disease, cystinosis, and uremic medullary cystic disease. Focal glomerulosclerosis is the most common glomerulopathy leading to renal failure in young children, but older children may suffer from many forms of chronic glomerulonephritis.

## ABNORMALITIES ASSOCIATED WITH LOSS OF RENAL FUNCTION

With progressive loss of renal function, many metabolic changes occur (Table 111-4). The inability of patients with CRI to tolerate excess protein or nitrogen intake is well recognized. The measure of blood urea nitrogen (BUN) is a function of dietary protein intake and renal clearance. Therefore, if protein intake remains constant as renal function declines, the BUN will increase. As blood urea concentration increases, urinary urea clearance will increase until a steady state is achieved. Therefore, the patient with a BUN of 60 mg/dL will remain in nitrogen balance. However, the cost of achieving nitrogen balance is a high blood concentration of urea and other nitrogenous wastes. When these levels become excessive, uremic symptoms occur. Uremia may lead to anorexia, with a subsequent reduction in protein intake and a fall in BUN. This change can lead less experienced physicians to think that the patient is improving when actually he or she is becoming malnourished, a condition that will further complicate the disease process. The BUN at which uremic symptoms occur depends on the patient's age, nutritional status, state of hydration, and the presence or absence of other metabolic abnormalities.

With further loss of renal function, phosphorus excretion falls. This may cause transient hyperphosphatemia and secondary hypocalcemia. The kidney produces 1,25-dihydroxycholecalciferol, the most active metabolite of vitamin D. Its synthesis is reduced in patients with renal insufficiency, which results in reduced intestinal calcium absorption and hypocalcemia. Hyperphosphatemia associated with reduced calcium absorption results in low serum calcium. The relative contribution of these two is unknown; however, the net result of both is a lowered level of serum calcium, which then stimulates secretion of parathyroid hormone (PTH). Increased serum PTH suppresses proximal tubular reabsorption of phosphorus and normalizes serum phosphorus, but also causes reabsorption of calcium and phosphorus from bone. This effect, coupled with decreased calcification of bone due to reduction in vitamin D activity, leads to renal osteodystrophy. Renal osteodystrophy in children is a combination of the pathologic changes seen with rickets and secondary hyperparathyroidism. Rickets occurs only in growing bone; therefore, the ricketic component of renal osteodystrophy is present only in children.

As reduction in renal function progresses, hydrogen ion balance becomes positive. Normally, more than half the hydrogen ion excreted by the kidney is in the form of ammonium. Ammonia is produced by renal tubular cells and excreted into the tubular lumen. When hydrogen ion is available, ammonia ($NH_3$) becomes ammonium ($NH_4$). This positively charged polar molecule resists reabsorption and is excreted in the urine. With further loss of nephron mass, there is less and less ammonia produced, thereby decreasing hydrogen ion excretion. Thus, early in the course of renal failure, the patient may maintain a urinary pH that is acid while having reduced hydrogen ion excretion.

The second major buffer involved in acid excretion is phosphate. Because phosphate balance is maintained until relatively late in the course of renal failure, hydrogen ion excretion by this mechanism continues until the end-stage of the disease. As residual renal function decreases, there is a greater need to increase sodium excretion through the few remaining nephrons. This may be accomplished in some patients only by suppressing proximal tubular sodium reabsorption. If suppression occurs, then bicarbonate reabsorption from the proximal tubules also must be reduced, resulting in increased bicarbonate excretion, an alkaline urine pH, and worsening of acidosis.

Sodium intolerance in patients with CRF is well recognized. However, some children with CRF secondary to obstructive uropathy or cystic diseases may not be able to conserve sodium. Children with loss of renal function must maintain sodium intake within a narrow range. A normal adult may tolerate a dietary sodium intake of 2 to 1000 mEq per day. A patient with CRF and only 10% residual renal function may become sodium-depleted if dietary intake is less than 40 mEq per day. Conversely,

---

**TABLE 111-3. Etiology of CRF in Children\***

Obstructive uropathy, including reflux nephropathy or renal dysplasia secondary to obstruction

Renal hypoplasia/dysplasia

Glomerulopathy/glomerulonephritis (all forms)

Hereditary disease, including hereditary nephritis or renal cystic diseases

\* In order of frequency

---

**TABLE 111-4. Metabolic Abnormalities Associated with CRF**

Elevated BUN–protein intolerance

Decreased phosphate excretion

Decreased sodium excretion

Reduced ability to conserve sodium

Decreased hydrogen ion excretion

Decreased potassium excretion

Reduced production of 1,25-dihydroxycholecalciferol

Reduced production of erythropoietin

the same patient may become hypertensive if sodium intake exceeds 80 mEq per day.

Potassium balance can become positive in patients with CRF. Hyperkalemia usually is not seen until residual renal function is well below 10% of normal. Hyperkalemia may be seen earlier in the course of CRF if the patient is sodium-depleted. Hyperkalemia may occur with greater than 10% residual function in the rare patient who has defective renin release secondary to renal damage. Hypokalemia can occur in some patients with CRF because of renal potassium wasting, but usually results from anorexia, emesis, and inadequate potassium intake.

Anemia, a well-known consequence of CRF, is the result of defective erythropoietin production by the damaged kidney. Patients with renal failure also have reduced GI absorption of iron. Therefore, when evaluating these patients, iron deficiency as a cause for anemia must be considered. Exogenous erythropoietin is now available; through its use and avoidance of iron deficiency, the anemia of CRF can be reversed.

Neuropathy is a recognized part of the uremic syndrome. In children, especially infants, this consequence of CRF is of special importance. CRF early in life may delay brain development and lead to permanent neurologic impairment. Careful neurologic and frequent developmental evaluation of these children is required. Decisions concerning the timing of dialysis or transplantation may depend on the results of these examinations.

## TREATMENT

Once CRF is recognized and the physiology of lost renal function is understood, treatment is required. The nondialytic treatment of a child with renal insufficiency is in a state of flux. Numerous changes in recommended therapy have been made over the past few years and will continue to be made as more information becomes available about the metabolic abnormalities and the requirements for growth in these children (Table 111-5).

Changing dietary intake is one of the more important therapeutic interventions in children with CRF. However, these changes are very difficult to implement and almost impossible to monitor. Two of the earliest signs of CRF are lethargy and reduced exercise tolerance. These symptoms may be a primary manifestation of retained uremic toxins or may result from anorexia, poor caloric intake, and an energy deficit. In children with CRF,

### TABLE 111-5.  Nondialytic Therapy of CRI/CRF

**Diet**
Provide at least 100% RDA caloric intake
Protein intake controversial; range 0.5–1.5 g/kg/d

**Renal Osteodystrophy**
1,25-dihydroxycholecalciferol (dose variable)
Calcium carbonate (as a calcium supplement and PO₄ binder)

**Anemia**
May require iron
Erythropoietin

**Hypertension**
Control sodium intake
If hyperreninemic, consider ACE inhibitor

**Acidosis**
May improve with reduced protein intake
Sodium citrate or NaHCO₃, 2–4 mEq/kg/d

it is difficult to differentiate symptoms of uremia from those that may be secondary to poor nutrition. Caloric intake of at least 100% of the recommended dietary allowance (RDA) for age should be provided to children with CRF. Dietary supplements may be required to reach this goal. Although increased caloric intake is recommended, it may not be used properly. Many dietary supplements used in the treatment of CRF contain glucose or simple carbohydrates. A relative glucose intolerance secondary to peripheral resistance to insulin may develop as renal failure progresses. Early in renal insufficiency, this defect is overcome by an enhanced insulin production; thus, hyperglycemia is avoided at the expense of hyperinsulinemia. Later in the course of the disease, hyperglycemia may develop, since even high levels of insulin cannot overcome the peripheral insensitivity to insulin. Serum glucose levels should be monitored when carbohydrate supplements are given. This relative glucose intolerance also may cause hypertriglyceridemia.

Patients with CRF may develop hyperlipidemia if fats are used as a caloric supplement instead of glucose. Whether this causes increased morbidity in infants and children is unknown.

Dietary protein intake is the most controversial aspect of nutritional therapy of patients with chronic renal disease. Patients with CRF do not use protein normally; therefore, one could argue that they require a greater protein intake than children without renal failure to sustain normal growth and development. However, increased protein intake can accelerate the loss of residual renal function and the need for renal replacement therapy. The optimum dietary protein intake for a child with renal failure may be very low (0.3 g/kg/day), and this quantity may need to be supplemented with an essential amino acid mixture to sustain nitrogen balance. From a practical standpoint, this is difficult to accomplish and can be expensive. Until studies provide answers to this dilemma, we recommend a diet containing proteins of high biological value providing 0.5 to 1.5 g/kg/day.

The management of renal osteodystrophy in children with CRI is extremely important. If left untreated, these children will develop severe limb deformities and certainly will grow poorly. They may develop symptomatic bone pain and metaphyseal fractures. In the past 15 years, there has been a significant advancement in the understanding of vitamin D metabolism. Two very important steps in the synthesis of active vitamin D metabolites are known to occur in the kidney. Vitamin D can undergo hydroxalation at both the 1 and 24 position in the renal interstitium. Renal hydroxalation leads to the formation of 1,25-dihydroxycholecalciferol, which recently has been synthesized and is available for use in patients with CRF. Its availability has made the treatment of renal osteodystrophy safer and more effective. In the past, both adults and children with CRI were treated with aluminum hydroxide gels to bind dietary phosphates and reduce absorption in an attempt to maintain phosphate balance. However, intake of aluminum by children with renal insufficiency has recently been shown to cause toxicity. Aluminum toxicity should be suspected in patients who have had significant intake and develop unusual, unexplained neurologic symptoms, or in children who have unexpected worsening of renal osteodystrophy. Aluminum toxicity should also be suspected in children with CRF who become hypercalcemic with therapeutic doses of vitamin D. Aluminum-containing phosphate binders are no longer recommended for use in this setting. Many authors now recommend the use of calcium carbonate, which can serve both as a phosphate binder and a source of additional dietary calcium; the latter is deficient in the diets of most patients with CRF. With the timely initiation of therapy with 1,25-dihydroxycholecalciferol and calcium carbonate, many of the adverse effects of renal osteodystrophy can be minimized.

Treatment of the anemia associated with chronic renal disease is difficult, and a cure may be impossible. As stated before, many children with CRF become iron-deficient secondary to persistent microscopic blood loss in stools and to low dietary iron intake. If iron deficiency is present, it should be corrected; however, the anemia usually persists despite iron therapy. One of the many functions of the kidney is to produce erythropoietin, and this is lost in patients with severe renal damage. Without this hormone, erythrocyte production is reduced and a hypoplastic anemia results. Recombinant human erythropoietin is now available for the treatment of children with CRF. This agent corrects the anemia in patients with CRF and thus eliminates the need for costly and potentially dangerous blood transfusions.

Hypertension is a common sign of progressive loss of renal function and most often results from excessive blood volume. The most effective treatment is to reduce sodium intake or to increase sodium excretion. Patients with renal failure become intolerant of both excessively high and low sodium intakes. If sodium restriction is too rigid, the patient may become hypovolemic, and this can exacerbate other signs of CRF. Sodium intake must be adjusted carefully to avoid both of these extremes. Occasionally, patients with CRF develop hypertension that is not volume-related but is due rather to an excessive production of renin. These children can be treated successfully with an angiotensin-converting enzyme inhibitor that will block the conversion of angiotensin I to angiotensin II, lower peripheral resistance, and normalize blood pressure. When the patient with CRF develops hypertension, especially because of excessive blood volume, it may mean the child will soon require dialysis.

Patients with progressive loss of renal function frequently develop metabolic acidosis. This can occur early in the course when obstructive uropathy is the cause of CRF. Acidosis may cause anorexia, vomiting, lethargy, growth failure, and other symptoms that mimic uremia. Correction with alkali therapy may reverse many of the above symptoms and delay the need for renal replacement therapy. The base can be given as sodium bicarbonate or sodium citrate, usually in a dosage of 1 to 2 mEq/kg/day. Potassium salts may be used occasionally in the rare patient with CRF who also loses potassium. When the child with CRF can no longer tolerate the use of sodium buffers and, therefore, acidosis cannot be corrected, renal replacement therapy may be indicated.

Classical uremic neuropathy is rarely seen in children. If it is noted, vigorous protein restriction may give temporary relief; however, this finding would surely indicate the need for renal replacement therapy.

## GROWTH FAILURE

Growth failure is a common and often untreatable consequence of CRF in children. Growth failure is particularly severe in children who develop renal insufficiency in the first year of life. Infants with CRF grow poorly between birth and age 2. Even if normal growth velocity can be achieved from age 2 onward, so much growth potential has been lost that dwarfism is the result. Growth retardation could be avoided if catch-up growth were achieved after successful renal replacement therapy. However, accelerated growth only rarely occurs after a successful renal transplant. To affect growth in this population, early recognition of CRF is essential.

To correct growth failure, one must attempt to correct all the metabolic abnormalities mentioned. Adequate dietary intake is important, especially in infants with renal failure. Recently, several infants with CRF were identified early in life and aggressive nutritional therapy was initiated. Dietary intake was given by tube feedings (either nasogastric or transpyloric) in an amount to provide at least 100% of the RDA for calories and 1 to 2 g/kg/day of protein. Although data are sparse, near-normal growth

has been achieved in some patients. Providing adequate nutrition to older dialysis patients has also affected growth favorably.

Many children with CRF cannot conserve sodium. If sodium is restricted in these patients, poor growth may result; conversely, greater sodium intake by these patients will improve growth. Acidosis is often a complication of CRF, and correction and control of the acidosis is essential to normal growth in this population. Early and aggressive therapy of renal osteodystrophy with vitamin D metabolites and calcium carbonate is required for optimal growth in these children. The anemia seen secondary to CRF may slow growth in these patients. Growth potential can be improved by careful attention to maintaining acid–base, electrolyte, and water balance in these patients. Treating renal osteodystrophy and providing adequate nutrition are essential in maintaining normal growth velocity. It has been suggested that children with CRF may have improved growth when given supraphysiologic doses of recombinant human growth hormone, and early published results of the use of this therapy are encouraging.

## Selected Readings

Andreoli SP, Bergstein JM, Sheppard DJ. Aluminum intoxication from aluminum containing phosphate binders in children with azotemia not undergoing dialysis. New Engl J Med 1984;310:1079.

Betts PR, McGrath G. Growth pattern and dietary intake in children with chronic renal insufficiency. Br Med J 1972;2:189.

Chantler C, Holliday M. Progressive loss of renal function. In: Holliday MA, Barratt TM, Vernier RL, eds. Pediatric nephrology, ed 2. Baltimore: Williams & Wilkins, 1987:773.

Chesney RW, Mehls O, Anast CS, et al. Renal osteodystrophy in children: the role of vitamin D, phosphorus, and parathyroid hormone. Am J Kidney Dis 1986;7:275.

Polinsky MS, Kaiser BA, Stover JB, Frankenfield M, Baluarte HJ. Neurologic development of children with severe chronic renal failure from infancy. Pediatr Nephrol 1987;1:157.

Rizzoni G, Broyer M, Guest G, Fine R, Holliday MA. Growth retardation in children with chronic renal disease: scope of the problem. Am J Kidney Dis 1986;7:256.

Wassner SJ, Abitbol C, Alexander S, et al. Nutritional requirements for infants with renal failure. Am J Kidney Dis 1986;7:300.

*Principles and Practice of Pediatrics, Second Edition.*
edited by Frank A. Oski et al. J. B. Lippincott Company, Philadelphia © 1994.

## CHAPTER 112
# *End-Stage Renal Disease*

### Edward C. Kohaut

## DIALYSIS

It is often difficult to decide when to initiate dialytic therapy in the child with chronic renal failure. There is no given level of serum creatinine or creatinine clearance used as an absolute guide to the need for dialysis. Most children who require dialysis will have residual renal functions of less than 10% of normal. However, even within this group there is a variable need for dialytic therapy. When the child nearing end-stage renal disease (ESRD) no longer can function normally, is lethargic, cannot attend school, and has a poorer quality of life, dialytic therapy is indicated. Poor or absent growth may be an indication for considering dialysis, although growth may not normalize after dialysis is initiated. If it is found that the use of supraphysiologic doses of recombinant human growth hormone will normalize growth velocity in children with ESRD, then poor growth velocity will no longer be an indication for dialysis. Indications for infant dialysis may be different and will be discussed separately.

## Hemodialysis

Hemodialysis is a process by which blood is passed over an artificial semipermeable membrane, allowing the transfer of small molecules from the blood into surrounding dialysate. The rate of solute transfer depends on the concentration gradient of the solute, the blood flow over the membrane, and the permeability of the membrane to the solute. Water movement across the membrane is a function of hydraulic pressure. Hemodialysis is a relatively efficient process. Blood flows of 100 mL/minute through the dialyzer are possible, even in small patients. At that rate, using modern dialyzers, urea can be cleared at 70 to 80 mL/minute. Thus, during the treatment the patient will have almost normal renal function. However, it is impractical to hemodialyze a child for more than 4 to 5 hours, three times a week. Aggressive hemodialysis performed for 15 hours a week would be equivalent to only 10% of normal renal function. This is an important point and should be stressed to children with renal failure and their parents. There is often the expectation that once placed on dialysis, everything will return to normal; that certainly is not the case.

### Vascular Access

Vascular access has always been a particular problem for children undergoing hemodialysis. The blood vessel used must be large enough to permit the blood flow necessary for effective dialysis. In the small, frequently malnourished child with renal failure, femoral vessels are often the only option for vascular access. A Scribner shunt placed in the femoral vessels until recently had been the most common form of access in small children; large vessels were used and high blood flows could be obtained. With this means of treatment, an external shunt with polyethylene tubing runs from the blood vessel through the skin, and it can be a chronic source of infection and irritation. These shunts often malfunction because of clots, require revision, and rarely function more than a few months. However, they were useful because many children require only a few months of dialysis before renal transplantation.

Subclavian catheters have been used recently for semipermanent vascular access. This advance, coupled with the development of single-needle dialysis technology, has reduced the need for external shunts. Although the possibility of infection is still present, these newer catheters can be removed easily and a new one inserted at another site if infection is suspected. With this method there is no loss of vascular integrity. Some programs have even used subclavian catheters to hemodialyze infants. If it is suspected that the patient will require long-term hemodialysis, then a subcutaneous access should be created. This usually is done by forming an arteriovenous fistula (the anastomosis of an artery directly to a vein) or by placing a graft (using a foreign material, usually polytetrafluoroethylene, to connect an artery to a vein). Either procedure usually provides many years of access for hemodialysis. Ideally, these procedures should be performed in the upper extremity, usually the forearm, but in smaller children grafts may have to be placed in the femoral vessels to achieve adequate blood flow.

Some of the major complications of hemodialysis are related to access devices. External shunts can be displaced by an active child, and this may result in massive bleeding. Even subcutaneous access devices can bleed from trauma, although trauma more often causes hematomas around the vessels, which may lead to compression and loss of flow or thrombosis. Infection was a common complication in patients with transcutaneous (Scribner) shunts, and it remains a problem with subclavian catheter access. Infection is uncommon when subcutaneous access is used, but strict sterile technique must be used when entering the vessels. These devices also may become infected when a patient becomes bacteremic. It may be wise to give prophylactic antibiotics before procedures when bacteremia can be expected (eg, dental procedures). Despite our best efforts, shunts and fistulas thrombose more frequently in children than in adults. This difference presumably is related to the smaller vessels and relatively lower blood flow in children. The pediatrician caring for these children should always examine these access devices and be aware of the frequent complications associated with them.

### Procedure

The hemodialysis procedure itself is technically more demanding in children than in adults. The size of the dialyzer and blood tubing should be determined by the patient's blood volume. Ideally no more than 10% of the child's blood volume should be in the extracorporeal circuit. Unfortunately, dialysis equipment and supplies are produced for the larger adult market, and compromises or innovations are required to meet the requirements for small children.

Another major complication of hemodialysis is a result of its efficiency. The child may begin dialysis with an elevated blood urea nitrogen (BUN) level that, with a large, efficient dialyzer, is lowered rapidly, leading to a sharp reduction in extracellular osmolality. If an equally rapid reduction in intracellular osmolality of brain cells does not follow, this will result in cerebral edema; this is termed *dysequilibrium syndrome*. This syndrome includes headache, abdominal pain, nausea, vomiting, and muscle cramps, followed by convulsions and coma. The syndrome can be avoided if urea clearances are restricted to 3 or, at the most, 4 mL/min/kg. Disequilibrium syndrome is seen more often in pediatric centers because of the availability of dialyzers that are more efficient than needed for the patient's size. Despite this, pediatric nephrologists have developed the required strategies to avoid this syndrome in even the smallest of patients.

Hypotension is a common complication of hemodialysis and occurs more frequently in children than in adults. During the hemodialysis procedure, excess fluid is removed from the extracellular fluid space, where it has accumulated since the last dialysis session. If blood volume is reduced rapidly and equilibration from the remaining extracellular fluid space is slow, hypovolemia will usually result. Normally, this would be compensated for by an increase in peripheral vascular resistance, thus maintaining a normal blood pressure. However, vascular tone is deficient during dialysis and hypotension often results. The lack of response of peripheral vessels to hypovolemia is thought to be due to activation of certain vasoactive substances by exposure of blood to the dialysis membrane. Less biologically active dialysis membranes are being studied. The incidence of hypotension can be limited by slow, regular removal of fluid.

There are many other complications of the dialysis procedure, including sudden death from many causes. The incidence of mechanical complication can be lowered by careful equipment maintenance and an ever-vigilant nursing staff. This supervision is especially important when dialyzing small children whose inquiring minds and busy fingers may not be aware of the dangers surrounding them.

At an experienced pediatric dialysis center, symptom-free dialysis of even the smallest child is possible. It is more difficult to achieve this goal if interdialytic salt and water intake have caused such excessive changes in body composition that vigorous dialysis cannot be avoided. Most centers limit the protein intake of children treated with hemodialysis to 1 g/kg/day, with variability based on age and the needs of individual patients. Sodium intake is restricted to less than 1.5 mEq/kg/day. This may be too low for some patients with residual function and salt wasting. High-potassium foods should be avoided, and specific potassium restrictions are sometimes required. Some children treated with hemodialysis chronically have large water intakes. They should be encouraged to limit fluids to 1 to 1.5 L/m²/day.

### Adjunctive Therapy

Many of the therapeutic recommendations discussed in Chapter 111 for children with chronic renal failure who do not yet require dialysis also apply to children treated with hemodialysis. As has already been discussed, certain dietary restrictions are required in the management of these patients, but more of the chronic complications noted in these children are related to malnutrition than to dietary noncompliance. After a vigorous hemodialysis treatment, children may be anorexic secondary to the disequilibrium syndrome; then, as the concentration of uremic toxins rises before the next dialysis, they may become anorexic from uremia. This anorexic cycle leads to malnutrition, which may perpetuate poor intake. Poor dietary protein intake can cause a fall in the BUN, which may lead a less experienced physician to think that the patient is getting improved dialysis when actually the child is becoming malnourished. Malnutrition causes muscle wasting and a reduction in creatinine, which again can suggest improved dialysis when actually the patient's health is failing. Careful and frequent dietary assessments must be made and caloric dietary supplements encouraged if energy intake falls below 100% of recommended dietary allowance (RDA). Protein supplements are occasionally needed in severely anorexic patients. Too little protein intake is as harmful as too much in children treated with hemodialysis.

Dietary phosphate intake must also be reduced. In the past, phosphate absorption was decreased by the use of aluminum hydroxide phosphate binders. This is no longer recommended, because patients receiving dialysis may develop aluminum toxicity, manifested by dementia or worsening of renal osteodystrophy. Calcium carbonate, now recommended as a replacement for aluminum hydroxide, acts as both a phosphate binder and a calcium supplement. Vitamin supplements are required by children with ESRD who are treated with hemodialysis, including the need for 1,25-dihydroxycholecalciferol supplementation. Folate and other water-soluble vitamins are removed by hemodialysis; therefore, intake of a daily multivitamin supplement with folate is recommended.

### Results

The treatment of the larger child with hemodialysis is usually successful. Dialyzing small infants remains difficult, although limited data suggest success. The mortality rate associated with hemodialysis is very low in children weighing more than 15 kg who are treated at a pediatric dialysis center. However, this is not to say that improvement is unnecessary. Children treated with hemodialysis rarely grow normally and have great difficulty maintaining a reasonably normal life. Children have not been recommended for home hemodialysis treatment in the past, and hemodialysis performed in a specialized center results in a disrupted school schedule and reduced peer interaction. However, when this therapy is performed in a pediatric unit dedicated to the needs of chronically ill children, patients who for medical or social reasons cannot be treated with home therapy can thrive while being treated with hemodialysis.

## Peritoneal Dialysis

The use of peritoneal dialysis as a renal replacement therapy for children has a relatively short history. In the 1950s and 1960s peritoneal dialysis was used to treat acute renal failure. Treatment of chronic renal failure with peritoneal dialysis was unsuccessful until reliable peritoneal access was developed in the late 1960s. At that time, several pediatric programs using intermittent peritoneal dialysis were developed. Because of the parallel development of a more efficient therapy (hemodialysis), intermittent peritoneal dialysis never was used widely to treat chronic renal failure in either children or adults.

### CAPD and CCPD

In 1976, a new form of peritoneal dialysis that later became known as continuous ambulatory peritoneal dialysis (CAPD) was described. CAPD overcomes the relative inefficiency of the peritoneal membrane by exposing it continually to dialysate. In the early 1980s, this form of dialysis was introduced as a form of therapy for children with chronic renal failure. In 1981, another form of continuous peritoneal dialysis was introduced and subsequently was named continuous cycling peritoneal dialysis (CCPD). CCPD has been adapted more recently to children with ESRD. The descriptions of CAPD and CCPD have rekindled the interest of many pediatric nephrologists in peritoneal dialysis.

Both CAPD and CCPD are forms of dialysis that can be done at home. CAPD is a manual process. The patient or caretaker attaches a bag of sterile dialysate to a tube and it enters the peritoneal cavity. This fluid remains there for 3 to 5 hours and then is drained into the same bag, which is discarded, and a new bag is aseptically attached to the tubing. This procedure is repeated three or four times a day and a single 8-hour session is performed at night. CCPD is very similar, except that the rapid filling and emptying is performed by a cycling device at night and there is a single long dwell during the day. The patient is fully ambulatory during the daytime with either procedure.

These two forms of continuous peritoneal dialysis have been a major advance in the treatment of children with ESRD. They have provided forms of therapy that can be implemented at home, permitting the patient to attend school and have relatively normal peer interactions. Both forms of therapy are less costly than in-center hemodialysis, and either one can be used to treat even the smallest infant. The major disadvantage of CAPD is that it is labor-intensive. The caretaker, usually a parent, must be available to exchange a bag of dialysate every 4 to 5 hours during the day. Each bag exchange may take from 20 to 40 minutes, depending on how rapidly the fluid drains from the abdomen. Many parents may tire of this procedure after a period of time. CCPD is less demanding, and the caretaker must do only two procedures: at bedtime, attaching the tubing from the patient's peritoneal cavity to the cycling device, and in the morning, disconnecting the patient from the cycling device.

CAPD and CCPD are comparable in their efficacy of controlling the abnormal metabolic values associated with ESRD. Clearances of low-molecular-weight substances are similar with CAPD and CCPD. Clearance of middle molecules and higher-molecular-weight toxins may be slightly improved with CAPD. The major disadvantage of CCPD is the fact that the patient must have a cycling device available, and this decreases mobility because the device is not portable. Since CAPD and CCPD are so similar, there is no reason why both procedures cannot be taught to the same patient or parent. One may, on some days, take advantage of decreased labor involved in CCPD, and on other days use the mobility provided by CAPD. The rest of this discussion will treat these two forms of therapy as interchangeable, since most of the complications and problems associated with them are similar.

Both therapies require peritoneal access, usually by surgical placement of a Tenckhoff catheter. The catheter usually enters the peritoneal cavity at the lateral edge of the rectus muscle. A purse-string suture is placed around the peritoneal membrane, making as watertight a seal as possible. A Dacron cuff is placed at the entrance site of the peritoneal membrane. The catheter is then tunneled under the skin, exiting through the skin at some distance from where the catheter enters the peritoneum. The catheter should be placed by a surgeon who understands the unique problems of children with ESRD, because the procedure differs in many respects from that performed on adults.

As with other forms of dialysis, access is more of a problem in children than adults. Children have more omentum than adults. A possible complication resulting from this difference is outflow obstruction caused by a piece of omentum wrapping around the catheter. To avoid this complication, many pediatric programs advise partial or even total removal of the omentum at the time of catheter placement. Dialysate leakage is another complication seen at a higher rate in children than adults, and this is thought to be caused by a relative decrease in the quantity of subcutaneous tissue in children. Leakage of dialysate has been minimized by using the peritoneal purse-string suture and by placing the catheter at the lateral edge of the rectus muscle.

### Complications

Hernias may occur when patients begin therapy with continuous dialysis, or they may develop later in the course of therapy due to persistently increased intra-abdominal pressure. These hernias usually can be repaired, and although patients may need to receive hemodialysis for a short period, they can return to peritoneal dialysis. Some programs advise that the abdomen be left empty during the day if hernias recur. This causes a significant reduction in total clearance.

The most common complication of peritoneal dialysis is peritonitis. It usually is diagnosed by the caretaker, who notes cloudy effluent dialysate. Most often the patient is infected with coagulase-negative staphylococcus, is rarely seriously ill, and is treated at home with intraperitoneal antibiotics. If peritonitis is not diagnosed and treated quickly, or if the patient is infected with a gram-negative organism, then a more serious illness may result. If antibiotics cannot sterilize the peritoneal fluid, or if the patient develops recurrent infection, then removal of the peritoneal catheter may become necessary. Frequent peritonitis may cause the patient to choose another form of dialysis. Some nephrologists may advise patients to seek another means of therapy if the incidence of peritonitis is high.

### Adjunctive Therapy

Adjunctive therapy for the child treated with peritoneal dialysis is similar to that advised for patients treated with hemodialysis. One of the advantages of peritoneal dialysis is a relatively high clearance of middle- and high-molecular-weight toxins. Unfortunately, the peritoneal membrane is not selective, and loss of vital large molecules such as protein also occurs. Therefore, when patients are treated with peritoneal dialysis, protein intake must be increased. Water-soluble vitamins and vitamin D metabolites are lost through the peritoneal membrane, and patients sustained by these forms of dialysis must supplement their diets with the active form of vitamin D and multivitamins.

### Results

Many children have been treated with various forms of peritoneal dialysis. The advantages and disadvantages of each method are

| TABLE 112-1.    Advantages of CAPD and CCPD | |
|---|---|
| **CAPD** | **CCPD** |
| Mobility | Less time-consuming |
| No machine | No daytime pass |
| Simple procedure | Reduced protein loss? |
| Less costly | Reduced incidence of hernia and peritoneal leaks? |
| Higher solute clearances | |

listed in Table 112-1. No one form of dialysis can be recommended for all patients, and each potential method of therapy must be judged according to how it can benefit each individual patient. The goal for every child with ESRD is to have a well-functioning renal allograft. The treatments described are both a means to reach that goal and a support when circumstances make transplantation impossible.

## Treatment of the Small Infant With ESRD

Aggressive treatment of a young infant with renal insufficiency may stimulate as many emotional, ethical, and economic issues as questions pertinent to medical therapy. Until recently the approach to the young infant was to provide nondialytic therapy of variable aggressiveness until the infant survived to a certain age or size when dialysis or renal transplantation were thought possible. Unfortunately, this approach has led to certain problems. The first is that normal infants achieve 30% of their growth potential during the first 2 years of life. Infants with renal insufficiency, unless optimally treated, grow poorly during this critical period. If the patient is growth-retarded by age 2 and therapy is initiated, catch-up growth rarely occurs; the patient will never be of normal height. Of greater concern is that rapid brain growth also occurs during the first 2 years of life. Children with renal insufficiency during infancy may develop permanent and progressive neurologic complications. Because of the availability of CAPD, CCPD, and improved nutritional support, many investigators now believe that early and aggressive therapy of infants with chronic renal insufficiency is indicated.

Infants should receive aggressive medical management even before initiating dialysis. This treatment should include attempts to correct acid–base abnormalities, normalize calcium and phosphorus metabolism, and, most importantly, ensure adequate nutrition. The abnormalities seen in infants with renal insufficiency are similar to those seen in babies who have been malnourished during the first year of life. If patients will not or cannot ingest adequate calories due to the anorexia of chronic renal insufficiency, then possibly nutritional supplements using enteral feedings may be indicated. If, despite adequate nutrition and correction of metabolic abnormalities, the infant still fails to thrive as indicated by poor linear growth, poor head growth, and weight gain, dialysis should be considered.

One approach to this situation may be to treat the infant with hemodialysis, then perform a renal transplant as soon as possible. Until recently, renal transplantation in infants has been associated with a high mortality rate, but recent results have demonstrated success in a limited number of patients. This approach requires specialized hemodialysis techniques and well-motivated parents. Another approach to treating these patients may be to use peritoneal dialysis and then to perform renal transplantation when the patient is older and the procedure is better tolerated. This method now has been used by several groups with some success.

# RENAL TRANSPLANTATION

Renal transplantation is the goal of therapy for children with ESRD. A well-functioning renal allograft is superior to dialysis in its ability to effect psychosocial and physical rehabilitation. However, successful transplantation may be difficult to achieve.

## Criteria for Acceptance for Transplantation

The criteria for accepting a patient for transplantation are constantly changing. Until recently, children under age 5 were rarely considered candidates for transplantation. The initial results in this age group were disappointing. However, more modern experience would indicate that children between ages 1 and 5 who received live, related-donor (LRD) renal allografts had acceptable outcomes. Most authors would not recommend transplantation for the infant less than 1 year of age who is thriving while being treated with a form of peritoneal dialysis. If an LRD renal allograft is available, transplantation may be the best option for the child between ages 1 and 5. If an LRD kidney is unavailable and the child is thriving on dialysis, then cadaveric transplantation might be delayed until the patient is older. Cadaveric transplantation may be the only option for the young child who fails to thrive while being treated with dialysis.

Uremia may cause severe neurologic complications, including developmental delay. This may be permanent, but it also may improve with treatment. Therefore, decisions as to whether a child is an acceptable transplant candidate based on mental function can be difficult. Parents of these children should be made fully aware of these complications and should be active participants in all decisions concerning transplantation. If the decision is made not to pursue transplantation, then support from the renal program should be provided.

All children with chronic illness have some difficulty with psychosocial adaptation to their disease. This often is made most manifest during adolescence and results in rebellion and noncompliance. Nonadherence to treatment regimens by the transplant patient often will result in allograft rejection. If predisposing factors for noncompliance are recognized in a patient, transplantation could be delayed until counseling to reduce this risk is done.

Malignancy is a contraindication to transplantation for many adult patients. In children with bilateral Wilms' tumor, transplantation is considered if the patient is followed for a year on dialysis and no recurrence or metastasis is noted.

Obstructive uropathy is the most common single cause of ESRD in children. Many of these patients have abnormal bladders. Experience suggests that in most cases these bladders can be used for transplantation. Careful evaluation of the bladder is suggested, but only rarely will it be found lacking. Even patients with neurogenic bladders can be transplanted and urine drained by intermittent catheterization.

Many immunologically mediated glomerulopathies that cause ESRD may recur in the transplanted kidney (Table 112-2). Although the disease recurrence rate is significant, the number of grafts lost due to recurrent disease is small. Patients who develop renal failure secondary to these glomerulopathies may still be transplanted, but the risk of recurrence should be made clear to them and their families. If the patient were to lose a graft from disease recurrence, a second transplant would not be recommended.

In summary, there are very few absolute contraindications to transplantation. Any child with ESRD deserves to be evaluated for renal transplantation.

## Donor Selection

The best renal allograft survival rates are reached when a live, related, human leukocyte antigen (HLA) identical kidney is transplanted. When an HLA-identical sibling donates an organ, the graft survival rate at 1 year exceeds 90%. Unfortunately, many younger children do not have siblings old enough to be considered as donors. Children often receive LRD renal allografts from a parent instead of a sibling. By definition, parents are a one-haplotype match with their children. Success of transplantation among one-haplotype-matched pairs exceeds 80% at 1 year. When an LRD kidney is unavailable, use of a cadaveric donor is necessary. At this writing, both patient and graft survival rates are less than those quoted for LRD transplantation. It is hoped that as our knowledge of immunologic tolerance advances, cadaveric donor renal transplantation will become as successful as LRD.

There always have been more patients waiting for cadaveric organs than there are organs available. The recent formation of a national organ bank will increase the chances that a child will be offered an immunologically acceptable cadaveric renal allograft.

## Immunosuppression

Current commonly used immunosuppressive drugs are listed in Table 112-3.

Corticosteroids have been used to treat and prevent graft rejection. The exact mechanism of action is unknown. Prednisone is the most commonly used corticosteroid, but there are no data to suggest that it is superior to other forms. Dosage regimens during the first few months after the transplant vary widely among transplant programs. Most dedicated pediatric transplant centers agree that a low maintenance dose should be the goal. Some programs advise very low daily doses of prednisone, but most prefer alternate-day steroids at a dose of 0.3 to 0.5 mg/kg. A daily dose of prednisone of 8.5 mg/m$^2$/day or greater will

---

**TABLE 112-2.    Glomerulopathies That May Recur in a Transplanted Kidney**

Focal glomeruloscerosis
Goodpasture syndrome (anti-GBM disease)
Membranoproliferative glomerulonephritis types I and II
Rapidly progressive glomerulonephritis
Henoch-Schönlein purpura, IgA nephropathy
Systemic lupus erythematosus
Membranous glomerulonephritis

---

**TABLE 112-3.    Commonly Used Immunosuppressants**

**Maintenance Therapy**
Azathioprine
Prednisone
Cyclosporine
Antilymphocyte globulin

**Treatment of Rejection**
Methylprednisolone
Antilymphocyte globulin
OKT3, monoclonal antibody to T cells

cause growth failure. Other complications of chronic steroid usage include hypertension, hypercholesterolemia, cushingoid appearance, aseptic necrosis of the femoral head, and an increased incidence of specific infections. Large doses of steroids (20/mg/kg/day) may be used for 3 or 4 days to reverse acute rejection.

Azathioprine (Imuran) may prevent rejection but will not reverse it. It affects many functions within the immune system. The dose varies in the early post-transplant period, but most programs advise a maintenance dosage of 1 to 2 mg/kg/day. Because the most common complication of azathioprine is myelosuppression, the white blood cell count, platelet count, and hematocrit should be monitored during therapy. This drug also may be hepatotoxic; the dose should be reduced if liver enzymes become elevated. Azathioprine contributes to the increased incidence of infection noted in these patients.

Cyclosporine is a newer agent that is more specific in its effect on the immune system than the drugs previously mentioned. It is only weakly suppressive to the bone marrow but is a potent inhibitor of many T lymphocyte functions. It prevents the generation of cytotoxic T lymphocytes, thought to be the cells mainly responsible for acute rejection. The dose of cyclosporine varies from patient to patient, and drug levels must be followed to ensure effect and avoid toxicity. Unfortunately, cyclosporine is nephrotoxic. There appears to be an acute toxicity, associated with high serum drug levels, that is reversible when the dose is lowered.

Many pediatric programs now advise the use of all three of these drugs together. The use of azathioprine with low-dose prednisone may allow the use of lower doses of cyclosporine. It is hoped that at these lower doses, cyclosporine's effect would be present but its toxicity minimal.

Another class of agents used in treating or controlling rejection are the antibodies that are directed against lymphocytes. Antilymphocyte globulin (ALG) and antithymocyte globulin (ATG) have been used extensively in human transplantation. ATG or ALG may be useful immediately after a transplant in the patient with a nonfunctioning graft due to acute tubular necrosis. Because acute tubular necrosis may be worsened with cyclosporine, ATG or ALG could be used until the graft begins to function, and then cyclosporine could be started. ATG and ALG are effective in the treatment of acute rejection. They are potent immunosuppressives, and their long-term use will increase the risk of viral and fungal infections.

These agents are polyclonal antibodies directed against lymphocytes. Recently monoclonal antibodies directed to specific antigens present on all T lymphocytes have been produced, and the first of these is OKT3. Early reports suggest that this agent can reverse acute rejection even when the rejection episode did not respond to steroids. Whether its use will extend beyond treatment of transplant rejection is speculative. Many newer antirejection therapies are currently under study, but none have replaced those mentioned above at this time.

## Monitoring the Patient After Transplant

Follow-up of the child who has had a successful renal transplant should be a rewarding experience for the pediatrician. Often the previously shy, lethargic, chronically ill patient emerges into an outgoing, energetic, "normal" child. It is a rare transformation that we have the privilege to observe. At the same time, the patient's very happy parents must be cautioned that rejection can occur. Without careful follow-up, many problems may develop, including serious and life-threatening infections.

Classically, acute rejection of the renal allograft presents with systemic symptoms such as fever, lethargy, anorexia, chills, and joint pain. The graft should be tender and swollen. Unfortunately,

with modern immunosuppressive protocols, acute rejection, especially if it occurs after the first month post-transplant, is rarely classical. Patients may have acute rejection made manifest only by a rising serum creatinine level, a mildly elevated blood pressure, and a renal allograft that is slightly swollen. Obviously, careful and frequent observation of these patients is required to detect these changes. Sometimes the graft may need to be biopsied to confirm the diagnosis. If detected early, most episodes of acute rejection can be reversed. Acute rejection, if it occurs, usually is seen within 6 months of transplantation and is rarely diagnosed after that time. However, acute rejection can be seen at any time if immunosuppressive therapy is discontinued by the noncompliant patient.

Chronic rejection can start anytime in the post-transplant patient. It usually is associated with a slowly increasing creatinine level accompanied by hypertension. Allograft biopsy is needed to confirm the diagnosis. Chronic rejection cannot be treated. However, with continued immunosuppression and, most importantly, control of hypertension, it may be years before the patient needs to return to dialysis.

Blood pressure must be monitored in the post-transplant patient. Hypertension may be seen not only secondary to rejection, but also as a consequence of prednisone, cyclosporine, and (rarely) stenosis at the anastomosis of the graft renal artery. Significant elevations in blood pressure must be evaluated and treated, since hypertension from any cause may damage the allograft.

Fever in the immunosuppressed patient is an emergency that should alert the pediatrician to the possibility of a life-threatening infection. A complete evaluation is indicated, even if the patient does not appear very ill. Steroids often mask symptoms of serious disease in these patients. The possibility of fungal and serious viral infections must be considered. Hospitalization may seem unnecessary, but often is advised when the transplanted child develops fever.

## Prognosis

Available data would suggest that at least 60% of children who receive LRD allografts and 50% of children who receive cadaveric transplants would be free of dialysis at 10 years post-transplant. However, graft survival curves have not yet flattened. There is a slow but constant incidence of graft failure even 15 years post-transplant. It is hoped that patients currently undergoing renal transplantation will have an even higher long-term success rate.

The long-term outlook for the child with chronic renal failure is unfolding. Ideally we might hope to prevent those diseases and birth defects that cause the child to be devastated with chronic renal failure; until then, we must deal with these problems. In two decades, not only have the lives of these children been lengthened, but the quality of their lives improved.

## Selected Readings

Alliapoulos JC, Salusky JB, Hall T, et al. Comparison of continuous cycling peritoneal dialysis with continuous ambulatory peritoneal dialysis in children. J Pediatr 1984;105:721.

Baum D, Powell D, Calvin S, et al. Continuous ambulatory peritoneal dialysis in children: comparison with hemodialysis. New Engl J Med 1982;307:1537.

Diaz-Buxo JA, Walker PJ, Farmer CD, et al. Continuous cyclic peritoneal dialysis. Trans Am Soc Artif Intern Organs 1981;27:51.

Donckerwolcke RA, Chantler C. Hemodialysis. In: Holliday MA, Barratt TM, Vernier RL, eds. Pediatric nephrology, ed 2. Baltimore: Williams & Wilkins, 1987:799.

Ettenger RB, Fine RN. Renal transplantation. In: Holliday MA, Barratt TM, Vernier RL, eds. Pediatric nephrology, ed 2. Baltimore: Williams & Wilkins, 1987:828.

Kohaut EC, Whelchel J, Waldo FB, Diethelm AG. Aggressive therapy of infants with renal failure. Pediatr Nephrol 1987;1:150.

Nevins TE. Transplantation in infants less than 1 year of age. Pediatr Nephrol 1987;1:154.

Popovich RP, Moncrief JW, Nolph KD, et al. Continuous ambulatory peritoneal dialysis. Ann Intern Med 1978;88:449.

*Principles and Practice of Pediatrics, Second Edition.*
edited by Frank A. Oski et al. J. B. Lippincott Company, Philadelphia © 1994.

# CHAPTER 113
# *Renal Malformations*

## Edith P. Hawkins

Malformations of the kidney are classified conventionally as primary developmental or secondary nondevelopmental anomalies. Developmental (primary) anomalies are defined as malformations resulting from alterations in growth, migration, nephrogenesis, and blastemal differentiation. Nondevelopmental (secondary) anomalies are changes superimposed on a kidney in which the underlying architecture appears to have developed normally. These changes may be related to a variety of factors such as maternal disease, vascular injury, and teratogens. Malformations related to genetic determinants may be primary (eg, ectopies) or secondary (eg, cysts).

Abnormalities of migration and fusion lead to such anomalies as ectopia, crossed ectopia (the ureter arising from the contralateral side), horseshoe kidney, and pelvic "cake" kidney. Abnormalities of ureteric budding may lead to double ureters, crossed ectopia, or bilateral displacement of the vesicoureteral insertions. These anomalies are generally asymptomatic but may be associated with an increased incidence of infection and occasionally with symptoms of obstruction.

## HYPOPLASIA

Hypoplasia is an anomaly in which insufficient renal parenchyma is formed. It is generally sporadic, rarely familial. There may be a decrease in the number of normal or enlarged nephrons (frequently in association with a decrease in the number of lobules), suggesting a decreased number of ureteric bud divisions, or there may be a decrease in the size of nephrons that are normal in number. This latter condition represents an abnormality of growth and is seen in children with mental retardation syndromes.

Hypoplasia is a rare malformation requiring morphologic confirmation. It often is confused clinically with atrophy, which can be differentiated by the presence of scarring or alterations in the architectural pattern of the kidney. Radiographic diagnosis is difficult and never certain. Evidence of reflux or recurrent infection suggests atrophy rather than hypoplasia. Unilateral and segmental renal hypoplasias are now considered to be atrophic rather than primary developmental anomalies.

Bilateral renal hypoplasia ranks fourth as a cause of renal failure in children. The common form, oligomeganephronia, is an isolated, sporadic malformation characterized by extremely small kidneys that have decreased numbers of enlarged nephrons. The glomeruli may be twice the norm in diameter, area, and volume. The tubules are even larger, have frequent diverticuli, and are cystically dilated. Clinically there is a male/female ratio of 3:1. The major defect is in tubular concentration, leading to polyuria and dehydration. Growth retardation and moderate proteinuria are common when renal failure ensues. These children are good candidates for transplantation, since the renal anomaly is usually an isolated malformation. A second, rare form of bilateral hypoplasia leading to renal failure is characterized by decreased numbers of normal nephrons.

## DYSPLASIA

Dysplasia is defined as altered differentiation of metanephric blastema. It is seen with obstruction occurring before the completion of nephrogenesis, in association with several multiple malformation syndromes, or sporadically as an isolated event. The term is limited to kidneys showing the characteristic histologic changes: collecting ducts lined by primitive epithelial cells with hyperchromatic nuclei; differentiated fibromuscular collars surrounding the ducts; and a loose, undifferentiated mesenchymal stroma. Metaplastic cartilage is often present in the cortex but is not an essential feature. There is always some metanephric differentiation, and primitive glomeruli and tubules are seen in varying numbers. Cysts, primarily involving tubules and ducts, are common (Fig 113-1).

About 90% of dysplastic kidneys that are not part of a malformation syndrome are accompanied by additional urinary anomalies, usually obstructive. The most common of these anomalies is obstruction of the prostatic urethra in males. This condition is designated as posterior urethral valves, but in reality is more likely to be urethral stenosis of varying degrees of severity. When the obstruction is complete, there is severe bilateral dysplasia. Lesser degrees of obstruction may not affect the kidney during the period of active nephrogenesis but may cause hydronephrosis or scarring later. Ureteral anomalies and malpositions,

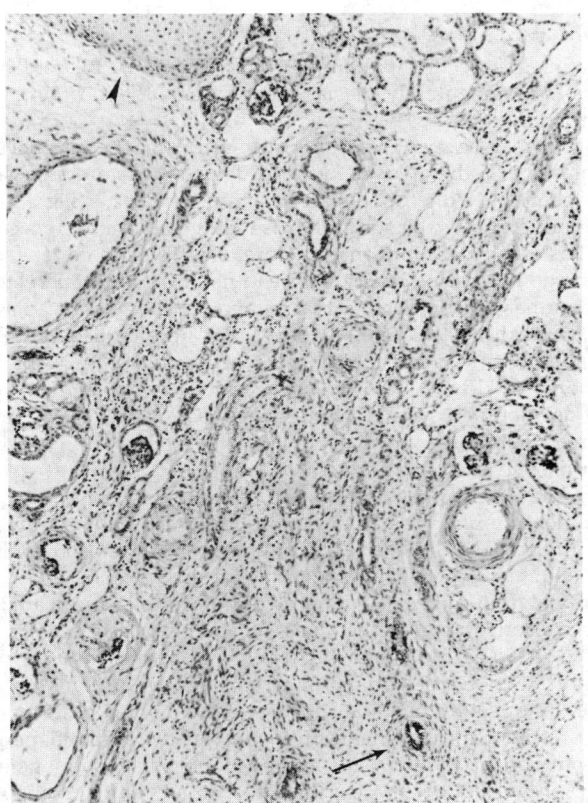

**Figure 113-1.** In this section from a cystic dysplastic kidney, primitive tubules surrounded by fibromuscular collars (*arrow*) are seen embedded in a loose mesenchymal stroma. Microscopic cysts and a few primitive glomeruli are present. One focus of metaplastic cartilage (*arrowhead*) can also be identified. (Masson's trichrome, magnification ×60)

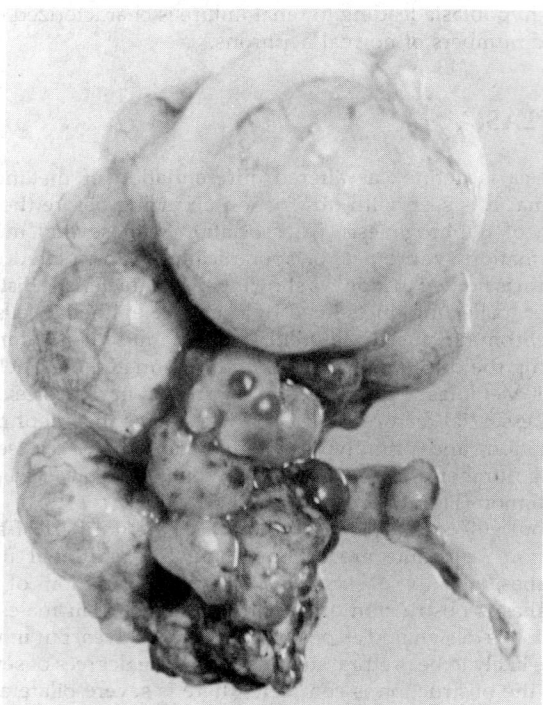

**Figure 113-2.** This multicystic dysplastic kidney is composed of multiple cysts of various sizes. No normal renal parenchyma can be identified. The ureter is cystically dilated at its junction with the renal pelvis and atretic distally.

sometimes associated with ureteroceles, may cause bilateral, unilateral, or segmental dysplasia, depending on the location of the obstruction.

The most severe forms of dysplasia are the multicystic-dysplastic and the aplastic kidneys. These forms are associated with complete ureteropelvic obstruction or aplasia (Fig 113-2). The multicystic-dysplastic kidney is enlarged, has multiple cysts, and has an absent reniform structure. It appears to be related to obstruction occurring relatively late in nephrogenesis and usually has an inner core of more normal renal parenchyma. The aplastic-dysplastic kidney is quite small and has little corticomedullary development. Microscopically most of the tissue is dysplastic. This type of kidney seems to be a result of obstruction early in fetal development. Renal agenesis may sometimes be the most severe form of this condition, but it may also occur as an anomaly secondary to a vascular or genetic event.

In bilateral complete dysplasia, there is maternal oligohydramnios and placental amnion nosodum related to fetal anuria. The infants have low-set ears, prominent infracanthal folds, a flattened, beaked nose, micrognathia, creased skin, and varying positional deformities of the limbs. All of these changes are features of Potter's syndrome. This syndrome was originally described in association with bilateral renal agenesis but is now recognized to result from prolonged oligohydramnios of any cause. Infants with bilateral severe dysplasia or agenesis tend to die of respiratory insufficiency in the immediate postnatal period. The pulmonary hypoplasia seen in infants with renal agenesis or dysplasia has been considered to be the result of oligohydramnios, but some studies suggest that, in addition to being hypoplastic, the lungs of these infants are dysplastic.

The sporadic form of diffuse bilateral dysplasia is unassociated with obstruction and varies in severity, but several infants follow the same course as those with severe dysplasia related to obstruction. It is thought that dysplasia unassociated with mechanical

obstruction is related to a disruption of normal epithelial-mesenchymal interaction during tubular induction. Recent experimental studies showing that abnormal protein glycosylation is associated with the development of dysplasia in the chick embryo support this theory.

The unilateral multicystic-dysplastic kidney is the most common cause of a palpable abdominal mass in an infant and is generally discovered early. Lesser forms of unilateral or segmental dysplasia may remain asymptomatic for varying periods of time. These kidneys are said to be more susceptible to infection and occasionally cause pain. Hypertension often occurs and may be alleviated by excision of the affected kidney.

## RENAL CYSTIC MALFORMATIONS

### Polycystic Disease

Polycystic disease of the kidney is hereditary and occurs in two forms: an autosomal recessive condition, infantile polycystic disease (IPCD), and an autosomal dominant condition, adult polycystic disease (APCD). Cysts arise after birth in APCD and may not appear until late childhood in IPCD as well. In both types, the underlying renal architecture is normal. Thus, cyst formation in these cases may be considered secondary to the congenital genetic determinant.

IPCD, which is rare, is always accompanied by diffuse biliary dysgenesis (congenital hepatic fibrosis) and has three distinct presentations. The most common presentation is in the neonatal period. The infant is born with greatly enlarged, cystic, reniform kidneys (Fig 113-3), but the mechanism of cyst formation is still unclear. Papillary hyperplasia of the tubular epithelium with secondary tubular obstruction, delayed tubular canalization, structural alterations in the tubular basement membranes, and changes secondary to toxic metabolites have all been suggested as causes of cyst formation. Epithelial hyperplasia, possibly due to overexpression of growth factors or oncogenes or loss of suppressor genes, is now considered the most likely primary mechanism, perhaps associated with one or more of the other factors. The cysts are fusiform dilatations of the collecting ducts, which radiate from the medulla through the cortex to the subcapsular

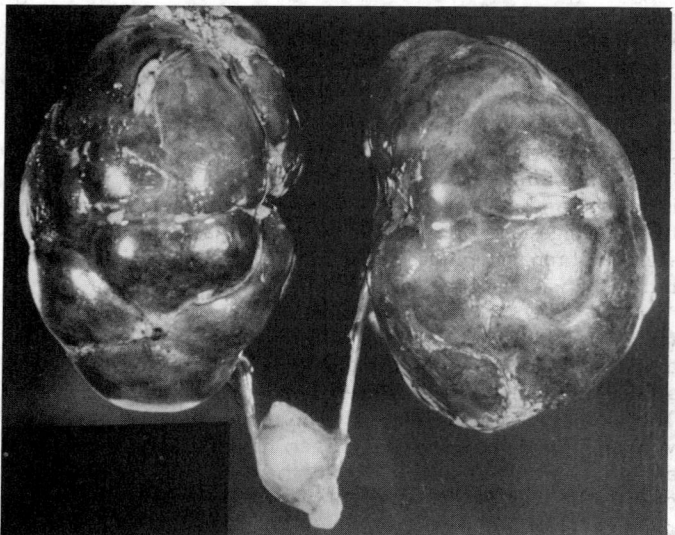

**Figure 113-3.** The massive enlargement of these kidneys from a neonate with infantile polycystic kidney disease can be appreciated when they are compared with the bladder, which is of normal size. Small cysts can be seen throughout both kidneys.

region. Normal renal parenchyma is present in the areas between cysts. The liver is occasionally enlarged, and each portal area has increased peripheral bile ducts that appear to ring the portal region and actually represent three-dimensional, flattened sacs. A slight increase in portal fibrous tissue is also present. The infants are oliguric and usually die within a few days of pulmonary insufficiency due to lung hypoplasia. Maternal oligohydramnios is considered to be the major factor contributing to the hypoplasia, although compression of the thoracic cage by the massively enlarged kidneys has also been suggested. A few infants survive and merge clinically and morphologically with the second type of presentation.

Infants past the neonatal period and young children with IPCD present with flank masses and hepatosplenomegaly. The renal cysts are more rounded and less prominent than in the neonatal form of disease, and medullary duct ectasia is a constant and prominent feature. Portal fibrosis is increased, and varying degrees of bile duct ectasia are seen. Small pancreatic cysts may be present. Clinically the patients have a concentrating defect, which places them at risk to develop dehydration. They may also have renal tubular acidosis. The creatinine clearance is usually somewhat decreased for age, but renal function may remain stable for several years before progressing to renal failure. Transplantation is the treatment of choice, since the disease does not recur in the transplanted kidney. Hypertension, which tends to develop early, is a common problem and requires aggressive therapy. Some children develop portal hypertension, which occasionally results in bleeding esophageal varices. This complication responds to portacaval shunting.

Some children and young adults who present with portal hypertension and progressive hepatic fibrosis associated with biliary dysgenesis have mild renal involvement consisting of the same type of cystic dilatation of collecting ducts and tubules as seen with IPCD in infants and young children. Most investigators believe that this subset of patients has a milder version of IPCD.

APCD usually presents in the fourth or fifth decade of life. In about 90% of the patients in North America, the disease is due to a mutation in a gene on the short arm of chromosome 16. However, there are some families in which the causative gene has not yet been localized. About 8% of the adults who enter dialysis programs each year have APCD, but a smaller number of infants and children also may develop symptomatic APCD. The disease is always bilateral, but it may occur asynchronously in the two kidneys. The kidneys may be large or small. They have variable numbers of cysts involving all portions of the nephron and collecting ducts (Fig 113-4). Scattered cysts may be present in the liver and pancreas, but hepatosplenomegaly, portal fibrosis, and biliary dysgenesis are not features of APCD. Maternal oligohydramnios and neonatal pulmonary insufficiency are also not seen in APCD. The absence of these findings or the presence of berry aneurysms, which are rare in IPCD, aid in the differentiation between APCD and IPCD. Ultrasound of children with APCD may occasionally show medullary striations suggestive of IPCD. The definitive diagnosis of APCD in childhood rests on molecular diagnostic studies in a child with a positive family history or the demonstration of asymptomatic cystic disease in one of the parents. Since there is a relatively high incidence of spontaneous mutations, a negative family history does not rule out the diagnosis.

Clinically, children with APCD may have recurrent urinary tract infections. Occasional patients require dialysis early in the course of the disease, but most maintain stable renal function for 10 years after the onset of symptoms before progressing to renal failure. Tubular defects are not seen. Hypertension tends to occur less often and later in children with APCD than in those with IPCD. These children are also good candidates for renal transplantation.

## Glomerulocystic Disease

Glomerulocystic disease, another form of renal cystic malformation, includes a heterogenous group of disorders. It is generally sporadic or associated with other congenital malformations, but has been reported to be familial, and a possible autosomal dominant pattern of inheritance has been suggested. The kidneys may be grossly enlarged or small; those in patients with familial disease are always small. Microscopically there are diffuse cysts of Bowman's space, particularly in the subcortical region. In some instances there is medullary fibrosis and varying degrees of collecting duct ectasia, suggesting intrarenal obstruction as a possible mechanism of formation. I have seen one infant with radiologically normal kidneys at birth who at age 5 months developed massively enlarged kidneys. Microscopically, there were diffuse glomerular cysts and significant medullary duct ectasia and fibrosis.

Infants with glomerulocystic disease usually present in the newborn period with abdominal masses and decreased renal function and frequently die from associated malformations. Infants who survive tend to have chronic but stable renal insufficiency. A few show improved function with time, and a few progress to renal failure. The recent report of a family in which several adult members were found to have asymptomatic glomerulocystic disease supports the suggestion that some forms may have an autosomal dominant pattern of inheritance and good renal function.

## Other Cystic Diseases

Medullary cystic disease (MCD) and familial juvenile nephrophthisis (FJN) are also hereditary forms of renal cystic malformation in which cysts are present only in the medulla.

MCD usually occurs in adults, has an autosomal dominant pattern of inheritance, and is rarely associated with renal symp-

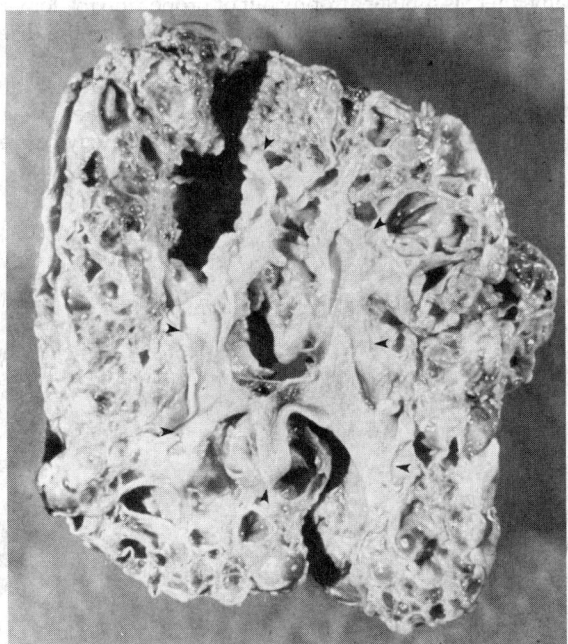

**Figure 113-4.** The cut surface of this bisected kidney from a patient with adult polycystic kidney disease shows cysts of various sizes. These cysts are present throughout the parenchyma and obliterate normal renal architecture. There is no separation between cortex and medulla, and the usual reniform shape has been lost. The pelvis can be seen in the middle of the specimen (*arrowheads*).

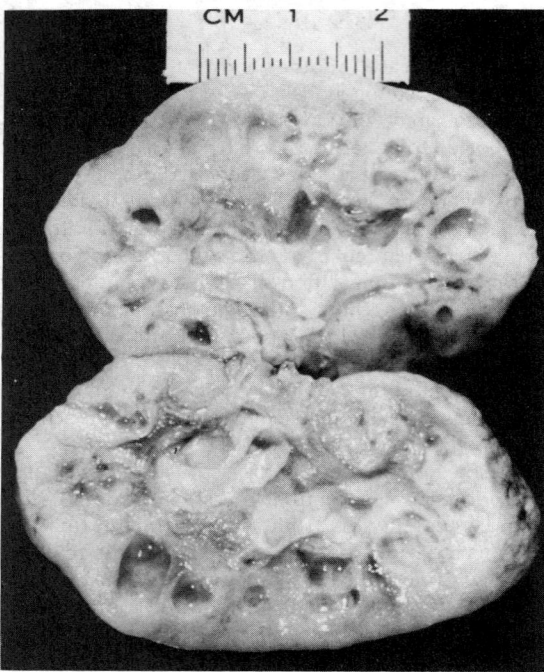

**Figure 113-5.** This kidney from an 11-year-old girl with juvenile nephronophthisis is small and pale. The cortex is somewhat thin and there are multiple medullary cysts of various sizes.

toms, although occasionally these patients present with renal colic related to the passage of blood clots.

FJN has an autosomal recessive pattern of inheritance and a high incidence of consanguinity and leads to renal failure in childhood. After the onset of symptoms, the kidneys are small and pale; cysts are present in the medulla (Fig 113-5). Microscopically, there is tubular atrophy out of proportion to glomerular damage and frequent large medullary cysts. Late in the disease, there is also impressive interstitial fibrosis and thinning of the cortex. Clinically, children with FJN exhibit a tubular defect characterized by inability to concentrate the urine, polyuria, polydipsia, growth retardation, and anemia, which may be greater

than predicted from the degree of renal failure. Similar clinical and morphologic findings are seen in association with a number of malformation syndromes.

A newly identified renal malformation, identified as congenital tubular dysgenesis or congenital renal tubular immaturity, is characterized by tubular hypoplasia and a failure of development beyond the primitive undifferentiated stage. This malformation has been described in several families. Consanguinity has been present in most instances, and in at least one family enlarged kidneys with increased numbers of glomeruli have been described. The infants have been stillborn or anuric and have died in the early neonatal period. An autosomal recessive mode of inheritance with some alteration in perfusion and glomerular filtration or abnormalities of fetal growth factors has been suggested. Similar tubular abnormalities have been described in the kidneys of the donor twin in the twin-twin transfusion syndrome.

Other inherited renal diseases, such as Alport and nail-patella syndromes, are associated with abnormalities in the development of the glomerular basement membrane.

## ASSOCIATED ANOMALIES

A wide variety of renal anomalies are seen in association with malformation syndromes, and the list continues to increase. Liver, pancreas, and CNS anomalies frequently accompany renal malformations. Renal dysplasia and cortical cysts are prominent in such syndromes as Meckel's, Jeune's, Zellweger, prune belly, and VATER. Small cortical cysts, alone or in association with dysplasia, are seen in many of these syndromes, as well as in several of the trisomies. Medullary cysts and interstitial nephritis occur in Jeune's, Laurence-Moon-Bardet-Biedl, and renal-retinal syndromes, and diffuse cysts may be seen in the syndromes of Ehlers-Danlos, tuberous sclerosis, and von Hippel-Lindau. Diffuse cystic disease in tuberous sclerosis is rare but may be the first evidence of disease. The cysts are lined by a hyperplastic, eosinophilic epithelium that is quite distinct and virtually diagnostic (Fig 113-6). The only other conditions in which somewhat similar, but less distinctive, epithelium is seen are the von Hippel-Lindau syndrome, in which the epithelial cytoplasm tends to be clear and the associated malformations dominate the clinical picture, and acquired cystic disease in the kidneys of patients on chronic dialysis.

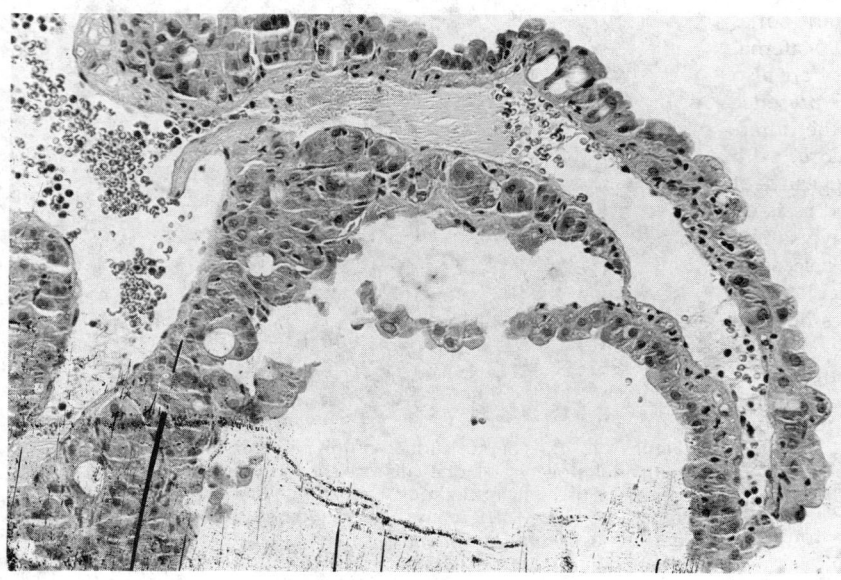

**Figure 113-6.** Cysts associated with tuberous sclerosis are quite distinctive. The epithelium is hyperplastic and often papillary. It is deeply eosinophilic and has an apocrine-like appearance (hematoxylin and eosin, magnification ×160). (Slide courtesy of Dr. E. Wilson, Children's Hospital, Birmingham, AL.)

## Selected Readings

Avner ED. Renal cystic disease: insights from recent experimental investigations. Nephron 1988;48:89.

Bernstein J. Hepatic and renal involvement in malformation syndromes. Mt Sinai J Med 1986;53:421.

Carson RW, Deepak B, Cavallo T, DuBose D Jr. Familial adult glomerulocystic kidney disease. Am J Kidney Dis 1987;9:154.

Hawkins EP, Page ML, Langston C. Twin-twin transfusion; effects on organ maturation. Lab Invest 1989;60:3P.

Herrera GA. C-erb B-2 amplification in cystic renal disease. Kidney Int 1991;40: 509.

Reeders ST, Germino GG. The molecular genetics of autosomal dominant polycystic kidney disease. Sem Nephrol 1989;9:122.

Risdon RA. Development, developmental defects, and cystic diseases of the kidney. In: Heptinstall RH, ed. Pathology of the kidney, ed 4. Boston: Little, Brown, 1992:93.

Schwartz BR, Lage JM, Pober BR, et at. Isolated congenital renal tubular immaturity in siblings. Human Pathol 1986;17:1259.

Spencer Jr, Maizels M. Inhibition of protein glycosylation causes renal dysplasia in the chick embryo. J Urol 1987;138:984.

Voland Jr, Hawkins EP, Wells TR, et al. Congenital hypernephronic nephromegaly with tubular dysgenesis. Pediatr Pathol 1985;4:231.

*Principles and Practice of Pediatrics, Second Edition.*
edited by Frank A. Oski et al. J. B. Lippincott Company, Philadelphia © 1994.

## CHAPTER 114
# *Glomerulonephritis and Nephrotic Syndrome*

## Phillip L. Berry and Eileen D. Brewer

## GLOMERULONEPHRITIS

Glomerulonephritis (GN) is the result of an immune process that injures the glomeruli of the kidney. This heterogenous group of diseases appears to be mediated primarily by immune mechanisms that invoke inflammatory reactions that cause alteration of glomerular structure and function throughout both kidneys. Impairment of tubular function may be present but is not predominant and results from either glomerular injury itself or direct immunologic injury similar to that affecting the glomeruli.

## Pathogenesis

The pathogenesis of GN has been actively studied since the 1950s but is not yet fully understood. Injury induced by nephritogenic immune complexes, coagulation factors, and reaction to exogenous toxins may all contribute to the complex pathology of these disorders.

### Immunologic Injury to the Glomerulus

Immunofluorescence and electron microscopic examination of renal biopsies from most patients with GN reveal immune complex deposits in the glomerular basement membrane (GBM) or mesangium, suggesting that immune complexes play a key role in pathogenesis. The location of immune complexes within the glomerulus depends mostly on their size and charge, and whether they are deposited as preformed complexes or are formed in situ.

It is now believed that immune complex deposits in the *subepithelial* region of the GBM form in situ. The nidus of immune complex growth may involve either a fixed glomerular antigen or a soluble exogenous antigen that binds to the glomerulus in a subepithelial location and recruits new layers of host antibody. Patients with circulating anti-GBM antibody and rapidly progressive GN (type I idiopathic, Goodpasture syndrome) are human analogues of experimental renal disease in which autoantibody reacts with native fixed GBM antigens. In other experimental animal models, injection of anti-GBM antibody produces a pathologic lesion similar to that observed in human membranous GN. Because no autoantibody to native glomerular antigen has yet been identified in patients with membranous GN, this disease is thought to begin with the adherence of exogenous antigens to the GBM, rendering it immunogenic.

Subepithelial deposits of immune proteins are now well known to be induced by exogenous antigens. These antigens are "planted" in the GBM by interaction with negatively charged GBM sites or by charge-independent processes. The charge-dependent mechanism may be important in the pathogenesis of poststreptococcal GN. Nephritogenic streptococci produce positively charged extracellular proteins that have been localized in the subepithelial GBM deposits of some patients. Positively charged IgG, possibly derived from desialation of IgG by neuraminidase-producing streptococci, has also been identified in subepithelial deposits in some patients.

Trapping of preformed circulating immune complexes in the subepithelial region of the GBM, originally thought to be the likely mechanism of immune complex deposition there, has not been persuasively demonstrated in human disease.

Immune complex deposits in the *subendothelial* region of the GBM and in the mesangium are probably also formed in situ, either from reaction to endogenous antigens or to exogenous antigens trapped in these regions during filtration. Endogenous subendothelial antigens may be the nidus for in situ immune complex formation in lupus nephritis. Exogenous antigens retained in the subendothelial or mesangial regions probably combine in situ with circulating antibodies to form the large immune complexes associated with the proliferative GNs of lupus, IgA nephropathy, and Henoch-Schönlein purpura (HSP) nephritis. In experimental animal models, subendothelial and mesangial deposits also originate from the trapping of preformed circulating immune complexes during glomerular filtration, but evidence is not convincing that this mechanism is pathogenetic in human GN.

### Mediators of Immune Complex Glomerular Injury

Immune complexes induce glomerular injury indirectly by activating cellular and humoral mediators. Neutrophils, T cells, and macrophages are attracted to glomerular immunoglobulin deposits. Once present and activated, they produce tissue injury by releasing toxic products such as proteolytic enzymes and reactive oxygen species, which digest the GBM.

IgG-containing immune complexes may also recruit humoral mediators such as the complement components. The complement terminal membrane attack complex (C5-C9) has direct membranolytic activity. In addition, the chemotactic and vasoactive properties of complement fragments (C3a, C5a) may attract more neutrophils to the site and alter glomerular permeability.

### Coagulation Factors

Coagulation factors are important, if not primary, contributing factors to the pathogenesis of GN. In patients with rapidly progressive GN, deposition of fibrin and its derivatives at sites of glomerular injury is critical to the formation of glomerular crescents. Platelet activation occurs in many renal diseases, even those without microangiopathy, and results in elaboration of substances potentially injurious to the kidney. Platelet cationic proteins neutralize the glomerular negative charge, resulting in proteinuria. Platelet-activating factor (PAF) produces a decline in renal vascular resistance, mesangial cell contraction, and subsequent reduction of the glomerular filtration rate (GFR). PAF also promotes glomerular monocyte accumulation, fibrin deposition, and crescent formation. Platelet-derived growth factor (PDGF) has properties similar to PAF and may also promote glomerulosclerosis. Increased production of PDGF may be important in stimulating mesangial and endothelial cell proliferation in proliferative forms of GN.

### Toxic Factors

A few exogenous nephrotoxins affect the glomerulus primarily. These include the drugs D-penicillamine, trimethadione, probenecid, and captopril, and a few of the heavy metals, such as mercury and gold. The mechanism of injury may be direct GBM injury, as occurs with trimethadione and mercury, or by induction of immune complexes, as occurs with D-penicillamine. The histopathology induced by these toxins is usually membranous GN. Increased glomerular permeability to protein and subsequent moderate to heavy proteinuria occurs. Proteinuria per se may contribute to alterations in the metabolism of the GBM that further glomerular injury.

### Clinical Presentations

GN may present clinically in a variety of ways. Classification by clinical presentation (Table 114-1) is helpful in narrowing the differential diagnosis and directing the diagnostic evaluation.

The *acute nephritic syndrome* is the sudden onset of hematuria, either gross or microscopic, proteinuria, decreased GFR, occasionally oliguria and retention of salt and water, which may be associated with edema, circulatory volume overload, and hypertension. The hallmark of this syndrome is hematuria and red blood cell casts in the urine, with only minimal to moderate proteinuria. Acutely decreased GFR may result from decreased filtration surface area caused by cellular proliferation, endothelial swelling, and neutrophil infiltration, as well as from inflammation-mediated local vascular changes that decrease net filtration pressure and from obstruction of Bowman's space by fibrin deposition and crescent formation. The mechanism for salt and water retention is poorly understood. It may occur without changes in serum albumin concentration and is often out of proportion to the decrease in GFR. Volume overload leads to suppression of aldosterone and impaired potassium and hydrogen ion excretion, which contributes to the hyperkalemia and acidosis observed in some acutely nephritic patients.

Some patients with *chronic GN* have few overt symptoms. Asymptomatic hematuria or proteinuria discovered on routine urinalysis may be the presenting signs. Malaise, fatigue, anemia,

---

**TABLE 114-1. Clinical Presentation of Glomerulonephritis**

Acute nephritis syndrome
Chronic glomerulonephritis
  Asymptomatic hematuria or proteinuria
  Chronic renal failure
Rapidly progressive glomerulonephritis
Nephrotic syndrome

---

and failure to grow normally may be the only signs of slowly progressive chronic GN with chronic renal failure.

If the clinical course is one of nephritis with rapid decline in renal function to uremia and often permanent loss of renal function, the presentation is termed *rapidly progressive GN*. Renal biopsies from these patients frequently show glomerular crescent formation alone or in addition to identifying characteristics of a specific histopathologic type of GN.

Patients with the *nephrotic syndrome* have massive proteinuria (in excess of 40 mg/m$^2$/hour in children), hypoproteinemia, hyperlipidemia, and edema. Hematuria, either gross or microscopic, may be present but is not the prominent feature.

This chapter will discuss the many kinds of GN of children and adolescents under the major headings of these clinical presentations. Since most of the disease entities that present with the acute nephritic syndrome may also have an insidious onset characteristic of chronic GN, acute and chronic GN are grouped together.

## ACUTE AND CHRONIC GN OF CHILDHOOD

The disorders that may present primarily with hematuria and red blood cells casts, whether in an acute or chronic fashion, include IgA nephropathy, HSP nephritis, lupus nephritis, the nephritis of chronic bacteremia, and membranoproliferative GN. Patients with membranoproliferative GN usually present with the nephrotic syndrome, so this disease entity will be discussed in detail under the heading of the nephrotic syndrome. Patients with acute poststreptococcal GN always present acutely, although occasionally the signs and symptoms may be so mild that patients do not seek medical attention.

### Acute Poststreptococcal GN

Acute poststreptococcal GN (APSGN) is the most common form of immune-mediated nephritis in children. It is by far the most common form of postinfectious nephritis, although infection with a variety of other bacterial, viral, parasitic, rickettsial, and fungal agents may be followed by an acute nephritic syndrome similar to that following infections with nephritogenic strains of group A beta-hemolytic streptococci. Historically, most cases of APSGN were related to type 12 group A streptococci, but the current list of nephritogenic types has been expanded to include types 1, 2, 3, 4, 18, 25, 49, 55, 57, 60, and perhaps 31, 52, 56, 59, and 61. In contrast to "rheumatogenic" strains of group A streptococci, which cause acute rheumatic fever associated with pharyngeal infection, nephritogenic strains of group A streptococci may cause either pharyngeal or skin infections. APSGN may occur in epidemics but is more often encountered sporadically. The attack rate in epidemics has been estimated at about 10% to 12%. Incidence figures are extremely unreliable, however, because many cases of APSGN are mild and do not come to medical attention. In fact, APSGN may occur without any accompanying identifiable urinary abnormalities.

Susceptibility to APSGN may be genetically determined as well as dependent on favorable host factors. The disease occurs most often in elementary-school children (mean age 7 years), affects twice as many males as females, and is quite rare before age 3 years. An episode of group A streptococcal throat or skin infection precedes all cases of APSGN. In most instances, the interval between the infection and the onset of clinical GN is about 8 to 14 days, although both longer and shorter intervals have been reported.

Proof of the previous infection by culture is seldom available, but serologic evidence of streptococcal infection (ie, an elevated specific antibody titer) should be present at the time of presentation. Serum antistreptolysin O (ASO) titer is elevated in 80% of cases associated with antecedent pharyngitis. The characteristic rise in the ASO titer is blunted by antimicrobial therapy, and the ASO titer is seldom elevated following skin infection. When antihyaluronidase (AHT) and antideoxyribonuclease B (anti-DNase B) titers are also measured, proof of preceding infection nears 100%. The latter titers are particularly important if the preceding infection was a pyoderma. Elevation of serum antistreptococcal titers is essential to diagnose APSGN with certainty, but the magnitude of the titers is of no prognostic significance. The absence of serologic confirmation of a recent streptococcal infection renders the diagnosis of APSGN suspect, and other forms of nephritis should be considered (see Differential Diagnosis below).

## Clinical Features

The clinical expression of APSGN is quite variable and extends from a completely asymptomatic form to the most severe manifestations of acute renal failure, including edema, oliguria, congestive heart failure, hypertension, and encephalopathy. The most common presenting symptoms are hematuria, proteinuria, and edema, often accompanied by rather nonspecific findings of lethargy, anorexia, vomiting, fever, abdominal pain, or headache.

Gross hematuria is present in only 30% to 50% of children with APSGN. The urine is usually described as smoky, tea-colored, cola-colored, or occasionally dirty greenish-colored. At least two thirds of hospitalized patients have edema, which is initially mild and may be noted only periorbitally, but can become quite marked, especially if normal fluid intake occurs over several days at the height of the disease. Evidence of circulatory congestion such as orthopnea, dyspnea, cough, auscultatory rales, and gallop rhythms are apparent on physical examination in many children with edema. The chest x-ray usually shows cardiomegaly and pulmonary edema of varying degrees. Severe congestive heart failure is very rare. Hypertension is quite common in inpatients (50% to 90%), but hypertensive encephalopathy, characterized by headache, somnolence, convulsions, coma, confusion, aphasia, transient blindness, agitation, or combativeness, occurs in only a few (5%).

## Laboratory Features

Laboratory investigation should begin with a careful analysis of the urine. The specimen may be yellow, slightly discolored, or grossly bloody, and usually has a high specific gravity and a low pH. Microscopic hematuria with predominantly dysmorphic erythrocytes in the centrifuged urinary sediment is present in virtually all cases, and leukocyturia is almost as common. Red blood cell casts are found very often (60% to 85%) in centrifuged specimens where the resuspended sediment is freshly examined and is of acid pH. Leukocyte casts as well as hyaline and granular casts are often seen. The presence of leukocytes and leukocyte casts should not be considered evidence of superimposed urinary tract infection, but rather of glomerular inflammation. Proteinuria occurs in most cases and correlates qualitatively with the amount of blood in the urine, reaching nephrotic proportions in less than 5% of patients.

A laboratory evaluation for streptococcal infection is mandatory. Serum ASO, AHT, and anti-DNase B titers as described above are most helpful for confirming previous recent infection. Throat and skin lesion cultures may also be positive at the time of nephritis and should be treated with appropriate antibiotics. Asymptomatic family members may also have positive cultures. Family screening for subclinical streptococcal disease and nephritis has been recommended.

One of the most important diagnostic laboratory findings in APSGN is a depressed serum concentration of C3. Activation of the alternative pathway of complement occurs in most cases, resulting in reduced serum C3 levels in at least 90% of patients

examined in the early phase of their nephritis. Serum C4 is occasionally also depressed. Serum C3 returns to normal concentrations 10 days to 8 weeks after the onset of the nephritis. If the serum C3 is not measured within the first few days of presentation of the nephritis, the concentration may already have returned to normal, and its depression will have been missed. Prior treatment of the streptococcal infection with penicillin may attenuate the period of depression of serum C3 so that serum C3 appears normal at the time of presentation of the nephritis. The degree of serum C3 depression bears no relationship to the severity of the disease. A follow-up serum C3 must be obtained 6 to 8 weeks after the onset of the acute episode to document the return of a normal concentration. If the concentration remains low, other kinds of nephritis, such as membranoproliferative GN or lupus, are more likely, and renal biopsy confirmation of the diagnosis should be sought.

GFR is usually depressed in hospitalized patients during the acute stage of moderate to severe nephritis. Serum urea nitrogen may be elevated disproportionately to serum creatinine. Even when GFR is normal or only slightly decreased, severe salt and water retention may occur. Urine volume is usually reduced, but severe oliguria is uncommon. Urine concentrating ability is well preserved. The fractional excretion of sodium is usually less than 1%, even in the presence of reduced GFR. The acutely inflamed kidney of APSGN retains sodium even in the face of acute renal failure, unlike the high fractional excretion of sodium that occurs in acute tubular necrosis. If a child with APSGN is allowed free access to fluids, dilutional hyponatremia may develop. When acidosis and hyperkalemia occur, they are the result of aldosterone suppression caused by extracellular volume expansion, as well as of reduced GFR, if severe.

## Pathology

Although patients with APSGN rarely undergo a renal biopsy today, many were assessed by biopsy in previous decades, giving us a comprehensive understanding of the histologic spectrum of the disease. By light microscopy the glomeruli are enlarged and hypercellular, filling Bowman's space. The glomeruli are relatively bloodless because of the occlusion of capillary lumina by proliferating mesangial and endothelial cells accompanied by a variable amount of infiltration by polymorphonuclear leukocytes, monocytes, and eosinophils within the capillary lumina and mesangium. Crescents are uncommon but may be extensive and are associated with a poorer prognosis. The renal tubules are normal in appearance but may be abnormally separated by interstitial edema. The blood vessels are usually normal. Electron microscopy reveals typical electron-dense "humps" between the glomerular capillary basement membrane and the epithelial cells. The humps are present on immunofluorescence studies, showing up as bright granular deposits containing predominantly IgG and C3. Other immune reactants, such as IgM, IgA, fibrin, and other components of the alternative pathway of complement, may be found along the capillary walls and in the mesangium.

## Pathogenesis

Based on morphologic, serologic, and clinical parameters, it is widely accepted that APSGN is immune complex-mediated, although the precise mechanism is unknown. Immune complexes containing IgG and C3 have been identified in the serum of these patients; however, attempts to identify streptococcal antigens within these complexes, either in the circulation or fixed in glomeruli, have been negative, inconclusive, or difficult to repeat. It is possible that streptococcal antigens bind to the glomerular capillary wall, forming the nidus for in situ immune complex formation. It is also speculated that streptococci themselves may produce glomerular injury and set the stage for inflammatory changes, or that streptococci induce autologous IgG/anti-IgG complexes through neuraminidase desialation of host IgG and neoantigen formation.

## Differential Diagnosis

Many renal disorders may at their onset mimic APSGN, but only a few do so commonly and with great synonymity. The absence of proof of preceding streptococcal infection or the simultaneous occurrence of infection plus nephritis tends to discount the diagnosis of APSGN. GN caused by infectious agents other than streptococci (staphylococci, viruses) is usually coincident with the infection and often lacks the telltale sign of hypocomplementemia. The course of other infection-associated GN depends on the natural history of that infection more often than on the renal manifestations.

Other disorders frequently confused with APSGN include benign hematuria, IgA nephropathy, hereditary nephritis, idiopathic hypercalciuria, and resolving episodes of previously undiagnosed postinfectious GN. Episodic hematuria coincident with an upper respiratory tract infection and normal serum complement levels help distinguish these disorders. In contrast, membranoproliferative GN may present as an acute nephritic syndrome during a streptococcal infection, but with hypocomplementemia, which, when reassessed at a later date, does not resolve.

The nephritis of HSP may precisely mimic APSGN if associated with mild extrarenal manifestations and an evanescent rash. A careful history and physical examination may uncover the true diagnosis in such cases. Preceding streptococcal infection and hypocomplementemia are rare.

The exacerbation of a chronic, previously unrecognized GN must also be excluded. These patients may exhibit episodic gross hematuria, hypertension, or azotemia at the time of an intercurrent infection. A prior history of renal symptoms or features of chronic renal failure, such as growth retardation or renal osteodystrophy, should be carefully sought to help distinguish these from APSGN.

## Treatment

No specific or general therapy is effective in ameliorating the inflammatory lesion of APSGN. All therapy is supportive and directed toward treating the clinical manifestations of acute nephritis. Hypertension, although usually only mild to moderate in severity, may be severe and require emergency treatment. Severe hypertension with encephalopathy demands immediate treatment. Fast-acting vasodilators such as intravenous diazoxide (3 to 5 mg/kg/dose), intravenous hydralazine (0.15 mg/kg/dose), or sublingual nifedipine (0.25 to 0.5 mg/kg/dose) are suitable choices for initial therapy. If multiple doses are required, maintenance antihypertensive therapy should be started. Loop diuretics and fluid restriction are important adjunct therapies and usually suffice alone for mild hypertension, as well as relieving edema and circulatory congestion. Restricting fluid intake to an amount equal to insensible water loss may obviate the need for diuretic therapy. On the other hand, the use of diuretics may allow the patient to have a more palatable diet and avoid the psychological tension associated with severe fluid restriction. Patients with oligoanuria may respond poorly to diuretics and thus require strict fluid restriction for control of edema and hypervolemia. In these patients, hyperkalemia should be anticipated and treated with dietary potassium restriction, binding resins, or dialysis as needed.

All patients should receive a course of penicillin or other antistreptococcal antibiotic if there is evidence of ongoing throat or skin infection. This in no way influences the course or prognosis of the nephritis. Unless the disease is particularly severe and the child chooses to rest, bed rest is no longer recommended during the course of APSGN. Dietary limitations of sodium, potassium, and water may be necessary during hospitalization but are usually liberalized before the patient is discharged from the hospital.

Those who require maintenance antihypertensive therapy should continue to have dietary sodium restriction at home.

## Prognosis

Overall, the prognosis of APSGN is excellent, with full recovery expected in more than 98% of affected children. The resolution must be documented at follow-up office visits over time. Most children spend no more than 5 days in the hospital, but the disease resolves quite slowly over many months. Few children develop chronic renal failure. Hypertension usually resolves within three weeks, as does gross hematuria. The latter may be exacerbated by exercise or intercurrent infections, but its reappearance is of no prognostic significance. Microscopic hematuria persists for many months and has been documented for as long as 3 years in a few patients. Proteinuria resolves within a few months; its persistence should raise concern regarding the possibility of an incorrect diagnosis or chronicity. The serum C3 concentration must be measured again 6 to 8 weeks after the acute episode. Failure of C3 to increase into the normal range during this period of time strongly suggests the diagnosis of membranoproliferative GN, and a renal biopsy should be done for confirmation.

## IgA Nephropathy

IgA nephropathy is characterized histologically by the presence of mesangial IgA deposits and clinically by chronic hematuria and normal renal function early in the course. Once considered a benign disease, IgA nephropathy is now known to progress to chronic renal failure in adulthood in as many as 40% of patients.

### Clinical Features

Almost three fourths of the children who present with IgA nephropathy are males. The mean age of presentation for both sexes combined is 9 years. Hematuria is the most common initial sign, occurring microscopically in 100% and macroscopically in 85% of the children with biopsy-proven IgA nephropathy. Gross hematuria may be a constant feature or it may occur episodically, usually in association with a febrile illness unrelated to the urinary tract. Proteinuria unrelated to gross hematuria occurs in about 40% to 50% of the affected children, reaching the nephrotic range in some. Isolated proteinuria is not a sign of IgA nephropathy in children. Patients with moderate to severe proteinuria are at greater risk of developing renal insufficiency. Hypertension, found in about 10%, is not a prominent feature, even when patients are followed for many years; its occurrence usually coincides with the development of chronic renal failure. About 20% of the patients have a mild decrease in GFR during episodic gross hematuria. Complaints of fever, malaise, and loin or abdominal pain are common at that time as well. Renal function usually returns to normal after the acute episode.

### Laboratory Features

Laboratory studies, other than a renal biopsy examination, will not confirm the diagnosis of IgA nephropathy. Serum IgA levels are elevated in no more than half of the patients and appear to bear no relationship to the disease severity or activity. Serum IgG, IgM, and C3 concentrations are seldom abnormal.

### Pathology

The diagnosis of IgA nephropathy requires demonstration of dominant IgA or IgA codominant with IgG deposition in the mesangium of glomeruli in the absence of clinical or laboratory evidence of systemic lupus erythematosus, HSP, or chronic liver disease. IgA may be found in glomeruli in several other nephropathies but is not the dominant immune reactant, nor is it confined to the mesangium. Intense immunofluorescence staining for IgG is found in biopsies of IgA nephropathy, but the intensity never exceeds that of IgA. IgM, C3, and properdin often accompany IgA in the same pattern as the IgA distribution, but with much less intensity. Electron microscopy confirms the presence of electron-dense deposits in the mesangium and rarely in adjacent subepithelial or intramembranous spaces of the GBM.

Although immunofluorescence defines the glomerulopathy, light microscopy predicts the prognosis. Biopsies have been classified into three groups according to the severity of glomerular proliferative changes. About one fourth of the biopsies show histologically normal glomeruli with little or no interstitial disease. The rest are about evenly divided between those showing mesangial hypercellularity and those showing focal and segmental mesangial proliferation as well as areas of necrosis, synechiae, crescent formation, or glomerular capillary wall collapse and sclerosis.

### Pathogenesis

The presence of IgA in the mesangium, the recurrence of IgA nephropathy in renal allografts, and the observations that serum IgA concentrations are increased in some patients and that IgA-containing circulating immune complexes are found in nearly half the patients studied strongly suggest that systemic IgA plays a role in the pathogenesis of this disease. Controversy exists regarding which type of IgA may be important in the development of the renal pathology. The predominant form of IgA found in renal biopsies from affected patients is polymeric $IgA_1$, reflecting the increased serum concentration of polymeric $IgA_1$ found by numerous investigators. Secretory IgA has been studied but to date does not appear to play a major role in the immunogenesis of IgA nephropathy occurring in the absence of gastrointestinal disorders.

Cellular immune mechanisms are also under investigation, but no consistent abnormalities have been found. A genetic predisposition to IgA nephropathy is suggested by the white male preponderance of patients, the association of HLA-BW35 and IgA nephropathy, and the occurrence of the disease in multiple members of the same family and in HLA-identical twins.

### Differential Diagnosis

The presence of microscopic hematuria with or without mild proteinuria between episodes of gross hematuria also occurs in hereditary nephritis (Alport syndrome), in benign hematuria, and in idiopathic hypercalciuria, occasionally in membranoproliferative GN (MPGN), and rarely in membranous GN. Hereditary nephritis can be distinguished from IgA nephropathy clinically if there is a positive family history or associated deafness. MPGN usually is associated with a decreased serum C3 level and heavier proteinuria. Membranous GN is usually associated with the nephrotic syndrome as well as microscopic and less often gross hematuria. Benign hematuria occurs without proteinuria or other signs or symptoms of renal disease. Proteinuria is also absent in idiopathic hypercalciuria, which can be diagnosed by the presence of abnormally high calcium excretion in a 24-hour urine collection.

IgA nephropathy is easily confused with acute poststreptococcal GN, especially if the initial presentation is an episode of gross hematuria and mild systemic complaints. In IgA nephropathy, unlike acute poststreptococcal GN, there is no latent period between the infection and the onset of hematuria, and the serum C3 concentration is normal. Gross hematuria persists only a few days in patients with IgA nephropathy, usually resolving when the associated fever remits.

The nephritis of HSP is even more difficult to distinguish from IgA nephropathy. If the rash is transient and not obviously purpuric and if the extrarenal manifestations of HSP are mild, the clinical syndrome is identical to IgA nephropathy. Furthermore, the renal biopsy findings of HSP nephritis are virtually identical to those of IgA nephropathy. These similarities have led some to speculate that IgA nephropathy is a monosymptomatic form of HSP.

### Therapy

The potential for progression of IgA nephropathy to chronic renal failure and end-stage renal disease has led to uncontrolled trials of prednisone and even cytotoxic drug therapy in patients with severe symptoms, advanced renal biopsy lesions, heavy proteinuria, or already apparent renal failure. Prednisone therapy appears to improve urinary findings in some patients, a few of whom also appear to have had improvement or stabilization of histopathologic lesions in subsequent renal biopsies. Data are too limited to determine if the progression of renal failure can be retarded by therapy. Until controlled therapeutic trials are done, no specific drug therapy can be recommended. Medical management of hypertension and chronic renal failure, when it occurs, are the treatment measures of choice.

### Prognosis

Most children with IgA nephropathy have either a very slowly progressive or completely benign course until adulthood. Predicting which 5% to 10% will develop end-stage renal disease in childhood or adolescence is difficult. Heavy proteinuria, hypertension, and a renal biopsy showing glomerular proliferative lesions with crescents, sclerosis, or GBM alterations suggest a poor prognosis.

## HSP Nephritis

HSP is a systemic vasculitis that typically affects children and presents as a triad of purpuric rash, crampy abdominal pain, and arthritis. Signs and symptoms of nephritis may not appear until days or several weeks into the course of the disease. Because of the unproven assumption that these children are allergic to drugs, food, microorganisms, or some other unidentified antigens, the term *anaphylactoid purpura* has been applied to this disease. Although children with HSP do not appear to be more allergic than others, the term has persisted.

HSP is probably mediated by IgA, which can be identified by immunofluorescence staining of renal and skin biopsies from affected patients. The renal lesion is identical to that seen in IgA nephropathy, raising the question of whether IgA nephropathy and HSP may be a spectrum of the same disease.

### Clinical Features

Most affected children are white boys between the ages of 3 and 10 years. Two thirds of patients report the onset of an upper respiratory tract infection 1 to 3 weeks before the onset of purpura. The incidence of HSP is seasonal, with its peak in winter.

The disease usually begins with an acute erythematous macular rash, most often on the ankles and spreading to the dorsum of the legs, the buttocks, and the ulnar surfaces of the arms. The trunk is spared. Within a day, the lesions become purpuric and may coalesce. The skin lesions disappear in about 2 weeks, although in some children the rash comes and goes over a period of days to weeks. Many patients experience edema of the scalp, face, and dorsum of the hands and feet with the rash. Joint pain, with or without edema, occurs in 60% to 75% of cases. Colicky abdominal pain with melena or bloody diarrhea occurs in one half of the affected children and mimics other gastrointestinal diseases. Severe vasculitis of the bowel may result in gastrointestinal hemorrhage, perforation, or intussusception.

The renal manifestations of HSP are clinically important in a few patients, but if the urine is examined over the duration of the disease, abnormalities will be found in almost every case. The spectrum of renal disease in HSP is broad, ranging from asymptomatic hematuria and proteinuria to full-blown acute nephritic syndrome with the nephrotic syndrome. Hypertension is uncommon.

### Laboratory Features

No laboratory test is diagnostic of HSP. Leukocytosis occurs early in the course. Hemoglobin, hematocrit, and the peripheral blood smear are normal, as are the platelet count, bleeding time, and coagulation studies. The erythrocyte sedimentation rate may be elevated. Microscopic hematuria and proteinuria are often present in the urinalysis. Gross hematuria may be seen in 20% to 30% of cases. Azotemia occurs in up to 20% but is usually transient. Uremia requiring acute dialysis for a short time is very rare.

Serum IgA concentration is elevated in 50% of the children with HSP. The elevation often occurs during the acute phase only, with levels returning to normal as symptoms resolve. Serum C3 concentration is normal, but breakdown products of complement are increased in the serum, indicating complement activation, presumably by circulating immune complexes or cryoglobulins, which have been identified in many patients.

### Pathology

If the clinical signs and symptoms of HSP are atypical, the diagnosis can be confirmed by microscopic examination of skin and renal biopsy specimens. Skin lesions typically show a leukocytoclastic vasculitis, characterized by transmural and perivascular infiltration with polymorphonuclear leukocytes, histiocytes, and sometimes eosinophils. The renal lesion is identical to that seen in IgA nephropathy (see above) and ranges from no identifiable abnormalities by light microscopy to mesangial proliferation, focal and segmental proliferative lesions, and diffuse proliferative lesions with or without crescents. Brightly staining deposits of IgA are always found in the mesangium by immunofluorescence. Electron microscopic examination shows dense deposits in the same location.

### Pathogenesis

The pathogenesis of HSP may involve a primary immune defect of IgA activity. The systemic nature of HSP, the appearance of IgA in extrarenal blood vessels, and the presence of IgA-containing circulating immune complexes in the serum of most patients suggest this possibility. It has been assumed that an immune response is triggered by the presentation of offending antigen(s) to the surface of either the respiratory or gastrointestinal tract, which then leads to the production of IgA antibodies, which may form immune complexes in the blood. The complexes then make their way to various sites, including the kidney, where an inflammatory response ensues. For years, antigenic stimuli for the IgA response have been intensively sought, and although many allergens have been implicated, specific relationships have never been substantiated.

### Differential Diagnosis

The purpuric nature and distribution of the skin lesions of HSP can be quite characteristic. If the rash is atypical in distribution, other causes of purpura such as leukemia, septicemia, hemolytic-uremic syndrome, systemic lupus erythematosus, and idiopathic thrombocytopenic purpura must be considered. The abdominal symptoms mimic many infectious and inflammatory bowel diseases. HSP may actually cause an acute surgical emergency secondary to bowel perforation or intussusception. Pancreatitis is uncommon. Vasculitis of the testis may resemble torsion of the testis, orchitis, or incarcerated hernia. Joint symptoms are difficult to distinguish from those seen in rheumatoid arthritis, lupus, and acute rheumatic fever. The renal manifestations of HSP may appear identical to those seen in acute poststreptococcal GN, bacterial endocarditis, systematic lupus erythematosus, polyarteritis, and membranoproliferative GN.

### Clinical Course and Therapy

The clinical course varies from very mild to severe. Most patients have several bouts of rash and abdominal pain over the first month of disease. Recurrences over a longer period of time may be associated with a poorer prognosis. The main determinant of the overall prognosis is the persistence and severity of the renal disease. Children with minor urinary abnormalities have an excellent prognosis for complete recovery, whereas those who present with a severe acute nephritic syndrome or the nephrotic syndrome may develop chronic renal failure and even end-stage renal disease. Patients who have renal disease should have long-term follow-up until the urinalysis is normal for several years. Those showing persistent urinary abnormalities or evidence of progressive renal failure should be seen by a pediatric nephrologist.

Therapy is limited to supportive measures. Careful monitoring to detect serious abdominal complications is of paramount importance in patients with abdominal pain. When abdominal pain is severe and incapacitating even after administration of analgesics, corticosteroids may provide relief. The use of analgesics and steroids is not without risk, as they may mask symptoms of gastrointestinal perforation. There is no evidence that corticosteroids have any beneficial effect on the clinical course of the renal disease.

## GN of Systemic Lupus Erythematosus

The full spectrum of disease caused by systemic lupus erythematosus (SLE) is described in Chapter 15. Only the renal and urinary tract manifestations will be described here.

The percentage of patients with SLE who have renal disease varies between 35% and 90%, depending on the clinical criteria used to diagnose SLE nephritis. If a renal biopsy examination is done and includes immunofluorescence and electron microscopy as well as light microscopy, almost 100% of the patients show some abnormality.

### Clinical and Laboratory Features

The nephritis of SLE, like the extrarenal manifestations of SLE, presents in a variety of ways with varying levels of intensity. Rarely, patients with known SLE may have no symptoms of renal disease and a completely normal urinalysis, but show the most active renal lesion by renal biopsy. Some patients have only renal disease without extrarenal signs of SLE initially. Most patients have enough signs and symptoms to meet criteria diagnostic of SLE, whether or not their renal disease is prominent initially.

SLE usually presents in young adulthood, primarily in females (8 : 1 female/male ratio). However, 20% to 25% of the cases are diagnosed in the first two decades of life, even occurring rarely in infants. Renal disease seems to be equally common among adults and children. All World Health Organization (WHO) classes of nephritis occur in childhood (Table 114-2).

The laboratory diagnosis of SLE is reviewed in detail in Chapter 15. The serum C3 and C4 concentrations are usually depressed, and antinuclear antibody and anti-double-stranded DNA antibody titers are elevated at the time of diagnosis of SLE nephritis. If not, and if extrarenal manifestations of SLE are minimal, the diagnosis may be in question until these serologic tests become abnormal later in the course of the disease, sometimes even months or years after presentation with nephritis. SLE nephritis is suggested by the presence of urinary abnormalities, including hematuria, proteinuria, or casts (red cell, white cell, hyaline, or broad/waxy). Proteinuria may be mild or moderate or in the nephrotic range. Heavy proteinuria is usually associated with more severe disease on renal biopsy. Sometime during their course, three fourths of all patients with SLE have either urinary

**TABLE 114-2. World Health Organization (WHO) Classification of SLE Nephritis**

| Class | Histopathology | Description |
|---|---|---|
| Class I | Normal kidneys | Slight or no detectable changes by LM, EM, or IF |
| Class II | Mesangial changes | |
| IIA | Minimal alteration | Normal LM, mesangial deposits of immunoglobulin and complement by IF, mesangial deposits by EM |
| IIB | Mesangial glomerulitis | Same as IIA but also mesangial hypercellularity (>3 cells per mesangial area away from vascular pole in 2 to 4-mcm sections) or increased mesangial matrix. Minimal tubular or interstitial changes. |
| Class III | Focal and segmental proliferative glomerulonephritis | In addition to any finding(s) in Class II, less than 50% of glomeruli involved with focal areas of intra- and extracapillary cell proliferation, necrosis, karyorrhexis, and leukocytic infiltration. EM and IF can show subendothelial as well as mesangial deposits. Tubular and interstitial changes usually focal. |
| Class IV | Diffuse proliferative glomerulonephritis | Similar to Class III but involving more glomerular surface area and >50% of the glomeruli. IF and EM often show abundant subendothelial deposits. Interstitial involvement more marked. Membranoproliferative variant has prominent mesangial cell proliferation and capillary wall thickening by mesangial extensions. |
| Class V | Membranous glomerulonephritis | No mesangial, endothelial, or epithelial cell proliferation. Capillary walls diffusely and uniformly thickened. IF and EM show mesangial and subepithelial deposits. Minimal interstitial involvement like Class II. |

*EM,* electron microscopy; *IF,* immunofluorescence; *LM,* light microscopy

abnormalities or depressed GFR, as noted either by an elevated serum creatinine level or by a decreased creatinine clearance.

In patients with renal interstitial disease, renal tubular disorders, such as type IV renal tubular acidosis or glucosuria, may occur. Ureteral vasculitis and noninfectious cystitis have been described in patients with SLE and may be responsible for obstructive uropathy and lower urinary tract symptoms, respectively.

**Pathology and Clinicopathologic Correlations**

Over the years, several classifications of lupus nephritis have been proposed. The most widely accepted is that of WHO (see Table 114-2). The classification is a useful investigational tool, but because not every biopsy fits neatly into one of these classes, the use of the WHO classification for predicting the prognosis for an individual patient may not be helpful.

Biopsies from 6% of the patients show normal kidneys (class I), although minimal electron-dense deposits associated with IgG and complement found exclusively in the mesangium are allowed in this class. Urinary abnormalities and renal failure almost never occur in this group.

Mesangial proliferative lupus GN accounts for 20% of biopsies (class II). Varying degrees of mesangial hypercellularity and mesangial deposition of IgG or IgM and C1q, C4, C3, and properdin are found in these biopsies. Clinically, asymptomatic urinary abnormalities most commonly characterize patients with class II disease.

Renal biopsies of focal and segmental proliferative lupus GN (class III) are characterized by the finding of additional deposits of C1q, C4, C3, and properdin in the capillary walls, but with fewer than 50% of glomeruli being involved by the disease process. This lesion is similar to that found in severe IgA nephropathy and HSP nephritis. Hematuria and proteinuria are present in most patients, but nephrotic syndrome and renal failure are uncommon. About 23% of biopsies are class III.

Diffuse proliferative GN (class IV) is found in 40% of biopsies. The pathology is similar to class III, but more than 50% of glomeruli are affected, making the lesion more severe. Electron microscopic and immunofluorescence studies show heavy deposits of immunoglobulin and complement, especially in the subendothelial space of the capillary wall. When these deposits are circumferential, the capillary loop has a "wire loop" appearance. Mesangial and epimembranous deposits are numerous. Crescent formation is variable but may be severe and correlates with the clinical course of rapidly progressive GN. Hematuria is almost always present in patients with class IV nephritis. Most patients with nephrotic syndrome and renal failure also have biopsies that fall into this category. Class IV lupus nephritis is associated with progressive uremia and a high mortality rate.

Membranous lupus GN (class V) accounts for 9% of renal biopsies. This lesion is characterized by subepithelial deposits of IgG and C3, as well as mesangial hypercellularity and mesangial and subendothelial immune deposits. Membranous lupus nephritis may precede extrarenal manifestations of SLE by many years and may be diagnosed initially as idiopathic membranous GN.

A few patients have predominantly interstitial disease, vascular disease, or severe sclerosis. Tubulointerstitial disease frequently accompanies glomerular involvement, especially in class III and IV nephritis. Rarely, tubulointerstitial disease occurs alone. Interstitial inflammatory infiltrates are usually focal and associated with interstitial fibrosis and tubular atrophy. Vasculitis involving the larger blood vessels of the kidney sometimes leads to vascular necrosis, hypertension, and renal failure in patients with SLE.

## Therapy and Prognosis

Although the beneficial effect of corticosteroid therapy for the extrarenal manifestations of SLE is well accepted, no controlled trial of this therapy for lupus nephritis in children has ever been done. Long-term controlled studies of adults with various WHO classes of disease are in progress. Results so far suggest that intermittent bolus intravenous cyclophosphamide therapy in combination with corticosteroids may be most effective in preserving renal function and reducing the risk of progression to end-stage renal disease with the fewest side effects.

Overall, survival of children with SLE is good, with 75% alive at 10 years and 65% surviving 15 years after diagnosis. Most deaths are caused by infection.

## Nephritis of Chronic Bacteremia

An immune complex-mediated proliferative GN may occur in the course of acute and subacute bacterial endocarditis, chronically infected ventriculoatrial shunts, and osteomyelitis. All have in common the presence of chronic bacteremia, usually with coagulase-positive or -negative staphylococci or streptococci. Patients with visceral abscesses (pulmonary, sinus, intra-abdominal), with and without documented bacteremia, rarely have presented with a similar picture. When bacteremia is documented, the pathogens are usually coagulase-positive staphylococci, but sometimes are gram-negative organisms.

### Clinical and Laboratory Features

The diagnosis should be suspected in patients with a source of chronic bacteremia who develop hematuria and proteinuria or red blood cell casts. Hydrocephalic children with "shunt nephritis" from chronically infected ventriculoatrial shunts present with the nephrotic syndrome in 30% to 50% of cases. In all patients, blood cultures are usually positive for the inciting organism. Most patients also have decreased serum C3 concentrations, positive rheumatoid factor, and the presence of circulating cryoglobulins and immune complexes. The serum level of other components of complement (C4 and C1q) may be depressed. Acute renal failure with oliguria occurs, especially with bacterial endocarditis or a visceral abscess that is occult for a long time before diagnosis. The incidence of acute renal failure is high in intravenous drug abusers, who often present late for treatment and may be infected with resistant organisms or have right-sided valvular disease with initially negative blood cultures.

### Pathology and Pathogenesis

The renal lesion in these patients is mesangial proliferation or mesangiocapillary proliferation, like type I membranoproliferative GN. The lesion may be focal or diffuse; it usually is more severe when the underlying illness is unsuspected and goes untreated for some duration. Such patients may also develop chronic pathologic changes with focal or diffuse scarring of the glomeruli. Extensive crescent formation and the clinical course of rapidly progressive GN occurs rarely. Immunofluorescence staining usually shows mesangial and capillary loop granular deposits of IgG, IgM, and C3. Soluble antigens of the infecting organism, with and without their specific antibodies, have been demonstrated in glomeruli, suggesting a direct role for immune complexes in the pathogenesis of this lesion, either by deposition of circulating complexes or antigen-induced GBM injury with in situ immune complex formation.

### Prognosis and Therapy

Specific antibiotic therapy for the underlying infection usually results in resolution or inactivation of the GN over a few weeks,

although in some cases GN persists for years after apparent eradication of the infection. As part of therapy, infected ventriculoatrial shunts should be removed and later replaced. Visceral abscesses should be surgically drained. If an infection is ineffectively treated, the GN may progress to chronic renal failure and end-stage renal disease, but this is rare thanks to currently available antibiotic therapy.

## RAPIDLY PROGRESSIVE GN

Rapidly progressive GN (RPGN) is a designation given to the group of disease processes characterized clinically by a rapid deterioration in renal function to uremia and often end-stage, irreversible renal failure within a few weeks to months (Table 114-3). The term RPGN has also been used to describe the pathologic lesion of diffuse glomerular extracapillary crescent formation that is common to many of the disorders that cause clinical RPGN. The terms *crescentic GN* and *extracapillary proliferative GN*, which describe the usual but not invariable pathologic lesion of clinical RPGN, are now used by many instead of the term RPGN. Other pathologic lesions, such as the necrotizing GN of Wegener's granulomatosis, can also result in clinical RPGN. The term RPGN in this section will include all forms of clinical RPGN. The discussion of pathology and pathogenesis will focus only on crescent formation, the most common histopathologic lesion associated with clinical forms of RPGN.

## Clinical and Laboratory Features

RPGN, either idiopathic or associated with any of the disorders in Table 114-3, usually presents with symptoms of acute GN, often gross hematuria, edema, hypertension, and oliguria/anuria. Most patients have severe anemia, out of proportion to their degree of azotemia or the apparent duration of their symptoms. Other symptoms may be those of the associated disorder, such

---

**TABLE 114-3. Disorders Associated with RPGN and Usually Glomerular Crescent Formation**

**Primary Renal Disorders**
IgA nephropathy
Membranoproliferative glomerulonephritis types I and II
Membranous glomerulonephritis
Alport syndrome (hereditary nephritis)
Idiopathic: Type I—Anti-GBM disease without pulmonary hemorrhage
          Type II—Immune complex disease
          Type III—No immune complexes, ANCA-associated

**Disorders Associated With Infection**
Poststreptococcal glomerulonephritis
Bacterial endocarditis
Hepatitis B
Other infection (pulmonary, sinus, or intra-abdominal abscess)

**Disorders Associated With Systemic Disease**
Systemic lupus erythematosus
Henoch-Schönlein syndrome (anaphylactoid purpura)
Goodpasture syndrome (anti-GBM disease with pulmonary hemorrhage)
Wegener's granulomatosis, polyarteritis nodosa, and other ANCA-associated vasculitides
Mixed cryoglobulinemia
Neoplasm (lymphoma, carcinoma)

as the purpuric rash of HSP or hemoptysis from the pulmonary hemorrhage associated with Goodpasture syndrome or Wegener's granulomatosis. Goodpasture syndrome includes the triad of nephritis (usually RPGN), pulmonary hemorrhage, and anti-GBM antibody formation demonstrable in the circulation or in renal or lung tissue. Wegener's granulomatosis is a systemic necrotizing vasculitis that involves the kidney, nasal mucosa, tracheobronchial tree, and lungs. Vasculitic skin lesions, sinusitis, serous otitis media, epistaxis, saddle-nose deformity, cough, eye lesions, and cardiac and neurologic symptoms may be present.

Antineutrophil cytoplasmic autoantibodies (ANCA), either cytoplasmic staining (C-ANCA) or perinuclear or nuclear staining (P-ANCA), are important serologic markers useful for differentiating the underlying disease and assessing the activity of some forms of RPGN. When ANCA are present in the serum, the glomerular lesion is always pauci-immune necrotizing and crescentic GN. Ninety percent of the patients with untreated active Wegener's granulomatosis are C-ANCA positive and 80% of the patients with pauci-immune polyarteritis nodosa are either C-ANCA or P-ANCA positive, while patients with immune complex-mediated polyarteritis are ANCA negative. Patients with the pauci-immune subtype of idiopathic RPGN (type III) are usually P-ANCA positive.

## Pathology and Pathogenesis

Glomerular crescents are believed to be derived from proliferation and epithelioid transformation of blood-borne monocytes (macrophages) that migrate from the glomerular capillary into the urinary space through breaks or gaps in an injured GBM. Leakage of fibrinogen and other intravascular contents through the pathologic gaps leads to fibrin polymerization, which probably acts as a nidus for the crescent formation. The increasing size of the proliferating crescent compresses the functional glomerulus to a smaller and smaller mass. Eventually, fibroblasts from the renal interstitium may migrate into the crescent and convert the crescent into a sclerotic or fibrous scar. Predominance of fibrous crescents, global glomerular sclerosis, interstitial fibrosis, and tubular atrophy in a renal biopsy specimen portends a poor clinical prognosis. Unpredictably, some crescents may resolve without permanent injury. The latter is more common in RPGN associated with infectious disorders, such as poststreptococcal GN.

Multiple disease processes can lead to severe GBM injury with gaps and subsequent development of crescents and RPGN (see Table 114-3). Most of these disorders are discussed in detail elsewhere in this chapter.

When no other primary glomerular disease can be diagnosed, and when crescents can be identified in 50% or more of the glomeruli sampled by a renal biopsy, the disorder is called idiopathic RPGN. Subtypes of idiopathic RPGN are classified according to the etiology of the GBM injury. In *Type I*, antibody to GBM antigen (anti-GBM) is formed secondary to an unknown stimulus and results in linear deposition of IgG along the GBM, readily identifiable by immunofluorescent staining of a renal biopsy. The glomerular endocapillary cells may show little if any proliferation. Most of these patients have measurable circulating anti-GBM antibody, although in some it is not detectable until after nephrectomy. In *Type II*, circulating immune complexes of unknown etiology are deposited in the mesangium and subendothelial portions of the GBM. These deposits are recognized as a granular pattern of IgG or IgM by immunofluorescent staining, and as electron-dense deposits by electron microscopic examination of a renal biopsy. The circulating immune complexes may be measurable, and serum C3 may be decreased if it is also present in the deposits. *Type III* (pauci-immune) is characterized by the sparsity or absence of any immune deposits, either linear or granular, in the glomeruli. The renal biopsy usually has features of necrotizing GN similar to that of Wegener's granulomatosis

or polyarteritis nodosa, suggesting that type III may not be a distinct idiopathic RPGN subtype, but a renal-limited variant of a systemic necrotizing vasculitis. In addition, since 80% of the patients with type III RPGN are ANCA positive, ANCA may participate directly in the pathogenesis of the glomerular lesion by activating neutrophils and monocytes within glomerular capillaries, resulting in necrotizing inflammatory injury and subsequent crescent formation.

## Therapy

Therapy for RPGN has been aimed at stopping glomerular injury to prevent progression of or further crescent formation. If indicated, therapy should be started as early as possible after diagnosis if it is to be of any value. Because RPGN is rare and is associated with many disorders of diverse etiology, no good, large, controlled therapeutic trials have been or may ever be done to document the efficacy of a given drug regimen. High-dose steroids alone or in combination with cytotoxic agents such as cyclophosphamide have not significantly altered the clinical outcome in small controlled studies. Anticoagulant therapy (heparin, warfarin, or dipyridamole) has theoretic appeal in preventing fibrin polymerization as a nidus for crescent formation. However, such therapy is dangerous in uremic patients, especially in those at risk for pulmonary hemorrhage, and not even a small controlled study has been done to confirm its efficacy. At present, anticoagulant therapy alone or in combination cannot be recommended. Plasmapheresis in combination with high-dose steroids and cytotoxic agents may be advantageous in the treatment of patients with anti-GBM disorders or vasculitis (ANCA-associated such as Wegener's granulomatosis or lupus). Children with RPGN associated with poststreptococcal GN probably need only supportive care, as they will often improve with or without drug therapy.

## Prognosis

Hospitalization may be prolonged for children with RPGN. Most require dialysis and have complications of therapy such as severe hypertension. About half the children with RPGN and crescents in over 50% of their glomeruli by renal biopsy will progress to end-stage renal disease and require chronic dialysis or a renal transplant. The recurrence rate of RPGN in the transplanted kidney is 10% to 30%, depending on the underlying disorder.

## NEPHROTIC SYNDROME

The nephrotic syndrome (NS) is a clinical condition resulting from the loss of large amounts of protein from the blood into the urine. The amount of proteinuria is usually sufficient to cause hypoproteinemia and consequent edema. Hyperlipidemia and lipiduria are also part of the fully expressed NS.

The NS may be a feature of any form of childhood GN or may be secondary to other systemic diseases, nephrotoxins, or allergic reactions (Table 114-4). The discussion in this section will concentrate on GN, specifically those histopathologic types that occur in children, whose clinical presentation is primarily that of the NS itself and not of the nephritic syndrome. Various names, including lipoid nephrosis, idiopathic NS of childhood, childhood nephrosis, nil lesion syndrome, and foot process disease, have been used to identify this condition, but none provides insight into the nature of the underlying pathogenesis. In this chapter, we have chosen to use the term *primary NS* instead of idiopathic NS or any of the other names, to avoid confusion between the clinical NS and the variety of pathologic entities associated with it. The specific disorders to be discussed are minimal change disease (MCNS), diffuse mesangial proliferative GN, focal segmental

## TABLE 114-4. Causes of the Nephrotic Syndrome

**Primary Nephrotic Syndrome**
Minimal change disease
Diffuse mesangial proliferative glomerulonephritis
Focal segmental glomerulosclerosis
Membranoproliferative glomerulonephritis
Membranous glomerulonephritis

**Secondary Nephrotic Syndrome**
*Other Renal Diseases*
Hemolytic-uremic syndrome, anti-GBM disease, IgA nephropathy, idiopathic RPGN, diffuse mesangial sclerosis

*Infectious*
Bacterial (poststreptococcal, infective endocarditis, shunt nephritis, leprosy, syphilis), viral (hepatitis B, cytomegalovirus, Epstein-Barr, varicella, HIV), protozoal (malaria, toxoplasmosis), parasitic (schistosomiasis, filariasis)

*Neoplasia*
Lymphoma leukemia, Wilms' tumor, pheochromocytoma, others

*Medications*
Mercurials, gold, penicillamine, trimethadione, mephenytoin

*Systemic Diseases*
Systemic lupus erythematosus, Henoch-Schönlein purpura, polyarteritis nodosa, Takayasu syndrome, dermatitis herpetiformis, sarcoidosis, Sjögren syndrome, amyloidosis, diabetes mellitus

*Allergic Reactions*
Insect stings, poison oak and ivy, serum sickness

*Familial Disorders*
Alport syndrome, Fabry disease, nail-patella syndrome, sickle-cell disease, Finnish nephrosis

*Circulatory Disorders*
Constrictive pericarditis, congestive heart failure, renal vein thrombosis

*Miscellaneous*
Chronic renal allograft rejection, preeclampsia, malignant hypertension

glomerulosclerosis (FSGS), membranoproliferative GN (MPGN), membranous GN (MGN), and the NS of infants.

## Overview

Primary NS has been reported to occur with an annual incidence as high as seven cases per 100,000 children under age 16 years, but an incidence of two per 100,000, the figure determined in a 16-year population survey in Erie County, New York, seems more likely to represent the usual incidence rate.

In early childhood, about 80% of the children with primary NS have MCNS. Of these, 60% are between ages 2 and 6 years. MCNS is quite uncommon in infants under age 1 year and accounts for only 30% of adolescent and 15% to 20% of adult cases. Because older children are more likely to have underlying histopathologic types of GN other than MCNS, a diagnostic renal biopsy is usually performed early in their disease course. The histopathologic type, more than age at onset or any other feature of the NS, determines the clinical outcome.

About 3.5% of the children with primary NS have affected siblings. Affected monozygotic but not dizygotic twins have been reported. No specific pattern of inheritance has been associated with any histopathologic subtype, although familial incidence has been reported more often for FSGS. Vertical transmission of primary NS has not been documented. Suggested associations of primary NS with specific HLA antigens, complement deficiencies, and atopy have been suggested but not substantiated.

## Structural Basis of Proteinuria

The GBM is composed of collagens, glycoproteins, and a variety of negatively charged glycosaminoglycans. Negative charge is enhanced by sialic acid residues on the visceral epithelial cells covering the GBM. The whole structure is an effective barrier to the passage of plasma proteins, which are for the most part too large and too negatively charged to cross into the urinary space. Using quantitative clearance studies of neutral, anionic, and cationic dextrans of differing molecular radii in normal humans, investigators have demonstrated that small molecules easily pass into the urine, large molecules are hindered, positively charged molecules pass by facilitated clearance, and negatively charged molecules are repelled and remain in the capillary blood.

Pathologic alterations of the glomerular barrier allow proteinuria to occur. Three types of alteration have been identified. The first is a loss of negative charge along the GBM and the epithelial cell surface, without obvious structural damage. This type of change occurs in MCNS. A second type, commonly found in FSGS, is separation of the epithelial cell from the GBM. The third type is the appearance of gaps in the GBM through which elements of blood, including cells, may pass. A combination of these alterations occurs when immune proteins are deposited along the inner (subendothelial) or outer (subepithelial) aspect of the GBM. Such deposits occur most often in MPGN and MGN. Lesions that begin as negative-charge loss may progress to loss of structural integrity and eventually to sclerosis. Progressive sclerosis and subsequent loss of GFR may be sufficient to decrease protein excretion, so that the NS appears to improve.

## Clinical Consequences of Proteinuria

Many proteins appear in the urine of nephrotic patients, but albumin is found in greatest abundance. Albuminuria is the primary cause of hypoalbuminemia, which is the main determinant of reduced plasma colloid oncotic pressure in primary NS. Reduction of oncotic pressure causes a shift of fluid from the intravascular compartment to the interstitial space, with consequent edema. In response to a loss of vascular volume, the kidney increases its reabsorption of sodium and water and worsens the edema.

Historically, nephrotic patients were thought to reabsorb sodium avidly via the renin-angiotensin-aldosterone axis in response to decreased intravascular volume associated with low plasma oncotic pressure. Recently, investigators have shown that some nephrotic patients actually have increased or normal plasma volume and normal or suppressed serum renin and aldosterone levels, suggesting that salt and water retention may be a primary renal disturbance, as in acute GN. Each explanation may be valid for some patients with NS, depending on their underlying renal disease or the stage of their disease at the time of study.

## Laboratory Features

Proteinuria is the hallmark of NS. The urinalysis shows qualitatively large amounts of protein (2 to 4+ by dipstick), a high specific gravity, and hyaline and granular casts. To be classified as nephrotic-range proteinuria, the protein excretion rate should exceed 40 mg/m$^2$/hr in a 24-hour urine collection. In children, especially the very young, reliable 24-hour urine collections are difficult to obtain. Alternative measurements, such as a random urine protein/creatinine ratio of above 1.0, may be substituted. A low serum albumin concentration correlated with a series of strongly positive (2+ or more) dipstick tests for albumin in random urinalyses may also suffice.

Urinary protein selectivity (ie, the relative clearance of albumin versus proteins of larger molecular weight) has been useful to some clinicians for differential diagnosis and for predicting steroid responsiveness in a given patient. Patients with MCNS usually selectively excrete albumin; in contrast, patients with focal sclerosis or proliferative lesions excrete albumin and larger-molecular-weight proteins, such as IgG, equally. A comparison of albumin to IgG clearance can be calculated by the following formula:

$$\%\text{Selectivity} = (U_{IgG})(P_{alb})/(P_{IgG})(U_{alb}) \times 100$$

where $U_{IgG}$ and $P_{IgG}$ = urine and plasma concentrations of IgG, and $U_{alb}$ and $P_{alb}$ = urine and plasma concentrations of albumin. If the percentage selectivity is less than 10%, patients are usually steroid-responsive; a ratio greater than 10% has been associated with a poor response to steroid therapy. Unfortunately, the percentage selectivity is not always accurate and should be used only as one of many clinical and laboratory aids in planning therapy.

The massive proteinuria of NS usually causes hypoalbuminemia. Hypoalbuminemia becomes clinically significant when the serum albumin is 2.5 g/dL or less and edema occurs. Studies of hepatic albumin synthesis in nephrotics have shown an insufficient increase in albumin synthesis to replace ongoing albumin losses. The albumin synthesis rates in nephrotics, especially those with poor dietary protein intake, are considerably less than might be expected from the normal hepatic potential for increased albumin synthesis, which is about three times the baseline rate. Renal tubular catabolism of albumin also increases by three to five times the normal rate in nephrotics.

Like albumin, the concentration of other plasma proteins, such as coagulation inhibitors and vitamin D-binding globulin (Table 114-5), are decreased because of increased urinary losses, decreased synthesis, or increased catabolism. Some plasma protein levels, including those of coagulation factors and lipoproteins, are actually increased in NS. The increased levels probably result from an increased and relatively unregulated hepatic production of protein in response to hypoalbuminemia. The significance of these aberrations is discussed below in the section on extrarenal complications.

Serum cholesterol, triglycerides, and total lipids are elevated in most cases of primary NS of childhood. Serum concentrations of low-density lipoproteins and very-low-density lipoproteins are increased, but high-density lipoproteins may be normal, increased, or reduced, depending on the severity of the proteinuria and the type of underlying renal lesion. Total cholesterol levels are usually very elevated, exceeding 400 mg/dL in two thirds of the children with MCNS. The degree of hypercholesterolemia is inversely related to the serum albumin concentration. The serum concentration of triglycerides is more variable and may remain normal in some patients until the NS is quite severe. The pathogenesis of hyperlipidemia is incompletely understood. A marked increase in hepatic synthesis of lipoproteins and a reduction in catabolic removal occurs in the NS. These abnormalities are correlated with the renal clearance of albumin and not the rate of albumin synthesis.

Lipiduria, a common urinary abnormality, is best appreciated by polarized light microscopy. Oval fat bodies, which are lipid-laden renal tubular cells sloughed into the urine, may be easily identified in the urinary sediment, even without a polarized microscope.

Hematuria occurs in some children with primary NS, and it may be helpful in narrowing the differential diagnosis. Transient microscopic hematuria occurs in only 25% of the children with MCNS, and gross hematuria is almost never encountered. In children with other forms of primary NS, either gross or microscopic hematuria is present more than half the time.

Renal function measured by creatinine or inulin clearance is normal or increased in most patients with NS, although one third of the children with MCNS show transient depression of GFR at the onset of their disease, probably due to hypovolemia and poor renal perfusion. If GFR remains low after NS has been treated and the affected child has improved clinically, the child should be evaluated for an underlying diagnosis other than MCNS. Renal tubular wasting of glucose, bicarbonate, amino acids, or phosphate, typical of partial or complete Fanconi syndrome, is extremely uncommon and suggests the diagnosis of FSGS.

### Extrarenal Complications and General Management

Each protein abnormality of NS causes specific clinical consequences. Hypoalbuminemia causes edema, which usually begins insidiously with unexpected weight gain and early morning periorbital swelling that shifts during the day to the lower legs and feet. In time, anasarca may occur, occasionally associated with an inability to open the eyes, respiratory distress from ascites or pleural effusions, and scrotal or labial edema that prevents walking. Therapy for severe edema includes intravenous or oral furosemide, alone or in combination with intravenous albumin infusions or oral metolazone. These therapies should be used judiciously, as they may produce profound electrolyte disturbances and cause hypovolemic shock or venous thromboses in patients already predisposed to these complications. Intravenous albumin infusions should be reserved for children with severe hypovolemia who may develop orthostatic hypotension, prerenal azotemia, or shock, or for those with severe and refractory edema.

Other potential adverse affects of hypoalbuminemia include enhanced platelet aggregability, increased stimulation of lipoprotein production, and enhanced drug toxicity due to higher circulating free drug concentrations of drugs that are normally protein-bound.

Protein-calorie malnutrition is a rare complication of chronic NS, seen only in children with unremitting proteinuria. These children tend to eat poorly, preventing the compensatory production of protein that can occur in well-nourished nephrotics. Urinary losses of proteins other than albumin may lead to clinically significant problems in some patients with chronic, unremitting NS. Increased urinary losses of vitamin D-binding globulin and of the 25-hydroxyvitamin D bound to it may be a principal cause of the osteomalacia sometimes seen in these patients. Clinical hypothyroidism is a rare problem caused by loss of thyroid-binding proteins as well as free thyroxine, with resultant depression of serum total and free thyroxine and total triiodothyronine and a compensatory increase in serum thyroid-stimulating hormone.

Decreased serum concentrations of immunoproteins are thought to be the basis of the predisposition of nephrotic patients to infection with encapsulated bacteria. The exact mechanism for serum IgG depression, an almost universal finding in patients with primary NS, is unknown and cannot be accounted for by urinary loss of IgG alone. The sluggish activity of the alternate pathway of complement is probably the result of urinary loss of factor B, which plays a pivotal role in the production of C3b, the

---

**TABLE 114-5.  Common Plasma Protein Concentration Derangements in Patients with the Nephrotic Syndrome**

| Increased Levels | Decreased Levels |
|---|---|
| Alpha-2 globulins | Albumin |
| Beta globulins | Alpha-1 globulins |
| Coagulation factors | IgG |
| Antifibrinolysins | Coagulation inhibitors |
| Most lipoproteins | Transferrin |
| | Transcortin |
| | Thyroxine-binding globulin |
| | Vitamin D-binding globulin |

principal opsonin of *Escherichia coli*, *Streptococcus pneumoniae*, and *Haemophilus influenzae*. Infections with these organisms are the main cause of death in nephrotic children. Primary peritonitis is a particular problem: 6% of nephrotic children suffer at least one episode of bacterial peritonitis. Aggressive antibiotic therapy, specific for the common bacterial pathogens listed above, should be given at the first suspicion of systemic or peritoneal infection. Pneumococcal and *H. influenzae* B vaccines may be effective long-term deterrents to infection, but can be given only to patients who are in remission and on no immunosuppressive medications at the time of vaccination to achieve an effective antibody response. The use of prophylactic antibiotics during relapses is controversial but advocated by some clinicians. Nephrotic patients ordinarily tolerate viral infections well, unless they are receiving high-dose immunosuppressants.

The incidence of thrombotic events in nephrotic children is low (1.8%), but the consequences are sometimes fatal. Sites of thrombosis include the inferior vena cava, renal veins, hepatic veins, pulmonary artery, pulmonary veins, femoral arteries, deep leg veins, and the sagittal sinus. Arterial thromboses are more common in children than in adults with NS. Renal vein thrombosis is more common in older children and adults with the NS of MGN.

Numerous defects in hemostasis occur in NS. Alterations in almost every coagulation factor and clotting inhibitor, as well as increased platelet adhesiveness and defects in the fibrinolytic system, have been reported. Systemic anticoagulation is indicated for all patients who develop thromboembolic disease and for those at high risk because of immobilization. Avoidance of bed rest, volume depletion, diuretics, and deep venous or arterial punctures are important aspects of the management of patients at risk for thrombosis.

The clinical significance of hyperlipidemia in children with NS is unknown. Epidemiologic studies of nonnephrotic patients who have decreased ratios of high-density to low-density cholesterol have shown an increased risk of developing arteriosclerotic coronary heart disease in those patients. Studies in a few patients with chronic NS suggest that these children are similarly at risk. Hyperlipidemia plays a role in the hypercoagulable state of nephrotic patients and may play a role in the progression of glomerulosclerosis.

### Pathogenesis of Primary NS

It is widely held that diseases giving rise to primary NS are immune-mediated. In MCNS, and perhaps mesangial proliferative GN and FSGS, abnormalities of immunoglobulin synthesis, lymphocyte function, and lymphokine production occur. In MPGN and MGN, immune complexes deposited in the GBM cause local damage, and massive proteinuria ensues. Further details of pathogenesis will be reviewed for each disease below.

## Minimal Change Disease

MCNS is characterized by the onset of NS without systemic disease, hypocomplementemia, or other serious signs of renal disease. Although nephritic features (hematuria, azotemia, and hypertension) occur in 10% to 30% of children with MCNS, these signs seldom occur together and are almost never severe or persistent. Patients with MCNS are notably young—two thirds of them present between ages 2 and 6 years. For this reason, preadolescents with NS and no nephritic signs, hypocomplementemia, or signs of systemic disease do not need a kidney biopsy before the initiation of therapy. Steroid therapy effectively induces a remission in most patients. Prompt and sustained remissions correlate well with minimal changes of glomerular morphology.

Clinical and laboratory features and pathophysiology are those of NS described above.

### Pathology

Renal biopsies of patients with MCNS either appear normal by light microscopy or show no more than a mild, focal increase in mesangial cellularity and mesangial matrix. Tubular atrophy, interstitial fibrosis, and vascular changes are absent. Electron microscopic findings include effacement of epithelial cell foot processes, normal GBM thickness, and no more than an occasional small paramesangial electron-dense deposit. Immunofluorescence staining may be negative or slightly positive for IgM and rarely IgG and C3 in the mesangium.

### Pathogenesis

In 1974, Shalhoub hypothesized that MCNS may be caused by an abnormal clone of T cells that produces a lymphokine that damages the GBM. His hypothesis was based on four well-recognized clinical observations indicative of T-cell activity: remissions of NS are induced by rubeola infection, patients with NS have increased susceptibility to pneumococcal infection, remissions of NS are induced by steroids and cyclophosphamide, and MCNS occurs in some patients with Hodgkin's disease. Many studies have been performed to investigate a potential role of lymphocytes in the pathogenesis of MCNS. Although no consistent abnormalities of T- or B-cell numbers have been found, abnormalities of lymphocyte function are present in patients with MCNS.

Serum from patients in relapse, but not those in remission, inhibits lymphocyte growth in vitro, either because it contains inhibitory substances or lacks certain factors necessary for growth. This finding may not be specific for MCNS, however, because serum from patients with FSGS and MGN also inhibits in vitro lymphocyte growth. Several recent experiments have shown that products of stimulated lymphocytes from nephrotic patients reduce glomerular polyanionic charge of rat glomeruli. Foot process effacement was induced in some of the animals. Consistent production of proteinuria in these animals did not occur. Cellular immunity is altered in relapse, so that affected patients have markedly reduced response to tuberculin and other skin tests.

Although not specific for MCNS and apparently unrelated to glomerular injury, consistent abnormalities of immunoglobulins are found in NS. Serum IgG concentrations are decreased in relapse but usually return to normal in remission. Serum IgM concentration is often increased in relapse and may continue to be high or return to normal in remission. Low serum levels of IgG result in part from urinary loss, but decreased production has also been demonstrated. The mechanisms controlling the observed abnormalities of serum IgG and IgM are unknown.

### Differential Diagnosis

Differentiating MCNS from the rest of the disorders causing primary NS (see Table 114-4) has been made easier by reports of the International Study of Kidney Disease in Children (ISKDC). By examining clinical and laboratory features of patients with biopsy-proven primary NS, these investigators identified certain clinical patterns suggestive of the underlying renal histopathology. Patients with MCNS usually present before age 6 years; those with MPGN rarely present before age 8 years. Hypertension is less common in MCNS (13%) than in FSGS (33%). Hematuria is transient and uncommon in MCNS (25%), but occurs in more than half the patients with other diseases. Decreased serum C3 concentration occurs in three fourths of the patients with MPGN, but serum C3 is almost always normal in other forms of primary NS. Patients with MCNS almost always respond to steroid therapy, so when the diagnosis of MCNS is suspected clinically but no remission of the NS is induced after 8 weeks of steroid therapy, another diagnosis is likely, and a diagnostic renal biopsy should be performed.

### Therapy and Outcome

The diagnosis of NS is usually first suspected in the outpatient setting. Hospitalization for a new nephrotic is strongly recommended for dietary and if needed diuretic management of edema, for initiation of steroid therapy, and for parent and patient education about the disease. At least 24 hours before starting steroid therapy, a tuberculin skin test should be done; if the result is negative, treatment may be safely started.

Recommendations for steroid therapy have been made by the ISKDC and others. A usually adequate steroid regimen consists of prednisone 60 mg/m²/day in three equally divided doses for 4 weeks, followed by 40 to 60 mg/m²/day as a single dose given every other day in the morning for an additional 4 to 12 weeks. A maximum dose of 80 mg of prednisone per day is advisable. This standard approach was recently challenged by the German collaborative study, which showed that an initial 6-week course of daily prednisone followed by 6 weeks of alternate-day therapy resulted in a 50% reduction in the number of patients who relapsed during the subsequent 12 months, when compared with the relapse rate of patients treated with a shorter course of steroids. The typically responsive patient loses the proteinuria within the first 3 weeks of therapy. During the period of alternate-day prednisone, the dose of prednisone is gradually decreased and discontinued about 3 to 4 months after initiating therapy.

Relapses occur in 80% of affected children, often during the period of slow prednisone tapering. During this time, the urine should be checked routinely at home for protein, using a dipstick daily or at least three times a week to screen for early signs of relapse, before the onset of edema. Patients who have fewer than two relapses in a 6-month period may be treated as described above for each relapse. Those who have more than two relapses in a 6-month period are called frequent relapsers and may do well on longer courses of alternate-day prednisone. Patients who cannot tolerate cessation of steroid therapy without a relapse are called steroid-dependent. Steroid toxicity may become a major problem for either frequent relapsers or steroid-dependent patients, who receive high dosages of daily steroids for a long period of time.

Frequent relapsers and steroid-dependent patients may require a diagnostic renal biopsy. If the biopsy shows MCNS and additional therapy to control the NS is desirable, a 2-month course of chlorambucil (0.2 mg/kg/day) or cyclophosphamide (2.5 mg/kg/day) may produce a sustained remission. Patients with frequently relapsing NS have more prolonged remissions than steroid-dependent patients after cytotoxic therapy. During therapy, patients should have a weekly complete blood count to monitor for signs of bone marrow depression that might require altering or stopping the drug dosage. Before beginning therapy with cytotoxic drugs, patients and parents should also be warned of other potential drug side effects, such as sterility in males after long-term cyclophosphamide therapy. Cyclosporine has also been effective in inducing a remission in steroid-dependent patients, but the relapse rate after discontinuation of this drug has been substantial.

Most patients with MCNS are hospitalized for no more than a week at the time of diagnosis, and most never require hospitalization again. When feeling well, patients should attend school as usual, without any special physical restrictions. A sodium-restricted diet is mandatory during relapses and while the patient is taking prednisone. Maintaining a low-sodium diet during remissions may be psychologically helpful if the child is a frequent relapser. Immunizations are usually withheld until the child is in remission and has been off steroids for at least 3 months. No live-virus vaccine should be given to a patient or his or her siblings while the patient is taking high-dose daily steroids or cytotoxic drugs.

The long-term prognosis for MCNS is excellent. Most patients (80%) enter a sustained remission during adolescence. The overall death rate in a large group of patients with MCNS followed by the ISKDC for 5 to 15 years was 2.6%.

## Diffuse Mesangial Proliferative GN

A few children, probably less than 3%, presenting with primary NS have diffuse mesangial hypercellularity with or without mesangial electron-dense deposits on renal biopsy. By immunofluorescence, the deposits are frequently IgM, occasionally associated with C3, and are located in the mesangium and rarely in the capillary loop. Biopsies with predominantly IgM deposits have been classified by some as IgM mesangial nephropathy, but patients with this lesion have been found to have no distinguishing clinical features compared with other children with idiopathic NS. The significance of IgM deposits, like the pathogenesis of diffuse mesangial proliferation, is unknown. Some patients who have had serial biopsies have been noted to develop FSGS, which usually heralds a poor prognosis.

Clinically, children with NS and diffuse mesangial proliferative GN are more likely to have microscopic hematuria (90%), hypertension (50%), reduced renal function (25%), and poor initial response to steroid therapy (35% to 70%). Despite their steroid resistance, patients generally have a good prognosis, with some undergoing spontaneous remission of NS and less than 10% progressing to severe renal failure. For those who do progress to end-stage renal disease, the recurrence rate of diffuse mesangial proliferative GN in a renal transplant has been reported to be as high as 40%.

## Focal Segmental Glomerulosclerosis

FSGS is the pathologic description of a lesion that results from several etiologies (Table 114-6). The idiopathic form may also represent several different etiologic insults to the kidney, but our current knowledge does not allow differentiation as yet.

### Clinical and Laboratory Features

About 10% of the children presenting with primary NS are found to have FSGS by renal biopsy, but not all patients with FSGS present this way. Twenty percent of the cases are diagnosed after

---

**TABLE 114-6. Etiology of Focal Segmental Glomerulosclerosis**

**Primary Renal**
Idiopathic, with or without mesangial hypercellularity

**Secondary**
Reflux nephropathy
Reduced renal mass (single kidney, partial nephrectomy)
Heroin abuse nephropathy
Analgesic abuse nephropathy
Sickle-cell disease
Alport syndrome
Late stage of nephritis of chronic bacteremia
Chronic rejection of renal transplant
HIV-associated nephropathy

asymptomatic proteinuria has been found; these patients usually develop NS at a later date. Microscopic hematuria occurs in more than half the affected children at presentation, but gross hematuria is rare. Renal tubular defects, including renal glucosuria, generalized ammoaciduria, renal tubular acidosis, partial or complete Fanconi syndrome, and concentrating defects, occur occasionally and portend future progression to renal failure. Patients who are hypertensive at presentation (40%) do not have a significantly worse prognosis for progression to renal failure.

### Pathology

Early in the disease, the renal lesions of FSGS are quite focal and predominantly are located in the juxtamedullary glomeruli, so that affected glomeruli may not be obtained at the initial or even one or two subsequent percutaneous renal biopsies. The renal lesion of FSGS has characteristic features by light microscopy. The glomeruli are usually enlarged, with segmental capillary loop collapse and increased mesangial matrix. The visceral epithelial cells are often vacuolated and may be lifted off the GBM or may form caps over sclerotic areas. Foam cells, which are foamy-appearing lipid-laden histiocytes, are sometimes associated with the segmental lesions. Mesangial hypercellularity occurs in 50% of the biopsies of affected children. Tubulointerstitial disease is almost always present. IgM, often accompanied by C3, can be identified by immunofluorescence microscopy in the mesangium or focally along the GBM of affected capillary loops. Fibrin staining occurs in areas of sclerosis. Electron microscopic examination demonstrates endothelial cell swelling, effacement of visceral epithelial cell podocytes, sclerosis, and scattered immune deposits.

### Clinical Course and Therapy

Whether or not the diagnosis of FSGS is made on the initial renal biopsy or a subsequent biopsy, affected children have a similar clinical course. Only 20% of children with FSGS initially respond to prednisone with a complete remission. Most of these relapse, and some progress to end-stage renal disease. Cytotoxic drugs and cyclosporine are not of proven value but are still used by many clinicians in selected patients in an attempt to control severe NS. Pulse intravenous methylprednisolone therapy for 8 to 12 weeks in conjunction with alternate-day oral prednisone has been used successfully in a few patients; further trials evaluating the efficacy of this therapy are still in progress.

Renal failure is present initially in almost half of the affected children. Progression to end-stage renal disease occurs in 20% to 30% within 5 years and in almost 60% within 10 years. Persistent NS and an increase in globally sclerotic glomeruli in follow-up biopsies have been associated with progressive disease. No other clinical or pathologic markers of progressive disease have been confirmed. FSGS recurs frequently (25%) in renal transplants, unfortunately sometimes with massive proteinuria and NS within the first 24 hours and renal allograft loss within days to weeks.

## Membranoproliferative GN

The evolution of classifications of chronic GN has resulted in a confusing list of historical names for MPGN. MPGN has been called *lobular* or *mixed membranous and proliferative GN* and *hypocomplementemic GN*, and is still sometimes called *mesangiocapillary GN*. The name MPGN is derived from the glomerular histopathologic lesion of patients with this disorder. Microscopic examination of renal biopsies of affected patients shows a marked increase in mesangial cellularity and extension of mesangial cells into the capillary wall, causing the GBM to appear thickened and reduplicated.

MPGN is a chronic disease of children and adults that may be idiopathic or occasionally associated with other systemic dis-

eases. The age of onset in most patients is between 8 and 20 years. The male to female sex ratio is equal. A genetic predisposition to MPGN is suggested by the association of MPGN with an inherited deficiency of several complement components, an association with the extended haplotype HLA-B8, DR3, SC01, GL02, the occurrence of the disease in some siblings, and the rarity of the disease in blacks.

### Clinical Features

About 10% of the cases of primary NS in childhood are caused by MPGN, but only about half of the children with MPGN present with NS. Another quarter present with the acute nephritic syndrome, and about one fourth with asymptomatic proteinuria or hematuria. Gross hematuria, hypertension, and azotemia each occur in 30% of patients. When these signs appear together, MPGN is easily confused with acute poststreptococcal GN. Most patients have microscopic or gross hematuria at onset, and almost all have proteinuria. In those presenting without proteinuria, a low serum C3 may be the only clue to the diagnosis.

### Laboratory Features

Laboratory features of primary NS occur in most patients. In these patients and in those with nonnephrotic proteinuria, the urine is usually positive for blood and often contains cellular casts. Anemia is common and often disproportionate to the degree of renal failure. Serum C3 concentrations are decreased in 60% to 75% of patients at the time of diagnosis. Thus, the absence of this abnormality does not rule out the diagnosis of MPGN.

### Pathology

There are two well-defined subtypes of MPGN and a controversial third subtype. *Type I* is characterized by enlarged, lobular glomeruli with obliteration of capillary lumens and marked mesangial proliferation. Mesangial proliferation may be so marked that mesangial cells wedge between the GBM and the endothelium, resulting in an apparent reduplication of GBM material and a "tram track" appearance. Electron microscopy shows mesangial and subendothelial deposits, which are positive for IgG and C3 by immunofluorescence staining. *Type II* shares many of the same light microscopic findings as type I, but mesangial proliferation is less. Electron microscopy shows characteristic very dense material within the GBM that gives type II MPGN its other common designation, *dense deposit disease*. The origin of this dense material is unknown; it is not immune complex material. Positive immunofluorescence staining, mainly for C3, outlines the GBM around the dense deposits but does not occur within them. C3 also occurs in the mesangium and sparsely in the subendothelial and subepithelial spaces. Children with *type III* disease have mesangial, subendothelial, subepithelial, and transmembranous deposition of IgG and C3, with extensive disruption of the GBM.

Some investigators have described further subtypes of MPGN in which the location and composition of the immune deposits differ slightly from those seen in type I. These additional subtypes have not proven to be useful classifications for prediction of clinical outcome, since identical clinical disease has been associated with each subtype.

### Pathogenesis

The morphologic diversity of renal biopsies from patients with MPGN suggests heterogeneity of pathogenesis. Immune complex deposition is a prominent feature of all types of MPGN. Circulating immune complexes have been measured in patients with all types of MPGN, but their presence does not correlate with the severity of disease activity or the degree of hypocomplementemia. The stimulus for immune complex formation is unknown.

Complement activation occurs by at least two mechanisms in MPGN. In type I MPGN, immune complexes stimulate the classical pathway, depleting serum concentration of C1q, C2, and C4 along with C3 and C5. Low serum C3 levels may retard the normal clearing of immune complexes from the circulation. As mentioned previously, inherited deficiencies of complement have been associated with MPGN types I and III. In type II disease, alternate pathway activation by C3 nephritic factor ($NF_a$) reduces the serum concentration of C3, whereas C4 remains normal and C5 is normal or minimally depressed. This type of C3 nephritic factor is an IgG autoantibody that increases alternate pathway degradation of C3. The presence of C3 nephritic factor does not appear to affect the outcome of patients with MPGN. Another recently described nephritic factor, $NF_t$, causes complement activation in type III MPGN and results in markedly depressed serum C3 and C5 levels with normal C4 concentration.

### Course and Therapy

A few patients have spontaneous remissions of NS that may last for years. The only evidence of disease activity during this "silent phase" may be persistent hypocomplementemia. The natural history of patients with MPGN is to progress slowly toward end-stage renal disease. About half of the patients reach end-stage disease 10 years after diagnosis. If the serum creatinine exceeds 2 mg/dL at presentation, dialysis will probably be required within 3 years. Hypertension, gross hematuria, and unremitting NS with edema predict a poor prognosis.

Historically, many treatments for MPGN have been tried, including steroids, other immunosuppressants, anticoagulants, and nonsteroidal anti-inflammatories. Recently a double-blind, prospective, controlled trial of daily aspirin and dipyridamole therapy was associated with maintenance of a higher GFR, but had no effect on proteinuria in affected adults followed up for many years. The ISKDC showed beneficial results of long-term alternate-day prednisone for maintaining renal function in children with all types of MPGN, but aggressive management of steroid-induced hypertension was required in some.

Renal transplantation is successful in patients with MPGN, although types I and II may both recur in the allograft. The recurrence rate may be as high as 50% in type II MPGN. However, graft loss to recurrent disease is insufficient to consider withholding transplantation.

## Membranous GN

MGN is a rare disorder of children, accounting for less than 6% of the cases presenting with primary NS. The frequency of occurrence increases in adolescence (10% to 20%), and the disorder is common in adults with NS (20% to 40%). MGN occurs as a primary renal disease (idiopathic MGN) in 65% to 80% of affected children, but is associated with systemic diseases or exposure to drugs and toxins in the rest (Table 114-7). The presentation of MGN may antedate the appearance of associated disorders, such as SLE, hepatitis B infection, or neoplasm, by months or years and may be confused with idiopathic MGN. MGN rarely recurs in renal transplants, but it often does arise de novo for reasons that are unclear, unless its occurrence is facilitated by glomerular changes of rejection.

### Clinical and Laboratory Features

Symptoms of MGN are usually gradual in onset. About one third of the cases are discovered on routine screening urinalysis by the presence of proteinuria. The other two thirds present with edema and NS. Proteinuria may be selective or nonselective. Hypertension occurs in 30% or fewer. Microscopic hematuria is common in children with MGN (roughly 80% in some series) and gross hematuria occurs in up to 20%. Renal function is usually normal at presentation. Serum C3 is normal, except in lupus and hepatitis B-associated MGN, in which it is usually low. Patients with hep-

| TABLE 114-7. Etiology of Membranous Glomerulonephritis |
|---|
| **Primary Renal** |
| Idiopathic (no identifiable associated condition) |
| **Associated With Infectious Disorders** |
| Hepatitis B (chronic presence of hepatitis B surface antigen) |
| Syphilis (congenital or secondary) |
| Poststreptococcal disease |
| Hydatid disease |
| Leprosy |
| Malaria |
| **Associated with Systemic Disorders** |
| Systemic lupus erythematosus |
| Thyroiditis (with thyroglobulin antibodies) |
| Fanconi syndrome (with anti-tubular basement membrane or anti-renal tubular epithelial antibodies) |
| Sickle-cell disease |
| Neoplasm (carcinoma, leukemia, Wilms' tumor) |
| Other (Sjögren syndrome, Gardner-Diamond syndrome, Kimura disease, celiac disease, diabetes mellitus) |
| **Associated With Drugs or Toxins** |
| Heavy metals (gold, mercury, bismuth, silver) |
| D-penicillamine |
| Trimethadione |
| Probenecid |
| Captopril |
| **De Novo in Renal Transplant** |

atitis B-associated MGN are usually younger (less than 10 years old), male, often black or Oriental, and without overt clinical manifestations of hepatitis. Their serum aspartate aminotransferase (AST) is mildly to moderately elevated. Liver biopsies, when done, have shown evidence of chronic hepatitis. Hepatitis B surface antigen has been demonstrated in glomeruli in some of these patients, as well as in the circulation of all. Appearance of hepatitis B core antibody in the serum has correlated with remission of NS in a few patients.

### Pathology

The characteristic pathologic lesion of MGN is diffuse thickening of the glomerular capillary wall by deposition of small immune complexes on the subepithelial side of the GBM without significant cellular proliferation. The deposits always contain IgG and often C3 by immunofluorescence staining. Silver staining of light microscopic sections shows spikes of argyrophilic GBM projecting outward around the subepithelial deposits toward the urinary space. With progression of the lesion, the deposits become incorporated into a very thickened GBM; the spikes then appear elongated, and some even join together to form silver-positive circles or domes around the deposits. In advanced lesions, focal and segmental glomerular sclerosis develops.

Stages of MGN are classified by the light and electron microscopic appearance of the deposits in renal biopsy specimens. *Stage I* refers to small, discrete subepithelial deposits in a GBM of normal thickness. *Stage II* deposits are larger, with intervening well-developed spikes of GBM in a uniformly thickened capillary wall. *Stage III* deposits are larger still, often completely engulfed by spikes to give a railroad-track appearance on silver stain, in an irregularly thickened capillary wall with narrowed capillary lumen. In *stage IV*, the deposits are almost entirely intramembranous and in various stages of dissolution; areas of glomerular sclerosis and tubular atrophy are present. *Stage V* is a healing stage noted in some patients that consists of regression of the capillary wall changes and electron-dense deposits with decreased intensity or disappearance of IgG by immunofluorescence staining. In general, the stage of MGN correlates with the duration of illness, although in some cases the lesion remains stable over years.

### Pathogenesis

The pathogenesis of MGN in humans is poorly understood, although it has been well studied in laboratory models. A likely possibility suggested by experimental models is that circulating antibodies react with intrinsic GBM antigens (or extrinsic antigens with an affinity for deposition in the GBM), resulting in formation of in situ immune complexes and the evolution of the events described above. Alternatively, deposition of preformed circulating immune complexes with an affinity for the GBM may be the initial event. Such deposits might be formed from a variety of stimuli, either endogenous (tissue antigens) or environmental (infectious agents, drugs, toxins). The rarity of measurable circulating immune complexes in affected patients, however, makes this possibility unlikely.

### Prognosis and Therapy

The course of idiopathic MGN is slowly progressive over years, resulting in chronic renal failure within a decade in only about 10% of children presenting under 10 years of age and in 20% of adolescents. Remissions of proteinuria are spontaneous in up to 30%. Whether any treatment should be given for children is uncertain, but for those with unremitting NS, a trial course of 8 weeks of alternate-day high-dose prednisone, followed by a tapering dose for a few weeks, seems to have little risk of toxicity. Currently, there are no criteria to identify children at risk of developing renal failure who might benefit from therapy, and no studies to suggest what treatment might be effective with the least side effects. Adults with MGN fare worse, so they are usually treated. What treatment if any should be given remains controversial. A well-controlled randomized trial of 6 months of alternate-day, moderately high-dose prednisone therapy showed no benefit of treatment during 4 years of follow-up in 158 Canadian adults with MGN, NS, and near-normal renal function before therapy. In contrast, another study of 81 similar adults in Italy followed for 2 to 11 years after a well-controlled randomized trial of 6 months of high-dose daily methylprednisolone, alternating monthly with daily chlorambucil, showed a significant remission of NS and better preservation of renal function for treated patients. More clinical trials must be done to confirm that dual therapy with steroids and a cytotoxic agent is desirable for all.

Treatment of patients with MGN and associated disorders is dictated by the underlying disorder. In children with MGN and congenital or secondary syphilis, early treatment with penicillin leads to rapid recovery. MGN associated with drugs or toxins usually is diagnosed after 6 to 12 months of exposure. Withdrawal of the inciting agent usually leads to recovery after several more months.

## NS in Infants

Onset of NS within the first 6 months of life must be considered separately because a different group of underlying disorders occurs in infants than in children and adolescents. The most common disorder presents at birth or in the first few weeks of life, often in infants of Finnish ancestry, leading to the designation congenital NS (CNS) or CNS of the Finnish type. Various other diseases, both primary renal and secondary to other disorders, either congenital or acquired, present in early infancy and may be confused with CNS (Table 114-8).

### Primary Renal

Unfortunately, the primary renal disorders are not easily separated by either clinical presentation or pathologic appearance of the kidney. All patients have proteinuria, hypoalbuminemia, hyperlipidemia, hypogammaglobulinemia, and normal renal function. Edema may not occur initially, but appears within a few weeks. Hematuria is uncommon. Renal biopsies show effacement of foot processes, diffuse epithelial cell proliferation, mesangial cell proliferation, and increased mesangial matrix, no electron-dense or immunofluorescent-positive deposits, persistence of fetal glomeruli, and microcysts. The microcysts represent dilated proximal tubules, once thought to be a diagnostic feature of CNS, but now known to be a nonspecific finding of infants with NS. Focal segmental sclerosis progressing to global sclerosis with tubular atrophy and interstitial fibrosis occurs with advancing age in patients with CNS, diffuse mesangial sclerosis (DMS), and FSGS.

Family history, clinical outcome, and response to immunosuppressive therapy may be the only way to arrive at a final diagnosis in infants with primary renal disease. MCNS is rare in early infancy but has been reported in infants as young as 3 weeks, is quite responsive to steroid therapy, and does not progress to end-stage renal disease. MCNS should be suspected if the renal biopsy shows no chronic changes and the family history is negative. FSGS, also rare, may be responsive to steroid therapy. Because of the risk of severe infectious complications in the immunocompromised infant with CNS, steroid therapy should not be undertaken routinely. DMS is a very rare disorder that is clinically indistinguishable from CNS. It occurs in siblings but not parents, suggesting autosomal recessive genetic transmission. It is nonresponsive to steroid therapy and progresses to end-stage renal disease before age 3 years. DMS is distinguishable pathologically from CNS by the predominance of mesangial matrix expansion without mesangial hypercellularity, The pathologic lesion progresses to sclerosis of the capillary loops.

CNS is the most common cause of NS in infants. With or without Finnish ancestry, CNS is genetically transmitted in an autosomal recessive fashion. The incidence in Finland is about 1.2 cases per 10,000 births. Most cases seen in North America have no apparent Finnish ancestry, but are otherwise not different

---

**TABLE 114-8. Causes of Nephrotic Syndrome in Infants**

**Primary Renal**

Congenital nephrotic syndrome (with or without Finnish ancestry)
Diffuse mesangial sclerosis
Minimal change nephrotic syndrome
Focal segmental glomerulosclerosis

**Secondary to Other Disorders**

Congenital infection (syphilis, toxoplasmosis, cytomegalovirus, rubella, hepatitis B, malaria)
Toxins (mercury, drugs)
Systemic lupus erythematosus
Neoplasm (Wilms' tumor)
Drash syndrome (ambiguous genitalia, Wilms' tumor, nephropathy)
XY gonadal dysgenesis
Lowe syndrome
Nail-patella syndrome
Renal vein thrombosis
Hemolytic-uremic syndrome

from the Finnish cases. The pathogenesis of CNS may be related to defects in the genes controlling GBM heparan sulfate-rich proteoglycan synthesis or degradation. Decreased synthesis or increased degradation could account for the decreased number of heparan sulfate-rich anionic sites observed in the lamina rara externa of the GBM of infants and children with CNS. The lack of anionic sites diminishes the effectiveness of the GBM as an electrostatic barrier. Proteinuria then occurs, and progressive glomerular damage ensues with time, as suggested by other experimental models of NS.

CNS may be identified in utero by elevation of amniotic fluid and maternal serum alpha-fetoprotein and in fetal renal tissue by foot process effacement with diffuse epithelial proliferation. In pregnancies known to be at risk, prenatal diagnosis is possible, but a normal amniotic fluid alpha-fetoprotein does not exclude the presence of the disease in the fetus. The placenta is usually quite large, often weighing more than 25% of the infant's birth weight.

Infants with CNS are usually small for gestational age and born prematurely. Umbilical hernias are often prominent. Edema is present at birth in at least half the patients. Even when edema is not present, proteinuria significant enough to cause hypoalbuminemia and hypoimmunoglobulinemia is present. The infants are rendered immunocompromised and highly susceptible to severe bacterial infections; these may occur in more than 85% of patients and should be treated with supplemental immunoglobulins as well as specific antibiotics. Thyroxine ($T_4$) is lost in the urine and usually leads to hypothyroidism that requires supplemental therapy. Newborn thyroid screening may detect low blood levels of $T_4$ before the clinical diagnosis of CNS. Thyroid-stimulating hormone concentration may still be normal at that time, but a decreased serum thyroid-binding globulin concentration due to its urinary loss will suggest the correct diagnosis. Later in infancy, sufficient loss of transferrin and iron or protein-bound 25-hydroxyvitamin D may cause iron deficiency anemia or vitamin D deficiency, respectively. Thromboembolic complications may occur from the hypercoagulability associated with severe chronic NS.

Renal function is normal initially but progressively deteriorates to end-stage renal disease, usually by age 3 years. Delayed growth and development and malnutrition from excessive protein losses, anorexia, and poor feeding occur in all affected infants. Untreated infants die before age 4 years. Good survival (80%) has been attained only by early aggressive medical therapy with dialysis and early renal transplantation. Catch-up growth and development is common after transplant. CNS does not recur in the renal transplant. Aggressive medical management should include nutritional supplementation, diuretics to control edema, anticoagulants (aspirin or dipyridamole) if indicated to control thromboembolism, and prophylactic penicillin to prevent infection. Bilateral nephrectomy and dialysis may be indicated before the onset of end-stage renal disease, even when renal function is still greater than 50% of normal, to treat severe growth failure, malnutrition, and other unresponsive complications of chronic NS. The diagnosis of CNS should be certain before nephrectomy, dialysis, and renal transplantation are contemplated.

### Secondary to Other Disorders

Secondary causes of NS in infancy (see Table 114-8) may be identified by signs and symptoms of the underlying disorder, such as the stigmata of congenital syphilis or nail-patella syndrome, by a history of exposure to toxic drugs (mercury teething solution), or by specific diagnostic laboratory tests. The renal pathologic lesions vary from classic membranous nephropathy associated with congenital syphilis to immune complex proliferative GN associated with other congenital infections and lupus to the unique GBM nephropathy associated with nail-patella

syndrome. Therapy is directed at the underlying disorder. Recovery may be rapid in congenital syphilis treated with penicillin and lupus treated with corticosteroids. Drash syndrome, a rare genetic disorder characterized by ambiguous genitalia, gonadoblastomas, Wilms' tumor, and progressive nephropathy, has no specific therapy. The proteinuria is unresponsive to steroids and renal failure occurs early, reaching end stage between ages 1 and 3 years.

## Selected Readings

### General

Glassock RJ, Adler SG, Ward HJ, Cohen AH. Primary glomerular diseases. In: Brenner BM, Rector FC, eds. The kidney, ed 4. Philadelphia: WB Saunders, 1991:1182.
Rodriguez-Iturbe B, Garcia J, West CD, et al. Isolated glomerular diseases. In: Holliday MA, Barrett TM, Vernier RL, eds. Pediatric nephrology, ed 2. Baltimore: Williams & Wilkins, 1987:407.

### Immune Mechanisms

Couser WG. Mediation of immune glomerular injury. J Am Soc Nephrol 1990;1: 13.
Oliveira DB, Peters DK. Autoimmunity and the pathogenesis of GN. Pediatr Nephrol 1990;4:185.

### Acute Poststreptococcal GN

Clark G, White RHR, Glasgow EF, et al. Poststreptococcal GN in children: clinicopathologic correlations and long term prognosis. Pediatr Nephrol 1988;2:381.
Potter EV, Lipschultz SA, Abidh S, et al. 12- to 17-year follow-up of patients with poststreptococcal acute GN in Trinidad. N Engl J Med 1982;307:725.

### IgA Nephropathy

Andreoli SP, Bergstein JM. Treatment of severe IgA nephropathy in children. Pediatr Nephrol 1989;3:248.
Hogg RJ, Silva FG. IgA nephropathy. Natural history and prognostic indices in children. In: Berlyne G, Giovannetti P, eds. Contributions to nephrology. Basel: S. Karger, 1984:214.
Levy M, Gonzales-Burchard G, Broyer M, et al. Berger's disease in children. Natural history and outcome. Medicine 1985;64:157.
Linne T, Berg V, Bohman O, Sigstrom L. Course and long-term outcome of idiopathic IgA nephropathy in children. Pediatr Nephrol 1991;5:383.
Southwest Pediatric Nephrology Study Group. A multicenter study of IgA nephropathy in children. Kidney Internat 1982;22:643.
Waldo FB, Alexander R, Wyatt RJ, Kohaut EC. Alternate-day prednisone therapy in children with IgA-associated nephritis. Am J Kidney Dis 1989;13:55.

### Henoch-Schönlein Purpura Nephritis

Van Es LA, Kauffman RH, Valentijn RM. Henoch-Schönlein purpura. In: Holliday M, Barrett M, Vernier R, eds. Pediatric nephrology, ed 2. Baltimore: Williams & Wilkins, 1987:492.

### GN of Systemic Lupus Erythematosus

Austin HA, Klippel JH, Balow JE, et al. Therapy of lupus nephritis. Controlled trial of prednisone and cytotoxic drugs. N Engl J Med 1986;314:614.
McCurdy DK, Lehman JA, Bernstein B, et al. Lupus nephritis. Prognostic factors in children. Pediatrics 1992;89:240.
Southwest Pediatric Nephrology Study Group. Comparison of idiopathic and systemic lupus erythematosus-associated membranous glomerulopathy in children. Am J Kidney Dis 1986;7:115.

### Nephritis of Chronic Bacteremia

Arze RS, Rashid H, Morley R, et al. Shunt nephritis: report of two cases and review of the literature. Clin Nephrol 1983;20:27.
Beaufils M, Morel-Maroger L, Sraer J-D, et al. Acute renal failure of glomerular origin during visceral abscesses. N Engl J Med 1976;295:185.
Neugarten J, Gallo GR, Baldwin DS. GN in bacterial endocarditis. Am J Kidney Dis 1984;3:371.

### Rapidly Progressive GN

Bruns FJ, Adler S, Fraley DS, et al. Long-term follow-up of aggressively treated idiopathic rapidly progressive GN. Am J Med 1989;86:400.
Jeanette JC, Falk RJ. Antineutrophil cytoplasmic autoantibodies and associated diseases: a review. Am J Kidney Dis 1990;15:517.
Southwest Pediatric Nephrology Study Group. A clinicopathologic study of crescentic GN in 50 children. Kidney Internat 1985;27:450.

### NS in Childhood

Bernare DB. Extrarenal complications of the NS. Kidney Internat 1988;33:1184.

International study of kidney disease in children. The NS in children: prediction of histopathology from clinical and laboratory characteristics at the time of diagnosis. Kidney Internat 1978;13:43.

Mavichak V, Dirks JH. Pathophysiology of the NS: mechanisms of edema. In: Cameron IS, Glassock R, eds. The NS. New York: Marcel Dekker, 1988:251.

### Minimal Change NS

International study of kidney disease in children. Minimal change NS in children: deaths during the first 5 to 15 years' observation. Pediatrics 1984;73:497.

Nash MA, Edelmann CM, Bernstein J, Barnett HL. Minimal change NS, diffuse mesangial hypercellularity and focal glomerular sclerosis. In: Edelmann CM, ed. Pediatric kidney disease, ed 2. Boston: Little, Brown, 1992:1267.

Niaudet P and the French Society of Paediatric Nephrology. Comparison of cyclosporin and chlorambucil in the treatment of steroid-dependent idiopathic NS: a multicentre randomized controlled trial. Pediatr Nephrol 1992;6:1.

### Diffuse Mesangial Proliferative GN

Silva F, Hogg R. Minimal change NS-focal sclerosis complex (including IgM nephropathy and diffuse mesangial hypercellularity). In: Tisher C, Brenner B, eds. Renal pathology with clinical and functional correlations. Philadelphia: JB Lippincott, 1989:265.

Southwest Pediatric Nephrology Study Group. Childhood NS associated with diffuse mesangial hypercellularity. Kidney Internat 1983;23:87.

Yang JY, Melvin T, Sibley R, et al. No evidence for a specific role of IgM in mesangial proliferation of idiopathic NS. Kidney Internat 1984;25:100.

### Focal Segmental Glomerulosclerosis

Arbus GS, Poucell S, Bacheyie GS, et al. Focal segmental glomerulosclerosis with idiopathic NS: three types of clinical response. J Pediatr 1982;101:40.

Mendoza SA, Reznik VM, Griswold WR, et al. Treatment of steroid-resistant focal segmental glomerulosclerosis with pulse methylprednisolone and alkylating agents. Pediatr Nephrol 1990;4:303.

Southwest Pediatric Nephrology Study Group. Focal segmental glomerulosclerosis in children with idiopathic NS. Kidney Internat 1985;27:442.

### Membranoproliferative GN

Habib R, Kleinknecht MC, Levy M. Idiopathic membranoproliferative GN in children. Report of 105 cases. Clin Nephrol 1973;1:194.

Tarshish P, Bernstein J, Tobin J, Edelmann C. Treatment of mesangiocapillary GN with alternative day prednisone: a report of the International Study of Kidney Disease in Children. Pediatr Nephrol 1992;6:123.

Watson AR, Poucell S, Thorner P, et al. Membranoproliferative GN type I in children: correlation of clinical features with pathologic subtypes. Am J Kidney Dis 1984;4:141.

West CD. Idiopathic membranoproliferative GN in childhood. Pediatr Nephrol 1992;6:96.

### Membranous GN

Cameron JS. Membranous nephropathy—still a treatment dilemma. N Engl J Med 1992;327:638.

Cattran DC, Delmore T, Roscoe J, et al. The Toronto GN Study Group: a randomized controlled trial of prednisone in patients with idiopathic membranous nephropathy. N Engl J Med 1989;320:210.

Kerjaschki D. Molecular pathogenesis of membranous nephropathy. Kidney Internat 1992;41:1090.

Ponticelli C, Zucchelli P, Passerini P, et al. A randomized trial of methylprednisolone and chlorambucil in idiopathic membranous nephropathy. N Engl J Med 1989;320:8.

Southwest Pediatric Nephrology Study Group. Comparison of idiopathic and systemic lupus erythematosus-associated membranous GN in children. Am J Kidney Dis 1986;7:115.

### Congenital NS

Jensen JC, Ehrlich RM, Hanna MK, et al. A report of four patients with the Drash syndrome and a review of the literature. J Urol 1989;141:1174.

Mahan JD, Mauer SM, Sibley RK, et al. Congenital NS: evolution of medical management and results of renal transplantation. J Pediatr 1984;105:549.

Steffensen GK, Nielsen KF. NS in the first 3 months of life. Child Nephrol Urol 1990;10:1.

*Principles and Practice of Pediatrics, Second Edition.*
edited by Frank A. Oski et al. J. B. Lippincott Company, Philadelphia © 1994.

## CHAPTER 115
# *Hereditary Renal Disorders*

## 115.1 *Progressive Hereditary Nephritis*

### David R. Powell

Many progressive hereditary nephritis syndromes have been described. This chapter will focus on a phenotypically heterogenous group of kindreds who exhibit a similar ultrastructural abnormality of the glomerular basement membrane (GBM) in affected family members, and who share the clinical findings of persistent hematuric nephritis in multiple family members with progression of renal involvement to chronic renal failure in at least one of these affected individuals. Based on the classification system of Atkin and colleagues (see Selected Readings), all of these kindreds have types of Alport syndrome. Individual kindreds have their own phenotypes; progression of renal failure may proceed at a similar rate in affected individuals of the same kindred, and these individuals may share certain nonrenal features that other kindreds do not display. These unique phenotypes would best be classified, and will eventually be understood, by the nature of their specific genetic defect. However, at present such a classification approach is possible for only a few Alport syndrome kindreds.

## CLASSIFICATION

Classification of Alport syndrome by phenotype is useful for research and in providing prognostic information to family members. The classification system of Atkin and colleagues is based on three major characteristics of Alport syndrome kindreds. First, affected males nearly always develop end-stage renal disease (ESRD); in some kindreds, these males reach ESRD during childhood or adolescence, while in others they are middle-aged before they reach ESRD. When intrakindred mean ages of ESRD in affected males are pooled from many kindreds, a clear bimodal distribution exists, with an intrakindred mean age of roughly 31 years separating juvenile from adult types. Second, in some kindreds but not in others, affected individuals may develop hearing loss. Third, Alport syndrome is inherited as an X-linked dominant trait in many kindreds but as an autosomal dominant trait in others.

These characteristics led to the following classification system. *Type I Alport syndrome* is juvenile-type nephritis with deafness but an unclear mode of inheritance. These kindreds may ultimately be reclassified if affected males have offspring or with identification of specific gene mutations. *Type II* is an X-linked dominant, juvenile-type nephritis with deafness. *Type III* is an X-linked dominant, adult-type nephritis with deafness. *Type IV* is an X-linked dominant, adult-type nephritis without deafness or other nonrenal findings. *Type V* is an autosomal dominant nephritis with deafness, thrombocytopenia, giant platelets, and impaired platelet aggregation; platelet studies are normal in relatives free of renal and audiometric abnormality. *Type VI* is an autosomal dominant, juvenile-type nephritis with deafness. The predominant forms of Alport syndrome are the X-linked types II, III, and IV.

## CLINICAL CHARACTERISTICS

Among progressive hereditary nephritis syndromes, Alport syndrome is the most common, with an estimated gene frequency of one in 5000 in the United States. This diagnosis accounts for as much as 3% of all childhood chronic renal failure and for 0.6% of all patients in Europe who are starting renal replacement therapy. Patients with Alport syndrome come from all geographic and racial backgrounds. The vast majority present with microscopic or macroscopic hematuria, but patients may rarely present with deafness, hypertension, proteinuria, edema, or renal failure.

Individuals with a gene for Alport syndrome are considered to be affected only if they exhibit hematuria. Hematuria is present in most affected family members by the time they reach 6 years of age. Microscopic hematuria may be found at birth, it may be intermittent in females and younger males, and it may not be discovered until adulthood in some females. Episodes of macroscopic hematuria are frequent; they usually appear a few days after the onset of an upper respiratory infection and rarely last longer than 1 to 2 weeks. Proteinuria may appear during the first decade of life; it is often intermittent in young males and in females of all ages. The onset of proteinuria is considered a poor prognostic sign because it is often present and progressive in patients who eventually develop renal failure, and since it can result in nephrotic syndrome in young adults (usually males).

Virtually all males with Alport syndrome develop chronic renal failure. In affected males with adult types of Alport syndrome, early chronic renal failure progresses steadily to ESRD over the course of a few years. Affected females are less likely to develop chronic renal failure. The exception is kindreds with type V Alport Syndrome, in which ESRD may be as frequent in males as females due to autosomal dominant inheritance. Data on 600 patients with Alport syndrome who required renal replacement therapy have been reported to the European Dialysis and Transplant Association Registry since 1975. Analysis of these data found that only 20% of all patients who reached ESRD were female, and that these females reached ESRD at a median age of 32 years, significantly older than for men (median age 25 years, range 6 to 72 years). Thus, the renal disease of Alport syndrome was milder in females.

Kindreds with type IV Alport syndrome have normal hearing, but kindreds with all other types of Alport syndrome exhibit bilateral cochlear deafness. Affected individuals have hearing loss at frequencies between 2 and 8 kHz, which is easily demonstrated by audiometric screening. The use of this screening tool shows that up to 85% of males and 18% of females with Alport syndrome have significant hearing loss by 15 years of age. Hearing loss is often progressive and is more severe in males. In some kindreds, progression of hearing loss portends progression of renal failure. Although some affected individuals with ESRD have so-

cially normal hearing, most patients with milder hearing loss have less severe renal involvement.

Ocular defects are found in individuals with Alport syndrome. Lenticonus anterior, a protrusion of the anterior lens into the chamber, may occur in these patients and can lead to significant visual impairment; it is sometimes present with cataracts. Other patients have bilateral, multiple whitish spots surrounding the fovea. Some authors associate these perimacular spots with more severe renal involvement.

Other syndromes of progressive hereditary nephritis are less well characterized. A syndrome of progressive hereditary nephritis without deafness has been described in which GBM changes differ from those in Alport syndrome. In these kindreds, inheritance is autosomal dominant, affected individuals may develop hematuria during childhood, and females are more likely than males to develop renal failure. Chronic glomerulonephritis and deafness coexist in kindreds with Charcot-Marie-Tooth disease, hyperprolinemia, and hereditary interstitial nephritis. Familial occurrence has been described for both IgA nephropathy and focal segmental glomerulosclerosis, but such kindreds are rare and it is unclear whether familial and nonfamilial forms of these diseases differ in clinical course and prognosis.

## PATHOLOGY

Renal biopsy specimens from young children with Alport syndrome may appear normal, but abnormalities are usually found in specimens from patients over 5 years of age. Light microscopic findings are usually nonspecific, but immature or fetal glomeruli may be found. Biopsies from patients with renal failure show segmental glomerular sclerosis, tubular atrophy, and interstitial fibrosis with foam cells; these foam cells are seen in kidneys with chronic glomerulonephritis from many causes. Immunofluorescent studies of renal biopsy tissue from these patients are either negative or nonspecific.

The GBM of patients with Alport syndrome has a distinct appearance by electron microscopy. In some areas, the GBM is thin, measuring 50 to 150 nm wide compared with the normal 200 to 350 nm. In other areas, the membrane is thick, measuring 300 to 550 nm wide. These thick areas have a characteristic split appearance formed by a crisscrossing network of 100-nm-wide bands of lamina densa. Lucent areas between these bands often contain multiple, small, dark particles. Some capillary loops have only thin segments, some only thick segments, and others have both. The frequency of thin segments seems to decrease with age, while thick segments increase. Split, thick segments may be found as early as 1 year of age but are sometimes absent from the first biopsy specimen. Segments of thick and split GBM are more frequent in males but occur in both sexes. Some investigators argue that an increase in thick segments on biopsy correlates clinically with increased proteinuria. The observation that strongly suggests the diagnosis of Alport syndrome is the finding of thin, normal, and thickened segments of GBM in the same biopsy specimen.

Basement membranes in nonrenal tissues are also abnormal in affected individuals. In the cochlea, the stria vascularis shows thickening and splitting of the capillary basement membrane, similar to the changes seen in the glomerulus. In anterior lenticonus, the basement membrane forming the anterior lens capsule is thinned, allowing protrusion of the anterior lens.

## PATHOGENESIS

The GBM of individuals with Alport syndrome is attenuated and apparently ruptures easily. In theory, repeat episodes of rupture and healing may account for areas of focal thickening and ultimately account for the impaired glomerular filtration. Such observations suggest that Alport syndrome results from a primary abnormality of basement membrane glycoproteins. Early evidence that the GBM of these patients had an abnormal glycoprotein composition was obtained from studies showing that polyclonal and monoclonal antibodies directed against GBM components failed to recognize at least two antigens from the noncollagenous regions of basement membrane collagen in some Alport syndrome patients. It seemed likely that a mutation in one of these antigens, which made it unavailable or unrecognizable to the antibodies, also was primarily responsible for Alport syndrome.

Gene linkage studies have mapped the three X-linked Alport syndrome types (types II, III, and IV) to a single area on the X chromosome, within region Xq21.2–22.1 near the centromere. Thus, these three phenotypes appear to result from different mutations of a single genetic locus. However, genes for the two main structural proteins of basement membrane, the alpha-1 and alpha-2 chains of type IV collagen, do not seem to be involved, since both are located on chromosome 13.

Recently, three new type IV collagen chains have been identified. One of these proteins, the alpha-5 chain of type IV collagen (COL4A5), is encoded by a gene located in the q22 region of chromosome X, the same locus as Alport syndrome. In the kidney, this protein is localized almost exclusively in the GBM. Several mutations of the COL4A5 gene have now been identified in patients with Alport syndrome; to date, each mutation is unique to a specific kindred, suggesting that hundreds of mutations may ultimately be found. Almost certainly, COL4A5 is the gene involved in X-linked types of Alport syndrome, with different mutations of the COL4A5 gene being responsible for the different Alport syndrome phenotypes. Interestingly, one patient with profound deafness was found to have a large deletion mutation resulting in a loss of the COL4A5 region required for assembling the collagen network; it is possible that the profound nature of the hearing deficit is related to the severe nature of this mutation.

## DIAGNOSIS AND DIFFERENTIAL DIAGNOSIS

Children found to have hematuria in multiple urine samples over an interval of a few weeks should be evaluated for the possibility of a progressive hereditary nephritis. Personal and extended family histories of hematuria, proteinuria, hypertension, ophthalmologic abnormalities, deafness, renal failure, and bleeding tendencies must be thoroughly documented. Physical examination and laboratory evaluation should seek evidence for renal failure, hearing loss, lenticonus anterior, perimacular spots, and thrombocytopenia. In addition, all family members should be tested on multiple occasions for hematuria. If the workup suggests the presence of familial hematuria, the differential diagnosis would include epidemic acute poststreptococcal glomerulonephritis (APSGN), familial idiopathic hypercalciuria, Alport syndrome, other progressive hereditary nephritis syndromes, IgA nephropathy, and familial benign hematuria. APSGN should be evaluated by careful history, appropriate serologic testing, and serum complement levels; hypercalciuria is evaluated by the measurement of 24-hour urinary calcium excretion. The possibility of Alport syndrome may be evaluated by screening affected family members with audiometry and, if necessary, by ophthalmologic consultation. Renal biopsy is usually reserved for patients with proteinuria or renal insufficiency, but it can be justified for prognostic purposes, since biopsy evaluation can be diagnostic for IgA nephropathy and strongly suggestive of Alport syndrome. New kindreds with Alport syndrome are still diagnosed using the criteria outlined at the beginning of this chapter. Other progressive hereditary nephritis syndromes have a family history of

renal failure in affected individuals but do not meet the criteria for Alport syndrome. In contrast, familial benign hematuria is a diagnosis of exclusion, and family members must be followed for the development of proteinuria, renal failure, and deafness. Patients with persistent hematuria but without evidence of familial involvement must also be followed closely, since Alport syndrome is associated with a new mutation rate of 17% and since 7% of female obligate carriers do not have hematuria. Tests designed to detect mutations in the Alport syndrome COL4A5 gene are on the horizon and will probably be used in the near future as part of the workup for persistent hematuria.

Prenatal diagnosis is not yet routinely available for any of the progressive hereditary nephritis syndromes, although it can potentially be performed now for a few Alport syndrome kindreds with known COL4A5 gene mutations.

## TREATMENT

No specific therapy is available for patients with hereditary nephritis. Hearing aids temporarily benefit patients with Alport syndrome and hearing loss. Chronic renal failure is treated with dialysis or renal transplantation. Some patients with Alport syndrome develop anti-GBM antibodies after receiving a renal transplant, presumably because the donor kidney contains the COL4A5 antigen that is absent in the host. However, severe anti-GBM nephritis is rare, and graft survival in patients with Alport syndrome is not different from that of patients without Alport syndrome.

## Selected Readings

Atkin CL, Gregory MC, Border WA. Alport syndrome. In: Schrier RW, Gottschalk CW, eds. Diseases of the kidney, ed 4. Boston: Little, Brown, 1988:617.

Gretz N, Broyer M, Brunner FP, et al. Alport's syndrome as a cause of renal failure in Europe. Pediatr Nephrol 1987;1:411.

Grunfeld JP. The clinical spectrum of hereditary nephritis. Kidney Internat 1985;27:83.

Kashtan CE, Kleppel MM, Butkowski RJ, Michael AF, Fish AJ. Alport syndrome, basement membranes and collagen. Pediatr Nephrol 1990;4:523.

Tryggvason K. Cloning of Alport syndrome gene. Ann Med 1991;23:237.

*Principles and Practice of Pediatrics, Second Edition.*
edited by Frank A. Oski et al. J. B. Lippincott Company, Philadelphia © 1994.

## 115.2 *Familial Benign Hematuria*

David R. Powell

The syndrome of familial benign hematuria (FBH) has been variously referred to as benign, essential, primary, idiopathic, persistent, or recurrent hematuria. Affected individuals usually present with persistent or intermittent microscopic hematuria detected on routine urinalysis, or with gross hematuria brought on by a febrile illness. Significant proteinuria is absent. Physical examination is normal, and no abnormalities are noted with audiometric and ophthalmologic examinations. Laboratory evaluation reveals normal renal function and platelet count. Family history is negative for deafness, renal failure, or significant proteinuria. Screening typically identifies hematuria in other family members from multiple generations, but these individuals fail to demonstrate hearing loss, renal failure, or proteinuria.

Renal biopsies from affected individuals are normal by light microscopy and immunofluorescence; segmental glomerular sclerosis, interstitial foam cells, and persistence of fetal glomeruli are not found. Electron microscopy reveals the characteristic finding of focal or widespread thinning of the glomerular basement membrane (GBM); however, these thin segments are not interspersed with segments of thick and split GBM typical of Alport syndrome.

The inheritance pattern of FBH is probably autosomal dominant in some kindreds, but data are scarce and a stricter definition of this syndrome is needed. This definition should include the finding of persistent microscopic hematuria and biopsy evidence of thin, but not thick and split, GBM in affected family members. Also, no affected family member should exhibit deafness, significant proteinuria, chronic renal failure, or abnormal kidney tissue by light microscopy or immunofluorescence.

The diagnosis and the differential diagnosis of FBH are the same as those for progressive hereditary nephritis (see Chap. 115.1). FBH is a diagnosis of exclusion. Affected males in some Alport syndrome kindreds do not develop chronic renal failure until 50 years of age; since these individuals may not have typical electron microscopic findings of Alport syndrome at a young age, their syndrome may be misdiagnosed as FBH. At present, the only way to diagnose FBH in a kindred is by obtaining a characteristic renal biopsy from one affected family member, and by documenting that several affected males lived a long life free of chronic renal failure. Thus, affected individuals of kindreds with the diagnosis of FBH should be monitored regularly for the development of proteinuria, renal failure, hearing loss, and hypertension. The appearance of chronic renal failure in any family member requires careful reevaluation of the original diagnosis. On the other hand, firmly establishing the diagnosis of FBH in a kindred may prevent unnecessary future investigations in affected family members.

## Selected Readings

Atkin CL, Gregory MC, Border WA. Alport syndrome. In: Schrier RW, Gottschalk CW, eds. Diseases of the kidney, ed 4. Boston: Little, Brown, 1988:617.

Rogers PW, Kurtzman NA, Bunn SM Jr, White MG. Familial benign essential hematuria. Arch Intern Med 1973;131:257.

Yoshikawa N, Matsuyama S, Iijima K, Maehara K, Okada S, Matsuo T. Benign familial hematuria. Arch Pathol Lab Med 1988;112:794.

*Principles and Practice of Pediatrics, Second Edition.*
edited by Frank A. Oski et al. J. B. Lippincott Company, Philadelphia © 1994.

# 115.3 *Familial Juvenile Nephronophthisis*

## David R. Powell

Familial juvenile nephronophthisis (FJN) is characterized clinically by polyuria, anemia, growth failure, and progressive renal failure, and pathologically by chronic tubulointerstitial nephritis and medullary cysts. It accounts for 1% of end-stage renal disease (ESRD) in the United States, and may be more common in Europe.

The renal pathology, clinical findings, and course of patients with this disorder are indistinguishable from those found in patients with medullary cystic kidneys; in fact, the two disorders are considered a single disease by some investigators. Careful genetic studies, however, have established the presence of two distinct syndromes. Nephronophthisis is the diagnosis when the inheritance pattern is autosomal recessive. Patients are age 10 on average at the disease onset but may present as infants. They often have associated nonrenal anomalies, and have an unusually frequent family history of consanguineous marriages. In contrast, medullary cystic kidney disease is the diagnosis when the inheritance pattern is autosomal dominant; patients are age 28 on average at the disease onset and rarely have nonrenal anomalies.

Children with FJN present with polydipsia, polyuria, weakness, anemia, and azotemia. Less than half of the affected children have significant growth failure at presentation, and edema and hypertension are unusual. Patients may be hypokalemic and have renal tubular acidosis. Urinalysis is usually unremarkable except for mild tubular proteinuria. The tubular damage present in this disease usually causes a urine-concentrating defect with subsequent polyuria and polydipsia. In fact, an inability to maximally concentrate the urine may precede azotemia and may be the first sign of the disease in an asymptomatic patient. Hypokalemia may contribute to this hyposthenuric state and also to the weakness exhibited by many patients. Tubular damage may also lead to a salt-wasting state, which could explain the lack of hypertension and edema in these patients. Renal failure progresses to ESRD within 1 to 10 years and contributes to growth failure and anemia. However, many investigators think that the severity of anemia is out of proportion to the degree of renal failure; decreased erythropoietin production by the damaged renal medulla may be a contributing factor, but hard data in support of this claim are lacking.

Children with FJN may have other findings such as ophthalmologic and skeletal abnormalities, cerebellar ataxia, mental retardation, and hepatic fibrosis. The most common ophthalmologic disorders in these patients are tapetoretinal degeneration and retinitis pigmentosa, associated with blindness; however, colobomas, nystagmus, amblyopia, myopia, strabismus, and optic nerve atrophy also occur in these children. The combination of nephronophthisis and retinal abnormalities, known as the renal-retinal syndrome, is quite heterogeneous. The nature of the retinal lesion and the age of onset of retinal abnormalities are highly variable. Patients in some kindreds develop hepatic fibrosis, while patients in other kindreds develop cerebellar ataxia, mental retardation, and cone-shaped epiphyses. Some asymptomatic family members heterozygous for the renal-retinal syndrome demonstrate electroretinographic abnormalities but have normal renal function. At present, the genetic link between renal-retinal syndrome and FJN is unknown.

Kidney biopsy specimens show little change early in the disease. Later, light microscopy studies show tubular atrophy with marked interstitial lymphocytic infiltrate and fibrosis; glomeruli are relatively spared until significant renal failure develops. Small medullary cysts are found in up to 75% of patients. Epithelial cells lining these cysts are flattened and surrounded by thick basement membrane. Microdissection studies show that medullary cysts arise from both the distal convoluted tubules and the collecting tubules. The observation that medullary cysts may not be present in affected kidneys, or that they may be few in number or appear late in the disease course, suggests that these cysts arise secondary to progressive interstitial inflammation and fibrosis and that they are not responsible for the functional defects or clinical findings of FJN. However, ultrastructural studies show regions of thick, lamellated, and duplicated tubular basement membrane interspersed with regions where this membrane is thin or absent, suggesting that a defect in the tubular basement membrane structure may be primarily responsible for cyst formation and the nephronophthisis syndrome. At present, firm evidence is lacking to implicate any pathogenic mechanism as primary in this disorder.

Patients presenting with the typical signs and symptoms of FJN are easily diagnosed when siblings have the disease. However, family history of sibling involvement is lacking in 50% of the patients. In these cases, a demonstration of renal insufficiency, small kidneys, and medullary cysts in the same patient strongly suggests nephronophthisis; the small kidneys and medullary cysts are best demonstrated by ultrasound or CT scanning. Laurence-Moon syndrome can have similar findings, but its other clinical characteristics prevent confusion with nephronophthisis. Sporadic cases of medullary cystic disease occurring in younger patients may be impossible to distinguish from nephronophthisis unless the pattern of inheritance becomes clear later. Kidney size and cyst size usually differentiate between nephronophthisis and infantile or adult polycystic kidney disease; late onset, infantile polycystic kidney disease with hepatic fibrosis, however, can be confused with nephronophthisis, and renal biopsy may be required for diagnosis. Large medullary cysts in a teenager suggest the diagnosis of medullary sponge kidney, but these patients do not develop renal failure. The demonstration of medullary cysts makes the diagnosis of dysplastic or hypoplastic kidneys unlikely.

Radiologic studies must be performed to rule out obstructive uropathy as a cause of tubular damage.

Occasionally, the diagnosis of nephronophthisis is not established even after radiologic evaluation, ultrasound, and biopsy of the kidney. In these cases, an effort should be made to establish the diagnosis if renal tissue becomes available postmortem.

The therapy for patients with FJN is symptomatic. Salt wasting is treated with salt supplements, metabolic acidosis with alkali, hypokalemia with potassium, polyuria with free access to water, and chronic renal failure with the usual supportive therapy. Patients tolerate dialysis and transplantation well, and there is currently no evidence of disease recurrence in transplanted kidneys.

## Selected Readings

Gardner KD Jr. Medullary and miscellaneous renal cystic disorders. In: Schrier RW, Gottschalk CW, eds. Diseases of the kidney, ed 4. Boston: Little, Brown, 1988: 559.

Noel LH, Gubler MC, Bobrie G, Savage COS, Lockwood CM, Grunfeld JP. Inherited defects of renal basement membranes. Adv Nephrol 1989;18:77.

Resnick J, Vernier R. Renal cystic diseases and renal dysplasia. In: Holliday MA, Barratt TM, Vernier RL, eds. Pediatric nephrology, ed 2. Baltimore: Williams & Wilkins, 1987:371.

Waldherr R, Lennert T, Weber H-P, Fodisch HJ, Scharer K. The nephronophthisis complex: a clinicopathologic study in children. Virch Arch 1982;394:235.

*Principles and Practice of Pediatrics, Second Edition.*
edited by Frank A. Oski et al. J. B. Lippincott Company, Philadelphia © 1994.

# 115.4 *Nephropathy of Diabetes Mellitus*

L. Leighton Hill and Seth Paul Kravitz

Renal failure is the leading cause of death in patients with insulin-dependent diabetes mellitus (IDDM). Of the patients with IDDM, 30% to 50% will ultimately develop end-stage renal disease (ESRD). Diabetes mellitus is a major cause of renal failure worldwide and accounts for over 25% of the patients entering dialysis and transplantation programs in the United States. The development of ESRD is rarely seen in the second decade of life but is common in the third, fourth, and fifth decades. Of extreme interest and largely unexplained at this time is the fact that one half to two thirds of the patients with IDDM do not develop significant nephropathy, regardless of duration.

## NATURAL HISTORY

The development of significant dipstick-positive proteinuria is usually the first clinical sign of the nephropathy of diabetes mellitus. However, before the development of proteinuria, several hemodynamic and morphologic changes occur in the kidney. At the time of diagnosis, there is usually evidence of increased glomerular filtration rate, renal blood flow, and filtration fraction. Renal size is often increased, and microalbuminuria may be present. These early functional changes appear to be related to glycemic control, since improvement in metabolic control is associated with a return toward normal of these parameters. The

disappearance of microalbuminuria is usually followed by many years of normal albuminuria. After only 18 months to 2 years duration of diabetes, thickening of the basement membrane and mesangial expansion develop and tend to increase over time. By 5 to 15 years duration, 30% to 40% of the patients with diabetes mellitus develop persistent microalbuminuria. The definition of microalbuminuria varies significantly depending on the method of collection and assay used. Mogensen uses a rate between 20 and 200 $\mu$g/min, with less than 20 $\mu$g/min being normoalbuminuria and more than 200 $\mu$g/min being clinical or overt proteinuria. Many investigators believe that microalbuminuria is a reliable predictor of later overt clinical proteinuria, chronic renal insufficiency, and other microvascular complications.

Clinically detectable overt proteinuria is generally found between 10 and 30 years after the diagnosis of IDDM, with the peak occurring 15 to 20 years after diagnosis. Azotemia usually occurs within 5 to 10 years of the onset of clinically significant proteinuria, and ESRD usually ensues within 1 to 2 years of the development of azotemia. Hypertension is almost invariably present in patients with significant nephropathy, and the nephrotic syndrome occurs in 5% to 10%. However, this sequence and the timing are not invariable, and extensive nephropathy can occur without proteinuria. Several therapeutic interventions have been tried in an attempt to alter the natural course of this disease.

## PATHOLOGY

The most common pathologic lesion seen in diabetic nephropathy is diffuse glomerular sclerosis, a generalized widening of the glomerular mesangium with matrix material, which ultimately invades the subendothelial space, occludes the capillary lumina, and reduces filtration surface. Other pathologic changes include nodular glomerulosclerosis (Kimmelstiel-Wilson lesion), glomerular basement membrane thickening, afferent and efferent glomerular arteriolar hyalinosis, tubulointerstitial changes, and "capsular drops" in the parietal Bowman's capsule.

## PATHOGENESIS OF VASCULAR COMPLICATIONS

There has been an ongoing controversy over the years concerning the pathogenesis of the vascular complications in IDDM. Most investigators have considered the microangiopathic changes to be related to the metabolic, hormonal, and physiologic disturbances resulting from insulin deficiency (metabolic theory). Others, however, believe that diabetic-linked genetic determinants of vascular disease exist more or less independently of hyperglycemia and other metabolic abnormalities (co-inherited genetic theory).

Arguments favoring the metabolic theory include the presence of typical pathologic changes of diabetic nephropathy in individuals with secondary diabetes of multiple causes; the development of typical lesions in normal kidneys transplanted into patients with diabetes; regression of typical lesions in diabetic kidneys transplanted into persons without diabetes; the occurrence of similar pathologic lesions in the kidneys of animals with experimental diabetes; and the reversibility of experimental lesions in animals with excellent glycemic control. However, proponents of the co-inherited genetic theory cite the overall lack of good clinical correlation between microangiopathic disease, including kidney disease, and the degree of metabolic control of diabetes, and the finding that 50% to 70% of patients with IDDM do not develop significant nephropathy. Nevertheless, the preponderance of scientific data seems to suggest that insulin deficiency, with the associated metabolic, hormonal, and physiologic disturbances, is the principal cause of diabetic nephropathy and other microangiopathy.

Just how insulin deficiency causes renal damage is unclear. Hormonal alterations (growth hormone, glucagon, kinins, renin, prostaglandins) may be important. Recent evidence suggests a correlation between nonenzymatic glycosylation of tissue and long term complications in diabetes. Diminution of fixed negative charges (eg, glycoaminoglycans) in the basement membrane may reduce the repulsive electrostatic interaction with negatively charged plasma proteins and thereby increase the filtration and excretion of proteins. Over the past decade, evidence has accumulated that suggests a role for functional hemodynamic changes in the generation of diabetic nephropathy. Hostetter and colleagues have proposed that there is microvascular dilatation in the diabetic kidney with increased glomerular blood flow, glomerular hyperfiltration, and an increase in mean glomerular transcapillary hydraulic pressure difference. They point out that the pathologic lesion of diabetic nephropathy (diffuse glomerular sclerosis) is the same lesion that occurs in other entities associated with whole-kidney and single-nephron hyperfiltration states, such as in high-protein feeding and reduction in renal mass. Elevated glomerular capillary pressure may be the principal cause of the mesangial expansion and sclerosis. It is likely that both hemodynamic factors and biochemical changes contribute to the development of renal damage.

## PREVENTION AND TREATMENT OF NEPHROPATHY

Despite conflicting evidence, more and more studies appear to suggest that good to excellent metabolic control of IDDM, especially early in the course of the disease, may be beneficial in the prevention or at least the postponement of the microangiopathy of IDDM. Once nephropathy is clinically manifest by proteinuria, metabolic control is unlikely to have an influence. Nevertheless, most clinicians experienced in the care of IDDM continue to attempt to achieve good control of blood sugar, even in patients with established nephropathy. Patients with IDDM should be routinely tested for proteinuria at each visit. Once proteinuria is discovered by dipstick testing (30 mg/dL or greater), it should be quantitated over a 24-hour period, and these quantitative measurements should then be repeated once or twice a year along with serum creatinine determinations. Some diabetologists and nephrologists advocate screening diabetics after 5 years' duration for microalbuminuria, because these individuals with microalbuminuria may be at increased risk for later complications and should receive increased attention and perhaps therapeutic intervention. After 10 years' duration of diabetes, a serum creatinine should be done yearly, even in the absence of proteinuria.

Blood pressure measurements should be routinely taken at each visit. Control of blood pressure in the patient with diabetes is extremely important at any stage of renal involvement. Evidence exists that progression of renal disease can be retarded by adequate blood pressure control. Therefore, good to excellent blood pressure control is mandatory in the patient with IDDM. Several antihypertensive agents can be used successfully, but the most promising are the angiotensin-converting enzyme inhibitors. These drugs not only lower systemic blood pressure, but also appear to reduce intrarenal hypertension. Therefore, they may affect directly, at least to some degree, one of the factors thought to contribute to diabetic nephropathy. This category of antihypertensive drugs produces a decrease in urinary protein excretion in patients with and without hypertension. Current research is focused on whether this class of drugs can be beneficial when only microalbuminuria is present.

The management of ESRD in patients with diabetes includes comprehensive medical management, dialysis, and transplantation (see Chap. 112).

## Selected Readings

Brown DM, Mauer SM. Diabetes mellitus. In: Holliday MA, Barratt TM, Vernier RL, eds. Pediatric nephrology, ed 2. Baltimore: Williams & Wilkins, 1985:513.

Hostetter TH, Rennke HG, Brenner BM. The case for intrarenal hypertension in the initiation and progression of diabetic and other glomerulopathies. Am J Med 1982;72:375.

Mogensen CE. Microalbuminuria as a predictor of clinical diabetic nephropathy. Kidney Internat 1987;31:673.

Taguma Y, Kitamoto Y, Futaki G. Effect of captopril on heavy proteinuria in azotemic diabetics. N Engl J Med 1985;313:1617.

Viberti G, Keen H. The patterns of proteinuria in diabetes mellitus: relevance to pathogenesis and prevention of diabetic nephropathy. Diabetes 1984;33:686.

*Principles and Practice of Pediatrics, Second Edition.*
edited by Frank A. Oski et al. J. B. Lippincott Company, Philadelphia © 1994.

# 115.5 *Sickle Cell Nephropathy*

David R. Powell

Children with sickle cell anemia and often those with sickle cell trait may present with a wide spectrum of significant urinary tract disorders, including hyposthenuria, acidosis, hematuria, proteinuria, nephrotic syndrome, chronic renal failure, and urinary tract infection.

Most patients with sickle cell disease cannot maximally concentrate their urine, probably because of chronic damage to the renal medulla. Medullary blood vessels—in particular the vasa recta—participate with the long loops of Henle in a countercurrent multiplication and exchange system that maintains medullary hyperosmolality and allows urine to be concentrated. This process normally results in a medullary environment that is hyperosmolar, acidotic, and hypoxic, all of which predispose to the sickling of red blood cells in children with this disease. Sickle cells may obstruct blood flow in these medullary vessels, leading to infarction and interstitial fibrosis and ultimately to the disruption of the normal concentrating mechanism. Hyposthenuria first appears in young children, and at this age is reversible by administering multiple blood transfusions. However, by adolescence, hyposthenuria is irreversible, and maximal urine concentration is in the range of 450 mOsm/L. Patients with sickle cell trait gradually follow the same course; by middle age, they develop a similar degree of irreversible hyposthenuria. Clinically, children with sickle cell disease and hyposthenuria may present with enuresis and are at greater risk than normal for dehydration; however, hyposthenuria is rarely a life-threatening complication.

A mild defect in maximal urinary acidification and potassium excretion by the distal tubule has been found in many patients with sickle cell anemia. The pathogenesis of this defect appears to be similar to that for hyposthenuria. Clinically significant hyperchloremic metabolic acidosis and hyperkalemia are rarely seen in these patients, even during sickle cell crises.

Hematuria is common in children with sickle cell disease or trait. The onset is usually sudden and unprovoked, although some cases are associated with trauma, exercise, upper respiratory infection, or sickle cell crisis. Bleeding is usually painless, unless accompanied by papillary necrosis. Hematuria may be microscopic or macroscopic, and episodes can last from days to months; gross hematuria occurs in up to one third of the patients. Massive, life-threatening hematuria can occur, usually in adult males but sometimes in children; it originates from the left kidney in three fourths of the cases. Most cases occur in patients with sickle cell trait, probably because many more individuals are hemizygous than homozygous for the sickle hemoglobin gene. As with hyposthenuria, hematuria probably results from sickling of red blood cells in the renal medulla. This causes obstruction to blood flow, with subsequent infarction, interstitial hemorrhage, and hematuria; papillary necrosis may be present. Radiologic studies, including intravenous pyelography and renal arteriography, often do not pinpoint the site of bleeding. Membranoproliferative glomerulonephritis (MPGN), renal artery thrombosis, and renal vein thrombosis are other complications of sickle hemoglobinopathy that can lead to hematuria. Since hematuria secondary to sickle hemoglobinopathy is a diagnosis of exclusion, children with sickle cell anemia or trait should be evaluated for other causes of hematuria that are unrelated to this disease.

Children with sickle cell anemia may develop persistent proteinuria or frank nephrotic syndrome; focal segmental glomerulosclerosis (FSGS) is often seen on renal biopsy. Less common findings include MPGN, isolated mesangial hypercellularity, membranous glomerulopathy, and a picture consistent with minimal lesion nephrosis. Renal vein thrombosis is a rare cause of nephrotic syndrome in these children. Circulating immune complexes are found in children with sickle cell anemia and MPGN, and similar complexes are seen in the glomerular basement membranes of these children. Renal tubular epithelial antigens have been found in these complexes; hypothetically, these antigens enter the circulation during renal ischemic episodes and subsequently stimulate the production of specific antibodies.

Of much greater concern is the possibility that the pathogenesis of FSGS is related to a similar lesion found in the remnant kidney model. In this model, the removal of one kidney results in increased blood flow and glomerular filtration rate (GFR) in the remaining kidney. In rats, this hyperfiltration leads to proteinuria,

mesangial hypercellularity followed by FSGS, and eventually chronic renal failure. Children with sickle cell anemia have renal blood flows and GFRs much higher than normal. Among other possibilities, an increased excretion of the vasodilating prostaglandin $E_2$ may be responsible for these hemodynamic changes. The high GFR of children and young adults with sickle cell disease may eventually lead to glomerular damage in many of these patients, presenting histologically as mesangial hypercellularity followed by FSGS, and clinically as proteinuria followed by chronic renal failure.

In support of this hypothesis, a recent prospective study found that 4.2% of 725 patients with sickle cell anemia developed chronic renal failure. In these patients, the predominant renal lesion was glomerulosclerosis, and the pre-azotemic findings of hypertension, proteinuria, nephrotic syndrome, hematuria, and worsening anemia were significant risk factors for developing chronic renal failure. Interestingly, the Central African Republic $\beta^s$-gene cluster haplotype was found in many of the patients with chronic renal failure.

Children with sickle cell anemia and trait are at increased risk for urinary tract infection and pyelonephritis, presumably due to their immunologic defects. It is unclear whether these infections result in an increased incidence of renal scarring in children with sickle cell disease.

The management of sickle cell nephropathy requires, first and foremost, aggressive therapy of dehydration, acidosis, hypoxia, hyperosmolarity, infection, and severe anemia. The consequences of hyposthenuria are minimal if affected children have free access to water and drink fluids liberally. Increased urinary free water losses must be replaced during episodes of dehydration and crisis. Nephrotic syndrome is usually treated symptomatically; prednisone therapy is unlikely to be of benefit unless biopsy findings are consistent with minimal lesion nephrosis.

The gross hematuria of sickle cell nephropathy is usually self-limited if the child is kept at bed rest until significant bleeding stops and is then restricted to quiet activities for the next 3 to 4 weeks; however, a recurrence of bleeding is not unusual. Other reported therapies for gross hematuria in these patients are of uncertain value because of a lack of controlled studies. These therapies include diuresis; urine alkalinization; transfusions, including partial exchange transfusion; hyperbaric oxygen; triglycyl vasopressin; oral urea to inhibit sickling; epsilon-aminocaproic acid, which inhibits potentiators of urinary tract bleeding such as urokinase; selective renal embolization in coordination with cystoscopy; and urologic procedures, including calyceal tamponade with bougie, pelvic lavage with silver nitrate or oxychlorosene, and unilateral nephrectomy.

Since conservative measures usually succeed and since heavy bleeding from the remaining kidney can occur after unilateral nephrectomy, a conservative approach is recommended that first exhausts medical management options before urologic consultation is obtained.

Although the appearance of chronic renal failure increases the mortality rate in adults with sickle cell disease, this increased rate may not be that much higher than in adults with chronic renal failure from other causes. Some patients with sickle cell anemia and end-stage renal disease tolerate maintenance hemodialysis well, while others suffer from severe anemia and hyperkalemia. Peritoneal dialysis may be preferred in patients with a past history of stroke who are being treated with frequent transfusions, since deferoxamine removes iron more efficiently and without significant toxicity when peritoneal dialysis rather than hemodialysis is used.

Preliminary data suggest that survival of kidneys transplanted into patients with sickle cell anemia or trait is similar to that of kidneys transplanted into other patients with chronic renal failure. Although experience with renal transplantation in children with sickle cell disease is limited, an aggressive approach toward providing these children with renal transplants is warranted at this time.

## Selected Readings

Allon M. Renal abnormalities in sickle cell disease. Arch Intern Med 1990;150:501.

De Jong PE, Statius van Eps LW. Sickle cell nephropathy: new insights into its pathophysiology. Kidney Internat 1985;27:711.

Nissenson AR, Port FK. Outcome of end-stage renal disease in patients with rare causes of renal failure. I. Inherited and metabolic disorders. Q J Med 1989;73:1055.

Powars DR, Elliott-Mills DD, Chan L, et al. Chronic renal failure in sickle cell disease: risk factors, clinical course, and mortality. Ann Intern Med 1991;115:614.

Tejani A, Phadke K, Adamson O, Nicastri A, Chen CK, Sen D. Renal lesions in sickle cell nephropathy in children. Nephron 1985;39:352.

*Principles and Practice of Pediatrics, Second Edition.*
edited by Frank A. Oski et al. J. B. Lippincott Company, Philadelphia © 1994.

# 115.6 *Oxalosis (Primary Hyperoxaluria)*

### David R. Powell

Oxalosis is the name for two rare autosomal recessive disorders associated with excess production and excretion of oxalic acid. It is characterized clinically by a progression to renal failure secondary to nephrocalcinosis or recurrent calcium oxalate nephrolithiasis. In oxalosis type I, the increase in urinary oxalate is accompanied by an increase in glycolate excretion; in oxalosis type II, L-glycerate excretion is increased. Since oxalosis type II is quite rare, this discussion will concentrate on oxalosis type I.

Patients with oxalosis type I lack an active form of the enzyme alanine:glyoxylate aminotransferase (AGT1) in their liver peroxisomes. This disease has three known phenotypes: hepatocytes lack AGT1 protein, have enzymatically inactive AGT1 protein in peroxisomes, or have enzymatically active AGT1 protein mistargeted to mitochondria instead of peroxisomes. Recently, patients with the latter two phenotypes were found to have specific point mutations in the AGT1 gene. In the absence of peroxisomal AGT1, glyoxylate is not adequately converted to less toxic metabolites and instead is metabolized to oxalate and glycolate. Oxalate is removed from the body by renal excretion; in oxalosis, the urine is oversaturated with oxalate in an attempt to compensate for excessive oxalate production. Calcium oxalate crystals then precipitate in renal tubules and collecting ducts, leading to chronic renal injury.

The onset and severity of renal involvement is variable in patients with oxalosis. Two thirds of the patients are symptomatic before age 5, and most present with recurrent episodes of abdominal pain, gross hematuria, and other evidence of urolithiasis. Renal insufficiency, growth failure, and renal tubular acidosis may be present at the time of diagnosis. Abdominal roentgenograms demonstrate urolithiasis and nephrocalcinosis, and renal ultrasounds reveal diffuse, exaggerated echogenicity; the kidney size is usually normal. Although there are more common causes than oxalosis for urolithiasis in children, this diagnosis makes up 1% to 2% of total cases and must be ruled out. A few patients with oxalosis present in infancy with renal failure. The evaluation of any infant with renal failure should include abdominal roentgenogram and ultrasound examinations. These will demonstrate the same findings in infants with oxalosis as in older children, except that urolithiasis is absent. In infants with cortical nephrocalcinosis and renal failure, the possible causes are oxalosis, chronic glomerulonephritis, and renal cortical necrosis.

To document the presence or absence of oxalosis, patients with urolithiasis or nephrocalcinosis should collect a 24-hour urine sample for oxalate, or a spot urine sample for an oxalate/creatinine ratio in the younger child. High urinary oxalate levels in two collections confirms the diagnosis of hyperoxaluria. The diagnosis of primary oxalosis type I is best made by characterizing AGT1 abnormalities in liver tissue, but also may be made by demonstrating high levels of urinary glycolate in the absence of secondary causes of hyperoxaluria such as ethylene glycol ingestion or disease or resection of the distal ileum. In children presenting with chronic renal failure and oliguria or anuria, hyperoxaluria may be impossible to document; due to limitations of available assays, measuring serum oxalate cannot make the diagnosis. However, support for the diagnosis can come from an analysis of the AGT1 profile in the liver, or by demonstrating calcium oxalate deposits in the kidney and other organs. Extrarenal sites that may be evaluated for these deposits include skin, retina, joints, and bone. A kidney biopsy is usually striking because birefringent, pyramid-shaped crystals form rosettes within proximal tubular lumina; positive staining with alazarin red suggests that these are calcium oxalate crystals. Findings elsewhere in the kidney are nonspecific; glomeruli appear normal, but tubular epithelium is destroyed, and severe interstitial inflammation and fibrosis are often present.

The natural history of untreated oxalosis is a gradual progression to a uremic death. In the past, over 80% of the patients died of renal failure by age 20; 90% were dead within 10 years of diagnosis. The emphasis now is on early diagnosis of oxalosis before significant renal damage has occurred and on avoiding further renal injury by preventing calcium oxalate precipitation in the kidneys. Early diagnosis of affected siblings of an index case is possible, because urinary oxalate levels and renal echogenicity by ultrasound can be increased in the first month of life. However, chorionic villus and amniotic fluid sampling have not been helpful in the prenatal diagnosis of oxalosis, because AGT1 is not expressed in these villi and because oxalate readily diffuses across the placenta. At present, a fetal liver biopsy is required for prenatal diagnosis of oxalosis; it is hoped that DNA probe analysis will soon allow a diagnosis to be made at less risk.

Certain measures may prevent stone formation and renal damage in oxalosis patients who are not yet uremic. These include increasing urine output with liberal fluid and sodium intake and with calcium-sparing diuretics such as thiazides. Also, increased magnesium and phosphate intakes lead to their increased levels in urine and subsequent inhibition of calcium oxalate crystallization. The body oxalate burden can be lowered by avoiding oxalate-rich foods and ascorbic acid. Treatment with pyridoxine, a cofactor for AGT activity, may increase glyoxalate metabolism by this enzyme; the decreased oxalate production that results can lead to a gradual decrease in urinary oxalate excretion over weeks to months.

Patients with oxalosis and chronic renal failure continue to overproduce oxalate. Oxalate is no longer removed through the kidneys, and the body burden increases. No form of dialysis adequately removes oxalate from the body, and extrarenal deposits accumulate, leading to disabling bone disease, cardiac dysrhythmias, and peripheral vascular insufficiency. The disease also rapidly recurs in transplanted kidneys, returning patients to their uremic state and all of its complications. Scheinman and co-workers have found that patients with oxalosis and renal failure can be transplanted successfully if their body burden of oxalate is not too large at the time of transplant, if episodes of graft rejection are minimized, and if the measures noted above that inhibit ongoing calcium oxalate precipitation in the kidney are instituted. Nevertheless, even patients who are successfully transplanted initially are at great risk for long-term complications and loss of graft function due to their underlying oxalosis. This experience has led others to perform combined liver/kidney transplants as the only means available to eliminate oxalate overproduction. This approach has succeeded in some patients who were not too debilitated at the time of transplant, but long-term follow-up is lacking. At present, aggressive management of children with oxalosis and renal failure is justifiable, but therapy must be individualized.

## Selected Readings

Hillman RE. Primary hyperoxalurias. In: Scrive CR, Beaudet AL, Sly SW, Valle D, eds. The metabolic basis of inherited disease, ed 6. New York: McGraw-Hill, 1989:933.

Leumann EP, Niederwieser A, Fanconi A. New aspects of infantile oxalosis. Pediatr Nephrol 1987;1:531.

Purdue PE, Lumb MJ, Allsop J, Minatogawa Y, Danpure CJ. A glycine-to-glutamate substitution abolishes alanine: glyoxalate aminotransferase catalytic activity in a subset of patients with primary hyperoxaluria type 1. Genomics 1992;13:215.

Scheinman JI. Primary hyperoxaluria: therapeutic strategies for the 1990s. Kidney Internat 1991;40:389.

Watts RWE, Morgan SH, Danpure CJ, et al. Combined hepatic and renal transplantation in primary hyperoxaluria type I: clinical report of 9 cases. Am J Med 1991;90:179.

*Principles and Practice of Pediatrics, Second Edition.*
edited by Frank A. Oski et al. J. B. Lippincott Company, Philadelphia © 1994.

# 115.7 *Nail-Patella Syndrome (Hereditary Onycho-Osteodysplasia)*

David R. Powell

The cardinal features of the nail-patella syndrome (NPS) are dysplastic nails and hypoplastic patellae; some patients have iliac horns, knee and elbow abnormalities, cataracts, and renal disease. NPS is inherited as an autosomal dominant disorder, probably with full penetrance but variable expressivity. The locus for NPS is located on chromosome 9, linked to the loci for both adenylate kinase 1 and the ABO blood group.

Nephropathic and nonnephropathic forms of NPS apparently exist, because renal disease aggregates in some NPS kindreds while sparing others. In kindreds with a history of nephropathy, 48% of the family members develop renal disease and 14% go on to renal failure; interestingly, the presence of nephropathy or renal failure in parents with NPS does not appear to increase the risk of the same complication in their children. Most patients present with proteinuria, which may lead to nephrotic syndrome, and occasionally NPS is associated with congenital nephrosis. Chronic renal failure has been reported in children under age 10 years but usually develops in teenagers and young adults, sometimes after years of asymptomatic proteinuria.

Kidney biopsy specimens from NPS patients have characteristic findings by electron microscopy. The glomerular basement membrane is irregularly thickened with electron lucent areas in the lamina rara externa and interna, and fibrillar or periodic collagen-like material is present in these membranes and in mesangial matrix. This collagen-like material was not found in a biopsy specimen from a relative free of NPS. Recent work suggests that some of these patients have an abnormal antigenicity of the glomerular basement membrane similar to that found in patients with Alport syndrome. These findings suggest that the basic abnormality of NPS involves disordered connective tissue metabolism, but how this leads to renal failure is unclear.

The degree of electron microscopic abnormality does not seem to correlate with a loss of kidney function in NPS, since changes were present in biopsy specimens of some NPS patients who had no clinical evidence of renal dysfunction. Patients with NPS and a normal glomerular filtration rate, including those with nephrosis, do not demonstrate significant findings by light microscopy. However, patients with renal failure often demonstrate the nonspecific changes of proliferative and chronic glomerulonephritis.

Patients with NPS, especially those from kindreds with a history of renal disease, must be monitored periodically for the development of nephrosis and renal failure. No specific therapy exists for renal involvement in NPS; treatment of nephrosis and renal insufficiency are symptomatic.

## Selected Readings

Bennett WM, Musgrave JE, Campbell RA, et al. The nephropathy of NPS. Am J Med 1973;54:304.

Looij BJ Jr, Te Slaa RL, Hogewind BL, van de Kamp JJP. Genetic counseling in hereditary osteo-onychodysplasia with nephropathy. J Med Genet 1988;25:682.

*Principles and Practice of Pediatrics, Second Edition.*
edited by Frank A. Oski et al. J. B. Lippincott Company, Philadelphia © 1994.

CHAPTER 116
# *Disorders of Renal Tubular Transport*

# 116.1 *Renal Tubular Acidosis*

L. Leighton Hill and Myra Chiang

Renal tubular acidosis (RTA) is a biochemical syndrome characterized by a persistent hyperchloremic (non-anion gap) metabolic acidosis and is caused by abnormalities in the renal regulation of bicarbonate concentration. The glomerular filtration rate (GFR) is usually normal: it may be mildly to moderately depressed but is never severely abnormal. Clinical manifestations suggesting the possibility of RTA include unexplained acidosis, failure to thrive and grow, profound weakness, polyuria, nephrolithiasis, nephrocalcinosis, and rickets.

An understanding of the normal renal mechanisms for maintaining bicarbonate concentrations at appropriate levels is essential for understanding the various types of RTA. In normal individuals, urinary net acid excretion (that is, the hydrogen excreted as titratable acid and as ammonium ions minus any urinary bicarbonate) *equals* the quantity of acid added to extracellular fluids from the diet plus metabolism plus any fecal losses of alkali. RTA is due to an upset in this hydrogen ion balance because of abnormal losses of bicarbonate in the urine, or insufficient hydrogen ion excretion in the urinary buffers, or both. These RTA syndromes have a wide variety of pathogenetic mechanisms and causes.

## CLASSIFICATION AND PATHOGENESIS

A classification of RTA is shown in Table 116-1.

Proximal RTA is a defect in the proximal tubular reabsorption of filtered bicarbonate. Ordinarily about 85% (somewhat less in infants) of filtered bicarbonate is reabsorbed in the proximal tubule and 15% (somewhat more in infants) in the distal nephron. In proximal RTA, the tubular maximum for bicarbonate reabsorption is abnormally low, so that at normal plasma levels of bicarbonate more than 15% of filtered bicarbonate is delivered to the distal nephron for reabsorption, resulting in the urinary excretion and lowering of the bicarbonate concentration in the body fluids. Proximal RTA represents a defect in the sodium/hydrogen ion exchange mechanism in this segment of the nephron.

The mechanisms of transport impairment in proximal RTA have not been defined. Possibilities include a defective sodium/potassium ATPase activity in the basolateral membrane, which normally provides the gradient for maximal efficiency of the luminal sodium/potassium antiporter; a defect in the sodium/hydrogen antiporter itself; or deficiency or inhibition of carbonic anhydrase activity.

Patients with proximal RTA spill bicarbonate into the urine at lower-than-normal plasma bicarbonate concentrations (ie, the renal threshold for bicarbonate is reduced). The fractional excretion of filtered bicarbonate ($^{Fe}HCO_3^-$) is increased. Since the amount of bicarbonate filtered per day varies from hundreds to thousands of milliequivalents, depending on the patient's size, there is the potential for very large losses of this most important

buffer from the body stores. In proximal RTA, the distal mechanisms of acidification are intact.

Distal RTA (see Table 116-1) is seen in two major forms. Type 1 is usually associated with hypokalemia or normokalemia (secretory defect or gradient defect) or rarely with hyperkalemia (voltage-dependent defect). Type 4 RTA is always associated with hyperkalemia. Distal RTA type 1 results from a reduced rate of hydrogen ion secretion by the distal nephron, which may be due to a primary disorder of the hydrogen ion secretory pump (classic distal RTA), increased back-leak of secreted hydrogen ion from lumen to cell (gradient defect), or a decrease in the lumen-negative electrical potential difference that normally promotes hydrogen ion secretion (voltage-dependent RTA). Patients with distal type 1 cannot lower their urine pH below 5.5 regardless of the degree of the acidosis. Patients have also reduced total acid excretion, principally because of a low rate of ammonium secretion. Hypokalemic distal RTA most likely involves reduced function or inhibition of H,K-ATPase.

In the other type of distal RTA, hyperkalemic type 4 RTA, the acidification defect is probably related to impaired renal ammoniagenesis because of hyperkalemia. These patients usually can produce an acid urine (pH <5.5) but cannot excrete the necessary amounts of hydrogen ion in urinary buffers (eg, ammonium) to avoid a metabolic acidosis, and cannot excrete potassium normally. Type 4 RTA is usually observed in children with either a deficiency in circulating aldosterone or unresponsiveness of the renal tubular transport sites to aldosterone.

Distal RTA type 1 may be seen in an incomplete or partial form. This is probably true of the other types, but clinical descriptions of partial defects have been limited to distal type 1. Transient instances of RTA have been described for all three major types of RTA. RTA may be inherited (eg, type 1 autosomal dominant trait) or acquired. Disorders associated with RTA types 2 and 1 are shown in Tables 116-2 and 116-3. Proximal RTA can occur as an isolated abnormality either sporadically or as an inherited disorder. However, it is much more common for proximal RTA to be seen as part of the Fanconi syndrome with associated glycosuria, aminoaciduria, hyperphosphaturia, and so forth.

## CLINICAL CHARACTERISTICS

### Proximal RTA Type 2

Most patients with proximal RTA type 2 manifest this tubular abnormality as part of the Fanconi syndrome, a syndrome of

| TABLE 116-1. Pathophysiologic Classification of RTA | |
|---|---|
| Type | Pathophysiology |
| Proximal RTA (type 2) | Impaired proximal tubular $HCO_3^-$ reabsorption |
| Distal RTA (type 1) | Impaired distal tubular $H^+$ secretion |
|    Secretory defect ("classic distal RTA") |    $H^+$ pump failure |
|    Gradient defect |    Increased back-leak of secreted $H^+$ |
|    Voltage-dependent defect |    Reduced luminal electronegativity |
| Hyperkalemic distal RTA (type 4) | Impaired ammoniagenesis |
|    Hypoaldosteronism | |
|       Primary | |
|       Secondary | |
|    Pseudohypoaldosteronism | |
|       Total | |
|       Partial | Increased NaCl reabsorption in ascending |
|    Chloride shunt | loop of Henle |

## TABLE 116-2. Disorders Associated with RTA Type 2

**Isolated Defect**
Sporadic
Hereditary
Use of carbonic anhydrase inhibitors

**Fanconi Syndrome**
Primary, Secondary
*Inherited*
Cystinosis
Tyrosinemia
Lowe syndrome
Hereditary fructose intolerance
Wilson disease
Glycogen storage disease
Metachromatic leukodystrophy
Osteopetrosis with carbonic anhydrase deficiency
Cytochrome-c-oxidase deficiency
*Defect in Calcium Metabolism*
Hyperparathyroidism
  Primary
  Secondary
*Dysproteinemic States*
Multiple myeloma
Light chain diseases
Monoclonal gammopathy
Amyloidosis
*Interstitial Renal Disease*
Sjögren disease
Medullary cystic disease
Renal transplant rejection
Chronic renal vein thrombosis
Balkan nephropathy
*Drugs and Toxins*
Outdated tetracycline
Maleic acid
Cadmium
Lead
Mercury
*Miscellaneous*
Malignancy
Chronic nephrotic syndrome
Congenital heart disease

## TABLE 116-3. Disorders Associated with Distal RTA Type I

**Primary**
Sporadic
Hereditary

**Secondary (Acquired)**
*Genetic Diseases*
Ehlers-Danlos
Wilson disease
Hereditary elliptocytosis
Fabry disease
Sickle-cell nephropathy
Osteopetrosis with carbonic anhydrase deficiency
Medullary cystic disease
Hereditary hypercalciuria
Marfan syndrome
Sensorineural deafness
*Disorders Causing Nephrocalcinosis*
Idiopathic hypercalciuria
Medullary sponge kidney
Primary hyperparathyroidism
Hyperthyroidism
Vitamin D intoxication
*Autoimmune Diseases*
Sjögren syndrome
Systemic lupus erythematosus
Chronic active hepatitis
Fibrosing alveolitis
Primary biliary cirrhosis
Hyperglobulinemic purpura
Thyroiditis
Cryoglobulinemia
*Tubulointerstitial Diseases*
Obstructive uropathy
Balkan nephropathy
Chronic pyelonephritis
Leprosy
Transplant rejection
*Drugs and Toxins*
Amphotericin B
Lithium
Toluene
*Miscellaneous*
Hepatic cirrhosis
Malnutrition

multiple proximal tubular dysfunctions (see Chap. 116.2). The clinical manifestations in these instances may be related to the condition causing the Fanconi syndrome or to some of the other tubular abnormalities that are a part of the syndrome. Patients with proximal RTA type 2 as an isolated disorder usually present either with unexplained acidosis or with failure to thrive and grow properly. The acidosis, as with all types of RTA, is a hyperchloremic metabolic acidosis. Usually at presentation the patient is in a reasonably steady-state condition; the extent of lowering of the plasma bicarbonate is determined by the severity of the proximal tubular defect in bicarbonate reabsorption. This steady state has been reached because the filtered load of bicarbonate (GFR $\times$ PHCO$_3^-$) has decreased to a point at which the amount that escapes reabsorption by the impaired proximal tubule is small enough to be completely reabsorbed by the distal nephron. Therefore, on presentation there is usually no bicarbonate in the urine, and since the distal acidification mechanisms are intact in proximal RTA, the urine is acid (pH <5.5). During the

acidosis, total acid excretion (titratable acid + ammonium − bicarbonate) is appropriately elevated (>60 $\mu$Eq/1.73 m$^2$/min) and the urine anion gap is negative (chloride > sodium plus potassium). If the patient with proximal RTA type 2 is then treated with sufficient base, the plasma bicarbonate will increase and the amount of bicarbonate filtered will increase. This will overwhelm the impaired proximal tubules with bicarbonate, resulting in a large increase in delivery of bicarbonate to the distal nephron. The urine will therefore contain increasing amounts of bicarbonate as the plasma level increases and the urine becomes alkaline, even though the plasma bicarbonate may still be below normal. The fractional excretion of bicarbonate ($^{Fe}$HCO$_3^-$) is increased despite the fact that the plasma bicarbonate level is still abnormally low. Under these circumstances, total acid excretion would decrease to abnormally low levels, since the bicarbonate in the urine would be increased and the increased bicarbonate delivery to the distal nephron would interfere with proper use of the titratable acid buffers (principally phosphate buffer) and the ammonia buffer.

In summary, patients with proximal RTA type 2 have severe bicarbonate wasting when plasma bicarbonate levels are normal, but during the untreated or acidotic state, their bicarbonaturia ceases, urinary pH becomes acid, and urinary net acid excretion approximates net acid production. Patients with proximal RTA type 2 often have hypokalemia, but serum potassium levels may be normal. The low potassium levels have been attributed to increased delivery of sodium to the distal nephron, where, under the stimulus of aldosterone (aldosterone increases because of the sodium losses and mild volume depletion), sodium is reabsorbed in exchange for potassium ions, which are then excreted. Patients with proximal RTA type 2 do not usually have hypercalciuria, and urinary citrate excretion is normal. Patients with this form of RTA seldom manifest the complications of nephrocalcinosis, nephrolithiasis, or rickets, which are common manifestations in patients with untreated distal RTA type 1. They may, however, manifest with muscle weakness and polyuria, both caused by hypokalemia.

## Distal RTA Type 1

Patients with this type of RTA may present with unexplained acidosis or with failure to thrive and grow, hypokalemia, or one or more of the complications of RTA such as nephrolithiasis, nephrocalcinosis, rickets, or polyuria. The urine pH in distal RTA type 1 is never very acid (pH 5.5 or greater), the total acid excretion is always abnormally low, and the urine anion gap is positive despite the degree of acidosis. Hypokalemia is common and may be severe. Hypercalciuria is also common and urinary citrate excretion is low. These abnormalities, along with the persistently alkaline urine, are instrumental in the development of nephrocalcinosis and nephrolithiasis in these patients. It is unknown whether the low urinary citrate excretion is primary or is secondary to the prolonged metabolic acidosis. In the inherited variety of distal RTA type 1, metabolic acidosis may occur in the first few months of life. Most preadolescent children with distal RTA type 1 waste bicarbonate and have a significantly higher fractional excretion of bicarbonate than do adults with this type

of RTA. In cases inherited as an autosomal dominant trait, the affected child usually wastes bicarbonate, while the affected parent does not. Proximal tubular functions in patients with type 1 RTA are normal. A voltage-dependent type of distal RTA type 1 is rare and is associated with hyperkalemia; however, the urine pH is always 5.5 or greater. Most patients with distal RTA type 1 have either hypokalemia or normokalemia.

## Distal RTA Type 4 (Hyperkalemic)

Hyperkalemic distal RTA (type 4) is thought to be the most common type of RTA in both children and adults. It represents an abnormality of distal tubular function in regard to the renal handling of hydrogen and potassium ions. It manifests with a persistent hyperchloremic (non-anion gap) metabolic acidosis and hyperkalemia. The hyperkalemia is probably the most distinctive clinical characteristic of this type of RTA when compared with types 1 and 2, since both of these types usually have either normal, or quite frequently low, serum potassium concentrations. Patients with type 4 RTA usually can make an acid urine (pH <5.5), but total acid excretion is low due to very low rates of ammonia excretion, the urine anion gap is positive, and the renal excretion of potassium is inappropriate to the serum concentration of potassium. The defects in urinary potassium and hydrogen ion excretion appear to be secondary to hypoaldosteronism or to end-organ resistance to aldosterone (pseudohypoaldosteronism). Hypoaldosteronism can be primary or secondary (Table 116-4).

Primary hypoaldosteronism is seen in patients with acute adrenal insufficiency, Addison's disease, and salt-losing congenital adrenal hyperplasia. Patients may show all the signs of adrenal insufficiency, including salt wasting, tendency to low blood volume and low blood pressures, metabolic acidosis, hyponatremia, and hyperkalemia. Peripheral renin activity (PRA) is usually increased, but there is a virtual absence of circulating aldosterone. Renal function in these patients, including renal tubular function, is within normal limits.

Secondary hypoaldosteronism results from decreased production or release of the active form of renin due to destruction of the cells of the juxtaglomerular apparatus, as seen in patients with intrinsic renal disease such as lupus nephropathy, diabetic nephropathy, obstructive uropathy, and interstitial nephritis. Reduction in overall renal function can be demonstrated, but the

**TABLE 116-4.   Clinical Spectrum of Distal Type IV Hyperkalemic RTA**

| Mechanism Designation | PRA | Aldo | Plasma | | Salt Wasting |
| --- | --- | --- | --- | --- | --- |
| | | | BV | BP | |
| Hypoaldosteronism | | | | | |
| Primary mineralocorticoid deficiency, no intrinsic renal disease | Increase | Decrease | Nor/decr. | Nor/decr. | Yes |
| Primary hyporeninemic, secondary hypoaldosteronism due to intrinsic renal disease | Decrease | Decrease | Nor/incr. | Nor/incr. | No |
| Pseudohypoaldosteronism, end-organ resistant to aldosterone | | | | | |
| Total resistance | Increase | Increase | Decrease | Nor/decr. | Yes |
| Partial resistance associated with renal immaturity | Nor/incr. | Nor/incr. | Normal | Normal | No |
| Chloride shunt or Gordon syndrome | Decrease | Decrease | Increase | Increase | No |

*PRA*, plasma renin activity; *Aldo*, aldosterone; *BV*, blood volume; *BP*, blood pressure; *Nor/incr.*, normal or increased; *Nor/decr.*, normal or decreased.

*Modified from McSherry E. Renal tubular acidosis in childhood. Kidney Internat 1981;20:799*

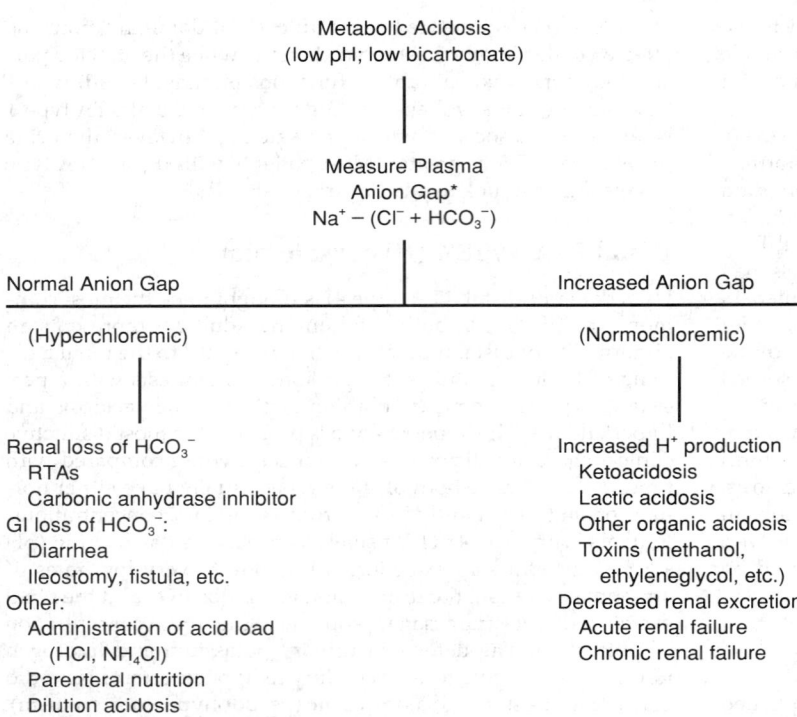

Metabolic Acidosis
(low pH; low bicarbonate)

Measure Plasma
Anion Gap*
$Na^+ - (Cl^- + HCO_3^-)$

| Normal Anion Gap | Increased Anion Gap |
|---|---|
| (Hyperchloremic) | (Normochloremic) |
| Renal loss of $HCO_3^-$ | Increased $H^+$ production |
| RTAs | Ketoacidosis |
| Carbonic anhydrase inhibitor | Lactic acidosis |
| GI loss of $HCO_3^-$: | Other organic acidosis |
| Diarrhea | Toxins (methanol, |
| Ileostomy, fistula, etc. | ethyleneglycol, etc.) |
| Other: | Decreased renal excretion |
| Administration of acid load | Acute renal failure |
| (HCl, NH₄Cl) | Chronic renal failure |
| Parenteral nutrition | |
| Dilution acidosis | |

*Normals: Neonates—18 or less, older infants and children—16 or less, adolescents—14 or less.

**Figure 116-1.** The differentiation of metabolic acidosis into hyperchloremic and normochloremic types.

hyperkalemia and metabolic acidosis are out of proportion in severity to the degree of renal insufficiency. These patients do not demonstrate salt wasting or tendency to low blood volume, and their blood pressure may be either normal or elevated.

Pseudohypoaldosteronism (end-organ resistance to aldosterone) resembles primary hypoaldosteronism except that the aldosterone level is either normal or elevated. The aldosterone resistance may be total or partial. Total resistance to aldosterone results in salt wasting, hyponatremia, and hyperkalemia. Patients have a marked tendency to develop low blood volume and hypotension, just like patients with true hypoaldosteronism; however, the PRA and plasma aldosterone levels are markedly elevated. Aldosterone receptors have been found to be missing in mononuclear leukocytes of patients with pseudohypoaldosteronism. The severity of the renal salt wasting and potassium ion retention diminishes after infancy in most patients, permitting discontinuation of salt supplements. However, the disordered renal handling of sodium and potassium appears to persist, although less severely.

Partial resistance to aldosterone may be seen in infants and young children. These patients have hyperkalemia and metabolic acidosis but do not have salt wasting. The PRA and plasma aldosterone levels may be normal or only slightly elevated. The abnormalities are transient in many patients, leading to the postulation that renal immaturity may be a factor. Several of these patients have had unilateral anomalies of the kidneys or urinary system.

Another form of type 4 RTA occurs in both children and adults and is associated with salt retention. Its pathogenesis has been attributed to an abnormally increased reabsorption of sodium chloride in the thick ascending limb of Henle (chloride shunt), which causes salt retention, tendency to increase blood volume, and hypertension. This entity has also been called Gordon syndrome, and seems to be in many ways a mirror image of Bartter's syndrome. Short stature is common, and most patients appear

to have inherited the syndrome via an autosomal dominant mode of transmission. The PRA and plasma aldosterone levels are both reduced.

## DIAGNOSIS

Patients with all forms of RTA have a hyperchloremic metabolic acidosis. This type of acidosis must be differentiated from an anion-gap type of acidosis by measuring the plasma undetermined anion gap* (Fig 116-1). Once a hyperchloremic (non-anion gap) metabolic acidosis has been demonstrated, it is important to rule out other causes of this type of acidosis before making a diagnosis of RTA. The chief differential diagnosis is usually diarrhea with bicarbonate loss in the stools, since this is by far the most common cause of hyperchloremic metabolic acidosis. In patients with consistently alkaline urine, it is wise to consider the possibility of a urinary tract infection with a urea-splitting organism. If there is any suspicion of a urinary tract infection, a urine culture should be done. The plasma pH, partial pressure of carbon dioxide ($PCO_2$), and total carbon dioxide must be measured several times to document the persistence of the acidosis. All urine passed should be tested for pH; at least some of these should be done with a pH meter, which is more accurate than dipsticks.

Although the ability to acidify is very important, very little hydrogen ion is actually excreted as free hydrogen ion. Most hydrogen ion is excreted as titratable acid or as ammonium, both components of the total acid excretion. Ammonium excretion is by far the most important of the two, principally because it is the one that increases so significantly in chronic metabolic acidosis. Many clinical laboratories do not provide the measurement

* Undetermined anion gap = $Na^+ - (Cl^- + HCO_3^-)$ (Normals: Neonates, 18 or less; older infants and children, 16 or less; adolescents and adults, 14 or less)

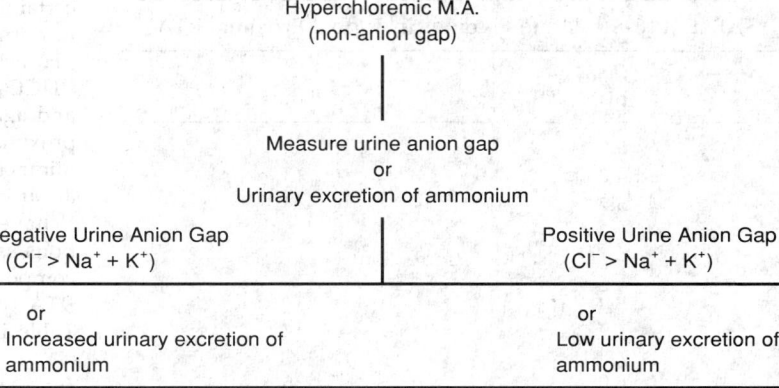

**Figure 116-2.** First step in the workup of a patient with hyperchloremic (non-anion gap) metabolic acidosis. Ammonium can be measured directly or indirectly using the urinary anion gap. A negative urine anion gap indicates adequate urinary ammonium excretion. A positive urine anion gap indicates low excretion of ammonium and suggests a distal tubular acidification defect.

of urinary ammonium to the clinician, so indirect means of predicting ammonium excretion have been used (eg, the urinary anion gap). It is best to measure urinary ammonium directly if this test is available; if not, then the urinary anion gap will suffice and should be determined several times using spot (untimed) urines (Fig 116-2).

The urine anion gap is calculated using the measured concentration of electrolytes in the urine: sodium + potassium − chloride. If the chloride concentration exceeds the sum of sodium and potassium concentrations, the anion gap is said to be negative. If the chloride concentration is less than the sum of the sodium and potassium, then the urine anion gap is said to be positive. A negative value for urine anion gap suggests adequate ammonium excretion and can be seen in hyperchloremic metabolic acidosis secondary to diarrhea, untreated proximal RTA, prior administration of an acid load, or urinary tract infection with a urea-splitting organism (Fig 116-3). In contrast, a positive urine anion gap suggests a distal acidification defect.

Again, the urine anion gap is a good way to estimate urinary ammonium excretion—the most important component of total acid excretion—but direct measurement of $NH_4$ is better. The urine anion gap is obviously not as reliable if the urine contains large amounts of unmeasured anions such as ketoacids, penicillin, and salicylates, which will lead to underestimation of urinary ammonium excretion. Glomerular function should be evaluated with a serum creatinine, and several serum potassium concentrations should be done.

## Proximal RTA Type 2

A urine anion gap measurement provides rapid distinction between proximal and distal RTA. Diagnosis of proximal RTA is established when other disorders producing a negative anion gap have been excluded (see Fig 116-3). Definitive diagnosis of proximal RTA is made by the demonstration of an acid urine (pH <5.5) during periods of acidosis but only a mildly acid or alkaline

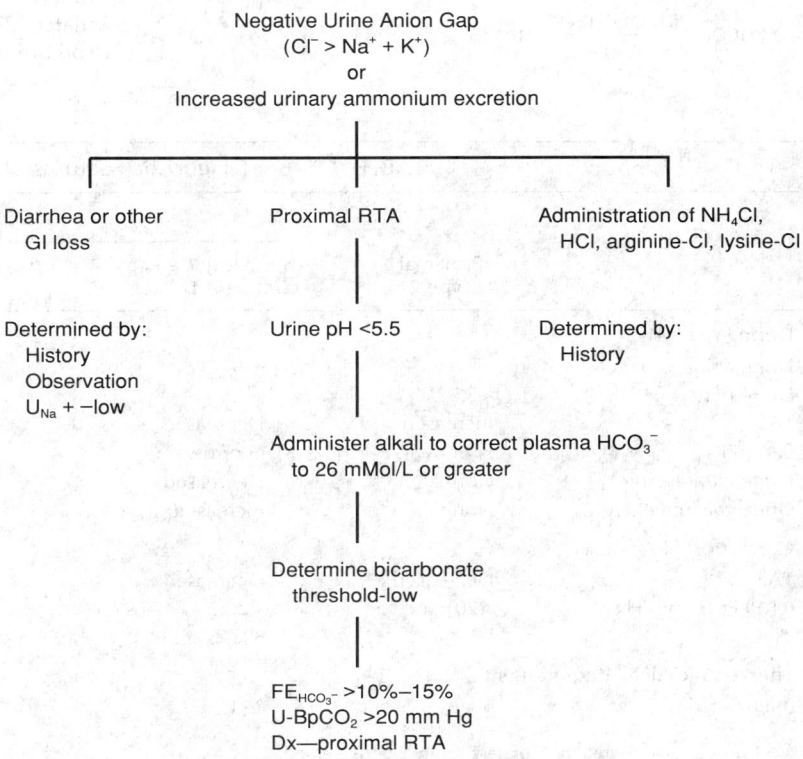

**Figure 116-3.** Workup of untreated patient with hyperchloremic metabolic acidosis and a negative urine anion gap or a high urinary ammonium excretion. (Modified from Rodriguez-Soriano J, Vallo A. Renal tubular acidosis. Pediatr Nephrol 1990;4:268.)

TABLE 116-5.  Urine Findings in Type 2 Proximal RTA

| Urine pH | Plasma |
|---|---|
| 5.0 | 14 |
| 4.8 | 13 |
| 5.2 | 14 |
| NaHCO₃ Correction | |
| 6.5 | 17 |
| 7.0 | 19 |
| 7.4 | 21 |
| 8.0 | 26 |

urine (pH >6.0) with partial correction of acidosis. In the patient data shown in Table 116-5, the plasma bicarbonate is still in the range of 17 to 19 mEq/L after treatment, yet the urine pH has jumped almost two pH units to the 6.5 to 7.0 range. Similarly, in RTA type 2, the total acid excretion (principally accounted for by ammonium) is in the normal range (>60 $\mu$Eq/1.73 m²/min) during the untreated period of acidosis, but drops to abnormally low levels with partial correction of the acidosis. The urine anion gap is also negative during untreated acidosis, implying adequate urinary ammonium concentration, but with treatment the urine anion gap becomes positive.

Bicarbonate is virtually absent from the urine during the period of maximal untreated acidosis but is present in large amounts with partial correction, demonstrating a low threshold for bicarbonate excretion (see Fig 116-3). Fractional excretion of bicarbonate ($^{Fe}HCO_3^-$)* is low during acidosis, but with partial correction (eg, to the 17 to 19 mEq/L range, as in Table 116-5), the $^{Fe}HCO_3^-$ will probably be found to exceed 10% to 15% and would

$$ ^{*\,Fe}HCO_3^- = \frac{^{U}HCO_3^-/^{P}HCO_3^-}{U_{cr}/P_{cr}} \times 100 $$

certainly exceed 10% to 15% if the plasma bicarbonate is brought to normal levels by treatment (see Fig 116-3). Measurement of pH, urinary anion gap (or ammonium excretion), $^{U}HCO_3^-$, and $^{Fe}HCO_3^-$ during acidosis, with partial correction of the acidosis and again with full correction, should demonstrate a defect in proximal tubular bicarbonate reabsorption if present. The urine minus blood $P_{CO_2}$ is normal in proximal RTA (see Fig 116-3), as are urinary calcium and citrate excretions. Any patient proven to have proximal RTA should have other proximal tubular functions assessed, since this type of RTA is most often found as a component of the Fanconi syndrome. The diagnostic features of RTA type 2 are contrasted with the other varieties of RTA in Table 116-6.

## Distal RTA Type 1

The patient with a positive urine anion gap (that is, the urine chloride concentration is less than the sum of concentrations of sodium and potassium) or with abnormal total acid excretion (titratable acid + ammonium − bicarbonate) probably has a distal type of RTA (Fig 116-4). The next step is to measure the plasma potassium concentration (see Fig 116-4). If the potassium is normal or low, along with inability to acidify properly and a positive urinary anion gap, then a diagnosis of distal RTA type 1 seems appropriate.

Occasionally patients, such as those with partial RTA, do not have plasma bicarbonate levels that are clearly low. In such cases, a provocative challenge may be indicated. Most commonly used in this situation is the ammonium chloride load. A dose of 75 mEq (4 g NH₄Cl) per square meter body surface area, or 0.15 g/kg of NH₄Cl, can be given orally, by nasogastric tube, or intravenously and should lower the bicarbonate level to the range of 12 to 16 mEq/L, which is, of course, clearly low. In distal RTA type 1, the urine pH will remain at 5.5 or greater, the total acid excretion will remain abnormally low, and the urine anion gap will remain positive despite this acid challenge. If there is a reluctance to use ammonium chloride because of the patient's condition, a furosemide challenge can be used. This normally stimulates distal acidification mechanisms by greatly increasing sodium delivery to the cortical and medullary collecting ducts.

TABLE 116-6.  Diagnostic Features of the Types of RTA

| | Proximal Type 2 | Distal Type 1 Secretory Defect Gradient Defect | Distal Type 1 Voltage-Dependent Defect | Distal Type 1 With HCO₃⁻ Wasting | Distal Type 4 |
|---|---|---|---|---|---|
| **During Acidosis** | | | | | |
| Urine anion gap | − | + | + | + | + |
| Urine pH | <5.5 | >5.5 | >5.5 | >5.5 | <5.5 |
| TAE | Increased | Decreased | Decreased | Decreased | Decreased |
| Serum K⁺ | N or decr. | N or decr. | Increased | N or decr. | Increased |
| Urine citrate excret. | Normal | Decreased | Decreased | Decreased | Normal |
| Urine calcium excret. | Normal | Increased | Increased | Increased | |
| **Correction of Acidosis** | | | | | |
| TAE | Decreased | Decreased | Decreased | Decreased | Decreased |
| (U-B) PCO₂ mm Hg | >20 | <20 | <20 | <20 | variable |
| $^{Fe}HCO_3$ | >15% | 3%–5% | 3%–5% | 5%–15% | 5%–10% |
| **Therapeutic Alkali Requirement** | | | | | |
| (mEq/Kg/day) | 5–20 | 1–4 | 1–4 | 4–15 | 1–5 |

*TAE*, total acid excretion; *N or decr.*, normal or decreased.

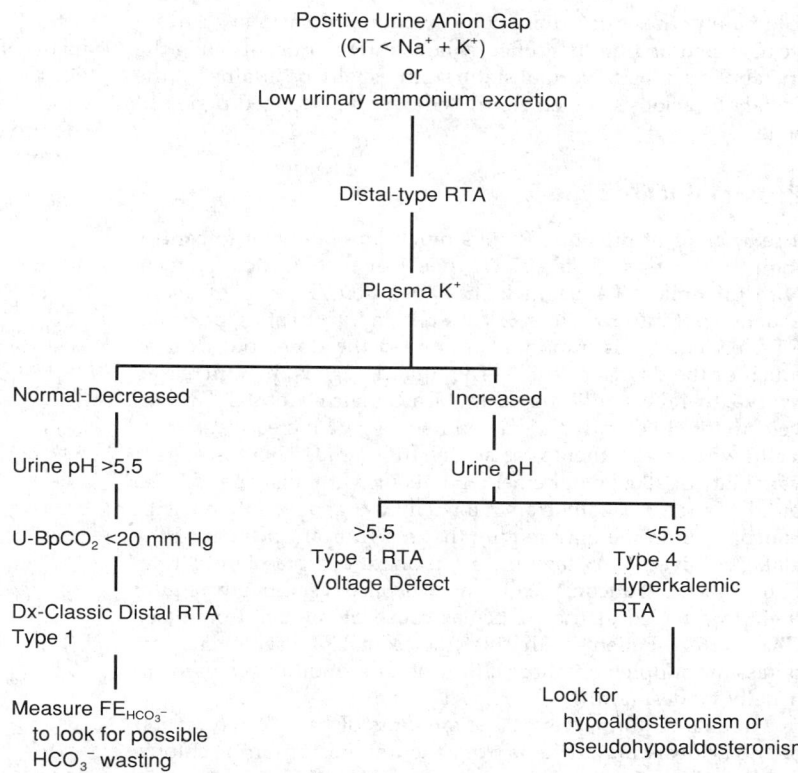

Positive Urine Anion Gap
($Cl^- < Na^+ + K^+$)
or
Low urinary ammonium excretion

Distal-type RTA

Plasma $K^+$

Normal-Decreased

Urine pH >5.5

$U-BpCO_2$ <20 mm Hg

Dx-Classic Distal RTA
Type 1

Measure $FE_{HCO_3^-}$
to look for possible
$HCO_3^-$ wasting

Increased

Urine pH

>5.5
Type 1 RTA
Voltage Defect

<5.5
Type 4
Hyperkalemic
RTA

Look for
hypoaldosteronism or
pseudohypoaldosteronism

**Figure 116-4.** Outline of the approach to a patient with hyperchloremic metabolic acidosis who has a positive urine anion gap or low urinary ammonium excretion and, presumably, a distal renal defect.

Furosemide should not be used in patients with low serum potassium concentrations. A sodium sulfate infusion can also be used to study distal acidification mechanisms. If the plasma potassium concentration is elevated and the urine pH remains above 5.5 after the acid load, the diagnosis of distal RTA type 1 due to a voltage-dependent defect (reduced luminal electronegativity) is established (see Fig 116-4).

Urine minus blood $Pco_2$ remains a controversial test in assessing acidification mechanisms, but it is often low in distal RTA type 1 and may help to differentiate the different pathogenetic mechanisms in distal RTA type 1. This measurement is done by first loading the patient with bicarbonate (either orally or intravenously) until the plasma bicarbonate exceeds 24 mEq/L and the urine pH exceeds 7.6, and then by measuring the $Pco_2$ in a spot urine and blood specimen obtained nearly simultaneously. A measurement of less than 20 mm Hg strongly suggests distal RTA type 1. This test is a reliable evaluation of the exchange of hydrogen ions for sodium ions in the distal nephron because of the absence of carbonic anhydrase on the luminal surface of the collecting tubules. The carbonic acid formed in the lumen after the exchange of the sodium ion in $NaHCO_3$ for a hydrogen ion is then not immediately broken down to carbon dioxide and water. Since the carbon dioxide remains hydrated, it cannot diffuse back into the cells and blood, and therefore is delivered to the urinary bladder as $H_2CO_3$; the voided urine can then be measured for $Pco_2$. Urine calcium is frequently increased (>4 mg/kg/day) and urinary citrate excretion is low.

Patients with distal RTA type 1 should also have a timed quantitative measure of urinary bicarbonate excretion or a measurement of $^{Fe}HCO_3^-$ to determine if bicarbonate wastage is part of the clinical picture, since this is common in young children with distal RTA and has strong therapeutic implications. If the patient with distal RTA type 1 is not an $HCO_3^-$ waster, then the $^{Fe}HCO_3^-$ should be less than 5%. Type 1 patients who waste $HCO_3^-$ may have an $^{Fe}HCO_3^-$ in the 5% to 15% range, but it should not exceed 15%.

## Distal RTA Type 4 (Hyperkalemic)

Patients with distal RTA type 4 have a positive urine anion gap and low total acid excretion (<60 $\mu$Eq/1.73 m²/min), similar to that of distal RTA type 1. However, the presence of hyperkalemia and acid urine pH (<5.5) distinguishes type 4 from type 1 distal RTA (see Fig 116-4).

Once the diagnosis of distal type 4 hyperkalemic RTA is established, the underlying pathophysiology should be determined if possible. At least some of the clinical determinants are shown in Table 116-4. A careful physical examination in regard to the status of the extracellular and blood vascular volume is essential, as are repeated measurements of the blood pressure. In addition, a PRA, plasma aldosterone, and urinary electrolytes are indicated in most instances. On the basis of these tests plus a detailed history, serum creatinine, ultrasound studies of the kidneys, and routine urine examinations, a diagnosis of the particular variety of type 4 RTA can usually be made (see Table 116-4).

## THERAPY

### General

Administration of alkali is common to the therapy of almost all types of RTA. The most frequently used alkalies are sodium bicarbonate and sodium citrate, the latter usually given as Shohl's solution. Each gram of $NaHCO_3$ provides 12 mEq of bicarbonate, and Shohl's solution contains 1 mEq of citrate per milliliter of solution. In patients with hypokalemic types of RTA, a percentage of alkali can be given as the potassium salt. Plasma bicarbonate, either direct or indirect (from pH and $Pco_2$), and serum potassium determinations should be performed every 2 to 4 days during alkali dosage adjustment. After correction of the acidosis, bicarbonate and potassium levels should be measured every 2 weeks for 1 to 2 months and then monthly for several more months.

Ultimately, these determinations are done three to six times a year, depending on the difficulty encountered in controlling the metabolic acidosis. Normal stature can usually be attained if the metabolic acidosis is well controlled over a prolonged period of time.

## Proximal RTA Type 2

The acidosis of proximal RTA is much more difficult to control than the acidosis of distal RTA type 1 or type 4. Most patients with proximal RTA begin with 4 to 6 mEq/kg/day of alkali, usually split into four to six doses per day. In treating proximal RTA patients, it is important to spread the doses out over as much of the day as possible. The total dosage is then increased every 2 to 4 days until the serum bicarbonate is normal. Growth velocity of children with isolated RTA type 2 increases dramatically when alkali therapy is successfully used. There is a great variability of alkali requirement in patients with this type of RTA, but the range is usually from 5 to 20 mEq/kg/day. Patients with Fanconi syndrome may require that a significant portion of the alkali be given as potassium bicarbonate or potassium citrate. Patients with Fanconi syndrome will also very likely require therapy directed at the particular cause of the syndrome (see Chap. 116.2). Patients with isolated proximal RTA seldom require potassium supplementation; if they do, the amounts required are usually modest (1 to 3 mEq/Kg/day).

Patients requiring very large amounts of base for correction of the acidosis may benefit from the administration of chlorothiazide (10 to 20 mg/kg/day), dietary sodium chloride restriction, or both. The thiazide diuretics tend to increase the proximal tubular reabsorption of bicarbonate by inducing a mild contraction of the extracellular fluid space.

## Distal RTA Type 1

Alkali therapy in these patients is usually initiated at a dose of 1 to 2 mEq/kg/day if there is no evidence of bicarbonate wasting and at 4 to 6 mEq/kg/day if there is bicarbonate wasting. The successful dosage in the patient without bicarbonate wasting is usually in the range of 1 to 4 mEq/kg/day. The distal RTA type 1 patient with bicarbonate wasting usually requires doses of from 4 to 15 mEq/kg/day. Total doses can be split into two or three administrations per day. Type 1 patients with particularly severe problems with potassium homeostasis may require that 20% to 50% of the total base be given as potassium citrate. Successful correction of the acidosis will result in a return to normal of the urinary calcium and citrate excretions and will greatly lessen the chances of the development of such complications as nephrolithiasis, nephrocalcinosis, and rickets.

## Distal RTA Type 4 (Hyperkalemic)

Doses of base in the range of 1 to 5 mEq/kg/day are usually sufficient to correct the acidosis and may also correct the hyperkalemia of distal RTA type 4. Obviously, potassium containing alkali should be avoided. Furosemide is also effective in returning serum potassium levels to normal, but it should not be used in patients demonstrating a salt-wasting defect. Rarely it is necessary to resort temporarily to the use of exchange resins (Kayexalate or sodium polystyrene sulfonate) to control the hyperkalemia.

RTA type 4 has many etiologies, and often the principal therapeutic efforts are directed toward the underlying disease causing the RTA, whether this be lupus, diabetes, interstitial nephritis, obstructive uropathy, unilateral renal disease, or others. If the problem results primarily from mineralocorticoid deficiency, then hormonal replacement therapy will very likely be quite effective.

If the patient has pseudohypoaldosteronism, then large supplements of sodium chloride may be required for successful therapy. On the other hand, patients with the chloride shunt (Gordon syndrome) usually benefit greatly from salt restriction and from the use of furosemide or other loop diuretics. Other antihypertensives may also be necessary to control the hypertension.

## Selected Readings

Battle DC, Hizon M, Cohen E, et al. The use of the urinary anion gap in the diagnosis of hyperchloremic metabolic acidosis. N Engl J Med 1988;318:594.

Carlisle EJ, Donnelly SM, Halperin ML. Renal tubular acidosis (RTA): recognize the ammonium defect and pHorget the urine pH. Pediatr Nephrol 1991;5:242.

McSherry E. Renal tubular acidosis in childhood (nephrology forum). Kidney Internat 1981;20:799.

Rodriguez-Soriano J. Renal tubular acidosis. In: Edelmann CM Jr., ed. Pediatric kidney disease, ed 2. Boston: Little, Brown, 1992:1737.

Rodriguez-Soriano J, Vallo A. Renal tubular acidosis. Pediatr Nephrol 1990;4:268.

Sabatini S, Kurtzman NA. Pathophysiology of the renal tubular acidosis. Sem Nephrol 1991;11;202.

*Principles and Practice of Pediatrics, Second Edition.*
edited by Frank A. Oski et al. J. B. Lippincott Company, Philadelphia © 1994.

# 116.2 *Pan-Proximal Tubular Dysfunction (Fanconi Syndrome)*

Eileen D. Brewer and David R. Powell

The Fanconi syndrome (FS) is the result of generalized transport dysfunction of the proximal renal tubule. It is characterized classically by excessive urinary losses of amino acids, glucose, bicarbonate, and phosphate, and also calcium, magnesium, uric acid, and other organic acids, low-molecular-weight (tubular) proteins, sodium, potassium, and water. The urinary losses can result in metabolic acidosis, dehydration, hypokalemia, hypophosphatemia, rickets, and growth retardation in children. Many inherited and acquired disorders can lead to FS in adults and children (Table 116-7). When FS occurs in childhood, however, the cause is usually hereditary and related to an inborn error of metabolism.

## PATHOPHYSIOLOGY

Basic abnormalities underlying renal tubular transport dysfunction in FS are incompletely understood. Since a variety of inherited, acquired, and experimentally induced conditions can cause FS, specific pathologic mechanisms operative in one disorder may not necessarily be present in another, although each could lead to a final common pathway that results in the expression of FS. Suggested possibilities for a final common pathway include defective generation of energy to drive the transport processes, increased back-leak of reabsorbed solutes across the cell membrane into the tubular lumen, and abnormal action or location of carriers that normally transport solutes across the cell membrane from the tubular lumen into the intracellular space.

## TABLE 116-7. Causes of the Fanconi Syndrome

**Hereditary**

*Primary*
Idiopathic

*Secondary*
Cystinosis
Lowe syndrome
Tyrosinemia type 1
Galactosemia
Hereditary fructose intolerance
Glycogen storage disease
Wilson disease
Other (cytochrome-c-oxidase deficiency, metachromatic leukodystrophy, Alport syndrome)

**Acquired**

*Intoxications*
Drugs
 Gentamicin and other aminoglycosides
 Outdated tetracycline
 Cephalothin
 Valproic acid
 Streptozotocin
 6-Mercaptopurine
 Azathioprine
 Cis-platinum
Toxins
 Heavy metals (lead, mercury, cadmium, uranium, platinum)
 Glue (toluene) sniffing
 Paraquat
 Maleic acid (experimental in animals)

*Disease states*
Nephrotic syndrome
Sjögren syndrome
Multiple myeloma
Light chain nephropathy
Hypergammaglobulinemia
Amyloidosis
Interstitial nephritis with anti-tubular basement membrane antibody
Renal vein thrombosis
Malignancy (lymphoma, carcinoma)
Renal transplantation

## CLINICAL AND LABORATORY FINDINGS

The general clinical manifestations of FS depend on the patient's age and the type and chronicity of the underlying disease. Infants and children most often present with failure to thrive. Many features of FS, including chronic acidosis, volume contraction, hypokalemia, hypophosphatemia, and abnormal vitamin D metabolism, contribute to impaired linear growth. However, in some cases, especially in patients with cystinosis, these factors alone are not sufficient to explain the severity of the growth retardation. Rachitic bone changes may be a presenting or accompanying clinical sign in some children with FS. If the child has been walking, bowing deformities of the legs may be noticed first. A child who does not yet bear weight may have straight legs but noticeable metaphyseal widening at the wrists, knees, or ankles and radiographic changes classic for rickets at these sites. Infants less than 5 months old rarely have the clinical findings of rickets.

Episodic vomiting, anorexia, polydipsia and polyuria, chronic constipation, and unexplained fevers are nonspecific symptoms of chronic FS. Constipation probably results from chronic volume depletion associated with the polyuria, hypokalemia, and chronic metabolic acidosis of untreated FS. Unexplained fevers, which occur especially frequently in infants and young children with cystinosis, may reflect episodic dehydration.

The laboratory findings of FS mostly reflect abnormal proximal renal tubular function. In normal children, more than 98% of the filtered amino acids are reabsorbed in the proximal renal tubule. In FS, hyperaminoaciduria occurs in the presence of normal plasma amino acid levels and is an exaggeration of the normal excretory pattern of each amino acid, with the percentage of tubular reabsorption of each amino acid decreased below normal. Since urinary losses are trivial compared to intake, hyperaminoaciduria is not clinically significant, but it is an important clinical marker for FS. Plasma and urinary amino acids should be sampled simultaneously as part of the clinical evaluation of patients with FS.

Urinalysis often reveals characteristic abnormalities, including glucosuria in the presence of a normal blood sugar concentration; abnormally high urine pH ($>5.5$) in the presence of mild to moderate hyperchloremic metabolic acidosis, but appropriately low with severe acidosis (type 2 renal tubular acidosis); specific gravity 1.010 to 1.015, even in the presence of dehydration; and mild albuminuria (1 to 2+ or 30 to 100 mg/dL) with normal serum protein and albumin.

Glucosuria, which is often intermittent, rarely exceeds 2+ (500 mg/dL) on the dipstick and is clinically insignificant except as a marker of FS. Patients who present with severe hyperchloremic metabolic acidosis (plasma bicarbonate 10 to 15 mEq/L) usually have a urinary pH less than 5.5, characteristic of type 2 (proximal) renal tubular acidosis. When their acidosis is treated and the plasma bicarbonate concentration is kept in the normal range by supplemental alkali therapy, the excretion of bicarbonate will exceed 15% of the bicarbonate filtered by the glomerulus, a value typical of proximal renal tubular acidosis. The urinary pH usually exceeds 7.0. Fractional excretions of bicarbonate as high as 30% have been reported. If a patient is severely volume depleted, paradoxical metabolic alkalosis can actually occur, but it will change to metabolic acidosis after volume expansion. Volume depletion in affected patients is the result of obligatory polyuria, which is mainly due to the wasting of sodium, amino acids, glucose, and other osmotically active solutes from the proximal tubule. Polyuria may be worse in the presence of chronic hypokalemia, which can impair urinary concentration in the distal rental tubule and stimulate thirst and polydipsia. In patients with FS, the urine specific gravity rarely exceeds 1.015 to 1.020, even in the presence of severe dehydration; thus, urine specific gravity should not be used as an indicator of hydration status.

Mild albuminuria (2+ or less, or 100 mg/dL or less by urinalysis dipstick) usually indicates tubular proteinuria. Tubular proteinuria is characterized by the predominance of low-molecular-weight species such as lysozyme (molecular weight 15,000 daltons) and beta$_2$ microglobulin (molecular weight 11,800 daltons), but also albumin (molecular weight 40,000 daltons). Proteins of about 40,000 daltons or less, including a small amount of albumin, are normally filtered by the glomerulus, then reabsorbed and catabolized in the proximal tubule. In FS, proximal tubular transport dysfunction presumably results in tubular proteinuria. Like glucosuria and generalized amino aciduria, tubular proteinuria is of no clinical significance except as a marker of FS. Proteinuria may be more pronounced in Lowe syndrome, occasionally exceeding 1 g/m$^2$/day, but has never been associated with the clinical nephrotic syndrome.

Serum chemistries are often abnormal in fully expressed FS.

Besides hyperchloremic metabolic acidosis with a normal anion gap, patients may have hyponatremia, hypokalemia, hypophosphatemia, and in some cases hypouricemia. Serum calcium and magnesium are usually normal, despite increased losses of calcium and magnesium in the urine. Excessive sodium loss in the urine without sufficient sodium intake can eventually result in hyponatremia, although increased delivery of sodium to the distal renal tubule and high levels of renin and aldosterone caused by volume depletion will increase distal tubular sodium reabsorption to avoid hyponatremia. The preferential distal reabsorption of sodium worsens hypokalemia, because potassium is exchanged for sodium in the reabsorption process when bicarbonate is also present in excess in the distal nephron. The combination of excessive distal tubular secretion of potassium and increased proximal tubular rejection of potassium creates obligatory loss of large amounts of potassium in the urine, usually leading to hypokalemia and severe total body potassium depletion. This can cause weakness, poor growth, and fatal cardiac arrhythmias. Treatment of acidosis with sodium bicarbonate without potassium supplementation can result in death.

Hypophosphatemia results from excessive urinary wasting of phosphate and reduced tubular reabsorption of phosphate, even at low serum phosphate concentrations. Serum parathyroid hormone concentration is usually normal. Serum levels of 1,25-dihydroxyvitamin D, which is made in the proximal renal tubule by 1-hydroxylation of 25-hydroxyvitamin D, are often reduced or lower than expected for the degree of hypophosphatemia, which is a major stimulus for 1,25-dihydroxyvitamin D production. Hypophosphatemia, impaired renal tubular vitamin D metabolism, excessive urinary calcium excretion, and chronic acidosis all contribute to the chronic bone disease (ie, rickets and osteomalacia) of patients with FS.

Most patients with FS waste uric acid in the urine and have hypouricemia. Patients with hereditary fructose intolerance exposed to fructose have transient hyperuricemia instead, because of the abnormal biochemical pathways underlying this disease.

Some affected patients, especially those with cystinosis and some with Lowe syndrome, may have decreased carnitine reabsorption in the proximal tubule and carnitine deficiency. Carnitine is required to transport free fatty acids into mitochondria for subsequent energy production. Carnitine deficiency may contribute to muscle weakness and delayed development.

## CAUSES

Table 116-7 lists many of the causes of FS. Most of these disorders are discussed elsewhere in this text. The rest of this section will focus on diseases associated with FS that occur in childhood and lead to progressive chronic renal failure.

### Cystinosis (Nephropathic Cystinosis)

Cystinosis is a rare lysosomal storage disease in which intracellular cystine accumulation is associated with FS, chronic renal failure, growth failure, corneal opacities, photophobia, and hypothyroidism. It is not related to the disease cystinuria, which is a genetically transmitted defect for transport of the dibasic amino acids in the renal tubule and intestine, resulting in massive urinary cystine and cystine nephrolithiasis. In cystinosis, plasma cystine concentration is normal, and urinary cystine concentration is elevated only to a degree consistent with the generalized hyperaminoaciduria of FS.

Three types of cystinosis are recognized: infantile nephropathic, adolescent or juvenile onset, and a benign adult form, in which intracellular cystine is only moderately increased (30 to 50 times normal, compared with 100 to 1000 times normal for

nephropathic cystinosis) and FS is absent. Only cornea, bone marrow, peripheral leukocytes, and skin fibroblasts exhibit significant cystine crystals in these adult patients; retinal depigmentation and renal involvement are noticeably absent. Adolescent cystinosis is similar to infantile nephropathic cystinosis, except for the later age of onset of recognizable symptoms and the slower progression to end-stage renal failure. Both the adolescent and adult forms of cystinosis are extremely rare. This discussion will focus on infantile nephropathic cystinosis, the most common and most severe presentation of this disease.

Cystinosis is inherited as an autosomal recessive trait and occurs in one of every 200,000 live births in North America. The carrier frequency approximates one in 225 people. This disease usually occurs in blond, light-complexioned children of European descent, but has been diagnosed in African-Americans, Hispanics, and people from the Middle East. The chromosomal locus of the gene responsible for cystinosis is unknown. The biochemical basis of this disease is defective carrier-mediated transport of cystine out of intracellular lysosomes. Cystine is the disulfide of the amino acid cysteine and is very insoluble in water. Cystine transport out of lysosomes is greatly diminished in patients homozygous for cystinosis and moderately diminished for heterozygote carriers. Accumulation of 100 to 1000 times the normal amount of cystine often leads to crystal formation within affected cells. Birefringent, hexagonal, or rectangular crystals may be identified by slit-lamp examination of the cornea and conjunctiva or by microscopic examination of alcohol-fixed sections of kidney, rectal mucosa, thyroid follicles, liver, spleen, or bone marrow.

How intralysosomal accumulation of cystine results in FS is not yet understood. In vitro studies of rabbit proximal tubules that were intracellularly loaded with cystine by using cystine dimethyl ester have demonstrated that excess cystine decreases energy (ATP) generation. Reduction of ATP necessary to drive transport processes could be the primary event leading to inhibition of transtubular transport in this disorder.

Patients with infantile nephropathic cystinosis appear normal for the first 6 to 18 months of life and then develop symptoms of FS, including dehydration, electrolyte disturbances, failure to thrive, and rickets. An impaired ability to sweat contributes to frequent episodes of fever, flushing, and vomiting during excessive heat exposure. Characteristic corneal crystals are not present at birth, but are usually evident by 6 to 12 months of age. The crystals do not reduce visual acuity, but may be the main cause of photophobia, which begins within the first few years of life and worsens with age. Older patients may experience the continuous feeling of foreign-body irritation and may even develop corneal ulceration and blepharospasm. A generalized patchy depigmentation at the periphery of the retina, characteristic for cystinosis, has been identified as early as age 5 weeks in affected patients. Visual acuity remains unaffected until at least after 10 years of age. The cause of declining vision is uncertain, but extensive cystine accumulation has been identified in the retinal pigment epithelium of a 22-year-old patient and might be the primary cause. Hepatosplenomegaly may be noted before the age of 5 years but is clinically insignificant. Whether liver disease will be part of the later clinical manifestations of cystinosis remains to be seen, since the oldest patients with infantile nephropathic cystinosis are now only in their twenties.

In most patients, hypothyroidism occurs from destruction of the thyroid follicles by cystine crystal accumulation. Screening thyroid function studies reveal elevated serum levels of thyroid-stimulating hormone before symptoms of hypothyroidism occur. The mean age for initiation of thyroid supplementation is 10 years, but therapy has been necessary as early as age 3 years.

Renal manifestations of cystinosis are initially the most serious. In the first years of life, electrolyte abnormalities resulting from FS may be quite severe and difficult to normalize with oral supplementation of alkali, potassium, phosphorus, and 1,25-dihydroxyvitamin D. Progressive renal failure, characterized by a slowly rising serum creatinine, is usually noticeable by age 5 years. Virtually all patients not treated with cysteamine develop end-stage renal disease by age 10 years. Renal biopsy specimens show little change until renal failure appears, at which time light microscopy may reveal interstitial fibrosis and glomerular sclerosis, and electron microscopy may demonstrate characteristic crystals in the interstitium and proximal tubular cells.

As renal failure progresses, the electrolyte abnormalities of FS sometimes become easier to manage because of the reduced filtered load presented to the abnormal tubule. Successful renal transplantation from either a living related donor, including a heterozygote parent, or a cadaver donor is possible and has altered the natural course of cystinosis. Patients are now surviving into the second and third decades of life. FS does not recur in the transplanted kidney. Cystine may accumulate in the interstitium and occasionally in the mesangium of the glomeruli of the transplanted kidney, but not in the tubular cells.

After renal transplantation, cystine continues to accumulate in tissues other than the kidney. Of most concern is the finding that about 30% of patients over age 10 years have decreased visual acuity and 15% have corneal ulceration. Some patients have also developed pancreatic exocrine insufficiency and insulin-dependent diabetes mellitus. Almost all patients continue to have growth failure and delayed sexual maturation. Cystine accumulates in testicular tissue, and so far no male fertility in cystinosis has been demonstrated. Primary ovarian failure has been described, but the delivery of a healthy infant to a 20-year-old female cystinotic has also been reported. Stunted height remains an emotional and social problem for most older adolescents and adults with cystinosis. Neurologic and muscular dysfunction may become important late manifestations of cystinosis in long-term survivors. Several cases of neurologic and muscular problems, including dementia, spasticity, swallowing difficulty, and muscle wasting, have now been reported. Postmortem examinations have shown extensive crystal accumulation in dura, meninges, and perivascular spaces of the brain and in muscle.

The diagnosis of cystinosis can be made clinically by the presence of FS and the demonstration by slit-lamp examination of pathognomonic crystals in the cornea. In vitro measurement of accumulated cystine in peripheral leukocytes or skin fibroblasts is the definitive way to diagnose cystinosis. Procurement of bone marrow or kidney tissues is no longer necessary to make the diagnosis. Prenatal diagnosis is possible by demonstrating increased levels of cystine in cultured amniotic cells obtained by amniocentesis at 16 weeks' gestation. Diagnosis as early as 9 weeks' gestation has been possible with chorionic villus sampling and measurement of elevated cystine levels in this tissue.

The treatment of cystinosis, besides symptomatic treatment of FS and progressive renal failure, is directed at depletion of intracellular cystine in affected tissues. The most effective agent to date has been cysteamine, which can enter lysosomes and react with cystine to form a mixed disulfide of cysteamine and cysteine. This compound is a structural congener of lysine that can be transported out of the lysosome by an unaffected carrier-mediated mechanism. The result is a reduction in the accumulation of intracellular cystine. When oral therapy is started early in life, progression of renal failure may be slowed or halted and linear growth improved, but FS is not reversed. The need for dosing every 6 hours and the unacceptable smell and taste of cysteamine may limit its long-term effectiveness in some patients. Phosphocysteamine, which lacks the foul smell and taste, has been more acceptable to some patients, but since it is rapidly metabolized by the gut to cysteamine, it does not completely avoid cysteamine's unacceptable features. Newer, more palatable, and longer-acting therapeutic compounds are desirable but not apparent at this time. Cysteamine therapy may be of particular benefit in preserving the function of extrarenal organs in long-term survivors after renal transplantation. Oral cysteamine therapy has not been effective in reducing corneal cystine crystal accumulation, but topical cysteamine applied 10 to 12 times daily has been effective in some after months of consistent therapy. Penetrating keratoplasty may be required in severe cases of corneal erosion.

The severe short stature of cystinotic patients may be improved by treatment with recombinant human growth hormone; clinical studies evaluating this therapy are currently in progress.

## Lowe Syndrome (Oculocerebrorenal Syndrome)

Lowe syndrome is an X-linked recessive disorder that characteristically occurs in males who present in early infancy with dense congenital cataracts and often glaucoma, followed later in the first year of life by the appearance of renal tubular dysfunction, mental retardation, muscular hypotonia, and areflexia. Seizures are uncommon. Growth failure becomes evident in some after age 1 year and usually in all by age 3 years. In surviving adults, final heights are less than the third percentile for normal men. Bone age lags behind height age after age 3 years until growth is complete. Noninflammatory arthritis has occurred in some after the first decade of life.

The gene for Lowe syndrome has recently been mapped to the Xq25-q26 locus of the X chromosome. The gene encodes a protein highly homologous to inositol polyphosphate-5-phosphatase, an enzyme involved in the structure of cell membranes. The pathogenesis of Lowe syndrome is unknown, but an inborn error of inositol phosphate metabolism is a likely possibility.

The diagnosis of Lowe syndrome is made clinically, usually by the appearance of renal dysfunction during the first year of life in a male with congenital cataracts. Tubular proteinuria (including albuminuria identifiable by urinary dipstick screening), polyuria, and generalized hyperaminoaciduria appear first, usually within the first few months of life. Excretion of the branched-chain amino acids (valine, isoleucine, and leucine) may be relatively spared compared with other amino acids. Albuminuria may reach nephrotic proportions in later childhood, but has not been associated with decreased serum albumin or other features of the clinical nephrotic syndrome.

Other manifestations of FS are quite variable. Glucosuria is an intermittent, inconstant finding by urine dipstick evaluation and of small magnitude when evaluated quantitatively. Most patients have some degree of hyperphosphaturia, but not all develop hypophosphatemia or require phosphate supplementation. Rickets and osteomalacia may occur in early childhood and require therapy with 1,25-dihydroxyvitamin D and phosphate supplements. Type 2 renal tubular acidosis may occur within the first year of life, at a much later age in the first decade, or not at all. Potassium wasting, when present, has been mild and easy to treat with potassium supplements.

Renal failure is a late manifestation, usually starting after age 3 years and in most not progressing to end stage through the third decade. Since the oldest patient reported is only 41 years old, it is difficult to know what the late renal history of most patients will be. Renal biopsies from young children with Lowe syndrome may be normal or show tubular dilatation, atrophy, and interstitial fibrosis, with the earliest injury identified in the proximal tubules. Electron microscopy may reveal shortening of the brush border and disruption of mitochondria in the tubular cells. When the glomeruli become involved, the earliest findings are nodular thickening and splitting of the glomerular basement membrane and effacement of the foot processes. Renal biopsies from older children may show only nonspecific changes associated with chronic renal failure from any cause.

Other laboratory findings of Lowe syndrome include elevation of the erythrocyte sedimentation rate for unknown reasons; elevation of the serum creatine kinase, aspartate aminotransferase, and lactate dehydrogenase, probably related to direct muscle involvement by Lowe syndrome; and elevation of serum total and HDL cholesterol, with normal serum triglycerides. Urinary carnitine excretion is increased, and plasma free carnitine has been low in some patients.

Therapy for Lowe syndrome is entirely symptomatic and directed at ophthalmologic intervention for cataracts and glaucoma, electrolyte and vitamin D metabolite supplementation as needed for FS, and physical therapy and special education for neurologic problems. Most children have died in late childhood or early adulthood from intercurrent infections or renal failure.

## Idiopathic FS

The diagnosis of idiopathic FS is one of exclusion and no doubt includes cases with a variety of as yet unidentified etiologies. Idiopathic FS can develop at any age. Most cases are sporadic, but genetic transmission also has been identified, most often in an autosomal dominant fashion. In some cases, only hyperaminoaciduria or tubular proteinuria appears in childhood, with the complete FS not becoming manifest until as late as the third or fourth decade of life. Therapy is symptomatic. Patients with both the sporadic and familial forms of idiopathic FS are at risk for developing chronic renal failure within 10 to 30 years of diagnosis. Some progress to end-stage disease and require dialysis or transplantation. Recurrence of FS in the absence of allograft rejection has been reported in at least one case.

## DIAGNOSIS

FS is rarely idiopathic, and an underlying condition should always be sought in children. The possibility of toxin exposure exists at any age, although toxins are a more common cause of FS in adults than in children. Past history of drug therapy should be reviewed, and the possibility of drug ingestion or of heavy metal contamination from the environment must be considered.

The age at which a child becomes symptomatic with FS often aids in correctly diagnosing the underlying disease. When a patient presents with FS in the first few months of life, an inborn error of metabolism should be suspected. Infants with galactosemia or hereditary fructose intolerance can be acutely symptomatic within the first few days of life if exposed to formula or foods containing galactose or fructose, respectively. Later in infancy or childhood, patients with galactosemia, hereditary fructose intolerance, or tyrosinemia usually exhibit failure to thrive, vomiting, jaundice, and hepatomegaly and only intermittent FS, depending on the severity of the disease or, in the case of galactosemia or hereditary fructose intolerance, whether exposure to galactose or fructose is repeated but intermittent. The diagnosis of galactosemia is suggested by the findings of galactosuria and cataracts in an infant chronically fed lactose- or galactose-containing formulas. Punctate cataracts in the fetal lens nucleus may be identifiable at birth. A definitive diagnosis requires the demonstration of deficiency of galactose-1-phosphate uridyl-transferase in red blood cells, fibroblasts, leukocytes, or hepatocytes. Symptoms of hereditary fructose intolerance, which include convulsions and coma, appear only after the introduction of foods containing fructose or sucrose. Diagnosis is established by an intravenous fructose tolerance test and by demonstrating deficiency of aldolase B activity in liver biopsy tissue. Patients with tyrosinemia type 1 have elevated plasma and urinary concentrations of tyrosine and methionine and increased urinary excretion of the hydroxyphenolic acids. Diagnosis is made by demonstrating large amounts of succinylacetone in the urine and a deficiency of fumarylacetoacetate fumaryl hydrolase in lymphocytes, fibroblasts, or liver biopsy tissue.

Infants and toddlers presenting with FS may have any of the above illnesses but are most likely to have cystinosis. Children with nephropathic cystinosis generally do not show their first signs and symptoms before age 6 months or after age 2 to 3 years. The presence of corneal cystine crystals by slit-lamp examination and the measurement of increased levels of cystine in peripheral leukocytes or skin fibroblasts makes the diagnosis. If the patient is male and has congenital cataracts and developmental delay, Lowe syndrome is likely. Rarely, infants with FS have hepatomegaly, abnormal glucose tolerance, ketonuria, ketonemia, and glycogenosis on liver biopsy, similar to type I (von Gierke) glycogen storage disease, but usually without a deficiency of hepatic glucose-6-phosphatase activity. Partial or complete FS may also be associated with cytochrome-c-oxidase deficiency. The major clinical symptoms are hypotonia and progressive weakness. The diagnosis is made by measurement of reduced cytochrome-c-oxidase activity in muscle biopsy tissue.

In early childhood, some cases of FS are discovered incidentally when a urinalysis obtained for another reason reveals dipstick-positive glucose in the presence of a normal blood glucose. Dipstick-positive albuminuria in a patient with congenital cataracts may be the first sign of renal tubular dysfunction that will lead to the correct diagnosis of Lowe syndrome.

Older children presenting with FS usually have an acquired form of FS, although Wilson disease, a rare inborn error of copper metabolism, may not be diagnosed until the end of the first decade of life. These patients usually present with hepatic, neurologic, or psychiatric abnormalities rather than FS, which may be found incidentally during the evaluation. Hepatic cirrhosis, Kayser-Fleischer rings (greenish-brown deposits of copper in the Descemet membrane of the cornea), and neurologic symptoms ranging from behavioral and psychiatric disorders to flapping tremors and dystonia are characteristic of Wilson disease. Serum ceruloplasmin concentration is decreased to below 20 mg/dL. Failure to incorporate radioactive copper into serum ceruloplasmin after an oral tracer dose makes the definitive diagnosis.

Acquired FS should be suspected in the presence of conditions such as nephrotic syndrome, renal transplantation, renal vein thrombosis, glue (toluene) sniffing, lead or other heavy metal intoxication, or exposure to drugs such as gentamicin or valproic acid (see Table 116-7). The dysproteinemias and amyloidosis occur almost exclusively in adults. Idiopathic FS is the diagnosis used when all other causes have been excluded.

## TREATMENT

Identification of the underlying cause for FS is crucial to direct therapy. In some cases, specific therapy or withdrawal of an offending substance may normalize the tubular dysfunction. When no specific therapy exits, symptomatic treatment of the electrolyte disturbances and bone disease of FS is the only alternative.

Proximal renal tubular acidosis may be severe, requiring large amounts of alkali therapy divided into four to six daily doses. Potassium supplementation is almost always necessary when alkali therapy is given. Administration of the potassium salt of citrate, bicarbonate, or acetate fulfills the dual purpose of treating acidosis and preventing hypokalemia. Mixtures of sodium and potassium citrate or potassium citrate alone are available commercially for oral use. Sodium wasting and dehydration are treated with combinations of sodium bicarbonate, citrate, and chloride, depending on the degree of acidosis. Prevention of dehydration from obligatory polyuria is best handled by allowing the patient free access to fluids. If the patient is vomiting and cannot readily ingest adequate fluid, dehydration may occur rapidly and will require early intervention with intravenous replacement therapy.

Hypophosphatemia and impaired renal vitamin D metabolism are the factors leading to rickets and other bone complications. Phosphate supplementation is usually given as neutral phosphate solution, 1 to 3 g divided into four to six daily doses. Diarrhea is a side effect of excessive oral phosphate therapy. The simultaneous administration of phosphate and alkali supplements may lead to tetany from acute hypocalcemia, so phosphate supplements should be added with caution in patients receiving alkali therapy. In some patients, supplementation with 1,25-dihydroxyvitamin D or dihydrotachysterol, neither of which requires further renal metabolism for biological activity, is necessary to heal and sustain healing of rickets and osteomalacia. Hypercalciuria and transient hypercalcemia are toxic side effects of excessive vitamin D metabolite therapy.

Chronic dialysis and renal transplantation are viable alternatives for the management of end-stage renal disease in most patients. However, prolonged survival by renal replacement therapy in patients with rare inborn errors of metabolism is now revealing important nonrenal late manifestations of these diseases.

## Selected Readings

Attree O, Olivos IM, Okabe I, et al. The Lowe's oculocerebrorenal syndrome gene encodes a protein highly homologous to inositol polyphosphate-5-phosphatase. Nature 1992;358:239.

Brewer ED. Fanconi syndrome: clinical disorders. In: Goncik HC, Buckalew VM, ed. Renal tubular disorders. New York: Marcel Dekker, 1985:475.

Charnas LR, Bernardini I, Rader D, Hoeg JM, Gahl WA. Clinical and laboratory findings in the oculocerebrorenal syndrome of Lowe, with special reference to growth and renal function. N Engl J Med 1991;324:1318.

Gahl WA, Schneider JA, Schulman JD, Thoene JG, Reed GF. Predicted reciprocal serum creatinine at age 10 years as a measure of renal function in children with nephropathic cystinosis treated with oral cysteamine. Pediatr Nephrol 1990;4:129.

Gahl WA, Thoene JG, Schneider JA, O'Regan S, Kaiser-Kupfer MI, Kuwabara T. Cystinosis: Progress in a prototypic disease. Ann Intern Med 1988;109:557.

Smith ML, Pellett OL, Cass MM, et al. Prenatal diagnosis of cystinosis utilizing chorionic villus sampling. Prenat Diag 1987;7:23.

Wilson DP, Jelley D, Stratton R, Coldwell JG. Nephropathic cystinosis: improved linear growth after treatment with recombinant human growth hormone. J Pediatr 1989;115:758.

*Principles and Practice of Pediatrics, Second Edition.*
edited by Frank A. Oski et al. J. B. Lippincott Company, Philadelphia © 1994.

## 116.3 *Disorders of Renal Glucose Transport*

### L. Leighton Hill

Primary renal glucosuria is a selective defect of proximal tubular glucose transport in which glucose is excreted in the urine at normal concentrations of blood glucose. The handling of all other filtered substances by the proximal tubules is normal. The pattern of inheritance in some pedigrees has been interpreted to be autosomal dominant; however, the pattern in most families seems most consistent with that of an autosomal recessive defect. There are thought to be at least two types of renal glucosuria, although the distinction is not always clear and some investigators question the validity of separation into types. In one type, the maximum

tubular reabsorptive capacity for glucose is low; that is, there is a reduced ability of almost all tubules to transport glucose. In another type, the maximum tubular reabsorptive capacity for glucose is normal, but there is apparently a wide spectrum in the ability of individual nephrons to reabsorb glucose so that some glucose is spilled despite the normal overall capacity of the proximal tubules to reabsorb glucose.

Primary renal glucosuria is clinically benign and asymptomatic and needs no therapy. However, it must be differentiated from diabetes mellitus. This is done by measuring glucose in near-simultaneously obtained blood and urine via several random simultaneous tests or through a 3-hour glucose tolerance test. If the patient has renal glucosuria, the blood sugars should be within normal range, although the glucose tolerance curve may be somewhat flat if the urinary glucose loss is considerable. The patient usually spills in each urine specimen obtained despite the normal blood glucose levels.

It is very important to ensure that the renal glucosuria is not an expression of pan-proximal tubular dysfunction (Fanconi syndrome). Pan-proximal tubular dysfunction syndromes may be hereditary or acquired. Renal glucosuria may also be seen with other tubular defects that are not part of the Fanconi syndrome. In addition, transient renal glucosuria has been described in such conditions as acute pyelonephritis and exposure to renal toxins and is also seen in the late stages of chronic renal insufficiency.

*Principles and Practice of Pediatrics, Second Edition.*
edited by Frank A. Oski et al. J. B. Lippincott Company, Philadelphia © 1994.

## 116.4 *Disorders of Renal Phosphate Transport*

### Myra L. Chiang

Since the original report of vitamin D-resistant rickets by Fuller Albright and his group in 1937, several forms of hereditary rickets with differing modes of inheritance have been recognized (Table 116-8).

| TABLE 116-8.   Hereditary Forms of So-called Vitamin-D Resistant Rickets |
|---|
| **Phosphopenic Mechanisms (Primary Hypophosphatemia)** |
| X-linked hypophosphatemia |
| Hypophosphatemic bone disease |
| Hereditary hypophosphatemia with hypercalciuria |
| **Calcipenic Mechanisms (Secondary Hypophosphatemia)** |
| Vitamin D dependency type I (defective synthesis of hormone) |
| Vitamin D dependency type II (defective hormone receptor function) |

*Modified from Scriver CR, Tenenhouse HS, Glorieux FH. X-linked hypophosphatemia: an appreciation of a classic paper and a survey of progress since 1958. Medicine 1991;70:218*

# X-LINKED HYPOPHOSPHATEMIA

X-linked hypophosphatemia (XLH) is the most common type of hereditary rickets, with an incidence of one in 20,000 births. Molecular genetic research in the Hyp mouse, the murine homologue of the human disease, has led to the localization of the gene defect at the Xp22 region of the X chromosome. The primary defect is an inability to reabsorb filtered phosphate and resides in the proximal renal tubular brush border membrane, resulting in phosphate wasting and severe hypophosphatemia. In addition, there is impaired regulation of the renal 1-alpha-hydroxylase activity, resulting in an inappropriately low 1,25-dihydroxyvitamin $D_3$ level relative to the degree of hypophosphatemia. This suggests that the X-linked mutation may also perturb the regulation of vitamin D metabolism. The possibility of a humoral circulating factor affecting the proximal tubular cells was recently demonstrated in the Hyp mouse.

## Clinical and Radiologic Findings

Males are more severely affected than females. The most striking clinical manifestation is short stature, with the characteristic lateral bowing of the lower extremities usually apparent when the child begins to walk. Genu varum is more common than genu valgum, and there is a waddling gait. Craniosynostosis of the sutures is common, which leads to a frontal bossing. Extraskeletal ossification and deafness may be present. Dentin formation is defective and spontaneous tooth abscesses are not uncommon. Craniotabes, rachitic rosary, and deformity of the upper extremities and pelvis occur less frequently than in vitamin D deficiency and vitamin D dependency rickets. In addition, patients with XLH do not have myopathy or seizures, which may occur in the other two forms of rickets. Growth retardation is marked in untreated males, who seldom reach a height of 5 feet. Degenerative painful joint disease often develops in adult life.

Radiologic features include the loss of the provisional zone of calcification, abnormal widening of the epiphyseal plate, and cupping and fraying of the metaphyses. Coarse trabeculation is also seen, most notably at the distal ends of long bones. All the radiologic findings are more pronounced in the lower extremities.

## Laboratory Findings

The age at which hypophosphatemia first appears is variable. Some patients have consistently low serum phosphorus values from birth, while others develop them at about 6 to 8 months of age. This delay has been attributed to the normally low glomerular filtration rate (GFR) in newborns. The age-related variations in normal serum phosphorus level must be considered in interpreting abnormal values. Serum phosphorus concentrations between 1 and 2.5 mg/dL are characteristic in older children with the disease, but levels may be as high as 4 mg/dL in infants with this condition. In contrast to the other forms of rickets (Table 116-9), serum calcium is normal or low-normal. Parathyroid hormone (PTH) concentration is usually normal, and aminoaciduria is absent. Serum concentration of 25-hydroxyvitamin $D_3$ is usually normal and that of 1,25-dihydroxyvitamin $D_3$ (calcitriol) is slightly low or normal, despite the prevailing hypophosphatemia that is normally a stimulator of renal 1-alpha-hydroxylase.

The main biochemical feature of XLH is the low tubular reabsorption of filtered phosphate in the presence of a low serum phosphate and the absence of secondary hyperparathyroidism. The percent tubular reabsorption of phosphate (%TRP) can be calculated from the creatinine and phosphate concentrations on a near-simultaneously obtained random urine and serum sample:

$$\%TRP = 1 - \frac{U\,po_4}{S\,po_4} \times \frac{Scr}{Ucr} \times 100$$

Normal %TRP in children ranges from 80% to 95%. The mean %TRP in patients with XLH is reduced to the 40% to 70% range. Since changes in GFR affect the TRP, a more appropriate measure of the maximum tubular phosphate transport (TmP) is TmP/GFR. The TmP can be obtained from Bijvoet's normogram by plotting the known values of TRP and creatinine clearance.

## Treatment

The goals of treatment are to prevent or correct rickets or osteomalacia and to achieve normal adult height. The most effective treatment consists of a combination of 1 to 4 g of oral elemental phosphate, preferably the potassium salt (Neutra-Phos-K), in five or six divided doses per day and 1,25-dihydroxyvitamin $D_3$ (Rocaltrol) at an initial dose of 0.025 to 0.05 µg/kg/day, with the dose increased gradually to attain a maximal suppression of PTH without inducing hypercalcemia or hypercalciuria. High-dose oral phosphate therapy can cause diarrhea, so that it is wise to start with a lower dose and advance slowly. The concomitant use of 1,25-dihydroxyvitamin $D_3$ enhances the intestinal absorption of calcium and phosphate. This enhanced calcium absorption prevents secondary hyperparathyroidism, which may occur with phosphate therapy alone. However, treatment with vitamin D is not without risks: it can lead to hypercalcemia, hypercalciuria, nephrocalcinosis, and renal damage. Nephrocalcinosis has been reported in up to 47% of a large series of children with XLH treated with 1,25-dihydroxyvitamin $D_3$. The use of new vitamin D analogues with low calcemic activity such as 22-oxacalcitriol, which is still in an experimental stage, may ameliorate this problem in the future. To monitor for vitamin D toxicity, serum calcium, serum creatinine, the spot urinary calcium/creatinine ratio

### TABLE 116-9.  Biochemical Findings in Rickets

| Type | Calcium | Phosphate | Alkaline Phosphatase | iPTH | 25-(OH)D$_3$ | 1,25-(OH)$_2$D$_3$ | Urine Calcium |
|---|---|---|---|---|---|---|---|
| Vitamin D-deficient | ↓ or N | ↓ or N | ↑ | ↑ | ↓ | ↓ or N | ↓ or N |
| Vitamin D-dependent type 1 | ↓ | ↓ or N | ↑↑ | ↑ | N | ↓↓ | ↓ |
| Vitamin D-dependent type 2 | ↓ | ↓ or N | ↑↑ | ↑ | N | ↑↑ | ↓ |
| X-linked hypophosphatemia | N | ↓↓ | ↑ | N | N | N or ↓ | ↓ |
| Hypophosphatemic bone disease | N | ↓↓ | ↑ | N | N | N | N |
| Hereditary hypophosphatemic rickets with hypercalciuria | N | ↓↓ | ↑ | N or ↓ | N | ↑ | ↑ |

↑, increased; ↓, decreased; N, normal

(normal, <0.21) should be checked regularly. Renal ultrasound should be obtained yearly for early detection of nephrocalcinosis.

Although long-term therapy with phosphate and 1,25-dihydroxyvitamin $D_3$ has led to increased serum phosphate concentration, decreased serum alkaline phosphatase activity, healing of rickets, and increased growth velocity, the renal tubular phosphate leak is unchanged, and most patients fail to achieve expected adult height. Exogenous growth hormone has recently been shown to be effective in promoting tubular reabsorption of phosphate alone or in conjunction with 1,25-dihydroxyvitamin $D_3$ and phosphate therapies, leading to normalization of serum phosphate, bone healing, and acceleration of linear growth without the significant morbidity associated with exogenous high-dose calcitriol and phosphate. At present, the data are too limited to recommend growth hormone therapy for routine treatment of XLH. The remarkable advances in molecular biology may soon reveal the gene defect in X-linked hypophosphatemia and lead the way to gene therapy, which will be the definitive treatment.

## HYPOPHOSPHATEMIC BONE DISEASE

Hypophosphatemic bone disease (HBD) is an inherited disorder of phosphate homeostasis that resembles XLH. Both are characterized by low TmP/GFR, low serum phosphorus, normal serum calcium, and normal PTH level. However, there are important differences between the two conditions. HBD is inherited in autosomal dominant fashion if not sporadic. While osteomalacia of the long bones is present in both conditions, active rickets is not present in HBD. Fractional renal excretion of filtered phosphate is normal in the fasting phosphatemic state in HBD, and patients with HBD have a normal serum level of 1,25-dihydroxyvitamin $D_3$. Children with HBD are successfully treated with 1,25-dihydroxyvitamin $D_3$ alone, leading to an increase in serum phosphate to normal, improved tubular reabsorption of phosphate, and a fall in plasma alkaline phosphatase activity with bone healing.

## HEREDITARY HYPOPHOSPHATEMIC RICKETS WITH HYPERCALCIURIA

Hereditary hypophosphatemic rickets with hypercalciuria (HHRH) was first described by Tieder and colleagues in 1985. Although it has similarities with XLH and HBD, it differs from the other two hereditary conditions in ways that have important therapeutic implications. The mode of inheritance is autosomal recessive or autosomal dominant. The clinical and radiologic findings are similar to those of XLH. The outstanding difference between HHRH and the other two entities is the presence in HHRH of elevated 1,25-dihydroxyvitamin $D_3$, leading to hypercalciuria. The pivotal defect in HHRH is severe renal phosphate leak resulting in hypophosphatemia, which in turn stimulates renal 1-alpha-hydroxylase, leading to increased synthesis of 1,25-dihydroxyvitamin $D_3$. Consequently, intestinal calcium and phosphorus absorption are augmented, with a resulting increase in the renal filtered calcium load and hypercalciuria. A second effect of enhanced intestinal calcium absorption is suppression of PTH secretion; this in turn brings about a further increase in calciuria.

Urinary calcium excretion should be determined in any patient presenting with hereditary rickets before treatment is initiated. Patients with HHRH respond to phosphorus therapy alone with no risk of secondary hyperparathyroidism developing. Vitamin D is contraindicated because it may further increase intestinal absorption of calcium, increasing the risk of nephrocalcinosis and renal damage.

## VITAMIN D-DEPENDENT RICKETS

Vitamin D-dependent rickets is an inborn error of vitamin D metabolism transmitted as autosomal recessive and is divided into types 1 and 2.

### Type 1

Vitamin D-dependent rickets type 1 is secondary to a defect in the renal 1-alpha-hydroxylase responsible for the synthesis of 1,25-dihydroxyvitamin $D_3$ from 25-hydroxyvitamin $D_3$. The precise intracellular location of the defect is unclear. The onset of symptoms is usually within the first year of life, with hypocalcemic tetany, convulsions, muscle weakness, and growth failure. A history of adequate vitamin D intake is usually obtained. Physical examination reveals a small, hypotonic child with findings similar to those in children with vitamin D-deficient rickets, including thickening of the wrists and ankles, frontal bossing with wide anterior fontanelle, costochondral beading, and bowing of extremities. Severe tooth enamel hypoplasia is common. Trousseau and Chvostek signs are frequently positive. These children demonstrate the classic radiologic features of rickets, which are indistinguishable from vitamin D-deficient rickets. Hypocalcemia (often <8 mg/dL) is a cardinal feature. Serum phosphate is usually low but may be near normal. Alkaline phosphatase and PTH levels are elevated and aminoaciduria is present. The diagnosis is made by demonstrating a normal serum 25-hydroxyvitamin $D_3$ level and a low or undetectable serum 1,25-dihydroxyvitamin $D_3$ level. Treatment with 0.5 to 4 $\mu$g/day of 1,25-dihydroxyvitamin $D_3$ is effective in most cases, followed by a maintenance dose usually in the range of 0.25 to 2 $\mu$g/day.

### Type 2

Vitamin D-dependent rickets type 2 appears to result from an end-organ resistance to the effect of 1,25-dihydroxyvitamin $D_3$. The defect appears to be in the binding of the metabolite. The clinical and radiologic findings are almost identical to those in type 1 disease, except that alopecia is present in about half the patients with vitamin D-dependent rickets type 2. The alopecia is seen in patients with the most severe resistance to 1,25-dihydroxyvitamin $D_3$ and probably reflects dysfunction in 1,25-dihydroxyvitamin $D_3$ target cells in the hair follicles. Biochemically, type 2 differs from type 1 in that the level of 1,25-dihydroxyvitamin $D_3$ is very high.

Treatment of this form of rickets is difficult, and response to therapy appears to be related to the presence or absence of alopecia. Most patients require a much higher dose of vitamin D (5 to 60 $\mu$g/day of 1,25-dihydroxyvitamin $D_3$). Long-term administration of parenteral calcium may be required to maintain normal serum calcium in some patients.

## PSEUDOHYPOPARATHYROIDISM

Pseudohypoparathyroidism is a heterogenous group of disorders characterized by target cell (renal tubular and osseous) unresponsiveness to PTH. The unresponsiveness results in increased tubular reabsorption of phosphate, leading to increased %TRP and hyperphosphatemia and a defect in the PTH-driven mobilization of bone calcium that results in hypocalcemia. The renal resistance of PTH can be due to several mechanisms and forms the basis for differentiating the disease into several types.

### Type 1

Pseudohypoparathyroidism type 1 is caused by the failure of PTH to activate adenylcyclase in the renal cell membrane, which results in deficient production of cyclic adenosine monophosphate (cAMP). Pseudohypoparathyroidism type 1 is further subclassified into types 1a and 1b.

Type 1a is the most common form. The molecular defect is in the alpha subunit of a guanine nucleotide binding protein ($\alpha$Gs) that couples hormone receptors to stimulation of adenylate cyclase. This defect appears to be inherited in an autosomal dominant fashion. Because the same $\alpha$Gs is involved in generating cAMP response to other hormones, hypothyroidism, gonadal dysfunction, and other endocrinopathies have been associated with pseudohypoparathyroidism type 1a. These patients usually show a combination of distinctive skeletal and developmental features collectively called Albright hereditary osteodystrophy (AHO), including short stature; thick-set, stocky, or obese body habitus with round facies and short neck; and brachydactyly (short metacarpals, metatarsals, or phalanges, particularly involving the fourth and fifth). They may manifest increased bone density by x-ray, particularly in the skull. Cutaneous, subcutaneous, and perivascular calcifications in the basal ganglia region, subcapsular cataracts, and dental anomalies are common. Mental retardation may be present. Most patients present with symptoms of increased muscular excitability secondary to hypocalcemia; these include tetany, seizures, muscle cramps, and episodes of laryngeal spasm.

In type 1b, the $\alpha$Gs activity is normal, the resistance is limited to PTH, and the physical appearance is normal. The molecular defect is likely to involve the signal transduction component of the PTH receptor. The disease may be sporadic or familial. The mode of inheritance has not been defined.

Treatment is directed at normalizing the serum calcium concentration. Excellent response has been reported to therapy with 1,25-dihydroxyvitamin $D_3$ or dihydrotachysterol. Calcium carbonate or calcium acetate may be necessary to bind phosphate in the intestinal lumen and decrease its absorption, thereby lowering its serum concentration.

## Type 2

Pseudohypoparathyroidism type 2 results from the inability of cAMP to initiate the PTH-directed metabolic events. These patients show a rise in cAMP excretion, but there is no phosphaturic response. The disease is rarely familial. Patients with this subtype do not have the skeletal anomalies of AHO. Treatment is the same as for type 1.

## Other

Pseudopseudohypoparathyroidism is the term used to describe patients with the anatomical stigmata of AHO but normal serum levels of calcium and phosphate. It is seen in relatives of patients with pseudohypoparathyroidism type 1a and may represent a variant in the expression of the disease.

Another variant of pseudohypoparathyroidism is pseudohypohyperparathyroidism. In these patients, the resistance to PTH appears to be limited to the renal tubular cells. The bone cells respond normally to the elevated levels of PTH; as a result, these patients exhibit subperiosteal resorption and osteitis fibrosa cystica.

## Selected Readings

Brown AJ, Finch JL, Hilker SL, et al. New active analogues of vitamin D with low calcemic activity. Kidney Internat 1990;38(S29):S22.

Hanna JD, Kazuhiko N, Chan JC. X-linked hypophosphatemia, genetic and clinical correlates. Am J Dis Child 1991;145:865.

Marx SJ. Vitamin D and other calciferols. In: Scriver CR, Beaudet AL, Sly WS, et al., eds. The metabolic basis of inherited disease. New York: McGraw-Hill, 1989:2029.

Rasmussen H, Tenenhouse HS. Hypophosphatemias. In: Scriver CR, Beaudet AL, Sly WS, et al., eds. The metabolic basis of inherited disease. New York: McGraw-Hill, 1989:2581.

Scriver CR, Reade T, Halal F, Costa R, Cole DE. Autosomal hypophosphatemic bone disease responds to 1,25-$(OH)_2$ $D_3$. Arch Dis Child 1981;56:203.

Scriver CR, Tenenhouse HS, Glorieux FH. X-linked hypophosphatemia: an appreciation of a classic paper and a survey of progress since 1958. Medicine 1991;70:218.

Spiegel AL. Pseudohypoparathyroidism. In: Scriver CR, Beaudet AL, Sly WS, et al., eds. The metabolic basis of inherited disease. New York: McGraw-Hill, 1989:2013.

Tieder M, Modai D, Samuel R, et al. Hereditary hypophosphatemic rickets with hypercalciuria. New Engl J Med 1985;312:611.

Walton RJ, Bijvoet OL. Normogram for derivation of renal threshold phosphate concentration. Lancet 1975;2:309.

Wilson DM, Lee PD, Morris AH, et al. Growth hormone therapy in hypophosphatemic rickets. Am J Dis Child 1991;145:1165.

*Principles and Practice of Pediatrics, Second Edition.*
edited by Frank A. Oski et al. J. B. Lippincott Company, Philadelphia © 1994.

# 116.5 *Nephrogenic Diabetes Insipidus*

## L. Leighton Hill

Nephrogenic diabetes insipidus (NDI) is a hereditary or acquired disorder characterized by renal tubular resistance to antidiuretic hormone (ADH). The inability to concentrate the urine because of this tubular disease leads to marked polyuria with compensatory polydipsia. The pattern of inheritance in the great majority of cases is consistent with a sex-linked dominant transmission with complete expression only in the afflicted male and variable penetrance in the female. The gene responsible for this entity has been localized to a small region of the human X chromosome (Xq28). However, other patterns of transmission have been suggested, and transmission from father to son has been described in some families. In the X-linked cases, females usually show a limited tubular response to vasopressin. Even in males there may be variation in the degree of severity of the defect; most are diagnosed in early infancy because of a severe defect, but some have a mild enough disease to escape detection until the second or third decade of life.

The defect in hereditary NDI, at least in males with the severe defect, usually is more severe than that seen in the acquired types. There are two general causes of the acquired types. The first is the loss of the concentration gradient in the medullary interstitial tissues as a result of the tissue destruction occurring with obstructive uropathy, vesicoureteral reflux, sickle-cell nephropathy, cystic disease, pyelonephritis, interstitial nephritis, and nephrocalcinosis. The second cause is the decreased responsiveness to ADH by the distal tubules and collecting ducts, although the concentration gradient in the medullary interstitial tissues remains intact. Conditions that cause this alteration include hypokalemic states, hypercalcemia, amyloidosis, sarcoidosis, and various drugs that interfere with the action of ADH, such as lithium, demeclocycline, cisplatinum, vinblastine, methoxyflurane, amphotericin B, colchicine, and propoxyphene. This second group of conditions more closely resembles hereditary NDI than does the first group. NDI can also be seen as part of the Fanconi syndrome, most likely because of the chronic hypokalemia that often occurs.

## PATHOPHYSIOLOGY

In normals, the antidiuretic action of arginine vasopressin (ADH) is mediated by the sequential steps of ADH binding to its cell surface receptor, followed by receptor-mediated stimulation of adenylate cyclase. Accumulation of cyclic AMP in distal tubular and collecting duct cells results, and there is an increase in plasma cyclic AMP but no consistent change in urinary cyclic AMP excretion. In the distal nephron, cyclic AMP is believed to increase the rate of water transport, possibly by increasing the number of water-specific channels in luminal membranes. Normal levels of arginine vasopressin are found in patients with NDI as measured by radioimmunoassay.

ADH is thought to act on at least two distinct types of receptors. The $V_1$ (platelet/vascular/hepatic) receptor is cyclase-independent and is linked to the hydrolysis of phosphatidyl inositol. The $V_2$ or renal receptor is linked to adenylate cyclase, is phosphatidyl inositol independent, and mediates distal tubular and collecting duct water reabsorption. There are also extrarenal vasopressin $V_2$-like receptors that mediate vasodilatation and an increase in plasma renin activity and stimulate the release of Factor VIIIc and von Willebrand factor.

In NDI, $V_1$ receptor responses appear to remain intact, but renal $V_2$ receptor responses are abnormal because an antidiuretic response to the administration of either arginine vasopressin or to the antidiuretic $V_2$-specific agonist 1-desamino-8-D-arginine vasopressin (DDAVP) is not obtained and there is no increase in plasma cyclic AMP concentration. In NDI, $V_2$ receptor abnormality may be generalized (renal and extrarenal) or may be limited to the kidney, suggesting heterogeneity in the congenital form of this disease.

## CLINICAL FEATURES

The most common clinical manifestations of NDI are shown in Table 116-10. Polyuria is constant even during periods of dehydration. Elevated body temperature, a consequence of the dehydration, often leads to multiple investigations attempting to identify possible bacterial, viral, or parasitic infections. The large fluid ingestion may interfere with attaining adequate calorie intake; this, along with the deleterious effects of the chronic hypernatremia, leads to failure to thrive. The constant need for intake of liquids interferes with normal sleep patterns. Chronic severe constipation is another result of the constant tendency to negative water balance that characterizes NDI. When a child with NDI is well hydrated, a dramatic reversal in the condition is seen: the signs and symptoms of dehydration disappear, the fever abates, and the vomiting, irritability, and other manifestations disappear until dehydration recurs.

| TABLE 116-10.   Clinical Manifestations |
| --- |
| Polyuria and polydipsia |
| Growth and developmental failure |
| Recurrent bouts of dehydration |
| Unexplained fever |
| Thirst |
| Vomiting |
| Constipation |
| Onset during infancy |
| Positive family history |
| Irritability |

## LABORATORY FINDINGS

Hypernatremia and hyperchloremia are commonly seen when the patient has been in negative water balance. The urinalysis is usually normal, except for being inappropriately dilute (ie, specific gravity <1.006 and urine osmolality <200 mOsm/kg) despite evidence of dehydration. Small amounts of protein and a few red blood cells may be found in the urine, and the blood urea nitrogen (BUN) may be elevated during dehydration. With rehydration, the sodium, chloride, BUN, and creatinine levels return to normal and, although the urine remains dilute, the protein and red blood cells disappear. When the patient is in water balance, the glomerular filtration rate and all other renal function tests, aside from the inability to conserve water, are normal.

In the infant with NDI, the serum sodium is often elevated early in the morning because of insufficient fluid intake during the night, but may return to normal during the day concomitant with adequate fluid intake. Ultrasound examination may reveal marked dilatation of the urinary tract in NDI because of extremely high water turnover. This is usually minimal at the time of diagnosis in very young infants, but it may be found to be massive later if control of water balance is not good. Marked dilatation of the urinary tract may also be seen in patients not identified as having NDI until later in childhood.

## DIAGNOSIS

The diagnosis of NDI is suspected because of polyuria, polydipsia, bouts of dehydration, hypernatremia, dilute urines, and a positive family history. The differential diagnosis includes other causes of polyuria such as central diabetes insipidus, diabetes mellitus, psychogenic water drinking, and chronic renal insufficiency. Patients with diabetes mellitus have elevated blood and urine sugars and seldom have hypernatremia. Patients with primary polydipsia have normal to low-normal serum sodium concentrations. Patients with chronic renal insufficiency have azotemia even when hydrated, usually demonstrate isosthenuria rather than hyposthenuria, and generally have a much milder degree of polyuria than patients with diabetes insipidus.

The chief differential is often between central (ADH-deficient) diabetes insipidus and nephrogenic (vasopressin-resistant) diabetes insipidus. An attempt to assess and document the magnitude of the polyuria and polydipsia by measuring intakes and outputs is essential. The most important test is a well-controlled water deprivation or concentration test in the hospital during the day and under close medical supervision (Table 116-11). The patient should not be allowed to lose more than 5% of body weight before terminating the study. Careful weights are essential, as are periodic observations of vital signs and urine and serum osmolalities and sodiums. A urine/plasma osmolality ratio of 2.0 or more is sufficient to rule out both nephrogenic diabetes insipidus and central (ADH-deficient) diabetes insipidus. If the polyuria continues and the urine is not concentrated despite a 4% to 5% body weight loss or the completion of the whole time course of the water deprivation test, then these two diagnoses remain strong possibilities.

The next step in the diagnostic process is to test the renal tubular response to antidiuretic substances. The testing substance of choice is desmopressin acetate (DDAVP), a synthetic analogue of 8-arginine vasopressin. The DDAVP should be given intranasally at a dosage of 10 $\mu$g in infants and 20 $\mu$g in older children. Urines should be measured for volume and for concentration (specific gravity and osmolality) at 1- to 2-hour intervals after administration. If there is no response in terms of decrease in volume of urine and increase in the osmolality of the urine, then a second dose should be given and additional urine samples col-

### TABLE 116-11. Water Deprivation Test

1. Conduct the test in the hospital, during the day with close observation.
2. Give breakfast or formula feeding early (eg, 5:45 a.m.) with usual liquids.
3. At starting time (eg, 6 a.m.) have the patient void and discard. With an infant, record time of spontaneous voiding and use this as starting time.
4. Weigh the patient carefully at starting time and record.
5. NPO from start time.
6. Obtain serum sodium and osmolality in vicinity of starting time.
7. Measure each urine voided for volume, specific gravity, and osmolality. Record time of each voiding.
8. Weigh, take temperature, and measure pulse rate every 2 hours × 3 then every hour × 6.
9. Repeat serum sodium and osmolality after 4 hours and then every 2 hours × 4 and also at conclusion of test.
10. Terminate the test when one or more of the following conditions is met:
    a. The specific gravity is 1.020 or more and urine osmolality is 600 mOsm/kg or more.
    b. The patient has lost 4%–5% of body weight or has definite clinical signs of dehydration.
    c. The period of water deprivation reaches 6 hours for a young infant (<6 months), 8 hours for the child between 6 months and 2 years, and 12 hours for the child over age 2.
11. It is crucial to make the following observations at the time the test is stopped: body weight, vital signs including temperature, serum sodium, serum osmolality, and urine specific gravity, osmolality, and volume.

lected for volume and concentration. Serum sodium and osmolality should be obtained before and 4 hours after the administration of the DDAVP. The infant is allowed to take in fluid during this test. An alternative test would be to give aqueous vasopressin USP (Pitressin) at a dosage of 2 units/m² body surface area intravenously over a 1-hour period in 20 mL of isotonic saline. Urines should be obtained during the aqueous vasopressin USP (Pitressin) infusion, at the conclusion of the infusion, and 1 hour and 2 hours after the infusion for measurement of volume, specific gravity, and osmolality.

With either of these stimulation tests (DDAVP or aqueous vasopressin USP [Pitressin]), a urine/plasma ratio for osmolality of 1.5 or greater would indicate an adequate tubular response to antidiuretic substances. If the patient fails to concentrate the urine with the water deprivation test and also after DDAVP or aqueous vasopressin USP (Pitressin) stimulation, then a diagnosis of NDI is indicated. If the patient fails to concentrate with the water deprivation test but does respond to DDAVP or aqueous vasopressin USP (Pitressin) stimulation by decreasing urine volume

to less than 20 mL/m²/hr and by raising the urine/plasma ratio for osmolality to at least 1.5, then a diagnosis of central (ADH-deficient) diabetes insipidus is indicated.

Once a diagnosis of NDI is made, it must be determined whether the defect is hereditary or acquired. Onset at an early age and a family history of polyuria and bouts of dehydration in infancy would strongly suggest that the defect is hereditary. The workup would include a thorough drug exposure history, ultrasound studies of the kidneys and urinary tract, serum electrolytes, BUN, creatinine, serum calcium, and possibly a cystogram. These studies should be sufficient to rule in or out the causes of secondary or acquired NDI mentioned above.

## THERAPY OF HEREDITARY NDI

The daily water turnover of infants and children with NDI can be enormous, equalling half or more of the patient's total body water each day. The intake of volumes of this magnitude may be very difficult to achieve purely from a mechanical point of view. Fluid intake as high as 300 to 400 mL/kg/day may be required just to maintain water balance. This high free water intake should be spaced fairly evenly over the 24-hour period, even at night to prevent early-morning dehydration and hypernatremia. A diet that will result in a low renal solute load is of major importance in reducing the obligatory renal water requirement. Such a diet is reasonably low in protein and sodium chloride. In the infant, breast milk is preferable, but if it is unavailable, a low-protein, low-electrolyte commercial formula will suffice. Roughly 6% of the total calories should come from protein, and the daily sodium intake should not exceed 1 mEq/kg of body weight. In older children, the daily protein intake should be about 2 g/kg, and the total daily sodium content should be in the range of 1 to 2 g.

The importance of a low renal solute load in determining the volume of obligatory urine water is shown in Table 116-12. Two disease states, chronic renal insufficiency and NDI, are compared with the normal patient. The same diet is assumed for each of these three children (that is, a diet yielding about 600 mOsm of solute for renal excretion per day). The normal child should be able to concentrate to 1200 mOsm/L of urine water, the patient with chronic renal failure can usually concentrate to about 300 mOsm/L, and the patient with NDI can concentrate in the vicinity of 100 mOsm/L. The obligatory urine volume is determined by dividing the total solute load for excretion by the maximum ability to concentrate. As can be seen in this theoretical example, the person with no disease would have an obligatory renal water requirement of 0.5 L; the patient with chronic renal insufficiency would have a mild polyuria, with an obligatory water excretion of 2 L/day; and the patient with NDI would have severe polyuria,

### TABLE 116-12. Water Turnover Related to Inability to Concentrate Urine

| Disease | Solute Load (SL)* | Maximum Ability to Concentrate (c) | V = SL/C† | Obligatory Renal Water in Liters (V) | Degree of Polyuria |
|---|---|---|---|---|---|
| None | 600 | 1200 mOsm/kg | V = 600/1200 | 0.5 | None |
| Chronic renal failure | 600 | 300 mOsm/kg | V = 600/300 | 2.0 | Mild |
| NDI | 600 | 100 mOsm/kg | V = 600/100 | 6.0 | Severe |
| NDI | 300 | 100 mOsm/kg | V = 300/100 | 3.0 | Moderate |

* Average diet might yield 600 mOsm of solute/m² to be excreted by kidney (principally urea, electrolytes, and other nitrogenous products.)

† V = SL/C where V = obligatory urine volume in liters; SL = 24-hour renal solute load, and C = concentration of urine in mOsm/kg of water.

with an obligatory renal water excretion of 6 L/day. If the diet of the patient with NDI were reduced in protein and sodium chloride content so that the renal solute load was decreased to 300 mOsm/day, then the obligatory renal water excretion would be only 3 L/day instead of 6 L/day, a dramatic decrease.

The thiazide diuretics can be used to diminish the polyuria further. The thiazide diuretics increase sodium excretion, thereby producing a borderline low blood volume. As a result, increased proximal tubular reabsorption of salt and water occurs, and there is less delivery of water to the concentrating sites in the kidney. With a slower flow rate through the collecting ducts, some water diffuses from the collecting duct lumen to the medullary interstitial tissues despite the lack of effect of ADH. The thiazide may decrease urine volume by as much as 20% to 40%. Therefore, these drugs are valuable in the very young infant who has a great physical problem in taking in the volume of free water required to stay in water balance. The decrease in urine volume also prevents or lessens the degree of dilatation of the urinary tract, which is almost inevitable at the high water turnover rates these patients experience when untreated. Since the effect of the thiazide is almost completely nullified by a high sodium intake, sodium restriction to the level previously recommended is vital.

The other agents that appear to be helpful in the management of NDI are prostaglandin synthetase inhibitors (eg, indomethacin). The effects of prostaglandins on renal function are quite complex and appear to vary with the particular prostaglandin involved and the particular situation under which it is tested. In general, however, it appears that prostaglandin synthetase inhibitors usually inhibit water excretion.

Obviously, the treatment of the acquired types of NDI varies depending on the therapy necessary to treat the underlying disease causing the secondary tubular defect. However, many of the principles outlined for the therapy of hereditary NDI also apply to patients with the acquired variety. In particular, these patients benefit from the provision of extra free water and a diet that will yield a low renal solute load.

## Selected Readings

Bichet DG, Arthus MF, Lonergan M. Platelet vasopressin receptors in patients with congenital nephrogenic diabetes insipidus. N Engl J Med 1988;318:881.

Bichet DG, Arthus MF, Lonergan M. Platelet vasopressin receptors in patients with congenital nephrogenic diabetes insipidus. Kidney Internat 1991;39:693.

Bichet DG, Razi M, Lonergan M, et al. Hemodynamic and coagulation responses to 1-desamino-8-D-arginine vasopressin in a patient with congenital nephrogenic diabetes insipidus. N Engl J Med 1988;318:881.

Brennan B, Seligsohn U, Aochberg Z. Normal response of factor VIII and von Willebrand factor to 1-desamino-8-D-arginine vasopressin in nephrogenic diabetes insipidus. J Clin Endocrinol Metab 1988;67:191.

Monn E. Prostaglandin synthetase inhibitors in the treatment of nephrogenic diabetes insipidus. Acta Pediatr Scand 1981;70:39.

Williams RH, Henry C. Nephrogenic diabetes insipidus transmitted by females and appearing during infancy in males. Ann Intern Med 1947;27:84.

*Principles and Practice of Pediatrics, Second Edition.*
edited by Frank A. Oski et al. J. B. Lippincott Company, Philadelphia © 1994.

# 116.6 *Bartter's Syndrome*

Myra L. Chiang

Bartter's syndrome is a renal tubular disorder characterized by hypokalemic metabolic alkalosis, hyperreninemia with secondary hyperaldosteronism, normal blood pressure with pressor resistance to angiotensin II and norepinephrine, increased prostaglandin $E_2$, and juxtaglomerular apparatus hyperplasia on renal biopsy. It can occur sporadically or as an autosomal recessive disorder.

## PATHOGENESIS

The underlying abnormality in this syndrome is unclear. Various hypotheses have been proposed and challenged. Currently, a defect in chloride reabsorption in the ascending limb of the loop of Henle is thought to be the primary disturbance. This abnormal chloride transport leads to increased urinary potassium excretion by decreasing potassium reabsorption in the thick ascending limb and by stimulating potassium secretion in the distal nephron through an increase in the rate of distal delivery of tubular fluid. The induced hypokalemia leads to decreased cAMP generation in the collecting duct, which, along with the decreased medullary hypertonicity from the decreased NaCl reabsorption in the ascending limb of the loop of Henle and the increased distal tubular flow, explains the abnormal concentrating ability seen in this disorder. The defect in chloride transport may also account for the increased magnesium and calcium excretion. Hypokalemia stimulates the synthesis of vasodilator prostaglandins (which may account for the pressor resistance); these in turn activate the renin-angiotensin-aldosterone system and sympathetic nervous system to maintain blood pressure.

## CLINICAL CHARACTERISTICS

Most patients present with failure to thrive, vomiting, dehydration, weakness, and constipation. The onset of symptoms usually occurs between age 6 and 12 months. There may be a preceding history of premature delivery and maternal hydramnios with elevated chloride concentration in the amniotic fluid. Complaints of fatigue, muscle cramps, salt craving, polydipsia, and polyuria with varying severity are common. Developmental delay is variable. Physical examination is often unremarkable except for short stature. Some patients have a distinctive facial appearance characterized by prominence of forehead, triangular facies, drooping mouth, and large eyes and pinnae.

## LABORATORY FINDINGS

Characteristic laboratory abnormalities are hypokalemia, hypochloremia, metabolic alkalosis, and increased fractional excretion of potassium and chloride. Evidence of urinary sodium wasting may be present. Magnesium depletion is common, and hypercalciuria is seen in over 50% of the cases; this may be associated with an elevated serum 1,25-dihydroxyvitamin D level. Elevated plasma renin activity is consistently present. Plasma aldosterone levels are often increased but may be normal due to the suppressive effect of hypokalemia. Additional findings may include hyposthenuria; mild glycosuria and aminoaciduria; phosphaturia leading to hypophosphatemia and rickets; elevated urinary prostaglandins; elevated plasma bradykinin; hyperuricemia; defects in platelet aggregation; and abnormalities in cation content of red blood cells. A renal sonogram or CT scan may show nephrocalcinosis. Juxtaglomerular apparatus hypertrophy and hyperplasia is the most striking histologic abnormality on renal biopsy. However, this is not a consistent finding and is not unique to Bartter's syndrome.

## DIAGNOSIS

The diagnosis of Bartter's syndrome is made when the following criteria are present: hypokalemic, hypochloremic metabolic alkalosis with elevated urinary potassium and chloride ions; hyperreninemia in the presence of normal blood pressure; and exclusion of covert use of loop diuretics by history and appropriate tests.

If the diagnosis is uncertain, the most definitive test is to measure the distal fractional chloride reabsorption during hypotonic saline or dextrose water infusion. However, this is not an easy test to perform and is not routinely done even by nephrologists.

The major differential diagnosis for Bartter's syndrome is Gitelman syndrome (primary magnesium-losing tubulopathy), which closely resembles Bartter's syndrome with hypomagnesemia. These two disorders can be distinguished clinically by the fewer, milder, and later onset of symptoms and by the absence of urinary concentrating defect and the tendency to hypocalciuria in patients with Gitelman syndrome.

Other differential diagnoses for Bartter's syndrome include Fanconi syndrome, cystinosis, cystic fibrosis, chloride-deficient diets, familial chloride diarrhea, surreptitious vomiting, pyloric stenosis, and covert laxative abuse.

## TREATMENT

The goals of therapy are to correct hypokalemia; to improve the associated symptoms of tiredness, easy fatigability, muscle weakness, and muscle cramps; to foster normal growth and development; and to forestall the development of renal insufficiency. This is usually best achieved by a combination of oral potassium ion supplementation, potassium-ion-sparing diuretics, and prostaglandin synthetase inhibitors. Response to therapy is variable. Hypomagnesemia when present should be corrected to correct hypokalemia, since magnesium ion depletion aggravates kaliuresis. The use of angiotensin-converting enzyme inhibitors may be successful in ameliorating the clinical symptoms in some patients.

## Selected Readings

Bettinelli A, Bianchetti MG, Girardin E, et al. Use of calcium excretion values to distinguish two forms of primary renal tubular hypokalemic alkalosis: Bartter and Gitelman syndromes. J Pediatr 1992;120:38.

Dillon MJ. Disorders of renal tubular handling of sodium and potassium. In: Holliday MA, Barratt TM, Vernier RL, eds. Pediatric nephrology. Baltimore: Williams & Wilkins, 1987:598.

Gill JR. Bartter's syndrome. In: Gonick HC, Buckalew VM, eds. Renal tubular disorders: pathophysiology, diagnosis and management. New York: Marcel Dekker, 1985:457.

Hene RJ, Koomans HA, Dorhout Mees EJ, et al. Correction of hypokalemia in Bartter's syndrome by enalapril. Am J Kidney Dis 1987;9:200.

Rovetto CR, Welch TR, Hug G, Clark KE, Bergstrom W. Hypercalciuria with Bartter syndrome: evidence for an abnormality of vitamin D metabolism. J Pediatr 1989;15:397.

*Principles and Practice of Pediatrics, Second Edition.*
edited by Frank A. Oski et al. J. B. Lippincott Company, Philadelphia © 1994.

# CHAPTER 117
# *Circulatory Disturbances*

## *117.1 Renal Hypertension*

### L. Leighton Hill and Seth Paul Kravitz

Transient hypertension may be seen during the course of several acute renal diseases, such as acute glomerulonephritis, anaphylactoid purpura nephritis, hemolytic-uremic syndrome, and acute renal failure, and after urologic surgery. The hypertension associated with these diseases is usually volume-dependent, but also may be renin-dependent or both. More sustained renal hypertension is seen with slowly progressive forms of glomerulonephritis such as membranoproliferative or epimembranous glomerulonephritis. Hypertension (predominantly volume-dependent) is seen with chronic renal failure and with end-stage renal disease (see Chaps. 111 and 112). This discussion is limited to renin-dependent hypertension, which in most cases involves disturbances of the circulation to the kidney.

## RENIN-DEPENDENT HYPERTENSION

The renal hypertension associated with activation of the renin-angiotensin-aldosterone system is usually severe. Although renovascular hypertension is considered the prototypical lesion causing renin-dependent hypertension, several renal diseases may have hypertension based on local obliteration of vessels with increased renin production. Probably the most common of these is the hypertension associated with renal scarring resulting from reflux and urinary tract infections. Renin-induced hypertension may be seen as a late complication of renal vein thrombosis. Dysplastic kidneys, hypoplastic kidneys (general or segmental), polycystic kidneys, obstructive uropathy, and radiation nephritis may be associated with renin-induced hypertension.

Some tumors of the kidney directly produce renin and cause hypertension without altering renal circulation. Juxtaglomerular cell tumors and nephroblastomas may cause hypertension through this mechanism. Nephroblastomas and hamartomas may also block the arterial supply to areas of the kidney, resulting in ischemia and renin production.

Diagnostic studies necessary to differentiate these renal parenchymal diseases may include urinalysis, urine cultures, renal ultrasonography or intravenous urograms, and voiding cystourethrograms. Arteriography and divided renal vein renins usually are not done except in unusual situations when a surgical approach is contemplated.

# RENOVASCULAR HYPERTENSION

Renovascular hypertension (RVH) results from the impairment of blood flow to part or all of one or both kidneys and accounts for between 4.5% and 11.5% of sustained secondary hypertension during childhood. Main renal arteries or smaller intrarenal arteries may be affected. The incidence of RVH is substantially lower in black than in white patients.

## Etiology

RVH is second only to coarctation as a cause of surgically remediable hypertension in children. Obstruction of blood flow to the kidneys can be extrinsic (eg, para-aortic tumor, para-aortic lymph nodes) or intrinsic (Table 117-1). Of the intrinsic lesions listed, fibromuscular dysplasia is the one seen most often in children. Fibromuscular dysplasia is usually limited to the renal arteries but it may involve multiple arteries, including the cerebral, mesenteric, hepatic, and splenic arteries. Renal artery stenosis may be seen with neurofibromatosis, William syndrome, Marfan syndrome, abdominal coarctation, Takayasu disease, and congenital rubella syndrome.

## Pathogenesis

The decrease in renal perfusion brought about by the arterial obstruction leads to renal ischemia, which stimulates increased renin secretion. The resultant increase in angiotensin II causes generalized vasoconstriction and hypertension. Angiotensin II also stimulates aldosterone production (secondary hyperaldosteronism), which through its action on the distal nephron leads to increased sodium chloride reabsorption and extracellular volume expansion, as well as to potassium wasting by the kidney. The volume expansion may suppress renin release to some extent. In unilateral RVH, there is suppression of renin release from the contralateral kidney.

## Clinical Findings

Table 117-2 contains clinical clues that suggest a renovascular origin for hypertension. RVH should be considered in any case of severe or refractory hypertension in a child, especially in the first decade of life. The presence of retinopathy, signs of secondary hyperaldosteronism (hypokalemia, mild metabolic alkalosis), and an abdominal bruit should lead to a consideration of RVH. Hypertension associated with a unilateral small kidney and an excellent response to angiotensin-converting enzyme inhibitors also merits consideration of RVH.

The preliminary workup should include a urinalysis, serum creatinine, serum calcium, and electrolytes. An ECG and chest radiograph can be obtained to look for evidence of left ventricular hypertrophy. Many nephrologists recommend an echocardiogram

**TABLE 117-1. Intrinsic Renal Artery Disease**

Fibromuscular lesions:
  Intimal
  Medial
  Perimedial
Arteritic lesions
Thrombotic and embolic lesions
Aneurysms
Arteriovenous malformations (fistulas)
Neurofibromatosis (intimal lesion, nodular lesion)
Abdominal coarctation with renal artery involvement
Arteriosclerotic lesions

**TABLE 117-2. Clinical Clues That Suggest Renovascular Hypertension**

Abrupt onset of severe hypertension
Epigastric, subcostal, or flank bruit
Progression to malignant-phase hypertension
Retinopathy
Hypokalemia
Plasma bicarbonate high-normal to elevated
Hypertension refractory to intensive antihypertensive regimen
Hypertension with unilateral small kidney
Excellent response to angiotensin-converting enzyme inhibitors
Transient impairment in renal function in response to angiotensin-converting enzyme inhibitor

for evaluating cardiac status since it is more sensitive in demonstrating left ventricular hypertrophy. Either ultrasonography (preferred) or an intravenous urogram should be part of the preliminary workup to search for abnormalities such as obstructive uropathy, mass lesions, renal scarring, cystic disease, and abnormal renal size. Renal scans are helpful in screening for renal scarring.

## Diagnostic Studies

Diagnostic studies that evaluate for evidence of renovascular hypertension may be classified as either screening tests or confirmatory tests. The ultimate confirmation of renovascular hypertension is the resolution of the hypertension with correction of the lesion.

Before describing the tests used to evaluate patients for renovascular hypertension, we must briefly discuss some of the limitations of these tests. Many of the screening tests reported in the literature have a high sensitivity and specificity when looking at patients with renovascular hypertension. However, when these tests are used in the general population, they have relatively low predictive values. The reason for this discrepancy is that the incidence of renovascular hypertension is low in the population. In that situation, the number of false-positive patients in the general population will lower the positive predictive value of any test. This must be considered when evaluating test results.

### Screening Tests

*Peripheral Renin Activity.* The measurement of a peripheral vein renin activity (PRA) is of little value as a screening test or as a diagnostic test for RVH. PRA has been reported to have a sensitivity of 57% and a specificity of only 66%. Several drugs may stimulate or suppress renin activity, and several conditions, including adrenal insufficiency, salt-wasting renal disease, pheochromocytoma, and hyperthyroidism, may stimulate PRA. Indexing the renin activity to urine sodium excretion improves the measurement's usefulness to some degree.

*Renal Imaging Studies.* Ultrasonography provides accurate information on renal location, size, volume, and contour and should be done as part of the preliminary workup to rule out some of the renal parenchymal diseases mentioned previously. However, it gives no information as to renal function. In newborns, it may be useful in visualizing aortic thrombosis associated with umbilical artery catheters.

Doppler imaging of renal arterial flow at the time of ultrasonography is currently being evaluated. Preliminary figures in adults are encouraging, but there are limitations in the ability to get an adequate study. There are insufficient data in children to evaluate its potential usefulness.

Intravenous urograms are preferred over sonograms by some, but "rapid sequence urograms" are no longer performed routinely because of a high rate of false-positive results.

Radionuclide imaging techniques have not proved to be any more accurate than hypertensive urograms in screening for renovascular disease. To improve the accuracy of the test, isotopic renography after angiotensin-converting enzyme (ACE) inhibition has been developed (see below). CT scanning and MRI have not proved to be useful in diagnosing renal artery stenosis.

Digital subtraction angiography is less invasive than renal arteriography, but visualization of the main renal arteries does not compare with arteriography, and the branches of the renal artery seldom are visualized adequately. Some clinicians find digital subtraction angiography useful, and improvements in this technique can be expected in the future.

ACE inhibitors have been used with serum renin levels, radionuclide imaging, and renal vein renin determinations to improve the predictive values of these tests. Renal function in a kidney that has renal artery stenosis depends on an elevated efferent arteriole tone that is maintained by high renin levels. This tone is depressed when an ACE inhibitor is given. With radionuclide imaging, there is a decreased uptake and clearance of the isotope from the kidney after captopril (one of the ACE inhibitors) is given. This test has been useful in improving sensitivity and specificity in adults, but the experience in children has been limited. The captopril challenge test measures the rise in peripheral renin after the administration of oral captopril. Positive predictive values in adults have ranged from 32% to 92%, with one study in children having a positive predictive value of 43%. Captopril has also been given before obtaining renal vein renins. The ultimate usefulness of the captopril challenge test and captopril renography in children is yet to be determined, but it appears that a negative captopril challenge test or captopril renography will provide strong evidence against renal vascular hypertension.

### Confirmatory Tests

Renal arteriography with renal vein renins remains the gold standard in the diagnosis of renovascular hypertension. These studies are usually done concomitantly and provide both anatomical and functional information. The purpose of these studies is to visualize a functionally significant lesion. The presence of collateral vessels with a stenotic lesion implies a significant lesion. Recognizing a branch lesion may be helpful in renal vein sampling.

Differential renal vein renins are obtained from effluent venous blood from each renal vein and from the inferior vena cava. In unilateral RVH, the affected (ischemic) kidney should have a renal vein renin activity at least 1.5 times greater than that from the renal vein of the contralateral kidney. In addition, a renal/systemic index should be calculated, looking at the renal vein renin levels in comparison to the inferior vena cava (IVC). Obviously, sampling errors can occur that will negate the value of the study. Because higher renal vein renin activities increase the reliability of the study, the differential renal vein studies usually are done after some maneuver designed to stimulate renin production, such as sodium depletion, the administration of loop diuretics, or the administration of ACE inhibitors. The presence of a significant difference in renal vein activity predicts benefit of surgery in 90% of the patients; however, a significant number of patients with negative studies also will benefit from surgery.

## Clinical Management

The major objectives of management are to prevent the complications of hypertension by controlling blood pressure and preventing or slowing the loss of renal function. Control of moderate to severe hypertension is essential while diagnostic studies are being performed. Long-term therapy of renovascular hypertension may be medical, using pharmacologic agents, or surgical. Surgical options include nephrectomy, partial nephrectomy, revascularization by reconstructive vascular surgery, and autotransplantation.

An additional therapeutic option is the use of percutaneous transluminal renal angioplasty (PTRA). In this technique, a balloon catheter is used to dilate the constricted portion of the renal artery. PTRA is especially valuable in RVH associated with fibromuscular dysplasia. Since children have fibromuscular dysplasias as the cause of their RVH much more often than arteriosclerotic lesions, children appear to be good candidates for this therapy. PTRA has a beneficial effect in 85% to 100% of the patients with fibromuscular dysplasia, as opposed to 65% to 94% of lesions due to atherosclerosis. The lesions of neurofibromatosis, developmental anomalies of the abdominal aorta, and lesions secondary to arteritis are less likely to have a successful outcome. The restenosis rates after PTRA vary from 13% to 30%. Advantages of PTRA over surgery include less anesthesia, minimal patient morbidity, shorter hospital stays, and lower costs when PTRA is successful. In some medical centers, PTRA is attempted at the time of renal arteriography. Complications of the procedure include hemorrhage at the puncture site, embolization to the kidney, thrombus formation, renal infarction, and dissection or rupture of the renal vasculature. The procedure should not be performed unless a vascular surgeon is available, and it may be attempted before surgical revascularization.

Factors favoring surgical over medical therapy for RVH include younger age, hypertension refractory to medication, a general medical status suitable for surgery, and a decrease in renal function because of progressive arterial disease. In children who would otherwise face a lifetime of medical therapy, a surgical approach should be strongly considered. In bilateral disease, it seems prudent to attempt revascularization by reconstructive vascular surgery, with one kidney done at a time. PTRA has been attempted with bilateral disease.

Pharmacologic management of the blood pressure in RVH has improved greatly with the introduction of the beta blockers in the 1970s and the ACE inhibitors in the 1980s. ACE inhibitors block the conversion of angiotensin I to angiotensin II, thereby lowering angiotensin II concentration and reducing the degree of vasoconstriction and the secretion of aldosterone. An ACE inhibitor is usually the drug of choice in RVH. ACE inhibitors must be used with extreme caution if there is bilateral renal artery stenosis or evidence of stenosis in a solitary kidney: patients have presented with renal failure subsequent to initiating ACE inhibitor therapy in these circumstances. Because ACE inhibitor therapy is frequently initiated before bilateral renal artery stenosis is diagnosed, a cautious approach is prudent. The patient should be monitored for evidence of azotemia or hyperkalemia after beginning therapy with captopril, enalapril, or lisinopril (ACE inhibitors). There is some concern about the long-term effects of ACE inhibitor therapy for renovascular disease because these drugs decrease systemic blood pressure at the expense of decreased perfusion to the stenotic kidney.

Long-term medical therapy is indicated in the patient whose vascular lesion is not amenable to surgical correction. Medical therapy also may be useful in other situations, such as in very young children to allow the renal vasculature to grow sufficiently to permit revascularization procedures. Under these circumstances, renal function must be followed closely because it may deteriorate from progressive arterial disease, even though blood pressure control is successful. If renal function does deteriorate, then reconsideration must be given to surgery or to PTRA.

## Selected Readings

Chevalier RL, Tegtmeyer CJ, Gomez RA. Percutaneous transluminal angioplasty for renovascular hypertension in children. Pediatr Nephrol 1987;1:89.

Gauthier B, Trachtman H, Frank R, et al. Inadequacy of captopril challenge test for diagnosing renovascular hypertension in children and adolescents. Pediatr Nephrol 1991;5:42.

Idrissi A, Fournier A, Boudailliez B, et al. The captopril challenge test as a screening test for renovascular hypertension. Kidney Internat 1988;34(suppl 25):S138.

Kohler TR, Zierler RE, Martin RL, et al. Noninvasive diagnosis of renal artery stenosis by ultrasonic duplex scanning. J Vasc Surg 1986;4:450.

Sfakianakis GN, Jaffe DJ, Bourgoignie JJ. Captopril scintigraphy in the diagnosis of renovascular hypertension. Kidney Internat 1988;34(suppl 25):S142.

Textor SC. ACE inhibitors in renovascular hypertension. Cardiovasc Drug Ther 1990;4:229.

Willems CD, Shah V, Uchiyama M, et al. Captopril as an aid to diagnosis in childhood hypertension. Clin Exper Theory Pract 1986;A8:747.

*Principles and Practice of Pediatrics, Second Edition.*
edited by Frank A. Oski et al. J. B. Lippincott Company, Philadelphia © 1994.

# 117.2 *Renal Vascular Thrombosis*

## L. Leighton Hill

The kidney of the newborn infant appears to be particularly at risk for the development of vascular thromboses. The vessels are small, renal blood flow is relatively low, the neonate is relatively polycythemic, vascular resistance is high, and fibrinolytic mechanisms may be immature. Over two thirds of the children with this disorder are under 1 month of age. The ratio of males to females in reported series has ranged from 1.4 : 1 to 1.9 : 1 in the newborn period. Not all cases are diagnosed antemortem, and routine postmortem examinations have revealed the presence of renal venous thrombosis (RVT) in as many as 1.9% to 2.7% of neonatal deaths.

## RENAL VENOUS THROMBOSIS

RVT may be unilateral (most common) or bilateral. It is a rare condition in children past the neonatal period.

## Etiology

In neonates and young infants, RVT is seen with dehydration, shock, increased tonicity of body fluids, and polycythemia. Infants with RVT frequently have endured perinatal asphyxia, prenatal or postnatal stress, or septicemia. There is a high incidence of preceding diarrhea. Not uncommonly, these infants have been exposed to radiographic contrast media. Additional predisposing factors in the newborn period include congenital renal anomalies, congenital nephrosis, severe pyelonephritis, and maternal diabetes. RVT can be primary, first involving the veins of the kidney, or secondary, extending into the renal veins from a thrombus in the inferior vena cava.

RVT seen after infancy is usually associated with the nephrotic syndrome or with cyanotic congenital heart disease (either spontaneously or following angiography). RVT does not cause the nephrotic syndrome; rather, patients with the nephrotic syndrome have a predisposition for the development of RVT because plasma proteins involved in the coagulation pathways are lost in the urine. RVT can also be seen as a complication of burns in children.

## Pathogenesis

During conditions of hypovolemia, hemoconcentration, hyperviscosity, hyperosmolarity, sepsis, and asphyxia, local microthrombi may occur peripherally in venous radicals, and the thrombus formation may then progress through the arcuate and interlobular veins toward the main renal vein. Much more rarely, the clotting process moves in the opposite direction. The overwhelming majority of cases represent intraluminal thrombosis, but rarely there can be extraluminal interference with the normal pattern of flow of venous channels in the kidney. Intraluminal thrombus formation may be initiated by vascular endothelial cell injury. RVT causes renal congestion and occasionally infarction.

## Signs and Symptoms

There may be sudden enlargement of one or both kidneys. About 60% of the patients with RVT have a palpably enlarged renal mass. Most patients have hematuria, which may be gross but more often is microscopic and may be absent. Renal enlargement may occur without other symptoms, but more often there are associated symptoms and signs, including one or more of the following: pallor, tachypnea, vomiting, abdominal distention, shock, fever, and oliguria or anuria. Many of the signs and symptoms noted are due to the underlying disorder causing the RVT rather than to the vascular catastrophe itself. Physical examination most often reveals abdominal distention and unilateral or bilateral flank masses. Hypertension is uncommon.

## Laboratory Findings

Proteinuria is common, although in some instances it may be due to the physical presence of gross blood in the urine. Over 50% of the infants with RVT demonstrate evidence of a microangiopathic hemolytic anemia with red cell fragmentation; thrombocytopenia; low levels of fibrinogen, Factor V, and plasminogen; and an increase in fibrin degradation products. These findings reflect the presence of an active disseminated intravascular coagulation. Depending on the severity and whether the thrombosis is unilateral or bilateral, azotemia and other biochemical evidence of acute renal failure may be present.

Intravenous urograms should not be done. The most useful imaging studies include sonography of the urinary tract, which may reveal enlarged size, altered echogenicity, loss of corticomedullary definition, and a decrease in the size of the central sinus echo, and Doppler evaluation of renal arterial and renal venous blood flow. Isotope renography may also be useful. Selective venography may provide precise delineation of the vascular thrombosis but must be considered risky and is usually unnecessary.

## Differential Diagnosis

The many causes of hematuria must be considered. The common presence of a microangiopathic hemolytic anemia in RVT makes hemolytic-uremic syndrome an important differential diagnosis. Other causes of renal enlargement such as perirenal hematoma, abscess, hydronephrosis, cystic renal disease, and renal tumors should also be considered in the differential diagnosis.

## Treatment

For the most part, therapy should be conservative and supportive. Correction of underlying pathophysiologic abnormalities should be attempted. If oliguria and azotemia occur, medical management of acute renal failure may be required; in some instances dialysis is needed. The efficacy of anticoagulant therapy (heparin) has not been documented by controlled studies and should be considered only if there is laboratory evidence of continuing intravascular coagulation. A surgical approach in the acute phase is rarely indicated. The mortality rate is substantial and relates more to the underlying disease process itself than to the RVT. Recovery of function in affected kidneys may occur, but progressive atrophy may result in small, scarred kidneys. Hypertension may be a late complication. Chronic renal failure can be the outcome in some patients who have bilateral RVT. Other patients may show predominantly tubular dysfunction as the sequela of RVT.

## RENAL ARTERIAL THROMBOSIS

Renal arterial occlusions, formerly very rare, are now being seen more often, probably because of the extensive use of umbilical artery catheters. The kidney may be enlarged but usually not to the extent that a mass is palpable. Abdominal distention and vomiting are common. Hypertension is seen more often than with renal venous thrombosis and may be difficult to control despite aggressive pharmacologic therapy. Hematuria, proteinuria, oliguria or anuria, and azotemia are often seen. The presence of renal failure depends on whether the thrombosis is unilateral or bilateral. Ultrasound and radionuclide imaging are important diagnostic studies.

Treatment is largely supportive. Attempts at thrombectomy usually are contraindicated. Persistent abnormalities in renal size and function are common, and acute or chronic management of renal failure including dialysis may be necessary. The renovascular hypertension may persist, requiring continued therapy; fortunately, in many instances the hypertension resolves.

## Selected Readings

Adelman RD. Long-term follow-up of neonatal renovascular hypertension. Pediatr Nephrol 1987;1:35.
Kaplan BS, Chesney RW, Drummond KN. The nephrotic syndrome and renal vein thrombosis. Am J Dis Child 1978;132:367.
Renfield ML, Kraybill EN. Consumptive coagulopathy with renal vein thrombosis. J Pediatr 1973;82:1054.
Stringer DA, Krysl J, Manson D, Babiak C, Daneman A, Liu P. The value of Doppler sonography in the detection of major vessel thrombosis in the neonatal abdomen. Pediatr Radiol 1990;21:30.

*Principles and Practice of Pediatrics, Second Edition.*
edited by Frank A. Oski et al. J. B. Lippincott Company, Philadelphia © 1994.

## CHAPTER 118
# *Urolithiasis*

### L. Leighton Hill

There is a marked variation worldwide in the incidence of stones in children. In some countries, such as Turkey and Thailand, urolithiasis is endemic; bladder stones predominate and dietary factors are postulated to play a causative role. In contrast, stones are uncommon in children in the United States, where less than 1% of all renal stones occur in children under age 10 and less than 3% in children under age 19, and where most stones have a metabolic origin. In the United States boys with stones outnumber girls by 2 : 1, stones are very uncommon in black children, and bladder stones are much less common than upper tract stones. Although the two conditions may coexist, a distinction should be made between urolithiasis (stones in the urinary tract) and nephrocalcinosis, which is an increase in the calcium content of the renal tissue itself.

## FORMATION OF STONES

Urinary calculi consist of a very small glycoprotein matrix with surrounding organic or inorganic crystals. Urinary crystalloids capable of being crystallized include calcium, phosphorus, oxalates, cystine, uric acid, xanthine, and ammonium. Supersaturation of the urine with various ionic species eventually leads to precipitation, with subsequent crystal growth. Two products appear to be important in this process: the solubility product and the formation product. Below the solubility product for a given ionic pair (eg, calcium and oxalate), the solution is undersaturated and crystal formation does not occur. Above the formation product for a given ionic pair, the solution is supersaturated and spontaneous precipitation occurs. Between the solubility product and the formation product lies the metastable region in which precipitation does not occur unless the system is disturbed.

Urine volume, through its effect on dilution and concentration, obviously plays a critical role in determining the degree of saturation. Urine pH is an important factor in determining solubility. Crystalline nuclei rarely form in free solution but rather on existing surfaces. Theoretically, any factor that increases the number of nuclei in tubular fluid or urine, such as epithelial injury, could lower the metastable limit, the supersaturation at which crystals first form.

There are also inhibitor substances that inhibit crystallization. Inhibitor absence has been suggested to explain calculus formation in patients with normal excretion of urinary crystalloids. Inhibitor substances are believed to include citrate, pyrophosphate, urinary glycoprotein crystallization inhibitors, Tamm-Horsfall mucoprotein, uropontin, and magnesium/calcium and sodium/calcium ratios in the urine. There are undoubtedly many other as yet unidentified inhibitors. The physicochemical principles underlying the formation of renal stones remain poorly defined.

A classification of stones according to their composition is shown in Table 118-1. Calcium is a constituent of 90% of calculi. Calcium phosphate, the principal constituent of the calcium stones listed in part I of Table 118-1, is also found in struvite and other stones listed in the table. The hypercalciuric stones are divided into hypercalcemic hypercalciuria and normocalcemic hypercalciuria, but there is some overlapping of these two groups. The struvite stones (magnesium ammonium phosphate) often are called "infection stones."

## CLINICAL FEATURES

The presentation in children, especially young children and infants, may be very nonspecific. Gross or microscopic hematuria may be the only manifestation, or hematuria may be accompanied by nonspecific abdominal pain or by fever, pyuria, and abdominal pain. Signs and symptoms might be those of a urinary tract infection (UTI). Typical renal colic is unusual in the small child but can be present in the older child. In some instances, the stone or gravel already has been passed spontaneously. Frequently the patient has a family history of stones. Urinary stones can cause

## TABLE 118-1. Urolithiasis Classification Based on Stone Composition

I. Calcium stones (calcium oxalate and calcium phosphate)
  A. Hypercalciuria
    1. Hypercalcemic hypercalciuria
      Hyperparathyroidism
      Thyrotoxicosis
      Vitamin D intoxication
      Idiopathic infantile hypercalcemia
      Sarcoidosis
      Neoplastic deposits in bones
      Immobilization
    2. Normocalcemic hypercalciuria
      Idiopathic or familial hypercalciuria
        Absorptive
        Renal
        1,25-dihydroxycholecalciferol-induced
      Distal RTA (type 1)
      Acetazolamide use
      Loop diuretic use
      Immobilization
      Vitamin D excess
      Cushing's syndrome
  B. Hyperoxaluria (calcium oxalate)
    1. Primary hyperoxaluria types 1 & 2
    2. Secondary hyperoxaluria
      Inflammatory bowel disease
      Pyridoxine deficiency
      Massive doses of vitamin C
  C. Hyperglycinuria (calcium oxalate stones)
  D. Idiopathic urolithiasis
II. Magnesium ammonium phosphate (struvite) plus basic calcium phosphate (apatite)
  A. Urinary tract infection with urea-splitting organisms (mostly *Proteus* species)
  B. Foreign body plus urinary stasis plus infection
III. Uric acid stones*
  A. Hyperuricosuria
    1. Gout
    2. Lesch-Nyhan syndrome
    3. High purine diet
    4. Type I glycogen storage disease
    5. Leukemia-lymphoma
    6. Leukemia-lymphoma cytotoxic prescription
IV. Xanthine stones*
  A. Primary xanthinuria
  B. Allopurinol therapy
V. Dihydroxyadenine stones*
VI. Cystine stones
  A. Cystinuria

\* Disorders of purine metabolism

The diagnosis of urolithiasis also can be made by the proven passage of a stone, gravel, or sludge. Whenever urolithiasis is considered, any passed material must be saved and the urine must be strained, whether at home or in the hospital, in an attempt to obtain a stone.

The formation of a stone within the urinary tract is not a specific disease but instead is a complication of many highly varied disorders. The next step must be to determine which of the disorders caused the stone. Therefore, all passed stones or stonelike material must be tested completely for composition. The stone should be solubilized and analyzed qualitatively and quantitatively for its main contents. This should be done in a laboratory experienced in stone analysis. Children with the diagnosis of urolithiasis should have radiologic investigation of the urinary tract to evaluate for a possible anatomical abnormality of the genitourinary tract, to assess for the presence of and degree of obstruction caused by the stone, to search for other stones, and to determine if nephrocalcinosis is also present. This will usually include either an ultrasound study of the urinary tract or an intravenous urogram and occasionally a cystourethrogram.

The laboratory workup is suggested in Table 118-2. The metabolic evaluation of stone formers should begin 4 to 6 weeks after stone diagnosis and passage, as passage itself may cause transient changes in urinary chemistry. The serum calcium determines the possible presence of hypercalcemia. Serum phosphorus may be low in hyperparathyroidism, in one type of hypercalciuria, and in renal tubular acidosis (RTA), and may be elevated in the tumor lysis syndrome. Serum creatinine estimates glomerular function. The electrolytes, pH, $Pco_2$, and urine pH are used to investigate the possibility of RTA. All children with stones should have a spot chemical urine test for cystine to rule out cystinuria and a quantitative amino acid analysis if the spot test is positive. A timed urine sample (at 6, 8, 12, or preferably 24 hours) is collected for quantitative measurement of calcium and uric acid. Because of the present difficulty in measuring oxalate, it is not quantified routinely. Quantitative urinary calcium excretion or a spot urine for calcium/creatinine ratio will provide information as to the possible presence of hypercalciuria. Hyperuricosuria can occur without hyperuricemia.

These mostly routine tests frequently will provide a diagnosis

obstruction of the urinary flow, dilatation of the urinary tract, and ultimately renal parenchymal damage. Stones can predispose to UTIs; conversely, UTIs can be important in the formation of stones.

## DIAGNOSIS

A high index of suspicion frequently is required to make the diagnosis of urolithiasis. Demonstration of the stone can be done by imaging techniques such as a plain radiograph of the abdomen, intravenous urograms, an ultrasound study of the urinary tract, or tomograms. All stones containing calcium are radiopaque. Cystine stones are slightly radiopaque because of the sulfur present in cystine. Struvite stones also are radiopaque. The stones that are most frequently radiolucent are those resulting from disorders of purine metabolism (see Table 118-1).

## TABLE 118-2. Laboratory Workup

**Blood Determinations**
Calcium, repeat 2 or 3 times
Phosphorus
Alkaline phosphatase
Creatinine
Electrolytes
pH and $Pco_2$
Uric acid

**Urine Studies**
Urinalysis, repeat 2 or 3 times
Urine culture
Spot urine for cystine (cyanide-nitroprusside test)
Urine pHs, repeat 4–6 times
Spot urine for calcium/creatinine ratio
24-hour urine for calcium, creatinine, oxalate, and uric acid. Add xanthine if patient has hypouricemia and quantitative amino acids if spot test for cystine is positive.

**Other Studies**
Ammonium chloride loading test may be necessary to assess renal ability to acidify.

as to the etiology of the stone. Sometimes leads from the routine tests may suggest more sophisticated studies. An accurate chemical analysis of the stone itself will greatly enhance the possibility of a correct diagnosis.

## CLASSIFICATION

### Calcium Stones

#### Hypercalciuria

The diverse conditions causing hypercalcemia (see Table 118-1) are discussed in Chapter 140. Hypercalcemia is more apt to cause nephrocalcinosis than urolithiasis. The normocalcemic hypercalciurias include distal RTA type 1, discussed in Chapter 116.1. The use of acetazolamide can cause a picture identical to that of RTA type 1. Loop diuretic administration, especially in preterm infants, has caused nephrocalcinosis and urolithiasis. Immobilization can cause hypercalciuria whether or not the serum calcium is elevated.

#### Idiopathic or Familial Hypercalciuria

One of the most common causes of stones at any age is idiopathic or familial hypercalciuria, a normocalcemic form of hypercalciuria. Familial hypercalciuria may account for up to 50% of stones in children. Urinary calcium excretion exceeds 4 mg/kg/day, or the calcium/creatinine ratio exceeds 0.21. Calcium excretion studies should be done several times while the patient is free of infection or obstruction and on an unrestricted diet (except for the fasting studies).

At least three mechanisms have been invoked to explain the familial normocalcemic type of hypercalciuria. The first—absorptive hypercalciuria—is a primary intestinal epithelial defect that permits excessive intestinal absorption of calcium. Parathyroid hormone (PTH) function is normal or suppressed, and urinary calcium excretion returns to normal during fasting. A second type of hypercalciuria is called renal hypercalciuria because of apparently defective calcium reabsorption by the renal tubules. The renal loss of calcium results temporarily in a lower serum calcium level, which stimulates PTH production, bringing the serum calcium back to normal. Renal hypercalciuria is characterized by elevated PTH levels, which stimulate increased production of 1,25-dihydroxycholecalciferol, which then enhances the intestinal absorption of calcium and increases the filtered load of calcium in the kidney. Children with renal hypercalciuria continue to put out calcium in abnormal amounts (>4 mg/kg/day) during fasting. A third type of hypercalciuria—1,25-dihydroxycholecalciferol-induced hypercalciuria—is recognized by some investigators. It is hypothesized that the defect may be a renal tubular leak of phosphate. The ensuing hypophosphatemia is thought to stimulate the renal synthesis of 1,25-dihydroxycholecalciferol, which then enhances intestinal absorption of calcium, which in turn provides extra calcium for renal excretion.

Many experts in calcium physiology argue that dividing the hypercalciurias into several pathogenetic entities is unjustified. They offer instead a unifying hypothesis that the various forms of hypercalciuria result from the same generalized defect, possibly a disordered regulation of 1,25-dihydroxycholecalciferol production.

Children with idiopathic hypercalciuria also may have hematuria (either gross or microscopic), even though no stones have been detected. Hypercalciuria also should be in the differential diagnosis of isolated hematuria. Patients with hypercalciuric hematuria may later develop stones. Many patients with biochemical evidence of hypercalciuria never experience problems with stone formation.

#### Hyperoxaluria

Primary hyperoxaluria is a general term for two rare genetic disorders that result in recurrent calcium oxalate urolithiasis and nephrocalcinosis. Nephrocalcinosis is a greater problem than urolithiasis because the deposition of calcium oxalate in the renal parenchyma ultimately leads to tissue destruction, fibrosis, and chronic renal failure. The renal calculi are extremely radiopaque and homogenous. Secondary hyperoxaluria with stone formation also can occur, most often due to chronic inflammatory bowel disease such as Crohn's disease or to ileal bypass. There apparently is increased intestinal oxalate absorption in enteric types of secondary hyperoxaluria.

#### Idiopathic Urolithiasis

Idiopathic urolithiasis refers to the finding of a stone in a patient whose workup, including urine cultures, urologic evaluation, and metabolic evaluation, is entirely negative. The number of children in this group is small, since a cause for stones usually can be found.

### Struvite Stones

Struvite (magnesium ammonium phosphate) stones occur as the result of UTIs with urease-containing bacteria. These organisms, most commonly *Proteus* species, can split urinary urea into ammonia ions, which buffer hydrogen ions to form ammonium molecules, thereby producing a strongly alkaline urine loaded with ammonium compounds. The persistently alkaline urine favors the crystallization of calcium phosphate (apatite), and the increase in ammonium concentration raises the magnesium ammonium phosphate product. Seventy-five percent of struvite stones in children are seen below age 5, and 80% are in boys. Children with struvite stones frequently have vesicoureteral reflux or other urologic abnormalities. The UTIs associated with struvite stones can be quite resistant to therapy, and organisms have been cultured from the interior of the stone. Complete removal of these stones is mandatory.

### Cystinuria

Cystinuria is a hereditary disorder of amino acid transport affecting the epithelial cells of both the renal tubule and the gastrointestinal tract. The gastrointestinal defect apparently causes no clinical problems. However, the renal tubular abnormality results in hyperexcretion in the urine of the neutral amino acid cystine and the cationic amino acids lysine, ornithine, and arginine. The diagnosis is proved by demonstrating abnormal quantities of these amino acids in a timed urine specimen. The only clinical expression of cystinuria is urolithiasis; otherwise, those with this disorder can live a normal life. It is unknown whether urolithiasis will eventually develop in every person with cystinuria.

### Uric Acid Stones

Uric acid stones resulting from primary gout are extremely rare in children. Hyperuricemia with uric acid calculi is seen as part of the Lesch-Nyhan syndrome, a rare inborn error of metabolism. Uric acid stones also may be seen as a consequence of the hyperuricosuria of type 1 glycogen storage disease. Hyperuricemia with uric acid stones or gravel in the urinary tracts of both kidneys is occasionally the presenting feature of leukemia. More commonly, the calculi occur after cytotoxic chemotherapy of leukemia or lymphoma (tumor lysis syndrome). Urine flow may be blocked, resulting in acute renal failure. High uric acid levels also can be nephrotoxic and produce renal parenchymal damage directly.

## TREATMENT

One of the most important measures in preventing the formation or further growth of any stone regardless of etiology is to increase urine volume, which reduces the urinary concentrations of calcium, phosphorus, oxalates, cystine, uric acid, and other possible constituents of stones. This dilution of the urine can be accomplished by raising the fluid intake to 1.5 to two times normal ($2400 \text{ mL/m}^2$/day or more). The high fluid intake should be distributed as much as possible throughout the 24 hours, including at bedtime and during the night if the patient awakens. Early morning urines should be kept at a specific gravity of less than 1.014. UTI, if present, must be treated and a search for anatomical abnormalities completed. Any urologic abnormalities predisposing to infections or stones should be corrected.

### Stone Removal

Many stones will pass through and out of the urinary tract spontaneously. Others may dissolve slowly (eg, uric acid stones) or at least not grow as a result of medical treatment. Some stones must be removed: struvite stones, stones causing prolonged obstruction with obstructive nephropathy, and stones causing significant chronic pain or resistant UTI. The traditional surgical management of patients with calculus disease in the past consisted of endoscopic manipulation with stone baskets or loops for stones in the lower part of the ureter (below the pelvic brim) or open surgical procedures for calculi higher in the urinary tract. These traditional methods of stone removal are being replaced by a variety of new modalities, including extracorporeal shock-wave lithotripsy, percutaneous nephrostolithotomy, and the use of percutaneously placed endoscopes to fragment calculi with ultrasound waves or lasers. These techniques, used first in adults, are now finding widespread application in children and represent a dramatic advance in medical therapy.

### Specific Therapeutic Measures

The treatment for pediatric hypercalciuria and stones due to hypercalcemia is elimination of the cause of the hypercalcemia; that is, parathyroidectomy (for patients with hyperparathyroidism), treatment of thyrotoxicosis or Cushing's disease, withdrawal of vitamin D therapy, at least partially mobilizing immobilized patients, and so on. Distal RTA, a form of normocalcemic hypercalciuria, can be treated with appropriate amounts of sodium bicarbonate or sodium citrate plus potassium citrate, striving to keep the serum bicarbonate concentration in the range of 22 to 28 mEq/L (see Chap. 116).

The therapy of urolithiasis due to familial or idiopathic hypercalciuria is controversial. It is probably no longer necessary to try to distinguish the various types of hypercalciuria in regards to therapy; rather, all patients with stones from idiopathic or familial hypercalciuria should be treated similarly, with increased fluid intake and reduced calcium intake and sodium intake. Thiazide diuretics, which enhance renal tubular reabsorption of calcium, are quite effective in reducing calcium excretion and preventing recurrent stone formation. Since high sodium chloride intakes tend to negate this effect of thiazides, restriction of sodium intake to a maximum of 2 g/day is indicated. The addition of potassium citrate to this regimen (1 to 2 mEq/kg/day) is advised. Whether or not to use thiazide drugs for long-term therapy depends on the number of recurrences of stones and the complications encountered. Dietary calcium restriction can be tried but must be used cautiously in a growing child. The use of phosphate compounds (cellulose phosphate, orthophosphate) in children is poorly tolerated and has generally been abandoned.

Of these therapies for familial hypercalciuria, the thiazide diuretics have been the most successful, but long-term use of a thiazide would be considered only in those patients with recurrent stones. The therapy of familial hypercalciuria is not completely clear at this time. Thiazides reduce stone formation in patients with recurrent idiopathic urolithiasis, even though urinary calcium before treatment was normal.

There is no effective therapy for the primary hyperoxalurias. A few patients with type I appear to respond partially to pyridoxine therapy. Salts of phosphate, citrate, and magnesium, aimed at increasing the solubility of calcium oxalate, have been used with some success.

All fragments of struvite stones must be removed, since failure to do so may result in persistent infection and recurrence of stones. Complete eradication of infection and the correction of any anatomical abnormality causing urinary stasis is essential.

Allopurinol therapy is very effective in patients with uric acid and dihydroxyadenine stones. A high urine output is also valuable in treating these two types of stones. Alkalinization of the urine to a pH of 6.5 with sodium bicarbonate or sodium citrate is important in treating and preventing uric acid calculi. Hemodialysis may be necessary to control the extreme hyperuricemia seen in patients with the tumor lysis syndrome.

Dilution of the urine decreases the saturation of cystine, and alkalinization will increase the solubility of cystine. The alkali therapy must be divided over the entire day and night so as to ensure a pH above 7 (ideally above 7.4). Of these two treatments, increasing the fluid intake is much more important. D-penicillamine is another effective therapy, but it is seldom used because it is expensive and has many side effects.

### Selected Readings

Barratt TM. Urolithiasis and nephrocalcinosis. In: Holliday MA, Barratt TM, Vernier RL, eds. Pediatric nephrology, ed 2. Baltimore: Williams & Wilkins, 1987:700.

Bleyer A, Angus ZS. Approach to nephrolithiasis. Kidney 1992;25:1.

Coe F. Treatment of hypercalciuria. N Engl J Med 1984;311:116.

Coe FL, Parks JH, Asplin JR. The pathogenesis and treatment of kidney stones. N Engl J Med 1992;327:1141.

Hufnagle KG, Khan SN, Penn D, et al. Renal calcifications: a complication of long-term furosemide therapy in preterm infants. Pediatrics 1982;70:360.

Hulbert JC, Reddy PK, Gonzales R, et al. Percutaneous nephrostolithotomy: an alternative approach to the management of pediatric calculus disease. Pediatrics 1985;73:610.

Mulley AG Jr. Shock-wave lithotripsy. N Engl J Med 1986;314:845.

Pak CYC, Peters P, Hurt G, et al. Is selective therapy of recurrent nephrolithiasis possible? Am J Med 1981;71:615.

# SECTION VIII

# The Gastrointestinal System

*Principles and Practice of Pediatrics, Second Edition.*
edited by Frank A. Oski et al. J. B. Lippincott Company, Philadelphia © 1994.

## CHAPTER 119

# Normal Gastrointestinal Function

### Mark A. Gilger

The primary functions of the gastrointestinal (GI) tract include the intake, digestion, and absorption of nutrients and fluids, the exclusion and processing of oral pathogens and allergens, and the elimination of waste.

## DEGLUTITION

The normal swallow has three phases—oral, pharyngeal, and esophageal. The oral and pharyngeal phases are voluntary; the esophageal phase is reflexive. In feeding infants, sucking is accomplished by a rhythmic lowering of the tongue and compression of the nipple or areola. The bolus of milk is propelled backward by a rolling action of the tongue posteriorly. The nasopharynx is then sealed off by the soft palate, and the larynx is brought upward and forward as the epiglottis covers the trachea. The esophageal phase begins with a relaxation of the upper esophageal sphincter, allowing the bolus to enter the esophagus. A primary peristaltic wave is initiated, which then transports the bolus to the stomach. A secondary peristaltic wave within the body of the esophagus may be initiated by distention and frequently occurs as a result of esophageal reflux.

Peristalsis is also initiated in the esophagus by migrating motor complexes. These rhythmic involuntary complexes originate independently of swallow or distention and sweep through the entire GI tract, terminating in the rectum.

The ability to swallow solid foods, while partially present at birth, is completely functional by age 4 to 6 months. Children who have not been fed solids by age 15 months have difficulty swallowing them. This suggests that infancy is a critical time in the development of the ability to handle solid foods.

## THE ESOPHAGUS

The esophagus develops from the embryonic foregut. During elongation, the luminal surface differentiates into stratified squa-

mous epithelium. The esophagus and respiratory tract begin as a single tube, which divides by 2 months' gestation. Incomplete division of the tube into two separate organs results in a variety of tracheoesophageal anomalies.

The esophagus is a collapsed hollow tube, lying posterior to the trachea. Unlike the rest of the GI tract, it has no serosal surface. The upper third of the esophagus is striated or skeletal muscle, while the lower esophagus is smooth muscle. The luminal surface is covered with stratified squamous epithelium. Blood is supplied to the upper third of the esophagus by the inferior thyroid artery, while branches of the descending thoracic aorta supply the body. The left gastric artery supplies blood to the lower third of the esophagus. Venous drainage is to the superior vena cava superiorly, the azygos vein from the body, and the gastric veins from the lower esophagus. The gastric veins drain to the portal venous system. In cases of portal hypertension, venous flow can reverse, resulting in esophageal varices. The esophagus is innervated by the spinal accessory nerve and the vagus nerve.

Functionally, the esophagus is divided into three zones: the upper esophageal sphincter, the body, and the lower esophageal sphincter (LES). The upper esophageal sphincter has a resting pressure of about 100 mm Hg and normally is closed. Swallowing results in relaxation and dilation of the upper esophageal sphincter

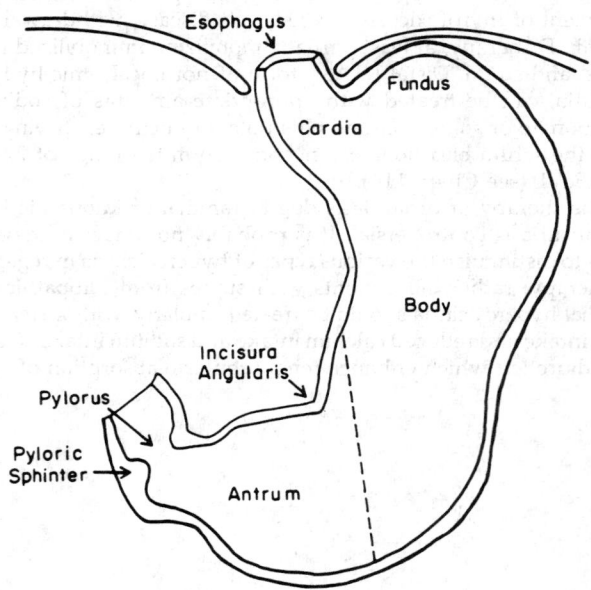

**Figure 119-1.** Anatomical regions of the stomach. (Sleisenger MH, Fordtran JS. Gastrointestinal disease: pathophysiology, diagnosis, and management. ed 3. Philadelphia: WB Saunders, 1983:506. Reproduced by permission.)

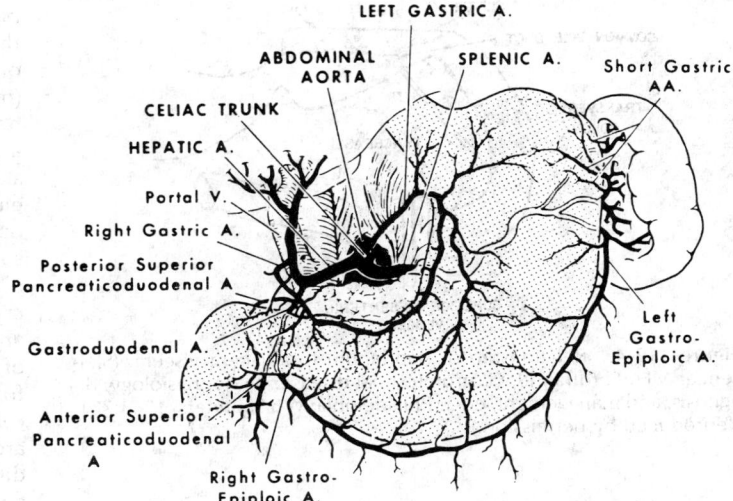

**Figure 119-2.** Blood supply to the stomach and duodenum. Each of the three major branches of the celiac axis supplying the stomach and the anastomotic connections to the superior mesenteric artery near the duodenum is illustrated. (Sleisenger MH, Fordtran JS. Gastrointestinal disease: pathophysiology, diagnosis, and management. ed 3. Philadelphia: WB Saunders, 1983:1544. Reproduced by permission.)

and initiates a primary peristaltic wave that passes through the body of the esophagus. The LES has a resting manometric pressure of about 20 mm Hg and also is normally contracted. The primary peristaltic wave opens the LES for about 7 seconds to allow passage of material into the stomach. The LES then returns to its resting state, which prevents reflux of acidic gastric contents into the esophagus.

## THE STOMACH

The stomach develops from the primitive foregut and is evident by 4 weeks' gestation. Gastric glands appear by about 11 weeks' gestation. Structurally, the stomach is divided into four parts: the cardia, fundus, body, and antrum, terminating with the pyloric sphincter (Fig 119-1). Gastric glands present in the lining of the stomach are composed of four cell types: chief cells (zymogen cells), which contain zymogen granules and secrete pepsinogen; parietal cells (oxyntic cells), which secrete hydrochloric acid and intrinsic factor; mucous neck cells; and endocrine-like cells. Hydrochloric acid production is present at birth and increases in amount until reaching normal adult levels by about 1 month of age. Pepsin production is evident at 16 weeks' gestation and reaches adult levels by age 2 years.

Blood supply is provided by the left and right gastric branches of the celiac artery (Fig 119-2). Venous drainage is through the left and right gastric veins into the portal vein. The stomach is innervated by the vagus nerve.

The stomach has at least four major functions: storing meals, mixing and grinding foods, controlling the emptying of food into the duodenum, and acting as the initial barrier to pathogens and allergens entering the GI tract. The fundus provides most of the storage capacity and responds to the ingestion of food by relaxing and increasing gastric volume. Mixing and grinding of food is accomplished by the phasic gastric contractions and the cone shape of the antrum. The gastric pacemaker, located in the body, generates three-per-second depolarization waves, which initiate contractions that push food toward the antrum (Fig 119-3). These contractions increase in strength at the antrum, forcing the smaller food particles, usually about 1 mm in size, into the duodenum. The emptying of food is controlled by the pylorus, which allows a relatively constant flow of nutrients into the duodenum. Liquids tend to empty more quickly, and factors such as high fat content and high osmolarity of the meal tend to delay gastric emptying.

Gastric acid plays an important role in destroying or damaging intestinal pathogens. This acid barrier is the first of a series of

nonimmunologic mechanisms to eradicate pathogens and other noxious agents.

## THE SMALL INTESTINE

The small intestine develops from the midgut portion of the fetal archenteron or primitive gut. Initial growth occurs out of the

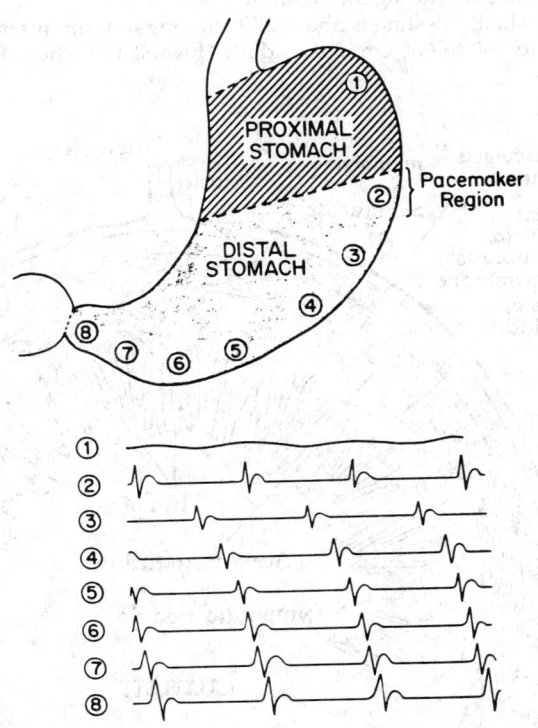

**Figure 119-3.** Electrical regions of the stomach and typical extracellular electrical recordings. The proximal stomach, consisting of the fundus and the proximal third of the corpus, is electrically silent (tracing 1). The distal stomach shows cyclic triphasic potentials, the gastric slow waves, which originate in the pacemaker region along the greater curvature and then sweep distally toward the pylorus. The gastric slow waves organize distal gastric contractions temporally and spatially, since action potentials (not shown) can occur only during the slow wave. (Sleisenger MH, Fordtran JS. Gastrointestinal disease: pathophysiology, diagnosis, and management. ed 3. Philadelphia: WB Saunders, 1983: 526. Reproduced by permission.)

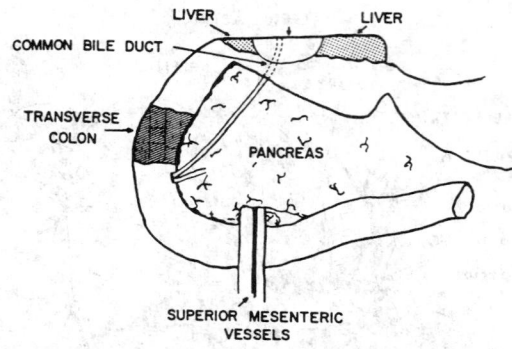

**Figure 119-4.** Relationship of duodenum to adjacent viscera. (Sleisenger MH, Fordtran JS. Gastrointestinal disease: pathophysiology, diagnosis, and management, ed 3. Philadelphia: WB Saunders, 1983:781. Reproduced by permission.)

abdominal cavity, within the vitelline stalk of the umbilicus. It returns into the abdominal cavity by 10 weeks' gestation due to the fixation of the cecum to the right lower quadrant of the abdomen. Failure of this fixation rotation results in the common malrotation syndromes. Villous formation is first apparent at 8 weeks' gestation and proceeds in a proximal to distal fashion. By 12 weeks, the entire small bowel has both villi and crypts, and the enzymatic activities of pepsin, trypsin, and lipase have been documented by 18 weeks' gestation. The small intestine immune apparatus, M cells, and Peyer's patches appear at 2 weeks' gestation. The number of Peyer's patches increases until puberty, then decreases throughout adult life.

The small intestine is about 250 cm long in term infants and grows to 360 to 660 cm in the adult. The first 10 inches of small bowel or duodenum is fixed to the peritoneum (Fig 119-4). Beyond the ligament of Treitz, the intestine is freely mobile, supported only by the mesentery. The small intestine is covered by serosa (mesentery) beginning at the ligament of Treitz (Fig 119-5). Beneath the serosa lie two muscular layers, an outer longitudinal and an inner circular layer, which act in concert to provide peristalsis. Within the submucosa, the next layer, lie numerous cellular elements, including lymphocytes, plasma cells, mast cells, eosinophils, and macrophages. Brunner's glands are present in the submucosa of the duodenum.

The mucosal or luminal surface is covered with the villi and crypts, which increase the surface area available for digestion and absorption of nutrients (Fig 119-6). The villi are composed of at least four cell types: absorptive cells; goblet cells, responsible for mucus production; endocrine cells; and the specialized M cells, the major site of antigen absorption and processing. Crypts are composed of four cell types: Paneth's cells; goblet cells; undifferentiated or principal cells, responsible for cellular proliferation; and endocrine (argentaffin, enterochromaffin) cells, responsible for the production of gut hormones such as gastrin, secretin, cholecystokinin, somatostatin, enteroglucagon, motilin, neurotensin, serotonin, gastric inhibitory peptide, and vasoactive inhibitory peptide.

The two major functions of the small bowel are to digest and absorb nutrients, water, vitamins, and minerals and to recognize and process antigenic and noxious substances. The small intestine absorbs 80% of the water ingested daily, and the colon absorbs the rest (Fig 119-7). Minerals are absorbed either passively, by diffusion, convection, or solvent drag, or by active transport. The absorption of sodium is facilitated by the sodium-potassium pump (Na-K-ATPase) (Fig 119-8).

Digestion begins in the stomach with the action of pepsin on protein. This action is not essential, and most protein digestion

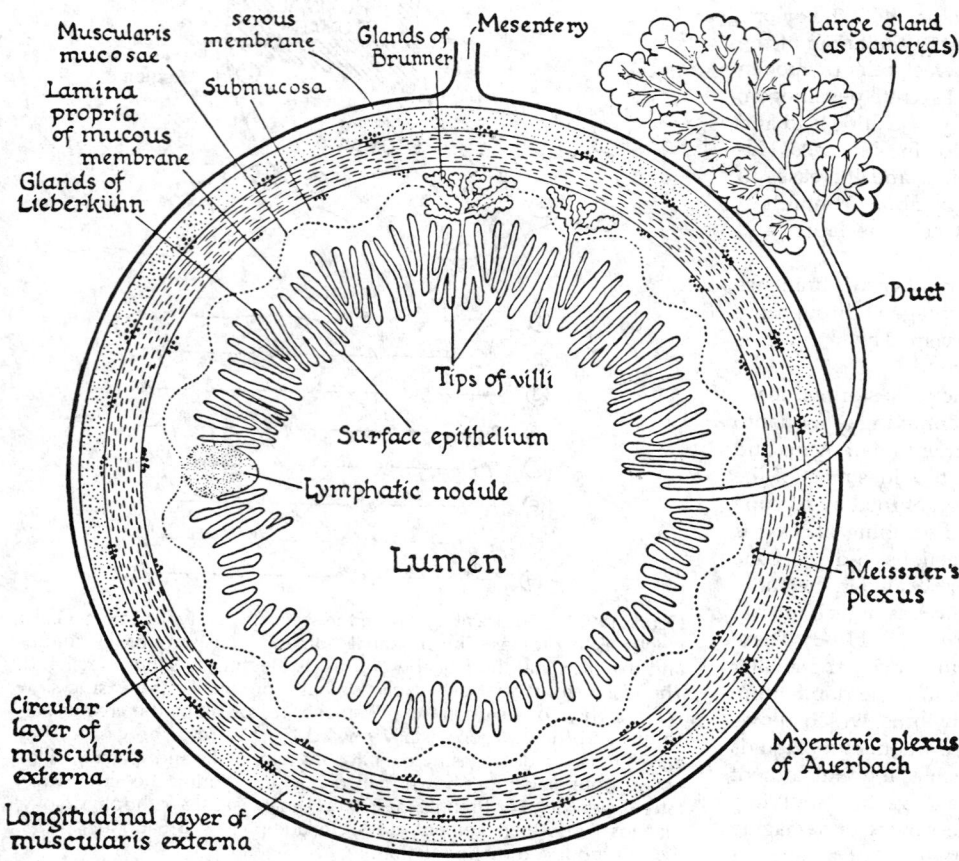

**Figure 119-5.** Schematic cross section of the intestinal tract. (Bloom WN, Fawcett DW. A textbook of histology. Philadelphia: WB Saunders, 1968. Reproduced by permission.)

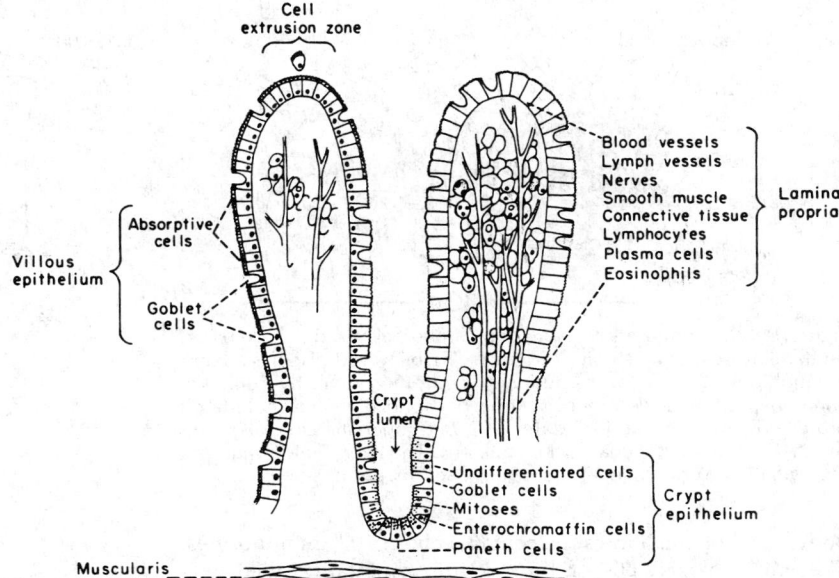

**Figure 119-6.** Diagram of two sectioned villi and a crypt illustrates the histologic organization of the small intestinal mucosa. (Sleisenger MH, Fordtran JS. Gastrointestinal disease: pathophysiology, diagnosis, and management, ed 3. Philadelphia: WB Saunders, 1983:783. Reproduced by permission.)

occurs in the proximal small intestine by the hydrolytic action of the pancreatic enzymes, trypsin and chymotrypsin. Carbohydrate is digested by pancreatic amylase and intestinal brush border enzymes such as galactosidase (lactase), glucosidase (maltase), and sucrase-isomaltase. Salivary amylase contributes little to starch digestion since it is degraded by gastric acid. Fat digestion is accomplished by the action of pancreatic lipase and colipase, which hydrolyze triglyceride to long-chain fatty acids and monoglycerides. Bile salts solubilize fatty acids and monoglycerides through the formation of micelles (Fig 119-9).

The small bowel is sterile at birth but rapidly acquires microflora by both oral and anal routes shortly after birth. The flora become adultlike by 3 years of age, with anaerobes predominating. These microflora remain quite constant through adult life and act as a barrier to bacterial pathogens by preventing their colonization.

## IMMUNOLOGY OF GUT

The small intestinal mucosa contains more immunocytes (plasma cells, lymphocytes, and so forth) than any other organ in the

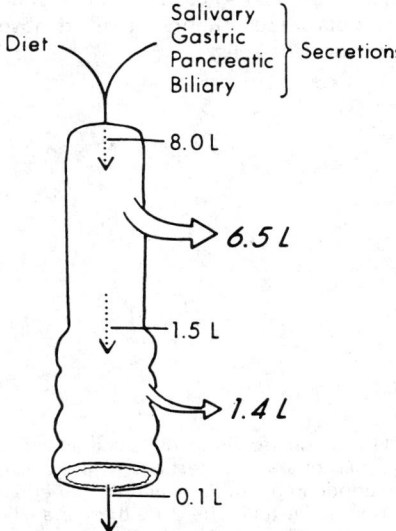

**Figure 119-7.** Approximate values for the volume of fluid entering the small intestine and colon and the small intestinal and colonic water absorption each day in healthy adults. (Sleisenger MH, Fordtran JS. Gastrointestinal disease: pathophysiology, diagnosis, and management, ed 3. Philadelphia: WB Saunders, 1983:812. Reproduced by permission.)

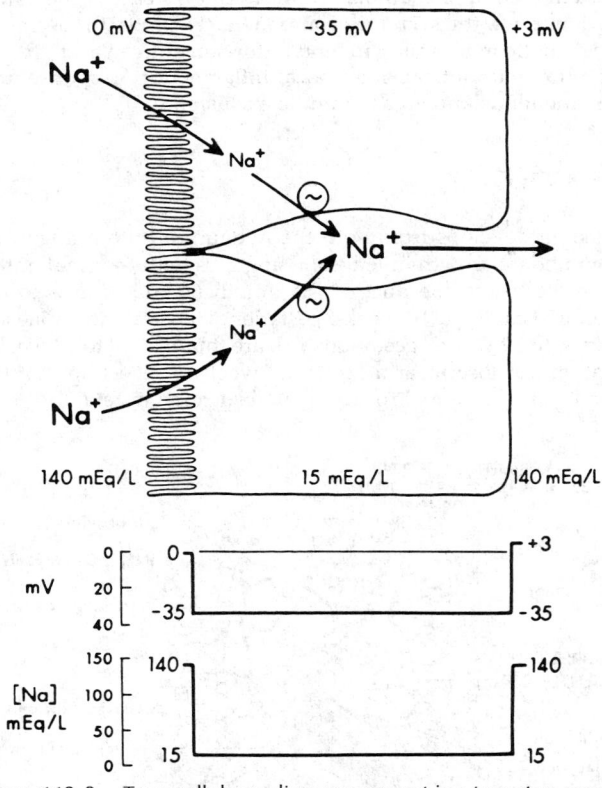

**Figure 119-8.** Transcellular sodium movement is a two-step process. The basolateral sodium pump (Na-K-ATPase) is the driving force for sodium extrusion from the epithelial cell. Intracellular sodium activity is about 15 mEq/L, and the potential difference across the luminal membrane is about 35 mV. Although transcellular sodium movement is against an electrochemical concentration gradient, sodium movement into the epithelial cell is down an electrochemical concentration gradient, as emphasized by the two bottom panels. (Sleisenger MH, Fordtran JS. Gastrointestinal disease: pathophysiology, diagnosis, and management, ed 3. Philadelphia: WB Saunders, 1983:814. Reproduced by permission.)

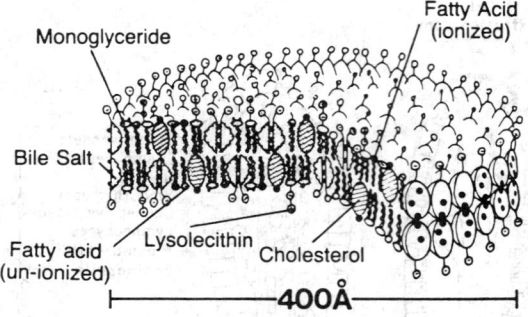

**Figure 119-9.** Proposed structure of the intestinal mixed micelle based on the light-scattering studies of Carey. The bilayered disc has a band of amphiphilic bile salt at its periphery and other, more hydrophobic components (fatty acids, monoglyceride, phospholipids, and cholesterol) protected within its interior. (Carey MC. Enterohepatic circulation. In: Arias AM, Popper H, Schacter D, et al, eds. The liver: biology and pathology. New York: Raven Press, 1982. Used by permission.)

body: 1 cm of small intestine contains about $10^{10}$ immunocytes. The immunologic cells of the gut are commonly called gut-associated lymphoid tissue (GALT). The GALT has four basic components: intraepithelial lymphocytes, solitary lymphoid follicles, lamina propria lymphocytes and plasma cells, and Peyer's patches. Peyer's patches contain M cells (membranous cells). The M cell has no villi and is thought to be the prime site for antigen recognition and absorption. Immunoglobulin A (IgA) in its dimeric form is the predominant antibody of the gut. It is produced locally by plasma cells in the lamina propria and secreted into the lumen after joining to the secretory component (Fig 119-10). Secretory IgA is unique in its ability to bind to foreign antigen and prevent absorption without causing a local inflammatory response; this phenomenon is known as immune exclusion.

## THE COLON

The colon develops from both the midgut and the hindgut. To accommodate growth in length, it migrates with the small intestine into the vitelline duct of the umbilicus and returns to the abdominal cavity at 10 weeks' gestation. Haustra and teniae appear at 8 to 12 weeks' gestation. Villi are found at 10 to 12 weeks' gestation but disappear at 24 to 28 weeks, suggesting that the colon has the potential for nutrient absorption in fetal life.

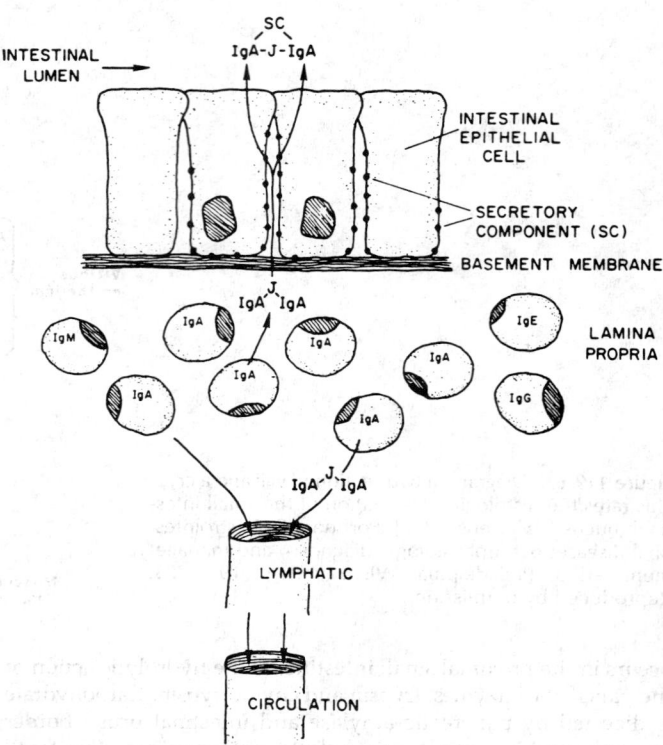

**Figure 119-10.** Transport of IgA into intestinal secretions. Dimer IgA containing J chain is secreted by plasma cells in the lamina propria. This molecule may couple with secretory component (SC) on the basal or lateral surface of the epithelial cell. The sIgA molecule then is transported through the cell and into the intestinal lumen. IgA produced in the lamina propria also can enter the draining lymphatics and circulation. (Adapted from Kagnoff MF. Immunology of the digestive system. In: Johnson LR, ed. Physiology of the gastrointestinal tract. New York: Raven Press, 1981. Used by permission.)

The structure of the colon is similar to that of the small intestine, except the villi are replaced by a flat columnar epithelium and the outer longitudinal muscle is separated into three distinct bands, the teniae coli. Between the teniae are outpouchings, termed haustra, separated by folds. The colonic mucosa is characterized by the crypts of Lieberkühn, lined with absorptive cells, goblet cells, and endocrine cells.

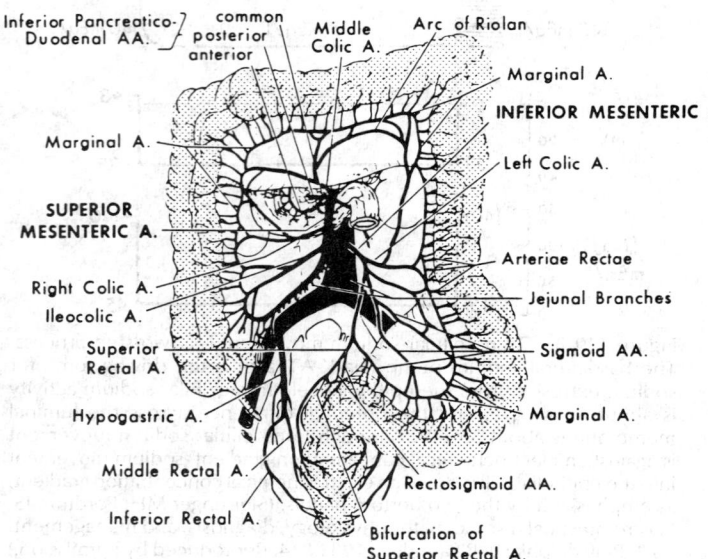

**Figure 119-11.** Blood supply to the small and large intestines. Figure shows anastomotic connections to the celiac axis in the region of the duodenum, and between the superior and inferior mesenteric arteries. Illustrated here are those branches of the left and middle colic arteries that in many patients connect directly (and apart from the marginal artery) to form the arc of Riolan, or "meandering mesenteric" artery. (Sleisenger MH, Fordtran JS. Gastrointestinal disease: pathophysiology, diagnosis, and management, ed 3. Philadelphia: WB Saunders, 1983:1544. Reproduced by permission.)

The blood supply to the colon is via branches of the superior and inferior mesenteric arteries, with associated venous and lymphatic structures (Fig 119-11).

The colon has two basic functions, the absorption of water and electrolytes and the storage and elimination of feces. The colon absorbs all but about 19% of the water left after passage through the small intestine (see Fig 119-7). Colonic microflora can metabolize unabsorbed nutrients, particularly carbohydrate, which can then be absorbed. This process, termed colonic salvaging, may represent a vestigial nutritive function. Fecal material is stored in the distal colon and excreted via a complex series of neural stimuli, addressed in the following chapter.

## Selected Readings

Arey LB. Developmental anatomy. Philadelphia: WB Saunders, 1974.

Brandtzaeg P, Baklien K. Immunohistochemical studies of the formation and epithelial transport of immunoglobulins in normal and diseased human intestinal mucosa. Scand J Gastroenterol 1976;36:1.

Bustamante S, Koldovsky O. Synopsis of development of the main morphological structures of the human GI tract. In: Lebenthal E, ed. Textbook of gastroenterology and nutrition in infancy. New York: Raven Press, 1981:49.

Christie DL. Development of gastric function during the first month of life. In: Lebenthal E, ed. Textbook of gastroenterology and nutrition in infancy. New York: Raven Press, 1981:118.

Estrada RL. Anomalies of intestinal rotation and fixation. Springfield, Ill.: CV Mosby, 1958.

Gray GM, Cooper HL. Protein digestion and absorption. Gastroenterology 1971;61:535.

Herbst JJ. Development of suck and swallow. J Pediatr Gastroenterol Nutr 1981;2(suppl 1):131.

Hofmann AF, Small DM. Detergent properties of bile salts: correlation with physiological function. Annu Rev Med 1967;18:333.

Israel EJ, Walker WA. Host defense development in gut and related disorders. Pediatr Clin North Am 1988;35:1.

Koldovsky O. Development of the functions of the small intestine in mammals and man. Basel: S Karger, 1969.

Scammon RE, Kittleson JA. The growth of the GI tract of the human fetus. Proc Soc Exp Biol Med 1926;24:303.

Siegal M, Lebenthal E. Development of GI motility and gastric emptying during fetal and newborn periods. In: Lebenthal E, ed. Textbook of gastroenterology and nutrition in infancy. New York: Raven Press, 1981:136.

Sleisenger MH, Fordtran JS. GI disease: pathophysiology, diagnosis, and management, ed 3. Philadelphia: WB Saunders, 1983.

Solcia E, Capella C, Buffa R, et al. Endocrine cells of the digestive system. In: Johnson LR, Christensen J, Grossman MI, et al., eds. Physiology of the GI tract. New York: Raven Press, 1981:39.

Tomasi TB Jr. Mechanisms of immune regulation at mucosal surfaces. Rev Infect Dis 1983;5:784.

*Principles and Practice of Pediatrics, Second Edition.*
edited by Frank A. Oski et al. J. B. Lippincott Company, Philadelphia © 1994.

# CHAPTER 120
# *Functional Constipation and Encopresis*

## William J. Klish

Constipation is a common complaint in children and is one of the problems most frequently referred to the pediatric gastroenterologist. Since stool habits are a major concern of many parents, the physician or health-care worker should become familiar with both normal and abnormal patterns of defecation to properly advise parents.

*Constipation* refers to both the frequency of defecation and the consistency of the stool. Both of these parameters change with age and diet, enhancing concern among parents who compulsively monitor their children's stool habits. The normal infant tends to pass a stool after each feeding, but this varies considerably. Breast-fed infants and those fed elemental diets have less frequent stools than infants fed conventional formulas. Children older than 6 months of age tend to pass a stool at least once a day. Less frequent stools should be of concern if they are hard, dry, unusually large, or difficult to pass.

*Encopresis* denotes the syndrome of fecal soiling or incontinence secondary to constipation. Although psychological symptoms are often present in children with this problem, they should not be considered the primary cause of the soiling. Psychogenic incontinence should be a diagnosis reserved for older and previously toilet-trained children who have full bowel movements in their pants on a regular basis.

Many general causes exist for constipation. It is often a familial complaint, and the parents of constipated children often report being constipated when they were children. This implies a genetic component to constipation and may be the result of an increased efficiency of water extraction from fecal material due to either a congenitally long or hypomotile large bowel. Diet plays a role in the volume and hardness of fecal material throughout life. Some dietary residue such as plant fiber tends to make stools soft, whereas other residue, such as the calcium salts in cow's milk, tends to make stools firm. Elemental and chemically defined diets decrease dietary residue and thus decrease stool frequency.

Hospitalized children may become constipated due to a decreased stimulus for defecation resulting from inactivity. Diseases associated with fever may result in acute constipation. Some chronic diseases, such as hypothyroidism, are associated with constipation. The differential diagnosis of constipation is discussed below.

## PATHOPHYSIOLOGY

For defecation to proceed, a normal rectum and puborectalis muscle, normal internal and external anal sphincters, and normal innervation of these structures through both the autonomic and somatic nervous systems must be present. The rectum functions not as a storage area for fecal material but rather as a sensing organ that initiates the process of defecation. When stool moves into the rectum from the sigmoid colon, pressure is put on the wall and the rectal valves. This pressure initiates an impulse within the intrinsic nervous system of the rectum, resulting in relaxation of the internal anal sphincter, which is experienced as the urgency felt just before defecation. If it is inconvenient to defecate, contraction of the external sphincter is initiated first by reflex and then intentionally. The external sphincter is assisted by contraction of the puborectalis muscle, which helps constrict the anal canal. If the external sphincter is held contracted long enough, the reflex to the internal sphincter wanes and the urge to defecate disappears. When it is convenient to defecate, the external sphincter is consciously relaxed and stool is propelled by colonic peristalsis through the open anal canal. As stool enters the anal canal, a secondary reflex is initiated via the somatic nervous system that results in contraction of the abdominal musculature and assists in emptying the lower colon.

Children who develop functional constipation associate discomfort with defecation. The most common reason for discomfort is an anal fissure resulting from either hard stool or the use of suppositories, enemas, or a rectal thermometer. Occasionally, the sense of discomfort results from a bad toilet-training experience. Whatever the cause, the result is the same. Whenever the child feels the sensation associated with relaxation of the internal anal sphincter, he or she aggressively contracts the external sphincter to prevent expulsion of stool and the pain it is expected to bring. Stool collects in the rectum, and over a period of months the rectum gradually dilates. As it enlarges it becomes less capable of propulsive peristaltic activity, resulting in more stool retention. As the rectal volume increases, its sensory capacity diminishes, making retention easier. Eventually, the constipation becomes self-perpetuating.

Encopresis develops when the rectal vault enlarges sufficiently to exert pressure on the structures of the floor of the pelvis, including the levator muscle. This muscle interdigitates with the anal sphincters. As it is pushed downward, the anal sphincters become distorted and the anal canal shortened. If the external anal sphincter is allowed to relax, it assumes a slightly open position. During activity, loose or mushy stool can then flow around firmer stool present in the rectum and leak out. Affected children instinctively know they have little control over the leakage at this point, so they often adopt a casual attitude that is frustrating to their parents. They constantly smell of fecal material, which may result in ridicule by their peers and secondary psychological problems.

## CLINICAL FINDINGS

The most common symptom associated with constipation is chronic recurrent abdominal pain, which occurs in about 60% of the patients. The pains are intermittent and localized to the periumbilical region and resemble functional abdominal pain. Enuresis is reported in about 30% of the children with encopresis. Many have daytime as well as nocturnal enuresis, which resolves when the constipation is treated.

Stools of very large caliber are another associated symptom. Parents often must break up stools mechanically to flush the toilet. The size of the stool is a function of the size of the colon.

Fecal incontinence in children with encopresis tends to occur in the late afternoon and early evening, but can occur at any time of the day or night. The pattern of incontinence tends to parallel the child's activity, with less soiling occurring when the child is sedentary. Most children insist that they do not feel the stools coming and do not perceive the sensation of impending soiling until they actually feel stool in their underwear.

Poor appetite and poor growth are occasionally seen in association with constipation. This may result from early satiety due to the feeling of fullness of the colon. Parents frequently describe their constipated children as lethargic.

## DIAGNOSIS

The diagnosis of functional constipation or encopresis is made from the history and physical examination. Stool is often palpable

in the abdomen, particularly in the left lower quadrant. Rectal examination reveals a short anal canal associated with a large dilated rectum, full of stool. The external sphincter is intact, and the child can squeeze the examiner's finger. The anus should be properly positioned about midway between the scrotum and tip of the coccyx in males and about one-third the distance from the vaginal fourchette in females. It should also be centered within the perianal skin pigmentation.

If a barium enema is done, no bowel preparation should be used so that the large rectum dilated with stool can be appreciated. Dilatation of the rectum to the anal verge is diagnostic of functional constipation and rules out Hirschsprung's disease.

Rectal manometry can be helpful in distinguishing functional constipation from Hirschsprung's disease and sacral nerve abnormalities. Functional constipation is associated with normal relaxation of the internal anal sphincter and no contraction of the external anal sphincter in response to considerable distention of the rectal ampulla. Normal contraction of the external anal sphincter should be elicited by stimulation of the perianal skin to rule out abnormalities of sensory input.

## DIFFERENTIAL DIAGNOSIS

Functional constipation must be differentiated from Hirschsprung's disease, anterior displacement of the anus, and sacral nerve abnormalities (usually associated with spina bifida occulta). Other causes of constipation are listed in Table 120-1.

## TREATMENT

Simple constipation in the neonate is best treated with a nonabsorbable carbohydrate such as that present in dark corn syrup or Maltsupex. Maltsupex is usually given at a dose of 1 teaspoon added to the formula three times a day. In older children and adolescents with simple constipation, stool softeners such as Colace or bulk agents are suggested.

In children with long-standing functional constipation or encopresis associated with a megarectum, a laxative program is required. Treatment is initiated by emptying the rectal vault with an enema. A large-volume enema preparation such as soapsuds is usually more effective than a small-volume enema such as phospho-soda (Fleet enema). If stool in the rectal vault is firm, a preliminary mineral-oil enema will act as a softener and lubricant.

Once the rectum has been cleared of stool, a program of daily laxatives should be initiated to prevent reaccumulation of fecal material and to allow the rectum to return to normal size. Laxatives should be taken only once a day, preferably in the morning so that the day's activity can enhance the effect. The preferred laxative is concentrated, flavored milk of magnesia, starting at a dose of ½ teaspoon for children less than 2 years old, 1 teaspoon for children age 2 to 5 years, and 2 teaspoons for children older than 5 years. The dose is titrated up or down in increments of ½ to 1 teaspoon, depending on the daily response. If a bowel movement did not occur in the previous 24 hours, the dose is increased; if diarrhea occurred in the previous 24 hours, the dose is decreased. Adjustments are made daily until a dose is found that stimulates one or two normal bowel movements per day. It may take 3 to 4 weeks to establish the proper dose of laxative. Other laxatives shown to be effective include senna, given along with mineral oil and lactulose. Whatever laxative is used, the parents should be instructed on how to manage the dose themselves.

Patients should be reexamined at 1- to 2-month intervals, and a rectal examination should be done to determine rectal vault size. Laxatives can be tapered when the rectal vault returns to

Lemoh JN, Brooke OG. Frequency and weight of normal stools in infancy. Arch Dis Child 1979;54:719.
Levine MD. Children with encopresis: a descriptive study. Pediatrics 1975;56:412.
Silverberg M. Constipation in infants and children. Pract Gastroenterol 1987;11:43.
Silverman A, Roy C. Constipation, fecal incontinence, and proctologic conditions. In: Pediatric gastroenterology, ed 3. St. Louis: CV Mosby, 1983.

*Principles and Practice of Pediatrics, Second Edition.*
edited by Frank A. Oski et al. J. B. Lippincott Company, Philadelphia © 1994.

## CHAPTER 121
# *Chronic Nonspecific Diarrhea of Childhood*

### William J. Klish

Chronic nonspecific diarrhea of childhood (also called protracted diarrhea or irritable bowel syndrome) is a common and often frustrating problem seen in children between 6 and 36 months of age. It is characterized by a pattern of two or more loose, voluminous stools per day lasting for more than 4 weeks, unassociated with other symptoms such as pain or growth failure. Children with this syndrome usually are not bothered by the diarrhea. Their parents, however, have difficulty dealing with this symptom since most of the affected children are still in diapers and the stool volume is so great that it spills from the diapers, making a mess.

## ETIOLOGY

Although chronic nonspecific diarrhea of childhood is the most common form of chronic diarrhea without failure to thrive in young children, the etiology remains unknown. Since malabsorption of nutrients is not a factor in this disease, the cause of the diarrhea is either enhanced secretion of fluid in the distal bowel or interference with absorption of water and electrolytes from the colon. Chronic nonspecific diarrhea is frequently initiated by an acute infection that is usually treated with a broad-spectrum antibiotic such as ampicillin, so alteration of bacterial flora in the colon may play a role in the etiology of the diarrhea.

Some investigators have thought that the diarrhea might be induced by the increased intake of fluids observed in these children. However, the increased thirst is more likely to be the effect rather than the cause of the diarrhea. Some children drink large amounts of fruit juice, such as apple juice. This undoubtedly plays some role in the perpetuation of the diarrhea, since apple juice contains enough nonabsorbable carbohydrate such as sorbitol to induce colonic fermentation, resulting in the stimulus for diarrhea, as seen in other forms of carbohydrate intolerance.

A low dietary fat intake has been hypothesized to play a role in the persistence of the diarrhea, but this observation has not

---

**TABLE 120-1. Causes of Constipation**

**Functional Constipation and Encopresis**

**Dietary Causes**
Protracted vomiting
Excessive intake of cow's milk
Lack of bulk in diet

**Drugs That Affect Motility**

**Structural Defects of the Anus or Rectum**
Anterior displacement of the anus
Anal or rectal stenosis
Presacral teratoma
Rectal prolapse

**Smooth Muscle Disease**
Scleroderma
Dermatomyositis
Systemic lupus erythematosus
Primary chronic intestinal pseudo-obstruction

**Abnormal Myenteric Ganglion Cells**
Hirschsprung disease
Chagas' disease
von Recklinghausen disease
Multiple endocrine neoplasia type 2B

**Absence of Abdominal Musculature**

**Spinal Cord Defects**
Spina bifida occulta
Myelomeningocele
Meningocele
Diastematomyelia
Paraplegia
Cauda equina tumor
"Tethered cord" syndrome

**Metabolic and Endocrine Disorders**
Hypothyroidism
Hypoparathyroidism
Renal tubular acidosis
Diabetes insipidus
Vitamin D intoxication
Idiopathic hypercalcemia
Hypokalemia

**Neurologic and Psychiatric Conditions**
Myotonic dystrophy
Amyotonia congenita
Mental retardation
Psychosis

---

normal size, which may take 6 months to 1 year. At that time, parents and children should be instructed about proper diet and the use of bulk agents to avoid hard stools. During laxative therapy, attempts should be made to establish a bowel habit. Once the parent determines when the laxative begins to stimulate, the child should be asked to sit on the toilet at that approximate time each day. This behavior should continue after the laxative has been discontinued.

## Selected Readings

Davidson M, Kugler MM, Bauer CH. Diagnosis and management in children with severe and protracted constipation and obstipation. J Pediatr 1963;62:261.

held up under scrutiny. However, since many of these children eventually are placed on strict elimination diets, dietary restriction of fiber and other residue may help perpetuate the loose stools.

One group of investigators has suggested that disordered small intestine motility plays a role in the etiology of chronic nonspecific diarrhea of childhood. They showed that the migrating motor complex of the duodenum was not suppressed as it normally should be with the introduction of glucose into the bowel. This implies that children with this disorder have relative hypermotility of the intestine during meals.

## DIFFERENTIAL DIAGNOSIS

The diagnosis of chronic nonspecific diarrhea of childhood should be suspected if the following criteria are met: child's age between 6 and 36 months; two or more loose, voluminous stools per day, frequently containing undigested food particles; diarrhea lasting for more than 4 weeks; absence of abdominal pain; absence of failure to thrive; and absence of a definable cause for the chronic diarrhea.

Disaccharide intolerance, infection, protein hypersensitivity, and occasionally inflammatory bowel disease can mimic chronic nonspecific diarrhea in presenting symptoms. Carbohydrate intolerance can be diagnosed by placing the patient on a totally unrestricted diet with milk and testing several stools for the presence of sugar or acid. Unabsorbed disaccharide (lactose or sucrose) will appear in the stool either unchanged or partially fermented to the monosaccharides, including glucose. Their presence can be determined through the use of Clinitest tablets or glucose test tape. Completely fermented sugars result in the production of organic acids such as acetic and butyric acids. Their presence can be found by testing the stool pH with nitrazine paper. A pH of less than 5.5 is considered suggestive of carbohydrate intolerance.

Stools should be cultured for bacteria. Most pathogenic bacteria cannot produce diarrhea for longer than several weeks. However, *Campylobacter jejuni* has been implicated in several cases of chronic diarrhea and must be ruled out. The presenting symptoms of *Giardia lamblia* infection can be identical to those of chronic nonspecific diarrhea, and this infection must also be ruled out.

A complete blood count with differential, reticulocyte count, and a stool guaiac test might give a clue to the presence of either protein hypersensitivity or inflammatory bowel disease. Eosinophilia is occasionally present in protein hypersensitivity. If this diagnosis is suspected, a carefully constructed elimination diet should be initiated, making certain that the child receives adequate intake to thrive.

## TREATMENT

Before initiating treatment, it is important to stress that although the diarrhea is hard for the parents to deal with, it does not threaten the child's well-being. Treatment fails in 10% to 20% of children regardless of the form of therapy. The syndrome improves with age, and most children have outgrown it by age 3 years.

Therapy should be initiated by placing the child on a normal diet for his or her age. If the diet has been restricted, many children will normalize their stool pattern due to an increase in dietary residue. If large amounts of fruit juices are being given, attempts should be made to substitute other liquids.

Psyllium bulk agents are very effective at minimizing the diarrhea. A dose of 2 to 3 g of psyllium fiber should be given twice a day for 2 weeks. It can be mixed with other foods for palatability. If a good response is obtained, the psyllium can usually be dis-

continued without return of the diarrhea. If no response is seen in 7 to 10 days, there is no need to persist with psyllium therapy. Other bulk agents do not appear to be as effective as psyllium.

Cholestyramine has been used successfully to treat this syndrome. A dose of between 7.5 and 20 g/day, divided into four doses, should be given for 2 weeks. Since there is some potential for side effects from cholestyramine, this should not be tried until after psyllium therapy fails.

Occasional children will respond to a 7- to 10-day course of metronidazole. The recommended amount is 15 mg/kg/day, divided into three doses.

## Selected Readings

Boyne LJ, Kerzner B, McClung HJ. Chronic nonspecific diarrhea: the value of a preliminary observation period to assess diet therapy. Pediatrics 1985; 79:557.

Cohen SA, Hendricks KM, Eastham EJ, et al. Chronic nonspecific diarrhea. Am J Dis Child 1979;133:490.

Fenton TR, Harries JT, Milla PJ. Disordered small intestinal motility: a rational basis for toddlers' diarrhea. Gut 1983;24:897.

Smally JR, Klish WJ, Campbell MA, Brown MR. Use of psyllium in the management of chronic nonspecific diarrhea of childhood. J Pediatr Gastroenterol Nutr 1982;1: 361.

Walker WA. Benign chronic diarrhea of infancy. Pediatr Rev 1981;3:153.

*Principles and Practice of Pediatrics, Second Edition.*
edited by Frank A. Oski et al. J. B. Lippincott Company, Philadelphia © 1994.

## CHAPTER 122
# *Gastrointestinal Bleeding*

### Marilyn R. Brown

Gastrointestinal (GI) bleeding in children is common, and occasionally it is life-threatening. The physician first should determine if the child has bled. Therapy may need to be instituted before the site of bleeding is determined. The physician should attempt to find out whether the bleeding is from the upper (originating above the ligament of Treitz) or lower GI tract. The etiology and specific site of bleeding should be determined, if possible. Twenty years ago, a definite cause could be found in only about half the cases, but current diagnostic techniques, including fiberoptic endoscopy, radiography, scintigraphy, and angiography, allow localization of the site of bleeding in most cases.

Some causes of bleeding are more likely to occur at different ages, and some causes are associated with different rates of bleeding, varying from slow loss of small amounts to rapid loss of large amounts. Minor bleeding may be due to esophagitis, infective and allergic enterocolitis, Crohn disease, colonic polyps, and anal fissures. Slow chronic bleeding can result from chronic esophagitis, chronic inflammatory bowel disease, and sometimes from colonic polyps. Acute significant losses may be due to esophageal varices, hemorrhagic gastritis, peptic and stress ulcers, Meckel's diverticulum, ulcerative colitis, and vascular malformations. Passage of a "currant jelly" stool (mixed blood and mucus, of light-red color) often indicates an acute intestinal obstruction such as midgut volvulus or intussusception (the telescoping of one part of the intestine into another).

## ESTABLISHING BLOOD LOSS

It must first be determined if blood loss has occurred. Many substances ingested by children may be mistaken for blood. Red food coloring, fruit-flavored drinks, fruit juices, and beets may color the vomitus or stool reddish. Stools can acquire a black color from ingested iron, bismuth subsalicylate, grape juice, spinach, and blueberries. The vomitus is tested by Gastroccult (pH-buffered) and the stool by guaiac, Hemoccult, or Hematest for the presence of blood. If a child presents in the office with anemia for which there is no clear explanation, several stools should be tested for occult blood.

## TYPE OF BLEEDING

A description of the color, location, and amount of blood is usually helpful. Did the child cough up blood (hemoptysis) or vomit up blood (hematemesis) following epistaxis? Gastric acid will turn the blood a brown color. Bright-red blood (hematochezia) or blood streaking in the stool is most often due to polyps, proctitis, or constipation with anal fissures or hemorrhoids. Bright-red blood on the outside of the stool accompanied by pain on passage of the stool is usually from an anal fissure. Bright-red blood mixed with mucus in a loose stool is typical of chronic ulcerative colitis. The classic currant jelly stool occurs from ileocolic intussusception and may occur with midgut volvulus. Melena (black or dark-maroon stool) suggests a lesion proximal to the right colon, such as a Meckel's diverticulum. A bleeding duodenal ulcer may present with red bloody stools instead of melena because of rapid transit through the GI tract.

If the patient enters the emergency department with melena or hematochezia with evidence of anemia or hypotension, gastric contents must be aspirated to look for evidence of upper GI bleeding.

The magnitude of the blood loss is important in formulating the therapeutic and diagnostic plan, as is the patient's age. Severe life-threatening hemorrhage is rare in children, but the cause is usually found; in contrast, the cause of chronic slow blood loss is sometimes difficult to determine.

## AGE-INDEPENDENT ETIOLOGIES

Certain causes of GI bleeding are more common in specific age groups, but there is considerable overlap (Table 122-1). At all ages, stress (burns, CNS trauma) and aspirin ingestion may lead to gastric stress erosions and ulcerations. Thrombocytopenia and coagulopathies must be considered. Intestinal bleeding is not uncommon in children with cancer who develop thrombocytopenia secondary to chemotherapy. Chemotherapy may be followed by esophagitis, gastritis, and enterocolitis. Although primary tumors of the GI tract are rare, they must be considered in the differential diagnosis at any age. Giardiasis is rarely accompanied by blood in the stool, but this is common in amebiasis.

## AGE-ASSOCIATED ETIOLOGIES

### Neonatal

In the first few days of life, hematemesis or the passage of bloody stools in a healthy newborn is most likely due to swallowed ma-

**TABLE 122-1. Etiologies of GI Bleeding**

**Neonate**
Swallowed maternal blood
Hemorrhagic disease of the newborn
Anal fissure
Hemorrhagic gastritis
Stress ulcers
Infective enterocolitis
Protein-sensitive enterocolitis
Hirschsprung enterocolitis
Duplication cysts
Midgut volvulus
Vascular malformations

**The First 6 Months of Life**
Nonspecific colitis
Anal fissure
Esophagitis
Infective enterocolitis
Protein-sensitive enterocolitis
Intussusception
Lymphonodular hyperplasia
Duplication cysts
Hirschsprung enterocolitis
Vascular malformations

**6 Months to 5 Years**
Epistaxis
Esophagitis
Esophageal varices
Gastritis
Infective enterocolitis
C difficile colitis
Lymphonodular hyperplasia
Intussusception
Meckel's diverticulum
Vascular malformations
Henoch-Schönlein purpura
Hemolytic-uremic syndrome
Neutropenic typhlitis
Polyps
Anal fissure

**5 to 18 Years**
Same as 6 mo–5 yr, plus
Mallor-Weiss tear
Gastritis
Peptic ulcer
Chronic ulcerative colitis
Crohn disease
Hemorrhoids

ternal blood, which can be differentiated from fetal hemoglobin by the Apt alkali denaturation test. If the red blood denatures with alkali to a brown color, the hemoglobin is of adult origin.

Hemorrhagic disease of the newborn with prolongation of the prothrombin time must be considered when vitamin K has not been given. Breast-fed infants are particularly susceptible to this complication.

An anal fissure is a common cause of bleeding, usually initiated by the passage of a firm stool that makes a small tear along the anal canal.

Significant bleeding in the neonate, particularly the stressed newborn and premature infant, may occur from hemorrhagic gastritis, gastric erosions, or gastric stress ulcers. Necrotizing enterocolitis (ischemic damage to the bowel wall) may begin with mild diarrhea, which is positive for reducing substances, and with increased gastric residuals after feeding, followed by the appearance of abdominal distention, pneumatosis intestinalis, and blood in the stool. Hirschsprung enterocolitis, midgut volvulus, and intestinal duplication cysts may also present with bleeding and must be kept in mind.

Irritation from nasogastric tube feedings is a common cause of small amounts of blood in the gastric aspirate or stool.

## The First 6 Months

Nonspecific colitis has recently been shown to be a common cause of hematochezia in infants younger than 6 months old. Gastroesophageal reflux in the infant is very common and may cause reflux esophagitis with blood loss.

Of the bacterial etiologies, shigellosis or salmonellosis may cause small amounts of blood in diarrheal stool, but *Campylobacter jejuni* is a more common cause. Enteroinvasive, enterotoxic, and enteropathogenic *Escherichia coli* infections can cause bloody diarrhea, but tests for diagnosis are not readily available. Recently, testing for *Escherichia coli* serotype 0157: H7 which causes bloody diarrhea and hemolytic-uremic syndrome has become more widely available. Antibiotic-associated diarrhea is common, but blood loss in the stool is not common. The presence of *Clostridium difficile* organisms and toxin is fairly common in the asymptomatic infant, but the association of antibiotic usage and subsequent diarrhea with blood in the stools may signify a causative role. Viral diarrheas are less often associated with blood in the stool.

Milk- or soy protein-induced enteropathy is a common cause of blood-streaked stools early in infancy. This may also occur in breast-fed infants, and the mother may be tried on a milk- or soy-free diet.

Lymphonodular hyperplasia of the colon is characterized by multiple tiny yellowish nodules, which are enlarged lymphoid follicles with mucosal inflammation and thin epithelial lining overlying them. These nodules are thought to be secondary to infection and are often associated with the appearance of blood in the stool.

Intestinal arteriovenous malformations, hemangiomas, or telangiectasias will occasionally bleed.

## 6 Months to 5 Years

Epistaxis must always be considered as a cause of blood in vomitus. The blood loss from gastroesophageal reflux associated esophagitis may be associated with "coffee grounds" (dark brown) emesis, but is generally occult; it may cause chronic anemia.

Extrahepatic portal hypertension from extrahepatic blockage of the portal vein may occur early in life, and the associated esophageal varices may first bleed during the second year of life. Bleeding from esophageal varices secondary to liver disease may occur at any age.

Intussusception occurs most often during the first 2 years of life and usually presents with brief, frequent spasms of severe abdominal pain. The process may progress to vomiting, lethargy, currant jelly stools, and complete intestinal obstruction. A sausage-shaped mass may be felt in the abdomen. Diagnosis is confirmed by barium enema or ultrasound, and reduction with air, water, or barium under mild pressure is successful in most cases. In patients over age 2, a mass acting as a lead point is often present.

Meckel's diverticulum, a remnant of the oomphalomesenteric duct located about 30 cm from the ileocecal valve, is often asymptomatic; however, when it contains gastric mucosa, acid secretion can cause ulceration of the adjacent ileum with subsequent painless bleeding presenting as black or maroon stools and anemia. The diagnosis is made by $^{99m}$Tc pertechnetate radionuclide scan. Some radiologists use intravenous histamine-2 receptor blockers (H2 blocker) to enhance visualization. Pertechnetate is taken up by epithelial cells of the gastric mucosa. Surgery is indicated for bleeding. A Meckel's diverticulum may act as a lead point for intussusception.

Henoch-Schönlein purpura is a systemic vasculitis in which abdominal cramps and intestinal bleeding may precede the purpuric skin manifestations. Hemolytic-uremic syndrome may follow a variety of infections such as *E coli* 0157:H7, causing a severe colitis with frequent bloody stools before the onset of uremia and anemia. Neutropenic typhlitis is a necrotizing enterocolitis involving the cecum and right colon in immunosuppressed patients.

Juvenile colonic polyps (inflammatory hamartomas) are the most common cause of intermittent painless hematochezia in children 2 to 5 years old. Most polyps are solitary and located within 30 cm of the anus. The diagnosis is made by digital rectal examination, barium enema, sigmoidoscopy, or colonoscopy. Snare cauterization polypectomy through the colonoscope is appropriate.

## 5 to 18 Years of age

Although the following diagnoses may be made before a patient is 5 years old, these diagnoses are more common afterwards.

Epistaxis is more common in older children. An episode of forceful vomiting may cause a small linear (Mallory-Weiss) tear at the gastroesophageal junction, with minimal or moderate blood loss. Ingestion of caustic medications may irritate the esophageal mucosa.

Gastric erosions from aspirin ingestion are less common today because of the decreasing use of aspirin in children. The increased use of nonsteroidal anti-inflammatory drugs has been associated with increased abdominal pain and evidence of gastritis and bleeding.

The spiral gram-negative organism *Helicobacter pylori* (formerly known as *Campylobacter pylori*) may inhabit the surface of antral mucosal epithelial cells. Its presence is always associated with local inflammation (chronic gastritis). Children with *H pylori* gastritis may present with recurrent epigastric pain, nausea, vomiting, hematemesis, and occult blood in the stools. Most children with duodenal ulcers have *Helicobacter* infection. If the organism can be eradicated, the relapse rate after treatment of the ulcer is 20%; if the organism is not eradicated, the relapse rate is about 80%. The organism can be detected by testing an endoscopic antral biopsy for urease activity, or by observing the organism microscopically in the antral biopsy specimen. A C13 urea breath test is a noninvasive diagnostic test for urease activity. Positive antibody titers indicate past or present infection. The organism is sensitive to bismuth subcitrate, amoxicillin, tinidazole, and metronidazole. The highest rate of eradication with drugs available in the United States is with combination therapy, usually bismuth subsalicylate, amoxicillin, metronidazole, and an $H_2$ blocker for 4 to 6 weeks.

The inflammatory bowel diseases—Crohn disease and chronic ulcerative colitis—are of unknown etiology and are characterized by a remitting–relapsing symptom pattern. In mild stages of Crohn disease, chronic ulcerative colitis, or ulcerative proctitis, there may be only occult blood or small amounts of visible blood in the stool. Crohn disease that involves only the small intestine may be accompanied only by occult blood in the stool. The nearer the lesions are to the anus, the more likely it is that hematochezia will occur. Tenesmus is more common in ulcerative colitis, whereas Crohn disease may present with painless bright-red bleeding. Severe blood loss is more common in ulcerative colitis, but occurs in both. Both usually have other signs and symptoms, including diarrhea, weight loss, fever, abdominal pain, anorexia, malaise, joint pain, and decreased growth. Diagnosis is suspected by history, physical examination, the presence of microcytic anemia, thrombocytosis, elevated erythrocyte sedimentation rate, or hypoalbuminemia, and is confirmed by intestinal radiographs, colonoscopy, and biopsy. Sulfasalazine (or the newer acetylsalicylate derivatives) and corticosteroids are the mainstays of treatment.

Peutz-Jeghers syndrome consists of diffuse GI hamartomas, most marked in the small bowel, associated with melanotic areas on the buccal mucosa and lips. Other chronic polyposes include juvenile polyposis coli, familial adenomatous polyposis, and Gardner's syndrome (familial adenomatous polyposis associated with bony lesions, subcutaneous tumors, and cysts). The latter two conditions have clear malignant potential, and colectomy in late childhood is advised.

Vascular lesions take a variety of forms. Telangiectasias may be associated with Turner syndrome. Small angiodysplasias, hemangiomas, or arteriovenous malformations may occur, and arteriography may be helpful in diagnosis. Hemorrhoids are relatively uncommon in children, so portal hypertension should be considered. A rare cause of monthly bleeding in an adolescent female is ectopic endometrium in the GI tract.

## DIAGNOSIS

A careful history and physical examination will be helpful in most cases (Fig 122-1). The child's condition will determine the rapidity of the approach to diagnosis. If the child is pale and weak with tachycardia and hypotension, immediate stabilization of the cardiovascular status is paramount, and history, physical examination, diagnosis, and therapy must be done rapidly.

Important elements of the history include the child's age, amount and character of the bleeding in vomitus or stool, associated abdominal or rectal pain, diarrhea, drug ingestion, fever, systemic symptoms such as joint pain or aphthous ulcerations, growth pattern, recent illnesses, foreign travel, and family history of GI or bleeding disorders.

Important components of the physical examination are general appearance; vital signs; examination of skin for telangiectasias,

purpura, or melanotic spots on lips; evidence of epistaxis, abdominal organomegaly, tenderness, or masses; and anorectal examination to verify the presence of blood in the stool and to identify fissures, fistulas, and distal polyps.

If there is upper GI bleeding on gastric aspiration, upper endoscopy is attempted when the gastric aspirate following lavage is almost clear. Small-diameter endoscopes allow examination of infants. If upper GI bleeding has stopped or has been minimal, an upper GI radiologic exam or upper endoscopy may be done. Upper GI bleeding usually is accompanied by melena; however, if the bleeding has been abrupt, the stool guaiac may still be negative. Also, bleeding from a duodenal ulcer may result in red blood in the stools if the transit through the intestinal tract is rapid.

Upper GI bleeding is more likely to be massive than is lower GI bleeding. Massive lower GI bleeding may come from a Meckel's diverticulum, arteriovenous malformation, or intestinal duplication, but occasionally occurs with the inflammatory bowel diseases. Currant jelly stool with abdominal pain and tenderness suggests infarction of the bowel secondary to intussusception. Similar findings may be present secondary to intestinal volvulus or an incarcerated internal hernia, which are also surgical emergencies.

Melena may signify upper or lower GI bleeding. Meckel's diverticulum commonly presents as painless melena in a healthy 18- to 24-month-old child who has a significant decrease in hematocrit. If bleeding is ongoing, visualization through the colonoscope may be hindered by the blood. In these situations, a $^{99m}$Tc sulfur colloid-labeled red cell scan or angiography may be helpful in identifying a site of bleeding. If these do not identify a lesion, colonoscopy can be attempted following a large-volume cleansing electrolyte lavage. CT or MRI scanning is helpful only when the bleeding is from an identifiable mass.

If hematochezia is accompanied by diarrhea, a sigmoidoscopy is helpful in determining friability or visualizing the pseudomembranes associated with *C difficile* infection. Biopsies may reveal amebae or distinguish between chronic and acute inflammatory changes. Stool cultures for *Shigella, Salmonella, C jejuni, Yersinia, E coli* 0157: H7, and *C difficile* toxin should be considered.

Colonoscopy is most helpful in the diagnosis of inflammatory bowel disease, arteriovenous malformations visible through the mucosal surface, lymphonodular hyperplasia, and polyps. Barium enemas are valuable for detecting polyps, inflammatory bowel disease, lymphonodular hyperplasia, Hirschsprung disease, and

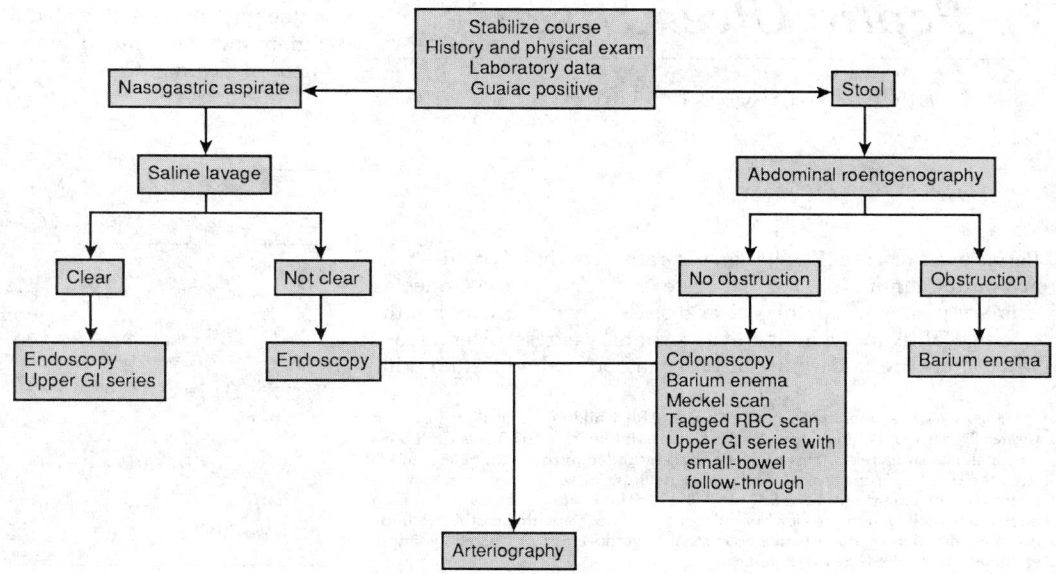

**Figure 122-1.** Approach to acute GI bleeding.

colonic duplication, and for the diagnosis and treatment of intussusception.

## THERAPY

Therapy of a massive GI hemorrhage is aimed at resuscitating the patient, localizing the site of bleeding, and deciding on a treatment plan to stop the hemorrhage. If orthostatic or frank hypotension is present, an intravenous catheter is inserted to obtain blood for laboratory studies and for the infusion of normal saline or colloid until properly typed and crossmatched blood is available. Blood is sent for complete blood count, type and crossmatch, erythrocyte sedimentation rate, platelet count, clotting functions, liver function tests, blood urea nitrogen, and serum electrolytes. A large-bore nasogastric tube is placed into the stomach and gastric contents are aspirated. An aspirate of red blood or "coffee grounds" material from the stomach indicates bleeding above the ligament of Treitz, although absence of blood does not rule out bleeding just distal to the pylorus. If fresh blood is present, saline lavage is done until bleeding ceases. Abdominal roentgenograms taken in the upright, supine, and cross-table lateral positions are taken to look for signs of obstruction and air outside the GI tract.

Further therapy for severe upper GI bleeding consists of blood replacement and neutralization of gastric acid. An intravenous infusion of an $H_2$-receptor antagonist such as cimetidine (10 mg/kg q 6 hr) may be used to decrease gastric acidity.

After endoscopy and intravenous administration of an $H_2$ blocker, antacids and sucralfate may be given through the nasogastric tube to keep the gastric pH above 5 and to coat the irritated mucosal surfaces. If bleeding esophageal varices are seen, or if the bleeding site cannot be identified and bleeding continues, intravenous vasopressin (2.5 units/kg over 20 minutes followed by 0.01 units/kg/minute continuously for 24–48 hours) is given. Currently the use of a somatostatin analogue and nitroglycerine is being evaluated.

If bleeding cannot be controlled, sclerotherapy or rubberbanding for varices, endoscopic heater probe (or laser) coagulation of bleeding sites, selective angiography with embolization, or surgery is the next step.

Therapy for mild bleeding depends on the lesions found.

In an intensive care unit, GI bleeding occurs in 5% to 10% of the children. Significant bleeding requiring transfusion occurs most often in children with coagulopathy.

## Selected Readings

Chang MH, Wang TH, Hsu JY, et al. Endoscopic examination of the upper GI tract in infancy. Gastrointest Endosc 1983;29:15.

Drumm B, Sherman P, Cutz E, et al. Association of *Campylobacter pylori* on the gastric mucosa with antral gastritis in children. N Engl J Med 1987;316:1557.

Hillemeier C, Gryboski JD. GI bleeding in the pediatric patient. Yale J Biol Med 1984;57:135.

Hyams JS, Leichtner AM, Schwartz AN. Recent advances in diagnosis and treatment of GI hemorrhage in infants and children. J Pediatr 1985;106:1

Killbridge PM, Dahms BB, Czinn SJ. *Campylobacter pylori*-associated gastritis and peptic ulcer disease in children. Am J Dis Child 1988;142:1149

Liebman WM. Diagnosis and management of upper GI hemorrhage in children. Pediatr Ann 1976;5:690.

Oldham KT, Lobe TE. GI hemorrhage in children. Pediatr Clin North Am 1985;32:1247.

Sherman NJ, Clatworthy HW Jr. GI bleeding in neonates. A study of 94 cases. Surgery 1967;62:614.

Silber GH, Klish WJ. Hematochezia in infants less than 6 months of age. Am J Dis Child 1986;140:1097.

Spencer R. GI hemorrhage in infancy and childhood: 476 cases. Surgery 1964;55:718.

*Principles and Practice of Pediatrics, Second Edition.*
edited by Frank A. Oski et al. J. B. Lippincott Company, Philadelphia © 1994.

# CHAPTER 123
# *Peptic Ulcer Disease*

## Kathleen J. Motil

Peptic ulcer disease (PUD) is an ulcerative condition of the stomach or duodenum that may be acute or chronic. It is classified as primary peptic (idiopathic) ulcer disease when it occurs in otherwise healthy individuals and as secondary (stress) ulcer disease when there are underlying disorders associated with injury, illness, or drug therapy. Most primary peptic ulcers are chronic and more often duodenal in origin; most stress ulcers are acute and more often gastric in location (Table 123-1).

Although PUD is thought to be relatively uncommon in children, recent advances in fiberoptic endoscopy and $H_2$-receptor antagonist therapy have led to increased awareness of the condition, more accurate diagnoses, and an aggressive approach to medical treatment.

This work is a publication of the USDA/ARS Children's Nutrition Research Center, Department of Pediatrics, Baylor College of Medicine and Texas Children's Hospital, Houston, Texas. This project has been funded in part with federal funds from the U.S. Department of Agriculture, Agricultural Research Service under Cooperative Agreement number 58-7-MN1-6-100. The contents of this publication do not necessarily reflect the views or policies of the U.S. Department of Agriculture, nor does mention of trade names, commercial products, or organizations imply endorsement by the U.S. Government.

| TABLE 123-1. Patterns of PUD and Their Frequency in Children | | |
|---|---|---|
| | Frequency (%) | |
| Clinical Feature | *Primary Peptic Ulcer* | *Secondary Stress Ulcer* |
| Duration of symptoms | | |
| Acute | 17 | 96 |
| Chronic | 83 | 4 |
| Location of ulcer | | |
| Gastric | 16 | 30 |
| Duodenal | 33 | 21 |

# ETIOLOGY AND PATHOGENESIS

The etiology of PUD in children is unknown, but the heterogeneity of its manifestations suggests that different mechanisms may account for its development.

The pathogenesis of PUD is thought to relate to an imbalance between destructive and defensive factors in the gastrointestinal (GI) tract (Table 123-2). The destructive factors of the gastric mucosa include endogenous and exogenous factors, such as hydrochloric acid, pepsin, bile salts, ethanol, drugs, and stress, while the defensive factors include the unstirred mucous layer, bicarbonate secretion, mucosal blood flow, prostaglandins, and epithelial cell renewal.

Acid is essential in the development of primary PUD. Oxidative phosphorylation of glucose and fatty acids within the gastric parietal cells produces hydrogen ions that are actively secreted across a concentration gradient into the gastric lumen. There is good correlation between the number of parietal cells in the stomach and acid output. When intraluminal acid concentrations are twice normal, the gastric barrier may be broken. When other substances such as pepsin, bile or its metabolites, alcohol, salicylates, or urea are placed in the stomach, further disruption of the barrier may occur. Disruption of the mucosal barrier allows increased back-diffusion of hydrogen ions from the gastric lumen into the mucosal cells, further damaging the gastric tissue. This destruction is associated with release of histamine, which in turn leads to vasodilation and stimulates the parietal and chief cells to produce more acid and pepsin, respectively. Protection against mucosal destruction is provided by the secretion of the surface mucous layer, the active transport of bicarbonate for buffering capacity, prostaglandin synthesis, and mucosal blood flow containing an adequate oxygen and nutrient supply for epithelial cell function and renewal.

The regulation of acid secretion is accomplished by several factors, including the parasympathetic fibers of the nervous system, gastrin, and histamine. Vagal innervation stimulates the parietal cell mass directly through the release of acetylcholine and indirectly through the release of gastrin from antral G cells. Gastrin is the most important stimulant of gastric acid secretion and is released in the presence of an alkaline antrum, by direct contact with ingested peptides and amino acids, and by the intravenous administration of calcium. Histamine is thought to exert a permissive effect on acid secretion by sensitizing parietal cells to other stimuli.

The most important factor in the development of PUD in children is the production of hydrochloric acid and gastrin. Acid secretion in infancy begins after 48 hours of life and achieves adult levels by age 6 months (Table 123-3). Basal acid production in children with primary PUD generally is higher than in healthy individuals (Table 123-4). Maximal and peak acid production

| TABLE 123-3. Gastric Acid Secretion in Infants and Children After Stimulation | | |
|---|---|---|
| Age | Volume (mL/hr) | Acid Output (mEq/kg/hr) |
| 4 wk | 3 | 0.02 |
| 12 wk | 13 | 0.10 |
| 24 wk | 64 | 0.17 |
| 4–9 yr | 42 | 0.24 |
| >11 yr | 143 | 0.19 |

during pentagastrin stimulation also is greater in children with PUD, although there is overlap with normal values.

Serum gastrin concentrations are normal in children with primary or secondary gastric ulcers and may be normal or moderately elevated (100 to 120 pg/mL) with primary duodenal ulcers (Table 123-5). Hypergastrinemia may be seen in other entities, such as the Zollinger-Ellison syndrome, antral G-cell hyperplasia, long-standing pyloric obstruction, renal failure, short-gut syndrome, hyperparathyroidism, multiple endocrine neoplasias, pheochromocytoma, neurofibromatosis, primary pernicious anemia, and atrophic gastritis.

# PATHOLOGY

Primary peptic ulcers usually are solitary lesions located in the duodenum and less commonly in the gastric antrum (Table 123-6). The lesions are round or oval, less than 2 cm in size, and have a sharply punched-out defect. The ulcer may be superficial, may erode into the muscularis mucosa, or may penetrate the entire wall into adjacent organs. Chronic ulcers underlying scarred mucosa may cause puckering of the gastric folds and result in a spoke-like appearance on gross examination. The histologic appearance in PUD is that of active necrosis. The base and margins of the ulcer have fibrinoid debris overlying an acute inflammatory infiltrate. In the base of the ulcer, granulation tissue infiltrated with mononuclear cells is present and rests on a more solid collagenous scar. With re-epithelialization, the glands of the mucosal margins become mucus-secreting, a change called intestinalization.

Secondary stress ulcers occur as single or multiple lesions and are found primarily in the stomach. The lesions tend to be circular, less than 1 cm in diameter, and involve the mucosa or superficial epithelium. The ulcer base appears brown due to acid digestion of superficial bleeding, but the lesion is not indurated. An acute inflammatory infiltrate may be found in the margins and base of the ulcer, but scarring of the blood vessel walls is absent. Re-epithelialization is rapid and demonstrates many mitotic nuclei.

| TABLE 123-2. Pathophysiology of PUD Disease | |
|---|---|
| Destructive Factors | Defensive Factors |
| Endogenous | Endogenous |
|   Hydrochloric acid |   Unstirred mucous layer |
|   Pepsin |   Bicarbonate secretion |
|   Bile salts |   Mucosal blood flow |
| Exogenous |   Prostaglandins |
|   Ethanol |   Epithelial cell renewal |
|   Drugs | |
|   Stress | |

| TABLE 123-4. Gastric Acid Production in Children With Peptic Ulcer Disease | | | |
|---|---|---|---|
| | Hydrochloric Acid Output (mEq/kg/hr) | | |
| Group | Basal | Maximal | Peak |
| Ulcer disease | | | |
|   Duodenal | 0.12 ± 0.04 | 0.51 ± 0.05 | 0.57 ± 0.04 |
|   Gastric | 0.06 ± 0.02 | 0.47 ± 0.08 | 0.52 ± 0.10 |
| Healthy | 0.07 ± 0.02 | 0.30 ± 0.05 | 0.36 ± 0.05 |

| TABLE 123-5. Serum Gastric Levels in Children With Peptic Ulcer Disease | | | |
|---|---|---|---|
| | Serum Gastrin (pg/mL) | | |
| | | Protein Meal Stimulation | |
| Group | Basal | (1 h Postprandial) | (2 h Postprandial) |
| Ulcer disease | | | |
| Duodenal | 40 ± 7 | 69 ± 11 | 57 ± 9 |
| Gastric | 44 ± 7 | 50 ± 7 | 46 ± 6 |
| Healthy | 34 ± 6 | 45 ± 6 | 39 ± 7 |

## EPIDEMIOLOGY

The incidence of PUD in children is unknown (Table 123-7). The prevalence is estimated to be 1.7% in large general pediatric practices and 3.4 per 10,000 pediatric hospital admissions. The male/female ratio is 1.5 : 1. Primary PUD occurs at any age, but its frequency is higher in older children and adolescents. Primary and stress ulcers occur in a ratio of 7:1 in children more than 6 years old. Secondary stress ulcers are more common in infants less than 6 months old and are equal in frequency to primary peptic ulcers in children aged 6 months to 6 years.

## PREDISPOSING FACTORS

Several entities have been implicated as predisposing factors for PUD in children (Table 123-8). The genetic influence is important: a family history of ulcers can be elicited in at least 30% of children with primary peptic disease. Studies of twins also suggest a greater frequency of concordance in identical than in fraternal twins. Patients are more often HLA-B5 positive, and complications of PUD occur more frequently in individuals with blood group type O. Two thirds of the patients with PUD have elevated pepsinogen I levels. This pattern of pepsinogen is inherited in an autosomal dominant manner and is thought to be a useful marker for the genetic predisposition to PUD. Genetic factors do not play a role in secondary stress ulcers.

The role of emotional stress in the development of primary PUD is controversial. Children who have ulcers try hard to please, are described as "nervous" and perfectionists, tend to excel in schoolwork, often experience family discord, and may have experienced recent separation or loss within the family. Emotional disturbances can be identified in nearly 40% of the children with PUD.

Exogenous factors such as alcohol use, cigarette smoking, and caffeine use increase the incidence of ulcer formation. Alcohol and caffeine stimulate the production of acid, while cigarette smoking decreases pancreatic secretions and alkalinity in the duodenum.

Drugs and systemic illnesses have been associated with the production of secondary ulcers. Corticosteroid therapy often is complicated by the appearance or reactivation of stress ulcers, presumably due to the inhibition of phospholipase A and prostaglandin synthesis. Similarly, aspirin and nonsteroidal anti-inflammatory agents inhibit prostaglandin synthesis, thereby increasing the risk of ulcer formation. Stress ulcers in children can occur in conjunction with systemic illnesses such as sepsis, hypotension, respiratory distress, extensive burns (Curling's ulcer), and brain injury (Cushing's ulcer). These ulcers may result from a low-flow state (ie, a shunting of blood from the superficial epithelium during stress, leading to a relative hypoxemia and depletion of nutrients necessary for the energetics of cellular metabolism).

Recently a spiral, urease-producing bacterium, *Helicobacter pylori*, has been associated with primary antral gastritis and peptic ulcerations in children. The gastritis is characterized by infiltrates of polymorphonuclear leukocytes in the acute stage, followed by infiltrates of lymphocytes and plasma cells in the chronic stage. *H pylori* is not present in secondary gastritis associated with disorders such as Crohn disease or eosinophilic gastroenteritis. The organism may be found in ulcers located in the esophagus or duodenum, but only in the presence of gastric metaplasia. *H pylori* is a major predisposing factor to PUD, but infection alone is insufficient to cause ulcer formation. Little is known about the source and spread of *H pylori*, but transmission from infected family contacts has been suggested. The eradication of *H pylori* results in a rapid resolution of the acute inflammatory component of the gastritis, but the chronic inflammatory component may persist for as long as 1 year. The eradication of the organism also is associated with a pronounced reduction in the relapse rate of duodenal ulcers. Ulcer relapse is associated with either reinfection or recrudescence of *H pylori* infection.

## CLINICAL FEATURES

The clinical picture of PUD in children is variable and depends on the classification of the ulcer and the patient's age. Abdominal pain, generally localized to the epigastric or periumbilical area, is the most common presenting symptom (Table 123-9). Typical ulcer pain that worsens with fasting, is relieved with meals, and wakens the patient at night is uncommon in children. Nausea, vomiting, and anorexia occur in 25% or less of the children with ulcer disease, and hematemesis and melena in less than 20%. Frontal headaches are present in about 10% of children. Failure to thrive is rarely associated with PUD.

Abdominal tenderness and overt GI bleeding are found on physical examination in at least half the children with PUD. An

| TABLE 123-6. Pathologic Features of Peptic Ulcer Disease | | |
|---|---|---|
| Type of Ulcer | Macroscopic Features | Microscopic Features |
| Primary peptic | Solitary | Fibrinoid crater base |
| | Located in duodenum | Acute inflammation |
| | Superficial or erosive | Granulation tissue |
| | | Collagenous scarring of blood vessels |
| Secondary stress | Multiple | Shallow hemorrhagic base |
| | Located in stomach | Acute inflammation |
| | Superficial | |

**TABLE 123-7. Epidemiology of Peptic Ulcer Disease in Children**

| Feature | Occurrence |
|---|---|
| Incidence | ? |
| Prevalence (%) | 1.7 |
| Sex (male/female) ratio | 1.5:1 |
| Age distribution (%) | |
| Birth to 6 mo | 14 |
| 6 mo to 2 yr | 8 |
| 2 to 5 yr | 17 |
| 5 to 10 yr | 30 |
| 10 to 15 yr | 31 |

**TABLE 123-9. Presenting Features of Peptic Ulcer Disease in Children**

| Clinical Feature | Frequency (%) |
|---|---|
| **Symptom** | |
| Abdominal pain | 71 |
| Epigastric | 57 |
| Periumbilical | 32 |
| "Typical" | 9 |
| Nausea | 25 |
| Vomiting | 18 |
| Hematemesis | 18 |
| Melena | 13 |
| Anorexia | 17 |
| Headache | 11 |
| Failure to thrive | 3 |
| **Sign** | |
| Abdominal tenderness | 58 |
| GI bleeding | 53 |
| Acute abdomen | 22 |
| Perforation | 18 |
| Obstruction | 7 |
| Anemia | 11 |

acute abdomen with features of abdominal distention, decreased bowel sounds, and peritoneal irritation, consistent with the diagnosis of intestinal perforation or obstruction, occurs in nearly one fourth of children at presentation.

In general, infants and children less than 6 years old are more likely to have an acute secondary ulcer in conjunction with illness, surgery, or trauma; older children and adolescents tend to display features of primary PUD. The features of primary PUD generally are chronic symptoms of abdominal pain and vomiting, while secondary ulcers are more frequently associated with acute GI bleeding and vomiting.

In the neonate, perforation of a gastric ulcer usually is the first manifestation of the disease, although bleeding also occurs. The neonate commonly has a history of prematurity, respiratory distress, sepsis, hypoglycemia, or an intraventricular hemorrhage. Infants less than 3 years old may present with chronic symptoms consistent with the diagnosis of primary PUD. However, ulcers in this age group usually are acute; manifest with hematemesis, melena, or perforation; and are associated with underlying illness or injuries. Secondary ulcers in this age group are located equally in the stomach or duodenum, while primary ulcers tend to occur in the stomach. In children between 3 and 6 years of age, periumbilical pain and vomiting are the more common presenting symptoms characteristic of primary disease, although hematemesis and melena associated with stress ulcers may be seen. The stomach and duodenum are affected equally.

In children more than 6 years old and in adolescents, the clinical findings are comparable to those in adults with primary PUD. Epigastric abdominal pain that awakens the child at night or is relieved with food is typical. In other instances, the pain

**TABLE 123-8. Factors Predisposing to Peptic Ulcer Disease in Children**

**Primary Peptic Ulcer**
Genetic factors
Psychological factors
Alcohol
Caffeine
Cigarette smoking
*Helicobacter pylori*

**Secondary Stress Ulcer**
Drugs (corticosteroids, aspirin, nonsteroidal agents)
Complications of systemic illness (sepsis, hypotension, respiratory distress)
Injury (burns, brain injuries)

may be a vague abdominal discomfort with little relief from food, or may radiate to the back or upper quadrants if penetration of a viscus occurs. Hematemesis, melena, and anemia may be noted frequently.

Despite the presence of typical complaints, the interval between the onset of symptoms and the establishment of a diagnosis may exceed 10 months. Duodenal ulcers are more common in primary PUD. However, secondary ulcers, when present, may be found equally in the stomach and the duodenum and usually are associated with chronic diseases of the lungs, kidneys, liver, or joints.

## LABORATORY AND RADIOLOGIC STUDIES

Laboratory studies in PUD generally are normal unless overt or occult bleeding is a prominent feature. About 10% of children with PUD have an iron-deficiency anemia. Hemoglobin, hematocrit, serum iron, and ferritin levels may be low, while the reticulocyte count and total iron-binding capacity may be elevated with chronic blood loss. Red blood cell smears may show hypochromic, microcytic morphology, and stool smears may be positive for occult blood.

Gastric acid analysis shows higher maximal and peak acid outputs after pentagastrin stimulation in PUD, although there is overlap with normal values (see Table 123-4). Fasting serum gastrin levels in children with ulcers may be within the normal range or elevated; however, the response of serum gastrin levels to a protein meal is higher than normal in children with primary PUD (see Table 123-5). Neither of these tests is performed routinely unless the patient remains symptomatic despite appropriate medical management or the diagnosis of Zollinger-Ellison syndrome is entertained. In the presence of antral gastritis and PUD, *H pylori* may be detected by an *H pylori*-specific IgG antibody serologic test or a $^{13}$C-urea breath test. Pepsinogen I levels also may be useful to predict which children with PUD will relapse after attaining ulcer healing in conjunction with $H_2$-receptor antagonist or *H pylori* therapy. Serum pepsinogen I levels also are elevated (>90 mg/mL) in PUD and may serve as a reliable marker of the genetic predisposition to primary PUD.

An upper GI series is the most readily available test for the diagnosis of PUD in children. Roentgenographic signs of PUD in the duodenum are characterized by a filling defect or a deformity of the duodenal bulb. In some instances, duodenal irritability may be the only finding because the barium moves too rapidly out of the bulb or a fibrin clot covers the ulcer. Ulcer craters also may be found in the pyloric region, leading to outlet obstruction. The diagnosis of PUD should not be made unless a persistent crater is demonstrated. Deformity of the duodenal bulb with scar formation suggests the presence of a previous ulcer and does not imply the presence of currently active disease.

Primary gastric ulcers usually are located on the lesser curvature of the stomach. The crater is sharply delimited and surrounded by edematous, radiating gastric folds that may obstruct the pyloric channel. In contrast, stress ulcer craters are shallow and often multiple, and may be present in both the stomach and duodenum.

Overall, upper GI series detect PUD in 70% of the children who are studied. The frequency of detection for duodenal ulcer, however, is 89%, compared with 50% for gastric ulcers. Air contrast imaging may enhance the features of primary and secondary PUD and lead to more accurate diagnosis.

Other roentgenographic studies may be necessary to document the presence of complications of PUD. Abdominal films in the upright or lateral decubitus position may demonstrate free air in the abdomen if perforation has occurred. Similarly, celiac axis angiography may be useful to identify the source of persistent upper GI bleeding caused by PUD.

## Endoscopy

Fiberoptic endoscopy has become the diagnostic procedure of choice for the detection of PUD in children. Gastroesophagoduodenoscopy is indicated to determine the source of upper GI bleeding and to make the initial diagnosis of PUD, or when roentgenographic findings are absent in symptomatic patients. Endoscopy confirms the diagnosis of PUD in 97% of the patients examined for this purpose. Detection of *H pylori* requires cultures, measurement of urease activity (CLO test, Delta West, Australia), or Warthin-Starry silver stains of the antral biopsy tissue specimens.

## DIFFERENTIAL DIAGNOSIS

The diagnosis of PUD in children may be difficult to make because the symptoms often mimic those of other diseases. Indeed, errors in diagnosis may be as high as 12%; the most common incorrect diagnoses are appendicitis and Meckel's diverticulum. The principal conditions to consider in the differential diagnosis are gastroduodenitis, Zollinger-Ellison syndrome, chronic recurrent (functional) abdominal pain, gastroesophageal reflux, esophagitis, pancreatitis, cholelithiasis, appendicitis, Meckel's diverticulum, intussusception, inflammatory bowel disease, and infectious diarrhea (Table 123-10). The symptoms of abdominal pain, vomiting, and rectal bleeding may be common to all of these entities and lead to a significant diagnostic dilemma. Therefore, the diagnosis of PUD depends primarily on the physician's awareness and should be considered early in the differential diagnosis of abdominal pain.

*Nonulcer peptic disease*, or *gastroduodenitis*, may present with the classic manifestations of PUD or with atypical features characterized by poorly localized, periodic abdominal pain and tenderness, nausea, vomiting, belching, bloating, flatus, and anorexia.

| TABLE 123-10. Differential Diagnosis of Peptic Ulcer Disease | |
|---|---|
| Gastroduodenitis | Cholelithiasis |
| Zollinger-Ellison syndrome | Appendicitis |
| Chronic recurrent abdominal pain | Meckel's diverticulum |
| Gastroesophageal reflux | Intussusception |
| Esophagitis | Infectious diarrhea |
| Pancreatitis | Inflammatory bowel disease |

The condition is clinically indistinguishable from PUD and the diagnosis must be confirmed by endoscopy and biopsies.

*Zollinger-Ellison syndrome*, an uncommon diagnosis in children, is characterized by hypersecretion of gastric acid, intractable ulcer disease, and intestinal malabsorption due to a gastrin-secreting tumor (gastrinoma) of the pancreas. Fasting serum gastrin levels usually are increased and may assist in the differential diagnosis. In some instances, secretin stimulation studies and CT scanning of the abdomen are necessary to differentiate between PUD and this entity.

*Chronic recurrent abdominal pain* occurs in about 10% of school-aged children and may be difficult to distinguish from PUD. The precipitating factors associated with chronic recurrent abdominal pain often are vague or have a psychosocial overlay in an otherwise well child. The diagnosis of functional abdominal pain usually is made by excluding organic illness through appropriate diagnostic studies, including endoscopy if necessary.

*Gastroesophageal reflux, esophagitis, pancreatitis, cholecystitis,* and *appendicitis* may be confused with primary PUD because these illnesses have similar clinical features, including epigastric or periumbilical abdominal pain, nausea, and vomiting. Similarly, *Meckel's diverticulum, intussusception, inflammatory bowel disease,* and *infectious diarrhea* may manifest with rectal bleeding and can mimic the pattern of secondary stress ulcers. Multiple diagnostic studies, including serum amylase determinations, liver function studies, stool cultures for pathogenic bacteria and smears for parasites, ultrasonography, roentgenographic studies, radionuclide imaging, and upper or lower endoscopy, may be necessary to delineate the cause of the illness and eliminate the possibility of PUD (Table 123-11).

## TREATMENT

The goal of medical therapy in PUD is to promote ulcer healing, relieve pain, and prevent complications. The control of gastric acid production by drugs, diet, and the avoidance of factors that stimulate acid secretion is essential (Table 123-12).

The mainstay of medical management includes antacids (Maalox II, Mylanta II) and $H_2$-receptor antagonists (cimetidine, ranitidine, famotidine). Antacids promote the healing of ulcers and provide relief of symptoms by neutralizing gastric acid. The recommended oral dosage for primary PUD is 0.5 mL/kg of a liquid preparation (30 mL/1.73 m²) 1 and 3 hours after meals and at bedtime for 6 weeks. In the presence of stress ulcers, acute bleeding can be controlled by a nasogastric drip of antacids, 1.0 mL/kg/hr (60 to 80 mL/1.73 m²/hr), adjusted to maintain the gastric pH above 4. The side effects of antacid therapy—diarrhea and constipation—can be ameliorated by adjusting the proportion of magnesium and aluminum in the dosing regimen. Calcium antacids and sodium bicarbonate are unsuitable for chronic use because of the potential for increased acid secretion after buffering capacity ceases or systemic alkaline and sodium loading, respectively.

TABLE 123-11. Diagnostic Studies
for Peptic Ulcer Disease in Children

**Laboratory Studies**
Complete blood cell count and differential
Reticulocyte and platelet counts
Prothrombin time, partial thromboplastin time
Serum iron, total iron-binding capacity, ferritin
Fasting serum gastrin
Serum amylase
Liver function studies
Serum bilirubin, alkaline phosphatase
Stool guaiac, culture, smears
*H pylori*-specific IgG, IgA antibodies
$^{13}$C-urea breath test

**Radiologic Studies**
Upper GI series
Meckel scan
$^{99m}$Tc-tagged red blood cell scan
Angiography

**Special Studies**
Gastric acid analysis
Duodenoscopy and biopsy

TABLE 123-12. Treatment of Peptic Ulcer
Disease in Children

**Medical**
Hospitalization
Nasogastric suction and lavage
Blood transfusion
Medications (antacids, H$_2$-receptor antagonists, anticholinergics)
Diet (avoid snacks)
Abstinence (cigarette smoking, alcohol, aspirin)

**Surgical**
Truncal or selective vagotomy
Pyloroplasty
Antrectomy

H$_2$-receptor antagonists are potent inhibitors of basal and food-stimulated acid production. Their use is associated with a healing rate of 90% in children with PUD. The oral regimens for cimetidine and ranitidine are 30 to 40 mg/kg/day in four divided doses and 6 mg/kg/day in three divided doses, respectively, for 6 to 8 weeks. H$_2$-receptor antagonist therapy may be a useful nighttime adjunct to antacid therapy if night pain occurs. In the presence of complications of PUD, cimetidine (20 to 30 mg/kg/day in six divided doses) or ranitidine (2 to 3 mg/kg/day in four divided doses) may be given intravenously to minimize acid production. H$_2$-receptor therapy also is effective in the prophylaxis of GI bleeding after critical illness, brain injury, or surgery. Side effects associated with these drugs are uncommon; rebound hypersecretion of hydrochloric acid may occur after discontinuation of the medication. Compliance with H$_2$-receptor antagonist therapy has been better than compliance with antacids alone. Maintenance therapy with H$_2$-receptor antagonists does not protect entirely against a recurrence of primary PUD. Therapy with these drugs beyond 1 year is not recommended, although serious long-term side effects have not been documented.

Other medications such as sucralfate and anticholinergic drugs may be added to the therapeutic regimen. Sucralfate binds to the erosive surface of the ulcer and protects the mucosa from further damage. Anticholinergics such as propantheline bromide (0.25 mg/kg/dose) decrease acid secretion, but the effective dose often produces side effects such as blurred vision and dry mouth. Cytoprotective drugs have not been studied sufficiently in children to warrant their use.

Dietary intervention also may promote ulcer healing. Milk feedings have been found to raise the gastric pH and to prevent GI bleeding in hospitalized children. The factors responsible for the reduction of gastric acidity are unknown, although several peptides and hormones found in bovine and human milk have been implicated. Frequent snacks should be avoided to minimize food-stimulated acid secretion. Alcoholic beverages, cigarette smoking, aspirin, and other drugs that damage the gastric mucosal barrier are contraindicated.

The treatment of *H pylori*-associated PUD is controversial. H$_2$-receptor antagonist therapy is associated with healing of the acute ulcerations in the duodenum, but it does not resolve the antritis nor eradicate *H pylori*. The most effective treatment against the organism requires a course of triple-drug therapy, including bismuth salts (Pepto-Bismol), amoxicillin, and metronidazole for 6 weeks. Combination therapy results in the successful eradication of *H pylori* in 80% of the cases. *H pylori*-specific IgG antibodies or pepsinogen I levels can be used to monitor the success of therapy; levels of these markers increase with the exacerbation of *H pylori* and decrease with its eradication.

The surgical management of PUD is reserved for patients with complications of ulcers, including intractable pain, perforation, hemorrhage, and obstruction. Truncal or selective vagotomy with pyloroplasty, or in some instances antrectomy, is the most common procedure performed in children with PUD.

## COMPLICATIONS

Hospitalization for PUD usually is unnecessary unless the complications of intractable pain, obstruction, active bleeding, or perforation are present. If signs of gastric outlet obstruction are found, food should be withheld and nasogastric suction applied for several days. Surgical intervention should be considered if the obstruction does not resolve within 72 hours of nasogastric drainage. If GI bleeding is present, a large-bore nasogastric tube should be inserted and the stomach lavaged repeatedly with ice-cold normal saline. Vital signs, central venous pressure, and hematocrit values should be monitored carefully to determine whether blood transfusions are necessary. During severe hemorrhage, selective abdominal angiography may be necessary to identify the site of bleeding. Intravenous vasopressin, 0.3 to 0.4 units/1.73 m$^2$/min for 48 hours, may control active bleeding. Surgical intervention should be considered when one third to one half of the total blood volume has been replaced.

## PROGNOSIS

The prognosis of primary PUD in children and adolescents is less than optimal. Disease recurs within 1 year in 35% to 50% of all patients, and at least two thirds have repeated relapses over the years. About 60% of children with recurrences require surgery, although the availability of H$_2$-receptor antagonists may reduce this rate. However, the benefits of safe and effective surgical intervention may outweigh the long-term inconvenience, cost, and disability associated with chronic relapsing PUD.

The prognosis of secondary stress ulcers is affected by the precipitating illness or injury. The outcome in the neonate with gastric hemorrhage and perforation is poor. Healing generally occurs in infants and children who develop an acute ulcer, although emergency surgery may be necessary for hemorrhage or perforation. Recurrences of stress ulcers are unlikely with resolution of the underlying illness.

## Selected Readings

Blumer JL, Rothstein FC, Kaplan BS, et al. Pharmacokinetic determination of ranitidine pharmacodynamics in pediatric ulcer disease. J Pediatr 1985;107:301.

DeGiacomo C, Lisato L, Negrini R, et al. Serum immune response to *Helicobacter pylori* in children: epidemiologic and clinical implications. J Pediatr 1991;119:205.

Drumm B, O'Brien A, Cutz E, et al. *Campylobacter pyloridis*-associated primary gastritis in children. Pediatrics 1987;80:192.

Drumm B, Rhoads JM, Stringer DA, et al. Peptic ulcer disease in children: etiology, clinical findings, and clinical course. Pediatrics 1988;82:410.

Drumm B, Sherman P, Chiasson D, et al. Treatment of *Campylobacter pylori*-associated antral gastritis in children with bismuth subsalicylate and ampicillin. J Pediatr 1988;113:908.

Gryboski JD. Peptic ulcer disease in children. Med Clin North Am 1991;75:899.

Nord KS, Rossi TM, Lebanthal E. Peptic ulcer in children. Am J Gastroenterol 1981;75:153.

Tam PKH. Hypergastrinemia in children with duodenal ulcer. J Pediatr Surg 1988;23:331.

Tam PKH, Saing H. Gastric acid secretion and emptying rates in children with duodenal ulcer. J Pediatr Surg 1986;21:129.

Tam PKH, Saing H, Lau JTK. Diagnosis of peptic ulcer in children: the past and present. J Pediatr Surg 1986;21:15.

*Principles and Practice of Pediatrics, Second Edition.*
edited by Frank A. Oski et al. J. B. Lippincott Company, Philadelphia © 1994.

# CHAPTER 124
# *Intussusception*

## William J. Pokorny

Intussusception is the most common cause of intestinal obstruction in infants aged 3 months to 1 year. It is rare in the first month of life. There is great regional variation in the incidence of intussusception, from less than 0.5 to four per 1000 live births.

## PATHOPHYSIOLOGY

Intussusception is the result of invagination or telescoping of a portion of the bowel into the more distal bowel (Fig 124-1). The portion of the bowel that invaginates into the more distal bowel, the *intussusceptum*, is pulled along with its mesentery by peristaltic waves. As the proximal bowel is pulled into the lumen of the *intussuscipiens*, or distal bowel, the mesentery is compressed and angled, resulting initially in lymphatic obstruction and subsequently in venous obstruction. The intussuscepted mass quickly obstructs the intestinal lumen, with resulting distention and peristaltic rushes proximal to the obstructing mass. With each peri-

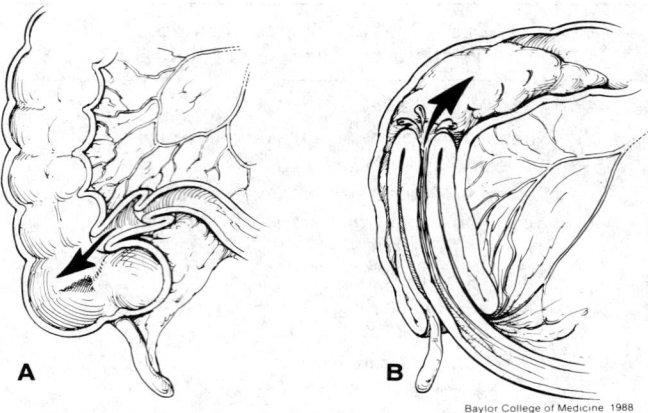

**Figure 124-1.** The development of an ileocolic intussusception. (**A**) The invagination typically begins several centimeters proximal to the ileocecal valve. As the ileum is drawn into the more distal bowel, the lumen is obstructed and the mesenteric vessels become compressed. (**B**) Edema and venous engorgement develop, with accumulation of blood and mucus ("currant jelly") in the lumen of the colon. If not reduced, infarction of the intussusceptum occurs.

staltic rush the patient experiences colicky pain. Early in the course of illness, the affected infant will reflexively evacuate the distal colon and pass several partially formed stools. As reflex ileus and pylorospasm develop, the infant begins to vomit. Initially the vomitus is clear, but as signs of intestinal obstruction develop, the vomitus becomes bile-stained and eventually fecaloid. The peristaltic rushes and colicky pain first occur at intervals of several minutes and last only a few seconds. During the intervals between peristaltic rushes, the infant appears to be in no discomfort, and the abdomen is soft and scaphoid.

At this time a mass is almost always palpable. Since 95% of the cases of intussusception are ileocolic, with the invaginating bowel beginning just proximal to the ileocecal valve, the sausage-shaped mass can be found in the distribution of the colon, commonly in the area of the hepatic flexure but occasionally more distally. In 3% of the cases, the intussuscepting intestine prolapses through the rectum.

As the edema from lymphatic obstruction and venous engorgement increases, the hydrostatic pressure within the intussusception increases until it equals the arterial pressure, at which time arterial inflow ceases. During this process, the intestinal mucosa becomes ischemic, with a transition of the endothelial cells to goblet cells and an outpouring of mucus into the intestinal lumen. Venous engorgement results in leakage of blood into the intestinal lumen, and the blood and mucus form "currant jelly" stools. Currant jelly stools are a fairly late sign of intussusception, usually requiring several hours to develop. They have been reported in 85% of the patients in some series and are more common in younger patients.

If complete intestinal obstruction ensues, the child may develop abdominal distention, fluid loss from vomiting and sequestration of intraluminal fluid, and continuous abdominal pain. If there is a further delay in diagnosis and treatment, infarction of the intussusceptum will occur. In most cases this is associated with generalized peritonitis; if untreated, death of the patient occurs within 2 to 5 days.

## ETIOLOGY

Most infants who develop intussusception are healthy and well-nourished. About 10% have a previous history of diarrhea, and many have signs and symptoms of respiratory tract infections.

Some 65% of intussusceptions occur before the patient's first birthday. In almost all patients less than 1 year old, no clear cause of the intussusception can be identified. Studies have been performed in an attempt to identify a viral etiology for intussusception. Adenoviruses and rotaviruses have been found in the stools of some patients. Hypertrophic lymphoid tissue of the bowel, including hypertrophied Peyer's patches and enlarged mesenteric lymph nodes, often is found in young patients with intussusception. The enlarged collection of lymphoid tissue in the ileal wall may act as a lead point for the development of the intussusception. At the lead point of the intussusception there appears to be a thumbprint in the thickened, edematous ileal wall. The ileum at this point is usually several millimeters thick; an inexperienced surgeon may confuse this with tumor formation and request a biopsy.

About 2% to 3% of older children with intussusception have a recognizable lesion as the lead point, including polyps, Meckel's diverticulum, nodular or ectopic pancreas, small enterogenous cysts, lymphomas, and benign tumors of the ileal wall. The base of the appendix also may act as a lead point. Localized edema or hemorrhage such as that seen in patients with Henoch-Schönlein purpura, abdominal trauma, hemophilia, and leukemia also may act as a lead point. Altered intestinal motility or uncoordinated peristalsis (such as that following head injuries, use of anticholinergic medication, or enteritis associated with AIDS) also has been associated with the development of intussusception. Postoperative intussusception occurs most often after retroperitoneal dissections, particularly for tumors, and after fundoplication, presumably as a result of vagal manipulation. Nearly all intussusceptions associated with altered motility are located in the small bowel. Patients with cystic fibrosis may develop intussusception as a result of mucus-laden hypertrophied mucosal glands, which act as lead points, and as a result of the thick, tenacious fecal material associated with enzymatic insufficiency. Most of these cases occur in children age 4 years or older. Chronic indwelling tubes may be associated with intussusception; edema of the bowel wall caused by the tube serves as the intussuscepting point.

## CLINICAL PRESENTATION

Nearly all affected infants present with vomiting and colicky pain. However, because these two symptoms are nonspecific and common, they are less likely to prompt a visit to the physician. Infants typically are seen later in the course of illness, at which time they are more likely to have currant jelly stools and high fever. Intussusception in infants less than 3 months old is less likely to be reduced by barium enema.

## DIAGNOSIS

The diagnosis of intussusception frequently is made from a clinical history of intermittent, colicky pain lasting only a few seconds and extending over the course of several hours, after which the patient becomes lethargic, vomits, and shows signs and symptoms of intestinal obstruction. On physical examination, a palpable sausage-shaped mass in the distribution of the colon, typically in the area of the transverse colon, confirms the diagnosis. If currant jelly stools are noted in association with a sausage-shaped mass and intermittent colicky pain, the diagnosis is no longer in doubt. At times, the intussusception mass will be located medial to the lateral edge of the rectus abdominis muscle and below the edge of the liver, making palpation difficult. This is particularly true when some degree of intestinal obstruction and abdominal distention has developed. In addition, only 65% of infants with

intussusception will have currant jelly stools. For these reasons, any infant or young child with signs and symptoms of distal small bowel or colonic obstruction, intermittent colicky pain, currant jelly or guaiac-positive stools, or a sausage-shaped mass in the distribution of the colon should undergo a diagnostic barium enema examination. The diagnosis will be confirmed in 100% of the patients in whom the intussusceptum extends through the ileocecal valve into the colon.

## DIFFERENTIAL DIAGNOSIS

Intussusception should be included in the differential diagnosis of any condition characterized by abdominal pain, blood in the stool, or an intra-abdominal mass. Intussusception is often confused with gastroenteritis. Although intermittent colicky abdominal pain is typical of both, the pain associated with intussusception is more constantly episodic. Early in the illness, the infant with intussusception appears well between paroxysms of pain.

Intussusception, particularly cecal-colic intussusception, occasionally results in partial intestinal obstruction and presents with liquid, blood-streaked, loose stools similar to those seen with infectious enterocolitis. Guaiac-positive and blood-streaked stools are common in infants with gastroenteritis. The bloody-mucoid or currant jelly stools are the result of venous-congested, vascularly compromised intestine; they may also be seen in other processes such as volvulus and incarcerated internal hernia.

## TREATMENT

The modern treatment protocol and guidelines for the use of barium enema are described in Table 124-1. The primary concern is rapid resuscitation of the volume-depleted child. This requires placement of a large intravenous plastic catheter for intravenous administration of fluids and, if necessary, of blood products. Gastric aspiration through a nasogastric tube prevents further vomiting and enteric accumulation of fluid. Antibiotics are reserved for patients with peritoneal signs or evidence of compromised bowel. As soon as the diagnosis is made, the operating room should be prepared for emergency surgery, as it would be in the case of an incarcerated hernia. If the patient's hemoglobin

---

**TABLE 124-1.  Principles of Barium Enema Reduction of Intussusception**

1. Notify OR to prepare for emergency operation if barium reduction is not successful.
2. Initiate resuscitation with intravenous fluids and nasogastric suction.
3. Insert ungreased Foley catheter in rectum, distend balloon, and pull down against levators. Tape catheter in place and hold buttocks tightly together. Wrap legs.
4. Let barium run from a height of 3'6" above the table while intermittently fluoroscoping the patient.
5. Abandon procedure if barium column is stationary and its outline is unchanged for 10 minutes.
6. Reducation is marked by:
   Free flow of barium well into ileum;
   Expulsion of feces and flatus with the barium;
   Disappearance of the mass on physical examination; and
   Clinical improvement of the child.
7. Failure to reduce the intussusception requires prompt operative intervention.

*(Modified from Ravitch MM. Intussusception. In: Welch KJ, Randolph JG, Ravitch MM, et al, eds. Pediatric surgery. Chicago: Year Book Medical Publishers, 1987:868)*

is low, blood should be typed and crossmatched, because bowel resection may be necessary.

Only after resuscitation has been initiated should the patient be taken to the radiology suite for a diagnostic and therapeutic contrast enema examination with fluoroscopy. At present, contrast materials used include air, water-soluble contrast, and barium. If the risk of perforation is increased, air or water-soluble contrast is a better choice than barium.

Once the diagnosis is confirmed by contrast enema, a decision must be made whether to attempt hydrostatic reduction (Fig 124-2). The only absolute contraindications to hydrostatic reduction are free intraperitoneal air or peritoneal signs and systemic signs of compromised intestine. Relative contraindications include intestinal obstruction as evidenced by multiple air-fluid levels with dilated segments of small bowel. Several cases have been reported in which patients with high-grade bowel obstruction developed perforation and barium spillage during attempted hydrostatic reduction. If a filling defect suggesting a lead point is seen after reduction, laparotomy should be done.

At present, 30% to 70% of the patients with intussusception are successfully treated by hydrostatic reduction of the intussusception. The recurrence rate after both hydrostatic reduction and surgical reduction is close to 5%; recurrences usually occur shortly after the successful reduction.

Patients with free air or peritoneal signs and patients in whom hydrostatic reduction is unsuccessful should be taken directly to the operating room for operative reduction. Because the intussusceptum causes vascular compromise, these are true surgical emergencies. Successful operative reduction is possible in most patients; however, nearly 25% of infants requiring surgery require resection because reduction is impossible or the intestine is nonviable. The compromised bowel may be excised and a primary ileocolostomy performed.

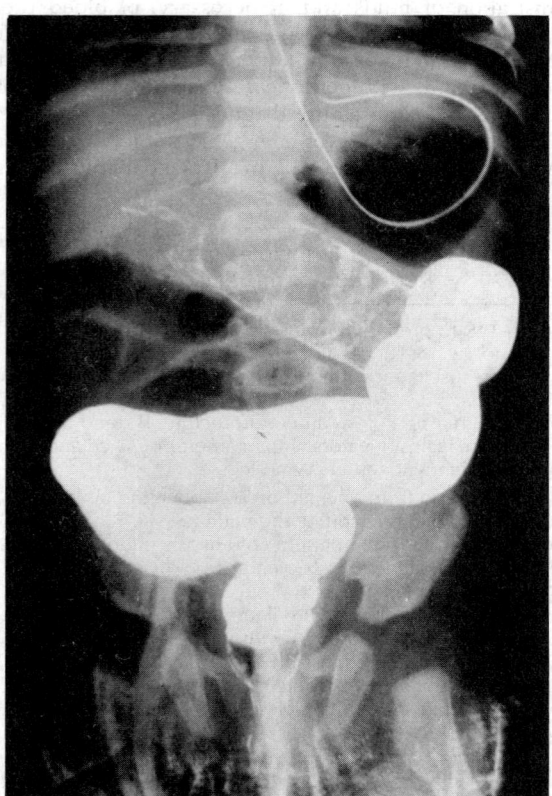

**Figure 124-2.** Barium enema study showing the coiled-spring pattern of barium around the intussusceptum in the transverse colon.

## Selected Readings

Blane CE, DiPietro ME, White SJ, et al. An analysis of bowel perforation in patients with intussusception. J Can Assoc Radiol 1984;35:113.

Ein SH, Ferguson JM. Intussusception: the forgotten postoperative obstruction. Arch Dis Child 1982;57:788.

Ein SH, Shandling B, Reilly BJ, Stringer DA. Hydrostatic reduction of intussusceptions caused by lead points. J Pediatr Surg 1986;21:883.

Fishman MC, Borden S, Cooper A. The dissection sign of nonreducible ileocolic intussusception. AJR 1984;143:5.

Guo JZ, Ma XY, Zhou QH. Results of air pressure enema reduction of intussusception: 6396 cases in 13 years. J Pediatr Surg 1986;21:1201.

Jennings C, Kelleher J. Intussusception: influence of age on reducibility. Pediatr Radiol 1984;14:292.

Liu KW, MacCarthy J, Guiney EJ, Fitzgerald RJ. Intussusception: current trends in management. Arch Dis Child 1986;61:75.

Palder SB, Ein SH, Stringer DA, Alton D: Intussusception: barium or air? J Pediatr Surg 1991;26:271.

Pokorny WJ, Suggs N, Harberg FJ. Factors leading to surgical treatment of intussusception. Surg Gynecol Obstet 1978;147:574.

Pokorny WJ, Wagner ML, Harberg FJ. Lateral wall cecal filling defects following successful hydrostatic reduction of cecal-colic intussusceptions. J Pediatr Surg 1980;15:156.

Ravitch MM. Intussusception. In: Welch KJ, Randolph JG, Ravitch MM, et al., eds. Pediatric surgery. Chicago: Year Book Medical Publishers, 1987;868.

Turner D, Rickwood AM, Brereton RJ. Intussusception in older children. Arch Dis Child 1980;55:544.

*Principles and Practice of Pediatrics, Second Edition.*
edited by Frank A. Oski et al. J. B. Lippincott Company, Philadelphia © 1994.

## CHAPTER 125
# *Motility Disorders*

### Ellen L. Blank

Common gastrointestinal (GI) complaints such as dysphagia, anorexia, heartburn, nausea, vomiting, chest pain, abdominal bloating, abdominal pain, diarrhea, or constipation comprise the presentation of GI motility disorders. These symptoms may occur acutely as a reversible ileus with infections or as a mechanical bowel obstruction. Postsurgical syndromes such as ileus, dumping, postvagotomy gastropathy, and duodenogastric (bile) reflux also are commonly regarded as disorders of GI motility. Disease states involving intestinal stenoses or pathologic changes in enteric muscles or nerves have been shown to impair GI function sufficiently to produce chronic clinical symptoms. These include collagen vascular diseases, amyloidosis, muscular dystrophy, hypothyroidism, diabetes mellitus, hypoparathyroidism, pheochromocytoma, Hirschsprung's disease, and familial autonomic dysautonomia.

Recurrent signs and symptoms of intestinal dysfunction without any demonstrable obstructing lesion present a diagnostic dilemma. When secondary collagen vascular, neurologic, hormonal, or drug-induced causes are absent, the diagnosis of primary intestinal pseudo-obstruction is suggested. New histologic and physiologic tests can differentiate some cases to be either disorders of enteric neurons or smooth muscle.

Pseudo-obstruction may occur sporadically or as part of a familial syndrome; about 20% of the cases are familial. Involvement may also occur in other organs containing smooth muscle such as the urinary bladder, gallbladder, and eyes. The onset of symptoms may occur in infancy or in a previously healthy child.

Barium radiographic studies are helpful in locating areas of intestinal dilatation. Contrast or ultrasound studies of the gallbladder and urinary bladder demonstrate any associated anomalies. If full-thickness intestinal biopsy specimens are available, enteric nervous system abnormalities may be identified using Smith's method of silver staining, and smooth muscle abnormalities can be seen with hemotoxylin-eosin or Masson trichrome stains.

Manometric studies have shown abnormalities in the esophagus and small intestine of patients with chronic intestinal pseudo-obstruction. Esophageal motility studies have demonstrated decreased resting lower esophageal sphincter pressure, failure of lower esophageal sphincter relaxation normally seen with swallowing, and disordered muscle contractile patterns through the esophagus. Antroduodenal motility studies have demonstrated at least three types of abnormalities: absent migrating myoelectric complexes, usually found during fasting; abnormal postprandial motility, and lower-than-normal amplitude of intestinal smooth muscle contractions.

Vigorous nutritional support with enteral tube feeding or parenteral nutrition has decreased the morbidity and mortality of pseudo-obstruction syndromes in children. This therapy allows most affected children to grow and develop normally. Specific prokinetic agents aimed at improving motility have been unsuccessful. Cisapride has had limited success in relieving GI complaints. Conservative management of obstructive episodes should be used as much as possible to avoid repeated laparotomies.

## Selected Readings

Anuras S, Mitros FA, Soper RT, et al. Chronic intestinal pseudo-obstruction in young children. Gastroenterology 1986;91:62.

Hyman PE, McDiarmid SV, Napolitano J, Abrams CE, Tomomasa T. Antroduodenal motility in children with chronic intestinal pseudo-obstruction. J Pediatr 1988;112:899.

Navarro J, Sonsino E, Boige N, et al. Visceral neuropathies responsible for chronic intestinal pseudo-obstruction syndrome in pediatric practice: analysis of 26 cases. J Pediatr Gastroenterol Nutr 1990;11:179.

Vargas JH, Sachs P, Ament ME. Chronic intestinal pseudo-obstruction syndrome in pediatrics. J Pediatr Gastroenterol Nutr 1988;7:323.

*Principles and Practice of Pediatrics, Second Edition.*
edited by Frank A. Oski et al. J. B. Lippincott Company, Philadelphia © 1994.

## CHAPTER 126
# Anorectal Malformations

### William J. Pokorny

Embryonic development of the anus and rectum with separation from the urogenital tract primarily occurs between the 4-mm (4th week) and 16-mm (6th week) stage of embryonic development but continues to the 56-mm stage. Major anorectal malformations occur in one per 5000 live births, with minor anomalies

**TABLE 126-1. Classification of Anorectal Malformations**

| Female | Male |
|---|---|
| High | High |
|   Anorectal agenesis |   Anorectal agenesis |
|     With rectovaginal fistula |     With rectourethral fistula |
|     Without fistula |     Without fistula |
|   Rectal atresia |   Rectal atresia |
| Intermediate | Intermediate |
|   Rectovaginal fistula |   Anorectal agenesis |
|   Rectovestibular fistula |   Rectourethral fistula |
|   Anal agenesis without a fistula |   Anal agenesis without a fistula |
| Low | Low |
|   Anovestibular fistula |   Anocutaneous fistula |
|   Anocutaneous fistula |   Anal stenosis |
|   Anal stenosis |   Rare malformations |
| Cloacal malformations | |
| Rare malformations | |

reported in as many as one per 1500 live births. Imperforate anus has been reported in siblings and in members of one family over three generations.

Table 126-1 lists types of anorectal malformations according to sex, the level of rectal descent, and the presence or absence of a fistula. The level of rectal descent is determined clinically by reviewing the invertogram (Wangensteen-Rice radiograph) and by identifying the level of the rectum in relation to a line drawn between the pubis and coccyx (pubococcygeal line) and the lowest quarter of the ossified ischium (I point). With high lesions, the rectum does not penetrate the levator muscle and is above the pubococcygeal line. An intermediate lesion partially traverses the levator muscle and ends below the pubococcygeal line but above the I point. A low imperforate anus is above the level of the translevator muscle and below the I point.

Lesions close to the anus are more common than high and intermediate lesions in girls; high lesions are more common in boys. Nearly 80% of the boys with a high lesion have a fistula to the urinary tract, and nearly all girls with a high lesion have a fistula to the vagina, bladder, or cloaca (Figs 126-1, 126-2).

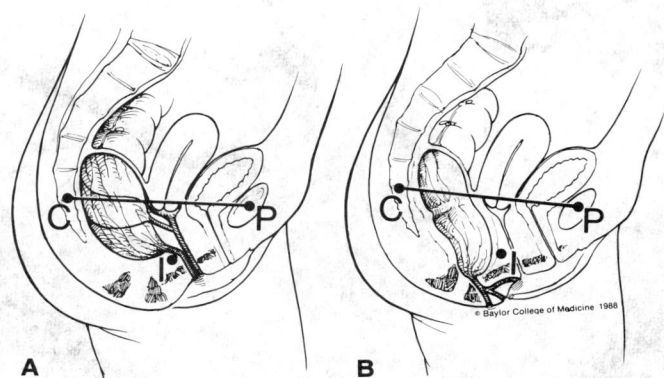

**Figure 126-1.** Anorectal anomalies in the female. (**A**) High lesions usually have a fistula to the vagina, whereas intermediate lesions may have a fistula to the vagina or outside the hymen at the vestibule. (**B**) Low lesions may also have a fistula to the vestibule or to the fourchette or perineum.

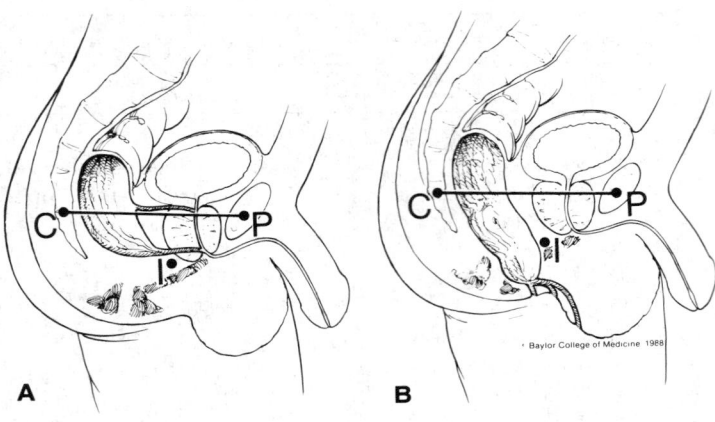

**Figure 126-2.** Anorectal anomalies in the male. (**A**) 80% of high and intermediate lesions have fistulas to the bulbar or membranous urethra. (**B**) 90% of males with low lesions have a fistula to the perineum or median raphe.

## DIAGNOSIS

The level of the anorectal anomaly cannot be predicted from the appearance of the perineum. However, several findings on physical examination suggest the level of an imperforate anus. A flat bottom with no crease or anal dimple and no evidence of an external sphincter predicts a high imperforate anus (Fig 126-3). On the other hand, a well-developed anal dimple is not always associated with a low anomaly. Nevertheless, a well-developed raphe, anal dimple, and bucket-handle raphe suggest a low lesion. Ninety percent of the boys with a low lesion have a fistula to the perineum. Whitish inspissated mucus (perineal pearls) or meconium-stained material may be expressed from the fistula in the subcuticular tract along the raphe of the perineum, scrotum, or even ventral surface of the penis (Fig 126-4). Often the perineal fistula is not obvious at birth but becomes evident with the passage of a small fleck of meconium during the first 24 hours of life (Fig 126-5). The passage of flatus or meconium in the urine is diagnostic of a high or intermediate anomaly with a fistula to the urethra or bladder.

In most girls, the lesion is low (Fig 126-6). Nearly all of these girls have a fistula to the perineum, as an anterior or ectopic anus (Fig 126-7) to the fourchette or to the vestibule, which is between the posterior fourchette and the hymenal ring (Fig 126-8). Openings into the vestibule may be associated with low lesions or high lesions with long fistulas. The complete absence of an external fistula indicates a high or intermediate lesion. Most girls with high lesions have a fistula to the vagina; fistulas to the urinary tract are rare. In patients with a single opening, a cloacal anomaly must be considered.

Initial diagnostic studies are designed to identify the level of descent of the rectum and to detect associated anomalies, including fistulas. Ultrasound is useful to evaluate the anatomical integrity of the urinary tract. If there is no evidence of a genitourinary anomaly at birth, intravenous pyelography and voiding cystourethrography should be done before discharge or when the child is 6 weeks old and better able to concentrate the dye.

The urine should be examined for meconium or squamous epithelial cells. A chest radiograph may be obtained with a nasogastric tube in place to rule out esophageal, cardiac, and vertebral anomalies. If cardiomegaly is present, cardiac evaluation should be done. An abdominal-pelvic radiograph may reveal anomalies of the gastrointestinal tract as well as of the lumbosacral spine.

If the patient exhibits no evidence of a fistula to the perineum, a Wangensteen-Rice radiograph (invertogram) should be obtained after 12 hours of life; this allows sufficient time for air to reach the rectum.

## ASSOCIATED MALFORMATIONS

Associated anomalies are reported in 40% to 50% of the patients with imperforate anus. Associated anomalies must be sought in infants with all forms of anorectal malformations. The genitourinary, gastrointestinal, skeletal, and cardiovascular systems may

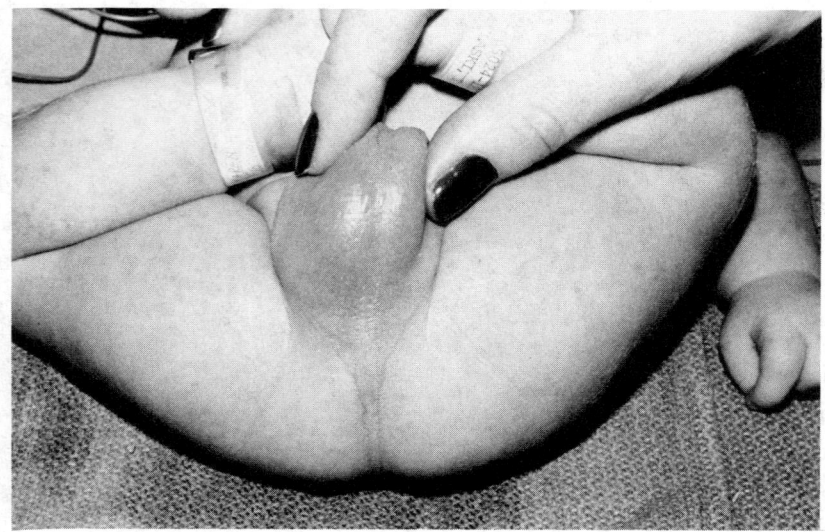

**Figure 126-3.** Perineum of a male with a high lesion and a rectourethral fistula. After 24 hours there is no evidence of a fistula to the perineum or raphe. A colostomy was done on the second day of life, and reconstruction of the anus and rectum at 1 year.

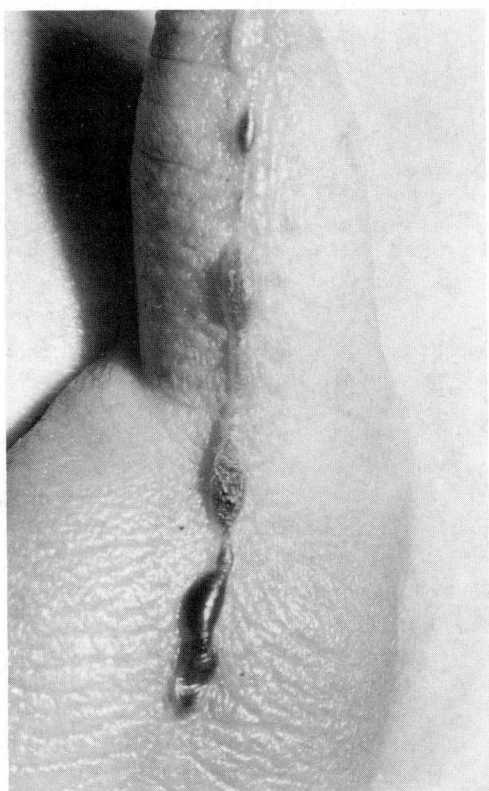

**Figure 126-4.** Male with a low lesion and fistula to the median raphe. Note meconium along the median raphe. A perineal anoplasty was done shortly after birth.

be affected. In addition to imperforate anus, esophageal atresia, vertebral anomalies, and radial and renal anomalies make up the VATER association. The association has been expanded to VACTERL, where "C" represents cardiac lesions and "L" represents limb deformities. When one of these anomalies is seen, the others should be sought.

Nearly 40% of the infants with imperforate anus have genitourinary anomalies, ranging from minor genital anomalies such as hypospadias to renal agenesis. Unilateral renal agenesis is the most common defect, occurring in 8% to 25% of the patients with imperforate anus.

Gastrointestinal anomalies occur in 10% to 15% of the children with imperforate anus. Esophageal atresia is the most common anomaly of this kind and is often associated with maternal polyhydramnios. Although uncommon, Hirschsprung's disease is occasionally seen with imperforate anus and may complicate the postoperative course.

Cardiovascular anomalies are reported in 7% to 12% of the patients with imperforate anus. Ventricular septal defect and tetralogy of Fallot are two of the more common anomalies.

Skeletal anomalies are found in 6% to 20% of the patients with anorectal malformations. Vertebral anomalies, usually sacral, are the most common defect. As many as 50% of the patients with high lesions have sacral vertebral anomalies. The development of the sacrum, levator musculature, and sacral nerves is closely related. Neurologic control of both the rectum and bladder is provided by nerves arising from the second, third, and fourth sacral segments. Normal innervation and levator musculature development may occur with deficiencies of the fourth and fifth sacral vertebrae. Loss of the second through fifth sacral segments usually results in uncorrectable fecal and urinary incontinence.

In addition to the absence of the sacral vertebrae, other spinal abnormalities that result from improper midline fusion of bony, mesenchymal, and neural structures have been reported with anorectal malformations. These abnormalities, referred to as spinal dysraphism, include intraspinal masses, lipomyelomeningoceles, tethered cord, and occult meningocele. These abnormalities may cause a progressive neurologic deficit and impaired continence. Once neurologic function is lost, it often does not return to normal despite neurosurgical intervention. All patients with anorectal malformations should be evaluated by ultrasonography, CT, or MRI to identify lesions of the lumbosacral spine and cord.

## TREATMENT

The treatment of imperforate anus depends on the level of descent of the rectum and on the presence or absence of a fistula to the urinary tract, vagina, or perineum. Children with ectopic or anterior anus are usually asymptomatic during infancy but become constipated when their diet changes and their stools become more formed and solid. At that time, the anus should be surgically moved posteriorly to its normal location.

Infants with low lesions and perineal fistulas may require only dilation of the tract to allow fecal evacuation. If the tract is small,

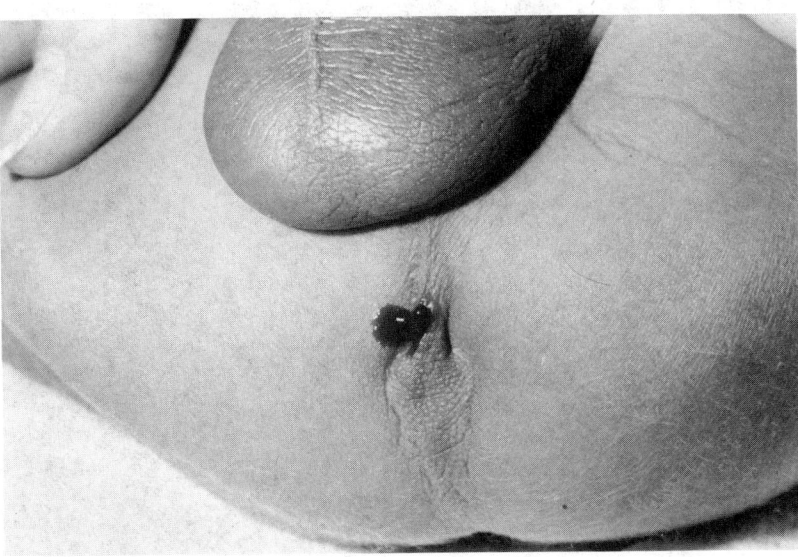

**Figure 126-5.** Male with anoperineal fistula. Meconium did not appear until 18 hours after birth. A perineal anoplasty was done on the second day of life.

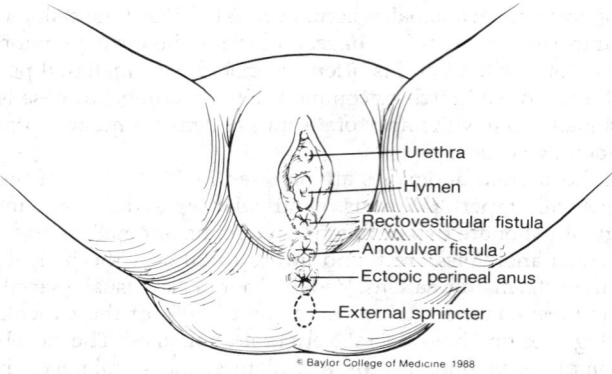

Urethra
Hymen
Rectovestibular fistula
Anovulvar fistula
Ectopic perineal anus
External sphincter

© Baylor College of Medicine 1988

**Figure 126-6.** Appearance of fistulas on the female perineum.

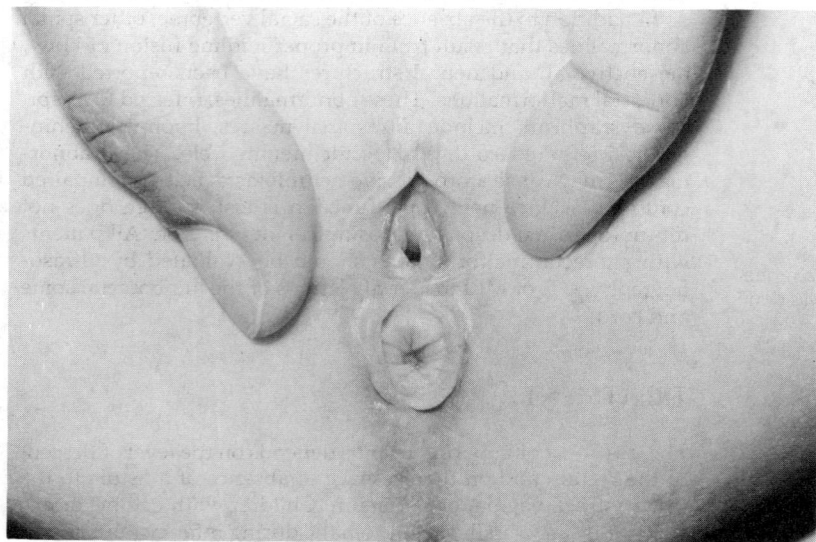

**Figure 126-7.** Ectopic perineal anus located posterior to the fourchette but anterior to the external sphincter. The patient did well with dilations until 6 months of age, when the anus was moved to the normal location.

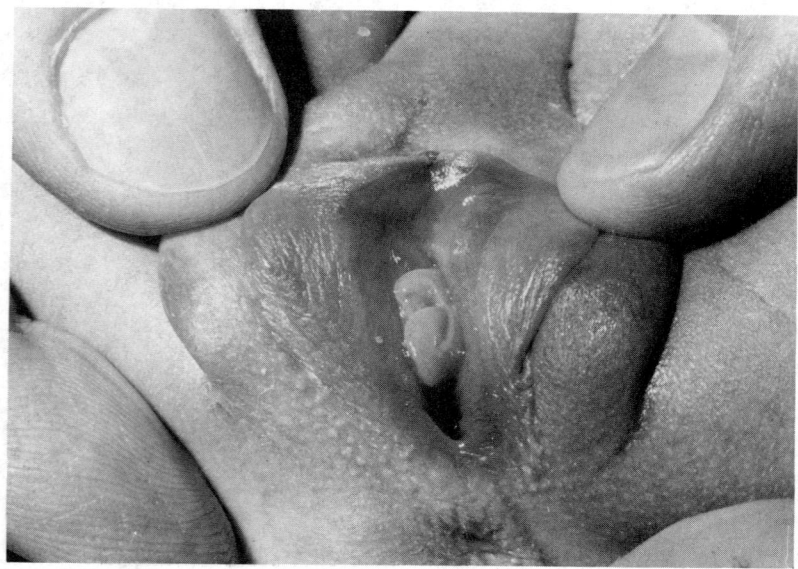

**Figure 126-8.** Rectovestibular fistula located between the hymen and fourchette in the fossa navicularis. A colostomy was done on the second day of life, and anorectal reconstruction at 1 year.

a perineal anoplasty must be done to enlarge the anal opening and to prevent rectal and colonic dilation. Girls with a fistula to the fourchette may need only dilation until they are older and can undergo surgical translocation of the anus to its normal location on the perineum.

Openings into the vestibule in girls may be either high with a long fistula or low. Low openings may be treated by dilatation and, at age 6 months, by translocation of the anus to its normal position. High lesions with a long fistula require a diverting colostomy. Repeated dilations are usually inadequate to prevent chronic constipation with rectal dilation, and dilations may injure the septum between the rectal fistula and vagina, resulting in a rectovaginal fistula.

Children with high and intermediate lesions should undergo diverting colostomies as soon as the diagnosis is confirmed. This is particularly important in patients with fistulas to the urinary tract. Failure to completely divert the feces from the fistula will result in recurrent urinary tract infections. Hyperchloremic acidosis may result from the passage of urine through the rectourinary fistula, where it is absorbed from the colon. This leads to elevated serum chloride levels and hyperchloremic acidosis. Closure of the fistula will eliminate this problem. Occasionally a girl with a cloacal anomaly is encountered in whom the urine empties into a dilated, poorly emptying vagina. This leads to recurrent urinary tract infections. In these patients, the urinary tract must be decompressed to divert the urine, and the vagina must be adequately drained. Immediate primary repair to reconstruct the urogenital sinus may be done.

Patients with high lesions undergo a colostomy at birth, and the condition is corrected by a sacral-perineal or abdomino-sacral-perineal pull-through operation after the infant has attained a size of about 10 kg and 1 year of age.

## PROGNOSIS

Nearly all patients with low malformations have normal rectal function. The outcome of patients with high and intermediate malformations varies: a good outcome has been reported in 33% to 80% of the patients. The outcome depends on operative technique, anatomical development or maldevelopment, and patient cooperation. A significant number (up to 50%) of the patients with high anomalies have sacral vertebral defects. Patients with anomalies of S3 have varying degrees of neurologic deficit to the perineum, including the rectal and bladder sphincters. Patients with absence of S2–S5 have a complete neurologic loss to the perineum. These patients may develop fecal or urinary incontinence. Finally, it is rare for a child with a high anomaly to have perfect rectal function. Toilet training may be difficult until the child is older, often 5 or 6 years of age. The rectal function and fecal continence continue to improve into early adolescence. If the patient and his or her family can be supported through the early postoperative years, rectal function nearly always improves to an acceptable level.

In the early postoperative period, constipation may be due to stenosis and, rarely, to Hirschsprung's disease, but it is more often due to a lack of rectal sensation for fecal material, which leads to fecal impaction. Attention must be given to regular evacuations to prevent impactions. Once impaction develops, the rectum and distal colon become overdistended and lose their muscular tone and peristaltic function. This must be prevented. In some instances, daily laxatives or enemas are required.

### Selected Readings

Czeizel A, Ludanyi I. An aetiological study of the VACTERL association. J Pediatr 1985;144:331.

deVries PA. The surgery of anorectal anomalies: its evolution, with evaluations of procedures. Curr Probl Surg 1984;21(5):1.
deVries PA, Cox KL. Surgery of anorectal anomalies. Surg Clin North Am 1985;65:1139.
deVries PA, Pena A. Posterior sagittal anorectoplasty. J Pediatr Surg 1983;17:638.
Karrer FM, Flannery AM, Nelson MD, McLone DG, Raffensperger JG. Anorectal malformations: evaluation of associated spinal dysraphic syndromes. J Pediatr Surg 1988;23:45.
Khoury MJ, Cordero JF, Greenberg F, et al. A population study of the VACTERL association. Pediatrics 1983;71:815.
Kottmeier PK, Dizadiw R. Complete release of the levator ani sling in fecal incontinence. J Pediatr Surg 1967;2:111.
Mollard P, Marechal JM, deBeaujeu MJ. Surgical treatment of high imperforate anus with definition of the pubo-rectalis sling by an anterior perineal approach. J Pediatr Surg 1978;13:499.
Pena A. Posterior sagittal anorectoplasty as a secondary operation for the treatment of fecal incontinence. J Pediatr Surg 1983;18:762.
Smith EI, Tunell WP, Williams GR. A clinical evaluation of the surgical treatment of anorectal malformations. Ann Surg 1978;187:583.
Soave F. Endorectal pull-through: 20 years' experience. J Pediatr Surg 1985;20:568.
Tunnell WP, Austin JC, Barnes PD, Reynolds A. Neuroradiologic evaluation of sacral abnormalities in imperforate anus complex. J Pediatr Surg 1987;22:58.
Weaver DD, Mapstone CL, Yu PL. The VATER association: analysis of 46 patients. Am J Dis Child 1986;140:225.

*Principles and Practice of Pediatrics, Second Edition.*
edited by Frank A. Oski et al. J. B. Lippincott Company, Philadelphia © 1994.

## CHAPTER 127
# *Ulcerative Colitis*

## W. Daniel Jackson and Richard J. Grand

Ulcerative colitis (UC) is a chronic relapsing inflammatory disease of the colon and rectum of unknown etiology. It was first described in 1875 as a chronic inflammatory bowel disease distinct from infectious colitis. In 1960, criteria differentiating UC from Crohn's colitis were established, but some cases of inflammatory bowel disease remain indeterminate.

## PATHOLOGY

The inflammation in UC is limited to the colon and rectum. Table 127-1 contrasts the patterns of pathologic involvement in UC and Crohn's disease. Based on these patterns, a distinction between the two entities can usually be made. The distal colon is most severely affected, and the rectum is involved in most patients with UC. Inflammation is limited primarily to the mucosa and consists of continuous involvement along the length of the bowel with varying degrees of ulceration, hemorrhage, edema, and regenerating epithelium. Although considered to be limited to the colon, inflammation may extend uninterrupted to the cecum and up to 25 cm into the terminal ileum as "backwash" ileitis without stenosis or distortion. In severe disease where the mucosal epithelium has been destroyed, inflammation may extend beyond the muscularis mucosae into the submucosa. Intervening areas of granulation tissue and regenerating epithelium may form islands of tissue, termed pseudopolyps. Thickening of the bowel

TABLE 127-1. Comparative Features of Ulcerative Colitis and Crohn's Disease

| | UC | Crohn's Disease |
|---|---|---|
| Site of disease | | |
| Upper GI | 0% | 20% |
| Ileum alone | 0% | 19 |
| Ileum and colon | Backwash ileitis | 52% |
| Colon alone | 90% (distal colon predominant) | 9% (proximal colon predominant) |
| Rectum | ~100% | Rare (<5%); perianal disease in 25% |
| Gross pathology/radiology | Hemorrhagic mucosa, diffuse continuous inflammation, pseudopolyps, loss of haustra, no perirenal disease | Segmental involvement, skip regions, focal aphthae, thickened bowel wall, serosal fat, narrow separate bowel loops, anal tags, fistulas |
| Histology | Mucosal and submucosal inflammation, cryptitis, crypt abscess and distortion, depletion of goblet cells | Transmural inflammation, noncaseating granulomas, prominent lymphoid tissue, preserved goblet cells, fibrosis |

wall and fibrosis are rare, although shortening of the colon and focal colonic strictures may occur in long-standing disease.

The histology of UC lesions demonstrates continuous acute and chronic inflammation with mucosal and submucosal infiltration by polymorphonuclear leukocytes and mononuclear cells (Fig 127-1). The colonic crypts show the most characteristic changes. Cryptitis and crypt abscesses characterize acute inflammation, which may lead to chronic changes of crypt distortion with branching and dropout, diminished goblet mucous cells, and Paneth cell metaplasia. There are no granulomas and little fibrosis.

## ETIOLOGY

The cause of UC is unknown. No infective agent has been found, although the lesions resemble changes seen with infectious colitis. There is evidence of autoimmunity in terms of serum antibodies, immune-complex complement activation, and lymphocytes directed against colonic epithelium, but these phenomena are not consistently observed and do not correlate with disease activity. The therapeutic efficacy of glucocorticoids and immunosuppressants in controlling the activity of UC may be due to effects of suppression of immunologic mediators of inflammation. The association of UC with a high familial prevalence of atopic diseases and extraintestinal manifestations of erythema nodosum, arthritis, uveitis, and vasculitis supports the presence of genetic immunologic factors in the pathogenesis. However, there are insufficient

data at present to determine whether immune mechanisms have a primary or secondary role. Although allergic colitis occurs, it is rarely seen after infancy and is usually transient. There is insufficient evidence for an allergic etiology for UC. No specific dietary practices have been unequivocally implicated in the etiology or as risk factors. Nonsmokers are overrepresented relative to Crohn's disease. There are no data to support a psychosomatic etiology in terms of stress, personality type, or psychiatric illness, although emotional and other psychosocial factors may affect the presentation and course of the disease.

Although there are no specific heritable patterns, 15% to 40% of the patients may have other family members with inflammatory bowel disease, with an incidence about 10 times greater when there is a positive family history. However, concordance between monozygotic twins is low, and HLA patterns have not been specific.

## EPIDEMIOLOGY

The incidence of UC in children has gradually increased. The incidence in the general population ranges from 3.9 to 7.3 cases per 100,000, with a prevalence ranging from 41.1 to 79.9 cases per 100,000 population. The disease is more prevalent in Caucasians, with increased representation among those of Jewish backgrounds. UC occurs more commonly in Northern Europe and North America, with an urban predominance. Affected females outnumber affected males by about 50%. The distribution

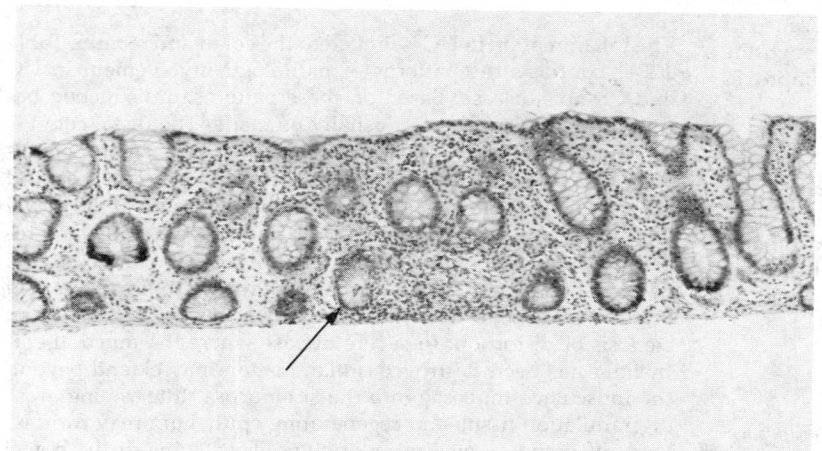

Figure 127-1. Rectal biopsy specimen of an adolescent girl with ulcerative colitis. Note the increased acute and chronic inflammatory cells in the lamina propria with invasion of the crypts, producing cryptitis and a crypt abscess (*arrow*). There is mild distortion of the crypt architecture consistent with chronic disease.

of age at onset is bimodal, with the major peak in the second and third decades and a second peak in the fifth and sixth decades. Between 15% and 40% of all the patients with UC present before age 20 years, with a peak onset in adolescence. The disease is rare in children less than 2 years old, although cases in infants have been reported. Most cases of infantile colitis are due to cow's milk or soy protein allergy and are transient. In the 10- to 19-year-old age group, the incidence has been estimated at 2.3 cases per 100,000 population.

## CLINICAL PRESENTATION

There are at least four patterns of presentation of UC, differing in the extent of mucosal inflammation and systemic disturbance (Table 127-2). Extraintestinal manifestations of disease, including growth disturbance, may be presenting features and may precede the manifestations of overt colitis. The first sign of disease may be growth disturbance characterized by decreased linear-growth velocity due to subtle chronic dietary caloric deficits attributed to relative anorexia or to the increased metabolic demands of inflammation. Nondestructive arthritis involving peripheral large joints may precede and may not correlate with intestinal symptoms. The skin lesions of erythema nodosum may be seen on the extensor surfaces of the arms and legs before recognition of colitis. In all of these patients, the erythrocyte sedimentation rate may be elevated, suggesting a systemic inflammatory process, or stool examination may reveal occult blood and leukocytes due to the underlying colitis. Biochemical signs of liver involvement are uncommon. About 4% of the patients have presented with or have been complicated by sclerosing cholangitis, characterized by fatigue, pruritus, and the gradual appearance of jaundice.

The most common presentation is the insidious onset of diarrhea and hematochezia (overt rectal bleeding), usually without systemic signs of fever, weight loss, or hypoalbuminemia. In these patients, the disease is often confined to the distal colon and rectum; the physical examination is normal, without abdominal tenderness; and the course remains mild, with intermittent exacerbations.

About 30% of the patients have moderate signs of systemic disturbance and present with bloody diarrhea, cramps, urgency, anorexia and weight loss, malaise, mild anemia, and low-grade or intermittent fever. Physical examination may reveal abdominal tenderness, and stool will show varying amounts of blood and leukocytes.

Severe colitis occurs in about 10% of the patients and is characterized by more than six bloody stools per day, significant anemia, hypoalbuminemia, fever, tachycardia, and weight loss. The abdomen may be diffusely tender or distended. A subgroup of patients with severe colitis may not respond to medical therapy and may require early colectomy. Criteria for recognizing these patients have been proposed.

## COMPLICATIONS

The most serious complication of UC, toxic megacolon, occurs in less than 5% of the patients and is a medical and surgical emergency. In this entity, dilatation of the diseased colon is accompanied by fever, tachycardia, hypokalemia, hypoalbuminemia, and dehydration. A leukocytosis with a predominance of immature neutrophils may be present. Some of these signs, particularly fever and tenderness, may be masked by high-dose steroid treatment. The patient with toxic megacolon is at risk for colonic perforation, gram-negative sepsis, and massive hemorrhage. Effective monitoring requires supine and upright radiographs to assess colonic caliber and exclude the presence of intra-abdominal free air, which would indicate perforation. Management should include stool bacterial culture, assay for *Clostridium difficile* toxin, broad-spectrum antibiotics, and high-dose steroids. Since most distention occurs in the anteriorly located transverse colon, positioning the patient in the prone position and careful colonic decompression with a rectal tube may be helpful. Patients who fail to respond promptly to these aggressive medical measures will require colectomy.

With long-standing disease, a colonic stricture may occur. In adults, this may be due to carcinoma; in children, benign postinflammatory fibrotic stricture is more likely. Intra-abdominal and hepatic abscesses occur less often than with Crohn's disease, except after perforation or colectomy.

## DIAGNOSIS

The diagnosis of UC is based on clinical presentation, radiologic findings, mucosal appearance, and histology, as well as on the exclusion of other known etiologies of colitis. A complete history should be obtained, with attention to family history, exposure to infectious agents or antibiotic treatment, retardation in growth or sexual development, and extraintestinal manifestations. The physical examination should include assessment of hydration, nutritional status, and systemic and extraintestinal signs of chronic disease. The presence of fever, orthostasis, tachycardia, abdominal tenderness, distention, or masses indicates moderate to severe disease and the need for hospitalization.

### Laboratory Evaluation

A complete blood cell count will disclose leukocytosis or anemia. The erythrocyte sedimentation rate is elevated in about 70% of the patients and is a marker of inflammatory activity. Electrolyte disturbances are uncommon except with dehydration, but serum protein and albumin levels may be low. Due to either poor intake or losses from colonic inflammation and bleeding, serum iron and magnesium levels may be low. Elevated serum transaminases and alkaline phosphatase may signify sclerosing cholangitis. Stool should be examined for blood, leukocytes, and ova and parasites. Culture of fresh stool should allow exclusion of *Salmonella, Shigella, Campylobacter*, toxigenic or hemorrhagic *Escherichia coli, Aeromonas hydrophila*, and *Yersinia*. Serologic titers may help exclude *Entamoeba histolytica*. The colitis due to the toxins of *C difficile* may resemble the lesions in UC or Crohn's disease or

---

| TABLE 127-2. UC Patterns of Presentation |
| --- |
| **Extraintestinal (<5%)** |
| Growth failure, arthropathy, erythema nodosum, occult fecal blood, elevated sedimentation rate, nonspecific abdominal pain, altered bowel pattern, cholangitis |
| **Mild Disease (50%–60%)** |
| Diarrhea, mild rectal bleeding, abdominal pain |
| No systemic disturbance |
| **Moderate Disease (30%)** |
| Bloody diarrhea, cramps, urgency, abdominal tenderness |
| Systemic disturbance: anorexia, weight loss, mild fever, mild anemia |
| **Severe Disease (10%)** |
| More than six bloody stools per day, abdominal tenderness, ±distention, tachycardia, fever, weight loss, significant anemia, leukocytosis, hypoalbuminemia |

may complicate underlying inflammatory bowel disease. An assay for *C difficile* toxin should be obtained on all patients regardless of prior antibiotic treatment. Finding a pathogen does not exclude underlying inflammatory bowel disease in which the incidence of secondary infections is increased.

## Radiology

Chest and abdominal radiographs, both upright and supine, will show the extent of colonic dilatation and help exclude obstruction due to stricture and pneumoperitoneum from perforation. These films form a baseline for later comparisons. A barium enema examination can be used to assess the character and extent of colonic disease but should never be performed in patients with acute, active colitis. In cases of mild to moderate colitis without dilatation, an air contrast barium enema study will reveal the mucosal detail necessary to detect ulcerations. Even without air contrast, a barium enema may reveal the chronic changes of foreshortening, loss of haustrations, pseudopolyps, and strictures as well as spasm (Fig 127-2). However, direct inspection by flexible sigmoidoscopy may be safer and more informative. Unless defined on barium enema with reflux into the terminal ileum, an upper GI barium series and small bowel follow-through with fluoroscopic study of the terminal ileum is necessary to define small bowel involvement. The most sensitive and specific study of the small intestine is obtained with a barium enteroclysis. In Crohn's colitis the ileum may be stiffened, nodular, and contracted, while in the "backwash" ileitis of UC the ileum is dilated and mucosal detail is effaced. In UC there should be no other signs of small bowel involvement. In moderately to severely ill patients with

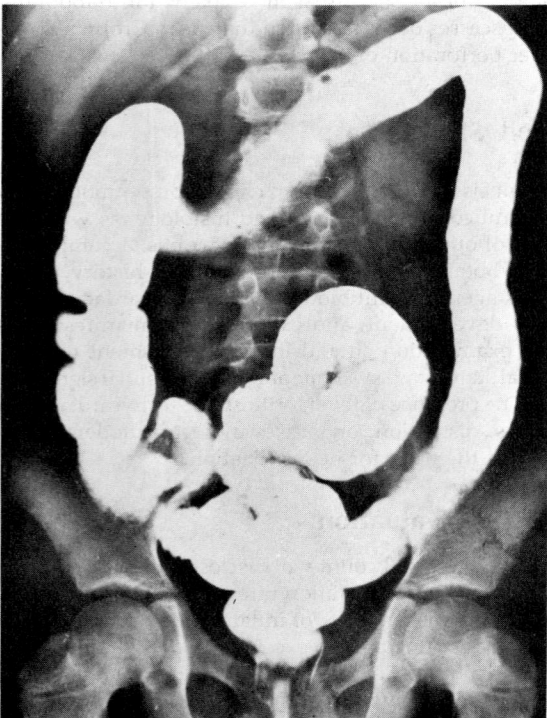

**Figure 127-2.** Single-contrast barium enema study in a 10-year-old boy with ulcerative colitis. There is continuous involvement of the entire colon with reflux of barium into the terminal ileum through a normal ileocecal valve. The small caliber, shortening and loss of haustra of the transverse and distal colon indicate long-standing disease. The irregular mucosal margins of the cecum and transverse colon suggest active ulceration. The poor coating and dilatation of the terminal ileum may represent backwash ileitis. There are no strictures or signs of obstruction.

dilated bowel, extensive bleeding, persistent fever, or an abdominal mass, abdominal ultrasound or CT scanning may demonstrate abscesses. Radionuclide studies are rarely helpful unless barium studies cannot be safely done.

## Endoscopy

Flexible sigmoidoscopic or colonoscopic inspection of the colon and ileum, in conjunction with mucosal biopsies, is the most sensitive and specific means of evaluating intestinal inflammation. In many cases it may make barium contrast studies unnecessary. Active disease is characterized by diffuse continuous involvement of the mucosa with edema, erythema, and friability. Erosions may be seen in the acute stages, followed by mucosal regeneration forming pseudopolyps in the atrophic mucosa of chronic disease. In UC, proctitis is usually present and, although the entire colon may be involved, the distal colon usually is affected more severely. Focal, segmental, or right-sided colonic inflammation with rectal sparing suggests Crohn's disease, and small bowel involvement should be excluded. Biopsies should be obtained from multiple colonic levels, including the rectum.

## DIFFERENTIAL DIAGNOSIS

GI complaints are prevalent in children: up to 10% of children, particularly those aged 7 to 11 years, may seek medical attention for the complaint of recurrent abdominal pain, usually periumbilical in location. In most of these cases, extensive evaluation for inflammatory bowel disease is contraindicated unless there are associated features of fever, diarrhea, growth disturbance, or other extraintestinal manifestations. On the other hand, the periumbilical location of the pain is nonspecific and should not be considered pathognomonic for functional abdominal pain, because it is also characteristic of most cases of inflammatory bowel disease. In cases of uncomplicated recurrent abdominal pain, constipation, lactose intolerance, urinary tract infection, peptic disease, or psychosocial causes should be considered.

Rectal bleeding may be due to Meckel's diverticulum, hemolytic-uremic syndrome, polyposis, hemorrhoids, or anal fissures. The bleeding from Meckel's diverticulum is usually painless, copious, and without fecal leukocytes. Hemolytic-uremic syndrome can often be excluded by inspecting the blood smear and measuring the blood urea nitrogen. Polyps may be detected by sigmoidoscopy or barium enema. Fissures may be secondary to constipation or may be the perianal manifestations of Crohn's disease, particularly if inflammation is prominent.

Colitis, characterized by fecal leukocytes accompanying the bleeding and sigmoidoscopic evidence of inflammation, may be caused by infection or allergy. Infection with *Salmonella, Shigella, Campylobacter, Yersinia, Aeromonas,* certain strains of *E coli,* and *E histolytica* may resemble UC and should be excluded. *C difficile* pseudomembranous colitis may be present even in the absence of a history of antibiotic treatment and seems to be more prevalent in patients with inflammatory bowel disease. Food proteins, usually cow's milk or soy protein in infancy, may produce an allergic colitis distinguished from UC only by histology, which in allergic disease reveals a predominant eosinophilic infiltration of the mucosa. Except for rare eosinophilic gastroenteritis, such a response occurs only in infancy and responds promptly to exclusion of the allergenic protein.

Before the onset of overt GI manifestations of UC, the patient may be followed for prodromal growth retardation or extraintestinal disease. For example, extraintestinal signs of UC may be mistaken for primary endocrine disorders, rheumatologic diseases, or anorexia nervosa.

## THERAPY

Since UC is confined to the colon, total proctocolectomy is curative. However, because of the potential complications of surgery and the difficulties in adapting to an ileostomy and life without a colon, medical management is attempted initially. Surgery is reserved for failure to respond, severe complications, chronic steroid dependence, or excessive risk of carcinoma in long-standing disease.

## Medical Therapy

The goals of medical therapy of UC in children are to control inflammation and symptoms and to prevent relapses. The choice of therapy depends on the severity of the inflammation.

*Mild cases* of colitis unaccompanied by systemic signs can be managed on an outpatient basis with rest, low-residue diet, and the gradual introduction of sulfasalazine or a non-sulfa 5-aminosalicylate alternative (Table 127-3). Response to treatment is expected within 2 weeks, with reduction in stool frequency, bleeding, and cramps. Subsequently, activity and diet may be liberalized as tolerated.

*Moderate disease*, when colitis is accompanied by systemic signs, requires hospitalization for proper evaluation, observation for complications, and management. In addition to bed rest and a low-residue diet, corticosteroids are given. Sulfasalazine or a non-sulfa 5-aminosalicylate alternative may be used as an adjunct, although additional benefits have not been proved in disease of moderate or greater activity. Hypoalbuminemia and anemia may require transfusion to optimize recovery. Failure to respond to this regimen warrants a trial of bowel rest with nutritional support by elemental formula or parenteral nutrition. The immunosuppressant azathioprine or its active metabolite 6-mercaptopurine are useful in refractory disease dependent on chronic steroid therapy.

---

### TABLE 127-3. Pharmacologic Therapy for UC

**Moderate to Severe Colitis**

Methylprednisolone or prednisone: 1–2 mg/kg/day divided bid for 2 weeks; taper to 1–2 mg/kg/day qd over 4–6 weeks, depending on clincial response. When clinical remission is achieved, taper to qod and discontinue over another 4 weeks

Sulfasalazine: 40–50 mg/kg/day divided bid to qid initiated gradually during steroid taper in daily 250-mg increments until full dose is achieved (maximum, 3–4 g/day).

Non-sulfa 5-amino salicylates (dose varies according to product used)

Folate supplementation: 1 mg/kg

**Mild or Localized Distal Colitis**

Sulfasalazine: 40–50 mg/kg/day divided bid to qid

Non-sulfa 5-amino salicylates (dose varies according to product used)

Folate: 1 mg/day

Hydrocortisone enemas

**Refractory Disease**

Azathioprine: 2 mg/kg/day

6-Mercaptopurine: 1 mg/kg/day

**Preventive Maintenance**

Sulfasalazine: 40–50 mg/kg/day divided bid to qid

Non-sulfa 5-amino salicylates (dose varies according to product used)

Folate: 1 mg/day

---

*Severe disease* with copious bloody diarrhea, weight loss, fever, abdominal tenderness or distention, leukocytosis, anemia, and hypoalbuminemia indicates loss of homeostasis and should be treated as an emergency, with hospitalization and surgical consultation. Some of these patients will eventually require colectomy for failure to respond to medical therapy or because of the emergence of life-threatening complications such as toxic megacolon, hemorrhage, or perforation. Central venous access is helpful in the management of these cases and ultimately will be necessary to provide adequate parenteral nutritional support, because complete bowel rest is mandatory. Anemia and hypoalbuminemia should be corrected with blood and albumin transfusions. Dehydration and electrolyte disturbances should be anticipated and reversed. Magnesium is essential to colonic function and is often depleted, a fact reflected in low urinary magnesium excretion after a parenteral challenge dose of magnesium sulfate, even in the presence of normal serum magnesium levels. After blood has been drawn for culture and stool obtained for bacterial culture, parasite examination, and *C difficile* toxin assay, broad-spectrum antibiotic coverage should be instituted. Intravenous adrenocorticotropin or high-dose steroid treatment is essential. Serial abdominal radiographs should be obtained for surveillance of complications, which may be masked by steroid treatment. CT, radionuclide-labeled leukocyte scans, or ultrasound examination to search for abscesses is indicated in patients who fail to respond to treatment. Most patients who fail to respond to a maximal medical regimen within 2 weeks ultimately will require colectomy. Prolonging medical treatment and postponing surgery in these cases increases the risk of complications due to immunosuppression, steroid therapy, central venous catheters, transfusions, and hospitalization. Current research trials suggest that cyclosporin A may be effective in controlling severe colitis until the slow-acting immunosuppressive agents (azathioprine or 6-mercaptopurine) exert their steroid-sparing effects.

## Pharmacologic Agents

Sulfasalazine and steroids are the principal therapeutic agents for UC (see Table 127-3). Sulfasalazine has proved efficacious in controlling mild disease and in reducing the frequency of relapses once disease remission has been obtained. Sulfasalazine is an azo-bonded combination of 5-aminosalicylate and sulfapyridine. The parent compound is split by colonic flora to the two constituents. The 5-aminosalicylate is poorly absorbed and is considered to be the active anti-inflammatory moiety, presumably through inhibition of prostaglandin synthesis. Among the effects attributed to 5-aminosalicylic acid are inhibition of lipoxygenase activity, which mediates migration of polymorphonuclear leukocytes; inhibition of prostaglandin $E_2$ synthesis; reduction in the levels of thromboxane $B_2$ and 6-keto-prostaglandin $F_1$; and antisecretory effects. The sulfapyridine is absorbed and excreted in the urine. It is responsible for the side effects of allergy, hemolytic anemia, rash, headaches, and nausea. These effects are relatively common, often dose-dependent, and transient. Oligospermia has been reported and is considered reversible. The principal role of the azo-bonded sulfapyridine seems to be to prevent small intestine absorption of the salicylate, since very little of the parent compound is transported across the intestinal mucosa. Alternative unabsorbable salicylate preparations have been formulated to avoid the sulfapyridine complications, including a diazo-bonded dimer of 5-aminosalicylic acid (Dipentum) and other forms of 5-aminosalicylic acid (Asacol, Pentasa). Children at risk for G6PD deficiency should be screened before sulfasalazine treatment. Because of the potential for intolerance, the sulfasalazine dosage should be gradually increased from 10 mg/kg/day over 1 week to a maximum dosage of 40 to 50 mg/kg in two to four divided doses. Symptoms and blood cell counts should be monitored closely. Because sulfasalazine impairs folate absorption, folate supplements, 1 mg/day, are given.

Corticosteroids are effective in the control of moderate to severe UC. In this context, steroids do not seem to adversely affect surgical outcome, should surgery become necessary. Treatment is begun with a relatively high dosage of prednisone or methylprednisolone (1 to 2 mg/kg/day) in divided doses and is sustained until disease is controlled, usually within 2 weeks, and then maintained in a single daily dose of at least 1 mg/kg/day for another 2 to 4 weeks. Subsequently, with adjunctive use of sulfasalazine or 5-aminosalicylate, the dose is tapered gradually by 5-mg decrements weekly to an alternate-day dosage of 0.3 to 1 mg/kg, followed by gradual withdrawal. If exacerbation of disease activity prevents the withdrawal of steroids, chronic alternate-day steroid therapy may be necessary. Although the alternate-day steroid regimen causes less adrenal suppression and less severe side effects of hirsutism and altered body composition, patients receiving doses of more than 0.3 mg/kg/day may remain at increased risk for osteoporosis, hypertension, and diabetes. Effects on growth are equivocal because disease activity itself may cause growth retardation. Some patients resume normal growth velocity only after steroid suppression of their disease activity. Other patients whose disease remains in remission may show catch-up growth velocity only after steroid withdrawal.

Topical nonsystemic corticosteroid therapy may be possible when disease is limited to the distal colon and rectum. Recent studies have confirmed the efficacy of 5-aminosalicylic acid enemas in the control of left-sided or distal colitis and maintenance of remission. Hydrocortisone enemas and foam have been used in an attempt to reduce the dose of systemic steroids necessary to control distal disease. Nonabsorbable topical steroid enemas currently are undergoing clinical trials.

Immunosuppressants such as azathioprine and its active metabolite 6-mercaptopurine have been useful in the control of steroid-dependent inflammatory bowel disease but have not been approved for pediatric use in UC. These agents have at least a 3-month lag in steroid-sparing efficacy and are not useful in acute disease. However, cyclosporin A has been effective, in limited research series, in arresting fulminant colitis. To date, indications for its use and its safety and ultimate efficacy have not been established. The major risks are the consequences of immunosuppression and bone marrow suppression, including leukopenia and opportunistic infection. Lymphoproliferative malignancy, previously thought to be a complication of these agents, is extremely rare. As with prolonged steroid treatment, the potential benefits and risks of these agents must be weighed against the curative benefits and surgical risks of colectomy.

## Nutritional Therapy

The goals of nutritional therapy are to restore metabolic homeostasis by correcting nutrient deficits and replacing ongoing losses, to provide sufficient energy and protein for positive nitrogen balance or net protein synthesis, and to promote catch-up growth toward premorbid percentiles. The provision of adequate nutrients is essential for optimal healing. In UC, where malabsorption is unlikely and increased metabolic requirements are small or unproved, the undernutrition is caused by a reduced voluntary intake of calories and protein. On the basis of diet diary analysis of current intake, oral protein and calorie supplements are prescribed to make up calorie and protein deficits. Guidelines for supplementation are to provide at least 140% of the recommended daily allowance for height and age for both energy and protein. Continuous nocturnal nasogastric infusions of enteral formula through a soft Silastic catheter may be necessary for patients who cannot voluntarily increase their intake. For severe disease, when bowel rest is desired as an adjunct to medical treatment,

parenteral nutrition through a central venous catheter or elemental diet is necessary to achieve nutritional goals.

Nutritional support in patients with UC is less likely to help establish a remission than in patients with Crohn's disease. Nevertheless, correcting nutrient deficiencies and maintaining adequate nutritional status are valuable in preventing deterioration of the patient's medical condition and in preparing patients for surgery. Common mineral deficiencies include magnesium and zinc, and these should be corrected.

## Surgery

Surgery is indicated when medical and nutritional therapies fail to control the disease or prevent significant morbidity due to either disease or treatment. Although in most cases medical management is successful in controlling UC and prolonged remissions are possible, a cure can be obtained only by surgical excision.

Indications for colectomy in acute UC include uncontrolled hemorrhage, severe colitis that fails to respond within 2 weeks to intensive treatment (including corticosteroids, antibiotics, bowel rest, and nutritional support), and complications of toxic megacolon, stricture, or perforation. Elective colectomy is indicated in patients with prolonged steroid dependence or steroid-induced complications due to treatment of chronic active disease; retardation of growth and sexual maturation despite nutritional support; and long-standing disease or epithelial dysplasia of rectal or colonic mucosa, which increases the risk of carcinoma. The morbidity and mortality of elective colectomy in a patient whose disease activity is controlled and whose nutritional status has been optimized are much less than in the acutely ill patient, whose risk of mortality can be up to 23% and who faces a greater prospect of postoperative complications.

There are several surgical options. A partial colectomy is often performed, leaving a rectal stump as a blind or Hartmann pouch and creating a terminal ileostomy. If the rectal disease cannot be controlled or if ileostomy is preferred, proctectomy should be performed. The risks of extraintestinal complications and carcinoma remain as long as there is residual diseased mucosa. If the disease in the rectal segment can be controlled with a combination of topical and systemic steroids, it is possible to perform a careful and complete rectal mucosectomy, preserving the pelvic nerves and the rectal musculature and sphincters, through which the ileum may be pulled and anastomosed to the anus. A variety of pouches may be constructed to create a reservoir, aiding continence, but this may be unnecessary because the ileum can dilate. Inflammation of the neorectum or ileal pouch, termed pouchitis, suggests stasis, possible Crohn's disease (which must be excluded by biopsy), or failure of complete dissection of the rectal mucosa before ileal pull-through. Metronidazole has been the most effective agent in the treatment of pouchitis. With the ileoanal pull-through and the use of antimotility agents such as loperamide, the patient often can achieve complete continence with relatively few bowel movements per day. Perianal irritation is treated topically with sitz baths, careful hygiene, and cholestyramine ointment, which may absorb irritating bile acids.

Before surgery, psychological preparation and the involvement of an enterostomal specialist can ease the child's transition to life with an ileostomy.

## PROSPECTIVE MANAGEMENT AND PROGNOSIS

UC is a chronic disease requiring careful surveillance, patient education, and expert management by a team consisting of a pediatrician, gastroenterologist, nutritionist, psychiatrist or psychologist, social worker, and nurse. An alliance with a pediatric surgeon familiar with inflammatory bowel disease is essential for the management of potential complications. The success of management depends on the degree to which the patient and family understand and participate in the treatment. Nutrition and growth, sexual maturation, psychosocial adjustment to disease, and compliance with therapy should all be monitored as carefully as one monitors the clinical signs and symptoms of disease activity outlined above.

The frequency of follow-up depends on the course and on activity, but intervals should be no greater than 6 months. Most children have the potential for a full active life with good general health. Ten percent of the patients will experience only the presenting episode of colitis but must be followed carefully because of the risk of cancer in later life. Some 20% of the patients will have intermittent symptoms, 50% will have chronic disease, and the remaining 20% will have chronic, active, incapacitating disease.

The risk of colonic carcinoma in pediatric-onset UC increases by an estimated 10% to 20% per decade after the first 10 years of disease, depending on the extent of involvement. Because the risk is cumulative, patients with persistent symptoms and pancolitis of early onset in youth are at greatest risk. The risk of carcinoma appears to be less in patients with left-sided colitis or proctitis. Most tumors arise in the distal colon and rectum and may be preceded by histologic signs of dysplasia. Histologic evidence of dysplasia warrants consideration of proctocolectomy.

Sigmoidoscopy and rectal biopsy to detect dysplasia or polyps have been recommended every 6 months for patients with disease of more than 10 years' duration, in conjunction with an annual colonoscopy. However, such surveillance is costly, fallible, and not without morbidity, and the efficacy of surveillance in preventing lethal cancer is unproved. These considerations have led some to advocate prophylactic colectomy in patients with longstanding disease that began in childhood or adolescence. More study is needed to determine the optimal management of carcinoma risk.

The advent of steroids and potent immunosuppressants has dramatically altered the prognosis for medical management of UC, with fewer patients requiring surgery to control the disease. Most patients can resume full activities, including school attendance and athletics. UC has no specific effect on fertility and poses no risk to the fetus. However, poor nutritional status and medical treatment, especially with 6-mercaptopurine and azathioprine, pose risks for pregnant women, and sulfasalazine may produce reversible oligospermia. UC that manifests during pregnancy may be more severe. About 30% to 50% of the patients with preexisting disease may experience exacerbations during pregnancy.

Despite the successes of medical management, there is no medical cure. The medications used to control the disease have potential morbidity, and the risk of colonic carcinoma is significant and cumulative, warranting careful surveillance. Confronting a chronic disease that entails frequent medical visits and frustrating relapses, or the prospects of surgery in childhood and adolescence, is a tremendous emotional burden for both the patient and family and requires ongoing psychosocial support. Colectomy both cures the disease and eliminates the risk of colorectal carcinoma but carries its own risk of potential morbidity, discomfort, and mortality. All of these factors must be considered and reconciled by the patient, family, and medical team in the long-term management of children with UC.

## Selected Readings

Binder SC, Patterson JF, Glotzer DJ. Toxic megacolon in UC. Gastroenterology 1974;66:1088.

Chong SKF, Blackshaw AJ, Morson BC, et al. Prospective study of colitis in infancy and early childhood. J Pediatr Gastroenterol Nutr 1986;5:352.

Classen M, Götze H, Richter H-J, Bender S. Primary sclerosing cholangitis in children. J Pediatr Gastroenterol Nutr 1987;6:197.

Collins RH, Feldman M, Fordtran JS. Colon cancer, dysplasia, and surveillance in patients with UC. N Engl J Med 1987;316:1654.

Kelts DG, Grand RJ. Inflammatory bowel disease in children and adolescents. Curr Probl Pediatr 1980;10:5.

Kirschner BS, Voinchet O, Rosenberg IH. Growth retardation in children with inflammatory bowel disease. Gastroenterology 1978;75:504.

Lichtiger S, Present DH. Preliminary report: cyclosporine in treatment of severe active UC. Lancet 1990;336:16.

Lindsley CB, Schaller JG. Arthritis associated with inflammatory bowel disease. J Pediatr 1974;84:6.

Martin LW, LeCoultre C, Schubert WK, et al. Total colectomy and mucosal proctectomy with preservation of continence in UC. Ann Surg 1977;186:477.

Motil KJ, Grand RJ. Nutritional management of inflammatory bowel disease. Pediatr Clin North Am 1985;32:44.

Motil K, Grand R. UC and Crohn's disease in children. Pediatr Rev 1987;9:109.

Podolsky DK. Inflammatory bowel disease. N Engl J Med 1991;325:928 and 1008.

Powell G. Milk- and soy-induced enterocolitis of infancy. J Pediatr 1978;93:553.

Price AB, Morson BC. Inflammatory bowel disease: the surgical pathology of Crohn's disease and UC. Hum Pathol 1975;6:7.

Trnka YM, LaMont JT. Association of Clostridium difficile toxin with symptomatic relapse of chronic inflammatory bowel disease. Gastroenterology 1981;80:693.

Verhave M, Winter HS, Grand RJ. Azathioprine in the treatment of children with inflammatory bowel disease. J Pediatr 1990;117:809.

Werlin SL, Grand RJ. Severe colitis in children and adolescents: diagnosis, course and treatment. Gastroenterology 1977;73:838.

*Principles and Practice of Pediatrics, Second Edition.*
edited by Frank A. Oski et al. J. B. Lippincott Company, Philadelphia © 1994.

# CHAPTER 128
# *Crohn's Disease*

## W. Daniel Jackson and Richard J. Grand

Crohn's disease is a transmural inflammatory process that may affect any segment of the gastrointestinal (GI) tract from mouth to anus in a discontinuous fashion. The small bowel is involved in 91% of the cases, particularly the distal ileum (71%), usually (52%) in combination with colitis (ie, ileocolitis). Isolated colonic disease without clinical or radiologic evidence of small bowel involvement occurs in 9% of patients. The small bowel involvement is responsible for many of the specific nutritional complications of Crohn's disease, while the colonic involvement poses the greatest challenge for differentiation from other infectious and inflammatory bowel diseases. Although Crohn's disease shares many features with ulcerative colitis, several features allow differentiation of the two disorders (see Table 127-1).

## PATHOLOGY

Unlike the findings in ulcerative colitis, the inflammation in Crohn's disease usually does not involve a continuous segment of bowel and often appears as discrete focal ulcerations (ie, aphthae) with relatively intact intervening mucosa. As the disease progresses, in the 61% of cases involving the colon, right-sided inflammation predominates, with relative sparing of the rectum.

| TABLE 128-1. Crohn's Disease: Patterns of Involvement |
| --- |
| **Extraintestinal Signs and Growth Retardation** |
| Anorexia, malaise, fatigue |
| Perianal disease, stomatitis |
| Erythema nodosum, pyoderma gangrenosum |
| Anemia, hepatitis, renolithiasis, arthritis, clubbing |
| **Small Bowel Involvement** |
| Diarrhea |
| Abdominal mass, postprandial cramps, nausea |
| Malabsorption |
| Mineral and vitamin deficiencies (Fe, Zn, Mg, folate, vitamin B$_{12}$) |
| **Colonic Features** |
| Diarrhea, ugency |
| Rectal bleeding, fecal leukocytes |
| Perianal fistula, abscess |

Anal involvement, in the form of skin tags, anal fissures, abscesses, and fistulas, is more common in Crohn's disease than in ulcerative colitis and occurs in approximately 25% of the patients, often preceding intestinal symptoms. The inflammation is usually transmural and is recognized as mesenteric inflammation, fat encroachment on the serosal surface, stiffening of the small bowel loops due to fibrosis, and adhesions, stricture formation, and fistulas to other loops of bowel, bladder, vagina, or skin.

The histology of the lesions in Crohn's disease reveals the transmural nature of the acute and chronic inflammation, often showing edema, lymphoid aggregates, and significant fibrosis. Mucosal changes may resemble those of ulcerative or infectious colitis, with cryptitis, crypt abscesses, and distortion of crypt architecture. Some areas of the bowel may be normal or may show only mild chronic inflammation. Noncaseating granulomas may be found in as many as 50% of the patients, and coupled with the transmural inflammation, disease distribution, and clinical presentation, they provide strong support for the diagnosis of Crohn's disease (Figs 128-1, 128-2).

## ETIOLOGY

As in ulcerative colitis, the cause of Crohn's disease is unknown. The familial clustering of Crohn's disease supports a genetic predisposition. It is possible that different mechanisms are responsible for the initial insult and for the chronic inflammatory response. The pathogenesis of the chronic inflammation may involve abnormalities in the regulation of the immune response to intestinal antigens including infections agents. Autoimmune or inappropriate immune or cytokine responses have been implicated on the basis of the favorable response to corticosteroids and other immunosuppressive agents. Dietary factors implicated in the cause are decreased dietary fiber and excessive consumption of refined carbohydrates and food additives. However, many putative causes, such as psychosomatic causes, smoking, dietary factors, or immunocompromise, are not consistently observed and usually are better considered consequences of the stresses of chronic illness or undernutrition accompanying the disease.

## EPIDEMIOLOGY

The incidence of Crohn's disease has risen to an estimated 3.5 new cases per 100,000 population per year, making Crohn's disease more common than ulcerative colitis in pediatric practice. The epidemiology is similar to that of ulcerative colitis, with an increased prevalence among Caucasians (especially in the Jewish population), approximately equal male and female representation, and a bimodal age at onset, with peaks in the second and third and again in the sixth decades of life. Although there is an increased prevalence of Crohn's disease among first-degree relatives, there is no specific heritable pattern.

## CLINICAL PRESENTATION

The presentation of Crohn's disease in children depends on the location and extent of inflammation. In many cases, the onset is insidious with nonspecific features of GI involvement or extraintestinal manifestations leading to delayed or incorrect diagnosis. There is an average delay of 13 months from the onset of symptoms to diagnosis. Diarrhea, abdominal pain (most frequently postprandial periumbilical cramping), fever, and weight loss are the most common presenting features. Rectal bleeding, seen in 30% Crohn's disease cases, is much less common than in ulcerative colitis and usually signifies colonic involvement.

The three general patterns of clinical presentation based on anatomical involvement show considerable overlap. Patients with the first pattern present with nonspecific extraintestinal manifestations and growth retardation (see Table 128-1). Overt clinical signs of GI involvement may not appear for years, although this inflammation may be extensive enough to cause early satiety, nausea, poor feeding, and malabsorption syndromes. Over time, net energy and protein deficits are reflected in decreased weight velocity followed by decreased height velocity and delayed skel-

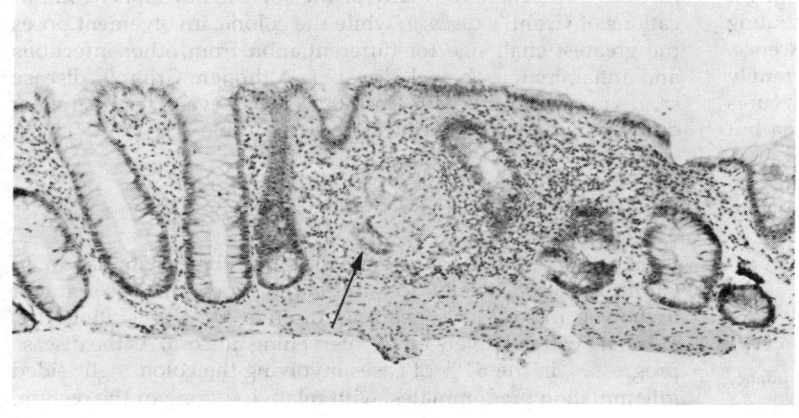

**Figure 128-1.** Colonic biopsy of an adolescent girl with active Crohn's disease. Note the distortion of the crypt architecture with a prominent noncaseating granuloma and giant cells (*arrow*) amid increased acute and chronic inflammation of the lamina propria.

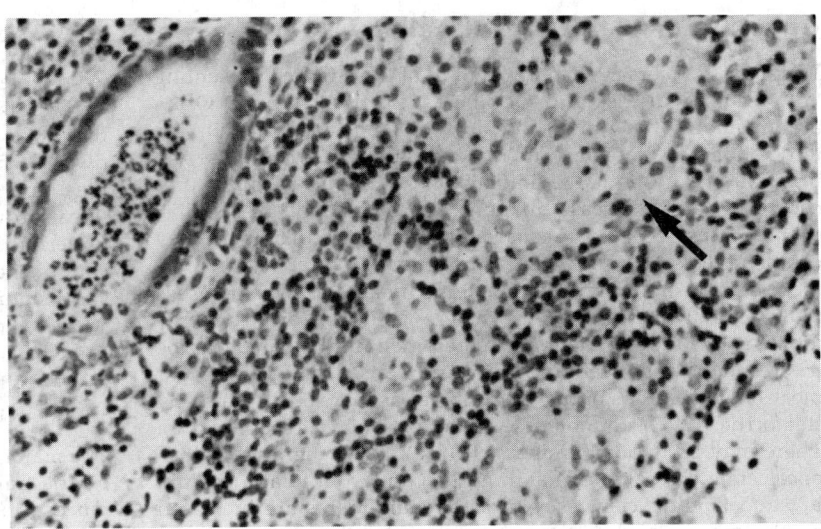

**Figure 128-2.** High-power view of a large crypt abscess adjacent to a granuloma (*arrow*) in a patient with Crohn's disease.

etal and sexual maturation. As a consequence of nutritional, growth, and maturational problems, patients may be referred to specialists in endocrinology for assessment of short stature and hypogonadism or to psychiatrists for evaluation of anorexia or poor feeding. Certain extraintestinal features that may be clues indicating the presence of Crohn's disease include perianal disease, oral aphthae, erythema nodosum, arthritis, uveitis, and digital clubbing. The blood smear may show a microcytic anemia, and there may be an elevated white blood cell and platelet count and an inexplicably elevated erythrocyte sedimentation rate. Abdominal radiographs may show an unusual gas pattern with some small bowel dilatation. Recognizing this insidious mode of presentation leads to timely use of specific tests to confirm the diagnosis.

Another pattern of presentation is produced by small bowel involvement, which probably is responsible for much of the postprandial cramping, early satiety, nausea, and poor feeding that patients report. Rarely, the esophagus or stomach may be affected. Diarrhea may occur and, in the absence of colitis, most likely signifies a malabsorption syndrome. Estimates of the prevalence of malabsorption in children with Crohn's disease depends on the nutrient that is malabsorbed but range from 17% for lactose and 29% for fat to 70% for protein. The frequency of lactose malabsorption is normal when adjusted for that expected for the ethnic distribution of Crohn's patients and may not be a consequence of small bowel inflammation. Deficiencies of iron, folate, and vitamin $B_{12}$ may be more pronounced in patients with small bowel disease, particularly those with terminal ileum involvement.

Colonic involvement may present as diarrhea, often associated with cramps and urgency to defecate after any distention of the inflamed colon by the fecal stream. Other signs of colitis may be indistinguishable from those seen in ulcerative colitis and consist of an inflammatory exudate of neutrophils into the lumen and occult or overt rectal bleeding. Perianal disease and relative sparing of the rectum is more frequent in Crohn's colitis than in ulcerative colitis and may be the only differentiating features. A rare complication, toxic dilatation with risk of perforation and sepsis, known as toxic megacolon, has been reported in Crohn's colitis; treatment is the same as outlined for toxic megacolon complicating severe ulcerative colitis (see Chap. 127).

With Crohn's disease, these three patterns of anatomical involvement overlap to produce a clinical presentation unique for each patient, and a clinical diagnosis alone usually is not possible or sufficient.

## Extraintestinal Signs

The systemic nature of Crohn's disease is apparent in the range of potential involvement of extraintestinal organs. Arthritis and arthralgias may occur in as many as 11% of cases and usually present as a seronegative monoarticular arthritis of a knee or ankle or as a migratory polyarthritis. Arthritis is more common in patients with colonic involvement (eg, colitis, ileocolitis) and seems to parallel disease activity, although occasionally it precedes overt GI signs. Sacroiliitis and ankylosing spondylitis are rare and occur predominantly in patients with histocompatibility gene HLA-B27.

Approximately 5% of the patients develop cutaneous lesions of erythema nodosum, erythema multiforme, or pyoderma gangrenosum. The latter condition is a severe deep ulceration of the skin, often preceded by minor trauma or associated with surgical incisions or stoma sites. Management requires control of the underlying bowel disease, often with the addition of metronidazole, topical cromolyn sulfate, and occasional skin grafting.

Signs of liver disease occur in fewer than 8% of patients with Crohn's disease. Mild histologic abnormalities of steatosis may be more common. Liver involvement correlates with bowel disease activity but rarely progresses to cirrhosis or chronic active hepatitis. Sclerosing cholangitis has been reported in two adolescents with Crohn's colitis. Cholelithiasis, usually asymptomatic, may follow ileal dysfunction or resection, which interrupts the enterohepatic circulation of bile acids, leading to decreased cholesterol solubility characteristic of lithogenic bile. Prolonged periods of bowel rest without meal-stimulated gallbladder contraction allows stasis of bile in the gallbladder, which contributes to sludge and stone formation.

Urologic manifestations include calcium oxalate renal calculi due to increased intestinal oxalate absorption accompanying steatorrhea and subsequent increased renal excretion. Ureteral inflammation may develop from adjacent transmural bowel inflammation and lead to pyuria, obstruction, and infection. Hydroureter or hydronephrosis may result from renal stones, inflammation, or external compression from adjacent intestinal masses. Recurrent urinary tract infections and pneumaturia may herald enterovesical fistulas. Other signs include uveitis, acutely symptomatic in fewer than 3% and asymptomatic in as many as 30% of the patients; aphthous stomatitis; osteoporosis; anemias of chronic disease, iron deficiency, vitamin $B_{12}$ and folate deficiencies; or zinc deficiency, implicated in taste dysfunction, acrodermatitis, poor healing, and growth failure.

## Undernutrition and Growth Failure

Weight loss occurs in as many as 87% of the children presenting with Crohn's disease and may be as much as 12.5 kg. Often accompanying the weight loss are impaired linear growth, retarded bone development and mineralization, and delayed sexual maturation. These changes initially may be subtle and often precede overt bowel disease by months or years (Fig 128-3). Most of these effects seem to be caused by undernutrition because they can be reversed by nutritional supplementation.

The cause of undernutrition in inflammatory bowel disease is multifactorial. In most patients with growth failure, dietary energy intake is less than the average requirement for age and may be the result of poor feeding from altered taste, early satiety, or meal-related cramps or diarrhea. Some cases are complicated by steatorrhea (29%) and increased enteric protein excretion (70%). There may be hypoalbuminemia (50%), hypomagnesemia, hypocalcemia, fat-soluble vitamin losses, and iron, folate, vitamin $B_{12}$, and zinc deficiencies. Nutrient requirements are increased by the metabolic demands of fever and inflammation, losses through fistulas, and demands for repletion of lean body mass and fat deficits beyond those normally imposed by growth, especially in adolescents.

Most endocrine tests are normal in patients with growth retardation and short stature associated with Crohn's disease. Although bone age may be delayed and serum insulin-like growth factor-1 levels depressed, both respond to nutritional therapy, and pituitary, thyroid, adrenal, and growth hormone studies are normal. Similarly, arrested sexual maturation, with delayed puberty and menarche, responds to nutritional therapy and control of the disease.

Growth failure may occur with or without steroid therapy. Although there is evidence that corticosteroids may suppress linear growth, their use in controlling Crohn's disease often permits growth to resume at normal rates. Whether accelerated or "catch-up" growth sufficient to reach the premorbid growth percentiles is possible during high-dose steroid treatment is unclear.

Over time, the patient with long-standing disease may adapt to a state of chronic undernutrition and become a "nutritional dwarf," characterized by height stunted below expected percentiles, appropriate weight for height, and normal to subnormal linear growth velocity. The consequences of untreated chronic undernutrition in a child with Crohn's disease are poor disease control, increased complications, delayed puberty, and permanent short stature.

## COMPLICATIONS

The major intestinal complications of Crohn's disease are caused by the transmural nature of the inflammation, extending from mucosa to serosa. Contiguous loops of bowel or other organs may be enveloped in inflammation. Adhesions, strictures, and abscesses may develop, with a risk of obstruction or bacterial overgrowth. Fistulas may form to any abdominal or pelvic structure and should be suspected to underlie any chronic draining ulcer or sinus. Enterocutaneous, enteroenteric, perirectal, labial, enterovaginal, and enterovesical fistulas may pose a nutritional hazard, because they are conduits for major losses of protein and other nutrients. Perianal disease occurs in 25% of the patients with Crohn's disease, most often in the context of colonic inflammation and fistula formation. Skin tags, anal fissures, and perianal or perirectal abscesses may precede other signs of intestinal Crohn's disease or develop during an exacerbation of colitis. Although often minor in appearance, these lesions can create severe discomfort and be quite refractory to treatment. Massive hemorrhage and toxic megacolon, which are potential

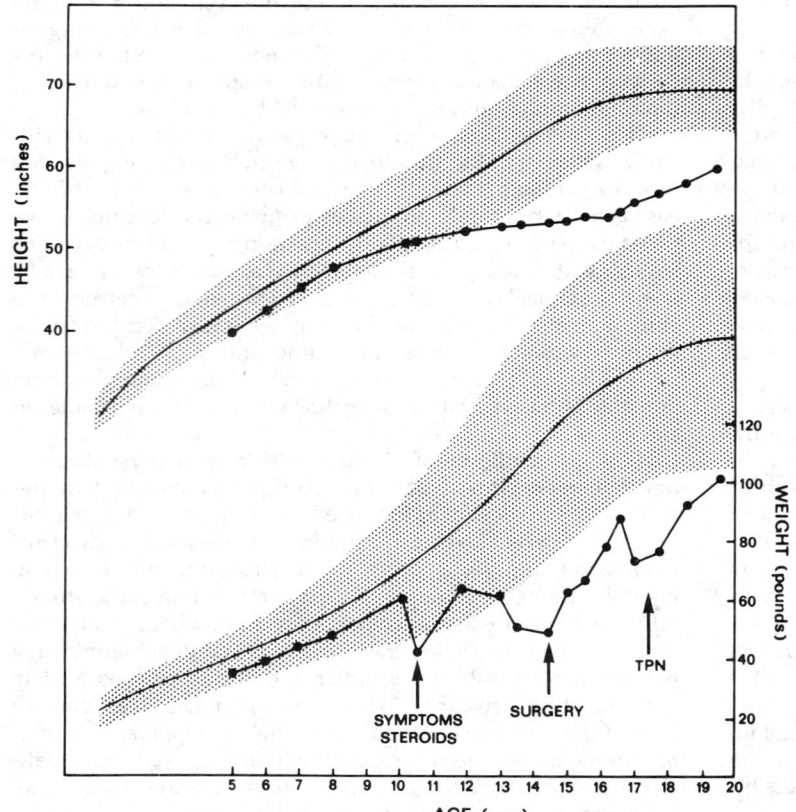

**Figure 128-3.** Growth curve of an adolescent with Crohn's disease. The reduction in linear growth preceded the acute weight loss and onset of symptoms. Although growth accelerated after steroid treatment, limited surgical resection, and parenteral nutrition, premorbid percentiles were not achieved.

complications of ulcerative colitis, occur only rarely in Crohn's disease.

The risk of malignancy of all types appears to be increased in patients with Crohn's disease, estimated as 20 times greater than normal for patients with Crohn's disease diagnosed before the age of 21 years. Nevertheless, the incidence of small bowel carcinoma is low, and the rates of colonic carcinoma are much lower than in patients with ulcerative colitis. However, rates of colorectal cancer approach those of ulcerative colitis when adjusted for the extent of colonic involvement in Crohn's colitis. The association of colonic mucosal dysplasia with carcinoma in Crohn's disease is not sufficiently established to recommend prophylactic colectomy, although surveillance colonoscopy and biopsies are prudent in patients with long-standing Crohn's colitis.

## DIAGNOSIS

The diagnosis of Crohn's disease is based on clinical presentation, radiologic findings, and mucosal appearance and histology and on exclusion of alternative causes. A complete history should be obtained, with attention to family history, exposure to infectious agents or antibiotic treatment, extraintestinal manifestations, and retardation in growth rate or in sexual development. Physical examination should include assessment of hydration, nutritional status, signs of peritoneal inflammation, and signs of systemic chronic disease. Features suggesting Crohn's disease are stomatitis, perianal skin tags or inflammation, and clubbing. Fever, orthostasis, tachycardia, and abdominal tenderness, distention, or mass should be considered indications for admission to the hospital.

### Laboratory Evaluation

A complete blood cell count can detect leukocytosis or identify anemia. The erythrocyte sedimentation rate is elevated in 90% of the patients and may be useful as a marker of inflammatory activity. Serum total protein and albumin levels may be low as a consequence of severe undernutrition and enteric protein losses. Serum magnesium, iron, and plasma zinc levels may be low due to poor intake coupled with cumulative losses from sloughed intestinal epithelial cells or bleeding. Ileal dysfunction may be revealed by a low vitamin $B_{12}$ and low fat-soluble vitamin levels. Urinalysis may reveal pyuria. Fresh stool should be obtained for examination of blood, leukocytes, and parasites and cultured for infectious pathogens. Microbiologic studies should include culture for *Yersinia enterocolitica* and assay for *Clostridium difficile* toxin. Serologic titers may help exclude *Entamoeba histolytica*. Detection of pathogens may not exclude the existence of underlying Crohn's disease, but the infections must be treated first.

### Radiology

Although the extent of radiographic involvement has not correlated with clinical disease activity, radiologic studies are often essential to diagnosis and management.

Upright and supine radiographs of the abdomen and a chest x-ray will demonstrate the extent of bowel dilatation and help exclude ileus, intestinal obstruction, or pneumoperitoneum, signifying perforation. If clinical colitis is present and colonoscopy is unavailable, a barium enema study with air contrast to reveal mucosal detail may demonstrate characteristic aphthous lesions and show cecal or segmental involvement or right-sided predominance (Figs 128-4, 128-5), although the ileum may not be adequately defined. An upper GI series with small bowel follow-through and careful fluoroscopic study of the terminal ileum is essential to define the small bowel involvement, which affects

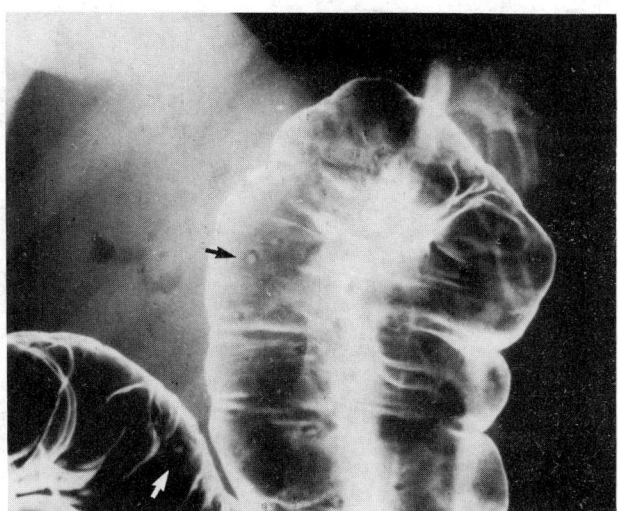

**Figure 128-4.** Air contrast barium enema in a patient with Crohn's disease demonstrating aphthae (*arrows*) in the splenic flexure.

more than 90% of the patients with Crohn's disease (Fig 128-6). A small bowel enteroclysis study provides the best definition of small bowel lesions and fistulas. The terminal ileum or other loops may be relatively rigid, constricted, and nodular, with fixed deformities despite fluoroscopic manipulation, features due to the transmural nature of the inflammation in Crohn's disease. This appearance may be contrasted with that of the "backwash" ileitis seen in ulcerative colitis, in which mucosal detail is effaced and dilatation occurs without signs of bowel wall thickening. An

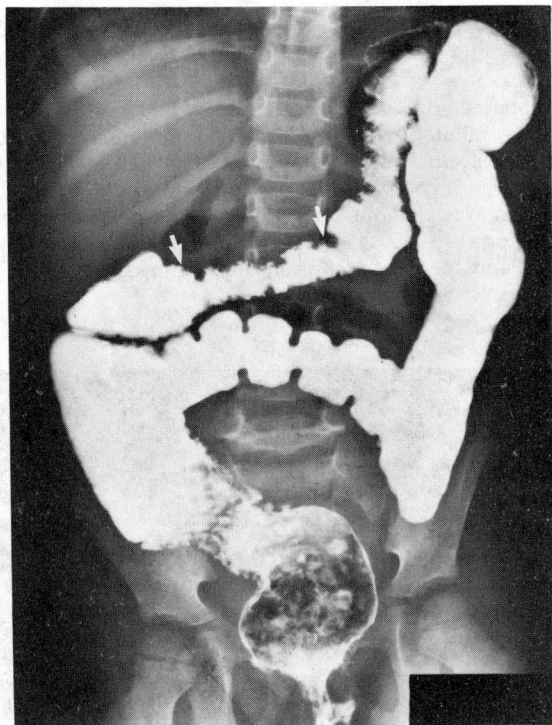

**Figure 128-5.** Barium enema study in an 8-year-old girl with Crohn's disease reveals segmental colitis involving discrete regions of the transverse colon (*between arrows*). Notice the irregular mucosal margins consistent with active ulceration and edema. The rectum, shown with residual stool, was spared.

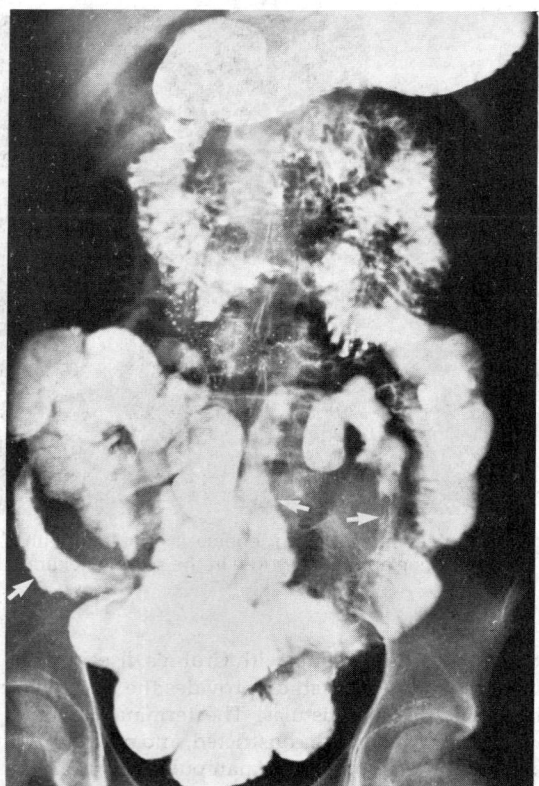

**Figure 128-6.** Small bowel follow-through of an upper GI series in a 16-year-old girl after treatment with prednisone for Crohn's disease presenting initially with marked small bowel obstruction and growth failure. Notice the separation of bowel loops and the long S-shaped segment of constricted nodular terminal ileum (*arrows*). The cecum is elevated, suggesting a contracted ascending colon. Despite the narrowed lumen, there is no obstruction.

abdominal mass, persistent focal tenderness, fever, or obstruction should be evaluated by ultrasound or computed tomography to exclude abscess. If Crohn's disease is suspected but difficult to demonstrate or if complications are suspected, computed tomography often can demonstrate the bowel wall thickening, fat wrapping, or abscesses (Fig 128-7). Radionuclide scans lack the resolution and specificity required for diagnosis.

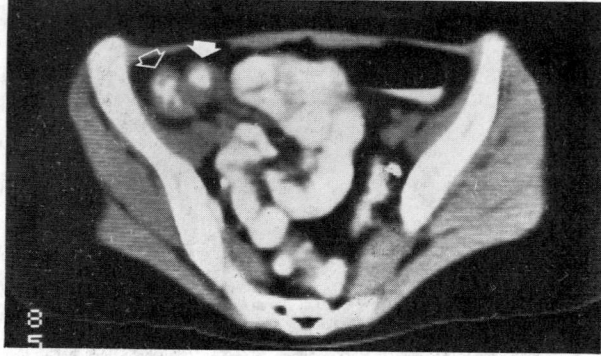

**Figure 128-7.** Computed tomogram of the lower abdomen of a 12-year-old girl with Crohn's ileocolitis. Notice the thickened bowel wall of terminal ileum (*solid arrow*) and cecum (*open arrow*), and thickened mesentery. No abscesses or fistulas were demonstrated.

## Endoscopy

Colonoscopy with biopsy of the colon and terminal ileum is the most sensitive and specific test for evaluating Crohn's ileocolitis. As reflected in its pathology, the lesions of Crohn's disease may appear as discrete ulcerations or aphthae of the mucosa, often with a central exudate and corona of erythema. Intervening areas may be normal in appearance and histologic characteristics. In more than 60% of the patients with colonic involvement, disease is more active in the proximal colon and cecum. Although perianal disease may be present, the rectum is often spared. Because the histology of regions that appear grossly normal may show signs of nonspecific chronic inflammation, biopsies must be obtained from multiple sites, regardless of gross endoscopic appearance. Endoscopy to explore the esophagus, stomach, and duodenum is indicated when involvement is suspected on clinical or radiologic grounds.

## DIFFERENTIAL DIAGNOSIS

Crohn's disease appears in many forms, which makes diagnosis and differentiation from other entities challenging. Signs of inflammation (eg, fever, abdominal cramps, tenderness), extraintestinal lesions, or an elevated sedimentation rate can often differentiate inflammatory causes of growth failure from endocrine or psychogenic syndromes such as growth hormone deficiency, hypopituitarism, and anorexia nervosa. Signs of colitis on stool examination, barium study, or colonoscopy with biopsy or the presence of oral aphthae or perianal disease can localize the inflammation to the GI tract. The presence of extracolonic disease or granulomas on biopsy favors Crohn's disease over ulcerative colitis, although in the absence of such features, Crohn's disease cannot be excluded. In some cases, Crohn's colitis clinically and histologically may be indistinguishable from ulcerative colitis until extracolonic or histologic features appear. There is even a report of the co-occurrence of the two disease patterns. Occasionally, evidence of Crohn's disease does not appear until inflammation develops in the ileostomy or ileoanal pouch of patient who has had a colectomy for what was presumed to be ulcerative colitis.

GI disorders are common in pediatric patients, with as many as 10% of children between the ages of 7 and 11 years seeking medical attention for the complaint of recurrent abdominal pain, usually periumbilical in location. Unless there are signs of inflammation or growth disturbance, extensive evaluation for inflammatory bowel disease is contraindicated. Nevertheless, the periumbilical nature of the pain is nonspecific and not pathognomonic for functional abdominal pain because it is characteristic of most children presenting with inflammatory bowel disease. In uncomplicated recurrent abdominal pain, discomfort due to stool retention, lactose intolerance, peptic disease, urinary tract infection, pelvic inflammatory disease, or psychosocial causes should be considered and eliminated.

Rectal bleeding is more common in ulcerative colitis than in Crohn's disease and has many causes in addition to colitis, such as Meckel's diverticulum, hemolytic-uremic syndrome, Henoch-Schönlein purpura, intestinal polyps, or hemorrhoids. Anal fissures secondary to constipation usually present without signs of colitis or chronic perianal inflammation and skin tags.

Pathogens such as *C difficile, Y enterocolitica,* enteropathogenic *Escherichia coli, Aeromonas hydrophila, Giardia lamblia,* and *Entamoeba histolytica* must be excluded, along with the customary *Salmonella, Shigella,* and *Campylobacter* cultured in the setting of enterocolitis. These agents are often overlooked in the initial evaluation and may produce a chronic inflammatory picture resembling Crohn's ileocolitis. Tuberculosis, *Yersinia,* and lymphoma may involve the small bowel, predominantly the terminal ileum, which is rich in lymphoid tissue, and may resemble Crohn's disease clinically and radiographically.

Unlike most other rheumatologic diseases of childhood, the arthritis of inflammatory bowel disease is usually asymmetric, involving large joints of the lower extremities without deformity.

## THERAPY

Because no pharmacologic regimen has been shown to alter the long-term outcome of Crohn's disease, the goals of treatment are to minimize the morbidity of disease exacerbations without introducing iatrogenic morbidity.

### Pharmacologic Therapy

Corticosteroids can effect short-term remissions of active small bowel disease in 70% of the patients. Unfortunately, symptoms may recur with reduction of the dosage such that 70% of these patients suffer relapse within 1 year. Continuous low-dose treatment does not seem to prevent relapse, but higher-dose, alternate-day steroids may allow control of symptoms with a minimum of side effects and a lower risk of growth retardation. Indications for steroid therapy are limited to symptoms refractory to other agents, extensive small bowel disease, severe or persistent systemic and extraintestinal complications, and postoperative recurrences.

In active disease, induction of remission is achieved with a dosage of 1 to 2 mg/kg/day of prednisone or methylprednisolone (up to 60 mg/day), tapered after 2 to 3 weeks by 5-mg weekly decrements over 4 to 6 weeks. The steroid is then tapered to an alternate-day regimen and discontinued as allowed by the patient's symptoms (Table 128-2).

Potential morbidity of high-dose steroid therapy includes adrenal suppression, hypertension, osteoporosis, glaucoma, cataracts, masking of symptoms, pseudotumor cerebri, hirsutism, cutaneous striae, and altered body composition. An alternate-day regimen may minimize these effects and should be used when possible. However, steroid therapy should always be initiated using a daily dose regimen. The effects on growth are equivocal, because the disease activity itself may cause growth retardation.

Some patients resume normal growth velocity only after steroid suppression of their disease activity. Other patients, whose disease is quiescent, may show catch-up growth velocity only after steroid withdrawal. A general principle is to use the least corticosteroid necessary to control disease activity and allow growth and full function.

In as many as 75% of the patients who cannot be managed without high-dose or prolonged corticosteroids or who are at risk for complications of steroid therapy, immunosuppressive agents (eg, azathioprine, 6-mercaptopurine) are useful in maintaining remission and allowing reduction in steroid dosage. Although bone marrow suppression and opportunistic infection are potential risks, current evidence from clinical trials suggests that these complications are rare and can be weighed against the known morbidity of chronic steroid treatment. Lymphoid malignancy is an extraordinarily rare complication of immunosuppressive therapy. These agents do not seem to be useful in acute management, and several months of treatment may be required before clinical efficacy in terms of steroid-sparing, perianal disease, or fistula healing.

The role of cyclosporine in acute exacerbations of Crohn's disease has not been determined decisively, but early experience suggests that short-term benefits may be achieved.

Sulfasalazine, administered in a dosage of 40 to 50 mg/kg/day (maximum, 3 to 4 g/day), is useful in the management of Crohn's colitis. In conjunction with steroid treatment, it is better than placebo in ileocolitis. Although it has not been proved effective in preventing relapse or in treating small bowel disease, it is often continued as a chronic regimen. Sulfasalazine usually is introduced gradually, depending on patient tolerance. It often can be renewed after dosage reduction because of side effects of headache, nausea, vomiting, or bloody diarrhea. Neutropenia and oligospermia are reversible side effects. Folate malabsorption due to competitive inhibition of absorption is treated with 1 mg/day supplements. Because the side effects of sulfasalazine are caused primarily by the sulfapyridine moiety and the anti-inflammatory effects are caused by the topical activity of the relatively poorly absorbed 5-aminosalicylate moiety, alternative oral non-sulfa preparations of 5-aminosalicylic acid (5-ASA; Asacol, Pentasa, Dipentum) have been created to prevent proximal GI absorption . There is evidence that all these agents are effective in colitis, though data for Crohn's disease are preliminary. Pentasa and Asacol are forms of 5-ASA allowing some release in the small intestine and ileum with theoretical efficacy in ileitis.

Metronidazole is an antimicrobial agent effective against anaerobic bacteria, including *C difficile*, *E histolytica*, and *G lamblia*, that is indicated in patients with Crohn's colitis unresponsive to sulfasalazine or with complications of perianal disease or small intestinal bacterial overgrowth. Clinical series support its role in healing perineal fistulas with up to a 70% response rate for children with perianal disease. Potential morbidity includes reversible peripheral neuropathy with chronic use and a potential increased risk of malignancy.

Antimotility agents such as loperamide (0.1 mg/kg/dose twice or three times daily; maximum dose, 4 mg) may be used to prolong intestinal transit time and facilitate fluid absorption, providing relief from diarrhea at night and at social functions. These agents should be used with caution and discontinued if there are symptoms of cramping distention, or fever. Agents that bind bile acids, such as cholestyramine, may be useful in reducing the choleraic diarrhea that follows ileal dysfunction or resection.

### Nutritional Therapy

Because of the limitations and morbidity of medical treatment and the nutritional impact of Crohn's disease, increased emphasis

---

**TABLE 128-2. Pharmacologic Therapy of Crohn's Disease**

**Acute Exacerbation**

Methylprednisolone or prednisone: 1–2 mg/kg/day divided bid, taper to 1 mg/kg/day qd and then to qod over 4 to 6 weeks, depending on clinical response. When remission is achieved, taper and discontinue.

**Remission**

Sulfasalazine: 40–50 mg/kg/day divided bid to qid (maximum, 3–4 g/day)
Non-sulfa 5-aminosalicylates
Folate supplement: 1 mg/day

**Perianal Disease or Fistula**

Metronidazole: 15 mg/kg/day divided q 8 h

**Refractory Disease**

Azathioprine: 2 mg/kg/day divided bid
6-Mercaptopurine: 1.5 mg/kg/day divided bid

has been placed on nutritional rehabilitation and therapy as a way of altering the course of Crohn's disease. Optimal prospective management in patients with inflammatory bowel disease should include regular assessment of growth and nutritional status. Data to follow are height by stadiometer, body weight, triceps skin fold, mid-arm muscle circumference, and serum levels of protein, albumin, and transferrin. A reduction in growth velocity over an interval may presage or contribute to an exacerbation of Crohn's disease activity. Maintenance of optimal nutritional status with aggressive support of energy and protein intake may prolong remission or allow reduced corticosteroid treatment. The goals of nutritional therapy in Crohn's disease must include recovery of metabolic homeostasis by correcting specific nutrient deficits and replacing ongoing losses; provision of sufficient energy and protein for positive nitrogen balance (ie, protein synthesis) and healing; and promotion of catch-up growth toward premorbid percentiles.

Deficiencies in iron, folate, or vitamin $B_{12}$ should be corrected with appropriate supplements. Magnesium depletion, better reflected in low urinary excretion after a challenge dose than in plasma concentration, should be corrected by parenteral magnesium sulfate. Low plasma zinc levels suggest low dietary intake, redistribution to circulating hepatic pools as a consequence of chronic inflammation, or depletion due to active mucosal inflammation and enteric losses. Treatment consists of supplements of zinc sulfate (1 to 2 mg/kg/day of elemental zinc). Oral protein and calorie supplements are prescribed to make up deficits revealed by dietary analysis of voluntary intake. The guidelines for supplementation suggest providing at least 140% of the recommended daily allowance for height-age for energy and protein intake. Continuous nocturnal nasogastric infusions through a soft Silastic catheter may be necessary in patients who cannot voluntarily increase their intake. An elemental formula may be necessary if there is significant malabsorption, symptoms from partial obstruction, or a goal of reducing the antigen load to an inflamed colon. A gastrostomy tube is an option for those who cannot tolerate a nasogastric tube yet who need chronic supplementation. In severe or complicated Crohn's disease, in which enteral feeding is not possible or bowel rest is desired, parenteral nutrition through a central venous catheter is necessary to achieve nutritional goals.

The optimal nutritional therapy serves as an adjunct to medical therapy in controlling symptoms and inducing remission. Short-term remissions have been achieved by aggressive elemental enteral or parenteral nutritional support alone. Elemental diets have been advocated as primary initial therapy to induce remission until immunosuppressive agents become effective. They have been variably ineffective in closing fistulas, but most eventually require surgery. After nutritional rehabilitation and disease remission have been achieved, efforts should continue to ensure catch-up growth rates of at least 0.5 cm each month and 1 kg each month toward premorbid percentiles.

## Surgery

Unlike ulcerative colitis, in which disease is limited to the colon and can be cured by total colectomy, there is no definitive surgical cure for Crohn's disease. For these reasons and because of the high incidence of complications requiring repeat operation, surgery is reserved for the acute and chronic complications of Crohn's disease refractory to medical or nutritional therapy. Indications include intestinal obstruction, fistula, abscess, uncontrolled hemorrhage, toxic megacolon, perforation, and growth failure in the setting of localized disease. Local resection is more successful in isolated small bowel disease than in the presence of colitis. Intractable colitis is managed by total proctocolectomy or segmental colectomy with anastomosis. The endorectal pull-through operation used for intractable ulcerative colitis never should be used for Crohn's disease because of the risk of perirectal or pelvic abscess or perianal disease. Perianal abscesses often need draining with probing or contrast agent injection to exclude underlying fistulas; proctectomy is rarely required to control perianal disease; and anal tags should not be excised.

## PROSPECTIVE MANAGEMENT AND PROGNOSIS

Crohn's disease is a chronic incurable disease requiring careful surveillance, patient education, and expert management by a team consisting of a pediatrician, gastroenterologist, nutritionist, psychiatrist or psychologist, social worker, and nurse. An alliance with a pediatric surgeon familiar with inflammatory bowel disease is essential for management of potential complications. The success of long-term management is determined in part by the degree to which the patient and family understand and participate in the treatment.

Nutritional status, growth, sexual maturation, psychosocial adjustment to disease, and compliance with therapy should be monitored as carefully as one monitors the clinical signs and symptoms of disease activity. The frequency of follow-up depends on the course of disease activity, but intervals should be no longer than 6 months. Most children with Crohn's disease can expect to live full, productive lives with good general health. Mortality is low, but morbidity is high, especially in patients with colonic involvement. Fertility is unaffected in Crohn's disease unless there is malnutrition or inflammatory damage to reproductive organs. Disease activity often remains stable or improves during pregnancy, although an exacerbation may follow delivery. There seems to be no increased risk to the fetus. Although the incidence of colorectal carcinoma is increased in Crohn's disease, the risk is poorly defined and seems too low to warrant prophylactic colectomy.

The management of Crohn's disease in children is complex and requires adaptation of the patient to the lifelong unpredictable nature of this disease, the morbidity of chronic medication and hospital visits, and the demands of adolescent development. A willingness to become active in the management of his or her condition and to work with the team involved in each case is probably the patient's best prognostic feature.

## Selected Readings

Beeken WL. Absorptive defects in young people with regional enteritis. Pediatrics 1974;52:69.

Bernstein L. Complications of inflammatory bowel disease. Pract Gastroenterol 1987;11:35.

Gryboski J, Spiro HD. Prognosis in children with Crohn's disease. Gastroenterology 1978;74:87.

Homer DR, Grand RJ, Colodny AH. Growth, course and prognosis after surgery for Crohn's colitis. Pediatrics 1977;59:717.

Kelts DG, Grand RJ. Inflammatory bowel disease in children and adolescents. Curr Probl Pediatr 1980;10:5.

Kirschner BS, Voincher O, Rosenberg IH. Growth retardation in inflammatory bowel disease. Gastroenterology 1978;75:5048.

Markowitz J, Daum F, Aiges M, et al. Perianal disease in children and adolescents with Crohn's disease. Gastroenterology 1984;86:829.

Motil K, Grand RJ. Nutritional management of inflammatory bowel disease. Pediatr Clin North Am 1985;32:447.

Motil K, Grand RJ. Ulcerative colitis and Crohn's disease in children. Pediatr Rev 1987;9:109.

Podolsky DK. Inflammatory bowel disease (two parts). N Engl J Med 1991;325:928.

Price AB, Morson BC. Inflammatory bowel disease: the surgical pathology of Crohn's disease and ulcerative colitis. Hum Pathol 1975;6:7.

Seidman E, LeLeiko N, Ament M, Berman W, Caplan D, et al. Nutritional issues in pediatric inflammatory bowel disease. J Pediatr Gastroenterol Nutr 12:424.

Verhave M, Winter HS, Grand RJ. Azathioprine in the treatment of children with inflammatory bowel disease. J Pediatr 1990;117:809.

*Principles and Practice of Pediatrics, Second Edition.*
edited by Frank A. Oski et al. J. B. Lippincott Company, Philadelphia © 1994.

CHAPTER 129
# Antibiotic-Associated Colitis and Diarrhea

W. Daniel Jackson and Richard J. Grand

A spectrum of gastrointestinal (GI) disturbances ranging from frank pseudomembranous colitis to chronic diarrhea has been associated with antibiotic treatment in adults and children. Studies have identified cytopathic toxins elaborated by *Clostridium difficile* as the cause of most cases of antibiotic-associated pseudomembranous colitis and many cases of antibiotic-associated diarrhea.

## PATHOLOGY

Pseudomembranous colitis is a term denoting the characteristic endoscopic and pathologic features found in antibiotic-associated colitis. The rectal mucosa is erythematous and friable with small (<5 mm), raised, yellowish plaques that may be discrete or confluent. Histologically, these lesions are superficial mucosal erosions surmounted by a tenacious pseudomembrane consisting of fibrin, mucus, polymorphonuclear leukocytes, and necrotic epithelium. The submucosa is edematous with acute and chronic inflammatory infiltrates and mucus-congested glands and goblet cells. Although typically involved in pseudomembranous colitis, the rectum may be spared. Cases have been reported in which significant disease was recognized only on small bowel biopsy or colonoscopy to the proximal colon.

## MICROBIOLOGY AND ETIOLOGY

Most cases of antibiotic-associated enterocolitis have been attributed to overgrowth of *C difficile* in the context of antibiotic suppression of normal competitive bowel flora.

*C difficile* is a gram-positive anaerobic bacillus resistant to most antibiotics. It may be isolated from blood agar culture and inoculated into chopped meat broth media made selective by the addition of cycloserine and cefoxitin. *C difficile* produces two exotoxins implicated in the secretory and inflammatory features of enterocolitis. Toxin A is a potent enterotoxin and chemotactic agent causing inflammation and secretion of a hemorrhagic exudate in ligated rabbit ileal loops but having little effect on cultured fibroblast cells used for cytopathic assay. Conversely, toxin B is one of the most potent cytotoxins in cultured fibroblast assays but has no activity against intact animal intestinal epithelium. Although toxin B has been the traditional diagnostic marker, toxin A is now considered the principal agent in the pathogenesis of *C difficile*-related diarrhea and colitis. No strains of *C difficile* have been described that produce toxin B without also producing toxin A, although the converse has not been excluded.

*C difficile* is considered part of the normal flora of infants younger than 1 year of age and has been isolated from 25% to 50% of neonates and 45% of infants. Significant toxin B titers may be measured in 25% to 50% of asymptomatic infants. The reasons for asymptomatic carriage in infancy are unknown but

may include the absence of toxin receptors, maternal antitoxin, or immature inflammatory responses. *C difficile* colonization occurs in only 4% to 18% of older children and is rarely isolated from the stools of adults, although it is a common vaginal species. In one study of self-limited mild diarrhea associated with antibiotic treatment in a group of young children, most of whom were infants younger than 1 year of age, no correlation of symptoms with *C difficile* colonization or toxin was found. Culture and toxin assay for *C difficile* therefore may not be clinically valid in children younger than 1 year of age.

*C difficile* is more frequently implicated in chronic or colitic diarrhea. In a study of adults with antibiotic-associated diarrheal states, 27% had demonstrable *C difficile* toxin. In adults and children, *C difficile* colonization with toxin production is responsible for at least 95% of antibiotic-associated pseudomembranous colitis. Pseudomembranous colitis due to *C difficile* has been rarely reported in settings where antibiotics have not been used. In addition, there are rare reports of pseudomembranous enterocolitis attributed to other organisms such as *Clostridium perfringens* and *Staphylococcus aureus*.

## PATHOGENESIS

The indigenous, mixed bowel flora form an important host defense mechanism limiting proliferation and colonization of potential bacterial pathogens. The composition of the bowel flora is kept remarkably constant with a thousandfold predominance of anaerobic bacteria, despite a great variety of dietary and physiological changes. The ability of the indigenous flora to limit proliferation or exclude colonization of pathogenic bacteria is called *colonization resistance* and is important in protecting the host at the gut interface with the environment.

Oral or intravenous antibiotic agents that produce fecal levels sufficient to alter the bowel flora, particularly antibiotics active against the indigenous anaerobic population, reduce the colonization resistance of the intestinal lumen to *C difficile*. *C difficile* may be harbored normally in limited numbers or may be introduced from environmental reservoirs, vaginal sources, other colonized contacts, or environmental surfaces. The relative resistance of *C difficile* to most conventional antibiotics allows it to proliferate and elaborate its cytopathic and enterotoxic toxins associated with invasiveness, inflammation, and secretion. The superficial inflammation may progress to mucosal necrosis and exudation of protein and leukocytes, continuing until the conditions are poor for *C difficile* proliferation because of competition with other bowel flora or the introduction of specific antibiotic therapy. Because the toxins are responsible for the inflammation, agents that bind or eliminate toxins, such as cholestyramine or other resins, may have some efficacy.

## CLINICAL PRESENTATION

Diarrhea is a common, often expected, side effect of antibiotic treatment in children and is usually a self-limited, dose-related, and mild consequence, resolving after the course of treatment is completed. These uncomplicated sporadic cases are unlikely to be caused by *C difficile* proliferation. In a subset of patients, however, a severe chronic enterocolitis may develop, with profuse watery diarrhea beginning 4 to 10 days after initiation or as late as 4 weeks after discontinuation of antibiotic treatment. The diarrhea may be associated with dehydration, electrolyte depletion, vomiting, and abdominal distention. Hypokalemia, hypoalbuminemia, and metabolic acidosis may occur. The onset of fever, crampy abdominal pain, tenesmus or urgency, and neutrophilic leukocytosis, with or without hematochezia, suggests inflammation of the colon. Significant hypoproteinemia with edema, ascites, and pleural effusion complicates only the most severe cases of pseudomembranous colitis and is ominous. Dilation of the colon may produce toxic megacolon. Because of the risks of perforation, peritonitis, and sepsis, this is a medical and surgical emergency.

Another pattern of antibiotic-associated enterocolitis is diarrhea of variable severity without evolution of signs of frank colitis. The diagnosis in this situation may be delayed for months until colitis develops or *C difficile* is considered in the cause and the toxin assay is performed. Despite lack of clinical signs of overt pseudomembranous colitis, focal colitis may be found on colonoscopy. Chronic *C difficile* diarrhea may resemble other malabsorptive syndromes and contribute to growth failure in children.

Most cases of antibiotic-associated enterocolitis occur in patients without underlying GI disorders who are treated with antibiotics for other conditions (eg, respiratory illness, often with questionable indication) or have undergone bowel preparation for surgery. Virtually every antibiotic has been implicated in the cause of *C difficile* enterocolitis, but the most commonly cited are ampicillin and amoxicillin, clindamycin, and cephalosporins, all potent in suppressing normal bowel anaerobic flora but with relatively less activity against *C difficile*. The prevalence of ampicillin- and cephalosporin-associated enterocolitis in children reflects the prevalence of administration of these drugs by pediatricians. Clindamycin, administered relatively infrequently to children, is less frequently associated with diarrhea and enterocolitis in children than it is in adults. Other antibiotics implicated include penicillins, sulfonamides, and trimethoprim-sulfamethoxazole (Table 129-1). The relation of antibiotic-associated enterocolitis to combinations, dosage, or duration of antibiotic therapies is unknown.

## DIAGNOSIS

*C difficile*-associated enterocolitis should be suspected in any patient with acute onset of severe diarrhea or colitis with concomitant or prior oral or intravenous antibiotic treatment; chronic diarrhea of unknown cause, with or without a history of prior antibiotic treatment; and exacerbation of suspected or previously documented inflammatory bowel disease.

In addition to antibiotic treatment, the history should elicit details regarding fever, vomiting, pain, tenesmus, urgency, and rectal bleeding. Physical examination should assess hydration status, hemodynamic stability, and abdominal tenderness or distention, the latter suggesting toxic dilatation. Laboratory findings typically show a neutrophilic leukocytosis, which can be impressive ($>30,000/mm^3$) in pseudomembranous colitis or minimal in mild chronic *C difficile*-induced diarrhea. Hypoproteinemia is common in pseudomembranous enterocolitis but rare in chronic diarrhea. Stool examination for occult blood and leukocytes may confirm colitis. An isolation of *C difficile* should be requested with the routine stool cultures for *Salmonella*, *Shigella*, *Campylobacter*,

toxigenic *Escherichia coli*, and *Yersinia* species and examination for parasites.

However, the most specific test for *C difficile* disease is the cytotoxic assay for toxin B in serially diluted stool samples, measuring cytopathic effects in cultured fibroblasts. The cytopathic activity is specifically neutralized by an antitoxin derived from another *Clostridium* species, *C sordellii*. After infancy, the presence of toxin B is usually associated with clinical disease, although cytotoxic titers do not correlate with severity. Unfortunately, the assay requires 18 to 24 hours and laboratory tissue culture technology. Most efforts have been directed toward the development of a rapid, sensitive, and specific assay for toxin A. Latex agglutination assays have proved to be too low in specificity and sensitivity for clinical reliability. More promising are enzyme-linked immunoassays and dot immunobinding assays. These assays can produce results within several hours, allowing early initiation of specific therapy.

Flat and upright abdominal radiographs may show signs of ileus with small bowel dilatation and air–fluid levels but are nonspecific. Barium enema examination may show edema, ulcerations, and "thumbprinting" or nodular contour defects due to edema and pseudomembranes, but this study is unnecessary for diagnosis and increases the risk of bowel perforation. Sigmoidoscopy or colonoscopy should be done as soon as the diagnosis of pseudomembranous colitis is entertained and may reveal characteristic findings of discrete or confluent pseudomembranous inflammation of the rectum and colon. Disease may occur more proximally in the presence of an unimpressive sigmoidoscopic examination. Colonoscopy is usually negative in cases of chronic diarrhea when there are no other signs of colitis, although biopsies may show signs of focal inflammation. The availability of a rapid *C difficile* toxin assay may make diagnosis by endoscopy unnecessary except in severe or equivocal cases in which immediate treatment is necessary.

## DIFFERENTIAL DIAGNOSIS

Chronic diarrhea may be caused by a variety of viral and bacterial pathogens. Susceptibility to the more common enteric bacterial pathogens, *Shigella, Salmonella, Campylobacter, E coli* and *Yersinia*, is also increased in the host whose intestinal flora have been altered or eradicated by broad-spectrum antibiotic treatment. Cytomegalovirus, *Entamoeba histolytica*, and other pathogens may cause chronic diarrheal states and focal colitis. Lactose intolerance, celiac disease, cystic fibrosis, acquired immunodeficiency, and other disorders associated with malabsorption should be entertained in the differential diagnosis of chronic diarrhea. Inflammatory bowel disease may present similarly or may be complicated by *C difficile* enterocolitis. There is evidence that patients with inflammatory bowel disease are more susceptible to colonization by *C difficile*. The sigmoidoscopic appearance may resemble the focal inflammation with relative rectal sparing encountered in Crohn's colitis.

Pseudomembranous colitis unassociated with antibiotic treatment has been observed in necrotizing enterocolitis of neonates, in the diversion colitis after bowel surgery, in Hirschsprung's enterocolitis, in uremic colitis, in hemolytic-uremic syndrome, and in congenital heart disease with bowel ischemia related to congestive heart failure.

## TREATMENT

Hemodynamic homeostasis should be established using vigorous rehydration, correction of electrolyte disturbances, and albumin infusions as indicated by clinical findings, such as orthostasis,

---

**TABLE 129-1. Antibiotics Most Commonly Associated With *C difficile* Enterocolitis in Children**

Ampicillin, amoxicillin
Cephalosporin
Penicillin G, V
Clindamycin, lincomycin
Erythromycin
Trimethoprim-sulfamethoxasole

dehydration, and edema (Table 129-2). If possible, antibiotics should be discontinued or changed to an intravenous preparation known to be less frequently associated with anaerobic bacterial suppression and pseudomembranous colitis. Antimotility agents such as Lomotil, paregoric, or loperamide should be discontinued because of the risk of stasis and the induction of toxic megacolon. Enteric precautions should be instituted to prevent the spread of *C difficile* to other patients or family members at risk, especially those being treated with antibiotics.

After the diagnosis is sufficiently supported by clinical and sigmoidoscopy findings or confirmed by demonstration of *C difficile* toxin, metronidazole, administered as 15 mg/kg/day in three divided doses, up to 250 mg per dose, should be administered for 14 days. An alternative is oral vancomycin, administered as 125 mg four times daily for 7 to 14 days. Metronidazole and vancomycin are equally efficacious against *C difficile*, with clinical response expected in 2 to 10 days. The advantages of metronidazole include its minimal suppression of normal aerobic fecal flora and its low cost. The rate of relapse may also be lower, based on its limited suppression of normal fecal flora, allowing recovery of normal colonization resistance. Metronidazole is the drug of choice for parenteral therapy. Bacitracin, miconazole, and tetracycline have been used successfully to eradicate *C difficile* but have no advantages over metronidazole in efficacy or cost. Cholestyramine has been used to bind the toxin and has been reported helpful in mild disease. However, because of its limited efficacy and its potential for binding the antibiotics used in specific treatment, it is no longer recommended.

Relapses associated with the reappearance of symptoms and toxin production are relatively common and may occur after apparent eradication of *C difficile* toxin in as many as 14% of the patients within 21 days after vancomycin treatment of pseudomembranous colitis and in as many as 67% of the children with chronic diarrhea. *C difficile* may be cultured from the stools of some patients who are toxin free and asymptomatic after treatment. Toxin B may be detectable in a subset of patients after clinical resolution but does not imply nor predict relapse. Although some patients suffer recurrent relapses with any antibiotic treatment, others may harbor the organism without disease during subsequent antibiotic treatment. Multiple relapses warrant evaluation for underlying chronic inflammatory bowel disease. The reasons for variable resistance to antibiotic-associated enterocolitis are undoubtedly complex but probably are related to factors such

as the composition of the indigenous bowel flora, transit time, presence of receptors for toxins, and immunologic mucosal defenses. Bacterial spores may survive therapy and repopulate the colon, or organisms may be acquired from environmental exposures. Clusters of occurrence in hospital settings have been reported from direct patient contact and indirectly from environmental surfaces. Family and day-care contacts, including adults, frequently harbor the organism and may be sources of reinfection. *C difficile* is also part of the normal vaginal flora, which may account for the high rates of colonization in neonates.

## PREVENTION

Prophylactic administration of broad-spectrum antibiotics should be used only when strictly indicated, particularly the antibiotics such as ampicillin or amoxicillin commonly implicated in *C difficile*-associated enterocolitis. The risk of suppression of bowel flora and increased susceptibility to *C difficile* enterocolitis should be weighed in the selection of antibiotic treatment. Hospitalized patients with documented disease should be strictly isolated from other susceptible antibiotic-treated patients and hospital rooms thoroughly disinfected. Asymptomatic family contacts may be screened and treated in cases of recurrent relapses, but there is no evidence that vancomycin or metronidazole eliminate the carrier state. There is interest but no scientific support for altering bowel flora with *Lactobacillus* preparations as an adjunct to therapy for relapses or for prevention.

## PROGNOSIS

Before recognition of the association of pseudomembranous colitis or chronic antibiotic-associated diarrhea with the toxins of *C difficile* and the option of therapy with oral vancomycin, the mortality rate from pseudomembranous colitis in children was as high as 28%. The availability of safe and efficacious treatment, coupled with the recognition of the spectrum of presentation of antibiotic-associated enterocolitis and its propensity for relapse, has dramatically improved the prognosis, and severe complications and death are now rare.

## Selected Readings

Bartlett JG, Tedesco FJ, Shull S, et al. Symptomatic relapse after oral vancomycin therapy of antibiotic associated pseudomembranous colitis. Gastroenterology 1980;78:431.
Chang T, Gorbach SL. Rapid identification of *Clostridium difficile* by toxin detection. J Clin Microbiol 1982;15:465.
Cherry RD, Portnoy D, Fabbari M, et al. Metronidazole: an alternate therapy for antibiotic-associated colitis. Gastroenterology 1982;82:849.
Elstner CL, Lindsay AN, Book LS, Matsen JM. Lack of relationship of *Clostridium difficile* to antibiotic-associated diarrhea in children. Pediatr Infect Dis 1983;2:364.
Feigin RD. Antimicrobial agent-induced pseudomembranous colitis. Pediatr Rev 1981;3:147.
Finegold SM. Intestinal microbial changes and disease as a result of antimicrobial use. Pediatr Infect Dis 1986;5:S88.
George WL, Rolfe RD, Finegold SM. Treatment and prevention of antimicrobial agent-induced colitis and diarrhea. Gastroenterology 1980;79:366.
Hentges DJ. The protective function of the indigenous intestinal flora. Pediatr Infect Dis 1986;5:S17.
Kim K, Dupont HL, Pickering LK. Outbreak of diarrhea associated with *Clostridium difficile* and its toxin in day-care centers: evidence of person-to-person spread. J Pediatr 1983;102:376.
Laughon BE, Viscidi RP, Gdovin SL, Yolken RH, Bartlett JG. Enzyme immunoassays for detection of *Clostridium difficile* toxins A and B in fecal specimens. J Infect Dis 1984;149:781.
Sutphen JL, Grand RJ, Flores A, et al. Chronic diarrhea associated with *Clostridium difficile* in children. Am J Dis Child 1983;137:275.
Tedesco FJ. Antibiotic-associated pseudomembranous colitis with negative proctosigmoidoscopy examination. Gastroenterology 1979;77:295.
Thompson CM, Gilligan PH, Fisher MC, Long SS. *Clostridium difficile* cytotoxin in the pediatric population. Am J Dis Child 1983;137:271.

**TABLE 129-2. Therapeutic Strategy for Suspected *C difficile* Enterocolitis in Children**

1. Ensure hemodynamic homeostasis.
2. Discontinue antibiotics or substitute intravenous alternative.
3. Discontinue antimotility agents (eg, Lomotil, paregoric, loperamide).
4. Institute enteric precautions.
5. Obtain abdominal radiographs for baseline and to exclude toxic dilatation.
6. Perform sigmoidoscopy and biopsy.
7. Obtain stool for bacterial culture, ova and parasite examination, occult blood, leukocytes.
8. Perform *C difficile* toxin assay on liquid stool.
9. Oral agents:
   Metronidazole: 15 mg/kg/day divided tid for 7–14 days
   Vancomycin: 125 mg qid for 7–14 days
   Parenteral (if unable to tolerate oral) metronidazole: 7.5 mg/kg q 6 h
10. Monitor clinical response.

Triadafilopoulos A, Pothoulakis C, O'Brien MJ, LaMont T. Differential effects of *Clostridium difficile* toxins A and B on rabbit ileum. Gastroenterology 1987;93: 273.

Trnka YM, Lamont JT. Association of *Clostridium difficile* toxin with symptomatic relapse of chronic inflammatory bowel disease. Gastroenterology 1981;80:693.

Tucker KD, Carrig PE, Wilkins TD. Toxin A of *Clostridium difficile* is a potent cytotoxin. J Clin Microbiol 1990;28:869.

Viscidi RP, Bartlett JG. Antibiotic-associated pseudomembranous colitis in children. Pediatrics 1981;67:381.

*Principles and Practice of Pediatrics, Second Edition.*
edited by Frank A. Oski et al. J. B. Lippincott Company, Philadelphia © 1994.

## CHAPTER 130
# *Chronic Recurrent Abdominal Pain*

### William J. Klish

Chronic, recurrent abdominal pain is undoubtedly the most frustrating problem a pediatrician must manage. It is also common. Unless the diagnosis is dealt with in a positive manner and the parents develop confidence in that diagnosis, they will constantly seek medical advice and frequently shop around for answers.

The symptom of abdominal pain is frightening to the average parent. It conjures up images of life-threatening problems such as appendicitis or obstruction. Many children who experience chronic recurrent abdominal pain of any cause are obviously in great discomfort. They grip their stomachs, frequently become pale, and are not interested in play. If the physician casually writes off the symptom as functional or psychologic, he or she will lose the confidence of the parents, who observe their child in pain and know that the symptom is not "in the child's head." Physicians themselves frequently worry about missing a diagnosis in these cases, and this self-doubt may be subtly conveyed to the parents.

It is imperative that the physician approach the diagnosis of chronic recurrent abdominal pain with confidence. The pediatrician must never doubt that the child is in actual pain and must build a trusting relationship with the parents. He or she should discuss the differential diagnosis with the parents at the beginning and rule out potential diagnoses in a logical manner. If the diagnosis of functional pain is made, the pediatrician should discuss it at length, emphasizing that the pain is not life threatening. These measures usually allay the fears of the parents sufficiently that they can deal with the symptom effectively. Occasionally, the child's fear of going to school or some other phobia may be so deep seated that removal of the pain as a defense mechanism may only lead to its replacement with something else. These children should be referred for psychologic therapy.

## PATHOGENESIS OF VISCERAL PAIN

When Aristotle described the five senses, he omitted the sensation of pain. The ancient Greeks considered pain to be an emotion or something unpleasant, the opposite of pleasure. For centuries, arguments have raged over whether pain is a separate, distinct sensation or a psychologic reaction to a complex feeling. Even though pain perception is now assigned to a specific sensory faculty, the chronic recurrent abdominal pain of childhood, more than any other form of pain, exemplifies this historic uncertainty.

Receptors for transmitting pain are described morphologically as undifferentiated nerve endings. They can be stimulated by mechanical, chemical, or thermal stimuli. In the case of the viscera, these receptors are most sensitive to mechanical stimuli. Receptor substance is contained within vesicles at the nerve ending and is released on stimulation, causing depolarization of the nerve when it combines with receptors on the external surface. This action is terminated by a specific hydrolytic enzyme surrounding the nerve terminal. In severe trauma to tissue, this hydrolytic enzyme may be destroyed, resulting in prolonged depolarization of the nerve cells by the receptor substance and persistent pain. One of the receptor substances thought to be active in pain fibers is substance P, an 11-amino acid peptide, but other substances have also been postulated.

The afferent nerve fibers involved in the transmission of pain follow a course through the sympathetic ganglion chain and enter the dorsal horn of the spinal cord, where they synapse. Afferents from the viscera enter the dorsal horn with afferents from cutaneous structures of the corresponding dermatome. There is overlap at the synaptic junctions between these two sources of nerve impulses. This gives rise to the phenomenon of referred pain. As the input from visceral structures increases, more impulses are received by the fibers, which share their input between visceral and cutaneous structures. This input eventually is perceived by the brain as arising from cutaneous structures.

Another mechanism that may play a role in the cutaneous localization of visceral pain is the peritoneocutaneous reflex of Morley. Certain somatic nerve endings in the parietal peritoneum may extend into the roots of the mesentery and posterior portion of the diaphragm. When these nerves are stimulated, pain is referred to the corresponding skin area. This reflex is usually the result of inflammation from peritonitis.

Neurons that synapse with afferents from the viscera in the dorsal horn of the spinal cord cross to the opposite side and ascend through the lateral spinothalamic tract to the thalamus. A third neuron then carries the sensation by means of the internal capsule to the cerebral cortex.

A satisfactory theory of pain must account for the evidence that local factors in the spinal cord and events occurring in the cerebral cortex (eg, anxiety) may influence the perception or threshold of pain. The gate theory is an attempt to explain this. It proposes that pain fibers are subject to the influence of larger-diameter afferents that originate in the substantia gelatinosa of the spinal cord. These neurons interact through an axoaxonic synapse that, under normal conditions, is dominant, and the gate is closed. As excitation from the viscera increases, this modulating effect is overcome, and pain is felt. Feedback from the brain may alter the transmission from this interneuron. In functional abdominal pain, anxiety may decrease the modulating effect to the point that normal intestinal sensations are perceived as pain. The interneuronal receptors in the system are opiate receptors that are normally activated by the endogenously produced opiates, enkephalins, and endorphins.

Under normal circumstances, the only stimulus that is adequate to initiate pure visceral pain is increased intravisceral pressure caused by stretching, distention, or contraction of the viscus. Inflammation decreases the visceral threshold for pain. With the exception of colonic pain, true visceral pain is felt at or near the midline of the body; colonic pain tends to be referred to the area directly above the point of stimulation. Pain referred away from the midline suggests several possibilities: inflammation of a viscus rather than a simple disturbance of motor function, which lowers the pain threshold and gives rise to referred pain; a stimulus of extreme severity, such as the passage of a calculus, which refers pain because of its high-intensity stimulus; or extension of the disease process to the peritoneum, which stimulates somatic nerve endings.

## DIFFERENTIAL DIAGNOSIS

Most children who have chronic recurrent abdominal pain unassociated with other significant symptoms have functional pain. However, this diagnosis is one of exclusion, because no specific diagnostic test is available. It is important to discuss this diagnosis with the parents before evaluation so that, if other potential diagnoses are excluded, the parents do not attribute the diagnosis of functional pain to the physician's inability to diagnose something more serious.

The common entities that cause chronic recurrent abdominal pain of childhood, listed in their approximate order of frequency, are functional abdominal pain, lactose intolerance, simple constipation, musculoskeletal pain, parasitic infection, reflux esophagitis, peptic ulcer disease, and inflammatory bowel disease. Most of these diagnoses can be screened without a multitude of laboratory and x-ray examinations.

*Lactose intolerance* is probably the second most common cause of abdominal pain in childhood. If a child is genetically programmed to become lactase deficient, the activity of this enzyme gradually begins to decrease around 4 to 6 years of age. If milk drinking continues at a constant rate, the enzyme activity eventually will not be sufficient to hydrolyze the entire amount of lactose ingested; as a result, some lactose spills into the distal small bowel and colon, where it is fermented by bacteria, and gases such as hydrogen and carbon dioxide are produced. This gas production, if great enough, may cause intestinal dilatation and pain. As the syndrome progresses, diarrhea results from the osmotic effect of the unabsorbed sugar and its fermentive products. Early in the development of lactose intolerance, pain may be the sole symptom.

Diagnosing lactose intolerance as a cause of abdominal pain is sometimes difficult because the laboratory tests (eg, breath hydrogen production, lactose tolerance test) tend to be too sensitive, and the condition is overdiagnosed as a result. It is also difficult to establish cause and effect from these tests. Dietary restriction may be the easiest way to establish lactose intolerance as a cause of abdominal pain. The child should be given a lactose-free diet for about 2 weeks. If the abdominal pain disappears, the diagnosis can be suspected. However, it should be confirmed by giving the child lactose again and observing for reexacerbation of symptoms. This cycle should be completed twice to ensure that lactose intolerance is present. After the diagnosis is established, the parents can be counseled intelligently. Because lactose intolerance is a dose-related phenomenon, most children can tolerate some lactose-containing foods. Low-lactose dairy products (eg, cheese) should be reintroduced as tolerated. This would preclude the need for calcium supplementation.

Children with *simple constipation* frequently complain of abdominal pain. The parents and children do not make the association between the number of bowel movements and the pain. Unless the physician asks specifically about the frequency of bowel movements, the diagnosis may go unrecognized for a long time. Rectal examination is helpful in establishing this diagnosis, but a trial of a mild stimulant may be necessary to establish cause.

*Musculoskeletal pain* arising from the abdominal muscles is a diagnosis that can be overlooked easily. School-aged children are frequently engaged in competitive sports and subjected to intensive exercise training programs. These can result in strained muscles and chronic myositis of specific muscle bundles. The pain is usually described as sharp or knife-like and may be triggered by various activities or body positions. It is usually located at or near the insertion of the rectus or oblique muscles into the costal margin or iliac crest. Palpating along these insertions with a fair degree of pressure may locate a trigger point that reproduces the pain and establishes the diagnosis. If the abdominal muscles are tightened during the physical examination and the pain still is reproduced by palpation, the origin is undoubtedly musculoskeletal.

Occasionally, *intestinal parasites* (eg, *Giardia*, pinworms) may cause only abdominal pain. Stool should be examined for ova and parasites as part of the evaluation of all children with this problem.

*Inflammatory bowel disease* and *peptic ulcers* usually cause enough symptoms that their diagnosis is apparent. However, an occasional patient may complain initially of nonspecific abdominal pain and nothing else. It is helpful to obtain a complete blood count, reticulocyte count, sedimentation rate, and stool guaiac test to screen for these diagnoses. If the child is anemic, has an elevated reticulocyte count or positive results on the stool guaiac test, or has an elevated sedimentation rate, additional studies (eg, endoscopy, x-ray examinations) should be obtained.

Many other diseases can cause abdominal pain in children, but most of the other diagnoses are associated with other symptoms. If the child complains only of abdominal pain and results of all of the tests suggested earlier are negative, the physician should feel comfortable in making the diagnosis of functional abdominal pain.

## TREATMENT

The treatment for most of the diagnoses previously discussed is obvious. Lactose intolerance requires restriction of dairy products in the diet, and simple constipation is best treated by a bulk agent (eg, psyllium) or a mild stimulant (eg, senna). Salicylate used for 1 week as an anti-inflammatory agent frequently is enough to allow musculoskeletal pain to subside.

If the diagnosis of functional abdominal pain is made, it is helpful to discuss this diagnosis with the parents in the same manner as organic disease. The physician must convey the message that the pain is real but is not caused by a process that will become progressively worse and threaten the life of the child. The analogy of a headache in an adult is useful. The pain of a headache is real, but it is treated only as pain, and under normal circumstances, it is not allowed to interfere with daily responsibilities. A child's responsibility is to go to school, and pain should not prevent this from happening. If the pain is severe, it should be treated with medications, such as acetaminophen. Antimotility agents are usually ineffective. Using a hot pad or hot water bottle as a counterirritant is sometimes helpful. Above all, the physician should instill confidence in parents that the pain is not threatening to their child's well-being and will disappear as the child matures.

## Selected Readings

Bishop B. Pain: its physiology and rationale for management. Phys Ther 1980;60: 13.

Bowsher D. Pain pathways and mechanisms. Anesthesia 1978;30:935.

Klish WJ. Visceral pain. In: Chey WY, ed. Functional disorders of the digestive tract. New York: Raven Press, 1983:237.

Ness TJ, Gebhart GF. Visceral pain: a review of experimental studies. Pain 1990;41: 167.

Wordhouse CRJ, Bockner S. Chronic abdominal pain: a surgical or psychiatric symptom? Br J Surg 1979;66:348.

*Principles and Practice of Pediatrics, Second Edition.*
edited by Frank A. Oski et al. J. B. Lippincott Company, Philadelphia © 1994.

# CHAPTER 131
# *Henoch-Schönlein Syndrome*

### Steven R. Martin, David A. Bross and W. Allan Walker

Henoch-Schönlein syndrome, also known as anaphylactoid, allergic, or rheumatoid purpura, Henoch-Schönlein purpura, and the Schönlein-Henoch syndrome, is primarily a disorder of childhood. It was first described more than 150 years ago, and the diagnosis still relies on a constellation of clinical signs affecting principally the skin, joints, kidneys, and gastrointestinal (GI) tract.

The cause remains unknown, but a genetic predisposition is likely. Familial clustering has occasionally been reported, although family members may have common environmental exposures. However in end-stage renal failure after Henoch-Schönlein syndrome, 75% of children receiving allografts from living-related donors develop recurrent disease, compared with no disease recurrence in those receiving cadaveric donor kidneys. Abnormalities in the major histocompatibility (MHC) locus have been associated with Henoch-Schönlein syndrome. Weak associations with HLA-B35 and HLA-DR4 and strong associations with failure of expression of genes coding for complement components C4a and C4b, which also map to the MHC locus, have been described. The search for specific precipitating factors has been unsuccessful despite many cases being preceded by an upper respiratory infection and peak incidence in winter months. Clustering of cases has occurred but in the largest series of patients no clustering that would suggest a common infectious agent was observed. In rare cases, dietary allergens or drugs have been implicated, but more systematic examinations have not supported a dietary cause.

## PATHOPHYSIOLOGY

The pathologic lesions seen in Henoch-Schönlein syndrome are probably mediated by immunologic mechanisms. Demonstrated abnormalities include raised serum IgA concentrations, increased rates of IgA synthesis, and in patients with Henoch-Schönlein syndrome and their first-degree relatives, increased numbers of IgA-committed B lymphocytes. High spontaneous IgA production occurs in B lymphocytes from those with Henoch-Schönlein syndrome. In the presence of T lymphocytes, suppression of immunoglobulin synthesis is enhanced by pokeweed mitogen and inhibited by concanavalin A, which is the reverse of the effect normally seen. Circulating IgA and IgG immune complexes and IgA rheumatoid factor have been described, although data supporting the presence of classic antigen-antibody complexes has been questioned; possibly, IgA aggregates or complexes of IgA with complement are being detected. Complement C2 deficiency has been associated with Henoch-Schönlein syndrome, but low levels of C3 and C4 have not been consistently found. The C3 breakdown product, C3d, is elevated. Monocyte and macrophage Fc-receptor function may be depressed during active disease. It

appears that IgA interaction with IgG and other plasma proteins may form large aggregates that activate the alternate pathway of complement associated with low properdin levels. Complement activation and the deposition of IgA in target organs results in the elaboration of mediators of inflammation, including vascular prostaglandins such as prostacyclin, which may play a central role in the pathogenesis of the vasculitis.

Despite the absence of thrombocytopenia and normal coagulation studies, bleeding into target organs occurs. Fibrin-stabilizing factor (Factor XIII) is depleted in Henoch-Schönlein syndrome, correlating particularly with intestinal symptoms. The gene for factor XIIIB subunit is part of the "regulator of complement activation" gene cluster on chromosome 6, possibly accounting for the observed associations among the MHC, complement, and Factor XIII in Henoch-Schönlein syndrome. It is also postulated that proteases released during the inflammatory response degrade Factor XIII, resulting in tissue fibrin deposition and the development of vasculitis.

Skin lesions characteristically show a leukocytoclastic vasculitis with accumulation of neutrophils and erythrocytes around small vessels. Electron microscopic and immunofluorescence studies demonstrate simultaneous deposition of immunoglobulins, especially IgA, C3, and fibrin or fibrinogen within the vessel walls. Similar deposits have been found in lesions of the gastrointestinal tract and the glomerular mesangium of the kidney.

Renal biopsies usually reveal an endocapillary proliferative glomerulonephritis, accompanied by extracapillary cell proliferation of varying degrees, resulting in crescent formation. The extent of crescent formation has been used to determine prognosis with respect to progression to chronic renal disease.

Cerebral and meningeal vessels show a fibrinoid necrotizing arteriolitis, but no studies examining immune deposition have appeared.

## CLINICAL MANIFESTATIONS

Most cases of Henoch-Schönlein syndrome occur in children younger than 7 years of age, although adult cases have been reported. The entity is uncommon in infants younger than 1 year of age. Males are affected more frequently than females in most reported series. Although all races are susceptible, Caucasians predominate in most series.

The syndrome usually presents in a previously healthy child. The onset may be acute, with many features appearing at once, or gradual, with symptoms appearing over days to several weeks. The frequency of signs and symptoms is listed in Table 131-1. Low-grade fever and malaise are common early in the illness. Half of the patients present with a skin rash, which is central to the diagnosis. Occasionally, the rash appears several weeks after other signs are noticed. The time of appearance of other features varies, although in most cases, involvement of the joints, gastrointestinal tract, and skin occur within several days of onset.

Skin lesions, which occur in all patients, may be urticarial at the onset, occasionally developing hemorrhagic centers similar to erythema multiforme. More often, a reddish, nonpruritic, maculopapular rash subsequently appears, frequently coalescing to form larger purpuric areas. Scattered petechial lesions may be seen. The rash is typically located on the lower extremities and buttocks, but may involve the trunk, face, and upper extremities. The lesions arise in crops and follow the usual evolution of ecchymoses, turning brown, then yellow, and fading over several days. Ulceration and scarring are rarely seen.

Subcutaneous edema of the dorsum of the hands, feet, scalp, ears, and periorbital region occurs in as many as half of the patients. This nonpitting, localized swelling may be quite tender

## TABLE 131-1. Frequency of Signs and Symptoms in Henoch-Schönlein Syndrome

| Manifestation | % of Patients |
| --- | --- |
| Rash | 100 |
| Abdominal pain | 70 |
| Joint pain | 60–90 |
| Guaiac-positive stools | 56 |
| Subcutaneous edema | 50 |
| Fever | 50 |
| Ileus | 40 |
| Hematuria | 30–40 |
| Vomiting | 25 |
| Proteinuria | 10–20 |
| Scrotal involvement | 10–15 of males |
| Hematemesis | 10 |
| Hepatomegaly | 10 |
| CNS involvement | 2–8 |
| GI hemorrhage | 5 |
| Intussusception | 3 |

and distorting. It is more common in children younger than 3 years of age.

GI involvement occurs in as many as 85% of patients (see Table 131-1). Colicky abdominal pain occurs in as many as 70% of patients and in 14% of patients may precede other symptoms by several weeks. The diagnostic difficulties may prompt a laparotomy. Other common symptoms are melena or guaiac-positive stools (56%), ileus (40%), vomiting (25%), and hematemesis (10%). Life-threatening complications such as massive gastrointestinal hemorrhage and intussusception may occur in 5% and 3% of cases, respectively. Hemorrhage from the stomach has been reported frequently and may require surgical intervention. In Henoch-Schönlein syndrome, intussusception is more common in older children and is frequently ileoileal; the lead point may be formed by submucosal hemorrhages. Surgical reduction is usually recommended. The more usual presentation seen in children younger than 3 years of age is ileocolic intussusception. Other, less common modes of GI involvement include pancreatitis, intestinal perforation, vasculitis of the gallbladder, and protein-losing enteropathy. Hepatomegaly of uncertain cause has been described in as many as 10% of patients.

Joint pains with periarticular swelling occur in two thirds of patients with Henoch-Schönlein syndrome. In approximately 25%, joint symptoms may precede the rash. Large joints are most frequently affected; less commonly, fingers and wrists may be involved. The joint space is normal, and warmth and effusions are rare. Joint involvement is the most transient feature of Henoch-Schönlein syndrome and resolves without residual damage. The incidence of renal disease varies from 40% to 60% in different studies. The spectrum of findings ranges from microscopic hematuria in 50% of those with renal involvement to gross hematuria (40%), nephrotic syndrome (30%), mild proteinuria (25%), and acute nephritis with hypertension (15%); in 5% of patients, the renal disease progresses to chronic renal failure.

Renal involvement appears before other symptoms in only 3% of patients. In some cases, renal disease occurs as the other manifestations are resolving; this pattern is thought by some to herald a more complicated renal course. More severe renal disease seems to occur in older children and is often associated with the increased severity of other symptoms.

The clinical course is favorable if microscopic hematuria alone is noticed. If diffuse involvement with crescent formation in more than 50% of glomeruli occurs, the clinical manifestations are more severe, and the frequency of progression to chronic renal failure is higher.

Acute scrotal involvement is seen in 10% to 15% of males. Scrotal involvement occasionally is severe enough to suggest testicular torsion, but surgical exploration usually reveals local hemorrhage or hematoma of the scrotum and its contents. Technetium 99m pertechnetate imaging has been used to differentiate the two entities. Hyperemia is seen in Henoch-Schönlein syndrome, but the tracer activity is absent in testicular torsion.

The incidence of neurologic symptoms varies with the definition used. It has been estimated at 2% to 8% in most series, but if behavioral changes and headaches are included, as many as 43% of patients may be affected. Other manifestations of central nervous system (CNS) involvement include seizures in half of patients with neurologic symptoms, focal neurologic deficits in a third, and peripheral nerve involvement in only a few.

Seizures may be associated with cerebral ischemia secondary to the vasculitis, or with subarachnoid, subdural, cortical or intraparenchymal hemorrhages. Hypertension associated with renal disease is an additional complication. Most symptoms are transient, although permanent deficits can result from hemorrhage or rarely from infarction.

Rare complications attributed to Henoch-Schönlein syndrome have included pulmonary hemorrhages, cardiac involvement, intramuscular hemorrhage, and ureteral vasculitis with stenosis.

## LABORATORY DATA

No pathognomonic laboratory tests are available for Henoch-Schönlein syndrome. There is usually a leukocytosis of 10,000 to 20,000/mm$^3$ with a left shift. Normochromic anemia is frequent, possibly reflecting intestinal blood loss. The erythrocyte sedimentation rate is mildly elevated in as many as 75% of patients. Platelet counts are usually normal although thrombocytosis has been reported; coagulation studies are normal.

The total hemolytic complement levels are low in a third of patients, associated with normal C3 and C4 but with low properdin levels. Serum immunoglobulins are raised early in the course and return to normal after several months. Assays for antinuclear antibodies and IgG rheumatoid factors are negative. Factor XIII (ie, fibrin-stabilizing factor) is lower in Henoch-Schönlein syndrome than other types of vasculitis. Concentrations lower than 50% of normal reportedly heralds complications, and levels normalize with resolution of the disease. Abdominal symptoms are particularly associated with low Factor XIII levels.

Renal disease may be implicated on urinary microscopy by the demonstration of blood, casts, and protein in the urine. Serum creatinine and blood urea nitrogen levels may be elevated, and electrolyte alterations and hypoalbuminemia may be found. In more severe cases of nephritis or nephrotic syndrome, a renal biopsy may be indicated.

Radiologic studies with contrast agents show abnormalities most often in the small intestine, predominantly the duodenum and jejunum. Hypomotility, thickened folds, pseudotumors, and "thumbprinting" characteristic of submucosal hemorrhages may be seen. The terminal ileum may show changes resembling those of Crohn's ileitis. Residual damage may later manifest as small intestinal strictures. Colonic involvement is unusual. Intussusception is sometimes demonstrated. Ultrasound has been advocated for the diagnosis intussusception; the bowel forms a characteristic "Swiss roll" pattern.

Endoscopy may reveal erosive gastritis and duodenitis, and punctate, erythematous lesions may coalesce, giving rise to purpuric lesions. Colonic aphthoid ulcers and rectal ulcers have been observed. Sigmoid biopsies have shown only nonspecific acute and chronic inflammatory changes that are most prominent around the vessels.

## DIFFERENTIAL DIAGNOSIS

For the complete syndrome, the diagnosis is rarely in question. Because single manifestations can appear before the characteristic rash, other causes of acute abdominal pain must be considered, and the child must be evaluated for nephritis or arthritis.

Similar rashes may be seen with septicemia, coagulopathies, systemic lupus erythematosus, hemolytic uremic syndrome, and after streptococcal glomerulonephritis. Blood cultures, low C3 levels, and positive assays for antinuclear antibodies, abnormal platelet counts, and clotting studies can differentiate these entities from Henoch-Schönlein syndrome.

Nephritis with mesangial IgA deposits may be seen in Iga nephropathy (ie, Berger's disease), systemic lupus erythematosus, and cirrhosis. More severe renal involvement usually occurs after other manifestations have appeared, readily differentiating Henoch-Schönlein syndrome from other causes of glomerulonephritis. However, some authorities think that Henoch-Schönlein syndrome is the systemic form of IgA nephropathy. This view is supported by the observations that both diseases may occur in the same patient, within the same family or in identical twins of which one developed IgA nephropathy and the other Henoch-Schönlein syndrome. Immunologic and genetic differences and different clinical courses of the two diseases suggest that they are distinct disorders with common renal pathology.

Rheumatoid arthritis and rheumatic fever may cause joint pains with skin rashes but are easily differentiated from Henoch-Schönlein syndrome. Polyarteritis nodosa involving skin, kidneys, joints, and GI tract may be difficult to differentiate from Henoch-Schönlein syndrome. Muscles are often involved, and cardiac involvement should be sought.

## TREATMENT

Treatment is supportive. In acute cases, adequate hydration should be provided, and the patient should be monitored for possible complications. Frequent assessment of vital signs and hematocrit, stool examination for blood, and abdominal examinations are important. Any sudden increase in abdominal symptoms may be secondary to intussusception or perforation of the bowel or to pancreatitis. Because the location of intussusception in Henoch-Schönlein syndrome is more commonly in the small bowel, surgical intervention is usually required. Intracranial complications may be manifested by sudden changes in behavior or level of consciousness. The nephropathy is treated with attention to fluid balance, electrolyte status, salt intake, and the possibility of hypertension.

Optimal nutrition should be maintained, especially during more prolonged courses. Salicylates may alleviate joint discomfort, but they should be used with caution if abdominal symptoms appear prominent, especially if the possibility of gastrointestinal bleeding exists.

Considerable controversy has surrounded the use of corticosteroids, particularly for abdominal pain. Anecdotal evidence suggests a role for a short course of prednisone in a dose of 1 to 2 mg/kg/day for 5 to 7 days to hasten resolution of pain. Steroid administration has been advocated by some to reduce the likelihood of intussusception. The response in individual cases has been striking and no ill effects of use of prednisone in this manner have been reported. No controlled, prospective trials have been performed to address this problem, and retrospective studies leave the optimal management in doubt. Many patients improve without specific intervention, and corticosteroids are not recommended for skin rash, edema, joint pains, or renal disease. Major manifestations of localized vasculitis in the lungs, testes, and CNS should be treated with corticosteroids.

Severe renal involvement has been treated with azathioprine or cyclophosphamide in combination with prednisone to reduce long-term renal disease. However, the usefulness of this therapy has not been established by a controlled study. The clinical manifestations of Henoch-Schönlein syndrome, especially abdominal symptoms, were significantly improved between 1 and 3 days after administration of Factor XIII concentrate. Relapse of abdominal symptoms was associated with a subsequent fall in plasma Factor XIII levels.

## CLINICAL COURSE AND PROGNOSIS

In the absence of renal disease and major CNS involvement, the prognosis is excellent. The illness lasts for 4 to 6 weeks in most cases, although approximately half of the patients have one or more recurrences, usually within 6 weeks but sometimes as late as 7 years after the onset of illness. Children younger than 3 years of age tend to have a shorter, milder course and fewer recurrences.

In rare cases, long-term morbidity is accounted for by residual CNS damage. Chronic renal disease develops in 10% to 25% of those who have nephritis initially (5% of all patients). Long-term follow-up is usually necessary in patients with renal involvement, because progression of renal disease may not occur for many years. Microscopic hematuria alone is associated with good long-term prognosis. The outcome of more severe renal involvement is less predictable. Although nephrotic syndrome with crescent formation in more than 50% of glomeruli is more often associated with a poor outcome, as many as 40% of these patients may have normal long-term renal function.

## Selected Readings

Al Rasheed SA, Abdurrahman MB, Al Mugeiren MM, Al Fawaz IM. Henoch-Schönlein syndrome in Saudi Arabia. J Trop Pediatr 1991;37(3):127.

Bomelberg T, Claasen U, Von Lengerke HJ. Intestinal ultrasonographic findings in Schönlein-Henoch syndrome. Eur J Pediatr 1991;150(3):158.

Case records of the Massachusetts General Hospital. Weekly clinicopathologic exercises. Case 35-1991. A 59 year-old man with abdominal pain, microscopic hematuria, and a jejunal abnormality shown on a CT scan. N Eng J Med 1991;325(9):643.

Cull DL, Rosario V, Lally KP, Ratner I, Mahour GH. Surgical Implications of Henoch-Schönlein purpura. J Pediatr Surg 1990;25:741.

Dalens B, Travade P, Labbe A, Bezou MJ. Diagnostic and prognostic value of fibrin stabilizing factor in Schönlein-Henoch syndrome. Arch Dis Child 1983;58(1):12.

Davin JC, Foidart JB, Mahieu PR. Fc-receptor function in Henoch-Schönlein disease of childhood. Proc Eur Dial Transplant Assoc 1983;19:590.

Fukui H, Kamisuji H, Nagao T, Yamada K, et al. Clinical evaluation of a pasteurized factor XIII concentrate administration in Henoch-Schönlein purpura by the Japanese Pediatric Group. Thromb Res 1989;56:667.

Garcia-Fuentes M, Martin A, Chantler C, Williams DG. Serum complement components in Henoch-Schönlein purpura. Arch Dis Child 1978;53(5):417.

Glasier CM, Siegel MJ, McAlister WH, Shackelford GD. Henoch-Schönlein syndrome in children: gastrointestinal manifestations. AJR 1981;136(6):1081.

Hasegawa A, Kawamura T, Ito H, Hasegawa O, Ogawa O, Honda M, Ohara T, Hajikano H. Fate of renal grafts with recurrent Henoch-Schönlein purpura nephritis in children (part 1). Transplant Proc 1989;21:2130.

Hu SC, Feeney MS, McNicholas M, O'Halpin D, Fitzgerald RJ. Ultrasonography to diagnose and exclude intussusception in Henoch-Schönlein purpura. Arch Dis Child 1991;66:1065.

Kamitsuji H, Tani K, Taniguchi A, Taira K, Iida Y, Kanki H, Fukui H. Activity of blood coagulation factor XIII as a prognostic indicator in patients with Henoch-Schönlein purpura. Eur J Pediatr 1987;146:519.

Katz S, Borst M, Seekri I, Grosfeld JL. Surgical Evaluation of Henoch-Schönlein purpura. Experience with 110 children. Arch Surg 1991;126:849.

Knight JF. The rheumatic poison: a survey of some published investigations of the immunopathogenesis of Henoch-Schönlein purpura. Pediatr Nephrol 1990;4:533.

McLean RH, Wyatt RJ, Julian BA. Complement phenotypes in glomerulonephritis: increased frequency of homozygous null C4 phenotypes in IgA nephropathy and Henoch-Schönlein purpura. Kidney Int 1984;26:855.

Meadow SR, Scott DG. Berger disease: Henoch-Schönlein syndrome without the rash. J Pediatr 1985;106:27.

Nielsen HE. Epidemiology of Schönlein-Henoch purpura. Acta Paediatr Scand 1988;77:125.

Ostergaard JR, Storm K. Neurologic manifestations of Schönlein-Henoch purpura. Acta Pediatr Scand 1991;80(3):339.

Reif S, Jain A, Santiago J, Rossi T. Protein losing enteropathy as a manifestation of Henoch-Schönlein purpura. Acta Pediatr Scand 1991;80(4):482.

Sharief N, Ward HC, Wood CB. Functional intestinal obstruction in Henoch-Schönlein purpura. J Pediatr Gastroenterol Nutr 1991;12(2):272.

Stevenson JA, Leong LA, Cohen AH, et al. Henoch-Schönlein purpura: simultaneous demonstration of IgA deposits in involved skin,intestine and kidney. Arch Pathol Lab Med 1982;106:192.

Tomomasa T, Hsu JY, Itoh K, Kuroume T. Endoscopic findings in pediatric patients with Henoch-Schönlein purpura and gastrointestinal symptoms. J Pediatr Gastroenterol Nutr 1987;6:725.

Turi S, Belch JJ, Beattie TJ, Forbes CD. Abnormalities of vascular prostoglandins in Henoch-Schönlein purpura. Arch Dis Child 1986;61(2):173.

Utani A, Ohta M, Shinya A et al. Successful treatment of adult Henoch-Schönlein purpura with factor XIII concentrate. J Am Acad Dermatol 1991;24(3):438.

*Principles and Practice of Pediatrics, Second Edition.*
edited by Frank A. Oski et al. J. B. Lippincott Company, Philadelphia © 1994.

**TABLE 132-1. Established Causes of Protein-Losing Enteropathy in Children**

Epithelial alteration
  Celiac disease
  Gastrointestinal allergy
  Graft-versus-host disease
  Parasitic infestations
Mucosal ulceration
  Crohn's disease
  Ulcerative colitis
  Enterocolitis (eg, necrotizing, allergic, vasculitic, infectious, radiation, toxic)
Impaired lymphatic flow
  Primary lymphangiectasia
  Secondary lymphangiectasia
    Lymphoma
    Graft-versus-host disease
    Radiation enteritis
    Crohn's disease
    Parasitic infestation
    Scleroderma
    Abdominal tuberculosis
    Congestive heart failure or constrictive pericarditis
    Venous obstruction

*From Thomas DW. Protein-losing enteropathy. In: Gryboski J, ed. Pediatric case reports in gastrointestinal disease, vol 7, no. 2 Newtown, PA: Associates in Medical Marketing Co, 1987*

# CHAPTER 132
# *Protein-Losing Enteropathy*

## Dan W. Thomas and Frank R. Sinatra

Numerous disorders can result in excessive loss of serum proteins from the gastrointestinal (GI) tract. This form of intestinal dysfunction is called protein-losing enteropathy (PLE). PLE indicates an underlying GI disturbance but is not pathognomonic of a specific disorder. The more common maladies associated with PLE in children are listed in Table 132-1.

## PATHOPHYSIOLOGY

The exact mechanism of serum protein exudation is not known in all instances of PLE. Three basic causes have been proposed: mucosal ulceration, epithelial alteration, and impaired lymphatic flow. Impaired lymphatic flow is probably the most frequent cause of protracted PLE. By a similar mechanism, impeded systemic venous return, such as that found with cardiac failure or constrictive pericarditis, can indirectly lead to PLE by compromising lymph flow through the thoracic duct into the systemic circulation. Bowel wall edema is an additional potential contributing factor when portal venous flow is hindered. Perturbed systemic venous return and bowel wall edema may be responsible for the PLE

that results in children who have undergone Fontan operations for congenital heart disease.

PLE appears to be a nonselective process. Cellular elements, usually lymphocytes, may also be lost from the bowel wall, especially in patients with impaired intestinal lymphatic drainage. Levels of serum proteins with short half-lives, such as fibrinogen, are less affected than those with long turnover times, such as albumin. Hypoproteinemia does not occur in every case of PLE, because increased synthesis of serum proteins can compensate for ongoing losses. This is possible because of the efficiency of intraluminal digestion and reabsorption of protein exuded from the bowel and the capacity of the liver to increase its rate of protein synthesis if nutritional status is adequate. Disproportionate protein loss occurs in patients with GI bleeding from generalized intestinal mucosal diseases, such as chronic inflammatory bowel disease.

Many other primary GI disturbances can be associated with PLE. Generalized malabsorption frequently occurs with PLE if the bowel wall lymphatics or mucosal surface are involved (eg, gluten-induced enteropathy, lymphangiectasia). Children with fat malabsorption, as manifested by steatorrhea or low serum levels of fat-soluble vitamins, without concomitant PLE are likely to have a primary disorder of intraluminal digestion (eg, pancreatic insufficiency due to cystic fibrosis). The finding of gross or occult blood in the stool may also help localize the site of dysfunction to the intestinal mucosal surface.

## CLINICAL FINDINGS

In most cases of PLE, the clinical findings of the primary underlying disorder dominate the clinical picture. The associated PLE is suggested by edema or hypoproteinemia. Occasionally, these findings are the primary presenting manifestations of the un-

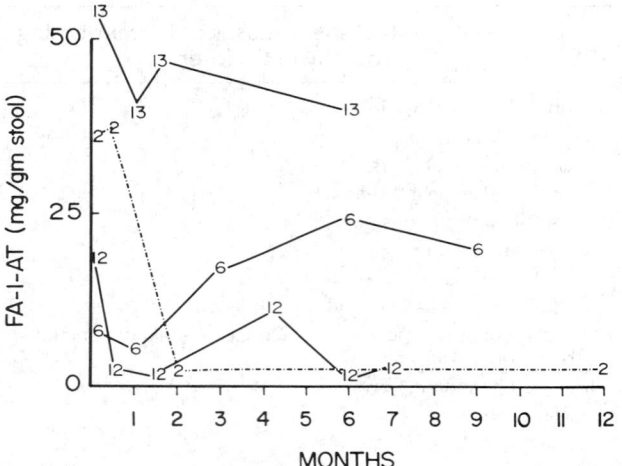

**Figure 132-1.** Serial random fecal $\alpha_1$-antitrypsin concentrations. Line 2 represents a 5-year-old girl with celiac disease. Her symptoms and steatorrhea resolved after beginning a gluten-free diet. Line 6 represents a 15-year-old boy with short stature, hypoproteinemia, and allergic enteropathy. Temporary clinical improvement occurred on an elemental diet. Line 12 represents a 15-year-old boy with ileal Crohn's disease. He was well after resection of a diseased ileal segment. Disease activity flared soon after and was eventually controlled by medical therapy. Line 13 represents a 6-year-old boy with secondary lymphangiectasia, chylothorax, and chylous ascites after cardiovascular surgery; all three conditions persisted despite all therapeutic efforts. (Thomas DW. Random fecal alpha-1-antitrypsin concentration in children with gastrointestinal disease. Gastroenterology 1981;80:776.)

derlying disorder. PLE should be considered in all cases of unexplained edema or hypoproteinemia. Anemia and lymphocytopenia can occur concomitantly with PLE. A young child with asymmetric limb edema may have congenital lymphatic obstruction (ie, primary lymphangiectasia), in which peripheral and intestinal lymphatics are often involved.

## DIAGNOSIS

Methods for detecting PLE were unavailable until the 1960s, when radiolabeled protein excretion tests were developed. Before this time, a large percentage of patients diagnosed as having "idiopathic hypercatabolic hypoproteinemia" probably had unrecognized PLE. The technique used most frequently was the quantitation of excreted radioactivity after the intravenous injection of $^{51}$Cr-albumin. Normal persons excrete less than 1% of the administered radioactive dose over a 2- to 4-day collection period. These studies contributed to our understanding of normal GI protein catabolism and demonstrated the frequent association of PLE with a wide variety of bowel disorders. Studies involving the use of $^{131}$I-albumin indicated that as much as 10% of daily protein catabolism occurs in the gut in healthy persons. Widespread use of these techniques was not possible in pediatric patients. These studies were difficult to perform, required a 3- to 4-day hospitalization, used radioactive agents, and were relatively expensive. The radiolabeled proteins used for these studies are not generally available in the United States for clinical purposes.

Attempts to measure protein loss in the stool were unsuccessful because of intraluminal protein digestion. Losses were consistently underestimated because of the efficiency of protein digestion and reabsorption. Fecal nitrogen quantitation was an inaccurate method of diagnosing PLE. Malabsorption of dietary nitrogen may significantly alter the results of these studies. Children with

cystic fibrosis typically have azotorrhea and steatorrhea without PLE, and patients with Crohn's disease may have PLE and normal fecal nitrogen excretion.

A practical technique for screening for PLE now exists. The screening test is the measurement of the fecal $\alpha_1$-antitrypsin ($\alpha_1$-AT) excretion. The properties of this protein make it uniquely suited as a natural marker of PLE. $\alpha_1$-Antitrypsin is normally a major serum protein component, accounting for approximately 4% of the total serum protein content, and has a molecular weight similar to that of albumin. It is relatively resistant to intestinal and bacterial proteolytic enzymes and therefore is excreted immunologically intact in the stool. These properties allow for the quantitation of fecal, $\alpha_1$-AT to serve as a marker for excessive serum protein loss from the bowel. Clinical studies have shown that determination of fecal $\alpha_1$-AT is a simple and reliable screening test for PLE. Most disorders known to result in PLE are associated with increased fecal $\alpha_1$-AT excretion. An exception appears to be PLE associated with the loss of serum protein from the gastric mucosa. In these cases, $\alpha_1$-AT appears to be degraded in the acid environment of the stomach.

Fecal $\alpha_1$-AT excretion may be expressed as stool concentration, intestinal clearance, or total daily output. Normal intestinal clearance is considered to be 13 to 40 mL/day and is calculated by the formula: clearance = fecal $\alpha_1$-AT × daily stool output/serum $\alpha_1$-AT. In most clinical situations, a single $\alpha_1$-AT determination on a random specimen appears adequate. Healthy persons excrete approximately 1 to 2 mg of $\alpha_1$-AT per 1 g of dry stool. Young, exclusively breast-fed or formula-fed infants appear to have higher fecal $\alpha_1$-AT concentrations, but total daily excretion is not increased because of the decreased total stool volume in breast-fed and formula-fed infants.

Human $^{99m}$Tc-labeled albumin imaging has been used to detect PLE. This technique may help to localize the site of bowel protein loss in difficult cases.

Screening for PLE by the determination of fecal $\alpha_1$-AT can be used to identify and follow the clinical course of various GI disorders associated with PLE. In children with Crohn's disease, PLE is the most common functional abnormality. Screening for PLE can therefore be used to aid in the diagnosis of Crohn's disease and to follow disease activity. The value of serial fecal $\alpha_1$-AT values in monitoring the disease activity of various GI disorders is illustrated in Figure 132-1.

The evaluation of the child with suspected protein-losing en-

---

**TABLE 132-2.   Evaluation for Hypoalbuminemia**

Estimate protein intake
Evaluate hypercatabolic stress
Initial laboratoy tests
  Serum total protein
  Liver function tests
  Prothrombin time
  Urinalysis
  Complete blood count
  Erythrocyte sedimentation rate
Screening tests for digestive dysfunction
  72-hour fecal fat
  Fecal $\alpha_1$-antitrypsin
  Fecal smear for occult blood

*From Thomas DW. Protein-losing enteropathy. In: Gryboski J, ed. Pediatric case reports in gastrointestinal disease, vol. 7, no. 2. Newtown, PA: Associated in Medical Marketing Co, 1987.*

teropathy is usually prompted by the finding of hypoproteinemia. An approach to the evaluation of a hypoproteinemic child is given in Table 132-2.

## TREATMENT

Management of children with PLE depends on the successful treatment of the primary underlying condition. In the case of protein sensitivity disorders, such as gluten-induced enteropathy and GI allergy, elimination of the inciting protein is curative. The treatment of specific GI and non-GI disorders associated with PLE is discussed elsewhere in this book.

## Selected Readings

Bhan MK, Khoshoo V, Chowdhary D, et al. Increased fecal alpha-1-antitrypsin excretion in children with persistent diarrhea associated with enteric pathogens. Acta Paediatr Scand 1989;78:265.

Colon AR, Sandberg DH. Protein-losing enteropathy in children. South Med J 1973;66:641.

Dinari G, Rosenbach Y, Zahavi I, et al. Random fecal alpha-1-antitrypsin excretion in children with intestinal disorders. Am J Dis Child 1984;138:971.

Hess J, Kruizinga K, Bijleveld CMA, et al. Protein-losing enteropathy after Fontan operation. J Thorac Cardiovasc Surg 1984;88:606.

Karbach U, Ewe K. Enteric protein loss in various gastrointestinal diseases determined by intestinal alpha-1-antitrypsin clearance. Z Gastroenterol 1989;27:362.

Lan JA, Chervu LR, Marans Z, et al. Protein-losing enteropathy detected by [99m]Tc-labeled human serum albumin abdominal scintigraphy. J Pediatr Gastroenterol Nutr 1988;7:872.

Thomas DW, McGilligan KM, Carlson M, et al. Fecal alpha-1-antitrypsin and hemoglobin excretion in healthy human milk-, formula-, or cow's milk-fed infants. Pediatrics 1986;78:305.

Thomas DW, Sinatra FR, Merritt RJ. Random fecal alpha-1-antitrypsin concentration in children with gastrointestinal disease. Gastroenterology 1981;80:776.

Thomas DW, Sinatra FR, Merritt RJ. Fecal alpha-1-antitrypsin excretion in young people with Crohn's disease. J Pediatr Gastroenterol Nutr 1983;2:491.

Waldman TA. Protein-losing enteropathy. Gastroenterology 1966;50:422.

*Principles and Practice of Pediatrics, Second Edition.*
edited by Frank A. Oski et al. J. B. Lippincott Company, Philadelphia © 1994.

## CHAPTER 133
# *Protein Intolerance*

## Christopher Duggan and W. Allan Walker

Ever since Lucretius (95–55 B.C.) pointed out that "one man's food might be another's poison," the concept of adverse reactions to food has captured the attention of the lay and medical communities. The modern manifestations of this phenomenon are reflected in advertising campaigns for "hypoallergenic" products designed for "sensitive" persons and in widespread dietary manipulations for children and adults with untoward nutritional consequences. Rational consideration of the gastrointestinal and systemic side effects of foods requires agreement on the terms of discussion and on the limits of our knowledge in this challenging field.

An *adverse reaction* to food is a general term implying any abnormal response to food or food additives. *Food intolerance* means any physiologic abnormality attributed to food ingestion, including immunologic and nonimmunologic (eg, toxic, metabolic, or pharmacologic) mechanisms. *Food allergy, food hypersensitivity,* or *protein intolerance* imply an immunologic reaction to a protein component of the diet that can be reproduced in food challenges. *Food anaphylaxis* is a subset of food allergies in which an IgE-mediated (type I) hypersensitivity reaction occurs. This chapter focuses on the latter two categories, with emphasis on the allergic enteropathies likely to come to the attention of pediatricians; allergic processes causing systemic reactions are described elsewhere in this book.

## COMMON FOOD ANTIGENS

Whether because of the widespread use of cow's milk-based formulas or because of the antigenic potential of their proteins, allergic reactions to cow's milk proteins are clearly the most clinically important in infancy. Formerly, the whey protein $\beta$-lactoglobulin, a dimer of 24 kd, was thought to be the prime allergen, but subsequent studies have shown that patients with cow's milk allergy react to multiple milk proteins, of which more than 20 have been identified. Food processing techniques, such as pasteurization and homogenization, can alter protein structure and the antigenicity of these proteins.

Soy proteins can induce allergic disease, with clinical symptoms and intestinal biopsies resembling those of cow's milk allergy. Soy allergy is especially common in Japan, paralleling the frequent exposure to soy proteins during infancy. Other notable antigens in food include those in eggs, peanuts and other legumes, nuts, fish, citrus fruits, and yeast. In Scandinavian countries, allergy to fish proteins is common. The enteropathy associated with gluten sensitivity (ie, celiac disease) is a special type of food intolerance and is discussed in Chapter 135.3.

## ANTIGEN HANDLING BY THE GASTROINTESTINAL TRACT

For antigens ingested in the diet to cause symptoms, they must cross the gastrointestinal mucosal barrier to be recognized by the systemic or local immune system. Antigens can take several routes: specialized M cells overlying Peyer's patches are able to process antigens and present them to the gut-associated lymphoid tissue (GALT); enterocytes can take up antigens directly by endocytosis or exocytosis; and some antigens can move through intercellular gaps.

Several impediments limit the amount of foreign antigens gaining access to the immune system. Nonspecific barriers to this process include proteolytic enzymes of the stomach and pancreas, which degrade complex proteins into smaller peptides and amino acids; gastrointestinal peristalsis, which leads to fewer antigens presented per unit time; mucous secretions overlying the enterocyte; and lysosomal enzymes of the intestinal epithelial cells. Specific immunologic components of antigen handling include the aforementioned GALT—the large number of phagocytes, eosinophils, mast cells, and T and B lymphocytes found in the lamina propria, Peyer's patches, and among the epithelial cells (intraepithelial lymphocytes) throughout the gastrointestinal tract. IgA is made and secreted in response to certain food antigens and plays a crucial role in host defense.

An important aspect of this complex system is its alteration with age and illness. Young infants have lower levels of intestinal IgA and fewer intraepithelial lymphocytes than do older ones.

Immaturity seems to favor priming the systemic immune response in the face of antigen uptake instead of the development of tolerance, which is a more mature response. In states of intestinal inflammation, ulceration, immunodeficiency, or malnutrition, intact proteins more readily cross the intestinal mucosa barrier. The immature or damaged barriers allow increased antigen uptake, with the risk of sensitization and subsequent allergic response.

# COW'S MILK PROTEIN INTOLERANCE

Allergy to cow's milk proteins was first described early in this century after advances in food technology led to the development of artificial infant formulas. By 1906, anaphylaxis to cow's milk was described, serum precipitins were found in animal models, and successful prevention with desensitizing injections of bovine serum was performed. Advances in our understanding of immunopathophysiology plus a finer appreciation for the wide range of symptoms due to cow's milk allergy have expanded our knowledge since then.

Several prospective studies with a variety of clinical and laboratory definitions of milk allergy have placed the prevalence of this disorder at 0.5% to 7.5% among European and North American infants. Risk factors include a family history of atopy and early dietary exposure to cow's milk. The age of onset is directly correlated with the time of introduction of artificial formulas. Even exclusively breast-fed infants can develop symptoms of protein intolerance, which may respond to elimination of the offending agent from the mother's diet.

## Gastrointestinal Manifestations

Symptoms referable to the gastrointestinal tract are among the most common in cow's milk allergy, occurring in 50% to 80% of patients. Several clinical entities have been described. These are probably related to a variety of immune responses other than type I, IgE-mediated disease (eg, Arthus reactions, T-cell cytotoxic reactions).

### Colitis

The presentation of milk-induced colitis can range from asymptomatic gastrointestinal blood loss with anemia to explosive bloody diarrhea and hypovolemic shock. Depending on the clinical setting, the differential diagnosis is broad and can include infectious gastroenteritis (eg, *Salmonella, Shigella, Yersinia, Campylobacter, Clostridium difficile*), necrotizing enterocolitis, sepsis, inflammatory bowel disease, intussusception, volvulus, and bowel infarction. Structural causes of gastrointestinal bleeding such as polyps, Meckel's diverticulum, and arteriovenous malformations may need to be considered. Historic features suggesting allergic colitis include recent ingestion of cow's milk and a family history of allergic disease.

Evaluation of these infants should include a thorough search for infectious agents, a complete blood count with a differential count, and coagulation studies. Peripheral eosinophilia is often seen, and a Wright's stain of the stool can reveal eosinophils. The diagnosis can be confirmed by flexible sigmoidoscopy. Endoscopic findings include patchy erythema and occasional ulcerations alternating with normal mucosa. Biopsies reveal eosinophils and plasma cells throughout the lamina propria, with infiltration of the crypts and surface epithelium by eosinophils. Although the histologic appearance may be similar to that of an acute infectious colitis, it is usually without the characteristic features of idiopathic ulcerative colitis. Children with milk-induced colitis are not predisposed to the later development of ulcerative colitis or Crohn's disease.

Further diagnostic confirmation of cow's milk colitis is often achieved by eliminating milk products and introducing a formula without cow's milk proteins. Because of the high rate of cross-reactivity to soy proteins, we recommend beginning a casein hydrolysate formula (eg, Nutramigen, Pregestimil) for severe symptoms of colitis. Depending on the clinical severity on presentation, additional milk challenges should be delayed until the child is 1 year of age.

### Malabsorption Syndrome

In an infant with poor growth and chronic diarrhea, a small bowel enteropathy secondary to milk allergy should be suspected. Although hypersensitivity to cow's milk antigens is the most frequent cause of an allergic enteropathy, reactions against other dietary proteins can produce similar findings. Stools may show evidence of carbohydrate and fat malabsorption, and there may be accompanying symptoms suggesting an allergic process (eg, eczema, recurrent wheezing). Small bowel biopsy reveals various degrees of villous atrophy with a patchy distribution; severe enteropathy can resemble the total villous atrophy of celiac disease. In addition to gluten sensitivity, other causes of malabsorption in infancy should be considered: immune deficiency (including acquired immune deficiency syndrome), chronic infectious enteritis (eg, *Giardia*), chronic protein malnutrition, bacterial overgrowth, primary or secondary lactase deficiency, and chronic diseases of the liver and pancreas (including cystic fibrosis).

Dietary management of protein intolerance enteropathy includes elimination of the offending antigen or antigens. Cow's milk enteropathy in an infant is treated by using a formula with casein hydrolysate as its protein source. In an older child with a more varied diet, strict attention is necessary to avoid ingestion of foods that may contain small but clinically important amounts of the relevant protein. Because the mucosal lesion may take several months to heal, reintroduction of milk proteins should take place only after adequate growth and nutritional repletion has been demonstrated.

### Eosinophilic Enteritis

Controversy exists about the role of protein intolerance in the pathogenesis of eosinophilic enteritis, a clinicopathologic entity distinct from allergic enterocolitis and the enteropathy described earlier. These patients often respond to treatment similar to that given to children with milk-induced colitis or enteropathy. This syndrome is discussed fully in Chapter 134.

### Other Gastrointestinal Symptoms

Symptoms and syndromes ranging from irritable bowel syndrome, abdominal migraine, gastroesophageal reflux, and chronic aphthous ulcerations have been ascribed to protein intolerance, but usually without convincing proof of an immunologic basis. Colic is often treated by dietary manipulation, although its relation to true protein intolerance is rarely documented. Food intolerance or allergy may be the cause of colic in 10% to 12% of otherwise healthy infants, and a change of formulas may improve symptoms. The resolution of colic coincident with a change in formula is a necessary but not sufficient condition to prove an allergic cause for these symptoms. Because frequent formula changes during infancy can convince the parents that their children are particularly susceptible to allergies and other illnesses, any treatment of colic by a formula change should be done with the reassurance that food allergy in infants is usually a short-lived phenomenon and that many factors may contribute to colic.

## Nongastrointestinal Manifestations

Shock due to anaphylactic reactions to food represents a true type I hypersensitivity reaction, although it is the least common form of all food allergies. Unlike the enteropathies described earlier, whose clinical expressions uniformly lessen with advancing age, a small percentage of patients with IgE-mediated reactions retain their allergy for life. Because anaphylaxis can occur with ingestion of minute amounts of antigen, any diagnostic challenge of a patient with purported allergens must occur with venous access assured and epinephrine, antihistamines, and steroids available. Other immediate reactions include urticarial rashes, lip swelling, and laryngeal edema. A study of a series of 13 fatal or near-fatal anaphylactic reactions to food found that two thirds of the fatal but none of the nonfatal reactions occurred at school, emphasizing the need for heightened public awareness of and preparedness for these emergencies.

Atopic dermatitis has been linked to food allergy. Sampson and colleagues (1985) found evidence of food hypersensitivity in 63 of 113 patients with severe eczema; egg, peanut, and milk proteins accounted for 72% of the reactions. However, only those children who fail standard medical therapy (eg, topical steroids, emollients) have a sufficiently high incidence of food allergy to warrant evaluation along these lines.

Respiratory symptoms, including wheezing, have been attributed to food protein allergy, and many infants who exhibit dermatologic findings also have acute bronchospasm. In the older child, asthma can be a manifestation of protein allergy, although symptoms often take hours to days to occur and are therefore difficult to diagnose. Heiner's syndrome refers to the symptom complex of pulmonary hemosiderosis, wheezing, chronic rhinitis, otitis media, and anemia, all of which resolve on dietary elimination of cow's milk proteins. The incidence of this syndrome seems to be declining with the practice of limiting infants' exposure to cow's milk.

## EVALUATION OF SUSPECTED FOOD ALLERGY

Part of the controversy surrounding the topic of food allergy lies in the difficulty with which the diagnosis is made. This difficulty probably reflects the multiple immunologic mechanisms that may be operative in protein intolerance, particularly among the allergic enteropathies. Immediate hypersensitivity reactions may be detected by IgE antibodies and be readily apparent clinically; reactions associated with circulating immune complexes or cell-mediated immune response may follow hours to days after ingestion of certain antigens, and laboratory evidence for their occurrence may be difficult to obtain. Multiple diagnostic tests are frequently employed in the diagnosis of food allergies, including dietary elimination, radioactive immunosorbent tests (RASTs), skin tests, and open or blinded food challenges.

If parents or patients suspect food allergy, they often perform some type of dietary elimination before seeking medical advice. These diets may not completely eliminate the purported agent unless careful attention is paid in examining all food labels. A milk avoidance diet, for instance, must exclude cow's milk and all dairy products. An empiric use of an elimination diet is usually not helpful because of these reasons. On the other extreme, self-imposed elimination diets can be so strict as to endanger the intake of calories and proteins necessary for growth and development. Care must be taken in the design of exclusionary diets so that they remain palatable and nutritionally adequate. The input of a skilled pediatric nutritionist is crucial.

The utility of RAST testing to detect food allergy is limited by the technique's measurement of IgE antibodies, which are the immunologic mediators in only a select group of patients. In patients with acute-onset dermatologic or respiratory manifestations of cow's milk allergy, the sensitivity and specificity of RAST testing are approximately 80%. In patients with gastrointestinal symptoms, RAST testing is usually much less helpful. Other serum immunoglobulins (eg, IgG, IgA) directed toward certain food antigens are found in healthy controls and merely represent exposure, not a pathologic reaction, to food proteins.

Skin tests in the assessment of food allergy have similar degrees of sensitivity and specificity as RASTs, but they are usually cheaper than RAST testing. However, skin testing can be technically difficult when performed on infants and is more reliable in children older than 3 years of age. A negative skin test in older children is helpful in ruling out disease, although a positive test does not confirm the diagnosis.

The use of food challenges has greatly aided the scientific study of protein intolerance, and double-blind, placebo-controlled challenges have become the gold standard for diagnosis. Many studies have shown that relying on parental history alone greatly overestimates the incidence of food allergy as diagnosed by a double-blind food challenge. In patients with a history of severe reactions, food challenges may be contraindicated. All challenges, especially in the very young, should be done under close medical supervision. Bock and colleagues (1988) produced guidelines for office-based food challenges.

## TREATMENT OF PROTEIN INTOLERANCE

The therapeutic mainstay in protein intolerance is strict dietary avoidance of the offending antigen. In the case of cow's milk intolerance, soy-based or casein hydrolysate formulas may be used, although as many as 25% of the infants who exhibit intolerance to cow's milk protein are intolerant of soy. Casein hydrolysate formulas, in which the in vitro breakdown of casein leads to small peptides with molecular weights less than 1200, are recommended by the American Academy of Pediatrics Committee on Nutrition for the treatment of protein intolerance. Unfortunately, these formulas are expensive and unpalatable, two factors that detract from their effectiveness. Whey hydrolysate formulas contain slightly larger peptides and may be less suitable for dietary management of food allergy. Case reports of allergic reactions to a whey hydrolysate formula originally advertised as "hypoallergenic" have been published.

In the rare case of intolerance to protein hydrolysates, formulas whose protein source is free amino acids are available (eg, Vivonex), but they usually have high osmolarities. Indiscriminate use of wide-ranging elimination diets should be discouraged, and objective evidence supporting specific protein intolerance symptoms should be sought and documented, especially for patients presenting with a history of multiple food allergies. Any child whose intake has been restricted for any reason should be monitored for the nutritional sufficiency of his or her diet.

Drug therapy for food allergies, including the use of prostaglandin synthetase inhibitors and oral cromolyn, has not proven beneficial. Rarely, low-dose systemic steroids are used for infantile colitis if strict adherence to an elemental diet has produced no benefit.

## PREVENTION

Because many of the symptoms of cow's milk protein intolerance occur most frequently in the first year of life, exclusive breast-feeding during this time, with delayed introduction of solid foods until 4 to 6 months of age, helps to prevent the onset of this food allergy. This advice should be given to parents of infants with a strong family history of atopy, and it is in keeping with the American Academy of Pediatrics recommendations for infant nutrition. Whether exclusive breast-feeding early in infancy protects against the development of other allergic diseases or merely delays their onset remains controversial.

The finding of an elevated cord Ige level is an accurate predictor of the newborn infant's chances of subsequent development of allergic disease. Studies have been undertaken to assess whether altering the maternal diet during pregnancy would change the incidence of allergies in their infants. Two controlled, prospective studies of Swedish women with a family history of atopy failed to show any effect, despite dietary restriction or inclusion of purported allergens and lengthy follow-up.

## Selected Readings

Anderson JA. The establishment of common language concerning adverse reactions to foods and food additives. J Allergy Clin Immunol 1986;78:140.

Bishop J, Hill DJ, Hosking CS. Natural history of cow milk allergy: clinical outcome. J Pediatr 1990;116:862.

Bock SA, Sampson HA, Atkins FM, et al. Double-blind, placebo-controlled food challenge (DBPCFC) as an office procedure: a manual. J Allergy Clin Immunol 1988;82:986.

Chandra RK, Hamed A. Cumulative incidence of atopic disorders in high risk infants fed whey hydrolysate, soy, and conventional cow's milk formula (2 parts). Ann Allergy 1991;67:129.

David TJ. Anaphylactic shock during elimination diets for severe atopic eczema. Arch Dis Child 1984;59:983.

Gern JE, Yang E, Evrard HM, et al. Allergic reactions to milk-contaminated "nondairy" products. N Engl J Med 1991;324:976.

James JM, Sampson HA. An overview of food hypersensitivity. Pediatr Allerg Immunol 1992;3:

Jenkins HR, Pincott JR, Soothill JF, et al. Food allergy: the major cause of infantile colitis. Arch Dis Child 1984;59:326.

Lake AM, Whitington PF, Hamilton SR. Dietary protein-induced colitis in breast-fed infants. J Pediatr 1982;101:906.

Metcalfe DD, Sampson HA, Simon RA, eds. Food allergy: adverse reactions to foods and food additives. Boston: Blackwell Scientific, 1991.

Sampson HA, McCaskill CC. Food hypersensitivity and atopic dermatitis: evaluation of 113 patients. J Pediatr 1985;107:669.

Sampson HA, Mendelson L, Rosen JP. Fatal and near-fatal anaphylactic reactions to food in children and adolescents. N Engl J Med 1992;327:380.

Stern M, Walker WA. Food allergy and intolerance. Pediatr Clin North Am 1985;32:471.

Walker WA. Pathophysiology of intestinal uptake and absorption of antigens in food allergy. Ann Allergy 1987;59:7.

*Principles and Practice of Pediatrics, Second Edition.*
edited by Frank A. Oski et al. J. B. Lippincott Company, Philadelphia © 1994.

CHAPTER 134
# Eosinophilic Gastroenteritis

## Glenn T. Furuta and W. Allan Walker

Eosinophilic gastroenteritis is a rare clinicopathologic entity that occurs during infancy, childhood, and adolescence. The clinical manifestations include vomiting, abdominal pain, malabsorption, gastrointestinal obstruction, and ascites. The cause is unknown, but the disease has been associated with allergic symptoms. In the appropriate clinical setting, the diagnosis of eosinophilic gastroenteritis requires a histologic demonstration of markedly increased numbers of eosinophils in the gastrointestinal tract.

## HISTOPATHOLOGY

The infiltration of eosinophils in the gastrointestinal tissues can occur in a circumscribed or diffuse manner. Circumscribed infiltration produces a polypoid lesion, and diffuse infiltration may involve multiple anatomical compartments in the gastrointestinal tract. Some investigators classify the diffuse form of eosinophilic gastroenteritis into categories based on the major area of involvement (eg, mucosal, muscular, serosal). Although this classification is clinically useful, it does not reflect the fact that many patients may have multiple areas of involvement (Table 134-1).

Mucosal involvement is the most common pediatric form of eosinophilic gastroenteritis and usually presents with vomiting, diarrhea, failure to thrive, and protein-losing enteropathy. Thickening of the bowel wall with subsequent obstructive symptoms is commonly seen if muscular involvement is predominant. Serosal infiltration may cause an exudative ascites that is rich in eosinophils and protein.

The gastric antrum and small intestine are the principle sites of involvement, although esophageal and colonic abnormalities have been reported. The gastric antrum is most commonly affected, and patchy involvement may occur. A small bowel biopsy can show partial or complete villous atrophy with a massive infiltration of the lamina propria with eosinophils.

Many clinical presentations have been reported. Two infants with symptoms suggesting pyloric stenosis were found to have marked antral eosinophilia. Several children with occult blood loss and another patient with presumed functional abdominal pain were found to have eosinophilic gastroenteritis.

## PATHOGENESIS

The pathogenesis of eosinophilic gastroenteritis is unknown. Evidence suggesting the role of food intolerance is conflicting. Infants seem to display a clinical course more consistent with milk allergy, and some older patients are found to have proven food allergies. Between 20% and 50% of patients have an allergic condition such as asthma or rhinitis.

The causative role of the eosinophil in tissue destruction and symptoms is not clear. Eosinophils produce a variety of proteins that are thought to be involved in parasite killing and in vitro cytotoxicity. The extent of eosinophil activation has been correlated with the degree of histologic damage, strongly suggesting a primary role of the eosinophil in the pathology seen in this disease. Inflammatory cells such as mast cells also have been implicated in the pathogenesis of eosinophilic gastroenteritis.

## DIAGNOSIS

Physical findings are usually nonspecific. Hepatosplenomegaly and lymphadenopathy have been reported, and long-standing disease may produce malnutrition.

Peripheral eosinophilia is an inconsistent finding, occurring in 13% to 85% of patients. Eosinophilia usually does not occur in circumscribed disease. IgE levels appear to be elevated in patients with more severe disease but not consistently. Charcot Leyden crystals, derived from eosinophils, can sometimes be found in the stool. In diffuse disease, malabsorption may occur, and the bone marrow may be infiltrated with eosinophils.

Radiographic bowel abnormalities are nonspecific. The small bowel may appear normal or demonstrate mucosal thickening with coarsening and nodularity of the folds. In mucosal disease, air contrast studies of the antrum may reveal an irregular lacy antral surface instead of the normal smooth, bald surface. If the

**TABLE 134-1.   Eosinophilic Gastroenteritis: Relation Between Histopathologic Type and Clinical Manifestations**

| Type | Clinical Manifestations | Age |
|---|---|---|
| Circumscribed | Obstruction, intussusception, bleeding | Adolescence |
| Diffuse | | |
| Mucosal disease | Vomiting, diarrhea, bleeding, protein-losing enteropathy, failure to thrive, malabsorption | >6 mo to adolescence |
| Muscle layer disease | Obstructive symptoms, gastric outlet obstruction | >3 mo |
| Serosal infiltration | Exudative eosinophilic ascites | >5 y<br>>5 y |

colon is involved, a cobblestone pattern similar to that of granulomatous colitis may be seen.

Gastrointestinal biopsies, usually obtained at endoscopy, are the cornerstone of diagnosis. Involved tissue may appear erythematous, granular, nodular, or ulcerated but often look normal. Because the lesions may appear normal and involvement is often patchy, it is essential to obtain multiple biopsy specimens, which include the antrum, for histologic evaluation. Occasionally, the diagnosis is made at exploratory laparotomy; serosal disease may present with an acute abdomen or if muscular disease causes complete obstruction.

## DIFFERENTIAL DIAGNOSIS

The nonspecific symptoms seen in cases of eosinophilic gastroenteritis make the diagnosis difficult unless a high index of suspicion is maintained. Peripheral eosinophilia may be helpful, but other conditions such as collagen vascular diseases, especially polyarteritis nodose, and enteroinvasive parasitic infestation should be excluded.

The radiographic abnormalities may be seen in the antrum of other types of gastritis, such as aspirin ingestion, peptic ulcer disease, early granulomatous disease, and in infections, such as histoplasmosis and tuberculosis.

Gastric tumors (eg, carcinoma, lymphoma, leiomyoma, leiomyosarcoma), which are rare in children, may exhibit nodular radiographic abnormalities. Enlarged gastric folds may be seen in Zollinger-Ellison syndrome and Ménétrier's disease.

The combination of gastric lesions and small bowel radiographic abnormalities suggests the diagnosis of eosinophilic gastroenteritis, but Crohn's disease and granulomatous infections may have similar findings.

Tissue eosinophilia can be seen in inflammatory bowel disease, peptic disease, amoebiasis, or other parasitic infections. Eosinophilic granulomatous disease, tropical sprue, chronic granulomatous disease usually have less eosinophilia and other clinical signs and symptoms.

## TREATMENT

No specific treatment or consistently effective diet is available. An elimination diet should be attempted if the clinical symptoms are mild and the allergen can be identified. If a clear association between the disease and the ingestion of specific foods has been demonstrated, symptoms can improve markedly after the offending agents are discontinued. The use of elimination diets in patients without a clear precipitant has not been particularly use-

ful, although there are reports of long-lasting responses. If elimination diets are used for prolonged periods, care should be taken to ensure a complete and well-balanced diet.

Corticosteroids can be used if the response to an elimination diet is not satisfactory or if the patient is extremely ill. In some cases, steroids have improved the histologic abnormalities within 2 months of initiation of therapy. Prednisone (1 to 2 mg/kg/day for 7 days to 3 months) has been used. Clinical improvement generally is prompt, and patients can be quickly weaned off steroids. Some patients may need long courses of therapy that require an alternate-day dosing schedule. Other therapies, including sodium cromolyn and ketotifen, have been used with varying results. Although surgery is needed for lesions producing complete obstruction, corticosteroid therapy has relieved the symptoms of some patients.

## PROGNOSIS

The prognosis varies according to the type and extent of eosinophilic infiltration. For circumscribed and muscle layer disease, the prognosis is excellent, particularly if surgical intervention alleviates the symptoms.

For diffuse mucosal disease, the prognosis varies. Some patients have long-term remissions, but others have chronic disease requiring prolonged steroid therapy. Complications include small bowel bacterial overgrowth, hemorrhage, and perforation. No malignant transformation has been reported.

## Selected Readings

Caldwell JH, Mekhijan HS, Hurtubise PE, et al. Eosinophilic gastroenteritis with obstruction: immunologic studies of seven patients. Gastroenterology 1978;74:825.

Caldwell JH, Sharma HM, Hurtubise PE, et al. Eosinophilic gastroenteritis in extreme allergy: immunopathologic comparison with non allergic gastrointestinal disease. Gastroenterology 1979;77,560.

Colon AR, Sorkin LF, Stern WR, et al. Eosinophilic gastroenteritis. J Pediatr Gastroenterol Nutr 1983;2:187.

Goldman H, Proujansky R. Allergic proctitis and gastroenteritis in children: clinical and mucosal biopsy features in 53 cases. Am J Surg Pathol 1986;10:75.

Katz AJ, Goldman H, Grand RJ. Gastric mucosal biopsy in eosinophilic (allergic) gastroenteritis. Gastroenterology 1977;73:705.

Katz AJ, Twarog FJ, Zeiger RS, Falchuk ZM. Milk-sensitive and eosinophilic gastroenteropathy: similar clinical features with contrasting mechanism and clinical course. J Allergy Clin Immunol 1984;74:72.

Kershavarzian A, Saverymuttu SH, Tai PC, et al. Activated eosinophils in familial eosinophilic gastroenteritis. Gastroenterology 1985;88:1041.

Melamed I, Feanny SJ, Sherman PM, Roifman C. Benefit of ketotifen in patients with eosinophilic gastroenteritis. Am J Med 1991;90:310.

Moore D, Lichtman S, Lentz J, et al. Eosinophilic gastroenteritis presenting in an adolescent with isolated colonic involvement. Gut 1986;27:1219.

Scully RE. Case records of the Massachusetts General Hospital: case 20-1992. N Engl J Med 1992;326:1342.

Snyder JS, Rosenblum N, Wershil BK, et al. Pyloric stenosis and eosinophilic gastroenteritis in infants. J Pediatr Gastroenterol Nutr 1987;6:543.

Steffan RM, Wyllie R, Petras RE, et al. The spectrum of eosinophilic gastroenteritis-report of six pediatric cases and a review of the literature. Clin Pediatr 1991;30:404.

Talley NJ, Shorter RG, Phillips SF, Zinsmeister AR. Eosinophilic gastroenteritis: a clinicopathological study of patients with disease of the mucosa, muscle layer and subserosa tissues. Gut 1990;31:54.

Wershil BK, Walker WA. The mucosal barrier, IgE-mediated gastrointestinal events, and eosinophilic gastroenteritis. Gastroenterol Clin North Am 1992;21:387.

Whittington PF, Whittington GL. Eosinophilic gastroenteropathy in childhood. J Pediatr Gastroenterol Nutr 1988;7:379.

*Principles and Practice of Pediatrics, Second Edition.*
edited by Frank A. Oski et al. J. B. Lippincott Company, Philadelphia © 1994.

# CHAPTER 135
# *Malabsorption States*

Impaired intestinal absorption of nutrients may result from several clinical conditions, including short bowel syndrome, small bowel bacterial overgrowth, celiac disease, and various immunodeficiency states. Malabsorption of carbohydrate can result in failure to thrive, diarrhea, and weight loss, but unlike malabsorption of essential amino acids, fatty acids, vitamins, or minerals, it does not lead to specific nutrient deficiencies.

*Principles and Practice of Pediatrics, Second Edition.*
edited by Frank A. Oski et al. J. B. Lippincott Company, Philadelphia © 1994.

## 135.1 *Short Bowel Syndrome*

### Carlos H. Lifschitz

Short bowel syndrome can be caused by prenatal events, such as congenital short bowel, volvulus, small bowel atresia, or gastroschisis. Acquired causes of the syndrome include volvulus, necrotizing enterocolitis, meconium ileus, and Crohn's disease. Because most cases occur in the perinatal period, the remaining length of bowel must be sufficient to allow the nutrient absorption required for growth. Despite the compensatory intestinal growth, dominated by villous hyperplasia, that usually occurs, various degrees of nutrient malabsorption may persist.

The adaptation phase that follows massive resection of the intestine can last as long as 3 years. Total oral or enteral nutrition ultimately may be feasible if at least 20 to 30 cm of small bowel remains and the ileocecal valve is intact. During the adaptation period and sometimes during periods of accelerated growth, in-travenous nutrition may be mandatory. When a patient is being weaned from intravenous nutrition, prolonged enteral feedings administered as a constant infusion through a nasogastric tube or a gastrostomy may be necessary. The degree of nutrient malabsorption that results from a short bowel is related to the extent of the resection, the segment of bowel resected, and the existence of the ileocecal valve.

Although disaccharidases are more abundant in the jejunum, they also occur in the ileum, and carbohydrate malabsorption may not be severe if the jejunum is resected, particularly if the ileocecal valve has not been removed. Carbohydrate malabsorption can be secondary to decreased surface absorptive area and diminished disaccharidase activity as a result of diminished bowel length, mucosal irritation resulting from gastric hypersecretion (frequently observed in extensive small bowel resections), or accelerated transit time. Small bowel bacterial overgrowth can occur in patients with short bowel syndrome. The bacteria may use the carbohydrate before it is absorbed, causing gas formation and diarrhea.

Protein is malabsorbed to a lesser extent than are other nutrients. The decreased absorption of protein is in proportion to the amount of intestine resected, but small bowel bacterial overgrowth may lead to enteric protein losses and protein malabsorption.

The degree of impairment of fat absorption is related to the segment and length of bowel resected. Because fat cannot be absorbed in the jejunum, severe fat malabsorption occurs in cases of extensive ileal resection. The ileum is the site for bile salt reabsorption; removal of this segment of bowel causes bile salts to be malabsorbed and the bile acid pool to decrease, which impairs micelle formation and malabsorption of fat and fat-soluble vitamins. Vitamin $B_{12}$ malabsorption also occurs with ileal resection.

After proximal small bowel resection, iron, zinc, and folate deficiency may occur in addition to decreased absorption of calcium, magnesium, and phosphorus. Resection of the colon may result in water and sodium losses. The small bowel may compensate for the absence of the colon through an increased capacity to reabsorb water and electrolytes. Calcium and magnesium soaps may form in the lumen of the bowel in cases of fat malabsorption and lead to hypocalcemia and hypomagnesemia. Pancreatic secretions may be decreased after a proximal resection because of the loss of stimulation by cholecystokinin.

The treatment of short bowel syndrome includes the use of lactose-free, elemental diets with low osmolality. Resins to bind bile acids (eg, cholestyramine) may be helpful in bile acid-induced diarrhea, which usually occurs after shorter resections. A low-fat diet is indicated after extensive resections, particularly those that include the distal ileum. The use of medium-chain triglycerides may be advantageous, because micelle formation is not necessary for their absorption. However, essential fatty acid deficiency may occur with the use of low-fat diets that contain predominantly medium-chain triglycerides. If gastric hypersecretion develops, it may be controlled by therapy with $H_2$-receptor blockers. If small bowel bacterial overgrowth occurs, it must be treated (see Chap 135.2).

## Selected Readings

Biller JA. Short small-bowel syndrome. In: Grand RJ, Sutphen JL, Dietz WH, eds. Pediatric nutrition: theory and practice. Boston: Butterworths, 1987:481.

Dorney SFA, Ament ME, Berquist WE, Vargas JH, Hassall E. Improved survival in very short small bowel of infancy with use of long-term parenteral nutrition. J Pediatr 1985;107:521.

Williamson RC. Intestinal adaptation. Part I. N Engl J Med 1978;25:1393.

Williamson RC. Intestinal adaptation. Part II. N Engl J Med 1978;26:1444.

Wilson SE. Pediatric enteral feeding. In: Grand RJ, Sutphen JL, Dietz WH, eds. Pediatric nutrition: theory and practice. Boston: Butterworths, 1987:771.

*Principles and Practice of Pediatrics, Second Edition.*
edited by Frank A. Oski et al. J. B. Lippincott Company, Philadelphia © 1994.

# 135.2 Small Bowel Bacterial Overgrowth

## Carlos H. Lifschitz

In healthy persons, the stomach, duodenum, and upper small bowel are sterile or the number of organisms never surpasses $10^5$ colony-forming units per 1 mL (CFU/mL). The organisms commonly found are lactobacilli, streptococci, *Haemophilus influenzae*, *Haemophilus parainfluenzae*, *Veillonella*, and *Propionibacterium acnes*. Mechanisms such as gastric acidity, secretions of the intestine and pancreas, immunoglobulins, and especially intestinal peristalsis aid in maintaining a low bacterial count. The distal ileum contains as many as $10^9$ CFU/mL, including gram-negative bacilli and anaerobes. The ileocecal valve is important in preventing an anaerobic, colonic-type flora in the distal small bowel. Impairment of any of these mechanisms may result in small bowel bacterial overgrowth. The clinical entities in which bacterial overgrowth may occur are listed in Table 135-1.

Small bowel bacterial overgrowth frequently leads to malabsorption of carbohydrate because of intraluminal use by bacteria. Presenting symptoms are abdominal distention as a result of gas formation, vomiting, and diarrhea. Diarrhea can result from bacterial degradation of brush border disaccharidases and from a decrease in small bowel villous height and a consequent decrease in the transport of monosaccharides.

Hypoproteinemia, which usually occurs in patients with small bowel bacterial overgrowth, can be the result of protein loss due to mucosal injury by the bacteria or of altered absorption of dietary protein due to luminal bacterial degradation.

Bile acids, acted on by anaerobic bacteria in the upper portion of the small bowel, are deconjugated. Deconjugated bile acids cannot be reabsorbed in the distal small bowel and can cause diarrhea when they reach the colon. The lack of reabsorption of bile acids results in a diminished bile acid pool and impaired fat absorption. Small bowel bacterial overgrowth can also produce intestinal mucosal changes that interfere with the formation of chylomicrons. Colonic bacteria act on malabsorbed fat and transform it into hydroxylated fatty acids, which can cause diarrhea.

The absorption of fat-soluble vitamins can be impaired by a similar mechanism. Patients with small bowel bacterial overgrowth are at risk for bleeding disorders that result from vitamin K deficiency, night blindness due to vitamin A malabsorption, and rickets due to vitamin D deficiency. Vitamin $B_{12}$ deficiency also occurs in patients with small bowel bacterial overgrowth, and the deficiency appears to result from bacterial use of vitamin $B_{12}$.

The diagnosis of small bowel bacterial overgrowth is made by intestinal intubation, aspiration, culture, and colony count of intestinal fluid. High fasting breath hydrogen levels may herald bacterial overgrowth. Treatment includes the correction of the underlying abnormality by resection of intestinal strictures or adhesions or the use of sulfonamides or oral antibiotics, such as kanamycin, neomycin, or gentamicin. In older children, metronidazole or tetracyclines may be used. An ion exchange resin such as cholestyramine may help bind bacterial products such as bile acids.

## Selected Readings

Heyman MB, Perman JA. Nutrition in bacterial overgrowth syndromes of the gastrointestinal tract. Grand RJ, Sutphen JL, Dietz WH, eds. Pediatric nutrition: theory and practice. Boston: Butterworths, 1987:445.
Toskes PP, Donaldson RM. The blind loop syndrome. In: Sleisenger MH, Fordtran JS, eds. Gastrointestinal disease. Philadelphia: WB Saunders, 1983:1023.

*Principles and Practice of Pediatrics, Second Edition.*
edited by Frank A. Oski et al. J. B. Lippincott Company, Philadelphia © 1994.

# 135.3 Celiac Disease

## Carlos H. Lifschitz

Celiac disease is characterized by villous atrophy of the proximal small bowel, and it responds to the withdrawal of gluten from the diet. The fraction of gluten called gliadin has been identified as the agent responsible for the disease. The relation between celiac disease and intolerance to dietary wheat and rye was recognized by Dicke in 1950. The highest rate of celiac disease occurs in Ireland, where 1 in 300 persons is affected. The prevalence in some areas of the United States is estimated to be 1 in 2000. For unknown reasons, the prevalence of this disease is slowly decreasing.

The age at which cereal is introduced into the diet and the amount and type of cereal ingested may affect the presentation of the disease. Precocious presentation may occur between 10 to 18 months of age with frothy, liquid, foul-smelling stools. The child acquires the celiac aspect, characterized by wasting and severe abdominal distention, at approximately 1 year of age. The other form of presentation occurs at 2 to 3 years of age with poor feeding, lack of weight gain for several months or actual weight

### TABLE 135-1. Factors Predisposing to Small Bowel Bacterial Overgrowth

| | |
|---|---|
| **Congenital Bowel Abnormalities** | **Changes in Peristalsis** |
| Gastroschisis | Chronic diarrhea |
| Small bowel atresia | Pseudo-obstruction |
| Meconium ileus | Scleroderma |
| Malrotation | Diabetes |
| Duodenal webs | |
| | **Nutritional Factors** |
| **Abdominal Surgery** | Celiac disease |
| Postoperative adhesions | Malnutrition (severe) |
| Intestinal bypass surgery | Hypokalemia |
| Roux-en-Y procedures | |
| Short bowel | **Hypochlorhydria** |
| Gastrectomy | |
| Vagotomy | **Other** |
| | Nasojejunal tubes |
| **Acquired Bowel Abnormalities** | Antacids, $H_2$-receptor blockers |
| Crohn's disease | Cystic fibrosis |
| Tumors | |
| Fistulas | |

loss, irritability, and diarrhea consisting of foul-smelling, bulky stools. Monosymptomatic forms may present with constipation or severe, recurrent abdominal pain. The disease has been diagnosed in adolescents with no major gastrointestinal complaints but who consulted a physician because of short stature. The disease is more prevalent among persons who carry the HLA-B8, HLA-DR3, or HLA-DR7 antigens.

Laboratory analyses are nonspecific, and serum abnormalities, such as low hemoglobin, iron, albumin, cholesterol, calcium, phosphate, vitamin A, or carotene levels, are related to the malabsorption but are nonspecific for the disease. Fat globules may be identified in a stool smear, and fat malabsorption can be quantified by means of a 72-hour stool collection (ie, normal absorption >95% of ingested fat). After ingestion of D-xylose, the serum level 1 hour later remains low. However, this test is not sensitive and is not specific for celiac disease. Intestinal permeability tests using small-molecular-weight sugars can detect alteration of the small bowel mucosa. Although elevated serum levels of antigliadin antibodies and antireticulin antibodies may indicate the disease, the diagnosis requires a peroral small bowel biopsy. Endomysial antibodies seem to be the most sensitive and specific of the noninvasive tests for the diagnosis of celiac disease.

A small bowel biopsy can demonstrate moderate to severe villous atrophy and a chronic inflammatory infiltrate of the lamina propia. If the biopsy results support the clinical and laboratory findings, the patient is placed on a gluten-free diet for 6 to 12 months. Small bowel biopsy repeated at the end of this period should demonstrate normalization of the villous architecture. To confirm the diagnosis, the patient is reexposed to gluten for 2 years or until symptoms recur, at which time a third biopsy is recommended. This biopsy should demonstrate recurrence of villous atrophy and chronic inflammatory infiltrate. The strict diagnostic criteria have been revised.

Although small bowel villous atrophy in conjunction with the clinical picture described is characteristic of celiac disease, other abnormalities, such as dietary protein intolerance, can present in a similar manner. Lactose malabsorption is frequently observed in patients with celiac disease as a result of decreased lactase activity. In these patients, lactose-free or lactose-hydrolyzed milk is recommended. Fat and fat-soluble vitamin malabsorption is also seen in patients with celiac disease. The inability to absorb fat probably is not related solely to a mucosal defect, because fat is absorbed primarily in the distal ileum, which is the less affected part of the small bowel in celiac disease. A decreased contraction of the gallbladder, probably due to a lack of cholecystokinin secretion by the damaged enterocytes of the proximal small bowel, may explain the lack of bile acid secretion and consequent fat malabsorption. In patients with prolonged malnutrition, potassium deficiency may result in muscle dysfunction, which may lead to bowel distention, stasis, and small bowel bacterial overgrowth.

The celiac crisis is a medical emergency that can occur in a patient in whom exposure to gluten has been prolonged or who is intentionally or inadvertently reexposed to gluten. Intercurrent illnesses may precipitate a celiac crisis.

Treatment entails the complete removal of gluten from the diet and caloric supplementation during the period of catch-up growth; vitamin and mineral supplements are recommended during this time. The recommendation that patients remain on a gluten-free diet for life is questioned by some investigators.

## Selected Readings

Falchuk ZM. Update on gluten-sensitive enteropathy. Am J Med 1979;67:1085.
McNeish AS, Harms HK, Rey J, et al. The diagnosis of celiac disease. Arch Dis Child 1979;54:783.
Unsworth DJ, Walker-Smith JA, Holborow EJ. Gliadin and reticulin antibodies in childhood coeliac disease. Lancet 1983;1:874.
Working Group of the European Society for Pediatric Gastroenterology and Nutrition. Revised criteria for the diagnosis of celiac disease. Arch Dis Child 1990;65:909.

*Principles and Practice of Pediatrics, Second Edition.*
edited by Frank A. Oski et al. J. B. Lippincott Company, Philadelphia © 1994.

# 135.4 *Immunodeficiency States*

Carlos H. Lifschitz

## ACQUIRED IMMUNE DEFICIENCY SYNDROME

The acquired immune deficiency syndrome (AIDS) has been reported in children since 1983 and may be found among hemophiliacs, transfusion recipients, and infants born to high-risk parents. The gastrointestinal (GI) manifestations observed in patients with AIDS include esophagitis and diarrhea with or without parasitic, viral, or bacterial infections. Nutrient malabsorption is not always a factor in the illness, although children may have nutrient malabsorption even if they do not have overt symptoms.

Organisms commonly associated with the diarrhea in AIDS patients are *Candida albicans, Cryptosporidium,* cytomegalovirus, atypical mycobacteria, and *Salmonella typhimurium.* Even in the absence of systemic or enteric infections or malignancy, many adult and pediatric AIDS patients suffer from chronic diarrhea, anorexia, and weight loss. *Mycobacterium avium-intracellulare* has been found in the small bowel of patients with AIDS and has been associated with diarrhea. The organism is an acid-fast bacillus that has been found in macrophages of the lamina propria of the small bowel. Patients with cytomegalovirus infections may have diarrhea, and viral inclusions can be found at different levels of the GI tract. Ileitis or colitis together with esophageal and colonic ulcers from which the virus can be cultured have been reported.

The GI symptoms of AIDS can mimic those of other diseases. The symptoms of AIDS patients, who suffer from chronic diarrhea and have marked abdominal distention and malnutrition, have been compared with the symptoms of celiac disease. The histologic picture of the small bowel mucosa is compatible with partially treated celiac disease in that it has patchy atrophy alternating with more normal segments of mucosa. In other patients, the clinical symptoms are similar to those of inflammatory bowel disease. These patients complain of abdominal pain, weight loss, diarrhea, and fever. AIDS in children may also manifest as pseudomembranous necrotizing jejunitis.

AIDS may be expressed as a failure to thrive, with or without diarrhea. Diarrhea and malabsorption are more prevalent in patients with documented GI infections. Increased fecal fat, diminished appetite, and weight loss are frequently observed in these patients. A small bowel biopsy can identify infiltration of the lamina propria with chronic inflammatory cells and occasional subtle villous atrophy. Nonspecific inflammatory cell infiltrate can also be seen in the colon. These histologic and functional abnormalities have been referred to as AIDS enteropathy. The evaluation of patients with AIDS who present with GI symptoms should include a careful search for bowel pathogens. However, in many patients in whom pathogens can be identified, diarrhea often persists despite a variety of therapeutic interventions, including systemic treatment for fungal or mycobacterial disease and intravenous antibiotics for other infections. Feedings can be administered through a nasogastric tube if children are too debilitated to take food orally. This technique may also facilitate gastric emptying and formula tolerance.

## IGA DEFICIENCY

Selective IgA deficiency is the most common of the primary immunodeficiency states, affecting approximately 1 in 700 of the population. Because other immunoglobulins, such as IgM, may compensate for the deficiency, only 13% of the patients have significant GI symptoms. The GI manifestations of IgA deficiency are chronic diarrhea, steatorrhea, lactose malabsorption, milk-protein intolerance, and those secondary to infestation by *Giardia lamblia*. The relation between serum or secretory IgA deficiencies and GI symptoms has not been clarified completely, but a secretory IgA deficiency appears to be the form associated with malabsorption. Celiac disease, lymphonodular hyperplasia, ulcerative colitis, Crohn's disease, and disaccharidase deficiencies have been associated with IgA deficiency. Moreover, small bowel villous atrophy has been observed in patients with IgA deficiency and giardiasis. Diarrhea and malabsorption usually improve after treatment for *G lamblia*.

## PANHYPOGAMMAGLOBULINEMIA

Approximately 60% of the patients with the common variable form of immunoglobulin deficiency have chronic or recurrent diarrhea; most of these patients also have malabsorption. Infestation by *G lamblia* is common, and secondary disaccharidase deficiencies and clinical carbohydrate intolerance may occur. However, malabsorption can also occur in patients in whom *Giardia* cannot be found. The intestinal mucosa may reveal altered villous architecture, although malabsorption may occur although the small bowel histology is normal. Small bowel bacterial overgrowth can complicate the clinical picture in some patients, but treatment of this condition does not necessarily resolve the symptoms. Malabsorption can also result from the development of gastric achlorhydria and deficiency of intrinsic factor leading to vitamin $B_{12}$ malabsorption and myeloblastic anemia. In rare cases, the syndrome can include neutropenia and pancreatic exocrine insufficiency. A rare condition, ulcerative jejunoileitis, may complicate common variable hypogammaglobulinemia and result in severe nutrient malabsorption.

## X-LINKED HYPOGAMMAGLOBULINEMIA

Patients with X-linked hypogammaglobulinemia suffer from diarrhea and malabsorption less often than do those with common variable hypogammaglobulinemia. Diarrhea usually resolves after 2 years of age. Giardiasis occurs frequently and can lead to malabsorption.

## COMBINED IMMUNODEFICIENCIES

Patients with rare conditions such as Wiskott-Aldrich syndrome usually have a history of chronic blood-tinged diarrhea early in infancy.

The second most common primary immunodeficiency syndrome is severe combined immunodeficiency. Diarrhea and malabsorption are common in infants who have deficient humoral and cellular immune mechanisms. Few studies have traced the pathogenesis of the malabsorption state. The villi of the jejunal mucosa are stunted, and marked mucosal edema and a large number of vacuolated macrophages can be seen. Malabsorption may be limited initially to lactose, but it eventually encompasses other nutrients. Treatment by bone marrow grafting may cause a graft-versus-host reaction and result in marked villous shortening, diarrhea, enteral protein loss, and nutrient malabsorption. Small bowel bacterial overgrowth may aggravate malabsorption.

## T-CELL DEFICIENCY

Patients with DiGeorge syndrome frequently have oral and esophageal candidiasis and prolonged diarrhea.

## TREATMENT FOR MALABSORPTION IN IMMUNODEFICIENCY STATES

Metronidazole or quinacrine hydrochloride (Atabrine) can be used to eradicate *Giardia*. Treatment for *Cryptosporidium* and *Mycobacterium avium-intracellulare* has not been successful. Nutritional support should include a lactose-free diet and preferably the use of hydrolyzed proteins. Elimination of fresh vegetables and fruits may reduce the risk of introducing pathogenic bacteria to immunosuppressed persons.

## Selected Readings

Ament ME. Immunodeficiency syndromes and gastrointestinal disease. Pediatr Clin North Am 1975;22:807.
Doe WF, Hapel AJ. Intestinal immunity and malabsorption. Clin Gastroenterol 1983;12:415.
Kotler DP. Gastrointestinal and nutritional manifestations of the acquired immunodeficiency syndrome. New York: Raven Press, 1991.
Shannon KM, Ammann AJ. Acquired immune deficiency syndrome in childhood. J Pediatr 1985;106:332.

*Principles and Practice of Pediatrics, Second Edition.*
edited by Frank A. Oski et al. J. B. Lippincott Company, Philadelphia © 1994.

# 135.5 *Enzyme and Transport Defects*

Robert J. Shulman

## CARBOHYDRATE MALABSORPTION

### Pathophysiology and Clinical Findings

Disorders of carbohydrate absorption are integrally linked with dysfunction of the small intestinal mucosal carbohydrate-digesting enzymes, lactase, sucrase, $\alpha$-dextrinase, and glucoamylase. Lactase activity increases substantially between 35 weeks' gestation and birth. Lactase is the only enzyme capable of hydrolyzing lactose. Sucrase and $\alpha$-dextrinase are two enzymes that are covalently linked in the intestinal brush border and develop full activity in early fetal life. Sucrase can hydrolyze sucrose, maltose, and the 1,4 bonds in glucose polymers and starches. α-Dextrinase can hydrolyze maltose but not sucrose, and it is the only enzyme that can hydrolyze the 1,6 bonds found in starches. Glucoamylase activity also is developed early in gestation and can hydrolyze maltose and the 1,4 linkages from the nonreducing ends of starches (ie, glucose polymers, complex starches).

If lactose, sucrose, and maltose are not hydrolyzed and absorbed, they remain as osmotically active molecules in the lumen of the bowel. Nonabsorbed glucose polymers and starches have a similar but smaller effect inversely proportional to molecular size. All disorders associated with significant carbohydrate malabsorption can induce a net secretion of water that increases the rate of intestinal transit and can decrease the absorptive capacity for other nutrients. The result is watery diarrhea and cramping that ceases if patients are not fed.

Malabsorbed carbohydrate passes into the colon, where it is converted by bacterial fermentation to fatty acids, which also are osmotically active, and to hydrogen gas. These conversion products are partially absorbed; some of the hydrogen gas is excreted in breath. When carbohydrate is malabsorbed beyond the capacity of bacterial fermentation, the result is acid stools (pH <6) and fecal carbohydrate loss (ie, stools positive for reducing substances, such as glucose).

Disorders of carbohydrate digestion or absorption may or may not be associated with failure to thrive in infancy, depending on the degree of exposure to the offending carbohydrate. Nutritional or growth abnormalities do not result if the diet is nutritionally adequate and contains little or no offending carbohydrate.

## Primary Disorders

Infants with the rare condition of congenital lactase deficiency are symptomatic at birth if a lactose-containing diet (eg, breast milk, formula) is fed. Lactose tolerance appears to increase during childhood for reasons that are not entirely understood. Late-onset lactase deficiency, an autosomal recessive trait, develops between 3 and 5 years of age. It occurs in 5% to 20% of white Caucasian and 70% to 75% of African-American children in North America, in 74% of Hispanic children, and in 55% of Filipino children. Lactase activity appears to be regulated at the level of gene transcription. Although lactose malabsorption also occurs in late-onset deficiency, lactose intolerance, characterized by watery diarrhea, abdominal pain, and cramping, may not be present because symptoms depend in part on the patient's subjective response to gas and pain, the lactose load, the rate of gastric emptying, and in some cases, the residual lactase activity.

In North America, the incidence of sucrase and α-dextrinase deficiency is 0.2%. In this autosomal recessive disorder, patients have a defect in the posttranslational processing of the enzymes; sucrase activity is absent and dextrinase activity is partially or completely absent. Patients usually become symptomatic in infancy when a sucrose-containing diet is introduced. As with congenital lactase deficiency, patients appear to develop tolerance to sucrose with age.

In glucose and galactose malabsorption, an autosomal recessive disease, hydrolysis of carbohydrates proceeds normally, but patients lack the ability to absorb glucose or galactose, carbohydrates that appear to have a common transport mechanism. The defect appears to be a mutation in the sodium glucose cotransporter gene. The disorder is often associated with abnormal renal tubular glucose transport, which results in a decreased threshold for glucose reabsorption. Symptoms occur if the diet contains lactose, sucrose, maltose, or starches.

Isolated fructose malabsorption has been described. Symptoms of abdominal pain, bloating, and diarrhea often follow the malabsorption of fructose-containing foods such as fruits and fruit juices. Symptoms do not develop after the ingestion of sucrose.

## Secondary Disorders

All the entities described must be differentiated from secondary carbohydrate intolerance, which results from damage to the enzyme-containing villous epithelial cells. Lactase usually is the most severely affected enzyme because of its normally low activity and the slow rate of recovery compared with that of the other enzymes. In contrast to sucrose and maltose, the rate-limiting step in lactose absorption is hydrolysis, not absorption. Lactase deficiency in infancy results commonly from enteric virus infections (eg, rotavirus) or small intestinal bacterial pathogens. A clinically significant deficiency may last from 3 to 4 weeks after an episode of acute gastroenteritis. Celiac disease and iron deficiency are other disorders that may be associated with lactase deficiency in older infants and children. If mucosal injury is severe, sucrase, α-dextrinase, and glucoamylase can be affected. In the worst cases, glucose absorption is impaired as a consequence of the reduced surface area available for absorption resulting from blunted and damaged villi.

## Diagnosis and Treatment

An accurate diet history is critical in the diagnosis of carbohydrate intolerance. The diagnosis often can be confirmed by exclusion of the suspected carbohydrate from the diet, followed by rapid abatement of the symptoms (Fig 135-1). Confirmatory evidence of carbohydrate malabsorption includes acid stools (ie, pH <6, measured with nitrazine paper on a fresh stool sample) and, in severe cases, stools positive for reducing substances (ie, glucose, measured with Clinitest tablets or Tes-Tape paper). Although sucrose is not a reducing sugar, bacterial degradation usually hydrolyzes the sugar to glucose and fructose and yields a positive test.

The diagnosis of carbohydrate malabsorption can be confirmed with an oral tolerance test, but this is neither sensitive nor specific. The hydrogen breath test is a more useful diagnostic tool. In the oral tolerance and the breath hydrogen tests, a 2 g load of the carbohydrate per 1 kg of body weight is administered as a 20% solution. A rise in blood glucose of less than 25 mg/dL in response to the oral tolerance test is presumptive evidence of carbohydrate malabsorption, as is a rise in breath hydrogen greater than 10 parts per million over baseline. A definitive diagnosis is achieved when normal (in the primary disorders) or abnormal (in the secondary deficiencies) histology is found and enzyme activity is absent in a small intestinal biopsy specimen obtained perorally.

The treatment of choice for the primary disorders is exclusion of the offending carbohydrate from the diet, presumably for life. However, tolerance generally improves with age, and small amounts of the carbohydrate can be consumed without clinical symptoms. Lactose intolerance can be overcome when the meal is supplemented with the lactase enzyme obtained from the fungus Aspergillus oryzae (Lactrase, Lactaid). Recent evidence suggests that sucrase and α-dextrinase intolerance can be improved by adding fresh bakers' yeast (Saccharomyces cerevisiae) to the meal. Glucose and galactose malabsorption requires the use of fructose as the dietary carbohydrate, because fructose transport by facilitated diffusion is unaffected in this disorder. Fructose malabsorption requires the removal of free fructose from the diet.

## PROTEIN AND AMINO ACIDS

Enterokinase deficiency is a rare disorder in which pancreatic proenzymes are not activated. It must be differentiated from pancreatic insufficiency, cystic fibrosis, and celiac disease in infants who present with diarrhea, failure to thrive, hypoprotei-

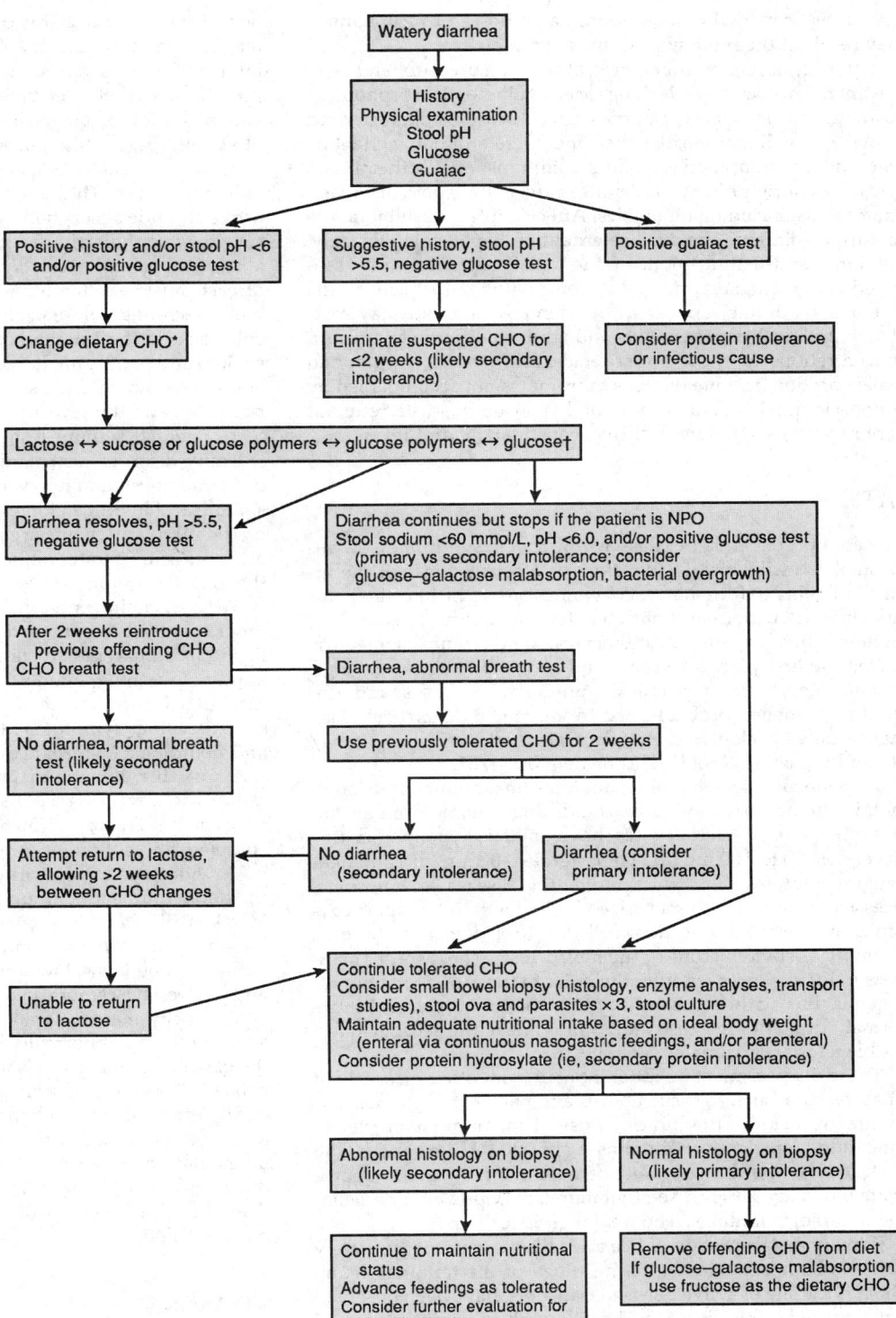

Figure 135-1. Scheme for diagnosing and treating primary and secondary carbohydrate malabsorption. This general outline may have to be individualized. It is important to make only one change at a time in the feeding regimen (eg, carbohydrate concentration, volume of the feeding) and to allow adequate time between changes to assess the results.

nemia, and steatorrhea. Treatment with pancreatic supplements has been successful, and the condition tends to improve as patients mature.

Many autosomal recessive disorders characterized by aminoaciduria have associated defects in intestinal amino acid transport. A lack of sodium-dependent (at least for lysine) transport leads to malabsorption of cystine, lysine, arginine, and ornithine in cystinuria. Infants with Hartnup's disease have decreased uptake of tryptophan, methionine, and to a lesser degree, lysine and glycine. Dipeptides and tripeptides can still be absorbed in these disorders and account for the absence of a nutritional deficiency. The conversion of malabsorbed tryptophan to amines and indoles by colonic bacteria and their subsequent absorption may account for some of the symptoms of the disease, such as dermatitis or mental deterioration. Large doses of nicotinamide may result in the remission of these symptoms.

Other disorders of amino acid absorption are rare, and clear treatment protocols are lacking. Methionine malabsorption (ie, oasthouse urine disease, Smith-Strang disease) is characterized by sweet-smelling urine, diarrhea, mental retardation, and white hair, and it is associated with defects in transport of other amino acids. Lysinuric protein intolerance affects transport of dibasic amino acids, including dipeptides. Affected infants exhibit failure to thrive, diarrhea, mental retardation, hepatosplenomegaly, vomiting, and malnutrition. Lysine malabsorption also is associated with mental retardation. Patients with iminoglycinuria (ie, Joseph's syndrome) appear to be asymptomatic but may malabsorb proline, hydroxyproline, and glycine. Nevertheless, serum concentrations of these amino acids are normal. Tryptophan malabsorption (ie, blue diaper syndrome) is not accompanied by aminoaciduria, but patients develop hypercalcemia with resultant nephrocalcinosis, failure to thrive, constipation, and fever.

## FATS

Abetalipoproteinemia (ie, Bassen-Kornzweig syndrome), an autosomal recessive disease, develops as a consequence of the infant's inability to form normal chylomicrons in the intestinal mucosa. Infants are normal at birth but develop diarrhea, steatorrhea, failure to thrive, anemia, acanthocytosis, and retinitis pigmentosa during the first year. Between 5 and 10 years of age, neurologic findings (eg, ataxia, hyporeflexia, muscular weakness, and athetoid movements, probably due to vitamin E deficiency) characteristically develop. Serum triglyceride levels are below 10 mg/dL, and the cholesterol level is below 50 mg/dL.

Hypobetalipoproteinemia is an autosomal dominant disorder that, in the homozygous form, is indistinguishable from abetalipoproteinemia. Heterozygotes have milder hypolipemia (triglycerides, 50 to 100 mg/dL; cholesterol <100 mg/dL) and neurologic symptoms. Chylomicron retention disease, an autosomal recessive disorder, is characterized by inability to transport chylomicrons from the intestinal cell due to a defect in the final assembly of chylomicrons or their exocytosis. The disorder manifests in infancy with symptoms similar to those of abetalipoproteinemia but without acanthocytosis. Serum triglycerides are normal but do not increase after a fatty meal; the serum cholesterol level is approximately 65 mg/dL.

These diseases must be differentiated from other disorders of fat absorption, such as cystic fibrosis and pancreatic insufficiency. Treatment includes the judicious use of medium-chain triglycerides and large doses of vitamins A (15,000 IU/day) and E (100 IU/kg/day). The dosages must be adjusted to maintain appropriate blood levels. The use of vitamin E may prevent or ameliorate neurologic findings. The treatment is for life.

Primary malabsorption of bile acids results in nonfatty, watery diarrhea. Abnormalities in the histology of the terminal ileum, which is the site of active bile acid transport, have been observed in patients with this disorder. The villous atrophy in the terminal ileum may diminish the number of bile acid receptors. The diarrhea results from bile acid-induced colonic water secretion. Although most patients present with numerous watery stools and weight loss, milder forms have been described. Patients generally respond to treatment with the bile acid-binding agent cholestyramine. The dose must be titrated for the individual patient, but the usual dosage range is 50 to 100 mg/kg/day.

## MINERALS

Congenital magnesium malabsorption is an autosomal recessive disease characterized by a defect in the carrier-mediated absorption of magnesium that is partly overcome by high intraluminal magnesium concentrations. Convulsions and tetany begin in early infancy. Serum magnesium and calcium levels are low, and the phosphorus level is elevated. Treatment entails the continued administration of magnesium (60 mg/kg/day). Administration of vitamin $B_6$ (1 g/day) promotes magnesium absorption.

Congenital chloride-losing diarrhea is associated with maternal polyhydramnios. The symptoms are the consequence of impaired active chloride absorption in the ileum and colon. The infant has severe, watery diarrhea soon after birth and develops metabolic alkalosis, hypochloremia, hyponatremia, and hypokalemia. The disease must be differentiated from bile acid malabsorption, hormone-secreting tumors, and intestinal obstruction. The stool chloride is in the 150 mEq/L range and exceeds the sum of fecal sodium and potassium. If treated adequately with sodium chloride and potassium chloride supplements, infants grow and develop normally, and the severity of the disorder decreases with age.

Congenital sodium-losing diarrhea, another rare autosomal recessive disorder, also manifests with polyhydramnios. Patients develop acidosis and hypokalemia because of a defect in intestinal sodium and hydrogen ion exchange. Stool sodium is in the range of 100 mEq/L. Patients are treated for the disorder with sodium and potassium citrate solutions. Although treated patients thrive, the long-term prognosis is unknown.

Acrodermatitis enteropathica is an autosomal recessive disorder that leads to zinc deficiency due to zinc malabsorption. A ligand in human milk facilitates zinc absorption, and symptoms appear at weaning. Infants develop diarrhea and a red, excoriated rash that begins in the perioral and perianal areas and then spreads. Other symptoms include alopecia, recurrent infections, and neurologic disturbances. Patients usually have low plasma levels of zinc, but the diagnosis is confirmed most easily by a rapid (1 to 2 weeks) response to zinc sulfate (25 mg orally three times daily). Treatment (50 mg/day) is continued indefinitely for complete and continued resolution of the symptoms.

A widespread defect in copper transport that also involves the duodenum and jejunum causes Menkes' disease, a recessive X-linked disorder. It is characterized by broken, stubbly hair, hypopigmentation, osteoporosis, flared metaphyses, pudgy facies with drooping jowls, low serum copper and ceruloplasmin levels, and progressive cerebral degeneration. No treatment is available.

Hemochromatosis is an autosomal recessive disorder characterized by an abnormally increased rate of iron absorption by the gastrointestinal tract. The metabolic defect has not been elucidated. The increased iron absorption and the reduced iron storage by the reticuloendothelial system lead to systemic iron overload with resulting cirrhosis, diabetes, heart failure, and skin pigmentation. Because iron accumulation takes many years, the disease is rare in children. The amount of iron in the diet probably determines the onset of the disease. The treatment of choice is routine phlebotomy.

## VITAMINS

Cobalamin (vitamin $B_{12}$) malabsorption (ie, Imerslund-Graesbeck syndrome) is an autosomal recessive disorder that may be caused by a decrease in the number or function of ileal receptors for cobalamin or by a defect in cobalamin intracellular transport. Patients usually present in the first 2 years of life, but sometimes later, with megaloblastic anemia, poor feeding, ataxia, paresthesia, and low serum levels of cobalamin. This disorder must be differentiated from others of cobalamin metabolism: lack of intrinsic factor, inactive or rapidly degraded intrinsic factor, ineffective splitting of R binders from cobalamin due to pancreatic insufficiency, or binding of cobalamin by intestinal bacteria in bacterial overgrowth syndromes. Except for the associated proteinuria, other symptoms resolve with cobalamin administration (200 to 1000 μg/month, given intramuscularly).

Congenital folate malabsorption occurs almost exclusively in girls and manifests with a megaloblastic anemia and anorexia between 2 and 3 months of age in association with mental impairment. Whether treatment completely prevents the central nervous system disease is unclear, because patients appear to have impaired uptake of folate into cerebrospinal fluid. Treatment with folinic acid (1.5 mg/day given intramuscularly) is probably necessary throughout life.

## Selected Readings

Barr RG, Perman JA, Schoeller DA, et al. Breath tests in pediatric gastrointestinal disorders: new diagnostic opportunities. Pediatrics 1978;62:393.

Bondy PK, Rosenberg LE, eds. Metabolic control and disease. Philadelphia: WB Saunders, 1980.

Cooper BA, Rosenblatt DS. Inherited defects of vitamin $B_{12}$ metabolism. Ann Rev Nutr 1987;7:291.

Danks DM. Inborn errors of trace mineral metabolism. Clin Endocrinol Metab 1985;14:591.

Davis RE. Clinical chemistry of folic acid. Adv Clin Chem 1985;25:233.

Gishan FK, Lee PC, Lebenthal E, et al. Isolated congenital enterokinase deficiency: recent findings and review of the literature. Gastroenterology 1983;85:727.

Holmberg C. Congenital chloride diarrhoea. Clin Gastroenterol 1986;15:583.

Popovic OS, Kostic KM, Milovic VB, et al. Primary bile acid malabsorption. Gastroenterology 1987;92:1851.

Roy CC, Levy E, Green PHR, et al. Malabsorption, hypocholesterolemia, and fat-filled enterocytes with increased intestinal apoprotein B: chylomicron retention disease. Gastroenterology 1987;92:390.

Scriver CR, Beaudet AL, Sly WS, et al, eds. The metabolic basis of inherited disease. New York: McGraw-Hill 1989

*Principles and Practice of Pediatrics, Second Edition.*
edited by Frank A. Oski et al. J. B. Lippincott Company, Philadelphia © 1994.

# CHAPTER 136
# *Appendicitis*

## William J. Pokorny

Appendicitis is the most common illness in childhood for which emergency surgical consultation is sought. In older children, the signs and symptoms are frequently typical and the diagnosis quickly made. However, the classic syndrome may not be evident and the correct diagnosis may be obscure in the preschool-aged population, in whom a delay in diagnosis results in an incidence of rupture at the time of surgery approaching 65%, and in adolescent girls, 40% of whom may have a normal appendix at laparotomy despite a preoperative diagnosis of appendicitis or acute right lower quadrant pain. The presentation of appendicitis varies with age, and the incidence of other illnesses whose presentation may be confused with this diagnosis varies with age. The annual incidence of appendicitis is 4 per 1000 children, and it is diagnosed two to three times per week on the pediatric surgical services of large city or county hospitals and children's hospitals. Appendicitis is most common in adolescents and young adults but is also reported during infancy.

## PATHOGENESIS

Inflammation of the appendix uniformly results from the obstruction of the appendiceal lumen. This occurs most frequently as a result of a fecal concretion and lymphoid hyperplasia of the appendiceal wall. Only fecal concretions that calcify appear on radiographs as fecaliths; they are found in approximately 5% of patients with appendicitis. The recognition of a fecalith on an abdominal radiograph of a child with abdominal pain confirms the diagnosis of appendicitis. A fecalith is associated with a high incidence of perforation of the appendix.

As mucus is secreted into the obstructed appendiceal lumen in the presence of coliform organisms, the appendix becomes distended and secondarily infected. Distention of the hollow viscus results in pain, which is transmitted by the autonomic nerve to thoracic nerve roots 10 and 11 and is interpreted as coming from the periumbilical area. The pain usually is colicky as the appendix contracts against the obstruction, but as the inflammation and distention increase, the pain becomes constant. As the inflammation process progresses, a localized ileus develops in the area of the cecum, and the patient then develops a reflex ileus with associated pylorospasm, loss of appetite, and vomiting. It is an important diagnostic consideration that the vomiting follows the onset of periumbilical pain. Although children with appendicitis rarely eat, preadolescents must be carefully questioned about eating, because they may say they are hungry and ask for food but, when presented with food, do not eat.

As the visceral and parietal peritoneum becomes involved by the inflammatory process, the pain localizes to the right lower quadrant. By this time, the pain is steady, and the patient exhibits peritoneal signs, including tenderness, guarding, and rebound. The inflammatory process begins intraluminally with ulceration of the mucosa and breakdown of normal defense mechanisms with migration of leukocytes and bacteria through the muscular and serosal layers of the appendiceal wall. Frank necrosis and rupture of the appendiceal wall eventually occur. The process then becomes localized as a para-appendiceal abscess, or generalized peritonitis develops. Patients with a para-appendiceal abscess typically continue to have localized pain, usually with a palpable mass discovered in the right lower quadrant or found on rectal examination. In patients with generalized peritonitis, the localized abdominal pain progresses to general peritonitis with generalized peritoneal signs and poor localization.

The progression of appendicitis to necrosis and perforation occurs in only 10% of the patients by 24 hours but in almost 50% by 48 hours. To avoid a high incidence of perforation, it is important that the diagnosis be made and the patient operated on in the first 24 hours.

## DIAGNOSIS

### Course and Symptoms

The diagnosis of appendicitis depends on an understanding of the pathogenesis and progression of the disease. In the first few hours after onset, the child may have only umbilical pain and tenderness poorly localized to the right lower quadrant. Pylorospasm may not have developed, and bowel sounds may be normal. Because there is no ileus, abdominal radiographs may be normal, as may the leukocyte count and temperature. By 12 hours, reflex ileus and pylorospasm typically have developed with loss of appetite, vomiting, and decreased bowel sounds. The inflammatory process typically reaches the peritoneum, and the pain and tenderness become localized to the right lower quadrant. The leukocyte count and temperature are mildly increased. Early in the syndrome, abdominal radiographs typically show scoliosis with curvature of the spine concave to the right due to muscle spasm and a dilated cecum containing an air–fluid level. By 24 hours, the full syndrome has developed in most patients, and 10% have progressed to perforation. By 48 hours after onset, 50% have perforated appendixes. These children appear ill, and they do not like to move or even cry because of the peritoneal irritation. They are most comfortable lying on their sides with hips and knees flexed. When asked to walk, they do so slowly with a shuffling gait and in a bent-over position. By this time, the leukocyte count is above 15,000/mm$^3$, and the temperature is elevated. After perforation occurs, abdominal radiographs show a paucity of bowel gas in the right lower quadrant and the development of generalized ileus with multiple small bowel air–fluid levels.

The location of the appendix in the abdomen explains the variation of symptoms seen with appendicitis. If the appendix is anterior and in contact with the anterior abdominal wall, very early localization to the right lower quadrant occurs. A distended, firm appendix often can be palpated if the child is seen early before abdominal guarding due to pain and intestinal distention due to ileus develop. If the appendix is retrocecal or located in the posterior portion of the abdomen, localization of the pain and tenderness on examination occur late if at all. If the appendix is posterior in the pelvis, the pain may localize only to the lower abdomen, and tenderness to palpation is poorly localized. However, point tenderness can be elicited, and a palpable appendix or mass may be found on rectal examination. The psoas sign, elicited by extension of the hip to stretch the psoas muscle, is positive if the appendix is posterior and in contact with the psoas muscle.

The most confusing symptom attributed to appendicitis is diarrhea. Many instances of delay in obtaining surgical consultation have occurred because the child had "diarrhea" and was considered to have gastroenteritis. Almost 15% of children with appendicitis have diarrhea, but it is a specific form of diarrhea and should not be confused with that seen with gastroenteritis. During the early stages of appendicitis, before the development of ileus, patients may reflexively evacuate the distal colon. Parents may give a child with "stomach pain" laxatives, which can also cause frequent soft or liquid stools. The diarrhea of appendicitis is most common in patients with a low-lying appendix in proximity to the sigmoid colon and rectum. The inflammatory process extends to the muscular wall of the sigmoid colon, and any distention of the sigmoid colon by fluid or gas may cause tenesmus; the child goes to the toilet and passes gas and small amounts of stool. This relieves the symptoms until the sigmoid colon again becomes distended with gas or fluid a few minutes later. In contrast, the child with gastroenteritis typically has voluminous liquid stools. If the child or parent is asked only about the frequency of stools and not about the volume and character, the two conditions may be confused. The child with frequent stools due to sigmoid colon irritation and a pelvic appendix typically has tenderness on rectal examination; the child with gastroenteritis does not.

Processes in the urinary tract, including infection and ureteral stones, can mimic appendicitis, and appendicitis can manifest with signs and symptoms of urinary tract infection and pain. This may occur when the inflamed retrocecal appendix lies over the right ureter, causing partial obstruction and inflammation of the ureter. Dilatation of the right collecting system, right flank and back pain, and leukocytes in the urine are observed. The inflamed appendix may also lie against the bladder and cause inflammation of the bladder wall. As the bladder contracts, the patient experiences pain that may be referred to the groin or penis; the child stops voiding after evacuating only a small volume of urine. The bladder refills, the child again has a sense of urgency, and the cycle repeats. This results in urgency and frequency with only small amounts of urine voided. Inflammation of the bladder wall is associated with pyuria, but the leukocytes are not as numerous as in cystitis. Exquisite anterior tenderness may be elicited on rectal examination, and the condition can be confused with acute prostatitis. However, acute prostatitis is rare in childhood.

Approximately 65% of preschool-aged children have perforated appendixes at surgery. Perforation may result from a delay in diagnosis because the young child does not exhibit the symptom complex typical of appendicitis in older children and adults. Pain localizes poorly in young children, and periumbilical generalized pain and tenderness, rather than right lower quadrant pain, may be reported. Vomiting is a nonspecific symptom in a young child and frequently is associated with gastroenteritis. Because appendicitis is not common in the young child, but vomiting and abdominal pain associated with gastroenteritis are common, appendicitis often is not considered. This may delay diagnosis. In our own experience with preschool-aged children, if the correct diagnosis was considered at initial medical consultation, the perforation rate was 35%. In children diagnosed and treated for some other disease during the first medical consultation, the perforation rate was 83%. This indicates the importance of maintaining a high index of suspicion when treating children with abdominal pain. Any child in whom appendicitis is a possibility should be admitted for observation. Young children with perforation of the appendix more commonly present with generalized peritonitis, and older children and adults commonly have a localized inflammatory process and develop a para-appendiceal abscess.

Although constipation may occur at any age and cause abdominal pain, it is most often confused with appendicitis in children 4 to 10 years of age. A report of a bowel movement on the day of admission does not exclude this diagnosis, because children of this age frequently are unwilling to describe their bowel function. This diagnosis usually can be confirmed on rectal examination, but some children have a normal rectal examination with evidence of fecal accumulation on an abdominal radiograph. The pain associated with constipation usually is colicky but may be dull and steady. The pain tends to vary in intensity to a much greater extent than the pain of appendicitis, which is usually persistent and progressively worsening. On physical examination, the child with constipation may exhibit mild voluntary guarding and tenderness, but often the tenderness is poorly localized to the periumbilical area. Depending on the amount of voluntary guarding, a fecal mass may be palpable. An enema given in the emergency center can relieve symptoms. However, the distention and peristalsis of the colon and cecum associated with an enema in a child with appendicitis increases abdominal pain.

Appendicitis in adolescent girls is sometimes difficult to diagnose because other causes of abdominal pain, including ovarian cyst, menstrual and ovulatory pain, and pelvic inflammatory disease, may mimic appendicitis. Although not proved, it is generally accepted that perforation of the appendix in a young adolescent girl may be associated with scarring of the fimbriae and fallopian tubes, increasing the likelihood of infertility.

The syndromes associated with ovarian cyst typically are of abrupt onset and initially localized to the right or left lower quadrant. Vomiting is uncommon in this group of disorders, and the leukocyte count typically is less than 11,000/mm$^3$. Adolescent girls with right lower quadrant abdominal pain in whom the differential diagnosis includes ovarian pathology should undergo preoperative ultrasound. Ultrasound findings associated with an ovarian source of pain include an ovarian cyst greater than 3 cm in diameter and fluid in the cul-de-sac, suggesting rupture of the ovarian cyst. The surgeon must be cautious, because adolescent girls usually have some cystic changes of the ovary demonstrable with ultrasonography. Patients with menstrual cramps typically have a recurrent history of cramps associated with menstrual flow. Ovulatory pain (ie, mittelschmerz) is of sudden onset and is localized to the right or left lower quadrant. It is associated with copious tenacious mucoid vaginal discharge and mild GI symptoms without an increased leukocyte count or fever. Pain of minor dysmenorrhea or mittelschmerz typically persists for less than 24 to 36 hours. Pelvic inflammatory disease can be excluded by the absence of leukocytes in the vaginal secretions.

The differential diagnosis of appendicitis includes viral syndromes, which usually present with fever and systemic symptoms, including headache and malaise, before the onset of abdominal pain and vomiting. Gastroenteritis may be confused with appendicitis in very young children, but typically presents with voluminous liquid stools and persistent crampy abdominal pain that does not localize. Peritoneal signs usually are absent. Mesenteric adenitis has been associated with abdominal pain. Because many children normally have large mesenteric lymph nodes, large nodes are not evidence of mesenteric adenitis. Right lower lobe pneumonia may be associated with phrenic nerve irritation, which may cause muscular spasm, ileus, and pain referred to the right lower quadrant. Typically, the degree of pain is out of proportion to the amount of abdominal tenderness. In addition, the leukocyte counts in pneumonia typically are higher than in early appendicitis. A subphrenic inflammatory process due to ruptured appendicitis may be associated with pleural effusion and pulmonary consolidation that mimics a primary pulmonary process. Meckel's diverticulitis, although uncommon, can present in a manner identical to appendicitis, although the pain may not localize to the right lower quadrant. Free intraperitoneal air may be seen on upright abdominal radiographs in Meckel's diverticulitis but rarely in appendicitis. Approximately 10% of the patients with Crohn's disease have an acute illness that is misdiagnosed preoperatively and is treated surgically as appendicitis. If this occurs, the otherwise normal appendix should be removed unless the base of the appendix is involved in the inflammatory process. The terminal ileum should be left in place if it is not obstructed.

## Laboratory Findings

The diagnosis of appendicitis depends primarily on the history and physical findings. The leukocyte count, hematocrit, and hemoglobin should be determined and a urinalysis performed before a child with suspected appendicitis is taken to the operating room. The leukocyte count can be normal in early appendicitis, but usually it is increased. If neutropenia is detected, a viral syndrome must be ruled out. Neutropenia that develops late in the course of appendicitis and is associated with generalized peritonitis is a poor prognostic sign. Urinalysis is helpful in excluding urinary tract infection. Serum electrolytes, blood urea nitrogen, and serum creatinine levels should be determined in any patient with persistent vomiting or peritonitis to help assess the general state of hydration and electrolyte balance. Any patient in whom the diagnosis is uncertain should undergo further diagnostic evaluation, including abdominal and chest radiography and abdominal ultrasound examination. In the child with classic signs and symptoms of appendicitis, these studies need not be done.

Abdominal ultrasound examination commonly reveals an enlarged, inflamed appendix, periappendiceal abscess, or phlegmon, but a normal appendix cannot be identified. Many centers rely on ultrasound to diagnose difficult cases. Barium enema examinations may be helpful in a patient with persistent abdominal pain but without a typical history or physical findings of appendicitis and for whom the diagnosis remains in doubt. The appendix may fill in 80% of the normal patients who are examined by barium enema. The radiographic findings in appendicitis include cecal spasm, partial filling of the appendix with a paracecal mass, and a cut-off of the contrast within the appendix. Although the proximal appendix may fill even in the setting of a distal obstruction and appendicitis, an astute radiologist usually can identify the exact location of the appendix, and tenderness to palpation can be elicited at that location.

## TREATMENT

The treatment of appendicitis is appendectomy. Patients with appendicitis and no evidence of metabolic derangement should be taken directly to the operating room. Patients with significant fluid losses due to vomiting or sequestration of intraluminal or intraperitoneal fluid should be given intravenous fluids containing 5% dextrose in 0.5 N saline or lactated Ringer's solution. The fluid losses of persistent vomiting should be replaced with 0.5 N saline. A volume of 20 mL/kg can be infused rapidly and is usually sufficient to reestablish urine output and increase intravascular volume. The calculated fluid deficit should be replaced in the operating room and during the postoperative period. No patient with a significant fluid deficit should be taken to the operating room before adequate urinary output and an adequate intravascular volume have been established. A patient with evidence of a perforated appendix should be given appropriate antibiotics preoperatively to ensure adequate tissue antibiotic concentrations during surgery. Gentamicin, ampicillin, and clindamycin commonly are used, but other combinations of antibiotics that provide adequate coverage for anaerobic and aerobic microorganisms can be used. Peritoneal fluid should be routinely cultured for aerobic and anaerobic microorganisms in patients with gangrenous or perforated appendixes.

We operate on all patients with appendicitis as promptly as possible. Some surgeons recommend nonoperative treatment of a child with a localized para-appendiceal abscess, if the course is one of progressive resolution of the para-appendiceal abscess and improvement of symptoms with antibiotic therapy; the patients undergo surgery 8 to 12 weeks later as an interval appendectomy. In most centers, primary surgical drainage of the abscess with initial appendectomy is preferred. Most patients with simple acute appendicitis can be cared for with intravenous fluids and without a nasogastric tube for approximately 12 to 24 hours, at which time oral intake can be resumed. Most patients can be discharged within 3 days of surgery. Patients with a perforated appendix typically have ileus that lasts 3 to 5 days, requiring continuous nasogastric drainage. They commonly receive a 4- to 7-day course of intravenous antibiotic therapy that resolves the symptoms. Although postoperative intra-abdominal infections and wound infections are rare in patients with acute appendicitis, almost 5% of the patients with ruptured appendixes develop postoperative intra-abdominal sepsis and form an abscess, and 3% to 7% develop wound infections if the wounds are closed primarily. Many surgeons close only the fascia in the case of a perforated appendix, which virtually eliminates the problem of wound infection, but care of the open wound is more difficult for the patient's family. Most patients with ruptured appendixes are discharged from the hospital 5 to 10 days after surgery.

## Selected Readings

Bower RJ, Bell MJ, Ternberg JL. Controversial aspects of appendicitis management in children. Arch Surg 1981;116:885.

David IB, Buck JR, Filler RM. Rational use of antibiotics for perforated appendicitis in childhood. J Pediatr Surg 1982;17:494.

Graham JM, Pokorny WJ, Harberg FJ. Acute appendicitis in preschool age children. Am J Surg 1980;139:247.

Janik JS, Ein SH, Shandling B, et al. Nonsurgical management of appendiceal mass in late presenting children. J Pediatr Surg 1980;15:574.

Janik JS, Firor HV. Pediatric appendicitis: 20-year study of 1640 children at Cook County (Illinois) Hospital. Arch Surg 1979;114:717.

Karp MP, Caldarola VA, Cooney DR, et al. The avoidable excesses in the management of perforated appendicitis in children. J Pediatr Surg 1986;21:506.

King DR, Browne AF, Birken GA, et al. Antibiotic management of complicated appendicitis. J Pediatr Surg 1983;18:945.

Marchildon MB, Dudgeon DL. Perforated appendicitis: current experience in a children's hospital. Ann Surg 1977;185:84.

Rubin SZ, Martin DJ. Ultrasonography in the management of possible appendicitis in childhood. J Pediatr Surg 1990;25:737.

*Principles and Practice of Pediatrics, Second Edition.*
edited by Frank A. Oski et al. J. B. Lippincott Company, Philadelphia © 1994.

CHAPTER 137

# *Ascites*

## William J. Cochran

Ascites is the accumulation of fluid in the peritoneal cavity. Ascites is a manifestation of an underlying disorder, such as cirrhosis, congestive heart failure, nephrotic syndrome, protein-losing enteropathy, or malnutrition associated with hypoalbuminemia. Ascites has been a recognized entity since the time of Hippocrates, who stated, "When the liver is full of fluid and this overflows into the peritoneal cavity so that the belly becomes full of water, death follows." Although the predicted outcome is less bleak today, much controversy remains about the pathogenesis and treatment of ascites.

## PATHOGENESIS

The presumed initiating factor in the development of ascites in cases of congestive heart failure is increased hydrostatic pressure. In patients with the nephrotic syndrome, protein-losing enteropathy, or malnutrition, the associated hypoalbuminemia results in a decreased oncotic pressure. These alterations in Starling forces cause fluid to move from the intravascular space to the extravascular space. When the rate of extravascular fluid production exceeds the ability of the lymphatic system to reabsorb this fluid and transport it back to the vascular system, the fluid accumulates in the peritoneal cavity resulting in ascites.

The exact role of hypoalbuminemia in the development and maintenance of ascites is controversial, because many patients with hypoalbuminemia or analbuminemia do not have ascites. Approximately 50% of patients with serum albumin concentrations less than 2.5 g/dL develop ascites. The pathogenesis of ascites in cirrhosis is less well defined and remains an area of active research.

Two major theories have been proposed to explain the formation of ascites: the underfill theory and the overflow theory. According to the underfill theory, ascitic fluid accumulates in the peritoneal cavity secondary to the alterations in Starling forces. Intrahepatic venous obstruction, caused by hepatic inflammation, scarring, and regenerative nodules, increases hydrostatic pressure in the hepatosplanchnic venous system. Increased hydrostatic pressure, in conjunction with a low oncotic pressure due to decreased hepatic protein synthesis, forces fluid out of the hepa-

tosplanchnic vascular space into the peritoneal cavity. The intravascular volume is decreased, which stimulates the renin-angiotensin-aldosterone system to retain renal sodium to replenish the intravascular volume. Sodium retention increases the hydrostatic pressure in the hepatosplanchnic circulation, which promotes the accumulation of more ascitic fluid, establishing a vicious cycle.

The overflow theory proposes that the primary cause of ascitic fluid accumulations is renal sodium retention and subsequent plasma volume expansion through an unknown mechanism. The sodium retention causes an expansion of the intravascular space, which increases the hydrostatic pressure in the hepatosplanchnic circulation and results in fluid extravasation into the peritoneal cavity. Experimental evidence suggests that sodium retention occurs before the development of ascites.

The integrated theory incorporates aspects from both of the two traditional theories. The integrated theory proposes that peripheral arterial vasodilation decreases the effective blood volume, which initiates sodium and water retention. This increases the total blood volume, increasing the hepatosplanchnic circulation and its hydrostatic pressure, resulting in fluid extravasation. The peripheral vasodilation occurs relatively early in the course of chronic liver disease. It is manifested clinically by a resting tachycardia and a wide pulse pressure found in persons with cirrhosis without ascites. Theoretically, diminished hepatic function results in decreased inactivation of endogenous vasodilators such as glucagon, vasoactive intestinal polypeptide, or substance P. The accumulation of endogenous vasodilators decreases the systemic vascular resistance, which decreases the effective blood volume, leading to the activation of the renin-angiotensin-aldosterone system and the sympathetic nervous system. Activation of the renin-angiotensin-aldosterone system increases renal vascular resistance and promotes the proximal and distal tubular reabsorption of sodium. In addition to increasing renal vascular resistance, activation of the sympathetic nervous system also promotes proximal tubular reabsorption of sodium directly and increases renin secretion.

Although the integrated theory does not account for all the complex cardiovascular and renal changes in patients with cirrhosis and ascites, it is the most commonly accepted explanation. Additional research is needed to elucidate the pathogenesis of ascites in these patients.

## DIFFERENTIAL DIAGNOSIS

The differential diagnosis of ascites is subdivided into eight major categories: portal hypertension, hypoalbuminemia, infectious, chylous, urinary, gastrointestinal, miscellaneous, and pseudoascites (Table 137-1). Portal hypertension, the most common cause of ascites in North America, can have a prehepatic, hepatic, or posthepatic origin. The major cause of prehepatic portal hypertension is portal vein thrombosis or occlusion, which can result in the development of esophageal varices but rarely causes ascites. Hepatic-origin portal hypertension is often secondary to hepatic fibrosis or cirrhosis. These disorders can result from congenital hepatic fibrosis, neonatal hepatitis, biliary atresia, $\alpha_1$-antitrypsin deficiency, cystic fibrosis, chronic active hepatitis, or one of several storage diseases. Although primary and metastatic hepatic tumors may cause portal hypertension and ascites, the incidence is rare. Hepatic cysts, which may result in ascites, commonly occur with polycystic kidney disease. Posthepatic causes of portal hypertension include the Budd-Chiari syndrome (ie, hepatic vein thrombosis), constrictive pericarditis, or congestive heart failure. The latter two possibilities emphasize the importance of a thorough cardiac examination when evaluating a patient with ascites.

Hypoalbuminemia may be associated with ascites. The most

## TABLE 137-1. Categories in the Differential Diagnosis of Ascites

Portal hypertension
  Prehepatic
    Portal vein thrombosis or occlusion
  Hepatic
    Fibrosis
    Cirrhosis
    Tumors
    Cysts
  Posthepatic
    Budd-Chiari syndrome
    Constrictive pericarditis
    Congestive heart failure
Hypoalbuminemia
  Nephrotic syndrome
  Protein-losing enteropathy
  Malnutrition
  Hydrops fetalis
Infectious causes
  Bacterial peritonitis
  Fungal peritonitis
  Tuberculous peritonitis
  Cytomegalovirus
  Toxoplasmosis
  Syphilis
Chylous
  Traumatic
  Lymphatic obstruction
  Lymphatic abnormalities
Urinary causes
  Posterior urethral valves
  Bladder perforation
  Ureteral stenosis
  Urethral stenosis
  Neurogenic bladder
Gastrointestinal causes
  Pancreatic causes
  Intestinal atresia
  Meconium peritonitis
  Bile peritonitis
Miscellaneous causes
  Gynecologic disorders
  Ventriculoperitoneal shunts
  Eosinophilic peritonitis
  Hypothyroidism
Pseudoascites
  Omental cysts
  Mesenteric cysts
  Enteric duplication

common disorder associated with hypoalbuminemia and ascites is the nephrotic syndrome, although protein-losing enteropathy, malnutrition, and hydrops fetalis can also be responsible.

Ascites caused by infectious agents require prompt diagnosis and treatment. The infections may be bacterial, fungal, or secondary to tuberculosis. Congenital cytomegalovirus, toxoplasmosis, or syphilis infections may be associated with significant ascites.

Chylous ascites can be associated with trauma, lymphatic obstruction, or lymphatic abnormalities. Traumatic chylous ascites can result from a surgical procedure, an accidental blunt or penetrating injury, or child abuse. The most common cause of lymphatic obstruction that produces chylous ascites is lymphadenopathy. Neoplasms are a rare cause of chylous ascites in children, although they are the most common cause of chylous ascites in adults. The major lymphatic abnormalities associated with chylous ascites are lymphangiectasia, lymphangiomatosis, and congenital "leaky lymphatics." The latter disorder occurs in infants

younger than 2 months of age who have chylous ascites of unknown cause. The disorder is thought to result from delayed maturation of the lacteals, allowing chyle to leak into the peritoneal cavity.

Urinary ascites is responsible for approximately 50% of the neonatal cases. Posterior urethral valves cause approximately 60% of cases, and bladder perforation is responsible for 20%. Less common causes of urinary ascites are ureteral stenosis, urethral stenosis, and neurogenic bladder.

Gastrointestinal disorders are an uncommon cause of ascites. Pancreatic ascites can be associated with pancreatitis or pancreatic pseudocysts. Rarely, neonatal ascites has a pancreatic origin. Other potential gastrointestinal causes of neonatal ascites are intestinal atresia, meconium peritonitis, and bile peritonitis.

Ascites rarely result from gynecologic disorders, such as ovarian cysts or pelvic inflammatory disease. Ventriculoperitoneal shunts are infrequently associated with ascites. Eosinophilic peritonitis is a rare cause of ascites in children but is readily diagnosed from a markedly elevated eosinophil count in the ascitic fluid. Hypothyroidism may be associated with ascites, which resolves with thyroid replacement therapy.

Disorders that can mimic ascites or pseudoascites include omental cysts, mesenteric cysts, and enteric duplication. Failure to differentiate pseudoascites from true ascites before performing a paracentesis may be detrimental to the patient.

## Physical Examination

The clinical hallmark of ascites is abdominal distention (Fig 137-1). Other potential physical findings of ascites include bulging flanks, protrusion of the umbilicus, and scrotal swelling. Patients with portal hypertension may have a prominent abdominal venous pattern (Fig 137-2).

When there is massive ascites (see Fig 137-1), the patient's condition is obvious. In less dramatic presentations, three physical signs can help detect ascites: flank dullness, shifting dullness, and fluid wave. Flank dullness is verified with the patient in the supine position. In patients with ascites, the gas-filled loops of bowel float to the center of the abdomen on top of the ascitic fluid. When the physician percusses the abdomen, it is tympanitic at the umbilicus and dull below the level of fluid into the flanks. Shifting dullness can be assessed by percussing the abdomen while the patient is in the supine position and then in the right and left lateral decubitus positions. Ascites is suggested if the point of dullness shifts with the changes in position. A fluid wave is elicited by having the patient place the lateral aspect of his or her hands longitudinally on the abdomen. The examiner taps the lateral abdominal wall lightly while feeling the opposite wall for a fluid wave. Flank dullness and shifting dullness have the greatest sensitivity, and the fluid wave has the greatest specificity.

The puddle sign is a test previously advocated to test for ascites. After being been prone for 5 minutes, the patient rises on his or her hands and knees while the examiner lightly taps the flanks, auscultating the most dependent portion of the abdomen. The test is positive for ascites if a sloshing sound or change in the percussive sound occurs with lateral movement of the stethoscope. This test has a very low sensitivity and need not be done.

The physical examination alone is not sufficiently accurate or sensitive enough to detect ascites. In one study of patients with equivocal ascites, the physical examination alone had an accuracy rate of only 56%.

Patients in whom ascites is secondary to cirrhosis may have physical signs of chronic liver disease, such as large hemorrhoids, peripheral edema, scleral icterus, spider telangiectasia, and splenomegaly. Other aspects of a physical examination that require particular attention in patients with ascites are the cardiac and chest examination. There are several potential cardiac causes

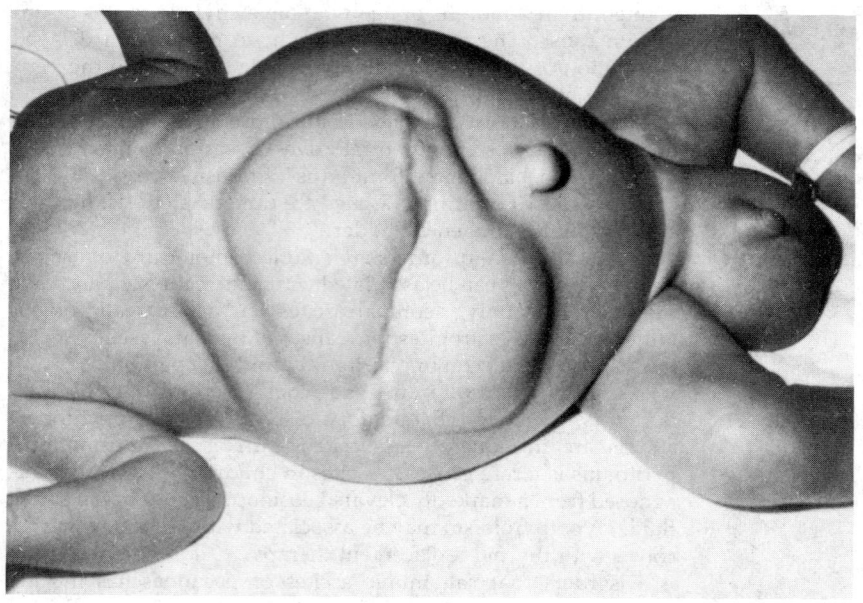

**Figure 137-1.**   A 6-month-old infant with severe neonatal hepatitis. Note the marked abdominal distention, bulging of the flanks, wound and umbilical herniation, and scrotal swelling.

of ascites. Patients with massive ascites may be tachypneic due to compromised intrathoracic volume. Some patients may develop sympathetic pleural effusions.

A physical assessment of nutritional status should be performed. Patients with ascites may be compromised nutritionally because of the underlying disorder that caused the ascites. Patients with massive ascites may experience early satiety, resulting in inadequate intake, or they may have malabsorption secondary to an edematous intestinal tract; both of these conditions can adversely affect their nutritional status. Patients with cirrhosis also may develop deficiencies of fat-soluble vitamins or essential fatty acids, nutritional signs for which the physician must be alert.

## Radiologic Evaluation

Because physical examination is not sensitive enough for detecting submassive ascites, other means are required. Plain radiographs

of the abdomen may be helpful. The classic radiographic findings of ascites include separation of and floating bowel loops; abdominal haziness; indistinct psoas muscle shadows; and increased pelvic density in the upright position. These nonspecific signs are not sufficiently sensitive to detect ascites. More reliable signs include an increased distance (>2 mm) between the properitoneal fat stripe and the right colon (ie, McCort or flank stripe sign), a radiolucent shadow between the lateral wall of the liver and the abdominal wall (ie, Hellmen sign), radiodensity superior and lateral to the bladder (ie, dog's ear sign), and obliteration of the lower lateral hepatic angle. Of these four signs, the flank stripe sign and obliteration of the lower hepatic angle are the most sensitive and reliable indicators of ascites in 55% and 85% of patients, respectively.

Ultrasound, unlike plain radiography, is sensitive and specific for ascites. Ultrasound can demonstrate as little as 150 mL of fluid in vivo. Ultrasound can differentiate free from loculated fluid or detect causes of pseudoascites such as an omental cyst.

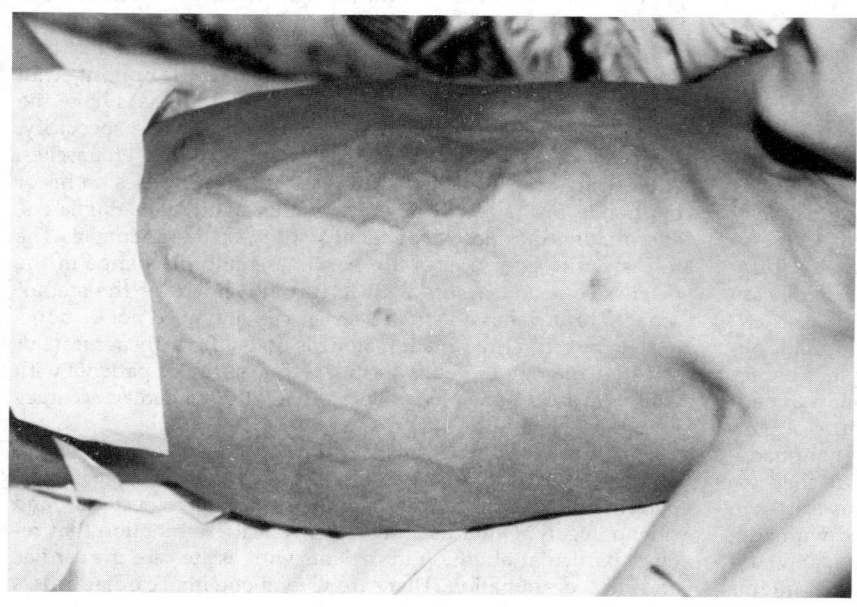

**Figure 137-2.**   An 11-year-old child with portal vein obstruction. Note the prominent abdominal vasculature.

Abdominal ultrasound scans should be obtained during the initial evaluation of every patient with ascites before paracentesis. This helps to differentiate true ascites from pseudoascites, for which paracentesis may be detrimental. Ultrasound is the diagnostic procedure of choice because of its sensitivity, specificity, and noninvasive nature.

Computed tomography is extremely sensitive in the detection of ascites, but it should be performed only in special circumstances, because of the expense and exposure to radiation.

## Analysis of Ascitic Fluid

Ascitic fluid for diagnostic evaluation is obtained by abdominal paracentesis. Paracentesis is indicated in patients who present with new onset of ascites after performing an abdominal ultrasound, in those with suspected peritonitis, in patients with cirrhosis and ascites who deteriorate suddenly, and possibly in the assessment of patients with blunt abdominal trauma. Paracentesis also can be used therapeutically in certain situations.

Paracentesis is performed with the patient in a supine position. The preferred sites of needle insertion are the avascular linea alba midway between the umbilicus and the pubic symphysis or either lower quadrant lateral to the abdominal rectus muscle. To minimize leakage, the latter site may be preferable in patients with tense ascites. The needle should not be placed through a scar because of the increased possibility of bowel perforation. The patient should void or be catheterized before paracentesis to avoid puncture of a distended bladder. Care should be taken to avoid any distended abdominal vessels. After the site is prepared aseptically and local anesthesia is administered, a 23-gauge needle is inserted at an angle until ascitic fluid is obtained. Insertion of the needle in a Z-track fashion minimizes fluid leakage. Approximately 20 to 50 mL of fluid should be removed for diagnostic evaluation.

Paracentesis is a safe procedure with a complication rate of 1% to 3%. Potential complications include persistent leakage, bladder or intestinal perforation, scrotal swelling, pneumoperitoneum and bleeding. Paracentesis is not contraindicated for patients with coagulopathies. It has been estimated that the risk of bleeding, which would require a transfusion, from paracentesis is less than the risk of acquiring hepatitis from a transfusion of fresh-frozen plasma, which does not need to be given to a patient with a coagulopathy before paracentesis.

Various tests can be performed to classify the ascitic fluid further and determine its cause. Traditionally, peritoneal fluid had been separated into transudative and exudative categories. Most often, ascitic fluid is a transudate and is associated with an increased hydrostatic pressure in the portal system or with decreased serum oncotic pressure. Typically, transudative ascitic fluid is clear or straw colored, with total protein concentrations less than 2.5 to 3.0 g/dL or less than one half the plasma total protein concentration. The concentrations of electrolytes, urea, creatinine, glucose, triglycerides, cholesterol, and hydrogen ions are almost identical to plasma levels. Trace elements tend to be present in lower concentrations than in plasma. There may be an increased level of fibrin split products in ascitic fluid relative to plasma. The leukocyte count is less than 250 to 500 cells/mm$^3$; less than one third of the cells are neutrophils. Gram stain and cultures reveal no organisms.

Exudative ascitic fluid is secondary to inflammation of the peritoneum or abdominal viscera (ie, peritonitis, pancreatitis) or caused by leakage of lymph or chyle into the peritoneal cavity. Exudative peritoneal fluid is usually turbid or cloudy. Characteristically, the protein content is elevated, with the total protein concentration typically above 3 g/dL. The protein content may be less in patients with hypoproteinemia. The ratio of ascitic protein to plasma protein can be determined in these patients and

tends to be greater than 0.5 with exudative ascites. Lactate dehydrogenase (LDH) is elevated relative to plasma; the ratio of ascitic fluid LDH to plasma LDH is greater than 0.6. An elevated leukocyte count is common in patients with peritonitis; the count is greater than 500 leukocytes/mm$^3$, and more than 50% of the cells are neutrophils (ie, absolute neutrophil count of >250/mm$^3$). Initial studies found that the pH of ascitic fluid from a patient with peritonitis tended to be low, less than 7.31, and the lactate level elevated. It was proposed that a pH gradient of greater than 0.1 between arterial blood and ascitic fluid indicated peritonitis. However, ascitic fluid pH and lactate levels and their gradients between blood and ascitic fluid are not sensitive predictors of peritonitis, although they are specific. A low ascitic fluid pH is associated with a high mortality rate. The single best predictor of peritonitis is a neutrophil count greater than 250 cells/mm$^3$. The leukocyte count in ascites can increase during diuretic treatment but the neutrophil count does not. Peripheral leukocytosis does not affect the leukocyte or neutrophil count of ascites.

Classification of ascites into transudative and exudative categories based on total protein and LDH levels is suboptimal. Many patients with cirrhosis and ascites have elevated protein concentrations in their ascitic fluid. The protein concentration can be increased in the ascitic fluid by diuretic therapy. It has been proposed that the serum–ascites albumin gradient is superior in differentiating transudative and exudative ascites. If the serum–ascites albumin concentration is greater than 1.1 g/dL, transudative ascites is likely. Exudative ascites typically has a serum–ascites albumin concentration gradient less than 1.1 g/dL. It is important to simultaneously measure the serum and ascites albumin concentration. The physician should always obtain a Gram stain and culture of the ascitic fluid when a paracentesis is performed. The sensitivity of ascitic fluid cultures are greatly increased if 10 mL of fluid is placed into aerobic and anaerobic blood culture bottles at the bedside. If tuberculosis is a consideration, the sensitivity is increased if a greater amount of fluid is obtained, centrifuged, and then appropriately cultured.

Chylous fluid usually appears milky. Fat globules, which can be seen with Sudan stain, produce the milky appearance, and the fluid may be clear or yellowish if the patient has not ingested fat for an extended period, in which case lymph ascites may be a more appropriate term. The leukocyte count is higher in chylous ascites than in ascites of other causes, with the exception of infectious peritonitis. The average leukocyte count is 1000 to 5000 cells/mm$^3$, with lymphocytes constituting the majority of cells. The concentration of triglycerides in chylous fluid is much greater than in serum.

Pancreatic ascitic fluid has exudative characteristics, with an elevated protein level and leukocyte count. Pancreatic ascites can develop in cases of acute pancreatitis, chronic pancreatitis, or pancreatic pseudocyst. The gross appearance of pancreatic ascitic fluid is usually turbid, but it may be bloody with hemorrhagic pancreatitis. The hallmark of pancreatic ascites is elevated amylase and lipase levels in the peritoneal fluid, which are greater than those in serum. Infants younger than 4 to 6 months of age are relatively amylase deficient, and in an infant with pancreatic ascites, the amylase level in the ascitic fluid may be low, making it imperative to determine the lipase level.

Urinary ascites is typified by increased creatinine and urea levels in the peritoneal fluid, higher than serum levels. Sodium and chloride levels tend to be less than those in serum, and potassium levels tend to be higher.

Bile ascites is a rare disorder that occurs in neonates secondary to spontaneous perforation of the bile ducts. The ascitic fluid is bile stained, just as in a patient with ascites and cholestasis; unlike the latter condition, bile ascites is associated with levels of total and direct bilirubin, which are greater in the peritoneal fluid than in serum.

Malignant ascites, rare in children, is characterized by elevated protein and LDH levels. The serum–ascites albumin concentration gradient is less than 1.1 g/dL in 93% of these patients. The glucose level may be low, and the fluid may be bloody. Ascitic fluid secondary to the nephrotic syndrome has the characteristics of ascitic fluid associated with cirrhosis. It is straw colored with a total protein concentration less than 2.5 g/dL and an albumin gradient of greater than 1.1 g/dL.

## TREATMENT

Several medical and surgical therapeutic modalities can be used to treat ascites. The initial therapy must be directed at the underlying disorder, after which the ascites may be treated. The mere presence of ascites does not mandate therapy. Therapy should be instituted if secondary complications develop, such as patient discomfort, reduced mobility, or impaired respiratory, cardiovascular, or gastrointestinal function. The treatment of patients should focus on reducing symptoms with a minimum of complications induced by the treatment.

Medical treatment consists primarily of nutritional and diuretic therapies. Bed rest is recommended frequently for adults with ascites, because of the theoretical possibility that an upright position activates the renin-angiotensin-aldosterone and sympathetic nervous systems, which increases tubular reabsorption of sodium. Prolonged bed rest for pediatric patients is not a practical therapeutic modality, and the goal of normalizing the lives of pediatric patients to promote sound psychologic development is poorly served by enforced bed rest.

Salt restriction is the mainstay of nutritional therapy in the treatment of ascites and should be instituted immediately. Sodium retention, whether primary or secondary, is responsible for maintaining ascites. Moderate to marked salt restriction alone can result in significant diuresis in 10% to 20% of patients. Sodium intake should be restricted to 1 to 2 mEq/kg/day, even if diuretics are prescribed; sodium restriction may reduce diuretic requirements. Indeed, inadequate sodium restriction is a relatively common cause of diuretic resistant ascites. More severe sodium restriction can result in a large negative sodium balance; ascites is decreased at the expense of growth.

Therapy must be directed at the normalization and maintenance of nutritional status. Patients with massive ascites may have early satiety because of gastric compression, or they may have gastroesophageal reflux, which can limit intake, ultimately producing malnutrition. Patients with ascites and hypoalbuminemia may have an edematous intestinal tract, which causes malabsorption and a deterioration in their nutritional status. Patients with ascites caused by liver disease may malabsorb fat and fat-soluble vitamins and require specific therapy.

Although water intake may have to be restricted in some patients with cirrhosis, water intake need not be a concern for most of those who can excrete the amount of fluid normally consumed. Excessive fluid intake should be discouraged. Fluid restriction of 50% to 70% of maintenance should be instituted if the serum sodium decreases much below 130 mEq/L. Diuretics are frequently used in the management of patients with ascites. Rational use of these agents requires a thorough understanding of the pathophysiology of ascites and knowledge of the diuretics themselves. Spironolactone, the first diuretic to be employed, inhibits sodium reabsorption in the distal and collecting tubules by inhibiting the effect of aldosterone. It is a weak natriuretic agent that increases sodium excretion by only 2%; it does not cause hypokalemia. The initial starting dose is 2 to 3 mg/kg/day administered in divided doses. If there is no significant diuresis after 4 days, the dose should be doubled to a maximum of 400 mg/day. Potential side effects include hyperkalemia, gyneco-

mastia, and metabolic acidosis. The latter complication develops as a result of spironolactone inhibition of renal hydrogen ion secretion.

If sodium restriction and spironolactone do not result in adequate diuresis, furosemide should be added. Furosemide is a potent natriuretic agent that increases sodium excretion by 20% to 25% by inhibiting sodium reabsorption in the ascending limb of the loop of Henle. Furosemide should be used only in conjunction with spironolactone, because without the latter agent, the sodium not absorbed in the loop of Henle would be absorbed in the distal and collecting tubules because of the hyperaldosteronemia of these patients. Furosemide therapy can be started at 1 to 2 mg/kg/day in divided doses. The major complication associated with furosemide is a marked kaluresis, which can cause hypokalemia and metabolic alkalosis. Hypokalemia may result in arrhythmias and growth failure. Hypokalemia may precipitate hepatic encephalopathy, because hypokalemia causes increased renal production of ammonium. Other potential complications of furosemide use include hyponatremia, hypochloremia, and azotemia.

Diuresis should be induced gradually. After diuretic therapy is begun, fluid comes initially from the intravascular space and then is replaced by edema or ascitic fluid. Edema fluid is mobilized more readily than ascitic fluid, which can be mobilized at a maximal rate of 900 mL/day in adults. Patients with ascites and edema can be diuresed aggressively as long as edema is present. Patients without edema probably should not be diuresed more than 300 to 500 mL/day. Aggressive diuresis should be avoided in patients with decreased renal function because of the possible development of hypovolemia, further reduction in renal function, and development of the hepatorenal syndrome. All patients who receive diuretic therapy should be monitored closely for electrolyte, urea, and creatinine levels.

Albumin can be infused intravenously in conjunction with furosemide to achieve a more rapid diuresis in patients who are acutely symptomatic. Albumin is administered in a dose of 0.5 to 1 g/kg over 1 to 2 hours, and 1 mg of furosemide per 1 kg is given intravenously halfway through the infusion. Because albumin enters the peritoneal fluid, the effect is transient. This therapy is expensive, may result in increased portal pressure, and may cause variceal bleeding. Autogenous ascitic infusion has been done with variable success and has limited applicability.

Nonsteroidal anti-inflammatory agents should be used with caution in patients with cirrhosis and ascites. These agents inhibit renal prostaglandin synthesis, which causes a marked reduction in renal blood flow, glomerular filtration rate, and free water clearance. These agents also reduce the natriuretic activity of furosemide.

Many patients do not respond to nutritional and diuretic therapy and are referred to as having diuretic resistant ascites; they physician must consider surgical therapy for this group. Surgical therapy consists of paracentesis or insertion of a peritoneovenous shunt. Until recently, the removal of a large amount of ascitic fluid was strongly discouraged because of potential electrolyte abnormalities, renal impairment, and hypovolemia. However, large-volume paracentesis can be performed safely and without adversely affecting hemodynamic or renal functions if it is done in conjunction with intravenous administration of albumin; 8 g/L of ascitic fluid are removed over 1 to 2 hours. The mobilization of ascitic fluid by therapeutic paracentesis with albumin infusion is more effective and safer than conventional diuretic therapy and is considered the treatment of choice by many persons for the management of tense ascites. Chronic paracentesis without albumin infusion is associated with loss of a large amount of protein, which can further reduce serum protein levels and adversely affect the patient's nutritional status.

Two peritoneovenous shunts are used: the LeVeen and Denver

shunts. The LeVeen shunt, which has been the shunt of choice, consists of a perforated tube connected to another tube with a one-way, pressure-sensitive valve. The perforated portion is placed in the abdominal cavity; the other end is tunneled subcutaneously over the chest and inserted into the superior vena cava. When abdominal pressure exceeds superior vena cava pressure, ascitic fluid is drawn into the circulatory system. The Denver shunt is similar except that it has a bulb that can be pumped to transfer ascitic fluid to the circulatory system. Although experience with these shunts in children has been limited, the results have been successful.

Both types of shunts are associated with a high rate of complications. Patients with peritoneovenous shunts may develop infections, most commonly *Staphylococcus*, which cannot be eradicated from the shunt, requiring the shunt to be removed. The incidence of bacterial infections can be decreased by giving prophylactic antibiotics before procedures. Intravascular coagulation occurs in approximately 25% of persons with shunts, probably because of the large amount of fibrin split products and other clotting factors in the ascitic fluid transported to the vascular system. This high incidence of intravascular coagulation can be decreased by removing all of the ascites at the time of shunt surgery. The postoperative use of aspirin decreases the incidence of this significant complication. The shunts also frequently become occluded: 40% at 3 months and 80% at 2 years. Other potential complications include pulmonary embolism, congestive heart failure, bleeding varices, and small bowel obstruction. The high incidence of complications and occlusion limit the usefulness of the shunts.

# COMPLICATIONS

Complications associated with ascites can be secondary to the presence of ascites itself or to the therapeutic modalities used to treat the ascites. Massive ascites can impair respiratory function by pushing up the diaphragm, decreasing intrathoracic volume, or by the presence of pleural effusions. Ascites can increase intraabdominal pressure, resulting in gastroesophageal reflux or early satiety. Massive ascites can cause patient discomfort and reduce mobility. The multiple complications of diuretic therapy, paracentesis, and peritoneovenous shunt were discussed in the previous section.

Spontaneous bacterial peritonitis (SBP) is a complication that occurs when the ascitic fluid becomes infected (ie, peritonitis) in the absence of a local source of infection such as a perforation. The incidence of SBP is approximately 15%, but it occurs most commonly in patients with cirrhosis and ascites and occurs much less frequently when the ascites is caused by the nephrotic syndrome or congestive heart failure. The reticuloendothelial system phagocytic activity is decreased in cirrhosis, accounting for the increased incidence of SBP. The ascitic fluid of these persons has lower total protein and complement levels, which predispose them to developing SBP. Aerobic gram-negative organisms are most commonly recovered and are responsible for approximately

72% of cases. *Escherichia coli* is the most common aerobic gram-negative organism, followed by *Klebsiella*. Aerobic gram-positive organisms are detected in 29% of patients, with *Streptococcus* and enterococcal species accounting for most of these infections. Anaerobes are responsible for fewer than 8% of SBP cases. If multiple organisms are recovered from the ascitic fluid, a secondary cause for the infection should be sought.

Patients with SBP most commonly present with fever, abdominal pain, and no other source of infection. They may also present with hypotension, diarrhea, portosystemic encephalopathy, or unexplained deterioration despite previously stable cirrhosis. Ten percent of patients with SBP are totally asymptomatic at the time of presentation. The key to making the correct diagnosis is to be alert to the possibility and perform paracentesis if the patient has any symptoms compatible with SBP.

Therapy should be instituted for any patient if the neutrophil count of the ascitic fluid is greater than 500 cells/mm$^3$ or if the clinical condition is compatible with SBP and the neutrophil count is greater than 250 cells/mm$^3$. Treatment should not wait until cultures are positive, because patients with SBP deteriorate rapidly if appropriate treatment is not instituted promptly. Ampicillin and an aminoglycoside provide good coverage, but it may not be advisable to give a patient with cirrhosis and diminished renal function a nephrotoxic drug. Cefotaxime is considered the drug of choice for presumed SBP. Therapy should be continued for 10 to 14 days. Blood and urine cultures should be obtained before starting therapy, because 50% and 40%, respectively, are positive.

SBP is associated with a mortality rate of 25% to 50%. There is a high recurrence rate of SBP in those who survive the initial episode, with the probability of recurrence of 70% within 1 year. Because of the high mortality rate and frequent recurrence of SBP, patients with cirrhosis who recover from the initial episode of SBP should be considered for liver transplantation after the infection has resolved.

## Selected Readings

Arroyo V, Gines P, Planas R. Treatment of ascites in cirrhosis: diuretic, peritoneovenous shunt, and large-volume paracentesis. Gastroenterol Clin North Am 1992;21:237.

Athow AC, Wilkinson ML, Saunders AJ, et al. Pancreatic ascites presenting in infancy, with review of the literature. Dig Dis Sci 1991; 36:245.

Bundrick TJ, Cho SR, Brewer WH, et al. Ascites: Comparison of plain film radiographs with ultrasound. Radiology 1984; 152:503.

Churchill RJ. CT of intra-abdominal fluid collections. Radiol Clin North Am 1989;27: 653.

Cochran WJ, Klish WJ, Brown MR, et al. Chylous ascites in infants and children: a case report and literature review. J Pediatr Gastroenterol Nutr 1985;4:668.

Dudley FJ. Pathophysiology of ascites formation. Gastroenterol Clin North Am 1992;21:215.

Fiedorek SC, Casteel HB, Reddy G, et al. The etiology and clinical significance of pseudoascites. J Gen Intern Med 1991;6:77.

Garcia-Tsao G. Spontaneous bacterial peritonitis. Gastroenterol Clin North Am 1992;21:257.

Herrera JL. Current medical management of cirrhotic ascites. Am J Med Sci 1991;302: 31.

Machin GA. Diseases causing fetal and neonatal ascites. Pediatr Pathol 1985;4:195.

Moskovitz M. The peritoneovenous shunt: expectations and reality. Am J Gastroenterol 1990;85:917.

Williams JW, Simel DL. Does this patient have ascites? How to divine fluid in the abdomen. JAMA 1992;267:2645.

*Principles and Practice of Pediatrics, Second Edition.*
edited by Frank A. Oski et al. J. B. Lippincott Company, Philadelphia © 1994.

# CHAPTER 138
# *Pancreatitis*

## Steven L. Werlin

## ACUTE PANCREATITIS

Acute pancreatitis is the second-most common pancreatic disorder in children after cystic fibrosis. Blunt abdominal trauma and viral infections, especially mumps, account for most cases. Other causes are much less common (Table 138-1). Child abuse is a major cause of traumatic pancreatitis in young children. More recently defined causes of pancreatitis include refeeding after starvation, Kawasaki disease, and Reye's syndrome. Improved techniques have enabled increased the recognition of congenital abnormalities associated with pancreatitis.

**TABLE 138-1. Causes of Acute Pancreatitis in Children**

| | |
|---|---|
| Drugs and toxins | Complication of endoscopic |
|   Alcohol |   retrograde |
|   Azathioprine |   cholangiopancreatography |
|   L-Asparaginase |   Pancreas divisum |
|   Corticosteroids |   Pancreatic ductal abnormalities |
|   Estrogen |   Pancreatic pseudocyst |
|   Furosemide |   Postoperative |
|   6-Mercaptopurine |   Tumor |
|   Methyldopa | Systemic disease |
|   Pentamidine |   Bone marrow transplantation |
|   Scorpion bites |   Cystic fibrosis |
|   Sulfasalazine |   Diabetes |
|   Tetracycline |   Head trauma |
|   Thiazides |   Hemolytic uremic syndrome |
|   Valproic acid |   Hyperlipoproteinemia types |
| Hereditary pancreatitis |   I and IV |
|   Idiopathic causes |   Hyperparathyroidism |
| Infectious causes |   Kawasaki disease |
|   Coxsackievirus B |   Malnutrition |
|   Epstein-Barr virus |   Periarteritis nodosa |
|   Hepatitis A virus |   Peptic ulcer |
|   Influenza A virus |   Refeeding after malnutrition |
|   Measles |   Systemic lupus erythematosus |
|   Mumps | Traumatic causes |
|   *Mycoplasma* |   Blunt injury |
|   Rubella |   Child abuse |
|   Reye's syndrome |   Scoliosis surgery |
| Obstructive |   Surgical trauma |
|   Ampullary disease | |
|   Ascariasis | |
|   Biliary tract malformations | |
|   Cholelithiasis and | |
|     choledocholithiasis | |
|   Duplication cyst | |

The sequence of events leading to pancreatitis has not been adequately defined. Many investigators think that activation of proteolytic pancreatic proenzymes after co-localization with lysosomal hydrolases within the acinar cell leads to autodigestion and further activation and release of active proteases. Lecithin is activated by phospholipase $A_2$ into the toxic lysolecithin. Prophospholipase is unstable and can be activated by minute quantities of trypsin. The healthy pancreas is protected by three factors: pancreatic proteases are synthesized as inactive proenzymes; digestive enzymes are segregated into secretory granules; and the presence of protease inhibitors.

The histopathologic findings of acute pancreatitis are related to the release of activated proteolytic and lipolytic enzymes. Interstitial edema appears early. As the episode of pancreatitis progresses, localized and confluent necrosis, blood vessel disruption leading to hemorrhage, and an inflammatory response in the peritoneum may develop.

The definition of acute pancreatitis and its differentiation from chronic pancreatitis have been subjects of much dispute. The most widely accepted definition holds that acute pancreatitis is an isolated episode with complete morphologic and histologic resolution. Acute pancreatitis may recur, but unless structural damage occurs, it rarely becomes chronic.

### Clinical Manifestations

The child with acute pancreatitis has continuous midepigastric and periumbilical abdominal pain, often radiating to the back, with vomiting and, frequently, fever. He appears acutely ill and is restless and uncomfortable. He may lie on his side. The pain increases in severity for 24 to 48 hours. During this interval, vomiting may increase, and the patient may require hospitalization for fluid and electrolyte therapy. The acute case is usually self-limited, and the prognosis is excellent.

In more severe cases, jaundice, ascites, and pleural effusions may occur. Acute hemorrhagic pancreatitis, the most severe form of acute pancreatitis, is rare in children. In this life-threatening condition, the child is severely ill with intractable nausea, vomiting, and abdominal pain. The pancreas may become necrotic and transformed into an infected, inflammatory, hemorrhagic mass or phlegmon. The mortality rate from shock, renal failure, infection, massive gastrointestinal bleeding, and other complications approaches 50%. Several classification systems have been devised to predict the outcome of pancreatitis, but none is relevant for pediatric patients.

### Laboratory Findings

Because no test is accepted as a reference standard for the diagnosis of pancreatitis, many tests have been recommended. The most widely used tests are determinations of serum amylase and lipase activities. The serum amylase level is typically elevated for 4 to 5 days, and the lipase is elevated longer. False-positive and false-negative results occur. Many nonpancreatic conditions have been associated with hyperamylasemia. False-positive results may occur in testing patients with diabetic ketoacidosis, renal failure, burns, and an elevation of salivary amylase, as occurs in mumps. Fractionation of serum amylase into the salivary and pancreatic components can be readily done in most clinical laboratories. We prefer to determine the serum lipase, which may be more specific than amylase for acute pancreatitis. Its use in the past was limited by technical difficulties that have been overcome.

The levels of another serum enzyme, immunoreactive cationic trypsin (IRT), increase in acute pancreatitis and decrease in pancreatic insufficiency. Experience with this technique in children is still limited. Newer tests, such as those for serum pancreatic elastase 1 and phospholipase $A_2$, are being studied.

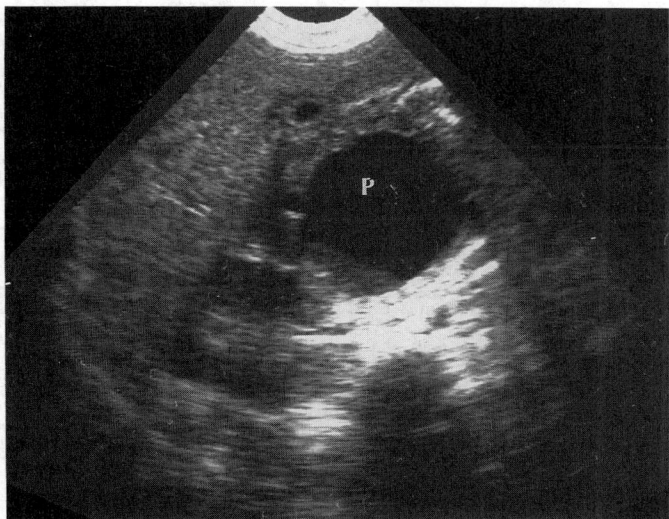

**Figure 138-1.** Pancreatic pseudocyst (*P*). This 5-cm pseudocyst developed in a 16-year-old boy 2 weeks after recovery from an episode of acute pancreatitis. (Courtesy of John Sty, M.D., Children's Hospital of Wisconsin, Milwaukee, WI.)

Commonly found laboratory abnormalities include leukocytosis, hyperglycemia, glucosuria, hypocalcemia, and hyperbilirubinemia. Radiologic findings are usually nonspecific. A sentinel loop of small bowel or a segmental ileus may be seen. Ultrasonography and computed tomography (CT) are cornerstones in the diagnosis and management of pancreatitis. These studies may demonstrate diffuse pancreatic enlargement, indeterminate pancreatic masses, pancreatic and extrapancreatic fluid collections, and peripancreatic abscesses, but at least 20% of patients with acute pancreatitis have normal CT examinations.

## Treatment

Treatment of mild and moderate episodes of acute pancreatitis is supportive and expectant. The aims of therapy are to relieve pain and restore homeostasis. Meperidine is given as necessary for pain control. Fluid and electrolyte balance is maintained. Nasogastric suction is useful to control vomiting but does not speed resolution of the underlying pancreatitis. Antibiotics are used only for the treatment of a specific infection. Improvement usually occurs in 2 to 4 days. The patient with acute pancreatitis may be refed after clinical symptoms have resolved and the serum amylase and lipase have returned to near normal. Surgery is rarely required. The treatment of severe acute pancreatitis usually is prolonged and may require total parenteral nutrition and surgical drainage.

## PANCREATIC PSEUDOCYST

Pancreatic pseudocyst formation is an uncommon sequela of pancreatitis. Pseudocysts are delineated by a fibrous wall in the lesser peritoneal sac, which may enlarge or extend in almost any direction, producing a variety of symptoms. A pseudocyst is suggested if an episode of pancreatitis fails to resolve, an abdominal mass develops after an episode of pancreatitis, or pancreatitis relapses shortly after resolution. Clinical features may include pain, nausea, vomiting, and jaundice.

The most useful diagnostic techniques are ultrasound scans (Fig 138-1), CT scanning, and endoscopic retrograde cholangiopancreatography (ERCP). Because of its ease, availability, and low cost, ultrasonography is the test of first choice. Sequential studies of patients with pancreatitis have demonstrated that pancreatic pseudocyst formation is more common than previously thought. Many are completely asymptomatic and resolve spontaneously. Most gastroenterologists recommend that ultrasound scans be routinely be performed 2 weeks after an episode of pancreatitis for evaluation of possible pseudocyst formation.

Pseudocysts smaller than 4 cm usually resolve spontaneously. Until recently, the treatment of nonresolving and large pseudocysts was surgical. Percutaneous drainage of pancreatic pseudocysts with a pig-tailed catheter is an accepted nonoperative treatment. If surgery is required, the pseudocyst must be allowed to mature for 4 to 6 weeks before surgical drainage is performed. A delay is not required before percutaneous drainage.

## CHRONIC PANCREATITIS

The cause of chronic or recurrent pancreatitis in children is usually hereditary, traumatic, or anomalies of the pancreatic or biliary

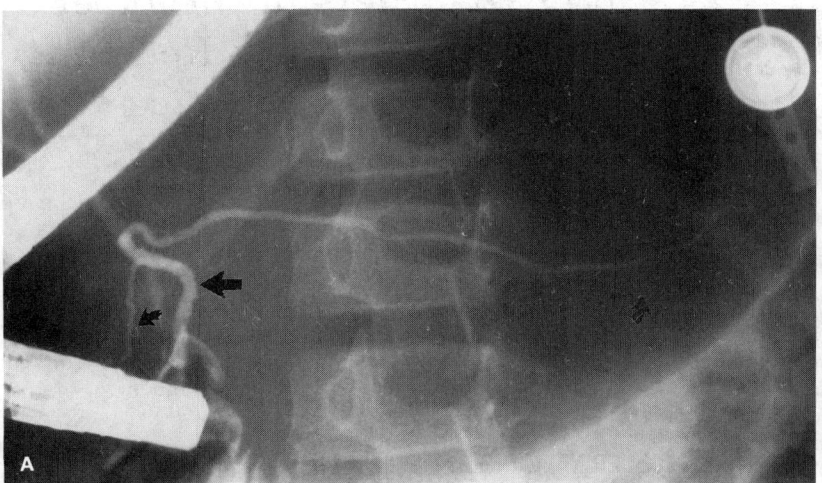
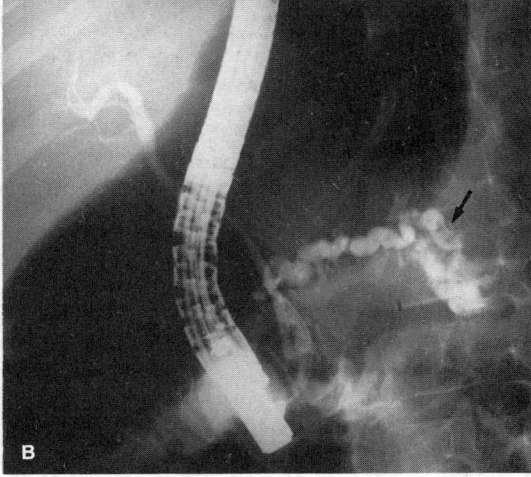

**Figure 138-2.** (**A**) Normal pancreatogram. Notice the excellent visualization of the side branches (*small arrows*) and the main pancreatic duct (*large arrow*). (Courtesy of Anthony Bohorfoush, M.D., Medical College of Wisconsin, Milwaukee, WI.) (**B**) Chronic pancreatitis. Notice the dilatation and tortuosity of the main pancreatic duct. Filling defects represent intraductal stones (*arrow*).

ductal systems. Many kindreds have been described in which the disease is transmitted as an autosomal dominant trait with incomplete penetrance. Symptoms frequently begin in the first decade but are usually mild at onset. Although spontaneous recovery from each attack occurs in 4 to 7 days, episodes become progressively more severe. Hereditary pancreatitis is diagnosed if the disease affects successive generations of a family. Evaluation during symptom-free intervals may be unrewarding until calcifications, pseudocysts, or pancreatic insufficiency develop. Other conditions associated with chronic relapsing pancreatitis are hyperlipoproteinemia (ie, types I and V), hyperparathyroidism, ascariasis, and cystic fibrosis. Most cases of recurrent pancreatitis in childhood are associated with anatomical abnormalities.

Every child who has experienced more than one episode of pancreatitis must be thoroughly evaluated. Serum lipid, calcium, and phosphorus levels are determined. In the appropriate clinical setting, stools are evaluated for *Ascaris*. A sweat test is performed. Plain abdominal films are evaluated for the presence of pancreatic calcifications. Ultrasound or CT scans are performed to detect a pseudocyst. The biliary tract is evaluated for the presence of stones.

Experience with ERCP in children is growing. ERCP, which defines the anatomy of the gland, should be considered in the evaluation of children with idiopathic, nonresolving, or recurrent pancreatitis and before surgery in patients with pseudocysts. In these cases, ERCP may detect unsuspected anatomical defects that are amenable to surgical therapy (Fig 138-2). This technique is useful and safe even in very young children if performed by experienced investigators. Pancreatograms from a normal child and from a child with chronic pancreatitis are shown in Figure 138-2.

## DISORDERS OF THE DUCTS AND SPHINCTER

Although a variety of anatomical defects leading to pancreatitis have been described in case reports, only two, choledochal cysts and pancreas divisum, are commonly seen in practice.

### Choledochal Cysts

A choledochal cyst is a congenital dilatation of the extrahepatic biliary tract and usually causes symptoms of biliary tract obstruction, such as nausea, vomiting, and fever, with the classic triad of pain, jaundice, and an abdominal mass. These features are thought to be caused by an anomalous long common channel of the pancreatic and common bile ducts. The presentation sometimes may be that of pancreatitis. The diagnosis is usually easily made by ultrasound or CT scans.

A choledochocele, an intraduodenal choledochal cyst, frequently can only be diagnosed by ERCP. The symptoms of choledochocele may be those of pancreatitis or biliary tract obstruction. The treatment of all forms of choledochal cyst is surgical resection.

### Pancreas Divisum

In normal embryologic development, the dorsal and ventral pancreatic anlage fuse by the end of the sixth week of gestation. Incomplete fusion may lead to pancreas divisum, a condition in which the dorsal and ventral portions of the pancreas drain into the duodenum independently, and a variety of other anomalies. A large body of literature has developed about whether these anomalies predispose the patient to pancreatitis. Various anomalies of the ductal system exist in 30% to 40% of normal persons, and pancreas divisum is seen in 5% to 15%. Although the controversy is not settled, the consensus opinion is that pancreas

divisum predisposes to pancreatitis only when it is associated with an anomaly, such as stenosis of the accessory sphincter. Several surgical and therapeutic endoscopic procedures have been recommended with only mixed success.

## Selected Readings

Agarwal N, Pitchumoni CS. Simplified prognostic criteria in acute pancreatitis. Pancreas 1986;1:69.

Brown CW, Werlin SL, Geenen JE, Schmalz M. The diagnostic and therapeutic role of endoscopic retrograde cholangiography in children. J Pediatr Gastro Nutr 1993;17:19.

Ghishan FK, Greene HL, Avant G, et al. Chronic relapsing pancreatitis in childhood. J Pediatr 1983;102:514.

Jaffe RB, Arata JA, Matlak ME. Percutaneous drainage of traumatic pancreatic pseudocysts in children. AJR 1989;152:591.

Kattwinkel J, Lapey A, diSant'Agnese PA, et al. Hereditary pancreatitis: three new kindreds and a critical review of the literature. Pediatrics 1973;51:55.

Lankisch PG. Acute and chronic pancreatitis, an update on management. Drugs 1984;28:554.

Lott JA. Inflammatory diseases of the pancreas. Crit Rev Clin Lab Sci 1982;17:201.

Ranson JHC. The role of surgery in the management of acute pancreatitis. Ann Surg 1990;211:382.

Warshaw AL. Dominant dorsal duct syndrome: pancreas divisum redefined. J Pediatr Gastroenterol Nutr 1990;10;281.

Weizman Z, Durie PR. Acute pancreatitis in childhood J Pediatr 1988;113:24.

*Principles and Practice of Pediatrics, Second Edition,*
edited by Frank A. Oski et al. J. B. Lippincott Company, Philadelphia © 1994.

# CHAPTER 139
# *Disorders of the Liver and Biliary System*

# *139.1 Disorders of the Liver and Biliary System Relevant to Clinical Practice*

Donald A. Novak, Frederick J. Suchy,
and William F. Balistreri

Significant changes in hepatic anatomy and physiology occur in the neonate. These rapid maturational alterations are required for the infant to cope with its changing environment.

## ALTERATIONS IN HEPATIC ANATOMY IN EARLY LIFE

Postnatally, the liver grows in proportion to the infant's height, weight, and age; there is, in addition, a change in the proportions of the liver. The liver may account for as much as 10% of the total body volume in the fetus, but this organ constitutes approximately 5% of body weight at birth and only 2% of the adult human.

## Clinical Assessment of Liver Size

The standard clinical indices of liver size are the degree of projection of the liver edge below the costal margin, the span of dullness on percussion, and the length of the vertical axis of the liver, estimated radiographically. Several studies have provided a baseline of age-related values. In 1957, McNicholl's study of 317 healthy infants and children established values for the projection of the liver edge below the costal margin and emphasized that a projection of greater than 3.5 cm in the midclavicular line (MCL) in the newborn indicated hepatic enlargement. The measurement of liver span may be subject to less variability than the degree of projection. Younoszai and Mueller measured liver span (vertical height) by percussing the upper margin and palpating the lower edge in the right MCL in older patients. A linear increase in the span, similar in both sexes, correlated with body weight and age. Lawson and colleagues determined the liver span in the MCL in 350 infants and children by percussion of the upper and lower borders. The mean liver span was found to be curvilinearly related to age (Table 139-1); by extrapolation, the range was estimated to be 1.9 cm at 1 week of age to 7.7 cm (males) and 6.3 cm (females) at 20 years of age. The major factors correlating liver size in children with normal growth patterns were age and sex. The expected span of liver dullness in the MCL in children between 12 and 20 years of age can be obtained by the following equations:

Boys: Span (cm) = (0.032 × weight [lb]) + (0.18 × height [in]) − 7.86
Girls: Span (cm) = (0.027 × weight [lb]) + (0.22 × height [in]) − 10.75

Reiff and Osborn determined in 100 healthy newborns that the mean liver span was 5.9 ± 0.8 cm by percussion; this value, much larger than that cited earlier, suggests that extrapolation of the curve of Lawson and associates may not be accurate for the neonatal age range. There was a poor correlation of span with measurement of liver projection below the costal margin. Reiff and Osborn emphasized the clinical utility of the assessment of liver span.

Liver volume may more accurately reflect liver size, because a change in shape may not necessarily be distributed equally. Liver volume as assessed by ultrasound, a reproducible and noninvasive method, correlated inversely ($r = -0.79$) with age. The relative volume (expressed per unit body weight) in the first year of life (~48 mL/kg) was almost twice the volume at 15 years of age (~25 mL/kg).

## Clinical Assessment of Gallbladder Size

The gallbladder is readily visualized in children, even neonates, with high-frequency real-time ultrasound imaging. Because the gallbladder may be distended in sick infants, often in conjunction with sepsis, it is important to define criteria useful in differentiating a normal gallbladder in a newborn from a gallbladder or biliary tract that is pathologically enlarged or atretic (see Table 139-1). In a study of children between the ages of 1 month and 16 years, ultrasound scans showed a gradual age-related increase in the size of the gallbladder. Wall thickness was never more than 3 mm; the lumen of the common hepatic duct increased with age but was never greater than 4 mm.

## Functional Alterations During Development

Functional deficiencies have been repeatedly observed in normal, healthy newborn infants, and this has led to extensive investigation of the alterations in the quantitative pattern of various enzymes during embryonic development. Despite marked intraspecies differences, several general concepts can be stated.

During late fetal and early postnatal development, the differentiation of tissue function depends on de novo synthesis of enzymes, not on activation of enzymes already present in the embryonic tissue. Greengard documented the quantitative pattern of enzymatic differentiation in early life and observed that the increase in their concentrations (ie, emergence) occurs in clusters that correlate with the changing functional requirements of the developing organism. Substrate and hormonal flow across the placenta and dietary and hormonal input in the postnatal period modulate the development of these enzymatic processes. The lipid composition of various cell and organelle membranes changes rapidly in response to alterations in the composition of dietary lipids. The role of genetic preprogramming (ie, effect of the biologic clock) also must be considered in understanding the ontogeny of enzyme activities.

## Age-Related Differences in Standard Biochemical Assays

There are well-defined age-related changes in the biochemical parameters of hepatic function. For example, serum ceruloplasmin and $\alpha_1$-antitrypsin values appear not to vary significantly with age after the immediate perinatal period. Kattwinkel and colleagues determined that serum levels of aspartate aminotransferase, $\gamma$-glutamyltransferase, 5'-nucleotidase, and total alkaline phosphatase and its bone isoenzymes exhibit significant age dependency in normal children. Throughout early life, cholesterol concentrations increase rapidly. The normal reference values cited in Table 139-1 for the analytes have various origins; the ranges cited are based on the mean ±2 SD. It is important for researchers at each institution to establish a working range using their instrumentation.

### Alkaline Phosphatase

The total activity of alkaline phosphatase in human serum varies considerably with age and to some degree with sex. The largest proportion of these age-dependent differences is caused by an increased isoenzyme originating in bone; these fluctuations are most significant during periods of accelerated bone growth. Values must be interpreted in the context of these known physiological changes. In the newborn, the reference normal values may be as much as four times the adult values; throughout the remainder of childhood, alkaline phosphatase activity may be three times the adult value, with a decline after puberty.

### Ammonia Nitrogen

Except for a transient increase in the ammonia content of peripheral blood in the normal neonate, ammonia nitrogen values during early life are similar to adult values. The "transient hyperammonemia" in early life is multifactorial, possibly because of shunting of blood through the ductus venosus and immaturity of metabolic processes.

### $\alpha$-Fetoprotein

The concentrations of $\alpha$-fetoprotein (AFP), a glycoprotein synthesized by embryonic tissues (eg, liver, yolk sac), are highest in serum during the 10th to 14th weeks of fetal life. Concentrations decrease rapidly, especially in the perinatal period.

| TABLE 139-1. Liver Morphology and Biochemistry by Age | | | | | | | | |
|---|---|---|---|---|---|---|---|---|
| | **Newborn** | | | | | | | |
| | *Birth* | *1–7 Days* | 1 Mo | 2 Mo | 3 Mo | 4 Mo | 5 Mo | 6 Mo |
| **Morphology** | | | | | | | | |
| Liver size | | | | | | | | |
| Weight (g) | FT = 125 | | M = 300 | → | → | → | → | → |
| | | | F = 240 | → | → | → | → | → |
| Distance below | | x̄ = 1.8 | 1.5 | → | → | → | → | 1.8 |
| LCM (cm) | | R = 1–2.5 | | | | | | |
| Span (cm) | | 5.9 ± 0.8 (18) | | | | | | M = 2.4 |
| | | | | | | | | F = 2.8 |
| Gallbladder | | | | | | | | |
| Width (cm) | | | x̄ = 0.9 | → | → | → | → | → |
| | | | R = 0.4–1.6 | → | → | → | → | → |
| Length (cm) | | | x̄ = 2.5 | → | → | → | → | → |
| | | | R = 1.1–5.8 | → | → | → | → | → |
| W:L ratio | | | 0.37 | | | | | |
| **Biochemistry** | | | | | | | | |
| ALT (U/L) | 0–23 | 0–53 | 3–37 | 3–30 | | | | |
| AST (U/L) | 22–38 | 14–70 | | | | | | |
| Albumin (g/dL) | Cord = 3.6–4.4 | | | | | | | |
| | FT = 2.4–4.8 | 2.4–5.5 | | 3.0–4.5 | | | | |
| Alkaline phosphatase (U/L) | Cord = 83–183 | | | | | | | |
| | FT = 62–368 | | ← | 80–270 | → | → | → | → |
| 5'-nucleotidase (U/L) | <10 | | | → | → | → | → | |
| AFP (ng/mL) | P = 134,700 | | | | | | | |
| | FT = 48,406 | 33,100 | 2,650 | 323 | 88 | 74 | 47 | 13 |
| Bile acids (μM) | | | | | | | | |
| Cholylglycine† | Cord = <1.0 | Day 1 = 2.0 | | | | | | |
| | | Day 4 = 9.5 | 5.5 | | 4.2 | 4.0 | 3.5 | 3.5 |
| Total bilirubin (mg/dL) | Cord = up to 2.8 | <48 h = 6 | • Total up to 1.5 | | throughout life after 1 mo of age | | | |
| | P = <24 h = 1–6 | P = 3–5 d = 10–12 | | | | | | |
| | FT = <24 h = 2–6 | FT = 4–6 | • Direct <0.4 | | | | | |
| Cholesterol (mg/dL) | Cord = 47–98 | | | | | | | |
| | FT = 50–167 | 65–175 | ← | ← | 80 | 184 | | |
| γ-Glutamyl-transferase | Cord = 19–270 | 13–198 | 4–120→ | → | → | ← | ← | M 5–65 |
| | | | | | | | | F 5–35 |

Abbreviations: x̄, mean; R, range; P, premature; FT, full-term newborns; M, males; F, females; AFP, α-fetoprotein; ALT, alanine aminotransferase; AST, aspartate aminotransferase.
* Bowers-McComb method (37°C).
† Fasting.
Arrows indicate that information does not differ from that in nearest column.

## γ-Glutamyltransferase

γ-Glutamyltransferase (γ-glutamyl transpeptidase; γ-GTP) is a multifunctional, membrane-bound glycoprotein that serves catalytic and detoxification functions. Because of the difficulty in interpreting alkaline phosphatase values, measurement of γ-GTP may be of benefit in the pediatric population; activity is high at birth and declines rapidly with maturation.

## 5'-Nucleotidase

Serum 5'-nucleotidase activity is usually elevated in hepatobiliary diseases, but unlike serum alkaline phosphatase, its activity is not increased in infancy, childhood, skeletal disorders, or pregnancy.

# CONGENITAL ANOMALIES AND ABERRATIONS OF HEPATIC PHYSIOLOGY IN EARLY LIFE

Hepatic structural and functional abnormalities due to congenital or acquired defects can manifest in the perinatal period. The response of the neonatal liver to injury from a variety of insults may be stereotypic: for example, the formation of giant cells.

## Anomalies

Reductions or increases in the external lobation of the liver are rare. More frequent are abnormalities of the hepatic ducts and gallbladder, such as partial or complete duplication or congenital

| 12 Mo | 2 Y | 3 Y | 4 Y | 5 Y | 6–9 Y | 10 Y | 15 Y | Adult |
|---|---|---|---|---|---|---|---|---|
| → | 400 | 460 | 510 | 555 | 665 | 770 | 1150 | 1630 |
| → | 390 | 450 | 500 | 550 | 685 | 810 | 1180 | 1415 |
| → | 1.1 | 1.0 | 0.6 | 1.0 | 0.9 | 1.0 | 0.9 | |
| 2.8 | 3.5 | 4.0 | 4.4 | 4.8 | 5.1–6.1 | 6.1 | 6.8–7.1 | 7.7 |
| 3.1 | 3.6 | 4.0 | 4.3 | 4.5 | 4.8–5.4 | 5.4 | 5.8–6.0 | 6.3 |
| → | $\bar{x} = 1.7$ | → | → | → | $\bar{x} = 1.8$ | $\bar{x} = 1.9$ | $\bar{x} = 2.0$ | $\bar{x} = 2.5$ |
| → | $R = 1.4–2.3$ | → | → | → | $R = 1.0–2.4$ | $R = 1.2–3.2$ | $R = 1.3–2.8$ | |
| → | $\bar{x} = 4.2$ | → | → | → | $\bar{x} = 5.6$ | $\bar{x} = 5.5$ | $\bar{x} = 6.1$ | $\bar{x} = 9.0$ |
| → | $R = 2.9–5.2$ | → | → | → | $R = 4.4–7.4$ | $R = 3.4–6.5$ | $R = 3.8–8.0$ | |
| | 0.40 | | | | 0.32 | 0.34 | 0.33 | |
| | | | | | | 3–28 | | M = 7–46 |
| | | | | | | | | F = 4–35 |
| 13–64 | | 16–46 | | | 20–45 | 15–40 | 15–30 | M = 8–46 |
| | | | | | | | | F = 7–34 |
| | | | | | | | | F = 3.7–5.3 |
| 3.5–4.8 | | 3.8–5.0 | | 4.0–5.6 | | 3.0–5.5 | 3.5–4.9 | M = 4.2–5.5 |
| → | → | 80–390 | → | → | 115–460 | 60–280 | 30–250 | 30–115 |
| 9 | → | → | → | → | → | → | → | → |
| 1.5 | ← | ← | ← | <1.0 | → | → | → | → |
| → | → | → | → | → | → | → | → | M = 9–69 |
| | | | | | | | | F = 3–33 |

absence of the gallbladder. Riedel's lobe, a tongue-shaped mass of normal liver tissue that projects downward from the right lobe, is a common anatomical variation.

## Hepatomegaly

In the evaluation of unexplained hepatomegaly (Table 139-2), ultrasound can demonstrate hepatic size and consistency. A hyperechogenic (bright) appearance of the hepatic parenchyma is common in children and can be caused by metabolic disease (eg, glycogen storage disease) or a fatty liver (eg, malnutrition, hyperalimentation, steroid therapy). This ultrasound finding in children can guide further evaluation, such as liver biopsy with quantitative and qualitative assays for fat or specific enzyme assays.

## Cholestasis

### Chronic Cholestasis

Infants and children with hepatobiliary dysfunction, regardless of the cause, are at risk for the sequelae of prolonged cholestasis, including retention of endogenous compounds (eg, bilirubin, bile acids) that are usually excreted by the liver and malabsorption of fats and fat-soluble vitamins secondary to diminished intestinal bile acid concentrations. Chronic liver disease with resultant impairment of hepatic function may alter nutrient metabolism.

TABLE 139-2.  Pathophysiology and Differential
Diagnosis of Liver Enlargement

I. Increased number or *size* of cells in the liver
  A. Inflammation (hepatocyte or Kupffer cell enlargement, inflammatory cells)
    1. Viral acute and chronic
    2. Bacterial (sepsis, abscess, cholangitis)
    3. Toxic
  B. Storage disease
    1. Fat
      a. Reye's syndrome
      b. Malnutrition
      c. Obesity
      d. Metabolic liver disease
      e. Lipid infusion (eg, TPN)
      f. Cystic fibrosis
      g. Diabetes mellitus
    2. Glycogen (eg, multiple forms of glycogen storage disease)
    3. Specific lipid storage disease
      a. Gaucher's disease
      b. Neimann-Pick disease
      c. Wolman disease
    4. Miscellaneous
      a. $\alpha_1$-Antitrypsin deficiency
      b. Wilson's disease
      c. Hypervitaminosis A
  C. Infiltration
    1. Primary tumors
      a. Hepatoblastoma
      b. Hepatocellular carcinoma
      c. Hemangioma
      d. Focal nodular hyperplasia
    2. Secondary or metastatic tumors
      a. Lymphoma
      b. Leukemia
      c. Histiocytosis
      d. Neuroblastoma
      e. Wilms' tumor
II. Increased size of *vascular space*
  A. Intrahepatic obstruction to hepatic vein outflow
    1. Veno-occlusive disease
    2. Hepatic vein thrombosis (eg, Budd-Chiari)
    3. Hepatic vein web
  B. Suprahepatic
    1. Congestive heart failure
    2. Pericardial disease
      a. Tamponade
      b. Constrictive pericarditis
III. Increased size of biliary space
  A. Congenital hepatic fibrosis
  B. Caroli's disease
IV. Idiopathic (? benign)

Growth failure may result from aberrations in hormonal balance. Hepatic disease may progress, with the eventual development of hepatic cirrhosis, portal hypertension, and liver failure. Therapy is largely symptomatic, and in most cases, progression of the underlying hepatic disease cannot be halted. General recommendations for therapy are given in Table 139-3.

A patient with chronic cholestasis may develop intense pruritus, occasionally before the first birthday. Xanthomas also may develop. The cause of pruritus remains obscure, but it may be related to an accumulation of abnormal forms of bile acids in serum and tissue. Xanthoma formation may be relates to the elevated serum lipid values found in chronic cholestasis. Therapy for both complications is aimed at more efficient excretion of these endogenous compounds. Cholestyramine resin (8 to 16 g/day) and phenobarbital (3 to 5 mg/kg/day) may be given to stimulate bile excretion. The usefulness of these agents is limited by the extent of residual bile flow, and both drugs have side effects. Cholestyramine is unpalatable, difficult to administer, and may cause constipation and fat-soluble vitamin deficiency. Phenobarbital may cause sedation, paradoxic hyperexcitability, and addiction.

Rifampin in a dose of 10 mg/kg/day (maximum, 300 mg/day) has been evaluated in a few pediatric patients with pruritus and found efficacious, as has partial biliary diversion. Transplantation may be indicated for some children with severe pruritus. Therapy with ultraviolet B light has proved useful in the control of pruritus in adults. Plasma perfusion and therapy with carbamazepine or hydroxyzine have been used in adults, but their usefulness in children must be evaluated.

Nutritional inadequacies are often a problem in the child with chronic cholestasis. Fat malabsorption is common because of diminished intestinal bile acid concentrations. Provision of adequate calories and supplements containing medium-chain triglycerides, which are more readily absorbed, as orally administered formula or through nasogastric drip is essential. Fat-soluble vitamin (eg, A, D, E, K) deficiency is common in children with chronic cholestasis. Vitamin D deficiency may cause rickets; vitamin K deficiency may be responsible for catastrophic hemorrhage; and vitamin E deficiency may be responsible for a progressive neuromuscular syndrome once thought to be an inherent feature of multiple cholestatic diseases. Deficiency (ie, malabsorption) of vitamin E causes a neuropathy characterized by progressive loss of myelinated axons of peripheral nerves and degeneration of spinal cord posterior columns; the neuronal tocopherol content may be low. Clinically, areflexia, cerebellar ataxia, ophthalmoplegia, and peripheral neuropathies are seen. Because these lesions appear to be partly reversible in young children, careful monitoring of fat-soluble vitamin levels is necessary. Vitamin E levels may be falsely elevated because of elevated serum lipid levels, and the ratio of serum vitamin E to total serum lipids (normal ratio, <0.6 mg/g in children <12 years) should be followed. Oral supplementation should be given as necessary, but intramuscular administration has been required in some patients. D-$\alpha$-Tocopheryl polyethylene glycol-1000 succinate is a water-soluble form of vitamin E that is well adsorbed after oral administration and is safe and effective for the prevention and correction of the vitamin E deficiency of chronic cholestasis.

Despite careful attention to caloric intake, mineral balance, and vitamin status, poor hepatic synthetic function may limit growth. At this point, the patient may become a candidate for orthotopic liver transplantation. Survival rates of 70% to 90% are reported for this procedure, which may be curative. The success rates and degree of organ availability increase significantly as the infant attains adequate size (>10 kg), although use of hepatic size reduction techniques have made transplantation more available to smaller children, as may use of living, related donors.

## Total Parenteral Nutrition-Related Cholestasis

Parenteral nutrition is a life-saving form of therapy in the neonate, child, or adult who is unable to receive enteral nutrition. Unfortunately, serious complications are frequent, among which total parenteral nutrition (TPN)-related cholestasis is second in incidence only to catheter-related sepsis.

Cholestasis associated with parenteral nutrition occurs primarily in premature infants, although hepatobiliary lesions have been described in older children and adults. In an early report, the incidence of cholestasis in children receiving TPN was 50% of infants with birth weights below 1000 g and 18% of infants with birth weights of 1000 to 1500 g. Other investigators have confirmed the inverse relation between gestational age and the incidence of TPN-related cholestasis. The onset of cholestasis appears to be related to the duration of infusion, usually occurring after at least 2 weeks of therapy. TPN-related hepatic disease

**TABLE 139-3.    Suggested Medical Management
of the Consequences of Persistent Cholestasis**

| Effect | Management |
|---|---|
| A. Malnutrition due to: | |
| 1. Malabsorption of dietary long-chain triglyceride (LCT) | 1. Replace with dietary formula or supplement containing medium-chain triglyceride (MCT) |
| | a. Adequate protein (vegetable sources) |
| | b. Adequate calories (complex starch) |
| 2. Fat-soluble vitamin deficiency | 2. Supplement/monitor |
| a. Vitamin A (eg, night blindness, thick skin) | a. Replace with 5000–25,000 IU/day as Aquasol A |
| b. Vitamin E (eg, neuromuscular degeneration) | b. Replace with 50–400 IU/kg/day as $\alpha$-tocopherol; |
| c. Vitamin D (eg, metabolic bone disease) | c. Replace with 5000–8000 IU/d of $D_2$ or 3–5 $\mu$g/kg/d of 25-hydroxycholecalciferol |
| d. Vitamin K (eg, hypoprothrombinemia) | d. Replace with 2.5–5.0 mg every day as water-soluble derivative of menadione |
| 3. Micronutrient deficiency | 3. Calcium/phosphate/zinc supplementation |
| 4. Deficiency of water-soluble vitamins | 4. Supplement with twice the recommended daily allowance |
| B. Retention of biliary constituents: | |
| 1. Bile acids and cholesterol (itch/xanthomas) | 1. Remove/chelate: |
| | a. Bile acid binders (cholestyramine, 8–16 g/d) |
| | b. Choleretics (phenobarbital, 3–5 mg/kg/d) |
| | c. Rifampin (10 mg/kg/d) |
| | d. Ursodeoxychocic acid 15 mg/kg/d |
| | e. Potential therapies include: |
| | 1. UV-B light |
| | 2. Carbamazepine |
| | 3. Plasmaperfusion |
| 2. Trace elements, such as copper (eg, hepatotoxicity) | 2. Role of avoidance of food enriched in copper (?); potential role of chelating agents |
| C. Progressive liver disease: | |
| 1. Variceal hemorrhage | 1. Management of variceal bleeding: |
| | a. Acute: |
| | 1. Lavage |
| | 2. Vasopressin |
| | 3. Balloon tamponade |
| | 4. Endoscopic sclerotherapy |
| | b. Chronic |
| | 1. Sclerotherapy |
| | 2. $\beta$ blockade |
| | 3. Surgical (ie, shunt vs variceal ligation) |
| 2. Ascites | 2. Ascites management |
| | a. Sodium restriction (1–2 mEq/kg/d) |
| | b. Spironolactone (2–3 mg/kg/d in divided doses); if diuresis inadequate after 2–4 days, double dose; follow urine and serum electrolyte concentrations |
| | c. Further diuretic therapy (ie, furosemide or thiazides) with albumin |
| 3. End-stage liver disease | 3. Transplantation |

frequently occurs in sick, premature infants, typically those undergoing episodes of sepsis, shock, abdominal surgery, and necrotizing enterocolitis.

TPN-related cholestasis has an insidious onset. Jaundice may be observed but is attributed to "physiological" hyperbilirubinemia. The diagnosis is often entertained first when routine parenteral nutrition-related surveillance laboratory tests reveal elevated serum levels of conjugated bilirubin. Serum bile acids levels are usually elevated; an increase in serum bile acid levels is often the earliest biochemical abnormality associated with TPN-related cholestasis. Later in the disease course, serum aminotransferase and serum alkaline phosphatase levels may become abnormal. Hepatic synthetic function typically remains normal.

The differential diagnosis of TPN-related cholestasis includes the many causes of neonatal cholestasis and is a diagnosis of exclusion. The possibility of transfusion-related hepatitis must, in the proper clinical setting, be entertained, as must the risk of hepatic drug toxicity. The evaluation should concentrate on identifying other potentially treatable causes of cholestasis, including infectious, metabolic, or anatomical disorders that may be detected in as many as 10% of infants evaluated for possible TPN-related liver dysfunction. This exercise is imperative, because alternative therapy may be available.

The hepatic pathology of TPN-related cholestasis is nonspecific. Early changes include hepatocyte and canalicular cholestasis, extramedullary hematopoiesis, giant cell transformation, and pseudoacinar formation. Later changes reflect worsening disease, with inflammatory infiltrates, ductular proliferation, and fibrosis. Although hepatic fibrosis, cirrhosis, and hepatic failure have been documented in patients receiving long-term TPN, milder changes, including ductular proliferation and inflammation, can reverse with discontinuation of TPN and resumption of oral feedings.

The cause of TPN-related cholestasis is unknown. In early life, the infant has a period during which hepatic uptake and presumably excretion of bile acids and other organic anions is diminished. The premature infant may be unusually susceptible to cholestasis. Elevated serum concentrations of the potentially toxic bile acid lithocholate occur during prolonged TPN administration and may potentiate cholestasis. Fasting alone may predispose the infant to cholestasis through lack of hormonal stimulation of bile secretion. Sepsis, common in the infant on TPN, is known to cause cholestasis. Amino acids are often implicated in the cause of TPN-associated cholestasis, and there is indirect evidence that amino acid infusions may influence the development of cholestasis. In rat pups, intraperitoneal injection of the amino acid tryptophan causes an elevation in serum bile acid levels. Certain amino acids have been shown to inhibit bile acid uptake into isolated hepatocytes. The amino acid composition of TPN infusates is capable of altering bile flow rates in animals. Conversely, there is little evidence to suggest that intravenous fat or glucose are associated with cholestasis. Other possible factors in the genesis of TPN-related cholestasis include deficiencies or excesses of various minerals or trace elements and of carnitine.

Management of the patient with TPN-related cholestasis is difficult. Continuation of TPN may result in worsening hepatic disease. Conversely, complete withdrawal of TPN may result in a catabolic state and poor growth. A prudent approach is to attempt slow introduction of enteral feeding, stimulating gastrointestinal (GI) hormone release and bile flow. The protein infusion should be limited to the lowest amount required for growth, and ratios of more than 250 calories per gram of nitrogen should be avoided. Improved solutions (eg, taurine supplementation) or altered infusion schedules (eg, cyclic TPN) may offer promise. The use of minimal enteral feedings (ie, oral administration of approximately 10% of the daily caloric needs) may prevent or ameliorate TPN-related cholestasis.

The prognosis for infants who develop TPN-related cholestasis appears to be generally good, but long-term follow-up studies are not available.

TPN-related cholelithiasis occurs primarily in preterm infants. Patients may be asymptomatic or may present with signs and symptoms of acute cholecystitis, including emesis, rapid rise of serum bilirubin, fever, and sepsis. Diagnosis depends on clinical suspicion and ultrasonography. Factors important in the genesis of TPN-related cholestasis may also play a role in the causation of cholelithiasis; in particular, fasting may be associated with gallbladder stasis. With continued fasting and TPN administra-

tion, biliary sludge, composed of thick bile intermixed with pigment granules, calcium bilirubinate, and cholesterol crystals, may form. Sludge, identifiable by ultrasound, appears to be the precursor of stone formation, and prolonged gallbladder stasis may predispose to stone formation. The administration of furosemide and of TPN solutions may increase calcium secretion into bile, increasing its lithogenicity. Gallbladder sludge resolves spontaneously with the resumption of enteral feedings. Gallstones rarely have been reported to clear with feeding. Cycling of TPN administration does not appear to be helpful.

### Total Parenteral Nutrition-Associated Hepatobiliary Dysfunction in Older Patients

Although hepatic dysfunction with TPN is most often reported in infants, some reports describe the development of cholestasis, associated with bile ductular proliferation, periportal inflammation, and fibrosis, in older patients who have undergone massive intestinal resection, requiring prolonged parenteral nutrition. Less severe abnormalities, including steatosis without cholestasis, have been observed in adults with GI dysfunction requiring TPN. It is unclear whether these cases share a similar pathogenesis with TPN-related cholestasis of infancy.

## METABOLIC DISEASE OF THE LIVER

The liver plays a central role in carbohydrate, lipid, and amino acid synthesis and degradation. It is not surprising that the liver is primarily or secondarily involved in many states of metabolic derangement. For example, the absence of a crucial enzyme may cause a build-up of toxic metabolites; this is found in patients with tyrosinemia. Conversely, sequestration of a synthesized product within the liver may lead to hepatic and systemic damage, as is seen in $\alpha_1$-antitrypsin deficiency.

Hepatic metabolic disease may be suggested by the family history or by the pattern of symptom onset. For example, liver injury after the initiation of fructose ingestion should suggest the diagnosis of fructosemia. Clinical features of liver-based metabolic diseases are nonspecific but include jaundice, hepatosplenomegaly, failure to thrive, dysmorphism, developmental delay, hypotonia, seizures, and progressive neuromuscular dysfunction. Screening laboratory data may reveal hypoglycemia, hyperammonemia, increased transaminase levels, acidosis, and hypoprothrombinemia. The metabolic disease can be confirmed in a variety of ways. Percutaneous hepatic biopsy allows histologic examination and measurement of specific enzyme activities or substrate accumulation. The physician must remain alert to the possibility of metabolic disease.

### Disorders of Amino Acid Metabolism

#### Hereditary Tyrosinemia

Tyrosine is an amino acid important in the synthesis of melanin, thyroid hormones, and catecholamines. Metabolism of tyrosine to fumaric acid and acetoacetic acid proceeds down a pathway with several intermediates. Deficiency or immaturity of any of the enzymes catalyzing these steps may lead to hypertyrosinemia. Transient neonatal tyrosinemia is a self-limiting condition of premature neonates, presumably caused by an immaturity of tyrosine aminotransferase activity. Vitamin C may be effective in enhancing enzyme activity in these patients. Hypertyrosinemia may also occur in any form of severe hepatic injury, typically in concert with high serum methionine levels.

Type 1 hereditary tyrosinemia is an autosomal recessive disorder. The acute form manifests in infancy with symptoms of jaundice, failure to thrive, anorexia, hepatosplenomegaly, ascites, hypoprothrombinemia, clinical bleeding, rickets, and hepatic failure or cirrhosis. The chronic form usually is seen later in life with cirrhosis or hepatocellular carcinoma. Episodic, severe, acute peripheral neuropathy is common in patients surviving infancy and is an important cause of morbidity and mortality.

Laboratory features include diminished hepatic synthetic function, including decreased vitamin K-dependent clotting factors and hypoalbuminemia. Serum aminotransferase levels are mildly to moderately elevated, as is serum bilirubin. Hemolytic anemia or hypoglycemia may occur.

Fanconi's syndrome, with attendant hyperphosphaturia, glycosuria, proteinuria, and aminoaciduria, is often evident. Rickets, presumably secondary to hypophosphatemia, may complicate the picture. Serum tyrosine values are extraordinarily high, as may be serum methionine levels. The phenolic acid by-products of tyrosine metabolism (ie, *p*-hydroxyphenyl lactic, *p*-hydroxyphenyl pyruvic, and *p*-hydroxyphenyl acetic acids) are excreted in the urine, as are succinyl acetone and succinyl acetoacetate.

*Pathogenesis.* The enzymatic defect in type 1 tyrosinemia appears to be at the level of fumaryl acetoacetase. The gene responsible for this activity has been mapped to human chromosome 15. This deficiency causes a build-up of potentially toxic metabolites, including succinyl acetone and succinyl acetoacetate. These intermediates are toxic reactive metabolites that may cause renal and hepatic damage as a result of binding to sulfhydryl groups of proteins.

*Hepatic Pathology.* The hepatic injury in tyrosinemia presumably begins in utero, as illustrated by elevated cord blood α-fetoprotein (AFP) levels with normal serum tyrosine levels. The liver exhibits nodular cirrhosis and extensive fibrosis. Pseudoacinar formation, fatty infiltration, and iron deposition may occur. Hepatocellular carcinoma may be found in the older patients with cirrhosis.

*Therapy.* There is no specific therapy for the acute form of type 1 tyrosinemia, which is typically fatal in the first year of life. Dietary modifications to limit intake of phenylalanine, tyrosine, and methionine appear to improve renal dysfunction, but the effects on the hepatic disease are unclear. Proper diagnosis is important for genetic counseling, and prenatal diagnosis is available. Liver transplantation can correct most of the biochemical abnormalities of hereditary tyrosinemia. Liver transplantation is the treatment of choice for infants with liver failure. In patients surviving with chronic liver disease, the timing of transplantation may be difficult. Because of the great risk of developing hepatocellular carcinoma, liver transplantation is recommended for all tyrosinemic children with cirrhotic nodules demonstrated on computed tomography (CT) or ultrasound examinations. Neurologic crises provide an additional reason to consider early liver transplantation.

## Disorders of Carbohydrate Metabolism

### Galactosemia

Classic galactosemia is a clinical syndrome resulting from deficient galactose-1-phosphate uridyltransferase activity. Affected infants typically present in the neonatal period shortly after the initiation of feedings containing galactose (eg, lactose-containing formulas, breast milk). Symptoms vary, but affected infants may present with vomiting, failure to thrive, diarrhea, poor feeding behavior, abdominal distention, and hypoglycemia. Hepatomegaly and jaundice are common and may be followed by ascites, edema, and aminoaciduria. Cataracts may be present at birth. Later findings may include persistently elevated conjugated bilirubin levels, cirrhosis, and mental retardation. If patients receive a lactose-

free formula only in infancy, they may present later in life with cataract formation, mental retardation, and hepatic disease. There is a strong association between galactosemia and *Escherichia coli* sepsis, which may be a presenting feature of affected infants.

Laboratory features include the presence of reducing substance (ie, galactose) in the urine, suggested by a positive Clinitest in the absence of a positive urine glucose oxidase reaction (Clinistix). Galactosuria may be confirmed by chromatography. These tests may be negative despite the presence of galactosemia if the infant is receiving galactose-free formula or is vomiting. Additional abnormalities include signs of hepatic injury, elevated aminotransferase levels, prolonged prothrombin time, hyperchloremic acidosis, hypoglycemia, albuminuria, and aminoaciduria.

*Pathogenesis.* Classic galactosemia due to deficiency of galactose-1-phosphate uridyltransferase produces an accumulation of galactose-1-phosphate and galactose in various organs with resultant toxicity. Cataracts are caused by the accumulation of galactitol, with resultant alterations of water content and metabolism in the lens. Galactose-1-phosphate may inhibit phosphoglucomutase, preventing glucose release from glycogen. Liver disease may be secondary to the build-up of another metabolite, galactosamine, although this remains uncertain. Deficiency of galactokinase and perhaps of galactose-4-epimerase activity have been reported to cause a syndrome similar to classic galactosemia.

*Pathology.* Tissue damage in galactosemia correlates with ingested galactose. Early findings typically include cholestasis and fatty change. Later changes may include bile ductular proliferation and pseudoacinar formation. Cirrhosis may eventually occur.

*Diagnosis.* The presence of urine-reducing substances in the absence of urine glucose suggests the diagnosis. An assay of galactose-1-phosphate uridyltransferase activity should be performed in all suspected cases, using the erythrocyte uridine diphosphate (UDP) glucose consumption test. The possible variants include total absence of activity; the Duarte variant, consisting of decreased enzyme activity in clinically normal persons; and a third variant, found primarily in the African-American population, in which approximately 10% of residual enzyme activity exists. Many states now routinely perform postnatal screening for galactosemia, and prenatal diagnosis is available for this autosomal recessive disease.

*Therapy.* Therapy for classic galactosemia is total elimination of dietary galactose. In the perinatal period, lactose-containing formula should be replaced with soy formula, which contains small amounts of galactose in unusable form, or with Pregestimil or Nutramigen, also essentially galactose free. Women at risk for the delivery of galactosemic infants should restrict milk intake through pregnancy to reduce in utero toxicity.

*Prognosis.* Galactosemia usually is fatal if untreated. Institution of dietary therapy, although life saving, may not prevent all complications of classic galactosemia, including delayed neurologic development and premature ovarian failure. Dietary therapy is more efficacious in patients with galactokinase deficiency.

### Glycogen Storage Diseases

The glycogen storage diseases are a heterogeneous group of disorders in which there are alterations in glycogen synthesis or degradation. Hepatomegaly is a frequent but not universal finding (Table 139-4).

Type 1 glycogen storage disease (ie, von Gierke's disease) is the most commonly recognized glycogenosis. The presentation usually includes hepatomegaly and profound hypoglycemia, with

### TABLE 139-4. Inborn Errors of Metabolism Involving the Liver

| | Enzyme Deficiency | Clinical Manifestations | Laboratory Features | Management |
|---|---|---|---|---|
| **Carbohydrate Metabolism** | | | | |
| *Disorders of Fructose Metabolism* | | | | |
| Hereditary fructose intolerance | Fructose-1-phosphate aldolase | *Acute*: vomiting, seizures, etc. *Chronic*: jaundice, hepatomegaly, failure to thrive (FTT) | Hypoglycemia, ↓$PO_4$, ↑uric acid, ↑SGOT, renal tubular dysfunction | Fructose- (and sucrose-) free diet |
| F-1,6-DP deficiency | F-1,6-diphosphatase | Hyperventilation, coma, hepatomegaly | Hypoglycemia, ketosis, lactic acidosis | Fructose- (and sucrose-) free diet |
| Essential fructosuria | Fructokinase | Alimentary hyperfructosemia | Fructosuria | None required |
| *Disorders of Galactose Metabolism* | | | | |
| Galactosemia | Galactose-1-phosphate uridyl transferase | Vomiting, jaundice, hepatomegaly, failure to thrive | Hypoglycemia, reducing substances in the urine, abnormal liver function tests, renal tubular dysfunction | Galactose- (and lactose-) free diet |
| Galactokinase deficiency | Galactokinase | Cataracts | Galactosuria | Dietary restriction |
| Epimerase deficiency | UDP-galactose-4-epimerase | None | ↑Gal-1-$PO_4$ | None |
| *Glycogen Storage Disease* | | | | |
| Type I (von Gierke's) (A, B, C) | Glucose-6-phosphatase or translocases | Hepatomegaly, growth failure, bleeding tendency | Hypoglycemia, hyperlipemia, lactic acidosis, ↑uric acid | Nocturnal (nasogastric) feeding; corn starch |
| Type III (Cori/Forbes) | Amylo-1,6-glucosidase (debrancher) | Hepatomegaly, growth failure, muscle weakness (progressive) | Hypoglycemia, hyperlipemia, ↑transaminases (No renal impairment) | Frequent feeding, high protein diet |
| Type IV (Andersen) | α-1,4-glucan 6-glycosyl transferase (brancher) | Vomiting, diarrhea, FTT, hepatosplenomegaly (±cirrhosis) | Abnormal, liver function tests, acidosis | None specific |
| Type IV (Hers) | Hepatic phosphorylase | Hepatomegaly | | |
| **Protein Metabolism** | | | | |
| *Disorders of Tyrosine Metabolism* | | | | |
| Transient (Neonatal) | Tyrosine aminotransferase (TAT) | | | Vitamin C-responsive |
| *Nontransient* | | | | |
| Hereditary tyrosinemia (type I) | Fumaryl acetoacetase | FTT, jaundice, hepatosplenomegaly, rickets | Abnormal liver function tests, acidosis, renal dysfunction | Low phenylalanine, low tyrosine diet, transplantation |
| Tyrosinemia (type II) | | | | |
| Richner-Hanhart | TAT (?) | | | |
| "Medes case" | p-hydroxyphenyl oxidase | | | |
| Atypical forms: | | | | |
| Endo et al | 4-Hydroxyphenyl-pyruvate oxidase (4-HPPA oxidase) | | | |
| Giardi et al | 4-HPPA dioxygenase | Acute intermittent ataxia | | |
| "Hawkinsinuria" | "Defect in rearrangement," p-HPPA →homogentisic | | | |
| *Inherited Urea Cycle Enzyme Defects* | | | | |
| CPS deficiency | Carbamyl phosphate synthetase I (*1* in Fig 139-2) | Lethargy, coma, episodic vomiting, ketoacidosis (provoked by ingestion) | Hyperammonemia ↓BUN, ↑SGOT/SGPT | *For all types*: Protein restriction (essential AA/keto analogues) |
| OTC deficiency (X-linked dominant) | Ornithine carbamyltransferase (*2* in Fig 139-2) | Lethargy, coma, episodic vomiting, ketoacidosis (provoked by ingestion) | Hyperammonemia ↓BUN, ↑SGOT/SGPT (low or absent plasma citrulline) (↑urine orotate) | Elimination of exogenous ammonia and urea precursors; exchange, dialysis; alternate pathways of excretion (eg, sodium benzoate) |

## TABLE 139-4. *(Continued)*

| | Enzyme Deficiency | Clinical Manifestations | Laboratory Features | Management |
|---|---|---|---|---|
| Citrullinemia | Argininosuccinate synthetase (*3 in Fig 139-2*) | Mental retardation | ↑plasma citrulline; ↑$NH_3$ after meals | |
| Argininosuccinic aciduria | Argininosuccinate lyase (*4 in Fig 139-2*) | Mental retardation, seizures, ataxia | Postprandial hyperammonemia; arginosuccinic acid (ASA) in urine | Variable success Open liver biopsy may be associated with catastrophic course (hyperammonemic crises) secondary to catabolic stress |
| Argininemia | Arginase (*5 in Fig 139-2*) | Spastic diplegia, seizures, mental retardation | ↑Blood and cerebrospinal fluid (CSF) levels of arginine | |
| N-AGS deficiency | *N*-acetylglutamate synthetase (*10 in Fig 139-2*) | Ataxia, mental retardation | Hyperammonemia, hyperaminoacidemia (↑serum glutamate), ↑lactate | |
| **Lysosomal Enzymes** | | | | |
| Wolman disease | Lysosomal acid lipase | Infancy (fatal before 12 mo); vomiting, diarrhea, hepatosplenomegaly, FTT, steatorrhea (grossly, liver is yellow) | Symmetric calcification of adrenals, anemia; vacuolation of lymphocytes, deposition of triglycerides and cholesterol ester in various organs | None |
| Cholesterol ester storage disease | Lysosomal acid lipase | More benign; hepatosplenomegaly (liver, yellow-orange) | Deposition of triglyceride and cholesterol ester in various organs, portal hypertension; hyper-$\beta$-lipoproteinemia | None |
| **Disorders of Bile Acid Metabolism** | | | | |
| *Primary (?)* | | | | |
| Cerebrotendinous xanthomatosis | Hepatic sterol-hydroxylase (block in bile acid synthesis) | Tendon xanthomas, cataracts, progressive neurologic dysfunction, premature atherosclerosis | Cholesterol and cholestanol in tissues, bile acid deficiency (cholic and cheno) | Bile acid (cheno) replacement |
| Clayton et al (JCI, 1987) | 3$\beta$-OH-$\Delta^5$-steroid dehydrogenase-isomerase | Familial giant cell hepatitis | Cholestasis | Bile acid replacement |
| Setchell et al (JCI, 1988) | $\Delta$4-3-oxosteroid 5$\beta$-reductase | Familial giant cell hepatitis | Cholestasis | Bile acid replacmenet |
| "Eyssen" syndrome | Deficiency of 26-hydroxylating system (?) | Neonatal cholestasis | ↑Trihydroxycoprostanic acid (THCA), ↓cholate | None |
| *Secondary* | | | | |
| Zellweger's (Cerebrohepatorenal) | Defective formation of C-27 bile acids (peroxisomal defect) | Hypotonia, FTT, mental retardation, renal cortical cysts | ↑Serum iron, ↑Urine excretion of pipecolic acid ↑Dihydroxycoprostanic acid (DHCA) and THCA in bile | None |
| **Disorders of Metal Metabolism** | | | | |
| Wilson's disease (copper toxicosis) | ? | Hepatic dysfunction, neurologic disease | Hypoceruloplasminemia | Copper chelation, copper restriction |
| Menkes (steely hair; copper deficiency of nature) | ? X-linked recessive | Abnormal hair, progressive CNS degeneration, hypopigmentation, bone changes, arterial changes | Low serum copper, low ceruloplasmin; liver Cu ↓↓; intestinal Cu↓↓ | Copper administration has not been successful |
| Idiopathic hemochromatosis | ? | (Rarely presents in children) Weakness and malaise, diabetes, pigmentation, hepatomegaly (±cirrhosis) | ↑plasma iron, ↑chelatable iron (urine), ↑↑plasma ferritin, ↑hepatic iron | Iron chelation (venesection) |

*(continued)*

TABLE 139-4. *(Continued)*

| | Enzyme Deficiency | Clinical Manifestations | Laboratory Features | Management |
|---|---|---|---|---|
| Neonatal iron storage disease | ? | Jaundice, apnea, rapid deterioration (fatal); cirrhosis | Iron accumulation (lysosomal) in various organs | ? Iron chelation |
| **Disorders of Bilirubin Metabolism** | | | | |
| Crigler-Najjar (type I) | UDP-glucuronyl transferase | Marked jaundice (onset in first days of life); bilirubin encephalopathy (fatal); kernicterus | Severe unconjugated hyperbilirubinemia, normal liver function tests | Phototherapy Exchange (?) Transplantation |
| Crigler-Najjar (type II) | (Partial) UDP-glucuronyl transferase | Jaundice; rare encephalopathy | Moderate ↑ unconjugated bilirubin in serum | Phenobarbital |
| Gilbert | ? | Scleral icterus (fluctuating) | Fasting → ↑bilirubin, pigment in liver (centrizonal) | None |
| Dubin-Johnson | ? | Chronic, intermittent jaundice (liver grossly black) | Fasting → ↑bilirubin pigment in liver (centrizonal) | None |
| Rotor | ? | Intermittent jaundice | Marked ↑ in urinary coproporphyrin (isomer type I) | None |
| **Miscellaneous** | | | | |
| $\alpha_1$-Antitrypsin deficiency | Not known (missense mutation glutamic acid → lysine) | Neonatal cholestasis, hepatomegaly | ↓Serum $\alpha_1$-antitrypsin (phenotype PiZZ) | None specific |
| Cystic fibrosis | Cystic fibrosis transmembrane conductance regulatory protein | Pancreatic insufficiency, pulmonary infection, neonatal cholestasis, jaundice, hepatomegaly, portal hyertension | ↑Sweat Cl, steatorrhea, possibly abnormal liver function tests | None specific Ursodeoxcholic acid (?) |
| Erythropoietic protoporphyria (EPP) | Ferrochelatase (autosomal dominant) | Solar urticaria, eczema, progressive hepatic damage | Excess protoporphyrinuria (red cells and feces) and liver (+ cholestasis) | Avoid sunlight $\beta$-carotene (?) |

the onset usually but not invariably within the first month of life. The kidneys may be enlarged. Older patients typically present with growth failure.

*Pathophysiology.* The enzymatic defect in type I glycogenosis is the absence of glucose-1-phosphatase activity in the liver and kidney. This enzyme is key in allowing release of glucose from the hepatocyte after glycogenolysis. The severe and life-threatening hypoglycemia (as low as 5 to 10 mg/dL) found in glycogen storage disease type I is a result of this defect and occurs after short periods of fasting. During hypoglycemia, serum glucagon levels in glycogen storage disease type I are high, and insulin levels are low, resulting in glycogen breakdown without a concomitant rise in serum glucose (Fig 139-1). The glucose-6-phosphate formed by means of glycolysis cannot be hydrolyzed to glucose and is shunted through the glycolytic pathway, resulting in increased serum lactate concentrations and subsequent lactic acidosis. Excess glucose-6-phosphate enters the hexose monophosphate shunt, resulting in the formation of NADPH. Excess pyruvate may be oxidized to acetyl CoA, with the formation of excess NADH. The accumulation of these components may be important in the genesis of the hyperlipidemia found in glycogen storage disease type I. Hyperuricemia appears to result from an elevated rate of purine synthesis, secondary to a decrease in hepatic adenosine triphosphate (ATP) levels, which is caused by a lack of phosphatase activity. Hypophosphatemia may occur because of the cellular retention of inorganic phosphorus as glucose-6-phosphate. Platelet dysfunction, recurrent fever, and the development of hepatic adenomas have been found.

Glycogen storage disease type I has been subdivided. Type IB glycogenosis is a disorder that is clinically similar to type I glycogen storage disease, but when the enzyme assay is carried out with frozen hepatic tissue, the activity is found to be normal. However, glucose-6-phosphatase activity in fresh tissue is absent. These features suggest enzyme latency (ie, release of active enzyme by freezing) and indicate that the enzyme is active but in vivo is not accessible to the substrate. Further studies have documented the deficiency of the carrier protein that transports glucose-6-phosphate across the smooth endoplasmic reticulum to the enzyme. Neutropenia and recurrent infections may occur in glycogen storage disease type IB.

*Pathology.* The hepatocytes in either form of glycogen storage disease type I are loaded with glycogen. Hepatic nuclear hyperglycogenosis is present, as is steatosis; there is no associated fibrosis. Adenoma formation may occur late in the untreated illness.

*Diagnosis.* The patient with glycogen storage disease type I has fasting hypoglycemia; there is no rise in serum glucose values after glucagon or epinephrine administration. The definitive diagnosis is made through determination of glucose-6-phosphatase activity in hepatic biopsy tissue, fresh and frozen if possible. The inheritance pattern is autosomal recessive.

*Therapy.* The treatment of patients with glycogen storage disease type I consists of maintaining adequate serum glucose levels, minimizing the stimuli for hepatic glycogenolysis. Initial

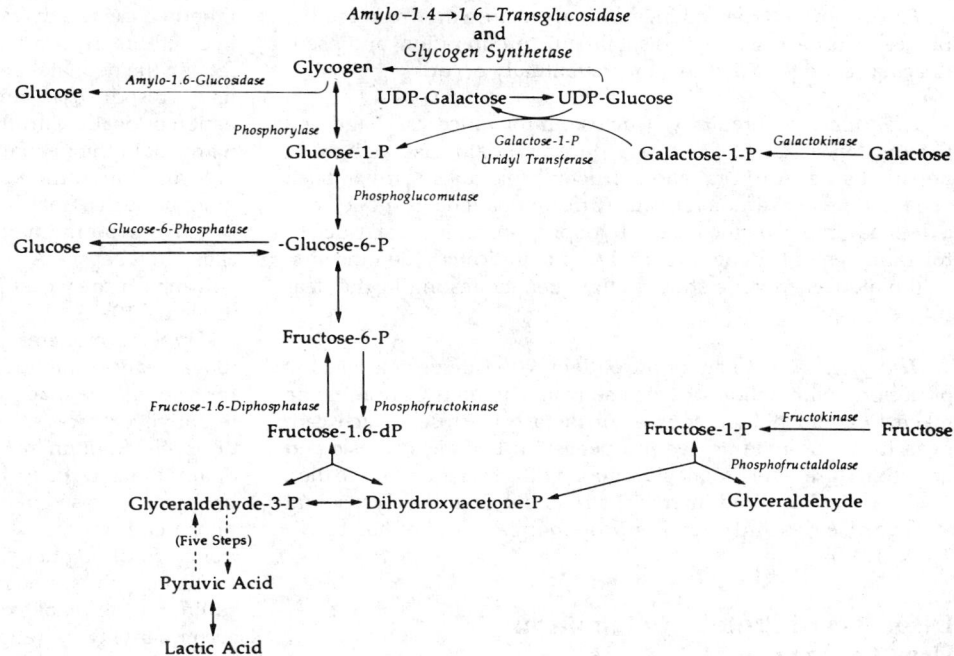

**Figure 139-1.** Embden-Meyerhof-Parnas-Cori pathway of anaerobic glycolysis.

attempts included the use of portacaval shunts to increase the glucose supply to the systemic circulation. Subsequent attempts focused on the use of frequent daytime feedings, with continuous nocturnal carbohydrate infusion, to inhibit excessive glycogenolysis. An infusion rate of approximately 8.5 mg of carbohydrate per minute appears to completely suppress endogenous glucose production. Concern exists that provision of carbohydrate at this rate may lead to continued glycogen synthesis and eliminate alternate sources of fuel vital to cerebral metabolism. However, provision of carbohydrates through nocturnal drip infusion has been demonstrated to improve biochemical abnormalities, decrease hepatomegaly, and enhance catch-up growth. The preferred method of therapy for older children consists of the provision of carbohydrate in the form of uncooked cornstarch in a water suspension served at room temperature. Cornstarch administration every 6 hours in this form produces a relatively stable blood glucose response.

*Prognosis.* The prognosis for patients with type I glycogen storage disease appears to be good with adequate therapy. Long-term follow-up studies of patients treated with nocturnal infusion or cornstarch therapy are not yet available.

### Other Glycogenoses

Type III glycogenosis (ie, Cori's disease) is caused by deficiency of the debrancher enzyme, amylo-1,6-glucosidase. Affected patients may present in a fashion similar to that observed in glycogen storage disease type I, with hepatomegaly and growth failure. Hypoglycemia typically is less severe than in type I disease. Muscular weakness and cardiomegaly are often seen. The hepatic pathology is similar to that in type I glycogen storage disease, but hepatic fibrosis, progressing rarely to cirrhosis, may occur. The severity of the disease may lessen at the time of puberty. Proper therapy remains unclear, although success in ameliorating muscle weakness has been reported with the use of high-protein enteral feedings; cornstarch therapy may also be considered under carefully scrutinized clinical conditions.

Type IV glycogen storage disease typically appears within the first year of life with failure to thrive, gastroenteritis, and hepatosplenomegaly. The hepatic disease is rapidly progressive, with development of ascites and portal hypertension, often within the second year of life. This rare disease is caused by diminished levels of amylo-1:4 → 1:6-transglucosidase (ie, brancher enzyme). Death is usually the result of hepatic failure, although cardiomyopathy has been reported as a terminal event. Micronodular cirrhosis is found on pathologic examination of the liver. Liver transplantation may be curative.

### Hereditary Fructose Intolerance

Of the three identified defects in fructose metabolism, only hereditary fructose intolerance (aldolase deficiency) is capable of causing permanent liver disease. The other forms of altered fructose metabolism include fructose-1,6-diphosphatase deficiency, which is associated with hepatomegaly, hypoglycemia, and acidosis (ie, liver biopsy reveals steatosis) and essential fructosuria, which is caused by a deficiency of hepatic fructokinase and is a benign disorder.

The symptoms of fructose-1-phosphate aldolase deficiency (ie, hereditary fructose intolerance) become apparent only when fructose is added to the diet in the form of fructose-containing foods or through ingestion of milk containing sucrose (ie, glucose-fructose). Children with this autosomal recessive disorder present with vomiting, hepatomegaly, diarrhea, and failure to thrive. Younger infants may present with jaundice, bleeding disorders, ascites, edema, dehydration, sepsis, and shock. Postprandial hypoglycemia and seizures may occur. Aversion to ingestion of sweet foods is common. The hepatic disease may progress to cirrhosis or hepatic failure.

Deficiency in fructose-1-phosphate aldolase results in accumulation of fructose and fructose-1-phosphate within hepatocytes. Fructose-1-phosphate appears to impair glycogenolysis and gluconeogenesis, causing hypoglycemia. Inorganic phosphorus is "trapped" in the form of fructose-1-phosphate, resulting in hypophosphatemia, and in depletion of ATP with resultant hyperuricemia. Serum aminotransferase levels and serum conjugated bilirubin levels may rise. Hepatic synthetic defects may manifest as coagulopathy. Hypokalemia, hyperlactatemia, and hypochloremic acidosis may occur. Fructosuria may occur, sometimes in conjunction with renal tubular acidosis and Fanconi's syndrome.

*Pathology.* Repeated ingestion of fructose may result in hepatocellular necrosis, steatosis, bile duct proliferation, and pseudoacinar changes. Cirrhosis may eventually occur.

*Diagnosis.* Hereditary fructose intolerance is diagnosed through an assay of fructose-1-phosphate aldolase activity in hepatic tissue. An intravenous fructose tolerance test has been used, but it is hazardous because affected patients respond with a decrease in blood glucose and hypophosphatemia. Oral fructose tolerance tests are dangerous and are not indicated. Identification of the aldolase β gene should allow genetic testing in the near future.

*Therapy.* Treatment of the patient with fructosemia consists of lifelong elimination of fructose from the diet. Care must be taken to avoid hidden sources of dietary fructose, which can, even in small amounts, lead to persistent hepatic steatosis and growth failure. The prognosis is good with strict attention to diet.

Disorders of lipid metabolism, including the lysosomal storage diseases and abetalipoproteinemia, are summarized in Table 139-4.

## Disorders of Protein Metabolism: Urea Cycle Enzyme Defects

### Hyperammonemia

The differential diagnosis of hyperammonemia in childhood includes disorders of the urea cycle, organic acidemias, disorders of fatty acid oxidation, transient hyperammonemia of the neonate, Reye's syndrome, drug toxicity (eg, secondary to valproate), and hepatic failure. Differentiation of these situations is important because specific therapy is available for certain disorders.

Ammonia is eliminated from the body through the formation of urea in the liver (Fig 139-2). Accumulation of this potentially toxic substrate can be ascribed to primary or acquired alterations in any of the enzymatic steps in this cycle. Episodes of hyperammonemia may depress consciousness and eventually produce permanent impairment of neurologic function. Death may occur.

Hyperammonemia in the newborn is most often secondary to inherited defects in urea cycle enzymes. If untreated, deficiency in ornithine transcarbamylase, a sex-linked recessive disorder, is fatal in the neonatal period. Affected heterozygous girls may also have episodic hyperammonemia with subsequent mental retardation or death. Citrullinemia and argininosuccinic acidemia may manifest in the neonatal period with hyperammonemic coma or in a subacute form with mental retardation. Patients with argininemia suffer from hyperammonemia and spastic diplegia. Affected newborns may have a clinical picture resembling that caused by sepsis. A high index of suspicion is required. An algorithm for the workup of infants with hyperammonia is shown in Figure 139-3.

Hyperammonemia may be reduced through the use of peritoneal dialysis, hemodialysis, or venovenous hemofiltration. Efforts should be made to induce ammonia excretion through alternative pathways. Therapy should be tailored to individual disorders. Sodium benzoate is often given to allow the excretion of ammonia in the form of hippurate. Arginine or citrulline may be given in cases of ornithine transcarbamylase or carbamylphosphate synthetase deficiency to enhance the excretion of nitrogen. Sodium phenylacetate may be given in argininosuccinase deficiency; glutamine may be conjugated with phenylacetate, resulting in the renal excretion of phenylacetylglutamine and the accompanying excretion of nitrogen. These steps have allowed successful management of many episodes of hyperammonemia, with longer survival of affected patients. Catastrophic episodes, however, still may occur despite adequate therapy. Efforts at identification of carriers and prenatal diagnosis are critical. Specific prenatal diagnosis of ornithine transcarbamylase deficiency has been described, and early prospective treatment of at-risk infants may result in a more favorable outcome.

Organic acidemias such as propionic acidemia, isovaleric acidemia, methylmalonic acidemia, glutaric acidemia, and multiple carboxylase deficiencies may also manifest with hyperammonemia in the newborn. Typically, serum ammonia levels are elevated to a lesser degree than that observed in urea cycle defects, and acidosis and ketosis are usually evident. Evaluation includes careful analysis of the pattern of urinary organic acid excretion. Therapy focuses on correcting specific defects including acidosis and removal of ammonia through the use of dialysis.

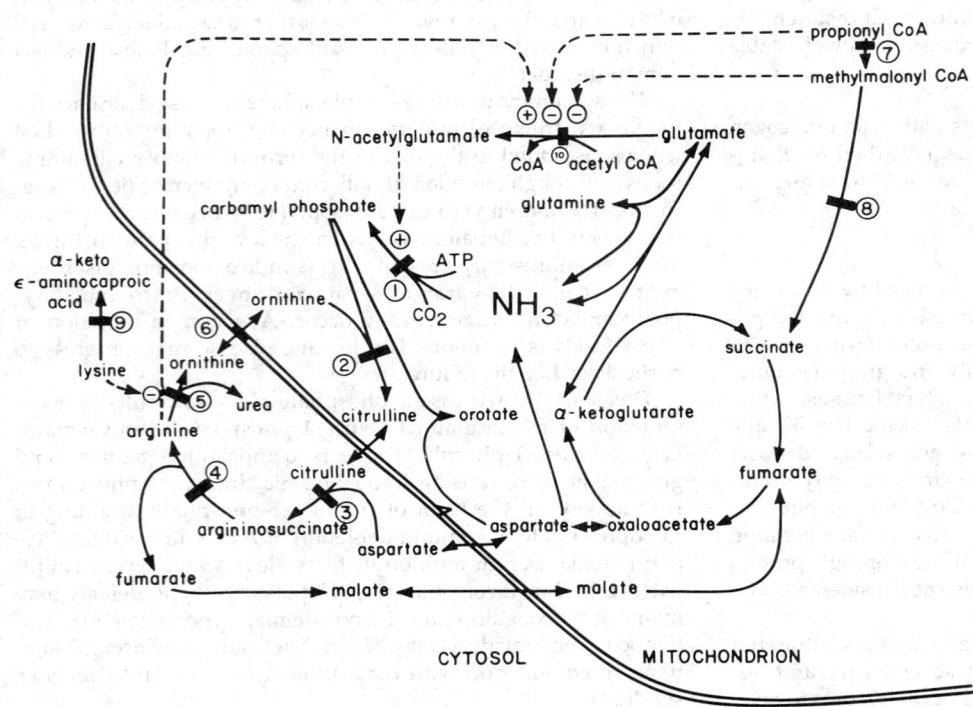

**Figure 139-2.** Urea cycle. Major metabolic pathways for the use of ammonia. Solid bars indicate the sites of primary enzyme defects (or suspected sites of primary enzyme defects) in various inherited metabolic disorders associated with hyperammonemia. (*1*) CPS I; (*2*) OTC; (*3*) argininosuccinate synthetase; (*4*) argininosuccinate lyase; (*5*) arginase; (*6*) mitochondrial ornithine transport; (*7*) propionyl CoA carboxylase; (*8*) methylmalonyl CoA mutase; (*9*) L-lysine dehydrogenase; (*10*) N-acetylglutamate synthetase. Dotted lines indicate sites of pathway activation (⊕) or inhibition (⊖). (Flannery DB, Hsia VE, Wolf B. Current status of hyperammonemic syndromes. Hepatology 1982;2:495.)

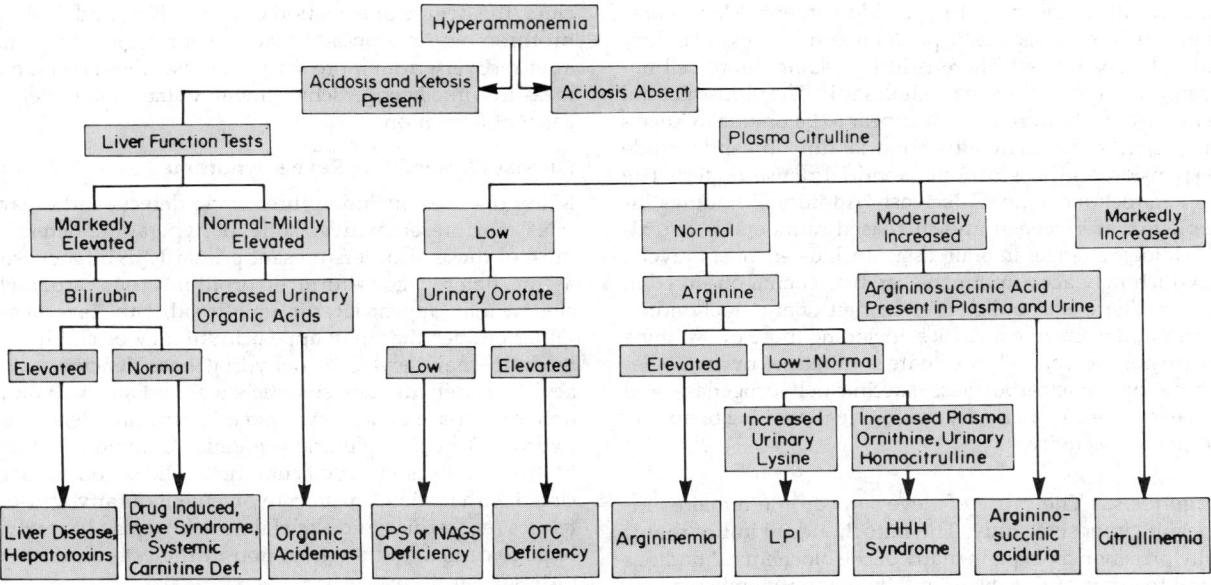

**Figure 139-3.** Differential diagnosis of hyperammonemia. LPI, lysinuric protein intolerance. (Batshaw ML. Hyperammonemia. Curr Probl Pediatr 1984;14:1.)

Transient hyperammonemia of infancy is a disorder primarily found in premature infants, often in conjunction with respiratory distress. Typically, ammonia levels rise rapidly during the first days of life, producing central nervous system (CNS) depression and coma in the second and third days of life. Family history is negative, unlike that often found for infants with urea cycle defects or organic acidemias. The cause of this disorder is unknown, although diminished hepatic blood flow in the neonatal period has been postulated. Therapy is aimed at reducing serum ammonia levels, and dialysis has been used. Prognosis appears to be good for aggressively treated patients surviving the neonatal period.

### Reye's Syndrome

Reye's syndrome became a topic of widespread interest in the mid-1970s, when a dramatic increase in incidence was observed. Although the ensuing years have brought a better understanding of the epidemiology and therapy of Reye's syndrome, the cause remains unclear.

*Clinical and Laboratory Features.* Reye's syndrome, or acute encephalopathy and fatty degeneration of the viscera, follows a biphasic course. Typically, a mild prodromal upper respiratory tract illness occurs. Reye's syndrome after varicella and other viral illnesses has also been described. Recovery from the prodromal illness seems initially uneventful, but within a week, pernicious vomiting occurs. There is usually no fever. Irritability and lethargy may be present initially. Most patients do not progress from this point. Some, however, may display delirium and stupor followed by progression to seizure, coma, or death due to brain stem herniation. Focal neurologic findings are absent. These features have been incorporated into a clinical staging scheme (Table 139-5). Mild hepatic enlargement occurs, although jaundice does not. The cerebrospinal fluid is normal. The encephalopathy may continue for 24 to 96 hours, by which time gradual improvement in neurologic function begins to occur in patients who eventually recover or progression is obvious.

The laboratory features of this syndrome are well known. Diagnostic criteria include serum aminotransferase level elevation to at least threefold above normal. Initial serum aminotransferase levels appear to have no prognostic significance. Serum ammonia may be normal or elevated at presentation, as may the prothrom-

bin time. Prognostic information may be gained through measurement of these two parameters. Serum ammonia levels above 100 mg/dL and a corrected prothrombin time of 3 seconds or longer than control levels on admission are harbingers of progression to deeper coma grades. Hypoglycemia may affect primarily infants and younger children. The differential diagnosis of a child presenting with a Reye-like picture includes CNS infections, salicylate toxicity, valproate and other drug toxicity, urea cycle disorders, disorders of fatty acid oxidation, and organic acidemias.

*Epidemiology.* The incidence of Reye's syndrome rose dramatically in the early mid-1970s, to a peak of 555 nationally from 1979 to 1980. The number of cases reported has declined steadily since then; only 91 new cases were reported in 1985. The yearly incidence typically rose in conjunction with influenza epidemics. The typical age at onset of Reye's syndrome is 6 to 8 years, but adult cases have been reported. The parallel decline in the incidence of Reye's syndrome and in aspirin use needs definitive explanation.

*Pathology.* The liver biopsy is useful in confirming the diagnosis of Reye's syndrome. Grossly, the liver may be yellow or

| TABLE 139-5. | Clinical Grades of Reye's Syndrome at Time of Admission | |
|---|---|---|
| Clinical Grade | | Symptoms |
| I | Mild-moderate | Unusually quiet or mild lethargy |
| II | | Deep lethargy, confusion; possibly brief unconsciousness |
| III | | Extreme lethargy or light coma lasting <3 hours; possibly seizures or agitation |
| IV | Severe | Seizures; possibly, agitation and combativeness; usually protracted deep coma lasting >3 hours; intermittent decerebrate posturing |
| V | | Seizures; deep coma; decerebrate posturing; fixed pupils. |

white as a result of the high triglyceride content. Microscopic findings include the characteristic panlobular microvesicular fatty infiltration of hepatocytes. There is little inflammation, cell necrosis is rare, and there is little or no cholestasis. The ultrastructural changes in the mitochondria, which appear to be unique to Reye's syndrome, reflect changes in mitochondrial function and include matrix expansion and loss of mitochondrial dense bodies. The number of mitochondria may decrease. Additional findings include depletion of glycogen and increased numbers of peroxisomes. Histologic changes in brain tissue include edema of myelin sheaths, which may account for the cerebral edema observed in this disorder. There is also distortion of neuronal mitochondria. Intramitochondrial enzyme activities, including those of ornithine transcarbamylase, carbamylphosphate synthetase, pyruvate dehydrogenase, pyruvate carboxylase, succinic dehydrogenase, and cytochrome oxidase, are markedly reduced in the setting of normal cytosolic enzyme activity.

*Pathogenesis.* The cause of Reye's syndrome remains unknown despite intensive study. The mitochondrial injury that is universally present may explain many of the biochemical findings and clinical features of this disorder. Hyperammonemia may result from the reduction of activity of mitochondrial urea cycle enzymes in the presence of protein catabolism. As evidenced by the clinical course of patients with congenital urea cycle defects, hyperammonemia may be associated with vomiting, coma, hyperventilation, and cerebral edema. Reye's syndrome is also associated with excessive lipolysis from adipocytes. Subsequent elevation of serum free fatty acids, ketopenia, and increased serum long-chain and urinary medium-chain dicarboxylic acids suggests impairment of fatty acid β-oxidation. The accumulation of dicarboxylic acids and fatty acids in serum may further potentiate mitochondrial damage, causing uncoupling of oxidative phosphorylation.

The cause of the mitochondrial dysfunction is unknown, although viral infection is related to disease onset. Influenza A and B viruses, varicella, reovirus, echoviruses, coxsackieviruses A and B, adenovirus, Epstein-Barr virus, herpes simplex and herpes zoster, rubeola, and mumps have all been associated with Reye's syndrome. Because these viruses typically cause characteristic self-limited disease separate from Reye's syndrome, multiple additional factors have been postulated to play a role. A variety of toxins, including drugs (eg, valproic acid, salicylates) and insecticides, have been associated with Reye-like illnesses. An interesting analogy is the illness caused by ingestion of hypoglycin A, a toxin found in the unripe fruit of the ackee tree, which may induce Jamaican vomiting sickness, characterized by vomiting, hypoglycemia, fatty infiltration of the liver, and coma, often resulting in death.

Salicylates have been implicated in the pathogenesis of Reye's syndrome. Although Reye's syndrome does not represent acute salicylate toxicity, multiple studies have suggested a higher incidence of aspirin use in patients developing Reye's syndrome compared with age-matched and antecedent illness-matched controls. Children with connective tissue disease requiring chronic aspirin therapy appear to be at higher risk for Reye's syndrome than the general population. Current recommendations are to withhold aspirin use in children during periods of increased varicella and influenza activity.

*Therapy.* Treatment of Reye's syndrome, which involves careful monitoring for progression in the early, less severe stages and intensive care addressing increased intracranial pressure in the more severe stages, is discussed in Chapter 156.

*Prognosis.* The prognosis for patients with grade I disease is excellent, with rapid recovery expected. Prognostic indices include the degree of elevation of serum $NH_3$ and prolongation of prothrombin time on admission. Neurologic deficits may occur after recovery from more severe disease; these include deficits in measured intelligence, achievement, visual-motor integration, and concept formation.

### Diseases Resembling Reye's Syndrome

Many diseases, including urea cycle defects and organic acidemias, may present with episodes of hyperammonemia. Although most of these disorders present primarily in infancy, some, such as the heterozygous form of ornithine transcarbamylase deficiency, may appear later in childhood with Reye-like illnesses. Other entities that may appear in infancy or childhood include medium-chain acyl CoA dehydrogenase deficiency, long-chain acyl CoA dehydrogenase deficiency, and short-chain acyl CoA dehydrogenase deficiency; systemic carnitine deficiency; and 3-hydroxy-3-methyl glutaric acidemia. Common features shared by these defects include acute metabolic decompensation associated with fasting, chronic involvement of fatty acid-dependent tissues (eg, cardiac and skeletal muscle), episodes of hypoketotic hypoglycemia, and an alteration in the esterification of plasma or tissue carnitine.

Carnitine aids in the transfer of long-chain fatty acids across the inner mitochondrial membrane, where they undergo β-oxidation. Mixed, myopathic, and systemic forms of carnitine deficiency have been postulated. All forms are associated with hypoglycemia, lipid accumulation in liver, skeletal muscle, and heart, and low serum carnitine levels. Replacement therapy may be of use, primarily in the therapy of myopathic carnitine deficiency.

Deficiencies of enzymes involved in intramitochondrial fatty acid β-oxidation pathways have been described. Medium- and long-chain acyl CoA dehydrogenase deficiencies may manifest with episodes of nonketotic coma, usually provoked by fasting. Vomiting, hypoglycemia, and hyperammonemia are frequently observed features. Liver biopsy in long-chain acyl CoA dehydrogenase deficiency (LCAD) reveals large amounts of microvesicular fat. Similar changes are found in medium-chain acyl CoA dehydrogenase deficiency (MCAD). These defects in fatty acid oxidation should be suspected in any child with a history of recurrent episodes of vomiting, lethargy, coma, and hypoglycemia. There are no ketones in the urine. The presentation of MCAD deficiency is in early childhood, although that of LCAD deficiency is primarily in young infants (<4 months). LCAD deficiency appears to be the more severe form and may be associated with hypotonia, hepatomegaly, cardiomyopathy, developmental delay, and death. MCAD deficiency has been associated with sudden infant death syndrome.

Diagnostic efforts should include a search for characteristic patterns of urine dicarboxylic acid excretion during acute episodes of illness or after fasts. A total plasma carnitine concentration less than 30 $\mu$mol/L suggests a fatty acid oxidation disorder. Other diagnostic measures may include measurement of acyl CoA dehydrogenase activity in liver or in fibroblasts. Postnatal DNA screening for MCAD deficiency has been advocated. Treatment modalities are unproven and therefore remain speculative, but they have included high-carbohydrate, low-fat diets and carnitine supplementation. Avoidance of fasting is recommended. In the acutely ill child, glucose should be administered at rates sufficient to prevent fatty acid mobilization ($\sim$10 mg/kg/minute) until oral feeding can be resumed.

## Disorders of Metal Metabolism

### Wilson's Disease

Wilson's disease (ie, hepatolenticular degeneration) is an autosomal recessive disorder of copper metabolism. The clinical presentation is highly variable, but symptoms are rarely evident before 5 years of age. Patients younger than 20 years of age tend to present with predominantly hepatic manifestations, such as asymptomatic hepatomegaly, an illness mimicking acute hepatitis, and with a picture similar to other forms of chronic active hepatitis. Hepatic insufficiency associated with cirrhosis may develop slowly and manifest with signs of portal hypertension, including ascites, edema, and variceal hemorrhage. Conversely, patients may present with fulminant hepatic failure associated with a brisk hemolytic anemia; this specific presentation is almost uniformly fatal. Older patients present with predominantly neurologic and psychiatric disturbances. These disorders are often initially subtle and include deterioration in school or job performance, behavioral changes, slurred speech, and tremors. If untreated, severe dysarthria and dystonia result, often leading to psychiatric hospitalization or institutionalization. Kayser-Fleischer rings (ie, copper deposits on the inner surface of Descemet's membrane) are invariably found if neurologic disease exists, but they may be absent in the younger patient with liver disease only. Hemolysis, presumably secondary to release of copper from the liver, may be present, as may calcified, pigmented gallstones. Other clinical features may include Fanconi's syndrome, with progressive renal disease and arthritis.

*Pathogenesis.* Although the molecular basis for Wilson's disease is unknown, its manifestations are thought to result from excessive accumulation of copper in the liver, eyes, CNS, and kidneys. The reason for copper accumulation is unknown, but the most likely explanation may be defective excretion of copper from hepatocytes into the bile, presumably secondary to an undefined lysosomal defect. A mutation closely linked to Wilson's disease has been mapped to the long arm of chromosome 13; the inheritance pattern is autosomal recessive. Data indicate a defective synthesis of the copper-binding protein, ceruloplasmin. The defect appears to reside at the level of messenger RNA production. The precise cause of copper hepatotoxicity is unclear, but a postulated mechanism is the oxidation of sulfhydryl groups, depleting stores of reduced glutathione. Copper also may inhibit a variety of enzymatic processes.

The natural history of Wilson's disease begins with the asymptomatic storage of copper in hepatocytes. As saturation occurs, hepatocyte necrosis occurs, with the stored copper released into the circulation. This may result in hemolysis and copper deposition in the eye, kidney, and CNS. Hepatic fibrosis and cirrhosis occur in conjunction with the progressive deposition of copper in other tissues.

Laboratory features of Wilson's disease usually include a low serum ceruloplasmin level. Serum copper may be elevated, particularly during episodes of hemolysis, and urinary copper excretion is markedly increased. Examination of urine copper excretion after a dose of D-penicillamine may be of particular value. Hepatic copper content is invariably increased to over 250 µg/g dry weight. Liver tissue may contain fatty infiltration, glycogen granules, and enlarged Kupffer's cells. A lesion indistinguishable from that observed in chronic active hepatitis may be observed in some patients. Advanced cases may demonstrate hepatic fibrosis and cirrhosis.

*Diagnosis.* The diagnosis of Wilson's disease should be considered in every child with unexplained hepatic disease. A high level of clinical suspicion must be maintained. Kayser-Fleischer rings should be sought with a careful slit lamp examination. Signs of chronic liver disease must be sought. Neurologic signs, especially in the older patient, may be found. CNS lesions may be demonstrated with CT or magnetic resonance (MRI) scans. Helpful laboratory features include decreased serum ceruloplasmin levels and an elevated serum copper level; the 24-hour urinary copper excretion rate, normally less than 40 µg/24 hours,

may be over 100 µg/24 hour in Wilson's disease. This finding, however, may be present in other forms of chronic liver disease. To discriminate, a dose of oral D-penicillamine increases urinary copper excretion in Wilson's disease to levels of 1200 to 2000 µg/day. Hepatic biopsy, when assessed for histology change and hepatic copper content, is the reference standard for diagnosis of Wilson's disease. In patients exhibiting the fulminant presentation of Wilson's disease, serum alkaline phosphatase and serum aminotransferase levels are often disproportionately low, but the serum and urine copper content is markedly elevated.

*Therapy.* Untreated, Wilson's disease is uniformly fatal. Adequate therapy is available in the form of D-penicillamine, a copper-chelating agent. D-Penicillamine ($\beta,\beta$-dimethylcysteine) is given orally in initially low doses, increasing to 1 g/day for adults and 0.5 to 0.75 g/day for younger children. Urinary copper excretion increases initially during D-penicillamine therapy, leading to "decoppering" of the patient. Urinary copper levels later stabilize, reflecting the maintenance of copper balance. In conjunction with this therapy, a diet low in copper must be instituted; foods with a high copper content such as liver, chocolate, nuts, and shellfish should be avoided. These restrictions should maintain the daily copper intake below 1 mg/day. Water sources should be analyzed for copper content. With the institution of therapy, an improvement in hepatic and neurologic function is usually found, and the Kayser-Fleischer rings regress. This therapeutic program must be adhered to for life. One study found that patients who discontinue therapy often die within 3 years. For patients unable to take D-penicillamine, therapy with Trien (triethylene tetramine dihydrochloride), an alternative chelating agent, is equally effective. Studies have suggested that zinc, administered orally, may maintain a negative copper balance in some patients with Wilson's disease, but zinc should be considered as primary therapy only for patients unable to tolerate D-penicillamine and Trien.

For patients with Wilson's disease who present with fulminant hepatic failure associated with hemolysis, intensive support is indicated; plasma perfusion, hemodialysis, and peritoneal dialysis may be efficacious in lowering the serum copper and in decreasing the copper burden. However, the hepatic injury is apparently irreversible, and after stabilization, efforts should be directed toward rapid diagnosis and referral of the patient for liver transplantation, which is curative.

*Prognosis.* Untreated, Wilson's disease is uniformly fatal. Death may occur from hepatic, neurologic, renal, or hematologic complications. The prognosis for patients presenting with fulminant hepatic failure and hemolysis is uniformly poor without liver transplantation. With proper therapy, the prognosis for most patients with Wilson's disease is usually good, although individual differences in response to chelation therapy exist. Siblings of patients with Wilson's disease should be carefully screened for the disease, and D-penicillamine therapy instituted in asymptomatic patients.

### Indian Childhood Cirrhosis

Indian childhood cirrhosis is a form of familial childhood cirrhosis that occurs primarily in Indian Hindu families but has also been described in Central American, Middle Eastern, and West African children, and studies suggest the presence of a similar disorder in children in the United States. Onset of the disease typically occurs in children younger than 3 years of age. Patients present with hepatomegaly, pale stools, fever, and behavioral changes. Jaundice may be evident. The hepatic disease typically progresses rapidly. Hepatic biopsy confirms progression from a nonspecific early stage to one with progressive fibrosis and subsequently to widespread necrosis and cirrhosis. The disease is usually fatal within the first 5 years of life. Suggested causes include excessive dietary intake of copper, perhaps through the use of copper and brass cooking and storage vessels. It is possible that a genetically determined disorder of copper metabolism exists, especially in the North American variety. Therapy with D-penicillamine may allow complete recovery, especially if started early in the disease course.

### Neonatal Hemochromatosis

Neonatal hemochromatosis is a poorly characterized and extremely rare disorder in which hepatic insufficiency develops within the first 4 to 7 days of life. Typically, affected infants are born prematurely, and there appears to be an increased familial incidence. A hemorrhagic diathesis is often prominent. Affected patients may die within the first week of life. Pathologic examination reveals increased iron deposition in multiple organs, including the liver, pancreas, heart, and thyroid glands. The patients have no evidence of hemolytic disease. Although the respective roles of extrinsic iron, infection, and genetic predisposition remain obscure, neonatal hemochromatosis does not appear to be genetically related to hereditary hemochromatosis. Diagnosis may be made by finding hemosiderosis in minor salivary glands on biopsy of oral mucosa. There is no documented treatment except for liver transplantation, which is difficult at this age.

## Miscellaneous Errors of Metabolism Affecting the Liver

### Inborn Errors of Bile Acid Metabolism

Inherited defects in the biosynthetic pathway can cause cholestasis and progressive liver injury. Novel analytic techniques, including fast atom bombardment ionization with mass spectrometry (FAB-MS), have allowed the diagnosis of these disorders, which previously might have been characterized as one of the idiopathic, familial syndromes of cholestasis, such as Byler's disease or neonatal hepatitis. The mechanism of cholestasis in these conditions may be related to a failure to synthesize adequate amounts of primary bile acids, which are essential for bile formation and the increased production of unusual bile acids with hepatotoxic potential.

Two inborn errors involving the bile acid steroid nucleus have been associated with familial neonatal cholestasis and giant cell hepatitis. The disorders were associated with severe cholestatic jaundice from birth, progressive liver injury, and if untreated, death from hepatic failure early in life. A $3\beta$-hydroxysteroid dehydrogenase or isomerase deficiency has been confirmed in several patients by the failure to synthesize primary bile acids with the concomitant production and accumulation of increased quantities of $3\beta$-hydroxy-$\Delta^5$-sterol intermediates. The FAB-MS technique has allowed the diagnosis of $\Delta^4$-3-oxosteroid-5$\beta$-reductase deficiency in infants with cholestatic liver disease. This defect resulted in markedly reduced primary bile acid synthesis and the accumulation of potentially toxic bile acid precursors, $\Delta^4$-3-oxo- and allo-bile acids.

The experience with the use of oral bile acid administration to treat inborn errors of bile acid metabolism has been extremely promising. The rational for this therapeutic approach is that bile acid replacement can provide a stimulus for bile secretion and inhibit endogenous synthesis and accumulation of potentially toxic bile acids produced in response to the enzyme deficiency. For example, in patients with the $\Delta^4$-3-oxosteroid-5$\beta$-reductase deficiency, combined treatment with cholic acid (to inhibit endogenous bile acid synthesis) and ursodeoxycholic acid (to stimulate bile flow) has been successful in completely suppressing $\Delta^4$-3-oxo and allo-bile acid production and in normalizing or improving markedly liver tests and hepatic histology.

### Cystic Fibrosis

The hepatobiliary system is involved in 20% to 50% of patients with cystic fibrosis. In most cases, this involvement is clinically insignificant, but with improved life expectancies in this disorder, more hepatobiliary complications are being reported. Scott-Jupp and associates observed a progressive rise in the prevalence of clinically apparent liver disease among 1100 patients with cystic fibrosis from 0.3% in a 0- to 5-year-old group to a peak of 8.7% among those between the ages of 16 and 20.

Infants with cystic fibrosis may present with persistent neonatal cholestasis, often in association with meconium ileus. Infants with this syndrome may appear to have a hypoplastic extrahepatic biliary tract at operative cholangiography, and hepatoportoenterostomy has been performed because of misdiagnosis. In nonoperated patients, bile flow spontaneously resumes in time. Cystic fibrosis should be considered in all infants with neonatal cholestasis.

Liver pathology of affected infants reflects biliary ductal obstruction, presumably by inspissated secretions. Excessive biliary mucus is associated with periportal inflammation and mild intrahepatic bile ductular hyperplasia. Older patients with cystic fibrosis may develop steatosis of the liver. Tender hepatomegaly may occur with right ventricular heart failure. Focal biliary cirrhosis may occur in early childhood, but it becomes more prominent in adulthood. Approximately 24% of patients who die of cystic fibrosis have changes consistent with focal biliary cirrhosis found during autopsy. A small percentage of patients with focal biliary cirrhosis subsequently develop multilobular biliary cirrhosis associated with jaundice, portal hypertension, and hepatic failure. Variceal hemorrhage may occur in this condition.

Management of patients with cystic fibrosis with significant hepatic disease has included sclerotherapy, shunting, and occasionally orthotopic liver transplantation. Administration of ursodeoxycholic acid (15 mg/kg/day) may result in biochemical and functional improvement in the hepatic disease associated with cystic fibrosis. Long-term effects and prognosis are uncertain.

Biliary complications of cystic fibrosis include microgallbladder in 15% to 20% of patients and gallstones in as many as 15% of patients. Gallstone formation may involve abnormal gallbladder size and motility, excessive amount and viscosity of gallbladder and biliary mucus, and diminished bile acid output lithogenic bile and probable cholesterol supersaturation of bile.

Stenosis of the common bile duct may occur in some patients with cystic fibrosis and liver disease.

### $\alpha_1$-Antitrypsin Deficiency

$\alpha_1$-Antitrypsin, a 50-kd glycoprotein that is synthesized in the liver, functions as a protease inhibitor to neutralize a broad spectrum of proteolytic enzymes, although its major target protease is leukocyte elastase. $\alpha_1$-Antitrypsin accounts for approximately 80% of the serum $\alpha_1$-globulin fraction. Homozygous deficiency of $\alpha_1$-antitrypsin is associated with neonatal cholestasis and with childhood and adulthood cirrhosis, and an increased incidence of primary liver cancer has been proposed. Homozygous and heterozygous deficient persons are at risk for pulmonary disease.

$\alpha_1$-Antitrypsin occurs in more than 75 variant forms, designated as Pi phenotypes, each inherited in a codominant fashion. The normal phenotype is MM; the type most often associated with hepatic disease is ZZ. Patients with ZZ phenotypes have low serum $\alpha_1$-antitrypsin levels, usually 10% to 15% of normal. A Pi null/null phenotype has been described in which no $\alpha_1$-antitrypsin is present in the serum. Adults with cirrhosis have also been described in conjunction with MZ, M Malton, and M Duarte phenotypes.

The incidence of the PiZZ (homozygous deficient) phenotype is estimated to be 1 in 2000 to 4000. The clinical manifestations of the PiZZ phenotype in children vary. Approximately 10% of these patients present with clinical evidence of neonatal hepatic disease. Another 40% to 50%, although asymptomatic, have hepatic biochemical abnormalities when tested at 3 months of age. Patients presenting with neonatal cholestasis may be jaundiced in the first week of life, and acholic stools and hepatomegaly may be observed. Jaundice often clears by the fourth month of life. Approximately equal proportions of these infants continue to have abnormal liver function and, if untreated, die by age 10 of complications related to hepatic cirrhosis; have persistently abnormal hepatic function with slow progression to cirrhosis; have continued mild hepatic dysfunction and fibrosis, with survival into adulthood; or have resolving hepatic disease with a return to normal function.

Pathologic findings in the liver may correlate with any of the previously described clinical conditions. In the neonatal period, the hepatic lesion may be indistinguishable from that usually found in neonatal hepatitis. Cirrhosis has been reported in neonates and in the preterm infant. Variable degrees of bile duct proliferation may occur early in the disease; this specific histologic feature portends a more severe course. The characteristic hepatic lesion in $\alpha_1$-antitrypsin deficiency is the presence of periodic acid-Schiff–positive, diastase-resistant hepatocyte inclusions. These globules, antigenically related to $\alpha_1$-antitrypsin, occur predominantly in periportal hepatocytes. These inclusions may not be visible before 4 months of age, but their size increases with age. In more advanced disease, biopsy findings may reveal extensive fibrosis, and few intrahepatic bile ducts may be found.

The pathophysiology of the hepatic disease observed in $\alpha_1$-antitrypsin deficiency is unclear. Patients with the PiZZ phenotype produce, because of a point mutation, an abnormal $\alpha_1$-antitrypsin protein characterized by the substitution of lysine for glutamate at position 342. Electron microscopic findings suggest that the secretion of $\alpha_1$-antitrypsin from the hepatocyte may be blocked at the step before entrance into the Golgi apparatus, resulting in accumulations of abnormal proteins within the hepatocyte. These deposits also occur in the absence of hepatic disease; thus it is unclear whether retained $\alpha_1$-antitrypsin is toxic to the liver. Studies in transgenic mice suggest that this is the case. Breast-feeding does not appear to favorably influence prognosis.

Diagnosis involves ascertaining the patient's $\alpha_1$-antitrypsin phenotype; measurement of $\alpha_1$-antitrypsin levels is less reliable. Characteristic hepatic biopsy findings are confirmatory. Family members of affected patients should be screened.

Treatment of hepatic disease associated with $\alpha_1$-antitrypsin deficiency is supportive. Hepatic transplantation, if required, is curative. Replacement therapy using enzyme derived from human donors is being evaluated as therapy for the pulmonary disease of $\alpha_1$-antitrypsin deficiency. The utility of replacement therapy in hepatic disease is unknown but may be detrimental. Future therapy may involve modulation of gene expression to turn off protein production.

## VIRAL HEPATITIS

Viral hepatitis in children is a major health concern throughout the world. Multiple hepatotropic viruses causing disease in humans have been identified. These include hepatitis A, hepatitis B, the delta agent (ie, hepatitis D), and the more recently described hepatitis C and E. Other viruses capable of causing hepatitis include Epstein-Barr virus (EBV), cytomegalovirus (CMV), varicella

virus, herpes simplex virus, rubella, and coxsackievirus B; typically these organisms cause hepatitis as part of a multisystem presentation, and they are discussed in other chapters.

## Hepatitis A

Hepatitis A virus (HAV), a member of the picornavirus family, is an RNA virus. Hepatitis A accounts for as many as 25% of cases of hepatitis in the developing world. Transmission is usually through the fecal-oral route, although parenteral transmission has been recorded. Consumption of contaminated food or water is usually implicated. There is no known carrier state, and transmission is by person-to-person spread during the preicteric stage of disease. Fecal viral shedding is maximal during the late incubation period (28 days), immediately before or after symptom onset. As a result of this method of spread, infants may be ideal vectors of HAV infection, with spread to other family members or to other children at day-care centers. Institutionalized children are also at high risk for disease acquisition.

Clinical symptoms of HAV infection may be absent or, especially in children younger than 2 years of age, may consist of nausea, vomiting, and diarrhea. The patient is often anicteric. In adults, symptoms of acute hepatitis predominate. Approximately two thirds of those with symptoms become jaundiced. Prodromal symptoms of fever, headache, and anorexia may occur. In most patients, HAV infection has a mild course and clinical improvement occurs rapidly. Aminotransferase levels, which peak within 1 week of disease onset, usually normalize within several weeks but may remain elevated for several months (Fig 139-4). Diagnosis may be made through the demonstration of anti-HAV IgM in serum; anti-HAV IgG develops later and persists for life. The disorder invariably resolves. There is no evidence of chronic hepatitis due to HAV. A small percentage of patients may develop fulminant hepatitis due to HAV, accounting for a fatality rate for those infected with HAV of less than 1%.

Treatment of HAV infection is symptomatic, and hospitalization is rarely required. Dietary therapy has no proven role. Prevention of disease spread is a major goal of therapy. Infected infants should not return to their day-care center until 2 weeks after onset of symptoms to minimize the exposure of others to fecal shedding. If HAV is documented in a day-care center attendee, parent, or employee, 0.02 mL/kg of immune globulin should be given to all employees and children. Standard immune globulin is effective in modifying the clinical manifestations of HAV infection but must be given within 2 weeks of exposure. Immune globulin prophylaxis is not required for casual contacts of patients with HAV infection outside of the day-care center. A prototype inactivated hepatitis A vaccine was well tolerated by children in a controlled trial, and a single dose was highly protective against clinically apparent hepatitis A.

## Hepatitis B

The hepatitis B virus (HBV) is a DNA virus of the hepadnavirus family. HBV-related viral particles can be found in serum and tissue of infected persons. Contained within the virion is the core protein (HBcAg), within which is the viral DNA. Also present are the surface antigen (HBsAg), DNA polymerase, and the e antigen (HBeAg). Diagnostic efforts focus on identification of antigens HBsAg or HBeAg, antibodies generated in response to them (eg, anti-HBs, anti-HBe, anti-HBc), or viral DNA in serum.

Transmission of HBV usually occurs by the parenteral route, through exchange of blood or body secretions. The virus has been demonstrated in blood, semen, saliva, and breast milk. Transmission may occur through intimate contact of any type and through vertical (ie, mother to infant) transmission. Persons

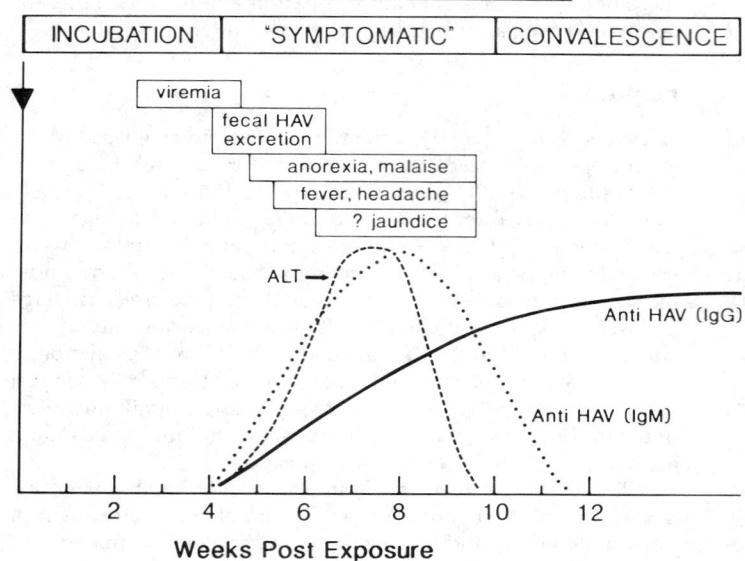

**PHASES OF HAV INFECTION**

| INCUBATION | "SYMPTOMATIC" | CONVALESCENCE |

**Figure 139-4.** Typical course of hepatitis A infection. The period of viremia, which occurs during the incubation phase, is brief. The duration of fecal excretion overlaps this prodromal phase and is present early in the symptomatic phase. Jaundice may occur up to 6 weeks after exposure but is not present in all cases. The aminotransferase ALT (SGPT) elevation also precedes the development of clinical symptoms; values usually remain abnormal after serum bilirubin returns to normal. Anti-HAV is detectable early in the acute "symptomatic" phase of the illness; the initial response is anti-HAV IgM, which peaks shortly after the onset of symptoms and progressively declines. This is succeeded by a gradual rise in anti-HAV of the IgG class, which peaks after the symptomatic phase and remains detectable indefinitely (arrow = exposure). (From Balistreri WF. Viral hepatitis. Pediatr Clin North Am 1988;35:640.)

at high risk include those with frequent exposure to blood or blood products. Children at greatest risk in the United States include those born to mothers who had acute hepatitis B in the third trimester or are chronic HBsAg carriers. Institutionalized children, hemophiliacs, hemodialysis patients, and intravenous drug abusers are at risk for disease. The prevalence of the HBsAg carrier state in the United States is approximately 0.1%.

The incubation period of HBV is estimated at 60 to 180 days, and the subsequent infection is often subclinical, but symptoms occur in 25% to 30% of patients (Fig 139-5). Early symptoms may be systemic and include fever, symmetric arthropathy, and skin eruptions, and urticarial or, in some children, a papular acrodermatitis known as Gianotti-Crosti syndrome. The disease is often anicteric. Malaise, right upper quadrant pain, and a variety of nonspecific GI complaints may occur. Diagnosis of acute hepatitis B is made in the proper clinical setting through the demonstration of HBsAg and anti-HBc IgM in serum. HBsAg positivity in the absence of anti-HBc IgM suggests chronic infection.

The outcome of HBV infection varies. Adults and older children infected with HBV typically have a benign course with complete resolution. Approximately 1% of patients may suffer from fulminant hepatitis. A chronic carrier state may ensue after HBV infection in fewer than 1% to 10% of older patients. At least 20% of preschool-aged children with acute HBV infection become chronic carriers. Virtually all infants born to HBsAg-positive mothers contract HBV unless intervention is initiated; of these, approximately 90% become chronic carriers. Transmission in the neonatal period may occur at delivery when the infant is in contact with large amounts of maternal blood. Infants may become infected postnatally from the mother or from infected siblings. In each case, development of the chronic carrier state is common. Infection acquired during the neonatal period is typically asymptomatic. Less commonly, a mild icteric hepatitis may occur. In rare cases, fulminant hepatic failure may occur, particularly after infection with a precore defective variant of HBV.

Children who are chronic HBsAg carriers are often asymptomatic and seldom have a history of previous hepatitis. Problems inherent in the chronic carrier state include risk of disease transmission to others and increased risk for the development of cirrhosis and of hepatocellular carcinoma. Chronic infection may be associated with asymptomatic infection, chronic persistent hepatitis, or chronic active hepatitis. The diagnosis of chronic HBV infection rests on the demonstration of elevated transami-

nases and HBsAg positivity, often accompanied by HBV DNA or HBeAg seropositivity. Patients with HBeAg positivity are in the "replicative" phase of disease, during which active viral replication and hepatic inflammation occur. Eventually, the viral genome is inserted into the hepatocytic genome of the patient; integration of the viral genome may form the basis of future malignant transformation. Subsequently, the patient may become

**PHASES OF HEPATITIS B INFECTION**

| INCUBATION | "SYMPTOMATIC" | CONVALESCENCE |

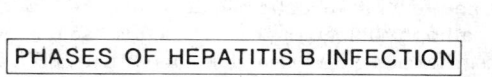

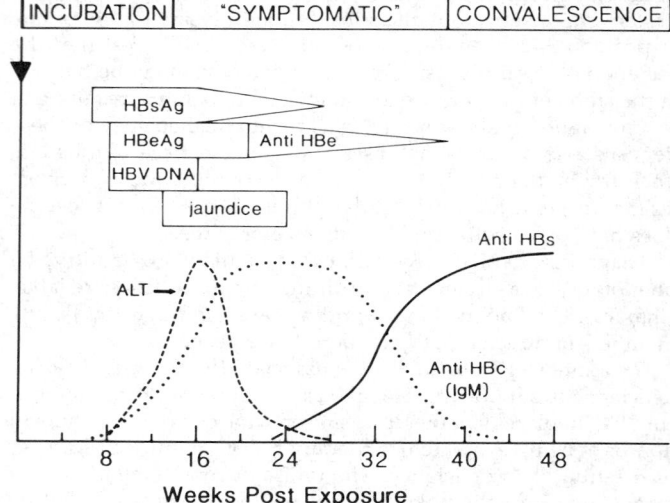

**Figure 139-5.** Typical course of hepatitis B infection. After exposure to HBV (arrow), the earliest detectable serum marker is a rise in HBsAg, which may appear at any time (weeks 1–10) postexposure; HBV DNA and HBeAg follow closely. HBsAg is detectable 2 to 8 weeks before the onset of the symptomatic phase, which is heralded by an increase in aminotransferase (ALT) levels, serum bilirubin concentrations, and constitutional signs. Clearance of HBsAg by immune aggregation with anti-HBc occurs by 6 to 8 months postinfection; those who fail to clear are termed HBsAg carriers. Anti-HBc, which appears just prior to the symptomatic phase, is the first detectable host-induced immunologic marker of hepatitis B infection. Anti-HBc of the IgM class may be the only marker of HBV infection in serum after clearance of HBsAg, and before a rise in anti-HBs. Anti-HBc is not a neutralizing antibody and therefore, in contrast to anti-HBs, is not protective. (From Balistreri WF. Pediatr Clin North Am 1988;35:647.)

anti-HBe positive, indicating a low or absent level of viral replication. Seroconversion to anti-HBe positivity is usually associated with a remission of chronic liver disease. This seroconversion, however, is frequently preceded by a period in which viral replication increases, often accompanied by a flare of hepatic disease. The transformation from HBeAg positivity to anti-HBe positivity occurs spontaneously at a rate of 5% to 15% annually in infected children. Inactivation is not permanent in all cases, and reactivation of disease with resumption of HBeAg positivity may occur. Approximately 30% of patients who lose HBeAg revert to HBeAg positivity. These reversions are also associated with exacerbations of hepatic disease. As many as 15% of patients with HBsAg positivity may spontaneously become HBsAg negative.

Studies of adults and children suggest a role for interferon-$\alpha$ in the treatment of chronic hepatitis B virus infection. Specifically, 37% of adults with chronic, replicative hepatitis B infection given 5 million units of interferon daily for 16 weeks had a sustained loss of hepatitis B viral replication, defined as a loss of HBeAg and HBV DNA. Although the mechanism is not certain, early data suggest an enhancement of cytolytic T-cell recognition and function. Patients most likely to respond include those with HBV DNA levels below 100 pg/mL and those with pretreatment alanine aminotransferase values above 100 U/L. The results of treating some groups of children have been promising. Although standard doses have not been established, the loss of viral replication has been suggested in 30% to 50% of Hispanic children treated with 5 to 10 million units/m² given three times per week. Response rates may be lower in perinatally infected patients and in children of Asian ancestry. It is likely that the poor response in these children was the result of the profound immunologic tolerance to HBV induced by exposure to the virus early in life. The duration of interferon therapy is usually 6 months; side effects include fever (predominantly in the first month of therapy), malaise, autoimmune phenomena, and bone marrow suppression. Patients with decompensated HBsAg-positive liver disease may develop hepatic failure during treatment.

Because of the limitations of treatment, attention must continue to focus on disease prevention. Infants of infected mothers should be given hepatitis B immune globulin and hepatitis B vaccine. Universal vaccination of children against hepatitis B virus has been recommended by the American Academy of Pediatrics. Despite current uncertainty concerning optimal immunization schedules and the duration of protection, this step should dramatically decrease new cases of hepatitis B virus infection and its complications, including hepatocellular carcinoma, in the years to come.

## Hepatitis Delta Infection

The hepatitis delta virus (HDV) is a defective RNA virus that requires the hepatitis B virus to cause infection. The virion, a 36-nm particle enclosing HDV RNA, is encased within an HBsAg coat. HDV infection does not occur without acute or chronic hepatitis B infection. The modes of transmission of the delta agent appear to be similar to those discussed for hepatitis B. Endemic areas include the Amazon Basin (ie, Labrea hepatitis), the Mediterranean basin, areas of European Russia, and developing tropical areas. In the United States, risk factors for HDV infection are those associated with HBV infection, especially percutaneous transmissions.

Infection with HDV can occur as a simultaneous coinfection with acute hepatitis B or as a superinfection with HDV in the HBsAg chronic carrier. Because HDV depends on the presence of HBV, replication of the delta agent is limited to the number of hepatocytes infected with hepatitis B. The presence of delta virus coinfection usually does not modify the underlying severity of the HBV infection. In most cases, the disease is self-limited, but coinfection may be associated with a higher rate of fulminant hepatitis. HBV and HDV coinfection is responsible for as much as 30% of fulminant hepatitis worldwide; in this specific form of infection, there are frequently two peaks of serum aminotransferase activity, usually a few weeks apart. Presumably, the first peak corresponds to HDV and HBV infection and the second to HBV replication, which is no longer inhibited by HDV replication.

Superinfection with HDV occurs in chronic carriers of HBV subsequently exposed to HDV. In these patients, the presence of HBV-colonized hepatocytes allows the rapid establishment of HDV infection, with a resultant increase in disease severity. Fulminant hepatitis frequently occurs in HBV infected persons who are then superinfected with HDV. Chronic active hepatitis occurs in as many as 60% of HBV patients with HDV superinfection. The outcome varies. A chronic HDV carrier state may develop, usually associated with severe progressive chronic liver disease. Conversely, HDV or HBV infection may resolve.

The diagnosis of HDV infection rests on a high level clinical suspicion; all patients with fulminant hepatic failure and patients known to be carriers of HBsAg who suffer acute exacerbation of disease activity must be studied serologically. The presence of delta antigen or of IgM antibodies to HDV (anti-HDV) is evidence of infection. There has been no specific treatment for this disease, but data suggest a role for interferon therapy. Preventive measures are aimed at the prevention of HBV infection.

## Non-A, Non-B Hepatitis

Non-A, non-B (NANB) hepatitis refers to hepatitis for which no other cause (ie, viral hepatitis type A, B, or D; CMV; EBV; drug reactions) can be documented. It is likely that several NANB viral agents exist. Two have been delineated: hepatitis C and E.

### Epidemic Non-A, Non-B Hepatitis: Hepatitis E

The E form of hepatitis appears to be enterically transmitted, probably through fecally contaminated water supplies. Epidemics may involve large numbers of cases. Outbreaks have occurred in Asia, Africa, and Russia. The incubation period appears to be 35 to 45 days, with a peak age of incidence between 15 and 40 years. The disease may be mild to severe in intensity, with an approximately 20% incidence of fatality in pregnant women. The responsible agent appears to be a 32- to 34-nm virus-like particle that is also transmissible to animals.

The viral genome of these particles, designated hepatitis E, has been partially cloned and suggests that hepatitis E may be a member of the calicivirus family. No commercial serologic assays for this agent are available. There is no evidence to suggest that hepatitis E causes chronic infection. No treatment is available.

### Parenteral Non-A, Non-B Hepatitis: Hepatitis C

Hepatitis C virus [HCV] is the major cause of post-transfusion and community-acquired non-A, non-B hepatitis. The virus consists of a single-stranded RNA genome and shares some similarities in nonstructural proteins with the flavivirus family. Cloning of the agent and ongoing refinement of HCV-specific serologic assays have led to rapid advances in our understanding of the clinical course of acute and chronic infection and in the seroepidemiology of the virus. The overall prevalence in the United States of antibody against HCV is about 0.6%. Transmission has occurred primarily by blood or blood products. Serologic screening of blood donors has led to a dramatic decrease in cases associated with blood transfusion, but transmission by intravenous drug use and sexual contact remain important. Vertical transmission from mother to infant may occur, particularly in the setting of maternal human immunodeficiency virus infection, but probably much less often than with hepatitis B. Household spread is not frequent.

The clinical manifestations of acute HCV infection are usually mild and may be missed unless tests of liver dysfunction are serially evaluated after a possible exposure. The virus does not appear to be an important cause of fulminant hepatitis, but chronic infection develops in more than 50% of the patients. The illness in these patients is often characterized by a fluctuating pattern of aminotransferase elevations and few symptoms, but as many as 25% of these patients ultimately develop cirrhosis. There is also a strong association between HCV infection and the development of hepatocellular carcinoma.

The serodiagnosis of HCV infection relies on a second-generation enzyme immunoassay (ie, ELISA-2) and recombinant immunoblot assay (ie, RIBA-2), which detect antibody against several viral antigens. A polymerase chain reaction-based assay has been used as a research tool to detect HCV RNA. In patients with acute transfusion-associated or sporadic hepatitis, the new serologic assays may detect antibody within 8 weeks; most patients test positive by 20 weeks after exposure. Serial measurement of anti-HCV antibodies may be required to exclude infection. Moreover, 90% to 95% of the patients with chronic non-A, non-B hepatitis have anti-HCV antibodies using the second-generation assays.

Treatment of chronic hepatitis C infection with interferon-$\alpha$ for 6 months improves liver tests and histopathologic abnormalities in about 50% of adults. Half of these patients can be expected to relapse after discontinuation of therapy, but they usually respond to retreatment. There is little information on the treatment of chronic HCV infection in children.

The efficacy of prophylaxis against hepatitis C with standard immune globulin is unproven. However, a single injection of immune globulin may be reasonable after percutaneous exposure to anti-HCV–positive blood.

# CHRONIC HEPATITIS

Chronic hepatitis may occur as a result of persistent hepatic viral infection, as seen in conjunction with hepatitis B, D, and C. Drugs that have been cited as the cause of chronic hepatitis include oxyphenisatin, nitrofurantoin, methyldopa, isoniazid (INH), dantrolene, and acetaminophen. Chronic lupoid or autoimmune chronic hepatitis, first described by Waldenström, may be responsible for chronic hepatitis with rapid progression to cirrhosis. Metabolic disorders such as Wilson's disease and $\alpha_1$-antitrypsin deficiency may present with clinical and histologic features similar to those found in chronic hepatitis. Biliary tract disease, particularly primary sclerosing cholangitis, must be considered in the differential diagnosis.

Chronic hepatitis is a prolonged necroinflammatory process involving the liver. The clinical manifestations have an insidious onset. The diagnosis rests on the finding of abnormally elevated serum aminotransferase levels, typically for a period of at least 6 months. Other investigators suggest the appropriateness of applying the label "chronic" to hepatic disease after a shorter observation period, perhaps 4 months, particularly if signs of chronic hepatic disease are present. Between 30% and 50% of pediatric patients present with acute illness. The onset of ascites, encephalopathy, hypoalbuminemia, hypergammaglobulinemia, and hypoprothrombinemia may be sudden.

Regardless of the mode of onset, a liver biopsy is required to establish the diagnosis of chronic hepatitis and the severity of the underlying histopathologic process, which are essential to establish for appropriate treatment. The biopsy may reveal changes consistent with chronic persistent hepatitis, chronic lobular hepatitis, or chronic active hepatitis, each of which implies

a different prognosis. Characteristic pathologic findings of specific disease entities may be found. In infection secondary to HBV, hepatocytes have a "ground glass" appearance with orcein-positive inclusions. Biopsies from hepatitis C patients may exhibit fatty infiltration, acidophilic bodies, bile duct damage, and lymphoid aggregates. Hepatitis due to drug toxicity histologically resembles viral disease, and the biopsy specimen in autoimmune hepatitis frequently contains an infiltrate of plasma cells.

## Chronic Persistent Hepatitis

Chronic persistent hepatitis is most often observed after episodes of HBV or NANB viral infection. Patients are asymptomatic or may have vague complaints such as fatigue and anorexia. Hepatomegaly and right upper quadrant tenderness may be minimal. The patient may have a history of drug abuse. Serum aminotransferase values remain mildly increased after an acute episode of hepatitis. Other tests of liver function, including alkaline phosphatase, bilirubin, albumin, and serum globulin, usually are normal. If serum aminotransferase values remain elevated for more than 6 months, a liver biopsy should be performed. Findings suggestive of chronic persistent hepatitis include infiltration of the portal tracts with lymphocytes and a lack of significant fibrosis. The "limiting plate" of hepatocytes about the portal area remains intact.

## Chronic Lobular Hepatitis

Chronic lobular hepatitis is a histologic pattern often seen in the biopsy specimens of patients with resolving acute viral hepatitis. In this disorder, spotty necrosis and inflammatory infiltration with lymphocytes may be seen in the lobule, although the portal tracts are relatively spared.

Hepatic disease associated with these biopsy findings is typically mild and does not appear to progress to hepatic failure or cirrhosis. No therapy is available. A precautionary statement is in order. Before the diagnosis of chronic persistent hepatitis is made, the adequacy of biopsy specimens must be ensured so as not to miss portal area involvement suggestive of active hepatitis. Patients with chronic active hepatitis treated with immunosuppressive therapy may develop histologic findings similar to those of chronic persistent hepatitis. After therapy is discontinued, the biopsy of these patients may revert to histologic findings consistent with chronic active hepatitis.

## Chronic Active Hepatitis

Chronic active hepatitis is characterized by hepatic inflammation, necrosis, and fibrosis, which may progress to cirrhosis and eventually liver failure. Prolonged HBV infection accounts for 15% to 20% of cases of chronic active hepatitis. In addition, 30% to 50% of cases of hepatitis C infection may result in chronic active hepatitis.

Up to 20% of chronic active hepatitis cases are ascribed to autoimmune chronic hepatitis, a disorder most frequently diagnosed in young women aged 15 to 25 years. The disease may be associated with other disorders of presumably immunologic origin, including thyroiditis, arthritis, rash, and Coombs-positive hemolytic anemia. Presenting features commonly resemble those of acute viral hepatitis and may include weakness, nausea, vomiting, behavioral changes, malaise, and jaundice. Conversely, and less commonly, patients may be asymptomatic, and the disease may be discovered when liver function abnormalities are uncovered in the course of routine evaluations. Laboratory features include elevated serum aminotransferases, often in the range of 500 to 1000 IU. Coagulation defects and hypergammaglobulinemia usually exist. Serologic abnormalities include positive LE cell tests in approximately 15% of cases, and antinuclear and anti-smooth muscle antibodies in 70%. In addition, some cases of chronic active hepatitis in children and adults are associated with the presence of anti-liver-kidney microsome (anti-ER) antibodies. These patients may form a distinct subset of patients with autoimmune chronic hepatitis, characterized by early age at onset and rapidly progressive hepatic disease. HLA types B8 and DRW3 appear to be associated with the development of autoimmune chronic active hepatitis. Findings on physical examination often include jaundice, mild hepatomegaly, and splenomegaly. Signs of chronic liver disease, including spider telangiectasias and palmar erythema, may be present. In advanced cases, findings may reflect underlying hepatic cirrhosis and may include edema, ascites, variceal hemorrhage, and hepatic encephalopathy.

Pathologic findings in chronic active hepatitis, regardless of cause, include the characteristic finding of piecemeal necrosis. In this histopathologic process, portal inflammation breeches the portal-parenchymal interface (limiting plate), and necrosis of bordering hepatocytes is present. In more severe disease, bands of necrosis may spread from portal area to portal area, central area to portal area, or central area to central area (bridging necrosis). Fibrosis extends into the lobule, eventually causing cirrhosis. Bridging or of multilobular necrosis usually denotes severe, progressive disease. Cirrhosis may be present at the time of diagnosis.

## Pathophysiology

Because chronic active hepatitis may be the end result of several disease entities, including viral infection, autoimmune phenomena, and drug toxicity, it is unlikely that only one mechanism for the production of chronic active hepatitis exists. In autoimmune chronic active hepatitis, a generalized increase in immune system activity is observed. Serum $\gamma$-globulin levels are elevated and autoantibodies are present. Autoimmune chronic active hepatitis is associated with non–T-cell-mediated, antibody-dependent, and cell-mediated cytotoxic reactions against hepatocytes. Decreased suppressor T-cell function has been found. Corticosteroids appear to improve suppressor T-cell function in autoimmune chronic active hepatitis. Conversely, in HBsAg-positive chronic active hepatitis, suppressor T-cell function, although abnormal, is not altered by corticosteroids. HBsAg-associated chronic active hepatitis has been associated with cytotoxic T-cell responses against infected hepatocytes bearing viral antigens. The associations of these changes to disease suppression and activity continue to be explored.

## Natural History, Prognosis, and Therapy

*Drug-Associated Chronic Active Hepatitis.* Removal of the offending drug usually results in arrest of hepatic inflammation and, in most cases, complete recovery. Corticosteroids are not of value. Hepatic failure may ensue if the involved agent is not rapidly identified and discontinued. Rechallenge with a drug suspected of causing this form of liver injury is not justified because fulminant liver failure may occur.

*Virus-Associated Chronic Active Hepatitis.* The outcome and potential therapy of these disorders were discussed earlier. Steroid therapy is of little benefit and may be harmful. Antiviral therapy continues to be developed. The incidence of primary hepatocellular carcinoma is increased in patients with chronic hepatitis B or C infection; these tumors have occurred in young children with chronic HBsAg positivity. The effectiveness of early screening programs for hepatocellular carcinoma, including serial AFP determinations and high-resolution ultrasound, must be verified.

*Autoimmune Chronic Active Hepatitis.* Controlled studies of the therapy of autoimmune chronic active hepatitis and the natural history of the untreated condition have been performed only in adults; typically, untreated patients had a 5-year mortality rate of 30% to 50%. Children and adults respond to immunosuppressive therapy. Corticosteroid therapy, with or without the addition of azathioprine, improves the clinical, biochemical, and histologic features of chronic active hepatitis and prolongs life in most patients, but progression to cirrhosis may not be prevented.

The decision to treat depends on the patient's clinical status and on histologic findings. Patients with extreme elevations of serum aminotransferase values and $\gamma$-globulin levels and those with bridging or multilobular necrosis on hepatic biopsy carry a high risk of rapid progression to cirrhosis and deserve therapy. Prednisone usually is begun with a dosage of 1 to 2 mg/kg/day; this dosage is continued until clinical and biochemical remission (ie, aminotransferase values less than twice normal) is achieved, usually within the first 3 months of therapy. Subsequently, the dosage is lowered in decrements of 5 mg every 4 to 6 weeks until a maintenance dosage of 10 to 20 mg/day is achieved. Evidence of biochemical or clinical relapse necessitates a return to the starting dose. For patients who cannot be maintained on low-dose steroids or who develop serious side effects, azathioprine (1 to 2 mg/kg/day) should be considered. Monitoring for bone marrow suppression is essential. Because daily steroid use may suppress linear growth in children, anecdotal reports suggest the use of alternate-day steroids in the long-term management of autoimmune chronic active hepatitis. This form of therapy, although capable of normalizing aminotransferase values, has not produced sustained histologic remission in adults. Despite the reported salutary effect of an alternate-day steroid regimen on growth of children with autoimmune chronic active hepatitis, this form of therapy should be used only with caution.

Therapy should be assessed at 6 to 12 months after initiation with a repeat percutaneous liver biopsy to ensure histologic resolution. Disappearance of symptoms, normalization of biochemical abnormalities, and regression of histologic findings justify attempts at slow withdrawal of the medication.

Response to steroid therapy is generally good. Approximately 70% of treated patients respond initially to therapy, but many of these patients relapse shortly (within 6 months) after discontinuation of medication and again require immunosuppressive therapy. Patients who relapse do not appear to have a higher morbidity or mortality rate from hepatic disease than do those in whom remission is sustained. However, the incidence of medication-related side effects may limit future therapy. Chronic active hepatitis associated with anti-endoplasmic reticulum antibody positivity may represent a particularly aggressive form of disease, requiring rapid diagnosis and aggressive therapy for adequate outcome. Orthotopic liver transplantation is a therapeutic option for patients who progress to end-stage liver disease.

# DRUG-INDUCED LIVER DISEASES

Drug-related hepatotoxicity occurs in children less often than in adults, presumably because children receive fewer drugs than adults. Age-related differences in hepatic metabolism probably also play a role. For example, halothane hepatotoxicity rarely occurs in children, but sodium valproate hepatotoxicity has been described almost exclusively in children. In the former instance, immaturity of hepatic metabolic processes may limit the production of toxic metabolites; in the latter situation, degradation of toxic compounds may be limited by immaturity, with resultant hepatotoxicity.

Many agents are capable of producing hepatotoxicity. These

include environmental and "natural" hepatotoxins (ie, *Amanita*) and medicinal agents. Most drug reactions affecting the liver in children are the result of exposure to analgesics, steroids, or anti-inflammatory, anti-infective, or antineoplastic drugs. The liver is uniquely sensitive to toxic agents, presumably because of its central role in the metabolism and detoxification of xenobiotics. The liver is capable of detoxifying potentially toxic compounds through its mixed function oxidase system (MFOS); inducers such as phenobarbital may stimulate the hepatic metabolism of drugs. The MFOS is also capable of transforming nontoxic agents into toxic metabolites, potentiating hepatic damage. Genetic factors, sex, age, nutritional status, and other systemic illnesses can influence the hepatotoxic potential of a given substance.

## Pathogenesis

Agents that produce hepatic disease may do so in several ways. Direct hepatotoxins injure the hepatocyte through peroxidation of membrane lipids, with subsequent cell necrosis. Carbon tetrachloride is a direct hepatotoxin. Indirect hepatotoxins interfere with specific cellular metabolic pathways. These agents may be cytotoxic (eg, galactosamine, tetracycline, 6-mercaptopurine) or cholestatic (eg, estrogenic steroids). Direct and indirect hepatotoxins cause predictable liver injury with effects are generally dose dependent. Idiosyncratic hepatotoxins cause hepatic disease in an unpredictable fashion that is generally not dose related. In some cases, drug-related hypersensitivity may play a role. These cases are typically accompanied by rash, fever, and eosinophilia, and they require prior exposure to the offending agent, usually 1 to 5 weeks before reaction onset. Other idiosyncratic reactions include those dependent on the presence of specific metabolic defects. These patients may produce and be unable to metabolize specific toxic intermediates of drug metabolism. In these instances, the systemic features of hypersensitivity are not present, and hepatotoxicity may occur after various periods of drug exposure. Cases of phenytoin, sodium valproate, and some isoniazid toxicity may be secondary to this mechanism.

## Pathology

The pathologic findings of drug-related hepatotoxicity vary. In general, predictable reactions are associated with characteristic patterns of hepatic damage. Examples include carbon tetrachloride and acetaminophen, which cause centrilobular hepatocyte damage. Idiosyncratic toxins often cause diffuse changes of necrosis or cholestasis. Inflammation may be prominent, and the hepatic lesion produced may be similar to that seen in acute viral hepatitis. Steatosis is observed with tetracycline toxicity (microvesicular) and with ethanol toxicity (macrovesicular). Cholestatic changes with inflammatory infiltrates may be found with the injury associated with erythromycin estolate and chlorpromazine. Cholestasis without inflammation is usually seen with estrogenic and androgenic steroids. Androgenic steroids also affect the development of peliosis hepatis. Hepatic vein thrombosis has been linked to oral contraceptive use, and hepatic veno-occlusive disease may be observed after the use of antineoplastic drugs. Hepatic tumors have been associated with anabolic steroid and oral contraceptive use. Chronic active hepatitis may be the result of drug administration.

## Clinical and Laboratory Findings

Clinical manifestations of drug-related toxicity are often mild and nonspecific. In the case of hypersensitivity, fever, rash, and arthralgia may be present. Because many cases of drug-related hepatotoxicity occur in ill, hospitalized patients, it may be difficult to separate symptoms of underlying illness from those related to drug toxicity. Similarly, elevated hepatic enzyme levels may be attributed to the underlying illness. Other causes of hepatic dysfunction must be considered, including, in the appropriate clinical setting, viral- and transfusion-related hepatitis, biliary tract disease, sepsis, and hypoxia.

Laboratory features of drug-related hepatotoxicity are variable and nonspecific. Hepatocellular necrosis leads to marked increases in serum aminotransferase levels. Serum alkaline phosphatase and 5'-nucleotidase values may also increase, although usually to a lesser degree. The prothrombin time may be prolonged in the presence of extensive hepatic necrosis, serum albumin values may be depressed, and jaundice may develop. Hyperammonemia may be found in sodium valproate hepatotoxicity or in acute hepatic failure. Milder elevation of serum aminotransferase levels may occur in microvesicular steatosis or with the use of drugs that stimulate the cytochrome P-450 enzyme system (ie, MFOS). The diagnosis of drug hepatotoxicity syndromes depends on a high level of clinical suspicion and an appropriate clinical history. In some cases, such as in acetaminophen toxicity, serum drug levels may be useful in predicting hepatotoxicity. A hepatic biopsy may help to identify characteristic patterns of hepatic injury attributable to specific drugs.

## Treatment

The treatment of drug-related hepatotoxicity usually rests on withdrawal of the offending agent. In some cases, specific therapy is available. Examples include the use of N-acetylcysteine in acetaminophen overdose and chelation therapy in toxicity due to iron overload. Generally, therapy is supportive. The prognosis of drug-related hepatotoxicity is good after the involved drug is withdrawn. The prognosis of fulminant hepatic failure is poor, with survival rates below 50%. If recovery occurs, it usually is complete. Continued use or rechallenge with the hepatotoxic drug may be associated with fatal liver injury.

## FULMINANT HEPATIC FAILURE

Fulminant hepatic failure (FHF) results from acute, massive hepatocellular necrosis or from sudden, severe impairment of hepatocellular function. Patients typically have no evidence of prior hepatic dysfunction. Hepatic encephalopathy is a prerequisite for the diagnosis of FHF. In cases of viral hepatitis, encephalopathy must occur within 8 weeks of onset. Hepatic failure complicating chronic liver disease may present with similar clinical and laboratory features. In FHF, all hepatic functions are usually impaired, including hepatic synthetic, excretory, and detoxifying functions.

## Etiology

Approximately 50% of FHF cases are caused by acute viral hepatitis. Hepatitis A, B, C, D, and E may all cause FHF, as may Epstein-Barr virus, herpes simplex virus, and enteroviral infections. Other non-A, non-B agents may be involved as well. Hepatotoxic drugs may be responsible for 25% of cases of FHF. Acetaminophen toxicity is a common cause. Less commonly associated agents include intravenous tetracycline, halothane, sodium valproate, ethanol, carbon tetrachloride, methyldopa, and isoniazid. Poisoning due to ingestion of the mushroom *Amanita phalloides* may be responsible. Hepatic ischemia due to endotoxic shock, vascular occlusion, or congenital heart disease may result in massive necrosis. In childhood, metabolic disorders including galactosemia, tyrosinemia, hereditary fructose intolerance, and Wilson's disease may cause FHF.

## Clinical Features

The patient may have had a recent episode of viral hepatitis or recent drug and toxin ingestion. Patients or their parents may report the onset of lethargy, nausea, vomiting, fever, lack of appetite, and abdominal pain. Jaundice may have developed. Hepatic encephalopathy may initially manifest with minor behavioral or motor disturbances. Infants may become irritable, eat poorly, and exhibit disturbed sleep patterns; older children may be confused and exhibit slurred speech. Asterixis, elicited through dorsiflexion of the hand at the wrist, may be demonstrable. Hepatic encephalopathy may progress to deep coma. Fetor hepaticus is often present. Ascites may develop, and there may be frequent episodes of bleeding. Hyperventilation may be an early sign, with hypoventilation becoming a problem in more advanced stages of disease. Cardiac arrhythmias (eg, tachycardia, bradycardia) and hypotension often occur. Hepatomegaly may occur, and a rapidly decreasing hepatic size is an ominous sign.

## Laboratory Features

Laboratory features include elevation of conjugated and unconjugated serum bilirubin. Serum aminotransferases may be dramatically elevated initially, although a subsequent decrease may occur as the patient's condition worsens. Indices of hepatic synthetic function are commonly altered. Serum albumin concentrations may be normal at presentation but decrease with time. The prothrombin time is markedly elevated and usually does not improve with vitamin K administration; values over 50 seconds have been associated with poor outcome. The serum concentrations of clotting factors synthesized in the liver (ie, Factors I, II, V, VII, IX, and X) are usually low, and Factor VIII levels are normal or increased. Levels of Factor VII, which has a short plasma half-life, below 8% of normal have been associated with a very poor outcome. Platelet concentrations may be diminished secondary to bone marrow suppression, disseminated intravascular coagulation, or hypersplenism. Platelet function may also be abnormal.

Serum ammonia may be elevated, but the onset of encephalopathy may precede this rise, which presumably is caused by an inadequacy of urea cycle function. Serum sodium values are frequently diminished in the setting of renal resorption of sodium and elevated total-body sodium values. Hypokalemia may result from increased renal excretion of potassium. Hypoglycemia may occur, particularly in children, presumably because of depletion of hepatic glycogen, inadequacy of gluconeogenesis, and hormonal dysfunction. Azotemia may occur; serum creatinine values rise, and blood urea nitrogen values may remain stable or fall because of deficient urea synthesis. Hypophosphatemia, hypocalcemia, and hypomagnesemia may occur. Hyperventilation may cause systemic alkalosis, but cell necrosis may result in systemic acidosis. Hepatic biopsy, which is seldom possible in patients with FHF because of marked coagulopathy, reveals massive hepatocellular necrosis, which may be patchy or zonal. Bridging necrosis and sparse inflammation may also be seen. In cases of tetracycline toxicity or of acute fatty liver of pregnancy, microvesicular fatty infiltration of hepatocytes occurs. Hepatic failure in these cases is presumably secondary to hepatocyte organelle dysfunction.

## Pathogenesis

The pathogenesis of acute hepatic failure is poorly understood. Anoxia or hypoxia of the liver may lead to hepatocellular necrosis, and multiple drugs may cause hepatocyte necrosis through direct hepatocellular membrane damage, through formation of toxic intermediate products of metabolism, or through interference with cell metabolic pathways. Less well understood is the mechanism through which viral hepatitis produces FHF in some patients and mild self-limiting infection in others. The direct effects of viral infection and individual systemic immune responses to that infection presumably play a role. The final common pathway is hepatic necrosis, with effects on hepatic synthetic, excretory, and detoxifying functions. Other factors that may contribute to FHF include infection, endotoxemia, tissue hypoxia, and individual differences in hepatocyte regenerative capabilities.

The cause of hepatic encephalopathy is unknown. Several theories have attempted to correlate observed biochemical abnormalities with hepatic encephalopathy. These include the ammonia theory, the synergism theory, the false neurotransmitter theory, and the GABA-ergic neurotransmission theory.

The ammonia theory proposes that hepatic encephalopathy is caused by elevated serum ammonia levels due to colonic production of free ammonia ion and to failure of the liver to convert ammonia to urea. Patients with inherited disorders of the urea cycle suffer neurologic dysfunction, including lethargy and coma. Contradicting this theory is the finding that hepatic encephalopathy may occur before elevation of serum ammonia levels. Moreover, elevated serum ammonia levels in animals do not produce changes consistent with those of hepatic encephalopathy on electroencephalograms or visual evoked potential testing.

The synergism theory proposes that hyperammonemia, in conjunction with methionine derivatives (ie, mercaptans produced by intestinal bacteria) and short-chain fatty acids, is capable of causing hepatic encephalopathy.

The false neurotransmitter theory proposes that compounds such as octopamine are produced by intestinal bacteria during episodes of hepatic encephalopathy. These false neurotransmitter substances may reach the brain because of disordered blood–brain barrier function and cause cerebral dysfunction. The plasma levels of amino acids are increased in hepatic encephalopathy. These substances may enter the CNS and become false neurotransmitters through $\beta$-hydroxylation. It is unclear whether these substances are capable of producing behavioral and neurologic changes consistent with hepatic encephalopathy.

$\gamma$-Aminobutyric acid (GABA), also produced by colonic bacteria, may play a role in the production of hepatic encephalopathy. GABA receptors possess binding sites for benzodiazepines and barbiturates, which appear to enhance the inhibitory response to GABA. Specific benzodiazepine antagonists may partially and temporarily reverse the effects of hepatic encephalopathy.

Cerebral edema, observed in many cases of FHF, may occur because of disruption of the blood–brain barrier, expansion of the interstitial space, or failure of cellular autoregulatory (eg, osmotic regulation) mechanisms. Attempts at control of cerebral edema have included steroid and mannitol administration. Steroids do not appear to help, but mannitol may be effective in diminishing intracranial pressure. The therapy for FHF was previously discussed.

## Prognosis

If recovery from FHF occurs, it is usually complete, with no residual hepatic dysfunction. Patients with FHF due to HBV and especially those (45%) HBV with HDV coinfection may have chronic active hepatitis after recovery.

The survival rate is best for patients with FHF due to HAV (60% to 70%) and acetaminophen intoxication (50%). Lowest survival rates are found for those with FHF secondary to non-A, non-B hepatitis and idiosyncratic reactions to halothane (10% to 20%). Multiple prognostic indicators have been proposed. The following factors are associated with a poor prognosis:

Acetaminophen toxicity associated with a pH less than 7.3 (95% mortality), prothrombin time of more than 100 seconds, and a creatinine level of more than 300 $\mu$mol/L with grade 3 encephalopathy (77% mortality)

Viral hepatitis and drug reactions associated with an age of less than 11 or more than 40 years, jaundice more than 7 days before onset of encephalopathy, bilirubin levels higher than 300 $\mu$mol/L, and a prothrombin times greater than 50 seconds

Other proposed variables have included Factor 5 levels less than 20% or Factor 7 levels of less than 8% of controls. Grade 4 coma, renal failure, and major episodes of GI bleeding have been identified as poor prognostic signs in the pediatric population. The decision to transplant is a difficult one and must be based on relative outcomes of FHF and of transplantation. Twenty-eight percent of transplantation candidates die awaiting organs. For those who receive organs, the survival rate is approximately 60%. Transplantation is usually curative. Although patients transplanted secondary to fulminant hepatitis B infection may remain serologically positive, they rarely have clinical disease, unlike those transplanted for chronic HBV. One group suggested the need for transplantation be determined by grade 4 encephalopathy and the need for continued FFP infusions to keep the prothrombin time within 10 seconds of control values.

Hepatocellular failure is the cause of death of 20% of the patients with FHF, and 80% of the deaths are caused by complications, including cerebral edema, GI hemorrhage, and sepsis.

## PORTAL HYPERTENSION

### Etiology and Clinical Presentation

Portal hypertension occurs in children because of obstruction to blood flow at one of several sites. An extrahepatic or presinusoidal block most often occurs in children as a result of obstruction to blood flow in the portal vein or one of its branches. In approximately 40% of children with this lesion, a history of portal vein injury may be elicited. Causes of injury include umbilical vein catheterization, neonatal omphalitis, or surgical trauma. Older children may have a history of abdominal trauma or pancreatitis. Clinical signs at presentation may include abdominal pain, diarrhea, and abdominal distention. Splenomegaly is usually found, although the liver size is normal. Ascites and GI hemorrhage, usually from esophageal varices, may occur. Multiple congenital anomalies, including biliary, cardiovascular, and urinary tract abnormalities, have been associated with this syndrome. Laboratory findings are consistent with hypersplenism: thrombocytopenia, neutropenia, or anemia. Abnormalities of coagulation factors may be detected.

### Diagnosis

Diagnosis is by ultrasound, angiography of the portal venous system, and MRI, all of which are useful in demonstrating the anatomy of the portal venous system. Because intrinsic liver disease must be excluded, hepatic biopsy may be required.

### Prognosis

Hemorrhage from esophageal varices is frequently observed in cases of extrahepatic portal hypertension; in one series, the incidence was 79% of children. Presumably because of relatively intact hepatocellular function, most of these bleeding episodes are well tolerated and may be treated conservatively and with endoscopic sclerotherapy. Portosystemic shunt procedures have also been used, but shunt surgery in young children carries a high rate of failure because of shunt thrombosis. In addition, the long-term risk of encephalopathy exists. In affected children, bleeding episodes usually decrease in frequency with age, often

ceasing entirely in the third decade of life, presumably because of the development of effective collateral circulation.

### Alternate Forms

Other forms of portal hypertension include those caused by intrahepatic sinusoidal lesions and those secondary to postsinusoidal defects. Examples of the former include portal hypertension associated with hepatic cirrhosis due to $\alpha_1$-antitrypsin deficiency, congenital hepatic fibrosis, or Wilson's disease. Examples of the latter include Budd-Chiari-like syndromes (eg, obstruction of the inferior vena cava at the level of the diaphragm, hepatic venous occlusion due to vasculitis, tumor, masses, or polycythemia). Other causes of postsinusoidal block include hepatic veno-occlusive disease, typically associated with bone marrow transplantation, and constrictive pericarditis with resultant relative obstruction to vena caval flow.

## VARICEAL HEMORRHAGE

Anastomoses between the systemic and splanchnic venous circulations occur throughout the abdomen. These include connections between the spleen and kidneys and between the mesenteric and gonadal veins. Other connections are found in the areas of the rectum and, most important clinically, in the region of the gastroesophageal junction. Esophageal varices are submucosal veins that connect the azygos and hemiazygos veins to the portal circulation. When portal hypertension occurs, flow develops from the high-pressure portal venous system through these vessels with resultant vessel dilation. Factors predisposing to variceal hemorrhage include portal venous pressure gradients of at least 12 mm Hg, decreasing thickness of varix walls, increasing variceal transmural pressure, and increasing varix radii. Large, thin-walled vessels are more likely to bleed than small varices. Not all patients with these varices have episodes of hemorrhage. Other risk factors for variceal hemorrhage include ingestion of salicylate- and ethanol-containing products.

### Clinical Manifestations

The clinical manifestations of portal hypertension include splenomegaly and, in some cases, hepatomegaly. Caput medusae (ie, dilated abdominal wall veins) may develop. Variceal hemorrhage typically manifests as painless, massive hematemesis. Blood may be passed rectally as hematochezia or as melena. The patient may be known through prior studies, including barium swallow or upper endoscopy, to have esophageal varices. The precise diagnosis in the patient who presents with acute upper GI tract bleeding must await hemodynamic stabilization. After this has been accomplished, the site of bleeding should be ascertained through endoscopy of the esophagus, stomach, and duodenum. Endoscopy should be performed on an emergency basis, but only in a well-controlled environment, such as an intensive care unit or an operating room. Airway protection may be necessary. The differential diagnosis includes gastritis, Mallory-Weiss tears, and peptic ulcer disease.

### Treatment

Gastric lavage is performed before and after endoscopy, usually with saline to remove large blood clots. There is no clear advantage to lavage with chilled fluids, and this procedure may result in significant hypothermia in the pediatric patient. Intravascular volume replacement is administered as needed, with care taken to avoid overadministration of sodium or of volume, which can worsen the variceal hemorrhage. Monitoring the central venous pressure may be useful in this regard. Replacement of erythrocytes, clotting factors, and platelets may be required. Vital signs must be checked frequently.

These measures are sufficient to control variceal hemorrhage in most children. If hemorrhage continues, vasopressin should be administered intravenously. Vasopressin is a nonspecific vasoconstrictor that reduces blood flow through splenic, gastric, and intestinal arterioles; portal venous pressure is reduced. Vasopressin can be administered as a bolus dose initially; subsequently, a continuous infusion is administered for 12 to 24 hours, and the dosage is slowly tapered. Intra-arterial administration of vasopressin has no advantage over intravenous administration. Side effects, more common in adults than in children, include myocardial infarction and ischemic bowel disease.

Another pharmacologic agent that has been proposed in the management of variceal hemorrhage is nitroglycerin, which, given in concert with vasopressin, may further decrease portal pressure and ameliorate the side effects of vasopressin therapy. There are few data on this combination in pediatric patients. Somatostatin may reduce splanchnic blood flow in man and has minimal systemic side effects but has not been used in children. Propranolol has been used to prevent initial and recurrent variceal hemorrhage in adults. Limited data suggest that this agent may be effective in decreasing portal pressure in children with portal hypertension. However, during acute hemorrhage, propranolol decreases cardiac output and heart rate and is contraindicated.

Continuing hemorrhage after vasopressin administration is an indication for balloon tamponade of varices with the Sengstaken-Blakemore tube. This form of therapy controls hemorrhage in 40% to 80% of patients. In some cases, hemorrhage is controlled with inflation of only the gastric balloon in conjunction with traction on the tube. Balloon tamponade is associated with a relatively high incidence of rebleeding, as high as 60% in some series. Potential side effects of therapy include pulmonary aspiration if the airway is left unprotected, esophageal rupture, and suffocation.

Sclerotherapy, a technique in which a sclerosing agent such as ethanol or sodium tetradecyl sulfate is injected into or around esophageal varices through an endoscope, is most often performed after the patient's medical condition has stabilized. Variceal hemorrhage is controlled in 80% to 95% of patients treated. Subsequent injections are required to obliterate varices. Rebleeding may occur in as many as one third of patients during the course of sclerotherapy. Studies comparing sclerotherapy with shunt surgery in adults suggest that the two modalities are similar in terms of patient survival; those receiving shunts appear more likely to develop hepatic encephalopathy, and those receiving sclerotherapy are more likely to have repeated episodes of variceal hemorrhage, some requiring shunt procedures. Studies suggest that sclerotherapy is safe and effective in children; sclerosant volumes are lower than those used in adults. Emergent sclerotherapy as a method of bleeding control may also be indicated. Prophylactic sclerotherapy has also been used in adults before the first episode of variceal hemorrhage, but this procedure is not recommended. Sclerotherapy, although generally safe, may cause esophageal perforation and stricture. Long-term control of bleeding from gastric varices may not be achieved by this technique.

Other methods of controlling variceal hemorrhage include the nsurgical creation of a portal-systemic shunt and transthoracic ligation of esophageal varices. Although portosystemic shunts have occasionally been successfully used in children, they are technically difficult to perform in young children. Success rates are limited by the small vessel size, and shunt surgery carries a high mortality rate, especially when performed as an emergency procedure. Hepatic encephalopathy may occur in the postoperative period, even with a technically successful shunt. Shunt surgery may make future attempts at hepatic transplantation more difficult. Percutaneously placed intrahepatic shunts may alleviate this difficulty, although relatively few have been performed in children.

Good results have been reported with the Sigiura and modified Sigiura procedures, consisting of esophageal transection with devascularization. Rebleeding episodes appear to be rare (approximately 2%) and encephalopathy does not occur. This procedure may be an option for children with variceal bleeding, but large series in the United States have not been reported.

## ASCITES

Ascites, a collection of free fluid within the peritoneal cavity, is frequently seen in patients with cirrhosis and portal hypertension. Physical examination findings consistent with ascites include recent enlargement of abdominal girth, protuberance of the umbilicus, and shifting dullness of physical examination; a "fluid wave" may be detected.

### Pathophysiology

Multiple factors interplay in the cause of ascites in patients with portal hypertension. The underfill theory of ascites formation suggests that, in the presence of portal hypertension, an imbalance of Starling forces develops in the splanchnic circulation and in the hepatic sinusoids, leading to excess production of lymph. This fluid may accumulate in the peritoneal cavity in the form of ascites. The plasma volume is redistributed out of the vascular space, with a resultant decrease in the effective circulating volume. The diminished effective volume causes renal sodium and water resorption in an effort to augment circulating volume, perpetuating the process and resulting in further accumulation of ascites. An alternative hypothesis, the overflow theory of ascites, postulates that the primary defect is impaired renal excretion of sodium with subsequent expansion of plasma volume before the formation of ascites. In this scenario, a combination of increased portal pressure and decreased plasma oncotic pressure (decreased serum albumin) leads to an imbalance of Starling forces, with the subsequent accumulation of ascites. These mechanisms are not mutually exclusive, and the cause of the avid sodium retention seen in patients with advanced hepatic disease is presumably multifactorial. Increased urine and serum levels of aldosterone may be found in patients with chronic liver disease. Prostaglandin E metabolism may be altered in cirrhotic patients with resultant sodium retention. Increased sympathetic nervous system activity may lead to sodium retention. Abnormalities in atrial natriuretic factor excretion or metabolism may play a role.

### Diagnosis

Ascites may be diagnosed from historic evidence of chronic liver disease associated with compatible physical examination findings. Radiographic signs of ascites may include diffuse "haziness" of the abdomen, displacement of bowel loops medially, indistinct hepatic margins, and displacement of the lateral liver border medially. Abdominal ultrasound or CT scans may confirm the presence of ascites. Diagnostic paracentesis should be performed in all patients with new-onset ascites to rule out acute peritonitis. Useful studies include peritoneal fluid polymorphonuclear cell count (ie, >500 cells/U suggest peritonitis), Gram stain, and total protein, glucose, and lactate dehydrogenase levels.

### Treatment

Ascites is difficult to treat in children with liver disease. Marked accumulation of ascites may be associated with discomfort, dyspnea, anorexia, and gastroesophageal reflux. Control of ascites, although not shown to prolong life, may result in improved patient comfort. Effective therapy must be aimed at the altered renal handling of salt and water in liver disease. Dietary sodium intake usually is limited to 1 to 2 mEq/kg/day as a first step, but the restriction of dietary sodium must be tempered by the necessity of maintaining adequate caloric intake. Fluid restriction typically is not required in patients with adequate urine output and in whom there is no hyponatremia.

If sodium restriction is insufficient to produce diuresis, pharmacologic therapy may be required. The goal of diuretic therapy is to inhibit renal sodium retention and produce a gradual diuresis without simultaneously decreasing circulating plasma volume. In adults, the maximal rate of peritoneal ascitic fluid absorption is approximately 700 to 900 mL/day. Diuresis of more than 900 mL/day results in volume contraction, with the attendant risks of renal insufficiency and hyperkalemia. Accompanying edema may allow more rapid diuresis. Similar data are unavailable in children. Therapy usually is initiated with spironolactone, an inhibitor of aldosterone, which is begun in a dosage of 2 to 3 mg/kg/day. Spironolactone acts on the distal tubule and is potassium sparing. Diuresis usually occurs within 3 to 5 days of therapy initiation; adequate response may be confirmed by achievement of an elevation of the urine sodium to potassium ratio above 1. If the response is inadequate, the dose may be doubled, or an additional diuretic agent with a proximal tubular site of action, such as a thiazide, furosemide, or ethacrynic acid, may be added. Complications of diuretic agents include hypokalemia, hyponatremia, and if circulating vascular volume is decreased, renal insufficiency and encephalopathy. Urine and serum electrolyte concentrations must be followed carefully.

Paracentesis is usually not recommended except as a diagnostic measure. However, large-volume paracentesis followed by intravenous colloid (ie, albumin) infusion is a safe and effective method of removing ascites in adults. Until similar data have been accrued for the pediatric age group, this method cannot be recommended for children, except for relief of significant respiratory compromise.

## HEPATORENAL SYNDROME

The hepatorenal syndrome denotes the occurrence of unexplained progressive renal disease in patients with hepatic disease. The hepatorenal syndrome occurs in patients with ascites and portal hypertension after a precipitating event, most often one producing a decrease in circulating plasma volume. Laboratory features include a low urine sodium in conjunction with azotemia. The differential diagnosis of oliguria in the cirrhotic patient also includes prerenal causes and acute tubular necrosis; if acute tubular necrosis is present, support with dialysis is necessary until renal function returns.

There is no specific therapy for hepatorenal syndrome, but sodium and fluid intake should be limited. Dialysis may be useful for patients with acute hepatic dysfunction in whom adequate hepatic function is expected to return. The prognosis of the patient with hepatorenal syndrome and chronic liver disease is poor, and transplantation should be considered.

## HEPATIC TRANSPLANTATION

With the availability of the immunosuppressive agent cyclosporine, liver transplantation has become a viable option for many patients with acute fulminant hepatic failure and chronic hepatic disease. Potential candidates for liver transplantation include those with the following conditions.

Diseases after a progressive, irreversible, downhill course, such as biliary atresia after a failed Kasai procedure

Decompensated hepatic disease, especially if accompanied by life-threatening complications, such as ascites with spontaneous bacterial peritonitis and variceal hemorrhage

Intractable pruritus or severe metabolic bone disease with resultant social invalidism

Diseases for which no alternative therapy is available, such as the type I Crigler-Najjar syndrome.

Contraindications to liver transplantation include unresectable extrahepatic primary malignancy, malignancy metastatic to the liver, or terminal disease uncorrectable by liver transplantation. Disorders in children for which liver transplantation may be required include biliary atresia, tyrosinemia, $\alpha_1$-antitrypsin deficiency, neonatal hepatitis (rarely), fulminant hepatic failure, and Wilson's disease with fulminant hepatic failure.

Survival rates after liver transplantation range from 60% to 90%. Slightly lower rates of survival are reported for infants younger than 1 year of age and weighing 5 to 10 kg. Size is a major limiting factor in transplantation because of technical difficulties and because of the lack of donors weighing less than 10 kg. Newer technologies, including split liver transplants and the use of living related donors, are partially ameliorating the problem.

Potential complications of liver transplantation include hepatic artery thrombosis, graft necrosis, biliary anastomotic leakage, GI bleeding, and GI perforation. Viral and bacterial sepsis may occur. Despite immunosuppression with cyclosporine, episodes of rejection may occur. Treatment of these episodes includes bolus administration of corticosteroids and, if needed, additional immunosuppressive agents, including monoclonal antilymphocyte antibody preparations.

Despite these limitations, liver transplantation is a lifesaving and potentially curative procedure for many patients with hepatic disease. Follow-up of children who have undergone liver transplantation entails careful monitoring of cyclosporine levels and hypertension, which often occurs after liver transplantation. Episodes of rejection must be quickly differentiated from episodes of viral hepatitis, ordinarily by percutaneous hepatic biopsy. Additional psychosocial issues arise as the patient and his or her family returns to their social environment. The use of newer immunosuppressive agents, including FK506, may further enhance the success of hepatic transplantation and allow multiple organ (ie, gut and liver) transplantation.

## BILIARY TRACT DISEASE

Primary sclerosing cholangitis (PSC) is a disorder characterized by inflammation and subsequent fibrosis of the hepatobiliary system. The term implies the absence of other biliary lesions, including postsurgical abnormalities, choledocholithiasis, and bile duct carcinoma. Reports suggest that PSC is much more common in children and in adults than was previously recognized.

The epidemiology of PSC in childhood is uncertain. In adults, 50% to 80% of patients with PSC have idiopathic inflammatory bowel disease, usually chronic ulcerative colitis, and approximately 4% to 5% of patients with inflammatory bowel disease have PSC. Young men are most commonly affected. The limited experience in children suggests a slight male predominance and an association with chronic ulcerative colitis.

### Clinical Presentation

The clinical features at presentation vary widely. In adults, the insidious onset of fatigue and pruritus is followed by jaundice. In children, abdominal pain, fever, jaundice, and pruritus all have been reported as presenting features. PSC has been diagnosed before the onset of symptoms through abnormal hepatic function tests in the setting of inflammatory bowel disease. Patients may present with hepatomegaly or hepatosplenomegaly with or without jaundice. One or more of these findings usually are seen in 50% to 75% of patients at presentation.

## Laboratory Features

Children and adults with PSC usually have elevated serum alkaline phosphatase and γ-GTP levels; both are markers of cholestasis. The serum bilirubin level may or may not be elevated. Serum aminotransferase levels often are only moderately increased. In children, serum immunoglobulin levels may be elevated, and serum antinuclear antibodies and anti-smooth muscle antibodies are more commonly found in children with PSC than in adults. Hepatic copper levels usually are elevated in adults with PSC, as are urinary copper excretion, serum ceruloplasmin levels, and serum copper levels. These biochemical features have not been sufficiently studied in children with PSC.

## Radiologic Features

The radiologic features of PSC reflect the progressive injury of bile ducts that is characteristic of this disorder. Endoscopic retrograde cholangiography is usually performed to visualize the biliary tree. Other potentially useful techniques include percutaneous transhepatic cholangiography and, in rare cases, operative cholangiography. Typical radiographic features of PSC include diffuse, 1- to 2-cm strictures of the intrahepatic and extrahepatic biliary systems, often with intervening, slightly dilated segments, producing a beaded appearance. Narrow band-like strictures may be seen, as may diverticulum-like outpouchings. Similar changes may be found in immunodeficient patients and those with histiocytosis.

## Hepatic Pathology

Histologic abnormalities in PSC include periductal fibrosis and inflammation with subsequent ductal obliteration. The course of PSC can be divided into four stages:

1. Enlargement of portal tracts, with edema, increased connective tissue and bile duct proliferation; mild inflammation may be present
2. Growth of fibrous tissue into the periportal parenchyma
3. Formation of fibrotic septa
4. Biliary cirrhosis.

It is thought that the finding of "pericholangitis" on hepatic biopsy in a patient with inflammatory bowel disease represents PSC of the small bile ducts. Pathologically, the liver of children with PSC may exhibit inflammation and piecemeal necrosis, and the condition may be mistaken for chronic active hepatitis. Histologic cholestasis may be less common in children than in adults.

## Pathogenesis

Theories proposing a role for bacterial or viral infections or for specific bile duct toxins are not supported by the evidence. However, an immunologic cause is strongly suggested by the elevated serum IgG levels and autoantibody positivity in childhood PSC. Supportive evidence includes a positive association with HLA-B8 and HLA-DR3, the presence of circulating immune complexes, and the apparent T-lymphocyte-mediated destruction of bile ducts observed in PSC. The precise mechanism of pathogenicity is unknown.

## Therapy

No specific therapy for PSC is available. In patients with associated chronic ulcerative colitis, proctocolectomy does not appear to favorably influence the course of PSC, and peristomal varices may form in patients so treated. Penicillamine, a copper-chelating agent, proved to be of no benefit in a controlled trial. Limited experience using ursodeoxycholic acid therapy suggests at least a transient improvement in symptoms and biochemical abnormalities.

The usefulness of other immunosuppressive agents (eg, corticosteroids, azathioprine, cyclosporine) and of antifibrogenic agents (eg, colchicine) has not been prospectively evaluated. Episodes of cholangitis may occur and should be vigorously treated. Dominant stricture formation may occur, accompanied by increases in serum bilirubin levels and episodes of cholangitis. Conservative management of these strictures in adult patients has included transhepatic or endoscopic balloon dilation. Cholangiocarcinoma may occur in 10% to 15% of patients with PSC. Orthotopic liver transplantation is a viable alternative for patients with advanced disease. PSC usually does not appear to recur in recipients of liver transplants.

The prognosis for patients with PSC is highly variable. Early studies showed PSC to be a relentlessly progressive disorder, with a mean period of 57 months from diagnosis to death. Later studies suggest the existence of a subgroup of patients who do well, with a 9-year survival rate of 75%. The prognosis of children with PSC is unknown.

Other hepatobiliary disorders associated with inflammatory bowel disease include steatosis, chronic active hepatitis, hepatic granulomas, cholelithiasis, and occlusion of the portal or hepatic veins.

## SPONTANEOUS PERFORATION OF THE COMMON BILE DUCT

Spontaneous perforation of the common bile duct typically is detected in the first 3 months of life. Symptoms of infants at and before diagnosis include failure to thrive, irritability, vomiting, and acholic stools. Physical examination may reveal jaundice and sometimes find abdominal distention, often with bile-stained hydrocele and hernia sacs secondary to the bile-stained ascites. Laboratory features may include leukocytosis and conjugated hyperbilirubinemia. Serum aminotransferase values may be mildly elevated. The diagnosis may be suggested by hepatobiliary scintigraphy, which demonstrates tracer activity outside the biliary tract. Paracentesis may yield bile-stained ascitic fluid.

The diagnosis depends on demonstration of a bile duct perforation at the time of operative cholangiography. The perforation typically is at the junction of the cystic and common bile ducts, which suggest an area of developmental weakness at this site. The hepatic pathology is nonspecific in this condition: cholestasis may be present, portal tracts may be edematous, and bile duct proliferation is occasionally found.

Surgical therapy is required; drainage with or without suture closure of the perforation has been recommended. Alternatively, internal drainage through a roux-en-Y loop anastomosis to the gallbladder has been recommended in some infants.

## CYSTIC DISEASES OF THE LIVER

Cystic diseases of the liver include choledochal cysts, autosomal recessive and dominant forms of polycystic kidney disease, congenital hepatic fibrosis, and Caroli's disease. Although similar pathologic features may occur in several of these disorders, differences in the manner of inheritance and distinct morphometric and clinical features suggest that the disorders have separate causes.

## Choledochal Cysts

Choledochal cysts occur in as many as 2% of infants with obstructive jaundice. This potentially correctable lesion must be sought in all cholestatic infants.

### Clinical Features

Choledochal cysts may manifest at any age. There is a 3 : 1 female predominance. The infantile form usually presents in the first few months of age with jaundice and acholic stools; hepatomegaly may develop. A palpable abdominal mass may be found in as many as 60% of these patients. Approximately 50% of infants experience vomiting and failure to thrive. Infants with choledochal cysts have various degrees of hepatic impairment at diagnosis. Those with cirrhosis and portal hypertension usually have a poor prognosis despite cyst resection.

Children older than 2 years of age may present with the classic signs of abdominal pain (often secondary to pancreatitis), jaundice, and an abdominal mass, but all three findings are present in fewer than 25% of affected patients. Episodes of recurrent cholangitis may also occur. Hepatic injury due to obstruction caused by the cyst is usually less severe in patients who are first seen at an older age; their prognosis is better. Abnormalities of the pancreatic duct are common in patients with late-onset choledochal cysts, as are coexisting hepatic and biliary anomalies, including double common duct, double gallbladder, and accessory hepatic ducts. Biliary and pancreatic calculi may be detected.

### Pathology

Five types of choledochal cysts have been described (Fig 139-6). Type I cysts (93%) represent fusiform dilation of the extrahepatic bile ducts. Type II cysts (6%) are diverticula of the extrahepatic bile duct. Type III cysts (2%) are choledochoceles of the distal common duct. Type IV cysts are similar to type I cysts, but in addition to fusiform dilation of the extrahepatic duct, intrahepatic and extrahepatic duct cysts or extrahepatic cysts are present. In type V cysts, there may be one or more cystic dilatations of the intrahepatic bile ducts. Hepatic pathology depends in part on age at diagnosis. In infants, the hepatic pathology resembles that seen in biliary atresia. Prolonged obstruction may result in cirrhosis with portal hypertension or recurrent pancreatitis.

### Pathogenesis

The pathogenesis of choledochal cysts is unknown. Theories formulated to explain the features of this disorder include the possibility that the cysts are congenital malformations or that they are acquired as a result of injury to bile duct walls from infection or pancreatic enzymes. Choledochal cysts may also be part of the spectrum of idiopathic neonatal cholangiopathy.

### Diagnosis

The diagnosis of choledochal cysts is usually made with ultrasonography, which has demonstrated choledochal cysts in utero. Other potentially useful techniques include radionuclide scintigraphy, CT scans, endoscopic retrograde cholangiopancreatography, and percutaneous transhepatic cholangiography.

### Therapy

Therapy usually involves surgical excision of the cyst. A Roux-en-Y loop of jejunum is used to drain the proximal duct system. Cholangitis may occur postoperatively, and the development of malignancy in retained cystic tissue is a risk.

## Infantile Polycystic Disease

The infantile form of polycystic liver disease is inherited in an autosomal recessive fashion. Affected infants may present with bilateral flank masses, hepatomegaly, splenomegaly, oligohydramnios, pulmonary hypoplasia, proteinuria, and hematuria. The kidneys are massively enlarged, and there are cystic dilatations of the collecting tubules. Renal fibrosis, scant at first, increases with time. Hepatic changes parallel those in the kidney. Macroscopic cysts are rarely observed. Microscopic examination reveals cystic dilation of ductules in the periphery of the portal zone and portal fibrosis that increases with age. The number of bile ducts is increased. This lesion appears to be distinct from that seen in congenital hepatic fibrosis.

Infantile polycystic disease of the liver and kidney is diagnosed from the ultrasound appearance or with excretory urography. Liver biopsy and renal biopsy may also be useful. Survival usually is limited by the presence of severe pulmonary or renal disease.

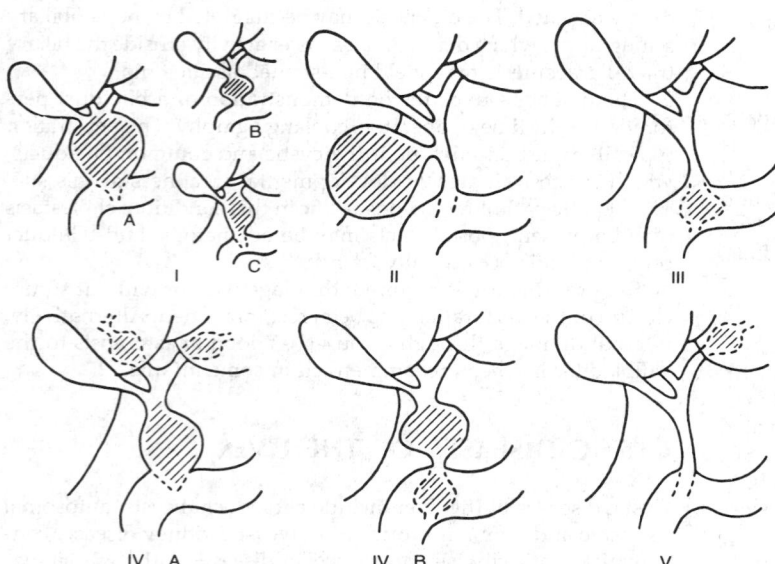

**Figure 139-6.**   Classification of choledochal cysts.

Hepatic function is typically well maintained. Portal hypertension may occur in long-term survivors.

## Congenital Hepatic Fibrosis

Congenital hepatic fibrosis appears to be inherited in an autosomal recessive fashion, although sporadic cases occur. The hepatic lesion is characterized by broad bands of periportal or perilobular fibrous tissue surrounding irregularly shaped islands of normal hepatocytes. These bands of fibrous tissue may contain clusters of distorted biliary duct elements, sometimes described as bile duct hamartomas, that appear to communicate with the biliary tree. Portal venous anomalies may exist. Renal anomalies occur frequently in this disorder. The most common associated lesion is renal tubular ectasia. Another associated lesion resembles that seen in adult polycystic kidney disease. Nephronophthisis may be associated with hepatic findings of congenital hepatic fibrosis; these patients have severe, progressive renal disease.

The signs and symptoms of congenital hepatic fibrosis usually begin in childhood and include hepatomegaly and splenomegaly. Indices of hepatic function, including serum albumin levels and prothrombin time, are normal, as are serum bilirubin and aminotransferase values. Portal hypertension is common, and hemorrhage from esophageal varices may occur. A subset of patients with congenital hepatic fibrosis and associated bile duct dilation may experience repeated episodes of cholangitis and microabscess formation. Biliary calculi may form.

Medical management of patients with congenital hepatic fibrosis is directed toward the consequences of portal hypertension. For example, endoscopic sclerotherapy is used in those with variceal hemorrhage. Vigorous treatment of episodes of cholangitis is necessary.

Syndromes associated with hepatic lesions similar to those in congenital hepatic fibrosis include Meckel's syndrome (ie, encephalocele, polydactyly, cystic renal disease), Jeune syndrome, Ellis-van Creveld syndrome, Ivemark syndrome, and tuberous sclerosis.

## Caroli's Disease

Caroli's disease is characterized by saccular dilation of the intrahepatic bile ducts, absence of portal hypertension or cirrhosis, and a high incidence of cholangitis and lithiasis. Renal cystic disease may be associated with the liver disease. Overlap exists between Caroli's disease and congenital hepatic fibrosis with intrahepatic biliary duct dilation, and type IV and V choledochal cysts may share certain features.

Patients with Caroli's disease often present in childhood with episodes of abdominal pain, fever, jaundice, and tender hepatomegaly, attributable to episodes of cholangitis. Laboratory features include elevated serum alkaline phosphatase and conjugated bilirubin levels. Ultrasound or CT scans may suggest the diagnosis. Percutaneous transhepatic cholangiography is useful in determining the extent of disease.

Episodes of cholangitis require antibiotic therapy. Biliary calculi may necessitate surgery. Disease localized to a single lobe of the liver may be treated by partial hepatectomy. Other surgical drainage procedures have been used, with variable results. Cholangiocarcinoma has been reported in patients with Caroli's disease.

## GALLBLADDER DISEASE

### Hydrops

Hydrops of the gallbladder denotes noninflammatory, noncalculous distention of the gallbladder, often associated with illnesses such as scarlet fever, familial Mediterranean fever, polyarteritis nodosa, leptospirosis, and Kawasaki disease. Patients receiving long-term parenteral nutrition may have acute distention of the gallbladder, presumably secondary to prolonged fasting. Affected children present with abdominal pain (100%), vomiting (75%), right upper quadrant tenderness (93%), and a palpable mass (55%); fever rarely occurs. The differential diagnosis includes intussusception, appendiceal abscess, and acute acalculous cholecystitis. The diagnosis is confirmed with ultrasound.

### Pathogenesis

Postulated causes of hydrops include vasculitis or serositis of the gallbladder, aggravated by bile stasis. In other cases, enlarged mesenteric lymph nodes may obstruct the cystic duct. Hydrops in the newborn may be related to transient plugging of the ductal system.

### Therapy

Conservative therapy is indicated in most cases of mucocutaneous lymph node syndrome and cases of parenteral nutrition-related gallbladder dilation. In other cases, cholecystotomy or cholecystectomy has been necessary because of impending gallbladder perforation. Typically, green, black, or white bile is drained from the acutely dilated gallbladder; no stones are found, and bile cultures are sterile. The lack of inflammation in the gallbladder wall differentiates this disorder from acute acalculous cholecystitis.

## Acute Acalculous Cholecystitis

Acute acalculous cholecystitis accounts for 5% to 15% of cases of cholecystitis in adults and 5% to 30% of cases in children. Clinical features include jaundice (approximately 30%), abdominal pain (95%), fever, anorexia, nausea, and vomiting. The acute onset of right-sided abdominal tenderness suggests this diagnosis. The differential diagnosis includes appendicitis, intussusception, calculous cholecystitis, and peritonitis. Laboratory features include hyperbilirubinemia, leukocytosis, and elevated serum alkaline phosphatase levels.

Acute acalculous cholecystitis has been associated with severe trauma and has been seen in postoperative patients. Associated autoimmune disorders include systemic lupus erythematosus, diabetes mellitus, and rheumatoid arthritis, which suggests that vasculitis underlies the lesion. Anatomical anomalies of the cystic duct may also be associated with hydrops. Acalculous cholecystitis has also been related to TPN, but most cases appear to be associated with infection. Specific organisms include *Salmonella*, group A and B streptococci, parasites such as *Giardia lamblia* and *Ascaris*, and tuberculosis.

Ultrasound scans can confirm the diagnosis of acute acalculous cholecystitis. Radionuclide scintigraphy and CT scans may be useful.

Treatment of this disorder involves cholecystectomy and the treatment of any systemic infection. The gallbladder mucosa is edematous and demonstrates an inflammatory infiltrate. The gallbladder bile is usually sterile on culture.

## Cholelithiasis

Cholelithiasis is less common in children than in adults, and in many affected children, a specific cause can be identified. The clinical presentation varies, and gallstones often are discovered in asymptomatic patients undergoing abdominal examination for other reasons. Symptoms of gallstone disease include abdominal pain, nausea, vomiting, and in older patients, fatty food intolerance. The abdominal pain may resemble colic, may radiate to the right scapula, or in older patients, may localize to the right upper quadrant. Dark urine or jaundice, perhaps secondary to hemolytic anemia, may be noticed; fever rarely occurs.

Pigment stones, composed primarily of calcium bilirubinate in polymeric or monomeric forms, or cholesterol stones may be identified. Several factors may contribute to pigment stone formation, including increased secretion of unconjugated bilirubin into bile or deconjugation of conjugated bilirubin in bile, probably by bacterial $\beta$-glucuronidase.

Hemolytic anemias are associated with pigment stone formation in children. Sickle cell disease is associated with an incidence of gallstone formation of approximately 42% by 18 years of age. Wilson's disease may be associated with stone formation, as may other erythrocyte hemoglobinopathies and enzymopathies. Children receiving long-term TPN may develop pigment stones.

Cholesterol gallstones form in three stages. In stage I, bile becomes supersaturated with cholesterol because of increased biliary secretion of cholesterol or diminished biliary bile acid secretion, perhaps because of increased fecal bile acid losses. The cholesterol-saturated bile must then undergo nucleation or cholesterol crystallization from a saturated solution. Factors that probably add to the risk of cholesterol stone formation include gallbladder stasis, absence of putative inhibitors of gallstone nucleation, including apolipoprotein AI and AII, and the presence of promoters of gallstone nucleation, including mucous glycoproteins.

Cholesterol gallstones in the pediatric population usually occur in adolescent girls; obesity and parity correlate with the incidence of cholelithiasis in these patients. Children with cystic fibrosis, ileal Crohn's disease, and ileal resections have excessive fecal bile acid loss and may form gallstones. Chronic cholestasis also increases the risk of gallstone formation.

### Radiologic Findings

Plain abdominal roentgenograms may reveal pigment (ie, radiopaque) stones. Cholesterol stones are radiolucent. Ultrasound is the method of choice for detecting gallstones, but radionuclide scintigraphy may aid in assessing gallbladder function.

### Therapy

Cholecystectomy is the method of choice for treating symptomatic gallstone disease in children. Operative cholangiography usually is performed at the time of surgery to exclude common duct stones. Laparoscopic cholecystectomy is being used with increasing frequency in children and adolescents. The role of surgery in the child with asymptomatic cholelithiasis is controversial. The course of children with asymptomatic gallstones has not yet been defined, and there are no alternative therapeutic methods available for children. Nonoperative gallstone dissolution with oral chenodeoxycholic acid, fragmentation of stones with extracorporeal shock waves, and biliary tract perfusion with solvents are methods untried in children. The prognosis after gallstone removal is excellent.

## LIVER DYSFUNCTION IN HEART DISEASE

Children and adults with congenital or acquired cardiac disease may have secondary hepatic dysfunction. Congestive heart failure may cause diminished hepatic blood flow and elevated hepatic venous pressure. Midzonal distention, atrophy, and necrosis may then result. Left-sided heart failure leads to diminished cardiac output with resultant decreases in hepatic blood flow. Central zonal hypoxia and necrosis may then follow. Clinical findings include tender hepatomegaly, especially in cases of venous congestion. Laboratory features include prolongation of the pro-

thrombin time, unresponsiveness to vitamin K, and markedly increased aminotransferase and serum bilirubin levels. Hypoglycemia may be severe. Autopsy studies of children with hypoplastic left-sided heart syndrome and coarctation of the aorta have shown a high incidence of hepatic necrosis compared with other forms of congenital heart disease.

## SICKLE CELL DISEASE

Patients with sickle cell anemia are at high risk for hepatic abnormalities. Autopsy studies reveal cirrhosis in 10% of patients with sickle cell disease. The postulated causes of injury include hypoxic injury from sickling, viral hepatitis, gallstones, right-sided heart failure, iron overload, and alcohol and drug abuse. Hepatic sickle cell crisis may occur in as many as 10% of patients admitted to the hospital with sickle cell disease. Manifestations include jaundice, nausea, abdominal pain, and fever. Tender hepatomegaly is often found. Serum aminotransferase and bilirubin values are elevated. Viral hepatitis, fulminant hepatic failure, and gallbladder disease may also occur in patients with sickle cell disease. Children with sickle cell disease may develop extreme hyperbilirubinemia with total serum bilirubin values of 20 mg/dL, presumably due to intrahepatic sickling. These markedly increased levels are not associated with extreme pain, fever, or hemolytic or veno-occlusive crisis. The clinical course of these patients is benign, with gradual resolution of bilirubin values.

## Selected Readings

### Aspects of Hepatic Development

Arey LB. Developmental anatomy, ed 2. Philadelphia: WB Saunders, 1965.

Balistreri WF, Heubi JE, Suchy FJ. Immaturity of the enterohepatic circulation in early life: factors predisposing to ''physiologic'' maldigestion and cholestasis. J Pediatr Gastroenterol Nutr 1983;2:346.

Balistreri WF, Schubert WK. Liver disease in infancy and childhood. In: Schiff L, Schiff ER, eds. Diseases of the liver, ed 6. Philadelphia: JB Lippincott, 1987: 1337–1426.

Carroll BA, Oppenheimer DA, Muller HH. High-frequency real-time ultrasound of the neonatal biliary system. Radiology 1982;145:437.

Castell DO, O'Brien KD, Muench H, et al. Estimation of liver size by percussion in normal individuals. Ann Intern Med 1969;70:1183.

Coppoletta JM, Wolbach SB. Body length and organ weights of infants and children: a study of the body length and normal weights of the more important vital organs of the body between birth and 12 years of age. Am J Pathol 1933;9:55.

Dawkins MJR. The hazards of birth. Adv Reprod Physiol 1966;1:217.

Greengard O. Enzymic differentiation of human liver: comparison with the rat model. Pediatr Res 1977;11:669.

Henning SJ. Postnatal development: coordination of feeding, digestion and metabolism. Am J Physiol 1981;241:G199.

Henschke CI, Goldman H, Teele RL. The hyperechogenic liver in children: cause and sonographic appearance. AJR 1982;138:841.

Kattwinkel J, Taussig LM, Statland BE, Verter JI. The effects of age on alkaline phosphatase and other serologic liver function tests in normal subjects and patients with cystic fibrosis. J Pediatr 1973;82:234.

Knight JA, Haymond RE. γ-Glutamyltransferase and alkaline phosphatase activities compared in serum of normal children and children with liver disease. Clin Chem 1981;27:48.

Lawson EE, Grand RJ, Neff RK, Cohen LF. Clinical estimation of liver span in infants and children. Am J Dis Child 1978;132:474.

McGahan JP, Phillips HE, Cox KL. Sonography of the normal pediatric gallbladder and biliary tract. Radiology 1982;144:873.

McNicholl B. Palpability of the liver and spleen in infants and children. Arch Dis Child 1957;32:438.

Meites S, ed. Pediatric clinical chemistry: a survey of reference (normal) values, methods, and instrumentation, with commentary, ed 3. Washington, DC: American Association for Clinical Chemistry, 1988.

Reiff MI, Osborn LM. Clinical estimation of liver size in newborn infants. Pediatrics 1983;71:46.

Rylance GW, Moreland TA, Cowan MD, Clark DC. Liver volume estimation using ultrasound scanning. Arch Dis Child 1982;57:283.

Soyka LF, Redmond GP, eds. Drug metabolism in the immature human. New York: Raven Press, 1981.

Wu JT, Book L, Sudar K. Serum alpha-fetoprotein (AFP) levels in normal infants. Pediatr Res 1981;15:50.

Younoszai MK, Mueller S. Clinical assessment of liver size in normal children. Clin Pediatr 1975;14:378.

## Parenteral Nutrition-Related Cholestasis

Balistreri WF, Novak DA, Farrel MK. Bile acid metabolism, total parenteral nutrition and cholestasis. In: Lebenthal E, ed. Total parenteral nutrition in children: indications, complications, and pathophysiologic considerations. New York: Raven Press, 1986:319.

Farrell MK, Balistreri WF. Parenteral nutrition and hepatobiliary dysfunction. Clin Perinatol 1986;13:197.

Merritt RJ, TPN-associated cholestasis. J Pediatr Gastroenterol Nutr 1986;5:12.

## Metabolic Disease

Berger R, Smith GPA, Stoker-de Vries SA, et al. Deficiency of fumarylacetoacetase in a patient with hereditary tyrosinemia. Clin Chim Acta 1981;114:37.

Burton BK. Inborn errors of metabolism: the clinical diagnosis in early infancy. Pediatrics 1987;79:359.

Glew RH, Basu A, Prence EM, et al. Biology of disease: lysosomal storage diseases. Lab Invest 1985;53:250.

Hostetter MK, Levy HL, Winter HS, et al. Evidence for liver disease preceding amino acid abnormalities in hereditary tyrosinemia. N Engl J Med 1983;308:1265.

Mock DM, Perman JA, Thaler MM, et al. Chronic fructose intoxication after infancy in children with hereditary fructose intolerance; a cause of growth retardation. N Engl J Med 193;309:764.

Odievre M, Gentile C, Gautier M, et al. Hereditary fructose intolerance in children: diagnosis, management and course in 55 patients. Am J Dis Child 1978;132:605.

## Glycogen Storage Disease

Chen Y, Cornblath M, Sidbury J. Cornstarch therapy in type 1 glycogen storage disease. N Engl J Med 1984;310:171.

Greene HL. Glycogen storage disease. Semin Liver Dis 1982;2:291.

Schwenk W, Haymond M. Optimal rate of enteral glucose administration in children with glycogen storage disease type 1. N Engl J Med 1986;314:682.

Williams JC. Nutritional goals in glycogen storage diseases. N Engl J Med 1986;314:709.

## Wilson's Disease

Czaja MJ, Weiner FR, Schwarzenberg SJ, et al. Molecular studies of ceruloplasmin deficiency in Wilson's disease. J Clin Invest 1987;80:1200.

Gollan JL. Treatment of Wilson's disease: in D-penicillamine we trust—what about zinc? Hepatology 1987;7:593.

Riely CA. Wilson's disease. Pediatr Rev 1984;5:217.

Scheinberg IH, Jaffe ME, Sternlieb I. The use of trientine in preventing the effects of interrupting penicillamine therapy in Wilson's disease. N Engl J Med 1987;317:209.

Walshe JM. The liver in Wilson's disease. In: Schiff L, Schiff ER, eds. Diseases of the liver. ed 6. Philadelphia: JB Lippincott, 1987;1037.

## Cystic Fibrosis

Isenberg JN. Cystic fibrosis: its influence on the liver, biliary tree, and bile salt metabolism. Semin Liver Dis 1982;2:302.

Park RW, Grand RJ. Gastrointenstinal manifestations of cystic fibrosis: a review. Gastroenterology 1981;81:1143.

## $\alpha_1$-Antitrypsin Deficiency

Garver RI, Mornex J, Nukiwa T, et al. Alpha-1-antitrypsin deficiency and emphysema caused by homozygous inheritance of nonexpressing alpha-1-antitrypsin genes. N Engl J Med 1986;314:762.

Sveger T. Liver disease in alpha-1-antitrypsin deficiency detected by screening of 200,000 infants. N Engl J Med 1976;294:1316.

Udall JN, Dixon M, Newman AP, et al. Liver disease in alpha-1-antitrypsin deficiency: a retrospective analysis of the influence of early breast vs. bottle feeding. JAMA 1985;253:2679.

Wewers MD, Casolaro A, Sellers SE, et al. Replacement therapy for alpha-1-antitrypsin deficiency associated with emphysema. N Engl J Med 1987;316:1005.

## Hyperammonemia

Brusilow SW, Batshaw ML, Waber L. Neonatal hyperammonemic coma. Adv Pediatr 1982;29:69.

Brusilow SW, Danney M, Waber LJ, et al. Treatment of episodic hyperammonemia in children with inborn errors of urea synthesis. N Engl J Med 1984;310:1630.

Flannery DB, Hsia VE, Wolf B. Current status of hyperammonemic syndromes. Hepatology 1982;2:495.

Hudak ML, Jones MD, Brusilow SW. Differentiation of transient hyperammonemia of the newborn and urea cycle enzyme defects by clinical presentation. J Pediatr 1985;107:712.

## Reye's Syndrome and Mimickers

Heubi JE, Daugherty CC, Partin JS, et al. Grade 1 Reye's syndrome: outcome and predictors of progression to deeper coma grades. N Engl J Med 1984;331:1539.

Heubi JE, Partin JC, Partin JS, et al. Reye's syndrome: current concepts. Hepatology 1987;7:155.

Hurwitz ES, Barrett MJ, Bregman D, et al. Public Health Service Study of Reye's syndrome and medications: report of the main study. JAMA 1987;257:1905.

Stanley CA. New genetic defects in mitochondrial fatty acid oxidation and carnitine deficiency. Adv Pediatr 1987;34:59.

Vianey-Liaud C, Divry P, Gregersen N, et al. The inborn errors of mitochondrial fatty acid oxidation. J Inherit Metab Dis 1987;10:159.

## Hepatitis

Balistreri WF. Viral hepatitis. Pediatr Clin North Am 1988;35:637.

Chang M-H, Hwang L-Y, Hsu H-C, et al. Prospective study of asymptomatic HBsAg carrier children infected in the perinatal period: clinical and liver histologic studies. Hepatology 1988;8:374.

Chen D-S, Hsu N H-M, Sung J-L, et al. A mass vaccination program in Taiwan against hepatitis B virus infection in infants of hepatitis B surface antigen-carrier mothers. JAMA 1987;257:2597.

Davis GL, Hoofnagle JH. Reactivation of chronic hepatitis B virus infection. Gastroenterology 1987;92:2028.

DiBisceglie AM, Rustigi VK, Hoofnagel JH, et al. Hepatocellular carcinoma. Ann Intern Med 1988;108:390.

Hoofnagle JH, Mullen KD, Jones DB, et al. Treatment of chronic non-A, non-B hepatitis with recombinant human alpha interferon. N Engl J Med 1986;315:1575.

Hoofnagle JH, Shafritz DA, Popper H. Chronic type B hepatitis and the "healthy" HBsAg carrier state. Hepatology 1987;7:758.

Koff RS. Natural history of acute hepatitis B in adults reexamined. Gastroenterology 1987;92:2035.

Lemon SM. Type A viral hepatitis. N Engl J Med 1985;313:1059.

Shih W, Esteban JI, Alter HJ. Non-A, non-B hepatitis: advances and unfulfilled expectations of the first decade. Prog Liver Dis 1986;8:433.

Smedile A, Rizzetto M. The hepatitis delta virus and its disease. Viewpoints Dig Dis 1987;19:1.

Stevens CE, Taylor PE, Tong MJ, et al. Yeast-recombinant hepatitis B vaccine: efficacy with hepatitis B immune globulin in prevention of perinatal hepatitis B virus transmission. JAMA 1987;257:2612.

## Chronic Hepatitis

Arasu TS, Wyllie R, Hatch TF, et al. Management of chronic aggressive hepatitis in children and adolescents. J Pediatr 1979;95:514.

Czaja AJ, Beaver SJ, Shiels MT. Sustained remission after corticosteroid therapy of severe hepatitis B surface antigen-negative chronic active hepatitis. Gastroenterology 1987;92:215.

Fitzgerald JF. Chronic hepatitis. J Pediatr 1984;104:893.

Maggiore G, Bernard O, Hadchovel M, et al. Treatment of autoimmune chronic active hepatitis in childhood. J Pediatr 1984;104:839.

Maggiore G, Bernard O, Hanberg J, et al. Liver disease associated with anti-liver-kidney microsome antibody in children. J Pediatr 1986;108:399.

Schaffner F. Autoimmune chronic active hepatitis: three decades of progress. Prog Liver Dis 1986;8:485.

## Drug-Induced Liver Disease

Zimmerman HJ, Maddrey WC. Toxic and drug induced hepatitis. In: Schiff L, Schiff ER, eds. Diseases of the liver, ed 6. Philadelphia: JB Lippincott, 1987.

## Fulminant Hepatic Failure

Bismuth H, Samuel D, Gugenheim J, et al. Emergency liver transplantation for fulminant hepatitis. Ann Intern Med 1987;107:337.

Fraser CL, Arieff AL. Hepatic encephalopathy. N Engl J Med 1985;313:865.

Jones EA. Hepatic encephalopathy: an update. Viewpoints Dig Dis 1986;18:1.

Peleman RR, Gavaler JS, Van Thiel DH, et al. Orthotopic liver transplantation for acute and subacute hepatic failure in adults. Hepatology 1987;7:484.

Psacharopoulos HT, Mowat AD, Davies M, et al. Fulminant hepatic failure in childhood: analysis of 31 cases. Arch Dis Child 1980;55:252.

Russel GJ, Fitzgerald JF, Clark JH. Fulminant hepatic failure. J Pediatr 1987;111:313.

## Portal Hypertension

Alvarez F, Bernard O, Brunelle F, et al. Portal obstruction in children. 1. Clinical investigation and hemorrhage risk. 2. Results of surgical portosystemic shunts. J Pediatr 1983;103:696.

Bass NM. Preventing hemorrhage from esophageal varices. N Engl J Med 1987;317:893.

Cello JP, Crass RA, Grendell JH, et al. Management of the patient with hemorrhaging esophageal varices. JAMA 1986;256:1480.

Cello JP, Grendell JH, Crass RA, et al. Endoscopic sclerotherapy versus portacaval shunt in patients with severe cirrhosis and acute variceal hemorrhage. N Engl J Med 1987;316:11.

Fonkalsrud EW. Shunt operations for portal hypertension in children. J Pediatr 1983;103:741.

Terblanche J, Bornman PC, Kahn D, et al. The management of acute variceal bleeding. Prog Liver Dis 1986;8:541.

Williams R, Westoby D. Endoscopic sclerotherapy for esophageal varices. Dig Dis Sci 1986;31:1085.

## Ascites

Epstein M. Renal complications in liver disease. In: Schiff L, Schiff ER, eds. Disease of the liver, ed 6. Philadelphia: JB Lippincott, 1987:903.

Pockros PJ, Reynolds TB. Rapid diuresis in patients with ascites from chronic liver disease: the importance of peripheral edema. Gastroenterology 1986;90:1827.

Simon DM, McCain JR, Bonkouwsky HC. Effects of therapeutic paracentesis on systemic and hepatic hemodynamics and on renal and hormonal function. Hepatology 1987;7:423.

Wyllie R, Arasu TS, Fitzgerald JF. Ascites: pathophysiology and management. J Pediatr 1980;97:167.

## Hepatic Transplantation

Esquivel CO, Koneru B, Karrer F, et al. Liver transplantation before 1 year of age. J Pediatr 1987;110:545.

Gartner JL, Zitelli BJ, Malatack JJ, et al. Orthotopic liver transplantation in children: two year experience with 47 patients. Pediatrics 1984;74:140.

Malatack JJ, Schnaid DJ, Urbach AH, et al. Choosing a pediatric recipient for orthotopic liver transplantation. J Pediatr 1987;111:479.

## Primary Sclerosing Cholangitis

Classen M, Gotze H, Richter H, et al. Primary sclerosing cholangitis in children. J Pediatr Gastroenterol Nutr 1987;6:197.

Helzberg JH, Petersen JM, Boyer JL. Improved survival with primary sclerosing cholangitis. Gastroenterology 1987;92:1869.

LaRusso NF, Weisner RH, Ludwig J, McCarthy RL. Primary sclerosing cholangitis. N Engl J Med 1984;310:899.

Lefkowitch JH, Martin EC. Primary sclerosing cholangitis. Prog Liver Dis 1986;II:557.

El-Shabrawl M, Wilkinson ML, Portmann B, et al. Primary sclerosing cholangitis in childhood. Gastroenterology 1987;92:1226.

Sisto A, Feldman P, Garel L, et al. Primary sclerosing cholangitis in children: study of five cases and review of the literature. Pediatrics 1987;80:918.

## Abnormalities of the Biliary Tract

Alvarez F, Bernard O, Brunelle F, et al. Congenital hepatic fibrosis in children. J Pediatr 1981;99:370.

Cole BR, Conley SB, Stapleton FB. Polycystic kidney disease in the first year of life. J Pediatr 1987;111:693.

Hermansen MC, Starshak RJ, Werlin SL. Caroli disease: the diagnostic approach. J Pediatr 1979;94:879.

Magilavy DB, Speert DP, Silver TM, et al. Mucocutaneous lymph node syndrome: report of two cases complicated by gallbladder hydrops and diagnosed by ultrasound. Pediatrics 1978;61:199.

Ryckman FC, Noseworthy J. Neonatal cholestatic conditions requiring surgical reconstruction. Semin Liver Dis 1987;7:134.

Todani T, Watanabe Y, Toki A, et al. Reoperation for congenital choledochal cyst. Ann Surg 1988;207:142.

## Cholelithiasis

Honore LH. Cholesterol cholelithiases in adolescent females. Arch Surg 1980;115:62.

Mok HY, Druffel ER, Rampone WM. Chronology of cholelithiasis. N Engl J Med 1986;314:1075.

Sarnaik S, Slovis TL, Corbett DP, et al. Incidence of cholelithiasis in sickle cell anemia using the ultrasonic gray-scale technique. J Pediatr 1980;96:1005.

Takiff H, Fonkalsrud EW. Gallbladder disease in childhood. Am J Dis Child 1984;138:565.

## Chronic Cholestasis

Sokol RJ. Medical management of the infant or child with chronic liver disease. Semin Liver Dis 1987;7:155.

Cynamon HA, Andres JM, Iafrate RP. Rifampin relieves pruritus in children with cholestatic liver disease. Gastroenterology 1990;98:1013.

Whitington PF, Whitington GL. Partial external diversion of bile for the treatment of pruritus associated with intrahepatic cholestasis. Gastroenterology 1988;95:130.

## Parenteral Nutrition

Balistreri WF, Bove KE. Hepatobiliary consequences of parenteral alimentation. Prog Liver Dis 1990;9:567.

## Metabolic Disease

Cross NCP, Cox TM. Hereditary fructose intolerance. Int J Biochem 1990;22:685.

Freese DK, Tuchman M, Schwarzenberg SJ, et al. Early liver transplantation is indicated for tyrosinemia type 1. J Pediatr Gastroenterol Nutr 1991;13:10.

Levy HL. Nutritional therapy for selected inborn errors of metabolism. J Am Coll Nutr 1989;8:549.

Mitchell G, Larochelle J, Lambert M, et al. Neurologic crises in hereditary tyrosinemia. N Engl J Med 1990;322:432.

Odievre M. Clinical presentation of metabolic liver disease. J Inherit Metab Dis 1991;14:256.

Phaneuf D, Labelle Y, Berube D, et al. Cloning and expression of the cDNA encoding human fumarylacetoacetate hydrolase, the enzyme deficient in hereditary tyrosinemia: assignment of the gene to chromosome 15. Am J Hum Genet 1991;48:525.

Waggoner DD, Buist NRM, Donnell GN. Long-term prognosis in galactosemia. J Inherit Metab Dis 1990;13:802.

## Defects in Bile Acid Synthesis

Buchman MS, Kvittington EA, Nazer H, Gunasekaran T, Clayton PT, Sjovall J, Bjorkhem I. Lack of 3-beta-hydroxy-delta⁵-C27-steroid dehydrogenase/isomerase in fibroblasts from a child with urinary excretion of 3-beta-hydroxy-delta⁵-bile acids. J Clin Invest 1990;86:2034.

Ichimaya H, Nazer H, Gunasekaran T, Clayton P, Sjovall J. Treatment of chronic liver disease caused by 3-beta-hydroxy-delta⁵-C27-steroid dehydrogenase deficiency with chenodeoxycholic acid. Arch Dis Child 1990;65;1121.

Setchell KD, Suchy FJ, Welsh MB, Zimmer-Nechemias L, Heubi J, Balistreri WF. Delta⁴-3-oxosteroid-5-beta-reductase deficiency described in identical twins with neonatal hepatitis. J Clin Invest 1988;82:2148.

## Hyperammonemia

Batshaw ML. Inherited hyperammonemia: an algorithm for diagnosis. Hepatology 1987;7:1381.

Maestri NE, Hauser ER, Bartholomew D, Brusilow SW. Prospective treatment of urea cycle disorders. J Pediatr 1991;119:923.

## Reye's Syndrome and Mimickers

Hale DE, Bennett MJ. Fatty acid oxidation disorders: a new class of metabolic diseases. J Pediatr 1992;121:1.

## Wilson's Disease and Presumed Defects of Metal Metabolism

Barnard JA, Manci E Idiopathic neonatal iron storage disease. Gastroenterol 1991;101:1420.

Brewer GJ, Yuzbasiyan-Gurkan V. Wilson's disease. Medicine (Baltimore) 1992;71;139.

Schilsky ML, Scheinberg IH, Sternlieb I. Prognosis of Wilsonian chronic active hepatitis. Gastroenterology 1991;100:762.

Tanner MS, Bhave SA, Pradhan AM, Pandit AN. Clinical trails of penicillamine in Indian childhood cirrhosis. Arch Dis Child 1987;62:1118.

## Cystic Fibrosis

Columbo C, Castellani MR, Balistreri WF, et al. Scintigraphic documentation of an improvement in hepatobiliary excretory function after treatment with ursodeoxycholic acid in patients with cystic fibrosis and associated liver disease. Hepatology 1992;15:677.

Columbo C, Setchell KD, Podda M, et al. Effects of ursodeoxycholic acid therapy for liver disease associated with cystic fibrosis. J Pediatr 1990;117:482.

Scott-Jupp R, Lama M, Tanner MS. Prevalence of liver disease in cystic fibrosis. Arch Dis Child 1991;66:698.

## $\alpha_1$-Antitrypsin Deficiency

Brantly M, Courtney M, Crystal RG. Repair of the secretion defect in the Z form of $\alpha_1$-antitrypsin by the addition of a second mutation. Science 1988;242:1700.

Ibarguen E, Gross CR, Savik SK, Sharp HL. Liver disease in $\alpha_1$-antitrypsin deficiency: prognostic indicators. J Pediatr 1990;117:864.

Perlmutter DH. The cellular basis for liver injury in $\alpha_1$-antitrypsin deficiency. Hepatology 1991;13:172.

## Hepatitis B

Margolis HS, Alter MJ, Hadler SC. Hepatitis B: evolving epidemiology and implications for control. Semin Liver Dis 1991;11:84.

Perillo RP, Schiff ER, Davis GL, et al. A randomized controlled trail of interferon alpha-2B alone and after prednisone withdrawal for the treatment of chronic hepatitis B. N Engl J Med 1990;323:295.

Ruiz-Moreno M, Rua MJ, Molina J, et al. Prospective, randomized controlled trail of interferon-alpha in children with chronic hepatitis B. Hepatology 1991;13:1035.

Utili R, Sagnelli E, Galanti B, et al. Prolonged treatment of children with chronic hepatitis B with recombinant alpha 2a-interferon: a controlled, randomized study. Am J Gastroenterol 1991;86:327.

## Hepatitis C

Davis GL, Balart LA, Schiff ER, et al. Treatment of chronic hepatitis C with recombinant interferon alpha. A multicenter randomized controlled trail. N Engl J Med 1989;321:1501.

Genesca J, Esteban JI, Alter HJ. Blood-borne non-A, non-B hepatitis: hepatitis C. Semin Liver Dis 1991;11:147.

Thaler MM, Park CK, Landers DV, et al. Vertical transmission of hepatitis C virus. Lancet 1991;338:17.

## Hepatitis A

Werzberger A, Mensch B, Kuten B, et al. A controlled trail of a formalin-inactivated hepatitis A vaccine in healthy children. N Engl J Med 1992;327:453.

## Hepatitis E

Reyes GR, Purdy MA, Kim JP, et al. Isolation of a cDNA from the virus responsible for enterically transmitted non-A, non-B hepatitis. Science 1990;247:1335.

## Hepatitis—General

Hoofnagle JH, Di Bisceglie AM. Serologic diagnosis of acute and chronic viral hepatitis. Semin Liver Dis 1991;11:73.
Katkov WN, Dienstag JL. Prevention and therapy of viral hepatitis. Semin Liver Dis 1991;11:165.
Bradley DW, Krawczynski K, Beach MJ, Purdy MA. Non-A, non-B hepatitis: toward the discovery of hepatitis C and E viruses. Semin Liver Dis 1991;11:128.
Alter HJ. NewKit on the block: evaluation of second generation assays for detection of antibody to the hepatitis C virus. Hepatology 1992;15:350.

## Chronic Hepatitis

Johnson PJ, McFarlane IG, Eddleston ALWF. The natural course and heterogeneity of autoimmune-type chronic active hepatitis. Seminars in liver disease 1991;11:187.
Maddrey WC, Combes B. Therapeutic concepts for the management of idiopathic Autoimmune Chronic Hepatitis. Seminars in liver disease 1991;11:248.

## Portal Hypertension

Hassall E, Berquist WE, Ament ME, Vargas J, Dorney S. Sclerotherapy for extrahepatic portal hypertension in childhood. J Pediatr 1989;115:69.
Sokal EM, Van Hoorebeeck N, Van Obbergh L, et al. Upper gastrointestinal tract bleeding in cirrhotic children candidates for liver transplantation. Eur J Pediatr 1992;151:326.
Thapa BR, Mehta S. Endoscopic sclerotherapy of esophageal varices in infants and children. J Pediatr Gastroenterol Nutr 1990;10:430.
Westaby D, Hayes PC, Gimson AES, Polson RJ, Williams R. Controlled clinical trail of injection sclerotherapy for active variceal bleeding. Hepatology 1989;9:274.

## Ascites

Hoefs JC. Diagnostic paracentesis. Gastroenterology 1990;98:230.

## Hepatic Transplantation

Lloyd-Still JD. Impact of hepatic transplantation on mortality from pediatric liver disease. J Pediatr Gastroenterol Nutr 1991;12:305.
Whitington PF, Balistreri WF. Liver transplantation in pediatrics: indications, contraindications, and pretransplant management. J Pediatr 1991;118:169.
Zitelli BJ, Gartner C, Malatack JJ, Urbach AH, Zamberlain K. Liver transplantation in children: a pediatrician's perspective. Pediatr Ann 1991;20:691.

## Primary Sclerosing Cholangitis

Goldberg E, Gerdes H. Primary sclerosing cholangitis: is medical therapy on the way? Gastroenterology 1992;102:729.
Lindor KD, Wiesner RH, MacCarty RL, Ludwig J, LaRusso NF. Advances in primary sclerosing cholangitis. Am J Med 1990;11:56.

## Abnormalities of the Biliary Tract

Forbes A, Murray-Lyon IM. Cystic disease of the liver and biliary tract. Gut 1991; Sept. (Suppl):S116.
Karrer FM, Hall RJ, Stewart BA, Lilly JR. Congenital biliary tract disease. Surg Clin North Am 1990;70:1403.
Stephenson BM, Rees BI. Choledochal cysts: their management revisited. Br J Clin Pract 1990;44:447.

## Cholelithiasis

Friesen CA, Roberts CC. Cholelithiasis. Clinical characteristics in children. Clin Pediatr (Phila) 1989;28:294.
Holcomb GW Jr, Holcomb GW III. Cholelithiasis in infants, children and adolescents. Pediatr Rev 1990;11:26B.
Ware RE, Kinney TR, Casey JR, Pappas TN, Meyers WC. Laparoscopic cholecystectomy in young patients with sickle hemoglobinopathies. J Pediatr 1992;120:58.

*Principles and Practice of Pediatrics, Second Edition.*
edited by Frank A. Oski et al. J. B. Lippincott Company, Philadelphia © 1994.

# 139.2 *Liver Abscess*

Prathiba Nanjundiah and William J. Klish

Because the liver has systemic and portal circulations, it is surprising that liver abscess is an unusual problem in infants and children. The low incidence is partly attributable to the extensive network of reticuloendothelial cells that line the sinusoids, which are capable of clearing bacteria. Early use of antibiotics and improved medical and surgical care have reduced bacterial exposure to the liver and account for the infrequency of this disorder.

The exact incidence of hepatic abscess in children is unknown. Dehner and Kissane reported a 0.38% incidence at autopsy in patients younger than 15 years of age. In this large series studied from 1917 to 1967, 41% of the patients were younger than 2 years and 67% were 2 to 5 years of age. The incidence was estimated to be 3 per 100,000 admissions to a large pediatric hospital. In another review, the incidence was 25 per 100,000 pediatric hospital admissions. This suggests an increase in the incidence of this disorder, which may be related to the use of advanced diagnostic techniques. The prolonged lifespan of patients with primary and secondary immune defects could also account for older children with pyogenic liver abscess.

Hepatic abscess in the neonatal period is rare. However, liver abscess in children of all age groups have been reported. There is no definite sex predilection except in patients with chronic granulomatous disease, which is seen in boys.

## PATHOGENESIS

Infectious agents may reach the liver by direct invasion from contiguous structures, through the portal vein, by systemic (hematogenous) bacteremia, or by direct inoculation during surgery or through traumatic events. Cases in which the mode of transmission is obscure are described as cryptogenic.

Systemic bacteremia with hematogenous spread to the liver through the hepatic artery appears to be the most common source of liver abscess in children. In Dehner and Kissane's series, the hematogenous route was responsible for 78% of the cases.

The portal system is the second most common route by which bacteria may reach the liver, and it accounts for most of the hepatic abscesses in the neonate. In the newborn period, solitary liver abscesses (usually due to gram-negative organisms) have been reported as a complication of umbilical venous catheterization or omphalitis. However, most liver abscesses in the neonate are multiple. Portal vein inflammation and bacteremia can be associated with infections of the abdominal cavity. The development of hepatic abscess as a complication of Crohn's disease is rare and has been described in only two adolescents. Liver abscess in Crohn's disease may be secondary to seeding of the mesenteric vessels with portal bacteremia from the inflamed loops of bowel.

Direct extension of infection from contiguous structures has accounted for 11% of the liver abscesses in children. Ascending cholangitis is a frequent complication of hepatic portoenterostomy in patients with biliary atresia and may lead to abscesses of the liver in these patients.

Penetrating and nonpenetrating trauma to the liver may lead to liver abscesses, presumably from the proliferation of bacteria within the localized hematomas or biliary collection that may result from trauma. This mode of infection is rare in children.

Cryptogenic hepatic abscess has been reported in children with fever of unknown origin and accounts for a smaller percentage of patients. Hepatic abscesses also have been reported in patients with cat-scratch disease.

There is an increased incidence of hepatic abscess in immunocompromised children. Children with chronic granulomatous disease and acute leukemia are at increased risk. The pathophysiology may be related to chronic, low-grade intestinal infection or the small number of viable granulocytes and monocytes. Patients on steroid therapy are at risk because of suppression of the natural host defenses.

Pyogenic liver abscess has been reported as a complication of anaerobic bacterial invasion of hepatic infarcts in patients with sickle cell anemia. These patients have other abnormalities that may contribute to their increased risk, such as splenic dysfunction and increased gut permeability to certain bacteria from microinfarcts.

Liver abscesses can result from infection of central parenteral nutrition catheters or ventriculoperitoneal shunts. Biliary tract disease predisposes the patient to the development of multiple liver abscess, and portal vein inflammation usually results in a single abscess. Solitary abscess is most common in the right lobe of the liver.

## ETIOLOGY

*Staphylococcus aureus* accounted for 33% of the liver abscesses in children in a review by Dehner and Kissane. Two or more organisms were recovered in 52% of the children, and 32% of the patients were colonized by gram-negative organisms. Gram-negative organisms such as *Escherichia coli, Aerobacter, Pseudomonas* and *Proteus* species have been isolated frequently from liver abscesses in neonates. With improvement in culture techniques, anaerobes (eg, *Actinomyces, Fusobacterium,* and *Bacteroides* species) and mycobacteria (ie, typical and atypical in human immunodeficiency virus-infected patients) have been described in children. Fungi, especially *Candida albicans,* have been isolated from liver abscesses in neonates and leukemic patients on total parenteral alimentation. *Entamoeba histolytica* is a well-known cause of liver abscess.

## PATHOLOGY

Microscopically, liver abscesses are characterized by an area of necrosis surrounded by polymorphonuclear leukocytes, large mononuclear cells, and lymphocytes. Adjacent to the inflammatory cell infiltrate, fibrous tissue intermingled with hepatocytes may be seen. Microorganisms may be seen in the necrotic center or at the periphery of the abscess cavity.

## CLINICAL FEATURES

The signs and symptoms of hepatic abscess are nonspecific and frequently are related to the underlying disease, especially in the neonate. A history of recent travel to endemic areas of amebiasis, previous abdominal surgery, trauma, immunodeficiency, or inflammatory bowel disease may be elicited. Fever, abdominal pain, nausea, vomiting, loss of appetite, weakness, and malaise are the

most constant and prominent symptoms. Weight loss, diarrhea, and pleuritic pain occur less frequently. A history of fever of unknown cause, with or without abdominal pain, in an otherwise healthy child should suggest the diagnosis of liver abscess. Patients with multiple abscesses generally experience a more acute illness, and patients with solitary abscesses usually have a subacute or chronic course.

Hepatomegaly occurs in 40% to 80% of the patients. Tenderness on percussion of the right upper quadrant of the abdomen is usually elicited but may not be appreciated unless the physician specifically examines this region. Jaundice is not a clinical feature of liver abscess unless there is associated biliary tract disease. Other physical findings include abdominal distention and decreased breath sounds or rales from pulmonary involvement due to pleural effusion or fixed hemidiaphragm.

## DIAGNOSIS

The initial laboratory studies may show some degree of anemia and leukocytosis. The erythrocyte sedimentation rate may be elevated. Nonspecific elevations of transaminases, glutamine peptidase, and alkaline phosphatase may be seen in some patients. If the abscesses are secondary to biliary tract disease, bilirubin and alkaline phosphatase levels may be elevated.

Blood cultures are frequently positive in patients with multiple liver abscesses. Chest radiographs may reveal a pleural effusion or a fixed hemidiaphragm. Ileus and air in the liver abscess may be seen on abdominal roentgenograms.

Abdominal imaging techniques are particularly useful in younger children, who are unable to localize pain. Ultrasound is a sensitive technique that does not require exposure to radiation and is recommended as the first imaging modality in children. However, new imaging techniques such as magnetic resonance imaging (MRI) and computed tomography (CT) are considerably more sensitive and have improved the diagnosis of these infections. Although both of these techniques are expensive, they provide accurate information about the number, size, and location of abscesses within the liver parenchyma, and lesions of approximately 1 cm in diameter can be detected. With intravenous contrast studies, hypodense abscesses are demonstrated readily and can be differentiated from vascular lesions and tumors of the liver.

## DIFFERENTIAL DIAGNOSIS

The differential diagnosis of fever, abdominal pain, vomiting, and malaise in young children often includes hepatitis, appendicitis, tuberculosis, pyelonephritis, bowel obstruction, occult trauma, and liver tumors. In adolescents, choledochal disease is possible, and gonorrheal or chlamydial perihepatitis or Fitzhugh-Curtis syndrome should be considered in girls.

The differentiation of amebic abscess from pyogenic liver abscess is difficult. In one large pediatric series, many patients with amebic abscesses had traveled to an endemic area. The most common presenting symptoms included fever, cough, or difficulty breathing, abdominal pain, loss of appetite, and weight loss. Diarrhea was not a constant symptom. Seventy-seven percent of the patients had an isolated mass in the right hepatic lobe, and 81% had hepatomegaly on physical examination.

Examination of stool specimens for cysts and trophozoites of *E histolytica* is positive in only 10% to 30% of the patients with amebic abscess. The presence of *E histolytica* trophozoites in the abscess is diagnostic, but they are usually found only in the wall of an abscess cavity. Counterimmunoelectrophoresis of serum for the detection of antibody to *E histolytica* is a rapid test and establishes a presumptive diagnosis. A positive titer (>1:128) on the indirect hemagglutination assay of serum is confirmatory and has an 85% to 95% accuracy.

## TREATMENT

Untreated and undiagnosed liver abscess is fatal. Although surgical drainage of the solitary pyogenic abscess is mandatory, a percutaneous aspiration with ultrasound or CT guidance can be performed. A catheter is placed into the abscess cavity under CT or ultrasound guidance, the contents are aspirated, and a draining catheter is placed. Surgical support is essential for this procedure, because spillage of abscess material into the peritoneal or pleural cavity, hemorrhage, and other complications may occur. More data must be generated for children before this treatment can be widely recommended.

Except in amebic abscess, percutaneous aspiration is useful in all cases of liver abscesses as a guide to proper antibiotic therapy. Antibiotic therapy should be based on information gained from Gram stain of the abscess material, culture, and antibiotic susceptibility. A combination of a semisynthetic penicillin or a cephalosporin plus an aminoglycoside has been recommended for initial therapy of liver abscess in children. Third-generation cephalosporins have better penetration into the abscess cavity and may work in the acidic environment produced by bacteria and necrotic debris. Clindamycin, cefoxitin, or metronidazole should be administered for anaerobic isolates, depending on susceptibility. The optimal duration and route of administration of antibiotics for children with drained solitary liver abscess has not been determined. A regimen of 2 to 4 weeks of parenteral antibiotic therapy followed by 1 to 2 weeks of an appropriate oral antibiotic is recommended by most physicians. The combination of amphotericin B and 5-fluorocytosine is recommended in the treatment of fungal liver abscesses.

The aspirate should be evaluated cytologically, particularly in patients who fail to respond to treatment or who have negative ameba titers, to exclude malignant lesions. Multiple liver abscesses are difficult to treat and are not amenable to surgical therapy. Prolonged antibiotic therapy plus treatment of any underlying illness is crucial for effective management.

## COMPLICATIONS AND PROGNOSIS

The complications of hepatic abscesses are relatively common. Pleural and pulmonary inflammation, peritonitis, subphrenic or subhepatic abscesses, and hemobilia are a few of the complications.

Polymicrobial bacteremia, hypoalbuminemia, multiple liver abscesses, or any complication is associated with an increased mortality. Mortality rates as high as 80% have been reported. A high index of suspicion of liver abscess, in conjunction with better imaging modalities, advanced microbial isolation techniques, and newer antibiotics, should significantly reduce the mortality of this disease.

### Selected Readings

Donovan AJ, Yellin AE, Ralls PW. Hepatic abscess. World J Surg 1991;15:162.
Chusid MJ. Pyogenic hepatic abscess in infancy and childhood. Pediatrics 1978;62: 554.
Dehner LP, Kissane JM. Pyogenic hepatic abscess in infancy and childhood. J Pediatr 1969;74:763.
Goldenring JM, Flores M. Primary liver abscesses in children and adolescents. Clin Pediatr 1986;25:153.
Greenstein AJ, Lowenthal D, Hammer GS, et al. Continuing changing patterns of disease in pyogenic liver abscess: a study of 38 patients. Am J Gastroenterol 1984;79:226.
Haffer A, Boland F, Edwards MS. Amebic liver abscess in children. Pediatr Infect Dis 1982;1:5.
Puck JM. Bacterial, parasitic, and other infections of the liver. In: Walker WA, Durie PR, Hamilton JR, et al, eds. Pediatric gastrointestinal disease, ed 1st. Philadelphia: BC Dekker, 1991;2:890.
Kaplan SL. Pyogenic liver abscess. In: Feigin RD, Cherry JD, eds. Textbook of pediatric infectious diseases, ed 2. Philadelphia: WB Saunders, 1987:749.
Laurin S, Kaude JV. Diagnosis of liver-spleen abscesses in children with emphasis on ultrasound for the initial and follow-up examination. Pediatr Radiol 1984;14: 198.
Moss TJ, Pysher JT. Hepatic abscess in neonates. Am J Dis Child 1981;135:726.
Nolan JP. Bacteria and the liver. N Engl J Med 1978;299:1069.
Vachon L, Diament MJ, Stanley P. Percutaneous drainage of hepatic abscesses in children. J Pediatr Surg 1986;21:366.
Weinberg RJ, Klish WJ, Brown MR, et al. Hepatic abscess as a complication of Crohn's disease. J Pediatr Gastroenterol Nutr 1983;2:174.
Pineiro-Carrero VM, Andres JM. Morbidity and mortality in children with pyogenic liver abscess. Am J Dis Child 1989;143:1424.

*Principles and Practice of Pediatrics, Second Edition.*
edited by Frank A. Oski et al. J. B. Lippincott Company, Philadelphia © 1994.

## 139.3 *Cholecystitis*

Kathleen J. Motil

Cholecystitis is an inflammatory disease of the gallbladder that may be acute or chronic. In some instances, acute cholecystitis may be superimposed on the preexisting chronic form of the disease. Acute and chronic cholecystitis may be classified further as calculous or acalculous, based on the presence or absence of gallstones, which, if present, occur in 80% to 85% of children who have this disorder. Chronic cholecystitis with cholelithiasis is the most common pattern, occurring in almost two thirds of children with this diagnosis. The frequencies of the patterns of cholecystitis are shown in Table 139-6.

## ETIOLOGY AND PATHOGENESIS

Acute cholecystitis may result from any of three primary events in the gallbladder: bile stasis, an inflammatory response, or ischemia (Table 139-7). Stasis usually results from obstruction of the cystic duct due to gallstones but may occur secondary to the edema produced by stones, hyperplastic lymph nodes, or a neoplasm. Starvation, dehydration, and immobilization are associated with stasis due to interruption of gallbladder contraction and

TABLE 139-6. Patterns of Cholecystitis and Their Frequency

| Type | Frequency (%) |
| --- | --- |
| **Acute Cholecystitis** | |
| Calculous | 19 |
| Acalculous | 5 |
| **Chronic Cholecystitis** | |
| Calculous | 64 |
| Acalculous | 12 |

TABLE 139-7. Pathophysiology of Cholecystitis

**Acute Cholecystitis**
Bile stasis
    Obstruction (gallstones, lymph nodes, tumor)
    Starvation
    Immobilization
Inflammation
    Bile salts
    Lysolecithin
    Pancreatic juice
    Bacteria
Ischemia
    Torsion
    Systemic vascular disease
**Chronic Cholecystitis**
Recurrent obstruction and inflammation

emptying. Bile salts, lysolecithin, pancreatic juice, and bacteria have been implicated as agents responsible for inciting the inflammatory response. Torsion of the gallbladder or systemic vascular disease may lead to ischemic changes of the biliary tract. After the initial attack subsides, the mucosal surface of the biliary tract heals, and the wall becomes scarred. If the inflammation subsides but the cystic duct remains obstructed, the gallbladder may become distended (ie, hydrops). Recurrent attacks of obstruction and inflammation lead to progressive scarring of the gallbladder with loss of function and additional gallstone formation.

## PATHOLOGY

The pathologic features of acute cholecystitis include an enlarged gallbladder that is filled with turbid bile, fine sandy gravel, or gallstones (Table 139-8). The gallbladder wall is thickened and may be ulcerated or perforated. The inflammatory response is characterized by edema, polymorphonuclear cell infiltration, vascular congestion, and necrosis.

The features of chronic cholecystitis vary. The gallbladder may be contracted or enlarged. The gallbladder wall is thickened, and the mucosal folds may be flattened. The lumen contains clear, mucoid bile; stones usually are formed. Microscopic features include increased subepithelial fibrosis and an infiltrate of lymphocytes, plasma cells, macrophages, and mononuclear cells. Cholesterolosis occurs when crystals of cholesterol are deposited in the submucosal macrophages of the gallbladder.

Ninety percent of all gallstones are made of calcium bilirubinate and calcium carbonate. Rarely, gallstones consist primarily of cholesterol.

## EPIDEMIOLOGY

The incidence of cholecystitis in children ranges from less than 1% to 4%. Although this disorder is less common in children than in adults, its frequency in childhood appears to be increasing. Girls are affected more commonly than boys after adolescence. Both sexes are affected equally before this age (Table 139-9). The occurrence of cholecystitis in the white population is almost twice that in the black and Hispanic populations. Acute and chronic cholecystitis, with or without gallstones, has been reported in all age ranges and may even occur in the fetus. Acalculous cholecystitis affects younger children more commonly, and calculous cholecystitis occurs more frequently in adolescents. The age distribution of acute and chronic cholecystitis is shown in Table 139-9.

## PREDISPOSING FACTORS

Several entities have been implicated as predisposing factors for cholecystitis in children (Table 139-10). Hemolytic disease, including congenital spherocytosis, sickle cell anemia, and thalassemia, has been found in more than one third of children with cholecystitis and gallstones. Children who are maintained on total parenteral nutrition for more than 4 weeks are at risk of developing biliary tract disease due to bile stasis. Ileal abnormalities, particularly ileal resection and the loss of the ileocecal valve associated with necrotizing enterocolitis, intestinal atresia, short gut syndrome, or Crohn's disease, further aggravate the development of biliary tract disease and gallstone formation. Pregnancy, with its attendant hormonal alterations, and obesity are each associated with approximately 30% of the cases of cholecystitis and cholelithiasis.

Bacterial enteric infections (eg, *Salmonella, Shigella, Pseudomonas, Leptospira, Escherichia coli, Clostridium welchii*), parasitic infestations (eg, *Giardia, Ascaris*), viral gastroenteritis, infectious hepatitis (eg, type A), urinary tract infections, Kawasaki syndrome, scarlet fever, respiratory infections, and pneumonia have been implicated as infectious causes of cholecystitis in 12% of the patients.

A family history of biliary or hepatic disease may be identified in 12% of the children with cholecystitis. Previous abdominal

TABLE 139-8. Pathologic Features of Cholecystitis

| Macroscopic Features | Microscopic Features |
|---|---|
| **Acute Cholecystitis** | |
| Enlarged gallbladder | Perforation |
| Thickened walls | Edema |
| Turbid bile | Polymorphonuclear cell infiltrate |
| Gravel or gallstones | |
| Ulceration | Vascular congestion |
| **Chronic Cholecystitis** | |
| Enlarged or contracted gallbladder | Subepithelial fibrosis |
| Thickened walls | Infiltrate of polymorphonuclear and plasma cells, macrophages, and morphonuclear cells |
| Clear, mucoid bile | |

TABLE 139-9. Epidemiology of Cholecystitis in Childhood

| | |
|---|---|
| Sex distrubtion | |
| Female–male ratio | 2:1 |
| Race distribution | |
| White–black–Hispanic ratio | 2:1:1 |
| Age distribution (% of cases) | |
| Birth–5 y | 22 |
| 6–10 y | 19 |
| 11–15 y | 30 |
| 16–20 y | 29 |

TABLE 139-10. Factors Associated With Cholecystits in Childhood

| Factors | Frequency (% of Cases) |
|---|---|
| Hemolytic disease | 37 |
| Ileal abnormalities | 37 |
| Pregnancy | 31 |
| Obesity | 27 |
| Total parenteral nutrition | 19 |
| Infection | 12 |
| Family history of biliary disease | 12 |
| Previous abdominal surgery | 9 |
| Cystic fibrosis | 7 |
| Biliary tract anomalies | 6 |
| Cirrhosis | 4 |
| Trauma | 1 |
| Other (congenital anomalies, drugs, ventilatory support) | <1 |

TABLE 139-11. Clinical Features of Cholecystitis in Childhood

| Finding | Frequency (% of Cases) |
|---|---|
| **Symptom** | |
| Abdominal pain | 67 |
| Right upper quadrant | 79 |
| Epigastrium | 19 |
| Radiation to back, shoulder | 38 |
| Vomiting | 41 |
| Dietary fat intolerance | 33 |
| **Sign** | |
| Abdominal tenderness | 68 |
| Jaundice | 35 |
| Fever | 27 |
| Mass | 17 |

surgery with adhesions or inflammation around the biliary tract and abdominal trauma may have pathologic significance. Congenital or acquired malformations of the biliary tract (eg, choledochal cyst, stenosis of the cystic duct) have been implicated in the development of cholecystitis. Anomalies of other organs (eg, exstrophy of the bladder, rectal atresia, hypospadias, tracheoesophageal fistula, pulmonary stenosis, skeletal anomalies) have been noted in children with cholecystitis. The surgical treatment of scoliosis has been associated with cholelithiasis because of the postoperative bilirubin load and altered calcium homeostasis associated with immobilization. Cystic fibrosis and cirrhosis have been associated with gallbladder disease. Other factors such as drugs (eg, furosemide, narcotics) and ventilatory support have been associated with cholecystitis.

## CLINICAL FEATURES

The clinical presentation of cholecystitis varies from total absence of symptoms to florid illness. The symptoms of cholecystitis in children are similar to those in adults and are summarized in Table 139-11. Episodic abdominal pain localized to the right upper quadrant and epigastrium or radiating to the back or shoulder is the most common complaint and occurs in two thirds of the children with cholecystitis. Abdominal tenderness, generalized or localized to the right upper quadrant, is found on examination in at least two thirds of the children with cholecystitis. Vomiting and dietary fat intolerance affect 30% to 40%. Jaundice develops in at least one third of the patients and is more common in children than in adults. Jaundice usually is attributed to inflammation around the common duct rather than to obstruction secondary to choledocholithiasis. Fever occurs in at least one fourth of the patients. Infrequently, a mass may be palpated and usually is associated with acute acalculous cholecystitis. Symptoms may be noticed for only a few days, but they may be present as long as 10 years before the correct diagnosis of cholecystitis is made.

## LABORATORY AND RADIOGRAPHIC STUDIES

Although leukocytosis and elevated serum bilirubin and alkaline phosphatase levels may be found in many patients, laboratory studies, including liver function tests, are of limited diagnostic

value (Table 139-12). A complete blood cell count and hemoglobin electrophoresis may be indicated to determine the presence of an underlying hemolytic disorder.

Abdominal ultrasonography is the most effective, noninvasive method of delineating gallbladder dilation, thickened walls, and the presence of stones in the gallbladder or common bile and hepatic ducts. Significant abnormalities can be demonstrated in at least 90% of the children tested.

Hepatobiliary imaging with a $^{99m}$Tc-labeled iminodiacetic acid derivative may be useful to demonstrate a nonfunctioning gallbladder in acute cholecystitis. Although performed infrequently, endoscopic retrograde cholangiopancreatography may suggest cystic or common bile duct obstruction in the absence of visualization of the gallbladder.

An oral cholecystogram may not aid in the diagnosis of acute cholecystitis, because the gallbladder cannot be visualized during acute disease. The oral cholecystogram is most useful if acute cholecystitis is thought to be unlikely and the test supports the clinical impression. In chronic cholecystitis, approximately 60% of oral cholecystograms in children opacify and are sufficient to detect gallstones. If the gallbladder cannot be visualized, the study must be repeated.

TABLE 139-12. Diagnostic Studies for Cholecystitis in Childhood

**Laboratory**
Complete blood count and differential
Urinalysis
Serum bilirubin, alkaline phosphatase
Liver function tests
Serum amylase
Hemoglobin electrophoresis

**Sonography and Radiography**
Abdominal ultrasound
$^{99m}$Tc-iminodiacetic acid derivative scan
Endoscopic retrograde cholangiopancreatography
Oral/intravenous cholecystography
Intraoperative cholangiography

**Other Studies**
Gastroesophageal endoscopy/biopsy

Intravenous cholangiography may be more useful than oral cholecystography in acute cholecystitis. If the bile ducts opacify but the gallbladder does not, the diagnosis of acute cholecystitis is likely. However, if serum bilirubin levels are greater than 3.0 mg/dL, the gallbladder and bile ducts do not opacify on intravenous cholangiography. An intravenous cholecystogram is of little practical value in chronic cholecystitis because of the high frequency of false-negative studies.

An abdominal flat plate serendipitously may show asymptomatic calcified gallstones. Because gallstones are not calcified in at least 50% of children, they will not be seen on a plain roentgenogram of the abdomen. Moreover, calcifications constitute a nonspecific finding that is consistent with other diagnoses, including tuberculosis, bacterial or amebic abscesses, intrahepatic calculi, hemangioma, echinococcal cysts, neuroblastomas, or hepatic neoplasms.

## DIFFERENTIAL DIAGNOSIS

Cholecystitis may mimic other diseases and cause a significant delay in the correct diagnosis. In various studies, 13% of the children with cholecystitis were given the preoperative diagnosis of appendicitis, and 21% with sickle cell disease were diagnosed initially as having a sickle cell crisis. Cholecystitis should be considered early in the differential diagnosis of abdominal pain.

The principal conditions to consider in the differential diagnosis of cholecystitis are appendicitis, pancreatitis, gastroesophageal reflux, esophagitis, peptic ulcer disease, hepatitis, hepatic abscess or tumor, intussusception, pyelonephritis or nephrolithiasis, and pneumonitis (Table 139-13). Acute appendicitis is the disease most often confused with acute cholecystitis. Generally, abdominal tenderness, fever, and leukocytosis progress more relentlessly in appendicitis than in cholecystitis. Laparotomy can resolve the diagnostic dilemma.

Acute pancreatitis may be difficult to differentiate from cholecystitis because these illnesses have similar clinical features and because serum amylase levels may be elevated in acute cholecystitis although the pancreas is normal. Pancreatitis may occur in conjunction with acute cholecystitis. Cholelithiasis may cause acute pancreatitis as stones traverse the common bile duct and ampulla of Vater. Abdominal ultrasound scans may aid in the differential diagnosis of pancreatitis and cholecystitis. Gastroesophageal reflux, esophagitis, or peptic ulcer disease may be confused with cholecystitis. Gastroesophageal endoscopy with biopsies is an appropriate first test to differentiate among these entities.

The spectrum of diseases that may affect the liver (eg, hepatitis, abscess, tumor) is broad. Multiple diagnostic modalities such as liver function tests, ultrasound, computed tomography, or liver biopsy may be necessary to delineate the cause of the illness and eliminate the possibility of cholecystitis. Intussusception should be considered in the child with acute abdominal pain. Contrast roentgenography may be necessary to rule out gastrointestinal obstruction. Renal and pulmonary disease may also be associated with abdominal pain. Abnormalities on the auscultation of lungs, urinalysis, and appropriate radiographic studies should clarify these issues.

## TREATMENT

The treatment of acute cholecystitis includes hospitalization, hydration with intravenous fluids, correction of electrolyte abnormalities, discontinuation of oral feedings, and insertion of a nasogastric tube for suction (Table 139-14). Medications (eg, meperidine, morphine) should be considered for pain relief. Antibiotics have no therapeutic value in early acute cholecystitis, because the illness has an uncomplicated course, but if the clinical condition worsens (eg, fever, chills, increased pain, abdominal mass), antibiotic therapy is recommended. Ampicillin, gentamicin, and clindamycin or chloramphenicol combined are the drugs advocated for the treatment of biliary infections, because they are excreted in bile or provide adequate coverage for enteric organisms. Second- or third-generation cephalosporins (eg, cefoperazone, cefoxitin, cefotaxime) may be an alternate choice, particularly in protracted biliary disease.

Although the management of uncomplicated acute cholecystitis is controversial, cholecystectomy is the treatment of choice. If the child appears seriously ill or complications of cholecystitis are apparent, laparotomy must be performed immediately. Cholecystectomy can be performed safely and without delay even in children who are seriously ill. If the child's condition is precarious, cholecystostomy may be the preferred temporary procedure. One exception to this treatment plan is the child with sickle cell anemia whose course is complicated by acute cholecystitis or an abdominal pain crisis. Urgent cholecystectomy under these circumstances has been associated with a high rate of surgical complications. Elective cholecystectomy is advocated after the patient with hemolytic disease has been stabilized and treated with preoperative partial exchange transfusions. Laparoscopic cholecystectomy recently has been shown to be a safe and efficacious surgical procedure for the management of biliary tract disease in children with sickle cell hemoglobinopathies. Lithotripsy with oral bile acid therapy is not a satisfactory alternative to cholecystectomy because of the lifelong tendency toward gallstone formation in these children.

Surgery is the preferred treatment for chronic cholecystitis, particularly in the case of cholelithiasis. Controversy exists about the treatment of asymptomatic cholelithiasis in children. Because spontaneous disappearance of gallstones in infancy has been reported, a period of observation for 2 to 3 months of the asymptomatic patient who has sludge or noncalcified stones in the gallbladder may be warranted. However, elective cholecystectomy is advised for all symptomatic patients, those with calcified stones,

---

**TABLE 139-13. Differential Diagnosis of Cholecystitis in Childhood**

| | |
|---|---|
| Appendicitis | Hepatic abscess, tumor |
| Pancreatitis | Intussusception |
| Gastroesophageal reflux | Pyelonephritis |
| Esophagitis | Nephrolithiasis |
| Peptic ulcer disease | Pneumonitis |
| Hepatitis | |

**TABLE 139-14. Treatment of Cholecystitis in Childhood**

| Medical | Surgical |
|---|---|
| Hospitalization | Cholecystectomy |
| Intravenous hydration | Exploration of the common duct |
| Correction of electrolyte abnormalities | |
| Nasogastric suction | |
| Analgesics | |
| Antibiotics | |

and those asymptomatic patients in whom sludge or noncalcified stones do not resolve after 2 to 3 months. The operative mortality rate for this procedure is less than 1% for children. Operative cholangiography and exploration of the common duct are indicated for choledochal stones, recurrent pancreatitis, a history of jaundice, serum bilirubin levels greater than 6 mg/dL, or dilatation of the common bile duct. However, ductular stones have been identified in only 6% of the children who have undergone cholecystectomy. The use of pharmacologic agents that dissolve gallstones or procedures that desiccate gallstones in situ require further study.

## COMPLICATIONS

The major complication of acute cholecystitis is perforation, which may manifest as a localized pericholecystic abscess, an extension into the peritoneal cavity with generalized peritonitis, or the formation of a cholecystenteric fistula, primarily with the duodenum or the hepatic flexure of the colon. Surgical intervention is indicated for these complications. Less frequently, ascending cholangitis, liver abscess, or sepsis may complicate the clinical course of acute cholecystitis.

The complications of chronic cholecystitis in the absence of cholelithiasis are minimal. Patients with gallstones are at risk for recurrent bouts of acute cholecystitis, pancreatitis, perforation, bile peritonitis, biliary obstruction, biliary cirrhosis, and cancer of the gallbladder.

## PROGNOSIS

The prognosis after surgery for children with cholecystitis but without underlying hemolytic disease is excellent. The overall mortality rate for acute and chronic cholecystitis is less than 2% for children. Ten-year follow-up of children with gallbladder disease detected no further illness after cholecystectomy in 97% of patients. In children with hemolytic disorders, 82% had resolution of their episodes of abdominal pain and jaundice for as long as 6 years after cholecystectomy.

## Selected Readings

Bailey PV, Connors RH, Tracy TF, et al. Changing spectrum of cholelithiasis and cholecystitis in infants and children. Am J Surg 1989;158:585.

Cheng ERY, Matthias MI. Cholecystitis and cholelithiasis in children and adolescents. J Natl Med Assoc 1986;78:1073.

Holcomb GW Jr, O'Neill JA Jr, Holcomb GW III. Cholecystitis, cholelithiasis and common duct stenosis in children and adolescents. Ann Surg 1980;191:626.

King DR, Ginn-Pease ME, Lloyd TV, et al. Parenteral nutrition with associated cholelithiasis: another iatrogenic disease of infants and children. J Pediatr Surg 1987;22:593.

Pokorny WJ, Saleem M, O'Gorman RB, et al. Cholelithiasis and cholecystitis in childhood. Am J Surg 1984;148:742.

Reif S, Sloven D, Lebenthal E. Gallstones in children. Am J Dis Child 1991;145:105.

Roslyn JJ, Berquist WE, Pitt HA, et al. Increased risk of gallstones in children receiving total parenteral nutrition. Pediatrics 1983;71:784.

Stephens CG, Scott RB. Cholelithiasis in sickle cell anemia: surgical or medical management. Arch Intern Med 1980;140:648.

Takiff H, Fonkalsrud EW. Gallbladder disease in childhood. Am J Dis Child 1984;138:565.

Ware RE, Kinney TR, Casey JR, et al. Laparoscopic cholecystectomy in young patients with sickle hemoglobinopathies. J Pediatr 1992;120:58.

*Principles and Practice of Pediatrics, Second Edition.*
edited by Frank A. Oski et al. J. B. Lippincott Company, Philadelphia © 1994.

# 139.4 *Cirrhosis*

### William J. Cochran

Cirrhosis is a chronic liver disease characterized by a marked increase in connective tissue and by diffuse destruction and regeneration of hepatic parenchymal cells. The word cirrhosis comes from the Greek word *kirrhos*, which means tawny. This term was used because the liver was a tawny color in the first recognized type of cirrhosis, alcoholic cirrhosis. Secondary to many different causes, cirrhosis is an irreversible end stage of chronic liver disease. Because the number of children with cirrhosis is increasing, those involved in the health care of children should have some knowledge of this disorder and its inevitable complications. This chapter reviews the classification, causes, complications, and treatment of cirrhosis.

## CLASSIFICATION

Cirrhosis has been classified according to morphologic, histologic, and etiologic findings. Unfortunately, there is little correlation between the cause and pathology, because the liver reacts to insults in a limited number of ways, and cirrhosis is the final stage of response. The etiologic classification is probably the most practical for clinicians, although others are discussed briefly in deference to their frequent mention in the literature.

The morphologic classification characterizes the gross appearance of the liver according to size of nodule and consists of three major groups: micronodular, macronodular, and mixed micronodular and macronodular. Micronodular cirrhosis consists of diffuse, small nodules less than 3 mm in diameter and is commonly found in alcohol-induced cirrhosis. Patients with biliary atresia, Indian childhood cirrhosis, and hemochromatosis may have micronodular cirrhosis.

Macronodular cirrhosis consists of different-sized nodules, most greater than 3 mm in diameter, up to several centimeters in diameter. Wilson's disease (ie, hepatolenticular degeneration) is an example of macronodular cirrhosis. Other disorders that initially appear micronodular may progress to macronodular cirrhosis if the patient lives long enough.

In mixed micronodular and macronodular cirrhosis, both types of nodules occur in equal numbers. The cirrhosis that results from autoimmune hepatitis is characterized by this mixed type of morphology.

The histologic classification divides cirrhosis into portal, postnecrotic, posthepatic, biliary, and obstructive cirrhosis. Unlike the morphologic description, which is nonspecific, the histologic classification may enable precise determination of the cause of the disease, such as Wilson's disease with increased copper deposition, hemochromatosis with excessive iron deposition, $\alpha_1$-antitrypsin deficiency with periodic acid-Schiff–positive, diastase-resistant granules, and biliary atresia with its bile duct proliferation.

## ETIOLOGY

Numerous pediatric disorders can lead to cirrhosis (Table 139-15), in part because the liver responds to injury in a limited man-

| TABLE 139-15. Causes of Cirrhosis |
|---|
| Biliary tract disorders |
|    Biliary atresia |
|    Choledochal cyst |
|    Intrahepatic bile duct paucity |
|    Segmental dilatation of the intrahepatic biliary tree |
|    Congenital hepatic fibrosis |
|    Cystic fibrosis |
|    Sclerosing cholangitis |
| Genetic and metabolic causes |
|    $\alpha_1$-Antitrypsin deficiency |
|    Wilson's disease |
|    Hemochromatosis |
|    Galactosemia |
|    Hereditary fructose intolerance |
|    Glycogen storage disease |
|    Wolman's disease |
|    Niemann-Pick disease |
|    Gaucher's disease |
|    Tyrosinemia |
|    Osler-Weber-Rendu disease |
| Infection |
|    Hepatitis B |
|    Hepatitis C |
|    Cytomegalovirus |
|    Syphilis |
| Cardiac cirrhosis |
| Autoimmune diseases |
| Nutritional factors |
| Drugs and toxins |
| Miscellaneous causes |
|    Indian childhood cirrhosis |
|    Zellweger syndrome |
|    Neonatal hepatitis |

ner and cirrhosis is the final common pathway. The exact mechanism of the development of cirrhosis is unknown. The major etiologic categories of pediatric cirrhosis include biliary tract disorders; genetic and metabolic disorders; infectious, cardiac, immune, nutritional, drug, and toxin disorders; and miscellaneous diseases. Because many cases represent inherited diseases, it is important to determine the cause and provide appropriate genetic counseling. In most cases, determination of the cause of cirrhosis does not alter the therapeutic plan for the affected child.

## Biliary Tract Disorders

Biliary tract disorders are responsible for the greatest number of cases of cirrhosis in the pediatric population; extrahepatic biliary atresia is most common. The incidence of biliary atresia is from 1 in 8000 to 20,000 live births. The disorder appears to be acquired rather than a result of abnormal development, as evidenced by the rare occurrence of biliary atresia in autopsied fetuses and premature newborns.

One causative factor in the development of biliary atresia is reovirus type 3. Infants with biliary atresia have antibodies to reovirus type 3 (62%) more frequently than infants with neonatal hepatitis (52%) and normal infants (12%). Mice injected intraperitoneally with reovirus type 3 develop a lesion similar to biliary atresia.

Biliary atresia manifests as cholestasis in the newborn period. Unfortunately, there are no laboratory tests or radiographic studies that accurately differentiate biliary atresia from other cholestatic disorders of the newborn, such as neonatal hepatitis. A hepatobiliary scan can be helpful in ruling out the diagnosis of biliary atresia by demonstrating excretion of the tracer by the liver into the intestinal tract. Lack of excretion, however, is a nonspecific finding. The best diagnostic test, other than exploratory laparotomy, is percutaneous needle liver biopsy. The histologic hallmark of biliary atresia is bile duct proliferation and a widened portal area. The liver biopsy is a sensitive diagnostic test, and if the described findings are evident, exploratory laparotomy and intraoperative cholangiography are indicated.

If biliary atresia is found during laparotomy, a Kasai procedure (ie, portoenterostomy) should be performed. If the infant is older than 3 months of age and advanced fibrosis exists, performance of a Kasai procedure is controversial. The controversy results from the poor prognosis of patients with biliary atresia who undergo surgery after the age of 3 months. These infants have a 5-year survival rate of approximately 10%, compared with 70% to 90% if surgery is performed before the age of 3 months. Moreover, if liver transplantation is required, the surgical procedure may be more difficult if abdominal surgery was performed previously.

Choledochal cysts are a relatively uncommon cause of cirrhosis; the incidence is 1 in 13,000 to 15,000 live births. The cysts may be a congenital dilatation of the hepatic or common bile duct or may be an actual diverticulum of one of the ducts. Some patients may present in infancy with cholestasis; others are seen later in life with the classic triad of jaundice, abdominal pain, and a right upper quadrant mass. A choledochal cyst can be diagnosed with abdominal ultrasound, which may reveal cystic dilatation of the extrahepatic biliary tree. A hepatobiliary scan can aid in the diagnosis by showing a rounded extrahepatic structure that retains the tracer and is distinguishable from the gallbladder. Treatment consists of excision of the cyst and performance of a choledochojejunostomy. Untreated patients develop cirrhosis. There may be a higher incidence of cholangiocarcinoma in this patient population.

Intrahepatic bile duct paucity refers to a group of disorders characterized by a reduction or absence of bile ductules in the portal triads of the liver. Unlike the one to two bile ductules usually found per portal triad, the paucity syndromes are characterized by less than one-half bile duct per triad. This group of disorders can be subdivided into two major categories: syndromatic and nonsyndromatic. The syndromatic form comprises Alagille syndrome (ie, arteriohepatic dysplasia) and Byler syndrome (ie, progressive intrahepatic cholestasis). Alagille syndrome, in addition to the paucity of intrahepatic bile ducts, is characterized by vertebral arch defects, growth retardation, mental retardation, hypogonadism, and congenital heart disease, most frequently with peripheral pulmonary stenosis. Affected patients also have a typical facial pattern characterized by a broad forehead, mild hypertelorism, a straight nose, and a small pointed chin. Treatment is supportive. Approximately 12% of these patients develop cirrhosis.

Byler syndrome is a rare disorder that was first observed in an Amish kindred but has now been reported in other parts of the world. It is believed to be an autosomal recessive disorder and is characterized by intrahepatic bile duct paucity, mental and physical retardation, and areflexia. The prognosis is worse than that of patients with Alagille syndrome, because most patients develop cirrhosis resulting in death during the first or second decade of life.

The nonsyndromatic form of intrahepatic bile duct paucity is not associated with other anomalies. These patients typically have pruritus and hyperlipidemia. Their prognosis is intermediate between that of patients with Alagille and Byler syndromes, with approximately 40% developing cirrhosis.

Congenital segmental dilatation of the intrahepatic biliary tree may progress to cirrhosis. Caroli's disease, an autosomal recessive disorder, is characterized by hepatomegaly and dilated intrahepatic ducts that contain bile. There is a significant potential for the formation of stones within these dilated ducts and for the development of cholangitis. Although affected patients tend not to develop cirrhosis, a subset of patients have severe periportal fibrosis and do develop cirrhosis.

Congenital hepatic fibrosis is a rare autosomal recessive disorder characterized by multiple bands of fibrous tissue that run throughout the liver and by dysmorphic bile ducts within the fibrous tissue. The exact cause is unknown, but the condition is thought to be secondary to abnormal development of the bile ducts. Affected patients tend to present with hepatosplenomegaly and portal hypertension and may develop cholangitis, biliary calculi, and intrahepatic abscesses. Most patients have associated renal disease in the form of renal tubular ectasia or polycystic kidney disease.

Cystic fibrosis is the most common lethal genetic disease affecting Caucasians. It is inherited in an autosomal recessive pattern and affects approximately 1 in 2000 live births. The lungs and pancreas are the primary organs affected, although multiple organ systems are involved. Hepatobiliary disorders occur in 20% to 60% of patients with cystic fibrosis, and the incidence increases with age. About 16% to 30% of patients have microgallbladders, and 6% to 24% have cholelithiasis. Hepatic steatosis is the most common liver abnormality, occurring in at least one third of patients with cystic fibrosis. This complication is in part secondary to the malnutrition, which is prevalent in these patients. Some infants with cystic fibrosis present with cholestasis secondary to sludge in the biliary tree. Patients with cystic fibrosis may develop focal biliary cirrhosis or multilobular cirrhosis, although cirrhosis rarely is the presenting manifestation of cystic fibrosis. Focal biliary cirrhosis occurs in 10% of infants dying in the first 3 months of life and then increases to 27% after the first year. This lesion histologically is characterized by inspissation of eosinophilic microprotein in the bile ducts, bile duct proliferation, chronic inflammation, and portal fibrosis. As with other liver diseases associated with cystic fibrosis, the incidence of multilobular cirrhosis increases with age; it is approximately 5% among patients older than 12 years of age and 10% among those older than 25 years of age.

Primary sclerosing cholangitis is a chronic inflammatory disease of unknown cause that rarely occurs in children. It is characterized by progressive fibrosis of the intrahepatic and extrahepatic biliary ducts. These ducts are best visualized by endoscopic retrograde cholangiopancreatography (ERCP), which reveals multiple focal areas of stricture and irregularities. Sclerosing cholangitis most commonly is associated with inflammatory bowel disease, histiocytosis X, or immunodeficiency states. About 24% of cases in children are not associated with an underlying disorder. Patients commonly present with abdominal pain, jaundice, and hepatomegaly. Liver enzyme levels are almost always elevated. Liver biopsy reveals portal fibrosis and pericholangitis. The progression to frank cirrhosis is variable, although it tends to occur 5 to 10 years after diagnosis. There is no effective therapy other than liver transplantation.

## Genetic and Metabolic Disorders

$\alpha_1$-Antitrypsin deficiency is the prototypic genetic and metabolic disorder resulting in cirrhosis in pediatric patients. $\alpha_1$-Antitrypsin is an acute-phase reactant that is synthesized in the liver and is the major antiproteolytic agent in the body. $\alpha_1$-Antitrypsin de-

ficiency is an inherited disorder of glycoprotein metabolism, with a prevalence of 1 in 1500 to 34,000 persons. The phenotype is determined by Pi (protease inhibitor) typing. The normal person is PiMM, and the homozygote-deficient person is PiZZ. PiZZ persons have approximately 15% to 20% of the normal $\alpha_1$-antitrypsin levels, and PiMZ and PiSS persons have levels, respectively, 60% and 65% of normal. The disorder can manifest with cholestasis in infancy, cirrhosis in childhood, or chronic obstructive pulmonary disease in early adulthood. The diagnosis is made from a low $\alpha_1$-antitrypsin level, abnormal Pi typing, and finding cytoplasmic granules of $\alpha_1$-antitrypsin on liver biopsy.

Treatment is primarily supportive unless severe liver disease ensues, in which case liver transplantation is curative. Intermittent intravenous infusion of purified $\alpha_1$-antitrypsin from plasma has normalized serum $\alpha_1$-antitrypsin levels and halted the progression of lung disease in adults. There is no experience with this treatment in children with liver disease. The prognosis of pediatric patients with liver disease is variable. Approximately 25% develop cirrhosis and die in the first decade of life, another 25% die in the second decade of live, 25% have persistent abnormalities in liver function but survive into adulthood, and in another 25%, the liver disease appears to resolve.

Wilson's disease (ie, hepatolenticular degeneration) is an inherited disorder of copper metabolism. Wilson's disease is thought to be an autosomal recessive disorder; the gene responsible for the defect in copper metabolism is on chromosome 13. The prevalence of Wilson's disease ranges from 1 to 30 per million live births. The exact defect in copper metabolism is uncertain, although it results in deposition of copper in most organs, especially the liver, brain, and kidneys. Patients with Wilson's disease usually are seen after 5 years of age; one patient was diagnosed at the age of 2 years.

Many presentations are possible, although younger patients usually present with liver disease and older patients with neurologic symptoms. The liver disease can manifest as acute or chronic hepatitis, cholestasis, portal hypertension, cirrhosis, or liver failure. The neurologic symptoms range from deterioration in handwriting and personality changes to athetoid movements and a parkinsonian-like state. Patients with Wilson's disease may have a hemolytic anemia, arthropathy, skeletal fractures, hematuria, or Fanconi's syndrome.

The diagnosis of Wilson's disease is based on increased urinary copper excretion and decreased serum copper and ceruloplasmin levels. The copper content of the liver is significantly elevated. Kayser-Fleischer rings result from the deposition of copper in Descemet's membrane of the cornea. These rings increase in size with the duration of the disease and resolve over time with appropriate therapy. The finding of Kayser-Fleischer rings is essentially diagnostic.

Therapy is directed toward achieving and maintaining a negative copper balance for life. Therapy consists of a reduction in dietary copper and the use of D-penicillamine, which chelates copper. Other potential agents that can be used are triethylene tetramine and zinc sulfate. Although the prognosis of untreated patients is dismal (ie, death is essentially universal), patients who are diagnosed early enough and treated appropriately have a normal life expectancy.

Hemosiderosis, a condition in which iron stores are increased within the liver, is associated with such disorders as hemochromatosis, neonatal iron overload syndrome, transfusional iron overload (which can occur with thalassemia and sickle cell disease), alcoholic liver disease, and excessive dietary iron intake. Primary hemochromatosis is an inherited disorder of iron metabolism resulting in an increase in total body levels of iron of 20 to 50 times that normally present. This condition presents most commonly in adulthood. The iron is deposited in all organs of the body, particularly the liver, pancreas, skin, and heart. Most persons with hemosiderosis have a marked increases in hepatic fibrous tissue or frank cirrhosis. Diabetes, congestive heart failure, arrhythmias, and abnormal skin pigmentation are relatively frequent. Plasma iron is elevated, and transferrin is saturated or nearly saturated, although the transferrin level itself is low because of the severity of the liver disease. The level of ferritin which reflects iron stores is elevated, usually in the range of several thousand micrograms per deciliter. The amount of iron excreted in the urine after administration of desferrioxamine is significantly increased and correlates relatively well with the quantity of excess iron stores.

Treatment of hemochromatosis is aimed at removing iron from the body. Iron removal can be achieved with repeated phlebotomy or with chelation therapy. Because each pint of blood contains approximately 200 mg of iron, repeated phlebotomy for prolonged periods can remove significant quantities of iron. Chelation therapy is most commonly done with desferrioxamine, which can result in the loss of 10 or 20 mg/day. Continuous subcutaneous infusion may be more effective. Untreated patients die of cirrhosis or heart failure.

Galactosemia is an inherited disorder of galactose metabolism that results in severe liver disease in infancy that progresses to cirrhosis if left untreated. It is an autosomal recessive disorder that occurs with a frequency of 1 in 10,000 to 30,000 live births. There is a deficiency of galactose-1-phosphate uridyltransferase, which causes an accumulation of galactose-1-phosphate in the liver, brain, lens, kidney, and adrenal. These infants, if fed lactose, which consists of glucose and galactose, present in infancy with vomiting, diarrhea, failure to thrive, developmental delay or retardation, cataracts, cholestasis, or cirrhosis. The liver biopsy is nonspecific and reveals hepatic steatosis, fibrosis, necrosis, and pseudoacinar formation. The latter is a nonspecific finding in several metabolic disorders. A preliminary diagnosis is made when reducing substances and no glucose are found in the urine. The definitive diagnosis is made by finding low levels of galactose-1-phosphate uridyltransferase in erythrocytes. Treatment consists of excluding galactose from the diet; if instituted sufficiently early, symptoms resolve, and the patient will have a normal life expectancy.

Hereditary fructose intolerance is an autosomal recessive disorder with a prevalence of 1 in 40,000. Affected patients have a deficiency in the enzyme fructose-1-phosphate aldolase, which results in the hepatic accumulation of fructose-1-phosphate. This latter compound is a competitive inhibitor of phosphorylase and interferes with the breakdown of glycogen to glucose. The reduction in glycolysis results in hypoglycemia and lactic acidosis. Patients with this disorder usually present in infancy with vomiting, irritability, diarrhea, cholestasis, hepatomegaly, seizures of hypoglycemia after ingesting the disaccharide sucrose, which is composed of glucose and fructose.

Laboratory evaluation reveals fructose in the urine, elevated liver enzymes, and elevated bilirubin. The liver biopsy is nondiagnostic but reveals hepatic steatosis, necrosis, cholestasis, and pseudoacinar formation. Eventually, fibrosis and cirrhosis develop. The definitive diagnosis can be made by performing a fructose tolerance test; blood glucose and phosphorus levels fall and lactate levels increase in patients with heredity fructose intolerance. Fructose tolerance tests should be administered in a controlled setting, because hypoglycemia and shock may occur. The level of enzyme can also be determined in a liver biopsy specimen. Treatment consists of the elimination of fructose from the diet. If instituted early, symptoms resolve, and the patient will have a normal life expectancy.

Hereditary tyrosinemia is a rare disorder of tyrosine metabolism that is inherited in an autosomal recessive pattern. It appears to be the result of a deficiency of fumarylacetoacetate hydrolase (ie, fumarylhydrolase), the last enzyme in the degradation of tyrosine. As a result, the serum levels of tyrosine and other intermediates, such as succinylacetone, become elevated, and these substances appear to be responsible for the tissue injury. These patients develop severe liver disease and frequently die of liver failure in the first year of life. They may also present with cirrhosis, renal tubular dysfunction (including Fanconi's syndrome), or vitamin D-resistant rickets. Tyrosinemia is diagnosed if elevated blood levels of tyrosine and methionine are found and if succinylacetone is detected. A diet low in tyrosine and methionine may help normalize the serum amino acid pattern, but the liver disease frequently progresses. Liver transplantation has been performed successfully in patients with tyrosinemia and is the only hope for survival in patients with severe progressive liver disease.

Glycogen storage diseases are rare inherited disorders of glycogen metabolism; each type is the result of a specific enzyme deficiency. Almost all types of glycogen storage diseases are associated with glycogen accumulation and subsequently with some degree of hepatomegaly, except those that involve only skeletal muscle. Types I, II, III, and IV are those in which the untreated patient can develop significant liver disease, cirrhosis, or liver failure. Type IV glycogen storage disease is the type most frequently associated with cirrhosis.

Liver biopsy can be extremely useful in making the diagnosis of glycogen storage disease. The histology of the liver is different in the various types and can often be differentiated by electron microscopy. Type I is associated with significant hepatic steatosis and nuclear hyperglycogenosis and may be associated with the development of hepatic adenomas. Type II disease is associated with glycogen-filled lysosomes without significant steatosis or nuclear glycogenosis. Type III has nuclear glycogenosis similar to type I, but no steatosis. There is prominent fibrosis, which typically does not occur in type I. Type IV has broad bands of fibrous tissue or frank cirrhosis. The hepatocytes have eccentric nuclei and glycogen-filled lysosomes.

Treatment is directed toward avoidance of hypoglycemia and its associated hormonal disruption, which is thought to contribute to the complications of glycogen storage disease. Treatment entails providing frequent high-starch meals during the day and continuous nasogastric or gastrostomy feedings at night. This regimen has resulted in a reduction in liver size, improved liver function, normalization of liver enzymes, and decreased levels of liver glycogen.

Several lipid storage disorders associated with hepatic fibrosis or cirrhosis include cholesterol ester storage disease, Wolman's disease, Niemann-Pick disease, and Gaucher's disease. Cholesterol ester storage disease is an inherited disorder associated with a decrease in acid lipase. The cholesterol esters and triglycerides accumulate in the liver. Fibrosis occurs and varies in severity. Patients present with hepatosplenomegaly and an elevated serum cholesterol. There is no specific therapy, although liver transplantation may be required and appears to "cure" the disease.

Wolman's disease, an autosomal recessive disorder, is secondary to acid lipase deficiency, as is cholesterol ester storage disease. Wolman's disease, however, is associated with deposition of cholesterol esters and triglycerides in the liver, small intestine, bone marrow, lymph nodes, kidney, thymus, brain, and adrenal glands. The adrenal glands are calcified. The liver, in addition to having deposits of cholesterol esters and triglycerides, demonstrates periportal fibrosis. These patients usually present in infancy with diarrhea, failure to thrive, icterus, and hepatosplenomegaly. There is no effective treatment, and the patients usually die during the first year of life.

Niemann-Pick disease is an autosomal recessive disorder secondary to lysosomal sphingomyelinase deficiency. As a result of this enzymatic deficiency, sphingomyelin and cholesterol accumulate in the reticuloendothelial cells, especially in the liver, spleen, and bone marrow. Hepatocytes are vacuolated and Niemann-Pick foam cells are seen in liver biopsy specimens. Periportal fibrosis is evident. Of the five major types, the most common is the acute neuropathic infantile form, manifesting in infancy with hepatosplenomegaly and neurologic deterioration. There is no effective therapy, and the prognosis for patients with infantile type Niemann-Pick disease is poor.

Gaucher's disease appears to be an autosomal recessive disorder that results from a deficiency in $\beta$-glucosidase and causes an accumulation of glycosyl ceramide in the reticuloendothelial cells. Liver biopsy reveals the lipid-filled Gaucher cells with a typical "wrinkled tissue paper" appearance. These cells are located around the central vein and the sinusoids. Although some fibrosis may occur, patients rarely develop cirrhosis and portal hypertension. Serum acid phosphatase levels are elevated. There are three major classifications of this disease: infantile, juvenile, and adult, although the age of presentation does not correspond to the type of disease. Patients with the infantile type of disease present with hepatosplenomegaly, thrombocytopenia, and neurologic deterioration and die within the first year of life. Those who present with the juvenile type also have hepatosplenomegaly, but neurologic involvement is less severe and the prognosis is much better than for the infantile type. The adult type also has hepatosplenomegaly and thrombocytopenia, but without neurologic involvement. Recent studies indicate that macrophage-targeted glucocerebrosidase may be helpful.

Osler-Weber-Rendu disease (hereditary hemorrhagic telangiectasia) is an autosomal dominant disorder characterized by telangiectasia that can involve the skin, mucous membranes, gastrointestinal tract, liver, lung, and brain. The lesions develop during puberty and have significant potential for bleeding; surgical therapy may be required. Infrequently, these patients develop fibrosis or cirrhosis.

## Infection

Many different organisms can infect the liver and cause hepatitis, including hepatitis A, hepatitis B, hepatitis C, delta hepatitis, Epstein-Barr virus, cytomegalovirus, rubella, and syphilis. Chronic hepatitis tends to occur only after infections with hepatitis B, delta hepatitis, hepatitis C, or syphilis. There are two major types of chronic hepatitis, chronic persistent hepatitis (CPH) and chronic active hepatitis (CAH). Ten percent of patients with acute hepatitis B remain positive for HBsAg; 70% of these patients develop CPH and 30% develop CAH. Superinfection with delta hepatitis results in an increased frequency of chronic hepatitis. CPH is characterized by mild portal inflammation, which is considered relatively benign and requires no specific therapy. CAH is characterized by extension of the inflammatory response out of the portal area into the lobule and is associated with piecemeal necrosis. CAH has the potential to progress to cirrhosis and liver failure. The occurrence is 20% in adults and approximately 4% in infants and children.

Steroids, alone or in conjunction with azathioprine, have been used successfully to treat some patients, although their use remains controversial. Preliminary research indicates that $\alpha$-interferon may induce remissions in 30% to 40% of patients with CAH due to hepatitis B, but further evaluation is required before recommending it for clinical use.

After acute hepatitis C, a significant number of patients develop chronic hepatitis. The frequency ranges from 7% in sporadic cases to 80% in immunosuppressed patients. On average, 50% of patients acutely infected with hepatitis C develop chronic hepatitis, and 20% develop cirrhosis.

Cirrhosis is a rare complication of congenital syphilis and cytomegalovirus infections. With appropriate therapy, the hepatitis resolves, and cirrhosis does not develop.

## Cardiac Cirrhosis

Cirrhosis may develop secondary to congenital heart disease or congestive heart failure as the result of passive congestion and ischemia of long duration. The signs and symptoms of the heart disease are prominent, with few or none referable to the liver disease other than hepatosplenomegaly. The initial lesion consists of dilatation of the central vein and the sinusoids. As time passes, centrilobular hemorrhage, necrosis, and fibrosis occur. Liver enzymes are elevated, with minimal elevation in bilirubin except in severe cases. As cardiac failure persists, the centrilobular fibrosis extends into the lobule, and if the patient survives long enough, cirrhosis develops. If cardiac function is normalized before cirrhosis develops, liver disease can stabilize or resolve, depending on its stage.

Budd-Chiari syndrome (ie, obstruction or thrombosis of the hepatic vein) and constrictive pericarditis result in similar hepatic lesions, which improve after appropriate treatment of the underlying disorder is administered.

## Autoimmune

Autoimmune chronic active hepatitis is a rare disorder in the pediatric population, but it has potentially severe consequences. Autoimmune hepatitis initially presents as any other hepatitis with nonspecific symptoms, hepatomegaly, and jaundice. Evaluation fails to produce evidence of hepatitis A, B, or other viral infections or evidence of other causes of liver disease, such as Wilson's disease or $\alpha_1$-antitrypsin deficiency. With autoimmune hepatitis, the erythrocyte sedimentation rate and immunoglobulins are elevated. Autoantibodies, such as anti-smooth muscle antibody, antinuclear antibody, liver-kidney microsomal antibody (ie, endoplasmic reticulum antibody), or antiactin antibodies may be found in as many as 80% of patients.

Treatment of this disorder remains controversial. Institution of therapy with prednisone is generally agreed on. Some physicians also recommend instituting therapy with azathioprine at the onset, but others use such therapy only when prednisone therapy alone has been unsuccessful. Cyclosporin A has been tried in patients who do not respond to the other therapies. Inadequate response to therapy results in progression of the liver disease or the development of cirrhosis. Reports indicate that most patients with autoimmune chronic hepatitis have cirrhosis at the time of presentation.

## Nutritional Disorders

Malnutrition in the forms of undernutrition and overnutrition is a worldwide problem. The most common hepatic abnormality in infants and children suffering from malnutrition is hepatic steatosis. This disorder occurs in most children with severe protein-calorie malnutrition. The frequency of hepatic steatosis in obese patients ranges from 66% to 99%. Some investigators believe that hepatic steatosis can progress to cirrhosis, although this remains controversial.

Total parenteral nutrition (TPN) is a commonly used therapeutic modality. Cholestasis is often encountered when TPN is used, especially in premature infants. Hepatic fibrosis and cirrhosis occur rarely as a consequence of TPN, but they do occur if TPN is administered for prolonged periods of time.

Jejunoileal bypass surgery was a relatively commonly performed operation for the treatment of the morbidly obese in the 1960s and 1970s. The surgery is used today in some institutions to treat severe hypercholesterolemia. Unfortunately, approximately one third of these patients develop liver disease, including fibrosis, hepatitis, and micronodular cirrhosis. Approximately 10% of these patients develop cirrhosis over a period of many years. There are numerous theories about to the cause of cirrhosis in these patients, although the exact mechanism is unknown.

Vitamin A, a fat-soluble vitamin, is an essential nutrient required for many metabolic processes. Hypervitaminosis A, however, can result in pseudotumor cerebri and liver disease. Ingestion of over 40,000 IU of vitamin A for prolonged periods of time can result in cirrhosis.

## Drugs and Toxins

Although many drugs are hepatotoxic, relatively few of these drugs contribute to the development of cirrhosis. Alcohol is the primary cause of drug-induced cirrhosis. Alcohol abuse results in micronodular cirrhosis. Approximately 75% of patients who consume 1 pint of alcohol per day for 15 years have significant liver disease. Methotrexate can cause portal cirrhosis, and the potential for development of cirrhosis is increased by alcohol intake, daily use of methotrexate, prior liver disease, and obesity. Patients with long-term methotrexate therapy probably should undergo a liver biopsy after each 1 to 1.5 g is administered. Approximately 1% to 2% of patients taking chlorpromazine become jaundiced after 1 to 2 months of therapy. The liver disease in most of these patients resolves over 1 year. A small percentage develop biliary cirrhosis. Other drugs that can potentially result in cirrhosis are amiodarone and perhexiline maleate.

Among toxins that can cause cirrhosis are carbon tetrachloride, dimethylnitrosamine, vinyl chloride, arsenic, and aflatoxin.

## Miscellaneous

There are three main disorders in the miscellaneous category of cirrhosis: Indican childhood cirrhosis, Zellweger syndrome, and neonatal hepatitis. Indian childhood cirrhosis is a chronic inflammatory liver disease of unknown cause that occurs predominantly in India and Southeast Asia, although a few cases have been reported in the United States and Great Britain. The disorder affects children as young as 1 month to 10 years of age, with a peak incidence between 1 and 3 years. A family history can be obtained in 30% of cases. Early in the course of the disease, the liver histology is characterized by a diffuse inflammatory process with ballooning degeneration, Mallory bodies, and fibrosis. A large amount of copper is deposited in the liver, as in Wilson's disease; however, patients with Indian childhood cirrhosis do not have low ceruloplasmin levels and do not develop Kayser-Fleischer rings. Until recently no specific therapy was available for this disorder, but it appears that therapy with D-penicillamine may be beneficial. Death frequently occurs within 8 months of the onset if no treatment is provided.

Zellweger syndrome (ie, cerebrohepatorenal syndrome) is a rare autosomal recessive disorder that appears to be secondary to deficiencies of several peroxisomal enzymes. This syndrome is characterized by central nervous system deficits (eg, developmental delay, hypotonia, seizures), facial dysmorphic features, cortical cysts of the kidney, and cirrhosis. Hepatomegaly is normally present at birth along with cholestasis. As the disease progresses, a micronodular cirrhosis develops, and iron deposition increases. There is no specific therapy for this disorder, and death usually occurs in the first year of life.

Neonatal hepatitis is a relatively common disorder of unknown cause initially presenting as cholestasis in the newborn period. Other causes for cholestasis, such as infections and biliary atresia, need to be ruled out. Histologically, there is lobular disarray, inflammation, necrosis, and multinucleated giant cells. Unlike biliary atresia, there is no bile duct proliferation. Nonfamilial

hepatitis has a mortality rate of 30%; 2% of patients develop cirrhosis. The prognosis is worse if there is a family history of neonatal hepatitis, in which case the mortality approximates 60%, and 10% develop cirrhosis.

## CLINICAL MANIFESTATIONS

The clinical manifestations of cirrhosis are the same regardless of the cause of the disease. Patients with certain disorders have manifestations of that specific disorder (eg, Kayser-Fleischer rings in Wilson's disease), but the manifestations of cirrhosis itself are the same.

Children with cirrhosis fail to thrive and become malnourished unless aggressive nutritional support is provided. The cause of the malnutrition is multifactorial and includes decreased hepatic protein synthesis, malabsorption of fat and fat-soluble vitamins due to a reduction in enteric bile salts, anorexia secondary to chronic disease, and early satiety as a result of ascites. The fat malabsorption and edema of the intestinal tract can result in chronic diarrhea.

Portal hypertension develops as a result of cirrhosis, and these children have hepatosplenomegaly. Late in the course of cirrhosis, liver size can decrease secondary to a loss of hepatocytes. The spleen can become significantly enlarged and cause hypersplenism with its associated thrombocytopenia and possible leukopenia and anemia. Patients with portal hypertension may also have prominent abdominal vessels.

Patients with cirrhosis frequently are edematous because of decreased serum albumin and increased total body level of water, which is primarily caused by increased extracellular fluid volume. Cirrhotic patients have various degrees of jaundice. If jaundice occurs during the time in which the teeth are developing, the teeth become a greenish color. As a result of decreased ability to excrete bile salts, the serum bile acid level is elevated and can result in pruritus. When severe, excoriations and lichenification are noticed. Other potential physical findings in cirrhosis include palmar erythema, spider angiomas, digital clubbing, and delayed sexual maturation.

## COMPLICATIONS

There are many potentially serious complications of cirrhosis. Failure to thrive, delayed sexual development, and hypersplenism have been discussed briefly. Ascites, peritonitis, portal hypertension, and gastrointestinal hemorrhage frequently accompany cirrhosis and are discussed in Chapters 122, 137, and 139.5. Other potential complications of cirrhosis are hematologic abnormalities, coagulation disorders, hepatic encephalopathy, hepatorenal syndrome, liver failure, and cholelithiasis.

Hematologic abnormalities include thrombocytopenia, leukopenia, and anemia. Thrombocytopenia and leukopenia are secondary to hypersplenism. Hypersplenism results in platelet counts in the range of 50,000 to 100,000 cells/mm$^3$. If the platelet count is less than 20,000 cells/mm$^3$, another cause for thrombocytopenia should be sought. The cause of anemia in patients with cirrhosis is multifactorial and includes hypersplenism, iron deficiency due to gastrointestinal bleeding, and hemolytic anemia, which can be associated with chronic active hepatitis. Anemia also can be caused by vitamin E deficiency or to alterations in erythrocyte membrane lipid component. Malabsorption of fats and fat-soluble vitamins can lead to alterations in the fatty acid component and the cholesterol-phospholipid ratio in the erythrocyte membrane and can cause decreased erythrocyte survival. Elevated serum lithocholic acid levels can induce spur cell anemia, and lithocholic acid may be elevated in patients with cirrhosis.

Coagulation disorders are common in patients with cirrhosis. These patients may be deficient in vitamin K and have a reduction in the vitamin K-dependent clotting Factors II, VII, IX, and X. Factor VII has the shortest half-life and is the first to become reduced when vitamin K levels are deficient. The prothrombin time is the most sensitive coagulation indicator of vitamin K deficiency. The potential for the reduction in all hepatic clotting factors exists in advanced stages of cirrhosis, because hepatocyte mass and its synthetic capabilities are reduced.

Patients with severe liver disease may have findings consistent with disseminated intravascular coagulation (DIC). These findings consist of thrombocytopenia, elevated prothrombin and partial thromboplastin times, decreased fibrinogen, and elevated fibrin split products. The cause of the thrombocytopenia and reduced clotting factors has been discussed. Fibrin split products are normally cleared by the liver; if the clearance is impaired by severe liver disease, the result is increased fibrin split products. Finding these abnormalities in a patient with severe liver disease does not necessarily indicate true DIC.

Hepatic encephalopathy is a complex neuropsychiatric disorder thought to be caused by the metabolic alterations associated with hepatocellular failure. The elevation in serum ammonia that occurs with liver failure had long been thought to cause hepatic encephalopathy. It is now known that hyperammonemia is not solely responsible and that the cause of hepatic encephalopathy is multifactorial. Other contributory factors include alterations in the permeability of the blood–brain barrier, other neurotoxins (eg, mercaptans, short-chain fatty acids), false neurotransmitters (eg, octopamine and GABA), and alterations in serum amino acid pattern (eg, decreased ratio of branched-chain amino acids to aromatic amino acids). Initially, patients have impaired intellectual functioning, followed by lethargy, coma, and seizures. They manifest asterixis, hyperreflexia, and decerebrate posturing.

There is controversy about the treatment of hepatic encephalopathy. Therapy generally is directed toward improving hepatocellular function and decreasing potential aggravating factors. Unfortunately, except for liver transplantation, little can be done to improve hepatocellular function other than to discontinue any potential hepatotoxic drug. Attempts should be made to reduce production and absorption of ammonia. Neomycin therapy has long been used in this disorder to decrease bacterial formation of ammonia. Lactulose helps prevent the absorption of ammonia by decreasing intraluminal pH and retaining the ammonium ion in the gut, which subsequently is excreted. Whether these agents should be used alone or together remains a subject for debate. Other potential therapeutic modalities include a reduction in protein intake in an attempt to reduce endogenous ammonia production. Protein intake should not be curtailed totally, because the result is increased catabolism of endogenous protein and subsequent ammonia production. The use of branched-chain amino acid and TPN formulas has been relatively successful.

Other neurologic problems can develop in children with chronic cholestasis secondary to vitamin E deficiency. Vitamin E deficiency is encountered in 50% to 75% of children with chronic cholestasis. The first neurologic deficit to develop is areflexia, followed by ataxia, peripheral neuropathy, and ophthalmoplegia. These abnormalities can be prevented or reversed with the institution of vitamin therapy and the normalization of vitamin E status.

Patients with cirrhosis develop the hepatorenal syndrome relatively commonly; this disorder is one of the primary causes of death in cirrhosis. The exact cause of the syndromes is unknown, but it appears to be related in part to marked renal vasoconstriction, which appears to be related to a decrease in effective arterial blood volume. Marked humoral disturbances, which mediate renal vasoconstriction, occur as a result of the reduced blood volume. Several factors can predispose the cirrhotic patient to develop the hepatorenal syndrome, such as gastrointestinal bleeding, therapeutic abdominal paracentesis, and vigorous diuresis. The net effect of all three of these factors is to compromise blood volume further. The initial presentation is similar to prerenal azotemia with reduced urine output, low urine sodium concentration, high urine osmolality, and a relatively benign urinary sediment. Unlike true prerenal azotemia, patients with the hepatorenal syndrome do not respond well to extracellular fluid volume.

Therapy for the hepatorenal syndrome is not effective, and this disorder frequently is fatal. True prerenal azotemia may be differentiated from the hepatorenal syndrome by monitoring central venous pressure and normalizing it with volume expanders. Portacaval shunting or placement of a LeVeen or Denver shunt has been used to improve intravascular volume and has been relatively successful. Other therapies, such as dopamine, have met with limited success. The best approach in the treatment of the hepatorenal syndrome is prevention. The syndrome can be prevented if nephrotoxic drugs are avoided, gastrointestinal bleeding is treated aggressively, rigorous diuretic therapy is avoided, and large quantities of ascitic fluid are not removed at one time.

Acute hepatic failure can occur after viral hepatitis, Reye's syndrome, or drug exposure, or it can result from progressive cirrhosis. Acute hepatic failure is associated with a mortality of approximately 70%, and hepatic failure secondary to end-stage cirrhosis is uniformly fatal unless a liver transplant is performed.

The biochemical hallmark of hepatic failure in cirrhotic patients is reduced levels of the transaminases with a progressive increase in bilirubin levels, prothrombin and partial thromboplastin times, and ammonia. The blood urea nitrogen may decrease secondary to inability of the liver to manufacture urea, or it may increase in response to the development of the hepatorenal syndrome. Treatment is primarily supportive and directed at maintaining cerebral, renal, cardiac, and hepatic function. The complications of hepatic failure, such as encephalopathy, hepatorenal syndrome, and bleeding disorder, should be anticipated and attempts made to prevent their occurrence. Nutritional support for these patients is complicated because of the need to restrict protein intake and because of potential fluid and electrolyte problems.

There is an increased incidence of cholelithiasis in patients with cirrhosis. Gallstones occur more frequently in patients with decompensated cirrhosis (35%) compared with those with compensated cirrhosis (7%). It is important to consider cholelithiasis in the differential diagnosis of increasing jaundice in cirrhotic patients.

## TREATMENT

Prevention of cirrhosis is the ultimate goal. After cirrhosis is established, there is no specific therapy other than liver transplantation. The disorders in which cirrhosis is potentially preventable and the specific preventive steps were discussed earlier. Supportive therapy for patients with cirrhosis is directed toward the improvement and maintenance of nutritional status. The aim is to support growth, prevent gastrointestinal bleeding, avoid hepatotoxic drugs and toxins, and treat any of the potential complications encountered aggressively.

Nutritional support is the major therapy, especially because most patients with cirrhosis are malnourished. The cause of malnutrition in these patients is multifactorial and includes anorexia secondary to chronic disease, early satiety due to ascites, and malabsorption of nutrients, especially fats and fat-soluble vitamins, due to decreased intraluminal bile acids. Other potential nutrient deficiencies include folic acid, riboflavin, and iron.

A nutritional assessment should be performed at the initial

visit, and various anthropometric measurements and laboratory tests should be administered periodically. Of the anthropometric measurements readily obtainable—weight, height, weight for height, and skinfold thickness—weight is the most variable and is not necessarily a good index of nutritional status. Without any significant change in nutritional status, the patient's weight can increase or decrease significantly as a result of alterations in the amount of ascitic fluid present. Measurement of the triceps skinfold thickness (TSF) can yield some information about fat stores, which usually are depleted in these patients. Determination of arm muscle circumference (ie, mid-arm circumference − [3.14 × TSF]) can provide information about the patient's muscle mass. In addition to checking liver function and liver enzymes, other laboratory tests that provide information about the patient's nutritional status should be performed periodically, including determination of serum albumin, transferrin, calcium, phosphorous, iron, vitamin E, 1,25-dihydroxyvitamin D, and prothrombin time.

Patients in the early stage of cirrhosis should consume high-protein, high-calorie diets. Protein intake may range from 2.5 to 3 g/kg/day. Care must be taken to avoid precipitation of hepatic encephalopathy. Administration of a formula with medium-chain triglyceride (MCT; Portagen, Pregestamil, Alimentum) may help improve fat absorption; MCT absorption has a low requirement for bile salts relative to long-chain triglycerides. Because of the anorexia and early frequently reported in cirrhotic patients, nighttime nasogastric feedings may be required to ensure adequate intake.

Fat-soluble vitamins should be supplemented and their levels monitored because of the potential for malabsorption in cirrhotic patients. Supplementation should include Aquasal A (10,000 to 25,000 IU/day), Aquamephyton, 25-hydroxyvitamin D (3 to 5 µg/kg/day), and vitamin E (50 to 400 IU/day). These patients may reasonably be supplemented with a daily multiple vitamin. Calcium supplements also may be necessary because of the loss of calcium from saponification with malabsorbed fats.

Patients with cirrhosis frequently have pruritus, which can be treated by the administration of choleretic agents such as phenobarbital, ursodeoxycholic acid, or cholestyramine. Antipruritic agents (eg, diphenhydramine, hydroxyzine) can provide significant relief. The patient's nails should be trimmed to avoid excoriation and possible infection.

Other potential complications of cirrhosis, such as ascites, peritonitis, gastrointestinal bleeding, hepatic encephalopathy, and the hepatorenal syndrome, are discussed elsewhere in this book. Liver transplantation has been a major advance in the treatment of cirrhosis. The procedure is performed successfully in infants and children. The introduction of cyclosporine has significantly improved the survival rate of transplant patients; the current 1-year survival rate ranges from 75% to 90%. This procedure, however, is difficult and expensive, and postoperative complications are frequent. Transplantation is extremely stressful for the patient and family. Nevertheless, for a patient with end-stage cirrhosis of the liver, transplantation is the only hope for survival.

## Selected Readings

Acalovschi M, Badea R, Pascu M. Incidence of gallstones in cirrhosis. Am J Gastroenterol 1991;86:1179.

Alagille D, Estrada A, Hadchouel M, et al. Syndromatic paucity of interlobular bile ducts (Alagille's syndrome or arteriohepatic dysplasia): review of eighty cases. J Pediatr 1987;110:195.

Alvarez F, Bernard O, Brunelle F, et al. Congenital hepatic fibrosis in children. J Pediatr 1981;99:370.

Balistreri WF, Bove KE. Hepatobiliary consequences of parenteral alimentation. Prog Liver Dis 1990;567.

Barton NW, Brady RO, Dambrosia JM, et al. Dose-dependent response to macrophage-targeted glucocerebrosidase in a child with Gaucher disease. J Pediatr 1992;120:227.

Bass NM, Ockner RK. Drug induced liver disease. In: Zakim D, Boyer TD, eds. Hepatology: a textbook of liver disease. Philadelphia: WB Saunders, 1990.

Bhusnusmath SR, Walia BN, Singh S, et al. Sequential histopathologic alterations in Indian childhood cirrhosis treated with D-penicillamine. Hum Pathol 1991;22:653.

Butterworth RF. Pathogenesis and treatment of portal-systemic encephalopathy: an update. Dig Dis Sci 1992;37:321.

Dehner LP, Snover DC, Sharp HL, et al. Hereditary tyrosinemia type I (chronic forms): pathologic findings in the liver. Hum Pathol 1989;20:149.

Epstein M. The hepatorenal syndrome. Hosp Pract 1989;24:65.

Ferry GD, Whisennand HH, Finegold MJ, et al. Liver transplantation for cholesterol ester storage disease. J Pediatr Gastroenterol Nutr 1991;7:376.

Forbes A, Murray-Lyons IM. Cystic diseases of the liver and biliary tract. Gut 1991;32:S118.

Huges RD, Wendon J, Gimson AES. Acute liver failure. Gut 1991;32:S86.

Ibarguen E, Gross CR, Savik SK, et al. Liver disease in alpha-1-antitrypsin deficiency: prognostic indicators. J Pediatr 1990;117:864.

Iwai N, Yanagihara J, Tokiwa K, et al. Congenital choledochal dilatation with emphasis on pathophysiology of the biliary tract. Ann Surg 1992;215:27.

Kaplan MM. Medical approaches to primary sclerosing cholangitis. Semin Liver Dis 1991;11:56.

Karrer FM, Lilly JR, Stewart BA, et al. Biliary atresia registry, 1976 to 1989. J Pediatr Surg 1990;25:1076.

Krugman S. Viral hepatitis: A, B, C, D and E infection. Pediatr Rev 1992;203.

Moses SW. Pathophysiology and dietary treatment of glycogen storage disease. J Pediatr Gastroenterol Nutr 1990;11:155.

Rutledge JC. Progressive neonatal liver failure due to type C Niemann-Pick disease. Pediatr Pathol 1989;9:779.

Sarles J, Scheiner C, Sarran M, et al. Hepatic hypervitaminosis A: a familial observation. J Pediatr Gastroenterol Nutr 1990;10:71.

Shabrawi E, Wilkinson M, Portmann B, et al. Primary sclerosing cholangitis in childhood. Gastroenterol 1987;92:1226.

Silk DBA, O'Keefe SJD, Wicks C. Nutritional support in liver disease. Gut 1991;32:S29.

Singh I, Johnson GH, et al. Peroxisomal disorders: biochemical and clinical diagnostic considerations. Am J Dis Child 1988;142:1297.

Thaler MM. Cirrhosis. In: Walker WA, Durie PR, et al, eds. Pediatric gastrointestinal disease: pathophysiology, diagnosis, management. Philadelphia: BC Dekker, 1991.

Whitington PF, Balistrer WF: Liver transplantation in pediatrics: indications, contraindications, and pretransplant management. J Pediatr 1991;118:169.

*Principles and Practice of Pediatrics, Second Edition.*
edited by Frank A. Oski et al. J. B. Lippincott Company, Philadelphia © 1994.

## 139.5 *Portal Hypertension*

### William J. Cochran

Portal hypertension is an abnormal condition of sustained elevated pressure in the portal venous system. Normal portal vein pressure is between 5 and 10 mm Hg. Portal vein pressure measurements rarely are made in clinical practice, because they are difficult to do and are invasive. Several studies have documented that the complications of portal hypertension do not occur until the portal pressure gradient (ie, gradient between the portal vein and the hepatic veins or the inferior vena cava) exceeds 12 mm Hg. Normal is less than 5 mm Hg. Above this threshold value, the absolute portal pressure correlates poorly with the complications associated with portal hypertension. The increased portal pressure prompts the formation of portosystemic collaterals, which divert portal blood to the systemic circulation. In severe cases of cirrhosis, as much as 90% of the portal blood enters the systemic circulation through these collaterals and bypasses the liver.

## ETIOLOGY

Several factors contribute to the development and maintenance of portal hypertension. An increased vascular resistance to portal blood flow is the initiating factor responsible for the development of portal hypertension. Blood flow into the portal circulation increases because of splanchnic arteriolar vasodilation. This splanchnic vasodilation is secondary to an increase in several circulating vasodilators, including vasoactive intestinal polypeptide, glucagon, and prostacyclin, due to reduced metabolism by the liver. An increased plasma volume is the result of renal sodium retention.

There are three major sites of increased vascular resistance: prehepatic, intrahepatic, and posthepatic (Table 139-16). Within the prehepatic category, portal vein thrombosis is the most common cause of portal hypertension in pediatric populations. Portal vein thrombosis can develop as a result of sepsis, pancreatitis, umbilical vein catheterization, or omphalitis. When this condition evolves, many small collateral veins develop and transport portal blood to the liver. This condition is referred to as cavernomatous transformation of the portal vein, in which the normal vein is replaced by many small tortuous veins.

Intrahepatic portal hypertension can be presinusoidal, sinusoidal, or postsinusoidal in origin. Hepatic schistosomiasis is an example of presinusoidal portal hypertension and is second only to cirrhosis as the most common cause of portal hypertension on a worldwide basis, although this infection is exceedingly rare in North America. Portal hypertension develops in patients with hepatic schistosomiasis as the result of ova deposited in the portal venules and the subsequent periportal granulomatous reaction. Neoplasms and hepatic cysts, as seen in polycystic disease or Caroli's disease, may compress the portal venules and cause portal hypertension. Cirrhosis is the primary cause of sinusoidal portal hypertension in children and adults. The most common causes of cirrhosis in children include biliary atresia, neonatal hepatitis, and $\alpha_1$-antitrypsin deficiency. Intrahepatic postsinusoidal portal hypertension is rare in children. In adults, it is most often secondary to veno-occlusive disease.

The classic cause of posthepatic portal hypertension is the Budd-Chiari syndrome, which is a thrombus in the hepatic vein at the entry to the inferior vena cava. Posthepatic portal hypertension also can develop as the result of severe right heart failure or constrictive pericarditis.

## Diagnosis

Portal hypertension can be determined by several modalities (Table 139-17), but it is diagnosed most frequently by physical ex-

---

**TABLE 139-16.  Causes of Portal Hypertension**

Prehepatic origin
    Portal vein thrombosis
Intrahepatic origin
    Presinusoidal
        Schistosomiasis
        Neoplasms
        Hepatic cysts
    Sinusoidal
        Cirrhosis
    Postsinusoidal
        Veno-occlusive disease
Posthepatic origin
    Thrombosis
        Budd-Chiari syndrome
    Cardiac
        Right-sided ventricular heart failure
        Constrictive pericarditis

---

**TABLE 139-17.  Diagnosis of Portal Hypertension**

Physical Examination
    Splenomegaly
    Ascites
    Prominent abdominal vessels
    Esophageal varices
    Hemorrhoids/rectal varices
    Evidence of chronic liver disease
Invasive techniques
    Direct measurement of portal pressure
    Measurement of hepatic venous pressure gradient
    Angiography
    Splenoportography
Endoscopy
Noninvasive techniques
    Barium swallow
    Ultrasonography

---

amination. The physical manifestations of portal hypertension may include splenomegaly, ascites, prominent abdominal vessels, esophageal varices, and hemorrhoids or rectal varices. Splenomegaly and ascites often develop in patients with portal hypertension, although ascites usually is found when the condition is of sinusoidal or postsinusoidal, and rarely, presinusoidal origin. Other physical manifestations of chronic liver disease include icterus, spider hemangiomas, asterixis, encephalopathy, and malnutrition.

Several invasive and noninvasive techniques can be used to document portal hypertension. The invasive techniques include direct measurement of portal pressure, measurement of the hepatic venous pressure gradient, angiography, splenoportography, and endoscopy. Direct measurement of portal pressure can be done by puncturing an intrahepatic branch of the portal vein percutaneously or during abdominal surgery by inserting a needle directly into the portal vein. The former procedure is difficult to do, especially in small children, and the latter is an unacceptable procedure just to diagnose portal hypertension.

Measurement of the hepatic venous pressure gradient is being used for adults with increasing frequency. A catheter is placed in the hepatic vein under fluoroscopic control, and the free hepatic venous pressure is obtained. The catheter then is advanced until the catheter occludes a small hepatic vein, and the wedged hepatic venous pressure is measured. The hepatic venous pressure gradient is the difference between the wedged hepatic venous pressure and the free hepatic venous pressure. Normally, the gradient is less than 5 mm Hg, and greater than 10 mm Hg is indicative of portal hypertension. It is elevated in patients with hepatic-origin portal hypertension but normal in those with hypertension due to extrahepatic causes such as portal vein thrombosis. It is the diagnostic modality most often used in adult studies assessing the efficacy of pharmacologic agents to reduce portal pressure. Experience with this measurement in the pediatric population is limited.

Angiography is helpful in detecting portal hypertension by documenting the portosystemic collateral circulation, and it can define the vascular anatomy if surgery is contemplated. Selective superior mesenteric angiography is performed after catheterization of the femoral artery. After injection, films are obtained to demonstrate the arterial and venous phases. In cases of portal vein thrombosis, the portal vein does not fill, although normally it is visualized after 10 to 20 seconds. Many fine collateral channels can be demonstrated around the occluded portal vein in patients with cavernomatous transformation of the portal vein.

Another angiographic feature of patients with portal hypertension is antegrade (reversed) portal flow.

Splenoportography has been used to demonstrate the portal venous system, but this procedure was associated with a significant risk of splenic injury and bleeding. It should not be used unless surgery can be performed immediately if complications occur. There is little indication for splenoportography, because the portal system can be visualized with the less invasive digital subtraction techniques.

Endoscopy is the diagnostic modality used most commonly to detect esophageal, gastric, or duodenal varices. Fiberoptic endoscopy can be performed rapidly and safely in infants and children. This method is more sensitive in the detection of varices than barium swallow or ultrasonography. Endoscopy allows the visual inspection of the varices to determine their size and color, which is helpful in predicting the risk of bleeding.

There are two noninvasive techniques for detecting portal hypertension: the barium swallow and ultrasonography. Before the advent of flexible endoscopy, the barium swallow was the test performed most commonly to detect portal hypertension. Most patients in whom the condition is of long duration have esophageal varices, which can be identified by barium swallow. The worm-like varices are shown in Figure 139-7.

Ultrasonography has been useful in evaluating children with portal hypertension. In addition to predicting the presence of portal hypertension, ultrasonography is helpful in evaluating the cause of the portal hypertension such as cirrhosis, hepatic cysts, or portal vein thrombosis. Ultrasound can determine the diameter of the portal vein, which increases with age. In adults, an enlarged portal vein diameter suggests portal hypertension. In children, it is more helpful to determine the ratio of portal vein diameter (in mm) to surface area (in m²). If this ratio exceeds 12, esophageal varices are likely. The ratio of the lesser omentum thickness to aortic diameter is another useful parameter to assess, because the lesser omentum increases in thickness with portal hypertension. A ratio greater than 1.9 is associated with the presence of esophageal varices. In healthy persons, the portal vein increases in diameter with inspiration. This increase does not occur with inspiration in patients with portal hypertension and is thought to be a more reliable indicator of the condition than the actual diameter of the portal vein. Another reliable marker of portal hypertension is reversal of portal vein flow by Doppler exami-

nation. Ultrasound may enable evaluation of the patency of portosystemic shunts.

## Complications and Treatment

There are four major potential complications of portal hypertension: ascites, variceal bleeding, portosystemic encephalopathy (PSE), and splenomegaly with its associated hypersplenism. Ascites, a frequent problem in patients with sinusoidal and postsinusoidal portal hypertension, is uncommon in patients with presinusoidal portal hypertension. Potential complications of ascites include spontaneous bacterial peritonitis, compromised respiratory status, and discomfort.

Variceal bleeding is the most frequent and potentially lifethreatening complication of portal hypertension. Approximately 25% to 40% of adult patients eventually have active bleeding from their varices. The mortality rate among adults with esophageal variceal bleeding may be as high as 50%. Among children, the mortality rate is lower, but remains significant at 12% to 21%. Bleeding occurs most commonly from esophageal varices but may be secondary to gastric, small intestinal, or colonic varices.

Patients with portal hypertension who present with an acute upper gastrointestinal (GI) hemorrhage are evaluated and treated initially in a manner similar to any patient with upper GI hemorrhage. The first efforts are devoted to the ABCs of resuscitation: airway, breathing, and circulation. Most patients with GI bleeding are stable from a respiratory standpoint unless they have massive bleeding with shock or if they are vomiting large amounts of blood with clots and aspirate. It is imperative that patients with GI bleeding have adequate intravenous access to allow rapid restoration of their blood volume. Care should be taken not to overexpand their blood volume, because this could elevate portal pressure, worsening the variceal bleeding.

The initial evaluation of upper GI bleeding should include a complete blood cell count, liver function tests including coagulation studies, serum electrolytes, renal function tests, and a blood type for crossmatching blood products. A nasogastric tube should be placed and gastric lavage performed. Iced saline is the classic recommendation, although there is no evidence to support its use over saline at room temperature, and the use of iced saline in infants may cause hypothermia. Gastric lavage enables the

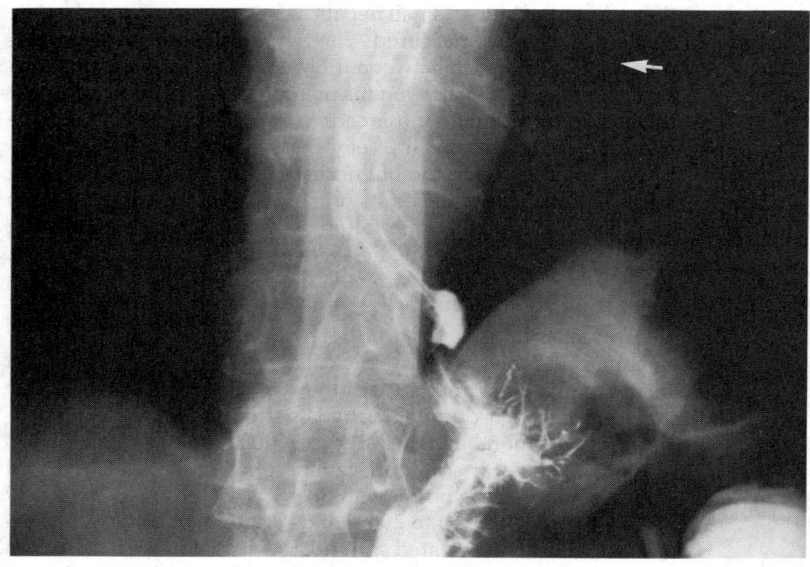

**Figure 139-7.** A barium swallow in a patient with portal hypertension and esophageal varices. The linear structures (*arrow*) in the esophagus indicate esophageal varices. (Courtesy of Thomas Colley, M.D., Geisinger Clinic, Danville, PA.)

physician to document upper GI hemorrhage, assess the degree of bleeding, and prepare the patient for endoscopy. There is no evidence that placement of a nasogastric tube precipitates variceal bleeding. If large clots preclude lavage, a large-bore oral gastric tube such as an Ewald or Edlich tube should be used, and the physician may consider elective intubation to prevent aspiration.

When patients with known portal hypertension and esophageal varices present with an acute upper GI hemorrhage, the physician cannot assume that the bleeding is from the varices. After the patient has been stabilized, upper endoscopy should be performed to determine the bleeding source. In approximately 40% to 50% of the patients, the bleeding is from a source other than esophageal varices. Administration of appropriate therapy depends on the cause of bleeding. Frequently, these patients will bleed from gastric or duodenal ulcers. In these cases, therapy with $H_2$-receptor blockers or sucralfate should be instituted. These agents, however, exert no beneficial effect on bleeding esophageal varices. Patients with upper GI hemorrhage should not have barium swallows performed in an attempt to diagnose the cause of bleeding. Although this study may detect esophageal varices, it does not prove that the patients are bleeding from the varices. Gastric blood and clots make interpretation of the gastric component of an upper GI series challenging, and it is difficult to perform an endoscopy on a patient who recently had an upper GI series.

Endoscopy is the best method for determining the cause of upper GI hemorrhage, and it can be therapeutic in terms of performing sclerotherapy for bleeding varices or using the heater probe on bleeding ulcers. Sclerotherapy is performed by means of the endoscope by injecting a sclerosing agent, usually sodium morrhuate, directly into or adjacent to the varix. This therapeutic modality has been effective in children and in adults and is considered to be the procedure of choice for control of bleeding esophageal varices. This procedure is not risk free; complications occur in 10% to 40% of the patients, and there is a mortality rate of less than 1%. The most common complications are fever, retrosternal chest pain, esophageal ulceration, bleeding, perforation, and stricture formation.

The mainstay of pharmacologic therapy for esophageal variceal bleeding is vasopressin. Vasopressin is a short-acting vasoconstrictor that increases splanchnic vascular resistance, thereby decreasing splanchnic blood flow and portal pressure. Vasopressin increases the lower esophageal sphincter pressure, which may compress the submucosal blood vessels, decreasing variceal blood flow. Vasopressin is administered intravenously because no benefit is derived from selective administration, and the latter is associated with a high frequency of complications. Controversy persists in the question of bolus therapy (0.3 U/kg over 20 minutes) usage before continuous infusion (0.2 to 0.4 U/1.73 $m^2$/minute) of vasopressin is begun. Therapy should be started at the lower dose and increased as needed to control the bleeding. The maximal dose is 1 U/minute. Above this, there is a high incidence of side effects with little further reduction in portal pressure. The major side effects are related to vasoconstriction and include bowel ischemia, myocardial ischemia, decreased cardiac output, bradycardia, cerebrovascular accidents, and diarrhea. It may exert an antidiuretic effect, resulting in hyponatremia. After bleeding ceases, the vasopressin is continued for an additional 12 hours before the administration is tapered and discontinued, diminishing the likelihood of rebound bleeding.

Nitroglycerin is a vasodilator that is used in adult patients in conjunction with vasopressin therapy. The systemic vasodilation caused by nitroglycerin results in reflex splanchnic vasoconstriction, decreasing portal pressure. The major side effects of vasopressin are from its systemic vasoconstrictive effects, which are reduced by the systemic vasodilatory effects of nitroglycerin. The combination of vasopressin and nitroglycerin is more effective than vasopressin alone in controlling bleeding in adult patients. Studies in pediatric patients have yet to be performed.

The use of somatostatin in controlling GI bleeding in adult patients is under investigation. This agent decreases splanchnic blood flow by inhibiting the release of various vasodilatory GI peptides, such as vasoactive intestinal polypeptide. Its role in the treatment of acute variceal hemorrhage is yet to be determined.

Another therapeutic modality that has been used in cases of resistant bleeding esophageal varices is balloon tamponade. There are several tubes available for use. The Sengstaken-Blakemore tube has a gastric and esophageal balloon with a gastric lumen. The Minnesota tube is similar but has gastric and esophageal lumens in addition to the two balloons. The ability to suction esophageal contents makes the Minnesota tube preferable. The tube is inserted, and the gastric balloon is inflated and then pulled back, applying pressure on the gastroesophageal junction. A radiograph of the abdomen confirms its position. If the bleeding does not stop, the esophageal balloon is inflated. The gastric and esophageal lumens should be suctioned continuously. Esophageal balloon inflation should not exceed 24 hours. The use of this therapy is limited, because it is associated with a high rate of complications, including esophageal rupture and aspiration, and because sclerotherapy is available and effective. Balloon tamponade is associated with a 50% rebleeding rate.

If aggressive medical management fails to control variceal bleeding, several surgical procedures can be considered, such as devascularization of the stomach and distal esophagus, portosystemic shunt surgery, and liver transplantation. There are several portosystemic shunts that can be performed. Nonselective shunts are portacaval and splenorenal shunts. Due to the diversion of blood flow away from the liver, these shunts are associated with a high rate of postoperative encephalopathy that occurs in approximately 15% of the patients. Selective shunts, such as the distal splenorenal shunt, attempt to decompress the gastric and esophageal venous component of the portal system while maintaining blood flow to the liver. As a result of maintaining hepatic blood flow, these shunts are associated with a lower incidence of postoperative encephalopathy and are therefore preferred over the nonselective shunts. Transjugular intrahepatic portacaval shunts have been proposed as an alternative to traditional shunts but further investigation is required. Shunt surgery should be considered in patients with portal hypertension who continue to bleed despite medical therapy or in patients who reside a long distance from a facility capable of treating variceal bleeding.

Liver transplantation has become an effective means of treating resistant variceal bleeding in patients with end-stage liver disease. These surgical therapeutic modalities are extensive procedures and are associated with high rates of complications when performed in an emergency situation. They should be considered as a last resort.

PSE is a neuropsychiatric disorder characterized by alterations in consciousness, impaired intellectual abilities, and several abnormal neuromuscular signs such as asterixis. Laboratory evaluation of affected patients reveals elevated ammonia levels, and an electroencephalogram demonstrates diffuse slowing. This condition develops most often in patients with severe liver disease who have developed portosystemic shunts. PSE may develop in patients with portal hypertension in whom portosystemic shunts have been created surgically. Although multiple theories have tried to explain its pathogenesis, the exact cause of PSE is unknown. Therapy is directed toward a reduction in serum ammonia levels by decreasing dietary protein, controlling any ongoing GI hemorrhaging, and removing blood from the GI tract. Neomycin can be administered to decrease enteric bacterial ammonia production, and lactulose is used to trap ammonia in the gut. Any precipitating cause of PSE, such as a bacterial infection, should be treated.

Splenomegaly and associated hyperglycemia is a frequent problem in patients with portal hypertension. The patients may have massive splenomegaly, predisposing them to splenic rupture after blunt abdominal trauma. The patient's symptoms vary from moderate left upper quadrant pain or left shoulder pain to overt shock. Patients with hypersplenism have a reduction in one or more hematologic components. If the condition is severe, treatment consists of splenectomy. If splenectomy is performed, patients should receive prophylactic treatment with pneumococcal vaccine.

## Prevention

Preventive measures can reduce the incidence of variceal bleeding in patients with portal hypertension. Although several medical and surgical therapeutic modalities are available, their applications remain controversial.

Products that can precipitate or worsen variceal bleeding should be avoided by children with portal hypertension. Aspirin is a potentially aggravating factor in variceal bleeding. Because aspirin is part of several medications, patients should be taught to read the label of medications to avoid inadvertent consumption of aspirin. Prophylaxis with cimetidine or ranitidine has not helped to prevent variceal bleeding. Their use should be limited to patients with peptic ulcer disease or gastroesophageal reflux.

Several agents have been used to reduce portal venous pressure in an attempt to diminish the likelihood of variceal bleeding. Propranolol is the agent most often employed. Propranolol is a nonselective beta blocker that reduces splanchnic blood flow and portal pressure by blocking vasodilatory splanchnic $\beta$-adrenergic receptors and by decreasing cardiac output. This results in a reduction in gastroesophageal collateral blood flow, decreasing the risk of variceal bleeding. Several studies have documented the efficacy of propranolol in reducing the risk of variceal bleeding. The dose administered is that required to decrease the heart rate by 25%. One study found that abrupt discontinuation of propranolol resulted in a relatively rapid onset of a high rate of variceal bleeding. No controlled study has assessed propranolol use in children with portal hypertension, although it has been used in pediatric patients with an apparent beneficial response. Its use should be determined on an individual basis, and if used, patients should be cautioned not to discontinue usage abruptly so that rebound bleeding can be avoided.

Other cardioselective beta blockers, atenolol and metoprolol, have been used to reduce portal pressure and the incidence of variceal bleeding, but these agents seem to be less effective than propranolol.

In a study in adult patients, propranolol used in conjunction with a vasodilator, isosorbide-5-mononitrate, was more effective than propranolol alone in decreasing portal pressure without any increased adverse effects. Clinical trials are under way to assess the efficacy of combination pharmacologic therapy compared with propranolol alone at preventing variceal bleeding.

There are three potential surgical modalities available to prevent variceal bleeding: endoscopic sclerosis of the varices, portosystemic shunting, and liver transplantation. Prophylactic endoscopic sclerotherapy is probably the surgical procedure of choice at this time for preventing recurrent variceal hemorrhage. Several controlled studies of adult populations have shown that endoscopic sclerotherapy significantly reduces the incidence of recurrent variceal bleeding. The limited experience with sclerotherapy in pediatric patients suggests the efficacy of the procedure. Patients with extrahepatic portal hypertension appear to have a better response to sclerotherapy than patients with intrahepatic portal hypertension. In one study, the transfusion requirement was reduced by 85% in those with extrahepatic portal hypertension and by only 43% in the intrahepatic group. Sclerotherapy is a safe procedure, but there are several potential complications associated with its use.

Portosystemic shunting was the first surgical modality used to prevent variceal hemorrhage. Shunt surgery effectively reduces portal pressure and the recurrence of variceal bleeding, and splenomegaly and hypersplenism may resolve with shunting. Of the many types of shunting procedures, the distal splenorenal shunt is the one most commonly performed. The major problems associated with shunt surgery are the thromboses of the shunts and development of PSE.

Liver transplantation is an accepted therapeutic modality for the treatment of end-stage liver disease and its associated complications, including variceal bleeding. The use of cyclosporine has been the major factor in improving the survival rate for pediatric liver transplantation to 85%, but transplantation should be reserved for those with end-stage liver disease.

The therapeutic modality used for preventing variceal hemorrhage depends on several factors, including whether it is to be used for the prevention of initial variceal hemorrhage or the prevention of recurrent hemorrhage. The risk of variceal hemorrhage for patients with esophageal varices is between 25% and 40%. Due to the frequency of variceal hemorrhage, the high morbidity and mortality rates associated with variceal hemorrhage, and the high rate of rebleeding, the physician should attempt to prevent initial hemorrhage. Propranolol administration is the therapeutic modality of choice for the prevention of initial variceal hemorrhage. Prospective, randomized controlled studies of adult patients have shown propranolol to be effective at reducing the rate of initial bleeding and improved survival compared with placebo or sclerotherapy. Propranolol is a relatively safe drug even when used chronically, as in this situation.

Studies assessing the efficacy of portosystemic shunt surgery revealed that the incidence of initial variceal hemorrhage was reduced. However, shunt surgery was associated with a high incidence of PSE, and survival was not as good as for medically treated patients. Portosystemic shunt surgery should not be used to prevent initial variceal hemorrhage.

Sclerotherapy is the primary therapeutic modality for acute variceal bleeding, but its role in preventing initial hemorrhage is unclear. The results of studies evaluating the effectiveness of sclerotherapy in preventing initial variceal hemorrhage are conflicting, with some showing benefit and others showing no benefit. A potential reason why sclerotherapy may not be beneficial is that even if esophageal varices are obliterated, varices may develop elsewhere, such as the stomach or duodenum, that may bleed. Further studies are required before sclerotherapy can be recommended for the prevention of initial variceal hemorrhage.

After variceal bleeding has occurred, the risk of rebleeding is between 50% and 80%, making it imperative to try to prevent rebleeding. Propranolol has little effect on the rate of early rebleeding (ie, first 6 weeks after a bleed), but it does appear to reduce the incidence of late rebleeding. Therapy with propranolol does not improve long-term survival in this group of patients. Theoretically, combination therapy with propranolol and isosorbide mononitrate may be more effective than propranolol alone, but the results of clinical trials are not yet available.

Portosystemic shunt surgery appears to be the most effective means of decreasing the risk of rebleeding to between 5% and 25%, but shunt surgery is invasive, associated with a high incidence of PSE, and may make subsequent liver transplantation more difficult. The distal splenorenal shunt is as effective as nonselective shunts in reducing the incidence of rebleeding, it is associated with a lower frequency of encephalopathy, and it does not have as much impact on subsequent liver transplantation, making it the preferred shunting procedure. This may be the preferred therapeutic modality for patients who do not have ready access to centers with the ability to perform sclerotherapy for acute variceal bleeding.

Sclerotherapy reduces the incidence of rebleeding by as much as 50% and improves survival compared with no prophylactic therapy. Even after complete eradication of esophageal varices, varices may reappear. Repeat endoscopic evaluation and repeat sclerosis should be performed on a regular basis. Portosystemic shunt surgery is more effective than sclerotherapy at reducing the incidence of rebleeding, but shunt surgery is more invasive and carries with it the risk of encephalopathy. Sclerotherapy reduces the incidence of rebleeding to a greater extent than does propranolol. The decision about whether to use sclerotherapy or portosystemic shunt surgery has to be made on an individual basis.

Devascularization surgery should be reserved for patients who are not candidates for sclerotherapy or shunt surgery. Liver transplantation should be considered for patients with recurrent variceal bleeding and end-stage liver disease.

Bleeding esophageal varices are the major complication of portal hypertension. The decision to employ prophylactic therapy and the particular therapeutic modality to employ must be individualized and depends on the patient's underlying disease, proximity to a medical facility where variceal bleeding can be treated, and the physician's personal experiences. All patients should wear a bracelet or chain that states that they have portal hypertension and that indicates their blood type.

## Selected Readings

Alvarez F, Bernard O, Brunelle F, et al. Portal obstruction in children. I. Clinical investigation and hemorrhage risk. J Pediatr 1983;103:696.
Alvarez F, Bernard O, Brunelle F, et al. Portal obstruction in children. II. Results of surgical portosystemic shunts. J Pediatr 1983;103:703.
Boles ET, Wise WE, Birken G. Extrahepatic portal hypertension in children. Am J Surg 1986;151:734.
Bosch JB, Pizcueta P, Feu F, et al. Pathophysiology of portal hypertension. Gastroenterol Clin North Am 1992;21:1.
Burroughs AK, McCormick PA. Prevention of variceal rebleeding. Gastroenterol Clin North Am 1992;21:119.
Gentil-Kocher S, Bernard O, Brunelle F, et al. Budd-Chiari syndrome in children: Report of 22 cases. J Pediatr 1988;113:30.
Grace ND. Prevention of initial variceal hemorrhage. Gastroenterol Clin North Am 1992;21:149.
Henderson JM. Liver transplantation for portal hypertension. Gastroenterol Clin North Am 1992;21:197.
Hill ID, Bowie MD. Endoscopic sclerotherapy for control of bleeding varices in children. Am J Gastroenterol 1991;86:472.
Hyams JS, Leichtner AM, Schwartz AN. Recent advances in diagnosis and treatment of gastrointestinal hemorrhage in infants and children. J Pediatr 1985;106:1.
Lebrec D. Methods to evaluate portal hypertension. Gastroenterol Clin North Am 1992;21:41.
Matloff DS. Treatment of acute variceal bleeding. Gastroenterol Clin North Am 1992;21:103.
Rabinowitz SS, Norton KI, Benkov KJ, et al. Sonographic evaluation of portal hypertension in children. J Pediatr Gastroenterol Nutr 1990;10:395.
Rikkers LF, Sorrell WT, Jin G. Which portosystemic shunt is best? Gastroenterol Clin North Am 1992;21:179.
Rodriguez-Perez F, Groszmann RJ. Pharmacologic treatment of portal hypertension. Gastroenterol Clin North Am 1992;21:15.

*Principles and Practice of Pediatrics, Second Edition.*
edited by Frank A. Oski et al. J. B. Lippincott Company, Philadelphia © 1994.

## *139.6 Hepatic Steatosis*

William J. Cochran

Hepatic steatosis, a common entity that frequently goes unrecognized, is a morphologic description of excessive fat in the liver. It is not a primary disease process and can occur in many situations. Fat normally accounts for less than 5% of the weight of the liver, but it may account for as much as 50% in conditions such as severe malnutrition.

## PATHOPHYSIOLOGY

Fat accumulates in the liver in a complex and, in certain situations, unknown manner. Although a complete discussion of hepatic lipid metabolism is beyond the scope of this chapter, several excellent reviews exist. Fat accumulation usually results from increased uptake, increased synthesis, decreased oxidation, or decreased secretion of fat by the liver. The uptake of free fatty acids by the liver is proportional to the amount of free fatty acids to which the liver is exposed. An increased uptake of free fatty acids promotes hepatic triglyceride synthesis. If the triglyceride release in the form of lipoproteins does not increase proportionally, fat accumulates in the liver. Several factors are associated with increased plasma free fatty acid levels: acute starvation, elevation of several hormones (eg, adrenocorticotropic hormone, thyrotropin, thyroid hormone, growth hormone), and drugs (eg, corticosteroids, epinephrine).

Hepatic triglyceride synthesis is increased in several disorders, but the condition secondary to alcoholism is best known. Metabolism of alcohol by the liver increases the NADH/NAD ratio, which promotes hepatic triglyceride synthesis. Ingestion of carbohydrates, especially glucose and fructose, also promotes hepatic triglyceride synthesis.

Fatty acids normally undergo $\beta$-oxidation in hepatic mitochondria. A reduction in the oxidation of fatty acids may result in the development of hepatic steatosis. This can occur secondary to chemicals such as hypoglycine A or amanitotoxin. Reduction of mitochondrial fatty acid oxidation also may contribute to the hepatic steatosis in patients with Reye's syndrome.

Decreased apoprotein synthesis by the liver results in decreased secretion of triglyceride from the liver. This process is believed to cause the hepatic steatosis that occurs in protein-calorie malnutrition. Drugs such as tetracycline, in large doses, can reduce hepatic protein synthesis and impair hepatic lipoprotein secretion. Carbon tetrachloride decreases apolipoprotein synthesis and impairs the transport of lipoprotein across cell membrane, resulting in hepatic steatosis.

## DISORDERS ASSOCIATED WITH HEPATIC STEATOSIS

The various disorders often associated with hepatic steatosis can be divided into several broad categories: nutritional, toxin- or drug-induced, metabolic, endocrine, infectious, and idiopathic (Table 139-18).

| TABLE 139-18. Disorders Associated With Hepatic Steatosis |
|---|
| **Nutritional** |
| Undernutrition (kwashiorkor) |
| Obesity |
| |
| **Toxin- or Drug-Induced** |
| Alcohol |
| Tetracycline |
| Valproic acid |
| Methotrexate |
| L-asparaginase |
| Actinomycin-D |
| Mitomycin C |
| Bleomycin |
| Corticosteroids |
| Vitamin A |
| Aflatoxin |
| Amanita toxin |
| Hypoglycine A |
| Total parenteral nutrition |
| Carbon tetrachloride |
| |
| **Metabolic** |
| Glycogen storage disease |
| Galactosemia |
| Fructose 1,6-diphosphatase deficiency |
| Congenital lactic acidosis |
| Methylmalonic acidemia |
| Tyrosinemia |
| Hyperlipoproteinemia |
| Gangliosidoses |
| Fucosidosis |
| Wolman disease |
| Cholesterol ester storage disease |
| Neimann-Pick disease |
| Medium chain acyl CoA dehydrogenase deficiency |
| Wilson's disease |
| $\alpha$-1 antitrypsin deficiency |
| |
| **Endocrine** |
| Cushing's disease |
| Diabetes mellitus |
| |
| **Infectious** |
| Hepatitis C |
| |
| **Idiopathic** |
| Reye's syndrome |
| Fatty liver of pregnancy |
| Fulminant hepatic failure |
| Inflammatory bowel disease |

Hepatic steatosis is associated with several nutritional disorders, the first of which, protein-calorie malnutrition, was noticed by Williams in 1933. Hepatic steatosis is uncommon in patients with marasmus (ie, protein and calorie deprivation) but common in patients with kwashiorkor (ie, protein deprivation), in whom fat can account for 50% of the weight of the liver. These patients frequently develop hepatomegaly, and their liver enzyme levels may be mildly elevated. Fat deposition begins first in the periportal area and progresses out to the central veins. With appropriate nutritional therapy, the fat disappears first from the central area and last from the periportal area. Although uncommon, other isolated nutritional deficiencies, such as pyridoxine or riboflavin deficiency, may be associated with hepatic steatosis. Hepatic steatosis is also common in patients suffering from overnutrition. Twelve percent of obese children in one study had elevated liver enzyme levels. All such patients who underwent liver biopsy had various degrees of hepatic steatosis. In studies of adult obesity, the frequency of hepatic steatosis ranges from 66% to 99%. In addition to hepatic steatosis, some obese patients have an increased amount of fibrous tissue. Although several investigators believe that this condition can progress to cirrhosis, this remains controversial.

Hepatic steatosis can be caused by multiple toxins and drugs, the most common of which is alcohol. As many as one third of asymptomatic alcoholics have hepatic steatosis. Acute deposition of hepatic fat actually can occur after just one alcoholic binge. Other drugs associated with hepatic steatosis include tetracycline, valproic acid, steroids, and in excessive doses, vitamin A. Antineoplastic agents associated with the development of hepatic steatosis include methotrexate, L-asparaginase, dactinomycin, mitomycin C, and bleomycin. Although the exact mechanism is uncertain, total parenteral nutrition can be associated with hepatic steatosis. In adults, the condition appears to develop secondary to the delivery of excessive calories, and in children, it appears to be a toxic reaction.

Food contaminated with *Aspergillus flavus* can result in the development of hepatic steatosis. This fungus produces aflatoxin, which inhibits the incorporation of thymidine into DNA and RNA polymerase, resulting in hepatic steatosis. Consumption of *Amanita phalloides*, which produces *Amanita* toxin, also is associated with acute fatty liver and with other gastrointestinal, renal, and central nervous system disturbances. Jamaican vomiting sickness, once common in the Caribbean, is now rare. The illness resulted from the consumption of unripe akee fruit (*Blighia sapida*), which contains hypoglycine A. In addition to other severe disturbances, hypoglycine A can cause hepatic steatosis.

Inborn errors of carbohydrate, protein, and lipid metabolism may have hepatic steatosis as a morphologic component of the disease. Disorders of carbohydrate metabolism associated with hepatic steatosis include glycogen storage disease, galactosemia, fructose 1,6-diphosphatase deficiency, and congenital lactic acidosis. Methylmalonic acidemia and tyrosinemia are disorders of protein metabolism that may involve increased amounts of hepatic fat, although this is a relatively minor histologic component of the latter disorder. Defects in lipid metabolism that involve hepatomegaly and increased hepatic fat include hyperlipoproteinemia, the gangliosidoses, fucosidosis, Wolman disease, cholesterol ester storage disease, and Niemann-Pick disease. In most disorders that result in hepatic steatosis, the excess fat occurs as triglycerides. Although this is true for patients with hyperlipoproteinemia, the excess fat occurs as cholesterol esters in those with Wolman disease and cholesterol ester storage disease. Glycolipids accumulate in patients with gangliosidoses, glycosphingolipids in those with fucosidosis, and cholesterol and glycosphingolipids in those with Niemann-Pick disease. Other metabolic disorders associated with liver disease and excessive hepatic fat include Wilson's disease and $\alpha_1$-antitrypsin deficiency.

The endocrine disorders that result in excessive hepatic fat are Cushing's disease and diabetes mellitus. The frequency of fatty liver is 50% in diabetic adults and less than 5% in juvenile-onset diabetics. The reason for this difference is unclear but may be related to the higher frequency of obesity in adult diabetics.

Most infections of the liver result in inflammation with little accumulation of fat. The single infection that can result in a fatty liver is hepatitis C.

The idiopathic category of hepatic steatosis includes Reye's syndrome (see Chap. 156), fatty liver of pregnancy, and inflammatory bowel disease. Fatty liver of pregnancy usually occurs during the third trimester of the first pregnancy. The patients have a sudden onset of vomiting and abdominal pain, after which jaundice develops and hematemesis and premature labor occur. Laboratory evaluation reveals hyperbilirubinemia, elevated liver enzymes, and leukocytosis. This disorder is not readily differentiated from viral hepatitis unless a liver biopsy is performed; the biopsy reveals a fatty liver with little or no inflammation or necrosis. Fatty liver of pregnancy has a mortality rate greater than 20% and is treated with supportive therapy and rapid delivery of the infant.

Hepatic steatosis occurs in approximately 33% of patients with inflammatory bowel disease, making it the most common hepatobiliary disorder associated with inflammatory bowel disease. The cause of hepatic steatosis in inflammatory bowel disease is unknown but is most likely multifactorial. Malnutrition, corticosteroids, and bacterial toxins have been implicated in the pathogenesis.

## DIAGNOSIS

Liver biopsy is the definitive means for identifying hepatic steatosis. Percutaneous liver biopsies can be performed in children easily and safely. The major potential complications associated with liver biopsy are bleeding, pneumothorax, and perforation of the gallbladder. An ultrasonographic examination of the liver should be obtained before performing a liver biopsy to rule out liver pathology, such as a hemangioma of the liver, which may be a contraindication for performing this procedure.

There are two general histologic patterns of hepatic steatosis: macrovesicular and microvesicular. Macrovesicular hepatic steatosis is the term applied if large lipid vacuoles fill the hepatocyte, displacing the nucleus to the cell's periphery (Fig 139-8A). Macrovesicular steatosis is associated with alcohol, corticosteroids, nutritional, and metabolic disorders and diabetes. Liver function is relatively well preserved in this type of steatosis. Microvesicular hepatic steatosis is characterized by small lipid vacuoles, which are dispersed throughout the cytoplasm, with the nucleus remaining in the center of the hepatocyte (Fig 139-8B). This pattern of fatty deposition is associated with different toxins or drugs such as hypoglycine A and tetracycline, fatty liver of pregnancy, and Reye's syndrome. Unlike entities associated with macrovesicular steatosis, disorders associated with microvesicular steatosis are characterized by clinical and laboratory evidence of liver dysfunction.

Noninvasive means of detecting hepatic steatosis include ultrasonography and computed tomography (CT). Hepatic steatosis

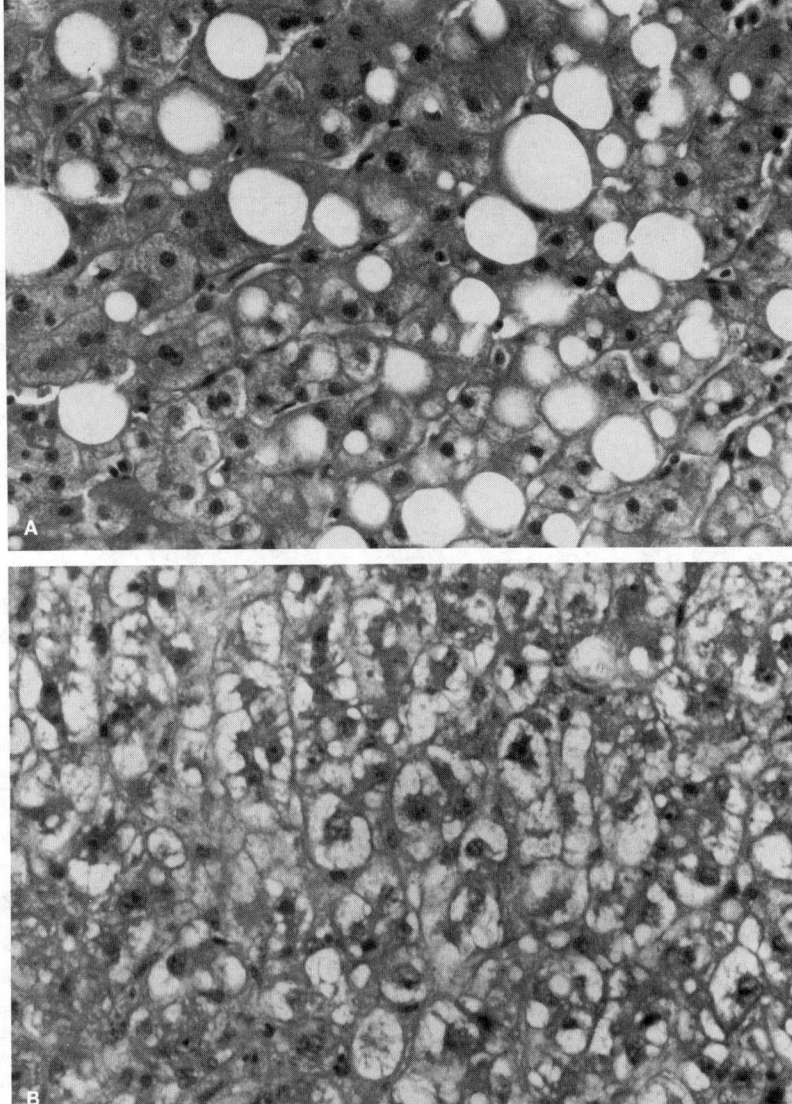

**Figure 139-8.** (**A**) Macrovesicular hepatic steatosis in alcoholic liver disease. Large lipid vacuoles are evident, and in some hepatocytes, the nucleus is displaced to the cell's periphery. (Original magnification ×312.5.) (**B**) Microvesicular hepatic steatosis in a fatal case of fatty liver in pregnancy. Coalescing lipid vacuoles within the hepatocytes distort the cell outlines and render a foamy appearance. The nucleus remains in the center of the cell. (Original magnification ×312.5; courtesy of P. Cera, M.D., Geisinger Clinic, Danville, PA.)

results in brightly reflective ultrasound echo pattern. This pattern is fairly specific for hepatic steatosis. Hepatic steatosis is more readily identified by CT. CT examination of a fatty liver demonstrates that the liver parenchyma is of lower density than the spleen, and CT can help in differentiating focal fatty infiltrates from tumor. Focal hepatic infiltration is more difficult to evaluate by means of ultrasonography.

## TREATMENT AND PROGNOSIS

Hepatic steatosis is a nonspecific finding in many disorders. Treatment should address the underlying disorder that has caused the hepatic steatosis. There is no specific therapy for hepatic steatosis itself.

The prognosis of patients with hepatic steatosis depends on the primary process responsible for the disease. Although some investigators think that hepatic steatosis itself is not detrimental, accumulating evidence supports the theory that hepatic steatosis may progress to cirrhosis.

## Selected Readings

Adkins MC, Halvorsen RA, duCret PP. CT evaluation of atypical hepatic fatty metamorphosis. J Comput Assist Tomogr 1990;14:1013.

Alpers DH, Sabesin SM. Fatty liver: biochemical and clinical aspects. In: Schiff L, Schiff ER, eds. Diseases of the liver. New York: JB Lippincott, 1987.

Colon AR. Hepatic steatosis in children. Am J Gastroenterol 1977;68:260.

Doherty JF, Golden MH, Brooks SE. Peroxisomes and the fatty liver of malnutrition: a hypothesis. Am J Clin Nutr 1991;54:674.

Hautekeete ML, Degott C, Benhamou JP. Microvesicular steatosis of the liver. Acta Clin Belg 1990;45:311.

Kinugasa A, Tsunamoto K, Farukawa N, et al. Fatty liver and its fibrous changes found in simple obesity of children. J Pediatr Gastroenterol Nutr 1984;3:408.

Mabie WC. Acute fatty liver of pregnancy. Crit Care Clin 1991;7:799.

Nussbaum MS, Fischer JE. Pathogenesis of hepatic steatosis during total parenteral nutrition, part 2. Surg Annu 1991;23:1.

Powell EE, Cooksley WG, Hanson R, et al. The natural history of nonalcoholic steatahepatitis: a follow-up study of forty-two patients for up to 21 years. Hepatology 1990;11:74.

Scataridge JC, Scott WW, Donovan PJ, et al. Fatty infiltration of the liver: ultrasonographic and computed tomographic correlation. J Ultrasound Med 1984;3:9.

Vierling JM. Hepatobiliary complications of ulcerative colitis and Crohn's disease. In: Zakim D, Boyer TD, eds. Hepatology: a textbook of liver disease. Philadelphia: WB Saunders, 1990.

# Endocrine Abnormalities

*Principles and Practice of Pediatrics, Second Edition.*
edited by Frank A. Oski et al. J. B. Lippincott Company, Philadelphia © 1994.

CHAPTER 140

# The Parathyroid Glands

## John L. Kirkland

Recent advances in understanding calcium homeostasis have revealed a rigidly controlled system involving the liver, bone, intestines, kidneys, and parathyroid glands. This system is remarkable for its inherent stability, but diseases of the parathyroid gland or the other organs in this system may cause significant clinical and metabolic disorders in children. Transient parathyroid gland dysfunction in the neonate is discussed elsewhere in this book.

## PHYSIOLOGY

Parathyroid hormone (PTH) is secreted from the cell as an 84-amino acid peptide with a half-life of 5 to 8 minutes. PTH is degraded by the Kupffer cells of the liver into midregion and carboxy-terminal fragments, which have no biologic activity but remain in the blood. Previous methods used to measure PTH were complicated by these inactive components. Newer assays using two-site immunoradiometric and immunoaffinity-extraction bioassays have facilitated an understanding of PTH dynamics in health and diseases. A combination of plasma membrane calcium sensors and calcium selective transmembrane channels may signal the cell to produce and secrete PTH. PTH exerts its major actions by binding to receptors in the bone and kidney. PTH indirectly activates the osteoclasts in the bone and increases resorption of mineralized bone, which mobilizes calcium and phosphorus. PTH activates the proximal and distal tubular cells in the kidney to promote calcium resorption and to inhibit phosphorus resorption. PTH stimulates the production of 1,25-dihydroxyvitamin $D_3$ in the kidney.

In the bone and renal cells, PTH acts through two membrane receptor systems. The first system activates adenylate cyclase, with subsequent production of cAMP. cAMP acts as a second messenger to mobilize intracellular calcium and increase protein phosphorylation. The second system stimulates the breakdown of phosphoinositide to diacylglycerol products. These products

stimulate protein kinase C activation. These two systems promote genomic activation.

PTH regulates closely the concentration of calcium in the extracellular fluids. The concentration of calcium throughout the day is stable, but variations exist in the calcium concentration secondary to changes in the concentrations of serum proteins. The usual daily variation of total calcium concentrations is less than 2%. The extracellular concentration of calcium is $10^{-3}$ M, with three major components. The unbound component, or free calcium, composes approximately 50% of the total amount of calcium and is the most important regulator of physiological processes. The bound components compose the other 50%, with protein binding accounting for approximately 40% and anion binding for approximately 10%.

Albumin is the most significant protein binding calcium, with each albumin molecule capable of binding 12 calcium molecules, depending on the extracellular pH. Acidosis decreases the binding capacity and increases the free extracellular concentration of calcium, and alkalosis increases the binding capacity and decreases the free extracellular concentrations of calcium. These alterations in binding capacity explain the variations in clinical signs that occur with disturbances in acid–base regulation. Bicarbonate, citrate, and phosphate complexes compose the anion binding system. The intracellular concentration of calcium is approximately $10^{-6}$ M and is maintained by three intracellular pump-leak transport systems.

The calcium concentration is rigidly controlled because of the important role that calcium ions assume in numerous metabolic processes, including the permeability of plasma membranes in neural tissue, the mineralization of developing bone, the promotion of coagulation, and the intracellular role as a second messenger for transmembrane hormone signals. The calcium-selective transmembrane channels may play a role in this process. The low levels of intracellular calcium promote a release of PTH, and high levels of serum calcium depress the release of PTH. The increased levels of PTH stimulate important compensatory mechanisms as discussed earlier.

An understanding of calcium homeostasis must include an explanation of the actions of vitamin D. Vitamin D has two entry points into the body: from the skin and from dietary supplementation. The skin contains a previtamin D compound, 7-dehydrocholesterol. Ultraviolet energy from the sun or other sources convert this substance to a previtamin D compound, which is converted by heat-sensitive reactions to vitamin D. Vitamin D is transferred by a serum binding protein to the liver. Dietary sources may include irradiated ergosterol, vitamin $D_2$, or vitamin $D_3$. Vitamin $D_2$ and $D_3$ differ slightly in their structure, but they have similar functions.

Vitamin $D_2$ and $D_3$ are hydroxylated in the liver at the 25 position by a 25-hydroxylase enzyme. Diseases of the liver and pharmacologic agents, including phenytoin and phenobarbital, have been reported to interfere with this important hydroxylation step. Interference in this step may result in vitamin D deficiency. The 25-hydroxyvitamin D is transported to the kidney, where another hydroxylation step occurs at the 1 position. 1,25-Dihydroxyvitamin $D_3$ is the most active metabolite and is responsible for most actions of vitamin D. The 1 hydroxylation is stimulated through the actions of PTH, estrogen, growth hormone, prolactin, and insulin.

Vitamin D exerts its effects by binding to intracellular proteins, which have been discovered in most of the body tissues examined. The proteins undoubtedly have numerous important roles other than the control of calcium metabolism. After the vitamin D molecule has bound to the intracellular vitamin D receptors, the receptor–vitamin D complex attaches to a specific part of the DNA, the responsive element, through a DNA-binding domain. Binding to the DNA allows stimulatory regions of the gene to initiate important translational events. For example, the intestinal cells are stimulated to produce calbindin-D, a calcium-binding protein that facilitates the transport of calcium from the intraluminal space of the intestines to the extracellular compartment. Another role is the generation of osteoclasts from progenitor cells. The osteoclasts enhance the release of calcium from the bone, providing the body with a method to compensate for acute hypocalcemia.

The pathophysiology of the system is remarkable in that perturbations can occur with predictable consequences to calcium homeostasis at each level of control. The disturbances of the parathyroid glands are described in this chapter.

# HYPOPARATHYROIDISM

Hypoparathyroidism in children is a rare entity, excluding transient hypoparathyroidism in neonates. This disease is recognized clinically by its accompanying hypocalcemia. The clinical manifestations of hypocalcemia are secondary to neuromuscular instability. The most common presentation is a seizure, which may be preceded by numbness and tingling sensations in the extremities. Chvostek's sign (ie, stimulation of the upper lip by tapping the facial nerve in front of the ear), Trousseau's sign (ie, carpopedal spasm produced by inflation of the blood pressure cuff greater than the systolic blood pressure for 2 minutes), laryngospasm, bronchospasm, and prolonged QT intervals on the electrocardiogram (ECG) can occur.

## Etiology

### Autoimmune Hypoparathyroidism

Hypoparathyroidism occurring as a part of an autoimmune complex is a well-described entity. The basic disease process is known as the polyglandular autoimmune syndrome type I or as the autoimmune polyendocrinopathy-candidiasis-ectodermal dystrophy (APECED) syndrome. The consistent feature is a failure of the parathyroid glands to secrete PTH because of an immunologic destruction of the hormone-producing cells.

These children usually present with acute signs of hypocalcemia, such as tetany, seizures, and neuromuscular irritability. Mucocutaneous candidiasis may precede the hypoparathyroidism. Other endocrinopathies include hypoadrenalism, hypogonadism, hypothyroidism, and diabetes mellitus. The pathologic findings signaling glandular failure include lymphocytic infiltration of the parathyroid glands.

Treatment for this type of hypoparathyroidism is discussed later in this chapter. A child with this clinical entity should be examined frequently for other endocrinopathies. Many cases are

secondary to an autosomal recessive gene and appropriate genetic counseling should be considered.

### DiGeorge Syndrome

DiGeorge syndrome was described originally in infants with congenital absence of the thymus, absence of the parathyroid glands, and deficient cell-mediated immunity. Later descriptions included cardiovascular malformations, including truncus arteriosus and aortic arch syndromes. Typical dysmorphic features of the face have been reported. These include low-set ears, short philtrum, micrognathia, and a small fish-like mouth. Pathologic findings include absent, aplastic, and hypoplastic parathyroid glands.

### Acute Illnesses

Acute illnesses in children, such as gram-negative sepsis, have been associated with hypocalcemia secondary to a relative hypoparathyroidism. The cause of the relative hypoparathyroidism in critically ill children is unknown, but it may be related to macrophage-generated interleukins, which may act as calcium ionophores. The critically ill child admitted to an intensive care unit is a prime candidate. Recognition may be delayed in some severe illnesses because of the concern for the primary problem. However, correction of the hypocalcemia is a requisite for patient improvement, because many cardiovascular agents require appropriate concentrations of calcium. Ionized calcium levels rather than total serum calcium levels reflect the child's true status, because disturbances in total calcium determination from hypoalbuminemia, fluctuations in the bicarbonate ion, and radiographic contrast media may complicate total serum calcium measurements.

### Isolated Hypoparathyroidism

Isolated hypoparathyroidism unassociated with other endocrine diseases or as a result of thyroid surgery can occur. The cause of isolated hypoparathyroidism is unknown, but its clinical and laboratory findings and its treatment is identical to other forms of hypoparathyroidism. The familial forms may be caused by gene mutations near the PTH gene, located on the short arm of chromosome 11.

### Hypomagnesemia

Congenital or acquired magnesium deficiency produces hypocalcemia secondary to the diminished production and effectiveness of PTH. Congenital hypomagnesemia is caused by urinary or gastrointestinal losses from unknown cellular defects. Infants and children have other metabolic disturbances, such as hypokalemia. Acquired hypomagnesemia is usually secondary to another disease. The clinical manifestations usually consist of tetany, carpopedal spasms, or seizures. The laboratory findings consist of serum levels of magnesium less than 1.5 mEq/L. Treatment consists of replacement with magnesium intravenously, intramuscularly, or orally. Magnesium levels should be determined frequently to avoid overdosage with parenteral solutions of magnesium. Diarrhea may result from oral administration of magnesium. The replacement amount should be decreased accordingly and then retried at a higher dosage.

## Laboratory Findings

The characteristic laboratory findings of hypoparathyroidism include hypocalcemia and hyperphosphatemia. The PTH level is low in most of the situations described earlier. Radiographs of bones do not usually show any diagnostic features. The differential diagnosis includes hypocalcemia for other reasons, such as phosphate-induced hypocalcemia, renal failure, and hypocalcemic rickets. The clinical history, laboratory assessment, and radiographs can facilitate the evaluation. Children with pseudohypoparathyroidism present with hypocalcemia and hyperphosphatemia, but their PTH levels are elevated.

## Treatment

The immediate treatment of hypoparathyroidism can be generalized if modifications are made for each specific cause. All untreated patients with hypoparathyroidism have hypocalcemia, which requires immediate medical intervention. The hypocalcemia is treated with intravenous calcium. Numerous preparations exist, and each has its own benefits. Pediatricians frequently use 10% calcium gluconate initially as an intravenous solution. One milliliter of this solution supplies 9 mg of elemental calcium. A neonate with seizures and laryngospasm may require an initial dosage of 1 to 2 mL/kg. Older children may require a total volume of 5 to 10 mL. The infusion of calcium should be slow, with strict attention paid to the heart rate or an ECG monitor. Bradycardia is an indication to discontinue temporarily the infusion of calcium. Subsequent intravenous calcium is administered at a rate of 25 to 100 mg of elemental calcium per kilogram of body weight per day, depending on the severity of the hypocalcemia.

The intravenous use of calcium may result in skin necrosis if extravasation occurs. This complication may develop despite the continuous monitoring of intravenous sites, prompting some physicians to administer intravenous calcium only as an intermittent bolus. A 10% calcium chloride solution can be used for intravenous treatment, but it is more irritating to the veins than calcium gluconate. One milliliter of this solution contains 27.3 mg of elemental calcium.

Oral treatment with calcium supplementation may be initiated when the patient becomes stable. One milliliter of calcium glubionate (Neo-Calglucon) contains 23 mg of elemental calcium, and calcium lactate power is 13% elemental calcium (100 mg of calcium lactate = 13 mg of elemental calcium). Other commercial preparations are available with various amounts of elemental calcium. The amount of calcium supplementation administered should be regulated closely by serum calcium determinations. The amount of elemental calcium administered to maintain eucalcemia usually is 50 to 150 mg/kg/day. The physician should remember that calcium administration through the gastrointestinal system depends on the presence of 1,25-dihydroxyvitamin $D_3$ or its analogues.

Treatment with various forms of vitamin D is the only method available to treat chronic hypocalcemic states such as hypoparathyroidism, because PTH is unavailable in a pharmacologic preparation. Most vitamin D supplementation is undertaken with dihydrotachysterol, 25-hydroxyvitamin D (Calderol), or 1,25-dihydroxyvitamin $D_3$ (Rocaltrol). Vitamin D itself was used previously in very large amounts, but its long half-life made corrections in dosage to maintain eucalcemia difficult. Dihydrotachysterol is administered in a dose of 0.05 mg to 0.5 mg/day. A solution facilitates small changes in the dosage required to maintain eucalcemia. 25-Hydroxyvitamin D is administered as 20 μg on a daily or alternate-day basis and increased slowly. Experience in infants and children is limited. 1,25-Dihydroxyvitamin $D_3$ is initiated with a dose of 0.25 μg/day and increased to several micrograms each day, depending on the response of the serum calcium level and the size of the child. Rocaltrol has a more rapid onset of action than dihydrotachysterol, and therapeutic manipulation is easier. The gelatinous material in Rocaltrol can be removed from the capsule to administer smaller amounts to neonates and infants. 1,25-dihydroxyvitamin $D_3$ may be administered intravenously (Calcijex), but its use in children is limited.

The optimal goal of long-term management is to maintain eucalcemia and eucalciuria. Patients with the best control are those who obtain monthly tests of calcium levels and submit 24-hour urine collections twice yearly for calcium content analysis. The optimal serum calcium level is one that is in the low range of normal. The optimal urinary calcium level should be less than 4 mg/kg/day or less than 0.3 mg of calcium per 1 mg of creatinine. Older children and adolescents may require serum calcium levels less than the normal range to avoid hypercalcuria.

## HYPERPARATHYROIDISM

Hyperparathyroidism is an uncommon disorder among pediatric patients, but it is important because an aggressive approach must be undertaken to prevent chronic renal diseases from nephrocalcinosis. The clinical manifestations of hypercalcemia from any cause are similar. The neuromuscular and gastrointestinal organs are affected initially. Muscle weakness, paralysis, hyporeflexia, constipation, anorexia, and vomiting may be observed. The kidney may be affected adversely with resulting polyuria and polydipsia. Nephrocalcinosis may occur later. The cardiovascular symptoms may reveal bradycardia and a reduced QT interval.

## Etiology

### Neonatal Hyperparathyroidism

A rare form of hypercalcemia in neonates is primary hyperparathyroidism. The cause is hyperplasia of the parathyroid glands. The PTH levels are increased, and the resorption of bones with demineralization produces hypercalcemia. Phosphate levels are low. Medical treatment as outlined later is frequently inadequate to manage the hypercalcemia, and total parathyroidectomy may be required. Parathyroid gland autotransplantation to the extremity appears to be successful in some case reports. The parathyroid tissue can be removed from the extremity as required to maintain eucalcemia. Subtotal parathyroidectomy has a significant risk for the continuation or recurrence of hypercalcemia in neonates.

### Parathyroid Adenoma

Hypercalcemia later in childhood is most likely secondary to hyperparathyroidism from parathyroid adenomas. The presenting clinical signs may include paralytic ileus and personality changes, or the child may be asymptomatic. The adenoma may be detected when biochemical screening tests are performed for routine physical examinations. The diagnosis can be confirmed biochemically by hypercalcemia, hypophosphatemia, and elevated PTH levels. Hypercalcuria may occur. Radiographic findings may consist of osteitis fibrosa cystica. Sonographic techniques enable presurgical localization of the lesion. Hypocalcemia may occur after surgery, but it resolves as the remaining parathyroid glands recover.

### Multiple Endocrine Neoplasia Type I

Multiple endocrine neoplasia type I (MEN I) or Wermer's syndrome is an autosomal dominant form of an inherited disease in which hyperparathyroidism, pancreatic tumors, and pituitary adenomas occur. Almost all affected patients have hyperparathyroidism secondary to enlargement and hyperplasia of all parathyroid tissue. The cause is unknown, but studies using restriction fragment link polymorphisms have located a potential MEN I gene on chromosome 11. Some cases have been reported among neonates and children. The diagnosis is confirmed by hypercalcemia, elevated levels of PTH, and the familial incidence. Treatment consists of subtotal parathyroidectomy (3½ glands) with autotransplantation of a small amount of parathyroid tissue to the muscles of one of the extremities.

### Familial Hypercalcemic Hypocalciuria

Familial hypercalcemic hypocalciuria is an autosomal dominant form of hypercalcemia that was known previously as familial benign hypercalcemia. The diagnosis is unsuspected in most children unless other family members are known to have hypercalcemia. The cause of this disorder is unknown. Numerous investigators have postulated causes, but none has explained all of the biochemical findings.

The cardinal finding is hypercalcemia, occurring from the neonatal period, with relative hypocalciuria for the degree of hypercalcemia. The serum calcium levels are usually in the range of 11 to 12 mg/dL, with few levels greater than 14 mg/dL. Urinary calcium expressed in terms of milligrams of calcium per 1 mg of creatinine is normal or elevated slightly, but it is less than would be expected from primary hyperparathyroidism. (The normal levels of urinary calcium are less than 4 mg/kg/day, and the calcium-creatinine ratio is usually less than 0.3). Nephrocalcinosis does not occur. PTH levels are normal but elevated for the degree of hypercalcemia. Serum magnesium levels are elevated in some children. Other biochemical studies related to calcium and vitamin D metabolism such as 1,25-dihydroxyvitamin $D_3$, calcitonin, and urinary cyclic AMP levels and radiographic examination of the skeleton do not reveal consistent abnormalities, or they are normal. The diagnosis can be corroborated by the asymptomatic nature of the disorder, unlike the signs and symptoms of hypercalcemia secondary to hyperparathyroidism.

Surgical removal of all parathyroid tissue results in hypoparathyroidism. Removal of only parts of the parathyroid gland doesn't improve the hypercalcemia. No treatment of the hypercalcemia is recommended.

### Laboratory Findings

Hyperparathyroidism from any cause can be recognized by elevated levels of PTH concomitant with hypercalcemia and hypophosphatemia. The newer assays for the intact (1-84) PTH molecule have facilitated the measurements that previously were difficult to obtain. However, most PTH assays are more helpful if calcium levels are incorporated. The negative feedback system between calcium and PTH allows other causes of hypercalcemia, such as hypervitaminosis D, to be differentiated. Ultrasound evaluation of the parathyroid gland can identify hyperplasia and adenomas. The diagnosis of familial hypercalcemic hypocalciuria usually is based on a normal level of PTH, relative hypocalciuria (frequently the urinary calcium levels are normal), and modest hypercalcemia, with the same biochemical findings in other family members.

### Treatment

Treatment of hypercalcemia secondary to hyperparathyroidism must include treatment of the underlying disorder. The immediate treatment requires hydration, which can be done orally in cooperative children or by intravenous methods in uncooperative ones. Twice maintenance fluid rates or greater are used. Dehydration secondary to nausea, vomiting, and polyuria can occur with hypercalcemia, and definite amounts to correct the dehydration should be added to the total fluid replacement volume. The administration of intravenous saline after rehydration offers an added benefit, because calcium excretion is enhanced by sodium excretion. Furosemide or other loop diuretics may be used, because they increase sodium excretion and calcium excretion. Glucocorticoids such as prednisone in pharmacologic amounts have been used because they decrease intestinal absorption of calcium, but their effects are minimal in hypercalcemia due to hyperparathyroidism. Sunlight, any form of vitamin D, and dairy products should be avoided during hypercalcemia. These treatments usually suffice in children, but additional treatment can be undertaken with calcitonin, phosphorus, mithramycin, peritoneal dialysis, and bisphosphonates. The latter forms of treatment have been used in adults, and the experience in treating children is nonexistent or limited.

### Selected Readings

Favus MJ. Primer on the metabolic bone diseases and disorders of mineral metabolism. Richmond: William Byrd Press, 1990.

Harrison HE, Harrison HC. Disorders of calcium and phosphorus metabolism in childhood and adolescence. Philadelphia: WB Saunders, 1979.

*Principles and Practice of Pediatrics, Second Edition.*
edited by Frank A. Oski et al. J. B. Lippincott Company, Philadelphia © 1994.

## CHAPTER 141
# *Puberty and Gonadal Disorders*

### Leslie P. Plotnick

## PUBERTY

Because the range of normal onset and progression of puberty is broad and different in boys and girls, pediatricians must have a solid grasp of normal pubertal events to assess when a child falls outside the normal range and is in need of evaluation or treatment.

Puberty is initiated by changes in the sensitive negative feedback system between the gonads and the hypothalamus and pituitary in the prepubertal child. Puberty involves an increase in gonadal steroid production (ie, gonadarche) and an increase in adrenal steroid production (ie, adrenarche).

In most girls, puberty begins between 8 and 13 years of age and is completed, on average, in 4.2 years (range, 1.5 to 6 years). The time from the onset of breast buds to menarche is 2.3 ± 1.0 years. In 99% of boys, puberty begins between 9 and 14 years of age and is completed, on average, in 3.5 years (range, 2 to 4.5 years).

If a girl shows signs of pubertal maturation before 8 years of age or a boy shows signs before 9 years of age, the child should be evaluated for precocious puberty. If no signs of pubertal development occur by 13 years of age in girls or by 14 years of age in boys, the child should be evaluated for pubertal delay.

The timing of progression of puberty is also important. Pubertal changes that progress too rapidly or arrest in progression require evaluation.

## HYPOTHALAMIC-PITUITARY-GONADAL PHYSIOLOGY

Pituitary release of luteinizing hormone (LH) and follicle-stimulating hormone (FSH) is regulated by the hypothalamic factor, gonadotropin-releasing hormone (GnRH; also called luteinizing hormone-releasing hormone or factor). The hypothalamic secretion of this peptide is controlled by various neurotransmitters, which can be influenced by higher signals, such as visual and olfactory stimuli and stress. GnRH is secreted in pulses, the frequency of which is important for pituitary LH and FSH secretion. LH and FSH stimulate the testes to produce testosterone and the ovaries to produce estrogen and stimulate ovulation. The gonadal sex steroids feed back centrally. The feedback usually is negative, except that positive feedback of estrogens is needed to produce the LH surge required for ovulation.

## PRECOCIOUS SEXUAL DEVELOPMENT

Causes of precocious or inappropriate sexual development are listed in Table 141-1. In evaluating a child for sexual precocity, a careful medical and family history is imperative. Does the child have any history of a central nervous system (CNS) disorder? What is the child's growth pattern? Is there evidence of linear growth acceleration? Previous growth measurements are valuable. When did the various pubertal changes begin? How fast have

---

### TABLE 141-1. Precocious or Inappropriate Sexual Development

**True or Central Precocious Puberty (Central Gonadotropin Secretion)**
Idiopathic
Central nervous system (CNS) tumors: hamartomas, other
Other CNS disorders: trauma, postinfectious, hydrocephalus
Severe primary hypothyroidism

**Precocious Puberty Independent of Pituitary Gonadotropins**
Girls
  Exogenous estrogen exposure
  Estrogen-secreting tumors (adrenals or ovaries)
  Ovarian cysts
  McCune-Albright syndrome
Boys
  Exogenous adrogen exposure
  Adrenal androgen secretion
    Congenital adrenal hyperplasia
    Adrenal tumors
  Testicular androgen secretion
    Tumors
    Familial Leydig cell hyperplasia
  Gonadotropin-secreting tumors
  McCune-Albright syndrome

**Heterosexual Development**
Virilization in girls
  Congenital adrenal hyperplasia
  Adrenal tumors
  Ovarian tumors
Feminization in boys
  Adrenal tumor
  Testicular tumor
  Increased peripheral conversion of androgens to estrogens

**Variations of Normal Puberty**
Premature thelarche
Premature adrenarche
Pubertal gynecomastia

---

these changes progressed? Is the child outgrowing clothes and shoes rapidly? Has the child's appetite increased? When did the parents and siblings have pubertal changes? Is there a history of early sexual development in any relatives? Questions regarding exposure to any exogenous source of sex steroids must be asked. Creams and pills can contain sex steroids, especially estrogens, and oral contraceptives are readily found in many homes. Are any athletes in the home taking anabolic steroids?

The physical examination should include a careful examination of the fundi. The child's skin should be inspected for signs of oiliness, acne, and café au lait spots. The thyroid should be palpated. The presence of axillary hair and odor, the amount of breast tissue, and whether the nipples and areolae are enlarging and thinning should be evaluated. The abdomen should be carefully palpated for masses. The amount, location, and character of pubic hair should be noted.

In girls, the clitoris, labia, and vaginal orifice should be examined carefully. Is there evidence of maturation of the labia minora? Does the vaginal mucosa look red and shiny (prepubertal) or pink and dull (estrogenized)? Is the clitoris of normal size? Are vaginal secretions evident on the genitalia or on the child's underwear?

In boys, the stretched length and width of the penis should be measured. Careful palpation and measurement of the testes is key. Are the testes prepubertal in length (<2.5 cm), or are they enlarging? Is there a difference in size and consistency of the two testes, suggesting a unilateral mass? Transillumination of the testes may be helpful, especially if there are size discrepancies. Is the scrotum thinning, or does it look thick and nonvascular (ie, prepubertal)? Are the results of the neurologic examination normal?

### True or Central Precocious Puberty

True or central precocious puberty is caused by early maturation of hypothalamic GnRH secretion. This form of precocious puberty is much more common in girls than in boys.

In many cases, no definable CNS abnormality can be found, and the problem falls into the idiopathic category, which occurs more frequently in girls than in boys. In idiopathic precocious puberty, although the onset is at an early age, the pattern and timing of progression of pubertal events are normal.

A search for an underlying CNS abnormality should be made by imaging of the CNS with computed tomography (CT) or magnetic resonance imaging (MRI). CNS tumors, especially hypothalamic hamartomas, are known causes of central precocious puberty. Neurofibromas, gliomas, and other tumors have been found with some frequency. Other CNS lesions, such as hydrocephalus, post-trauma, and postinfectious encephalitis or meningitis, are associated with precocious puberty.

Children with central precocious puberty have accelerated linear growth, advanced bone ages, and pubertal levels of LH, FSH, and the sex steroids, estradiol and testosterone. Because LH and FSH levels fluctuate, single samples may be inadequate to make this diagnosis. Multiple samples, which may be taken at 20-minute intervals for 1 or more hours, are helpful. A GnRH infusion with LH and FSH levels determined at regular intervals can help clarify this diagnosis.

In boys, the finding of bilateral pubertal-sized testes almost always indicates central precocious puberty. This is an extremely important point in the physical examination, because it determines the diagnostic workup.

Early attempts to treat central precocious puberty with medroxyprogesterone (Provera) and the weak androgen, danazol, successfully reversed some secondary sex characteristics but did not prevent bone age acceleration and compromise of adult stature. Cyproterone acetate, an antiandrogen, has been used with some success in Europe but is not available in the United States.

The discovery that the pulse frequency of endogenous GnRH is important for pituitary LH and FSH secretion has had a major impact in designing treatments for blocking LH and FSH release. GnRH agonists that provide consistent, not fluctuating, GnRH levels lower LH and FSH levels. Long-acting GnRH analogues have been successful in inhibiting pituitary LH and FSH release and in stopping the progression of puberty. In many cases, secondary sex characteristics have regressed.

Treatment with GnRH analogues produces a prepubertal hormonal state, and growth acceleration, bone age advancement, and the progression of secondary sex characteristics cease. The first GnRH analogue to treat precocious puberty was approved by the Food and Drug Administration in the early 1990s, with others following.

The decision to treat should depend on several factors. First, the age of the child and his or her adjustment to the pubertal changes must be considered. A 2-year-old child is in need of treatment, but a 7-year-old child may psychologically handle the changes well. The rapidity of pubertal progression as well as chronologic age must be considered. In the older child with precocious puberty, the major issues in deciding whether to treat are the magnitude of bone age advancement and the rapidity of its progression, the degree of compromise of adult stature, and the decreases in predicted adult height.

Any form of pituitary gonadotropin-independent precocious sex hormone exposure causes accelerated linear growth and advanced bone age. If the bone age is advanced enough after the pathologic cause is removed, the child may experience spontaneous gonadotropin-dependent puberty. This puberty, although precocious for the chronologic age, is not precocious for bone age. This situation is typically seen in a boy in whom the diagnosis of congenital adrenal hyperplasia was made late and treatment with glucocorticoids was begun at an advanced bone age. In this situation, treatment with a GnRH analogue may be indicated.

In some patients with severe prolonged untreated primary hypothyroidism, precocious sexual development may be seen and is associated with pubertal levels of LH and FSH. These patients exhibit poor linear growth and usually delayed bone age. If the TSH overproduction is suppressed by exogenous thyroxine, the LH and FSH concentrations decrease to prepubertal levels, and the pubertal changes regress.

## Precocious Puberty Independent of Pituitary Gonadotropins

### Girls

Girls with precocious puberty independent of pituitary gonadotropins have a non–gonadotropin-stimulated or independent source of estrogens producing their pubertal changes. An exogenous source of estrogens must be sought. The use of skin creams and medications must be pursued and the labels read to see whether they contain estrogen. Birth control pills are widely used, and although they may not be in the child's home, grandparents, friends, and baby-sitters may keep them in unprotected locations. In some cases, ingestion of animal protein, especially poultry, has been reported to produce estrogenization in a child if the animal received estrogens.

Estrogen-producing tumors of the ovary and adrenal gland must be considered. Adrenal estrogen-producing tumors are rare and are associated with high estradiol levels and increased levels of other adrenal sex hormones. They should be visible with abdominal CT or MRI scans. Estrogen-producing ovarian tumors are more common and may be palpable during careful bimanual examination. As with adrenal tumors, estradiol levels are usually high. Ultrasound and CT scans usually demonstrate the ovarian mass. Ovarian cysts, associated with high levels of estradiol, are another cause of gonadotropin-independent precocious puberty and are demonstrable with imaging. Sometimes ovarian cysts are recurrent.

Treatment entails removal of the estrogen source if exogenous exposure is the cause. If an adrenal or ovarian tumor is found, surgical excision and, if the tumor is malignant, additional treatment is indicated. Ovarian cysts are difficult to treat because they may recur, and surgical excision may make no difference in the patient's long-term clinical course.

McCune-Albright syndrome is an unusual syndrome of irregular café au lait spots, polyostotic fibrous dysplasia, and precocious puberty. It is seen in both sexes. Excessive hormone production by other glands (eg, thyroid) may be present. The cause is likely to be an abnormality in a subunit of the G-protein of the receptor. In most cases, the gonadal activation is gonadotropin independent.

### Boys

Boys with gonadotropin-independent precocious puberty have a source of androgens independent of central gonadotropin secretion. Exogenous androgen exposure must be considered. With the widespread abuse of androgens (ie, anabolic steroids) by athletes, young children are at risk for exposure.

An adrenal source of androgens, including an adrenal tumor or an adrenal biosynthetic defect (eg, 21-hydroxylase deficiency, 11-hydroxylase deficiency) causes precocious puberty in boys. Those with an adrenal or exogenous androgen source show clinical virilization, including linear growth acceleration and bone age advancement, but have prepubertal testes on examination.

Adrenal tumors are associated with high levels of adrenal androgens that are not suppressed with glucocorticoid administration. CT or MRI is important in establishing the diagnosis. Adrenal enzyme deficiencies show characteristic precursor and androgen patterns, and the elevated androgen levels are suppressible with exogenous glucocorticoids.

Testicular tumors may produce elevated androgens and cause precocious puberty. On examination, the testes show a size discrepancy; the testis with the tumor is larger and often has an irregular consistency.

The syndrome of premature Leydig cell maturation or "familial testotoxicosis" is gonadotropin independent, but there is premature Leydig cell maturation with pubertal levels of testosterone despite prepubertal LH patterns. Because maturation of spermatogenesis occurs, these patients are fertile.

Treatment of gonadotropin-independent precocious puberty in boys entails removal of the androgen source in exogenous exposure. Excision of adrenal or testicular tumors is indicated, with additional treatment if the lesions are malignant. Adrenal enzyme deficiencies require appropriate glucocorticoid replacement.

GnRH analogue treatment is not useful in familial Leydig cell hyperplasia. Recent reports indicate that ketoconazole, which inhibits enzymes in the testosterone biosynthetic pathway, may be a useful treatment.

An additional cause of precocious puberty in boys is human chorionic gonadotropin (hCG)-producing tumors. These tumors may be in the CNS (ie, germinomas) or elsewhere in the body (eg, hepatoma, hepatoblastoma, teratoma, chorioepithelioma). Because some LH assay antibodies cross-react with hCG, laboratory tests may show factitiously elevated LH and prepubertal FSH levels. Specific assays document that the gonadotropin is hCG. Because a gonadotropin is being secreted, the testes are enlarged, and boys with this problem may clinically resemble those with central precocious puberty.

# Heterosexual Development

Heterosexual development is defined as virilization in girls and feminization in boys. When it occurs before the normal age of puberty, it can be called heterosexual precocity. But whether it occurs at a prepubertal age or later, the diagnostic causes, evaluation, and treatment are the same.

Virilization in girls can be caused by adrenal and ovarian lesions. Adrenal enzyme deficiencies (eg, 21-hydroxylase, 11-hydroxylase, and 3β-hydroxysteroid dehydrogenase deficiencies) produce virilization. Typically, girls with these enzyme deficiencies have genital ambiguity as neonates, but other manifestations may occur later, sometimes as subtle as hirsutism or acne in a teenager or adult. Adrenal or ovarian androgen-producing tumors must be sought in any female with virilization by measuring plasma levels of sex steroids and by diagnostic imaging with ultrasound, CT, or MRI.

Boys with signs of feminization may have an adrenal estrogen-producing tumor, a testicular tumor, or increased peripheral conversion of androgens to estrogens, as with a familial increase in aromatase activity or certain tumors such as hepatomas.

Measurement of sex hormone levels, diagnostic imaging, tests of suppression with glucocorticoids, and adrenocorticotropin (ACTH) stimulation tests are helpful in defining the cause.

# VARIATIONS OF NORMAL PUBERTY

Three variations of normal pubertal development occur frequently and must be differentiated from progressive and pathologic processes. These are premature thelarche (in girls), premature adrenarche (in girls and boys), and pubertal gynecomastia (in boys).

## Premature Thelarche

Premature thelarche is a common entity in which there is clinical evidence of mild estrogenization in girls, typically between 1 and 4 years of age. Breast enlargement occurs, often without nipple and areolar development. No sexual hair develops, and there is no linear growth acceleration. This is an isolated phenomenon, and lack of progression is the hallmark. Laboratory tests show incomplete estrogenization of the vaginal mucosa, a normal bone age, and prepubertal gonadotropin patterns. Estradiol levels are usually prepubertal but may be slightly increased.

Postulated causes include ovarian cysts and transient pituitary gonadotropin secretion. No treatment is necessary. Close follow-up is important, because the early stages of precocious puberty may be clinically indistinguishable from premature thelarche.

## Premature Adrenarche

Premature adrenarche is caused by early activation of adrenal androgens, producing pubic and axillary hair development and axillary odor. In girls, the pubic hair often begins on the labia. There are no other signs of pubertal changes and no signs of abnormal virilization. If signs of gonadarche are observed, an evaluation for precocious puberty is indicated. If virilization occurs, a workup for virilizing lesions is necessary. Some children with this diagnosis may have mild neurologic problems. Height and bone age are often slightly greater than the mean but fall within two standard deviations. Plasma adrenal androgens and urinary androgen metabolites (17-ketosteroids) are increased to the early pubertal range.

Typically, premature adrenarche occurs in 6- to 8-year-old children, but it may be seen in much younger children. The sexual hair gradually increases. Evidence suggests that a substantial percentage of children with this diagnosis may have mild 21-hydroxylase deficiency, and an ACTH stimulation test may be useful for diagnosing some patients.

## Pubertal Gynecomastia

Pubertal gynecomastia is common in teenage boys, typically beginning in Tanner stage 2 or 3 and lasting for about 2 years. In some boys, the ratio of estradiol to testosterone may be elevated. Severely affected boys may require surgical reduction.

Tamoxifen and testolactone may be effective for treating gynecomastia in moderate cases.

Pathologic causes of gynecomastia must be considered. Hypogonadism (eg, Klinefelter's syndrome [47XXY]); partial androgen insensitivity; partial blocks in testosterone biosynthesis; hyperthyroidism; adrenal, testicular, or LH and hCG-producing tumors; liver tumors or disease; and chronic debilitating illness causing malnutrition have all been associated with gynecomastia. A variety of drugs can cause gynecomastia: androgens, estrogens, hCG, psychoactive drugs (eg, phenothiazines), street drugs and alcohol, testosterone antagonists (eg, ketoconazole, cimetidine, spironolactone), and antituberculosis and cytotoxic agents.

Obese teenage boys may present with large breasts that are only adipose tissue and of no pathologic consequence. However, determining whether glandular breast tissue exists in an extremely obese boy may be difficult.

# DELAYED PUBERTY

The causes of delayed puberty are listed in Table 141-2. An evaluation for pubertal delay is indicated if no signs of puberty are observed in a girl by 13 years of age or in a boy by 14 years of age. Evaluation is also indicated if there is an arrest in pubertal maturation.

The differential diagnosis of delayed or absent puberty rests on the initial gonadotropin levels. If LH and FSH levels are high, a primary gonadal abnormality exists. If LH and FSH levels are normal or low, a search for central hormonal abnormalities or chronic disease must be undertaken.

---

**TABLE 141-2.   Causes of Delayed Puberty**

**Elevated Gonadotropin Levels**

Gonadal failure: autoimmune, chemotherapy or radiation, traumatic, infectious, postsurgical, torsion, "vanishing testes," pure gonadal dysgenesis, myotonic dystrophy

Complete androgen insensitivity syndrome

Complete 17α-hydroxylase deficiency

Chromosomal abnormalities
  Turner's syndrome
  Klinefelter's syndrome

**Normal or Low Gonadotropin Levels**

Constitutional delay of growth and adolescence

Hypopituitarism
  Isolated LH/FSH deficiency
  associated with hyposmia or anosmia (Kallmann's syndrome)
  Multiple hormone deficiencies

Chronic disease

Syndromes
  Prader-Willi
  Laurence-Moon-Biedl

## Elevated Gonadotropin Levels

Patients with elevated LH and FSH levels have evidence of bilateral gonadal failure and lack of appropriate sex steroid levels to feed back centrally. After LH and FSH levels are found to be elevated, a karyotype should be determined. Common causes of delayed puberty are chemotherapy, radiation therapy, and autoimmune glandular failure.

Girls with the XY karyotype who have complete androgen insensitivity develop breasts at the appropriate age, but no sexual hair develops, and no menses occur. Girls with the XY karyotype and complete 17-hydroxylase deficiency (ie, no sex steroids can be formed) have no secondary sex characteristics. If these syndromes are partial, enough androgen is present to cause genital ambiguity in the neonate or virilization during puberty.

*Turner's syndrome* is a common cause of delayed breast development and elevated gonadotropin levels. It is invariably associated with short stature and often with other anomalies, including webbed neck, increased nevi, high-arched palate, shield chest, coarctation of the aorta, renal anomalies, an increased arm-carrying angle, and edema of the hands and feet. Most girls with this syndrome have a 45X karyotype, but many have a mosaic pattern (45X/46XX) or an X-chromosomal structural abnormality (eg, ring or isochrome). Buccal smears are not adequate for this diagnosis. Sexual hair develops in girls with Turner's syndrome because adrenal androgens are not affected.

Boys with *Klinefelter's syndrome* (47XXY) usually come to attention because of gynecomastia and small testes (ie, inadequate masculinization). They are usually clinically normal at birth, and throughout childhood, they are tall with slim builds and long limbs. They may also have mosaic chromosome patterns (eg, 46XY/47XXY) or multiple X chromosomes.

Treatment of patients with gonadal failure involves replacing sex steroids. Depending on the age of the patient and whether or not height is an issue, this can be done gradually over several years or more abruptly.

In young teenage boys, injectable testosterone can be used. A typical regimen is testosterone enanthate administered intramuscularly in a dose of 50 mg/month initially and gradually increased to full adult doses of 300 mg every 3 weeks. Long-term replacement therapy with oral testosterone preparations is not recommended because of the hepatotoxicity of 17$\alpha$-alkylated steroids.

In girls, conjugated estrogens can be started at 0.3 mg/day, with doses increased gradually until satisfactory breast development is achieved. After 1 to 2 years of estrogen treatment or if vaginal spotting occurs, treatment with estrogens in cycles of about 25 days per month, with a progestational agent overlapping for about the last 10 days of each cycle, should be started. Estradiol can also be given in gradually increasing doses. Depot estrogen preparations given monthly have been used. New transdermal estrogen patches may be useful in long-term treatment. After adequate estrogenization has occurred, long-term treatment can be achieved with a combination oral contraceptive pill.

## Normal or Low Gonadotropin Levels

The most common cause of pubertal delay is *constitutional delay*, discussed in the next chapter. Usually, a careful physical examination in a mid-teenaged boy reveals early signs of puberty, which progress on follow-up examinations. Reassurance may be all that is necessary. However, more severely affected boys may be psychologically disabled by this problem, and a short course

of exogenous testosterone (eg, testosterone enanthate given intramuscularly as 50 to 100 mg/month for 4 to 6 months) should be seriously considered. Short courses of modest doses do not appear to adversely affect ultimate stature. Bone age should be monitored whenever androgens are used.

*Isolated gonadotropin deficiency* may or may not be associated with anosmia or hyposmia (ie, Kallmann's syndrome). It may be difficult to differentiate from constitutional delay in certain cases, and overnight gonadotropin sampling or GnRH testing may be helpful. Baseline LH and FSH levels do not differentiate prepubertal or hypogonadotropic from early pubertal levels. Search for an organic cause requires CNS imaging. Prolactin-secreting pituitary adenomas may produce gonadotropin deficiency. LH and FSH deficiency is more commonly associated with other pituitary hormone deficiencies, especially GH deficiency. The differential diagnosis of hypopituitarism is discussed in Chapter 142. Induction and maintenance of puberty in these patients must be coordinated with other hormonal replacement therapy. Traditionally, puberty has been induced and maintained with exogenous sex steroids, as discussed earlier in this chapter. Gonadotropin injections can be used to induce fertility in patients with central gonadotropin deficiency. GnRH has been given in pulsatile fashion to induce puberty and to produce fertility.

Some adolescent girls may develop normally, but because they lack normal central cyclic function, they do not have normal menses. Any chronic disease during childhood and adolescence may delay puberty and growth. Particular attention must be paid to the possibility of subtle gastrointestinal disease, especially inflammatory bowel disease, and to the patient's nutritional status. Inadequate caloric intake or excessive exercise can delay puberty and cause amenorrhea.

Certain syndromes are associated with central gonadotropin deficiency, particularly the Prader-Willi and Laurence-Moon-Biedl syndromes. Hypothyroidism can cause delayed puberty or precocious puberty.

Blind children may have pubertal delay, and associated pituitary-hypothalamic dysfunction must be considered in these children.

In virtually all patients with primary gonadal failure or central gonadotropin deficiency, treatment with sex steroids can induce and maintain satisfactory sexual maturation and satisfactory sexual functioning. Patients with central gonadotropin deficiency have hope for fertility with the use of gonadotropins or GnRH preparations.

## Selected Readings

Kaplan SL, Grumbach MM. Pathophysiology and treatment of sexual precocity. J Clin Endocrinol Metab 1990;71:785.

Kritzler RK, Plotnick LP, Migeon CJ. Sexual development alterations. In: Hoekelman RA, ed. Primary pediatric care. St Louis: CV Mosby, 1992:1063.

Lee PA, O'Dea L StL. Primary and secondary testicular insufficiency. Pediatr Clin North Am 1990;37:1359.

Mahoney CP. Adolescent gynecomastia; differential diagnosis and management. Pediatr Clin North Am 1990;37:1389.

Pescovitz OH. Precocious puberty. Pediatr Rev 1990;11:229.

Plotnick LP. Precocious puberty. In: Carpenter, Rock, eds. Pediatric and adolescent gynecology. New York: Raven Press:1992;153.

Rosenfield RL. Diagnosis and management of delayed puberty. J Clin Endocrinol Metab 1990;70:559.

Rosenfield RL. The ovary and female sexual maturation. In: Kaplan SA, ed. Clinical pediatric endocrinology. Philadelphia: WB Saunders, 1990:259.

Styne DM. The testes: disorders of sexual differentiation and puberty. In: Kaplan SA, ed. Clinical pediatric endocrinology. Philadelphia: WB Saunders, 1990:367

Wheeler MD, Styne DM. Diagnosis and management of precocious puberty. Pediatr Clin North Am 1990;37:1255.

Wilson DM, Rosenfeld RG. Treatment of short stature and delayed adolescence. Pediatr Clin North Am 1987;34:865.

*Principles and Practice of Pediatrics, Second Edition.*
edited by Frank A. Oski et al. J. B. Lippincott Company, Philadelphia © 1994.

# CHAPTER 142
# *Growth, Growth Hormone, and Pituitary Disorders*

## Leslie P. Plotnick

## GROWTH

Problems related to normal or abnormal growth are common in pediatric practice. Short stature can be defined as height more than two standard deviations (2 SD) below the mean and tall stature as height more than 2 SD above the mean. Three percent of children are at or more than 2 SD below the mean, and 3% are at or more than 2 SD above the mean.

In addition to actual height and weight at any one time, the rate of growth over time is essential in deciding which children may have pathologic growth and which do not. A child may have normal height and weight but an extremely subnormal rate of growth, indicating the need for an evaluation. The importance of regular height and weight measurements and of plotting these measurements on growth curves, so that deviations from normal velocities can be detected early, cannot be overemphasized (see Figs 6-8 through 6-13 in Chap. 6 for height and weight curves for girls and boys, birth to 36 months, and 2 to 18 years.)

Because the timing of puberty affects growth rate, Tanner has modified the growth curves to include curves for early and late developers. These curves are useful in adolescents with early-normal and late-normal onset of puberty and should be used to assess the normalcy of growth in these children (Fig 142-1).

Growth velocity curves are important to use when evaluating children for disorders of growth. These curves are shown in Figure 142-2. Velocities for children with early-normal and late-normal puberty are superimposed on the curves.

Bone age is also important in evaluating a child for a growth problem. Children with normal bone ages are unlikely to have a systemic chronic disease or a hormonal abnormality as the cause of the growth problem. Significantly delayed or advanced bone ages (ie, >2 SD from the mean) may indicate pathology and require evaluation.

## SHORT STATURE OR POOR LINEAR GROWTH

A child with a height below the third percentile or whose growth curve has been crossing percentiles downward should be carefully examined for a pathologic cause of poor growth (Table 142-1).

Probably the largest category of causes of poor growth is *major organ system disease.* Most patients in this category have a disorder that is not subtle, and the history and physical examination disclose the problem without extensive laboratory testing. However, some disorders may not be evident from history and physical examination and require laboratory studies for diagnosis. Renal disorders, particularly renal tubular acidosis, require evaluation by electrolytes, chemistries, and urinalysis. Particularly difficult

to define are patients with gastrointestinal (GI) abnormalities. Patients with inflammatory bowel disease, especially Crohn's disease, may have growth failure for several years before GI symptoms become evident. A complete blood cell count with an erythrocyte sedimentation rate test may be helpful, but GI contrast studies and endoscopy are required to make the diagnosis. Patients with celiac disease may not have the classic history of malabsorption stools and hyperphagia. These children often are thin and have poor appetites. Certain laboratory tests (eg, erythrocyte folate, carotene, and antigliadin antibodies) may help with this diagnosis, but the only definitive diagnostic test is a small bowel biopsy. The decision of when to do the more extensive GI studies (eg, radiologic, endoscopic) rests on the persistence of a poor growth rate over time, with other laboratory tests remaining normal and no other diagnosis being made, especially if the child's weight is more affected than the height. Malnutrition of any cause, including malabsorption or inadequate caloric intake, is associated with poor growth.

*Chromosomal disorders* are often associated with poor growth. These usually are evident from characteristic dysmorphic features and developmental delay. Turner's syndrome and its variants (ie, absence or structural abnormalities of one X chromosome or a mosaic pattern) may manifest with classic phenotypic features or may have only minor clinical features. Girls with non-45X karyotypes (ie, mosaics, rings, isochromes or partial X deletions) are more likely to lack the classic phenotypic features. All short girls with subnormal growth rates should have banded karyotyping as part of the laboratory evaluation. Buccal smears are not adequate, because they do not reveal structural abnormalities or mosaic patterns. Banded karyotyping is expensive and adds considerably to the cost of the evaluation. However, Turner's syndrome may be as common as growth hormone (GH) deficiency and should be considered in all short girls. Growth curves for girls with Turner's syndrome are available.

Growth retardation is often seen as part of the clinical picture in children with a variety of inborn *metabolic errors.*

*Intrauterine growth retardation* (IUGR) is another category associated with short stature. Children who are severely small for gestational age at birth often have poor postnatal growth. These children may have dysmorphic features, indicating a specific syndrome associated with IUGR. They may be nondysmorphic but thin, especially with very thin extremities, minimal body fat, and thin, narrow faces. Bone ages may be delayed or normal.

*Familial or genetic short stature* is a common cause of short stature in children. Usually the parents' heights are in the lower normal percentiles for adults. This is not a disorder, because these children are entirely normal. Their heights are usually at or slightly below the third percentile but not at or more than 3 SD below the mean. They have normal growth velocities, and their height curve parallels the third percentile. Their bone ages are normal, and their pubertal growth spurt is normal in timing and magnitude.

One or both of the parents may be short for a pathologic reason, which the child may have inherited, such as familial GH deficiency or mild chondrodysplasias. If a parent's height is more than 2 SD below the mean (ie, less than third percentile) or if the parent is disproportionately short for the family, both parent and child may have pathologic short stature.

Constitutional slow growth with delayed adolescence, called *constitutional delay,* is another common diagnostic category. This variant of normal growth is seen much more frequently in boys than in girls. Typically, affected children lag 2 to 4 years behind average in height, bone age, and pubertal development. There is often a positive family history in parents, older siblings, or other family members.

If growth rate is normal, the height is at or slightly below the third percentile, there is a positive family history, and the bone

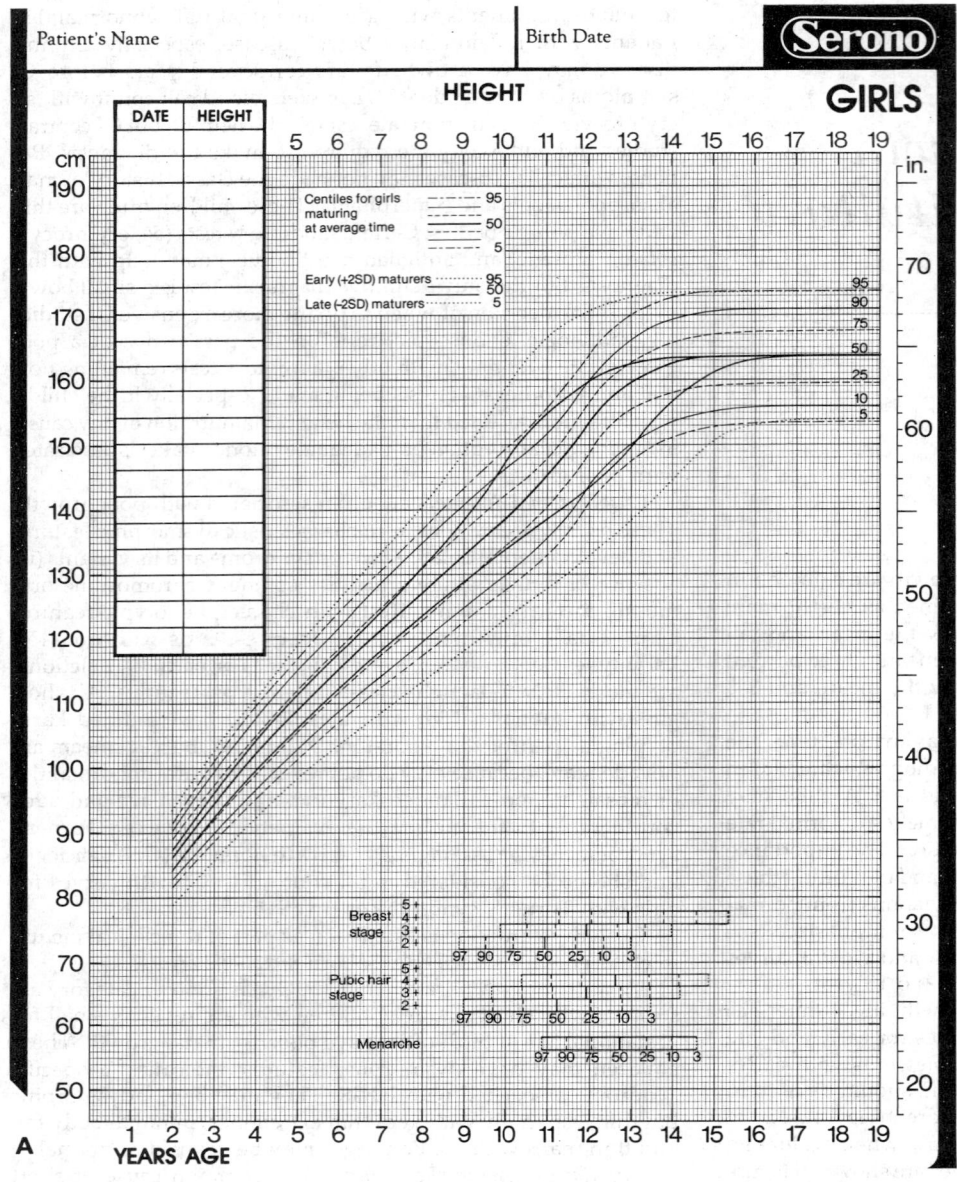

**Figure 142-1.** Early and late puberty curves for girls **(A)** and boys **(B)**, superimposed on the average curve. (North American growth & development longitudinal standards. Height: distance and velocity for girls and boys. From Tanner JM. J Pediatr 1985;107. Distributed by Serono Laboratories, Randolph, MA.)

age is delayed by 2 to 4 years, no additional evaluation is needed. However, if there is any concern about a subnormal growth velocity, further evaluation is indicated. Patients with early inflammatory bowel disease or with milder degrees of GH deficiency may initially resemble children with constitutional delay. Because growth velocity gradually drops with age and is at its lowest just before the pubertal growth spurt begins (see Fig 142-2), teenagers with constitutional delay may spend a prolonged time at this low rate. Growth velocity should be assessed in relation to bone age and chronologic age.

*Endocrine abnormalities* are another diagnostic category of short stature. Cortisol excess (ie, cortisol in greater amounts than physiologic needs) produces short stature, whether the excess cortisol is exogenous, due to oral, topical, or inhalant glucocorticoids, or endogenous, as in Cushing's disease. Children with cortisol excess have a subnormal linear growth rate, delayed bone age, and typical cushingoid clinical features: round, plethoric "moon" face, centripetal obesity, increased dorsal fat pad ("buffalo hump"), and proximal muscle weakness. When the source of excess glucocorticoids is removed, the growth rate increases, but the ultimate height can be compromised by years of glucocorticoid excess.

Hypothyroidism is a distinct endocrine cause of short stature, characterized by a subnormal linear growth rate, increased weight gain, and a delayed bone age. When the diagnosis is made and appropriate treatment given, children undergo catch-up growth. The threshold for performing thyroid function tests should be low for a child with a question of poor growth rate, because the diagnostic tests and treatment are of minimal risk, inexpensive, and effective. Treatment often has dramatic effects on clinical signs and symptoms and growth. Patients with pseudohypoparathyroidism have a characteristic phenotype that includes short stature.

Poorly controlled insulin-dependent diabetes mellitus may be associated with short stature and poor linear growth rate. The growth retardation in poorly controlled diabetes can be severe. Improving metabolic control usually normalizes the growth rate.

*GH deficiency* is a diagnostic category that has undergone considerable flux in recent years. GH deficiency may be idiopathic, organic, or familial; it is occasionally psychosocial and reversible. It may occur alone or with other pituitary hormone deficiencies. Children with classic GH deficiency have short stature, poor linear growth rate, and delayed bone age, and they are usually chubby.

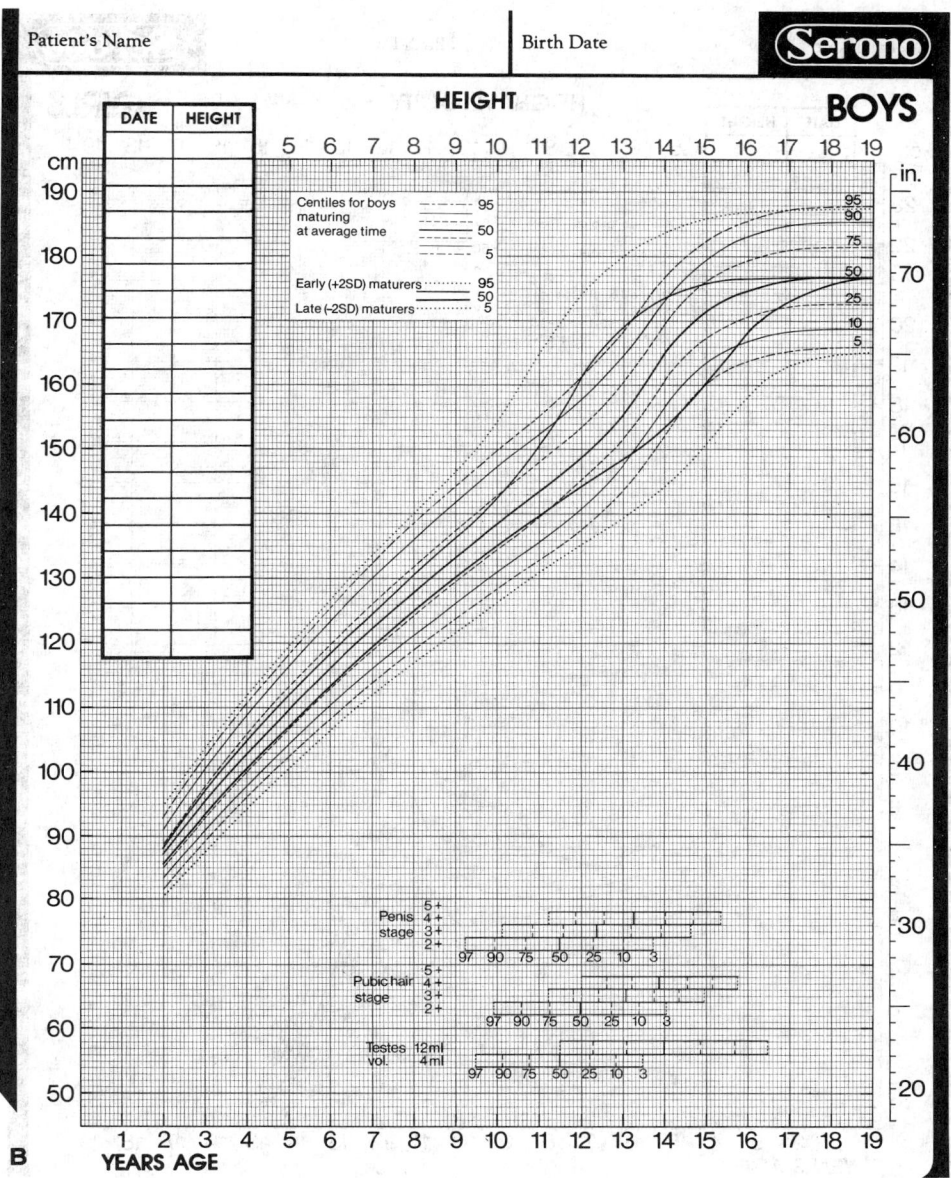

**Figure 142-1.** (Continued)

They may have fasting hypoglycemia, and boys may have small penises. They fail to release normal amounts of GH in response to certain standard pharmacologic stimuli.

Various degrees of GH deficiency occur; there is a continuum from normal GH secretion to classic GH deficiency, and where a physician draws the line between normal and abnormal is arbitrary. Some patients respond normally to pharmacologic tests but have low physiologic 24-hour GH secretion, and some have borderline responses to pharmacologic tests; both groups of patients have partial GH deficiency or neurosecretory defects. Other patients secrete normal amounts of immunologically active GH that is biologically subactive. Patients in these categories may have been previously classified as having constitutional delay. The level of somatomedin-C in some of these patients may be borderline or low.

The diagnosis of classic GH deficiency remains clear-cut, but the standards of diagnosis of the lesser degrees of GH compromise or of biologically subactive GH are in flux. Because some or many of these patients may benefit from treatment with exogenous GH, this is an important question for pediatric endocrinologists.

Specific causes of GH deficiency, isolated or associated with other pituitary hormone deficiencies, are congenital abnormalities (including septo-optic dysplasia), trauma, CNS infections, vascular abnormalities, irradiation for malignancies, tumors (eg, craniopharyngiomas), and infiltrative processes such as histiocytosis.

*Craniopharyngiomas* are the most common tumors associated with pituitary and hypothalamic deficiencies. They are tumors of the Rathke pouch and are usually suprasellar but may be entirely intrasellar. Patients with craniopharyngiomas usually present with headache, visual abnormalities and neurologic symptoms. They may also have symptoms of diabetes insipidus and growth failure.

On physical examination, they may have visual defects (eg, field cuts, optic atrophy, papilledema) and signs of pituitary hormone deficiencies. CNS imaging shows calcifications in most patients and identifies the tumors. Treatment is surgical excision, often followed by radiation therapy, and appropriate hormonal replacement therapy.

Some children who are born smaller or larger than their genetic growth potential gradually *shift percentiles*, up or down, for height and weight. A typical example is a child who at birth is in the

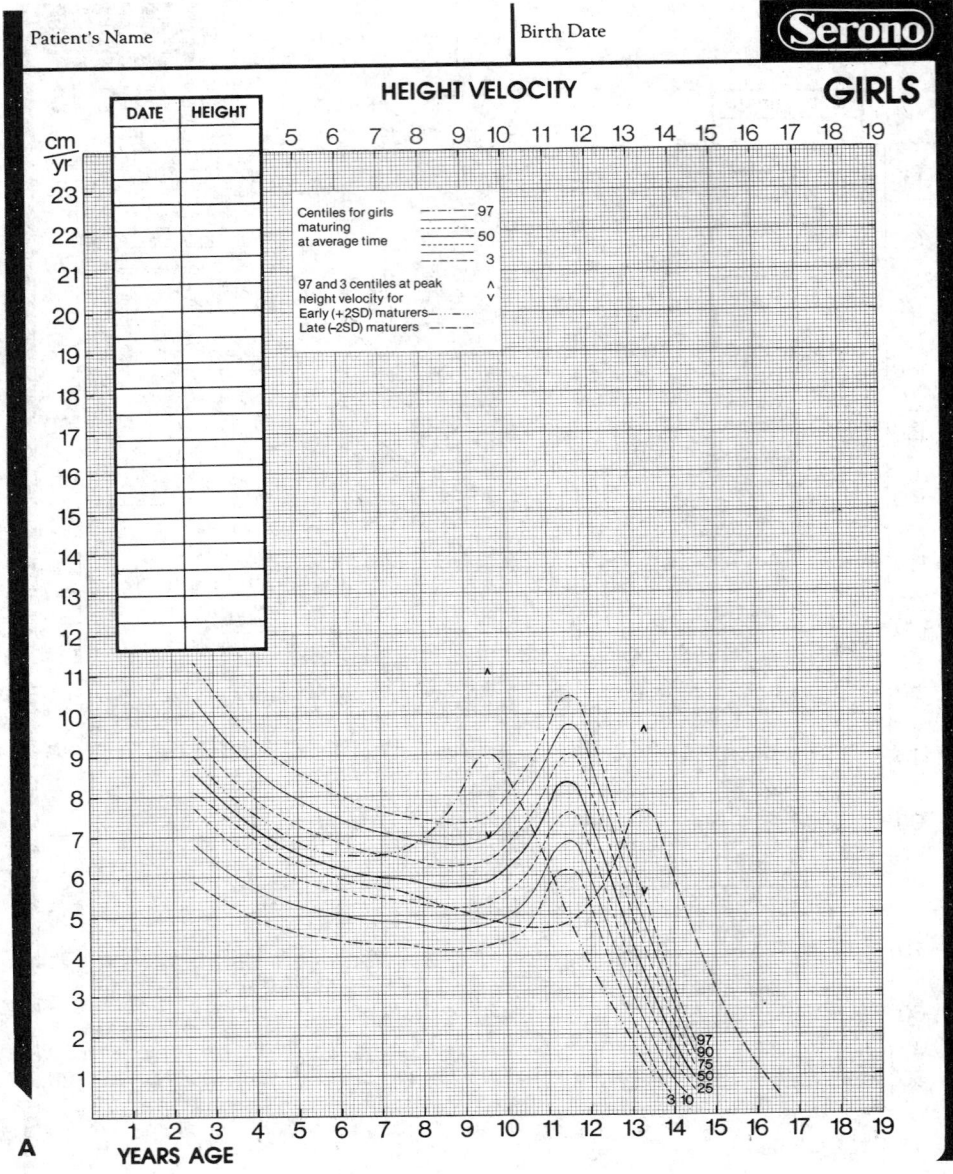

Patient's Name

Birth Date

**Serono**

**HEIGHT VELOCITY**

**GIRLS**

Centiles for girls maturing at average time ———— 97 / 50 / 3

97 and 3 centiles at peak height velocity for
Early (+2SD) maturers ————
Late (−2SD) maturers ————

**A**  **YEARS AGE**

**Figure 142-2.** Growth velocity curves for girls (**A**) and boys (**B**), including early and late pubertal patterns. (North American growth & development longitudinal standards. Height: distance and velocity for girls and boys. From Tanner JM. J Pediatr 1985;107. Distributed by Serono Laboratories, Randolph, MA.)

90th percentile for length and weight but whose parents are in the 10th percentile for height. During the first 1 to 2 years of life, this child gradually decelerates to approximately the 10th percentile. Sometimes it is difficult to differentiate this pattern from pathologic growth. The key points are a gradual deceleration of height and weight proportionally, deceleration not below the genetically anticipated percentile, and once the percentile is reached, velocities normalizing and height and weight remaining at that percentile. If the deceleration is abrupt and falls to less than the fifth percentile or to a percentile below the parents' percentile, further evaluation is needed.

*Skeletal dysplasias*, including rickets, are obvious causes of poor growth. The skeletal abnormalities are usually evident on physical examination, as are abnormal arm spans and upper and lower segment ratios. Radiologic studies can help identify the specific abnormalities.

*Psychologic factors* have been associated with poor growth. The growth abnormality can be caused by severe deprivation of caloric intake. Children in disturbed families may have psychosocial dwarfism, with disturbed eating and sleeping behaviors and transient pituitary hormone deficiencies, especially of GH

and ACTH. When the child is removed from the adverse home environment, catch-up growth occurs, and the hormonal levels normalize.

Various *medications* may produce poor growth. Glucocorticoids were discussed earlier in this chapter. Stimulants such as amphetamines and methylphenidate, especially in high doses, have been associated with impairment of weight and height.

## TALL STATURE AND EXCESSIVE LINEAR GROWTH

Most children with tall stature (ie, heights more than 2 SD above the mean) have familial or genetic tall stature; their parents or other family members are tall. This, like familial short stature, is not pathologic. These children grow above the 95th percentile, but their growth curves are parallel to it. Their linear growth velocities are normal, and their bone ages are normal. Their pubertal growth spurt is normal in timing and magnitude, although they tend to grow in the upper normal velocity percentiles.

Certain syndromes are associated with tall stature and should

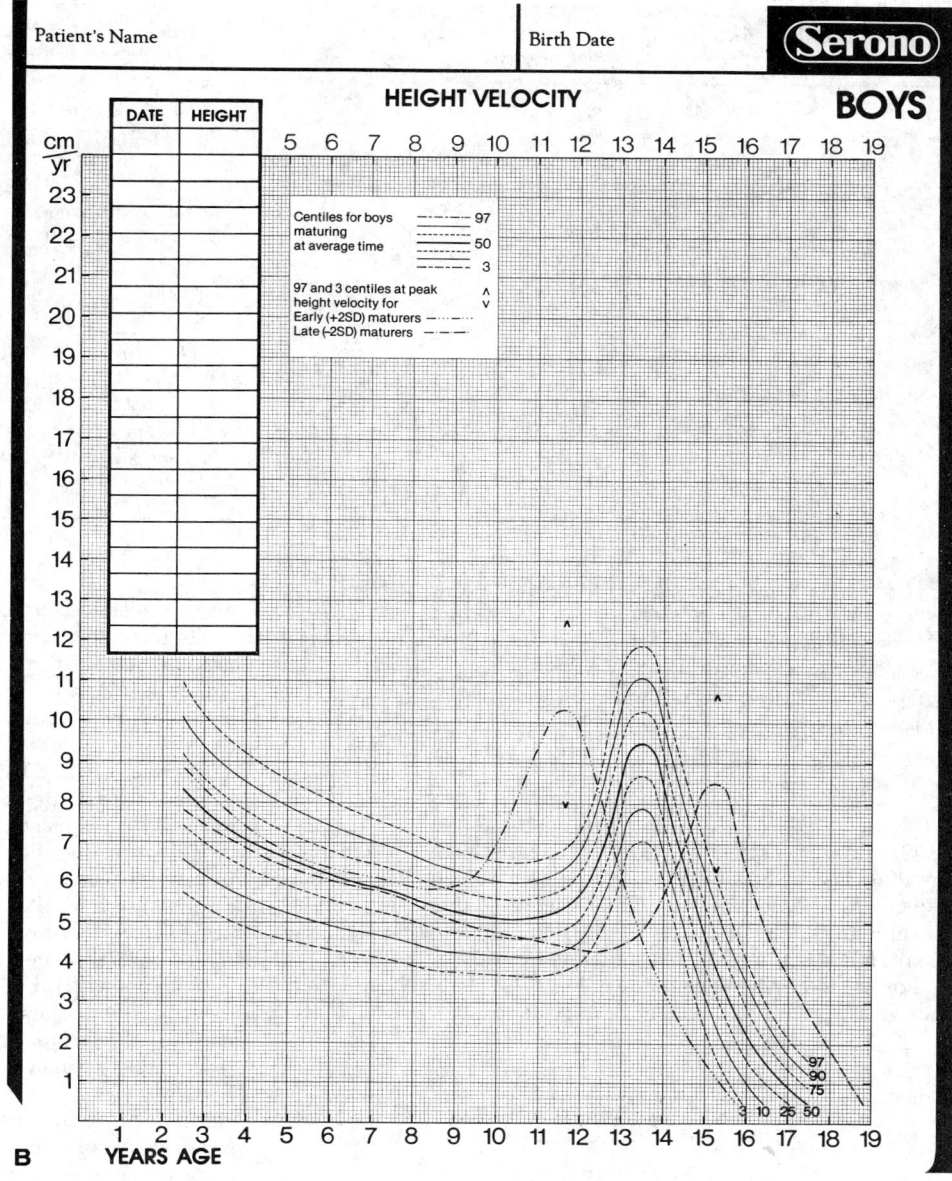

Figure 142-2.   (*Continued*)   **B**

be sought on examination. Marfan syndrome, cerebral gigantism, homocystinuria, Klinefelter's syndrome (XXY), and XYY karyotypes are associated with tall stature.

Nutritional obesity is often associated with tall stature. Obese children typically show linear growth in the upper normal percentiles and may also have bone ages at the upper limits of normal (ie, approximately 1 to 2 SD above the mean). This is in contrast to the weight gain associated with endocrine abnormalities such as hypothyroidism, Cushing's disease, and GH deficiency, in which linear growth rate is subnormal and bone age is delayed.

Endocrine abnormalities can cause tall stature. Children with hyperthyroidism may have an excessive linear growth rate during the hyperthyroid period, but this finding is usually not a presenting complaint.

GH excess (ie, pituitary gigantism) causes excessive linear growth rates. GH excess is rare in childhood and adolescence and is usually caused by a pituitary GH-producing tumor or sometimes by excess GH-releasing factor production from a hypothalamic or peripheral tumor, such as a pancreatic tumor.

Many children with tall stature and excessive linear growth rates probably have precocious sex hormone secretion due to central precocious puberty or a variety of gonadal or adrenal abnormalities (see Chap. 141). Children with precocious sex hormone secretion have excessive linear growth rates initially. However, the hormones also cause rapid bone age advancement and early epiphyseal fusion, which compromise adult stature.

High doses of sex steroids can be used to treat tall stature if the predicted adult height is excessive.

## HYPOTHALAMIC-PITUITARY-GROWTH HORMONE PHYSIOLOGY

The regulation of GH secretion is shown in Figure 142-3. Pituitary release of GH is controlled by two hypothalamic factors, a GH-releasing factor and an inhibiting factor, somatostatin. Hypothalamic release of these factors is controlled by neurotransmitters secreted by higher neurons that respond to factors such as sleep, exercise, and physical and emotional stress.

GH is released in bursts, and the levels fluctuate markedly during the day and night, with higher values usually occurring during the early hours of sleep.

## TABLE 142-1. Causes of Short Stature or Poor Linear Growth

Major organ system disease
  Central nervous system
  Cardiac
  Pulmonary
  Hematologic
  Renal
  Gastrointestinal or nutritional
Chromosomal disorders: Turner's syndrome
Inborn errors of metabolism
Intrauterine growth retardation
Familial or genetic short stature
Constitutional delay of growth and adolescence
Endocrine disorders
  Cortisol excess (exogenous or endogenous)
  Hypothyroidism
  Pseudohypoparathyroidism
  Poorly controlled diabetes
  Growth hormone deficiency (eg, idiopathic, organic, familial, psychosocial)
Shifting linear percentiles
Skeletal disorders
Deprivation or psychosocial dwarfism
Medications

## TABLE 142-2. Tests for Growth Hormone Deficiency

Screening tests
  Exercise: before and after 20 minutes of jogging on a level surface or up and down stairs
  Sleep: useful for inpatients; measure GH approximately 45 minutes after onset of nighttime sleep
Definitive pharmacologic tests ("arginine" through "glucagon" in the following list measure ability of the hypothalamic-pituitary unit to secrete GH)
  Arginine
  L-Dopa
  Insulin hypoglycemia
  Clonidine
  Glucagon
  GRF (ie, measures only pituitary GH function)
Physiologic tests: sampling every 20 to 30 minutes, intermittently or with a continuous blood withdrawal pump

GH produces linear growth by generating the formation of another class of hormones called the somatomedins or insulin-like growth factors, of which somatomedin-C, also called insulin-like growth factor-I (IGF-I), is the predominant growth-promoting factor. IGF-I is thought to be generated mostly in the liver.

For GH to be able to generate IGF-I, the GH must be normally biologically active and able to bind to its receptor. The receptor and all postreceptor steps must be intact. Once generated, IGF-I acts through its receptors on target tissues to produce linear growth. A defect anywhere in the GH-IGF-I axis can produce short stature and a clinical picture identical to that of GH deficiency. Only laboratory studies are able to differentiate one kind of defect from another. IGF-I and GH also exert negative feedback at the pituitary and hypothalamic levels, affecting GH secretion.

Tests for GH deficiency are summarized in Table 142-2. An inadequate response to a screening test indicates the need for definitive testing. For classic GH deficiency to be diagnosed, a patient must fail two definitive pharmacologic tests. Most laboratories use a level of 7 to 10 ng/mL peak value as the cut-off point between normal and subnormal. Different assays have different normal ranges.

Patients with other disorders of the GH–IGF-I axis have been described. A biologically subactive GH molecule or an abnormality in the GH receptor (ie, Laron dwarfism) causes an inability to generate normal amounts of IGF-I. A group of patients in Equador with a GH receptor defect has been described. Administration of exogenous GH can help differentiate patients with biologically subactive GH from those with Laron dwarfism, because a response of an increase in IGF-I and an increase in growth rate is seen only in patients with biologically subactive GH and not in those with Laron dwarfism. Patients with peripheral resistance to IGF-I also have been described.

Partial GH deficiency can be difficult to diagnose. A subnormal growth rate, delayed bone age, and low or low-normal IGF-I levels are clues. Twenty-four-hour physiologic GH monitoring may help with this diagnosis. Ultimately, a trial of GH therapy may be useful.

Newer methods include the measurement of GH-binding proteins (GHBP). GHBP correlate inversely with 24-hour GH secretion and directly with the increase in IGF-I and increase in growth velocity on GH therapy. GHBPs reflect the cellular expression of the GH receptor. The levels of IGF-binding proteins, mainly IGF-BP3, correlate with GH production and may be a screening tool for GH deficiency.

## WORKUP FOR SHORT STATURE OR POOR LINEAR GROWTH VELOCITY

The evaluation of a child with poor growth begins with a careful history. Height and growth patterns and the timing of puberty in parents, siblings, and other relatives should be asked about.

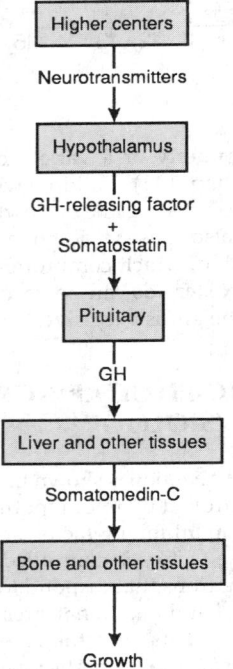

**Figure 142-3.** Regulation of growth hormone secretion.

Gestational age and length and weight at birth are important. Anything in the history to suggest major organ system pathology should be heeded, remembering that renal and GI disorders can be quite subtle. The child's psychologic adjustment to his stature should be investigated, as should the overall family functioning. Nutritional issues should be discussed.

The child's growth curve should be carefully evaluated. If no previous growth data are available, questions about changes in shoe and clothing sizes and about how the child's growth compares with that of siblings and peers can be helpful. For example, "He used to be a head taller than his sister, who's 3 years younger, but now they're the same height," is revealing information. Every effort should be made to obtain previous growth data.

The entire complete physical examination is important. Any features of chronic disease should be elicited. Accurate height and weight measurements are mandatory. Careful fundoscopic examination looking for evidence of optic nerve abnormalities, and confrontation visual fields, should be done. Because dentition reflects bone age, the age appropriateness of primary and secondary teeth should be assessed. Are there any dysmorphic features of the face or body habitus or extremities? The thyroid should be carefully palpated. Are there signs of sexual maturation? In boys, is the penis abnormally small? Are there any clinical features of cortisol excess or of Turner's syndrome? Is the child's appearance proportionate or disproportionate for arm span and for upper and lower segment ratios?

If there are clues to a specific diagnosis, a complete laboratory workup is unnecessary. For example, if the child appears normal on examination and the history and growth curve strongly suggest familial short stature, no workup is necessary. Perhaps only a bone age evaluation to assess predicted height should be done. If the child is clearly cushingoid, the specific cause of this should be pursued.

In the many children in whom no clear cause is evident after history and physical examination, we recommend the following starting laboratory workup: complete blood count with erythrocyte sedimentation rate, chemistry panel including electrolytes, urinalysis with specific gravity and pH (urine culture if any signs of infection are present), bone age, thyroid hormone levels (ie, $T_4$, $T_3RU$, TSH), screening GH test (eg, exercise), IGF-I, and banded karyotyping for girls.

Any specific abnormalities found should be investigated further, but if nothing abnormal is seen other than perhaps a significant bone age delay, the next step depends on the clinical impression and on the child's growth curve and current growth rate. Growth is an ongoing dynamic process, and evaluation over time is useful. If a child's growth rate is persistently subnormal such that he or she gradually or abruptly falls away from a normal curve, a repeat investigation or a more detailed look (eg, 24-hour GH monitoring, repeat definitive GH testing, pursuit of subtle GI pathology) may be indicated.

Despite the sophisticated diagnostic testing available, some children have clearly negative workup results, do not fit the diagnosis of constitutional delay, and are left with a diagnosis of idiopathic short stature. Children in this category need careful follow-up, because a specific cause may become evident with time.

## TREATMENT OF SHORT STATURE

If a specific diagnosis is made, the condition is treated appropriately. For example, if primary hypothyroidism is found, thyroid replacement therapy is indicated. This section discusses treatment with exogenous GH, anabolic steroids, and androgens for children with GH disorders, IUGR, Turner's syndrome, familial short stature, constitutional delay, and idiopathic short stature.

Until the spring of 1985, GH in the United States and elsewhere was obtained exclusively from cadaver pituitaries. In the United States, it was distributed by the National Hormone and Pituitary Program for patients in research protocols and, starting in the mid-1970s, through several commercial companies by prescription. The supply was limited. Most children treated were GH deficient. In 1985, pituitary GH was withdrawn because a few young men treated with pituitary GH in the 1960s and 1970s died of Creutzfeldt-Jakob disease, a slow virus disease similar to kuru and scrapie. It seemed likely that the slow virus particles had contaminated some pituitary GH preparations in the past, and because it was impossible to ensure that this could not occur with later preparations, the hormone was withdrawn from use. Fortunately, studies with recombinant DNA-produced biosynthetic GH were already under way. In October 1985, the first of these was approved for use in GH-deficient children, and in May 1987, a second preparation became available.

Pituitary GH and biosynthetic GH have identical effects. Patients taking biosynthetic GH may have measurable antibodies to GH in low titers. This does not appear to be clinically significant; no effect on growth rate has been seen.

A GH-deficient child usually grows 3 to 4 inches in the first year of treatment and 2 to 3 inches in each successive year. Catch-up growth to the normal range may be gradual. Recommended doses are different for different preparations, but they are 0.06 or 0.10 mg/kg/dose given on alternate days, three times a week. Daily treatment (approximately 0.20 to 0.30 mg/kg/week divided into six or seven injections) has supplanted thrice-weekly therapy for many patients because of data documenting better growth rates on daily treatment regimens. Dose-response questions are being studied. The intramuscular route has been replaced by subcutaneous injections.

The use of GH for other diagnostic categories is investigational. GH treatment has been effective to a modest degree in helping some children with IUGR grow faster. There is evidence that GH, the anabolic steroid oxandrolone, and low-dose estrogens, when used alone, can increase the growth rate of girls with Turner's syndrome. In one large study, treatment with GH alone or in combination with oxandrolone in Turner's syndrome produced a sustained increase in growth rate for at least 6 years. For the girls who completed treatment, their mean height was 8.1 cm above their initial projected final height (151.9 versus 143.8 cm). However, the cost of this treatment option must be considered.

Boys with constitutional delay clearly may benefit from treatment with androgens during their teenage years. Low-dose testosterone given by monthly injection for 4 to 6 months can gently accelerate growth, bone age, and spontaneous puberty. Anabolic steroids may be helpful in younger children with constitutional delay.

Some children with mild deficiencies in GH secretion may clinically resemble patients with constitutional delay. Because these patients may benefit from GH treatment, a trial of GH should be considered for patients with subnormal growth velocities and low-normal IGF-I levels, perhaps before androgen treatment is considered.

Children with familial short stature grow at normal velocities and do not need any treatment to help them achieve a genetically appropriate height. There is often tremendous pressure to intervene in some way and put the child on GH treatment. In some families, the focus on being taller as a cure for all ills suggests the need for psychiatric intervention. It has not yet been demonstrated that GH treatment can increase the adult height of non–GH-deficient normal children.

Idiopathic short stature is a leftover diagnostic label for short children who do not fall into any specific diagnostic category. A child who is inappropriately small for the family; who has a negative history, physical examination, and laboratory evaluation;

and who does not fit the category of constitutional delay is considered to have idiopathic short stature.

The use of GH treatment in children with constitutional delay, familial short stature, and idiopathic short stature has been studied by several investigators. A national study is under way. In some published studies, as many as 50% of treated children had significant increases in their growth rates. After GH treatment is stopped, the growth rate in many patients decelerates, sometimes to or below the pretreatment growth rate. There are no data available to indicate the persistence of the increased growth rate nor to show whether ultimate adult stature is affected. However, for a child who is very short (ie, height >2.5 to 3 SD below normal) and especially one with a subnormal growth rate, a trial of GH treatment may be considered, although this is controversial.

The side effects of biosynthetic GH treatment include development of various degrees of insulin resistance (although hyperglycemia is rare), mild sodium and water retention that is not clinically significant, development of anti-GH antibodies that is not clinically significant, lowering of thyroxine levels, and increased basal metabolic rate, which is possibly a desirable effect. Occasionally, slipped capital femoral epiphyses has been reported, but it is not clear if this is related to GH treatment.

The major concern about GH therapy is its oncogenic potential. Growth hormone treatment has been associated with an increased risk of leukemia, but in the United States, it is mostly in patients who were previously treated for brain tumors and who were probably at greater risk of developing a second malignancy. It has been estimated that the overall annual increased risk may be in the range of 1 in 40,000. More epidemiologic research should be done to answer this important question.

The side effects of anabolic steroids include virilization, bone age advancement, and, rarely, hepatotoxicity.

GH-releasing factor, through pulsatile infusion pump or bolus injections, has been shown to stimulate linear growth velocity in GH-deficient children with a hypothalamic defect. Whether this is equal to or better than GH treatment in effect, ease of administration, and cost is being studied. Trials with IGF-I are beginning in patients with GH receptor defects.

# DISORDERS OF ANTIDIURETIC HORMONE

Antidiuretic hormone (ADH, vasopressin) is released from the posterior pituitary by neurons originating in the hypothalamic supraoptic and periventricular nuclei. ADH release is mediated through osmoreceptors and baroreceptors, and secretion increases in response to hypovolemia and hyperosmolality. ADH acts by means of the kidney to reabsorb water, which decreases urine volume and increases urine osmolality.

## Diabetes Insipidus

Diabetes insipidus is a disorder of subnormal ADH secretion or reduced kidney responsiveness to ADH. Renal responsiveness can be established by monitoring the response to exogenous vasopressin. ADH deficiency may be genetic but more often is caused by lesions in the hypothalamic area, commonly tumors and infiltrative disorders, such as histiocytosis. Trauma, inflammatory processes, and vascular abnormalities are also causes of ADH deficiency.

ADH deficiency manifests with symptoms of polyuria and polydipsia with large volumes of dilute urine. Symptoms are often dramatic and may be abrupt in onset. The search for an organic cause requires head CT or MRI scans, a search for histiocytosis, and an evaluation for dysfunctions of other areas of the hypothalamic-pituitary axis.

The best diagnostic test is water deprivation. This test should be done under careful observation in a well-hydrated child. Body weight, urine and serum sodium and osmolality, urine volumes, and ADH levels should be measured at baseline, frequently during the test, and at the end of the test. The ADH level is not essential for the diagnosis. If serum osmolality and serum sodium values rise above normal in the context of poor urine concentration, the diagnosis of diabetes insipidus is made. A weight loss of a maximum of 5% is allowed. At the end of the water deprivation test, exogenous ADH (ie, injection of aqueous vasopressin) is given to assess renal responsiveness.

Children with psychogenic or neurogenic polydipsia as the primary problem must be differentiated from those with diabetes insipidus. These children usually have low serum sodium and osmolality.

Diabetes insipidus due to ADH deficiency is treated with exogenous ADH. The best mode of treatment is with intranasal DDAVP, a long-acting analogue of arginine vasopressin. To eliminate nighttime awakening to urinate and drink, treatment is begun with low doses initially that are gradually increased. DDAVP can also be given parenterally. In most patients, DDAVP can be given every 12 hours. A long-acting preparation given by injection (ie, pitressin tannate in oil, duration 2 to 4 days) was successful before DDAVP became available and can still be used in the rare patient unable to take DDAVP. Because infant diets have a low solute load, their urine should remain dilute, and long-acting ADH preparations are contraindicated. A shorter-acting spray (ie, lysine vasopressin, duration 4 to 6 hours) can be given before bedtime to produce short-lasting antidiuresis during the night.

An intact thirst mechanism allows patients on ADH preparations to easily regulate their fluid balance on their own as long as they have free access to water. In the unusual patient with abnormal thirst, regulation becomes difficult, and strict prescriptions of fluid intake must be given.

## Syndrome of Inappropriate Antidiuretic Hormone Secretion

Excess endogenous or exogenous ADH without fluid restriction leads to water intoxication: water retention and weight gain, hyponatremia, and production of a small amount of concentrated urine. The typical symptoms are lethargy, weakness, nausea, vomiting, headaches, and seizures.

In children, the most likely causes of the syndrome of inappropriate antidiuretic hormone secretion are intracranial disease (eg, meningitis), neurosurgery, head trauma, and pulmonary disease. Malignancies producing excess ADH are uncommon in children.

The treatment is fluid restriction. In severe cases, use of hypertonic saline with diuretic therapy (eg, furosemide) may be indicated. Slow and steady correction is required.

## PROLACTIN

Prolactin is the one pituitary hormone whose major physiologic control is an inhibiting factor, dopamine. Pathologic processes occur when prolactin is secreted in excess amounts because of a pituitary prolactin-secreting adenoma or to a loss of hypothalamic dopamine inhibition due to interruption of normal pathways, especially by trauma, tumors, or infiltrative processes in the hypothalamus. Certain drugs (eg, phenothiazines, cimetidine, opiates) can cause hyperprolactinemia. Excess prolactin suppresses pituitary LH and FSH secretion and is associated with galactorrhea. The decrease in LH and FSH leads to impotence, oligomenorrhea, amenorrhea, infertility, and delayed puberty.

The diagnosis of excess prolactin secretion is made by finding an elevated prolactin level in a euthyroid, nonpregnant patient. CNS imaging with CT or MRI scans and a workup for evidence of other dysfunction of the hypothalamic-pituitary unit are necessary. Very high prolactin levels are usually associated with large tumors.

Treatment options include careful observation, medical therapy with dopamine agonists, and surgery. Bromocriptine is the major therapeutic option. It is a dopamine agonist, and the response to treatment is rapid. In some cases, bromocriptine therapy has been associated with regression in tumor size. Surgery, especially transsphenoidal for microadenomas, is not uniformly successful, and recurrences are frequent. For patients who do not respond well to bromocriptine or surgery, radiation therapy may be indicated.

## Selected Readings

Allen DB, Fost N, Blizzard RM, eds. Access to treatment with human growth hormone: medical, ethical and social issues. Growth Genet Horm 1992;8(suppl 1): 1.

Cara FJ, Johanson AJ. Growth hormone for short stature not due to classic GH deficiency. Pediatr Clin North Am 1990;37:1229.

Daughaday WH. Growth hormone deficient-like syndromes and their etiologies. Growth Genet Horm 1992;8:1.

Gertner JM. Adverse effects of growth hormone treatment. Growth Genet Horm 1992;8(suppl 1):18).

Kaplan SA. Growth and growth hormone: disorders of the anterior pituitary. In: Kaplan SA, ed. Clinical pediatric endocrinology. Philadelphia: WB Saunders, 1990:1.

Kritzler RK, Plotnick LP. The short child: a matter of time or cause for concern? Postgrad Med 1985;78:51.

Lyon AJ, Preece MA, Grant DB. Growth curve for girls with Turner syndrome. Arch Dis Child 1985;60:932.

Mahoney CP. Evaluating the child with short stature. Pediatr Clin North Am 1987;34: 825.

Raiti S, Kaplan SL, Van Vliet G, et al. Short-term treatment of short stature and subnormal growth rate with hGH. J Pediatr 1987;110:357.

Ranke MB, et al. Turner syndrome: spontaneous growth in 150 cases and review of the literature. Eur J Pediatr 1983;141:81.

Rogol AD. Growth hormone physiology and pathophysiology. Growth Genet Horm 1991;7:1.

Root AW, Diamond FB, Bercu BB. Short stature: when is growth hormone indicated? Contemp Pediatr 1987;4:26.

Rosenfeld RG, Frane J, Attie KM, et al. Six year results of a randomized, prospective trial of human growth hormone and oxandrolone in Turner syndrome. J Pediatr 1992;121:49.

Rosenfeld RG, Hintz RL, Johanson AJ, et al. Results from the first 2 years of a clinical trial with recombinant DNA derived hGH in Turner syndrome. Acta Paediatr Scand (Suppl) 1987;331:59.

Rosenfield RL. Low-dose testosterone effect on somatic growth. Pediatrics 1986;77: 853.

Saenger P: Use of growth hormone in the treatment of short stature: boon or abuse? Pediatr Rev 1991;12:355.

Underwood LE. Growth hormone therapy for short stature: yes or no? Hosp Pract 1992;192.

Wilson DM, Rosenfeld RG. Treatment of short stature and delayed adolescence. Pediatr Clin North Am 1987;34:865.

*Principles and Practice of Pediatrics, Second Edition.*
edited by Frank A. Oski et al. J. B. Lippincott Company, Philadelphia © 1994.

# CHAPTER 143
# *Insulin-Dependent Diabetes Mellitus*

## Leslie P. Plotnick

Insulin-dependent diabetes mellitus (IDDM) is a common, serious disease of childhood and adolescence. The diagnosis is usually straightforward, but long-term management is a major challenge for the child, the family, and the health care team. Developments in the past decade have made the attainment of metabolic control a technical possibility, but diabetes management is stressful to the family, and psychologic and behavioral issues often interfere with the goal of metabolic control. Few other diseases require the extensive self-care management needed to care for IDDM.

## DEFINITION AND DIAGNOSTIC CRITERIA

Since the statement from the National Diabetes Data Group in 1979, diabetes has been classified as two main types. Type I or IDDM is the type most commonly found in children and adolescents. This type has also been called juvenile-onset, ketosis-prone, or brittle diabetes. Patients with IDDM are insulinopenic and need exogenous insulin to prevent ketosis and to preserve life.

Type II or non–insulin-dependent diabetes mellitus (NIDDM) is most commonly found in adults and in obese persons. This type has also been called adult-onset, maturity-onset, ketosis-resistant, or stable diabetes. Affected patients are not insulin dependent or ketosis prone, but they may use exogenous insulin, and they can develop ketosis in certain situations. Some patients with type II diabetes have insulin resistance and hyperinsulinemia.

For diabetes to be diagnosed, a child must have the classic symptoms with a random plasma glucose level above 200 mg/dL (11.1 mmol/L), or if asymptomatic, an oral glucose tolerance test must show elevated fasting values ($\geq$140 mg/dL in venous plasma or $\geq$120 mg/dL in venous whole blood) and elevated postglucose values on more than one occasion. After a dose of 1.75 g of glucose per 1 kg of ideal body weight (maximum, 75 g), the 2-hour glucose value and an intervening value must be elevated ($\geq$200 mg/dL in venous plasma; $\geq$180 mg/dL in venous whole blood).

The diagnosis of IDDM in a child is rarely subtle. Most present with the classic symptoms of polyuria, polydipsia, polyphagia, weight loss, and lethargy. Glucose tolerance testing is rarely necessary for diagnosis.

## EPIDEMIOLOGY

The prevalence of IDDM in the United States in children and adolescents varies somewhat according to different sources, with most studies reporting a rate of 1.2 to 1.9 cases per 1000 members of the population of this age group.

There are major worldwide variations in incidence, with the United States having an intermediate incidence. Incidence increases with age and peaks in early to middle puberty. There is also a seasonal distribution of newly diagnosed cases: for unknown reasons, more cases are diagnosed in the cooler months. Males and females are about equally affected.

## GENETICS, ETIOLOGY, AND PATHOGENESIS

Our understanding of the genetics, cause, and pathogenesis of IDDM has increased greatly. No one diabetes gene exists. Instead, certain genetic alterations raise or lower the risk of $\beta$-cell damage. Inheritance of HLA antigens DR3 and DR4 is associated with an increased risk of developing IDDM. Inheritance of one of these HLA antigens confers a 3- to 5-fold risk of developing IDDM; inheritance of both confers a 10- to 20-fold risk. DR3 or DR4 occurs in about 95% of persons with IDDM. Variations on the DQ antigen also may account for changes in the risk of developing IDDM. For example, on the DQ $\beta$ chain, an amino acid variation at position 57, nonaspartic acid, is associated with a marked increase in risk.

The chance of IDDM developing in a second sibling is summarized in Table 143-1 and is directly related to the shared HLA haplotypes. Approximately 5% of the diabetic patients' siblings develop IDDM.

Certain genetic alterations raise or lower the risk of $\beta$-cell damage. Fewer than 50% of identical twins are concordant for IDDM, indicating that a susceptibility to IDDM, rather than the disease itself, is inherited. This inherited susceptibility appears to place the $\beta$ cell at unusual risk for immunologic, inflammatory damage. The less than 50% concordance in identical twins and the marked geographic variation in incidence of IDDM support the significance of external factors in the process of $\beta$-cell damage.

Beta cell destruction occurs in genetically susceptible people. At least 80% of the functional $\beta$-cell mass must be destroyed before overt glucose intolerance occurs. The process of $\beta$-cell destruction in most cases, is immune mediated, probably takes months or years, and may be initiated by external, environmental factors. It is controversial whether this is a relentless, progressive process inevitably producing IDDM or whether the process may wax and wane over time and sometimes enter remission. One hypothesis is that the exposure to the environmental factors may be recurrent and intermittent or continuous (eg, viral infections, dietary factors, environmental toxins, stress) rather than a single triggering event. The damaged $\beta$ cell presents to the immune system an antigen recognized as nonself. The ability of macrophages to present these antigens to helper T cells depends on the class II (D) HLA molecules and on their three-dimensional structure, which is determined by the amino acid sequence of the HLA molecules' $\alpha$ and $\beta$ chains. Another hypothesis suggests that certain HLA types may bind the antigens intracellularly, preventing their exposure to the immune system and protecting against the development of IDDM.

The autoimmune processes release cytokines that are destructive in the $\beta$ cells directly or that destroy tissue by generating free radicals, because $\beta$ cells have low levels of antioxidants. Interleukin-1, tissue necrosis factor-$\alpha$, and interferon-$\gamma$ have roles

in this destructive process. There are probably two phases in the process of $\beta$-cell destruction: an early cytokine-dependent initiation phase and a later phase with antigen-specific T-lymphocyte proliferation, which amplifies and perpetuates $\beta$-cell destruction. $\beta$-Cell protective mechanisms, specifically the production of heat shock proteins, can help $\beta$ cells resist immunologic damage.

IDDM susceptibility is probably conferred by unfavorable combinations of common gene alleles for HLA and $\beta$-cell destructive and $\beta$-cell protective mechanisms. Specific HLA types appear necessary for IDDM development, but they are not sufficient.

Most newly diagnosed patients with IDDM have measurable immunologic markers: islet cell antibodies and insulin autoantibodies. Islet cell antibodies (ICA) may be cytoplasmic or surface antibodies. High-titer ICAs confer a greater risk of subsequently developing IDDM than low titers. ICAs are probably more predictive in children, as is the persistence of positivity.

Another important immunologic marker is insulin autoantibodies (IAAs). IAAs in combination with ICAs and high-titer IAAs are associated with an increased risk of developing IDDM. Antibodies to a 64-kd islet antigen have also been associated with subsequent development of IDDM. This 64-kd protein appears to be glutamate decarboxylase.

## PATHOPHYSIOLOGY

Insulin is the body's major anabolic hormone. In the fed state, it stimulates energy storage in the forms of glycogen, protein, and adipose tissue. When insulin levels are low or deficient, mobilization of stored substrate occurs (ie, glycogenolysis, proteolysis, lipolysis) and tissue uptake of glucose is inhibited. Because insulin is a potent antilipolytic hormone, a greater degree of insulin deficiency is required for lipolysis than for glucose intolerance to occur. In the early stages of insulin deficiency, hyperglycemia predominates, and a more severe degree of insulin deficiency is necessary for ketonuria, ketonemia, and acidosis to develop.

In addition to insulin deficiency, a relative excess of counterregulatory hormones (eg, growth hormone, cortisol, glucagon, catecholamines) must exist to produce the picture of diabetic ketoacidosis (DKA). Hyperglycemia produces an osmotic diuresis causing the symptoms of polyuria and polydipsia. Passive electrolyte loss occurs along with the osmotic diuresis. Weight loss is caused by the general catabolic state and the osmotic diuresis. Eventually, dehydration results and is especially severe if the child cannot drink enough fluid to compensate for the diuresis, as in the case of vomiting or a decreased level of consciousness. Lipolysis results in ketone production, causing metabolic acidosis.

## CLINICAL PRESENTATION

Most children with IDDM present with the classic symptoms of polyuria, polydipsia, polyphagia, and weight loss; many also complain of lethargy. If the diagnosis is not made and treatment is not begun, further metabolic decompensation occurs, with worsening DKA.

In young children and infants, the diagnosis is more likely to be missed in its early stages because of difficulty in recognizing early symptoms, and children of these ages are more likely to present with severe ketoacidosis. If pediatricians inquire specifically about the classic symptoms in patients with nonspecific signs of illness and weight loss, this diagnosis is more likely to be made quickly. Early diagnosis avoids further metabolic decompensation and the risks of DKA.

Most children with new-onset IDDM have symptoms of less than 1 month's duration, but some have had mild to moderate

| TABLE 143-1. Risk of Developing IDDM if One Sibling is Affected | |
|---|---|
| Identical twins | <50% |
| HLA identical | 1 in 5 |
| HLA haploidentical | 1 in 20 |
| HLA nonidentical | 1 in 100 |

symptoms for several months. Questions about bed-wetting, nocturia, number of diapers used, or leaving class to use the bathroom may help uncover polyuria.

IDDM must be considered in any child with clinical dehydration who continues to urinate regularly. Too often, frequent urination leads the parent or physician to incorrectly conclude that the child is not dehydrated. Routine dipstick testing for urine glucose and ketones in patients with nonspecific symptoms such as lethargy, weight loss, nausea, and vomiting and in those with specific IDDM symptoms could greatly enhance the early diagnosis of this disease before severe metabolic decompensation has occurred.

New-onset IDDM may be managed in an inpatient or outpatient setting, depending on the severity of the patient's metabolic abnormalities and the health care resources available.

## CLINICAL COURSE

After the initial presentation, most newly diagnosed children with IDDM undergo a honeymoon period or remission phase. During this period, the remaining functional $\beta$ cells regain the ability to produce insulin, possibly as a result of elimination of hyperglycemia. Measurement of C-peptide levels has demonstrated that improved insulin secretion occurs during this phase. Because endogenous insulin secretion increases, requirements for exogenous insulin decrease, usually dropping to less than 0.5 U/kg/day. Hypoglycemia becomes a potential problem. This phase usually begins within 1 to 3 months after diagnosis and lasts for several months, sometimes as long as 12 to 24 months. It is a period of relative well-being, with metabolic normalcy as indicated by normal glycosylated hemoglobin (HbA$_{1C}$) levels. Education about the honeymoon period must be included in the education of the newly diagnosed patient, because denial of disease and subsequent failure to monitor are likely to occur unless patients and families learn about this phase and expect its occurrence and its end.

As this phase ends, the remaining $\beta$ cells lose their capacity to secrete insulin, and requirements for exogenous insulin rise. This usually occurs gradually but, as in cases of acute infection, it may be abrupt. Careful monitoring and frequent dose adjustments are extremely important during the end of the remission phase, and close contact between the patient and physician is necessary.

## GOALS OF TREATMENT

### Normal Development

Normal growth in height and weight and normal timing of adolescent pubertal development are important goals of long-term management. Chronically undertreated children with poorly controlled IDDM often fail to grow normally and have delayed skeletal maturation (ie, bone age) and delayed sexual maturation. The growth retardation can be severe. Growth is an important factor to follow, and height, weight, and pubertal development should be monitored carefully. The causes for deviations from normal velocities should be sought.

Children receiving excessive insulin doses may gain weight too rapidly. Excessive insulin doses, which can cause rebound hyperglycemia and ketosis, can produce the same degree of growth retardation as chronically inadequate doses. Mauriac syndrome (ie, IDDM, growth retardation, and hepatomegaly) is caused by poor diabetic control, and although patients with this syndrome are usually receiving inadequate insulin doses, excessive doses have also been associated with this clinical picture.

## Management of Insulin-Dependent Diabetes Mellitus

Education of the patient and family with the goal of independent management of IDDM at home is important. Some families achieve independence quickly. Others require intensive and repeated education on a one-to-one basis or in group programs. Independent decision making by patients and families who are well educated about diabetes and its management enhances independence, feelings of control, and self-esteem, and it is important for long-term psychologic success. Most day-to-day decisions regarding hyperglycemia, hypoglycemia, illness, ketonuria, unusual activities, or eating schedules can be handled appropriately by knowledgeable families. Frequent blood glucose monitoring, which is discussed later in this chapter, is the cornerstone of management.

Children and adolescents with IDDM should be encouraged to participate in any activities that are appropriate to their age and interest. An adolescent with sports practice three times a week after school can learn how to increase calories or decrease insulin doses and to keep her blood glucose levels in an acceptable range during the activity. Certain precautions must be taken. For example, a source of calories must be readily available during a physical activity. When adolescents drive, a readily available glucose source must be in easy reach, not locked in the glove compartment. Medic-Alert bracelets or necklaces should be worn.

The diet should be designed around the child's and family's food preferences and habits using sound nutritional principles. It is important that families participate in the planning of the diet and that the amount of food be adequate for satiety to maximize adherence.

### Avoiding Metabolic Abnormalities

Avoidance of metabolic abnormalities is another important goal. Blood glucose monitoring several times a day along with urinary ketone checks are mainstays of management. Significant hyperglycemia and hypoglycemia should be avoided. In young children, especially preschoolers, blood glucose levels vary widely. To avoid serious hypoglycemia in this age group, compromises may have to be made in tolerating hyperglycemia.

HbA$_{1C}$ levels should be monitored regularly usually every 3 to 4 months with a goal of achieving a level in or near the normal range. Normal values vary depending on the laboratory method used. Blood lipids should be monitored and dietary modifications made if hyperlipidemia occurs.

Ketonuria should be treated early. In most patients who monitor regularly, DKA can be avoided by responding to hyperglycemia, ketosis, and periods of illness by adjusting insulin doses.

The demands of the diabetes management regimen are high and require care and understanding on the part of the families and the health care team to maximize the child's chances for successful emotional development.

## MANAGEMENT

### Insulin

Several insulin preparations are available. Standard beef and pork mixes are still available but have the disadvantage of containing a beef component that is more antigenic than pork or human insulin. The standard preparations usually are less expensive. Purified pork insulin and human insulin, produced by recombinant DNA technology or by changing the different amino acid in pork insulin, are the insulin preparations most commonly used. Human insulin may be less antigenic than pork insulin, and the recombinant DNA product is available in unlimited quantities. Human insulin may have a shorter duration of action than pork insulin in some children. Recent anecdotal reports suggest an increase in hypoglycemia unawareness when using human insulin, but this has not been supported in other reports.

Regular insulin is rapid acting and is the insulin used to rapidly treat hyperglycemia, ketosis, and DKA. Semilente is another short-acting insulin. NPH or Lente are intermediate in peak and duration of action. Ultralente is a long-acting insulin with duration of more than 24 to 36 hours. However, human Ultralente may have a much shorter duration of action (Table 143-2).

Most children and adolescents require two injections per day of short- and intermediate-acting insulin to achieve satisfactory metabolic control; the injections are administered shortly before breakfast and dinner. During the honeymoon period, when insulin requirements are at a minimum, one injection per day may be satisfactory for control. Except for this period, it is difficult in most patients to achieve control with a single daily injection. Absorption may vary from different injection sites and is more rapid in exercised sites and at higher temperatures. Injection into hypertrophied sites may slow absorption.

Frequent blood glucose monitoring is necessary so that patients can respond to the levels by adjusting their insulin doses. For example, if an occasional fasting blood glucose level falls above the target range, the morning regular insulin dose should be increased. If the fasting blood glucose level is increased for several consecutive days, the evening NPH dose should be increased.

During the honeymoon period, dose requirements may drop below 0.5 U/kg/day. Except during this period, most preadolescent children need about 0.75 to 1.0 U/kg/day. Teenagers usually require about 1 to 1.2 U/kg/day after the first few years of the disease.

Patients on a twice-daily dosage regimen typically need about two thirds of the total dose in the morning and one third before dinner. The doses usually are split between one-third regular and two-thirds NPH to one-half regular and one-half NPH. More regular insulin usually is required in the morning because of an early morning glucose rise. This early morning glucose increase (ie, dawn phenomenon) may be caused by normal nocturnal increases in some counter-regulatory hormones.

Other insulin regimens may be needed to achieve adequate control. Sometimes the evening dose must be separated, with regular insulin given before dinner and NPH at bedtime to maintain adequate insulin levels throughout the entire night. Sometimes additional regular insulin is needed before lunch, but this is difficult to arrange in a school-aged child without interfering with her school schedule.

Ultralente can be used to provide a continuous, fairly steady insulin level with a single daily dose, with regular insulin given before each meal. The use of continuous subcutaneous insulin infusion pumps can be considered in highly motivated and conscientious patients. Regular insulin is used for continuous subcutaneous infusion to achieve a continuous basal rate, with bolus doses given before meals.

When insulin doses are above 1.5 U/kg/day and especially when they are at or above 2 U/kg/day, overtreatment must be considered. Excess insulin doses can worsen control and produce a clinical picture of widely variable blood glucose values. The Somogyi phenomenon is rebound hyperglycemia after hypoglycemia, which may be asymptomatic. This is caused by release of counter-regulatory hormones (eg, catecholamines, cortisol, glucagon, growth hormone) in response to hypoglycemia.

During the last decade, improvements in the purity of insulin preparations have markedly decreased local and systemic allergic reactions. Lipoatrophy, the loss of subcutaneous adipose tissue, is rare. Lipohypertrophy, increased deposits of adipose tissue, still occurs and may be related to poor injection technique. Proper site rotation is important in preventing lipohypertrophy.

## Dietary Management

Diet is a cornerstone of diabetes management. Children and adolescents with IDDM require a nutritionally balanced diet with adequate calories and nutrients for normal growth. The recommended diet usually contains 50% to 55% carbohydrate calories, 20% protein, and approximately 30% fat. Most carbohydrate calories are complex carbohydrates, and the fat portion should emphasize low levels of cholesterol and saturated fats. Timing of meals and snacks should minimize blood glucose variability. In addition to the usual three meals, midafternoon snacks are necessary, particularly because they are timed to coincide with the typical peak of the morning NPH insulin dose and with most after-school sports activities. Bedtime snacks are important for most children receiving evening NPH doses. Midmorning snacks are useful in preschool-aged children, but most school-aged children find them disruptive to their school routine. This snack usually is not recommended after a child begins elementary school.

Occasional treats should be allowed by the diet plan, and patients and families should learn how to adjust insulin doses for times of increased caloric intake, such as holidays and birthdays. Calorie control with avoidance of obesity is necessary for certain patients. A sense of satiety and a diet that fits with the family's food preferences are necessary for maximum and realistic adherence to dietary recommendations. The diet should be individualized for each child and family.

Some centers have reported an increased frequency of eating disorders, particularly in adolescent girls with IDDM. When this occurs, it's metabolic consequences can be devastating, and aggressive intervention (eg, admission to an eating disorders unit) is indicated.

## Exercise

Physical fitness and regular exercise are important for all patients with IDDM. Insulin requirements may be lower, metabolic control improved, and self-esteem and body image better in the physically fit child. During periods of exercise, extra calories or lower insulin doses may be needed to prevent hypoglycemia. Blood glucose monitoring to assess the effects of exercise on blood glucose and the response to these therapeutic maneuvers should be done to arrive at an effective regimen for the individual patient. Regular

| TABLE 143-2. | Timing of Action of Available Insulins | | |
|---|---|---|---|
| Insulin | Onset (hours) | Peak (hours) | Usual Duration (hours) |
| Regular | | | |
| Human | 0.5–1.0 | 2–3 | 3–6 |
| Pork | 0.5–2.0 | 3–4 | 4–6 |
| NPH/Lente | | | |
| Human | 2–4 | 4–10 | 10–16 |
| Pork | 4–6 | 8–14 | 16–20 |
| Ultralente | | | |
| Human | 6–10 | Minimal (?) | 18–20 |
| Animal | 8–14 | Minimal | 24–36 |
| Mixed (70% NPH, 30% regular) | | | |
| Human | 0.5 | 2–12 | 24 |

exercise is to be encouraged at any age, because it then can become part of the child's health care regimen.

When metabolic control is poor (eg, the child has hyperglycemia with or without ketosis), the stress of exercise may worsen metabolic control. Some patients have a delayed hypoglycemic response to exercise, and if this occurs, adjustments in insulin dose and calories become necessary.

## Monitoring

One of the major advances of the last decade has been the technique of self-monitoring of blood glucose. Numerous reagent strips, glucose meters, and finger puncture devices are available. Current glucose meters are small, portable, and accurate. Improvements and advances include memory storage at 300 readings with the date and time of the reading. A noninvasive blood glucose meter is expected to become available in the future.

Blood glucose is traditionally monitored before meals, before snacks (eg, midmorning, midafternoon, bedtime), and in the middle of the night at approximately 3:00 a.m., the anticipated lowest nighttime point, if evening NPH is used. Two to four recorded readings a day usually provide enough information to assess and achieve control. During a period of metabolic instability, more frequent monitoring is necessary. Fasting and preprandial blood glucose readings in the 70 to 150 mg/dL range, postprandial levels below 180 to 200 mg/dL, and 3:00 a.m. values above 65 mg/dL indicate good control.

A specified insulin dose is appropriate when the blood glucose values are in this target range. Doses of regular insulin can be changed using a sliding scale (Table 143-3) when a specific blood glucose level is outside the target range. For example, if the fasting blood glucose is 50 mg/dL one day, less regular insulin is needed that morning. When patterns outside the target range occur, NPH doses can be adjusted to achieve blood glucose levels in the target range. For example, if fasting values are around 50 mg/dL for several consecutive days, the evening NPH dose should be reduced. Most physicians increase the target ranges for infants and small children and accept blood glucose values less than 200 mg/dL. Blood glucose determinations before lunch and bedtime snacks are necessary to fine tune regular insulin doses.

The measurement of HbA$_{1C}$ levels is another major advance in diabetes management. This is an objective level that measures an average blood glucose reading over approximately the previous 2 months. Various methods are available, and normal ranges vary. The upper limit of normal in our hospital laboratory is 7.9%. Levels below 9% are considered very good control, and levels below 10% are reasonable.

Some patients can achieve values in the normal or near-normal range with relative ease. These children may have some residual endogenous insulin secretion. Diabetes management teams can be successful in helping patients achieve improved HbA$_{1C}$ levels, but some patients may not achieve levels in the goal range. Studies linking chronic complications of IDDM to specific HbA$_{1C}$ levels can be related to a particular laboratory's results if the physician is aware of the differences in the normal ranges.

Urinary ketones also should be monitored. Even patients who do accurate and regular blood glucose monitoring need to check urinary ketones, particularly when the blood glucose levels are above 250 mg/dL, when they have a fever, when they feel nauseous or are vomiting, or when they are just not feeling well. This is important in achieving the goal of aborting DKA episodes by treating early ketosis.

Some patients do not monitor blood glucose levels frequently enough, or their reported blood glucose levels do not fit with their HbA$_{1C}$ levels. In these patients, 24-hour fractionated urine glucose patterns may provide information on which to base insulin dose adjustments.

Blood lipids should be monitored at least yearly. Because IDDM is associated with other autoimmune diseases, especially thyroid disease, periodic monitoring should be done (eg, thyroid antibodies, thyroid-stimulating hormone, thyroxine). Patients should be seen by the health care team about every 3 months. Regular monitoring for ophthalmologic complications and for nephropathy are discussed later in this chapter.

## Education

Education is fundamental to diabetes management and control. Patients and families need to understand all aspects of diabetes, including acute and long-term complications. They must understand details of insulin action, including duration and timing, injection techniques, dietary information, blood glucose monitoring, and urinary ketone checks. They must gain skills in integrating the demanding clinical regimen into their schedules so that they can achieve emotional stability and ongoing psychologic growth.

Education must be appropriate to the child's age and the family's educational background, and it must be ongoing. Shifting responsibility from parent to child for diabetes self-care skills (eg, insulin injections) should be done gradually and when the child shows interest and readiness to do so. Premature shifting of responsibility may be a cause of deterioration in metabolic control.

The life of the entire family is affected by having a child with IDDM. Sharing responsibilities and attending support groups and camps for IDDM children can help with psychologic adjustment.

Teaching about and managing diabetes are best handled by a diabetes management team, including a physician, nurse educator, dietitian, and psychologist or psychiatric social worker.

## Prediction of Insulin-Dependent Diabetes Mellitus

If the onset of IDDM could be predicted and if persons who will eventually develop IDDM could be accurately identified, the strategies to prevent onset of IDDM could be effectively tested. The measurement of the immunologic markers, ICAs and IAAs, in first-degree relatives of IDDM patients is being done at certain institutions. In those with positive immune markers, intravenous glucose infusions can be used to assess the first-phase insulin response. The combination of positive ICA, positive IAA, and defective first-phase insulin release is strongly suggestive of development of IDDM in several years. Testing of $\beta$-cell function should become more standardized before more accurate predictions are available.

| | Sliding Scale Regular Dose | |
| TABLE 143-3. Example of an Insulin Regimen for a 30-kg Child | | |
| Blood Glucose | AM (before breakfast) 12 NPH | PM (before dinner) 6 NPH |
|---|---|---|
| <50: | 3 | 2 |
| 50–100 | 5 | 3 |
| 100–150 | 6 | 4 |
| 150–200 | 7 | 4 |
| 200–250 | 8 | 5 |
| 250–300 | 9 | 6 |
| >300 | 10 | 7 |

## Experimental Interventions in New-Onset Diabetes

The most successful agent used to preserve remaining $\beta$-cell function in newly diagnosed IDDM is cyclosporine. The effects of treatment with cyclosporine, when given shortly after diagnosis of IDDM, have strongly supported the immune hypothesis of IDDM's cause and have shown that it is possible to alter, for a time, the natural history of relentless $\beta$-cell destruction.

These studies showed that the rate of $\beta$-cell loss could be slowed, but that ongoing decline in $\beta$-cell function occurred, indicating continuous activity of the destructive process. The studies also showed that stopping cyclosporine therapy was associated with rapid progression to clinical IDDM and that the side effects of cyclosporine are of concern, especially its nephrotoxic effects. Pancreatic transplantation in identical twins discordant for IDDM indicate that the immunologic destructive potential probably is lifelong, with a need for lifelong immunosuppression.

Other agents that have shown some preliminary benefit used in clinical trials of new-onset IDDM are azathioprine and nicotinamide. Another approach is high-dose insulin infusion, using an external artificial pancreas for 1 to 2 weeks after diagnosis of IDDM in patients with measurable C-peptide. One study showed better $\beta$-cell function in the experimental group than in conventionally treated controls, suggesting that $\beta$-cell rest may help preserve $\beta$-cell function, perhaps by ameliorating the autoimmune destructive process.

One goal of these studies may be "cure." However, another important goal is maintaining some $\beta$-cell function to produce a less severe and easier-to-manage diabetes, which should allow a significant reduction in acute and chronic diabetic complications.

## Prevention

The rationale behind preventing IDDM is to intervene at an earlier time than at its diagnosis, at a time when a greater percentage of $\beta$-cell mass remains intact. First-degree relatives of patients with IDDM can be screened for markers (eg, ICAs, IAAs, first-phase insulin response to intravenous glucose) and may enter clinical prevention trials taking place at a few centers. The problems of taking screening techniques into the general population are great, and the predictive ability must be improved before clinical prevention trials can be done accurately.

Pharmacologic intervention in newly diagnosed IDDM or as a preventive measure in genetically susceptible people with positive immune markers should be done only in carefully controlled trials by qualified investigators. Treatment of individual patients with these new methods outside of clinical trials should not be done.

## Transplantation

Whole or partial pancreas transplants have been successful in IDDM but require lifelong immunosuppression. These transplants usually are done only in patients with IDDM who are already receiving or will need immunosuppressive treatment for a kidney transplant. Patients with severe diabetic complications have received solo pancreatic transplants if it was deemed that the risk of immunosuppressive treatment was outweighed by the risk of the diabetic complications.

Newer immunosuppressive agents under study (eg, FK506) may be less toxic than cyclosporine and may perhaps broaden the criteria for pancreatic transplantation in the future.

Another approach to transplantation has been to use isolated $\beta$ cells. Novel ways being tried include placing the islets in the thymus and creating permselective membranes to encapsulate the $\beta$ cells. These membranes should allow insulin and glucose to pass through the membranes but be impermeable to antibodies, protecting transplanted $\beta$ cells from detection and rejection by the immune system. This latter approach has been successful across animal species lines and is an active area of research that holds great hope for the future.

"Camouflaging" islets with a protein that blocks T-cell binding by masking the donor HLA class I antigens with antibody fragments is being investigated. An additional problem that remains is the source of islets. There are not enough brain-dead cadaver donors in the United States to provide pancreas tissue for all the established and newly diagnosed patients with IDDM.

The risk-benefit ratio of chronic immunosuppressive therapy does not warrant pancreatic transplantation in children and adolescents with IDDM.

## Control to Prevent Complications

The Diabetes Control and Complications Trial (DCCT) is a national study to assess the relation between metabolic control and microvascular, macrovascular, and neurologic complications. The primary prevention part addressed the question of whether good metabolic control can prevent the onset of diabetic complications. The secondary intervention part addressed whether improved metabolic control can prevent progression or cause regression of early complications. Released in 1993, study results show a significant improvement in time of onset and rate of progression of microvascular complications in patients with "intensive" compared to "standard" diabetes control. One worrisome complication of intensive control is a threefold greater incidence of severe hypoglycemia (requiring assistance from another person).

Several other studies have shown that diabetic complications, background retinopathy, proliferative retinopathy, and nephropathy occur more frequently in patients with poorer diabetic control.

The duration of IDDM correlates with the incidence of complications. The duration of disease after puberty, rather than the entire duration, is the important factor.

The physician should aim for the best possible level of metabolic control. Hypoglycemia is a major risk, and the methods of insulin delivery (ie, two to three injections per day or the basal and bolus approach with insulin infusion pumps) are not truly physiologic.

Blood glucose targets are about 70 to 150 preprandially, less than 180 to 200 postprandially, and greater than 65 during the night (usually 2:00 to 3:00 a.m.). Even with these targets, grouped data generally show $HbA_{1C}$ levels 1.5 to 2 times the nondiabetic mean, and even with this level of control, the frequency of hypoglycemia can be high. Although insulin infusion pumps have been successful in lowering and maintaining improved $HbA_{1C}$ levels in highly motivated adults, results in children and teenagers have not been as successful and may not yield any sustained improvement in control. It may be that the attention and motivation given to metabolic control is more important than the actual insulin delivery regimen. It seems prudent to try to achieve the best possible metabolic control for each patient, tempered by the frequency and severity of hypoglycemia, concerns about excessive weight gain, and the degree of metabolic vigilance tolerable to that particular child and family.

The underlying cause of the microvascular complications may be chronic protein glycosylation intracellularly and extracellularly and the accumulation of these advanced glycosylation end products. The experimental use of a medication (eg, aminoguanidine) to prevent glycosylation can prevent the eye, kidney, and nerve complications in diabetic laboratory animals.

# COMPLICATIONS

## Acute Effects

### Hypoglycemia

Hypoglycemia (ie, blood glucose less than 50 to 60 mg/dL) occurs in patients on insulin whether they are or are not in tight metabolic control, but it occurs more frequently when blood glucose levels are kept close to normal. Hypoglycemic symptoms may be mild (ie, adrenergic symptoms of tremors, sweating, hunger, palpitations); moderate (ie, adrenergic plus neuroglycopenic symptoms of headache, irritability or other mood change, sleepiness, confusion, inattentiveness, impaired judgment, weakness), or severe (ie, unresponsiveness, coma, convulsions). Mild and moderate reactions can be treated by ingesting simple sugars (ie, 10 to 15 g of glucose). Moderate reactions may require assistance by another person and additional carbohydrate. Severe reactions require treatment with intravenous glucose or parenteral glucagon (0.1 mg/kg to a maximum of 1.0 mg IM or subcutaneously). All patients' families and day-care providers, teachers, coaches, and others should learn the signs and symptoms of hypoglycemia, have a readily available source of glucose to treat it (eg, a tube of cake frosting), and ideally have and know how to use glucagon injections to treat severe reactions. Recent evidence suggests that a longer duration of disease and tight metabolic control are associated with a diminished counter-regulatory hormone response to hypoglycemia, and some patients have hypoglycemic unawareness. These factors increase the risk of severe hypoglycemia. Young children often cannot notify their parents of hypoglycemic symptoms, and goals for metabolic control may need to be loosened. There is also concern that hypoglycemia may have deleterious effects on learning. Fear of hypoglycemia, particularly after a severe reaction, may cause long-lasting acceptance by patients and families of unacceptably high blood glucose levels (>200 mg/dL).

### Hyperglycemia and Ketosis

Patients with IDDM and their families must learn how to adjust insulin doses to treat the inevitable hyperglycemia that occurs with IDDM or when to call their health care provider for assistance with this. Ketosis may occur occasionally or more frequently, and patients must know how to respond.

### Diabetic Ketoacidosis

DKA is a common and potentially life-threatening, acute complication of IDDM. It is the most common cause of death in patients with IDDM younger than their mid-twenties. Mortality rates may be as high as 6% to 10%. DKA can be defined as a blood glucose level usually greater than 250 mg/dL, pH less than 7.2 or 7.3, and plasma bicarbonate level of 15 or less. Severe DKA is defined as a pH of 7.1 or less and a bicarbonate level of 10 or less; milder forms may be seen. Careful monitoring of blood glucose and urinary ketones and appropriate treatment responses to early metabolic abnormalities can prevent a significant number of DKA episodes in established IDDM patients. In new-onset IDDM, attention to early signs and symptoms of diabetes by the primary health care providers and families may help lower the number of newly diagnosed patients presenting with severe DKA.

The basic cause of DKA is absolute or relative insulin deficiency. There are also elevated levels of counter-regulatory or stress hormones (eg, glucagon, cortisol, growth hormone, catecholamines) that antagonize insulin. These hormonal abnormalities produce hyperglycemia (by increased glucose production and decreased use), which leads to an osmotic diuresis and dehydra- tion, lipolysis and hyperlipidemia, acidosis due to the production of ketones (ie, acetoacetate, $\beta$-hydroxybutyate) from fatty acids, and electrolyte abnormalities due to intracellular-extracellular shifts and urinary losses. Table 143-4 lists the common errors in DKA diagnosis and management.

### Presentation and Definition

The usual manifestations of DKA include a history of classic signs and symptoms of polyuria, polydipsia, and weight loss. After patients are sufficiently ketotic and acidotic, they have the fruity breath odor of ketosis. Many also exhibit nausea, vomiting, and lethargy. State of consciousness may vary from awake and alert (with mild DKA) to drowsiness or coma. Hyperventilation and dehydration also occur. Abdominal pain and an elevation in leukocytes may be due solely to DKA and be confused with an acute abdomen. These clinical findings usually resolve with therapy of DKA, but if not, an underlying cause (eg, appendicitis) must be sought. DKA must be considered in children who are vomiting and appear dehydrated but who continue to urinate excessively.

In a known diabetic patient, DKA may be precipitated by an acute infection but is usually caused by omission of insulin. This may be deliberate or be based on a misconception that insulin doses should be eliminated or significantly decreased because of anorexia or vomiting. Careful monitoring of blood glucose levels and urinary ketones and appropriate therapeutic response can help avoid many DKA episodes.

Recurrent DKA in most cases is now thought to be caused by deliberate insulin omission, sometimes by a child without the parents' knowledge and sometimes by the child and parents in collusion. Putting a responsible adult in charge of the insulin injections and using a simplified regimen (eg, one or two shots per day) may be successful in lowering the number of or eliminating the DKA episodes.

The degree of hyperglycemia does not correlate with the degree of acidosis, and patients may be severely acidotic but only minimally hyperglycemic. The diagnosis of DKA can be rapidly established at the bedside with a meter glucose reading and a urinary or serum ketone determination using strips or tablets.

---

**TABLE 143-4. Common Errors in Diabetic Ketoacidosis Diagnosis and Management**

Using good urine output to mean the patient is not significantly dehydrated (usually occurs with new-onset IDDM)

Delay in starting insulin: waiting for all laboratory values to be done or waiting for infusion pump

Letting the blood glucose drop too low by not adding enough glucose to the intravenous fluids

Too aggressive fluid intake (too rapid or too much)

Feeding patient too early, causing nausea and vomiting before gastric peristalsis normalizes

Decreasing the intravenous insulin rate or discontinuing intravenous insulin when the blood glucose has decreased but the patient is still acidotic

Not anticipating cerebral edema

Not heeding and treating symptoms of cerebral edema (eg, worsened sensorium, severe headache)

Not carefully reviewing clinical and laboratory data and adjusting the treatment plan as needed (ie, rigidly adhering to a predetermined treatment regimen)

Stopping the intravenous insulin before starting subcutaneous insulin

Not giving subcutaneous insulin before a meal or snack

*Treatment*

The basic components of DKA treatment are fluid and electrolyte replacement (with careful attention to potassium) and insulin. This must be done with frequent monitoring of clinical and laboratory factors, using a flow sheet (Table 143-5) and paying careful attention to details and trends.

*Fluid Replacement.* Dehydration affects virtually all patients with DKA. Water and electrolyte losses occur because of polyuria caused by the osmotic diuresis produced by glycosuria, hyperventilation, vomiting, and diarrhea. The best measure of dehydration is the patient's current weight compared with a recent, healthy weight. Dry mucous membranes, poor skin turgor, and orthostatic hypotension are clinical indications of dehydration. Most patients with DKA are 5% to 10% dehydrated. Patients in shock may have greater degrees of dehydration.

Adequate intravenous fluid replacement is extremely important and should begin as soon as the diagnosis of DKA is established. Normal saline (NS) or Ringer's lactate, an isotonic solution, is recommended initially because they help to restore the intravascular volume and therefore maintain blood pressure and kidney perfusion, which enhances glucose loss through the kidney, resulting in a lower blood glucose level.

For initial rehydration, 20 mL/kg of normal saline is recommended in the first hour. Some clinicians prefer Ringer's lactate. Rarely, colloid (ie, albumin) is needed for patients in shock. After about the first hour, the patient's state of hydration should be reassessed to determine if another infusion of normal saline (10 to 20 mL/kg) is needed in the second hour.

After this initial reexpansion, half isotonic saline (0.45% NS = ½ NS) should be used unless the patient is significantly hyperosmolar, when NS should continue. The amount is based on the calculated deficit and usually is about 1.5 times maintenance.

A variety of published recommendations are given for the rate of fluid replacement:

Administer 50% of the deficit in the first 8 to 10 hours and then the remaining 50% over the next 14 to 16 hours plus ongoing losses (eg, urine output, vomitus).

Use NS, 500 mg/m²/hour, for first 2 hours and then 250 mL/ m²/hour of ½ NS in the third hour, with later adjustments as indicated.

Administer 50% of the deficit over 12 hours and then give the remaining 50% over the next 24 to 36 hours plus maintenance and ongoing losses.

For a 30-kg child with 10% dehydration (ie, 3-L deficit), use 300 mL/hour for the first 2 hours using NS, 150 mL/hour for the next 8 hours using ½ NS, 75 mL/hour for the next 16 hours using ½ NS plus ongoing losses; replace the urine output hourly with ½ NS, and replace insensible losses with 40 mL of ½ NS/hour.

Recommendations for a maximum of 4 L/m²/day of fluid also have been made.

Urinary catheters are rarely needed. Nasogastric tubes may be needed in obtunded, vomiting patients; for patients in shock, monitoring central venous pressure may be needed.

*Insulin.* For more than a decade, continuous low-dose insulin infusion has been the method of choice. Short-acting (regular) insulin is the only type used. The advantages of a continuous intravenous insulin infusion are the elimination of the problem of poor absorption from subcutaneous and intramuscular sites in a dehydrated patient and rapid clearance, allowing easy dose adjustment, which makes management more controllable.

The usual recommended dose is 0.1 U/kg/hour. Sometimes a bolus of the same dose is given before starting the insulin infusion. Running the infusate (30 to 50 mL) through the tubing to saturate binding sites on the tubing is recommended.

The insulin infusion is best given separately from the replacement fluids so the rates can be independently adjusted, and it is best to use an infusion pump.

If no improvement in acidosis is seen within about 2 hours, the intravenous insulin rate should be increased to 0.15 U/kg/ hour or 0.20 μ/kg/hour.

A decrease in glucose should occur at a rate of about 75 to 100 mg/dL/hour. In the first hour or two of treatment, there is a decrease in glucose level from the initial rehydration fluids as intravascular volume expands.

The blood glucose level corrects to normal levels more quickly than the acidosis, and it is necessary to continue intravenous insulin until the acidosis is cleared. Continuing the intravenous insulin infusion until urinary ketones are cleared may enable easier management after the infusion is discontinued and subcutaneous insulin is started. If the blood glucose level decreases to 250 mg/dL and acidosis is still detected, glucose should be added to intravenous fluids, starting with 5% dextrose and increasing as needed to 7.5% or 10% dextrose to keep the blood glucose approximately 250 mg/dL. If the blood glucose level is less than 300 at the onset of treatment, it is useful to add 5% dextrose at the onset of therapy. In some patients, despite the use of 10% dextrose, the blood glucose may fall too low (perhaps <100 mg/dL), and it becomes necessary to decrease (not discontinue) the intravenous insulin infusion rate.

*Potassium.* Patients with DKA have total-body potassium depletion, but the measured serum potassium may be high, normal, or low. There is an exchange of intracellular potassium ions for extracellular hydrogen ions. Treatment with insulin causes potassium to move intracellularly, causing a decrease in serum potassium. Both hypokalemia and hyperkalemia are potential causes of death, and the serum potassium therefore must be monitored every 1 to 2 hours, and potassium should not be added to the intravenous fluids until the serum potassium level is known and the patient is voiding. An electrocardiogram can help assess whether hypokalemia or hyperkalemia is present while awaiting the potassium level.

If serum potassium is elevated at the onset of treatment, adding potassium to the intravenous fluids should not be done until the

| TABLE 143-5. Diabetic Ketoacidosis Flow Sheet | |
|---|---|
| Feature | Monitoring Schedule |
| Clinical data | |
| Weight | Onset of treatment and every 1–2 h initially |
| Vital signs | |
| State of consciousness | |
| Laboratory data | |
| Electrolytes (Na, K, Cl, HCO₃), venous pH | Every 1–2 h for the first 4–8 h and then every 2–4 h until DKA is cleared |
| Glucose | Hourly |
| Blood urea nitrogen, creatinine, calcium, phosphate levels | Every 4–8 h depending on initial levels and type of fluids used |
| Urinary ketone level | Every void |
| Fluids | Type and rate; record hourly input |
| Urine output | Record every void |
| Potassium, phosphate, bicarbonate | Record amounts added to fluid |
| Insulin | Dose, rate, and route |

serum potassium has fallen into the normal range. If the potassium is normal or low, potassium should be added to the intravenous fluids unless there is renal failure. Generally, 40 mEq/L is used. If the serum potassium is low, more than 40 mEq/L may be needed and careful monitoring (eg, electrocardiograms, frequent blood determinations) is therefore required. Potassium chloride, potassium phosphate, or potassium acetate may be used.

*Sodium.*    Patients with DKA have lost sodium through the urine and have a total-body sodium loss. Most have low serum sodium levels, probably due to hyperglycemia, which has osmotic pressure and causes dilution of the extracellular sodium. Lipemic serum falsely lowers the sodium level.

During DKA treatment, serum sodium levels should be monitored closely to ensure the sodium concentration is not decreasing. A failure of serum sodium to increase as glucose levels decrease, may be a marker for excess free water (see Cerebral Edema below). A rise in serum sodium as the glucose level falls, helps prevent rapid osmolality changes. It is useful to calculate the osmolality ($2[Na] + [glucose]/18$) to ensure it remains in the normal (not low) range.

Sodium replacement involves intravenous normal saline, 20 mL/kg during the first hour and 10 to 20 mL/kg during the second hour, if indicated. After this initial volume reexpansion, ½ NS is recommended. If serum osmolality drops, normal saline (instead of ½ NS) is needed.

*Phosphate.*    Phosphate depletion occurs in DKA because of poor food intake, the catabolic state, and urinary losses. Insulin treatment cause phosphate to move intracellularly lowering serum phosphate levels. In clinical studies, routine phosphate administration has not been demonstrated to have any advantage in DKA treatment. There are potential theoretical benefits for phosphate use; phosphate depletion can impair CNS and myocardial function and cause insulin resistance and shift the hemoglobin-oxygen dissociation curve to impair oxygen delivery to the tissues.

Phosphate replacement is indicated when the serum phosphate is very low, less than 2 mEq/L. Many clinicians recommend some phosphate replacement (not above 1.5 mEq/kg/day) for approximately 8 to 12 hours after the initial fluid reexpansion, with potassium added half as potassium chloride and half as potassium phosphate. One advantage of using part potassium phosphate instead of all potassium chloride is that less chloride is given. When phosphate is given, there is a risk of hypocalcemia, and calcium levels must be monitored.

*Bicarbonate.*    Treatment of DKA with bicarbonate to help correct acidosis has been controversial. The treatment of DKA with insulin generates bicarbonate as ketones are metabolized, and there is no need to use bicarbonate in mild or moderate DKA. These patients gradually correct their acidosis as insulin and fluid treatment proceed. Potential risks of bicarbonate include overtreatment producing a metabolic alkalosis, greater risks of hypokalemia and paradoxic cerebrospinal fluid acidosis. Clinical trials of bicarbonate in severe DKA have not shown improvement in DKA outcome whether or not bicarbonate was used.

Bicarbonate use should be reserved for patients who are severely acidotic if the acidosis may threaten respiratory or cardiac function (eg, pH ≤7.0 to 7.1 and bicarbonate ≤5) and to administer enough bicarbonate only for a small partial correction (eg, to raise the pH to 7.2, maximum). Generally, 1 to 2 mEq/kg of bicarbonate given over approximately 2 hours and added to the first bottle of ½ NS (not NS) can be given. The pH should be rechecked approximately 30 minutes after the infusion. Do not give bicarbonate to hypokalemic patients until treatment with potassium is ongoing.

*Converting to Subcutaneous Insulin.*    Patients should be continued on intravenous fluids and an intravenous insulin infusion until they are clinically stable with normal sensorium and normal vital signs, until the acidosis is cleared (ie, normal venous pH and bicarbonate), and until they can take fluids and food orally without vomiting. Any identified precipitating factor (eg, infection) should have been treated.

Regular insulin is used for the first day or so after a DKA episode. Subcutaneous insulin takes time to take effect, and the intravenous insulin infusion must be continued for 30 to 60 minutes after the first subcutaneous dose of insulin is given. This prevents insulin levels from becoming too low, which would allow recurrence of lipolysis and ketogenesis. A dose between 0.10 to 0.25 U/kg is given before a meal.

The switch from intravenous to subcutaneous insulin is best done during the daytime. The subcutaneous insulin doses should all be followed within approximately 0.5 hour by a meal or snack, and doses of regular insulin are needed about every 4 to 6 hours. During this period of dose adjustment, frequent blood glucose measurements and urinary ketone checks are important. Dose adjustment depends on the patient's blood glucose response to previous subcutaneous doses. When the patient's usual insulin requirement is known and the precipitating factor of the DKA is cleared, the patient may be able to resume his or her usual dose of insulin as soon as normal caloric intake is reestablished. For example, a well-controlled child who had an episode of moderate DKA due to a skipped insulin dose with a viral gastroenteritis could probably resume the usual insulin schedule fairly soon after her DKA has cleared and she can eat normally; DKA is cleared at approximately 1 a.m., the intravenous fluids and intravenous insulin are continued through the night, vomiting has ceased and the child can eat and drink without nausea. The usual a.m. dose may be satisfactory before breakfast. Some patients may need lower insulin doses after a DKA episode due to decreased caloric intake, but some may need more. Frequent monitoring of blood glucose and urinary ketones is imperative. Newly diagnosed patients need to have their current insulin requirements established.

There are two common errors that occur during this transition period. First, the intravenous insulin infusion is discontinued without giving subcutaneous insulin, and the patient becomes hyperglycemic, ketotic, and even acidotic within several hours. This is done because the blood glucose is normal or low and the acidosis is cleared. If this condition occurs during the night, it may be 4 to 8 hours before it is appreciated that the patient's metabolic control has deteriorated. The second common error is to withhold regular insulin before a meal because the blood glucose is normal or low. When this is done, the blood glucose increases to high levels after eating, and the general response is then to give regular insulin to lower the blood glucose level, which may fluctuate over a wide range during the remainder of the day. The best approach is to give regular insulin before eating to prevent a postprandial glucose rise.

*Prevention.*    Many episodes of DKA can be prevented by vigilance and careful monitoring of blood glucose and urinary ketones. Urinary ketones should be checked whenever blood glucose is elevated to approximately 250 mg/dL or higher and if the patient is feeling ill. This cannot be overemphasized. When ketone tests become positive (moderate to large), extra regular insulin can be given until the ketones are clear. Failure to monitor, failure to recognize or pay attention to symptoms of illness, and failure to contact the health care team early may lead to episodes of DKA that could have been prevented. Proper sick-day management can prevent DKA.

Recurrent DKA is uniformly caused by deliberate insulin omission, often in dysfunctional families, but it may be also caused by putting too much responsibility for IDDM management on a child or adolescent without adequate parental supervision.

*Sick-Day Management.*    Deterioration of metabolic control during infections in children is due in part to the increase in stress or counter-regulatory hormones, which have hyperglycemic and lipolytic effects and which produce relative insulin deficiency and requirements for increased insulin occur. Alternatively, because decreases in caloric intake occur with illness in children, especially with nausea and vomiting, insulin requirements may drop, and hypoglycemia may occur.

The goals of sick-day management are the prevention and treatment of hypoglycemia and significant hyperglycemia and the prevention of DKA. The physician's advice is essential, as is parental supervision. Sick-day management should not be left to a child or teenager. The underlying illness needs to be diagnosed and treated (eg, infection). The basis of management includes frequent blood glucose and urinary ketone checks (at least every 4 hours for blood glucose and every void for urinary ketones); insulin adjustment (using regular) based on blood glucose levels and urinary ketones; and substituting equivalent calories of sugar-containing fluids (eg, soda, fruit juice, Jell-O, popsicles) if the child cannot or will not eat solids. Depending on the type of illness, the insulin dose may be the usual NPH or Lente dose, with regular insulin doses adjusted up or down for blood glucose levels; a decrease in the NPH or Lente with regular insulin adjusted for blood glucose levels; or only regular insulin given about every 4 hours. Persistent vomiting (ie, several times in a row so that no calories are retained) or refusal to take fluids orally or food requires an emergency room or clinic visit. Glucagon must be available in the home.

Supplemental regular insulin at doses of 10% to 20% of the 24-hour requirement given every 4 to 6 hours are often effective in preventing significant hyperglycemia and in clearing or preventing ketosis.

*Other Management Topics.* Ketones (eg, acetoacetate) interfere with creatinine measurements. A child with DKA may have an elevated creatinine suggesting he or she is in renal failure when this is a spurious measurement. Creatinine should be rechecked as the ketoacidosis clears.

Use of Acetest tablets to determine the presence of serum ketones is useful to rapidly establish a diagnosis of DKA. However, serum dilutions (titers) on acetest tablets are not useful in establishing the severity of the acidosis. Acetest tablets (ie, nitroprusside reaction) do not measure $\beta$-hydroxybutyrate, which is the major ketone in DKA. Because DKA treatment causes a shift toward acetoacetate from $\beta$-hydroxybutyrate, using this qualitative ketone method may suggest the patient is worsening although total ketones and acidosis are improving, and this method is not useful in following the course of DKA treatment.

It is not necessary to wait for the pump to arrive to start intravenous insulin. One hour's worth of insulin can be put in an intravenous solution and infused over 1 hour. If the timing is not exact, no harm occurs. Delay in starting fluids and insulin leads to worsening of the patient's clinical status.

The diagnosis of DKA can be established rapidly at the bedside by a meter blood glucose reading and a rapid assessment of serum ketones (ie, Acetest method). Usually, a venous pH measure will be rapidly available. The initial fluid reexpansion can then be started. Insulin can be started immediately or delayed by 1 to 2 hours. It is not necessary to wait for all the laboratory results before starting treatment if the diagnosis of DKA is evident. However, potassium should not be added to the intravenous fluids until the serum potassium level is known. An electrocardiogram can help establish rapidly whether the serum potassium level is low, normal, or high.

*Complications*

Cerebral edema is an unpredictable, often fatal, and uniformly feared complication of treating DKA. It usually occurs when biochemical abnormalities are improving. Cerebral edema probably accounts for half or more of DKA-associated deaths. Subclinical brain swelling occurs often during DKA treatment. Factors implicated but not pinpointed as possible causes of cerebral edema are too rapid a drop in blood glucose, dropping the blood glucose to an excessively low level, excessive fluid administration, tonicity of intravenous fluids, failure of the serum sodium to rise during treatment, and the use of bicarbonate.

A comprehensive review of 69 cases of intracerebral complications in DKA found that infants and children younger than 5 years of age and new-onset IDDM patients made up an excessive proportion of cases. Neither rate or tonicity of hydration fluids, rate of blood glucose decrease, amount of sodium given, degree of decrease in serum sodium concentration, nor the use of bicarbonate could be implicated as causes of cerebral edema. Half of the patients had histories suggesting dramatic changes in neurologic status before respiratory arrest occurred, and treatment before respiratory arrest had a better outcome. This review indicated that close neurologic monitoring and treatment to decrease raised intracranial pressure, when definite signs of neurologic deterioration occur, could improve outcome. "However, treatment appears to be successful in only 50% of patients who give sufficient warning for such intervention, and they comprised half of the study population" (Rosenbloom, 1990).

DKA prevention is essential. Other studies have shown that fluid intakes above 4.0 L/m²/day are associated with more cases of cerebral edema. Failure of serum sodium to rise in the face of decreasing glucose levels may indicate excess free water administration and occurs more frequently in patients with complications attributable to brain edema.

Until the causes of cerebral edema are better defined, it seems prudent to pay attention to all of these factors in DKA treatment but most importantly to anticipate cerebral edema, knowing it occurs more commonly in infants and young children and with new-onset IDDM. Be prepared to recognize its signs and symptoms of increased intracranial pressure, such as severe headache, arousal and sensorium or behavior changes, changes in blood pressure, dilated pupils, problems with temperature regulation, slow pulse, and onset of incontinence. Careful clinical monitoring is essential.

Treatment involves intubation and hyperventilation to lower increased intracranial pressure, and mannitol (probably 1 g/kg by intravenous bolus) and fluid restriction. Mannitol should be located by the bedside or nearby for the first 24 hours of treatment. However, even early treatment did not prevent severe or fatal CNS damage in almost half of the patients in one study.

## Chronic Effects

### Autoimmune Disease

Associated autoimmune disease, particularly thyroid dysfunction, occurs with greater frequency with IDDM. Thyroid function should be monitored periodically (every few years at a minimum) in IDDM patients.

### Joint Dysfunction

Limited joint mobility, perhaps due to glycosylation of tissue proteins, is a marker for long-term poor control and is associated with other complications (eg, retinopathy, nephropathy and neuropathy). The hands and other joints should be examined.

### Growth Disturbances

Linear growth is negatively affected by poor diabetic control. Decreased growth velocity, crossing percentiles downward for height and weight, eventual short stature, and delayed skeletal and sexual maturation are associated with chronic undertreatment with insulin. An extreme form of this, the Mauriac syndrome or diabetic dwarfism, occurs rarely and is usually associated with hepatomegaly. Careful height and weight measurements should be obtained every 3 to 4 months and plotted on growth curves so that deviations from normal velocities can be detected early. Alternatively, treatment with excessive insulin doses often leads to excessive weight gain, causing the weight curve to cross percentiles upward. The maintenance of normal growth curves for height and weight is an important goal of diabetes management.

## Retinopathy

Most patients with IDDM develop background retinopathy after 15 to 20 years of the disease. The percentage of patients developing proliferative retinopathy is less, with studies reporting incidences of 20% to 50%. About 5% to 10% of IDDM patients become blind. Early treatment with laser photocoagulation can significantly reduce the rate of progression to blindness. All patients with IDDM should be evaluated yearly by an ophthalmologist, with regular-interval eye examinations by the child's pediatrician and diabetes physician. These yearly examinations should begin within 5 years of the onset of the disease. The DCCT showed that intensive blood glucose control delayed onset and slowed progression of retenopathy.

## Nephropathy

About 30% to 40% of patients with IDDM eventually develop end-stage renal disease and need dialysis or transplantation. End-stage renal disease is an important cause of morbidity and mortality. Diabetic nephropathy is characterized by proteinuria, which may be severe, producing a nephrotic syndrome, hypertension, initial hyperfiltration (ie, increased glomerular filtrate rate [GFR]), and progressive renal insufficiency (ie, increasing serum creatinine and urea nitrogen, decreasing GRF). Glomerular damage, especially mesangial expansion and basement membrane thickening, is the most characteristic histologic finding. The importance of tight metabolic control to prevent nephropathy or slow its progression has been shown recently by the DCCT.

A genetic predisposition may be an important underlying factor. All patients with IDDM should be monitored by urinalysis, with a check for protein, serum creatinine, and blood urea nitrogen at least annually for the first few years of the disease. Twenty-four-hour urine samples for quantitative protein and, if possible, tests for microalbuminuria should be done at lease yearly, preferable starting in the first year after the diagnosis. Blood pressure should be monitored accurately several times a year. After hypertension, overt proteinuria, or elevation in serum creatinine or urea nitrogen is found, monitoring of renal function several times each year and consultation with a nephrologist is warranted. Microalbuminuria (<200 to 250 mg/day) may be a marker for the early stages of nephropathy. Low-protein diets have been successful in slowing or preventing progression of renal insufficiency in IDDM, but there are concerns about their use in growing children.

Hypertension is an extremely important factor that is known to accelerate the progression of nephropathy. It should be aggressively treated. Angiotensin-converting enzyme (ACE) inhibitors are recommended. It is not known whether using ACE inhibitors to lower blood pressures already in the normal range are useful in preventing or retarding nephropathy. It is also important for patients to avoid other risk factors, such as smoking.

## Neuropathy

Symptomatic diabetic neuropathy, peripheral or autonomic, is uncommon in children and adolescents with IDDM, although changes in nerve conduction may be measured after 4 to 5 years of the disease. Overall, neuropathy is a common IDDM complication, and its frequency increases with the duration of disease and degree of hyperglycemia. Improvements in glycemic control may help neuropathic symptoms. Clinical trials of aldose reductase inhibitors have reported serious side effects.

## Macrovascular Complications

Patients with IDDM tend to have coronary artery, cerebrovascular, and peripheral vascular disease more often, at an earlier age, and more extensively than the nondiabetic population. Hypertension, elevated blood lipid levels, and cigarette smoking are other risk factors for developing macrovascular complications. Risk factor assessment, including lipid panels, blood pressure measurements, and determining if the patient smokes, should be done, and treatment should be instituted as indicated. A strong admonition against smoking and referral to an appropriate program for patients who are already smokers is indicated.

## Selected Readings

Allen DB, MacDonald MJ. Pancreas and islet cell transplantation for type I diabetes mellitus. Does it have a role for children? Adv Pediatr 1990;37:391.

Arieff AL. Proteinuria and microalbuminuria as predictors of nephropathy. Hosp Pract 1992;27(Suppl 1):51.

Bhatia V, Wolfsdorf J. Severe hypoglycemia in youth with IDDM: frequency and causative factors. Pediatrics 1991;88:1187.

Bottazzo GF, Foulis AK, Bosi E, Todd I, Pujol-Borell R. Pancreatic β-cell damage: in search of novel pathogenic factors. Diabetes Care 1988;11(Suppl 1):24.

Brink SJ. Pediatric and adolescent diabetes mellitus. Chicago: Year Book Medical Publishers, 1987.

Brownlee M. Glycosylation of proteins and microangiopathy. Hosp Pract 1992;27(suppl 1):46.

Chase P, Gorg S, Jelley D. DKA in children: role of outpatient management. Pediatr Rev 1990;11:297.

Chase PH. Avoiding the short- and long-term complications of juvenile diabetes. Pediatr Rev 1985;7:140.

Drash AL. Clinical care of the diabetic child. Chicago: Year Book Medical Publishers, 1987.

Drash AL, Arslenian SA. Can IDDM be cured or prevented? A status report on immunomodulatory strategies and pancreas transplantation Pediatr Clin North Am 1990;37:1467.

Duck SC, Wyatt DT. Factors associated with brain herniation in the treatment of DKA. J Pediatr 1988;113:10.

Ellis EN. Concepts of fluid restriction in DKA and HHNC. Pediatr Clin North Am 1990;37:313.

Faustman D, Coe C. Prevention of xenograft rejection by marking donor HLA class I antigens. Science 1991;252:1700.

Gerich JE, Mokan M, Veneman T, et al. Hypoglycemia unawareness. Endocrinol Rev 1991;12:356.

Ginsberg-Fellner F. Insulin-dependent diabetes mellitus. Pediatr Rev 1990, 11:239.

Harris GD, Fiordalisi I, Harris WL, Mosovich LL, Finberg L. Minimizing the risk of brain herniation during treatment of DKA: a retrospective and prospective study. J Pediatr 1990;117:22.

Hellerstrom C, Anderson A, Groth G, et al. Experimental pancreatic transplantation in diabetes. Diabetes Care 1988;11(suppl 1):45.

Johnston JM. Management of DKA. In: Clinical diabetes reviews, vol 1. : American Diabetes Association, 1987;119.

Krane EJ. DKA: biochemistry, physiology, treatment and prevention. Pediatr Clin North Am 1987;34:935.

Lacy PE, Hegre OD, Gerasimidin-Vazeou A, et al. Maintenance of normoglycemia in diabetic mice by subcutaneous xenografts of encapsulated islets. Science 1991;254:1782.

Lanza RP, Butler DHA, Borland M, et al. Xenotransplantation of canine, bovine and porcine islets in diabetic rats without immunosuppression. Proc Natl Acad Sci U S A 1991;88:11100.

Lorenz R, Wysocki T. The family and childhood diabetes: conclusions. Diabetes Spectrum 1991;4:290.

Nerup J, Mandrup-Poulsen T, Molvig J, Helgvist S. Wogengen L, Egeberg J. Mechanisms of pancreatic beta cell destruction in type I diabetes. Diabetes Care 1988;11(suppl 1):16.

Palmer JP, McCullock DK. Prediction and prevention of IDDM—1991. Diabetes 1991;40:943.

Raskin P. Is tight blood sugar control effective and justified? Negative. Hosp Pract 1992;27(suppl 1):21.

Rosenbloom AL. Intracerebral crises during treatment of DKA. Diabetes Care 1990;13:22.

Skyler J. Is tight blood sugar control effective and justified? Affirmative. Hosp Pract 1992;27(suppl 1):17.

Sperling M, ed. DKA. In: Physician's guide to insulin-dependent (type 1) diabetes mellitus: diagnosis and treatment. : American Diabetes Association, 1988:63.

Sperling M, ed. Pathogenesis. In: Physician's guide to insulin- dependent (type I) diabetes: diagnosis and treatment. : American Diabetes Association, 1988:9.

Sperling MA. Diabetes mellitus. In: Kaplan SA, ed. Clinical pediatric and adolescent endocrinology. Philadelphia: WB Saunders, 1982:131.

Sperling MA. Outpatient management of diabetes mellitus. Pediatr Clin North Am 1987;34:917.

Travis LB, Brouhard BH, Schreiner BJ. Diabetes mellitus in children and adolescents. Philadelphia: WB Saunders, 1987.

Travis LB. An instructional aid on insulin-dependent diabetes mellitus, ed 7. Fort Worth, TX: Stafford-Lowdon, 1985.

Zeller K, Whittaker E, Sullivan L, et al. Effects of restricting dietary protein on the progression of renal failure in patients with IDDM. N Engl J Med 1991;324:78.

Ziegler AG, Herskowitz RD, Jackson RA, Soeldner JS, Eisenbarth GS. Predicting type I diabetes. Diabetes Care 1990;13,762.

*Principles and Practice of Pediatrics, Second Edition.*
edited by Frank A. Oski et al. J. B. Lippincott Company, Philadelphia © 1994.

# CHAPTER 144
# *The Thyroid Gland*

## Patricia A. Donohoue

## NORMAL THYROID DEVELOPMENT AND THYROID HORMONE SYNTHESIS

The thyroid gland first appears in the fourth week of gestation as an epithelial proliferation and invagination of the endoderm of the foregut, and at this time, the synthesis of thyroglobulin begins. The thyroid then penetrates the mesoderm and migrates downward but remains connected to the floor of the foregut by means of the thyroglossal duct. This duct eventually becomes solid and normally disappears completely. By the seventh week of development, the now bilobed gland reaches its normal position in front of the trachea. By the 10th to 11th week, the fetal thyroid begins to trap and organify (oxidize) iodide, and by the 12th week, colloid formation is detectable. By the 11th week of gestation, the thyroid gland secretes thyroxine ($T_4$), but the timing of the onset of secretion of triiodothyronine ($T_3$) is unknown. Maturation of the fetal hypothalamic-pituitary-thyroid axis occurs by the 20th week, and thyroid-stimulating hormone (TSH) is detectable by the 13th week.

The synthesis of thyroid hormone is regulated through a central biologic feedback system. Under the stimulatory influence of the hypothalamic tripeptide thyrotropin-releasing hormone (TRH), also known as thyrotropin-releasing factor (TRF), the pituitary thyrotrophs secrete TSH. TSH enters the circulation and binds to specific receptors on the thyroid gland to stimulate $T_4$ production. This stimulation occurs within the cell through a second messenger, cyclic adenosine monophosphate (cAMP), a mechanism common to many peptide hormones. The circulating levels of $T_4$ and $T_3$ feed back at the level of the pituitary and the hypothalamus to regulate the release of TSH.

Thyroid hormone synthesis is a multistep procedure that begins when circulating iodide is trapped by the iodine pump and is organified by thyroperoxidase. Organic iodide binds to the tyrosine residues of thyroglobulin, resulting in the formation of monoiodotyrosine (MIT) and diiodotyrosine (DIT). MIT and DIT condense to form $T_3$ and $T_4$, the major thyroid hormones produced. $T_3$ and $T_4$ are stored on the thyroglobulin molecule in the form of colloid or released from the thyroglobulin molecule into the circulation. Thyroglobulin itself is not normally released into the plasma and, if detected, may indicate a thyroid cell abnormality, such as carcinoma. Although the major thyroid hormone produced in and secreted by the thyroid gland is $T_4$, its effects are exerted in peripheral tissues through its deiodination to the much more potent $T_3$. The amount of $T_3$ secreted by the thyroid gland itself adds a minimal fraction to the total circulating $T_3$ under physiological conditions. Inborn errors in thyroid hormone metabolism have been described for all of these steps.

The thyroid gland produces a third thyroid hormone, reverse $T_3$ ($rT_3$), which is synthesized from $T_4$ by a deiodinase different from that which produces $T_3$. The $rT_3$ levels are high during fetal life, when $T_3$ levels are quite low. After birth, $rT_3$ levels decrease markedly, and $T_3$ levels rise into the normal range. In certain conditions, such as the euthyroid sick syndrome, the levels of circulating $rT_3$ may be elevated.

$T_4$ and $T_3$ are transported in the plasma bound to the thyroid hormone-binding proteins thyroxine-binding globulin (TBG), the major binding protein, and thyroxine-binding prealbumin. Albumin also binds thyroid hormone with low affinity. The protein-bound fractions of circulating $T_4$ and $T_3$ account for more than 99% of the total hormone, and more than 70% of the total is bound to TBG. Even minor changes in the levels of the thyroid hormone-binding proteins can result in a significant change in the level of total circulating hormone, although the free (ie, metabolically available, non–protein-bound) hormone remains the same. For the same reason, TBG acts as a buffer to protect the tissues from fluctuations in $T_4$ levels. As with inborn errors of thyroid hormone synthesis, many disorders of thyroid hormone-binding proteins have been described, the most common of which is the X-linked condition of TBG deficiency.

The physiological effects of thyroid hormone are protean, accounting for the myriad symptoms seen in thyroid disorders. These effects include protein synthesis, cell growth and differentiation, critical effects on the maturation of the central nervous system and skeleton, maintenance of oxidative metabolism and heat production, and maintenance of cardiovascular function. The circulating levels of thyroid hormone affect muscle tone, deep tendon reflexes, and maturation of the epidermis.

The thyroid gland is also the source of calcitonin, produced by the so-called C cells. These cells are embryologically derived from the neural crest and are not truly thyroid in origin. The physiological effects calcitonin oppose those of parathyroid hormone.

## THYROID FUNCTION TESTS

### Static Tests

The static tests of thyroid function include measurement of plasma levels of the various components of the thyroid system. Normal values for many of these components are given in Table 144-1.

Total $T_4$ concentration is determined by radioimmunoassay (RIA). It is the most widely used test of thyroid function and reflects the total of the protein-bound and free hormone. Free $T_4$ is measured by RIA or by equilibrium dialysis. The RIA may use a single or double antibody techniques, the choice of which greatly effects the levels obtained (see Table 144-1).

Total and free $T_3$ concentrations are determined using the methods described for $T_4$. Two thirds of the $T_3$ measured in plasma arises from peripheral deiodination of $T_4$, and only one third arises from direct secretion from the thyroid gland.

The $T_3$ resin uptake ($T_3RU$) is commonly employed to estimate the number of thyroid hormone-binding protein sites and reflects the circulating level of free $T_4$. It is not a measure of plasma $T_3$ concentration. Radiolabeled $T_3$ is added to an aliquot of the patient's serum and binds to all available (ie, unoccupied) TBG

TABLE 144-1. Thyroid Function Tests in Infancy, Childhood, and Adulthood

| Age | Thyroxine (μg/dL) | Triiodothyronine (ng/dL) | Thyroxine-Binding Globulin (mg/dL) | Thyroid-Stimulating Hormone* (μU/mL) |
|---|---|---|---|---|
| Cord Blood | 10.8 | 50 | 2.7 | 9.0 |
| | (6.5–17.5) | (15–85) | (0.7–4.7) | (<2.5–17.4) |
| 1–3 d | 16.5 | 240 | | 8.0 |
| | (11.0–21.5) | (100–380) | | (<2.5–13.3) |
| 1–4 wk | 13.0 | 175 | 2.5 | 4.0 |
| | (8.0–17.0) | (100–300) | (0.5–4.5) | (0.6–10.0) |
| 1–12 mo | 11.0 | 175 | 2.6 | 2.1 |
| | (7.0–15.5) | (100–260) | (1.6–3.6) | (0.6–6.3) |
| 1–5 y | 10.5 | 165 | 2.1 | 2.0 |
| | (7.0–15.0) | (95–250) | (1.3–2.8) | (0.6–6.3) |
| 6–10 y | 9.3 | 150 | 2.0 | 2.0 |
| | (6.5–13.5) | (95–240) | (1.4–2.6) | (0.6–6.3) |
| 11–15 y | 8.1 | 133 | 2.0 | 1.9 |
| | (5.0–11.8) | (80–215) | (1.4–2.6) | (0.6–6.3) |
| 16–20 y | 8.1 | 130 | 2.0 | 1.8 |
| | (4.5–11.7) | (80–210) | (1.4–2.6) | (0.2–7.6) |
| 21–50 y | 7.3 | 123 | 1.8 | 1.8 |
| | (4.3–12.5) | (70–204) | (1.2–2.4) | (0.2–7.6) |

Thyroid-stimulating hormone levels in term and premature infants rise rapidly postpartum to reach a peak of 60 to 100 μU/mL within the first hours of life and then decrease to normal by 16 to 24 hours.

Values given represent mean; normal ranges are in parentheses below the mean values.

*Data adapted from Fisher DA. The thyroid. In: Rudolph AM, ed. Pediatrics. Norwalk, CT: Appleton & Lange, 1987:1504 and Fisher DA. The thyroid. In: Kaplan SA, ed. Clinical pediatric endocrinology. Philadelphia: WB Saunders, 1990:95. TSH data are adapted from LaFranchi SH. Hypothyroidism, congenital and acquired. In: Kaplan SA, ed. Clinical pediatric and adolescent endocrinology. Philadelphia: WB Saunders, 1982:82. For normal values in premature infants, the reader is referred to Delange F, Dalhem A, Bourdoux P, et al. Increased risk of primary hypothyroidism in preterm infants. J Pediatr 1984;105:462; Ballabio M, Nicolini U, Jowett T, et al. Maturation of thyroid function in normal human fetuses. Clin Endocrinol 1989;31:565; and Thorpe-Beeston JG, Nicolaides KH, Felton CV, et al. Maturation of the secretion of thyroid hormone and thyroid stimulating hormone in the fetus. N Engl J Med 1991;324: 532. The appropriate normal range for free thyroxine must be based on the type of assay employed by the reference laboratory.*

binding sites. Because TBG has a greater affinity for $T_4$ than $T_3$, the radioactive $T_3$ does not displace the patient's $T_4$ from the TBG molecule. A resin that binds $T_3$ is added, and the unbound radioactive $T_3$ taken up by the resin. This percentage increases as the number of available TBG binding sites decreases. The $T_3RU$ test is useful only if the total $T_4$ concentration is known.

The free thyroxine index (FTI), an estimation of the free $T_4$ concentration, is calculated from the total $T_4$ concentration and the $T_3RU$ using the following formula: FTI = $T_4 \times T_3RU$ (patient)/$T_3RU$ (average for laboratory).

TSH levels are determined by RIA and are helpful in the interpretation of thyroid hormone levels. The pituitary gland is sensitive to changes in thyroid hormone levels, and elevated levels may indicate early thyroid gland failure or inadequate thyroid hormone replacement therapy before plasma thyroxine concentrations decrease.

TBG levels can now be determined reliably in most laboratories and are useful in the interpretation of abnormal thyroid hormone levels. TBG levels may be altered by a variety of conditions and medications (Table 144-2).

Many drugs may affect thyroid function tests because of interactions at various levels of thyroid hormone synthesis, release, and metabolism (Table 144-3). A thorough history of medications is essential in the evaluation of a patient with a thyroid abnormality. Immunoglobulin measurements helpful in the evaluation of thyroid disorders include antithyroglobulin and antimicrosomal antibodies, which may be present in autoimmune disorders of the gland, and thyroid-stimulating immunoglobulin (TSI), which

is important in the pathogenesis of hyperthyroidism. TSH-blocking antibodies can be measured at some centers.

## Dynamic Tests

The TRH stimulation test of TSH release is a helpful tool in the evaluation of patients whose thyroid hormone and TSH levels do not establish a diagnosis. In response to an intravenous infusion of TRH, the normal person has a brisk rise in serum TSH,

TABLE 144-2. Factors that Influence Thyroid-Binding Globulin Levels

| Increased TBG | Decreased TBG |
|---|---|
| Congenital (X-linked) | Congenital (X-linked) |
| Hepatitis | Hepatic cirrhosis |
| Porphyria | Nephrosis |
| Heroin, methadone | Androgens |
| Estrogens, pregnancy (oral contraceptives) | Antiestrogens |
| 5-Fluorouracil | Glucocorticoids |
| Perphenazine (Trilafon) | Acromegaly |
| | Protein-losing enteropathy |
| | Protein-calorie malnutrition |
| | Hyperthyroidism |

TABLE 144-3. Drugs That Influence Thyroid Hormone Levels

| Characteristic | Drug | Effect |
| --- | --- | --- |
| Drugs that have a CNS effect to alter thyroid hormone levels; glucocorticoids may inhibit the conversion of $T_4$ to $T_3$ | Dopamine, L-dopa | Decreased TSH causes decreased $T_4$ |
| | Glucocorticoids | Decreased TSH causes decreased $T_4$ |
| | Metoclopramide | Increased TSH (transient) |
| Drugs that directly decrease thyroid hormone synthesis, most often by decreasing iodide organification; exceptions are nitroprusside, which inhibits iodide trapping, and lithium carbonate, which inhibits release of $T_4$ and $T_3$ from thyroglobulin | p-Aminosalicylate, phenylbutazone, sulfonamides, aminoglutethimide, nitroprusside, lithium carbonate | All: decreased $T_4$, decreased free $T_4$ and increased TSH |
| Compounds that decrease the gut absorption of orally administered tyroxine | Cholestyramine, soybean flour | Decreased $T_4$, free $T_4$ and thus increased TSH |
| Drugs that inhibit the binding of $T_4$ and $T_3$ to TBG; phenytoin also acts to increase cellular uptake of $T_4$, which decreases the free $T_4$ concentration | Salicylates | Decreased $T_4$, normal free $T_4$ and TSH |
| | Phenylbutazone | Decreased $T_4$, normal free $T_4$ and TSH |
| | Phenytoin | Decreased $T_4$, decreased free $T_4$, normal $T_3$ and TSH |
| Drugs that change uptake or metabolism of thyroid hormones, | Heparin | Normal $T_4$, increased free $T_4$, normal $T_3$ and TSH |
| | Phenytoin | Decreased $T_4$, decreased free $T_4$, normal $T_3$, and TSH |
| | Glucocorticoids | Decreased $T_4$, decreased free $T_4$, decreased $T_3$, normal TSH |
| | Propanolol | Decreased $T_3$ (only in hyperthyroidism) |
| Drugs that induce hepatic mixed function oxidases and enhance clearance of thyroxine; effect may be accompanied by increased $T_4 \rightarrow T_3$ conversion | Diphenylhydantoin, phenobarbital, carbamazepine, rifampicin | All: Decreased $T_4$ and free $T_4$ with normal $T_3$ and TSH due to combined effects |
| Drugs that enhance $T_4 \rightarrow T_3$ conversion | Exogenous growth hormone | Decreased $T_4$ and free $T_4$, normal $T_3$ and TSH |

$T_3$, triiodothyonine; $T_4$, thyroxine; TBG, thyroxine-binding hormone; TSH, thyroid-stimulating hormone.

*Adapted from Kaplan MM. Interactions between drugs and thyroid hormones. Thyroid Today 1981;4:5; and Burger AG. Effects of certain pharmacologic agents on the peripheral metabolism of thyroxine. In: Ingbar SH, Braverman LE, ed. Werner's The thyroid: a fundamental and clinical text. Philadelphia: JB Lippincott, 1986:351.*

followed by a slower return to the normal range. This is accompanied by a similar rise and fall in the serum prolactin level. The magnitude and timing of the TSH response to TRH help to differentiate normal from abnormal thyroid function. Examples include an exaggerated TSH response in hypothyroidism and a blunted response in hyperthyroidism.

The $T_3$ suppression test is helpful in differentiating hyperthyroidism due to autonomous gland hyperfunction (ie, TSI stimulation) from other causes. After a baseline determination of early radioactive iodine uptake, the patient is treated with exogenous $T_3$ for 1 week, at which time the radioactive iodine uptake test is repeated. An autonomously hyperfunctioning gland does not show the normal decrease in radioiodine uptake.

## Radiologic Studies

Radiologic studies of the thyroid gland involve the administration of radioactive isotopes, which are taken up by the thyroid gland and, to some extent, by other tissues. Because the percentage of administered radioactivity taken up by the gland is higher in infants and children than in adults and because the radiation

risk to the thyroid gland is cumulative, the use of these studies for infants and children should be minimized. The commonly accepted indications for performing these studies in children include the evaluation of thyroid nodules, as an adjunctive test elucidating the cause of hyperthyroidism, localizing ectopic thyroid tissue, evaluation of dyshormonogenesis, and as a last resort when the combination of other static and dynamic tests of thyroid function are inconclusive.

Three radioactive isotopes are commonly used for thyroid studies. [131]I results in the highest absorbed dose of radioactivity and has the longest half-life; its use is reserved for thyroid ablative therapy. [123]I emits much less $\beta$-radiation and is usually the isotope for iodine uptake studies. [99m]Tc pertechnetate results in the lowest dose of radioactivity, but once taken up by the thyroid gland, it is not further metabolized and is not useful in studies of thyroid hormone metabolism and release. However, it can be used in the evaluation of thyroid nodules (ie, hot versus cold) and goiters (eg, homogeneous versus nonhomogeneous uptake; increased versus decreased uptake).

The 24-hour uptake of radioactive iodine is a common method of assessing the daily iodine turnover of the thyroid gland. It reflects the cumulative effect of thyroid clearance, renal clearance, thyroid retention, and dietary intake, and it is reported as the percentage of the total dose given.

In the early or 20-minute uptake test, the percentage of uptake for 20 minutes after the intravenous dose of isotope is cumulatively measured. This uptake reflects thyroid uptake and organification of the circulating iodine load and is less affected by factors that modify the 24-hour uptake. Some patients are advised to consume a diet low in iodine before evaluation by the uptake test.

The perchlorate or thiocyanate discharge test is performed after the 20-minute uptake and is a measure of the amount of radioactive iodine that can be released from the gland after uptake. This test is useful in the evaluation of suspected dyshormonogenesis.

The $T_3$ suppression test described earlier is helpful in the diagnosis of hyperthyroidism. It can also be used as a method to detect relapses in Graves' disease without an interruption in the patient's therapy.

Ultrasound of the thyroid gland can be used to differentiate solid from the more rare cystic nodules and may be as useful as a low-risk screening procedure for this purpose.

## ABNORMAL THYROID CONDITIONS

Abnormalities of the thyroid gland may result from altered function (eg, hypothyroidism, hyperthyroidism), altered structure (eg, enlargement, nodule), or nonthyroidal causes (eg, drugs, other illnesses).

### Hypothyroidism

Hypothyroidism is defined as a state in which the thyroid gland fails to secrete sufficient quantities of thyroid hormone. Primary hypothyroidism results from a problem inherent to the gland itself, and secondary or central hypothyroidism results from the failure of pituitary stimulation of the thyroid gland. Primary and central hypothyroidism can be congenital or acquired.

#### Congenital Hypothyroidism

Congenital hypothyroidism is a disease with an overall prevalence of 1 of 4000 live births, including 1 of 2000 persons of Far Eastern or Hispanic descent, 1 of 5500 persons of European descent, and 1 of 32,000 persons of African descent. Ninety-five percent of all cases are sporadic, and 5% are genetic, most often reflecting a dyshormonogenesis. There is a 2 : 1 female to male predominance, and associations with specific human lymphocyte antigen (HLA) types have been reported in certain populations. Newborn screening for congenital hypothyroidism is carried out in all 50 states in the Unites States, but the methods of screening vary. Healthy, premature infants have lower $T_4$ concentrations than term infants of the same chronologic age. This must be kept in mind when evaluating the results of the newborn screen. If the newborn screen blood sample is obtained within the first day of life, and the TSH level may be falsely elevated because of the peripartum TSH surge.

*Etiology.* The causes of congenital hypothyroidism are considered here according to the types of hypothyroidism they produce.

*Permanent primary hypothyroidism* denotes irreversible failure of the thyroid gland to produce sufficient thyroid hormone. The most common cause is an ectopic thyroid gland, which results from improper migration during fetal development. It accounts for over two thirds of all cases detected by newborn screening

worldwide. The ectopic thyroid tissue often can be demonstrated by $^{99m}$Tc scanning, and it is most commonly found at the base of the tongue (ie, lingual thyroid). These aberrantly located glands do not function properly and do not produce an adequate amount of thyroid hormone.

The next most common cause of congenital primary hypothyroidism is hypoplasia or aplasia of the gland, and this thyroid dysgenesis may result from the same pathophysiologic process as ectopy of the gland. In some cases, immunoglobulins have been implicated in the pathogenesis. A TSH-binding inhibitor immunoglobulin (TBII) has been described in sibling cases of nongoitrous neonatal hypothyroidism and in association with maternal chronic lymphocytic thyroiditis (CLT). TBII may be associated with a transient form of hypothyroidism in the newborn. TBII is detectable in maternal and infant sera. Another antibody known as thyroid growth-blocking immunoglobulin has been associated with thyroid dysgenesis. It can block the growth of thyroid cells in vitro. Antithyroglobulin and antimicrosomal antibodies are not known to play a direct role in the pathogenesis of congenital hypothyroidism.

The third most common cause of congenital primary hypothyroidism is dyshormonogenesis, an inborn error of thyroid hormone synthesis, secretion, or metabolism. It is responsible for most of the familial cases of congenital hypothyroidism. The most common form is a defect in the organification of iodide. Other causes of familial congenital hypothyroidism include deiodination defects, abnormal thyroglobulin, iodide trapping defects, TSH receptor abnormalities (eg, familial unresponsiveness to TSH), and failure of thyroid hormone secretion. A rare peripheral resistance to thyroid hormone has been described in which affected patients have clinical hypothyroidism, but elevated $T_4$ levels and normal TSH levels prevent neonatal recognition of the disease.

Congenital hypothyroidism may result from maternal radioactive iodine treatment if it has been given after the 8th week of gestation, when fetal iodide trapping has begun.

*Transient primary hypothyroidism* is a self-limited process, and the cause is determined by a careful history. The causes include maternal iodine deficiency (eg, endemic goiter), fetal or neonatal exposure to iodine (eg, maternal medications, amniofetography, painting of the cervix, painting of the umbilical stump), maternal antithyroid drugs, maternal antibodies (eg, TBII), and rarely, association with the nephrotic syndrome (ie, urinary loss of iodine). This condition is more likely to occur in premature than in full-term infants (Delange et al, 1984). Although transient, these conditions may require temporary treatment with thyroid hormone.

*Permanent central hypothyroidism* is generally associated with congenital hypopituitarism and may account for as many as 5% of cases of congenital hypothyroidism. Hypopituitarism may be associated with midline cranial defects (eg, septo-optic dysplasia, cleft lip or palate), pituitary aplasia, idiopathic hypopituitarism, and in association with other severe central nervous system (CNS) malformations.

*Low $T_4$ level without hypothyroidism* is most commonly caused by TBG deficiency, an X-linked disorder with a frequency similar to that of central hypothyroidism. It is easily differentiated from true hypothyroidism, because the level of free $T_4$ is normal, the $T_3$RU is high, and the TBG level is low. This condition does not require treatment. Low $T_4$ levels may be seen in ill neonates as a manifestation of the euthyroid sick syndrome (ie, nonthyroidal illness), which is discussed later.

*Diagnosis.* Congenital hypothyroidism rarely is diagnosed from clinical abnormalities. These children have normal birth weight and length and a slightly larger than average head circumference at birth, and one third of them have longer than average gestation. Most cases are detected as a result of newborn screening tests, which must be confirmed by thyroid function

**TABLE 144-4. Signs and Symptoms of Congenital Hypothyroidism**

| | |
|---|---|
| Large fontanelles | Prolonged jaundice |
| Umbilical hernia | Constipation |
| Macroglossia | Lethargy |
| Mottled, dry skin | Difficulty feeding |
| Hypotonia | Cool skin |
| Abdominal distention | Sleeps through night (newborn period) |
| Hoarse cry | Hypothermia |
| Respiratory distress | Goiter (rare) |

tests using a venous blood sample. The dried filter paper test does not suffice as the confirmatory test.

Certain clinical features of hypothyroidism, listed in Table 144-4, may suggest the diagnosis before the results of the newborn screening tests are available. Features that suggest the possibility of hypopituitarism (eg, midline defects, hypoglycemia, micropenis) should lead to an evaluation for central hypothyroidism. Goiters are rarely present in patients with congenital hypothyroidism, even in cases of dyshormonogenesis. They may be seen in cases of placental transmission of a goitrogen, and they may be large enough to produce upper airway obstruction.

The hormonal patterns found in congenital hypothyroxinemia are summarized in Table 144-5. In true hypothyroidism, other tests may be helpful in determining the cause of the disease, including thyroid scanning; urinary iodine if iodine toxicity or deficiency is suspected; bone age, which may be quite delayed in long-standing hypothyroidism; thyroglobulin level, which may help differentiate ectopic from dysplastic glands; and $\alpha$-fetoprotein levels, which may be elevated in long-standing disease.

*Treatment.* The treatment of congenital hypothyroidism consists of replacement of thyroid hormone with oral levothyroxine in a singe daily dose of 8 to 10 $\mu$g/kg/day. The total replacement dose may be used at the outset of therapy unless there is evidence of cardiac disease, in which case a stepwise increase in dosage is recommended. Breast-feeding is not a substitute for replacement therapy, because thyroid hormones, although measurable in breast milk, do not provide adequate serum levels in the infant. The goals of treatment include maintenance of the $T_4$ level in the upper half of the normal range for the age,

being careful to avoid overtreatment because of the complications of neonatal hyperthyroidism. In primary hypothyroidism, several months of treatment may be necessary before the TSH level normalizes. Rarely, the pituitary set point for TSH release may be elevated in these patients, causing the TSH level to remain high despite normal free $T_4$ and $T_3$ levels.

With prompt and adequate treatment, children with congenital hypothyroidism have the potential for normal somatic and intellectual growth and development. If left untreated, severe mental retardation and neurologic dysfunction ensues, which is more severe in children with primary than with central hypothyroidism. Patients in whom treatment is begun before 6 weeks of age have an average IQ of 100. If treatment is begun at 6 weeks to 3 months, the average IQ decreases to 95; if begun at 3 to 6 months, the average IQ is 75. After 6 months the average IQ is 55 or less.

A variety of other neurologic and learning disorders have been associated with untreated congenital hypothyroidism, including hearing loss, ataxia, attention deficit disorder, abnormalities of muscle tone, and speech defects. Somatic growth and skeletal development are also impaired, and other clinical manifestations become apparent (see Table 144-4). With severe hypothyroidism, cardiac failure may develop. The sequelae of untreated congenital hypothyroidism are devastating. If an infant has evidence of congenital hypothyroidism on the basis of the newborn screen and a speedy diagnosis cannot be made after the confirmatory tests have been obtained, therapy should be initiated before establishing the diagnosis. The treatment is inexpensive and has low risk if thyroid hormone levels are measured frequently. In these cases, the child should be treated until 3 years of age, when the medication can be temporarily discontinued for 1 to 2 months without risk while a diagnosis is established.

### Acquired Hypothyroidism

Acquired hypothyroidism appears after the newborn period in a child who did not have congenital hypothyroidism. The estimated prevalence is 1 per 500 to 1000 school-aged children, with a female to male preponderance of 4 : 1. Certain types of acquired hypothyroidism are familial.

*Etiology.* As with congenital hypothyroidism, the causes of acquired hypothyroidism can be divided into those that produce primary or those that produce central hypothyroidism. Patients who are critically ill with a nonthyroidal illness may appear to have chemical hypothyroidism, a condition known as the euthyroid sick syndrome.

**TABLE 144-5. Hormonal Patterns in Congenital Hypothyroxinemia**

| Cause | First Newborn Screen | | Follow-up Confirmation | | | |
|---|---|---|---|---|---|---|
| | $T_4$ | TSH | $T_4$ | $T_3$RU | TSH | Free $T_4$ |
| Primary hypothyroidism | Low | High | Low | Low/Nl | High | Low |
| Central hypothyroidism | Low | Nl* | Low | Low/Nl | Nl* | Low |
| Transient hypothyroidism | Low | High | Nl | Nl | Nl | Nl |
| Thyroid-binding globulin deficiency† | Low | Nl | Low | High | Nl | Nl |

Nl, normal; $T_4$, thyroxine; TSH, thyroid-stimulating hormone; $T_3$RU, triiodothyronine resin uptake.
* The normal level of TSH seen in central hypothyroidism is inappropriately low for the decreased levels of $T_4$ and free $T_4$.
† The diagnosis of thyroid-binding globulin (TBG) deficiency is most accurately made by demonstration of a low TBG level.

*Primary acquired hypothyroidism* in childhood is characterized by low $T_4$ levels, elevated TSH, and a variety of clinical manifestations. It most often results from immunologic destruction of the thyroid gland, but many nonimmunologic causes are known.

The most common cause is CLT, also known as Hashimoto's thyroiditis. A defect in cell-mediated immunity results in lymphocytic infiltration and enlargement of the thyroid gland. Titers of antithyroglobulin and antimicrosomal antibodies are elevated in more than 80% of patients. Patients with CLT present with nontender enlargement of the gland, which may be asymmetric. The patients are often euthyroid, but some may present with transient hyperthyroidism or have signs and symptoms of hypothyroidism.

CLT may occur alone or in association with other autoimmune endocrine diseases known as the autoimmune polyglandular syndromes types I and II (Table 144-6). Because of this association, the diagnosis of CLT should lead to a search for these other autoimmune processes, some of which may result in severe illness, such as Addison's disease and diabetes mellitus. There is an increased incidence of CLT among patients with chromosomal abnormalities, including Down syndrome, Turner syndrome, and Klinefelter syndrome. This is particularly important in patients with Down syndrome, because many of the clinical manifestations of hypothyroidism are seen in this syndrome and may lead to a delay in the diagnosis of hypothyroidism.

Subacute thyroiditis may produce hypothyroidism. Environmental causes of primary hypothyroidism include goitrogen ingestion (eg, iodides, antithyroid drugs, other medications; see Table 144-3), thyroidectomy, and radioactive iodine ablative therapy. Infiltrative diseases that can cause hypothyroidism include histiocytosis and cystinosis.

Some of the causes of congenital hypothyroidism (eg, ectopic gland, dyshormonogenesis) may not result in thyroid decompensation and the inability to meet metabolic demands until later in childhood.

*Central acquired hypothyroidism* is caused by pituitary or hypothalamic dysfunction. This central process may itself be primary (ie, idiopathic) or may be the result of another disease process. Idiopathic hypopituitarism is manifested by deficiencies of some or all of the anterior pituitary hormones, including TSH, growth hormone, adrenocorticotropin hormone, luteinizing hormone (LH), and follicle-stimulating hormone (FSH). Hypopituitarism can be secondary to infiltrative disease (eg, histiocytosis), tumor (eg, craniopharyngioma), head trauma, surgery, and radiation

### TABLE 144-7. Signs and Symptoms of Acquired Hypothyroidism

Short stature, decreased growth velocity
Obesity, myxedema
Goiter (primary hypothyroidism)
Delayed skeletal and dental age
Cold intolerance
Constipation
Dry, cool skin
Thinning of hair
Lethargy
Delayed reflex return
Bradycardia
Delayed puberty
Abnormal menses
Precocious puberty (rare)
Muscular pseudohypertrophy (rare)
Galactorrhea (rare)*

* Hypothalamic thyroid-releasing hormone (TRH) stimulates prolactin release from the posterior pituitary. In primary hypothyroidism, increased TRH may produce hyperprolactinemia and galactorrhea.

therapy. There is a greater chance of posterior pituitary involvement in secondary hypopituitarism than in idiopathic hypopituitarism. Posterior pituitary involvement is most often evident as diabetes insipidus (ie, vasopressin deficiency).

TSH deficiency is usually associated with generalized pituitary or hypothalamic dysfunction. Isolated TSH deficiency is rare and may be caused by a lack of TRH stimulation (eg, receptor defects in the pituitary, tumor invasion of the critical hypothalamic nuclei), or it may be idiopathic.

*Diagnosis.* The diagnosis of hypothyroidism is usually straightforward. The clinical features are listed in Table 144-7. The earliest sign of hypothyroidism in a child is often a slowing of the linear growth rate, as skeletal growth is sensitive to thyroid hormone levels. This is reflected in a delayed bone age and often in delayed puberty. In some cases of primary hypothyroidism, there is precocious puberty due to "spillover" release of LH and FSH in addition to increased TSH release. These children may have normal or relatively advanced bone ages due to the effects of sex steroids, buy they do not have the associated pubertal growth spurt. There may be a severe loss of height potential.

Except in the rare cases of peripheral resistance to thyroid hormone, circulating levels of $T_4$ and $T_3$ are low in hypothyroidism. Tests that assess concentrations of thyroid hormone-binding proteins (eg, $T_3RU$, TBG level) or free $T_4$ levels must be performed before therapy is initiated. TSH levels help differentiate primary from secondary hypothyroidism. The cause of primary hypothyroidism often can be determined by careful history of goitrogen exposure, surgery, or radiation exposure or from assessment of antithyroid antibody levels. A determination of the cause of secondary hypothyroidism must involve an assessment of the hypothalamic-pituitary system, and radiologic studies of the brain may be necessary to rule out tumor or infiltrative disease.

*Treatment.* The treatment of acquired hypothyroidism is thyroid hormone replacement with a single daily dose of oral levothyroxine (3 to 5 $\mu$g/kg/day for children, decreasing to 1 to 3 $\mu$g/kg/day for adults). In cases of hypothyroidism due to goitrogen exposure, it may be possible to treat the hypothyroidism by removing exposure to the goitrogen.

### TABLE 144-6. Clinical Features of Autoimmune Polyglandular Syndromes

| Type I | Type II |
| --- | --- |
| Primary hypothyroidism | Primary hypothyroidism |
| Primary hypogonadism | Primary hypogonadism |
| Vitiligo | Vitiligo |
| Pernicious anemia | Pernicious anemia |
| Alopecia | Alopecia |
| Malabsorption | Malabsorption |
| Adrenal insufficiency | Adrenal insufficiency |
| Mucocutaneous candidiasis | Myasthenia gravis |
| Chronic active hepatitis | Type I diabetes mellitus |
| Hypoparathyroidism | Hyperthyroidism |
| Onset in infancy or childhood | Onset in adults |
| Probably autosomal recessive | Autosomal dominant |
| No HLA association | HLA-B8, DR3 associated |

It is important to monitor the growth rate and $T_4$ levels in all patients and TSH levels in patients with primary hypothyroidism. Many children who commence treatment after long-standing hypothyroidism may experience school and behavioral problems, which may be related to a decrease in attention span and an increase in energy level as they become euthyroid.

The *euthyroid sick syndrome*, also known as the low $T_3$ syndrome, is a condition seen in patients with nonthyroidal illness in whom the total $T_3$ level is below normal, the total $T_4$ level is often low, and the TSH level is in the normal range. The $rT_3$ levels may be elevated or normal. Impaired conversion of $T_4$ to $T_3$ results in low $T_3$ levels. The patient's illness may cause increased metabolic clearance of $T_4$ and a decreased ability of the pituitary to secrete TSH. As a result, total $T_4$ concentration may decrease, but free $T_4$ may remain normal due to the presence of a circulating inhibitor of $T_4$ binding to TBG. In cases of a low level of free $T_4$, there is some evidence to suggest that tissue hypothyroidism does exist in this syndrome, but this may be adaptive and even beneficial in severe illness. If the patient recovers from the underlying illness, serum TSH levels increase and may become elevated before the $T_3$ and $T_4$ levels return to normal. Replacement therapy with $T_4$ is not recommended.

## Hyperthyroidism

Hyperthyroidism occurs when the thyroid gland secretes excessive amounts of thyroid hormone. The clinical manifestation is called thyrotoxicosis. Like hypothyroidism, hyperthyroidism may be congenital or acquired. Hyperthyroidism in childhood is rare and accounts for fewer than 5% of all cases of hyperthyroidism.

### Congenital Hyperthyroidism

Congenital hyperthyroidism, more often called neonatal thyrotoxicosis, is seen almost exclusively in infants of mothers with Graves' disease. Neonatal thyrotoxicosis may be transient, lasting up to several weeks, or prolonged, lasting over 6 months. It is a serious illness requiring prompt and aggressive management. This disease occurs in as many as 1 of 70 infants of mothers with Graves' disease. It has an equal sex distribution, unlike the later-onset form of thyrotoxicosis, which has a female preponderance. If maternal TSI titers are more than five times the normal values, regardless of whether she has had ablative thyroid therapy, the risk of neonatal thyrotoxicosis is greatly increased. Neonatal thyrotoxicosis accounts for about 1% of all cases of pediatric thyrotoxicosis.

*Etiology.* The cause of the transient form of neonatal thyrotoxicosis is probably transplacental passage of TSI (ie, maternal IgG). The prolonged or persistent form of the disease may be caused by endogenously produced TSI from the infant's own lymphocytes or from transplacentally acquired maternal lymphocytes.

*Diagnosis.* The diagnosis is made on the basis of clinical findings combined with elevated levels of $T_4$, free $T_4$, and $T_3$. The diagnosis may sometimes be available prenatally through cordocentesis for fetal thyroid hormone levels. Fetal tachycardia and intrauterine growth retardation may suggest the diagnosis. Affected patients often have low birth weight and microcephaly. They also exhibit marked irritability and hyperactivity, tachycardia, tachypnea, prominent eyes, thyroid enlargement, and a failure to gain weight despite marked hyperphagia. The glandular enlargement may be so marked that it causes respiratory distress requiring endotracheal intubation. Other features include vomiting, severe diarrhea, hepatosplenomegaly, jaundice, thrombocytopenia, and cardiac failure. The mortality rate in untreated cases is 15% to 25%, and death is most often caused by cardiac

failure. The severity of the disease does not correlate with the size of the goiter, but it may be related to maternal TSI levels.

*Treatment.* The treatment of neonatal thyrotoxicosis is directed toward immediate management of the symptoms and reduction in the amount of thyroid hormone produced. This treatment must be initiated in the newborn or intensive care nursery with adequate cardiopulmonary monitoring and venous access.

Therapy consists of a combination of Lugol's solution (5% iodine and 10% potassium iodide), given as one drop every 8 hours; propylthiouracil, administered as 5 to 10 mg/kg/day; and propranolol, given at a rate of 2 mg/kg/day. Treatment with dexamethasone is helpful in some cases. If no improvement occurs within 24 hours, the doses of Lugol's solution and propylthiouracil should be increased by at least 50%. If evidence of cardiac failure arises, the infant should be digitalized promptly. Adequate caloric intake is vital in these hypermetabolic infants. Serum levels of thyroid hormone must be carefully monitored to ensure adequate therapy and to avoid hypothyroidism. In milder cases, Lugol's solution and propranolol may not be needed.

Long-term complications of neonatal thyrotoxicosis can occur even in patients who receive prompt and adequate treatment. These include premature craniosynostosis and neurodevelopmental defects, particularly intellectual impairment; both may be caused by intrauterine thyrotoxicosis. The intellectual impairment usually correlates with premature craniosynostosis, but a direct effect of thyrotoxicosis on the developing brain cannot be ruled out.

### Acquired Hyperthyroidism

Acquired hyperthyroidism is most often due to Graves' disease (ie, autoimmune thyrotoxicosis). The female to male ratio ranges from 3 : 1 to 5 : 1. There is a familial tendency and an association with HLA types B8 and DR3. Emotional stress as a precipitating factor of thyrotoxicosis has been described frequently.

*Etiology.* The cause of Graves' disease is autonomous hyperfunction of the thyroid gland, stimulated by TSI. TSI levels are elevated in most patients. TSI binds to the TSH receptors on the thyroid cells, producing the stimulatory effect. Graves disease is serologically related to CLT in that antithyroid antibodies may be elevated in patients with Graves' disease and in their unaffected family members. The events that stimulate the production of TSI and their relation to antithyroid antibodies are unknown.

*Diagnosis.* The diagnosis of Graves' disease is based on the combination of clinical findings (Table 144-8) and the characteristic elevations of thyroid hormone levels. The thyroid gland

| TABLE 144-8. Signs and Symptoms of Hyperthyroidism |
|---|
| Goiter |
| Anxiousness, nervousness |
| Tachycardia |
| Widened pulse pressure |
| Increased appetite |
| Weight loss or gain |
| Tremor |
| Proptosis |
| Heat intolerance |
| Increased growth velocity |
| Diarrhea |
| Sleep disturbances |

is almost invariably enlarged, and tachycardia, nervousness, and widened pulse pressure are seen in more than 80% of patients. Most patients experience weight loss, although weight gain may occur because of a significantly increased appetite. Proptosis or exophthalmos is a common finding, but the Graves' ophthalmopathy in children usually is less severe than in adults.

The thyroid hormone profile characteristically shows elevated total $T_4$, free $T_4$, and $T_3$ levels, accompanied by very low or undetectable levels of TSH. In some cases, the $T_3$ level is elevated with a normal level of $T_4$ (ie, $T_3$ toxicosis). The source of $T_3$ in patients with $T_3$ toxicosis is direct secretion by the gland. In these patients, the contribution of $T_3$ secreted by the gland may equal or exceed that of peripheral $T_4$ deiodination to the total circulating $T_3$.

In patients with hyperthyroidism without exophthalmos, it may be difficult to differentiate among early CLT, subacute thyroiditis, and Graves' disease. If TSI levels are not elevated, a radioactive iodine uptake scan aids in the diagnosis. Characteristically, patients with Graves' disease have elevated uptake that is not suppressed with administration of $T_3$. Patients with CLT or subacute thyroiditis generally have normal or decreased uptake of $^{123}I$.

*Treatment.* The three forms of treatment for Graves' disease are medical, surgical, and radioactive iodine ablation. The mainstay of medical management is antithyroid medication, with methimazole (Tapazole) or propylthiouracil. Both are equally effective in decreasing the production of $T_4$ and $T_3$ by the thyroid gland, but propylthiouracil also blocks the peripheral deiodination of $T_4$ to $T_3$. propylthiouracil is not known to significantly decrease thyroid gland secretion of $T_3$ and may therefore not provide significant advantage over methimazole in patients with $T_3$ toxicosis. The dose of propylthiouracil is 5 to 10 mg/kg/day, divided equally into three doses. The dose of methimazole is approximately one-tenth the propylthiouracil dose, and it has the advantage of a longer serum half-life, allowing twice-daily or even single-daily doses. If the symptoms of thyrotoxicosis are particularly bothersome to the patient, they may be alleviated by treatment with propranolol concomitantly with antithyroid medication until the symptoms improve. The patient should become euthyroid within 6 weeks.

The medical therapy of thyrotoxicosis is somewhat controversial. In some centers, the dose of antithyroid medication is increased until the patient becomes hypothyroid, at which time thyroid hormone replacement is added to the regimen. This gives the theoretical advantage of maximal suppression of the gland, minimizing the likelihood of relapse. This theory has been supported by clinical trials (Hashizume, et al, 1991). In other centers, the dose of antithyroid medication is titrated to maintain the patient in a euthyroid state. After the patient becomes euthyroid, treatment is continued for a period of time, usually not less than 1 year, before the child is assessed for remission by a $T_3$ suppression test or by discontinuing antithyroid medication. If relapse occurs, the antithyroid medication can be restarted or alternative treatment instituted.

Approximately 5% to 10% of patients treated with antithyroid medication experience side effects from the medication. Most of these side effects are minor, and include erythematous skin rashes, urticaria, and arthralgias. Granulocytopenia is the most frequently seen serious side effect and is generally heralded by a fever or sore throat. Vasculitis, at times severe, is another serious side effect. If side effects occur, discontinuation of the drug generally reverses the problem. The patient may then be treated with a different antithyroid preparation; however, the same reaction may occur.

If medical treatment must be discontinued because of side effects, frequent relapses, or inability to comply with the treatment schedule, thyroid ablative therapy should be implemented. Sur-

gical subtotal thyroidectomy is effective and has low morbidity when performed by an experienced surgeon. The patient must be euthyroid for surgery, and preoperative treatment with iodides such as Lugol's solution is often recommended to decrease vascularity of the gland. The risks include hypothyroidism (up to 50%), transient hypocalcemia (10% to 20%), and rarely, hypoparathyroidism, recurrent laryngeal nerve damage, or recurrence of thyrotoxicosis. $^{131}I$ ablation has been widely used to treat thyrotoxicosis in adults. Its use in children has been limited because of a theoretical risk of the later development of thyroid or other malignancies. However, the data currently available suggest that $^{131}I$ treatment in childhood or adolescence does not affect the risk of developing thyroidal or nonthyroidal cancers or leukemia and does not increase the risk of birth defects in the patient's offspring. Remission from thyrotoxicosis should occur within several weeks, and it is often followed by permanent hypothyroidism after several months or years.

*Prognosis.* The prognosis for children with Graves' disease is generally good. Evidence suggests that with antithyroid medication alone, remission of Graves' disease, defined as being euthyroid for 1 year after stopping medication, occurs at a rate of approximately 25% every 2 years. In some cases, relapse of hyperthyroidism or spontaneous hypothyroidism may occur after remission.

A rare but life-threatening complication of Graves' disease is thyroid storm, also called thyrotoxic crisis. This is a clinical diagnosis based on the manifestations of exaggerated and uncontrolled hyperthyroidism. Patients generally present with marked hyperthermia and tachycardia and may develop cardiac failure, vomiting, diarrhea, and CNS abnormalities, including confusion, apathy, and coma. Thyroid storm can be precipitated by many events but most often is associated with infection, surgery, or trauma. The therapy includes aggressive antithyroid treatment including propylthiouracil or Tapazole, Lugol's solution, or lithium carbonate; prevention of thyroid hormone action with $\beta$-blockade; antipyretics; support of life-threatening conditions using intravenous hydration, oxygen, and digitalis; and treatment of any underlying infection.

Other causes of hyperthyroxinemia are rare. They include subacute thyroiditis, pituitary resistance to thyroid hormone, familial dysalbuminemias, TBG excess, factitious hyperthyroidism from excessive intake of exogenous thyroid hormone, and TSH-secreting pituitary tumors.

## Thyromegaly

Thyromegaly, which is enlargement of the thyroid gland or goiter, is uncommon in children. Causes include infiltration, inflammation, or stimulation of the gland. The enlargement may be diffuse or nodular (Table 144-9). Enlargement of certain nonthyroidal structures may mimic thyromegaly.

### Diffuse Thyromegaly

Diffuse thyromegaly is most often caused by autoimmune thyroid diseases, including Hashimoto's thyroiditis (ie, CLT) and Graves' disease. Autoimmune thyroid disease accounts for more than 90% of the patients with diffuse thyromegaly. There is a female preponderance among children with diffuse thyromegaly. The cause, diagnosis, and treatment of these two diseases were discussed previously.

Two rarer forms of thyroiditis may also produce diffuse thyromegaly. *Subacute thyroiditis,* presumably caused by a virus, is seen much less frequently in children than in adults. It usually presents with firm, tender enlargement of the gland during or immediately after a viral syndrome involving pharyngitis, fever, myalgia, and fatigue. A painless enlargement of the thyroid gland has been described in this disease. At the time of presentation, thyroid function tests often suggest thyrotoxicosis, with elevated thyroid hormone levels and undetectable TSH levels due to inflammatory destruction of the gland and release of $T_4$ and $T_3$ into the circulation. However, in contrast to Graves' disease, the 24-hour uptake of radioactive iodine is very low.

After the hyperthyroid phase of several weeks to months, there is a recovery phase that may last several months. During this phase, the thyroid function tests reveal chemical hypothyroidism, with decreased serum $T_4$ and elevated TSH levels and an abnormally high radioactive iodine uptake. After the hypothyroid phase, the patient usually recovers completely with normal thyroid function tests and a gland of normal size and consistency. In rare cases, permanent hypothyroidism has been described. Antithyroid antibodies may be measurable during the acute and hypothyroid phases but generally disappear after recovery.

Treatment includes anti-inflammatory therapy, including aspirin and possibly glucocorticoids, during the acute phase. If the patient is disturbed by the symptoms of hyperthyroidism, propranolol may be added, but treatment with antithyroid medication is not indicated. During the recovery phase, hypothyroidism should be treated with Synthroid for several months, at which time the dose is tapered and serum $T_4$ and TSH levels are remeasured.

*Acute (suppurative) thyroiditis* is a rare cause of diffuse thyromegaly, especially in the Unites States. It is caused by a bacterial infection of the gland and may be unilateral or bilateral. Most cases occur during or after an upper respiratory tract infection. The most common organisms cultured from an acutely infected thyroid gland are *Staphylococcus aureus* and *Streptococcus hemolyticus* or *S pneumoniae*.

The patient presents with acute onset of fever, chills, sore throat, and dysphagia and with an extremely tender and enlarged gland. Thyroid function tests are usually normal, including radioactive iodine uptake, and antithyroid antibodies are undetectable. Early treatment with parenteral antibiotics, after aspiration for culture, is necessary to avoid abscess formation and rupture. With prompt and aggressive treatment, full recovery is expected. In some children, acute thyroiditis has been associated with a fistula of the piriform sinus. In these patients, the left lobe of the gland is more often involved. In certain parts of the world diffuse thyromegaly due to iodine deficiency (ie, endemic goiter) is still common, but supplementation of dietary salt with iodine has made iodine deficiency a rare problem in North America.

In some cases of diffuse thyromegaly, particularly in adolescent girls, no cause can be determined and the diagnosis of *idiopathic (simple) goiter* is made. Other causes of enlargement of the thyroid gland (see Table 144-9) are ingestion of a goitrogen including antithyroid medication, other drugs, and certain foods, familial dyshormonogenesis, and rare pituitary abnormalities, such as pituitary resistance to thyroid hormone or a TSH-secreting pituitary adenoma.

## Nodular Thyromegaly

Nodular thyromegaly, an enlargement of one or more areas of the thyroid gland, may be unilateral or bilateral and is usually nontender. Some causes of nodular thyromegaly are listed in Table 144-9. Certain nonthyroidal tissues may present with an enlargement in the area of the thyroid gland, including lymphadenopathy, cysts (eg, thyroglossal duct, branchial cleft), neurofibroma, hemangioma, and lymphangioma.

Thyroid nodules are rare in children. The most common cause of asymmetric enlargement of the thyroid gland is Hashimoto's thyroiditis. However, the incidence of malignant neoplasms is higher in children's nodules than in adults' nodules. A compre-

### TABLE 144-9. Causes of Thyromegaly

| Diffuse | Nodular |
|---|---|
| Hashimoto's thyroiditis | Hashimoto's thyroiditis |
| Thyrotoxicosis | Thyroid cyst |
|   Graves' disease | Thyroid adenoma |
|   Thyroiditis |   Hyperfunctional (hot) |
|   TSH-secreting adenoma |   Hypofunctional (cold) |
|   Pituitary resistance | Thyroid carcinoma |
| Goitrogen exposure |   Papillary |
| Dyshormonogenesis |   Follicular |
| Iodine deficiency |   Mixed papillary or follicular |
| (endemic) |   Anaplastic |
| Idiopathic (simple) goiter |   Medullary |
| Acute, subacute thyroiditis | Nonthyroidal masses |

*TSH*, thyroid-stimulating hormone.

hensive and rapid diagnostic evaluation of solitary or multiple thyroid nodules is imperative.

The history should include questions about previous irradiation to the head, neck, or thorax for any reason, because this has been shown to increase the risk for later development of thyroid neoplasia. This risk is proportional to the dose of irradiation, and the neoplasm may appear anywhere between 3 and 35 years later. Rapid and painless enlargement of the nodule may suggest neoplasia. If the nodule is tender or intermittently painful, it is more likely to be caused by acute or subacute thyroiditis or a hemorrhagic cyst. The risk of malignancy is higher in solitary than in multiple nodules. Symptoms that suggest hypothyroidism or hyperthyroidism are less likely to occur with malignant than with benign lesions.

Family history is especially important in the case of multiple endocrine neoplasia syndromes, which are associated with medullary carcinoma of the thyroid gland, multiple mucosal neuromas, pheochromocytoma, and hyperparathyroidism.

Physical examination of the neck must include careful palpation of the gland and its surrounding structures, including local lymph nodes. Consistency, movability, and tenderness of the nodule must be evaluated.

The diagnostic evaluation of thyroid nodularity must include blood and radiologic tests of thyroid function. Blood tests should include thyroid hormone and TSH levels (most often normal in malignant lesions), antithyroid and antibodies (in CLT), and calcitonin levels before and after pentagastrin stimulation if medullary carcinoma of the thyroid is suspected. Thyroglobulin levels, although helpful in the follow-up of treated thyroid carcinoma as a marker for recurrence, are not always helpful in the initial evaluation.

Radiologic studies are of prime importance in the evaluation of thyroid nodules. Radiographs may show calcification of the gland or local lymph nodes or demonstrate pulmonary metastases. Ultrasound can differentiate solid from cystic nodules. Radioisotope scanning can assess the functional activity of the nodule. A hyperfunctional (hot) nodule is more likely to be caused by an adenoma, thyroiditis, or thyrotoxicosis than by a carcinoma. A hypofunctional (cold) nodule is more likely to be malignant or nonthyroidal. A solitary isofunctional (warm) nodule is more likely to be benign than malignant.

In most pediatric centers, a definite tissue diagnosis, made by needle biopsy or surgical excision, is recommended for all thyroid nodules. In the case of warm nodules, a trial of thyroid hormone suppression may be undertaken in an attempt to shrink the nodule. If the nodule enlarges or fails to decrease in size, surgical exploration is necessary.

The prognosis for children with differentiated thyroid carcinomas is generally good, but because of the slow tumor growth and sometimes delayed appearance of metastases, life-long follow-up is mandatory. The survival time of patients with undifferentiated (ie, anaplastic) thyroid carcinomas is usually only 6 to 12 months. The clinical course of medullary carcinoma of the thyroid varies widely and is difficult to predict at the time of diagnosis.

## Selected Readings

Ballabio M, Nicolini U, Jowett T, et al. Maturation of thyroid function in normal human fetuses. Clin Endocrinol 1989;31:565.

Burger AG. Effects of certain pharmacologic agents on the peripheral metabolism of thyroxine. In: Ingbar SH, Braverman LE, eds. Werner's The Thyroid: a fundamental and clinical text. Philadelphia: JB Lippincott, 1986:351.

Delange F, Dalhem A, Bourdoux P, et al. Increased risk of primary hypothyroidism in preterm infants. J Pediatr 1984;105:462.

Fisher DA. The thyroid. In: Rudolph AM, ed. Pediatrics. Norwalk, CT: Appleton & Lange, 1987:1504.

Fisher DA. The thyroid. In: Kaplan SA, ed. Clinical pediatric endocrinology. Philadelphia: WB Saunders, 1990:95.

Fisher DA, Vanderschueran-Lodeweyckx M. Laboratory tests for thyroid diagnosis in infants and children. In: Delange F, Fisher DA, Malvaux P, eds. Pediatric thyroidology. Basel: S Karger, 1985:127.

Hashizume K, Ichikawa K, Sakurai A, et al. Administration of thyroxine in treated Graves' disease: effects on the level of antibodies to thyroid-stimulating hormone receptors and on the risk of recurrence of hyperthyroidism. N Engl J Med 1991;324:947.

Hung W. Thyroid nodules and thyroid cancer. In: Delange F, Fisher DA, Malvaux P, eds. Pediatric thyroidology. Basel: S Karger, 1985:271.

Kaplan MM. Interactions between drugs and thyroid hormones. Thyroid Today 1981;4:5.

LaFranchi SH. Hypothyroidism, congenital and acquired. In: Kaplan SA, ed. Clinical pediatric and adolescent endocrinology. Philadelphia: WB Saunders, 1982:82.

Lippe BM, Landaw EM, Kaplan SA. Hyperthyroidism in children treated with long term medical therapy: twenty-five percent remission every two years. J Clin Endocrinol Metab 1987;64:1241.

Thorpe-Beeston JG, Nicolaides KH, Felton CV, et al. Maturation of the secretion of thyroid hormone and thyroid stimulating hormone in the fetus. N Engl J Med 1991;324:532.

*Principles and Practice of Pediatrics, Second Edition.*
edited by Frank A. Oski et al. J. B. Lippincott Company, Philadelphia © 1994.

## CHAPTER 145
# *The Adrenal Cortex*

Patricia A. Donohoue

## NORMAL ADRENAL DEVELOPMENT AND STEROID HORMONE SYNTHESIS

The fetal adrenal cortex develops from coelomic mesothelium near the developing gonads. The cortex then separates from the gonads, which migrate to their adult positions. For this reason, rests of adrenal cortical tissue may appear along the paths of migration or near the gonads in adults. By the 6th week of gestation, steroid-producing cells appear in the cortex, and by the 10th week, the fetal zone (comprising 80% of the total volume) and the adult (definitive) zone are producing steroid hormones in response to adrenocorticotropic hormone (ACTH) stimulation. The fetal zone, whose major products are estrogen and androgen precursors, begins to degenerate by the 8th month of gestation. At that time, the adult zone begins to differentiate into a mature adult cortex that secretes three families of steroid hormones: mineralocorticoids, glucocorticoids, and androgens. This process of differentiation is not completed until approximately 3 years of age.

The adult adrenal cortex constitutes about 90% of the mature gland and is composed of three zones. The outermost zone, the zona glomerulosa, accounts for 15% of the cortical volume and is the site of mineralocorticoid synthesis. The zona fasciculata constitutes 75% of the cortex, and the reticularis, the innermost zone, constitutes 10%. The zona fasciculata and zona reticularis are one functional unit, involved in glucocorticoid and androgen biosynthesis. The zona reticularis secretes steroids under basal conditions, and the zona fasciculata stores lipids for stress steroidogenesis.

All three groups of steroid hormones are produced from cholesterol, which is supplied by the circulation or produced endogenously. Under the stimulation of the anterior pituitary hormone ACTH, cholesterol is converted to pregnenolone. This is the rate-limiting step in steroid hormone biosynthesis. Pregnenolone serves as the precursor for all three families of adrenal steroid hormones (Fig 145-1).

ACTH release is controlled centrally by the hypothalamic hormone, corticotropin-releasing hormone (CRH). ACTH secretion may also be under the influence of immune system. Normal ACTH secretion occurs in a diurnal pattern, which results in the normal diurnal fluctuation in serum cortisol levels: highest in the early morning and lowest in the evening. The serum cortisol level completes the feedback loop by controlling hypothalamic CRH secretion and pituitary ACTH secretion. Serotonin stimulates and norepinephrine inhibits hypothalamic CRH secretion. The daily cortisol secretion rate is approximately $12.1 \pm 3$ mg/m$^2$ of body surface area. The total daily cortisol production increases with growth. Based on the daily average production of cortisol and the potencies of various pharmacologic glucocorticoid preparations, recommendations can be made about the average daily dose of each that would be required for physiological replacement (Table 145-1). Many preparations also have a mineralocorticoid effect. In times of physiological stress, it is recommended that cortisol replacement doses be increased.

Most cortisol circulates in the blood bound to cortisol-binding globulin (CBG), also known as transcortin, an $\alpha$-globulin secreted by the liver. It is the free fraction of cortisol that is biologically active. Estrogens increase CBG levels, and liver disease and the nephrotic syndrome are associated with decreased CBG levels. However, free cortisol levels are unaffected by these conditions.

The major physiological metabolic effects of cortisol are glycogen synthesis, gluconeogenesis, fat catabolism, and protein catabolism. At high levels, glucocorticoids induce a wide variety of metabolic changes, including immunosuppression, osteoporosis, glucose intolerance, increased gastric secretion, and altered central nervous system (CNS) function.

Glucocorticoid (eg, cortisol) secretion plays a central role in the hypothalamic-pituitary-adrenal axis, and mineralocorticoid (eg, aldosterone) secretion is controlled mainly by the renin-angiotensin system. This is mediated through the cells of the zona glomerulosa, which have specific membrane receptors for angiotensin II. Stimulation of the adrenal with ACTH produces only a transient increase in aldosterone levels. The average daily al-

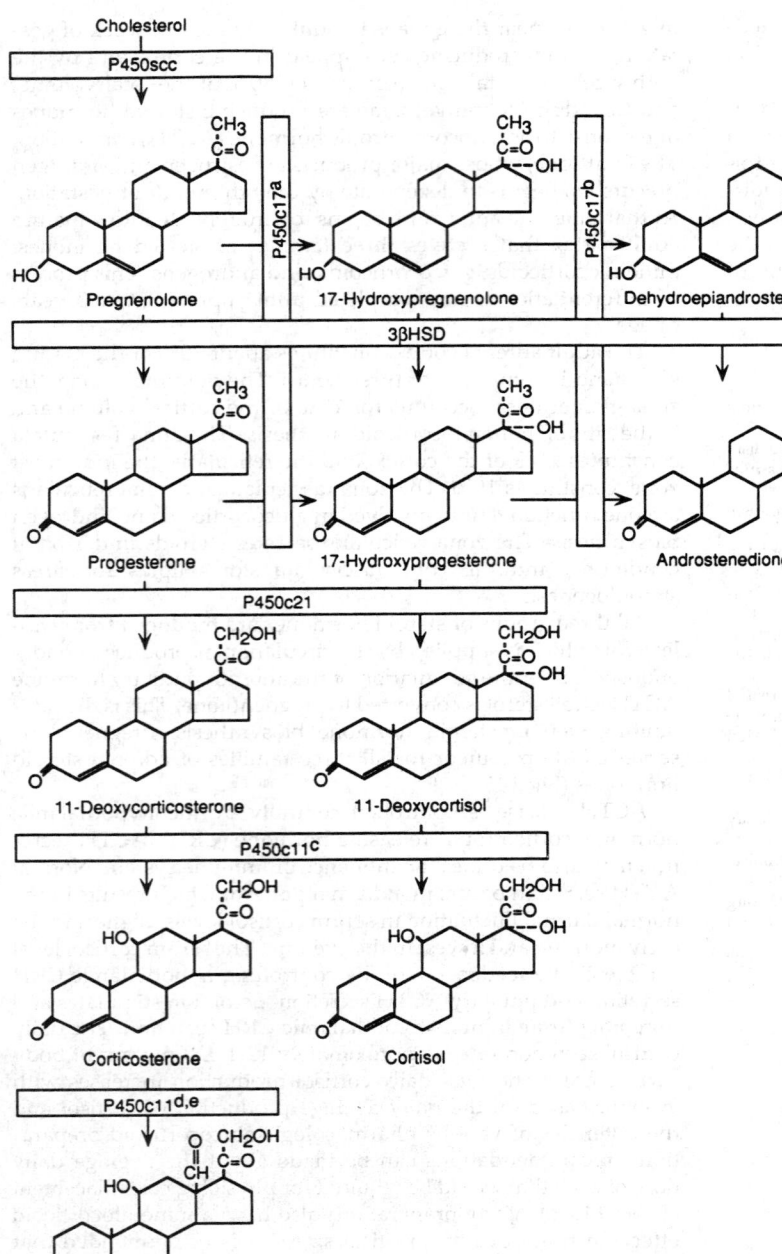

**Figure 145-1.** Adrenal steroid biosynthetic pathways. Enzyme names: P450scc, 20-hydroxylase, 22-hydroxylase, 20,22-desmolase; P450c17, [a]17α-hydroxylase, [b]17,20-desmolase (lyase); 3β-HSD, 3β-hydroxysteroid dehydrogenase, $\Delta^5\Delta^4$-isomerase; P45c21, 21-hydroxylase; P45c11, [c]11β-hydroxylase, [d]18-hydroxylase (CMOI), [e]18-dehydrogenase (oxidase) (CMOII); CMOI, corticosterone methyl oxidase I; CMOII, corticosterone methyl oxidase II. The 20-hydroxylase, 22-hydroxylase, and 20,22-desmolase are activities of the same P450scc enzyme. Both 17α-hydroxylase and 17,20-desmolase activities are properties of the same P450c17 enzyme. However, 11β-hydroxylase and CMO activities are properties of two different isozymes of P450c11, encoded by different genes. In addition, several isoforms of 3β-HSD exist.

dosterone secretion rate is not related to body surface area and is similar for infants and adults (approximately 100 μg/day). The major physiological effect of mineralocorticoids is exerted at the level of the distal convoluted tubule, where they promote sodium retention and potassium excretion.

The factors that control adrenal androgen secretion are less well understood. In prepubertal children, the production of adrenal androgens is very low. At puberty, their production increases, and normal adrenarche occurs. The most potent adrenal androgen is androstenedione, which is converted outside the adrenal gland to the more potent androgen, testosterone. At very high levels, dehydroepiandrosterone, a weak androgen, may exert androgenic effects. In pubertal and adult males, the adrenal gland contributes little to the total androgen production. However, in pubertal and adult females, at least 50% of the circulating testosterone is derived from adrenal androstenedione.

## TESTS OF ADRENOCORTICAL FUNCTION

### Static Tests

The static tests of adrenocortical function provide a limited amount of information and usually must be accompanied by dynamic testing in the diagnostic evaluation of adrenal disorders. Normal values for some adrenal steroid levels and responses to dynamic tests are given in Table 145-2.

The *serum cortisol level* is measured by radioimmunoassay and is interpretable only if the time of day that the sample was obtained is known. If the cortisol level is subnormal at 8 a.m., the time of a normal peak, hypocortisolism is suspected. However, this test does not discriminate among primary adrenal failure, ACTH deficiency, or defect in the biosynthesis of cortisol. A low cortisol level late in the day is normal and is of little value in the

### TABLE 145-1. Glucocorticoid Dosages and Relative Potencies

| Preparation | Physiologic Replacement Dose* |
|---|---|
| Hydrocortisone | 12.5 mg/m²/day, IM or IV |
| | 25.0 mg/m²/day, PO |
| Cortisone acetate | 16 mg/m²/day, IM or IV |
| | 32 mg/m²/day, PO |

| Steroid Preparation | Effect† Glucocorticoid (mg) | Mineralocorticoid (mg) |
|---|---|---|
| Cortisone | 100 | 100 |
| Hydrocortisone | 80 | 80 |
| Prednisone | 20 | 100 |
| Prednisolone | 20 | 100 |
| Methylprednisolone | 16 | No effect |
| 9α-Fluorocortisol | 5 | 0.2 |
| Dexamethasone | 2 | No effect |

\* Recommended doses for daily physiological replacement of glucocorticoid. The actual optimal dose must be titrated for each patient.

† Relative glucocorticoid and mineralocorticoid potencies. The dose given for each preparation represents that which has anti-inflammatory effect equivalent to 100 mg of cortisone.

assessment of adrenal failure. However, if elevated in a nonstressed patient, it may indicate absence of the normal pattern of diurnal variation, which is often seen in Cushing's syndrome. Because the serum cortisol level rises briskly in response to stress such as fever, trauma, surgery, fear, or anxiety, single determinations of cortisol levels cannot reliably be used to diagnose hypercortisolism.

Determination of the *serum ACTH level* is useful only if accompanied by other tests of adrenal function. The diurnal variation in cortisol levels is preceded by similar fluctuations in ACTH levels. An extremely elevated ACTH level in the setting of subnormal serum cortisol levels suggests primary adrenal failure. However, because ACTH mediates the rise in serum cortisol in response to stress, its levels are highly variable.

Mineralocorticoid status is assessed by measurement of *plasma renin activity* (PRA), which is elevated in mineralocorticoid deficiency. PRA is a measure of the rate of conversion of angiotensinogen to angiotensin I. Factors such as blood pressure, posture, sodium intake, and renal function affect PRA and must be considered in the interpretation of the test result. However, the PRA assay may be useful in monitoring the adequacy of mineralocorticoid replacement therapy. Plasma levels or urinary excretion of aldosterone and deoxycorticosterone also are useful for assessing mineralocorticoid secretion.

Plasma *adrenal androgen levels* are less affected by physiological conditions such as stress and state of hydration than are other static tests of adrenocortical function. They are useful in the evaluation of hyperandrogenic states due to a variety of causes, such

### TABLE 145-2. Normal Plasma and Urinary Steroid Hormone Levels With Static and Dynamic Tests

| Test | Values |
|---|---|
| **Resting Levels** | |
| Plasma cortisol* | 8 a.m.: 11 ± 2.5 µg/dL; 8 p.m.: 3.5 ± 1.5 µg/dL |
| Urinary 17-hydroxycorticosteroids (17-OHCS) | 2.9 ± 1.2 mg/m²/24 h |
| Urinary free cortisol | 25–65 µg/m²/24 h |
| **Adrenal Capacity** | |
| IV test: 25 USP U Acthar over 6 h | Plasma cortisol: 40 ± 5 µg/dL at 6 h |
| IV test: 0.25 mg Cortrosyn stat | Plasma cortisol: 32 ± 4 µg/dL at 2 h |
| IM test: 20 U/m² Acthar gel every 8 h for 3 days | Urinary 17-OHCS: 85 ± 15 mg/m²/24 h after 3 days |
| **ACTH Capacity†** | |
| Oral metyrapone: 300 mg/m² every 4 h for 24 h | Urinary 17-OHCS increase >9 mg/m²/24 h |
| Oral metyrapone: 300 mg/m² at midnight | 8 a.m.: 11-deoxycortisol, 7–22 µg/dL |
| IV metyrapone: 500 mg/m² (max, 1 g) over 4 h | Plasma 11-deoxycortisol: 5–15 µg/dL at 5 h, with plasma cortisol level decreasing to near zero |
| Regular insulin 0.1 U/kg iv or glucagon 0.1 mg/kg im | Rise in serum cortisol >20 µg/dL, or a two-fold increase from baseline |
| **Pituitary Suppression Test** | |
| Low-dose dexamethasone: 1.25 mg/m²/24 h (in 3 divided doses) for 3 d | Urinary 17-OHCS <1 mg/m²/24 h or decrease in plasma or urinary androgens in hyperandrogenic states |
| High-dose dexamethasone: same, with 3.75 mg/m²/24 h | Same |

\* Stress or anxiety may cause elevation of cortisol levels far above the stated normal range.

† Metyrapone will no longer be available for diagnostic testing in the near future. Insulin-induced hypoglycemia or glucagon stimulation will be the tests of choice for ACTH capacity. The specifics of these tests are detailed in Vandershueren-Lodenweyck M, et al. J Pediatr 1974;85:182.

as adrenal tumors and adrenal enzyme deficiencies. However, elevated levels must be investigated further with the appropriate stimulation or suppression tests.

Plasma levels of a number of *steroid precursors and adrenal androgens* are helpful in the diagnosis and therapeutic management of the inherited steroidogenic enzyme deficiencies (eg, congenital adrenal hyperplasia). Normal values for these levels depend on the reference laboratory, but age and gender differences are reflected in the representative set of normal values provided in Table 145-3.

Measurement of urinary steroids and their metabolites is a helpful adjunct to determination of plasma steroid levels. The 24-hour excretion of *urinary 17-hydroxycorticosteroids* is a measure of daily glucocorticoid production. The 24-hour *urinary free cortisol* is widely used in the assessment of Cushing's syndrome. The 24-hour excretion of *urinary 17-ketosteroids* reflects the total daily adrenal androgen production and is useful in the diagnostic evaluation and assessment of treatment adequacy in hyperandrogenic states.

## Dynamic Tests

### ACTH Stimulation Test

The ACTH stimulation test is used to evaluate the adrenal gland's response to pharmacologic levels of ACTH. The intravenous short ACTH test is used for assessing cortisol production by a failing adrenal gland. Serum cortisol levels are measured 60 and sometimes 120 minutes after the rapid intravenous infusion of synthetic 0.25 to 0.5 mg ACTH (Cortrosyn) or during and after an 8-hour infusion. A subnormal response in a patient who has not received glucocorticoid therapy may indicate primary adrenal failure (ie, Addison's disease) and must be followed by a prolonged stimulation test with intramuscular ACTH. A patient who fails to respond to a 2-week course of long-acting intramuscular ACTH (ACTHAR gel) has primary adrenal failure and is committed to life-long glucocorticoid replacement therapy in addition to mineralocorticoid therapy, because all steroid-producing cells in the adrenal gland are ultimately affected in this disease.

The intravenous ACTH test is used to assess the adrenal gland's recovery after a prolonged course (>1 month) of pharmacologic doses of glucocorticoids. A subnormal response reflects the loss of ability to respond to ACTH stimulation after prolonged suppression of ACTH secretion. Unlike patients with Addison's disease, these patients should have normal mineralocorticoid production, and they should have a normal cortisol response to a 2-week course of ACTHAR gel.

The intravenous ACTH test is also useful in the assessment of adrenal enzyme deficiencies, especially 21-hydroxylase deficiency. The cortisol precursors progesterone and 17-hydroxyprogesterone are measured before and 30 minutes (and sometimes 60 minutes) after a rapid infusion of ACTH. The rate of rise is calculated and compared with normal ranges according to age, gender, and stage of the menstrual cycle. This test should be preformed during the follicular phase of the cycle in menstruating females.

### ACTH Secretion Tests

Several dynamic tests are available for the assessment of ACTH secretion in patients with suspected hypopituitarism. Perhaps the most sensitive test of ACTH release is *insulin-induced hypoglycemia*. After an intravenous bolus of regular insulin, serial measurements of blood glucose, cortisol, and growth hormone levels are made. Symptomatic hypoglycemia is the desired end point, but changes in level of consciousness must be treated with prompt administration of intravenous dextrose. The test is not recommended for infants because of the risk of CNS damage from hypoglycemia.

The *glucagon stimulation test* is more appropriate in the younger age group. After an intramuscular injection of glucagon, the blood glucose level initially rises and then drops rapidly because of the release of endogenous insulin. Serum cortisol and growth hormone levels should increase in response to this fall in blood glucose.

The *metyrapone test* may be used in the assessment of ACTH secretory ability. Metyrapone blocks the activity of the enzyme 11-hydroxylase, which is needed to convert 11-deoxycortisol to cortisol (see Fig 145-1). When cortisol levels drop, ACTH secretion is stimulated, increasing the production of cortisol precursors. This can be measured by a rise in serum levels of ACTH and 11-deoxycortisol and in urinary 17-hydroxycorticosteroids. The ACTH-stimulated gland eventually overrides the enzymatic block, allowing cortisol production to occur. However, patients must be closely observed during this test, because acute adrenal insufficiency may be precipitated if there is marked ACTH deficiency.

In patients who have overproduction of glucocorticoids or adrenal androgens, it is important to assess whether there is autonomous or suppressible hypersecretion. The *dexamethasone suppression test* is useful in these cases and can be administered as a low-dose or a high-dose test. After oral administration of dexamethasone, a potent glucocorticoid, pituitary ACTH secretion should be inhibited. Patients with elevated adrenal androgen levels secondary to biosynthetic block have decreased androgen production while ACTH stimulation is suppressed. In patient with Cushing's syndrome due to an autonomous ACTH-producing tumor, such as a pulmonary carcinoma, hypercortisolism does not respond to dexamethasone.

---

**TABLE 145-3.** Normal Values for Adrenal Androgens and Commonly Measured Cortisol Precursors

| Hormone | Adult Males* | Adult Females | Pregnant Females | Females at Delivery | Umbilical Cord | Prepubertal Children (<7 y) |
|---|---|---|---|---|---|---|
| Androstenedione | 114 ± 21 | 180 ± 58 | 249 ± 82 | 387 ± 176 | 126 ± 58 | 21 ± 12 |
| Dehydroepiandrosterone | 553 ± 178 | 534 ± 157 | 363 ± 233 | 1,016 ± 806 | 350 ± 150 | 39 ± 28 |
| 17-OH-progesterone | 95 ± 30 | 60 ± 20† / 270 ± 60‡ | 350 ± 70 | 550 ± 75 | 1,520 ± 350 | 35 ± 25 |
| Progesterone | 35 ± 5 | 58 ± 22† / 1,330 ± 550‡ | 2,800 ± 1,100 | | | 22 ± 5 (m) / 23 ± 6 (f) |

\* Values (ng/dL) in mean ± SD.
† Follicular phase.
‡ Luteal phase.

## ADRENOCORTICAL ABNORMALITIES

### Congenital Adrenal Hyperplasia

Congenital adrenal hyperplasia (CAH) is a family of diseases caused by an inherited deficiency of any of the enzymes necessary for the biosynthesis of cortisol (see Fig 145-1). These enzymes, with the exception of 3β-hydroxysteroid dehydrogenase, are members of the cytochrome P-450 family. The cytochromes P-450 are microsomal or mitochondrial terminal oxidases involved in electron transport and require NAD and flavoproteins as co-factors. Deficiency of any one of these enzymes results in decreased production of cortisol and increased secretion of ACTH. With stimulation by ACTH, the adrenal cortex becomes hyperplastic, and steroid precursors preceding the enzymatic block accumulate. These accumulated precursors are shunted, if possible, to a steroidogenic pathway that is unaffected by the enzymatic block. Each particular form of CAH is manifested by the clinical features produced by deficient end products (eg, glucocorticoid, mineralocorticoid, androgen) and by accumulated or shunted precursors (eg, mineralocorticoid or androgen excess). CAH is inherited as an autosomal recessive disorder and has an equal sex distribution. A summary of these diseases and their clinical features is given in Table 145-4. The severity of the clinical features varies among families.

The most common form of CAH is caused by 21-hydroxylase (21-OH) deficiency, accounting for more than 90% of the cases. The most severe form, the salt-losing form, is caused by complete absence of 21-OH activity and results in cortisol and mineralocorticoid deficiencies. Affected girls have ambiguous genitalia at birth due to hypersecretion of adrenal androgens, which are converted to testosterone. Affected and untreated girls and boys usually present with symptoms of acute adrenal insufficiency, known as a salt-losing crisis, at 1 to 3 weeks of age.

The simple virilizing form is caused by a partial 21-OH deficiency. Patients with this disease produce adequate amounts of cortisol and aldosterone under the stimulation of excess ACTH and elevated PRA levels, but at the expense of excess androgen production. Girls may present with ambiguous genitalia or post-natal virilization, and boys may present with suspected isosexual precocious puberty, although the testes remain prepubertal in size. The combined frequencies of the salt-losing and simple virilizing forms approximates 1 in 10,000 to 13,000 births among Caucasians. The incidence among Asian and black populations is somewhat lower.

A mild degree of 21-OH deficiency, the attenuated form, manifests as hirsutism or menstrual irregularities in adolescent or adult females. In an asymptomatic form, there are biochemical abnormalities consistent with 21-OH deficiency, but no clinical features are evident.

### Diagnosis

The diagnosis of CAH due to 21-OH deficiency is made when elevated levels of hormones preceding the enzymatic block (see Fig 145-1) are demonstrated in a child with the typical clinical findings. A female infant with virilization of the external genitalia or a male infant with a salt-losing crisis (dehydration with hyponatremia, hyperkalemia, and acidosis) has elevated plasma 17-hydroxyprogesterone, progesterone, and androstenedione levels, increased urinary 17-ketosteroids, elevated PRA and ACTH levels, and low or undetectable serum cortisol. Older children who present with inappropriate virilization (ie, simple virilizing form) have normal cortisol and electrolyte levels, but with the same elevated hormone levels as described for the younger group. These children also have growth acceleration and advanced skeletal age due to the effects of sex steroids.

In the salt-losing form, treatment is first directed at correcting the life-threatening metabolic abnormalities of adrenal crisis by correction of dehydration with intravenous saline and dextrose, correction of hyperkalemia with insulin and glucose if necessary, and after a blood sample is obtained for steroid hormone measurements, glucocorticoid replacement with the rapidly acting

**TABLE 145-4. Clinical Features of the Different Forms of Congenital Adrenal Hyperplasia at Diagnosis**

| Deficient Enzyme | Clinical Form | Elevated Levels | Abnormal Sexual Development |
|---|---|---|---|
| **21-Hydroxylase** Complete deficiency | Salt-losing | Urinary 17-ketosteroids, plasma 17-hydroxyprogesterone, plasma androstenedione, plasma renin activity (PRA), ACTH | Females: ambiguous genitalia |
| Partial deficiency | Simple virilizing | Same as above | Females: ambiguous genitalia Males and females: postnatal virilization |
| Mild deficiency | Attenuated | Same, but milder elevations | Female adolescents: hirsutism, menstrual irregularities |
| **11-Hydroxylase** | Hypertensive | Urinary 17-hydroxycorticosteroids, urinary 17-ketosteroids, plasma 11-deoxycorticosterone (DOC), plasma 11-deoxycortisol, plasma androstenedione | Females: ambiguous genitalia Males and females: postnatal virilization |
| **17-Hydroxylase** | Hypertensive | Plasma DOC, plasma corticosterone | Males: absent or incomplete virilization |
| **3β-Hydroxysteroid dehydrogenase** Complete deficiency | Salt-losing | Plasma dehydroepiandrosterone (DHA), 17-hydroxypregnenolone, PRA, ACTH | Males and females: ambiguous genitalia |
| Partial deficiency | Mild | Plasma DHA, 17-hydroxypregnenolone | Female adolescents: hirsutism |
| **Cholesterol side-chain cleavage** | Salt-losing, "lipoid" | No steroids produced | Males: absent virilization |

intravenous glucocorticoid, hydrocortisone, at a "stress" dosage, which is three times the calculated dose for daily physiological replacement. Because parenteral mineralocorticoid preparations are no longer available, prolonged treatment with high-dose glucocorticoids is necessary until oral mineralocorticoids can be tolerated. This allows enough mineralocorticoid effect from the glucocorticoid preparation to achieve a lowering of the serum potassium concentration and adequate urinary sodium retention. In many cases, supplemental sodium chloride must be added for infants to maintain normal serum electrolyte levels.

### Treatment

Treatment with glucocorticoids promptly decreases the ACTH level and the excess androgen production. Children with the salt-losing form of CAH have a lifelong requirement for glucocorticoid replacement but may tolerate discontinuation of daily mineralocorticoid therapy when they reach adulthood. Careful titration of glucocorticoid therapy is necessary, because the balance between undertreatment (ie, androgen excess) and overtreatment (ie, cushingoid features) may be within a narrow dosage range and varies significantly from patient to patient.

For the simple virilizing form of 21-OH deficiency, mineralocorticoid therapy is not needed. However, mineralocorticoid supplementation has been successfully employed to decrease the required glucocorticoid dose for adequate suppression of adrenal androgen levels. Glucocorticoid therapy must be titrated for optimal results, as in the salt-losing form.

In treating both forms of this disease, as for all children receiving glucocorticoid therapy, the dosage must be increased during times of stress and the parents must be trained to administer intramuscular hydrocortisone during times when the child cannot take the medication orally.

### Prognosis

The prognosis for children with 21-OH deficiency is good with careful follow-up and titration of hormonal replacement therapy. Some degree of morbidity is associated with surgical correction of the external genitalia in girls, and this may be significant if multiple surgical procedures are needed. Fertility is normal in males with the salt-losing form, but females with this form may have decreased fertility, for unknown reasons. In the simple virilizing form, fertility is unaffected in adequately treated males and females.

### Prenatal Diagnosis

The prenatal diagnosis of 21-OH deficiency is available for families at risk. The diagnosis is based on the presence of elevated amniotic fluid levels of 17-hydroxyprogesterone combined with HLA typing of fetal cells. The genes for 21-OH lie within the HLA complex on chromosome 6 and are inherited with the HLA complex. If the HLA haplotypes of a previously affected sibling are known and no HLA recombination has occurred, the 21-OH status of the fetus can be determined by the HLA type. In some centers, chorionic villus biopsy specimens can be analyzed for HLA and by hybridization with DNA probes for the HLA and 21-OH genes, allowing prenatal diagnosis much earlier in pregnancy.

### Prenatal Treatment

Prenatal treatment has proved effective in preventing the development of ambiguous genitalia in females, but only if it is instituted early in the first trimester. A mother at risk is treated with dexamethasone until amniocentesis can provide information about the genetic sex and HLA type of the fetus. The dose of dexamethasone required for adequate suppression of amniotic fluid levels of 17-hydroxyprogesterone may produce maternal cushingoid features.

It is possible to test unaffected siblings for 21-OH deficiency carrier status to provide genetic counseling. In response to an intravenous ACTH stimulation test, heterozygotes have normal baseline levels with an exaggerated increase in levels of the steroid precursors progesterone and 17-hydroxyprogesterone. Determination of HLA types confirms the biochemical findings.

Other causes of CAH occur rarely and are not discussed here in detail. Some features of these forms are listed in Table 145-4. The principles of treatment are similar, although the clinical presentations vary widely from salt-losing to hypertensive and from abnormal virilization in females to inadequate virilization in males. Although prenatal diagnosis based on biochemical testing is available for other forms of CAH, 21-OH deficiency is the only HLA-linked form.

## Hypofunction of the Adrenal Cortex

Hypofunction of the adrenal cortex is rare in childhood and may be primary or secondary to ACTH deficiency. Adrenal insufficiency due to enzymatic defects in cortisol biosynthesis was discussed earlier in the section on congenital adrenal hyperplasia.

### Primary Adrenal Insufficiency

Primary adrenal insufficiency or failure is most often due to Addison's disease. The most common cause of Addison's disease is autoimmune destruction of the adrenal cortex, as is seen in the autoimmune polyglandular syndromes. Approximately 45% of patients with autoimmune Addison's disease (ie, caused by antiadrenal antibodies) develop one or more other autoimmune endocrinopathies, most often thyroid disease. Other, rarer causes of primary adrenal failure are congenital adrenal hypoplasia, bilateral adrenal hemorrhage (as in the Waterhouse-Friderichsen syndrome), trauma, thrombosis, infection (eg, tuberculosis), destruction due to tumor metastases, or degeneration, as is seen in adrenoleukodystrophy.

In primary adrenal failure, there is decreased or absent production of all three groups of adrenal steroid hormones. In most cases, the signs and symptoms of adrenal insufficiency develop slowly, particularly the hyperpigmentation associated with increased ACTH. These features are listed in Table 145-5.

The diagnosis is based on demonstration of elevated ACTH levels combined with decreased or absent cortisol and mineralocorticoid production. The fasting 8 a.m. cortisol level is low and fails to rise with ACTH stimulation. The fasting glucose value may be low, and hyponatremia with hyperkalemia may be present. PRA is usually elevated. Adrenal androgen levels may be below normal in adolescent patients. Antiadrenal antibody levels should be measured, and antibodies to other endocrine glands.

Treatment includes physiological replacement with glucocorticoid and mineralocorticoid. Glucocorticoid dosage must be increased during times of stress.

### Secondary Adrenocortical Insufficiency

Secondary adrenocortical insufficiency is most often due to ACTH deficiency. Rarely, resistance to ACTH may occur.

ACTH deficiency may be due to idiopathic hypopituitarism (congenital), congenital malformations of the pituitary or hypothalamus, destruction of the pituitary or hypothalamus (infection, hemorrhage, tumor, irradiation, infiltrative disease), or iatrogenic causes (glucocorticoid treatment of the mother prenatally or pharmacologic glucocorticoid treatment postnatally).

In the absence of primary adrenal disease, ACTH deficiency does not result in mineralocorticoid deficiency. Therefore, hyponatremia, hyperkalemia, and dehydration are not seen as manifestations of ACTH deficiency. In fact, cortisol deficiency may result in decreased renal clearance of free water, resulting in fluid retention. This is often apparent in patients with diabetes

TABLE 145-5. Signs and Symptoms of Adrenal Insufficiency

**Glucocorticoid Deficiency**
Fasting hypoglycemia
Increased insulin sensitivity
Decreased gastric acidity
Gastrointestinal symptoms (eg, nausea, vomiting)
Fatigue

**Mineralocorticoid Deficiency**
Muscle weakness
Weight loss
Fatigue
Nausea, vomiting, anorexia
Salt craving
Hypotension
Hyperkalemia, hyponatremia, acidosis

**Androgen Deficiency (ie, older children, adults)**
Decreased pubic and axillary hair
Decreased libido

**Increased ACTH and $\beta$-Lipotropin**
Hyperpigmentation

TABLE 145-6. Causes of Cushing Syndrome

**ACTH Independent**
Iatrogenic (eg, glucocorticoid therapy)
Andrenocortical tumors (eg, adenoma, carcinoma, micronodular disease)

**ACTH Dependent**
Hypothalamic CRF-producing tumor
Pituitary ACTH-producing tumor
Ectopic CRF-producing tumor (eg, pancreas, lung)
Ectopic ACTH-producing tumor (eg, lung, bronchus, gut)
Iatrogenic (eg, ACTH therapy)
Increased serotonin levels (eg, idiopathic)

insipidus, who may appear to have improvement of their disease if ACTH deficiency develops.

The diagnosis of ACTH deficiency is based on absence of the 8 a.m. peak in serum cortisol and on lack of response to tests of ACTH secretion (insulin-induced hypoglycemia, glucagon stimulation, metyrapone). In cases of partial ACTH deficiency, the patient may produce enough ACTH for normal daily physiological needs (normal 8 a.m. cortisol, normal 24-hour urinary 17-hydroxycorticosteroids) but be unable to respond to stress and fail the tests of stimulated ACTH secretion. In any child with ACTH deficiency, the secretion of other anterior and posterior pituitary hormones must be carefully assessed.

ACTH deficiency is treated with glucocorticoid at physiological replacement doses. The dosage must be carefully titrated to prevent overtreatment, which seems to occur at lower doses in children with ACTH deficiency than in those with primary adrenal failure. Mineralocorticoid treatment is unnecessary.

## Adrenocortical Hyperfunction

Adrenocortical hyperfunction is most often manifested by the effects of glucocorticoid excess, called Cushing's syndrome.

### Etiology

The most common cause of Cushing's syndrome is iatrogenic administration of pharmacologic doses of a glucocorticoid as an anti-inflammatory or immunosuppressive agent. Other causes of Cushing's syndrome are rare in childhood (Table 145-6). These include ACTH-dependent hypercortisolism (Cushing's disease) and primary adrenal hypercortisolism. Among children with hypercortisolism who are not receiving exogenous glucocorticoids, those who are less than 7 years old are more likely to have a primary adrenal cause. Those over 7 years old are more likely to have ACTH-dependent hypercortisolism. The clinical features of hypercortisolism are listed in Table 145-7.

### Diagnosis

The diagnosis of Cushing's syndrome is based on demonstration of hypercortisolism and determination of its source in patients not receiving glucocorticoid treatment.

Measurement of serum cortisol levels at 8 a.m. and in the evening may fail to show the normal diurnal variation. However, the diurnal pattern may not mature in normal children until after 3 years of age. Serum ACTH levels are of some value. Low levels do not rule out the possibility of an ACTH-producing tumor, but high levels usually rule out a primary adrenal cause. The 24-hour urinary 17-hydroxycorticosteroid levels and free cortisol levels are usually elevated, as are 17-ketosteroids in some cases.

In children with equivocal clinical features and baseline static test results, an overnight dexamethasone suppression test may be the most advantageous dynamic screening test. After a single dose of dexamethasone (0.6 mg/m² given orally at 11 p.m.), the 8 a.m. serum cortisol should be less than 5 $\mu$g/dL in a normal child. If the child fails the overnight test, a low-dose and then a high-dose dexamethasone suppression test (see Table 145-2) should be performed. Failure to respond to the low-dose test in conjunction with appropriate suppression on the high-dose test suggests an ACTH-producing pituitary adenoma. Failure to respond to the high-dose dexamethasone test suggests an ectopic ACTH producing tumor or an adrenal tumor.

If a pituitary, adrenal, or ectopic ACTH-producing tumor is suspected, radiologic imaging studies must be performed to visualize the tumor. Many ACTH-producing pituitary tumors are microadenomas, visible only at the time of transsphenoidal pituitary exploration.

TABLE 145-7. Clinical Features of Hypercortisolism

Obesity with violaceous striae
  Generalized in infants
  Truncal in older children with moon facies or buffalo hump
Decreased height velocity
  Short stature
  Delayed bone age
Plethora, increased hematocrit
Easy bruisability
Hypertension
Osteoporosis
Glucose intolerance
Poor wound healing
Increased frequency of infections
Renal stones, hypercalciuria
Weakness, muscle wasting (unusual in infants)
Depression

**Treatment**

The treatment of Cushing's syndrome is removal of the cause of hypercortisolism. In iatrogenic disease, this is not always possible, because of the nature of the disorder, which requires glucocorticoid treatment.

In ACTH-dependent disease the source of ACTH production usually must be removed surgically. In pituitary Cushing's disease, medications such as cyproheptadine and bromocriptine have been more effective in lowering ACTH levels in adults than in children. Bilateral adrenalectomy was once the only treatment for ACTH-dependent disease, but most patients then developed Nelson's disease (ie, pituitary enlargement, hyperplasia of ACTH producing cells).

In primary adrenal disease, adrenalectomy, unilateral in the case of a tumor and bilateral in micronodular disease, is the treatment of choice.

The most commonly encountered side effect of these treatments is adrenal insufficiency, due to ACTH deficiency or to adrenalectomy. In the case of unilateral adrenalectomy, the contralateral adrenal gland will need time to recover from prolonged lack of ACTH stimulation. Patients who undergo pituitary exploration have a small risk of developing panhypopituitarism.

**Prognosis**

The prognosis for patients with Cushing's syndrome is based on the underlying cause. Patients with adrenal or pituitary adenomas have a good prognosis after adequate surgical resection. Those who have adrenal or ectopic ACTH-producing carcinomas have a poorer prognosis.

Hypersecretion of adrenal androgens may be caused by CAH or to an adrenal tumor. In addition, feminizing adrenocortical tumors have been described. Adrenal tumors, including adenomas and carcinomas, are rare in childhood; they are treated by surgical resection and in some cases, adjunctive therapies.

Hypersecretion of mineralocorticoids may be caused by the hypertensive form of CAH (see Table 145-4) or to primary hyperaldosteronism. In 11-OH or 17-OH deficiency, glucocorticoid replacement therapy results in lowering of mineralocorticoid levels. Hyperaldosteronism is exceedingly rare in childhood and is treated with the aldosterone inhibitor, spironolactone.

Rare causes of apparent mineralocorticoid excess include an inherited defect in the conversion of cortisol to cortisone and licorice ingestion.

## Selected Readings

Donohoue PA, Berkovitz GD. Female pseudohermaphroditism. Semin Reprod Endocrinol 1987;5:233.

Migeon CJ. Adrenal cortex. In: Rudolph AM, ed. Pediatrics. Norwalk, CT: Appleton & Lange, 1987:1471.

Migeon CJ, Donohoue PA. Congenital adrenal hyperplasia caused by 21-hydroxylase deficiency: its molecular basis and its remaining therapeutic problems. Endocrinol Metab Clin North Am 1991;20:277.

Migeon CJ, Donohoue PA: Adrenal disorders. In: Kappy MS, ed. Wilkins' diagnosis and treatment of endocrine disorders in childhood and adolescence, ed 4. Springfield, IL: Charles C. Thomas, in press.

*Principles and Practice of Pediatrics, Second Edition.*
edited by Frank A. Oski et al. J. B. Lippincott Company, Philadelphia © 1994.

# CHAPTER 146
# *The Adrenal Medulla*

### Patricia A. Donohoue

## NORMAL ADRENAL MEDULLARY DEVELOPMENT AND SECRETIONS

Early in embryogenesis, primitive sympathetic nervous system ganglion cells migrate from neural ectoderm, differentiate into pheochromoblasts, and penetrate the adrenal cortex. These pheochromoblasts develop into the chromaffin cells of the adrenal medulla.

The adrenal medulla is innervated by sympathetic nerves that originate in the splanchnic system. This sympathoadrenal system is controlled by a complex set of central neural connections and is involved in the production, storage, and secretion of catecholamines. The adrenal medulla is exposed to the relatively high concentrations of glucocorticoids found in the venous drainage of the adrenal cortex.

The major catecholamines in humans are dopamine, norepinephrine, and epinephrine, all of which are synthesized in nerve endings. Epinephrine is the major product of the adrenal medulla. Tyrosine is hydroxylated to form dopa, which is then converted to dopamine, a neurotransmitter within the central nervous system (CNS). Dopamine also acts as the precursor for synthesis of norepinephrine, the principal neurotransmitter of the sympathetic nervous system. Norepinephrine is then converted to epinephrine in the adrenal medulla, in an enzymatic step controlled by glucocorticoid. Epinephrine exerts its physiologic effects by interaction with $\alpha$- and $\beta$-adrenergic receptors. The physiological effects of epinephrine are widespread and are separated into the $\alpha$- and $\beta$-receptor effects (Table 146-1).

## TESTS OF ADRENAL MEDULLARY PRODUCTS

Measurement of single catecholamine levels, such as norepinephrine and epinephrine, are rarely helpful, because patients who have excess production may have periods of low blood levels and persons with normal production have high levels in response to stress. Persons with symptoms of catecholamine excess are best evaluated by measurement of catecholamines and their me-

**TABLE 146-1. Physiologic Effects of Epinephrine**

| $\alpha$ Effects | $\beta$ Effects |
|---|---|
| | Vasodilation |
| Vasoconstriction | Cardiac stimulation |
| Sweating | Lipolysis |
| Uterine contraction | Gluconeogenesis |
| Pupillary dilation | Uterine relaxation |
| Inhibition of insulin release | Bronchodilation |
| Intestinal relaxation | Intestinal |
| Norepinephrine release | relaxation |

**TABLE 146-2. The Multiple Endocrine Neoplasia Syndromes**

| Neoplasia | MEN Type I* | MEN Type IIa† | MEN Type IIb |
|---|---|---|---|
| Pheochromocytoma | | +‡ | + |
| Medullary thyroid carcinoma | | + | + |
| Multiple neural tumors | | | + |
| Parathyroid or hyperplasia | + | + | |
| Pancreatic islet tumors | + | | |
| Anterior pituitary tumors | + | | |

* Also known as Wermer's syndrome.
† Also known as Sipple's syndrome.
‡ The + indicates that the tumor is associated with the syndrome.

**TABLE 146-3. Signs and Symptoms of Pheochromocytoma**

Hypertension
Sweating and flushing
Palpitations and tachycardia
Emotional lability
Headache
Nausea and vomiting
Constipation
Polyuria and polydipsia

tabolites normetanephrine, metanephrine, homovanillic acid (HVA), and vanillylmandelic acid (VMA) in a 24-hour urine sample. Serial measurements of these compounds in blood and urine after paroxysmal attacks of catecholamine release may also be informative.

## ABNORMALITIES OF THE ADRENAL MEDULLA

Abnormalities of the adrenal medulla are caused by benign or malignant tumors that secrete catecholamines.

## Pheochromocytoma

Pheochromocytoma is rare in childhood but must be considered in a child with hypertension or other symptoms of catecholamine excess. This tumor may arise from any chromaffin tissue, but it is most often found in the adrenal medulla. Bilateral adrenal or extra-adrenal tumors are a more common feature in pediatric pheochromocytomas than adult pheochromocytomas, and they are often associated with the familial multiple endocrine neoplasia (MEN) syndromes. The neoplasias associated with the various MEN syndromes are listed in Table 146-2. Features consistent with these associated tumors (eg, medullary carcinoma of the thyroid) should be sought in any patient with pheochromocytoma. The MEN syndromes are inherited in an autosomal dominant manner and have variable expression. Pheochromocytomas are also associated with neuroectodermal dysplasias (eg, neurofibromatosis).

Pheochromocytoma is benign in more than 90% of pediatric patients. There is a male preponderance among children with this tumor, but the sex ratio is reversed in adults. The peak incidence occurs between 9 and 12 years in the pediatric group.

The signs and symptoms of pheochromocytoma are those of catecholamine excess (Table 146-3). These features are highly variable and are likely to be paroxysmal, but the hypertension may be sustained. Hypertensive crisis may occur during anesthesia.

### Diagnosis

The diagnosis of pheochromocytoma is based on demonstration of increased catecholamines and their metabolites in a 24-hour urine sample and in blood. These substances urinary free epinephrine and norepinephrine, metanephrine, and VMA. Urinary VMA levels may be falsely elevated with certain drugs such as aspirin, penicillin, and sulfa preparations. If these test results are inconclusive, a clonidine suppression test may be useful. Clonidine causes a decrease in blood catecholamine levels only if they are not elevated due to secretion from an autonomous source. If suspected from the biochemical tests, the tumor can usually be localized by ultrasound, computed tomography, magnetic resonance imaging, or intravenous pyelography. Venography to demonstrate elevated levels of catecholamines should only be performed after adequate $\alpha$-blockade with Regitine to prevent a hypertensive crisis. Scintigraphic imaging with [131]I-metaiodobenzylguanidine (MIBG scan) has been used to demonstrate the presence of a pheochromocytoma. MIBG is similar in structure to norepinephrine and is concentrated in tissues that are synthesizing catecholamines by means of norepinephrine in storage granules.

### Treatment

The treatment of pheochromocytoma is surgical excision. This requires extensive preoperative treatment with $\alpha$- and $\beta$-blockade and with $\alpha$-methyltyrosine if needed. If bilateral adrenalectomy is necessary, treatment for primary adrenal insufficiency must be promptly instituted. Postoperative recording of blood pressure and catecholamine levels is needed to monitor for tumor recurrence. Malignant tumors are diagnosed on the basis of functional tumor in nonchromaffin tissue areas. Benign tumors may cause blood vessel or capsular invasion but do not spread beyond chromaffin tissue areas. Malignant tumors grow slowly and are resistant to irradiation and chemotherapy; symptoms are treated medically, with various degrees of success.

## Neuroblastoma

Neuroblastoma is one of the most common solid tumors of childhood and may arise from the adrenal medulla. It can be sporadic or familial. The diagnosis is based on demonstration of elevated HVA or VMA levels in the urine and on radiologic localization. The treatment and prognosis of neuroblastoma are discussed elsewhere in this book.

## Other Tumors

Other tumors of the adrenal medulla include ganglioneuroblastoma and ganglioneuroma. These tumors may manifest with chronic watery diarrhea due to tumor secretion of vasoactive intestinal peptide. The diarrhea resolves after excision of the tumor.

### Selected Readings

Bravo EL, Gifford RW Jr. Pheochromocytoma: diagnosis, localization and management. N Engl J Med 1984;311:1298.

Reckler JM, Vaughan ED Jr, Tjeuw M, Carey RM. Pheochromocytoma. In: Vaughan ED Jr, Carey RM, eds. Adrenal disorders. New York: Thieme Medical Publishers, 1989:259.

Voorhess ML. Adrenal medulla, sympathetic nervous system and multiple endocrine adenomatosis. In: Rudolph AM, ed. Pediatrics. Norwalk, CT: Appleton and Lange, 1987:1497.

# The Nervous System

Principles and Practice of Pediatrics, Second Edition.
edited by Frank A. Oski et al. J. B. Lippincott Company, Philadelphia © 1994.

## CHAPTER 147
# Evaluation of the Child With Neurologic Disease

### Marvin A. Fishman

## PATIENT HISTORY AND NEUROLOGIC EXAMINATION

The most important parts of the evaluation of a child with neurologic symptoms are the history and physical examination. Principles used during the general portion of the evaluation are applicable to the child with a neurologic problem. Slight modification of the approach can increase the amount of information obtained. The purpose of the history is to obtain information that enables a tentative diagnosis to be made. With a tentative diagnosis in mind, the neurologic examination is performed to see if the findings are consistent with the postulated diagnosis. For example, if a patient is thought to have idiopathic epilepsy but has an abnormal neurologic examination, the possibility of a structural lesion causing the seizures should be considered. In the case of the child with a complaint of weakness, cerebellar dysfunction should be considered, as well as disease of nerve or muscle, because unsteadiness may be interpreted as weakness. Tests of coordination, power of individual muscle groups, reflexes, and sensation can help differentiate the cause of the symptom.

Information obtained from the history should allow the tempo of the illness to be assessed and the findings to be interpreted in accord with neuroanatomic and neurophysiologic principles. The physician should determine if the disease process is acute or chronic and whether the onset was abrupt or insidious. Occasionally, an event such as intercurrent illness or trauma results in closer than usual observation of a child and discovery of a preexisting problem; a history dating the beginning of neurologic symptoms may not always be accurate. A decrease in the rate of acquisition of new developmental skills or loss of previously acquired skills suggests a degenerative process. Specific questions should be asked to help clarify the meaning of terms used by the historian. Dizziness may indicate vertigo or light-headedness. Weakness may refer to loss of muscle power, fatigue, or unsteadiness. Blurred vision may indicate diplopia, decreased acuity, a visual field defect, or scotomata. Each of these would have different importance in terms of localizing the area of dysfunction. The physician has to decide if the symptoms can be explained by dysfunction of one part of the nervous system or if the process is diffuse or multifocal. Different physical findings correlate with each of these possibilities.

Information obtained during the history should include details of the mother's pregnancy, labor, and delivery. These are times when insults may affect the nervous system of the fetus or neonate and produce immediate or subsequent neurologic problems. Particular attention to the schedule of acquisition of motor and language developmental milestones yields information about the onset of the disease and whether the problem involves specific areas of function. A summary of normal developmental milestones is shown in Table 147-1.

Many neurologic illnesses are familial, and important clues to the child's illness may be obtained from careful review of the family history. Family members may not know the specific name of the disease being considered but may be familiar with symptoms and signs. This is particularly true with familial diseases involving the cerebellum, peripheral nerves, or muscle. Subtle manifestations of neurocutaneous syndromes may not have been appreciated previously, and the finding of tuberous sclerosis or neurofibromatosis in the child can result in identifying other affected relatives. Occasionally, diseases are diagnosed erroneously by family members. Any severe headache may be mistakenly referred to as migraine. It is important to elicit a detailed history in family members to see if the symptoms do suggest migraine.

The physical examination begins when the child enters the examining room; observations continue during the history taking. Significant information about the cranial nerves and cerebellar and motor function can be obtained by watching an infant crawl, walk, or play with toys. The general physical examination should include measurement of head size. Transillumination of the skull may be informative in children younger than 1 year of age and may help detect lesions such as chronic subdural hematomas, porencephalic cysts, and Dandy-Walker malformations. Dysmorphic features or cutaneous abnormalities may help establish a diagnosis. A Wood's lamp examination may be necessary to detect the depigmented ash-leaf lesion seen in tuberous sclerosis. Metabolic disorders resulting in the accumulation of excessive amounts of lipids or other materials may result in enlargement of the liver and spleen. Cardiac murmurs may predispose to neurologic complications such as embolic strokes and cerebral abscesses. A cranial bruit may suggest a large intracranial vascular malformation. Cutaneous abnormalities, dimples, vascular malformations, and tufts of hair over the lower back may be associated with occult spinal dysraphism. Limb growth asymmetry suggests a chronic hemiparesis.

## TABLE 147-1.    Normal Developmental Milestones

| Newborn | 8 Weeks | 12 Weeks |
|---|---|---|
| In ventral suspension, head hangs down<br>When prone, pelvis raised and knees under abdomen<br>Complete head lag on traction<br>Walking reflex<br>Grasp reflex | In ventral suspension, head in same plane as rest of body<br>When prone, chin lifts off couch<br>Hands held open part of the time<br>Fixes and follows object through arc greater than 90°<br>Smiles and makes sounds | In ventral suspension, head held above rest of body<br>Head bobs when supported sitting<br>No grasp reflex<br>Turns head to sound, notices hands, follows object through 180° arc<br>Recognizes mother |

| 20 Weeks | 28 Weeks | 40 Weeks |
|---|---|---|
| When prone, chest off couch and weight on forearms<br>No head lag on traction<br>Can grasp objects and bring them to mouth<br>Smiles at mirror<br>Excites with feeding<br>Laughs aloud | When prone, can support upper trunk with weight on hands and arms extended<br>Rolls prone to supine<br>Sites on floor with support of hands<br>Bears weight on legs in standing position<br>Transfers objects<br>Imitates sounds<br>Responds to name<br>Drinks from cup<br>States syllables | Creeps on abdomen<br>Achieves sitting position independently<br>Pincer grasp<br>Waves bye-bye |

| 52 Weeks | 15 Months | 18 Months |
|---|---|---|
| Walks like bear<br>May walk independently<br>Releases toys<br>Plays simple games<br>Interest in picture books<br>Uses 2 to 3 words with meaning<br>Understands simple phrases | Creeps upstairs<br>Can sit in chair<br>Achieves standing position independently<br>Stacks 2 to 3 cubes<br>Uses cup, rotates spoon<br>Knows some body parts | Pulls toys when walking<br>Takes off shoes and socks<br>Uses jargon and normal language<br>Imitates mother<br>Follows simple request<br>Turns pages in groups |

| 2 Years | 2½ Years | 3 Years |
|---|---|---|
| Walks up stairs placing both feet on each step<br>Kicks ball<br>Stacks more than 5 cubes<br>Puts on socks<br>Some dressing skills<br>Uses phrases<br>Names common objects<br>Turns pages singly<br>Places objects in formboard puzzles | Jumps with both feet<br>Holds crayon in hand<br>Toilet trained<br>Knows name and sex<br>Follows instructions<br>Identifies objects<br>May name a color | Rides tricycle<br>Draws circles and tries to imitate cross<br>Independent dressing skills except for buttons<br>Normal speech<br>Goes upstairs one foot at a time<br>May know nursery rhymes<br>Beginning to understand prepositions |

| 4 Years | 5 Years | 6 Years |
|---|---|---|
| Walks downstairs with one foot on each step<br>Copies cross<br>Asks numerous questions<br>Imaginative play | Skips on both feet<br>Can tie shoelace<br>Copies square<br>Knows age<br>Distinguishes morning from afternoon<br>Beginning to draw a man | Copies a diamond<br>Repeats digits<br>Counts<br>Knows number of fingers |

The formal neurologic examination is used to confirm the information obtained by observation and to corroborate the suspected diagnosis based on the history. It is often easier to proceed with the infant seated in his mother's lap rather than seated or lying on an examining table. Beginning the examination with the legs and working upward results in better cooperation than if more unpleasant aspects of the examination, such as funduscopy, are performed first.

Cranial nerve testing is easy to perform. Cranial nerve I, the olfactory nerve, often is not tested unless there is a specific indication for doing so. Cranial nerve II, the optic nerve, can be inspected and tested. Vision can be assessed by several methods in children who are too young to cooperate for formal testing with visual charts. Various drums or tapes can be used to elicit opticokinetic nystagmus in young infants. With infants older than 6 months, various small objects, even a fleck of paper, can be placed in front of them, and their attempts to pick it up can be observed. Each eye can be tested separately. Cranial nerves III, IV, and VI are responsible for eye movements, pupillary responses, and lid opening. They can be tested by observing spontaneous eye movements and by having the child watch toys such as puppets. Facial sensation, governed by cranial nerve V, can be tested with a wisp of cotton. The motor branch of cranial nerve V supplies the muscles of mastication. These can be tested by having the child open his jaw against resistance and by palpating the masseter muscles as the teeth are clenched. Facial movements, orchestrated by cranial nerve VII, can be assessed when the child smiles and laughs and with volitional movements. Asking the child to smile allows observations of the symmetry of the nasolabial folds; the symmetry of burying of eyelashes can be observed as the eyes are closed. The symmetry of the strength of the eyelids can be tested as attempts to open the upper lids are made when the child attempts to keep his eyes tightly closed. Auditory acuity, controlled by cranial nerve VIII, can be tested by using a tuning fork or watch or by giving whispered instructions out of sight of the child. Lower cranial nerves IX, X, XI, and XII can be tested by eliciting a gag reflex, watching the palate contract, and observing movements of the tongue.

The assessment of motor function in preschool children is made while watching the child play, crawl, climb, or walk. Activities can be designed to test upper or lower extremity function. Lifting a child with the examiner's hands placed in the patient's axillae tests shoulder girdle function. Lifting a child off the ground while he holds the examiner's thumbs tests hand strength. Tone is tested by passively moving the child's limbs.

Deep tendon reflexes are elicited in children by similar techniques used in adults. Infants have developmental reflexes in the newborn period that disappear with normal development. The more common developmental reflexes are listed in Table 147-2. The abnormal persistence of these reflexes usually is accompanied by other abnormalities of the neurologic examination or a lack of appropriate developmental skills. The isolated persistence of one of these reflexes should be interpreted cautiously because of the significant variation in normal age ranges during which they disappear.

Cerebellar function can be assessed in young infants and preschool children by watching them play. This is particularly useful for observing upper extremity function and balance. The skill with which young children perform fine motor tasks is age dependent, and the assessment of normalcy must take this into consideration. Infants often can be coaxed into reaching for small objects, and during these maneuvers, fine motor coordination and hand function are observed. The presence of adventitial or associated movements can be evaluated at this time. Watching a child walk or run is helpful in determining cerebellar function and motor strength, peripheral nerve function, and abnormalities of tone.

The sensory examination often is difficult to perform and to interpret accurately in infants and preschool children. When performed near the end of a history taking and examination session, attention and cooperation may be lacking. Under these circumstances, completing the sensory examination at a later time may yield more useful information. Engaging the child to "play games" often enhances effort and interest. Testing of cortical or sensory modalities such as double simultaneous stimulation, stereognosis, or graphesthesia requires accurate reporting by the examinee. Reliable information often cannot be obtained until the child is of school age.

## LABORATORY INVESTIGATIONS

The laboratory tests frequently used in the evaluation of children with neurologic problems are discussed briefly. A few indications are given for each test, but the discussion is neither complete nor comprehensive. Readers can refer to other sections of this book in which the use of laboratory tests are discussed in conjunction with specific diseases or problems.

### Electroencephalogram

The electroencephalogram (EEG) is a useful tool but may have limitations based on the technical quality of the record, skill of the interpreter, and ability of the test to provide specific answers to questions raised by clinicians. For example, the diagnosis of a seizure disorder is primarily a clinical one, and an interictal tracing may not be accurate enough to diagnose epilepsy. The EEG pattern changes with age and may be used to assess maturation in premature infants. The pattern also may depend on the region or the location from which it is recorded, and it is modified by alertness, drowsiness, and sleep. A skilled and experienced interpreter should be able to recognize these normal variations.

EEG abnormalities may be transient. The usual 30- to 60-minute clinical recording is adequate to detect most abnormalities, but under certain circumstances, longer recordings may be helpful, particularly when trying to document epileptic discharges. Activating techniques such as sleep and hyperventilation may be helpful in eliciting abnormalities. Occasionally, longer monitoring records combined with simultaneous videotaping are helpful in the diagnosis and classification of difficult seizure disorders. The technology is available to perform ambulatory monitoring, but this technique has some limitations compared with routine multichannel recordings. During routine recording, the EEG may be accompanied by other physiologic monitoring such as heart rate, air flow, chest wall movement, and percutaneous blood gas analyses to gain more information about neonatal seizures, apnea problems, sleep disturbances, or other disorders.

The most common application of the EEG is in the study of seizure disorders. The EEG may help decide if paroxysmal behavioral events are seizure manifestations. Epileptic discharges on a interictal record does not prove that the clinical event in question was a cortical seizure, even though it may suggest this diagnosis. If clinical events occur with sufficient frequency, the physician may try to "capture" the behavior by simultaneous EEG and video recording. The EEG may help differentiate certain seizure types. Complex partial seizures may be similar to certain types of absence seizures. Clinical differentiation may not be

---

| TABLE 147-2. Common Newborn Reflexes |
|---|
| *Moro reflex*—Present in normal newborns and disappears by 3 months of age |
| *Grasp reflexes (palmar and plantar)*—Present in normal newborns and disappear by 3 months of age |
| *Lower extremity crossed extension reflex*—Present at birth and disappears by 1 month of age |
| *Extensor plantar response*—Variably present in normal newborns and disappears by 8–12 months of age |
| *Placing reflex*—Present at birth and disappears by 1–2 months of age |
| *Stepping reflex*—Present at birth and disappears by 1–2 months of age |
| *Asymmetric tonic neck reflex*—Variably present in normal newborns and disappears by 3 months of age |

possible, but the distinction is important, because each type of seizure responds to different antiepileptic medication (Fig 147-1). The EEG helps in this type of differentiation and is helpful in differentiating pseudoseizures from real seizures and infantile spasms from other types of myoclonic seizures in infancy. It may be used to help gauge the response to therapy for infantile spasms and absence epilepsy. Children who develop new types of seizures or have worsening of their epilepsy should have EEGs repeated as part of the evaluation. This may help with decisions regarding therapy and may suggest a progressive disorder. The decision to discontinue medication after a seizure-free period is a clinical one, but an EEG can be an aid in making that decision.

The EEG is used in the evaluation of apneic episodes and sleep problems. This is best done as part of a polygraphic recording, which also measures additional physiological parameters. The EEG is useful in evaluating patients in coma, particularly if the cause is unknown. Certain drugs, such as barbiturates and benzodiazepines, may cause changes in the EEG pattern that strongly suggest drug effect. The EEG may be helpful in suggesting a diffuse metabolic insult as a cause of unresponsiveness. It can differentiate focal lesions from generalized abnormalities and may suggest brain stem dysfunction as a cause of coma. Patients with subacute sclerosing panencephalitis, herpes simplex encephalitis, and various degenerative diseases may have characteristic patterns on their tracings. Serial EEGs performed after significant head trauma may have prognostic value regarding recovery and the potential for developing epilepsy; they also may help determine the cause of some post-traumatic symptoms.

## Electromyography and Nerve Conduction Velocities

Electrodiagnostic techniques are most useful for studying diseases of the motor unit (ie, anterior horn cell, peripheral nerve, neuromuscular junction, and muscle). They play little or no role in studying diseases of the central nervous system for routine clinical purposes. Their value is in localizing areas of dysfunction rather than providing specific etiologic diagnoses. Certain patterns on the electromyogram (EMG) tend to suggest "neurogenic" or "myopathic" processes. A definitive diagnosis cannot be made by this test alone; it must be combined with clinical impressions,

neurologic examination, and other laboratory tests, including muscle biopsies. The EMG is helpful for studying diseases affecting the neuromuscular junction, such as myasthenia gravis and botulism.

Nerve conduction velocities, motor and sensory, are helpful in detecting diseases of the peripheral nerves and particularly for demyelinating neuropathies. In the latter case, there are significant reductions in conduction velocities. In diseases affecting primarily the axon of the peripheral nerve, the conduction velocities may be only mildly reduced. Certain techniques can be used to measure the conduction through the proximal portion of the nerve, which may be helpful in diagnosing the Guillain-Barré syndrome.

## Evoked Potentials

The measurement of evoked potentials is a useful neurophysiologic technique. The evoked potential is an electrical manifestation of the brain's response to a stimulus. This electrical response to a specific stimulus cannot be measured in a routine EEG because its very low amplitude is overshadowed by the background brain wave activity. The evoked potential is time-locked to the stimulus and can be extracted from the background activity by the technique of computer signal averaging. The computer averages the response to many repetitive similar stimuli, such as auditory clicks or visual patterns, and is able to generate a set of waves corresponding to signals generated by specific anatomic structures along pathways conducting the impulse within the nervous system.

*Visual evoked potentials* are most helpful in detecting lesions anterior to the optic chiasm. Pattern-shift visual evoked potentials are more useful and sensitive than flash evoked responses. The visual evoked potential can be used to follow certain diseases of the retina, optic nerves, and chiasm, but it generally is not a sensitive test of cortical blindness and may not correlate well with the clinical examination of vision.

*Brain stem auditory evoked potentials* can test the peripheral auditory apparatus, including cranial nerve VIII and the various relay stations conducting the impulse through brain stem structures. It is a sensitive test of hearing and can be used in children who cannot cooperate for audiograms.

*Somatosensory evoked potentials* are elicited by stimulating a peripheral nerve and then recording over the spine and scalp as the stimulus travels toward the brain. Somatosensory evoked potentials may be used to test the integrity of the spinal cord ascending sensory pathways and peripheral nerves and is helpful for detecting lesions in spinal roots, cauda equina, spinal cord, or brain stem. The technique has been used during spinal surgery to avoid injury to the spinal cord itself.

## Neuroimaging

Ultrasonography, computed tomography (CT), and magnetic resonance imaging (MRI) are used to visualize the nervous system.

### Ultrasonography

Ultrasonography is an extremely useful procedure that often is used for examining neonates and young infants. Its advantages include portability; it can be done at the bedside, obviating the need to transport critically ill infants to a radiology suite. Moreover, it is relatively inexpensive compared with other imaging procedures. Ultrasonography can be performed serially to follow the course of an intracranial problem.

The best definition of the intracranial anatomy is obtained when the transducer is placed over the anterior fontanelle. This approach permits coronal and sagittal views of the brain. Axial views are possible by scanning through the temporoparietal bone, but this is rarely done because scanning through bone decreases

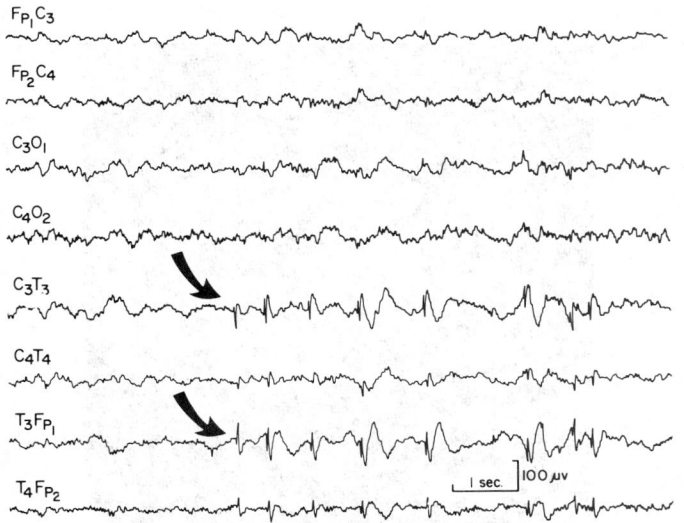

**Figure 147-1.** Electroencephalogram (EEG) of a child with complex partial seizures, which shows left temporal spikes (*arrows*). This EEG pattern in a child with brief lapses and automatisms indicates that the seizures do not represent absence spells. (Courtesy of Peter Kellaway, PhD., Baylor College of Medicine, Houston, TX.)

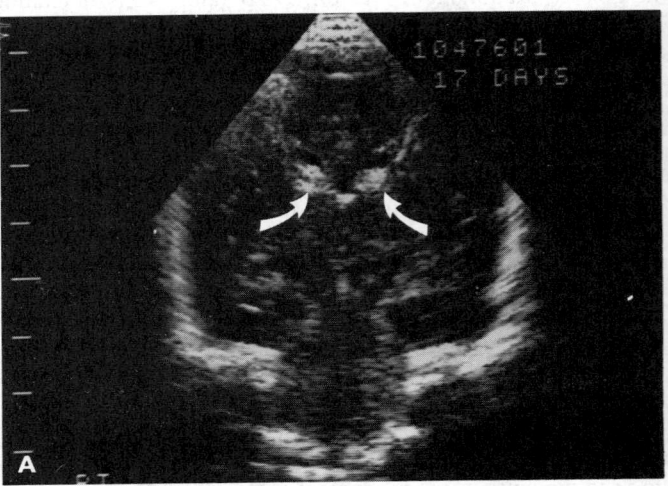
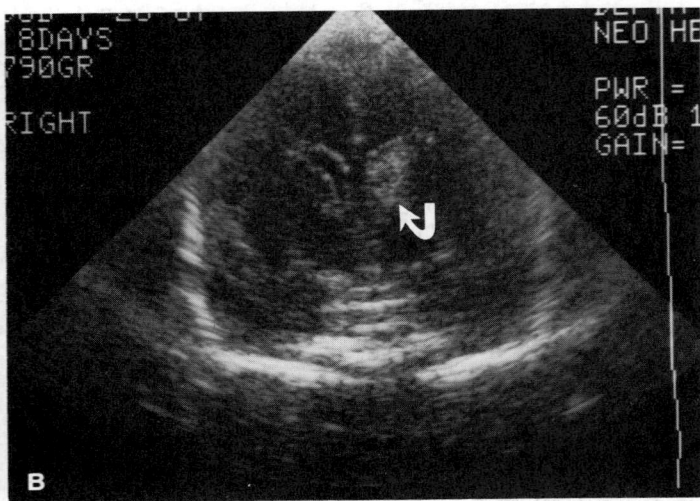

**Figure 147-2.** (**A**) Ultrasound examination reveals bilateral subependymal hemorrhages (*arrows*). (**B**) Hemorrhage fills one frontal horn (*arrow*) and is associated with slight dilatation of the contralateral ventricle. (Courtesy of Robert Dutton, MD., Texas Children's Hospital, Houston, TX.)

the definition. This technical problem limits scanning to children whose anterior fontanelles are patent.

Ultrasonography is most often used to study intracranial hemorrhage in premature infants. Periventricular hemorrhage, the most common form of intracranial bleeding in this age group, can be detected readily by ultrasonography (Fig 147-2). The consequences associated with these hemorrhages, including post-hemorrhagic ventricular dilatation, intracerebral hemorrhage, porencephaly, and subependymal pseudocyst formation, can be detected by this technique. Subarachnoid, parenchymal, thalamic, choroid plexus, and intracerebellar hemorrhage also can be diagnosed. Ischemic lesions in the preterm and full-term infant initially appear as areas of increased echo density. Some of these lesions become cystic as they resolve.

Ultrasonography is useful in diagnosing and following the course of congenital abnormalities that affect the ventricular system, such as hydranencephaly, Dandy-Walker cyst, arachnoid cyst, porencephalic cyst, and various forms of hydrocephalus. Other congenital anomalies, such as holoprosencephaly, agenesis of the corpus callosum, and various cerebellar malformations, may be detected. The complications of meningitis in infants, such as the development of hydrocephalus, infarction, and abscesses, can be followed by ultrasonography. Abnormalities primarily involving the parenchyma, including acquired and congenital lesions, often are visualized with greater definition by other imaging techniques. Examples include heterotopias, gyral malformations, tumors, focal infarcts, lesions associated with surrounding edema, and small calcifications.

## Computed Tomography

Cranial CT, a commonly used noninvasive imaging procedure, provides useful information about acquired and congenital lesions. The question has arisen whether cranial CT examinations should be performed if the results will not affect therapy, such as in the child with microcephaly. Because the information obtained may be useful in determining the cause and pathogenesis of the child's neurologic dysfunction, there may be indications for this procedure even if the results will not be followed by active intervention. Some indications for performing cranial CT scanning include suspected developmental abnormalities of the brain, which may be associated with abnormalities in head size and dysmorphic features involving the cranium and face, and neurocutaneous disorders, such as tuberous sclerosis, neurofibromatosis, and Sturge-Weber disease. Other indications are ab-

normal increases in head size, focal neurologic signs or symptoms, increased intracranial pressure, and coma of unknown origin.

Cranial CT scans are helpful in diagnosing primary or metastatic brain tumors and for following the results of therapy. The complications of infectious processes (eg, meningitis, encephalitis, abscesses) involving the nervous system and complications of significant acute head injuries may be diagnosed by CT. CT is also sensitive in detecting intracranial calcifications; it often shows abnormalities although plain skull radiographs are normal. When studying metabolic or infectious problems associated with intracranial calcifications, a CT scan should be performed instead of plain skull radiographs.

## Magnetic Resonance Imaging

MRI is a noninvasive procedure that has great potential. The patient receives no radiation, and it appears to be more sensitive than CT to white matter diseases. It is particularly helpful in diagnosing posterior fossa problems, because there is no attenuation related to bone and fewer artifacts are created. Recon-

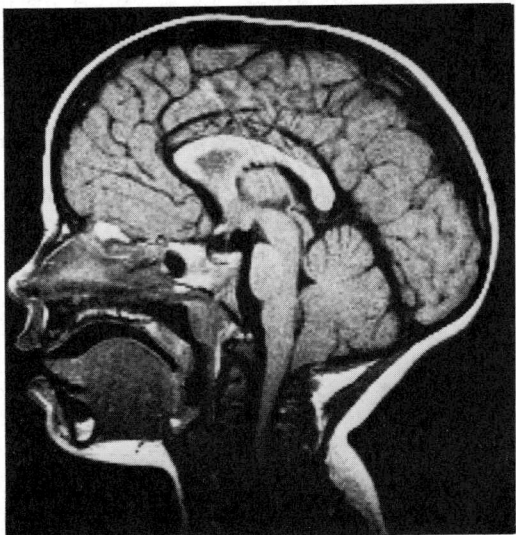

**Figure 147-3.** Magnetic resonance scan of the brain in a sagittal midline view. (Courtesy of Clark Carrol, MD., Texas Children's Hospital, Houston, TX.)

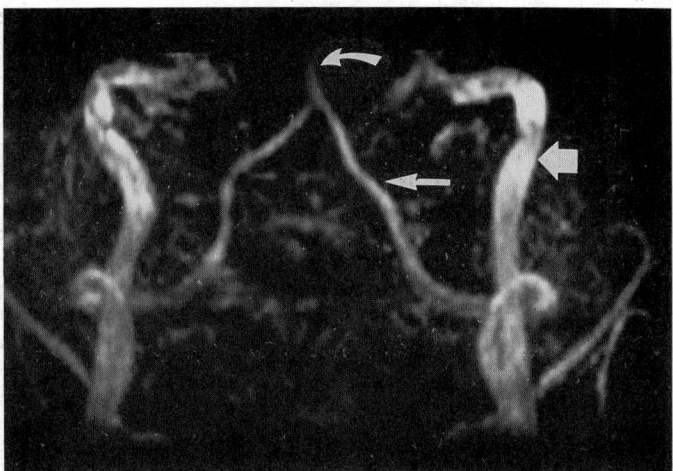

**Figure 147-4.** The magnetic resonance angiographic image demonstrates the carotid artery (*arrow head*), vertebral artery (*straight arrow*), and basilar artery (*curved arrow*).

struction of the images in multiple planes is accomplished more readily with MRI than CT (Fig 147-3). Compared with CT, MRI is more costly and less able to demonstrate small calcifications. Another problem is not being able to use ferromagnetic metals in the region of the scanner because of the powerful magnet; all equipment, including ventilators, must not contain this type of metal. Special equipment is available but is not commonly used. CT remains the more practical procedure for emergency problems.

Magnetic resonance angiography can be used to visualize large and medium-sized intracranial vessels (Fig. 147-4). This is done without the injection of contrast material and uses sophisticated software for producing the images. Both the arterial and venous systems can be imaged.

## Other Diagnostic Procedures

Cerebral angiography is not discussed in this chapter because of its limited applicability. The reader should refer to those diseases for which this procedure is helpful. Discussion of the examination of the cerebrospinal fluid has been omitted from this chapter and readers should refer to individual disease processes for which this is a helpful diagnostic procedure.

## Selected Readings

Aminoff MJ. Evoked potentials in clinical medicine. J Med 1986;59:345.
Chiappa KH, Ropper AH. Part one: Evoked potentials in clinical medicine. N Engl J Med 1982;306:1140, 1205.
Ferry PC. Computed cranial tomography in children. J Pediatr 1980;96:961.
Fishman MA, ed. Pediatric neurology. Orlando, FL: Grune & Stratton, 1986.
Han JS, Benson JE, Kaufman B, et al. MR imaging of pediatric cerebral abnormalities. J Comput Assist Tomogr 1985;9:103.
Hecox KE, Cone B, Blaw ME. Brain stem auditory evoked response in the diagnosis of pediatric neurologic diseases. Neurology 1981;31:832.
Johnson MA, Pennock JM, Bydder GM, et al. Clinical NMR imaging of the brain in children: normal and neurologic disease. AJNR 1983;4:1013.
Kellaway P, Hrachovy RA. Electroencephalography. In: Swaiman KF, Wright FS, eds. The practice of pediatric neurology. St. Louis: CV Mosby, 1982.
Levene MI, Williams JL, Fawer C. Ultrasound of the infant brain. London: Blackwell Scientific Publications, 1985.
Mizrahi EM, Dorfman LJ. Sensory evoked potentials: clinical applications in pediatrics. J Pediatr 1980;97:1.

*Principles and Practice of Pediatrics, Second Edition.*
edited by Frank A. Oski et al. J. B. Lippincott Company, Philadelphia © 1994.

# CHAPTER 148
# *Developmental Defects*

### Marvin A. Fishman

## HYDROCEPHALY

Hydrocephaly is a congenital or acquired disorder in which there is an excessive amount of cerebrospinal fluid (CSF) within the cerebral ventricles. More CSF is produced than can be reabsorbed. Increased pressure within the ventricular system may be transitory or persistent. Enlarged cerebral ventricles due to the loss of brain tissue (formerly called hydrocephalus ex vacuo) is excluded from consideration in this chapter, because it does not meet the definition of inadequate absorption of CSF and increased pressure. Noncommunicating hydrocephaly refers to conditions in which the ventricular fluid does not communicate with the fluid in the basal cisterns or spinal subarachnoid spaces. This implies a block of the CSF flow within the ventricular system. In communicating hydrocephaly, the block is outside the ventricular system or its exit foramina.

CSF is formed within the ventricular system, mainly by the choroid plexus through the processes of active secretion and diffusion. The fluid exits the ventricular system by way of foramina in the fourth ventricle and circulates into the lumbar and subarachnoid spaces. Most CSF absorption takes place at the arachnoid villi leading to venous channels of the sagittal sinus. In adults, the total CSF volume is approximately 150 mL, and only 25% is within the ventricular system. The rate of formation is approximately 20 mL/hour, and the CSF turns over three to four times per day.

## Pathogenesis

Impaired absorption of CSF due to obstruction of flow or dysfunction of absorptive mechanisms is the most common mechanism for producing hydrocephalus. If flow is blocked within the ventricular system, there is a disproportionate dilatation of the ventricles proximal to the block. In aqueductal stenosis, the lateral and third ventricles are disproportionately dilated compared with the fourth ventricle. If the block is extraventricular, there is a relatively proportionate increase in size of all ventricles.

Hydrocephalus secondary to excessive secretion of CSF is rare, and when it occurs, it usually is associated with a functioning choroid plexus papilloma. Mechanical obstruction by the tumor or fibrosis of the subarachnoid spaces secondary to bleeding from the tumor may contribute to the hydrocephalus. Thrombosis of the superior sagittal sinus can interfere with absorption of the CSF, but with venous sinus thrombosis, usually there is cerebral edema or infarction of the cerebral cortex; hydrocephalus only occurs late in the illness.

With obstruction to the flow of CSF, compensatory mechanisms of absorption may develop. One of these is increased movement of CSF across the ependymal lining of the ventricular system, usually occurring when there is a significant increase in CSF pressure; it is detected as periventricular low-density areas by computed tomography (CT) or increased periventricular water by magnetic resonance imaging (MRI). The ventricular dilatation usually begins in the frontal and occipital horns of the lateral ventricles and is followed by more symmetric dilatation of the remainder of the ventricles. With an intraventricular block, the subarachnoid space over the cerebral hemispheres becomes obliterated, and the vascular system becomes compressed, resulting in increased venous pressure in the dural sinuses. Eventually, the cerebral mantle becomes thinner to accommodate the increased CSF volume. If the cranial sutures have not fused, abnormal increases in head size occur in infants. In older children, this compensatory mechanism is not available; intracranial pressure increases, and symptoms develop more readily than in young infants. The rapidity and severity of the process depends on the imbalance between CSF production and absorption. The greater the imbalance, the faster symptoms and signs develop, and the more severe they are. Complete obstruction to absorption is not compatible with life. With only a slight imbalance between production and absorption, the process is slower and more insidious. The imbalance may become compensated as alternative mechanisms of CSF absorption develop, but at the expense of an increased ventricular size.

## Etiology

Congenital hydrocephalus may result from congenital malformations of the nervous system, including isolated aqueductal stenosis, or may be associated with other malformations, including the Dandy-Walker malformation, which consists of a large cyst in the posterior fossa continuous with the fourth ventricle and partial or complete absence of the cerebellar vermis. A common associated malformation syndrome is that of meningomyelocele with Arnold-Chiari malformation. Other syndromes include a sex-linked form of aqueductal stenosis and chromosomal anomalies resulting in syndromes with additional multiple congenital malformations. Arachnoid cysts or congenital tumors may obstruct the ventricular system. Congenital hydrocephalus may be caused by intrauterine infections, which cause inflammation of the ependymal lining of the ventricular system or the meninges in the subarachnoid space, subsequently occluding the CSF pathways. Among the more common infections causing congenital hydrocephalus are rubella, cytomegalovirus, toxoplasmosis, and syphilis.

Hydrocephalus may be acquired postnatally secondary to infections of the nervous system (eg, bacterial meningitis), brain tumors, and arachnoiditis secondary to bleeding into the subarachnoid space from a ruptured arteriovenous malformation, aneurysm, or trauma. Premature infants may develop hydrocephalus secondary to intraventricular hemorrhage.

## Symptoms and Signs

The primary process (eg, tumor, infection, bleeding) and the symptoms and signs caused by increased intracranial pressure secondary to the hydrocephalus may contribute to the clinical picture. The severity of the findings is influenced by the rate at which the hydrocephalus develops and the development of alternate pathways of CSF absorption. Nonspecific symptoms include headaches of various locations and intensities; they occasionally occur early in the morning and are associated with vomiting. Personality and behavior changes, including irritability

or indifference, sometimes occur. Lethargy and drowsiness are relatively late symptoms. Nausea and vomiting are secondary to increased intracranial pressure, particularly in the posterior fossa. Nonspecific signs include third and sixth cranial nerve deficits, which result in paresis of extraocular muscles and may lead to diplopia. Papilledema may be a late finding if the intracranial pressure is not markedly elevated and the process is a slow, chronic one. Changes in vital signs occur relatively late and indicate distortion of the brain stem. In young children, the anterior fontanelle may become full or distended; this is accompanied by excessive head growth and dilatation of scalp veins. The setting sun sign is produced by paralysis of upward gaze and results in the sclera being visible above the iris. Spasticity develops first in the lower extremities and then in the arms and results from stretching of motor fibers around the bodies of the lateral ventricles. Dilatation of the third ventricle may cause pressure on the hypothalamus, resulting in disturbances in sexual development and in fluid and electrolyte imbalance.

## Diagnosis and Therapy

The advent of noninvasive neuroimaging techniques such as CT or MRI has made the diagnosis of hydrocephalus relatively straightforward. The pattern of ventricular dilatation, the presence of interstitial edema (ie, CSF in the white matter surrounding the ventricles), and an underlying cause for obstruction of CSF flow are usually readily apparent (Fig 148-1). Examination of the CSF should be undertaken if there is suspicion of a relatively recent infection or if there is a clinical suspicion of subarachnoid bleeding but no evidence of such on neuroimaging studies. In infancy, chronic subdural hematomas may present in a similar fashion and can be detected by neuroimaging procedures.

Treatment includes specific therapy for any underlying condition associated with the hydrocephalus, such as brain tumor, abscess, and chronic meningitis. Surgery is the most effective means of treating progressive hydrocephalus, and a shunt system between the cerebral ventricles and the peritoneal cavity is the most commonly employed technique. The shunt, which allows diversion of the CSF into the peritoneal cavity where it is absorbed, is a palliative measure and not a cure. The complication rate is relatively high, and problems encountered include mechanical obstruction of the shunt system and infections within it, which may produce meningitis or ventriculitis. Shunt infections may be indolent and often are caused by organisms that usually are not considered pathogens, such as *Staphylococcus epidermidis*. Medical therapy designed to decrease CSF production may be used when the hydrocephalus is slowly progressive and perhaps transitory. This includes the ventricular enlargement that is sometimes seen after subarachnoid hemorrhage, meningitis, or intraventricular hemorrhage in premature infants. The therapeutic agents used include acetazolamide, furosemide, and glycerol. These agents also may be used in the interim period when an infected shunt system has to be removed and before a new system can be reinserted.

## Prognosis

Intellectual and motor function of the hydrocephalic child are determined by the problem causing the hydrocephalus rather than by the ventricular dilatation itself. The natural history of intrauterine infections, meningitis, brain tumors, or other disorders determines the prognosis. The disabilities produced by the hydrocephalus include motor problems related to spasticity or coordination deficits, visual impairment secondary to optic atrophy from long-standing increased intracranial pressure, and intellectual impairment. Intellectual ability is usually less signifi-

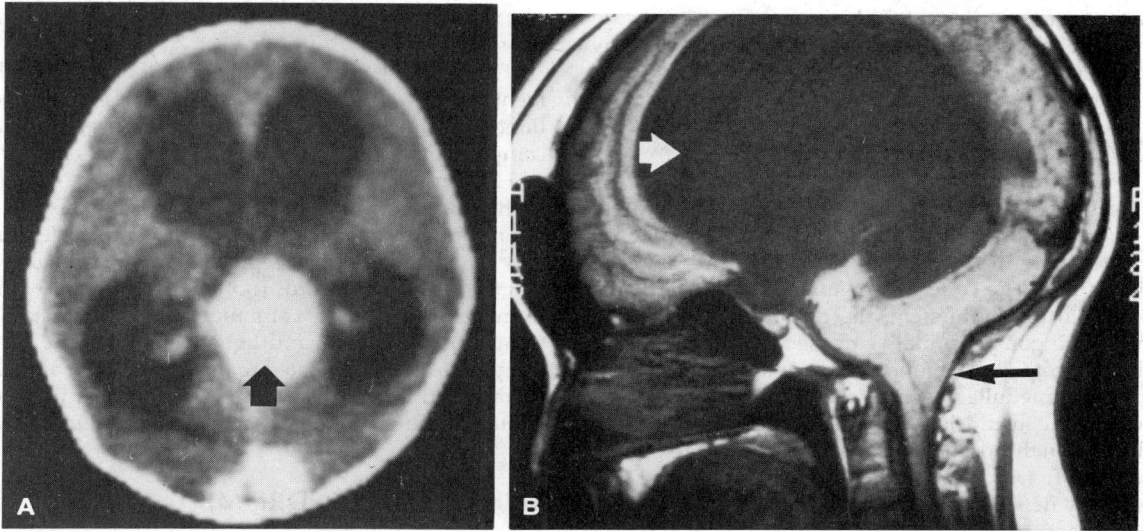

**Figure 148-1.** (**A**) CT scan with contrast enhancement demonstrating hydrocephalus secondary to an aneurysm of the vein of Galen (*arrow*). (**B**) MRI, sagittal plane, demonstrating hydrocephalus (*white arrow*) and an Arnold-Chiari type II malformation (*black arrow*) with downward displacement of the brain stem into the cervical canal. (Courtesy of Clark Carrol, M.D., Texas Children's Hospital, Houston, TX.)

cantly affected than motor performance, because the gray matter of the brain is less affected by the hydrocephalus than the white matter.

## ARNOLD-CHIARI MALFORMATION

The Arnold-Chiari malformation involves the brain stem and lower portion of the cerebellum. These structures are displaced downward into the cervical canal. There are various degrees of the malformation. In type I, the medulla is displaced downward into the spinal canal with tongue-like processes of the cerebellum. In type II, in addition to the type I findings, the fourth ventricle is elongated and extends into the spinal canal. The downward displacement may be such that the cervical cord is kinked on itself and the foramen magnum and upper cervical canal may be packed tightly with the displaced tissue. In the rare type III malformation, there is an associated cervical spina bifida with herniation of brain tissue through the defect. As a result of the distal displacement, lower cranial nerves and cervical spinal nerve roots may be stretched. There often are associated nervous system abnormalities. Children with meningomyeloceles and hydrocephalus usually have an associated Arnold-Chiari malformation. It also may be associated with hydromyelia and syringomyelia. Other minor malformations include beaking of the tectal plate and large massa intermedia.

Arnold-Chiari malformations usually occur in children with spina bifida and hydrocephalus. The symptoms and signs are those caused by the malformations. With significant downward displacement of the hind brain, there may be stretching of the lower cranial nerves, which can produce facial paralysis, hoarseness or stridor, or difficulty with swallowing. If the upper segments of the spinal cord are involved, there may be motor deficits in the arms. Cerebellar ataxia and vertical nystagmus also have been described in patients with Arnold-Chiari malformation.

The symptoms related to Chiari type I malformation include neck pain, back pain, scoliosis, torticollis, motor dysfunction, and apnea. The ages of the patients ranged from 1 month to 14 years. Several children had associated syringomyelia.

The downward displacement of the hind brain can be detected by neuroimaging procedures (see Fig 148-1B). In addition to CT or MRI of the posterior fossa, MRI of the spinal cord may be necessary to detect the associated malformations.

Shunting of an associated hydrocephalus would be the first procedure attempted in treating these patients. If this does not

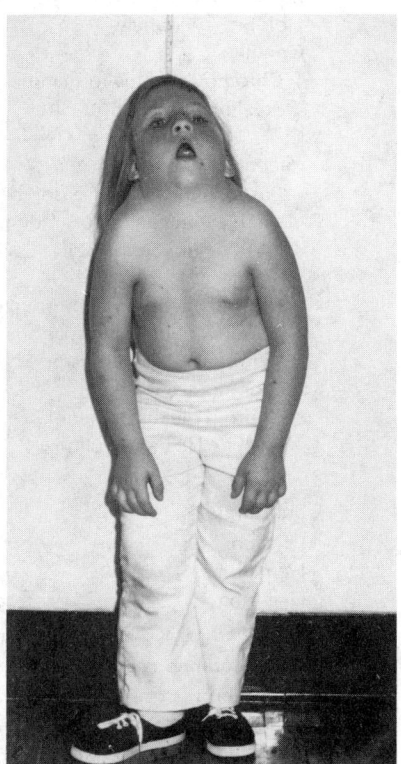

**Figure 148-2.** Girl with Klippel-Feil syndrome has a short neck and retrocollis due to limited neck flexion. The lateral neck rotation is also limited. Her low occipital hairline is not visible in this photograph.

improve the symptoms attributable to hind brain or cervical cord dysfunction, occipital decompression and cervical laminectomy should be considered.

## SYRINGOMYELIA AND HYDROMYELIA

Syringomyelia is a rare condition in children. It describes a cavity within the spinal cord lined by glial elements that is paracentral in location. The cavity may extend over many segments or be isolated to just a few. The cervical area often is involved. If the syrinx extends into the brain stem, the condition is known as syringobulbia. Syringomyelia may be associated with abnormalities of the cervicomedullary junction, including Arnold-Chiari malformation, intramedullary spinal cord tumors, spinal cord trauma, and arterial insufficiency to the cord. The signs and symptoms depend on the location of the syrinx and any associated condition. There often is wasting of the small muscles of the hands and sensory deficits involving the arms. Deep tendon reflexes may be absent. Involvement of the descending tracts may cause spasticity in the lower extremities. There may be a dissociated sensory disturbance with loss of pain and temperature but preservation of touch; this may occur in a segmental distribution and is caused by the cavity destroying the commissural fibers of the spinal cord.

The diagnosis may be made by MRI of the spinal cord. Treatment consists of therapy for the primary lesion, such as associated tumor or the cervical medullary junction abnormality and decompression of the syrinx itself in some patients.

Hydromyelia involves symmetric dilatation of the central canal of the spinal cord. The enlarged canal is lined by ependyma and often communicates with the fourth ventricle. The enlargement may extend over many segments and may include the entire length of the spinal cord. It often is associated with other malformations, including communicating hydrocephaly, Arnold-Chiari malformation, and aqueductal stenosis. The signs and symptoms often are related to the associated malformations, and therapy is directed toward them. It is unclear if any findings are related to the dilatation of the central canal itself.

## KLIPPEL-FEIL SYNDROME

The characteristic three clinical findings of Klippel-Feil syndrome are short neck, limited neck motion, and low occipital hairline (Fig 148-2). The type I form of the syndrome consists of fusions

---

### TABLE 148-1. Large Head Syndromes

**Hydrocephaly**

Congenital
  Aqueductal stenosis ⎤ with or without meningomyelocele
  Communicating ⎦ and Arnold-Chiari malformation
Dandy-Walker syndrome
Hydranencephaly
Porencephaly
Holoprosencephaly
Genetic:
  Chromosomal malformation
  Sex-linked
Cysts
Infectious
  Postinflammatory disease (meningitis)
  Viral (cytomegalovirus, mumps, other)
  Parasitic (toxoplasmosis)
Vascular
  Postsubarachnoid hemorrhage
  Arteriovenous malformation
  Vein of Galen aneurysm
Tumor
  Choroid plexus papilloma
  Posterior fossa neoplasm
  Other

**Subdurals**

Effusion
Hematoma
Hygroma
Empyema

**Neurocutaneous Disorders**

Neurofibromatosis
Tuberous sclerosis
Multiple hemangiomatosis
Incontinentia pigmenti
Basal cell nevus syndrome
Neurocutaneous melanosis

**Toxic-Metabolic Causes**

Benign increased intracranial hypertension associated with antibiotics, vitamins, endocrine disorders, "catch-up" growth after malnutrition, galactosemia, anemias

**Cranioskeletal Dysplasias**

Anemias
Achondroplasia
Osteogenesis imperfecta
Osteopetrosis
Metaphyseal dysplasia
Platybasia
Fibrous dysplasia (Albright's syndrome)

**Storage and Degenerative Disease**

Leukodystrophies
  Canavan's spongy degenerative
  Alexander's
Lysosomal disease
  Tay-Sachs
  Generalized gangliosidosis
  Mucopolysaccharidosis
  Metachromatic leukodystrophy
Peroxisomal disorders
  Neonatal adrenoleukodystrophy
Amino acid disorders
  Maple syrup urine disease

**Unknown Causes**

Cerebral gigantism
Megalencephaly
  Familial
  Dominant
Wiedemann-Beckwith syndrome

involving the cervical and upper thoracic vertebrae. In type II, only the cervical vertebrae are involved, and there may be fusion of several segments. In type III, lesions similar to those found in types I and II occur, but there also is involvement of lower thoracic and lumbar vertebrae. Various forms of the syndrome have been transmitted as autosomal dominant and autosomal recessive traits. Malformations in other organ systems are common. These include extraocular palsies, deafness, macrocephaly, hydrocephaly, and meningoceles. Neurologic abnormalities, including mirror movements, nystagmus, and mental retardation, have been described. Musculoskeletal anomalies include thoracic scoliosis, spina bifida occulta, abnormalities of ribs, and Sprengel's deformity. Webbing of the neck and facial asymmetry may be evident. Less commonly, congenital heart disease and genitourinary anomalies are found. Cleft lip and palate and abnormalities of the gastrointestinal tract, lungs, and skin also have been reported.

## MACROCEPHALY AND MICROCEPHALY

### Macrocephaly

Macrocephaly refers to a head size two standard deviations above the mean. There are many causes for large heads. Table 148-1 lists the more common conditions associated with large head size. In some children, a large brain (ie, megalencephaly) may be the underlying condition. This may be familial and not accompanied by any additional symptoms and signs or there may be an associated mental deficiency and other neurologic abnormalities such as hypotonia.

Infants have been described who are macrocephalic and whose head growth parallels a normal growth pattern but is above the 95th percentile. CT reveals slight ventricular dilation and increased width of the subarachnoid space over the convexities of the hemispheres. The development of most of these children is normal or only slightly delayed. If head growth continues parallel to the 95th percentile, no intervention is necessary. The exact cause of this condition is uncertain. It has been referred to as extraventricular obstructive hydrocephalus or external hydrocephalus. Another possibility is that the fluid over the convexities represents small subdural hematomas with secondary hydrocephalus. The diagnosis can be established by CT or MRI, and the children can be followed with serial head circumference measurements. Any deviation from the anticipated growth pattern warrants repeat neuroimaging studies. Usually by the preschool years, the head size deviates less from the 95th percentile, and the fluid collections remain stable or decrease.

### Microcephaly

Microcephaly indicates a head size less than two standard deviations below the mean. This indicates an accompanying small brain (ie, microencephaly). The causes are multiple. In primary microcephaly, there is no identifiable insult to the developing brain that subsequently inhibits its growth. The primary microcephalies include familial forms and the cases that seem to occur in isolation. Newborn infants often do not exhibit striking deficits, unlike the infants who have sustained a major insult in utero. Eventually, intellectual impairment becomes apparent, and some children develop motor deficits and epilepsy.

Other anomalies sometimes associated with microcephaly include agyria, lissencephaly, micropolygyri, schizencephaly, macrogyri, and heterotopia. These infants usually have severe deficits that are apparent in the neonatal period.

Microcephaly can be seen in a variety of chromosomal anomalies, intrauterine infections secondary to inherited metabolic disorders, intrauterine anoxia or vascular events, and insults in the perinatal period.

## Selected Readings

Barnett HJM, Foster JB, Hudgson P. Syringomyelia. In: Walton JH, ed. Major problems in neurology. Philadelphia: WB Saunders, 1973.

DeMyer W. Megalencephaly in children. Clinical syndromes, genetic patterns and differential diagnosis from hydrocephalus. Neurology 1972;22:634.

Dure LS, Percy AK, Check WR, Laurent JP. Chiari type I malformation in children. J Pediatr 1989;115:573.

Edwards JH. The syndrome of sex-linked hydrocephalus. Arch Dis Child 1961;36:486.

Fishman MA. Hydrocephalus. In: Eliasson SG, Prensky AL, Hardin WB, eds. Neurological pathophysiology. New York: Oxford University Press, 1978.

Forward KR, Fewer D, Stiver HG. Cerebrospinal fluid shunt infections. J Neurosurg 1983;59:389.

Foster JB, Hudgson P, Pearce GW. The association of syringomyelia and congenital cervico-medullary anomalies: pathological evidence. Brain 1969;92:25.

Gunderson CH, Greenspan RH, Glaser GH, Lubs HA. The Klippel-Feil syndrome: genetic and clinical re-evaluation of cervical fusion. Medicine (Baltimore) 1967;46:491.

Guthkelch AN, Riley NA. Influence of aetiology on prognosis in surgically treated infantile hydrocephalus. Arch Dis Child 1969;44:29.

Lorber J, Priestley BL. Children with large heads: a practical approach to diagnosis in 557 children, with special reference to 109 children with megalencephaly. Dev Med Child Neurol 1981;23:531.

Portnoy HD, Croissant PD. Megalencephaly in infants and children. Arch Neurol 1978;35:306.

Pryor H, Thelander H. Abnormally small head size and intellect in children. J Pediatr 1968;73:593.

*Principles and Practice of Pediatrics, Second Edition.*
edited by Frank A. Oski et al. J. B. Lippincott Company, Philadelphia © 1994.

## CHAPTER 149
# *Acute Encephalopathies*

Julie Thorne Parke

The term *encephalopathy* refers to a diffuse disturbance of brain function, resulting in behavioral changes, altered consciousness, or seizures. The term is usually reserved for noninfective causes of brain dysfunction. The term *encephalitis* refers to brain dysfunction resulting from an infectious process. Clinically, it may be difficult to differentiate the two, and an infectious process must always be considered in a patient with evidence of an acute disturbance of brain function.

Many conditions can cause acute brain dysfunction in children, resulting in progressive alterations of consciousness (Table 149-1). Many of these conditions are treatable and may have a favorable outcome if an accurate diagnosis is made and appropriate therapy instituted.

## PATHOPHYSIOLOGY

To function normally, the brain must be adequately supplied with substrates and cofactors for energy production and for synthesis of structural components. There must be adequate blood flow to deliver the substrates and to remove waste products. Many encephalopathies are caused by cytotoxic injury, which occurs if energy production is disrupted by a lack of oxygen or glucose or

TABLE 149-1. Causes of Acute Encephalopathy in Childhood

| Oxygen, Substrate, or Cofactor Deprivation | Metabolic and Endocrinologic Disturbance | Postinfectious Disorders |
|---|---|---|
| Hypoxia | Fluid/electrolyte imbalance | Acute disseminated encephalomyelitis |
|   Pulmonary disease |   Water intoxication | Reye's syndrome |
|   Alveolar hypoventilation |   Hypo- or hypernatremia | **Exogenous Toxins** |
|   Carbon monoxide poisoning |   Hypo- or hypermagnesemia | Drugs (sedatives, anticholinergics, psychotropics, salicylates) |
|   Methemoglobinemia |   Hypo- or hypercalcemia | Insecticides/pesticides |
|   Anemia |   Hypo- or hyperphosphatemia | Heavy metals, lead |
| Anoxia or ischemia |   Acidosis or alkalosis | **Abnormal Temperature Regulation** |
|   "Near-miss" sudden infant death syndrome |   Trace metal deficiency | Hypothermia |
|   Cardiac arrest |   "Scalds" encephalopathy | Heat stroke |
|   Near-drowning | Endocrinologic disturbance | |
|   Cardiac dysrhythmia |   Diabetes mellitus | |
|   Congestive heart failure |   Hypo- or hyperthyroidism | |
|   Hypotension |   Hypo- or hyperparathyroidism | |
|   Diffuse intravascular coagulation |   Hypopituitarism | |
| Hypoglycemia | Organ failure | |
| Vitamin or cofactor deficiency |   Hepatic | |
|   Thiamine |   Renal | |
|   Niacin |   Pancreatic | |
|   Pyridoxin |   Intussusception or volvulus | |
|   $B_{12}$ |   Hypertensive encephalopathy | |
| Folate | Inborn errors of metabolism | |
| |   Aminoacidurias (branched chain ketoacidosis) | |
| |   Organic acidurias (propionic, methylmalonic, isovaleric acidemias, $\beta$-ketothiolase deficiency) | |
| |   Urea cycle defects | |
| |   Systemic carnitine deficiency | |

*Adapted from Plum F, Posner JB. The diagnosis of stupor and coma, ed. 3. Philadelphia: FA Davis, 1982.*

by inadequate cerebral blood flow. Cytotoxic injury may also occur with direct poisoning of the neuron by exogenous toxins or drugs or by endogenous toxins arising from an error of metabolism or from inadequate removal of toxic wastes by the kidneys or liver. Cytotoxic injury is frequently accompanied by cerebral edema and increased intracranial pressure, amplifying cerebral ischemia.

Other encephalopathies may be caused by interference with neurotransmission rather than actual cytotoxic injury. Severe electrolyte disturbances may alter the electrical properties of cellular membranes. Various toxins and drugs may similarly interfere with membrane polarization or may alter neurotransmitters, interfering with neuronal activity.

## CLINICAL PRESENTATION

The earliest signs of an acute encephalopathy may be subtle, including personality disturbances, a shortened attention span, and changes in mentation. Cognitive deficits, such as difficulty in processing new information and perceptual and memory deficits, are common in the initial stages. Abnormal movements, particularly fine tremors, asterixis, or myoclonus, may be present. Primitive reflexes, such as the grasp, snout, sucking, and rooting responses, may be elicited on examination. With increasing severity of brain dysfunction, alteration in the level of consciousness occurs, progressing from lethargy and obtundation to stupor and coma. Some patients retain their alert appearance but become increasingly disoriented and agitated. Other patients have alternating periods of hyperalertness and drowsiness, gradually pro-

gressing to longer periods of unresponsiveness. Seizures occur frequently and may be generalized or focal.

Diffuse symmetric abnormalities in motor tone and strength are common. Focal motor abnormalities are uncommon and, if present, tend to fluctuate in severity or change in location. The pupillary examination may be helpful in determining the cause of the encephalopathy. Preservation of the pupillary light reflexes in the presence of respiratory depression and deep coma suggests a metabolic coma. The absence of pupillary light reflexes suggests asphyxia, anticholinergic drug or glutethimide ingestion, or structural disease as the cause of coma. Alterations in the respiratory pattern are common in acute encephalopathies and may facilitate an accurate diagnosis if used in conjunction with direct determinations of the arterial blood pH, partial pressures of oxygen and carbon dioxide, and bicarbonate concentration (Table 149-2).

## ETIOLOGY

### Hypoxic-Ischemic Encephalopathy

Oxygen and glucose are the two major substrates needed for energy production in the brain. The supply of these two substrates and the cofactors necessary to allow usage of the substrates depends on an adequate cerebral blood flow. The brain is particularly vulnerable to even brief interruptions of blood flow or oxygen supply, because it possesses almost no reserves of nutrients and metabolizes at one of the highest rates of any organ in the body. If the brain's oxygen supply is insufficient, whether because of decreased availability or decreased delivery, con-

TABLE 149-2.  Some Causes of Abnormal Ventilation in Unresponsive Patients

| Hyperventilation | Hypoventilation |
|---|---|
| *Metabolic Acidosis* | *Respiratory Acidosis* |
| Anion gap | Acute (uncompensated) |
|    Diabetic ketoacidosis* |    Sedative drugs* |
|    Diabetic hyperosmolar coma* |    Brain stem injury |
|    Lactic acidosis |    Neuromuscular disorders |
|    Uremia* |    Chest injury |
|    Alcoholic ketoacidosis |    Acute pulmonary disease |
|    Acidic poisons* | Chronic pulmonary disease* |
|    Ethylene glycol | *Metabolic Alkalosis* |
|    Methyl alcohol | Vomiting or gastric drainage |
| Paraldehyde | Diuretic therapy |
|    Salicylism (primarily in children) | Adrenal steroid excess (Cushing's syndrome) |
| No anion gap | Primary aldosteronism |
|    Diarrhea | Bartter's syndrome |
|    Pancreatic drainage | |
|    Carbonic anhydrase inhibitors | |
|    $NH_4Cl$ ingestion | |
|    Renal tubular acidosis | |
|    Ureteroenterostomy | |
| *Respiratory Alkalosis* | |
| Hepatic failure* | |
| Sepsis* | |
| Pneumonia | |
| Anxiety (hyperventilation syndrome) | |
| *Mixed Acid-Base Disorders (Metabolic Acidosis and Respiratory Alkalosis)* | |
| Salicylism | |
|    Sepsis* | |
|    Hepatic failure* | |

\* Common causes of stupor or coma.
Plum F, Posner JB. *The diagnosis of stupor and coma, ed. 3. Philadelphia: FA Davis, 1982;186.*

sciousness is lost rapidly. If oxygenation is restored immediately, consciousness returns without sequelae. However, if oxygen deprivation lasts longer than 1 or 2 minutes, signs of an encephalopathy may persist for hours or permanently. Total ischemic anoxia lasting longer than about 4 minutes usually results in severe irreversible brain damage. In rare instances, especially near-drowning events, recovery of brain function occurs despite more prolonged periods of anoxia.

Major causes leading to hypoxic-ischemic encephalopathy include obstruction of the airway, as in drowning, choking, or suffocation, and a sudden decrease in cardiac output, as in cardiorespiratory arrest, severe dysrhythmias, severe hypotension, or massive systemic hemorrhage. Carbon monoxide poisoning may produce a hypoxic encephalopathy because carbon monoxide binds tightly to hemoglobin, diminishing its oxygen-carrying capacity. Subacute chronic hypoxia, as occurs in congestive heart failure, severe anemia, or pulmonary disease, may also cause an encephalopathy. However, severe neurologic changes usually occur only after a prolonged period of chronic hypoxia, and the cause of hypoxia is generally evident. Cerebral edema is a consistent feature in patients who have had an acute anoxic-ischemic event, and may be quite severe. Some patients may show a "lucent" interval of 12 to 24 hours before lapsing into coma with signs of cerebral edema. Occasionally, patients who have had oxygen deprivation or carbon monoxide intoxication develop a delayed postanoxic encephalopathy characterized by rapid neurologic deterioration several weeks after the initial insult.

The treatment of hypoxic-ischemic encephalopathy includes adequate oxygenation, rapid restoration of perfusion, and good fluid and electrolyte balance. Hyperosmolar agents and controlled hyperventilation may be necessary to reduce intracranial pressure. Anticonvulsants may also be necessary. The prognosis is difficult to determine early in the course, because patients may remain comatose for days, eventually recovering with few sequelae. Early evidence of brain stem dysfunction is a poor prognostic sign.

## Metabolic and Endocrinologic Disturbances

### Hypoglycemia

Hypoglycemia is a serious, correctable cause of metabolic encephalopathy. The tolerance to hypoglycemia varies, but symptoms usually occur when blood glucose levels fall below 40 mg/dL. The severity of symptoms is determined by the availability of alternative substrates for cerebral metabolism. Patients with hypoglycemic encephalopathy may present with a variety of neurologic symptoms, including simple confusion, delirium, abrupt focal neurologic signs resembling a stroke, focal or generalized seizures, or coma. Because the spectrum of clinical presentations is so wide, hypoglycemia should be suspected in every patient with acute neurologic dysfunction. Blood should be drawn immediately for a glucose determination, and glucose should be administered. If treated promptly, neurologic symptoms are reversible. Persistent deficits may occur with prolonged or recurrent hypoglycemic attacks.

The most common symptomatic hypoglycemia in childhood is ketotic hypoglycemia. This disorder is most frequently seen in thin, young children who have a mild infectious illness, which precipitates vomiting, altered mental status, and seizures, accompanied by hypoglycemia and ketosis. The cause of ketotic hypoglycemia is not clear, but it may be the result of limited liver glycogen stores and an inability to mobilize gluconeogenic precursors. Patients with this disorder should be treated immediately with glucose and then should be maintained on dietary therapy of frequent feedings during the day and bedtime snacks. Another common cause of hypoglycemia is an excessive dosage of insulin. Less common causes of hypoglycemia include hereditary defects in gluconeogenesis, insulin-secreting pancreatic tumors, deficiency of growth hormone or of cortisol, hepatitis, and Reye's syndrome. Excessive ingestion of alcohol may also produce hypoglycemia.

### Diabetic Ketoacidosis

Diabetes mellitus is the most common endocrinologic disease presenting as an acute encephalopathy, although pituitary, adrenal, parathyroid, and thyroid disorders occasionally present with similar symptoms. Diabetic ketoacidosis typically occurs in patients with relatively severe diabetes who neglect to take their insulin or who have an associated acute infection. Polyuria, polydipsia, and fatigue lead to a dehydrated state with metabolic acidosis. Nausea, vomiting, and acute abdominal pain may be prominent early in the course. Hyperventilation is common and reflects the body's attempt to compensate for the metabolic acidosis. The neurologic examination is nonfocal, and brain stem function is usually intact.

The treatment of diabetic ketoacidosis may have serious neurologic consequences. Sudden lowering of serum osmolality may produce a shift of water into the brain, causing marked cerebral edema. This should be suspected when patients recovering from diabetic ketoacidosis complain of headache or become increasingly lethargic. Profound hypophosphatemia may occur as dehydration is corrected and the serum glucose level is lowered, causing further neurologic dysfunction. In addition to ketoacidosis, hypoglycemia, uremia, hypertension, and cerebral infarction should be considered in the diabetic presenting with an acute encephalopathy.

## Disorders of Fluid and Electrolyte Balance

Disturbances in water and sodium metabolism can cause a spectrum of neurologic signs and symptoms, ranging from confusion and seizures to deep coma with increased intracranial pressure. Neuronal function depends on a correct ionic environment and can be altered by any changes in composition or volume of body fluids. Electrolyte disturbances occur fairly frequently in young children because their cutaneous water losses are relatively higher than those of an adult, and renal conservation of water is less efficient than in adults. The young child has a reduced tolerance for water deprivation or abnormal water loss. Disorders of electrolytes and serum osmolality are common causes of acute encephalopathy in childhood. Consciousness is altered if serum osmolality is less than 260 mOsm/kg or greater than 330 mOsm/kg. The total concentration of osmotically active materials in the interstitial and intracellular fluids is equal, because there is free diffusion of water across the cell membranes. A decrease in extracellular osmolality leads to cellular overhydration, and an increase in extracellular osmolality leads to cellular dehydration.

### Hyponatremia

Hyponatremia or water intoxication may be caused by a sudden hypotonic water load, a disproportionate loss of sodium, or inappropriate retention of water. Numerous neurologic disorders stimulate antidiuretic hormone release in excess of the amount required to maintain a normal concentration of serum sodium. Meningitis, head trauma, brain neoplasms, and acute or subacute peripheral neuropathy have been associated with the syndrome of inappropriate antidiuretic hormone. A variety of endocrine disorders, pulmonary disorders, and drug ingestions increase antidiuretic hormone secretion and predispose the patient to hyponatremia. Chronic hyponatremia, which may occur in chronic renal disease, is better tolerated than acute changes in sodium balance. Clinical symptoms are caused by the accumulation of water within the cells, which is related in some way to altered excitability of the neural membrane. Moderately severe hyponatremia may cause confusion, delirium, and multifocal myoclonus. Seizures and coma are usually associated with severe hyponatremia and may be life threatening. Seizures may be multifocal or generalized and typically occur with serum sodium concentrations between 95 to 110 mEq/L.

The treatment of hyponatremia depends on the cause. Infants with hyponatremic dehydration are rehydrated with isotonic solutions. Patients with water intoxication due to antidiuretic hormone excess or a free-water load can often be treated with fluid restriction. Hypertonic saline solutions should be reserved for patients with severe hyponatremia manifested by seizures or coma.

### Hypernatremia

Acute hypernatremia is most commonly caused by severe water depletion in children with diarrhea. It may also occur in patients receiving excessively concentrated solutions by tube feeding or in patients with diabetes insipidus. Symptoms of encephalopathy usually occur with serum sodium levels in excess of 160 mEq/L or total osmolalities of 340 or more mOsm/kg. Most of the dehydration in hypertonic states is intracellular. Because circulatory volume is relatively well maintained, clinical signs of dehydration such as tachycardia and poor skin turgor are less prominent than in hyponatremic or isotonic dehydration. Brain shrinkage predisposes the child to petechial brain hemorrhages and to extraaxial hemorrhage. Venous sinus thrombosis and cerebral infarctions may also occur. There is a high mortality rate, and many of the survivors have permanent neurologic sequelae, including hemiparesis, seizure disorders, and mental retardation.

The treatment of hypernatremic dehydration involves the slow replacement of fluids. Rapid rehydration predisposes to cerebral edema with seizures and other manifestations of water intoxication.

### Hypocalcemia

Hypocalcemia produces hyperexcitability of the peripheral and central nervous systems. Headaches and muscular cramping and twitching are early signs. Positive Chvostek and Trousseau signs are easily elicited, and carpopedal spasm may be prominent. Seizures are common and may be generalized, focal, or multifocal. Management consists of correction of the metabolic disturbance with intravenous administration of calcium gluconate. Chronic oral administration of calcium and vitamin D may be necessary, depending on the underlying cause.

### Hypercalcemia

Neurologic manifestations of hypercalcemia include headaches, hallucinations, rigidity, tremor, and psychotic behavior. Some patients present with a slowly progressive dementia. Treatment depends on the cause. Severe hypercalcemia may require the use of a chelating agent.

### Hypomagnesemia

Symptoms of hypomagnesemia, which occur when serum magnesium drops below 1 mEq/L, include confusion, irritability, hallucinations, and coma. Muscle twitching, myoclonic jerks, and tremors are common. Generalized seizures may occur. Examination shows increased muscle tone, carpopedal spasm, and positive Chvostek and Trousseau signs. Treatment consists of slow intravenous administration of magnesium sulfate.

### Hypermagnesemia

Severe hypermagnesemia causes somnolence, lethargy, coma, and respiratory failure. There is a peripheral neuromuscular paralysis with loss of the deep tendon reflexes. Treatment is difficult. It may include the administration of calcium and neostigmine, and hemodialysis may be necessary in severe cases.

## Organ Failure

### Hepatic Encephalopathy

There are numerous causes of acute hepatic failure during childhood, including inborn errors of metabolism, acute viral hepatitis, ascending cholangitis, Reye's syndrome, and ingestion of hepatotoxic substances. Other disorders, including Wilson's disease, chronic heart failure, and biliary atresia, are more likely to cause symptoms of chronic hepatic failure. Acute hepatic encephalopathy may be precipitated in these patients by intercurrent infection, excessive protein intake, or gastrointestinal hemorrhage. Numerous metabolic disturbances occur in hepatic failure, many of which may contribute to the encephalopathic state. Hypokalemia, hypomagnesemia, and alkalosis are common. Short-chain and medium-chain fatty acids and $\beta$-hydroxylated phenylethylamines accumulate and may act as toxins or false neurotransmitters. Ammonia combines with $\alpha$-ketoglutaric acid in the brain to form glutamic acid, leading to $\alpha$-ketoglutarate depletion, which interferes with the activity of the tricarboxylic acid cycle. Alterations in the pattern of serum amino acids also occur.

Patients may show initial apathy, confusion, or lethargy. Some patients have visual hallucinations and become extremely agitated. A coarse, flapping tremor of the hands (ie, asterixis) frequently occurs. Grimacing, jerking, and other motor disturbances are common. The level of consciousness may fluctuate dramatically from confusion to reversible decerebrate or decorticate posturing. The laboratory examination is helpful in making the diagnosis of hepatic coma, because many of the liver function tests are abnormal and the arterial blood ammonia level is usually markedly elevated. A bleeding diathesis may predispose the patient to intracranial hemorrhage. The electroencephalogram shows diffuse slowing in the early stages, progressing to an unusual pattern of triphasic waves as the patient becomes stuporous.

Treatment of acute hepatic encephalopathy focuses on correction of multiple metabolic abnormalities. High concentrations of glucose prevent hypoglycemia and possibly decrease the accumulation of short-chain fatty acids. Protein intake should be severely limited. Broad-spectrum antibiotics and lactulose administered by nasogastric tube or enema may help reduce ammonia accumulation. Attention should be given to gastroesophageal bleeding and intercurrent infections. Exchange blood transfusions or hemodialysis can be used to correct metabolic abnormalities and improve clotting functions. Cerebral edema may be massive, requiring controlled hyperventilation, hyperosmolar agents, and possibly corticosteroids. Although hepatic coma may be reversible, the mortality rate is high.

### Uremic Encephalopathy

Acute and chronic renal failure are associated with numerous neurologic complications, including uremic encephalopathy, peripheral neuropathy, hypertensive encephalopathy, hemorrhagic complications, and dialysis dysequilibrium syndrome. The precise cause of the encephalopathy associated with uremia has not been determined. Urea is not the sole toxin, because urea infusions do not reproduce the encephalopathy and because hemodialysis reverses the encephalopathy even when urea is added to the dialyzing bath. The severity of neurologic symptoms does not correlate well with the level of azotemia. Encephalopathic features have been reported in patients with blood urea nitrogen (BUN) values as low as 48 mg/100 mL but have been absent in others with BUN values exceeding 200 mg/100 mL. Some investigators have suggested that increased permeability of cell membranes allows access to the brain of normally excluded neurotoxic compounds such as organic acids.

The clinical picture of uremic encephalopathy is nonspecific, as are most of the metabolic encephalopathies. Early symptoms include lethargy or agitation, tremulousness, asterixis, and myoclonic jerks. Tetany, which is unresponsive to calcium administration, may occur. Muscle tone is usually increased. Generalized or focal seizures may occur, and meningeal irritation with nuchal rigidity has been described. Myokymic twitching of muscles, cramps, and intractable hiccups may occur.

Treatment of uremia by dialysis may lead to an encephalopathy known as the *dialysis dysequilibrium syndrome*. This syndrome is characterized by the abrupt onset of lethargy, visual hallucinations, and generalized seizures progressing to a comatose state, which occurs at the end of dialysis or up to 24 hours later. Papilledema and other signs of increased intracranial pressure may be observed. These symptoms are secondary to cellular overhydration, which occurs when urea is removed from the circulation and extracellular space but remains high in the intracellular space.

### Hypertensive Encephalopathy

An acute encephalopathy with seizures or coma may be the initial symptom of hypertensive disease. Neurologic symptoms may begin abruptly with severe headache, vomiting, and seizures, which tend to be focal, progressing to obtundation and coma. Patients frequently have focal weakness or focal neurologic signs on examination. Visual obscurations may occur. Most patients with hypertensive encephalopathy have abnormal funduscopic examinations with retinal artery spasm, retinal exudates, or papilledema, although the fundi may be normal. Hypertensive encephalopathy is usually associated with a sustained diastolic pressure of 120 mm Hg or greater. Initially, neurologic signs tend to be focal and fleeting in duration, because they are caused by vasoconstriction. In the later stages, the patient experiences focal increases in vascular permeability, focal edema, and necrosis. Neurologic signs become more persistent, typically lasting a few minutes to several days but then disappearing, leaving little residual deficit. Spinal fluid pressure is usually elevated, as is cerebrospinal fluid protein. Treatment focuses on cautious lowering of blood pressure, because rapid decreases in blood pressure may cause cerebral ischemia.

### Pancreatic Encephalopathy

Acute pancreatitis may cause an encephalopathy, and chronic relapsing pancreatitis may cause episodic stupor or coma. The encephalopathy usually begins several days after the onset of pancreatitis and is characterized by agitation or stupor, focal or generalized convulsions, and signs of bilateral corticospinal tract dysfunction. The pathogenesis is not understood, although postmortem evidence of patchy demyelination of white matter in the brain has led to the hypothesis that enzymes liberated from the pancreas play a role. Biochemical complications of acute pancreatitis, such as hyperosmolality, acidosis, and hypocalcemia, may also contribute to the encephalopathy.

## Inborn Errors of Metabolism

Several inborn errors of metabolism may cause acute, often recurrent encephalopathic symptoms. In many patients, the enzyme deficiency is incomplete. The encephalopathic episodes are usually triggered by minor illnesses with an associated increase in catabolism. Urea cycle defects, carnitine deficiency syndromes, and a number of aminoacidopathies and organic acidurias may cause recurrent episodes of vomiting and ataxia, followed by alterations in sensorium.

A history of similar episodes or a family history of consanguinity or a previously affected sibling strongly suggests an inherited defect in metabolism. It is important to collect laboratory samples at the time of presentation, because laboratory abnormalities may correct rapidly with intravenous fluids. Diagnostic studies should include blood ammonia, lactate, glucose, serum amino acids, and urine organic acids.

## Intoxications

Drug-induced encephalopathy must always be considered in the child presenting with unexplained seizures or an alteration in mental status, particularly if there is evidence of involvement of other organ systems. Drug-induced encephalopathy may be caused by accidental ingestion, therapeutic overdosage, or deliberate abuse. Many drugs in common use are capable of producing agitation, delirium, stupor, and coma when taken in large amounts (Table 149-3).

### Sedatives

Sedatives, such as barbiturates, benzodiazepines, glutethimide, and alcohol produce coma if taken in large enough amounts. Nystagmus, ataxia, and dysarthria frequently precede signs of impaired consciousness in sedative overdosage. In larger amounts, most sedatives selectively depress the level of consciousness and respiratory function while sparing pupillary light reflexes. The pupils may remain small and reactive even with large ingestions that produce coma, hypotension, respiratory failure, and flaccid paralysis with areflexia. A notable exception is glutethimide (Doriden), which characteristically produces midposition or moderately dilated pupils that are unequal and fixed to light. Glutethimide tends to cause prolonged coma with marked fluctuations in the level of consciousness. Treatment is primarily supportive, but dialysis may be of use in severe cases.

### Anticholinergics

Intoxication with antihistamines and anticholinergic agents such as tricyclic antidepressants and scopolamine causes central nervous system excitation with confusion, anxiety, hallucinations, and delirium. Hyperpyrexia, seizures, and coma may occur. Anticholinergic intoxication may be reversed by repetitive intravenous administration of physostigmine. Cardiac dysrhythmias frequently occur with overdosage of tricyclic antidepressants and may require aggressive therapy.

### Salicylates

Encephalopathic symptoms may occur with acute or chronic salicylate intoxication. Initial symptoms include hyperpnea, vomiting, tinnitus, restlessness, and delirium. Lethargy, convulsions, and coma with respiratory failure and cardiovascular collapse may follow. Salicylate ingestion must be differentiated from Reye's syndrome and organic acidurias that cause metabolic acidosis. Treatment consists of intravenous fluid replacement with correction of acidosis. Acetazolamide increases the excretion of salicylates. Exchange transfusion, peritoneal dialysis, or hemodialysis may be necessary in severe cases. The neurologic symptoms are potentially reversible, although severe poisoning may be fatal.

### Environmental Toxins

Numerous environmental toxins can cause acute encephalopathic symptoms. Chlorinated insecticides may cause a period of excitability with disorientation, tremor, muscle twitching, and headache, which is followed by seizures and respiratory failure.

Inorganic lead poisoning occurs with chronic ingestion of the metal from lead-containing paint or putty or from exposure to smelters. Nonspecific symptoms of systemic involvement precede the encephalopathy. Initial symptoms may include irritability, anorexia, failure to gain weight, constipation, vomiting, and anemia. The onset of the encephalopathy is often abrupt, with a brief period of ataxia and persistent vomiting followed by intractable seizures and signs of massive cerebral edema. Papilledema and cranial nerve VI palsies are common. Focal motor signs and focal or multifocal seizures may suggest a mass lesion rather than a diffuse encephalopathy. Lumbar puncture is generally contraindicated because of the likelihood of herniation. However, if performed to rule out infection, it may show an elevated protein concentration and a mild mononuclear pleocytosis.

Initial management involves treatment of cerebral edema and control of seizure activity. Pharmacologic treatment with dimercaprol (BAL) in combination with calcium-EDTA should be initiated as soon as possible. The prognosis for patients with acute lead encephalopathy is poor. The mortality rate is high, and the patients who recover have a high incidence of permanent neurologic deficits, including mental retardation, behavioral disorders, motor disabilities, and persistent seizure disorders.

## Parainfectious Neurologic Syndromes

Symptoms of an acute encephalopathy occasionally occur after or in conjunction with a systemic illness. In some cases, the encephalopathy is caused by direct viral invasion of the nervous system. However, other instances appear to be due to an indirect, immune-mediated reaction to the infection. Parainfectious encephalomyelitis, also called acute disseminated encephalomyelitis, is an acute demyelinating disease that follows a viral illness or some immunizations. The demyelination is believed to occur as a result of an acquired, delayed hypersensitivity to myelin and a direct attack on the myelin sheath by sensitized lymphocytes. Alternatively, it has been suggested that damage to small vessels may be the primary event in the pathogenesis of the illness with a secondary loss of myelin.

Clinical evidence of neurologic deterioration appears in a few days to 3 weeks after a vaccination or a viral illness. Initial symptoms include nonspecific signs such as fever, headache, vomiting,

**TABLE 149-3. Exogenous Toxins Causing Acute Encephalopathy**

| Pharmacotherapeutic Agents | Drugs of Abuse |
| --- | --- |
| Sedative/hypnotics (barbiturates, glutethimide, benzodiazepines) | Alcohol |
| | Amphetamines |
| Narcotic analgesics | Narcotics |
| Antihistamines | Cannabis |
| Anticholinergics | LSD |
| Anticonvulsants | Mescaline |
| Phenothiazines | Psilocybin |
| Tricyclic antidepressants | Phencyclidine |
| Salicylates | Solvents |
| Iron | **Environmental Toxins** |
| Penicillin | Carbon monoxide |
| Cimetidine | Lead and heavy metals |
| Steroids | Organophosphates |
| | DDT |
| | Hydrocarbons |
| | Solvents |

anorexia, and meningism. The nonspecific symptoms may be followed by the acute onset of seizures with a rapid progression to confusion, lethargy, and coma. Other patients develop motor deficits, visual field defects, aphasia, ataxia, movement disorders, or cranial nerve abnormalities. The disease is usually acute, progressing to maximal severity within 1 week. The duration varies, with some patients showing a rapid improvement within days and others improving slowly over several weeks. There are no pathognomonic laboratory findings in acute disseminated encephalomyelitis. The cerebrospinal fluid protein may be mildly elevated, and there may be a lymphocytic pleocytosis. The electroencephalogram is usually abnormal, showing diffuse, nonspecific slowing. Magnetic resonance imaging is helpful diagnostically, showing multiple areas of involvement in most patients. The mortality rate is high, with death occurring in 10% to 30% of patients. Approximately one third of the survivors have neurologic sequelae.

The clinical and pathologic features in young children with parainfectious encephalopathy are somewhat different from those in older children. Children younger than 2 years of age develop generalized seizures and evidence of elevated intracranial pressure rather than multifocal signs. Instead of foci of demyelination, there are nonspecific pathologic changes similar to those found in anoxia, including gross brain edema and acute neuronal vacuolization and degeneration. There is no evidence of inflammation or infection. The cause of this acute encephalopathy in young infants is obscure, and its relation to immune-mediated acute disseminated encephalomyelitis is not clear. Treatment focuses on the reduction of cerebral edema and aggressive management of seizures.

## Reye's Syndrome

Reye's syndrome, an encephalopathy with fatty degeneration of the viscera, may occur after a number of viral infections, but it most commonly follows influenza B viral infections and varicella. However, no virus has been recovered from brain tissue, and the disease is not caused by active viral invasion. This syndrome may occur in persons of all ages, but it is most common among children and adolescents.

Several environmental toxins and drugs have been implicated in the pathogenesis of Reye's syndrome. Interest in recent years has centered on salicylates. The current opinion is that the primary pathologic abnormality in Reye's syndrome lies in the mitochondria, and that salicylates exacerbate the preexisting metabolic abnormality. Characteristically, profuse vomiting and confusion occur several days after an upper respiratory infection or varicella. A phase of hyperexcitability with restlessness, disorientation, and combativeness follows. The more severely affected children become comatose with decorticate or decerebrate posturing. Classic signs of rostrocaudal deterioration with progressive loss of brain stem reflexes may occur. Numerous laboratory abnormalities occur, the most significant of which are elevated serum transaminases, hyperammonemia, and hypoprothrombinemia. Bilirubin is normal. Hypoglycemia occurs in 40% of patients, most often in children younger than 2 years of age. Creatine phosphokinase, lipase, amylase, and lactate dehydrogenase are elevated. Uric acid, lactate, pyruvate, $\beta$-hydroxybutyric acid, acetoacetic acid, and several other organic acids are also elevated. The serum cholesterol concentration is decreased, as are several serum proteins, including lipoproteins, clotting factors, and components of the complement system. The plasma cortisol and prolactin levels are elevated. The histopathologic features in the liver are characteristic, showing microvesicular steatosis, glycogen depletion, and abnormal mitochondria. Mitochondrial abnormalities have been seen in neurons, renal tubular cells, and other organs. The most prominent neuropathologic feature is marked cytotoxic cerebral edema.

The treatment of Reye's syndrome is directed at supportive care and management of cerebral edema, which may be massive. Hypertonic solutions of glucose and mannitol, early elective intubation, hyperventilation, and intracranial pressure monitoring have roles in the standard treatment of Reye's syndrome. Other treatment modalities that remain controversial include corticosteroid therapy, pentobarbital-induced coma, deep hypothermia, and exchange transfusions. The mortality rate has been markedly reduced by aggressive supportive care and management of intracranial pressure. Many patients recover without significant neurologic sequelae.

## Selected Readings

Blisard S, Davis L. Neuropathologic findings in Reye syndrome. J Child Neurol 1991;6:41.

Brown J, Habel A. Toxic encephalopathy and acute brain-swelling in children. Dev Med Child Neurol 1975;17:659.

DeVivo D. Reye syndrome and associated metabolic encephalopathies. In: Fishman M, ed. Pediatric neurology. Orlando, FL: Grune & Stratton, 1986:203.

Forbes G, McCormick K. Disturbances of water and electrolytes. In: Farmer T, ed. Pediatric neurology, ed. 3. Philadelphia: Harper & Row, 1983:265.

Garrettson L. Poisoning. In: Pellock J, Myer E, eds. Neurologic emergencies in infancy and childhood. Philadelphia: Harper & Row, 1984:155.

Marks N, Bodensteiner J, Bobele G, et al. Parainflammatory leukoencephalomyelitis: clinical and magnetic resonance imaging findings. J Child Neurol 1988;3:205.

Parke J. Para-infectious neurologic syndromes. In: Fishman M, ed. Pediatric neurology. Orlando, FL: Grune & Stratton, 1986:219.

Piomelli S, Rosen J, Chisolm J, Graif J. Management of childhood lead poisoning. J Pediatr 1984;105:523.

Plum F, Posner J. Multifocal, diffuse, and metabolic brain diseases causing stupor and coma. In: Plum F, Posner J. The diagnosis of stupor and coma, ed. 3. Philadelphia: FA Davis, 1982:177.

Rebouche C, Engel A. Carnitine metabolism and deficiency syndromes. Mayo Clin Proc 1983;58:533.

Sparling MA. Diabetic ketoacidosis. Pediatr Clin North Am 1984;31:591.

*Principles and Practice of Pediatrics, Second Edition.*
edited by Frank A. Oski et al. J. B. Lippincott Company, Philadelphia © 1994.

CHAPTER 150

# Static Encephalopathy

## Alan K. Percy

Static encephalopathy is a disorder of motor function against a background of a static or nonprogressive brain injury, usually as a result of a prenatal or perinatal event. The term encompasses a heterogeneous group of disorders whose causes are diverse and is synonymous with the term *cerebral palsy*. The motor dysfunction of the person with static encephalopathy clearly signifies to others the presence of a handicapping condition. In addition to the motor dysfunction, which may range from mild to severe, associated neurologic difficulties include mental retardation, seizures, communication dysfunction, and visual and hearing deficits. Individuals with static encephalopathy are, as a group, among the most handicapped in our society. In the United States, as many as 500,000 children may be affected and, thus, represent an important public health responsibility.

The classification of static encephalopathy has changed little from Freud's description of a century ago and represents the involvement, individually or in combination, of cerebral hemispheres, leading to upper motor neuron signs including spasticity; of basal ganglia, leading to extrapyramidal signs; and of the cerebellum, leading to hypotonia and ataxia. The resulting classification includes spastic forms (hemiplegia, tetraplegia, or diplegia); extrapyramidal forms (choreoathetosis or dystonia); and a cerebellar form (ataxia). Mixed forms also have been described. The comparative frequency of each form of static encephalopathy as determined from Swedish and American studies is shown in Table 150-1. The preponderance of spastic forms is evident. In general, males outnumber females at a ratio of 1.2 : 1. The increasing prominence of diplegic forms (symmetric lower extremity involvement greater than that in the upper extremities) is the result of increased survival of low–birth-weight infants with predominantly periventricular lesions.

The incidence of static encephalopathy has changed substantially over the last 30 years (Table 150-2). The declining incidence seen in the 1960s was attributed to improved prenatal and perinatal care. In particular, better treatment of Rh incompatibility states, with a resulting decrease in damage to the basal ganglia from kernicterus, has led to a reduction in the extrapyramidal form. The increasing incidence noted in the past 2 decades also is related to better perinatal care, especially of low–birth-weight infants. Thus, the changing incidence pattern is felt to reflect improved survival yielding an apparent increase in incidence.

## RISK FACTORS

Risk factors for static encephalopathy vary with the period or timing of the insult. More than a century ago, Little described cerebral palsy (static encephalopathy) and related it causally to difficulties in the birth process. Data from several large population-based studies confirmed the subsequent notion, first advanced by Freud, that static encephalopathy in the vast majority of children *cannot* be attributed to birth asphyxia, and that "difficult birth in itself is merely a symptom of deeper effects that influenced the development of the fetus." In fact, no specific cause can be identified for more than 50% of infants in whom the condition develops. Congenital disorders appear to account for 30% to 40% of the total and infections of the central nervous system account for another 5% to 10%. In addition, multiple births (ie, twins) represent an increased risk for static encephalopathy. Neonatal events previously associated with asphyxia are at least as likely to occur with congenital disease. These include

**TABLE 150-1.   Comparative Percentage Distribution of Static Encephalopathy**

| Type | Swedish Series* | Boston Children's Hospital† |
|---|---|---|
| Hemiplegia | 37 | 41 |
| Tetraplegia | 7 | 19 |
| Diplegia | 41 | 5 |
| Ataxia | 5 | — |
| Dyskinesia | 10 | 22 |
| Mixed | — | 13 |

* 1979–1982.
† 1959.

**TABLE 150-2.   Comparative Incidence Pattern of Static Encephalopathy**

| Rochester, Minnesota | | Sweden | |
|---|---|---|---|
| Period | Incidence* | Period | Incidence* |
| 1950–1958 | 2.3 | 1959–1962 | 1.9 |
| | | 1963–1966 | 1.7 |
| | | 1967–1970 | 1.3 |
| 1968–1976 | 1.6 | 1971–1974 | 1.6 |
| | | 1975–1978 | 2.0 |
| | | 1979–1982 | 2.2 |
| | | 1983–1986† | 2.5 |

* Incidence per 1000 live births.
† Preliminary

meconium in the amniotic fluid, low 10-minute Apgar scores, neonatal seizures, apnea, newborn neurologic abnormalities, and slow head growth. Furthermore, epilepsy and mental retardation alone do not follow birth asphyxia. Prematurity, low birth weight, and placental dysfunction are increasingly important factors in the genesis of static encephalopathy. The infant with low Apgar scores from a late asphyxial event, who does not show signs of newborn encephalopathy, will not have cerebral palsy.

Spastic diplegia most commonly is the result of prematurity and postnatal complications of premature birth. When seen in the full-term infant, it usually is the result of a complicated pregnancy and delivery. Spastic diplegia is not seen in the term infant whose only insult at birth is late asphyxia. That is, antenatal risk factors must have been present.

During the past 3 decades, infant mortality rates have fallen dramatically in the developed countries of the world. This has been attributed to improved prenatal and perinatal care. The fact that these improvements have not had a favorable impact on the incidence of static encephalopathy provides further support for causative factors other than the birth process itself in this disorder. Extensive evaluation of electronic fetal monitoring revealed that this technique did not improve the outcome in terms of neurologic development in either term or preterm infants. In addition, birth asphyxia that is significant enough to produce brain injury also damages the kidneys, liver, lungs, and heart. Finally, infants with neurologic sequelae that are secondary to a significant perinatal asphyxial event always have signs of newborn encephalopathy. Those infants injured sometime during the prenatal period may have had time to recover before parturition and may not have perinatal encephalopathy. Thus, their static problems can be assigned clearly to insults occurring at a time other than birth.

Static encephalopathy may result from postnatal events such as infection, trauma, or cardiac disease as well, although only 10% to 20% of cases have this origin. Less commonly, systemic disease (hematologic, immunologic, or metabolic), neoplasm, vascular malformation, or demyelinating disease are responsible. Postnatal events leading to static encephalopathy may occur throughout infancy and childhood. Of these, infection and trauma are the most significant.

## THE PATHOPHYSIOLOGY OF MOTOR DYSFUNCTION

The abnormalities of motor function that accompany static encephalopathy represent disorders of tone, disorders of balance, and disorders of involuntary movement. Disorders of tone include diplegia, which often is the result of prematurity. When static encephalopathy occurs in premature infants, 80% have a diplegic form. Disorders of balance reflect cerebellar involvement and are characterized by ataxia and, to some extent, hypotonia. Disorders of involuntary movement are accompanied by dystonia and choreoathetosis, and indicate an insult to the basal ganglia.

Neuropathologic evaluation of static encephalopathy demonstrates a fixed, nonprogressive lesion. The motor dysfunction hardly is static, however. The spastic disorders, particularly the diplegic form, commonly present with hypotonia, and only over the course of weeks or months does the pattern of spasticity develop. Similarly, the movements of choreoathetosis that signify extrapyramidal involvement seldom are present in early infancy and often begin to emerge after the child's first birthday. The evolution of motor involvement reflects the interplay of maturing normal neural elements and impaired or abnormal neural elements on movement.

The pathophysiology of these motor disorders may be divided into six major categories. The categories may overlap in some patients, and not every individual will display the full array of abnormalities, except possibly those who are impaired most severely. This classification provides a useful framework, however, for understanding the pathophysiology of motor difficulties in patients with static encephalopathy.

Disorders of postural fixation result in an inability to orient the trunk and extremities to attain a vertical posture and are caused by spasticity in the limbs and hypotonia of the trunk.

Failure to suppress brain-stem postural reflexes similarly disrupts proper orientation to the environment. These reflex centers rely on labyrinthine (vestibular) input to modulate extensor tone, increasing extensor tone in the supine position and flexor tone in the prone position. In neither position can the child interact effectively with his or her external surroundings.

Disorders of tone are associated with increased tone (spasticity) in the antigravity muscles. These are the flexor muscles of the upper extremities and the extensor muscles of the lower extremities. The end result is flexed upper extremities and extended lower extremities, which prevent the performance of both individual and integrated motor activities, ultimately leading to fixed postural deformities.

Disorders of voluntary movement are characterized by a lack of motor planning and integrated motor activities, which can be noted most easily in walking, running, or hand dexterity.

Disorders of involuntary movement encompass dystonia and choreoathetosis. Such movements often are exacerbated by attempts to initiate voluntary motor acts and may be heightened by anxiety or tension. In some children, these involuntary movements may progress over time to rigidity, in effect lessening involuntary movements and virtually prohibiting voluntary acts.

Failure of development of cortical reactions results in the inability of a child to generate appropriate self-protection mechanisms or to suppress certain primitive reflexes such as the palmar and plantar grasps.

## ASSOCIATED ABNORMALITIES

Associated neurologic abnormalities may be seen in patients with each form of static encephalopathy. These include mental retardation, visual deficits, and seizures. About 50% of affected children have strabismus. Among the spastic forms of the disorder, those children with tetraplegia generally have profound retardation, cortical blindness, and seizures. In addition, they are likely to have swallowing difficulties as a manifestation of pseudobulbar palsy and to be at greater risk for aspiration and its attendant problems. The hemiplegic and diplegic forms of static encephalopathy are accompanied by retardation and seizures in one third of affected children. A hemianopia (visual field deficit) may occur in one third of all patients with hemiplegia. Children with choreoathetosis may have normal intellect and rarely have seizures. Their severe motor disorder limits meaningful interaction, however.

## DIFFERENTIAL DIAGNOSIS

Static encephalopathy must be distinguished from progressive disorders and from familial disorders of similar appearance. A progressive static encephalopathy is a contradiction and should prompt careful review of the diagnosis. As an acquired disorder, static encephalopathy does not exhibit a familial pattern. It often presents with hypotonia and must be distinguished from other causes of hypotonia. In patients with static encephalopathy, the degree of hypotonia exceeds the degree of weakness, and the deep tendon reflexes usually are brisk. Injury to the spinal cord may produce weakness and hypotonia initially. Spinal muscular atrophy or anterior horn cell disease (Werdnig-Hoffmann disease) is characterized by weakness, hypotonia, and areflexia. Disorders of peripheral nerve and muscle cause weakness and hypotonia that are proportional and, in the case of peripheral nerve disease, hyporeflexia also is present.

The spastic forms of static encephalopathy must be differentiated from other neurologic disorders that are associated with upper motor neuron signs, including intracranial mass lesions such as a neoplasm, brain abscess, or subdural fluid collection; hydrocephalus; cerebrovascular disease such as vasculitis or arteriovenous malformation; and disorders of white matter such as multiple sclerosis or the various types of leukodystrophy. The clinical presentation of these disorders should be readily distinguishable from that of static encephalopathy.

The extrapyramidal forms of static encephalopathy must be differentiated from other extrapyramidal disorders of childhood, including the different forms of dystonia, benign familial chorea, and Huntington disease.

## TREATMENT AND PROGNOSIS

Treatment goals for patients with static encephalopathy include optimizing the motor and intellectual capabilities of each child and providing for realistic social interaction. Motor dysfunction requires an individualized physical and occupational therapy program and an appropriate educational curriculum. Physical therapy is essential to minimize contractures and orthopedic deformities from muscle imbalance. In some instances, surgical intervention may be required; in others, orthotic devices may be sufficient to treat these problems.

Regular reassessment is essential for the child with static encephalopathy to evaluate the status of the therapeutic and educational regimen and provide for appropriate modifications. In some instances, deterioration or apparent deterioration will occur and must be assessed carefully. Possible explanations for apparent deterioration are inaccurate initial assessment; inappropriate expectations of parents and therapists; an inadequate or inappropriate treatment program; depression; intoxication with anticonvulsant medications; medical-surgical problems such as excessive weight gain, dislocated hips, or fixed joint deformities; or unrecognized, slowly progressive disorders such as muscular dystrophy, spinal muscular atrophy, leukodystrophy, neuronal storage disease, or a neoplasm. The possible role of depression deserves emphasis. Children with static encephalopathy can be identified readily by their motor dysfunction. By preschool age, these children are capable of recognizing the fact that they are different, and appropriate attention must be given to their mental health as well.

The prognosis for a child with static encephalopathy depends on a number of factors, including the extent of the motor dysfunction, the extent of associated abnormalities, and the availability of appropriate educational and therapeutic programs. A child with spastic tetraplegia is least likely to demonstrate significant progress, whereas a child with mild spastic hemiplegia or diplegia has a very favorable prognosis. In either case, the role of the family and society will be a major determinant.

## FUTURE CONSIDERATIONS

The prevention of static encephalopathy should be a long-term goal of research in this area. Improved prenatal and perinatal care is responsible for previously improved incidence rates, and advances in the treatment of Rh incompatibility states have reduced the occurrence of extrapyramidal forms of the disorder. Improved perinatal care also has led to increased survival, however, especially of preterm infants, thereby increasing the group that is at risk for spastic diplegia. Effective strategies are required to minimize this possibility. Similarly effective strategies must be developed to promote the treatment and education of these children and to integrate them into their families and society. Recent advances made in brain imaging and spectroscopy (nuclear magnetic resonance and single photon emission computed tomography) may provide fundamental information regarding the

functional capabilities of the brain in neonates who are at risk for static encephalopathy as well as guide treatment strategies during their later years.

## Selected Readings

Bax M. Terminology and classification of cerebral palsy. Dev Med Child Neurol 1964;6:295.

Blair E, Stanley FJ. Intrapartum asphyxia: A rare cause of cerebral palsy. J Pediatr 1988;112:515.

Davies PA, Drillien CM, Foley J, et al. Cerebral palsy. In: Drillien CM, Drummond MB, eds. Neurodevelopmental problems in early childhood. Oxford: Blackwell Scientific Publications, 1977:259.

Grant A, Joy M-T, O'Brien N, Hennessy E, MacDonald D. Cerebral palsy among children born during the Dublin randomised trial of intrapartum monitoring. Lancet 1989;2:1233.

Hagberg B, Hagberg G, Olow I. The changing panorama of cerebral palsy in Sweden. IV. Epidemiological trends 1959-1978. Acta Paediatr Scand 1984;73:433.

Kudrjavcev T, Schoenberg BS, Kurland LT, Groover RV. Cerebral palsy (CP)—trends in incidence and changes in concurrent neonatal mortality: Rochester, Minnesota, 1950-1976. Neurology 1983;33:1433.

Naeye RL, Peters EC, Bartholomew M, Landis JR. Origins of cerebral palsy. Am J Dis Child 1989;143:1154.

Nelson KB. What proportion of cerebral palsy is related to birth asphyxia? J Pediatr 1988;112:572.

Percy AK. Neonatal asphyxia and static encephalopathies. In: Fishman MA, ed. Pediatric neurology. Orlando, Fla: Grune & Stratton, 1986:57.

Teplin SW, Howard JA, O'Connor MJ. Self-concept of young children with cerebral palsy. Dev Med Child Neurol 1981;23:730.

Torfs CP, van den Berg BJ, Oechsli FW, Cummins S. Prenatal and perinatal factors in the etiology of cerebral palsy. J Pediatr 1990;116:615.

*Principles and Practice of Pediatrics, Second Edition.*
edited by Frank A. Oski et al. J. B. Lippincott Company, Philadelphia © 1994.

# CHAPTER 151
# *Benign Intracranial Hypertension*

## Marvin A. Fishman

Benign intracranial hypertension is a syndrome in which there is increased intracranial pressure in patients who have no history of an acute insult to the nervous system such as hypoxic ischemic disease, no acute encephalopathy such as Reye's syndrome, no focal or lateralizing neurologic signs, no evidence of intracranial tumor or obstruction to cerebrospinal fluid (CSF) flow, and normal results of CSF analyses except for increased pressure. This syndrome has occurred in children of all ages. There is no sex predilection as there is in adults, in whom there is a significant preponderance of females. The syndrome has been recognized for more than 80 years. Most of the earlier reported cases were associated with otitis media, mastoiditis, and lateral sinus thrombosis. The condition then was described as otitic hydrocephalus. Complications of otitis media have become less frequent precipitating factors, presumably related to the more aggressive use of antibiotics in the treatment of middle ear infections. A variety of conditions have been associated with this syndrome (Table 151-1). The most common cause now is "catch-up growth," which

is confined to pediatric patients in some series. This may be seen in patients with a number of conditions, such as cystic fibrosis and nutritional deprivation syndromes, and after the correction of underlying chronic conditions such as patent ductus arteriosus and complications of prematurity. Rarely, a familial form of the syndrome has been reported.

## PATHOGENESIS

The exact pathogenesis of increased intracranial pressure is not known. Different mechanisms may be operative in the various causes. Obstruction of the dural venous sinus system by thromboses resulting in increased intracranial venous pressure may cause decreased CSF absorption and intracranial hypertension. Alternatively, the increase in intracranial venous pressure may be transmitted directly to the CSF compartment. In other situations, the mechanism is less clear. Additional possibilities include an increased rate of CSF formation, a rise in brain volume secondary to an increase in interstitial fluid volume or cerebral blood volume, or a decreased rate of CSF absorption by arachnoid villi. Increased CSF production in the absence of a choroid plexus papilloma is highly unlikely. Studies using positron emission tomography have demonstrated that the intracerebral blood volume does not increase sufficiently to account for the rise in intracranial pressure. In addition, no evidence exists to support the presence of either vasogenic or cytotoxic brain edema to account for an increase in brain volume, which could produce intracranial hypertension. The most attractive hypothesis is that of altered absorption of CSF. Supporting evidence for this hypothesis has been derived from CSF perfusion studies in patients with benign intracranial hypertension, which have demonstrated reduced conductance to CSF outflow. Studies of the transport of intrathecal iodine 131 human serum albumin have revealed decreased

### TABLE 151-1.   Causes of Benign Intracranial Hypertension

**Circulatory–Hematologic**
Gastrointestinal hemorrhage
Polycythemia
Iron deficiency anemia
Hemophilia
Dural sinus thrombosis
Hypercoagulable state
Pernicious anemia
Obstruction of superior vena cava
Sickle cell anemia
Cryofibrinogenemia

**Drugs**
Tetracycline
Nalidixic acid
Steroid administration
Steroid withdrawal
Progestational agents
Indomethacin
Sulfamethoxazole
Oral contraceptives
Lithium carbonate
Thyroid hormone
Penicillin
Minocycline
Gentamicin

**Endocrine**
Hyperparathyroidism
Hypoparathyroidism
Adrenal insufficiency
Hyperadrenalism
Menarche
Obesity
Menstrual abnormalities
Pregnancy
Hyperthyroidism

**Infection**
Infectious mononucleosis
Mastoiditis
Lyme disease
Postinfectious states

**Neurologic Conditions**
Guillain-Barré syndrome
Recurrent polyneuritis
Head trauma

**Systemic Conditions**
Lupus erythematosus
Sarcoidosis
Paget's disease
Chronic hypoxia
Pulmonary hypoventilation
Serum sickness
Cryoglobulinemia
Catch-up growth
Nephrotic syndrome
Allergies
Connective tissues syndromes
Wiskott-Aldrich syndrome
Galactosemia

plasma absorption of intrathecally injected isotope and abnormal transport of the material within the CSF pathways, thus indicating stasis and decreased absorption.

## SYMPTOMS AND SIGNS

The onset of symptoms in patients with benign intracranial hypertension may be insidious or abrupt. The most common complaint is headache. Nausea, vomiting, and visual disturbances also are noted frequently. The visual complaints have included double vision, blurred vision, soreness of the eyes, and transient obscurations. Occasional complaints have included dizziness, vertiginous sensations, tinnitus, neck pain, paresthesias, radicular pain, and facial pain. The level of consciousness is relatively unimpaired.

The neurologic examination reveals no focal deficits. Occasionally, minor tremors and alterations in tone and reflexes have been noted. Abnormalities have been related primarily to the eyes and visual system. Papilledema has been noted in the vast majority of cases. Young infants whose fontanelles and cranial sutures are open may not have disc edema. Occasional cases

have been reported in adults without papilledema, but they have met the diagnostic criteria and had documented increased intracranial pressure by lumbar puncture. The papilledema almost always is bilateral. Sometimes, unilateral or asymmetric involvement has been reported. In children old enough to cooperate for examination, visual field defects may be noted. The most common finding is an enlarged blind spot. Other findings include generally constricted visual fields, altitudinal defects, and nasal defects, often in the inferior quadrant. Decreased visual acuity is a late finding.

## DIAGNOSIS

The diagnosis of benign intracranial hypertension has been facilitated by the development of noninvasive neuroimaging techniques, mainly computed tomography (CT) and magnetic resonance imaging (MRI). The diagnosis is one of exclusion. Clinically, the patient has a relatively normal neurologic examination, normal spinal fluid except for increased intracranial pressure, and an imaging procedure (CT or MRI) that shows no evidence of a mass lesion or obstruction to CSF flow. The majority of patients have one of the underlying conditions listed in Table 150-1. In some patients, however, no precipitating event can be identified. If all the diagnostic criteria are met, an overlooked cause of intracranial hypertension is unlikely. Before today's sophisticated imaging techniques were available, a midline neoplasm occasionally would go undiagnosed at the time of the initial evaluation. Other conditions that may be difficult to diagnose and may mimic benign intracranial hypertension include carcinomatous meningitis, fungal meningitis, and diffuse gliomatosis cerebri.

## TREATMENT

Approaches to lowering intracranial pressure are applicable to all patients. In those children in whom a specific cause is identified (eg, iron deficiency anemia), treatment of the underlying disorder may result in resolution of the intracranial hypertension. Similarly, discontinuation of an antibiotic that is thought to precipitate the syndrome often will result in improvement. In those patients in whom no precipitating event or other identifying condition can be treated, symptomatic therapy is instituted. No reliable data are available regarding the effectiveness of any proposed method of therapy; in about 25% of patients, the problem resolves after the initial diagnostic lumbar puncture is performed.

Suggested treatment includes performing a lumbar puncture after obtaining a normal neuroimaging study. The lumbar puncture confirms the diagnosis of benign intracranial hypertension and is the first therapeutic intervention. Many patients experience relief of symptoms after the removal of CSF. A second lumbar puncture should be done several days later, even in an asymptomatic patient, to measure the CSF pressure again. If the pressure remains elevated after several additional examinations, pharmacologic intervention is indicated. Treatment with acetazolamide may help to decrease CSF formation and, thus, lower intracranial pressure. Fairly large dosages, about 50 mg/kg/d in children, are needed to achieve a concentration that is sufficient to inhibit CSF forming enzymes in the choroid plexus. Other agents, such as glycerol, 1 to 2 g/kg every 6 hours, have been used. Raising the serum osmolality has been shown to decrease CSF production, and this may be the mechanism whereby these agents reduce increased intracranial pressure when they are administered on a long-term basis. If this approach does not result in resolution of the increased intracranial pressure, a course of steroids can be attempted. In children in whom the pressure remains elevated despite pharmacologic therapy, surgical intervention should be considered. CSF diversion procedures, optic nerve sheath decompression, and thecoperitoneal shunts have been used effectively.

The resolution of symptoms after the initiation of therapy does not necessarily indicate that the pressure has been relieved. Papilledema may take weeks to months to resolve and, therefore, is not a good parameter by which to judge the immediate effectiveness of therapy. Direct measurement of CSF pressure is necessary to monitor treatment. The goal of therapy is to relieve symptoms and avoid permanent visual disabilities. Therefore, whenever possible, visual fields and the blind spot should be assessed in patients who do not respond promptly to treatment. Deterioration in the results of this examination is an indication for more aggressive therapy.

The main concern during treatment is the persistence of visual disabilities. The clinical findings early in the course of the disease do not differentiate those patients who are likely to have sequelae. Persistent impaired visual acuity is not related to the presence of transient visual obscurations or the degree of papilledema. Fortunately, only a minority of patients have persistent visual defects or diminished acuity. Loss of visual acuity and visual fields may be reversed with rapid, vigorous therapy, with good functional recovery. Therefore, close observation is extremely important.

A rare complication of benign intracranial hypertension is the development of the empty-sella syndrome. This is thought to occur in patients with congenital absence of the diaphragmatic sella. Continued pressure on the pituitary is thought to compress the gland and result in the eventual appearance of the sella being empty. There usually are no associated endocrine symptoms, but growth hormone deficiency may occur.

Recurrent episodes of benign intracranial hypertension have been noted. This is unusual and thought to occur in about 10% of all patients.

The papilledema usually resolves within 3 to 6 months. Symptoms in patients who have been treated effectively usually disappear before this time. Rarely, papilledema may persist for more than 12 months. Some patients have spontaneous resolution of the syndrome and, in many others, the increased intracranial pressure remits as soon as any type of therapy is initiated.

## Selected Readings

Amacher AL, Spence JD. Spectrum of benign intracranial hypertension in children and adolescents. Child's Nervous System 1985;1:81.

Baker RS, Baumann RJ, Buncic JR. Idiopathic intracranial hypertension (pseudotumor cerebri) in pediatric patients. Pediatr Neurol 1989;5:5.

Baker RS, Carter D, Hendrick EB, Buncic JR. Visual loss in pseudotumor cerebri of childhood. Arch Ophthalmol 1985;103:1681.

Brooks DJ, Beaney RP, Leenders KL, et al. Regional cerebral oxygen utilization, blood flow, and blood volume in benign intracranial hypertension studied by positron emission tomography. Neurology 1985;35:1030.

Buchheit WA, Burton C, Haag B, Shaw D. Papilledema and idiopathic intracranial hypertension. N Engl J Med 1969;280:938.

Corbett JJ, Savino PJ, Thompson S, et al. Visual loss in pseudotumor cerebri. Arch Neurol 1982;39:461.

Corbett JJ, Thompson HS. The rational management of idiopathic intracranial hypertension. Arch Neurol 1989;46:1049.

Couch R, Camfield PR, Tibbles JAR. The changing picture of pseudotumor cerebri in children. Can J Neurol Sci 1985;12:48.

Fishman RA. The pathophysiology of pseudotumor cerebri. Arch Neurol 1984;41:257.

Grant DN. Benign intracranial hypertension. Arch Dis Child 1971;46:651.

Raichle ME, Grubb RL, Phelps ME, et al. Cerebral hemodynamics and metabolism in pseudotumor cerebri. Ann Neurol 1978;4:104.

Rose A, Matson DD. Benign intracranial hypertension in children. Pediatrics 1967;39:227.

Weisberg LA. Benign intracranial hypertension. Medicine (Baltimore) 1975;54:197.

*Principles and Practice of Pediatrics, Second Edition.*
edited by Frank A. Oski et al. J. B. Lippincott Company, Philadelphia © 1994.

## CHAPTER 152
# Cerebrovascular Disease in Childhood

## Andrew J. Kornberg and Arthur L. Prensky

Cerebrovascular disease can be divided broadly into two primary pathophysiologic processes: occlusion and hemorrhage. In occlusive vascular disease, blood vessels are occluded by the formation of clot (thrombosis) or the migration of clotted material via other vessels from the heart, vessels, or other organs (embolism). In hemorrhagic vascular disease, there is rupture of blood vessels with bleeding into cerebral parenchyma and subarachnoid, subdural, and epidural spaces.

Both these broad processes have in common reduced blood flow to brain tissue and consequent ischemia of neural tissue. If the ischemia is severe enough, there is death of nerve cells and surrounding tissue, which is defined more properly as infarction or stroke. In addition, hemorrhage may cause pressure on parenchyma and consequent ischemia and infarction by further obstruction to blood flow locally and generally by the effects of pressure alone.

## PATHOPHYSIOLOGY

The type and extent of damage caused by cerebrovascular disease are dependent on the vascular supply to an area and the metabolic needs of the area supplied. The brain receives its blood supply from the carotid and vertebrobasilar circulations, and, to a lesser degree, from small blood vessels from the leptomeninges. The two circulations are essentially separate, but numerous anastomoses exist at the level of the circle of Willis and the leptomeninges. The significance of these anastomoses is variable, but their importance in preventing hypoperfusion is dependent on how quickly flow is interrupted to an area. The more slowly the occlusion occurs, the more likely it is that an area of brain will be perfused adequately by these anastomoses and that ischemia and subsequent damage will be prevented. Certain areas of the brain are supplied by end arteries that have few or ineffective anastomoses. The occlusion of end arteries is likely to result in infarction of the tissue they supply. Some areas of the brain lie between the most distal portions of two circulations, such as those from the anterior and middle cerebral arteries. These are supplied to some degree by both circulations and, consequently, are somewhat protected from the occlusion of one or the other vessel. These areas, however, the so-called watershed areas, are vulnerable to damage from a decrease in the cerebral perfusion pressure.

Just as stroke can be caused by a lack of arterial blood flow, it also can result from obstruction of outflow from the brain, the veins, and the venous sinuses. The pathophysiology of this entity is related to "back pressure," which causes stasis and subsequent ischemia, as well as raises intracranial pressure and decreases perfusion of the brain. This type of "back pressure" also may cause the rupture of smaller vessels that feed the venous sinuses.

A transient ischemic attack is defined as a loss of neurologic function lasting less than 24 hours. It is related to ischemia of tissue, whereas stroke is related to infarction of tissue. The presentation of cerebrovascular disease is related to damage occurring in the specific areas of the brain supplied by the ischemic vessel and the functions that these areas perform. Thus, strokes in the carotid system usually present with hemiplegia, hemispheric sensory loss, aphasia, or hemianopsia, whereas events in the vertebrobasilar circulation typically present with brain stem dysfunction, such as vertigo, disturbances in balance, and bilateral motor, sensory, and visual disturbances.

Stroke is relatively rare in childhood. In a population-based study from Rochester, Minnesota, the annual incidence rate was 2.52 cases per 100,000, or about one half the incidence of primary intracranial neoplasm. Of these, 0.63 of every 100,000 cases was an ischemic stroke and 1.89 of every 100,000 cases was a hemorrhage. This study did not include patients with sickle cell anemia, however, which is a risk factor of some magnitude. Thus, the actual incidence of cerebrovascular disease may be much higher. Adult series report between 90 and 110 cerebrovascular accidents per 100,000 adults per year. Of these, the greatest majority are thrombotic strokes related to occlusive vascular disease.

Many strokes in children are without a known cause, or else are related to a complication of a disease originating outside the central nervous system. Congenital heart disease, sickle-cell disease, vasculitis, infection, and trauma are the usual causes of childhood stroke. Although these diseases frequently are evident before the stroke occurs, stroke sometimes is the presenting problem. Atherosclerosis and hypertension, the major systemic disorders that are associated with occlusive vascular disease in adults, are rare causes of thrombosis in the pediatric population.

## OCCLUSIVE CEREBROVASCULAR DISEASE
(Table 152-1)

More than three fourths of all thrombotic events occur in the carotid artery or branches of the middle cerebral artery. A specific cause can be identified in about 50% to 60% of patients and an arterial occlusion without a specific cause can be identified in a further 20% of patients. The cause of the event should be sought aggressively, as treatment of the primary disorder may prevent recurrent episodes of stroke.

### Atherosclerosis

When atherosclerosis occurs in children, it generally is the result of an inherited disorder of lipid or lipoprotein metabolism. Hyperlipoproteinemia types 1, 2, and 4 are associated with premature atherosclerosis in children, including plaques in the major cerebral vessels. The same problem can be found in children with hypercholesterolemia with low levels of high-density lipoproteins, and in children with hyperlipidemia associated with juvenile diabetes. Treatment of these children involves lowering their blood

**TABLE 152-1. Occlusive Cerebrovascular Diseases in Children and Adolescents**

Thrombosis
Abnormalities of the arterial wall
   Atherosclerosis
      Lipid abnormalities
      Down syndrome
      Progeria
   Arteritis
      Systemic lupus erythematosus
      Polyarteritis nodosa
      Takayasu disease
      Henoch-Schönlein purpura
      Radiation
      Infection
         Meningitis
         Mastoiditis
      Other
   Trauma
      External and internal trauma
      Dissection
   Congenital and hereditary disorders
      Kinking and tortuosity of vessels
      Fibromuscular dysplasia
      Neuroectodermal disorders
         Sturge-Weber syndrome
         Neurofibromatosis 1
         Tuberous sclerosis
      Sickle cell disease
      Metabolic disorders
         Homocystinuria
         MELAS syndrome (mitochondrial encephalomyopathy and stroke)
         Menke's disease
         Fabry's disease
         Other
   Moyamoya syndrome
      Moyamoya disease
   Migraine
Acute infantile hemiplegia
Hypercoagulable states
   Dehydration
   Hemolytic-uremic syndrome
   Nephrotic syndrome
   Cryoglobulinemia
   Polycythemia
   Leukemia and its treatment
   Thrombocytosis
   Antithrombin III deficiency
   Protein C deficiency
   Protein S deficiency

Embolism
Cardiac disease
   Cyanotic heart disease
   Valvular disease
   Bacterial endocarditis
   Arrhythmia's
   Tumor
Peripheral thrombosis and embolism

lipid levels with dietary manipulation or medication. Disorders that predispose to accelerated atherosclerosis, such as Down syndrome and progeria, also may predispose to stroke.

## Arteritis

The term *arteritis* refers to inflammatory changes in vessel walls. The arteritides affect vessels of many different sizes, with certain disorders typically affecting smaller vessels. The arteritides usually are associated with systemic symptoms such as fever, myalgia, arthralgia, and weight loss. Multiple organ systems, particularly the kidneys and lungs, often are involved. Significant laboratory findings include an elevated sedimentation rate, decreased serum complement levels, and increased antinuclear antibody titers. If the arteritis is limited to the central nervous system, however, these laboratory abnormalities may be absent. Treatment usually is with immunosuppressive agents such as corticosteroids.

Systemic lupus erythematosus (SLE) is one of the most common collagen vascular diseases in childhood. Between 13% and 30% of children with SLE have neurologic complications from their disease. In some series, cerebrovascular occlusive disease is reported to develop in 3% of children with SLE, with most of them having significant multi-system disease at the onset of complications.

Takayasu's disease is an arteritis of unknown cause that involves primarily the aorta and its branches. The disorder is most common in females between the second and fifth decade of life, but it has been reported in infants. Claudication in the upper extremities and loss of pulses with bruits usually are noted. Left untreated, the disorder is progressive and may be fatal. Stroke is uncommon, occurring in about 10% of patients.

Other causes of arteritis, such as polyarteritis nodosa and Henoch-Schönlein purpura, are unusual in childhood. Angiography in patients with these disorders may reveal evidence of one or more areas of stenosis or vessel occlusion. Recent improvements in magnetic resonance (MR) angiography may allow ready evaluation of these disorders without the risks associated with angiography.

Spasm or thrombosis of arteries at the base of the brain occurs in association with severe meningitic infections. This type of occlusive vascular disease is more common with chronic fungal and tuberculous meningitides, but also can be seen with acute bacterial meningitis in children, particularly if treatment is delayed. The chances of a full recovery are poor. Major strokes rarely occur when bacterial meningitis is treated rapidly.

Radiation therapy for a variety of brain tumors may predispose a patient to the development of arteritis of both small and larger vessels. Radiation therapy has been associated with moyamoya disease (see below).

## Trauma

Trauma probably is the single most common cause of occlusion of the extracranial portions of the carotid system in children. The pathophysiology associated with trauma initially is an intimal tear, then the formation of a dissecting aneurysm of the involved vessel, and subsequent occlusion of the vessel by thrombosis. The thrombus may extend distally, or an embolus can arise from the thrombus and occlude more distal vessels. The putative pathophysiology agrees well with the clinical syndromes seen with this type of injury. The neurologic deficit may be acute or associated with a delay in the onset of symptoms and a subsequent progressive stuttering course. Trauma may occur to the carotid artery externally in the neck or internally as a result of intraoral injury, such as results from a fall onto a pencil or stick. Vertebral artery dissections associated with twisting of the neck, such as can occur in chiropractic manipulations, have been described in adults and children.

## Congenital and Hereditary Disorders

Extracranial vessels (the carotid arteries in particular) sometimes are extremely tortuous. They may form kinks and interrupt blood flow, and have been associated with transient ischemic episodes and stroke.

Fibromuscular dysplasia is a disorder that involves predominantly medium-sized arteries and usually affects females in their second to fifth decades. Pathologically, segmental hyperplasia with intervening saccular dilatation is noted. This appears as a "string of beads" on angiography. It usually involves extracranial vessels, but has been seen in intracranial vessels and is an uncommon cause of stroke in children.

A variety of neuroectodermal disorders have been associated with stroke in childhood. Sturge-Weber syndrome is a congenital malformation of the venous vasculature that manifests with a facial angioma (port-wine stain) involving the first or second division of the trigeminal nerve, and with an associated leptomeningeal angioma on the ipsilateral side of the port-wine stain. The disorder commonly presents with progressive hemiparesis, focal seizures, retardation, and, on occasion, cerebral hemorrhage. The pathophysiology is primarily that of abnormal venous return through the vessels of the angioma, stagnation of blood, and local hypoxemia with subsequent damage to neurons. Diagnosis is made on the basis of the clinical features and the typical calcifications seen on computed tomography (CT) scan that resemble a railroad track. Neurofibromatosis type 1 has been associated with moyamoya syndrome (see below), particularly after cranial irradiation for an optic glioma or other intracranial tumors early in life. Tuberous sclerosis has been associated with embolic stroke, possibly related to emboli from cardiac rhabdomyomas.

## Sickle-Cell Disease

Sickle-cell disease is a recessively inherited hemoglobinopathy in which hemoglobin S (HbS) comprises more than 50% of the hemoglobin in red cells. It is the most common hemoglobinopathy in the United States, and about 8% of the black population has the trait. The prevalence of stroke in individuals with sickle-cell disease ranges from 5% to 17% in different series. Most of these patients have the complications before they reach 15 years of age. Ischemic strokes tend to occur in younger individuals, whereas intracranial hemorrhage typically occurs in young adults.

HbS forms intracellular polymers, especially under conditions of low oxygen tension, and leads to a rigid, deformed red blood cell surface or membrane (the sickle cell). Initially, the sickling is reversible on reoxygenation, but with repeated episodes, the membrane is damaged and remains sickled. The abnormal shape of the red cell may impede movement though the microvasculature and cause regional hypoperfusion. Although this mechanism long has been presumed to be the cause of stroke, radiologic and pathologic studies have provided evidence that the mechanism actually is a large-vessel occlusive vasculopathy. The vessels primarily involved include the supraclinoid internal carotid artery and the proximal areas of the middle and anterior cerebral arteries. The stenosis or occlusion of large intracranial vessels at the base of the skull can lead to the angiographic appearance of moyamoya syndrome (see below), and emboli from proximal vessels may cause distal hypoxia and further exacerbation of sickling and obstruction. The clinical features are similar to those that accompany other cerebrovascular events, but focal or generalized seizures commonly herald the onset of the stroke. The prognosis of a patient with an acute stroke in association with sickle-cell disease is poor. About 75% have permanent deficits, and seizures develop in 50% to 60%. Treatment involves providing adequate oxygenation and hydration, and instituting hypertransfusion therapy to maintain HbS levels less than 20%.

The use of anticoagulation may be indicated in patients who have thrombotic events. Recurrent events are common, but a recent study showing the predictive value of transcranial ultrasonography in individuals with sickle-cell disease may enable hypertransfusion therapy to be used to prevent subsequent strokes in individuals who are at high risk.

## Metabolic Disorders

The prototype metabolic disorder associated with stroke in childhood is homocystinuria. In this recessively inherited disorder, the amino acid homocystine accumulates in the body. Homocystine has been thought to increase platelet stickiness and possibly damage the intima of vessels, predisposing to intravascular thrombosis. Thrombi and emboli can be seen in all types and sizes of vessels of the central nervous system, including the veins (see below). The disorder is characterized by a somewhat marfanoid habitus, mild to moderate retardation, and ectopic lenses. Homocystinuria is diagnosed by the finding of homocystine in the blood or excessive amounts in the urine. The phenotype can be produced by different enzymatic abnormalities, with the most common type being responsive to pyridoxine (vitamin $B_6$) as a result of the activation of cystathionine synthase. Other metabolic disorders associated with stroke include the mitochondrial disorders, particularly mitochondrial myopathy, encephalopathy, lactic acidosis, and stroke-like episodes (MELAS syndrome), but also Leigh disease and Menkes' syndrome; organic acidurias such as methylmalonic, propionic, and isovaleric acidemias, and glutaric aciduria type 1; Fabry's disease; sulfite oxidase deficiency; and ornithine-transcarbamylase deficiency. Laboratory diagnosis of these conditions in a child with stroke involves blood and urine evaluation to determine amino acid, serum ammonia, copper, and arterial lactate and pyruvate levels (which are increased in patients with mitochondrial disorders). Treatment of the underlying disorder may prevent the recurrence of stroke.

## Moyamoya Syndrome

Moyamoya disease is a chronic, progressive, arterial disease of unknown cause that is characterized by progressive stenosis and occlusion of the intracranial portion of the internal carotid arteries and other vessels that comprise the circle of Willis. The slow progression of the disorder allows collaterals to form from the external carotid circulation as well as the vertebrobasilar system. Other collaterals from transdural and leptomeningeal vessels occur and predispose to subdural bleeds. The disease is named after the angiographic appearance of the collateral vessels that supply the distal internal carotid and the middle and anterior cerebral arteries from the external carotid circulation. The Japanese term *moyamoya*, meaning "something hazy, like a puff of smoke drifting in the air," describes the distinctive angiographic appearance of the disorder (Fig 152-1A). No specific cause of moyamoya disease is identifiable. A variety of conditions appear similar to moyamoya disease on angiography, including sickle-cell disease, neurofibromatosis type 1, cranial irradiation, fibromuscular dysplasia, Down syndrome, tuberculous meningitis, and Fanconi's anemia.

Symptoms occur in childhood and affect females more commonly. A variety of clinical patterns have been identified, the most common of which is that of multiple transient ischemic events with some of the transient episodes followed by permanent residual neurologic abnormalities (see Fig 152-1B). Less common presentations include acute stroke, transient ischemic attacks without permanent residual abnormalities, and acute intracranial hemorrhage related to the rupture of thin-walled collateral vessels. The disorder is progressive and is associated with declining intelligence and focal seizures. The diagnosis is based on the clinical

presentation and characteristic findings on angiography. MR imaging and MR angiography demonstrate the abnormalities as well (see Fig 152-1C). The availability of a noninvasive technique such as MR angiography is particularly important in children because considerable technical difficulties are associated with formal angiography (see new methods of investigation below).

The treatment of moyamoya syndrome is primarily surgical, as a variety of medical therapies have failed to retard the progression of this disorder. Surgical techniques directed at improving perfusion to partially ischemic areas of the brain have improved the prognosis of children with this disorder in long-term follow-up.

## Migraine

Migraine headaches occur in 10% to 25% of the population, with a significant percentage beginning in childhood or young adulthood. Complicated migraine (ie, migraine that is associated with neurologic deficits such as hemiplegia) has been estimated to occur in 1% of the population. Most migraine-related neurologic events are brief, last less than 1 hour, and are associated with a full recovery. Events of longer duration and permanent deficits are seen occasionally, however. Based on a review of 34 years of the literature, Featherstone defined individuals who are at risk of having a stroke associated with migraine as being more commonly female, with a history of classic or complicated migraine, and usually less than 40 years of age. Only about 15% of patients who have a stroke in connection with migraine are children. The prognosis for migraine-related stroke may be slightly better than for stroke of other causes. The diagnosis is based on other causes of stroke being excluded, the event occurring during a migraine attack, and the patient having a definite history consistent with migraine. Treatment is supportive, and vasodilators or anticoagulation given at the onset of a neurologic abnormality have not been shown to be of definite benefit. Prophylactic treatment of migraine reduces the frequency and severity of headache, and may decrease the risk of stroke.

## Acute Infantile Hemiplegia

*Acute infantile hemiplegia* is a term that has been used in a variety of ways. It has been used to describe the sudden onset of a stroke with hemiplegia when no specific cause is found, and also to describe a particular syndrome of fever and partial seizures of acute onset with subsequent hemiparesis. The seizures are difficult to control, typically last for many hours, and leave the child with a flaccid hemiparesis. The hemiparesis may improve, but 80% of the children have significant disability, including retardation. Within a year, epilepsy supervenes. On CT or MR imaging, evidence of acute infarction can be seen, but on angiography, often no occlusions can be demonstrated. No cause has been identified for this syndrome, but some investigators believe that it may be the result of a local arteritis.

## Hypercoagulable States

Hypercoagulability, or the tendency for circulating blood spontaneously to form a thrombus, is a potential cause of stroke in young patients. The site of clot formation varies and can include both the arterial and the venous sides of the circulation. As mentioned previously, the pathophysiology of venous thrombosis is that of "back pressure" causing vessel rupture and bleeding. Local pressure on parenchyma and perfusing vessels compounds the ischemia and causes further damage. With extensive venous thrombosis, raised intracranial pressure occurs, with subsequent hypoperfusion of the brain. Clinically, venous thrombosis pre-

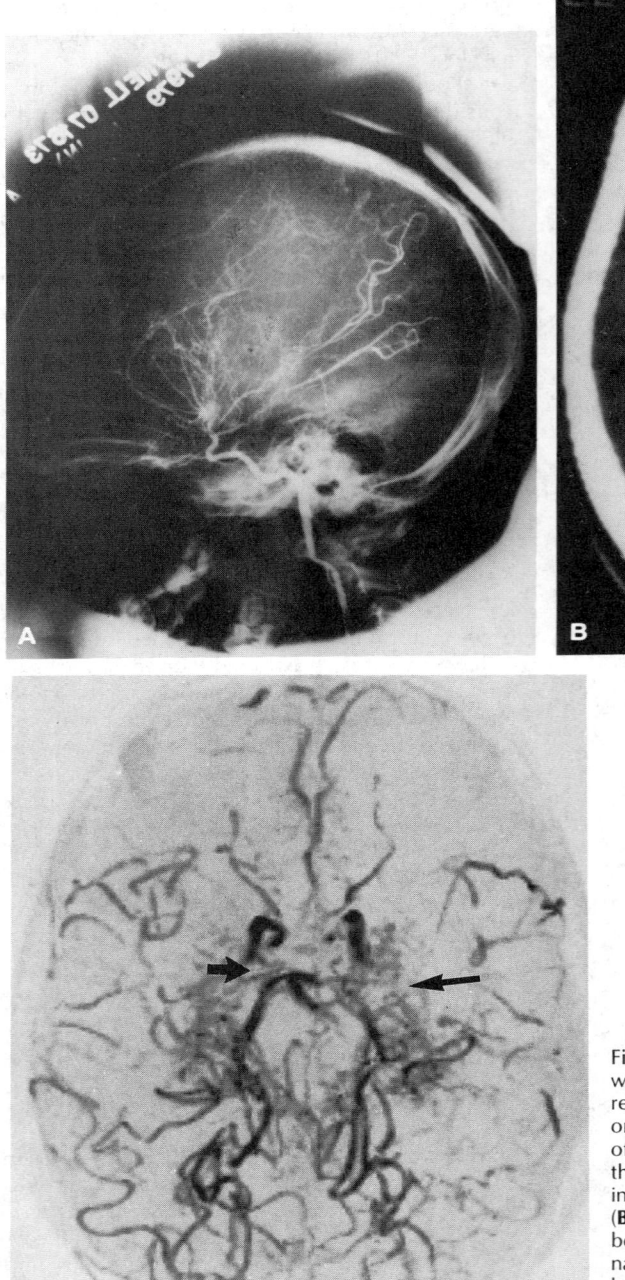
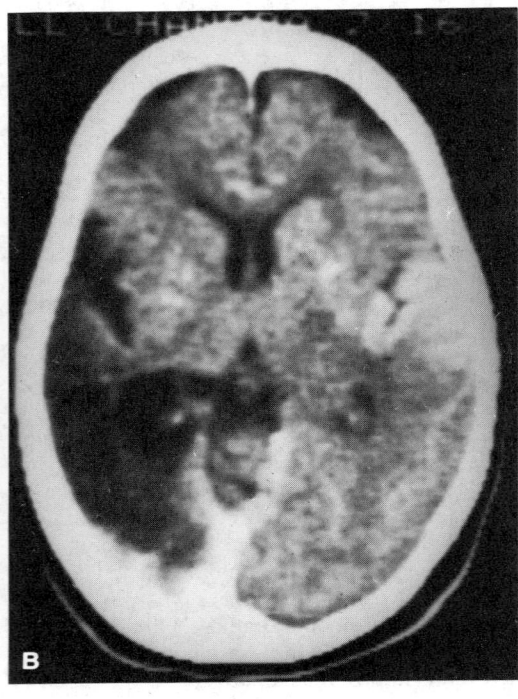

**Figure 152-1.** Moyamoya disease. (**A**) A network of fine collaterals is seen deep in the cerebrum lateral to the sella turcica. The vessels originate, for the most part, from the branches of the external carotid artery and help to supply the internal circulation. A tortuous leptomeningeal anastomosis also helps to supply the brain. (**B**) Multiple strokes of different ages are seen in both cerebral hemispheres. (**C**) Magnetic resonance angiography demonstrates the fine collaterals deep in the cerebrum (*arrow*) and the cut-off of intracranial vessels around the circle of Willis (*arrowhead*).

sents with partial seizures or focal neurologic findings such as a hemiparesis. Signs or symptoms of raised intracranial pressure may be seen, such as headache, vomiting, lethargy, visual disturbances, and papilledema. Diagnosis can be difficult and previously has relied on particular patterns seen on CT scan, angiography (particularly the venous phase), and radionuclide studies. The difficulty of diagnosing the state in live patients was pointed out by Banker when, in a study of patients examined postmortem for occlusive cerebrovascular disease, she demonstrated pathology that affected primarily the venous system in more than 50% of patients. Recent improvement in MR imaging and MR angiography (see below) may make diagnosis simpler.

Hypercoagulable states may be divided into those with primary and secondary causes. The primary causes include states in which there is absence or dysfunction of a substance(s) that usually is present to prevent thrombus formation. These disorders commonly are inherited and occur early in life. A history of recurrent thrombosis or a family history of thrombosis frequently is present. Primary causes of hypercoagulability include protein C, protein S, and antithrombin III deficiencies, and fibrinogen pathway abnormalities. The secondary causes include a group of diseases or drugs that result in intravascular thrombosis, either by depleting substances that prevent thrombosis, increasing the propensity of the blood to clot, or damaging the endothelium of blood vessels. Some of these causes are listed in Table 152-1. The underlying cause of the hypercoagulability must be treated, and heparin recently has been shown to be beneficial in patients with sinus vein thrombosis.

## Embolism

There are several causes of embolic occlusive vascular disease in children, including paradoxic emboli from the venous system, phlebitis of pulmonary veins resulting from lung infections, cardiac disease, and lesions of the aorta and great vessels in the neck. For practical purposes, almost all embolic occlusions that occur in children after the perinatal period are the result of congenital or acquired heart disease. The vast majority of these emboli are associated with cyanotic congenital heart disease, particularly the tetralogy of Fallot and truncus arteriosus. Clinical studies suggest that embolic occlusions may occur in 5% to 10% of children with these two disorders. About three fourths of these strokes occur within the first 2 years of life. Pathologic studies of children who die with congenital heart disease before or after surgical correction of these disorders suggest that the incidence of emboli may be as high as 15% to 20%, and that many emboli occur after catheterization and surgical attempts to correct the cardiac deformity.

Other cardiac lesions also can be a source of emboli. Disease of the mitral or aortic valves can result in cerebral emboli. Since the decline in the incidence of rheumatic fever, however, this is a relatively unusual cause of embolization. Prolapsed mitral valves have been associated with an increased risk of embolization, particularly in the first or second decade of life. Other cardiac disorders that can cause brain emboli include subendocardial fibroelastosis, various types of cardiomyopathy, tumors of the heart such as atrial myxomas and rhabdomyomas, bacterial endocarditis, and cardiac dysrhythmias.

On rare occasions, cerebral emboli also can arise from lesions in the walls of the great vessels of the thorax and neck. Coarctation of the aorta may be a source of emboli to the brain.

It is not always possible to distinguish an embolic from a thrombotic cerebrovascular event. Strokes caused by emboli are said to be more sudden in onset, often accompanied by focal seizures or headache, and a cause of more limited deficits. At times, the deficit may be complete, but it improves rapidly as the clot breaks up and the area is reperfused. Unfortunately, no combination of these clinical parameters allows successful differentiation between embolization and thrombosis. If a child has a disorder in which the incidence of embolization is high, that fact becomes extremely important in establishing the diagnosis. When the source of a cerebral embolus cannot be removed, the patient may benefit from treatment with platelet antiaggregants or anticoagulants.

## INTRACRANIAL HEMORRHAGE (Table 152-2)

### Abnormalities of the Clotting Mechanism

Deficiency of clotting factors, such as in hemophilia (factor VIII deficiency), factor IX deficiency (Christmas disease), von Willebrand's disease, thrombocytopenia (particularly idiopathic thrombocytopenic purpura), and disseminated intravascular coagulation, can be associated with spontaneous or post-traumatic intracerebral hemorrhage.

The presenting symptoms and signs of intracranial hemorrhage are seizures, focal neurologic signs, or evidence of increased intracranial pressure. The underlying disease responsible for abnormalities in the clotting mechanism need to be corrected to ensure recovery and prevent recurrence. Occasionally, the clot may need to be evacuated surgically if control of the raised intracranial pressure cannot be achieved medically.

**TABLE 152-2.   Causes of Hemorrhagic Vascular Disease**

Abnormalities of the clotting mechanism
   Decreased clotting factors
   Thrombocytopenia
   Disseminated intravascular coagulation
Vascular malformation
   Arteriovenous malformation
   Cerebral aneurysm
     Congenital
     Acquired: mycotic, traumatic, embolic
Hypertensive cerebrovascular disease
Intracranial neoplasm
Trauma

## Vascular Malformations

Congenital abnormalities of cerebral blood vessels are the most common cause of intracranial bleeding. These malformations include arteriovenous malformations (AVMs), angiomas, and aneurysms.

AVM is the most common abnormality and consists pathologically of normal and abnormal veins and arteries. These usually are found in the distribution of the internal carotid and middle cerebral arteries, but also occur in the posterior circulation and posterior fossa. They may present clinically as an intracranial mass, a focal or generalized seizure disorder, or an acute hemorrhage. Presentation as a mass lesion is unusual, but symptoms of raised intracranial pressure and slowly progressive neurologic symptoms or signs typically occur. Between 50% and 70% of children with AVMs have intracranial hemorrhage, and about 25% to 40% have seizures. Of those who do have hemorrhage, the great majority have blood within the subarachnoid space. Some have blood within the brain substance, which produces acute focal signs.

At the time of acute rupture, blood mixed in the cerebrospinal fluid may result in nuchal rigidity, severe headache, nausea, and vomiting. Excessive numbers of red blood cells or xanthochromia

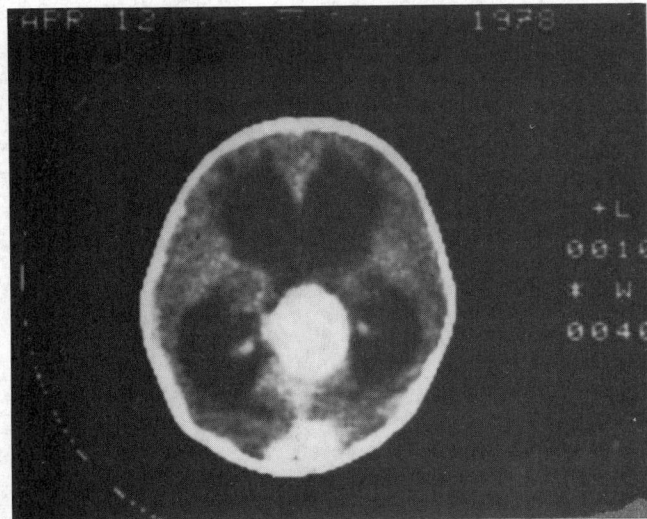

**Figure 152-2.** Aneurysm of the vein of Galen. A large aneurysm of the vein of Galen in a 6-week-old infant. The aneurysm compromises the aqueduct of Sylvius, resulting in severe hydrocephalus.

in the cerebrospinal fluid may raise suspicion that a hemorrhage has occurred. Bruits can be heard over the cranial vault in about 25% of patients with symptomatic AVMs. The larger the malformation, the more likely it is that a bruit will be heard. Most AVMs are large enough to be identified by the radiographic scanning techniques now in use, but improvements in imaging techniques may improve diagnosis further. Occasionally, a small malformation will not be picked up by scanning if there is no surrounding hemorrhage or if the AVM is obliterated by the blood. If an AVM is suspected, arteriography is the most useful diagnostic procedure available. It also is needed to determine which vessels feed and drain the malformation, and to decide whether the lesion can be treated surgically. If the lesion is too extensive to be operated on, it may be possible to reduce its size by introducing artificial emboli to obstruct the arteries that feed it.

Telangiectasias are the second most common vascular malformation in children. They essentially are capillary angiomas. The vessels that make up the lesion look like widely dilated capillaries. These lesions occur anywhere in the brain, but are seen frequently in the posterior fossa and in the bases pontis. Such

malformations often are asymptomatic throughout life and can be inherited (Osler-Weber-Rendu disease). When they produce symptoms, it is almost always the result of intracerebral hemorrhage. Occasionally, these hemorrhages are large enough to produce elevated intracranial pressure, either by acting as a mass or by obstructing the flow of cerebrospinal fluid and producing hydrocephalus. The most common presentation, however, is the acute onset of focal symptoms and signs without elevated intracranial pressure. The hemorrhage often can be seen on CT scan. Usually, these hemorrhages are not large enough to require surgical evacuation. In many instances, the associated malformation is obliterated by the bleeding.

An aneurysm of the vein of Galen (Fig 152-2) is in reality a vascular malformation involving both arteries and veins. It lies above the tectum of the midbrain and can obstruct the aqueduct of Sylvius and produce hydrocephalus. Similar to any other very large vascular malformation, an aneurysm of the vein of Galen may present with marked shunting of blood between arteries and veins, causing high-output congestive heart failure. This presentation is common in the neonate. Less severely involved

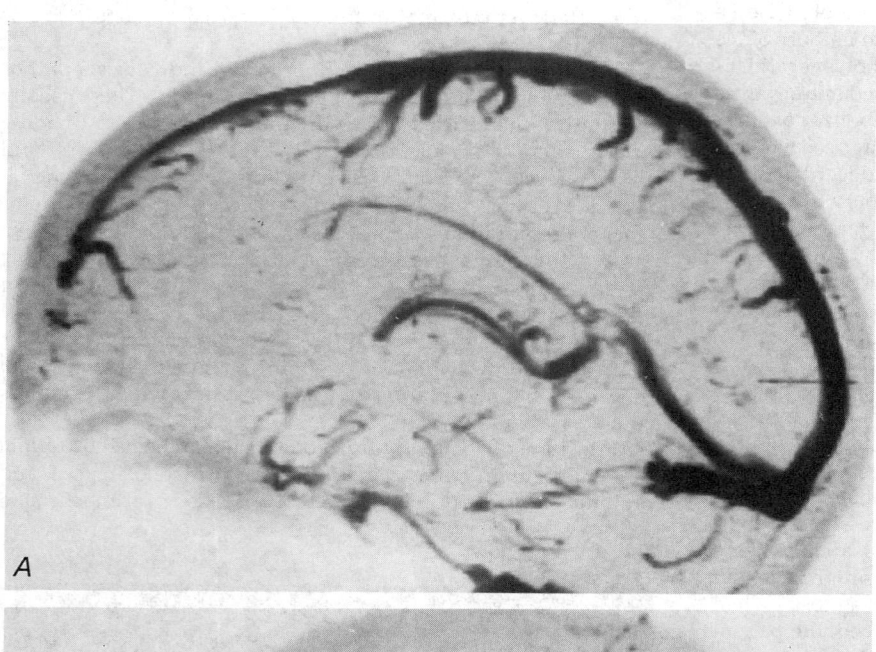

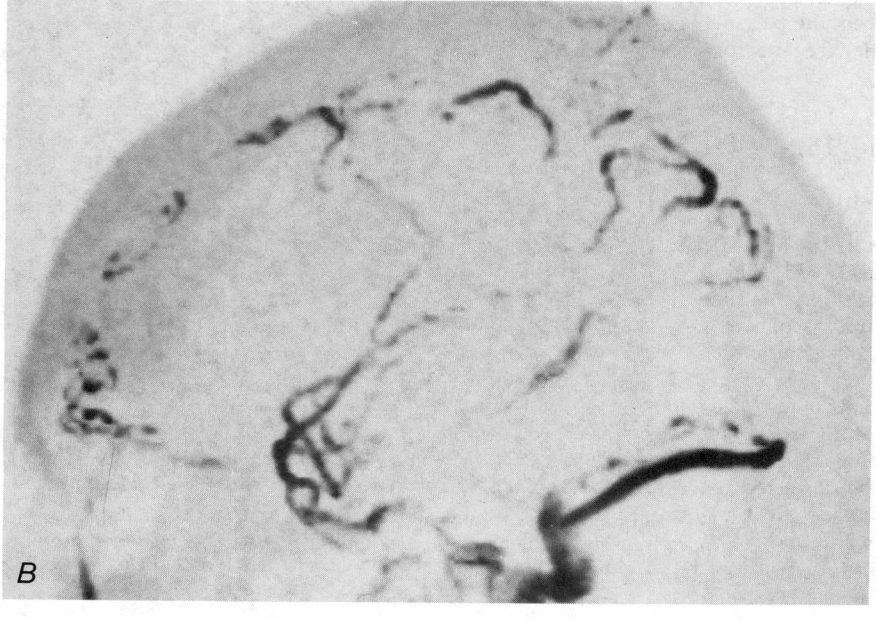

**Figure 152-3.** Sinus vein thrombosis. (**A**) A magnetic resonance venogram demonstrates patent sinus veins. (**B**) Sagittal sinus vein thrombosis is readily demonstrated by magnetic resonance venography, with a void in the signal in the sagittal sinus.

infants may have increased heart size and macrocephaly because of hydrocephalus. The accepted treatment of this malformation is to occlude the feeding vessels, if possible, either by clipping the arteries or by therapeutic embolization with metal coils. The prognosis is poor for patients with a massive aneurysm or congestive cardiac failure.

## Arterial Aneurysms

Aneurysms are rare in children. Less than 2% of all aneurysms become symptomatic in patients less than 19 years of age. About 90% of the aneurysms that become symptomatic during childhood are located in the anterior or middle cranial fossa. The majority are congenital in origin, that is, there is a defect in the arterial wall and the internal elastic lamina and the media are missing. An increased proportion of symptomatic aneurysms in children, however, are caused by infection (particularly emboli from bacterial endocarditis), trauma, and, in rare instances, tumor. Congenital aneurysms in children occur most frequently at the distal portion of the internal carotid and the proximal middle cerebral arteries, as well as in the anterior and posterior communicating vessels. Although most aneurysms in children do cause subarachnoid and, less frequently, intracerebral hemorrhage, some act as masses and cause primarily compression of the oculomotor or other cranial nerves. A higher incidence of congenital aneurysms is associated with fibromuscular dysplasia, kinking and coiling of carotid vessels, coarctation of the aorta, and polycystic kidney disease than with other diseases that affect blood vessels.

Mycotic aneurysms can result from embolization from the heart as well as from bacterial and fungal disorders affecting the meninges. Mycotic and traumatic aneurysms are present less frequently at the bifurcation of the major intracranial vessels and are seen more often distally in the middle and anterior cerebral arteries. Mycotic aneurysms are more likely to be multiple than are aneurysms that result from trauma or those that are congenital. They also are more likely to rupture, especially with anticoagulation.

Cerebral arteriography is the procedure of choice for the diagnosis of an aneurysm. MR angiography also has been refined to such a degree that aneurysms may be seen. About two thirds of symptomatic children do have abnormalities on CT scan, however, including evidence of intracerebral or subarachnoid hemorrhage or a focal enhancing lesion. Because congenital aneurysms in children frequently are larger than those seen in adults, they are more likely to be detected by conventional scanning techniques before rupture occurs.

The treatment of aneurysms in children is surgical and does not differ appreciably from that in adults. Vasospasm does occur in the presence of subarachnoid bleeding in children, and treatment with volume expansion to produce mild hypertension and calcium channel blockers such as nimodipine may be useful.

## Other Causes of Intracranial Hemorrhage

A cerebral hemorrhage can be a manifestation of both leukemia and the drugs used to treat it.

Hypertension is a much less frequent cause of hemorrhage in children than in adults, but such catastrophes can occur because of elevated blood pressure levels in conjunction with renal, cardiovascular, or endocrine disorders.

Trauma certainly is the most common cause of subarachnoid hemorrhage in infants and young children, and is associated with accidental and non-accidental injury.

Bleeding into a preexisting tumor may be responsible for an intracerebral accumulation of blood. An area of marked surrounding cerebral edema may indicate this diagnosis.

## NEW TECHNIQUES IN THE DIAGNOSIS OF CEREBROVASCULAR DISEASE

A variety of new imaging techniques have been developed recently and are especially important in the diagnostic workup of pediatric patients with cerebrovascular disease. MR imaging has

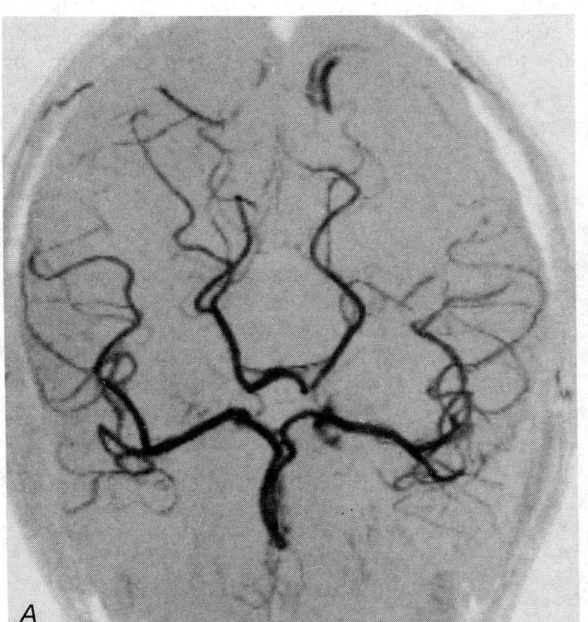
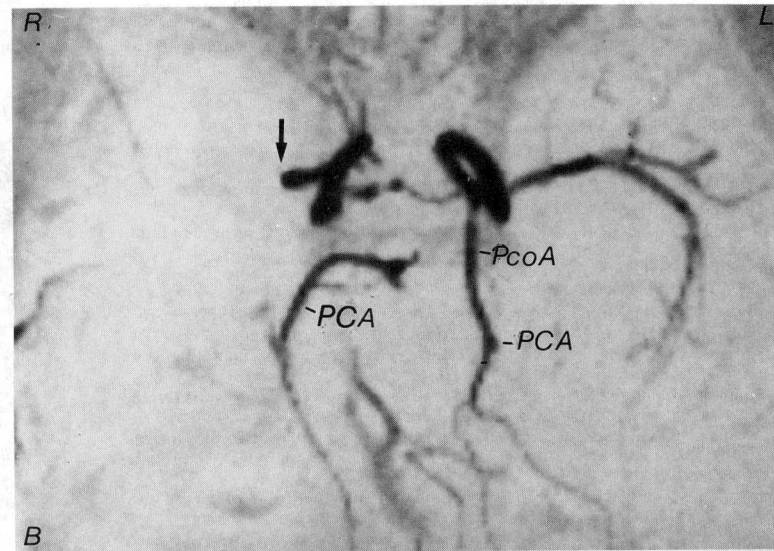

**Figure 152-4.** Magnetic resonance angiography. (**A**) A normal magnetic resonance angiogram. Clear, accurate images of cerebral vessels are readily obtained. (**B**) An occlusion of the right middle cerebral artery is readily demonstrated (*arrow*). *PCA*, posterior cerebral artery; *PCoA*, posterior communicating artery.

evolved over the years to the point that it now provides considerable information to the clinician. It produces superb images with little or no artifact related to bone. It can demonstrate abnormalities before any can be seen on CT, provides excellent images of the venous sinuses, and allows the diagnosis of sinus vein thrombosis to be made readily (Fig 152-3). It has the advantage of not requiring the radiation that conventional CT does. The major disadvantage of MR imaging is that data acquisition takes a considerable amount of time (although it is decreasing), and that the images are degraded by movement. For this reason, many pediatric patients require some sort of sedation or anesthesia for optimal images to be obtained. MR angiography also provides information both on the arterial side (Fig 152-4) and on the venous side (see Fig 152-3) of the cerebrovascular system. The images are of high quality and the procedure is not invasive. The gold standard examination is formal angiography, however, and, until studies comparing the two techniques show MR angiography to be as sensitive, formal angiography will remain the preferred procedure.

## APPROACH TO THE PATIENT

The approach to a patient with cerebrovascular disease is twofold. First, general support and then specific treatment of the event is necessary. An excellent review by Oppenheimer and colleagues of the complications of acute stroke is recommended reading. Second, the importance of making an etiologic diagnosis cannot be overstated. Finding a cause may allow the administration of a specific treatment and enable the clinician to prevent recurrence and provide prognostic information.

## Selected Readings

Aicardi J, Amsili J, Chevrie JJ. Acute hemiplegia in infancy and childhood. Dev Med Child Neurol 1969;11:162.

Banker BQ. Cerebral vascular disease in infancy and childhood. I. Occlusive vascular disease. J Neuropathol Exp Neurol 1961;20:127.

Barron TF, Gusnard DA, Zimmerman RA, Clancy RR. Cerebral venous thrombosis in neonates and children. Pediatr Neurol 1992;8:112.

Baumann RJ, Carr WA, Shuman RM. Patterns of cerebral arterial injury in children with neurological disabilities. J Child Neurol 1987;2:298.

Dusser A, Goutiéres F, Aicardi J. Ischemic strokes in children. J Child Neurol 1986;1:131.

Einhäupl KM, Villringer A, Meister W, et al. Heparin treatment in sinus venous thrombosis. Lancet 1991;338:597.

Featherstone HJ. Clinical features of stroke in migraine: A review. Headache 1986;26:128.

Golden GS. Stroke syndromes in childhood. Neurol Clin 1985;3:59.

Gordon N, Isler W. Childhood moyamoya disease. Dev Med Child Neurol 1989;31:98.

Hess DC, Adams RJ, Nichols FT III. Sickle cell anemia and other hemoglobinopathies. Semin Neurol 1991;11:314.

Israels SJ, Seshia SS. Childhood stroke associated with protein C or protein S deficiency. J Pediatr 1987;111:562.

Lagos JC, Riley HD Jr. Congenital intracranial vascular malformations in children. Arch Dis Child 1971;46:285.

Natowicz M, Kelley RI. Mendelian etiologies of stroke. Ann Neurol 1987;22:175.

Oppenheimer S, Hachinski V. Complications of acute stroke. Lancet 1992;339:721.

Packer RJ, Rorke LB, Lange BJ, Siegel KR, Evans AE. Cerebrovascular accidents in children with cancer. Pediatrics 1985;76:194.

Rothman SM, Fulling KH, Nelson JS. Sickle cell anemia and central nervous system infarction: A neuropathological study. Ann Neurol 1986;20:684.

Schoenberg BS, Mellinger JF, Schoenberg DG. Cerebrovascular disease in infants and children: A study of incidence, clinical features, and survival. Neurology 1978;28:763.

Thrush AL, Marano GD. Infantile intracranial aneurysm: Report of a case and review of the literature. AJNR 1988;9:903.

van Hellenberg Hubar JLM, Gabreëls FJM, Ruitenbeek W, et al. MELAS syndrome. Report of two patients, and comparison with data of 24 patients derived from the literature. Neuropediatrics 1991;22:10.

Zee C-S, Segall HD, McComb JG, et al. Intracranial arterial aneurysms in childhood: More recent considerations. J Child Neurol 1986;1:99.

Principles and Practice of Pediatrics, Second Edition.
edited by Frank A. Oski et al. J. B. Lippincott Company, Philadelphia © 1994.

# CHAPTER 153
# Acute Head Trauma

## N. Paul Rosman

Pediatric head injuries are a very important cause of childhood morbidity and mortality. Each year in the United States, nearly 5 million children sustain a head injury; of these, about 200,000 are hospitalized. Such injuries, which are twice as frequent in boys as in girls, have many different causes: motor vehicle accidents, falls, bicycling and other recreational activities, competitive sports, and assaults (including child abuse). In 1986 in the United States, about 150,000 children suffered a traumatic brain injury. About 80% of these injuries were mild, 15% were moderate to severe, and 5% were fatal. Seven thousand of the children died from the direct effects of the trauma or from secondary complications or associated injuries, accounting for 30% of all childhood deaths from trauma that year. Each year in this country, almost 30,000 individuals 19 years of age and younger are left with permanent disabilities from moderate or severe head trauma, including post-traumatic epilepsy (PTE), motor handicaps, cognitive impairment, learning difficulties, and behavioral and emotional problems.

This chapter presents an approach to the diagnosis and treatment of acute head injuries in children, with consideration given to the clinical syndromes that are encountered most frequently. In addition, the prognosis of acute brain injuries in children is discussed. The scalp, skull, and brain all can suffer injury as a result of head trauma. Figure 153-1 depicts the brain, its surrounding structures, and the main associated pathologies that can complicate head trauma. The scalp, which is highly vascular, lies outermost, bounded on its inner surface by the galea aponeurotica, a tendinous sheath connecting the frontalis and oc-

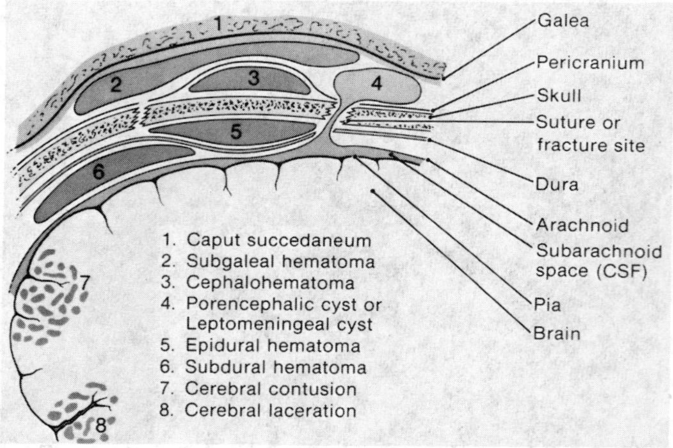

1. Caput succedaneum
2. Subgaleal hematoma
3. Cephalohematoma
4. Porencephalic cyst or Leptomeningeal cyst
5. Epidural hematoma
6. Subdural hematoma
7. Cerebral contusion
8. Cerebral laceration

Galea
Pericranium
Skull
Suture or fracture site
Dura
Arachnoid
Subarachnoid space (CSF)
Pia
Brain

Figure 153-1. The brain, surrounding structures, and major types of pathology following acute head injury. (Rosman NP, Herskowitz J, Carter AP, et al. Acute head trauma in infancy and childhood. Pediatr Clin North Am 1979;26:708.)

cipitalis muscles. Beneath the galea is the subgaleal compartment. Immediately below this lies the skull, the outermost portion of which is the pericranium, or external periosteum. The outer and inner tables of the skull are separated by the diploic space, which is traversed by small veins. The dura, lying immediately below the inner table of the skull, contains few blood vessels (in contrast to the highly vascular leptomeninges, which are closely approximated to the brain). Small-caliber veins from the leptomeninges cross the subdural space to drain into dural sinuses. The brain is bathed in and protected by cerebrospinal fluid (CSF), which is located in the cerebral subarachnoid spaces, cisterns at the base of the brain, ventricular cavities, interconnecting channels, and foramina.

Intracranial pressure (ICP) is the sum total of pressures exerted by intracranial structures: brain tissue, the intracranial vascular tree, and the CSF. The skull of the newborn and infant is not a rigid box; rather, it consists of membranous bones, with fontanelles and unfused bony structures providing outlets for the increases in ICP that are seen so commonly in head-injured children. In older children, in whom the cranial sutures have fused, however, the foramen magnum provides the only major outlet through which increases in ICP can be accommodated.

## MANAGEMENT

### Patient History

It is essential that the specific circumstances of an episode of head trauma be determined and that predisposing factors be identified. Such information should be sought directly from the injured child whenever possible, and also from any observers. Attention should be paid to memory loss, perseverative questioning (persisting repetition of a question with no memory of having asked it before), confusion, visual disturbance, and symptoms of increased ICP such as irritability, altered consciousness, repeated vomiting, and severe headache.

### General Physical Examination

The patient's vital signs demand immediate attention and, at times, emergency intervention. Alterations may indicate shock (decreased blood pressure, increased pulse rate) or intracranial hypertension (increased blood pressure, decreased or increased pulse rate, slowed or irregular respirations). Systemic hypotension in the head-injured child usually is caused by an injury outside the central nervous system, as with intra-abdominal bleeding (eg, from a ruptured spleen) or bleeding into soft tissues (eg, associated with a long-bone fracture or a major scalp laceration). Occasionally, however, systemic hypotension can be of intracranial origin (eg, from an epidural hematoma).

The child's entire body should be checked for signs of trauma. The neck should be examined with particular care because of possible injury that often is unsuspected. Neck injury is suggested by cervical abrasions, cervical spine tenderness, or meningism. The latter also can result from subarachnoid bleeding or cerebellar tonsillar herniation. Initial assessment may be limited because of immobilization of the neck by a collar or sandbags. The scalp should be inspected and all scalp lacerations examined. The skull should be palpated for areas of tenderness or loss of anatomic integrity. Tension of the anterior fontanelle should be assessed in the young child. Periorbital hemorrhage ("raccoon eyes" sign), ecchymosis behind the ear (Battle's sign) or behind the eardrum (hemotympanum), or bleeding from the ears or nose should be noted. These signs, along with CSF otorrhea or rhinorrhea, are indications of basal skull fracture.

## Neurologic Examination

The neurologic examination should assess the child's alertness, orientation, and memory. The presence and extent of retrograde and anterograde (post-traumatic) amnesia should be determined. A child's repeated asking of the same question is reflective of a post-traumatic memory disturbance of anterograde type. The level of consciousness may range widely. The Glasgow Coma Scale (GCS, Table 153-1), with scores ranging from 3 (worst) to 15 (best), provides a useful and reproducible scoring system for quantifying the level of consciousness. Although most studies have reported a low GCS score to correlate with severe neurologic morbidity and substantial mortality, it recently has been shown that many children with a GCS score of 3 to 5 can do surprisingly well if their head injury has not been complicated by a hypoxic-ischemic insult.

The neuro-ophthalmologic evaluation should include pupil size and reactivity. Small pupils are seen with diencephalic and pontine injuries; a unilateral dilated pupil suggests temporal lobe herniation on the same side. The fundi should be examined carefully, and evidence of retinal and pre-retinal (subhyaloid) hemorrhages and papilledema should be sought. Abnormalities of ocular gaze and position should be observed. If there is no neck injury, the oculocephalic ("doll's head") maneuver can be used to assess any apparent limitation of eye movements. With the child supine, the head is rotated to one side and then to the other. When the head is moved to the left, the eyes should deviate to the right (and vice versa) if brain stem pathways controlling eye movements are functioning normally. Lateral gaze also can be tested in the comatose patient by means of caloric stimulation. In this case, the child's head is elevated 30° above the horizontal and one external auditory canal is irrigated with about 5 mL of ice water. If brain stem function is normal, the eyes should turn toward the ear being irrigated. It is important to be certain that the auditory canal is clear and the eardrum is intact before performing this test.

---

**TABLE 153-1.  Glasgow Coma Scale**

| Response | Score |
|---|---|
| **Best Motor Response** | |
| Obeys | 6 |
| Localizes pain | 5 |
| Withdraws | 4 |
| Flexion to pain | 3 |
| Extension to pain | 2 |
| Nil | 1 |
| **Best Verbal Response** | |
| Oriented | 5 |
| Confused conversation | 4 |
| Inappropriate words | 3 |
| Incomprehensible sounds | 2 |
| Nil | 1 |
| **Eye Opening** | |
| Spontaneously | 4 |
| To speech | 3 |
| To pain | 2 |
| Nil | 1 |

Rosman NP, Oppenheimer EY, O'Connor JF. Emergency management of pediatric head injuries. Emerg Med Clin North Am 1983;1:144.

The extent to which the motor system can be examined depends on the child's alertness. Decorticate, decerebrate, and other abnormal posturing should be noted. Also, the distribution (hemiparetic or paraparetic) of any muscular flaccidity or spasticity should be observed. In the responsive child, more detailed motor, sensory, and coordinative testing is possible. Testing for abnormal reflexes (such as palmar grasp, suck, or rooting reflexes), eliciting deep tendon reflexes, and checking for plantar responses complete this portion of the examination.

## Investigative Studies

### Plain Radiographs

The need for radiologic examination of the child with a head injury is dictated by the severity of the head trauma, as reflected by the patient's state of consciousness and the presence or absence of focal neurologic signs. Severe head injury, with significant loss of consciousness and focal neurologic signs (GCS score 3 to 8), requires plain radiographs and further radiologic workup. The initial examination in a child with severe head trauma should include anteroposterior and lateral views of the cervical spine, as well as anteroposterior, inclined anteroposterior (Towne projection), and lateral views of the skull; the last is taken with a horizontal beam (cross table) to demonstrate any air–fluid levels in the cranial cavity or paranasal sinuses indicative of compound or basal fracture. With extensive head or facial trauma, radiographs should include a Waters projection of the facial bones and films of the orbits.

In a patient with moderate head trauma with localizing neurologic signs or a history of loss of consciousness (GCS score 9 to 12), routine skull radiographs alone usually suffice. If there is no history of neck injury, cervical spine films probably are unnecessary. In a child with mild head trauma without focal neurologic signs or loss of consciousness (GCS score 13 to 15), skull and spine films usually are not needed. If a depressed skull fracture is suspected, tangential views of the area should be obtained in addition to standard views.

### Cranial Computed Tomography

In patients with severe head trauma or those with localizing neurologic signs regardless of the severity of the injury, the most helpful and least invasive imaging modality is the cranial computed tomography (CT) scan. Unilateral intracranial hemorrhage usually is readily evident on CT scan as a relatively dense mass in the immediate post-traumatic period, a time when the scan does not require the infusion of contrast medium. After several days, however, extravasated blood that is broken down incompletely may be of the same density as contiguous brain; thus, scans at that time should be done with and without contrast enhancement. In addition to disclosing blood within brain parenchyma (as in contusion) or outside the brain (as with subdural hematoma), cranial CT scanning can demonstrate brain edema, loss of brain tissue, hydrocephalus, midline displacements and other mass effects, and skull fractures. Some treatment centers have recommended that routine skull radiography be abandoned in favor of immediate cranial CT scanning with bone windows. Although it frequently is true that clinical decisions can be made on the basis of the findings on CT scanning alone, the scan may fail to demonstrate focal skull depressions, as well as stellate, facial, basal, and other fractures.

In selected cases of spinal trauma (ie, with fractures that are suspected, but undetected, on plain films), CT scanning of the spine is a useful adjunct to standard radiography.

### Ultrasonography

In the newborn or young infant with open fontanelles and sutures, real-time ultrasonography may be very helpful in demonstrating displacement or obstruction of the ventricular system and the presence of intraventricular, parenchymal, and subarachnoid blood. Thus, ultrasonography should be performed in all newborns who have suffered traumatic births, as well as in premature newborns (with or without a history of trauma), because the latter infants are at high risk for periventricular/intraventricular hemorrhage.

### Magnetic Resonance Imaging

Magnetic resonance imaging (MRI), which provides a detailed demonstration of brain anatomy without exposing the patient to ionizing radiation, has become an increasingly valuable diagnostic tool. Advantages of MRI include safety (no known biologic hazards and no reported side effects), the ability to image in any plane, excellent depiction of normal and pathologic anatomy, the ability to identify vessels without contrast injections, and superiority to cranial CT in demonstrating the posterior fossa, where bone artifacts interfere with CT imaging. In cases of head trauma, however, MRI is of greatest assistance in evaluating injuries that are subacute or chronic, rather than ones that are acute.

Acute bleeding (ie, that occurring within the first 1 to 3 days after the injury), whether it is extra-axial (as with subdural and subarachnoid hemorrhage) or intra-axial (as with cerebral contusion), frequently is more difficult to recognize with MRI than with CT, because the deoxyhemoglobin in such lesions gives rise to a signal that is iso-intense with brain on T1-weighted images and of low or hypo-intensity on T2-weighted images. By contrast, edema surrounding areas of acute parenchymal hemorrhage is seen well with MRI, because T2-weighted images of edema have high signal intensity. Also, because of the ease with which sections can be obtained in multiple planes with MRI, and because no MRI signal is transmitted by bone, small collections of blood (for example, a thin convexity extra-axial hematoma) may be visualized more easily with MRI than with CT. It is because of this that MRI is more useful than CT in imaging the posterior fossa. MRI is especially useful for detecting lesions that are iso-dense on CT, such as subacute (3 to 14 days) and chronic (more than 14 days) extra-axial hematomas, which show high signal intensity on both T1- and T2-weighted images as a result of the formation of methemoglobin in subacute hematomas and increased protein content in chronic hematomas. Diffuse white matter shearing injuries are seen very well with MRI, because these lesions show increased signal intensity on T2-weighted images. A disadvantage of MRI compared to CT is the longer imaging time needed and its unsuitability for critically ill patients with life support systems that require continuous monitoring.

### Cerebral Angiography

Except for rare patients (such as one in whom it is important to try to demonstrate a vascular injury in the head or neck), cerebral angiography largely has been replaced by CT and MRI in the assessment of individuals with acute head trauma.

### Lumbar Puncture

Lumbar puncture should not be performed in a child with a head injury unless complicating central nervous system infection is suspected. It usually is contraindicated in the presence of significantly elevated ICP and is absolutely contraindicated in the presence of an intracranial mass. Lumbar puncture may show evidence of central nervous system infection, recent or older subarachnoid bleeding, and elevated ICP.

### Subdural Taps

Subdural taps may be indicated as a diagnostic measure, a therapeutic measure, or both. A maximum of 15 mL of fluid is removed from each subdural space, without aspiration; within a day or two, the taps can be repeated.

## Other Studies

In moderately and severely injured children, and in those in whom the cause or circumstances of the injury are unknown, additional studies may be indicated. These include a complete blood count; determination of the serum amylase level; urinalysis; platelet and clotting studies; toxic screens on blood, urine, and gastric aspirate; and a skeletal survey for old and recent fractures.

## TREATMENT

### General Support

Treatment of the child with head injury must be directed toward the entire patient. The head and neck must be stabilized and, if neck trauma is suspected, a firm cervical collar or sandbags applied. The airway must be cleared by proper positioning and gentle suction, and patency ensured by inserting an oral airway. If needed, ventilatory support, including orotracheal or nasotracheal intubation, should be provided. One hundred percent oxygen (at 3 to 10 L/min) is administered by means of a bag and mask or by nasal prongs, with the arterial oxygen tension ($PaO_2$) maintained at 90 to 100 mm Hg.

An intravenous line should be established and circulatory support provided. Active bleeding should be stopped. With infrequent exceptions, shock is not a sign of head injury in childhood and is caused by associated injury, such as rupture of an abdominal viscus (eg, the liver) or bleeding into extracranial soft tissues (eg, next to a long-bone fracture). Occasionally, however, rapid intracranial bleeding into the epidural space or even a large amount of extracranial bleeding into the scalp can cause a child to go into shock. In all children with severe head injury, a central venous line should be placed for fluid management and an arterial line should be inserted to monitor blood pressures and facilitate measurements of blood gases. In patients with severe head trauma, especially when concern exists about the child's cardiac or pulmonary status or when hemodynamic abnormalities are not responding to treatment, a Swan-Ganz catheter should be inserted. Hypovolemia (loss of more than 20% of the blood volume) is corrected by the intravenous administration of lactated Ringer's solution, fresh-frozen plasma, 5% albumin in normal saline solution, or blood. Circulatory failure can be treated with epinephrine, dobutamine, or dopamine. With frank cardiac arrest, the child should be given intravenous epinephrine, which, if ineffective, should be repeated in double dose. Intravenous atropine also can be given during asystole, although its usefulness in children has not been documented. If asystole is prolonged or if metabolic acidosis is confirmed, intravenous sodium bicarbonate should be administered.

Accompanying injuries, such as those to the scalp, chest, abdomen, limbs, or spine, may require specific treatment. With suspected abdominal bleeding or intestinal perforation, CT scanning of the abdomen should be done. Limb fractures should be splinted. The stomach should be emptied by nasogastric intubation to prevent vomiting and aspiration, and to keep pressure on the diaphragm from causing secondary respiratory compromise. The bladder should be catheterized and a urinary output of at least 1 mL/kg/h should be maintained. Fever should be controlled by sponging the patient and administering antipyretic agents. If the child's circulatory status is adequate, fluid intake should be restricted to two-thirds maintenance to avoid overload. Electrolyte abnormalities and coagulation defects should be corrected. Vital signs should be observed with care. Elevation of the systolic blood pressure, slowing or speeding of the pulse, and slowed or irregular respirations are indicative of intracranial hypertension. In most children with severe head injuries (GCS scores of 5 or less), the ICP should be monitored continuously (see be-

low). If seizures occur, anticonvulsant drugs should be given (see below).

### Post-Traumatic Seizures

Early post-traumatic seizures (ie, those occurring within the first week after head injury) develop in about 5% of children who are hospitalized after sustaining head trauma. Of these children, about one in four has additional seizures after the first week.

The immediate treatment of post-traumatic seizures in children is essentially the same as the treatment of nontraumatic seizures. Phenytoin sodium (Dilantin) is the drug of choice because of its rapid entry into the brain and lack of prominent sedative effect. It should be given intravenously at a dosage of 15 to 18 mg/kg (at a rate of 25 to 50 mg/min) while the pulse and electrocardiogram are monitored. The maximum dose is 1000 mg. If seizures do not subside fully one half hour after phenytoin has been administered, paraldehyde at a dosage of 0.10 to 0.25 mL/kg, or 1.0 to 1.5 mL per year of age (maximum dose 7 mL), mixed with an equal volume of mineral oil, can be given rectally. If necessary, the same dose can be repeated in 1 hour and every 2 to 4 hours thereafter. Paraldehyde also can be given by nasogastric tube or deep intramuscular injection. If seizure activity continues, intravenous diazepam (Valium) can be used as an alternative or adjunct to paraldehyde at a dosage of 0.2 to 0.5 mg/kg (at a maximum rate of 1 to 2 mg/min), with a total dose not greater than 2 to 4 mg in the infant or 5 to 10 mg in the older child. This dose of diazepam can be repeated every 15 to 30 minutes, to a total of three doses if necessary. A benzodiazepine that is structurally similar to diazepam but has a much longer duration of action is lorazepam (Ativan). It is given by intravenous injection at a dosage of 0.05 to 0.10 mg/kg (at a maximum rate of 1 mg/min). If needed, an additional 0.05 mg/kg can be given 10 minutes later. The maximum total dose is 4 mg. Phenobarbital is another drug that can be used. It, too, should be given intravenously at a dosage of 15 to 20 mg/kg (at a rate of 30 to 100 mg/min). If needed, one half the initial dose can be given 1 hour later and then every 4 to 6 hours thereafter. The maximum total dose is 300 mg. Phenobarbital and benzodiazepines (such as diazepam and lorazepam) given together may act synergistically to cause respiratory and cardiovascular depression.

In studies to date, the use of prophylactic anticonvulsant agents has not been shown to prevent the later development of epilepsy in the head-injured patient who has not had a seizure. A review of seven randomized, double-blind, controlled studies of head-injured adults and children given phenytoin, phenobarbital, or both to prevent post-traumatic seizures has shown phenytoin to reduce seizures in the first week after the head injury, but not beyond this point.

### Raised Intracranial Pressure

ICP, the summation of pressures derived from structures within the cranium, is determined by pressures exerted by the brain, the cerebral blood vessels, and the CSF. ICP is elevated if it measures greater than 15 mm Hg in children, or greater than 7 mm Hg in newborns and infants. In patients with acute head trauma, causes of raised ICP include bleeding into the epidural, subdural, or subarachnoid spaces, or into the brain; brain hyperemia causing diffuse cerebral swelling (from days 1 to 3); brain edema accompanying brain contusion or hematoma (from days 2 to 10); acute hydrocephalus from subarachnoid bleeding; and pseudotumor cerebri.

The individual can adapt temporarily to increased ICP by displacing CSF through the foramen magnum into the distensible lumbar subarachnoid space; some adaptation also is accomplished by compression of the low-pressure intracranial venous system.

The major adaptive mechanism, however, is an increase in the rate of CSF resorption, which can rise to as much as 2 mL/min, or six times its rate of formation. When these mechanisms no longer can compensate adequately for the rise in ICP, clinical signs of raised ICP become evident. The clinical symptoms and signs of acutely raised ICP are shown in Table 153-2. There is no single therapy for raised ICP. Therapeutic modalities employed include supportive measures and medical and surgical treatment.

### Supportive Measures

When a patient's ICP is raised, respiratory and circulatory support must be provided. The head should be elevated to 30° above the horizontal and stabilized in the midline. Fluids should be restricted to 1000 mL/m$_2$/d (two thirds of daily maintenance). Urine output should be maintained at 1 mL/kg/h. Elevated temperature should be reduced.

### Monitoring of Intracranial Pressure

Continuous monitoring of ICP has been especially valuable in poorly responsive head-injured patients, because they are difficult to monitor by clinical parameters alone. Although criteria for monitoring ICP in patients with head trauma have not been established firmly, most advocate its use in those with a GCS score of 5 or less, or a GCS score of 8 or less with cranial CT scan evidence of a mass lesion or brain injury such as contusion or diffuse cerebral swelling. Additionally, monitoring is indicated in any head-injured child who is unconscious, who is in shock, who has deteriorating results of neurologic examination, or whose cranial CT scan shows distortion or displacement of the brain.

Advantages of ICP monitoring include the ability to assess the need for treatment, the efficacy of treatment, and whether treatment should be continued (to maintain, if possible, a CSF pressure of less than 20 mm Hg). ICP can be monitored by devices that can be placed in several intracranial sites (the ventricular system, brain parenchyma, or cerebral subarachnoid, subdural, or epidural spaces), in the spinal subarachnoid space, or in an extracranial position overlying a patent anterior fontanelle. Patients who are being monitored also should have arterial and central venous lines placed, and their vital signs should be monitored continuously. Such patients need to be cared for in an intensive care unit.

Although the many advantages provided by ICP monitoring are undeniable, including guidance of therapy and assistance in prediction of clinical outcome, there are associated risks (such as the introduction of infection), technical problems (mechanical), and situations in which monitoring can be falsely reassuring (as with temporal lobe or posterior fossa lesions that can cause local increases in pressure that are undetected by conventionally placed monitors, or when the monitor is placed contralateral to the side of a supratentorial mass, which tends to give a falsely low ICP reading). Furthermore, such monitoring has not been shown to improve neurologic outcome in head-injured children.

### Medical Management

A number of medical measures are useful in the treatment of patients with elevated ICP in association with acute head trauma (Table 153-3). When considering therapeutic alternatives, it is important to recall that brain swelling occurring during the first 2 to 3 days after a head injury usually is the result of an increase in cerebral blood volume. Between days 3 and 5, the ICP may rise as a result of true cerebral edema. Elevation of the ICP often is seen on about day 9 or 10, probably secondary to an increase in the volume of CSF caused by disturbance in its reabsorption.

Passive hyperventilation works very quickly and does not potentiate intracranial bleeding or lead to secondary increase in the ICP ("rebound"). Thus, it is the most appropriate initial, nonsurgical treatment of intracranial hypertension occurring after head injury. Its efficacy does decrease over time, however. Passive hyperventilation lowers ICP by reducing arterial carbon dioxide tension (PaCO$_2$), thereby inducing vasoconstriction. An immediate reduction in arterial PaCO$_2$ of 5 to 10 mm Hg lowers the ICP by 25% to 30% in most patients. The PaCO$_2$ should not be brought to less than 20 mm Hg unless the jugular bulb PaO$_2$ is monitored (to ensure that cerebral blood flow continues to be adequate). Otherwise, complicating cerebral ischemia may ensue. In the head-injured patient, inability to reduce the ICP by passive hyperventilation usually indicates a grave prognosis.

Administering mannitol is another highly effective means of rapidly lowering elevated ICP. Because there is no transport carrier for mannitol in brain capillaries (the site of the blood–brain barrier), when it is given intravenously, the drug remains in plasma and creates an osmotic gradient, causing water to move from the brain through capillary walls into their lumina, thereby reducing ICP. Mannitol does not reduce brain swelling in regions where the blood–brain barrier is defective. It also slows the production of CSF, which reduces ICP further. Additionally, mannitol may withdraw CSF from the subarachnoid spaces. When mannitol is given repeatedly, fluid and electrolyte imbalances and accompanying dehydration may result. Thus, when it is used, the patient's serum osmolality should be kept between 300 and 320 mOsm/L. Fluid and electrolyte problems, along with the potential development of rebound, limit mannitol's long-term use. Mannitol also increases cerebral blood flow and, therefore, may potentiate intracranial bleeding, although this risk probably is small once hyperventilation is established. Thus, mannitol should be given with some caution during the first 2 to 3 days after a head injury, when brain swelling is caused primarily by hyperemia.

Glycerol is useful in both the immediate and long-term treatment of intracranial hypertension complicating head trauma. For immediate management, it can be administered intravenously. For long-term treatment, it usually is given orally. Its mechanisms of action and limitations of use are the same as those of mannitol. Additionally, when it is used for long periods, glycerol often causes excessive weight gain. Because glycerol is metabolized by the liver, nephrotoxicity, which is a potential concern with excessive mannitol use, is not a problem.

The induction of coma with barbiturates has been helpful in the treatment of intracranial hypertension after severe head injury in patients in whom other measures have failed. Pentobarbital has been the barbiturate used most often. Barbiturates, like hyperventilation, reduce intracranial hypertension by causing cerebral vasoconstriction, thereby decreasing cerebral blood flow. They also reduce cerebral metabolism by as much as 50%, which further enhances their clinical effect. Serum pentobarbital levels

---

**TABLE 153-2. Clinical Symptoms and Signs of Acutely Raised Intracranial Pressure**

| Infants | Children | Both |
|---|---|---|
| Full fontanelle | Headache | Altered mental state |
| Separated sutures | Papilledema | Vomiting |
| (Macrocrania) | | Strabismus (CN VI, (III) palsies); "setting sun" sign |
| (Papilledema) | | Altered vital signs (increased blood pressure, decreased or increased pulse rate, decreased respirations) |
| | | (Signs of herniation) |

*After Rosman NP, Oppenheimer EY, O'Connor JF. Emergency management of pediatric head injuries. Emerg Med Clin North Am 1983;1:149.*

TABLE 153-3.  Medical Treatment of Acutely Elevated Intracranial Pressure in Patients With Head Trauma

| Agent | Dose | Administration | Onset of Action | Peak Action | Advantages | Side Effects or Limitations |
|---|---|---|---|---|---|---|
| Passive hyperventilation | Reduce $Paco_2$ from 40 to 20 mm Hg | Continuous | Seconds to minutes | 2–30 min | Very prompt action | Effect may not be sustained; cerebral ischemia |
| Mannitol | 0.25–1.50 g/kg | Every 1–4 h IV | 5–30 min | 15–90 min | Prompt action | Fluid/electrolyte imbalances; renal failure; intracranial bleeding; possible rebound |
| Glycerol | 0.25–1.00 g/kg | Every 2–8 h IV or PO | 15–30 min | 30 min (IV); 60–80 min (PO) | Prompt action PO or IV | Fluid/electrolyte imbalances; intracranial bleeding; possible rebound |
| Pentobarbital | 1–3 mg/kg (loading dose 5–20 mg/kg) | Every 1–3 h IV | 1–2 min | Minutes | Prompt action; no rebound | Hypotension; renal failure; need for careful monitoring |
| Hypothermia | 27°C–31°C | Continuous | Approximately 1 h | 2–3 h | No rebound | Cardiac arrhythmias; need for careful monitoring |
| Dexamethasone | 0.2 mg/kg (loading dose 1.5 mg/kg) | Every 6 h IV | 18–24 h | 12–24 h | No rebound | Slow onset of action; apparent lack of efficacy in head injury; gastrointestinal hemorrhage |

*IV*, intravenously; *PO*, orally.

of 3 to 4.5 mg/dL should be maintained. Advantages of barbiturate coma include rapidity of action and absence of rebound. Also, it does not potentiate intracranial bleeding. This treatment necessitates careful monitoring of the patient in an intensive care facility. In the treatment of head-injured patients, failure of barbiturate coma to reduce the ICP, as with passive hyperventilation, usually is an ominous sign.

Induced hypothermia is an additional means of treating raised ICP. With lowering of the body temperature to 30°C, the cerebral metabolic rate is decreased by almost 50%. The mechanisms of action, advantages, and limitations of hypothermia are very similar to those of barbiturate coma, with about a 6% reduction in cerebral blood flow observed for each degree (Celsius) that the temperature is lowered. Reduction in ICP is more rapid with pentobarbital than with hypothermia, and hypothermia probably never is adequate as a sole means of treating intracranial hypertension.

Steroids, such as dexamethasone (Decadron), act more slowly than do hyperosmolar agents in reducing increased ICP. It has been suggested that they stabilize the blood–brain barrier, enhance brain energy supplies, promote renal excretion of electrolytes and water, reduce CSF formation, and stabilize lysosomal and other cell membranes. They also may facilitate CSF absorption that is impaired by inflammatory changes in the subarachnoid space or arachnoid villi. Steroids do not produce rebound and do not potentiate intracranial bleeding, although gastrointestinal hemorrhage may occur. Despite their widespread use in the treatment of head injuries, when studied in controlled clinical trials, steroids, even in "megadoses," have not been demonstrated to be effective for this use.

Diuretic agents have been shown to reduce brain water and to decrease the formation of CSF and, therefore, have been used to treat increased ICP. These agents include acetazolamide (Diamox), ethacrynic acid (Edecrin), and furosemide (Lasix), the last of which appears to be the most potent of the three. The furosemide dosage is 0.5 to 1.0 mg/kg every 3 to 6 hours. Diuretics

alone are not very effective in rapidly reducing major elevations in ICP, but may be effective in long-term treatment when only a moderate reduction in pressure is needed. Acetazolamide probably should not be used because of its central vasodilator effect.

### Surgical Management

On occasion, elevations in ICP cannot be reversed adequately by specific interventions or by the empiric medical means just discussed. In such circumstances, surgical management may be indicated. Aspiration of the subdural spaces may be helpful therapeutically. When there is a marked elevation in ICP, with signs of impending or evolving brain herniation, a ventricular tap with slow withdrawal of CSF may be lifesaving. If the raised ICP continues in an unremitting fashion, decompression craniotomy may be needed.

Although no definite evidence exists that the control of ICP alters outcome in the head-injured child, anyone who has seen a substantial number of such patients can remember children in whom the control of intracranial hypertension was lifesaving.

## CLINICAL SYNDROMES IN CHILDREN WITH ACUTE HEAD INJURIES

### Scalp Injuries and Swellings

Contusions and lacerations are the most frequent complications of head injury. Lacerations should be cleaned thoroughly and sutured if necessary. An underlying (depressed) skull fracture should be sought. Tetanus prophylaxis may be needed.

In the older child, most scalp swellings after head trauma are caused by subgaleal hematomas, but in infants, particularly newborns, other causes also exist. In neonates, diffuse scalp swelling with decreased transillumination suggests a subgaleal hematoma, whereas diffuse scalp swelling with increased transillumination indicates a caput succedaneum. If the scalp swelling is focal, particularly in the parietal region, and transillumination is decreased, the newborn very likely has a cephalhematoma (with an underlying skull fracture in 5% to 25% of cases). If the swelling is focal and transillumination is increased, a porencephalic or leptomeningeal cyst with an associated "growing" skull fracture is suggested. The clinical approach to the diagnosis of post-traumatic scalp swellings in childhood is summarized in Figure 153-2.

No treatment is required for subgaleal hematoma, caput succedaneum, or cephalhematoma; in fact, aspiration of fluid from the scalp is contraindicated because of the risk of complicating infection. A leptomeningeal cyst must be treated surgically, however, by removing or replacing the protruding arachnoid and repairing the dural tear.

## Skull Fractures

There are six major kinds of skull fractures that occur in childhood: (1) linear, (2) depressed, (3) compound, (4) basal, (5) diastatic, and (6) "growing." Linear fractures constitute about 75% of all skull fractures. They are especially frequent in children less than 2 years of age and occur most often in the temporoparietal region. Although these fractures need not be treated themselves, they may overlie serious intracranial conditions, such as epidural hemorrhage, for which treatment is urgently required. Linear fracture in the infant or young child should raise the possibility of neglect or inflicted injury. Linear fractures heal within 1 to 2 months.

In depressed skull fractures, either continuity of the bony calvarium is disrupted or, particularly in the newborn, the skull simply may be indented, causing a so-called "ping-pong ball" or "pond" fracture, unaccompanied by a break in the cranial vault. Depressed skull fractures can be missed easily if tangential skull films, which usually demonstrate a double density (bone on bone) at the fracture site, are not obtained. Although depressed skull fractures are best seen with plain radiographs, many also can be seen on CT, particularly when a bone fragment is displaced. Depressed skull fractures are of particular concern because the underlying brain may be bruised or lacerated. Some clinicians advocate surgical elevation of depressed fractures if the depression is more than 5 mm or if the depressed fragment extends below the inner table of the skull, but such elevation does not appear to reduce the risk of PTE, presumably because of brain injury sustained at impact.

Compound or open skull fractures, with laceration of the scalp extending to the fracture site, are of urgent concern because of the danger of complicating infection. Treatment involves metic-

ulous debridement of the wound, search for a foreign body, copious irrigation with a sterile solution, and the administration of parenteral antibiotics and, if needed, tetanus prophylaxis. When a compound depressed fracture is found, the fracture should be elevated promptly to minimize the risk of complicating infection.

Only about 20% of basal skull fractures can be recognized on standard skull radiographs because of the anatomic complexity of the base of the skull. Although the addition of multiplanar tomography and thin-section cranial CT scanning appreciably increases the frequency with which such fractures can be seen on radiography, firm diagnosis frequently is dependent on the recognition of coexisting signs. These include hemorrhage in the nose, nasopharynx, middle ear, over the mastoid bone (Battle's sign), or about the eyes ("raccoon eyes" sign). Cranial nerve palsies sometimes occur, most frequently affecting cranial nerves I, VII, and VIII. CSF rhinorrhea and otorrhea, reflecting fractures of the cribriform plate or petrous temporal bone, respectively, are worrisome signs of basal skull fracture because of the risk of complicating bacterial meningitis, usually caused by *Streptococcus pneumoniae*. No clear evidence exists that prophylactic antibiotic therapy diminishes the frequency of this complication. Metrizamide CT cisternography can be very useful in identifying the location of a CSF leak complicating a fracture of the skull base. Hemorrhage into the cranial sinuses can cause an appearance on x-ray film simulating sinusitis. Skull films may show intracranial air (pneumocephalus), indicating continuity between a paranasal or mastoid sinus and the inside of the skull. Occipital fractures involving the foramen magnum may be accompanied by tachycardia, hypotension, and irregular respirations.

Diastatic skull fractures are traumatic separations of cranial bones at a suture site. They most frequently affect the lambdoid suture and are seen most often in the first 4 years of life. Diastatic fractures should be monitored closely in children younger than 3 years of age because they can become sites of "growing" fractures.

"Growing" skull fractures are caused by the herniation of tissue through torn dura and an associated fracture (linear or diastatic) into the overlying scalp. Such fractures occur most often in the parietal region (Fig 153-3). The herniating tissue either is solid brain or is cystic in nature, usually a porencephalic cyst (communicating with a lateral ventricle) or a leptomeningeal cyst. It is the pulsating, herniating tissue and associated scarring that prevents fusion of the fracture margins and causes the fracture to "grow." Although such fractures occasionally evolve immediately, they develop more often within weeks or months of the head injury. Only rarely do they occur in children older than 3 years of age.

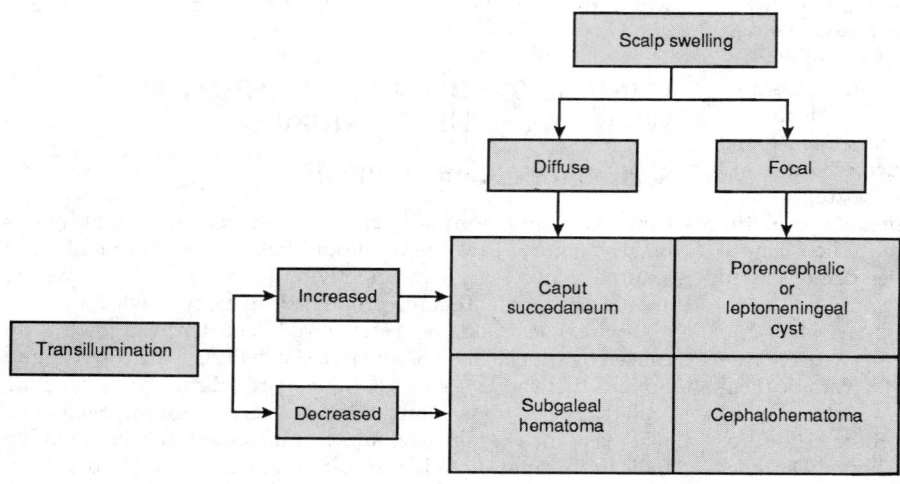

**Figure 153-2.** Clinical approach to the diagnosis of scalp swellings in childhood. (Rosman NP. Managing acute head trauma. Contemp Pediatr 1986;3:34.)

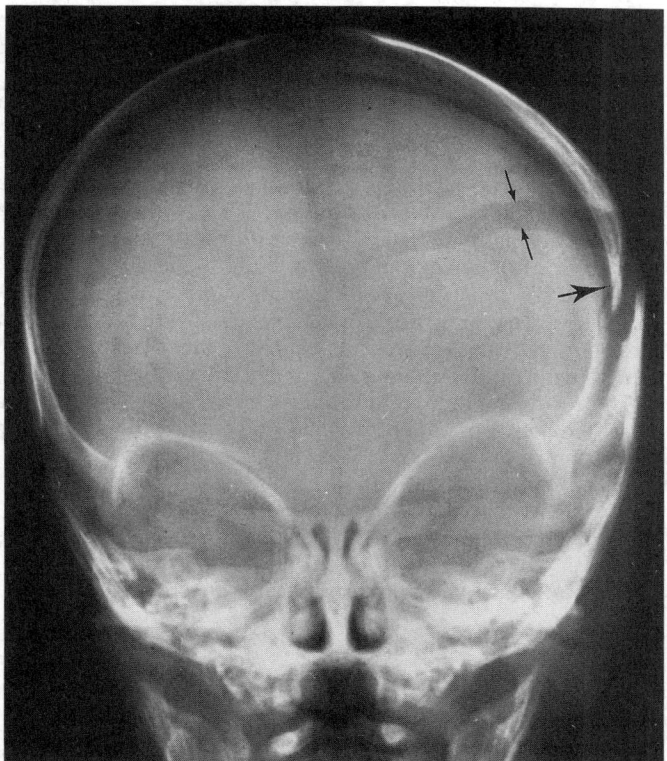

**Figure 153-3.** Posteroanterior radiograph of the skull shows a "growing" parietal skull fracture (*small arrows*) in a 9-week-old infant with an adjacent depressed parietal fracture; the depressed fragment (*large arrow*) lies beneath the squamous temporal bone.

## Cerebral Concussion

Cerebral concussion is a clinical state characterized by a transient impairment of consciousness with loss of awareness and responsiveness immediately after a head injury and persisting for seconds, minutes, or, occasionally, hours. The force of injury needed to cause a concussion is somewhat less than that required to cause a skull fracture. The causative trauma usually is blunt. Concussion is much more likely to occur when the head moves freely after the impact (acceleration/deceleration) than when it is held firmly in place (compression). Concussive injuries cause an increase in ICP followed by a temporary shear strain on the upper brain stem, resulting in loss of consciousness. The concussed brain does not have any consistent morphologic abnormality. It seems likely that the clinical state is caused by suddenly increased and unmet energy demands of the brain.

Concussion is associated with three types of amnesia: a temporary retrograde amnesia that extends back to events predating the head injury by some years, a permanent retrograde amnesia that encompasses the few seconds or minutes that immediately preceded the injury, and a temporary post-traumatic (anterograde) amnesia that is characterized by an impaired ability to form new memories that usually lasts for some hours. In the absence of a history of definite loss of consciousness, demonstration of these types of amnesia is exceedingly useful in establishing the diagnosis of concussion. Also, the duration of the amnesia serves as a useful indicator of the severity of the head injury.

Children who have had a concussion should be observed closely for at least 24 hours; almost all recover uneventfully. A few, however, can be quite disabled by the development of a postconcussional syndrome, which is characterized by headache, dizziness, irritability, nervousness, inability to concentrate, and, occasionally, behavioral and cognitive impairment. The patho-

genesis of the postconcussional syndrome is unsettled. Organic, environmental, and emotional factors each have been cited, with evidence for an organic basis mounting.

A triad of symptoms that often follows minor head injury in young children includes lethargy, irritability, and vomiting, unaccompanied by loss of consciousness. These symptoms, which are attributed to torsion of the brain stem, usually subside within 48 to 72 hours.

## Cerebral Contusion and Laceration

In contusion and laceration, in contrast to concussion, there is a bruising (contusion) or tearing (laceration) of the brain. A blunt head injury predisposes a patient to contusion, whereas a penetrating injury predisposes a patient to laceration. In addition to direct brain injury, the brain can be damaged from an external source causing forceful impact against dural septa or irregular bony projections, particularly in the anterior and middle cranial fossae. Brain lesions can occur directly beneath the site of impact (coup injury) or more remotely, opposite the site of impact (contrecoup injury). The poles and undersurfaces of the frontal and temporal lobes are especially vulnerable. The diagnosis of contusion or laceration is established clinically by the demonstration of focal neurologic signs, including seizures, that are known or presumed to have been absent before the head injury occurred. The cranial CT scan or MRI often provides important radiologic confirmation.

One complication of special concern in patients with cerebral contusion and laceration is PTE. PTE occurs more often with laceration than with contusion. With complicating skull fracture, PTE is more likely when the fracture is depressed than when it is linear (Fig 153-4). When a concussion also has occurred, PTE is more likely to develop when the duration of unconsciousness was more than 1 hour and when the post-traumatic amnesia was longer than 24 hours. The electroencephalogram has been disappointingly unhelpful in predicting the occurrence of PTE in head-injured children. About 5% of children who are hospitalized

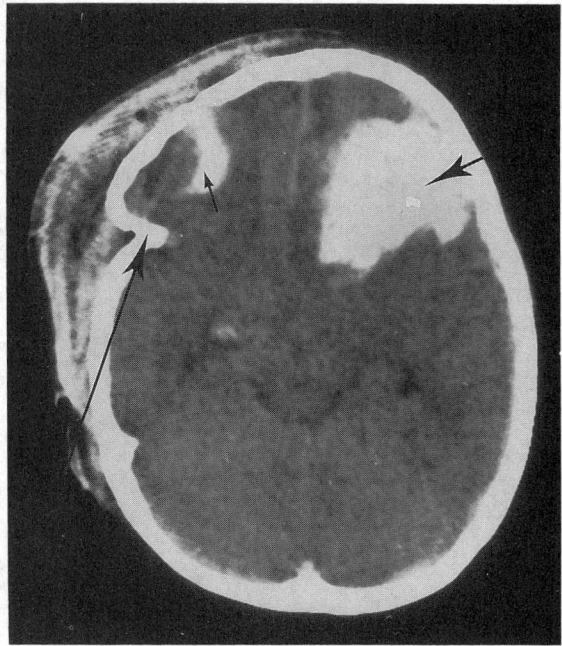

**Figure 153-4.** Cranial CT scan shows a depressed skull fracture (*long arrow*) in a 4-year-old child with an overlying subgaleal hematoma and an underlying cerebral contusion (*small arrow*) with a contralateral cerebral hematoma (*large arrow*).

after sustaining head trauma suffer a seizure within the first week after their injury (early PTE). Although early PTE is common in children who have had a mild head injury, particularly those less than 5 years of age, in general, the more severe the head injury, the more likely early PTE is to occur. In 20% to 30% of cases of early PTE, seizures continue beyond the first week. Another 5% of children who are hospitalized because of head trauma have seizures more than a week after the injury (late PTE). As with early PTE, late PTE is more likely to occur when the head injury has been more severe. Of those patients who have late PTE, about half eventually cease having attacks, about 25% continue to experience 10 to 15 seizures per year, and another 25% have further seizures, but only rarely.

## Acute Epidural and Subdural Hematomas

The clinical points that aid in the diagnosis of and distinction between acute epidural and subdural hematoma are outlined in Table 153-4. Both types of hematoma are located much more frequently above the tentorium (supratentorial hemorrhage) than in the posterior fossa (infratentorial hemorrhage). Of the supratentorial hematomas, the subdural variety is 5 to 10 times more frequent than its epidural counterpart. An acute epidural hematoma most often is temporoparietal in location and is associated with a fracture of the squamous temporal bone in about 70% of cases. Although they usually are caused by laceration of the underlying middle meningeal artery, at least 25% of epidural hematomas in children are of venous origin (from dural sinuses, middle meningeal veins, emissary and diploic veins). Acute subdural hematomas characteristically are of venous origin, resulting from tearing of bridging meningeal veins; occasionally, they are arterial in origin. They usually are frontoparietal in location, with an accompanying skull fracture seen in only 30% of cases. Underlying brain contusion frequently is associated.

Acute subdural hemorrhages are seen most often in infancy, with a peak frequency at the age of 6 months, whereas acute epidural hematomas tend to occur in older children (when the dura is less firmly adherent to the inner table of the skull). In both types of hematomas, the degree of antecedent head trauma may be quite mild. Acute epidural hematomas usually are unilateral, whereas at least 75% of acute subdural hematomas are bilateral. Seizures occur in less than 25% of children with acute epidural hematomas, but in 60% to 90% of those with acute subdural hematomas. Retinal and pre-retinal hemorrhages are found frequently in association with acute subdural hematomas, but are uncommon with acute epidural hemorrhage. The "biphasic course" (impaired consciousness/alertness/impaired consciousness) that is said to be characteristic of acute epidural hematoma in adults is seen rarely in children.

The relatively large volumes of extravasated blood that are present in both types of hematoma produce symptoms and signs of intracranial hypertension. These include irritability or lethargy, vomiting, fullness of the anterior fontanelle, headache, papilledema, and elevation of the systolic blood pressure with a decreased or increased pulse rate and slowed, irregular respirations (see Table 153-2). With sufficient elevation of pressure in the supratentorial compartment, unilateral transtentorial herniation may occur.

The cranial CT scan is particularly valuable in differentiating acute epidural and subdural hematomas above the tentorium. The former tends to assume a lenticular configuration, whereas the latter characteristically is curvilinear or crescentic in appearance. The mortality rate in children with acute epidural hematoma has varied from 9% to 17%, but the survivors tend to be relatively free of neurologic sequelae. Although mortality with acute subdural hematoma often has been less than that with acute epidural hematoma, it has been as high as 17% to 20% in some series. Neurologic morbidity (motor deficits, seizures, cognitive impairment) is greater with acute subdural hematoma than with acute epidural hematoma because of the frequency with which the

TABLE 153-4.　Clinical Features of Acute Epidural and Subdural Hematomas

| Clinical Feature | Epidural | Subdural |
| --- | --- | --- |
| **Supratentorial** | | |
| Frequency | Less | 5–10 times greater |
| Skull fracture | 70% | 30% |
| Source of hemorrhage | Arterial or venous | Almost always venous |
| Age | Usually older than 2 y | Usually younger than 1 y |
| Location | Usually temporoparietal | Usually frontoparietal |
| Laterality | Usually unilateral | 75% bilateral |
| Seizures | Less than 25% | 75% |
| Preretinal and retinal hemorrhages | Uncommon | Very frequent |
| Increased intracranial pressure | Present | Present |
| Computed cranial tomography (CCT) configuration | Usually lenticular | Curvilinear or crescentic |
| Mortality | Relatively high | Usually lower |
| Morbidity | Low | High |
| **Infratentorial** | | |
| Frequency | 2–3 times greater | Less |
| Skull fracture | Almost always | Frequent |
| Source of hemorrhage | Venous | Venous |
| Impaired consciousness | Frequent | Frequent |
| Acute hydrocephalus/medullary compression | Variable | Variable |
| Other posterior fossa signs | Variable | Variable |

more deeply situated subdural hematoma is accompanied by injury to the underlying brain.

Epidural and subdural hemorrhages also can occur in the posterior fossa after head injury, but they are much less frequent in this infratentorial location than they are above the tentorium. Here, in contrast to their relative frequencies above the tentorium, acute epidural hematomas are 2 to 3 times more frequent than are acute subdural hematomas. Occipital skull fractures are common with both types of infratentorial hematoma, particularly those that are epidural. In both types of infratentorial hematoma, the bleeding is venous. Clinical signs include impaired consciousness, headache, vomiting, and altered respirations. Only about half of the children have posterior fossa signs such as ataxia, nystagmus, and cranial nerve palsies. These posterior fossa hemorrhages may be complicated by upward herniation of the cerebellum through the tentorial notch or, more often, by downward displacement of the cerebellar tonsils through the foramen magnum.

If acute epidural hemorrhage is suspected clinically, the diagnosis should be confirmed promptly by a cranial CT scan; these hematomas sometimes enlarge so rapidly, with accompanying signs of acutely elevated ICP and progressive hemiparesis, that immediate neurosurgical treatment is usually required (craniotomy, surgical removal of blood clot, and attention to the bleeding source).

If acute subdural hemorrhage is suspected clinically, neurosurgical intervention rarely is needed before the diagnosis is confirmed by cranial CT scan. On occasion, however, with acutely elevated ICP in infants in whom a subdural hematoma is suspected, the subdural space should be tapped as a combined diagnostic and therapeutic measure.

## Subacute and Chronic Subdural Hematomas

In addition to their acute presentation (with symptoms appearing within 48 hours of head injury), subdural hematomas also can be subacute (with the onset of symptoms between 3 and 21 days) or chronic (with symptoms appearing after 21 days). Unlike acute subdural hematomas, which are most common in infancy, most chronic subdural hematomas occur in older children and adolescents. In these less acute hematomas, recurrent vomiting from intracranial hypertension still can be seen. Macrocrania, reflecting a longer lasting increase in ICP, often is present, and the head may have a box-like appearance. Transillumination of the skull characteristically shows a diffuse increase in spread of the light. The anterior fontanelle may be excessively large or full. Funduscopy may disclose well-established papilledema. Seizures are frequent. Motor abnormalities, including hypertonicity and agitation, can be found. Systemic signs, such as irritability, vomiting, fever, anemia, and poor weight gain, are seen commonly. MRI is the ideal imaging modality to demonstrate these non-acute hematomas.

Methods of treating subacute and chronic subdural hematomas include subdural taps with aspiration of subdural fluid, external drainage with shunting of subdural fluid to the peritoneum or to a pleural cavity, and bur holes (or occasionally craniotomy) with aspiration or surgical removal of subdural clots.

## PROGNOSIS IN PATIENTS WITH ACUTE BRAIN INJURY

Most children who are hospitalized after head injury with loss of consciousness, skull fracture, or cerebral contusion recover completely, usually within 24 to 48 hours. A small number of these children have a postconcussional syndrome or post-traumatic seizures. A smaller group still has severe head injury resulting in prolonged coma, with persisting cognitive, behavioral, or motor deficits.

## Severe Head Injuries and Neurologic Outcome

The GCS has proved useful in assisting in the prediction of mortality and neurologic morbidity after head injury. With this scale, head injuries can be classified as mild (GCS score 13 to 15), moderate (GCS score 9 to 12), or severe (GCS score 3 to 8). In the absence of accompanying systemic injury, children with a GCS score of 6, 7, or 8 rarely, if ever, die after head trauma, those with a GCS score of 4 or 5 are unlikely to die, but those with a GCS score of 3 face a mortality rate of 50% to 60% (usually within the first 2 to 3 days after injury). Children with a GCS score of 6 or more have an 80% to 90% chance of recovering with independent function and minimal neurologic deficit. With a GCS score of 4 or 5, cognitive, academic, and other neurologic deficits can be anticipated in 50% to 60% of cases. Children with a GCS score of 3 who survive their head injury have a high incidence of significant cognitive and other neurologic residua. In most such cases, cognitive deficits (attention, intelligence, memory, language), personality change, emotional upset, and social maladjustment are more disabling than is any residual motor handicap.

## Duration of Post-Traumatic Coma and Neurologic Outcome

Coma lasting less than 24 hours rarely is associated with permanent neuropsychologic sequelae, except when there has been accompanying focal injury of the brain. Coma of less than 6 weeks in duration is associated with return to independent function in more than 90% of children. Coma lasting 6 weeks to 3 months also is followed by return to independent function, with moderate disability or good recovery in 90% of patients. With coma lasting longer than 3 months, recovery of normal neurologic and psychologic function is seen less often. Such benchmarks notwithstanding, children and adolescents have a greater capacity than do adults to recover from severe head injury, and their cognitive and social skills can continue to improve for more than 3 years.

## Neurologic Outcome in Patients With Milder Head Injuries

Outcome data on neurologic sequelae after mild head injuries have varied considerably in different series. Most such children appear to recover quickly and completely, although later neurologic deficits (often quite subtle) sometimes are found. These include symptoms of postconcussional syndrome, temporary cognitive difficulties, behavioral changes, and occasional post-traumatic seizures.

## Age as a Factor in Neurologic Outcome

Of the many factors that influence outcome after head injury, the severity of the injury is the most significant. Next in importance is patient age. Numerous studies have shown that, after head injuries of comparable severity, children usually recover more fully than do adults. With regard to mortality in the head-injured child, the highest rates are seen in the first 2 years of life. After that point, mortality declines steadily throughout childhood, with the lowest rate seen at 12 years of age. Mortality then rises again, with the steepest increase occurring between the ages of 15 and 24 years (when motor vehicle accidents surpass both falls and bicycle accidents as the major cause of head injury).

## Selected Readings

Adams JH. The neuropathology of head injuries. In: Vinken PJ, Bruyn GW, eds. Handbook of clinical neurology, vol 23. Amsterdam: North Holland, 1975:35.

Barnett GH, Chapman PH. Insertion and care of intracranial pressure monitoring devices. In: Ropper AH, Kennedy SK, eds. Neurological and neurosurgical intensive care, 2nd ed. Rockville: Aspen, 1988:43.

Chestnut RM, Marshall LF. Treatment of abnormal intracranial pressure. Neurosurgery Clinics of North America 1991;2:267.

Choux M, Lena G, Genitori L, et al. Pediatric head injuries. In: Braakman R, ed. Handbook of clinical neurology, vol 57. Amsterdam: North Holland, 1990:327.

Crowe W. Aspects of neuroradiology of head injury. Neurosurgery Clinics of North America 1991;2:321.

Levin HS, Hamilton WJ, Grossman RG. Outcome after head injury. In: Braakman R, ed. Handbook of clinical neurology, vol 57. Amsterdam: North Holland, 1990:367.

Lipper MH, Kishore PRS. Radiological investigation of acute head trauma. In: Becker DP, Gudeman SK, eds. Textbook of head injury. Philadelphia: WB Saunders, 1989:102.

Rodriguez JG, Brown ST. Childhood injuries in the United States. Am J Dis Child 1990;144:627.

Ropper AH, Rockoff MA. Treatment of intracranial hypertension. In: Ropper AH, Kennedy SK, eds. Neurological and neurosurgical intensive care, 2nd ed. Rockville: Aspen, 1988:23.

Rosman NP. Traumatic brain injury. In: Miller G, Ramer JC, eds. Static encephalopathies of infancy and childhood. New York: Raven Press, 1992:283.

Rosman NP, Oppenheimer EY. Post-traumatic epilepsy. Pediatr Rev 1982;3:221.

Rosman NP, Oppenheimer EY, O'Connor JF. Emergency management of pediatric head injuries. Emerg Med Clin North Am 1983;1:141.

Temkin NR, Dikmen SS, Winn HR. Posttraumatic seizures. Neurosurgery Clinics of North America 1991;2:425.

*Principles and Practice of Pediatrics, Second Edition.*
edited by Frank A. Oski et al. J. B. Lippincott Company, Philadelphia © 1994.

# CHAPTER 154
# *Seizure Disorders in Infants and Children*

## 154.1 *Epilepsy*

### Daniel G. Glaze

Epilepsy is the symptomatic expression of underlying brain pathology or disordered brain function, not a disease in the usual sense. The incidence of epilepsy has been reported to range from 0.8% to 1.1%. It is the most common neurologic disorder seen in children, and about 50% of all cases of epilepsy start in childhood. Epilepsy is defined as a randomly recurring symptom complex resulting from an episodic disturbance of central nervous system function, associated with an excessive, self-limited, neuronal discharge. Variation in clinical manifestations is accounted for by variation in the portion of the brain involved.

Epilepsy can have many causes; in general, any event having the potential to produce insult to the brain can result in epilepsy. In many children, the cause is a static or nonprogressive en-cephalopathy secondary to historical antecedents such as hypoxia, hemorrhage, central nervous system infection, head trauma, and developmental defects of the brain. Cerebral insult as a consequence of labor and delivery complications is a much less common cause than previously thought. Although specific entities such as tuberous sclerosis, neurofibromatosis, brain tumors, some degenerative diseases, and certain inborn errors of metabolism can present initially with recurrent seizures, these diagnoses are suggested by other signs and symptoms revealed by the history and physical examination. For certain seizure disorders, familial neonatal convulsions, classic absence seizures, and certain partial seizure disorders (eg, benign epilepsy of childhood with rolandic spikes), there may be historical evidence of a genetic predisposition. In about half of all children with recurrent seizures, the workup will not disclose a specific cause. Isolated seizures can occur as a consequence of hypoglycemia or other acute metabolic derangements. Such seizures do not constitute epilepsy, because specific therapy for the primary disorder obviates the necessity of maintenance therapy with antiepileptic drugs.

## CLASSIFICATION AND DESCRIPTION OF SEIZURE TYPES

Diagnostic accuracy and treatment options have improved greatly during the past decade as a consequence of advances made in many areas. These include the adoption of a universally accepted descriptive classification system, the increased availability of serum drug monitoring, the development of new antiepileptic drugs, advances in video-electroencephalogram (EEG) monitoring and neuroimaging techniques, and improved knowledge of drug interactions. Nonetheless, a carefully detailed history and physical examination remain of prime importance to diagnosis.

Epilepsy is a clinical, not a laboratory, diagnosis, and errors in diagnosis, seizure classification, and subsequent treatment are most often the consequence of an inadequate history and physical examination. A number of relatively benign, episodic spells often are misdiagnosed and even treated as seizures. These include breath-holding spells, benign paroxysmal vertigo, syncope, tics, and even masturbation. The physician rarely has the opportunity actually to witness a clinical seizure and usually must rely on a description provided by the parents. A seizure often is a very frightening experience for parents and it is understandable that their ability to recall details, time relationships, and the sequence of events can be limited. Frequently, the parents may not have witnessed the event and can report only what they were told by a teacher or other witness. It often is worthwhile to obtain a description by telephone from the actual witness. When the available clinical description is vague and unconvincing, it may be appropriate to delay definitive diagnosis and treatment and to instruct parents in what to look for should attacks recur.

The classification system for epileptic seizures currently in use (Table 154-1) is based on both clinical and EEG features. It divides seizures into two major categories, generalized and partial. Generalized seizures are those in which the clinical features indicate the involvement of both cerebral hemispheres from the start. Consciousness usually is impaired and, when motor involvement is present, it is bilateral and relatively symmetric from the very beginning. Conversely, partial seizures are characterized by clinical features suggesting that only a limited or functional area of one cerebral hemisphere is involved. They begin focally, although they may become generalized. Partial seizures are divided further into those with elementary or simple symptomatology and those with complex symptomatology. In children, elementary partial seizures most commonly are focal motor or focal sensory phenomena, and consciousness is preserved unless there is secondary generalization. Complex partial seizures usually have their origin

---

TABLE 154-1. Classification of Epileptic Seizures

Generalized Seizures
Tonic-clonic
Clonic
Tonic
Atonic
Myoclonic
Absence

Partial Seizures
Elementary symptomatology
  With motor symptoms
  With sensory symptoms
Complex symptomatology
  With impairment of consciousness only
  With cognitive symptomatology
  With affective symptomatology
  With psychosensory symptomatology
  Compound forms
Partial seizures secondarily generalized

*Commission on Classification and Terminology of the International League Against Epilepsy. Proposal for revised clinical and electroencephalographic classification of epileptic seizures. Epilepsia 1981;22:489*

---

in temporal or frontal lobe structures and the clinical features encompass a spectrum of complex phenomena, including behavioral automatisms, alterations of perception, hallucinations, changes in affect and memory, and ideational distortions.

## Generalized Seizures

Generalized tonic-clonic seizures are characterized clinically by an abrupt arrest of activity and an immediate loss of consciousness. The tonic phase, consisting of sustained, generalized contraction of flexor or extensor muscles, usually lasts only a few seconds. The clonic phase that follows is characterized by symmetric, rhythmic, clonic activity consisting of alternating contraction and relaxation of major appendicular or axial muscle groups. The clonic phase is longer in duration than the tonic phase, but often terminates spontaneously in less than 5 minutes. Respiration may be irregular and stridulous, and sphincter incontinence may or may not be present. The clonic phase usually is followed by a variable period of confusion and lethargy, which may persist from minutes to hours, and sleep is common.

Clonic seizures are identical to the clonic phase of tonic-clonic seizures. Generalized tonic seizures are characterized by sustained contraction of flexor or extensor muscle groups, giving the child a stiff or rigid appearance. A coarse tremor may be superimposed, but it should not be confused with the rhythmic, alternating muscle contraction and relaxation of clonic activity. A distinction often can be made by asking the parents to supplement their verbal description with a demonstration of what they observed. Both clonic and tonic seizures also will be followed by postictal signs and symptoms similar to those seen with generalized tonic-clonic seizures.

Atonic seizures are characterized by the abrupt loss of postural tone and limpness. In contrast to akinetic seizures, the loss of consciousness lasts for several minutes, and there usually is postictal confusion and lethargy or sleep.

Myoclonic seizures are characterized by very brief, random contractions of a muscle or group of muscles occurring unilaterally or bilaterally, and either singly or in clusters. Consciousness usually is preserved. Myoclonic seizures are seen most often with progressive or degenerative types of encephalopathy accompanied by intellectual deficits as well as other overt abnormalities on neurologic examination. Akinetic or "drop attacks" are a subclass of myoclonic seizures and are characterized by a precipitous loss of postural tone. The child abruptly becomes limp and drops to the floor. With nonambulatory infants, there may be precipitous loss of tone resulting in head nodding or slumping forward. The duration of myoclonic seizures is only a few seconds, and there is immediate resumption of normal activity with no postictal lethargy or confusion.

Absence seizures are characterized clinically by very brief episodes of altered awareness during which there is transient arrest of activity and the child appears to stare blankly. The duration of these episodes seldom is longer than 5 to 10 seconds, but they can recur many times a day. They rarely are seen in children less than 3 years of age, and most have their onset before 10 years of age. The child commonly is not aware that a seizure has occurred and frequently is assumed to be daydreaming. A child who is daydreaming, however, is aware of doing so and usually responds when his or her name is called or he or she is touched. In contrast, a child with absence seizures usually denies awareness of any lapse and does not respond to verbal or physical stimuli. Subtle motor activity such as rhythmic eye blinking, drooping of the head, or slight movements of the arms may accompany the staring episodes. The seizure is terminated by the immediate return of environmental awareness, and the child may resume an activity at the point where it was interrupted. A generalized, symmetric three-per-second spike and wave pattern is the EEG hallmark of absence seizures.

## Partial Seizures

The initial features of a partial seizure are especially important. Tonic deviation of the head and eyes to one side, or some other localized motor or sensory feature preceding a secondarily generalized tonic-clonic seizure may be a clue to focal cortical origin of the attack. In children, elementary partial seizures usually are focal motor or sensory. The initial feature may be focal twitching involving the distal portion of an extremity, which may remain localized or spread to become a hemiconvulsion. Similarly, focal sensory seizures may be initiated by the appearance of a sensation of numbness or tingling in an extremity, which may remain confined to that area or spread to involve the entire side of the body. Consciousness often is preserved, but will be lost if there is secondary generalization.

Complex partial seizures have a variety of clinical expressions and are subclassified on this basis. One form in which there is impairment of consciousness only is characterized by transient, blank staring or confusion. These episodes can be mistaken for absence seizures, but the attacks usually last 30 seconds or longer, whereas absence episodes commonly last less than 10 seconds. An EEG can be helpful in distinguishing between the two forms, because a three-per-second generalized spike and wave pattern is the hallmark of absence seizures, whereas focal discharge from temporal or frontal areas is anticipated with complex partial seizures. Another form of partial complex seizure involves "cognitive symptomatology." This form is characterized clinically by an abrupt alteration in mental state that involves disruption of time relationships and memory. Older children sometimes describe feelings of unreality, remoteness, detachment, or depersonalization. Forced thinking, a deluge of thoughts, or perseveration of a thought also have been described. Déjà vu or jamais vu, the impression of an inappropriate familiarity or unfamiliarity with a place or situation, occasionally may be reported. Attacks characterized by "affective symptomatology" may be described as inexplicable feelings of fear or dread, or other emotional experiences that intrude abruptly on the patient's prevailing affective state. Attacks characterized by "somatosensory disturbances" are notable for distortions of perception or hallucinations. Some children report transient distortions of perception concerning the size of objects (micropsia or macropsia), and others describe hallucinations involving taste or smell as well as formed visual hallucinations.

Probably the most familiar complex partial seizure is the psychomotor attack that is characterized by semi-purposeful motor automatisms. The stereotyped automatisms may be perseverative in nature, and the child will exhibit continuing repetition of the activity in which he was engaged before the onset of the seizure. For example, if the child was walking, he may continue to walk, but without purposeful direction. If the child was writing, he may continue to move the pencil across the page without producing decipherable script. The simplest type of automatisms are masticatory, sucking, and lip-pursing movements. Patting, scratching, or picking at clothing also may be seen. More complex behaviors such as fumbling with clothing as if to undress or turning about as if searching for something are less common. Finally, "compound forms" may be seen that incorporate various elements of the several varieties just described. In an individual child, the form taken usually is stereotyped from one attack to another.

## Epileptic Syndromes

The international classification of epileptic seizures is confined to a description of individual seizure types. An increasing number of distinct epileptic syndromes are recognized and the terminology used in daily communication consists of descriptions of syndromes. The Commission on Classification and Terminology of the International League Against Epilepsy has proposed a classification system for the epileptic syndromes. This system initially divides all epileptic syndromes according to whether the epilepsy is partial, generalized, or uncertain, and then subdivides these categories according to the presence or absence of presumed cause. The epilepsy is considered to be secondary (or symptomatic) if obvious pathology is demonstrable, the patient has a history of or demonstrates neurologic or mental impairment, or if the causes are presumed on the basis of studies of previous patients with the same seizure type and location. A modified summary of the epileptic syndromes is shown in Table 154-2.

Several epileptic syndromes are unique to childhood and contain certain features that distinguish them from the more typical primary or secondary types of epilepsy. Infantile spasms or infantile massive spasms are peculiar to infancy and early childhood, with a peak incidence of onset between 2 and 7 months of age. They have been described as occurring in three clinical forms. Flexor spasms consist of sudden flexion of the neck, trunk, and extremities, which may be so violent that the torso will "jackknife" at the waist. Extensor spasms consist of abrupt extension of the neck and trunk with adduction or abduction of the extremities. The predominant form is a mixed flexor-extensor spasm most commonly consisting of flexion of the neck, trunk, and arms, with extension of the legs and, less commonly, flexion of the legs and extension of the arms. Infantile spasms tend to occur in clusters, with each cluster consisting of 2 to 125 individual spasms. Each individual spasm lasts only a few seconds, although a cluster may extend over several minutes. Spasms rarely occur during actual sleep, but frequently occur on arousal. In most instances, the EEG shows the distinctive pattern of hypsarrhythmia.

Infantile spasms must be distinguished from benign myoclonus of early infancy and benign neonatal sleep myoclonus, which are characterized by normal EEG results, normal development, and occurrence during sleep. Massive spasms frequently are misinterpreted as startle responses or attacks of colic. A careful history usually will elicit the absence of a preceding startle stimulus or

---

**TABLE 154-2.   Modified Classification of Epileptic Syndromes**

1. Localization-related (focal, local, partial) epilepsies and syndrome
   1.1 Idiopathic with age-related onset
      Benign childhood epilepsy with centrotemporal spike
      Childhood epilepsy with occipital paroxysms
      Primary reading epilepsy
   1.2 Symptomatic, all other partial epilepsies consequent to a known or suspected disorder of the central nervous system.
2. Generalized epilepsies and syndromes
   2.1 Idiopathic with age-related onset
      Benign neonatal familial convulsions
      Benign neonatal convulsions
      Benign myoclonic epilepsy in infancy
      Childhood absence epilepsy
      Juvenile absence epilepsy
      Juvenile myoclonic epilepsy
   2.2 Cryptogenic or symptomatic
      West syndrome (infantile spasms)
      Lennox-Gastaut syndrome
   2.3 Symptomatic
      2.3.1 Nonspecific etiology
         Early myoclonic encephalopathy
      2.3.2 Specific syndromes such as those associated with inborn-error metabolisms, malformations
3. Epilepsies and syndromes undetermined, whether focal or generalized
   3.1 With both generalized and focal seizures
      Neonatal seizures
      Severe myoclonic epilepsy in infancy
      Acquired epileptic aphasia (Landau-Kleffner sydnrome)
   3.2 Without unequivocal generalized or focal features
4. Special syndromes
   4.1 Situation-related seizures
      Febrile convulsions
      Isolated seizures
      Seizures occurring only when there is an acute metabolic or toxic event

*Commission on Classification and Terminology of the International League Against Epilepsy. Proposal for revised classification of epilepsies and epileptic syndromes. Epilepsia 1989;30:389.*

---

the information that the episodes are too precipitous in onset and offset, and too short in duration to fit the usual clinical picture of colic. Although crying may follow an infantile spasm, it is not the inconsolable crying that is encountered in infants with cramping abdominal pain.

Infantile spasms have occurred in association with numerous and seemingly unrelated pathologic states, and no one specific factor or circumscribed group of factors has been identified as a common etiologic abnormality. Etiologic associations provide the basis for division of these spasms into two broad groups. In the idiopathic or cryptogenic group, there is no demonstrable cause, the child's development usually has been normal until the onset of spasms, and the results of computed tomography (CT) scans of the brain are normal. In the symptomatic group, a specific etiologic factor can be identified, developmental or neurologic abnormalities have preceded the onset of spasms, and the results of CT scans of the brain often are abnormal. The cryptogenic group represents no more than 10% to 15% of the total, and they have a better prognosis than does the symptomatic group.

Causes associated with the symptomatic group of infantile spasms include cerebral dysgenesis, intrauterine infections, and genetic disorders. Two syndromes of cerebral dysgenesis that have been associated with infantile spasms are the Miller-Dieker syndrome (lissencephaly with or without a chromosome 17 abnormality) and Aicardi's syndrome (females with agenesis of the corpus callosum, distinctive chorioretinopathy, and mental retardation).

The relationship of pertussis immunization to the onset of infantile spasms has generated interest and concern for many years. The Child Neurology Society and the American Academy of Neurology have reviewed this subject, reached similar conclusions, and issued position papers based on the scientific data available. These organizations concluded that there is no specific clinical or neuropathologic syndrome associated with diphtheria-tetanus-pertussis (DTP) vaccine and no means by which a diagnosis of brain damage resulting from DTP immunization can be established in an individual case. Well-designed, controlled epidemiologic studies have failed to prove an association between DTP immunization and infantile spasms. Children receive their initial DTP immunizations at an age when infantile spasms have their onset. The administration of pertussis vaccine is associated with a short-term increase in the risk of seizures (mostly febrile seizures) and complete recovery is expected. Children whose neurologic problems begin soon after immunization warrant a full diagnostic work-up.

The Lennox-Gastaut syndrome is one type of symptomatic generalized epilepsy and it is age-dependent. The Lennox-Gastaut syndrome is characterized by the onset in early childhood of mixed seizures (including tonic, tonic-clonic, atonic, akinetic or myoclonic, and absence), refractoriness to common antiepileptic drugs, an abnormal EEG (generalized, slow spike and slow wave activity), and a high incidence of developmental and mental retardation. This syndrome frequently is preceded by infantile spasms. Etiologic factors are similar to those outlined with infantile spasms. In 30% of the cases, the Lennox-Gastaut syndrome appears in children who have no antecedents, previous epilepsy, or clinical or neurologic evidence of brain damage, and who have had previously normal development.

Benign focal epilepsy of childhood (also called benign epilepsy of childhood with rolandic or centrotemporal spikes) is a form of partial epilepsy that is characterized by an onset between the ages of 4 and 10 years. The seizures typically occur during sleep, although daytime seizures also may be seen. The seizures most frequently begin with clonic twitching of one side of the face. There may be involvement of the tongue or upper extremity, and secondary generalization. If the child is awake, he or she may experience paresthesias involving the mouth and throat. The child usually appears well immediately after the seizure. The occurrence of seizures during sleep may cause uncertainty as to whether the child has had a nightmare or a seizure. The children are otherwise well and have a history of normal development. Neuroimaging studies in these children have been unremarkable. The EEG is characterized by independent spike discharges occurring focally in one or both central ("rolandic") regions. Focal spike activity is enhanced during sleep and may occur only at this time. EEG background activity is otherwise normal. Both the seizures and the spike focus typically have a short natural history and usually are resolved by puberty or soon after. It is this natural history, in addition to normal development of the child and normal results of neuroimaging studies, that suggests the terminology of benign focal epilepsy. There is evidence that the EEG trait (the central spike with a normal background) is inherited as an autosomal dominant gene with a particular age penetrance. The inheritance pattern of the seizures is familial, but appears to be multifactorial. Similar varieties of benign focal epilepsy have been identified in association with temporal, parietal, and occipital spike foci.

Childhood epilepsy with occipital paroxysms is associated with an EEG pattern that is characterized by unilateral or bilateral occipital spike or sharp waves and seizures that are hemiclonic or consist of automatisms and that typically are preceded by visual symptoms (amaurosis, phosphenes, illusions, or hallucinations).

In 25% of the cases, the seizures are followed immediately by migraine-like headaches.

## ANCILLARY LABORATORY STUDIES

In approaching the laboratory evaluation, the physician must recall that epilepsy is primarily a clinical diagnosis. Some laboratory studies are necessary to establish a baseline for future comparison, and others can help with formulating medical treatment and prognosis. Indications for laboratory studies should be based on information extracted from the history and physical examination. If specific disease entities such as hypocalcemia, hypoglycemia, or other metabolic, toxic, or degenerative disorders are valid considerations, additional studies relevant to the particular entity are, of course, appropriate.

### Electroencephalography

An EEG has value only when it is interpreted in the context of the child's age, the history, and the physical findings. The quality of information gained from an EEG is related directly to the standards of the laboratory and the training and experience of the personnel. A routine EEG always should be recorded during wakefulness and sleep, and, in older children, during hyperventilation and photic stimulation. Because normal organizational and frequency characteristics change rapidly with advancing age and cerebral maturation, it is particularly important that the interpretation of EEGs in infants and young children be done by an electroencephalographer who has had specific training and experience with this age group. EEGs in many laboratories are interpreted by adult neurologists with little or no experience with infants and young children.

The duration of a routine EEG recording in most laboratories is about 1 hour. This 1-hour "sample" is taken to be representative of the patient's cerebral electrical activity during any average 24-hour period. An obvious potential exists for sampling to take place at a time when no epileptiform activity is present. A sleep-deprived EEG or a routine EEG obtained at a subsequent date may demonstrate abnormalities that were not evident in the initial "sample." The yield of useful information is enhanced when the EEG can be scheduled in particular relationship to a clinical seizure. The EEG should be recorded as soon as possible after any seizures that occur in neonates and infants up to 6 months of age. If an EEG is recorded in children with febrile seizures who are 6 to 36 months of age, it should be delayed until 5 to 10 days after the seizure, because the child's postictal brain wave activity may be transiently and diffusely slow for several days and its significance misinterpreted. In patients with nonfebrile seizures, the EEG should be recorded as soon as possible after the event.

Normal EEG results should not necessarily dissuade a physician from making a diagnosis of epilepsy in the face of a convincing clinical description. The initial EEG often does not contain epileptiform discharges. Investigators have found that the initial EEG in 25% to 58% of affected children may be normal or borderline without epileptiform abnormalities. Similarly, abnormal EEG results do not necessarily confirm a clinical suspicion of epilepsy. The type and location of an abnormality is expected to correlate with the clinical data. When available clinical and EEG data do not provide a basis for confident classification regarding seizure type, or in cases in which pseudo-seizures are suspected, video-EEG monitoring may be justified. Protracted monitoring can be relatively expensive, however, and should be undertaken only when the frequency of the seizures suggests a reasonable probability that a clinical event will be captured during a 6- to 24-hour recording.

## Neuroimaging

Routine skull radiographs seldom are indicated or helpful except when overt bony pathology is detected by physical examination. Neuroimaging studies may be indicated in cases of partial seizures or if the history and physical examination suggest structural lesions, degenerative diseases, or a congenital structural abnormality. There is no justification, however, for the routine use of these relatively expensive procedures.

## Hematologic and Hepatic Tests

Because most of the antiepileptic drugs in use have the potential to produce hematologic or hepatic side effects, a baseline complete blood count, platelet count, and liver enzyme analysis should be obtained, dependent on the known toxic effects of the drug to be used.

## MEDICAL TREATMENT

Successful treatment of a child with epilepsy demands more than just preventing recurrent seizures. The sensitive physician must adopt both an educational and an advocacy position, assuring acceptance of the child's epilepsy by the family, by teachers and classmates, and by the community. Misconceptions about epilepsy still abound and often have an adverse impact on a child's self-esteem and psychosocial development. Time invested in providing a clear explanation, in lay language, of the nature of epilepsy, the objectives of treatment, and the simple fundamentals of pharmacokinetics can allay apprehensions, dispel misconceptions, and promote compliance with the prescribed drug regimen.

Population studies suggest that about 70% of patients in whom epilepsy is diagnosed ultimately will become seizure-free, and that the majority can expect to discontinue anticonvulsant medication. A higher likelihood of remission has been reported in children than in adults. Children with epilepsy in association with mental retardation or cerebral palsy, however, have very low rates of remission. The literature does not reflect universal agreement on the optimal duration of anticonvulsant therapy. In most instances, a seizure-free period of at least 2 to 3 consecutive years is a conservative objective before the gradual withdrawal of medication should be considered. Monitoring of serum drug levels at reasonable intervals can provide a guideline for the adjustment of drug dosages as the child grows. Complete seizure control is not possible in some children and, in those instances, the occurrence of an occasional seizure is preferable to an increase in the dosage of anticonvulsants to levels that produce sedation and dysequilibrium, compromising both cognitive function and social interaction.

## Treatment After the Nonfebrile First Seizure

The initiation of antiepileptic drug therapy after an initial, nonfebrile seizure in otherwise well children continues to be controversial. It may be argued that some children have a benign developmental disorder of seizure threshold that they will outgrow. These include children whose generalized tonic-clonic seizures begin between 1 and 10 years of age, and who have normal neurologic examinations and normal or nonspecific abnormal EEG results, and children with benign epilepsy with rolandic spikes. Some physicians feel that the stigma attached to the diagnosis of epilepsy and the potential adverse side effects of antiepileptic drugs, especially on behavior and cognitive function, outweigh the risk of recurrent seizures. The risk for recurrence in children with a first, nonfebrile seizure has been addressed in only a few studies and has been reported to vary from 52% to 61%. Recur-

rence rates are much higher after a second seizure (79% to 90%), and most seizures recur within 6 months of the first (70% to 74%). Recurrence rates are highest in patients with abnormal results on neurologic examination, focal spikes in the EEG, and complex partial seizures. Recurrence rates in otherwise normal children, who have normal EEG results after the first, nonfebrile, generalized tonic-clonic seizure, range from 10% to 30%. As yet, there is no universally accepted consensus regarding withholding treatment after the occurrence of a first such seizure during childhood. A clinician who sees a child after a single seizure—especially a child who is neurologically and mentally normal, and who has normal EEG results—may consider, after discussion with the patient and parents, withholding therapy pending the occurrence of a second seizure.

## Antiepileptic Drugs

Optimal response to drug therapy and control of seizures can be obtained in about 70% of children if a few general principles are observed carefully:

1. Initiate therapy with a drug that is known to be effective for the specific type of seizure disorder being treated. If several drugs are equally effective, start with the one that is least toxic, least expensive, and requires the least amount of laboratory monitoring.
2. Always initiate therapy with a single drug. The introduction of more than one variable complicates the assessment of side effects and therapeutic efficacy.
3. Start with a dosage that falls near the lower end of the known therapeutic range (Table 154-3).
4. Dosage intervals should be based on the half-life of the drug being used (Table 154-4). It may be necessary to administer drugs with relatively short half-lives 2 to 3 times a day. Even though drugs with long half-lives, such as phenobarbital, can be delivered in a single daily dose, transient sedation may be noted at peak levels or sluggishness may be seen during the early morning hours when the total dose is delivered at bedtime.
5. Maintain the initial dosage for an interval that is sufficient to achieve a steady state before assessing therapeutic efficacy or checking blood levels. Drug metabolism and excretion begin almost immediately after absorption, and the drug continues to accumulate in the body until the elimination rate is in equilibrium with the daily intake. As a general rule, long-term oral administration for about five times the half-life of the drug is required to achieve a steady state.
6. If the initial dosage does not produce satisfactory seizure control, advance it incrementally until seizure control is obtained or the patient exhibits dose-related side effects (sedation, ataxia, etc.). Serum concentrations of anticonvulsants can be measured as a guideline for adjusting the administered dosage (see Table 154-4).
7. If the addition of a second drug becomes necessary, add only one drug at a time. If little or no improvement was seen with the initial drug, consideration should be given to withdrawing it gradually after the second drug has reached therapeutic blood levels and seizures are improved significantly or are controlled.
8. There is no logic to support the simultaneous administration of two drugs in the same chemical group.
9. Periodic laboratory monitoring is indicated when drugs that are known to have a significant incidence of hematologic or hepatic side effects are being used.
10. The withdrawal of antiepileptic drugs always should be gradual to avoid the precipitation of status epilepticus.

TABLE 154-3. Commonly Used Antiepileptic Drugs: Dosage and Side Effects

| Drug | Oral Dosage (mg/kg/d) | How Supplied | Side Effects |
|---|---|---|---|
| Carbamazepine (Tegretol) | 10–30 | 100-, 200-mg tablets 100-mg/5-ml suspension | Diplopia, vertigo, ataxia, sedation, nausea and vomiting, thrombocytopenia, leukopenia, and agranulocytosis |
| Ethosuximide (Zarontin) | 20–40 | 250-mg capsules; 250-mg/5-mL syrup | Abdominal pain, anorexia, nausea and vomiting, headache, dizziness, photophobia, aplastic anemia, leukopenia, agranulocytosis |
| Phenobarbital | 3–8 | Tablets in 8, 15, 16, 30, 32, 65, and 100 mg; 20-mg/5-mL elixir | Sedation, hyperkinesis, ataxia, nystagmus |
| Phenytoin (Dilantin) | 3–8 | 50-mg tablets; 30- and 100-mg capsules; 30-mg/5-mL suspension; 125-mg/5-mL suspension | Nystagmus, ataxia, sedation, hypertrichosis, gum hyperplasia, leukopenia, agranulocytosis |
| Primidone (Mysoline) | 5–30 | 50-, 250-mg tablets; 250-mg/5-mL suspension | Sedation, hyperkinesis, ataxia, nystagmus |
| Valproic acid (Depakene, Depakote) | 10–40 | 250-mg/5-mL syrup; 250-, 500-mg capsules; 125-, 250-, 500-mg tablets 125-mg "sprinkles" | Nausea and vomiting, increased appetite with weight gain, anorexia with weight loss, transient alopecia, hepatic failure, anemia, leukopenia, thrombocytopenia, acute pancreatitis |

## Pharmacokinetics

A basic understanding of pharmacokinetics is required if antiepileptic drugs are to be used successfully. Familiarity with the absorption and distribution characteristics of the drug, the degree to which it is bound to plasma proteins, and the way in which it is metabolized and excreted is essential if blood concentrations are to be maintained at therapeutic levels with minimal fluctuation between doses. Most antiepileptic drugs are weak acids and are absorbed slowly from the small intestine. Absorption can be influenced by antacids, rapid gut transit time, malabsorption syndromes, and variations in solubility characteristics between generic preparations.

By the time most antiepileptic drugs reach the bloodstream, they are bound (to varying degrees) to plasma proteins (see Table 154-4). The protein-bound fraction of the drug does not cross the blood–brain barrier and, thus, does not reach the site of intended biologic action. Both therapeutic effectiveness and clinical symptoms of dose-related toxicity are accounted for by the "free" or unbound fraction. The routine blood levels that are used as a guide in clinical practice reflect the total drug concentration, including both the free and the protein-bound fractions. In most instances, the extent of protein binding of a given drug is relatively stable from patient to patient. A small number of patients can be characterized as being inherently high or low binders, but the most common cause of clinically significant alteration of protein binding is drug interactions. The following clinical situations might produce suspicion of altered protein binding. The child who exhibits clinical signs and symptoms of drug intoxication in the context of a blood level that is within the therapeutic range may have an elevated concentration of free drug as a result of some drug interaction. This also might be seen in the rare child who has an inherently low protein-binding capacity. Conversely, the child who seems to require large doses and "super-therapeutic" levels to achieve seizure control, but who exhibits no clinical symptoms of toxicity, may have a higher than average binding capacity. In both of these clinical situations, the determination of "free" levels may serve as a better guideline for dosage adjustment. Most laboratories are capable of measuring free drug in plasma ultrafiltrate. Because protein-bound drug does not cross into saliva or tears, these body fluids also can be used to assay free drug concentrations.

TABLE 154-4. Commonly Used Antiepileptic Drugs

| Drug | Half-life* (h) | Protein Bound (%) | Blood Levels (μg/mL) |
|---|---|---|---|
| Phenytoin (Dilantin) | N 30–60 C 20 ± 2 A 24 ± 12 | 90 | 10–20 |
| Phenobarbital | N 70–100 C 55 ± 15 A 96 ± 12 | 50–60 | 15–40 |
| Ethosuximide (Zarontin) | C 30 ± 6 A 55 ± 5 | 0 | 40–150 |
| Valproic acid (Depakene) | 12 ± 6 | 90 | 50–100 |
| Primidone (Mysoline) | 12 ± 6 | 3 | 5–15 |
| Carbamazepine (Tegretol) | C 14 ± 5 A 17 ± 7 | 60–80 | 4–12 |

* N, newborn; C, child; A, adult.

## Blood Level Monitoring

In recent years, blood level monitoring has permitted the dosage requirement of anticonvulsant medications to be tailored to the individual needs of a given patient. Ideally, dosage adjustment should be made on the basis of "trough" drug levels. This may not always be practical, however, because families have difficulty coming in to have blood specimens drawn before the child takes the morning dose of medication. In actual practice, most blood levels probably are obtained during return office visits at varying times of the day. It can be useful, however, to make note of the interval between collection of the blood specimen and ingestion of the most recent dose. This makes it possible to estimate whether the measurement more nearly approximates a peak or a trough level based on the known half-life and peak time of the drug being used.

The blood levels of antiepileptic drugs that define a therapeutic range (see Table 154-4) are intended to be used as general guidelines, always in the context of the clinical state of the child. The lower limit of the range identifies the minimal level that is required to produce seizure control in the average patient. The upper limit identifies the level at which the average patient exhibits clinical symptoms of dose-related toxicity. Seizures will be controlled in a few children with blood levels somewhat lower than the minimal range, but others will require and tolerate levels somewhat above the maximum. The circumstances in which blood levels can be useful in clinical decision making are as follows: 5 to 14 days (five times the drug half-life) after treatment has been initiated at a given dosage, or after a change is made in the dosage (levels drawn before a steady state is achieved will not reflect accurately the optimal concentrations that can be achieved with the dose being used); when previously controlled seizures begin to recur (the most common explanation for this circumstance is noncompliance, but, occasionally, a child will have been allowed to outgrow a dosage); when clinical symptoms of toxicity become evident or when suspected drug interactions need assessment; and every 6 to 8 months in a rapidly growing child, especially one whose seizures have been controlled easily at low therapeutic levels.

## Commonly Used Drugs

Currently, 18 drugs approved by the United States Food and Drug Administration are available for the treatment of seizures. Six of these, either alone or in some combination, are used for seizure control in the majority of children who are responsive to medical therapy. These six are phenobarbital, phenytoin, carbamazepine, ethosuximide, valproic acid (VPA), and primidone (see Tables 154-3, 154-4). Evidence indicates that therapy with a single agent suffices for the majority of children, but a significant number require more than one drug. Phenobarbital, phenytoin, carbamazepine, and VPA have been used successfully in the control of generalized tonic-clonic, clonic, and tonic seizures. Ethosuximide is the usual drug of choice in the treatment of absence seizures, and VPA appears to be equally effective. VPA, ethosuximide, and clonazepam have been useful in patients with myoclonic and akinetic seizures. Adrenocorticotropic hormone and prednisone are the only agents proven to be effective in infantile spasms. Some studies have suggested that VPA may have efficacy in the treatment of infantile spasms; however, these observations have not been verified in a controlled trial. Clonazepam has limited usefulness because of sedative side effects and the development of drug tolerance. Elementary partial seizures have responded to carbamazepine, phenytoin, and phenobarbital. Carbamazepine is the drug of choice in the treatment of complex partial seizures; phenytoin, primidone, and phenobarbital are effective second choices.

## Common Problems and Drug Side Effects

Many of the common problems associated with the use of antiepileptic drugs can be avoided easily. Liquid preparations should not be used, except when absolutely necessary. Elixir of phenobarbital is a strong-tasting, alcoholic solution that frequently induces a fit of spitting and sputtering, resulting in an indeterminate loss of part of the dose. Phenobarbital is available in both 8-mg and 16-mg tablets that can be crushed easily and added to a teaspoon of food. Phenytoin suspension must be shaken vigorously to avoid delivering a weak dose of supernatant from a relatively full bottle or a concentrated dose from an almost empty bottle. The 50-mg, scored, chewable tablet is an alternative dosage form for infants and young children. Other liquid preparations (carbamazepine, ethosuximide, valproic acid) are more tolerable and may be used to maintain effective anticonvulsant blood levels. If liquid preparations must be used, they should be dispensed with a calibrated measuring device and the dosage should be specified in cubic centimeters rather than teaspoons. The nausea and vomiting that sometimes is caused by VPA can be avoided by using the sprinkle preparation or by using the enteric-coated tablets in a child who is old enough to swallow. The gastric irritation that occasionally is seen with ethosuximide can be avoided by scheduling doses after meals. The use of pill boxes and dosage schedules that coincide with the daily habits of individual patients can help reduce the problems of noncompliance.

Paradoxic hyperkinesis is a well-known, common side effect of phenobarbital in young children. When phenobarbital is prescribed, the parents should be forewarned of this side effect and reassured that it is not hazardous. Because hyperkinesis can alter school performance and patient and parent interactions, however, another medication probably should be substituted. Although behavioral side effects are reported infrequently with other drugs, the physician should not dismiss complaints of consistent irritability in a particular child when there appears to be a strong temporal relationship between its appearance and initiation of the drug. Frank psychosis has been reported rarely with ethosuximide and carbamazepine, usually in the context of preexisting psychiatric disturbance. Behavioral side effects usually cease when the offending drug is withdrawn. Gingival hyperplasia and hypertrichosis are relatively well known potential side effects of phenytoin. Parental supervision of oral hygiene can reduce the problem of gingival hyperplasia significantly, and a small amount of excess body hair usually is not a contraindication to the use of phenytoin if the drug appears to be essential to seizure control in a given patient. Involuntary movement disorders are uncommon side effects of antiepileptic drugs, but tremor has been reported with VPA, chorea with phenytoin, and dystonia with carbamazepine.

Sedation and dysequilibrium are perhaps the most common dose-related side effects of antiepileptic drugs. Although these symptoms may be seen more often with phenobarbital and phenytoin toxicity, they also have been encountered with carbamazepine, primidone, and VPA. Hematologic changes, including aplastic anemia, neutropenia, and thrombocytopenia, have been reported in association with the use of most of the commonly prescribed anticonvulsants. A spectrum of hypersensitivity states also has been seen with the majority of the drugs currently in use. These have included rash, diffuse lymphadenopathy, and Stevens-Johnson syndrome. These toxic effects are relatively rare, but many clinicians have made it a practice to obtain a complete blood count every 2 to 3 weeks during drug induction and every 3 to 4 months thereafter. The incidence of fatal VPA-induced hepatotoxicity has been found to be highest in children less than 2 years of age and in patients of any age who are receiving multiple anticonvulsant therapy. The use of VPA is not encouraged in children less than 2 years of age; if the agent is used, close monitoring of the patient is prudent. Typically, the onset of hepatic failure has occurred within the first 6 months of treatment, with a latent period than has been as long as 1 to 3 years. In most cases, though not all, serum enzyme levels become normal after the dosage of VPA is reduced or discontinued. The apparent distinct hepatotoxic reaction that leads to irreversible liver failure probably represents a rare idiosyncratic response to VPA and cannot be predicted reliably from liver function test results. Initial symptoms of toxicity include nausea, vomiting, anorexia, lethargy, edema, loss of seizure control followed by jaundice with or without ascites, coma, hemorrhagic phenomena, hypoglycemia, renal failure, and death. Because hepatic dysfunction in patients with asymptomatic elevations in hepatic enzyme levels during VPA therapy typically does not progress to hepatic failure, such symptomatic elevations may have an apparently benign prognosis. The natural history of this effect remains unknown, however, because significant elevations in hepatic enzyme levels consistently have led to changes in the drug regimen. Normal serum glutamine oxaloacetic levels reportedly are neither sensitive nor discriminative for the early detection of serious hepatotoxicity caused by VPA. Close clinical monitoring of the patient is prudent. Changes in the drug regimen should be considered, however, for elevations in the aspartate aminotransferase level to values greater than three times normal. Hyperammonemia associated with altered consciousness, but without other abnormalities of liver function, has been reported in a few young children who have responded to withdrawal of the drug. It has been reported that routine monitoring of any of the antiepileptic drugs rarely identifies and protects patients who are at risk for antiepileptic-associated life-threatening reactions. Screening laboratory studies, including routine determinations such as complete blood count and serum chemistries, as well as specialized studies in high-risk patients such as serum lactate, pyruvate, ammonia, and carnitine levels, can yield information regarding the child's general health. Patients who need subsequent blood monitoring, especially if they are receiving VPA therapy, are those in high-risk groups, including patients with biochemical disorders, altered health status, neurodegenerative disease, or a history of significant adverse drug reaction, and infants who are receiving multiple drug therapy.

## Drug Interactions

Drug interactions with other drugs can inhibit metabolism, induce metabolism, or cause displacement from protein-binding sites. The resulting alteration of serum concentrations or of the ratio of free drug to bound drug can account for symptoms of clinical intoxication or the recurrence of seizures. The concomitant administration of VPA and one or more antiepileptic drugs such as carbamazepine, phenobarbital, or phenytoin will accelerate markedly the metabolic conversion of VPA, resulting in the need for a larger VPA dosage. During multiple drug therapy, the half-life of VPA is shorter. These differences have been attributed to the induction of hepatic enzymes by other antiepileptic drugs. VPA appears to act as a metabolic inhibitor, frequently making it necessary to reduce phenobarbital dosages after VPA is added. VPA appears to increase concentrations of the active epoxide metabolite of carbamazepine by inhibiting elimination of the carbamazepine epoxide. VPA can increase the free fraction of phenytoin by displacing it from protein-binding sites, although metabolic inhibition also may play a role in increasing phenytoin levels. Reportedly, in the presence of VPA, total phenytoin concentrations in the so-called therapeutic range may be associated with clinical toxicity. Determining the free fraction of phenytoin may be necessary. In addition, because VPA plasma concentra-

tions may have wide diurnal fluctuations, the protein-binding interaction of VPA and phenytoin may vary during the day. Chlorpromazine, prochlorperazine, chlordiazepoxide, anticoagulants, estrogens, chloramphenicol, cimetidine, and isoniazid may elevate blood levels of phenytoin by impairing its metabolism. Antacids taken in close proximity to a dose can impair the absorption of phenytoin almost completely. Carbamazepine levels are increased by troleandomycin, erythromycin, cimetidine, and isoniazid. Carbamazepine accelerates theophylline metabolism.

## Discontinuing Antiepileptic Drugs

A number of studies have attempted to address the question of when to terminate antiepileptic drug therapy. A clear consensus has not yet emerged. There is agreement that a large number of children who have remained seizure-free for 2 to 5 consecutive years will not experience a recurrence after medication is withdrawn. For other children, it may be necessary to continue medication indefinitely, particularly in those who have fixed, major neurologic deficits in addition to seizures. In general, children in whom seizures came under prompt control and no other significant neurologic deficits exist tend to remain seizure-free when medication is discontinued. There is no agreement regarding whether age at seizure onset or particular EEG characteristics are significant risk factors for recurrence. Some clinicians obtain an EEG at the initiation or conclusion of drug withdrawal and will prolong treatment in the face of markedly abnormal EEG results, including very active epileptiform abnormalities. Seizures in children are most likely to recur during the period of drug withdrawal.

We believe that children should be maintained seizure-free for 2 to 3 consecutive years before drug withdrawal is considered. Antiepileptic drugs always should be discontinued gradually, usually over a period of 4 to 6 weeks. Only one drug should be withdrawn at a time if the child has been taking multiple drugs. In the case of adolescents, it seems reasonable to exercise extra caution regarding driving during the period of drug withdrawal.

## Cognitive and Behavioral Effects of Drugs

Many factors may have adverse effects on cognitive function and behavior in children with epilepsy. These include seizure type and frequency, cause, accompanying neurologic deficits, basic intellectual endowment, and the psychosocial milieu. Learning difficulties appear to be more frequent in children with epilepsy than in the general population. Many studies have attempted to assess the adverse effects of antiepileptic drugs on cognitive function. Cross-study comparison has been difficult for a number of reasons, including variability in patient age, drug regimens, drug levels, seizure type and frequency, psychologic/educational test instruments employed, and bias inherent in data obtained from parent and teacher questionnaires. There is no question that phenobarbital can produce paradoxic hyperkinesis in some children, and common sense suggests that drug dosages that are sufficient to produce lethargy or sedation will affect learning and social interaction.

Although suggestive evidence exists that many, if not all, antiepileptic drugs have adverse effects on behavior or cognition in certain children, more well-controlled studies are required to resolve this issue. Physicians should heed the reports of parents and teachers in assessing the potential effects of antiepileptic drugs on the cognitive skills and behavior of individual children. If it appears highly probable that a given drug is producing adverse effects, then the physician should consider altering the dose or substituting another drug.

## COUNSELING PATIENTS AND PARENTS

Diagnosing the condition and initiating appropriate drug therapy are only the initial steps in caring for a child with a seizure disorder. Parents and children often have many questions, misconceptions, and fears. They always want to know if the child will "outgrow" seizures, what to do during a seizure, and how seizures may influence participation in school and sports. Dispelling misconceptions and providing guidance is just as important as dispensing medication. Anxious and overprotective parents or overly solicitous teachers and peers can affect the child's psychosocial development adversely. Parents and older children should have a clear understanding that epilepsy is not a disease entity per se, but is the symptomatic expression of disordered cerebral function, and that the prognosis for seizure control is dependent on underlying etiologic factors and may vary significantly from one child to another. On the basis of specific etiologic factors, or the absence thereof, the physician can provide the family with an individualized understanding and prognosis.

Frequently, parents are very concerned that their child might die during a seizure. It should be emphasized that the objective of maintenance drug therapy is to prevent seizure recurrence and that a period of observation is required to optimize the medication dosage. If further seizures occur, they most likely will be brief in duration. Most seizures terminate spontaneously within 5 minutes, and death as a result of seizures is exceedingly rare. Indeed, fatalities usually are the consequence of the patient being engaged in a potentially hazardous activity when a seizure occurs (swimming unattended, operating a motorized vehicle, or climbing to some high place).

Parents should be reassured that the brevity of most seizures obviates the necessity of making a dash for the emergency department. If a seizure persists beyond 10 to 15 minutes, it is appropriate to seek medical assistance. Teachers and school nurses also should be advised that it is not necessary to send a child home after a brief, uncomplicated seizure. Excessive zeal in this regard can only diminish self-esteem, raise anxiety levels, and alter social interaction with classmates. The family should be fully informed of the rationale for drug choice and use, and of the potential dose-related and non–dose-related side effects. Compliance can be enhanced by advising the use of an inexpensive pillbox that is compartmentalized to hold daily medications for 1 week.

## Precautions

In general, the child with epilepsy should be treated as a normal child, with a few notable precautions. As with all children, swimming always should be supervised. Until seizures are well controlled, bicycle riding should be restricted to low-traffic residential areas, and climbing to rooftops should be discouraged. Sports and athletic activities often are extremely important to young people, and decisions regarding participation should involve the parents, patient, and physician in an open discussion. In most instances, epilepsy should not exclude a child from participation in sports activities. Situations in which a seizure could cause a dangerous fall, such as rope climbing, activities on parallel bars, and high diving, should be avoided. It is suggested that competitive underwater swimming also be avoided. Participation in contact collision sports should be given individual consideration. Common sense suggests, however, that contact or collision sports might pose significant risks to a patient who is continuing to have several seizures per month.

## Immunizations

Current recommendations state that pertussis immunization may affect seizure risk adversely and should be deferred in children with a personal history of seizures and in those with certain neurologic conditions such as tuberous sclerosis, certain inherited metabolic disorders, or other conditions predisposing them to seizures. The pertussis component of DTP vaccine should be eliminated from subsequent immunizations in the child who has had a seizure within 48 hours of a prior DTP immunization.

## Puberty

Puberty traditionally has been considered to have an adverse effect on the course of epilepsy, especially in females. An increase, decrease, or no change in seizure frequency during puberty has been reported. Physicians have been cautioned against withdrawing antiepileptic drugs during this period, even when the patient has met currently accepted criteria for discontinuing therapy. This attitude is not supported by the evidence, however.

## Teratogenesis

Physicians have a special obligation to adolescents and potentially sexually active girls and their parents in making them aware of the potential teratogenic effects of antiepileptic drugs. No woman should receive antiepileptic drugs unnecessarily and, in the girl who has been seizure-free for several years, consideration should be given to gradual withdrawal of medication before a pregnancy is planned. The discontinuation of antiepileptic drugs in pregnant women who have required medication to control seizures is not recommended, because prolonged seizures could cause serious harm to both the woman and the fetus.

Most antiepileptic drugs in current use have been reported to produce congenital malformations, ranging from minimal defects such as cleft lip (amenable to satisfactory cosmetic repair) to major cardiac defects and spinal dysraphism. In general, however, the pregnant woman with epilepsy who requires drugs for seizure control has about a 90% chance of delivering a normal child.

## Driver's Licensure

The restriction imposed by epilepsy on eligibility for a driver's license is a major concern for adolescents and teenagers. In some instances, the aspiration for licensure can be a potent motivation for compliance with medication regimens. Legal requirements and the duration of restrictions vary from state to state and physicians must be acquainted with the regulations of the state in which they practice. In general, it is recommended that patients be seizure-free for at least 9 to 12 consecutive months before being licensed to drive. The physician may be required to attest to the seizure-free interval and to the patient's compliance with the prescribed drug regimen. For medical-legal purposes, it may be useful for the physician to document by an entry in the clinical record that the patient and the parents have been advised of the relevant regulations.

## Selected Readings

Ad Hoc Committee for the Child Neurology Society Consensus Statement on Pertussis Immunization and the Central Nervous System. Pertussis immunization and the central nervous system. Ann Neurol 1991;29:458.
Bourgeois BFD. Pharmacologic interaction between valproate and other drugs. Am J Med 1988;84:29.
Camfield C, Camfield P, Smith E, et al. Asymptomatic children with epilepsy: Little

benefit from screening for anticonvulsant-induced liver, blood, or renal damage. Neurology 1986;36:838.

Camfield PR, Camfield CS, Dooley JM, et al. Epilepsy after a first unprovoked seizure in childhood. Neurology 1985;35:1657.

Commission on Classification and Terminology of the International League Against Epilepsy. Proposal for revised classification of epilepsies and epileptic syndromes. Epilepsia 1989;30:389.

Commission on Classification and Terminology of the International League Against Epilepsy. Proposal for revised clinical and electroencephalographic classification of epileptic seizures. Epilepsia 1981;22:489.

Committee on Drugs of the American Academy of Pediatrics. Behavioral and cognitive effects of anticonvulsant therapy. Pediatrics 1985;76:644.

Committee on Infectious Diseases 1983–1984 of the American Academy of Pediatrics. Pertussis vaccine. Pediatrics 1984;74:303.

Dalessio DJ. Seizure disorders and pregnancy. N Engl J Med 1985;312:559.

Diamantopoulos N, Crumrine PK. The effect of puberty on the course of epilepsy. Arch Neurol 1986;43:873.

Dodson WE, Tasch V. Pharmacology of valproate acid in children with severe epilepsy: Clearance and hepatotoxicity. Neurology 1981;31:1047.

Ferry PC, Banner W Jr, Wolf RA. Seizure disorders in children. Philadelphia: JB Lippincott, 1986.

Gomez MR, Klass DW. Epilepsies of infancy and childhood. Ann Neurol 1983;13:113.

Hauser WA, Nelson KB. Epidemiology of epilepsy in children. Cleve Clin J Med 1991;56(Suppl):S185.

Pellock JM, Willmore LJ. A rational guide to routine blood monitoring in patients receiving antiepileptic drugs. Neurology 1991;41:961.

Shinnar S, Vining EPG, Mellitis EO, et al. Discontinuing antiepileptic medication in children with epilepsy after two years without seizures. N Engl J Med 1985;313:976.

Tharp BR. An overview of pediatric seizure disorders and epileptic syndrome. Epilepsia 1987;28(Suppl 1):S36.

Therapeutics and Technology Assessment Subcommittee. Assessment: DTP vaccination. Neurology 1991;42:47.

Wylie E, Wylie R. Routine laboratory monitoring for serious adverse effects of antiepileptic medications: The controversy. Epilepsia 1991;32(Suppl 5):S74.

*Principles and Practice of Pediatrics, Second Edition.*
edited by Frank A. Oski et al. J. B. Lippincott Company, Philadelphia © 1994.

# 154.2 *Status Epilepticus*

Daniel G. Glaze

## DEFINITION

Status epilepticus may be defined as seizure activity that lasts longer than 15 to 30 minutes or repeated seizures between which the child does not return to the baseline level of consciousness. In convulsive status, the child has a prolonged, generalized tonic-clonic seizure or the repetition of such seizures without a return to full consciousness between episodes. In nonconvulsive status, such as absence status and complex partial status, the clinical presentation is a prolonged "twilight" or semicoma state. In epilepsia partialis continua, consciousness is preserved in the face of continuous, focal motor activity.

About 12% of patients with newly diagnosed epilepsy will have a seizure lasting 30 minutes or longer. The greatest proportion of cases of status epilepticus occur in children, and less than 25% occur as an idiopathic event. The occurrence of status epilepticus should prompt a full diagnostic workup. Previously, overall mortality figures as high as 30% were reported, but recent investigators have reported a mortality rate of 3% to 6% in chil-

dren. This decrease in mortality is the result of more rapid diagnosis and support, combined with better medical treatment and improved intensive care. Death usually is attributable to the underlying cause of status epilepticus rather than to a prolonged seizure. When this information is considered, mortality related to prolonged seizures per se has been reported to be as low as 1% to 2%.

## TREATMENT

Tonic-clonic status epilepticus is a life-threatening situation and represents a neurologic emergency. Prolonged seizures can lead to a series of metabolic derangements that potentially can cause neuronal damage. Tonic-clonic status epilepticus that progresses beyond 60 minutes may be associated with severe, permanent brain damage or death. The longer the seizure lasts, the more difficult it will be to stop. The therapeutic measures outlined here are appropriate in those cases in which a seizure or repeated seizures continue unabated for 15 to 30 minutes. Some clinicians consider almost any tonic-clonic seizure to be an episode of status epilepticus and intervene with both supportive and drug therapy. In children, infectious processes, toxic or metabolic disorders, and chronic forms of encephalopathy, as well as the sudden withdrawal of antiepileptic drugs may underlie or precipitate this condition.

Therapy must address the immediate problem of stopping the seizure, providing supportive measures (supplemental oxygen, a clear airway, an intravenous glucose source, etc.), detecting and correcting any predisposing or precipitating factors, and incorporating a drug with a long half-life to prevent the recurrence of seizures once they have been arrested.

### Supportive Measures

The preservation of vital functions takes precedence:

1. Blood pressure, respiration, and cardiac function are maintained to avoid hypoxic-ischemic damage to the brain. Resuscitation equipment should be available.
2. Blood samples are obtained for electrolyte, glucose, blood urea nitrogen, calcium, and magnesium measurements, and for antiepileptic drug level determinations if the patient has been treated previously for seizures.
3. An intravenous line is inserted for the infusion of a glucose solution to maintain the blood sugar level at about 150 mg/dL. Fluids should be limited initially to 1000 to 1200 mL/m$^2$.
4. Increased intracranial pressure is treated if evident.

### Drug Therapy

Excluding infants who are less than 2 to 3 months of age, diazepam in an intravenous dose of 0.25 to 0.30 mg/kg may be given (maximum dose 5 mg in children less than 5 years old and 10 mg in children 5 to 10 years old). In children who are 5 to 10 years old, an alternative method of calculating the dose is 1 mg per year of age to a maximum of 10 mg.

Because of its short half-life and characteristic distribution within body tissues, the effect of diazepam is very short. The duration of action of intravenous diazepam is less than 1 hour. Seizures may recur within 20 to 30 minutes. Therefore, if seizures are arrested, an antiepileptic drug with a longer duration of action must be given. Phenytoin administered in a glucose-free intravenous fluid such as normal saline, at an initial dose of 15 to 20 mg/kg, is suggested. The danger of inducing cardiac dysrhythmia is minimized by using a slow infusion rate of 0.5 to 1.0 mg/kg/min, or a maximum of 50 mg/min. An advantage associated with the use of phenytoin is the general absence of sedation and respiratory depression. If seizures persist after the initial doses of diazepam and phenytoin are given, this combination may be repeated. If seizures continue after about 20 to 30 minutes, phenobarbital at a dose of 10 mg/kg at a rate of 50 to 100 mg/min may be used. If this regimen is unsuccessful, neurologic consultation is appropriate.

In neonates and very young infants, intravenous phenobarbital at a dose of about 20 mg/kg is advised. The dose may be repeated up to a maximum of 40 mg/kg. If necessary, this may be followed by phenytoin given intravenously in doses starting at 10 mg/kg, at rates of 1 mg/kg/min. A dose of 10 mg/kg may be repeated if seizures continue.

The use of lorazepam, a long-acting benzodiazepine, as the initial drug in the treatment of status epilepticus appears promising. Lorazepam has a rapid onset and a more prolonged duration of anticonvulsant action than does diazepam. Although its half-life of 10 to 15 hours is less than that of diazepam, lorazepam continues to achieve effective brain levels for 8 to 24 hours. The suggested dose is 0.05 to 0.1 mg/kg (maximum dose 4 mg) given intravenously and repeated one or two times as needed. At this time, lorazepam has not been approved by the United States Food and Drug Administration for use in children for this purpose. After additional clinical trials, it may be approved eventually and replace diazepam as the drug of choice for patients with status epilepticus.

## Selected Readings

Crawford TO, Mitchell WG, Snodgrass SR. Lorazepam in childhood status epilepticus and serial seizures. Neurology 1987;37:190.
Crawford TO, Mitchell WG, Fishman LS, et al. Very high dose phenobarbital for refractory status epilepticus in children. Neurology 1988;38:1035.
Cruse RP. Treatment of status epilepticus. Cleve Clin J Med 1989;56(Suppl 2):S-254.
Curless RG, Holzman BH, Ramsay RE. Paraldehyde therapy in childhood status epilepticus. Arch Neurol 1983;40:477.
Giang DW, McBride MC. Lorazepam versus diazepam for the treatment of status epilepticus. Pediatr Neurol 1988;4:358.
Hauser WA. Status epilepticus: Epidemiological considerations. Neurology 1990;5(Suppl 2):9.
Holmes GL. Do seizures cause brain damage? International Pediatrics 1988;3:158.
Lockman LA. Treatment of status epilepticus in children. Neurology 1990;5(Suppl 2):43.
Pellock JM. Recent advances concerning status epilepticus. International Pediatrics 1990;5:189.
Phillips SA, Shanahan RJ. Etiology and mortality of status epilepticus in children: A recent update. Arch Neurol 1989;46:74.

*Principles and Practice of Pediatrics, Second Edition.*
edited by Frank A. Oski et al. J. B. Lippincott Company, Philadelphia © 1994.

# *154.3 Febrile Seizures*

### Marvin A. Fishman

Febrile seizures are a worldwide problem and occur in 2% to 4% of children less than 5 years of age. In some populations in the Pacific, the incidence is as high as 15%. This may be the result of closer living arrangements among family members, making detection more likely, as well as racial or geographic differences. A febrile seizure is defined as a convulsion that is associated with an elevated temperature greater than 38°C occurring in a child who is less than 6 years of age. Exclusions to the diagnosis include a history of a previous afebrile seizure, central nervous system infection or inflammation, or acute systemic metabolic abnormalities that may produce convulsions. Febrile seizures are classified into two groups based on their clinical features. Simple (benign) febrile seizures are those that last less than 15 minutes, do not have focal features, and, if they occur in a series, have a total duration of less than 30 minutes. Complex febrile seizures include those that last more than 15 minutes, have focal features or postictal paresis, and occur in series with a total duration greater than 30 minutes.

## PATHOGENESIS

The reason that febrile seizures occur only in infants and young children is still unclear, as are the mechanism whereby fever induces the seizure and the exact factors that appear to be under hereditary influence.

Febrile seizures occur during both bacterial and viral infections, and may occur more frequently in patients with illnesses that are accompanied by severe constitutional symptoms. The convulsion often takes place as the temperature is increasing rapidly, but may occur as it is declining. Febrile seizures are an age-related phenomenon in that they appear in children between the ages of 6 months and 6 years.

Attempts have been made to link susceptibility to febrile seizures with abnormalities of neurotransmitters. The concentration of γ-aminobutyric acid, an inhibitory transmitter, was found to be reduced in the cerebrospinal fluid (CSF) of children who were studied after their first or second febrile seizure. No correlation was found between the duration of the seizure and the concentration of γ-aminobutyric acid; however, because the samples were obtained after the convulsion, it still is possible that the abnormality was a secondary phenomenon rather than a primary event.

Genetic factors appear to be important in the expression of the condition. An increased incidence of febrile seizures exists among first-degree relatives of children with febrile seizures. These events are estimated to occur in 10% to 20% of parents and siblings (a rate that is at least 2.5 times higher than would be anticipated in a random population). The concordance rate for febrile seizures in monozygotic twins is much higher than that in dizygotic twins, in whom the rate is similar to that of other siblings. A complex segregation analysis of febrile seizures occurring in more than 450 families during a 30-year period recently was completed. Different models explained the rate of occurrence based on the frequency of febrile convulsions in the proband. In children who had a single febrile convulsion, a polygenic (common familial environment) model was most appropriate. If the proband had experienced multiple febrile convulsions, however, the most consistent model was that of a single major locus with nearly dominant seizure susceptibility.

There also appears to be a relationship between febrile seizures and an increased incidence of epilepsy in families of the proband.

Siblings and parents of patients with febrile seizures have a 4% to 10% incidence of epilepsy. Also, siblings of patients with epilepsy are at increased risk for febrile seizures.

## SIGNS AND SYMPTOMS

The vast majority of febrile seizures are simple. Prolonged convulsions occur in less than 10% of children with febrile seizures, and focal features are seen in less than 5%. Generalized seizures are mainly clonic, but both atonic and tonic episodes have been noted. Involvement of the facial and respiratory muscles is noted frequently. Complex febrile seizures occur as the initial convulsion in the majority of children who experience them. An initial simple febrile seizure can be followed by a subsequent complex febrile seizure, however, and vice versa. Children usually have a significantly elevated body temperature, but about 25% of febrile convulsions occur in children whose temperatures are between 38°C and 39°C. Children who have repeated febrile seizures do not always experience them with the same degree of fever. Also, they do not occur every time the child has a temperature elevation similar to the one that was associated with the preceding febrile seizure. The majority of febrile seizures are seen on the first day of illness, and, in some children, they are the first sign of the accompanying infection.

## DIFFERENTIAL DIAGNOSIS

The main concern in evaluating an infant or child with a febrile convulsion is the possibility of underlying meningitis or encephalitis. Thorough evaluation by an experienced clinician almost always will detect the child with meningitis. If the only indication for performing a lumbar puncture is a febrile seizure, meningitis will be found in less than 1% of patients. Less than half of these will have bacterial meningitis. In children who have meningitis presenting with seizures, as many as 40% (particularly younger infants) may not have meningeal signs. They may have other symptoms and findings, however, that strongly suggest the presence of meningitis. Thus, it is exceedingly rare for bacterial meningitis to be diagnosed solely on the basis of a "routine" evaluation of CSF after a febrile seizure.

Seizures usually are distinguished easily from other types of involuntary movements occurring in sick infants. Chills usually consist of fine rhythmic oscillatory movements about a joint and are not clonic in nature. They rarely involve facial or respiratory muscles. Also, chills are not accompanied by a loss of consciousness, which does occur during a generalized seizure.

The detection of an underlying metabolic disorder presenting as a seizure in a febrile child is rare. A careful review of the history usually provides other clues suggesting the likelihood of an underlying problem.

## DIAGNOSTIC TESTS

The routine performance of lumbar punctures in all children with febrile seizures does not seem warranted. Those children who might be considered candidates for examination of the CSF include young infants, children whose febrile seizure occurs after the second day of illness, cases in which the clinician is unsure of his or her judgment regarding the presence or absence of meningitis, and situations in which it is not possible to observe the patient.

The routine performance of skull radiographs in children with febrile seizures is useless. Information obtained from this study is not helpful in the immediate treatment of the child. If imaging of the brain is indicated (by abnormal head size, an abnormal neurologic examination [especially with focal features], or signs or symptoms of increased intracranial pressure), computed tomography or magnetic resonance imaging should be done. Serum electrolyte, blood sugar, calcium, and urea nitrogen level determinations are of very low yield and need not be performed routinely. They should be done when the results of the history or physical examination indicate a need for them. Patients with significant vomiting, diarrhea, and abnormal fluid intake may be suspected of having acute metabolic disturbances, and routine serum chemistries should be performed in these children. The routine use of electroencephalography (EEG) in all children with febrile seizures is not warranted. A tracing obtained within 1 week or less of the seizure is abnormal in at least one third of these children. Febrile convulsions of long duration or with focal features increase the likelihood that abnormalities will be found. Abnormal EEG results do not identify those children in whom epilepsy subsequently will develop and should not be used as the basis for deciding which children need anticonvulsant therapy.

## TREATMENT OPTIONS

### Short-Term Treatment

A child who is convulsing actively needs to be treated urgently, especially if the seizure has been present for 10 minutes or longer and shows no signs of abating. Immediate attention should be directed toward assuring that the patient has an adequate airway, is breathing well, and has satisfactory perfusion and circulatory status. Blood should be obtained for the determination of electrolyte and glucose levels, if the latter is indicated. At this point, antiepileptic drugs should be administered, intravenously if possible. One strategy is to give a short-acting anticonvulsant such as diazepam (0.2 to 0.3 mg/kg) followed immediately by phenytoin (about 10 mg/kg). These agents should be administered slowly to avoid the development of cardiac dysrhythmias and hypotension. If seizures persist, doses of the medications can be repeated. The clinician should be ready to intubate the child if respirations become inadequate. Rarely, a third drug, such as phenobarbital (about 10 mg/kg), may need to be given if seizures persist and are unresponsive to doses of phenytoin that are adequate to produce high therapeutic blood levels. Phenobarbital may need to be administered a second time if seizures persist.

Alternatively, phenobarbital can be given as the initial drug. Disadvantages of this approach, however, include delay in onset of action in comparison to diazepam, production of lethargy, and risk of producing respiratory depression or arrest if the seizures are uncontrolled and diazepam has to be used as a second drug.

Rectally administered diazepam, at a dosage of 0.5 mg/kg (maximum 5 mg), has been used in other countries for the control of febrile seizures. It is effective in about 80% of patients. Preparations for rectal use are not available in the United States, so this form of the drug has not been used widely here.

After the seizures are under control, the fever should be treated with antipyretic agents such as acetaminophen or aspirin and with physical methods such as sponging with tepid water and using a cooling mattress, if necessary.

### Prophylactic Treatment

Controversy exists regarding which children should be treated with continuous antiepileptic drug therapy to prevent recurrent febrile seizures. Continuous administration of phenobarbital and maintenance of a serum level of at least 15 $\mu g/mL$ reduces the risk of recurrence to about one third of what might be expected with no treatment (about 10% to 15% versus 30% to 40%). Although the incidence of recurrent febrile seizures can be reduced, no data prove that treatment decreases the incidence of sequelae associated with prolonged seizures or the development of epilepsy, which occurs at greater frequency in children who have febrile seizures than in the general population. Because febrile seizures have so few sequelae and such a good prognosis in the vast majority of children, the benefits of therapy must be considered carefully and compared to the side effects of the medication. Changes in behavior and sleep patterns are noted in about 30% to 40% of children who are given phenobarbital and are severe enough to require discontinuation of the drug in 20%. Phenobarbital does not appear to have a significant negative impact on intellectual development and cognitive function in children, although some studies have reported adverse effects. A recent study demonstrated a very mild reduction in the intelligence quotient (IQ) of children who took phenobarbital for 2 years. This was noted particularly in the group of children who were expected to have the lowest IQ levels.

In the decision-making process, risk factors for predicting recurrence, sequelae, and the development of epilepsy, as well as the psychologic and emotional makeup of the family need to be considered. The family's attitudes regarding drug administration should be ascertained. Poor compliance may result if the family does not understand the risks and benefits of therapy. Children who are very young (less than 12 months old) at the time of the first episode are at highest risk for recurrent seizures. Complex febrile seizures are risk factors for the development of sequelae, and complex febrile seizures and abnormal neurologic or developmental status are risk factors for the development of epilepsy.

Of the three aspects of the natural history—recurrence rate, development of sequelae, and development of epilepsy—only the recurrence rate can be modified with antiepileptic drug therapy. Patients at risk for other sequelae can be identified, and this is helpful in terms of counseling families. Once a population is identified that has a 50% likelihood of epilepsy development, the decision still must be made whether to institute therapy at the time of the febrile seizures or to wait until the epilepsy actually develops.

The prophylactic use of other anticonvulsant agents (Table 154-5), such as primidone and valproic acid, has been shown to be effective in reducing the incidence of recurrent febrile seizures.

Primidone is equal in efficacy to phenobarbital and may have fewer side effects. Valproate is effective, but the cost and toxicity associated with its use may outweigh its benefits in the majority of cases. Carbamazepine has not been effective when used either in initial therapy or in the treatment of children in whom phenobarbital has failed. Phenytoin has not been demonstrated to be effective. This may be explained in part by the difficulty inherent in achieving consistent therapeutic phenytoin levels in young infants, and possibly by poor compliance.

The intermittent use of rapidly acting agents such as nitrazepam and the suppository form of diazepam has been shown to be as effective as the continuous administration of phenobarbital in preventing recurrent febrile seizures. Neither nitrazepam nor the suppository form of diazepam is available in the United States, however.

Recently, a double-blind randomized trial of diazepam versus placebo for the prevention of recurrent febrile seizures failed to demonstrate the efficacy of orally administered diazepam. The reason for the treatment failure may have been poor compliance, however, rather than lack of effectiveness of diazepam.

Because fever is the precipitating event in febrile seizures, attempts at reducing elevated temperature are a logical approach. Attempts at parent education have been made, however, including detailed written and oral instructions regarding the use of antipyretics, without success. The recurrence rate among patients whose parents were so instructed was 25%, which is similar to that of an untreated population.

## PROGNOSIS

The prognosis for children with febrile seizures can be divided into three categories: recurrence rate for febrile seizures, development of neurologic sequelae, and development of epilepsy. The major factor influencing the recurrence of febrile seizures is the age of the infant at the time of the first seizure. The younger the child, the more likely it is that febrile convulsions will recur. If the first seizure occurs at less than 1 year of age, the recurrence rate is about 50% to 65%, in contrast to a rate of 28% if the first seizure occurs after that point. If the first seizure does not occur until at least 2½ years of age, the recurrence rate is reduced to about 20%. Other factors that have been shown in some studies to influence the recurrence rate have been abnormal development before the first febrile seizure, a history of afebrile seizures in parents and siblings, and the number of subsequent febrile illnesses. About 50% to 75% of recurrences take place within 1 year of the initial seizure, and about 90% occur within 2½ years. This recurrence rate can be influenced by the intermittent use of rapidly acting antiepileptic drugs or continuous prophylactic treatment.

Neurologic sequelae reported as a result of febrile seizures include death, status epilepticus, motor coordination deficits, mental retardation, and learning and behavioral problems. The exact incidence of these complications is uncertain, but appears to be exceedingly low. They occur only in children who have experienced complex febrile seizures. Many of the reports documenting these complications have been anecdotal and derived from biased populations consisting of children who were evaluated at hospitals or clinics. In population-based studies, the incidence of these complications is very low. In the National Collaborative Perinatal Project, about 5% of children who had febrile seizures had episodes lasting longer than 30 minutes. No children in that study sustained permanent motor deficits, and none of the patients had impaired mental development unless afebrile seizures developed subsequently.

Another study has confirmed that status epilepticus as a result of febrile seizures does not cause new neurologic deficits. Children

### TABLE 154-5. Antiepileptic Drug Treatment and Seizure Recurrence

| | Percentage of Patients With Recurrent Febrile Seizures | |
| --- | --- | --- |
| | Treated | Control or Inadequate Treatment |
| Carbamazepine | 18.5 | 25 |
| | 81.3* | — |
| Diazepam | 12† | 42 |
| Phenobarbital | 13 | 34 |
| Phenytoin | 32 | 34 |
| Primidone | 10 | 57 |
| Valproate | 13 | 47 |

\* Phenobarbital failures.
† Intermittent treatment.

with prior neurologic abnormalities do have a higher risk of subsequent febrile as well as afebrile seizures than do normal children after an episode of status epilepticus. In other studies, some children who have had long-term neurologic abnormalities may have been expressing preexisting developmental deviations rather than the sequelae that follow febrile seizures in otherwise normal children.

Children who have febrile seizures are at increased risk for the development of epilepsy. In a normal child who has a simple febrile seizure, this risk may be twice that of the general population, or 1.0% versus 0.5%. Abnormal neurologic development in the presence of complex febrile seizures, particularly focal seizures, greatly increases the risk, by as much as 30- to 50-fold. In the National Collaborative Perinatal Project, children who were neurologically abnormal and had a focal seizure had a 15.4% incidence of afebrile seizures by 7 years of age. In a population-based study in Rochester, Minnesota, in which patients were observed into adulthood, the risk ranged from 2.4% among children with simple febrile convulsions to as high as 49% among children with focal, prolonged, and repeated episodes within 24 hours. These risk factors often were associated with partial unprovoked seizures, whereas subsequent unprovoked generalized seizures were more likely to be associated with the number of febrile convulsions experienced and a family history of unprovoked seizures. In the National Collaborative Perinatal Project, half the children who had nonfebrile seizures never had recurrent febrile seizures. Thus, recurrence does not appear to be a prerequisite for the development of epilepsy.

## Selected Readings

Annegers JF, Hauser WA, Shirts SB, Kurland CT. Factors prognostic of unprovoked seizures after febrile convulsions. N Engl J Med 1987;316:493.

Autret E, Billard C, Bertrand P, Motte J, Pouplard F, Jonville AP. Double-blind, randomized trial of diazepam versus placebo for prevention of recurrence of febrile seizures. J Pediatr 1990;117:490.

Camfield PR, Camfield CS, Shapiro SH, Cummings C. The first febrile seizure—antipyretic instruction plus either phenobarbital or placebo to prevent recurrence. J Pediatr 1980;97:16.

Ellenberg JH, Nelson KB. Febrile seizures and later intellectual performance. Arch Neurol 1978;35:17.

Farwell JR, Lee YJ, Hirtz D, Sulzbacher SI, Ellenberg JH, Nelson KB. Phenobarbital for febrile seizures—effects on intelligence and on seizure recurrence. N Engl J Med 1990;322:364.

Fishman MA. Febrile seizures. In: Fishman MA, ed. Pediatric neurology. Orlando: Grune & Stratton, 1986.

Gerber MA, Berliner BC. The child with a "simple" febrile seizure—appropriate diagnostic evaluation. Am J Dis Child 1981;135:431.

Knudsen FU. Intermittent diazepam prophylaxis in febrile convulsions. Acta Neurol Scand 1991;83:1.

Maytal J, Shinnar S. Febrile status epilepticus. Pediatrics 1990;86:611.

Nelson KB, Ellenberg JH. Predictors of epilepsy in children who have experienced febrile seizures. N Engl J Med 1976;295:1029.

Nelson KB, Ellenberg JH. Prognosis in children with febrile seizures. Pediatrics 1978;61:720.

Rich SS, Annegers JF, Hauser WA, Anderson VE. Complex segregation analysis of febrile convulsions. Am J Hum Genet 1987;41:249.

Rutter N, Smales ORC. Role of routine investigations in children presenting with their first febrile convulsions. Arch Dis Child 1977;52:188.

Wolf SM, Forsythe A. Behavior disturbance, phenobarbital and febrile seizures. Pediatrics 1978;61:728.

Wolf SM, Forsythe A. Epilepsy and mental retardation following febrile seizures in childhood. Acta Paediatr Scand 1989;78:291.

Wolf SM, Forsythe A, Stunder AA, et al. Long-term effect of phenobarbital on cognitive function in children with febrile convulsions. Pediatrics 1981;68:820.

*Principles and Practice of Pediatrics, Second Edition.*
edited by Frank A. Oski et al. J. B. Lippincott Company, Philadelphia © 1994.

CHAPTER 155

# The Comatose Child

## Daniel G. Glaze

## DEFINITION AND PATHOPHYSIOLOGY

Coma is not a specific disorder, but a sign of central nervous system (CNS) dysfunction. It may be caused by either a primary or a systemic condition affecting the CNS. A patient in a coma is unresponsive to any environmental stimuli. Coma is a medical emergency and represents a life-threatening situation requiring prompt supportive therapy to prevent hypoxia and rapid etiologic diagnosis to ensure that proper specific therapy is initiated.

The term *coma* often is used inappropriately to describe virtually any state of altered consciousness. The terms used in this chapter to describe altered states of consciousness are defined below. The correct use of these terms in clinical practice and publications is recommended.

Coma: A state of altered consciousness in which the patient is unresponsive to any environmental stimuli.

Stupor: A state in which the patient appears to be awake or in light sleep, can be aroused by mild external stimulation, and will respond to questions or commands, but lapses into an immobile or sleep-like state when stimulus is removed.

Persistent vegetative state: A persistent state of wakefulness without awareness; patient response is limited to primitive postural and reflex movements.

Locked-in syndrome: Quadriplegia and mutism with preserved consciousness demonstrated by communication by intact vertical eye movements.

Brain death: Irreversible cessation of all brain functions, including the brain stem; a state that is characterized by no CNS function above the level of the spinal cord.

The standardized Glasgow Coma Scale is used widely in evaluating a patient's responsiveness after traumatic coma and, more recently, nontraumatic coma (Table 155-1). This scale, which depends only on a clinical examination performed at the bedside, allows staging by serial examinations of the patient and has permitted comparative study of patients in different centers. Its usefulness in young children is limited somewhat, however, by the fact that some of the parameters depend on the patient understanding and responding to language.

In general, the underlying pathophysiology of coma is accounted for by two types of lesions or processes: those that affect the reticular formation of the brain stem (which also may involve centers maintaining respiratory and circulatory integrity) and those that affect the brain diffusely (bilateral hemispheric dysfunction). The latter category includes CNS lesions, systemic infections, and toxic or metabolic disturbances. These disturbances also may be associated with brain edema and prolonged seizures, which in themselves may cause brain damage.

**TABLE 155-1. Glasgow Coma Scale**

| Response | Form of Occurrence | Score |
|----------|-------------------|-------|
| Eye opening | Spontaneous | 4 |
| | To speech | 3 |
| | To pain | 2 |
| | None | 1 |
| Verbal | Oriented | 5 |
| | Confused conversation | 4 |
| | Inappropriate words | 3 |
| | Incomprehensible sounds | 2 |
| | None | 1 |
| Best motor | Obeys commands | 6 |
| | Localizes pain | 5 |
| | Withdraws | 4 |
| | Abnormal flexion | 3 |
| | Extension response | 2 |
| | None | 1 |

*Modified from Jennett B, Teasdale G, Braakman R, et al. Predicting outcome in individual patients after severe head injury. Lancet 1976;1:1031.*

## EVALUATION AND TREATMENT

### Short-Term Treatment

The evaluation and treatment of the comatose child falls into two phases. During the immediate phase, treatment precedes diagnosis and its most important aspects include stabilizing the child and protecting him or her from sustaining further brain damage. This is followed by an evaluation of etiologic possibilities for the coma. After immediate treatment of the comatose child, the physician must be ready to manage the potential complications of a prolonged altered state of consciousness. Knowledge of the probable prognosis for recovery or long-term impairment will facilitate patient care and improve communication with the child's parents.

During the initial phase of treatment, the physician must ensure that the patient's brain is receiving adequate substrate for energy production. The airway must be maintained and sufficient oxygen and ventilation provided; a child with inadequate respiratory effort needs intubation and respirator assistance. The patient's cardiac output must be evaluated and cardiac dysrhythmias and hypotension treated appropriately. Treatment also should include control of the body temperature, especially in children with hyperthermia (temperature greater than 42°C), to prevent irreversible damage to the CNS. The possibility of reversible hypoglycemic encephalopathy should be considered and immediate treatment of the patient (after blood is obtained for determination of the serum glucose level) should include the administration of 1 mg/kg of concentrated glucose solution (50% dextrose).

Recurrent or prolonged seizures can produce brain damage; iatrogenic paralysis and ventilation do not protect against this damage. Therefore, status epilepticus requires emergency treatment (see Chapter 154.2).

During the initial treatment period, a rapid physical examination should be done to search for signs of trauma that might necessitate immediate laboratory testing and surgical or neurosurgical intervention. The child should be evaluated for signs of increased intracranial pressure, keeping in mind that papilledema may not be apparent for hours after the onset of increased intracranial pressure. Loss of venous pulsations may be helpful in the early identification of increased intracranial pressure. If intracranial hypertension is present, immediate therapy should be initiated, including hyperventilation to reduce the $PCO_2$ to 25 to 30 mm Hg and elevation of the head. (For further therapeutic measures for intracranial hypertension, see Chapter 151.)

After immediate assessment and treatment has been performed, further historical information should be obtained. The diagnostic workup should include measurement of serum electrolyte, arterial blood gas, and serum calcium levels, along with liver and renal function tests and a complete white blood cell count. Lumbar puncture should be considered in the presence of signs of meningeal irritation, such as nuchal rigidity, to evaluate for such possibilities as meningitis or subarachnoid hemorrhage. It should be remembered that signs of meningeal irritation may be absent in young children or infants. When the history is suggestive or the cause of coma is not clear, blood and urine evaluation for toxicologic studies should be done.

### Physical Examination

The general physical examination can provide clues to the cause of coma. Of particular importance are signs of trauma and vital signs, including respiratory pattern, heart rate and rhythm, and blood pressure. The neurologic examination must include particular attention to pupillary size and reactivity, ocular motility, respiratory rate and pattern, and motor response to pain.

*Pupils.* Metabolic coma or early stage rostral-caudal herniation with interruption of descending sympathetic pathways is associated with small but reactive pupils; midbrain involvement is associated with nonreactive, mid-position, or mildly dilated (5 to 7 mm) pupils; intoxication or poisoning by organophosphates, phenothiazines, or opiates is associated with miosis (pupils less than 2 mm in diameter). Less frequently, small pupils may be seen with pontine lesions.

*Extraocular Motility.* In a comatose child, intact brain stem function is suggested by full-reflex eye movements in response to the doll's eyes maneuver, which is performed by holding the patient's eyes open and rocking the head from side to side multiple times. If the eyes remain in the primary position or straight ahead during this maneuver, brain stem function is compromised. Caloric stimulation is a more sensitive test that may be performed after the tympanic membrane is determined to be intact. The head is positioned in the midline and is raised 30° from the horizontal. Then, 50 mL of ice water is instilled into the external auditory canal against the tympanic membrane. Tonic deviation of the eyes to the side in which the ice water was instilled indicates an intact brain stem; any asymmetry or absence of eye deviation implies a structural or metabolic brain stem lesion.

*Respiration.* Bilateral cortical damage may result in Cheyne-Stokes respiration, which is characterized by periodically alternating episodes of hyperventilation and apnea. Metabolic disturbances such as respiratory alkalosis or metabolic acidosis, or a midbrain lesion may cause central neurogenic hyperventilation characterized by rapid regular breathing.

True neurogenic hyperventilation is rare; the tachypneic hypocapnia that is observed commonly in unconscious individuals probably is the result of stimulation by pulmonary congestion of afferent peripheral reflexes arising in the lung and chest wall. Pontomedullary damage may be associated with an atactic or irregular respiratory pattern.

*Motor Response.* The quality of the patient's motor response may be assessed after the administration of a painful stimulus such as supraorbital ridge compression. Purposeful movement with localization of the stimulus by the patient suggests a high level of intact brain function. Lesions compressing the brain at the thalamic level may be associated with decorticate posturing, which is characterized by flexion of the upper extremities at the elbow and extension with internal rotation of the lower extremities. Midbrain lesions may be associated with decerebrate posturing, which is characterized by extension and internal rotation of both the upper and lower extremities. Pontomedullary lesions frequently are associated with no response to pain.

### Etiologic Factors

Once the child has been stabilized, a more exhaustive search for an etiology may be necessary. In general, the causes of coma can be divided into two major categories: traumatic and nontraumatic. Blunt trauma to the head is a common occurrence in childhood. Alteration of consciousness that lasts less than 24 hours after blunt trauma is termed *concussion*. The neuropathologic implication of concussion is that no microscopic or gross change in the brain has resulted. If the period of unresponsiveness lasts longer than 24 hours, the clinical diagnosis is contusion of the brain. The neuropathologic changes associated with contusion include focal hemorrhage and necrosis of brain tissue. The magnitude of alteration caused in brain function after blunt trauma is dependent on several variables, including the amount of force exerted on the skull, the area of skull struck, the direction of force against the skull, the relative mobility of the skull, and the angular velocity of the brain after the trauma. The frontal, temporal, and occipital lobes are especially prone to injury caused by rotational acceleration forces when there has been rotation and flexion of the skull on the neck. Flexion and rotational acceleration may cause brain stem injury.

The evaluation of head trauma may include skull films if the clinician finds or suspects depressed skull fractures, or fractures across the middle meningeal artery groove or through the base of the skull. Depressed skull fractures may be associated with laceration of the brain and dura, and should be identified and evaluated quickly. Fractures across the middle meningeal artery groove may be associated with tearing of the meningeal artery and subsequent epidural hemorrhage. Epidural hematoma frequently is associated with a biphasic clinical presentation, with an initial episode of coma immediately after the injury, followed by a lucid interval, after which loss of consciousness ensues as the hematoma enlarges. Periorbital ecchymosis, cerebrospinal fluid (CSF) rhinorrhea, and hemorrhage behind the tympanic membrane are signs of basilar skull fracture. Acute subdural hematoma may follow laceration of the dura associated with depressed skull fracture.

Chronic subdural hematoma may follow closed head injury, which causes tearing of the bridging veins. Subarachnoid hemorrhage in children most commonly is the result of head trauma or ruptured arteriovenous malformations. Subarachnoid hemorrhage may be suggested by an abnormal funduscopic examination showing subhyaloid (pre-retinal) hemorrhages, signs of meningeal irritation (which may be absent in comatose children), and xanthochromic CSF. A history of trauma dictates that injury to visceral organs or long bones be searched for. These injuries may be associated with hemorrhage and hypovolemic shock, or with fat embolism from long-bone fractures.

The nontraumatic causes of coma in children fall into four categories: mass lesions, toxic/metabolic disorders, infections, and seizures. Toxic/metabolic abnormalities affect the CNS diffusely and are characterized by a history of progressive CNS dysfunction leading to coma. Neurologic findings usually are symmetric, although motor signs that vary from one side to the other may be present at times. Typically, the pupillary light reflex is preserved; in cases of glutethimide intoxication, anoxia, profound hypothermia, atropine intoxication, or barbiturate intoxication leading to apnea, however, the pupillary light reflex may be absent. More typically, drug ingestion is associated with miotic pupils. In cases of narcotic overdose, administration of the narcotic antagonist

naloxone hydrochloride (initial dose, 0.01 mg/kg IV) is diagnostic and associated with arousal of the patient and pupillary dilatation. Coma may occur if the serum osmolality is less than 260 mOsm/kg or greater than 330 to 350 mOsm/kg. Blood sodium levels less than 120 mEq/L, and especially levels less than 100 mEq/L, may be associated with coma. Arterial blood gas and acid–base abnormalities may occur in comatose children and provide clues to the underlying etiologic factors. For example, diabetic ketoacidosis, uremic encephalopathy, and lactic acidosis are associated with metabolic acidosis; hepatic encephalopathy and salicylate intoxication are associated with respiratory alkalosis; and respiratory-depressant drugs or acute or chronic pulmonary failure may be associated with respiratory acidosis. A history of severe vomiting, rapidly developing coma, and laboratory signs of hepatic dysfunction after a minor illness should suggest the possibility of Reye's syndrome. This disorder may be associated with hypoglycemia caused by hepatic failure and significant increased intracranial pressure. Coma may occur in children with diabetes mellitus either secondary to osmotic diuresis with glycosuria, dehydration, ketoacidosis, and depletion of salt, or as a result of an overdose of insulin and associated hypoglycemia because of either miscalculation or failure to consume sufficient carbohydrates in relation to the insulin administered. Other endocrine disorders, including thyrotoxicosis, myxedema, adrenal insufficiency, and Cushing's disease, may lead to coma, although systemic signs of endocrine dysfunction usually are evident in these cases before coma supervenes.

In evaluating the comatose child, it is critical to determine whether the condition has been caused by an intracranial mass lesion. Such lesions may require neurosurgical intervention, in contrast to toxic/metabolic disorders, infections, or seizures, for which medical treatment is indicated. Intracranial mass lesions that may be associated with coma include intracerebral hemorrhage, subdural and epidural hematomas, brain abscesses, brain tumors, and cerebral infarction with edema. Usually, supratentorial mass lesions initially are associated with focal or lateralizing signs and symptoms, such as hemiparesis or hemispheric sensory deficits, before they produce coma. With progressive involvement, coma may occur, and deterioration proceeds in a rostral-caudal manner, beginning with hemispheric dysfunction and followed by impaired function of the thalamus, the midbrain pons, and then the medulla. This progressive deterioration usually is reflected by changes in reflex eye movements, pupillary size and reactivity, motor response to pain, and respiratory pattern. Recognition of these signs of transtentorial herniation is important, because immediate neurosurgical intervention may be indicated. Other supratentorial lesions may be so placed as to cause herniation of the medial portion of the temporal lobe (the uncus) and produce midbrain compression and signs of midbrain compromise, including ipsilateral pupillary dilatation, before coma supervenes.

Although they are infrequent, arterial thrombosis and intracranial hemorrhages may occur in association with inborn errors of metabolism such as homocystinuria, with collagen vascular diseases, with deficiencies of plasma clotting factors such as factor VIII, with disorders giving rise to thrombocytopenia such as leukemia, and with types of hemoglobinopathy such as sickle-cell disease. Venous thrombosis occurs more commonly than does arterial thrombosis and may follow severe dehydration and pyogenic infection of the middle ear or mastoid or paranasal sinuses.

Infratentorial lesions that involve the brain stem may alter consciousness early, and the typical rostral-caudal progression of signs may not occur. Impairment in eye movements and pupillary function may be early localizing signs. Midbrain lesions usually are associated with mid-positional pupils that are nonreactive to light stimulus; pontine lesions may be associated with "pinpoint" pupils. Dysconjugate eye movements or conjugate deviation of the eyes away from the side of the lesion and the side of the hemiparesis are suggestive of an infratentorial lesion involving the brain stem.

Infections of the CNS and the meninges must be suspected in every comatose child, and a lumbar puncture for CSF analysis should be performed in all cases except those in which there is strong evidence of an intracranial mass lesion that might be associated with herniation. Signs of meningeal irritation may not be present in infants and young children. The differential diagnosis of infections involving the CNS should include not only acute bacterial meningitis, but also tuberculous meningitis, viral encephalitis, and fungal and rickettsial diseases. Any severe systemic infection may lead to coma, and common childhood illnesses may be followed by symptoms similar to those of encephalomyelitis. Acute hemorrhagic leukoencephalopathy may follow a course much like that of parainfectious encephalomyelitis and may be associated with abnormal CSF findings, including elevated pressure, pleocytosis of mononuclear cells and red cells, and elevated protein levels.

Seizures may be associated with impaired consciousness. Usually, the duration of postictal unresponsiveness is brief, but prolonged postictal coma may occur after status epilepticus or in some children with underlying head trauma, CNS infections, or severe forms of metabolic encephalopathy.

### Laboratory Evaluation

In addition to blood tests and CSF examination, two other tests may be particularly helpful in the evaluation of the comatose child. Computed tomography of the head is indicated in certain cases of head injury, including those associated with coma, and when an intracranial mass is suspected. An electroencephalogram (EEG) performed at the time of presentation may provide information on the underlying pathophysiology responsible for coma: bilateral hemispheric involvement versus brain stem lesion, diffuse versus lateralized lesions or processes, and the occurrence of seizures. Characteristics of the EEG may suggest a specific category of disorders, such as metabolic aberrations or drug intoxications. Serial EEG examinations may be helpful in monitoring the patient's recovery.

## Long-Term Treatment and Complications

The physician must be aware that, after the initial immediate treatment of the comatose child, a number of late complications may occur, including seizures. In the case of head injury, most children who have seizures will evidence them early on.

Of children who are hospitalized after head injury, about 5% have seizures within the first week after the event. Among children surviving severe head injury, 20% to 25% have unprovoked seizures. In head-injured patients who have not had a seizure, prophylactic antiepileptic drug therapy has not proven beneficial in preventing subsequent epilepsy. Some children may relapse into an encephalopathic state during the first few days after apparent partial or complete recovery from anoxic or hypoglycemic insults. The prognosis in these instances is variable, and some patients may not recover or may die.

A number of systemic problems may complicate a patient's course after brain injury associated with coma. Inappropriate secretion of antidiuretic hormone (ADH) may complicate the initial phase of treatment. Central diabetes insipidus may occur as a late sequela of brain injury and require treatment with ADH analogues. Elevated blood pressure is frequent in the acute phase of injury and may persist as a difficult treatment problem. Propranolol has been suggested as the most effective drug if therapy is required. A significant number of children with severe brain injury require prolonged intubation or tracheostomy because of aspiration, apnea, or hypoventilation. These patients may have difficulty handling secretions and be at risk for atelectasis and pneumonia. These children also are at increased risk for various infections (including ventriculitis if intracranial pressure monitoring or ventriculoperitoneal shunt devices have been required), aspiration pneumonia, or urinary tract infections. In addition, they are at risk for decubitus ulcers. An increased incidence of sinusitis and otitis media has been observed in children with nasogastric or nasotracheal tubes. These infections usually are caused by nosocomial flora, which may be resistant to commonly used antimicrobial agents.

## PROGNOSIS AND OUTCOME

It frequently is very difficult to predict the outcome of a comatose child. Of all the factors that might bear on prognosis, the cause of the coma probably is the most important. For example, the prognosis for children whose comas are consequent to drug overdose or a toxic/metabolic disorder appears to be much more favorable than the prognosis for those with coma resulting from most other causes. Coma caused by hypoxic-ischemic insults has a very poor prognosis in most cases. After coma caused by head trauma, infants and children appear to have better outcomes than do adults. There are no data, however, that allow more precise age delineation between younger and older children.

The relationship of the Glasgow Coma Scale to the outcome in children with traumatic brain injury has been examined. Except for patients who have had prolonged hypoxemia, it appears that all children, including those with Glasgow Coma Scale scores of 3 to 5, can have a satisfactory outcome. Mortality is higher among those with Glasgow Coma Scale scores of 3 to 5 than among those with scores of 6 or greater. Death occurs predominantly in children with Glasgow Coma Scale scores of 3. Nonsurvivors have an increased incidence of shock, a need for cardiopulmonary resuscitation, and higher intracranial pressure. Most deaths occur in those patients who have no heart rate at the scene. Survivors with Glasgow Coma Scale scores of 3 to 5 have longer intensive care unit stays and longer intervals before recovery of cognition than do those with scores of 6 or greater. Of all survivors, 17% to 37% may have a deficit in either memory, speech and language, or motor function, or an attention-deficit disorder. A hypoxic-ischemic insult at the time of the accident appears to be a devastating and confounding variable in patients with head injury. In the absence of hypoxic-ischemic injury, children with traumatic brain injury and Glasgow Coma Scale scores of 3 to 5 may recover independent function. Aggressive treatment is warranted for children with severe head injury, even if the Glasgow Coma Scale scores are low. The duration of the coma may have prognostic significance.

The majority of children who are comatose or in a vegetative state longer than 1 month in the case of nontraumatic coma, or longer than 3 months in the case of traumatic coma, appear to have little hope for recovery. A number of studies have attempted to evaluate the effectiveness of laboratory tests such as the EEG and evoked potentials in formulating a prognosis. EEGs showing no evidence of brain activity may be recorded in patients with drug overdoses who experience complete recovery. Repeatedly abnormal EEG results (eg, no detectable brain activity or burst suppression pattern) during coma that is not associated with an uncomplicated drug overdose or a reversible toxic/metabolic disorder indicate an extremely poor prognosis for significant recovery.

A few studies have been done of the outcome and prognosis for children whose coma is secondary to nontraumatic disorders in which a number of influential or predictive factors have been noted. Coma caused by hypoxia-ischemia appears to have a poorer outcome than does coma resulting from other factors.

Also, the need for assisted ventilation, increased intracranial pressure for longer than 2 days, and the duration of the coma (especially if it is more than 2 weeks) appear to be associated with a very poor prognosis. In children whose coma is secondary to trauma, certain features of the examination, including absence of the pupillary light reflex, absent or impaired spontaneous eye movements, and absent motor responses or posturing, have been noted to be associated with a very poor prognosis for recovery or with death. These observations have not been confirmed in a study of children whose comas resulted from nontraumatic disorders.

## Persistent Vegetative State

The term *persistent vegetative state* is used to describe a clinical syndrome following brain damage in which, after the initial period of coma, patients seem to be in a state of wakefulness without awareness. As many as 12% of patients who survive coma remain in a persistent vegetative state. Those patients who make a reasonable recovery after sustaining brain damage associated with coma usually do not pass through this state. It has been suggested that this term be applied to any patient who fails to regain functional awareness of his or her environment after at least 1 month in a coma. Recent observations, however, suggest that patients may enter this state very early, and that certain features (including decerebrate or decorticate responses, roving eye movements, and spontaneous blinking) may be early clues to its occurrence.

Though a persistent vegetative state may follow a coma resulting from any one of many causes, it appears to follow hypoxia/ischemia most commonly. Although the pathologic features of a persistent vegetative state vary with the underlying etiologic factors, findings usually include diffuse neuronal damage in the cerebral hemispheres. The few studies that have been done of persistent vegetative states in children indicate that they have an extremely poor prognosis for recovery. It has been suggested that, if a vegetative state persists for more than 1 month after the acute brain injury, parents can be advised that there is little chance for any meaningful neurologic recovery.

## Locked-In Syndrome

The term *locked-in syndrome* is used to denote the clinical state of quadriplegia and mutism with preserved consciousness, which usually is demonstrated by communication by intact vertical eye movements. These patients are entirely awake and responsive, although their repertoire of responses is limited to blinking and sometimes to jaw and eye movement. The locked-in syndrome commonly results from bilateral ventral pontine infarction after basilar artery occlusion, but it has been reported with other conditions, such as tumors, drug overdose, trauma, brain stem encephalitis, and hemorrhage. EEG results that indicate reactivity to external stimuli may be useful in confirming the diagnosis. In most adults and children, the prognosis for recovery is poor, but recognition of the locked-in syndrome is important for humane patient care.

## Brain Death

Brain death is the irreversible cessation of all functions of the entire brain, including the brain stem. Medical standards for the determination of brain death in children recently have been reported. The report emphasizes the need to determine and ensure the absence of remediable or reversible factors, including toxic and metabolic disorders, sedative-hypnotic drugs, paralytic agents, hypothermia, hypotension, and surgically remediable conditions, and sets forth the following physical examination criteria:

1. Coma and apnea must coexist. The patient must exhibit complete loss of consciousness, vocalization, and volitional activity.
2. The absence of brain stem function must be indicated by midposition or fully dilated pupils that do not respond to light; the absence of spontaneous eye movements and those induced by oculocephalic and caloric (oculovestibular) testing; and the absence of movement of bulbar musculature, including facial and oropharyngeal muscles. The corneal, gag, cough, sucking, and rooting reflexes are absent; respiratory movements are absent with the patient off the respirator.
3. The patient must not be significantly hypothermic or hypotensive for his or her age.
4. The tone should be flaccid and spontaneous or induced movements absent, excluding spinal cord events such as reflex withdrawal or spinal myoclonus.
5. The examination should remain consistent with brain death throughout the observation and testing.

The required duration of these clinical criteria varies with the age of the patient and the laboratory tests used. In patients between 7 days and 2 months of age, the task force recommends that two examinations and EEGs be done at least 48 hours apart. In patients between 2 months and 1 year of age, the recommendation is for two examinations and EEGs to be performed at least 24 hours apart, although a second examination and EEG are not necessary if a concomitant radionuclide angiographic study demonstrates no cerebral arteries. In patients greater than 1 year of age, laboratory testing is not required; the task force recommends an observation period of at least 12 hours. They also suggested that if it is difficult to assess the extent and irreversibility of brain damage, a more prolonged period of observation lasting at least 24 hours should be undertaken, although this could be reduced if the EEG demonstrates cerebral electrical silence or the concomitant radionuclide angiographic study does not reveal cerebral arteries.

## Hysterical Nonorganic Coma

Hysterical coma, although rare in young children, may be seen in adolescents. Episodes of feigned or hysterical coma may be precipitated by some stressful, emotional situation and usually begin with observers present. The neurologic examination is normal. Lateral eye movements after oculocephalic testing may be absent, because visual fixation can suppress this reflex. Other maneuvers, however, such as placing the patient on his or her side and then turning the patient to the opposite side may demonstrate lateral eye movements. The eyes usually are closed tightly and, if opened by force, will close again rapidly. If cold caloric testing demonstrates nystagmus, this virtually proves that the coma is feigned or hysterical.

## Selected Readings

Antony JH. Relapsing encephalopathy after hypoxia. J Pediatr 1978;72:433.

Facco E, Zuccarello M, Pittoni G, et al. Early outcome prediction in severe head injury: Comparison between children and adults. Childs Nerv Syst 1986;2:67.

Feinberg WM, Ferry PC. A fate worse than death: The persistent vegetative state in childhood. Am J Dis Child 1984;138:128.

Gillies JD, Seshia SS. Vegetative state following coma in childhood: Evolution and outcome. Dev Med Child Neurol 1980;22:642.

Golden GS, Leeds N, Kremenitzer MW, et al. The "locked-in" syndrome in children. J Pediatr 1976;89:596.

Hauser WA, Nelson KB. Epidemiology of epilepsy in children. Cleve Clin J Med 1991;56(Suppl):S185.

Jennett B, Teasdale G, Braakman R, et al. Predicting outcome in individual patients after severe head injury. Lancet 1976;1:1031.

Johnston RB, Mellits ED. Pediatric coma: Prognosis and outcome. Dev Med Child Neurol 1980;22:3.

Lieh-Lai MW, Theodorou AA, Sarnaik AP, et al. Limitations of the Glasgow Coma Scale in predicting outcome in children with traumatic brain injury. J Pediatr 1992;120:195.

Mahoney WJ, D'Souza BJ, Haller JA, et al. Long-term outcome of children with severe head trauma and prolonged coma. Pediatrics 1983;71:756.

Margolis LH, Shaywitz BA. The outcome of prolonged coma in childhood. Pediatrics 1980;65:477.

Plum F, Posner JB. The diagnosis of stupor and coma, ed 3. Philadelphia: FA Davis Co, 1982.

Task Force for the Determination of Brain Death in Children. Guidelines for the determination of brain death in children. Ann Neurol 1987;22:616.

*Principles and Practice of Pediatrics, Second Edition.*
edited by Frank A. Oski et al. J. B. Lippincott Company, Philadelphia © 1994.

# CHAPTER 156
# *Reye Syndrome*

Penelope Terhune Louis

Reye syndrome, first described in 1963, is an acute, life-threatening, postinfectious, metabolic encephalopathy that affects predominantly school-age children, occasionally infants, and rarely adults. Over the years, the disease and its clinical manifestations have received widespread recognition.

Characteristically, a prodromal illness—most often influenza or varicella infection—is followed in 3 to 5 days by the onset of persistent and intractable vomiting. Initially, patients are well oriented, but irritable and lethargic. Some patients have no change in consciousness and remain only lethargic with no progression to unconsciousness. The serum glutamic-oxaloacetic transaminase (SGOT) and serum glutamate pyruvate transaminase (SGPT) levels are 3 to 30 times normal. The serum bilirubin level rarely exceeds 1 mg/dL. Serum ammonia concentrations are variable at presentation. With encephalopathy worsening to a hyperexcitable state, the patient is intermittently out of contact with the environment. Further progression to a deeper comatose state is characterized by decerebrate and decorticate posturing, hyperventilation, and, finally, flaccid paralysis with loss of involuntary ventilatory control. The comatose patient uniformly has an elevated ammonia concentration ranging from 3 to 20 times normal. The encephalopathy typically persists for 24 to 96 hours, with gradual improvement in survivors. Recovery of consciousness in patients with permanent neurologic impairment may require weeks.

Criteria for the case definition of Reye syndrome include the following: an acute, noninflammatory encephalopathy documented clinically by an alteration in consciousness and, if available, cerebrospinal fluid containing less than eight leukocytes per cubic millimeter; hepatopathy documented by liver biopsy on autopsy or a threefold or greater rise in the SGOT, SGPT, or serum ammonia level; and no more reasonable explanation for the cerebral or hepatic abnormalities.

It is important to assess accurately the severity of the illness, because the therapies for severely affected children are aggressive, invasive, and dangerous. Several staging systems have been developed, culminating in the National Institutes of Health (NIH) Staging System. The most extensively used system includes electroencephalographic (EEG) information that previously was believed to have prognostic value. The EEG criteria have been replaced and the resulting NIH Staging System consists of the following five stages:

Stage I: Lethargy; follows verbal commands; normal posture; purposeful response to pain; brisk pupillary light reflex; and normal oculocephalic reflex.

Stage II: Combative or stuporous; inappropriate verbalizing; normal posture; purposeful or nonpurposeful response to pain; sluggish pupillary reflexes; and conjugate deviation on doll's eyes maneuver.

Stage III: Comatose; decorticate posture; decorticate response to pain; sluggish pupillary reaction; and conjugate deviation on doll's eyes maneuver.

Stage IV: Comatose; decerebrate posture and decerebrate response to pain; sluggish pupillary reflexes; and inconsistent or absent oculocephalic reflex.

Stage V: Comatose; flaccid; no response to pain; no pupillary response; no oculocephalic reflex.

During the last 22 years, more than 3000 cases of Reye syndrome have been reported to the United States Centers for Disease Control, with a case fatality rate varying from 26% to 42%. From 1967 to 1973, between 11 and 83 cases were reported annually. Between 1974 and 1983, the reporting frequency increased to a peak of 555 cases in 1979–1980. Thereafter, there has been a steady decline in cases, such that Reye syndrome now is a rare disease. In addition, there has been a trend in recent years toward diagnosis in earlier coma stages.

## PATHOGENESIS

Despite intensive study, the pathogenesis of Reye syndrome remains incompletely defined. It is unclear whether the pathogenesis can be explained by a primary injury to the mitochondria of multiple organs, including the brain, liver, and muscle, with its metabolic consequences, or whether a primary hepatic injury leads to metabolic consequences that produce the biochemical abnormalities and encephalopathy. Morphologic and biochemical studies have confirmed the presence of a characteristic injury. Pleomorphic, enlarged mitochondria with disrupted cristae, electron-lucent matrices, and reduced numbers of dense bodies are characteristic of the hepatic pathology of Reye syndrome. Associated reductions in mitochondrial enzymes involved in ureagenesi and gluconeogenesis, and in enzymes associated with the citric acid cycle have been observed. Further evidence of mitochondrial injury is suggested by the finding of dicarboxylic acids in the urine and serum.

Morphologic and biochemical study of the brain in patients with Reye syndrome has revealed swollen astrocytes and myelin blebs. Alterations in the morphology of the mitochondria have been identified only in neurons. Despite these morphologic changes, mitochondrial enzyme activities in the brain are not reduced as they are in the liver. This is somewhat inconsistent, because it suggests that brain mitochondrial injury may play an unimportant role in the observed encephalopathy of Reye syndrome.

The role of salicylates in the pathogenesis remains unclear. Salicylate use commonly precedes the onset of Reye syndrome. Serum salicylate concentrations are increased in patients with Reye syndrome compared to control patients; however, no correlation has been found between coma grade and serum concentration. Salicylates are known to stimulate macrophages that are activated by a viral infection, endotoxin, and phagocytosis. The stimulation of macrophages results in the release of tumor necrosis factor and interleukin-1. Tumor necrosis factor and interleukin-1 are mediators of the toxic and metabolic effects that are similar to those observed in Reye syndrome.

In 1982, the Committee on Infectious Disease of the American Academy of Pediatrics issued a statement warning against the use of salicylates in children with possible varicella or influenza infection, and a program of public education was initiated. Some authors have cited the reduction in aspirin use and the decrease in the occurrence of Reye syndrome as an argument to support the association between aspirin administration and this disorder. Other authors dispute these conclusions, stating that even the prospective, controlled, epidemiologic study performed by the United States Public Health Service showed histologic support for the diagnosis of Reye syndrome in only 27% of the patients, and no electron microscopic evidence was presented.

Based on available evidence, it appears that a primary mitochondrial injury stimulates multiple metabolic disturbances, and hyperammonemia, free fatty acidemia, lactic acidosis, and dicarboxylic acidemia are the results. Synergistically, the metabolic abnormalities and the underlying mitochondrial injury lead to the observed pathophysiology through incompletely understood mechanisms. Fatty acids, dicarboxylic acids, salicylates, and other factors may inhibit mitochondrial ureagenesis and potentiate their individual metabolic effects. Alternatively, they may inhibit adenosine triphosphate synthesis and lead to profound reductions in high-energy phosphate, which is required to catalyze an array of enzymatic reactions.

## TREATMENT

The treatment of children with Reye syndrome ranges from relatively simple provision of glucose to children with stage I findings to extremely complex neurologic intensive care for children with more severe stages of the disease. Therapy is significantly dependent on the stage of the disease in patients with Reye syndrome.

Children who are in stage I require close neurologic evaluation, frequent glucose level determinations, and daily measurements of ammonia, transaminase, and electrolyte levels. Hypoglycemia is avoided by the provision of intravenous glucose, coupled with close monitoring of the glucose level. Children with stage I Reye syndrome have an excellent prognosis if they undergo observation in the hospital and receive glucose and electrolyte intravenous therapy.

Children who have disease of stage II or higher require significantly more care and must be treated in the hospital's intensive care facility.

In all patients with stage III disease or stage II disease progressing toward stage III, aggressive therapy consisting of intubation, hemodynamic monitoring, intracranial pressure monitoring and control, and ammonia reduction therapies should be practiced.

## FLUID AND ELECTROLYTES

Several types of electrolyte disturbances are seen in patients with Reye syndrome, the most well recognized of which is hypoglycemia. There also may be abnormalities of potassium, calcium, and phosphorus. In the presence of inappropriate antidiuretic hormone secretion or diabetes insipidus, fluid balance is disordered.

## RESPIRATORY SUPPORT

Patients with stage I disease do not require respiratory support, but adequate oxygenation must be ensured. Those with more severe stages of Reye syndrome need aggressive support to prevent hypoxia and hypercapnia. All children with stage III Reye syndrome should undergo intubation and hyperventilation electively.

## HEMODYNAMIC MONITORING AND SUPPORT

Arterial and central venous pressure lines are placed to monitor meticulously the fluid and cardiovascular status.

## COAGULOPATHY

Most of these patients have a bleeding diathesis, which should be treated with the necessary blood products when clinical bleeding is noted.

## TEMPERATURE CONTROL

It is important to control the temperature in children with Reye syndrome, because decreases may contribute to hemodynamic instability and increases will cause a rise in the cerebral metabolic rate.

## INTRACRANIAL PRESSURE MANAGEMENT

The most significant advances in the care of children with this disease appear to be in the areas of supportive care and management of intracranial hypertension. Measures to decrease intracranial pressure include elevating the head of the bed, administering controlled mechanical hyperventilation, and using osmotic diuretics. The use of high doses of barbiturates in the treatment of elevated intracranial pressure in patients with Reye syndrome is controversial. Although this pharmacologic treatment seems to be effective in reducing intracranial pressure, it also is associated with significant complications.

### Selected Readings

Chesney PJ. Pediatric infectious disease—associated syndromes. In: Fuhrman BP, Zimmerman JJ, eds. Pediatric critical care, ed 1. St Louis: Mosby-Year Book, 1992:1030.

Dean JM, Rogers MC. Reye syndrome. In: Rogers MC, ed. Textbook of pediatric critical care, ed 1. Baltimore: Williams & Wilkins, 1987:629.

Forsyth BW, Horwitz RI, Acampora D, et al. New epidemiologic evidence confirming that bias does not explain the aspirin/Reye's syndrome association. JAMA 1989;261:2517.

Heubi JE, Partin JC, Partin JS, et al. Reye's syndrome: Current concepts. Hepatology 1987;7:255.

Hurwitz ES, Barret MJ, Bergman D, et al. Public health study of Reye's syndrome and medications. JAMA 1987;257:1905.

Mickell JJ. Reye's syndrome. In: Shoemaker WC, Ayres S, Grenvik A, et al, eds. The Society of Critical Care Medicine textbook of critical care, ed 2. Philadelphia: WB Saunders, 1989:1041.

Morens DM, Sullivan-Bolyai JZ, Slater JE, et al. Surveillance of Reye syndrome in the United States, 1977. Am J Epidemiol 1981;114:406.

Orlowski JP, Gillis J, Kilham HA. A catch in the rye. Pediatrics 1987;80:638.

Trauner DA. What is the best treatment for Reye's syndrome? Arch Neurol 1986;43:729.

*Principles and Practice of Pediatrics, Second Edition.*
edited by Frank A. Oski et al. J. B. Lippincott Company, Philadelphia © 1994.

# CHAPTER 157
# *Childhood Neuropathies*

## 157.1 *Disorders of the Anterior Horn Cell*

Julie Thorne Parke

The anterior horn cells may be involved selectively in a number of acquired and inherited diseases. Certain viruses, particularly poliomyelitis, demonstrate a specific affinity for these nerve cells. Herpes zoster and coxsackievirus also occasionally affect anterior horn cells. Inherited conditions influencing the anterior horn cells include the spinal muscular atrophies (SMAs) and a number of metabolic disorders. Damage to the anterior horn cells is characterized clinically by weakness, atrophy, and hyporeflexia. Fasciculations are common. Because the dorsal sensory root is not involved in these disorders, sensory abnormalities are not present. Motor nuclei in the brain stem are involved commonly, so bulbar involvement is seen frequently.

## PROGRESSIVE SPINAL MUSCULAR ATROPHY

Progressive SMA is a degenerative disease affecting the anterior horn cells of the spinal cord and the motor cells of cranial nerve nuclei. It usually is inherited as an autosomal recessive trait, but autosomal dominant and X-linked recessive inheritance patterns also have been reported. Several classifications of the disease have been proposed based on patient age at the onset of symptoms, severity of the symptoms, and length of survival. Several distinct clinical presentations exist (Table 157-1). Within any individual family, there usually is a high level of concordance, so that affected siblings often have similar forms of the disease. A number of reports have described both mild and severe forms occurring within the same family, however, supporting the view that the different phenotypes are part of the same genotypic spectrum. In 1990, the genetic abnormality was localized to chromosome 5q11. The abnormality appears to be the same in both the acute and the chronic form of the disease, indicating phenotypic heterogeneity with genetic homogeneity. Pathologically, there is a loss of anterior horn cells in the spinal cord. Surviving neurons show changes of chromatolysis and pyknosis. There is no sign of inflammation.

## Acute Infantile Spinal Muscular Atrophy (Acute Werdnig-Hoffmann Disease, Spinal Muscular Atrophy Type 1)

Patients with the most severe form of SMA present a stereotypic picture, with the onset of symptoms occurring within the first 6 months of life. In one third of cases, the onset is in utero, with a notable decrease in fetal movements during the last months of pregnancy. These children are hypotonic and weak in the neonatal period, and they have significant feeding difficulties and respiratory distress. Other children may appear normal for the first few weeks of life while generalized weakness of the extremities, trunk, and bulbar muscles gradually develops. A typical "frog leg" posture, characterized by abduction of the arms with flexion at the elbows, and abduction of the legs with flexion at the knees, is seen in the early stages of the disease.

Physical examination reveals marked hypotonia and generalized and symmetric weakness. Movements may be limited to flickering of the fingers and toes. The tendon reflexes almost invariably are absent. The child is unable to support the head and

**TABLE 157-1.    Progressive Spinal Muscular Atrophies (SMAs)**

| Disorder | Inheritance | Age of Onset | Clinical Features |
|---|---|---|---|
| Acute infantile SMA (Werdnig-Hoffmann disease, SMA type 1) | Autosomal recessive | In utero to 6 months | Frog-leg posture<br>Severe weakness with some movements of fingers and toes; most are unable to sit<br>Areflexia<br>Tongue atrophy and fasciculations<br>Progressive swallowing and respiratory problems<br>Survival less than 3 years |
| Intermediate SMA (chronic Werdnig-Hoffmann disease, SMA type 2) | Autosomal recessive; rarely autosomal dominant | 3 months to 15 years | Proximal weakness; most sit, some walk until teens<br>Decreased or absent reflexes<br>Long periods of apparent arrest<br>High incidence of scoliosis, contractures<br>Unusual tremor (minipolymyoclonus)<br>Survival varies several years to third decade |
| Kugelberg-Welander disease | Autosomal recessive; rarely autosomal dominant | 5 years to 15 years | May be part of continuous disease spectrum of SMA type II<br>Proximal weakness with hip and shoulder atrophy<br>Calf hypertrophy<br>Decreased or absent reflexes<br>May remain ambulatory into fourth decade |

cannot straighten the trunk when held in ventral suspension. Respirations are shallow and chest movements may be paradoxic. Feeding difficulties occur early, and secretions pool in the mouth as swallowing becomes impaired further. There may be visible atrophy and fasciculations of the tongue. The extraocular muscles are not affected. The child appears alert and attentive, and development is normal with the exception of motor skills. Contractures are not common in the early stages of the disease, although a small percentage of patients have congenital contractures or dislocation of the hip. The natural course is one of gradually increasing weakness, with feeding difficulties and respiratory compromise. In most cases, death occurs from a pulmonary infection with respiratory failure before the patient reaches 3 years of age.

The two most useful diagnostic studies are electromyography and muscle biopsy. Serum creatine phosphokinase and aldolase levels may be increased slightly, but more often are normal. Electromyography typically reveals fibrillations at rest, suggestive of active denervation, and a marked reduction of motor unit potentials on voluntary effort. Regular, repetitive, involuntary firing of single motor units appears to be unique to the acute form of SMA. The large, complex, polyphasic motor unit potentials that are characteristic of chronic denervation are not seen in young infants with this disorder. The muscle biopsy findings in infantile SMA are diagnostic, revealing large numbers of round, atrophic fibers intermingled with clumps of hypertrophic fibers of uniform histochemical type (Fig 157-1).

The treatment of acute infantile SMA is limited to supportive care. Respiratory insufficiency frequently becomes a problem before 1 year of age, and survival beyond 2 years of age is rare. Because of the poor prognosis of these children, artificial ventilation rarely, if ever, is justifiable. Appropriate genetic counseling is mandatory.

## Intermediate Spinal Muscular Atrophy (Chronic Werdnig-Hoffmann Disease, Spinal Muscular Atrophy Type 2)

Intermediate SMA usually presents in the middle of the first year of life. Development is appropriate until about 6 months of age, when motor milestones become delayed. The child may learn to sit independently and to stand, but independent walking usually is not achieved. Weakness is symmetric and proximal muscles tend to be involved more severely than are distal muscles. In-

volvement of the truncal muscles often is prominent, leading to kyphoscoliosis. There usually is a fine tremor of the hands. Tongue fasciculations and atrophy are noted in about half of the patients, but chewing and swallowing difficulties are rare. The deep tendon reflexes are absent or diminished. As in patients with the acute form of the disease, intelligence is normal. The course of the illness is variable, and there may be long periods in which the disease appears to be static. Many patients have a stable course after the initial months of progressive weakness and may survive until adult life.

Results of the electromyographic examination differ somewhat from those found in patients with the acute form of intermediate SMA in that fibrillation potentials are not prominent and motor unit action potentials tend to be polyphasic and large in amplitude. Examination of muscle biopsy samples reveals features similar to those found in acute infantile SMA, although large sheets of atrophic fibers usually are not seen. The muscle biopsy is helpful in making the diagnosis, but is not a reliable indicator of the prognosis and, at times, may reveal findings indistinguishable from those seen in acute infantile SMA.

No specific treatment is available for this disorder. Therapy should be directed toward preventing contractures by a combination of physiotherapy, bracing, and orthopedic procedures. Attention should be paid to maintaining correct posture of the spine, because scoliosis may be rapidly progressive and can cause severe thoracic distortion, adding to the respiratory impairment.

## Juvenile Spinal Muscular Atrophy (Kugelberg-Welander Disease, Juvenile Proximal Hereditary Muscular Atrophy)

Typically, juvenile SMA begins between 5 and 15 years of age, although earlier and later times of onset have been described. Weakness frequently starts in the hip girdle, causing difficulty in walking, climbing stairs, and rising from a seated position. As pelvic girdle weakness progresses, the child may use the hands to push off the knee when rising from the floor (Gowers' maneuver). The calf muscles may appear hypertrophied in comparison with the atrophic thigh muscles, leading to the erroneous diagnosis of Duchenne or Becker's muscular dystrophy. Involvement of the shoulder and arm muscles becomes apparent in the later stages of the illness. Facial weakness and bulbar symptoms are rare. Most patients remain ambulatory until their third or fourth decade, at which time severe hip weakness necessitates

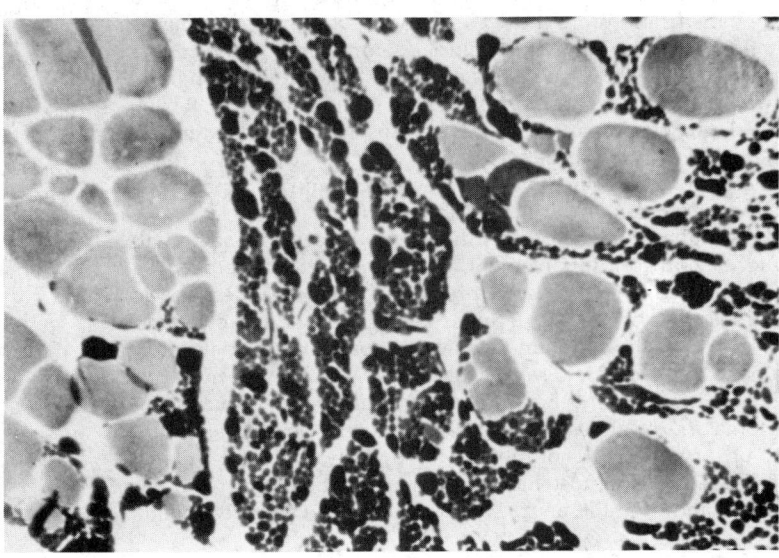

**Figure 157-1.** Muscle biopsy sample of a patient with Werdnig-Hoffman disease showing characteristic groups of rounded, atrophic type II (*dark*) muscle fibers adjacent to groups of normal-size or hypertrophic type I (*light*) muscle fibers.

the use of a wheelchair. Skeletal deformities are not common early in the disease, but kyphoscoliosis and contractures may occur when the patient becomes wheelchair bound.

Laboratory studies are very important in this disorder, as it may be indistinguishable clinically from a number of other types of myopathy. The serum creatine phosphokinase level is elevated in about half of the patients, but rarely is as high as that seen in individuals with Duchenne dystrophy. Electromyography reveals evidence of denervation and reinnervation, with fibrillations, fasciculations, and large-amplitude polyphasic potentials. Muscle biopsy samples show signs of denervation, with angular, atrophic fibers and fiber type grouping. The biopsy is of utmost importance in juvenile SMA, because the disorder may be mistaken for a number of illnesses that cause slowly progressive proximal weakness. In the early stages of the disease, juvenile SMA may resemble Duchenne muscular dystrophy, particularly if significant calf hypertrophy is present. The absence of toe walking and heel cord tightening may help differentiate SMA from Duchenne dystrophy. Facioscapulohumeral muscular dystrophy, limb-girdle dystrophy, and inflammatory myopathies also are included in the differential diagnosis.

## OTHER HEREDITARY DISORDERS OF THE ANTERIOR HORN CELL

A number of less common diseases can affect the anterior horn cell. A rare disorder, progressive juvenile bulbar palsy (Fazio-Londe disease), causes progressive weakness of the facial, ocular, and bulbar muscles, starting in the first decade. As the disease advances, the trunk and limb muscles also become involved. Death occurs within several years. Pathologically, there is loss of motor nuclei throughout the brain stem and of anterior horn cells in the spinal cord. The cause of the disease is unknown. There have been a number of descriptions of children with progressive weakness and atrophy of the shoulder girdle and peroneal muscles. Some of these cases of scapuloperoneal or facioscapulohumeral muscular atrophy appear to be caused by anterior horn cell disease, although others seem to have a myopathic basis.

Arthrogryposis multiplex congenita is a syndrome consisting of multiple contractures of the joints of the arms and legs that are present at birth. This syndrome may be caused by pathology in the anterior horn cell, peripheral nerve, neuromuscular junction, muscle, or joints and joint capsules. The anterior horn cell type is most common and results from a marked decrease in the number of anterior horn cells in the cervical and lumbar cord. The patients are profoundly weak and have decreased range of motion of the joints with multiple contractures. Deep tendon reflexes are absent. The typical posture is one of extension of the arms with internal rotation of the forearms and finger flexion. The thighs usually are flexed at the hips and rotated externally, and the feet have a talipes equinovarus deformity. Weakness generally is not progressive in these patients and orthopedic procedures may improve function of the joints.

A number of metabolic conditions have been associated with anterior horn cell involvement. Several patients have been described who have progressive proximal muscle weakness, fasciculations, cramps, and hyperreflexia suggestive of motor neuron disease, but who are found to have hexosaminidase deficiency. In patients with classic Tay-Sachs disease, the anterior horn cells may be involved by the storage of ganglioside, producing hypotonia and weakness. The disease picture is dominated by pathology in other parts of the nervous system, however. Anterior horn cell pathology also has been noted in patients with Pompe's disease and infantile neuroaxonal dystrophy. Hyperglycinemia,

B-hydroxyisovaleric aciduria, and $\beta$-methylcrotonylglycinuria also have been associated with clinical conditions similar to SMA.

## INFECTIOUS DISEASES INVOLVING THE ANTERIOR HORN CELL

Poliomyelitis is an acute viral disease that exhibits a specific predilection for the anterior horn cells. The illness begins with fever, malaise, and, frequently, gastrointestinal symptoms. These symptoms are followed by a meningitic illness, with stiffness and pain in the neck and pain in the back muscles. In a small percentage of infections, paralysis develops during the acute meningeal illness. Occasionally, paralysis may be delayed for 1 to 2 weeks after the meningeal symptoms. The legs usually are more involved than the arms, but weakness may occur in any muscle group. The muscular weakness may be associated with fasciculations and pain initially, and then progress to a flaccid paralysis. Muscular involvement may be asymmetric and restricted to muscles in one extremity, or it may involve the trunk and all the extremities. Bulbar involvement occurs in 10% to 30% of children with paralytic poliomyelitis, causing difficulty in swallowing or breathing. Examination of the cerebrospinal fluid reveals a lymphocytosis, with a normal glucose level and a normal or slightly elevated protein level. The virus cannot be isolated from the cerebrospinal fluid, but may be recovered from stool suspensions or throat washings. Electromyography reveals evidence of denervation (fibrillation potentials) after a period of about 3 weeks. As recovery progresses, polyphasic motor unit action potentials of increasingly large amplitude are recorded, indicating reinnervation.

The prognosis of patients with paralytic poliomyelitis varies depending on the site and severity of the paralysis. The mortality rate in bulbar disease is about 10%, with death usually resulting from respiratory failure. The mortality rate associated with spinal poliomyelitis is about 1%. Gradual improvement occurs in most cases, but many patients are left with residual weakness. Occasionally, further progression of muscle weakness occurs many years after the acute paralytic illness. The neurologic findings are similar to those of amyotrophic lateral sclerosis, but the relationship of the previous infection to the later development of classic motor neuron disease is unclear. Poliomyelitis has become a rare disease since the advent of widespread immunization, but sporadic cases still occur.

Coxsackievirus infections occasionally show an affinity for anterior horn cells, causing a paralytic illness similar to poliomyelitis. Numerous other viruses and immunizations have been associated with the development of transverse myelitis with anterior horn cell involvement. Transverse myelitis begins abruptly 1 to 3 weeks after a viral illness. Severe back or root pain usually is the initial symptom, and may be accompanied by fever, malaise, neck stiffness, and diffuse muscular aching. Disruption of the anterior horn cells in the cervical or lumbar enlargements causes a flaccid paralysis of the extremities. Because involvement of the cord is not limited to the anterior horn cells, but involves corticospinal tracts as well, the flaccidity may change gradually to spasticity. A sensory loss extending to the level of cord impairment is detectable, and bowel and bladder dysfunction occurs in almost all patients.

## Selected Readings

Alexander M, Emery E, Koerner F. Progressive bulbar paresis in childhood. Arch Neurol 1976;33:66.

Brooke M. Diseases of the motor neurons. In: Brooke M, ed. A clinician's view of neuromuscular diseases, ed 2. Baltimore: Williams & Wilkins, 1986.

Brzustowicz L, Lehner T, Castilla L, et al. Genetic mapping of chronic childhood-onset spinal muscular atrophy to chromosome. Nature 1990;344:540.

Darwish H, Sarnat H, Archer C, et al. Congenital cervical spinal atrophy. Muscle Nerve 1981;4:106.

Dyck PJ, Thomas PK, Lambert E, Bunge R, eds. Peripheral neuropathy, vol II. Philadelphia: WB Saunders, 1984.

Gordon N. The spinal muscular atrophies. Dev Med Child Neurol 1991;33:930.Greenberg F, Fenolio K, Hejtmancik F, et al. X-linked infantile spinal muscular atrophy. Am J Dis Child 1988;142:217.

Pearn J, Carter C, Wilson J. The genetic identity of acute infantile spinal muscular atrophy. Brain 1973;96:463.

Pearn J, Gardner-Medwin D, Wilson J. A clinical study of chronic childhood spinal muscular atrophy: A review of 141 cases. J Neurol Sci 1978;38:23.

Russman B, Iannacone S, Buncher C, et al. Spinal muscular atrophy: New thoughts on the pathogenesis and classification schema. J Child Neurol 1992;7:347.

*Principles and Practice of Pediatrics, Second Edition.*
edited by Frank A. Oski et al. J. B. Lippincott Company, Philadelphia © 1994.

# 157.2 *Peripheral Neuropathy*

## Julie Thorne Parke

Involvement of the peripheral nerves may occur in a variety of different disorders, including systemic diseases, infections, and poisonings. In addition, there are a number of hereditary diseases in which degeneration of the peripheral nerves is a major feature. Diseases of the peripheral nerve have been classified in a number of different ways. They may be categorized according to type of functional impairment (motor, sensory, autonomic, or mixed), site of pathologic involvement (primary involvement of axon or myelin), clinical course and tempo (acute, subacute, or chronic), or presumed etiology. None of these systems of classification is entirely satisfactory, and combinations of clinical, electrophysiologic, and pathologic features usually are employed to determine the etiology. Despite a thorough diagnostic search, the cause of polyneuropathy remains obscure in more than half of all cases.

## CLINICAL FEATURES

The term *polyneuropathy* signifies a generalized disorder of nerve function that usually is symmetric; *mononeuropathy* implies a disorder of a single peripheral nerve; and *mononeuropathy multiplex* refers to the dysfunction of multiple single nerves. The clinical signs of a neuropathy reflect the function of the peripheral nerves involved. The characteristic symptoms of a polyneuropathy are weakness and sensory impairment. The weakness usually is more pronounced distally and often is more severe in the lower extremities than in the upper extremities. A gait disturbance may be an early feature of the disorder. Patients with primarily motor involvement commonly have a "high stepping gait" that is used to overcome their bilateral footdrop. The distal tendon reflexes usually are absent. In long-standing diseases, such as the hereditary types of neuropathy, there may be wasting of the affected distal musculature, producing an "inverted champagne bottle" or "stork leg" appearance of the legs. In a few forms of polyneuropathy, notably the Guillain-Barré syndrome (GBS), weakness tends to be proximal and may be attributed mistakenly to a myopathic process. The sensory abnormalities in most neuropathies, similar to the weakness, tend to be distal, becoming gradually less severe in more proximal parts of the limbs. Thus, sensory loss appears to be in a "glove and stocking" distribution on examination. In infants and young children, profound sensory loss may lead to self-mutilation, with injury to the insensitive areas. In certain diseases, such as Friedreich's ataxia, there is selective involvement of the posterior column of the spinal cord, resulting in marked impairment of proprioceptive and vibratory sensation, with less impairment of pain and temperature sensation.

Pure motor or sensory forms of neuropathy occur, but most disorders cause a combination of motor and sensory symptoms. Polyneuropathies that are predominantly motor include GBS and the neuropathy of porphyria. Types of neuropathy with severe sensory disturbances but little motor disability include the hereditary sensory neuropathies and some drug-induced neuropathies. If autonomic nerves are affected, abnormalities of pupillary reaction, impaired sweating, impaired bladder and bowel control, and postural hypotension may be noted. Autonomic involvement is a constant feature of the polyneuropathy that is associated with diabetes mellitus and of one form of hereditary sensory neuropathy, the Riley-Day syndrome.

Several physical signs are helpful in the diagnosis of polyneuropathy. Skeletal deformities, such as pes cavus and "hammer-toe" deformities, are suggestive of long-standing disorders beginning in infancy and usually are caused by hereditary neuropathies (Fig 157-2). If scoliosis is present, it also is suggestive of a long-standing hereditary neuropathy. Associated retinitis pigmentosa, sensorineural deafness, cerebellar ataxia, or cardiomyopathy suggests a hereditary rather than acquired disorder. The peripheral nerves usually are normal to palpation, but may be enlarged in patients with some forms of hypertrophic neuropathy. Enlargement of the peripheral nerves occurs predominantly in patients with demyelinating neuropathies and may be found in those with chronic inflammatory neuropathies and some hereditary neuropathies, such as Charcot-Marie-Tooth disease and Refsum disease.

Electrodiagnostic studies are particularly helpful in the diagnosis of peripheral neuropathy. Motor and sensory conduction velocities are slowed to varying degrees in patients with most forms of polyneuropathy. In contrast, nerve conduction velocities in patients with anterior horn cell disease or types of myopathy usually are normal. Nerve conduction velocities may be normal or slowed only slightly in patients with primarily axonal neuropathies, but the amplitude of the compound motor action potential is reduced markedly in these patients. Specialized studies of proximal nerve conduction velocity may be necessary to demonstrate proximal lesions, such as occur in GBS. Biopsy of the sural nerve may be useful in making the diagnosis by revealing evidence of either an axonal or a demyelinating process. The specific cause of the neuropathy, however, rarely is established by biopsy alone.

## SPECIFIC ETIOLOGIES

### Inflammatory Polyradiculoneuropathy (Guillain-Barré Syndrome)

The most common cause of acute weakness from peripheral nerve involvement is GBS. This syndrome is characterized by the acute or subacute development of a polyradiculoneuropathy, usually after an upper respiratory tract infection or an episode of gastroenteritis. A number of infectious agents have been associated with the illness, including Epstein-Barr virus, coxsackievirus, influenza viruses, echoviruses, cytomegalovirus, and *Mycoplasma*

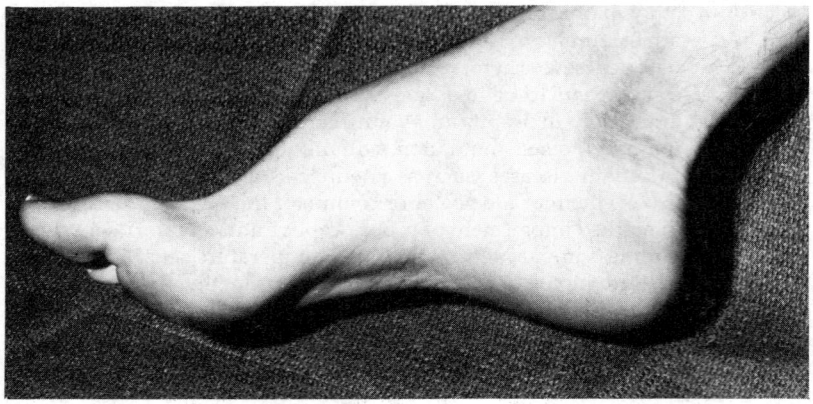

Figure 157-2.    Pes cavus in a child with a hereditary hypertrophic neuropathy.

*pneumoniae.* GBS also may follow immunization. Pathologically, the disorder is characterized by the presence of inflammatory lesions, with segmental demyelination scattered throughout the peripheral nervous system. The most severely involved segments are the rootlets and the proximal portions of the peripheral nerves.

Much evidence supports an immunologic basis for this disease. The neuropathologic and clinical features are very similar to those of an experimental condition known as experimental allergic neuritis, which is induced in animals by the injection of peripheral nerve tissue with Freund adjuvant. Experimental allergic neuritis can be transferred passively between animals by sensitized lymphocytes, but not by serum, suggesting that it is mediated by a delayed hypersensitivity mechanism. The prevailing opinion is that demyelination in GBS is secondary to a cell-mediated immune response that is directed against a component of peripheral myelin. Humoral immunity also has been found to be altered in patients with GBS, and may contribute to the pathogenesis of the disorder.

Clinical symptoms typically follow an antecedent infection after a latent period that varies in length from several days to several weeks. The most common initial symptoms are numbness and paresthesias of the hands and feet, followed by progressive weakness involving all four extremities. Motor impairment usually begins in the lower extremities and progresses in an ascending pattern to involve the upper extremities, trunk, and cranial nerves. A descending pattern of weakness also has been observed. Occasionally, the onset is abrupt, with simultaneous involvement of all extremities. The weakness usually is symmetric, although minor differences between the sides may occur.

There is a spectrum of motor involvement, varying from mild weakness to a complete flaccid quadriplegia. Muscle stretch reflexes are markedly reduced or absent. Involvement of the cranial nerves is common, with facial diplegia occurring in 50% of patients. Lower cranial nerve dysfunction may give rise to dysarthria and difficulty in swallowing and coughing. Significant respiratory muscle weakness occurs in 20% of patients and may necessitate artificial ventilation. Sensory symptoms are much less prominent than is weakness, but a distal sensory loss, particularly involving proprioception and vibratory sensation, may be present.

The autonomic nervous system is involved frequently, with episodes of paroxysmal hypertension or hypotension, tachycardia or bradycardia, and facial flushing, and sweating abnormalities. Bowel and bladder function may be impaired early in the course of the disease, but sphincter dysfunction usually is short-lived. The neurologic symptoms evolve fairly rapidly over the first few days, with maximum disability reached within 1 week in most cases. There is a stable period of 1 to 3 weeks, after which recovery begins. The recovery may be rapid, taking place in 6 to 8 weeks, or it may be slow, lasting many months.

Many patients with GBS have some variation in clinical presentation or laboratory test results. The currently accepted criteria for the diagnosis of this syndrome are listed in Table 157-2. Several variants of GBS are recognized. The most common of the variants occurring in childhood is a syndrome of acute external ophthalmoplegia, ataxia, and areflexia known as the Miller-Fisher syndrome. The ophthalmoplegia often is bilateral and may be complete with pupillary involvement. The course usually is benign, with recovery taking place within 3 to 6 months.

The most important laboratory finding in patients with GBS is an elevated cerebrospinal fluid protein content without a pleocytosis (albuminocytologic disproportion). The total cerebrospinal fluid protein level may be normal in the early stages of the illness, but is elevated in almost all patients after an interval of several days. The protein content continues to increase after the disease stabilizes, reaching a peak 2 to 4 weeks after the onset of the disease and ranging from 45 to 800 mg/dL.

Electrophysiologic studies also are helpful in the diagnosis of GBS, with abnormalities of motor and sensory conduction occurring in 90% of patients. Characteristic electrodiagnostic features include marked slowing of conduction velocities, prolonged distal latencies, and dispersion of the evoked responses. Proximal nerve conduction is characteristically slow and can be measured by studying the latency of the F response. This may be the only abnormal electrophysiologic finding in the early stages of the disease. In later stages of the disease, electromyographic studies may show denervation potentials indicating axonal damage, which is associated with a poor prognosis for complete recovery.

The treatment of GBS is largely supportive. Careful monitoring of respiratory function is very important during the early stages of the illness to prevent death as a result of respiratory failure. Elective intubation and mechanical ventilation should be used aggressively in patients with any evidence of respiratory compromise, because respiratory failure may occur abruptly if they become fatigued. Good nursing care and physiotherapy are important in severely affected patients. Most children with GBS recover completely, although the convalescence may be prolonged. The value of corticosteroids in the treatment of GBS has been debated, but no convincing evidence exists to support their use. Plasmapheresis has been shown to be beneficial both in shortening the length of the illness and in lessening the associated long-term disability. Recent studies suggest that treatment with high-dose intravenous immunoglobulin is similar in efficacy to plasmapheresis, but has fewer adverse effects.

A number of entities may produce a clinical picture similar to that of GBS. The ascending form of acute transverse myelitis and early cord compression may be difficult to distinguish from GBS initially. The presence of pyramidal tract signs, a clear sensory level, and persistent sphincter disturbances support involvement

## TABLE 157-2.   Criteria for Diagnosis of Guillain-Barré Syndrome

**Required**

Progressive motor weakness in more than one extremity
Areflexia (or distal areflexia with hyporeflexia of biceps and knee jerks)

**Strongly Supportive**

Clinical features (in order of importance):
   Progression up to 4 weeks into illness
   Relative symmetry
   Mild sensory symptoms or signs
   Cranial nerve involvement (facial weakness in 50%)
   Recovery beginning 2 to 4 weeks after progression ceases
   Autonomic dysfunction
   Absence of fever at onset of symptoms
Cerebrospinal fluid (CSF) features:
   Protein level elevated after first week of symptoms
   Ten or fewer mononuclear leukocytes per mm$^3$
Electrodiagnostic features:
   Nerve conduction slowing or block (80%)
   Prolongation of F-wave latencies

**Casting Doubt**

Marked, persistent asymmetry of weakness
Persistent bowel or bladder dysfunction
Bowel or bladder dysfunction at onset
More than 50 mononuclear leukocytes per mm$^3$ in CSF
Presence of polymorphonuclear leukocytes in CSF
Sharp sensory level

**Rule Out the Diagnosis**

Current history of hexacarbon abuse
Abnormal porphyrin metabolism
Recent diphtheritic infection
Evidence of lead neuropathy or intoxication
Purely sensory syndrome
Definite diagnosis of poliomyelitis, botulism, hysterical paralysis, or toxic neuropathy

*Adapted from Asbury AK. Diagnostic considerations in Guillai-Barré syndrome. Ann Neurol 1981;9(Suppl):1.*

of the spinal cord rather than the root and peripheral nerve. Acute paralytic poliomyelitis may present with weakness simulating GBS, but there generally are more systemic symptoms, more marked meningeal signs, and a cellular response in the cerebrospinal fluid. Uncommon conditions that may cause acute symmetric weakness include porphyria, diphtheritic polyneuropathy, heavy metal intoxication, systemic lupus erythematosus, periodic paralysis, tick paralysis, rabies, and botulism.

## Postinfectious Neuropathies

Bell's palsy, an acute paralysis of the face, is the most common postinfectious neuropathy. It frequently occurs after mild upper respiratory tract infections or episodes of otitis media. Patients often complain of pain localized in the ear, which is followed by the rapid development of weakness of the entire side of the face. The nasolabial fold on the affected side is flattened, and the child may be unable to close the eye. Taste sensation may be altered, and there may be hyperacusis as a result of involvement of the nerve to the stapedius muscle.

The prognosis for recovery is good, particularly if the paralysis is not complete. Convalescence begins within a few days to several weeks. Some evidence suggests that treatment with corticosteroids may be beneficial if it is started within 2 to 3 days of the onset of weakness. Therapy should include measures to protect the exposed cornea of the affected eye by taping and using artificial tears. The differential diagnosis of an acute facial palsy includes demyelinating disease, brain stem tumor, otitis media, and mastoiditis.

A painless abducens nerve paralysis also may occur after a nonspecific viral illness. The prognosis for this type of cranial nerve VI palsy is excellent, with improvement beginning in 3 to 6 weeks and total recovery seen in most children by 3 months. Isolated oculomotor, glossopharyngeal, and hypoglossal nerve palsies occur much less commonly.

## Brachial Plexopathy

An acute brachial plexopathy may occur in children after acute febrile illnesses or immunizations. The disorder is characterized by the sudden onset of pain in the shoulder and upper arm, followed by the rapid development of flaccid weakness involving primarily the muscles that are innervated by the upper roots of the brachial plexus. The paralysis may be severe, and atrophy of the affected muscles occurs. Sensory loss is minimal or absent. Electrophysiologic studies reveal slowing of nerve conduction velocities, low-amplitude evoked responses, and evidence of denervation. Physiotherapy is required to prevent contractures, because recovery tends to be very slow, occurring over many months.

## Genetically Determined Neuropathies

The genetically determined neuropathies tend to be slowly progressive, symmetric disorders that may be inherited as either an autosomal dominant or a recessive trait (Table 157-3). These forms of neuropathy are predominantly motor and usually are associated with deformities of the feet, such as pes cavus and hammer toe. The foot deformities may precede the development of weakness by many years and, in some cases, may be the only manifestation of the disease. The hereditary neuropathies are classified on the basis of clinical, electrophysiologic, genetic, and pathologic features. The specific metabolic defects are known in only a minority of the disorders (Table 157-4).

### Hereditary Motor and Sensory Neuropathy Type I (Hypertrophic Peroneal Muscular Atrophy, Charcot-Marie-Tooth Disease)

Hereditary motor and sensory neuropathy (HMSN) type I is the most common of the hereditary neuropathies. This type of peroneal muscular atrophy usually is inherited in an autosomal dominant manner, but autosomal recessive and X-linked recessive modes of inheritance have been reported. The most common form of the disease is associated with a large, submicroscopic DNA duplication on the proximal 17p chromosome. There is marked variability in the clinical features among different family members. The onset is in childhood and the disorder is characterized by progressive weakness and atrophy beginning in the intrinsic foot muscles and the peroneal muscles. There often is a history of foot abnormalities such as pes cavus or hammer toe, and some family members with foot deformities do not have apparent weakness. The progressive footdrop causes the child to become progressively more clumsy and to trip frequently. The small muscles of the feet and the distal leg become atrophic, giving a "stork leg" or "inverted champagne bottle" appearance to the legs. As the disease progresses, intrinsic hand muscles and

TABLE 157-3.    The Hereditary Motor and Sensory Neuropathies (HMSN)

| Disorder | Inheritance | Age of Onset | Clinical Features |
|---|---|---|---|
| HMSN I (peroneal muscular atrophy) | Autosomal dominant | Childhood | Awkward gait, weakness and atrophy of anterior tibial and peroneal muscles; later hand involvement; sensory loss minimal; slow nerve conduction velocities |
| HMSN II (neuronal form of peroneal muscular atrophy) | Autosomal dominant | Late childhood | Normal or near-normal nerve conductions with low amplitude response |
| HMSN III (Dejerine-Sottas disease) | Autosomal recessive | Infancy | Delayed motor development; marked sensory loss; small stature with skeletal deformities; cranial nerve involvement; deafness; nerve conductions markedly reduced; elevated cerebrospinal fluid protein level |
| HMSN IV (Refsum disease) | Autosomal recessive | Early childhood to second decade | Abnormal gait, sensory deficits, exacerbations and remissions of weakness; ataxia; retinitis pigmentosa; progressive deafness; cardiomyopathy; ichthyosis; elevated cerebrospinal fluid protein level; abnormal electroretinogram; slow nerve conduction velocities; accumulation of phytanic acid |

muscles of the proximal legs may become involved. Stretch reflexes are decreased or absent. Sensory function is normal or impaired only slightly. Peripheral nerves may be hypertrophic on palpation.

Reduced motor nerve conduction velocities are a hallmark of HMSN type I. Conduction velocities usually are less than one half of normal in the upper extremities and may be slowed profoundly in the lower extremities. Pathologically, there is a pre-dominant loss of myelinated fibers in the peripheral nerves, with evidence of attempted remyelinization. Whorls of Schwann cells and multiple layers of poorly formed regenerating myelin cause a characteristic "onion bulb" appearance (Fig 157-3).

No specific treatment exists for HMSN type I, although ankle orthoses may help to alleviate the footdrop and improve the gait. Life expectancy is not reduced significantly, and patients usually remain ambulatory throughout life.

TABLE 157-4.    Hereditary Neuropathies With Known Biochemical Abnormality

| Disorder | Inheritance | Biochemical Defect | Associated Clinical Features |
|---|---|---|---|
| Acute intermittent porphyria | Autosomal dominant | Uroporphyrinogen 1 synthetase deficiency | Abdominal pain; acute psychosis; progressive weakness; tachycardia; hypertension. |
| Krabbe's disease | Autosomal recessive | Galactocerebroside β-galactosidase deficiency | Irritability; spasticity; loss of milestones in early infancy; elevated cerebrospinal fluid protein level. Death within 1–2 years. |
| Metachromatic leukodystrophy | Autosomal recessive | Arylsulfatase A deficiency | Ataxia; spasticity; intellectual regression; loss of reflexes age 2–3 years; elevated cerebrospinal fluid protein level. Slower juvenile form. |
| Adrenoleukodystrophy | X-linked recessive | Peroxisomal defect in fatty acid oxidation (very long chain fatty acid accumulation) | Behavior changes; gait disturbance; visual loss; adrenal insufficiency between ages 5–10 years. Later-onset forms occur. |
| Refsum disease | Autosomal recessive | Peroxisomal defect (alpha-oxidation of long chain fatty acids, phytanic acid accumulation) | Ataxia; ichthyosis; deafness; retinitis pigmentosa; progressive sensorimotor neuropathy. |
| Fabry's disease | X-linked recessive | α-Galactosidase A deficiency | Painful sensory neuropathy (burning feet); angiokeratomas in bathing suit distribution; renal failure; stroke. |
| Bassen-Kornzweig disease (abetalipoproteinemia) | Autosomal recessive | β-Lipoprotein deficiency | Fat malabsorption; vitamins A, E, and K deficiencies; progressive ataxia; retinitis pigmentosa; developmental retardation; acanthocytosis; low cholesterol level. |
| Tangier disease | Autosomal recessive | α-Lipoprotein deficiency | Yellow tonsils; hepatosplenomegaly; sensory neuropathy. |

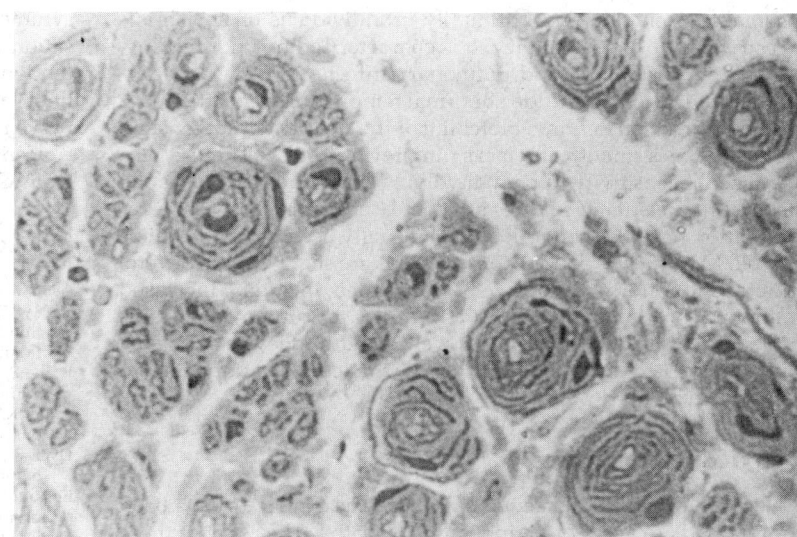

**Figure 157-3.** Sural nerve biopsy sample in a patient with hereditary motor and sensory neuropathy type I (Charcot-Marie-Tooth disease) shows multiple laminations of Schwann cells producing a characteristic "onion-bulb" formation.

## Hereditary Motor and Sensory Neuropathy Type II (Neuronal Form of Peroneal Muscular Atrophy)

HMSN type II differs pathologically from HMSN type I in that nerves show the degeneration of axons and much less evidence of demyelination and remyelinization. Clinically, this disorder is similar to HMSN type I, although the onset may be later and there is less involvement of the hand muscles. Sensory involvement is more common. Autosomal dominant and less common congenital or early onset autosomal recessive forms have been described. Motor nerve conduction velocities are normal or slowed only slightly, but the amplitude of the compound muscle action potential is reduced and there is evidence of denervation on electromyography, indicating an axonal process.

## Hereditary Motor and Sensory Neuropathy Type III (Dejerine-Sottas Disease, Hypertrophic Neuropathy of Infancy)

Dejerine-Sottas disease is an uncommon disorder that is inherited in an autosomal recessive manner. Pathologically, there is severe disruption of the myelin in many different nerves, with marked onion bulb formation and hypertrophy of the nerve. The onset of clinical features is in infancy, with delayed motor development. Affected children have both proximal and distal muscular weakness. Walking is impaired and these patients may never learn to run. Weakness increases in severity during the second decade. Skeletal deformities, such as pes cavus and kyphoscoliosis, are common. Sensory loss may be notable. Nerves are markedly hypertrophic to palpation. Pupillary responses and lower cranial nerve function also may be affected. Motor nerve conduction velocities are reduced markedly, consistent with a severe demyelinating disorder. Cerebrospinal fluid protein values may be elevated significantly.

The motor disability of Dejerine-Sottas disease is progressive, and patients usually are confined to a wheelchair by the time they reach adult life. Milder cases occur in the siblings of children with the typical disorder. Because the onset commonly is in infancy, other infantile demyelinating neuropathies must be excluded, including metachromatic leukodystrophy and Krabbe's disease.

## Hereditary Motor and Sensory Neuropathy Type IV (Refsum Disease)

Refsum disease is a recessively inherited disorder that is characterized by a diffuse polyneuropathy, ataxia, and retinitis pig-

mentosa. Additional features include progressive deafness, cardiomyopathy, ichthyosis, and night blindness. Skeletal malformations occur frequently and include pes cavus and shortened metacarpal bones. The onset varies from early childhood to the second decade. The peripheral neuropathy is progressive and symmetric. There may be episodes of acute exacerbation of weakness from which the patient may recover. These exacerbations may resemble closely inflammatory polyradiculoneuropathy. Sensory deficits are present. The cardiomyopathy may be clinically important, with the development of left ventricular failure or cardiac dysrhythmias.

Numerous laboratory test abnormalities are detected in patients with Refsum disease. The cerebrospinal fluid protein level may be elevated significantly. The electroretinogram may be severely altered. Both motor and sensory nerve conduction velocities are prolonged. Sural nerve biopsy reveals demyelination with onion bulb formation. The Schwann cells often contain sudanophilic and metachromatic droplets, which may represent phytanic acid deposition. The diagnosis of this disorder can be confirmed by measurement of the serum phytanic acid level. Patients with Refsum disease are unable to metabolize phytanic acid by $\alpha$-oxidation, so the substance accumulates in the tissues.

The treatment of Refsum disease focuses on the exclusion of dietary phytanic acid. Phytanic acid is found in dairy products, vegetables, fatty meats, fish, chocolate, and nuts. Improvement in muscular strength and nerve conduction velocities has been seen to follow adherence to a strict diet. Plasmapheresis has been helpful in patients with severe, life-threatening episodes.

### Hereditary Sensory Autonomic Neuropathies

Hereditary sensory neuropathies occur much less frequently than do sensorimotor neuropathies. The major feature of both type I and type II forms of these conditions is distal sensory loss with painless ulceration of the feet. The severity varies widely. Type I is inherited dominantly; type II is a recessive trait. Type II sensory neuropathy usually presents in infancy or early childhood with severe sensory loss and may affect the hands and trunk as well as the feet. Progressive and nonprogressive types occur. Autonomic disorders are seen frequently. Pathologically, either the number of myelinated fibers is decreased or the fibers are totally absent.

Familial dysautonomia (Riley-Day syndrome) is a sensory neuropathy notable for its involvement of the autonomic nervous system. It is a rare familial disorder that is inherited in an autosomal recessive manner, primarily in individuals of Jewish ancestry, with onset in infancy. It is characterized by poor feeding, vomiting, irritability, and pulmonary infections. Signs of autonomic dysfunction include abnormal temperature regulation, decreased or absent tearing, blotching of the skin, and hypotension. The tongue is smooth and lacks fungiform papillae. There is generalized insensitivity to pain, involving the cornea as well as the skin. Muscle stretch reflexes are decreased or absent. Mental retardation has been reported. Death usually occurs in early childhood. Motor nerve conduction velocities are slightly slow. Several metabolic abnormalities have been reported, including increased amounts of homovanillic acid and decreased amounts of vanillylmandelic acid in the urine, as well as reduced levels of plasma dopamine $\beta$-hydroxylase, the enzyme that converts dopamine to norepinephrine.

## Toxic Neuropathies

Many pharmaceutical agents as well as toxic chemicals have been implicated as causes of peripheral neuropathy. The onset of these polyneuropathies usually is insidious after prolonged exposure to the toxin. A careful history of drug use and environmental exposure to toxins is of utmost importance in making a diagnosis. Some of the more common agents causing toxic neuropathies are listed in Table 157-5.

Lead poisoning in children typically produces symptoms similar to those of encephalopathy. On occasion, however, a peripheral neuropathy may precede the development of encephalopathic symptoms. Lead usually causes a motor neuropathy with only mild sensory impairment. The distribution of weakness is distal, with patients having either footdrop or wristdrop. The diagnosis is suggested by a history of pica and may be confirmed by an elevated lead concentration in the blood. Treatment consists of removal of the source of lead and administration of a chelating agent. Long-term arsenic intoxication may cause paresthesias and symmetric distal weakness, primarily in the feet and legs. Sensation is decreased in a glove and stocking distribution, and the tendon reflexes are depressed. Transverse white striae (Mees' lines) are seen in the fingernails 6 weeks after exposure. Cranial nerve involvement is unusual, and the cerebrospinal fluid protein concentration is normal, helping to differentiate arsenic poisoning from GBS.

## Selected Readings

Asbury A. Diagnostic considerations in Guillain-Barré syndrome. Ann Neurol 1981;9(Suppl):1.
Axelrod F, Pearson J. Congenital sensory neuropathies. Diagnostic distinction from familial dysautonomia. Am J Dis Child 1984;138:947.
Brune P, McKusick V. Familial dysautonomia. Report of genetic and clinical studies with a review of the literature. Medicine (Baltimore) 1970;49:343.
Colan R, Snead O, Or S, et al. Steroid-responsive polyneuropathy with subacute onset in childhood. J Pediatr 1980;97:374.
Dyck PJ, Thomas PK, Lambert EH, Bunge R. Peripheral neuropathy, ed 2. Philadelphia: WB Saunders, 1981.
Epstein M, Sladky J. The role of plasmapheresis in childhood Guillain-Barré syndrome. Ann Neurol 1990;28:65.
Ferrière G, Guzzetta F, Kulakowski S. Nonprogressive type II hereditary sensory autonomic neuropathy. J Child Neurol 1992;7:364.
Gabreels-Festen A, Joosten E, Gabreels F, et al. Hereditary and sensory neuropathy of neuronal type with onset in early childhood. Brain 1991;114:1855.
Guillain-Barré Syndrome Study Group. Plasmapheresis and acute Guillain-Barré syndrome. Neurology 1985;35:1096.
Hobson A. Peripheral neuropathy in childhood: An update in diagnosis and management. Pediatr Ann 1983;12:814.
Lupski J, de Oca-Luna R, Slaughenhaupt S, et al. DNA duplication associated with Charcot-Marie-Tooth disease type 1A. Cell 1991;66:219.
Vanasse M, Dubowitz V. Dominantly inherited peroneal muscular atrophy (hereditary motor and sensory neuropathy Type 1) in infancy and childhood. Muscle Nerve 1981;4:26.
Vedanaryanan V, Kandt R, Lewis D, et al. Chronic inflammatory demyelinating polyradiculoneuropathy of childhood: Treatment with high dose intravenous immunoglobulin. Neurology 1991;41:828.

---

TABLE 157-5.  Toxic Neuropathies

**Industrial Chemicals and Insecticides**
Acrylamide
Carbon disulfide
Cyanide
n-Hexane
Organophosphates (cholinergic symptoms with delayed-onset neuropathy)
Trichloroethylene (facial numbness)
Tri-orthocresylphosphate

**Metals**
Lead (especially neuropathy of radial nerve, causing wrist drop)
Arsenic (Mees' lines, sensory deficit)
Mercury
Thallium (ataxia, alopecia, seizures)

**Pharmaceutical Agents**
Chloramphenicol
Cisplatin
Diphenylhydantoin
Disulfiram
Gold (may be acute)
Hydralazine
Isoniazid
Metronidazole
Vincristine

*Principles and Practice of Pediatrics, Second Edition.*
edited by Frank A. Oski et al. J. B. Lippincott Company, Philadelphia © 1994.

CHAPTER 158
# *Diseases of the Neuromuscular Junction*

Julie Thorne Parke

A number of different conditions may interfere with the transmission of the electrical impulse across the neuromuscular junction. The neuromuscular junction consists of the terminal portion of the motor nerve, the synaptic cleft, and the end plate region of the muscle. The nerve impulse originates in the anterior horn cell and is propagated down the axon of the motor nerve into the motor nerve terminals. Depolarization of the nerve terminals opens calcium channels, causing the release of acetylcholine into the synaptic cleft. Acetylcholine binds to receptors on the muscle end plate, altering the permeability to ions and causing localized depolarization of the end plate (the end plate potential). If the amplitude of the end plate potential reaches threshold, a muscle fiber action potential is generated. The muscle action potential is propagated along the muscle fiber and into the interior of the muscle fiber by the T tubules, initiating muscle fiber contraction. Acetylcholine acts at the postsynaptic membrane for only a brief period before it is broken down by an enzyme, cholinesterase, into two inactive components, choline and acetic acid. The choline is taken up by the presynaptic nerve terminal, where choline acetyltransferase catalyzes the re-synthesis of acetylcholine.

Neuromuscular transmission can fail if insufficient acetylcholine is released (presynaptic process) or if the number of acetylcholine receptors is insufficient to interact with the acetylcholine (postsynaptic disorder). Conditions interfering with the presynaptic events include some forms of congenital myasthenia gravis, botulism, hypocalcemia, hypermagnesemia, and neuromuscular blockade from antibiotics. Disorders affecting the postsynaptic events include autoimmune myasthenia gravis, some types of congenital myasthenia gravis, organophosphate poisoning, and iatrogenic neuromuscular blockade with curare (Table 158-1). Neuromuscular transmission failure also may occur if there is inhibition of or a deficiency in acetylcholinesterase, causing a depolarization block.

Disorders of neuromuscular transmission are manifested clinically by muscle weakness, which is exacerbated by exercise and improved by rest. Defects in neuromuscular transmission can be documented by pharmacologic tests and by electrophysiologic studies, including repetitive nerve stimulation and single-fiber electromyography.

## JUVENILE MYASTHENIA GRAVIS

### Pathophysiology

The juvenile and adult forms of myasthenia gravis are autoimmune disorders that are characterized by an autoimmune attack on the acetylcholine receptor. Circulating antibodies to the acetylcholine receptor bind to the receptor on the muscle end plate, blocking its function. Morphologic studies show a simplified postsynaptic membrane with poorly developed folds and clefts, and a loss of functional acetylcholine receptor sites. Antibody can be demonstrated on the postsynaptic membrane, further im-

plicating an immunologic process in its destruction. Circulating acetylcholine receptor antibodies can be measured, but the titer does not correlate well with the clinical condition of the patient. A lymphocyte-mediated immune response to acetylcholine receptors also has been identified. The thymus plays a role in the disease, possibly by sensitizing specific lymphocytes to produce acetylcholine receptor antibodies.

### Clinical Features

The onset of juvenile myasthenia gravis usually is after 10 years of age, although it can be much earlier. Girls are affected more commonly than are boys. The cardinal feature of the disease is easy fatigability. The onset usually is gradual, with symptoms most apparent in the afternoon or evening when the patient is tired. Occasionally, the onset is quite sudden and may appear to have been precipitated by an infectious illness. The weakness characteristically improves with rest and is made worse with sustained effort. In about one half of patients, weakness first appears in the ocular muscles, causing ptosis or diplopia (Fig 158-1). Ptosis frequently is asymmetric and may be unilateral. It tends to fluctuate during the day and to vary from day to day. Involvement of the ocular muscles is variable, but may be quite severe, causing a total ophthalmoplegia. About one fourth of patients have weakness of the bulbar musculature, resulting in difficulties speaking, swallowing, or chewing. The facial muscles are involved in most patients. Weakness of the palate and tongue may make speech unintelligible. The child's voice may be strong initially, becoming softer and less distinct during continued conversation. Difficulty chewing food is a common problem, and many patients support their jaw in one hand to assist with chewing. Swallowing difficulties and choking spells may occur. Weakness of the muscles of the neck, particularly the neck extensors, causes the head to fall forward. Patients with predominantly bulbar symptoms are

| TABLE 158-1. Disorders of Neuromuscular Transmission |
|---|
| **Presynaptic** |
| Botulism |
| Eaton-Lambert syndrome |
| Hypermagnesemia |
| Hypocalcemia |
| Snake bite |
| Antibiotics |
| Congenital myasthenia gravis |
| ? Tick paralysis |
| **Inhibition or Deficiency of Acetylcholinesterase** |
| Organophosphates |
| Congenital myasthenia gravis |
| **Postsynaptic** |
| Autoimmune myasthenia gravis |
| Curare (d-tubocurarine) |
| α-Bungarotoxin |
| Congenital myasthenia gravis |

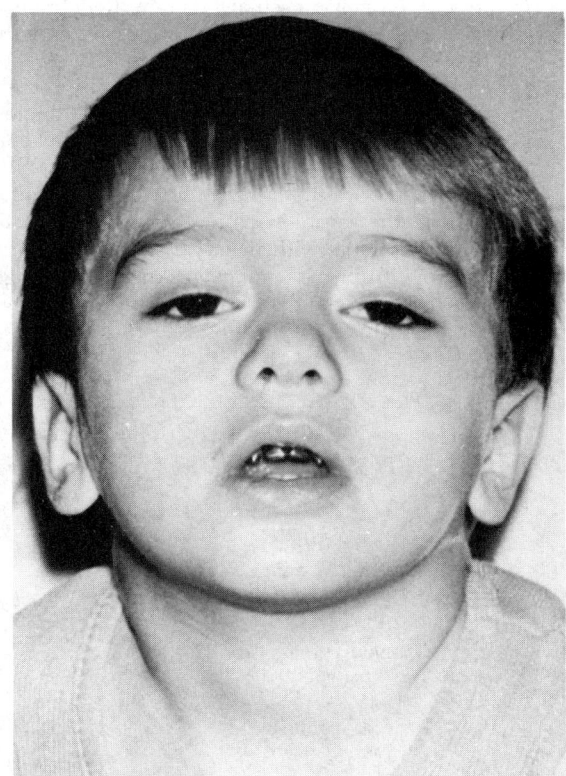

**Figure 158-1.** Four-year-old child with juvenile myasthenia gravis, exhibiting fluctuating ptosis and bilateral facial weakness.

at risk of the development of respiratory failure, particularly during an intercurrent infection.

A smaller number of children (about 20%) have generalized weakness of the extremities. Fatigability may be demonstrated in younger children by having them climb stairs or hold their arms outstretched for an interval. In older children, repetitive testing of deltoid strength or performance of multiple deep knee bends may help disclose the weakness. Regardless of the distribution of weakness, the principal features are a fluctuating quality to the weakness and susceptibility to fatigue. These features differ from those of other neuromuscular disorders, which produce relatively constant symptoms.

## Diagnostic Studies

The diagnosis of myasthenia gravis usually can be made on the basis of the history and physical examination, and may be confirmed by pharmacologic tests. A small dose of an anticholinesterase drug produces a dramatic improvement in strength. Edrophonium chloride (Tensilon) is preferred because of its rapid onset and short duration of action. The availability of acetylcholine is increased by inhibiting the enzyme cholinesterase, thereby improving neuromuscular transmission. A placebo injection of normal saline should be given before the edrophonium. A test dose of one tenth of the total dose is given initially. If no complications occur with the test dose, then the full dosage of 0.2 mg/kg, with a maximum dosage of 10 mg, is given intravenously. The patient's heart rate and blood pressure must be monitored throughout the test and atropine sulfate should be immediately available, because a cholinergic crisis develops in occasional patients that is manifest by extreme bradycardia or transient respiratory weakness requiring ventilatory support. A marked but short-lived improvement in weakness usually is seen in patients with myasthenia. Neostigmine may be used if a longer effect is necessary to evaluate limb strength.

Electrophysiologic studies are helpful in documenting transmission failure at the neuromuscular junction. Repetitive nerve stimulation produces a characteristic fall in amplitude between the first and the fourth or fifth responses (decremental response). It may be necessary to test several muscles, because the abnormality may not be present in all muscles. Selective single-fiber electromyography is possible in some patients and may confirm the variability in synaptic transmission time in patients with rather mild disease. Antibodies to the human muscle acetylcholine receptor are found in the serum of as many as 90% of patients. Unfortunately, the patients with negative antibody test results typically are those with purely ocular weakness or mild generalized weakness in whom the diagnosis is uncertain. A negative test result does not exclude the diagnosis.

## Treatment and Prognosis

A number of different therapeutic modalities are available for the treatment of myasthenia gravis. The approach selected should take into consideration the age of the patient, the severity of the disease, and the potential benefits and risks of each form of therapy. Cholinesterase inhibitors improve neuromuscular transmission by inhibiting the enzymatic degradation of acetylcholine, prolonging its effect on the muscle end plate. These agents result in symptomatic improvement in strength in most patients with myasthenia gravis and may be sufficient to produce normal or near-normal strength in some. Pyridostigmine bromide (Mestinon) and neostigmine bromide (Prostigmin) are the most commonly used agents (Table 158-2). The dosage of cholinesterase inhibitor used and the dosing interval must be adjusted carefully based on close clinical observation. The dosage required by a given individual may vary during the day and from one day to the next. A cholinergic crisis may result from excessive anticholinesterase dosing as a result of the accumulation of acetylcholine at the neuromuscular junction. Both nicotinic symptoms, such as increased muscle weakness and fasciculations, and muscarinic symptoms, such as diarrhea, pallor, sweating, increased salivation, cardiovascular disturbances, and visual blurring, may occur (Table 158-3). An overdose of anticholinesterase medications producing weakness of respiratory muscles and respiratory distress may be difficult to distinguish from myasthenic crisis causing respiratory insufficiency. Close monitoring of the patient's muscle strength, pulmonary function, and ability to cough adequately is critical during these periods. Elective intubation and ventilatory support should be instituted before respiratory insufficiency occurs.

Other treatment modalities, including thymectomy, corticosteroid therapy, and immunosuppressive agents, are aimed more directly at the basic immunologic mechanism of the disease. Corticosteroid therapy, given on an alternate-day schedule, is effective in many patients who have an incomplete response to anticholinesterase drugs. Unfortunately, the complications of corticosteroid therapy in young children may make their long-term use unsatisfactory. The importance of the thymus gland in myasthenia gravis long has been recognized, and thymectomy has been accepted as a successful method of treatment. The beneficial effects of thymectomy are not fully understood, but it is likely that the thymus sensitizes lymphocytes to form antibodies directed at the acetylcholine receptors in the postsynaptic membrane. A sternotomy is the accepted surgical approach for thymectomy, although some surgeons prefer a transcervical approach. Total removal of the thymus gland is essential for maximal benefit. The postoperative care of these children often is complex, and careful monitoring and observation in an intensive care setting is required. The efficacy of thymectomy appears to be greatest

| | Equivalent Doses* | | | Starting Oral Dosages | | |
|---|---|---|---|---|---|---|
| Drug | Oral | IM | IV | Infant | Older Child | Adult |
| Pyridostigmine bromide (Mestinon) | 60 | 2 | 0.7 | 4–10 mg every 4 hours | 30 mg every 4 hours | 60 mg every 4 hours |
| Neostigmine bromide (Prostigmin) | 15 | | | 1–2 mg every 4 hours | 7.5–10 mg every 4 hours | 15 mg every 4 hours |
| Neostigmine methylsulfate | | 0.5 | 0.5 | | | |

**TABLE 158-2.   Cholinesterase Inhibitors in the Treatment of Myasthenia Gravis**

*IM, intramuscular; IV, intravenous.

| TABLE  158-3.    Side Effects of Cholinesterase Inhibitors |
| --- |
| **Muscarinic** |
| Abdominal cramps |
| Diarrhea |
| Nausea |
| Vomiting |
| Increased salivation |
| Increased bronchial secretions |
| Irritability |
| Anxiety |
| Sleep disturbances |
| Coma |
| Seizures |
| **Nicotinic** |
| Muscle fasciculations |
| Muscle weakness |

in patients with primarily bulbar symptoms. It is less effective and generally not recommended for patients with solely ocular symptoms. Plasmapheresis has been used as an intensive, short-term intervention in patients with myasthenia. It is helpful in patients who have had a short-term exacerbation of weakness during myasthenic crisis or after a thymectomy. It also is used to produce rapid improvement in strength in preparation for thymectomy.

The prognosis of patients with juvenile myasthenia gravis is relatively good, in that complete or partial remissions occur in 25% within 2 years of onset of the disease. The disease often is characterized by a fluctuating course of remissions and exacerbations, however. The severity of symptoms is variable, and some children have severe disease necessitating frequent hospitalizations and mechanical ventilatory support. About 80% of children improve after thymectomy.

## TRANSIENT NEONATAL MYASTHENIA GRAVIS

The syndrome of transient neonatal myasthenia gravis is found in infants born of mothers with myasthenia gravis. The disease is caused by the transplacental passage of the IgG acetylcholine receptor antibodies and occurs in about 15% of the newborn children of affected mothers. Symptoms usually appear in the first few hours after birth, although the onset may be delayed for several days. Initial symptoms include hypotonia, diffuse muscle weakness, respiratory distress, and feeding difficulties. Ptosis or ocular motility problems may occur. Symptoms usually last for several weeks, but may persist for several months. The child then recovers fully and has no greater incidence of the later onset of myasthenia gravis than does the general population. The severity of the mother's illness is not correlated with the occurrence or severity of the infant's myasthenia. The diagnosis of neonatal myasthenia may be made with repetitive nerve stimulation studies, by documentation of the presence of circulating antibody to acetylcholine receptors, and by the response to short-acting anticholinesterase medication. Supportive care and anticholinesterase agents are necessary in about 80% of patients.

## CONGENITAL MYASTHENIA GRAVIS

There are several rare varieties of congenital myasthenia gravis with onset at birth or in early childhood and persistent symptoms. The disorders usually are familial, with autosomal recessive inheritance occurring most frequently. Similar to other disorders of neuromuscular transmission, the syndromes are characterized by fluctuating weakness. Recurrent episodes of apnea may occur. Severe ocular muscle weakness is characteristic of several of the syndromes. Congenital myasthenia gravis differs from acquired myasthenia gravis in that there is no evidence of an autoimmune etiology. Detailed physiologic and morphologic studies have identified specific abnormalities in the neuromuscular junction in patients with several of the syndromes (Table 158-4). Patients with these disorders do not respond to immunosuppressive therapy or to thymectomy. The response to cholinesterase inhibitors is variable.

## BOTULISM

### Pathophysiology

The exotoxin of *Clostridium botulinum* is one of the most potent neurotoxins known. It is absorbed from the intestine or an infected wound and is distributed in a hematogenous manner to peripheral cholinergic nerve synapses, such as the neuromuscular junction. The toxin irreversibly blocks acetylcholine release from the presynaptic nerve terminals. Recovery occurs by sprouting of terminal motor neurons and the formation of new motor end plates.

In children and adults, poisoning may occur after ingestion of the toxin in inadequately cooked or improperly canned food. The anaerobic bacillus and the exotoxin it produces are destroyed by heat, so proper cooking of food should eliminate outbreaks. At high altitudes, water boils at a lower temperature and the

| TABLE  158-4.    Distinguishing Features of Congenital Myasthenic Syndromes | | | | |
| --- | --- | --- | --- | --- |
| Features | Defect in ACh Synthesis or Mobilization | End-Plate AChE Deficiency | Slow-Channel Syndrome | End-Plate AChR Deficiency |
| Inheritance | Recessive | Recessive | Dominant | Recessive |
| Abnormal fatigability | + | + | + | + |
| Reduced muscle bulk | − | + | + | Occasionally + |
| Hyporeflexia | − | + | +, − | − |
| Age at onset of symptoms | At birth | At birth | Variable | At birth |
| Response to anticholinesterase drugs | + | − | +, − | + |
| Circulating AChR antibodies | − | − | − | − |

*AChR, acetylcholine; AChE, acetylcholinesterase; AChR, acetylcholine receptor.*
*After Engel A. Myasthenia gravis and myasthenic syndromes. Ann Neurol 1984;16:519.*

exotoxin is not destroyed during boiling, accounting for the greater frequency of botulism in mountain locales. The majority of outbreaks of botulism can be traced to home-canned foods, particularly vegetables, fruits, fish, and condiments. Wound botulism results from infection of traumatized tissue by the organism, with subsequent toxin production. Most cases occur subsequent to wounds sustained in open fields or on farms, particularly compound extremity fractures. A third type of botulism, infant botulism, differs from food-borne and wound botulism because it is caused by ingestion of the spores of *C botulinum* rather than the exotoxin. It occurs almost exclusively in children in the first year of life, usually in those between 5 and 12 weeks of age. The ingested spores colonize the intestinal tract and produce the *C botulinum* toxin. The source of the spores frequently is not found. Honey has been implicated as the source in about 20% of patients, however, and environmental sources, such as yard soil, have been implicated in other cases.

Seven antigenically distinct types of *C botulinum* toxin have been identified. Disease in humans is caused primarily by toxin types A, B, E, and F. Type E botulism almost always can be traced to fish and fish products. Almost all cases of infant botulism have been caused by toxin types A or B.

## Clinical Features

Clinical symptoms appear within 1 to 2 days after the consumption of contaminated food or within 1 to 2 weeks after wound inoculation. The initial symptoms of food-borne infection may resemble those of food poisoning: vomiting, diarrhea, and abdominal pain. Commonly, similar symptoms develop in several members of a family. Weakness of the extraocular muscles occurs, causing blurred vision and diplopia. Failure of convergence may be the first symptom. Visual problems often are accompanied by other bulbar symptoms, including dizziness, dysarthria, and dysphagia. Some patients have only bulbar symptoms; others have varying degrees of extremity weakness. Weakness may occur quite rapidly after the ingestion of large amounts of toxin, causing a flaccid paralysis and respiratory failure. In wound botulism, the toxin is released slowly into the circulation so that the onset of symptoms and the progression of weakness is slower. Examination reveals involvement of the extraocular muscles. Pupillary responses may or may not be affected. Tendon reflexes typically are absent, but may be present. Sensory abnormalities are not seen. In patients with milder disease, fatigability is not as prominent as in patients with myasthenia gravis.

The clinical appearance of infant botulism is quite different from that of food-borne or wound botulism. Constipation is the first sign of illness, although this symptom frequently may be overlooked. Infants gradually become listless and weak over a period of days to weeks. As the bulbar muscles become involved, there is difficulty feeding and the cry becomes weaker. Drooling and pooling of food and secretions in the posterior pharynx may occur. Ptosis, ophthalmoplegia, and diminished facial expression are present. Hypotonia and generalized muscle weakness most often are manifest initially as a loss of head control. Respiratory arrest may occur abruptly in patients with severe disease. Botulism may be responsible for some cases of unexpected sudden death in infancy.

## Diagnostic Studies

Electrophysiologic studies are helpful in demonstrating a disturbance in neuromuscular transmission in patients with botulism. The compound muscle action potential elicited by a single stimulus to the nerve is small, and the amplitude declines with repetitive stimulation at a slow rate. Repetitive stimulation at fast rates produces an increase in the amplitude of muscle action po-

tentials. Needle examination demonstrates a distinctive pattern of brief, small, abundant motor unit potentials that may be diagnostic of botulism in the context of the clinical syndrome. Confirmation of the diagnosis of botulism depends on detection of the toxin or the organism in the patient or the implicated food. In infant botulism, the organism may be isolated from stool culture.

## Differential Diagnosis

Botulism in children must be distinguished from myasthenia gravis, Guillain-Barré syndrome, tick paralysis, and chemical intoxications. Patients with myasthenia gravis typically have preserved pupillary reactions and usually do not have areflexia. Fatigability is much more prominent in myasthenia gravis, and the edrophonium chloride (Tensilon) test result is dramatically positive. Clinical differentiation from Guillain-Barré syndrome may be difficult. Patients with Guillain-Barré syndrome usually have ascending weakness, with a later onset of cranial nerve involvement. Frequent paresthesias and elevated cerebrospinal fluid protein content also help to distinguish this disorder. Electromyography is helpful in differentiating both Guillain-Barré syndrome and myasthenia gravis from botulism.

In addition to these disorders, the differential diagnosis of infant botulism includes Werdnig-Hoffmann disease, poliomyelitis, and diphtheria. The early extraocular muscle and pupillary involvement, the symmetry of weakness, and the absence of fever or pharyngitis, as well as the characteristic electrophysiologic findings, should increase the suspicion of botulism.

## Treatment and Prognosis

The treatment of all forms of botulism is directed toward aggressive supportive care, with particular attention paid to respiratory support. The prognosis generally is good if the patient is supported adequately, although recovery may be very slow, taking weeks to many months in severely affected individuals. In cases of food-borne botulism, if the patient is seen early, emetics and gastric lavage should be used to reduce the amount of unabsorbed toxin. Antitoxin may be given, although evidence of its efficacy once neurologic manifestations have occurred is lacking. If food-borne botulism is suspected, state and federal health officials should be notified immediately. The treatment of wound botulism includes exploration and debridement of the site, in conjunction with antitoxin and antibiotic therapy. Guanidine may be of some value in improving muscle strength in mild or moderately severe cases of food-borne or wound botulism. Infant botulism is a self-limiting disease, generally lasting 2 to 6 weeks. The use of antitoxin and antibiotics has not been shown to influence its course. Antibiotics are not used because bacterial death may liberate *C botulinum* toxin, increasing the amount of toxin in the gastrointestinal tract. Aggressive supportive care is required throughout the period of hypotonia and weakness, and many infants require prolonged ventilator support. Constipation may persist for months and may improve with the use of stool softeners and adequate hydration. The mortality with botulism is 20% to 25% in cases of food-borne or wound botulism. The mortality of recognized cases of infant botulism is about 3%. Relapse of infant botulism after apparent resolution of clinical symptoms may occur, making close follow-up necessary.

## TICK PARALYSIS

### Pathophysiology

A progressive, ascending flaccid paralysis may be caused by the attachment of certain species of ticks. In North America, the disease is caused most commonly by *Dermacentor andersoni* (wood tick) or *Dermacentor variabilis* (dog tick). *Ixodes holocyclus* (scrub tick) is the cause of the disease in Australia. Most cases of tick paralysis occur in the spring or summer and involve young children, especially girls with long hair. The tick frequently attaches near the hairline, where it remains unnoticed. Clinical symptoms begin within several days after the tick attaches. Tick paralysis is thought to be caused by a toxin released by the ticks, but the exact mechanism and site of the toxin's action are not known. It has been postulated that the toxin prevents depolarization in the terminal portions of the motor neurons.

## Clinical Features

Tick paralysis may begin with general symptoms such as irritability and diarrhea. Initial neurologic signs include gait ataxia and areflexia. Weakness of the legs then becomes apparent and advances in an ascending, symmetric pattern to involve the trunk and upper extremities. If the tick remains attached, the weakness may progress to involve the bulbar musculature, producing dysarthria, dysphagia, blurred vision, and facial weakness. Respiratory compromise may occur. Patients may complain of numbness and tingling of the extremities, but objective sensory abnormalities are rare.

## Diagnostic Studies

Routine laboratory studies are not helpful in establishing the diagnosis of tick paralysis. The cerebrospinal fluid protein level is normal, which helps to distinguish tick paralysis from Guillain-Barré syndrome. Electrophysiologic studies usually reveal a reduced amplitude of the compound muscle action potential, with no significant incremental or decremental response with repetitive stimulation. Motor and sensory nerve conduction velocities are decreased slightly in the distal segments.

## Treatment and Prognosis

Recovery occurs within 1 to 5 days after removal of the tick. Intensive supportive care with assisted ventilation for respiratory failure may be required during this period. The tick must be removed for recovery to occur. Removal is achieved best by covering the tick with petrolatum to cause it to withdraw before removing it with forceps. Care should be taken to remove the entire tick so that secondary infection does not occur.

## NEUROMUSCULAR TOXINS

A number of pharmacologic and environmental agents may interfere with neuromuscular transmission (Table 158-5). Organophosphates, such as parathion, cause irreversible inhibition of acetylcholinesterase, resulting in an accumulation of acetylcholine in the synaptic cleft. These insecticides cause muscle paralysis

| TABLE 158-5. Drugs Affecting Neuromuscular Transmission |
| --- |
| Antibiotics (tetracyclines, trimethoprim, polymyxins, aminoglycosides, lincomycin, clindamycin) |
| β-Adrenergic blockers (propranolol) |
| Phenytoin |
| Procainamide |
| Quinidine |
| Chloroquine |
| Lithium |
| Phenothiazines |
| Succinylcholine |
| Pancuronium bromide |
| Anticholinesterases |
| Adrenocorticotropic hormone |
| Corticosteroids |

with prominent autonomic symptoms. Common neuromuscular blocking agents used in anesthesia, such as succinylcholine, may cause prolonged paralysis in patients with clinical or subclinical myasthenia gravis. A number of antibiotics, such as neomycin, streptomycin, kanamycin, colistin, and tetracycline, interfere with the release of acetylcholine, aggravating preexisting neuromuscular transmission problems. Several other drugs, including propranolol, phenytoin, and corticosteroids, may have a similar effect on neuromuscular transmission. The treatment of drug-induced neuromuscular blockade consists of supportive care and the substitution of a different drug.

## Selected Readings

Engel A. Myasthenia gravis and myasthenic syndromes. Ann Neurol 1984;16:519.

Glauser T, Maguire H, Sladky J. Relapse of infant botulism. Ann Neurol 1990;28:187.

Johnson R, Clay S, Arnon S. Diagnosis and management of infant botulism. Am J Dis Child 1979;133:586.

Lefvert A, Osterman P. Newborn infants to myasthenic mothers: A clinical study and an investigation of acetylcholine receptor antibodies in 17 children. Neurology 1983;33:133.

Long S. Botulism in infancy. Pediatr Infect Dis J 1984;3:266.

Matthes J, Kenna A, Fawcett P. Familial infantile myasthenia: A diagnostic problem. Dev Med Child Neurol 1991;33:924.

Papazian O. Transient neonatal myasthenia gravis. J Child Neurol 1992;7:135.

Pickett J, Berg B, Chaplin E, et al. Syndrome of botulism in infancy: Clinical and electrophysiological study. N Engl J Med 1976;295:770.

Roach E, Buono G, McLean W, et al. Early onset myasthenia gravis. J Pediatr 1986;108:193.

Rodriquez M, Gomez M, Howard F, Taylor W. Myasthenia gravis in children: Long-term follow-up. Ann Neurol 1983;13:504.

Snead V, Benton J, Dwyer D, et al. Juvenile myasthenia gravis. Neurology 1980;30:732.

Swaiman K, Wright F. The practice of pediatric neurology, ed 2. St Louis: Mosby-Year Book, 1982.

Swift TR. Disorders of neuromuscular transmission other than myasthenia gravis. Muscle Nerve 1981;4:334.

Vincent A, Cull-Candy S, Newsom-Davis J, et al. Congenital myasthenia: Endplate acetylcholine receptors and electrophysiology in five cases. Muscle Nerve 1981;4:306.

*Principles and Practice of Pediatrics, Second Edition.*
edited by Frank A. Oski et al. J. B. Lippincott Company, Philadelphia © 1994.

## CHAPTER 159
# *Hereditary and Acquired Types of Myopathy*

## Darryl C. De Vivo and Salvatore DiMauro

Molecular genetics has revolutionized our current understanding of neuromuscular diseases. The inherited conditions embrace all patterns of heredity, both mendelian and non-mendelian. The term *muscular dystrophy* is used to describe a group of conditions that are inherited, progressive, and characterized by myodegeneration. Other conditions are referred to as types of *myopathy,* such as congenital myopathy (eg, central core disease) or metabolic myopathy. In general, forms of metabolic myopathy are classified according to the involved pathway (eg, types of glycogenosis, forms of mitochondrial myopathy), and the specific biochemical defect often is known. Whenever possible, these diseases are classified according to the molecular, genetic, or biochemical defect, because the phenotypic expression of one molecular defect may be quite heterogenous. Thus, Duchenne type muscular dystrophy (DMD) and Becker's muscular dystrophy (BMD) are locus diseases, as are McLeod syndrome and the dystrophy that is associated with glycerol kinase deficiency. We now know that the heterogenous phenotypes associated with a specific genetic defect may result from variable involvement of contiguous genes, depending on the size of the deleted genetic segment.

The acquired muscle disorders are classified according to etiologic factors whenever possible or by the characteristics of the tissue reaction. Hence, we use the terms inflammatory, toxic, nutritional, and endocrinologic to describe these diverse conditions.

## HEREDITARY TYPES OF DYSTROPHY

### X-Linked Diseases

#### Duchenne Type Muscular Dystrophy

DMD is the most severe form of progressive primary muscular degeneration and is associated with a genetic abnormality in band 1 of region 2 of the short (p) arm of the X chromosome. This genetic locus is designated Xp2.1. About 1:3000 liveborn males have this condition, with one third of all cases representing new mutations. The dystrophy is manifest at birth, becomes clinically evident between 3 and 5 years of age, and progresses inexorably over the next 2 decades before culminating in the death of the patient. Most patients become wheelchair dependent between 10 and 12 years of age. Complications result from cardiac involvement, nervous system involvement, musculoskeletal deformities, and failing respiratory function. Levels of serum enzymes that originate from skeletal muscle are elevated, most notably creatine kinase (CK). The CK value is very high after birth and remains remarkably elevated during the presymptomatic phase, permitting early diagnosis of siblings at risk. Rarely, the infant is affected clinically. Infant macroglossia has been noted on occasion and motor milestones may be delayed. One third of patients with DMD are late walkers, that is, they do not walk in-

dependently until after 15 to 18 months of age. Parents retrospectively report developmental clumsiness and motor sluggishness in running, climbing stairs, rising from the ground after falling, and pedaling a tricycle. Abnormalities of gait and posture appear in middle childhood with the emergence of increasing lumbar lordosis, pelvic waddling, frequent falling, and Gowers' sign. Although it is distinctive in DMD, Gowers' sign may be seen in patients with any condition that causes pelvic girdle weakness. Enlargement of the musculature becomes evident, with characteristic involvement of calf, gluteal, lateral vastus, deltoid, and infraspinatus groups. Weakness is more evident in the proximal muscles, and tendon reflexes are diminished at the knees, biceps, and triceps. Only in the preterminal phase are the distal tendon reflexes noticeably affected. Contractures of the iliotibial bands, hip flexors, and heel cords develop before ambulation is lost. After ambulation is lost, the muscles decrease in size, contractures progress with loss of joint mobility, and kyphoscoliosis develops with further compromise of respiratory function.

Cardiac involvement is evident in all patients with DMD, but rarely is the cause of death. Similarly, cardiac abnormalities may be noted in female carriers of DMD, even when the serum CK values are normal. Degenerating muscle fibers and small foci of fibrosis are scattered throughout the myocardium and conduction systems. The posterobasal region and adjacent lateral wall of the left ventricle are involved commonly and prominently. The electrocardiographic (ECG) changes are distinctive: tall right precordial R waves and deep Q waves in the left precordial and limb leads.

Nervous system involvement has been recognized since the earliest descriptions of DMD. It is a nonprogressive process and may be associated with "atrophy" of the brain on computed tomography (CT). Some patients also have macrocephaly. The mean intelligence quotient (IQ) is about 80, and the individual IQ values correspond to a gaussian, bell-shaped distribution curve. It is not known whether the associated mental retardation is another example of a contiguous gene syndrome.

The electromyogram (EMG) is distinctively myopathic, with decreases in the amplitude and duration of the compound action potential and enrichment of the interference pattern. A large number of the motor units are polyphasic, and occasional sparse fibrillation potentials are observed consistently. Sensory and motor conduction velocities are normal.

The histopathologic abnormalities seen in the various types of muscular dystrophy are distinctive, but are not specific for any entity. Necrosis and regeneration dominate the histopathologic findings in biopsy samples from young patients with DMD, and end-stage biopsy samples obtained from patients with preterminal disease reveal replacement with fat cells and fibrous tissue. Groups of necrotic degenerating fibers are the most prominent early features in DMD. These clusters of necrotic cells are invaded by phagocytes, and the infiltration is followed by active regeneration. A variation in fiber size becomes evident, with small atrophic fibers adjacent to hypertrophied elements. Some of the large fibers are hypercontracted or have undergone hyalinization. Endomysial and perimysial connective tissue gradually increases with disease progression. Plasma membrane defects have been seen by electron microscopy in non-necrotic muscle fibers and are thought to represent an early or possibly basic change in DMD. The basal lamina overlying the plasma membrane defect is normal.

The etiology of DMD is genetic, but the pathophysiology remains obscure. This will not be the case much longer, however, because antibodies now are available for the gene product. The protein, termed *dystrophin,* has a molecular weight of 440 kd, and its structure and function are expected to be elucidated in the near future. DMD and its allelic variants then will be definable by immunochemical methods, and more rational therapeutic interventions can be contemplated. The traditional methods of care will remain applicable until the disease can be prevented from appearing or progressing. Family counseling, physical therapy, proper use of orthotic devices, selective surgical interventions to treat joint contractures and spinal deformities, and dietary management are important interventions that will improve the quality and length of life for patients with DMD. Clinical trials of promising therapeutic regimens have been conducted during the past several years by the Collaborative Investigation of Duchenne Dystrophy (CIDD) group sponsored by the Muscular Dystrophy Association. The CIDD group has documented carefully the clinical course of DMD and has developed rigorous protocols to assess the efficacy of various drugs and hormones in its treatment.

The differential diagnosis of DMD includes autosomal recessive limb-girdle dystrophy presenting in early life (Tunisian form), BMD, Emery-Dreifuss dystrophy, congenital muscular dystrophy, muscle carnitine deficiency, the childhood form of acid maltase deficiency, and juvenile spinal muscular atrophy (Kugelberg-Welander syndrome). Females with clinical features of DMD must undergo genetic and cardiologic examination. These patients may represent sporadic cases of autosomal recessive limb-girdle dystrophy, manifesting carriers of DMD or genuine examples of DMD resulting from selective chromosomal aberrations. These aberrations include Turner's syndrome (*XO* karyotype), mosaic states (*X/XX* or *X/XX/XXX*), a structurally abnormal X chromosome, or an X-autosomal translocation.

The diagnosis of DMD can be made reliably in virtually every case with currently available information. The clinical presentation and course are constant in most instances. The CK value is very high in the preclinical phase and falls gradually as the muscle mass disappears in later years. The EMG and ECG findings are distinctive, and the morphologic findings on biopsy of the skeletal muscle are characteristic. Dystrophic immunoreactivity of muscle obtained on biopsy and analysis of blood DNA finalize the diagnosis. This constellation of clinical and laboratory findings permits the exclusion of those diseases that masquerade clinically as DMD in almost every case. The emerging molecular and biochemical advances should add measurably to our understanding of the phenotypic expressions of diseases associated with a genetic defect at the Xp2.1 locus, collectively referred to as dystrophinopathies.

### Becker's Muscular Dystrophy

Two other disorders share a genetic defect at or near the Xp2.1 locus: BMD and the McLeod syndrome. BMD represents a more benign version of DMD. Current information indicates that BMD and DMD are allelic gene abnormalities. BMD is similar to DMD, but the age of onset is later and the progression is slower (Table 159-1).

Pseudohypertrophy is striking and pes cavus deformities are present frequently in patients with BMD. Unlike in DMD, cardiac and nervous system involvement are unusual. Patients with BMD may have children, although infertility is higher in this population. All female progeny are obligate carriers and all sons are unaffected.

The EMG in patients with BMD is distinctly myopathic, but neurogenic features also may be present. Results of muscle biopsy are compatible with a dystrophic process, but neurogenic atrophy may be seen in half the cases. It is believed that the neurogenic features could result from muscle fiber splitting. Dystrophic immunoreactivity is present in muscle obtained on biopsy, but there are discontinuities in the subsarcolemmic staining pattern. DNA deletions or point mutations are "inframe," allowing for the synthesis of a truncated mutant protein. The serum CK values are elevated, but to a less striking degree than in patients with DMD.

Differentiating between BMD and limb-girdle muscular dystrophy may be difficult in sporadic cases. Calf hypertrophy often is more marked and persistent in patients with BMD. Loss of ambulation is the single best discriminator between DMD and BMD (see Table 159-1). Contractures, a rigid spine, and the absence of pseudohypertrophy help to distinguish Emery-Dreifuss muscular dystrophy from BMD. The treatment approaches and genetic counseling are similar to those for DMD.

### McLeod Syndrome

The McLeod syndrome has been viewed by some as the minimal expression of the Xp2.1 gene abnormality. The gene encoding the Kx antigens in the Kell red blood cell antigen system is contiguous to the DMD locus. McLeod syndrome is manifested by absence of the Kx antigens, hemolytic anemia, acanthocytosis, elevated serum CK activity, and a benign, nonprogressive myopathy. The skeletal muscle biopsy reveals muscle fiber necrosis and regeneration. One classic patient had the genetic misfortune of suffering from chronic granulomatous disease, McLeod red cell phenotype, DMD, retinitis pigmentosa, idiopathic intestinal pseudo-obstruction, and mental retardation. The McLeod syndrome may be confused with polymyositis.

### Emery-Dreifuss Syndrome

Emery-Dreifuss syndrome also is inherited as an X-linked recessive condition. This disease begins in early childhood and progresses very slowly. Weakness is evident first in the legs, with later involvement of the pectoral girdle. Contractures of the elbows and heel cords are prominent, and early features and rigidity of the spine also may be present. Distal muscles are spared and there is no pseudohypertrophy. Atrial conduction abnormalities may occur and, ultimately, the cardiac involvement may result in sudden death. The serum CK values are elevated moderately. Scoliosis and hyperextension of the cervical vertebrae are conspicuous features in the rigid spine syndrome, a form of congenital muscular dystrophy. It is not certain that Emery-Dreifuss syndrome and rigid spine syndrome differ genetically, but the gene defect for Emery-Dreifuss syndrome is being cloned, and the answer to this question should be forthcoming.

## Autosomal Types of Dystrophy

The generalized types of dystrophy that are inherited in an autosomal manner include the various forms of myotonia, periodic paralysis, and congenital dystrophy.

### Types of Myotonia

The types of myotonia are divided into two groups: progressive and nonprogressive. Myotonic dystrophy is the only progressive disorder. The nonprogressive disorders include myotonia congenita, paramyotonia, and a number of atypical myotonic disorders.

Myotonic dystrophy follows a pattern of autosomal dominant inheritance. Gene mapping studies have localized the defect to the long arm of chromosome 19. The unstable gene mutation is an expanding trinucleotide sequence. This amplification correlates with the clinical phenomenon of anticipation. The gene product

| TABLE 159-1. | Age (y) of Onset, Loss of Ambulation, and Death in BMD and DMD | |
|---|---|---|
| Clinical Event | DMD | BMD |
| Onset | 3–5 | 12 |
| Loss of ambulation | 9.0 ± 2.3 | 30.5 ± 12.0 |
| Death | 16.2 ± 3.7 | 42.0 ± 15.9 |

is unknown, but the molecular basis for the myotonia appears to involve abnormal sodium channel function. In general, patients with myotonic dystrophy do not complain of their myotonia, and infants with congenital myotonic dystrophy have no clinical or electrical evidence of the disorder. In contrast, patients with the nonprogressive forms of myotonia are aware of their disease and are bothered by this symptom, and myotonia can be demonstrated in infancy. The clinical manifestations of myotonic dystrophy are protean, and this disorder is viewed more properly as a systemic disorder with muscle involvement. Virtually all systems are involved in this condition. Severe brain involvement may occur in the congenital form and adults have mental deterioration. Smooth, striated, and cardiac muscle tissues are affected. Myotonia involves striated muscle and anal sphincter; smooth muscle involvement has been seen in the gastrointestinal tract, gallbladder, uterus, ureter, and ciliary body of the eye. Endocrine disturbances include testicular tubular atrophy, pituitary dysfunction, and diabetes mellitus associated with peripheral insulin resistance. Baldness and cataracts are common, as is hypogammaglobulinemia. Cataracts are represented as multicolored subcapsular opacities that are visualized best by slit lamp examination.

Virtually all affected infants with congenital myotonic dystrophy have their mother as the affected parent, despite the fact that the gene is transmitted as an autosomal dominant trait. Numerous complications of pregnancy have been recognized, including an increased rate of spontaneous abortion, reduced fetal movements, polyhydramnios, uterine inertia during labor, and postpartum hemorrhage (often associated with retained placental fragments). Neonatal mortality is increased and the infant displays numerous abnormal features. Neonatal respiratory distress, paralyzed diaphragm, hypotonia, bilateral facial weakness, talipes, and delayed motor and mental retardation are common clinical features. Myotonia is conspicuously absent and is not clinically evident until later in the first decade of life. Congenital hip dislocation and hernias are the result of muscular laxity. Mild mental retardation is evident in most, if not all, affected children, and hydrocephalus has been reported in some instances. The correlation between maternal myotonic dystrophy and the congenital form of the disease is overwhelming, but unexplained. An expansion of the CTG triplet repeat at the 3′ end of the gene located on chromosome 19q 13.3 is the molecular basis for this disease. Clinical anticipation in successive generations is associated with an increasing number of nucleotide triplet repeats.

The muscle histopathology of myotonic dystrophy is distinctive. Type I fiber atrophy and centrally placed nuclei are characteristic, even in the congenital form. These and other findings suggest an arrest in muscle development: hypoplasia rather than active degeneration. Other common features include ringed fibers, sarcoplasmic masses, and nuclear chains.

The nonprogressive types of myotonia as a group are rare, and the symptomatology is limited to skeletal muscle, unlike myotonic muscular dystrophy. Myotonia congenita is an autosomal dominant trait first described in detail by Thomsen in 1876. Thomsen himself and his affected relatives were particularly troubled by myotonic involvement of the hands, legs, and eyelids. Myotonia appears in infancy and muscular hypertrophy is evident. Becker later sorted out the autosomal dominant (Thomsen) form of nonprogressive myotonia from the recessive form, in which generalized myotonia first appears in early to middle childhood. Muscular hypertrophy is even more striking in the recessive form of the disease. Subtle weakness also may be present. The results of laboratory studies are unremarkable in patients with the nonprogressive types of myotonia, with only occasional minor histopathologic changes evident in skeletal muscle obtained on biopsy. Absence of the muscle fiber 2B subpopulation has been reported. The muscle changes may be more obvious in par-

amyotonia, a rare, autosomal dominant, myotonic condition that is exacerbated by cold exposure.

Treatment of the various types of myotonia is directed toward their symptoms, and toward the debilitating features of myotonic dystrophy specifically. The myotonia may be relieved with quinine sulfate, procainamide, or phenytoin. Fortunately, patients with myotonic muscular dystrophy seldom complain of the myotonia, and treatment of the condition is indicated less frequently. Quinine sulfate and procainamide may be hazardous when given to patients with cardiac conduction disturbances. Patients with the nonprogressive types of myotonia do not have cardiac involvement, but are very troubled and disabled by the myotonia.

Patients with myotonic dystrophy need general medical supervision and support. Cardiac conduction disturbances and sensitivity to various anesthetics may be life-threatening. Medical and rehabilitative intervention, insertion of cardiac pacemakers, treatment of respiratory problems, and the use of various orthotic devices are helpful.

## The Periodic Paralyses

Numerous conditions of diverse etiology may result in periodic paralysis. High or low serum potassium values often are associated with this syndrome. The primary periodic paralyses are inherited as an autosomal dominant trait, whereas the secondary disorders result from acquired conditions that perturb body water and electrolyte status or thyroid function. The genetically determined conditions are associated with modest disturbances of potassium homeostasis, in contrast to the nongenetic conditions. Thyrotoxic periodic paralysis resembles hypokalemic periodic paralysis. It is remarkably more common in males (6 : 1) and Asians (3 : 1). The condition is sporadic and resolves with effective treatment of the hyperthyroidism.

The primary periodic paralyses are hypokalemic, hyperkalemic, and normokalemic. A fourth, and rarer, form of periodic paralysis is associated with a bidirectional ventricular tachycardic dysrhythmia.

The hypokalemic form presents in middle to late childhood. During the attack, there is a modest fall in the serum potassium level and in urinary retention of sodium, potassium, chloride, and water. These electrolyte changes can produce a characteristic ECG change. The attacks may be provoked by the ingestion of carbohydrate or sodium, or by excitement. The attacks initially are infrequent, but daily attacks may occur during early adulthood. The episodes decrease in frequency in late adulthood, but older patients may have a fixed limb weakness. Glucose-insulin infusion may provoke an attack, and oral potassium salts attenuate the episode. These findings are diagnostic of the condition.

The hyperkalemic form also is inherited as an autosomal dominant trait with initial presentation during the first or second decade of life. There is a modest rise in the serum potassium value during the attack, accompanied by a kaliuresis. Some patients have myotonia involving facial, lingual, thenar, or finger extensor muscles; others do not. The presence of myotonia in a subset of patients with hyperkalemic periodic paralysis suggests genetic linkage with paramyotonia congenita. This apparent association will be resolved when the genetic basis of these clinically diverse conditions is understood. Primary hyperkalemic periodic paralysis can be provoked by the oral administration of potassium chloride.

The normokalemic form is more debatable as a distinct nosologic entity. Again, as with the other primary forms, it is transmitted as an autosomal dominant trait with onset in childhood. It is provoked by potassium loading (in some families, but not others), exposure to cold, alcohol, and rest after physical activity. Glucose administration has no effect, but sodium loading may improve the weakness.

The periodic paralysis that is associated with cardiac tachycardic dysrhythmias also has some heterogenous elements. It is inherited, possibly as a dominant trait, but the total number of reported cases is only six. Three cases were thought to be hyperkalemic, one normokalemic, and one hypokalemic. Dysmorphic features have been described, including short stature, clinodactyly, microcephaly, midfacial hypoplasia, low-set ears, and cryptorchidism. The cardiac dysrhythmia potentially is fatal. Two patients have died suddenly.

The muscle biopsy sample often reveals few or no abnormalities in patients with the periodic paralyses during the early symptomatic years, even during a paralytic episode. Later, a distinctive vacuolar myopathy develops. These biopsy changes often correlate with fixed limb weakness.

Lack of electrical excitability of the muscle fiber surface membrane is common to the various forms of primary periodic paralysis, and an abnormality of the sodium channel characterizes the electrophysiologic study results in patients with paramyotonia congenita and those with hyperkalemic periodic paralysis. The resting membrane potential, studied in vitro, is reduced in patients with primary hypokalemic periodic paralysis and in those with the acquired form associated with thyrotoxicosis. It is known that both insulin and thyroid hormone increase the activity of the sodium-potassium pump, but this information does not facilitate an understanding of the clinical symptomatology associated with modest decreases in serum potassium values.

Treatment begins with accurate diagnosis of the syndrome. Aggravating environmental factors must be avoided to minimize the frequency and intensity of the attacks. Acetazolamide is the preferred drug for both the hypokalemic and hyperkalemic forms of primary periodic paralysis; it also may be useful in the paralysis that is associated with cardiac dysrhythmias. Treatment of the paralysis, however, may worsen the cardiac disturbance. Imipramine has been useful in one patient in controlling the dysrhythmia. Acetazolamide is ineffective in treating the paralysis that is associated with hyperthyroidism. Propranolol is helpful, but control of the thyroid disease is more important.

### Congenital Types of Muscular Dystrophy

Many primary diseases of muscle may present in early infancy, but only a few are referred to as congenital types of muscular dystrophy. This distinction, therefore, is arbitrary, and to some degree confusing. The conditions discussed here are two syndromes that cause dystrophic changes in skeletal muscle examined by biopsy. These syndromes are distinguished by the presence or absence of nervous system pathology.

Congenital muscular dystrophy without nervous system involvement appears to be inherited as an autosomal recessive trait, although many cases are sporadic. The infants are weak at birth and hypotonia is present often, although not invariably. Similarly, joint contractures frequently accompany the weakness. Respiratory difficulties may be present and largely determine the outcome. The "dystrophic" process itself is rather stationary, in part controverting the use of the term. The infants do reasonably well if they survive past infancy. Weakness does not progress in any measurable way, but orthopedic complications may supervene and require therapeutic intervention. The laboratory abnormalities are variable. The CK values often are elevated, but only modestly in most cases. The EMG is distinctly myopathic and fibrillations are scarce. The muscle tissue is abnormal, with fiber diameter variability and an abundance of endomysial and perimysial connective tissue. Necrosis of single muscle fibers is quite unusual.

The clinical course of the patient is influenced largely by the respiratory complications that develop. The muscle disease appears to be primarily nonprogressive in most patients, and many of these children are very bright. Aggressive support and orthopedic corrective surgery is warranted in any child who has survived past infancy. The pathophysiology underlying this genetic disorder is unknown.

Congenital muscular dystrophy with nervous system pathology has a less favorable prognosis. Fukuyama and associates emphasized this disorder in 1960, and it often is referred to as the Fukuyama syndrome. In Japan, the birth incidence of Fukuyama congenital dystrophy is about half that of DMD. Mothers of affected infants report decreased fetal movements and the newborn is weak and hypotonic. Sucking efforts and crying are weak, and there is decreased facial expression. The calves may be enlarged and contractures of the knee joints and elbows are common; tendon reflexes are decreased or absent. Generalized convulsions may occur in half of the patients, and motor retardation is evident during later development. Many children eventually sit or crawl, but few are able to walk. Atrophy of limb muscles is increasingly evident, and most children die within the first decade.

The serum CK values are elevated 10- to 50-fold in most instances and the EMG is distinctly myopathic. The skeletal muscle examined at biopsy is abnormal, with variation of fiber type diameter, necrosis of fibers, scattered foci of inflammation, and increased endomysial and perimysial connective tissue. The neuropathology is equally remarkable and descriptive of altered neuronal migration and cortical sulcation. The cortex is thick and smooth, particularly in the temporal and occipital regions. These findings are indicative of lissencephaly or polymicrogyria. There is reduced central white matter and associated cerebral ventricular enlargement. The pathogenesis of this autosomal recessive condition is unknown. Therapy is largely supportive, with anticonvulsant drugs being necessary to control the seizures.

## Localized Types of Dystrophy

A number of forms of muscular dystrophy are characterized by localized muscular involvement. These syndromes may preferentially involve the limb girdle musculature, the facioscapulohumeral (FSH) groups, the scapular and peroneal groups, the distal limb musculature, the extraocular muscles, or the oropharyngeal muscles. Most of these categories are quite heterogenous and phenotypic features are varied.

### Limb-Girdle Syndromes

Walton and Nattrass, in 1954, introduced the term *limb-girdle muscular dystrophy* to describe a number of patients who did not fulfill the clinical criteria for DMD or FSH dystrophy. The patients were either male or female, often were in middle to late childhood, and had serum enzyme, EMG, and skeletal muscle biopsy abnormalities of the type commonly encountered in patients with a muscular dystrophy. This large and ill-defined group of patients has been whittled down in the past 4 decades to a much smaller group as newer entities have been identified. We now recognize juvenile spinal muscular atrophy, congenital types of myopathy (eg, central core disease), and metabolic forms of myopathy, all of which previously were classified as limb-girdle muscular dystrophy. A small group of patients still exists who have a dystrophic process that is inherited as an autosomal recessive trait, however, justifying continued use of the term. Some of these patients will prove to have Xp2.1 locus genetic defects presenting in males or females. The availability of a biochemical probe for various types of dystrophy will help sort out these issues in the near future. For the moment, the term *limb-girdle* represents a convenient diagnostic pigeonhole when other diagnostic explanations fall short.

### Facioscapulohumeral Dystrophy

The syndrome of FSH dystrophy and its variants are inherited as autosomal dominant traits, and their expression may be quite variable, even among family members. As the term implies, facial, periscapular, and humeral muscle groups are affected. Unlike most forms of dystrophy, involvement may be asymmetric and an isolated congenital absence of a muscle may occur. The condition generally is benign, presenting in adolescence and progressing slowly over decades, often with periods of clinical arrest. A few cases have started in infancy with a more malignant course. Initial presentation as Möbius' syndrome with congenital facial weakness also has been described. Early childhood onset may be associated with a sensorineural hearing loss or an exudative telangiectasia of the retina (Coats' disease). The clinical presentation in childhood, however, usually is more subtle. Patients may sleep with their eyes partially open and have difficulty whistling or sipping through a straw. One variant is known as the scapuloperoneal syndrome; scapular winging and footdrop are common signs. Subtle weakness of the facial muscles may coexist or develop later.

The pathogenesis of these syndromes is obscure. Some cases seem to have myopathic elements and others are distinctly neurogenic. The biopsy samples also may have some prominent inflammatory features, raising the question of an inflammatory myopathy and justifying a clinical trial with corticosteroids. In some patients, surgical fixation of the scapulae to the posterior thoracic wall improves shoulder-girdle function.

### Distal Limb Syndromes

Distal muscle syndromes are distinctly rare at all ages and particularly so in children. Welander described a Swedish family with distal weakness in several generations that was transmitted as an autosomal dominant trait. Symptoms became manifest in adulthood, although onset in early childhood has been described. The hands and forearms are affected primarily. Progression of the disorder is slow and serum enzyme values are normal.

### Ocular Syndromes

Eye involvement may be isolated (ocular myopathy) or combined with pharyngeal dysfunction (oculopharyngeal dystrophy). Many other conditions, such as thyroid disease, inflammatory disorders, myasthenia gravis, and mitochondrial disorders, also cause ocular muscle dysfunction. The two genetic forms of ocular dystrophy usually are transmitted as autosomal dominant traits. The onset typically is in middle adulthood and progression of the disease is slow. Serum CK values are normal. Ocular dystrophy is manifested by ptosis and weakness of facial and proximal limb musculature. Early manifestations may be evident in late childhood. Oculopharyngeal dystrophy develops much later, with ptosis and dysphagia. Eye, facial, and limb-girdle muscles are less involved. These conditions are distinctly rare and should not be confused with congenital ptosis, which is benign, nonprogressive, and often unilateral.

## HEREDITARY TYPES OF MYOPATHY

### Congenital Types of Myopathy

A group of neuromuscular diseases exists that present in early infancy, are inherited as mendelian traits, and are recognized by distinctive histochemical abnormalities. These disorders often are referred to as benign, nonprogressive forms of myopathy. They are not invariably nonprogressive, however, and it is not certain that the defect is intrinsic to the muscle fiber. As a group of disorders, there is considerable overlap in phenotypic expression. Congenital hip dislocation, kyphoscoliosis, infantile hypotonia, and decreased responsiveness of tendon reflexes are common clinical features. The distinctive histochemical abnormality involves the type I muscle fiber exclusively or preferentially. CK values and nerve conduction velocities are normal, and the EMG shows brief, abundant, polyphasic potentials of short duration and low amplitude.

Central core disease was the first entity to be described in this group of disorders. Shy and Magee, in 1956, studied five family members who had been slow in learning to walk and continued to have mild weakness throughout life. Several members had congenital dislocation of the hips. The genetic pattern was consistent with an autosomal dominant trait. The muscle biopsy in all five individuals revealed a unique alteration. The central core of myofibrils was compacted and amorphous, and the results of oxidative enzyme stains were negative in this region. Electron microscopy demonstrated relatively normal-appearing myofibrils, with no mitochondria in the central core region. This disorder increases the risk of malignant hyperthermia.

Multicore (minicore) disease also has been described in a few cases. Fibers of both types contain the multicore pattern. Siblings and male twins also have been described with these histologic abnormalities.

Nemaline myopathy was the second entity to be described in this group of diseases. In 1963, Shy, Engel, Somers, and Wanko reported a clinical syndrome of infantile hypotonia, muscular hypoplasia, mild weakness, reduced or absent tendon reflexes, and relative sparing of intelligence. Subsarcolemmic accumulations of rod-like structures were present and were seen more commonly in the type I fibers. The rods were similar to Z disk material, from which they presumably are derived. Females are affected more often, but the genetic pattern is autosomal dominant or recessive. The weakness is relatively nonprogressive, but death may result from respiratory failure. Dysmorphic features are more characteristic in nemaline myopathy, including elongated facial features, high-arched palate, kyphoscoliosis, pectus excavatum, and pes cavus.

Myotubular (centronuclear) myopathy was the third of these diseases to be described. Several investigators have suggested that this disorder may represent an arrest in embryonic muscle development. Rows of centrally placed nuclei are characteristic, predominantly in type I fibers. Type I fiber predominance and hypotrophy also may coexist.

The clinical syndrome is more varied in myotubular myopathy and can be life-threatening. Prenatal onset of the disorder is suggested by diminished fetal movements. The postnatal presentation may vary, with one group of patients being weak at birth. Motor development is slow, respiratory effort may be compromised, and death may occur before the child reaches 3 years of age. Generalized weakness is evident, with preferential involvement of eye, facial, and neck muscles. A second group of patients is detected in early childhood with a gait abnormality and difficulty in climbing stairs. Focal or generalized seizures may coexist in this group. Other patients may not have symptoms until the second or third decade of life.

The combination of ophthalmoparesis and facial diplegia is distinctive in children with myotubular myopathy. Genetic transmission is variable from one family to another, including autosomal dominant or X-linked recessive patterns. Some have segregated type I muscle fiber hypotrophy with central nuclei from myotubular myopathy as a separate entity, but the distinctions may be only apparent.

Since 1966, numerous abnormalities have been added to the list of disorders, all based on distinctive histochemical features. This list includes sarcotubular myopathy, fingerprint body myopathy, reducing body myopathy, cytoplasmic body myopathy, zebra body myopathy, trilaminar body myopathy, congenital fiber-type disproportion, lysis of myofibrils and type I fibers, and myopathy with peripheral crescents. The difficulty with these diseases is the fact that more clinical features are shared than not. Therefore, it is difficult to make a diagnosis on clinical grounds alone, and a muscle biopsy is essential to characterize the distinctive histopathologic features. EMG is of limited value, and the findings generally are nonspecific. Serum enzyme values and nerve conduction velocities usually are normal.

Rehabilitative efforts should be undertaken and respiratory function should be protected, particularly during intercurrent illnesses. A cuirass may be helpful in compromised patients during pulmonary infection. The patient may use the cuirass at night to obtain adequate rest. Some patients may have difficulty with negative pressure units because of laxity of pharyngeal muscles and resulting obstructive apnea. Oximetry used in conjunction with the cuirass is an effective way to monitor airway patency under these circumstances. Annual vaccination for the influenza viruses is an important preventive measure.

## Metabolic Types of Myopathy

### Types of Glycogenoses

Eleven distinct enzyme defects are known to affect glycogen metabolism (Fig 159-1). Nine of these defects affect muscle directly: type II, acid maltase deficiency (Pompe's disease); type III, debrancher deficiency (Cori-Forbes disease); type IV, brancher deficiency (Andersen's disease); type V, myophosphorylase deficiency (McArdle's disease); type VII, muscle phosphofructokinase (PFK) deficiency (Tarui disease); type VIII, the autosomal recessive form of phosphorylase kinase deficiency; type IX, phosphogly-

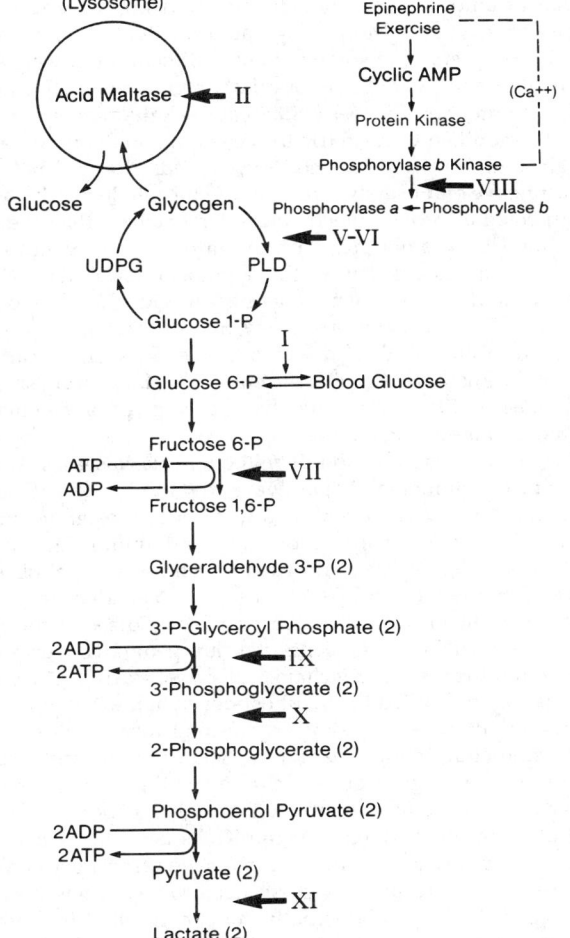

**Figure 159-1.** Schematic representation of glycogen metabolism and glycolysis. The Roman numerals indicate the sites of documented enzyme defects. *I,* glucose-6-phosphatase; *II,* acid maltase; *III,* debranching, *IV,* branching; *V,* muscle phosphorylase kinase; *IX,* phosphoglycerate kinase; *X,* phosphoglycerate mutase; *XI,* lactate dehydrogenase. *PLD,* phosphorylase-limit dextrin; *UDPG,* uridine diphosphate glucose; *AMP,* adenosine monophosphate; *ATP,* adenosine triphosphate; *ADP,* adenosine diphosphate.

cerate kinase (PGK) deficiency; type X, phosphoglycerate mutase (PGAM) deficiency; and type XI, lactic dehydrogenase (LDH) deficiency.

*Type II: Acid Maltase Deficiency.*    Two major clinical syndromes are associated with acid maltase deficiency. The first syndrome (Pompe's disease) presents in early infancy and is associated with death before 1 year of age. The clinical picture is distinctive, with infantile hypotonia, weakness, areflexia, macroglossia, massive cardiomegaly, and moderate hepatomegaly. The infant is alert and there is little clinical measure of central nervous system dysfunction. Death results from cardiac and pulmonary failure. The peripheral lymphocytes contain vacuoles that are positive on periodic acid–Schiff staining, and acid maltase activity is virtually absent in all tissues. The condition is transmitted as an autosomal recessive trait. The glycogen content is increased in all tissues, with the predominant accumulation occurring within lysosomes. The presence of much free glycogen in tissues also has been noted, however.

The serum CK values are elevated moderately and the EMG is myopathic, with bizarre high-frequency pseudomyotonic discharges. The potentials are polyphasic and the interference pattern is reduced. Chest radiographs reveal massive cardiomegaly. The ECG demonstrates a shortened PR interval, depressed ST segments, and inverted T waves. Muscle biopsy reveals a severe vacuolar myopathy with material that is positive on periodic acid–Schiff staining stored in lysosomes and increased free glycogen particles present in the cytoplasm. In the nervous system, glycogen accumulates in glial and neuronal cell bodies. The anterior horn cells are engorged with glycogen. Severe involvement of brain stem and spinal motor neurons contributes to the clinical appearance of spinal muscular atrophy with weakness, hypotonia, and areflexia. There is no effective treatment, but prenatal diagnosis and genetic counseling are available.

The second syndrome associated with acid maltase deficiency is a more benign neuromuscular disorder that presents in childhood or early adulthood. This syndrome usually is limited to skeletal muscle, with progressive weakness and respiratory insufficiency. The condition in early childhood simulates DMD, with calf enlargement and Gowers' sign. The serum CK values may range from 200 to 2000 IU/L and the EMG results are distinctly abnormal. In the adult form, the clinical appearance may be confused with that of limb-girdle dystrophy or chronic polymyositis. Cardiac function is normal in patients with the childhood and adult versions of acid maltase deficiency. Mental retardation coexists occasionally in the childhood form.

*Type III: Debrancher Deficiency.*    Type III deficiency results from a deficiency of amylo-1,6-glucosidase. The classic presentation in infancy is one of fasting hypoglycemia, ketonuria, growth retardation, and hepatomegaly. Patients are weak and hypotonic, and have poor head control. These signs usually remit gradually around the time of puberty, although a few patients exhibit slowly progressive weakness into adult life. The muscle biopsy sample reveals a severe vacuolar myopathy with storage of glycogen. Weakness commonly is more evident in the proximal groups, but distal wasting may be quite noticeable and suggestive of a motor neuron disease or chronic neuropathy. Motor nerve conduction velocities actually may be decreased, and the EMG may contain a mixed pattern, including fibrillations, positive sharp waves, and myotonic discharges. The nervous system and heart are spared clinically in this disease. No effective treatment is available for this autosomal recessive condition.

*Type IV: Brancher Deficiency.*    Type IV deficiency is the result of a deficiency of the enzyme amylo-1,4-1-6-transglucosidase. It is a rapidly progressive, fatal condition that is manifested by hepatosplenomegaly, progressive cirrhosis, and chronic liver failure. Death often occurs in late infancy or early childhood. Some of the patients may appear to have infantile spinal muscular atrophy with hypotonia, weakness, and areflexia. There is no effective therapy for this autosomal recessive condition.

*Type V: Myophosphorylase Deficiency.* Myophosphorylase deficiency was the first glycogenosis to be described. McArdle, in 1951, reported a syndrome associated with weakness, fatigue, and muscle cramping with pain after exercising. He also observed a lack of lactic acid production by the exercising muscle and proposed a defect in glycolysis. Intense exercise may lead to muscle necrosis and myoglobinuria in patients with myophosphorylase deficiency. Irreversible renal failure may ensue. Most patients recover muscle function between attacks, but about 25% have some fixed weakness. Serum CK values are elevated at rest and may increase dramatically during an attack of myoglobinuria. Rarely, the condition may present as a fatal, infantile myopathy. Heart function is normal in patients with McArdle's disease. The nervous system is not involved, although seizures are more common than would be expected. Hypoglycemia and hyperventilation may be the factors that contribute to convulsions in patients with this disorder. The diagnosis is suspected when a flat lactate response to ischemic exercise is obtained, and is confirmed by examination of tissue from skeletal muscle obtained at biopsy.

Dietary manipulations may be beneficial in attenuating the symptoms of myophosphorylase deficiency. Frequent carbohydrate snacks and high-protein and high-fat meals have been touted as beneficial in ameliorating symptoms in these patients and improving their exercise tolerance. Myoglobinuria can be minimized by avoiding strenuous, prolonged physical exercise. Moderate sustained exercise leads to a "second wind" phenomenon that presumably represents a metabolic conversion from carbohydrate to fatty acids as a fuel source for skeletal muscle. This condition is transmitted as an autosomal recessive trait.

*Type VII: Muscle Phosphofructokinase Deficiency.* Type VII deficiency was described by Tarui in 1965 and resembles McArdle's disease clinically. Symptoms typically begin in the second decade and include exercise intolerance, cramps, and myoglobinuria. Three cases of a severe infantile variant of PFK deficiency have been described. One infant died at 6 months of age with respiratory complications. A sibling was delayed developmentally at 14 months of age. The third patient was a female infant with developmental retardation and corneal ulcerations. Erythrocyte PFK activities are reduced 50% in this syndrome, and it is transmitted as an autosomal recessive trait. The partial PFK deficiency that occurs in red cells may cause erythrocytosis and mild hemolytic anemia.

*Type VIII: Myophosphorylase Kinase Deficiency.* Type VIII syndrome is a rare condition, resulting from a deficiency of the kinase that converts the inactive "b" form of myophosphorylase to the active "a" form. Total phosphorylase activity is normal, but the active form represents less than 10% of the total enzyme activity. The clinical profile is that of infantile hypotonia and delayed motor development. Four patients with otherwise typical McArdle's disease also have been shown to have an apparently autosomal recessive defect of phosphorylase kinase.

*Type IX: Phosphoglycerate Kinase Deficiency.* An X-linked recessive disease, PGK deficiency commonly presents with nonspherocytic hemolytic anemia and neurologic disturbances. Patients are mentally retarded, with language delay and behavioral abnormalities. Seizures also are common. Two patients have had an isolated myopathy, with exercise-induced myoglobinuria and renal insufficiency. As in patients with other glycolytic defects, no rise in the venous lactate level is observed after forearm ischemic exercise. PGK is a single polypeptide that is encoded by a gene located on the X chromosome. There are no known tissue-specific isoenzymes.

*Type X: Phosphoglycerate Mutase Deficiency.* Apparently an autosomal recessive disorder, type X deficiency is very rare and presents with recurrent attacks of exercise-induced myoglobinuria. Affected patients are clinically well and asymptomatic between attacks. The condition results from a deficiency of the muscle-specific (M) subunit of this dimeric enzyme, which is represented in adult muscle predominantly by the homodimer PGAM-MM.

*Type XI: Lactate Dehydrogenase Deficiency.* LDH deficiency is a rare condition that is caused by the absence of the muscle-specific (M) subunit and is associated with exercise-induced myoglobinuria. One Japanese family has been studied in detail, and the findings are compatible with an autosomal recessive pattern. The LDH muscle-specific (M) subunit has been assigned to a gene on chromosome 11. Forearm ischemic exercise produces a marked rise in the pyruvate level, with little or no rise in the lactate level.

## Mitochondrial Diseases

Defects of mitochondrial metabolism are being recognized with increasing frequency. Morphologic abnormalities of mitochondria have been observed in some patients. Mitochondria were either overly abundant, very large, or misshapen. A distinctive abnormality of mitochondria was evident at the light microscopic level with the modified Gomori trichrome stain, and fibers containing this abnormality were labeled "ragged-red." Ragged-red fibers are distinctive and usually represent the morphologic counterpart of suspected or proven biochemical defects that affect the inner mitochondrial membrane. Current information suggests that ragged red fibers are seen in those mitochondrial diseases that are associated with a defect involving intramitochondrial protein synthesis. The muscle morphology may be normal in patients with other mitochondrial diseases, however, such as carnitine palmitoyl transferase (CPT) deficiency. This fact emphasizes the need for a classification scheme that is predicated on biochemical and molecular genetic criteria.

The current classification of mitochondrial diseases is based on the principal metabolic pathways that are located in this organelle and on the dual genetic control of the respiratory chain (Fig 159-2). Organic acids, fatty acids, and amino acids are the principal sources of fuel, and each substrate is metabolized to acetylcoenzyme A (acetyl-CoA). Acetyl-CoA condenses with oxaloacetate to form citric acid. Citric acid is oxidized in the Krebs cycle. The reducing equivalents that are generated during oxidation enter the respiratory chain and are reoxidized. The energy of oxidation is coupled to the phosphorylation of adenosine diphosphate, ultimately yielding adenosine triphosphate.

The mitochondrial diseases of muscle or brain can be subdivided into five major groups according to the locus of the biochemical lesion: defects of mitochondrial transport, defects of substrate utilization, defects of the Krebs cycle, defects of oxidation-phosphorylation, and defects of the respiratory chain.

Defects of the respiratory chain need to be subclassified further, because this metabolic pathway is controlled by both the nuclear genome and the mitochondrial genome. The primary molecular defect is located in the nuclear DNA in some instances, and in the mitochondrial DNA in other instances. A third group involves a primary nuclear DNA defect with a secondary disturbance of mitochondrial DNA. These conditions have been called defects of intergenomic signaling.

Primary mitochondrial DNA defects occur sporadically, or are inherited as maternal, non-mendelian traits. Maternal inheritance resembles X-linked and autosomal dominant inheritance patterns

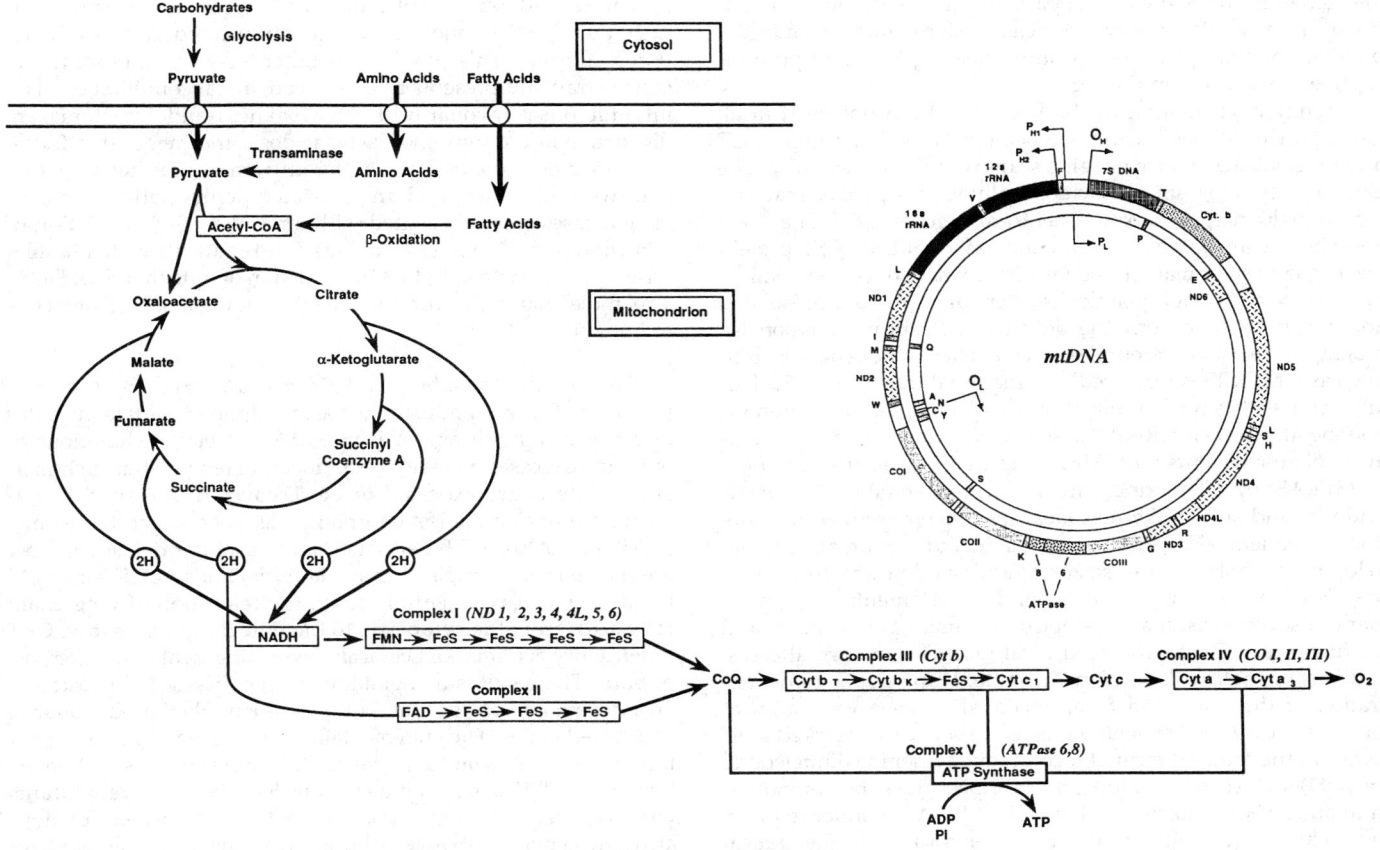

**Figure 159-2.** Pathways involved in the oxidative metabolism of mitochondrial fuels. The current classification of mitochondrial diseases is based on this scheme. Five events are important: (1) mitochondrial transport of substrates; (2) substrate utilization; (3) oxidation in the Krebs cycle; (4) oxidation-phosphorylation; and (5) cellular respiration. The mitochondrial genome is inserted in the diagram to signify its role in the respiratory chain. The 13 mtDNA-encoded subunits of the respiratory chain are shown in parentheses above complexes I, III, IV, and V. *NADH*, the reduced form of nicotinamide-adenine dinucleotide; *ATPase*, adenosine triphosphatase; *ATP*, adenosine triphosphate; *ADP*, adenosine diphosphate; *FMN*, flavin mononucleotide; *FAD*, flavin adenine dinucleotide; *CoQ*, coenzyme Q; *PI*, inorganic phosphate.

in that the maternally transmitted trait is passed from the mother to her children, and the disease appears in consecutive generations. The maternally inherited trait differs from the X-linked inherited trait because both male and female progeny inherit the condition from their mother. Similarly, the maternally inherited trait differs from the autosomal dominant trait because a higher percentage (theoretically, 100%) of the progeny are affected. The phenotypic expression of a maternally inherited trait is modulated by replicative segregation and the threshold effect. These two concepts are predicated on the fact that there are multiple mitochondrial DNA copies in each mitochondrion, and there are hundreds or thousands of mitochondria in each cell. As a result, the distribution of wild-type mitochondrial DNA and mutated mitochondrial DNA drifts randomly in each successive cell division. As the percentage of mutated mitochondrial DNA copies approaches a theoretic threshold, the cellular phenotype reflects the genotype and displays energy failure.

Kearns-Sayre syndrome is characterized by three fundamental criteria: pigmentary degeneration of the retina, ophthalmoplegia, and clinical onset before 20 years of age. Other signs often occur, including heart block, cerebellar syndrome, and an elevated cerebrospinal fluid (CSF) protein concentration in excess of 100 mg/dL. Ragged-red fibers are present in skeletal muscle obtained at biopsy and sensorineural hearing loss is frequent. Endocrine disturbances are associated with this syndrome, and short stature

is the most common problem. Diabetes mellitus and hypoparathyroidism may develop, and may contribute to fatal episodes of coma or to seizures, respectively. A spongy degeneration is seen without exception in the brain of all patients examined at autopsy. Basal ganglia calcification is observed in all patients with hypoparathyroidism. Folic acid levels are reduced in the CSF, and coenzyme Q10 concentrations in serum and muscle are decreased. Replacement therapy has been proposed on the basis of these observations. A cardiac pacemaker is necessary as therapy for heart block.

Virtually all reported cases of Kearns-Sayre syndrome have been sporadic, and about 98% of affected patients have major deletions of the mitochondrial genome. Sporadic cases of progressive external ophthalmoplegia also have been associated with these deletions, suggesting that this abnormality of ocular motility is the minimal clinical expression of Kearns-Sayre syndrome. Large mitochondrial DNA deletions also have been observed in infants with Pearson syndrome, a frequently fatal sporadic disease of infancy that is manifested by pancytopenia and pancreatic exocrine dysfunction. In addition, large mitochondrial DNA deletions have been described recently in a family with maternally inherited diabetes mellitus and deafness.

MERRF (myoclonus epilepsy and ragged-red fibers) is otherwise known as the Fukuhara syndrome. The clinical expression of this disease is dominated by myoclonus, ataxia, limb weakness, and generalized seizures. Most patients have symptoms in childhood or early adolescence. Associated signs often include dementia, optic atrophy, short stature, hearing loss, and proprioceptive sensory loss in the legs.

Spongy degeneration of the brain has been observed in all patients with MERRF who have been examined at autopsy. CT and magnetic resonance imaging scans reveal brain atrophy. The electroencephalogram characteristically shows paroxysmal epileptiform discharges that are either focal or generalized. The blood and CSF lactate values often are increased, but the CSF protein level usually is normal. Endocrine disturbances have been limited to one case of "hypothalamic disorder" and one case of isolated adrenocorticotropic hormone deficiency. Positron emission tomography revealed cerebral and cerebellar hypometabolism in one case. MERRF is inherited as a maternal trait. About 75% of affected patients have a mitochondrial DNA point mutation involving the transfer RNA *lys* gene. No effective treatment is available for patients with MERRF aside from seizure control.

MELAS (mitochondrial myopathy, encephalopathy, lactic acidosis, and stroke-like episodes) has been described in more than 70 patients. The original criteria included normal early development, short stature, seizures, and sudden onset of hemiparesis, hemianopsia, or cortical blindness. Dementia was prominent in several cases, as was episodic vomiting, headache, and hearing loss. CT scan revealed focal lucencies in several cases, and basal ganglia calcifications in some. Diffuse spongy degeneration of the brain and focal encephalomalacia were seen at autopsy. Acanthocytes were reported in one case. Marked deficiency of the reduced form of nicotinamide-adenine dinucleotide (NADH)–cytochrome c reductase (complex I) has been reported in about 35% of affected individuals. MELAS is inherited as a maternal trait, and about 80% of patients fulfilling the clinical criteria for this condition have a mitochondrial DNA point mutation involving the transfer RNA *leu(UUR)* gene. Coenzyme Q10 is beneficial in treatment, and vigorous attempts should be made to control seizure activity.

Several other conditions with mitochondrial DNA point mutations have been described. Leber's hereditary optic neuropathy (LHON), a maternally inherited condition, is associated with a mitochondrial DNA point mutation involving the ND4 subunit of complex I. About 6% of individuals carrying this single point mutation have LHON. Ten additional point mutations involving mitochondrial DNA have been reported. Patients with several of these point mutations accumulate an increasing risk for the development of LHON. A maternally inherited condition affecting skeletal muscle and the heart has been associated with a mitochondrial DNA point mutation influencing the transfer RNA *leu(UUR)* gene. A maternally inherited condition associated with neuropathy, ataxia, retinitis pigmentosa, and developmental delay has been linked with a mitochondrial DNA point mutation affecting the subunit 6 gene of adenosine triphosphate synthase (complex V). Patients with an abundance of this point mutation are seen in early infancy with the Leigh syndrome phenotype. Many additional mitochondrial DNA point mutations probably will be reported before this chapter appears in print, reflecting the explosive pace of new discoveries in this area.

Two genetically determined conditions have been reported recently in association with ragged-red fibers detected in skeletal muscle obtained at biopsy. The first is an autosomal dominant condition that is manifested by late-onset external ophthalmoparesis, progressive limb weakness, bilateral cataracts, and precocious death. Multiple mitochondrial DNA deletions have been noted in all affected family members. The nuclear gene defect apparently alters the biologic integrity of the mitochondrial genome and predisposes to multiple deletions. This condition originally was thought to have an adult onset, but it has been reported recently in children with optic atrophy and ptosis.

The second example of a nuclear DNA defect causing a mitochondrial DNA abnormality is the mitochondrial DNA depletion syndrome. This condition is inherited as an autosomal recessive trait and presents as a fatal congenital condition or as an infantile-onset myopathy. Limb weakness and hypotonia are distinctive in the setting of lactic acidosis and ragged-red fibers. Two affected patients have suffered from a fatal hepatopathy, and two others have had an associated nephropathy. The congenital cases were associated with an 83% to 98% depletion of mitochondrial DNA in skeletal muscle; the patients with infantile-onset disease had a 66% to 83% depletion of mitochondrial DNA. The molecular basis for the intergenomic signaling defect is unknown.

*Defects of Mitochondrial Transport.* Specific transport systems in the inner mitochondrial membrane facilitate the entry of molecules, as shown in Figure 159-2. Genetic alterations of these translocases have not been documented yet, but such metabolic defects are expected to be discovered. Impaired flavin-adenine dinucleotide (FAD) uptake has been suggested as one possibility. Also, CPT deficiency and carnitine deficiency now are classified as examples of mitochondrial transport defects. CPT I and CPT II play a central role in the relocation of long-chain fatty acids from the cytoplasm to the mitochondrial matrix. CPT II deficiency is unmasked clinically by fasting, prolonged exercise, or both. The result is myoglobinuria. The disease is inherited as an autosomal recessive trait, but there is a marked predominance of affected males. The enzyme deficiency is generalized, but only rarely are these symptoms referable to other organs. A hepatic form of CPT II deficiency has been described in a few infants who had recurrent hypoketotic hypoglycemia and encephalopathy. In general, however, the enzyme defect is tolerated remarkably well and treatment is based on the nutritional and exercise-related factors that are known to precipitate attacks of myoglobinuria.

Carnitine deficiency also represents an example of defective mitochondrial transport. Historically, two forms of carnitine deficiency have been discussed: one confined to muscle (myopathic) and the second involving a generalized defect in carnitine (systemic). The myopathic form involved a defect in the uptake of carnitine by muscle. Consequently, transport of long-chain fatty acids across the inner mitochondrial membrane is blocked, with resulting accumulation of neutral lipids in the cytoplasm. This lipid storage is associated with a progressive weakness that begins in childhood. The carnitine concentrations are decreased in muscle, but normal in blood and liver. A defect in the active transport of carnitine into muscle has been suspected, but never proven. More recently, patients with myopathic carnitine deficiency have been shown to have a skeletal muscle tissue–specific deficiency of short-chain acyl coenzyme A (acyl CoA) dehydrogenase. Some patients respond to carnitine supplementation or to prednisone. The mechanism of action of prednisone is unknown.

Systemic carnitine deficiency is manifested by recurrent encephalopathy that often is triggered by an intercurrent infection. This presentation is very similar to that of Reye's syndrome. Carnitine concentrations are decreased in the serum and tissues, and there is excessive urinary excretion of carnitine. The legitimacy of systemic carnitine deficiency has been questioned since its first description in 1975. Most investigators believe that other biochemical mechanisms are at play to account for the reduced body stores of carnitine. Carnitine deficiency may result from excessive urinary loss, impaired hepatic synthesis, or associated genetic defects. Secondary carnitine deficiency is recognized with organic acidurias, respiratory chain defects, and defects of beta oxidation. Carnitine depletion results from the esterification of acyl CoA compounds that accumulate in these syndromes. The acylcarnitine esters are water-soluble and are excreted in the urine, resulting in a net loss of carnitine (Fig 159-3). Several patients previously described as having systemic carnitine deficiency have been shown to have a deficiency of medium-chain acyl CoA dehydrogenase. Other patients have a genetically determined autosomal recessive carnitine-responsive cardiomyopathy resulting from a primary defect of the plasma membrane carnitine transporter system. Carnitine supplementation is lifesaving in these patients, and supplementation is recommended whenever carnitine deficiency is documented.

*Defects of Substrate Utilization.*   Pyruvate has two major metabolic fates: carboxylation to oxaloacetate or decarboxylation to acetyl-CoA. The carboxylation reaction is catalyzed by pyruvate carboxylase. A deficiency of pyruvate carboxylase is associated with failure to thrive, developmental retardation, seizures, generalized hypotonia, and lactic acidosis. The French phenotype is associated with hyperammonemia, citrullinemia, and hyperlysinemia. Patients with this phenotype synthesize no enzyme protein and die within the first 4 months of life. The North American phenotype is less severe, because a mutated enzyme protein is synthesized with some residual activity. These patients have severe mental and motor developmental delay, and die during infancy or early childhood. Only one patient with the North American phenotype developed normally with intermittent metabolic crises. Pyruvate carboxylase activity also may be impaired secondarily by a deficiency of holocarboxylase synthetase or biotinidase. Biotinidase deficiency is treated easily with large doses of biotin.

The pyruvate dehydrogenase complex (PDHC) is composed of five enzymes, two of which, a kinase and a phosphatase, regulate the activity of the complex by phosphorylation (deactivation) and dephosphorylation (activation) of the first enzyme component ($E_1$). The $E_1$ component is composed of an alpha subunit and a beta subunit. The genes for these two subunits have been cloned and their sequence determined. The alpha subunit is the site of phosphorylation involving three serine residues. The alpha subunit currently appears to be the most vulnerable genetic locus of the PDHC, and the gene for this subunit is located on the proximal portion of the short arm of the X chromosome. Syndromes of varying severity are associated with PDHC deficiency. These syndromes vary from a benign condition of intermittent ataxia to a devastating condition of congenital lactic acidosis, failure to thrive, developmental delay, generalized hypotonia, and death in early infancy. Males are affected predominantly with the fatal congenital form, whereas females exhibit primarily the chronic progressive form. These females represent manifesting carriers of an X-linked trait.

A distinctive facial dysmorphism has been described in some infants with PDHC deficiency. The dysmorphic features are similar to those described in patients with the fetal alcohol syndrome, and it has been suggested that elevated acid aldehyde levels may be a common pathogenetic mechanism linking these two disorders.

At least 13 defects of fatty acid and ketone body metabolism have been described, as shown in Figure 159-4. Some of the defects involving the carnitine cycle were discussed earlier in this section, including the membrane carnitine transporter defect and CPT II deficiency. A deficiency of CPT I has been described in about 10 patients. These patients have an illness similar to Reye's syndrome in infancy, and may have associated renal tubular acidosis. This symptom responds to treatment with medium-chain triglycerides. Only one patient has been described with a defect of the carnitine-acylcarnitine translocase. This patient and the several patients described with the membrane carnitine transporter defect have very low tissue carnitine concentrations. Patients with CPT II deficiency have normal tissue and plasma carnitine concentrations. Patients with CPT I deficiency may have normal or high carnitine concentrations. Patients with defects involving the carnitine cycle demonstrate little, if any, dicarboxylic aciduria.

In contrast, patients with defects involving beta oxidation have remarkable dicarboxylic aciduria and carnitine deficiency. Five of these defects involve the first step in beta oxidation involving the conversion of acyl CoA to alpha-, beta-unsaturated acyl CoA. Three different acyl CoA dehydrogenases have been identified acting on either long-chain, medium-chain, or short-chain activated fatty acids. All three dehydrogenases use FAD as a cofactor. Reoxidation of FAD is accomplished by two FAD-dependent electron carriers (electron transfer factor [ETF] and ETF-dehydrogenase). The electrons ultimately are transferred to coenzyme Q10, which is located centrally within the respiratory chain. Acetyl-CoA, resulting from the beta oxidation of fatty acids, enters the Krebs cycle or the HMG-CoA cycle that is important in the biosynthesis of ketone bodies.

Severe hypoglycemic hypoketotic crises developing during prolonged fasting, physical exercise, or intercurrent infections characterize the clinical presentation of most patients with defects of beta oxidation. Medium-chain acyl CoA dehydrogenase deficiency is the most common of these defects. About 150 cases of medium-chain acyl CoA dehydrogenase deficiency have been described since 1983. The clinical description is reasonably uniform, with a history of recurrent metabolic crises in infancy or childhood, often triggered by infectious episodes and poor feeding. Hypoglycemia, with or without hyperammonemia, and inappropriately low urinary ketone body excretion are highly suggestive of a fatty acid oxidation defect. Liver biopsy may reveal fatty metamorphosis. Lipid accumulation in skeletal muscle is evident with long-chain acyl CoA dehydrogenase deficiency. Cardiac involvement also is prominent with the latter disorder.

Short-chain acyl CoA dehydrogenase deficiency has been described in several cases, each with different clinical presentations. One patient suffered muscle weakness and lactic acidosis after exercising, suggesting a muscle-specific defect. She benefited from oral carnitine supplementation. Another patient had an infantile multi-system disorder characterized by failure to thrive, progressive muscle weakness, microcephaly, and psychomotor retardation.

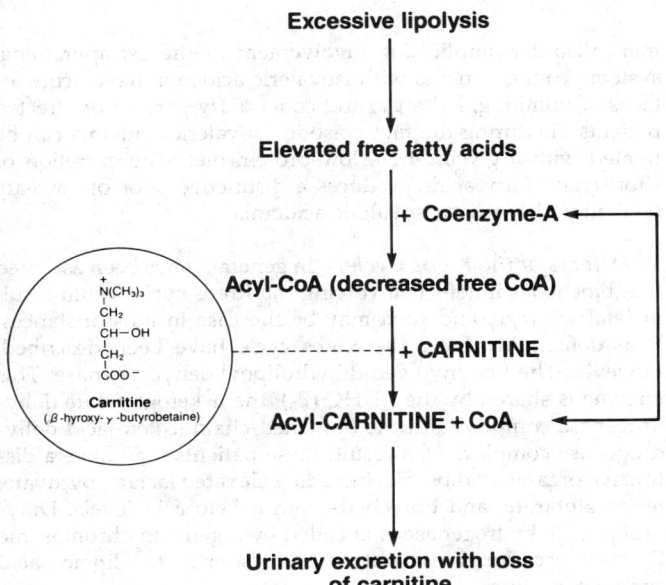

**Excessive lipolysis**

**Elevated free fatty acids**

**+ Coenzyme-A**

**Acyl-CoA (decreased free CoA)**

**+ CARNITINE**

**Acyl-CARNITINE + CoA**

$N(CH_3)_3$
$CH_2$
$CH-OH$
$CH_2$
$COO^-$

**Carnitine**
($\beta$-hyroxy-$\gamma$-butyrobetaine)

**Urinary excretion with loss of carnitine**

**Figure 159-3.**  Schematic representation of carnitine esterification of activated fatty acids and urinary excretion resulting in secondary carnitine depletion.

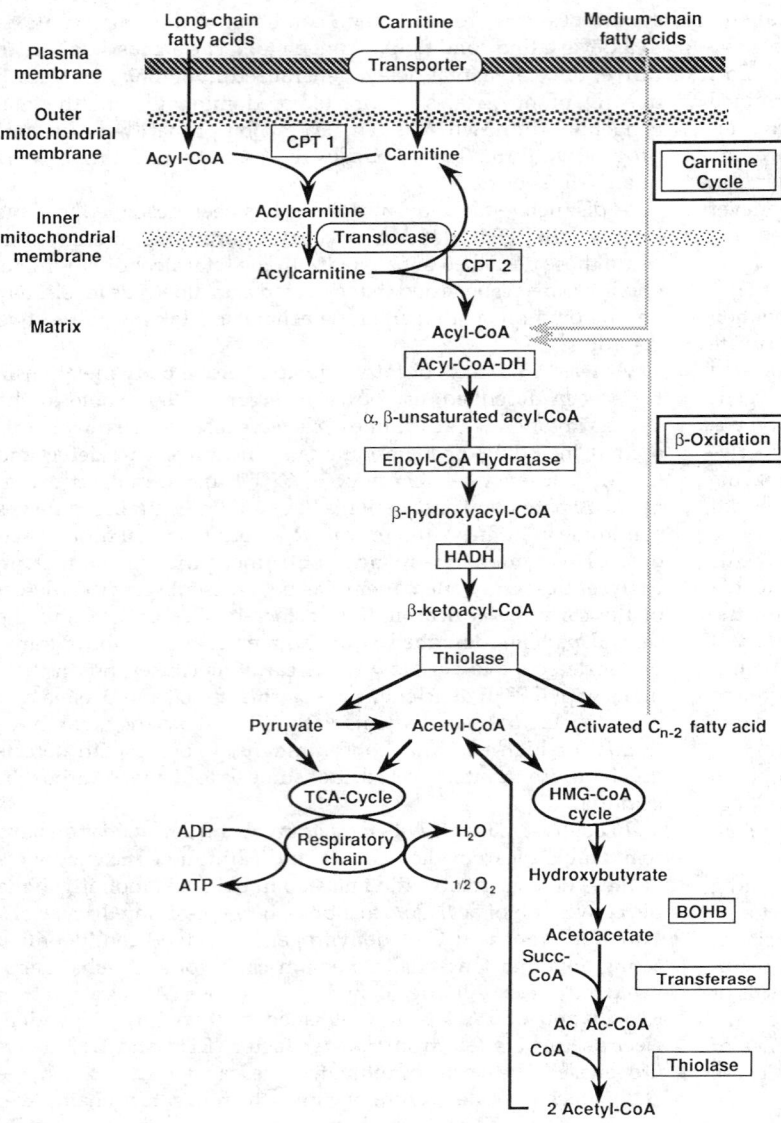

**Figure 159-4.** Schematic representation of fatty acid oxidation and ketone body synthesis. *ADP,* adenosine diphosphate; *ATP,* adenosine triphosphate.

Glutaric aciduria type II (multiple acyl CoA dehydrogenase deficiency) usually is associated with respiratory distress, hypoglycemia, hyperammonemia, generalized carnitine deficiency, and hypoketotic metabolic acidosis in the neonatal period, with death following within the first several weeks. A few patients, however, have become symptomatic in childhood or adulthood with findings of a lipid storage myopathy, weakness, or premature fatigue. The biochemical lesion of glutaric aciduria type II appears to affect the ETF or the ETF-dehydrogenase systems. As a result, all acyl CoA dehydrogenases are affected indirectly with a characteristic urinary organic acid pattern. A defect of ETF also is responsible for a milder disorder known as ethylmalonic-adipic aciduria. This disorder develops later in childhood and is characterized by recurrent episodes of vomiting, acidosis, and hypoglycemia. A few patients with the milder form of multiple acyl CoA dehydrogenase deficiency have responded to riboflavin supplementation.

The two remaining syndromes associated with the first step in beta oxidation include glutaric aciduria type I, which results from a specific defect of glutaryl-CoA dehydrogenase, and isovaleric acidemia, which results from a defect of isovaleryl-CoA dehydrogenase. Both conditions are transmitted as autosomal recessive disorders. Glutaric aciduria type I presents in early infancy as a pyramidal tract disorder. Later, these patients have a move-

ment disorder, implicating involvement of the extrapyramidal system. Young patients with isovaleric acidemia have acute attacks of vomiting, lethargy, and coma. Fifty percent of affected patients die during the first episode. Isovaleric acidemia can be treated with a glycine-rich, low-protein diet. The excretion of short-chain fatty acids produces a distinctive odor of "sweaty feet" in patients with isovaleric acidemia.

*Defects of the Krebs Cycle.* In general, it has been assumed that biochemical defects involving the Krebs cycle would result in fetal wastage, and such may be the case in most instances. Four defects involving the Krebs cycle have been described, however. The first involved dihydrolipoyl dehydrogenase. This enzyme is shared by the PDHC ($E_3$), the $\alpha$-ketoglutarate dehydrogenase complex, and the branched-chain $\alpha$-keto acid dehydrogenase complex. As a result, these patients may have a distinctive organic acid profile, including elevated lactate, pyruvate, $\alpha$-ketoglutarate, and branched-chain $\alpha$-keto acid levels. Dihydrolipoyl dehydrogenase is encoded by a gene on chromosome 7. An occasional patient may respond to lipoic acid supplementation.

The second Krebs cycle defect was described in 1986. These children had mental delay, microcephaly, hypotonia, and cerebral atrophy. The primary laboratory finding in this disorder is the excretion of large amounts of fumaric acid in the urine. The enzyme defect involves the mitochondrial and cytosolic isoforms of fumarase, both of which are encoded by the same gene located on chromosome 1. Fumarase deficiency has been documented in cultured skin fibroblasts, skeletal muscle, and liver.

A few patients have had a myopathy or encephalomyopathy resulting from a defect of succinate dehydrogenase (complex II). One patient had a muscle tissue–specific syndrome of limb weakness and myoglobinuria associated with combined deficiencies of aconitase and succinate dehydrogenase.

The most recent description of a Krebs cycle defect involves the α-ketoglutarate dehydrogenase complex. Patients with this disorder are seen in infancy with a severe encephalopathy and associated lactic acidosis.

*Defects of Oxidation-Phosphorylation Coupling.* As with the defects involving the Krebs cycle, defects of oxidation-phosphorylation coupling are rare and have been described in only two patients. The first patient was described by Luft and colleagues in 1962. Symptoms start in childhood or early adolescence, with fever, heat intolerance, profuse sweating, resting tachypnea and dyspnea, polydipsia, and polyphagia. The basal metabolic rate is decreased, but thyroid function test results are normal. Muscle biopsy samples demonstrate capillary proliferation and ragged-red fibers. Mitochondria are increased in number and greatly enlarged, with tightly packed cristae and paracrystalline or osmiophilic inclusions, as seen by electron microscopy. Respiratory control is lost in this syndrome, producing the biochemical state of loose coupling. Futile cycling of calcium between mitochondria and cytosol might explain the defect of oxidation-phosphorylation coupling, but the molecular basis for this observation remains unclear.

*Defects of the Respiratory Chain.* The respiratory chain is composed of five enzymatic complexes that are embedded in the mitochondrial membrane (see Fig 159-4). Complexes I, III, IV, and V represent genetic hybrids composed of polypeptides that are encoded by the nuclear DNA and the mitochondrial DNA; complex II is composed of polypeptides that are synthesized exclusively by nuclear DNA. The respiratory chain is composed of 67 polypeptides, 13 of which are encoded by mitochondrial DNA. Coenzyme Q and cytochrome c act as shuttling molecules between the respective complexes.

Respiratory chain disorders affect either muscle alone (myopathy), muscle and brain together (encephalomyopathy), or multiple systems, including variable involvement of the heart, kidney, liver, skeletal muscle, or brain (cytopathy). Lactic acidosis and serum carnitine deficiency are common laboratory correlates. Ragged-red fibers signify primary or secondary involvement of mitochondrial DNA with disturbance of intramitochondrial protein synthesis. The heterogenous clinical and laboratory features that are associated with defects of the respiratory chain are truly bewildering and complicate efforts to develop didactic generalizations that are useful to students of myology or neurology.

Complex I defects have been described in about 60 patients. One group has a pure myopathy manifested by exercise intolerance and myalgia starting in childhood or adulthood. A second group has symptoms of a multi-system disorder. Some of these patients have a fatal infantile form of the disease associated with severe congenital lactic acidosis, hypotonia, seizures, respiratory insufficiency, and death in early infancy. Other patients have a less severe encephalomyopathy that begins in childhood or adulthood and is manifested by exercise intolerance, weakness, ophthalmoplegia, pigmentary degeneration of the retina, optic atrophy, sensorineural hearing loss, dementia, cerebellar ataxia, and pyramidal tract signs. A defect in complex I also has been reported in patients with MELAS, progressive infantile polio-

dystrophy (Alpers' disease), and subacute necrotizing encephalomyelopathy (Leigh disease). Oral riboflavin treatment has been beneficial in one patient, but for the most part, no effective therapy is available for patients with defects in complex I.

Defects of complex II are the least well characterized syndromes that are associated with respiratory chain defects. Fatal infantile myopathy with lactic acidosis and encephalomyopathy are two disorders that have been attributed to a decrease in succinate-cytochrome reductase activity, but it remains unclear whether the observed defect of complex II represents a primary biochemical abnormality. One patient had a muscle tissue–specific combined defect of aconitase and succinate dehydrogenase associated with limb weakness and myoglobinuria.

Several patients have been described with defects of complex III. Again, the reported syndromes represent either a pure myopathy presenting in childhood or adolescence with occasional involvement of extraocular muscles, or a multi-system disorder with exercise intolerance, fixed limb weakness, pigmentary degeneration of the retina, sensorineural hearing loss, cerebellar ataxia, pyramidal tract signs, and dementia. Current information suggests the existence of tissue-specific isoforms for complex III. One patient had a pure myopathy, and the complex was normal in cultured skin fibroblasts and transformed lymphoid cells. Another patient had histiocytoid cardiomyopathy of infancy with markedly decreased complex III activity in cardiac muscle and normal activity in skeletal muscle and liver.

Numerous clinical syndromes have emerged in association with complex IV defects. The phenotypes of this complex are similar to the defects of complexes I and III in that they fall into two main categories: one associated with a pure myopathic syndrome and the other with prominent involvement of the brain and muscle.

The purely myopathic forms involve two strikingly different phenotypes. The first is a fatal infantile myopathy that is associated with generalized weakness, respiratory insufficiency, and death before 1 year of age. Lactic acidosis is prominent and renal dysfunction is manifested by glycosuria, phosphaturia, and aminoaciduria. Simultaneous involvement of the heart or liver has been described, but the nervous system has been spared. The second phenotype is a remarkable syndrome of muscle involvement termed "benign infantile mitochondrial myopathy" because the metabolic and biochemical abnormalities disappear during late infancy. These children have a severe neonatal myopathy and lactic acidosis. The clinical condition improves spontaneously and disappears by early childhood. The cytochrome oxidase deficiency is severe in skeletal muscle obtained at biopsy shortly after birth, but the enzyme activity increases to normal values by 1 or 2 years of life.

Infants with the fatal myopathic form of complex IV deficiency have no immunologically cross-reacting material in the tissue obtained at biopsy, in contrast to patients with the benign, reversible myopathic form, who have normal amounts of cross-reacting material in all muscle specimens, including those with very low catalytic enzyme activity.

The phenotype in a second group of patients with complex IV deficiency is dominated by central nervous system dysfunction. These patients have Leigh syndrome manifested by psychomotor retardation, brain stem abnormalities, and seizures. Although the brain is involved prominently clinically, the biochemical defect appears to be generalized, including cultured skin fibroblasts. Immunologic studies demonstrate the presence of cross-reacting material in all tissues. This condition is inherited as an autosomal recessive trait, but the basis for the biochemical defect remains unknown.

Two patients have been described with defects of complex V (mitochondrial adenosine triphosphatase). One patient had a congenital, slowly progressive myopathy. Muscle biopsy showed ragged-red fibers, and electron microscopy demonstrated paracrystalline inclusions in most mitochondria. The second patient was described to have muscle carnitine deficiency, but later exhibited a multi-system disorder characterized by weakness, dementia, ataxia, retinopathy, and peripheral neuropathy. Recently, a maternally inherited condition resulting from a mitochondrial DNA point mutation of the gene encoding subunit 6 of complex V was reported. This entity initially was described as a multi-system disorder with sensory neuropathy, ataxia, retinitis pigmentosa, dementia, seizures, and developmental delay. When the point mutation is abundant, the patients are affected in early infancy and have the neuropathologic features of Leigh disease.

## Malignant Hyperthermia

Malignant hyperthermia has occurred in association with several of the forms of myopathy discussed previously, including central core disease, various myotonic syndromes, and DMD. Most patients with malignant hyperthermia, however, have no obvious clinical symptoms of muscle disease, and the EMG and muscle histology results are normal or nonspecifically abnormal. These latter patients do have an underlying myopathy that may be manifested by increased serum CK values or in vitro studies that document sensitivity to caffeine or anesthetic agents. Malignant hyperthermia is inherited in most patients in an autosomal dominant pattern. Unfortunately, this condition may not be recognized until the patient is exposed to anesthetic agents such as halothane or succinylcholine, and such exposure may be catastrophic. The symptom complex is characterized by rapidly rising body temperature, tachycardia, tachypnea, cyanosis, and respiratory and metabolic acidosis. Usually, affected patients have rigidity and myoglobinuria. Unexplained fevers, muscle cramps, and increased serum CK values may represent clinical clues to the presence of malignant hyperthermia. A family history of an untoward anesthetic experience, recurrent myoglobinuria, or sudden death should suggest the possibility of this muscle condition. The clinical syndrome can be aborted by the intravenous administration of dantrolene. The molecular and biochemical basis for this autosomal dominant condition has been elucidated partially. Studies indicate that a single point mutation in the ryanodine receptor gene causes malignant hyperthermia in all breeds of pigs and some human families. This gene, encoding the calcium release channel, is localized on chromosome 19q 13.1. Linkage has been established between this gene and central core disease.

## Myoadenylate Deaminase Deficiency

Myoadenylate deaminase deficiency has failed to establish a firm basis in muscle nosology because the clinical manifestations are both protean and vague. Some patients, in fact, are asymptomatic; others demonstrate varying signs of weakness, hyporeflexia, periodic paralysis, paresthesias, and recurrent infections in childhood. The most common symptoms are muscle cramping and stiffness or pain after exercise. Myoglobinuria never has been reported, but serum CK values may be elevated slightly. Muscle specimens obtained at biopsy may appear normal or demonstrate nonspecific minor changes. The specific histochemical stain for myoadenylate deaminase has revealed that the enzyme deficiency is common, although the clinical appearance is not distinctive. This condition often is considered as a possible explanation for recurrent muscle cramps and easy fatigability. Some affected patients have had psychogenic disorders diagnosed.

# ACQUIRED DISORDERS

Muscle symptoms or frank weakness may be associated with numerous acquired illnesses in infancy or childhood, but in the aggregate, these conditions are rare compared to the hereditary disorders. The acquired disorders may be associated with three primary processes: inflammatory changes, toxic or nutritional insults to muscle, or various endocrinologic disturbances.

## Inflammatory Types of Myopathy

Inflammatory forms of myopathy are classified according to their diverse etiologic factors. Known infectious agents include viruses, bacteria, fungi, and parasites. Those disorders that result from viral processes may be subdivided into three groups: acute benign myositis (caused by influenza viruses A and B, parainfluenza virus, and adenovirus II), acute myoglobinuria (caused by influenza viruses A and B, coxsackievirus B5, echovirus 9, adenovirus 21, herpes simplex virus, and Epstein-Barr virus), and epidemic pleurodynia (caused by group B coxsackieviruses). Bacterial infections are less common and more localized. *Staphylococcus aureus* is the organism encountered most frequently in the subtropical and tropical regions of the world. Clostridial, tuberculous, syphilitic, and leprous infections of muscle are distinctly rare, but have been described in children. Fungal infections are rarer still, but parasitic infections may be encountered occasionally. Toxoplasmosis, cysticercosis, and trichinosis are the likely agents in this category of infections.

The most commonly encountered childhood inflammatory myopathic conditions are idiopathic and include the dermatomyositis-polymyositis complex. A child with dermatomyositis exhibits a rather stereotyped syndrome in most cases. Muscle tenderness, joint discomfort, and tissue edema are associated with the weakness. The child is extremely irritable and unhappy, and frequently cries when examined. Misery is the term often used to describe the clinical picture. Occasionally, the cutaneous features are subtle or absent, in which case the term polymyositis is appropriate. The annual incidence of dermatomyositis-polymyositis is about 3 to 5 cases per 1 million children. Females are affected more frequently, with a 3 : 2 female : male ratio. The onset usually is insidious, but fulminant presentations with severe weakness do occur.

Spontaneous exacerbations and remissions also occur, and death may result from gastrointestinal ulceration, perforation, or hemorrhage; cardiac dysrhythmias or myocarditis; respiratory failure; overwhelming sepsis; or suicide. Dystrophic calcification of soft tissues is a dreaded complication, often developing 2 or 3 years after the initial onset of clinical symptoms. The rash characteristically involves the upper eyelids, malar region of the face, ears, extensor regions of the limbs, and lateral aspects of the rib cage. Increased tortuosity of capillaries is evident in these regions and beneath the nail beds. These observations indicate that the target cell in this idiopathic condition is the endothelium, with prominent involvement of the intramuscular blood vessels. Immune complexes have been shown in venules within skeletal muscle of affected children.

The clinical picture is sufficiently distinctive to permit precise diagnosis in most cases. The laboratory findings, on the other hand, are variable. A leukocytosis and an elevated erythrocyte sedimentation rate may be detected in an acutely ill child, and serum enzyme levels, specifically those of CK and the transaminases, may be increased. Some patients have a positive antinuclear antibody test result, with the speckled pattern being the most common. The results of these blood studies may be normal in the presence of active muscle inflammation, however, and the degree to which the results are abnormal does not correlate very well with the patient's condition. The principal correlate with response to treatment, therefore, is the patient's clinical condition and perception of weakness.

The EMG is helpful in making the diagnosis. EMG findings include a mixture of neurogenic and myopathic features. Increased insertional activity indicates muscular irritability, fibrillations reflect the denervation of individual muscle fibers and fiber splitting, and decreased amplitude and duration of the compound action potential reflects direct injury to the muscle fiber. Some investigators have used the term *neuromyositis* to describe this mixed picture of muscle tissue involvement.

The results of muscle biopsy often are distinctive, with inflammatory infiltration, necrosis, phagocytosis, and gradual increase of endoneural connective tissue noted. Atrophy of muscle fibers at the periphery of the fascicle is the morphologic hallmark of this disease process. This distinctive finding has been termed *perifascicular atrophy,* and it suggests an ischemic mechanism as the explanation. Banker and Victor proposed the term *systemic angiopathy* instead of dermatomyositis, believing it to be a more accurate description of the disease process.

The clinical course of patients with dermatomyositis is variable. Some follow a monocyclic course, with full recovery in 6 to 24 months. Others experience a chronic polycyclic course, and a third group has a chronic continuous course. The prognosis for complete recovery was decidedly poor before the availability of corticosteroids and other therapeutic agents. Before 1960, about one third of patients died, one third survived with severe residual disability, and one third experienced a satisfactory recovery. Unfortunately, some patients have severe residual weakness, joint contractures, evidence of smoldering disease, and soft-tissue calcifications despite optimal therapeutic intervention. Calcinosis is more common in children than adults, ranging in incidence from 40% to 75%. Factors that correlate with the eventual development of calcinosis include severe disease at the outset, poor response to corticosteroids, persistent weakness, and severe generalized cutaneous vasculitis.

The mainstay of therapy in dermatomyositis is a corticosteroid agent. Prednisone is used commonly, and it is recommended that a high-dose regimen be started immediately and that treatment be projected over a long period, often 18 to 36 months. The recommended dosage is 60 to 100 mg/m$^2$/d, the equivalent of 2 to 3 mg/kg/day. Initially, the daily amount of medication should be divided into three or four doses to effect maximal suppression of the disease as quickly as possible. Within 2 to 6 weeks, an attempt should be made to adjust the regimen to a single dose each morning, and then to an alternate-day schedule if the drug continues to be effective. About two thirds of affected children respond to this regimen and recover satisfactorily. Treatment needs to be continued for 2 or 3 years in most patients. Therefore, it is essential that the side effects of prednisone be reviewed in detail with the child and the parents at the outset. Potassium supplementation, antacids, and proper dietary instruction are most important in this regard. A diet that is low in salt and carbohydrates and relatively high in protein appears to be beneficial and seems to be associated with less severe cushingoid features. Most series of patients described since the early 1960s indicate a significant reduction in mortality (5% to 10%) and a considerable improvement in satisfactory outcome (65% to 75%).

Unfortunately, there remains a subgroup of patients who do not do well. They often respond poorly to corticosteroids at the outset and exhibit prominent cutaneous manifestations of the disorder. A small number of patients may not absorb the orally administered steroids satisfactorily, but parenteral administration may be successful. It is more likely, however, that an alternative treatment regimen will be necessary using an antimetabolite, plasmapheresis, or cyclosporine. No statement can be made regarding the efficacy of these alternative therapies, because the total reported experience is limited and no controlled studies have been performed. Anecdotal experience with cyclosporine, limited as it is, is encouraging. It is the general belief that chemotherapy should be considered early in those children who are at risk for the development of calcinosis, particularly because there is no known therapy for this complication once it has occurred.

Physical therapy and rehabilitation are critical elements of treatment throughout the illness. Passive and active range of mo-

tion exercises and the proper use of assistive devices to facilitate ambulation are important for physical and psychologic well-being and for the restoration of good muscle function after the inflammatory process subsides.

The pathogenesis of dermatomyositis-polymyositis is unknown. An immunogenetic predisposition to a viral infection is suspected because 72% of affected patients have the HLA-B8 haplotype.

## Toxic and Nutritional Types of Myopathy

Toxic and nutritional forms of myopathy are distinctly rare in children and often are publishable as case reports when they are recognized. Muscle necrosis and fibrosis associated with contractures may result from intramuscular injections of certain drugs. Paraldehyde is notable in this regard.

Vincristine causes weakness affecting mainly the type 2 muscle fibers. This complaint is reversible when the drug is discontinued. Chloroquine and emetine also cause reversible types of myopathy.

Muscle necrosis and myoglobinuria may follow exposure to numerous drugs and toxins. Exogenous toxins include sea snake poisons, hornet poisons, and an unidentified myotoxic factor that has caused epidemic myoglobinuria in small fishing villages of northern Europe (Haff disease).

Hypokalemia from any cause may lead to muscle necrosis. Myoglobinuria has been reported after the administration of various kaliuretic agents, including amphotericin B and licorice. Succinylcholine may cause myoglobinuria in normal children. This phenomenon is to be distinguished from the myoglobinuria that follows the administration of anesthetic agents in children with the genetic trait for malignant hyperthermia, as discussed previously.

Malnutrition results from severe muscle wasting and weakness. Hypotonia may accompany rickets caused by vitamin D deficiency, and muscle weakness may result, rarely, from vitamin E deficiency.

## Endocrine Causes of Myopathy

Muscle weakness and atrophy may accompany several endocrine disorders. Perhaps most commonly seen is the weakness that accompanies corticosteroid therapy. This complication may contribute to the patient's disability when steroids are being used to treat a primary muscle disease such as dermatomyositis. Potassium wasting may compound this insult to muscle. The muscle biopsy sample characteristically reveals nonspecific atrophy of the type 2 fibers. This finding, however, is nondiagnostic and may be seen in nutritional and toxic states, disease atrophy, and infantile hypotonia resulting from cerebral factors. Proximal weakness is seen commonly in Cushing's syndrome.

Weakness and wasting of the pelvic girdle muscles is seen frequently with hyperparathyroidism, and the clinical syndrome may simulate a motor neuron syndrome. Serum CK values are normal. Muscle irritability and tetany may be the result of hypoparathyroidism and hypocalcemia.

Hyperthyroidism may cause several muscle disorders, but these conditions seldom are seen in children. Thyrotoxic periodic paralysis is similar to the familial hypokalemic form of this disorder, as discussed, and often is seen in Asian adult males. Thyrotoxic myopathy causes a slowly progressive weakness, and exophthalmic ophthalmoplegia may occur in the absence of clinically apparent hyperthyroidism. Congenital cretinism and childhood hypothyroidism can cause generalized muscular hypertrophy (Kocher-Debré-Sémélaigne syndrome). Hypothyroidism is associated with delayed contraction and relaxation of muscle fibers, increased CK values, and distinctive EMG abnormalities. These abnormalities have been termed *pseudo-*

*myotonic*, and include bizarre, high-frequency, polyphasic discharges.

The muscle symptoms in patients with these diverse forms of endocrinopathy generally revert to normal when the hormonal excess or deficiency is corrected.

## Selected Readings

Brooke MH, Carroll JE, Ringel SP. Congenital hypotonia revisited. Muscle Nerve 1979;2:84.

Brooke MH, Fenickel GM, Griggs RC, et al. Clinical investigations of Duchenne muscular dystrophy. Ann Neurol 1987;44:812.

DiMauro S, Bonilla E, Zeviani M, et al. Mitochondrial myopathies. J Inherited Metab Dis 1987;10(Suppl 1):113.

Emery AEH. X-linked muscular dystrophy with early contractures and cardiomyopathy (Emery-Dreifuss type). Clin Genet 1987;32:360.

Engel AG, Banker BQ. Myology. New York: McGraw-Hill, 1986.

Francke U, Ochs HD, de Martinville B, et al. Minor Xp21 chromosome deletion in a male associated with expression of Duchenne muscular dystrophy, chronic granulomatous disease, retinitis pigmentosa and McLeod syndrome. Am J Hum Genet 1985;37:250.

Gould RJ, Steeg CN, Eastwood AB, et al. Potentially fatal cardiac dysrhythmia and hyperkalemic period paralysis. Neurology 1985;35:1208.

Hale DE, Bennett MJ. Fatty acid oxidation disorders: A new class of metabolic diseases. J Pediatr 1992;121:1.

Hoffman EP, Brown RH Jr, Kunkel LM. Dystrophin: The protein product of the Duchenne muscular dystrophy locus. Cell 1987;51:919.

Koenig M, Hoffman EP, Bertelson CJ, et al. Complete cloning of the Duchenne muscular dystrophy (DMD) cDNA and preliminary genomic organization of the DMD gene in normal and affected individuals. Cell 1987;50:509.

MacLennan DH. The genetic basis of malignant hyperthermia. Trends in Pharmacological Science 1992;13:330.

Moraes CT, DiMauro S, Zeviani M. Mitochondrial DNA deletions in progressive external ophthalmoplegia and Kearns-Sayre syndrome. N Engl J Med 1989;320:1293.

Stanley CA, DeLeeuw S, Coates PM, et al. Chronic cardiomyopathy and weakness or acute coma in children with a defect in carnitine uptake. Ann Neurol 1991;30:709.

Tein I, DiMauro S, De Vivo DC. Recurrent childhood myoglobinuria. Adv Pediatr 1990;37:77.

Van Coster RN, Fernhoff PM, De Vivo DC: Pyruvate carboxylase deficiency: A benign variant with normal development. Pediatr Res 1991;30:1.

*Principles and Practice of Pediatrics, Second Edition.*
edited by Frank A. Oski et al. J. B. Lippincott Company, Philadelphia © 1994.

CHAPTER 160

# Slow Viruses Affecting the Central Nervous System

## John F. Griffith

Slow virus infections have in common a long incubation period, followed by progressive disease, which usually is limited to a single organ. The term refers only to the disease tempo and not to the biologic characteristics of the infectious agents. Some of these infections are caused by conventional viruses and others by unconventional agents that induce degenerative rather than inflammatory changes in brain tissue.

Diseases caused by conventional viruses include subacute sclerosing panencephalitis (SSPE), progressive multifocal leukoencephalopathy (PML), and chronic rubella encephalitis. Many now would include infection caused by human immunodeficiency virus (HIV) in the slow virus category because of its long incubation period and fatal outcome. In fact, the lentiviruses, which include HIV, derive their name from the slow course of the illnesses they cause. In the past few years, much has been learned about the nervous system manifestations of HIV infection. This subject is addressed in Chapter 14.1.6 as part of the general discussion of acquired immunodeficiency syndrome (AIDS).

## UNCONVENTIONAL VIRUSES

The unconventional viruses cause progressive, invariably fatal diseases with pathologic changes restricted to the central nervous system. The diseases, referred to as spongiform virus types of encephalopathy, include kuru and Creutzfeldt-Jakob disease (CJD) in humans, scrapie in sheep and goats, and transmissible mink encephalopathy. Pathologic features common to these disorders include nerve cell loss, gliosis, and vacuolar changes in neurons, giving the tissue a spongy appearance on histologic examination.

The original definition of slow virus infections is attributed to Sigurrdson, an Icelandic pathologist who worked primarily with diseases affecting sheep. One of these, a chronic encephalopathy called rida or scrapie, had been studied extensively for years. It was observed to have an incubation period of many months, followed by a progressive neurologic disease without any clinical, pathologic, or laboratory evidence to suggest infection. Proof that there was a filterable, transmissible agent causing scrapie was established decades before there was awareness that humans might be affected by the same type of disease process.

### Kuru

Observations in animals led ultimately to studies proving that certain degenerative brain diseases of humans also had an infectious basis. One of these, kuru, occurred in a tribe of New Guinea natives who practiced ritual cannibalism. The disease was characterized by progressive ataxia, tremors, motor disability, and dementia, which led to death in less than a year. It occurred predominantly in children and women, but all members of the tribe practicing cannibalism were at risk. The disease has been disappearing gradually since this practice has ceased.

Gajdusek demonstrated that a transmissible agent was responsible for this disease by inoculating brain tissue obtained from patients with kuru into chimpanzees. During the long incubation period, lasting from 16 to 38 months, the animals remained well. Once they became symptomatic, all died with clinical and pathologic features similar to those of kuru.

Most of what we know about the agent causing kuru and CJD has come from extensive studies of the scrapie agent. The virus(es) is extremely small and resistant to most viricidal agents, including heat, nucleases, and ionizing irradiation, and to antiseptics such as formaldehyde, ether, and alcohol. It is described best as a replicating agent without a nucleic acid core, protein capsid, lipid envelope, or other properties characteristic of viruses. It fails to stimulate immune responses or inflammatory reactions in the host. The term *prion* (proteinaceous infectious particle) now is used commonly to describe this agent; some think it represents a new class of microorganism.

### Creutzfeldt-Jakob Disease

CJD is a progressive degenerative disease that is characterized by dementia, ataxia, and signs referable to involvement of the pyramidal and extrapyramidal tracts. It usually occurs in the fifth and sixth decades of life, but a few cases recently have been identified in younger patients. Because the virus is resistant to most physicochemical agents known to inactivate viruses, it is not surprising that a few cases have occurred after contact with contaminated instruments and tissues. Two cases have been traced to the use of depth electrodes previously used in a patient with CJD. Other examples of human-to-human transmission have occurred after corneal and dural transplants. Recently, a small cluster of cases has occurred in young adults a number of years after treatment with brain-derived human growth hormone (HGH). Although these cases are few, considering the indeterminate length of the incubation period of this virus, concern remains for the larger group of HGH-treated patients who presently are asymptomatic.

It now is possible to make an etiologic diagnosis in some cases of CJD because of advances made in the characterization of the etiologic agent. The scrapie prion has been identified as a sialoglycoprotein with a known molecular weight. Antibodies developed against this protein have been used to detect its presence in the brain tissue of patients with CJD.

## CONVENTIONAL VIRUSES

### Subacute Sclerosing Panencephalitis

#### Clinical Features

SSPE is a slowly progressive measles encephalitis that occurs long after primary exposure to the virus. The initial measles infection, which usually is mild and uneventful, occurs in healthy infants and children, but at a statistically younger age than normal. After a number of months to years during which the patient is well, symptoms of SSPE develop. These usually appear between 5 and 9 years of age, but cases beginning in infancy and young adult life have been described. Males are affected more often than are females (3 : 1), and the disease has a tendency to occur more frequently in rural than in urban settings. Some temporal and geographic clustering of cases has been reported, but this is less certain. At one time, 200 to 300 new cases were reported annually in this country, but since the introduction of mass measles immunization in early infancy, SSPE has become a rare condition. This is not the case in developing countries, however, where measles continues to be a common childhood infection.

SSPE usually begins with minor behavioral changes, accompanied by deterioration in school performance. About this time, sudden involuntary movements develop that initially may not be recognized as myoclonic seizures. This sometimes is the first indication that medical attention is necessary. Other findings that may be present early in the disease course include chorioretinitis and focal cerebral signs such as dysphasia and apraxia. The subsequent disease course is variable, but commonly involves progressive deterioration over the course of 3 to 6 months, leading to coma, loss of speech, and marked motor dysfunction. Occasionally, the patient's condition will appear to stabilize or even improve for a time. This usually is attributable to reduction in seizure frequency or better control of infections or metabolic disturbances. Later in the disease, seizure frequency often diminishes. Blindness and decorticate rigidity are frequent late clinical features; death usually occurs as a result of infectious complications 6 to 12 months after the onset of symptoms.

#### Laboratory Findings

The cerebrospinal fluid (CSF) in patients with SSPE usually is normal, except for increased levels of IgG. This is the result of local measles antibody production rather than simply passive transfer of antibodies from the serum. The presence of anti-mea-

sles antibodies in the CSF is used to confirm the diagnosis. Brain biopsy no longer is indicated for diagnosis unless the clinical and laboratory findings are inconclusive. Recently, measles virus genomic sequences have been detected in the brain tissue of patients with SSPE by polymerase chain reaction, but this is not a practical or necessary diagnostic procedure, except in rare situations.

The electroencephalogram is an important diagnostic aid when synchronized bursts of spike suppression activity are present. This electrical pattern usually disappears as the disease progresses and myoclonic seizures subside. Occasionally, electroencephalographic findings are normal or only mildly abnormal when the disease process is most active.

#### Pathogenesis

The measles virus isolated from the brains of patients with SSPE has been studied extensively. It now is clear that complete replication of measles virus does not occur in nerve or glial cells. Electron microscopic studies of these cells show only densely packed viral nucleocapsids, not complete virions; final assembly and budding of virus does not occur. The reasons for this are not yet clear, but some recent studies seem to be relevant. The SSPE virus, which has been isolated in culture using cocultivation techniques, differs from measles virus in at least one important way. It lacks the M protein, which is responsible for virus assembly at the cell membrane. Why this occurs is unclear, but, presumably, brain cells inhibit expression of this antigen. Consequently, nucleocapsids replicate within cells, but are not assembled into complete viruses. The gradual accumulation of measles nucleocapsids within the cell over an extended period is thought to interfere with cellular function and cause disease.

#### Treatment

Treatment of SSPE has been attempted using most of the antiviral compounds developed in recent years. To date, no persuasive evidence exists that disease progression is altered by any specific therapy. Optimal supportive care, early treatment of infection, and attempts at seizure control remain the standard approaches. In SSPE, as with most viral infections, prevention is the goal, and the best way to accomplish this is with effective immunization programs for young children. New cases of SSPE are rare now in countries that have measles immunization programs.

### Progressive Rubella Encephalitis

Progressive rubella encephalitis (PRE) is similar to SSPE in certain respects. It is a progressive neurologic disorder that is characterized by motor and mental dysfunction and affects children who either had congenital rubella or were infected with the rubella virus in early childhood. It is a rare condition, presumably because rubella has been largely eliminated through effective immunization programs. PRE usually begins in the second decade of life with behavioral changes and motor disability characterized by incoordination, gait instability, and other signs of progressive pyramidal and extrapyramidal dysfunction. The brain pathology is characterized by perivascular infiltration of plasma cells and destructive lesions in the white matter.

Increased levels of antibodies to rubella virus are present in the serum and CSF of affected individuals. The virus has been cultured from both brain tissue and mononuclear cells, but little is known of the brain–virus interaction during the many years after primary infection occurs. Immune complexes containing IgG and rubella antigen have been identified in some patients, but their role in the pathogenesis of the disorder remains unclear.

There is no specific antiviral therapy of proven worth for PRE. The goal is to make the diagnosis early and to support patients and their parents during the course of rapid neurologic deterioration.

## Progressive Multifocal Leukoencephalopathy

### Clinical Features

PML is a condition that affects primarily immunocompromised adults in the fifth to seventh decades of life. Two cases have been described in young children with HIV infection, however, and it is reasonable to assume that PML will occur more frequently in the pediatric population as the AIDS epidemic accelerates. It is caused by viruses belonging to the *Papovaviridae* family, of which simian virus 40 (SV 40) is a member. The original virus recovered from the brain of a patient with PML was designated *JC virus*. It shared antigens in common with SV 40. Another brain isolate has been designated SV 40-PML virus because it is almost identical to SV 40 virus, even though it can be distinguished antigenically. PML is characterized by multifocal demyelinization and, thus, is the first example of virus-induced demyelinating disease in humans. Although it is rare and affects mainly older adults, it is relevant to pediatrics because a significant percentage of children have serum antibodies to the JC virus. The primary infection is nonspecific, and its relationship to the later onset of PML is not well understood. Presumably, the virus, which is latent in the host for years, is activated later as a result of altered immunity or other factors. It also is possible that PML occurs after primary infection in an immunocompromised host.

The disease usually is fatal within 3 to 6 months after the onset of symptoms. The clinical features vary depending on the primary location of brain lesions (widespread, patchy areas of demyelinization), but frequently include visual disturbances, progressive mental deterioration, and, sometimes, focal motor weakness, dysphasia, ataxia, and isolated cranial nerve dysfunction. The course commonly is progressive, but transient spontaneous improvement occurs occasionally. The CSF is normal and there are no other laboratory changes to suggest a progressive infection of the central nervous system.

### Laboratory Findings

The diagnosis of PML can be suspected on clinical grounds, but can be proved only by direct examination of tissue. Modern imaging techniques make it possible to identify focal lesions in the brain that are consistent with the diagnosis, but virus detection in brain tissue remains the only certain means of confirming the diagnosis.

### Treatment

There is no effective antiviral therapy of proven value in patients with PML. Occasional reports have suggested benefit from certain drugs, but, considering the variable course of this illness, transient improvement may be attributed to factors other than drug effect. At this time, the only recommended therapy is optimal supportive management. Although not all these patients are immunosuppressed, the association is frequent enough to suggest a cause-and-effect relationship.

### Selected Readings

Brockman JM, Kingsbury DT, McKinley MP, et al. Creutzfeldt-Jakob prion proteins in human brains. N Engl J Med 1985;312:73.

Brown P, Gajdusek DC, Gibbs CJ Jr, et al. Potential epidemic of Creutzfeldt-Jakob disease from human growth hormone therapy. N Engl J Med 1985;313:728.

Buchanan CR, Preece MA, Milner RDG. Mortality, neoplasia, and Creutzfeldt-Jakob disease in patients treated with human pituitary growth hormone in the United Kingdom. BMJ 1991;302:824.

Coyle PK, Wolinsky JS. Characterization of immune complexes in progressive rubella panencephalitis. Ann Neurol 1981;9:557.

Gajdusek DC. Unconventional viruses causing subacute spongiform encephalopathies. In: Fields BN, et al, eds. Virology. New York: Raven Press, 1985:1519.

Godec MS, Asher DM, Swoveland PT, et al. Detection of measles virus genomic sequences in SSPE brain tissue by the polymerase chain reaction. J Med Virol 1990;30:237.

Hall WW, Choppin PW. Measles-virus proteins in the brain tissue of patients with subacute sclerosing panencephalitis: Absence of the M protein. N Engl J Med 1981;304:1152.

Holman RC, Janssen RS, Buehler JW, et al. Epidemiology of progressive multifocal leukoencephalopathy in the United States: Analysis of national mortality and AIDS surveillance data. Neurology 1991;41:1733.

Johnson RT. Viral infections of the nervous system. New York: Raven Press, 1982.

*Principles and Practice of Pediatrics, Second Edition.*
edited by Frank A. Oski et al. J. B. Lippincott Company, Philadelphia © 1994.

# CHAPTER 161
# *Progressive Genetic Metabolic Disorders*

## 161.1 *The Leukodystrophies*

Alan K. Percy

## LEUKODYSTROPHY

The leukodystrophies are a group of progressive degenerative disorders involving myelin of the central and, in some instances, peripheral nervous systems. These disorders represent a fundamental abnormality in myelin formation and are referred to as *dysmyelinating conditions*, as opposed to demyelinating diseases, in which there is a loss of previously formed normal myelin. The clinical pattern of the leukodystrophies typically is characterized by the loss of previously acquired capabilities, whether motor or cognitive, signifying a degenerative disease. When this degenerative process occurs in early childhood, it often is possible to distinguish white matter or myelin dysfunction from gray matter or neuronal dysfunction based on the clinical appearance of the disorder. Patients with disorders of white matter display the loss of acquired motor capabilities such as ambulation or hand use, hypotonia, or ataxia, or signs of corticospinal tract involvement such as spasticity, hyperreflexia, or extensor plantar responses. Patients with disorders of gray matter demonstrate intellectual or cognitive deficits, such as the loss of language or communication skills, seizures, and blindness. Early in the course of the disease process, this formulation may guide the clinical and laboratory assessment. During later stages of these disorders, global nervous system involvement limits the effectiveness of this approach. In infants, a degenerative neurologic process is suggested by the loss of acquired developmental milestones. During childhood or adolescence, the usual presentation involves changes in behavior or school performance.

During infancy, the various types of leukodystrophy must be differentiated from a static encephalopathy. In the presence of rapid, clear-cut regression, this determination is straightforward. Subtle regression or a plateau in development, however, presents a greater diagnostic challenge. In the older child, consideration must be given to demyelinating processes such as multiple sclerosis or polyneuropathy (eg, Guillain-Barré syndrome). In addition, nutritional deficiency, a toxic encephalopathy (from heavy metal or drug intoxication with drugs such as neuroleptics, hypnotics, or anticonvulsants), a neoplasm of the central nervous system, an immunopathologic condition (systemic lupus erythematosus), or a chronic infectious process (human immunodeficiency virus/acquired immunodeficiency syndrome or subacute sclerosing panencephalitis) must be excluded.

Metachromatic leukodystrophy and globoid cell leukodystrophy (Krabbe disease) are autosomal recessive disorders of sphingolipid metabolism. The sphingolipids are a group of unique lipid compounds that are important constituents of biologic membranes. The tissue distribution of the individual sphingolipids differs dramatically. Some are prominent within neural elements and others are present in non-neural tissues. The sphingolipids galactocerebroside (galactosylceramide) and sulfatide are critical components of myelin, in both the central and peripheral nervous systems, whereas the group of sphingolipids called gangliosides are associated particularly with neurons and their axons and dendrites. Disorders of ganglioside metabolism are described in Chapter 12.7. Adrenoleukodystrophy is an X-linked disorder of very–long-chain fatty acid metabolism. Canavan disease, an autosomal recessive disorder, and Pelizaeus-Merzbacher disease, an X-linked disorder, are forms of leukodystrophy with recently described biochemical abnormalities. Alexander disease, an autosomal recessive disorder, lacks a precise explanation.

## Therapy

Effective therapy for the types of leukodystrophy is limited. Bone marrow transplantation is undergoing careful evaluation in patients with several of these disorders, and gene therapy strategies are under investigation. Significant hurdles must be cleared, however, before such therapies are available. Dietary therapy is being assessed in patients with adrenoleukodystrophy. Symptomatic therapy should be employed as indicated to treat infections, seizures, and other medical problems. The family should be provided with appropriate support, as the stress associated with caring for these children can be overwhelming.

Prenatal diagnosis is feasible for many of these disorders. Using amniotic fluid cells or chorionic villus samples, it is possible to provide accurate assessment of the fetus with regard to the relevant disorder.

## METACHROMATIC LEUKODYSTROPHY (SULFATIDE LIPIDOSIS)

Metachromatic leukodystrophy is an autosomal recessive disorder with an incidence of 1 per 40,000 whose biochemical basis is the inability to degrade the sphingolipid, sulfatide, or galactosyl-3 sulfate ceramide (Figs 161-1, 161-2). Sulfatide, along with galactosylceramide, is an important constituent of myelin. In this disorder, sulfatide sulfatase (arylsulfatase A), the lysosomal enzyme responsible for the degradation of sulfatide, is deficient. This deficiency results in the accumulation of sulfatide in both neural and non-neural (especially kidney and gallbladder) tissues, where it can be detected as metachromatic granules. Both central and peripheral myelin are abnormal, and excess sulfatide accumulates within neural elements. The neuropathology consists of widespread loss of myelin and oligodendroglia in the brain, and segmental demyelination of the peripheral nerves.

### Forms of the Disease

Metachromatic leukodystrophy occurs in three principal forms: late infantile (the most common), juvenile, and adult (Table 161-1). The distinction of separate phenotypes is arbitrary, because the variability reflects more a continuum of phenotypes than separate entities. The late infantile form appears at 1 to 2 years of age after the child has experienced normal early development, often including ambulation. Early signs are regression of motor skills, gait difficulties, ataxia, hypotonia, and extensor plantar responses. Deep tendon reflexes are diminished or absent as a result of peripheral nerve involvement. Optic atrophy is prominent early. The disorder progresses fairly rapidly, with the loss of motor and mental capabilities and of meaningful contact with the environment. Death by 6 years of age is usual.

Juvenile metachromatic leukodystrophy may actually represent two patterns of disease. An early juvenile form begins between 4 and 8 years of age with gait disturbance and intellectual decline. Ataxia and upper motor neuron signs are prominent, and deep tendon reflexes initially are increased and subsequently are lost. Clinical progression is less rapid than in the late infantile form. Extrapyramidal signs and seizures often appear, and death is common within 6 years of onset.

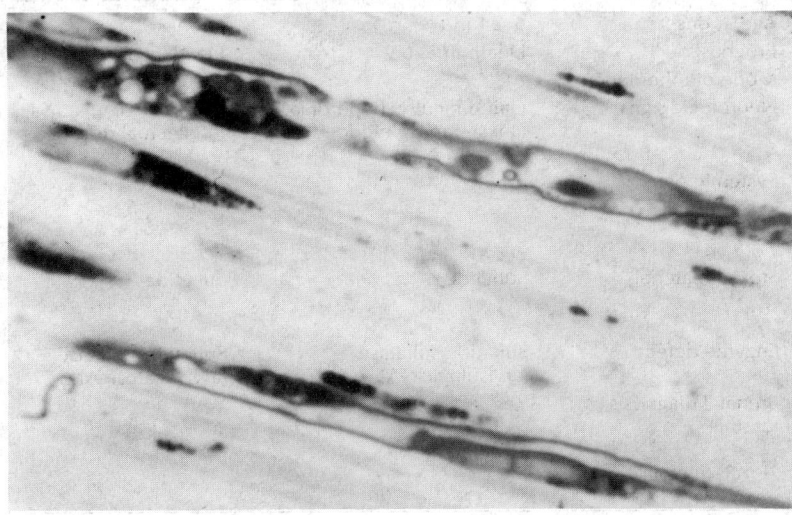

**Figure 161-1.** Light micrograph of peripheral nerve in longitudinal section from a patient with metachromatic leukodystrophy showing lipid inclusion material within the Schwann cell cytoplasm and in the interstitial space.

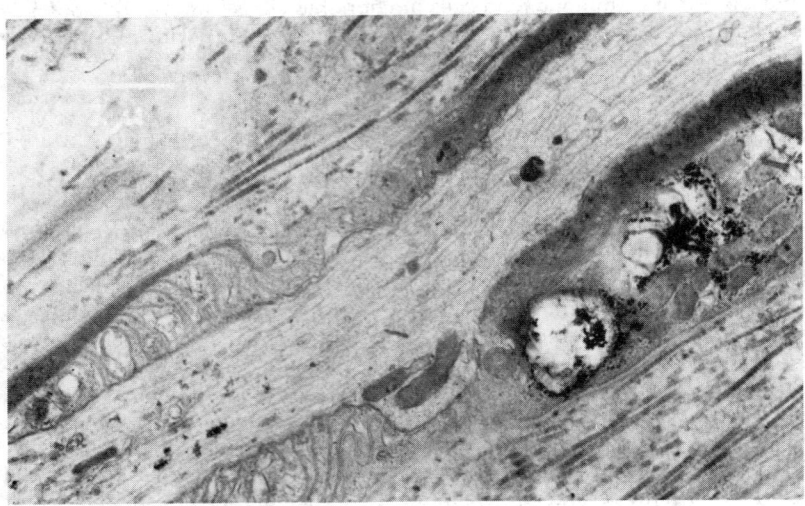

**Figure 161-2.** Electron micrograph of peripheral nerve in longitudinal section from a patient with metachromatic leukodystrophy shows densely staining inclusion material within the Schwann cell cytoplasm.

Alternatively, juvenile metachromatic leukodystrophy can begin between 6 and 16 years of age with personality and behavior changes and declining school performance. Seizures are common and motor dysfunction eventually ensues. The progression of this form is slower still, and survival is possible into late adolescence or early adulthood.

The adult form of metachromatic dystrophy presents as dementia or psychosis as early as 16 or as late as 60 years of age. Declining school or work performance often is the first sign of the disease. Motor dysfunction is inevitable, but its progression may be very slow.

Multiple sulfatase deficiency combines features of the late infantile form of metachromatic leukodystrophy, steroid sulfatase deficiency, and the mucopolysaccharidoses (see Table 161-1). Mucopolysaccharide storage is suggested by the presence of coarse facial features, hepatosplenomegaly, ichthyosis, and skeletal abnormalities. The tissue accumulation of sulfatides, mucopolysaccharides, and sulfated steroids reflects the pervasive deficiency of many different sulfatase activities.

## Diagnosis and Treatment

The diagnosis of metachromatic leukodystrophy is accomplished by careful clinical assessment and performance of appropriate laboratory studies. A history of regression and progressive deterioration of motor function, and signs of gait difficulties with weakness, hypotonia, hyporeflexia, and extensor plantar responses in the early forms, or behavioral and motor disability in older children or adolescents, suggests the diagnosis. Nerve conduction velocities are reduced as a reflection of peripheral nerve involvement. The cerebrospinal fluid (CSF) protein level is increased. Computed tomography (CT) or magnetic resonance imaging (MRI) reveals symmetric white matter lesions in the early forms of the disease and may demonstrate cortical atrophy in the later forms. Definitive diagnosis is made by establishing decreased activity of the enzyme, arylsulfatase A, preferably in leukocytes or skin fibroblast cultures. The availability of biochemical analysis has diminished greatly the role of peripheral nerve biopsy in detecting metachromatic granules.

**TABLE 161-1.  Characteristics of Sulfatide Lipidoses**

| Characteristic | Late Infantile | Juvenile | Adult | Multiple Sulfatase Deficiency |
|---|---|---|---|---|
| Age at onset | 6–24 mo | 4–8 y | 15 y or older | 6–18 mo |
| Prognosis | Death in 5–6 y | Death in 10–15 y | Slow progression | Death by age 10–12 y |
| Mode of inheritance | AR | AR | AR | AR |
| Neurologic signs | Gait difficulty, hypotonia, ataxia, rapid deterioration | Gait difficulty, ataxia, intellectual decline | Dementia, depression, psychosis, motor difficulty | Gait difficulty, hypotonia, ataxia, rapid deterioration |
| Systemic signs | | | | Coarse features, hepatosplenomegaly, skeletal deformity, ichthyosis |
| Stored material | Sulfatide | Sulfatide | Sulfatide | Sulfatide, cholesterol sulfate, mucopolysaccharide sulfate |
| Enzyme defect | Sulfatide sulfatase (arylsulfatase A) | Sulfatide sulfatase (arylsulfatase A) | Sulfatide sulfatase (arylsulfatase A) | Multiple sulfatases |
| Prenatal diagnosis feasible | Yes | Yes | Yes | Yes |

*AR,* autosomal recessive.

Arylsulfatase A activity in affected individuals usually measures less than 10% of control values, making this examination an ineffective means of differentiating the various clinical forms of the disorder. Fibroblast cultures may be used to distinguish the clinical types of metachromatic leukodystrophy based on their ability to degrade exogenous sulfatide, although this differentiation may not be straightforward in some cases. Cells from patients with the late infantile form metabolize little sulfatide. Cells from patients with the adult form have greater residual metabolic activity. Some individuals with the juvenile form of metachromatic leukodystrophy have normal levels of arylsulfatase A. These patients, instead, lack an activator protein that is necessary for sulfatide degradation. This can be demonstrated by abnormal catabolism of exogenous sulfatide in cultured fibroblasts and by the absence of the activator protein in leukocytes or fibroblast cultures using specific antibodies.

Recent advances in molecular genetics have identified two arylsulfatase alleles associated with metachromatic leukodystrophy, one detected exclusively in the late infantile form and the other in the juvenile and adult forms, thus providing a molecular basis for understanding the phenotypic heterogeneity of the disease. Additional mutant alleles undoubtedly will be identified.

Carrier detection is accomplished by measuring arylsulfatase A activity, and prenatal diagnosis is possible. Some normal individuals exhibit a pseudo-deficient arylsulfatase A state by biochemical assay, in which case, prenatal diagnosis could yield ambiguous results. Under these circumstances, it is necessary to evaluate the ability of the amniotic cells or trophoblasts to catabolize exogenous sulfatide in culture before deciding on the status of the fetus.

No effective treatment is available for metachromatic leukodystrophy. Enzyme replacement by tissue transplantation is under study. The recent use of bone marrow transplantation has suggested possible benefit in terms of improved arylsulfatase A activity and slowed disease progression, but convincing evidence of efficacy within the central nervous system is lacking. Careful consideration should be given to therapies that may modify the natural history in a way that would produce greater chronicity without effecting resolution. Supportive therapy is indicated to ensure proper nutrition and to treat medical problems, including seizures, as they occur.

## GLOBOID CELL LEUKODYSTROPHY (GALACTOSYLCERAMIDE LIPIDOSIS; KRABBE DISEASE)

Globoid cell leukodystrophy is an autosomal recessive disorder that has an incidence in Sweden of about 1 per 50,000, but apparently is less common outside Scandinavia. The biochemical abnormality involves the inability to degrade the sphingolipid, galactosylceramide, also called galactocerebroside. Galactocerebroside is an important component of myelin. Hence, both the central and peripheral nervous systems are affected in this disorder. Globoid cell leukodystrophy represents a fundamental failure in myelinogenesis. The small amount of myelin that is formed (less than 1% of normal) has a normal composition. Also, unlike metachromatic leukodystrophy, with its marked storage of sulfatide, there actually is a deficiency of galactocerebroside in this disorder. Globoid cells are multinucleate giant cells that occur in clusters throughout the brain and brain stem white matter, especially around venules, and apparently are elicited by the galactocerebroside. Indeed, the globoid cells contain excess quantities of this lipid. In addition, white matter is marked by the reduction or loss of oligodendroglia and by the presence of diffuse gliosis. Segmental demyelination is noted in peripheral nerves. The failure to synthesize myelin may be attributed to the

cytotoxic effect of galactosphingosine, or psychosine, on the oligodendrocyte. Psychosine, which is formed by removing the fatty acid from galactocerebroside, accumulates in the brains of these children in levels as high as 100 times normal.

### Forms of the Disease

Globoid cell leukodystrophy occurs in two principal forms: infantile (the more common) and late onset (Table 161-2). Infantile globoid cell leukodystrophy occurs early in the first year of life, usually by 6 months of age, and is characterized by extreme irritability, hypertonia, and developmental stagnation and regression. This is followed quickly by extensor posturing, rigidity, exaggerated startle response, optic atrophy, and cortical blindness. Deep tendon reflexes initially are prominent, but gradually are lost, and hypotonia replaces hypertonia, both of which are signs of peripheral nerve involvement. Death from intercurrent illness is usual by 12 months of age, although children occasionally survive to 18 to 24 months of age.

Late-onset globoid cell leukodystrophy appears after a period of normal development from 1.5 to 5 years of age. Typical features are gait abnormalities and ataxia with slower but relentless progression, including spasticity, visual loss with optic atrophy and cortical blindness, and profound psychomotor retardation.

### Diagnosis and Treatment

The definitive diagnosis of globoid cell leukodystrophy can be made by enzymatic assay. Galactocerebroside $\beta$-galactosidase activity, recently linked to chromosome 14, is deficient and can be assayed in leukocytes and fibroblast cultures. The need for enzyme analysis will be suggested by a careful history and physical assessment, and by the demonstration of reduced nerve conduction velocities and marked elevation of the CSF protein level (usually above 300 mg/dL). CT will show decreased white matter and increased density of the internal capsule, thalamus, and basal ganglia (Fig 161-3). MRI will reflect the failure of myelination by demonstrating reversal of the usual gray-white appearance.

Genetic counseling and prenatal diagnosis may be provided for potential carriers. The existence of a pseudo-deficiency state in carriers may cloud the picture, however, and necessitate assessment of the ability of amniotic cell or trophoblast cultures to degrade exogenous galactocerebroside. Caution must be exercised in the interpretation of such studies. Effective therapy for globoid cell leukodystrophy is lacking. Nevertheless, supportive care is important to assist the family during this difficult period.

## ADRENOLEUKODYSTROPHY

Adrenoleukodystrophy, first described as an X-linked disorder, now is recognized as a multifaceted complex including adrenoleukodystrophy and adrenomyeloneuropathy, both of which are X-linked, and an autosomal recessive form that appears in infancy (Table 161-3).

### Forms of the Disease

Adrenoleukodystrophy, the most common of the three disease forms, is a progressive disorder of young males 3 to 16 years of age (mean age, 8 years) that generally begins with personality changes or altered school performance and motor deficit. Seizures occur in 20% of children and occasionally signal the onset of the disorder. Motor involvement may be unilateral at first. Progression generally is relentless and results in profound psychomotor retardation, spasticity, and extensor posturing. Death occurs within 10 years of diagnosis. Adrenal insufficiency is important clinically

| TABLE 161-2. Globoid Cell Leukodystrophy | | |
| --- | --- | --- |
| Characteristic | Infantile | Late Infantile |
| Age at onset | Infancy | 1–5 y |
| Prognosis | Death by age 2 y | Death by age 10–12 y |
| Mode of inheritance | Autosomal recessive | Autosomal recessive |
| Neurologic signs | Irritability, extensor rigidity, optic atrophy, cortical blindness, rapid deterioration | Ataxia, gait difficulty, visual loss, psychomotor decline |
| Stored material | Galactosylceramide, galactosylsphingosine, (psychosine) | Galactosylceramide, galactosylsphingosine, (psychosine) |
| Enzyme defect | Galactosylceramide, β-galactosidase | Galactosylceramide, β-galactosidase |
| Prenatal diagnosis feasible | Yes | Yes |

in about 40% of children, although an equal number may have inadequate cortisol response to adrenocorticotropic hormone challenge. An "Addison disease only" phenotype of adrenoleukodystrophy is recognized now and may account for 40% of males with Addison disease.

Adrenomyeloneuropathy frequently is associated with adrenal insufficiency. This X-linked disorder usually appears in the third decade of life as a slowly progressive spastic paraparesis and a distal sensorimotor neuropathy. Bowel and bladder dysfunction accompany the motor disability. Adrenoleukodystrophy and adrenomyeloneuropathy may occur in the same family.

Neonatal adrenoleukodystrophy is a somewhat different entity and is the least often seen of the three types of disease. Beginning in early infancy, this autosomal recessive disorder represents a fundamental abnormality of the subcellular organelle known as the peroxisome and is related thereby to Zellweger syndrome and neonatal Refsum disease. Neonatal adrenoleukodystrophy is characterized by neonatal seizures, profound hypotonia, mild dysmorphic features, hepatomegaly with impaired function, and pigmentary abnormalities of the retina. Its progression is rapid, and death often occurs by the child's first birthday.

Neuropathologic evaluation of the adrenoleukodystrophy complex demonstrates a demyelinating process with a vigorous perivascular inflammatory response corresponding to the areas of clinical involvement. Adrenal atrophy is noted. The cortical cells are swollen, but the medullary cells are spared. In addition,

birefringent laminar inclusions are present in patients with adrenoleukodystrophy and adrenomyeloneuropathy, but not in those with the neonatal form of the disease. The characteristic pathologic feature of neonatal leukodystrophy is the absence or marked reduction and morphologic alteration of peroxisomes. Definitive diagnosis of each of these disorders depends on the demonstration of elevated levels of very–long-chain fatty acids (26-carbon chain) or an elevated ratio of C26:0/C22:0 fatty acids. Thus, the metabolic defect is a failure of very–long-chain fatty acid beta oxidation, a function that is located in the peroxisome and is distinct from mitochondrial fatty acid beta oxidation, probably caused by defective long-chain fatty acid activation by the peroxisomal enzyme, fatty acyl coenzyme A synthetase.

## Diagnosis and Treatment

The clinical diagnosis of adrenoleukodystrophy is based on results of the history and physical examination, characteristic changes seen on CT (confluent hypodensities in parieto-occipital white matter with contrast enhancement at the margins suggesting active demyelination; Fig 161-4) or MRI (symmetric periventricular signal increase) examination, normal nerve conduction velocities, abnormal brain stem auditory evoked responses (prolonged interpeak latency between waves I and V), and elevated CSF protein levels. Adrenomyeloneuropathy, in contrast, is characterized by normal CSF protein levels and normal results on CT of the brain (mild atrophy may be a late finding), but abnormal nerve conduction velocities and brain stem auditory evoked responses. Children with neonatal adrenoleukodystrophy, in addition to having elevated very–long-chain fatty acid levels and altered peroxisomes, demonstrate reduced plasmalogens and elevated phytanic acid and pipecolic acid levels in plasma. Marked abnormalities of brain stem auditory evoked responses, visual evoked responses, and electroretinography results also may assist in the clinical diagnosis.

Heterozygote detection may be accomplished reliably for adrenoleukodystrophy by combining the measurement of very–long-chain fatty acid levels and ratios with brain stem auditory evoked responses. As many as 15% of possible heterozygotes for adrenoleukodystrophy still may escape detection, however. With regard to the neonatal form, heterozygote detection is not possible. Nevertheless, prenatal diagnosis is feasible for each disorder in families that are known to be at risk.

Fifteen percent or more of female heterozygotes for adrenoleukodystrophy may have a generally mild form of the disease

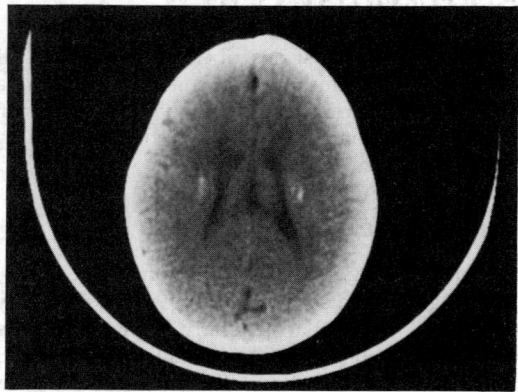

**Figure 161-3.** Nonenhanced brain CT scan of an infant with galactosylceramide lipidosis (Krabbe's disease) demonstrates lesions of increased density adjacent to the lateral ventricles.

| TABLE 161-3.  Adrenoleukodystrophy Complex |
| --- |

| Characteristic | Adrenoleukodystrophy | Adrenomyeloneuropathy | Neonatal Adrenoleukodystrophy |
| --- | --- | --- | --- |
| Age at onset | 3–16 y (mean age, 8 y) | 20–40 y | Infancy |
| Prognosis | Death in 1–10 y | Prolonged survival | Death in 1–4 y |
| Mode of inheritance | XLR | XLR | AR |
| Neurologic signs | Behavior problems, poor school performance, quadriparesis, blindness | Spastic paraparesis, distal neuropathy, urinary retention, impotence | Hypotonia, seizures, rapid deterioration, mild dysmorphism, hepatomegaly |
| Systemic signs | Hypoadrenalism in 50%, diminished response to ACTH, skin hyperpigmentation | Hypoadrenalism, hypogonadism | Normal adrenal function, hypoplastic adrenal glands |
| Stored material | Very–long-chain fatty acids | Very–long-chain fatty acids | Very–long-chain fatty acids, phytanic acid, bile acids, reduced plasmalogens |
| Enzyme defect | Peroxisomal fatty acyl-CoA synthetase | Peroxisomal fatty acyl-CoA synthetase | Absent or deficient peroxisomes |
| Prenatal diagnosis feasible | Yes | Yes | Yes |

*AR*, autosomal recessive; *XLR*, X-linked recessive; *ACTH*, adrenocorticotropic hormone; *acyl-CoA*, acyl coenzyme A.

that is characterized by a progressive spastic paraparesis, mild peripheral neuropathy, normal adrenal function, and elevated very–long-chain fatty acid levels in plasma or fibroblasts.

Effective therapy for the various forms of adrenoleukodystrophy is being sought actively. Bone marrow transplantation for enzyme replacement has not been helpful in neurologically impaired children with the disorder, but may retard disease onset in normal or mildly affected patients. Dietary therapy aimed at restricting the intake of long-chain fatty acids and modifying their endogenous formation seems to function similarly by restricting disease onset in presymptomatic individuals. Nevertheless, the treatment of progressive disease is ineffective.

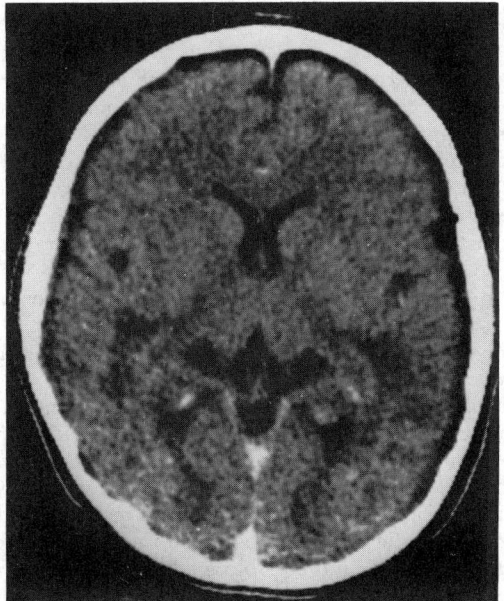

**Figure 161-4.**  Enhanced brain CT scan of a child with adrenoleukodystrophy indicates symmetric low-density lesions located posteriorly in the parieto-occipital regions with areas of contrast enhancement.

## ALEXANDER DISEASE

Alexander disease is a rare disorder that is thought to result from astrocyte dysfunction. This condition is characterized by psychomotor retardation, spasticity, seizures, and megalencephaly, usually occurring by 2 years of age. Progression to death is rapid. No metabolic defect has been defined and diagnosis is made by brain biopsy or at necropsy. The characteristic neuropathologic finding is the presence of eosinophilic bodies called Rosenthal fibers. These refractile bodies appear near astrocyte filaments and may represent degenerating filaments. Although Rosenthal fibers are seen in patients with numerous disorders (eg, glial tumors, multiple sclerosis, syringomyelia), their abundance in patients with Alexander disease is the diagnostic key. Demyelination is prominent in frontal white matter and in the brain stem.

In addition to the infantile form, juvenile and adult onset Alexander disease have been described much less frequently. In these forms, neurologic involvement appears to be confined to the brain stem and spinal cord, and mentation remains intact.

The clinical diagnosis of Alexander disease in the presence of psychomotor retardation, megencephaly, and seizures may be aided by CT or MRI, which demonstrate low-density lesions in cerebral white matter, particularly of the frontal region, and symmetric enhancement of caudate nuclei, the thalamus, and periventricular white matter after the administration of a contrast agent. Nevertheless, the diagnosis rests on the microscopic examination of brain tissue.

Treatment is supportive, with emphasis placed on the administration of appropriate anticonvulsant agents. Most cases have been sporadic, yielding no information regarding a possible genetic basis for this disorder.

## CANAVAN DISEASE

Canavan disease is an autosomal recessive leukodystrophy that is noted frequently in Ashkenazi Jews and is associated neuropathologically with spongy degeneration of the brain. Typically presenting in early infancy, this disorder usually causes death within the patient's first decade. Characteristic clinical features include psychomotor retardation, spasticity, blindness with optic atrophy, and macrocephaly. Seizures may occur in 25% to 50% of patients, but generally are not problematic. Brain imaging (CT or MRI) reveals diffuse white matter changes without ventriculomegaly. The recent revelation of increased N-acetylaspartic acid levels in the blood, urine, and CSF of affected patients led to the identification of aspartoacylase deficiency as the biochemical abnormality in Canavan disease and to the subsequent capability of prenatal diagnosis. The precise role of N-acetylaspartic acid in the pathogenesis of this disorder is unclear, but may involve the excitatory neurotransmitter system. No effective therapy is available.

## PELIZAEUS-MERZBACHER DISEASE

Pelizaeus-Merzbacher disease is a very rare and clinically heterogenous leukodystrophy of infancy that is characterized by rotatory nystagmus, slowly progressive psychomotor retardation, spasticity, ataxia, choreoathetosis, and X-linked recessive inheritance. The biochemical abnormality appears to be related to deletion or alteration of the proteolipid protein gene, which has been mapped to Xq22. Carrier detection has been achieved on this basis. The precise molecular defect varies between individual patients, however, indicating marked molecular heterogeneity as well. Definitive diagnosis was provided previously by matching the clinical pattern with neuropathologic study at brain biopsy or necropsy. Neuropathologic changes consist of diffuse demyelination, with intermingled islands of normal myelin, which yields the so-called tigroid appearance. MRI reveals high signal intensity of cerebral white matter and reversal of the usual gray-white matter appearance. These findings suggest a dysmyelinating process. In addition, the markedly abnormal visual, auditory,

and somatosensory evoked responses noted in patients with the disorder may aid in the clinical assessment. The disease progresses slowly and occasionally is misdiagnosed as static encephalopathy. Treatment is supportive.

Similar pathologic features have been described in male and female adolescents and adults, suggesting significant heterogeneity of Pelizaeus-Merzbacher disease. The availability of a biochemical marker may help to discriminate these variants.

## Selected Readings

Bridge PJ, MacLeod PM, Lillicrap DP. Carrier detection and prenatal diagnosis of Pelizaeus-Merzbacher disease using a combination of anonymous DNA polymorphisms and the proteolipid protein (PLP) gene cDNA. Am J Med Genet 1991;38:616.

Bruyn GW, Weenink HR, Bots GTAM. Pelizaeus-Merzbacher disease: The Lowenberg-Hill type. Acta Neuropathol (Berl) 1985;67:177.

Farrell K, Chuang S, Becker LE. Computed tomography in Alexander disease. Ann Neurol 1984;15:605.

Gieselmann V, von Figura K. Advances in the molecular genetics of metachromatic leukodystrophy. J Inherited Metab Dis 1990;13:560.

Matalon R, Michals K, Kaul R, Mafee M. Spongy degeneration of the brain, Canavan disease. International Pediatrics 1990;5:121.

Moser HW, Moser AB, Naidu S, Bergin A. Clinical aspects of adrenoleukodystrophy and adrenomyeloneuropathy. Dev Neurosci 1991;13:254.

Percy AK. The inherited neurodegenerative disorders of childhood: Clinical assessment. J Child Neurol 1987;2:82.

Polten A, Fluharty AL, Fluharty CB, Kappler J, von Figura K, Gieselmann V. Molecular basis of different forms of metachromatic leukodystrophy. N Engl J Med 1991;324:18.

Schuster V, Horwitz AE, Kreth HW. Alexander's disease: Cranial MRI and ultrasound findings. Pediatr Radiol 1991;21:133.

Stanbury JB, Wyngaarden JB, Fredrickson DS, et al. The metabolic basis of inherited disease, ed 6. New York: McGraw-Hill, 1989.

Svennerholm L, Vanier M-T, Månsson J-E. Krabbe disease: A galactosylsphingosine (psychosine) lipidosis. J Lipid Res 1980;21:53.

Uziel G, Bertini E, Bardelli P, Rimoldi M, Gambetti M. Experience on therapy of adrenoleukodystrophy and adrenomyeloneuropathy. Dev Neurosci 1991;13:274.

Zlotogora J, Chakraborty S, Knowlton RG, Wenger DA. Krabbe disease locus mapped to chromosome 14 by genetic linkage. Am J Hum Genet 1990;47:37.

*Principles and Practice of Pediatrics, Second Edition.*
edited by Frank A. Oski et al. J. B. Lippincott Company, Philadelphia © 1994.

# 161.2 The Metabolic Encephalopathies

### Edward R. B. McCabe

Many of the metabolic disorders include among their clinical features abnormalities of the central nervous system. Fortunately, a significant portion of these disorders can be treated to prevent progression of the encephalopathy. Because of the potential for treatment, it is extremely important that a definitive diagnosis be arrived at quickly, so that appropriate treatment may be instituted promptly. Rapid and definitive diagnosis also allows the family to plan realistically for the child's future, even if a specific treatment is not available. Genetic counseling is much more accurate and informative when the diagnosis is known, and it is important that family members have this information while they still are in their childbearing years. It is particularly unfortunate when the diagnosis is delayed until a subsequent pregnancy or birth of an affected sibling has occurred.

## DISORDERS OF CARBOHYDRATE METABOLISM

Hypoglycemia is a common cause of encephalopathy in children. Glucose is a critical substrate for energy production in the brain, and when its availability is interrupted, significant central nervous system dysfunction results. The signs and symptoms of central nervous system dysfunction include, at the extreme, convulsions and coma, but they may be less severe, involving confusion, irritability, listlessness, headache, eye rolling, and agitation. Night terrors also may accompany hypoglycemia in some patients. In addition, the child may evidence hunger, tachycardia, or sweating, the latter being especially noticeable on the brow and hands, which may be cold and clammy to the touch. Although the heart is dependent on fatty acids for its primary energy supply, glucose represents an important substrate; therefore, cardiomegaly, with or without overt cardiac failure, may be associated with hypoglycemia. Symptoms in the neonate and young infant may include poor feeding, a weak or high-pitched cry, limpness, cyanosis, and vomiting. Signs and symptoms should resolve rapidly with normalization of the blood glucose level unless the episode has been sufficiently profound or prolonged to result in dysfunction extending beyond the hypoglycemic episode. In these cases, the possibility of long-term sequelae is significant.

Hypoglycemia has been defined classically as a whole blood glucose level of less than 20 mg/dL or a serum or plasma glucose level of less than 25 mg/dL in the preterm or low–birth-weight infant during the first week of life; a blood glucose level of less than 30 mg/dL or a serum glucose level of less than 35 mg/dL in the full-size or term neonate from birth to 72 hours; and a blood glucose level of less than 40 mg/dL or a serum glucose level of less than 46 mg/dL thereafter. Others feel that these definitions represent population norms rather than physiologically acceptable glucose concentrations, and that a blood glucose level of less than 40 mg/dL or a serum glucose level of less than 45 to 50 mg/dL should be considered hypoglycemia regardless of the age of the individual. The differential diagnosis of hypoglycemia is extensive, but the history and clinical assessment can be helpful in narrowing the possibilities (Table 161-4). Specific biochemical or morphologic diagnostic testing is recommended for these disorders to tailor management, prevent recurrences, and treat the hypoglycemia effectively.

The primary complication of hypoglycemia is irreversible central nervous system damage. The goal of diagnosis and treatment is the prevention of acute and chronic hypoglycemia with attendant central nervous system compromise. A severe acute insult may result in respiratory compromise and death from status epilepticus or coma. The clinician must carry out the diagnostic evaluation with care and discretion so as to prevent hypoglycemia. For example, medium-chain acyl coenzyme A dehydrogenase deficiency may be diagnosed by the analysis of acyl carnitine levels in the urine after a carnitine challenge or by the measurement of oetanoylglycine and other organic acids without risk to the patient, whereas a fast or a fat challenge may lead to significant hypoglycemia and the risk of sequelae. If a definitive diagnosis has not been made and the risk of spontaneous or challenge-induced hypoglycemia exists, then the diagnostic plan should be worked out well ahead of time so that the necessary information may be obtained if the child becomes symptomatic, to avoid repeated hypoglycemic episodes. A secure intravenous line should be in place in any hospitalized patient who is at risk for iatrogenic or spontaneous hypoglycemia.

Treatment of an acute hypoglycemic episode involves the rapid restoration of normoglycemia to supply this substrate to the central nervous system. If venous access is readily available, the most rapid and effective therapy is intravenous glucose delivered at a rate of 0.5 to 1.0 g/kg, or 2 to 4 mL/kg of a 25-g/dL (25%) dextrose solution (D25) given at a rate of 1 mL/min. The glucose infusion should continue at a rate of 8 to 10 mg/kg/min, with frequent measurement of the blood glucose concentration and necessary adjustments made in the infusion rate to maintain a normal blood glucose level. If hypoglycemia persists despite increasing glucose infusion rates, hyperinsulinism should be considered. After the blood glucose level has stabilized and feeding has been reinitiated, the infusion rate may be decreased slowly, but never discontinued abruptly. Even in the absence of pathologic hyperinsulinemia, the insulin level will rise physiologically in response to the administration of glucose; therefore, the infusion must be tapered slowly (by decrements of 4 to 6 mg/kg/min at 4- to 6-hour intervals) to prevent rebound hypoglycemia.

Hypoglycemia is a medical emergency and, if percutaneous venous access is not achieved rapidly, a cutdown should be performed by someone who is skilled in this technique. Additional supportive measures may be necessary, including endotracheal intubation.

For the child with milder hypoglycemia, oral glucose may be beneficial, but care must be taken to protect against aspiration if the child is becoming obtunded. Glucagon (0.03 to 0.30 mg/kg, up to a maximum total dose of 1 mg intramuscularly) may be given, but with the knowledge that if it is effective, the benefit may be only transient, and, for patients with certain glycogen storage diseases, ketotic hypoglycemia, and other disorders in which glycogen has been depleted or is unavailable, it may have a minimal effect or none at all. Diazoxide, an antihypertensive

agent that also suppresses insulin release, may be useful in certain patients with hyperinsulinemia. The usual starting dosage of diazoxide is 8 to 12 mg/kg/d, given orally in divided doses every 8 to 12 hours, but the dosage may range between 5 and 20 mg/kg/d. Marked hypertrichosis is a prominent side effect that should be discussed with the parents at the time the drug is started, because this may become objectionable enough to them to interfere with compliance. The hypertrichosis is reversible when the drug is discontinued. Hemoglobin $A_{1c}$ may be used to monitor the magnitude of hyperglycemic excursions. Small, frequent feedings are useful for many patients with hypoglycemia, although the composition of the feedings differs according to the underlying disorder.

With severe and prolonged hypoglycemia, permanent encephalopathy is not unusual, particularly in young children. Learning disability, attention deficit disorder, developmental delay, ataxia, spasticity, or seizures may be seen. Seizures associated with normal blood glucose concentrations should be treated with the usual anticonvulsant medications. The family of a child with sequelae should be counseled regarding infant stimulation and special education. Most families have concerns regarding the genetic risk of recurrence, although they may not voice their concerns to the physician; therefore, this topic should be addressed with all families.

## DISEASES OF COPPER METABOLISM

### Menkes' Syndrome

Menkes' syndrome, also known as kinky hair disease or steely hair disease, is an X-linked disorder that is characterized by progressive neurologic deterioration beginning in the first 4 to 8 weeks of life, with apathy, somnolence, feeding difficulties, and myoclonic seizures. Many of these patients are born prematurely, fail to thrive, and have hypothermia. Patients also can be seen with acute sepsis. Their muscle tone varies from hypotonia and flaccidity to hypertonia and spasticity. The descriptive names for this disorder derive from the macroscopic dull, hypopigmented, sparse, and kinky appearance of the hair resembling steel wool. Microscopically, there are pili torti and monilethrix with friable, short hair. The child's face typically is pale, with pudgy cheeks, a bow-shaped upper lip, and microcephaly. The arteries are tortuous, with defective, fragmented elastic fibers. Generalized or focal cerebral and cerebellar degeneration may be seen, and may result from the vascular abnormalities. Low serum copper concentrations, low circulating ceruloplasmin levels, and decreased hepatic and brain copper content are observed. Copper absorption from the intestine is deficient, and elevated copper content in the intestinal mucosa, kidney, spleen, lung, muscle, pancreas, and placenta has suggested defective copper transport. The copper level is increased in cultured fibroblasts. Although progression followed by death in infancy or during the toddler years is typical, individuals with milder forms of this disorder have been described. Menkes' syndrome maps to chromosome xq13. Treatment with copper in the form of copper histidinate has been reported to prevent progression of the neurodegeneration, but this remains experimental, with considerable question regarding its general efficacy in patients with this disease.

### Wilson's Disease

Wilson's disease, or hepatolenticular degeneration, is a disorder with a variable clinical presentation, but typical features include neurologic manifestations, hepatocellular disease, Kayser-Fleischer rings of the cornea, a low serum ceruloplasmin level, and increased copper concentrations in the serum, urine, and

TABLE 161-4. Metabolic Disorders Associated With Hypoglycemia

| Metabolic Disorders | Diagnostic Comments |
|---|---|
| **Primary Disorders of Carbohydrate Metabolism** | |
| Glycogen storage disease: | Hepatomegaly and fasting hypoglycemia with: |
| IA. Glucose-6-phosphate deficiency | Prominent short stature, lactic acidemia |
| IB. Glucose-6-phosphate translocase deficiency | Neutropenia |
| III. Debrancher deficiency | Elevated red-cell glycogen |
| VI. Hepatic phosphorylase deficiency | Frequently a milder course |
| IX. Hepatic phosphorylase kinase deficiency | Mild course with X-linked inheritance |
| Fructose-1,6-diphosphatase deficiency | Profound hypoglycemia and acidemia |
| Hereditary fructose intolerance | |
| Fructose-1-phosphate aldolase deficiency | Jaundice and hepatomegaly develop after child begins sucrose/fructose intake; hypoglycemia and hypophosphatemia with fructose load |
| Galactosemia : galactose-1-phosphate uridyl transferase deficiency | Hypoglycemia rare, except with significant galactose load and more frequently a consequence of liver disease |
| Glycerol intolerance | Hypoglycemia associated with fat ingestion or glycerol challenge |
| **Disorders of Amino Acid and Organic Acid Metabolism** | |
| Organic acidemias including maple syrup urine disease, methylmalonic acidemia, propionic acidemia, isovaleric acidemia, glutaric acidemia, acetoacetyl-CoA thiolase deficiency, and others | Hypoglycemia associated with acidemia and, in some cases, with a "Reye's-like" syndrome with hyperammonemia, and cerebral edema |
| Congenital lactic acidoses | Lactic acidemia with disturbance of gluconeogenesis or energy metabolism |
| Biotinidase deficiency | Hypoglycemia associated with complex organic acidemia, ataxia progressing to seizures and coma, alopecia, and rash |
| **Disorders of Fat Metabolism** | |
| Medium chain acyl-CoA dehydrogenase deficiency (MCAD) | Fasting, nonketotic hypoglycemia assoicated with dicarboxylic acidemia; seen among patients with sudden infant death syndrome and acute life-threatening episodes |
| **Endocrine Disorders** | |
| Hyperinsulinism | Postprandial and postglucose infusion hypoglycemia; may be caused by increased islet cell mass (as with islet cell adenoma and nesidioblastosis) or functional hyperresponsiveness (as with leucine hypersensitivity); may be exogenous as in a diabetic who receives too much insulin or individuals with Munchausen or Munchausen-by-proxy syndrome |
| Infant of the diabetic mother | A specific form of hyperinsulinism found in large-for-gestational-age neonates with a history of maternal diabetes mellitus |
| Hypopituitarism | Hypothalamic or pituitary hormonal deficiencies resulting in the inability to mount a normal glycemic response to stress or to tolerate starvation; may include deficiencies of growth hormone adrenocorticotropic hormone or thyroid hormone |
| Adrenal insufficiency | Seen with the congenital adrenal hyperplasias and congenital adrenal hypoplasias as well as adrenal medullary unresponsiveness |
| **Limited Substrate Availability** | |
| Malnutrition | History of limited intake of protein or calories; signs and symptoms of kwashiokor or marasmus |
| Ketotic hypoglycemia | Fasting, ketotic hypoglycemia; frequently preceded by intercurrent illness; also known as accelerated starvation; typically seen between ages 1 and 7 years |
| **Infectious and Postinfectious** | |
| Sepsis | Hypoglycemia in all age groups, but must be particularly vigilant in neonatal period when signs and symptoms of hypoglycemia may be subtle |
| Reye's syndrome | History of chickenpox or flu-like illness; aspirin is an important risk factor |
| Neonatal | Must seek underlying etiology, especially sepsis, maternal diabetes; limited substrate availability makes neonates particularly vulnerable |
| Shock | Must consider hypoglycemia as possibly contributory in any individual with shock until glycemic status is determined |
| Liver disease | Must consider metabolic and nonmetabolic disorders as underlying etiologies |
| Toxic | Includes exogenous insulin; sulfonylurea salicylates, propranolol, L-asparaginase, and others |

liver. Two neurologic forms are recognized, although their signs and symptoms overlap. The dystonic form commonly is associated with liver disease in children, and symptoms include rigidity progressing to contractures. Choreiform or athetoid movements are manifestations of the lenticular degeneration. The pseudosclerotic form is typified by tremors and adult onset, with a more long-term progression than the dystonic form. The neurologic dysfunction associated with Wilson's disease is primarily motor, with no sensory component. Psychiatric manifestations may be seen and can be the primary complaint. Deterioration in school performance, alterations of mood, and acting out frequently are not recognized as manifestations of organic disease in these patients and are attributed to problems of preadolescent and adolescent socialization. The dementia caused by Wilson's disease may be severe, leading to the diagnosis of schizophrenia. Even if neurologic features are subtle or absent, the presence of Kayser-Fleischer rings by gross visual or slit lamp examination provides valuable clinical information. The corneal rings are present in virtually all patients with neurologic or psychiatric symptoms, but only in two thirds or less of those with hepatic abnormalities.

Additional features of Wilson's disease include acute or chronic hepatocellular disease, renal dysfunction, hemolytic anemia, neutropenia, thrombocytopenia, osteoporosis, osteomalacia, pathologic fractures, arthritis, cardiomyopathy, and hypoparathyroidism. Renal manifestations may range from generalized aminoaciduria to full renal Fanconi's syndrome, uricosuria with hypouricemia, renal lithiasis, nephrocalcinosis, and renal failure. In affected patients, the serum ceruloplasmin level generally is less than 20 mg/dL. Normal ceruloplasmin values are low in young infants (less than 3 months of age), however, and ceruloplasmin levels may be normal in as many as 5% of patients with Wilson's disease. An elevated copper content detected on liver biopsy is a particularly valuable measure. Although normal values vary between laboratories, the hepatic copper content of affected patients generally is at least 2½- to 5-fold above the upper limit of normal and frequently is elevated 10-fold or more. The serum copper concentration may be low, but overlap with normal levels makes this a less useful diagnostic test. Urinary copper excretion is increased from less than 40 $\mu$g/24 h in normal individuals to 100 to 1000 $\mu$g/24 h in affected patients. A test dose of penicillamine at 10 mg/kg results in an increase in copper excretion to 1200 to 3000 $\mu$g/24 h in patients with Wilson's disease. It is important that all containers, solutions, and equipment (including biopsy needles) that are used to collect tissue and fluids for copper determination be free of contaminating copper, because this could interfere with accurate measurement. The incorporation of intravenously administered radioactive copper into ceruloplasmin also has been used in diagnosing this condition.

Wilson's disease is an autosomal recessive disorder with linkage to retinoblastoma, esterase D, and other markers on chromosome 13 in the region of 13q14-21. Because the clinical features and age at onset of this disorder are so variable, physicians should subject siblings of affected patients to clinical and laboratory examination. Mildly symptomatic or presymptomatic individuals can be detected in this manner. Because of the variability in clinical expression of Wilson's disease, the differential diagnosis can be very broad, including acute viral hepatitis, chronic active hepatitis, $\alpha_1$-antitrypsin deficiency, and other causes of liver disease that are associated with progressive neurologic deterioration or dementia, including the porphyrias. The presence of Kayser-Fleischer rings, however, is a definitive sign. Specific laboratory testing is required.

Treatment of Wilson's disease with D-penicillamine (Cuprimine) for copper chelation should be instituted as early as possible in the course of the disease, with the best results obtained in patients in whom treatment has been started before symptoms

arise. The usual dosage is 100 mg/kg/d up to 500 to 750 mg/d in children less than 10 years of age and 1000 mg/d in older individuals, although dosages as high as 3000 mg/d have been used. D-penicillamine is given in 2 to 4 divided doses. It is an agent with a significant incidence of side effects, including allergic reactions, bone marrow suppression, and a variety of rashes. These may be prevented or minimized by starting the drug at a dosage of 200 to 250 mg/d and increasing the dosage at weekly intervals by increments of 200 to 250 mg/d. Restriction of copper intake should be considered, although strict restriction may be impractical. Zinc supplementation will prevent zinc deficiency from chelation and will decrease copper absorption by competition for uptake. Vitamin $B_6$ should be supplemented because penicillamine (particularly the L-isomer, but perhaps the D-isomer to a lesser extent) inhibits pyridoxine-dependent enzymes and can produce signs of pyridoxine deficiency.

The prognosis of patients with Wilson's disease and acute fulminant hepatitis is poor, but treatment should include peritoneal dialysis and possibly plasmapheresis. Aggressive and effective extraction of copper may not be successful in saving the life of such individuals. Liver transplantation has been effective in the treatment of patients with Wilson's disease, even those with acute disease, and should be considered in patients who do not respond to chelation, including those with acute, fulminant disease.

## THE PORPHYRIAS

The porphyrias are inborn errors of the heme biosynthetic pathway. Not all the porphyrias are associated with encephalopathy, but all are described here for the purposes of differential diagnosis and completeness. Those porphyrias with neuropsychiatric features are readily identifiable, as outlined in Table 161-5.

Heme biosynthesis is diagrammed in Figure 161-5. Of the eight enzymatic steps in this pathway, four are mitochondrial: δ-aminolevulinic acid (ALA) synthase (step 1), coproporphyrinogen (coprogen) oxidase (step 6), protoporphyrinogen (protogen) oxidase (step 7), and ferrochelatase (step 8). Four enzymes are cytoplasmic: ALA dehydratase (step 2), porphobilinogen (PBG) deaminase (step 3), uroporphyrinogen III (urogen III) cosynthase (step 4), and urogen decarboxylase (step 5). Clinical disorders are associated with all eight steps: step 1 with X-linked sideroblastic anemia and steps 2 through 8 with porphyrias. ALA and coprogen III move between the mitochondrial and cytoplasmic compartments, but no defects in the transport of these intermediates have been noted. There are eight clinically distinct porphyrias associated with seven enzymes (steps 2 to 8): porphyria cutanea tarda (PCT) is caused by the heterozygous deficiency of step 5 (urogen decarboxylase), and hepatoerythropoietic porphyria (HEP) is caused by the homozygous deficiency of this same enzyme. Table 161-5 details the clinical features of the porphyrias, listing them according to the enzyme sequence from step 2 through step 8. The disorders are discussed in the same sequence in the text.

ALA synthase is the initial and rate-limiting enzyme of heme biosynthesis, and it is regulated by negative feedback from the end product of the pathway heme. Two genes now are recognized for this enzyme: ALAS1 encodes the housekeeping gene and maps to 3p21, and ALAS2 is the erythroid-specific gene and maps to Xp11. A defect in ALAS2 results in X-linked sideroblastic anemia, which is characterized by hypochromic microcytic anemia that frequently is detected in childhood, hemochromatosis that leads to death at a relatively young age, hyperferricemia, increased peripheral siderocytes after splenectomy, and reduced protoporphyrin levels in the microcytes.

TABLE 161-5.    The Human Porphyrias

| Disease | Deficient Enzyme* | Genetics | Porphyria Classification | Major Symptoms | | |
|---|---|---|---|---|---|---|
| | | | | *Neuropsychiatric* | *Visceral* | *Photosensitivity* |
| ALAD porphyria | (2) ALA dehydratase | AR | Hepatic | + | + | − |
| Acute intermittent porphyria | (3) PBG deaminase | AD | Hepatic | + | + | − |
| Congenital erythropoietic porphyria | (4) Urogen III cosynthase | AR | Erythropoietic | − | − | + |
| Porphyria cutanea tarda | (5) Urogen decarboxylase | AD | Hepatic | − | − | + |
| Hepatoerythropoietic porphyria | (5) Urogen decarboxylase | AR | Hepatoerythropoietic | − | ± | + |
| Hereditary coproporphyria | (6) Coprogen oxidase | AD | Hepatic | + | + | ± |
| Variegate porphyria | (7) Protogen oxidase | AD | Hepatic | + | + | ± |
| Erythropoietic protoporphyria | (8) Ferrochelatase | AD | Erythropoietic | − | ± | + |

* Number in parentheses is enzyme sequence in the heme synthetic pathway.
† Enzymatic diganosis may be possible using other tissues, but has been well documented in those listed. Prenatal diagnosis at an enzymatic level is theoretically possible in all, but data are limited. In autosomal dominant disorders, family studies may be necessary in an attempt to evaluate heterozygous levels of activity.

## δ-Aminolevulinic Acid Dehydratase Porphyria

ALA dehydratase deficiency is an extremely rare autosomal recessive porphyria. Affected patients have varied from an infant with severe involvement and failure to thrive to a male in his seventh decade with minimal involvement. Hypotonia and paralysis may result in respiratory failure. Other features include vomiting and pain involving the extremities and abdomen. Remissions and exacerbations are typical, with exacerbations associated with inanition, stress, or ethanol intake. ALA dehydratase activity is decreased in erythrocytes to about 2% of normal levels. Intermediate ALA dehydratase activity to about 50% has been documented in parents and other relatives of affected individuals without associated symptomatology. The ALA dehydratase complementary DNA has been isolated and mutation analysis performed. The treatment of acute episodes with intravenous glucose may be helpful in some patients.

## Acute Intermittent Porphyria

Acute intermittent porphyria (AIP) is an autosomal dominant deficiency of PBG deaminase, which maps to the long arm of chromosome 11 (11q23-Hq23-ter). It is considered the most common of the inborn errors of porphyrin metabolism, with an estimated incidence of 5 to 10 per 100,000 in the United States, although as many as 90% of individuals with PBG deaminase deficiency are asymptomatic.

The characteristic features of acute episodes are severe abdominal pain and port-wine urine. Associated vomiting, constipation, abdominal distention, and ileus may lead to the diagnosis of surgical abdomen, but surgery should be avoided whenever possible during these attacks. Diarrhea and urinary retention or incontinence may be seen. Tachycardia, hypertension or hypotension, fever, leukocytosis, and seizures may accompany attacks, in addition to psychiatric disturbances, including disorientation, hallucinations, paranoia, anxiety, and depression. Motor neu-

ropathy is more common than is sensory neuropathy and is of extreme concern, because bulbar paralysis and respiratory insufficiency can occur and may be fatal.

Symptomatic AIP is rare before puberty, but has been reported. Acute attacks are precipitated by a variety of drugs, most of which induce ALA synthase. Prominent among these agents are barbiturates, phenytoin (Dilantin), oral contraceptives, sulfonamides, and valproic acid. AIP attacks also may occur with menstrual periods, decreased food intake, and stress. Stress factors include infections, ethanol intoxication, and surgery.

PBG and ALA levels frequently are elevated in the urine, but may be normal or minimally increased, especially in asymptomatic individuals with PBG deaminase deficiency. PBG deaminase activity in erythrocytes is reduced to about 50% of normal, but, as a result of wide variation in normal values leading to overlap of enzyme activity between patients with AIP and normal control individuals, enzyme activity should be measured in the parents of affected children and in other family members. Occasional patients have normal red cell PBG deaminase levels, and cultured fibroblasts may be used to measure enzyme activity. The enzyme deficiency also is expressed in amniotic fluid cells, liver, and lymphocytes. The PBG deaminase complementary DNA has been cloned and mutations analyzed.

The mainstay of treatment is prevention of attacks by avoidance of precipitating influences, including known exacerbating medications and stresses. Increased oral carbohydrate intake should be attempted early in an attack; if the patient does not respond to this treatment, then intravenous dextrose infusions should be used. These patients should be monitored for inappropriate antidiuretic hormone secretion. Propranolol has been used to control tachycardia and hypertension. The pain of an acute attack is severe, but may be treated with a narcotic analgesic (eg, morphine) and a phenothiazine (eg, chlorpromazine), although the narcotic analgesic increases the tendency toward constipation and urinary retention. Intravenous hematin should be considered when an attack continues for longer than 2 days

| Tissues for Enzyme Diagnosis† | Increased Intermediates in RBC | | | Increased Intermediates in Urine | | | | | Increased Intermediates in Stool | | |
|---|---|---|---|---|---|---|---|---|---|---|---|
| | Uro | Copro | Proto | ALA | PBG | Uro | Copro | 7-CP | Copro | Proto | IsoCP |
| RBCs | − | − | + | + | − | − | + | | − | − | − |
| RBCs, fibroblasts, liver, lymphocytes, amniotic fluid cells | − | − | − | + | + | − | − | − | − | − | − |
| RBCs, fibroblasts, amniocytes | + | ± | − | − | − | + | + | | + | − | − |
| RBCs, liver | − | − | − | − | − | + | ± | + | ± | − | + |
| RBCs, fibroblasts | − | − | + | − | − | + | − | + | − | − | + |
| Fibroblasts, leukocytes | − | − | − | + | + | + | + | − | + | − | − |
| Fibroblasts, lymphocytes | − | − | − | + | + | − | + | − | + | + | − |
| Erythrocytes, fibroblasts | − | − | + | − | − | − | − | − | ± | + | − |

or when there is rapid neurologic progression. The intravenous preparation may be given in a dosage of up to 4 mg/kg over 30 minutes or more, every 12 hours. Phlebitis and thrombophlebitis are seen frequently with intravenous hematin.

## Congenital Erythropoietic Porphyria

Congenital erythropoietic porphyria (CEP) is a rare autosomal recessive porphyria resulting from homozygous deficiency for urogen III cosynthase. Although its onset usually is in infancy, some patients are asymptomatic until adulthood. CEP frequently is suspected first on the basis of reddish to brown staining of the diapers in a neonate or infant. Photosensitivity is noted in an infant or young child, with vesicles and bullae in exposed areas of the skin that become crusted and superinfected. Scarring associated with hyperpigmentation and deformity is seen in some patients, with particular involvement of the phalanges, ears, and nose. Hypertrichosis in the form of fine, downy hair over the face and extremities is common. Porphyrin deposits in the teeth cause a reddish or brownish discoloration. The teeth and the serous vesicular fluid exhibit a red fluorescence under ultraviolet light because of the elevated porphyrin content. Other features include hemolytic anemia, splenomegaly, gallstones, and pathologic fractures.

Urogen III cosynthase activity can be measured in erythrocytes, fibroblasts, and amniocytes, and mutation analysis has been performed using the complementary DNA. Treatment involves protection from sunlight by limiting exposure and using sunscreen, administration of β-carotene, protection from trauma, and aggressive treatment of cutaneous infections to prevent scarring and deformity. Hypersplenism is an indication for total or subtotal splenectomy, and some patients are described to respond with reduced photosensitivity. Hematin infusions have been used successfully in patients with this disorder. Charcoal, which binds porphyrins, has been used orally with beneficial results: plasma and cutaneous porphyrin levels were reduced and symptoms abated.

## Porphyria Cutanea Tarda

PCT is a common porphyria that is subdivided into two types: type I, or sporadic, and type II, or familial. Urogen decarboxylase levels are decreased to 50% in both types, with the reduction found only in the liver in type I but generalized in the inherited type II. The sporadic form is seen in association with ethanol abuse, estrogen intake, or iron ingestion, as well as with other toxins or disorders. Type I PCT is seen more commonly in adults, whereas type II typically has its onset in childhood. Vesicles and bullae of the exposed skin, with crusting, scarring, and hyperpigmentation, are seen in both types, as is increased fragility of the skin. Hypertrichosis of the face may develop. Hepatic cirrhosis and siderosis are common findings, and there is an increased incidence of hepatocellular carcinoma.

Urogen decarboxylase deficiency may be documented in the liver in patients with types I and II PCT, and in the erythrocytes in patients with type II PCT. The urinary concentration of uroporphyrin exceeds that of coproporphyrin. The urogen decarboxylase locus maps to the short arm of chromosome 1 (1pter → p21). The urogen decarboxylase complementary DNA has been cloned and mutation analysis performed in familial PCT.

Treatment includes avoidance of precipitating exposures and protection from sunlight. Phlebotomy has been used and is presumed to work by decreasing total body iron levels. Chloroquine may be effective by forming a complex with porphyrins and improving their clearance, but its use has been associated with retinopathy.

## Hepatoerythropoietic Porphyria

HPT is a rare genetic disorder resulting from homozygous deficiency of urogen decarboxylase. Patients may be seen at any age, from infancy through adulthood. The porphyrins in this disorder have their origin in the liver and bone marrow. Clinical features include cutaneous photosensitivity, hypertrichosis, pigmentation of the urine and teeth, hemolytic anemia, and hepatospleno-

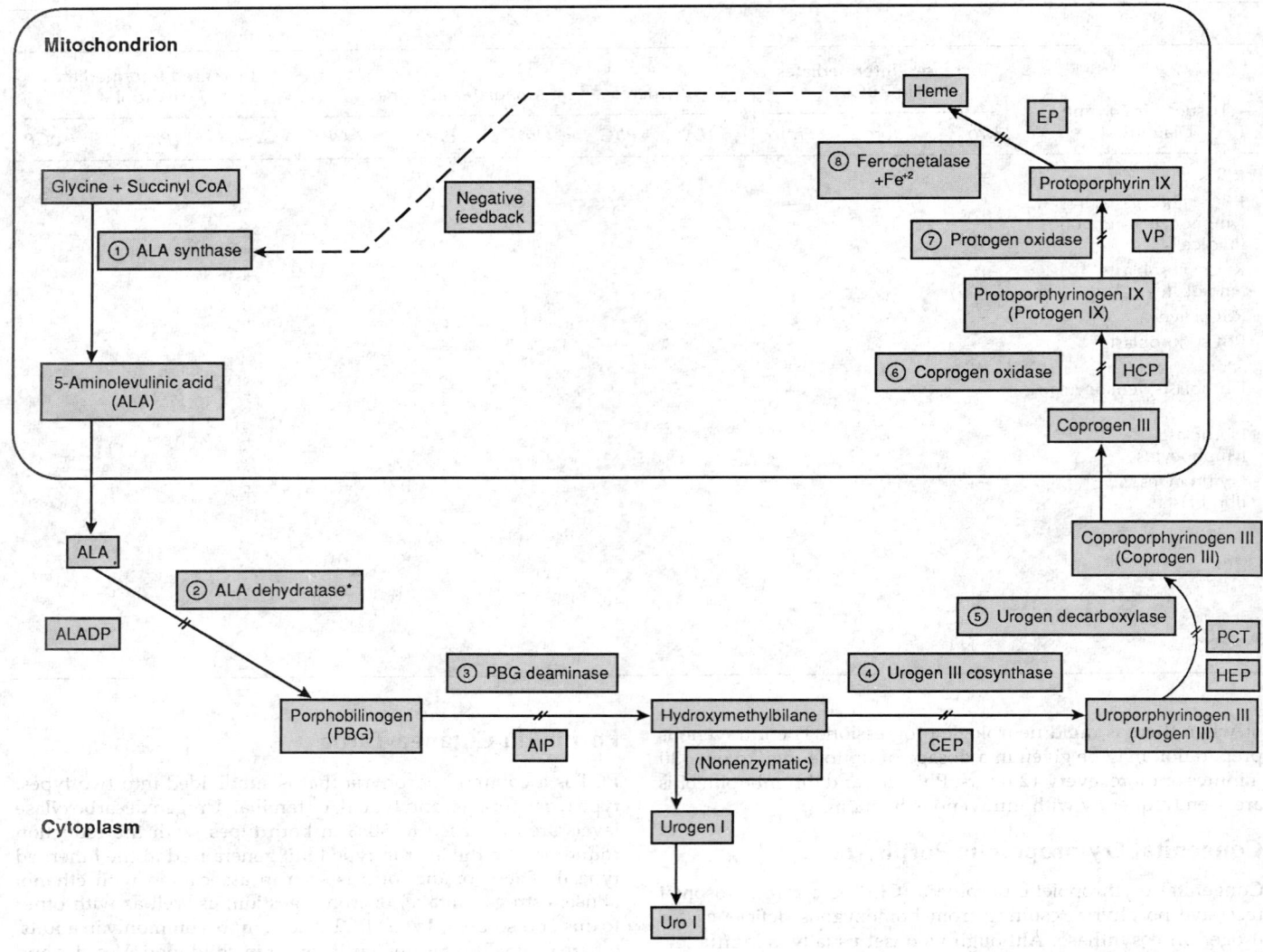

Figure 161-5.   Heme biosynthesis, showing the eight enzymatic steps.

megaly. The severity of the photosensitivity is similar to that seen in patients with CEP and more severe than that noted in individuals with erythropoietic protoporphyria (EP). Red cells and fibroblasts may be used for enzymatic diagnosis, and mutation analysis has been carried out. Current therapy relies on protection from sun exposure.

## Hereditary Coproporphyria

Hereditary coproporphyria (HCP) is an autosomal dominant disorder that is characterized by about 50% activity of coprogen oxidase, although several cases of homozygous HCP also have been seen. The clinical features of HCP are similar to those of AIP and include abdominal pain, gastrointestinal disturbances, and neuropsychiatric complaints, but about 30% of affected patients have photosensitivity as well. Paralysis, respiratory failure, and death have been reported. The disease has presented in the second decade of life and beyond. Precipitating features are similar to those of other porphyrias, with barbiturates being a common offender. Excessive urinary excretion of coproporphyrin is typical, with elevated excretion of ALA, PBG, and uroporphyrin during acute episodes. Coprogen oxidase can be assayed in fibroblasts and leukocytes of patients with the disease. A homo-

zygous HCP with an earlier onset also has been described. Treatment is similar to that for AIP.

## Variegate Porphyria

Variegate porphyria (VP) is the autosomal dominant heterozygous deficiency of protoporphyrinogen (protogen) oxidase. A relatively common disorder in South African whites, elsewhere it is somewhat less common than AIP. The disorder may present with neuropsychiatric and visceral features similar to those of AIP and HCP or with cutaneous photosensitivity. The skin findings are identical to those in patients with PCT, and the diagnosis of PCT may be made erroneously when the presentation is solely cutaneous. Precipitating factors are those of AIP and HCP. Homozygous VP is rare and presents clinically in childhood with more severe manifestations of the usual symptoms; it also may include mental retardation, prominent neurologic features, and growth delay. "Pseudoporphyria" has been described with porphyrin excretion resembling VP after the consumption of excessive quantities of porphyrin-containing brewers' yeast tablets. The plasma of patients with VP has a characteristic fluorescence emission at 626 nm. Protogen oxidase can be measured in lymphocytes and fibroblasts, and linkage to the $\alpha_1$-antitrypsin gene on chromosome 14 has been suggested. Treatment involves avoidance of factors associated with acute episodes, protection from the sun, and other measures described for AIP.

## Erythropoietic Protoporphyria

EP is the autosomal dominant heterozygous deficiency of ferrochelatase, the final enzymatic step in heme synthesis that involves the insertion of iron into protoporphyrin. EP is the most common of the erythropoietic porphyrias. Cutaneous photosensitivity is relatively mild and is noted first in childhood, usually before 6 years of age, with exposure to the sun or other bright light causing burning, edema, itching, and erythema. Lesions generally resolve after a few hours, although petechiae, purpura, vesicles, and crusting may develop and last several days before clearing. Scarring and disfigurement are not typical features of this porphyria, although mild scarring and hyperkeratosis may be seen after chronic eczematoid lesions have resolved. Anemia is rare and, when present, is non-hemolytic. Gallstones are relatively common. Hepatocellular disease is rare, but may be severe, progressing rapidly to cirrhosis and death. The presence of protoporphyrin in the red cells, plasma, and stool is characteristic of patients with EP. Ferrochelatase activity can be assayed in erythrocytes and fibroblasts. The ferrochelatase complementary DNA has been cloned and mapped to chromosome 18g22, and mutations have been analyzed. The primary cause of clinical problems in patients with EP is sunlight or strong artificial light. If exposure cannot be avoided, topical sunscreens may be of some help if they have a high "sun protection factor" of 26 or 34. Oral high-dose $\beta$-carotene is considered useful, but requires several weeks or months before tolerance to sunlight improves. In addition, the dosages necessary may lead to carotene discoloration of the skin. In the past, drugs and chemicals were not considered precipitating factors; with recognition of the potential severity of the associated liver disease, however, more attention is being paid to protecting patients from these agents. Iron, vitamin E, and cholestyramine have been recommended to prevent progression once hepatocellular disease is noted, but data on their efficacy are limited. There is a genetic animal model for EP, which is an autosomal recessive deficiency of ferrochelatase in cattle.

## DISORDERS OF AMINO AND ORGANIC ACID METABOLISM

### Hypoglycemia With or Without Hyperammonemia

Hypoglycemic disorders, including maple syrup urine disease, methylmalonic acidemia, propionic acidemia, isovaleric acidemia, glutaric acidemia, and acetoacetyl-CoA thiolase deficiency, generally present with acidemia that may be associated with a condition similar to Reye's syndrome and should be considered in any patient with Reye's syndrome, especially if there is a family history or a history of recurrence. Quantitative serum amino acids are diagnostic in patients with maple syrup urine disease and may be helpful, but are not diagnostic, in patients with the other organic acidemias that are characterized as ketotic hyperglycinemias. Urine organic acid analysis is diagnostic in the latter, and is indicated by the metabolic acidemia, odor (in patients with maple syrup urine disease and isovaleric acidemia, or "sweaty feet" disease), and neurologic symptoms. Acetoacetyl-CoA thiolase deficiency should be considered in the differential diagnosis of "idiopathic ketotic hypoglycemia." These patients have metabolic acidemia during hypoglycemic episodes. The urine organic

acid analysis may reveal only $\beta$-hydroxybutyrate, and measurement of enzyme activity may be required for diagnosis.

Medium-chain acyl coenzyme A dehydrogenase deficiency is characterized by nonketotic or hypoketotic fasting hypoglycemia. The urine organic acid analysis may show dicarboxylic aciduria, with adipic, suberic, and sebacic acids. These patients frequently evidence a reduced serum free-carnitine concentration, with an increased proportion of acyl carnitines. Urine collected during the first 6 hours after an oral carnitine load (100 mg/kg) shows typical acyl carnitine patterns by fast atom bombardment or tandem mass spectrometry analysis.

## Hyperammonemias

Hyperammonemia is characteristic of the urea cycle disorders, but also may be seen in patients with lysinuric protein intolerance, the hyperornithinemia-hyperammonemia-homocitrullinuria syndrome, transient hyperammonemia, and organic acidemias, as mentioned above. Neonates exhibit poor feeding, vomiting, and lethargy, which progresses to seizures, coma, and death. Patients with milder disease who are seen later in infancy or childhood may have episodic problems, including ataxia. Respiratory alkalosis from central stimulation, along with vomiting, are typical features of hyperammonemia. The determination of blood ammonia, quantitative serum amino acid (with particular attention to citrulline), and urine organic acid levels is important diagnostic testing that should be followed by specific enzymatic assays.

## Intractable Seizures

Hypsarrhythmia and myoclonus beginning early in life are typical of nonketotic hyperglycinemia. This autosomal recessive deficiency of the glycine cleavage enzyme can be diagnosed by the detection of elevated cerebrospinal fluid glycine levels; serum and urine glycine concentrations generally are increased as well. $\beta$-Alaninemia is an extremely rare disorder with a similar clinical presentation.

## Developmental Delay

Phenylketonuria (PKU) is the prototype among these amino acid disorders. Others, however, including variants of maple syrup urine disease and the organic acidemias, may have mental retardation as the main characteristic. Quantitative serum amino acid measurements, urine homocystine detection, and urine organic acid analyses are used to screen for these disorders.

## Autistic Behavior and Psychiatric Disturbances

Older patients with untreated PKU may evidence autistic behavior and schizophrenic symptoms. Schizophrenic behavior also has been described in some older patients with homocystinuria.

## OTHER DISORDERS

Other disorders that should be included in the differential diagnosis of the metabolic encephalopathies and that can be investigated by specific laboratory tests include many of the lysosomal storage diseases, certain of the peroxisomal disorders (especially Zellweger [cerebrohepatorenal] syndrome with elevated very–long-chain fatty acid levels), Lesch-Nyhan syndrome (hypoxanthine-guanine phosphoribosyltransferase deficiency), and primary or secondary hypophosphatemia.

## Selected Readings

Ampola MG. Metabolic diseases in pediatric practice. Boston: Little, Brown & Company, 1982.

Cotter PD, Baumann M, Bishop DF. Enzymatic defect in X-linked sideroblastic anemia: Molecular evidence for erythroid δ-aminolevulinate synthase deficiency. Proc Natl Acad Sci USA 1992;89(9):4028.

Delfau MH, Picat C, deRooij FW, et al. Two different point A to G mutations in exon 10 of the porphobilinogen deaminase gene are responsible for acute intermittent porphyria. J Clin Invest 1990;86:1511.

Kappas A, Sassa S, Galbraith RA, Nordmann Y. The porphyrias. In: Scriver CR, Beaudet AL, Sly WS, Valle D, eds. The metabolic basis of inherited disease, ed 6. New York: McGraw-Hill, 1989:1305.

Leonard JV, Middleton B, Seakins JWT. Acetoacetyl CoA thiolase deficiency presenting as ketotic hypoglycemia. Pediatr Res 1987;21:211.

Matsubara Y, Narisawa K, Tada K, et al. Prevalence of K329E mutation in medium-chain acyl-CoA dehydrogenase determined from Guthrie cards. Lancet 1991;338:552.

McKusick VA. Mendelian inheritance in man—catalogs of autosomal dominant, autosomal recessive and X-linked phenotypes, ed 9. Baltimore: The Johns Hopkins University Press, 1990.

Nyhan WL, Sakati NA. Diagnostic recognition of genetic disease. Philadelphia: Lea & Febiger, 1987.

Plewinska M, Thunell S, Holmberg L, Wetmur JG, Desnick RJ. δ-Aminolevulinate dehydratase deficient porphyria: Identification of the molecular lesions in a severely affected homozygote. Am J Hum Genet 1991;49:167.

Varga V, Hall BK, Wang SR, Johnson S, Higgins JV, Glover TW. Localization of the translocation breakpoint in a female with Menkes syndrome to Xq13.2–q13.3 proximal to PGK-1. Am J Hum Genet 1991;48:1133.

*Principles and Practice of Pediatrics, Second Edition.*
edited by Frank A. Oski et al. J. B. Lippincott Company, Philadelphia © 1994.

## *161.3 Rett Syndrome*

### Alan K. Percy

Rett syndrome is a pervasive developmental disorder affecting young females. After a period of apparently normal development, the patients reach a plateau and then experience a rapid decline in motor and cognitive function, usually beginning at 6 to 18 months of age. The principal clinical features consist of the loss of purposeful hand use; the development of stereotypic hand movements such as hand washing, hand wringing, or hand tapping (Fig 161-6); and the loss of communication skills. Generally, these children have developed the ability to speak a few words, but with the onset of the disorder, meaningful verbal communication is lost. In addition, affected individuals give very poor eye contact, which has led their behavior to be interpreted as autistic. An acquired-type deceleration of head growth is noted within the first 2 years of life; other features include periodic breathing while awake, with alternating periods of breath holding and hyperventilation. Seizures occur in many of these children, and may consist of both staring spells and generalized tonic-clonic episodes. Growth failure is evident, with short stature and small hand and foot size. In addition, the hands and feet tend to be markedly cooler than the remainder of the extremities, and the children seem to have diminished responses to pain.

Although the behavioral mannerisms (hand stereotypies and periodic breathing) of children with Rett syndrome are confined to wakefulness, sleep often is interrupted and periods of uncontrollable screaming are reported frequently by parents during the first few years of life. After the early period of decline, there is

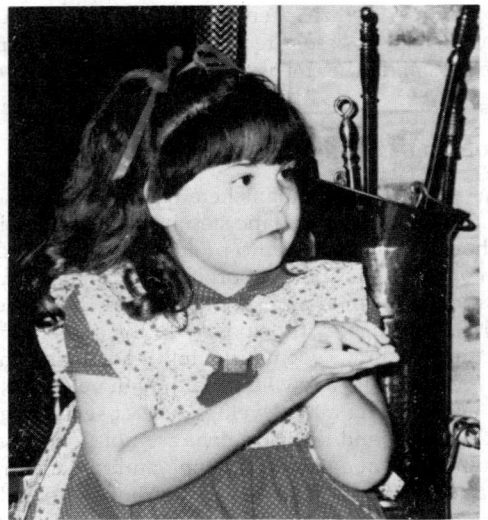

**Figure 161-6.** This photograph of a 5-year-old girl with Rett syndrome demonstrates the typical hand position associated with the disorder.

a rather long, relatively stable phase during which the episodes of screaming and the behavioral mannerisms may become milder. Attentiveness and eye contact improve to the extent that communication may occur through eye gaze or eye pointing. In later childhood and early adolescence, scoliosis is common. Affected individuals may survive well into adulthood. Because this disorder has been recognized only for about 25 years and accurate diagnosis has been possible only within the last decade, however, the natural history of Rett syndrome has not been fully elucidated.

The pathophysiology of Rett syndrome is poorly understood. The hyperammonemia that was described with the early cases no longer is considered to be characteristic. No biologic marker allows definitive diagnosis, which is based solely on clinical assessment. Clinical neurophysiologic studies have revealed progressive deterioration of function on electroencephalographic tracings, featuring slowing, loss of occipital dominant rhythm, and the appearance of multifocal spike and wave epileptiform activity. Previous reports of biogenic amine metabolite reduction in the cerebrospinal fluid have not been substantiated. Elevated cerebrospinal fluid β-endorphin levels have been noted in most instances, but this finding is not specific to Rett syndrome.

The occurrence of Rett syndrome exclusively in females has led to the suggestion that it is an X-linked disorder that is lethal in males. No affected males have been identified, and the precise genetic mechanism involved is unknown. It is possible, however, that nonrandom X-inactivation is occurring. The recurrence of Rett syndrome within individual families has been reported in less than 1% of cases. When recurrence has been described in more than one generation, the mode of transmission appears to be through the maternal side of the family. The prevalence rate of between 1 : 10,000 and 1 : 15,000 exceeds that of phenylketonuria in females.

The differential diagnosis of Rett syndrome includes infantile autism, with which it is confused most frequently. If the clinical criteria for autism and Rett syndrome are applied carefully, however, there should be no difficulty in making the distinction. In addition, any child with acquired deceleration of head growth and a diagnosis of progressive cerebral palsy should be evaluated carefully for the possibility of Rett syndrome. Angelman syndrome, which often is associated with a 15q deletion, should be excluded. Finally, other neurodegenerative disorders should be considered and appropriate diagnostic tests conducted. Periodic breathing has been described in patients with Joubert syndrome.

This condition can be differentiated from Rett syndrome, however, by the presence of cerebellar abnormalities on computed brain tomography of children with Joubert syndrome. The only imaging abnormality noted in patients with Rett syndrome is mild to moderate cortical atrophy, particularly during the later stages of the disorder. Neuropathologic assessment has revealed very few abnormalities besides reduced brain weight. The principal finding has been that of reduction in or lack of pigmentation within neurons of the substantia nigra.

No specific therapy is available for patients with Rett syndrome. The majority of children achieve independent walking, but lose this capability in later stages and are susceptible to the complications of relative immobility, including orthopedic deformities, particularly progressive scoliosis. Anticonvulsant agents are indicated if seizures occur; carbamazepine has been particularly effective. Programs involving physical and occupational therapy as well as early childhood education should be tailored to the individual child.

## Selected Readings

Ellison KA, Fill CP, Terwilliger J, et al. Examination of X chromosome markers in Rett syndrome: Exclusion mapping with a novel variation on multilocus linkage analysis. Am J Hum Genet 1992;50:278.

Glaze DG, Frost JD Jr, Zoghbi HY, Percy AK. Rett's syndrome: Correlation of electroencephalographic characteristics with clinical staging. Arch Neurol 1987;44:1053.

Hagberg B, Aicardi J, Dias K, Ramos O. A progressive syndrome of autism, dementia, ataxia, and loss of purposeful hand use in girls: Rett's syndrome: Report of 35 cases. Ann Neurol 1983;14:471.

Hagberg B, Witt-Engerstrom I. Rett syndrome: A suggested staging system for describing impairment profile with increasing age towards adolescence. Am J Med Genet 1986;24(Suppl 1):47.

Jellinger K, Seitelberger F. Neuropathology of Rett syndrome. Am J Med Genet 1986;24(Suppl 1):259.

Myer EC, Tripathi HL, Brase DA, Dewey WL. Elevated CSF beta-endorphin immunoreactivity in Rett's syndrome: Report of 158 cases and comparison with leukemic children. Neurology 1992;42:357.

Olsson B, Rett A. Autism and Rett syndrome: Behavioral investigations and differential diagnosis. Dev Med Child Neurol 1987;29:429.

Percy A, Gillberg C, Hagberg B, Witt-Enterström I. Rett syndrome and the autistic disorders. Neurol Clin 1990;8:659.

Rett A. Uber ein eigenartiges hirnatrophisches syndrome bei hyperammonamie im kindesalter. Wien Med Wochenschr 1966;116:723.

Zoghbi HY, Percy AK, Glaze DG, et al. Reduction of biogenic amine levels in the Rett syndrome. N Engl J Med 1985;313:921.

*Principles and Practice of Pediatrics, Second Edition.*
edited by Frank A. Oski et al. J. B. Lippincott Company, Philadelphia © 1994.

# *161.4 Basal Ganglia and Neurotransmitter Disorders*

### Joseph Jankovic

Biochemical or structural pathology in the basal ganglia may be manifested by movement disorders, groups of neurologic diseases or syndromes that are characterized either by slowness, paucity, and "freezing" of voluntary movement (bradykinesia, akinesia) or by excess abnormal involuntary movement (hyperkinesia, dyskinesia).

The basal ganglia seem to be important in the initiation, scaling, and controlling of the amplitude and direction of movement. This complex of deep nuclei is divided anatomically into the corpus striatum, the globus pallidus, and the substantia nigra (Fig 161-7). The corpus striatum, which includes the caudate nucleus and the putamen, receives input from the cerebral cortex and the thalamus, and, in turn, projects to the globus pallidus. The substantia nigra is divided into the dopamine-rich pars compacta, which is darkly pigmented because of a high content of neuromelanin, and the less dense pars reticularis. The pars reticularis is similar histologically and chemically to the medial segment of the globus pallidus, and both project by way of the thalamus to the pre-motor and motor cortex. The pars compacta gives rise to the nigral-striatal pathway, which is the main dopaminergic tract. The output of the basal ganglia, which once was thought to be in parallel with the pyramidal system (hence, the term "extra-pyramidal"), projects by way of the thalamus to the cerebral cortex and then to the pyramidal system. Integration of the basal ganglia with the cortex facilitates motor control.

The diagnosis of a particular movement disorder depends primarily on careful observation of the clinical phenomena. The bradykinetic movement disorders often are accompanied by rigidity, postural instability, and loss of automatic associated movements. The hyperkinetic involuntary movements are differentiated phenomenologically according to their characteristic clinical features, rapidity and duration of contractions, rhythmicity, pattern, and suppressibility (Table 161-6). In general, abnormal involuntary movements are exaggerated with stress and disappear during sleep; however, certain forms of myoclonus and tics may persist during all stages of sleep. In one clinic devoted to movement disorders, the most common hyperkinetic movements observed were tics, followed by dystonia, stereotypies, choreoathetosis, tremors, and myoclonus (Dure and Jankovic, 1988).

## PARKINSONISM

### Parkinson's Disease

Parkinson's disease (PD) usually is a condition of middle and late life, but the incidence of early onset (before 40 years of age) and juvenile (before 20 years of age) parkinsonism seems to be increasing. Although the rigid, akinetic form of parkinsonism appears to be more common in the juvenile cases, the typical resting tremor is present in many such patients. Dystonia (often involving the legs), levodopa-induced dyskinesias, and clinical fluctuations seem to be particularly common in the juvenile cases. Some patients with familial juvenile parkinsonism belong to group with the "hereditary dystonia-parkinsonism syndrome." Rare patients with juvenile parkinsonism who were examined at autopsy have been noted to have depigmentation of the substantia nigra, but Lewy bodies have not been detected. The absence of Lewy bodies does not indicate that these patients did not have PD, but probably reflects an age-related susceptibility of the neuronal cytoskeleton to develop the cytoplasmic inclusions. The neurotoxin 1-methyl-4-phenyl-1,2,3,6-tetrahydropyridine (MPTP) produces inclusions similar to Lewy bodies only in aged animals. Many other types of parkinsonism exist in addition to primary and MPTP-induced disease, some of which have their onset in childhood (Table 161-7).

### Wilson's Disease

Wilson's disease (WD) is one of the most important causes of juvenile parkinsonism and other movement disorders. Failure to diagnose this condition may have tragic consequences, including

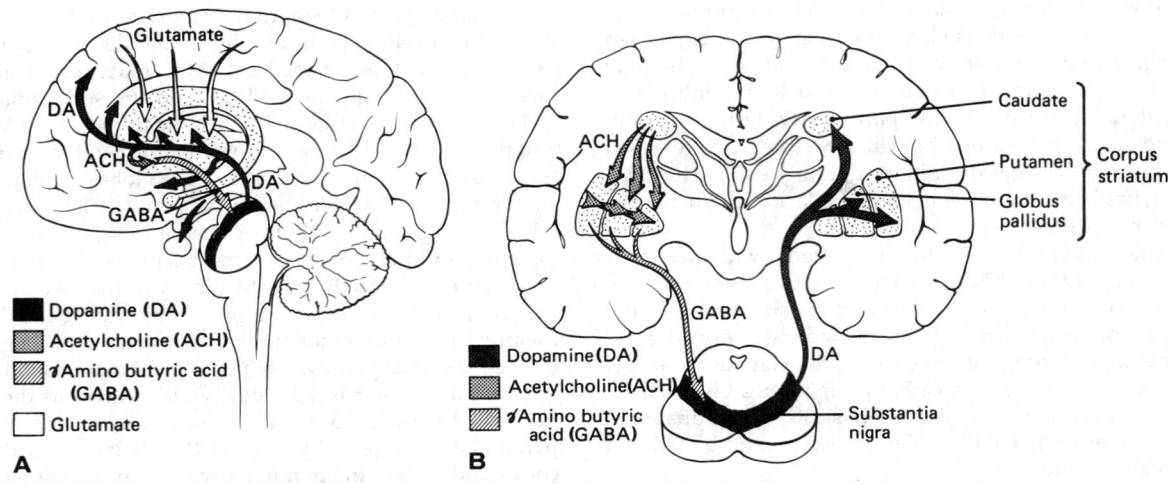

**Figure 161-7.** Schematic diagram of the brain showing some important neurotransmitter pathways involved in disorders of the basal ganglia. (**A**) Sagittal section. (**B**) Coronal section.

death as a result of irreversible liver cirrhosis and profound neurologic deficit. The gene for this autosomal recessive hepatolenticular degenerative disease has been linked to the esterase D locus on chromosome 13. The prevalence of the gene in the overall population is about 1%, although symptomatic WD is relatively rare (estimated prevalence, 30:1 million). The hepatic and neurologic dysfunction associated with WD is caused by a defect in

copper metabolism resulting from a reduction in the rate at which copper is incorporated into ceruloplasmin and a decrease in the rate at which it is excreted from the liver. Low ceruloplasmin levels usually are found in patients with WD, but do not seem to be the primary defect, because some patients with the disease and some heterozygotes have normal levels. Furthermore, the ceruloplasmin gene has been mapped to chromosome 3, not

**TABLE 161-6.   Differential Diagnosis of Hyperkinetic Movement Disorders**

| Clinical Features | Tremor | | | Chorea |
|---|---|---|---|---|
| | *At Rest* | *Postural* | *Kinetic* | |
| Characteristics | 3–7 Hz supination-pronation oscillatory ("pill rolling"): hands, legs, lips, jaw, (alternating contractions of antagonists) | 4–12 Hz flexion-extension oscillatory movement with arms outstretched: hands arms, head, voice, legs (simultaneous contractions of antagonists) | 3–5 Hz intention tremor on finger-to-nose and heel-to-shin test | Rapid, abrupt, flowing, unsustained, random, semi-purposeful, nonpatterned; *athetosis* is a slow chorea (writhing movement) |
| Associated features | Bradykinesia, rigidity (cogwheel), shuffling gait, postural instability, hypomimia, micrographia | Dystonia, parkinsonism, and hereditary peripheral neuropathy, torticollis, parkinsonism | Ataxia, titubation, dysdiadochokinesia, loss of check and other cerebellar or brain stem signs | "Milkmaid's grip," darting tongue," orofacial dyskinesia, hypotonia, pendular or "hung-up" reflexes, dementia in Huntington's disease, carditis in Sydenham's chorea |
| Etiology | Parkinson's disease, secondary parkinsonism, heterogenous disorders with parkinsonian features | Physiologic, accentuated physiologic, essential cerebellar outflow (midbrain rubral, wing beating) | Cerebellar disorders and tumors, multiple sclerosis, brain stem and cerebellar strokes | Huntington's disease, rheumatic fever (Sydenham), drug-induced hyperthyroidism, static encephalopathy, pregnancy, vasculitis, electrolyte metabolic imbalance |
| Treatment | Anticholinergics, amantadine, levodopa/carbidopa, dopamine agonists | Propranolol and other betablockers, benzodiazepines, phenobarbital, pyrimidine, clonazepam, amantadine, alcohol | No effective treatment, wrist-arm weights, thalamotomy | Treat underlying disorder, dopamine blocking or depleting agents, cholinergic agents |

chromosome 13. The excess copper not only accumulates in the liver and brain, but also can cause renal tubule damage, osteoporosis, and arthropathy. Kayser-Fleischer rings, the best-recognized ophthalmologic sign of WD, are caused by the deposition of copper in the cornea.

The onset of WD usually is between adolescence and 40 years of age, and its presentation seems to be age-dependent, with hepatic failure being more common in children and neurologic or psychiatric symptoms more frequent in adults. In a nonselected population of 31 patients with WD, the mean age at onset ($\pm$SD) was $21\pm5$ years. Sixty-one percent had neurologic symptoms, 13% had liver symptoms, and 10% had a combination of neurologic and liver problems. About one third of patients had psychiatric symptoms at disease onset, including depression, emotional lability, personality change, and slow mentation. Another one third had neurologic symptoms, particularly parkinsonism, pseudobulbar palsy, tremor, and dystonia; 14% had symptoms of liver disease, and 17% had their condition diagnosed by family screening. The most common neurologic findings at first evaluation were dysarthria (97%), dystonia (65%), dysdiadochokinesia (58%), rigidity (52%), gait and postural abnormalities (42%), tremor (32%), abnormal eye movements (32%), hyperreflexia (29%), drooling (23%), and bradykinesia (19%).

Because of its variable clinical expression, the diagnosis of WD often is delayed. Almost all patients with neurologic disease have Kayser-Fleischer rings, but this yellow-brown deposit at the limbus of the cornea also may be noted in patients with primary biliary cirrhosis and active hepatitis with cirrhosis. Occasionally,

a "sunflower cataract" may be seen as a result of copper deposition in the lens.

The diagnosis of WD usually is confirmed by the demonstration of low serum copper and ceruloplasmin levels, increased urine copper concentrations after a dose of penicillamine, and a rise in the level of copper in the liver (Table 161-8). The ratio of radioactivity in the plasma at 24 hours to that at 2 hours after the administration of an oral or intravenous dose of Cu-64 is less than 0.5 in patients with WD (the equivalent value is greater than 0.8 in normal individuals). Other laboratory abnormalities often detected in patients with WD include aminoaciduria, hypercalciuria, glycosuria, leukopenia, hemolytic anemia, thrombocytopenia, and renal tubal deficit. In about half of affected patients, computed tomography (CT) scanning of the brain reveals characteristic hypodense areas in the region of the basal ganglia, and magnetic resonance imaging (MRI) often reveals increased T2 signal intensity in the caudate and putamen bilaterally. Extensive degeneration of the corpus striatum, particularly the putamen, is seen at autopsy. Also, the cerebellum, brain stem, and subcortical white matter may be involved.

The goals of treatment in patients with WD are to reduce copper intake and create a negative copper balance by increasing copper output in the urine. D-penicillamine has been used successfully to chelate copper at dosages of 0.5 to 2.0 g/d. Penicillamine often produces considerable toxicity, however, including fever, urticaria, leukopenia, nephritis, thrombocytopenia, systemic lupus erythematosus, hemolytic anemia, Goodpasture's syndrome, pyridoxine deficiency, and a syndrome resembling myas-

| Stereotypy | Dystonia | Ballism | Mycoclonus Generalized | Mycoclonus Segmental | Tics |
|---|---|---|---|---|---|
| Repetitive, purposeless movements resembling normal voluntary movements | Sustained, twisting, usually low but may be rapid and may progress to fixed contractures (dystonic postures) | Abrupt, random, forceful, violent, flinging, usually proximal and unilateral, often spontaneously remits | Abrupt, irregular brief, jerk-like contractions of one or more muscles occuring sychronously or asynchronously, may be stimulus-sensitive | Rhythmic contraction of Agonists, not stimulus-sensitive, may persist during sleep | Rapid, sudden, unpredictable, coordinated jerks preceded by inner urge, waxing and waning, temporarily suppressible |
| Often associated with *akathisia* (sensory and motor restlessness) | Torticollis, writer's cramp, blepharospasm, spasmodic dysphonia, essential tremor, hypertrophy of contracted muscles | Initial hemiparesis, later choreoathetosis | Encephalopathy, seizures, dementia, periodic electroencephalogram, enhanced somatosensory evoked potentials | Palatal myoclonus may be associated with bulbar palsy; spinal myoclonus may be associated with myelopathy | Vocalizations, coprolalia, echolalia, copropraxia, echopraxia, obsessive-compulsive behavior, attention deficit disorder, sleep disturbance |
| Usually drug-induced (tardive dyskinesia) schizophrenia, autism, mental retardation, Rett syndrome | Dystonia musculorum deformans, adult-onset torsion dystonia, drug-induced | Lesion of contralateral subthalamic nucleus (hemorrhage, infarction, rarely tumor) | Postanoxic, uremic and other encephalopathies, Creutzfeldt-Jakob disease, subacute sclerosing panencephalitis, myoclonic epilepsy, Ramsay Hunt syndrome | Brain stem or spinal cord infarction, hemorrhage, myelitis, demyelinating disease | Gilles de la Tourette's syndrome, transient tic of childhood |
| May improve with dopamine blockers or depletors, beta blockers, opioid agonists or antagonists | Muscle relaxants, anticholinergics, tetrabenazine, baclofen, dopamine agonists, levodopa for diurnal dystonia, *C botulinum* toxin injections, thalamotomy | Dopamine blocking or depleting agents, thalamotomy | Clonazepam, 5-hydroxy-tryptophan, sodium valproate, piracetam, lisuride | Tetrabenzine, 5-hydroxy-tryptophan, clonazepam, anticholinergics | Dopamine blocking or depleting agents |

### TABLE 161-7.   Classification of Parkinsonism

**Primary Parkinson's Disease**

Idiopathic, dominated by:
  Tremor
  Postural-instability-gait-difficulty (PIGD)
  Akinesia (freezing)
  Dementia
  Depression
  Sensory disturbance
  Autonomic dysfunction
Inherited, associated with essential tremor, dystonia, or peripheral neuropathy
Young-onset, associated with dystonia or essential tremor

**Secondary Parkinsonism**

Drugs (dopamine blocking and depleting drugs, alpha-methyldopa, lithium, diazoxide, flunarizine, cinnarizine)
Toxins (manganese, mercury, carbon monoxide, cyanide, carbon disulfide, methanol, ethanol, MPTP)
Metabolic (parathyroid, acquired hepatocerebral degeneration, GM₁ gangliosidosis, Gaucher's disease)
Encephalitis and postencephalitic syndrome
Slow virus (Creutzfeldt-Jakob disease)
Vascular (multi-infarct, Binswanger's disease)
Brain tumor
Trauma and pugilistic encephalopathy
Hydrocephalus (normal and high pressure)
Syringomesencephalia

**Multiple System Degenerations (Parkinsonism Plus)**

Sporadic
  Progressive supranuclear palsy (ophthalmoparesis)
  Shy-Drager syndrome (dysautonomia)
  Olivopontocerebellar atrophy (ataxia)
  Parkinsonism-dementia-amyotrophic lateral sclerosis complex
  Striatonigral degeneration
  Corticodentonigra degeneration with neuronal achromasia
  Alzheimer's disease
Inherited
  Huntington's disease
  Wilson's disease
  Hallervorden-Spatz disease
  Familail parkinsonism-dementia syndrome
  Familial basal ganglia calcification
  Neuroacanthocytosis
  Spinocerebellar-nigral degeneration and Joseph disease
  Glutamate dehydrogenase deficiency

*Modified from Jankovic J. Parkinson's disease and related disorders of movements. In: Calne DB, ed. Handbook of experimental pharmacology. Berlin: Springer-Verlag, 1989:227.*

thenia gravis. Triethylene tetramine dihydrochloride (Trientine) in dosages of 400 to 800 mg three times a day before meals recently has been approved for the treatment of penicillamine-sensitive patients with WD. In addition to the chelating agents, zinc sulfate at a dosage of 300 to 1200 mg/d between meals may reduce copper absorption. When early diagnosis is made and dietary and chelating therapy are instituted, the progression of liver and neurologic dysfunction can be halted and even reversed. At least 2000 μg of copper should be excreted during the first 24 hours of penicillamine therapy. About one third of patients with WD experience deterioration despite penicillamine therapy, but most improve, sometimes after a latent period lasting several weeks or months. In patients with parkinsonian symptoms, levodopa and anticholinergic therapy may provide symptomatic relief.

Besides treating patients with symptomatic WD, it is of paramount importance to screen all their relatives and to institute therapy immediately if the disease is diagnosed in any of them. Patients who fail to improve with chelating or other pharmacologic therapy may experience marked relief of neurologic symptoms several months after liver transplantation.

## Huntington's Disease

The usual onset of Huntington's disease (HD) is in the fourth and fifth decades of life, but about 10% of patients are seen during childhood or adolescence. Both juvenile and adult-onset HD are autosomal dominant traits, with a defective gene mapped to a terminal band of the short arm of chromosome 4. The gene mutation was found to consist of an unstable enlargement of the CAG repeat sequence at 4p16.3 The majority of patients with juvenile HD have the akinetic-rigid syndrome termed the *Westphal variant*. Other features of juvenile HD include dementia, seizures, and ataxia. In addition, patients with juvenile HD are more likely to have inherited the abnormal gene from their father than from their mother, and they tend to segregate within families. Although the medium-sized spiny neurons (type I cells) usually are affected first in the adult form of HD, the large aspiny cells have been suggested to degenerate first in the juvenile form.

### TABLE 161-8.   Laboratory Tests in Wilson's Disease

| Laboratory Tests (units) | Normal | Wilson's Disease |
| --- | --- | --- |
| Serum copper (μg/100 mL) | 90–140 | <60 (10–100) |
| Serum ceruloplasmin (mg/100 mL) | 24–45 | <15 (0–30) |
| Urine copper (μg 24h ) | <40 | >200 (100–1000) |
| Urine copper after penicillamine (μg/6 h) | <400 | >800 |
| Liver copper (μg/g wet weight) | <10 | >30 |
| Liver uptake (Cu-64 at 24 h) | >60% | <50% |
| Plasma (Cu-64 24:2 h ratio) | >0.8 | <0.5 |

In contrast to the caudate nucleus, which typically is involved in the adult form of HD, the putamen seems to be most damaged in the juvenile form of the disease.

There are no pathognomonic neurodiagnostic tests for HD, but the diagnosis can be established with at least 95% accuracy when the DNA marker is identified. The psychologic and social impact of such testing in identifying presymptomatic individuals is being investigated. The combination of DNA polymorphism and positron emission tomography may be used in the future to detect HD in the preclinical phase.

The most remarkable biochemical change observed in the brains of adults with HD is a reduction in the activity of glutamic acid decarboxylase, particularly in the corpus striatum, substantia nigra, and other basal ganglia. In contrast, thyrotropin releasing hormone, neurotensin, somatostatin, and neuropeptide Y are increased in the corpus striatum. The depletion of $\tau$-aminobutyric acid in the corpus striatum may result in disinhibition of the nigral-striatal pathway. Coupled with the accumulation of somatostatin, the net result may be the release of striatal dopamine, which results in chorea. Dopamine-blocking drugs, such as haloperidol, and dopamine-depleting agents, including tetrabenazine, often are useful in controlling chorea. In patients with childhood HD, which usually is manifested by parkinsonian features, levodopa may provide symptomatic relief.

## Hallervorden-Spatz Disease

In contrast to WD, which is characterized by the abnormal deposition of copper, the hallmark of Hallervorden-Spatz disease (HSD) is the deposition of iron. This is most notable in the globus pallidus and substantia nigra. First described in 1922, the disease now is recognized as a specific clinical-pathologic entity. HSD usually starts between 4 and 12 years of age, but occasionally presents as parkinsonian dementia in adult life. Children with HSD have posture and gait abnormalities, bradykinesia, rigidity, and other parkinsonian features, including tremor. In addition, other hyperkinetic movement disorders, including dystonia and choreoathetosis, may be seen. Further symptoms include progressive dysarthria, dementia, ataxia, spasticity, seizure disorder, optic atrophy, and retinitis pigmentosa.

Most cases are inherited in an autosomal recessive pattern, but many occur sporadically and some phenotypically similar cases seem to be inherited by autosomal dominant transmission.

Laboratory studies usually are not helpful in diagnosing HSD, although the disease may be suspected when an MRI scan shows a central focus of increased T2 signal intensity surrounded by a zone of decreased signal in the region of the globus pallidus. Furthermore, increased iron uptake in the basal ganglia may be demonstrated by scintillation counting after the infusion of radioactive iron (Fe-59). Increased iron uptake also is confirmed by postmortem examination, which reveals pigmentary degeneration of the basal ganglia, particularly the internal segment of the globus pallidus and the zona reticularis of the substantia nigra. These pigmentary changes are due to a threefold to fourfold accumulation of iron in these areas. Another distinctive pathologic feature of HSD is marked neuroaxonal degeneration with the formation of spheroids. These glycoprotein-containing axonal swellings have been attributed to abnormal peroxidation. The abnormal accumulation of cysteine was demonstrated in one of our patients with HSD. This increased cysteine may chelate ferrous iron, which in turn promotes the generation of free radicals, causing the characteristic neuropathologic changes of the disease. Whether the primary defect is in the enzyme cysteine dioxyginase or some other metabolic pathway, it is possible that the pathologic abnormalities result from the damaging effect of lipid membrane peroxidation and hydroxyl radical formation accelerated in the presence of non–protein-bound iron. A similar mechanism has been proposed in patients with ceroid lipofuscinosis and those with HSD-like syndrome who have sea blue histiocytes in bone marrow and cytoplasmic inclusions in peripheral lymphocytes. HSD also resembles the neuraxonal types of dystrophy in that patients with both conditions have extrapyramidal signs and dementia, and axonal spheroids are seen on pathologic examination of their central and peripheral nervous systems.

Iron chelation with desferrioxamine and antioxidant therapy have been tried in patients with HSD, but no benefit has been demonstrated. Levodopa and anticholinergic drugs may provide modest symptomatic relief of parkinsonian symptoms.

## HYPERKINETIC MOVEMENT DISORDERS

### Tremor

Essential tremor (ET) probably is the most common cause of an oscillatory involuntary movement during childhood (Table 161-9). ET may start at any age, including infancy. One form of infantile ET is the hereditary chin tremor, which consists of rhythmic, three-per-second contractions of the chin that often are associated with deafness and are inherited in an autosomal dominant pattern. Another form of ET that begins during infancy or early childhood is so-called "shuddering attacks." Children may have more than 100 attacks a day, but symptom-free intervals may last as long as 2 weeks. The attacks are characterized by bursts of rapid trembling of the whole body, occasionally associated with head turning, involuntary sniffing, and throat clearing. During the attacks, the child usually sinks to the floor; the attacks may persist during sleep.

In addition to these forms of ET, the characteristic action-postural tremor also may be seen in children. The slower (about 6.5 Hz) tremor often involves the head and neck, whereas the more rapid tremor (8 to 12 Hz) tends to involve the hands. Many other variants of ET have been recognized, however. Although ET usually is "benign," it occasionally can progress to a very disabling movement disorder, interfering with writing, feeding, speaking, and other activities of daily living.

Although neurotransmitter abnormalities in the basal ganglia are suspected to underlie ET, no pathologic changes have been documented in the few brains that have been examined at autopsy. Besides the beta blockers, ET may improve with primidone, lorazepam, alprazolam, clonazepam, amantadine, clonidine, and ethanol.

Other oscillatory involuntary movements occasionally seen in infants and children are "head nodding," which often is associated with congenital nystagmus, including spasmus nutans; and the "bobble-headed doll's syndrome," which is seen with diencephalic lesions, including third-ventricle cysts or tumors, craniopharyngioma, hydrocephalus, and hypothalamic lesions.

### Chorea and Athetosis

Chorea consists of flowing, continuous, unsustained, rapid, abrupt, and random contractions, whereas athetosis consists of non-patterned, writhing movements that represent a form of "slow chorea." In contrast, ballism is a form of severe, coarse chorea; it usually is unilateral (hemiballism) and often is the result of a lesion in the contralateral subthalamic nucleus and adjacent structures. Many acquired and hereditary types of chorea can become manifest during childhood (Table 161-10). Almost all normal infants make movements that resemble chorea, but this physiologic chorea usually resolves by 8 months of age. Children with attention deficit disorder and hyperactivity have distal chorea called *chorea minima.*

## TABLE 161-9. Classification of Tremors

**Rest Tremors**

*Parkinson Tremor*
Parkinson's disease
Secondary parkinsonism
  Postencephalic
  Toxic: phenothiazines, butyrophenones, metoclopramide, reserpine, tetrabenazine, carbon monoxide, manganese, MPTP, carbon disulfide
  Tumor
  Trauma
  Vascular
  Metabolic: hypoparathyroidism, chronic hepatocerebral degeneration
Parkinsonism plus (heterogenous system degenerations)
Olivopontocerebellar atrophy
Progressive supranuclear palsy
Wilson's disease
Huntington's disease

*Spasmus Nutans*

*Hereditary Chin Quivering*

*Other*
Midbrain (rubral) tremor
Severe essential tremor
Roussy-Lévy syndrome

**Action Tremors**

*Postural Tremors*
Physiologic tremor
  Normal physiologic tremor
  Accentuated physiologic tremor
    Stress-induced: anxiety, fight, fatigue, fever
    Endocrine: thyrotoxicosis, hypoglycemia, pheochromocytoma
    Drugs, toxins: epinephrine, isoproterenol, caffeine, theophylline and other sympathomimetic agents, levodopa, amphetamines, lithium, tricyclic antidepressants, phenothiazines, butyrophenones, thyroxine, hypoglycemic agents, adrenocorticosteroids, alcohol withdrawal, mercury, lead, arsenic, bismuth, carbon monoxide, methylbromide, monosodium glutamate, sodium valproate, metrizamide, meperidine
Essential tremor
  Autosomal dominant
  With peripheral neuropathy: Charcot-Marie-Tooth disease (Roussy-Lévy syndrome)
  With other movement disorders (parkinsonism, torsion dystonia, spasmodic torticollis, myoclonus)
  Factors that accentuate physiologic tremor also enhance or unmask essential tremor
  Vitamin E deficiency

Action tremor of parkinsonism
Neuropathic tremor
  Peripheral neuropathies
  Motor neuron disease
Cerebellar postural hypotonic tremor (titubation)
Midbrain ("rubral") tremor
Dystonic (axial) tremor

*Kinetic (Intention) Tremor*
Cerebellar outflow tremor (superior cerebellar peduncle lesion)
  Multiple sclerosis
  Posterior circulation strokes
  Cerebellar degenerations
  Wilson's disease
  Drugs, toxins: phenytoin, barbiturates, lithium, meperidine, alcohol, mercury, 5-fluorouracil, vidarabine, amiodarone, cimetidine, tocainide
Midbrain ("rubral") tremor
Primary handwriting tremor
Dystonic (distal) tremor
Familial benign chorea and tremor

*Miscellaneous Tremors and Other Rhythmic Movements*
Idiopathic
Hysterical
Involuntary rhythmic movements not classified as tremors
  Cardiac and respiratory movements
  Convulsions
  Nystagmus
  Segmental myoclonus
  Oscillatory myoclonus
  Asterixis
  Fasciculations
  Clonus
  Minipolymyoclonus
  Shivering
  Shuddering
  Head flopping or nodding movements

*Modified from Jankovic J. Neurologic consultant. New York: Lawrence Della Corte Publications, 1984:1.*

## TABLE 161-10. Classification of Choreas

**Developmental Choreas**

*Physiologic Chorea of Infancy*
Kernicterus, cerebral palsy, "minimal cerebral dysfunction" (the choreiform syndrome)

**Hereditary Choreas**

*Amino Acid Disorders*
Glutaric acidemia, cystinuria, homocystinuria, phenylketonuria, Hartnup, argininosuccinicaciduia

*Carbohydrate Disorders*
Mucopolysaccharidoses, mucolipidoses, galactosemia, pyruvate dehydrogenase deficiency

*Lipid Disorders*
Sphingolipidosis (Krabbe's), globoid cell leukodystrophy, metachromatic leukodystrophy, Gaucher's, GM$_1$ and GM$_2$ gangliosidosis, ceroid lipofuscinosis

*Other Metabolic Disorders*
Lesch-Nyhan syndrome, Leigh disease, sulfite-oxidase deficiency, porphyria

*Heredodegenerative Disorders*
Hallervorden-Spatz, ataxia-telangiectasia, tuberous sclerosis, Sturge-Weber, Wilson's disease, myoclonus epilepsy, familial inverted choreoathetosis, hemoglobin SC disease, xeroderma pigmentosum, Pelizaeus-Merzbacher, familial striatal necrosis, Huntington's disease, benign familial chorea (hereditary chorea without dementia), choreoacanthocytosis (amyotrophic chorea), paroxysmal kinesigenic choreoathetosis, paroxysmal dystonic choreoathetosis (Mount-Reback), familial calcification of the basal ganglia, Joseph disease, olivopontocerebellar atrophies (hereditary ataxis)

**Drug-Induced and Toxic Choreas**

*Antipsychotic Neuroleptics*
Tardive dyskinesia

*Antiparkinsonian Drugs*
Dopaminergic (levodopa, bromocriptine, pergolide, lisuride), amantadine, anticholinergics

*Anticonvulsants*
Phenytoin, carbamazepine

*Noradrenergic Stimulants*
Amphetamines, methylphenidate, aminophylline, theophylline, caffeine, pemoline

*Steroids*
Oral contraceptives, anabolic steroids

*Opiates*
Methadone

*Miscellaneous Drugs*
Amoxapine, antihistamines, cimetidine, cyclizine, diazoxide, digoxin, isoniazid, lithium, methyldopa, metoclopramide, reserpine, triazolam, tricyclic antidepressants

*Toxins*
Alcohol intoxication and withdrawal, carbon monoxide, manganese, mercury, thallium, toluene, glue sniffing

*Metabolic*
Hyponatremia and hypernatremia, hypocalcemia, hypoglycemia and hyperglycemia, hypomagnesemia, hepatic encephalopathy (acquired hepatocerebral degeneration), renal encephalopathy

*Endocrine*
Hyperthyroidism, hypoparathyroidism, pseudohypoparathyroidism, hyperparathyroidism, chorea gravidarum (pregnancy). Addison's disease

*Nutritional*
Beriberi, pellagra, vitamin B$_{12}$ deficiency in infants

*Infectious*
Sydenham's chorea (post-streptococcal), scarlet fever (streptococcal erythrogenic toxin), diphtheria, pertussis, typhoid fever, viral encephalitis (mumps, measles, varicella, echo, influenza), postvaccinal, neurosyphilis, mononucleosis, legionnaires' disease, bacterial endocarditis, sarcoidosis, mycobacterium tuberculosis, bacterial meningitis

*Immunologically Mediated*
Systemic lupus erythematosus, periarteritis nodosa, Behçet's syndrome, Henoch-Schönlein purpura, multiple sclerosis

**Cerebrovascular Choreas**

Basal ganglia infarction, basal ganglia hemorrhage, arteriovenous malformation, polycythemia vera, migraine, transient cerebral ischemia

**Miscellaneous Choreas**

Posttraumatic, epidural hematoma, subdural hematoma, electrical injury to the nervous system, brain tumor, degeneration of nucleus centrum medianum of thalamus, hydrocephalus

*Modified from Kurlan R, Shoulson I. Facial choreas. In: Jankovic J, Tolosa E, eds. Advanced neurology, vol 49. Facial dyskinesias. New York: Raven Press, 1988.*

## Cerebral Palsy

Of the various causes of chorea that occur in childhood, static encephalopathy (cerebral palsy) probably is the most common (see Chapter 27.3). About one third of patients with cerebral palsy have chorea or athetosis (choreoathetosis) as the predominant motor disturbance, but dystonia also was seen in 70% of such patients in one study of dyskinetic cerebral palsy. The involuntary movements are notable in half of the patients during the first year and athetosis develops in the remainder over the subsequent 4 or 5 years. In one study, 82% of patients with athetotic cerebral palsy had jaundice, asphyxia, or both during the postnatal period, and about 60% had a history of premature birth.

Although the neurologic impairment in cerebral palsy usually is nonprogressive, patients have been described who have had delayed-onset progressive choreoathetosis and dystonia. These cases have been attributed to sprouting and denervation supersensitivity of receptors in the basal ganglia.

Kernicterus, a syndrome that usually is seen in premature infants with total serum bilirubin concentrations exceeding 10 mg/ dL, may be manifested by choreoathetosis, tremor, dystonia, rigidity, dysarthria, deafness, and limitation of upward gaze. Another cause of chorea that is seen in premature infants is severe bronchopulmonary aplasia. Mortality in these infants is about 30%, and there is evidence of neuronal loss in the basal ganglia at autopsy. Surviving infants generally have a good prognosis and the chorea usually resolves.

### Hereditary Chorea

Although the majority of children with HD have a parkinsonian syndrome, about one fourth have chorea. Another form of hereditary chorea is *benign hereditary chorea,* an autosomal dominant disorder that may present during infancy, childhood, or adolescence. Although it is benign, it may persist as a lifelong condition and rarely may be associated with intellectual impairment. Although caudate atrophy usually is not seen, 18-F-2-fluorodeoxyglucose positron emission tomography may indicate decreased cerebral glucose metabolism in the caudate nucleus.

Another cause of genetic childhood chorea is the Lesch-Nyhan syndrome. This complex motor-behavioral syndrome is inherited as an X-linked recessive trait and is a result of defective activity of the enzyme hypoxanthine-guanine phosphoribosyltransferase. The diagnosis is suspected when a young boy with delayed developmental milestones, spasticity, and choreoathetosis develops self-mutilatory behavior and is found to have sand-like deposits in his urine. Patients often have complications of hyperuricemia, including gouty arthritis, tophus formation, and obstructive nephropathy. Cerebrospinal fluid (CSF) studies of monoamine metabolites and postmortem biochemical assays have provided evidence for reduced dopamine and norepinephrine turnover in patients with this disorder.

### Sydenham's Chorea

The high frequency of complications of chronic rheumatic heart disease in patients with Sydenham's chorea (SC) suggests an association between rheumatic fever and this neurologic disorder. Further evidence is provided by the observation that children with SC have antistreptococcic antibodies, which react with neurons of the subthalamic and caudate nuclei. The pathology of SC has not been well studied, but some brains have had vasculitis, chiefly involving the basal ganglia, cortex, and cerebellum.

Coincident with a dramatic decline in cases of acute rheumatic fever, the incidence of SC also is decreasing rapidly. Of 240 patients admitted with the diagnosis of SC to the University of Chicago Hospital between 1951 and 1976, only 8% were seen after 1968. Irritability, emotional lability, and other behavioral problems usually accompany the involuntary movements of this disorder. In about 20% of cases, the chorea is strictly unilateral (hemichorea). Besides chorea, other clinical features of SC include the "milkmaid's grip," "spooning," and "hung-up" reflexes. In most cases, the chorea subsides within 5 to 15 weeks, but it may recur in as many as 30% of patients within 2 years. Recurrence is particularly likely during pregnancy (chorea gravidarum). Although the motor symptoms usually resolve completely, mental changes (particularly emotional lability) and cardiac problems may persist indefinitely. Persistent dopaminergic supersensitivity in affected individuals has been suggested by the high frequency of adverse reactions to central stimulants and to neuroleptics, together with psychotic features demonstrated on the Minnesota Multiphasic Personality Inventory test. Because there may be a latency period of about 1 to 6 months after the streptococcal infection before the onset of chorea, patients with SC may have normal erythrocyte sedimentation rates, and normal antistreptolysin and antistreptococcic antibody levels. In addition to an initial course of penicillin followed by the administration of prophylactic oral penicillin until the patient reaches 20 years of age,

a trial of corticosteroids, haloperidol, pimozide, reserpine, or tetrabenazine may be needed in severe cases. Besides SC, there are many other infectious causes of chorea, including meningitis.

## Dystonia

Dystonia consists of repetitive, patterned, twisting, and sustained movements that may be either slow or rapid. About 30% of all patients with dystonia have onset of the involuntary movements before they attain 20 years of age. The term *torsion dystonia* has replaced the old name of dystonia musculorum deformans and now is used to describe a dystonic state. Dystonic states may be classified according to their cause into primary idiopathic dystonia, secondary dystonia, or psychogenic dystonia (Table 161-11). Primary idiopathic torsion dystonia, whether sporadic or inherited, is not associated with intellectual, pyramidal, cerebellar, or sensory deficits. Most cases of primary childhood-onset dystonia are inherited as either an autosomal dominant or a recessive disorder, but no specific genetic markers have been identified thus far. Although autosomal recessive inheritance originally was proposed for Ashkenazi Jewish patients, recent studies suggest that autosomal dominant dystonia occurs with the same frequency in Jewish and non-Jewish patients. Autosomal dominant inheritance also is supported by the frequent coexistence of dystonia and ET within the same patient or the same kindred. Among 1000 patients with dystonia who were studied at the Baylor College of Medicine Movement Disorder Clinic, 20% had associated ET; conversely, about one third of patients with ET have dystonia. Cerebral palsy probably is the most common cause of secondary dystonia seen in children.

The distribution of dystonia seems to be age dependent; in children, it often starts distally, whereas in adults, a cranial-cervical distribution is more common. Furthermore, childhood dystonia tends to progress to generalized dystonia, but adult dystonia usually remains focal or segmental (Fig 161-8). Hemidystonia (unilateral dystonia) involving one half the body seems to be particularly common among children and young adults (Fig 161-9). About three fourths of patients with hemidystonia have evidence of a structural lesion in the contralateral basal ganglia, particularly the putamen. The causes include infarction or hemorrhage in one third and perinatal trauma in one fifth of cases. In many patients with secondary dystonia, particularly children, there often is a delay of several years after the acute event before the contralateral hemidystonia becomes manifest.

The severity of dystonia also varies. In some patients, it occurs only when they are participating in certain activities, the so-called *task-specific dystonias,* such as cramping during writing or typing, or "musician's hands." As the dystonia progresses, it often "overflows" to adjacent muscles and eventually becomes apparent even at rest. Rarely, the spasms become so severe as to cause cervical disk, nerve, or root problems, and muscle breakdown with myoglobinuria.

No specific morphologic changes have been noted at postmortem examination of the brains of patients with primary dystonia. A marked reduction in norepinephrine concentrations in the posterior and lateral hypothalamus, and an increase in the red nucleus have been reported, however, suggesting that the changes in norepinephrine levels resulted in the disinhibition of dopamine, serotonin, and cholinergic neurons. This may explain the beneficial effect of anticholinergic drugs in many patients with dystonia.

Certain orthopedic and musculoskeletal problems peculiar to the pediatric population may produce postural deformities that resemble dystonia. Congenital torticollis caused by contracture of the sternocleidomastoid muscle may produce a palpable mass and neck deformity in the first 6 to 8 months of life. Such congenital torticollis may be the result of local trauma during a breech

## TABLE 161-11.   Classification of Dystonic States

**Primary Idiopathic Dystonia**

*Inherited (Hereditary Torsion Dystonia, Dystonia Musculorum Deformans)*
Autosomal dominant
Autosomal recessive (pseudodominant)
X-linked recessive
Dystonia with marked diurnal variation*
Paroxysmal kinesigenic and nonkinesigenic dystonia*
Parkinsonism-dystonia*
*Sporadic (Idopathic Torsion Dystonia)*
Generalized
Segmental (usually secondary dystonias)
Hemidystonia
Multifocal
Focal: torticollis, occupational cramps, oromandibular dystonia, blepharospasm, spasmodic dysphonia

**Secondary Dystonia**

*Associated with Other Neurodegenerative Disorders*
Wilson's disease
Huntington's disease
Parkinsonism
Progressive supranuclear palsy
Progressive pallidal degeneration
Hallervorden-Spatz disease
Joseph disease
Ataxia-telangiectasia
Multiple sclerosis
Neuroacanthocytosis
Rett syndrome
Intraneuronal inclusion disease
Infantile bilateral striatal necrosis
Familial basal ganglia calcifications

*Associated with Metabolic Disorders*
Amino acid disorders
   Glutaric aciduria type I
   Methylmalonic acidemia
   Homocystinuria
   Hartnup disease
   Tyrosinosis

Lipid disorders
   Metachromatic leukodystrophy
   Ceroid lipofuscinosis
   Juvenile dystonic lipidosis ("sea blue" histiocytosis; gangliosidoses $GM_1$-, $GM_2$-variants: neurovisceral storage disease with supranuclear ophthalmoplegia)
Miscellaneous metabolic disorders
   Leigh disease
   Leber's disease and mitochondrial encephalopathies
   Lesch-Nyhan syndrome
   Triosephosphate isomerase deficiency
   Vitamin E deficiency

*Result of Known Specific Cause*
Perinatal cerebral injury and kernicterus (may be delayed in onset)
Infection
   Viral encephalitis, encephalitis lethargica, tuberculosis, Reye's syndrome, subacute sclerosing panencephalitis, Jakob-Creutzfeldt disease, acquired immunodeficiency syndrome; syphilis; acute infectious torticollis
Paraneoplastic brain stem encephalitis
Head trauma
Peripheral trauma
Atlantoaxial dislocation, subluxation, plagiocephaly
Gastroesophageal reflux (Sandifer's syndrome)
Cerebral vascular injury
Brain tumor
Arteriovenous malformation
Central pontine myelinolysis
Cerebral ectopia and syringomyelia
Tortiocular tilt
Toxins: MN, CO, $SC_2$, methane, wasp sting
Drugs: levodopa, bromocriptine, antipsychotics, metoclopramide, fenfluramine, ergots, anticonvulsants

**Psychogenic Dystonia**

* Also may occur sporadically.

*Modified from Jankovic J, Fahn S. Dystonic syndromes. In: Jankovic J, Tolosa E, eds. Parkinson's disease and movement disorders. Baltimore: Urban and Schwarzenberg, 1988:283.*

or difficult forceps delivery, spondylosis, asymmetric facet joint, basal impression, atlantoaxial dislocation, or other cervical-cranial anomaly. It is not known how many cases of infantile or juvenile scoliosis actually represent axial dystonia.

Dystonia usually consists of continual muscle contractions, although these may be modified by action, position, or stress. In some patients, dystonia fluctuates markedly in a paroxysmal or diurnal manner (Table 161-12). Diurnal dystonia usually occurs during the first decade of life. There is a 3:1 female preponderance, and familial clustering suggests an autosomal dominant pattern of inheritance. Patients usually are asymptomatic in the morning or after a daytime nap, but as the day progresses, they experience fatigability and dystonic movements, usually starting in the leg and later progressing to a more generalized dystonia. Some patients also have associated hyperreflexia, rigidity, and postural

tremor. The CSF homovanillic acid level often is low, and most patients improve with levodopa and anticholinergic therapy.

Another form of fluctuating dystonia is paroxysmal kinesigenic and nonkinesigenic dystonia. The chief difference is that the kinesigenic dystonia is precipitated by a sudden movement, such as arising rapidly from a chair or turning suddenly, whereas the nonkinesigenic dystonia occurs spontaneously. The kinesigenic form of paroxysmal dystonia is seen predominantly in boys, and has its onset between 5 and 15 years of age. The attacks usually last a few seconds and recur as many as 100 times a day, and the dystonia often is asymmetric and associated with choreoathetosis and epilepsy. Most patients with kinesigenic dystonia improve with anticonvulsant therapy, including phenytoin, carbamazepine, and barbiturates. The nonkinesigenic form of paroxysmal dystonia may begin in infancy, with the attacks lasting

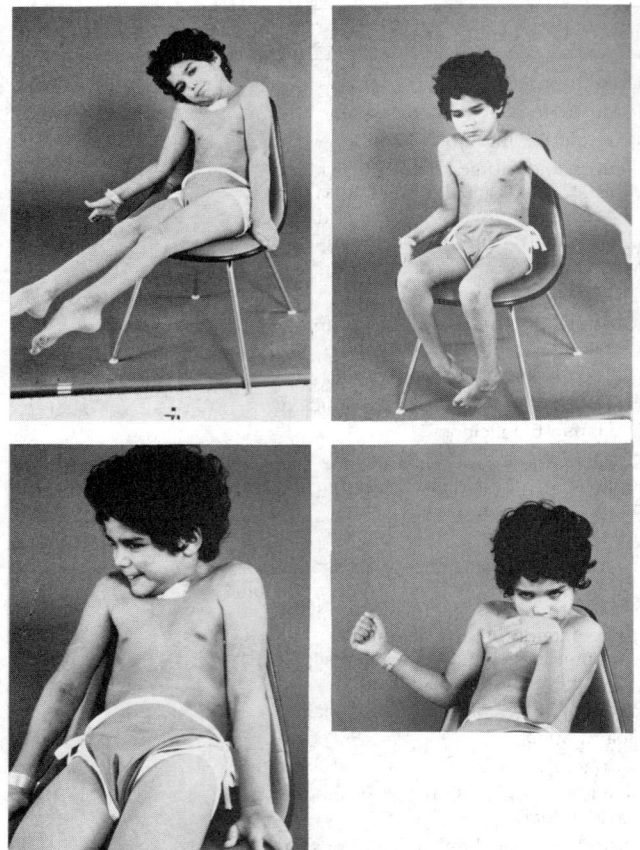

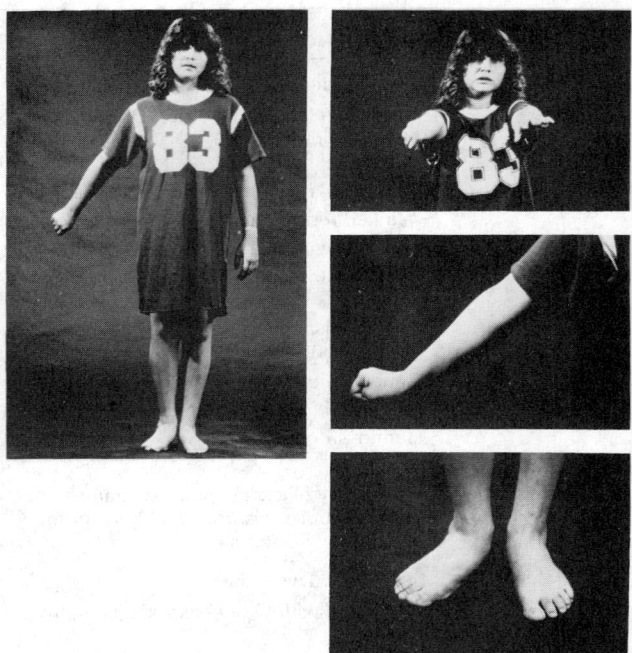

**Figure 161-9.** A 14-year-old girl with right hemidystonia as a result of left striatal injury at age 2 years. (Jankovic J, Fahn S. Dystonic syndromes. In: Jankovic J, Tolosa E, eds. Parkinson's disease and movement disorders. Baltimore: Urban & Schwarzenberg, 1988:283.)

**Figure 161-8.** An 8-year-old boy with autosomal dominant, generalized torsion dystonia. As a result of severe dystonic contractions, he had muscle breakdown, myoglobinuria, and renal failure requiring a temporary curarization and tracheostomy. (Jankovic J, Fahn S. Dystonic syndromes. In: Jankovic J, Tolosa E, eds. Parkinson's disease and movement disorders. Baltimore: Urban & Schwarzenberg, 1988:283.)

minutes to hours and recurring two or three times a month. The attacks may be precipitated by alcohol, coffee, fatigue, stress, exercise, or excitement. Besides dystonia, many patients with nonkinesigenic dystonia have choreoathetosis and ataxia, particularly during the attacks. This form of dystonia is resistant to pharmacologic therapy, but some patients improve with clonazepam, oxazepam, acetazolamide, valproate, carbamazepine, and haloperidol.

Another cause of paroxysmal dystonic postures occurring in infants and children, including torticollis and opisthotonos, is gastroesophageal reflux (Sandifer's syndrome). Multiple sclerosis, thyrotoxicosis, metabolic disorders such as Hartnup disease, paroxysmal dystonia in sleep (hypnogenic dystonia), and "infectious torticollis" also produce paroxysmal or fluctuating dystonia.

Accurate diagnosis is the first step in the treatment of patients with torsion dystonia. More extensive diagnostic investigation usually is prompted by the presence of atypical features such as impaired intellect, seizures, neuro-ophthalmologic abnormalities, ataxia, corticospinal tract signs, sensory deficits, severe speech disturbance, and unilateral distribution of the dystonia (Table 161-13). WD is one of the most important causes of dystonia, because it is curable. Another treatable, and possibly preventable, type of childhood dystonia is the drug-induced form. Dystonic movements may be caused by levodopa, bromocriptine, anticonvulsants, and ergots, but only the dopamine receptor blocking drugs such as the antipsychotics and antiemetics produce persistent tardive dystonia. Although acute transient dystonic reaction is a well-recognized complication of therapy with these

drugs, a small percentage of patients treated with the neuroleptics have persistent and often disabling dystonia. In such cases of tardive dystonia, the offending drug should be stopped and, if no spontaneous improvement occurs, the patient should be given trials of muscle relaxants, anticholinergic drugs, and tetrabenazine. About two thirds of children with idiopathic torsion dystonia obtain some benefit from high-dose anticholinergic therapy (30 to 60 mg of trihexyphenidyl per day). When trihexyphenidyl is used, it has to be introduced in small doses and increased gradually over a period of several weeks or months until symptomatic improvement is noted or side effects, such as mental dullness, blurring of vision, and other anticholinergic adverse reactions, prevent further increase in the dosage. In addition to anticholinergic drugs, we find that tetrabenazine, a monoamine-depleting agent, is effective in some patients with dystonia; occasionally, we combine it with pimozide, a postsynaptic dopamine receptor blocking drug. Other drugs that occasionally prove useful in the treatment of dystonia include carbamazepine, baclofen, valproate, primidone, lithium, lisuride, and bromocriptine. Patients with diurnal dystonia or dystonia in combination with parkinsonism often respond to levodopa. When pharmacologic therapy fails, *Clostridium botulinum* toxin injections may be tried, particularly for patients with focal dystonia. Stereotactic thalamotomy, cervical rhizotomy, and other surgical therapies usually are reserved for patients with disabling dystonia whose disease does not respond to pharmacologic therapy or chemodenervation with *C botulinum* toxin.

## Tics

About 25% of normal children have transient tics, making this the most frequent childhood-onset involuntary movement seen in a movement disorders clinic. One of the most common causes of pathologic tics in childhood is the Gilles de la Tourette's syndrome (TS). This motor-behavioral disorder is the expression of a genetic disturbance affecting the central nervous system. Its onset usually is between 2 and 15 years of age, and its expression is gender influenced; in boys, motor and vocal manifestations

**TABLE 161-12. Idiopathic Fluctuating or Paroxysmal Dystonias**

| Characteristic | Diurnal | Paroxysmal | |
| --- | --- | --- | --- |
| | | *Kinesigenic* | *Nonkinesigenic* |
| Male:female ratio | 1:1 | 4:1 | 3:2 |
| Age at onset (y) | <10 | 5–15 (1–35) | <5 (0–25) |
| Inheritance | AD, AR, sporadic | AD, sporadic | AD, sporadic |
| Duration of attacks | Hours | <5 min | Minutes to hours |
| Frequency of attacks | 1/d | 100/d | 3/mo |
| Associated features | Postural tremor, parkinsonism, hyperflexia | Choreoathetosis, epilepsy | Choreoathetosis, ataxia |
| Asymmetry | +++ | ++ | + |
| Ability to suppress attacks | 0 | +++ | +++ |
| Induced or precipitating factors | Afternoon and evening fatigue | Sudden movement, startle | Alcohol, coffee, fatigue, stress, exercise, excitement |
| Medical therapy | Levodopa, anticholinergics | Phenytoin, carbamazepine, barbiturates | Clonazepam, oxazepam, acetazolamide, valproate, carbamazepine, haloperidol |

AD, autosomal dominant; AR, autosomal recessive; +, occasionally; ++, usually; +++, almost always.

Modified from Jankovic J, Fahn S. Dystonic syndrome. In: Jankovic J, Tolosa Ed, eds. Parkinson's disease and movement disorders. Baltimore: Urban and Schwarzenberg, 1988:283.

seem to dominate, whereas in girls, behavioral problems such as obsessive-compulsive disorder seem more common.

In addition to simple tics such as blinking, facial grimacing, shoulder shrugging, and head jerking, many patients with TS have complex sequences of coordinated movements, including bizarre gait, kicking, jumping, body gyrations, scratching, and seductive or obscene gestures. The waxing and waning nature of tics, the irresistible urge before a tic and relief after a tic, the temporary suppressibility of the tics, and the recurrence of tics during sleep often result in the disorder being misdiagnosed as

**TABLE 161-13. Investigation of Patients With Atypical Dystonia**

**Blood Studies**

Ceruloplasmin, copper, creatine phosphokinase, myoglobin, glucose, lactate, pyruvate, uric acid, creatinine, workup for autoimmune disease

Examination of red cells for acanthocytosis or sickle-cell disease; lymphocytes for vacuolation (light microscopy) or inclusions (electromicroscopy)

Leukocytes: lysosomal enzymes, hypoxanthine guanine phosphoribosyltransferase (HPRT)

**Urine Studies**

Screening tests: amino acids, 24-h copper, column chromatography for oligosaccharides and mucopolysaccharides

**Cerebrospinal Fluid Studies**

Lactate, pyruvate

**Biopsies**

Liver: morphology, copper

Bone marrow: "sea blue" histiocytes, vacuolation

Skin: fibroblasts for lysosomal enzymes

Conjunctivae: neuronal inclusions

Rectal mucosa: neuronal inclusions

Muscle: mitochondrial abnormalities

Brain: neuronal inclusions or deposits

**Other Studies**

Slit lamp examination for Kayser-Fleischer ring, cataraacts, etc.

CT/MRI: basal ganglia calcifications or necrosis and other abnormalities

PET scan: glucose metaoblism, blood flow, $^{18}$F-L-dopa, receptor ligand studies

Spine radiographs or myelogram: atlantoaxial subluxation, Klippel-Feil deformity

Upper GI study: hiatal hernia in Sandifer-Kinsbourne sydnrome

Videotape: use quantitative rating scale and a polyelectromyograph for documentation

Electrophysiologic studies: electroencephalogram, electroretinogram, visual/brain stem, somatosensory, and cortical evoked responses, polysonnography, electromyography, nerve conduction tests; particularly useful in evaluation of paroxysmal and posttraumatic dystonia

CT, computed tomography; MRI, magnetic resonance imaging; GI, gatrointestinal; PET, positron emission tomography.

Modified from Jankovic J, Fahn S. Dystonic syndromes. In: Jankovic J, Tolosa Ed, eds. Parkinson's disease and movement disorders. Baltimore: Urban and Schwarzenberg, 1988:283.

having a psychogenic origin. The psychogenic nature of the condition also is suggested erroneously by the involuntary vocalizations that occur, which range from simple noises to coprolalia (obscene words), echolalia (repetition of words), and palilalia (repetition of a phrase or word with increasing rapidity). Coprolalia, although it is one of the most recognizable symptoms of TS, has been seen in only 40% of our patients thus far. Many patients also experience copropraxia, echopraxia, bizarre thoughts and ideas, thought fixation, compulsive ruminations, and perverse sexual fantasies. Sleep complaints, including restlessness, insomnia, enuresis, somnambulism, nightmares, and bruxism, have been noted in about half our patients, and about two thirds had evidence of motor tics recorded by polysomnography. If a broad spectrum of behavioral problems is included, then about 1% of all individuals manifest one or more aspects of the TS gene. Disturbance in the mesencephalic-mesolimbic system, which results

---

### TABLE 161-14. Classification of Myoclonus

**Physiologic Myoclonus (Normal Individuals)**
Sleep jerks (hypnic jerks)
Anxiety-induced
Exercise-induced
Hiccough (singultus)
Benign infantile myoclonus with feeding

**Essential Myoclonus (No Known Cause and No Other Gross Neurologic Deficits)**
Hereditary (autosomal dominant)
Sporadic
  Ballistic movement overflow myoclonus
  Oscillatory myoclonus
  Segmental myoclonus (rhythmic and non-rhythmic
  Nocturnal myoclonus
  Restless leg syndrome

**Epileptic Myoclonus (Seizures Dominant and No Encephalopathy, at Least Initially)**
Isolated epileptic myoclonic jerks
Cortical reflex myoclonus
Reticular reflex myoclonus
Primary generalized epileptic myoclonus
Epilepsia partialis continua
Photoconvulsive response
Infantile spasms
Childhood epileptic encephalopathy with slow spike and slow waves (Lennox-Gastaut syndrome, myoclonic-ataxic epilepsy, cryptogenic myoclonic epilepsy)
Familial myoclonic epilepsy (Janz)
Familial myoclonic epilepsy (Rabot)
Progressive myoclonus epilepsy: Baltic myoclonus (Unverricht-Lundborg)

**Symptomatic Myoclonus (Progressive or Static Encephalopathy Dominates)**
Progressive myoclonus epilepsy (PME)
  Lafora's body disease
  Neuronal ceroid lipofuscinosis
  Sialidosis (types I, II)
  Mitochondrial encephalopathy
  Noninfantile neuronopathic Gaucher's disease
  Biotin-responsive encephalopathy
  Lipidoses ($GM_2$ gangliosidosis, Tay-Sachs, Krabbe's)
Spinocerebellar degeneration
  Ramsay Hunt syndrome
  Friedreich's ataxia
  Ataxia-telangiectasia

Basal ganglia degenerations
  Wilson's disease
  Torsion dystonia
  Hallervorden-Spatz disease
  Progressive supranuclear palsy
  Huntington's disease
  Parkinson's disease
Dementias
  Creutzfeldt-Jakob disease
  Alzheimer's disease
Viral types of encephalopathy
  Subacute sclerosing panencephalitis
  Encephalitis lethargia
  Arbovirus encephalitis
  Herpes simplex encephalitis
  Postinfection encephalitis
Metabolic
  Hypoxic-ischemic encephalopathy
  Hepatic failure
  Renal failure
  Dialysis syndrome
  Hyponatremia
  Hypoglycemia
  Infantile myoclonic encephalopathy (polymyoclonus with or without neuroblastoma)
  Nonketotic hyperglycemia
Toxic types of encephalopathy
  Bismuth
  Heavy metal poisons
  Methyl bromide dichlorodiphenyltrichloroethane (DDT)
  Drugs, including levodopa
Physical types of encephalopathy
  Posttraumatic
  Heat stroke
  Electric shock
  Decompression injury
Focal central nervous system damage
  Post-stroke
  Post-thalamotomy
  Tumor
  Trauma
  Segmental myoclonus (branchial, spinal)

*Modified from Patel V, Jankovic J. Myoclonus. In: Appel SH, ed. Current neurology, vol 8. St. Louis: Mosby-YearBook, 1988:77.*

in disinhibition of the limbic system, has been suggested as the pathogenetic mechanism underlying TS.

Although haloperidol is recommended most frequently for TS, we find fluphenazine, pimozide, and tetrabenazine to be more effective and better tolerated. Patients with predominant behavioral symptoms may benefit from clonidine and fluoxetine. When TS is associated with attention deficit disorder and hyperactivity, central nervous system stimulants such as methylphenidate may be needed, but should be used cautiously.

## Myoclonus

In contrast to tics, myoclonus is a simple, jerk-like movement that is not coordinated or suppressible, and often is activated by volitional movement (Table 161-14). Benign neonatal sleep myoclonus, which is seen in the first month of life, usually is stimulus sensitive and occurs in the early stages of sleep. It should be differentiated from neonatal seizures and infantile spasms. Essential myoclonus usually begins before 20 years of age, is inherited in an autosomal dominant pattern, and may be associated with ET.

In patients with epileptic myoclonus, seizures often dominate the clinical presentation. Cortical reflex myoclonus is characterized by a time-locked electroencephalographic (EEG) event preceding the myoclonic movement and by enhanced amplitude of the somatosensory evoked potential. In contrast to the hyperexcitable sensorimotor cortex that underlies cortical myoclonus, reticular reflex myoclonus presumably is the result of hyperexcitable brain stem reticular formation, particularly the nucleus reticularis gigantocellularis. Progressive myoclonus epilepsy (PME) consists of myoclonus, seizures, and a progressive clinical course. One form of PME, Unverricht-Lundborg disease (also known as Baltic myoclonus), is characterized by stimulus-sensitive myoclonus that usually begins between 6 and 15 years of age. The patients also have dysarthria, ataxia, intention tremor, and mild intellectual decline, and most become bedridden within 5 years after onset of the disease. Epileptiform EEG findings may be seen as long as 3 years before the onset of clinical symptoms. The disease is inherited in an autosomal recessive pattern, and at least some cases may be associated with mitochondrial myopathy and encephalopathy. Another form of progressive myoclonus, Lafora's body disease, usually begins between 11 and 18 years of age, and is characterized by progressive dementia, apraxia, and cortical blindness, with total disability resulting within 5 to 8 years after onset. Biopsy of the skin (particularly the axillary skin), liver, muscle, or brain reveals typical inclusions (Lafora's bodies) that are positive on periodic acid–Schiff staining.

Ramsay Hunt syndrome is a group of heterogenous disorders that are dominated by a combination of progressive myoclonus and cerebellar ataxia. We recently studied a young girl with progressive myoclonus and blindness caused by neuronal ceroid lipofuscinosis. Myoclonus also may be a manifestation of viral encephalitis and typically is seen in patients with subacute sclerosing panencephalitis. In this subacute disorder, there is progressive dementia and "slow" myoclonus occurring about every second that is associated with periodic complexes on the EEG. Another form of myoclonic encephalopathy that occurs in young children is the opsoclonus–myoclonus syndrome or the "dancing eyes–dancing feet syndrome." This usually is seen after a febrile illness or in association with neuroblastoma, and marked improvement may be achieved with steroid therapy. Stimulus-sensitive myoclonus resembles another jerk-like movement disorder called "the startle disease" or hyperekplexia. Small myoclonic jerks (mini-polymyoclonus) also have been reported in children with chronic spinal muscular atrophy.

The idiopathic, generalized, or segmental forms of myoclonus may improve with treatment using clonazepam, sodium valproate, 5-hydroxytryptophan, tetrabenazine, reserpine, levodopa, and trihexyphenidyl. Recently, two new drugs (lisuride and piracetam) have shown promise in the treatment of patients with myoclonus.

## Stereotypies

Stereotypies are repetitive, purposeless, and seemingly voluntary movements such as chewing, rocking, and repetitive twirling or touching. These movements usually are seen in the setting of infantile autism or mental retardation. Attention recently has been directed toward another disorder that is characterized by marked stereotypy, namely Rett syndrome. This condition occurs only in girls, who have normal prenatal and perinatal growth and development. At the age of 6 to 18 months, they regress in their verbal and motor skills, lose purposeful use of their hands, and have jerky ataxia and typical stereotyped movements of the hands resembling hand washing and kneading. In addition to the motor manifestations, girls with Rett syndrome often have breath-holding spells, hyperventilation, loss of facial expression, poor eye contact, bruxism, dystonia, occasional seizures, apparent insensitivity to pain, and a variety of self-injurious and aggressive behaviors. The pathogenesis of Rett syndrome is unknown, and the vast majority of the cases occur sporadically, although some are familial.

## Selected Readings

Aron AM, Freeman JM, Carter S. The natural history of Sydenham's chorea. Am J Med 1965;38:83.

Berkovic SF, Andermann F, Carpenter S, Wolfe LS. Progressive myoclonus epilepsies: Specific causes and diagnosis. N Engl J Med 1986;315:296.

Brewer GJ, Yuzbasiyan-Gurkan V. Wilson disease. Medicine (Baltimore) 1992;71:139.

Dure L, Jankovic J. Childhood-onset movement disorders. In: Fahn S, Jankovic J, eds. Current opinion in neurology and neurosurgery, vol I. London: Gower Academic Journals, 1988:347.

Fitzgerald PM, Jankovic J, Glaze DG, et al. Extrapyramidal involvement in Rett's syndrome. Neurology 1990;40:293.

Gershanik OS. Parkinsonism of early onset. In: Jankovic J, Tolosa E, eds. Parkinson's disease and movement disorders. Baltimore: Williams & Wilkins, 1993:235.

Jankovic J. Diagnosis and classification of tics and Tourette syndrome. Adv Neurol 1992;58:14.

Jankovic J, Caskey TC, Stout JT, Butler I. Lesch-Nyhan syndrome: A study of motor behavior and CSF monoamine turnover. Ann Neurol 1988;23:466.

Jankovic J, Fahn S. Dystonic syndromes. In: Jankovic J, Tolosa E, eds. Parkinson's disease and movement disorders. Baltimore: Williams & Wilkins, 1993:337.

Lou J-S, Jankovic J. Essential tremor: Clinical correlates in 350 patients. Neurology 1991;41:234.

Patel VM, Jankovic J. Myoclonus. In: Appel SH, ed. Current neurology, vol 8. St Louis: Mosby-Year Book, 1988:77.

Stacy M, Jankovic J. Childhood dystonia. Pediatr Ann 1993:22.

Swaiman KF. Hallervorden-Spatz syndrome and brain iron metabolism. Arch Neurol 1991;48:1285.

Wexler NS, Rose EA, Housman DE. Molecular approaches to hereditary disease of the nervous system: Huntington's disease is a paradigm. Annu Rev Neurosci 1991;14:503.

*Principles and Practice of Pediatrics, Second Edition.*
edited by Frank A. Oski et al. J. B. Lippincott Company, Philadelphia © 1994.

# 161.5 *Diseases With Astrocyte Abnormalities*

Marvin A. Fishman

## ALEXANDER DISEASE

Alexander disease is a degenerative disorder of the nervous system in which no enzymatic or biochemical defects have yet been defined. The disease usually presents in infancy, but later-onset forms have been described.

### Pathogenesis

The pathogenesis of the disorder is unknown, but may reflect the dysfunction of astrocytes. This speculation is based in part on the finding of Rosenthal fibers in the brains of affected children. The fibers are the result of a conglutination of altered glial filaments, which form eosinophilic hyalin spheres in the cytoplasm of astrocytes. The spheres, which are thought not to result from the storage of abnormal material, are particularly prevalent beneath the pia mater and around blood vessels. In some cases, there is a loss of myelin, but this is thought to be a secondary event and not to represent a feature of the primary pathogenesis of the disease. Abnormally enlarged mitochondria have been noted, but it is unclear whether this is indicative of an abnormality of mitochondria metabolism.

### Pathology

The common feature of all the variants of Alexander disease is the presence of refractile eosinophilic bodies in relation to astrocytes. These bodies are most abundant in the subpial, subependymal, and perivascular areas, but may be found throughout the nervous system in both the white and gray matter, and may be seen in the spinal cord. The eosinophilic bodies are found in large, hypertrophied astrocytes, which have a perpendicular orientation to the surface of the brain in the subpial area and form a radial array around blood vessels. In the juvenile form of the disease, the brain stem may be involved predominantly and the medulla has been noted to be hypertrophied. Electron microscopy demonstrates filaments that form the Rosenthal fibers in the astrocytes of granular osmophilic material. Alpha B-crystallin is a major protein component of Rosenthal fibers, but its gene structure is normal.

There is a variable loss of myelin in patients with Alexander disease, which results in a soft and retracted appearance of the white matter. In infantile cases, this may be marked and present in a diffuse pattern. In patients with the juvenile and adult-onset forms of the disease, demyelination is more limited and patchy.

Rosenthal fibers are not specific for Alexander disease and have been noted in patients with a variety of disorders, including syringomyelia, astrocytic glioma, optic nerve glioma, multiple sclerosis, central pontine myelinolysis, disseminated cerebral gliomatosis, and neurofibromatosis.

### Symptoms and Signs

Three variants of Alexander disease have been described and are distinguished by their age of onset: infantile, juvenile, and adult.

They are grouped together under the term *Alexander disease* because they result in similar pathologic changes in various portions of the central nervous system, but it is not certain whether they are the same disease or different conditions with similar pathology.

The infantile form affects children between birth and 2 years of age, but the average onset of the illness is at 6 months of age. The course usually is 2 to 3 years, but variability exists; the duration of the disease varies from months to more than 5 years. Psychomotor retardation, megalencephaly (with or without hydrocephalus), spasticity, and seizures are the prominent features. The head may not be large at birth, but increases progressively in size during infancy. Increased intracranial pressure may be present, even without hydrocephalus. When hydrocephalus is present, it often is the result of partial obstruction of the aqueduct by proliferating astrocytes in the ependymal lining. Clinical examination does not disclose any abnormality of peripheral nervous system function.

The juvenile-onset form of the disease is much less common than the infantile form. This type is seen between 7 and 14 years of age, and its course is longer, varying between 1 and more than 10 years (average, 8 years). The intellect remains intact, unlike the infantile form. Findings are related to dysfunction of the brain stem, and include ptosis, nystagmus, facial diplegia, difficulty in swallowing, nasal speech, and tongue atrophy. Other features include generalized spasticity, weakness, and ataxia.

The adult-onset type of Alexander disease is rarest and occurs in young adulthood. The clinical syndrome resembles that of multiple sclerosis, and includes blurred vision, spasticity, nystagmus, dysarthria, and dysphagia.

### Diagnosis and Treatment

No specific tests are available to detect Alexander disease. The syndrome occurs in a sporadic fashion and familial cases are noted rarely. Therefore, the family history is not helpful.

Neuroimaging with computed tomography (CT) may be useful. Findings noted include low attenuation of the deep cerebral white matter, particularly in the frontal lobes. Similar areas of low attenuation have been noted in the subependymal regions of the ventricles. Early in the course of the disease, areas of increased density may be noted in some of the subependymal regions and in the basal ganglia, and these may show contrast enhancement. As the disease progresses, these features are lost. Serial cranial ultrasound studies have demonstrated enlarging subependymal cysts with evolving periventricular hyperechogenicity. Magnetic resonance imaging reveals an increased T2 signal in the cerebral white matter.

Thus, the diagnosis is based primarily on the clinical course of the disease after the exclusion of other degenerative diseases that have their onset in infancy, including other types of leukodystrophy and disorders associated with macrocephaly.

Supportive therapy is helpful in patients with Alexander disease. Antiepileptic drugs are used to treat the associated seizures. Attention to nutrition and control of infections with antibiotics is indicated. Psychosocial support of the family should be undertaken.

## CANAVAN DISEASE

Canavan disease is a spongy degeneration of the central nervous system that has several clinical variants. These are considered as one disorder only because similar pathologic changes in the brain have been noted. The clinical variants, which are categorized by age of onset into neonatal, infantile, and juvenile forms, may not represent a single entity, however, because they appear to have different inheritance patterns.

## Pathogenesis

The pathogenesis of Canavan disease is unknown, but may represent a metabolic disturbance of astrocytes. Astrocytes in affected individuals have been noted to have abnormal mitochondria and reduced levels of adenosine triphosphatase. The possible metabolic disturbance has been thought to result in excessive fluid accumulation, which produces vacuoles and gives the brain the spongy appearance that is the pathologic hallmark of the disease. The excessive fluid appears to occur within the cytoplasm of the astrocytes and also within myelin lamellae. It is unclear whether the changes noted in the mitochondria are primary or represent secondary effects of the disease. Recently, increased amounts of N-acetylaspartic acid have been noted in the urine and plasma of patients with Canavan disease. A corresponding deficiency of aspartoacylase was found in their cultured skin fibroblasts. In vivo nuclear magnetic resonance spectroscopy demonstrates an increased N-acetylaspartate signal and decreased signals from choline-containing compounds.

## Symptoms and Signs

The neonatal form of Canavan disease is seen extremely rarely. It is characterized by lethargy, crying, decreased spontaneous movement, and difficulty swallowing and sucking. Affected neonates are hypotonic and remain so. They have Cheyne-Stokes respiration and often die within a few weeks. The disease appears to occur in sporadic fashion; it is not clearly autosomal recessive or dominant, and no familial inheritance pattern has been reported.

The infantile form is the most common type of Canavan disease and occurs predominantly in Jews of northeastern European heritage, although patients with a variety of ethnic backgrounds have been described. The onset occurs within the first 6 months of life and the course usually is 3 to 4 years. At the onset, the infant appears sluggish and hypotonic, and has poor head control. Macrocephaly is present in the majority of infants. Development ceases and, in the second 6 months of life, the hypotonia changes to spasticity. When this occurs, auditory, visual, or tactile stimuli may precipitate decorticate or decerebrate posturing. Vision deteriorates with the development of optic atrophy and nystagmus. Occasionally, increased intracranial pressure has been noted, and this has not been caused by hydrocephalus. Focal and myoclonic seizures may develop, as well as other types of seizure activity. Occasionally, choreoathetosis may be present. In the end stages of the disease, paroxysmal episodes of sweating, hyperthermia, vomiting, and hypotension may occur.

The juvenile form of Canavan disease may have a long course, with onset occurring after 5 years of age and extending into adolescence. It is characterized by a progressive cerebellar syndrome in addition to dysarthria, dementia, and spasticity. Ataxia and tremor may be noted early in the course of the disease. Eventually, visual disturbances occur, which are characterized by loss of vision, optic atrophy, and abnormal retinal pigmentation. In contrast to the infantile form of the disease, the child's head size is not increased. Other features noted rarely have included partial deafness, hyporeflexia, and muscle wasting. Possible involvement of other organ systems has been suggested because of the presence of diabetes mellitus, probable hyperaldosteronism, and heart block.

## Pathology

In the infantile form of Canavan disease, the weight of the brain is increased. If the child survives more than 2 years, however, the brain weight tends to decline and return to the normal range. This often is accompanied by enlargement of the ventricular system secondary to the loss of brain substance rather than to the obstruction of cerebrospinal fluid flow. Vacuoles appear in the deep cortical layers and in the subcortical white matter. With long-standing disease, myelin, axons, and neurons are lost. Changes in the cerebellum are characterized by decreased numbers of Purkinje's cells and granular cells. Vacuoles also have been noted in the spinal cord.

Electron microscopy shows that the vacuoles are related to astrocytes swollen with watery cytoplasm and to split myelin lamellae at the intraperiod line. The mitochondria of the astrocytes are abnormal in appearance and elongated. The matrix and cristae are distended and distorted.

## Diagnosis and Treatment

There is a deficiency of aspartoacylase in the fibroblasts of patients with Canavan disease, and this is accompanied by an increased concentration of N-acetylaspartic acid in the urine. CT imaging of the brain has demonstrated diffuse attenuation of the white matter. The diagnosis usually is based on clinical criteria and on the exclusion of other degenerative and neurologic disorders that are associated with macrocephaly in infancy (eg, Alexander disease). A positive family history of a previous sibling with the infantile form of the disease obviously allows a premorbid diagnosis to be made.

No specific therapy is available for patients with Canavan disease. Symptomatic support includes nutritional therapy, antiepileptic drugs, and antibiotics as indicated. Psychosocial support for the family is important.

## Selected Readings

Adachi M, Schneck L, Cara J, et al. Spongy degeneration of the central nervous system (Van Bogaert and Bertrand type; Canavan's disease). Hum Pathol 1973;4: 331.

Austin SJ, Connelly A, Gadian DG, et al. Localized 1H NMR spectroscopy in Canavan's disease: A report of two cases. Magn Reson Med 1991;19:439.

Becker LE, Armstrong JB, Meloff KL. A large head in a 2-year-old boy. J Pediatr 1977;91:499.

Goebel HH, Bode G, Caesar R, et al. Bulbar palsy with Rosenthal fiber formation in the medulla of a 15-year-old girl. Localized form of Alexander's disease? Neuropediatrics 1981;12:382.

Goodhue WW Jr, Couch RD, Namiki H. Spongy degeneration of the CNS. Arch Neurol 1979;36:481.

Hess DC, Fischer AQ, Yaghmai F, et al. Comparative neuro-imaging with pathologic correlates in Alexander's disease. J Child Neurol 1990;5:248.

Hogan GR, Richardson EP Jr. Spongy degeneration of the nervous system (Canavan's disease). Report of a case in an Irish-American family. Pediatrics 1965;35:284.

Iwaki A, Iwaki T, Goldman JE, et al. Accumulation of alpha B-crystallin in brains of patients with Alexander disease is not due to an abnormality of the 5' flanking and coding sequence of genomic DNA. Neuroscience Letters 1992;140:89.

Jellinger K, Seitelberger F. Juvenile form of spongy degeneration of the CNS. Acta Neuropathol (Berl) 1969;13:276.

Matalon R, Kaul R, Casanova J, et al. Aspartoacylase deficiency: The enzyme defect in Canavan disease. J Inherited Metab Dis 1989;12:329.

Rushton AR, Shaywitz BA, Duncan CC, et al. Computed tomography in the diagnosis of Canavan's disease. Ann Neurol 1981;10:57.

Russo LS Jr, Aron A, Anderson PJ. Alexander's disease: A report and reappraisal. Neurology 1976;26:607.

Seil FJ, Schochet SS Jr, Earle KM. Alexander's disease in an adult. Arch Neurol 1968;19:494.

Sherwin RM, Berthrong M. Alexander's disease with sudanophilic leukodystrophy. Arch Pathol 1970;89:321.

Trommer BL, Naidich TP, Dal Canto MC, et al. Noninvasive CT diagnosis of infantile Alexander disease: Pathologic correlation. J Comput Assist Tomogr 1983;7:509.

*Principles and Practice of Pediatrics, Second Edition.*
edited by Frank A. Oski et al. J. B. Lippincott Company, Philadelphia © 1994.

# 161.6 *The Phakomatoses and Other Neurocutaneous Syndromes*

## Vincent M. Riccardi

## NEUROFIBROMATOSIS

Neurofibromatosis (NF) is more than one disorder. There are at least two specific types of NF, and perhaps as many as eight different forms of this disease. The most common type is von Recklinghausen's NF, or NF-1, which accounts for at least 85% of all patients with NF.

### NF-1: von Recklinghausen's Neurofibromatosis

NF-1 occurs with a frequency of about 1 in 4000 persons. It is an autosomal dominant trait, with about one half of the index cases representing new mutations, which means that a negative family history is common in the pediatric setting. The disorder is essentially the same whether it is inherited or results from a new mutation. NF-1 is highly variable in its expression, however, from one family to another, from one person to another within a family, and from one body part to another within a given person. On the other hand, its penetrance (ie, the likelihood that the mutant gene will express itself at all if it is present) is virtually 100%.

The gene for NF-1 resides on the proximal long arm of chromosome 17, specifically in band 17q11.2.

### Features

A checklist of the features that are characteristic of all types of NF, with an emphasis on NF-1, is provided in Table 161-15.

Café au lait spots (CLSs) are the hallmark of NF-1 and NF-6. They almost always are present in patients with NF-5, though in a segmental distribution, without crossing the body's midline. They are seen variably in patients with NF-2, NF-3, NF-4, and NF-NOS, but generally are absent in those with NF-7. In patients with NF-1, the hyperpigmented macules usually are larger than 15 mm in diameter and have sharply defined edges and a uniform intensity of coloration (Fig 161-10). CLSs are different from freckling, which is most likely to occur in regions of skin apposition; other than axillary freckling, the onset of freckling is later in childhood or adulthood.

Neurofibromas are of four types: cutaneous, subcutaneous, nodular plexiform, and diffuse plexiform. Cutaneous neurofibromas are the most common variety, eventually occurring in virtually all patients with NF-1. Often, they do not appear until just before or coincident with puberty. They are present in highest density over the trunk (Fig 161-11). Subcutaneous neurofibromas usually become apparent toward the end of the first decade of life or in early adulthood, and may be painful or tender. Nodular plexiform neurofibromas are complex clusters of subcutaneous-like neurofibromas along proximal nerve roots and major nerves. With continued growth along the spinal column, they often lead to spinal erosion and, eventually, spinal cord compression. Diffuse plexiform neurofibromas, with or without overlying hyperpigmentation, are congenital lesions that tend to enlarge steadily with age, at times perniciously (Fig 161-12).

---

**TABLE 161-15. A Checklist of Anatomic-Structural and Functional Features of Neurofibromatosis Type 1**

**Anatomic-Structural Features**

*Skin Pigmentation*
Café-au-lait spots; freckling: axillary, elsewhere; hyperpigmentation over a plexiform neurofibroma; other hyperpigmentation; hypopigmentation

*Discrete Neurofibromas*
Cutaneous: general, areola, nipple; subcutaneous; oral-pharynx-larynx; deep

*Plexiform Neurofibromas*
Craniofacial: orbital, other; chest wall; paraspinal: cervical, thoracic, lumbosacral; abdominal, retroperitoneal; limb; visceral

*Central Nervous System (CNS)*
Orbit: glioma, other; intracranial: chiasm, other; astrocytoma, schwannoma, meningioma, other; spinal

*Other Tumors*
Schwannoma (non-CNS); pheochromocytoma; carcinoid; other benign; malignancy

*Ocular*
Lisch nodules; hypertrophied corneal nerves; choroidal hamartomas; congenital glaucoma; eyelid ptosis; cataracts

*Skeletal*
Short stature; macrocephaly; craniofacial dysplasia; vertebral dysplasia; kyphoscoliosis/scoliosis; lumbar scalloping; pseudarthrosis: tibial, other; genu valgum/varum; pectus excavatum; other skeletal

*Miscellaneous*
Colon ganglioneuromatosis; xanthogranulomas (skin); vascular: angiomas, renal, cerebral, other; pulmonary fibrosis; cerebrospinal fluid: ventricle dilation, hydrocephalus, other abnormality; excess dental caries; electroencephalographic abnormality; other anatomic features

**Functional Features**

Cosmetic disfigurement; hypertrophic impairment; weakness/paralysis; incoordination; pain; seizures; other neurologic features; strabismus; visual impairment; hearing impairment; speech impediment; developmental delay; learning disability; school performance problems; mental retardation; psychosocial burden; psychiatric; headache; puberty disturbance; pruritus; constipation; gastrointestinal bleeding; hypertension; surgery; other functional features

---

Lisch nodules are relatively specific for NF-1. These lesions of the iris are found in less than 10% of patients with NF-1 who are younger than 6 years of age, but various investigators report their frequency to range from 90% to 100% in patients who are older than 10 years. If the nodules are large or are present in great number, they may be easy to see with an ordinary ophthalmoscope, but ruling out their presence requires careful examination with a slit lamp by an ophthalmologist who is familiar with these lesions.

Optic pathway gliomas are characteristic of NF-1, occurring in 15% of patients with this disorder. Ordinarily, an optic pathway glioma in the presence of CLSs will establish the diagnosis of NF-1. In addition, these lesions are an important cause of potentially preventable morbidity, including blindness. Therefore, in addition to having diagnostic utility, the detection of a presymptomatic optic pathway glioma also may help to decrease the likelihood of visual handicap or other complications among young patients with NF-1.

Pseudarthrosis, or bowing of the tibia, may occur as an independent lesion, but it often is one of the characteristic congenital lesions of NF-1. The congenital nature of the pseudarthrosis may be masked by a delay in diagnosis until weight bearing or walking

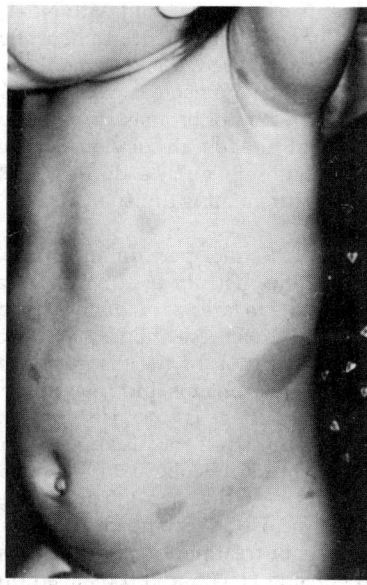

**Figure 161-10.** In patients with neurofibromatosis type 1, café au lait spots are usually larger than 15 mm in diameter, the edges are usually sharply defined, and the intensity of the coloration is uniform.

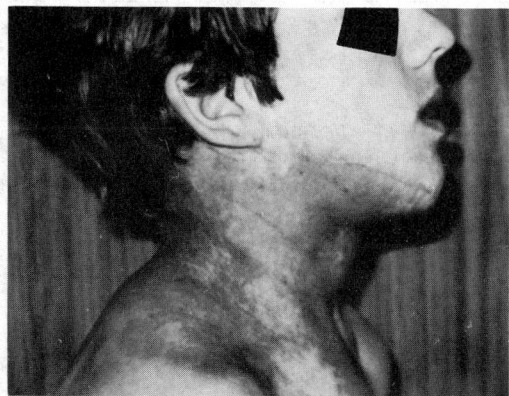

**Figure 161-12.** Plexiform neurofibromas, with or without overlying hyperpigmentation, are congenital lesions that tend to enlarge steadily with age.

is attempted. Any child with tibial pseudarthrosis should be presumed to have NF-1 until proven otherwise.

Sphenoid wing dysplasia is another congenital skeletal feature of NF-1. Similar to pseudarthrosis, it is a congenital primary bony dysplasia, although there sometimes may be an associated orbital/periorbital diffuse plexiform neurofibroma. Sphenoid wing dysplasia is a progressive lesion that occasionally leads to a pulsating enophthalmos, requiring surgical reconstruction of the posterior orbital wall.

The scoliosis that is typical of NF-1 usually involves the cervical and upper thoracic spine, and has an anterior angulation (kyphosis). It frequently becomes apparent between 6 and 10 years of age, although the presence of a hair whorl overlying an area

of vertebral dysplasia (Riccardi sign) at an earlier age may presage future problems.

Renovascular hypertension is one of the clinical problems of NF-1 that can be anticipated and treated effectively. All individuals who have NF-1 or are at risk for the disorder must receive regular blood pressure monitoring, regardless of their age, although adolescents and pregnant women are most likely to be affected.

Pheochromocytoma is another source of systemic hypertension, both intermittent and sustained, that is important because it is one of the preventable causes of untimely death among patients with NF-1.

Puberty disturbance probably is an overstated cause of morbidity among patients with NF-1. Premature or delayed puberty may indicate the presence of a chiasmal or hypothalamic glioma, however, which may be amenable to treatment (ie, with x-irradiation).

Short stature is seen in at least 16% of patients with NF-1, although no cogent pathophysiologic explanation has been forthcoming.

Macrocephaly also is present in 16% or more of affected patients. This finding is not always apparent in infancy, and is not correlated with any known functional compromise.

Although it occurs in only about 10% of patients with NF-1, pruritus that is associated with an actively growing neurofibroma may indicate that the lesion warrants close observation. Treatment approaches should respect the importance of mast cells as a primary component of neurofibromas.

Neurofibrosarcoma probably has an overall frequency of about 6% among patients with NF-1. Although the magnitude of this risk may be small, the relative risk is at least two orders of magnitude above that of the general population. Thus, the burden of proof in ruling out a neurofibrosarcoma rests with the clinician who elicits a history suggestive of such a lesion (ie, pain, a rapidly enlarging tumor, or an otherwise unexplained neurologic deficit).

**Natural History**

Although some investigators and clinicians continue to claim that NF-1 is a generally benign disorder, NF of any type (except, perhaps, NF-6) always is a progressive disorder, with a significant likelihood of serious morbidity and premature death.

At least for NF-1, the timing of onset of certain features is relatively well known (Table 161-16).

*Congenital Features.* Congenital glaucoma may occur in as many as 1% of infants with NF-1. Although buphthalmos may signal the presence of this potentially serious problem, its absence

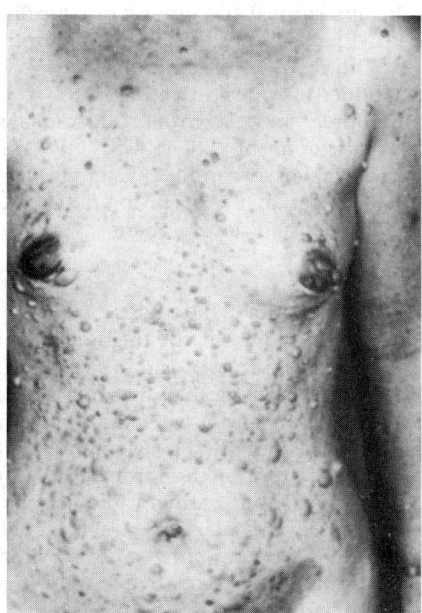

**Figure 161-11.** Cutaneous neurofibromas often are not apparent until puberty, and are present in highest density over the trunk.

**TABLE 161-16. Features of Neurofibromatosis Type 1 as a Function of Age**

**Congenital**

Glaucoma; plexiform neurofibromas; pseudoarthrosis; sphenoid wing dysplasia; vertebral dysplasia

**Infancy to Age 6 y**

Optic pathway glioma; learning disability; mental retardation; speech impediment; seizures

**Ages 6 Through 10 y**

School performance problems (including learning disability); scholiosis, with or without kyphosis; iris Lisch nodules

**Preadolescence and adolescence**

Cutaneous and subcutaneous neurofibromas; accelerated growth of plexiform neurofibromas; psychosocial burden; hypertention resulting from renovascular involvement; neurofibrosarcoma

**Adulthood**

Variable increase in the number and size of cutaneous and subcutaneous neurofibromas; hypertension resulting from renovascular involvement; neurofibrosarcoma; pheochromocytoma

does not eliminate the need for all infants with NF-1 to be observed closely for glaucoma. Tibial pseudarthrosis may be obvious by congenital bowing of the distal leg, or it may not become apparent until weight bearing or ambulation is attempted. Diffuse plexiform neurofibromas almost always are present at birth, but they may be subtle (ie, apparent only from associated overlying hyperpigmentation) or internal (ie, apparent only on radiographic studies). In view of the fact that diffuse plexiform neurofibromas of the superior mediastinum are a major cause of morbidity and even death in early childhood, it is reasonable to screen all newborns who have or are at risk for NF-1 with frontal and lateral chest radiographs. Sphenoid wing dysplasia sometimes is associated with an orbital/periorbital diffuse plexiform neurofibroma, but when it is not, the condition is unlikely to become symptomatic (ie, as a pulsating enophthalmos) until later in childhood. Similarly, vertebral dysplasia occasionally is associated with a diffuse plexiform neurofibroma, but is unlikely to be a source of concern until later in childhood.

*Infantile Features.* Optic pathway gliomas probably are congenital in origin, but in the absence of an orbital mass sufficient to cause proptosis, they usually are not apparent clinically until visual compromise can be appreciated by a parent or clinician. Some investigators have suggested screening all infants and young children who have NF-1 with cranial/orbital computed tomography (CT) scans or magnetic resonance imaging (MRI) scans in an attempt to detect optic pathway gliomas before the onset of visual loss.

Learning disabilities, distinct from mental retardation, are present in 40% to 60% of children with NF-1; these disabilities may be foreshadowed by infantile muscular hypotonia or a delay in attaining developmental milestones, but in any event usually are apparent by the time the child begins the first grade of school. Mental retardation occurs in about 8% of patients with NF-1, but its presence should not be presumed to be the result of NF-1 until an investigation for other causes has been completed and found to be negative or unrevealing. Speech impediments may involve articulation or language elements and usually are obvious by 3 years of age. Seizures of all types may occur at any time during childhood, although, as might be expected, those associated with hypsarrhythmia are seen early in infancy.

Often, the parents of a young child with NF-1 are concerned that he or she will have diffuse plexiform neurofibromas and, as a result, be seriously disfigured. It is reasonable to comfort these parents (and perhaps the youngster as well) with the information that diffuse plexiform neurofibromas do not have their onset during childhood, but already are obvious by early childhood. Moreover, even for children with a diffuse plexiform neurofibroma, extreme disfigurement is unusual.

*Later Childhood.* School performance problems resulting from learning disabilities usually become important in patients with NF-1 in the middle to later years of childhood (8 to 14 years of age). More than 50% of these children and their families are affected by this complication of the disorder. Lisch nodules in the iris cause no clinical problems, but their presence in patients with NF-1 after 6 years of age is so consistent that their absence after that age is a useful basis for discounting the diagnosis in individuals who are at risk. Scoliosis or kyphoscoliosis usually becomes apparent between the ages of 5 and 10 years, a fact that supports particularly close follow-up during this period. Early recognition and prompt treatment, almost always involving internal fixation (eg, using Harrington rods), can prevent or minimize serious deformities.

*Adolescence.* Cutaneous neurofibromas, subcutaneous neurofibromas, or both develop most often during adolescence, and their initial appearance tends to herald the onset of puberty rather than to follow it. Nodular plexiform neurofibromas may become apparent at this time. Previously appreciated diffuse plexiform neurofibromas irregularly undergo accelerated growth earlier in childhood, but are virtually certain to be aggravated during adolescence. In view of the increased activity of neurofibromas and the associated social stigmatization and personal emotional turmoil, it is not surprising that children with NF-1 may experience significant psychosocial difficulties during this stage of life. Renovascular hypertension and neurofibrosarcomas frequently become apparent in this age group.

*Adulthood.* Cutaneous or subcutaneous neurofibromas almost always increase significantly in number and size during all phases of adulthood, although there may be relative quiescence during the seventh and eighth decades. Pregnancy may initiate or aggravate the appearance and growth of neurofibromas. Pruritus associated with accelerated growth of neurofibromas may be a prominent and distressing symptom. Renovascular hypertension also continues to appear in young adulthood, particularly in women during pregnancy. Neurofibrosarcomas may develop in adult life and may occur in patients with NF-1 whose disease otherwise has been relatively mild. Pheochromocytomas associated with NF-1 almost always occur in adults, and pregnancy also may contribute to their development.

**Diagnosis**

According to a 1987 National Institutes of Health Consensus Development Conference on NF, the diagnostic criteria for NF-1 are met in an individual if two or more of the following are found: six or more CLSs greater than 5 mm in greatest diameter in prepubertal individuals and greater than 15 mm in greatest diameter in postpubertal individuals; two or more neurofibromas of any type, or one plexiform neurofibroma; freckling in the axillary or inguinal regions; optic pathway glioma; two or more iris Lisch nodules; a distinctive osseous lesion, such as sphenoid wing dysplasia or thinning of long-bone cortex, with or without pseudarthrosis; or a first-degree relative (parent, sibling, or offspring) with NF-1 diagnosed by the above criteria.

Establishing the diagnosis of NF-1 rarely is a problem in a child who is 1 year of age or older, because the requisite number of CLSs usually are obvious by that age, one or more additional features are likely to be present, and alternative diagnoses or either rare or otherwise apparent by virtue of their own unique features. At any age, given the presence of six or more CLSs that are 15 mm or greater in diameter, the likelihood of NF-1 is at or near 99%. Excluding the diagnosis of NF-1 in a child who is less than 1 year of age, however, may be difficult. Additional data to establish the diagnosis may be garnered using the evaluation protocol described later in this chapter, although the absence of other findings does not help to exclude the diagnosis of NF-1.

No laboratory tests are routinely available with which to confirm or exclude the diagnosis of NF-1. Although DNA-based genetic linkage data may be useful, clinical criteria usually suffice in patients older than 1 year of age. For cases of sporadic mutation, only 5% or so of the mutations are identifiable at the molecular level, making this test not feasible on a routine basis. Biopsies of CLSs and neurofibromas (or other tumors) cannot establish the diagnosis of NF-1; they can only confirm the type of lesion.

Ordinarily, by 1 year of age, the diagnosis of NF-1 can be established using the criteria noted. If the diagnosis is suspected but cannot be established after that age, an alternative form of NF should not be discounted categorically. The assistance of an established NF referral center should be sought. Once the diagnosis of NF-1 is made, the presence of any of its features that are likely to cause serious problems should be noted, even if they currently are asymptomatic (eg, optic pathway glioma, sphenoid wing dysplasia, vertebral dysplasia, diffuse plexiform neurofibroma), and should serve as a basis for close follow-up.

### Screening Evaluation

*Purpose.* The purpose of a screening evaluation is, first, to confirm the diagnosis of NF-1 by identifying features of the disease that are not apparent from the history and general physical examination. The second goal is to detect potentially compromising lesions before they become symptomatic, thereby minimizing the ultimate severity of the symptoms (ie, identifying an optic pathway glioma before it causes irreversible blindness).

*Elements.* Slit lamp ocular examination should be used to identify Lisch nodules, choroidal hamartomas, hypertrophied corneal nerves, and, perhaps, signs of an optic pathway glioma.

Cranial/orbital MRI scanning should be undertaken to detect presymptomatic optic pathway gliomas, cerebral gliomas, or posterior fossa gliomas.

Chest radiographs (frontal and lateral) are necessary to identify mediastinal neurofibromas and other tumors.

Spine radiographs (frontal and lateral) are required to locate vertebral dysplasia and larger paraspinal neurofibromas, and to serve as a baseline for potential subsequent screening for scoliosis.

Skull radiographs (frontal and lateral) are useful in screening for early sphenoid wing dysplasia and other craniofacial dysplasias.

An electroencephalogram (EEG) should be obtained to detect presymptomatic epileptogenic foci and to serve as a baseline for follow-up, recognizing the fact that about one of every eight patients with NF-1 has abnormal EEG findings in the absence of seizures.

Intelligence quotient determination and psychologic evaluation are useful to identify learning disabilities and facilitate special efforts on behalf of the youngster in school.

Audiogram/brain stem auditory evoked response testing is performed for two reasons: (1) to document normal hearing in the context of the high frequency of learning disabilities and speech impediments in these children; and (2) to detect acoustic neuromas, which, although they are rare, have been reported occasionally in patients with this disorder.

### Follow-up

If the results of a detailed history and physical examination and presymptomatic screening fail to reveal any potentially serious problems, routine follow-up visits are recommended at 6- to 18-month intervals. In the absence of new problems, follow-up efforts can be restricted to history-taking and physical examination; repeated routine screening is unnecessary. If there are new, evolving, or established clinical problems, appropriate follow-up intervals and the extent of evaluation are determined by the nature and severity of the clinical concerns. Relatively frequent consultation with various medical and surgical specialists, as well as with social workers and other health care specialists, often is necessary. Referral of the patient or family to a local chapter of Neurofibromatosis, Inc., the Texas NF Foundation, or the National NF Foundation for further information about the disorder and general support usually is helpful.

### Treatment

Medical therapy for NF-1 is similar to that used for the specific conditions seen in the absence of NF-1. Problems associated with NF-1 that are most likely to require medical treatment include constipation (ie, from colonic ganglioneuromatosis), seizures, headaches, hyperactivity and learning disabilities, anxiety, and renovascular hypertension. Pruritus in patients with NF is not treated effectively with histamine₁-blocking antihistamines, although some success has been obtained using the mast cell blocker, ketotifen. Mast cell blockers also may play a role in decreasing the rate of neurofibroma development. There is no absolute contraindication to the use of oral contraceptives in patients with NF-1, although evaluation on an individual basis obviously is appropriate. Antineoplastic chemotherapy has no role in the treatment of neurofibromas. Its role in the treatment of optic pathway gliomas still is investigational, and its utility in the treatment of neurofibrosarcomas is problematic. Radiotherapy for neurofibromas has no proven effect. It appears to be useful in the treatment of at least some optic pathway gliomas, although this is controversial.

Surgery is the mainstay of therapy for patients with NF-1, particularly for removing or debulking tumors (eg, neurofibromas, neurofibrosarcomas, pheochromocytomas), for treating skeletal dysplasia (eg, tibial pseudarthrosis, sphenoid wing dysplasia), for correcting scoliosis or kyphoscoliosis, and for treating at least some individuals with renovascular or other types of vascular compromise. In general, the surgical removal of neurofibromas is associated with suboptimal results; the tumors tend to recur and the possibility of a consequent neuropathy is significant. Surgical removal of a neurofibroma should be undertaken only if a specific major goal can be established beforehand.

Because 50% of the index cases of NF-1 represent new mutations, it is not surprising that the family history often fails to reveal another affected family member, especially if the index case (proband) is a child. For each offspring of a patient with NF-1, however, the recurrence risk is 50%. The severity of NF-1 in the offspring is unrelated to the severity of the disorder in the affected parent. Prenatal diagnosis is available relatively routinely for families with at least two or more affected or at-risk members. Prenatal diagnosis is not yet available for a patient with a new mutation who has not borne at least one offspring. Rapid progress is being made, however, and in each instance, consultation with a geneticist or NF specialist is warranted.

### Molecular Biology

DNA genetic linkage analysis of large numbers of families with NF-1, plus molecular analysis of the breakpoints in two patients with concordance of NF-1 and chromosome translocations involving chromosome band 17q11.2, have served as the basis for the rapid identification and cloning of the NF-1 gene. The NF-1 gene product, neurofibromin, is expressed in virtually all tissues studied, from both normal individuals and those with NF-1. It also is expressed in NF-1 neurofibromas, although its expression is lost in neurofibrosarcomas. Thus, it is unclear how the mutation actually leads to the NF lesions. On the other hand, neurofibromin is known to have an influence on guanosine nucleotide metabolism and *ras* oncoprotein function.

The enzyme cleaving a phosphate group from guanosine triphosphate (GTP) is guanosine triphosphatase (GTPase); the reaction product is guanosine diphosphate (GDP). GTPase activating protein (GAP) enhances the conversion of GTP to GDP. Neurofibromin functions, in part, as a GAP. Moreover, the gene product of the *ras* oncogene is in its active state only when it is coupled with GTP. Thus, enhanced conversion of GTP to GDP diminishes the ability of the *ras* oncoprotein to stimulate cell proliferation. This implies, in turn, that loss of GAP activities in mutant neurofibromin at key times in a cell's life may lead to abnormal growth promotion. It should be emphasized, however, that there is no way to show how an altered GAP-related function of neurofibromin accounts for the specific lesions of NF-1. Specifically, the discreteness of the lesions and their different times of appearance in the life of an affected patient are not accounted for.

It is of some interest that attempts to show loss of heterozygosity for the NF-1 gene in neurofibromas have met uniformly with failure; that is, it does not appear to occur. Although such loss may occur in neurofibrosarcomas, the data are conflicting. Neurofibrosarcomas, however, consistently do lose heterozygosity for the p53 gene on the short arm of chromosome 17, usually associated with a mutation on the remaining allele. This phenomenon is shared with numerous other malignancies, and is not unique to neurofibrosarcomas.

One other point of fascination exists about the NF-1 gene: rather uniquely, it contains three other genes sequestered on the antisense strand of its DNA nucleotide sequence. These genes include two forms of the ecotropic viral insertion site gene (EVI-1, EVI-2) and the gene for oligodendrocyte myelin glycoprotein. What the functions of these sequestered genes are, either under normal circumstances or as part of NF-1, is unclear.

Mutations in the mouse gene that is comparable (paralogous) to NF-1 have been constructed, and studies are under way to use them to gain insight into the function of the normal and mutant genes at this locus.

## NF-2: Bilateral Acoustic Neurofibromatosis

NF-2 is distinct from NF-1 both clinically and in terms of the gene locus. The NF-2 gene resides on the middle long arm of chromosome 22, specifically in the 22q11.2 band.

The definitive feature of NF-2 is the presence of bilateral acoustic neuromas, which actually are vestibular schwannomas. Intracranial and spinal cord meningiomas also occur frequently, as do spinal cord astrocytomas. Optic pathway gliomas do not occur in patients with this disorder. Paraspinal schwannomas and neurofibromas are common at all levels, but particularly in the cervical and lumbar regions. Cutaneous and subcutaneous neurofibromas generally are few in number and are present only infrequently. Plexiform neurofibromas of any type are rare. Cutaneous schwannomas are relatively common, even in early childhood; they may have the same coloration as the skin or be slightly hyperpigmented with or without associated hypertrichosis. Their size ranges from 3 to 8 mm. CLSs are few in number and relatively pale in color, and they tend to be somewhat less clearly demarcated and larger in size than those that are typical of NF-1. Although several patients with NF-2 have been reported with iris Lisch nodules, they are distinctly rare. On the other hand, posterior subcapsular cataracts are present consistently, even at a young age. Retinal hamartomas are another feature of NF-2. Both the cataracts and the retinal hamartomas may be particularly useful features for pursuing the diagnosis of NF-2 in a child. Other characteristics of patients with NF-1, such as skeletal and vascular dysplasias, short stature, macrocephaly, and learning disabilities, are not seen in patients with NF-2. Compared to NF-1, a larger proportion of index cases appear to represent new mutations. NF-2 is an autosomal dominant disorder, with a 50% risk for each offspring of an affected patient to bear the mutant gene and ultimately manifest the disorder. Recently, it has been suggested that there may be at least three forms of NF-2, each with a different level of overall severity.

### Diagnosis

In contrast to NF-1, the diagnosis of NF-2 may be difficult to establish in children, although the recent discovery that cutaneous schwannomas, cataracts, and retinal hamartomas occur in this age group may change this perception somewhat. The inclusive diagnostic criteria for NF-2 include the following:

Bilateral eighth cranial nerve masses seen with neuroimaging studies (CT scan, preferably, MRI scan), *or*
A first-degree relative with NF-2 and *either*
  A unilateral eighth cranial nerve mass, *or*
  Two of the following:
    Neurofibroma
    Meningioma
    Spinal astrocytoma
    Schwannoma
    Posterior subcapsular cataracts.

Often, the condition is asymptomatic through the first 15 years of life, although the cutaneous schwannomas, cataracts, and retinal hamartomas may be detectable during this period. The most frequent symptoms include headaches, hearing loss, and tinnitus, which most often are unilateral in the earliest stages of the disease. Once symptoms appear, however, progression generally is constant and relatively gradual, although rapid deterioration occurs occasionally. The progression of symptoms results from the appearance and growth of the various central nervous system (CNS) tumors. Pregnancy or, in some cases, the use of oral contraceptives leads to the onset of symptoms from meningiomas, acoustic neuromas, or both. Recognition of the disorder usually results from the development of symptoms from a CNS tumor or the presence of an affected first-degree relative. Occasionally, the detection of a paraspinal neurofibroma or schwannoma may lead to the correct diagnosis.

### Treatment

Surgery for the removal or debulking of intracranial, spinal, or paraspinal tumors is the mainstay of therapy for patients with NF-2. The consequences of surgical removal of an acoustic neuroma include further hearing loss and ipsilateral facial nerve palsy, although efforts are being made to use operative strategies that preserve hearing and facial nerve function. In addition, stereotactic radiation has been used with arguable success. Brain stem implants to restore some degree of hearing have been helpful for some patients. Because some acoustic neuromas have few or minor associated symptoms, even when they are quite large, the size of the tumor alone should not be used to time surgery. Women with NF-2 should be advised that pregnancy almost certainly will make the condition worse. In contrast to patients with NF-1, oral contraceptive use generally is contraindicated in individuals with NF-2, because it may seriously aggravate the growth and symptoms of the intracranial tumors. Severe disorientation may occur when patients are diving or swimming underwater, and drowning may result. All individuals who have or are at risk for NF-2 should be advised of this risk, and should be cautioned never to swim alone.

Genetic counseling is available as for NF-1, with two important differences. First, excluding the diagnosis in individuals who are at risk for NF-2 is much more difficult, especially in younger patients. Second, prenatal diagnosis is not as readily available, although it may be possible in some large families in collaboration with an NF-2 research group. Referral of the patient and family to the Acoustic Neuroma Association, Neurofibromatosis, Inc., or the National NF Foundation often is helpful.

### Molecular Biology

Meningiomas long have been known to lose a chromosome 22 (monosomy 22). Based on that knowledge, loss of all or portions of chromosome 22 was sought in meningiomas, schwannomas, and neurofibromas from patients with NF-2. The consistent loss of a portion of the 22q11.2 band in these tumors suggested that this might be the locus of the NF-2 gene. At least one large family with NF-2 has been studied by DNA linkage analysis, confirming the assignment of the NF-2 locus to 22q11.2, and other informative families have provided similar data. Cloning of the NF-2 gene has recently been accomplished, and the gene product is designated "schwannomin" by several research groups.

Although details of the function of the NF-2 gene are unknown, it does appear to function as a tumor suppressor gene, comparable to the retinoblastoma and p53 genes. This ultimately may provide a basis for gene replacement therapy as one approach to treating the tumors that are part of this disorder. The molecular data provide a basis for prenatal diagnosis using a genetic linkage strategy, however, in those families that are sufficiently large to be informative. To date, though, no instance of NF-2 prenatal diagnosis has been reported.

## TUBEROUS SCLEROSIS

Tuberous sclerosis (TS) is characterized by depigmented lesions of the skin, tumors of the CNS, ocular hamartomas, and an autosomal dominant pattern of inheritance. It is the combination of developmental abnormalities of the skin, nervous system, and eyes that traditionally has led to this disorder being grouped, along with the neurofibromatoses and von Hippel-Lindau disease (VHLD), in the category known as the phakomatoses. For a comprehensive review, the reader is referred to the publication by Gomez.

### Natural History

TS is a progressive disorder; the initial problems become worse and new lesions or complications appear with increasing patient age. There is marked variation in expression of the mutant gene. For a patient in whom the gene is expressed mildly, the natural history will be different than for a patient in whom the gene is expressed severely. The majority of patients have serious, compromising problems throughout their lives, most commonly mental retardation and seizures. Relatively few data are available to clarify the way in which patients with other problems (eg, renal angiomyolipomas, pulmonary interstitial fibrosis) fare over a lifetime. One exception may be the cardiac rhabdomyomas; these congenital cardiac tumors tend to regress at least to some degree with age. In any event, once the diagnosis of TS is made, the patient must be observed closely and the appropriate clinical, laboratory, and radiologic techniques used to identify new lesions and monitor the progression of those already identified. The malignant degeneration of benign tumors (eg, astrocytomas, fibromas) is not a feature of TS.

In view of the recent recognition that pertussis immunization

rarely can lead to a severe neurologic syndrome, the use of vaccines with a pertussis component is contraindicated in patients with TS. The point is not that we know that pertussis vaccination actually aggravates TS, but that the vaccine is at least a confounding factor in understanding the contributing factors if the child's course deteriorates after the vaccine is administered.

### Diagnosis

When multiple features of TS are present, the diagnosis is relatively easy to make. When only one feature is present, the diagnosis is likely to be considered only tentatively, if not overlooked entirely. Establishing the diagnosis of TS depends on detecting the presence of two or more of the following features:

Skin: Hypopigmented macules, usually elliptic in shape (ash-leaf spots); fibroadenomas (adenoma sebaceum), typically involving the malar regions of the face; periungual fibromas; shagreen patches, seen most commonly over the lower trunk; and a distinctive brown patch on the forehead. The latter lesion is especially important, as it may be the first and most readily recognized feature of TS to be appreciated on physical examination of neonates and infants with the disorder.
Teeth: Characteristic pits of the enamel
Eye: Choroidal hamartomas; hypopigmented defects of the iris
CNS: Periventricular tubers; cerebral astrocytomas; sacrococcygeal chordomas; nonspecific EEG abnormalities, including hypsarrhythmia
Cardiovascular: Cardiac rhabdomyomas; aortic and major artery constrictions
Kidney: Renal angiomyolipomas
Lungs: Diffuse interstitial fibrosis.

Seizures of all types, but particularly myoclonic jerks associated with hypsarrhythmia, and mental retardation are the most common symptoms leading to the consideration of the diagnosis of TS. MRI scans of the brain in patients with TS are virtually diagnostic and must be used in all individuals who are suspected of having the disorder. Heart failure or a cardiac murmur may indicate the presence of a cardiac rhabdomyoma, and deficient circulation or decreased pulses may indicate the presence of arterial tree involvement. Renal failure or an abdominal mass may lead to the recognition of hamartomatous kidney involvement. Dyspnea may indicate the presence of pulmonary involvement, but this anatomic feature of TS often is found coincidentally.

TS is the result of an autosomal dominant mutant gene. Precisely because new mutations are relatively common, a previously negative family history does not exclude the diagnosis. Moreover, once the diagnosis of TS has been established in the proband, all first-degree relatives must be evaluated carefully for subtle signs of the disorder before a new mutation is presumed. Anyone who bears the mutant gene for TS carries a 50% risk that each of his or her offspring will have the disorder.

### Treatment

No medical treatment is available for TS per se. The medical treatment used for seizures and other complications (eg, heart failure, renal failure) is the same as if TS were not present, unless surgery on the primary lesions is indicated. For example, surgical removal of a cardiac rhabdomyoma may be warranted, and some clinicians encourage an aggressive surgical approach to the renal angiomyolipomas, at least in advanced cases.

Because of the high frequency of new mutations and the variable expression of the disorder, counseling regarding recurrence among the siblings of an apparently sporadic case is difficult and is handled best by a center that specializes in TS. For an affected patient, the recurrence risk among offspring is 50%. Reliable prenatal diagnosis that relies on DNA genetic linkage data is not yet available (see below). There is broad worldwide experience, however, in identifying several manifestations of TS in fetuses using high-resolution ultrasound techniques. Cervical cystic tumors, renal cystic abnormalities, and cardiac rhabdomyomas all have been used to identify TS prenatally. The manifestation of cardiac rhabdomyoma is particularly susceptible to this approach. Thus, it is reasonable to subject to prenatal diagnosis using ultrasound technology all pregnancies of a parent with TS.

## Molecular Biology

The molecular biology approach to TS has focused thus far on genetic linkage and the association of one neonatal case with an associated translocation involving chromosomes 11 and 22. At the least, the data indicate genetic heterogeneity, with probably two, and perhaps three or more, loci. Genetic linkage data have established one TS locus on chromosome 9, specifically in band 9q23. The data from all families studied by genetic linkage provide clear evidence for genetic heterogeneity. The patient with the 11;22 translocation led to consideration of an 11q23 locus for TS. Additional linkage data have been consistent with this gene locus assignment, but they have not proven it. Moreover, there is a third group of families with data that are inconsistent with either a 9q or an 11q locus assignment. In view of these data, DNA molecular techniques should not be used for prenatal diagnosis unless the studies for the particular family are uniquely and unequivocally informative for the 9q34 locus.

# VON HIPPEL-LINDAU DISEASE

VHLD traditionally is grouped with the neurofibromatoses and TS as a phakomatosis on the basis of direct involvement of the CNS, vascular abnormalities, diffuse cystic changes in multiple organs, and malignant tumors of the kidney. It, too, is an autosomal dominant heritable condition.

## Natural History

VHLD is progressive. Regardless of the mode of presentation, patients with VHLD must be observed closely for the progression of prior lesions and the development of new ones. In particular, renal cell carcinoma or pheochromocytoma may develop at any time, and both are potentially curable. These same tumors may be malignant. CNS hemangioblastomas also may cause serious problems.

## Diagnosis

The diagnostically distinctive feature of VHLD is the retinal vascular hamartoma. In its presence, other features of the disorder add credence to the diagnosis. In the absence of retinal vascular hamartomas, establishing the diagnosis requires detecting a combination of the other features, or one of the other features plus an affected first-degree relative.

Retinal vascular hamartomas may be associated with visual disturbances and glaucoma; often they can be appreciated by direct ophthalmoscopy. They usually, but not always, are unilateral. CNS vascular hamartomas similar to those seen in the eye are another key feature of the disorder. Characteristic tumors include renal cell carcinoma, pheochromocytoma, epididymal cystadenoma, and pancreatic cysts. Diffuse cystic lesions throughout the kidneys may accompany the renal cell carcinomas. Other tumors may include oat cell carcinoma of the lung and hepatocellular carcinoma. Each of these features may be seen independently of VHLD, and biopsies merely contribute to describing the lesion and not to establishing the diagnosis of VHLD.

## Treatment

Medical treatment of VHLD is the same as that generally recommended for pheochromocytomas, renal cell carcinomas, or other tumors. The treatment approach to the vascular hamartomas is complex and must be tailored to the individual lesions.

Surgical removal of renal cell carcinomas and pheochromocytomas is the preferred treatment. In contrast to TS, a surgically conservative approach to the renal cysts usually is advised. The use of laser technology to treat the ocular angiomatosis has some merit and should be considered as one therapeutic approach.

Recurrence risk considerations for VHLD are as described for TS. The prospect for prenatal diagnosis is present, based on the assignment of the VHLD locus to the proximal long arm of chromosome 3.

## Molecular Biology

The loss of heterozygosity of chromosome 3 short arm markers in renal cell carcinomas, both from patients with VHLD and from those with isolated tumors, points to a locus for VHLD on the short arm of chromosome 3. Genetic linkage data from multiple medical centers have corroborated this finding and have pointed to a 3p25-26 locus for the VHLD gene. For a family with sufficient numbers of affected and at-risk individuals, the use of genetic linkage data should afford reasonably reliable prenatal diagnosis.

# STURGE-WEBER DISEASE

Sturge-Weber disease (SWD) also is referred to as encephalofacial angiomatosis and traditionally is known as the "fourth phakomatosis." It differs from the neurofibromatoses, TS, and VHLD by virtue of the absence of three features, however: cutaneous pigmentation defects, a clear excess of tumors, and heritability. In addition, the relatively large number of variant or atypical cases makes accurate comparisons difficult.

## Features

In addition to a facial port-wine stain and intracranial angiomatosis, primary involvement of the anterior chamber of the eye, specifically the trabecular network, and Schlemm's canal may lead to glaucoma (in either eye) in as many as 30% of patients with SWD. Macrocephaly and cutaneous xanthogranulomas also may be seen. No one feature is associated uniformly with any other, and histopathologic features cannot establish a diagnosis beyond confirming the type of lesion.

## Natural History

The anatomic features of SWD may be associated with mental retardation, seizures, hemiparesis, and visual deficits, including homonymous hemianopsia. The disorder is progressive, with worsening associated with continued development of calcifications in the vascular defects.

## Diagnosis

The diagnosis of SWD depends on the presence of a port-wine stain (nevus flammeus) of the face, primarily in the first division of the trigeminal nerve; leptomeningeal angiomatosis (including angiomatous involvement of the choroid plexus or choroid of the eye); or both.

## Treatment

No medical treatment is available for SWD, and the role of surgical treatment has yet to be defined. The use of lasers to treat the facial and ocular angioma lesions has been at least partially successful.

There is no precedent for SWD being recognized as a genetic or heritable disorder. Recurrence among siblings to the proband is unlikely. Caution is advised against prematurely discounting recurrence among offspring, however; the lack of precedence may reflect merely the lack of procreation of prior patients with SWD.

## ALBRIGHT'S SYNDROME

Albright's syndrome (AS) also is known as the McCune-Albright syndrome or polyostotic fibrous dysplasia. The cardinal features of the disorder are fibrous dysplasia of one or more bones, precocious puberty, and CLSs. Although some features of AS overlap with those of one or more of the neurofibromatoses, this rarely presents a diagnostic dilemma. At least one patient has been described for whom the original correct diagnosis was AS, but whose symptoms eventually progressed to satisfy the National Institutes of Health diagnostic criteria for NF-1. This case notwithstanding, a heritable element for AS remains to be established (see below).

## Features

The fibrous dysplasia of AS may involve any bone, but the most frequent sites are the femur, tibia, pelvis, phalanges, ribs, and humerus. Radiographically, there is a combination of radiolucent and radiopaque elements, except at the base of the skull, where diffuse sclerosis usually is seen. Precocious puberty or sexual precocity as it relates to this disorder more accurately is termed *pseudo-precocious puberty*; that is, blood levels of sex steroids are elevated, but levels of gonadotrophic hormones are normal. Early spermatogenesis and fertility can accompany these endocrine changes. CLSs, when they are present, usually are fewer in number and larger in size than are those seen in patients with NF (particularly NF-1). Hyperthyroidism may be seen in 30% or so of patients with AS. Much less frequently, other features, including acromegaly and elevated levels of growth hormone in the blood, intramuscular myxomas, hyperplastic reticuloendothelial tissues, and lymphoid or myeloid metaplasia also have been reported.

## Natural History

Progressive worsening of the osseous lesions in patients with AS is common, though they rarely become quiescent. Fractures may result, as well as shortening and deformity of the involved bones. Malignant degeneration apparently does occur, but only in less than 1% of patients with AS. The sexual precocity usually develops in the last half of the first decade of life, although it has been noted as early as 3 months of age. As mentioned, fertility may be part of the sexual precocity, although pregnancies are unusual. Adult fertility apparently is not affected. Hyperthyroidism may occur at any time in childhood and beyond.

## Treatment

Treatment of the premature puberty is carried out best under the auspices of a specialized pediatric endocrinology center. Bone grafting and subsequent surgical procedures to correct deformities may be indicated, depending on the extent and complications of the lesions. Close observation of the fibrous dysplasia lesions for malignant degeneration is warranted.

There is no clear precedent for a heritable component to AS, so recurrence risks among siblings and offspring probably are similar to the occurrence risks for the general population.

## Molecular Biology

Although heritability has not been an element of AS, it has been reasoned that a mutation of the alpha subunit of the G protein (Gs alpha) might be present in tumors and perhaps other tissues from patients with the disorder. Indeed, such a mutation has been found, but only in portions of the studied tissues. This finding is important for two reasons. First, it documents somatic mutation as a mechanism to account for human disease. Thus, the disorder has a genetic basis, but not a germ-cell or heritable basis. Second, the role of the G protein in determining the nature and availability of a nucleoside phosphate moiety (cyclic adenosine monophosphate) is similar to one of the functions of neurofibromin, the NF-1 gene product. Surely, the overlap of clinical features and this overlap at the genetic and cellular levels is instructive regarding the pathogenesis of both disorders.

## Selected Readings

Gomez MR. Tuberous sclerosis, 2nd ed. New York: Raven Press, 1988.
Riccardi VM. Neurofibromatosis: Phenotype, natural history and pathogenesis, 2nd ed. Baltimore: Johns Hopkins University Press, 1992.

*Principles and Practice of Pediatrics, Second Edition.*
edited by Frank A. Oski et al. J. B. Lippincott Company, Philadelphia © 1994.

## CHAPTER 162
# *Headache*

Arthur L. Prensky

Chronic and recurrent headaches are one of the most common neurologic complaints of children. Bille found that 2.5% of schoolchildren suffered from frequent headaches at 7 years of age and that 15.7% had similar complaints at 15 years of age. Other surveys indicate an even higher prevalence; in several Scandinavian countries, as many as 7% of all schoolchildren between 7 and 8 years of age have more than one headache each month. Ten percent to 20% of the adolescent population suffers from chronic headache syndromes.

The brain itself is insensitive to pain. Pain-sensitive fibers, however, are found on the walls of large intracranial arteries and veins, the dural sinuses, the periosteum of bone, extracranial vessels, the muscle and skin of the scalp, the mucosal surfaces of the nasal sinuses, the teeth and gums, and the temporomandibular joint. Inflammation, stretching, torsion, or contraction of innervated structures can activate these fibers and produce pain. As is true elsewhere in the body, pain derived from structures in the head or neck can be projected to other areas. For example, irritation or stretching of the undersurface of the tentorium cerebelli can project to the occipital region, whereas the superior surface projects to the frontal area because it is innervated by fibers of the first division of the fifth cranial nerve. Inflammation of the ethmoid sinuses may project to the frontal or temporal regions, whereas inflammation of the sphenoid sinuses can project to the frontal, temporal, parietal, or vertex regions of the skull. When confronted with a child who has acute, chronic, or recurrent severe headaches, it is the responsibility of the physician to determine the source of the pain, its cause, and the appropriate treatment.

## CHRONIC HEADACHE

There are many reasons why children get chronic or frequent recurrent headaches. The most common cause of headaches that are severe enough for a child to be brought to a physician is migraine, which accounts for at least 50% of chronic or recurrent headache syndromes. A large proportion of the remaining children have been felt to have headaches that result from stress, anxiety, or tension with resulting muscle contraction. Unfortunately, recent studies suggest that many individuals with so-called tension headaches do not have excessive contraction of scalp muscles at the time they are in pain. Nor is it clear any longer that migraine is primarily a vascular process. Olesen and his colleagues have noted no correlation between the locus and severity of pain and regional cerebral blood flow in patients with common migraine, or between neurologic symptoms and the area of reduction of cerebral blood flow in patients with classic migraine. The genesis of migraine may lie within the central nervous system (CNS) and not the vessels supplying it. Because the long-accepted pathophysiology of both these disorders is being questioned, it is not surprising that migraine headaches are difficult to distinguish from tension headaches in many children.

## MIGRAINE

The ad hoc Committee on Classification of Headache in 1962 described migraine headaches as "recurrent attacks of headache widely varied in intensity, frequency and duration." They divided this disorder into classic migraine, in which the headache was sharply defined and associated with transient visual or other sensory or motor prodromes, and "common" migraine, in which the headaches did not have a striking prodrome and were less likely to be well localized or unilateral. The committee also included "cluster" headaches, that is, headaches that occur in groups, are unilateral, and usually are associated with ipsilateral autonomic changes such as profuse tearing or nasal discharge. Hemiplegic and hemisensory migraines are disorders in which the headache is accompanied by sensory or motor phenomena that persist during and after the headache. Common migraine is by far the most frequent form of migraine headache in children. About 1 of every 10 young children with migraine has the classic form. This number increases during adolescence, although a distinct aura does not have to be present with each headache. Cluster headaches do occur in children, but are extremely rare. Ophthalmoplegic migraine also is rare, but is predominantly a pediatric disease; it has been reported in infants less than 1 year of age.

In 1988, the Classification Committee of the International Society for Headache redefined migraine. The diagnosis of common migraine required at least five attacks of headache lasting more than 4 hours accompanied by nausea, vomiting, photophobia, or phonophobia and two of the following: unilateral location,

pulsating quality, intensity that inhibits daily activities, or aggravation by routine physical activity. This is not a definition that is well suited to the diagnosis of migraine in children.

The generally accepted criteria for the diagnosis of migraine in childhood is repeated episodes of headache accompanied by at least three of the following symptoms: recurrent abdominal pain (with or without headache) or nausea or vomiting; an aura, which usually is visual, but may be sensory, motor, or vertiginous; throbbing or pounding pain; pain that is restricted to one side of the head (although it may shift sides from one headache to the next); relief of pain by brief periods of sleep; and a family history of migraine in one or more immediate relatives. Most children who have migraine have nausea or some type of abdominal distress, are helped by sleep, and have a family history of migraine. Localized, throbbing pain, and an aura are seen more frequently during and after puberty.

Migraine headaches in children differ from those in adults in that about 60% of the affected patients are male (this drops to about 33% in the adult population); unilateral headaches are less common before puberty; and a visual aura is much less frequent. The incidence of epilepsy with migraine varies from 5.4% to 12.3% in various series, but is less than 3% in adults. Nausea and vomiting occur in about the same percentage of individuals in both groups, and about 70% of children and adults have a strong family history of migraine.

Childhood migraine is more likely to vary in frequency than in severity. Children who otherwise fit the criteria for the diagnosis of migraine may have 1 headache per month and then begin gradually or abruptly to have 3 to 5 headaches per week. If they are not treated, these headaches will last for a period of weeks or months and can interfere with school and other usual activities. Occasionally, these exacerbations can be related to changes in mood, particularly depression or stress. Much of the time, however, no predisposing factor can be found to explain the increased headache frequency.

### Diagnosis

Migraine is a clinical diagnosis that is made by obtaining the patient's history. The physical examination generally is normal. Laboratory studies are not needed for confirmation unless there are physical signs or a doubtful history. In many published series of children with migraine headache, electroencephalogram (EEG) tracings often are abnormal and as many as 10% may be paroxysmal. Unless the abnormality seen on the EEG is focal, however, the tracing does not have any prognostic significance. Focal tracings do suggest the increased possibility of a lesion in the CNS and make it necessary to perform a computed tomography (CT) or magnetic resonance imaging (MRI) scan to rule out a mass lesion or vascular disorder. Occasionally, certain aspects of the clinical history should alert the physician to study the child further. These include a strong family history of cerebrovascular disease early in life or of intracranial hemorrhage, headaches that localize persistently to one side of the cranium without shifting, the onset of motor or sensory symptoms well after the headache has started, the failure of motor or sensory symptoms to clear within 24 hours after the headache has ceased, and the association of focal headaches with partial seizures involving the same hemisphere. Focal physical findings or evidence of increased intracranial pressure on examination also indicate the need for further evaluation or even hospitalization.

Many children have symptoms that are said to be "migraine variants." These patients may not have a headache with each attack. The relationship of migraine variants to migraine is based on one of two pieces of information: a strong family history of migraine or the known tendency of more typical forms of migraine to develop in children with these disorders later in life.

The most common and easily related of these variants is basilar migraine, which is most prevalent in adolescent girls. The symptoms that occur lie within the territory of the basilar circulation. Vertigo, syncope, unilateral or bilateral numbness, and dysarthria can be seen at the onset of the attack. Some children feel weak and unsteady, but do not faint. On recovery, there may be visual loss for a brief period and there usually is a pounding occipital headache. Confusion and memory loss also can occur. A small subgroup has generalized seizures, which sometimes are difficult to control.

Motion sickness is common in patients who have migraine, but it is not clear that recurrent attacks of paroxysmal vertigo are a migraine variant. Patients with migraine may experience isolated attacks of confusion or memory loss. They may have recurrent attacks of delirium. These patients may not complain of headaches, and there may be only a strong family history to suggest migraine.

Some children with recurrent episodes of abdominal pain have typical migraine later in life. Certainly, paroxysmal abdominal pain is more likely to be a migrainous than an epileptic syndrome, although paroxysmal EEG tracings are common with the disorder. Most children with recurrent abdominal pain do not suffer from either disorder.

Patients who have a genetic predisposition to migraine seem to react more severely to relatively minor head injuries. Sometimes, a minor episode of trauma is followed by the onset of common or classic migraine. Transient blindness or motor or sensory loss may occur without significant headache. These episodes are short-lived and this, as well as the absence of any evidence of intracranial injury on CT scan, suggests that the symptoms and signs are the response of a migraineur and not the result of a contusion.

## Treatment

Many migraine headaches can be relieved with simple analgesics such as aspirin or acetaminophen. In children less than 5 years of age, the usual dose is 1 grain per year of age; in those from 5 to 10 years of age, the dose is 5 grains; and in those more than 10 years of age, the dose is 10 grains. The medication should be taken as close to the onset of the headache as possible. The same dose may be repeated in 3 to 4 hours if needed. Because aspirin may be associated with Reye's syndrome, acetaminophen is recommended for younger children. If these mild analgesics are not effective, commercial preparations such as Fiorinal (butalbital, aspirin, and caffeine) or Midrin (a combination of isometheptene mucate, acetaminophen, and dichloralphenazone) may be used in older children. A tablet may be taken at the onset of the headache and again after 30 to 60 minutes. Adolescents can take two tablets at the onset of the headache and a third 60 minutes thereafter if indicated. Frequent, regular use of these analgesics may make prophylactic treatment more difficult. Older children with more severe migraines that occur less frequently (no more than twice a month) may benefit from the use of ergotamine tartrate at the onset of a headache. Children less than 12 years of age should take no more than 3 mg of ergot per headache, and older children should take no more than 6 mg. One milligram of ergotamine usually is taken at the onset of the headache and another milligram is taken every 30 minutes thereafter until the headache resolves, vomiting occurs, or the maximum amount of drug allowed has been taken. Frequently, the long-term use of ergots is associated with vascular disease. Intractable migraine headaches often can be relieved by the use of 5 to 10 mg of intravenous metoclopramide followed by 0.2 to 1.0 mg of intravenous dihydroergotamine every 8 hours for 2 to 3 days. A test dose of 0.1 to 0.3 mg of intravenous dihydroergotamine should be given initially. In older patients, dihydroergotamine can be administered subcutaneously at home. This frequently relieves the pain sufficiently to permit the patient to resume normal activities.

A novel new drug called sumatriptan, a serotonin agonist, soon will be available for the treatment of patients with acute migraine headaches. This agent is a selective agonist of 5-hydroxytryptamine–like receptors in the CNS. It can be administered orally or subcutaneously. It is not known when sumatriptan will be approved for use in children.

Migraine also may be treated prophylactically. This is particularly beneficial for children who tend to get frequent headaches and otherwise would require a large amount of analgesic medication or ergot for relief. Average doses of prophylactic medications include propranolol (1 to 2 mg/kg/d in three divided doses), cyproheptadine hydrochloride (0.3 mg/kg/d in three divided doses), phenobarbital or phenytoin (3 to 5 mg/kg/d), amitriptyline hydrochloride (1 to 2 mg/kg/d), or calcium channel blockers.

During the past decade, the most common forms of headache in children have begun to be treated with biofeedback and relaxation therapy. Initial studies were poorly controlled and involved very few children. Evidence is increasing, however, that pediatric as well as adult patients with common migraine and tension headaches do respond to this type of treatment. Of all children who can complete successfully a course of training in either biofeedback or relaxation techniques, 60% to 80% have a positive response consisting of reduction in the frequency and severity of their headaches. This compares favorably with the response obtained with medication. Follow-up studies suggest that the benefits of this training last for at least 1 year. Problems associated with these forms of behavioral therapy include limited facilities, cost, and failure of children to practice these learned techniques regularly.

The use of special diets to treat headaches generally is not successful, nor is desensitization to common allergens. No substantial evidence exists that migraine is an allergic disorder. Occasionally, some children have headaches after eating specific foods, such as chocolate, cheese, or other milk products. If the relationship of the headache to a specific food is well established, withdrawal of that particular food from the diet can be of help.

## TENSION HEADACHES

As noted earlier, it often is difficult to differentiate common migraine from tension headaches solely by the clinical description. No single factor in the history differentiates the two types. People who suffer from either type of headache tend to have a normal physical examination. A constellation of factors does help the physician to make a diagnosis, however. Tension headaches usually occur and are most severe during periods of obvious stress. This association is seen with migraine, but it is not as clear-cut. Migraine tends to involve the frontal and, to a lesser degree, temporal regions of the head, or to be localized retro-orbitally; tension headaches tend to involve the occipital or temporal regions bilaterally and often extend to the neck, or they are diffuse. Tension headaches often are continuous; they fluctuate throughout the day, but never disappear. Patients who have this constellation of features indicating a probable diagnosis of tension headaches are less likely to have immediate family members who have typical migraine. Nausea and vomiting occur with both types of headache when the pain is severe, but are much more common in children with migraine, as are isolated attacks of abdominal pain. The diagnosis is made by careful review of the history.

A subgroup of patients with tension headaches (as well as patients with migraine) suffer from an overt depression with a history of a clear-cut change in mood, self-image, interest in their usual day-to-day activities, appetite, and sleep habits. They often have multiple other somatic complaints. The headaches that these children have will not disappear until the underlying mood disorder is recognized and treated.

The pain resulting from tension headaches usually can be relieved with analgesics. Analgesics combined with codeine sometimes may be required, but the repeated use of codeine should be avoided. When tension headaches recur frequently, biofeedback and relaxation therapy is very useful. In that population of children whose headaches are related to depression, an anxiety neurosis, or a conversion reaction, however, referral to a psychiatrist is indicated.

## SINUS HEADACHES

Chronic or recurrent headaches occur in about 15% of children who have chronic sinusitis. Frequently, there is no increase in temperature. The most common accompanying symptoms or signs are rhinorrhea, postnasal drip, persistent cough, and recurrent ear infections. There may be pain with pressure over the frontal or maxillary sinuses, and these cavities can fail to transilluminate. (The frontal sinuses form later in childhood and are not developed fully in most children until the end of puberty.) Most sinus headaches in children result from infection of the sphenoid or ethmoid sinuses. There usually is no tenderness to palpation when these sinuses are inflamed, and signs of nasal congestion frequently are minimal. Pain usually is referred to the frontotemporal region, but it can occur over any part of the cranial vault. Sinus headaches often occur at the same time each day, build slowly, frequently have a throbbing quality, and vary markedly with change in position (because positional change may promote sinus drainage). The only certain means of diagnosing headaches that result from disease of one or more of the paranasal sinuses is by roentgenography. The diagnosis should be made only if the sinuses are clouded, exhibit a fluid level, or have a thickened mucosa.

Simple analgesics may help decrease the pain of sinus headaches, but sustained relief usually depends on long-term therapy with nasal decongestants and appropriate antibiotics. Surgical drainage is reserved for patients with intractable disease.

## OCULAR HEADACHES

Errors of refraction and strabismus are not associated with an increased incidence of headaches, other than perhaps hypermetropia or astigmatism, which usually produce a dull aching sensation in and around the eyes or, at worst, a mild frontal headache when the eyes are used for close work such as reading for a long period. Glaucoma, inflammation of orbital tissues, and masses within the orbit may produce severe eye pain that rarely is confused with headache. There usually are no other physical findings and treatment is as appropriate for the underlying disorder.

## EPILEPSY

Lateralized or generalized headaches frequently follow epileptic seizures and occasionally precede partial seizures as an aura. No consensus exists regarding whether headache can be the sole manifestation of an epileptic seizure. Headaches that often are diagnosed as migraine do occur more frequently in children who have epilepsy than they do in the general pediatric population. Children who have complex-partial seizures also tend to have headaches of brief duration and abrupt onset and termination. These headaches usually are relieved by anticonvulsants. It is possible, but not certain, that this form of cephalgia is a seizure.

## TRAUMA

Chronic and recurrent headaches frequently follow head trauma. As noted, trauma can be a triggering stimulus for the onset of worsening migraine. Headache is an integral part of the postconcussional syndrome, which also includes dizziness and personality changes. Fortunately, this syndrome is less common in children than in adults. When it does occur, it can persist for months. Postconcussional syndrome also is accompanied by anxiety, irritability, and, at times, frank depression. Traumatic injury to the soft tissue of the neck may be a cause of chronic headaches, which usually are referred to the occipital area of the head. On examination, the paraspinal muscles of the neck frequently are tender and the head may be restricted in its range of motion.

Trauma also may produce intracranial lesions that are associated with headache. Occasionally, patients with acute lesions, particularly intracerebral hemorrhage or acute subdural bleeding, may be alert enough to complain of headache. If so, the pain usually is severe and not throbbing. It often is localized on the same side as the site of the lesion, but sometimes is diffuse. Intracranial injuries also can be associated with chronic, increasingly severe headaches, which again may be localized or diffuse and have no special characteristics. This type of recurrent headache is seen with enlarging subdural hematomas. Regardless of the severity or location of the headache, there is no way to distinguish a severe cephalgia that follows cranial trauma resulting from extracranial contusion from one resulting from intracranial injury, or both. It is best to investigate a severe posttraumatic headache immediately by CT scan even if the patient does not have neurologic signs.

The treatment of posttraumatic headaches depends on their cause. Therapy for posttraumatic migraine does not differ from that for migraine in children who have not been traumatized. Analgesics are used to treat postconcussional headaches. These require time to disappear; if they persist over months and no associated structural lesion is discovered, the child may need a psychiatric evaluation. Headaches that result from intracranial lesions after head injury require that the underlying lesion be treated.

## OTHER EXTRACRANIAL CAUSES OF HEADACHE

Temporomandibular joint disease usually presents with pain that is maximal at the joint and extends into the face and the temporal region. In some patients, however, the pain occurs predominantly in the form of a temporal or frontotemporal headache, which can be unilateral or bilateral and usually does not throb. The diagnosis can be suspected by the child's history. The physical examination is especially helpful if there is limited movement of the temporomandibular joint, or if a click is palpated when the patient makes chewing movements. There also may be a noise that either the child or the examiner can hear when the joint is moved.

Inflammation of the vessels of the scalp and periodontal infections are other rare causes of chronic headache syndromes in children.

## INTRACRANIAL CAUSES OF HEADACHE

Headaches from intracranial lesions occur for one of two reasons: there is a localized or generalized increase in pressure within the skull, which stretches or distorts vessels at the surface of the brain or the arachnoid and dural membranes that cover the brain; or the pain-sensitive fibers in these brain coverings become irritated by infection or bleeding. Tumors or other masses such as abscess or hemorrhage usually are responsible for local distortion of the brain vessels or meninges. Nearly 80% of tumors in children, however, occur either in the posterior fossa or near the midline. Thus, they frequently obstruct the circulation of cerebrospinal fluid, with resulting hydrocephalus. When this occurs, the elevation in intracranial pressure is more diffuse and the headache often is bifrontal or generalized rather than localized over one part of the hemicranium.

It may not be possible to distinguish intracranial from extracranial causes of headache. Certain features, however, may suggest the likelihood of an intracranial mass, including severe occipital headache, headache that is made worse by straining or by sneezing or coughing, headache that awakens the patient from a deep sleep, headache that is exacerbated or improved markedly by a change in position, headache that is associated with projectile vomiting or vomiting without nausea, and headache with a history of focal seizures. If they are allowed to continue, these headaches usually increase in intensity and severity week after week. Patients who have headaches caused by intracranial mass lesions almost always have physical findings if the headaches have been present for several months. These findings include papilledema, unilateral or bilateral sixth nerve palsies, ataxia, and spasticity (particularly in the lower extremities), as well as more localized indications of brain dysfunction involving movement, vision, or language, depending on the site of the lesion.

Pseudotumor cerebri produces the same type of headache that is found in association with elevated intracranial pressure resulting from a mass lesion or hydrocephalus. Vomiting and blurred vision are frequent accompanying complaints, and papilledema, sixth nerve palsies, ataxia, and, less frequently, spasticity may be noted on physical examination. As the name implies, no mass is found with further laboratory studies. Pseudotumor cerebri probably is caused by the expansion of one or more intracranial fluid spaces, such as the vascular and extracellular fluid compartments.

Meningeal irritation usually results in an acute, diffuse, rapidly progressive headache that becomes so intense that it may be unbearable. If the cause is bleeding, then the onset may be explosive and the headache may become excruciating within only a minute or two. Such patients may have focal neurologic signs, but many do not. There frequently is a disturbance of orientation or consciousness. On physical examination, there may be nuchal rigidity caused by meningeal irritation. Occasionally, the examiner can see perivenous or subhyaloid hemorrhages in the eye, resulting from high intracranial pressure and the extravasation of subarachnoid blood.

It is the physician's first responsibility to rule out the possibility of an intracranial lesion. The association of any type of headache with a history of the recent onset or progression of neurologic signs warrants the performance of a CT or MRI scan. Focal headaches that are becoming increasingly frequent, more severe, or intractable to therapy also demand further investigation. Other situations indicating the need for an outpatient CT scan include the onset of chronic headaches after an episode of head trauma and the individual characteristics of the headache, such as a sudden change in its intensity accompanying a change in position.

The treatment of headaches resulting from intracranial catastrophies is not within the scope of this chapter. If the diagnosis of pseudotumor cerebri is made, the patient frequently may obtain relief from a single lumbar puncture performed for diagnostic reasons. If, as often is the case, symptoms recur and intracranial pressure returns to high levels within 3 to 4 days, dexamethasone (2 to 4 mg every 6 hours) may be used for 3 to 5 days and then withdrawn rapidly. Alternatively, acetazolamide (20 mg/kg/d) can be given in three divided doses. If this fails to relieve the patient's symptoms, then repeated lumbar punctures may be needed whenever symptoms recur, or glycerol can be used in gradually increasing dosages from 0.5 to 2.0 g/kg/d in three divided doses as tolerated. Obesity and chronic diarrhea are complications of oral glycerol therapy. Because long-term elevation of the intracranial pressure can affect the vision without causing other symptoms or signs, regular eye examinations should be performed in this group of children. Fenestration of the optic nerve sheath may preserve vision under these circumstances.

## ACUTE HEADACHE

A headache may be so severe that it brings a child to a doctor's office or to the emergency department seeking both a diagnosis and immediate relief of pain. Under these circumstances, it is extremely important that the physician distinguish between intracranial and extracranial causes of the headache, decide if admission to the hospital is necessary, and provide some plan to relieve the child's pain as quickly as possible. The basis of diagnosis still remains the history and physical examination, but, in the face of an acute cephalgia, it often is crucial to decide whether the child requires an immediate head scan or lumbar puncture to assist in the diagnosis and planning of immediate care.

Common intracranial causes of acute, severe headache are a mass lesion, infection, or intracranial hemorrhage. Extracranial causes include migraine, tension headaches, and, rarely, sinusitis. The most decisive factor in the history is whether this is the first such headache this child has experienced or whether it is another headache in an already established pattern of headaches that has been evaluated in the past. It also is important to know whether this particular headache has been associated with unusual antecedent events such as a head injury, seizure, fever, or change in sensory or motor function. Critical physical findings include meningismus, focal neurologic signs, papilledema or split sutures, evidence of cranial trauma (including blood in or behind the ear), and a depressed level of consciousness.

If this is the first attack of severe cephalgia without a significant prior headache history, immediate neural imaging is recommended if any of the following are present: a history of recent trauma, the recent onset of seizures, unusual behaviors predating the headache, fever, meningismus, papilledema, focal neurologic signs, or a depressed level of consciousness. The determination that it will be necessary to use drugs that will depress consciousness significantly to relieve the child's pain also may lead to early neural imaging. In the presence of a prior headache history with a presumed diagnosis, a recent history of trauma, unusual premorbid behaviors, meningismus, papilledema, and significant depression of consciousness indicate the need for immediate neural imaging, as do focal signs, unless they have been present in the past as part of a typical migraine syndrome.

A lumbar puncture should be considered if there is a fever without a cause accompanying the headache, meningismus, and new neurologic signs or abnormal behaviors in the presence of normal results on CT or MRI scanning.

The presence of abnormal results on lumbar puncture or an acute or subacute abnormality on brain scanning dictate that the child be hospitalized. The patient should be admitted to the hospital in the presence of normal test results, however, if there is clinical evidence of elevated intracranial pressure, new neurologic signs, or meningismus. In the face of pernicious vomiting, children also may have to be admitted for rehydration. Children require hospitalization at times for the treatment of intractable pain and, rarely, for short-term psychiatric care.

If the child has no evidence of an intracranial lesion, excruciating pain can be relieved by the intramuscular administration of 1 to 2 mg/kg of meperidine and 1 mg/kg of hydroxyzine. An alternate approach, which is particularly useful if the child is agitated, is to sedate him or her with pentobarbital or chloral hydrate. This usually requires hospital admission for observation.

If it is clear by the history that the child has migraine, the immediate intravenous administration of 5 to 10 mg of metoclopramide followed by 0.2 to 1.0 mg of dihydroergotamine (after a test dose of 0.1 to 0.3 mg), with the concomitant use of low-dose steroids may obviate hospitalization by relieving the headache rapidly in the emergency department. If this fails to relieve the pain over 2 to 3 hours, hospitalization for further parenteral therapy usually is indicated.

## Selected Readings

Baker RS, Baumann RJ, Buncic JR. Idiopathic intracranial hypertension (pseudotumor cerebri) in pediatric patients. Pediatr Neurol 1989;5:5.

Bille B. Migraine in school children. Acta Paediatr Scand 1962;51(Suppl 136):14.

Bille B, Ludvigsson J, Sanner G. Prophylaxis of migraine in children. Headache 1977;17:61.

Duckro PN, Cantwell-Simmons E. A review of studies evaluating biofeedback and relaxation training in the management of pediatric headache. Headache 1989;29:428.

Edmeads J. Emergency management of headache. Headache 1988;28:675.

Golden GS, French JH. Basilar artery migraine in young children. Pediatrics 1975;56:722.

Honig PJ, Charney EB. Children with brain tumor headaches: Distinguishing features. Am J Dis Child 1982;136:121.

Mindell JA, Andrasik F. Headache classification and factor analysis with a pediatric population. Headache 1987;27:96.

Olesen J. The ischemic hypotheses of migraine. Arch Neurol 1987;44:321.

Prensky AL. Migraine and migrainous variants in pediatric patients. Pediatr Clin North Am 1976;23:461.

Rapoport A. The diagnosis of migraine and tension-type headache, then and now. Neurology 1992;42(Suppl 2):11.

Raskin NH. Repetitive intravenous dihydroergotamine as therapy for intractable migraine. Neurology 1986;36:995.

Savoldi F, Tartara A, Manni R, et al. Headache and epilepsy: Two autonomous entities? Cephalalgia 1984;4:39.

Schulman EA, Silberstein SD. Symptomatic and prophylactic treatment of migraine and tension-type headache. Neurology 1992;42(Suppl 2):16.

*Principles and Practice of Pediatrics, Second Edition.*
edited by Frank A. Oski et al. J. B. Lippincott Company, Philadelphia © 1994.

## CHAPTER 163
# *Unclassified Nervous System Disorders: Alpers' Disease*

### Marvin A. Fishman

The term *Alpers' disease* (progressive poliodystrophy) traditionally has been used to refer to a progressive degenerative disease that begins in early infancy and is characterized by a rapidly deteriorating course associated with intractable seizures, loss of developmental skills, stupor, and death within several years of the onset. The diagnosis was based on the examination of brain tissue obtained at biopsy or necropsy. Therefore, it was unclear whether several different diseases could have similar pathology and be grouped together as Alpers' disease, or whether the pathology was specific and unique to a single disease entity.

## PATHOGENESIS

In the past, Alpers' disease had been considered to be of unknown etiology. A recent study of patients has begun to provide information, however, that points to a metabolic basis for the condition. Familial cases have been reported and the inheritance pattern has suggested an autosomal recessive disorder. The examination of tissues (including muscle and brain) has revealed the presence of abnormal mitochondria in some patients. Also, fatty infiltration of the liver has been noted in some children; this is believed not to result from the effects of antiepileptic drug therapy, but to be related to the primary disease.

Intermittent elevations in lactate and pyruvate levels have been found in the serum and, more importantly, in the cerebrospinal fluid (CSF) of some affected individuals. An increased ratio of lactate to pyruvate has been noted. The finding of increased concentrations of these metabolites in the CSF suggests an abnormality of pyruvate metabolism within the brain. The study of various tissues from involved patients has suggested various abnormalities in pyruvate metabolism. These have included disturbances in the pyruvate dehydrogenase complex, the second part of the citric acid cycle, oxidation of the reduced form of nicotinamide-adenine dinucleotide, cytochrome aa3, and pyruvate carboxylase. Thus, what previously was thought to be a degenerative disease of unknown etiology may represent an autosomal disorder associated with pyruvate dysmetabolism.

## PATHOLOGY

The hallmarks of Alpers' disease in the brain include status spongiosus with neuronal degeneration and loss. There often is glial proliferation resulting in an astrocytosis, and capillaries appear to be prominent and dilated. The disease involves primarily the cerebral gray matter and little, if any, change is found in the white matter. In severe cases, the thalamus, hippocampus, and cerebellum also may be involved. In patients in whom the liver is affected, the findings are those of subacute hepatitis with massive fatty degeneration, hepatocyte loss, bile duct proliferation, and fibrous scarring with or without cirrhosis. Changes in the muscle have included lipid infiltration, type grouping of fibers, or evidence of mitochondrial or lipid myopathies. Electron microscopy has revealed abnormal mitochondria in some cases.

## CLINICAL FEATURES

Two forms of Alpers' disease—infantile and juvenile—have been described. The infantile form usually has its onset between 1 and 3 years of age and occurs in children who are either normal or have had previous mild developmental delays. The course is rapid, and death occurs usually between 2 and 6 years of age. The initial symptoms may be vomiting and failure to thrive. These are followed by a severe seizure disorder that often presents with or is characterized by bouts of status epilepticus. The seizures may be focal or generalized, and myoclonus also is noted. Once the epilepsy becomes manifest, psychomotor development stops and previously mastered skills are lost. Affected children often have hypotonia and paresis, but this eventually may change to spasticity. Ataxia, visual disturbances, and deafness commonly develop. The clinical manifestations usually are exacerbated by intercurrent infections and stress. Clinical signs of liver disease, if they occur, develop late in the illness and may be manifest by hepatomegaly and ascites. Occasionally, the liver disease may progress rapidly and cause fatal hepatic failure.

The juvenile form of Alpers' disease has its onset between 4 and 10 years of age and follows a protracted slow course, with death occurring between 12 and 20 years of age. The findings are similar to those of the infantile form, but also involve muscle wasting and evidence of a polyneuropathy. The visual disturbances may include hemianopia as well as blindness. Optic atrophy and retinal pigmentary degeneration occur in some patients.

## DIAGNOSIS AND TREATMENT

The diagnosis of Alpers' disease is suggested on the basis of the clinical picture. Certain laboratory tests help to confirm the clinical suspicion. Examination of the CSF often reveals a significantly increased protein content, frequently greater than 200 mg/dL. The protein electrophoresis and oligoclonal banding patterns are normal. Lactate and pyruvate levels should be ascertained, and elevated levels or a lactate : pyruvate ratio greater than 15 in the CSF suggest an abnormality of pyruvate metabolism within the brain. Liver function test results often are abnormal even before antiepileptic drug therapy is initiated. The results of computed tomography (CT) may be normal or consist of slight generalized atrophy. The atrophy has been noted to be more prominent in the occipital region and hypodensity may be present in that area. The results of the electroencephalogram are abnormal, and high-amplitude slow activity often is seen together with polyspikes; evoked potentials often are abnormal. Muscle biopsies in some patients have demonstrated subsarcolemmic aggregation of mitochondria. The mitochondria frequently are enlarged and contain paracrystalline inclusions. In other patients, muscle biopsies have shown evidence of lipid myopathy or fiber type grouping.

Other diseases that involve brain and liver dysfunction include Wilson's disease, fructosemia, galactosemia, glycogen storage disease, Niemann-Pick disease, and Gaucher's disease. The clinical and laboratory features readily distinguish these entities from progressive poliodystrophy. Subacute necrotizing encephalomyelitis (Leigh disease) also may be associated with pyruvate dysmetabolism. The clinical symptoms of patients with Leigh disease are more diverse and progress at a variable rate. Brain stem signs, including nystagmus, abnormal eye movements, and abnormal respiratory patterns, are prominent. These are not major features of Alpers' disease. CT scans in Leigh disease may reveal abnormalities in the putamen.

No specific treatment is available for patients with Alpers' disease. The associated seizures often are refractory, and treatment with antiepileptic drugs may reduce their frequency, but rarely achieves complete control. No data are available regarding the efficacy of vitamins (including thiamine) or other dietary measures in the treatment of possible pyruvate dysmetabolism.

## Selected Readings

Bicknese AR, May W, Hickey WF, Dodson WE. Early childhood hepatocerebral degeneration misdiagnosed as valproate toxicity. Ann Neurol 1992; 32:767.

Boyd SG, Harden A, Egger J, Pampiglione G. Progressive neuronal degeneration of childhood with liver disease ("Alper's disease"): Characteristic neurophysiological features. Neuropediatrics 1986;17:75.

Gabreels FJM, Prick MJJ, Trijbels JMF, et al. Defects in citric acid cycle and the electron transport chain in progressive poliodystrophy. Acta Neurol Scand 1984;70:145.

Harding BN, Egger J, Portmann B, Erdohazi M. Progressive neuronal degeneration of childhood with liver disease. Brain 1986;109:181.

Huttenlocher PR, Solitare GB, Adams G. Infantile diffuse cerebral degeneration with hepatic cirrhosis. Arch Neurol 1976;33:186.

Narkewicz MR, Sokol RJ, Beckwith B, et al. Liver involvement in Alpers disease. J Pediatr 1991;119:260.

Prick MJJ, Gabreels FJM, Trijbels JMF, et al. Progressive poliodystrophy (Alper's disease) with a defect in cytochrome aa$_3$ in muscle: A report of two unrelated patients. Clin Neurol Neurosurg 1983;85:57.

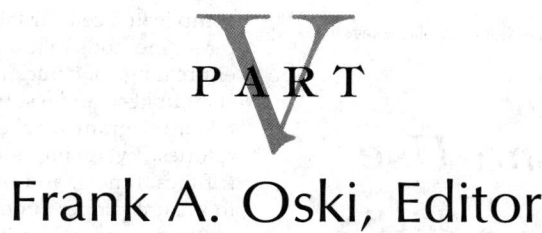

# PART V

Frank A. Oski, Editor

# The Pediatrician's Companion: Important Things You Forget to Remember

*Principles and Practice of Pediatrics, Second Edition.*
edited by Frank A. Oski et al. J. B. Lippincott Company, Philadelphia © 1994.

# CHAPTER 164
# *Evaluation and Use of Laboratory Tests*

## Lawrence S. Wissow

More than 10% of all health care spending in the United States pays for clinical laboratory services, a percentage that continues to increase as new and more complex laboratory tests are developed and aggressively marketed. Increasing equally is the concern that not all of this spending is in the best interests of good medical care. Laboratory tests can be powerful aides in diagnosis and patient management, but evidence shows that many physicians know little about the tests they commonly order. The result is often extra expense and, at times, avoidable morbidity.

It is one thing to prescribe what a physician should know about a test and another to find that information and make it available in clinically useful form. As with many medical technologies, the common use of most laboratory tests has preceded study of how well they perform and in what settings they should be used. Thus, this chapter has four goals:

- To list the characteristics of laboratory tests and how the clinician can use these characteristics to select the proper test for a given task
- To describe how laboratory tests fit into the larger process of medical diagnosis and screening
- To suggest ways in which clinicians can find information about test characteristics when that information is not generally available in popular texts or laboratory manuals
- To provide information about some laboratory tests commonly used by clinicians caring for children.

In this chapter, the term *test* means a laboratory or clinical procedure such as a determination of serum sodium level or a urinalysis. The concepts discussed here apply equally to most other procedures used to gather clinical information. For example, questions in a medical history or maneuvers in a physical examination can be considered tests for which performance characteristics can be defined and measured.

## CHARACTERISTICS OF TESTS

### Practical Considerations

One major class of decisions involved in choosing a test is practicality. Sometimes there is little choice; only one test or method offers the possibility of obtaining the needed information. Most times, however, a variety of tests is possible, and they vary in cost, availability, risk to the patient, and speed of obtaining results.

The skill or equipment required to perform the tests may vary, requiring the clinician to choose carefully which laboratory or machine to entrust with the analysis. Economic incentives often play a major role in this decision. For example, clinicians may help control costs, generate revenue for themselves, and obtain quicker answers by installing relatively simple laboratory equipment in their offices. These machines may measure the same parameters (eg, hemoglobin, blood protoporphyrin) as more complicated central-laboratory equipment, but they may use different methods that do not always yield parallel results over the entire range of clinically important values. They also require constant upkeep and testing using standard specimens, a task usually taken for granted when tests are performed in organized laboratories. Even simple office-laboratory equipment such as centrifuges, timers, and incubators must be monitored consistently to ensure proper functioning. Most texts on clinical laboratory methods suggest quality-control measures and programs suitable for office laboratories.

The importance of quality control and method-to-method variation cannot be overemphasized. For example, in 1985 the American College of Pathologists sent aliquots from a standardized blood sample for serum cholesterol determination to more than 5000 clinical laboratories. Reported results ranged from 197 to 379 mg/dL compared to a reference laboratory determination of 263. Wide variations, even among laboratories using identical autoanalyzers, suggested that uneven quality-control procedures rather than methodologic differences were mostly responsible for the discrepancies. Physicians should determine whether the laboratory to which they regularly send specimens participates in externally run quality-control programs and how closely quality is monitored internally.

The choices discussed below for detecting streptococci in cases of pharyngitis illustrate how practical aspects of test performance may influence the choice of test method. None of the tests is risky, but they vary in cost and, most importantly, in the speed with which results are obtained. Formal cost-benefit or cost-effectiveness analyses can help in this type of situation by clarifying the options involved and specifying information needed to make the decision.

## Performance Characteristics of Tests

How well a test performs can be described by several parameters, each of which is important in determining when the test may be useful.

A test's precision reflects how much difference to expect if the same specimen was tested repeatedly. For example, it is important for a clinician to know whether a change from 20% to 30% of neutrophils on a patient's differential white blood-cell count (WBC) reflects a resolution of the patient's neutropenia or is likely to be a variation in test performance.

A test's precision is not always related to its accuracy, that is, the relationship of test result to true value of the measured parameter. A machine may measure serum potassium with great precision, but values are meaningless if one does not recognize that hemolysis may render them inaccurate.

### The "Two-by-Two" Table

The following paragraphs refer to Figure 164-1, the standard "two-by-two" cross-tabulation frequently used to describe basic

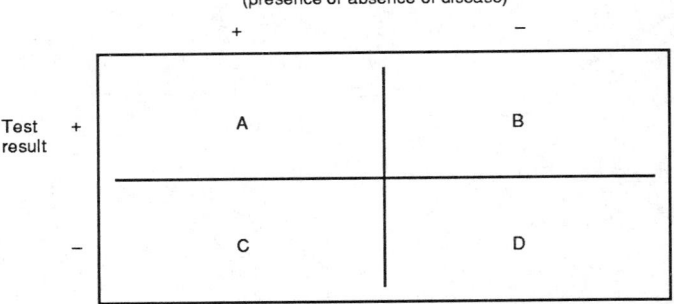

**Figure 164-1.** The "two-by two" cross-tabulation used to describe basic test characteristics.

test characteristics. Suppose test 1 is designed to detect disease X. The columns in Figure 164-1 represent two groups of individuals: those on the left (+) are known to have disease X; those on the right (−) are known to be free of the condition. The rows classify individuals based on results of test 1: the top row (+) counts all those whose test results were positive; the bottom row (−) counts all those whose test results were negative. Each cell (A, B, C, D) divides the group of tested individuals into four categories:

| Cell | Have disease X? | Test result | Label |
|------|-----------------|-------------|-------|
| A | yes | positive | true-positive |
| B | no | positive | false-positive |
| C | yes | negative | false-negative |
| D | no | negative | true-negative |

If the test worked perfectly, there would be 100% agreement between test results and true presence of disease (individuals only in cells A and D). This almost never occurs, which is a reminder in interpreting test results: a positive (or negative) test result does not guarantee that a disease is (or is not) present. The test only tells how great a chance there is that the disease is present.

### Sensitivity and Specificity

Test characteristics derived from sums and ratios of the four cell values (see Fig 164-1) determine how well a test performs a diagnostic task.

*Sensitivity* is the likelihood that a test will be positive in the presence of a targeted disease. Sensitivity is $A/(A + C)$, that is, the proportion of all individuals with disease X who have a positive result on test 1 (see Fig 164-1), or, sensitivity is the probability that test 1 will be positive in the presence of disease X. Test sensitivity is critical in screening for asymptomatic disease and ruling out specific diagnoses (discussed below). When A is large compared to C (eg, when $A/(A + C)$ is greater than .99), there is relative confidence that if test 1 is negative, an individual does not have disease X. This does not make any claims for what a positive test result means.

Specificity is the likelihood of a test to be negative in individuals who do not have the disease. Specificity is defined as $D/(B + D)$ (see Fig 164-1), the probability of a negative test result in an individual without disease X. Very specific tests often are used to confirm or "rule in" a suspected diagnosis. When D is very large compared to B ($D/(B + D)$ is close to 1), a positive result is unlikely to occur in an individual who truly does not have disease X. Based on specificity alone, this does not make any claims for what a negative test result means.

Sensitivity and specificity are further diagrammed in Figure 164-2 . The vertical axis corresponds to the columns of Figure 164-1. Counting up the axis represents persons from the (−) column, those without disease X, and counting down represents persons from the (+) column, persons with disease X. The horizontal axis corresponds to the rows of Figure 164-1. Test values considered to be positive are on the right, and test values considered to be negative are on the left. Areas beneath the two curves represent the number of individuals in each cell of Figure 164-1. Two important points about sensitivity and specificity follow.

First, for most tests, there is some range of results shared by individuals who have the disease and those who do not. Thus, if the definition of a positive and negative test changes, so do the relative sizes of A, B, C, and D and, consequently, the test's sensitivity and specificity. For most tests, a change in definition that benefits sensitivity does so at the expense of specificity, and vice versa. Only by changing the test, not the definition, is it likely to improve both simultaneously.

Second, how a test is used is determined by where the "cut points" are placed (dotted lines 1 and 2, see Fig 164-2). Test results below the value of line 1 define a population unlikely to have disease X, whereas results above line 2 indicate near certainty that X is present. The following example is modified from one developed by George Comstock.

During the development of the purified protein derivative (PPD) test for tuberculosis (TB), research was directed toward determining the optimal dose needed to detect infected individuals. Furcolow and coworkers (1941) tested increasing doses of PPD in known TB patients and in individuals who were presumed to be uninfected. A positive test was defined as a zone of induration 10 mm in diameter surrounding the site of PPD intradermal injection.

Table 164-1 shows the proportions of persons in each group testing positive at increasing doses of PPD. A dose of $10^{-4}$ mg appears to be a good dose for screening purposes; it identifies more than 99% of TB patients, while mistaking for positive only 8.5% of those uninfected. This dose is equivalent to the standard

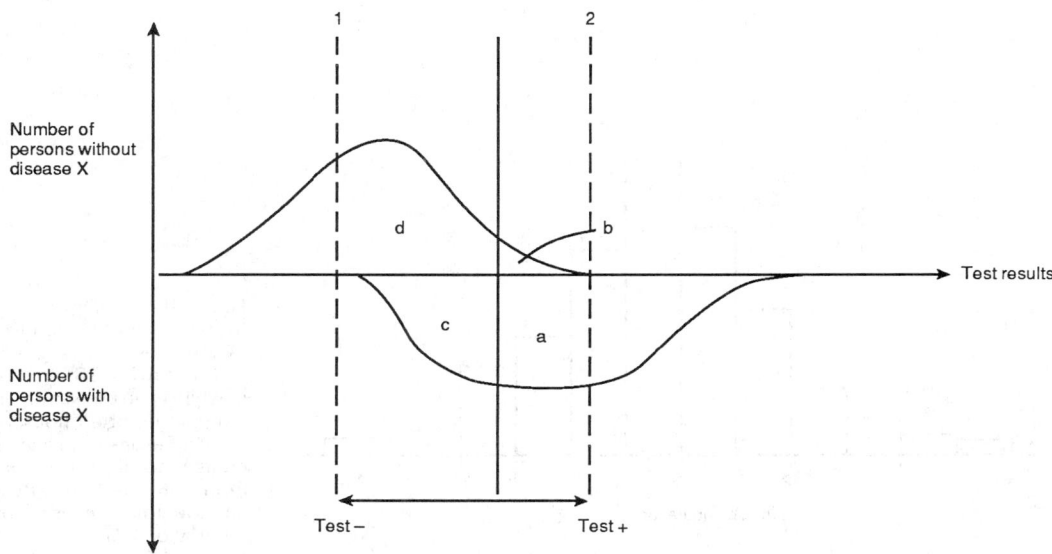

**Figure 164-2.** Sensitivity and specificity of tests (see Fig 164-1).

**TABLE 164-1.** Sensitivity and Specificity of Varying Doses of PPD Among Children With Active Tuberculosis and Those With No Known History of Exposure

| mg/dose PPD | Active TB* | | Not Exposed to TB | |
|---|---|---|---|---|
| | % + (Sensitivity) | % − (False −) | % + (False +) | % − (Specificity) |
| $10^{-9}$ | 3.3 | 96.7 | — | — |
| $10^{-8}$ | 15.0 | 85.0 | 0 | 100 |
| $10^{-7}$ | 21.7 | 78.3 | — | — |
| $10^{-6}$ | 65.0 | 35.0 | — | — |
| $10^{-5}$ | 93.3 | 6.7 | 6.5 | 93.5 |
| $10^{-4}$ | 100.0 | 0.0 | 8.5 | 91.5 |
| $10^{-3}$ | | | 26.6 | 73.4 |
| $10^{-2}$ | | | 53.6 | 46.4 |
| $10^{-1}$ | | | 84.7 | 15.3 |

\* Blanks indicate "not tested."
*Adapted from Furcolow ML, Hewell B, Nelson WE, Palmer CE. Quantitative studies of the tuberculin reaction. Public Health Rep 1941;56:1082.*

5-tuberculin-unit (TU) dose of PPD commonly used today for screening.

TB screening is more complicated, however, because in some parts of the world, false-positive PPD tests result from exposure to nontuberculous mycobacteria. In some parts of the southeastern United States, for example, more than 70% of persons tested have PPD reactions indicating such exposure. This could make diagnosing or screening for TB difficult in such an area. PPD reactions to nontuberculous mycobacteria, however, are usually smaller than reactions to TB. Thus, the use of different cut points for screening and for diagnosis has been workable.

Figure 164-3 shows the distribution of reaction sizes to 5-TU PPD testing in three populations. Figure 164-3A shows tests results in persons with culture-proven TB, Figure 164-3B shows results from Navy recruits who reported household contact with TB, and Figure 164-3C shows results from recruits who did not report contacts. Dotted line 1 is at a reaction size of 5 mm, the recommended cut point for confirmatory diagnosis in patients with a history of TB exposure or with an abnormal chest x-ray.

Applying this cut point to the population in Figure 164-3C, however, results in a large number of false positives, with the error rate increasing along with prevalence of nontuberculous mycobacteria. Thus, the recommended screening cut point is shown at dotted line 2, 10 mm, which may miss some real cases of TB, but greatly reduces the number of false positives. Some experts feel that cut points higher than 10 mm may be indicated in populations with high rates of nontuberculous infection and no history of exposure to TB.

**Predictive Value**

Usually, it is not enough to know that a test is very sensitive or very specific. What the clinician wants to know is how much confidence there is that a positive test result really means that disease is present or that a negative result really means that disease is absent. The most basic way to express this confidence is with two quantities, the test's positive and negative predictive values. Positive predictive value is the proportion of persons who test positive on test 1 who actually have disease X, or A/(A + B) (see Fig 164-1), or the probability that disease X will be present, given a positive test. The negative predictive value is D/(C + D) (see Fig 164-1), or the probability that disease is not present, given a negative test.

A test's positive and negative predictive values vary with the prevalence of the target disease in the studied population. This is illustrated by example—the use of enzyme-linked immunosorbent assays (ELISA) for human immunodeficiency virus (HIV). Although the characteristics of the HIV ELISA vary from manufacturer to manufacturer, in experienced hands, the test is felt to have a sensitivity that approaches 100% and a specificity of more than 99%. These are impressive statistics, and the tests yield impressive results when used in a high-prevalence population such as a group of hemophiliacs who received blood products before the use of treatments to inactivate HIV (Fig 164-4). With a prevalence of HIV antibodies approaching 50%, the positive and negative predictive values of the test are both nearly 100%. Figure 164-5 shows how the same test performs in a population of male Army recruits, in whom the prevalence of HIV positivity is reported to be 0.16%. The positive predictive value of the test is about 24%. In other words, for every true-positive result, there are about three that are false positive. Thus, HIV testing of low-prevalence populations requires sequential use of other tests, usually a repeat ELISA followed by a "western blot," to separate the true-positive from the false-positive results.

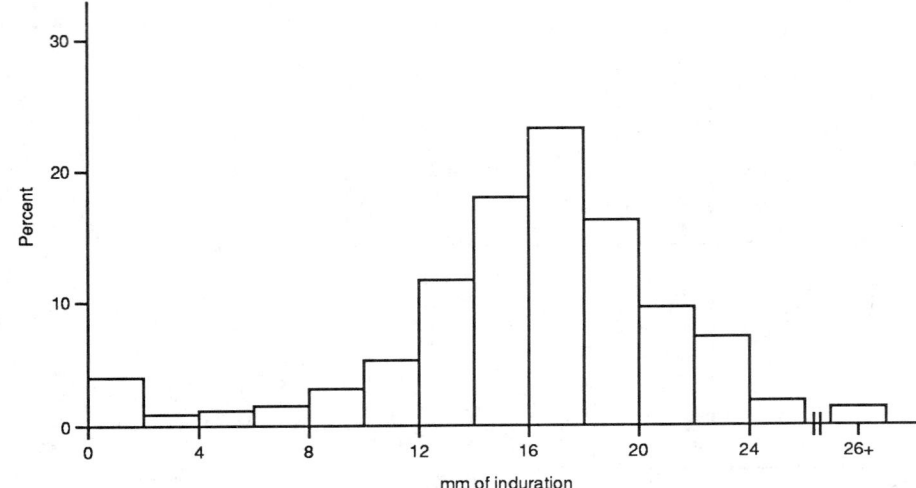

**Figure 164-3.** Distribution of reaction sizes to 5-TU PPD testing in three populations. (**A**) Test results in a group of persons with culture-proven TB. (**B**) Results from a group of white male US Navy recruits 17 to 21 years old who reported household contacts with TB. (**C**) Results from a group of US Navy recruits who did not report contacts, tested from 1961 to 1969. (Rust P, Thomas J. A method for estimating the prevalence of tuberculous infection. Am J Epidemiol 1975;101:311.)

**A**

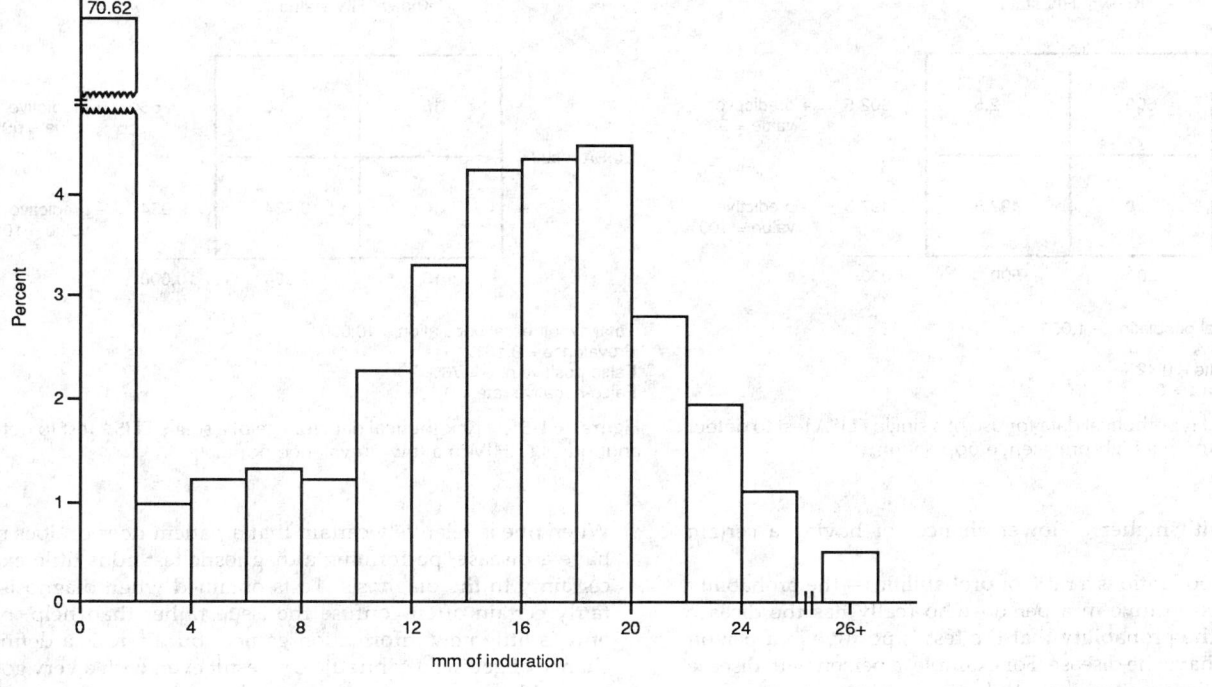

**B**

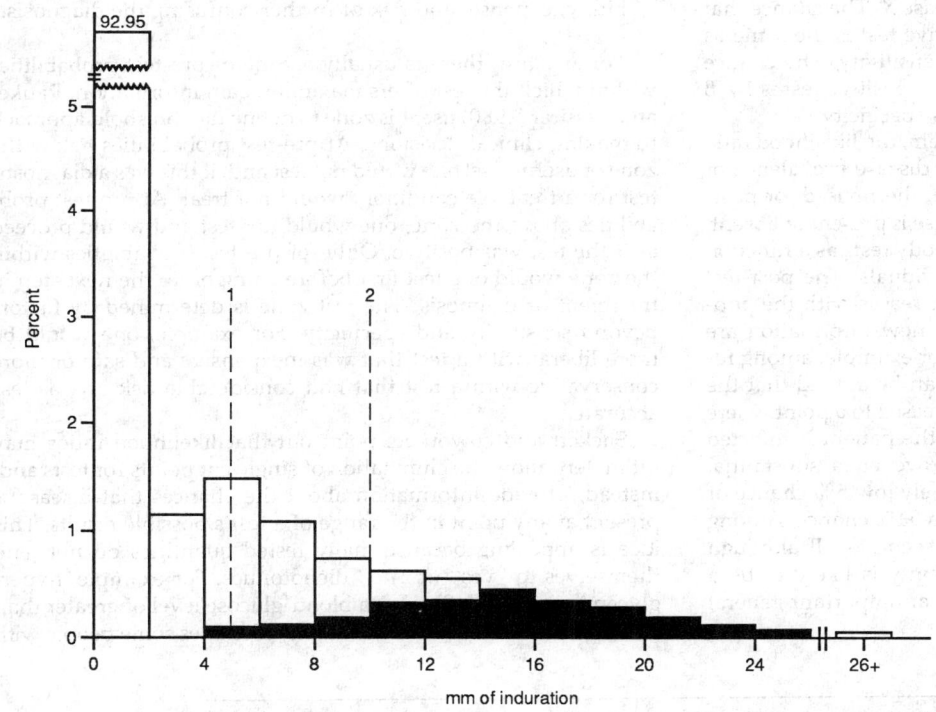

**C**

Figure 164-3. (*Continued*)

Even such a series of tests does not reduce the false-positive rate to zero; thus, many authorities question the utility and ethics of HIV and other testing in low-risk groups. In general, however, performing individual tests in series reduces the overall sensitivity and increases specificity. If all individuals who are positive on test 1 (true and false positives) are retested with test 2, there is no opportunity to learn more about individuals who were negative on test 1, but there is a chance to reduce the number of false positives.

## The Likelihood Ratio

An increasingly popular way of summarizing a test's capabilities is to state its positive or negative likelihood ratio. The likelihood ratio is similar to the predictive value in that it helps in assessing the diagnostic benefit of a positive or negative test result. Unlike the predictive value, the likelihood ratio is independent of the prevalence of disease. The likelihood ratio, then, is useful in assessing how well a test will do in different populations or for

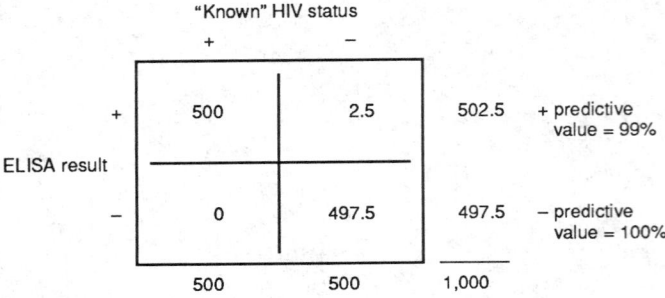

Total hypothetical population = 1,000
Prevalence = 50%
False-positive rate = 0.42%
False-negative rate = 0

**Figure 164-4.** Hypothetical data for use of a single ELISA test to detect antibodies to HIV in a high-prevalence population.

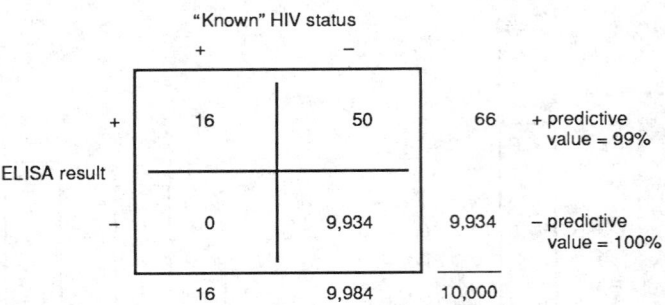

Total hypothetical population = 10,000
Prevalence = 0.16%
False-positive rate = 76%
False-negative rate = 0

**Figure 164-5.** Hypothetical data for use of a single ELISA test to detect antibodies to HIV in a low-prevalence population.

individuals with higher or lower chances of having a certain disease.

The likelihood ratio is a ratio of probabilities—the probability that the test is positive in a person who really has the disease compared to the probability that the test is positive in a person who does not have the disease. For example, a person with disease X is so many times more likely to have a positive result on test 1 than is a person who does not have disease X. The chance that a person with disease X will have a positive test is the same as A/(A + C) (see Fig 164-1), or the test's sensitivity. The chance that a person without disease X will have a positive test is B/(B + D) (see Fig 164-1), or 1 minus the test's specificity.

Using a formula known as Bayes' theorem, the likelihood ratio can be used to calculate, for any level of disease prevalence or pre-test chance that a patient has disease, the revised, or post-test chance, given the test results that disease is present or absent.

Table 164-2 shows results of HIV antibody tests as a function of population prevalence of positive individuals. The post-test chance that HIV antibodies are present increases with the population prevalence. Different amounts of new information are obtained depending on pre-test chance. For example, among female donors and male Army recruits, it can be argued that the post-test chance of HIV infection is not increased to a point where the clinician knows more about whether the patient is infected or not. Among transfusion recipients, however, a substantial amount of information is gained. A relatively low 5% chance of HIV positivity jumps to a practically certain 91% chance. Among the hemophiliacs, the information gain also seems to fall, although going from a 50–50 chance to near certainty is likely to be a clinically significant finding. This leads to an important general point:

When one is relatively certain that a patient does or does not have a disease, performing a diagnostic test adds little extra certainty to the diagnosis. Tests obtained when diagnosis is fairly certain often confuse the issue rather than help. Not only is little new information gained, but there is a definite chance of getting a contradictory result even with a very good test, which leads to further tests that carry significant morbidity, expense, and risk of further confusing the diagnosis.

For any test, there is usually a zone of pre-test probabilities within which the test offers maximum gain information. Pauker and Kassirer (1980) use this zone to define the threshold approach to making clinical decisions. At pre-test probabilities below the zone of usefulness, one would not test and, if this was a diagnostic test for a treatable condition, would not treat. At pre-test probabilities above the zone, one would not test and would proceed as if the test was positive. Only for pre-test probabilities within the zone would one test first before going on to the next step in treatment or diagnosis. The test zone is determined by factors beyond sensitivity and specificity. For example, one would be more liberal with a test that was inexpensive and safe or more conservative with a test that had considerable risk or was less accurate.

Sackett and coworkers point out that likelihood ratios may ultimately allow the elimination of single cut points for tests and, instead, provide information about the chances that disease is present at any point in the range of a test's possible results. This idea is appealing because many tested quantities do not lend themselves to "yes" or "no" dichotomies. For example, hyperglycemia may be defined as a blood-glucose level of greater than 130 mg/dL, but this definition falsely identifies some people with

| | **TABLE 164-2.** Post-Test Probabilities of HIV Seropositivity After a Single ELISA Test* | | | |
|---|---|---|---|---|
| **Population Group** | **Pre-Test Probability** | **Pre-Test Odds** | **Post-Test Odds** | **Post-Test Probability** |
| Hemophiliacs | 0.50 | 1:1 | 200:1 | .99 |
| Transfusion recipients | 0.05 | .05:1 | 10:1 | .91 |
| Male Army recruits | 0.0016 | .0016:1 | .32:1 | .24 |
| Female blood donors | 0.0001 | .0001:1 | .02:1 | .02 |

Based on a sensitivity of 100, a specificity of 99.5, and a likelihood ratio of 200.
*Pre-test probabilities from Meyer KB, Pauker SG. Screening for HIV: can we afford the false-positive rates? N Engl J Med 1987;317:238.*

diabetes as normal. Table 164-3 shows hypothetical post-test probabilities of diabetes for various blood-glucose levels and a range of pre-test probabilities of disease. It shows how a level of 130 mg/dL is more significant for a person with a 50–50 chance of having diabetes—someone giving a history of polyuria and polydypsia—than for a person with no symptoms and a low chance of having the disease. On the other hand, a level of 150 mg/dL has clinical significance for someone who is asymptomatic, and even a level of 100 mg/dL might be of concern in someone who had several clinical signs and symptoms and a high pre-test chance of illness.

### Measures of Agreement

Most evaluations of new tests are based on a comparison with some "gold standard," usually a more complicated but more accurate measure considered "the truth." In many situations, such as the evaluation of new tests for streptococcal pharyngitis discussed below, there is no readily available measure of truth. In these cases, rather than speak of a new test's sensitivity and specificity, we can more correctly speak of how well the new test agrees with the old one.

The simple way to compare agreement between two tests is to calculate the proportion of all cases tested in which the two tests give the same result. In Figure 164-6, this is the sum of A (the number of cases in which both tests are positive) plus D (the number of cases in which both tests are negative) divided by N (the total number of cases tested). This method breaks down, however, when most of the cases are labeled negative (or positive) by both tests. For example, data presented in Figure 164-7 show the agreement between an experienced physician (Observer 1) and a new student (Observer 2) carrying out auscultation of the heart. The experienced physician labels 10 of the 100 children tested as having a murmur; the student, who is not sure how a murmur sounds, labels all the children normal. Agreement between the tests is (0 + 90)/100 = .9, apparently very high, but it occurs by chance (or a combination of chance plus the fact that most of the children don't have murmurs).

Calculation of the kappa statistic separates the component of chance from the observed agreement. The first step in calculating kappa is similar to a chi-squared test. The two-by-two table is recreated with the values that would be obtained by chance alone. In the case of agreement, a new value for A (A') and D (D') should be calculated. The value expected for A, based on chance, is (A + C)/N × (A + B), while the value expected for D is (B + D)/N × (C + D). The expected degree of agreement based on chance alone is (A' + D')/N, which, in this example, is also 0.9.

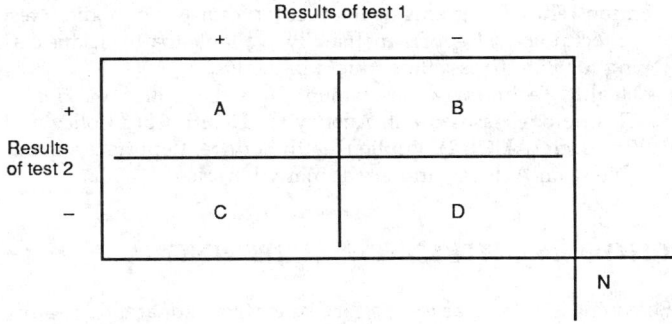

**Figure 164-6.** "Two-by-two" table for comparison of two tests.

Kappa is then calculated by taking:

$$\frac{\text{observed agreement} - \text{agreement expected by chance}}{1 - \text{agreement expected by chance}}$$

In the example, kappa is zero. Kappas of more than .75 indicate good agreement beyond what is expected by chance, whereas kappas of less than .40 suggest the two tests show poor agreement.

## Obtaining Information About Actual Tests

Clinicians often find it difficult to obtain data on the performance characteristics of tests. Laboratory tests, like many other medical technologies, are often put into widespread use before such data are developed or disseminated. Experimental data about laboratory tests may be available in published articles, although often in relatively specialized and technical journals. Haynes and coworkers (1981) provide a checklist for reading this type of article and for deciding if a new test is useful.

Other sources of information include journal reviews of test characteristics and reports from a variety of organizations that compile data about a range of medical technologies, including laboratory tests. These organizations usually combine an extensive literature review with the opinions of an expert panel. Their recommendations may be published in journals or ordered individually from the organization. Some of the larger technology assessment programs that examine diagnostic and screening tests include the following:

- Clinical Efficacy Assessment Project, American College of Physicians. These reports are often published in the *Annals of Internal Medicine*.
- Diagnostic and Therapeutic Technology Assessment Program, American Medical Association. These reports are often published in the *Journal of the American Medical Association*.
- Medical Necessity Program and the Technology Evaluation and Coverage Program, Blue Cross and Blue Shield Associ-

**TABLE 164-3.** Table of Hypothetical Post-Test Probabilities of Diabetes, Given Varying Pre-Test Probabilities and Different Cut Points of Defining Hyperglycemia

|  | Cutoff Glucose Levels (mg/dl) | | |
| --- | --- | --- | --- |
|  | *100* | *130* | *150* |
| Pre-Test Probabilities | | | |
| 0.1 | .12 | .35 | .64 |
| 0.5 | .56 | .83 | .94 |
| 0.9 | .92 | .98 | .99 |
| Hypothetical Likelihood Ratios | | | |
| 100 mg/dL—1.3 | | | |
| 130 mg/dL—5.0 | | | |
| 150 mg/dL—16.0 | | | |

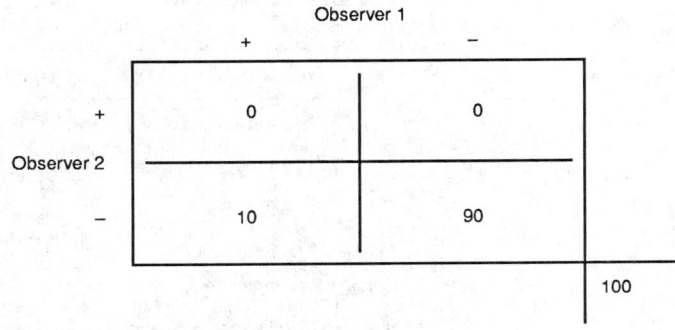

**Figure 164-7.** Hypothetical data for two observers in which observer 2 systematically calls all cases "negative."

ation. These programs develop criteria for use of a given test or technology. Reports are usually available to physicians caring for Blue Cross/Blue Shield patients.

- Health Technology Assessment Reports, Office of Health Technology Assessment, Agency for Health Care Policy and Research (AHCPR), Public Health Service. Reports are available from AHCPR and are at many libraries.

## CHOOSING TESTS FOR SCREENING

Screening is defined as testing for disease in an apparently healthy population or individual. Mainly because of test limitations, the goal of screening is not to detect disease in individuals but to identify persons who are at greater risk of having the disease and who warrant further testing. Commonly used pediatric screening tests include measurement of hematocrit to detect anemia, perinatal tests to detect inborn errors of metabolism and hemoglobinopathies, and tine tests to detect TB.

First, it is important to decide whether the target disease is a suitable candidate for detection by screening. Some important considerations follow:

- Is the disease serious enough to warrant the effort?
- Is the disease common enough, relative to its seriousness, to warrant mass testing of persons who show no signs of having it?
- Does the disease have a preclinical phase that allows it to be detected by a screening test?
- Is there any benefit, in terms of improved prognosis, ease of treatment, or risk of transmission to others, in detecting the disease in its preclinical phase?
- Are follow-up mechanisms available so persons who screen "positive" can be counseled and obtain rapid confirmatory testing or treatment?

If a disease is suitable for screening, a test must be identified. Some practical requirements for a screening test follow.

- The test must be easy to perform and interpret, including having relative immunity from subjectivity or minor variations in technique.
- The test should measure something definitely related to the condition under study rather than some epiphenomenon that might not be specific.
- The test must have acceptably low risk, morbidity, and cost to those being tested.

In addition, most screening tests are chosen or designed to be highly sensitive. That is, a negative result ideally indicates a very low chance that the tested individual is at risk of having the target disease. A positive result, however, may only mean that the individual is somewhat more likely to have the disease. Further testing is usually required because simple highly sensitive tests are not often very specific. The best screening tests are both highly sensitive and highly specific. Table 164-4 lists reported values of sensitivity and specificity for some tests commonly used to screen pediatric patients.

## THE ROLE OF LABORATORY TESTS IN MEDICAL DIAGNOSIS

As Sackett and coworkers (1985) point out, an optimal model of medical decision making involves the sequential formulation and testing of hypotheses about the nature of a patient's illness. The bulk of this process usually takes place during the history and physical examination. Laboratory tests, then, are used either to choose among competing hypotheses or to confirm suspicions before initiating treatment.

For example, a 6-month-old female infant is brought to a physician's office with a fever of 39°C and a 12-hour history of irritability. Even before taking the history and performing the physical examination, the physician generates a list of possible problems, then focuses the workup on maneuvers to support or dispute each problem on the list. Has the child been pulling at her ears or is there a previous history of otitis? Has there been a cough or is the respiratory rate increased?

At the end of the history and physical examination, two of the original hypotheses are discarded. The tympanic membranes move nicely, the chest is clear, and the respiratory rate and effort are normal, so otitis media and pneumonia are no longer strong possibilities. Although the child is somewhat fussy and prefers being held, she acts alert, smiles briefly, and shows some interest in her bottle of juice. She does not appear toxic; thus, she is relatively unlikely to have a major systemic illness.

The next three major hypotheses are a viral syndrome, a urinary tract infection (UTI), and meningitis, with the first two seeming most likely. What laboratory test or tests might the clinician order to differentiate among these conditions? Possibilities include performing a complete blood count (CBC), blood culture, urinalysis, or lumbar puncture, or performing no test at all.

One way to approach this problem is to look at the characteristics of the possible tests and determine how quickly these might make it possible to focus on the conditions that are most serious. Ideally, one chooses a single test capable of providing information about all the diagnoses being entertained rather than about just one. Usually, however, a series of disease-specific tests

### TABLE 164-4. Sensitivity and Specificity for Some Laboratory Tests Commonly Used in Pediatrics

| Test | Target Condition | Sensitivity | Specificity |
|------|------------------|-------------|-------------|
| Guthrie bacterial inhibition assay | Phenylketonuria (PKU) | About 100% | ⩾99%* |
| Tine (+ >2 mm) | Tuberculosis | 32% | 99%† |
| (+ >5 mm) | | 7% | 100% |
| VDRL | Syphilis | 86% | 97% |
| Hematocrit | Iron deficiency | 79% | 93%‡ |

* Test done at 48 hours of age, infant already feeding on milk; in populations with prevalence of about 1: 12,000, test has positive predictive value of 10% to 20%.
† Compared to PPD; specificity of PPD varies depending on prevalence of atypical mycobacterial infections.
‡ Derived from study of adult women; gold standard is positive response to trial of iron therapy.

must be performed, often in the order of the urgency of the illnesses.

The clinician's first decision might be whether to perform a lumbar puncture. Although the pre-test probability of meningitis is fairly low, it is the most serious of the conditions in the differential diagnosis. The lumbar puncture has fairly desirable characteristics for such a situation. Although it is invasive, it has a low complication rate in young patients and can be performed readily by most practitioners. Moreover, it is apparently a very sensitive (although not very specific) test for bacterial meningitis, just the characteristics desired for a screening or "rule out" test. Children with no cells in their cerebrospinal fluid are unlikely to have bacterial meningitis, although children with some cells may or may not have the disease. So, if the clinician's pre-test concern is high, a lumbar puncture might be performed. Although it may not establish the diagnosis, it is a major aid in assigning the patient to a risk category for urgent serious disease.

It is instructive to compare this outcome with the parallel approach of performing a urinalysis to evaluate the presumptive diagnosis of UTI. Again, even if a catheterized specimen is obtained, the test has a relatively low complication rate and can be performed quickly and reliably by most clinicians. The test's characteristics, however, are different from those of a lumbar puncture.

As discussed below, observations of white cells or bacteria on urinalysis provide fairly specific (but not very sensitive) indicators of UTI in infancy. These observations are much more reliable in older children. Positive findings are highly suggestive of UTI, but negative findings, especially from a female patient, probably warrant obtaining a urine culture.

Another approach is to use a test that, to some degree, provides information about all the possible hypotheses. In this case, the clinician might opt to order a complete blood count, looking especially at the total WBC. In one series of children with unexplained acute febrile illness, McGowan and coworkers (1973) found that more than 90% of febrile children with bacteremia had a WBC of greater than 10,000 (sensitivity), while about one third of children without bacteremia had a WBC of less than 10,000 (specificity). Thus, the WBC may be a good test to rule out bacteremia; that is, if the test is negative (between 5000 and 10,000), bacteremia is relatively unlikely. A positive test still requires follow-up diagnostic maneuvers to detect bacteremia or specific foci of infection.

## USING TESTS TO MONITOR THERAPY

A third major use of laboratory tests is to monitor therapy, either to measure the response of the illness or to check for unwanted side effects. The following are important characteristics of tests used for monitoring:

- Tests must have high precision or reproducibility. Test-to-test variation due to chance must be minimized so clinicians know when a new result reflects true physiologic change. Radiologic studies are particular examples in which variations in technique and interpretation occur from test to test.
- Tests should be noninvasive, atraumatic, and relatively inexpensive, so they can be used as often as necessary.
- Tests must accurately reflect changes in the disease being monitored. Multiple tests or tests from multiple sites may be required to assess adequately all relevant aspects of disease progression. Following the course of treatment for leukemia, for example, may require sampling of multiple sites for evidence of relapse. Alternatively, some disease markers, such as the sedimentation rate in collagen vascular disease, may be powerful enough that a single test can be used to follow a patient's progress.

- The test procedure or interpretation must control for other factors that could alter the test result. Many serum chemistry determinations, for example, can be altered falsely by hyperglycemia, hyperlipidemia, or hyperbilirubinemia, conditions that also may change during the course of therapy.

## ASSESSING INFORMATION ABOUT A TEST

Clinicians frequently must decide if a journal account of a new test warrants its use. The following questions, adapted from Haynes and coworkers (1981), may serve as guides to evaluating an account of a new or an old test.

*What gold standard did the authors use in their study of the new test?* In Figure 164-1, it was posited that the individuals in the left column really had the disease and those in the right column really did not. Usually, there is no such knowledge, and results of the new test are compared with results of another test that has its own degree of uncertainty. A variety of pitfalls can arise.

1. The old comparison test may not be performed properly. For example, an account of a new test that differentiates viral from streptococcal sore throats is compared with the goldstandard throat culture with its known susceptibility to falsenegative results when improperly performed. Were throat swabs performed consistently and meticulously, carried promptly to the laboratory, and plated by a competent technician? Was identification of the organism carried out with an accepted method? This type of problem often surfaces when a new test is put into use while old diagnostic procedures are used, rather than being tested in the context of a deliberate research project. This sort of problem makes it difficult to establish how well the new test really works.
2. Even if performed properly, the old test may not be worthy of gold-standard status. Sometimes, there is no better alternative, but often there is. Using the throat-swab example again, most research projects involving detection of streptococci in the pharynx use duplicate swabs as a gold standard because a single swab has been found to miss as many as 10% of truepositive cases.
3. Those performing the new test should be blind to how the patient is classified by the gold standard. Even relatively objective results can be swayed by biased observation.

*What population was used to study the new test?* As discussed, the population used to determine a test's characteristics can have profound influence on parameters such as positive and negative predictive values. Subtle problems also may arise as delineated by Ransohoff and Feinstein (1978) who have related these problems to the spectrum of disease among the studied patients.

1. All "disease-positive" patients may be individuals with advanced, unambiguous cases of the disease. It may be unknown how well the test will work in patients with earlier stages of illness or whose diagnosis is more debatable.
2. All control patients may be normal. The usual diagnostic task is not to differentiate persons with disease from those who are well but to choose who has a particular disease from among a group of people with similar symptoms. Thus, a test that separates children with rheumatoid arthritis from normal controls may not differentiate among those with collagen vascular disease, joint trauma secondary to overuse, and toxic synovitis.

*How is "normal" defined, either for the new test or for the gold standard?* Where a cut point divides normal and abnormal may influence greatly how a test performs and how it can be used. In most cases, the ideal way to define what is abnormal or normal is in terms of the target disease or body function being measured. For example, the best way to define an abnormally low hematocrit for diagnosing iron-deficiency anemia is to pick the point below which most individuals have a response to the administration of iron. Usually, however, cut points are calculated by performing a test on apparently normal individuals, then using statistical methods to define values of the test's results that are outside an expected normal range. In the hematocrit example, a large number of apparently healthy persons would be tested, and the lowest 5% of values would be declared too low. This method has a number of potential problems:

1. The population used to define normal may not be representative of all those on whom the test will be used. This is classically the case for tests developed in adult populations and for which normal values in children are not known. Similar problems can occur with race or sex differences.
2. The normal population may not be normal. It may contain persons who have the disease in question or other unrelated conditions that change the test's results.
3. The use of statistical techniques to define normal and abnormal (ie, greater than two standard deviations from the mean; less than the fifth percentile) automatically labels a fixed proportion of the tested population as abnormal, regardless of whether this degree of deviation from the average has any physiologic significance. Failure to recognize this phenomenon can lead to unnecessary evaluations for problems that do not exist. If a healthy individual undergoes 12 tests, such as on a standard 12-test chemistry panel that uses the plus-or-minus-two-standard-deviations rule for normalcy, the chance that all 12 results will be normal is only 54%.

*Is it clear how the new test is being used?* Whether the new test is used alone or in conjunction with other diagnostic information must be clear. An x-ray film, for example, may be read as is or the radiologist may be given clinical data to aid in interpretation. Both methods may be valid depending on the setting in which the test is used, but the latter method may require additional study of the relative weights given to the film and to the clinical information.

*Is the new test truly independent of the gold standard?* The new test should not incorporate any element of the gold standard. This occurs most often when the proposed test is a symptom complex used to identify a high-risk group of patients. Problems arise, for example, if a new test for UTI requires the presence of fever and dysuria while the gold-standard diagnosis was defined as fever and a positive urine culture. The authors of the new test would then conclude that fever is a useful tool for identifying children at risk for UTI.

# EXAMPLES OF COMMONLY USED PEDIATRIC TESTS

The following examples illustrate the use of tests in commonly occurring pediatric conditions. These examples are not thorough discussions of the medical decisions involved, but rather point out the importance of what information tests can and cannot provide.

## Tests for the Presence of Group A β-Hemolytic Streptococci

Tests to detect group A β-hemolytic streptococci (GABHS) are usually performed in the evaluation of patients with sore throat or other symptoms of pharyngitis. Symptomatic patients with positive tests are presumed to be infected with GABHS, although the test cannot differentiate actual infection from a temporary or chronic carrier state.

There are several clinical goals for detecting GABHS. Traditionally, the major goal is to prevent acute rheumatic fever by detecting active GABHS infection and eradicating the organism from the pharynx. Immediate identification of GABHS is not required because treatment within a few days of the onset of symptoms is adequate to prevent subsequent cardiac disease. Recent findings that early treatment of GABHS infection can reduce both morbidity and transmission of the organism have spurred interest in rapid diagnostic tests for GABHS, several of which are now available for clinical use.

### Gold Standards

The biggest problem in evaluating tests for GABHS is the lack of a clinically useful standard against which to judge test performance. This problem has two major aspects. First, the test is unable to determine actual GABHS infection. In the standard two-by-two table (see Fig 164-1), the ideal labels for the table's two columns in the case of GABHS infection are "patients with pharyngitis who truly have GABHS infection" and "patients with pharyngitis who do not have GABHS infection." There is no reliable way to make this differentiation, however, so most assessments of tests to detect GABHS use instead: "patients with pharyngitis who have GABHS present by the best available method" and "patients without symptoms" who are presumed not to be infected with GABHS or anything else. This may result in an overestimation of the test's performance, because it does not differentiate GABHS infections from other pharyngeal infections, or it may underestimate its performance if the prevalence of asymptomatic carriers is high.

Second, it is difficult to assess the sensitivity or specificity of a new test. All one can realistically state is how well the new test agrees with the results of the old one. This usually results in underestimating rather than overestimating the quality of the new test, if the new and old tests do not share common weaknesses. Both the standard culture techniques and the new rapid diagnostic methods have difficulties in detecting relatively light colonization with GABHS. When the two tests share weaknesses (or when they are not independent), it is impossible to predict whether the new test performs better or worse than it appears.

### Methods

*Obtaining Specimens From the Pharynx.* All methods for detecting GABHS share a common step, the use of a swab to obtain a sample of the flora from the mucosa of the posterior pharynx. This procedure has its own potential for error. Swabbing is reviewed here because of its clinical importance and because of its important role in the evaluation of tests for GABHS.

The recommended procedure for performing a throat swab is to make contact with both tonsils and the posterior pharynx while avoiding contact with the teeth, cheeks, gums, and tongue. It is important to actually swab these surfaces to remove adherent organisms rather than just to touch them. Swabbing exudates when they are observed can increase the chance of detecting GABHS. Cotton swabs can be used for culture methods, but synthetics are needed for rapid diagnostic tests. Studies using repeat swabbing, or subsequent culturing of tonsils swabbed prior to tonsillectomy, estimate that a single, well-done swab has between a 75% to 90% chance of finding GABHS if it is present. This success rate may be considerably lower in the typical uncooperative pediatric patient.

GABHS is a hardy organism. Swabs generally do not need to be placed in transport medium if a culture method is used and if swabs are plated within about 2 hours.

*Culturing to Detect GABHS.* Culture methods are the standard for detecting GABHS. Culturing involves three major steps: growing the organism on suitable media, isolating organisms that appear to be $\beta$-hemolytic, and showing that these organisms are in group A. Each step has opportunity for variation in technique and test performance.

GABHS grows on a variety of media, including trypticase soy and brain-heart infusion. Sheep red blood cells are added to the media to demonstrate hemolysis. Other red cells cannot be used because they may inhibit the growth of GABHS. Although it is controversial, some authors feel that the addition of certain antibiotics to the media makes it easier to identify light growths of GABHS.

The proper streak-stab technique must be used for beta hemolysis to be observed if GABHS is present. The original swab is rolled in a corner of the plate over a 1- to 2-cm area. This area is then streaked across the plate with a loop to spread the inoculum. The loop is then stabbed two or three times to the bottom of the plate to introduce organisms under the surface of the media. The plates are incubated upside-down for about 18 hours. Again, there is controversy about whether aerobic or anaerobic incubation is preferable.

$\beta$-Hemolytic streptococci appear as small (about 1 mm), non-pigmented colonies surrounded by a clear, colorless zone in which the red cells imbedded in the media are completely lysed. The zone around an isolated colony growing under good conditions should be clear enough for newsprint to be read through the culture medium. It is not always easy to separate beta from alpha hemolysis, in which the colonies are surrounded by a more indistinct zone that has a green or brown tint. On crowded plates, it may be necessary to use a microscope to look for the presence of unlysed cells, indicative of alpha hemolysis, in the zone around a suspicious colony.

Of the two major beta hemolysins, streptolysins O and S, only the latter is oxygen stable. Thus, it may be necessary to examine the stab site, usually with a microscope, to look for hemolysis around colonies that have grown anaerobically. The main risk of mistaking alpha for beta hemolysis is that some $\alpha$-hemolytic streptococci such as pneumococci, viridans, and group D may be sensitive to bacitracin and give false-positive reactions to sensitivity testing, the next step in the procedure.

Lancefield typing is the gold standard for grouping streptococci. Because it is a tedious procedure, a test for sensitivity to the antibiotic bacitracin is usually substituted in clinical laboratories. Group A streptococci are sensitive to bacitracin, while other groups generally are not. The bacitracin test ideally is performed by subculturing a $\beta$-hemolytic colony from an original plate onto a new plate on which has been placed a small paper disk impregnated with either 0.02 or 0.04 units of bacitracin. Subculturing is preferred because heavy growth is required to show definitively that a zone of inhibition, indicating sensitivity, is present around the disk. Using the disk on the original plate is reported to be only 70% as accurate as using two plates. The greatest risk is for false-positive results; that is, with light growth, some non-group A streptococci appear to be inhibited by the bacitracin. Using a second plate, however, adds an additional 18 to 24 hours to the time required to perform the test.

The bacitracin disk method does not have the accuracy of Lancefield typing, and most laboratories report bacitracin sensitivities as presumptive rather than definitive identification of GABHS. Assuming that one actually has a culture of GABHS, bacitracin sensitivity is about 95% to 99% sensitive and 83% specific compared to the Lancefield technique. In addition, from 1% to 6% of colonies of other kinds of streptococci may be bacitracin-sensitive. These problems are most likely to result in false-positive rather than false-negative results. Fluorescent antibody and latex agglutination tests are sometimes used in place of bacitracin sensitivity tests; they are more expensive, but are faster and perform slightly better.

A final issue in evaluating cultures involves the number of presumed GABHS colonies on an original plate. Some workers feel that light growth—fewer than 10 colonies—may be indicative of a carrier state rather than active infection. Given the variability in swabbing techniques, it seems prudent to consider any growth that is confidently identified as GABHS to be just as much evidence of infection as is heavier growth.

With all the variability, it seems reasonable to ask how well cultures can be performed in busy clinical settings where they are often performed by physicians rather than laboratory technicians. For example, when compared to tests in reference laboratories in state health departments, physician-office tests appear more likely to find false-negative than false-positive results. In one study by Rosenstein, Markowitz, and Gordis (1970), office physicians missed nearly 19% percent of $\beta$-hemolytic streptococci isolated by a state laboratory from duplicate specimens. The physicians missed more than 30% of $\beta$-hemolytic streptococci when there was only light growth of the organism. Despite these difficulties, culture techniques are the mainstay of GABHS diagnosis. Depending on the volume of testing, the cost of culturing ranges from about $2 to as little as 50 cents per patient, and culturing involves easily learned, simple technology.

*Rapid Diagnostic Tests for GABHS.* Several kinds of rapid tests for GABHS are available, and all are based on some technique for extracting and identifying group A antigen directly from throat swabs. Many of these tests have not been subjected to rigorous testing against carefully performed, paired throat swabs, so how well they perform is unknown. The advantage is that they produce results in 5 to 60 minutes, enabling treatment decisions to be made immediately.

Most rapid tests use either an acid solution or an enzyme to extract group A antigen. The tests then use a variety of methods, such as agglutination of latex particles coated with antibodies to group A protein or enzyme-linked colorimetric assays similar to ELISA techniques, to identify the antigen. In another type of rapid test, an enzyme produced by the GABHS cleaves a substrate, forming a fluorescent molecule that can be detected under ultraviolet light. These procedures, ranging from $2 to $4 per test, are more expensive than culture techniques and require varying levels of skill and special equipment. Another problem in assessing their clinical utility is that most published accounts have used laboratory technicians to perform the tests, even though they are made to be used by physicians in office settings. Latex agglutination tests, in particular, are difficult to interpret without a fair amount of supervised training.

Data on the performance of rapid tests vary greatly depending on the test used, the population studied, and the standard used for comparison. Pending studies using better culture standards and taking place in clinical settings, it is difficult to make firm recommendations on the use of rapid tests. Most authorities suggest a two-step approach. First, clinicians should select only tests that have been subjected to at least one carefully controlled study that has been published in a peer-reviewed journal. Second, clinicians should try the test in their own practice in parallel with the best culture techniques to which they have access, preferably duplicate cultures. Only after the test performs well in that setting should it be adopted for routine use.

*Using Tests for GABHS.* Most dilemmas involved in using tests for GABHS arise because microbiologic positivity on a test is not equivalent to clinical positivity. Thus, the clinician must combine an assessment of a patient's clinical picture with knowledge of the community's streptococci epidemiology to determine whether a test for GABHS is worth obtaining and, if so, to interpret the result. The decision to test is also influenced by the clinician's treatment goals. The following discussion is predicated on a desire both to treat acute morbidity and to prevent long-term complications.

No single symptom or group of symptoms has been identified to predict accurately which patients with pharyngitis have GABHS infection. With abrupt onset, symptoms such as fever, headache, abdominal pain, tender cervical adenopathy, tonsillar exudates, and scarlatiniform rash are highly suggestive of GABHS infection, and, in epidemic situations, may be highly predictive as well. In settings of endemic infection, however, many of these symptoms can be caused by other organisms as well as by GABHS, and their predictive value falls drastically. The presence of coryza, cough, and more generalized oropharyngeal or respiratory symptoms can be used to weigh against the possibility of GABHS. Physicians do not always agree on the presence of symptomatology. In one study (Wood, 1979), kappa scores for two physicians evaluating patients with sore throats were only .74 for whether the patient had a sore throat and .37 for whether the throat examination was abnormal.

The prevalence of GABHS carrier status in a community is an important part of interpreting test data. This varies from season to season and with the age of the child. Studies estimate that up to 50% of children have streptococci in their pharynx at some time during the year, with the prevalence of carriers peaking at the end of streptococci season. Thus, the clinical value of a positive test diminishes greatly at certain times of the year. At those times, physicians may find it more useful simply to treat patients with a high clinical likelihood of having GABHS infection.

Table 164-5 summarizes one approach to using tests for GABHS. It is divided into two sections, one for low-prevalence and one for high-prevalence periods, and further divided by the availability of culture or rapid diagnostic tests. Tests are used only in situations of relative uncertainty, such as when a patient's symptoms are relatively equivocal compared to the likelihood that GABHS is causing pharyngitis in the community. Testing is more useful if a reliable rapid test is available; otherwise, the priority is on alleviating acute symptoms without waiting for a test result in all but the most questionable cases.

## Screening for Iron-Deficiency Anemia

Traditionally, clinicians try to detect and treat iron-deficiency anemia both for its potential growth-limiting effects and as a marker for general poor nutritional status. There is increasing evidence, however, that clinically important effects of iron deficiency may occur before the onset of anemia.

### Methods

*Hematocrit.* Determination of the hematocrit is among the most common methods of screening for iron-deficiency anemia. The hematocrit is the percentage of blood volume occupied by the red blood cells. It can be measured in a number of ways, each of which has its own sources of error and its own clinical advantages.

The microcapillary tube method is one of the most common ways of determining a hematocrit. A fine capillary tube coated with anticoagulant is filled with blood, and the tube is centrifuged to pack the red blood cells to their minimum volume. Small office centrifuges capable of achieving the proper force cost less than $1000 and require a minimum of skill to operate. Well-mixed blood is added to the tubes until they are two thirds to three fourths filled. The tubes are plugged at one end with a claylike substance. The tubes are placed in the centrifuge with the stoppered end out and spun for at least 5 minutes, or 10 minutes if the hematocrit is thought to be greater than 50. Duplicate tubes should always be run, and results should agree to within 1 hematocrit point. Lack of agreement can indicate insufficient centrifugation or inadequate mixing of blood before filling the tubes. Sickle-cell disease and other conditions that interfere with cell packing can produce erroneously high results, while a centrifuge that has overheated from heavy use or high ambient temperatures can lyse red cells and give falsely low results.

Blood for microhematocrits frequently is obtained directly from a finger punctured with a lancet or other device. Careful technique is required. In infants, warming of an extremity is sometimes recommended to obtain adequate blood flow. Excessive squeezing risks extracting interstitial fluid and diluting the blood, yielding a falsely low hematocrit. The first drop of blood should be wiped away because it is more likely to be diluted than are later drops. Alternatively, constricting the blood flow to the area may falsely increase the measured hematocrit. In children younger than 1 week, fingerstick or heelstick hematocrits are generally higher than venous samples. By 1 year of age, a venous sample usually yields a higher hematocrit than one from a fingerstick.

Hematocrits can also be calculated from blood indices measured in automated counting devices. These machines can measure directly the average red-cell volume and the number of red cells per unit volume of blood. The product of these two measurements approximates the hematocrit. This calculated hematocrit often varies from the value obtained by spinning blood. Although this variation usually is small—a few percentage points—it can prove clinically significant if a fixed cut point is used to label patients as being anemic.

It is difficult to establish useful normal values for hematocrits and other red-cell indices. A first difficulty for any determination of normal is the establishment of some gold standard. When hematocrit is used to screen for iron deficiency, the gold standard most commonly accepted is response to a trial of iron therapy. Hematocrits are relatively poor predictors of response, with the result that cut points for low hematocrits are more indicative of screening goals than of physiologic differences between normal and abnormal populations.

For example, Garby and coworkers (1969) conducted a study of apparently healthy Swedish women with low to low–normal hematocrits. After an initial hematocrit level was established, the women were given a 3-month trial of iron; whether they responded with a rise in hematocrit from the initial value was determined. Choosing an optimum cut point in initial hematocrit to make the fewest errors in predicting whether an individual would respond to iron gave a sensitivity of only 79% and a specificity of 93%. Choosing a cut point that is better for screening could raise the sensitivity to 97%, but lower specificity to 47%. Put another way, the screening test would identify nearly all

TABLE 164-5. One Possible Approach to Decisions to Test or Treat for Streptococcal Pharyngitis

| Suspicion of Disease Based on Symptoms | Low | | High | |
|---|---|---|---|---|
| | Throat Culture | Rapid Test | Throat Culture | Rapid Test |
| Low | Test or do nothing | | Test | Test |
| Moderate | Test | Test | Treat | Test |
| High | Treat | Test | Treat | Treat |

The header spans: **Estimated Prevalence of Streptococcal Disease** over Low/High, and **Diagnostic Procedure** over the four columns.

The decision to test or treat is based on two assumptions:
1. A test can't tell disease from the carrier state, so the utility of the test is diminished in high-prevalence situations.
2. Clinical goals are both to treat acute symptoms and to prevent long-term sequelae.

persons who are iron deficient, but it would refer for further testing more than half of all persons who apparently had no need for supplemental iron.

Other difficulties in determining a normal range for hematocrits include variation by age, race, sex, time of day, the altitude at which an individual resides, and exposure to pollutants such as carbon monoxide. Age differences are of sufficient magnitude to require the use of age-specific tables or charts to interpret clinical results. Adolescent males present particular problems because increases in red-cell mass correlate with the onset of puberty rather than with chronologic age. Populations used to establish normal values also need to be carefully screened to exclude individuals with subclinical iron deficiency, lead poisoning, and hemoglobinopathies.

*Hemoglobin.* Measurement of hemoglobin is another method used widely to detect iron-deficiency anemia. Simple spectrophotometric methods measure hemoglobin as cyanmethemoglobin after reaction with certain reagents. These methods have good reliability, even in office laboratories, with 95% confidence limits within plus or minus 6%. As with determination of hematocrits, blood obtained from fingersticks or heelsticks may be diluted or concentrated with interstitial fluid, and additional error can take place when blood is pipetted and mixed with reagents. Hemoglobin concentrations also vary with a variety of patient and environmental factors. Blacks generally have hemoglobins about 0.5 g/dL lower than do whites, a phenomenon independent of age and not attributable to prevalence of poor nutritional status, thalassemia, or lead poisoning.

Hemoglobins and hematocrits do not always agree in reflecting a patient's iron status. The extent of disagreement varies with the cut points used to define anemia and with the laboratory techniques used. The following example illustrates how widely the two methods may diverge. In a study by Young and coworkers (1986), simultaneously obtained capillary microhematocrits and venous hemoglobins performed on 66 children had a kappa of only .26. Put another way, as a predictor of low hemoglobin, the capillary hematocrit was 90% sensitive (95% confidence limits 77% to 100%) and only 44% specific (95% confidence limits 29% to 57%).

*Red Blood-Cell Count.* By itself, the red blood-cell count is not often used as a screen for iron deficiency. Together with a spun hematocrit, the red blood-cell count (determined by simple, inexpensive electronic blood analyzers) can be used to calculate the mean corpuscular volume (MCV), a parameter that is very useful in screening. Otherwise, the MCV is not available except from more expensive machines.

*Mean Corpuscular Volume (MCV).* The MCV is among the most useful available blood indices. Its direct determination requires a Coulter-type cell counter, a relatively expensive piece of machinery for most physicians' offices. One advantage of MCVs over other indices is that the determination is relatively insensitive to dilutional problems that can result from improper fingerstick technique or inadequate mixing of venous blood that has settled in collection tubes. Artificially high MCVs can be caused by cold agglutinins that clump cells, a problem that can be avoided by warming the diluent to which the blood is added for counting, and by hyperglycemia, a problem that can be overcome by allowing the blood to incubate in diluent before measuring. Hyponatremia can produce a falsely low MCV, and thalassemia results in a truly low value.

When an individual becomes iron deficient, the MCV begins to fall at about the same time as the hematocrit. Pairing the MCV with either hematocrit or hemoglobin and considering a low value on either test to indicate a risk of iron deficiency can decrease the rate of false-negative screens found when hematocrit or hemoglobin are used alone. Again, care must be taken to use age- and sex-adjusted scales for normal values. The primary use of the MCV alone is to separate iron deficiency, lead poisoning, and thalassemic states from anemias due to blood loss, chronic disease, or decreased red-cell survival with increased production. In the former conditions, the MCV is usually low, while it may be normal or elevated in the latter conditions.

The range over which MCVs vary within a given individual's red cells can be measured and used, although more in diagnostic than in screening settings. The red-cell distribution width (RDW) is the coefficient of variation of the MCV (ie, the standard deviation of the measured MCVs divided by their mean). Larger RDWs indicate greater diversity in cell size. The most common use of the RDW is to differentiate thalassemia minor from iron deficiency. In the latter condition, larger numbers of reticulocytes, young red cells that are larger than mature cells, cause the RDW to be elevated.

*Erythrocyte Protoporphyrin (EP).* When iron deficiency slows the rate of hemoglobin synthesis, free molecules of protoporphyrins, precursor molecules in heme production, accumulate in red blood cells and remain in them during their lifetime in the circulation. Various processes that disrupt heme and porphyrin metabolism result in the accumulation of different types of porphyrins, with similar types being found in both iron deficiency and lead intoxication. These erythrocyte protoporphyrins can be measured readily and provide an additional means of screening. Zinc protoporphyrin (ZP) is particularly useful as a screening tool because its presence can be detected directly in whole blood with simple office equipment. Free erythrocyte protoporphyrin (FEP) also can be measured and provides equivalent clinical information, but its determination is more complicated and requires laboratory techniques.

FEP and ZP are useful tests because they are elevated in iron deficiency and lead poisoning but not in thalassemias. ZP is used increasingly as a part of hematologic screening in areas where lead poisoning is prevalent because it can help differentiate children with low-normal hematocrits who have thalassemia trait from those with iron deficiency or lead poisoning.

Both FEP and ZP values vary markedly with age. Both are high in infants younger than 2 months of age and remain at higher than adult levels throughout infancy. Both can also be elevated falsely, relative to the diagnosis of iron deficiency, in the presence of inflammatory conditions.

*Follow-Up Tests for Iron Deficiency.* The choice of follow-up tests after screening usually depends on the local prevalence of other conditions that must be differentiated from iron deficiency. Tests frequently performed include hemoglobin electrophoresis in areas with a high prevalence of sickle-cell disease and other hemoglobinopathies, blood lead determinations, a reticulocyte count, and examination of the peripheral blood smear. Economic factors also may play a role. In some situations, simply offering a therapeutic trial of iron to all children who screen positive may be indicated.

Other tests such as transferrin saturation, serum ferritin, and serum iron can be used in ambiguous situations, but they require relatively elaborate laboratory procedures and are subject to error due to inflammation or normal diurnal variation. In general, they are highly specific but not very sensitive tests for iron deficiency.

## The White Blood-Cell Count and Differential

Physicians offer many reasons for ordering a WBC, with or without a differential. Sometimes the WBC comes as part of a complete blood count (CBC) that has been ordered for another reason. In this case, the WBC may contain little useful information, or even be a cause for concern when one or more of the patient's white blood-cell lines is present in a slightly greater or lesser quantity than normal. In pediatric practice, most WBCs are ordered as part of evaluations for possible infection, or to follow the course of a patient who is being treated for infection. Other goals of the WBC and differential may be to diagnose hematologic malignancies or immunodeficiency states.

## Methods

*Total WBC.*   Manual WBCs are performed by first mixing a precise amount of blood with a combination diluent/stain/red-cell-lysing solution, usually acetic acid or 0.1N HCl with methylene blue added as a stain, to obtain a 1:20 dilution. A small amount of the mixture is placed on a hemocytometer, a precision-ground glass stage that, when fitted with a microscope cover slip, creates a chamber of known volume within which cells can be counted. Under a microscope with a 10× objective, cells are counted in five areas that are each 1-mm square. Because the counting chamber is 0.1 mm deep, this count gives the number of cells in 0.5 mm$^3$ of the diluted blood. Multiplying this figure by 40 gives the number of cells in 20 mm$^3$ of diluted blood, or in 1 mm$^3$ of the original sample.

This procedure is subject to error at many stages, the most common resulting from inaccurate pipetting during dilution, overfilling of the hemocytometer, and miscounting. These errors are then multiplied when calculating the actual WBC, with the result that most counts by this method are accurate to only plus or minus 15% to 25% of the measured value.

Most laboratories and many offices use electronic cell counters that are faster than manual methods and provide results that are accurate to about plus or minus 5%. Electronic counters also have their sources of error, however, among the most common being failure to count the diluent/lysing solution with which the blood is mixed. When it becomes contaminated, it can contain particles that the machine mistakenly identifies as cells.

*Differential Counts.*   White blood-cell differential counts often are performed manually. A thin smear of fresh, well-mixed, anticoagulated blood is made on a microscope slide or cover slip and stained with Wright's stain. The stained smear is then examined with an oil-immersion objective, and the frequency distribution of cell types in 100 to 200 consecutive white cells is tallied. This "differential count" can be reported as a frequency distribution. Alternatively, each frequency count converted into a fraction of the total cells counted can be multiplied by the total WBC to yield absolute counts for the various cell types present.

Manual differentials present two major problems for the clinician. They are time-consuming to perform and they require a skilled observer to differentiate properly the various cell types present. Both of these factors contribute to a relatively high cost per test. For these reasons, various automated methods of performing differential counts have been introduced. It is important that clinicians realize what sort of method is being used by the laboratory they use.

The most basic automated methods still use human observers for all cell identification, but they achieve increased efficiency by automatically focusing the slide under special high-resolution optics and allowing the technician to enter the differential directly into a computer reporting system. A next generation of machines uses computer image-recognition techniques to examine cells automatically, signaling an operator when the computer is unable to recognize a certain cell. Both methods provide results that are comparable in accuracy and information content to results of manual differentials.

Some clinical laboratories are introducing differential counts that no longer rely on optical imaging. Machines classify cells by size, color, and other parameters. These techniques do not produce conventional differential counts. Classification by size, for example, produces a three-part differential that sorts cells into small (mostly lymphocytes), medium (mostly monocytes, blasts, and immature neutrophils), and large (most granulocytes) categories. The machines are programmed to flag samples for manual examination if there is an unusual distribution of cell sizes or if unusual cell sizes appear.

The clinical utility of such devices remains to be assessed fully. In one study by Nelson and coworkers (1985), a three-part differential was about 57% sensitive and 88% specific in identifying abnormal smears compared to the results when technicians performed manual differential counts. On an adult general medical service, this led to a false-positive rate of 48% and a false-negative rate of 6%. The authors concluded that, even if half of the positive three-part counts had to be followed up manually as required in the study, the machine still could save money. The false-negative rate was comparable to that of 100-cell manual differential counts performed by technicians on routine samples. The study found that improperly obtained capillary blood specimens could generate bizarre three-part differentials, which, theoretically, are flagged by the machine.

## Sources of Error

All methods of performing differential counts are subject to at least one of the following sources of error. Along with the data below on clinical utility, the sources of error refine the indications for obtaining the test or a total WBC.

*Physiologic Variation.*   WBC counts and, to a lesser extent, differential counts vary among healthy individuals and from examination to examination of the same individual. This variation is manifested in the wide range of values usually quoted as normal. WBCs have been found to vary with time of day, smoking, stress, exercise, and administration of certain drugs. Age-specific variation, especially in neonates, is discussed below.

*Statistical Errors.*   The average adult human has more than 10$^9$ WBCs circulating in the blood. Thus, estimates of the number of five or six cell types, drawn from a sample of 100 or 200 cells, may contain a fairly large amount of error. Precise confidence limits for differential counts can be calculated using statistical theory. Rumke (1975) developed tables giving critical values below which a change in a component of a differential (the percentage of neutrophils, for example) was probably (95% confidence) due to chance. For a 100-cell differential and a cell-type frequency of between 20% and 80%, a difference of less than 10% on serial differentials is almost never statistically significant. For a 50-cell differential, frequently performed in leukopenic patients, a change of 16% or more is required to produce more variation on sequential differentials than is expected by chance.

*Errors in Technique.*   Differential counts also can be in error because of laboratory problems. Cells may not always be distributed uniformly on a smear, or they may be identified incorrectly. Band and mature neutrophils are often confused, as are monocytes, lymphocytes, and atypical lymphocytes.

## Clinical Uses of the WBC and Differential

As discussed in a previous example, no single test determines which patients have serious bacterial infections or septicemia. The total WBC, however, and, in some cases, the total number of neutrophils or the relative number of immature and mature neutrophils can help identify patients who, as a group, are at higher risk of having one of these conditions.

*Immediate Neonatal Period.* The total WBC, neutrophil count, and band count vary enormously in the first days of life, rising to a peak at 10 to 18 hours, then gradually declining toward values found later in infancy. Total WBCs reported during this period must be corrected for the presence of nucleated red blood cells that can be miscounted as white cells. The standard correction formula is to multiply the total number of nucleated cells (red and white) by $100/(NRBC + 100)$, where $NRBC$ = the number of nucleated red cells in a 100-cell differential count.

When age-specific (hour-by-hour) standards were used, Manroe and coworkers (1979) found that neutropenia was the single best predictor of sepsis in the immediate neonatal period. When three different white-cell indices—total neutrophils, total bands, and the band-to-neutrophil ratio—were combined, the study found no child who later proved to have sepsis to be normal on all three indices. In contrast, more than 98% of children who were sick with respiratory distress syndrome, asphyxia, or non-physiologic jaundice, but who did not develop infection, were normal on all three measures.

*Age of Less Than 1 Month.* When the infant is outside the neonatal period but younger than 1 month of age, the total WBC and neutrophil or band counts do not appear useful in predicting children who have bacteremia. In a study of febrile infants by Caspe and coworkers (1983), only two of seven infants at less than 1 month of age who developed bacteremia had elevated WBCs (more than $15,000/mm^3$) compared to three of four older infants.

*Over 1 Month of Age.* When the infant is older than 1 month of age, the total WBC appears to be the most helpful leukocyte index for identifying children at increased risk of bacteremia. As higher WBCs are used as a cutoff, the sensitivity of the test decreases, but the predictive value of a positive test increases. A cutoff of $10,000/mm^3$ as the upper limit of normal gives a sensitivity of about 90% and a specificity of about 38%. Given a 3.8% prevalence of bacteremia in sick infants without an apparent source of infection, the chance of bacteremia in a child with a WBC higher than 10,000 is 1 in 20, while a child with a count of less than 10,000 but more than 5000 has only 1 chance in 125 of being bacteremic (McLellan, 1986). Low WBCs, below 5000, occur less frequently but are considered an ominous sign of possibly overwhelming infection.

What use, then, is it to obtain a differential WBC, at least by conventional methods? It probably is true that serial differential white counts have little use in following the course of patients once they are found to be septic and receive treatment; small variations in the counts are difficult to interpret and changes in the total WBC are highly correlated with changes in the total neutrophil count. Thus, any monitoring may be limited to the total WBC.

On the other hand, examination of the smear by a trained observer can yield valuable information and is warranted for any patient in whom occult sepsis or a malignancy is in the differential diagnosis or when immunosuppression or bone marrow dysfunction is possible. Degenerative changes in neutrophils, especially vacuolization but also "toxic" granulations, appear to be fairly sensitive and specific indicators of bacteremia or significant infection (sensitivity 81%, specificity 93%), according to Liu and coworkers (1984). Vacuolization, however, usually does not occur in every neutrophil. In Liu's study, vacuoles were found in from 6% to 76% of neutrophils in any patient who had them. The technique used in the study was to examine 100 neutrophils, not 100 white cells, before concluding that vacuolization or toxic granules were present.

## Urinalysis and Culture to Detect Urinary Tract Infection

A urinalysis and culture comprise several tests, each of which may have a specific goal. The following paragraphs discuss the use of urinalysis to detect infection in the urinary tract.

How the urinalysis is performed and how its results are interpreted depend on the clinical setting or the nature of the patient's symptoms. Each setting involves different practical considerations and a different prevalence or pre-test probability of finding infection. Settings in which pediatricians frequently consider obtaining urine studies include the following:

- Screening asymptomatic individuals in both low- and high-risk populations
- Attempting to diagnose UTI in children who are ill but who have only generalized symptoms or have symptoms referable to other parts of the body
  - Testing individuals with symptoms suggestive of UTI. This group can be further divided as follows:
  - Individuals with symptoms of upper tract infection (ie, fever, chills, flank pain)
  - Individuals with symptoms of bladder involvement (ie, suprapubic pain, hematuria, frequency, dysuria)
  - Individuals with symptoms suggestive of urethritis, or the so-called frequency-dysuria syndrome. Many clinicians feel this category is more properly combined with the symptoms directly above and called "lower urinary tract" infection.

None of these symptom complexes, however, proves location of infection.

### Gold Standards

As with many commonly used clinical tests, it is difficult to define a gold standard against which to compare proposed methods of diagnosing UTIs. Commonly used standards include:

- Any bacterial growth from a urine specimen obtained directly from the bladder by catheterization or suprapubic aspiration
- A single culture with a colony count of $10^5$ or more organisms per milliliter of midstream urine obtained by the clean-catch method from symptomatic patients. As discussed below, this standard is probably high and misses many individuals who would have growth if a specimen were obtained directly from the bladder. Its applicability probably also is limited to infection with *Escherichia coli*, although this organism accounts for more than 80% of all UTIs.
- Two or more cultures obtained over several days with colony counts of $10^5$ or more organisms per milliliter of midstream, clean-catch urine from asymptomatic patients. This standard represents the controversy about the meaning and significance of isolated or persistent asymptomatic bacteriuria. Many clinicians feel bacteriuria without associated pyuria and symptoms represents a temporary state of urinary tract colonization rather than active infection.

Most techniques used in the diagnosis of UTI were developed originally for adult populations. It is generally assumed, but not known, that the results can be applied to children as well. It is especially likely that differences exist for children younger than 2 to 3 months of age, among whom the epidemiology of UTI is strikingly different from that of older children and adults. In the first months of infancy, male patients with UTIs outnumber females, while the opposite is true in later life. Infection in this age group may also result from hematogenous spread, whereas it is usually believed to ascend the urinary tract from outside sources in older individuals.

## Obtaining Urine for Analysis

The method by which urine is obtained for study influences the interpretation of urinalysis results. Urine that exits the urethra before being collected must cross potentially contaminated surfaces adjacent to the urethral meatus. Urine also may be contaminated by secretions from the vagina or from under the foreskin, so cells and bacteria from these sources must be distinguished from those present in the urine.

The suprapubic bladder tap is the method least likely to contain contaminants or introduce them into the urinary tract. Except for patients with genitourinary tract anomalies, the procedure has a low rate of complications, but it risks not obtaining a specimen if there is little urine in the bladder. Suprapubic taps are used best when a definitive specimen is needed urgently so therapy can be started.

Catheterization through the urethra obtains urine directly from the bladder. In very young children, catheterization carries a certain risk of trauma. In females, it may be difficult to visualize the urethra; in males, it may be difficult to thread the catheter into the bladder. The procedure should be stopped if the urethral meatus cannot be identified definitively or if resistance is encountered while the catheter is maneuvered.

Proper cleansing of the periurethral area before catheterization is imperative, both to avoid collection of a false-positive specimen and to reduce the risk of introducing bacteria into the urinary tract. In early studies of UTI microbiology, 2% of asymptomatic adult women who underwent urethral catheterization subsequently developed frequency and dysuria (Kass, 1956). Thus, antibiotic coverage is indicated after catheterization of very young children, who may not exhibit specific signs of UTI, or children suspected of having a urinary tract anomaly. Unless it is known that antibiotics will be administered subsequently, catheterization is contraindicated in very young, uncircumcised males whose foreskins cannot be retracted for adequate cleaning of the glans. The risk of contamination is high, and the lack of specific symptoms makes subsequent iatrogenic infection difficult to detect.

A midstream, clean-catch urine sample usually is sufficient when the patient's perineum can be adequately cleaned. Cleaning should be with a soap solution rather than a bactericidal substance so small amounts in the urine sample do not inhibit bacterial growth. In infants, a urine bag can provide good results if used properly. After the perineum is cleaned carefully and dried, the bag is applied, leaving as little room for leaks as possible. The bag must be removed promptly after the child urinates, and the urine must be removed from the bag using aseptic technique.

## Chemical Tests on Urine

After gross inspection for blood, pus, or abnormal pigmentation, the first step in most urinalyses is to perform a series of chemical tests to detect occult blood, ketones, glucose, bilirubin, and protein and to determine the urine's specific gravity and pH. Because this discussion involves the detection of UTIs, it focuses only on tests for blood, pH, and specific gravity.

Most clinicians test for occult blood in the urine with a dipstick. Hemoglobin and myoglobin in the urine react with a reagent in the dipstick to produce a color change that is matched against a standard printed on the dipstick's container. This matching can be performed best in natural or incandescent light. The test reveals intact erythrocytes, hemoglobin derived from intravascular hemolysis, and myoglobin. Microscopic examination of the urine for red cells and specific tests for myoglobin are often needed as follow-up for a positive test.

Some dipsticks available commercially reveal as little as 0.02 to 0.03 mg/dL of free hemoglobin or about 15 to 20 erythrocytes per microliter, both of which are felt to be below the threshold of clinical significance (Norman, 1987). Depending on the type of dipstick, indications of trace hemolyzed blood and levels of 1+, or greater than 50 erythrocytes per microliter, can be used as indicators of abnormally high levels of heme, myoglobin, or blood in the urine.

Several conditions may cause red cells to be present in the urine in varying quantities. Microscopic hematuria may follow trauma or vigorous exercise and is found without any accompanying symptoms in a small portion of apparently normal children. In combination with other findings, it may be indicative of anatomic anomalies, renal tumors, hemoglobinopathies, and nephritis. Hematuria associated with infection of the urogenital tract is usually accompanied by pyuria and symptoms such as suprapubic or flank pain and dysuria.

Urine pH also is usually measured with a dipstick. The measurement is useful in a variety of conditions. In the context of UTI, knowledge of pH is important in the evaluation of the urine sediment and as a predictor of the type of organism causing the infection. Elevations in urine pH can reduce drastically the survival of leukocytes. White cells remain intact in relatively acid urine (pH of less than 6.8) for as long as 48 to 72 hours, but at a more alkaline pH, their survival decreases markedly (Stansfeld, 1962). At a pH of 8.4, most white cells are no longer visible after a few minutes. A high pH, more than 7, is sometimes found in conjunction with UTIs caused by urea-splitting organisms such as *Proteus* species.

Urine specific gravity is most often measured with a refractometer, a device that indirectly measures a liquid's specific gravity by measuring the refraction of light as it passes through a small sample. It requires only a single drop of urine and the determination can be made in seconds. The disadvantage is that protein and glucose dissolved in the urine can give falsely elevated results. As with urine pH, determination of specific gravity is useful in many settings. Its main function in the setting of UTI is to signal a dilute urine in which bacterial colony counts may be falsely lowered.

## Examination of the Urinary Sediment

The term *sediment* suggests that particulates, cells, casts, crystals, and microorganisms suspended in the urine are only detected after centrifugation. Examination of both unspun and centrifuged urine may be required to diagnose UTI. Either examination may require quantifying what is observed. This has been accomplished traditionally by counting the number of objects per high-power field under a microscope, a method that lacks reproducibility. The size of a drop under a microscope slide can vary widely, even though it is usually about .05 mm$^3$, and the very small volume results in too great a sampling error for reliable diagnosis. The size of the field also makes it difficult to count more than a small number of objects.

More accurate and reproducible results are obtained by counting objects in urine with a hemocytometer. The hemocytometer allows counting of a fixed volume (ie, the central square contains 0.1 mm$^3$) and provides a smaller visual field with more uniform illumination so smaller objects can be seen more easily.

When tests call for centrifuged urine, a careful and reproducible procedure should be followed. A variety of procedures are recommended. The clinician should choose one and stick to it to develop experience with specimens prepared consistently. A fixed quantity of well-mixed urine (eg, 5 mL) is centrifuged at 2000 to 4000 rpm for 5 to 10 minutes in a conical-bottom tube. For non-quantitative tests, the supernatant is decanted by inverting the tube for 5 seconds, and the upright tube is shaken to suspend the pellet in the residual urine in the bottom of the tube. A Pasteur pipette can be used to remove one or two drops, which are then spread over a small (1 × 2 cm) area of a microscope slide (Jenkins, 1986). For quantitative work, the pellet is suspended in unspun urine to make a new volume of 1 mL; graduated tubes make this easier. The resulting concentration factor (ie, 5 if one starts with 5 mL of unspun urine) can be applied to observations in a hemocytometer to obtain results equivalent to concentrations in the unspun urine.

## Examination for White Blood Cells in Urine

White blood cells are continually excreted from the urinary tract. Under normal conditions, about 400,000 cells an hour leave the kidneys, or about 10 white cells per cubic millimeter of urine in an adult. When infection is present, the number of white cells in the urine increases, which can be used as an aid in diagnosis.

At least among adult patients, pyuria—defined as more than 10 WBC/mm$^3$—appears to be a very sensitive and specific indicator of infection (Stamm, 1983). It is found in more than 95% of symptomatic patients with bacteriuria of more than 10$^2$ colonies per milliliter, but in less than 1% of asymptomatic patients without bacteriuria. As discussed below, patients with pyuria but with urine bacterial counts of less than 10$^2$ colonies per milliliter on standard cultures are likely to have infection with *Chlamydia trachomatis, Neisseria gonorrhoeae,* or staphylococcus.

Pyuria appears to be a slightly less sensitive indicator of infection among children than it is among adults, although studies using equivalent cut points have not been conducted. Corman (1982) studied 100 children being evaluated for possible UTI in an outpatient setting. Using a cutoff of 50 WBC/mm$^3$ (five cells in the 0.1-mm$^3$ center area of a hemocytometer) in unspun urine to define infection gave a sensitivity of 64% and a specificity of 91% compared to culture results (positive defined as 10$^5$ or more colonies per milliliter). Ginsburg (1982), using a cutoff of 10 WBC in unspun urine per high-power dry microscope field, obtained a sensitivity of 70% among infants younger than 2 years who were hospitalized with culture-proven UTIs.

Examination of unspun urine with a hemocytometer is the best method for quantifying white cells. If a hemocytometer is not available, some estimates can be derived from examination of centrifuged urinary sediment, although they are much less reproducible. Stansfeld (1962) estimated that one white cell in spun sediment per high-powered field was equivalent to about five to six cells per cubic millimeter in unspun urine. Kusumi and coworkers (1981) found that counting white cells in centrifuged urine could miss individuals with small but significant degrees of pyuria. Twenty-eight percent of patients with 10 to 100 WBCs/mm$^3$ in their unspun urine had an average of less than 5 white cells per field when 10 fields of spun urine were examined. This rate of false-negative results fell, however, as the degree of pyuria increased.

Semiquantitative tests for leukocyte esterase in urine are gaining acceptance as a screening tool for pyuria that does not require microscopy. White cells contain esterases that are not otherwise present in urine, serum, or renal tissue. Reagents that react with these esterases and yield visible color changes have been incorporated into dipsticks. The dipstick is immersed in urine and then removed; within 15 to 30 minutes it can be compared against a color chart to determine if esterase is present.

The esterase test has proved to be highly specific (more than 94%) and moderately sensitive (75% to 95%, depending on the study). Intact white cells are not required for a positive test, so dilute or high-pH specimens in which white cells may no longer be visible can still be tested reliably.

## Counting Bacteria With Microscopy

Direct observation of urine for the presence of bacteria is another method frequently employed to determine rapidly the probability of UTI, and possibly to avoid the need for subsequent cultures. Several possible approaches vary in the ease with which they can be performed and the accuracy of their results (Jenkins, 1986).

*Observation of Unspun Urine.* Observation of unspun urine is probably best for specimens that have relatively high specific gravity, appear grossly cloudy, or are obtained from symptomatic individuals who do not give a history of urinary frequency. These are all situations in which the concentration of bacteria is likely to be high:

1. One drop of fresh, unstained urine, under a microscope coverslip. This method, although widely recommended, is probably not reliable enough to warrant routine use. Serious problems include wide variation in the size of the drop and difficulty in differentiating bacteria from crystals and amorphous debris.
2. A hemocytometer with fresh, unstained urine. The hemocytometer improves lighting and provides a uniform volume for counting organisms. It is still difficult to differentiate individual cocci from crystals and other objects. Using a cutoff of more than 5 organisms per 0.1 mm$^3$, the central area of a hemocytometer, and a culture with more than 10$^5$ colonies/mL as a gold standard, Corman (1982) obtained a sensitivity of 96% and a specificity of 89% among children being evaluated for possible UTI. The sensitivity fell to 65% and the specificity rose to 96% if 10$^3$ colonies/mL or more was used as a standard for infection. Thus, at least in a symptomatic population, positive results using this method predict a relatively high likelihood of infection. Negative results require follow-up tests such as a quantitative culture.
3. Gram stain of unspun urine: one or two drops of fresh, mixed urine are spread over a small area on a microscope slide, allowed to air dry, and Gram stained. Jenkins (1986) suggested looking at five fields with an oil-immersion objective. Although results obtained using this method are probably quite variable because the drops are not spread in a fixed area, several studies in adult patients suggest that finding any bacteria among the five fields searched is about 90% sensitive for a culture with 10$^5$ or more colonies/mL. Gram stain is superior to direct observation for identifying cocci and deciding whether a single organism or a mixture of flora is present. Its major disadvantages are the variability of quantification, which may be reduced if the clinician uses some reproducible technique, and the time and skill needed to perform the staining.

*Examination of Centrifuged Urine* Examination of centrifuged urine is probably best for individuals in whom low colony counts are expected, such as in patients with dilute urine or a history of urinary frequency. A consistent method of centrifugation must be used.

1. Examination of unstained sediment. This method has the advantage of concentrating the solid contents of the urine and allowing observation of casts and other cells in addition to bacteria. In a scan of five high-power (dry-objective) fields, finding an average of one or more bacteria per field has a sensitivity of about 95% for cultures of 10$^5$ or more colonies/mL. Using an average of 10 or more bacteria per field as a cut-off has a sensitivity of about 80% but a specificity of more than 95%. Thus, a positive test predicts a relatively high probability of significant bacteriuria.
2. Gram stain of spun sediment. This method is probably best for individuals in whom either contamination of the specimen or low concentrations of a true pathogen are expected. It provides the best opportunity to differentiate between various types of organisms and debris. Seeing any organisms, especially if there is one predominant morphology, on a scan of five oil-immersion fields has been reported to have a sensitivity of more than 95% and a specificity of about 66%. Specificity can be improved to more than 90%, with a cor-

responding drop in sensitivity, if the criteria for a positive test are raised to an average of two or more organisms per field.

One strategy for combining these methods is to use a hemocytometer and examination of unspun, unstained urine as an initial screen. If the test is positive, significant bacteriuria is likely. If it is negative and if there are symptoms or other positive tests suggestive of infection, a centrifuged, Gram-stained specimen can be examined. The chosen strategy depends on the population being examined, the cost and availability of quantitative cultures, and the need perceived for immediate treatment.

### Cultures to Diagnose Significant Bacteriuria

Quantitative culture, often followed by a determination of antimicrobial sensitivities, is the "standard" method of diagnosing significant bacteriuria and presumed UTI. These procedures most often are performed in central laboratories, but dipslide methods potentially permit nearly equivalent determinations of organism type and concentration in an office.

Standard quantitative cultures are performed by transporting a urine specimen to a laboratory and inoculating plates with a calibrated wire loop. The plates are read at 1 and 2 days to determine colony type and number. The so-called dipslide method uses a plastic slab or paddle coated on two sides with two different types of media. Each type permits or inhibits the growth of particular organisms while stains incorporated in the media are differentially taken up by various organisms and further help with identification. Materials packaged with the dipstick help identify colonies and enable estimates of the colony count per milliliter of urine.

Dipslides can be inoculated in the office or at the bedside simply by dipping them in a cup of urine or pouring the sample over each side of the slide. When this is done promptly, it circumvents the need to refrigerate specimens or use costly messenger services and reduces the chance of false-positive cultures. Once inoculated, dipslides can be stored at room temperature and either sent to a laboratory or retained in the office for reading. When read by experienced technicians, they can yield results equivalent or even superior to results of standard culture techniques. Their only major area of weakness is that the media used are relatively selective; thus, many contaminants and some less common pathogens such as streptococci do not grow well. Catheter or bladder tap specimens that may have low concentrations of organisms or that come from patients likely to have an unusual cause for their UTI should be cultured with standard procedures rather than with dipslides.

*Defining a Positive Culture.* The most common definition of a positive culture is one that has $10^5$ or more colonies or colony-forming units (CFU) per milliliter of urine. This figure was originally proposed by Kass (1956) in a study comparing asymptomatic adults with individuals who had symptoms suggestive of pyelonephritis. The $10^5$ cut point was 95% sensitive (ie, it identified 70 of 74 patients with pyelonephritis) and about 95% specific (ie, it labeled as positive about 4% of asymptomatic males and 6% of asymptomatic females). Even Kass pointed out that this cut point might not be appropriate in all settings. In particular, a lower level of growth might be expected when there is frequent voiding or rapid urine flow and organisms have less time to multiply in the bladder, the urine pH is low thereby inhibiting bacterial growth, or infection is caused by noncoliform pathogens that grow more slowly. Wide diurnal variations in colony counts have also been observed in patients with untreated UTI, with higher counts often obtained in first-voided morning urine that has stayed longest in the bladder. Some urinary or urethral pathogens, such as *C trachomatis* and *N gonorrhoeae*, do not grow at all under the processes normally used to culture urine.

Studies by Stamm and coworkers (1980, 1982) found that a cutoff of $10^2$ colonies/mL was appropriate to diagnose infection among symptomatic adult women in whom the prevalence of infection was about 50%. Using a positive culture from catheter or suprapubic specimens as a gold standard, Stamm found that half of symptomatic women with UTIs had colony counts of less than $10^3$/mL on a clean-catch specimen. The cut point of $10^2$ colonies/mL gave a sensitivity of 95% and a specificity of 85%. Importantly, Stamm did not find that patients with relatively low concentrations of organisms had more dilute urine than those with higher counts, or that they had voided more recently before giving a urine specimen. Thus, the lower cut point does not necessarily mean that symptomatic women have lower colony counts because they have greater urine flow or less time for their urine to incubate in the bladder.

Stamm's studies also demonstrated that finding multiple organisms on culture does not necessarily indicate that a clean-catch specimen has been contaminated with vaginal or perineal flora. Among symptomatic adult female patients who had $10^5$ or more coliform colonies/mL, nearly one third had other organisms cultured simultaneously from their urine. Among patients with $10^2$ to $10^5$ colonies/mL and confirmed infection by bladder tap or catheterization, nearly two thirds had more than one organism isolated from their urine.

### Rapid Tests to Detect Bacteriuria

A variety of tests have been developed to detect bacteria in the urine without standard culture techniques or microscopy. They have met with varying success, and their use probably is limited to certain settings that fit their characteristics.

The nitrite test is based on the ability of bacteria to reduce normally occurring urinary nitrate to nitrite. Dipstick versions of the test are available and are very specific but have shown varying sensitivity. Sensitivities as low as 50% have been found in symptomatic children, and as high as 80% have been found among those without symptoms (Powell, 1987). The most likely explanation for this variation in performance is that the reduction reaction takes time, from 4 to 6 hours in experimental conditions similar to those in UTIs. Thus, symptomatic children who void frequently may not retain urine in their bladder long enough for it to become positive. In addition, some bacteria, notably streptococci, do not have nitrate reductase and, thus, cannot be detected. This test seems best for screening or monitoring asymptomatic children, especially if first-voided morning urines can be obtained. Positive tests are highly suggestive of bacteriuria, but negative tests in the setting of symptoms need follow-up, probably with cultures.

Some central laboratories are also using ultrafiltration to detect bacteriuria. Urine is suctioned through a filter on which organisms are deposited and stained. Automated machinery can examine the filters and flag those that have apparently trapped organisms. In contrast to the nitrite test, filtration is very sensitive but not very specific. False positives are common when specimens are contaminated with urogenital flora or with white cells (McNeeley, 1987). In addition, from 5% to 13% of samples have been reported to clog the filters or cause abnormal staining, making the test uninterpretable.

### Using Symptoms, Bacteriuria, and Pyuria to Diagnose UTI

In practice, most clinicians use several tests in series or parallel to decide if a patient has a UTI. Among infants, data are relatively scant regarding the value of the tests described above. The lack of specific symptoms and the evidence that untreated infections at this stage in life can have especially severe consequences for later renal function suggest that systematic culturing be done with febrile children without other sources of infection and that

**TABLE 164-6. Possible Symptom- and Test-Based Approach to Diagnosis of Urinary Tract Infections in Adolescent/Adult Women**

| Symptoms/Urinalysis | | | | |
|---|---|---|---|---|
| "Urethral Syndrome"* | Cystitis† | Pyuria‡ | Culture Results | Possible Diagnosis |
| − | − | − | Not done | Normal |
| + | + | + | >$10^2$ coliforms | *Escherichia coli* UTI |
| + | − | + | <$10^5$ noncoliforms | Possible gram-positive UTI, possible GC or chlamydia |
| + | − | + | "Sterile" | Consider GC, chlamydia |
| − | − | + | >$10^5$ | Asymptomatic infection |
| − | − | − | >$10^5$ | "Colonization," significance unclear |

\* Frequency, urgency, dysuria.
† Sudden onset, suprapubic pain, gross or microscopic hematuria.
‡ Greater than 8–10 WBC/mm³ on unspun urine.
*Derived from Stamm, 1983; Stamm, et al, 1980, 1982—see references at end of chapter.*

early treatment be undertaken regardless of test results (Roberts, 1983).

Among older children and adults, it may be possible to use test results to decide on immediate or delayed treatment, or among various follow-up procedures such as quantitative urine culture and specific cultures for chlamydia or gonorrhea. Table 164-6, based on Stamm's work with adult patients, reflects two major premises: (1) that pyuria, when properly measured, is a reliable indicator of some sort of UTI and (2) that the presence of pyuria or symptoms should lower the diagnostic threshold for a positive quantitative culture below the usual $10^5$ cut point.

## Selected Readings

### Test Characteristics

Haynes RB and the Department of Clinical Epidemiology and Biostatistics. How to read clinical journals: II. To learn about a diagnostic test. Can Med Assoc J 1981;124:703.
Landis JR, Kock GG. The measurement of observer agreement for categorical data. Biometrics 1977;33:159.
Pauker SG, Kassirer JP. The threshold approach to clinical decision making. N Engl J Med 1980;302:1109.
Ransohoff DF, Feinstein AR. Problems of spectrum and bias in evaluating the efficacy of diagnostic tests. N Engl J Med 1978;299:926.
Sackett DL, Haynes RB, Tugwell P. Clinical epidemiology: a basic science for clinical medicine. Boston: Little, Brown & Co, 1985.

### Antibodies to HIV

Meyer KB, Pauker SG. Screening for HIV: can we afford the false-positive rate? N Engl J Med 1987;317:238.

### Chemistry Panels

Cebul RD, Beck RB. Biochemical profiles: applications in ambulatory screening and preadmission testing of adults. Ann Intern Med 1987;106:403.

### Iron-Deficiency Anemia

Dallman PR, Siimes M, Stekel A. Iron deficiency in infancy and childhood. Am J Clin Nutr 1980;33:86.
Evatt BL, Lewis SM, Lothe F, McArthur JR. Anemia: fundamental diagnostic hematology. Atlanta: Centers for Disease Control, United States Department of Health and Human Services, 1983.
Garby L, Irnell L, Werner I. Iron-deficiency anemia in women of fertile age in a Swedish community. III. Estimation of prevalence based on response to iron supplementation. Acta Medica Scandinavica 1969;185:113.
Young PC, Hamill B, Wasserman RC, Dickerman JD. Evaluation of the capillary microhematocrit as a screening test for anemia in pediatric practice. Pediatrics 1986;78:206.

### Streptococcal Pharyngitis

Centor RM, Meier FA, Dalton HP. Throat cultures and rapid tests for diagnosis of group A streptococcal pharyngitis. Ann Intern Med 1986;105:892.
Gerber MA, Spadaccini LJ, Wright LL, Deutsch L. Latex agglutination tests for rapid identification of group A streptococci directly from throat swabs. J Pediatr 1984;105:702.
Radetsky M, Wheeler RC, Roe M, Todd JK. Comparative evaluation of kits for rapid diagnosis of group A streptococcal disease. Pediatr Infect Dis J 1985;4:274.
Rosenstein BJ, Markowitz M, Gordis L. Accuracy of throat cultures processed in physicians' offices. J Pediatr 1970;76:606.
Todd JK. Throat cultures in the office laboratory. Pediatr Infect Dis J 1982;1:265.
Wood RW, Diehr P, Wolcott BW, et al. Reproducibility of clinical data and decisions in the management of upper respiratory illness: a comparison of physicians and nonphysician providers. Med Care 1979;27:767.

### Tuberculosis

American Thoracic Society. The tuberculin skin test. Am Rev Respir Dis 1981;123:343.
Furcolow ML, Hewell B, Nelson WE, Palmer CE. Quantitative studies of the tuberculin reaction. Pub Health Rep 1941;56:1082.

### Urinalysis

Corman LI. Simplified urinary microscopy to detect significant bacteriuria. Pediatrics 1982;70:133.
Ginsburg CM, McCracken GH. Urinary tract infections in young infants. Pediatrics 1982;69:409.
Jenkins RD, Fenn JP, Matsen JM. Review of urine microscopy for bacteriuria. JAMA 1986;255:3397.
Kass EH. Asymptomatic infections of the urinary tract. Trans Assoc Am Physicians 1956;69:56.
Kusumi RK, Grover PJ, Kunin CM. Rapid detection of pyuria by leukocyte esterase activity. JAMA 1981;245:1653.
McNeeley SG, Baselski VS, Ryan GM. An evaluation of two rapid bacteriuria screening procedures. Obstet Gynecol 1987;69:551.
Norman ME. An office approach to hematuria and proteinuria. Pediatr Clin North Am 1987;34:545.
Powell HR, McCredie DA, Ritchie MA. Urinary nitrite in symptomatic and asymptomatic urinary infection. Arch Dis Child 1987;62:138.
Roberts KB, Charney E, Sweren RJ, et al. Urinary tract infection in infants with unexplained fever: a collaborative study. J Pediatr 1983;103:864.
Stamm WE. Measurement of pyuria and its relation to bacteriuria. Am J Med 1983;75(1B):53.
Stamm WE, Counts GW, Running KR, et al. Diagnosis of coliform infection in acutely dysuric women. N Engl J Med 1982;307:463.
Stamm WE, Wagner KF, Amsel R, et al. Causes of the acute urethral syndrome in women. N Engl J Med 1980;303:409.
Stansfeld JM. The measurement and meaning of pyuria. Arch Dis Child 1962;37:257.

### White Blood-Cell Count and Differential

Caspe WB, Chamudes O, Louie B. The evaluation and treatment of the febrile infant. Pediatr Infect Dis J 1983;2:131.
Liu C-H, Lehan C, Speer ME, et al. Degenerative changes in neutrophils: an indicator of bacterial infection. Pediatrics 1984;74:823.
Manroe BL, Weinberg AG, Rosenfeld CR, Browne R. The neonatal blood count in health and disease. I. Reference values for neutrophilic cells. J Pediatr 1979;95:89.
McClellan D, Giebink GC. Perspectives on occult bacteremia in children. J Pediatr 1986;109:1.
McGowan JE, Bratton L, Klein JO, Finland M. Bacteremia in febrile children seen in a "walk-in" pediatric clinic. N Engl J Med 1973;288:1309.

Nelson L, Charache S, Keyser E, Metzger P. Laboratory evaluation of the Coulter "three-part electronic differential." Am J Clin Pathol 1985;83:547.

Rumke CL, Bezemer PD, Kuik DJ. Normal values and least significant differences for differential leukocyte counts. J Chronic Diseases 1975;28:661.

Shapiro MF, Greenfield S. The complete blood count and leukocyte differential count. An approach to their rational utilization. Ann Intern Med 1987;106:65.

*Principles and Practice of Pediatrics, Second Edition.*
edited by Frank A. Oski et al. J. B. Lippincott Company, Philadelphia © 1994.

# CHAPTER 165
# *Laboratory Values*

## Peter C. Rowe

The following reference values for laboratory tests have been drawn from the sources listed at the end of the chapter. They represent guidelines only, since the reference range from one institution to the next will vary, depending on the laboratory method used. To simplify the interpretation of laboratory results reported in International System (SI) units, conversion factors (from SI to conventional units) are provided. SI base units are the gram (g), the liter (L), and the mole (mol). Other abbreviations used throughout this chapter are listed below.

### SI Prefixes

| Factor | Prefix | Symbol |
|---|---|---|
| $10^3$ | kilo | k |
| $10^{-1}$ | deci | d |
| $10^{-2}$ | centi | c |
| $10^{-3}$ | milli | m |
| $10^{-6}$ | micro | $\mu$ |
| $10^{-9}$ | nano | n |
| $10^{-12}$ | pico | p |
| $10^{-15}$ | femto | f |

### Abbreviations

| | |
|---|---|
| CI | confidence interval |
| d | day |
| F | female |
| h | hour |
| Hb | hemoglobin |
| M | male |
| MCHC | mean corpuscular hemoglobin concentration |
| MCV | mean corpuscular volume |
| mEq | milliequivalent |
| min | minute |
| RBC | red blood cell |
| s | second |
| SD | standard deviation |
| U | unit |
| WBC | white blood cell |
| yr | year |

| BLOOD | | | |
|---|---|---|---|
| **Test** | **SI Reference Range** | **Conversion Factor** | **Conventional Units Reference Range** |
| Adrenocorticotropic hormone (ACTH) | Cord: 130–160 ng/L<br>1st week: 100–140<br>Adult 0800 h: 25–100<br>1800 h: <50 | | Cord: 130–160 pg/mL<br>1st week: 100–140<br>Adult 0800 h: 25–100<br>1800 h: <50 |
| Alanine aminotransferase (ALT) | <1 yr: 5–28 U/L<br>>1 yr: 8–20 | | Same as SI |
| Albumin | 35–50 g/L | | 3.5–5.0 g/dL |
| Aldolase | Newborn: <32 U/L<br>Child: <16<br>Adult: <8 | | Same as SI |
| Aldosterone | Newborn: 0.14–1.66 nmol/L<br>1 wk–1 yr: 0.03–4.43<br>1–3 yr: 0.14–1.66<br>3–5 yr: <0.14–2.22<br>5–7 yr: <0.14–1.39<br>7–11 yr: 0.14–1.94<br>11–15 yr: <0.14–1.39 | nmol/L × 36.1 = ng/dL | Newborn: 5–60 ng/dL<br>1 wk–1 yr: 1–160 ng/dL<br>1–3 yr: 5–60 ng/dL<br>3–5 yr: <5–80<br>5–7 yr: <5–50<br>7–11 yr: 5–70<br>11–15 yr: <5–50 |
| Alkaline phosphatase | Infant: 150–400 U/L<br>2–10 yr: 100–300<br>11–18 yr (M): 50–375<br>11–18 yr (F): 30–300<br>Adult: 30–100 | | Same as SI |
| $\alpha_1$-antitrypsin | 2–4 g/L | | 200–400 mg/dL |
| $\alpha$-fetoprotein | Fetal: peak of 2–4 g/L<br>Cord: <0.05 g/L<br>>1 yr: <30 $\mu$g/L | | Fetal: 200–400 mg/dL<br>Cord: <5<br>>1 yr: <30 |

## BLOOD (*Continued*)

| Test | SI Reference Range | Conversion Factor | Conventional Units Reference Range |
|---|---|---|---|
| Ammonia nitrogen | 9–34 µmol/L | µmol/L × 1.4 = µg/dL | 13–48 µg/dL |
| Amylase | Newborn: 5–65 U/L<br>>1 yr: 25–125 | | Same as SI |
| Androstenedione | Child: 0.17–1.7 nmol/L<br>Adult (M): 2.4–5.2<br>Adult (F): 2.7–8.0 | nmol/L × 28.7 = ng/dL | Child: 5–50 ng/dL<br>Adult (M): 70–150<br>Adult (F): 76–228 |
| Angiotensin-converting enzyme | <670 nmo l·L⁻¹·s⁻¹ | nmol·L⁻¹·s⁻¹ × 0.06 = nmol/mL/min | <40 nmol/mL/min |
| Anion gap [Na − (Cl + HCO₃)] | 7–14 mmol/L | | 7–14 mEq/L |
| Aspartate amino-transferase (AST) | <1 yr: 15–60 U/L<br>>1 yr: ≤20 U/L | | Same as SI |
| Bicarbonate | <2 yr: 20–25 mmol/L<br>>2 yr: 22–26 mmol/L | | <2 yr: 20–25 mEq/L<br>>2 yr: 22–26 |

| Bilirubin (total) | | *Preterm* | *Full Term* | µmol/L × 0.05848 = mg/dL | | *Preterm* | *Full Term* |
|---|---|---|---|---|---|---|---|
| | Cord: | <34 | <34 µmol/L | | Cord: | <2 | <2 mg/dL |
| | 0–1 d: | <137 | <103 | | 0–1 d: | <8 | <6 |
| | 1–2 d: | <205 | <137 | | 1–2 d: | <12 | <8 |
| | 3–5 d: | <274 | <205 | | 3–5 d: | <16 | <12 |
| | Thereafter: | <34 | <17 | | Thereafter: | <2 | <1 |

| Test | SI Reference Range | Conversion Factor | Conventional Units Reference Range |
|---|---|---|---|
| Bilirubin (conjugated) | 0–3.4 µmol/L | µmol/L × 0.05848 = mg/dL | 0–0.2 mg/dL |
| Calcium (ionized) | 1.12—1.23 mmol/L | mmol/L × 4 = mg/dL | 4.48–4.92 mg/dL |
| Calcium (total) | Preterm <1 wk: 1.5–2.5 mmol/L<br>Term: <1 wk: 1.75–3<br>Child: 2–2.6<br>Adult: 2.1–2.6 | mmol/L × 4 = mg/dL | 6–10 mg/dL<br>7–12<br>8–10.5<br>8.5–10.5 |
| Carbon dioxide (CO₂ content) | 22–26 mmol/L | | 22–26 mEq/L |

| Carbon monoxide (carboxyhemoglobin) | *% Total Hb* | | *Fraction of Hb Sat* |
|---|---|---|---|
| | Nonsmoker: <0.02 | | Nonsmoker: <2 |
| | Smoker: <0.01 | | Smoker: <10 |
| | Toxic: >0.20 | | Toxic: >20 |

| Test | SI Reference Range | Conversion Factor | Conventional Units Reference Range |
|---|---|---|---|
| Carotene | Infant: 0.37–1.30 µmol/L<br>Child: 0.74–2.42<br>Adult: 1.12–3.72 | µmol/L × 53.7 = µg/dL | Infant: 20–70 µg/dL<br>Child: 40–130<br>Adult: 60–200 |
| Ceruloplasmin | 1–12 yr: 300–650 mg/L<br>>12 yr: 150–600 mg/L | | 1–12 yr: 30–65 mg/dL<br>>12 yr: 15–60 |
| Chloride | 94–106 mmol/L | | 94–106 mEq/L |
| Cholesterol | Infant: 1.81–4.53 mmol/L<br>Child: 3.11–5.18<br>Adolescent: 3.11–5.44<br>Adult: 3.63–6.48 | mmol/L × 38.61 = mg/dL | Infant: 53–135 mg/dL<br>Child: 70–175<br>Adolescent: 120–200<br>Adult: 140–250 |
| Complement, C₃ | 1 mo: 0.61–1.30 g/L<br>6 mo: 0.87–1.36<br>Adult: 1.11–1.71 | | 1 mo: 61–130 mg/dL<br>6 mo: 87–136<br>Adult: 111–171 |
| Complement, C₄ | Newborn: 0.16–0.39 g/L<br>Adult: 0.15–0.45 g/L | | Newborn: 16–39 mg/dL<br>Adult: 15–45 |
| Complement, total hemolytic (CH 50) | 75–160 U/mL | | 75–160 U/mL |
| Copper | 0–6 mo: 3.1–11 µmol/L<br>6 yr: 14–30<br>12 yr: 12.6–25<br>Adult (M): 11–22<br>Adult (F): 12.6–24 | µmol/L × 6.353 = µg/dL | 0–6 mo: 20–70 µg/dL<br>6 yr: 90–190<br>12 yr: 80–160<br>Adult (M): 70–140<br>Adult (F): 80–155 |

(continued)

| BLOOD (*Continued*) | | | |
|---|---|---|---|
| **Test** | **SI Reference Range** | **Conversion Factor** | **Conventional Units Reference Range** |
| Cortisol | 0800 h (or pre-ACTH): 225–505 nmol/L<br>Post-ACTH: twice pre-ACTH value | nmol/L × 0.0362 = μg/dL | 0800 h (or pre-ACTH): 8–18 μg/dL<br>Post-ACTH: twice pre-ACTH value |
| Creatine kinase | Newborn: 76–600 U/L<br>Adult (M): 38–174<br>Adult (F): 96–140 | | Same as SI |
| Creatine kinase isoenzymes | *Fraction of Total Activity*<br>CK-BB (CK-1): absent or trace<br>CK-MB (CK-2): 0.04–0.06<br>CK-MM (CK-3): 0.94–0.96 | | *% Activity*<br>CK-BB (CK-1): absent or trace<br>CK-MB (CK-2): 4%–6%<br>CK-MM (CK-3): 94%–96% |
| Creatinine | Newborn: 27–88 μmol/L<br>Infant: 18–35<br>Child: 27–62<br>Adolescent: 44–88<br>Adult (M): 53–106<br>Adult (F): 44–97 | μmol/L × 0.0113 = mg/dL | Newborn: 0.3–1.0 mg/dL<br>Infant: 0.2–0.4<br>Child: 0.3–0.7<br>Adolescent: 0.5–1.0<br>Adult (M): 0.6–1.2<br>Adult (F): 0.5–1.1 |
| Dehydroepiandrosterone (DHEA) | Child: 3–10 nmol/L<br>Adult (M): 6–15<br>Adult (F): 7–18 | nmol/L × 0.2884 = μg/L | Child: 1–3 μg/L<br>Adult (M): 1.7–4.2<br>Adult (F): 2–5.2 |
| Dehydroepiandrosterone sulfate (DHEA-S) | 1–4 days: <52 μmol/L<br>Child: 1.6–6.6 | μmol/L × 0.37 × μg/mL | 1–4 days: <20 μg/mL<br>Child: 0.6–2.54 |
| Estradiol | *Male*<br>Pubertal stage I: 7–29 pmol/L<br>II: 40<br>III: >73<br>Adult: 29–132 | pmol/L × 0.2723 = pg/mL | 2–8 pg/mL<br>11<br>>20<br>8–36 |
| | *Female*<br>Pubertal stage I: 0–84 pmol/L<br>II: 0–242<br>III: 0–385<br>IV: 73–1101 | | 0–23 pg/mL<br>0–66<br>0–105<br>20–300 |
| | Follicular: 37–330<br>Midcycle: 367–1835<br>Luteal: 184–881 | | 10–90<br>100–500<br>50–240 |
| Free fatty acids | Child: <1.10 mmol/L<br>Adult: 0.3–0.9 | mmol/L × 28.25 = mg/dL | Child: <31 mg/dL<br>Adult: 8–25 |
| Ferritin | Child: 7–144 μg/L<br>Adult (M): 30–265<br>Adult (F): 10–110 | | Child: 7–144 ng/mL<br>Adult (M): 30–265<br>Adult (F): 10–110 |
| Fibrinogen | 2–4 g/L | | 200–400 mg/dL |
| Folate | 4–20 nmol/L | nmol/L × 0.4413 = ng/mL | 1.8–9.0 ng/mL |
| Folate (RBCs) | 340–1020 nmol/L packed cells | nmol/L × 0.4413 = ng/mL | 150–450 ng/mL |
| Follicle-stimulating hormone (FSH) | Prepubertal: <5 IU/L<br>Adult (M): 1.5–16<br>Adult (F): 2–17.2 | | Prepubertal: <5 mIU/mL<br>Adult (M): 1.5–16<br>Adult (F): 2–17.2 |
| Fructose | 55–330 μmol/L | μmol/L × 0.018 = mg/dL | 1–6 mg/dL |
| Galactose | Newborn: 0–1.11 mmol/L<br>Thereafter: <0.28 | mmol/L × 18.02 = mg/dL | Newborn: 0–20 mg/dL<br>Thereafter: <5 |

## BLOOD (*Continued*)

| Test | SI Reference Range | Conversion Factor | Conventional Units Reference Range |
|------|-------------------|-------------------|-----------------------------------|
| Gamma glutamyl transferase (GGT) | 0–3 wk: 0–130 U/L<br>3 wk–3 mo: 4–120<br>3 mo–1 yr (M): 5–65<br>3 mo–1 yr (F): 5–35<br>1–15 yr: 0–23<br>Adult: 0–35 | | Same as SI |
| Gastrin | <100 ng/L | | <100 pg/mL |
| Glucagon | 50–100 ng/L | | 50–100 pg/mL |
| Glucose | Preterm: 1.1–3.6 mmol/L<br>Full term: 1.1–6.1<br>1 wk–16 yr: 3.3–5.8<br>>16 yr: 3.9–6.4 | mmol/L × 18.02 = mg/dL | Preterm: 20–65 mg/dL<br>Full term: 20–110<br>1 wk–16 yr: 60–105<br>>16 yr: 70–115 |
| Haptoglobin | 0.4–1.8 g/L | | 40–180 mg/dL |
| Hemoglobin $A_{1c}$ | 0.039–0.077 fraction of total Hb | | 3.9%–7.7% of total Hb |
| $\beta$-Hydroxybutyrate | <100 $\mu$mol/L | $\mu$mol/L × 0.01041 = mg/dL | <1 mg/dL |
| 17-Hydroxyprogesterone | Prepubertal (M): 0.3–0.91 nmol/L<br><br>Prepubertal (F): 0.61–1.52<br>Adult (M): 0.61–5.45<br>Adult (F):<br>  Follicular: 0.61–2.42<br>  Luteal: 2.42–9.10 | nmol/L × 0.33 = ng/mL | Prepubertal (M): 0.1–0.3 ng/mL<br>Prepubertal (F): 0.2–0.5<br>Adult (M): 0.2–1.8<br>Adult (F):<br>  Follicular: 0.2–0.8<br>  Luteal: 0.8–3.0 |

| Immunoglobulins A, G, M | *IgA* | *IgG* | *IgM* |
|------|-------|-------|-------|
| | Newborn: 0–0.05 g/L | 6.4–16 g/L | 0.06–0.24 g/L |
| | 1–3 mo: 0.03–0.66 | 3.0–10.0 | 0.15–1.50 |
| | 3–6 mo: 0.04–0.90 | 1.4–10.0 | 0.15–1.10 |
| | 6–12 mo: 0.45–2.25 | 4.0–11.5 | 0.43–2.25 |
| | 1–2 yr: 0.35–2.40 | 3.5–12.0 | 0.36–2.40 |
| | 2–6 yr: 0.40–1.90 | 5.0–13.0 | 0.50–1.99 |
| | 6–12 yr: 0.40–2.70 | 7.0–16.5 | 0.50–2.60 |
| | 12–16 yr: 0.50–2.32 | 7.0–15.5 | 0.45–2.40 |
| | Adult: 0.70–3.90 | 6.5–15.0 | 0.40–3.4 |

| Test | SI Reference Range | Conversion Factor | Conventional Units Reference Range |
|------|-------------------|-------------------|-----------------------------------|
| Immunoglobulin E | Newborn: 0–24 $\mu$g/L<br>6–12 yr: 0–480<br>Adult: 0–960 | | Newborn: 0–10 U/mL<br>6–12 yr: 0–200<br>Adult: 0–400 |
| Insulin, fasting | 3–23 mU/L | | 3–23 $\mu$U/mL |
| Iron | Newborn: 20–48 $\mu$mol/L<br>4–10 mo: 5.4–12.5<br>3–10 yr: 9.5–27.0<br>Adult: 13.0–33.0 | $\mu$mol/L × 5.587 = $\mu$g/dL | Newborn: 110–270 $\mu$g/dL<br>4–10 mo: 30–70<br>3–10 yr: 53–119<br>Adult: 72–186 |
| Iron-binding capacity | Newborn: 10.6–31.3 $\mu$mol/L<br>Thereafter: 45–72 | $\mu$mol/L × 5.587 = $\mu$g/dL | Newborn: 59–175 $\mu$g/dL<br>Thereafter: 250–400 |
| Lactate | Venous: 0.5–2.0 mmol/L<br>Arterial: 0.3–0.8 | mmol/L × 9.01 = mg/dL | Venous: 5–18 mg/dL<br>Arterial: 3–7 |
| Lactate dehydrogenase | Newborn: 160–1500 U/L<br>Infant: 150–360<br>Child: 150–300<br>Adult: 100–250 | | Same as SI units |

(continued)

| | | BLOOD (*Continued*) | | |
|---|---|---|---|---|
| Test | SI Reference Range | Conversion Factor | | Conventional Units Reference Range |

| Lactate dehydrogenase isoenzymes | | *Fraction of Total* | | |
| | | LD 1 (heart): 0.24–0.34 | | |
| | | LD 2 (heart, RBCs): 0.35–0.45 | | |
| | | LD 3 (muscle): 0.15–0.25 | | |
| | | LD 4 (liver, muscle): 0.04–0.10 | | |
| | | LD 5 (liver, muscle): 0.01–0.09 | | |

**Lead**  <1.16 $\mu$mol/L  $\mu$mol/L $\times$ 20.7 = $\mu$g/dL  <24 $\mu$g/dL

**Lipids**

| | 95th %ile Values—mmol/L (mg/dL) | | 5th %ile Values—mmol/L (mg/dL) |
|---|---|---|---|
| | VLDL (Cholesterol) | LDL (Cholesterol) | HDL (Cholesterol) |
| | M / F | M / F | M / F |
| 5–9 yr: | 0.47 (18) / 0.62 (24) | 3.34 (129) / 3.62 (140) | 0.98 (38) / 0.93 (36) |
| 10–14 yr: | 0.57 (22) / 0.59 (23) | 3.41 (132) / 3.52 (136) | 0.96 (37) / 0.91 (35) |
| 15–19 yr: | 0.67 (26) / 0.62 (24) | 3.36 (130) / 3.49 (135) | 0.80 (31) / 0.91 (35) |

mmol/L $\times$ 38.61 = mg/dL

| Test | SI Reference Range | Conversion Factor | Conventional Units Reference Range |
|---|---|---|---|
| Luteinizing hormone | Prepubertal: <5 IU/L | | Prepubertal: <5 mIU/mL |
| | Adult (M): 3.9–18 | | Adult (M): 3.9–18 |
| | Adult (F): 2.0–22.6 | | Adult (F): 2.0–22.6 |
| Magnesium | 0.75–1.0 mmol/L | mmol/L $\times$ 2 = mEq/L | 1.5–2.0 mEq/L |
| Methemoglobin | <46 $\mu$mol/L | $\mu$mol/L $\times$ 0.0065 = g/dL | <0.3 g/dL |
| Osmolality | 285–295 mmol/kg | | 285–295 mOsm/kg |
| Phosphorus | Newborn: 1.36–2.91 mmol/L | mmol/L $\times$ 3.097 = mg/dL | Newborn: 4.2–9.0 mg/dL |
| | 1 yr: 1.23–2.00 | | 1 yr: 3.8–6.2 |
| | 2–5 yr: 1.13–2.20 | | 2–5 yr: 3.5–6.8 |
| | Adult: 0.97–1.45 | | Adult: 3.0–4.5 |
| Phytanic acid | <0.003 fraction of total serum fatty acids | | <0.3% of total serum fatty acids |
| Potassium | <10 days: 3.5–6.0 mmol/L | | <10 days: 3.5–6.0 mEq/L |
| | >10 days: 3.5–5.0 | | >10 days: 3.5–5.0 |

**Progesterone**

| *Male* | | |
|---|---|---|
| Prepubertal: 0.35–0.83 nmol/L | nmol/L $\times$ 0.314 = ng/mL | 0.11–0.26 ng/mL |
| Adult: 0.38–0.95 | | 0.12–0.30 |
| *Female* | | |
| Prepubertal: ≤0.95 | | ≤0.30 |
| Pubertal stage  II: ≤1.46 | | ≤0.46 |
| III: ≤1.91 | | ≤0.60 |
| IV: 0.16–41.34 | | 0.05–13.0 |
| Follicular: 0.06–2.86 | | 0.02–0.9 |
| Luteal: 19.08–95.40 | | 6.0–30.0 |

| Test | SI Reference Range | Conversion Factor | Conventional Units Reference Range |
|---|---|---|---|
| Prolactin | Newborn: <200 $\mu$g/L | | Newborn: <200 ng/mL |
| | Adult: <20 $\mu$g/L | | Adult: <20 ng/mL |
| Protein, total | Preterm: 40–70 g/L | | Preterm: 4.0–7.0 g/dL |
| | Term newborn: 50–71 | | Term newborn: 5.0–7.1 |
| | 1–3 mo: 47–74 | | 1–3 mo: 4.7–7.4 |
| | 3–12 mo: 50–75 | | 3–12 mo: 5.0–7.5 |
| | 1–15 yr: 65–86 | | 1–15 yr: 6.5–8.6 |
| Pyruvate | 0.03–0.10 mmol/L | mmol/L $\times$ 8.81 = mg/dL | 0.3–0.9 mg/dL |
| Renin | Adult: 0.30–1.14 ng$\cdot$L$^{-1}\cdot$s$^{-1}$ | ng$\cdot$L$^{-1}\cdot$s$^{-1}$ $\times$ 3.6 = ng/mL/h | Adult: 1.1–4.1 ng/mL/h |

## BLOOD (*Continued*)

| Test | SI Reference Range | Conversion Factor | Conventional Units Reference Range |
|------|-------------------|-------------------|-----------------------------------|
| Sodium | 135–145 mmol/L | | 135–145 mEq/L |
| Somatomedin C | 0–2 yr: 220–1000 IU/L | | 0–2 yr: 0.22–1.00 U/mL |
| | 3–5 yr: 270–1600 | | 3–5 yr: 0.27–1.60 |
| | 6–10 yr: 370–2100 | | 6–10 yr: 0.37–2.10 |
| | 11–12 yr: 450–2800 | | 11–12 yr: 0.45–2.80 |
| | 13–14 yr: 1100–4000 | | 13–14 yr: 1.10–4.00 |
| | 15–17 yr: 1000–2900 | | 15–17 yr: 1.00–2.90 |
| | Thereafter: 460–1500 | | Thereafter: 0.46–1.50 |
| Testosterone, free | Prepubertal: 2.08–13.19 pmol/L | | Prepubertal: 0.06–0.38 ng/dL |
| | Adult (M): 48.6–201 | | Adult (M): 1.40–5.79 |
| | Adult (F): 6.94–25 | | Adult (F): 0.20–0.73 |
| Testosterone, total | Prepubertal: 0.35–0.70 nmol/L | | Prepubertal: 10–20 ng/dL |
| | Adult (F): 0.8–2.6 | | Adult (F): 23–75 |
| | Adult (M): 9.5–30 | | Adult (M): 275–875 |
| Thyroid-stimulating hormone (TSH) | Cord: 0–17.4 μU/L | | Cord: 0–17.4 mIU/mL |
| | 1–3 days: 0–13.3 | | 1–3 days: 0–13.3 |
| | Thereafter: 0–5.5 | | Thereafter: 0–5.5 |
| Thyroxine ($T_4$), total | Cord: 95–168 nmol/L | nmol/L × 0.0775 = μg/dL | Cord: 7.4–13.0 μg/dL |
| | <1 mo: 90–292 | | <1 mo: 7.0–22.6 |
| | 1 mo–1 yr: 93–213 | | 1 mo–1 yr: 7.2–16.5 |
| | 1–5 yr: 94–194 | | 1–5 yr: 7.3–15.0 |
| | 5–10 yr: 83–172 | | 5–10 yr: 6.4–13.3 |
| | 10–15 yr: 72–151 | | 10–15 yr: 5.6–11.7 |
| | Adult: 55–161 | | Adult: 4.3–12.5 |
| Thyroxine $T_4$, free | 9–22 pmol/L | pmol/L × 0.0777 = ng/dL | 0.7–1.7 ng/dL |
| Transferrin | Newborn: 1.30–2.75 g/L | | Newborn: 130–275 mg/dL |
| | Adult: 2.20–4.00 | | Adult: 220–400 |

Triglycerides

**NORMAL UPPER LIMITS—MMOL/L (MG/DL)**

| | Male | Female |
|--|------|--------|
| | 0–4 yr: 1.12 (99) | 1.26 (112) |
| | 5–9 yr: 1.14 (101) | 1.19 (105) |
| | 10–14 yr: 1.41 (125) | 1.48 (131) |
| | 15–19 yr: 1.67 (148) | 1.40 (124) |
| | | mmol/L × 88.55 = mg/dL |

| Test | SI Reference Range | Conversion Factor | Conventional Units Reference Range |
|------|-------------------|-------------------|-----------------------------------|
| Triiodothyronine ($T_3$) | Cord: 0.23–1.16 nmol/L | nmol/L × 65.1 = ng/dL | Cord: 15–75 ng/dL |
| | <1 mo: 0.49–3.70 | | <1 mo: 32–240 |
| | 1 mo–1 yr: 1.70–4.31 | | 1 mo–1 yr: 110–280 |
| | 1–5 yr: 1.62–4.14 | | 1–5 yr: 105–269 |
| | 5–10 yr: 1.45–3.71 | | 5–10 yr: 94–241 |
| | 10–15 yr: 1.28–3.31 | | 10–15 yr: 83–215 |
| | Adult: 1.08–3.14 | | Adult: 70–204 |
| Triiodothyronine resin uptake | 0.25–0.35 | | 25%–35% |
| Urea nitrogen | 2–7 mmol/L | mmol/L × 2.8 = mg/dL | 5–20 mg/dL |
| Uric acid | 120–420 μmol/L | μmol/L × 0.0169 = mg/dL | 2–7 mg/dL |
| Vitamin A | Newborn: 1.22–2.62 μmol/L | μmol/L × 28.65 = μg/dL | Newborn: 35–75 μg/dL |
| | Child: 1.05–2.79 | | Child: 30–80 |
| | Adult: 1.05–2.27 | | Adult: 30–65 |
| Vitamin $B_6$ | 14.6–72.8 nmol/L | nmol/L × 0.247 = ng/mL | 3.6–18 ng/mL |
| Vitamin $B_{12}$ | 96–579 pmol/L | pmol/L × 1.355 = pg/mL | 130–785 pg/mL |
| Vitamin C | 11.4–113.6 μmol/L | μmol/L × 0.176 = mg/dL | 0.2–2.0 mg/dL |
| Vitamin $D_3$ (1,25 dihydroxy) | 60–108 pmol/L | pmol/L × 0.417 = pg/mL | 25–45 pg/mL |
| Vitamin E | 11.6–46.4 μmol/L | μmol/L × 0.043 = mg/dL | 0.5–2.0 mg/dL |
| Zinc | 10.7–22.9 μmol/L | μmol/L × 6.54 = μg/dL | 70–150 μg/dL |

## Hematology

| Age | HB (g/dL) Mean | HB (g/dL) −2 SD | Hematocrit (%) Mean | Hematocrit (%) −2 SD | MCV (fL) Mean | MCV (fL) −2 SD | MCHC (g/dL RBC) Mean | MCHC (g/dL RBC) −2 SD | Reticulocyte (%) | WBC (1000/mm³) Mean | WBC (1000/mm³) 95% CI | Platelets (1000/mm³) Mean (Range) |
|---|---|---|---|---|---|---|---|---|---|---|---|---|
| Term (cord blood) | 16.5 | 13.5 | 51 | 42 | 108 | 98 | 33.0 | 30.0 | 3.0–7.0 | 18.1 | 9.0–30.0 | 290 |
| 1–3 days | 18.5 | 14.5 | 56 | 45 | 108 | 95 | 33.0 | 29.0 | 1.8–4.6 | 18.9 | 9.4–34.0 | 192 |
| 2 weeks | 16.6 | 13.4 | 53 | 41 | 105 | 88 | 31.4 | 28.1 | | 11.4 | 5.0–20.0 | 252 |
| 1 month | 13.9 | 10.7 | 44 | 33 | 101 | 91 | 31.8 | 28.1 | 0.1–1.7 | 10.8 | 5.0–19.5 | |
| 2 months | 11.2 | 9.4 | 35 | 28 | 95 | 84 | 31.8 | 28.3 | | | | |
| 6 months | 12.6 | 11.1 | 36 | 31 | 76 | 68 | 35.0 | 32.7 | 0.7–2.3 | 11.9 | 6.0–17.5 | |
| 6–24 months | 12.0 | 10.5 | 36 | 33 | 78 | 70 | 33.0 | 30.0 | | 10.6 | 6.0–17.0 | (150–300) |
| 2–6 years | 12.5 | 11.5 | 37 | 34 | 81 | 75 | 34.0 | 31.0 | 0.5–1.0 | 8.5 | 5.0–15.5 | (150–300) |
| 6–12 years | 13.5 | 11.5 | 40 | 35 | 86 | 77 | 34.0 | 31.0 | 0.5–1.0 | 8.1 | 4.5–13.5 | (150–300) |
| 12–18 years (M) | 14.5 | 13.0 | 43 | 36 | 88 | 78 | 34.0 | 31.0 | 0.5–1.0 | 7.8 | 4.5–13.5 | (150–300) |
| 12–18 years (F) | 14.0 | 12.0 | 41 | 37 | 90 | 78 | 34.0 | 31.0 | 0.5–1.0 | 7.8 | 4.5–13.5 | (150–300) |

## URINE

| Test | SI Reference Range | Conversion Factor | Conventional Units Reference Range |
|---|---|---|---|
| Aminolevulinic acid | 8–53 μmol/d | μmol/d × 0.131 = mg/d | 1–7 mg/d |
| Calcium | <0.1 mmol/kg/d | mmol/d × 40 = mg/d | <4 mg/kg/d |
| Copper | <0.6 μmol/d | μmol/d × 63.7 = μg/d | <40 μg/d |
| Coproporphyrin | <300 nmol/d | nmol/d × 1.527 = μg/d | <200 μg/d |
| Cortisol, free | 70–340 nmol/d | nmol/d × 0.362 = μg/d | 25–125 μg/d |
| Creatinine | Infant: 71–177 μmol/kg/d | μmol/kg/d × 0.113 = mg/kg/d | Infant: 8–20 mg/kg/d |
| | Child: 71–194 | | Child: 8–22 |
| | Adolescent: 71–265 | | Adolescent: 8–30 |
| Cystine | 40–260 μmol/d | μmol/d × 0.12 = mg/d | 5–31 mg/d |
| Dehydroepiandrosterone (DHEA) | <5 yr: <0.3 μmol/d | μmol/d × 0.288 = mg/d | <5 yr: <0.1 mg/d |
| | 6–9 yr: <0.7 | | 6–9 yr: <0.2 |
| | 10–15 yr: <1.4 | | 10–15 yr: <0.4 |
| | Adult (M): <8.0 | | Adult (M): <2.3 |
| | Adult (F): <4.2 | | Adult (F): <1.2 |
| Epinephrine | <55 nmol/d | nmol/d × 0.183 = μg/d | <10 μg/d |
| Fluoride | <50 μmol/d | μmol/d × 0.019 = mg/d | <1 mg/d |
| Homovanillic acid (HVA) | *mmol/mol creatinine* | mmol/mol creatinine × 1.61 = μg/mg creatinine | *μg/mg creatinine* |
| | 1–12 mo: 0.75–21.7 | | 1–12 mo: 1.2–35.0 |
| | 1–2 yr: 2.5–14.3 | | 1–2 yr: 4.0–23.0 |
| | 2–5 yr: 0.43–8.4 | | 2–5 yr: 0.7–13.5 |
| | 5–10 yr: 0.31–5.6 | | 5–10 yr: 0.5–9.0 |
| | 10–15 yr: 0.15–7.4 | | 10–15 yr: 0.25–12.0 |
| | 15–18 yr: 0.31–1.24 | | 15–18 yr: 0.5–2.0 |
| Metanephrines | *mmol/mol creatinine* | mmol/mol creatinine × 1.74 = μg/mg creatinine | *μg/mg creatinine* |
| | <1 yr: 0.001–2.64 | | <1 yr: 0.001–4.6 |
| | 1–2 yr: 0.15–3.09 | | 1–2 yr: 0.27–5.38 |
| | 2–5 yr: 0.20–1.72 | | 2–5 yr: 0.35–2.99 |
| | 5–10 yr: 0.25–1.55 | | 5–10 yr: 0.43–2.70 |
| | 10–15 yr: 0.001–0.38 | | 10–15 yr: 0.001–1.87 |
| | 15–18 yr: 0.03–0.69 | | 15–18 yr: 0.001–0.67 |
| Norepinephrine | <590 nmol/d | nmol/d × 0.169 = μg/d | <100 μg/d |
| Osmolality | 50–1200 μmol/kg | | 50–1200 mOsm/kg |
| Oxalate | 110–440 μmol/d | μmol/d × 0.088 = mg/d | 10–40 mg/d |
| Porphobilinogen | 0–8.8 μmol/d | μmol/d × 0.226 = mg/d | 0–2 mg/d |

## URINE (*Continued*)

| Test | SI Reference Range | Conversion Factor | Conventional Units Reference Range |
|---|---|---|---|
| Potassium | 25–125 mmol/d (varies with diet) | | 25–125 mEq/d |
| Pregnanetriol | <7.4 μmol/d | μmol/d × 0.3365 = mg/d | <2.5 mg/d |
| Protein | 10–140 mg/L | | 1–14 mg/dL |
| Steroids: 17-hydroxy-corticosteroid | Prepubertal: 2.76–15.5 μmol/d | μmol/d × 0.3625 = mg/d | Prepubertal: 1–5.6 mg/d |
| | Adult (M): 11–33 | | Adult (M): 4–12 |
| | Adult (F): 11–22 | | Adult (F): 4–8 |
| Steroids: 17-ketosteroids | <1 mo: ≤6.9 μmol/d | μmol/d × 0.2884 = mg/d | <1 mo: ≤2 mg/d |
| | 1 mo–5 yr: <1.73 | | 1 mo–5 yr: <0.5 |
| | 6–8 yr: 3.47–6.9 | | 6–8 yr: 1–2 |
| | Adult (M): 21–62 | | Adult (M): 6–18 |
| | Adult (F): 14–45 | | Adult (F): 4–13 |
| Uric acid | 1.48–4.43 mmol/d | mmol/d × 169 = mg/d | 250–750 mg/d |
| Vanilylmandelic acid (VMA) | *mmol/mol creatinine* | mmol/mol creatinine × 1.75 = μg/mg | *μg/mg creatinine* |
| | 1–6 mo: 1.71–9.71 | | 1–6 mo: 3–7 |
| | 6–12 mo: 1.14–8.57 | | 6–12 mo: 2–15 |
| | 1–5 yr: 1.14–5.71 | | 1–5 yr: 2–10 |
| | 5–10 yr: 0.86–4.00 | | 5–10 yr: 1.5–7 |
| | 10–15 yr: 0.57–3.43 | | 10–15 yr: 1–6 |
| | >15 yr: 0.57–3.43 | | >15 yr: 1–6 |

## CEREBROSPINAL FLUID

### Cell Count Range

Preterm: 0–25 WBC × $10^6$ cells/L (57% polymorphonuclears)
Term: 0–22 WBC × $10^6$ cells/L (61% polymorphonuclears)
Child: 0–7 WBC × $10^6$ cells/L (0% polymorphonuclears)

### Cell Count Percentiles

| Age | Total WBC | | | Polymorphonuclears | | | Monocytes | | |
|---|---|---|---|---|---|---|---|---|---|
| | 25% | 50% | 75% | 25% | 50% | 75% | 25% | 50% | 75% |
| <6 wk | 0.50 | 2.57 | 5.16 | 0 | 0 | 2.42 | 0 | 0.83 | 2.71 |
| 6 wk–3 mo | 0.34 | 1.86 | 3.75 | 0 | 0 | 0.66 | 0 | 0.96 | 2.78 |
| 3–6 mo | 0.00 | 1.11 | 2.31 | 0 | 0 | 0.40 | 0 | 0.43 | 1.64 |
| 6–12 mo | 0.41 | 1.47 | 3.25 | 0 | 0 | 0.52 | 0.03 | 0.93 | 2.32 |
| >12 mo | 0.00 | 0.68 | 1.82 | 0 | 0 | 0 | 0 | 0.25 | 1.45 |

| Test | SI Reference Range | Conventional Units Reference Range |
|---|---|---|
| Glucose | Preterm: 1.3–3.5 mmol/L | Preterm: 24–63 mg/dL |
| | Term: 1.9–6.6 | Term: 34–119 |
| | Child: 2.2–4.4 | Child: 40–80 |
| Protein | Preterm: 0.65–1.50 g/L | Preterm: 65–150 mg/dL |
| | Term: 0.20–1.70 | Term: 20–170 |
| | Child: 0.05–0.40 | Child: 5–40 |
| Pressure | <200 mm $H_2O$ | <200 mm $H_2O$ |

## Selected Readings

Meites, S, ed. Pediatric clinical chemistry, ed. 2. Washington: American Association for Clinical Chemistry, 1981.

Metric Commission Canada Sector 9.10 Health and Welfare. SI manual in health care, ed. 2. Ottawa: Metric Commission Canada, 1982.

Rowe, PC, ed. The Harriet Lane handbook, ed. 11. Chicago: Year Book Medical Publishers, 1987.

Tietz, NB, ed. Clinical guide to laboratory tests. Philadelphia: WB Saunders, 1983.

*Principles and Practice of Pediatrics, Second Edition.*
edited by Frank A. Oski et al. J. B. Lippincott Company, Philadelphia © 1994.

CHAPTER 166
# Signs and Symptoms of Inborn Errors of Metabolism

Larry J. Shapiro

The typical newborn infant has a limited repertoire of reactions to use in response to adversity. Many of the signs and symptoms associated with inborn errors also may be typical of other more common disorders. It is essential, however, for the clinician to keep in mind that inborn errors do occur in infants and may cause problems. If appropriate laboratory tests are not pursued, the diagnosis may be missed and a treatable disorder could go unrecognized. Furthermore, failure to identify patients with inborn errors obviates the possibility of genetic counseling and prenatal diagnosis.

## EVALUATION

Vomiting, jaundice, diarrhea, seizures, lethargy, apnea, coma, abnormal hair, abnormal eyes, dysmorphic features, unusual odor, hypoglycemia, and metabolic acidosis may be seen in patients with inborn errors of metabolism (Table 166-1). Vomiting may reflect dietary protein or carbohydrate intolerance and is often seen in association with the adrenal failure of congenital adrenal hyperplasia. Vomiting may be projectile and mimic pyloric stenosis or may be attributed to gastroesophageal reflux. It is usually responsive to withdrawal of the offending nutrient. Jaundice is seen in a number of inborn error conditions and may be associated with intrinsic hepatocellular disease or may be due to increased production or decreased removal of bilirubin. Diarrhea is a relatively rare sign but may be a clue in those conditions indicated in Table 166-1. Seizures or altered mental status, which often produces notable and worrisome symptoms, is seen in many inborn errors. Trauma, asphyxia, intracranial hemorrhage, infection, and central nervous system malformations may be more common, but if these etiologies are not positively established, then metabolic disorders must be considered carefully. Abnormal hair or eyes or dysmorphic features are typical of some heritable defects of metabolism. Unusual odors are detected in some infants with inborn errors characterized by excretion of volatile organic acids. Such olfactory clues are enhanced by slightly acidifying a sample of urine or by smelling the patient's hair or the nape of his or her neck where sweat-derived organic acids may localize. Diagnosis of an inborn error should never be excluded based on absence of pathognomonic odor. A variety of physiologic and environmental factors may influence the ability to detect these odors. Finally, any unexplained biochemical alteration such as acidosis or hypoglycemia may be an indication for a more vigorous search for an underlying primary hereditary defect.

Initial laboratory evaluation of patients with suspected inborn errors of metabolism often include general measurements and spot tests indicated in Table 166-2. Hypoglycemia is a prominent feature of glycogen storage diseases types I and III as well as of defects of the gluconeogenic pathway. Secondary hypoglycemia is seen in maple syrup urine disease, organic acidemias, and disorders of fatty acid oxidation due to many mechanisms. Bilirubin levels, liver function studies, serum copper determinations, sweat chloride levels, and $\alpha_1$-antitrypsin quantitation or phenotyping may be clinically indicated. Blood pH should be assessed for evidence of metabolic acidosis. Many patients partially compensate for increased acid production with hyperpnea and lower $PCO_2$. Thus, plasma bicarbonate concentrations and calculated base deficit often need to be evaluated as well. Measuring electrolyte levels is also useful. Reduced serum sodium and elevated potassium values may reflect relative mineralocorticoid deficiency or resistance to mineralocorticoid activity. The most common of these disorders is 21 hydroxylase deficiency, a diagnosis of which usually can be established by finding elevated 17 hydroxyprogesterone levels. Such patients often present in adrenal crisis at 1 or 2 weeks of age. Girls with this disorder may have undergone some virilization of external genitalia, but affected boys are notoriously difficult to diagnose by physical examination alone unless there is already a high index of suspicion.

## METABOLIC ACIDOSIS

Metabolic acidosis is a frequent finding in sick newborn infants. Patients with hypoxemia, shock, poor perfusion, sepsis, and renal dysfunction, among others, may exhibit this laboratory finding. The magnitude of the anion gap is a useful measurement when determining etiology. Hyperchloremic acidosis without much expansion of the anion gap is often of renal origin. Identification of specific acids contributing to the gap is the most useful adjunct. Lactate levels are readily measured in most clinical laboratories. Results expressed as mEq/L can be used to estimate the extent to which lactate contributes to anions that are unaccounted for. Elevated lactate levels are seen secondary to hypoxemia or as a result of primary disturbances in lactate or pyruvate metabolism. Measurement of lactate-pyruvate ratios and plasma alanine levels may help in discriminating between these possibilities. A growing number of mitochondrial electron transport defects has been defined in recent years, but there is still a large number of infants with primary genetic lactic acidosis in whom specific etiologies are difficult to establish. If lactate does not account for most or all of the excessive anion gap, an organic acidemia should be pursued by measuring organic acid in urine by gas chromatography or volatile organic acids in plasma. A modest elevation of blood lactate level should be expected as a secondary event in many of the organic acidemias, but it usually does not account for the entire deficit of measured anions. When organic acidemia is suspected, urine and plasma samples should be frozen for subsequent analysis. These specimens should be obtained when the patient is acutely ill and likely to be excreting large amounts of abnormal metabolites.

## HYPERAMMONEMIA

Hyperammonemia is often a clinical sign of an underlying metabolic disturbance. Figure 166-1 shows elevated blood ammonia in a newborn is most often due to a primary genetic disorder of one of the urea cycle enzymes, transient hyperammonemia of the newborn, or some other inborn error that produces metabolites that interfere with waste nitrogen disposal. The latter conditions often can be suspected through detection of metabolic acidosis, which is usually not observed in primary urea cycle disturbances unless the patient develops shock or critical circulatory embarrassment. Plasma amino acids then provide useful data for subdividing the primary hyperammonemias. Elevated

## TABLE 166-1. Signs and Symptoms of Inborn Errors in Newborns

**Vomiting**
Disorders of steroid biosynthesis
Urea cycle disorders
Organic acidemias
Galactosemia
Hereditary fructose intolerance
Wolman's disease
Various amino acid disturbances

**Jaundice**
Galactosemia
Hereditary fructose intolerance
Tyrosinemia
$\alpha_1$-Antitrypsin deficiency
Hypothyroidism
Wolman's disease
Red blood cell membrane defects
Immune hemolytic anemias
Glycolytic defects
Crigler-Najjar syndrome

**Diarrhea**
Congenital disaccharidase deficiencies
Glucose-galactose malabsorption
Familial chloridorrhea
Wolman's disease
Tyrosinemia
Cystic fibrosis

**Hypoglycemia**
Branched-chain amino acid disorders
Organic acidemias
Fatty acyl-CoA dehydrogenase deficiencies
Galactosemia
Hereditary fructose intolerance
Gluconeogenic defects
Glycogen storage disease types I, III, VI

**Metabolic Acidosis**
Organic acidemias
Type I glycogen storage disease
Primary lactic acidoses
Pyruvate carboxylase deficiency
Gluconeogenic enzyme defects
Pyruvate dehydrogenase deficiency
Galactosemia
Hereditary fructose intolerance
Pyroglutamic aciduria

**Seizures, Lethargy, Apnea, Coma**
Nonketotic hyperglycinemia
$\beta$-Alaninemia
Organic acidemias
Other aminoacidopathies
Disorders producing hypoglycemia
Menke's syndrome
Urea cycle disorders
Fatty acyl-CoA dehydrogenase deficiency
Neonatal adrenoleukodystrophy

**Abnormal Hair**
Menkes' syndrome
Argininosuccinic aciduria
Phenylketonuria
Lysinuric protein intolerance

**Abnormal Odor**
Maple syrup urine disease
Isovaleric acidemia
Methionine malabsorption
Phenylketonuria
$\beta$-Methylcrotonyl-CoA carboxylase deficiency
Tyrosinemia

**Coarse or Dysmorphic Features**
$GM_1$ gangliosidosis
$\beta$-Glucuronidase deficiency
Fucosidosis
Neuraminidase deficiency
I cell disease
Glutaric acidemia II
Zellweger syndrome
Neonatal adrenoleukodystrophy

**Abnormal Eye Findings**
Galactosemia
Sulfite oxidase deficiency
$GM_1$ gangliosidosis
$\beta$-Glucuronidase deficiency
I cell disease
Neuraminidase deficiency
Zellweger syndrome

citrulline, argininosuccinic acid, or arginine levels are usually seen in citrullinemia, argininosuccinic acidemia, or hyperargininemia, respectively. Very low plasma citrulline values are found with blocks proximal to this metabolite in the urea cycle. Transient hyperammonemia of the newborn is probably a developmental defect in which elevated ammonia levels with normal levels of citrulline due to a maturational delay in expression of urea cycle enzymes are found.

## DISORDERS OF FATTY ACID OXIDATION

Abnormalities of fatty acid oxidation is a group of disorders recognized with increasing frequency. Patients with these disorders often present with alterations in mental status, hypoglycemia, fatty infiltration of the viscera, and a clinical picture reminiscent of Reye's syndrome. Disorders of fatty acid oxidation have been found in a significant proportion of victims of sudden infant death syndrome. Cellular oxidation of fatty acids requires their transport into mitochondria after the formation of acyl-carnitine esters, the production of acyl-CoA intermediates, and the subsequent activity of chain-length-specific acyl-CoA dehydrogenases. Finally, intact electron transport mediated by an electron transport flavoprotein (ETF) and ETF dehydrogenase is required. Defects in each of these steps have been recognized. In general, all result in an elevation of circulating free fatty acids, a relative inability to procedure $\beta$-hydroxybutyrate and acetoacetate (ketone bodies), even in response to fasting, and in a diversion of fatty acids from the

TABLE 166-2. Laboratory Evaluation of Patients With Suspected Inborn Errors of Metabolism

**General Methods**
Blood glucose
Lactate
pH
Electrolytes
Ammonia
Bilirubin
Liver function
Serum copper
Sweat chloride
$\alpha_1$-Antitrypsin
17 Hydroxyprogesterone
Ketone bodies
Free fatty acids

**Spot Tests**
Ferric chloride
Dinitrophenylhydrazine
Clinitest
Mucopolysaccharides
Cyanide nitroprusside
Methylmalonic acid

**Carbohydrates**
Reducing substances in urine
Oligosaccharide chromatography
Glycogen content of red blood cells, liver, or muscle
Mucopolysaccharide fractionation

**Amino Acid Chromatography**
Plasma
Urine

**Organic Acid Analysis**
Volatiles
Nonvolatiles

**Fatty Acid Chain Lengths**

**Specific Enzyme Assays**

**DNA-Based Diagnostic Tests**

detect glucose, galactose, or other reducing substances in urine. The cyanide nitroprusside test is positive in the presence of sulphur-containing amino acids such as homocystine or cystine. Caution must be used in the newborn period, because of the relatively reduced tubular reabsorptive capacity for cystine and the dibasic amino acids. Most inborn errors require sophisticated equipment and expertise for their definitive diagnosis. Gas chromatography, mass spectrometry, and specific enzyme assays may be needed. Increasingly, defects may be detected at a nucleic acid level, but the need for enzymatic activity assessment probably will persist in most of these conditions because of molecular heterogeneity.

Patients with inborn errors of metabolism may be detected via newborn screening. Most states mandate testing for phenylketonuria and hypothyroidism. Some states have more comprehensive programs that detect an array of conditions, potentially in a presymptomatic state. Implementation of these tests, however, differs according to regional priorities due to economic and other issues. For most inborn errors, screening tests of suitable sensitivity, specificity, and cost are not available, so clinical acumen is essential.

Treatment of hereditary metabolic disorders must be tailored to the clinical situation. Avoiding noxious nutrients, restricting dietary protein intake, and administering pharmacologic amounts of vitamins or cofactors may be beneficial. For a number of conditions, hepatic transplantation may be the only treatment consonant with a reasonable chance of success and an acceptable quality of life. Often, highly complex dietary manipulations are required. These depend on sophisticated nutritional and laboratory analytical services available at a limited number of centers. Acutely, in cases of suspected organic acidemias or urea cycle disorders, dietary protein should be restricted and sufficient calories provided to attempt to suppress endogenous tissue catabolism. If this treatment is continued, a protein-free intake cannot be maintained. Sufficient essential amino acids and nitrogen must be supplied to support growth and anabolism. This level of protein intake often must be determined empirically, but decisions are aided by careful measurement of relevant metabolites. Occasionally, dialysis may help in the emergent therapy of life-threatening inborn errors. In those conditions associated with hyperammonemia, alternative means of waste nitrogen excretion through administration of compounds such as sodium benzoate or sodium phenylacetate may be of considerable benefit. Many inborn errors of metabolism associated with cellular storage of bipolymers are not responsive to dietary therapy and await development of treatment such as gene replacement.

normal pathway of $\beta$ oxidation to $\omega$ oxidation, resulting in generation of measurable levels of dicarboxylic acids. Defects in ETF or ETF dehydrogenase may also produce accumulations of other organic acids such as glutaric acid or ethylmalonic adipic acid because their oxidation requires ETF-dependent acyl-CoA dehydrogenase as well.

## OTHER CONSIDERATIONS IN INBORN ERRORS

A number of spot tests (see Table 166-2) are used to detect inborn errors. They are useful but nonspecific and require more experience for accurate interpretation than is generally believed. Both false-positive and false-negative results are fairly frequent; thus, spot tests are relatively crude screening tests. The ferric chloride reaction may be positive in a number of disorders. The dinitrophenylhydrazine test yields a visible precipitate with urine containing significant amounts of $\alpha$ ketoacids such as in patients with maple syrup urine disease. Clinitest tablets can be used to

## CHROMOSOMAL DISORDERS

About 1 in 200 liveborn infants have detectable chromosomal disorders. Collectively, they account for a sizable fraction of malformations, morbidity, and mortality in the newborn period. Nearly all recognizable chromosomal defects are associated with aneuploidy for all or some segment of a chromosome. *Aneuploidy* means that some number of genes in a portion of the genome is present in other than the expected diploid complement. Duplications of chromosomal material produce trisomies (or, occasionally, tetrasomies, for example), and deletions or deficiencies produce monosomic conditions. In either event, the imbalance of gene expression created by these structural aberrations is presumed to produce clinical consequences. In few, if any, chromosomal disorders is it known which genes are implicated or even what number of genes is involved.

High-resolution banding procedures for karyotype analysis and molecular methods applied to clinical samples detect ever

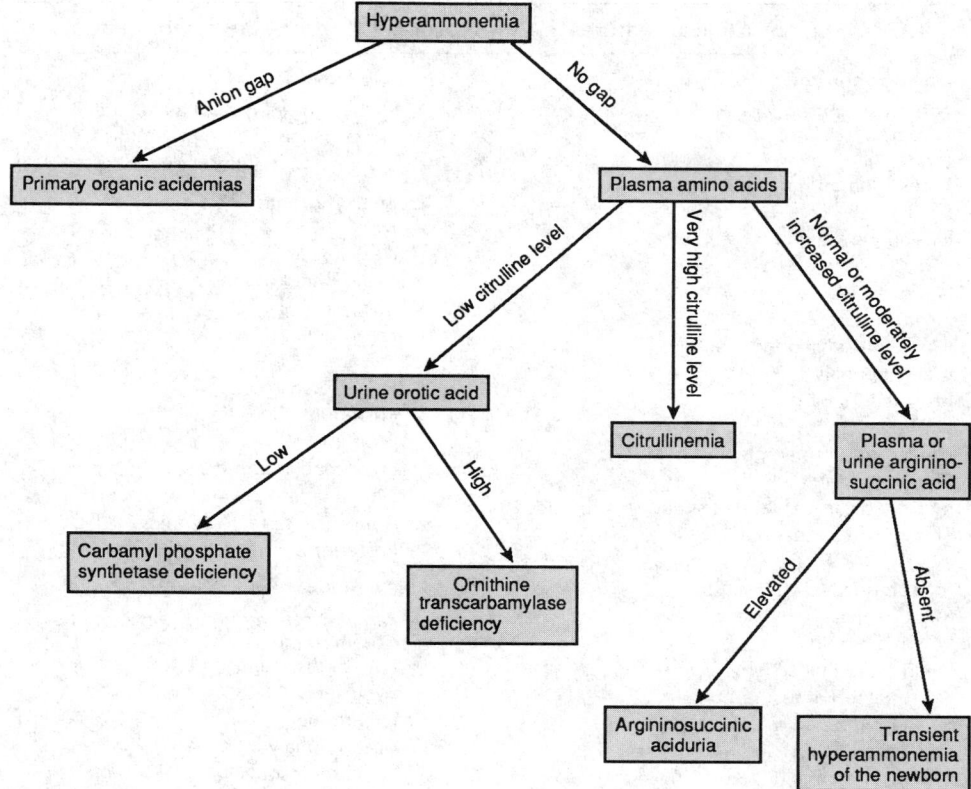

**Figure 166-1.** Hyperammonemia in the newborn. (Adapted from Batshaw, et al. Pediatrics 1981;68: 291.)

smaller degrees of abnormalities. Very small cytologically detectable deletions have been found in Prader-Willi syndrome, Miller-Dieker syndrome, DiGeorge syndrome, Langer-Giedion syndrome, aniridia-Wilms' tumor association, and retinoblastoma. The number of genes minimally needed to be deleted to produce these phenotypes is not known. Some monogenic disorders, however, clearly are associated with smaller intragenic deletions or loss of DNA that involves only a single gene (eg, some types of thalassemia). Thus, single-gene disorders and "chromosomal conditions" are likely to be considered simultaneously.

## Down Syndrome

The chromosome disorder most often observed in the newborn period is Down syndrome, which accounts for about one third of detected abnormalities. The constellation of facial, limb, and internal abnormalities found in this disorder is well known and virtually pathogenomic. Low birth weight, brachycephaly, small ears, upslanting palpebral fissures, redundant skin at the nape of the neck, Brushfield's spots, short and broad hands, clinodactyly of the fifth finger, simian creases, wide space between the first and second toes, and profound hypotonia are seen in most infants. As many as half of the children with Down syndrome have congenital heart defects. Ventricular septal defects and endocardial cushion defects account for two thirds of the abnormalities. About 5% of patients have gastrointestinal anomalies, including duodenal atresia and Hirschsprung's disease. Various immunologic abnormalities are detectable later in life with a high incidence of leukemias. In the newborn period, leukemoid reactions are frequently noted and may be associated with fetal hydrops. Mental retardation is an invariant concomitant of Down syndrome.

As with most other chromosome disorders, a presumptive diagnosis often may be made based on physical findings. Because of the lifelong and severe implication of these disorders, however, documentation with suitable cytogenetic studies should be carried out as soon as is feasible. This documentation confirms the diagnosis, assists in medical decision making, and rules out the possibility of a translocation, partial trisomy 21, or other unusual karyotypic constitution that might alter the recurrence risk. If rapid information is essential for making a therapeutic decision, bone marrow-derived chromosomes or cord blood lymphocyte chromosomes can be harvested after short-term culture, and slides can be prepared within hours. The morphologic findings and resolution of chromosomes studied with rapid harvesting may not permit detection of subtle abnormalities, but altered numbers of chromosomes should be readily recognizable.

---

### TABLE 166-3. Indications for Chromosome Studies

Features suggestive of a known chromosomal syndrome

Ambiguous genitalia

Stillborn infants or fetuses with no obvious cause of death or with multiple malformations

Infants with two or more major congenital abnormalities or multiple dysmorphic features

Neurologic defects with major or minor malformations

Parents, siblings, and other appropriate family members of infants found to have translocations, duplications, or deletions

Parents who have had multiple (three or more) spontaneous pregnancy losses of unknown etiology

**TABLE 166-4.   Clinical Features in Chromosome Disorders in Newborn Period**

**Down Syndrome**

*Trisomy 21; Trisomy for Part of 21; Mosaicism for Trisomy 21*
Hypotonia
Excess skin on back of neck
Flat facies
Upslanting palpebral fissures
Simian crease
Hip dysplasia
Heart disease
Gastrointestinal abnormalities
Brachycephaly
Brushfield's spots
Short hands
Ulnar loop dermatoglypia
Distal axial triradius
Increased gap between first and second toes

**Trisomy 18 Syndrome**

*Trisomy For All or Most of Chromosome 18*
Intrauterine growth retardation
Microcephaly
Polyhydramnios
Decreased fetal activity
Short palpebral fissures
Small mouth and mandible
Overlapping third and fifth fingers
Low-arch dermal ridge pattern
Hypoplasia of nails
Short sternum
Cryptorchidism
Cardiac defects
Renal abnormalities

**Trisomy 13 Syndrome**

*Trisomy for All or a Large Part of Chromosome 13*
Holoprosencephaly
Encephalocele
Microcephaly
Micropthalmia with coloboma
Cleft lip or palate
Capillary hemangiomas
Scalp defects
Polydactyly
Thin ribs
Cardiac defects
Cryptorchidism
Hypertonia or hypotonia

**Trisomy 8 Syndrome**

*Usually Mosaicism for Trisomy 8 or Partial Trisomy 8 Due to Translocation*
Thick lips
Deep-set eyes
Prominent ears
Camptodactyly

**Triploidy**

*69XXY or 69XXX Karyotype*
Placenta with hydatidiform changes
Prenatal growth retardation
Microphthalmia with coloboma
Syndactyly
Heart defects

**Triploidy** (*Continued*)

Stillborn or early neonatal death
Hypospadias and cryptorchidism
Brain malformations

**4p⁻ Syndrome**

*Partial Deletion of the Short Arm of Chromosome 4*
Marked intrauterine growth deficiency
Microcephaly
Hypotonia
Seizures
Hypertelorism
Posterior scalp defects
Cleft lip
Hypospadias and cryptorchidism
Simian crease
Abnormal dermatoglyphics
Posterior mouth

**Cri du Chat Syndrome**

*Partial Deletion of the Short Arm of Chromosome 5*
Low-birth-weight
Typical cry
Hypotonia
Microcephaly
Hypertelorism
Low-set ears
Abnormal facies
Congenital heart defects
Abnormal dermatoglyphics

**13q⁻ Syndrome**

*Deletion of Part of the Long Arm of Chromosome 13*
Intrauterine growth retardation
Microcephaly
Brain malformations
Prominent nasal bridge
Hypertelorism
Small or absent thumbs
Cardiac defects
Hypospadias and cryptorchidism
Retinoblastoma
Short neck

**18p⁻ Syndrome**

*Deletion of Part of the Short Arm of Chromosome 18*
Mild growth deficiency
Mild microcephaly
Ptosis
Hypertelorism
Micrognathia
Large ears
Small hands and feet

(continued)

## TABLE 166-4.  (Continued)

**18q⁻ Syndrome**

*Partial Deletion of the Long Arm of Chromosome 18*
Mild growth retardation
Hypotonia
Nystagmus
Microcephaly
Midface hypoplasia
Deep-set eyes
Abnormal dermatoglyphics
Cryptorchidism
Cardiac defects
Skin dimples at joints
Narrow or atretic ear canals
Long hands with tapering fingers

**21q⁻ Syndrome**

*Partial Deletion of the Long Arm of Chromosome 21*
Low-birth-weight
Hypertonia
Redundant eyelids
Large external ears
Micrognathia
Dysplastic nails
Delayed bony development

**Turner's Syndrome**

*XO Karyotype, but Many Patients Are
Mosaic for Some Other Cell Line
Including XO/XY; May Be Associated
With Structural Abnormalities of*
X Chromosome
Small stature
Ovarian dysgenesis
Lymphedema of hands and feet
Wide-spread nipples
Narrow maxilla
Low posterior hairline
Webbed neck
Short fourth metacarpal
Hyperconvex fingernails
Pigmented nevi
Renal anomalies
Cardiac defects
Cubitus valgus

**XXXXY Syndrome**

*Karyotype as Stated*
Hypotonia
Low-birth-weight
Abnormal facies
Radioulnar synostosis
Abnormal dermatoglyphics
Small penis and testes

---

The risk of Down syndrome and other aneuploidies increases with increasing maternal age, for reasons that are unclear. About half of all children with Down syndrome are born to mothers older than 35 years of age, although this group of women has only 5% to 7% of all liveborn infants. Trisomy 21 is present in 90% to 95% of patients with Down syndrome. The remainder have chromosomal translocations that may be de novo events in the infants examined or may represent the outcome of pregnancies of balanced translocation carrier parents. The latter group of parents may be at a significantly increased risk of having additional offspring with unbalanced karyotypes. Potential indications for undertaking cytogenetic analyses are listed in Table 166-3.

## Other Chromosomal Abnormalities

Trisomy 18 is often characterized by microcephaly, small palpebral fissures, overriding of the second and fifth fingers, and omphalocele (Table 166-4). Trisomy 13 should be suspected when a sloping forehead, holoprosencephaly, polydactyly, cleft lip and palate, and cystic kidneys are seen. Trisomy for all or parts of other chromosomes may be observed but much less frequently (see Table 166-4).

In addition to the disorders described here that are characterized by extra autosomal chromosomal material, partial deletions of autosomes are seen. Although many of these disorders have reasonably consistent phenotypes, there is, perhaps, more variability in clinical features because the precise extent of the deletion may differ from one individual to another. The features of some of the more commonly seen deletion syndromes are listed in Table 166-4.

Abnormality of structure or number of the sex chromosomes are particularly common. Based on karyotypes of early abortuses, Turner's syndrome due to an XO karyotype may be present in as many as 4% of all human conceptions. Despite the relatively mild phenotype of the syndrome postnatally, perhaps only 1 in 100 of these XO embryos survive. Those female fetuses who do make it to term often have lymphedema of the hands and feet with or without cystic hygromas. Also of consequence in the newborn period may be cardiac (coarctation of the aorta or aortic stenosis) or renal (eg, horseshoe kidneys) abnormalities. Later, typical features of short stature, gonadal dysgenesis, cubitus valgus, low posterior hairline, typical facies, widely spaced nipples, multiple pigmented nevi, hyperconvex fingernails, and short fourth metacarpals may become more apparent. Klinefelter's syndrome due to an XXY karyotype occurs in about 1 of 1000 newborn boys. Clinical detection in infancy of this syndrome or the equally frequent XYY syndrome is unusual. The greater the degree of aneuploidy, the more marked the dysmorphic features may be, rendering them more easily detectable in the newborn period. Thus, the XXXXY syndrome with its characteristic midface hypoplasia, genital abnormalities, and radioulnar synostosis may often be detected in infancy.

## Selected Readings

Barton BK. Inborn errors of metabolism: the clinical diagnosis in early infancy. Pediatrics 1987;79:359.

deGrouchy J, Turleau C. Clinical atlas of human chromosomes, ed 2. New York: John Wiley and Sons, 1984.

Jones KL. Smith's recognizable patterns of human malformation, ed 4. Philadelphia: WB Saunders, 1988.

Koch R, ed. Urea cycle symposium. Pediatrics 1981;68:271.

McKusick VA. Mendelian inheritance in man, ed 7. Baltimore: Johns Hopkins University Press, 1986.

Milunsky A. Genetic disorders and the fetus: diagnosis, prevention, and treatment, ed 2. New York: Plenum Press, 1986.

Scriver C, Beaudet AL, Sly WS, Valee D. The metabolic basis of inherited disease, ed 6. New York: McGraw-Hill, 1989.

*Principles and Practice of Pediatrics, Second Edition.*
edited by Frank A. Oski et al. J. B. Lippincott Company, Philadelphia © 1994.

# CHAPTER 167
# Common Syndromes With Morphologic Abnormalities

Walter W. Tunnessen, Jr.

A *syndrome* is a running together of symptoms (usually), which, taken as a whole, presents a picture of a disease or disorder. Morphologic abnormalities often recur in patterns that create a recognizable picture. In this chapter, 50 syndromes with morphologic abnormalities are presented in abbreviated form, along with a list of common (and some less common) features, comments regarding key associations and prevalence, information about performance and etiology, and references for further reading. Distinctive phenotypic features of syndromes are shown in accompanying figures. Syndromes are listed alphabetically below.

Aarskog's
Achondroplasia
AIDS embryopathy
Anhidrotic (hypohidrotic) ectodermal dysplasia
Aniridia-Wilms' tumor
Apert's
Beckwith-Wiedemann
Bloom's
Camptomelic dysplasia
Carpenter's
Cerebral gigantism
Cerebrohepatorenal (Zellweger)
CHARGE
Cockayne's
Cornelia de Lange's
Cri du chat
Crouzon's
Down
Fanconi's
Fetal alcohol
Fetal hydantoin
Hallermann-Streiff
Hurler's
Langer-Giedion
Larsen's

Leprechaunism
Marfan's
Menkes'
Morquio's
Mulibrey nanism
Noonan's
Oculoauriculovertebral
Oral-facial-digital
Prader-Willi
Progeria
Rothmund-Thomson
Rubinstein-Taybi
Russell-Silver
Saethre-Chotzen
Seckel's
Shprintzen's
Smith-Lemli-Opitz
Stickler's
TAR
Treacher Collins
Trisomy 13
Trisomy 18
Turner's
VATER
Williams

## Aarskog's Syndrome

### Key Features (Fig 167-1)

Round face
Hypertelorism
Small, short, broad nose—anteverted nostrils
Long philtrum
Short stature
Shawl scrotum—scrotal fold encircles base of phallus

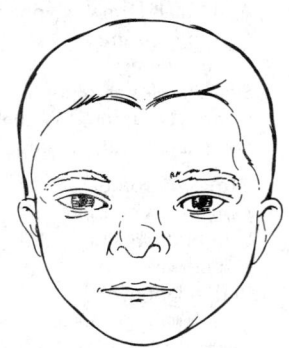

Figure 167-1.  Aarskog's syndrome.

### Other Findings

Ptosis of eyelids
Antimongoloid slant to eyes
Maxillary hypoplasia
Prominent metopic suture
Thin vermilion border of upper lip; pouting lower lip
Crease below lower lip
Widow's peak of hairline
Brachydactyly with clinodactyly of fifth fingers
Simian crease
Mild interdigital webbing
Mild pectus excavatum
Prominent umbilicus
Cryptorchidism
Low-set ears
Broad feet with bulbous toes
Proximal interphalangeal joint hyperextensibility with distal joint restriction

*Comments.*   Short stature is usually not evident until 2 to 4 years of age. With age, the round face becomes triangular.
The incidence of this syndrome is not known.

*Performance.*   Mild mental retardation is common.

*Etiology.*   X-linked recessive and autosomal dominant inheritance have been reported.

### Selected Reading

Berman P, DesJardins C, Fraser FC. The inheritance of the Aarskog facial-digital-genital syndrome. J Pediatr 1975;86:885.

## *Achondroplasia Syndrome*

### Key Features (Fig 167-2)

Short stature
Macrocephaly
Low, broad nasal bridge
Frontal bossing
Midfacial hypoplasia
Short limbs

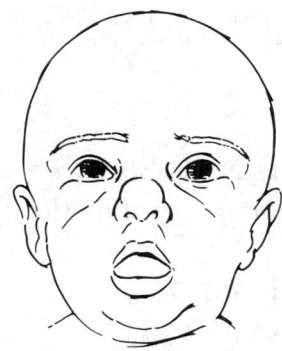

Figure 167-2.   Achondroplasia syndrome.

### Other Findings

Brachycephaly
Narrow nasal passages
Prominent mandible
Dental malocclusion; crowding of teeth
Small, cuboid-shaped vertebral bodies
Lumbar lordosis
Elbows lacking full extension
Short, stubby hands
Bowed legs
Small foramen magnum; occipitalization of C-1

*Comments.*   These infants have an early delay in motor development, particularly in walking and in head control because of its relatively large size. A narrow spinal canal and instability of C-1 and C-2 predispose to spinal cord injuries. Hydrocephalus occurs with increased frequency. Disorders of respiration are common, especially those caused by thoracic cage restriction or upper airway obstruction.
   The incidence is estimated at 1 : 10,000 to 1 : 20,000.

*Performance.*   Normal mental development is the rule unless there are central nervous system complications.

*Etiology.*   Inheritance is autosomal dominant, although 80% to 90% of cases represent fresh mutations.

### Selected Readings

Horton WA, Rotter JL, Rimoin DL, et al. Standard growth curves for achondroplasia. J Pediatr 1978;93:435.
Reid CS, Pyeritz RE, Kopits SE, et al. Cervicomedullary compression in young patients with achondroplasia: value of comprehensive neurologic and respiratory evaluation. J Pediatr 1987;110:522.

## *AIDS Embryopathy (Fetal AIDS Syndrome)*

### Key Features

Microcephaly
Prominent boxlike appearance of forehead
Flat nasal bridge
Mild upward or downward obliquity of eyes
Prominent palpebral fissures with blue sclerae
Ocular hypertelorism
Short nose with flattened columella
Well-formed triangular philtrum
Full vermilion border of lip
Patulous lips
Growth failure

*Comments.*   Whether maternal infection with human immunodeficiency virus (HIV) has distinct effects on the developing fetus is controversial.

### Selected Reading

Marion RW, Wiznia AA, Hutcheon RG, Rubinstein A. Fetal AIDS syndrome score. Am J Dis Child 1987;141:429.

## *Anhidrotic (Hypohidrotic) Ectodermal Dysplasia*

### Key Features (Fig 167-3)

Small, saddle-shaped nose
Frontal bossing
Prominent supraorbital ridges
Midface hypoplasia
Prominent, pouting lips
Small, conical, or missing teeth
Hyperthermia from inadequate sweating
Fine, dry, sparse hair

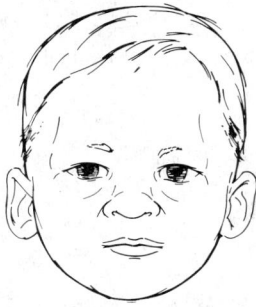

Figure 167-3.   Anhidrotic (hypohidrotic) ectodermal dysplasia.

## Other Findings

Wide cheekbones
Small, pointed, low-set ears
Soft, thin skin
Dystrophic nails
Chronic rhinorrhea
Thin, wrinkled eyelid skin
Hoarse voice
Scaling skin in neonates

*Comments.*   This disorder may be recognized first in infancy because of hyperthermia associated with the inability to sweat. The incidence of this form of ectodermal dysplasia is about 1 : 100,000 male births.

*Performance.*   Hyperthermia may result in mental and developmental delay.

*Etiology.*   Inheritance is X-linked recessive; carrier females may express some features.

## Aniridia-Wilms' Tumor Association

## Key Features (Fig 167-4)

Prominent lips
Micrognathia
Poorly formed, low-set ears
Aniridia
Microcephaly

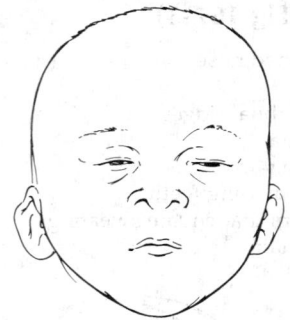

Figure 167-4.   Aniridia-Wilms' tumor.

## Other Findings

Poor growth
Ptosis of eyelids
Small palpebral fissures
Long, narrow face
High nasal bridge
Microcephaly
Cryptorchidism
Hypospadias
Kyphoscoliosis
Other ophthalmologic findings: congenital cataracts, nystagmus, blindness

*Comments.*   Infants with aniridia have an increased incidence of development of Wilms' tumors. Infants who have aniridia and the chromosomal deletion (11p13) have a 50% incidence of Wilms' tumor before age 4 years.
The prevalence of this association is not known.

*Performance.*   Moderate to severe mental retardation is usually present.

*Etiology.*   An interstitial deletion of the short arm of chromosome 11p13 is present in infants and children with the above constellation of findings. Not all infants with aniridia and associated Wilms' tumors have the chromosomal defect. Almost all cases are sporadic in occurrence, although a familial occurrence has been recorded due to balanced translocation.

## Selected Reading

Riccardi VM, Sujansky E, Smith AL, et al. Chromosomal imbalance in the aniridia-Wilms' tumor association: 11p interstitial deletion. Pediatrics 1978;61:604.

## Apert's Syndrome (Acrocephalosyndactyly)

## Key Features (Fig 167-5)

Craniosynostosis with flat occiput
Brachycephaly with high forehead
Midfacial hypoplasia—flat facies
Hypertelorism
Syndactyly, cutaneous or bony, of hands and feet

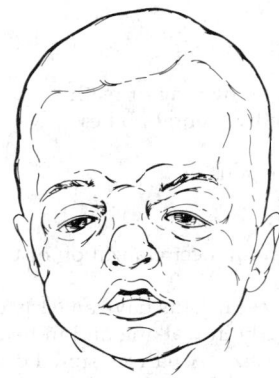

Figure 167-5.   Apert's syndrome (acrocephalosyndactyly).

## Other Findings

Shallow orbits with proptosis
Strabismus
Downslanting of palpebral fissures
Small nose, occasionally beaklike
Prominent mandible
High-arched palate; cleft soft palate in some cases
Ankylosis of elbow, shoulder, and hip
Hearing loss

*Comments.*   Mortality is increased in the neonatal period. Despite the craniosynostosis, increased intracranial pressure is not common. Acne vulgaris with extension to the forearm is found in most adolescents with this syndrome.
The incidence of this syndrome is estimated at 1 : 160,000.

*Performance.*   Mental development varies, although many have decreased mental capacity.

*Etiology.*   Apert's syndrome is autosomal dominant, with most cases representing fresh mutations.

# *Beckwith-Wiedemann Syndrome*

## Key Features (Fig 167-6)

Macrosomia—excessive postnatal growth
Macroglossia—large tongue
Prominent eyes
Capillary hemangioma (nevus flammeus) of the central forehead and eyelids
Abdominal wall defects: umbilical hernia, diastasis recti, omphalocele

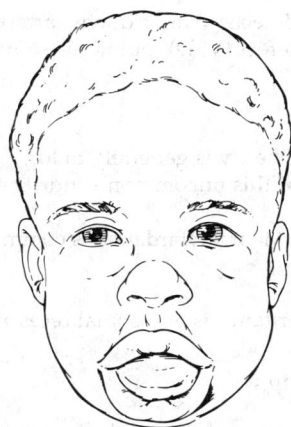

Figure 167-6.    Beckwith-Wiedemann syndrome.

## Other Findings

Large fontanelle
Linear creases in ear lobule
Prominent occiput
Visceromegaly: liver, kidneys, pancreas, uterus
Microcephaly
Midface hypoplasia
Large birth weight
Neonatal hypoglycemia
Advanced bone age

### Occasional Findings

Hemihypertrophy
Absent gonads
Clitoral hypertrophy
Diaphragm abnormalities: eventration, hernia
Muscular hypertrophy

*Comments.*    Although these infants are noted for their large size, they may not be abnormally large at birth. Phenotypic expression varies greatly. The neonatal hypoglycemia may be difficult to control. The enlarged tongue may result in significant feeding problems. An important association is the propensity to develop malignancies, particularly Wilms' tumor, adrenal carcinoma, and gonadoblastoma. Maternal hydramnios is common, and the incidence of prematurity is high.

The frequency of occurrence is estimated at 1 : 15,000 live births.

*Performance.*    Mild to moderate mental retardation may occur, although some researchers think retardation may be the result of hypoglycemia.

*Etiology.*    Most cases are sporadic in occurrence, but familial cases have been reported. Abnormalities of chromosome 11 have been reported in patients with features of this syndrome.

## Selected Readings

Pettenali MJ, Haines JL, Higgins RR, Wappner RS, Palmer CG, Weaver DD. Wiedemann-Beckwith syndrome: presentation of clinical and cytogenetic data on 22 new cases and review of the literature. Hum Genet 1986;74:143.
Sotelo-Avila C, Gonzalez-Crussi F, Fowler JW. Complete and incomplete forms of Beckwith-Wiedemann syndrome: their oncogenic potential. J Pediatr 1980;96:47.
Waziri M, Patil SR, Hanson JW, et al. Abnormality of chromosome 11 in patients with features of Beckwith-Wiedemann syndrome. J Pediatr 1983;102:873.

# *Bloom's Syndrome*

## Key Features (Fig 167-7)

Short stature of prenatal onset
Small, narrow facies with protruding ears
Mild microcephaly
Malar hypoplasia
Small nose
Facial erythematous rash over malar area, sun-induced

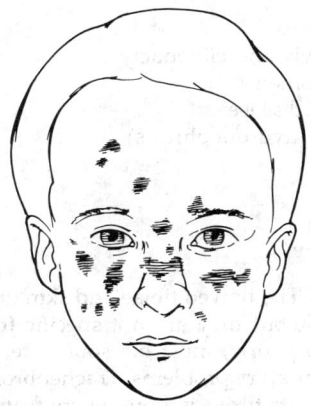

Figure 167-7.    Bloom's syndrome.

## Other Findings

High-pitched voice
Café-au-lait spots
Slender, delicate body build

*Comments.*    Patients with Bloom's syndrome have a remarkable resemblance to one another. The photosensitive dermatitis combined with poor growth usually suggests the diagnosis. The rash usually occurs over the nose, lips, malar area, forearms, and dorsa of the hands. Children with this disorder have a propensity for developing neoplasms, particularly lymphoreticular malignancies. Males may be sterile.

Slightly more than 100 cases have been described.

*Performance.*    Mild mental retardation may be present.

*Etiology.*    Almost half of the cases have been described in Ashkenazi Jews. Inheritance is autosomal recessive. On chromosomal analysis, a high incidence of sister chromatid exchange is found.

## Selected Reading

German J, Bloom D, Passarge E. Bloom's syndrome XI. Progress report for 1983. Clin Genet 1984;25:166.

## *Camptomelic Dysplasia Syndrome*

### Key Features

Anterior bowing of tibiae with pretibial skin dimple
Flat-appearing face
Low nasal bridge
Micrognathia
Short, narrow palpebral fissures
Dwarfism of prenatal onset
Small, bladeless scapulae

### Other Findings

Dolichocephalic head
Long philtrum
Cleft palate
Small mouth
Hypertelorism
Dysplastic ears
Lower extremities appear short compared to upper extremities
Small thoracic cage
Dislocated hips
Talipes equinovarus
Mild brachydactyly and clinodactyly
Protuberant abdomen
Congenital heart disease
Renal anomalies (hydronephrosis)
Hypotonia
Dislocated joints
Pterygium colli
Unruly hair

*Comments.* The bowed tibiae and skin dimple should suggest this disorder, but they are not specific for this syndrome. These infants do poorly; most die soon after birth or in early infancy from respiratory problems. Tracheobronchial hypoplasia is common. Failure to thrive is a prominent feature. A sex reversal phenomenon, male karyotype with female phenotype, has been reported in a number of cases.
The incidence is unknown.

*Performance.* Infants with this disorder have significant retardation.

*Etiology.* The inheritance pattern is not established, although some seem to fit an autosomal recessive pattern.

### Selected Reading

Hall BD, Spranger JW. Camptomelic dysplasia: further elucidation of a distinct entity. Am J Dis Child 1980;134:285.

## *Carpenter's Syndrome*

### Key Features

Obesity
Brachycephaly with variable synostosis of coronal, sagittal, and lambdoid sutures
Shallow supraorbital ridges
Flat nasal bridge
Lateral displacement of inner canthi
Short hands, stubby fingers
Partial syndactyly of third and fourth fingers
Preaxial polysyndactyly of the feet—duplication of first or second toe

### Occasional Abnormalities

Downslanting palpebral fissures
Epicanthal folds
Cranial asymmetry
Short neck
Postaxial polydactyly
Low-set ears
Congenital heart defects: patent ductus arteriosus (PDA), ventricular septal defect (VSD), pulmonic stenosis
Hypogenitalism
Small stature

*Comments.* Obesity is generally mild.
The incidence of this uncommon syndrome is unknown.

*Performance.* Mental retardation is common and of variable degree.

*Etiology.* Inheritance is autosomal recessive.

### Selected Readings

Cohen DM. Acrocephalopolysyndactyly type II-Carpenter syndrome: clinical spectrum, natural history, and an attempt at unification with Goodman and Summitt syndrome. Am J Med Genet 1987;28:311.
Temtamy SA. Carpenter's syndrome: acrocephalopolysyndactyly. An autosomal-recessive syndrome. J Pediatr 1966;69:111.

## *Cerebral Gigantism (Sotos Syndrome)*

### Key Features (Fig 167-8)

Prenatal onset of excessive size
Large hands and feet
Macrocephaly
Prominent forehead
Downslanting palpebral fissures
Hypertelorism
Prognathism (prominent jaw); narrow anterior mandible
Coarse-looking facies

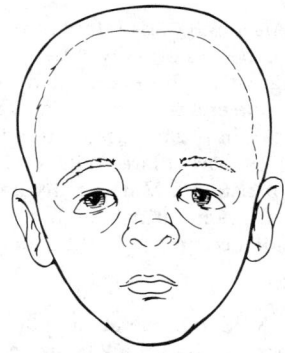

**Figure 167-8.** Cerebral gigantism (Sotos syndrome).

## Other Findings

Advanced osseous maturation
High, narrow palate
Poor coordination; clumsiness
Premature eruption of teeth
Seizures
Strabismus
Kyphoscoliosis

*Comments.* Hypotonia is almost invariable during the first year of life. Rapid growth occurs in the first 2 to 3 years of life, then proceeds at a fairly normal rate. In the neonatal period, feeding and respiratory problems are common. Behavior may be aggressive. An abnormal glucose tolerance test is found in more than 10% of cases.

The incidence of this uncommon syndrome is unknown.

*Performance.* Most children with this syndrome would be categorized as having a mild or borderline mental handicap. The perceived developmental and behavioral problems, however, may seem more severe than real because of expectations based on size rather than age.

*Etiology.* Sporadic occurrence, although a few families have been reported with parent and child affected.

## Selected Reading

Cole TRP, Hughes HE. Sotos Syndrome. J Med Genet 1990;27:571.
Sotos JF, Cutler EA, Dodge P. Cerebral gigantism. Am J Dis Child 1977;131:625.

# *Cerebrohepatorenal (Zellweger) Syndrome*

## Key Features (Fig 167-9)

Hypotonia
High forehead
Shallow, flat supraorbital ridges
Long, flat face
Inner epicanthal folds
Large fontanelle with open metopic suture
Micrognathia
Abnormal external ears

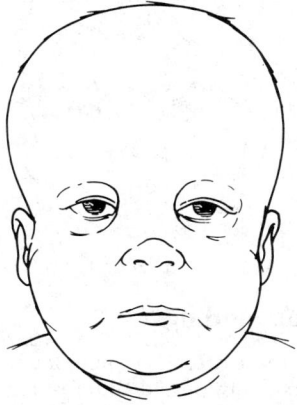

**Figure 167-9.** Cerebrohepatorenal (Zellweger) syndrome.

## Other Findings

Frontal bossing
Hepatomegaly; jaundice
Extra skin folds of the neck
Kidneys: albuminuria
Cardiac anomalies: patent ductus, septal defects
Simian crease
Contractures of joints, especially knee and fingers
Cryptorchidism
Corneal opacities, cataracts, glaucoma, Brushfield's spots
High-arched palate
Punctate epiphyseal calcifications of patellae, sternum, scapulae, and acetabulum
Talipes equinovarus

*Comments.* Infants with this syndrome do poorly from birth. Their suck is weak, failure to thrive occurs, and respiratory problems are common. Seizures occur in some infants. The generalized hypotonia is marked.

The incidence is estimated at 1 : 100,000, but identification of atypical cases and milder variants by biochemical means will result in a higher frequency. Early death is the rule.

*Performance.* Psychomotor development is retarded.

*Etiology.* Inheritance is autosomal recessive. In the classic syndrome, recognizable peroxisomes are missing from the liver and kidneys and are greatly reduced in skin fibroblasts. Elevated pipecolic acid concentrations in urine and plasma detected by routine amino acid chromatography are helpful but not diagnostic.

## Selected Readings

Kelley RI. Review: the cerebro-hepato-renal syndrome of Zellweger—morphologic and metabolic aspects. Am J Med Genet 1983;16:503.
Moser AE, Singh J, Brown FR, et al. The cerebrohepatorenal (Zellweger) syndrome: increased levels and impaired degradation of very long-chain fatty acids and their use in prenatal diagnosis. N Engl J Med 1984;310:1141.

# *CHARGE Association*

## Key Findings

Choanal atresia
Ear anomalies: small to cup-shaped lop ears
Deafness
Coloboma—retinal coloboma most common
Heart defects: tetralogy of Fallot, PDA, VSD, atrial septal defect (ASD)
Postnatal growth deficiency
Genital hypoplasia (males): microphallus, cryptorchidism

## Occasional Other Findings

Microcephaly
Facial asymmetry, palsy
Malar flattening
Long philtrum
Cleft lip/palate
Small mouth
Swallowing difficulties
Polyhydramnios in 50% of cases

*Comments.* This is not a specific disorder or diagnosis. Patients who have choanal atresia or colobomas of the eyes should be examined for other anomalies. The acronym is derived from C, coloboma; H, heart anomalies; A, atresia of the choanae; R, retardation—mental and somatic; G, genital hypoplasia; E, ear anomalies. Feeding problems are common in infancy, and early death occurs in some infants. Hypocalcemia may reflect the presence of abnormalities of the parathyroid gland and indicate thymic and major vessel abnormalities as well.

The incidence of this association is not known.

*Performance.* Mental retardation is present in almost all cases. Significant central nervous system malformations may be present.

*Etiology.* The occurrence seems sporadic. An insult to the developing embryo during the second month of pregnancy is postulated.

## Selected Readings

Cyran SE, Martinez R, Daniels S, et al. Spectrum of congenital heart disease in CHARGE association. J Pediatr 1987;110:576.

Pagon RA, Graham JM Jr, Zonana J, et al. Coloboma, congenital heart disease, and choanal atresia with multiple anomalies: CHARGE association. J Pediatr 1981;99: 223.

## *Cockayne's Syndrome*

### Key Features (Fig 167-10)

Microcephaly
Loss of facial adipose tissue; prominent facial bones
Slender nose
Sunken eyes
Large ears
Prominent chin
Growth deficiency, usually evident by age 2 years
Adipose tissue lost by mid-infancy to late infancy
Photosensitive, thin skin
Cool hands and feet—sometimes cyanotic

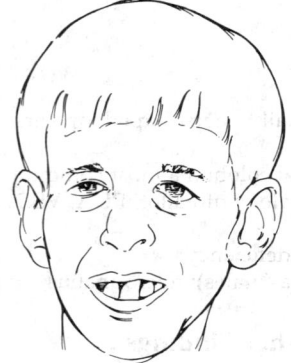

**Figure 167-10.** Cockayne's syndrome.

### Other Findings

Unsteady gait
Tremor
Corneal opacity, cataract; pigmentary retinal degeneration; optic atrophy

Mild to moderate joint limitation of knees, elbows, ankles
Limbs seem long; hands and feet seem large
Congenital absence of some teeth; increased dental caries
Dorsal kyphosis
Sensorineural deafness
Blindness
Scalp hair and eyebrows may be sparse
Cryptorchidism and small testes in males
Lack of normal breast development in females

*Comments.* Infants with this disorder appear normal at birth, but develop the loss of adipose tissue and growth failure rapidly in the first years of life. Radiographs of the skull reveal thickening and often intracranial calcifications.

Children with Cockayne's syndrome usually are unable to care for themselves by the late teenage years. Earlier in life, they are affected adversely by heat. Death often occurs in early adulthood from inanition and respiratory infections.

The incidence of this uncommon disorder is unknown.

*Performance.* There is moderate to severe mental retardation

*Etiology.* Inheritance is autosomal recessive.

## *Cornelia de Lange's Syndrome*

### Key Features (Fig 167-11)

Microbrachycephaly (small, round head)
Bushy eyebrows and synophrys (eyebrows run together)
Long, curly eyelashes
Small nose, anteverted nostrils
Thin lips with small midline beak of the upper lip and a corresponding notch in the lower lip
Downward curving angle of the mouth
Micrognathia
Long philtrum
Generalized hirsutism
Hypoplastic nipples
Low-pitched, weak, growling cry in infancy
Short stature
Micromelia of feet
Failure to thrive

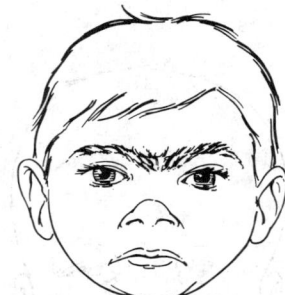

**Figure 167-11.** Cornelia de Lange's syndrome.

### Other Common Findings

Abnormalities of the extremities: micromelia, phocomelia, oligodactyly, proximally placed thumbs, simian crease, flexion contractures of the elbows, syndactyly of the second and third toes

High-arched palate
Undescended tests; hypospadias; genital hypoplasia
Congenital heart defects—VSD most common
Gastrointestinal tract anomalies—duplication most common

*Comments.* The facial appearance of infants is quite characteristic. They are difficult infants, are irritable, feed poorly, and have recurrent respiratory infections and gastrointestinal upsets. As they become older, autistic and self-destructive behavior may appear. Seizures occur in one fourth of cases.

The frequency of occurrence is estimated at 1 : 10,000 to 1 : 20,000.

*Performance.* The IQ of these infants is generally less than 50, and less than 35 in the majority of cases.

*Etiology.* The cause of this syndrome is unknown. Most cases are sporadic, with few familial cases reported. A similar appearance to that in Cornelia de Lange's syndrome has been described with two chromosomal abnormalities, duplication of 3q and duplication of 4p.

## Selected Reading

Hersh JH, Dale KS, Gerald PS, et al. Dup (4p) del (9p) in a familial mental retardation syndrome: resemblance to de Lange syndrome detected by high-resolution banding. Am J Dis Child 1985;139:81.

## *Cri du Chat Syndrome (5p—)*

## Key Features (Fig 167-12)

Microcephaly
Hypertelorism
Epicanthal folds
Downward slanting of palpebral fissures
High-pitched, shrill cry similar to that of a cat—reflects abnormal laryngeal development
Marked poor growth

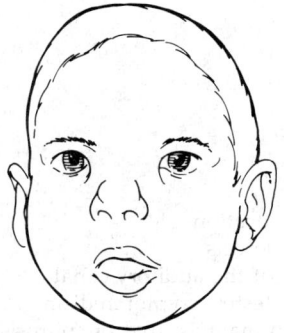

**Figure 167-12.** Cri du chat (5p–) syndrome.

## Other Common Features

Round face
Strabismus
Low-set or poorly formed ears; posteriorly rotated
Muscular hypotonia
Severe respiratory and feeding problems
Micrognathia
Prominent nasal bridge

Preauricular tags
Congenital heart defects of various types
Scoliosis
Transverse palmar creases
Low–birth-weight

### Less Common Features

Short philtrum
Cleft lip/palate
Bifid uvula
Facial asymmetry
Premature graying of hair

*Comments.* The characteristic catlike cry is not present in all cases, and it disappears in the first few years of life in those who have this clue. Facial features of affected infants change with age. Older children have a thin rather than round face.

The incidence has been estimated at 1 : 20,000 to 1 : 50,000 live births.

*Performance.* Affected infants are severely retarded.

*Etiology.* A deletion of the short arm of chromosome 5 is responsible for 85% of cases, while the remaining 15% are the result of an unbalanced translocation from a parental carrier.

## Selected Readings

Breg WR, Steele MW, Miller OJ, et al. The cri du chat syndrome in adolescents and adults: clinical findings in 13 older patients with partial deletion of the short arm of chromosome No 5 (5p—). J Pediatr 1970;77:782.
Wilkens LE, Brown JA, Nance WE, Wolf B. Clinical heterogeneity in 80 home-reared children with cri-du-chat syndrome. J Pediatr 1983;102:528.

## *Crouzon's Syndrome (Craniofacial Dysostosis)*

## Key Features (Fig 167-13)

Prominent eyes due to shallow orbits
Strabismus
Hypertelorism
Midfacial hypoplasia
Prognathism
Craniosynostosis—especially coronal and lambdoid sutures
Brachycephaly

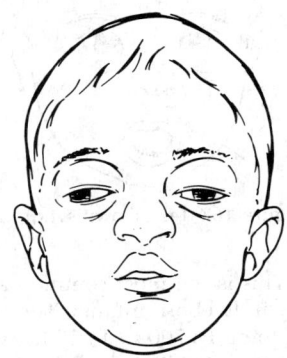

**Figure 167-13.** Crouzon's syndrome (craniofacial dysostosis).

## Other Findings

Flat nasal bridge
Nystagmus
Frontal bossing
Short upper lip
Drooping lower lip
High-arched palate
Crowded teeth, dental malocclusion
Bifid uvula, cleft palate
Atretic ear canals

*Comments.* Craniosynostosis occurs in the first year of life and may involve the sagittal as well as the coronal and lambdoidal sutures. Occasionally, increased intracranial pressure occurs. Headache and seizures may occur.

The incidence of this syndrome is not known.

*Etiology.* Inheritance is autosomal dominant, with 25% to 50% of cases representing new mutations.

## Down Syndrome

### Key Features (Fig 167-14)

Short stature
Typical craniofacial composite:
    Microcephaly-brachycephaly—small, round head; flat occiput
    Upslanting of palpebral fissures (mongolian slant)
    Inner epicanthal folds
    Speckling of the iris (Brushfield's spots)
    Small nose
    Low nasal bridge
    Small ears with small or absent ear lobes
    Flat facial profile
    Short neck
    Mouth held open, often with tongue protruding
Hypotonia
Brachydactyly—short hands and fingers
Single flexion crease on fifth finger
Congenital heart disease in one third to one half of cases—endocardial cushion defect and VSD most common

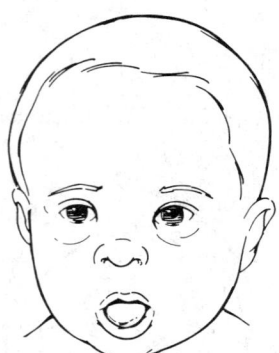

**Figure 167-14.** Down syndrome.

*Comments.* This is the most common autosomal chromosomal abnormality in liveborn infants. The frequency of occurrence is estimated to be 1 : 700 to 1 : 1000 live births.

In addition to the constellation of craniofacial findings, the newborn infant with Down syndrome is hypotonic and has hyperextensible joints and excess skin on the back of the neck. Transverse palmar lines (simian creases) are present in about 50%

of cases. Examination of dermatoglyphics reveals an increased number of ulnar loops.

There is significant morbidity and mortality in infancy and childhood due to congenital heart disease and an increased susceptibility to infection. One third of affected children die in the first year of life. Additional complications include an increased incidence of leukemia and, in newborns, a high incidence of duodenal atresia.

*Performance.* There is a wide range in IQ scores, but all are retarded in development.

*Etiology.* All children with this syndrome have an excess of chromosome 21 as either a trisomy or translocation. Mosaics may have a less severe phenotype. Trisomy 21 is the most common chromosomal abnormality, no matter what the maternal age. In infants with Down syndrome born to mothers younger than 30 years of age, about 92% have trisomy 21 and 8% are the result of translocations. If the mother is older than 30 years, 98% of infants show trisomy 21 and 2% show translocations. In D/G 21 translocations, one third are inherited and two thirds are sporadic, while in G/G 21 translocations only 10% are inherited and 90% are sporadic. The risk of having another child with trisomy 21 is about 1%. As maternal age increases so does the chance of having a child with trisomy 21. In mothers younger than 20 years of age, the incidence of Down syndrome is 1 : 2500 live births, while in mothers 45 years of age, it is about 1 : 50.

## Fanconi's Pancytopenia

### Key Features

Short stature
Microcephaly
Hypoplasia to aplasia of the thumb
Hyperpigmentation of skin—uneven
Pancytopenia develops at about 8 years of age

### Other Findings

Ptosis of the eyelid
Strabismus
Nystagmus
Microphthalmia
Aplasia of the radius
Clinodactyly
Syndactyly
Congenital hip dislocation
Rib and vertebral defects
Deafness—atresia of the auditory canal
Small penis, small testes, cryptorchidism
Urinary tract abnormalities: hydronephrosis, absent or ectopic kidneys

*Comments.* Some of these patients have no physical abnormalities. The first signs are those related to the pancytopenia—bleeding, pallor, and recurring infections. There is a higher incidence of leukemia and other cancers in these children. Most die late in the first decade of life.

A clue that helps separate this disorder from the TAR syndrome is that radial hypoplasia or aplasia occurs only with aplasia of the thumb in Fanconi's syndrome.

The incidence of this disorder is not known.

*Performance.*    Patients occasionally are mentally retarded.

*Etiology.*    Inheritance is autosomal recessive. Chromosomal fragility can be demonstrated on chromosomal examination.

## Selected Reading

Alter BP. Aplastic anemia in children: diagnosis and management. Pediatr Rev 1984;6:46.

# Fetal Alcohol Syndrome

## Key Features (Fig 167-15)

Mild to moderate microcephaly
Short palpebral fissures
Smooth philtrum
Thin vermilion border of upper lip

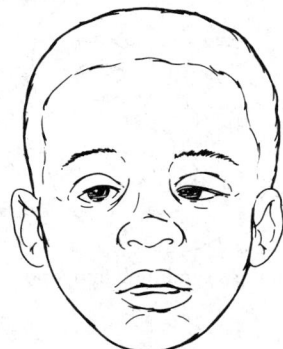

Figure 167-15.    Fetal alcohol syndrome.

## Other Findings

Maxillary hypoplasia
Short, upturned nose
Microphthalmia
Cleft lip or palate
Micrognathia
Short neck
Posteriorly rotated, prominent ears
Pectus excavatum
Clinodactyly
Small distal phalanges
Small fifth finger nails
Short stature
Hypotonia
Fine motor dysfunction
Cardiac murmurs: VSD, ASD usually gone by age 1 year

*Comments.*    The features of this syndrome vary, and, in part, are related to the amount of alcohol consumed by the mother during pregnancy. Two drinks per day may result in decreased birth weight, and four to six per day in subtle clinical findings. Hyperactivity in childhood is a common association. Affected infants are usually irritable and have a poor suck.

*Performance.*    Borderline to moderate retardation is present, depending on the severity of the association.

*Etiology.*    Ingestion of alcohol by the mother during pregnancy results in fetal alcohol syndrome.

## Selected Reading

Jones KL. Fetal alcohol syndrome. Pediatr Rev 1986;8:122.

# Fetal Hydantoin Syndrome

## Key Features (Fig 167-16)

Broad, depressed nasal bridge
Short, anteverted nose
Wide mouth with bowed upper lip
Broad alveolar ridge
Cleft lip and palate
Short neck
Congenital heart defects: VSD, ASD, coarctation of the aorta, tetralogy of Fallot
Hypoplastic distal phalanges with small nails
Poor growth, usually of prenatal onset

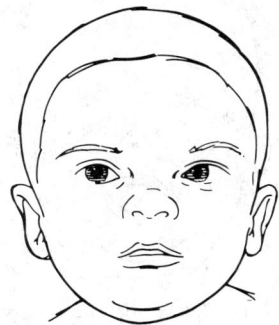

Figure 167-16.    Fetal hydantoin syndrome.

## Other Findings

Widely spaced small nipples
Coarse, profuse scalp hair
Hirsutism
Low-set hairline
Strabismus
Rib anomalies
Large anterior fontanelle; metopic suture ridging
Umbilical and inguinal hernias
Polydactyly; digitalized thumb
Microcephaly, brachycephaly
Coloboma, ptosis, glaucoma
Hypospadias

*Comments.*    Features occur in varying prominence and combination in exposed infants. It is estimated that 10% of infants born to mothers taking hydantoin present a full picture of the syndrome, while 30% have some of the features.

*Performance.*    Mild retardation occurs in many of these infants.

*Etiology.*    Exposure to hydantoin in utero results in fetal hydantoin syndrome. It may be possible to identify fetuses at risk for this syndrome by measuring the activity of epoxide hydrolase in amniocytes.

## Selected Readings

Buehler BA, Delimont D, Van Waer MV, Finnell RH. Prenatal prediction of risk of the fetal hydantoin syndrome. N Engl J Med 1990;322:1567.

Hanson JW, Smith DW. The fetal hydantoin syndrome. J Pediatr 1975;87:285.

## *Hallermann-Streiff Syndrome*

### Key Features (Fig 167-17)

Small stature
Brachycephaly
Frontal and parietal bossing
Malar hypoplasia
Micrognathia
Microphthalmia
Cataracts
Nose—thin, small, pointed, with hypoplastic cartilage
Microstomia—double chin

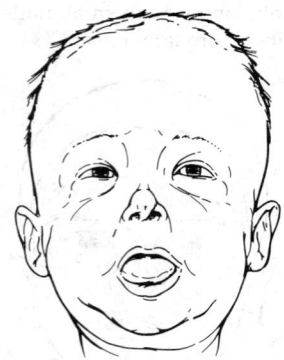

**Figure 167-17.**    Hallermann-Streiff syndrome.

### Other Findings

Hypoplastic and absent teeth, natal teeth, malocclusion
Atrophy of skin most prominent over nose and sutural areas of scalp
Thin, light hair with hypotrichosis; alopecia of frontal and occipital areas
Prominent scalp veins
Mild microcephaly
Delayed closure of fontanelles
High-arched, narrow palate
Cryptorchidism, hypogenitalism
Skeletal anomalies: syndactyly, spina bifida, lordosis, scoliosis
Cardiac defects—may have right-sided lesions

*Comments.*    Feeding and respiratory problems often occur in the neonatal period. The temporomandibular joint has a characteristic forward displacement on radiographic examination.

The incidence of this uncommon syndrome is unknown.

*Performance.*    Most children are developmentally normal, although 15% have mental retardation.

*Etiology.*    The disorder seems to be sporadic in occurrence.

## *Hurler's Syndrome (Mucopolysaccharidosis I)*

### Key Features (Fig 167-18)

Macrocephaly
Frontal prominence
Coarse facies
Wide, anteverted nostrils
Low, depressed nasal bridge
Hypertelorism
Corneal clouding
Enlarged lips
Claw hand
Hernias—umbilical, inguinal

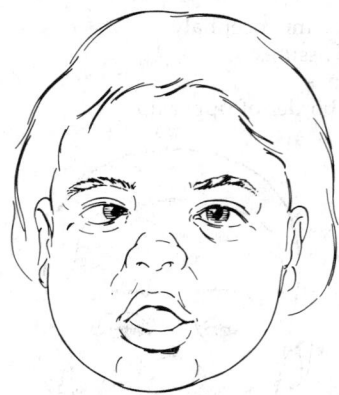

**Figure 167-18.**    Hurler's syndrome (mucopolysaccharidosis I).

### Other Findings

Open mouth
Chronic nasal discharge
Enlarged tongue
Thickened gums
Abnormally spaced teeth
Inner epicanthal folds
Kyphosis
Short neck
Gibbus secondary to anterior vertebral wedging
Hirsutism
Hepatosplenomegaly
Pectus carinatum and excavatum
Growth failure after infancy

*Comments.*    Infants with this syndrome appear normal at birth. During the first year of life, facial features become increasingly coarse and abnormalities become apparent. Recurrent respiratory infections are common. Death usually occurs before age 10 years from cardiorespiratory causes.

Radiographic changes that may help in the diagnosis include coarse bone trabeculation with sugarloafing of the bones of the hand, abnormal vertebral bodies, and wide ribs.

The incidence of Hurler's syndrome is estimated at 1 : 100,000.

*Performance.*    Increasingly severe developmental delay occurs with age. The children are markedly retarded.

*Etiology.*    Inheritance is autosomal recessive. A deficiency of $\alpha$-L-iduronidase allows for deposition of mucopolysaccharides in body tissues, leading to the typical picture. Dermatan sulfate and heparan sulfate are excreted in the urine.

# Langer-Giedion Type of the Trichorhinophalangeal Syndrome

## Key Features (Fig 167-19)

Large, bulbous, pear-shaped nose
Thickened alae nasi with tented nares
Sparse scalp hair
Mild micrognathia
Mild microcephaly
Large, laterally protruding ears
Multiple exostoses

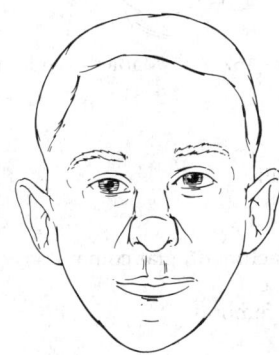

Figure 167-19. Langer-Giedion type of the trichorhinophalangeal syndrome.

## Other Findings

Heavy eyebrows
Long, prominent philtrum
Thin upper lip
Mild postnatal onset of growth deficiency
Tendency toward fractures
Loose skin early in life
Multiple nevi
Asymmetric limb growth
Scoliosis
Joint hypermobility
Winged scapulae
Exotropia
Hearing loss

*Comments.*   Recurrent respiratory tract infections are common. Coning of phalangeal epiphyses, evident by 3 or 4 years of age, is a helpful radiologic finding in addition to the exostoses. A significant delay in speech development is common.

The Langer-Giedion type of trichorhinophalangeal syndrome differs from other types by the presence of multiple exostoses, loose skin, joint hypermobility, microcephaly, nevi, and delayed speech.

The incidence of this uncommon disorder is not known.

*Performance.*   Mild to moderate mental retardation is found in many cases.

*Etiology.*   The occurrence of this syndrome is sporadic, with a deletion at 8q24 found in most cases.

## Selected Readings

Hall BD, Langer LO, Giedion A. Langer-Giedion syndrome. Birth Defects 1974;10(12):147.
Lüdecke H-J, Johnson C, Wagner MJ, et al. Molecular definition of the shortest region of deletion overlap in the Langer-Giedion syndrome. Am J Hum Genet 1991;49:1197.

# Larsen's Syndrome

## Key Features

Flat facies
Depressed, broad nasal bridge
Hypertelorism
Prominent forehead
Congenital dislocations of elbows, hips, and knees

## Other Findings

Broad thumbs
Long, nontapering, cylindrical fingers
Short metacarpals
Talipes equinovarus
Short stature
Cleft palate
Congenital heart disease—various types, particularly septal defects
Kyphoscoliosis

### Less Common Findings

Hydrocephalus
Hearing loss
Tracheomalacia and respiratory distress
Cervical spine instability

*Comments.*   The dislocations often create major orthopedic problems. Acquired cardiac lesions similar to those found in Marfan's syndrome occur, including mitral valve prolapse, aortic dilatation, aortic insufficiency, and dissecting aneurysms.

The incidence of this disorder is not known.

*Etiology.*   Inheritance is not known. Autosomal dominant and autosomal recessive cases have been reported.

## Selected Reading

Kiel EA, Frias JL, Victorica BE. Cardiovascular manifestations in the Larsen syndrome. Pediatrics 1983;71:942.

# Leprechaunism Syndrome

## Key Features (Fig 167-20)

Small face
Prominent eyes
Flat nasal bridge
Flared nostrils
Thick lips
Large, low-set ears
Body and facial hirsutism
Striking lack of subcutaneous tissue

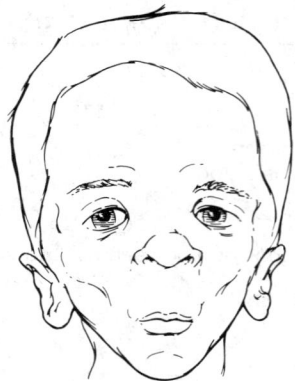

Figure 167-20.    Leprechaunism syndrome.

## Other Findings

Prenatal and postnatal growth deficiency
Gingival hypertrophy
Large mouth
Acanthosis nigracans
Large phallus
Breast hyperplasia
Clitoral and labia minora prominence
Hyperglycemia-hyperinsulinism
Microcephaly
Hypertelorism
Hernias—umbilical, inguinal
Hypotonia
Cryptorchidism
Large hands and feet

*Comments.*    These infants demonstrate marked failure to thrive, and most die in the second half of the first year.
The incidence of this rare syndrome is unknown.

*Performance.*    Mental and motor retardation is marked.

*Etiology.*    Inheritance seems autosomal recessive.

## Selected Reading

Rosenberg AM, Haworth JC, Degroot GW, et al. A case of leprechaunism with severe hyperinsulinemia. Am J Dis Child 1980;134:170.

## *Marfan's Syndrome*

## Key Features (Fig 167-21)

Tendency toward tall stature
Long, slender limbs
Subluxation of lens—usually upward
Dilatation of the aortic root

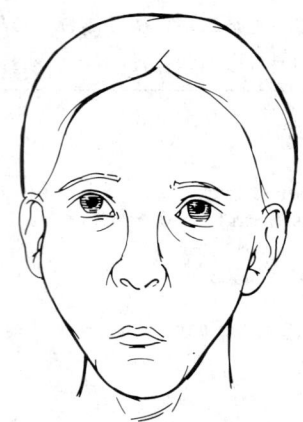

Figure 167-21.    Marfan's syndrome.

## Other Findings

Joint hyperextensibility
Scoliosis, kyphosis
Narrow face
Myopia, retinal detachment, glaucoma
Mitral valve prolapse
Hernias—inguinal, femoral
Large ears

*Comments.*    There is no characteristic facies associated with Marfan's syndrome. The lower segment of the body, symphysis pubis to heel, is longer than the upper segment. The arm span is greater than the height. Lifespan is shortened secondary to cardiovascular complications, particularly dissection of the aorta. Spontaneous pneumothoraces are another common problem.
The incidence is estimated at between 1 : 16,000 and 1 : 60,000.

*Performance.*    Mental retardation is not a characteristic of this disorder.

*Etiology.*    Inheritance is autosomal dominant. The fundamental defect is caused by mutations of the fibrillin gene on chromosome 15.

## Selected Readings

Chen S, Fagan LF, Nouri S, et al. Ventricular dysrhythmias in children with Marfan's syndrome. Am J Dis Child 1985;139:273.
Pyeritz RE, McKusick VA. The Marfan syndrome: diagnosis and management. N Engl J Med 1979;300:772.

## *Menkes' Syndrome*

## Key Features (Fig 167-22)

Pudgy, full cheeks with lack of facial expression
Coarse, light-colored, wiry hair that breaks easily
Thick, dry, pale skin
Short, broad, upturned nose
Marked failure to thrive after birth
Severe and progressive neurologic deterioration in the first few months of life with hypothermia, irritability, feeding difficulties, and seizures

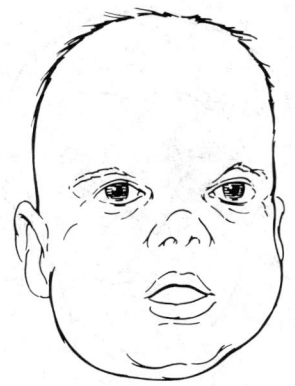

Figure 167-22.   Menkes' syndrome.

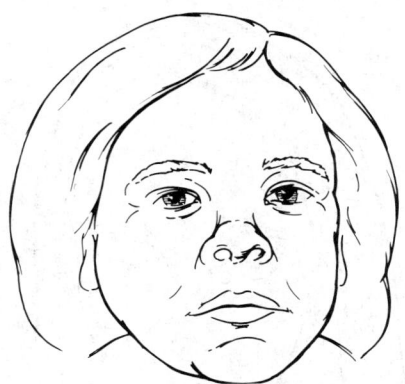

Figure 167-23.   Morquio's syndrome (mucopolysaccharidosis IV).

## Other Findings

Micrognathia
Premature birth
Susceptibility to infection
Thickened periosteum, suggesting child abuse
Loss of vision
Spasticity, hyperreflexia

*Comments.*   Infants with Menkes' syndrome appear normal at birth but rapidly deteriorate neurologically. The hair is normal at birth but becomes sparse, unruly, and light in color. Microscopically, the hair demonstrates a number of abnormalities, including twisting and beading.
   The incidence is estimated at 1 : 50,000 to 1 : 100,000 births. Ninety percent of these infants die by age 2 years.

*Performance.*   Severe retardation is progressive.

*Etiology.*   Menkes' syndrome is inherited as an X-linked recessive trait. The defect is one of copper transport. Serum, urine, liver, brain, and hair copper levels are low, while other tissues demonstrate an increased amount of copper. The serum ceruloplasmin is low to absent. There is no effective treatment for this disorder.

## Selected Readings

Hart DB. Menkes' syndrome: an updated review. J Am Acad Dermatol 1983;9:145.
Verga V, Hall BK, Wang S, et al. Localization of the translocation breakpoint in a female with Menkes' syndrome to Xq13.2–q13.3 proximal to PGK-1. Am J Hum Genet 1991;48:1133.

## Morquio's Syndrome (Mucopolysaccharidosis IV)

### Key Features (Fig 167-23)

Mild coarsening of facial features
Broad mouth
Short neck with restricted movement
Pectus carinatum
Short trunk
Short stature
Knocked knees

## Other Findings

Short, anteverted nose
Cloudy corneas (late in first decade)
Abnormal teeth with pitting and enamel hypoplasia
Hepatomegaly
Short, stubby hands
Joint laxity
Scoliosis, lumbar lordosis

*Comments.*   Not all of these children are coarse-featured. Generally, abnormalities begin to appear between ages 1 and 3 years. Neurologic complications occur secondary to spinal cord compression from C-1/C-2 dislocation. Aortic regurgitation is relatively common later in the course of the disorder. Progressive hearing loss is an additional feature.
   The incidence is estimated at 1 : 40,000. Lifespan is shortened.

*Performance.*   Affected children are normal mentally.

*Etiology.*   Inheritance is autosomal recessive. A marked excretion of keratan sulfate and chondroitin sulfate A can be found in the urine.

## Mulibrey Nanism

### Key Features (Fig 167-24)

Triangular facies
Forehead prominent and high
Growth deficiency—prenatal onset
Development of a thick adherent pericardium
Hepatomegaly and distended neck veins develop because of the constrictive pericarditis

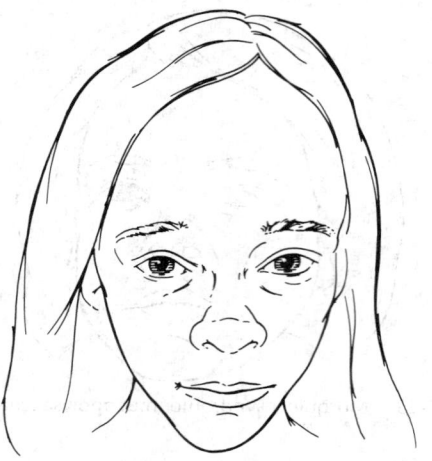

Figure 167-24.   Mulibrey nanism.

## Other Findings

Hands and feet appear relatively large
High-pitched voice
Skull appears enlarged
Strabismus
Yellow spots on the retina
Variable fibrous dysplasia

*Comments.*   This is an uncommon disorder, but it is important to diagnose early because of the constrictive pericarditis. True incidence is unknown.

*Performance.*   The intelligence is normal to mildly retarded.

*Etiology.*   Inheritance appears autosomal recessive.

## Selected Readings

Cumming GR, Kerr D, Ferguson CC. Constrictive pericarditis with dwarfism in two siblings (Mulibrey nanism). J Pediatr 1976;88:569.
Voorhess ML, Husson GS, Blackman MS. Growth failure with pericardial constriction. Am J Dis Child 1976;130:1146.

# *Noonan's Syndrome*

## Key Features (Fig 167-25)

Short stature in more than two thirds of cases
Broad forehead
Ptosis of eyelids
Low-set or malformed ears (fleshy folding of upper transverse portion of helix)
Low posterior hairline (webbed neck)

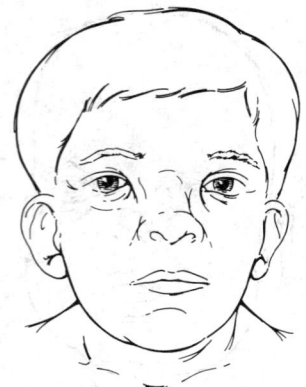

Figure 167-25.   Noonan's syndrome.

## Other Common Features

Cardiovascular abnormalities occur in almost half of cases. Right-sided defects are most common: valvular pulmonic stenosis, peripheral pulmonary artery stenosis, and PDA. ASDs and VSDs are less frequent. Coarctation of the aorta and Ebstein's anomaly occur occasionally.
Cryptorchidism
Epicanthal folds
Hypertelorism
Micrognathia
Flat nasal bridge—saddle nose
Deeply grooved philtrum
Mild antimongoloid slant to palpebral fissures
Dental malocclusion
High-arched palate
Bifid uvula
Shield chest
Pectus excavatum distally with proximal pectus carinatum
Lymphedema of lower extremities

### Less Common Findings

Hypoplastic nails
Hirsutism
Hemangiomas
Sensorineural deafness
Hydrocephaly
Seizures
Autoimmune thyroiditis
Hernias—umbilical, inguinal
Skeletal abnormalities: cubitus valgus, osteoporosis, retarded bone age, clinodactyly, polydactyly, scoliosis, kyphosis
Hypospadias, renal duplication

*Comments.*   Appearance of cases varies. Use of the term *male Turner's syndrome* is inappropriate and may lead to confusion. Although there is some resemblance to Turner's syndrome, a chromosomal abnormality has not been described in Noonan's syndrome.

If cardiac defects are not major, the prognosis for survival is generally good. Gonadal function may be compromised in some cases.

The prevalence of Noonan's syndrome is not established but may be as high as 1 : 1000.

*Performance.*   Mental retardation, usually mild, is present in almost half of cases.

*Etiology.* The basic defect resulting in Noonan's syndrome is unknown. Most cases are sporadic in occurrence, although several families with autosomal dominant or autosomal recessive inheritance have been reported.

## Selected Readings

Allanson JE. Noonan syndrome. J Med Genet 1987;24:9.
Duncan WJ, Fowler RS, Farkas LG, et al. A comprehensive scoring system for evaluation of Noonan syndrome. Am J Med Genet 1981;10:37.

# Oculoauriculovertebral Dysplasia (Goldenhar's Syndrome)

## Key Features (Fig 167-26)

Facial asymmetry with malar, maxillary, or mandibular hypoplasia
Macrostomia with cleftlike corner of mouth
Ear deformities: small, crumpled, complete absence, displaced
Preauricular tags or pits—most commonly in a line from the tragus to the corner of mouth

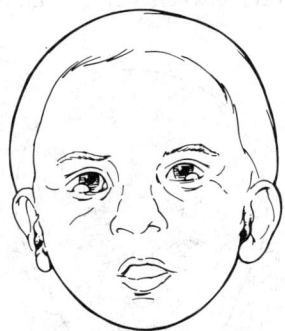

Figure 167-26. Oculoauriculovertebral dysplasia (Goldenhar's syndrome).

## Other Findings

Vertebral anomalies: hemivertebra, occipitalization of the atlas
Epibulbar dermoid at lower lateral margin of the eye
Lipodermoid at upper lateral margin of the eye
Notched upper eyelid
Low-set eye on side of asymmetry
Hearing loss
Frontal bossing

## Occasional Abnormalities

Coloboma of the iris or choroid
Rib anomalies
Talipes equinovarus
Cleft lip/palate
Ptosis
Congenital heart disease

*Comments.* The facial asymmetry is bilateral in 10% of cases.

The frequency of occurrence may be as high as 1 : 5600 live births.

*Performance.* A minority of these children are mentally retarded.

*Etiology.* Sporadic in occurrence. It is thought to represent an anomalous development of the first and second branchial arches.

## Selected Readings

Feingold M, Baum J. Goldenhar's syndrome. Am J Dis Child 1978;132:136.
Rollnick BR. Oculoauriculo-vertebral anomaly: variability and causal heterogeneity. Am J Med Genet 1988;4(suppl):41.

# Oral-Facial-Digital Syndrome (OFD)

## Key Features

Thin nose with hypoplasia of the alar cartilage
Flat midfacial region
Lateral placement of the inner canthi
Partial clefts in mid-upper lip, tongue, and alveolar ridges
Cleft of soft palate
Anomalous teeth
Webbing between buccal mucous membranes and alveolar ridge
Asymmetric shortening of digits with clinodactyly, with or without syndactyly
Dry, rough, sparse hair

## Other Findings

Hamartoma (lobules) of the tongue
Frontal bossing
Micrognathia
Flattened nasal tip
Dry skin
Polydactyly of the feet

*Comments.* This syndrome is often divided into two types, I and II. The description above best fits OFD I. In OFD II or Mohr syndrome, the tongue is cleft and polysyndactyly of the halluces, polydactyly of the hand, a broad nasal tip that may be bifid, ankyloglossia (bound-down tongue), and normal skin and hair are seen.

The incidence of OFD is estimated at 1 : 50,000. About one third of those with OFD I die in early infancy.

*Performance.* More than 50% of OFD I patients have mild mental retardation.

*Etiology.* OFD I is an X-linked dominant disorder, while OFD II has been described as both autosomal dominant and autosomal recessive.

## Selected Reading

Townes PL, Wood BP, McDonald JV. Further heterogeneity of the oral-facial-digital syndrome. Am J Dis Child 1976;130:548.

## *Prader-Willi Syndrome*

### Key Features (Fig 167-27)

Obesity—onset from infancy to 6 years (average 2 to 3 years)
Hypotonia—more severe in infancy
Hypogonadism—small penis and scrotum, cryptorchidism

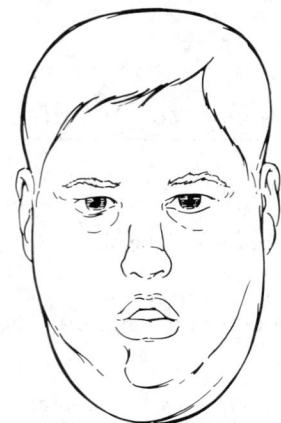

Figure 167-27.   Prader-Willi syndrome.

### Other Common Findings

Almond-shaped appearance of palpebral fissures
Narrow bifrontal diameter
Strabismus
Short stature
Small hands and feet
Fishlike mouth
Increased incidence of diabetes mellitus—nonketotic, insulin-resistant
Feeble fetal activity—often breech birth
Decreased oculocutaneous pigmentation

#### Less Common Findings

Congenital dislocated hips
Microcephaly
Clinodactyly
Syndactyly
Hyporeflexia, decreased Moro reflex
High-pitched voice
Primary amenorrhea or delayed menarche in females

*Comments.*   Feeding problems and hypotonia are often the initial clues in infancy. Later, increased appetite and obesity become problematic. Speech development is retarded. Although these children are usually happy, they are irritable when food is denied.

The incidence of this relatively common disorder is 1 : 16,000 live births. Life expectancy is shortened as a result of the obesity and its effects on the cardiac and respiratory systems.

*Performance.*   An IQ in the 40 to 60 range is most common.

*Etiology.*   Most children with this syndrome lack paternal inheritance of a segment of chromosome 15 q11.2–q12 or maternal disomy of the entire chromosome 15.

## Selected Readings

Butler MG, Meaney FJ. Standards for selected anthropometric measurements in Prader-Willi syndrome. Pediatrics 1991;88:853.
Cassidy SB. Prader-Willi syndrome. Curr Probl Pediatr 1984;14(1):1.
Robinson WP, Bottani A, Yagang X, et al. Molecular, cytogenetic, and clinical investigations of Prader-Willi syndrome patients. Am J Hum Genet 1991;49:1219.

## *Progeria (Hutchinson-Gilford Syndrome)*

### Key Features (Fig 167-28)

Alopecia—onset, birth to 18 months
Thin, warm, dry skin
Facial hypoplasia
Micrognathia (marked)
Thin nose—sculptured-appearing tip
Loss of subcutaneous fat (cheeks and pubic areas are last to be lost)
Head appears large for face
Fontanelles remain open
Stiff, partially flexed joints
Growth deceleration (between 6 and 18 months)
Slim bones

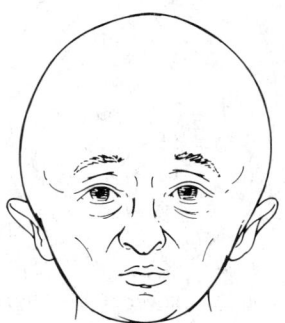

Figure 167-28.   Progeria (Hutchinson-Gilford syndrome).

### Other Findings

Delayed dentition
High-pitched voice
Prominent eyes
Thin lips
Dystrophic nails—thin, short, small
Skin develops increasing numbers of brownish spots and irregular pigmentation
Joints appear prominent

*Comments.*   This syndrome is often referred to as one of premature aging. Affected children look remarkably similar to one another. Adult height rarely exceeds 110 cm and weight, 15 kg. Three early features are midfacial cyanosis, skin resembling scleroderma (thick, inelastic), and a glyphic (pointed or sculptured) nasal tip.

The incidence of this disorder is estimated at 1 : 250,000 to 1 : 4,000,000. Average age at death is 12 to 13 years, usually the result of complications of atherosclerosis, myocardial infarction, congestive heart failure, or stroke.

*Etiology.*   The cause of this syndrome is not known.

## Selected Reading

Debusk FL. The Hutchinson-Gilford syndrome. J Pediatr 1972;60:697.

## *Rothmund-Thomson Syndrome*

### Key Features (Fig 167-29)

Skin—marblelike or reticulated appearance due to erythema and
    telangiectasia, pigmentation, and hypopigmentation
Photosensitivity
Cataract (develops rapidly, usually after age 2 years)
Sparse or absent eyebrows and eyelashes

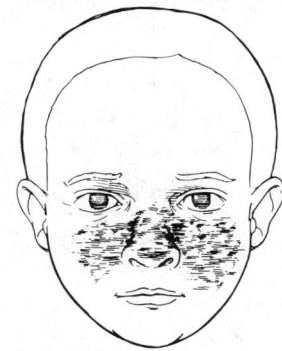

Figure 167-29.   Rothmund-Thomson syndrome.

### Other Findings

Short stature
Small hands and feet
Hypoplastic to absent thumbs; hypoplasia of radius, thumb, or
    ulna; absence of patella
Small saddle nose
Small dystrophic nails
Sparse hair—prematurely gray, occasional alopecia
Hyperkeratosis of palms and soles
Hypogonadism
Microcephaly
Frontal bossing
Defective dentition

    *Comments.*   Striking skin changes may be present at birth
or develop later. Photosensitivity is common. Skin cancer may
develop later in life.
    The incidence of this uncommon disorder is unknown.

    *Performance.*   Mental retardation occurs in some children.

    *Etiology.*   Inheritance appears autosomal recessive.

## Selected Reading

Berg E, Chuang T-Y, Cripps D. Rothmund-Thomson syndrome. J Am Acad Dermatol
    1987;17:332.

## *Rubinstein-Taybi Syndrome*

### Key Features (Fig 167-30)

Broad thumbs with radial angulation; broad great toes
Short stature
Microcephaly
Downslanting palpebral fissures
Hypoplastic maxilla with narrow palate
Beaked nose with nasal septum extending below alae nasi
Low-set or malformed auricles
Cryptorchidism

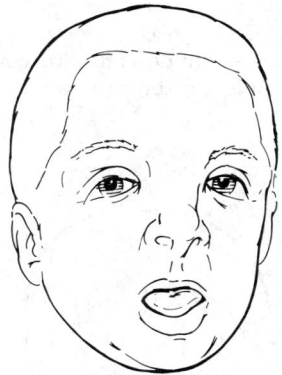

Figure 167-30.   Rubinstein-Taybi syndrome.

### Other Common Findings

Epicanthal folds
Strabismus
Nevus flammeus of forehead
Other fingers broad
Prominent forehead
Large anterior fontanelle
Congenital heart defect

#### Less Common Findings

Long eyelashes, heavy eyebrows
Mild micrognathia
Ptosis of eyelids
Cataracts, colobomas
Hypertelorism, broad nasal bridge
High-arched palate
Dental malocclusion
Overlapping toes
Polydactyly
Pectus excavatum
Kyphoscoliosis
Hypospadias
Hirsutism
Stiff gait
Hyperextensible joints

    *Comments.*   The broad thumbs and toes are usually the fea-
ture focuses attention on this diagnosis. Feeding and respiratory
problems are common in infancy. Patients with Rubinstein-Taybi
syndrome tend to form large keloids.
    The frequency of occurrence of this syndrome is not known,
but it is not uncommon.

    *Performance.*   All children affected with this disorder have
mental, motor, and social retardation. In most, IQ is less than 50.

*Etiology.* Occurrence is sporadic in almost all cases.

## Selected Reading

Johnson CF. Broad thumbs and broad great toes with facial abnormalities and mental retardation. J Pediatr 1966;68:942.

## Selected Readings

Oritz C, Cleveland RH, Jaramillo, D, Blickman JG, Crawford J. Urethral valves in Russell-Silver syndrome. J Pediatr 1991;119:776.
Saal HM, Pagon RA, Pepin MG. Reevaluation of Russell-Silver syndrome. J Pediatr 1985;107:733.
Tanner JM, Lejarraga H, Cameron N. The natural history of the Silver-Russell syndrome: a longitudinal study of 39 cases. Pediatr Res 1975;9:611.

# *Russell-Silver Syndrome*

## Key Features (Fig 167-31)

Short stature—prenatal in onset
Small, triangular facies with downturning corners of the mouth
Clinodactyly—short, incurved fifth fingers
Asymmetry—most commonly of the limbs
Cafè-au-lait spots
Head appears disproportionately large

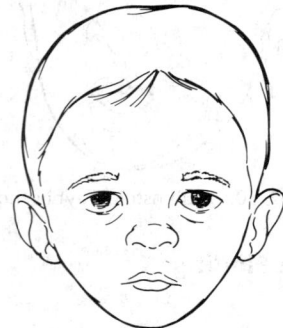

Figure 167-31.   Russell-Silver syndrome.

## Other Features

Liability to fasting hypoglycemia
Prominent eyes
Frontal bossing and mandibular hypoplasia on profile
Long eyelashes
Thin lips
Palate high and narrow
Crowded teeth
Poor muscular development
Syndactyly of second and third toes
Delayed closure of anterior fontanelle
Precocious puberty
Urogenital abnormalities: hypospadias, ambiguous genitalia, small testes, cryptorchidism, posterior and anterior urethral valves, ureteropelvic stenosis, vesicoureteral reflux, horseshoe kidney.

*Comments.*   Discussion continues whether there is one syndrome or two, Silver's and Russell's, the former with asymmetry.
Despite the short stature in infancy and childhood, Saal and colleagues reevaluated 15 patients later in life and found that 5 achieved normal adult height.
The incidence of this uncommon syndrome is not known.

*Performance*   Mild developmental delay occurs in about one third of cases.

*Etiology.*   The cause of this syndrome is not known. Hypopituitarism can closely mimic this disorder.

# *Saethre-Chotzen Syndrome (Acrocephalosyndactyly Type III)*

## Key Features (Fig 167-32)

Short anterior-posterior diameter of skull
High forehead
Flat occiput
Flat facies
Shallow orbits
Hypertelorism
Strabismus
Downslanting of palpebral fissures
Small ears
Facial asymmetry

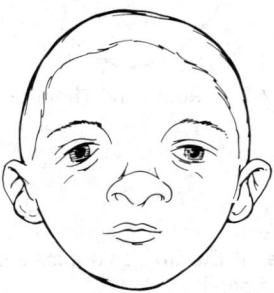

Figure 167-32.   Saethre-Chotzen syndrome (acrocephalosyndactyly type III).

## Other Findings

Small nose—often beaklike
Ptosis of eyelids
Large fontanelle
Microcephaly
Cutaneous syndactyly of second and third fingers, usually partial, and toes, usually third and fourth
Short fingers
Broad thumbs and great toes
Fingerlike thumbs
Limited elbow extension
Short clavicles
Cleft palate
Cryptorchidism
Short stature

*Comments.*   The abnormal head shape is felt to be the result of premature closure of the coronal suture. Some children develop increased intracranial pressure. Clinical expression varies.
The incidence of occurrence is not known, but this disorder may be the most common form of craniosynostosis.

*Performance.*   Most affected individuals are normal in mental development.

*Etiology.*    Inheritance is autosomal dominant.

## Selected Reading

Friedman JM. Saethre-Chotzen syndrome: a broad and variable pattern of skeletal malformation. J Pediatr 1977;91:929.

# Seckel's Syndrome

## Key Features (Fig 167-33)

Microcephaly—premature synostosis
Facial hypoplasia with prominent nose
Low-set, malformed ears—absent earlobes
Severe growth retardation

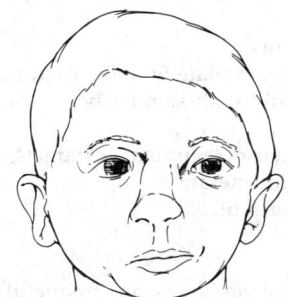

Figure 167-33.    Seckel's syndrome.

## Other Findings

Micrognathia
Facial asymmetry
Eyes appear prominent
Clinodactyly of fifth fingers
Simian crease
Dislocated hips
Cryptorchidism

### Occasional Findings

Strabismus
Partial adontia
Enamel hypoplasia
Sparse hair
Cleft lip
Scoliosis
Talipes equinovarus
Single flexion crease of fifth digit

*Comments.*    This syndrome is also known as the "bird-headed dwarf syndrome" because of the phenotypic features. Affected children may have 11 pairs of ribs and hypoplasia of the proximal radius, resulting in inability to extend the forearm. The incidence is unknown, but the syndrome is rare.

*Performance.*    All affected children have mental retardation.

*Etiology.*    Inheritance is probably autosomal recessive.

## Selected Reading

Majewski F, Goecke T. Studies of microcephalic primordial dwarfism: approach to a delineation of the Seckel syndrome. Am J Med Genet 1982;12:7.

# Shprintzen's (Velo-Cardio-Facial) Syndrome

## Key Features (Fig 167-34)

Cleft of soft palate—overt or occult (submucous)
Long nose with a broad squared nasal root
Narrow alae nasi
Mandible set back slightly
Learning disabilities
Cardiac abnormalities: VSD, right aortic arch, tetralogy of Fallot

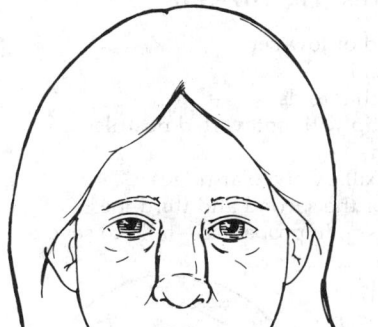

Figure 167-34.    Shprintzen's (velo-cardio-facial) syndrome.

## Other Findings

Narrow palpebral fissures
Long, myopathic facies
Malar flatness
Abundant scalp hair
Conductive hearing loss
Slender limbs, hyperextensible fingers
Hypotonia in infancy
Microcephaly
Inguinal hernia
Malformed auricles
Laryngeal web
Cryptorchidism
Hypospadias
Scoliosis
Small stature
Hypocalcemia

*Comments.*    Many of these children attend speech clinics because of cleft palate or hyponasal speech. Learning disabilities are present in almost all cases.

This diagnosis should be considered in any child with a conotruncal cardiac anomaly, particularly if associated with clefting.

The incidence of this disorder is not known.

*Performance.*    Mental retardation occurs in fewer than half of cases.

*Etiology.*    An autosomal dominant or X-linked dominant inheritance is postulated.

## Selected Readings

Lipson AH, Yuille D, Angel M, et al. Velocardiofacial (Shprintzen) syndrome: an important syndrome for the dysmorphologist to recognise. J Med Genet 1991;28: 596.

Shprintzen RJ, Goldberg RB, Young D, et al. The velo-cardio-facial syndrome: a clinical and genetic analysis. Pediatrics 1981;67:167.

# Smith-Lemli-Opitz Syndrome

## Key Features (Fig 167-35)

Ears—slanted or low-set
Ptosis of eyelids
Inner epicanthal folds
Broad nasal tip with anteverted nostrils
Micrognathia
Enlarged maxillary alveolar ridges
Syndactyly of the second and third toes
Cryptorchidism, hypospadias—mild to severe

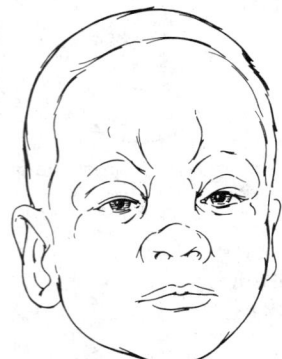

Figure 167-35.   Smith-Lemli-Opitz syndrome.

## Other Findings

Smallness for gestational age with failure to thrive postnatally
Microcephaly with narrow frontal area
Strabismus
Long philtrum
Simian crease
Congenital heart disease—various types
Variable muscle tone—hypotonia early and hypertonia later
Seizures
Cataract
Cleft palate
Skeletal defects: flexed fingers, polydactyly, vertical talus

*Comments.*   Feeding difficulties and vomiting are especially common in early infancy. Infants with this syndrome are usually irritable. Early death is common, with one of five dying within the first year of life and half by 18 months of age.

The incidence of this uncommon syndrome is unknown.

*Performance.*   There is moderate to severe mental retardation.

*Etiology.*   Inheritance is autosomal recessive.

# Stickler's Syndrome (Hereditary Arthro-Ophthalmopathy)

## Key Features

Flat facies
Depressed nasal bridge
Epicanthal folds
Maxillary hypoplasia
Micrognathia
Myopia—before 10 years of age

## Other Findings

Clefts of hard or soft palate
Long philtrum
Dental anomalies
Deafness—sensorineural, occurs in middle age
Hypotonia
Hyperextensible joints
Joint pains that may simulate juvenile rheumatoid arthritis
Marfanoid body build with slender body, long fingers, and increased arm span
Eye problems: retinal detachment, cataracts, strabismus, glaucoma, vitreous degeneration
Thoracic kyphosis or scoliosis
Pectus carinatum

*Comments.*   Eye problems are frequently the reason that patients are referred. A family history of early-onset myopia should always suggest this disorder. A progressive multiple epiphyseal dysplasia results in bony enlargement of the ankles, knees, and wrists, and joint pains may simulate juvenile rheumatoid arthritis. In the newborn period, the micrognathia may be life threatening. The phenotypic findings are extremely variable, however.

The incidence of this disorder is not known.

*Performance.*   Mental retardation is occasional.

*Etiology.*   Inheritance is thought to be autosomal dominant.

## Selected Readings

Liberfarb RM, Hirose T, Holmes LB. The Wagner-Stickler syndrome: a study of 22 families. J Pediatr 1981;99:394.

Temple IK. Stickler's syndrome. J Med Genet 1989;26:119.

# TAR (Radial Aplasia-Thrombocytopenia)

## Key Features

Aplasia or hypoplasia of radius—bilateral (thumbs are present, however)
Thrombocytopenia, present at birth
Leukemoid granulocytosis in the first year of life

## Other Findings

Defects of the hands: club hand, syndactyly
Defects of the legs and feet: dislocated hips, coxa valga, small feet, hypoplasia or aplasia of lower limbs
Congenital heart defects: tetralogy of Fallot, ASD
Rib anomalies: cervical rib, asymmetric first rib
Fused cervical vertebrae
Micrognathia, maxillary hypoplasia
Low-set ears
Excessive perspiration
Pedal edema

*Comments.* Thrombocytopenia is most severe in early infancy. Anemia and eosinophilia are common. Death occurs in almost half of these infants in early infancy due to hemorrhage. Diarrhea is common in the first year of life.

Thumbs are present with the radial aplasia in this disorder, but are absent or hypoplastic with the radial aplasia in Fanconi's syndrome.

The incidence of this disorder is not known.

*Performance.* Mental retardation has occurred in some patients, but was felt to be secondary to intracranial hemorrhage.

*Etiology.* Inheritance is autosomal recessive.

## Treacher Collins Syndrome

### Key Features (Fig 167-36)

Antimongoloid slant of palpebral fissures
Malar hypoplasia
Micrognathia
Lower lid coloboma

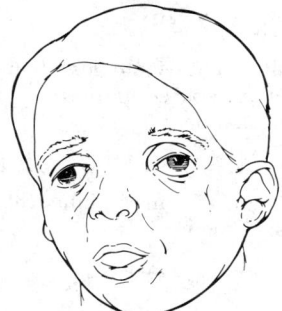

**Figure 167-36.** Treacher Collins syndrome.

## Other Findings

Partial to total absence of lower eyelashes
Malformed auricles—microtia, crumpled, absent auditory canal
Projection of scalp hair onto cheek
Beaklike nose
Deafness
Extra ear tags, blind fistulas
High-arched palate
Dental malocclusion
Macrostomia—unilateral

### Less Common Features

Cryptorchidism
Defects of cervical vertebrae
Congenital heart disease

*Comments.* Clinical expression varies. The incidence is 1 : 50,000 births.

*Performance.* Mental retardation is uncommon, and, if present, may be related to delayed detection of deafness.

*Etiology.* Inheritance is autosomal dominant, with as many as 50% of cases representing new mutations. The loci for the gene is thought to be in the region of 5q31–34.

## Selected Reading

Dixon MJ, Read AP, Donnai D, et al. The gene for Treacher-Collins syndrome maps to the long arm of chromosome 5. Am J Hum Genet 1991;49:17.

## Trisomy 13

### Key Features (Fig 167-37)

Microphthalmia (small eyes)
Cleft lip, cleft palate, or both
Moderate microcephaly with sloping forehead
Shallow supraorbital ridges
Localized scalp defects (cutis aplasia)
Broad, flat nose
Postaxial polydactyly of hands or feet
Congenital heart defects: VSD, ASD, PDA, dextrocardia
Micrognathia

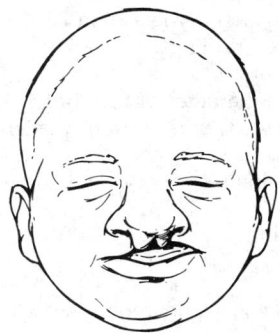

**Figure 167-37.** Trisomy 13.

### Less Common Findings

#### Head and Neck

Low-set, abnormally shaped ears
Loose skin of posterior neck
Short neck
Ocular hypotelorism or hypertelorism
Epicanthal folds
Capillary hemangioma of the glabella

#### Skeletal

Overlapping fingers
Short, dorsiflexed great toes
Rocker-bottom feet

## Neurologic

Hypertonia or hypotonia, seizures, agenesis of corpus callosum

## Ophthalmologic

Iris colobomas, cataracts, retinal detachment, retinal dysplasia

## Other

Omphalocele, malrotation of intestines, Meckel's diverticulum, renal anomalies, cryptorchidism

*Comments.* About 5% of affected infants exhibit some form of holoprosencephaly. The prognosis is extremely poor: 65% die in the first 3 months of life and 95% by age 3 years.

The incidence is estimated at 1 : 5000 live births.

*Performance.* All of these infants are severely developmentally delayed.

*Etiology.* An older maternal age seems to be a factor for development of trisomy 13. Nondisjunction accounts for 75% of the cases. Young mothers with trisomy 13 infants should have their chromosomes analyzed to detect translocations. If one parent is a translocation carrier, the recurrence risk is about 10%, while if the parents are normal, the risk is less than 1%.

## Selected Reading

Hodes ME, Cole J, Palmer CG, et al. Clinical experience with trisomies 18 and 13. J Med Genet 1978;15:48.

## *Trisomy 18 (Edward's Syndrome)*

## Key Features

Low–birth-weight, generally less than 2300 g
Common craniofacial findings:
    Prominent occiput
    Narrow bifrontal diameter of face-head
    Low-set malformed ears—often posteriorly rotated and flattened
    Short palpebral fissures
    Microphthalmia
    Small oral opening
    Small mandible
    Microcephaly
Congenital heart defects: VSD (90%), PDA (70%), ASD (20%)
Short sternum
Limited hip abduction
Short, dorsiflexed first toe
Clenched hand with overlapping fingers

## Other Common Features

Inner epicanthal folds
Ptosis of the eyelids
Narrow nasal bridge
Narrow palate
Mild hirsutism of the forehead
Large fontanelles
Short neck
Hypotonia followed by hypertonia
Hypoplastic nails
Wide-spaced nipples

Rocker-bottom feet
Hypoplastic or absent thumbs
Cleft lip/palate
Cryptorchidism, hypoplastic labia, prominent clitoris

*Comments.* This is a relatively distinctive syndrome. More than 100 abnormalities have been described.

Trisomy-18 infants have feeble movements in utero. Polyhydramnios is present in more than half of the pregnancies. The placenta is small, and the umbilical cord has a single umbilical artery.

Affected infants have severe developmental retardation with failure to thrive. A poor suck leads to feeding difficulties. Seizures and hydrocephalus occur relatively frequently. Hernias, including umbilical, inguinal, and diaphragmatic hernias, occur in almost one fourth of these infants. Tracheoesophageal fistulas may be found as well.

The prognosis is poor, with one third dying in the first month of life and one half by 2 months of age. Less than 10% of cases survive the first year.

The frequency of occurrence is estimated at 1 : 3500 to 1 : 7000 live births.

*Etiology.* Eighty percent of cases are caused by nondisjunction. About 10% are due to translocations. The mean maternal age is elevated.

## Selected Reading

Hodes ME, Cole J, Palmer CG, et al. Clinical experience with trisomies 18 and 13. J Med Genet 1978;15:48.

## *Turner's Syndrome*

**CAUTION:** Many patients with Turner's syndrome have minimal dysmorphic features.

## Key Features (Fig 167-38)

Short stature—adult height usually less than 144 cm
Broad chest with widely spaced nipples
Webbed posterior neck (about 50%)
Low posterior hairline
Short neck
Increased carrying angle of arms (cubitus valgus)
Primary or secondary amenorrhea

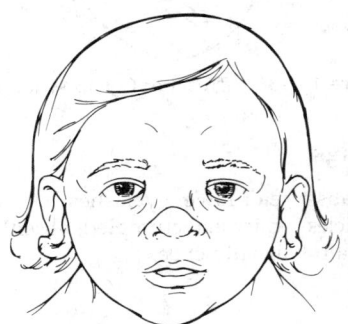

Figure 167-38.   Turner's syndrome.

## Neonatal Clue

Lymphedema of the dorsa of the hands and feet

## Other Phenotypic Clues

Abnormal ears—prominent
Epicanthal folds
Ptosis of the upper eyelids
Micrognathia
Downward and outward slant of palpebral fissures
Short fourth metacarpals
Toenails—hypoplastic, hyperconvex, deep set
Cutaneous nevi that increase with age
Sexual infantilism in postpubertal females

*Comments.* Congenital heart disease, particularly coarctation of the aorta, occurs in 15% to 30% of cases, and idiopathic hypertension in another 25%. Hearing loss occurs in 50% of cases, and various renal abnormalities in almost another 50%.

The prognosis is good for a normal lifespan if cardiovascular abnormalities and hypertension are absent.

The height of affected children is positively correlated with paternal height. Girls whose height is more than 2 STD below the mean for chronologic age should have a cytogenetic examination, even in the absence of dysmorphic features. Turner's syndrome should be considered in girls who develop lymphedema at any age.

The incidence of Turner's syndrome is estimated at 1 : 2500 to 1 : 6000 liveborn females, but about 20% of spontaneous abortions have a Turner karyotype.

*Performance.* Mental retardation is uncommon.

*Etiology.* The syndrome is the result of a partial or complete deletion of one X chromosome.

## Selected Readings

Massa GG, Vanderschuren-Lodeweyckk M. Age and height at diagnosis in Turner syndrome: influence of parental height. Pediatrics 1991;88:1148.
Simpson JL. Gonadal dysgenesis and abnormalities of the human sex chromosome: current status of phenotypic–karyotypic correlations. Birth Defects 1975;11(4): 23.

## *VATER Association*

## Key Features

No phenotypic facial abnormalities
Primary external abnormality is radial dysplasia
Anomalies that seem associated:
  Vertebral: hemivertebrae, sacral deformity
  Imperforate anus
  Esophageal atresia with tracheoesophageal fistula
  Radial dysplasia: thumb or radial hypoplasia, preaxial polydactyly, syndactyly
  Renal: aplasia, pelvic kidney, ureteropelvic obstruction
  Cardiac defects: VSD, ASD

## Less Common Findings

Prenatal growth deficiency
Ear anomalies
Large fontanelles
Lower limb defects
Rib anomalies
Inguinal hernia

Malformation of the small intestine
Choanal atresia
Cleft lip/palate
Scoliosis/kyphosis

*Comments.* The acronym is derived from V, vertebral or vascular; A, anal malformation; TE, tracheoesophageal fistula; R, radial limb or renal defects. Usually, three of the major components are necessary to use this diagnostic association. The presence of one or two anomalies should always lead to close inspection for others.

The incidence of VATER association is not known, but it is not uncommon.

*Etiology.* Occurrence of this syndrome is sporadic. It seems to be related to an intrauterine event occurring between the fourth and seventh week of gestation.

## Selected Reading

Weaver DD, Mapstone CL, Pao-lo Y. The VATER association: analysis of 46 patients. Am J Dis Child 1986;140:225.

## *Williams Syndrome*

## Key Features (Fig 167-39)

Depressed nasal bridge
Epicanthal folds
Periorbital fullness of subcutaneous tissues
Blue eyes with stellate pattern of iris
Anteverted nares
Long philtrum
Prominent thick lips with open mouth; drooping lower lip
Short stature
Husky (hoarse) voice

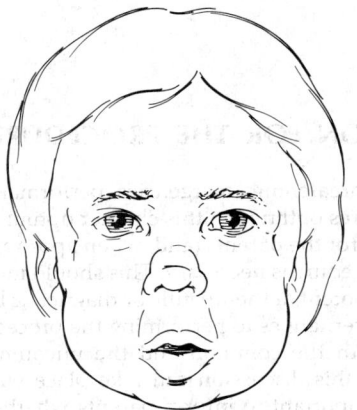

Figure 167-39.  Williams syndrome.

## Other Common Features

Mild microcephaly
Medial eyebrow flare
Full cheeks
Short palpebral fissures
Ocular hypotelorism
Strabismus

Mild antenatal growth deficiency
Friendly, loquacious personality
Hypoplastic nails (short, deep set, or brittle)
Cardiac defects: supravalvular aortic stenosis, valvular aortic stenosis, peripheral pulmonary artery stenosis, VSD, ASD, coarctation.
Renal artery stenosis (hypertension)
Pectus excavatum
Inguinal hernia
Partial adontia
Bladder diverticula
Nephrocalcinosis

*Comments.* The Williams syndrome was formerly called the syndrome of elfin facies, infantile hypercalcemia, supravalvular aortic stenosis, and failure to thrive. Evidence of infantile hypercalcemia is highly variable. In one series of patients, only 7 of 19 had supravalvular aortic stenosis, although murmurs were heard in 15 of 19. Children with this syndrome have a characteristic facial appearance. Their friendly, outgoing manner is often labeled as a cocktail-party personality.

As the children enter puberty, most attain heights above the fifth percentile. Normal sexual development occurs.

Renal or renovascular abnormalities occur in 50% of these patients.

The frequency of occurrence is not known, but this syndrome is not uncommon. The appearance is characteristic.

*Performance.* The average IQ is in the 50s. Testing reveals uneven developmental profiles compared to measured IQ, with reading abilities exceeding the expected level and visual motor skills lagging behind.

*Etiology.* The occurrence of this syndrome appears to be sporadic. There is some evidence of vitamin D sensitivity in many cases. Even patients who are normocalcemic and have no history of hypercalcemia have an abnormal response in levels of serum 25 OH vitamin D to pharmacologic doses of this vitamin.

## Selected Readings

Ingelfinger JR, Newburger JW. Spectrum of renal anomalies in patients with Williams syndrome. J Pediatr 1991;119:771.
Jones KL, Smith DW. The Williams elfin facies syndrome. J Pediatr 1975;86:718.
Pagon RA, Bennett FC, Laveck B, et al. Williams syndrome: features in late childhood and adolescence. Pediatrics 1987;80:85.

---

*Principles and Practice of Pediatrics, Second Edition.*
edited by Frank A. Oski et al. J. B. Lippincott Company, Philadelphia © 1994.

## CHAPTER 168
# *Pediatric Procedures*

### Peter C. Rowe

## PREPARATION FOR THE PROCEDURE

Except in life-threatening emergencies, performance of most pediatric procedures outlined in this chapter optimally begins with an explanation for the parents (and, when appropriate, the child) of why the procedure is necessary. This should include a realistic description of potential therapeutic or diagnostic benefits, a consideration of alternatives to performing the procedure, and a description of both the common and the uncommon associated risks. Much of this discussion can take place when requesting consent. It is important to inform parents whether they will be allowed in the room during the procedure. In this matter of personal preference for the physician and the family, there is only one clear rule: parents should be in the room to comfort and console, not to assist in a potentially painful experience for the child.

In talking about procedures with children, the language should be appropriate to their level of understanding, honest about the discomfort they are likely to experience, and relatively free of slang. The physician who announces "Before I stick you, I'm going to freeze your arm" is likely to have a more mobile patient than the one who says "Before I start your IV, we'll put some medicine in so that it won't hurt very much." Avoid presenting a child with the unrealistic suggestion that he or she has a choice in whether the procedure is performed. Virtually any healthy child will respond with a resounding "No" to the question "Would you like to have your bone marrow aspirated now?" In many instances, it is possible to offer the child appropriate choices: "Do you want the IV started in your left hand or in your right hand?" (The answer may still be "No.") Generally, it is helpful to set limits for what you expect from the child: "I don't mind if you yell, but your job is to be absolutely still." For excessively unruly older patients, contracts that increase the child's sense of control may be beneficial. A realistic (if limited) example follows: "If you agree to remain still for blood drawing, we will agree not to wake you between 2:00 and 7:00 a.m. to restart your IV." To avoid inadvertent breach of such agreements, they should be written, signed, and on display at the bedside.

A variety of behavioral strategies can decrease the child's anxiety. Simple ways to distract patients include asking them to squeeze an assistant's hand, count, describe someone's clothing, breathe deeply, and recall the details of a recent television program. Some children may respond to humor or to pleasing or vivid imagery in which they are urged to imagine themselves driving a car, riding a skateboard, or in the midst of a fantastic scene or adventure. For more cooperative patients, these strategies may be unnecessary, perhaps even insulting. It is always good to praise the child for a job well done.

After directing attention to the parents and the child, it is important to inform assistants of what is expected of them and to gather all necessary equipment beforehand so the procedure takes place smoothly. Finally, pediatric procedures may be a source of personal discomfort for the physician, and of frustration or anger when success is not immediate. In this regard, it is worth recalling a time-honored clinical rule. That is, if one individual has been unsuccessful in two or three attempts, it is time for another individual to try. Persistent efforts by a frustrated operator are unlikely to be rewarding and will certainly be stressful for the child.

# SEDATION AND ANESTHESIA

## Sedation

The need for sedation varies with the procedure and the age, developmental level, and temperament of the patient. With bone marrow aspirations, for example, some patients prefer not to be sedated so they can return to normal activities after the procedure, while others need mild sedation and a few require general anesthesia with ketamine. Table 168-1 lists common sedatives and analgesics used for pediatric procedures.

## Local Anesthetics

Lidocaine 1% is a suitable local anesthetic for most procedures in this chapter. It has a rapid onset of action, lasts 30 to 120 minutes, and causes minimal irritation of local tissues. To avoid systemic toxicity, no more than 4 mg/kg (0.4 mL/kg of a 1% solution without epinephrine) as a total dose should be infiltrated. Discomfort is minimized by using a 27- or 28-gauge needle (found on insulin syringes) and injecting the lidocaine slowly.

A new topical skin anesthetic, EMLA cream (an eutectic mixture of lidocaine and prilocaine), reduces discomfort with venipuncture, lumbar puncture, subcutaneous drug reservoir injections, even injection of local anesthetics. For optimal analgesia, the cream must be applied 60 minutes before the injection, then be covered with an occlusive dressing.

## Restraint

Manual restraint is the standard method of immobilization for most procedures, especially in infants. When assistants are un- available, restraint (or papoose) boards are a convenient means of safely stabilizing young children. If these are not available or if the patient is too large for the board, suitable restraints can be fashioned using hospital sheets (Fig 168-1).

# BLOOD SAMPLING AND INTRAVASCULAR ACCESS

## Skin-Puncture Sampling

In infants and children, skin-puncture blood sampling helps conserve sites of venous access, is usually less distressing for the patient than venipuncture, and is often more convenient. Warming the sampling site first to increase local blood flow improves the ease and validity of the collection. A cloth towel or disposable diaper soaked in warm water suffices for this purpose (water temperatures above 44°C may cause burns). Cleanse the puncture site with 70% alcohol and wipe dry with a sterile gauze pad (alcohol can cause hemolysis). Use either a short lancet (2.5 mm) or an automated lancet (eg, Autolet) to penetrate skin. Wipe away the first drop of blood, which may contain excessive interstitial and intracellular fluid. Hold the child's finger or heel below the level of the heart when possible and massage to express blood, allowing enough time for capillaries to refill. Avoid excessive squeezing of the area, which can increase interstitial and intracellular fluid content of the specimen. Samples may be inaccurate when the child is polycythemic, edematous, or poorly perfused.

Preferred sites for skin-puncture sampling are the palmar surface of the distal phalanx of the second, third, and fourth fingers, or the heel in infants. Avoid penetrating the calcaneus by using a lancet puncture smaller than 2.5 mm and by performing the puncture on the medial or lateral plantar surface (Fig 168-2).

## TABLE 168-1.  Sedatives and Analgesics

| Drug | Dose | Comments |
|---|---|---|
| Chloral hydrate | 25–100 mg/kg/dose as a single dose, PO or PR | Maximum dose 2 g. Contraindicated in marked hepatic or renal impairment. No amnestic or analgesic effect. |
| Diazepam | 0.04–0.2 mg/kg/dose PO, IV | Infuse slowly (no faster than 2 mg/min). Respiratory depression can occur, especially when given with a narcotic. Has an amnestic effect. |
| Lorazepam | 0.05 mg/kg/dose IM or slow IV | See comments under diazepam. |
| Midazolam | 0.035–0.15 mg/kg/dose IM or slow IV | See comments under diazepam. Use lower dose when administered with narcotics. |
| Pentobarbital | 2–6 mg/kg/dose PO, IM PR | Cardiovascular depression and hypotension can occur. |
| Fentanyl | 2 µg/kg/dose IM or slow IV | Short-acting (30–60 min) narcotic with a rapid onset of action. |
| Fentanyl and Midazolam | 1–2 µg/kg/dose IM or slow IV  0.035–0.15 mg/kg/dose IM or slow IV | This combination has sedative, analgesic, and amnestic effects. Both drugs are respiratory depressants. |
| Meperidine and Promethazine and Chlorpromazine | 1.0–1.5 mg/kg/dose IM (max 50 mg)  0.05–1.0 mg/kg/dose IM (max 25 mg)  0.5–1.0 mg/kg/dose IM (max 25 mg) | Give as a single IM injection. Begin with lower doses and titrate to the desired effect. Hypotension, respiratory depression, and prolonged sedation can occur. No amnestic effect. |

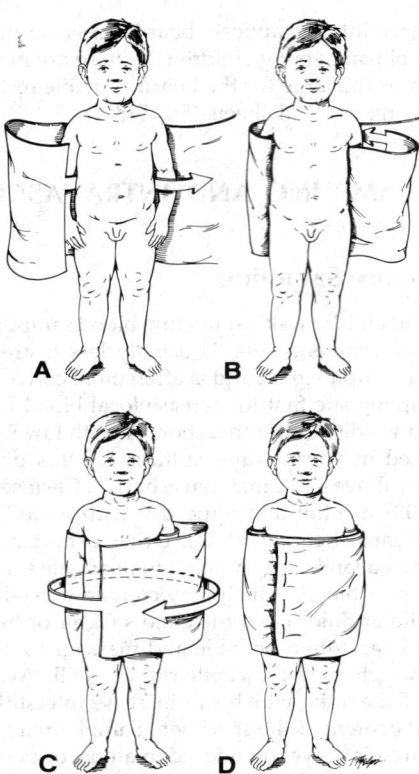

**Figure 168-1.**   Method for restraining the upper body using a hospital sheet.

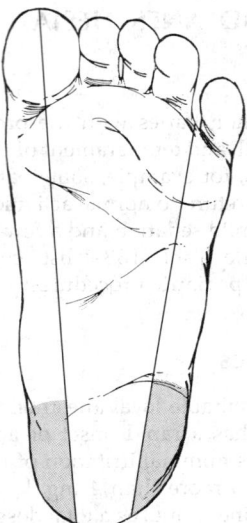

**Figure 168-2.**   Preferred sites for heel blood sampling in infants (hatched areas). The limits of the calcaneus are defined by two lines, one drawn parallel to the lateral margin of the heel from the space between the fourth and fifth toes and the other drawn parallel to the medial margin of the heel from the center of the great toe.

## Venipuncture and Conventional Venous Cannulation

Venipuncture for blood sampling is most successful when the patient is adequately immobilized, the vein is maximally distended, and all supplies for blood collection or intravenous infusion are arranged beforehand. Immobilization for simple venipuncture is preferably performed by an assistant, although with rambunctious children, the limb may need to be taped to an arm board. Maximal venous distention usually is achieved best by applying a tourniquet snugly enough to restrict venous return but not tightly enough to compromise arterial flow. Many children prefer a cloth or gauze pad under the tourniquet to prevent pinching of the skin. Other simple measures to increase distention and visibility of the vein include warming the site to increase blood flow, keeping the site dependent, tapping or flicking the vein, swabbing the vein with alcohol or iodine, or, if the site is in the arm, asking the patient to alternately make a fist and relax the hand. On a chronic basis, hand exercises may increase visibility of veins in the lower arm; acutely, application of 0.4% nitroglycerin ointment aids in venous cannulation.

The usual sites for venipuncture are in the hands and the antecubital fossa. Figure 168-3 shows the most accessible peripheral veins. If time permits, a survey of several sites for the most prominent vein may reduce the number of venipuncture attempts. Most venipunctures in children and adolescents can be performed using a 23-gauge butterfly needle, which allows ma-

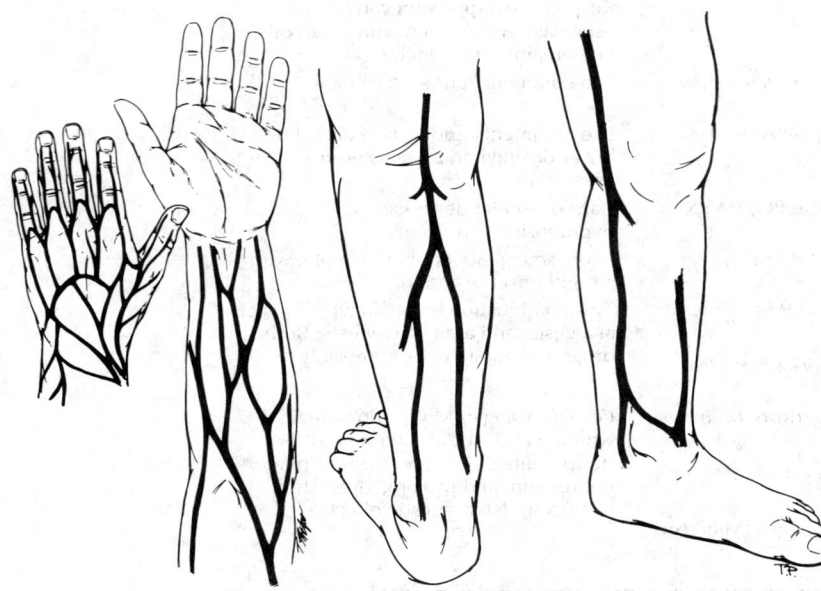

**Figure 168-3.**   Accessible peripheral veins for venipuncture and cannulation.

neuverability for the operator and causes minimal discomfort for the child.

The tourniquet should be applied as briefly as possible. The syringe can be attached to the butterfly tubing either before or after entering the vein. Once the vein is distended, cleanse the overlying skin with 70% alcohol, then allow this to dry. Apply traction to the skin to help immobilize the vessel. Warn the patient, then insert the needle into the skin at about a 30° angle with the bevel up. Enter the vein with a quick motion to prevent it from rolling. Slowly aspirate the required amount of blood; excessive suction can cause the vein to collapse. When blood flow is slow, some samples can be collected by removing the syringe and allowing blood to drip directly into the collection tube. When the collection is complete, release the tourniquet and remove the needle. Manual pressure with a gauze pad controls further bleeding.

## External Jugular Venipuncture

The external jugular vein occasionally is the most accessible site for venipuncture in young children. Special positioning ensures good visibility of the vein (Fig 168-4). With the patient supine, an assistant holds the child's head and neck over the edge of a table and rotates the head to one side to stretch the vein. An alternative to positioning the head over the edge of the table is to elevate the shoulders by placing pillows underneath them. To distend the external jugular vein, occlude the most proximal segment of the vein or provoke the infant to cry. It is essential to keep the syringe attached to the needle during venipuncture; otherwise, follow the general venipuncture technique described above. When the procedure is completed, apply manual pressure to the site with the child sitting upright.

## Intravenous Infusions

When selecting a site for intravenous infusions, consider the age and hand preference of the patient, whether there are underlying injuries, the degree of restraint required to keep the needle in place, whether the infusate burns or is damaging to surrounding tissues if extravasation occurs, and whether prolonged intravenous access is required. In general, select the most distal vein that is large enough to accommodate the catheter or needle, and spare the larger proximal veins for use if initial attempts fail or if prolonged intravenous access is anticipated. Veins are most easily cannulated if they are well anchored, such as at the site where two vessels meet (Fig 168-5A).

The procedure for inserting a butterfly needle for intravenous infusion is similar to that for venipuncture, except a padded restraint board for the limb usually is taped on first. After applying the tourniquet, visualizing the vessel, and cleansing the skin, insert the needle into the skin at a 30° angle several millimeters distal to the vein. This distance of subcutaneous tissue helps stabilize the needle in place. Enter the vein with a quick motion to prevent it from rolling. Advancing the needle too far can puncture the opposite wall of the vessel. When blood return is seen, stabilize the needle with one or two pieces of tape, remove the tourniquet, and test the patency of the line by flushing with 2 to 3 mL of normal saline. Apply a small dab of antibacterial ointment at the site at which the needle enters the skin and cover this with a small gauze tape. Securely padding and taping the butterfly enhances the longevity of intravenous access.

When using plastic over-the-needle catheters, several modifications of the foregoing are helpful. Some children prefer that the site be anesthetized with an intradermal bleb of 1% lidocaine. Check for local anesthesia, then pierce the skin distal to the vein with a needle larger than the gauge of the catheter (see Fig 168-5A). This prevents damage to the plastic sheaths, which can occur when the smaller 22- and 24-gauge catheters are inserted directly through the skin. Insert the catheter through the skin-puncture site and enter the vein with a quick stab (see Fig 168-5B). Blood should appear in the needle hub. Advance the catheter a few millimeters to ensure the plastic catheter tip sits inside the lumen (see Fig 168-5C). Then, holding the stylet needle in place, advance the catheter into the vein; it should advance completely without resistance. Remove the stylet, release the tourniquet, and flush with normal saline to assess patency. Do not return the stylet into the catheter when the catheter is in the vein, because the stylet can shear off fragments of plastic into the circulation.

If the catheter flushes normally, apply antibacterial ointment and secure the intravenous catheter as described above. Alternatively, transparent adhesives, which are often used in dressing central intravenous catheters, permit visualization of the skin entry site.

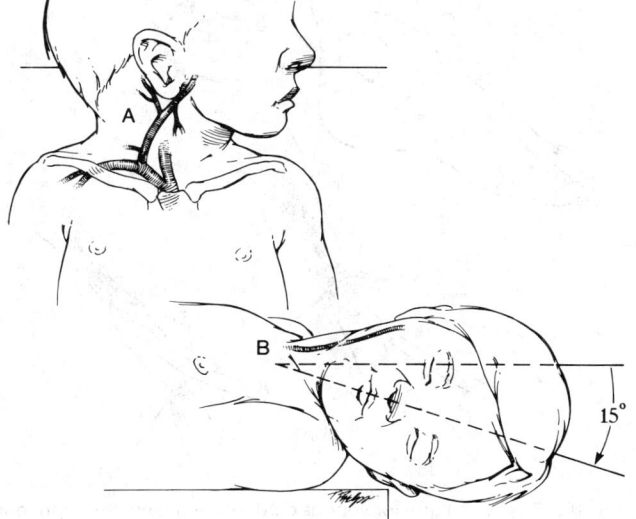

**Figure 168-4.** External jugular venipuncture. (**A**) Anatomy. (**B**) Visibility of the vein is improved if the head is turned to the opposite side and lowered 15° from the level of the table.

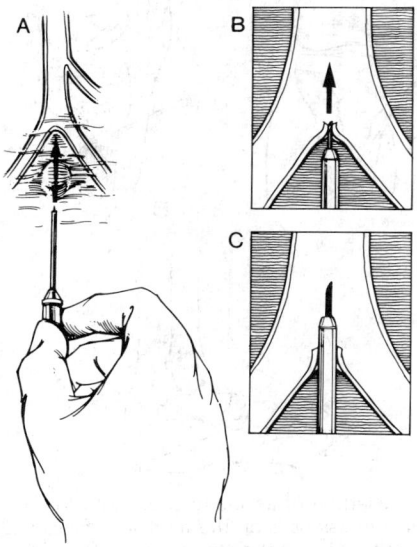

**Figure 168-5.** Insertion of a venous catheter.

## Intraosseous Infusions

In an emergency, intraosseous infusion provides quick access for fluids and most medications through the intramedullary veins to the general circulation. Three sites are commonly used in children: the proximal tibia, the distal tibia, and the distal femur. For infusions into the proximal tibia, insert the needle on the medial surface, 2 cm below the tibial tuberosity (Fig 168-6A). Direct the needle slightly inferiorly to avoid injuring the epiphysis (see Fig 168-6B). For infusions into the distal tibia, insert the needle on the medial surface proximal to the medial malleolus (see Fig 168-6C), directing the needle superiorly. For infusions into the distal femur, insert the needle in the midline anteriorly, 3 cm proximal to the lateral condyle. Direct the needle superiorly to avoid epiphyseal damage.

After determining the site to be used, cleanse the skin with povidone-iodine, then with 70% alcohol. If time permits, infiltrate the skin and down to the periosteum with 1% lidocaine. Use a bone-marrow needle with an obturator for intraosseous infusions. (Spinal needles and routine metal needles bend or become plugged with bone.) Insert the needle through the skin. When the needle reaches the periosteum, exert firm downward pressure, rotating the needle in a clockwise–counterclockwise manner. When the needle enters the marrow space, it becomes anchored in the bone and resistance suddenly drops. It is rarely necessary to advance the needle more than 1 cm. At this point, remove the inner stylet and flush with saline. Then, connect intravenous tubing to the needle and allow fluid to drip in. An infusion pump may be needed to infuse a large volume of fluid. The infusion site must be monitored for extravasation of fluids; hypertonic solutions should not be infused via this route. To reduce the small risk of osteomyelitis, remove the needle as soon as is feasible after secure intravenous access is obtained.

## Venous Cutdowns

When percutaneous venous cannulation or intraosseous infusions are unsuccessful, cutdowns provide a means of emergency venous access. The greater saphenous vein at the ankle is the preferred site for cutdown in infants and children. It is easily identified and placement of the cutdown at that site does not interfere with resuscitative measures around the neck and chest.

The vein is located midway between the anterior tibia and the medial malleolus. Immobilize the lower leg by taping the foot onto a padded restraint board with the ankle externally rotated. Apply a tourniquet to the calf to help distend the vein. After cleansing the area around the medial malleolus using aseptic technique, apply drapes and infiltrate the incision site and subcutaneous tissues with 1% lidocaine. Make a 1- to 2-cm transverse incision just anterior and proximal to the medial malleolus (Fig 168-7A). Using a curved mosquito hemostat, dissect bluntly down to the tibia in the direction of the vein. Lift the vein up and separate it from surrounding tissues (see Fig 168-7B), taking care to avoid the saphenous nerve, which runs just anterior to the vein. Pass 4-0 silk sutures under the most distal and proximal sites of exposed vessels. Tie the distal suture and use a distal clamp to exert traction. Leave the other suture untied and exert traction proximally. Using a number 11 blade with the cutting edge up, enter the vein laterally to create an incision through the upper third of the vessel. Cut the end of a silicone elastomer (eg, Silastic) catheter to create a 30° to 45° bevel. Insert an introducer into the venotomy incision and, while holding the catheter close to the tip with forceps, thread the catheter into the vein (see Fig 168-7C). Secure the catheter in place by tying the proximal suture around the cannulated vein (see Fig 168-7D). Remove the tourniquet before flushing with normal saline to test the patency of the catheter. Once patency is assured, suture the distal catheter to the skin, close the skin incision, apply antibiotic ointment and a sterile dressing, and tape the remaining tubing to the skin to protect against dislodgement.

Two modifications may enable faster cannulation in emergencies. One follows the procedure outlined above, except a standard plastic over-the-needle catheter replaces the more pliable Silastic catheter commonly used for cutdowns. This plastic catheter and needle can be inserted as soon as the vein is isolated,

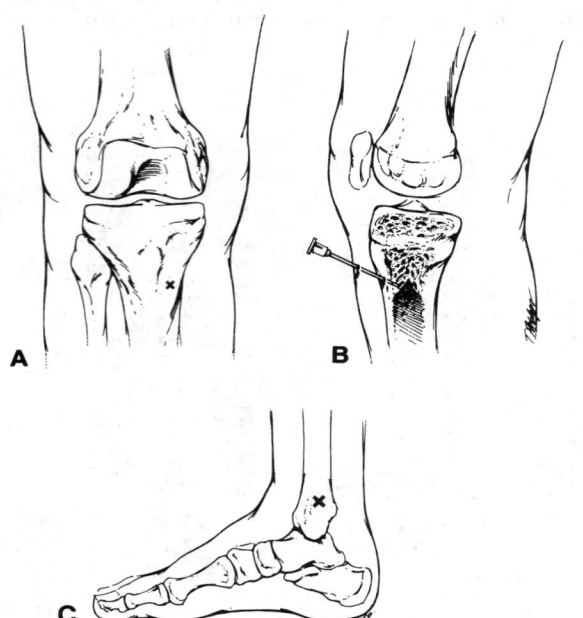

**Figure 168-6.** Insertion of an intraosseous infusion needle. The site for proximal tibia infusions is on the medial surface, 1 to 2 cm below the tibial tuberosity (**A**), orienting the needle inferiorly to avoid epiphyseal injury (**B**). (**C**) The site for needle insertion in the distal tibia.

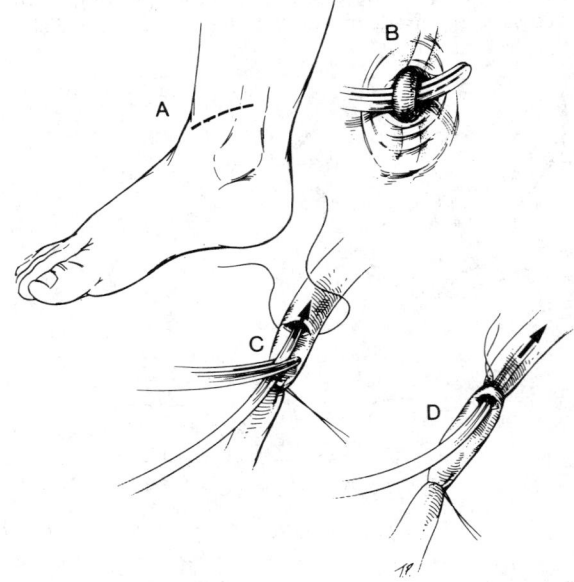

**Figure 168-7.** Technique for venous cutdown at the greater saphenous vein. A 1- to 2-cm incision is made anterior and proximal to the medial malleolus (**A**). After the vein is isolated (**B**) and a venotomy incision is made, the catheter is threaded into the vein (**C**). The proximal suture secures the catheter (**D**).

or the plastic catheter alone can be inserted through a small venotomy incision. A shorter catheter permits a higher rate of flow.

The second modification involves a different technique for isolating the vein. A larger incision is made, extending from the anterior crest of the tibia to the posterior border of the tibia just proximal to the medial malleolus. Using a closed hemostat with the point down, scrape along the tibia from anterior to posterior and pick up all the tissue within the incision. Turn the hemostat so the tip faces upward and open it widely to separate the tissues. Dissect the saphenous vein against the background of the hemostat. Then, follow the procedure outlined above.

## Femoral Venipuncture and Cannulation

With the patient positioned supine, an assistant holds the child's hips flexed and abducted (in a frog-leg position). The site for femoral vein puncture is 2 cm distal to the inguinal ligament and 0.5 cm medial to the femoral artery pulsation. The femoral artery is found by palpating along the inguinal ligament at a point midway between the symphysis pubis and the anterior superior iliac crest (Fig 168-8). Prepare the skin with povidone-iodine and 70% alcohol. With a syringe attached to a straight needle (21- to 23-gauge), enter the skin at a 30° angle and advance the needle while exerting negative pressure with the syringe. Once the desired volume of blood is obtained, exert pressure on the site with sterile gauze (for at least 5 minutes if the artery was punctured).

To insert a larger indwelling catheter at this site using the percutaneous Seldinger technique, prepare the site as above. Packaged kits for this procedure vary, so the operator is advised to refer to the instructions in the kit. Most kits supply a metal needle for initial insertion into the vein, a guide wire, and an infusion catheter. Using the landmarks described above, insert the metal needle attached to a syringe into the femoral vein. Stabilize the catheter with one hand, then detach the syringe. Blood should flow back freely. Insert the soft tip of the guide

wire through the metal needle and advance it several centimeters into the vein. There should be no resistance. While holding the guide wire in place, remove the metal needle. (Never remove the guide wire through the metal needle.) Next, advance the infusion catheter over the guide wire. It usually is necessary to enlarge the skin-puncture site with a small incision; do not cut the guide wire. To help the catheter pass through the skin, twist the catheter and advance it into the vein. Once the catheter is in place, withdraw the guide wire—this should be followed by free blood flow if the catheter is properly positioned.

## Percutaneous Arterial Puncture and Cannulation

The preferred site for percutaneous arterial puncture for blood-gas determinations is the radial artery at the wrist. It is easily located on the lateral aspect of the supinated wrist. Because the ulnar artery provides collateral flow to the hand through the palmar arch, ischemia distal to the site of arterial puncture is rare. The hazard of ischemia as a result of arterial spasm or vascular injury is the primary reason for avoiding the femoral and brachial arteries for routine arterial puncture. Septic arthritis of the hip, although uncommon, is another possible complication of femoral artery puncture.

To prepare for radial artery sampling, first check the adequacy of the ulnar blood flow to the entire hand. Compress both radial and ulnar arteries. After a brief period, release the ulnar artery compression. If the entire hand flushes while the radial artery is still compressed, the procedure can be performed safely. Next, secure the hand to a restraint board, with the wrist extended 20° to 30° by placing it over a gauze padding. Leave the fingers exposed so any color change is seen quickly. After cleansing the wrist area and the palpating fingers with povidone-iodine and wiping them with 70% alcohol, palpate the artery. In preterm infants, transillumination may help locate the artery. Using a 22- to 25-gauge needle, puncture the skin at a 30° to 45° angle (Fig 168-9A), then insert the needle just far enough to enter the lumen but not transfix the vessel. An alternative maneuver is to pierce through the artery to transfix it (see Fig 168-9B), then withdraw the needle slowly, observing for blood flow into the syringe or tubing (see Fig 168-9C). When the desired amount of blood has been withdrawn, apply pressure to the area for 5 minutes.

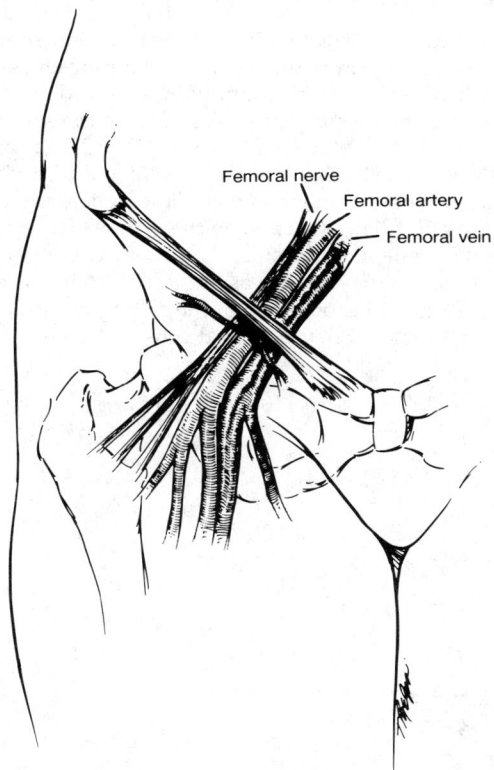

**Figure 168-8.** The femoral vessels.

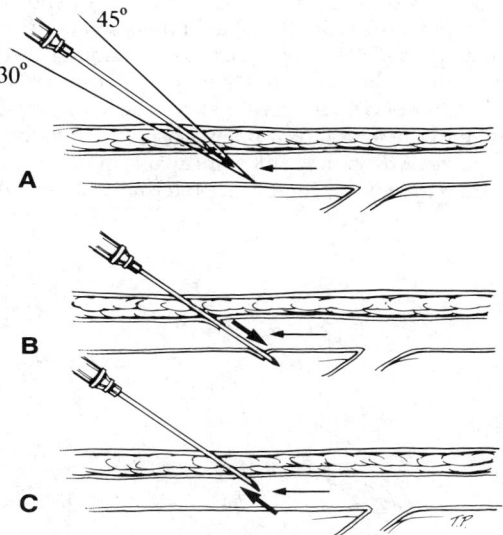

**Figure 168-9.** Percutaneous arterial puncture. Insert the needle or catheter at a 30° to 45° angle (**A**), just far enough to enter the lumen of the vessel. Alternatively, the needle can be advanced through the opposite wall of the artery (**B**), then withdrawn slowly as one watches for blood return (**C**).

For radial artery cannulation, only a few modifications are necessary. After infiltrating the area with 1% lidocaine, use a 20-gauge needle to puncture the skin over the point of maximal impulse (about 0.5-1 cm proximal to the distal wrist crease). Arterial puncture is then performed with a 22- to 24-gauge catheter. Radial artery cannulation can be performed like venous cannulation—after entering the vessel, rotate the catheter so the bevel faces down and advance the stylet and catheter 1 to 2 mm; then hold the stylet in place while advancing the catheter. Alternatively, insert the catheter through the skin-puncture site until it pierces through the artery. Remove the stylet and slowly withdraw the catheter. At the first sign of blood return, redirect the catheter toward the horizontal plane and advance the catheter to the hub. This maneuver is more difficult to perform with 24-gauge catheters, which tend to buckle. When it is advanced fully, the catheter should then be sutured in place. Apply antibiotic ointment and a dressing over the catheter site to prevent contamination.

## SELECTED DIAGNOSTIC AND THERAPEUTIC PROCEDURES

### Lumbar Puncture

Although lumbar puncture is generally a safe procedure, its performance under certain conditions is associated with serious complications. Children with thrombocytopenia or bleeding diathesis are at risk for epidural hematomas after lumbar puncture. Infants with compromised cardiorespiratory function may experience further deterioration when restrained for the procedure. Most important, cerebral herniation can occur after lumbar puncture in the setting of elevated intracranial pressure, even when the fontanelle is open. While it is important to examine the patient for evidence of papilledema, this physical finding may not be present despite substantial intracranial hypertension. Only needles with stylets should be used; use of open or butterfly needles is condemned because of the late development of intraspinal epidermoid tumors.

In the context of these important caveats, a key component of a successful lumbar puncture is adequate restraint of the patient. Children are most often restrained in the lateral recumbent position with their backs at the edge of and perpendicular to the examining table (Fig 168-10). The lumbar spine must be flexed as much as possible to maximize the interlaminar distance. The position of the child's head relative to the performer's dominant side is a matter of personal preference. The sitting position is an alternative to the lateral recumbent position when the patient is either capable of remaining still or incapable of offering resistance. This method may be preferable in preterm infants in whom neck

flexion and the knee-chest position are associated with hypoxemia.

A line connecting the superior portions of the posterior iliac crests passes through the spinous process of L-4, conveniently identifying the L3-4 and L4-5 interspaces, which are the preferred sites for lumbar puncture (see Fig 168-10). Once the child is positioned, don sterile gloves and cleanse the site three times with a povidone-iodine solution, starting at the site of skin puncture and working outward in a circular manner, and then once with 70% alcohol. Drape the area with a sterile towel. If local anesthesia is used, raise a wheal at the interspace with 1% lidocaine, then infiltrate the underlying tissues. Because this may distort local tissues, mark the insertion site by imprinting a fingernail beforehand, or keep a thumb on the spinous process above the intended interspace.

Using a 22-gauge needle with a stylet (the length of the needle depends on the size of the patient), puncture the skin midway between the spinous processes of the L3-4 or L4-5 interspace and aim slightly cephalad (toward the umbilicus). Ensure the needle enters directly in the midline and continues in the sagittal plane and advance it slowly, removing the stylet frequently to check for cerebrospinal fluid (CSF). This process is more important in smaller infants because one may not always feel a "pop" as the needle penetrates the dura. If the needle does not advance, withdraw it and redirect its angle. Once the needle enters the subarachnoid space and CSF is flowing freely, connect the manometer to measure CSF pressure (a worthless procedure when the patient is struggling and somewhat inaccurate when the neck and thighs are flexed). Collect the smallest volume of CSF necessary, controlling the rate of flow of CSF with the stylet. Allow the CSF to drip into collection tubes for diagnostic studies. Never aspirate CSF with a syringe, because enough negative pressure could cause herniation. Replace the stylet before withdrawing the needle, then cover the site with an adhesive bandage.

### Ventriculoperitoneal Shunt Tap

A pediatrician may be required to tap a ventriculoperitoneal shunt when a neurosurgeon is unavailable. The procedure can be lifesaving. The area over the shunt bulb is shaved with a straight razor. After donning surgical gloves, cleanse the skin with povidone-iodine and 70% alcohol. Insert a 23- or 25-gauge butterfly needle through the bulb of the shunt, holding the butterfly tubing as a makeshift pressure manometer. Fluid under pressure should flow out readily. Gentle suction on the syringe may be necessary if the ventricular end of the shunt is partially obstructed, whereas excessive suction may lead to aspiration of brain tissue into the catheter. If no fluid is obtained in the setting of intracranial hypertension, emergent neurosurgical consultation is necessary.

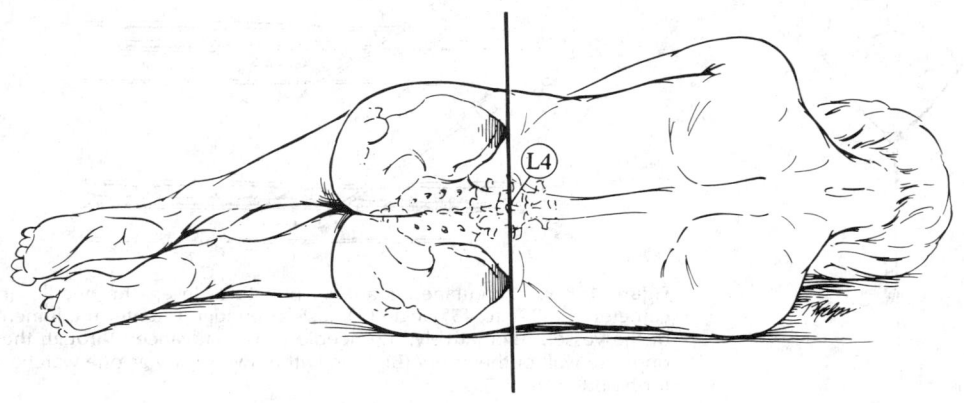

**Figure 168-10.**  Positioning of a child for lumbar puncture.

## Subdural Puncture

To obtain a diagnostic sample of subdural fluid or to drain an effusion, position the child supine with the head at the edge of the table. Shave the scalp and, after donning surgical gloves, cleanse the skin with povidone-iodine and 70% alcohol. The site of puncture is near the junction of the lateral aspect of the anterior fontanelle and the coronal suture. A helpful landmark for the site of puncture is the point at which a line drawn from the ipsilateral pupil would intersect the coronal suture at a perpendicular angle (Fig 168-11). Anesthetize the skin just anterior to the point of entry with a small wheal of 1% lidocaine. Insert an 18- to 20-gauge subdural needle (or a 20-gauge lumbar puncture needle) just through the skin, then pull the scalp posteriorly until the needle meets the coronal suture. This technique prevents fluid leakage after the needle is removed. Slowly insert the needle at a right angle to the surface. Brace the hand to prevent advancing the needle too far. Advance until resistance falls, signalling entry into the subdural space. This is usually no more than 5 to 10 mm below the skin surface. Remove the stylet and allow fluid to drain passively; never aspirate subdural fluid. To prevent hypotension, shift of the brain, or fresh hemorrhage, do not remove more than 15 to 20 mL at a time from each side. Once the needle is removed, the scalp returns to its original position. Apply collodion and cotton to the site.

## Tympanocentesis

Puncturing the tympanic membrane to aspirate fluid is a helpful procedure for determining which organism is causing otitis media. For this procedure, an otoscope with an operating head is required. Remove cerumen from the external canal with a curette or by irrigation (see below). Restrain and, if necessary, sedate the patient. Cleanse the external canal with 70% alcohol and remove any of this fluid before tympanocentesis. Bend a 22-gauge spinal needle as shown in Figure 168-12. Attach a 1-mL tuberculin syringe to the end of the spinal needle. An assistant can apply negative pressure with the syringe plunger, or the operator can connect a length of rubber tubing to the end of the tuberculin syringe, then apply negative pressure by mouth. Pass the needle just through the medial portion of the posterior inferior quadrant (see Fig 168-12). Apply negative pressure briefly, then withdraw the needle. The aspirate can be retrieved for culture and Gram staining by flushing the needle with a small volume of nonbacteriostatic saline.

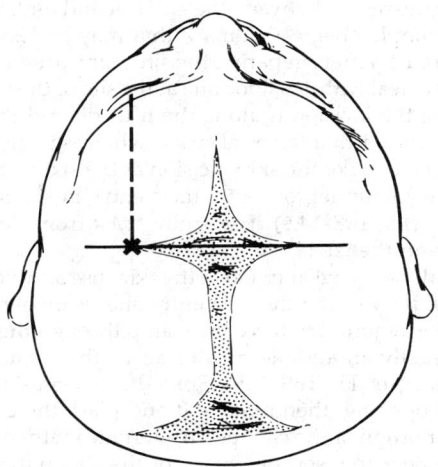

**Figure 168-11.** The site for subdural puncture.

## Removing Impacted Cerumen

A quick, painless method of removing excessive or impacted cerumen from the external auditory canal follows. After aspirating lukewarm water from a basin into a 20- or 30-mL syringe, attach the syringe to the tubing of a 23-gauge butterfly needle after the needle has been removed. Insert the tubing 1 to 2 cm into the external auditory canal and inject the water with a moderate force. The impacted cerumen usually flushes out after 60 to 90 mL of irrigation. If the patient experiences pain, discontinue irrigation because the tympanic membrane may be perforated.

## Nasogastric Tube Insertion

One can estimate the length required for a nasogastric (NG) tube by extending the tubing from the tip of the patient's nose to the earlobe to the xiphoid process. Small (5–8 Fr) tubes are used for continuous enteral alimentation in neonates; larger tubes (12–16 Fr in young children) are necessary for abdominal decompression.

Before inserting the NG tube, lubricate the tip to make passage through the nose less traumatic. Apply ice to the tube if it is excessively pliable. With the patient sitting upright, tilt the head back slightly and slide the tube into the nostril along the base of the nose, advancing the tube slowly in a horizontal plane. Once the NG tube has reached the nasopharynx, several maneuvers can be employed to ensure the tube is directed away from the trachea and into the esophagus. One maneuver is to tilt the head forward, thereby opening the esophagus. Another is to rotate the NG tube 180° so the curve in the tube faces the posterior pharynx. A third is to ask the patient to swallow or drink from a straw, since this maneuver closes the epiglottis. Once past the pharynx, advance the tube to the premeasured distance and check its position, either by attempting to aspirate gastric contents or by listening with a stethoscope over the stomach as a small volume of air is instilled into the tube. Tape the tube in place when the position is judged to be adequate. Withdraw the tube if excessive coughing or choking occurs during placement. To reduce the unpleasantness of NG tube removal, kink or clamp the tube and withdraw it slowly.

## Endotracheal Intubation

If intubation can be approached in a deliberate manner, complications from the procedure can be reduced. Ventilation of the apneic child should begin with efforts to clear the airway, followed by either mouth-to-mouth or bag-and-mask techniques.

As bag-and-mask ventilation with 100% oxygen proceeds, assemble all equipment necessary for intubation. This includes the following: one or, preferably, two laryngoscopes and blades (tested to ensure that batteries and lights are functional); endotracheal tubes, one larger and one smaller than the size estimated for the patient (see Table 168-2 for tube sizes); suction equipment of adequate size for the patient; precut tape and tincture of benzoin for securing the tube; and electrocardiogram (ECG) monitoring and secure venous access when possible. Optimally, the stomach contents should be evacuated before intubation begins.

Although endotracheal intubation in some emergency settings takes place without premedication, premedication is desirable in most urgent elective intubations. Drugs to use for rapid-sequence intubation are listed in Table 168-3. Atropine and a defasciculating dose of pancuronium are administered first, followed by about 3 minutes of bag-and-mask ventilation with 100% oxygen. An anesthetic agent, either thiopental sodium or ketamine, is then infused, followed immediately by succinylcholine or pancuronium for muscle relaxation. If succinylcholine is administered, ventilation with bag and mask is interrupted to reduce the risk of aspiration, and cricoid pressure is applied to occlude the

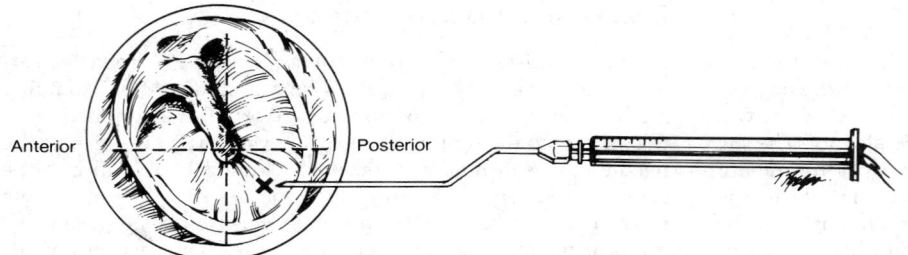

**Figure 168-12.**   Tympanocentesis of the left ear. A bent spinal needle allows a clearer view of the puncture site in the medial portion of the posterior inferior quadrant.

esophagus. Variations of this regimen frequently are dictated by clinical circumstances, and it is vital that the physician performing the intubation know the contraindications to the use of each drug.

At the start of the intubation, the patient should be positioned supine on a firm surface. Extend the patient's neck slightly and pull the jaw forward; a roll under the shoulder may assist in this maneuver. While an assistant applies cricoid pressure, hold the laryngoscope in the left hand and open the patient's mouth with your right hand. Introduce the laryngoscope blade on the right side of the mouth and push the tongue out of the line of vision. Two methods of visualizing the vocal cords can be used. The method used most often in infants is to advance the blade beyond the epiglottis and into the esophagus. The blade is then withdrawn slowly until the cords come into view. At this point, the epiglottis is anterior to the laryngoscope blade. The other method is to advance the blade into the vallecula, then lift the laryngoscope up and forward to visualize the vocal cords. Avoid bending the wrist, which creates a levering motion that can injure the gums and teeth.

Once the vocal cords are in view and pharyngeal secretions are suctioned, insert the endotracheal tube from the right side of the mouth and advance it 2 to 3 cm through the cords. Because the narrowest portion of the trachea in neonates is at the cricoid ring just distal to the cords, do not force a tube if resistance is encountered. Listen for symmetrical air entry into the chest and listen over the gastric area for signs of esophageal intubation. With some experience, the position of the tube can be palpated at the suprasternal notch in neonates. When satisfied with its position, secure the endotracheal tube with tape and obtain a chest x-ray to confirm positioning. If the patient develops bradycardia or cyanosis during the procedure, interrupt the intubation and resume bag-and-mask ventilation.

## Thoracentesis

In the cooperative child, aspiration of pleural fluid, or thoracentesis, is performed best with the patient sitting backward on a chair, with arms and head supported on a pillow. Uncooperative children may need to be sedated and restrained in this position. With arms elevated in this way, the lower tip of the scapula lies in the posterior axillary line just above the usual site for puncture—the seventh intercostal space (Fig 168-13A).

| TABLE  168-2.   Endotracheal Tube Size | |
| --- | --- |
| Age | Internal Diameter (mm) |
| Preterm infant | 2.5–3.0 |
| Term infant | 3.0–3.5 |
| 2 mo–1 yr | 3.5–4.0 |
| 2 yr | 4.0–4.5 |
| 2–15 yr | $\dfrac{16 + age\ (yr)}{4}$ |

After preparing the skin using standard sterile technique, raise a wheal with 1% lidocaine over the rib below the interspace selected for the thoracentesis. Anesthetize the underlying periosteum as well as the pleura in the interspace above that rib. Using a plastic catheter (16- to 20-gauge), penetrate the skin at the site of the wheal, then "walk" the needle over the superior edge of the rib (see Figure 168-13B). Gradually advance the needle until a "pop" is appreciated upon entry of the pleural space. Advance the catheter 2 to 3 mm to ensure the plastic sheath is in the pleural space. Remove the stylet, then attach a syringe with a stopcock to the hub of the catheter and slowly withdraw the desired volume of fluid. If no fluid is aspirated, the catheter may be advanced a few millimeters more or directed caudally if the effusion is in a more dependent area of the lung. An alternative method is to use a standard needle attached to a syringe via a stopcock. Advance the needle just into the pleural space and clamp it there with a hemostat to prevent lacerating the lung. At the end of the procedure, quickly withdraw the needle and apply a dressing to the site. Obtain a chest x-ray to assess for the presence of a pneumothorax.

## Chest-Tube Insertion for Pneumothorax

If the patient is hemodynamically compromised by a pneumothorax, the quickest way to evacuate air is by inserting a needle or plastic catheter into the second intercostal space in the midclavicular line anteriorly. A stopcock attached to the catheter then allows a release of further tension, if necessary. It is not advisable to evacuate all air in the pleural space before inserting a chest tube, because this removes the "cushion" of air between the chest wall and the lung and increases the risk of injury to the lung during the procedure.

For chest tube insertion, the patient is positioned supine with the arm restrained above the head. Positioning neonates with the affected side up may improve maneuverability. The site of chest tube insertion is in the fourth or fifth intercostal space at the level of the nipple between the anterior and midaxillary lines. Avoid the nipple area, a landmark that may be less obvious in preterm infants. After preparing the site using aseptic technique, raise a skin wheal with 1% lidocaine at the site of the skin incision. In neonates, the incision is along the fifth rib and the entry site is the adjacent fourth intercostal space, whereas in older children, it is desirable to make the skin incision at the sixth rib and create a subcutaneous tunnel to the thoracic entry in the fourth intercostal space (Fig 168-14A). The entire track from skin to pleura should be anesthetized.

After making a small incision in the skin, use a curved hemostat to dissect bluntly to the thoracic entry site. A moderate amount of pressure is required to force the clamp through the chest wall. There is usually an audible rush of air as the clamp enters the pleural space (see Fig 168-14B). Spread the hemostat to enlarge the pleural opening, then remove it and place the chest tube in the curved portion of the clamp. An alternate method for guiding the chest tube is to insert one blade of the clamp through a side hole in the tube. Appropriately sized chest tubes are 8 and 10 Fr for preterm infants, 12 Fr for term infants and children up to age

## TABLE 168-3. Drugs for Intubation

| Drug | Dosage | Comments |
|------|--------|----------|
| Atropine | 0.01–0.02 mg/kg | Minimum dose (0.1 mg; maximum dose 0.5 mg |
| Pancuronium (defasciculating dose) | 0.01 mg/kg | Not usually necessary in children younger than 4 years. May cause complete paralysis |
| Thiopental sodium | 4–6 mg/kg | Because of its hypotensive effects, this drug is contraindicated in hemodynamically unstable patients. |
| Ketamine | 1–2 mg/kg | Contraindicated in head trauma because it increases cerebral blood flow. Use with caution when propranolol or alpha blockers are used concurrently. |
| Succinylcholine | 1 mg/kg | Onset 30–45 sec; duration 3–10 min. Use a dose of 2 mg/kg in infants younger than 1 year. Contraindicated in burns, massive trauma, neuromuscular disease, and eye injuries (increases intraocular pressure). Its use can lead to hyperkalemia as well as bradycardia or dysrhythmias (always give atropine first). |
| Pancuronium | 0.04–0.1 mg/kg | Onset 1–2 min; duration 1 hr. Reversal drugs (reversal not possible until 40 min after administration): Atropine 0.02 mg/kg Neostigmine 0.07 mg/kg |

*Reproduced with permission from Peter C. Rowe, ed. Harriet Lane Handbook, ed 11. Chicago: Year Book Medical Publishers, 1987.*

3 years, 16 Fr for children 3 to 10 years of age, and 20 to 28 Fr for older children and adolescents.

Insert the clamp and chest tube through the subcutaneous tunnel created earlier and advance the tube into the pleural space (see Fig 168-14C). Condensation in the lumen of the tube indicates that it has entered the pleural space. Its entry site should be palpated to ensure that it is not in the subcutaneous tissues. In most instances, the tube should be directed anteriorly and superiorly, and advanced so all side holes are in the pleural space. Secure the chest tube with suture material or by wrapping a Band-Aid tab around the tube and suturing the tab to the skin. Close the incision site with a purse-string suture. Wrap petrolatum-soaked gauze around the tube at the skin entry site and cover with a sterile dressing and tape. Confirm the position of the chest tube with a chest x-ray.

## Pericardiocentesis

Aspiration of pericardial fluid, or pericardiocentesis, is at times an emergency lifesaving procedure. It is performed with the child sedated (if possible) and in a 30° sitting-up position. ECG monitoring during the procedure is essential. The preferred site for pericardiocentesis is just to the left of the xiphoid process, 1 cm inferior to the bottom rib. Infiltrate the puncture site with 1% lidocaine and prepare the skin using standard aseptic technique. Use an 18- to 20-gauge needle attached to a syringe via a stopcock. If time permits, attach the "V" lead of a surface ECG to the needle to observe for an injury pattern that indicates contact with the epicardium. Insert the needle inferior to the lowest rib at about a 60° angle to the skin. While gently aspirating, advance the needle toward the patient's left shoulder until pericardial fluid is obtained. Clamp a hemostat onto the needle at the skin entry site to prevent further advancement. Aspirate the pericardial fluid slowly. Repeated aspirations of fluid may be necessary, and can be simplified by insertion of a drainage catheter over a guide wire.

## Abdominal Paracentesis

Abdominal paracentesis is the removal of peritoneal fluid for therapeutic or diagnostic purposes. To minimize the risk of bladder puncture, it is important that the patient's bladder be empty before the procedure begins. Sedation may be necessary, but re-

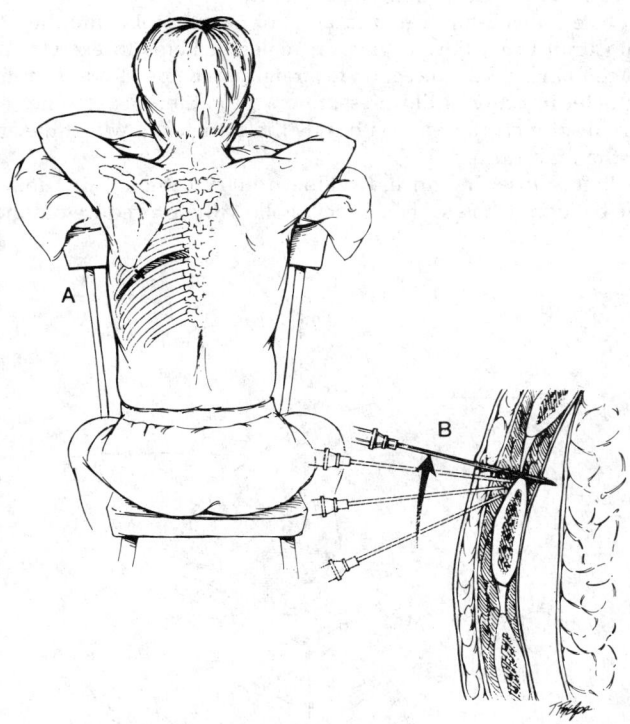

**Figure 168-13.** Positioning a child for thoracentesis. The customary site for needle insertion is in the seventh intercostal space, just inferior to the lower tip of the scapula (**A**). After the catheter is inserted through the skin overlying the body of the eighth rib, it is gradually advanced over the superior margin of the rib into the interspace (**B**).

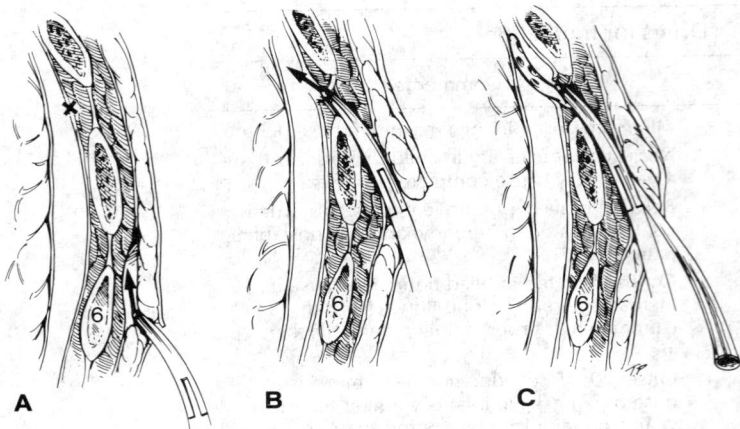

**Figure 168-14.** Chest tube insertion. A curved hemostat inserted through a skin incision (usually at the sixth rib) is advanced through the subcutaneous tissues to the thoracic entry site in the fourth intercostal space (**A**). The clamp is forced through the chest wall (**B**). The chest tube is guided into the pleural space by placing it in the curved portion of the clamp (**C**).

spiratory depressants should be used with extreme caution because most children with ascites have a degree of respiratory compromise due to elevation of the diaphragm.

Patients are most comfortable in a sitting or reclining position. Sites for paracentesis are in the midline, halfway between the umbilicus and the symphysis pubis, or in either lower quadrant several centimeters above the inguinal ligament, lateral to the rectus muscle and in a line with the nipples. Avoid scars from previous surgery, because bowel may adhere to the abdominal wall at these sites.

Cleanse the abdomen with povidone-iodine and 70% alcohol, then drape with sterile towels. Infiltrate the site of skin puncture with 1% lidocaine and puncture the skin with a 14- to 16-gauge needle. Use a 14- to 20-gauge intravascular plastic catheter for the paracentesis. Choose the gauge by considering the size of the patient and by estimating the viscosity of the peritoneal fluid (eg, pick a larger catheter when malignancy is suspected). Pull the skin to create a Z-track and, with a syringe attached to create negative pressure, insert the catheter through the puncture site, advancing just into the peritoneum. Remove the stylet and slowly withdraw the desired volume of fluid. Rapid removal of large volumes of ascitic fluids can lead to hypotension. When the collection is complete, remove the needle and apply a sterile dressing. Air aspirated from the peritoneal cavity is a sign of penetration of a hollow viscus and is an indication to remove the needle immediately.

## Suprapubic Bladder Puncture

Because the distended bladder is located intra-abdominally in infants, suprapubic aspiration is a common method of obtaining sterile urine specimens in patients younger than 2 years of age. The bladder must be distended for aspiration to be both safe and productive. The procedure should not be attempted until 30 to 60 minutes after the child's last void. It is important to obstruct urine outflow during the procedure by compressing the penile urethra in the male or by exerting anterior pressure on the female urethra by inserting a finger into the child's rectum. Because manual pressure is not always successful in preventing urination, attach a urine bag over the genitalia beforehand or have a sterile container available to catch a "midstream" specimen.

Position the child supine in a frog-leg position and palpate to determine the position of the bladder. After cleansing the suprapubic area with povidone-iodine and 70% alcohol, attach a syringe to a 22-gauge needle. Insert the needle in the midline, 1 to 2 cm above the symphysis pubis, directing it perpendicular to the horizontal axis of the child (Fig 168-15). Excessive inferior angulation can result in injury to the bladder neck. Exert gentle negative pressure on the syringe while advancing slowly to a

depth of no more than 2.5 cm. Urine appears in the syringe when the bladder is punctured. Once the specimen is collected, withdraw the needle and cover the site with an adhesive bandage. Transient hematuria is the most common complication of this procedure.

## Bladder Catheterization

Urinary catheterization is a safe, quick method of obtaining a sterile urine specimen. After explaining the procedure to the parents and child, position the patient supine. As with suprapubic bladder puncture, the child often may begin to urinate spontaneously before the catheter is inserted, so it is wise to have a sterile container on hand to collect a midstream specimen. The urethral opening in females is best visualized when the child holds her knees to her chest. Cleanse the urethral opening thoroughly with iodine. In females, swabbing in an anterior-posterior direction avoids fecal contamination. In males who have not been circumcised, retract the foreskin gently.

Insert a well-lubricated catheter or feeding tube into the urethra until urine flow begins. In males, it helps to exert gentle traction in a caudal direction to straighten the penis and simplify catheter insertion. Mild pressure on the catheter overcomes external sphincter spasm. Withdraw the catheter slowly at the end of the procedure.

Before inserting an indwelling urinary catheter, first inflate the balloon to assess its patency. Follow the procedure outlined

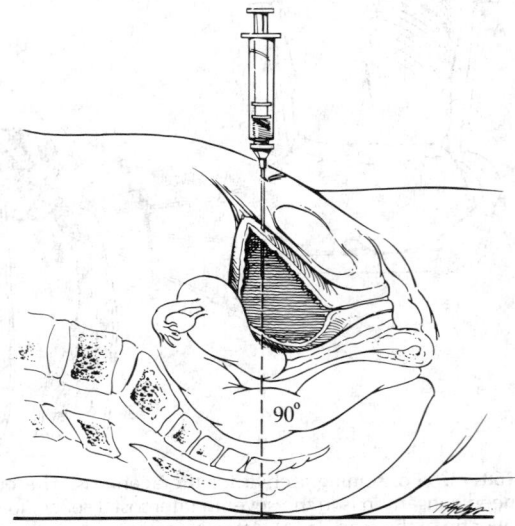

**Figure 168-15.** Suprapubic bladder puncture.

above for catheter insertion. Once urine flow begins, advance the catheter further before inflating the balloon to ensure the balloon is in the bladder and not in the proximal urethra. After the balloon is inflated, exert traction on the catheter to position the balloon at the trigone. Tape the catheter to the medial thigh, leaving sufficient slack so movement of the leg does not create tension on the catheter.

## Intramuscular Injections

Intramuscular (IM) injections are generally safe, but improper technique can lead to muscle contractures, abscess formation, intra-arterial injection, and nerve injury. For children who receive repeated injections, rotation of the injection sites protects against contractures. The safest sites in children are the anterolateral thigh

and ventrogluteal areas, followed by the deltoid and gluteal regions. The procedures for IM injection are similar regardless of the site. A 2.5-cm needle is used for all IM injections. The site is cleansed with alcohol, which is allowed to dry before the injection begins. Insert the needle using a quick motion. Always aspirate before injecting to avoid the serious consequences of intra-arterial injection. To prevent pain caused by tracking of the drug along the injection line, inject slowly into the muscle. After withdrawing the needle, rub the area for several seconds with a cotton ball or gauze pad. Figure 168-16 shows the sites for IM injection.

*Anterolateral Thigh (see Fig 168-16A).* The anterolateral thigh is popular for IM injections because the sciatic nerve and femoral vessels are distant from the injection site. The operator compresses a wide area of thigh muscle together to increase mus-

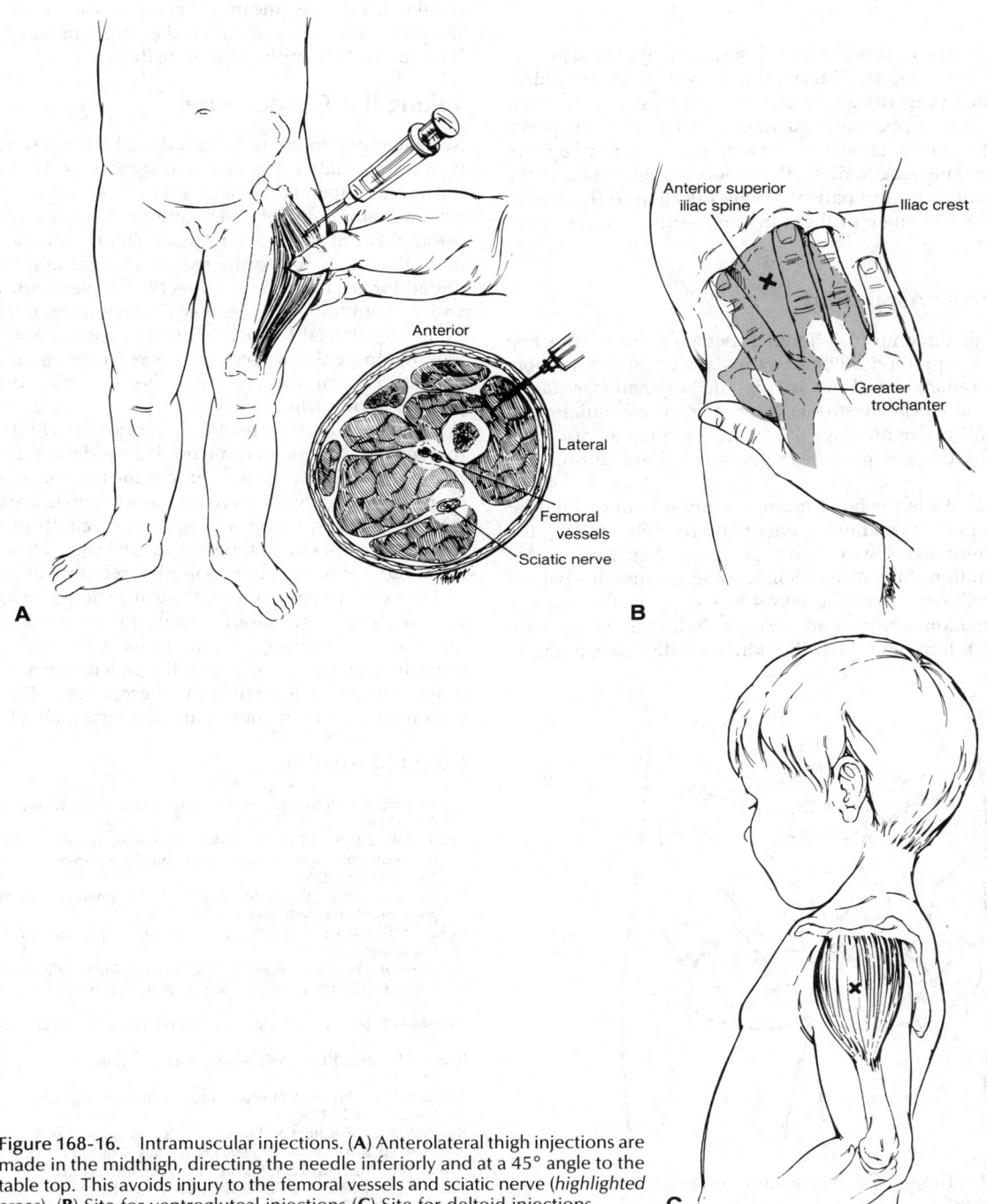

**Figure 168-16.** Intramuscular injections. (**A**) Anterolateral thigh injections are made in the midthigh, directing the needle inferiorly and at a 45° angle to the table top. This avoids injury to the femoral vessels and sciatic nerve (*highlighted areas*). (**B**) Site for ventrogluteal injections (**C**) Site for deltoid injections.

cle mass at the site. A 2.5-cm needle is inserted in the upper lateral quadrant of the midthigh. The needle is directed posteriorly at a 45° angle to the tabletop and inferiorly at a 45° angle to the long axis of the leg.

*Ventrogluteal Area (see Fig 168-16B).*   With the patient supine, the injection site is located by placing the operator's palm over the greater trochanter and the index finger over the anterior superior iliac spine, with the middle finger as close as possible to the tubercle of the iliac crest. The needle is inserted perpendicular to the skin, below the iliac crest in the center of this triangle, to a depth of 2.4 cm.

*Deltoid Area (see Fig 168-16C).*   The injection site in the deltoid muscle should be halfway between the acromion and the insertion of the deltoid muscle at the deltoid tuberosity of the humerus.

*Gluteal Area.*   Injection in the gluteal area involves a greater risk of sciatic nerve injury. This site should be avoided in children younger than 2 years of age, because muscle mass in this area is small. Inject in the upper outer quadrant, but lateral and superior to a line between the greater trochanter and posterior superior iliac spine, making sure to direct the needle perpendicular to the examining table with the patient prone. Injection in the medial direction (at a 90° angle to the skin) can result in sciatic nerve injury.

## Bone-Marrow Aspiration

The degree of discomfort children experience during the first bone-marrow aspiration influences the anxiety they feel before subsequent examinations. With appropriate explanation, sedation if necessary, and local anesthesia, bone-marrow aspiration need not be painful or frightening. Behavioral techniques discussed earlier in this chapter may be especially helpful during this procedure.

The standard site for bone-marrow aspiration in children of all ages is from the posterior superior iliac crest (Fig 168-17); the tibia is an alternative site in children younger than 3 months of age. For aspiration at the posterior iliac spine, position the patient prone with pillows under the pelvis to elevate it. Cleanse the skin with povidone-iodine and 70% alcohol, then raise a skin wheal with 1% lidocaine. After the skin is anesthetized, infiltrate

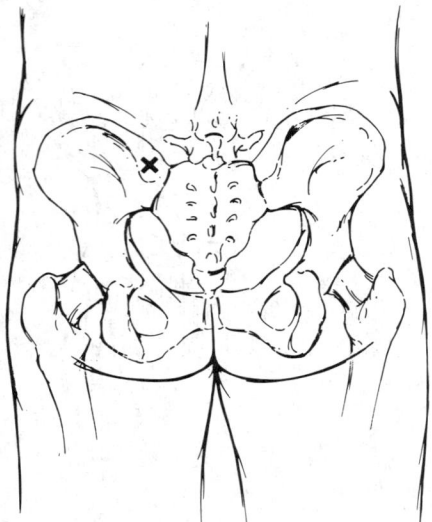

**Figure 168-17.**   The site for bone-marrow aspiration at the posterior superior iliac crest.

the subcutaneous tissues and gradually anesthetize a wide area of periosteum at the site of aspiration. Test the adequacy of the local anesthesia before proceeding.

A 16- or 18-gauge bone-marrow needle usually is used for the procedure, although some groups report success with a 22-gauge spinal needle. Steady but not excessive twisting pressure is exerted on the needle in a direction perpendicular to the surface of the bone. One hand should hold the needle in place over the bone. When the needle enters the marrow space, it becomes anchored in place, and decreased resistance may be felt. Remove the obturator and attach a 20-mL syringe. Aspirate rapidly for 1 to 2 seconds, taking care not to dilute the marrow specimen with sinusoidal blood (0.2 mL of marrow is sufficient). If no marrow is obtained, advance the needle further; change sites if this is not productive. The patient may complain of pain at the time of negative pressure on the syringe. Once the marrow specimen is obtained, prepare smears on glass slides. At the conclusion of the procedure, remove the needle, apply pressure to the site for 5 minutes, then apply a pressure dressing.

## Taking the Temperature

Rectal temperatures are the usual method of assessing body temperature in children younger than age 6 years. To position children for rectal temperatures, place them prone on the parent's lap or on the examining table. Separate the buttocks, then insert a lubricated rectal thermometer in a slightly anterior direction no more than 2.5 cm into the rectum (1.5 cm in infants). Time required for accurate measurements with electronic thermometers varies. Hold the older mercury thermometers in place for about 3 minutes. Rectal temperatures are contraindicated in children with neutropenia and rectal diseases. Insertion of thermometers beyond 2.5 cm increases the risk of rectal perforation and pneumoperitoneum.

Oral temperatures are more accurate once children understand they must keep the mouth closed around the thermometer. The thermometer is placed as far under the tongue as possible. While optimal readings with mercury thermometers are obtained after 8 to 10 minutes, this is an impractical length of time for most clinical settings. Oral temperatures are inaccurate in patients who have had hot or cold drinks in the preceding 20 minutes.

For axillary temperatures, the axilla should be patted dry (rubbing the skin may falsely elevate the temperature). The thermometer is placed high in the axilla with the end of the thermometer facing anteriorly, then the patient's arm is brought down to the patient's side against the thermometer. Optimal readings with mercury thermometers are obtained after 11 minutes.

## Selected Readings

Bergeson PS, Singer SA, Kaplan AM. Intramuscular injections in children. Pediatrics 1982;70:944.

Blumenfeld TA, Turi GK, Blanc WA. Recommended site and depth of newborn heel skin punctures based on anatomical measurements and histopathology. Lancet 1979;1:230.

Gleason CA, Martin RJ, Anderson JV, et al. Optimal position for a spinal tap in preterm infants. Pediatrics 1983;71:31.

Greene MG, ed. The Harriet Lane handbook, ed 12. Chicago: Year Book Medical Publishers, 1991.

Halperin DH, Koren G, Attias D, et al. Topical skin anesthesia for venous, subcutaneous drug reservoir and lumbar puncture in children. Pediatrics 1989;84:281.

Hughes WT, Buescher ES. Pediatric procedures, ed 2. Philadelphia: WB Saunders, 1980.

Kaplan SL, Feigin RD. Simplified technique for tympanocentesis. Pediatrics 1978;62:418.

Meites S, Levitt MJ. Skin-puncture and blood-collecting techniques for infants. Clin Chem 1979;25:183.

Ruddy RM. In: Fleisher GR, Ludwig S, eds. Textbook of pediatric emergency medicine, ed 2. Baltimore: Williams & Wilkins, 1988:1246.

Spivey WH. Intraosseous infusions. J Pediatr 1987;111:639.

Zeltzer LK, Jay SM, Fisher DM. The management of pain associated with pediatric procedures. Pediatr Clin North Am 1989;36:941.

*Principles and Practice of Pediatrics, Second Edition.*
edited by Frank A. Oski et al. J. B. Lippincott Company, Philadelphia © 1994.

CHAPTER 169

# Presenting Signs and Symptoms

Harry C. Dietz and Frank A. Oski

This chapter contains a group of common signs and symptoms. Each sign or symptom is followed by a list of possible causes, which are classified as common, uncommon, and rare. *Common causes* lists those diseases that, collectively, are responsible for the given sign or symptom in about 90% of patients who have it; the term is not meant to imply that the disease itself is necessarily common. *Uncommon causes* suggests that 1% to 10% of patients with the sign or symptom are found in that category. *Rare causes* lists the diseases that represent less than 1% of the causes of the symptom or sign under discussion. When confronted with a given symptom or sign, common causes should always be considered first.

## Abdominal Masses

### Common Causes

Appendiceal abscess
Bladder distention
Fecal collection
Hepatomegaly (any etiology)
Hydronephrosis
Multicystic dysplastic kidney
Neuroblastoma
Polycystic kidney disease (with or without liver involvement)
Pregnancy (with or without ectopic location)
Pyloric stenosis
Splenomegaly (any etiology)
Wilms' tumor

### Uncommon Causes

Adrenal hemorrhage
Hernia (with or without incarceration)
Intestinal duplication
Intussusception
Leukemia
Lymphadenopathy
Ovarian cyst
Renal vein thrombosis

### Rare Causes

Abscess
Anterior meningocele
Aortic aneurysm
Benign cystic causes
    Urachal cyst
    Mesenteric cyst
    Omental cyst
    Pancreatic cyst/pseudocyst
Bezoar

Hepatobiliary causes
    Cholecystitis/ascending cholangitis
    Choledochal cyst
    Hemangioendothelioma
    Hydrops of the gallbladder
Hydrometrocolpos
Intestinal causes
    Intestinal atresia (proximal dilatation)
    Malrotation with volvulus
    Meconium plug/ileus
    Regional enteritis
Retroperitoneal lymphangioma
Solid tumors
    Granulosa-theca cell tumor
    Hepatoblastoma
    Hepatocellular carcinoma
    Lymphoma
    Mesoblastic nephroma
    Nephroblastomatosis
    Rhabdomyosarcoma
    Teratoma (abdominal/ovarian)

## Selected Readings

Merten DF, Kirks DR. Diagnostic imaging of pediatric abdominal masses. Pediatr Clin North Am 1985;32:1397.
Wilson DA. Ultrasound screening for abdominal masses in the neonatal period. Am J Dis Child 1982;136:147.

## Abdominal Pain

### Acute

### Common Causes

Appendicitis
Bacterial enterocolitis
    *Campylobacter*
    Salmonella
    Shigella
    *Yersinia*
Dietary indiscretion
Food poisoning
Mesenteric lymphadenitis
Pharyngitis
Pregnancy (with or without ectopic location)
Urinary tract infection
Viral gastroenteritis

### Uncommon Causes

Cholecystitis/cholelithiasis
Diabetes mellitus
Hepatitis
Herpes zoster
Incarcerated hernia
Infectious mononucleosis
Intussusception
Meckel's diverticulum
Obstruction (adhesions)
Pelvic inflammatory disease
Peritonitis
    Post-trauma/instrumentation
    Spontaneous
Pneumonia
Sepsis

Trauma
  Bowel perforation
  Intramural hematoma
  Intraperitoneal blood
  Liver/spleen laceration or hematoma
  Musculocutaneous injury
  Pancreatic pseudocyst
Volvulus

## Rare Causes

Abdominal abscess
Acute arrhythmia
Acute rheumatic fever
Adynamic ileus
  Drugs
  Metabolic
  Postsurgery/trauma
Ascites
Eosinophilic gastroenteritis
Glomerulonephritis
Hemolysis
Malignancy
  Leukemia/lymphoma
  Solid tumor (with or without rupture/hemorrhage)
  Mesenteric arterial insufficiency/occlusion
  Nephrolithiasis
  Nephrotic syndrome
  Obstructive nephropathy
  Pancreatitis
  Testicular torsion
  Vasculitis
  Henoch-Schönlein purpura
  Kawasaki disease
  Polyarteritis nodosa
  Systemic lupus erythematosus

## Recurrent

### Common Causes

"Psychophysiologic"
  Conversion hysteria
  Depression
  Idiopathic recurrent pain
  Reaction anxiety
  Secondary gain
  Task-induced phobia (eg, school, sports)

### Uncommon Causes

Aerophagia
Constipation
Drugs
  Antibiotics
  Anticonvulsants
  Aspirin
  Bronchodilators
Dysmenorrhea
Enzymatic deficiency (eg, lactose intolerance)
Food allergy
Hepatosplenomegaly (any etiology)
Hiatal hernia
Inflammatory bowel disease
Irritable bowel syndrome
Mittelschmerz
Parisitic infection
  Ascariasis
  Giardiasis

Strongyloidiasis
Trichinelliasis
Peptic ulcerative disease
Sickle-cell anemia
Urinary tract infection

### Rare Causes

Abdominal epilepsy
Abdominal masses/malignancies
  Lymphoma
  Neuroblastoma
  Ovarian lesions
  Wilms' tumor
Abdominal migraine equivalent
Acute intermittent porphyria
Addison's disease
Angioneurotic edema
Bowel anomaly with obstruction
  Duplication
  Malrotation
  Stenosis
  Web
Choledochal cyst
Collagen vascular disease
Cystic fibrosis (meconium plug/ileus equivalent)
Endometriosis
Familial Mediterranean fever
Heavy metal intoxication
Hematocolpos
Hirschsprung's disease
Hyperlipoproteinemia
Hyperthyroidism
Hypoperfusion states
  Coarctation of the aorta
  Familial dysautonomia
  Superior mesenteric artery syndrome
Mesenteric cyst
Neurologic
  Central nervous system (CNS) mass lesion
  Radiculopathy
  Spinal cord injury/tumor
Recurrent/chronic arrhythmia
Recurrent pancreatitis
Wegener's granulomatosis

## Selected Readings

Alford BA, McIlhenny J. The child with acute abdominal pain and vomiting. Radiol Clin North Am 1992;30:441

Barr RG. Abdominal pain in the female adolescent. Pediatr Rev 1983;4:281.

Barr RG, Levine MD, Watkins JB. Recurrent abdominal pain of childhood due to lactose intolerance. N Engl J Med 1979;300:1449.

David EA, Werman HA, Rund DA. Use of leukocyte count and differential in the evaluation of abdominal pain. Am J Emerg Med 1986;4:482.

Dimson SB. Transit time related to clinical findings in children with recurrent abdominal pain. Pediatrics 1971;47:666.

Edwards NH. The accuracy of a Bayesian computer program for diagnosis and teaching in acute abdominal pain of childhood. Computer Methods Programs Biomed 1986;23:155.

Faro S, Maccato M. Pelvic pain and infections. Obstet Gynecol Clin North Am 1990;17:441.

Farrell MK. Abdominal pain. Pediatrics 1984;75(pt 2):955.

Feuerstein M, Barr RG, Francoeur TE, et al. Potential biobehavioral mechanisms of recurrent abdominal pain in children. Pain 1982;13:287.

Hatch EI. The acute abdomen in children. Pediatr Clin North Am 1985;32:1151.

Lake AM. Acute abdominal pain in childhood. Postgrad Med J 1979;65:119.

Lebenthal E. Recurrent abdominal pain in childhood. Am J Dis Child 1980;134:347.

Michener WM. An approach to recurrent abdominal pain in children. Primary Care 1981;8:277.

Muse KN. Cyclic pelvic pain. Obstet Gynecol Clin North Am 1990;17:427.

Poole SR. Recurrent abdominal pain in childhood and adolescence. Am Fam Physician 1984;30:131.

Ryan NM. Recurrent abdominal pain among school-aged children. MCN Am J Matern Child Nurs 1986;11:102.

# *Alopecia*

## Common Causes

Alopecia areata
Distal trichorrhexis nodosa
Physiologic (newborns)
   Temporal recession at puberty
Tinea capitis
Traction alopecia
Trichotillomania

## Uncommon Causes

Acute bacterial infections
   Cellulitis
   Folliculitis decalvans
   Pyoderma
Burns
Cancer therapy
   Antimetabolites
   Radiation
Chemical injury
Kerion
Proximal trichorrhexis nodosa
Psoriasis
Seborrhea
Viral infections
   Herpes simplex
   Varicella

## Rare Causes

Circumscribed alopecia
   Androgenic alopecia
   Aplasia cutis
   Conradi's disease
   Epidermal nevi—organoid
   Follicular aplasia
   Goltz's syndrome
   Hair follicle hamartoma
   Incontinentia pigmenti
   Infections
      Leprosy
      Tuberculosis
   Inflammatory etiologies
      Keratosis follicularis
      Lichen planus
      Morphea
      Porokeratosis of Mibelli
      Sarcoid
      Systemic lupus erythematosus
   Myotonic dystrophy
Diffuse alopecia
   Anagen effluvium
      Cytostatic agents in plants
         Mimosine
         Selemocystothionine
      Radium
      Thallium
   Anhidrotic ectodermal dysplasia
   Atrichia congenita

   Cartilage-hair hypoplasia
   Chondroectodermal dysplasia
   Crouston's syndrome
   Hair shaft deformities
      Monilethrix
      Pili torti
         Classic form
         Trichopoliodystrophy (Menkes' syndrome)
      Trichorrhexis invaginata
      Trichorrhexis nodosa
         Argininosuccinic aciduria
Hallermann-Streiff syndrome
Hidrotic ectodermal dysplasia
Langer-Giedion syndrome
Marinesco-Sjögren syndrome
Oculodentodigital dysplasia
Progeria
Rothmund-Thomson syndrome
Telogen effluvium
   Childbirth
   Chronic infection/illness
   Drugs
      Anticoagulants
      Anticonvulsants
      Antikeratinizing drugs
      Antithyroid drugs
      Heavy metals
      Hormones
   Excessive dieting
   High fever
   Hypothyroidism
   Stress
   Surgery

## Selected Readings

Atton AV, Tunnessen WW Jr. Alopecia in children: the most common causes. Pediatr Rev 1990;12:25.

Bergfeld WF. Hair disorders. Major Prob Clin Pediatr 1978;19:347.

Clore ER, Corey A. Hair loss in children and adolescents. J Pediatric Health Care 1991;5:245.

Levy ML. Disorders of the hair and scalp in children. Pediatr Clin North Am 1991;38:905.

Olsen EA. Alopecia: evaluation and management. Prim Care 1989;16:765.

Price VH. Office diagnosis of structural hair anomalies. Cutis 1975;15:231.

Price VH. Disorders of the hair in children. Pediatr Clin North Am 1978;25:305.

Stroud JD. Hair loss in children. Pediatr Clin North Am 1983;30:641.

# *Anorexia*

## Common Causes

Acute infection
Apparent anorexia
   Dieting/fear of obesity
   Manipulative behavior
   Unrealistic expectations of caretakers

## Uncommon Causes

Chronic infection
Drugs
   Aminophylline
   Amphetamines
   Anticonvulsants
   Antihistamines
   Antimetabolites

Digitalis
Narcotics
Esophagitis/gastroesophageal reflux
Food aversion in athletes
Iron deficiency
Irritable bowel syndrome
Pregnancy
Psychosocial deprivation (neglect/abuse)
Psychosocial factors
    Chronic mental/environmental stress
        Anxiety
        Fear
        Loneliness/boredom
    Depression
    Grief
    Mania

## Rare Causes

Acquired immune deficiency syndrome (AIDS)
Adrenogenital syndrome
Alcohol/drug abuse
Anorexia nervosa
Chronic disease
Collagen vascular disease
Congestive heart failure
Cyanotic heart disease
Electrolyte disturbances
    Hypercalcemia
    Hypochloremia
    Hypokalemia
Endocrine disease
    Addison's disease
    Diabetes insipidus
    Hyperparathyroidism
    Hypothyroidism
    Panhypopituitarism
Hypervitaminosis A
Inborn errors of metabolism
Kwashiorkor
Lead poisoning
Liver failure
Neurologic
    Congenital degenerative disease
    Diencephalic syndrome
    Hypothalamic lesions
    Increased intracranial pressure
    Mental retardation/cerebral palsy
Pain avoidance
    Appendicitis
    Constipation
    Gastrointestinal obstruction
    Inflammatory bowel disease
    Pancreatitis
    Superior mesenteric syndrome
Polycythemia
Postsurgery
Pulmonary insufficiency
Renal failure
Renal tubular acidosis
Schizophrenia
Zinc deficiency

## Selected Readings

Bernstein IL, Sigmundi RA. Tumor anorexia: a learned food aversion? Science 1980;209:416.
Brobeck JR. Nature of satiety signals. Am J Clin Nutr 1975;28:806.
Bryant-Waugh RJ, Lask BD, Shafran RL, Fosson AR. Do doctors recognize eating disorders in children? Arch Dis Child 1992;67:103.
Nussbaum MP, Shenker IR, Shaw H, Frank S. Differential diagnosis of anorexia nervosa. Pediatrician 1983;12:110.
Pugliese MT, Lifshitz F, Grad G, et al. Fear of obesity: a cause of short stature and delayed puberty. N Engl J Med 1983;309:513.
Smith NJ. Excessive weight loss and food aversion in athletes simulating anorexia nervosa. Pediatrics 1980;66:139.
Yates A, Leehey K, Shisslak CM. Running—an analogue of anorexia? N Engl J Med 1983;308:251.

# *Apnea*

## Common Causes

Breath-holding spells
Bronchiolitis
Extrinsic suffocation
Gastroesophageal reflux/aspiration
Idiopathic (? CNS immaturity)
Prematurity
Seizure

## Uncommon Causes

Arrhythmia
Asthma
Bronchopulmonary dysplasia "spells"
CNS hypoperfusion
CNS trauma/bleed
Congenital airway anomaly
Hypoglycemia
Hypoxemia/hypercarbia (severe)
Infection
    Croup
    Meningitis/encephalitis
    Epiglottitis
    Pertussis
    Pneumonia
    Sepsis
Laryngospasm
Laryngo-tracheo-bronchomalacia
Obstructive sleep apnea
Sudden infant death syndrome (SIDS)
Toxins/drugs

## Rare Causes

Anemia
Glossoptosis
Guillain-Barré syndrome
Hypocalcemia
Increased intracranial pressure
Infantile botulism
Intraventricular hemorrhage
Macroglossia
Metabolic disease
    Hyperammonemia
    Inborn errors
    Metabolic alkalosis
Micrognathia
Ondine's curse
Spinal cord injury
    Cervical spine instability
        Down syndrome
        Dwarfism
    Trauma
Tumor (CNS, airway)

## Selected Readings

Anders TF, Weinstein P. Sleep and its disorders in infants and children. A review. Pediatrics 1972;50:312.

Boltshauser E, Lange B, Dumermuth G. Differential diagnosis of syndromes with abnormal respiration (tachypnea-apnea). Brain Dev 1987;9:462.

Guilleminault C, Ariagno R, Korobkin R, et al. Mixed and obstructive sleep apnea and near-miss for sudden infant death syndrome: 2. Comparison of near-miss and normal control infants by age. Pediatrics 1979;64:882.

McBride JT. Infantile apnea. Pediatr Rev 1984;5:275.

Spitzer AR, Fox WW. Infant apnea. Pediatr Clin North Am 1986;33:561.

Torrey SB. Apnea. Pediatr Emerg Care 1985;1:219.

Valdes-Dapena MA. Sudden infant death syndrome: a review of the medical literature 1974–1979. Pediatrics 1980;66:597.

# Back Pain

## Common Causes

Mechanical derangement (muscle strain or poor posture)
Scheuermann's kyphosis
Scoliosis
Spondylolysis/spondylolisthesis

## Uncommon Causes

Disk space infection (diskitis)
Rheumatic disorders
Sacroiliac joint infections
Spina bifida occulta
Spinal cord tumors (lipomas, teratomas)
Vertebral osteomyelitis

## Rare Causes

Aneurysmal bone cyst
Aseptic necrosis of vertebrae
Benign osteoblastoma
Eosinophilic granuloma of vertebrae
Hemangioma of bone
Hematocolpos
Herniated nucleus pulposus
Herpes zoster
Malignancy involving bone (neuroblastoma, leukemia metastatic)
Osteomalacia of the spine
Paraspinal tumor or infection
Secondary hyperparathyroidism
Tuberculosis of the spine
Vertebral osteoid osteoma

## Selected Readings

Abram SR, Tedeschi AA, Partain CL, Blumenkopf B. Differential diagnosis of severe back pain using MRI, South Med J 1988;81:1487.

Aiken BM, Cohen BS. The role of congenital anomalies in low back pain. Maryland State Med J 1983;32:38.

Bunnell WP. Back pain in children. Orthop Clin North Am 1982;13:587.

Gonzales R, Marino RV. A diagnostic approach to childhood back pain. Journal of the American Osteopathic Association 1986;86:454.

Williams HJ, Pugh DG. Vertebral epiphysitis: a comparison of the clinical and roentgenologic findings. AJR 1963;90:1236.

# Chest Pain

## Common Causes

Costochondritic
    Arthritis
    Infectious costochondritis
    Tietze's syndrome
Cough
Herpes zoster
Idiopathic
Indigestion (heartburn, esophagitis)
Mitral valve prolapse
Musculoskeletal (strain, occult trauma)
Pneumonitis
Psychogenic
Reactive airway disease
Sickle-cell disease
Trauma

## Uncommon Causes

Arrhythmia
Congenital heart disease
Congestive heart failure
Esophageal (trauma associated with vomiting, foreign body)
Pleuritis/pleurisy
Pneumothorax
Precordial catch

## Rare Causes

Cholecystitis
Diaphragmatic irritation
    Abscess
    FitzHugh-Curtis syndrome
    Peritonitis
    Ruptured viscus
    Tumor
Endocarditis
Juvenile rheumatoid arthritis
Myocardial ischemia (eg, anomalous coronary artery)
Myocarditis
Osteomyelitis (vertebrae, ribs)
Peptic ulcerative disease
Pericarditis
Pneumomediastinum
Pulmonary embolism
Rheumatic fever

## Selected Readings

Asnes RS, Santulli R, Bemporad JR. Psychogenic chest pain in children. Clin Pediatr 1981;20:788.

Brenner JI, Berman MA. Chest pain in childhood and adolescence. J Adolesc Health Care 1983;3:271.

Calabro JJ, Jeghers H, Miller KA, Gordon RD. Classification of anterior chest wall syndromes. Letter. JAMA 1980;243:1420.

Calabro JJ, Marchesano JM. Tietze's syndrome: report of a case with juvenile onset. J Pediatr 1966;68:985.

Driscoll DJ, Glicklich LB, Gallen WJ. Chest pain in children: a prospective study. Pediatrics 1976;57:648.

Milov DE, Kantor RJ. Chest pain in teenagers. When is it significant? Postgrad Med 1990;88:145,153.

Selbst SM, Ruddy RM, Clark BJ, et al. Pediatric chest pain: a prospective study. Pediatrics 1988;82:319.

Sparrow MJ, Bird EL. "Precordial catch": a benign syndrome of chest pain in young persons. N Z Med J 1978;88:325.

# Coma

## Common Causes

CNS trauma
    Cerebral edema
    Concussion

Hemorrhage
  Epidural
  Subarachnoid
  Subdural
Increased intracranial pressure
Drug intoxication
  Analgesics
  Anticonvulsants
  Antihistamines
  Benzodiazepines
  Digoxin
  Ethanol
  Heavy metals
  Hydrocarbons
  Hypnotics
    Barbiturates
  Insulin
  Lithium
  Organophosphates
  Phencyclidine
  Phenothiazines
  Salicylate
  Tricyclic antidepressants

**Uncommon Causes**

Cardiorespiratory
  Cardiopulmonary arrest
  Hypercapnea
  Hypotension/shock
  Hypoxemia
Infection
  Abscess
  Encephalitis
  Meningitis
Metabolic
  Hypercalcemia/hypocalcemia
  Hypermagnesemia/hypomagnesemia
  Hypernatremia/hyponatremia
  Hypoglycemia
    Water intoxication
  Metabolic acidosis
  Metabolic alkalosis
Postictal state
Postoperative
  General anesthesia
  Hypotension/hypoxemia
Sepsis

**Rare Causes**

Cardiac
  Arrhythmia
  Hypertension
  Hypoperfusion
    Aortic stenosis
    Coarctation of the aorta
Cerebral tumors/metastases
Cerebrovascular
  Hemorrhage
  Thrombophlebitis
  Vasculitis
  Venous thrombosis
Dehydration
Diabetic ketoacidosis
Endocrine disorders
  Addison's disease
  Congenital adrenal hyperplasia
  Cushing's disease

Inborn errors of metabolism
  Hyperammonemia
  Hypoglycemia
Heat stroke
Hepatic failure
Hypothermia
Malignant hyperthermia
Porphyria
Postinfectious encephalomyelitis
  Measles
  Other viral infections
Psychiatric disturbances
  Fugue state
  Hysteria
Reye's syndrome
SIDS
Uremia

## Selected Readings

Dean JM, Kaufman ND. Prognostic indicators in pediatric near-drowning: the Glasgow coma scale. Crit Care Med 1981;9:536.

Helliwell M, Hampel G, Sinclair E, et al. Value of emergency toxicological investigations in differential diagnosis of coma. BMJ 1979;2:819.

Levy DE, Bates D, Caronna JJ, et al. Prognosis in nontraumatic coma. Ann Intern Med 1981;94:293.

Mickell JJ, Reigel DH, Cook DR, et al. Intracranial pressure: monitoring and normalization therapy in children. Pediatrics 1977;59:606.

Seshia SS, Seshia MMK, Sachdeva RK. Coma in childhood. Dev Med Child Neurol 1977;19:614.

## Constipation

Constipation is defined here as stools less frequent than expected by the caretaker.

**Common Causes**

Appendicitis
Breastfeeding (begins at about 6 weeks of age)
Cow's milk ingestion
Drugs
  Anticholinergics
  Antihistamines
  Narcotics
  Phenothiazines
Dysfunctional toilet training
Emotional disturbances
Functional ileus
Immobility
Inappropriate expectations of the caretaker
Intentional withholding
Intestinal abnormalities
  Atresia
  Hirschsprung's disease
  Microcolon
  Volvulus
  Web
Low dietary fiber
Meconium plug/ileus
Meningomyelocele
Mental retardation/cerebral palsy
Painful defecation (hemorrhoids, fissure, skin irritation)

**Uncommon Causes**

Diabetes mellitus
Electrolyte disturbances
    Hypercalcemia/hypocalcemia
    Hyperkalemia
Hypothyroidism
Imperforate anus/anal stenosis
Intestinal pseudo-obstruction
Lead poisoning
Salmonellosis
Spinal cord injury/tumor
Starvation

**Rare Causes**

Amyloidosis
Botulism
Dolichocolon
Multiple endocrine neoplasia
Myopathies/myotonias
Pheochromocytoma
Sacral malformations
Scleroderma
Tetanus
Tethered cord

## Selected Readings

Barr RG, Levine MD, Wilkinson RH, Mulvihill D. Chronic and occult stool retention: a clinical tool for its evaluation in school-aged children. Clin Pediatr 1979;18:674.
Bentley JFR. Constipation in infants and children. Gut 1971;12:85.
Davidson M, Kugler MM, Bauer CH. Diagnosis and management in children with severe and protracted constipation and obstipation. J Pediatr 1963;62:261.
Fleisher DR. Diagnosis and treatment of disorders of defecation in children. Pediatr Ann 1976;5:700.

# Cough

## Common Causes

Allergic disease
Aspiration (direct or indirect)
Atelectasis
Bacterial infection
    Bronchiectasis
    Bronchitis
    Pneumonia
    Sinusitis
    Tracheitis
Congestive heart failure
Environmental pollution
Foreign body
Gastroesophageal reflux
Infections, other
    Chlamydia
    Mycoplasma
    Pertussis
Postnasal drip
Reactive airway disease
Smoking/passive smoking
Viral infection
    Bronchiolitis
    Croup
    Pneumonitis
    Upper respiratory infection

**Uncommon Causes**

Cystic fibrosis
Malformation of the airway
Malignancy (primary or metastatic)
Mediastinal adenopathy
Psychogenic
Tracheobronchomalacia
Tracheoesophageal fistula
Tuberculosis
Vascular ring

**Rare Causes**

Allergic bronchopulmonary aspergillosis
Auricular nerve stimulation
Bronchogenic cyst
Congenital lobar emphysema
Immotile cilia syndrome
Lymphocytic interstitial pneumonitis
Opportunistic infections (pneumocystis carinii [PCP], cytomegalovirus [CMV], mycobacterium avium intracellulare [MAI], fungal)
Parasitic infection
Pulmonary embolism
Pulmonary hemosiderosis
Pulmonary sequestration
Sarcoidosis

## Selected Readings

Cloutier MM. Finding the cause of chronic cough in children. J Respir Dis 1980;1:20.
Cloutier MM, Loughlin GM. Chronic cough in children: a manifestation of airway hyperactivity. Pediatrics 1981;67:6.
Eigen H. The clinical evaluation of chronic cough. Pediatr Clin North Am 1982;29:67.
Godfrey RC. Diseases causing cough. European J Respiratory Diseases 1980;110(Suppl):57.
Irwin RS, Corrao WM, Pratter MR. Chronic persistent cough in the adult: the spectrum and frequency of causes and successful outcome of specific therapy. Am Rev Respir Dis 1981;123:413.
Irwin RS, Rosen MJ, Braman SS. Cough: a comprehensive review. Arch Intern Med 1977;137:1186.
Mellis CM. Evaluation and treatment of chronic cough in children. Pediatr Clin North Am 1979;26:553.
Stein MT. Chronic cough in infants younger than 3 months. West J Med 1982;136:505.
Wilmott RW. Pursuing the cause of persistent cough. Contemp Pediatr 1987;4:26.

# Cyanosis

## Common Causes

Acrocyanosis (especially cold stress)
Apnea of prematurity
Aspiration
    Direct (swallowing disorders, neuromuscular disease)
    Indirect (gastroesophageal reflux, emesis)
Atelectasis
Breath holding
Bronchiolitis
Congenital heart disease
    Decreased pulmonary blood flow (no pulmonary hypertension)
        Anomalous systemic venous return
        Ebstein's anomaly
        Hypoplastic right ventricle
        Pulmonary stenosis/atresia

Tetralogy of Fallot
Tricuspid stenosis/atresia/insufficiency
Eisenmenger's physiology
Increased pulmonary blood flow
Atrioventricular (AV) canal
Coarctation (preductal)
Hypoplastic left heart
Total anomalous pulmonary venous return (TAPVR)
Transposition
Truncus arteriosus
Ventricular septal defect (VSD) (large)
Pump failure
Aortic stenosis (severe)
Coarctation (postductal)
Patent ductus arteriosus
VSD
Croup
Crying
Drugs—respiratory depressants (eg, narcotics, benzodiazepines)
Hyaline membrane disease
Mucus plug
Nasal obstruction
Pneumonia
Pulmonary edema
Reactive airway disease
Seizures
Sepsis
Sleep apnea (tonsillar/adenoidal hypertrophy)

**Uncommon Causes**

Abdominal distention
Arterial thrombosis
Bronchopulmonary dysplasia
Chest wall abnormalities
Congenital bone/cartilage abnormalities
Pectus
Flail chest
Cystic fibrosis
Epiglottitis
Foreign body
Hypovolemia
Mediastinal mass
Persistent fetal circulation
Pickwickian syndrome
Pleural effusion
Pneumothorax
Polycythemia
Pulmonary hemorrhage
Retropharyngeal/peritonsillar abscess
Scoliosis
Tracheal compression
Abscess
Adenopathy
Hemorrhage
Tumor
Vascular ring
Tracheobronchomalacia/stenosis
Venous stasis

**Rare Causes**

Angioedema
Bronchogenic cyst
CNS disease
Edema
Hemorrhage
Infection
Trauma

Chylothorax
Diaphragmatic hernia
Factitious (blue paint/dyes/makeup)
Glossoptosis
Hemoglobinopathy (M, low oxygen affinity)
Hypoplastic lungs
Laryngeal web
Lobar emphysema
Methemoglobinemia
Methemoglobin reductase deficiency
Oxidant stress
Acetophenetidin
Antimalarials
Benzocaine
Crayons
Disinfectants
Ethylenediaminetetraacetic acid (EDTA)
Hydralazine
Marking dyes
Naphthalene
Nitrites
Amyl/butyl nitrate
Nitrate-contaminated well water
Nitrate food additives
Nitroglycerin
Plant nitrates (eg, carrots grown in contaminated soil)
Nitroprusside
Prilocaine
Pyridium
Sulfonamides
Vitamin K analogs
Ondine's curse
Primary pulmonary hypertension
Pulmonary AV malformation/fistula
Pulmonary embolism/thrombosis
Pulmonary hemosiderosis
Pulmonary sequestration
Pulmonary tumor (primary or metastatic)
Reflex sympathetic dystrophy
Respiratory muscle dysfunction
Botulism
Muscular dystrophy
Myasthenia gravis
Neuromuscular blockade
Phrenic nerve damage
Werdnig-Hoffmann disease
Superior vena cava (SVC) syndrome
Tracheoesophageal fistula
Tumor
Vocal cord paralysis

## Selected Readings

Engle MA. Cyanotic congenital heart disease. Am J Cardiol 1976;37:283.
Jaffe ER. Methemoglobinemia in the differential diagnosis of cyanosis. Hosp Pract (Off Ed) 1985;20:92,101,108.
Lees MH. Cyanosis of the newborn infant. J Pediatr 1970;77:484.
Levin AR. Management of the cyanotic newborn. Pediatr Ann 1981;10:16.

## Diarrhea, Chronic

### Common Causes

Antibiotic-induced
Carbohydrate malabsorption, hereditary
Lactose

Chemotherapy-induced
Cystic fibrosis
Dietary
    Allergy (milk, soy, other)
    Overfeeding
Infection
    Bacterial
    Human immunodeficiency virus (HIV)
    Parasitic
Postinfectious
    Carbohydrate malabsorption

## Uncommon Causes

Anatomic lesions
    Hirschsprung's disease
    Malrotation
Celiac disease
Gastrointestinal bleeding
Irritable bowel syndrome
Malnutrition, starvation
Necrotizing enterocolitis
Parenteral infections
    Otitis media
    Urinary tract infections
Regional enteritis
Ulcerative colitis

## Rare Causes

Abeta- and hypobetalipoproteinemia
Adrenal insufficiency
Biliary atresia
Blind loop syndrome
Carbohydrate malabsorption
    Sucrose, isomaltose, glucose, galactose
Chronic hepatitis
Enterokinase deficiency
Familial chloride diarrhea
Ganglioneuroma
Hyperthyroidism
Immune deficiency
    Combined immune deficiency
    Hypogammaglobulinemia
    IgA deficiency
Intestinal ischemia
Intestinal lymphangiectasia
Intestinal pseudo-obstruction
Liver abscess
Mesenteric artery insufficiency
Neuroblastoma
Pancreatic insufficiency and neutropenia (Schwachman-Diamond-Oski syndrome)
Pancreatic tumors
Radiation-induced
Short gut syndrome
Small bowel tumors; lymphosarcoma
Wolman's disease

## Selected Readings

Cohen SA, Hendricks KM, Mathis RK, et al. Chronic nonspecific diarrhea: dietary relationships. Pediatrics 1979;64:402.

Dewitt TG, Humphrey KF, McCarthy P. Clinical predictors of acute bacterial diarrhea in young children. Pediatrics 1985;76:551.

Drossman DA, Powell DW, Sessions JT Jr. The irritable bowel syndrome. Gastroenterol 1977;73:811.

Gall DG, Hamilton JR. Chronic diarrhea in childhood. Pediatr Clin North Am 1974;21:1001.

Gryboski JD. Chronic diarrhea. Curr Probl Pediatr 1979;9:5.

Hirschhorn N. The treatment of acute diarrhea in children: an historical and physiological perspective. Am J Clin Nutr 1980;33:637.

Larcher VF, Shepherd R, Francis DEM, Harries JT. Protracted diarrhoea in infancy. Arch Dis Child 1977;52:597.

Phillips SF. Diarrhea: a current view of the pathophysiology. Gastroenterol 1972;63:495.

# Dysphagia

## Common Causes

Chemical mucositis
    Caustic ingestion
    Gastroesophageal reflux with esophagitis
    Radiation/chemotherapy
Immature sucking/swallowing mechanism
Oropharyngeal infections
    Cervical adenitis
    Epiglottitis
    Gingivitis
    Herpetic stomatitis
    Peritonsillar abscess
    Pharyngitis
    Retropharyngeal abscess
    Tooth abscess
Physiologic expulsion reflux

## Uncommon Causes

Cerebral palsy
Cleft palate
Esophageal spasm
Esophageal stricture
External compression of the esophagus
    Esophageal diverticula
    Esophageal duplication
    Mediastinal masses/tumors
    Vascular anomalies
Foreign body
Infectious esophagitis
    *Candida*, herpes
Macroglossia (any cause)
Micrognathia
Pharyngeal diverticula
Physiologic (globus hystericus)
Submucosal cleft
Tracheoesophageal fistula

## Rare Causes

Choanal atresia
Collagen vascular disease
    Dermatomyositis
    Scleroderma
Diphtheria
Esophageal atresia, web, cyst
Laryngeal cyst, cleft
Muscular hypertrophy of the esophagus
Neuromuscular causes
    Botulism
    Bulbar and suprabulbar palsy
        Möbius' syndrome
    Chalasia/achalasia of the esophagus
    Congenital laryngeal stridor
    Cranial nerve palsy
    Demyelinating disease
    Guillain-Barré syndrome
    Hypotonias

Muscular dystrophy
Myasthenia gravis
Myotonic dystrophy
Pharyngeal or cricopharyngeal incoordination
Tetanus
Pharyngeal cyst, cleft
Rumination
Temporomandibular ankylosis/hypoplasia
Tumors (oropharynx, esophagus)

## Selected Readings

Eklof O, Ekstrom G, Eriksson BO, et al. Arterial anomalies causing compression of the trachea and/or oesophagus. Acta Paediatr Scand 1971;60:81.
Illingworth RS. Sucking and swallowing difficulties in infancy: diagnostic problem of dysphagia. Arch Dis Child 1969;44:655.
Kato S, Komatsu K, Haroda Y. Medication induced esophagitis in children. Gastroenterol Jpn 1990;25:485.

## Dysrhythmia

### Common Causes

Acidemia
Congenital heart disease
Drugs
    Antiarrhythmics
    Beta blockers
    Caffeine
    Cocaine
    Psychotropics
    Sympathomimetics
Hypoxemia
Idiopathic
Postoperative (cardiac procedures)

### Uncommon Causes

Cardiomyopathy (dilated, hypertrophic, infiltrative)
Electrolyte disturbances (especially K, Ca, Mg)
Myocarditis
Sickle-cell disease
Sick-sinus syndrome
Wolff-Parkinson-White syndrome (or other accessory bypass tracts)

### Rare Causes

Anomalous coronary artery
CNS
    Hemorrhage
    Infection
    Trauma
Collagen vascular disease
Complete congenital heart block
Endocrine (thyrotoxicosis, secondary electrolyte disturbance)
Kawasaki disease
Myocardial ischemia
Myocardial trauma
Myocardial tumors
Neonatal lupus
Prolonged QT syndrome
Rheumatic fever

## Selected Readings

Giardina ACV, Ehlers KH, Engle MA. Wolf-Parkinson-White syndrome in infants and children. Br Heart J 1972;34:839.

Morady F, Scheinman MM. Paroxysmal supraventricular tachycardia. Part I. Diagnosis. Modern Concepts Cardiovascular Disease 1982;51:107.
Morady F, Scheinman MM. Paroxysmal supraventricular tachycardia. Part II. Treatment. Modern Concepts Cardiovascular Disease 1982;51:113.

## Dysuria

### Common Causes

Candidal dermatitis/vaginitis
Chemical urethritis (bubble bath)
Contact dermatitis/vulvitis
Urethritis
Urinary tract infection
Viral cystitis

### Uncommon Causes

Foreign body
Herpes simplex
Meatitis
Pinworms
Urethral trauma

### Rare Causes

Appendicitis
Bladder diverticulum
Bladder outlet obstruction
    Posterior urethral valves
Bladder stones
Constipation
Drugs
    Amitriptyline
    Cytoxan
Hematospermia
Interstitial cystitis
Meatal stenosis
Posthitis
Prostatitis
Reiter's syndrome
Schistosomiasis
Stevens-Johnson syndrome
Tuberculosis
Urethral prolapse
Urethral stricture
Varicella

## Selected Readings

Brock WA, Kaplan GW. Voiding dysfunction in children. Curr Probl Pediatr 1980;10:4.
Spencer JR, Schaeffer AJ. Pediatric urinary tract infections. Urol Clin North Am 1986;13:661.

## Encopresis

### Common Causes

Chronic constipation
Diarrheal disorders
Emotional disturbance

### Uncommon Causes

Hirschsprung's disease

**Rare Causes**

Diastematomyelia
Epidural abscess
Poliomyelitis
Post–anorectal surgery
Osteomyelitis of the vertebral body
Sacral agenesis
Spinal cord tumor
Syringomyelia
Transverse myelitis

## Selected Readings

Bellman M. Studies on encopresis. Acta Paediatr Scand 1966;(Suppl 170):7.
Davidson M, Kugler MM, Bauer CH. Diagnosis and management in children with severe and protracted constipation and obstipation. J Pediatr 1963;62:261.
Johns C. Encopresis. Am J Nurs 1985;85:153.
Levine MD. Children with encopresis: a descriptive analysis. Pediatrics 1975;56:412.
Levine MD. The schoolchild with encopresis. Pediatr Rev 1981;2:285.
Levine MD. Encopresis: its potentiation, evaluation, and alleviation. Pediatr Clin North Am 1982;29:315.
Loening-Baucke VA, Cruikshank BM. Abnormal defecation dynamics in chronically constipated children with encopresis. J Pediatr 1986;108:562.
Rappaport LA, Levine MD. The prevention of constipation and encopresis: a developmental model and approach. Pediatr Clin North Am 1986;33:859.
Silber DL. Encopresis. Clin Pediatr 1969;8:225.

## Enuresis

**Common Causes**

Developmental delay of bladder function and capacity
Psychological

**Uncommon Causes**

Diabetes
Food allergy
Obstructive abnormalities of the urinary tract
Urinary tract infection

**Rare Causes**

Compulsive water drinking
Diabetes inspidus, central or nephrogenic
Lumbosacral anomalies
Seizure disorder
Sickle-cell anemia
Spinal cord tumors

## Selected Readings

Cohen MW. Enuresis. Pediatr Clin North Am 1975;22:545.
Friman PC. A preventive context for enuresis. Pediatr Clin North Am 1986;33:871.
Hinman F. Urinary tract damage in children who wet. Pediatrics 1974;54:142.
Maizels M, Firlit C. Guide to the history in enuretic children. Am Fam Physician 1986;33:205.
McLain LG. Childhood enuresis. Curr Probl Pediatr 1979;9:1.
Palmisano PA. Enuresis: causes, cures, and cautions. West J Med 1976;125:347.
Starfield B. Functional bladder capacity in enuretic and nonenuretic children. J Pediatr 1969;70:777.
Starfield B. Enuresis: its pathogenesis and management. Clin Pediatr 1972;11:343.
Werry JS. Enuresis—an etiologic and therapeutic study. J Pediatr 1965;67:423.

## Epistaxis

**Common Causes**

Allergic rhinitis
Repeated sneezing
Secondary to dryness and crusting over anterior portion of nasal septum
Trauma
External
Self-inflicted (nose picking)
Upper respiratory infection

**Uncommon Causes**

Factor XI deficiency
Hypertension
Platelet dysfunction syndromes
Sickle-cell anemia
Thrombocytopenia (any cause)
Von Willebrand's disease

**Rare Causes**

Angiofibroma
Ataxia-telangiectasia
Congenital syphilis
Ehlers-Danlos syndrome
Foreign body
Malaria
Measles
Nasal angiomas
Nasal diphtheria
Nasal polyp
Oral contraceptives
Osler-Weber-Rendu disease
Pertussis
Rheumatic fever
Scarlet fever
Scurvy
Typhoid fever
Varicella
Wegener's granulomatosis

## Selected Readings

Beran M, Petruson B. Occurrence of epistaxis in habitual nose-bleeders and analysis of some etiological factors. ORL 1986;48:297.
Juselius H. Epistaxis: a clinical study of 1,727 patients. J Laryngol Otol 1974;88:317.
McDonald TJ. Nosebleed in children: background and techniques to stop the flow. Postgrad Med 1987;81:217.
Okafor BC. Epistaxis: a clinical study of 540 cases. Ear Nose Throat J 1984;63:153.
Stevens M. Management of epistaxis. Aust Fam Physician 1986;15:707.

## Failure to Thrive

**Common Causes**

Neglect
Inadequate ingestion/metabolism of calories
Depression with anorexia
Manipulative behavior
Rumination as self-stimulation
Secondary malabsorption
Self-induced (vomiting, laxative abuse)
Specific deficiency (eg, zinc, biotin)
Starvation
Secondary neuroendocrine abnormalities
Abnormal cycling of growth hormone
Cortisol deficiency
Physical neglect/abuse
Psychosocial deprivation
Withholding of food as neglect/abuse

Intentional withholding of food
"Unintentional" withholding of food
　"Overwhelmed" caretaker
　　Lack of support systems (financial/social)
　　Primary personal needs (eg, drug/alcohol abuse)
　　Time constraints (eg, unsupervised eating, bottle propping)
　Psychotic or depressed caretaker
Nonorganic failure to thrive
　Inadequate volume of feeds
　　Too few feeds per day
　　Too little per feed
　　　Colic
　　　"Difficult" feeder
　　　Financial factors
　　　Ignorance
　　　Inexperienced/impatient caretaker with or without compounding child factors
　　Inappropriate foods for age
　　　Cultural factors
　　　Fad diets
　　　Financial factors
　　　Ignorance
　　Incorrect preparation of formula
　　　Chronic dilution
　　　　Financial factors
　　　　Ignorance
　　　　Prolonged use after gastroenteritis
　　　Inappropriate additives
Normal variants
　Delayed growth spurt
　Early-onset growth retardation
　Genetic "slightness"
Organic failure to thrive
　CNS etiologies
　　Mental retardation/cerebral palsy
　　Neurodevelopmental retardation
　Gastrointestinal etiologies
　　Chronic gastroenteritis
　　Gastroesophageal reflux
　　Pyloric stenosis
Prematurity
Small for gestational age

**Uncommon Causes**

Defective utilization of calories
　Chronic hypoxemia
　Diabetes mellitus
Defects in absorption
　Cystic fibrosis
　Enzymatic deficiencies
　Food sensitivity/intolerance
　Hepatitis
　HIV infection
　Inflammatory bowel disease
　Milk allergy
　Starvation
Inadequacy of food intake
　Cleft lip/palate
　Dyspnea of any cause
　　Congenital heart disease
　　Respiratory disease/insufficiency
　Immature suck/swallow
　Pharyngeal incoordination
Increased metabolism
　Chronic anemias
　Chronic/recurrent infections

Otitis, sinusitis, pneumonia
Parasites
Tuberculosis
Urinary tract infection
Chronic respiratory insufficiency
Congenital heart disease
HIV infection
Malignancies

**Rare Causes**

Defective utilization of calories
　Adrenal insufficiency
　Chromosomal syndromes
　Diabetes insipidus
　Diencephalic syndrome
　Drugs/toxins
　Dysmorphogenic syndromes
　Fetal exposure syndromes
　Hypopituitarism
　Hypothyroidism
　Metabolic disorders
　　Aminoacidopathies
　　Galactosemia
　　Organic acidurias
　　Storage diseases
　Parathyroid disorders
　Renal tubular acidosis
Defects in absorption
　Acrodermatitis enteropathica
　Biliary atresia/cirrhosis
　Celiac disease
　Hirschsprung's disease
　Immunologic deficiency
　Necrotizing enterocolitis
　Pancreatic insufficiency
　Short gut syndrome
Inadequacy of food intake
　Choanal atresia
　CNS disorders
　　Cerebral insults
　　Degenerative diseases
　　Drugs/toxins
　　Subdural hematoma
　Diaphragmatic hernia/hiatal hernia
　Esophageal atresia
　Generalized muscle weakness
　　Congenital hypotonia
　　Myasthenia gravis
　　Werdnig-Hoffmann disease
　Micrognathia/glossoptosis
　Tracheoesophageal fistula
Increased metabolism
　Acquired heart disease
　Adrenocortical excess
　Chronic inflammation (eg, juvenile rheumatoid arthritis, systemic lupus erythematosus)
　Chronic seizure disorder
　Drugs/toxins
　Hyperaldosteronism
　Hyperthyroidism

## Selected Readings

Baertl JM, Adrianzen B, Graham GG. Growth of previously well-nourished infants in poor homes. Am J Dis Child 1976;130:33.

Barbero GJ, Shaheen E. Environmental failure to thrive: a clinical view. J Pediatr 1967;77:639.

Berwick DM. Nonorganic failure-to-thrive. Pediatr Rev 1980;1:265.

Bithoney WG. Elevated lead levels in children with nonorganic failure to thrive. Pediatrics 1986;78:891.

Casey PH, Bradley R, Wortham B. Social and nonsocial home environments of infants with nonorganic failure-to-thrive. Pediatrics 1984;83:348.

Cupoli JM, Hallock JA, Barness LA. Failure to thrive. Curr Probl Pediatr 1980;10:5.

Ellerstein NS, Ostrov BE. Growth patterns in children hospitalized because of caloric-deprivation failure to thrive. Am J Dis Child 1985;139:164.

Hannaway PJ. Failure to thrive: a study of 100 infants and children. Clin Pediatr 1970;9:96.

Homer C, Ludwig S. Categorization of etiology of failure to thrive. Am J Dis Child 1981;135:848.

Mitchell WG, Gorrell RW, Greenberg RA. Failure-to-thrive: a study in a primary care setting. Epidemiology and follow-up. Pediatrics 1980;65:971.

Rosenn DW, Loeb LS, Jura MB. Differentiation of organic from nonorganic failure to thrive syndrome in infancy. Pediatrics 1980;66:698.

Sills RH. Failure to thrive. Am J Dis Child 1978;132:967.

Sills RH, Sills IN. Don't overlook environmental causes of failure to thrive. Contemp Pediatr 1986;3:25.

# *Fatigue*

## Common Causes

Acute recovery from surgery, trauma, most illnesses
Anemia
Chronic atopy
Eating disorders
    Excessive dieting (with or without anorexia nervosa, bulimia)
Excessive physical exertion
Mononucleosis (and most viral infections)
Obesity
Pregnancy
Psychosocial
    Chronic boredom
    Chronic depression/anxiety
    Grief
    Stress (prolonged and severe)
Sedentary lifestyle
Sleep disorders
    Insomnia
    Sleep pattern disruption (lack of REM sleep)

## Uncommon Causes

Acute bacterial infections
    Bacteremia
    Meningitis
Chronic hypoxemia
    Asthma
    Cardiomyopathy
    Chronic pulmonary disease
    Congenital heart disease
    Congestive heart failure
    Cystic fibrosis
    Heart disease
    Pericarditis
    Pulmonary hypertension
Chronic infections
    Brucellosis
    Cytomegalic inclusion disease
    Histoplasmosis
    Osteomyelitis
    Parasitic infestations
    Pyelonephritis
    Sinusitis
    Subacute bacterial endocarditis
    Toxoplasmosis
    Tuberculosis
    Urinary tract infection

Dehydration
Hepatitis
Upper airway obstruction (sleep apnea)
    Pickwickian syndrome
    Tonsillar-adenoidal hypertrophy

## Rare Causes

AIDS
Allergic tension fatigue syndrome
Connective tissue diseases
    Dermatomyositis
    Juvenile rheumatoid arthritis
    Mixed connective tissue disease
    Scleroderma
    Systemic lupus erythematosus
Endocrine disorders
    Diabetes insipidus
    Diabetes mellitus
    Hyperadrenalism/hypoadrenalism
    Hyperparathyroidism
    Hyperpituitarism/hypopituitarism
    Hyperthyroidism/hypothyroidism
Hepatic insufficiency
Hypoglycemia
Inborn errors of metabolism
Inflammatory bowel disease
Intussusception
Malignancy
    Leukemia
    Lymphoma
    Solid tumors
Metabolic disturbances
    Hypermagnesemia/hypomagnesemia
    Hypokalemia
    Hyponatremia
Neurologic
    Intracranial hematomas
    Myasthenia gravis
    Narcolepsy
Renal tubular acidosis
Toxins and drugs
    Alcohol
    Analgesics and salicylates
    Anticonvulsants
    Antihistamines
    Barbiturates
    Carbon monoxide
    Corticosteroids
    Digitalis
    Heavy metals
    Insulin
    Nicotine
    Pesticides
    Progesterones
    Sedatives
    Tetracycline
    Vitamin A
    Vitamin D
Uremia

## Selected Readings

Cavanaugh RM Jr. Evaluating adolescents with fatigue. Am Fam Physician 1987;35:163.

Rockwell DA, Burr BD. The tired patient. J Fam Pract 1977;5:853.

Solberg LI. Lassitude: a primary care evaluation. JAMA 1984;251:3272.

# Fever of Unknown Origin

Fever is defined here as a temperature higher than 38.5°C for more than 2 weeks.

## Common Causes

Collagen vascular disease
    Juvenile rheumatoid arthritis
    Lupus erythematosus
    Periarteritis nodosa
Factitious
Infections
    Atypical mycobacterial infections
    Epstein-Barr virus infections
    Osteomyelitis
    Sinusitis, mastoiditis
    Urinary tract infections
    "Viral syndromes"
Inflammatory bowel disease
    Regional enteritis
    Ulcerative colitis
Malignancy
    Acute lymphoblastic leukemia
    Neuroblastoma
    Hodgkin's disease
    Non-Hodgkin's lymphoma

## Uncommon Causes

Drug-induced
Infections
    Cat-scratch disease
    Cytomegalic inclusion disease
    Lung abscess
    Hepatitis
    Histoplasmosis
    Pelvic inflammatory disease
    Salmonellosis
Kawasaki disease
Lyme disease

## Rare Causes

Behçet's syndrome
Diabetes insipidus
    Central
    Nephrogenic
Diencephalic syndrome
Ectodermal dysplasia
Familial dysautonomia
Hepatoma
Infection
    Blastomycosis
    Brucellosis
    HIV infection
    Leptospirosis
    Liver abscess
    Lymphogranuloma venereum
    Malaria
    Perinephric abscess
    Psittacosis
    Q fever
    Rocky Mountain spotted fever
    Streptococcosis
    Subdiaphragmatic abscess
    Toxoplasmosis
    Tuberculosis
    Tularemia
    Viral encephalitis
    Visceral larva migrans
Myelogenous leukemia
Pancreatitis
Periodic disease (familial fever)
Reticulum-cell sarcoma
Sarcoidosis
Serum sickness
Thyrotoxicosis

## Selected Readings

Feigin RD, Shearer WT. Fever of unknown origin in children. Curr Probl Pediatr 1976;6:3.

Kleiman MB. The complaint of persistent fever: recognition and management of pseudo-fever of unknown origin. Pediatr Clin North Am 1982;29:201.

Lohr JA, Hendley JO. Prolonged fever of unknown origin: a record of experiences with 54 childhood patients. Clin Pediatr 1977;16:768.

McCarthy PL, Lembo RM, Baron MA, et al. Predictive value of abnormal physical examination findings in ill-appearing and well-appearing febrile children. Pediatrics 1985;76:167.

McClung HJ. Prolonged fever of unknown origin in children. Am J Dis Child 1972;124:544.

Musher DM, Fainstein V, Young EJ, Pruett TL. Fever patterns. Arch Intern Med 1979;139:1225.

Petersdorf RG, Beeson PB. Fever of unexplained origin: report on 100 cases. Medicine 1961;40:1.

Pizzo PA, Lovejoy FH, Smith DH. Prolonged fever in children: review of 100 cases. Pediatrics 1975;55:468.

# Gastrointestinal Bleeding

## In the Neonate

### Common Causes

Esophagitis
Gastritis
Ingested maternal blood
Necrotizing enterocolitis
Stress ulcer (gastric)

### Uncommon Causes

Acquired coagulopathy
Gastroenteritis (*Campylobacter* infections)
Hemophilia
Rectal trauma or gastrointestinal trauma
Thrombocytopenia
Vitamin K deficiency
Volvulus

### Rare Causes

Acute ulcerative colitis
Gastric polyp
Gastrointestinal duplication cyst
Intussusception
Leiomyoma
Milk allergy
Nasal or pharyngeal bleeding
Severe cyanotic congenital heart disease
Vascular malformation of the gut (hemangioma, telangiectasia, arteriovenous malformation)

## In Infancy

### Common Causes

Anal fissure
Cow's milk protein sensitivity
Esophagitis
Gastritis
Gastroenteritis

### Uncommon Causes

Acute intestinal ischemia
Drug ingestion, such as aspirin or caustic
Hemophilia
Intussusception
Meckel's diverticulum
Peptic ulcer
Thrombocytopenia

### Rare Causes

Duplication of the bowel
Gangrenous bowel
Hemangioma of the bowel
Henoch-Schönlein purpura
Polyps

## In Childhood

### Common Causes

Anal fissures
Esophagitis
Gastritis (possibly due to drug ingestion)
Gastroenteritis
Polyps

### Uncommon Causes

Acquired coagulation disturbance
Hemophilia
Henoch-Schönlein purpura
Inflammatory bowel disease
Meckel's diverticulum
Parasitism
Peptic ulcer
Thrombocytopenia

### Rare Causes

Chronic granulomatous disease
Diverticulitis
Ehlers Danlos syndrome
Esophageal varices
Hemangiomas and telangectasia
Hemolytic-uremic syndrome
Hemorrhoids
Intestinal foreign body
Lymphosarcoma
Peutz-Jeghers syndrome
Pseudoxanthoma elasticum
Scurvy

## Selected Readings

Berman WF, Holtzapple PG. Gastrointestinal hemorrhage. Pediatr Clin North Am 1975;22:885.
Cox K, Ament ME. Upper gastrointestinal bleeding in children and adolescents. Pediatrics 1979;63:408.
Hillemeier C, Gryboski JD. Gastrointestinal bleeding in the pediatric patient. Yale J Biol Med 1984;57:135.
Hyams JS, Leichtner AM, Schwartz AN. Recent advances in diagnosis and treatment of gastrointestinal hemorrhage in infants and children. J Pediatr 1985;106:1.
Oldham KT, Lobe TE. Gastrointestinal hemorrhage in children: a pragmatic update. Pediatr Clin North Am 1985;32:1247.
Silber G. Lower gastrointestinal bleeding. Pediatr Rev 1990;12:85.
Stanley-Brown EG, Stevenson SS. Massive gastrointestinal hemorrhage in the newborn infant. Pediatrics 1965;35:482.
Stevenson RJ. Gastrointestinal bleeding in children. Surg Clin North Am 1985;65:1455.
Wagner ML. Acute gastrointestinal bleeding in infants and children. Pediatr Ann 1975;4:663.

# Headache

## Common Causes

Extracranial infection
    Otitis/mastoiditis
    Pharyngitis
    Sinusitis
    Tooth abscess
Febrile illness
Migraine
Tension
    Anxiety
    Environmental stress

## Uncommon Causes

Depression
Eye strain
Meningitis/encephalitis
Temporomandibular joint disease
Trauma
    Concussion
    Occipital neuralgia

## Rare Causes

Allergy
Arnold-Chiari malformation
Cervical osteoarthritis
Chronic renal disease
Congenital erythropoietic porphyria
Cranial bone disease
Decreased intracranial pressure
    Post–lumbar puncture
Drugs
    Amphetamines
    Carbon monoxide
    Heavy metals
    Indomethacin
    Nalidixic acid
    Nitrates/nitrites
    Oral contraceptives
    Steroids
    Sulfa
    Tetracycline
    Vitamin A
Epilepsy
Hyperventilation
Increased intracranial pressure
    Hydrocephalus
    Mass/tumor/abscess
    Pseudotumor cerebri
Leukemia infiltration
Mastocytosis
Metabolic

Hyperammonemia
Hypercarbia
Hypoglycemia
Hyponatremia
Hypoxia
Metabolic acidosis
Myositis
Psychogenic
Conversion reaction
Mimicry
Secondary gain
Orbit
Glaucoma
Orbital tumor
Pheochromocytoma
Vascular
Anemia
Aneurysm
Arteritis
Giant cell
Periarteritis nodosa
Subacute bacterial endocarditis
Systemic lupus erythematosus
AV malformation
Cerebral infarct
Embolus
Thrombosis
Cluster headache
Hemorrhage
Epidural
Parenchymal
Subdural
Hypertension
Phlebitis
Venous sinus thrombosis

## Selected Readings

Diamond S. Severe headaches—understanding types and treatments. Drug Therapy 1975ȑrch:81.
Ferry PC. Diagnosis and office management of headaches in children. Clin Pediatr 1972;11:195.
Ferry PC. Office management of headaches in children. Drug Therapy 1973{n:78.
Hanson RR. Headaches in childhood. Semin Neurol 1988;8:51.
Honig PJ, Charney EB. Children with brain tumor headaches. Am J Dis Child 1982;136:121.
Ling W, Oftedal G, Weinberg W. Depressive illness in childhood presenting as severe headache. Am J Dis Child 1970;120:122.
MacDonald JT. Childhood migraine: differential diagnosis and treatment. Postgrad Med 1986;80:301.
Meloff KL. Headache in pediatric practice. Headache 1973;13:125.
Prensky AL. Migraine and migrainous variants in pediatric patients. Pediatr Clin North Am 1976;23:461.
Prensky AL. Differentiating and treating pediatric headaches. Contemp Pediatr 1984;1:12.
Rossi LN, Vassella F. Headache in children with brain tumors. Childs Nerv Syst 1989;5:307.
Swaiman KF, Frank Y. Seizure headaches in children. Dev Med Child Neurol 1978;20:580.

# Hematuria

## Common Causes

Benign causes
Benign recurrent hematuria
Familial hematuria
Idiopathic recurrent gross hematuria
Postural hematuria

Contamination
Menstrual
Munchausen's syndrome
Munchausen's syndrome by proxy
Pregnancy-related bleeding
Hemoglobinopathies
Hgb C
Hgb SC
Sickle-cell disease/trait (Hgb SS/SA)
Sickle-thalassemia trait
Hypercalciuria
Distal renal tubular acidosis
Diuretic therapy
Endocrine disorders
Diabetes mellitus
Hyperadrenocorticism
Hyperparathyroidism
Hypothyroidism
Hypercalcemia
Hyperphosphatemia
Hypertension
Immobilization
Juvenile rheumatoid arthritis
Medullary sponge kidney
Metabolic acidosis
Neoplasm
Renal tubular dysfunction
Sarcoidosis
Vitamin D excess
Hypoxia, asphyxia, and circulatory compromise
Acute tubular necrosis
Cortical and medullary necrosis
Infections
Cystitis (viral, bacterial)
Pyelonephritis
Urethritis
Meatal stenosis
Noninfectious cystitis
Cytoxan
Radiation
Perineal irritation
Phimosis
Post–infectious glomerulonephritis
Trauma
Fractured pelvis
Postcatheterization
Postcircumcision
Postsurgery
Renal contusion
Renal fracture
Urethral trauma
Urethral ulceration

## Uncommon Causes

Bladder diverticula/polyps
Coagulopathies
Drug-induced
Analgesic nephropathy
Cephalosporins
Cytoxan
Penicillin
Sulfonamides
Exercise
Glomerular disorders
Mesangioproliferative
Minimal change disease
Hydronephrosis

Infections
    Epididymitis
    Prostatitis
Masturbation
Periureteritis (appendicitis, ileitis)
Polycystic disease
Reflux nephropathy
Renal calculi
Renal vein thrombosis
Thrombocytopenia
Ureteropelvic junction (UPJ) obstruction
Urethral foreign body
Wilms' tumor

**Rare Causes**

Allergy
"Apparent"
    "Beeturia"
    Betadine
    Biliuria
    Desferoxamine
    Dyes
        Analine
        Congo red
    Hemoglobinuria
    Myoglobinuria
    Phenothiazines
    Porphyria
Diabetic nephropathy
Glomerular disorders
    Amyloidosis
    Crescentic glomerulonephritis (GN)
    Familial nephritis (Alport's)
    Focal segmental proliferative GN
    Focal segmental sclerosis
    Goodpasture's syndrome
    IgA nephropathy
    Membranous GN
    Mesangiocapillary GN
    Subacute bacterial endocarditis
    Systemic lupus erythematosus
    Wegener's granulomatosis
Hemangioma
Klippel-Trenaunay-Weber syndrome
Hematospermia
Immunologic
    Hemolytic-uremic syndrome
    Henoch-Schönlein purpura
    Polyarteritis nodosa
    Systemic lupus erythematosus
Infections
    Leptospirosis
    Malaria
    Schistosomiasis
    Toxoplasmosis
    Tuberculosis
    Varicella
Malignant hypertension
Medullary sponge kidney
Neoplasms
    Bladder cancer
    Prostatic cancer
Renal infarction
Retroperitoneal fibrosis
Vitamin deficiency
    Scurvy
    Vitamin K deficiency

## Selected Readings

Birch DF, Fairley KF. Haematuria: glomerular or nonglomerular? Letter. Lancet 1979;2:845.

Daeschner CW. Screening for renal diseases. J Pediatr 1976;88:369.

Dodge WF, West EF, Smith EH, Bunce H. Proteinuria and hematuria in school-children: epidemiology and early natural history. J Pediatr 1976;88:327.

Fassett RG, Horgan BA, Mathew TH. Detection of glomerular bleeding by phase-contrast microscopy. Lancet 1982;1:1432.

Given GZ. Hematuria in children. A guide in differential diagnosis. Urol Clin North Am 1974;1:561.

Ingelfinger JR, Davis AE, Grupe WE. Frequency and etiology of gross hematuria in a general pediatric setting. Pediatrics 1977;59:557.

James JA. Proteinuria and hematuria in children. Diagnosis and assessment. Pediatr Clin North Am 1976;23:807.

Jones DP, Stapleton FB. Hypercalciuria: an important cause of childhood hematuria. Contemp Pediatr 1987;4:69.

Lytton B. Bleeding from the urinary tract. Resident and Staff Physician 1978;June:50.

Lytton B. Bleeding from the urinary tract. II. When the bleeding is from the kidney. Resident and Staff Physician 1978;July:87.

Northway JD. Hematuria in children. J Pediatr 1971;78:381.

Vehaskari VM, Rapola J, Koskimies O, et al. Microscopic hematuria in schoolchildren: epidemiology and clinicopathologic evaluation. J Pediatr 1979;95:676.

West CD. Asymptomatic hematuria and proteinuria in children. Causes and appropriate diagnostic studies. J Pediatr 1976;89:173.

Wyatt RJ, McRoberts JW, Holland NH. Hematuria in childhood: significance and management. J Urol 1977;117:366.

## *Hemoptysis*

**Common Causes**

Aspiration
    Blood
        Epistaxis
        Gingivitis
        Tonsillitis
        Upper airway trauma (eg, intubation)
    Corrosives
    Foreign body
    Gastric contents
    Oral lesions
Cystic fibrosis
Pulmonary infection (bacterial)
    Bronchiectasis
    Bronchitis
    Pneumonia
    Tracheitis
Pulmonary infection (viral)
    Laryngitis
    Laryngotracheobronchitis
    Pneumonitis
Pulmonary trauma
    Contusion
    Penetrating injury

**Uncommon Causes**

Lung abscess
Pertussis
Pulmonary hemorrhage (barotrauma)
Pulmonary tuberculosis
Sickle-cell disease

**Rare Causes**

Arteriovenous malformation/fistula
    Rendu-Osler-Weber syndrome
Cardiac disease
    Endomyocardial fibrosis
    Mitral stenosis
    Pulmonary hypertension

Coagulopathy
Heiner's syndrome
Idiopathic pulmonary hemosiderosis
Munchhausen's syndrome
Munchhausen's syndrome by proxy
Pulmonary embolus
Pulmonary infection
    Aspergillosis
    Blastomycosis
    Coccidioidomycosis
    Hemorrhagic fevers
    Paragonimiasis
Pulmonary vasculitis
    Goodpasture's syndrome
    Polyarteritis nodosa
    Systemic lupus erythematosus
    Wegener's granulomatosis
Pulmonary venous thrombosis

## Selected Readings

Beckerman RC, Taussig LM, Pinnas JL. Familial idiopathic pulmonary hemosiderosis. Am J Dis Child 1979;133:609.
Smiddy JF, Elliott RC. The evaluation of hemoptysis with fiberoptic bronchoscopy. Chest 1973;64:158.
Tom LWC, Weisman RA, Handler SD. Hemoptysis in children. Ann Otol Rhinol Laryngol 1980;89:419.

# Hepatomegaly

## Common Causes

Benign cystic disease
Benign transient hepatomegaly (usually with gastrointestinal viral illness)
Biliary tract obstruction
    Alagille's disease
    Ascending cholangitis
    Biliary atresia
    Choledochal cyst
Congestive heart failure
Cystic fibrosis
Diabetes mellitus
Hyperalimentation
Iron-deficiency anemia
Leukemia, lymphoma
Malnutrition
Maternal diabetes
Neonatal hepatitis
Pulmonary hyperinflation ("apparent" hepatomegaly)
Septicemia
Sickle-cell anemia
Toxin/drug reactions (hepatitis, cholestasis, fatty infiltration)
    Acetaminophen
    Oral contraceptives
    Corticosteroids
    Hydantoins
    Phenobarbital
    Sulfonamides
    Tetracycline
Viral hepatitis
    Cytomegalovirus, Epstein-Barr virus, Coxsackie virus
    Hepatitis A; hepatitis B; non-A, non-B hepatitis

## Uncommon Causes

Chronic active hepatitis
Chronic anemias
Erythroblastosis fetalis
Hamartoma
Hemangioma
Klippel-Trenaunay-Weber syndrome
Hemolytic anemias
Hepatic abscess (pyogenic)
Hepatoblastoma
Inflammatory bowel disease
Liver hemorrhage
Metastatic tumors
Pericarditis
Reye's syndrome
Rocky Mountain spotted fever
Systemic inflammatory disease (eg, juvenile rheumatoid arthritis, systemic lupus erythematosus)
Visceral larva migrans

## Rare Causes

$\alpha_1$-Antitrypsin deficiency
Amyloidosis
Beckwith-Wiedemann syndrome
Brucellosis
Budd-Chiari syndrome
Candidiasis
Carnitine deficiency
Chédiak-Higashi syndrome
Crigler-Najjar syndrome
Farber's disease
Galactosemia
Gangliosidosis $M_1$
Gaucher's disease
Glycogen storage disease
Granulomatous hepatitis
    Chronic granulomatous disease
    Sarcoidosis
    Tuberculosis
Hemochromatosis
Hemophagocytic syndrome
Hepatic porphyrias
Hepatocellular carcinoma
Hereditary fructose intolerance
Histiocytic syndromes
Histoplasmosis
Homocystinuria
Hyperlipoproteinemia 1
Hypervitaminosis A
Infantile pyknocytosis
Infantile sialidosis
Klippel-Trenaunay-Weber syndrome
Leptospirosis
Lipodystrophy
Malaria
Mannosidosis
Methylmalonic acidemia
Moore-Federmann syndrome
Mucolipidosis
Mucopolysaccharidoses
Mulibrey nanism
Niemann-Pick disease
Parasitic infections
    Amebiasis
    Flukes
    Schistosomiasis

Rendu-Osler-Weber syndrome
Rickets
Tangier's disease
Tyrosinemia
Urea cycle defects
Veno-occlusive disease
Wilson's disease
Wolman disease
Zellweger syndrome

## Selected Readings

Goldenring JM, Flores M. Primary liver abscesses in children and adolescents. Review of 12 years' clinical experience. Clin Pediatr 1986;25:153.
Lawson EE, Grand RJ, Neff RK, Cohen LF. Clinical estimation of liver span in infants and children. Am J Dis Child 1978;132:474.
Reiff MI, Osborn LM. Clinical estimation of liver size in newborn infants. Pediatrics 1983;71:46.
Walker WA, Mathis RK. Hepatomegaly: an approach to differential diagnosis. Pediatr Clin North Am 1975;22:929.
Weisman LE, Cagle N, Mathis R, Merenstein GB. Clinical estimation of liver size in the normal neonate. Clin Pediatr 1982;21:596.
Younoszai MK, Mueller S. Clinical assessment of liver size in normal children. Clin Pediatr 1975;14:378.

## *Hirsutism*

### Common Causes

Familial or racial factors
Idiopathic hirsutism
Physiologic hirsutism
    Pregnancy
    Puberty

### Uncommon Causes

CNS injury
Drugs
    Anabolic steroids
    Oral contraceptives
    Cyclosporine
    Diazoxide
    Dilantin
    Minoxidil
    Progesterones
    Testosterone
Emotional stress (?)
Polycystic ovarian disease
Severe malnutrition

### Rare Causes

Achard-Thiers syndrome
Acromegaly
Adrenal disorders
    Adrenal carcinoma
    Congenital adrenal hyperplasia
    Cushing's syndrome
    Virilizing adrenal adenoma
Congenital erythropoietic porphyria
Dysmorphogenic syndromes (many)
Hypothyroidism
Male pseudohermaphroditism
Ovarian disorders
    Pure gonadal dysgenesis
    Virilizing ovarian tumors
        Arrhenoblastoma
        Granulosa-theca cell tumors

## Selected Readings

Bates GW. Hirsutism and androgen excess in childhood and adolescence. Pediatr Clin North Am 1981;28:513.
Bransome ED Jr. Hirsutism and virilization. Resident Staff Phys 1979;25:118.
Braunstein GD. Hirsutism in adolescents. West J Med 1979;131:522.
Givens JR. Hirsutism and hyperandrogenism. Adv Int Med 1976;21:221.
Greenblatt RB. Diagnosis and treatment of hirsutism. Hosp Pract 1973 June:91.
Hatch R, Rosenfield RL, Kim MH, Tredway D. Hirsutism: implications, etiology, and management. Am J Obstet Gynecol 1981;140:815.
Jones JR, Brandeis VT. Hirsutism in puberty—how serious is it? Contemp Pediatr 1985;2:47.
Rittmaster RS, Loriaux DL. Hirsutism. Ann Intern Med 1987;106:95.

## *Hoarseness*

### Common Causes

Allergy
Caustic ingestion
Excessive use of the voice
Foreign body
Infectious mononucleosis
Instrumentation (naso/orogastric tube)
Laryngitis
Laryngotracheitis
Laryngotracheobronchitis
Postintubation hoarseness
Postnasal drip
Vocal cord nodules
Vocal cord paralysis (postsurgical trauma)

### Uncommon Causes

Congenital vocal cord paralysis
Epiglottitis
Hypocalcemia (eg, hyperparathyroidism)
Hypothyroidism
Laryngeal trauma
Laryngomalacia
Sicca syndrome
Toxins (chemotherapy, lead, mercury, irradiation, smoke)
Tracheitis (bacterial)
Vocal cord polyps

### Rare Causes

Amyloidosis
Angioneurotic edema
Chromosomal abnormalities
    Achondroplasia
    Bloom's syndrome
    Cockayne's syndrome
    Cri du chat syndrome
    De Lange's syndrome
    Diastrophic dwarfism
    Dubowitz's syndrome
    Dysautonomia
    Williams' syndrome
Congenital abnormalities
    Arytenoid cartilage displacement
    Clefts
    Cysts
    Webs
Cricoarytenoid arthritis (juvenile rheumatoid arthritis)
Diphtheria
Recurrent laryngeal nerve impingement
    Aberrant great vessels

Cardiomegaly
Hemorrhage
Hilar adenopathy
Neoplasm
Recurrent laryngeal nerve dysfunction
  CNS disease
    Arnold-Chiari malformation
    Chédiak-Higashi disease
    Encephalitis
    Hallervorden-Spatz disease
    Huntington's chorea
    Infection
    Ischemia
    Kernicterus
    Meningitis
    Metabolic disease
    Multiple sclerosis
    Polyneuritis
    Pseudobulbar palsy
    Ramsay Hunt syndrome
    Storage disease
    Syphilis
    Syringobulbia
    Toxin
    Trauma
    Tumor
    Wilson's disease
  Motor unit dysfunction
    Botulism
    Muscular dystrophy
    Myasthenia gravis
    Toxins
    Werdnig-Hoffmann disease
Sarcoidosis
Storage diseases (eg, lysosomal)
Tetany
Tuberculosis
Tumors of the larynx
  Adenoma
  Carcinoma
  Chondroma
  Ectopic thyroid
  Fibroangioma
  Fibroma
  Fibrosarcoma
  Hamartoma
  Hemangioma
  Hygroma
  Leukemia
  Lymphoma
  Myoma
  Myxoma
  Neuroblastoma
  Neurofibroma
  Papilloma
  Rhabdomyosarcoma
  Xanthoma
Vocal cord hemorrhage (nontraumatic)
Wegener's granulomatosis

## Selected Readings

Baker BM, Baker CD, Le HT. Vocal quality, articulation, and audiological characteristics of children and young adults with diagnosed allergies. Ann Otol Rhinol Laryngol 1982;91:277.

Cohen SR, Geller KA, Birns JW, Thompson JW. Laryngeal paralysis in children: a long-term retrospective study. Ann Otol Rhinol Laryngol 1982;91:417.

Cohen SR, Thompson JW, Geller KA, Birns JW. Voice change in the pediatric patient: a differential diagnosis. Ann Otol Rhinol Laryngol 1983;92:437.

Cotton RT, Richardson MA. Congenital laryngeal anomalies. Otolaryngol Clin North Am 1981;14:203.

Newman B, Flom L, Rivero HJ, Oh KS. Vocal cord paralysis and cardiovascular disease in children. Ann Radiol 1986;29:697.

# Hyperhidrosis

## Common Causes

Emotional stimuli
Exercise
Fever, recovery from fever
Increased environmental temperature
Ingestion of spicy foods

## Uncommon Causes

Atopic predisposition
Chronic illness
  Brucellosis
  Pulmonary tuberculosis
Cluster headaches
Congestive heart failure
Drug withdrawal
Hypoglycemia
Respiratory failure
Salicylate intoxication

## Rare Causes

Acrodynia
Acromegaly
Auriculotemporal syndrome
Carbon monoxide poisoning
Carcinoid syndrome
Citrullinemia
Diencephalic syndrome
Familial dysautonomia
Familial periodic paralysis
Hyperthyroidism
Insulin overdose
Ipecac ingestion
Myocardial infarction
Organophosphate poisoning
Phenylketonuria
Pheochromocytoma
Pyridoxine deficiency
Spinal cord injury
Thrombocytopenia-absent radius (TAR) syndrome
Vasoactive intestinal peptide-secreting tumor

## Selected Readings

Cloward RB. Hyperhidrosis. J Neurosurg 1969;30:545.

O'Donoghue G, Finn D, Brady MP. Palmar primary hyperhidrosis in children. J Pediatr Surg 1980;15:172.

# Hyperkalemia

Hyperkalemia is defined here as a serum potassium level higher than 5.5 mEq/L.

## Common Causes

Artifactual
Hemolysis during venipuncture
Acidosis
Renal failure
Severe dehydration

## Uncommon Causes

Drugs
    Spironolactone
    Triamterene
Excessive potassium infusion
Shock

## Rare Causes

Addison's disease (adrenal insufficiency)
Cell lysis syndromes
Crush injury
Malignant hyperthermia
Renal tubular acidosis
Theophylline intoxication

# Hypernatremia

Hypernatremia is defined here as a serum sodium level higher than 145 mEq/L.

## Common Causes

Excessive loss of free water
    Diarrhea
    Diuretics
    High environmental temperature
    Hyperpnea
    Sweating
    Vomiting

## Uncommon Causes

Nephrogenic diabetes insipidus
Post–obstructive diuresis
Salt poisoning
Sickle-cell nephropathy

## Rare Causes

Cushing's disease
Diuretic phase of Acute tubular necrosis (ATN)
Hypercalcemic nephropathy

# Hypertension

## Common Causes

Agitation
Anxiety
Coarctation of the aorta
Essential hypertension
Immobilization
Obesity
Pain
Renal causes

Acute tubular necrosis
Congenital anomalies
    Hydronephrosis
    Nephrophthisis
    Polycystic kidneys
    Renal aplasia/hypoplasia/dysplasia
    Segmental hypoplasia
Glomerulonephritis (acute and chronic)
    Membranoproliferative, etc
    Postinfectious
Liddle's syndrome
Miscellaneous nephropathy
    Amyloidosis
    Diabetes mellitus
    Gout
Nephrolithiasis
Nephrotic syndrome
    Idiopathic
    Minimal change disease
Obstructive uropathy
Other nephritides
    Familial nephritis
    Hemolytic-uremic syndrome
    Henoch-Schönlein purpura
    Hypersensitivity/transfusion reaction
    Periarteritis nodosa
    Radiation
    Systemic lupus erythematosus
Pyelonephritis
Renal failure (acute and chronic)
Renal transplantation
Renal vascular disease
    Renal artery
        Aneurysm
        Arteritis
        Embolic disease
        External compression
    Fibromuscular dysplasia
    Fistula
    Stenosis
    Thrombosis
    Trauma
    Renal vein thrombosis
Retroperitoneal fibrosis
Trauma
Tumors
    Extrinsic tumors
        Adrenal carcinoma
        Neuroblastoma
    Renin-secreting tumors (J-G cell)
    Wilms' tumor
Small pressure-cuff size

## Uncommon Causes

Cardiovascular etiologies
    Anemia
    Aortic aneurysm/thrombosis
    Arteriovenous fistula
        Aortic insufficiency
        Aorticopulmonary window
        Patent ductus arteriosus
    Bacterial endocarditis
    Iatrogenic hypervolemia
    Polycythemia
    Pseudoxanthoma elasticum
    Radiation aortitis
    Takayasu's arteritis

Drugs and chemicals
  Glucocorticoids
  Glycyrrhizic acid (licorice)
  Heavy metals (lead, cadmium, mercury)
  Methysergide
  Mineralocorticoids
  Monoamine-oxidase inhibitors
  Oral contraceptives
  Phencyclidine
  Sodium salts
  Sympathomimetics (decongestants)
  Tricyclic antidepressants

### Rare Causes

Burns
CNS
  Dysautonomia (Riley-Day syndrome)
  Encephalitis
  Guillain-Barré syndrome
  Increased intracranial pressure
  Poliomyelitis
  Neurofibromatosis
Collagen vascular
  Dermatomyositis
  Scleroderma
Cystinosis
Endocrine
  Congenital adrenal hyperplasia
    11-β-hydroxylase deficiency
    17-hydroxylase deficiency
  Cushing's syndrome
  Hyperaldosteronism
    Primary
      Conn's syndrome
      Dexamethasone-suppressible
      Idiopathic nodular hyperplasia
    Secondary
  Hyperthyroidism
  Pheochromocytoma
Fabry's disease
Hypoxia
Malignant hyperthermia
Metabolic
  Hypercalcemia
  Hypernatremia
  Renal tubular acidosis (RTA) with nephrocalcinosis
Sickle-cell anemia
Stevens-Johnson syndrome

## Selected Readings

Bailie MD, Mattioli LF. Hypertension: relationships between pathophysiology and therapy. J Pediatr 1980;96:789.

Balfe JW, Rance CP. Recognition and management of hypertensive crises in childhood. Pediatr Clin North Am 1978;25:159.

de Swiet M, Fayers P, Shinebourne EA. Systolic blood pressure in a population of infants in the first year of life: the Brompton study. Pediatrics 1980;65:1028.

Hohn AR, Riopel DA, Loadholt B. Which blood pressure? J Pediatr 1984;104:89.

Hypertension: more than ever, a pediatric concern. Contemp Pediatr 1985;2:30.

Kaplan MR, Hernandez LG. The pathogenesis and diagnosis of hypertension in children. Pediatr Ann 1982;11:592.

Klein AA, McCrory WW, Engle MA. Hypertension in children. Cardiovasc Clin 1981;11:11.

Lauer RM, Burns TL, Clarke WR. Assessing children's blood pressure—considerations of age and body size: the Muscatine study. Pediatrics 1985;75:1081.

Lieberman E. Essential hypertension in children and youth: a pediatric perspective. J Pediatr 1974;85:1.

Loggie JMH, Horan MJ, Hohn AR, et al. Juvenile hypertension: highlights of a workshop. J Pediatr 1984;104:657.

Loggie JMH, New MI, Robson AM. Hypertension in the pediatric patient: a reappraisal. J Pediatr 1979;94:685.

Londe S. Causes of hypertension in the young. Pediatr Clin North Am 1978;25:55.

Londe S, Bourgoignie JJ, Robson AM, Goldring D. Hypertension in apparently normal children. J Pediatr 1971;78:569.

McCrory WW. Finding an elevated blood pressure—what does it mean? Pediatr Ann 1982;11:581.

McCrory WW. What should blood pressure be in healthy children? Pediatrics 1982;70:143.

Piazza SF, Chandra M, Harper RG, et al. Upper- vs lower-limb systolic blood pressure in full-term normal newborns. Am J Dis Child 1985;139:797.

Rosen PR, Treves S, Ingelfinger J. Hypertension in children. Am J Dis Child 1985;139:173.

Task Force on Blood Pressure Control in Children. Report of the Second Task Force on Blood Pressure Control in Children—1987. Pediatrics 1987;79:1.

## Hypokalemia

Hypokalemia defined here as a serum potassium level lower than 3.5 mEq/L.

### Common Causes

Chronic diarrhea
Diuretics
Malnutrition
Metabolic alkalosis
Vomiting/gastric suctioning

### Uncommon Causes

Excessive corticoids
Renal tubular disorders

### Rare Causes

Amphotericin B therapy
Bartter's syndrome
Colon cancer
Cushing's syndrome
Familial periodic paralysis
Laxative abuse
Primary aldosteronism
Pseudoaldosteronism
Ureterosigmoidostomy
Villous adenoma
Zollinger-Ellison syndrome

## Hyponatremia

Hyponatremia is defined here as a sodium level lower than 130 mEq/L.

### Common Causes

Diarrhea
Excessive salt-free infusions
Syndrome of inappropriate antidiuretic hormone (ADH) secretion
Water intoxication

### Uncommon Causes

Acute renal failure
Chronic renal failure
Congestive heart failure
High environmental temperatures

**Rare Causes**

Adrenal insufficiency
Cirrhosis
Cystic fibrosis and excessive sweating
Spurious
Hyperlipidemia
Hyperglycemia

# Hypotonia, Neonatal

## Common Causes

Asphyxia
Benign, congenital
Sepsis
Trauma

## Uncommon Causes

Congenital joint laxity
Down syndrome
"Hypermobility syndrome"
Hypothyroidism
Neonatal myasthenia
Spinal cord injury
Werdnig-Hoffmann disease

## Rare Causes

Achondroplasia
Cerebro-hepato-renal syndrome
Congenital lactic acidosis
Congenital myopathies
    Central core disease
    Myotubular myopathy
    Nemaline myopathy
Cri du chat syndrome
Ehlers-Danlos syndrome
Familial dysautonomia
Fetal warfarin syndrome
Generalized gangliosidosis
Glycogen storage disease (type II)
Hyperammonemia
Lidocaine toxicity
Mannosidosis
Maple-syrup urine disease
Marfan's syndrome
Myotonic dystrophy
Nonketotic hyperglycinemia
Osteogenesis imperfecta
Prader-Willi syndrome
Trisomy 13 syndrome
Williams' syndrome (idiopathic hypercalcemia)

## Selected Readings

Fishman MA, Finegold M. Progressive neurologic deterioration in a hypotonic infant. J Pediatr 1985;107:634.

Hanson PA. "Floppy baby" (Oppenheim's disease, amyotonia congenital). Pediatr Ann 1977;6:98.

Low NL. Spinal muscular atrophy syndromes. Pediatr Ann 1977;6:35.

Sarnat HB. Diagnostic value of the muscle biopsy in the neonatal period. Am J Dis Child 1978;132:782.

Slater GE, Swaiman KF. Muscular dystrophies of childhood. Pediatr Ann 1977;6: 50.

Spiro AJ. Approach to diagnosis in the child with muscle weakness. Pediatr Ann 1977;6:11.

Thompson CE. Pitfalls in muscle biopsies of hypotonic children. Dev Med Child Neurol 1985;27:675.

# Jaundice (Beyond the Neonatal Period)

## Common Causes

Acute or chronic hemolytic anemias
Gilbert's disease
Hepatitis A; hepatitis B; non-A, non-B hepatitis; Epstein-Barr virus

## Uncommon Causes

Cholelithiasis
Chronic active hepatitis
Cirrhosis
Cystic fibrosis
Drug-induced hepatitis
Total parenteral nutrition

## Rare Causes

Alagille's syndrome
$\alpha_1$-Antitrypsin deficiency
Benign recurrent cholestasis
Biliary atresia
Byler's disease
Chemical injury
Choledochal cyst
Dubin-Johnson syndrome
Fibrosing pancreatitis
Galactosemia
Glycogen storage disease
Hemophagocytic syndromes
Hereditary fructose intolerance
Niemann-Pick disease
Pheochromocytoma
Pyloric stenosis
Reye's syndrome
Rotor syndrome
Trisomy 18
rosinemia
Wilson's disease

## Selected Readings

Balistreri WF. Neonatal cholestasis. J Pediatr 1985;106:171.

Fung KP, Lau SP. Γ-Glutamyl transpeptidase activity and its serial measurement in differentiation between extrahepatic biliary atresia and neonatal hepatitis. J Pediatr Gastroenterol Nutr 1985;4:208.

Hirsig J, Rickham PP. Early differential diagnosis between neonatal hepatitis and biliary atresia. J Pediatr Surg 1980;15:13.

Johnston GS, Rosenbaum RC, Hill JL, Diaconis JN. Differentiation of jaundice in infancy: an application of radionuclide biliary studies. J Surg Oncol 1985;30: 206.

Lubin BH, Baehner RL, Schwartz E, et al. The red cell peroxide hemolysis test in the differential diagnosis of obstructive jaundice in the newborn period. Pediatrics 1971;48:562.

Maisels MJ. Bilirubin: on understanding and influencing its metabolism in the newborn infant. Pediatr Clin North Am 1972;19:447.

Mathis RK, Andres JM, Walker WA. Liver disease in infants. J Pediatr 1977;90:864.

Melhorn DK, Izant RJ Jr. The red cell hydrogen peroxide hemolysis test and vitamin E absorption in the differential diagnosis of jaundice in infancy. J Pediatr 1972;81: 1082.

Seligman JW. Recent and changing concepts of hyperbilirubinemia and its management in the newborn. Pediatr Clin North Am 1977;24:509.

Thaler MM. Jaundice in early infancy. Pediatr Ann 1977;6:286.

# Joint Pain

## Common Causes

Chondromalacia patellae
Growing pains

Osteomyelitis
Overuse
Septic arthritis
Sickle-cell disease
Sympathetic effusion
Tietze's syndrome
Transient synovitis
Trauma
    Contusion
    Fracture
    Hemarthrosis
    Sprain/strain
Viral arthritis
    Adenovirus
    Epstein-Barr virus
    Hepatitis
    Mumps
    Rubella
    Varicella

## Uncommon Causes

Attention-seeking behavior
Child abuse
Foreign body
Legg-Calvé-Perthes disease
Mycoplasma
Osgood-Schlatter disease
Osteochondritis dissecans
Popliteal cyst
Psoriatic arthritis
Reactive arthritis
    Brucella
    *Campylobacter*
    Salmonella
    Shigella
    *Yersinia*
Referred pain (retroperitoneal/intraperitoneal inflammation)
Slipped-capital femoral epiphysis
Subluxation of the patella

## Rare Causes

Bone tumors
Carpal-tarsal osteolysis
Congenital joint laxity
    Ehlers-Danlos syndrome
    Marfan's syndrome
    Stickler's syndrome
Cystic fibrosis
Fabry's disease
Gaucher's disease
*Giardia*
Gout
Hyperlipoproteinemia
Hyperparathyroidism
Idiopathic chondrolysis
Immunodeficiency
    Complement deficiency
    Hypogammaglobulinemia
Immunologic
    Acute rheumatic fever
    Ankylosing spondylitis
    Behçet's syndrome
    Dermatomyositis
    Giant-cell arteritis
    Henoch-Schönlein purpura
    Hepatitis

    Inflammatory bowel disease
    Juvenile rheumatoid arthritis
    Kawasaki disease
    Mixed connective tissue disease
    Polyarteritis nodosa
    Reiter's syndrome
    Scleroderma
    Serum sickness
    Sjögren's syndrome
    Systemic lupus erythematosus
Leukemia
Lipogranulomatosis
Lyme disease
Mucopolysaccharidosis
Mycobacterial disease
Psychogenic rheumatism
Reflex sympathetic dystrophy
Rickets
Sarcoidosis
Stevens-Johnson syndrome
Subacute bacterial endocarditis
Syphilis
    Charcot joint
    Infection
Thyroid disease
Villonodular synovitis
Whipple's disease

## Selected Readings

Fulkerson JP. The etiology of patellofemoral pain in young active patients: a prospective study. Clin Orthop 1983;179:129.

Kunnamo I, Kallio P, Pelkonen P, Hovi T. Clinical signs and laboratory tests in the differential diagnosis of arthritis in children. Am J Dis Child 1987;141:34.

Kunnamo I, Pelkonen P. Routine analysis of synovial fluid cells is of value in the differential diagnosis of arthritis in children. J Rheumatol 1986;13:1076.

Morrissy RT, Shore SL. Bone and joint sepsis. Pediatr Clin North Am 1986;33:1551.

Phillips PE. Viral arthritis in children. Arthritis Rheum 1977;20(Suppl; 2):584.

Schaller JG. Arthritis in children. Pediatr Clin North Am 1986;33:1565.

# Limb Pain

## Common Causes

Growing pains
Infection
    Cellulitis
    Osteitis
    Osteomyelitis
    Post–rubella vaccination
    Septic arthritis
    Soft-tissue abscess
    Toxic synovitis
    Viral myositis
Sickle-cell disease—vasoocclusive crisis
Trauma
    Chondromalacia patellae
    Compartment syndromes
    Dislocation and subluxation
    Fracture
    Hypermobility syndrome
    Joint strain, sprain, internal damage
    Myositis ossificans
    Pathologic fracture

Postimmunization
Shin splints
Soft-tissue contusion or hemorrhage
Stress fracture
Tendonitis, fasciitis, bursitis
Traumatic periostitis

## Uncommon Causes

Accessory tarsal ossicle
Collagen vascular disease (dermatomyositis, lupus)
Conversion reactions
Henoch-Schönlein purpura
Juvenile rheumatoid arthritis
Legg-Calvé-Perthes disease
Osgood-Schlatter disease
Osteochondritis dissecans
Rheumatic fever
Tarsal coalition

## Rare Causes

Bone tumors (osteogenic sarcoma, Ewing's sarcoma, chondrosarcoma)
Cushing's syndrome
Familial Mediterranean fever
Hemophilia
Histiocytosis X
Hyperparathyroidism
Hypervitaminosis A
Inflammatory bowel disease
Leukemia
Mucopolysaccharidosis
Myopathies
Neuroblastoma
Osteoporosis
Popliteal cyst
Rickets
Scurvy
Slipped-capital femoral epiphysis
Soft-tissue tumors (rhabdomyosarcoma, fibrosarcoma)
Sympathetic reflex dystrophy

## Selected Readings

Bowyer SL, Hollister JR. Limb pain in childhood. Pediatr Clin North Am 1984;31:1053.
Groshar D, Lam M, Even-Sapir E, et al. Stress fractures and bone pain: are they closely associated? Injury 1985;16:526.
Naish JM, Apley J. "Growing pains": a clinical study of non-arthritic limb pains in children. Arch Dis Child 1951;26:134.
Oster J, Nielsen A. Growing pains. Acta Paediatr Scand 1972;61:329.
Park H-M, Rothschild PA, Kernek CB. Scintigraphic evaluation of extremity pain in children: its efficacy and pitfalls. AJR 1985;145:1079.
Passo MH. Aches and limb pain. Pediatr Clin North Am 1982;29:209.
Peterson H. Growing pains. Pediatr Clin North Am 1986;33:1365.
Shapiro MJ. Differential diagnosis of nonrheumatic "growing pains" and subacute rheumatic fever. J Pediatr 1939;14:315.

# *Limp*

## Common Causes

Attention-seeking behavior (usually after minor trauma)
Calluses/corns/ingrown toenails
Chondromalacia patellae
Contusion
Foreign body (especially plantar surface)

Fracture (may be occult)
Growing pains
Hemophilia (hemarthrosis, soft-tissue bleed)
Immunization (local reaction)
Leg length discrepancy
Mimicry
Myositis (acute viral)
Poorly fitting shoes (tight or loose)
Shin splints
Sickle-cell disease (painful crisis/infarction)
Soft-tissue/cutaneous infection
Sprain/strain
Tendonitis
Torsion deformities
Transient synovitis

## Uncommon Causes

Arthritis (septic)
Baker's cyst
Blount's disease
Bone tumor (benign and malignant)
Calcaneal spurs
Child abuse
Congenital contractures
Coxa vera
Erythema nodosum
Legg-Calvé-Perthes disease
Leukemia
Neuromuscular disease
    Ataxia
    CNS bleed
    CNS infection
    Flaccid paralysis
    Migraine
    Muscular dystrophy
    Peripheral neuropathy
        Causalgia
        Diabetes mellitus
        Guillain-Barré syndrome
        Heavy metal intoxication
        Periodic paralysis
        Poliomyelitis
        Tick paralysis
    Radiculopathy
    Spastic paralysis
Osgood-Schlatter disease
Osteochondritis dissecans
Osteomyelitis
Phlebitis
Plantar wart
Referred pain
    Diskitis
    Epidural/paraspinal abscess
    Iliac adenitis
    Intraperitoneal infection/inflammation
    Pelvic inflammatory disease
    Retroperitoneal mass
Slipped-capital femoral epiphysis
Subluxation of the patella

## Rare Causes

Arthritis/arthralgia
    Acute rheumatic fever
    Dermatomyositis
    Henoch-Schönlein purpura

Inflammatory bowel disease
Juvenile rheumatoid arthritis
Kawasaki disease
Polyarteritis nodosa
Serum sickness
Systemic lupus erythematosus
Brucellosis
Caffey's disease
Congenital joint laxity (Ehlers-Danlos syndrome)
Erythromelalgia
Freiberg's disease
Hepatitis
Hypervitaminosis A
Hysteria
Intervertebral disk herniation
Köhler's disease
Larsen-Johansson disease
Neuroblastoma
Pott's disease
Psoas abscess
Pyomyositis
Rickets
Scurvy
Sever's disease
Sinding-Larsen disease
Trichinosis

## Selected Readings

Chung SMK. Identifying the cause of acute limp in childhood: some informal comments and observations. Clin Pediatr 1974;13:769.
Hensinger RN. Limp. Pediatr Clin North Am 1986;33:1355.
Illingworth CM. 128 limping children with no fracture, sprain, or obvious cause. Clin Pediatr 1978;17:139.
Phillips WA. The child with a limp. Orthop Clin North Am 1987;18:489.
Singer J, Towbin R. Occult fractures in the production of gait disturbances in childhood. Pediatrics 1979;64:192.

## *Lymphadenopathy (Generalized)*

### Common Causes

Infection (viral, fungal, spirochetal)
Juvenile rheumatoid arthritis
Serum sickness

### Uncommon Causes

Drug reactions
    Anticonvulsants, antithyroid, isoniazid
HIV infection
Hodgkin's disease
Infection, bacterial
Leukemia
Non-Hodgkin's disease
Systemic lupus erythematosus

### Rare Causes

Angioimmunoblastic lymphadenopathy
Dysgammaglobulinemia
Gaucher's disease
Hemophagocytic syndromes
Histiocytic medullary reticulosis
Histiocytosis
Hyperthyroidism
Metastatic neuroblastoma

Niemann-Pick disease
Sarcoidosis

## Selected Readings

Barton LL, Feigin RD. Childhood cervical lymphadenitis: a reappraisal. J Pediatr 1974;84:846.
Bedros A, Mann JP. Lymphadenopathy in children. Adv Pediatr 1981;28:341.
Canale VC, Smith CH. Chronic lymphadenopathy simulating malignant lymphoma. J Pediatr 1967;70:891.
Carithers HA. Lymphadenopathy. Am J Dis Child 1978;132:353. Correction: Am J Dis Child 1978;132:776.
Frizzera G, Moran EM, Rappaport H. Angio-immunoblastic lymphadenopathy. Am J Med 1975;59:803.
Herzog LW. Prevalence of lymphadenopathy of the head and neck in infants and children. Clin Pediatr 1983;22:485.
Kissane JM, Gephardt GN. Lymphadenopathy in childhood. Hum Pathol 1974;5: 431.
Knight PJ, Mulne AF, Vassy LE. When is lymph node biopsy indicated in children with enlarged peripheral nodes? Pediatrics 1982;69:391.
Lake AM, Oski FA. Peripheral lymphadenopathy in childhood. Am J Dis Child 1978;132:357.
Musiej-Nowakowska E, Rostropowicz-Denisiewicz K. Differential diagnosis of neoplastic and rheumatic diseases in children. Scand J Rheumatol 1986;15:124.
Rieger CHL, Lustig JV, Justman RA, Rothberg RM. Immunologic function of patients with chronic benign lymphadenopathy. Eur J Pediatr 1976;124:51.
Slap GB, Connor JL, Wigton RS, Schwartz S. Validation of a model to identify young patients for lymph node biopsy. JAMA 1986;255:2768.
Zuelzer WW, Kaplan J. The child with lymphadenopathy. Semin Hematol 1975;12: 323.

## *Odors of Disease*

### Common

| Disease | Odor |
|---|---|
| Diabetes | Fruity; acetonelike |
| Uremia | Fishy (trimethylamine ammonia) |

### Uncommon

| Disease | Odor |
|---|---|
| Intestinal obstruction | Feculent, foul |
| Intranasal foreign body | Fetid |
| Lung abscess | Foul, putrid |
| Vaginal foreign body | Foul |

### Rare

| Disease | Odor |
|---|---|
| Glutaric acidemia (type III) | Sweaty feet |
| Hypermethioninemia | Fish, rancid butter, boiled cabbage |
| Isovaleric acidemia | Sweaty feet |
| Maple-syrup urine disease | Maple syrup, caramel-like |
| Oasthouse syndrome (methionine malabsorption) | Dried malt or hops |
| Phenylketonuria | Musty, wolflike, stale |
| Trimethylaminuria | Rotting fish |
| Tyrosinemia | Rancid butter, fish |

## Selected Readings

Hayden GF. Olfactory diagnosis in medicine. Postgrad Med 1980;67:110.
Liddell K. Smell as a diagnostic marker. Postgrad Med J 1976;52:136.
Mace JW, Goodman SI, Centerwall WR, Chinnock RF. The child with an unusual odor. Clin Pediatr 1976;15:57.
Moriarty RA. Nasal foreign body presenting as an unusual odor. Am J Dis Child 1978;132:96.

## Polyuria

### Common Causes

Diabetes mellitus
Diuretic abuse
  Alcohol
  Caffeine
  Medications
Iatrogenic
  Aggressive parenteral hydration
  Diuretic use
Psychogenic polydipsia
Renal failure
Sickle-cell anemia
Urinary tract infection

### Uncommon Causes

Diabetes insipidus (central)
Interstitial nephritis
  Analgesic abuse
  Diphenylhydantoin
  Mercury poisoning
  Methicillin reaction
  Sulfonamides
Renal calculi/hypercalcemia
Renal tubular acidosis

### Rare Causes

Bartter's syndrome
Cystinosis
Medullary cystic disease of the kidney
Nephrogenic diabetes insipidus
Neuroblastoma/ganglioneuroblastoma
Pheochromocytoma

## Selected Readings

Czernichow P, Pomarede R, Basmaciogullari A, et al. Diabetes insipidus in children. III. Anterior pituitary dysfunction in idiopathic types. J Pediatr 1985;106:41.

Kohn B, Norman ME, Feldman H, et al. Hysterical polydipsia (compulsive water drinking) in children. Am J Dis Child 1976;130:210.

Scherbaum WA, Czernichow P, Bottazzo GF, Doniach D. Diabetes insipidus in children. IV. A possible autoimmune type with vasopressin cell antibodies. J Pediatr 1985;107:922.

## Proteinuria

### Common Causes

Chronic pyelonephritis
Isolated transient/intermittent proteinuria
  Cold exposure
  Congestive heart failure
  Exercise
  Febrile illness
  Idiopathic proteinuria
  Orthostatic proteinuria
  Pregnancy
  Trauma
  Urinary tract infection

### Uncommon Causes

Nephritic sediment
  Membranoproliferative glomerulonephritis
  Postinfectious glomerulonephritis
Nephrotic sediment
  Minimal change disease
  Preeclampsia
Tubular proteinuria
Acute tubular necrosis
Obstructive uropathy
Polycystic kidney disease

### Rare Causes

Drugs
  Captopril
  Fenoprofen
  Gold
  Penicillamine
  Probenecid
Nephritic sediment
  Hereditary nephritis
  IgA nephropathy
  Mixed cryoglobulinemia
  Rapidly progressive glomerulonephritis
  Subacute bacterial endocarditis
  Systemic lupus erythematosus
Nephrotic sediment
  Amyloidosis
  Diabetes mellitus
  Focal glomerulonephritis
  Membranous nephropathy
  Miscellaneous infections
    Hepatitis B
    Malaria
    Syphilis
Overflow proteinuria
  Bence Jones proteinuria
  Lysozymuria (in leukemia)
Tubular proteinuria
  Analgesic abuse
  Chronic hypertension
  Hypercalciuria
  Hyperuricemia
  Radiation nephritis

## Selected Readings

Burke EC, Stickler GB. Proteinuria in children. Clin Pediatr 1982;21:741.

Daeschner CW. Screening for renal diseases. J Pediatr 1976;88:369.

Dodge WF, West EF, Smith EH, Bunce H III. Proteinuria and hematuria in schoolchildren: epidemiology and early natural history. J Pediatr 1976;88:327.

Houser M. Assessment of proteinuria using random urine samples. J Pediatr 1984;104:845.

James JA. Proteinuria and hematuria in children: diagnosis and assessment. Pediatr Clin North Am 1976;23:807.

Pollak VE, Ooi BS. Just what is the significance of proteinuria? Resident Staff Phys 1971;Nov:89.

Robinson RR. Isolated proteinuria in asymptomatic patients. Kidney Int 1980;18:395.

Sinniah R, Law CH, Pwee HS. Glomerular lesions in patients with asymptomatic persistent and orthostatic proteinuria discovered on routine medical examination. Clin Nephrol 1977;7:1.

Stewart DW, Gordon JA, Schoolwerth AC. Evaluation of proteinuria. Am Fam Physician 1984;29:218.

Vehaskari VM, Rapola J. Isolated proteinuria: analysis of a school-age population. J Pediatr 1982;101:661.

West CD. Asymptomatic hematuria and proteinuria in children. Causes and appropriate diagnostic studies. J Pediatr 1976;89:173.

## Pruritus

### Common Causes

Atopic dermatitis
Cholestasis of pregnancy

Contact allergens (plants, cosmetics, dyes, medications)
Contact irritants (soaps, chemicals, excrement, wool)
Drugs
    Aminophylline
    Aspirin
    Barbiturates
    Erythromycin
    Gold
    Griseofulvin
    Isoniazid
    Opiates
    Phenothiazines
    Vitamin A
Dry skin
    Advanced age
    Excess bathing/strong detergents
    Low humidity
Foreign body
Hepatitis
High humidity
Insect bites/infestations
    Fleas, mosquitoes, scabies mites, lice, mites, chiggers
Iron-deficiency anemia
Parasitic infection
    Pinworms
    *Toxocara canis*
Pityriasis rosea
Psoriasis
Seborrheic dermatitis
Skin infections (bacterial/viral/fungal)
Urticaria

**Uncommon Causes**

Biliary obstruction
    Drug-induced
    Extrahepatic biliary obstruction
    Primary biliary cirrhosis
Chronic renal failure
Hematopoietic malignancies
    Hodgkin's disease
    Leukemia
    Lymphoma
Neurodermatitis
Parasitic infection
    Cercaria
    Hookworms
    Trichinosis

**Rare Causes**

Autoimmune (sytemic lupus erythematosus, juvenile rheumatoid
    arthritis)
Congenital ectodermal disorders
Endocrine diseases
    Carcinoid syndrome
    Diabetes mellitus
    Hyperthyroidism/hypothyroidism
    Hypoparathyroidism
Erythropoietic protoporphyria
Hematopoietic malignancies
    Mastocytosis
    Multiple myeloma
    Polycythemia vera
Malignant solid tumors
Neurologic syndromes
Psychosis

## Selected Readings

Edwards AE, Shellow WVR, Wright ET, Dignam TF. Pruritic skin disease, psychological stress, and the itch sensation. Arch Dermatol 1976;112:339.
Gilchrest BA. Pruritus: pathogenesis, therapy, and significance in systemic disease states. Arch Intern Med 1982;142:101.
Shelley WB, Arthur RP. The neurohistology and neurophysiology of the itch sensation in man. Arch Dermatol 1957;76:296.

# *Purpura (Petechial and Ecchymoses)*

**Common Causes**

Thrombocytopenia
Trauma
Viral infections

**Uncommon Causes**

Abnormal platelet function
Child abuse
Cupping and coin rubbing
Drug ingestion (aspirin)
Factitious
Henoch-Schönlein purpura
Hereditary coagulation disturbance
Infection
Septic emboli
Uremia
Vasculitis
Violent coughing

**Rare Causes**

Autoerythrocyte sensitization
Bernard-Soulier disease
Cushing's syndrome
Dysproteinemias
Exercise
Glanzmann's thrombasthenia
Hereditary hemorrhagic telangiectasia
Lyme disease
Macular cerulae
May-Hegglin anomaly
Osteogenesis imperfecta
Osteopetrosis
Platelet storage pool disease
Polyurethane exposure
Protein C deficiency
Protein S deficiency
Purpura fulminans
Schamberg's disease
Scurvy
Vitamin K deficiency

## Selected Readings

Rasmussen JE. Puzzling purpuras in children and young adults. J Am Acad Dermatol 1982;6:67.
Ratnoff OD. The psychogenic purpuras: a review of autoerythrocyte sensitization, autosensitization to DNA, "hysterical" and factitial bleeding, and the religious stigmata. Semin Hematol 1980;17:192.
Saulsbury FT, Hayden GF. Skin conditions simulating child abuse. Pediatr Emerg Care 1985;1:147.
Sorensen RU, Newman AJ, Gordon EM. Psychogenic purpura in adolescent patients. Clin Pediatr 1985;24:700.

## Scrotal Swelling

### Common Causes

Hernia
Hydrocele
Orchitis
Torsion of the cord
Torsion of the testicular appendage
Varicocele

### Uncommon Causes

Epididymitis
Henoch-Schönlein purpura
Idiopathic
Insect bites
Secondary to ascites

### Rare Causes

Angiomas
Cysts
Healed meconium peritonitis
Hypertriglyceridemia
Leukemia
Sarcoidosis
Scrotal cellulitis
Tumors

## Selected Readings

Bartsch G, Marberger FH, Mikuz G. Testicular torsion: late results with special regard to fertility and endocrine function. J Urol 1980;124:375.
Brosman SA. Testicular tumors in prepubertal children. Urology 1979;13:581.
Dresner ML. Torsed appendage. Urology 1973;1:63.
Kaplan GW. Acute idiopathic scrotal edema. J Pediatr Surg 1977;12:647.
Kaplan GW, King L. Acute scrotal swelling in children. J Urol 1970;104:219.
Pedersen JF, Holm HH, Hald T. Torsion of the testis diagnosed by ultrasound. J Urol 1975;113:66.
Skoglund RW, McRoberts JW, Ragde H. Torsion of testicular appendages: presentation of 43 new cases and a collective review. J Urol 1970;104:598.

## Seizures

### Common Causes

Febrile seizures
Idiopathic seizures

### Uncommon Causes

CNS infections
   Aseptic meningitis
   Bacterial meningitis
   Viral encephalitis
CNS injury
   Anoxic encephalopathy
   Child abuse
   Concussion
   Hemorrhage
Hypoglycemia

### Rare Causes

CNS infection
   Congenital infection
   Parasitic infection
   Syphilis
   Tetanus
   Tuberculosis
Congenital CNS malformation
   Agenesis/dysgenesis
      Holoprosencephaly
      Porencephaly
   Hydrocephalus
Drugs/toxins
   Aminophylline
   Amphetamines
   Antihistamines
   Atropine
   Camphor
   Carbon monoxide
   Drug withdrawal
   Heavy metals
   Hexachlorophine
   Hydrocarbons
   Local anesthetics
   Narcotics
   Organophosphates
   Penicillin
   Pertussis toxoid
   Phencyclidine
   Scabicides
   Steroids
   Tricyclic antidepressants
Inborn errors of metabolism
   Aminoacidopathy
   Galactosemia
   Organic aciduria
   Storage disease
Metabolic
   Hypernatremia
   Hypocalcemia
   Hypomagnesemia
   Hyponatremia
Miscellaneous
   Arrhythmia
   Dysmorphogenic syndromes (many)
   Kernicterus
   Metachromatic leukodystrophy
   Pyridoxine deficiency
   Rett syndrome
   Reye's syndrome
   Subacute sclerosing panencephalitis (SSPE)
Neurocutaneous syndromes
   Incontinentia pigmenti
   Linear sebaceous nevus
   Neurofibromatosis
   Sturge-Weber disease
   Tuberous sclerosis
Seizure mimics
   Breath-holding spells
   Hyperventilation
   Malingering
   Masturbation
   Migraine
   Myoclonus
   Narcolepsy
   Orthostatic hypotension
   Paroxysmal torticollis of infancy
   Pseudoseizures
   Sandifer's syndrome
   Shivering on urination
   Shuddering attacks

Syncope
Tics
Vertigo
Systemic infection
    Roseola
    Shigella
Tumors
Vascular
    Arteriovenous malformation
    Embolic phenomenon
    Hemorrhage
    Hypertension
    Sickle-cell disease
    Thrombosis
    Vasculitis

## Selected Readings

Rothner AD. "Not everything that shakes is epilepsy." The differential diagnosis of paroxysmal nonepileptiform disorders. Cleve Clin, J Med 1989;56(Suppl pt 2):PS206.
Snyder CH. Conditions that simulate epilepsy in children. Clin Pediatr 1972;11: 487.

## Splenomegaly

### Common Causes

Acute infections (bacterial, viral, rickettsial, protozoal, spirochetal, mycobacterial)
Congenital hemolytic anemias
    Hemoglobinopathies
    Hereditary spherocytosis
    Thalassemia major, thalassemia intermedia

### Uncommon Causes

Congestive splenomegaly
Cyanotic congenital heart disease
Hodgkin's disease
Juvenile rheumatoid arthritis
Leukemia
Lupus erythematosus
Non-Hodgkin's disease
Severe iron-deficiency anemia

### Rare Causes

Acquired autoimmune hemolytic anemia
Amyloidosis
Beckwith-Wiedemann syndrome
Brucellosis
Chronic granulomatous disease
Congenital erythropoietic porphyria
Dysgammaglobulinemia
Hemophagocytic syndromes
Histiocytosis
Hurler's syndrome and other mucopolysaccharide disorders
Malaria (in United States)
Metastatic neuroblastoma
Myelofibrosis
Osteopetrosis
Sarcoidosis
Serum sickness
Splenic cyst or hemangioma
Storage disease (eg, Gaucher's, Niemann-Pick)
Wolman's disease

## Selected Readings

Mimouni F, Merlob P, Ashkenazi S, et al. Palpable spleens in newborn term infants. Clin Pediatr 1985;24:197.
Silverstein MN, Maldonado JE. Asymptomatic splenomegaly. Postgrad Med 1970ğ: 80.

## Stridor

(Also see Hoarseness.)

### Common Causes

Allergic reaction
Croup
Foreign-body aspiration
Hypertrophied tonsils/adenoids
Peritonsillar abscess
Postinstrumentation edema
Retropharyngeal abscess
Secretions
Spasmotic croup
Subglottic stenosis (congenital, postintubation)
Vocal cord nodules

### Uncommon Causes

Corrosive ingestion
Epiglottitis
Granuloma (postintubation/tracheostomy)
Laryngeal trauma
Tracheitis (bacterial)
Vocal cord paralysis (congenital, postsurgical)
Vocal cord polyps

### Rare Causes

Angioneurotic edema
Bronchogenic cyst
Congenital goiter
Cricoarytenoid arthritis (juvenile rheumatoid arthritis)
Diphtheria
Ectopic thyroid
Esophageal foreign body
External tracheal compression
    Hemorrhage
    Infection
    Tumors
Farber's disease
Glossoptosis
Hemangioma
Hypoplastic larynx
Internal laryngocele
Laryngeal papilloma
Laryngeal tumors
Laryngismus stridulus (rickets)
Macroglossia
Opitz-Frias syndrome
Pierre Robin syndrome
Post-tracheostomy stricture
Psychogenic stridor
Sarcoidosis
Tetany
Thyroglossal duct cyst
Tracheoesophageal fistula

Tracheo-laryngo-esophageal cleft
Vascular ring

## Selected Readings

Frey EE, Smith WL, Grandgeorge S, et al. Chronic airway obstruction in children—evaluation with Cine-CT. AJR 1987;148:347.

Gonzales C, Reilly JS, Bluestone CD. Synchronous airway lesions in infancy. Ann Otol Rhinol Laryngol 1987;96:77.

McBride JT. Stridor in childhood. J Fam Pract 1984;19:782.

Milner AD. Acute stridor in the preschool child. BMJ 1984;1:811.

Quinn-Bogard AL, Potsic WP. Stridor in the first year of life. Clin Pediatr 1977;16:913.

Ryckman F, Rodgers BM. Obstructive airway disease in infants and children. Surg Clin North Am 1985;65:1663.

# Torticollis

## Common Causes

Congenital, muscular, or vertebral anomalies

## Uncommon Causes

Cervical adenopathy
Congenital nystagmus
Drug-induced (eg, phenothiazines, haloperidol, metoclopramide, trimethobenzamide)
Paroxysmal
Pharyngitis
Retropharyngeal abscess
Secondary to reflux esophagitis (Sandifer's syndrome)
Superior oblique muscle weakness

## Rare Causes

Calcification of intervertebral disks
Dystonia musculorum deformans
Eosinophilic granuloma of cervical vertebrae
Fibromyositis
Focal myositis
Hepatolenticular degeneration
Juvenile rheumatoid arthritis
Kernicterus
Osteomyelitis of the cervical vertebrae
Pneumonia of an upper lobe
Posterior fossa tumor
Spasmus nutans
Spinal tumor
Subluxation or dislocation of cervical vertebrae

## Selected Readings

Bray PF, Herbst JJ, Johnson DG, et al. Childhood gastroesophageal reflux: neurologic and psychiatric syndromes mimicked. JAMA 1977;237:1342.

Hanukoglu A, Somekh E, Fried D. Benign paroxysmal torticollis in infancy. Clin Pediatr 1984;23:272.

Hensinger RN. Orthopedic problems of the shoulder and neck. Pediatr Clin North Am 1986;33:1495.

Kiwak KJ. Establishing an etiology for torticollis. Postgrad Med 1984;75:126.

Klassen AC. Torticollis. Postgrad Med 1984;75:124.

Lipson EH, Robertson WC Jr. Paroxysmal torticollis of infancy: familial occurrence. Am J Dis Child 1978;132:422.

Murphy WJ, Gellis SS. Torticollis with hiatus hernia in infancy. Am J Dis Child 1977;131:564.

Plagiocephaly and torticollis in young infants. Editorial. Lancet 1986;2:789.

Sanner G, Bergstrom B. Benign paroxysmal torticollis in infancy. Acta Paediatr Scand 1979;68:219.

# Vertigo and Syncope

Vertigo (dizziness) and syncope (light-headedness, fainting) may be difficult symptoms for a child to distinguish with certainty. Many entities that are traditionally thought to cause syncope may also cause vertigo. Syncope, therefore, is discussed as a subheading of causes of vertigo.

## Common Causes

Benign paroxysmal vertigo
Drugs
    Alcohol
    Anticonvulsants
    Antihypertensives
    Aspirin
    Dilantin
    Gentamycin
    Narcotics
    Sedatives
    Streptomycin
Ear disease
    External canal impaction
        Cerumen
        Foreign body
    Inner ear disease
        Cholesteatoma (with extension)
        Fistula
        Mastoiditis (with extension)
        Suppurative labyrinthitis
        Vestibular neuronitis
        Viral (acute) labyrinthitis
    Middle ear disease
        Chronic suppurative otitis (with extension)
        Hemotympanum (basilar skull fracture)
        Otitis media (rare as isolated finding)
        Serous otitis media
        Tympanic membrane perforation
Headache
    Basilar artery migraine complex
    Migraine
Hyperventilation syndrome
Seizure
    Aura/recovery phase
    Reflex seizure
Visual impairment

## Uncommon Causes

CNS infection
    Abscess
    Encephalitis
    Meningitis
    Hypotension
    Trauma
    Basilar skull fracture
    Cerebellar lesion/hemorrhage
    Labyrinthine trauma
    Postconcussion syndrome

## Rare Causes

Adrenal insufficiency
Anemia
Arnold-Chiari malformation
Benign positional vertigo
Brain stem ischemia

Breath-holding spells
CNS tumors
    Acoustic neuroma
    Brain stem glioma
    Cerebellar glioma
    Ependymoma
    Medulloblastoma
Demyelinating disease
    Multiple sclerosis
Endocrine disorders
    Adrenal insufficiency
    Diabetes mellitus
    Thyrotoxicosis
Hypertension
Hypoglycemia
Increased intracranial pressure
Meniere's syndrome
Pellagra
Psychosomatic illness
Ramsay Hunt syndrome
Syncope (many causes previously discussed)
    Cardiovascular etiologies
        Arrhythmia
            Atrioventricular block
            Cardioauditory syndrome
            Emery-Dreifuss muscular dystrophy
            Mitral valve prolapse
            Paroxysmal atrial tachycardia
            Paroxysmal ventricular tachycardia
            Prolonged QT syndrome
            Sick-sinus syndrome
        Cardiac anomalies
            Aortic stenosis
            Pulmonary stenosis
            Tetralogy of Fallot
            Transposition
            Truncus arteriosus
        Carotid sinus syncope
        Coronary artery spasm
        Dysautonomia (Riley-Day syndrome)
        Idiopathic hypertrophic subaortic stenosis
        Left atrial myxoma
        Myocardial infarction
        Orthostatic hypotension
        Pulmonary hypertension
        Vasovagal stimulation
Vestibulocerebellar ataxia

## Selected Readings

Benditt DG, Remole S, Milsteins, Bailin S. Syncope: causes, clinical evaluation, and current therapy. Annu Rev Med 1992;43:283

Chang-Sing P, Peter CT. Syncope: evaluation and management. A review of current approaches to this multifaceted and complex clinical problem. Cardiol Clin 1991;9:641.

Drachman DA, Hart CW. An approach to the dizzy patient. Neurology 1972;22: 323.

Dunn D. Dizziness: when is it vertigo? Contemp Pediatr 1987;4:67.

Eviatar L, Eviatar A. Vertigo in children: differential diagnosis and treatment. Pediatrics 1977;59:833.

# Wheezing

## Common Causes

Aspiration
    Direct (eg, defective swallow, neuromuscular disease)
    Indirect (gastroesophageal reflux, emesis)
Asthma
Atopic disease
Bronchiectasis
Bronchiolitis
Bronchitis
Foreign-body aspiration
Pneumonitis

## Uncommon Causes

Bronchopulmonary dysplasia
Congestive heart failure
Cystic fibrosis
Hypersensitivity pneumonitis
    Allergic bronchopulmonary aspergillosis
Mediastinal mass/adenopathy
Pulmonary edema
Tracheobronchomalacia

## Rare Causes

$\alpha_1$-Antitrypsin deficiency
Angioneurotic edema
Carcinoid syndrome
Factitious wheezing
Lobar emphysema
Neoplasm/tumor
Psychogenic airway obstruction
Pulmonary hemosiderosis
Pulmonary sequestration
Pulmonary vasculitis
Sarcoidosis
Tracheobronchostenosis
Tracheoesophageal fistula
Vascular ring/sling
Visceral larva migrans

## Selected Readings

Barnes SD, Grob CS, Lachman BS, et al. Psychogenic upper airway obstruction presenting as refractory wheezing. J Pediatr 1986;109:1067.

Clayton D. Catching up with the ABCs of sneezing, wheezing, and itching. Can Med Assoc J 1984;130:1609.

Leffert F. Asthma: a modern perspective. Pediatrics 1978;62:1061.

Rachelefsky GS. The wheezing child. Pediatrics 1984;74(Suppl 5):941.

Richard W. Differential diagnosis of childhood asthma. Curr Probl Pediatr 1974;4: 3.

# Index

**Note:** Entry numbers followed by *t* or *f* refer to tables and figures, respectively. Roman numerals in **boldface** indicate color plates.

no definable cause, 1062
pneumograms in, 1060–1061
polysomnography in, 1061
seizures and, 1062
Appendectomy, 1901
Appendicitis, 1899–1901
adenovirus infection and, 1293
cholecystitis vs, 1948
clinical course and manifestations, 1899–1901
constipation vs, 1900
diagnosis, 1899–1901
differential diagnosis, 1900–1901
gynecologic pain vs, 1900–1901
incidence, 1899
laboratory findings, 1901
neonatal, necrotizing enterocolitis vs, 441
pathogenesis, 1899
peptic ulcer disease vs, 1854
perforation, 1900
treatment, 1901
*Yersinia pseudotuberculosis* infection vs, 1262
Appendix
carcinoid tumor, 1741
in cystic fibrosis, 1494
Apple juice, composition, 852t
Apraxia of speech, 692–693
Apt test, for fetal hemoglobin, 479t
Arachnoiditis, optic nerve, 1127
Arboviruses, 1266–1268
Argentine, Bolivian, and Venezuelan
hemorrhagic fever, 1271, 1275–1276
Australian (Murray Valley) encephalitis, 1276
California encephalitis, 1276–1277
chikungunya, 1277–1278
Colorado tick fever, 1278, 1347–1348
Congo-Crimean hemorrhagic fever, 1278
dengue fever, 1278–1279
eastern equine encephalitis, 1279–1280
filoviral hemorrhagic fevers, 1280
group C bunyavirus infections, 1280–1281
hemorrhagic fever with renal syndrome, 1281
infection. *See also specific infections*
DEET insect repellents in, 1271
guidelines for use, 1271
diagnosis, 1268–1269
differential diagnosis, 1269–1270
epidemiology, 1267–1268
geographic distribution, 1272t–1275t
isolation precautions, 1429t
prevention, 1270–1271, 1271t
reported cases, United states, 1267t
therapy, 1270
transmission, 1267–1268, 2168f
Japanese encephalitis, 1281–1282
Lassa fever, 1282
lymphocytic choriomeningitis, 1282–1283
monkeypox, 1283
Oropouche fever, 1283
phlebotomus (sandfly) fever, 1283
Rift Valley fever, 1283–1284
Rocio encephalitis, 1284
Ross River arthropathy, 1284
Sinbis virus infection, 1284–1285
St. Louis encephalitis, 1285
taxonomic and physical characteristics, 1267t
tick-borne encephalitis, 1285–1286
transmission, 1267–1268, 2168f
Venezuelan equine encephalitis, 1286
western equine encephalitis, 1286–1287
West Nile fever, 1286
yellow fever, 1287–1288
zoonosis, 1268, 2168f
Arcus juvenilis, inborn errors of metabolism and, 80t
Arenaviruses
Argentine, Bolivian, and Venezuelan
hemorrhagic fever, 1271, 1275–1276
lymphocytic choriomeningitis, 1282–1283
taxonomic and physical characteristics, 1267t
Argentine hemorrhagic fever, 1271, 1275–1276
Arginase deficiency, 90
Arginine, structure, 83f
Argininemia, 90, 1919t

Arginine vasopressin. *See also* Antidiuretic
hormone
fetal metabolism and, 286
inappropriate secretion
kidney failure and, 463–464
pathophysiology, 463f
receptors, in nephrogenic diabetes insipidus, 1827
in renal response to perinatal asphyxia, 461
synthetic analog. *See* Desmopressin
urine dilution/concentration, in fetus and
neonate, 459–460
Argininosuccinase deficiency, 90
Argininosuccinate lyase deficiency, 90, 1919t
Argininosuccinate synthetase deficiency, 90,
1919t
Argininosuccinic aciduria, 90, 1919t
Arnold-Chiari malformation, central
hypoventilation and, 1068
Arrhythmias, 1641–1645
in arrhythmogenic right ventricular dysplasia,
1613, 1613f
atrial, in rheumatic heart disease, 1637
atrial baffle procedures and, 1530
causes, 2222
complete AV block, 1643
ectopy, in neonate, 405
electrocardiography in, 1641–1645. *See also*
Electrocardiography, *specific
arrhythmia*
fetal, 399
heart block, in neonate, 404f, 405
junctional rhythm, 1642
in mitral valve prolapse, 1586
in myocarditis, 1601, 1605
in neonate, algorithm for management, 404f,
409
in oncocytic cardiomyopathy, 1613
poisoning and, 833–834
premature atrial contractions, 1643, 1644f
premature ventricular contractions, 1645
in rheumatic heart disease, 1637–1638
sinus, 1642
supraventricular, 1643–1645
supraventricular tachycardia, 1643–1645
in neonate, 404f, 404–405
vagal, 1642–1643
ventricular fibrillation, defibrillation for, 810
ventricular tachycardia, 1645, 1645f
bidirectional, periodic paralysis and, 2084
cardioversion for, 810
in neonate, 404f, 405
wandering pacemaker, 1642
Arsenic intoxication, peripheral neuropathy in,
2076
Arterial switch operation, for transposition of
great arteries, 566–567, 567f, 1530
Arteriohepatic dysplasia. *See* Alagille syndrome
Arteriovenous communications, retinal, 881
Arteriovenous fistula
congenital, 1748
pulmonary, 1649
systemic, echocardiography in, 1649
Arteriovenous malformation, 400
intracranial hemorrhage and, 2035–2036
Arteritis, 2032
cranial, 266
giant cell, 266
in Kawasaki disease, 1639
mesenteric, postcoarctectomy, 1577
Takayasu, 266
Arthralgia, 244
in acute lymphoblastic leukemia, 1704–1705
Lyme disease and, 250
Arthritis
in chikungunya, 1277–1278
in Crohn's disease, 1871
episodic, in cystic fibrosis, 1495
in erythema infectiosum, 1304
gonococcal, 1043, 1205
treatment, 1206t
gouty, 135
in Henoch-Schönlein purpura, 265

inborn errors of metabolism and, 81t
juvenile. *See also* Juvenile rheumatoid arthritis
classification, 243–244, 244t
in Kawasaki disease, 1425
in Lyme disease, 250, 1172
meningococcal infection and, 1202
in rheumatic fever, 1628
rheumatoid. *See* Rheumatoid arthritis
Ross River arthropathy, 1284
septic, 1042–1043
anaerobic bacteria in, 1166
arthrotomy in, 1043
aspiration in, 1043
differential diagnosis, 1043
etiologic agents, 1041f, 1043
fever of undetermined origin and, 1118
group B streptococcal, 535
*H influenzae*, 1189
in neonate, 529–530
in Sinbis virus infection, 1285
in SLE, 251
in sporotrichosis, 1381
in ulcerative colitis, 1865
in *Yersinia enterocolitica* infection, 1260
Arthritis-dermatitis syndrome, 787
Arthrogryposis, 342
fractures and, 502
Arthrogryposis multiplex congenita, 363, 2070
Arthro-ophthalmopathy, 507
inheritance and clinical features, 157t
morphologic abnormalities, 2196
Arthrotomy, in septic arthritis, 1043
Arthus reaction, 209
Articulation, 692
disorders, 692–693
functional, 693
error, 693
Arylsulfatase A deficiency, 125. *See also*
Metachromatic leukodystrophy
Arylsulfatase B deficiency, 119
Arylsulfatase C deficiency, 125
*Ascaris lumbricoides* infection, 1409–1410
isolation precautions, 1429t
Aschoff nodules, in rheumatic fever, 1627, 1627f
Ascites, 1902–1907, 1935–1936
bile, 1905
cholestasis and, treatment, 1915t
chylous, 432, 1903
fluid characteristics, 1905
complications, 1907
diagnosis, 1935
differential diagnosis, 1902–1903, 1903t
diuretic therapy, 1906, 1936
exudative, 1905
fluid analysis, 1905–1906, 1935
hypoalbuminemia and, 1902–1903
infection and, 1903, 1903t
malignant, 1906
in neonate, 431–432
causes, 431t, 431–432
delivery room resuscitation and, 317
evaluation, 432
treatment, 432
nutritional therapy, 1906
overflow theory, 1902, 1935
pancreatic, 1903
fluid characteristics, 1905
pathogenesis, 1902
pathophysiology, 1935
peritoneovenous shunts for, 1906–1907
physical examination in, 1903–1904, 1904f
in portal hypertension, 1902, 1935–1936, 1958
diagnosis, 1935
pathophysiology, 1935
treatment, 1935
radiologic evaluation, 1904–1905
spontaneous bacterial peritonitis and, 1907
transudative, 1905
treatment, 1906–1907, 1935–1936
underfill theory, 1902, 1935
urinary, 1903
fluid characteristics, 1905
in neonate, 431, 432, 460

nosocomial infections, 564, 1230
sepsis neonatorum, 517
endocarditis, 1621
*epidermidis*
endocarditis, 1621
infections, 1230
microbiology, 1228
folliculitis, 492
infections, 1228–1231
meningitis, 525
microbiology, 1228
Starvation, accelerated. *See* Hypoglycemia, ketotic
Statistics
childhood population of U.S., 6
actual and projected population, 6t
chi-squared test, 28
confidence limits, 27
in data analysis, 27–28
fertility rate, 6, 6f
live births, 6, 6f
mortality and morbidity, 6–7, 7t
neonatal, 7t, 7–8, 8f
Student's *t* test, 28
Status epilepticus, 827, 2057–2058
definition, 2057
treatment, 2057–2058
Steatorrhea
in cystic fibrosis, 1493, 1499
food allergy and, 229
in giardiasis, 1391–1392
''physiologic'', in neonate, 415
Stenosis
intracranial vessels. *See* Cerebrovascular disease, occlusive
laryngeal, 1480–1481
pulmonary, 1567–1571
intracavitary obstruction of right ventricle, 1570–1571
pulmonary artery, 1571
pulmonary valve, 1568–1570
in single ventricle, 1545
renal artery, 1094
subaortic, in single ventricle, 1545, 1546
Stensen's duct, 860
in parotitis, 994
Stents, intravascular, for stenosis, 1654
Stepping reflex. *See* Positive support reflex
Step-Two Diet, in familial hypercholesterolemia, 114
Stereotypy, 2125
Sterilization, in infant formula preparation, 604
Sternoclavicular sprain, 1006
Sternum, malformation, vascular dysplasia and, 911t
Steroid sulfatase deficiency, 125
Sterotypy, differential diagnosis, 2115t
Stevens-Johnson syndrome. *See also* Erythema multiforme bullosum
emphysema and, 1510
herpangina vs, 991t
Stickler's syndrome. *See* Arthro-ophthalmopathy
Stinging insects. *See* Bites and stings, insect sting allergy
Stomach
acid production, 1839, 1851
in infants and children, 1851t
in peptic ulcer disease, 1851t
anatomic regions, 1838f
anatomy, 1839
atresia, 418
biopsy, in *Helicobacter pylori* infection, 1177
blood supply, 1839f
cancer, 1741
*Helicobacter pylori* infection and, 1176
congenital malformations, obstruction and, 417–419
congenital webs, 418
diverticulum, 418
duplication, 423
electrical regions, 1839f
functions, 1839

hypoplastic, 418
nasogastric decompression, in neonate, 385
perforation, 418, 418f
ulcer. *See* Peptic ulcer disease
volvulus, 418
Stomatitis
aphthous. *See* Aphthous ulcers
herpetic, herpangina vs, 991t
Stomatocytosis, hereditary, 1664–1665
Stool. *See* Feces
''Stork bites.'' *See* Salmon patches
Stoxil. *See* Iododeoxyuridine
Strabismus, 888–890
evaluation for, 35
headache and, 896
incomitant, 889
in retinoblastoma, 1734
rubella and, 885
Straight leg raising test, in back pain, 1004
Strain, 1002–1003
grading, 1003
Strawberry hemangioma, 489
Streak gonad, 472
Streeter's bands, 1037
*Streptobacillus* spp., *moniliformis*, 1220. *See also* Rat-bite fever, streptobacillary
endocarditis, 1621
Streptococcosis, sinusitis vs, 953
*Streptococcus* spp.
*agalactiae. See Streptococcus*, group B
endocarditis, 1620–1621
enterococcus, 1621
extracellular products, 1627
*faecalis*, new terminology, 958t
*faecium*, new terminology, 958t
group A β-hemolytic
burn wound, isolation precautions, 1442t
carrier state, 1233
cervical adenitis, 984–989
endometritis, isolation precautions, 1433t, 1442t
erysipelas, 1233
funisitis, 564
impetigo, 1233
infection, 1231–1235
isolation precautions, 1442t
rheumatic fever and, 1626, 1628. *See also* Rheumatic fever
laboratory tests for, 2152–2154
microbiology, 1231–1232
nephritogenic, 1786. *See also* Glomerulonephritis, acute poststreptococcal
nosocomial infection, 564
omphalitis, 531
peritonsillar abscess and, 824
pharyngitis, 969–970, 1232–1233, 1234
diagnosis, 1234
herpangina vs, 991t
isolation precautions, 1442t
rapid diagnostic techniques, 1452
pneumonia, isolation precautions, 1442t
pyoderma, 1233
retropharyngeal abscess and, 824
scarlet fever, 1232, 1233, 1234
isolation precautions, 1442t
skin infection, isolation precautions, 1442t
streptotoccosis, sinusitis vs, 953
tonsillitis, 1232–1233, 1234
toxic shock syndrome, 1233
uvulitis, 978–979
wound infection, isolation precautions, 1442t
group B
antigenuria, 1452
bacteriology, 533–534
breast abscess, in neonate, 531
capsular polysaccharide antigens, 533
cellulitis-adenitis, 531, 986
colonization, 517
in pregnancy, 518, 534, 535
meningitis, 525–526, 527
necrotizing fasciitis, in neonate, 531

neonatal infection, 517. *See also* Infant, newborn, group B streptococcal disease; Meningitis, neonatal; Sepsis, neonatal
isolation precautions, 1442t
osteomyelitis, 529
pneumonia, 375, 376, 376f
polysaccharide vaccine, 524, 538
serotypes, 533
distribution of, 534
submandibular cellulitis/lymphadenitis, 531
transmission to neonate, 534
type III, capsular polysaccharide antigen, 519, 525–526, 535
virulence, 519, 535
group D
meningitis, 525
sepsis neonatorum, 517
α-hemolytic, sepsis neonatorum, 517
infections
isolation precautions, 1442t
streptococci other than groups A and B, 1235t, 1235–1236
Lancefield grouping, hemolytic reactions, human colonization, and disease, 1235t
microbiology, 1626–1627
*milleri*, new terminology, 958t
*mutans*, dental caries and, 867
pneumococcus, 1621
*pneumoniae*
infections, 1214–1217. *See also* Pneumococcal infection
meningitis, 1125. *See also* Meningitis, bacterial
microbiology, 1215
occult bacteremia, 1113–1114
penicillin-resistant, 1216
pneumonia, 1474
sepsis neonatorum, 517
sinusitis, 953
*pyogenes. See Streptococcus*, group A β-hemolytic
*sanguis*, aphthous ulers and, 865
structure, 1626f, 1626–1627
viridans
endocarditis and, 1621
infection, 1236
new terminology, 958t
Streptodornase, 1627
Streptokinase, 1627
Streptolysin O, 1627
Streptolysin S, 1627
Streptomycin
for infective endocarditis, 1623t
for opportunistic infection, 1147t
ototoxicity, 1239
for plague, 1214
prophylaxis, for plague, 1214
for rat-bite fever, spirillary, 1220
for tuberculosis, 1253t, 1254
for tularemia, 1239
Streptozyme agglutination test, 1234
Stress
amenorrhea and, 779
child's response to, 711
in chronic disease, 650
communicative, 694
development and, 702
in family, child abuse and, 651
hospitalization and, 710
illness and, 710–712
peptic ulcer disease and, 1850
protective factors against, 711
psychosocial stressors scale, 710t
resilience to, 710–711
tension headache and, 2137
ulcers, 1850
Stress fracture. *See* Fractures, stress
Stress reaction, acute, 711
Striae, 927

Symmers' fibrosis, 1417
Sympathomimetic agents, for allergic rhinitis, 238
Syncope
  atypical, 1641
  causes, 2243–2244
Syncytiotrophoblast, 275, 282
Synostosis, radioulnar, 1037
Synovial fluid, white cell count
  in juvenile rheumatoid arthritis, 247
  in Lyme disease, 250
  in septic arthritis, 1043
Synovitis, hip, transient (toxic), 1020
Syphilis, 1240–1244
  acquired, 1240
    incidence, 1240, 1240f
  in adolescent, 788–789
    clinical presentation, 788–789
    diagnosis, 789
    treatment, 789
  AIDS and, 1244
  clinical manifestations, 1241
  CNS involvement. See also Neurosyphilis
    cerebrospinal fluid findings, 1130t
  congenital, 548–552, 1240
    bullous lesions, 902, 902f
    cholestasis and, 425
    clinical manifestations, 541t, 548–550, 549f,
      550f, 1241
    diagnosis, 1243, 1243f
    early, 548
    epidemiology, 548
    incidence, 48f, 548, 1240f
    isolation precautions, 563
    late, 548
    mucocutaneous manifestations, 492
    ocular disorders, 885
    pathogenesis, 1241
    prevention, 551
    surveillance definition, 548
    transmission, 548
    treatment, 551–552, 1243–1244
  diagnosis, 1241–1243, 1242f, 1242t
  epidemiology, 1240
  incidence, 1240, 1240f
  incubation period, 788
  isolation precautions, 1442t
  late (latent), 789, 1241
    clinical manifestations, 1241
    treatment, 1243
  microbiology, 1240
  pathogenesis, 1240–1241
  in pregnancy, 548
  prevention, 1244
  primary, 788
    clinical manifestations, 1241
    ulcerative lesions, 790, 790t
  secondary, 789, 1240–1241
    annular lesions in, 939
    clinical manifestations, 1241
  sexual abuse and, 658
  tertiary. See Syphilis, late (latent)
  treatment, 1243–1244
Syringoma, 906
Syringomyelia, 2018
Systemic lupus erythematosus (SLE), 250–253
  C4A deficiency in, 189
  clinical manifestations, 245t, 251f, 251t, 251–
    252
  complications, 253
  course, 251t, 253
  cutaneous manifestations, 939
  diagnostic criteria, 253, 253t
  differential diagnosis, 253
  disorder resembling, in complement deficiency,
    189
  drug-induced, 253–254
  histopathology, 252–253
  laboratory findings, 252, 1790–1791
  maternal
    congenital heart block and, 254
    congenital heart disease and, 394t
  neonatal lupus phenomena, 254

nephritis in, 252, 252t. See also Lupus nephritis
occlusive cerebrovascular disease in, 2032
pathogenesis, 251
photosensitivity in, 935
prognosis, 253
treatment, 253

Tache cérébrale, 935
Tache noire, 1363
Tachycardia
  in congenital hyperthyroidism, 474
  in shock, 1082
  supraventricular, 1643–1645, 1644f
    in neonate, 403f, 404f, 404–405
  systemic perfusion and, 408–409
  ventricular, 1645, 1645f
    cardioversion, 810
    in neonate, 404f, 405
Tachypnea, 38
  in neonate, 303, 306, 369, 400
    transient, 374–375
      pneumonia vs, 376
  in shock, 1083
TAC solution, in wound care, 817t
Tahyna virus, 1276
Takayasu arteritis, 266, 2032
Talipes equinovarus. See Clubfoot
Tangier disease, 112–113, 2074t
Tanner stages, 766
  associated clinical processes/disorders, 771t
Tansy ragwort, ingestion of, 841
Tapeworm disease, isolation precautions, 1442t
Tar preparations, for atopic dermatitis, 235
TAR (radial aplasia-thrombocytopenia)
    syndrome, 1687–1688
  morphologic abnormalities, 2196–2197
Tarui disease (GSD VII), 107, 2088
Taussig, Helen, 4, 5
Taussig-Bing complex, 1539
Tauton agent, 1352
Tax Equity and Fiscal Responsibility Act
    (TEFRA), 17
Taxes, 703
Tay-Sachs disease, 121–122
  adult form, 122
  anterior horn cell involvement, 2070
  genetic mutation in, 173
  prenatal diagnosis, 298t
T cell(s). See T lymphocytes
T-cell leukemia/lymphoma, adult, 1349
Tear production, in dehydration, 63t
Teenager. See Adolescence
Teeth
  abscess. See Abscess, dental
  absence, congenital, 863
  avulsion, 873
  calculus formation, 870
  caries. See Dental caries
  cleaning and flossing, 877
  concussion, 872
  congenital anomalies, 863–864
    color, 863–864, 864t
    number, 863
    shape, 863, 863f
    size, 863
  in congenital syphilis, 550, 550f
  crazing, 872
  crown fractures, 872, 872f
  crown-root fracture, 872, 872f
  demineralization/remineralization, 867
  dentin and enamel fracture, 872, 872f
  discoloration, 863–864, 864t
  displacement, 873
  enamel fracture, 872, 872f
  enamel hypoplasia, 863, 863f
  eruption. See Dentition
  exfoliation, premature, 864
  extruded, 873
  fractures, 872, 872f
  grinding (bruxism), 875, 877
  intruded, 873

lateral displacement, 873
natal, 862
neonatal, 862, 862f
occlusion. See Malocclusion; Occlusion, dental
pulp necrosis, 868
reimplantation, 873
root fracture, 872, 872f
root resorption, 873
in skeletal dysplasias, 161t
subluxation, 872
supernumerary, 863
in tuberous sclerosis, 2133
Teething, 867
Tegretol. See Carbamazepine
Teichoic acid
  antibody levels, 1617
  S aureus, 1228
Telangiectasia
  hereditary hemorrhagic. See Rendu-Osler-
    Weber syndrome
  intracranial hemorrhage and, 2036
  in neonate, 305, 489
  oral, 864
  retinal, congenital. See Coats' disease
Telangiectasis, 898
  in scleroderma, 258
Telecanthus, 880
Telogen effluvium, hair loss and, 942–943
Temperature. See also Thermogenesis;
    Thermoregulation
  control
    cooling/heating blanket for, 1071
    devices for, 1071–1072
    radiant warming device, 1071
  decreased, 32
  elevated, 32
  of fetus, 326
  fluid loss and, 61
  measurement, 32, 2212
    axillary, 2212
    devices for, 1072
    oral, 2212
    rectal, 2212
  monitoring, in intensive care, 1072
  rectal
    in heat exhaustion, 999
    in heat stroke, 999
Temporomandibular joint disease, headache and,
    2138
Tendinitis, 1003
  Achilles, 1015
  flexor-pronator, 1008
  patellar, 1013, 1024
  posterior tibialis. See Shin splint syndrome
  quadriceps, 1024
  supraspinatus, 1007. See also Impingement
    syndrome
Tendon reflexes, examination, 43
Tennis elbow. See Elbow, lateral epicondylitis
Tenosynovitis, in juvenile rheumatoid arthritis,
    246
Tension-fatigue syndrome, 215
Teratogenicity
  anticonvulsant drugs, 2056
  hyperphenylalaninemia, 86
Teratogens, 278–279, 279t
  prenatal, cardiac risk, 394t
Teratoma. See also Germ cell tumors
  abdominal, in neonate, 434
  head and neck region, 1743
  in neonate, 574
    management, 575
  ovarian, 1744
  pathology, 1743
  sacrococcygeal, 1743
  testis, 1744
Terbutaline, for asthma, 217t, 825, 825t, 826t
Terminal care. See also Life support
  ethical issues, 14–15
Testicular regression syndrome, 471, 471f
Testis
  acute lymphoblastic leukemia, 1709

ISBN 0-397-51221-X

9 780397 512218

90000